Cardiovascular Medicine

James T. Willerson, M.D.
Edward Randall III Professor and Chairman
Department of Internal Medicine
University of Texas–Houston Medical School
Chief of Internal Medicine Service
Memorial-Hermann Hospital

Medical Director
Texas Heart Institute
Chief of Cardiology
St. Luke's Episcopal Hospital
Texas Medical Center
Houston, Texas
Editor of *Circulation*

Jay N. Cohn, M.D.
Professor of Medicine
Cardiovascular Division
University of Minnesota
Medical School
Minneapolis, Minnesota
Editor of the *Journal of Cardiac Failure*

Cardiovascular Medicine

SECOND EDITION

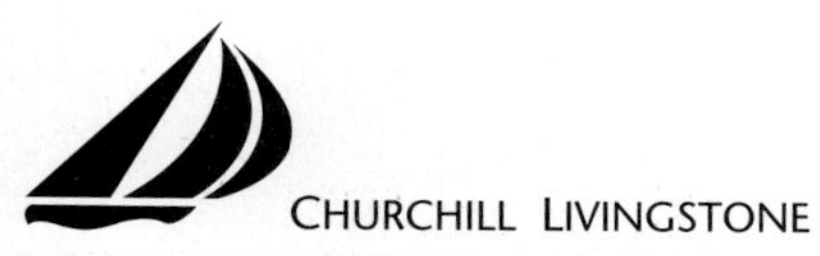

CHURCHILL LIVINGSTONE

A Harcourt Health Sciences Company
New York Edinburgh London Philadelphia

CHURCHILL LIVINGSTONE
A Harcourt Health Sciences Company

The Curtis Center
Independence Square West
Philadelphia, Pennsylvania 19106

Library of Congress Cataloging-in-Publication Data

Cardiovascular medicine / edited by James T. Willerson, Jay N. Cohn.—2nd ed.

p. cm.

Includes bibliographical references and index.

ISBN 0–443–07000–8

1. Cardiology. 2. Cardiovascular system—Diseases. I. Willerson, James T., Cohn, Jay N.

[DNLM: 1. Cardiovascular Diseases. WG 100 C26762 2000]

RC667.C395 2000

616.1—dc21 00–022728

Editor: Marc Strauss
Developmental Editor: Ann Ruzycka
Copy Editor: Mimi McGinnis
Production Manager: Linda Garber
Illustration Specialist: Rita Martello

CARDIOVASCULAR MEDICINE ISBN 0–443–07000–8

Printed in the United States of America.

Last digit is the print number: 9 8 7 6 5 4 3 2 1

CONTRIBUTORS

Leonard P. Adam, Ph.D.
Senior Research Investigator, Cardiovascular Drug Discovery, Bristol-Myers Squibb, Princeton, New Jersey
Molecular and Cellular Physiology of Differentiated Vascular Smooth Muscle

James K. Alexander, M.D.
Professor of Medicine (Cardiology), Baylor College of Medicine, Houston, Texas
Obesity

H. Vernon Anderson, M.D.
Professor of Medicine, University of Texas–Houston Medical School, Houston, Texas
Percutaneous Coronary Interventions for Stable Angina Pectoris

Stephen L. Archer, M.D., F.R.C.P.(C.)
Professor and Director, Division of Cardiology, Department of Medicine, University of Alberta Faculty of Medicine, Walter Mackenzie Health Science Center, Edmonton, Alberta, Canada
Pulmonary Hypertension

William F. Armstrong, M.D.
Professor of Internal Medicine, Division of Cardiology, University of Michigan Health System, Ann Arbor, Michigan
Echocardiography and Doppler Evaluation (Valvular Heart Disease)

Frank C. Arnett, M.D.
Professor of Internal Medicine and of Pathology and Laboratory Medicine, University of Texas–Houston Medical School; Chief, Rheumatology Service, Memorial Hermann Hospital and Lyndon B. Johnson General Hospital, Houston, Texas
Connective Tissue Diseases and the Heart

Jef Arnout, Ph.D.
Associate Professor, Faculty of Medicine, Center for Molecular and Vascular Biology, University of Leuven, Leuven, Belgium
Vascular Endothelial Cell Function and Thrombosis

David S. Bach, M.D.
Associate Professor of Medicine and Associate Director, Echocardiography Laboratory, University of Michigan Medical School, Ann Arbor, Michigan
Echocardiography (Congenital Heart Disease in the Adult)

Robert J. Bache, M.D.
Professor of Medicine, Cardiovascular Division, University of Minnesota Medical School–Minneapolis; Attending Physician, Fairview-University Medical Center, Minneapolis, Minnesota
Regulation of Coronary Blood Flow

Alan J. Bank, M.D.
Director of Research, St. Paul Heart Clinic, St. Paul; Associate Professor of Medicine, Cardiovascular Division, University of Minnesota Medical School–Minneapolis, Minneapolis, Minnesota
Arterial Compliance

Eddy Barasch, M.D.
Associate Professor of Medicine, University of Texas–Houston Medical School; Director, Echocardiography Laboratory, Memorial-Hermann Hospital, Houston, Texas
Echocardiography (Introduction: Cardiac Signs and Symptoms and Selected Noninvasive Diagnostic Methods) ▪ *Infective Endocarditis* ▪ *Echocardiography (Coronary Artery Disease)* ▪ *Echocardiography (Myocardial Disease)*

William H. Barry, M.D.
Nora Eccles Harrison Professor of Cardiology, University of Utah School of Medicine, Salt Lake City, Utah
Cardiac Hypertrophy: Physiologic and Clinical Considerations

Iris Baumgartner, M.D., Ph.D.
Head Physician, Division of Angiology, Swiss Cardiovascular Center, University Hospital, Bern, Switzerland
Gene Therapy (Vascular Medicine)

David G. Benditt, M.D.
Professor of Medicine, University of Minnesota Medical School–Minneapolis; Co-Director, Cardiac Arrhythmia Center, Fairview-University Medical Center, Minneapolis, Minnesota
Sinus Node Dysfunction ▪ *Syncope*

C. Gunnar Blomqvist, M.D., Ph.D.
Professor of Medicine, University of Texas Southwestern Medical Center at Dallas Southwestern Medical School, Dallas, Texas
Recognition and Physiologic Treatment of Cardiac Arrhythmias and Conduction Disturbances ▪ *Exercise*

Biykem Bozkurt, M.D., F.A.C.C.
Assistant Chief, Medical Services, VA Medical Center; Assistant Professor of Medicine, Cardiology Section, Baylor College of Medicine, Houston, Texas
Dilated Cardiomyopathy

Steven D. Brown, M.D.
Associate Professor and Interim Director, Division of Pulmonary and Critical Care Medicine, University of Texas–Houston Medical School; Chief of Internal Medicine and Vice Chief of Staff, Lyndon B. Johnson General Hospital, Houston, Texas
Chronic Obstructive Pulmonary Disease

Bruce H. Brundage, M.D.
Professor of Medicine and Radiological Sciences, and Chief, Division of Cardiology, Harbor–UCLA Medical Center, St. John's Cardiac Research Center, Torrance, California
Rapid-Speed Computed Tomography

Hans R. Brunner, M.D.
Professor, Faculty of Medicine, University of Lausanne; Chief, Division of Hypertension and Vascular Medicine, University Hospital, Lausanne, Switzerland
Hypertension (Vascular Medicine)

Matthew J. Budoff, M.D.
Division of Cardiology, University of California Medical Center, Los Angeles County Harbor, Los Angeles, California
Rapid-Speed Computed Tomography

Maximilian Buja, M.D.
Dean of the Medical School and Professor of Pathology and Laboratory Medicine, The University of Texas–Houston Medical School and Health Science Center, Affiliated with the Memorial-Hermann Healthcare System; Staff Member, Cardiovascular Pathology Laboratory, The Texas Heart Institute at St. Luke's Episcopal Hospital, Houston, Texas
Anatomic Abnormalities (Valvular Heart Disease) ▪ *Anatomic Abnormalities and Pathogenesis (Coronary Artery Disease)* ▪ *Anatomic Abnormalities (Myocardial Disease)* ▪ *Anatomic Abnormalities (Pericardial Disease)* ▪ *Atherosclerosis: Pathologic Anatomy*

Allen P. Burke, M.D.
Adjunct Professor of Pathology, Georgetown University School of Medicine; Staff Pathologist, Armed Forces Institute of Pathology, Washington, D.C.
Coronary Artery Disease in Women

Michel Burnier, M.D.
Associate Professor, Faculty of Medicine, University of Lausanne; Division of Hypertension and Vascular Medicine, University Hospital, Lausanne, Switzerland
Hypertension (Vascular Medicine)

Robert P. Byington, Ph.D.
Professor of Epidemiology, Department of Public Health Sciences, Wake Forest University School of Medicine, Winston-Salem, North Carolina
B-Mode Ultrasound: A Noninvasive Method for Assessing Atherosclerosis

Blase A. Carabello, M.D.
Professor of Medicine, Baylor College of Medicine; Chief of Medical Service, Veterans Affairs Medical Center, Houston, Texas
Aortic Valve Disease

C. Thomas Caskey, M.D.
Senior Vice President, Human Genetics and Vaccines Discovery, Merck & Co., Inc., West Point, Pennsylvania
Muscular Dystrophies Affecting the Heart

Ward Casscells, M.D.
O'Driscoll Levy Professor of Medicine, University of Texas–Houston Medical School; Chief of Cardiology, Department of Internal Medicine, and Associate Director, Cardiology Research, St. Luke's Episcopal Hospital–Texas Heart Institute, Houston, Texas
Homocysteine and Vascular Disease

Melvin D. Cheitlin, M.D.
Emeritus Professor of Medicine, University of California, San Francisco, School of Medicine; Former Chief of Cardiology, San Francisco General Hospital, San Francisco, California
Cardiovascular Involvement in AIDS

D. Chemla, M.D., Ph.D.
Lecturer, Faculty of Medicine, University of Paris XI; Staff Physician, Department of Cardiovascular Physiology, Hôpital de Bicetre, Le Kremlin Bicetre Cedex, France
Arrhythmogenic Right Ventricular Dysplasia

Elliot Chesler, M.D.
Professor of Medicine, University of Minnesota Medical School–Minneapolis; Chief, Cardiovascular Section, Veterans Affairs Medical Center, Minneapolis, Minnesota
Mitral Valve Disease ▪ *Mitral Valve Prolapse (Myxomatous Mitral Valve)*

Sandra K. Clapp, M.D.
Associate Professor of Pediatrics, Baylor College of Medicine, Houston, Texas
Interventional Therapy

Jay N. Cohn, M.D.
Professor of Medicine, Cardiovascular Division, University of Minnesota Medical School–Minneapolis, Minneapolis, Minnesota
Heart Failure: Pathophysiology and Recognition ▪ *The Management of Heart Failure* ▪ *Arterial Compliance* ▪ *Hypertension (Vascular Medicine)* ▪ *Shock*

Désiré Collen, M.D., Ph.D.
Professor, Faculty of Medicine, Center for Molecular and Vascular Biology, University of Leuven, Leuven, Belgium
Vascular Endothelial Cell Function and Thrombosis

Steven J. Compton, M.D.
Assistant Professor of Medicine, University of Utah School of Medicine; University Hospital, Salt Lake City, Utah
Long QT Syndromes

Denton A. Cooley, M.D.
Clinical Professor of Surgery, University of Texas–Houston Medical School; Surgeon-in-Chief, St. Luke's Episcopal Hospital–Texas Heart Institute, Houston, Texas
Surgical Treatment (Valvular Heart Disease) ■ Surgical Treatment (Coronary Artery Disease) ■ Surgical Treatment of Advanced Heart Failure ■ Diseases of the Aorta ■ Tumors of the Heart

John R. Cooper, Jr., M.D.
Associate Chief, Cardiovascular Anesthesiologist, Texas Heart Institute, Houston, Texas
Anesthesia for Cardiovascular Operations

Edouard Coraboeuf, Ph.D.†
Professor, University of Paris XII, Orsay, France
Cardiac Hypertrophy and Failure: Basic Aspects

James L. Cox, M.D.
Professor and Chairman, Department of Thoracic and Cardiovascular Surgery, Georgetown University School of Medicine, Washington, D.C.
Surgical Treatment of Arrhythmias

John R. Crouse, M.D.
Professor, Departments of Medicine and Public Health Sciences, Wake Forest University School of Medicine, Winston-Salem; Adjunct Professor of Epidemiology, School of Public Health, University of North Carolina at Chapel Hill, Chapel Hill, North Carolina
B-Mode Ultrasound: A Noninvasive Method for Assessing Atherosclerosis

Gladwin Das, M.D.
Assistant Professor of Medicine (Cardiology), University of Minnesota Medical School–Minneapolis; Attending Physician, Fairview-University Medical Center, Minneapolis, Minnesota
Pathophysiology, Clinical Recognition, and Treatment of Congenital Heart Disease ■ Cardiac Catheterization (Valvular Heart Disease)

Dominick S. D'Aunno, M.D.
Associate Professor, National Space Biomedical Research Institute, Baylor College of Medicine; Research Associate, Division of Space Life Sciences, Cardiovascular Laboratory, NASA, Johnson Space Center, Houston, Texas
Cardiovascular Changes Associated With Space Flight

Ali Denktas, M.D.
Cardiology Staff, University of Texas–Houston Medical School; Cardiologist, Hermann Hospital, Houston, Texas
Percutaneous Coronary Intervention for Acute Myocardial Infarction

Victor J. Dzau, M.D.
Professor and Chairman, Department of Medicine; Physician in Chief, Brigham and Women's Hospital, Harvard Medical School, Boston, Massachusetts
Circulatory Regulation: The Role of Vascular Remodeling

†Deceased.

Kim A. Eagle, M.D.
Professor of Internal Medicine and Senior Associate Chair, Department of Internal Medicine, Chief of Clinical Cardiology, The University of Michigan Medical Center, Ann Arbor, Michigan
Evaluation of Patients for Noncardiac Surgery

Jesse E. Edwards, M.D.
Professor, Laboratory Medicine and Pathology, University of Minnesota Medical School–Minneapolis, Minneapolis; Senior Consultant, JEE Cardiovascular Registry, United Hospital, St. Paul, Minnesota
Anatomic Abnormalities (Congenital Heart Disease in the Adult)

Eric J. Eichhorn, M.D.
Professor of Medicine, Cardiac Catheterization Laboratory, Department of Internal Medicine, University of Texas Southwestern Medical Center, Dallas, Texas
Substance Abuse and the Heart

Maurice Enriquez-Sarano, M.D.
Associate Professor of Medicine, Mayo Medical School; Consultant, Cardiovascular Diseases and Internal Medicine, Mayo Clinic, Rochester, Minnesota
Mitral Valve Disease

Charles D. Ericsson, M.D.
Professor of Medicine and Head, Clinical Infectious Diseases, Department of Internal Medicine, University of Texas–Houston Medical School, Houston, Texas
Prosthetic Valve Endocarditis

Rosa Maria Estrada y Martin, M.D.
Instructor, Division of Pulmonary and Critical Care Medicine, Department of Medicine, University of Texas–Houston Medical School, Houston, Texas
Chronic Obstructive Pulmonary Disease

William Fabian, M.D.
Assistant Professor of Medicine, Cardiovascular Division, Department of Medicine, University of Minnesota Medical School–Minneapolis, Minneapolis, Minnesota
Syncope

Andrew Farb, M.D.
Staff Cardiovascular Pathologist, Department of Cardiovascular Pathology, Armed Forces Institute of Pathology, Washington, D.C.
Coronary Artery Disease in Women

John Farmer, M.D.
Associate Professor, Sections of Cardiology and Atherosclerosis, Department of Medicine, Baylor College of Medicine; Chief of Cardiology, Ben Taub General Hospital, Houston, Texas
Atherosclerosis: Pathogenesis, Morphology, and Risk Factors

Diane Fatkin, M.D., B.Sc.(Med.), F.R.A.C.P.
Instructor in Medicine, Harvard Medical School; Research Fellow, Department of Genetics, Harvard Medical School and Howard Hughes Medical Institute; Physician, Department of Medicine, Brigham and Women's Hospital, Boston, Massachusetts
Hypertrophic Cardiomyopathy

James J. Ferguson, M.D.
Assistant Professor, Baylor College of Medicine; Clinical Assistant Professor, University of Texas–Houston Medical School; Associate Director, Cardiology Research, St. Luke's Episcopal Hospital–Texas Heart Institute, Houston, Texas
Coronary Artery Bypass Surgery and Percutaneous Coronary Intervention: Impact on Morbidity and Mortality in Patients With Coronary Artery Disease ▪ Cardiac Catheterization (Myocardial Disease) ▪ Intravascular Ultrasound: Clinical Applications

Victor J. Ferrans, M.D., Ph.D.
Chief, Pathology Section, National Heart, Lung, and Blood Institute, National Institutes of Health, Bethesda, Maryland
Anatomic Abnormalities (Valvular Heart Disease) ▪ Anatomic Abnormalities (Myocardial Disease) ▪ Anatomic Abnormalities (Pericardial Disease)

Pim J. de Feyter, M.D.
Interventional Cardiologist, University Hospital Rotterdam–Dijkzigt, Rotterdam, The Netherlands
Percutaneous Coronary Intervention for Unstable Coronary Artery Disease

Peter J. Fitzgerald, M.D., Ph.D.
Associate Professor of Medicine, and Co-Director, Center for Research in Cardiovascular Intervention, Stanford University Medical Center, Stanford, California
Intravascular Ultrasound

G. Fontaine, M.D., Ph.D.
Associate Professor of Cardiology, School of Medicine, University of Paris VI–Pitié Salpetrière; Research Director, Department of Cardiology, Jean Rostand Hospital, Ivry-sur-Seine, France
Arrhythmogenic Right Ventricular Dysplasia

F. Fontaliran, M.D.
Staff Physician, Department of Cardiology, Jean Rostand Hospital, Ivry-sur-Seine, France
Arrhythmogenic Right Ventricular Dysplasia

R. Frank, M.D.
Associate Professor of Cardiology, School of Medicine, University of Paris VI–Pitié Salpetrière; Chief, Department of Cardiology, Jean Rostand Hospital, Ivry-sur-Seine, France
Arrhythmogenic Right Ventricular Dysplasia

O. H. Frazier, M.D.
Professor of Surgery, University of Texas–Houston Medical School; Director, Surgical Research, and Chief, Cardiopulmonary Transplantation, St. Luke's Episcopal Hospital–Texas Heart Institute, Houston, Texas
Surgical Treatment (Valvular Heart Disease) ▪ Surgical Treatment (Coronary Artery Disease) ▪ Surgical Treatment of Advanced Heart Failure ▪ Diseases of the Aorta

Herbert L. Fred, M.D.
Professor of Medicine, University of Texas Health Science Center at Houston; Clinical Director, Department of Internal Medicine, Lyndon B. Johnson General Hospital, Houston, Texas
Pulmonary Embolism

Daniel B. Friedman, M.D.
Assistant Professor, Department of Internal Medicine, University of Texas Southwestern Medical Center at Dallas; Director, Cardiac Rehabilitation Program, Parkland Memorial Hospital, Dallas, Texas; Presbyterian Heart Group, Albuquerque, New Mexico
Exercise

Victor F. Froelicher, M.D.
Professor of Medicine, Stanford School of Medicine; Director-ECG/Exercise Laboratory, Cardiology Division, Veterans Affairs Palo Alto Health Care System, Palo Alto, California
Cardiac Rehabilitation

Robert L. Frye, M.D.
Rose M. and Morris Eisenberg Professor of Medicine and Chairman, Department of Internal Medicine, Mayo Medical School; Consultant, Cardiovascular Diseases, Mayo Clinic, Rochester, Minnesota
Aortic Valve Disease ▪ Mitral Valve Disease

Curt D. Furberg, M.D., Ph.D.
Professor, Department of Public Health Sciences, Wake Forest University School of Medicine, Winston-Salem, North Carolina
B-Mode Ultrasound: A Noninvasive Method for Assessing Atherosclerosis

Charles R. Garcia-Rodriguez, M.B.B.S.
Visiting Associate, Anesthesiology, Duke University Medical Center; Attending Anesthesiologist, Durham Veterans Affairs Medical Center, Durham, North Carolina
Intraoperative Hemodynamic Monitoring

Michael Gatzoulis, M.D., Ph.D., F.A.C.C.
Senior Lecturer, National Heart and Lung Institute, Imperial College of Medicine; Consultant Cardiologist, Royal Brompton Hospital, London, England
Surgical Treatment (Congenital Heart Disease in the Adult)

Gary Gerstenblith, M.D.
Professor of Medicine, and Director of Clinical Trials, Cardiology Division, Johns Hopkins School of Medicine, Baltimore, Maryland
Aging and the Cardiovascular System

N. Martin Giesecke, M.D.
Attending Anesthesiologist, Texas Heart Institute, Houston, Texas
Anesthesia for Cardiovascular Operations

Michael H. Gollob, M.D.
Cardiology Division, Baylor College of Medicine, Houston, Texas
Pacing and Defibrillation: Permanent Cardiac Pacing ▪ Pacing and Defibrillation: The Implantable Cardioverter-Defibrillator

John F. Goodwin, M.D., F.A.C.P.(Hon.), F.A.C.C., F.E.S.C.
Emeritus Professor, Department of Clinical Cardiology, Royal Postgraduate Medical School, London, United Kingdom
Restrictive Cardiomyopathy

Antonio M. Gotto, Jr., M.D., D.Phil.
The Stephen and Suzanne Weiss Dean, and Professor of Medicine, Weill Medical College of Cornell University, New York, New York
Atherosclerosis: Pathogenesis, Morphology, and Risk Factors

K. Lance Gould, M.D.
Martin Bucksbaum Distinguished University Chair, Professor of Medicine, University of Texas–Houston Medical School; Director, Weatherhead P.E.T. Center for Preventing and Reversing Atherosclerosis, Memorial-Hermann Hospital, Houston, Texas
Nuclear Imaging in Coronary Artery Disease

Paul A. Grayburn, M.D.
Professor of Medicine, Cardiac Catheterization Laboratory, Department of Internal Medicine, University of Texas Southwestern Medical Center, Dallas, Texas
Substance Abuse and the Heart

Scott M. Grundy, M.D., Ph.D.
Professor of Medicine, Center for Human Nutrition and the Departments of Clinical Nutrition and Internal Medicine, University of Texas Southwestern Medical Center, Dallas, Texas
Cholesterol Disorders

Peter G. Hagan, M.D.
Clinical Assistant Professor, Division of Cardiology, Internal Medicine Department, University of Michigan Medical School, Ann Arbor, Michigan
Echocardiography and Doppler Evaluation (Valvular Heart Disease)

Robert J. Hall, M.D.
Clinical Professor, Department of Medicine, Baylor College of Medicine; Clinical Professor of Medicine, University of Texas–Houston Medical School; Director, Cardiology Education, St. Luke's Episcopal Hospital–Texas Heart Institute, Houston, Texas
Coronary Artery Bypass Surgery and Percutaneous Coronary Intervention: Impact on Morbidity and Mortality in Patients With Coronary Artery Disease ▪ *Tumors of the Heart*

Ramesh Hariharan, M.D., M.R.C.P.(U.K.)
Assistant Professor of Medicine, Baylor College of Medicine; Staff Physician, Veterans Affairs Medical Center, Houston, Texas
Pulmonary Embolism

John H. Harris, Jr., M.D., D.Sc., F.R.A.C.A.(Hon.)
John S. Dunn Distinguished Professor in Radiology and Professor of Emergency Medicine, University of Texas–Houston Medical School; Radiologist and Chief, Emergency Radiology, Hermann Hospital, Houston, Texas
Principles of Chest Radiography

J. L. Hebert, M.D., Ph.D.
Lecturer, Faculty of Medicine, University of Paris XI; Staff Physician, Department of Cardiovascular Physiology, Hôpital de Bicetre, Le Kremlin Bicetre Cedex, France
Arrhythmogenic Right Ventricular Dysplasia

Craig R. Heim, M.D.
Former Associate Professor, Department of Medicine, Vanderbilt University School of Medicine, Nashville, Tennessee
Smoking

Otto M. Hess, M.D.
Professor of Cardiology, University of Bern; Swiss Cardiovascular Center, University Hospital, Bern, Switzerland
Aortic Valve Disease ▪ *Mitral Valve Disease* ▪ *Pulmonary and Tricuspid Valve Disease*

Andrew K. Hilton, M.D.
Assistant Professor of Anesthesiology, Duke University Medical Center; Attending Anesthesiologist, Durham Veterans Affairs Medical Center, Durham, North Carolina
Intraoperative Hemodynamic Monitoring

Alan T. Hirsch, M.D.
Associate Professor of Medicine and Radiology; Director, Vascular Medicine Program, Minnesota Vascular Diseases Center, University of Minnesota Medical School–Minneapolis, Minneapolis, Minnesotta
Peripheral Vascular Diseases

Jeffrey M. Isner, M.D.
Professor of Medicine and Pathology, Tufts University School of Medicine; Chief, Vascular Medicine and Cardiovascular Research, St. Elizabeth's Medical Center, Boston, Massachusetts
Gene Therapy (Vascular Medicine)

Grzegorz Kaluza, M.D., Ph.D.
Interventional Cardiology Research Fellow, Section of Cardiology, Department of Medicine, Baylor College of Medicine, Houston, Texas
Silent Ischemia

William B. Kannel, M.D.
Department of Medicine, Evans Memorial Research Foundation, Boston University Medical Center, Boston, Massachusetts
Coronary Risk Factors: An Overview

Norman M. Kaplan, M.D.
Clinical Professor of Internal Medicine, University of Texas Southwestern Medical Center, Dallas, Texas
Hypertension (Preventive Cardiology)

Arnold M. Katz, M.D., D.Med.(Hon.)
Professor of Medicine, University of Connecticut School of Medicine, Farmington, Connecticut
Regulation of Cardiac Contraction and Relaxation

Chuichi Kawai, M.D.
Professor Emeritus, Kyoto University, Kyoto, Japan
Natural History (Coronary Artery Disease)

Faisal Khan, M.D.
Cardiovascular Surgeon, St. Luke's Episcopal Hospital–Texas Heart Institute, Houston, Texas
Diseases of the Aorta

Neal S. Kleiman, M.D.
Associate Professor of Medicine, Baylor College of Medicine; Assistant Director of Cardiac Catheterization Laboratories, The Methodist Hospital, Houston, Texas
Silent Ischemia

Frank D. Kolodgie, Ph.D.
Research Scientist, Armed Forces Institute of Pathology, Washington, D.C.
Coronary Artery Disease in Women

Zvonimir Krajcer, M.D.
Clinical Professor, Baylor College of Medicine and University of Texas–Houston Medical School; Cardiologist and Program Co-Director, Peripheral Vascular Disease, St. Luke's Episcopal Hospital–Texas Heart Institute, Houston, Texas
Interventional Procedures for Vascular Disease

Edward G. Lakatta, M.D.
Chief, Laboratory and Cardiovascular Science, National Institute on Aging, Baltimore, Maryland
Aging and the Cardiovascular System

Victor R. Lavis, M.D.
Professor of Internal Medicine, Division of Endocrinology, University of Texas–Houston Medical School, Houston, Texas
Endocrine Disorders and the Heart

D. Richard Leachman, M.D.
Clinical Associate Professor of Medicine, University of Texas–Houston Medical School and Baylor College of Medicine; Director, Cardiac Catheterization Laboratory, Texas Heart Institute, St. Luke's Episcopal Hospital, Houston, Texas
Rheumatic Fever

Robert D. Leachman, M.D.†
Rheumatic Fever

Y. LeCarpentier, M.D., Ph.D.
Professor of Physiology, Faculty of Medicine, University of Paris XI; Chief of Cardiorespiratory Function Research, Hôpital de Bicetre, Le Kremlin Bicetre Cedex, France
Arrhythmogenic Right Ventricular Dysplasia

Joseph Lee, M.D.
Consultant in Cardiology, Baylor College of Medicine and Methodist Hospital, Houston, Texas
Neuromuscular Disorders and Heart Disease

Michael F. Lenis, M.D.
Cardiology Unit, Baylor College of Medicine and St. Luke's Episcopal Hospital, Houston, Texas
Pacing and Defibrillation: Permanent Cardiac Pacing

Benjamin D. Levine, M.D.
Associate Professor, Division of Cardiology, Department of Internal Medicine, University of Texas Southwestern Medical Center at Dallas; Director, Cardiac Rehabilitation, Presbyterian Hospital, Dallas, Texas
Exercise

†Deceased.

H. Roger Lijnen, Ph.D.
Professor, Faculty of Medicine, Center for Molecular and Vascular Biology, University of Leuven, Leuven, Belgium
Vascular Endothelial Cell Function and Thrombosis

Sheldon E. Litwin, M.D.
Associate Professor of Internal Medicine, Cardiovascular Division, University of Utah School of Medicine, Salt Lake City, Utah
Cardiac Hypertrophy: Physiologic and Clinical Considerations

Donald M. Lloyd-Jones, M.D.
Fellow, The National Heart, Lung, and Blood Institute's Framingham Heart Study, Boston University School of Medicine, Framingham, Massachusetts
Coronary Risk Factors: An Overview

Henry S. Loeb, M.D.
Professor of Medicine, Loyola University School of Medicine, Maywood; Chief of Cardiology, Edward Hines Veterans Administration Hospital, Hines, Illinois
Shock

Beverly H. Lorell, M.D.
Professor of Medicine, Harvard Medical School; Director, Hemodynamic and Molecular Physiology Laboratory, and Director, Program in Heart Failure, Beth Israel Deaconess Medical Center, Boston, Massachusetts
Clinical Abnormalities of Cardiac Relaxation

Thomas F. Lüscher, M.D.
Professor of Cardiology, Faculty of Medicine, University of Zurich; Head of Cardiology, University Hospital, Zurich, Switzerland
Circulatory Regulation: Basic Considerations

Michael P. Macris, M.D.
Medical Director, Cardiovascular Surgery, Spring Branch Medical Center, Houston, Texas
Surgical Treatment of Advanced Heart Failure

Giuseppe Mancia, M.D.
Professor of Medicine, University of Milan–Bicocca; Chairman, Department of Internal Medicine St. Gerardo Hospital, Monza (Milan), Italy
Circulatory Regulation: Basic Considerations

Douglas L. Mann, M.D.
Chief, Section of Cardiology, Baylor College of Medicine, Veterans Affairs Medical Center, Houston, Texas
Dilated Cardiomyopathy

Warren J. Manning, M.D.
Associate Professor of Medicine and Radiology, Harvard Medical School; Co-Director, Cardiac MR Center, Beth Israel Deaconess Medical Center, Boston, Massachusetts
Magnetic Resonance Imaging ▪ Transesophageal Echocardiography for Patients With Atrial Fibrillation

Keith L. March, M.D., Ph.D.
Associate Professor of Medicine and Physiology, Indiana University School of Medicine, Indianapolis, Indiana
Molecular and Cellular Physiology of Differentiated Vascular Smooth Muscle

Jonathan B. Mark, M.D.
Associate Professor of Anesthesiology, and Assistant Professor of Medicine, Duke University Medical Center; Chief, Anesthesiology Service, Veterans Affairs Medical Center, Durham, North Carolina
Intraoperative Hemodynamic Monitoring

Attilio Maseri, M.D.
Professor of Cardiology, Catholic University of the Sacred Heart; Director, Institute of Cardiology, Rome, Italy
Pathophysiology and Clinical Recognition of Coronary Artery Disease Syndromes

Jay W. Mason, M.D.
Professor and Chair, Department of Internal Medicine, University of Kentucky College of Medicine; Chair, Department of Internal Medicine, Kentucky Clinic, Lexington, Kentucky
Myocarditis ▪ *Long QT Syndromes*

Ali Massumi, M.D.
Clinical Professor of Medicine, Baylor College of Medicine; Program Director, Clinical Cardiac EPS, St. Luke's Episcopal Hospital and Texas Heart Institute, Houston, Texas
Sudden Cardiac Death

Christopher J. Mathias, D.Phil., D.Sc., F.R.C.P.
Professor of Neurovascular Medicine, University of London, at Imperial College School of Medicine, St. Mary's Campus, and Institute of Neurology, University College London; Consultant Physician and Director, Neurovascular Medicine Unit, St. Mary's Hospital, and Autonomic Unit, National Hospital for Neurology and Neurosurgery, Queen Square, London, England
Autonomic Dysfunction and Hypotension

Christian M. Matter, M.D.
Research Fellow, Harvard Medical School, and Cardiovascular Research, Department of Medicine, Brigham and Women's Hospital, Boston, Massachusetts
Circulatory Regulation: The Role of Vascular Remodeling

Wojciech Mazur, M.D.
Medical Resident, Division of Cardiology, Department of Medicine, Baylor College of Medicine, The Methodist Hospital, Houston, Texas
Silent Ischemia

Hugh A. McAllister, Jr., M.D.
Clinical Professor of Pathology, Baylor College of Medicine and University of Texas–Houston Medical School; Chief, Department of Pathology, St. Luke's Episcopal Hospital–Texas Heart Institute, Houston, Texas
Anatomic Abnormalities (Valvular Heart Disease) ▪ *Anatomic Abnormalities and Pathogenesis (Coronary Artery Disease)* ▪ *Anatomic Abnormalities (Myocardial Disease)* ▪ *Anatomic Abnormalities (Pericardial Disease)* ▪ *Tumors of the Heart*

A. Iain McGhie, M.D.
Clinical Assistant Professor of Medicine, University of Missouri–Kansas City School of Medicine; Staff Cardiologist, Mid-America Heart Institute, St. Luke's Hospital, Kansas City, Missouri
Nuclear Imaging ▪ *Radionuclide Techniques of Evaluation (Valvular Heart Disease)* ▪ *Exercise Testing* ▪ *Nuclear Imaging in Coronary Artery Disease* ▪ *Radionuclide Techniques in Cardiomyopathies and Myocarditis*

Gary E. McVeigh, M.D., Ph.D.
Senior Lecturer, The Queen's University Belfast; Consultant Physician, Belfast City Hospital, Belfast, Northern Ireland
Arterial Compliance

Rajendra H. Mehta, M.D.
Clinical Assistant Professor of Internal Medicine, University of Michigan Health System, Ann Arbor, Michigan
Evaluation of Patients for Noncardiac Surgery

Evangelos D. Michelakis, M.D.
Assistant Professor of Medicine, Department of Medicine, Division of Cardiology, University of Alberta, Edmonton, Alberta, Canada
Pulmonary Hypertension

Dianna Milewicz, M.D., Ph.D.
Associate Professor of Medicine, and Director, Division of Medical Genetics, University of Texas–Houston Medical School, Houston, Texas
Classification of Genetic Disorders ▪ *Inherited Disorders of Connective Tissue* ▪ *Genetic Aspects of Congenital Heart Disease*

Leslie W. Miller, M.D.
Professor of Medicine, and Director, Cardiovascular Division, University of Minnesota Medical School–Minneapolis; Attending Physician, Fairview-University Medical Center, Minneapolis, Minnesota
Heart Transplantation: Indications, Outcome, and Long-Term Complications ▪ *Heart Transplantation: Pathogenesis, Immunosuppression, and Diagnosis and Treatment of Rejection*

Jere H. Mitchell, M.D.
Professor of Medicine and Physiology and Director, Moss Heart Center, University of Texas Southwestern Medical Center at Dallas, Dallas, Texas
Exercise

Ali Moustapha, M.D.
Department of Internal Medicine, Division of Cardiology, University of Texas–Houston Medical School, Houston, Texas
Homocysteine and Vascular Disease

Susan D. Mueller, M.D.
Network Medical Director, Aetna US Healthcare, Houston, Texas
Pregnancy and the Heart

Charles E. Mullins, M.D.
Professor of Pediatrics, Baylor College of Medicine; Director Emeritus, Cardiac Catheterization Laboratories, Texas Children's Hospital, Houston, Texas
Interventional Therapy

Elizabeth G. Nabel, M.D.
Professor of Medicine, Division of Cardiology, University of Michigan Medical Center, Ann Arbor, Michigan; Scientific Director, Clinical Programs, National Institutes of Health National Heart, Lung, and Blood Institute, Bethesda, Maryland
Gene Therapy (Preventive Cardiology)

Gary J. Nabel, M.D., Ph.D.
Professor of Internal Medicine and Biological Chemistry, University of Michigan Medical Center, Ann Arbor, Michigan; Director, Vaccine Research Center, National Institutes of Medicine, Bethesda, Maryland
Gene Therapy (Preventive Cardiology)

Gerald V. Naccarelli, M.D.
Professor of Medicine, Pennsylvania State University College of Medicine; Chief, Division of Cardiology, and Director, Cardiovascular Center, Penn State Geisenger–Milton S. Hershey Medical Center, Hershey, Pennsylvania
Recognition and Physiologic Treatment of Cardiac Arrhythmias and Conduction Disturbances ■ Atrial Fibrillation/Flutter ■ Antiarrhythmic Drugs

Yasuyuki Nakamura, M.D.
Associate Professor, Shiga University of Medical Science, Otsu, Shiga, Japan
Natural History (Coronary Artery Disease)

Jagat Narula, M.B., M.D., D.M., Ph.D., F.A.C.C.
Associate Professor of Medicine, Division of Cardiovascular Diseases, Medical College of Pennsylvania and Hahnemann University Medical School; Director, Center for Molecular Cardiology, and Director, Center for Heart Failure and Transplantation Research, Hahnemann University Hospital, Philadelphia, Pennsylvania
Rheumatic Fever

Pascal Nicod, M.D.
Professor and Chairman, Department of Internal Medicine, University of Lausanne; University Hospital, Lausanne, Switzerland
Aortic Valve Disease ■ Pulmonary and Tricuspid Valve Disease ■ Mitral Valve Disease

John A. Oates, Jr., M.D.
Professor and Chairman Emeritus, Department of Medicine, Vanderbilt University School of Medicine, Nashville, Tennessee
Smoking

Eric N. Olson, Ph.D.
Professor and Chair, Department of Molecular Biology and Oncology, University of Texas Southwestern Medical Center at Dallas Southwestern Medical School, Dallas, Texas
Cardiac Development: Toward a Molecular Basis for Congenital Heart Disease

David Ott, M.D.
Clinical Professor of Surgery, University of Texas–Houston Medical School and Baylor College of Medicine; Cardiovascular Surgeon, St. Luke's Episcopal Hospital–Texas Heart Institute, Houston, Texas
Diseases of the Aorta

Igor F. Palacios, M.D.
Associate Professor of Internal Medicine, Harvard Medical School; Director, Interventional Cardiology, Cardiac Catheterization Laboratory, Massachusetts General Hospital, Boston, Massachusetts
Balloon Dilatation of the Cardiac Valves

Shilpesh Patel, M.D.
Cardiologist, Carolina Cardiology Associates, Rock Hill, South Carolina
Neuromuscular Disorders and Heart Disease

Martin D. Phillips, M.D.
Senior Medical Director, Aventis Behring, LLC, King of Prussia, Pennsylvania
Hematologic Disease and Heart Disease

Rosemary Radley-Smith, F.R.C.P., F.A.C.C.
Consultant Pediatric Cardiologist, Harefield Hospital, Harefield, England
Surgical Treatment (Congenital Heart Disease in the Adult)

Abdi Rasekh, M.D.
Staff Cardiologist, Center for Arrhythmia and Electrophysiology, St. Luke's Episcopal Hospital, Texas Heart Institute, Baylor College of Medicine, Houston, Texas
Sudden Cardiac Death

Bharat Raval, M.D.
Professor of Radiology University of Texas–Houston Medical School; Director of CT, Memorial-Hermann Hospital, Houston, Texas
Diseases of the Aorta

Dale G. Renlund, M.D.
Professor of Medicine, University of Utah School of Medicine; Division of Cardiology, LDS Hospital, Salt Lake City, Utah
Myocarditis

Ward A. Riley, Ph.D.
Professor of Neurology, Wake Forest University School of Medicine, Winston-Salem, North Carolina
B-Mode Ultrasound: A Noninvasive Method for Assessing Atherosclerosis

Killian Robinson, M.D.
Associate Professor of Medicine, Ohio State University College of Medicine and Public Health; Cardiology Staff, Cleveland Clinic Foundation, Cleveland, Ohio
Homocysteine and Vascular Disease

Luz Maria Rodriguez, M.D., Ph.D.
Associate Professor of Cardiology, Faculty of Medicine, University of Maastricht; Staff Physician, Department of Cardiology, University Hospital Maastricht, Maastricht, The Netherlands
Radiofrequency Catheter Ablation of Supraventricular and Ventricular Arrhythmias

Thom W. Rooke, M.D.
Professor of Medicine, Mayo Medical School; Head, Section of Vascular Medicine, Mayo Clinic, Rochester, Minnesota
Peripheral Vascular Diseases

Lewis J. Rubin, M.D.
Professor of Medicine, and Director, Pulmonary and Critical Care Medicine, University of California, San Diego, School of Medicine, San Diego, California
Pulmonary Hypertension

Mary E. Russell, M.D.
Adjunct Associate Professor, Harvard School of Public Health, Boston; Medical Director, Parexel International, Waltham, Massachusetts
Heart Transplantation: Indications, Outcome, and Long-Term Complications ▪ Heart Transplantation: Pathogenesis, Immunosuppression, and Diagnosis and Treatment of Rejection

Scott Sakaguchi, M.D.
Assistant Professor of Medicine and Director, Clinical Cardiac Electrophysiology Fellowship Program, University of Minnesota Medical School–Minneapolis, Minneapolis, Minnesota
Syncope

Merle A. Sande, M.D.
Clarence M. and Ruth N. Birrer Professor and Chairman, Department of Medicine, University of Utah School of Medicine, Salt Lake City, Utah
Cardiovascular Involvement in AIDS

Heinrich R. Schelbert, M.D.
Professor of Medicine, University of California, Los Angeles, UCLA School of Medicine; Attending Cardiologist, UCLA Medical Center, Los Angeles, California
Nuclear Imaging in Coronary Artery Disease

Urs Scherrer, M.D.
Professor of Cardiology and Internal Medicine, University of Lausanne; Cardiologist, University Hospital, Lausanne, Switzerland
Aortic Valve Disease ▪ Pulmonary and Tricuspid Valve Disease ▪ Mitral Valve Disease

Michael D. Schneider, M.D.
Professor of Medicine, Molecular and Cellular Biology, and Molecular Physiology and Biophysics, Baylor College of Medicine, Houston, Texas
Cardiac Development: Toward a Molecular Basis for Congenital Heart Disease

John J. Seger, M.D.
Clinical Associate Professor of Internal Medicine (Cardiology), Baylor College of Medicine, University of Texas–Houston Medical School; Electrophysiologist, Texas Heart Institute, St. Luke's Episcopal Hospital, Houston, Texas
Pacing and Defibrillation: Permanent Cardiac Pacing ▪ Pacing and Defibrillation: The Implantable Cardioverter-Defibrillator

Christine E. Seidman, M.D.
Professor of Medicine and Genetics, Harvard Medical School; Investigator, Howard Hughes Medical Institute and Brigham and Women's Hospital; Director, Cardiovascular Genetics Center, Department of Medicine, Cardiovascular Division, Brigham and Women's Hospital, Boston, Massachusetts
Hypertrophic Cardiomyopathy

J. G. Seidman, Ph.D.
Henrietta B. and Frederick H. Bugher Professor of Cardiovascular Genetics, Harvard Medical School; Investigator, Howard Hughes Medical Institute and Department of Genetics, Harvard Medical School, Boston, Massachusetts
Hypertrophic Cardiomyopathy

Ralph Shabetai, M.D., F.A.C.C.
Professor of Medicine Emeritus, University of California, San Diego, School of Medicine; Attending Physician VA Health Care System and UCSD Medical Center, La Jolla, California
Etiology, Pathophysiology, Clinical Recognition, and Treatment (Pericardial Disease)

John T. Shepherd, M.D., D.Sc., F.R.C.P.
Professor, Department of Physiology and Biophysics, Mayo Medical School, Rochester, Minnesota
Circulatory Regulation: Basic Considerations

Jürgen R. Sindermann, M.D.
Postdoctoral Research Fellow, Krannert Institute of Cardiology, Indianapolis, Indiana
Molecular and Cellular Physiology of Differentiated Vascular Smooth Muscle

Richard W. Smalling, M.D., Ph.D.
Professor, University of Texas–Houston Medical School; Medical Director, Cardiac Catheterization Laboratories, Memorial-Hermann Hospital, Houston, Texas
Percutaneous Coronary Intervention for Acute Myocardial Infection

Thomas Smitherman, M.D.
Professor of Medicine, University of Pittsburgh School of Medicine; Director, Coronary Care Unit, University of Pittsburgh Hospital, Pittsburgh, Pennsylvania
The History and Physical Examination

Burton E. Sobel, M.D.
E. L. Amidon Professor and Chair, Department of Medicine, University of Vermont College of Medicine; Physician-in-Chief, Department of Medicine, Fletcher Allen Health Care, Burlington, Vermont
Treatment of Acute Q Wave Myocardial Infarction

Michael S. Sweeney, M.D.
Consultant in Cardiovascular Surgery, Memorial-Hermann Hospital, Houston, Texas
Surgical Treatment (Valvular Heart Disease) ▪ Surgical Treatment (Coronary Artery Disease) ▪ Surgical Treatment of Advanced Heart Failure ▪ Diseases of the Aorta

Bernard Swynghedauw, Ph.D., M.D.
Director of Research, French National Institute of Health and Medical Research (INSERM), Lariboisière Hospital, Paris, France
Cardiac Hypertrophy and Failure: Basic Aspects

Heinrich Taegtmeyer, M.D., D.Phil.
Professor of Medicine, Division of Cardiology, University of Texas–Houston Medical School; Attending Physician, Memorial-Hermann Hospital, Houston, Texas
Fuels for the Heart

Paul S. Teirstein, M.D.
Director, Interventional Cardiology, Green Hospital of Scripps Clinic, La Jolla, California
Radiation Therapy

Francis T. Thandroyen, M.D., Ph.D.
Staff Cardiologist, Greenville Memorial Hospital and Bon Secours St. Francis Hospital; Cardiologist, Cardiovascular Associates, Greenville, South Carolina
Echocardiography (Coronary Artery Disease) ▪ Echocardiography (Myocardial Disease)

Andrew Thorburn, D.Phil.
Associate Professor, Department of Oncological Sciences, University of Utah School of Medicine, Salt Lake City, Utah
Cardiac Hypertrophy: Physiologic and Clinical Considerations

Sara Thorne, M.D., M.R.C.P.
Senior Lecturer, National Heart and Lung Institute, Imperial College of Medicine; Consultant Cardiologist, Royal Brompton Hospital, London, England
Surgical Treatment (Congenital Heart Disease in the Adult)

Carl Timmermans, M.D., Ph.D.
Associate Professor of Cardiology, Faculty of Medicine, University of Maastricht; Staff Physician, Department of Cardiology, University Hospital Maastricht, Maastricht, The Netherlands
Radiofrequency Catheter Ablation of Supraventricular and Ventricular Arrhythmias

Jack L. Titus, M.D.
Professor of Laboratory Medicine and Pathology, University of Minnesota Medical School–Minneapolis, Minneapolis; Adjunct Professor of Pathology, Baylor College of Medicine, Houston, Texas; Director, JEE Cardiovascular Registry, United Hospital, St. Paul, Minnesota
Anatomic Abnormalities (Congenital Heart Disease in the Adult)

Sanjeev Trehan, M.D.
Assistant Professor of Medicine, Division of Cardiology, University of Utah School of Medicine, Salt Lake City, Utah
Myocarditis

Naip Tuna, M.D., Ph.D.
Professor Emeritus, Department of Medicine, Cardiovascular Division, University of Minnesota Medical School–Minneapolis; Attending Physician, Department of Cardiology, Fairview-University Medical Center, Minneapolis, Minnesota
Electrocardiography

Renu Virmani, M.D.
Clinical Professor, Department of Pathology, Georgetown University School of Medicine, Washington, D.C.; Clinical Professor, Department of Pathology, University of Maryland School of Medicine, Baltimore; Clinical Professor, Department of Pathology, Uniformed University of Health Sciences F. Edward Hébert School of Medicine, Bethesda, Maryland; Clinical Professor, Department of Pathology, George Washington University School of Medicine and Health Sciences, Washington, D.C.; Clinical Research Professor, Department of Pathology, Vanderbilt University, School of Medicine, Nashville, Tennessee; Chairperson, Department of Cardiovascular Pathology, Armed Forces Institute of Pathology, Washington, D.C.
Coronary Artery Disease in Women

Bernard Waeber, M.D.
Professor, Faculty of Medicine, University of Lausanne; Chief, Division of Pathophysiology, University Hospital, Lausanne, Switzerland
Hypertension (Vascular Medicine)

Yang Wang, M.B., M.D.
Professor of Medicine (Cardiology) Emeritus, University of Minnesota Medical School–Minneapolis, Minneapolis, Minnesota
Pathophysiology, Clinical Recognition, and Treatment of Congenital Heart Disease ▪ Cardiac Catheterization (Valvular Heart Disease)

E. Kenneth Weir, M.D.
Professor of Medicine and Physiology, Department of Medicine, University of Minnesota Medical School–Minneapolis; Chief, Cardiology, Veterans Affairs Medical Center, Minneapolis, Minnesota
Pulmonary Hypertension, M.D.

Hein J. J. Wellens, M.D.
Professor of Cardiology, Faculty of Medicine, University of Maastricht; Chairman, Department of Cardiology, University Hospital Maastricht, Maastricht, The Netherlands
Atrioventricular Nodal and Subnodal Conduction Disturbances ▪ Supraventricular Tachycardias ▪ Preexcitation ▪ The Importance of Atrioventricular Dissociation ▪ Radiofrequency Catheter Ablation of Supraventricular and Ventricular Arrhythmias

Carl W. White, M.D.
Professor of Medicine, Cardiovascular Division, University of Minnesota Medical School–Minneapolis; Attending Physician, Fairview-University Medical Center, Minneapolis, Minnesota
Coronary Angiography

James T. Willerson, M.D.
Edward Randall III Professor and Chairman, Department of Internal Medicine, University of Texas–Houston Medical School; Chief of Internal Medicine Service, Memorial-Hermann Hospital; Medical Director, Texas Heart Institute; Chief of Cardiology, St. Luke's Episcopal Hospital, Texas Medical Center, Houston, Texas
The History and Physical Examination ▪ Pathophysiology and Clinical Recognition of Coronary Artery Disease Syndromes ▪ Exercise Testing ▪ Nuclear Imaging in Coronary Artery Disease ▪ Medical Treatment of Stable Angina ▪ Medical Treatment of Unstable Angina and Non–Q Wave Myocardial Infarction ▪ Treatment of Acute Q Wave Myocardial Infarction ▪ Restrictive Cardiomyopathy ▪ Other Cardiomyopathies ▪ Diseases of the Aorta ▪ Recognition and Physiologic Treatment of Cardiac Arrhythmias and Conduction Disturbances ▪ Endocrine Disorders and the Heart ▪ Connective Tissue Diseases and the Heart ▪ Neuromuscular Disorders and Heart Disease ▪ Hematologic Disease and Heart Disease ▪ Pregnancy and the Heart

James M. Wilson, M.D.
Clinical Associate Professor, Baylor College of Medicine; Staff Cardiologist, Texas Heart Institute and St. Luke's Episcopal Hospital, Houston, Texas
Coronary Artery Bypass Surgery and Percutaneous Coronary Intervention: Impact on Morbidity and Mortality in Patients With Coronary Artery Disease

Robert F. Wilson, M.D.
Associate Professor of Medicine, Cardiovascular Division, University of Minnesota Medical School–Minneapolis; Director, Catheterization Laboratory, Fairview-University Medical Center, Minneapolis, Minnesota
Coronary Angiography

Walter R. Wilson, M.D.
Professor, Department of Medicine, Mayo Medical School; Chief, Division of Infectious Diseases, Mayo Medical Clinic, Rochester, Minnesota
Infective Endocarditis

Michael D. Winniford, M.D.
Vice Chair and Professor of Medicine, Department of Internal Medicine, University of Iowa College of Medicine; Physician Director, UI Heart Care, Heart and Vascular Center, University of Iowa Hospital, Iowa City, Iowa
Smoking

Magdi Yacoub, F.R.C.S., F.R.S.
British Heart Foundation Professor of Cardiothoracic Surgery, Department of Cardiothoracic Surgery, National Heart and Lung Institute, Imperial College School of Science, Technology and Medicine; Royal Brompton and Hospital, London, England
Surgical Treatment (Congenital Heart Disease in the Adult)

Paul G. Yock, M.D.
Professor of Medicine, and Director, Center for Research in Cardiovascular Intervention, Stanford University Medical Center, Stanford, CA
Intravascular Ultrasound

Munir Zaqqa, M.D.
Staff Cardiologist, Texas Heart Institute and St. Luke's Episcopal Hospital, Houston, Texas
Sudden Cardiac Death

O. Zenati, M.D.
Fellow in Cardiology and Research, School of Medicine, University of Paris VI–Pitié Salpetrière, Jean Rostand Hospital, Department of Cardiology, Ivry-sur-Seine, France
Arrhythmogenic Right Ventricular Dysplasia

PREFACE

In developing the second edition of *Cardiovascular Medicine,* our goal has been to provide an authoritative and comprehensive review of important, clinically relevant topics pertaining to cardiovascular diseases. The rapid growth of new knowledge regarding mechanisms and management of these diseases has challenged the physician with a wide array of preventive, diagnostic, and therapeutic options. We hope this book will guide the interested physician to more knowledgeable and effective clinical management.

The specialty of cardiovascular medicine has become increasingly international. Recent achievements in basic science and clinical research have not respected national boundaries. Global interaction among scientists and physicians has rapidly expanded, thanks to major improvements in communications technology and to the growing recognition of our interdependence in advancing clinical science. We have therefore made it a priority to integrate in *Cardiovascular Medicine* contributions from American, European, and Asian-Pacific experts in order to provide a balanced discussion of topics and to summarize approaches and opinions from gifted physicians active worldwide in the care and treatment of patients with cardiovascular diseases.

The second edition of *Cardiovascular Medicine* includes discussions of anatomy, clinical and laboratory recognition, mechanisms responsible for cardiovascular abnormalities, and treatment of specific cardiovascular problems. Discussions of pertinent imaging and other noninvasive and invasive diagnostic methods are usually contained within chapters dealing with a particular cardiovascular abnormality, in addition to a new, distinct section on diagnostic testing in the beginning of the book.

We hope that our continued focus in this edition on relevant clinical problems; the organization of anatomic, diagnostic, mechanistic, clinical recognition, and treatment details for each topic within the same chapter; and the international scope of the contributors provides a book that is useful to all who care for patients with cardiovascular diseases. We are committed to a long-term effort to update and improve the book so that it approaches the very best possible contribution using the general theme we initiated in the first edition.

We wish to express our appreciation to our editors at Churchill Livingstone and at W.B. Saunders for the opportunity to undertake this project and for their outstanding help and patience in bringing it to fruition. Our heartfelt thanks go to our families and to our collaborators at the University of Texas Medical School at Houston, the Texas Heart Institute at Houston, and the University of Minnesota Medical School in Minneapolis, who assisted us in the development of this book. We are indeed grateful to our colleagues around the world who have contributed important chapters. Fnally, we express our appreciation to the teachers, students, and patients from whom we have learned so much. It is to them and to our families that we dedicate this book.

James T. Willerson, M.D.
Jay N. Cohn, M.D.

CONTENTS

Color plates follow frontmatter.

SECTION I INTRODUCTION: CARDIAC SIGNS AND SYMPTOMS AND SELECTED NONINVASIVE DIAGNOSTIC METHODS 1

1 The History and Physical Examination 3
James T. Willerson and Thomas Smitherman

2 Electrocardiography 29
Naip Tuna

3 Principles of Chest Radiography 65
John H. Harris, Jr.

4 Echocardiography 76
Eddy Barasch

5 Nuclear Imaging 99
A. Iain McGhie

6 Magnetic Resonance Imaging 133
Warren J. Manning

SECTION II CONGENITAL HEART DISEASE IN THE ADULT 145

7 Anatomic Abnormalities 147
Jack L. Titus and Jesse E. Edwards

8 Pathophysiology, Clinical Recognition, and Treatment of Congenital Heart Disease 179
Yang Wang and Gladwin Das

9 Echocardiography 237
David S. Bach

10 Interventional Therapy 257
Sandra K. Clapp and Charles E. Mullins

11 Surgical Treatment 285
Magdi Yacoub, Michael Gatzoulis, Sara Thorne, and Rosemary Radley-Smith

SECTION III VALVULAR HEART DISEASE 313

12 Anatomic Abnormalities 315
Hugh A. McAllister, Jr., L. Maximilian Buja, and Victor J. Ferrans

13 Aortic Valve Disease 325
Otto M. Hess, Urs Scherrer, Blase A. Carabello, Pascal Nicod, and Robert L. Frye

14 Pulmonary and Tricuspid Valve Disease 343
Otto M. Hess, Urs Scherrer, and Pascal Nicod

15 Mitral Valve Disease 347
Otto M. Hess, Urs Scherrer, Pascal Nicod, Elliot Chesler, Robert L. Frye, and Maurice Enriquez-Sarano

16 Mitral Valve Prolapse (Myxomatous Mitral Valve) 371
Elliot Chesler

17 Rheumatic Fever 386
Robert D. Leachman, D. Richard Leachman, and Jagat Narula

18 Infective Endocarditis 401
Walter R. Wilson and Eddy Barasch

19 Cardiac Catheterization 419
Yang Wang and Gladwin Das

20 Echocardiography and Doppler Evaluation 440
William F. Armstrong and Peter G. Hagan

21 Radionuclide Techniques of Evaluation 459
A. Iain McGhie

22 Balloon Dilatation of the Cardiac Valves 463
Igor F. Palacios

23 Surgical Treatment 485
Denton A. Cooley, O. H. Frazier, and Michael S. Sweeney

SECTION IV CORONARY ARTERY DISEASE ... 501

24 Anatomic Abnormalities and Pathogenesis 503
L. Maximilian Buja and Hugh A. McAllister, Jr.

25 Regulation of Coronary Blood Flow 521
Robert J. Bache

26 Pathophysiology and Clinical Recognition of Coronary Artery Disease Syndromes 528
James T. Willerson and Attilio Maseri

27 Silent Ischemia 569
Wojciech Mazur, Grzegorz Kaluza, and Neal S. Kleiman

28 Coronary Artery Disease in Women 579
Renu Virmani, Allen P. Burke, Andrew Farb, and Frank D. Kolodgie

29 Exercise Testing 586
A. Iain McGhie and James T. Willerson

30 Coronary Angiography 592
Robert F. Wilson and Carl W. White

31 Echocardiography 659
Francis T. Thandroyen and Eddy Barasch

32 Nuclear Imaging in Coronary Artery Disease 671
A. Iain McGhie, K. Lance Gould, Heinrich R. Schelbert, and James T. Willerson

33 Natural History 691
Chuichi Kawai and Yasuyuki Nakamura

34 Medical Treatment of Stable Angina 709
James T. Willerson

35 Medical Treatment of Unstable Angina and Non–Q Wave Myocardial Infarction 723
James T. Willerson

36 Treatment of Acute Q Wave Myocardial Infarction 742
Burton E. Sobel and James T. Willerson

37 Percutaneous Coronary Interventions for Stable Angina Pectoris 790
H. Vernon Anderson

38 Percutaneous Coronary Intervention for Unstable Coronary Artery Disease 802
Pim J. de Feyter

39 Percutaneous Coronary Intervention for Acute Myocardial Infarction 821
Richard W. Smalling and Ali Denktas

40 Radiation Therapy 827
Paul S. Teirstein

41 Surgical Treatment 839
Michael S. Sweeney, O. H. Frazier, and Denton A. Cooley

42 Coronary Artery Bypass Surgery and Percutaneous Coronary Intervention: Impact on Morbidity and Mortality in Patients With Coronary Artery Disease 859
James M. Wilson, James J. Ferguson, and Robert J. Hall

43 Cardiac Rehabilitation 893
Victor F. Froelicher

SECTION V BASIC ASPECTS OF MYOCARDIAL FUNCTION, GROWTH, AND DEVELOPMENT 913

44 Cardiac Development: Toward a Molecular Basis for Congenital Heart Disease 915
Michael D. Schneider and Eric N. Olson

45 Fuels for the Heart 936
Heinrich Taegtmeyer

46 Cardiac Hypertrophy and Failure: Basic Aspects 955
Bernard Swynghedauw and Edouard Coraboeuf

47 Cardiac Hypertrophy: Physiologic and Clinical Considerations 979
Sheldon E. Litwin, Andrew Thorburn, and William H. Barry

48 Regulation of Cardiac Contraction and Relaxation 989
Arnold M. Katz

49 Clinical Abnormalities of Cardiac Relaxation 1001
Beverly H. Lorell

SECTION VI MYOCARDIAL DISEASE 1019

50 Anatomic Abnormalities 1021
Hugh A. McAllister, Jr., L. Maximilian Buja, and Victor J. Ferrans

51 Dilated Cardiomyopathy 1034
Biykem Bozkurt and Douglas L. Mann

52 Hypertrophic Cardiomyopathy 1055
Diane Fatkin, J. G. Seidman, and Christine E. Seidman

53 Restrictive Cardiomyopathy 1075
James T. Willerson and John F. Goodwin

54 Other Cardiomyopathies 1090
James T. Willerson

55 Myocarditis 1096
Sanjeev Trehan, Dale G. Renlund, and Jay W. Mason

56 Cardiac Catheterization 1125
James J. Ferguson

57 Echocardiography 1135
Francis T. Thandroyen and Eddy Barasch

58 Radionuclide Techniques in Cardiomyopathies and Myocarditis 1143
A. Iain McGhie

59 Pathophysiology and Clinical Recognition of Heart Failure 1147
Jay N. Cohn

60 The Management of Heart Failure 1165
Jay N. Cohn

61 Heart Transplantation: Indications, Outcome, and Long-Term Complications 1185
Leslie W. Miller and Mary E. Russell

62 Heart Transplantation: Pathogenesis, Immunosuppression, and Diagnosis and Treatment of Rejection 1210
Mary E. Russell and Leslie W. Miller

63 Surgical Treatment of Advanced Heart Failure 1224
O. H. Frazier, Michael P. Macris, Denton A. Cooley, and Michael S. Sweeney

SECTION VII PERICARDIAL DISEASE 1239

64 Anatomic Abnormalities 1241
Hugh A. McAllister, Jr., L. Maximilian Buja, and Victor J. Ferrans

65 Etiology, Pathophysiology, Clinical Recognition, and Treatment 1245
Ralph Shabetai

SECTION VIII VASCULAR MEDICINE 1273

66 Molecular and Cellular Physiology of Differentiated Vascular Smooth Muscle 1275
Jürgen R. Sindermann, Leonard P. Adam, and Keith L. March

67 Circulatory Regulation: Basic Considerations 1286
John T. Shepherd, Thomas F. Lüscher, and Giuseppe Mancia

68 Circulatory Regulation: The Role of Vascular Remodeling 1299
Victor J. Dzau and Christian M. Matter

69 Vascular Endothelial Cell Function and Thrombosis 1311
H. Roger Lijnen, Jef Arnout, and Désiré Collen

70 Atherosclerosis: Pathologic Anatomy 1325
L. Maximilian Buja

71 Atherosclerosis: Pathogenesis, Morphology, and Risk Factors 1336
Antonio M. Gotto, Jr., and John Farmer

72 Diseases of the Aorta 1354
James T. Willerson, Bharat Raval, Michael S. Sweeney, O. H. Frazier, Faisal Khan, David Ott, and Denton A. Cooley

73 Peripheral Vascular Diseases 1399
Alan T. Hirsch and Thom W. Rooke

74 Gene Therapy 1417
Iris Baumgartner and Jeffrey M. Isner

75 Interventional Procedures for Treatment of Peripheral Vascular Disease 1426
Zvonimir Krajcer

76 B-Mode Ultrasound: A Noninvasive Method for Assessing Atherosclerosis 1446
John R. Crouse, Curt D. Furberg, Robert P. Byington, and Ward A. Riley

77 Intravascular Ultrasound 1454
Paul G. Yock and Peter J. Fitzgerald

78 Newer Imaging Modalities: Intravascular Ultrasound—Clinical Applications 1460
James J. Ferguson

79 Arterial Compliance 1479
Gary E. McVeigh, Alan J. Bank, and Jay N. Cohn

80 Hypertension 1496
Bernard Waeber, Hans R. Brunner, Michel Burnier, and Jay N. Cohn

81 Shock 1529
Henry S. Loeb and Jay N. Cohn

82 Autonomic Dysfunction and Hypotension 1537
Christopher J. Mathias

SECTION IX ELECTRICAL DISTURBANCES OF THE HEART 1561

83 Recognition and Physiologic Treatment of Cardiac Arrhythmias and Conduction Disturbances 1563
Gerald V. Naccarelli, C. Gunnar Blomqvist, and James T. Willerson

84 Sinus Node Dysfunction 1576
David G. Benditt

85 Atrioventricular Nodal and Subnodal Conduction Disturbances 1596
Hein J. J. Wellens

86 Supraventricular Tachycardias 1606
Hein J. J. Wellens

87 Preexcitation 1620
Hein J. J. Wellens

88 Atrial Fibrillation/Flutter 1632
Gerald V. Naccarelli

89 Transesophageal Echocardiography for Patients With Atrial Fibrillation 1650
Warren J. Manning

90 Long QT Syndromes 1656
Steven J. Compton and Jay W. Mason

91 Arrhythmogenic Right Ventricular Dysplasia 1665
G. Fontaine, F. Fontaliran, J. L. Hebert, D. Chemla, O. Zenati, Y. LeCarpentier, and R. Frank

92 The Importance of Atrioventricular Dissociation 1677
Hein J. J. Wellens

93 Syncope 1688
David G. Benditt, William Fabian, and Scott Sakaguchi

94 Sudden Cardiac Death 1710
Abdi Rasekh, Munir Zaqqa, and Ali Massumi

95 Antiarrhythmic Drugs 1739
Gerald V. Naccarelli

96 Pacing and Defibrillation 1758

Permanent Cardiac Pacing 1758
Michael H. Gollob, Michael F. Lenis, and John J. Seger

The Implantable Cardioverter-Defibrillator 1779
Michael H. Gollob and John J. Seger

97 Radiofrequency Catheter Ablation of Supraventricular and Ventricular Arrhythmias 1796
Luz Maria Rodriguez, Carl Timmermans, and Hein J. J. Wellens

98 Surgical Treatment of Arrhythmias 1815
James L. Cox

SECTION

X **CARDIAC EFFECTS OF SYSTEMIC DISORDERS, PREGNANCY, AGING, AND ENVIRONMENTAL CHANGE 1833**

99 Pulmonary Thromboembolism 1835
Herbert L. Fred and Ramesh Hariharan

100 Pulmonary Hypertension 1856
E. Kenneth Weir, Evangelos D. Michelakis, Stephen L. Archer, and Lewis J. Rubin

101 Chronic Obstructive Pulmonary Disease 1885
Steven D. Brown and Rosa Maria Estrada y Martin

102 Tumors of the Heart 1901
Robert J. Hall, Hugh A. McAllister, Jr., Denton A. Cooley, and L. Maximilian Buja

103 Endocrine Disorders and the Heart 1915
Victor R. Lavis and James T. Willerson

104 Connective Tissue Diseases and the Heart 1939
Frank C. Arnett and James T. Willerson

105 Substance Abuse and the Heart 1959
Eric J. Eichhorn and Paul A. Grayburn

106 Cardiovascular Involvement in AIDS 1973
Melvin D. Cheitlin and Merle A. Sande

107 Neuromuscular Disorders and Heart Disease 1985
Joseph Lee, Shilpesh Patel, and James T. Willerson

108 Hematologic Disease and Heart Disease 2001
Martin D. Phillips and James T. Willerson

109 Aging and the Cardiovascular System 2015
Gary Gerstenblith and Edward G. Lakatta

110 Pregnancy and the Heart 2025
Susan D. Mueller and James T. Willerson

111 Cardiovascular Changes Associated With Space Flight 2076
Dominick S. D'Aunno

SECTION

XI **SURGERY AND THE HEART 2089**

112 Evaluation of Patients for Noncardiac Surgery 2091
Rajendra H. Mehta and Kim A. Eagle

113 Anesthesia for Cardiovascular Operations 2104
N. Martin Giesecke and John R. Cooper, Jr.

114 Intraoperative Hemodynamic Monitoring 2116
Charles R. Garcia-Rodriguez, Andrew K. Hilton, and Jonathan B. Mark

SECTION XII **THE GENETIC BASIS FOR CARDIOVASCULAR DISEASE ... 2143**

115 Classification of Genetic Disorders 2145
Dianna Milewicz

116 Inherited Disorders of Connective Tissue 2150
Dianna Milewicz

117 Muscular Dystrophies Affecting the Heart 2160
C. Thomas Caskey

118 Genetic Aspects of Congenital Heart Disease 2170
Dianna Milewicz

SECTION XIII **NEWER IMAGING MODALITIES 2179**

119 Rapid-Speed Computed Tomography 2181
Matthew J. Budoff and Bruce H. Brundage

SECTION XIV **PREVENTIVE CARDIOLOGY 2191**

120 Coronary Risk Factors: An Overview 2193
Donald M. Lloyd-Jones and William B. Kannel

121 Exercise 2216
Benjamin D. Levine, Daniel B. Friedman, C. Gunnar Blomqvist, and Jere H. Mitchell

122 Smoking 2227
John A. Oates, Craig R. Heim, and Michael D. Winniford

123 Hypertension 2234
Norman M. Kaplan

124 Cholesterol Disorders 2244
Scott M. Grundy

125 Obesity 2259
James K. Alexander

126 Gene Therapy 2269
Elizabeth G. Nabel and Gary J. Nabel

127 Homocysteine and Vascular Disease 2277
Ali Moustapha, Ward Casscells, and Killian Robinson

APPENDIX 2286

Prosthetic Valve Endocarditis
Charles D. Ericsson

INDEX 2289

NOTICE

Cardiology is an ever-changing field. Standard safety precautions must be followed, but as new research and clinical experience broaden our knowledge, changes in treatment and drug therapy become necessary or appropriate. Readers are advised to check the product information currently provided by the manufacturer of each drug to be administered to verify the recommended dose, the method and duration of administration, and the contraindications. It is the responsibility of the treating physician, relying on experience and knowledge of the patient, to determine dosages and the best treatment for the patient. Neither the publisher nor the editor assumes any responsibility for any injury and/or damage to persons or property.

THE PUBLISHER

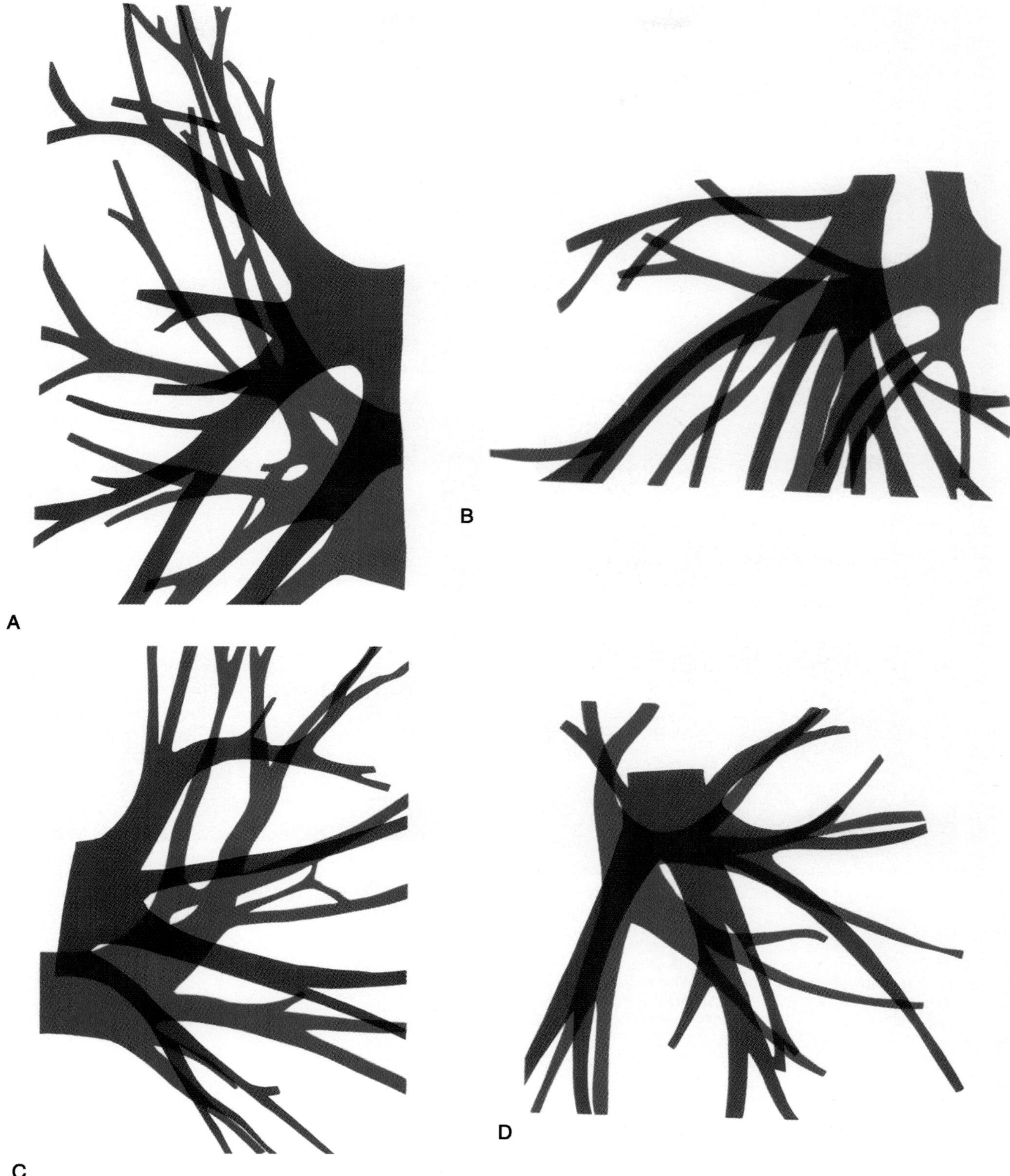

PLATE 3–1 Distribution and relation of pulmonary arteries (blue) and veins (red) in the right upper lobe **(A),** right lower lobe **(B),** left upper lobe **(C),** and left lower lobe **(D)** traced from a pulmonary arteriogram. **A** and **C,** In the upper lobes, the pulmonary arteries tend to be medial to the veins. The upper lobe veins cross the arteries toward the left atrium in a course that is inconsistent with the concept of arborization; for example, the upper lobe veins, if they were arterial in origin, would have a retrograde course from the main pulmonary arteries. **B** and **D,** In the lower lobes, the segmental arteries have an essentially oblique downward course and the veins are transversely oriented, leading to the left atrium.

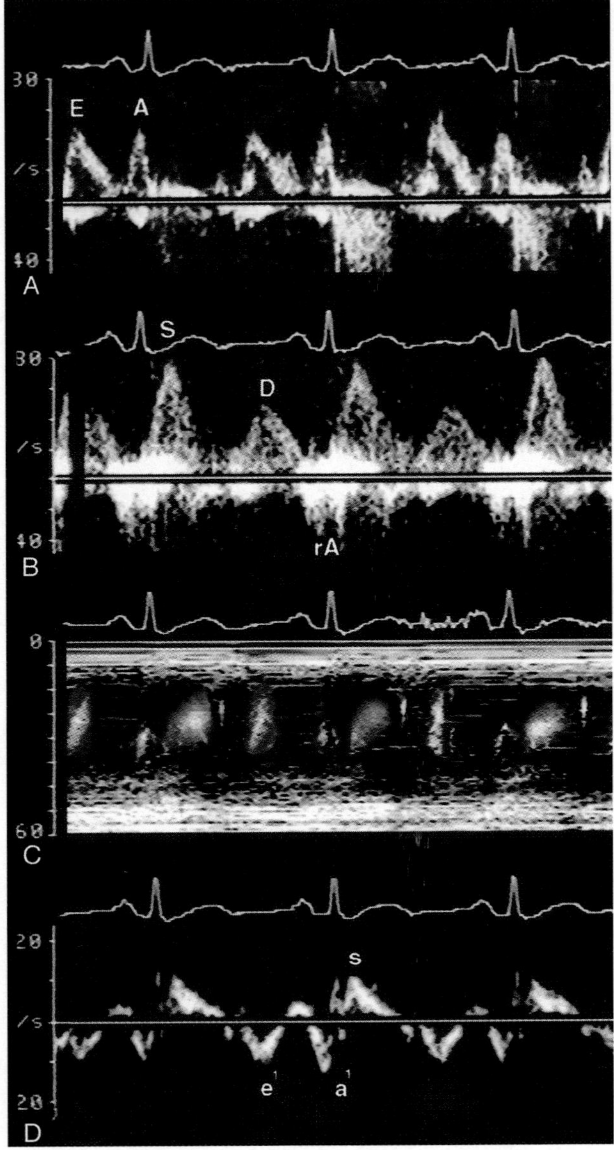

PLATE 4–1 Normal pulse-wave Doppler assessment of left ventricular diastolic function. **A,** Transmitral flow. A, late diastolic filling wave; E, early diastolic filling wave. **B,** Right upper pulmonic vein flow. D, diastolic wave; rA, reverse atrial wave; S, systolic wave. **C,** Transmitral color M-mode. **D,** Doppler tissue imaging interrogation of the lateral aspect of the mitral annulus. a[1], late diastolic wave of the mitral annulus motion; e[1], early diastolic wave of the mitral annulus motion; s, forward systolic wave of the mitral annulus motion.

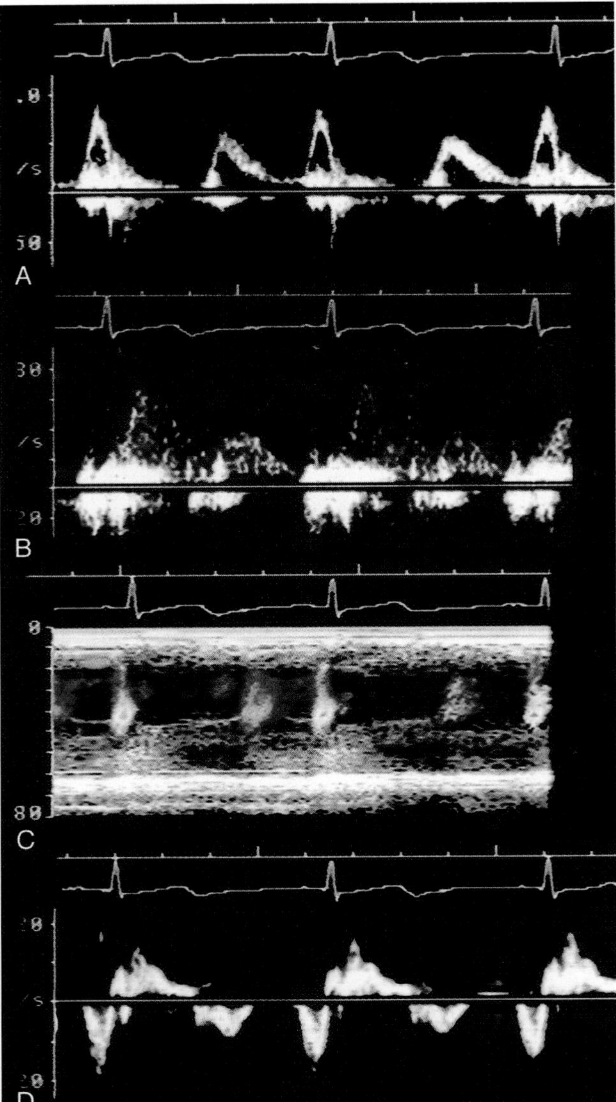

PLATE 4–2 Relaxation impairment pattern of left ventricular filling. The notations are similar to those in Plate 4–1A. **A,** Prolonged deceleration time of E wave, reverse, and E/A ratio. **B,** Predominance of systolic flow. **C,** A shallow slope (lower velocity) of the early transmitral flow. **D,** e′ peak velocity is <8 cm/s, with a more pronounced decrease of e′/a′ ratio than in normals.

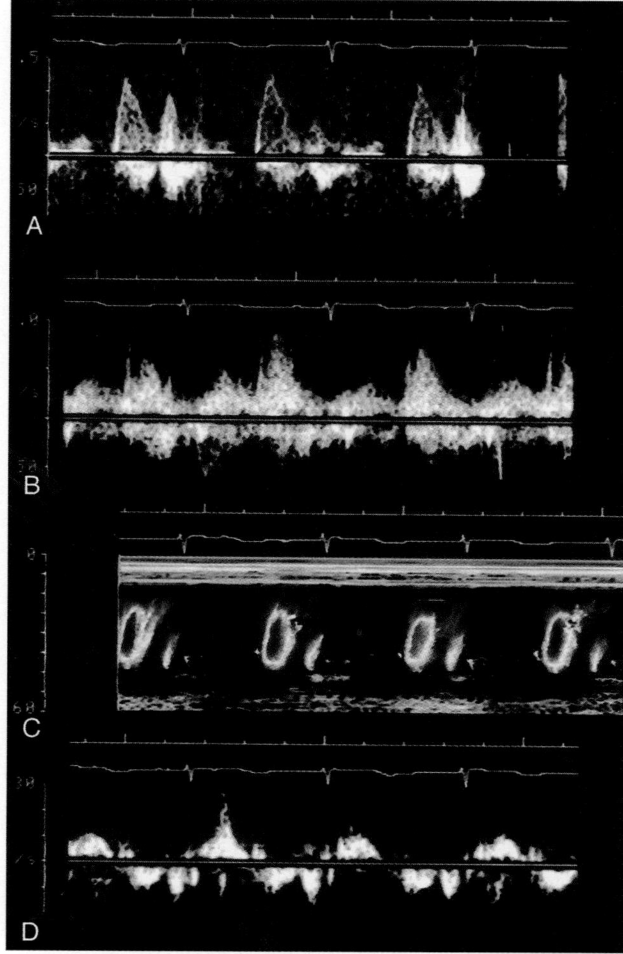

PLATE 4–3 Pseudonormalization pattern of left ventricular filling. An apparently normal transmitral flow **(A)** with a reverse systolic/diastolic (S/D) ratio in the right upper pulmonic vein flow **(B)** are the main Doppler features. **D,** Doppler tissue imaging shows reduced e velocity and e/a ratio.

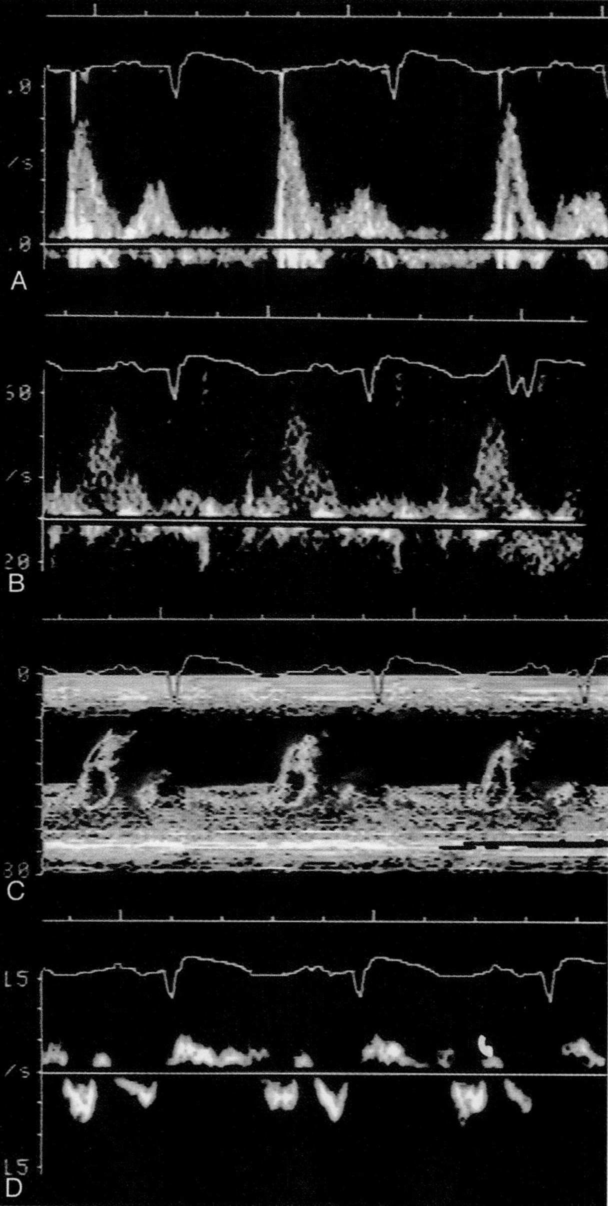

PLATE 4–4 Restriction pattern of left ventricular filling in a 55-year-old patient with dilated cardiomyopathy with severe left ventricular systolic dysfunction. **A,** High E/A ratio with short deceleration time. **B,** Reversed S/D ratio (rA wave not well shown). **C,** Delayed apical filling. **D,** Decrease e′ and s wave velocities (the last reflecting the poor left ventricular systolic function).

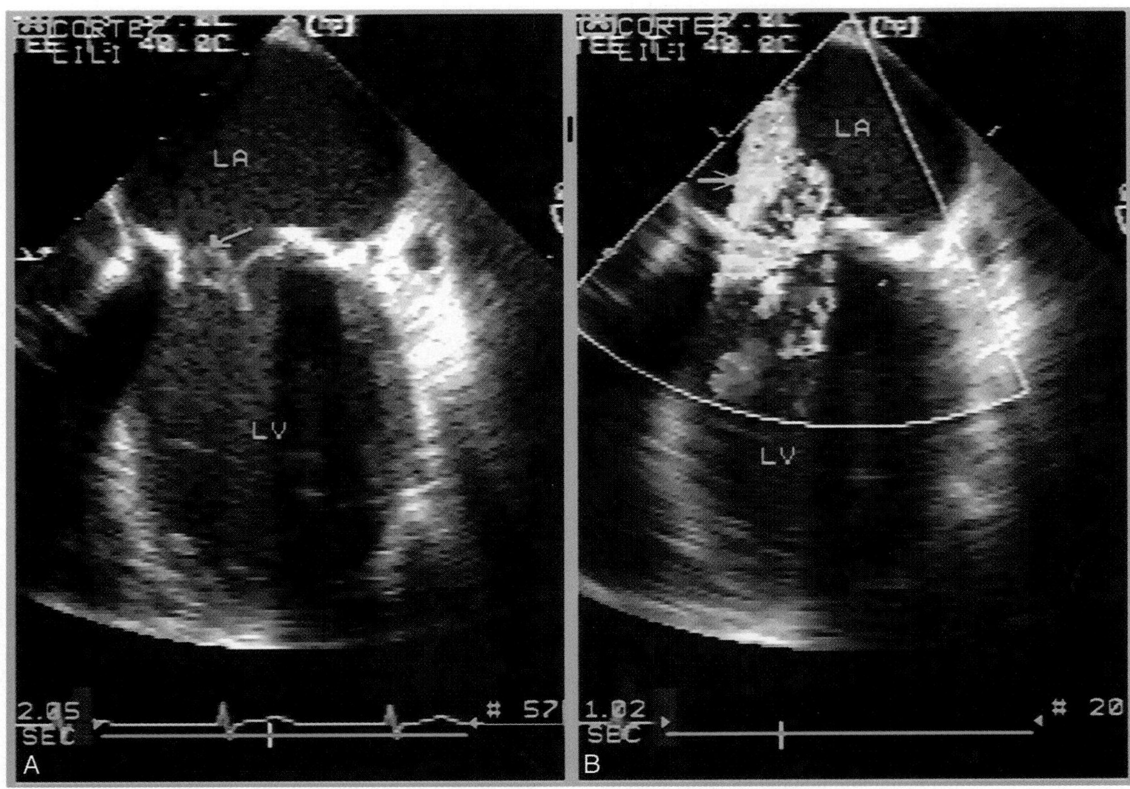

PLATE 4–5 Transesophageal echocardiography (TEE) horizontal plane view **(A)** shows a degenerated biologic prosthetic mitral valve (*arrows*), which explains the presence of moderate mitral regurgitation demonstrated by color-flow Doppler imaging **(B).** LA, left atrium; LV, left ventricle.

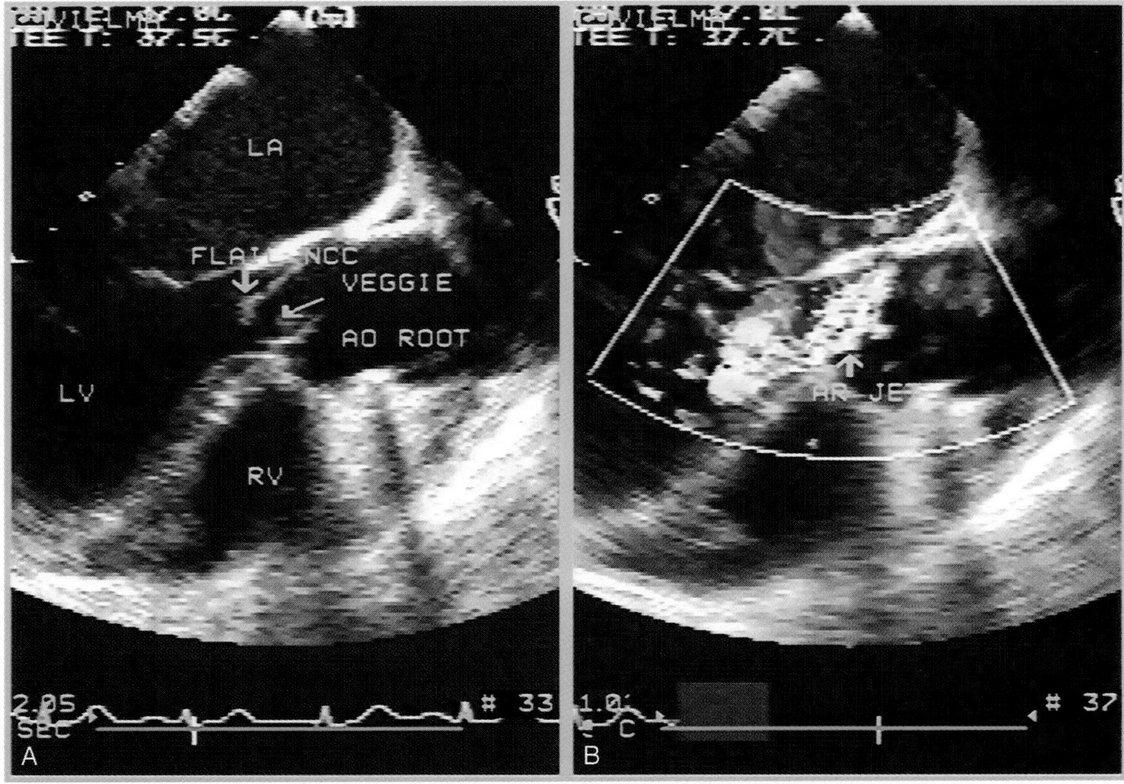

PLATE 4–6 A, TEE multiplane probe at 125 degrees shows a flail noncoronary cusp (NCC; *thick arrow*) and a small vegetation (*thin arrow*) attached to the right coronary cusp. AO root, aortic root; LA, left atrium; LV, left ventricle; RV, right ventricle. **B,** Color-flow Doppler imaging demonstrates the presence of significant aortic regurgitation (AR).

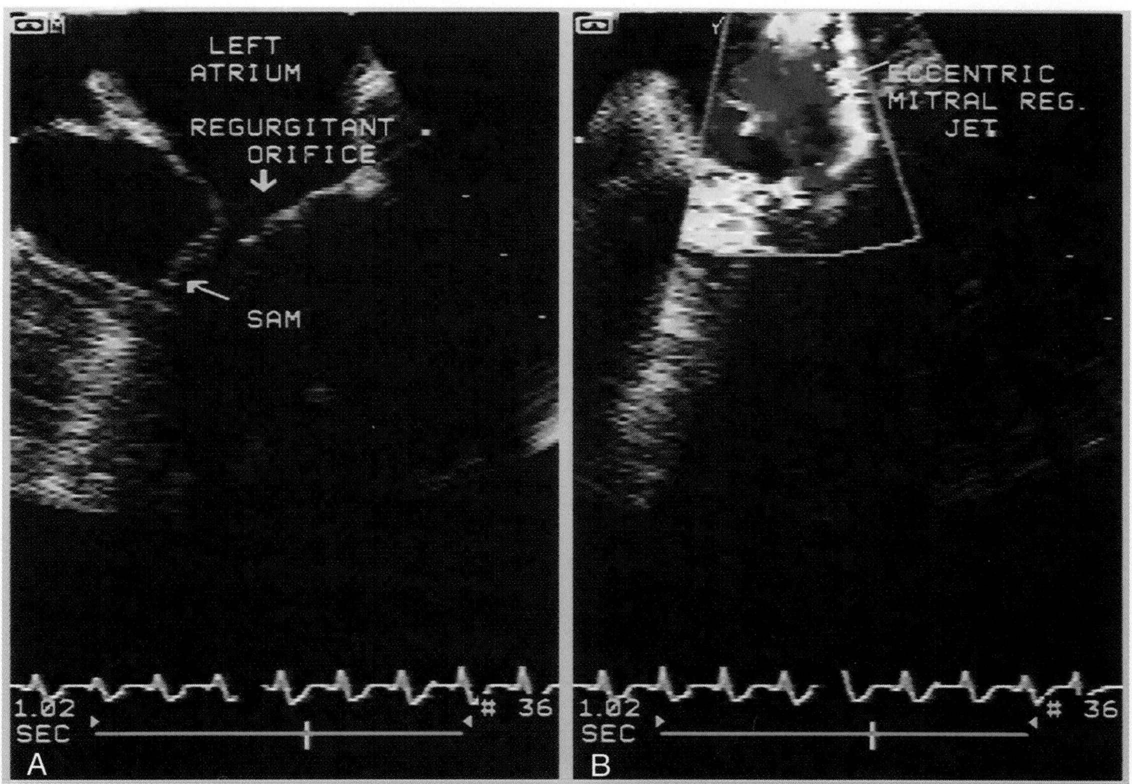

PLATE 4–7 A, TEE horizontal plane shows the systolic anterior motion (SAM) of the anterior mitral leaflet in a patient with hypertrophic obstructive cardiomyopathy. **B,** The presence of mitral regurgitation is shown with an eccentric jet directed toward the lateral wall of the left atrium, explained by SAM.

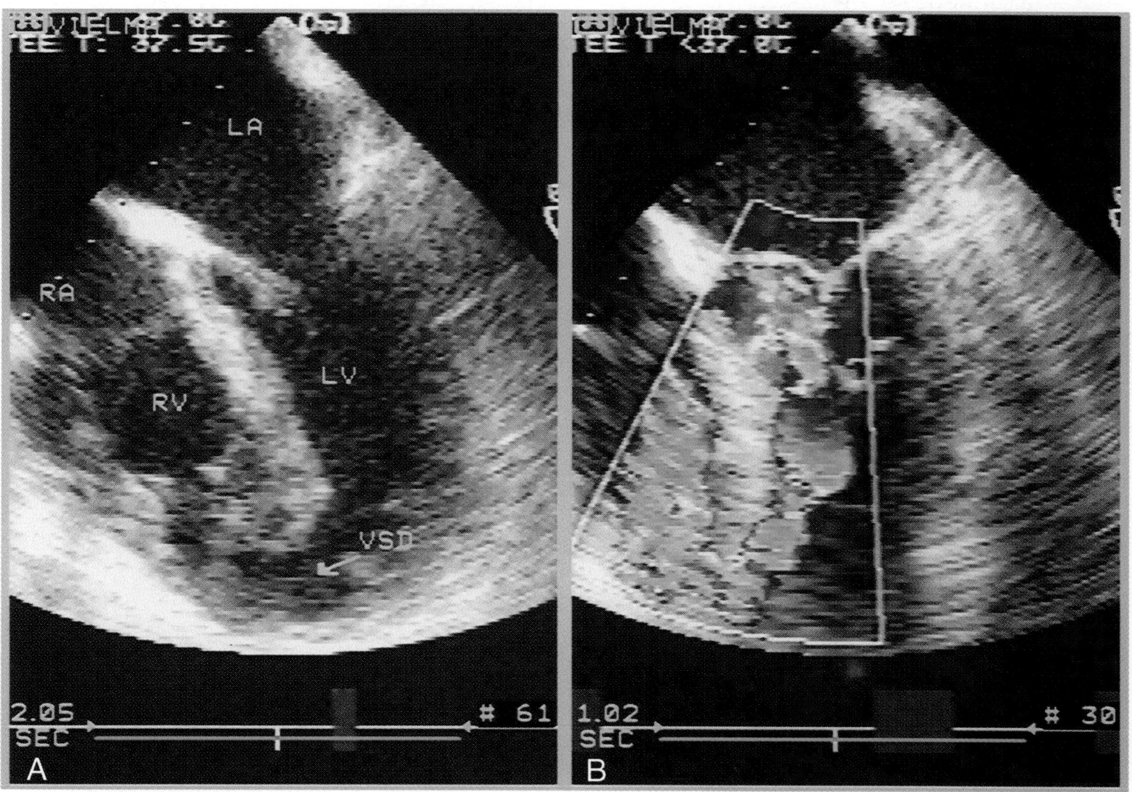

PLATE 4–8 A and **B,** TEE horizontal plane in a patient with an acquired ventricular septal defect (VSD) secondary to an anteroseptal myocardial infarction. LA, left atrium; LV, left ventricle; RA, right atrium; RV, right ventricle.

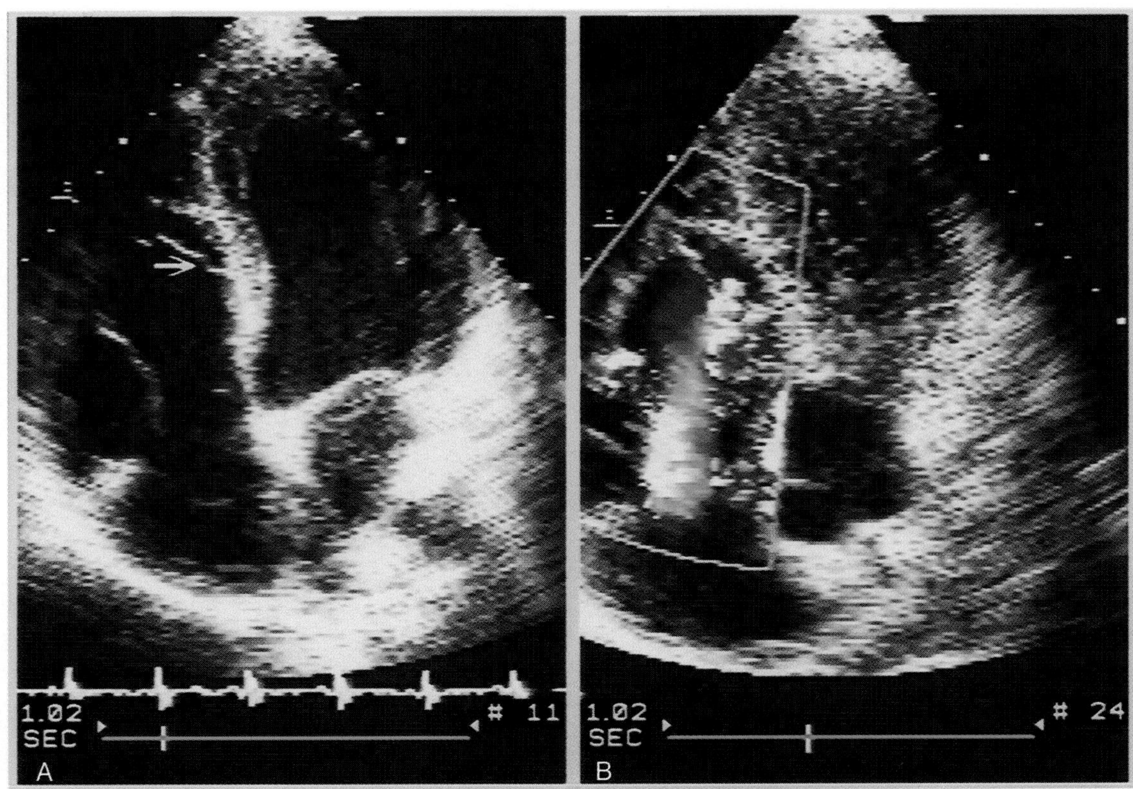

PLATE 4–9 TTE apical four-chamber **(A)** and five-chamber **(B)** views show the apical displacement (3.8 cm) of the septal leaflet of the tricuspid valve (*arrow* in **A**), with atrialization of the right ventricle consistent with Ebstein's anomaly. **B,** The color-flow Doppler image identifies the orifice of the regurgitant jet.

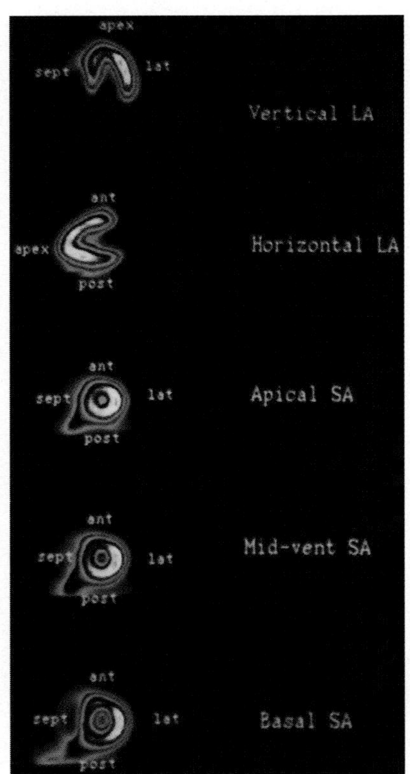

PLATE 5–1 Representative reconstructed tomograms from a myocardial perfusion study. Tomograms, from *top to bottom,* are the vertical long-axis (LA), horizontal long-axis (LA), apical short-axis (SA), midventricular (vent), and basal short-axis sections, respectively. ant, anterior wall; sept, interventricular septum; lat, lateral wall of left ventricle; post, posterior wall.

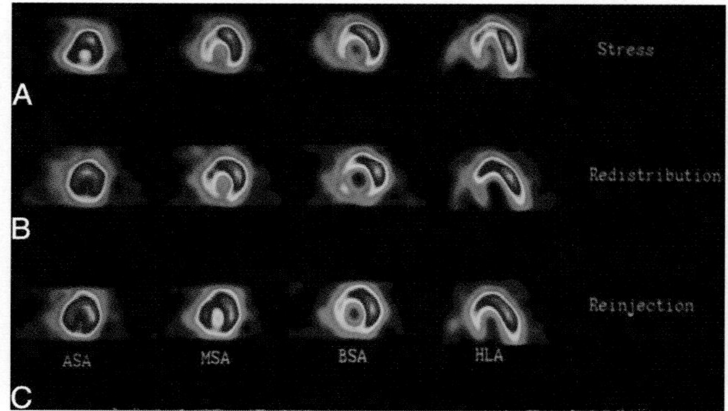

PLATE 5–2 Stress-redistribution-reinjection ^{201}Tl images. **A,** Stress images show areas of hypoperfusion involving the anteroseptal and inferoposterior portions of the left ventricle. **B,** There is minimal redistribution in these areas after 3 hours. **C,** However, following reinjection, there is evidence of significant reversibility in all areas. ASA, apical section; BSA, basal short-axis section; HLA, horizontal long-axis section; MSA, midventricular section.

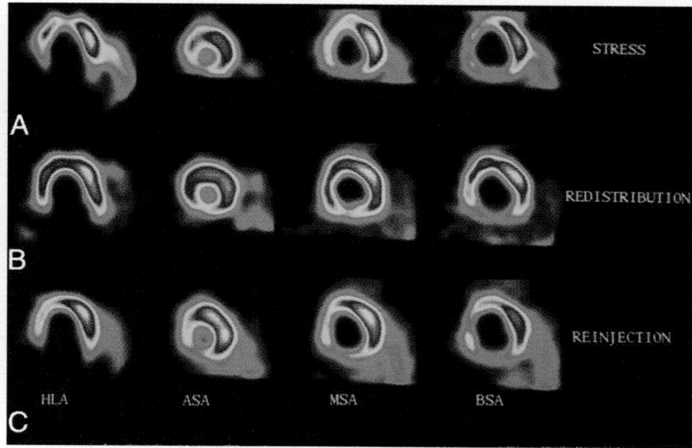

PLATE 5–3 Stress-redistribution-reinjection ^{201}Tl images. **A,** Stress images show severe perfusion defects involving the anteroseptal and inferoposterior aspects of the left ventricle. **B,** There is significant redistribution anteroseptally and inferiorly. **C,** After reinjection, there is significant worsening in these areas. ASA, apical section; BSA, basal short-axis section; HLA, horizontal long-axis section; MSA, midventricular section.

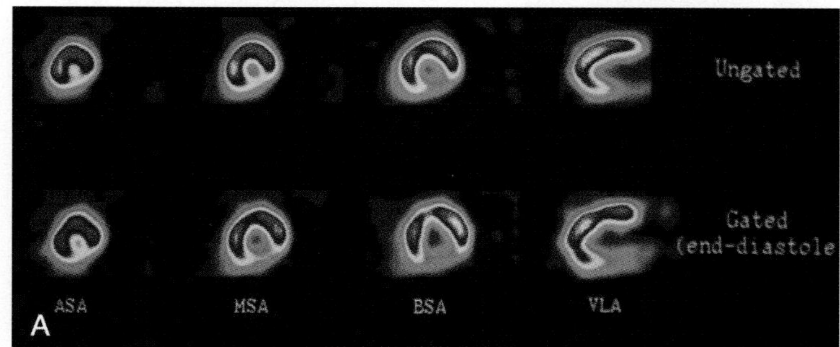

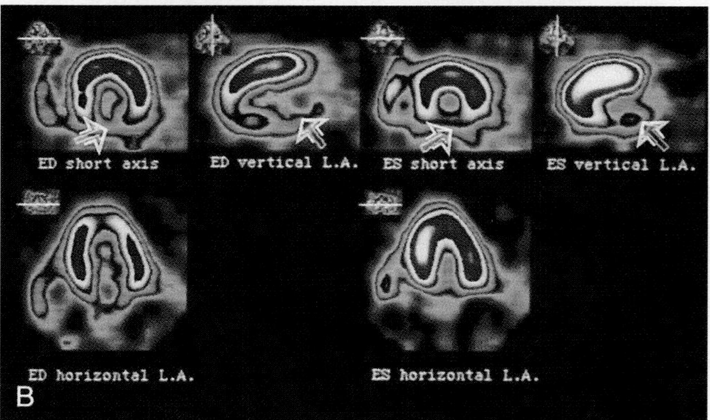

PLATE 5–4 Exercise sestaMIBI tomograms in a patient with right coronary artery disease and disease on the first diagonal branch of the left anterior descending coronary artery. **A,** Comparison of ungated (summed) and gated (end-diastolic) sestaMIBI tomograms. Both images reveal a severe inferior and posterior perfusion defect. In addition, there is an anterior perfusion defect clearly seen in the tomograms in end-diastole. ASA, apical section; BSA, basal short-axis section; MSA, midventricular section; VLA, vertical long-axis section. **B,** Gated postexercise sestaMIBI tomograms in end-diastole (ED) and end-systole (ES). There is a moderate-to-severe inferolateral and posterior perfusion defect (*arrow*) that shows evidence of systolic thickening indicating that the myocardium in this region remains viable. L.A., long axis.

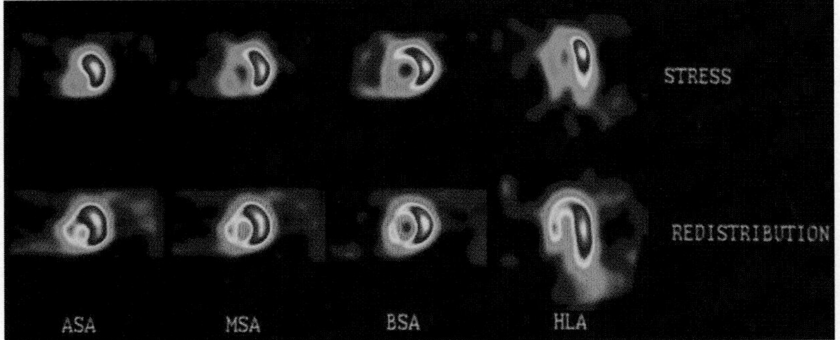

PLATE 5–5 ^{201}Tl tomograms of a patient with severe proximal disease of the left anterior descending coronary artery with no history of prior myocardial infarction. The stress images show a severe anteroseptal perfusion defect that extends inferiorly. Three hours later, redistribution images show evidence of reversibility. ASA, apical section; BSA, basal short-axis section; HLA, horizontal long-axis section; MSA, midventricular section.

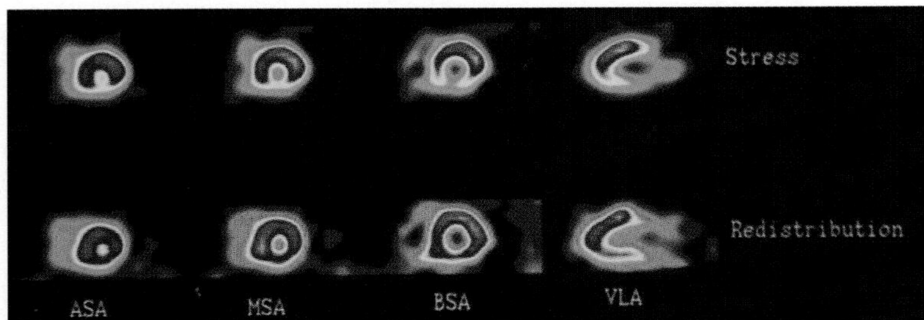

PLATE 5–6 ^{201}Tl tomograms from a patient with right coronary artery disease. The stress images reveal an inferior perfusion defect that extends posteriorly. Three hours later, the defect has almost totally reversed. ASA, apical section; BSA, basal short-axis section; VLA, vertical long-axis section; MSA, midventricular section.

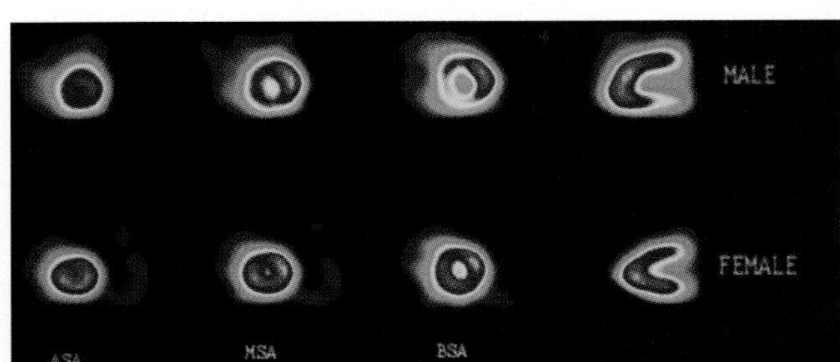

PLATE 5–7 Gender differences in normal ^{201}Tl tomograms. See text for further details. ASA, apical section; BSA, basal short-axis section; MSA, midventricular section.

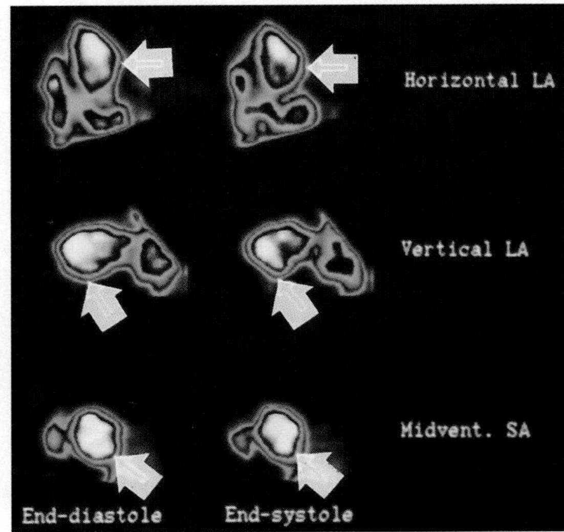

PLATE 5–8 Gated tomographic radionuclide ventriculogram, showing representative horizontal long-axis (LA), vertical LA, and a midventricular (midvent.) short-axis (SA) section. There is a posterolateral left ventricular aneurysm (*arrow*).

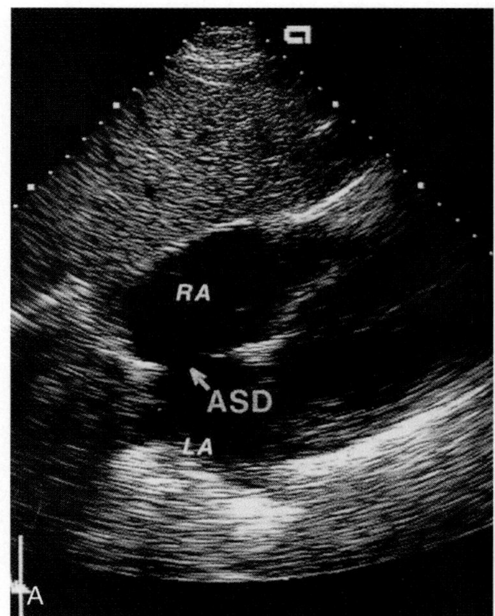

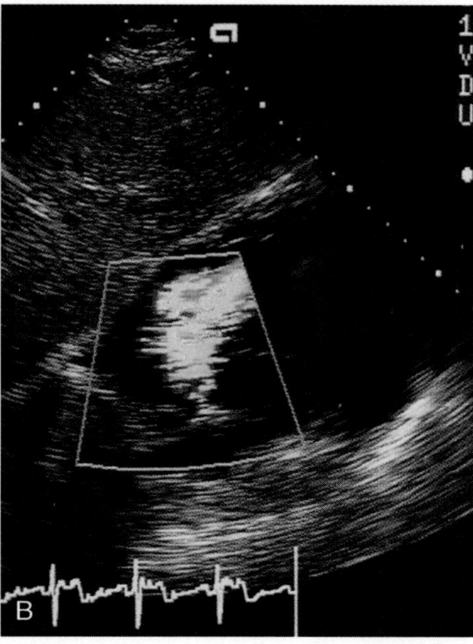

PLATE 9–1 Subcostal echocardiogram of a secundum-type atrial septal defect (ASD). **A,** Drop-out of echoes is noted between the right atrium (RA) and the left atrium (LA), demonstrating direct visualization of the ASD. **B,** Color-flow Doppler imaging demonstrates a predominant left-to-right shunt.

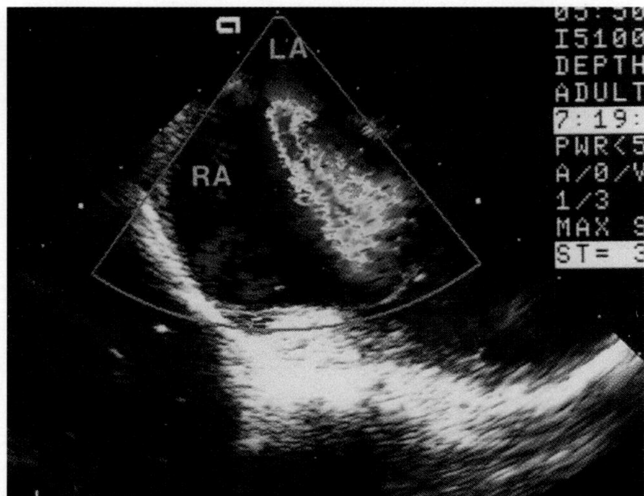

PLATE 9–2 Transesophageal echocardiogram of secundum-type atrial septal defect with color-flow Doppler imaging. A left-to-right shunt is demonstrated by the color jet in the right atrium (RA). A flow convergent zone is seen in the left atrium (LA), proximal to the flow through the atrial septal defect.

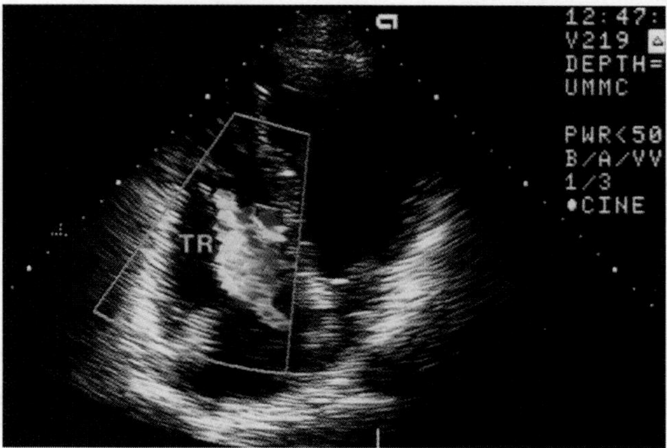

PLATE 9–3 Apical four-chamber echocardiogram in Ebstein's anomaly with color-flow Doppler imaging. Tricuspid regurgitation (TR) is demonstrated, with a color jet within the right atrium during systole. Note the apical displacement of the jet origin, correlating with the anomalous site of tricuspid valve leaflet coaptation within the body of the right ventricle.

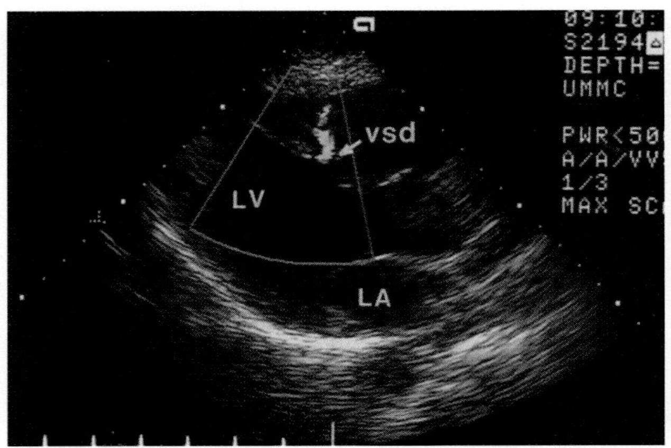

PLATE 9–4 Small muscular ventricular septal defect (vsd). From a parasternal long-axis view, a small shunt is detected through the ventricular septal defect with color-flow Doppler imaging. Small ventricular septal defects frequently are not directly visualized on echocardiographic imaging and are more reliably detected using Doppler techniques. LA, left atrium; LV, left ventricle.

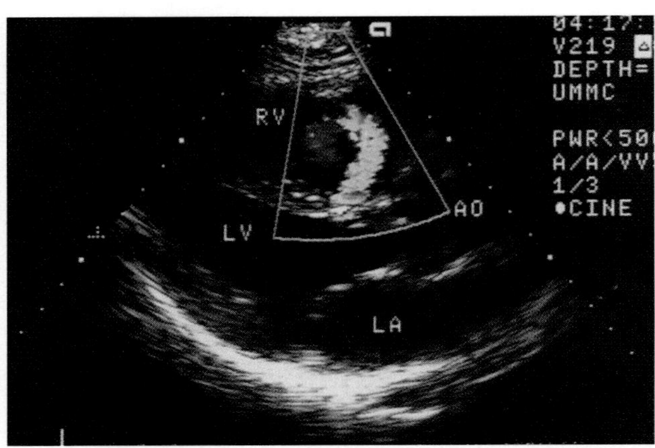

PLATE 9–6 Parasternal long-axis echocardiogram of a larger perimembranous ventricular septal defect with color-flow Doppler imaging. Prominent flow is demonstrated in the right ventricle (RV), with a relatively broad base at the interventricular septum. A flow convergent zone is seen in the left ventricle (LV), proximal to flow through the defect. AO, aortic root; LA, left atrium.

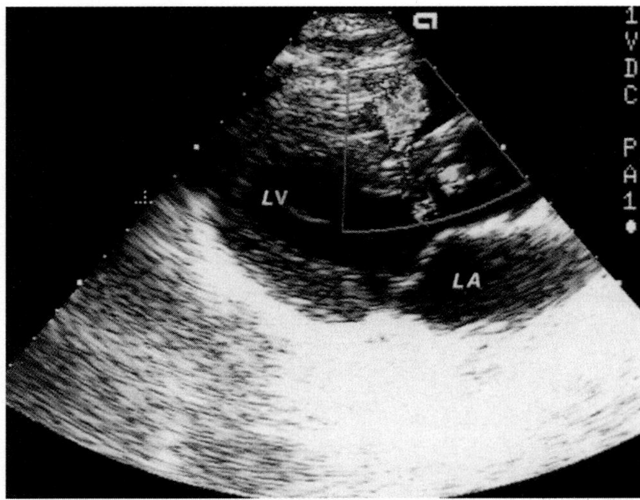

PLATE 9–5 Parasternal long-axis echocardiogram of small perimembranous ventricular septal defect. Color-flow Doppler imaging demonstrates prominent turbulent flow in the right ventricular outflow tract, with a narrow origin in the membranous portion of the interventricular septum. LA, left atrium; LV, left ventricle.

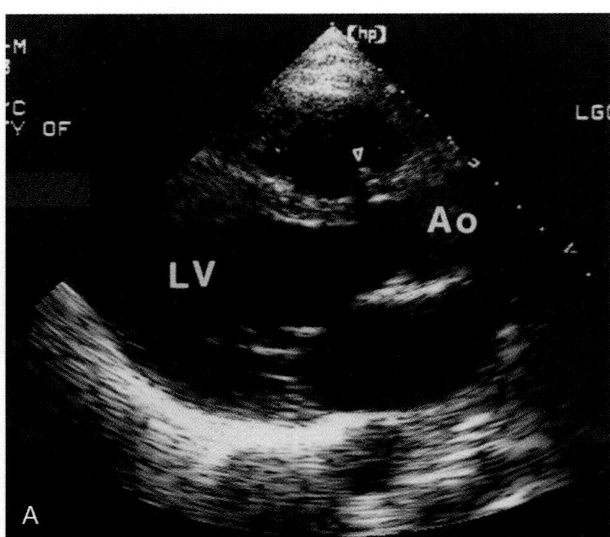

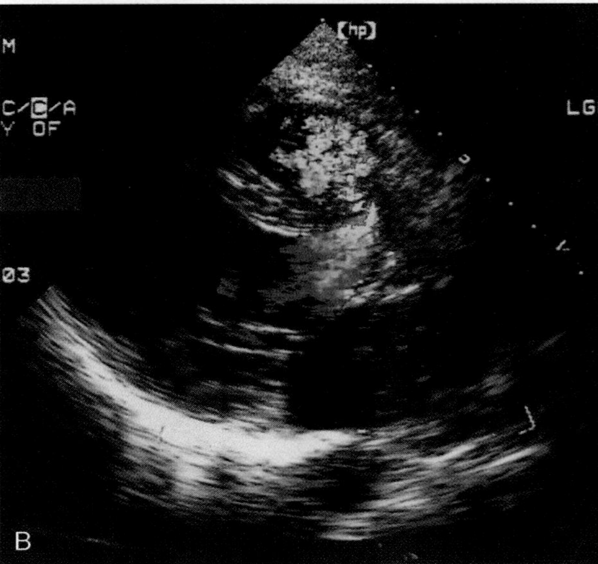

PLATE 9–7 Parasternal long-axis view of a ventricular septal aneurysm. **A,** A small aneurysm (*arrowhead*) is demonstrated, originating in the membranous portion of the interventricular and protruding into the right ventricular outflow tract. Ao, aortic root; LV, left ventricle. **B,** Color-flow Doppler imaging demonstrates shunting through a persistent defect.

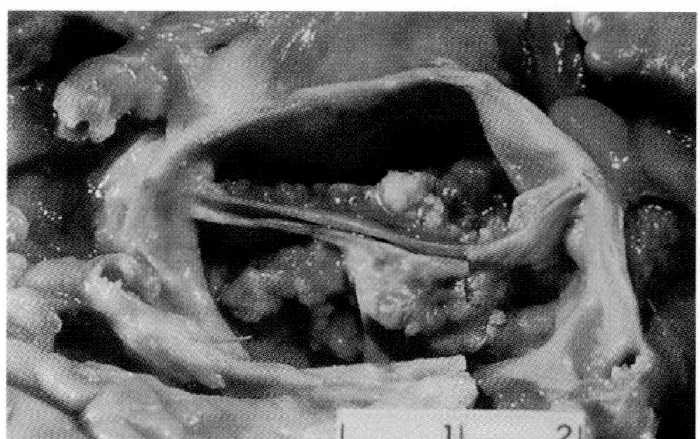

PLATE 12–1 Bicuspid aortic valve. Stenosis is secondary to fibrosis and calcification of the midportion and hinge of the cusps and usually not to fusion of the commissures, as is seen in rheumatic aortic stenosis.

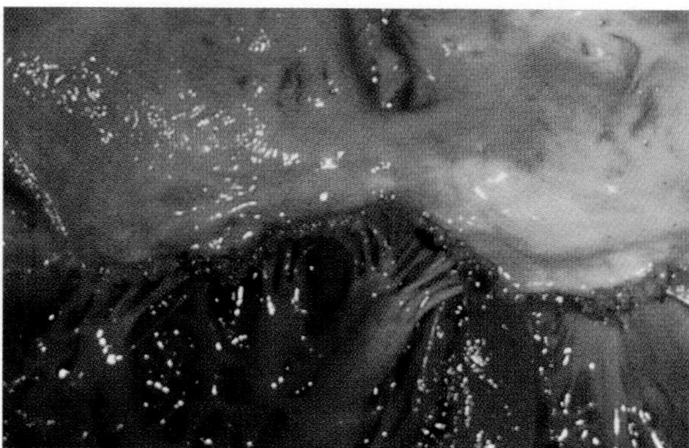

PLATE 12–2 Acute rheumatic valvulitis, mitral valve. Fibrinoid necrosis is represented by minute, translucent nodules (verrucae), 1 to 3 mm in diameter, along the lines of closure. Also see figure in Acute Rheumatic Fever chapter in this book, which illustrates acute rheumatic valvulitis of the aortic valve.

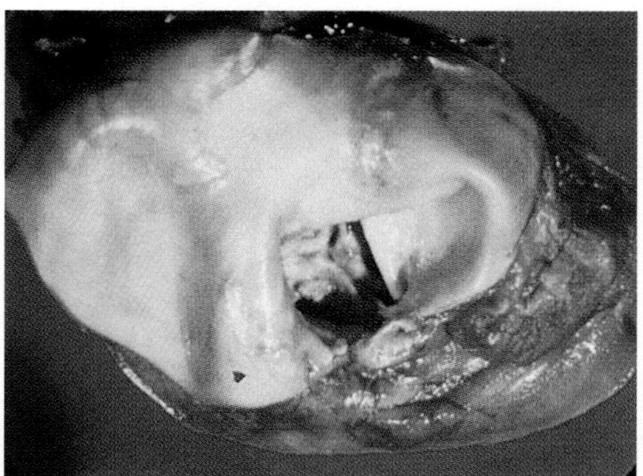

PLATE 12–3 Chronic rheumatic aortic stenosis. Diffuse thickening and fibrosis of the valves with commissural fusion resulting in marked aortic stenosis. Also note the extensive poststenotic dilatation of the ascending aorta.

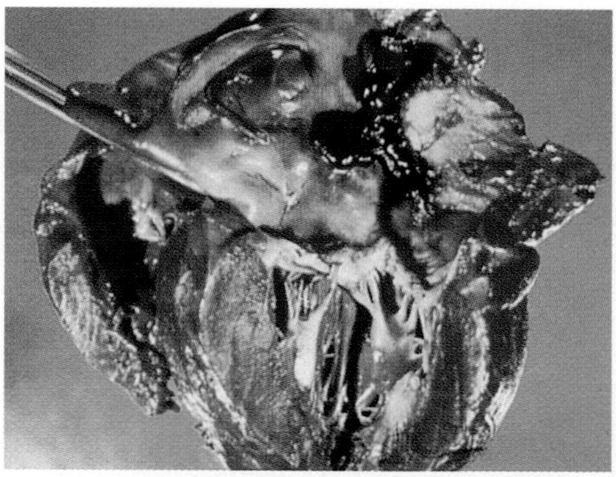

PLATE 12–4 Chronic rheumatic mitral stenosis. Note the thickening, fusion, and shortening of the chordae tendineae, as well as diffuse thickening and fibrosis of the valves, with commissural fusion. The left atrium is enlarged and contains a mural thrombus.

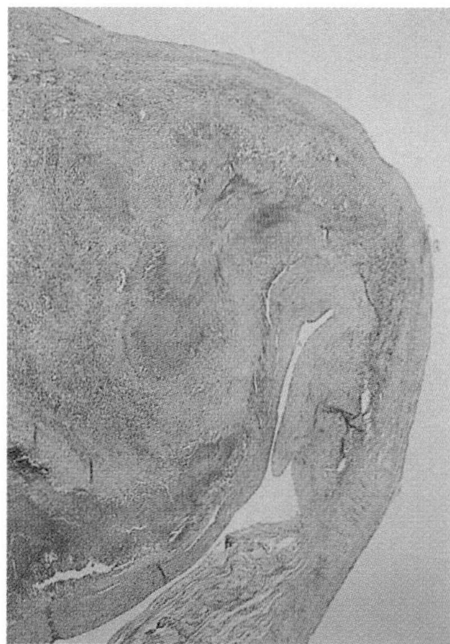

PLATE 12–5 Rheumatoid valve disease, mitral valve. Rheumatoid granulomas with extensive contiguous fibrosis involve the base and midportion of a mitral valve. Another rheumatoid granuloma is present in the adjacent subvalvular myocardium (H&E, ×75).

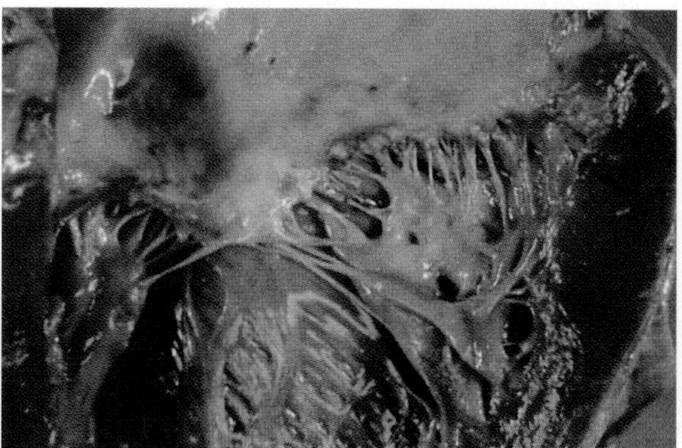

PLATE 12–6 Lupus erythematosus valvulitis (atypical verrucous endocarditis of Libman and Sacks), mitral valve. The lesions represent fibrinoid necrosis as sterile, dry, granular vegetations that may be single or multiple in conglomerates. They have no special tendency to occur along the free edge of the valves and may be scattered on the chordae tendineae and atrial or ventricular mural endocardium.

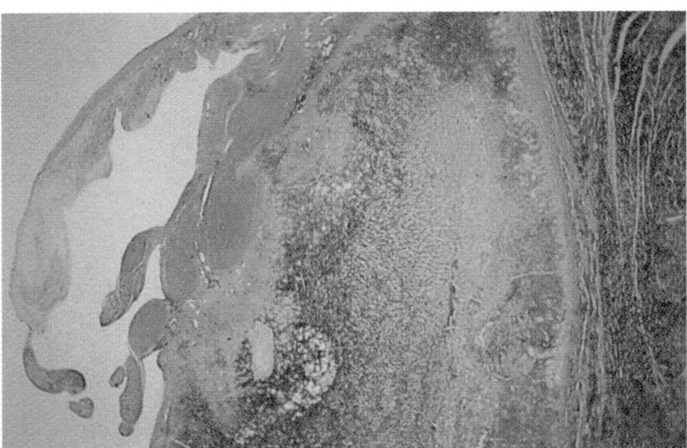

PLATE 12–7 Endomyocardial fibrosis with eosinophilia. The tricuspid valve and its chordae tendineae (blue at left) are separated from the subvalvular endocardium (blue at right) by an organizing thrombus containing numerous eosinophils (Masson trichrome, ×50).

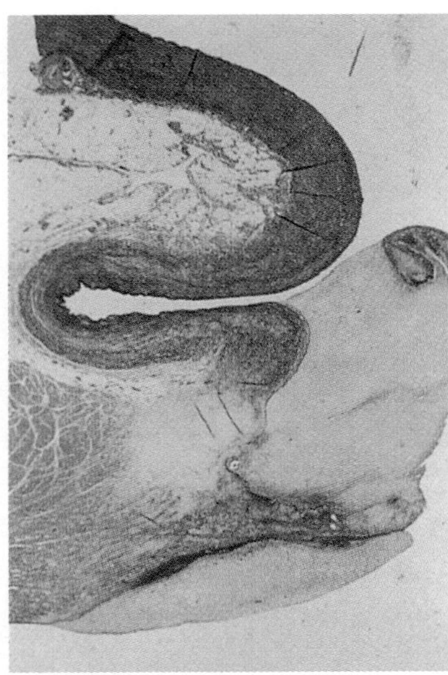

PLATE 12–8 Carcinoid heart disease, pulmonic valve. Heavy deposition of collagen, lacking in elastic fibers, occurs almost exclusively on the arterial aspect of the valve cusps, resulting in pulmonic stenosis (Movat pentachrome, ×25).

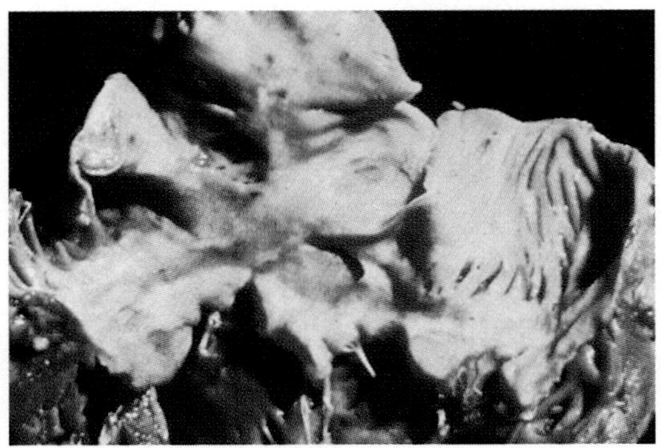

PLATE 12–9 Amyloid valve disease. Valvular involvement is usually minimal; however, diffuse involvement, as illustrated in this heart, can occur, resulting in thick, rigid cusps and stenotic or regurgitant orifices.

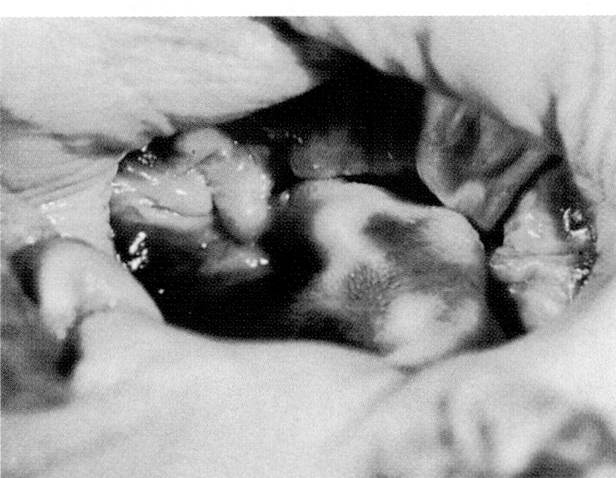

PLATE 12–10 Ochronotic valve disease, mitral valve. In ochronosis, the pigment deposition is most prominent at the base and midportion of the mitral and aortic valve cusps. The pigment deposition is associated with a contiguous fibroblastic response, resulting in dense fibrosis and stenotic or regurgitant valvular dysfunction.

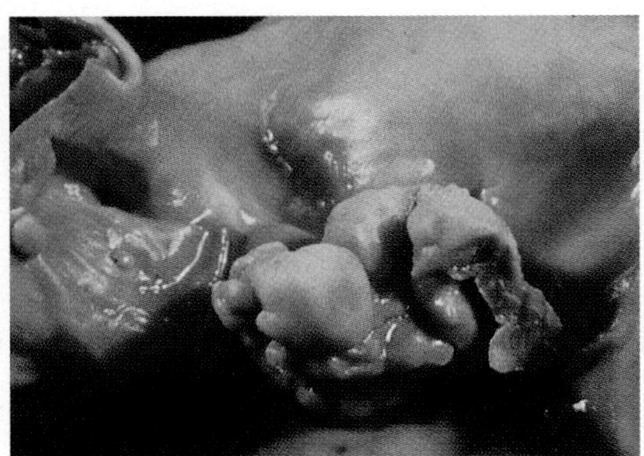

PLATE 12–11 Fungal vegetation, aortic valve. Fungal vegetations tend to be large and friable, with a tendency to embolization.

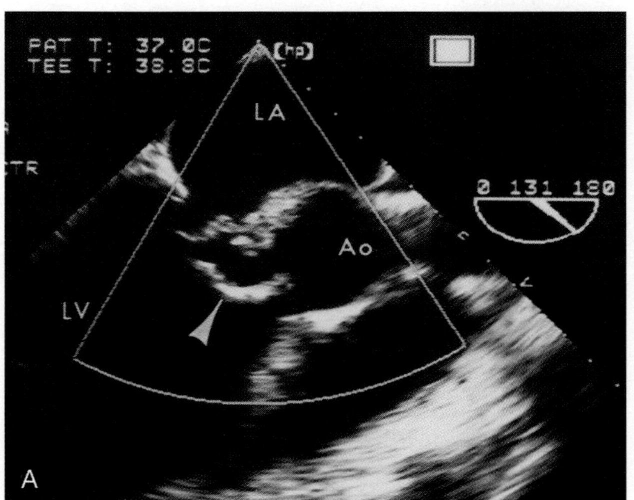

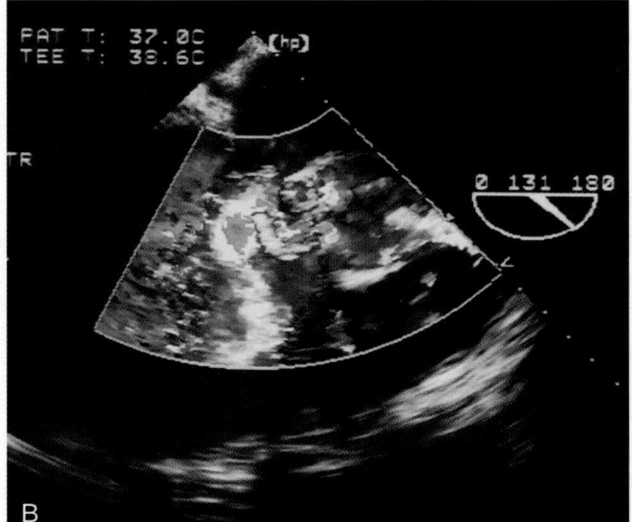

PLATE 20–1 Transesophageal echocardiogram (TEE) of a patient with an aortic valve vegetation. **A,** In diastole, the left atrium (LA), left ventricle (LV), and ascending aorta (Ao) are visible. Just below the aorta is a 1-cm mobile mass prolapsing into the left ventricular outflow tract (*arrowhead*), representing an acute aortic valve vegetation. **B,** In the same view, color-flow Doppler demonstrates severe aortic insufficiency, essentially filling the left ventricular outflow tract.

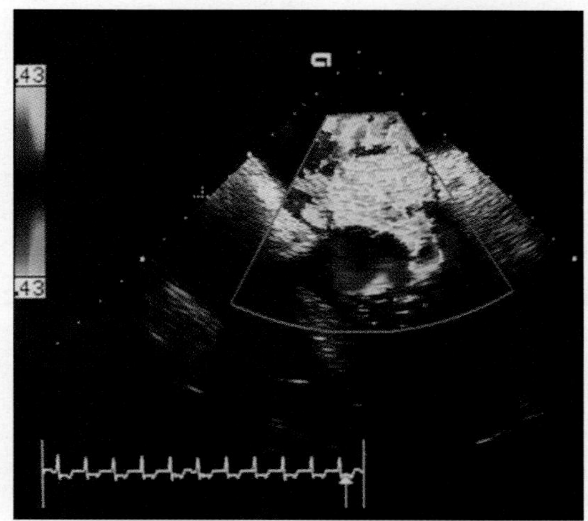

PLATE 20–2 Color Doppler echocardiogram from the same patient as presented in Fig. 20–15. Note the massive degree of mitral regurgitation, which fills the entire left atrial cavity.

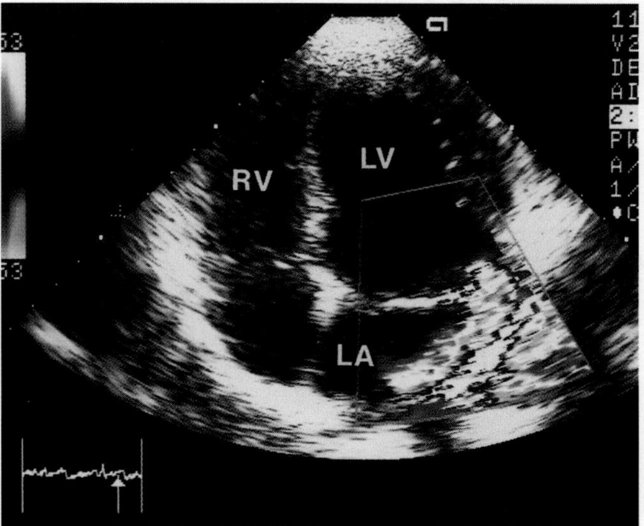

PLATE 20–3 Apical four-chamber view of a patient with mitral prolapse and moderate mitral regurgitation with an eccentric jet. Note the location of the jet, which appears to adhere to the lateral wall of the left atrium (LA). LV, left ventricle; RV, right ventricle.

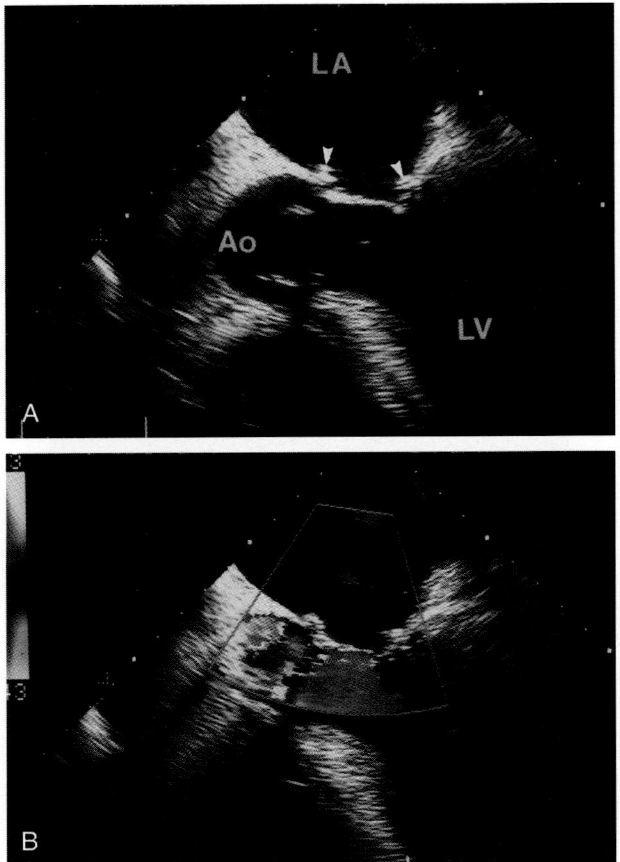

PLATE 20–4 Intraoperative TEE recorded in a patient after mitral valve repair. The repair was performed for severe mitral regurgitation due to a flail leaflet. Note the ring in the mitral annulus (*arrowheads*). **A,** Systolic frame (note the closed mitral valve and open aortic valve). Ao, aorta; LA, left atrium; LV, left ventricle. **B,** Color-flow Doppler examination in the same patient recorded in systole. Notice the absence of any mitral regurgitation after valve repair.

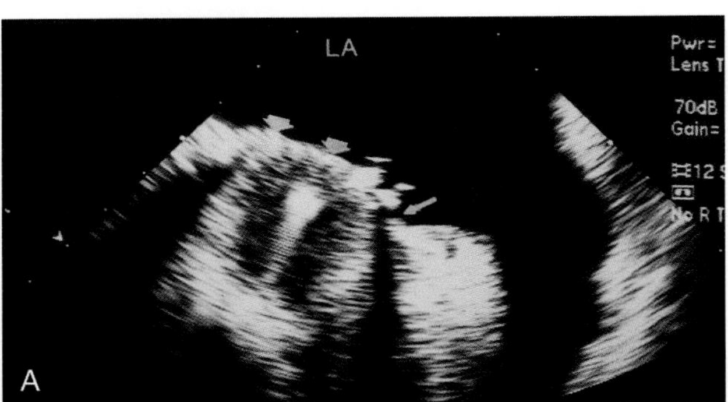

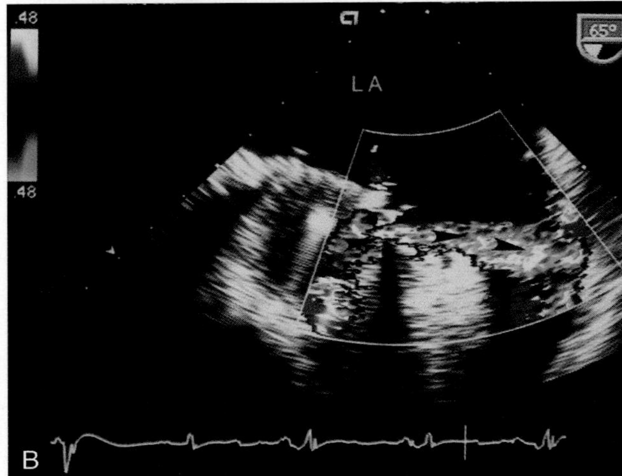

PLATE 20–5 TEE recorded in a patient with a Saint Jude mitral valve prosthesis and mitral regurgitation due to a paravalvar leak. **A,** In diastole, the two closed leaflets of the Saint Jude prosthesis can be seen (*thick arrows*). Additionally, immediately adjacent to the sewing ring is a communication between the left atrium (LA) and the left ventricle (*thin arrow*). This represents a partial valve dehiscence. **B,** The same view recorded with color-flow Doppler imaging. A mitral regurgitant jet is clearly visible traversing the area of the valve dehiscence.

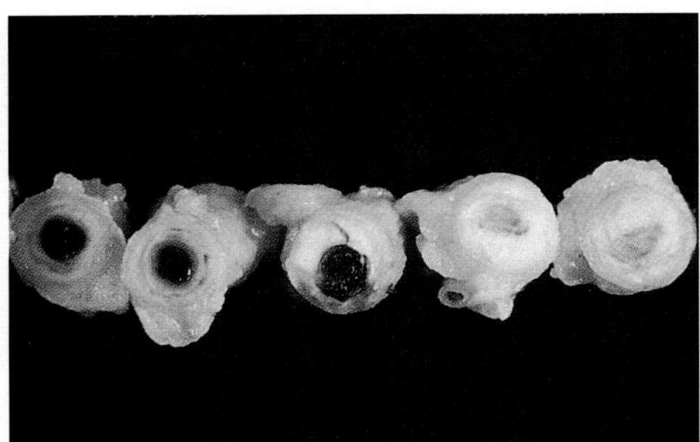

PLATE 24–1 Gross photograph of cross sections of a coronary artery shows atheromatous plaque, recent (dark) thrombus, and organized thrombus.

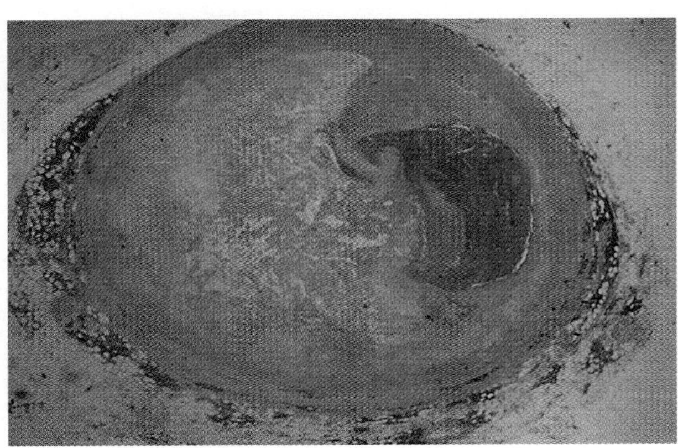

PLATE 24–2 Coronary artery with ruptured atheromatous plaque and occlusive thrombus. Low-power photomicrograph.

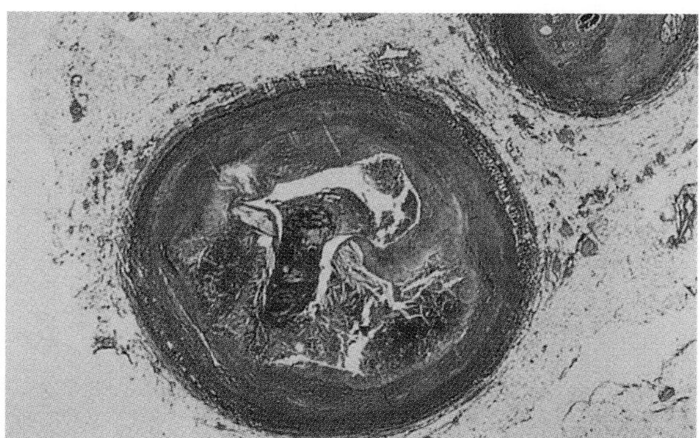

PLATE 24–3 Coronary artery shows a ruptured plaque with intraluminal and intraplaque thrombus. Low-power photomicrograph.

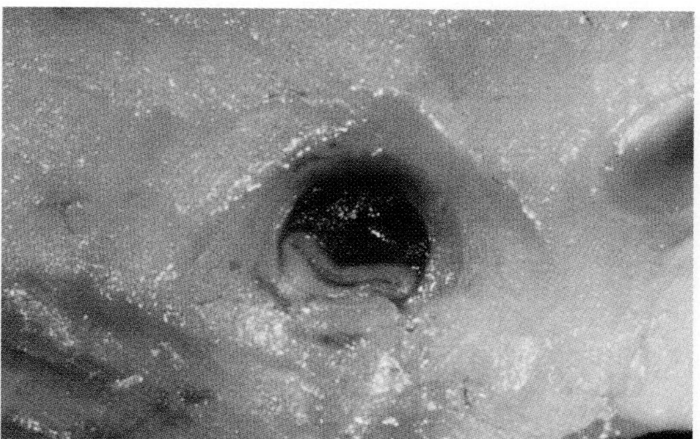

PLATE 24–4 Gross photograph of a spontaneously dissected coronary artery with mural hematoma.

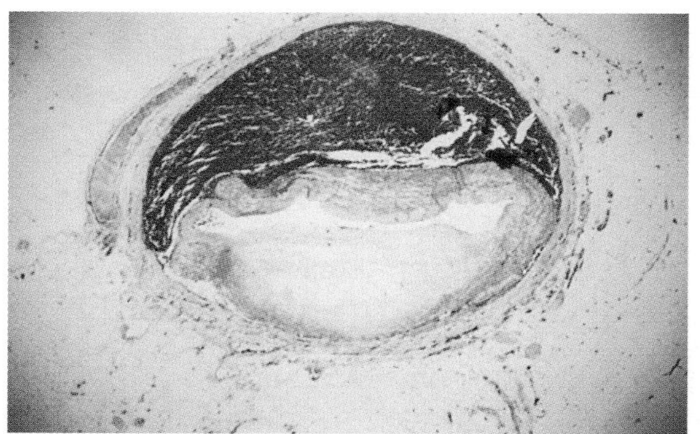

PLATE 24–5 Coronary artery with spontaneous dissection and mural hematoma.

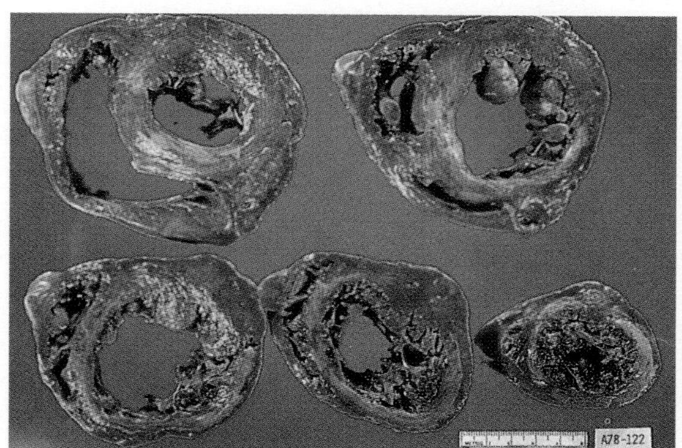

PLATE 24–6 Cross sections of the heart demonstrate a large acute transmural anteroseptal microcardial infarct (yellow area).

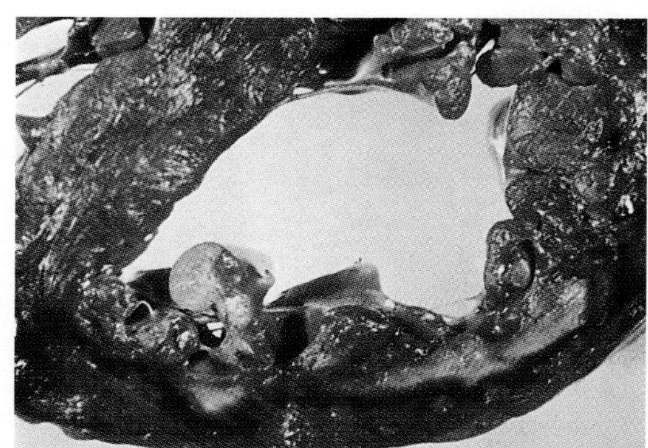

PLATE 24–7 Heart section demonstrates an acute subendocardial myocardial infarct.

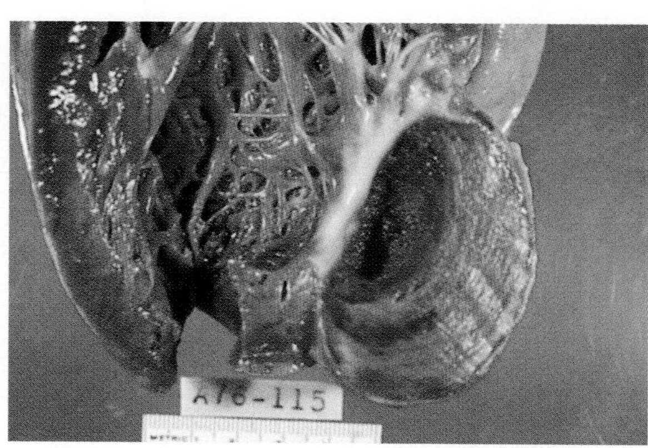

PLATE 24–8 Left ventricular aneurysm with mural thrombus resulting from healing of a transmural myocardial infarct.

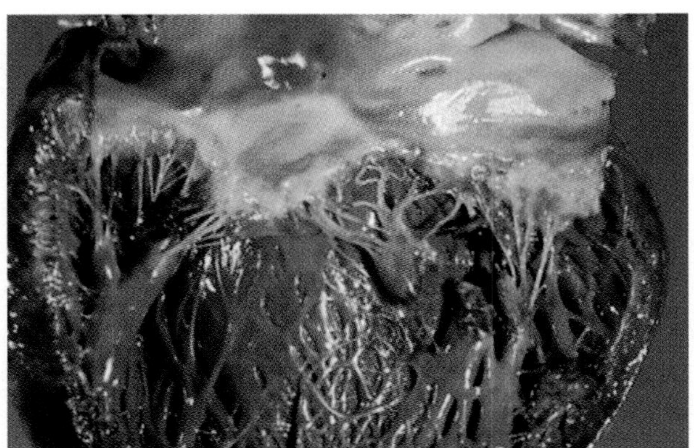

PLATE 24–9 Heart shows rupture of the posterior papillary muscle due to an acute myocardial infarct.

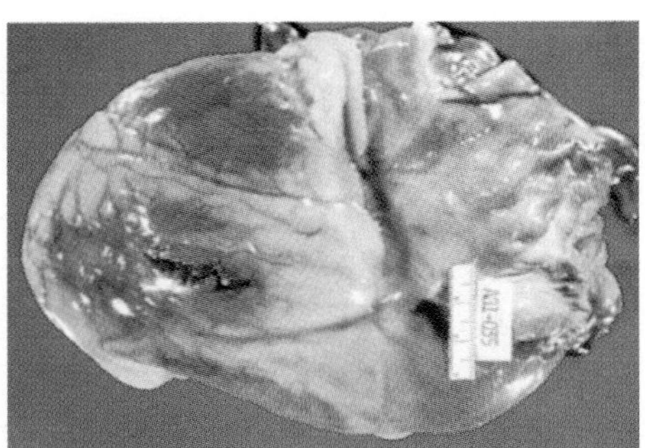

PLATE 24–10 Posterior surface of heart shows a laceration representing an external rupture site.

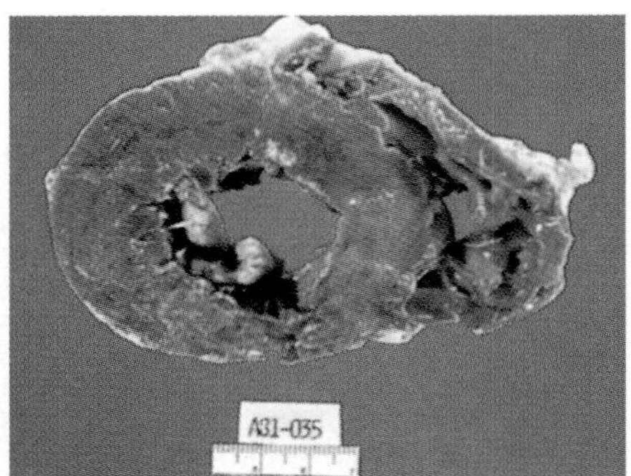

PLATE 24–11 Section of heart shows an acute transmural posterior myocardial infarct with an external rupture site.

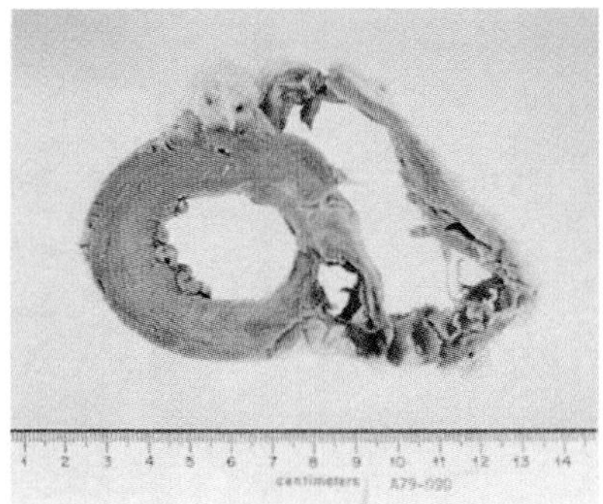

PLATE 24–12 Section of heart shows an acute transmural infarct of the posteroseptal left ventricle that has ruptured into the right ventricle, creating a ventricular septal defect.

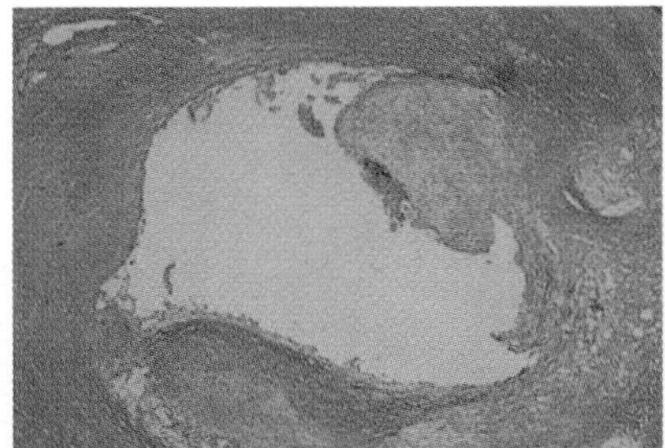

PLATE 24–13 Coronary artery after percutaneous transluminal coronary angioplasty shows platelet-rich microthrombi on the surface of a disrupted plaque.

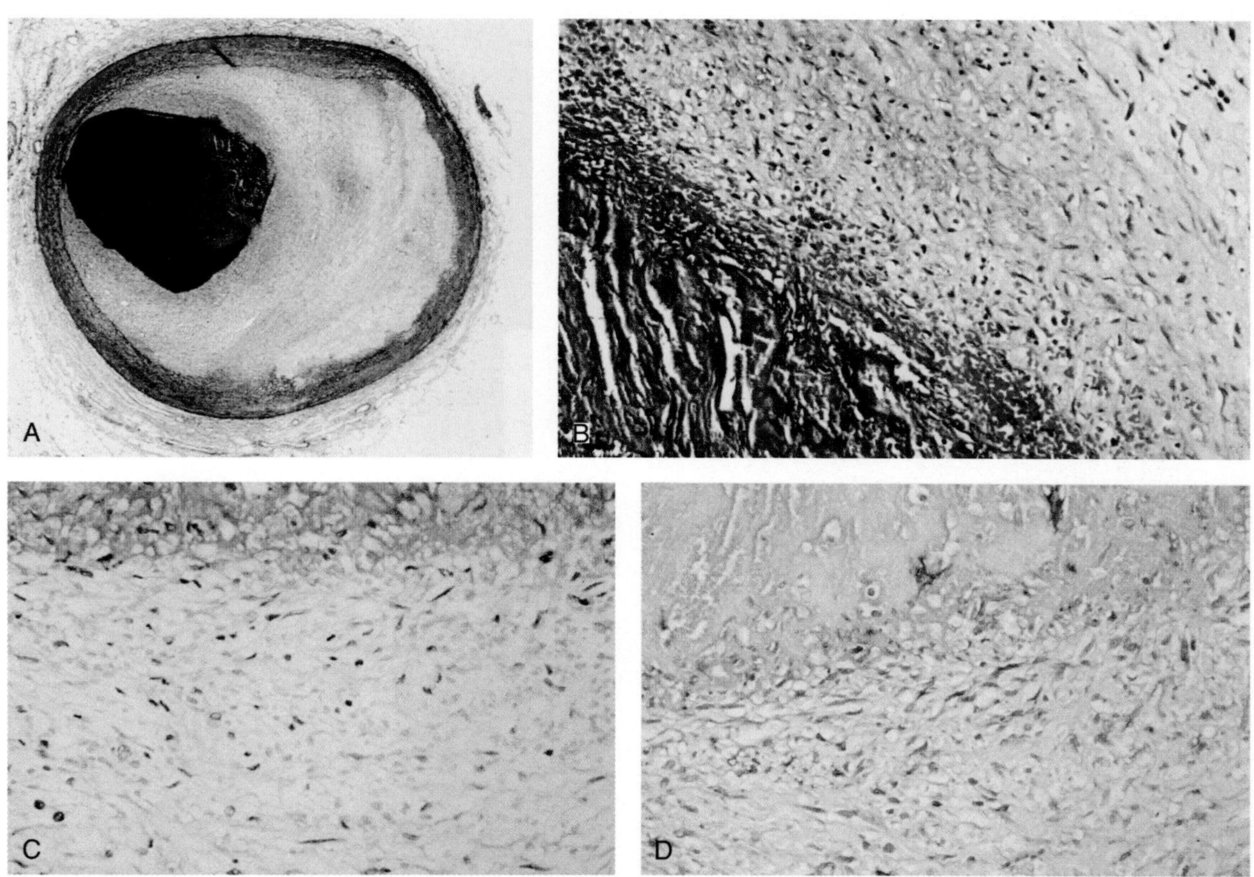

PLATE 28–1 A 33-year-old woman had sudden collapse and a witnessed cardiac arrest shortly after eating. Her risk factors for premature coronary artery disease included total serum cholesterol of 202 mg/dl, high-density lipoprotein cholesterol of 36 mg/dl, and smoking (serum thiocyanate, 119 mg/dl). Acute thrombosis of the left anterior descending coronary artery was found at autopsy. **A,** Low-power photomicrograph of an eccentric plaque with a superimposed nonocclusive thrombus. (Movat stain, ×15; the black area represents barium gelatin, the thrombus is red, and proteoglycans stain green). **B,** High-power view of the thrombus; the area underneath is composed mostly of smooth muscle cells and proteoglycans (green), and there is an absence of endothelial cells. (Movat stain, ×150). **C** and **D,** Immunohistochemical staining identified the spindle-shaped cells as anti–α-actin–positive smooth muscle cells **(D)** with occasional macrophages (anti–KP-1) **(C)** (×300).

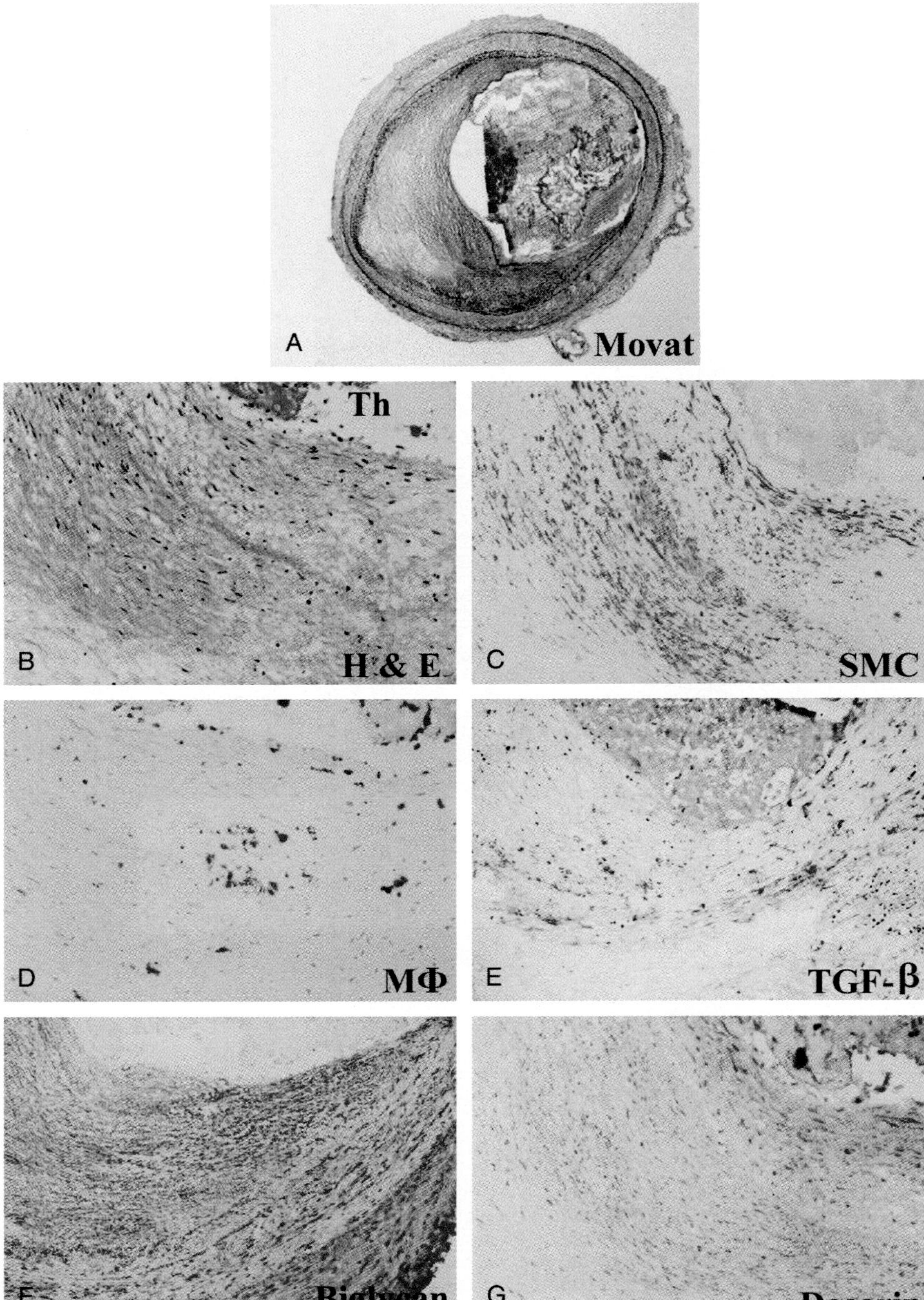

PLATE 28–2 A 48-year-old woman had a witnessed cardiac arrest. There was no previous medical history except for dysfunctional uterine bleeding. She had an acute transmural myocardial infarction of the anterior wall of the left ventricle with apical interventricular septal rupture. At autopsy, there was an acute occlusive thrombus in the mid–left anterior descending coronary artery at the left diagonal take-off; the right coronary artery was 70 percent narrowed proximally without any thrombus. **A,** Photo-micrograph of a left anterior descending coronary artery section shows plaque erosion. There is 60 percent cross-sectional luminal narrowing secondary to a plaque rich in smooth muscle cells and proteoglycans; the lumen is totally occluded by a thrombus. (Movat pentachrome, ×5). **B,** High-power view of the lesion near the thrombus (Th). (H&E, ×200). **C,** Immunostaining of smooth muscle cells (SMC) by HHF-35 antibody; note the high density of smooth muscle cells in the area of erosion. (×200). **D,** Rare CD68⁺ macrophages (Mϕ) were identified near the erosion site. (×200). **E,** Immunolocalization of TGF-β in an area rich in smooth muscle cells at the erosion site. (Antibody provided by Anita Roberts, National Cancer Institute, Bethesda, MD.) (×75). **F** and **G,** Photomicrographs of antibody staining against the proteoglycans biglycan and decorin; note the intense staining against biglycan. (Antibodies provided by Larry Fisher, National Institute of Dental Research, Bethesda, MD.) (×100).

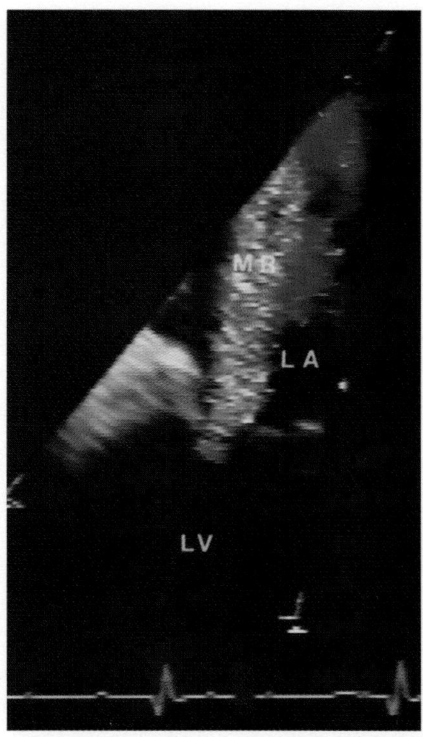

PLATE 31–1 Transesophageal imaging of the left atrium (LA) and left ventricle (LV) characterizes the origin of the jet of mitral regurgitation (MR) through the posterior leaflet of the mitral valve.

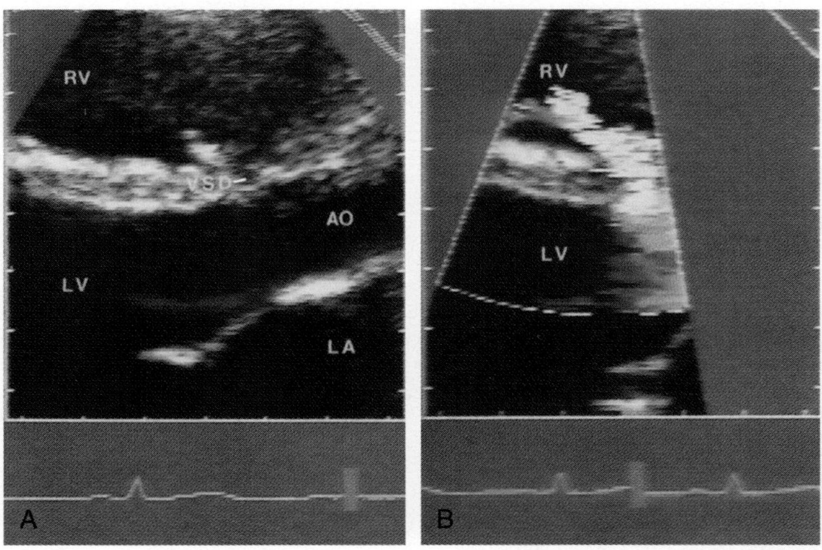

PLATE 31–2 **A,** Transthoracic parasternal long-axis view shows the left atrium (LA), left ventricle (LV), right ventricle (RV), and aorta (AO). VSD, ventricular septal defect. **B.** Color-flow Doppler demonstrates variance across the ventricular septum characteristic of a VSD.

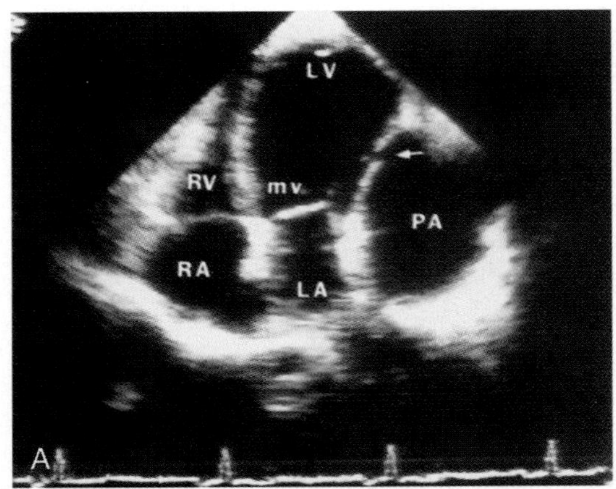

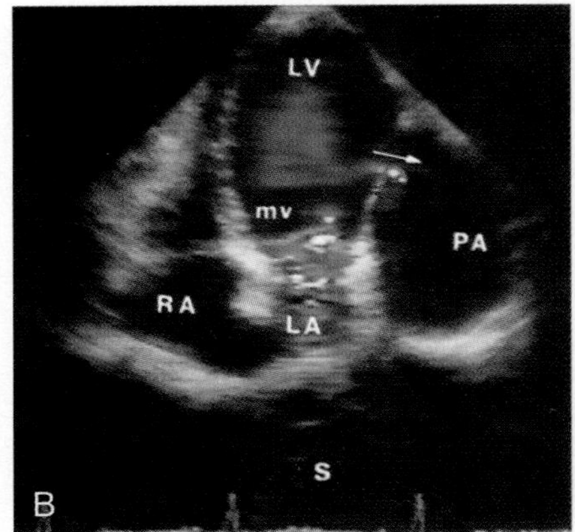

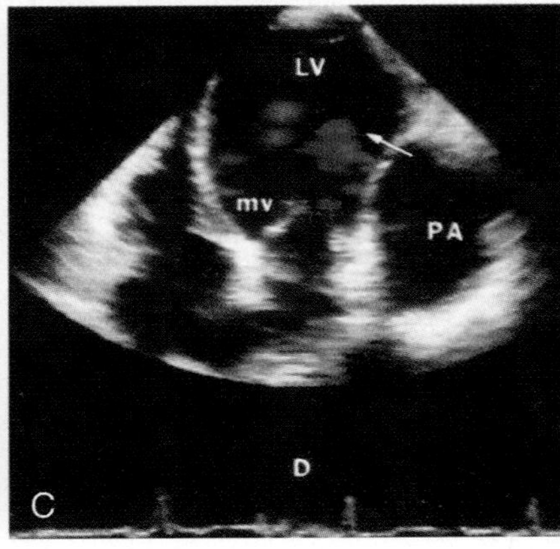

PLATE 31–3 A, Transthoracic apical view shows the left ventricle (LV), left atrium (LA), pseudoaneurysm (PA) of the LV, right ventricle (RV), and right atrium (RA). mv, mitral valve. **B** and **C,** Color-flow Doppler imaging shows the characteristic bidirectional flow in systole and diastole resulting from communication between the false aneurysm and the LV cavity. In systole (S) **(B),** the direction of flow is from the LV to the PA, whereas in diastole (D) **(C),** the direction of flow is from the PA to the LV. (**A–C,** From Gura GM: Video Atlas of Color Flow Doppler Echocardiography. Boston: Little, Brown, 1990.)

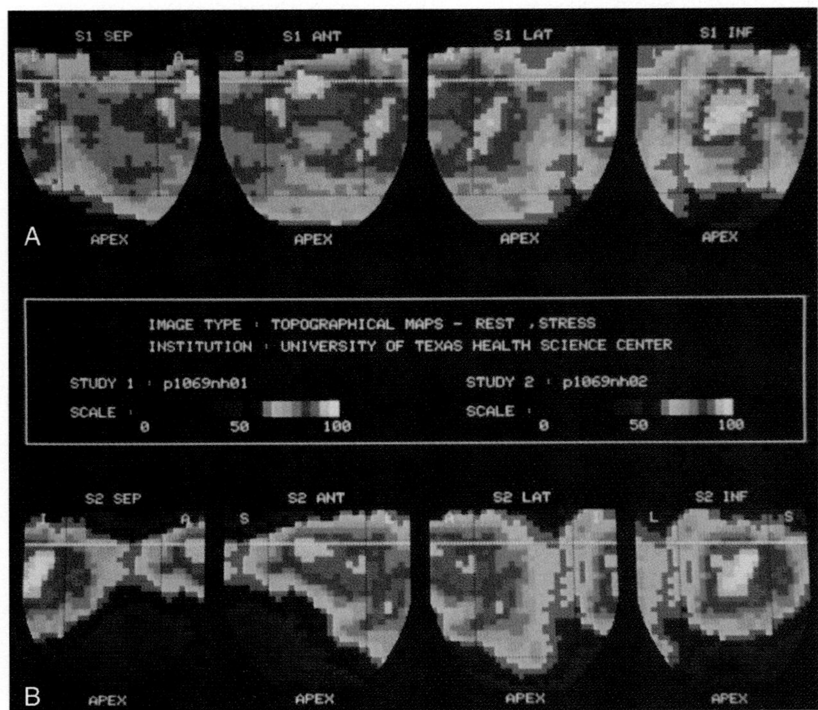

PLATE 32–1 Positron emission tomographic images in three-dimensional displays of the rest study **(A)** and dipyridamole study **(B)** of an asymptomatic patient with two normal thallium/treadmill stress tests before tomographic scanning. See text for details. (**A** and **B,** From Gould KL: Coronary Artery Stenosis. New York: Elsevier, 1990.)

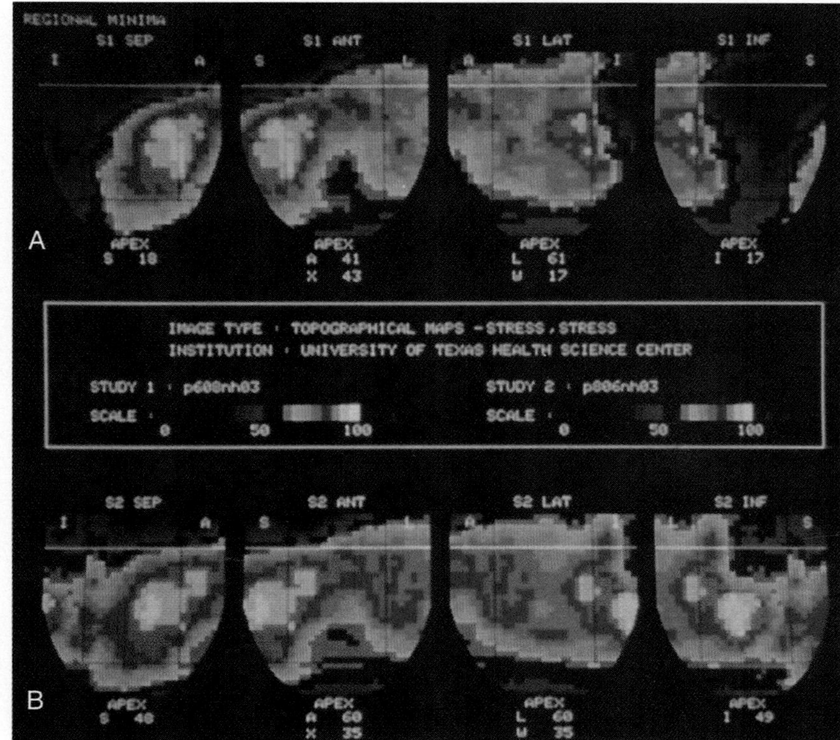

PLATE 32–2 Positron emission tomographic images after dipyridamole before **(A)** and after **(B)** 15 months on a vigorous risk modification program. (**A** and **B,** From Gould KL: Coronary Artery Stenosis. New York: Elsevier, 1990.)

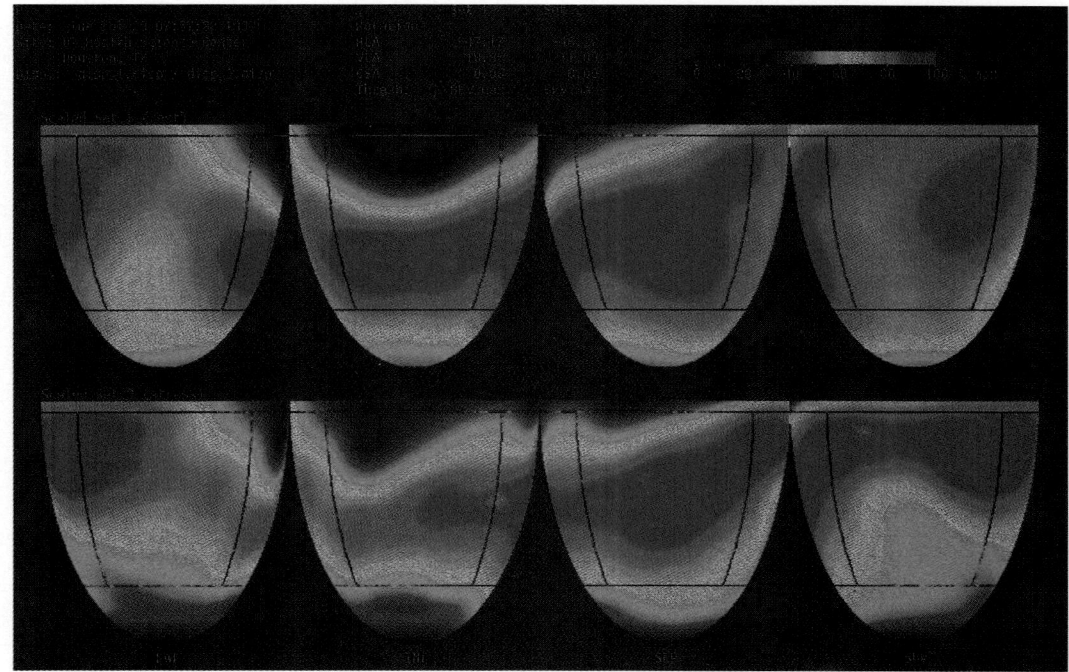

PLATE 32–3 Positron emission tomographic perfusion images show a normal resting perfusion image (*top*) but an abnormal longitudinal base-to-apex perfusion gradient after dipyridamole (*bottom*) from a patient with diffuse coronary atherosclerosis without segmental stenoses by coronary arteriography. The four three-dimensional views are (from left to right) lateral, inferior, septal, and anterior views. The color scale is from the highest perfusion (in red) decreasing through intermediate perfusion (in yellow) to the lowest perfusion (in blue). This abnormal perfusion pattern is not seen in normal subjects. Quantitative analysis of the entire coronary arteriographic tree showed the coronary arteries to be diffusely 20 to 30 percent smaller than normal in association with a total cholesterol level of 260 mg/dl and a strong family history of premature heart disease. (Adapted from Gould KL: Coronary Artery Stenosis and Reversing Heart Disease. 2nd ed. London: Arnold, 1998, distributed by Oxford University Press.)

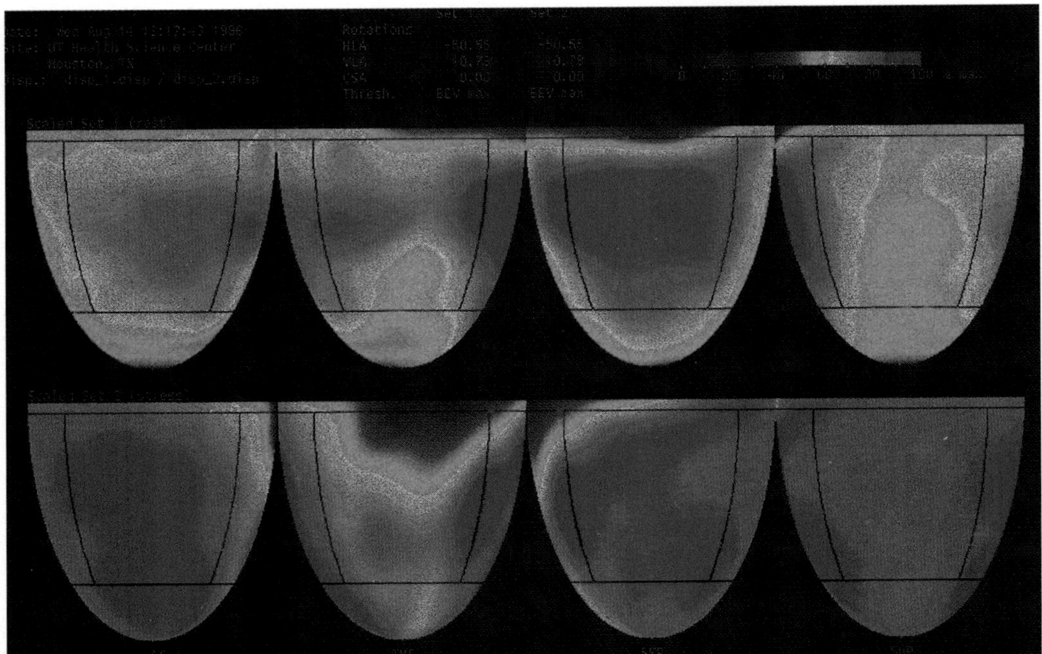

PLATE 32–4 Positron emission tomographic perfusion images show an abnormal, heterogeneous perfusion at rest (*top*) that improves after dipyridamole (*bottom*), reflecting heterogeneous endothelial dysfunction. There is a small, severe basal inferior segmental defect demonstrating myocardial steal, which indicates a small occluded, collateralized posterior artery without a scar. (From Gould KL: Coronary Artery Stenosis and Reversing Heart Disease. 2nd ed. London: Arnold, 1998, distributed by Oxford University Press.)

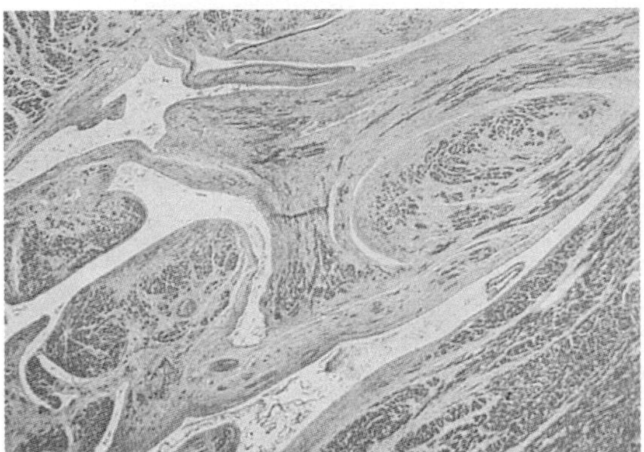

PLATE 50–1 Scleroderma. In contrast to polymyositis, there is no significant inflammatory cell infiltrate; rather, there is myocyte loss with replacement fibrosis and a diffuse interstitial increase in collagen deposition (H&E, ×250).

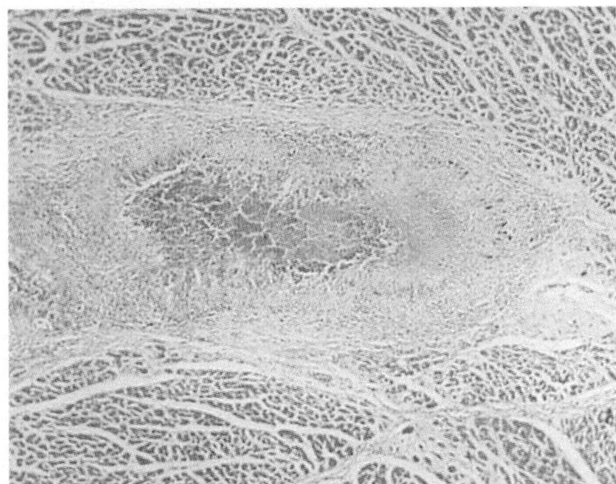

PLATE 50–2 Rheumatoid myocarditis. The myocardium contains a classic rheumatoid nodule with peripheral palisading histiocytes and central necrobiosis (H&E, ×250).

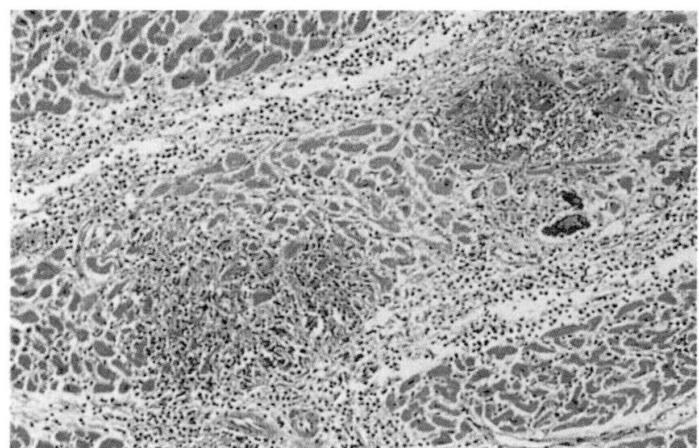

PLATE 50–3 Wegener's granulomatosis. There are extensive areas of myocyte necrosis associated with a mixed inflammatory cell infiltrate, including lymphocytes, eosinophils, and multinucleated giant cells (H&E, ×250).

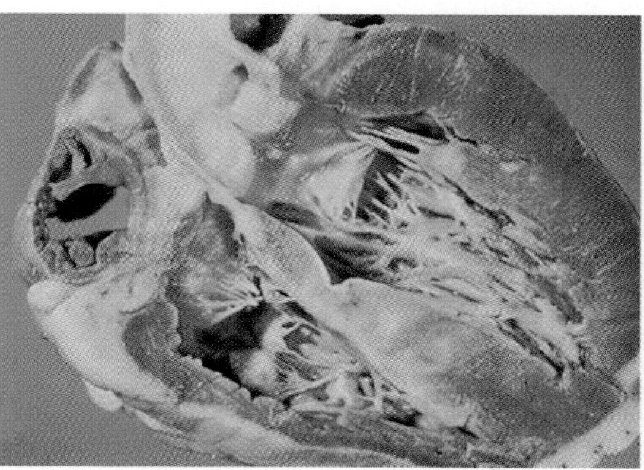

PLATE 50–4 Sarcoid. In cardiac sarcoid, the most common locations of granulomas are the mitral papillary muscles and the summit of the ventricular septum. The septal lesions are amenable to endomyocardial biopsy. Granulomas with associated fibrosis are noted here as mottled, white intramyocardial lesions.

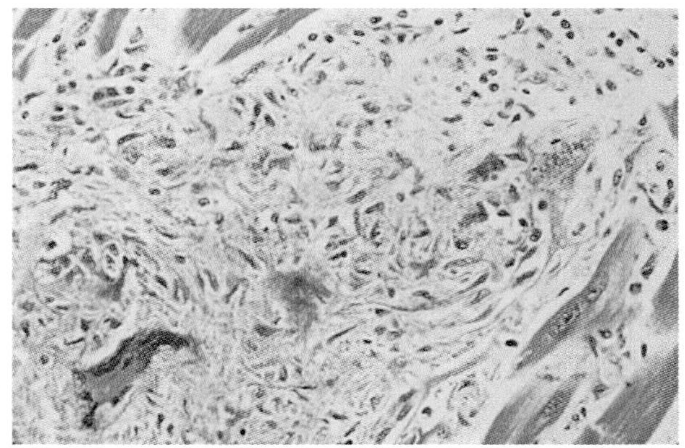

PLATE 50–5 Sarcoid. Microscopically, there is a granulomatous myocarditis, usually accompanied by dense fibrosis. Special stains for mycobacteria and fungi are negative (H&E, ×300).

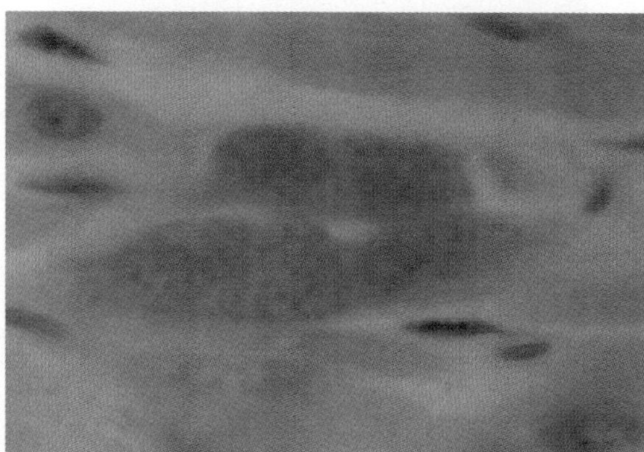

PLATE 50–6 Toxoplasmosis. Two cardiac myocytes with cysts containing *Toxoplasma* parasites. In cardiac toxoplasmosis, there is no inflammatory cell response until the cyst ruptures; therefore, if only areas of inflammation are examined microscopically, the diagnosis may be missed (H&E, ×400).

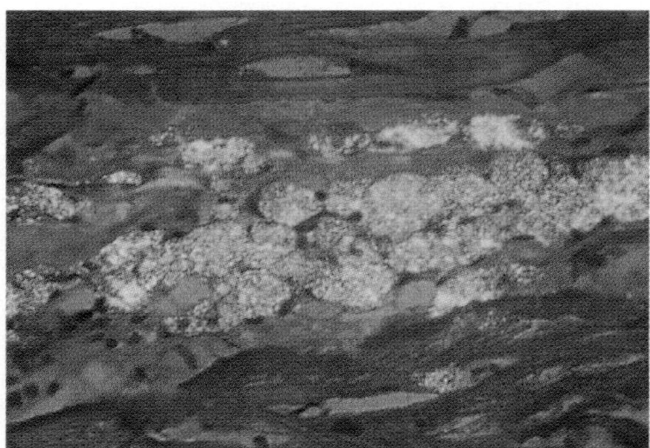

PLATE 50–7 Fabry's disease. Myocytes contain deposits of glycosphingolipid that show a strong birefringence in a frozen section preparation (H&E, ×150).

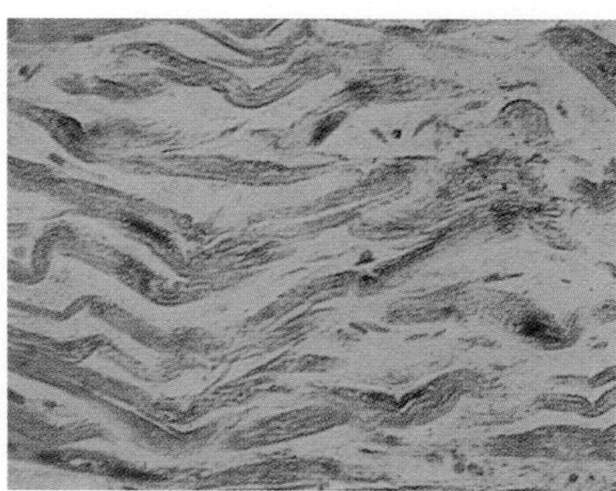

PLATE 50–8 Hemochromatosis. Cardiac myocytes contain deposits of iron, especially in the perinuclear area. The degree of cardiac failure is usually proportional to the amount of stainable iron (Prussian blue reaction, ×150).

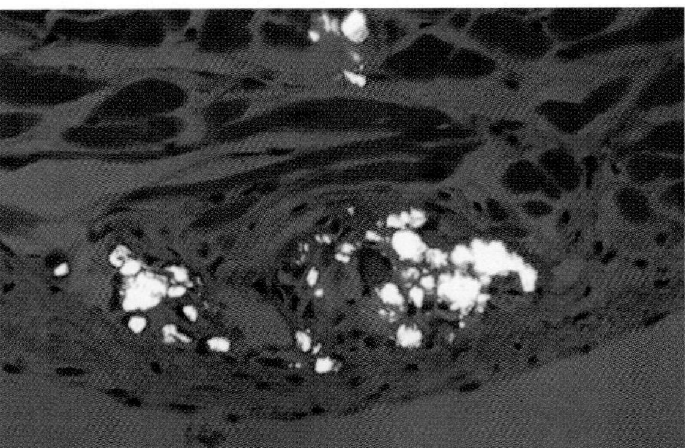

PLATE 50–9 Oxalosis. In contrast to hemochromatosis, where iron is deposited in the predominantly contractile myocytes, oxalate is deposited mainly in the conduction system. Therefore, these crystals are usually subendocardial, and the condition is associated with varying degrees of heart block (H&E, ×150, partially polarized light).

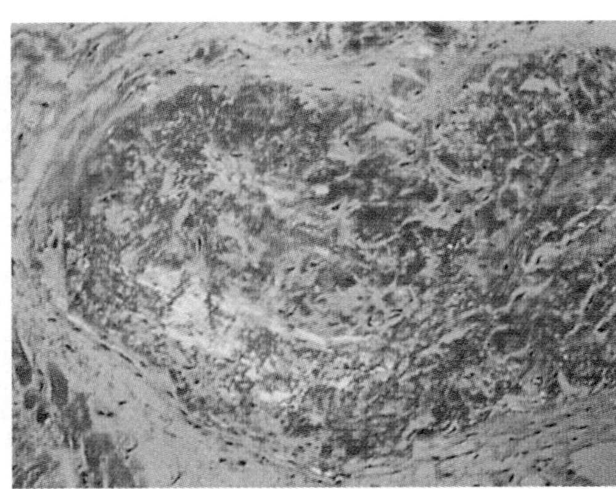

PLATE 50–10 Amyloid. The most common location for cardiac amyloid is in the myocardial interstitium; the next most common location is in the intramyocardial coronary arterioles. Interstitial amyloid is usually associated with myocyte loss and subsequent cardiac failure (Congo red, ×150).

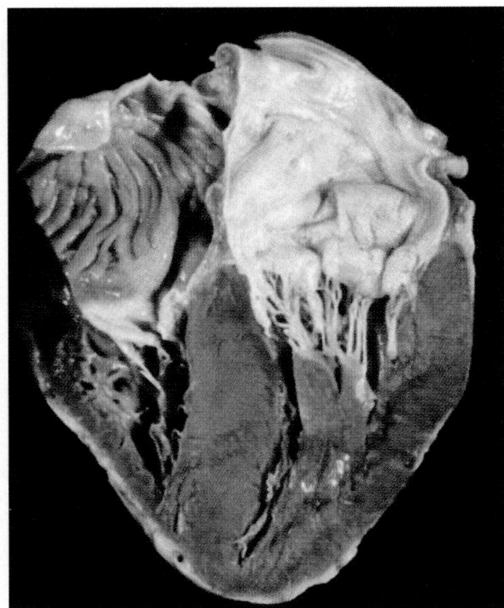

PLATE 52–1 Gross heart morphology in an individual who had hypertrophic cardiomyopathy (HCM). This section is cut in a longitudinal plane and shows the four cardiac chambers. The left ventricle is markedly hypertrophied with a reduced cavity size. An asymmetric pattern of hypertrophy is present, with predominant involvement of the interventricular septum. The left atrium is enlarged. The right ventricle and right atrium appear relatively normal.

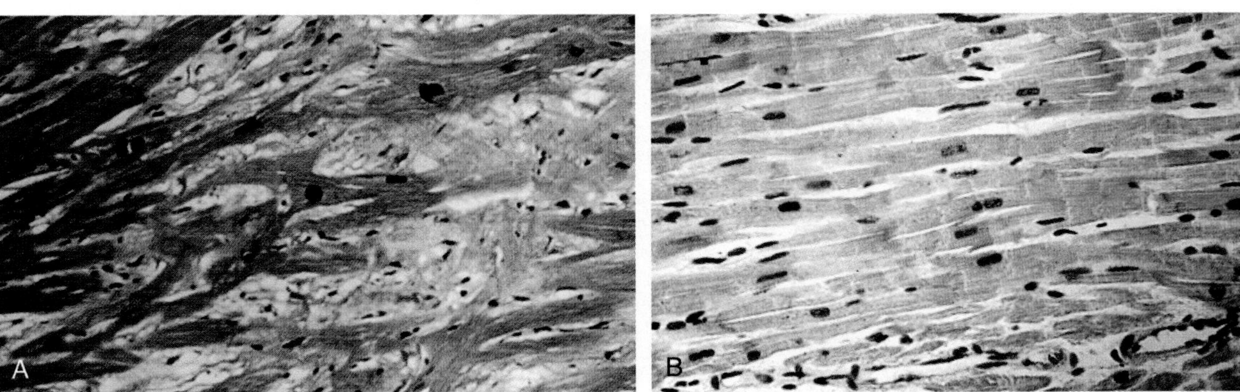

PLATE 52–2 Histologic specimens of left ventricular myocardium from an individual with HCM **(A)** and from a normal heart **(B)**. The myocardial sections are stained with H&E. Histopathologic findings in HCM are typified by myocyte hypertrophy with loss of the orderly alignment of sarcomeres (myofibrillar disarray). Myocyte nuclei are enlarged and hyperchromatic. An increased amount of loose intercellular connective tissue is present.

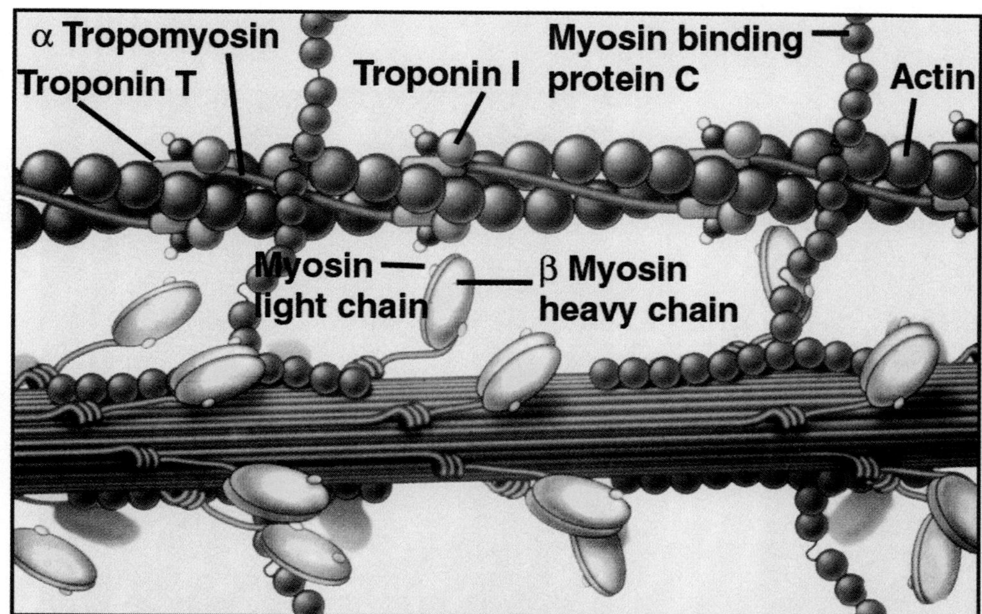

PLATE 52–3 HCM is caused by mutations in genes that encode sarcomere proteins. The components of the sarcomere in which HCM-causing mutations have been identified are shown: three thick filament proteins (*β* myosin heavy chain, regulatory myosin light chain, essential myosin light chain); four thin filament proteins (cardiac troponin T, cardiac troponin I, *α* tropomyosin, and cardiac actin); and cardiac myosin binding protein C. (Modified from Spirito P, Seidman CE, McKenna WJ, et al: The management of hypertrophic cardiomyopathy. N Engl J Med 336:775, 1997.)

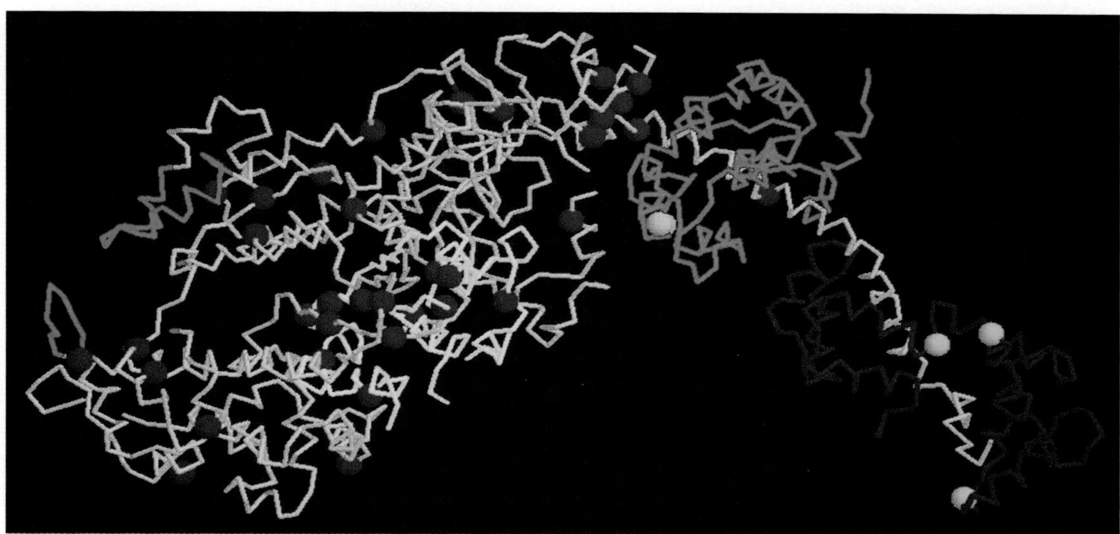

PLATE 52–4 Computer reconstruction of the three-dimensional crystal structure of myosin based on x-ray coordinates for chicken skeletal muscle myosin reported by Rayment et al.[226] The protein backbone is shown in white. Binding sites for myosin (green) and adenosine triphosphate (yellow) are indicated. Essential and regulatory myosin light chains are shown in blue and purple, respectively. HCM-causing mutations in the myosin heavy chain are denoted by red spheres; mutations in the essential and regulatory myosin light chains by orange spheres. Note the clustering of mutations in the adenosine triphosphate–binding domain. This image was generated using RasMol software.

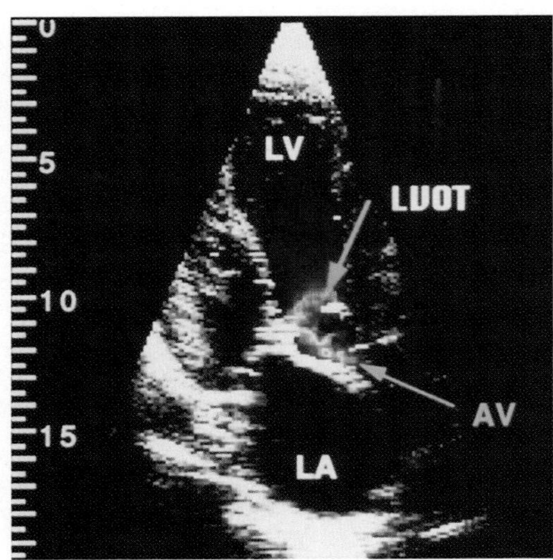

PLATE 57–1 Color-flow Doppler recording in a patient with dynamic left ventricular outflow tract (LVOT) obstruction. There is aliasing with a mosaic of color in the LVOT during systole indicative of marked turbulence of blood flow, thereby demarcating the site of obstruction. LA, left atrium; LV, left ventricle.

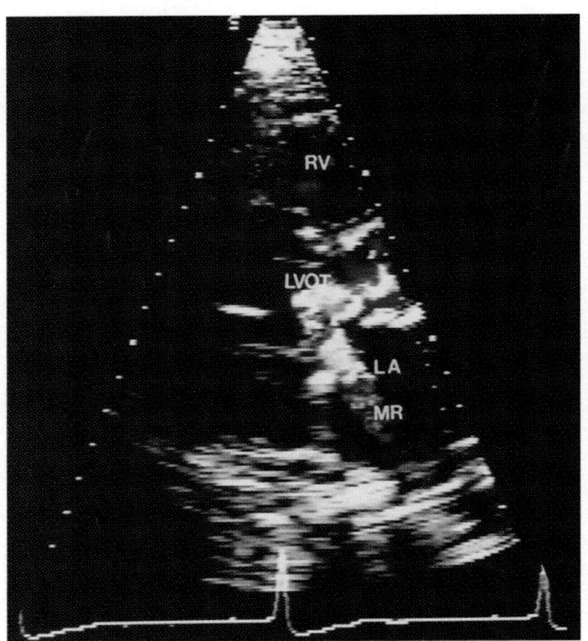

PLATE 57–2 Color-flow Doppler recording in a patient with dynamic left ventricular outflow tract (LVOT) obstruction. There is aliasing with a mosaic of color in the LVOT during systole indicative of marked turbulence of blood flow; concomitantly, there is a posteriorly directed jet of mitral regurgitation (MR) into the left atrium (LA). RV, right ventricle.

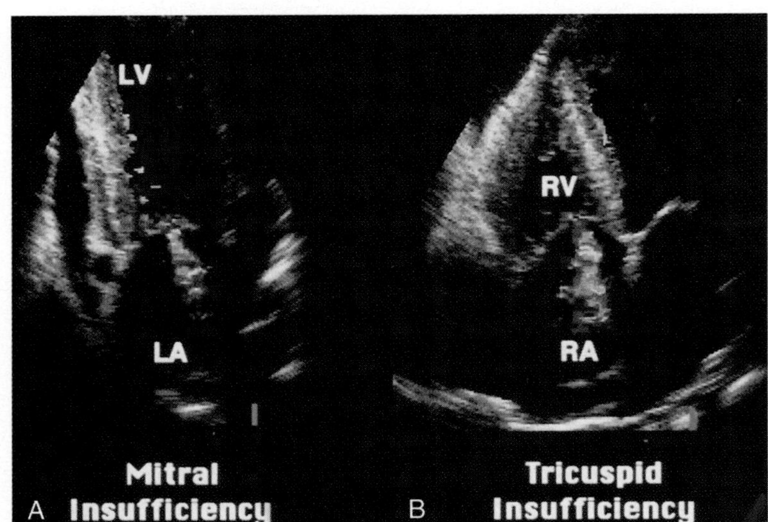

PLATE 57–3 Color-flow Doppler recording in a patient with amyloidosis. In these apical views, there is a mosaic of color in the left **(A)** and right **(B)** atria indicative of mild mitral regurgitation and mild tricuspid regurgitation, respectively. LA, left atrium; LV, left ventricle; RA, right atrium; RV, right ventricle.

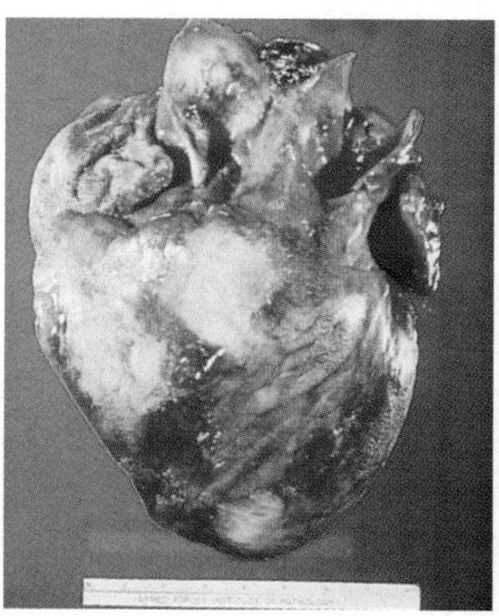

PLATE 64–1 Fibrinous pericarditis. In most types of pericarditis, the base of the heart is more involved than the apex; thus, a propensity for atrial arrhythmias exists in this condition.

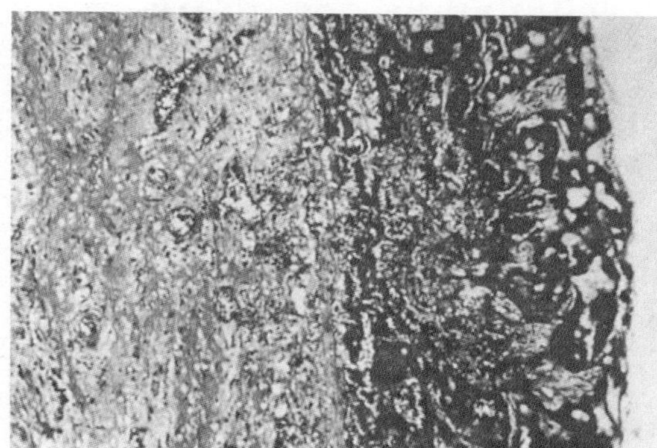

PLATE 64–2 Fibrinous pericarditis. Fibrin is deposited over the surface of the parietal and visceral pericardium. This fibrin layer may subsequently be organized by an ingrowth of fibroblasts, resulting in fibrous obliterative pericarditis. (H&E, ×120.)

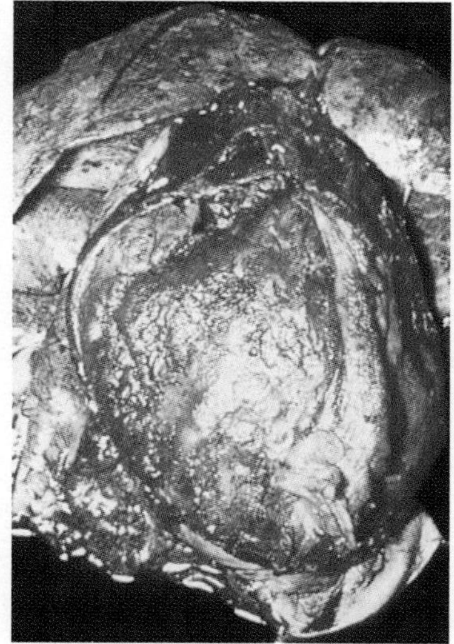

PLATE 64–3 Fibrous obliterative pericarditis. Note the thickened parietal and visceral pericardium.

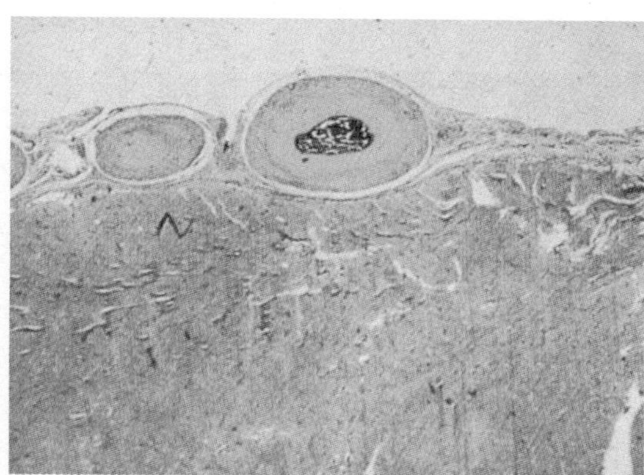

PLATE 64–4 Granulomatous pericarditis. The pericardium is thickened by dense fibrous tissue. Nonspecific fibrocalcific granulomas are present on the pericardial surface. (H&E, ×120.)

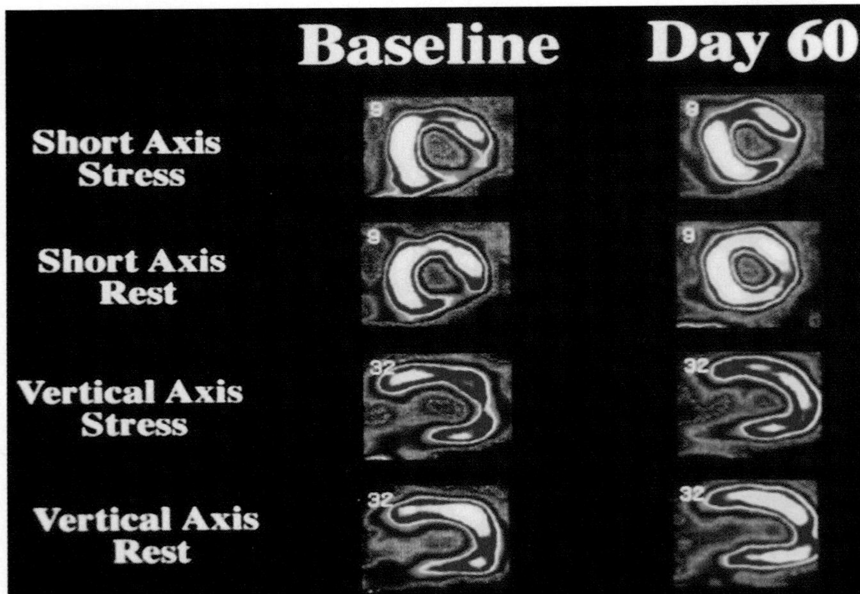

PLATE 74–1 Single-photon emission computed tomography–sestamibi perfusion scans show an improvement in perfusion to the inferolateral and anterior walls of the left ventricle both at rest and after exercise. Yellow, normal perfusion; red, ischemic. (From Losordo DW, Vale PR, Symes JF, et al: Gene therapy for myocardial angiogenesis: initial clinical results with direct myocardial injection of phVEGF165 as sole therapy for myocardial ischemia. Circulation 98:2800–2804,1998.)

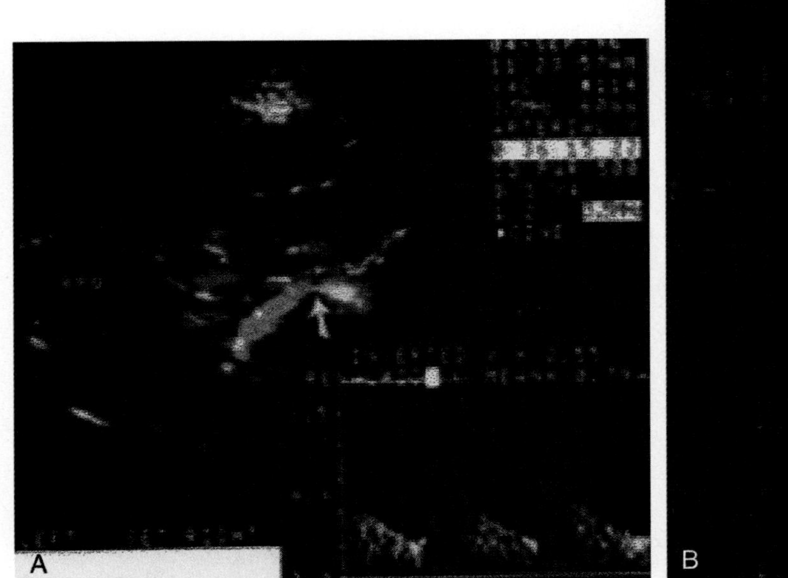

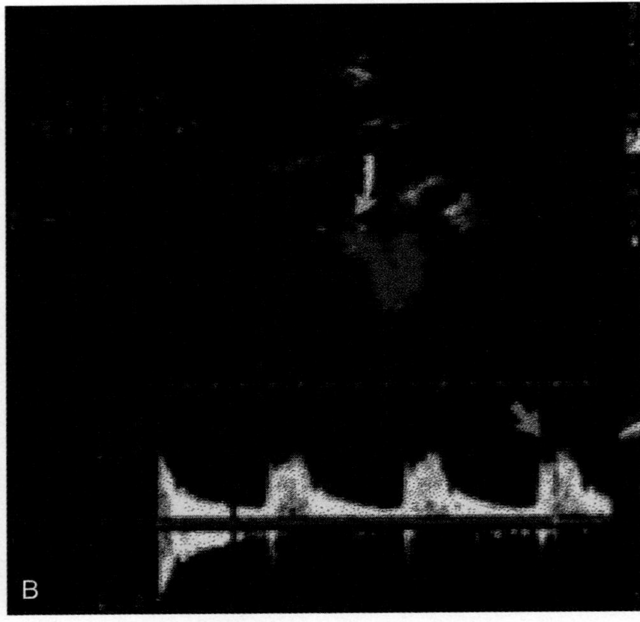

PLATE 75–1 A, Duplex ultrasound image of the right renal artery reveals ostial renal artery stenosis as indicated by high velocity (2.50 cm/sec) and mosaic pattern on color-flow image (*arrow*). **B,** Duplex ultrasound image of the same patient as in **A** reveals a stent in the right renal ostium (*curved arrow*), normal flow pattern, and normalization of renal flow velocity (100 cm/sec) after stent deployment (*straight arrow*).

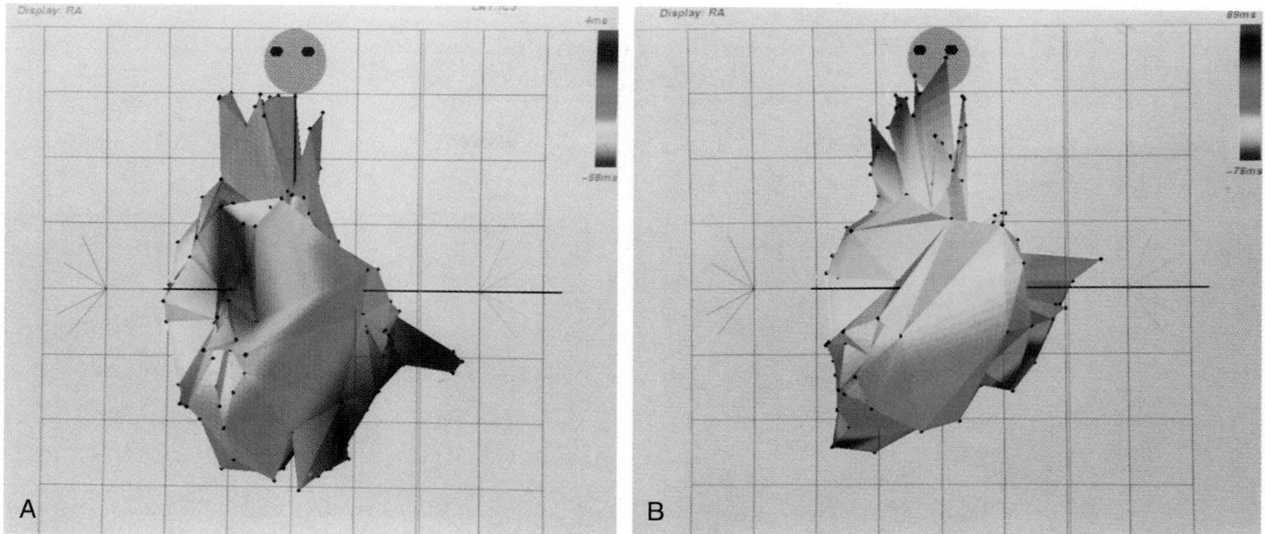

PLATE 97–1 A, Mapping of the right atrium during atrial tachycardia of the patient shown in Figure 97–13 using the CARTO system. The earliest atrial activation (−88 ms) was found high in the anterior wall of the right atrium. **B,** A new activation map of the right atrium was performed after successful radiofrequency ablation. Note that now the earliest atrial activation is in the sinus node region.

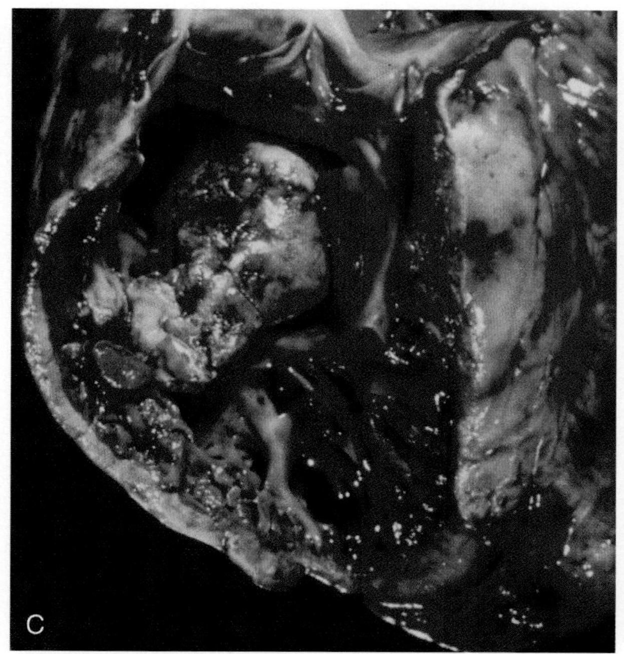

PLATE 99–1 A 47-year-old woman with unexplained shortness of breath had a referring diagnosis of Munchausen's syndrome. **C,** Autopsy view of a large thrombus in the right ventricle. Numerous old and new thromboemboli were present throughout the pulmonary arterial tree.

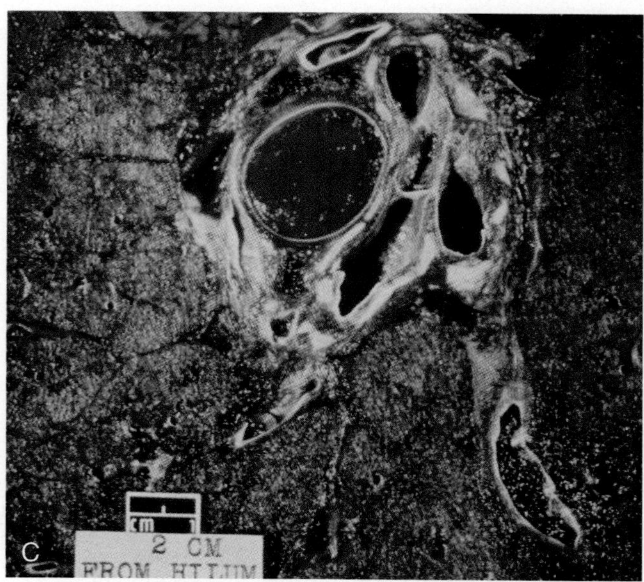

PLATE 99–6 A 68-year-old man had congestive heart failure, hemoptysis, and a right hilar mass thought to represent bronchogenic carcinoma. **C,** Sagittal section of the right lung shows an organized thrombus extending 8 cm from the hilum, totally occluding the right middle and lower lobe arteries, and accounting for the hilar mass seen on the chest radiograph.

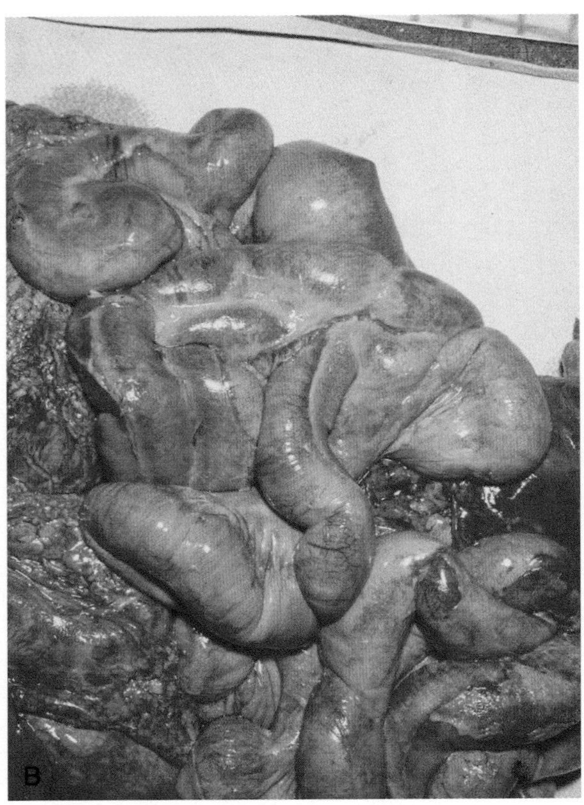

PLATE 99–8 A 55-year-old man underwent surgical correction of sigmoid volvulus. **B,** Autopsy view of the patient's intestines shows purulent peritonitis that resulted from disruption of the colon at the site of operative repair. There were no pulmonary thromboemboli.

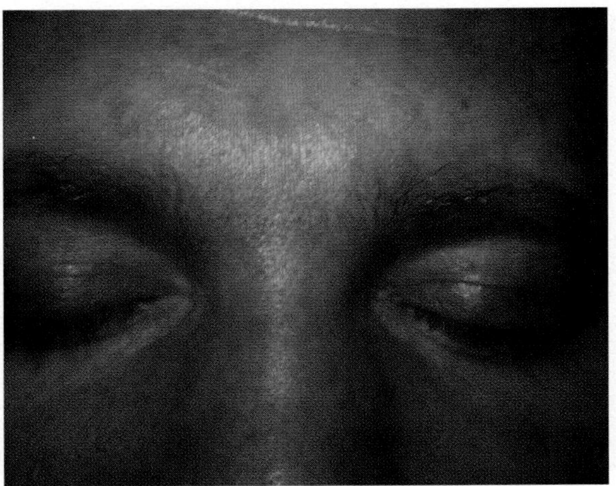

PLATE 104–1 Typical malar erythema (butterfly rash) of systemic lupus erythematosus.

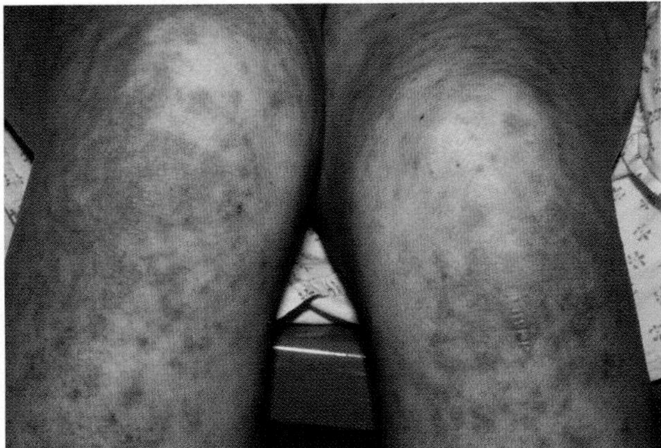

PLATE 104–2 Livedo reticularis in a patient with primary antiphospholipid syndrome. Biopsy of this skin rash would reveal thrombosis in capillaries and small vessels.

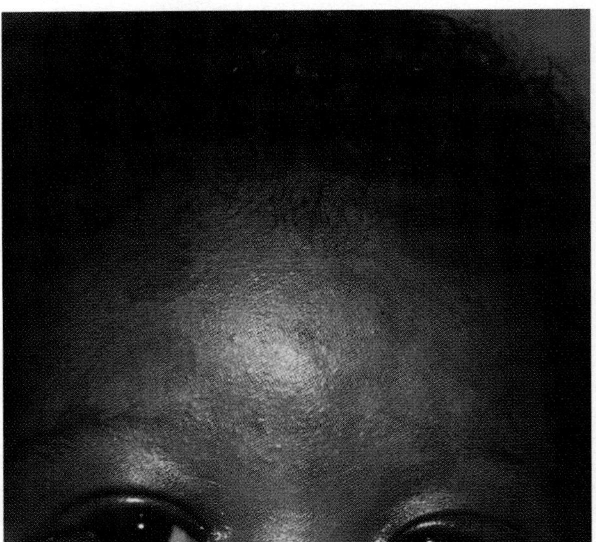

PLATE 104–3 Annular skin lesions of the neonatal lupus syndrome in an infant born of a mother with anti-Ro (SS-A) autoantibodies. The skin rash resolved concomitantly with disappearance of maternal antibodies at 5 to 6 months of age. Unlike neonatal lupus rash, congenital heart block due to anti-Ro (SS-A) antibodies is permanent.

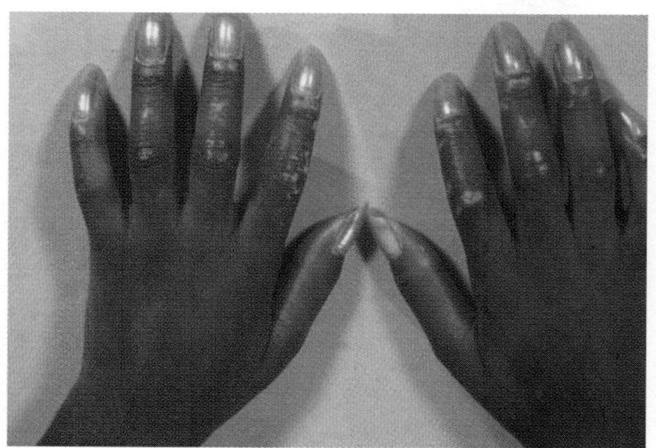

PLATE 104–4 Hands of a patient with scleroderma show tightening of the skin over the fingers (sclerodactyly) and areas of hypopigmentation.

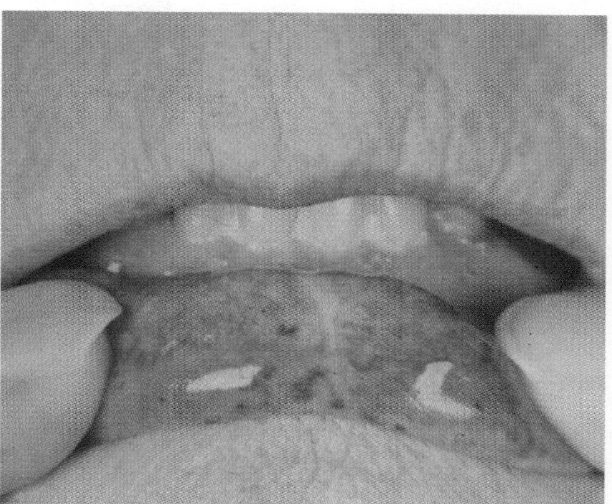

PLATE 104–5 Underside of the lower lip shows multiple telangiectasias in a patient with the CREST (calcinosis, Raynaud's phenomenon, esophageal dysmotility, sclerodactyly, and telangiectasia) variant of scleroderma.

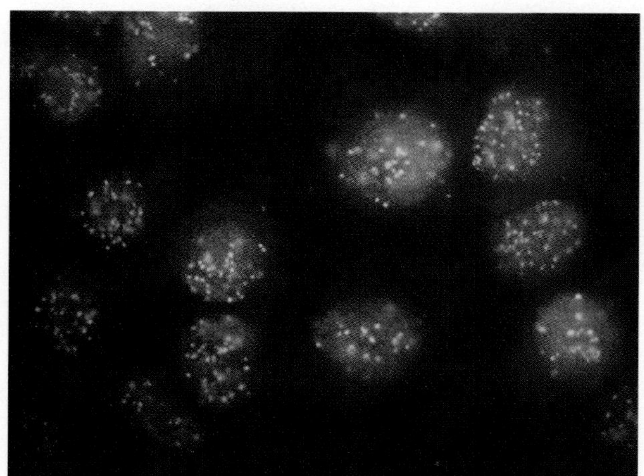

PLATE 104–6 Photomicrograph of an antinuclear antibody preparation shows immunofluorescence of discrete speckled nuclear pattern on HEp-2 cells, typical of serum anticentromere antibodies. These antibodies are usually found in mild scleroderma or the CREST variant.

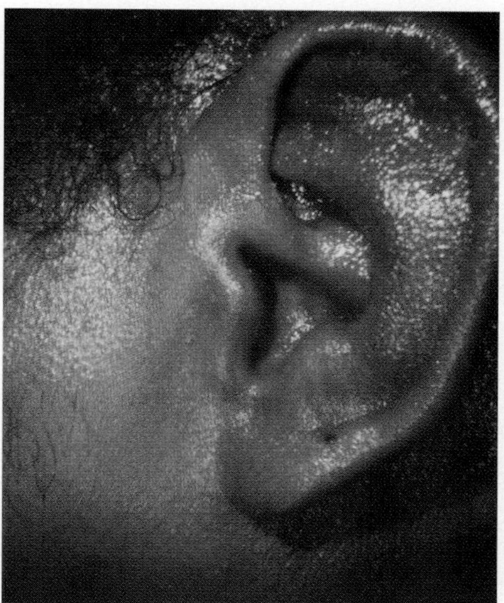

PLATE 104–7 Inflammation and partial collapse of auricular cartilage in a patient with relapsing polychondritis.

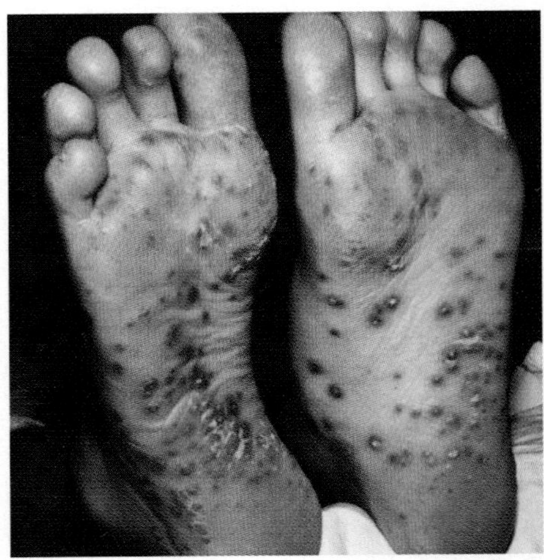

PLATE 104–8 The typical pustular rash (keratoderma blennorrhagica) of a patient with Reiter's disease.

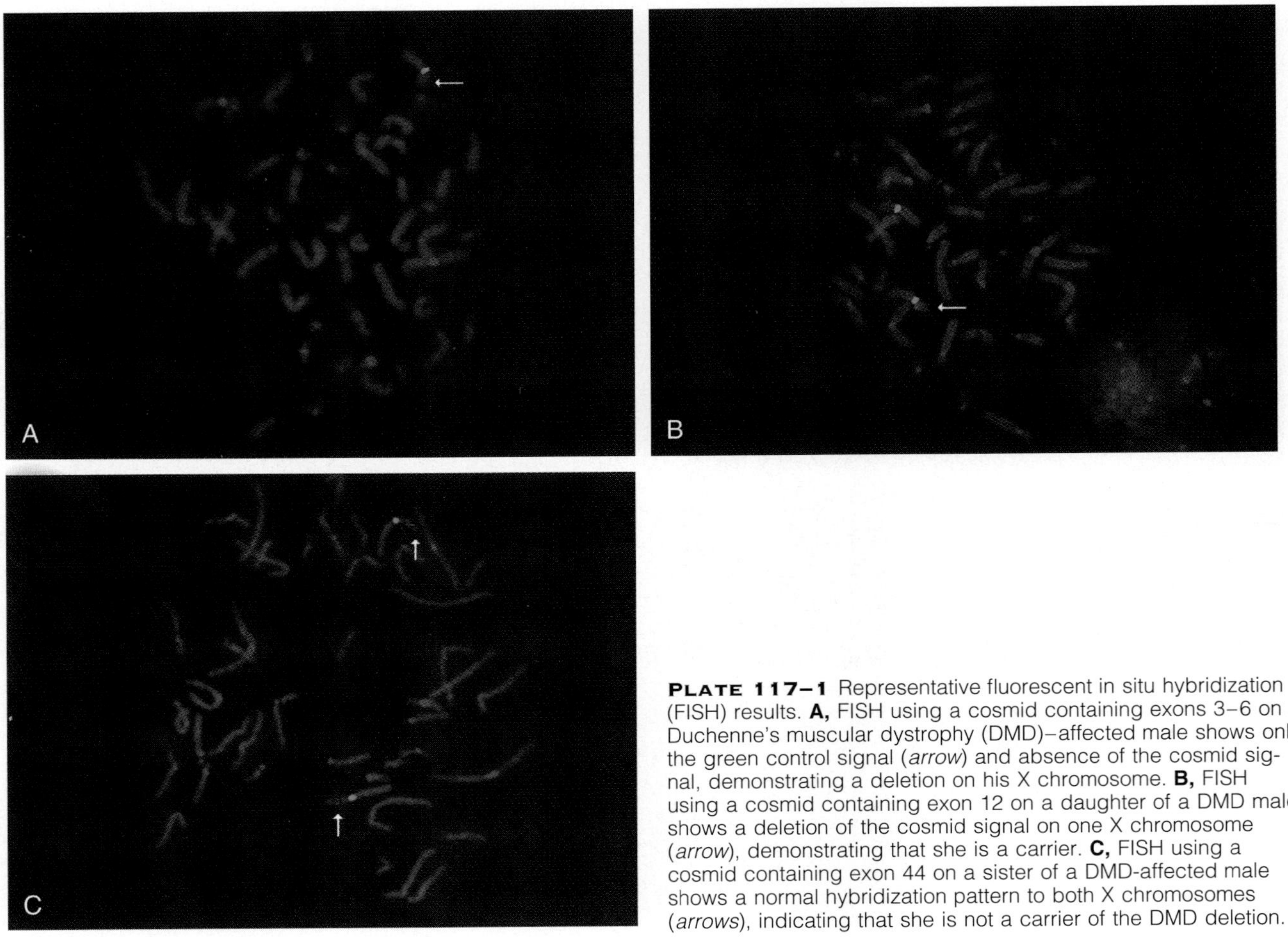

PLATE 117–1 Representative fluorescent in situ hybridization (FISH) results. **A,** FISH using a cosmid containing exons 3–6 on a Duchenne's muscular dystrophy (DMD)–affected male shows only the green control signal (*arrow*) and absence of the cosmid signal, demonstrating a deletion on his X chromosome. **B,** FISH using a cosmid containing exon 12 on a daughter of a DMD male shows a deletion of the cosmid signal on one X chromosome (*arrow*), demonstrating that she is a carrier. **C,** FISH using a cosmid containing exon 44 on a sister of a DMD-affected male shows a normal hybridization pattern to both X chromosomes (*arrows*), indicating that she is not a carrier of the DMD deletion.

SECTION I

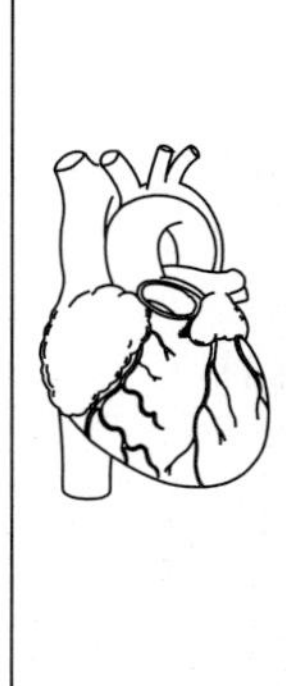

INTRODUCTION: CARDIAC SIGNS AND SYMPTOMS AND SELECTED NONINVASIVE DIAGNOSTIC METHODS

The History and Physical Examination

Electrocardiography

Chest Radiography

Echocardiography

Nuclear Cardiology

Magnetic Resonance Imaging

CHAPTER 1

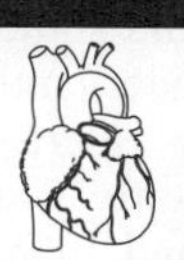

The History and Physical Examination

James T. Willerson and Thomas Smitherman

IMPORTANCE OF PATIENT HISTORY
Dyspnea
Chest Pain
Cough and Hemoptysis
Palpitation
Syncope
Cardiac Enlargement
Murmurs
Gallops
Edema
Rales
Pleural Effusion
Cyanosis
Clubbing
PHYSICAL EXAMINATION OF THE PATIENT WITH HEART DISEASE
Inspection
Blood Pressure Measurement
Regularity and Configuration of Pulses
Examination of the Jugular Venous Pulse
Inspection, Palpation, and Percussion of the Precordium
Auscultation
First Heart Sounds
Clicks
Murmurs
Gallop Sounds
Heart Sounds From Prosthetic Disc Heart Valves

Importance of Patient History

The importance of a carefully obtained and accurate history from the patient with cardiovascular disease cannot be overemphasized. In many instances, such a history enables one to recognize the etiology of the problem relatively rapidly. When a comprehensive and accurate history is not obtained, the physician is much less effective and definitive in assisting the patient.

The patient's general appearance often helps the well-trained physician to focus questions so as to obtain a meaningful history. The patient's family history may also assist the physician in the history-taking process, given that the genetic risks for cardiovascular disease are very important, especially when cardiovascular disease has occurred at a relatively young age in a patient's father, mother, siblings, or grandparents. Obvious risk factors for specific cardiovascular diseases enable the physician to elicit specific complaints related to the patient's cardiovascular problem. A history of substance abuse should lead to specific questions. Cardiovascular abnormalities detected on physical examination should also help the physician to elucidate a meaningful history from the patient.

We have found it useful to focus on a set of questions immediately directed at an apparent or a suspected cardiovascular abnormality during the first few minutes of interaction with the patient. General questions may be asked later, but we have found it helpful to focus on the seemingly most relevant questions first.

The physician must try to obtain both subjective and objective, even quantitative, answers to specific questions. Although it is necessary to know about the presence of chest pain, dyspnea, and easy fatigability, it is also necessary to determine the specific type of pain present and what provokes and relieves it. Similarly, learning the amount of effort required before dyspnea occurs or the amount of effort required before the patient tires is useful in determining specific etiologies for a particular cardiovascular problem and in determining the severity of the patient's limitation.

In evaluating the patient with chest pain, one must learn whether the pain is anginal or pleuritic in quality. Pleuritic pain raises questions concerning pulmonary or pericardial pain, whereas anginal pain suggests the presence of one of the coronary artery disease (CAD) syndromes or severe left ventricular (LV) outflow obstruction or severe LV hypertrophy. Dyspnea may be caused by pulmonary or cardiac problems but sometimes is simply a manifestation of anxiety. Easy fatigability can be caused by heart or lung disease or by extracardiac factors, such as anemia, thyrotoxicosis, obesity, renal disease, or a systemic malignancy.

A careful physical examination should elucidate the patient's family history, any substance abuse, any evidence of syncope, dyspnea, orthopnea, chest pain, abdominal pain, discomfort in the legs while walking, headaches, muscle weakness, hemoptysis, tiring unduly rapidly with physical effort, palpitations, fever, diaphoresis, loss of appetite, weight loss or gain, and history related to the presence or absence of risk factors for cardiovascular diseases.

A carefully obtained history from a patient with cardiovascular disease almost always leads the knowledgeable physician toward a more rapid and correct diagnosis of the patient's cardiovascular problem and the development of an effective treatment plan. When an accurate and careful history is not or cannot be obtained, it is often difficult to identify the correct etiology of a cardiovascular problem, and sometimes less than optimal diagnostic and therapeutic interventions are used.

Heart disease is manifested by various signs and symptoms. Cardiac dysfunction influences many organ systems, and many noncardiac illnesses are expressed in findings similar to those produced by cardiovascular diseases. The differential diagnosis of the signs and symptoms commonly seen in heart disease is addressed below.

Dyspnea

Dyspnea, the labored breathing usually referred to as *shortness of breath*, is a distressful sensation of air hunger. It is abnormal only when the sensation of breathlessness is inappropriate to the level of physical activity that provoked it. The major causes of dyspnea are listed in Table 1–1. Although substantial information is available on the normal control of ventilation, the mechanism of the uncomfortable breathlessness of dyspnea is unclear. It is notable that some causes of marked hyperpnea, such as metabolic acidosis, do not cause dyspnea. The same can be said of the hyperpneic phase of Cheyne-Stokes respiration. However, the examination can point to some abnormalities that may be responsible for initiation of the processes that eventually lead to dyspnea.

When left-sided congestive heart failure (CHF) and obstruction to filling of the left side of the heart develop, as occurs with mitral stenosis and left atrial myxoma, pulmonary venous and pulmonary capillary pressures are chronically elevated, causing interstitial and intra-alveolar edema. This interferes with normal pulmonary compliance and reduces airway size and oxygen diffusion. Disorders associated with intracardiac right-to-left shunts are accompanied by chronic systemic hypoxia. With uncomplicated right ventricular (RV) outflow obstruction, there is hypoperfusion of the pulmonary vasculature. In pulmonary diseases, ventilatory impairment is present; this can be attributed to either an obstructive or a restrictive phenomenon. Pulmonary embolization is followed by a reduction in pulmonary flow in the affected segments, with consequent ventilation-perfusion abnormalities. Bronchospasm may occur in the wake of a pulmonary embolus, probably mediated by the release of substances that lead to contraction of smooth muscle. The dyspnea that may occur with pulmonary hypertension with a normal cardiac output is not well understood but may be related in part to reflex-stimulated hyperventilation. There may be hypoxemia with severe anemia and at high altitudes, especially during exertion.

Cardiac and pulmonary disorders account for the vast majority of cases of dyspnea. When either system is involved in the absence of disease of the other, differentiation of the cause of dyspnea is usually not difficult. When both the heart and lungs are abnormal, differentiation of the etiology of the dyspnea is difficult but imperative. To differentiate cardiac from pulmonary dyspnea, associated signs and symptoms of heart disease should be sought. Progressive dyspnea over a relatively short time is usually an important clue to cardiac dyspnea, as opposed to the generally long-standing symptoms of pulmonary disease. The presence of pulmonary disease is usually obvious from the history and physical examination. Chronic progressive shortness of breath with a productive cough, chronic rhonchi and wheezes, diminished breath sounds, and respiratory capacity, with abnormal pulmonary function test values and the absence of evidence of heart disease, help to confirm pulmonary disease as the chief cause of dyspnea. Radiologic evidence of specific cardiac or pulmonary disease may provide cogent evidence for the cause of dyspnea.

Evidence of acute infection should be sought because this is frequently the cause of worsening symptoms in chronic lung diseases. Redistribution of pulmonary blood flow to the upper lung fields, usually a sign of increased pulmonary venous pressure and, hence, evidence of cardiac dyspnea, must be interpreted cautiously in the face of chronic obstructive lung disease, which may cause this radiologic change without raised pulmonary venous pressure.

Pulmonary emboli frequently cause dyspnea. The presence of conditions favoring venous thromboembolism or hemoptysis, pleuritic chest pain, fever, tachycardia, and jaundice from the history and physical examination, coupled with evidence of acute right heart strain on examination and electrocardiogram (ECG) and atelectasis or a pleural-based parenchymal radiodensity with a rounded profile toward the hilus (Hampton's lump) on chest radiography may provide clues to pulmonary emboli, especially large ones. If emboli are small, however, there may be insufficient clinical clues to establish the diagnosis, and lung scintigraphy or pulmonary arteriography may be necessary.

The characteristic features of disorders with an intracardiac right-to-left shunt (e.g., pulmonary stenosis, pulmonary hypertension, and severe anemia) usually facilitate establishment of the cause of dyspnea in patients with these disturbances. Patients with psychogenic dyspnea tend to demonstrate prominent sighing respiration with large and

TABLE 1–1 Important Causes of Dyspnea

- Heart disease
  - Left ventricular failure
  - Restrictive cardiomyopathy
  - Constrictive pericarditis
  - Pulmonary venous obstruction
    - Mitral stenosis
    - Cor triatriatum
    - Left atrial myxoma
    - Left atrial thrombus
    - Tamponade
- Lung disease
  - Obstructive airways disease
    - Chronic obstructive pulmonary disease
    - Asthma
  - Restrictive lung disease
    - Interstitial or diffuse alveolar lung disease
    - Disorders of chest wall and bellows function
    - Kyphoscoliosis
    - Arthritis
    - Neuromuscular disease
    - Obesity
  - Vascular disease
    - Pulmonary embolism
    - Primary pulmonary hypertension
- High-altitude exposure
- Anemia
- Anxiety (hyperventilation syndrome)

erratic tidal volumes. Other symptoms of hyperventilation and neurotic behavior may also be present.

Orthopnea is dyspnea during recumbent posture. It is usually due to LV failure or inflow obstruction. More of the lung is below the level of the heart during recumbency, and consequently pulmonary capillary pressure is further raised. Patients can often approximately quantify its severity on the basis of the number of pillows necessary to achieve relief. Reassumption of upright posture provides immediate relief. Similar symptoms may be encountered in patients with pulmonary disease. The mechanisms involved are probably the less efficient movement of the ventilatory apparatus and pooling of secretions in the recumbent position.

Paroxysmal nocturnal dyspnea occurs several hours after assumption of a recumbent position. It, too, is usually due to LV failure or inflow obstruction. Pulmonary venous pressure is raised by the lowered position of the lungs relative to the heart and by return of extravascular fluid to the intravascular space. Typically, the patient wakes, sits upright, and seeks "fresh air," often by opening a window. Pulmonary disease may cause a similar syndrome, probably for the same reason that it may cause orthopnea.

Chest Pain

Pain from different sources may be expressed as chest discomfort. Visceral pain is noted in the somatic area with which it shares a final common pathway. The demarcation of visceral pain, however, is less precise than that of somatic pain because of the distribution of visceral pain to several adjacent spinal cord segments. Chest pain due to cardiac disease consequently must be differentiated from that due to disorders of other thoracic viscera and the upper abdomen. Some of the important causes of chest pain are listed in Table 1–2.

TABLE 1–2 Common Causes of Chest Pain

- Heart disease
  - Angina pectoris
    - Atheromatous coronary artery disease
    - Nonatheromatous coronary artery disease
    - Aortic stenosis
    - Aortic insufficiency
    - Idiopathic hypertrophic subaortic stenosis (hypertrophic obstructive cardiomyopathy)
  - Myocardial infarction
  - Congestive cardiomyopathy
  - Pulmonary hypertension
  - Mitral valve prolapse (click-murmur) syndrome
  - Pericarditis
- Dissection of the aorta
- Pulmonary disease
  - Pulmonary embolism
  - Pleuritis
  - Pneumothorax
  - Pneumonia
  - Tumor
  - Collagen disease
  - Atelectasis
- Musculoskeletal disease
  - Arthritis
  - Costochondritis (Tietze's syndrome)
  - Bursitis
  - Intravertebral disc disease
  - Thoracic outlet syndrome
  - Muscle spasm
  - Fracture
  - Metastatic tumor or hematologic (leukemia) or plasma cell (myeloma) malignancy
- Neural disease
  - Intercostal neuritis
  - Herpes zoster
- Gastrointestinal disorders ("referred" chest pain)
  - Hiatal hernia
  - Cholecystitis
  - Pancreatitis
  - Ulcer disease
  - Bowel disease
- Neoplasm
- Emotional duress or anxiety (e.g., neurocirculatory asthenia, DaCosta's syndrome)

Angina Pectoris

Angina pectoris results from an imbalance between myocardial oxygen demand and oxygen delivery by coronary artery flow. It is most commonly due to a significant reduction in coronary blood flow. Coronary atherosclerosis is the most common cause of this reduction. However, angina may also be caused by disorders that increase myocardial oxygen demand, such as aortic stenosis and obstructive cardiomyopathy (hypertrophic obstructive cardiomyopathy), or by disorders that both increase myocardial oxygen demand and possibly decrease coronary artery flow, such as aortic regurgitation. Angina is typically described as substernal epigastric or left shoulder or jaw tightness, squeezing, pressure, heaviness, or a bursting sensation. The patient may describe it graphically with a clenched fist over the midchest (Levine's sign). It may also be described as a burning, sharp, stabbing, or numb sensation. Radiation of the pain occurs often and is usually projected to the left shoulder, neck, jaw, and ulnar distribution of the left arm. Radiation to the same areas on the right side and the epigastric area also occurs. Pain referral to the left scapular region of the back occurs but is less common.

Angina ordinarily is precipitated by exertion, emotional upsets, cold exposure, or eating and is usually relieved by rest or nitroglycerin within 5 minutes. It may be accompanied by dyspnea when myocardial ischemia is associated with LV dysfunction (diastolic, systolic, or both) or mitral regurgitation. Stable angina is usually predictable in both its frequency and ease of provocation. Unstable angina refers to pain that occurs at night (nocturnal angina), at rest (angina decubitus), with increasing frequency or duration, or with less predictable provocation and relief. It may be accompanied by either a normal ECG or one with manifestations of ischemia.

Acute Myocardial Infarction

With acute myocardial infarction (MI), the pain is similar to that of angina but is intense and prolonged, usually requiring medication (often opiates) for relief. It is usually accompanied by dyspnea, palpitations, and syncope when LV failure, cardiac rhythm, and conduction disturbances complicate the MI. The characteristic findings on physical examination and the ECG in patients with aortic valvular and subvalvular disease usually make it easy to differentiate angina complicating these disorders from angina caused by CAD. The chest pain that accompanies prolapse of the mitral valve (click-murmur syndrome), congestive cardiomyopathy, and pulmonary hypertension may mimic angina closely, but a carefully taken history will usually reveal atypical features for angina. The physical, radiographic, perfusion scintigraphy, and electrocardiographic examinations usually clarify the probable cause of the chest discomfort in these cases. Occasionally, however, only coronary arteriography will exclude the presence of significant coronary artery narrowing.

A small number of patients, mostly women, have typical angina pectoris with completely normal coronary arteriograms. Some have abnormal resting and exercise ECGs and inappropriate myocardial lactate production. The cause of this syndrome is not understood, but severe ventricular hypertrophy with limitation of coronary artery vasodilation, increased myocardial oxygen demand, and increases in coronary vascular resistance mediated by local increases in endothelin concentrations may be responsible on occasion. Coronary arteriography is sometimes necessary to differentiate it from atherosclerotic heart disease.

Chest pain resulting from pericarditis is usually pleuropericardial and increases in severity with coughing, deep breathing, movement, sometimes with swallowing, and usually with assumption of the supine position. A friction rub on examination and the typical electrocardiographic features usually serve to differentiate it from angina. Pain caused by a dissecting aneurysm of the thoracic aorta may also mimic angina, but it is characteristically of a tearing quality and may be most severe in the suprasternal notch, the neck, the back, or the lumbar region. It is often excruciatingly severe and requires narcotic analgesics for relief. Associated findings, such as pulse deficits, acute aortic regurgitation, a widened or disfigured aortic profile on chest radiography, or new neurologic deficits, should raise the index of suspicion for this disorder, especially in the patient with systemic arterial hypertension. Commonly, however, aortography or a noninvasive imaging procedure, such as magnetic resonance imaging (MRI), transesophageal echocardiography, or computed tomography (CT), will be necessary to establish the diagnosis with certainty.

Chest Pain of Noncardiac Origin

Patients with pulmonary problems may present with chest pain. When pain is a manifestation of pneumonia, pleurisy, pneumothorax, or pulmonary embolus, it is usually pleuritic. Gastrointestinal disorders, especially those of the esophagus, may be associated with referred pain to the chest. Although the pain of inflammation, diffuse spasm, rupture of the esophagus, peptic ulcer disease, pancreatitis, or cholecystitis may mimic angina, there are usually sufficiently specific complaints and atypical features for angina in a well-taken history to point to a gastrointestinal tract origin. Proper laboratory and radiologic examinations will reveal the source of the pain. It must be remembered that noncardiac disorders can act as a trigger for angina in the patient with CAD, and the confirmation of noncardiac diseases does not always eliminate the possibility that the patient's discomfort is angina.

A frequent cause of chest pain of noncardiac origin is associated with anxiety (DaCosta's syndrome, neurocirculatory asthenia, soldier's heart, cardiac neurosis). Although the pain may mimic angina, it is typically fleeting and lancinating or a prolonged aching pain; it usually occurs after rather than during effort. It is commonly associated with evidence of the hyperventilation syndrome. Unfortunately, the many problems and fears that accompany chronic heart disease often leave anxiety and a cardiac neurosis in their wake, so the symptoms of cardiac disease and neurosis coexist and must be carefully ferreted out by the physician.

Occasionally, costochondritis (Tietze's syndrome), the thoracic outlet syndrome, intercostal nerve herpes zoster, chest wall pain, and disorders of the thoracic and cervical spine may cause chest discomfort that must be differentiated from pain of cardiac origin; with herpes zoster infection and chest wall pain, the severe pain may precede the development of the characteristic skin rash by several days.

Cough and Hemoptysis

Coughing is a voluntary or reflex act to clear the tracheobronchial tree of secretions or particulate matter. The stimulus for coughing is usually produced by mucosal irritation from the larynx to second-order bronchi, which are responsive to inflammatory, mechanical, chemical, and thermal stimuli. The nature of the cough is an important factor in identifying its cause and the cough should be defined as productive or nonproductive, with characterization and quantification of the sputum.

Cough may be an early manifestation of pulmonary venous hypertension due to LV failure or pulmonary venous obstruction, as in mitral stenosis. It may be overlooked as a symptom of heart disease if respiratory infection precipitates cardiac decompensation. The cough of early heart failure is nonproductive or productive of only small amounts of whitish sputum. It most frequently is nocturnal, occurring soon after the patient becomes supine, and may continue as a prominent symptom interfering with sleep. It is related to bronchiolar edema and may be present without rales. Patients with mitral stenosis may also experience bouts of coughing, which may be confused with chronic bronchitis. Blood streaking of the sputum may occur after a paroxysm of coughing related to pulmonary venous congestion. Cough may also be a manifestation of CHF in children with large left-to-right shunts. A chronic nonproductive cough similar to that noted in early LV failure is common in patients with pulmonary fibrosis or infiltration and lesions that compress the trachea and bronchi, such as lung tumors and aortic aneurysms. Pulmonary infection produces a purulent, exudative cough. In chronic obstructive pulmonary disease (COPD), the cough is productive, with purulence dependent on the presence and severity of acute and chronic bronchitis. The sputum of patients with bronchiectasis is characteristically mucopurulent, malodorous, and copious.

Hemoptysis is a relatively rare manifestation of cardiac disease. The important causes of hemoptysis are itemized in Table 1–3. Occasionally, high pulmonary venous pressure resulting from chronic CHF or mitral stenosis may

TABLE 1-3 Causes of Hemoptysis

Cardiac
- Pulmonary venous hypertension
  - Left ventricular failure
  - Mitral stenosis
- Eisenmenger's syndrome

Pulmonary
- Infection
  - Pneumonitis
  - Bronchitis
  - Bronchiectasis
  - Abscess
- Tumor
- Trauma or foreign body

Vascular
- Rupture of atrioventricular fistula
- Thoracic aortic aneurysm
- Hereditary hemorrhagic telangiectasia (Osler-Weber-Rendu syndrome)

Primary pulmonary hypertension
Pulmonary embolism
Goodpasture's syndrome
Vasculitides
- Polyarteritis nodosa
- Systemic lupus erythematosus
- Wegener's granulomatosis

Bleeding diathesis

lead to the rupture of pulmonary capillaries and the production of blood-streaked sputum. Hemoptysis in mitral stenosis may be small in amount and recurrent or quite brisk when related to rupture of endobronchial bronchopulmonary venous varicosities. This is particularly likely when an abrupt increase in pulmonary venous pressure occurs with increased heart rate. Eisenmenger's syndrome also is sometimes associated with prominent hemoptysis; in these patients, hemoptysis presumably results from rupture of pulmonary arterioles as a consequence of increased pulmonary artery pressure and resistance. Encroachment on the tracheobronchial tree by an aortic aneurysm may lead to either a small amount of hemoptysis or fatal exsanguination.

Hemoptysis is usually due to disease in the lungs or the pulmonary vasculature. It is a relatively common manifestation of pulmonary infection, tumors, trauma, pulmonary embolism and infarction, and disorders affecting the pulmonary vasculature, such as Goodpasture's syndrome, hereditary hemorrhagic telangiectasia (Osler-Weber-Rendu syndrome), and several vasculitides (especially Wegener's granulomatosis, periarteritis nodosa, and systemic lupus erythematosus). Fortunately, these problems are usually easily differentiated from cardiac disease because of their characteristic features.

Palpitation

Palpitations are a subjective consciousness of the beating of the heart (Table 1–4). Alterations in heart rate, rhythm, or force of contraction may be experienced as palpitation. This sensation may be appreciated by the patient as a stopping, skipping, fluttering, jumping, pounding, or racing of the heart or as nervousness or uneasiness in the chest. With tachyarrhythmia, the patient may be able to describe the manner of onset and the rate and regularity of heartbeat. It is important to note associated symptoms related to the beating of the heart, particularly any change in the level of consciousness. Palpitations may be related to the occurrence of a cardiac arrhythmia but also can be experienced with no disturbance at all in rhythm or rate. Enhanced contractility or a heightened awareness of autonomic function with anxiety may sensitize the individual to the heartbeat.

Premature contractions of supraventricular or ventricular etiology may be experienced as an early beat, a pause or skipped beat, or "flopping" or "thudding" related to the intensely contractile beat after the premature beat.

Paroxysmal bouts of supraventricular tachycardia are often appreciated as being abrupt in onset. They may be irregular, as with atrial flutter/fibrillation, paroxysmal atrial tachycardia with block, multifocal atrial tachycardia, and atrial fibrillation, or regular, as with sinus tachycardia, paroxysmal atrial or atrioventricular (AV) junctional tachycardia, and atrial flutter. Cessation of these arrhythmias is likewise often abrupt. Ventricular tachycardia is more frequently manifested by its symptoms than as appreciation of palpitation. Other causes of palpitations include hyperkinetic states (e.g., intense exertion, fever, thyrotoxicosis, hypoglycemia, anemia, AV fistula, and pheochromocytoma).

Certain drugs that may be associated with the production of palpitations include amphetamines, ephedrine, aminophylline and other sympathomimetic agents, xanthine-containing beverages (coffee, tea, cola), alcohol, tobacco, and excessive digitalis glycosides or thyroid hormone. Hypokalemia, hypercalcemia, and hypoxia may produce palpitations by inducing atrial or ventricular rhythm disturbances. Anxiety states may be associated with palpitations because

TABLE 1-4 Causes of Palpitations

Extrasystoles
- Atrial premature beats
- Atrioventricular junctional (nodal) premature beats
- Ventricular premature beats

Tachyarrhythmias
- Supraventricular
  - Regular
    - Sinus tachycardia
    - Paroxysmal supraventricular tachycardia
    - Atrioventricular junctional tachycardia
    - Atrial flutter
  - Irregular
    - Atrial fibrillation
    - Paroxysmal supraventricular tachycardia or atrial flutter with block
    - Multifocal atrial tachycardia

Ventricular tachycardia
Bradycardia
- Sinus bradycardia
- Sinus arrest
- Second- or third-degree atrioventricular block

Conditions associated with increased force of cardiac contraction
- Thyrotoxicosis
- Anemia
- Fever
- Certain drugs, including catecholamines and cardiac glycosides

Anxiety states

of a heightened appreciation of cardiac function, emotional duress, hyperventilation, or tachycardia.

Determination of the cause of palpitations can be difficult. In addition to taking a careful history, performing the physical examination, and obtaining appropriate laboratory data, dynamic ECG (Holter) monitoring with a careful diary of the time and nature of symptoms can assist in the diagnosis and treatment. Event monitors and transtelephonic transmission of episodes of palpitations allow the correct diagnosis to be established. Exercise testing also may demonstrate the occurrence of arrhythmia during an increased workload or immediately after its cessation.

Syncope

Complete AV block is the most common cause of Stokes-Adams attacks, but fast or slow heart rates of any cause may be responsible. Unduly rapid or slow supraventricular or ventricular dysrhythmias or second-degree AV block produces fainting as a consequence of the inability of the heart to maintain normal cardiac output at these extremes of heart rate. The patient's ability to cope with cardiac dysrhythmia is influenced by the overall status of the heart and the presence of other forms of disease (e.g., cerebral vascular disease, anemia). Syncope may occur either at the onset of, during, or after the termination of the dysrhythmia. Bradyarrhythmias and, occasionally, advanced AV block are sometimes encountered with vasovagal episodes but also may occur with fainting associated with carotid sinus disease, traction on an esophageal diverticulum, mediastinal tumors, gallbladder disease, glossopharyngeal neuralgia, pleural and pulmonary irritation, and rapid decompression of pericardium, pleural, and peritoneal spaces by needle or catheter aspiration of fluid (Table 1–5).

Other forms of heart disease also may be associated with syncope. Effort syncope is one of the cardinal manifestations of hemodynamically significant aortic stenosis. Arteriolar vasodilatation during muscular work or as the result of activation of high-pressure baroreceptors in the left heart, with failure to increase cardiac output to balance this fall in peripheral vascular resistance, results in a reduction in systemic arterial blood pressure and diminished cerebral perfusion. Postexertional syncope occurs in hypertrophic obstructive cardiomyopathy due to an abrupt worsening of the muscular outflow obstruction that probably results from a rapid drop in LV filling and blood pressure in the face of a sustained increased inotropic state that occurs with cessation of exercise. Sudden and severe valvular obstruction occurring with left atrial myxoma or ball-valve thrombus or with thrombosis or malfunction of a prosthetic valve may also produce syncope. Tetralogy of Fallot is the most common form of congenital heart disease associated with syncope. Systemic vasodilatation with increased right-to-left shunting (probably associated with infundibular spasm) is likely the mechanism for fainting during "spells" in children with tetralogy of Fallot. Primary pulmonary hypertension may be associated with syncope.

The most common cause of fainting is vasodepressor or vasovagal syncope, which tends to occur in situations of emotional duress or, occasionally, in certain postures or positions. A marked reduction in systemic vascular resistance is associated with a fall in systemic arterial blood pressure without a compensatory increase in cardiac output; increased vagal activity with pronounced bradycardia then lowers cardiac output further, and loss of consciousness may ensue. Autonomic manifestations are prominent, with pallor, perspiration, epigastric distress or nausea, pupillary dilatation, yawning and hyperventilation, visual blurring, auditory diminution, weakness, confusion, and loss of consciousness.

TABLE 1–5 Causes of Syncope

- Cardiac
  - Decreased cerebral perfusion due to cardiac dysrhythmia or conduction defect
  - Left ventricular outflow obstruction
    - Valvular aortic stenosis
    - Supravalvular aortic stenosis
    - Discrete subvalvular aortic stenosis
    - Obstructive cardiomyopathy (hypertrophic obstructive)
  - Tetralogy of Fallot
- Orthostatic hypotension
- Vasovagal (vasodepressor, psychogenic)
- Micturition syncope
- Cough syncope
- Carotid sinus syncope
- Glossopharyngeal neuralgia
- Metabolic
  - Hypoglycemia
  - Hypoxia
  - Hyperventilation
- Central cerebral mechanisms
  - Cerebrovascular accident
  - Transient ischemic attacks
  - Subclavian steal syndrome
  - Migraine
  - Vasculitis
  - Tumor
  - Seizure disorder
- Hysteria

Orthostatic or postural hypotension with a significant fall in systemic arterial blood pressure is a result of a failure of adaptive reflexes or mechanical mechanisms to compensate in the upright posture. It may occur as a result of neuropathic disorders, such as diabetes mellitus, amyloidosis, tabes dorsalis, and alcoholic neuropathy. In primary autonomic insufficiency (Bradbury-Eggleston syndrome), there are associated defects in autonomic function, such as lack of sphincter control, tearing, salivation, or sweating, and in some patients, there is abnormal extrapyramidal activity (Shy-Drager syndrome). During upright posture, these patients, although hypotensive, have no compensatory tachycardia or other symptoms, such as sweating and nausea. Other causes of postural hypotension can include physical deconditioning or debilitation, sympathectomy, or the administration of antihypertensive agents.

In some patients, stimulation of the carotid sinus (*carotid sinus hypersensitivity*) leads to a profound decrease in systemic arterial pressure and a marked slowing of heart rate. Symptoms may be precipitated by relatively minor stimuli, such as head motion or a tight collar. Fainting is often precipitous, without presyncopal manifestations.

Cough syncope occurs usually in obese men with COPD and is rare in women or children. It is caused by the interaction of a number of mechanisms that lead to decreased cardiac output and central effects; among these are a rise in intrathoracic pressure with a fall in venous return, a marked increase in cerebrospinal fluid pressure and compression of intracranial vascular beds, a concussive effect produced by the sudden rise in intracranial cerebrospinal fluid pressure, an increase in cerebral vascular resistance induced by the hypocapnia of coughing, and increased vagal tone.

Micturition syncope is a sudden loss of consciousness after nocturnal voiding. It is probably caused by Valsalva maneuver–mediated reflex vagal tone and a fall in peripheral vascular resistance enhanced by the abrupt drop in intra-abdominal volume. It most commonly occurs after substantial alcohol consumption. Glossopharyngeal neuralgia may cause reflex stimulation of the vagus and result in fainting. Profound bradycardia is often associated with the disorder. In addition, there is often pain localized to the base of the tongue, pharynx, or larynx; tonsillar area; and ear, followed by syncope. Pressure in sensitive areas may also produce fainting.

Metabolic derangements that lead to hypoxia or hypoglycemia may cause fainting. Disturbances of the vascular supply within or leading to the cranial vault may produce syncope and certainly enhance the ability of other causes to produce a fainting spell. Vertebrobasilar transient ischemic attacks are a common cause of this form of syncope. Movement of the head into certain positions may cause obstruction of vertebral flow, particularly in certain spinal disorders. The subclavian steal syndrome is caused by major occlusion of the proximal subclavian artery with shunting of blood via the vertebral artery to the distal subclavian vessel during exercise as a result of vasodilatation and reduced resistance in the arterial vascular bed with exercise of the affected arm. A vascular bruit may be heard in the supraclavicular area, and there is reduced blood pressure on the affected side. Aortic arch syndrome (Takayasu's arteritis, Oriental pulseless disease) with involvement of the carotid vertebral system is frequently associated with blackout spells. Occasionally, cerebral vasospasm with migraine causes fainting.

Seizure disorders are not usually difficult to distinguish from syncope, with the exception of akinetic petit mal seizures. Assistance in differentiating this form of syncope from other varieties is provided by the presence of an aura, seizure activity, the lack of blood pressure and heart rhythm or rate disturbance, and the postictal state. Dysrhythmias that produce fainting may also produce convulsion. An electroencephalogram (EEG) can be helpful in establishing the cause of syncope in some patients.

Hysteria may express itself as fainting spells; these episodes often occur under dramatic circumstances. There usually is no change in pulse rate, systemic arterial blood pressure, or skin tone. The fainting occurs with grace and without injury, most frequently in young women. There often is a degree of detachment in the description of the event (*la belle indifférence*).

Differential assistance with the problem of syncope is provided by noting heart rate and rhythm, systemic arterial blood pressure, and respiration, as well as skin color and neck veins, during syncopal attacks. The type of onset, precipitating and alleviating factors, body position, and duration of symptoms are also helpful in establishing etiology. Fainting of cardiac etiology tends to produce pallor and cyanosis, jugular venous distention, and shortness of breath. Some abnormality of heart rate or rhythm is common. When peripheral mechanisms reduce cerebral flow, pallor is prominent but not usually accompanied by cyanosis or dyspnea, and jugular venous pressure is not elevated. Disturbance of primary cerebral flow often produces florid features and slow, stridorous respiration. Syncope related to Stokes-Adams attacks is abrupt and is not posturally related. Fainting with dysrhythmias most frequently occurs in a sitting or standing position. Although these characteristics of history and physical examination are helpful, dysrhythmias and transient heart block can at times be elusive to document. Dynamic electrocardiographic (Holter) monitoring and exercise stress testing may uncover these abnormalities when they are not present at rest.

Cardiac Enlargement

The most common cause of cardiac enlargement is CHF (Table 1–6). The heart enlarges as a compensatory mechanism in the face of volume or pressure overload. Cardiac muscle may hypertrophy and undergo dilatation as contractile efficiency and ability to do work decline. Valvular heart disease, pressure overload of the systemic or pulmonary circuit, and significant shunting of cardiac output are potential causes of cardiomegaly. Disease of the heart muscle itself due to ischemia or cardiomyopathy may also cause cardiac enlargement. There may be specific chamber enlargement, or the heart may be generally enlarged. Congestive cardiomyopathy typically produces four-chamber enlargement, or the heart may be generally enlarged. High-output states with heart failure due to beri-beri heart disease, AV fistula, anemia, and thyrotoxicosis may produce cardiac dilatation. Long-standing complete heart block with relatively large stroke volume is occasionally associated with enlargement of the heart without other evidence of heart disease. The heart of the normal, well-conditioned athlete may also enlarge. This normal compensatory dilatation and hypertrophy is associated with a large stroke volume and a relatively slow heart rate. The pericardium may be partly or completely absent on a congenital basis, which allows some expansion of the heart and may be mistaken for heart disease.

Pericardial effusion with apparent enlargement of the

TABLE 1–6 Causes of Cardiac Enlargement

Congestive heart failure
Valvular heart disease
Volume or pressure overload (e.g., left-to-right shunts, systemic arterial hypertension)
Heart muscle disease (ischemia or cardiomyopathy)
High-output failure
Ventricular aneurysm
Large stroke volume
Athlete's heart
Complete heart block
Pericardial effusion
Cardiac cysts and tumors
Absence of the pericardium

heart must be distinguished from cardiomegaly resulting from CHF. Evidence of significant valvular disease, hypertension, congenital heart disease, or cardiomyopathy is ordinarily absent. A history of pericarditis or of factors predisposing to pericarditis may be present. There is no definite specific chamber enlargement on chest radiography with pericardial effusions of modest size; globular cardiac enlargement ("water-bottle heart") occurs instead. The enlarged globular appearance of pericardial effusion most frequently must be differentiated radiographically from the cardiac enlargement associated with primary myocardial disease. With pericardial effusion, heart sounds are often distant, and a pericardial friction rub may be present. The echocardiogram or radionuclide blood pool scan is diagnostic of pericardial effusion when the effusion is large enough to allow its detection. In patients with primary myocardial disease, the heart sounds are usually of normal intensity, and prominent S_3 and S_4 gallops and murmurs of tricuspid or mitral regurgitation, or both, are often present.

Pericardial cysts most frequently produce a rounded or lobulated radiographic appearance and usually occur at the right cardiophrenic angle. Sometimes they are confused with cardiomegaly or ventricular aneurysm. They are not usually associated with symptoms. Tumors invading the pericardium are usually metastatic, but primary tumors occur rarely and may produce pericardial effusion.

Ventricular aneurysm may produce an abnormal bulge in the cardiac contour, especially along the anterolateral LV wall. Persistent ST-segment elevation on the ECG occurs in about 25 percent of these patients. Ventricular aneurysms may be associated with intractable CHF, recurrent ventricular dysrhythmias, and systemic embolic disease.

Murmurs

The generation of a murmur is caused by turbulence of blood flow within the heart or blood vessels. Murmurs occur due to the disruption of smooth laminar flow and production of eddies that generate vibrations. The presence of a murmur may reflect organic heart disease (Table 1–7). Murmurs may be physiologic, occurring without anatomic abnormalities, or may be observed in hyperdynamic circulatory states, as in anemia, fever, and thyrotoxicosis. Murmurs may be innocent (i.e., occurring without any significant anatomic or functional abnormality); these are most common in children and young adults. Murmurs must be distinguished from turbulent flow in veins (venous hum), increased flow during pregnancy (mammary souffle), bruits with AV fistulas or dilated intercostal arterial vessels, or friction rubs. Murmurs should be characterized in terms of their timing, quality, pitch and intensity, and point of maximal intensity and radiation and of the effect of various physiologic or pharmacologic maneuvers on their intensity. Grade 1 murmurs are faint and can be appreciated only with careful auscultation; grade 2 murmurs are relatively soft but readily audible; grade 3 murmurs are prominent and loud; grade 4 murmurs are associated with a thrill and are very loud; grade 5 are extremely loud murmurs; and grade 6 murmurs can be heard with the stethoscope held above the chest wall or even without a stethoscope.

Murmurs are classified on the basis of their duration or timing as being either systolic, diastolic, or continuous. Specific murmurs resulting from heart disease are discussed in other chapters in this book.

TABLE 1-7 Common Causes of Murmurs

- Valvular heart disease
  - Stenosis
  - Insufficiency of congenital or acquired etiology
- Nonvalvular outflow obstruction
  - Supravalvular and subvalvular outflow obstruction
  - Idiopathic hypertrophic subaortic stenosis (hypertrophic obstructive cardiomyopathy)
- Shunts (extracardiac and intracardiac)
- Complex congenital heart disease producing turbulence
- Physiologic murmurs
  - Hyperdynamic states
    - Anemia
    - Fever
    - Thyrotoxicosis
    - Pregnancy
    - Atrioventricular fistula
    - Excitement
  - Flow across normal valves in high-volume states
    - Diastolic rumble in mitral and tricuspid regurgitation, atrial and ventricular septal defect, patent ductus arteriosus
    - Complete heart block
    - Austin Flint murmur of aortic regurgitation
  - Innocent murmurs of childhood
- Anatomic distortion producing turbulence
  - Straight back syndrome
  - Pectus excavatum
  - Chest deformity
- High- to low-pressure communication
  - Ruptured sinus of Valsalva aneurysm
  - Coronary fistula
  - Anomalous origin of left coronary artery from pulmonary artery
  - Atrioventricular fistula
  - Arteriopulmonary connection
- Dilatation or stenosis of large or small vessels
  - Aneurysm or dilatation of aorta or pulmonary artery
  - Coarctation
  - Peripheral pulmonary stenosis
  - Atherosclerotic vascular narrowing
  - Pulmonary embolism
- Alteration of arterial or venous flow in nonconstricted vessels
  - Venous hum
  - Mammary souffle
  - High brachiocephalic flow in children
  - High flow in collateral vessels
    - Intercostal or bronchial collaterals in coarctation of aorta, pulmonic stenosis, or atresia
    - Aortic regurgitation
- Sounds resembling murmurs
  - Fusion of S_3 and S_4 gallops
  - Prolonged gallop sounds
  - Pericardial and pleural friction rubs

Gallops

Cardiac gallops are low-frequency vibrations that are best heard with light pressure with the bell of the stethoscope. Third heart sounds generally occur between 0.12 and 0.24 second after the aortic component of the second heart sound. Clinically, the third heart sound (S_3 gallop) may be a physiologic sound in children and young adults. It may be produced by factors that generate increased rate or volume of flow with high cardiac output or by conditions associated with cardiac dilatation and altered ventricular compliance, as in CHF. Fourth heart sounds (S_4 gallop) follow the P wave and precede the QRS complex. They occur with atrial contraction. Increased amplitude and audibility of these low-frequency vibrations are usually associated with increased ventricular stiffness (decreased compliance) from pressure or volume overload or with acute mitral regurgitation, systemic arterial hypertension, cardiomyopathy, or CAD. Audible fourth heart sounds may also be present during increased ventricular filling with normal compliance, as in high-output states and with first-degree heart block. Right-sided gallops are augmented by inspiration. During periods of rapid heart rate, third and fourth heart sounds may be superimposed to form a louder single "summation" gallop. Other diastolic sounds to be differentiated from S_3 and S_4 gallops are the opening snap of the mitral valve, the pericardial knock of constrictive pericarditis, and the "tumor plop" of atrial myxoma. The opening snap of the mitral (or tricuspid) valve occurs earlier than the S_3 gallop (0.02 to 0.12 second after the onset of the aortic component of the second heart sound). The sound is usually a high-pitched, brief, sharp event heard well with the diaphragm of the stethoscope, and the sound radiates widely over the left precordium. The tumor plop of atrial myxoma is an early diastolic sound of relatively low frequency that may be confused with an opening snap or third heart sound. Usually, it is of lower frequency and occurs later than most mitral valve opening snaps and slightly earlier than an S_3 gallop. The pericardial knock of constrictive pericarditis is ordinarily higher pitched, occurs earlier, and is louder than the S_3 gallop. Artificial pacemakers may also produce diastolic sounds that are extracardiac in origin. A sharp, high-frequency clicking or snapping sound may occur 0.08 to 0.12 second before the first heart sound and may be related to pacemaker-induced intercostal muscle contraction. In some instances, this sound signifies penetration of the electrode tip into or through the myocardium, but it also may be audible in normally positioned and normally functioning pacemakers.

Edema

Peripheral edema is a relatively late finding in the natural history of CHF. RV failure causes edema formation by elevation of systemic venous pressure. LV decompensation results in fluid and salt retention, producing edema as a result of reduced effective renal perfusion and the consequently increased renin production and subsequent aldosterone secretion. CHF is also associated with an inappropriately high secretion of antidiuretic hormone, which leads to water retention. Furthermore, chronic LV failure may lead to RV failure in the wake of chronic pulmonary venous and arterial hypertension. The resulting increased ventricular volumes that follow salt and water retention help to maintain cardiac output through the Frank-Starling mechanism but at the cost of an increase in the ventricular end-diastolic pressures and myocardial oxygen demand.

Peripheral edema formation should lead the physician to search for other evidence of LV or RV disease, or both. When these are not present, other etiologic factors must be sought. Constrictive pericarditis may be manifested by edema, and many patients have been followed mistakenly with the diagnosis of right-sided heart failure of uncertain cause or cryptogenic hepatic cirrhosis. Kussmaul's sign, pulsus paradoxus, a pericardial friction rub or knock, pericardial calcification, and a relatively small heart for the degree of edema point to the correct etiology.

In adults, edema formation occurs in dependent areas of the body. Some noncardiac diseases may lead to edema formation with a similar distribution; notable among these are chronic renal disease, profound hypoalbuminemia, Cushing's disease, and premenstrual edema.

Local obstruction of venous or lymphatic drainage usually causes asymmetric edema collection. In hepatic cirrhosis, ascites is usually large in volume relative to peripheral edema, except in the case of "cardiac" cirrhosis, in which peripheral edema may have been prominent before the onset of ascites.

Facial edema may occur with CHF, but it is more commonly caused by trichinosis, renal disease, and superior vena caval syndrome. It may also follow severe respiratory effort provoked by asthma or an upper respiratory obstruction.

Rales

Elevation of pulmonary capillary pressure to a level above the plasma oncotic pressure may be accompanied by transudation of fluid into the alveolar spaces, producing moist rales. LV decompensation and mitral stenosis are the most common causes. Pulmonary edema is characterized by excessive transudation of fluid and moist, bubbling inspiratory rales throughout the lung fields, whereas lesser degrees of decompensation are characterized by more localized physical findings with greater involvement of the lung bases. The main noncardiac causes of pulmonary edema are the adult respiratory distress syndrome ("shock lung"), pulmonary emboli, exposure to high altitudes, and certain drugs.

Many other disorders produce similar sounds. Atelectasis is characterized by fine, dry, crackling rales at the lung bases, which clear with deep breathing or coughing. Pulmonary infection with an inflammatory infiltrate produces evidence of consolidation in addition to rales. In COPD, somewhat coarser rales are typical and are usually accompanied by rhonchi, decreased breath sounds, wheezes, and prolongation of expiration. Pulmonary fibrosis is accompanied by distinctive dry, fine-to-medium inspiratory rales. Injury to pulmonary capillary endothelium in the respiratory distress syndrome, shock lung, or hypersensitivity reaction may produce noncardiac pulmonary edema with the characteristic moist rales of excess fluid in alveolar spaces.

Pleural Effusion

The surfaces of the visceral and parietal pleurae are normally separated by a thin layer of fluid generated by the visceral pleura. A number of factors may alter the balance between production and normal absorption of this fluid (Table 1–8). The visceral pleura is drained by the pulmo-

TABLE 1-8 **Important Causes of Pleural Effusions**

- Congestive heart failure
  - Left and right heart failure (if unilateral, usually right-sided effusion)
- Pulmonary venous hypertension with right heart failure
- Inflammation of pleura and/or lung
  - Infection
- Collagen disease with pulmonary involvement
  - Systemic lupus erythematosus
  - Rheumatoid arthritis
- Autoimmune phenomena after heart injury
  - Postpericardiotomy syndrome
  - Postmyocardial infarction syndrome (Dressler's syndrome)
- Tumor
  - Primary
  - Metastatic
- Pulmonary embolus with pulmonary infarction
- Abdominal ascites
- Subdiaphragmatic inflammatory processes
  - Pancreatitis
- Hypothyroidism
- Trauma
- Disruption of or damage to the thoracic duct
- Hypoalbuminemia

nary veins and lymphatics, and the parietal pleura is drained by systemic veins and lymphatics. Transudation of fluid into the pleural space may occur with marked elevation in pressure in either the systemic or the pulmonary venous beds because pleural drainage depends on both, but it occurs more frequently with elevation of both pressures. Therefore, although pleural effusion may occur with LV or RV failure alone, it is far more frequent with combined LV and RV decompensation. Failure-induced effusions are commonly bilateral. Unilateral pleural effusions caused by CHF are usually right-sided.

Pleural effusion related to CHF is usually accompanied by other signs and symptoms of cardiac decompensation. Factors that compromise lymphatic clearance may also result in pleural effusion. Inflammatory involvement of the pleura or adjacent pleural structures is a common cause of pleural effusion. In addition to an outpouring of fluid due to the inflammatory process, the lymphatic drainage may be compromised or obstructed by inflammation.

Bacterial, mycobacterial, and, occasionally, fungal and viral pulmonary and pleural infections produce pleural effusions, as may abdominal inflammatory processes. Lymphatic drainage from the abdomen passes through the diaphragm; therefore, direct communication may be present from abdominal to pleural spaces. Pancreatitis is occasionally associated with a left pleural effusion that has an increased amylase concentration. Hypoalbuminemia resulting from cirrhosis, the nephrotic syndrome, or other etiology may be associated with right-sided or bilateral pleural effusions. Tumors (primary or metastatic) to the lung or pleura are frequently associated with pleural effusions, often bloody and high in protein content and lactate dehydrogenase concentration. Hypothyroidism may produce large pleural (and pericardial) effusions that have low protein content.

Pulmonary infarction often produces a bloody pleural effusion, although a nonsanguineous effusion is also compatible with the diagnosis. Collagen vascular or connective tissue disease, especially systemic lupus erythematosus, may be accompanied by pleural effusion; the pleural effusion that occurs in some patients with rheumatoid arthritis typically has a low glucose content. The postpericardiotomy and post-MI (Dressler) syndromes are often associated with pleural effusions. Disruption of the thoracic duct by trauma or tumor produces a chylous effusion; bleeding from thoracic vascular structures may produce hemothorax or bloody pleural effusion.

Acute effusions and CHF-associated pleural effusions are generally transudates. Long-standing pleural effusions often have increased amounts of protein, regardless of the cause. Effusions with high specific gravity and increased protein content are characteristic of tumor and inflammation. The number and type of cells present in a pleural effusion can provide helpful information, as can measurements of lactate dehydrogenase and glucose.

Cyanosis

Desaturation of hemoglobin imparts a bluish coloration to the skin that is best appreciated in the mucous membranes, nail beds, conjunctiva, and earlobes. Cyanosis is recognized when 5 g/dl of unoxygenated hemoglobin is present, and arterial saturation has fallen to 75 to 85 percent. Because recognition of cyanosis depends on the absolute quantity of reduced hemoglobin present per 100 ml of blood, recognition of cyanosis in severely anemic patients can be difficult.

Cyanosis is divided into central and peripheral types (Table 1–9). *Central cyanosis* occurs with arterial desaturation because of inadequate oxygenation of hemoglobin owing to pulmonary dysfunction with ventilation-perfusion, oxygen diffusion, or ventilatory abnormalities; right-to-left shunting of desaturated venous blood into the systemic arterial circuit; ambient atmospheric hypoxia; or an abnormality of hemoglobin itself and its ability to transport oxygen. Patients with cyanotic congenital heart disease

TABLE 1-9 **Causes of Cyanosis**

- Peripheral cyanosis
  - Decreased blood flow in vasoconstricted states with oxygen extraction
    - Reduced cardiac output
    - Shock
    - Congestive heart failure
    - Cold exposure
    - Peripheral arterial and/or venous disease
- Central cyanosis
  - Arterial unsaturation due to impaired gas exchange in lungs
    - Hypoxia due to general hypoventilation with increased P_{CO_2} and decreased P_{aO_2}
    - Regional hypoventilation with respect to perfusion
    - Perfusion of unventilated regions of lung
    - Impaired diffusion
    - Low inspired oxygen tension
  - Right-to-left shunts
    - Intracardiac
    - Extracardiac
  - Hemoglobinopathy
- False cyanosis
  - Argyria

usually have a right-to-left shunt as a consequence of markedly increased pulmonary vascular resistance, RV outflow obstruction, or transposition of the great vessels. Differential cyanosis of hands and feet can be expected when venous and arterial mixing occurs after blood leaves the heart and pulmonary circuit. Toes, for example, are more cyanotic than fingers in a patent ductus arteriosus with right-to-left shunt; fingers may be more cyanotic than toes with transposition of the great vessels and a reversed shunt from a patent ductus arteriosus. The most common form of congenital cyanotic heart disease is tetralogy of Fallot. Cyanosis caused by intracardiac shunt lesions persists with oxygen administration, whereas that due to pulmonary etiology is often corrected. Abnormal hemoglobins may produce cyanosis.

Peripheral cyanosis unrelated to desaturation of central arterial blood may be observed in peripheral vascular beds in states of low flow or vasoconstriction. This is due to extensive local desaturation of hemoglobin in peripheral extremities and is commonly caused by exposure to cold, peripheral venous or arterial disease, or intense peripheral vasoconstriction. Clubbing often is found in association with long-standing central, but not peripheral, cyanosis. Central cyanosis due to hemoglobin abnormalities is not usually associated with clubbing.

The bluish skin color in argyria is sometimes mistaken for cyanosis. It is caused by silver deposition in skin and can be distinguished from cyanosis by the lack of involvement of mucosal membranes and failure of the skin to blanch with pressure. Patients with polycythemia may also exhibit true cyanosis with lesser degrees of arterial desaturation because of stagnation and sludging of blood flow in peripheral areas due to increased blood viscosity.

Clubbing

Clubbing is characterized by bulbous enlargement of the tips of the digits, spongy softening of the nail bed, and widening of the normal angle of entrance of the nail into the digit to 180 degrees or more. These changes are caused by edema and fibrous overgrowth of the digit tips and increased vascularization of the nail bed.

The changes may be familial, acquired, or associated with an underlying disorder, especially of the heart, lungs, liver, or alimentary tract. Familial clubbing can occur in otherwise healthy individuals. Clubbing has been reported to occur in association with certain occupations, such as jackhammer operation. It can be seen in patients with long-standing central cyanosis of either a cardiac or a pulmonary etiology. It rarely occurs with central cyanosis due to abnormal hemoglobin and does not occur with peripheral cyanosis. Asymmetric clubbing may be found in patients with shunts with unequal distribution of unsaturated blood, as in reversed shunting from patent ductus arteriosus. Clubbing without cyanosis is found in subacute bacterial endocarditis, in chronic suppurative pulmonary diseases, and in other intrathoracic disorders, especially lung tumor. One to 10 percent of patients with bronchogenic carcinomas have associated clubbing, as do patients with aneurysms of the aortic arch or the subclavian, innominate, or brachial artery and those with lymphangitis and the superior sulcus (Pancoast) syndrome.

Physical Examination of the Patient With Heart Disease

The examination of the patient with heart disease is approached in much the same way as a detective approaches a criminal problem. Rather than a single sign or symptom that provides the exact diagnosis, it is usually a combination of symptoms and physical signs or the absence of such that enables the examiner to suspect or recognize the presence of a particular abnormality. The examination is most efficient if the physician approaches the patient in a logical pattern, directing full attention to the solution of the problem at hand. One systematic pattern in which a patient may be examined is as follows:

1. Inspection of the patient
2. Measurement of systemic blood pressure, pulse rate, and pulse regularity
3. Examination of the carotid and peripheral arteries
4. Examination of the jugular venous pulse
5. Palpation and inspection of the precordium
6. Auscultation of the heart and lungs

Inspection

Inspection of the patient should include a careful, yet relatively rapid, appraisal of the patient from head to foot. One is specifically interested in the general appearance of the patient. Does he or she look ill? Is the patient dyspneic? Although general impressions can be erroneous, they are often helpful in corroborating the patient's previously elicited symptoms. In selected instances, one may be interested in continuing the inspection by asking the patient to perform such tasks as walking a certain distance or climbing a flight or two of stairs in the company of the examiner.

The initial inspection of the patient should assess the general body configuration. Is the patient abnormally tall or short? Is he or she obese, and is the typical mesomorphic, overly concerned appearance of some patients with CHD present? Does the appearance suggest the possibility of Marfan's syndrome? One should notice the color, pigmentation, and texture of the skin. Hemochromatosis can be recognized by the characteristic pigmentation, and scleroderma can be recognized by the thickening of the skin over the hands and fingers and around the mouth and eyes. The eyelids may be violaceous in dermatomyositis, and there may be a scaly erythematous eruption over the joints of the fingers. Episodic flushing of the skin is a hallmark of the carcinoid syndrome, which itself may cause tricuspid regurgitation and pulmonic stenosis. Systolic pulsation in the eyeballs or ear lobes is sometimes seen in severe tricuspid insufficiency. Xanthelasma, xanthomata, or both may be manifestations of hyperlipidemia and are seen in some patients with atherosclerotic vascular disease.

The presence or absence of a straight back, as well as sternal deformities, such as pectus excavatum, should be noted because sternal or spine deformities may distort or displace the heart and lead to erroneous signs of cardiac enlargement. Telangiectases of the lips, tongue, buccal mucosa, and fingertips are seen in patients with hereditary hemorrhagic telangiectasia (Osler-Weber-Rendu syndrome). Fine linear hemorrhages (splinter hemorrhages) under the fingernails may be the result of trauma in normal individuals but may also be a manifestation of bacterial endocarditis. Conjunctival petechiae also are present in some patients with bacterial endocarditis, but they may be seen in a high percentage of patients immediately after open heart surgery. In the latter situation, such petechiae usually are not a manifestation of endocarditis.

In female patients, a broad chest with widely spaced nipples and hypoplastic breast tissue in association with a webbed neck suggests Turner's syndrome; defects of the atrial and ventricular septa and coarctation are the usual cardiovascular abnormalities seen in these patients. Down's syndrome is recognized by the simian crease in the palms and by other typical physical features. Atrial septal defects, ventricular septal defects, AV canal defects, and patent ductus arteriosus are cardiac abnormalities commonly associated with this syndrome.

Clubbing of the fingers and toes has been defined as loss of the normal angle between the cuticle and the distal end of the fingers or toes through the proliferation of tissue in the subungual area. There often is associated sponginess of the proximal nail bed due to elevation of the entire nail by the tissue ingrowth. The pathogenesis of clubbing is not clear. Characteristically, it is associated with systemic arterial oxygen desaturation and therefore is most commonly seen in patients with cyanotic congenital heart disease or advanced pulmonary disease. Clubbing is also seen in a wide variety of other clinical conditions, including arteriovenous shunts, bacterial endocarditis, cirrhosis of the liver, ulcerative colitis, and certain malignant tumors. Sometimes clubbing occurs without any obvious underlying cause.

Abnormalities of the extremities may be a clue to the presence of heart disease in some patients. The Holt-Oram syndrome is characterized by a thumb resembling a finger (being hypoplastic and in the same plane as the remainder of the fingers), short forearms, and a forward thrust of the shoulders. Atrial septal defects are seen in some patients with this disorder. Flushing of the nail beds with each heartbeat (Quincke pulse) is a sign of a hyperkinetic circulation and is commonly seen in patients with severe aortic regurgitation. Anemia may be recognized by noting the pale color of the nail beds, the conjunctivae, or both.

Cyanosis, which is most easily visualized around the mouth or in the hands or fingernails, may not be detectable until the oxygen saturation of the blood has fallen to a level as low as 75 to 80 percent, although occasionally, particularly with polycythemia, it can be recognized at somewhat higher levels. It may exist as so-called central cyanosis, in which it is associated with excessive oxygen desaturation of the arterial blood, or as peripheral cyanosis, which results from localized oxygen desaturation of capillary blood and occurs in the presence of normal systemic arterial oxygen saturations. Central cyanosis is seen primarily in the nail beds, face, lips, and tongue; in contrast, peripheral cyanosis is encountered in areas where venous stasis is common, such as the ear lobes and lower extremities. Central cyanosis may result from intrapulmonary shunting due to abnormal ventilation-perfusion relationships or in association with venoarterial shunting of poorly oxygenated venous blood. The latter is characteristic of some congenital heart diseases, such as transposition of the great vessels and tetralogy of Fallot, but also may occur in patients with atrial and ventricular septal defects and patent ductus arteriosus when severe pulmonary hypertension causes shunting of blood from right to left. Peripheral cyanosis usually occurs with extreme peripheral stasis, such as in cardiogenic shock or severe CHF. It may also occur distal to sites of venous obstruction or in vasomotor abnormalities, such as Raynaud's disease.

In summary, a general inspection of the patient both at rest and, where applicable, under stress is of immense importance. Accuracy in diagnosing the etiology of the abnormality in a patient with cardiac disease depends largely on having thought of the appropriate possibilities on the basis of valuable clues obtained by a careful and thorough general inspection of the patient.

Blood Pressure Measurement

The current method of measuring blood pressure depends on auscultatory detection of the Korotkoff sounds over a peripheral artery (usually the brachial artery or the popliteal artery) at a point distal to the cuff compression of the vessel. The apparatus for measuring blood pressure consists of a compression cuff, a hand-operated bulb that allows inflation of the cuff, a valve that allows reduction of pressure in the cuff, and a manometer that measures pressure in the cuff. The cuff should be long enough to encompass at least half of the extremity being examined and should be 20 percent or greater in diameter than the extremity to which it is applied. When the cuff is too small for the extremity being examined, false elevations in the blood pressure recording will result. Measurement of blood pressure should be made with the patient as relaxed and comfortable as possible. The cuff is carefully deflated and then applied snugly. Before auscultation, one generally determines what cuff pressure obliterates the distal arterial pulse. The stethoscope is then positioned gently but firmly directly over the artery (either the brachial or popliteal) and the cuff is inflated to a level in excess of that required to obliterate the distal pulse. One then listens carefully as the cuff is deflated. The systolic blood pressure is recorded at the point at which the first tapping sound occurs for several consecutive beats. The diastolic pressure is that point at which definite muffling of the sounds occurs. One should also note and record the point at which the sounds totally disappear if it is different from the pressure level at which they become muffled. Blood pressure measurements should be made in both arms with the patient lying and standing. Differences in systolic blood pressures between the two arms in the supine position can be a valuable clue in diagnosing disorders, such as atherosclerotic vascular disease, involving the arterial supply of one of the upper extremities; dissecting aortic aneurysm, involving the blood supply to one of the arms; coarctation of the aorta, involving the origin of the left subclavian artery; or supravalvular aortic stenosis.

Blood pressure measurements should be made routinely

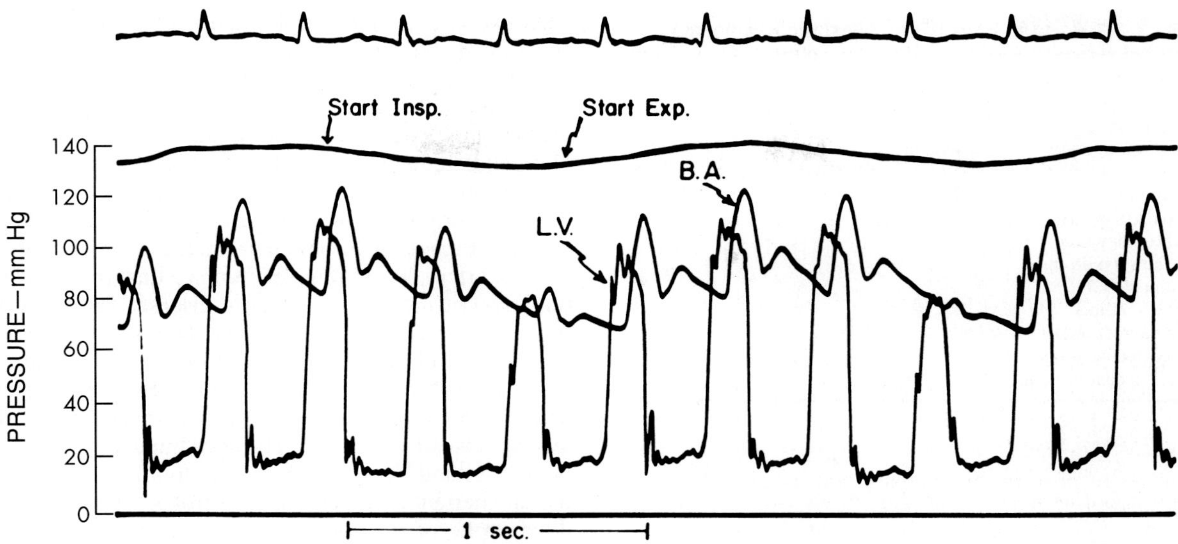

FIGURE 1–1 This paradoxical pulse was present in a patient with pericardial tamponade. Note the marked fall in brachial artery (B.A.) and left ventricular (L.V.) systolic pressure, with inspiration (Insp.) followed by a rise during expiration (Exp.).

in the legs of patients with hypertension, suspected coarctation of the aorta, aortic dissection, or peripheral vascular disease. In the adult, systolic blood pressure is usually 10 to 15 mm Hg higher in the legs compared with that in the arms. When there are marked pressure differences between the arms and legs, artifactual differences should always be excluded (e.g., those produced by improper cuff size). A significantly higher systolic blood pressure in the legs than in the arms is often found in patients with severe aortic regurgitation (Hill's sign). Lower systolic blood pressures are found in the legs of patients with coarctation of the aorta and severe aortoiliac disease.

One characteristic abnormality of blood pressure is the so-called paradoxical pulse or pulsus paradoxus (Fig. 1–1). This may be diagnosed when the systolic blood pressure falls more than the normal 10 mm Hg during inspiration. The mechanism of pulsus paradoxus is thought to be predominantly the result of pulmonary vascular pooling during inspiration and accentuated by conditions that

1. Limit the normal inspiratory increase in blood flow from the right ventricle to the pulmonary artery
2. Cause a greater-than-normal inspiratory pooling in the lungs
3. Cause wide extremes of intrathoracic pressure during inspiration and expiration
4. Interfere with venous return to the atrium relatively more during inspiration

Therefore, pulsus paradoxus is seen in patients with pericardial effusions of sufficient size to impede venous return to the heart during inspiration and in association with severe asthma, emphysema, superior vena caval obstruction, severe CHF, and constrictive pericarditis.

Normal blood pressure for adults less than 50 years old is considered to range between 100 and 140 mm Hg systolic and 60 to 90 mm Hg diastolic. In any individual patient, however, transient fluctuations above or below these normal values, especially in the systolic blood pressure, are a common occurrence and probably reflect changes in physiologic state. For example, systolic blood pressure rises with fever, anxiety, sudden fright, and exercise. However, with sedation and during sleep, both systolic and diastolic blood pressures tend to fall. Alterations in pulse pressure (the difference between systolic and diastolic pressures) may or may not be associated with cardiac disease (Table 1–10).

In some patients, systolic blood pressure may fall dramatically in the erect position, resulting in syncope. Such postural hypotension not uncommonly occurs even in a normal person initially arising from bed after a prolonged illness. In this instance, postural hypotension and syncope result from pooling of blood in the vessels in the lower extremities. At present, the most common cause of postural hypotension is the use of antihypertensive agents. Addi-

TABLE 1–10 Causes of Pulse Pressure Abnormalities

Increased Pulse Pressure	Narrow Pulse Pressure
Sinus bradycardia	Severe heart failure
Complete heart block	Shock
Emotion	Aortic stenosis (usually occurs but is not always present)
Exercise	Hypovolemia
Aortic regurgitation	Vasoconstrictive agents
Atrioventricular fistulas	
Fever	
Anemia	
Hyperthyroidism	
Beri-beri	
Inelastic aorta (elderly patients)	
Abnormal connections between aorta and pulmonary artery (patent ductus arteriosus, aorticopulmonary window)	
Rupture of sinus of Valsalva aneurysm	

TABLE 1–11 Causes of Orthostatic Hypotension

Idiopathic
Hyponatremia
Hypovolemia
Drugs (e.g., tranquilizers, vasodilators)
Central nervous system disease (e.g., syringomyelia, tabes dorsalis)
Addison's disease
Pheochromocytoma
Wernicke's syndrome
Amyloidosis
Diabetes mellitus
Primary autonomic insufficiency
After sympathectomy
Physical deconditioning

tional causes of postural hypotension are listed in Table 1–11.

Regularity and Configuration of Pulses

Pulse rate and regularity are determined by palpating the radial artery. The normal adult heart rate varies between 60 and 100 beats/min, although this is subject to the same physiologic influences as for systemic blood pressure. Sinus tachycardia implies a regular sinus rate of more than 100 beats/min, whereas sinus bradycardia refers to a regular sinus rate of less than 60 beats/min. It may be the result of either a slow sinus, an AV junction, or a ventricular pacemaker. Atrial fibrillation is a chaotic atrial rhythm recognized on physical examination by finding an abnormally irregular radial pulse. Occasional transient irregularity of the radial pulse may result from either atrial or ventricular premature beats. In this situation, the pause that follows the premature or early beat is short in the case of atrial extrasystoles and relatively long after ventricular extrasystoles. A bigeminal pulse is made up of coupled beats with regular alteration of the height of the pressure pulses. This occurs as the result of premature atrial or, more commonly, premature ventricular contractions. The height of the radial pulse varies because of the increased diastolic filling period after the premature ventricular beat, so the subsequent stroke output is greater than that associated with the ventricular extrasystole.

Pulsus alternans refers to a pulse pattern in which there is regular alternation between the height of the pressure pulses (Fig. 1–2). Such a finding may signify LV dysfunction, usually severe, and therefore may be associated with any disease leading to ventricular failure or with events, such as extreme tachycardia, that might impair ventricular function, if only temporarily. In the former circumstance, pulsus alternans is occasionally induced by a ventricular ectopic beat. The equality of pulses should be checked over the carotids and in both the upper and lower extremities. Unilateral reduction or absence of the pulse over one of these vessels suggests localized obstruction of that artery.

Pulse configuration may provide an important clue to cardiac disease. It is best determined by palpation of the carotid artery, providing, of course, that the patient does not have intrinsic carotid arterial disease. The carotid pulse is best examined with the patient reclining with the trunk of his body elevated at 15 to 45 degrees to the horizontal plane. The sternocleidomastoid muscles should be relaxed and the head either not rotated or rotated very slightly away from the examiner. The forefinger is generally used with light and then, if necessary, slightly heavier pressure in an attempt to assess the upstroke, the peak, and the downstroke of the carotid impulse. For precise separation of the various components of the carotid contour, one may also listen simultaneously to the heart sounds. The normal configuration of the carotid pulse consists of a smooth and rapid upstroke (Fig. 1–3). The summit of the carotid pulse is smooth and dome shaped. The descending limb from the systolic peak is less steep. The carotid incisura or dicrotic notch is not usually identifiable by palpation. Characteristic abnormalities of the carotid pulse are listed in Table 1–12. Examples of some of these abnormal carotid pulses are shown in Figure 1–3. An anacrotic carotid pulse is usually seen in patients who have isolated and hemodynamically significant valvular aortic stenosis. In these patients, the carotid pulse is of small volume and the anacrotic notch is palpable relatively low on the carotid upstroke. At the

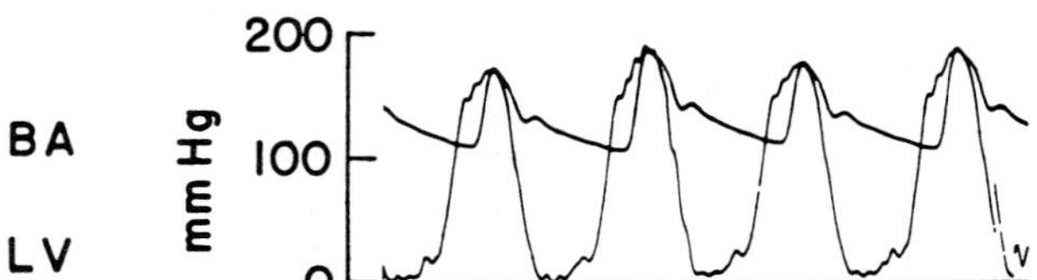

FIGURE 1–2 An example of pulsus alternans. The brachial arterial (BA) and left ventricular (LV) systolic pressures vary in a regular manner, such that every other pressure is reduced. Pressure is indicated on the vertical axis.

NORMAL CAROTID

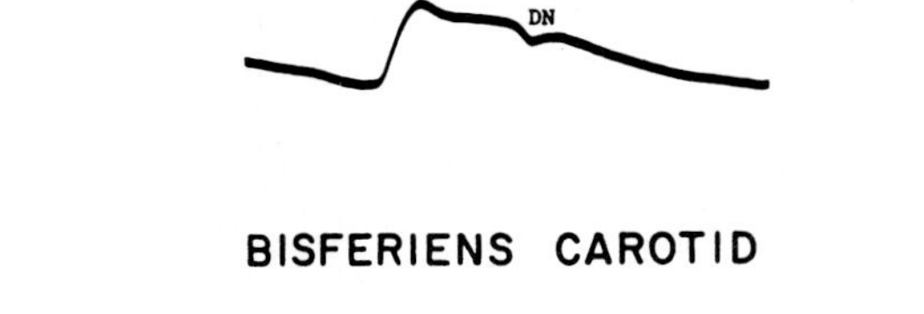

BISFERIENS CAROTID

DN

DN

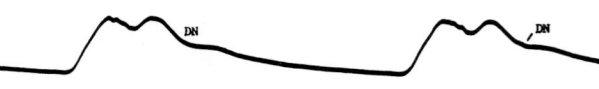

ANACROTIC CAROTID

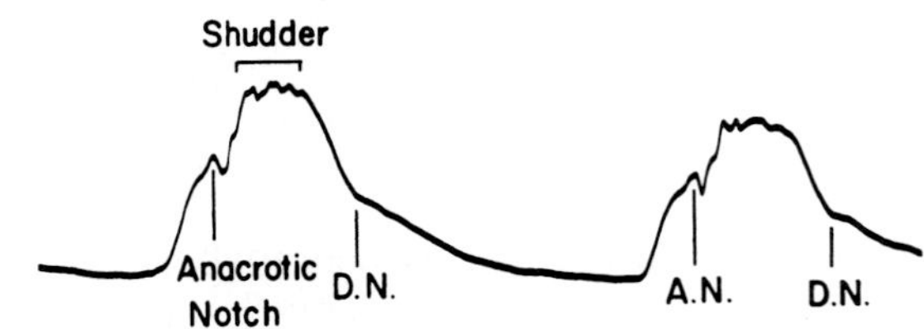

FIGURE 1–3 Examples of normal, bisferiens, and anacrotic carotid pulses. The anacrotic carotid pulse with the shudder was obtained from a patient with severe valvular aortic stenosis. AN, anacrotic notch; DN, dicrotic notch.

TABLE 1–12 **Arterial Pulse Abnormalities**

Abnormality	Description
Anacrotic pulse	A small, slowly rising pulse with a notch on the ascending limb, such that there are two deflections on the upstroke of the carotid
Bisferiens pulse	Two palpable systolic peaks of almost equal height
Dicrotic pulse	A second peak during diastole
Water-hammer pulse	Characterized by rapid and sudden systolic expansion
Idiopathic hypertrophic subaortic stenosis pulse	A carotid pulse with a very rapid upstroke, sometimes having a bisferiens quality

summit or peak of the carotid, one often feels a shudder. The entire carotid upstroke in these patients is markedly delayed. In the adult patient, assessment of the carotid upstroke is the single most valuable clue to the presence of hemodynamically significant valvular aortic stenosis, given the absence of intrinsic carotid arterial disease. In contrast, in aortic regurgitation, the carotid upstroke is extremely rapid and the pulse is sometimes described as a water-hammer pulse. The bisferiens pulse is found in some patients with severe aortic regurgitation, some with combined aortic stenosis and regurgitation, and some who have hypertrophic obstructive cardiomyopathy (HOCM). In the patients with HOCM or idiopathic hypertrophic subaortic stenosis, the carotid upstroke is typically rapid (Fig. 1–4).

A systolic thrill may be palpable over the carotid vessels. This vibration is produced by turbulent blood flow and represents the physical counterpart of a loud murmur heard on auscultation. In general, a thrill over the carotid is transmitted from the aortic root in patients with valvular heart disease, especially valvular aortic stenosis. Alternatively, a carotid thrill may represent local arterial disease, in which the thrill is usually unilateral and associated heart disease is absent. One should also listen with a stethoscope for bruits over the carotid vessels. A bruit over a carotid artery may represent a transmitted murmur from the precordium, as occurs in patients with valvular heart disease (especially aortic valve disease), or it may be a manifestation of intrinsic occlusive disease of the carotid vessel itself.

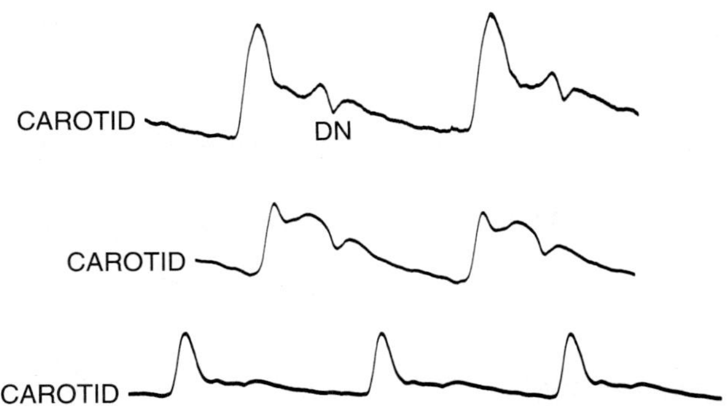

FIGURE 1–4 Three different examples of carotid pulses in patients with idiopathic hypertrophic subaortic stenosis. Note the characteristic rapid upstroke in all three and the "double hump" in the carotid downstroke in the top two examples. The systolic ejection period is prolonged in all three. DN, dicrotic notch.

Examination of the Jugular Venous Pulse

The information obtained from examination of the jugular venous pulse includes an estimation of the level of venous pressure and an evaluation of the individual components (Fig. 1–5). The external jugular vein is generally used to assess both the level and the waveform of venous pressure, although the internal jugular vein can also be used. The jugular veins reflect right atrial (RA) events with only a minimal delay, and venous pulsations can be differentiated from arterial pulsations in several ways. The pulsation seen at the anterior border of the sternocleidomastoid muscle is usually arterial, whereas pulsations at its posterior border are usually venous. Venous pulsations are influenced by respiration, tending generally to fall with inspiration and rise with expiration. Three separate pulsations can usually be identified in the venous pulse, in contrast to the single systolic pulsation noted in the arterial wave configuration (see Fig. 1–5). It is also possible to obliterate the venous pulsation by light pressure over the external jugular vein. Arterial pulsations are not as easily obliterated. In examining venous configuration, the position of the patient is of extreme importance. The higher the central venous pressure, the more vertical the subject should be so the venous waveform can be adequately examined. The patient is usually positioned with the trunk at an angle of 15 to 45 degrees to the horizontal plane, although if venous pressure is extremely high, it may be necessary to have the patient sit upright for adequate examination (Fig. 1–6). Lighting is also of extreme importance; either oblique or tangential lighting with respect to the vein is helpful. The right external jugular vein is usually the easiest to assess.

The sternal angle of Louis is used as a reference point for measurement of venous pressure because it is approxi-

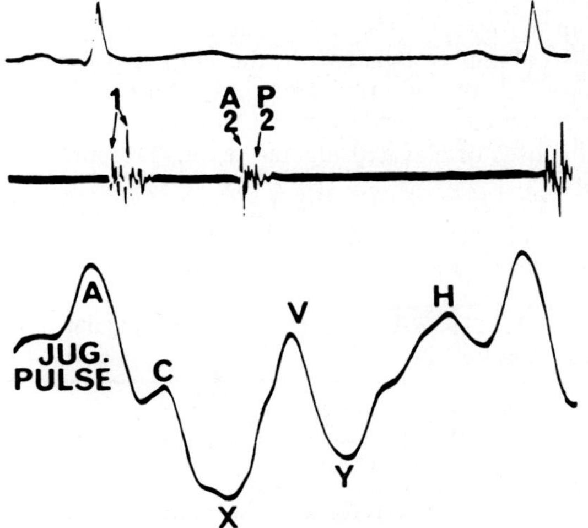

FIGURE 1–5 A normal jugular venous pulse configuration. Note the prominence of the A wave and that the X trough is deeper than the Y trough. A_2, aortic valve closing; P_2, pulmonary valve closing.

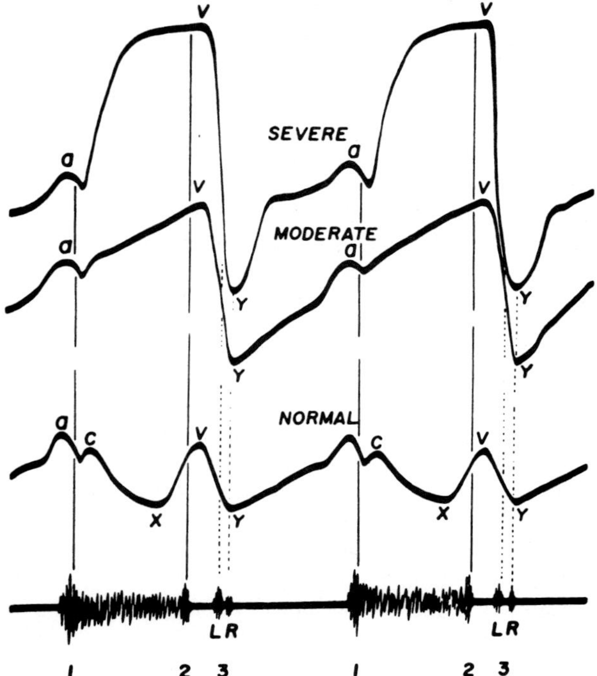

FIGURE 1–6 The jugular venous pulse configuration in a patient with severe tricuspid regurgitation, a patient with moderate tricuspid regurgitation, and a control patient. **Bottom,** Murmur of tricuspid regurgitation. Note the prominent V waves in the jugular venous pulse with severe and moderate tricuspid regurgitation. L and R, timing of left and right ventricular third heart sounds (S_3), respectively, in relation to the jugular venous pulse.

mately 5 cm above the level of the right atrium. After positioning the patient appropriately, such that the top of the level of the external jugular venous column can be identified, the vertical distance between the angle of Louis and the top of the venous column is measured. The addition of 5 cm to the value obtained provides an approximation of venous pressure. The normal venous pressure should be no more than 6 to 7 cm when it is measured in this way. In some patients, the venous pressure will be so high that even in the upright position, no definite upper level of the venous column is apparent. In the normal patient, venous pressure falls during inspiration, in contrast to the situation in some patients with cardiac tamponade or RV failure. Other causes of elevated jugular venous pressure are listed in Table 1–13.

The normal waveform of the external jugular vein is demonstrated (see Fig. 1–5). The A wave is the most prominent positive deflection in the external jugular pulse in the normal subject. It originates as a result of atrial contraction with a subsequent rise in RA pressure, which is reflected in the neck veins. It can be distinguished by its upstroke preceding that of the carotid arterial pulse palpated simultaneously on the opposite side of the neck. It is often easier, however, to time the jugular venous waveforms in conjunction with listening to the heart sounds. The A wave in the jugular venous pulse occurs almost simultaneously with the first heart sound. The size of the A wave depends on several factors, including the force of RA contraction, the resistance to RA emptying and RV filling, and the cardiac rhythm. Prominent A waves occur with tricuspid valve obstruction. Pulmonic stenosis and pulmonary hypertension in the presence of an intact septum also result in prominent A waves due to decreased ventricular compliance. In assessment of the A wave, the size and contractile strength of the right atrium must be considered (i.e., if it is large and dilated, it may have reduced contractile strength). In this situation, the A waves generated in the jugular venous pulse may not be impressive despite the presence of conditions such as significant tricuspid valve obstruction or pulmonary hypertension. When the right atrium contracts during ventricular systole with a closed tricuspid valve, "cannon A waves" are produced (Fig. 1–7). This is seen in complete AV block and occurs in other situations where AV dissociation exists (e.g., ventricular tachycardia or ventricular ectopic beats).

The X descent may be noticeable in other situations where AV dissociation exists, including ventricular tachycardia (and ventricular ectopic beats), as a result of the reduction in pressure in the jugular veins as blood flows into the right atrium. Its trough is usually deeper than that of the Y descent. In the normal jugular venous configuration, it is the most conspicuous wave. The generation of the X descent depends on three factors: atrial relaxation, the size of the RA cavity, and a decrease in intrathoracic pressure as a result of LV contractility. The X descent is usually exaggerated when RV stroke output is high, as occurs with a left-to-right shunt such as in atrial septal defect or with exercise, fever, or anxiety. The X descent may also be very sharp in constrictive pericarditis. In atrial

TABLE 1–13 Causes of Elevated Jugular Venous Pressure

Right ventricular failure
Vascular pulmonic stenosis
Infundibular pulmonary stenosis
Pulmonary hypertension
Tricuspid stenosis or insufficiency
Hypervolemia
Pericardial tamponade
Constrictive pericarditis
Superior vena caval obstruction

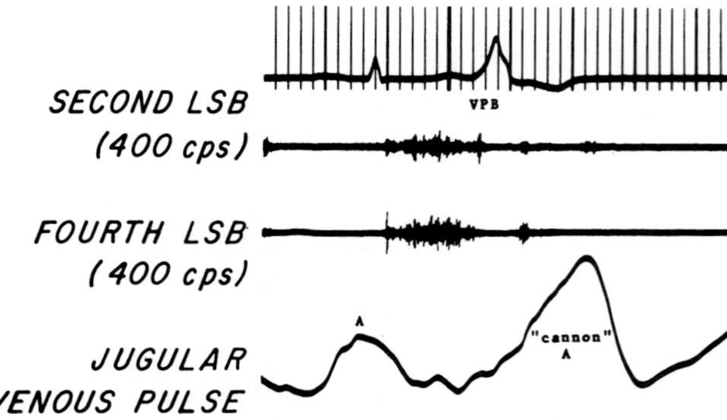

FIGURE 1–7 A "cannon" A wave is demonstrated. It occurs when the right atrium contracts on a closed tricuspid valve and is typically seen after a ventricular premature beat (VPB), as shown here, and in the patient with complete heart block. LSB, left sternal border.

fibrillation and with tricuspid regurgitation, the X descent either is not present or is partially abolished so that the Y trough is the deepest negative deflection.

The origin of the jugular C wave is still disputed. Although it may be a transmitted impulse from the underlying carotid artery, it most likely represents the rising up of the tricuspid valve cusps at the onset of RV systole.

The V wave begins during the period of ventricular contraction, and it is caused by passive filling of the right atrium via venous return in the presence of a closed tricuspid valve. The sudden termination of RA filling associated with opening of the tricuspid valve represents the descending limb of the V wave, or Y descent. The amplitude of the V wave depends on the amount of blood in the right atrium during ventricular systole. With tricuspid regurgitation (see Fig. 1–6), the systolic venous wave is due to actual regurgitation of blood from the right ventricle into the jugular venous system, so the V waves with significant tricuspid regurgitation are very large and in some instances larger than the A wave. Prominent V waves, equaling the A waves in amplitude, have also been noted in patients with atrial septal defects. The Y descent follows the pulmonary component of the second heart sound and begins with the opening of the tricuspid valve (see Fig. 1–5). Because the Y descent is a manifestation of ventricular filling, abnormalities in RV filling caused by changes in RV compliance will be reflected in the Y descent. Friedreich's sign refers to a prominent Y descent in the venous pulse; this is seen in constrictive pericarditis when the initial portion of RV filling is rapid after opening of the tricuspid valve, followed by subsequent sudden resistance to further filling as the expansion of the right ventricle is abruptly checked. This sign is not specific for constrictive pericarditis, however, but also may be seen in restrictive cardiomyopathies. The Y descent in tricuspid stenosis is markedly prolonged and damped due to the delayed RA emptying resulting from the tricuspid valve obstruction. The end of the steep Y descent corresponds to the point at which a third heart sound originating from the right ventricle would be heard. An LV third heart sound frequently occurs earlier than the end of the steep Y descent.

After the Y descent, there may be another rise in the venous pressure just before the A wave; this late positive wave is known as the *H wave* (see Fig. 1–5). This rise has been attributed to the inrushing of blood into the right ventricle, resulting in an upward movement of the tricuspid valve cusps. It is most likely to be noted with slow heart rates.

One further point must be made about examination of the cervical veins to warn the reader about venous hums. The *venous hum* is a continuous murmur heard over the cervical veins. It is commonly present in children and in many young adults, presumably reflecting a hyperkinetic cardiovascular system. From the clinical point of view, its importance is that it may be mistaken for a heart murmur. This hum tends to be of low or medium pitch. It may be heard over the anteroinferior cervical region and sometimes over the anterior chest. It tends to become slightly louder during diastole. The intensity of the hum is increased by placing the patient in the upright position, by inspiration, and by positioning the head in such a way that the cervical veins become attenuated. It is reduced in intensity or disappears entirely on assuming the supine position, during expiration, with the Valsalva maneuver, with direct compression of the veins, and with positioning the head such that the cervical veins become kinked or compressed.

Inspection, Palpation, and Percussion of the Precordium

Inspection and palpation of the precordium in the patient with cardiac disease are important and valuable parts of the physical examination. Percussion plays a less important role but can be used in an attempt to outline the borders of the left and right ventricles and to help in the identification of dextrocardia and dextroversion.

Inspection and palpation of the precordium can provide valuable clues to the underlying abnormality in the patient with heart disease. With the patient supine, one must carefully inspect and palpate the precordium, attempting to determine the presence and location of an LV and an RV impulse. The normal LV impulse is felt at the cardiac apex near the area of the left midclavicular line. It usually covers an area no greater than 3 cm in diameter, and the outward thrust is not sustained. With LV enlargement, the apex impulse may also become sustained, as in patients with significant aortic stenosis, or it may become more rapid, diffuse, and forceful, as in patients with significant aortic regurgitation. It may also consist of a double impulse, representing both a fourth heart sound and apical systolic thrust or regions of LV dyskinesis. A palpable fourth heart sound is present in some patients with LV outflow obstruction, CHD, systemic arterial hypertension, and myocardial disease of various causes. When palpable, the RV impulse is present in the fourth and fifth intercostal spaces immediately adjacent to the left sternal border. In most adults without RV enlargement, this impulse is not palpable, although in thin subjects it may be. The RV impulse is usually palpable in situations where RV hypertrophy or dilatation is present (e.g., in patients with mitral stenosis, myocardial disease, severe tricuspid regurgitation, or RV outflow obstruction).

Abnormal precordial pulsations should also be sought, such as those that occur after MI or during myocardial ischemia. These may be noted in any area between the pulmonary artery and the cardiac apex and are not uncommonly found in the left parasternal region, in the fourth and fifth intercostal spaces, sometimes making their differentiation from an RV impulse difficult.

The second and third left intercostal spaces should be carefully examined for the presence of a pulsation indicative of pulmonary artery enlargement. The pulmonary artery is usually not palpable in the absence of pulmonary artery enlargement except in very thin patients, pregnant patients, and some patients with the straight back syndrome. In the absence of these situations, however, a palpable pulmonary artery pulsation in adults without a hyperkinetic circulation usually means either a dilated pulmonary artery (secondary to an increase in pulmonary artery pressure and resistance) or increased pulmonary artery blood flow.

Heart sounds may be palpable. A loud second heart sound in association with pulmonary or systemic arterial hypertension may be palpable in the second and third left intercostal spaces just adjacent to the sternum. First heart sounds may be palpable at the cardiac apex in patients with mitral stenosis. As already noted, the fourth heart sound, or presystolic gallop, may be palpable in patients with reduced LV compliance. A third heart sound, or protodiastolic gallop, may also be palpable in some patients with conditions such as myocardial disease or significant mitral regurgitation.

Systolic and diastolic thrills associated with heart murmurs are detected by palpation. The finding of a systolic thrill indicates significant valvular heart disease and is usually associated with a loud systolic murmur. Systolic thrills palpable in the second and third intercostal spaces to the right of the sternum usually indicate hemodynamically significant valvular aortic stenosis. Those palpable in the same locations to the left of the sternum may indicate either hemodynamically significant valvular pulmonic or aortic stenosis. Systolic thrills along the lower left sternal border may occur as the result of severe tricuspid regurgitation, with ventricular septal defects, and occasionally in association with hypertrophic obstructive cardiomyopathy. Systolic thrills at the apex usually imply hemodynamically significant mitral regurgitation of LV outflow obstruction. Diastolic thrills along the lower left sternal border may occur with either tricuspid or mitral valve obstruction. A diastolic apical thrill best appreciated directly over the point of maximal impulse with the patient in the left lateral decubitus position ordinarily identifies the presence of hemodynamically significant mitral valve stenosis.

To accurately time a thrill, one may have to listen to the heart sounds or palpate a carotid artery, as well as the precordium, to determine whether the thrill occurs in systole or diastole.

Auscultation

Auscultation is never done in total isolation from the other features of the cardiac examination; rather, it is an integral part of the total examination, and when the information obtained from auscultation is combined with that obtained from general inspection, examination of the arteries and jugular veins, and inspection, palpation, and percussion of the precordium, a satisfactory hypothesis regarding the abnormality of the patient in question can usually be formulated.

Each examiner must choose a stethoscope that is individually comfortable. The ear pieces should fit the ear canal snugly without penetrating to a depth that is uncomfortable. The tubing of the stethoscope should allow maximal sound transmission, which occurs when the internal diameter of the tubing is approximately 3 mm. Double-tube stethoscopes are associated with less distortion of heart sounds than are single-tube models. The basic components of a stethoscope are a bell and a diaphragm, which are used, respectively, for low- and high-pitched sounds and murmurs.

During auscultation, the examiner should concentrate solely on listening to and analyzing heart sounds. Auscultation is most likely to be rewarding when both the physician and the patient are comfortable and the auscultation is done in either a relatively soundproof room or under very quiet circumstances. Strict attention should be paid to each of the various heart sound components audible during systole and diastole; therefore, one should listen for the first heart sound, for systolic murmurs and clicks, for the second heart sound and its splitting with respiration, for the presence of a third and fourth heart sound, and for diastolic murmurs and diastolic clicks, each in turn excluding the other events of the cardiac cycle as the physician pays strict attention to that portion of the cycle in which the sound in question is located. It is easy, unfortunately, to overlook the presence of gallops, clicks, and even murmurs unless one listens for them specifically. The listener must examine several different areas of the precordium with both the diaphragm and the bell and must have the patient in the ideal position to bring out heart sounds as the selective circumstances dictate.

The diaphragm of the stethoscope is most effective in identifying high-pitched sounds, such as systolic clicks, opening snaps of valves, splitting of the second heart sound, the first heart sound, certain systolic murmurs, and high-pitched diastolic murmurs, such as those of aortic and pulmonary regurgitation. The diaphragm should be firmly applied to the chest, and one should listen both to the right and left of the sternum in the second, third, and fourth intercostal spaces and at the cardiac apex.

The bell is used to hear low-frequency diastolic murmurs (i.e., tricuspid and mitral stenosis) and diastolic gallop sounds (S_3 and S_4) (Fig. 1–8). Diastolic gallop sounds are often best heard with the patient in the left lateral decubitus position and by listening with the bell in the third and fourth left parasternal intercostal spaces and over the apical impulse. Gallop sounds usually require the examiner to apply very light pressure with the bell to the precordium so that they can be easily heard; firm pressure with the bell may result in inability to hear an S_3 or S_4 even when it is present.

It is best to establish a routine for the sequence of areas in which one listens to the heart sounds; this ensures that each of the important areas will be auscultated. One can follow whatever pattern one finds easiest, but one approach is to listen with the diaphragm in the second and third intercostal spaces to the right of the sternum initially,

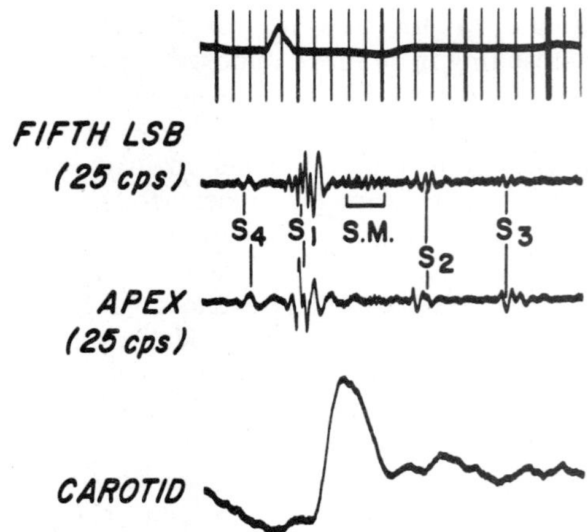

FIGURE 1–8 The low-frequency fourth (S_4) and third (S_3) heart sounds. The S_4 precedes the first heart sound (S_1), and the S_3 occurs in middiastole. S_2, second heart sound; LSB, left sternal border; SM, systolic murmur.

followed by listening to the same areas to the left of the sternum. One can then move the diaphragm down the sternal border to the fourth and fifth intercostal spaces. Finally, one moves to the apex and from there into the axilla to listen to heart sounds. One can then switch to the bell of the stethoscope and listen in the fourth and fifth intercostal spaces to the left of the sternum, followed by auscultation at the apex. We have found it easier to have the patient lie in the left lateral decubitus position at the end of the routine portion of the auscultatory examination so one can listen with the bell directly over the cardiac apex and along the left sternal border.

In appropriate situations, one must also examine a few additional areas. Specifically, the first and second intercostal spaces below the left midclavicular area should be auscultated when patent ductus arteriosus is suspected; a continuous murmur audible in this area may represent a patent ductus arteriosus. The systolic murmur of coarctation of the aorta may be heard well in the left infraclavicular region, in the suprasternal notch, or in the back in the midthoracic region at the level of the fourth or fifth spinous process. The systolic murmur of mitral regurgitation may radiate to the axilla and up the vertebral column so as to be audible even on the top of the head, or it may radiate toward the sternum and up along the left sternal border. Murmurs resulting from pulmonary arterial stenosis, a pulmonary embolus, pulmonary arterial stenosis, and pulmonary AV fistulas may be heard over the lungs. Scars should be examined for the presence of a continuous murmur suggestive of AV fistulas.

After completion of the routine auscultation in selected patients, one may want to determine how heart sounds change after mild exercise. This can be done by asking the patient to perform a few sit-ups and then listening to the heart sounds again. Not uncommonly, this will either bring out or make louder an S_3 and S_4. It may also help to accentuate the murmur of mitral stenosis when the obstruction across the mitral valve is not severe.

First Heart Sounds

Events in the left ventricle and aorta might be, at least in part, responsible for the genesis of the first heart sound; however, convincing evidence that mitral and tricuspid valve closure plays a major role in the production of the first heart sound has also been presented. First heart sounds are often initiated by a low-frequency component occurring immediately after the onset of rise in LV pressure. The first high-frequency component of the first heart sound occurs during the early phase of pressure rise in the left ventricle. The second high-frequency component occurs at the time of opening of the aortic valve. The next component occurs at the first peak of the aortic pulse, and the final component, when present, appears to coincide with maximal expansion of the aortic wall. The first heart sound may sound split to the examiner's ear or may sound as if it is single. It decreases in loudness with LV hypertrophy, with a dilated left ventricle, with a prolonged PR interval, and with reduced strength of contraction of the left ventricle. The first heart sound increases in amplitude when the LV cavity is small, when it is less compliant, when it is hypertrophied but the hypertrophy is predominantly the result of increased muscle mass rather than connective tissue, and when LV contractility occurs rapidly. The first heart sound is usually soft in the presence of aortic regurgitation and loud with mitral stenosis of hemodynamic significance. The first heart sound varies in intensity with atrial fibrillation, being somewhat softer after a long pause. Short PR intervals (the interval between atrial systole and ventricular systole) also result in increased intensity of the first heart sound. Where complete heart block or advanced AV block exists, the first heart sound varies in intensity on a beat-to-beat basis.

The second heart sound usually has two separate audible components; aortic valve closure provides one component and pulmonic valve closure contributes the second (Fig. 1–9). Splitting of the second heart sound is best heard in the second and third intercostal spaces to the left of the

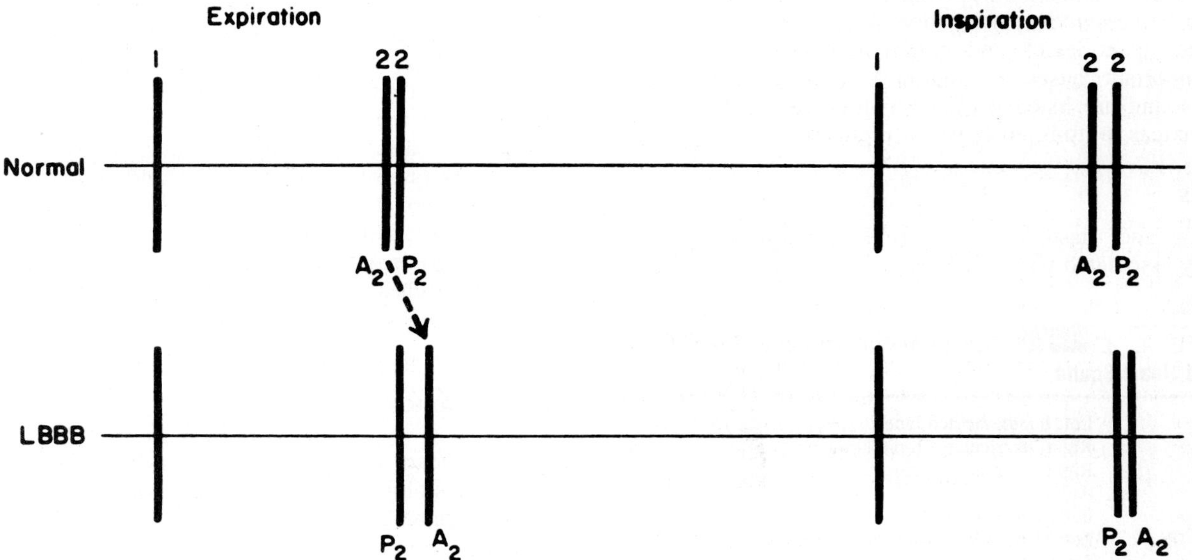

FIGURE 1–9 Top, Normal splitting of the second heart sound. **Bottom,** Paradoxical splitting. In normal splitting, pulmonary valve closure (P_2) follows aortic valve closure (A_2), and the splitting increases with inspiration. In paradoxical splitting, aortic valve closure follows pulmonic closure, and the splitting is widest during expiration. The paradoxical splitting of the second heart sound **(bottom)** occurred as the result of a left bundle branch block (LBBB).

sternum. The pulmonic component of the second heart sound is not usually heard low along the left sternal border or at the cardiac apex, except in situations where pulmonary artery pressure is significantly increased. In the normal situation, the widest splitting of the second heart sound occurs during inspiration (see Fig. 1–9). During expiration, the second sound becomes single, or the splitting between aortic and pulmonic components becomes narrower. The amplitude of the second heart sound is proportional to the peak value of the first derivative (dP/dt) of the pressure difference between the aorta or the pulmonary artery and the left or right ventricle. Increased pressure in the aorta or pulmonary artery is usually accompanied by a louder aortic or pulmonary component of the second heart sound. Systemic hypertension and coarctation cause loud aortic components, whereas pulmonary hypertension results in a loud pulmonary component of the second heart sound. LV and RV outflow obstruction, whether valvular, subvalvular, or supravalvular, usually results in fainter components of the second heart sound, and sometimes the aortic or pulmonary component of the second heart sound is absent.

Three general abnormalities can occur with respect to splitting of the second heart sound. The first is that the second heart sound may be a single sound, with neither audible nor detectable splitting. Second, the splitting may be wide during inspiration and may remain wide during expiration, so that the splitting sounds "fixed" to the ear. Third, paradoxical splitting (i.e., wider splitting of the second heart sound during expiration and narrowing during inspiration) may occur (see Fig. 1–9). Single second heart sounds (in some instances narrowly split sounds beneath the capability of the human ear to detect splitting) are heard in elderly people, in patients with truncus arteriosus (although split second heart sounds are occasionally heard in this abnormality), with ventricular septal defects complicated by severe pulmonary hypertension, and with severe pulmonary hypertension of any etiology. Fixed splitting of the second heart sound often but not invariably occurs with atrial septal defects. Apparent fixed splitting of the second heart sound is sometimes found in patients with right bundle branch block, partial anomalous venous return, ventricular septal defect, and mild pulmonary hypertension. The important causes of paradoxical splitting of the second heart sound are listed in Table 1–14, and an example of paradoxical splitting is shown in Figure 1–9.

Clicks

Systolic and diastolic clicks are high-frequency sounds usually associated with some form of cardiovascular abnormality. The different types of systolic and diastolic clicks and their distinguishing features and associated cardiovascular abnormalities are listed in Table 1–15. Examples of some of these are shown in Figures 1–10 and 1–11.

TABLE 1-14 Causes of Paradoxical Splitting of the Second Heart Sound

Left bundle branch block
Right ventricular ectopic beats
Right ventricular pacing
Angina pectoris
Left ventricular failure
Left ventricular outflow obstruction
Severe systemic hypertension

Paradoxical splitting occurs in some patients with these abnormalities but not in all of them.

Murmurs

Innocent or *functional* murmurs do not represent pathologic abnormalities. Innocent murmurs may occur as a result of increased velocity of blood flow across normal valves due to extracardiac factors. They are heard in patients with anemia or thyrotoxicosis and after exercise. Innocent murmurs are usually short, soft systolic murmurs that often change in intensity or disappear with changes in position, with rest, and/or with correction of an underlying abnormality, such as anemia. Diastolic murmurs are rarely, if ever, innocent murmurs. Innocent murmurs are common in children. Occasionally, the differentiation of an innocent or benign systolic murmur from one indicative of serious underlying cardiac pathology is difficult.

Systolic murmurs are classified as either systolic ejection murmurs or holosystolic murmurs. Systolic ejection murmurs terminate before the second heart sound and peak in intensity in early to midsystole, becoming softer thereafter. Valvular aortic and pulmonary stenosis (see Fig. 1–10) are characterized by systolic ejection murmurs. Holosystolic murmurs extend throughout systole, beginning immediately after the first heart sound and extending up to the second sound. The murmur of mitral regurgitation is an example of a holosystolic murmur (Fig. 1–12). The holosystolic murmur of tricuspid regurgitation typically (but not always) increases in intensity with inspiration (see Fig. 1–6).

Table 1–16 lists distinguishing features of the common systolic murmurs. One should remember that more than one murmur indicative of valvular heart disease can exist in a given patient. For example, it is not uncommon to find systolic and diastolic murmurs indicative of both valvular obstruction and regurgitation. The common types and locations of diastolic murmurs are listed in Table 1–17, and two examples are shown in Figure 1–11. The common types of continuous murmurs are listed in Table 1–18.

Pericardial friction rubs may be mistaken for cardiac murmurs, but they can be differentiated by their rough, harsh quality and by the fact that they have at least two components (systolic and diastolic) and sometimes three audible components (systolic, diastolic, and presystolic). They may be audible anywhere over the left precordium. They occur in some patients after MI or cardiac surgery, in uremia, after chest injury, and in association with systemic collagen diseases.

Gallop Sounds

The third heart sound, or *protodiastolic gallop* (S_3), although physiologic in children and young adults, is an abnormal sound in adults older than 30 years. Its origin is most likely from either the mitral or tricuspid valve leaflets, supporting structures, the ventricular myocardium, or a combination. It is found in patients with severe myocardial disease and in those with hemodynamically significant val-

TABLE 1-15 **Systolic and Diastolic Clicks**

Systolic Clicks		Diastolic Clicks
Early Systolic Clicks	***Mid- and Late Systolic Clicks***	***Opening Snaps***
Valvular aortic stenosis High-frequency sounds usually occurring 0.02–0.06 s from the initial high-frequency component of the first heart sound. These clicks do not change their timing with respect to the first heart sound, respiration, or change in position, nor does the intensity of the click fluctuate with respiration. The aortic valve ejection click either slightly precedes or occurs simultaneously with the carotid upstroke. This type of ejection click is commonly heard in the patient with a bicuspid aortic valve that is not heavily calcified. Valvular pulmonary stenosis An early systolic click with approximately the same timing as for the aortic click. These clicks become significantly softer or disappear during inspiration and become louder with expiration. One may also estimate the severity of the valvular pulmonary stenosis by the closeness of the pulmonary systolic click to the initial high-frequency deflection of S_1 with increasing severity. The click is closer to S_1. Dilated pulmonary artery or dilated aorta High-frequency clicks occurring with ejection timing are also heard in some patients with these abnormalities. The click occurring with a dilated pulmonary artery that either is due to pulmonary hypertension or is idiopathic usually is not significantly diminished in intensity during inspiration. Mitral valve prolapse Early systolic click or clicks occur in some patients with this entity. Typically, these clicks move closer to the first heart sound with inspiration, with assumption of the upright position, with the Valsalva maneuver, and with amyl nitrate administration. Their relationship to the carotid upstroke is variable in that they may precede, occur simultaneously with, or follow the carotid upstroke. Ebstein's anomaly Early systolic click is audible in some patients with this abnormality. Aneurysm of the membranous ventricular septum Some patients with this abnormality also have an early systolic click. Aortic valve prosthesis The intensity of the opening click of the Starr-Edwards aortic prosthesis should be approximately 50 percent or more of that of the closing click in the second right intercostal space. Abnormal function of the aortic prosthesis is suggested by gross reduction in the intensity of the opening click of the prosthesis.	Mitral valve prolapse The most common cause of a high-frequency click or clicks occurring in mid to late systole. Usually these clicks move closer to the first heart sound with inspiration, with assumption of the upright position, with amyl nitrate inhalation, and with the Valsalva maneuver. The click may be preceded by, enveloped by, or followed by a systolic murmur, or there may be no audible systolic murmur. Aortic regurgitation Mid- to late systolic clicks occur rarely in patients with significant aortic regurgitation.	Mitral valve A high-frequency sound audible along the left sternal border and at the cardiac apex in patients with mitral stenosis and in a rare patient without mitral valve disease. The presence of large amounts of calcium in the mitral valve apparatus may result in the absence of an opening snap even when significant mitral stenosis is present. The opening snap of the mitral valve usually occurs 0.03 to 0.14 s after the high-frequency component of aortic valve closure. In mitral stenosis, one can use the aortic closure and the mitral valve opening click as an indication of the severity of the mitral valve obstruction. With increasing severity of the mitral valve obstruction, this interval becomes progressively shorter. Mitral prosthesis Also a high-frequency sound, usually best heard along the left sternal border or at the cardiac apex. With malfunction of the prosthesis resulting from either tissue ingrowth, paravalvular regurgitation, or thrombus interference, the opening click may become markedly reduced in intensity. With severe mitral paravalvular regurgitation, the interval from aortic closure to mitral valve opening may become markedly reduced, whereas with tissue ingrowth or thrombus interference, this interval may be significantly prolonged. Tricuspid valve Some patients with tricuspid stenosis and patients with tricuspid prostheses have opening snaps of their tricuspid valve. This is also a high-frequency sound audible along the left sternal border and at the apex. Mitral valve prolapse Diastolic clicks have been recorded in some patients with this abnormality, but these clicks are extremely unusual.

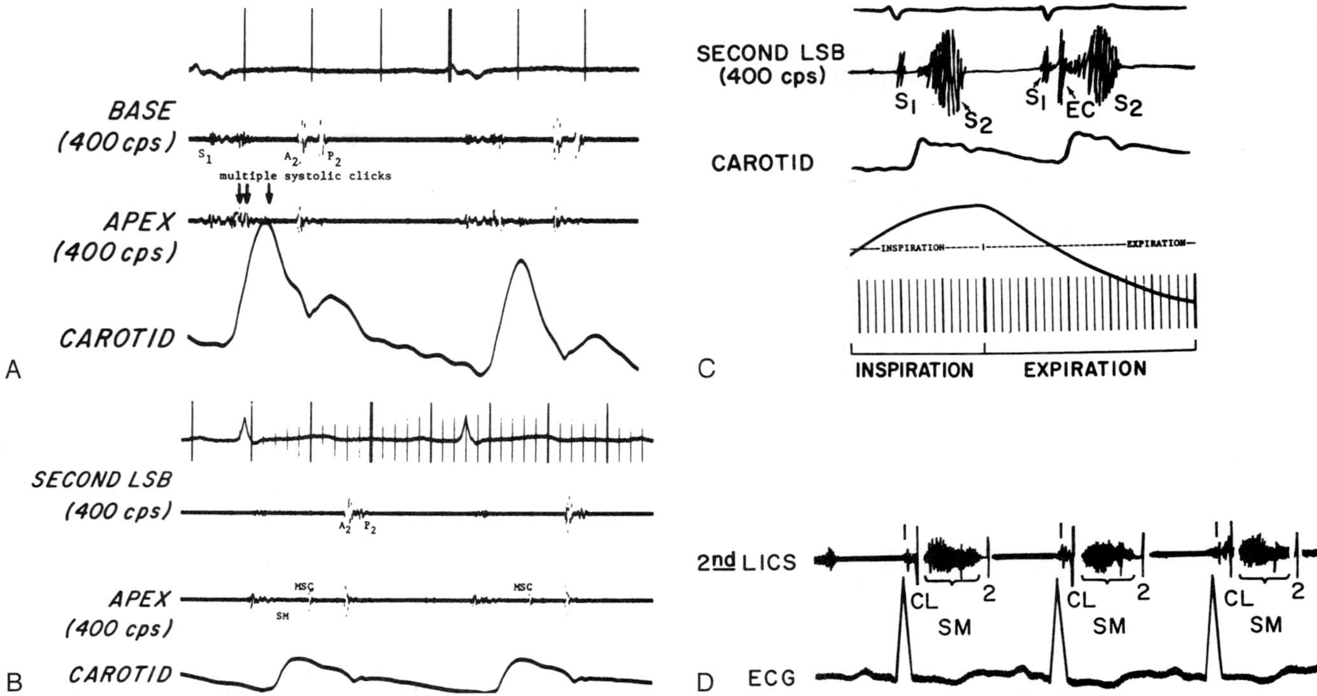

FIGURE 1–10 A, Midsystolic clicks in the recordings of the heart sounds at the base and apex of the left precordium in a patient with mitral valve prolapse. Typically, such a patient has a single midsystolic click (MSC) that moves closer to the first heart sound (S_1) with inspiration and with sitting and standing. However, as shown here, some patients with mitral valve prolapse have early systolic ejection clicks and multiple early and midsystolic ejection clicks. **B,** A mid-late systolic click in another patient with mitral valve prolapse. **C,** The early systolic click, ejection click (EC), in a patient with valvular pulmonary stenosis. This click is typically heard in the second left intercostal space. It becomes softer and disappears with inspiration and is easily audible during expiration. **D,** An early systolic ejection click in a patient with a bicuspid aortic valve. The intensity of this click does not change with respiration. The typical systolic ejection murmur in the patient with an obstructed bicuspid aortic valve is also shown. ECG, electrocardiogram; LICS, left intercostal space; LSB, left sternal border; SM, systolic murmur.

vular insufficiency, including aortic, mitral, tricuspid, and pulmonary valvular insufficiency. A third heart sound is demonstrated in Figure 1–8. The presence of a third heart sound is incompatible with a diagnosis of hemodynamically severe mitral obstruction in the absence of severe mitral insufficiency. However, an S_3 can be produced by significant aortic regurgitation or severe tricuspid regurgitation, even in the patient with severe mitral valve obstruction. One may be able to differentiate a third heart sound originating from the right or the left ventricle by recognizing that the S_3 is audible or becomes significantly more prominent during inspiration. This implies an RV origin

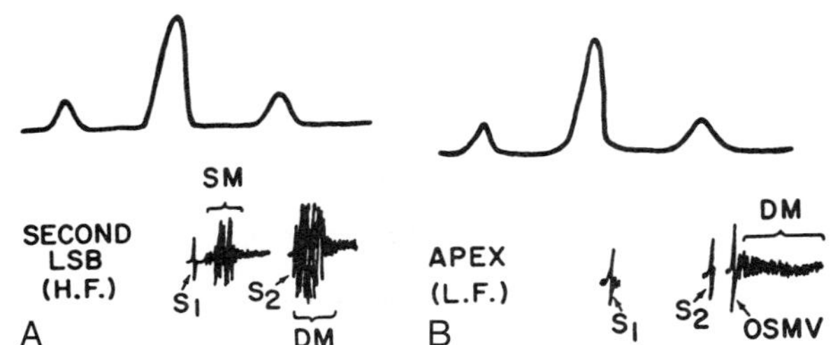

FIGURE 1–11 A and **B,** Two diastolic heart murmurs are demonstrated. **A,** A high-frequency (H.F.) diastolic decrescendo murmur (DM) in a patient with aortic regurgitation. **B,** A low-frequency (L.F.) diastolic rumble typical of mitral stenosis occurring immediately after an opening snap of the mitral valve (OSMV). LSB, left sternal border; SM, systolic murmur.

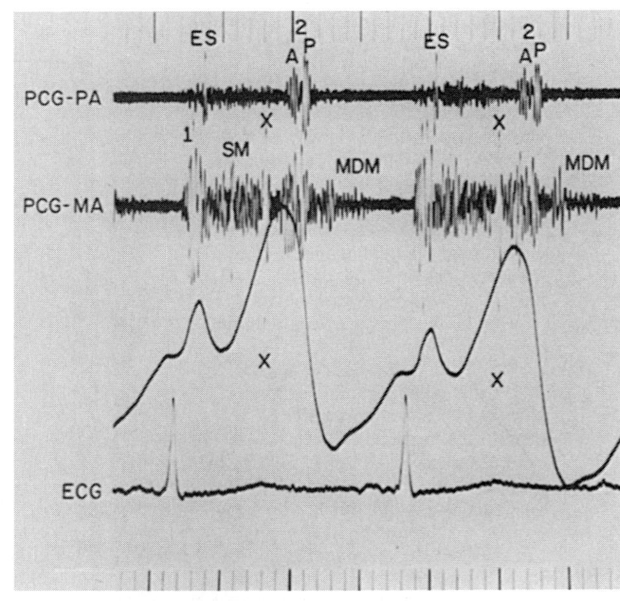

FIGURE 1–12 The holosystolic murmur typical of mitral insufficiency is demonstrated at the apex (second panel with heart sounds). The jugular venous pulse is shown in the third panel, and the patient's electrocardiogram (ECG) is shown in the bottom panel. A, aortic closure sound; ES, ejection sound; MA, mitral area; MDM, mid-diastolic murmur; P, pulmonic closure sound; PA, pulmonary artery position; PCG, phonocardiogram; SM, systolic murmur; X, descent of jugular venous pulse.

TABLE 1-16 **Systolic Ejection Murmurs**

Location	Differential Diagnosis
Second and third right and/or left intercostal spaces	A "flow" murmur indicative of either increased stroke volume or turbulence around the aortic valve but not hemodynamically significant aortic valve obstruction
	Valvular aortic stenosis. This murmur is audible anywhere over the left precordium and radiates up and toward the right shoulder and into both carotid arteries. If the obstruction is due to a bicuspid aortic valve that is not heavily calcified, there is usually an associated systolic ejection click
	Supravalvular aortic stenosis. Usually occurs in children or young adults and may have an associated characteristic physical appearance, namely elfin facies, and mental retardation. There is often a systolic blood pressure difference of greater than 15 mm Hg between the two arms, with blood pressure being higher in the right arm
	Subvalvular aortic stenosis (bar or diaphragm immediately beneath the aortic valve). In addition to the systolic murmur, there is often as associated diastolic murmur of aortic regurgitation. A systolic ejection click is usually not present
	Valvular pulmonary stenosis. This murmur is usually loudest to the left of the sternum. There is an associated systolic ejection click that decreases or disappears with inspiration and becomes prominent during expiration
	Coarctation of the aorta. This murmur may also be heard medial to the left scapula posteriorly and/or under the left clavicle anteriorly. The murmur is usually associated with systemic arterial hypertension and diminished or absent femoral pulses
	Atrial septal defect. Typically, a soft murmur caused by increased blood flow across the pulmonary valve and often associated with "fixed splitting" of the second heart sound
	Infundibular pulmonary stenosis. This murmur is best heard to the left of the sternum. There is usually no associated ejection click
	Peripheral pulmonary stenosis. This murmur may also be heard over the back
Second to fifth left intercostal spaces	Hypertrophic obstructive cardiopathy or idiopathic hypertrophic subaortic stenosis. This murmur usually does not radiate well into the carotid arteries. The murmur typically increases with Valsalva maneuver and upright position and in the beat following a ventricular premature beat. It characteristically decreases with squatting. On occasion, however, the Valsalva maneuver and squatting do not result in the expected changes in intensity of this murmur
Cardiac apex	Valvular aortic stenosis. On occasion this murmur may be loudest at the apex rather than at the base, making its differentiation from mitral regurgitation more difficult
	Mitral regurgitation resulting from papillary muscle dysfunction. This murmur often is of ejection type, beginning after the first heart sound, peaking in midsystole, and ending before the second sound. On occasion, however, this murmur is holosystolic rather than ejection
Holosystolic murmurs	
Fourth and fifth left intercostal spaces	Tricuspid regurgitation. This murmur typically increases with inspiration and is associated with prominent V waves in the jugular venous pulse. Occasionally the inspiratory increase in the murmur does not occur
	Ventricular septal defects. This murmur has no phasic respiratory change and is often associated with a systolic thrill along the left sternal border
Cardiac apex	Rheumatic mitral regurgitation and/or mitral regurgitation due to endocarditis
	Mitral regurgitation due to ruptured chordae tendineae
	Mitral regurgitation secondary to papillary muscle dysfunction. This murmur may have an ejection quality in some patients
	"Relative" mitral regurgitation. This is the mitral regurgitation due to left ventricular failure and an abnormal spatial relationship of the mitral leaflets and papillary muscles
	Mitral regurgitation associated with idiopathic hypertrophic subaortic stenosis or with left atrial myxoma

TABLE 1-17 Diastolic Murmurs

Location	Differential Diagnosis
High-pitched diastolic decrescendo murmurs Second to third left and right intercostal spaces	Aortic regurgitation. This is a blowing murmur that immediately follows the second heart sound. In general, valvular aortic regurgitation murmurs are best heard along the left sternal border in the second and third intercostal spaces, and aortic regurgitation due to aortic root disease (e.g., syphilis, spondylitis, dissection) is best heard along the right sternal border Pulmonary regurgitation. This murmur is usually best heard to the left of the sternum. Its timing and quality are similar to the murmur of aortic regurgitation
Low-pitched diastolic rumbles	
Third to fourth left intercostal spaces	Atrial septal defect. This murmur results from increased flow across the tricuspid valve
Fourth to fifth left intercostal spaces	Tricuspid stenosis. This murmur may become louder during inspiration and with maneuvers that increase venous return to the right atrium. Rheumatic fever or right atrial myxoma may be etiologies
Cardiac apex	Mitral stenosis. This low-pitched diastolic murmur follows immediately after the opening snap of the mitral valve when the latter is present. It is often best heard by having the patient lie on the left side and listening directly over the point of maximal impulse. The length of the diastolic murmur correlates directly with the severity of mitral obstruction Flow rumbles due to a large left-to-right shunt such as with large ventricular septal defects. These occur just after the second heart sound and are usually short in duration Austin Flint murmur. Apical diastolic rumble ordinarily of short length occurring in some patients with severe aortic regurgitation. This murmur usually results from vibration of the septal leaflet of the mitral valve due to the regurgitant aortic jet. The murmur may rarely result from late diastolic mitral regurgitation Carey-Coombs murmur. Short mid-diastolic rumble noted rarely in patients with acute rheumatic fever; murmur results from inflammation involving mitral valve leaflets "S_3 rumble complex." Some patients with hemodynamically important mitral regurgitation have a short diastolic rumble that follows the third heart sound. The rumble reflects a flow-related and relative mitral obstruction Left atrial myxoma may also produce a murmur that mimics mitral stenosis, except that it ordinarily is not associated with an opening snap of the mitral valve

TABLE 1-18 Continuous Murmurs

Location	Differential Diagnosis
First to second left intercostal spaces (and under left clavicle)	Patent ductus arteriosus
Second to fourth left intercostal spaces	Aorticopulmonary septal defect
Usually best heard in the second to third left intercostal spaces; occasionally may be best heard at the right of the sternum in the same area	Surgical shunts, such as aortopulmonary anastomoses
Usually best heard along the lower left sternal border, although it may be audible over the entire precordium	Rupture of sinus of Valsalva aneurysm
Audible over the left precordium	Coronary arteriovenous fistulae
May be audible anywhere that they occur	Atrioventricular fistulae

for the sound. The tumor plop sound of atrial myxoma is a high-frequency mid-diastolic sound that may be mistaken for an S_3.

The fourth heart sound, or *presystolic gallop* (S_4), is an abnormal sound (see Fig. 1–8). It is thought to originate within the left or right ventricle as a result of the left or right atrium being forced to contract more vigorously than normally due to reduced ventricular compliance in the ventricle from which it originates. It is almost always found in patients with severe CAD, LV outflow obstruction, or systemic arterial hypertension and in patients in sinus rhythm with important mitral regurgitation of recent onset. It is not present in patients with atrial fibrillation due to the absence of a discrete forceful atrial contraction.

A *summation gallop* is a prominent sound that occurs at rapid heart rates and represents the summation of both a presystolic and protodiastolic gallop sound. It is recognized with certainty by demonstrating a single loud gallop sound at relatively rapid heart rates, which at slower heart rates resolves into its individual components (i.e., S_3 and S_4).

Heart Sounds From Prosthetic Disc Heart Valves

The bioprosthetic disc cardiac valves normally produce clicks that identify their opening and closing. Figure 1–13 identifies the timing of these sounds for both aortic and mitral prosthetic valves. The opening and closing clicks of these valves are high-frequency sounds best heard with the diaphragm of the stethoscope. The opening click of the aortic prosthesis is best heard along the left sternal border and over the left precordium. The closing click of the aortic valve is best heard in the second and third left intercostal spaces. The opening and closing clicks of the mitral prosthesis are best heard at the lower left sternal border and the cardiac apex. With thrombosis, tissue ingrowth, or dehiscence of these valves, the opening clicks are often markedly reduced in amplitude. With tissue ingrowth or thrombosis of the aortic or mitral prosthesis, the S_1 opening click of the aortic valve and the S_2 opening click interval of the mitral valve may also be markedly prolonged.

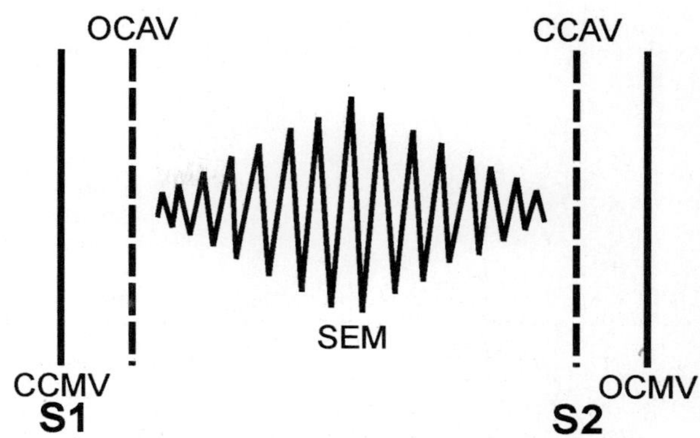

FIGURE 1–13 The prosthetic disc valve sounds for aortic and mitral valves are shown. AV, aortic valve; CC, closing click; MV, mitral valve; OC, opening click; SEM, systolic ejection murmur.

CHAPTER 2

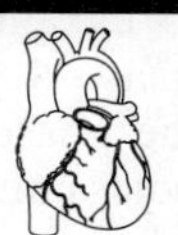

ELECTROCARDIOGRAPHY

Naip Tuna

BASIS OF THE ELECTROCARDIOGRAM
LEAD SYSTEMS
NORMAL ECG
P Wave
PR Segment
QRS Complex
ST-T Wave
Ventricular Gradient
QT Interval
U Wave
QRS Axis Determination
ABNORMAL ECG
P Wave Abnormalities
Left Atrial Enlargement (P Mitrale)
Right Atrial Enlargement (P Pulmonale)
Biatrial Enlargement
Atrial Infarction
Left Ventricular Hypertrophy
Biventricular Hypertrophy
Intraventricular Conduction Disturbances
Myocardial Ischemia and Injury
Acute MI
Old or Chronic MI
Diagnostic Criteria for MI
Localization of MI
Diagnosis of Anterior MI
Diagnosis of Inferior MI
Diagnosis of Posterolateral MI
Non–Q Wave MI
Noninfarction Q Waves
ST and T Wave Abnormalities
Electrolyte Abnormalities
Drug-Induced Electrocardiographic Changes
Miscellaneous Patterns
Improper Placement of Leads
SPECIAL CLINICAL PROBLEMS
Pericarditis
Myocarditis
Pulmonary Embolism
Central Nervous System Disorders (Neurogenic Repolarization Abnormalities)
Hypothermia
Cardiac Transplantation
INTERPRETATION OF THE ECG
Interpretation and Comments

BASIS OF THE ELECTROCARDIOGRAM

The electrocardiogram (ECG) is a record of cardiac electrical activity associated with the depolarization and repolarization of atrial and ventricular myocardium. During depolarization, when the cells are activated, their surface becomes negatively charged with respect to areas still in the resting state, which are positively charged. During the spread of activation, a flow of current from the negative to the positive areas can be represented as a dipole with positive charge in front of the negative charge. The dipole creates an electrical field that has a magnitude and orientation. During cardiac activation, dipoles from different locations with different orientations and strengths are present. The magnitude and direction of dipoles recorded from the body surface at any given moment represent the resultant of these individual dipoles. Thus, a large portion of the electrical activity of individual cells is canceled out.[1] In spite of the previously mentioned cancellations, the resultant ECG is a fair representation of the electrical activity of the heart and provides valuable information. The depolarization process of all cardiac tissues starts when transmembrane action potential reaches a critical threshold potential. At rest, a myocardial cell is polarized, the inside of the cell being negative (−90 mV) with respect to the outside. The resting transmembrane potential is mainly determined by the potassium gradient across the cell membrane. The intracellular potassium concentration is thirty to thirty-five times that of the extracellular concentration, and the extracellular concentration of sodium ion is about ten to fifteen times that of the intracellular concentration.

The movement of various ions across the cell membrane during depolarization (activation) and repolarization is complex and involves various ion channels, gates, and currents. Briefly, during depolarization of myocardial cell, there is rapid influx of sodium into the cell, accounting for phase zero of the action potential. During phase 1 of the action potential, the outward potassium current is activated, bringing the membrane potential from overshoot to 0 mV and to −20 mV. During phase 2, or plateau, the membrane potential remains relatively constant owing to the inward positive current carried by the calcium ions and the outward current carried by the potassium ions. Toward the end of phase 2 of the action potential, inward calcium current decreases progressively, and in phase 3, the completion of repolarization is achieved by inward movement of potassium. When the maximal negative voltage is reached, the phase 4 (resting membrane potential) is recorded.[2] The resting membrane potential of various cardiac tissues is as follows: sinoatrial (SA) node −50 to −60 mV; atrial muscle −80 to −90 mV; atrioventricular (AV) node −60 to −70 mV; Purkinje fiber −90 to −95 mV; and ventricular muscle −80 to −90 mV. In automatic cells, such as the SA node, the resting membrane potential rises gradually to the threshold level owing to spontaneous upsloping of phase 4 (diastolic depolarization). In nonautomatic cells, the phase 4 is constant and is maintained by the sodium potassium pump. The threshold of activation is reached when current from an adjacent depolarized cell excites them. The threshold potential for fast-response cells with Na channels is −60 to −70 mV, whereas for slow response cells with Ca channels, it is about −40 mV. Slow-response cells include the SA and the AV nodes.[3, 4]

When a cell is partially depolarized, to approximately −60 mV, there is a reduction in sodium current owing to inactivation of sodium channels. The resting membrane potential of partially depolarized cells is higher (less negative) than the potential that would permit activation of fast sodium channels. The action potentials of these cells have a slow rise of phase 0 and lower magnitude; thus, the electrophysiologic properties of SA node, atrial myocardial, AV node, His-Purkinje system, and the ventricular myocardium are different. Also, the electrophysiologic properties of ventricular myocardial cells close to the endocardium are different from those close to the epicardium or from those of the M (midmyocardial) cells. There are also differences between the action potentials of the myocardial cells of the left ventricle (LV) and the right ventricle (RV). The M cells of the RV have shorter action potential durations, deeper notches, and less prolongation of action potential duration on slowing the pacing rate. The differences appear to be related to the differences in K^+ currents between the M cells of the RV and the LV.[5–7]

The M cells of the ventricular wall represent at least 40% of the left ventricular free wall, have action potentials that are between those of the myocardial cells and those of the Purkinje cells, and have a significant role in determining the shape of the ECG. Under normal conditions, the activation process starts from the SA node and spreads rapidly into the atria. The activation is slowed in the AV node, which allows time for the atrial contraction to be completed before the start of ventricular contraction. The slowing in the AV node occurs because of cells whose activation is dependent on slow-channel calcium currents. The activation speeds up after it reaches the His-Purkinje system, which then is followed by the activation of ventricles.[8]

Lead Systems

The most commonly used lead system for the recording of cardiac potentials (voltages) is the 12-lead electrocardiographic system based on the original lead system developed by Einthoven and colleagues.[9] The 12-lead system assumes that the body is a homogeneous volume conductor, that there is a single dipole at the center of the volume conductor, and that the three limb leads represent an equilateral triangle. Precordial leads and augmented limb leads were later added to the original 3 bipolar limb leads. Currently the 12-lead system consists of 3 bipolar leads (lead I, lead II, and lead III), 3 unipolar augmented limb leads (aVR, aVL, aVF), and 6 unipolar precordial leads (V_1, V_2, V_3, V_4, V_5, V_6). Additional leads on the right side of the chest, such as V_3R, V_4R, V_5R, V_6R, or on the left side, such as V_7, V_8, and V_9, may be recorded as needed. The placement of electrodes is as follows: R (right arm), L (left arm), F (left leg), G (ground, right leg), V_1 (right sternal margin, fourth intercostal space), V_2 (left sternal margin, fourth intercostal space), V_3 (midway between electrodes V_2 and V_4), V_4 (left midclavicular line, fifth intercostal space), V_5 (left anterior axillary line, V_4 level), V_6 (midaxillary line, V_4 level), V_7 (posterior axillary line, V_4 level), V_8 (midscapular line, V_4 level), and V_9 (left paraspinal border, V_4 level). V_3R through V_6R represent locations similar to V leads, but on the right side. The bipolar leads record the potential difference between two limb electrodes: lead I between L positive and R negative; lead II between F positive and R negative, and lead III between F positive and L negative (positive and negative represent the positive and negative input). Augmented unipolar leads record the potential augmented by 50%[10]: aVR (augmented R potential) records the potential difference between R and (L + F)/2; aVL between L and (R + F)/2; and aVF between F and (R + L)/2. Unipolar precordial leads record the potential difference between V leads and the Wilson central terminal, which consists of inputs from right arm, left arm, and left leg electrodes, each connected through 5000-ohm resistors.[11] The potential at the central terminal is regarded as zero. The central terminal electrode is connected to the negative terminal on the ECG machine, and the precordial electrodes are connected to the positive terminal. Various leads used in electrocardiography record the potentials generated by the same dipole from various points on the body surface. Other electrocardiographic recording systems include the corrected and orthogonal vectorcardiographic leads X, Y, Z (the Frank lead system being the most widely used)[12] and the body surface mapping leads using multiple electrodes, up to 200.[13–15] The instantaneous vectors recorded by the X, Y, and Z leads are displayed as frontal plane (X and Y), sagittal plane (Y and Z), and horizontal plane (X and Z) loops, or their spatial magnitudes and orientations can be calculated and used in algorithms to diagnose various abnormalities. Vectorcardiography, which was quite popular in the past, is no longer used significantly in clinical practice because of economic considerations and questionable additional clinical benefit that it may provide beyond the 12-lead ECG.

Signal-averaged electrocardiography is another technique of recording cardiac potentials from the body surface. High-frequency, low-amplitude (about 20 μV or less) potentials located in the terminal 40 ms of the QRS are recorded after averaging 200 to 300 QRS complexes subjected to specific filtering and processing.[16, 17] This technique and intracardiac recordings are covered elsewhere in this book.

Normal ECG

This section covers the electrocardiographic wave forms, durations, intervals, and the electrical axis.[18, 19]

P Wave

The P wave, which is produced by the activation of the atria with impulses coming from the SA node (sinus

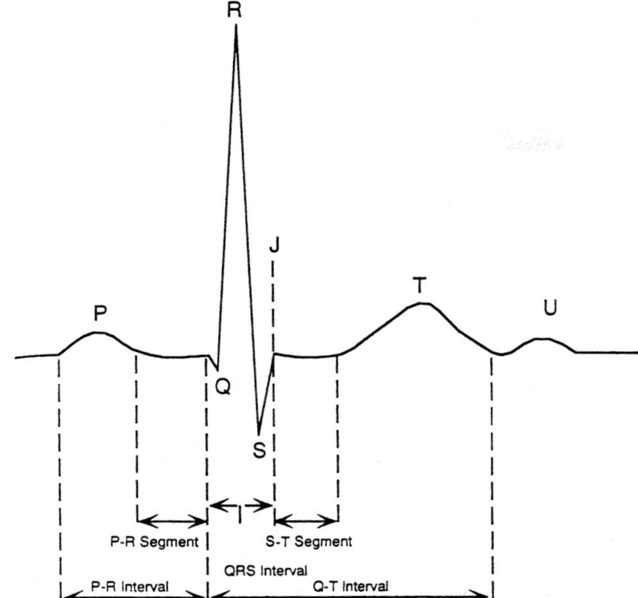

FIGURE 2–1 The major electrocardiographic waveforms. The measurement of P and QRS durations, PR and QT intervals, and PR and ST segments. (From Wagner GS [ed]: Marriott's Practical Electrocardiography. 9th ed. p. 13. Baltimore: Williams & Wilkins, 1994.)

rhythm) is the first wave form of the ECG. It is followed by the PR segment, which represents AV conduction. The QRS complex that follows it represents ventricular activation (depolarization), and the ST-T interval represents ventricular repolarization. The U wave that follows the T wave is most likely related to Purkinje tissue and M cell repolarization (Fig. 2–1).

James[20] described functionally and histologically discrete specialized pathways (anterior, middle, and posterior nodal pathways) in the atria connecting the sinus node and the AV node and the right and left atrium. Although both atria are simultaneously activated, the initial part of the P wave is dominated by the right atrial activation and the terminal part by the left atrial activation.[21, 22] In normal adults, the P duration is less than 120 ms. It is positive in leads I, II, and aVF, negative in lead aVR, and variable in leads aVL and III (positive or positive-negative). In V leads, it is generally upright, but it may be negative or biphasic (positive negative) in V_1 and biphasic in V_2 and, sometimes, in V_3. Usually, the P amplitude is less than 250 μV, and the negative component of P in V_1 is less than 0.04 mm/s. P wave morphology may change in ectopic atrial rhythms, wandering atrial pacemaker, atrial hypertrophy, dextrocardia, and lead placement errors. Changes in P wave morphology may lead one to suspect lead misplacement. Atrial repolarization is difficult to discern because it occurs during the PR segment and QRS. Atrial repolarization may cause PR segment depression in acute pericarditis and atrial infarction, and it may cause ST depression during exercise stress testing.

PR Segment

The PR segment includes activation of the AV node, the bundle of His, the bundle branches, and the Purkinje network. The PR interval measured from the beginning of the P wave to the beginning of QRS includes the PA, the AH, and the HV intervals and is 120 to 200 ms in duration. The PR interval influences ventricular filling and mitral valve closure, and if too long, it may cause early closure of the AV valve and interfere with diastolic filling of ventricles.[23]

QRS Complex

The activation wave coming from the AV node spreads through the bundle branches and the His-Purkinje system across the endocardium of both ventricles and then spreads across the ventricular walls.[24, 25] The left ventricular activation starts in the septum, left-side center, and anterior and posterior paraseptal regions of the LV, spreading to anterior and lateral walls and to the posterobasal LV—the last area to be activated. The right ventricular activation starts at the base of the anterior papillary muscle and then spreads to the septum and the free wall, the pulmonary conus, and the posterobasal regions, the last to be activated. Various parts of the LV and the RV are activated simultaneously. Septal depolarization produces the Q wave of the normal QRS, which has a width less than 20 to 30 ms. The R wave and the S wave are produced primarily by left ventricular activation, the RV contributing very little to the QRS in the normal ECG. The small r′ in V_1 through V_3 is usually caused by activation of the basal RV and LV during the final phases of ventricular activation. The QRS duration is usually 70 to 90 ms, less than 120 ms. The normal QRS axis in the frontal plane is −30 to +90 degrees. Left axis deviation is present when the axis is between −30 and −90 degrees, and right axis deviation is present when the axis is between +90 and ±180 degrees. QRS morphology is affected by electrical axis, position of heart in the chest cavity, chamber hypertrophies, myocardial infarctions (MIs), and myocardial diseases, as well as conduction abnormalities. The Q wave in limb leads and leads V_5 and V_6 is small, its duration is usually less than 30 ms, and its magnitude is less than 25% of the R wave in the same lead. In leads V_1 and V_2, the QRS morphology is a small r deep S; it is big R, big S (R = S) in V_3 ("transition"); big R small s in V_4; and big R with very small s in V_5 and V_6. The largest R or S in limb leads is between 0.5 and 1.6 mV, whereas in V leads, it is between 1.0 and 3.0 mV. In V_5 and V_6, the point at which R wave changes to S wave (intrinsicoid deflection) indicates the end of ventricular activation. The time from the beginning of QRS to the intrinsicoid deflection is called *ventricular activation time.* It is a measure of time of activation from the endocardium to the epicardium.

ST-T Wave

The ST-T wave is related to ventricular repolarization, which in normal individuals starts from the epicardium and progresses toward the endocardium. During ventricular repolarization, the epicardium recovers earlier than the endocardium because of shorter action potential duration of the epicardial myocardial cells as compared with the endocardial myocardial cells.[5, 26]

Ventricular Gradient[27]

The repolarization of the mammalian heart is different from the repolarization of an isolated muscle strip where the repolarization and depolarization are of equal duration and follow the same path, but have opposite polarity, resulting in an algebraic sum of zero (no gradient). In the mammalian heart, the repolarization starts from the epicardium rather than the endocardium (where the depolarization starts) and spreads toward the endocardium, giving rise to positive T, and the algebraic sum of QRS and T is no longer zero, indicating the presence of a "gradient."[27] The gradient has a magnitude and direction and can be determined from the area of QRS and T, each represented as a vector and using the Einthoven triangle. The normal gradient forms about a 30-degree angle with the QRS area vector.

Normally, the T wave is upright in leads I, II, aVF, and V_2 through V_6; variable in leads III and aVL; and inverted in lead aVR. The P and QRS also are normally inverted in lead aVR. The T can be inverted in leads V_1 and V_2, and in normal women, it can also be inverted in lead V_3. When T inversion in leads V_1 through V_3 is a normal variant, it is usually deepest in lead V_1 and its depth decreases in lead V_2 and more so in V_3. When the inversion in these leads is due to ischemia, the T wave depth is usually greater in lead V_3 than in leads V_2 or V_1. The T amplitude is about 20% of the QRS amplitude.

QT Interval

The QT interval is measured from the beginning of QRS to the end of the T wave, and it reflects the duration of activation (depolarization) and repolarization of ventricles and is a measure of action potential duration. Like the duration of action potential, the QT interval is also dependent on heart rate. Bazett[28] demonstrated the relation between the $\sqrt{R - R}$ cycle duration, the duration of ventricular systole, and the QT duration. The formula based on Bazett's concept is

$$\left(QT_c = \frac{QT}{\sqrt{R - R}}\right)$$

Although many equations better describing the relationship between the QT interval and the rate have been proposed, the formula based on Bazett's concept is the one that is most widely used clinically. Currently, the QT interval is measured in the lead with the longest QT, which is usually lead II; however, the QT interval may vary from lead to lead (QT dispersion) just like the action potential duration in the ventricular wall, which may vary according to location (endocardial, epicardial, M cells, LV, or RV). The U wave should not be included in the measurement of the QT interval. There is now interest in measuring the QT interval in all leads to obtain a value for the QT dispersion. Normally, the QT interval dispersion (the difference between the shortest and the longest QT interval) is about 50 ms.[29–32] However, there is considerable interobserver and intraobserver variability in the measurement of the QT interval as it is currently done, which makes the QT dispersion of questionable value.[33, 34]

U Wave

The U wave is about 0.1 mV in amplitude. It is best seen in the midprecordial leads and follows the T wave. The most prevalent view is that it is related to the repolarization of Purkinje fibers.[35] However, the mass of Purkinje tissue is relatively small, and it is questionable that this can account for the U wave. M cells, which compose at least 40% of the left ventricular free wall, have long action potential durations, have electrophysiologic properties between those of Purkinje fibers and those of myocytes, and have been proposed as a more likely candidate for the genesis of U waves.[36] The U wave is probably produced by the repolarization of both the Purkinje fibers and the M cells. The U wave corresponds to early after-depolarizations, but it can occur in their absence. Slow rate, hypokalemia, hypomagnesemia, and hypothermia—which prolong the action potential duration of Purkinje fibers and the M cells—are associated with prominent U waves and early after-depolarizations.

QRS Axis Determination

The QRS axis in the frontal plane can be determined by using the Einthoven equilateral triangle or the triaxial reference system derived from it (Fig. 2–2). The algebraic sums of positive and negative waves of QRS of any two

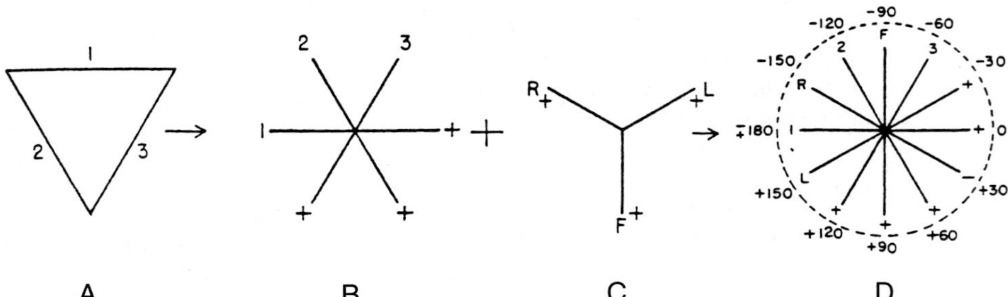

FIGURE 2–2 Constitution of the hexaxial reference system. **A,** Einthoven triangle, the sides of which represent the three standard limb leads. **B,** The triaxial reference system composed of the three sides of the Einthoven triangle rearranged so that they bisect one another. **C,** Lines of derivation of the three unipolar (aV) limb leads. **D,** The hexaxial reference system composed of the lines of derivation of the six limb leads (**B** + **C**) arranged so that they bisect each other. (**A–D,** From Marriott HJL [ed]: Practical Electrocardiography. 7th ed. p. 33. Baltimore: Williams & Wilkins, 1983.)

limb leads are plotted as vectors on respective leads, and lines perpendicular to the lead axis are dropped from their positive ends. A line is drawn from the center of the reference system to the point where the two perpendicular lines cross. The vector, which represents the QRS vector, has a magnitude and direction. The angle between lead I, which is assumed to be zero, and the QRS vector represents the QRS axis. Lead aVF represents +90 degrees and lead aVL −30 degrees. In normal individuals, the QRS axis ranges between −30 and +90 degrees. The axis between −90 and ±180 degrees is indeterminate. Most electrocardiographic computer programs use the area of QRS to determine the electrical axis. In some special situations, such as right bundle branch block (RBBB), in which there is a shallow but wide S wave in lead I together with a narrow, tall R wave, the QRS vector in lead I may have a negative value and the QRS axis can be misrepresented. The axis of P, T wave, and ventricular gradient can be determined in a similar manner. The electrical axis can also be determined by using the hexaxial reference system. The hexaxial reference system is constructed by adding the augmented limb leads aVR, aVL, and aVF to the triaxial system. The limb lead that demonstrates zero value for the algebraic sum of QRS represents the lead to which the QRS axis is perpendicular. Whether or not the axis is positive or negative can be determined by evaluating the QRS in other limb leads.

ABNORMAL ECG

P Wave Abnormalities

P wave morphology and orientation may change in various conditions. In ectopic atrial rhythms, the P wave is negative in leads III and aVF and positive in aVR. Although the exact location of ectopic focus in ectopic atrial rhythms cannot be determined from the ECG, it has been customary to diagnose "coronary sinus rhythm" when the P wave is inverted in leads III and aVF and positive in aVR, and the PR is normal; "left atrial rhythm" when the P is negative in leads I and V_6; and it is biphasic with "dome and dart" P in V_1; and "right atrial rhythm" when the P is positive in lead I but inverted in V_1 through V_3.

Left Atrial Enlargement (P Mitrale)

When there is left atrial enlargement (Fig. 2–3), the P is broad and notched in lead II, greater than 120 ms in duration, the internotch interval is 40 ms or greater, and in V_1, the P wave is biphasic with the width of negative portion (P terminal wave) exceeding 40 ms in duration and its depth exceeding 1 mm. The P axis is shifted leftward from its usual +30 to +60 degrees to about −30 degrees. The left atrial enlargement pattern is usually seen when there is increased left atrial volume and abnormal intra-atrial conduction associated with increased left atrial pressure with or without an increase in left atrial size. In left atrial enlargement, the ratio of P duration to PR segment is usually greater than 1.6 in lead II. Among electrocardiographic criteria for left atrial enlargement, P terminal area in lead V_1 greater than −0.04 mm/s has a sensitivity of 69 percent with a specificity of 93 percent; criteria related to P duration greater than 110 ms have a sensitivity of 33 percent and a specificity of 88 percent; and P notching has a sensitivity between 15 and 30 percent and a specificity of 64 to 100 percent.[37–41] There is a relatively high correlation between abnormal P terminal in lead V_1 and pulmonary capillary wedge pressure when the elevation is

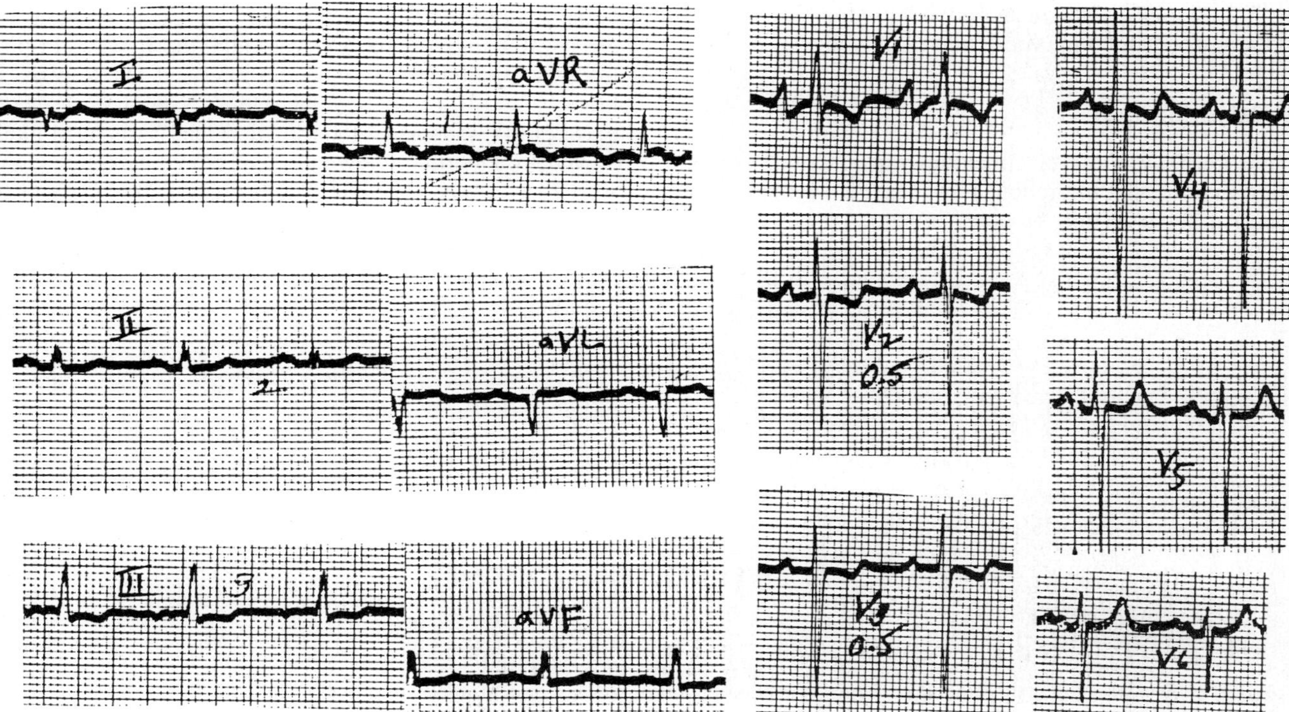

FIGURE 2–3 Left atrial enlargement. Right ventricular hypertrophy. Electrocardiogram (ECG) of a patient with severe mitral stenosis.

above 14 mm Hg.[42, 43] Intra-atrial conduction abnormality appears to be a common feature of left atrial enlargement regardless of the underlying etiology. Left atrial enlargement pattern also correlates with the development of atrial arrhythmias, atrial flutter, and atrial fibrillation.

Right Atrial Enlargement (P Pulmonale)

In right atrial enlargement (Fig. 2–4), the P duration is normal, there is rightward shift of the P axis to beyond +75 degrees, and there is peaked P with narrow base in lead II greater than 0.25 mV. In precordial leads, the initial positive part of P is peaked in V_1 with area greater than 0.06 mm/s. Right precordial QRS complexes may be influenced by right atrial enlargement, which may produce QR, Qr, qR, or qRS configurations.[44] Peaked P waves are most commonly seen in chronic obstructive pulmonary disease (COPD).[45] The correlation between P wave changes noted previously and right atrial enlargement is poor.[46–48] The correlation with QRS-based criteria is better than those based on P wave criteria.[44, 48, 49] Use of QRS axis greater than +0.90 degrees, R/S ratio in lead V_1 greater than 1 (in the absence of RBBB), and P amplitude in lead V_2 greater than 0.15 mV had a sensitivity of 49 percent and a specificity of 100 percent. Only 6 percent of patients with right atrial enlargement were diagnosed by using P criteria only.[49]

Pseudo–P pulmonale is considered when the P is tall in leads II, III, and aVF, suggesting P pulmonale, but there is abnormal terminal P in lead V_1. In this condition, the second peak of P in inferior leads is most prominent. Pseudo–P pulmonale is seen in left atrial enlargement.[49, 50]

Biatrial Enlargement

The diagnosis of biatrial enlargement is made when there are tall P waves with increased duration in leads II, III, and aVF and large biphasic P waves in lead V_1.

Atrial Infarction

There are no definite electrocardiographic criteria for the diagnosis of atrial infarction; however, PR segment elevation or depression may be noted in some cases.

Left Ventricular Hypertrophy

Left ventricular hypertrophy (LVH) and/or dilatation (Fig. 2–5) will in general result in an increase of QRS voltage and ST-T changes. The increase of QRS voltage has been attributed to increased left ventricular mass secondary to cellular hypertrophy and left ventricular enlargement.[48, 51] Left ventricular enlargement may cause increased activation fronts, and an increase in intracavitary blood mass may increase the ventricular potentials because of the Brody effect.[52] There are also changes in the relationship between the LV and the chest wall. In left ventricular enlargement, the LV is closer to the chest wall.[53] The QRS voltages are highest when there is an increase in left ventricular wall thickness associated with dilatation as compared with an increase in wall thickness alone.[54] The etiology of ST-T changes in LVH is unclear. It has been attributed to subendocardial ischemia secondary to hypertrophy, possibly associated coronary disease, mechanical forces, and abnormal repolarization owing to prolonged action potential of hypertrophied cells.[55] There is good correlation between the left ventricular mass determined by echocardiography and the ST-T changes.[56]

Electrocardiographic Criteria for the Diagnosis of LVH

Numerous criteria have been proposed for the electrocardiographic diagnosis of LVH based on voltage, ST-T changes, axis, QRS duration, and abnormal P terminal in lead V_1.[57] The sensitivity and specificity of criteria vary, with the sensitivity generally being low, between 10.6 and 55.6 percent, and the specificity varying between 88.5 and 100 percent.[57] The accuracy of electrocardiographic criteria will vary according to the prevalence of LVH in the population and the underlying cardiac disease.[58] In LVH, the voltage increase is noted primarily in leads reflecting the electrical activity of the left ventricle, the R wave in limb leads is usually greater than 2.0 mV, and the R wave in leads V_5 and V_6 or the S wave in leads V_1 and V_2 is greater than 2.5 mV. Abnormal P terminal in lead V_1 is most likely related to abnormal left ventricular compliance associated with LVH. Increased QRS voltage alone may be seen in normal individuals, particularly in those with thin chests.

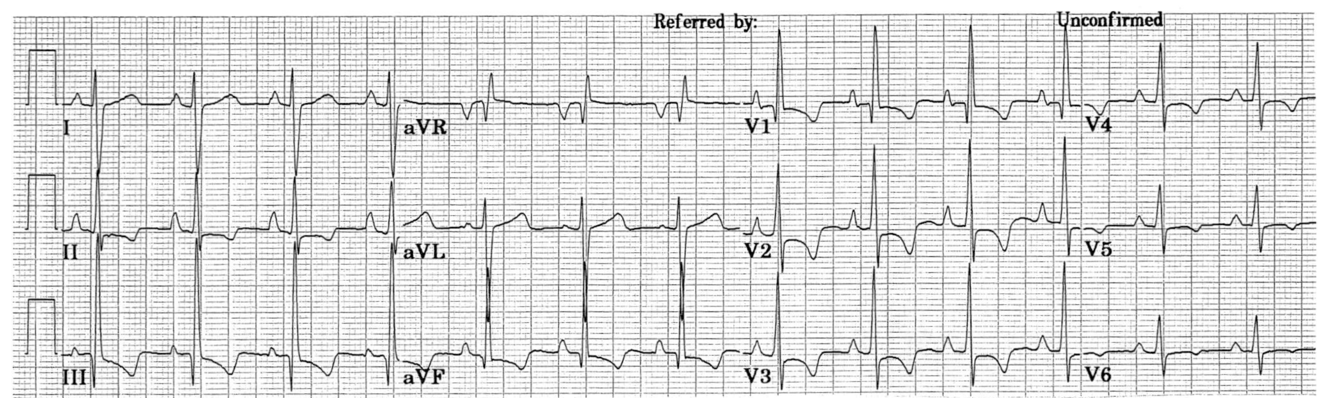

FIGURE 2–4 Right atrial enlargement and right ventricular hypertrophy with repolarization abnormality ("strain"). ECG obtained from a patient with primary pulmonary hypertension.

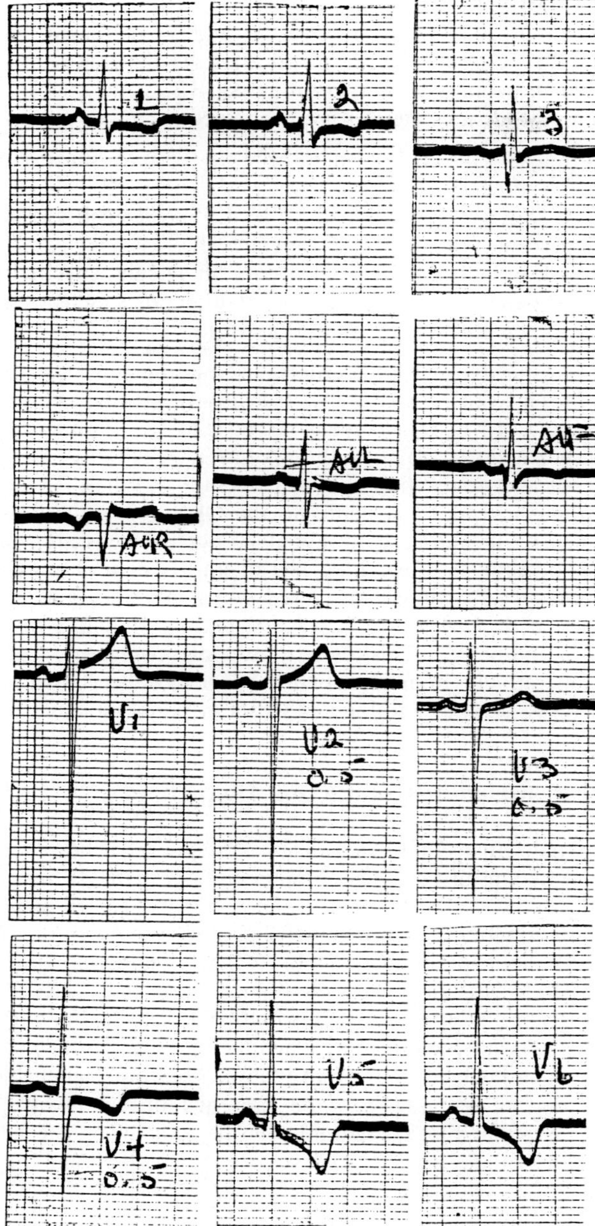

FIGURE 2–5 Left ventricular hypertrophy with ST-T abnormality ("strain").

However, the combination of increased voltage with ST-T abnormalities ("strain") in the absence of other causes for ST-T changes, such as ischemia, electrolyte abnormalities, or drug effects, makes the diagnosis of LVH much stronger.

SOKOLOW-LYON CRITERIA

1. Sum of S wave in V_1 and the greater of R wave in V_5 or $V_6 \geq 3.5$ mV or R wave in V_5 or $V_6 > 2.60$ mV.
2. R in lead I + S in lead III ≥ 2.5 mV.
3. R amplitude in lead aVL ≥ 1.1 mV.
4. R in lead aVF > 2.0 mV.
5. Ventricular activation time ≥ 0.06 s.

The sensitivity of Sokolow-Lyon criteria is 22 percent with a specificity of 83 to 90 percent.[59]

ROMHILT-ESTES POINT SCORE SYSTEM

1. Amplitude of R or S in any limb lead ≥ 2.0 mV, S in lead V_1 or $V_2 \geq 3.0$ mV, R in lead V_5 or $V_6 \geq 3.0$ mV is equal to 3 points.
2. ST-T typical of left ventricular strain is equal to 1 point if the patient is on digitalis, 3 points if the patient is not on digitalis.
3. P terminal in lead $V_1 \geq 0.1$ mV in depth and ≥ 0.04 s in duration is equal to 3 points.
4. Left axis deviation ≥ -30 degrees is equal to 2 points.
5. QRS duration ≥ 0.09 s is equal to 1 point.
6. Intrinsicoid deflection in lead V_5 or $V_6 \geq 0.05$ s is equal to 1 point.

A total of 5 points indicates definitive LVH, and 4 points indicates probable LVH. The sensitivity of Romhilt-Estes criteria is 54 percent with a specificity of 97 percent.[60]

CORNELL VOLTAGE CRITERIA[56, 61]

S in lead V_3 + R in lead aVL > 2.8 mV for men and > 2.0 mV for women. The QRS voltages in women are smaller than in men, most likely related to smaller left ventricular mass and possibly to the presence of breast tissue. The Cornell criteria, which are based on logistic regression models, have a sensitivity of 62 percent, a specificity of 92 percent, a positive predictive value of 90 percent, and a negative predictive value of 70 percent. The sensitivity of abnormal P terminal in lead V_1 for LVH is 57 percent with a specificity of 87 percent.[58]

Electrocardiographic Diagnosis of Right Ventricular Hypertrophy
(see Figs. 2–3 and 2–4)

Because the normal right ventricular mass is only about one third of the left ventricular mass, the RV contributes very little to the QRS. Most of the right ventricular forces are canceled by the dominant LV. When the right ventricular mass is increased sufficiently, the ECG will show tall R waves in lead $V_1 \geq 0.5$ mV, R/S ratio in lead $V_1 \geq 1$, abnormal S wave in lead V_5 or $V_6 \geq 0.7$ mV, and the frontal plane QRS axis will shift to the right, usually beyond +110 degrees. In the typical case of right ventricular hypertrophy (RVH), there is right axis deviation, prominent R in leads V_1 and V_2, with ST depression, inverted T, and deep S in leads V_5 and V_6.[62, 63] Right atrial enlargement (P pulmonale) also may be noted. The electrocardiographic criteria for RVH have poor sensitivity and moderate specificity.[48, 58, 64]

Biventricular Hypertrophy (Fig. 2–6)

The diagnosis of biventricular hypertrophy by ECG is difficult. The following may suggest biventricular hypertrophy[48, 58, 65]:

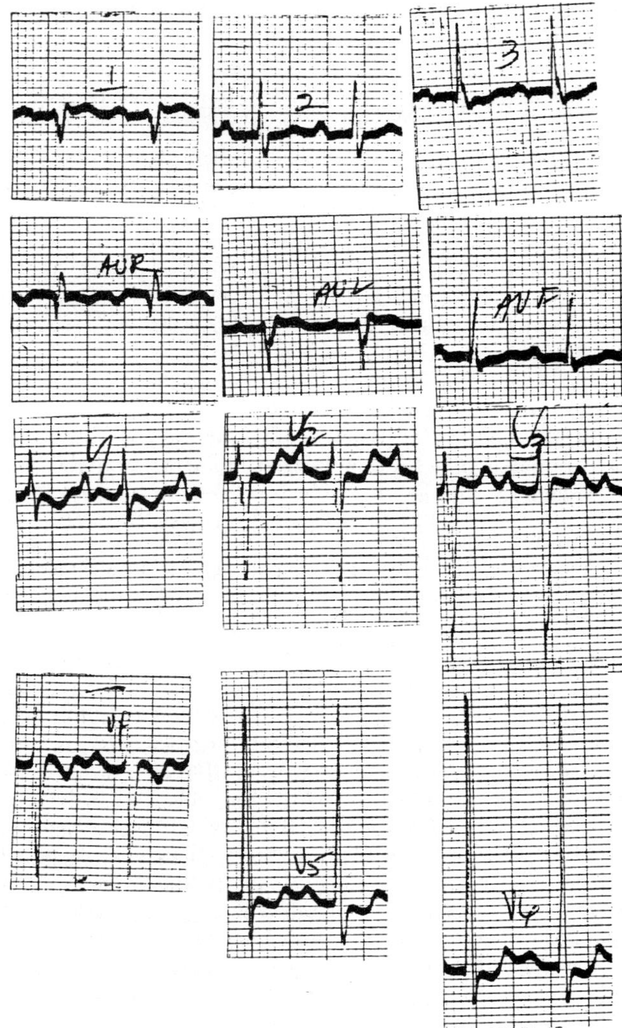

FIGURE 2–6 Biventricular hypertrophy. Note right axis deviation; tall R in V_1 with R/S ratio > 1.0; small R and deep S in V_2, V_3, V_4; and tall R in V_5, V_6.

1. Tall R and deep S in right and left precordial leads (Katz-Wachtel sign).[66]
2. Right axis deviation with LVH pattern in precordial leads.
3. Tall R in lead V_1 with small S < 1.0 mV or inverted T in V_1.
4. Transition zone shifted to the left in the presence of LVH.
5. Deep S in leads V_5 or V_6 > 0.7 mV with electrocardiographic criteria for LVH.

The sensitivity of these criteria is about 20 percent, and the specificity is 94 percent.[58]

Diagnosis of Left Ventricular Hypertrophy in the Presence of Conduction Defects

Numerous voltage criteria with various sensitivities and specificities have been used to diagnose LVH in the presence of left bundle branch block (LBBB).[67–69] There is significant correlation between the pre-LBBB and post-LBBB QRS voltages. The R voltages in leads I, V_5, and V_6 decrease, S voltage in leads V_1 and V_2 increases, and the QRS axis is shifted leftward after the development of LBBB in patients with intermittent LBBB.[70]

The following criteria have been used:

S in lead V_1 + R in lead V_5 or $V_6 \geq 3.5$ mV (sensitivity 74 percent).
S in lead V_2 + R in lead $V_6 \geq 4.5$ mV (sensitivity 86 percent, specificity 100 percent).
S in lead $V_3 \geq 2.5$ mV (sensitivity 56 percent, specificity 90 percent) and QRS axis < -40 degrees (sensitivity 30 percent, specificity 100 percent).[67–69]

The sensitivity of voltage criteria used to diagnose LVH in the presence of RBBB is low (sensitivity 2 to 68 percent, specificity 14 to 100 percent). S in lead III + (maximal precordial R + S) ≥ 3.0 mV has a sensitivity of 52 percent and a specificity of 84 percent.[71, 72] When P wave terminal in lead V_1 is added to the QRS voltage criteria, the sensitivity increases to about 70 percent with a specificity of about 80 percent.[73] The diagnosis of RVH in the presence of RBBB is considered when there is right axis deviation, R′ in lead V_1 > 1.5 mV, and prominent S wave in V_5 and/or V_6. This pattern is most commonly seen postoperatively in patients with congenital heart disease and RVH, such as tetralogy of Fallot or pulmonic stenosis.

Intraventricular Conduction Disturbances

Intraventricular conduction delay is diagnosed when there is a widening of the QRS complex greater than 110 ms. It can present itself as bundle branch blocks: LBBB when the abnormality involves the left bundle branch and, rarely, the AV node or bundle of His, where conduction tissue destined to become left bundle branch is affected[115]; RBBB when the right bundle branch is involved; nonspecific intraventricular conduction delay when the intramyocardial conduction is delayed; and preexcitation syndrome when the widening is secondary to the presence of delta waves. The fascicular blocks (hemiblocks) develop when the left anterior or the left posterior fasciculus is involved and may occur with wide QRS as well as with QRS with near-normal duration.

Left Bundle Branch Block

LBBB (Fig. 2–7) is in general due to damage of the left bundle branch at its origin, at the top of the interventricular septum, with disruption by fibrotic tissue or acute degeneration.

In LBBB, the activation starts in the RV and the left ventricular activation begins after near-completion of right ventricular activation by spread of excitation from the right to the left in the interventricular septum, with subsequent endocardial spread of activation in the LV through the distal branches of the left bundle branch. In LBBB, the normal septal Q wave in leads I, aVL, V_5, and V_6 is lost. The QRS duration is less than or equal to 120 ms. There is a broad-notched R wave in leads I, aVL, V_5, and V_6; the right-sided precordial leads V_1 and V_2 show small r and deep S with shift of transition zone to the left and an

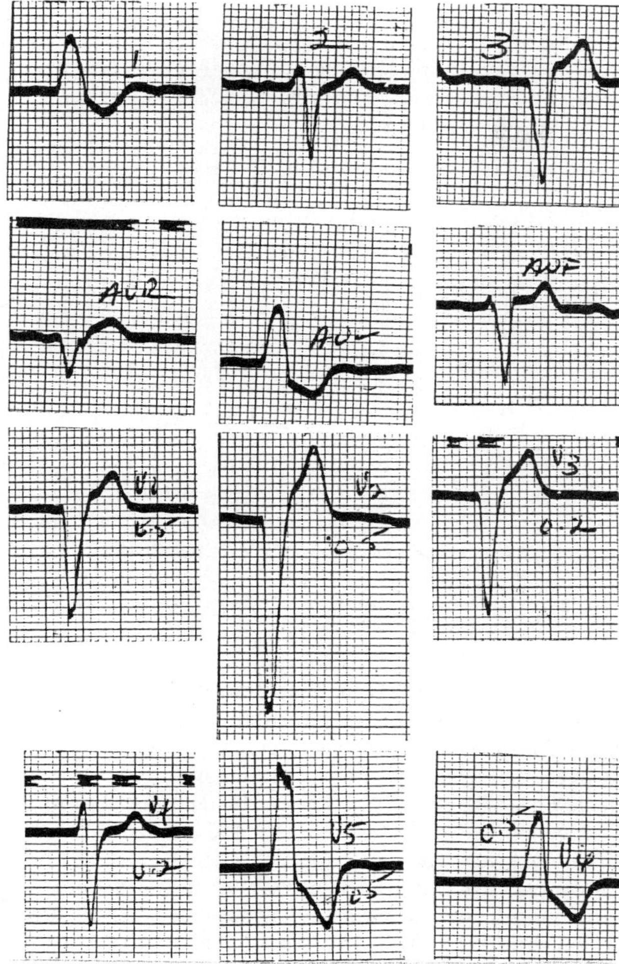

FIGURE 2–7 Left bundle branch block with left axis deviation and left ventricular hypertrophy. Atrial fibrillation. The patient had severe aortic stenosis.

increase of intrinsicoid deflection in leads V_5 and V_6 to 60 ms or longer. The ST-T is shifted in the opposite direction to the main deflection of QRS. ST-T is negative in leads I, aVL, V_5, and V_6 and is positive in leads V_1 and V_2 (secondary ST-T changes). The electrical axis in LBBB is normal or shifted leftward. Left axis deviation in the presence of LBBB is thought to be related to disease involving the left anterior fasciculus.[74, 75] However, in intermittent LBBB with left axis deviation, the majority of patients have normal axis during normally conducted beats.[76, 77]

LBBB and the Diagnosis of MI

The presence of Q in leads I, V_5, and V_6 is suggestive of MI with a sensitivity of 45 to 70 percent and a specificity over 80 percent. The presence of Q waves in inferior leads is highly suggestive of inferior MI; however, the sensitivity is less than 50 percent.[69, 78–80] Patients with idiopathic dilated cardiomyopathy with normal coronary arteries by angiography and no regional wall motion abnormalities by echocardiography whose ECGs show LBBB frequently have Q waves in leads I, aVL, and V_5 or V_6, suggesting anterolateral MI. Presence of Q in LBBB needs to be interpreted with caution because of false-positive findings. Criteria for the diagnosis of acute MI in the presence of LBBB include ST elevation $\geq$ 1 mm concordant with QRS polarity (5 points), ST depression $\geq$ 1 mm in leads V_1, V_2, or V_3 (3 points), and ST elevation $\geq$ 5 mm discordant with QRS polarity (2 points). A total score index of 3 or more points is associated with a specificity of 90 percent or greater.[81]

In LBBB, QRS and T are opposite in orientation (discordant). If they are concordant, then primary T wave abnormalities and ischemia should be considered (Fig. 2–8).[78]

Incomplete LBBB

In incomplete LBBB, the QRS morphology is similar to that of LBBB but the QRS duration is between 100 and 120 ms, the septal Q wave is absent, and there is notching or slurring of R with the delayed intrinsicoid deflection in leads V_5 and V_6.

In LBBB, the ventricular contraction is sequential, the left ventricular contraction follows the right ventricular contraction, and there is septal motion abnormality with its contraction being delayed.[82] In LBBB, the septal myocardial blood flow is decreased (septal perfusion abnormalities on thallium scan). This has been attributed to prolonged compression of septal arteries owing to asynchronous septal contraction.[83] LBBB is present in about 0.1 to 0.7 percent of the population.[84] LBBB can be congenital and may occur in the absence of cardiac disease when its course is benign. When acquired, its prognosis will depend on the underlying cardiac disease. In the Framingham study, over 50 percent of patients developing LBBB had coronary artery disease and/or heart failure.[85] Morbidity and mortality are higher in those patients with LBBB associated with left axis deviation, left atrial enlargement, and electrocardiographic abnormality before the development of LBBB.[86] LBBB in patients with coronary artery disease usually predicts more extensive disease and more severe left ventricular dysfunction.[87] In the Manitoba study,[88] 3983 pilots who served during World War II were followed for 29 years. Normal ECG was present in 54 percent before the development of LBBB. Fourteen percent showed LVH and 14 percent had ST-T abnormalities before the development of LBBB. None had heart disease at entry. Twenty-nine cases developed LBBB, and 17.2 percent of these died suddenly. Sudden death was ten times more frequent in subjects with LBBB than in those without. There was no difference in QRS duration or axis between sudden death and non–sudden death groups with LBBB. Also, there was no age difference. LBBB can be transient or persistent. It can alternate with RBBB, and it could be rate dependent. The clinical significance of rate-dependent LBBB is unclear.

Right Bundle Branch Block

RBBB (Fig. 2–9) is caused by disruption of conduction in the right bundle branch, which is a 4- to 5-cm-long and 1- to 2-mm-diameter structure that runs as a cable in the upper part of the septum on the right side until it reaches the base of the papillary muscle and then spreads as Pur-

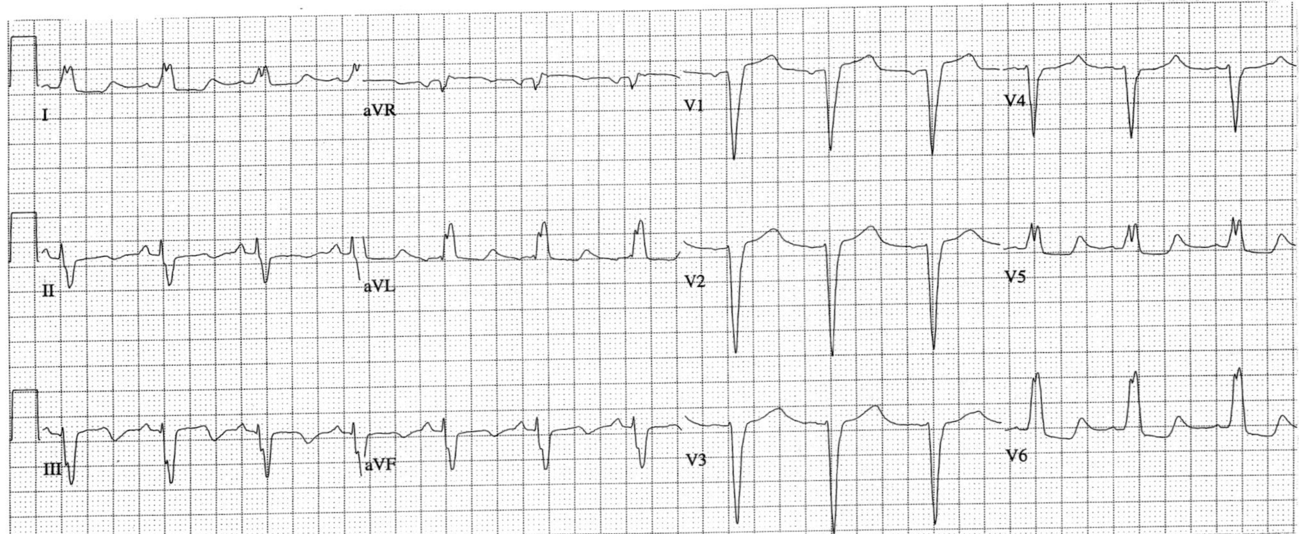

FIGURE 2–8 Left bundle branch block with primary T abnormality in a patient with ischemia (note T inversion in leads III and aVF and positive T in leads I, aVL, V_5, and V_6).

kinje network. In RBBB, the left side of septum and the LV are activated normally, and the right ventricular endocardial activation usually starts about 25 ms after the onset of QRS by slow spread of activation from left to right through the septum. The right ventricular activation continues after left ventricular activation is completed. In RBBB, the initial forces of ventricular depolarization are not altered. The terminal QRS forces are directed anteriorly and to the right. This will result in broad S waves in leads I, aVL, and V_6 and a large terminal R wave or R′ in V_1. The QRS duration is 120 ms or greater. The left precordial leads show wide S wave, wider than the preceding R wave. The right precordial leads V_1 and V_2 show delayed intrinsicoid deflection of greater than 50 ms with QRS morphology of rSR′ or rsR′. The ST-T orientation is opposite to the late R or wide S. The T is inverted in the right precordial leads and is upright in the left precordial leads. When primary T changes are present, such as in ischemia, the ST-T changes in leads V_1 and V_2 may be concordant, upright (Fig. 2–10).

The diagnosis of LVH in the presence of RBBB has low sensitivity but maintains high specificity. R′ amplitude in lead V_1 greater than 15 mm plus right axis deviation in the presence of RBBB has been interpreted as indicating RVH; however, the accuracy is low. The diagnosis of MI is not affected by RBBB except for posterolateral MI and for the presence of Q waves in leads V_1 and V_2 in acute right ventricular overload.

A special form of RBBB associated with persistent ST elevation in leads V_1 through V_3 in patients with no apparent structural heart disease, who have a propensity for life-threatening ventricular tachyarrhythmias, is known as *Brugada's syndrome* (Fig. 2–11).[89, 90] The unusual ST elevation has been described as coved, dome shaped, saddle-back, and triangular,[91, 92] and the R′ of QRS in leads V_1 through V_3 in many cases may actually represent a J wave. These changes are usually seen in the right precordial leads and appear to be related to the loss of action potential dome in right ventricular epicardium but not endocardium.[93] The electrical heterogeneity within the right ventricular epicar-

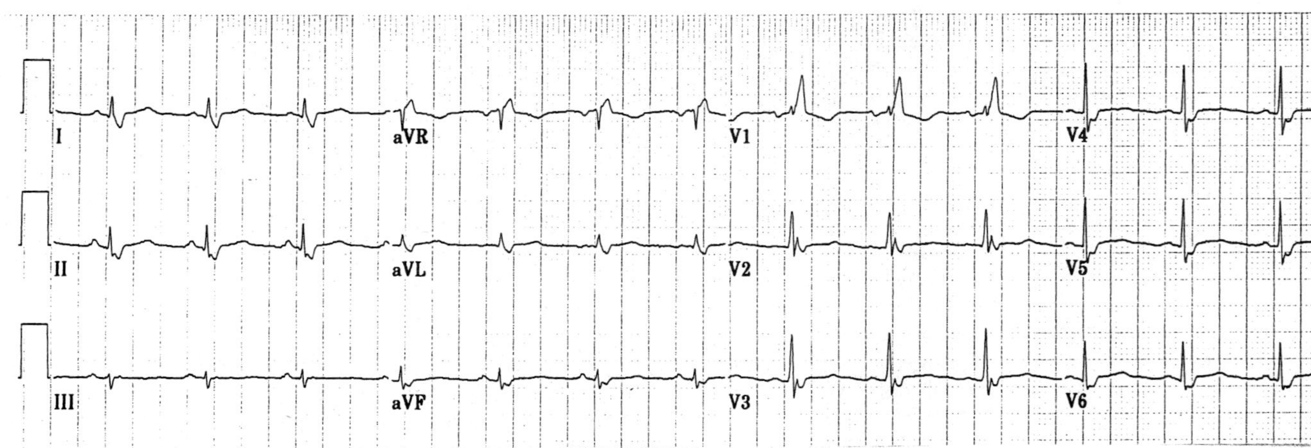

FIGURE 2–9 Right bundle branch block.

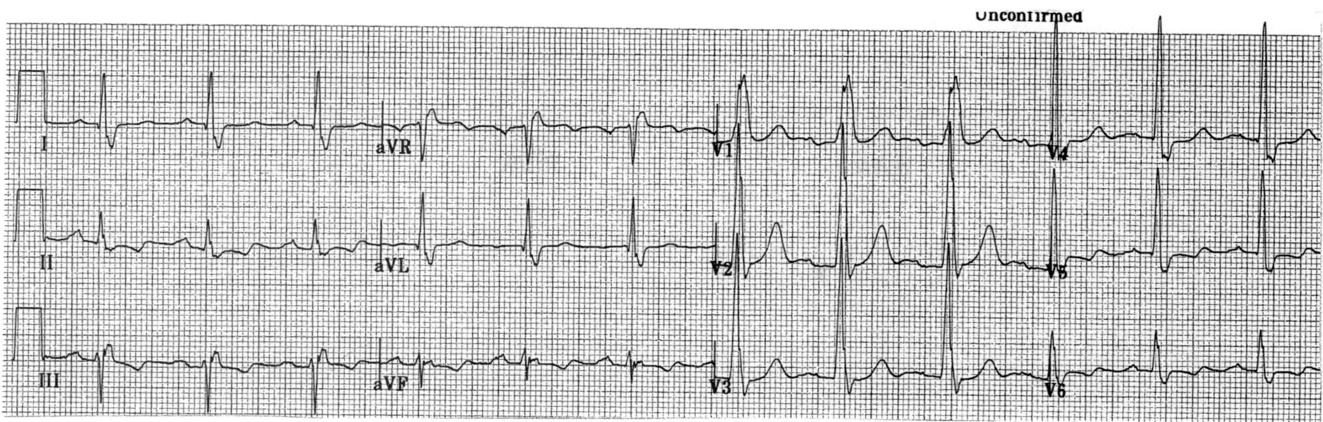

FIGURE 2–10 Right bundle branch block with primary T abnormality. Note positive T in leads V_1 to V_3 and inverted T in leads V_5 and V_6. ECG obtained from a patient with angina, severe coronary artery disease, and previous coronary artery bypass graft.

dium is thought to be responsible for ventricular tachyarrhythmias (VT/VF).[94–96] Recent data indicate that the Brugada syndrome is a primary electrical disease related to an ion channel gene mutation (*SCN5A*).[97] Another unusual form of RBBB in which there are two or more notches involving the R or R′ in lead V_1 or V_2 is seen in Ebstein's anomaly of the tricuspid valve, in arrhythmogenic right ventricular dysplasia, and after right ventriculotomy.

Incomplete Right Bundle Branch Block

Incomplete right bundle branch block (IRBBB) is similar to RBBB except the QRS duration is less than 120 ms. The QRS in lead V_1 may have an rSR′, rsR′, or rSr′ pattern. The etiology of IRBBB may be congenital, familial, or acquired. In 76 percent of 33 patients with IRBBB, pathologic studies revealed normal right bundle branch.[98] In the large majority of normal young persons, IRBBB is a variant of normal and does not represent conduction system disease. In these subjects, focal hypertrophy of the RV involving the basal and the pulmonary conus regions as a congenital developmental variant appears to be the cause of IRBBB.[98, 99] Thus, IRBBB represents a developmental variation in the thickness of the right ventricular free wall; it appears to have a genetic basis rather than being related to conduction system abnormality. Other causes of IRBBB are congenital or acquired heart disease with right ventricular dilatation or hypertrophy (atrial septal defect, pulmonic stenosis); injuries to the right bundle branch; and after open heart surgery, cardiac catheterization, coronary artery disease, and degenerative fibrotic processes involving the peripheral right bundle branch. In ostium secundum–type atrial septal defect, the IRBBB is associated with right axis deviation, whereas in ostium primum–type atrial septal defect and AV canal, the IRBBB is associated with left axis deviation. Epidemiologic studies in middle-aged men have demonstrated a progression of IRBBB to complete RBBB, suggesting abnormality in conduction as a cause of IRBBB. In a study of 1960 white males between the ages of 40 and 56 years, followed for 11 years, the incidence of IRBBB at entry was 6.8 percent. During follow-up, 222 men developed IRBBB (13.6 percent).[100] Left axis deviation greater than −30 degrees was present in 8.2 percent of subjects with IRBBB and in 2.4 percent of those without IRBBB at entry. Men developing IRBBB had a higher risk of development of left axis deviation, and this was not related to age or body weight. At baseline, 5.1 percent of men with IRBBB and only 0.7 percent of those without IRBBB developed complete RBBB during 11 years of follow-up. Over 20 years, subjects with IRBBB did not have increased mortality from coronary disease or cardiovascular disease, compared with controls without IRBBB.

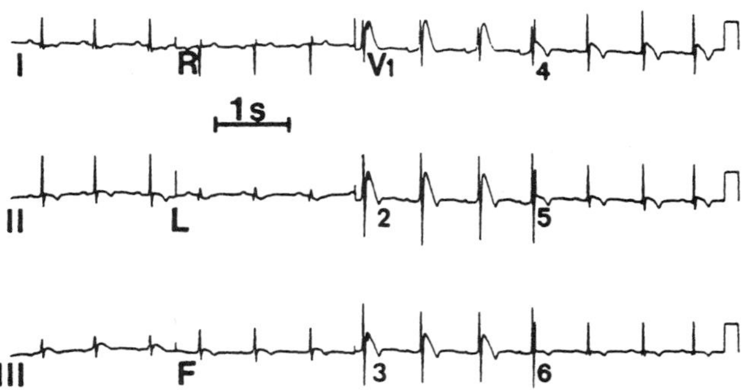

FIGURE 2–11 Patient with atypical right bundle branch block and ST elevation in leads V_1 to V_4. (From Brugada P, Brugada J: Right bundle branch block, persistent ST segment elevation and sudden cardiac death: a distinct clinical and electrocardiographic syndrome. A multicenter report. Reprinted with permission from the American College of Cardiology [J Am Coll Cardiol, 1992, Vol. 20, p. 1391].)

Prognostic Significance of RBBB and LBBB

The prognosis in both RBBB and LBBB in the absence of underlying cardiac disease is benign. There is no difference in prognosis between RBBB and LBBB in the absence of underlying heart disease.[101] The U.S. Air Force personnel studies on 237,000 subjects showed that RBBB was seen mostly in younger people below the age of 40 years, and it was eight times more frequent than LBBB. It was unusual to find a person below the age of 30 years with LBBB.[101] In another study involving 5204 subjects, average age 49.8 years, followed for 14 years, 123 had intraventricular conduction defect of RBBB, LBBB, left anterior hemiblock, and bifascicular block (RBBB + left anterior hemiblock).[102] Nineteen died. The incidence of RBBB in the young (18 to 32 years) was 0.15 to 0.29 percent, whereas in the older group, it was 2.4 percent. LBBB was 0.02 to 0.05 percent in the young and 1 to 1.2 percent in the old; and left anterior hemiblock was 0.2 to 1.2 percent in the young and 4.1 to 5.3 percent in the old. In other studies, RBBB was found in 0.2 percent of subjects in which 50 percent were under 20 years of age.[103] LBBB was extremely rare among young and healthy subjects. In another study involving 110,000 subjects screened, the incidence of RBBB was 0.18 percent and that of LBBB was 0.1 percent.[104] The incidence of RBBB is five to thirteen times more frequent than LBBB, depending on the population studied. Ischemic heart disease and hypertension are the most common causes of acquired RBBB.[104] Other etiologies include rheumatic heart disease, degenerative disease of the conduction system,[105, 106] myocarditis, congenital heart disease, and congenital bundle branch block. RBBB when congenital has an autosomal dominant trait with variable expression and penetration.[107, 108] Rate-dependent bundle branch block may be caused by tachycardia or bradycardia. RBBB is more frequently associated with tachycardia than is LBBB because of its longer refractory period as compared with the left bundle. With increasing rate, the bundle branch with the longest refractory period will fail to shorten the refractory period and will not conduct.[109, 110] Bradycardia-dependent bundle branch block results from either abnormal phase 4 spontaneous depolarization in the bundle branch or time-dependent reduction of responsiveness independent of resting membrane potential of the bundle.

Fascicular Blocks

Fascicular blocks (Figs. 2–12 and 2–13) develop when the conduction in the fascicles of the left bundle branch (anterior, septal, or middle, and posterior) is blocked. The anterior fascicle excites the anterior paraseptal ventricular wall, the posterior fascicle excites the posterior paraseptal area, and the septal fascicle excites the central area of the left side of the septum. In left anterior fascicular block, there is delay of activation of the superior anterior left ventricular free wall, which is activated by impulses spreading from the inferior wall. This results in mild prolongation of the QRS complex and shift of the frontal plane axis to the left between −45 and −90 degrees. There is a small r deep S in leads II, III, and aVF; small q large R pattern in lead aVL; and the intrinsicoid deflection in lead aVL is 45 ms or greater. The R/S ratio in lead II is less than 1. The QRS duration is 120 ms or less.[111] The peak of R wave in lead III precedes the peak of R in lead II and that in lead aVL precedes the R peak in lead aVR.[112, 113] When the left axis deviation is between −30 and −45 degrees, a diagnosis of possible left anterior fascicular block is made. Patients with no Q in leads aVL before the development of left anterior fascicular block will not develop it afterward. Thus, the presence of Q in lead aVL is not an absolute requirement for the diagnosis of left anterior fascicular block. In left posterior fascicular block, the frontal plane QRS axis is shifted to the right, +90 to ±180 degrees, there is a small r deep S pattern in leads I and aVL, small q and large R pattern in leads III and aVF, and the QRS duration is 120 ms or less.[111] This pattern can also be seen in RVH, COPD, and lateral MI. The diagnosis of left posterior fascicular block should be considered only in the absence of other conditions that can cause the same pattern. Although the incidence of left axis deviation greater than −30 degrees in the general population is 1.1 percent (2.4 percent over age 45 years), the incidence of left posterior fascicular block is 0.1 percent.[103, 114] The prognosis in fascicular block will depend on the underlying cardiac conditions. Isolated left anterior fascicular block in the absence of heart disease will not cause increased cardiac morbidity or mortality.[115a]

Septal fascicular block is suspected when there is prominent R in leads V_1 and V_2 with no axis shift in limb

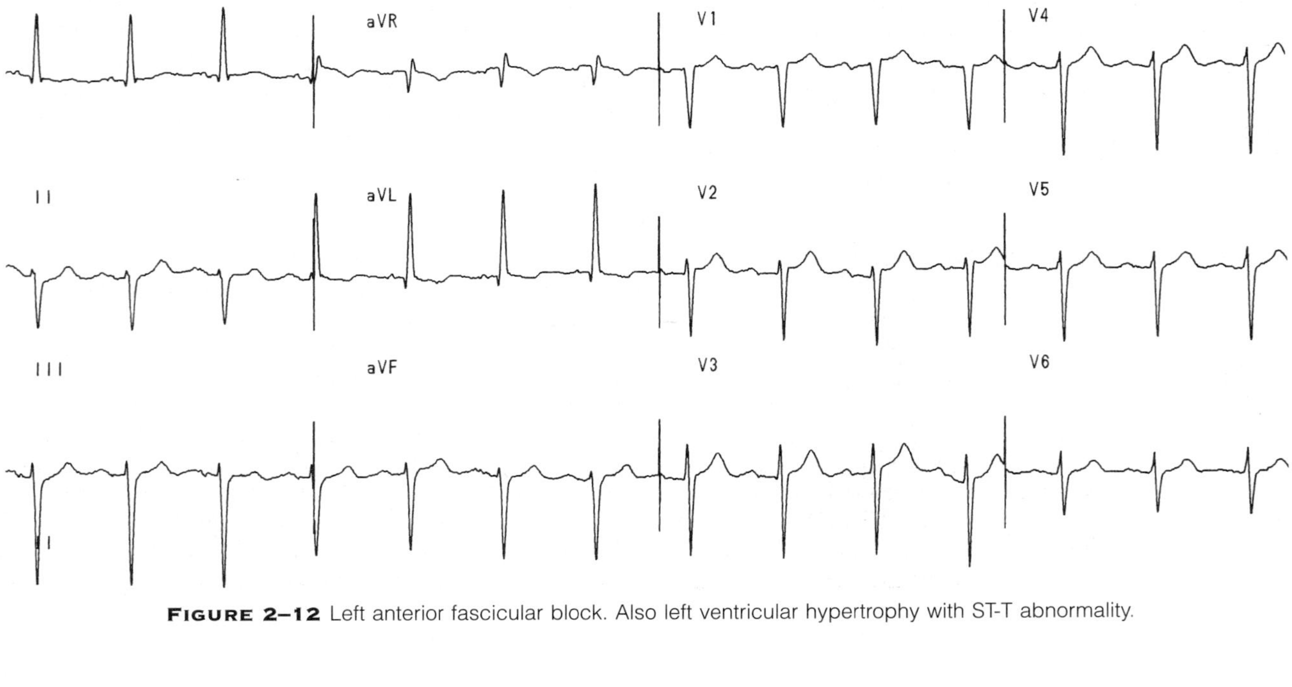

FIGURE 2–12 Left anterior fascicular block. Also left ventricular hypertrophy with ST-T abnormality.

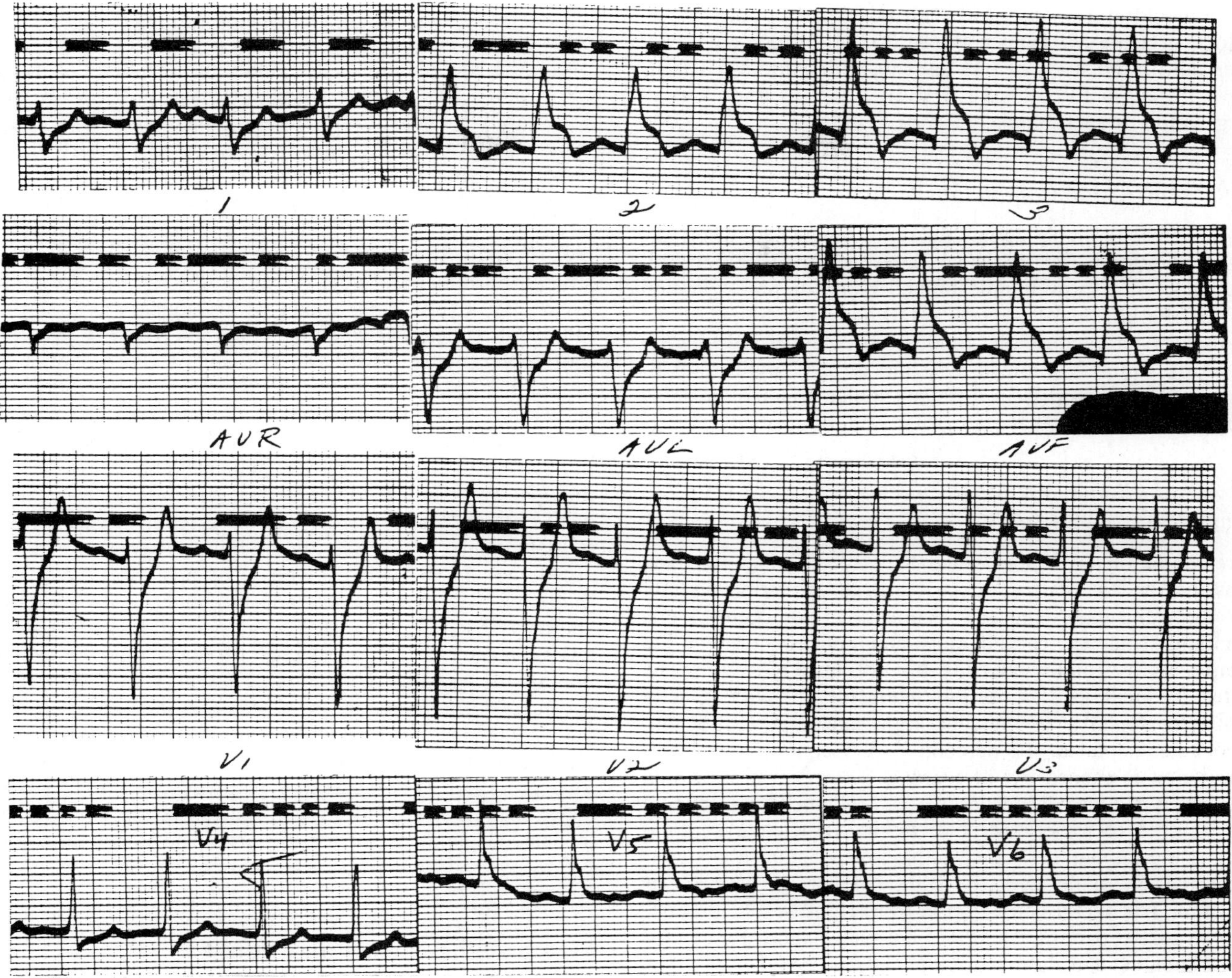

FIGURE 2–13 Left posterior fascicular block (it was transient). Acute inferior myocardial infarction (MI).

leads. The same QRS patterns can be seen in RVH or posterolateral MI or as a normal variant.

The left anterior fascicle is more susceptible to injury and consequently is more frequently involved than is the left posterior fascicle, which is less susceptible to injury. When left posterior fascicular block is associated with cardiac disease, usually the disease is more extensive than that seen with left anterior fascicular block.[111, 117]

Bifascicular Block

Bifascicular block is present when there is RBBB and block involving the anterior or the posterior fascicle of the left bundle branch. RBBB plus the left anterior fascicular block is the most common form, whereas RBBB plus left posterior fascicular block is less common.

Trifascicular block is suspected when there is bifascicular block or LBBB plus first-degree AV block. Trifascicular block is present only when the bifascicular block is associated with HV interval prolongation.[117] Up to 50 percent of subjects with bifascicular block and prolonged PR have prolongation of AH interval, giving rise to PR prolongation.[118] The prognosis in bifascicular and trifascicular blocks depends on the underlying heart disease. In patients with organic heart disease, the 5-year mortality is 35 percent, the most common cause of death being congestive heart failure.[119, 120] In patients without organic heart disease, the prognosis is better. Five-year mortality is 11 percent and development of complete heart block (CHB) is 1 percent.[120] In bifascicular block, even when HV is prolonged to above 75 ms, the development of complete heart block over 42 months of follow-up was low, 4.9 percent.[119]

The development of bundle branch block in MI is associated with lower left ventricular ejection fraction, higher creatine kinase, and more diseased vessels.[121] In one study involving patients with bundle branch block and acute MI, the mortality was 8.7 percent; in patients without bundle branch block, it was 3.7 percent. The bundle branch block was transient in 18.4 percent and persistent in 5.3 percent. The mortality in patients with persistent bundle branch block was 19.4 percent; with transient bundle branch block, it was 5.6 percent; and it was 3.7 percent when no bundle branch block was present. Thrombolytic therapy reduces the incidence of persistent bundle branch block and the overall mortality associated with persistent bundle branch block in acute MI from between 36 and 58 percent to 8.7 percent. In the study of 681 patients with acute MI, RBBB was present in 13 percent, LBBB in 7 percent, and alternating bundle branch block in 3.5 percent.[121]

Intraventricular Conduction Delay

Intraventricular conduction delay is diagnosed when the QRS duration is greater than 110 ms and the QRS morphology does not show bundle branch block or pre-excitation (Wolff-Parkinson-White [WPW] syndrome). Some of the causes of intraventricular conduction delay include hyperkalemia, antiarrhythmic drugs, and diffuse myocardial fibrosis. The prognosis in intraventricular conduction delay depends on the underlying cardiac abnormality.

Pre-excitation WPW Syndrome
(Figs. 2–14 and 2–15)[122]

Pre-excitation is present when accessory connections bypassing the AV node conduct the atrial excitation directly to the ventricles. The AV connections, or Kent fibers, contain usual myocardial cells and connect atria to the ventricles by running outside the AV fibrous ring.[123] The most frequent location is left lateral at 46 percent, with posterior septal at 26 percent, right lateral at 18 percent, and anteroseptal at 10 percent.[124] A second type of pre-excitation is caused by intracardiac connections, of which several types have been described. Mahaim fibers connect the middle or lower AV node to the ventricular septum, bypassing the bundle branches. Nodoventricular fibers connect the AV node with the right side of the ventricular septum. The septal activation is from right to left, producing an LBBB pattern. The PR is normal or short. Fasciculoventricular (ventriculoventricular) fibers connect the His bundle to either side of the ventricular septum. The QRS morphology varies according to which side of the septum it is connected to. The PR is normal. AV tracts connect the atria to the bundle of His or the bundle branches after bypassing the AV node. The QRS is not altered, but the PR is short. The AH interval is short and does not increase with rapid pacing. James fibers connect the atria to the lower third of the AV node or the proximal part of the bundle of His.

In pre-excitation, the ventricles are activated through both the bypass tract and the normal conduction through the AV node. The ventricular activation through the bypass structure occurs before the activation through the AV node, giving rise to the delta wave, which appears as a slurred initial QRS. The PR is short, less than 120 ms, whereas the QRS is wide. The ST-T segment is discordant, with inverted T in leads with tall R waves. The more the activation is conducted through the anomalous pathway, the shorter the PR interval, the wider the QRS, and the more abnormal the ST-T wave will be. The orientation of the delta wave and the QRS pattern depend on the location of the bypass tract.[125–127] In 5 to 15 percent of cases, there is more than one bypass tract. Multiple bypass tracts are noted, mostly in patients who have posterior septal and right free-wall bypass tracts and in patients with Ebstein's anomaly.[128] If not recognized, negative delta waves may be mistaken for MI. The prevalence of ventricular pre-excitation in the general population is about 1 to 3 per 1000 subjects.[129] The incidence is the same in the young and the old, suggesting a congenital basis. In Ebstein's anomaly, the bypass tract is always on the side of the anomalous tricuspid valve. The accessory pathway can conduct both antegrade and retrograde. When it conducts only retrograde (concealed conduction), it can participate in reciprocating AV tachycardia without pre-excitation of ventricles being present.

Myocardial Ischemia and Injury

Myocardial ischemia is diagnosed by electrocardiography when there is ST segment depression associated with de-

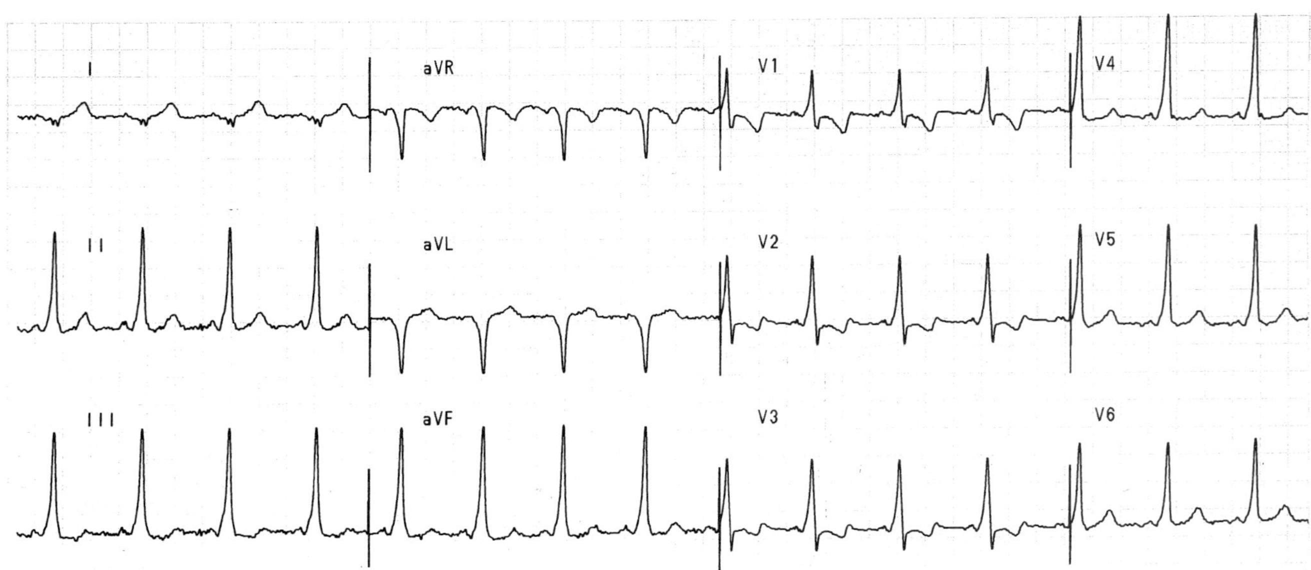

FIGURE 2–14 ECG from a patient with Wolff-Parkinson-White syndrome. Note negative delta waves in leads I and aVL consistent with left lateral anomalous connection.

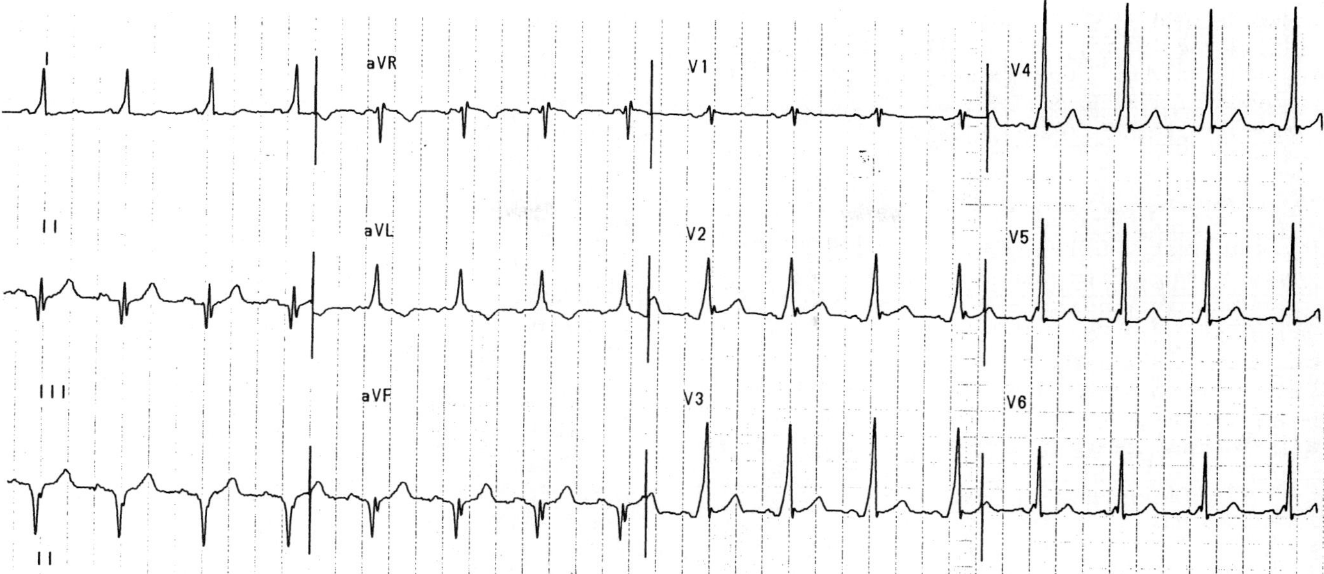

FIGURE 2–15 Pre-excitation (Wolff-Parkinson-White syndrome) with posteroseptal anomalous connection mimicking old inferior MI.

creased myocardial perfusion (ischemia) involving primarily the subendocardial layers of the myocardium. *Myocardial injury* is diagnosed when there is ST segment elevation seen with transmural ischemia, and it is usually seen with total occlusion of a coronary artery due to either a clot or a spasm. ST segment shifts in ischemia and injury are related to the cellular changes in the myocardium caused by ischemia. Ischemia results in injury currents between the ischemic and the normal myocardium. Ischemia will cause extracellular acidosis and a rise in extracellular potassium concentration, as well as increased lactate, fatty acids, and phosphate and an intracellular decrease of high-energy phosphates.[130–133] These will result in the rise of resting membrane potentials to −60 to −65 mV, reduced action potential amplitude and rate of rise of phase 0, and shortened action potential duration.[130, 134, 135] These changes in the ischemic area will produce potential gradients between the ischemic and the normal cells, giving rise to injury currents. During diastole (phase 4 of action potential), the injury current will flow from ischemic to normal cells (from the subendocardium toward the epicardium). This is called *diastolic injury current* and will cause a positive potential, resulting in elevation of the diastolic segment from end of T to the beginning of QRS when recorded by an epicardial electrode or a body surface electrode facing an ischemic area. During electrical systole, from the beginning of QRS to the end of T, the injury current flow will be from the normal to the ischemic area, resulting in ST depression. The diastolic injury current is abolished when the cell is activated and restarts after the recovery is complete at the end of T wave. The intracellular potential of ischemic cells during phases 2 and 3 of the action potential is more negative than that of normal cells, which results in the injury current flow from normal to ischemic area, opposite in direction to the diastolic injury current flow. This will result in ST depression. Capacitor-coupled electrocardiographic amplifiers that measure the amplitudes from the baseline level, which is the level of the TP segment, will record a depressed ST segment, which would be a summation of diastolic segment elevation plus the systolic ST segment depression. An ischemic ST depression is present when the ST is flat or downsloping and the depression is 1 mm or more, 80 ms after the J point (Figs. 2–16 and 2–17).

Electrocardiographic diagnosis of myocardial injury resulting from transmural ischemia related to cessation of flow in a coronary artery is based on ST elevation. ST elevation results from injury currents, diastolic and systolic, similar to those in myocardial ischemia. The ischemic cells are hypopolarized, the action potential duration is shortened, there is reduced upstroke velocity and reduced amplitude, and the cells in the center of ischemia may be inexcitable when the resting membrane potential increases to −65 mV or less. The diastolic injury current is directed from the injured to the normal tissue, whereas the systolic injury current, which results from shortened action potential duration of injured tissue, is directed from normal to injured tissue. Injury currents develop at the border between the injured and the normal cells. Diastolic current flow is from the injured tissue toward the normal tissue. An epicardial or body surface electrode facing the injured (infarcted) area will register a depressed diastolic segment. During electrical systole, the injury current will be directed from the normal to the injured tissue, resulting in ST elevation by an electrode facing the injured area. A capacitor-coupled electrocardiographic amplifier will record the summation of diastolic ST segment depression and systolic ST segment elevation as an augmented ST elevation. The shape and size of the boundary between the ischemic and the normal areas are the major determinant of ST segment elevation in transmural myocardial ischemia. The magnitude of the ST elevations may vary from 1 to 10 mm, and the ST configuration may be concave, convex, or flat (Fig. 2–18). The ST elevation can disappear rapidly after restoration of coronary flow in patients with coronary vasospasm or during coronary angioplasty when ischemia is caused

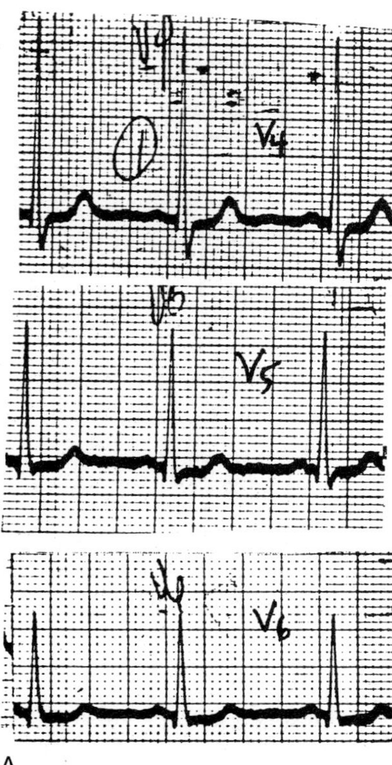

A

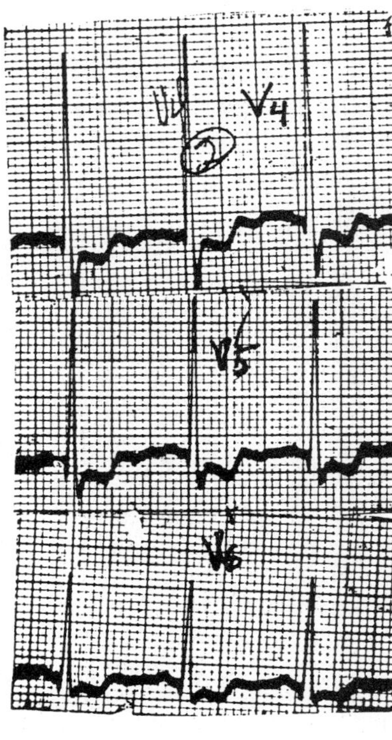

B

FIGURE 2–16 Ischemia. **A,** When the patient was asymptomatic. **B,** During angina precipitated by smoking cigarettes.

by balloon occlusion of a coronary artery.[136] ST elevation associated with coronary thrombosis resolves gradually after flow is restored by angioplasty or spontaneously.

The T wave inversions noted in ischemia are secondary to marked delay of recovery of injured cells as compared with normal cells. T inversions are not specific for ischemia.[137, 138]

Acute MI

The initial electrocardiographic findings in acute MI may be quite variable.[139, 140] Typically, the earliest changes, which may be transient, consist of large, peaked T waves (hyperacute T waves)[141] followed by symmetrically inverted T waves (coronary T waves), which are followed by ST segment elevation in leads facing the area of injury and ST segment depression in leads opposite to the area of injury (reciprocal ST depression).

ST elevation in the ECG is the usual initial manifestation of acute MI. Shortly thereafter, a Q wave will usually also develop. If there is no revascularization, with time, the ST segment elevation will gradually come down toward the baseline and the upright T wave becomes inverted, with the deepest T inversion being noticed at the time when the ST segment reaches the baseline. This will be achieved in about 2 weeks. T inversion is most likely related to increased duration of repolarization and its heterogeneity. The inverted T gradually becomes less inverted and finally may become upright. Lack of evolution of ST-T changes and maintenance of elevated ST segment after acute MI usually denote development of ventricular aneurysm or dyskinetic areas.[143–145] Secondary increases in the ST segment elevation while ST segment was decreasing indicate either development of pericarditis, expansion of acute MI, or development of new ischemia and extension of infarction. Revascularization of the culprit coronary artery can improve or abolish the ST segment elevation.[140] The majority of patients with ST segment elevation develop abnormal Q waves (Q wave infarct). Some patients with acute MI may have only ST segment depression or T inversion as the sole electrocardiographic manifestation of MI.[146, 147] These patients usually do not develop Q waves (non–Q wave MI), and their infarct size is generally smaller. They may have more collateral circulation, and the clinical course is more benign; however, the rate of recurrence of MI is higher.

About 20% of patients with symptoms suggesting MI but initially normal 12-lead ECGs will have confirmed MI.[139, 140] This is usually seen in patients with left circumflex occlusion. Additional electrocardiographic leads such as V_7, V_8, and V_9 may be helpful in these patients.[148] Thus, a normal 12-lead ECG cannot exclude acute MI.

ST segment elevation will help in localization of MI. When the ST segment elevation involves the anterior precordial leads, the acute MI is anterior,[149, 150] is related to left anterior descending coronary artery (LAD) occlusion, and involves the apical third of the septum and anterior wall (Fig. 2–19). When there is associated ST depression in inferior leads, the LAD occlusion is usually proximal.[151] Also, when the ST segment elevations involve leads I and aVL in addition to precordial V leads, usually there is proximal LAD occlusion. When ST segment elevation is present in leads II, III, and aVF, there is acute myocardial injury involving the middle and basal regions of the inferior LV, and it is usually associated with occlusion of the

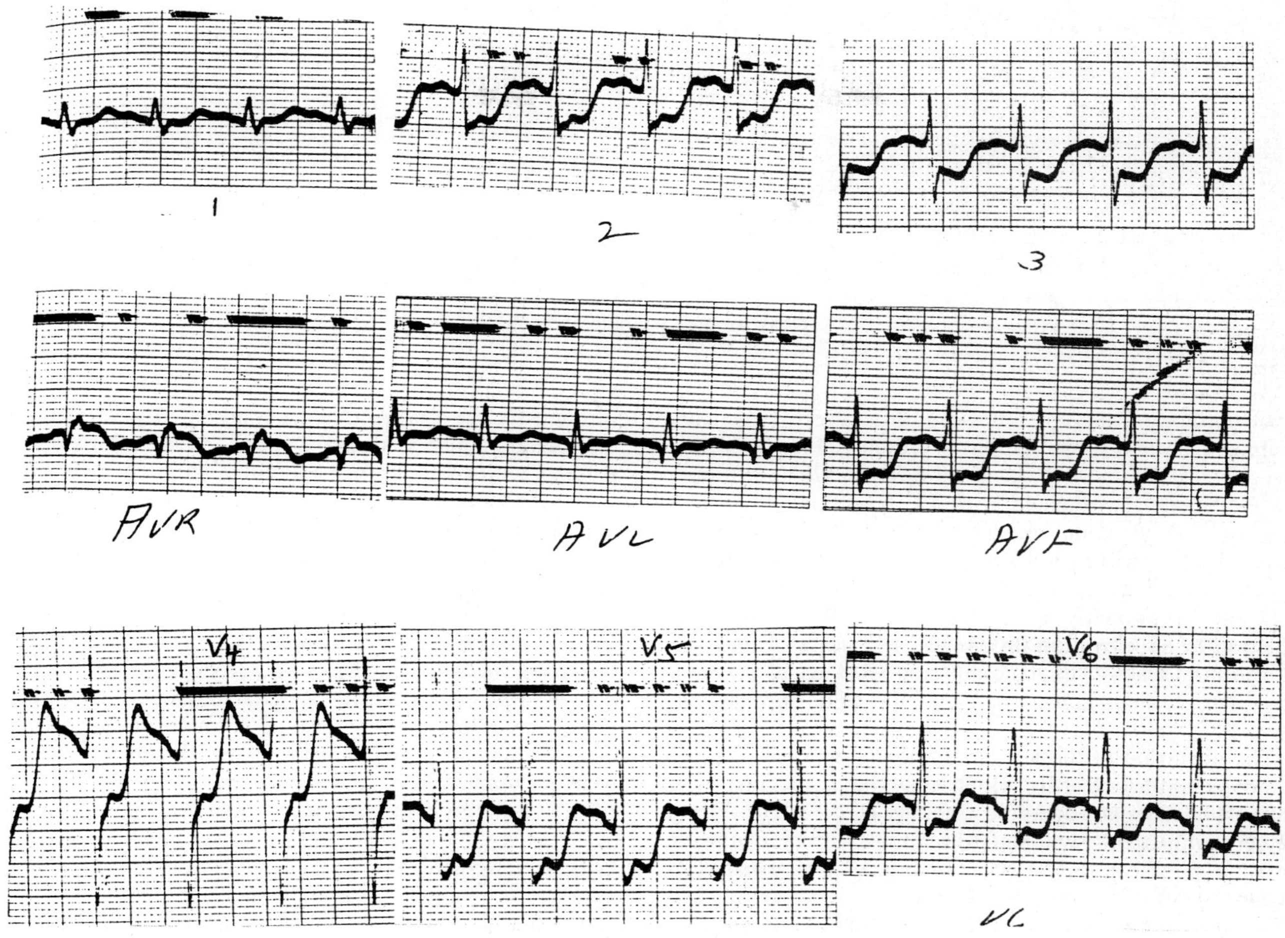

FIGURE 2–17 Ischemia.

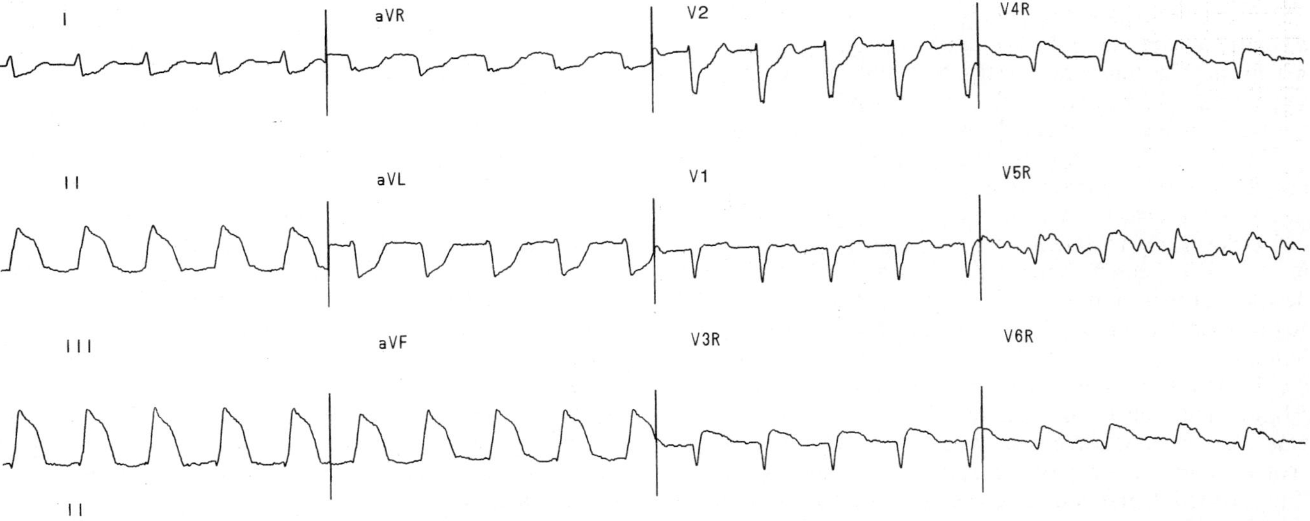

FIGURE 2–18 Acute inferior MI associated with right ventricular infarction. Note also ST elevation in leads V_3R to V_6R.

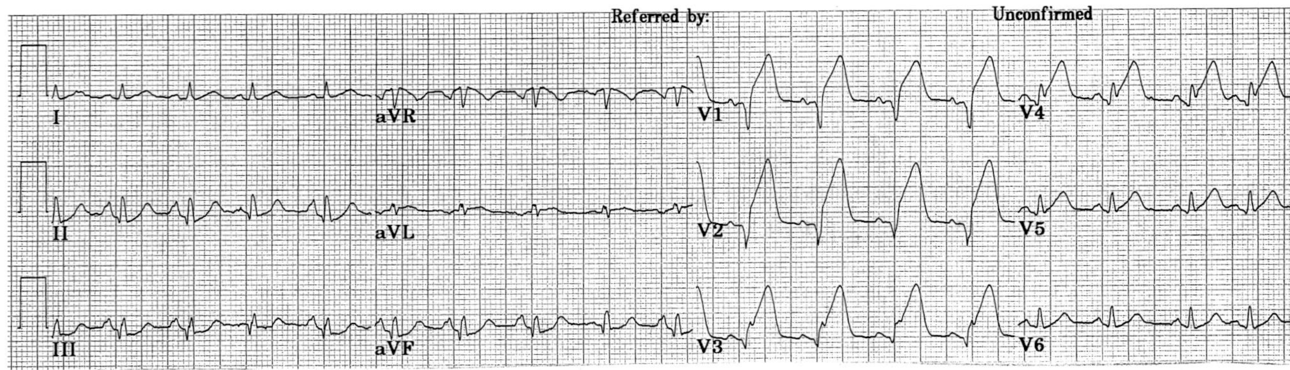

FIGURE 2–19 Acute anterior MI.

right coronary artery or left circumflex artery (when left dominant coronary circulation is present) (Fig. 2–20; see also Fig. 2–18).[149, 152, 153] In acute inferior MI, the inferior ST elevation is associated with ST depression in leads I and aVL. A proximal right coronary artery occlusion is present when there is additional RV infarction. RV infarction is associated with ST elevation in leads V_3R and V_4R and occasionally ST elevation in leads V_1 and V_2 in addition to ST elevation in leads II, III, and aVF.[154–157] ST elevation in lead V_1 in acute anterior MI is usually associated with a small conal branch of the right coronary artery.[158]

The occlusion of the left circumflex artery will result in acute posterolateral MI, which may be associated with variable electrocardiographic findings (Fig. 2–21). Thirty percent of patients with left circumflex artery occlusion have no significant ST segment change.[159] The usual electrocardiographic findings in acute posterolateral MI include ST segment elevation in leads II, III, aVF, V_5, and V_6; elevations in leads V_5 and V_6 as well as V_7, V_8, and V_9; or elevation only in leads V_5 and V_6 sometimes with ST depression in V_1 through V_4.[160–162] ST elevation in leads V_5 through V_6 associated with prominent U in leads V_1 through V_3 has a predictive accuracy of 87 percent for left circumflex artery occlusion.[149, 160] Ten to 20 percent of patients with acute inferior MI with additional ST elevation in leads V_5 and V_6 or ST depression in lead V_2 have isolated circumflex lesions.[152, 153] Acute right ventricular infarction is diagnosed by the presence of ST segment elevation in the right-side leads, V_3R through V_6R, with V_4R being the most valuable lead. ST elevation in lead V_4R predicts 85 percent of proximal right coronary artery occlusion in acute inferior MI. Reciprocal ST segment depressions in acute MIs associated with ST elevations usually predict more extensive coronary artery disease, larger infarct size, and higher mortality and incidence of heart failure.[163, 203]

Old or Chronic MI

Abnormal Q wave is the hallmark of old MI. Two mechanisms have been proposed for the development of abnormal Q wave. Window hypothesis assumes the infarct in the ventricular wall to be inert electrically, and the electrode facing the infarcted area will record negative potentials

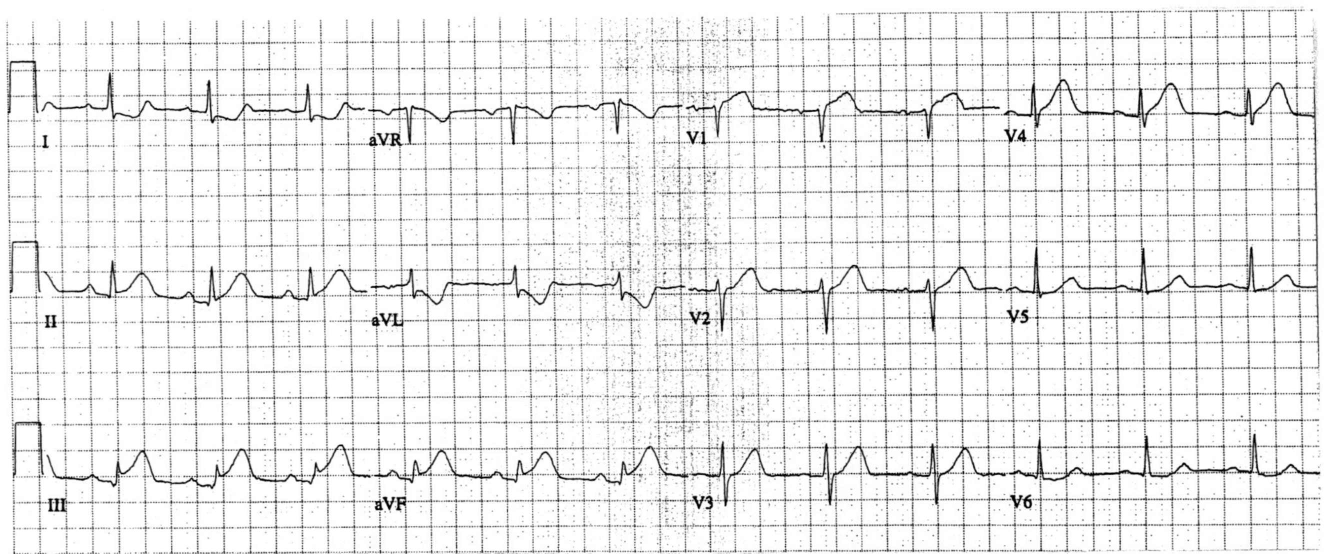

FIGURE 2–20 Acute inferior MI associated with right ventricular infarction (note ST elevation in V_1).

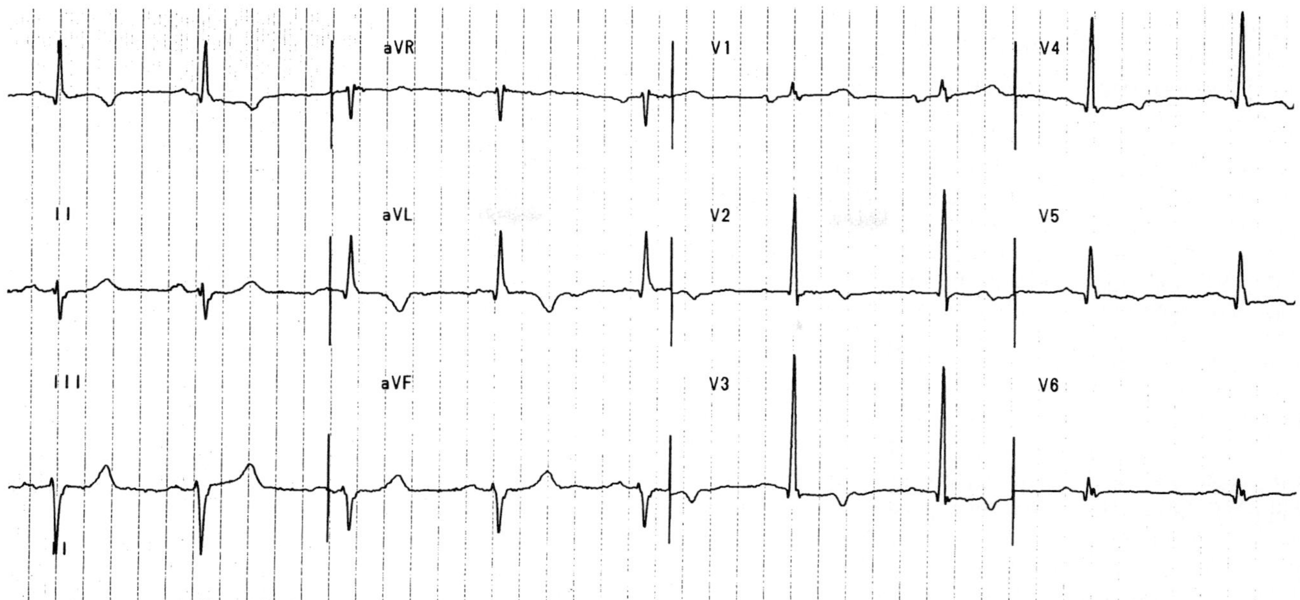

FIGURE 2–21 Posterolateral MI. Note prominent Q in leads I, aVL, V_6, and prominent R in leads V_1 to V_4 associated with T inversions in leads I, aVL, and V_2 to V_5.

generated in the remote areas of the heart during the initial part or during the entire QRS duration. The electrical silence during the inscription of the Q wave may be due to necrosis or severe ischemic injury of the infarct area without necrosis being present.[163] The other explanation is that the epicardial activation is markedly delayed because of the necrosis and the scar tissue that delay and alter the excitation pathway from the endocardium to the epicardium. During this period, the ventricular wall is electrically silent and the Q wave is produced. QS complexes are recorded if the electrical silence occurs throughout the QRS duration and small q large R or large Q small r complexes are recorded, depending on the magnitude of the delay in activation. For an abnormal Q wave to develop, the infarct size must be at least 3 to 4 cm in diameter and 5 to 7 mm thick and involve 50 percent or more of the left ventricular wall thickness and 10 percent of the left ventricular muscle mass.[164] Thus, an abnormal Q wave and old MI by ECG indicate large infarct size and extensive fibrotic involvement of infarcted area. Abnormal Q waves can develop in about 90 percent of anatomic transmural and 17 percent of anatomic subendocardial MIs.[165, 166] The infarcts should be classified as Q wave infarction or non–Q wave infarction. Presence or absence of Q wave cannot determine whether an infarction is transmural or subendocardial. The abnormal Q wave usually develops within 2 hours after the beginning of acute MI, and it reaches its maximal magnitude within 24 hours.[167–169] About 25 percent of abnormal Q waves revert to normal within 3 months and then nearly half within two decades.[170–174] The normalization of abnormal Q may be related to shrinking and reduction of volume of the infarcted tissue, recovery of electrically inert but viable tissue after reperfusion, and development of a new infarct opposite to the first one, canceling its manifestations. Transient Q waves may be seen in transient ischemia.[172, 173, 175–177] Hibernating or stunned myocardium may be electrically inert and produce abnormal Q waves, which may normalize after reperfusion is established.[172, 173, 175–178] Although the R wave amplitude may initially increase in acute MI, subsequently it will decrease secondary to loss of viable myocardium.[179, 180] Because of altered intramyocardial activation and conduction, slurred R or S waves may develop.[181, 182]

Diagnostic Criteria for MI

Abnormal Q waves exceeding 30 or 40 ms in duration are the hallmark of old MI. Their depth also is important, and the leads where they are present will help in localizing the MI. Autopsy studies have demonstrated the accuracy of Q wave criteria to be about 50 percent (30 to 88 percent).[183] In one study, 55 percent of patients with inferior Q and 29 percent of patients with anterior Q criteria had no MI at autopsy, whereas 13 percent with normal QRS and 45 percent with inferior Q criteria had MI at autopsy.[184] False-positive diagnosis is primarily due to the presence of abnormal Q waves related to other conditions in the absence of MI or to overlap between normal and abnormal Q waves, particularly in inferior leads. In patients with non–Q wave MI, Q criteria cannot be applied.

Localization of MI

The localization of MI can be made from lead groups with abnormal Q wave.[185–188] Three major groups can be identified: anterior MI, inferior MI, and posterolateral MI. In general, anterior MIs are associated with LAD occlusion, and the infarct usually involves the apical third of the anterior LV and septum. Inferior MI involves the right coronary artery when not left dominant, and the infarct affects the middle third and the basal portion of the inferior wall and the inferior septum. Posterolateral location is usually associated with left circumflex artery disease and involves the lateral wall of the LV.

Traditionally, the infarction localizations by electrocardiography have been quite detailed. A diagnosis of anteroseptal MI is made when Q wave is present in leads V_1 through V_4; anterior MI when abnormal Q is present in leads V_3 and V_4; lateral MI when abnormal Q is present in leads I, aVL, and V_6; anterolateral MI when abnormal Q is present in leads I, aVL, and V_4 through V_6; extensive anterior MI when abnormal Q is present in leads I, aVL, and V_1 through V_6; and high anterolateral MI when abnormal Q is present in leads I and aVL. Inferior (diaphragmatic) MI is diagnosed when abnormal Q is noted in leads II, III, and aVF; inferoanterior MI when abnormal Q is present in leads II, III, aVF, and V_4 through V_6; inferoposterior MI when abnormal Q is present in leads II, III, aVF and tall R is present in lead V_1; true posterior (posterobasal) MI is diagnosed when tall R is present in lead V_1; and posterolateral MI is diagnosed when abnormal Q is present in leads V_4 through V_6 and tall R in lead V_1. These MI localizations by electrocardiography are imprecise, and the simpler classification (anterior, inferior, posterolateral) is preferred.

Diagnosis of Anterior MI

The diagnosis of anterior MI is made when there are abnormal Q waves in two or more V leads, V_1 through V_6. When abnormal Q waves are also present in leads I and aVL, additional lateral MI may be present; and when abnormal Q waves are present in leads V_5 and V_6 apical MI may be present.[185] Other findings in anterior MI include narrow R wave with duration less than 10 to 20 ms in lead V_2[189]; poor R wave progression when the increase of R wave amplitude from leads V_1 to V_4 is reduced and does not show gradual increase of R amplitude and the R magnitude in lead $V_3 \leq 0.3$ mV; or abnormal R wave progression when the R amplitude in one of the leads from V_1 to V_4 is smaller than the preceding V lead, provided the R/S ratio in the same lead does not gradually increase. Diagnosis based on poor R wave progression or small r is weak[190] because other conditions may cause it, the most common one being misplacement of precordial electrodes one interspace or more above the usual level. LVH and left anterior fascicular block also may give rise to small R in leads V_1 through V_3. Other criteria to diagnose anterior MI have been proposed, including R wave in lead I < 0.4 mV without significant S wave, R wave in $V_3 < 0.15$ mV, or T inversion or ST elevations in leads V_2 and V_3 (sensitivity 85 percent, specificity 75 percent, positive predictive accuracy 69 percent).[190]

Diagnosis of Inferior MI

Inferior MI is associated with abnormal Q waves with duration longer than 30 ms, in inferior leads II, III, and aVF, with the most predictive finding being Q in lead aVF wider than 30 ms (sensitivity 90 percent, specificity 97 percent).[183] Lateral involvement is suspected when there is wide, greater than 40-ms duration R in leads V_1 and V_2 associated with increased R magnitude and R/S ratio $\geq$ 1.[186] The sensitivity of this finding is low, less than 50 percent. Apical involvement is suspected when, in addition to inferior leads, Q waves are present in leads V_5 and V_6. The sensitivity of this finding is also less than 50 percent.[186]

Diagnosis of Posterolateral MI

Posterolateral MI (Fig. 2–22) usually involves the middle third of the lateral left ventricular wall, but its location can be variable. The diagnostic criteria involve R wave duration in lead $V_1 \geq 40$ ms, R/S ratio in lead $V_1 \geq 1$, and R/S ratio in lead $V_2 \geq 1.5$. The sensitivity is about 35 percent, and the specificity is 95 percent.[188, 191] Septal fascicular block can mimic posterolateral MI.[192] Abnormal Q waves and ST-T changes are rare and, if present, involve mostly the inferior leads.

The ECG is good for identifying the location of MI; however, there are limitations, and it is poor for delineating the extent of MI.[193–195] In 15 to 30 percent of patients with Q wave MI, the abnormal Q will disappear with time or will become nonsignificant.[196] Abnormal Q in leads V_1 through V_3 correlates better with anteroapical rather than septal MI, abnormal Q in leads I, aVL, V_5, and V_6 correlates better with apical rather than lateral MI, and tall R in leads V_1 through V_2 (R/S > 1 and duration of R ≥ 40 ms) of "posterior MI" correlate better with basal lateral and lateral left ventricular MIs.[183, 188, 191, 197–199] Autopsy studies have shown that the ECG was accurate in predicting the full extent of MI in only 26 percent of cases. In 4 percent, the infarct size was smaller than expected, and in 70 percent of cases, the infarct extended into regions not indicated by the ECG.[193, 194] Efforts have been made to develop a scoring system to determine the infarct size. Scoring systems based on 54 criteria and 27 criteria have been developed.[186] The criteria include Q wave duration in various leads, R wave duration in leads V_1 through V_3, and R/Q and R/S ratios. Each criterion is assigned points from 1 to 3. Each point is equal to 3 to 4 percent of the LV.[185, 186, 189, 200] The correlation between the ECG and the measurement of infarct size during postmortem examination was greater than .70. The highest correlations are with anterior MI.[200]

Non–Q Wave MI

About 25 percent of acute MIs are non–Q wave MIs. Absence of Q wave in acute MI may be related to the smaller size of non–Q MI, early reperfusion, or the higher incidence of collaterals in non–Q MI. It may also be due to the location of infarct at the base of the heart, which is activated late during QRS; the Q may not have been sampled by the regular electrocardiographic leads, such as in posterolateral infarcts; the Q waves may have regressed; or the Q waves may disappear because of the development of MI in an area opposite the first lesion.[201] The most common ECG findings in non–Q MI consist of ST and T wave changes such as ST depression and T inversion.[146] Less frequently, ST elevation is noted.[202] Other findings include reduction of R wave size and development of R wave notches.[181, 182] The anterior non–Q MIs are usually associated with anterior precordial T inversions, whereas posterior non–Q MIs are associated with horizontal ST depression in leads V_1 through V_4.

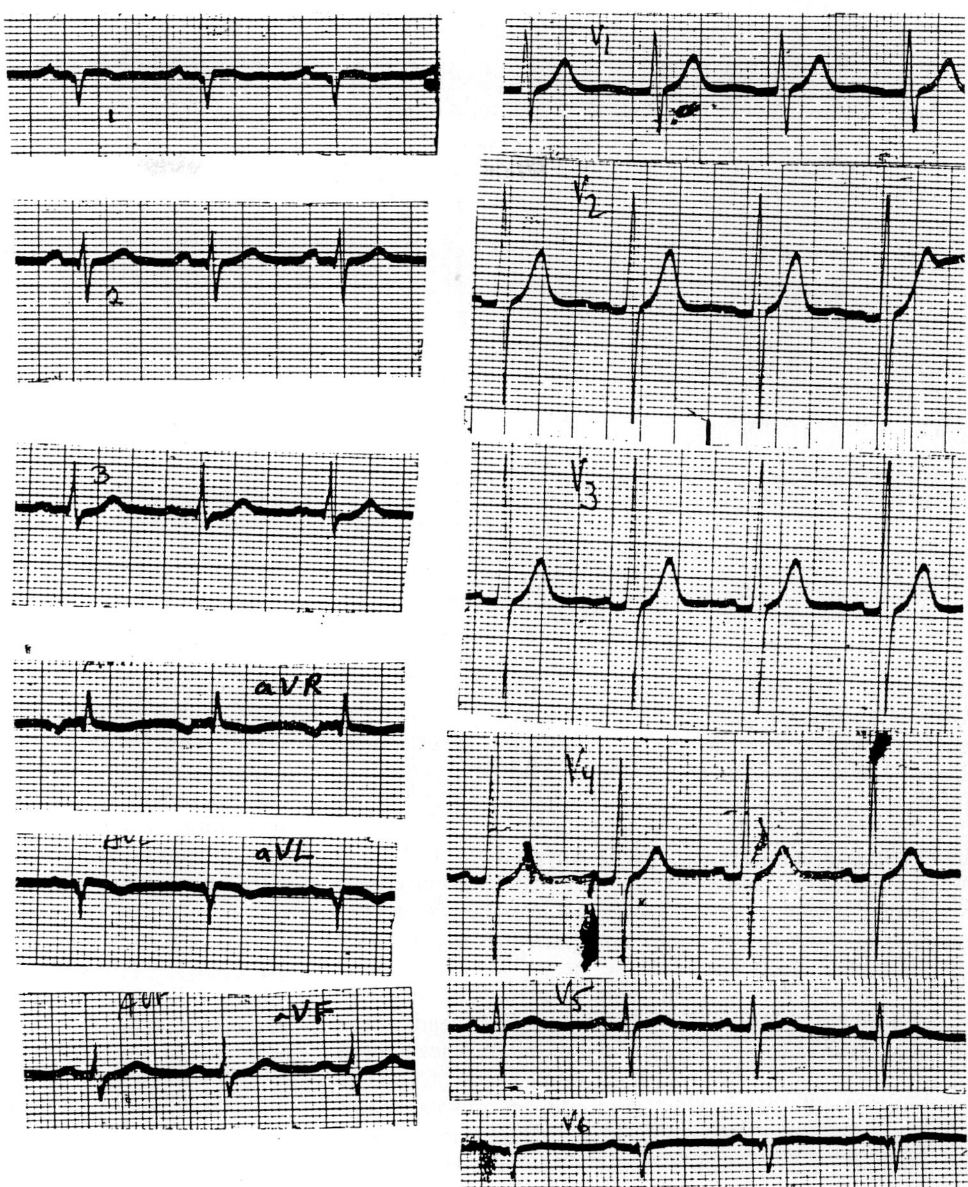

FIGURE 2–22 Posterolateral MI.

Coronary angiography in non–Q MI usually demonstrates a recanalized coronary artery.[204] If an occluded vessel is found, it usually involves the left circumflex artery.[205] The morbidity and mortality of patients with non–Q wave MI presenting with T inversion only are lower than those patients presenting with ST depression.[204, 206–208] Late mortality in non–Q wave MI is equal to that of Q wave MI; however, early mortality and cardiac enzyme levels are lower. Congestive heart failure, left ventricular wall abnormality, fresh thrombosis, and complete occlusion of an artery are noted less frequently in non–Q MI as compared with Q wave MI. Recurrent infarction is noted more frequently in non–Q MI.[209]

Noninfarction Q Waves

Although an abnormal Q wave is usually associated with MI, there are a number of situations in which an abnormal Q suggesting MI may be due to a totally different condition. Transient Q waves may develop in severe ischemia owing to transient inactivation of electrical activity of the myocardial cells. Q waves may also be seen in acute myocarditis and may be indistinguishable from MI. Other conditions affecting the myocardium, such as cardiac amyloidosis,[210] progressive muscular dystrophy,[211] Friedreich's ataxia, scleroderma, sarcoidosis, involvement of myocardium by malignancy, dilated cardiomyopathy of any cause, hypertrophic cardiomyopathy, particularly idiopathic hypertrophic subaortic stenosis, may all produce abnormal Q waves mimicking MI. In idiopathic hypertrophic subaortic stenosis, abnormal Q waves are usually associated with normal ST-T (Fig. 2–23). Abnormal precordial Q waves or low-amplitude R waves in leads V_1 and V_2 and also V_3 may be seen in COPD owing to low diaphragm and altered relationship between precordial V leads and the heart; in misplacement of precordial leads, one interspace or more

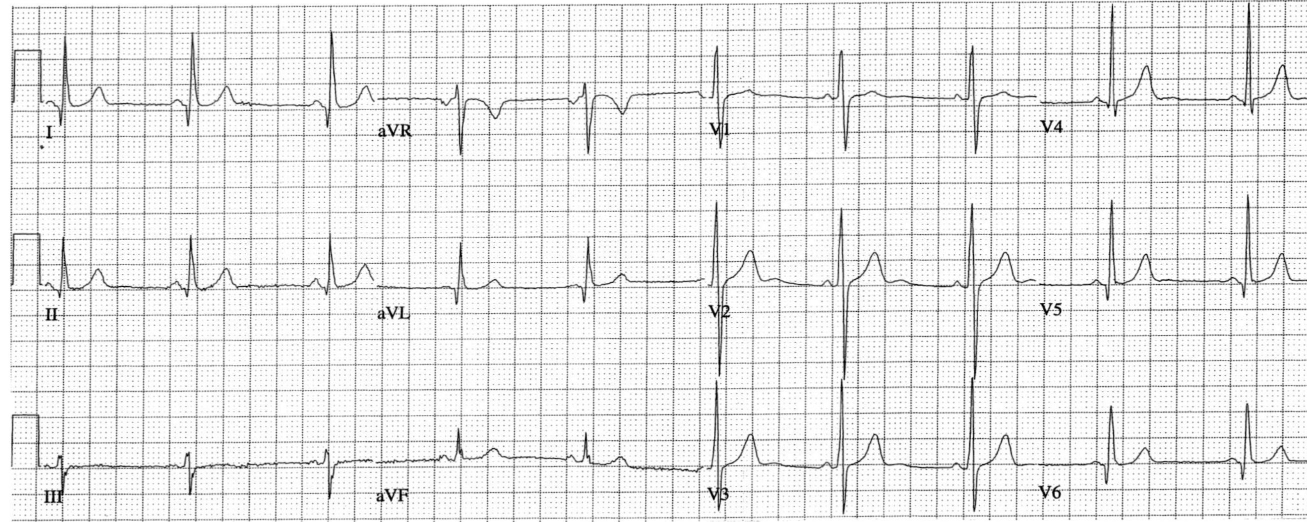

FIGURE 2–23 ECG from a 31-year-old man with idiopathic hypertrophic subaortic stenosis. Note prominent Q in leads I, aVL, V_5, and V_6 with normal ST-T.

above; in left anterior fascicular block, which will alter the orientation of initial QRS vectors; in marked LVH where QRS is shifted posteriorly and to the left; in LBBB; in chest deformity, such as pectus excavatum, pleural effusions,[212] and WPW. In pre-excitation (WPW) syndromes, inferior Q waves may be seen in posteroseptal anomalous connections, lateral Q waves in leads V_5, V_6, I, and aVL in left lateral connections, and Q waves in leads V_1 and V_2 in anteroseptal and right-sided anomalous connections. Precordial P waves could be used as a marker to identify misplacement of electrodes or mismatch between location of precordial electrodes and the heart. The P wave in lead V_1 is usually biphasic with positive and negative components, and it usually becomes positive in lead V_2 and remains positive in precordial leads when the placement of electrodes is appropriate and the patient has no COPD or chest deformity. If precordial electrodes are misplaced one interspace or more above, negative or biphasic P waves may be seen even in leads V_3 and V_4 where they should be positive. Abnormal Q waves mimicking MI can also be seen in switches involving various limb leads, severe hyperkalemia, acute pulmonary embolism, and pneumothorax.

ST and T Wave Abnormalities

ST and T wave changes are the most common findings in electrocardiography. When the ST-T changes are noted in the presence of conduction abnormalities such as LBBB, RBBB, and WPW syndrome, they are called *secondary ST-T changes* and result from altered activation of ventricles. Primary ST-T abnormalities are related to altered ventricular recovery and result from the changes in the slope of phase 2 or 3 of action potential and changes in the action potential duration. A large number of conditions may cause primary ST-T changes. Changes in the action potential duration of only 8 percent of the left ventricular myocardium will suffice to produce T wave abnormalities.[213] Myocardial ischemia is one of the most frequent causes of ST-T changes. Others include drugs such as digitalis, electrolyte abnormalities, pulmonary embolism, subacute and chronic phases of pericarditis, neurogenic ST-T abnormalities associated with cerebrovascular accident and central nervous system disorders, mitral valve prolapse, cocaine abuse, and rate-related causes such as postextrasystolic and post-tachycardia T wave changes. Because similar ST-T changes can be caused by various conditions, the term *nonspecific ST-T changes* has been adopted to describe them.

Electrolyte Abnormalities

Hyperkalemia

In hyperkalemia (Figs. 2–24 and 2–25), an increase in extracellular potassium concentration will affect the resting membrane potential and make it less negative (depolarization). When the cell membrane potential reaches a level above -60 mV, the cell becomes unresponsive. Hyperkalemia will cause a fall in action potential amplitude and V_{max} and will slow conduction, and the action potential duration will be shortened. Hyperkalemia will cause tall, peaked T waves with a narrow base, and the QT interval will shorten secondary to shortened action potential duration. At higher potassium concentrations above 6.5 mEq/L, the QRS will widen, the T waves may be more prominent, and there can be conduction abnormalities and changes in electrical axis. When the QRS starts to widen, the PR is also prolonged. With increasing serum potassium levels, the P amplitude will also decrease until it disappears.[214] At serum levels higher than 8.8 mEq/L, the P waves may disappear, the QRS may widen further, the ST segments may also disappear, and a sine wave (biphasic)–type QRS-T may develop. At these levels, the rhythm may be regular and the SA node may function and the sinus impulses may be conducted to the AV node through internodal pathways, which are more resistant to the depolarizing effect of elevated potassium without activating the atria (sinoventricular conduction). Usually, when the level

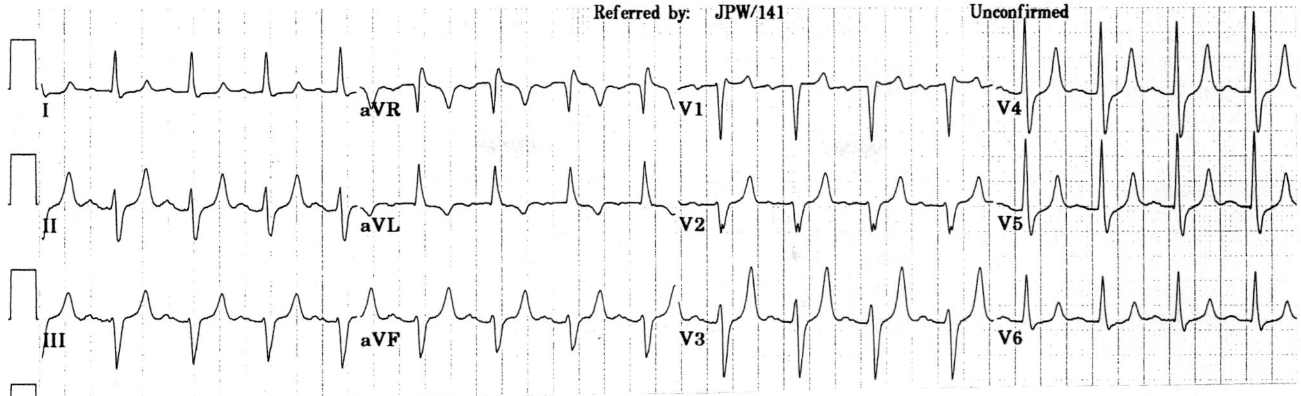

FIGURE 2–24 Hyperkalemia. Serum K = 6.8 mEq/L. Note intraventricular conduction delay, left anterior fascicular block, and prominent, pointed, narrow-base symmetric T waves. The patient's ECG was normal before the onset of hyperkalemia.

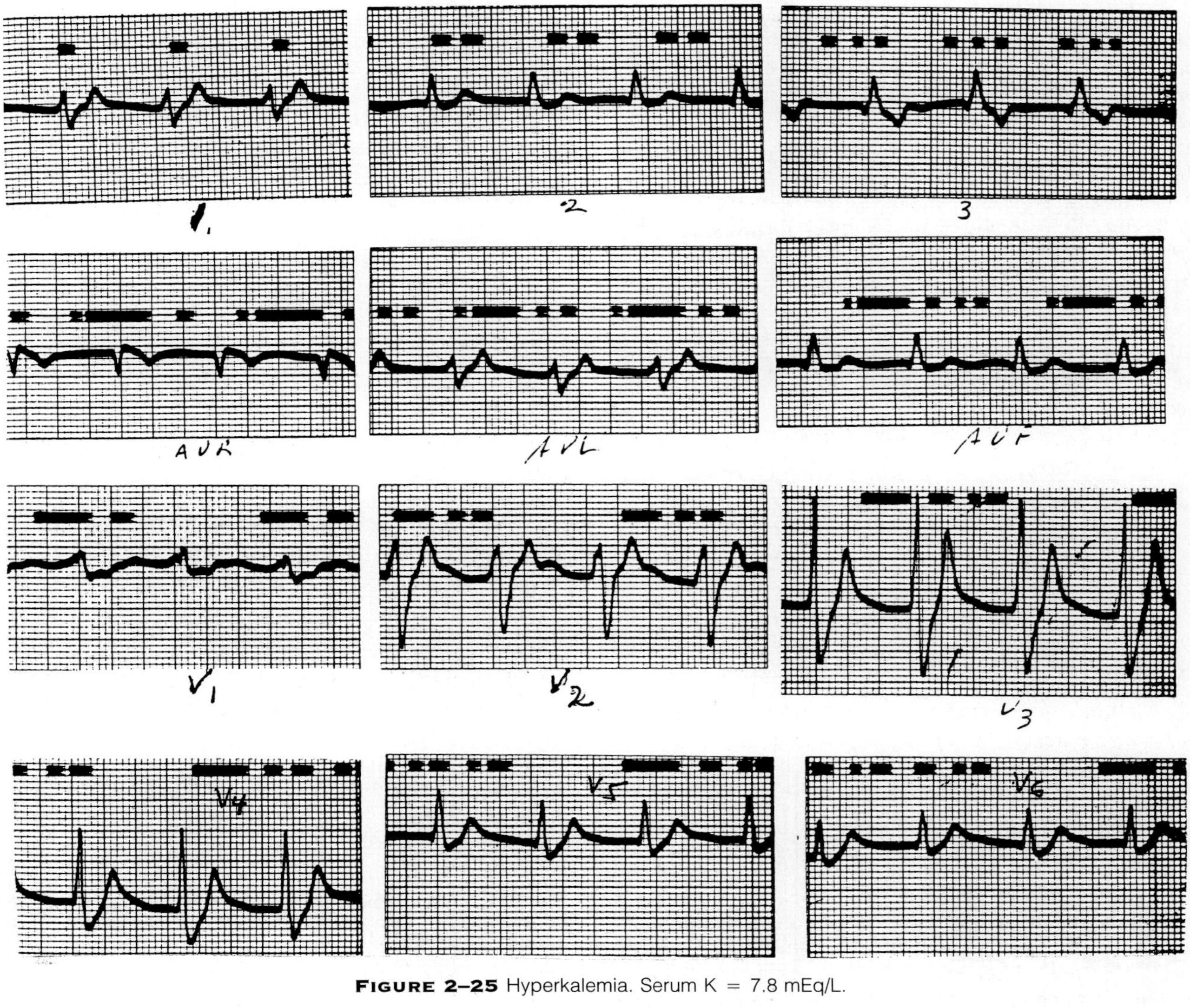

FIGURE 2–25 Hyperkalemia. Serum K = 7.8 mEq/L.

reaches 12 mEq/L or higher, the ventricles become unresponsive and ventricular fibrillation may develop. Hyperkalemia may occasionally cause ST elevation and Q waves mimicking acute MI. It may also cause intraventricular conduction abnormalities such as fascicular blocks, RBBB, or LBBB patterns.

Hypokalemia

Because of widespread use of diuretics, hypokalemia (Fig. 2–26) is a frequent cause of electrocardiographic abnormalities. Decreased extracellular potassium will result in hyperpolarized cells with increased action potential duration. These changes will result in prominent U waves and a decrease in T amplitude, and the U wave may become taller than the T wave. The ST segment becomes depressed. The QU interval is prolonged.[214–216] Although prominent U waves appear at potassium concentrations below 3.5 mEq/L, they become more obvious when the value drops below 3 mEq/L. Hypokalemia also is associated with atrial and ventricular extrasystoles as well as atrial tachycardia with block and ventricular tachyarrhythmias (torsades de pointes).

Other Electrolyte Abnormalities

Hypercalcemia will shorten the QT interval, which results from shortened phase 2 of action potential caused by an

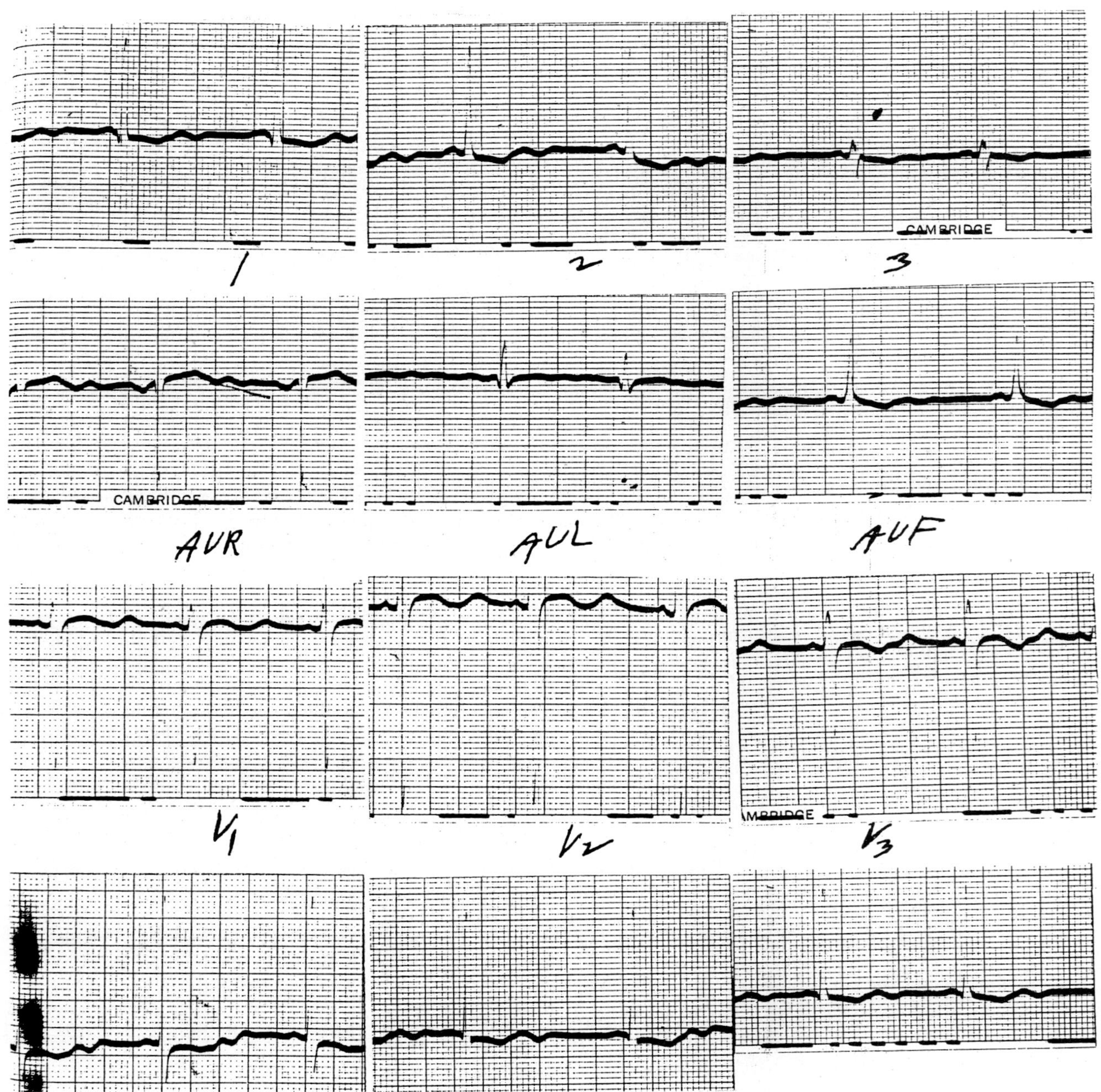

FIGURE 2–26 Hypokalemia. ST-T abnormality and prominent U waves.

increase of the outward potassium current, whereas *hypocalcemia* will prolong these measurements. Hypercalcemia may also produce depressed ST and inverted T,[214, 217, 218] such as that seen in digitalis effect. Severe hypercalcemia may cause second-degree and third-degree AV block.[216] There are no recognizable electrocardiographic changes associated with *hypermagnesemia* or *hypomagnesemia*.

Drug-Induced Electrocardiographic Changes

Digitalis will shorten the QT interval and cause ST segment depression and T inversion. The ST segment depression has an asymmetric shape and may have a scooped appearance. These changes are caused by shortening of phase 2 and a decrease of slope of phase 3 of ventricular action potential. Digitalis may also cause mild prolongation of the PR interval and slowing of ventricular response in atrial fibrillation or flutter when therapeutic levels of digitalis are achieved. Depression of SA node or depression of conduction from SA node to atria by digitalis will result in SA node arrest or SA block. The arrhythmias associated with digitalis excess include ectopic rhythms, such as atrial tachycardia with block, nonparoxysmal junctional tachycardia, ventricular premature contractions, ventricular tachycardia, bidirectional ventricular tachycardia, ventricular flutter and fibrillation, accelerated escape rhythms, and atrial fibrillation and flutter.[219] Excess digitalis may also cause AV block and AV dissociation with acceleration of a subsidiary pacemaker or lower junctional focus. Arrhythmias of digitalis toxicity appear to be related to delayed after-depolarizations and triggered activity.

Quinidine and other type I drugs, such as procainamide and disopyramide, widen the QRS by inhibiting the inward sodium current, slow the upstroke of phase 0 of action potential, and prolong the QT interval by increasing the duration of action potential, secondary to abnormal potassium conductance, reduced outward potassium flux, and increased inward calcium currents. There is depression of conduction in the atria, ventricles, and SA and AV nodes, as well as in the specialized cardiac conduction system. SA and AV block may result in sinus bradycardia, sinus arrest, SA block, prolongation of PR interval, or development of high-degree AV block. With higher doses, the electrocardiographic changes may increase, U waves may become more prominent, and patients may develop torsades de pointes. Torsades de pointes can also occur with low plasma levels of quinidine, when the QRS duration exceeds 25 percent of baseline, there is prolongation of the QT interval greater than 25 percent, and the QT_c is greater than 0.52 s.

The type IB drugs have minimal effect on the ECG. They will cause minimal shortening of the QT interval. The type IC drugs will prolong the PR and the QRS by slowing the myocardial conduction but will have minimal effect on the QT interval (prolongation). The beta and calcium channel blockers will slow conduction in the AV node and will prolong the PR interval. Amiodarone and sotalol will prolong the PR, QRS, and QT interval.

Phenothiazines and Tricyclic Antidepressants

Toxic effects on the ECG are similar to those produced by quinidine. They may cause prolongation of the QRS duration and the QT interval, may produce ST-T changes and prominent U waves, and may induce ventricular tachyarrhythmias. They can also cause AV block and bundle branch block. Lithium appears to affect primarily the SA node causing sinus bradycardia, SA node arrest, or exit block. Lithium can also produce T wave flattening or inversion. Other drugs associated with QT prolongation, torsades de pointes, and sudden death include the antibiotics erythromycin and ketoconazole, the antihistamines astemizole and terfenadine, and also terodiline.[220–222]

Miscellaneous Patterns

Juvenile T Wave Patterns

T inversions in leads V_1 through V_3 may be a normal finding in children and teens. In adults and older persons, the T waves in these leads become upright. Persistence of inverted T waves in leads V_1 through V_3 is called *juvenile T wave pattern,* and it is seen more commonly in women. The etiology is unclear. When present, the T inversion is usually more pronounced in lead V_1 than in lead V_3; whereas in ischemia or other abnormalities, the T inversion may be more pronounced in lead V_3 than in lead V_1.

"Memory" T Waves

Memory T waves are inverted T waves seen in normally conducted beats after cessation of ventricular pacing. These changes are transient, and their duration appears to be related to the length of ventricular pacing before cessation of pacing. They can also be seen in intermittent LBBB when normally conducted beats are recorded and after radiofrequency ablation of accessory pathways in WPW syndrome. The T inversion in postablation of accessory pathways is of the same polarity as the delta wave. It is assumed that the heart "remembers" the polarity of abnormal QRS (LBBB or paced QRS) or the delta wave.[223–227]

"Early Repolarization"

Early repolarization (Fig. 2–27) is a normal variant, and it consists of J point elevation and ST segment elevation, which is mostly concave. It is best noted in precordial leads and may be associated with a notch at the end of QRS and the beginning of the ST segment. It is more common in Africans, African Americans, and Eskimo children. This corresponds to the J wave or the Osborne wave, which was described in hypothermia, and it is common in baboons and dogs. There is evidence to link the J point elevation and the notch described previously to a notch of spike and dome morphology located at the end of phase 1 and the beginning of phase 2 of action potential recorded from epicardial-myocardial cells but not endocardial-myocardial cells. This notch appears to be related to transient outward current. Aminopyridine, which inhibits transient outward current, also inhibits the J wave.[95]

Electrical Alternans

This consists of alternation of QRS or T usually every other beat when their morphology and orientation change.

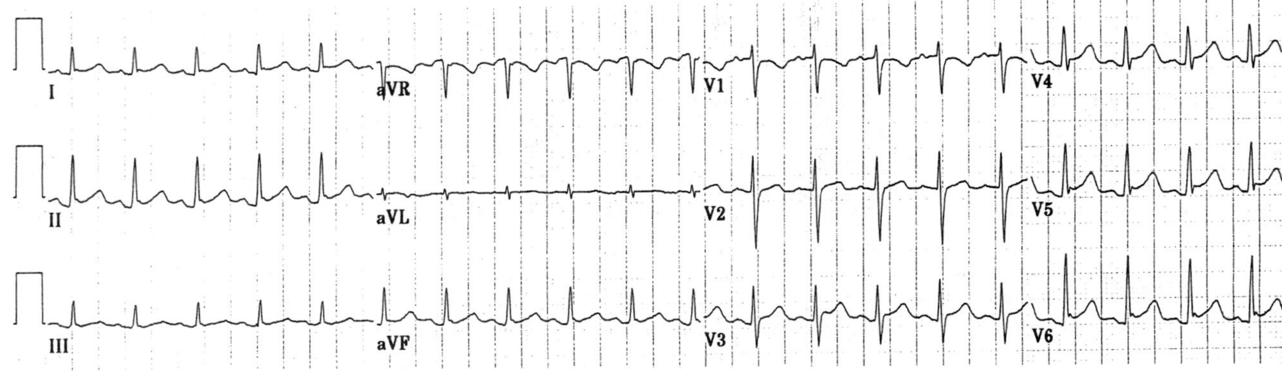

FIGURE 2–27 Sinus tachycardia with early repolarization. Note the notch at the J point.

Occasionally, the PR interval and the ST segment may also be involved. Electrical alternans has been noted in significant pericardial effusion with tamponade, ischemia, pulmonary embolism,[228, 229] and the congenital long QT syndrome.[230] Isolated T wave alternans has also been seen in hypocalcemia and patients on quinidine or amiodarone or with severe electrolyte disturbances, acute pulmonary embolism, advanced heart disease, and long QT syndrome.[230–235]

U Wave

The genesis of the U wave was discussed previously. Many factors affect the U wave, the most common one being hypokalemia. U wave inversion has been associated with myocardial ischemia, hypertension, LVH, RVH, aortic stenosis, aortic regurgitation, and mitral regurgitation.[236–238] U wave inversion during exercise stress testing has been associated with significant coronary artery disease and constitutes a positive stress test.[239]

Long QT Syndromes

The long QT may be acquired or congenital. Table 2–1 shows the acquired causes of long QT.[222] The congenital long QT syndromes may exhibit an autosomal dominant inheritance (Romano-Ward syndrome) or an autosomal recessive inheritance (Jervell and Lange-Nielson syndrome), which is associated with deafness. The congenital long QT syndromes represent a primary electrical disease caused by mutations involving specific ion channel genes.[240] They show genetic heterogeneity (*LQT1, LQT2, LQT3, LQT4, LQT5*) with various chromosome loci, gene mutation/protein, and current/channel involvement.[222] Both congenital and acquired forms of long QT syndrome are characterized by the prolongation of the QT interval. Patients with long QT syndromes are prone to ventricular tachycardia and torsades de pointes. The ventricular tachycardia may develop either during pauses or slow heart rates (pause dependent) or during sympathetic stimulation such as exercise or fright (adrenergic dependent). These patients usually have prominent U waves and abnormal T waves, sometimes associated with T wave alternans. The congenital long QT syndromes are adrenergic dependent, as are those related to intracranial disease, right radical neck dissection, right carotid endarterectomy, and mitral valve prolapse. In contrast, drug-induced long QT syndromes due to antiarrhythmic drugs, antibiotics (intravenous erythromycin), tricyclic antidepressants, phenothiazines, electrolyte abnormalities (hypokalemia, hypomagnesemia), and altered nutritional status such as starvation and use of liquid protein diets are pause dependent.[241]

Improper Placement of Leads

Improper placement of limb leads as well as precordial leads is a frequently encountered phenomenon that is not always recognized and may lead to misinterpretation of the ECG. Misplacement of limb leads involves not only the left arm, right arm, and left leg cables but also the right leg (ground) cable. The most common switch involves the right arm and left arm cables. Using the Einthoven equilateral triangle with proper polarity of leads (lead I = left arm positive, right arm negative; lead II = left leg positive, right arm negative; and lead III = left leg positive and left

TABLE 2–1 Secondary Causes of Acquired QT Prolongation

Antiarrhythmic Agents	*Lipid-Lowering Agents*
Class IA: quinidine, procainamide, *N*-acetyl-procainamide, disopyramide	Probucol
Class III: amiodarone, low risk of torsades de pointes	*Psychotropic Agents*
Class IV: bepridil, mibefradil	Tricyclic and tetracyclic antidepressants
Antihistamines	Haloperidol
Terfenadine	Phenothiazines
Astemizole	Risperidone
Antimicrobials	Selective serotonin reuptake inhibitors
Erythromycin	*Other Agents*
Trimethoprim-sulfamethoxazole	Organophosphates
Clarithromycin	Diuretics (reduced K^+, Mg^{2+})
Co-trimoxazole	Vasopressin (severe bradycardia)
Azithromycin	Chloral hydrate
Ketoconazole	Amantadine
Pentamidine	*Electrolyte Abnormalities*
Chloroquine	Hypokalemia
Gastrointestinal Causes	Hypomagnesemia
Cisapride	Hypocalcemia
Liquid protein diets	
Anorexia nervosa	

From Zipes DP, Wellens HJJ: Sudden cardiac death. Circulation 98[21]:2334–2351, 1998.

arm negative), the cable connection errors can be easily identified from the electrocardiographic morphology recorded in each lead.[242, 243] When there is left arm and right arm switch, lead I will have the mirror image of lead I, lead II will represent lead III, and lead III will represent lead II. Unipolar right arm cable will record from left arm (aVR = aVL), left arm cable will record from right arm (aVL = aVR), and left leg cable will remain unchanged. When the left foot and left arm cables are switched, lead I will represent lead II, lead II will represent lead I, and lead III will represent the mirror image of lead III. If the patient has a positive P and the QRS starts with an R wave and T is positive in lead III, the switch will result in inverted P, prominent Q wave, and inverted T. Lead aVF will represent lead aVL, and lead aVL will represent lead aVF. When the right arm and left leg cables are switched, lead I will represent the mirror image of lead III, lead II will represent the mirror image of lead II, and lead III will represent the mirror image of lead I; leads aVR and aVF will be switched. Switching the right leg (ground) cable with other extremity cables is not uncommon. Since the right leg and left leg are in close proximity as far as the equilateral triangle is concerned, the limb cable attached to the ground electrode will record the potential similar to lead aVF, but not identical. The most common switch is between the right arm and the right leg. This results in lead aVR that is quite similar to lead aVF. Leads aVL and aVF remain unchanged. Lead I would be like the mirror image of lead III. Lead II will be isoelectric and nearly a straight line because the potential difference between left leg and "right arm" cables would be minimal. Lead III will remain unchanged. When the switch involves the right leg and the left arm cables, lead I will be similar to lead II. Lead II will remain unchanged, and lead III would be isoelectric and like a straight line because of minimal potential difference between left leg and left arm cables. When the right leg and left leg are switched, there will be almost no difference from baseline. When arm and leg cables are switched (right arm with right leg and left leg with left arm), lead I will record a straight line, lead II will be a mirror image of lead III, lead III will be a mirror image of lead III, lead aVF will equal lead aVL. Switch of precordial cables will result in QRS and P morphology inappropriate for the V lead recorded. When the V_1 and V_3 cables are switched, the V_1 lead will show V_3 and V_3 will show V_1. Not only are the individual precordial electrodes switched, but sometimes the entire set of precordial leads is reversed with V_1 recording V_6 and V_6 recording V_1 characteristics. In addition to using the QRS morphology, using the P morphology is extremely helpful in identifying precordial lead misplacement. The P wave associated with V_1 and sometimes V_2 is usually biphasic whereas V_3 and other V leads will usually have a positive P wave. Changes also may occur when the precordial electrodes are misplaced one interspace or more above or below the correct level.

Special Clinical Problems

Pericarditis

The main electrocardiographic finding in early acute pericarditis (Fig. 2–28) is concave ST segment elevation with positive T waves in all leads except aVR and V_1. The PR segment is also depressed in the majority of cases. There are no reciprocal ST segment shifts as in acute myocardial injury. During recovery or the chronic phase of pericarditis, the ST segments return to baseline and the T waves become inverted. There is considerable variability in the extent of ST segment elevation and ST-T changes with time. In some cases, T inversions may remain for years as a marker of previous pericarditis. The ST and T segment shifts are related to subepicardial myocardial injury, which causes reduction in resting membrane potential and shortening of action potential duration. Systolic injury currents are directed toward the epicardium, and the diastolic injury currents are directed toward the endocardium. Acute pericardial tamponade may produce electrical alternans. This is most commonly seen during rapid accumulation of pericardial effusion secondary to malignancy. The alternans may involve the P, the QRS, and the T. Alternans results from swinging and rotation of the heart in the pericardial fluid with each heartbeat. In constrictive pericarditis, the QRS voltage is usually low and left atrial enlargement or atrial fibrillation are not uncommon. In pericardial effusion, the magnitude of electrocardiographic voltages is decreased.

Myocarditis

There are no specific electrocardiographic findings in myocarditis. When pericarditis is associated with acute myocarditis, ST segment elevations may be noted. Transient episodes of first-degree or second-degree AV block and nonspecific ST-T changes as well as intraventricular conduction delay or bundle branch blocks may be noted. Acute myocarditis can produce abnormal Q similar to that of MI.

Pulmonary Embolism

The electrocardiographic changes in pulmonary embolism (Fig. 2–29) are related to acute pulmonary hypertension and right ventricular and right atrial dilatation. The following ECG changes have been observed in pulmonary embolism: sinus tachycardia; shift of mean electrical axis to the right; inverted T waves in leads V_1 through V_3; development of right ventricular conduction delay IRBBB or RBBB; development of abnormal Q in leads III and aVF but not in lead II; QR or qR pattern in V_1, V_2, and V_3R; S_1, S_2, and S_3 pattern; or S_1, Q_3, T_3 pattern.[244, 245] Right atrial dilatation is probably responsible for abnormal Q in right precordial leads.[246] These findings are not specific for pulmonary embolism and need to be correlated with the clinical findings. Patients with pulmonary embolism also tend to develop atrial fibrillation or atrial ectopy.

Central Nervous System Disorders (Neurogenic Repolarization Abnormalities)

The electrocardiographic abnormalities consist of striking wide and deep T inversions in leads I, aVL, and V_4 through V_6, marked prolongation of QT interval, and ST segment elevation or depression (Fig. 2–30).[247] These changes are most commonly seen in subarachnoid hemorrhage[248] and

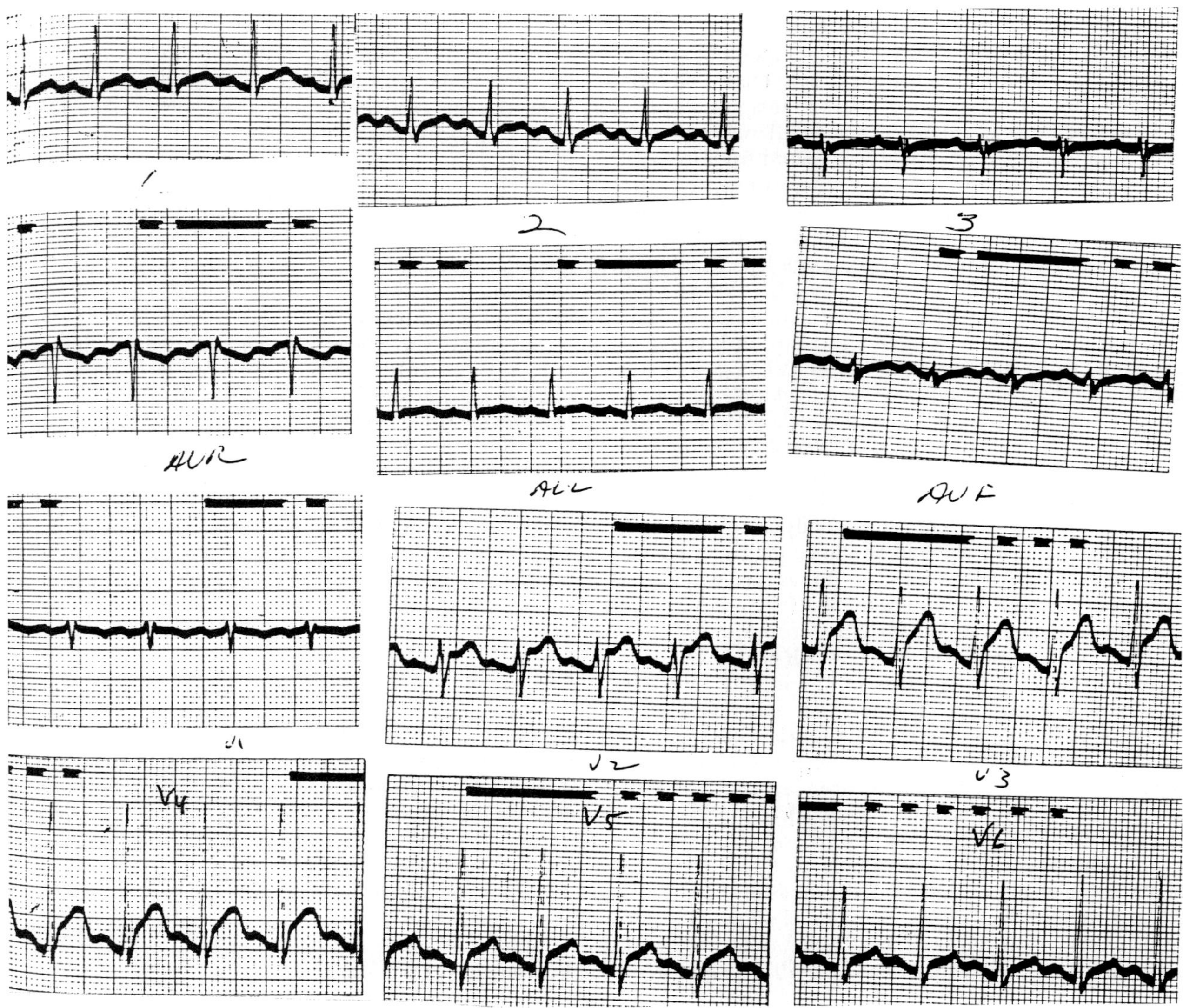

FIGURE 2–28 Acute pericarditis.

in patients with right cervical neck dissection with damage to the right sympathetic chain.[249] They also may be seen in head injuries, neoplasms, ischemic stroke, and electroconvulsive therapy.[250] The ST-T changes noted in central nervous system disorders are also called *neurogenic repolarization abnormalities*. If not recognized, they may be interpreted as showing myocardial ischemia or non–Q MI. These changes are most likely related to abnormal repolarization associated with the altered autonomic nervous system activation.

Hypothermia

In hypothermia (Fig. 2–31), when the body temperature becomes subnormal and drops to about 35°C or less, a notch or a wave appears at the end of QRS and the beginning of ST segment called the *J wave* or the *Osborne wave*. These subjects also have sinus bradycardia, prolonged PR and QRS, a long QT interval, and at times, atrial flutter or fibrillation. The J wave disappears after normothermia is restored.[251] The ionic basis of the J wave is not known. As mentioned previously, the Osborne wave is associated with the notch located between phases 1 and 2 of the action potential noted in the epicardial myocardial action potential but not endocardial myocardial action potential. It appears to be related to transient outward current and has a spike and dome morphology. The prominent action potential notch in epicardial but not endocardial myocardium provides a voltage gradient that manifests as the Osborne wave (J wave) or elevated J point.[95] Hypothermia and hypercalcemia accentuate the notch and the transient outward current. The effect of hypothermia is direct, and hypercalcemia sensitizes the high transient outward current of epicardial myocardium to increased calcium. Prominent notch may lead to phase 2 re-entry resulting in premature ventricular contractions, which may lead to ventricular tachycardia. The idiopathic J wave has been linked to life-threatening arrhythmia, such as in Brugada's syndrome. The Brugada syndrome is characterized by persistent ST elevation in leads V_1 through V_3, normal QT interval, and sudden cardiac death.[92, 93] RBBB is present in

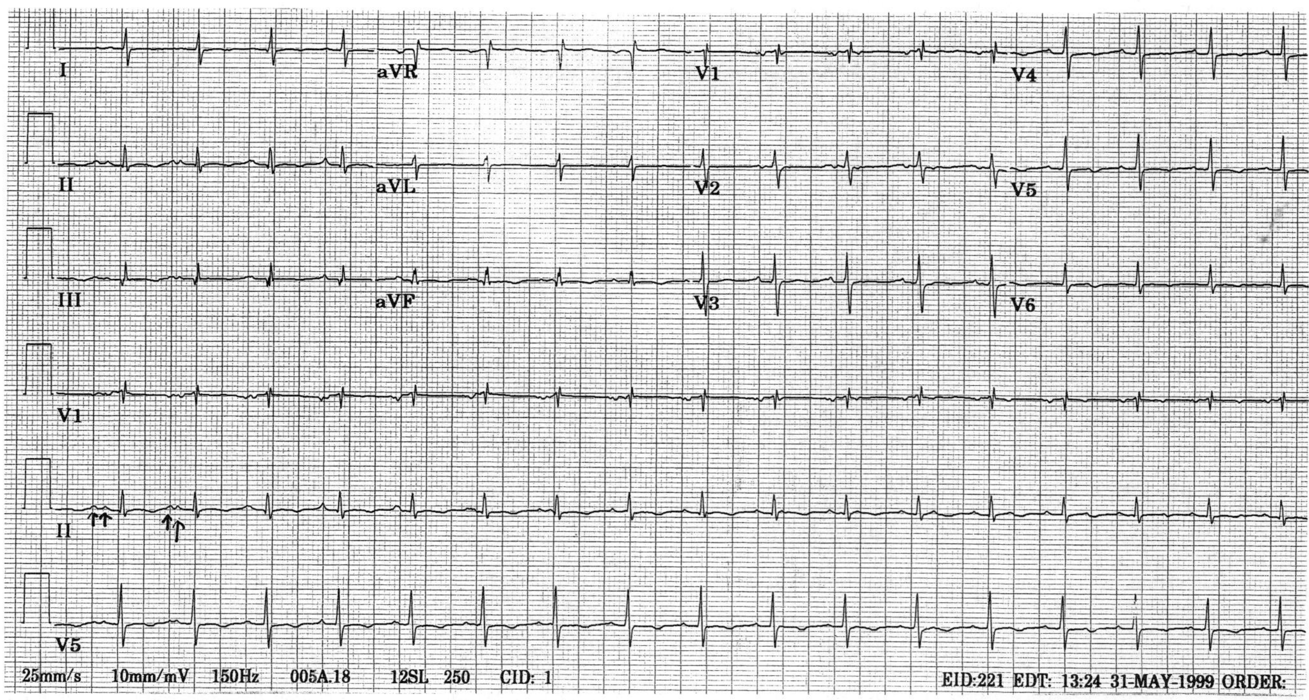

FIGURE 2–32 ECG of a patient with heart transplant. Sinus tachycardia, incomplete right bundle branch block, and nonspecific lateral T abnormality. Two P waves are present.

The computerized electrocardiographic interpretation that is now widely available is not yet reliable because of inaccuracies in the determination of intervals, in the recognition of all waveforms, and also in the interpretation of measured data. The problems arise mostly with the diagnosis of abnormalities, particularly rhythm abnormalities, including poor recognition of bipolar pacer spikes. Currently, computer-processed and computer-interpreted ECGs need to be overread by an experienced cardiologist.

References

1. Abildskov JA, Klein RM: Cancellation of electrocardiographic effects during ventricular excitation. Circ Res 11:247, 1962.
2. Hoffman BF, Cranefield PF: Electrophysiology of the Heart. New York: McGraw-Hill, 1960.
3. Cranefield PF: The Conduction of the Cardiac Impulse. Mt. Kisco, NY: Futura Publishing, 1975.
4. Sperelakis N: Origin of the cardiac resting potential. *In* Berne RM, Sperelakis N (eds): Handbook of Physiology, Sect. 2, The Cardiovascular System I. Bethesda, MD: American Physiological Society, 1979.
5. Antzelevitch C, Sicouri S, Lukas A, et al: Regional differences in the electrophysiology of ventricular cells: physiological and clinical implications. *In* Zipes DP, Jalife J (eds): Cardiac Electrophysiology: From Cell to Bedside. p. 228. Philadelphia: WB Saunders, 1995.
6. Drouin E, Charpentier F, Gauthier C, et al: Electrophysiologic characteristics of cells spanning the left ventricular wall of human heart: evidence for presence of M cells. J Am Coll Cardiol 26:185, 1995.
7. Volders PGA, Sipido KR, Carmeliet E, et al: Repolarizing K^+ currents I_{TO1} and IK_s are larger in right than left canine ventricular midmyocardium. Circulation 99:206, 1999.
8. Barr RC: Genesis of the electrocardiogram. *In* Macfarlane PW, Lawrie TDV (eds): Comprehensive Electrocardiography. New York: Pergamon, 1989.
9. Einthoven W, Fahr G, deWaart A: Über die Richtung und die manifeste Grösse der Potential-Schwankungen im Menschlichen Herzen und über den Einfluss der Herzlage auf die Form des Elektrokardiogramms. Arch Gesamte Physiol (Pflüger's) 150:275, 1913.
10. Goldberger E: A simple indifferent, electrocardiographic electrode of zero potential and a technique of obtaining augmented, unipolar extremity leads. Am Heart J 23:483, 1942.
11. Wilson FN, MacLeod AG, Barker PS: Electrocardiographic leads which record potential variations of the heart at a single point. Proc Soc Exp Biol Med 29:1011, 1932.
12. Frank E: An accurate, clinically practical system for spatial vectorcardiography. Circulation 13:737, 1956.
13. Taccardi B: Distribution of heart potentials on the thoracic surface of normal human subjects. Circ Res 12:341, 1963.
14. Vincent GM, Abildskov JA, Burgess MJ, et al: Diagnosis of old inferior myocardial infarction by body surface isopotential mapping. Am J Cardiol 39:510, 1977.
15. Lux RL, Burgess MJ, Wyatt RF, et al: Clinically practical lead systems for improved electrocardiography: comparison with precordial grids and conventional lead systems. Circulation 59:356, 1979.
16. Kuchar DL, Rosenbaum DS: Noninvasive recording of late potentials: current state of the art. Pacing Clin Electrophysiol 12:1538, 1989.
17. Simson MB: Signal averaging. Circulation 75(suppl III):III-69, 1987.
18. Macfarlane PW, Lawrie TDV (eds): Comprehensive Electrocardiology. Theory and Practice in Health and Disease. New York: Pergamon, 1989.
19. Mirvis DM: Electrocardiography. A Physiologic Approach. St. Louis: Mosby–Year Book, 1993.
20. James TN: The connecting pathways between the sinus node and the A-V node and between the right and left atrium in the human heart. Am Heart J 66:498, 1963.
21. Boineau JP, Canavan TE, Schuessler RB, et al: Demonstration of a widely distributed atrial pacemaker complex in the human heart. Circulation 77:1221, 1988.
22. Mirvis DM: Body surface distribution of electrical potential during atrial depolarization and repolarization. Circulation 62:167, 1980.
23. Janosik DL, Pearson AC, Buckingham TA, et al: The hemodynamic benefit of differential atrioventricular delay intervals for sensed and paced atrial events during physiologic pacing. J Am Coll Cardiol 14:499, 1989.

24. Durrer D, Van Dam RT, Freud GE, et al: Total excitation of the isolated human heart. Circulation 41:899, 1970.
25. Spach MS, Barr RC: Ventricular intramural and epicardial potential distributions during ventricular activation and repolarization in the intact dog. Circ Res 37:243, 1975.
26. Higuchi T, Nakaya J: T wave polarity related to the repolarization process of epicardial and endocardial ventricular surfaces. Am Heart J 108:290, 1984.
27. Wilson FN, MacLeod AG, Barker PS, et al: The determination and significance of the areas of the ventricular deflections of the electrocardiogram. Am Heart J 10:46, 1934.
28. Bazett HC: An analysis of the time relations of electrocardiograms. Heart 7:353, 1920.
29. Cowan JC, Yusoff K, Moore M, et al: Importance of lead selection in QT interval measurement. Am J Cardiol 61:83, 1988.
30. Garson A Jr: How to measure the QT interval. What is normal? Am J Cardiol 72:148, 1993.
31. Day CP, McComb JM, Campbell RWF: QT dispersion: an indication of arrhythmia risk in patients with long QT intervals. Br Heart J 63:342, 1990.
32. Higham PD, Campbell RWF: QT dispersion. Br Heart J 71:508, 1994.
33. Zabel M, Klingenheben T, Franz MR, et al: Assessment of QT duration for prediction of mortality or arrhythmic events after myocardial infarction: results of a prospective long-term follow-up study. Circulation 97:2543, 1998.
34. Coumel P, Maison-Blanche P, Badilini F: Dispersion of ventricular repolarization. Reality? Illusion? Significance? Circulation 97:2491, 1998.
35. Watanabe Y: Purkinje repolarization as a possible cause of the U wave in the electrocardiogram. Circulation 51:1030, 1975.
36. Antzelevitch C, Sicouri S: Clinical relevance of cardiac arrhythmias generated by after depolarizations: role of M cells in the generation of U waves, triggered activity and torsades de pointes. J Am Coll Cardiol 23:259, 1994.
37. Morris JJ, Estes EH, Whalen RE, et al: P-wave analysis in valvular heart disease. Circulation 29:242, 1964.
38. Romhilt DW, Bove KE, Conradi S, et al: Morphologic significance of left atrial involvement. Am Heart J 83:322, 1972.
39. Josephson ME, Kastor JA, Morganroth J: Electrocardiographic left atrial enlargement: electrophysiologic, echocardiographic and hemodynamic correlates. Am J Cardiol 39:967, 1977.
40. Miller DH, Eisenberg RR, Kligfield PD, et al: Electrocardiographic recognition of left atrial enlargement. J Electrocardiol 16:15, 1983.
41. Munnswamy K, Alpert MA, Martin RH, et al: Sensitivity and specificity of commonly used electrocardiographic criteria for left atrial enlargement determined by M-mode echocardiography. Am J Cardiol 53:829, 1984.
42. Chandraratna PAN, Hodges M: Electrocardiographic evidence of left atrial hypertension in acute myocardial infarction. Circulation 47:493, 1973.
43. DiBianco R, Gottdiener JS, Fletcher RD, et al: Left atrial overload: a hemodynamic, echocardiographic, electrocardiographic and vectorcardiographic study. Am Heart J 98:478, 1979.
44. Reeves WC, Hallahan W, Schwiter EJ, et al: Two-dimensional echocardiographic assessment of electrocardiographic criteria for right atrial enlargement. Circulation 64:387, 1981.
45. Ikeda K, Kubota I, Takahashi K, et al: P wave changes in obstructive and restrictive lung diseases. J Electrocardiol 18:233, 1985.
46. Kilcoyne MM, Davis AL, Ferrer MI: A dynamic electrocardiographic concept useful in the diagnosis of cor pulmonale: result of a survey of 200 patients with chronic obstructive pulmonary disease. Circulation 42:903, 1970.
47. Chou TC: Atrial abnormalities. *In* Chou TC (ed): Electrocardiography in Clinical Practice: Adult and Pediatric. p. 23. Philadelphia, WB Saunders, 1996.
48. Surawicz B: Electrocardiographic diagnosis of chamber enlargement. J Am Coll Cardiol 8:711, 1986.
49. Kaplan JD, Evans T Jr, Foster E, et al: Evaluation of electrocardiographic criteria for right atrial enlargement by quantitative two-dimensional echocardiography. J Am Coll Cardiol 23:747, 1994.
50. Chou TC, Helm RA: The pseudo P pulmonale. Circulation 32:96, 1965.
51. Thiry PS, Rosenberg RM, Abbott JA: A mechanism for the electrocardiogram response to left ventricular hypertrophy and acute ischemia. Circ Res 36:92, 1975.
52. Brody DA: A theoretic analysis of intracavitary blood mass influence on the electrocardiogram. Circ Res 4:731, 1956.
53. Feldman T, Childers RW, Borrow KM, et al: Change in ventricular cavity size: differential effects on QRS and T wave amplitude. Circulation 72:495, 1985.
54. Antman EM, Green LH, Grossman W: Physiologic determinants of the electrocardiographic diagnosis of left ventricular hypertrophy. Circulation 60:386, 1979.
55. Cameron JS, Myerburg RJ, Wong SS, et al: Electrophysiologic consequences of chronic experimentally induced left ventricular pressure overload. J Am Coll Cardiol 2:481, 1983.
56. Casale PN, Devereux RB, Kligfield P, et al: Electrocardiographic detection of left ventricular hypertrophy: development and validation of improved criteria. J Am Coll Cardiol 6:572, 1985.
57. Romhilt DW, Bove KE, Norris RJ, et al: A critical appraisal of the electrocardiographic criteria for the diagnosis of left ventricular hypertrophy. Circulation 60:185, 1969.
58. Murphy ML, Thenabadu PN, de Soyza N, et al: Re-evaluation of electrocardiographic criteria for left, right and combined cardiac ventricular hypertrophy. Am J Cardiol 53:1140, 1984.
59. Sokolow M, Lyon TP: The ventricular complex in left ventricular hypertrophy as obtained by unipolar precordial and limb leads. Am Heart J 37:161, 1949.
60. Romhilt DW, Estes EH: A point-score system for the ECG diagnosis of left ventricular hypertrophy. Am Heart J 75:752, 1968.
61. Casale PN, Devereux RB, Alonso DR, et al: Improved sex-specific criteria of left ventricular hypertrophy for clinical and computer interpretation of electrocardiograms: validation with autopsy findings. Circulation 75:565, 1987.
62. Sokolow M, Lyon TP: The ventricular complex in right ventricular hypertrophy as obtained by unipolar precordial and limb leads. Am Heart J 38:273, 1949.
63. Myers GB, Klein HA, Stoffer BE: The electrocardiographic diagnosis of right ventricular hypertrophy. Am Heart J 35:1, 1948.
64. Murphy ML, Thenabadu PN, Blue LR, et al: Descriptive characteristics of the electrocardiogram from autopsied men free of cardiopulmonary disease—a basis for evaluating criteria for ventricular hypertrophy. Am J Cardiol 52:1275, 1983.
65. Pagnoni A, Goodwin JF: The cardiographic diagnosis of combined ventricular hypertrophy. Br Heart J 14:451, 1952.
66. Katz LN, Wachtel H: The diphasic QRS type of electrocardiogram in congenital heart disease. Am Heart J 13:202, 1937.
67. Klein RC, Vera Z, DeMaria AN, et al: Electrocardiographic diagnosis of left ventricular hypertrophy in the presence of left bundle branch block. Am Heart J 108:502, 1984.
68. Kafka H, Burggraf GW, Milliken JA: Electrocardiographic diagnosis of left ventricular hypertrophy in the presence of left bundle branch block: an echocardiographic study. Am J Cardiol 55:103, 1985.
69. Haveld CJ, Sohi GS, Flowers NC, et al: The pathologic correlates of the electrocardiogram: complete left bundle branch block. Circulation 65:445, 1982.
70. Cokkinos DV, Demopoulas JN, Heimonas ET, et al: Electrocardiographic criteria of LVH in LBBB. Br Heart J 40:320, 1978.
71. Vandenberg B, Sagar K, Paulsen W, et al: Electrocardiographic criteria for diagnosis of left ventricular hypertrophy in the presence of complete right bundle branch block. Am J Cardiol 63:1080, 1989.
72. DeLeonardis V, Goldstein SA, Lindsay J Jr: Electrocardiographic diagnosis of left ventricular hypertrophy in the presence of complete right bundle branch block. Am J Cardiol 62:590, 1988.
73. Murphy ML, Thenabadu N, de Soyza N, et al: Left atrial abnormality as an electrocardiographic criterion for the diagnosis of left ventricular hypertrophy in the presence of left bundle branch block. Am J Cardiol 52:381, 1983.
74. Blondeau M: Complete left bundle branch block with marked left axis deviation of QRS: clinical and anatomic study. Adv Cardiol 14:25, 1975.
75. Dhingra RC, Amat-Y-Leon F, Wyndham C, et al: Significance of left axis deviation in patients with chronic left bundle branch block. Am J Cardiol 42:551, 1978.
76. Swiryn S, Abben R, Denes P, et al: Electrocardiographic determinants of axis during left bundle branch block: study in patients with intermittent left bundle branch block. Am J Cardiol 46:53, 1980.
77. Rosenbaum MB, Elizari MV, Lazzari JO: The Hemiblocks: New Concepts of Intraventricular Conduction Based on Human Anatomical, Physiological, and Clinical Studies. Oldsmar FL: Tampa Tracings, 1970.

78. Hands ME, Cook EF, Stone PH, et al: Electrocardiographic diagnosis of myocardial infarction in the presence of complete left bundle branch block. Am Heart J 116:23, 1988.
79. Rhoads DV, Edwards JE, Pruitt RD: The electrocardiogram in the presence of myocardial infarction and intraventricular block of the left bundle branch block type. Am Heart J 62:735, 1961.
80. Fesmire FM: ECG diagnosis of acute myocardial infarction in the presence of left bundle branch block in patients undergoing continuous ECG monitoring. Ann Emerg Med 26:69, 1995.
81. Sgarbossa EB, Pinski SL, Barbagelata A, et al: Electrocardiographic diagnosis of evolving acute myocardial infarction in the presence of left bundle branch block. N Engl J Med 334:481, 1996.
82. Grines CL, Bashore TM, Boudoulas H, et al: Functional abnormalities in isolated left bundle branch block. Circulation 79:845, 1989.
83. Hirzel HO, Senn M, Nuesch K, et al: Thallium-201 scintigraphy in complete left bundle branch block. Am J Cardiol 53:764, 1984.
84. Barrett PA, Peter CT, Swan HJC, et al: The frequency and prognostic significance of electrocardiographic abnormalities in clinically normal individuals. Prog Cardiovasc Dis 23:299, 1981.
85. Schneider JF, Thomas HE, McNamara PM, et al: Clinical-electrocardiographic correlates of newly acquired left bundle branch block: the Framingham study. Am J Cardiol 55:1332, 1985.
86. Schneider JF, Thomas HE, Kreger BE, et al: Newly acquired left bundle branch block: the Framingham study. Ann Intern Med 90:303, 1979.
87. Freedman RA, Alderman EL, Sheffield IT, et al: Bundle branch block in patients with chronic coronary artery disease: angiographic correlates and prognostic significance. J Am Coll Cardiol 10:73, 1987.
88. Rabkin SW, Mathewson FAL, Tate RB: Natural history of left bundle branch block. Br Heart J 43:164, 1980.
89. Brugada P, Brugada J: A distinct clinical and electrocardiographic syndrome: right bundle branch block, persistent ST segment elevation with normal QT interval and sudden cardiac death [abstract]. Pacing Clin Electrophysiol 14:746, 1991.
90. Brugada P, Brugada J: Right bundle branch block, persistent ST segment elevation and sudden cardiac death: a distinct clinical and electrocardiographic syndrome. A multicenter report. J Am Coll Cardiol 20:1391, 1992.
91. Brugada P, Geelen P, Brugada J: Further observations on the syndrome of a right bundle branch block with ST segment elevation and sudden cardiac death. N Trends Arrhythmias 9:333–334, 1993.
92. Fontaine G, Piot O, Sohal P, et al: Right precordial leads and sudden death. Relation with arrhythmogenic right ventricular dysplasia. Arch Mal Coeur Vaiss 89:1323, 1996.
93. Gussak I, Antzelevitch C, Bjerregaard P, et al: The Brugada syndrome: clinical, electrophysiologic, and genetic aspects. J Am Coll Cardiol 33:5, 1999.
94. Yan GX, Antzelevitch C: Cellular basis for idiopathic VT/VF syndrome [abstract]. Circulation 94:I-625, 1996.
95. Yan GX, Antzelevitch C: Cellular basis for the electrocardiographic J wave. Circulation 93:372, 1996.
96. Antzelevitch C, Nesterenko VV, Yan GX: Ionic processes underlying the action potential. *In* Liebman J (ed): Electrocardiology '96: From the Cell to the Body Surface. p. 219. Singapore: World Scientific, 1996.
97. Chen Q, Kirsch GE, Zhang D, et al: Genetic basis and molecular mechanisms for idiopathic ventricular fibrillation. Nature 392:293, 1998.
98. Massing GK, James TN: Conduction and block in the right bundle branch: real and imagined. Circulation 45:1, 1972.
99. Moore EN, Boineau JP, Patterson DF: Incomplete right bundle branch block: an electrocardiographic enigma and possible misnomer. Circulation 44:678, 1971.
100. Liao Y, Emidy LA, Dyer A, et al: Characteristics and prognosis of incomplete right bundle branch block: an epidemiologic study. J Am Coll Cardiol 7:492, 1986.
101. Rotman M, Triebwasser JH: A clinical and follow-up study of right and left bundle branch block. Circulation 51:477, 1975.
102. Siegman-Igra Y, Yahini JH, Goldbourt U, et al: Intraventricular conduction disturbances: a review of prevalence, etiology, and progression for ten years within a stable population of Israeli adult males. Am Heart J 96:669, 1978.
103. Ostrander LD: Bundle branch block. An epidemiologic study. Circulation 30:872, 1964.
104. Fahy GJ, Pinski SL, Miller DP, et al: Natural history of isolated bundle branch block. Am J Cardiol 77:1185, 1996.
105. Lev M: Anatomic basis for AV block. Am J Med 37:742, 1964.
106. Lenegre J: Etiology and pathology of bilateral bundle branch block in relation to complete heart block. Prog Cardiovasc Dis 6:409, 1964.
107. Stephan E, deMeeus A, Bouvagnet P: Hereditary bundle branch block: right bundle branch blocks of different causes have different morphologic characteristics. Am Heart J 133:249, 1997.
108. Esscher E, Hardell LI, Michaelsson M: Familial, isolated, complete right bundle branch block. Br Heart J 37:745, 1975.
109. Denes P, Wu D, Dhingra RC, et al: Electrophysiological observations in patients with rate dependent bundle branch block. Circulation 51:244, 1975.
110. El-Sherif N: Tachycardia-dependent versus bradycardia-dependent intermittent bundle branch block. Br Heart J 34:167, 1972.
111. Willems JL, Robles de Medina EO, Bernard R, et al: Criteria for intraventricular conduction disturbances and pre-excitation. J Am Coll Cardiol 5:1261, 1985.
112. Warner RA: Recent advances in the diagnosis of myocardial infarction. Cardiol Clin 5:381, 1987.
113. Castellanos A, Pina IL, Zaman L, et al: Recent advances in the diagnosis of fascicular blocks. Cardiol Clin 5:469, 1987.
114. Hiss RG, Lamb LE, Allen MF: Electrocardiographic findings in 67,375 asymptomatic subjects. X. Normal values. Am J Cardiol 6:200, 1960.
115. Narula OS: Longitudinal dissociation in the HIS bundle. Bundle branch block due to asynchronous conduction within the HIS bundle in man. Circulation 56:996, 1977.
115a. Ostrander Jr LD: Left axis deviation: prevalence, associated conditions, and prognosis. An epidemiologic study. Ann Intern Med 75:23, 1971.
116. Flowers NC: Left bundle branch block: a continuously evolving concept. J Am Coll Cardiol 9:684, 1987.
117. Barold SS: ACC/AHA guidelines for implantation of cardiac pacemakers: how accurate are the definitions of atrioventricular and intraventricular conduction blocks? Pacing Clin Electrophysiol 16:1221, 1993.
118. Denes P, Dhingra RC, Wu D, et al: H-V interval in patients with bifascicular block (right bundle branch block and left anterior hemiblock). Clinical, electrocardiographic and electrophysiologic correlations. Am J Cardiol 35:23, 1975.
119. McAnulty JH, Rahimtoola SH, Murphy E, et al: Natural history of "high risk" bundle branch block. N Engl J Med 307:137, 1982.
120. Dhingra RC, Wyndham C, Bauerfeind R, et al: Significance of chronic bifascicular block without apparent organic heart disease. Circulation 60:33, 1979.
121. Newby KH, Pisano E, Krucoff MW, et al: Incidence and clinical relevance of the occurrence of bundle branch block in patients treated with thrombolytic therapy. Circulation 94:2424, 1996.
122. Wolff L, Parkinson J, White PD: Bundle branch block with short PR interval in healthy young people prone to paroxysmal tachycardia. Am Heart J 5:685, 1930.
123. Becker AE, Anderson RH: The Wolff-Parkinson-White syndrome and its anatomical substrates. Anat Rec 201:169, 1981.
124. Reddy GV, Schamroth L: The localization of bypass tracts in the Wolff-Parkinson-White syndrome from the surface electrocardiogram. Am Heart J 113:984, 1987.
125. Milstein S, Sharma AD, Guiraudon GM, et al: An algorithm for the electrocardiographic localization of accessory pathways in the Wolff-Parkinson-White syndrome. Pacing Clin Electrophysiol 10:555, 1987.
126. Lindsay BD, Crossen KJ, Cain ME: Concordance of distinguishing electrocardiographic features during sinus rhythm with the location of accessory pathways in the Wolff-Parkinson-White syndrome. Am J Cardiol 59:1093, 1987.
127. Yuan S, Iwa T, Bando T, et al: Comparative study of eight sets of ECG criteria for the localization of the accessory pathway in Wolff-Parkinson-White syndrome. J Electrocardiol 25:203, 1992.
128. Colavita PG, Packer DL, Pressley GC, et al: Frequency, diagnosis, and clinical characteristics of patients with multiple accessory atrioventricular pathways. Am J Cardiol 59:601, 1987.
129. Gallagher JJ, Kasell J, Sealy WC, et al: The preexcitation syndromes. Prog Cardiovasc Dis 20:285, 1978.
130. Fozzard HA, Makielski JC: The electrophysiology of acute myocardial ischemia. Annu Rev Med 36:275, 1985.

131. Hill JL, Gettes LS: Effect of acute coronary artery occlusion on local myocardial extracellular K^+ activity in swine. Circulation 61:768, 1980.
132. Katz AM, Messiner FC: Lipid-membrane interactions and the pathogenesis of ischemic damage in the myocardium. Circ Res 48:1, 1981.
133. Kleber AG: Resting membrane potential, extracellular potassium activity and intracellular sodium activity during acute global ischemia in isolated perfused guinea pig hearts. Circ Res 52:242, 1983.
134. Prinzmetal M, Ishikawa K, Nakashima M, et al: Correlation between intracellular and surface electrograms in acute myocardial ischemia. J Electrocardiol 1:161, 1968.
135. Samson WE, Scher AM: Mechanism of ST segment alteration during acute myocardial injury. Circ Res 8:780, 1960.
136. Wagner NB, Sevilla DC, Krucoff MK, et al: Transient alterations of the QRS complex and ST segment during percutaneous transluminal balloon angioplasty of the left anterior descending coronary artery. Am J Cardiol 62:1038, 1988.
137. Surawicz B: Abnormalities of ventricular repolarization. *In* Electrophysiologic Basis of ECG and Cardiac Arrhythmias. p. 566. Baltimore: Williams & Wilkins, 1995.
138. Figueras J, Cinca J, Gutiérrez L, et al: Prolonged angina pectoris and persistent negative T waves in the precordial leads: response to atrial pacing and to methoxamine-induced hypertension. Am J Cardiol 51:1599, 1983.
139. Rude RE, Poole WK, Muller JE, et al: Electrocardiographic and clinical criteria for recognition of acute myocardial infarction based on analysis of 3,697 patients. Am J Cardiol 52:963, 1983.
140. Schwietzer P: The electrocardiographic diagnosis of acute myocardial infarction in the thrombolytic era. Am Heart J 119:642, 1990.
141. Madias JE: The "giant R waves" ECG pattern of hyperacute phase of myocardial infarction. J Electrocardiol 26:77, 1993.
142. Yusuf S, Lopez R, Maddison A, et al: Variability of electrocardiographic and enzyme evolution of myocardial infarction in man. Br Heart J 45:271, 1981.
143. Tzivoni D, Chenzbraun A: The significance of ST abnormalities in myocardial infarction. Cardiol Clin 5:419, 1987.
144. Mills RM, Young E, Gorlin R, et al: Natural history of S-T segment elevation after acute myocardial infarction. Am J Cardiol 35:609, 1975.
145. Arvan S, Varat MA: Persistent ST-segment elevation and left ventricular wall abnormalities. A 2-dimensional echocardiographic study. Am J Cardiol 53:1542, 1984.
146. Ogawa H, Hiramoor K, Haze K, et al: Classification of non–Q wave myocardial infarction according to electrocardiographic changes. Br Heart J 54:473, 1985.
147. Granborg J, Grande P, Pedersen A: Diagnostic and prognostic implications of transient, isolated negative T waves in suspected acute myocardial infarction. Am J Cardiol 57:203, 1986.
148. Zalenski RJ, Cooke D, Rydman R, et al: Assessing the diagnostic value of an ECG containing leads V_4R, V_8 and V_9: the 15-lead ECG. Ann Emerg Med 22:786, 1993.
149. Blanke H, Cohen M, Schlueter GU, et al: Electrocardiographic and coronary arteriographic correlations during acute myocardial infarction. Am J Cardiol 54:249, 1984.
150. Aldrich HR, Hindman NB, Hinoara T, et al: Identification of optimal electrocardiographic leads for detecting acute epicardial injury in acute myocardial infarction. Am J Cardiol 59:20, 1987.
151. Sgarbossa EB, Thompson T, Pinski SL, et al: Bedside identification of proximal LAD occlusion in patients with acute myocardial infarction [abstract]. Circulation 94:I-669, 1996.
152. Kontos MC, Desai PV, Jesse RL, et al: Usefulness of the admission electrocardiogram for identifying the infarct-related artery in inferior wall myocardial infarction. Am J Cardiol 79:182, 1997.
153. Braat SH, Brugada P, DenDulk K, et al: Value of lead V_4R for recognition of the infarct coronary in acute inferior myocardial infarction. Am J Cardiol 53:1538, 1984.
154. Andersen HR, Falk E, Nielsen D: Right ventricular infarction: diagnostic accuracy of electrocardiographic right chest leads V_3R to V_7R investigated prospectively in 43 consecutive fatal cases from a coronary care unit. Br Heart J 61:514, 1989.
155. Chou TC, van der Bel-Kahn J, Allen J: Electrocardiographic diagnosis of right ventricular infarction. Am J Med 70:1175, 1981.
156. Lopez-Sendon J, Coma-Canella I, Alcasena S, et al: Electrocardiographic findings in acute right ventricular infarction: sensitivity and specificity of electrocardiographic alterations in right precordial leads V_4R, V_3R, V_1, V_2, and V_3. J Am Coll Cardiol 6:1273, 1985.
157. Ilia R, Margulis G, Goldfarb B, et al: ST elevation in leads V_1 to V_4 caused by isolated right ventricular ischemia and infarction. Cardiology 74:396, 1987.
158. Ben-Gal T, Sclarovsky S, Herz I, et al: Importance of the conal branch of the right coronary artery in patients with acute anterior wall myocardial infarction: electrocardiographic and angiographic correlation. J Am Coll Cardiol 29:506, 1997.
159. Huey BL, Beller GA, Kaiser DL, et al: A comprehensive analysis of myocardial infarction due to left circumflex artery occlusion. Comparison with infarction due to right coronary artery and left anterior descending artery occlusion. J Am Coll Cardiol 12:1156, 1988.
160. Kulkarni AU, Brown R, Ayoubi M, et al: Clinical use of posterior electrocardiographic leads: a prospective electrocardiographic analysis during coronary occlusion. Am Heart J 131:736, 1996.
161. Boden WE, Kleiger RE, Gibson RS, et al: Electrocardiographic evolution of posterior myocardial infarction: importance of early precordial ST-depression. Am J Cardiol 59:782, 1987.
162. Mirvis DM: Physiologic bases for anterior ST segment depression in patients with acute inferior wall myocardial infarction. Am Heart J 116:1308, 1988.
163. Schamroth L (ed): Electrocardiology of Coronary Artery Disease. 2nd ed. Oxford: Blackwell Scientific, 1984.
164. Selvester RH, Wagner GS, Ideker RE: Myocardial infarction. *In* Macfarlane PW, Lawrie TDV (eds): Comprehensive Electrocardiology. Theory and Practice in Health and Disease. New York: Pergamon, 1989.
165. Freifeld AG, Schuster EH, Bulkley BH: Nontransmural versus transmural myocardial infarction. A morphologic study. Am J Med 75:423, 1983.
166. Raunio H, Rissanen V, Romppanen T, et al: Changes in the QRS complex and ST segment in transmural and subendocardial myocardial infarctions. A clinicopathologic study. Am Heart J 98:176, 1979.
167. Selwyn AP, Fox K, Welman E, et al: Natural history and evaluation of Q waves during acute myocardial infarction. Br Heart J 40:383, 1978.
168. Yusuf S, Lopez R, Maddison A, et al: Variability of electrocardiographic and enzyme evolution of myocardial infarction in man. Br Heart J 45:271, 1981.
169. Klainman E, Sclarovsky S, Lewin RF, et al: Natural course of electrocardiographic components and stages in the first twelve hours of acute myocardial infarction. J Electrocardiol 20:98, 1987.
170. Coll S, Betriu A, De Flores T, et al: Significance of Q-wave regression after transmural acute myocardial infarction. Am J Cardiol 61:739, 1988.
171. Montague TJ, Johnstone DE, Spencer CA, et al: Electrocardiographic and ventriculographic recovery pattern in Q wave myocardial infarction. J Am Coll Cardiol 8:521, 1986.
172. Barold SS, Falkoff MD, Ong LS, et al: Significance of transient electrocardiographic Q waves in coronary artery disease. Cardiol Clin 5:367, 1987.
173. Timmis GC: Electrocardiographic effects of reperfusion. Cardiol Clin 5:427, 1987.
174. Kaplan BM, Berkson DM: Serial electrocardiograms after myocardial infarction. Ann Intern Med 60:430, 1964.
175. Braunwald E, Kloner RA: The stunned myocardium: prolonged postischemic ventricular dysfunction. Circulation 66:1146, 1982.
176. Bashour TT, Kabbani SS, Brewster HP, et al: Transient Q waves and reversible cardiac failure during myocardial ischemia. Electrical and mechanical stunning of the heart. Am Heart J 106:780, 1983.
177. Haiat R, Chiche P: Transient abnormal Q waves in the course of ischemic heart disease. Chest 65:140, 1974.
178. Rahimtoola SH: The hibernating myocardium. Am Heart J 117:211, 1989.
179. Takatsu F, Kawai S, Okada R, et al: The presence of small q waves and decreased precordial r waves indicates a small amount of fibrosis of the anterior myocardial wall. J Electrocardiol 26:9, 1993.
180. Warner RA, Reger M, Hill NE, et al: Electrocardiographic criteria for the diagnosis of anterior myocardial infarction: importance of the duration of precordial R waves. Am J Cardiol 52:690, 1983.
181. Flowers NC, Horan LG, Johnson JC: Anterior infarctional changes occurring during mid and late ventricular activation detectable by surface mapping techniques. Circulation 54:906, 1976.
182. Flowers NC, Horan LG, Sohi GS, et al: New evidence for inferoposterior myocardial infarction on surface potential maps. Am J Cardiol 38:576, 1976.

183. Dwyer EM: The predictive accuracy of the electrocardiogram in identifying the presence and location of myocardial infarction and coronary artery disease. Ann N Y Acad Sci 601:67, 1990.
184. Horan LG, Flowers NC, Johnson JC: Significance of the diagnostic Q wave of myocardial infarction. Circulation 43:428, 1971.
185. Ideker RE, Wagner GS, Ruth WK, et al: Evaluation of a QRS scoring system for estimating myocardial infarct size. II. Correlation with quantitative anatomic findings for anterior infarcts. Am J Cardiol 49:1604, 1982.
186. Roark SF, Ideker RE, Wagner GS, et al: Evaluation of a QRS scoring system for estimating myocardial infarct size. III. Correlation with quantitative anatomic findings for inferior infarcts. Am J Cardiol 51:382, 1983.
187. Wagner GS, Freye CJ, Palmeri ST, et al: Evaluation of a QRS scoring system for estimating myocardial infarct size. I. Specificity and observer agreement. Circulation 65:342, 1982.
188. Ward RM, White RD, Ideker RE: Evaluation of a QRS scoring system for estimating myocardial infarct size. IV: Correlation with quantitative anatomic findings for posterolateral infarcts. Am J Cardiol 53:706, 1984.
189. Warner RA, Reger M, Hill NE, et al: Electrocardiographic criteria for the diagnosis of anterior myocardial infarction: importance of the duration of precordial R waves. Am J Cardiol 52:690, 1983.
190. Zema MJ, Collins M, Alonso DR, et al: Electrocardiographic poor R-wave progression: correlation with postmortem findings. Chest 79:195, 1981.
191. Bough EW, Boden WE, Korr KS, et al: Left ventricular asynergy in electrocardiographic "posterior" myocardial infarction. J Am Coll Cardiol 4:209, 1984.
192. Brembilla-Perrot B, Terrier de la Chaise A, Isaaz K, et al: The tall R wave in lead V_1 in posterior myocardial infarction: a reciprocal sign or a HIS-Purkinje conduction disturbance. Pacing Clin Electrophysiol 12:1650, 1989.
193. Savage RM, Wagner GS, Ideker RE, et al: Correlation of postmortem anatomic findings with electrocardiographic changes in patients with myocardial infarction. Circulation 55:279, 1977.
194. Sullivan W, Vlodaver Z, Tuna N, et al: Correlation of electrocardiographic and pathologic findings in healed myocardial infarction. Am J Cardiol 42:724, 1978.
195. Roberts WC, Cardin JM: Location of myocardial infarcts: a confusion of terms and definitions. Am J Cardiol 42:868, 1978.
196. Kaplan BM, Berkson DM: Serial electrocardiograms after myocardial infarction. Ann Intern Med 60:430, 1964.
197. Myers GB, Klein HA, Stoffer BE: Correlation of electrocardiographic and pathologic findings in anteroseptal infarction. Am Heart J 36:535, 1948.
198. Shalev T, Fogelman M, Oettinger M, et al: Does the electrocardiographic pattern of anteroseptal myocardial infarction correlate with the anatomic location of myocardial injury? Am J Cardiol 75:763, 1995.
199. Tamura A, Kataoka H, Mikuriya Y: Electrocardiographic findings in a patient with pure septal infarction. Br Heart J 65:166, 1991.
200. Palmeri ST, Harrison DG, Cobb FR, et al: A QRS scoring system for assessing left ventricular function after myocardial infarction. N Engl J Med 306:4, 1982.
201. Mirvis DM: Electrocardiography. A Physiologic Approach. St. Louis: Mosby–Year Book, 1993.
202. Boden WE, Gibdon RS, Schectman KB, et al: ST segment shifts are poor predictors of subsequent Q wave evolution in acute myocardial infarction. Circulation 79:537, 1989.
203. Willems JL, Willems RJ, Willems GM, et al: Significance of initial ST segment elevation and depression for the management of the thrombolytic therapy in acute myocardial infarction. European Cooperative Study Group for Recombinant Tissue Type Plasminogen Activator. Circulation 82:1147, 1990.
204. Park SE, Tani A, Minamino T, et al: Coronary angiographic features within 48 hours from onset of non–Q wave myocardial infarction with R wave regression and no ST segment depression. Cardiology 77:121, 1990.
205. Chamorro H, Barquin I, Gómez P, et al: Angiographic findings in non–Q wave infarction and their relation to ST-T changes. Rev Méd Chile 120:644, 1992.
206. Poehlman JH, Silverman ME: Clinical characteristics, electrocardiographic and enzyme correlations, and long-term prognosis of patients with chest pain associated with ST depression and/or T wave inversion. Am Heart J 99:173, 1980.
207. Sgarbossa EB, Topol EJ: Semantic ambiguity, the "non"-nosology and myocardial infarction. J Clin Epidemiol 47:441, 1994.
208. Maeda S: Different clinical implications for ST depression and T wave inversion in non–Q wave myocardial infarction. J Cardiol 24:357, 1994.
209. Spodick DH: Q-wave infarction versus S-T infarction. Nonspecificity of electrocardiographic criteria for differentiating transmural and nontransmural lesions. Am J Cardiol 52:913, 1983.
210. Hesse A, Altland K, Linke RP, et al: Cardiac amyloidosis: a review and report of a new transthyretin (prealbumin) variant. Br Heart J 70:111, 1993.
211. Yotsukura M, Miyagawa M, Tsuya T, et al: A 10-year follow-up study by orthogonal Frank lead ECG on patients with progressive muscular dystrophy of the Duchenne type. J Electrocardiol 25:345, 1992.
212. Manthous CA, Schmidt GA: Pleural effusion masquerading as myocardial infarction. Chest 103:1619, 1993.
213. Autenrieth G, Surawicz B, Kuo CS, et al: Primary T wave abnormalities caused by uniform and regional shortening of ventricular monophasic action potential in dog. Circulation 51:668, 1975.
214. VanderArk CR, Ballantyne F III, Reynolds EW Jr: Electrolytes and the electrocardiogram. Cardiovasc Clin 5:269, 1973.
215. Reddy GV, Schamroth L, Schamroth CL: Tall and peaked U waves in hypokalemia. Chest 91:605, 1987.
216. Surawicz B: Electrolytes, hormones, temperature and miscellaneous factors. *In* Electrophysiologic Basis of ECG and Cardiac Arrhythmias. p. 426. Baltimore: Williams & Wilkins, 1995.
217. Ahmed R, Yano K, Mitsuoka T, et al: Changes in T wave morphology during hypercalcemia and its relations to the severity of hypercalcemia. J Electrocardiol 22:125, 1989.
218. Lind L, Ljunghall S: Serum calcium and the ECG in patients with primary hyperparathyroidism. J Electrocardiol 27:99, 1994.
219. Vangt EJ, Wellens HJJ: The electrocardiogram in digitalis intoxication. *In* Wellens HJJ (ed): What's New in Electrocardiography? p. 315. Hingham, MA: Kluwer Academic, 1981.
220. Thomas SH: Drugs, QT interval abnormalities and ventricular arrhythmias. Adv Drug Reac Toxicol Rev 13:77, 1994.
221. Hanrahan JP, Choo PW, Carlson W, et al: Terfenadine-associated ventricular arrhythmias and QTc interval prolongation: a retrospective cohort comparison with other antihistamines among members of a health maintenance organization. Ann Epidemiol 5:201, 1995.
222. Zipes DP, Wellens HJJ: Sudden cardiac death. Circulation 98:2334, 1998.
223. Rosenbaum MB, Blanco HH, Elizari MV, et al: Electronic modulation of the T wave and cardiac memory. Am J Cardiol 50:213, 1982.
224. Engel JR, Shah R, De Podesta LA, et al: T wave abnormalities of intermittent left bundle branch block. Ann Intern Med 89:204, 1978.
225. Helguera ME, Pinski SL, Sterba R, et al: Memory T waves after radiofrequency ablation of accessory atrioventricular connections in the WPW syndrome. J Electrocardiol 27:243, 1994.
226. del Balzo U, Rosen MR: T wave changes persisting after ventricular pacing in canine heart are altered by 4-aminopyridine but not by lidocaine. Implications with respect to phenomenon of cardiac "memory." Circulation 85:1464, 1992.
227. Wood MA, DiMarco JP, Haines DE: Electrocardiographic abnormalities after radiofrequency catheter ablation of accessory bypass tracts in the Wolff-Parkinson-White syndrome. Am J Cardiol 70:200, 1992.
228. Surawicz B, Fisch C: Cardiac alternans: diverse mechanisms and clinical manifestations. J Am Coll Cardiol 20:483, 1992.
229. Tighe DA, Chung EK, Park CH: Electrical alternans associated with acute pulmonary embolism. Am Heart J 128:188, 1994.
230. Surawicz B: Abnormalities of ventricular repolarization. *In* Electrophysiologic Basis of ECG and Cardiac Arrhythmias. p. 566. Baltimore, Williams & Wilkins, 1995.
231. Navarro-Lòpez F, Cinca J, Sanz G, et al: Isolated T-wave alternans. Am Heart J 95:369, 1978.
232. Bardaji A, Vidal F, Richart C: T wave alternans associated with amiodarone. J Electrocardiol 26:155, 1993.
233. Verrier RL, Nearing BD: Electrophysiologic basis for T wave alternans as an index of vulnerability to ventricular fibrillation. J Cardiovasc Electrophysiol 5:445, 1994.
234. Rosenbaum DS, Jackson LE, Smith JM, et al: Electrical alternans and vulnerability to ventricular arrhythmias. N Engl J Med 330:235, 1994.

235. Zareba W, Moss AJ, le Cessie S, et al: T wave alternans in idiopathic long QT syndrome. J Am Coll Cardiol 23:1541, 1994.
236. Kishida H, Cole JS, Surawicz B: Negative U wave: a highly specific but poorly understood sign of heart disease. Am J Cardiol 49:2030, 1982.
237. Twidale N, Gallagher AW, Tonkin AM: Echocardiographic study of U wave inversion in the electrocardiograms of hypertensive patients. J Electrocardiol 22:365, 1989.
238. Miwa K, Miyagi Y, Fujita M, et al: Transient terminal U wave inversion as a wave specific marker for myocardial ischemia. Am Heart J 125:981, 1993.
239. Gerson MC, Phillips JF, Morris SN, et al: Exercise-induced U wave inversion as a marker of stenosis of the left anterior descending coronary artery. Circulation 60:1014, 1979.
240. Roden DM, Lazzara R, Rosen M, et al: Multiple mechanisms in the long-QT syndrome: current knowledge, gaps and future directions. Circulation 94:1996, 1996.
241. Jackman WM, Friday KJ, Anderson JI, et al: The long QT syndromes: a critical review, new clinical observations and unifying hypothesis. Prog Cardiovasc Dis 31:115, 1988.
242. Haisty WK, Pahlm O, Edenbrandt L, et al: Recognition of electrocardiographic electrode misplacements involving the ground (right leg) electrode. Am J Cardiol 71:1490, 1993.
243. Hedén B, Ohlsson M, Holst H, et al: Detection of frequently overlooked electrocardiographic lead reversals using artificial neural networks. Am J Cardiol 78:600, 1996.
244. Nielsen TT, Lund O, Kønne K, et al: Changing electrocardiographic findings in relation to vascular obstruction. Cardiology 76:274, 1989.
245. Sreeram N, Cheriex EC, Smeets JLRM, et al: Value of the 12-lead electrocardiogram at hospital admission in the diagnosis of pulmonary embolism. Am J Cardiol 73:298, 1994.
246. Sodi-Pallares D, Bisteni A, Hermann GR: Some views on the significance of qR and QR type complexes in right precordial leads in the absence of myocardial infarction. Am Heart J 43:716, 1952.
247. Burch GE, Meyers K, Abildskov JA: A new electrocardiographic pattern observed in cerebrovascular accidents. Circulation 9:719, 1954.
248. Yamour BJ, Sridharan MR, Rice JF, et al: Electrocardiographic changes in cerebrovascular hemorrhage. Am Heart J 99:294, 1980.
249. Hugenholz PG: Electrocardiographic changes typical for central nervous system after right radical neck dissection. Am Heart J 74:438, 1967.
250. Gould L, Gopalaswami C, Chandy F, et al: Electroconvulsive therapy–induced ECG changes simulating a myocardial infarction. Arch Intern Med 143:1786, 1983.
251. Clements SD, Hurst JW: Diagnostic value of electrocardiographic abnormalities observed in subjects accidentally exposed to cold. Am J Cardiol 29:729, 1972.
252. Gao S, Hunt SA, Widerhold V, et al: Characteristics of serial electrocardiograms in heart transplant recipients. Am Heart J 122:771, 1991.

CHAPTER 3

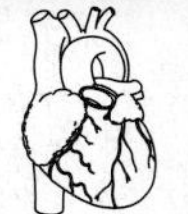

Principles of Chest Radiography

John H. Harris, Jr.

PRINCIPLES OF RADIOLOGIC TECHNIQUE
PRINCIPLES REGARDING THE CHEST X-RAY ITSELF
PRINCIPLES FOR ASSESSING THE RADIOGRAPHIC EXAMINATION
PATHOPHYSIOLOGIC PRINCIPLES PERTAINING TO THE RADIOGRAPHIC SIGNS OF CARDIOVASCULAR DISEASE
Heart
Aorta
Pulmonary Vasculature
Pulmonary Venous Hypertension
Pulmonary Arterial Hypertension
Pulmonary Embolism

Even in this age of high technological imaging, the conventional radiographic examination of the chest remains a cornerstone of clinical cardiology. Conventional chest radiography is universally available, relatively inexpensive, and cost-effective; it records cardiovascular abnormalities that are clinically silent as well as those that are not and provides an effective method of monitoring the status of cardiovascular disease and the effects of patient response to therapy. The static chest radiograph (CXR) does, indeed, reflect hemodynamic changes of pulmonary vasculature that occur secondary to cardiac disease.

The title of this chapter defines its contents. No attempt is made to describe in detail or in a definitive fashion any of the signs of cardiovascular disease as recorded by conventional chest radiography. For the purpose of discussion, the principles related to the interpretation of CXRs of patients with cardiovascular disease may be categorized into (1) those pertaining to radiographic technique, for example, radiologic technical factors that produce the image; (2) those regarding the radiographic examination itself, including routine and useful additional views, radiographic anatomy appropriate to cardiovascular disease, and nonpathologic conditions that effect the appearance of the cardiovascular system on chest radiography; (3) those that assess the radiographic examination; and finally, (4) pathophysiologic factors pertaining to the signs of cardiovascular disease as recorded on the CXR.

Principles of Radiologic Technique

A commonly misunderstood, or overlooked, platitude relative to chest radiography is that the purpose of the CXR is to enable one to clearly visualize the cardiomediastinal anatomy and the lungs (parenchyma, bronchi, and vessels) on the posteroanterior (PA) and lateral radiographs, for example, *image clarity,* defined as "the visibility of diagnostically important detail in the radiograph."[1] Optimal CXR images (Fig. 3–1) are the product of appropriate utilization of peak kilovoltage, amperage, and time, expressed as milliampere-seconds.[1] Equally important factors include the characteristics of the x-ray generator; the target film distance (72 inches); compatible film-screen combinations; the appropriate use of a "grid" (Potter-Bucky diaphragm), either stationary or reciprocating, to reduce scattered (secondary) radiation that commonly results from radiographic techniques required to obtain diagnostic chest examinations of patients with a large body habitus; and carefully controlled film processing. Matched film-screen systems are readily available from many manufacturers, including Kodak, 3-M, Agfa, and Sterling, to name a few.

It is a commonly held misconception[2] that the PA CXR is only "properly" exposed when the thoracic spine is visible through the cardiac shadow, thereby enabling one to see the lungs and diaphragm "behind the heart." To visualize the spine through the cardiac shadow requires a relatively "strong" (penetrating) x-ray beam, which usually results in either overexposure (Fig. 3–2) of the radiograph or secondary ("scattered," Compton) radiation "fog" (Fig. 3–3), both of which can obscure the pulmonary interstitium, bronchi, and pulmonary vessels. Radiation fog reduces image clarity by reducing image contrast.[3] Since the majority of radiographic chest examinations are obtained in both PA and lateral projections, the "lung behind the heart" is clearly demonstrated on the lateral radiograph. Overexposure of the CXR is appropriate in patients sustaining major blunt chest trauma in which it is critical to visualize the mediastinal soft tissue structures and the pulmonary parenchyma behind the heart, and in intensive care unit patients, where only a supine bedside examination is possible in order to enable some assessment of the lung base and the medial aspect of the diaphragm.

Principles Regarding the Chest X-Ray Itself

The routine radiographic examination of the chest includes the PA and lateral projections. Each is obtained with the patient erect and, whenever possible, in deep inspiration.

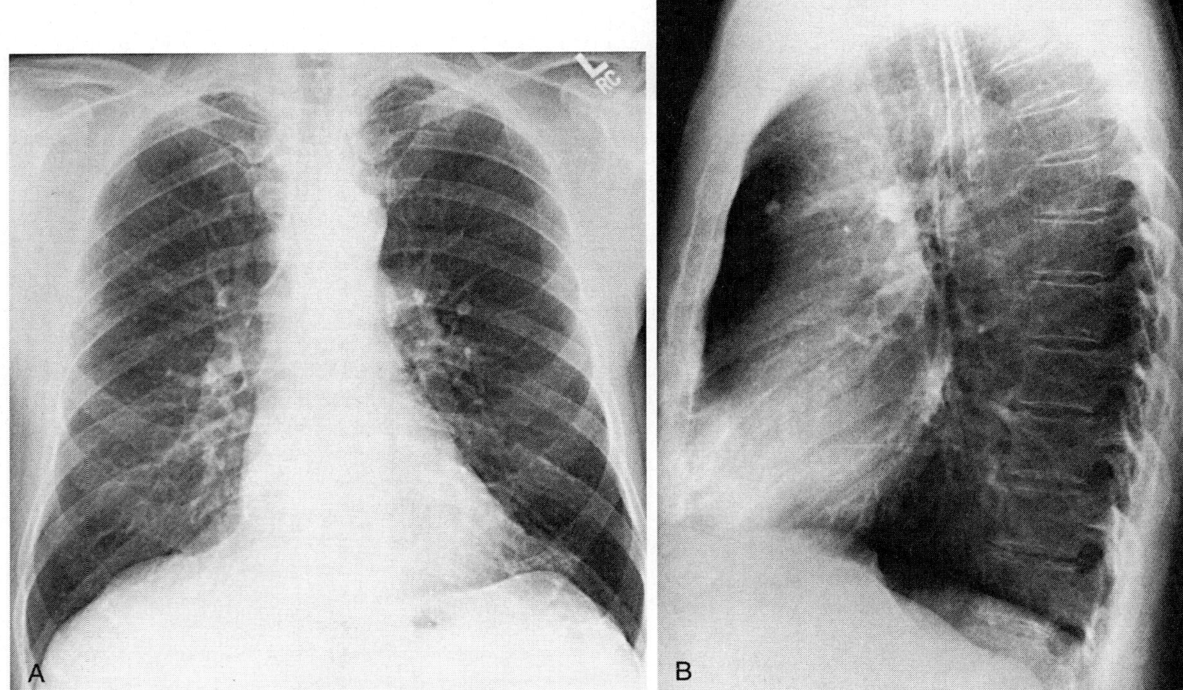

FIGURE 3–1 The cardiac silhouette, pulmonary vasculature, pulmonary parenchyma, diaphragmatic surfaces, and costrophenic angles should all be clearly visible without the use of a "bright" light in both the posteroanterior (PA) **(A)** and the lateral **(B)** projections. The technical factors used to obtain this PA radiograph **(A)** were 110 kVp and 1.6 mAs and, for the lateral **(B),** 110 kVp and 6.5 mAs.

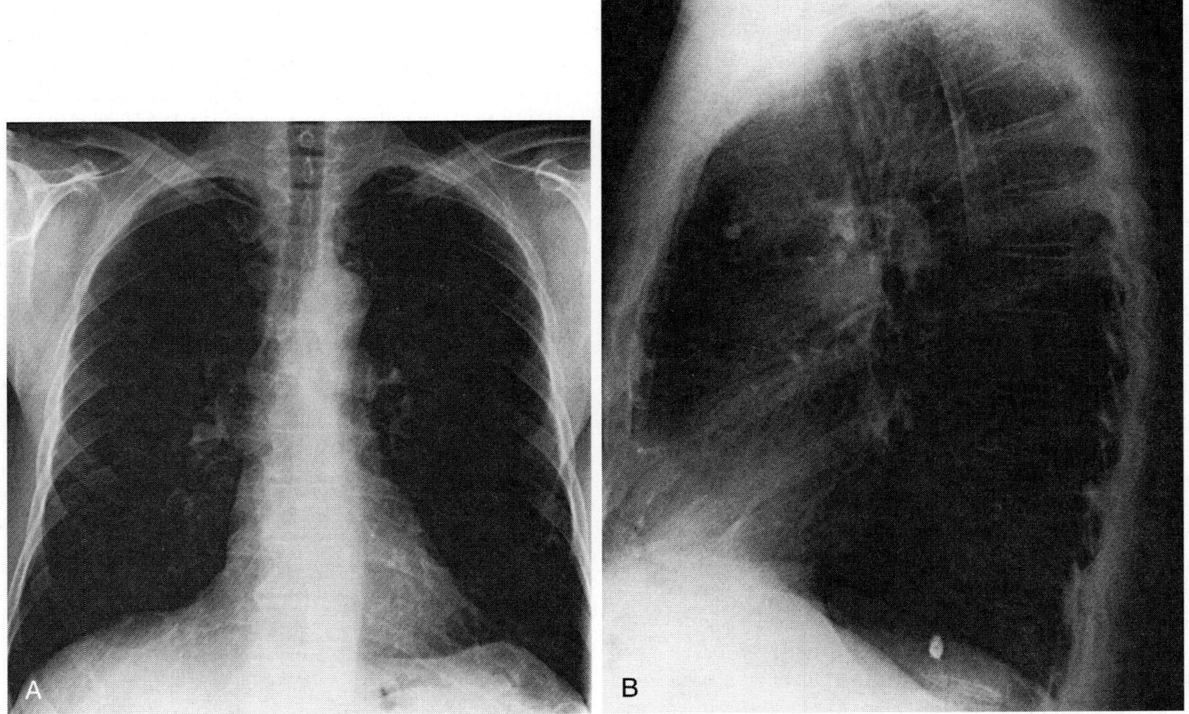

FIGURE 3–2 "Overpenetrated" PA **(A)** and lateral **(B)** chest x-rays (CXRs) of the same patient as in Fig. 3–1 obtained with 120 kVp and 3.0 mAs. This technique demonstrates the thoracic spine through the heart at the expense of "burning-out" the lungs, including the pulmonary vasculature.

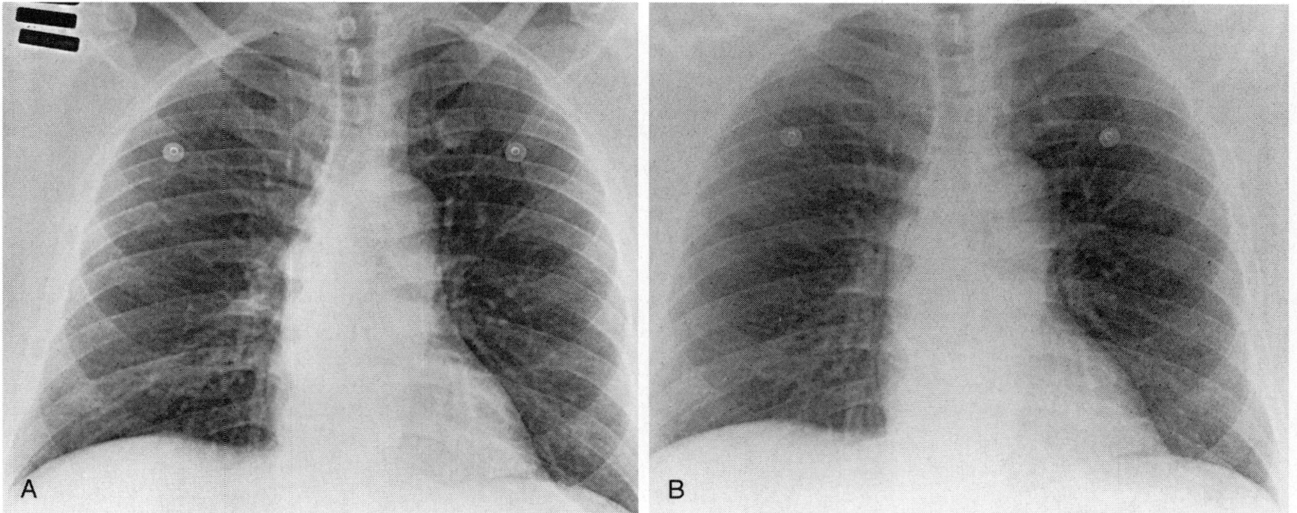

FIGURE 3–3 Effect of secondary (Compton) radiation "fog" on "image clarity" in the same patient: 110 kVp and 1.6 mAs **(A)**; 110 kVp and 6.9 mAs **(B)**. **A,** The image is "sharp" and the pulmonary parenchyma and vasculature are clearly demonstrated. **B,** Radiation "fog" diminishes image clarity, particularly as it relates to the lungs and the pulmonary vasculature.

Posteroanterior refers to the direction of penetration of the x-ray beam through, for example, the chest from posterior to anterior as the patient is positioned with the anterior chest wall closest to the film. The lateral CXR is obtained with the patient's left side close to the film. Such patient positioning, coupled with the x-ray target film distance of 6 ft, which includes the shortest possible subject-to-film distance relative to the heart, results in as accurate a representation of the cardiac size and configuration as is radiographically possible. Although the frontal CXR is obtained in the PA position, it is customarily displayed on the view box reversed right for left as though the patient were standing in front of the observer and with the right side of the image to the viewer's left.

The degree of inspiration is usually assessed by the relationship of the right hemidiaphragm to either the anterior or the posterior ends of the right ribs. Because the anterior rib ends have a greater respiratory range of excursion than do the posterior segments, the posterior rib segments are a more consistent landmark against which to estimate diaphragmatic excursion.

Since there is no objective radiographic measure of degree of inspiration, a "good" inspiratory effort is indicated by the right hemidiaphragm being in the right 8th posterior interspace or the level of the posterior segment of the 9th rib (see Fig. 3–1A). Patients with more compliant lungs may normally drive the right hemidiaphragm to the level of the posterior segment of the right 11th rib during maximal inspiration. In approximately 90 percent of patients, the right hemidiaphragm is normally approximately one interspace higher than the left.

The position and status of the aorta, the lateral margin of the left subclavian artery, the aorticopulmonary clear space ("window"), the main pulmonary artery, the lateral margin of the left auricular appendage, the lateral margin of the left ventricle, and on the right, the innominate artery, the superior vena cava, and the lateral margin of the right atrium are visible on the PA CXR (Fig. 3–4).

The right hilum is normally higher than the left. The hilar densities are composed mainly of right and left main pulmonary arteries and their primary divisions. On the right, the azygos vein is commonly visible as an almond-shaped, sharply marginated, homogeneous density at the junction of the trachea and the right stem bronchus.

It is important to identify the carina and the stem bronchi on the PA radiograph. The carinal angle is normally acute. An obtuse carinal angle, secondary to elevation of the left stem bronchus, is a reliable sign of left atrial dilatation due to either mitral stenosis or a component of cardiomyopathy.

Landmarks for assessing the degree of inspiration on the lateral CXR are not available, except that in a normal adult a "clear" space should be visible between the sternum and the anterior margin of the heart (retrosternal space) and between the posterior margin of the left ventricle and the spine (retrocardiac space). Diaphragmatic surfaces should be sharply defined and extend from relatively high anteriorly to low posteriorly in an arched contour and with acute posterior costophrenic angles. Diaphragmatic surfaces are normally not visible anteriorly because of the proximity of the base of the heart to each hemidiaphragm.

On the lateral CXR, the right hilum is anterior to the carina and more superiorly located than is the left hilum, which is posteroinferior to the carina. The anterior wall of the right atrium is substernal. Normally, the ascending aorta is not visible on the lateral CXR. The posterior segment of the aortic arch and the proximal descending aorta are usually visible, the latter normally superimposed on the upper or midthoracic vertebrae. The posterior margin of the cardiac silhouette is formed by the left atrium superiorly and the left ventricle inferiorly. Left atrial dilatation displaces the midthoracic esophagus posteriorly on swallowing function.

The inferior vena cava is usually visible extending through the diaphragm into the right atrium. Hoffman and Rigler[4] determined, in 1965, that if the distance between the posterior margin of the inferior vena cava and the posterior margin of the left ventricle exceeded 1.8 cm as

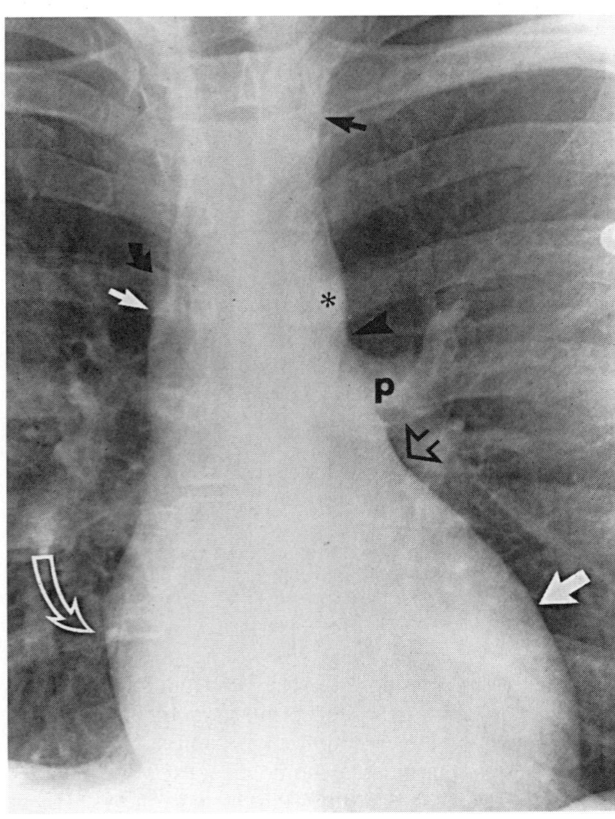

FIGURE 3–4 Normal PA CXR shows, along the left side of the cardiac silhouette, from superior to inferior, the lateral margin of the left subclavian artery *(straight black arrow)*, the aortic arch *(asterisk)*, the aorticopulmonary window *(arrowhead)*, the main pulmonary artery (p), the left auricular appendage *(open black arrow)*, and the lateral wall of the left ventricle *(large white arrow)*. On the right, the superior vena cava *(curved black arrow)*, the azygos vein *(small white arrow)*, and the wall of the right atrium *(curved open arrow)* are visible.

measured 2 cm above their crossing (Fig. 3–5), left ventricular preponderance was present.

The physician interpreting CXRs of patients with suspected or documented cardiovascular disease must be familiar with the normal and abnormal radiographic appearance of the pulmonary vasculature, particularly the upper lobe pulmonary arteries and veins.

The lobar pulmonary arteries arise from the right and left main pulmonary arteries, accompany the lobar and segmental bronchi[5–8] in the pattern of branches of a tree (arborization) radiating out from each hilum. In the upper lobes, the pulmonary arteries are vascular structures that extend upward and superolaterally from the superior portion of the hilum. The arterial margins are normally sharply

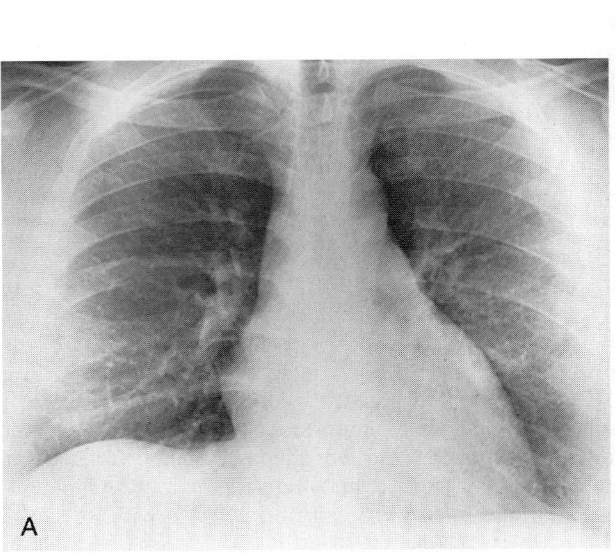

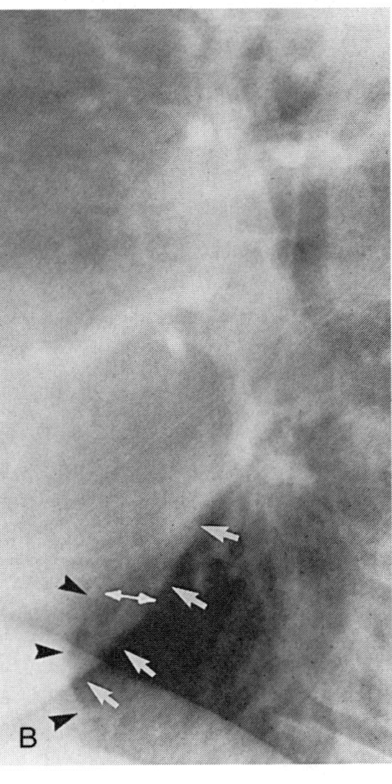

FIGURE 3–5 Relationship of the posterior wall of the left ventricle to the inferior vena cava on a lateral CXR as an estimate of cardiac size. **A,** On the erect PA CXR, the heart appears enlarged with left ventricular preponderance. **B,** However, on the lateral CXR, the distance between the inferior vena cava *(arrowheads)* and the posterior wall of the left ventricle *(arrows)* is less than 2 cm *(double-ended arrow)*, indicating that the heart is not enlarged.

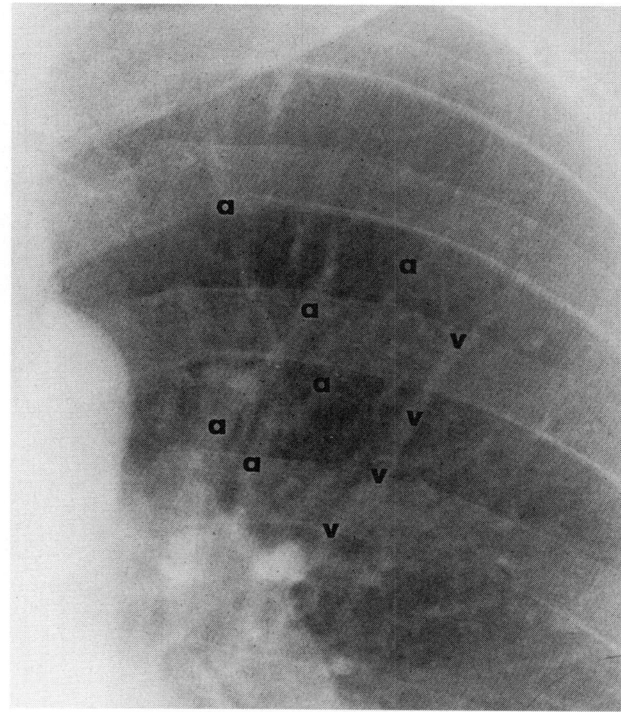

FIGURE 3–6 Normal left upper lobe pulmonary vasculature as seen on an erect PA CXR. The pulmonary arteries (a) extend upward from the superior aspect of the hilum in an arborizing pattern as they leave the hilum, the arteries are 3 to 4 mm in width with sharply defined margins. The arteries branch, taper, and gradually disappear as they approach the periphery of the lung. A left upper lobe vein (v) is visible in the second anterior interspace lateral to the arteries. It extends obliquely downward toward the left atrium in a course that is inconsistent with its arising from the pulmonary artery.

defined. The arteries branch and, gradually diminishing in caliber, become no longer visible approximately 2 cm from the pleura of the upper lobes[9] (Fig. 3–6).

On the erect PA CXR, upper lobe pulmonary veins are much less numerous than the pulmonary arteries. When visible, the upper lobe veins lie lateral to the arterial shadows. The most commonly visible upper lobe vein is found in the left first or second anterior rib interspace as a sharply defined vascular density formed by the junction of two tributary veins. The upper lobe vein curves downward in an inferomedial direction to "cross the hilum in a course that is inconsistent with it being an artery"[10] on its way to the left atrium (Plate 3–1; see also Fig. 3–6).

The lower lobe segmental arteries extend inferiorly and inferolaterally from the inferior aspect of the hila. Because the pulmonary circulation is a low-pressure system, the majority of the pulmonary blood volume is in the lung bases when the patient is erect. Consequently, on the erect CXR, the lower lobe segmental arteries are of greater caliber than those of the upper lobes in an approximate 3:1 ratio.[9] However, they branch and taper in caliber exactly as do the upper lobe arteries. Lower lobe segmental arteries are visible through the density of the heart, are commonly visible inferior to the dome of each hemidiaphragm, and should not be misinterpreted as subsegmental atelectasis.

Nonpathologic conditions that effect the cardiovascular silhouette include degree of inspiration, position (e.g., erect versus supine and PA versus AP [anteroposterior]), and less significantly, the cardiac cycle. The effect of inspiration and expiration on the heart, mediastinum, and pulmonary vasculature is demonstrated in Figure 3–7 and that of the erect and supine positions in Figure 3–8. The net result of expiration, recumbency, and the AP projection is to increase the transverse diameter of the heart. The change in cardiac size attributable to systole and diastole is approximately 1.0 cm and is, therefore, probably not recognizable and of no consequence in estimating cardiac size radiographically.[8]

Principles for Assessing the Radiographic Examination

The initial steps in assessing the CXR include being certain that the films are correctly identified with patient name, identification number, and date, and that the film is technically satisfactory relative to radiographic technique, positioning, degree of inspiration, and absence of motion artifacts, that is, that the examination is interpretable.

There is no "correct" or "right" way to assess the CXR for interpretation. One approach is to begin with the "corners of the film" and proceed from the shoulders to the thoracic cage, the abdominal upper quadrants, and the diaphragmatic surfaces, including the costophrenic angles, to the lungs, including the pulmonary vasculature, and finally, to the cardiac silhouette, aorta, and mediastinal structures.[2] The advantage of this system is that it forces the interpreter to evaluate areas of secondary interest first so that these important areas are not forgotten.

Another approach, preferred by the writer, is to begin with the cardiovascular silhouette, including the aorta, and proceed to the pulmonary vasculature, particularly the upper lobe vessels, since these are all anatomically, physiologically, and pathophysiologically related structures; then the lungs, including the trachea and stem bronchi; the diaphragmatic surfaces and costophrenic angles; the upper abdomen; and finally, the thoracic cage and shoulders. The logic to this "system" is that the observer's primary attention is directed to those structures principally involved

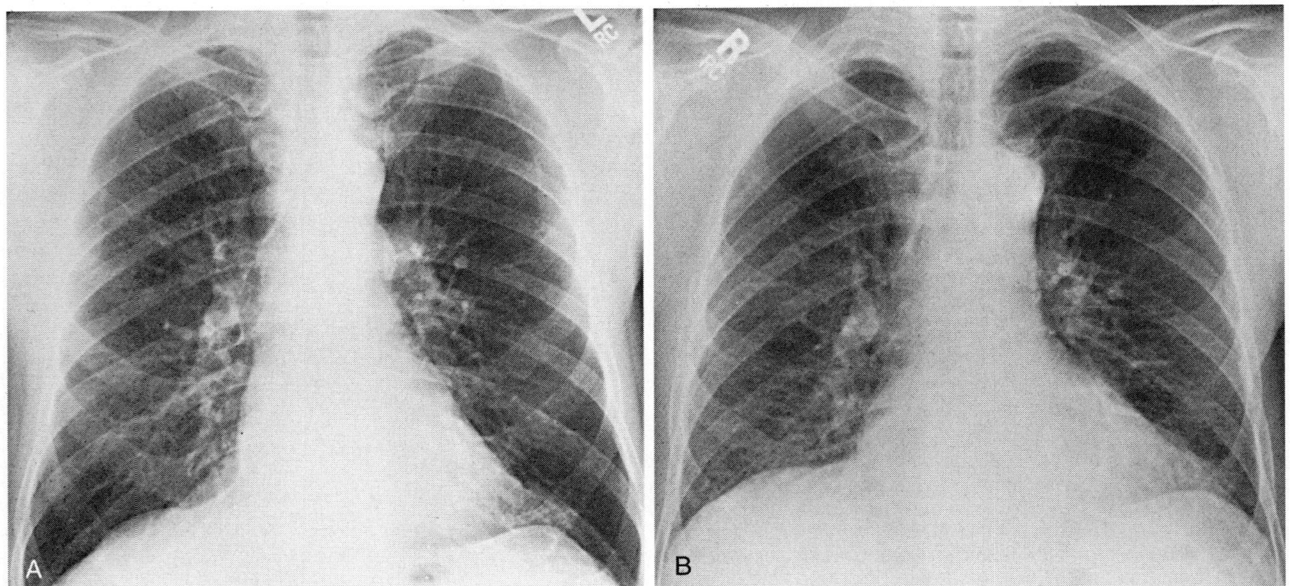

FIGURE 3–7 Effect of inspiration **(A)** and expiration **(B)** of the same patient obtained within minutes of each other. **B,** In expiration, both the superior mediastinum and the cardiac silhouette increased in transverse diameter.

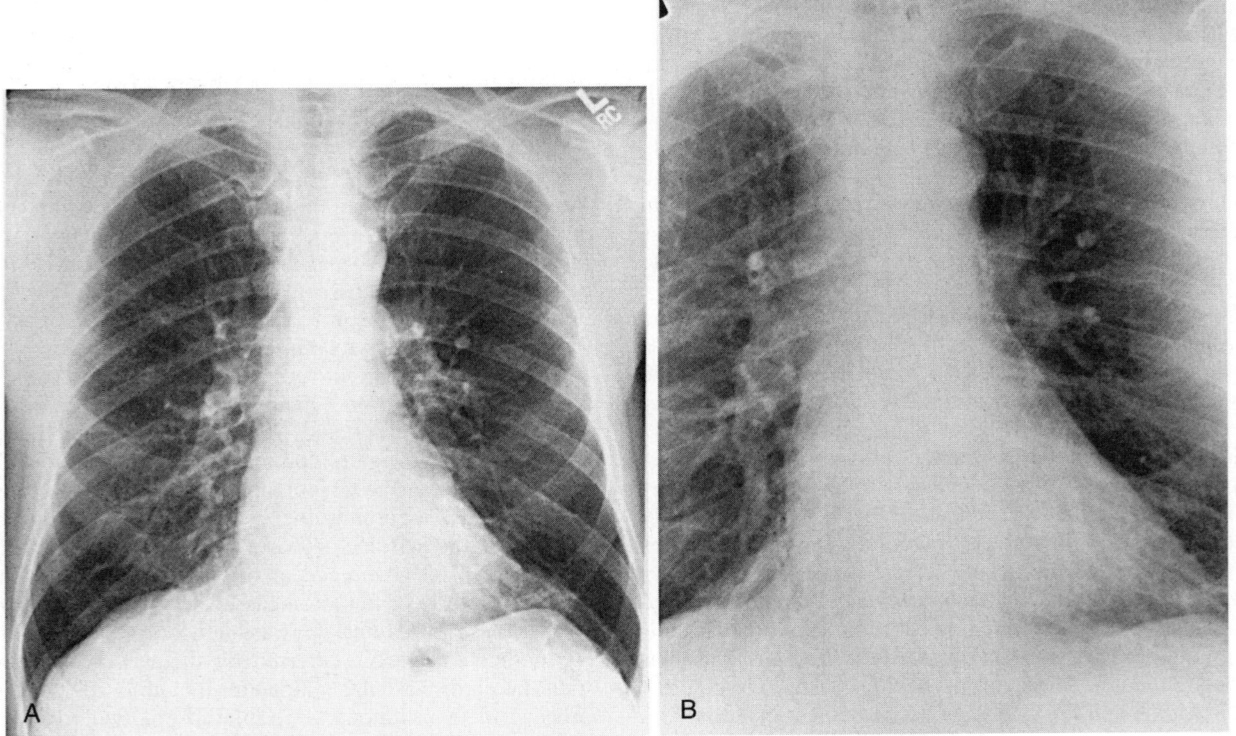

FIGURE 3–8 Effect of erect **(A)** and supine **(B)** posture on the PA CXR of the same patient obtained within minutes of each other. **A,** The erect PA CXR was obtained with a target film distance (TFD) of 72 inches and in deep inspiration. **B,** The supine CXR was obtained at a TFD of 46 inches and in deep inspiration. Recumbency produces positional redistribution of blood throughout the cardiovascular system, resulting in increased transverse diameter of the superior mediastinum and the cardiac silhouette as well as increased width of the upper lobe vessels.

in cardiovascular disease, namely, the heart and lungs. Whichever of these systems, or any modification, the observer chooses is really immaterial. What is important is that the observer develop his or her own system and follow that routine for the interpretation of every CXR examination.

Pathophysiologic Principles Pertaining to the Radiographic Signs of Cardiovascular Disease

Heart

The cardiovascular silhouette must be evaluated for cardiac size and configuration, including signs of isolated or diffuse chamber preponderance (the CXR does not distinguish between chamber dilatation and hypertrophy), cardiovascular disease, coronary calcification, and left ventricular aneurysm.

Cardiac size has traditionally been radiographically assessed by the cardiothoracic ratio,[11] the average value of which in a 70-kg adult is approximately 0.45. Limitations of the cardiothoracic ratio are that whereas all enlarged hearts are abnormal, the ratio can be falsely negative (e.g., the small heart of Addison's disease); the volume of the left ventricle must increase approximately 66 percent in order to produce an abnormal cardiothoracic ratio[12]; the right ventricle does not contribute to the cardiac silhouette on the PA CXR and, therefore, can be dilated without affecting the cardiothoracic ratio; and the transverse diameter of the heart is normally increased in expiration and recumbency. As previously described and illustrated, the more accurate CXR assessment of cardiac size is obtained from the inferior vena cava–left ventricular wall distance (see Fig. 3–5).

Left atrial dilatation may be first evidenced on the PA CXR by a change in the contour of the left auricular appendage from concave to convex prior to elevation of the left stem bronchus and/or the presence of the "double-outline" sign of the right heart border is noted. On the lateral CXR, early left atrial dilatation is reflected by posterior displacement of the contrast-filled esophagus; marked dilatation by posterior and superior displacement of the left stem bronchus.

Annular calcification most commonly involves the mitral or aortic valve. On the PA CXR, aortic valve calcification is best located by following the ascending aorta downward to its origin at the valve. On the lateral CXR, a line drawn from the junction of the sternum and diaphragm to the carina will pass through the aortic valve (Fig. 3–9).[13] (The mitral valve and its annulus lie posterior and inferior to that diagonal.)

Calcification of the annulus of the mitral valve is broad,

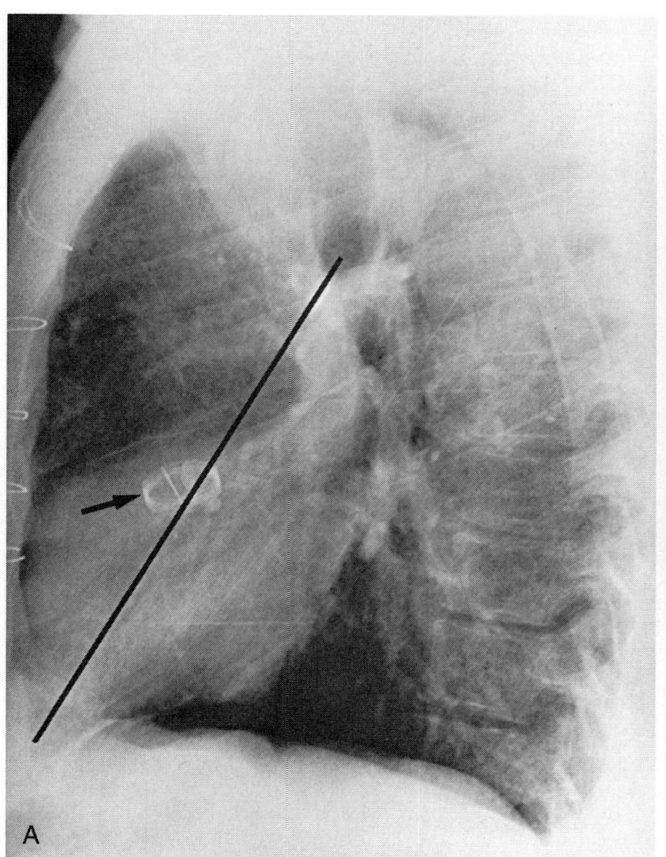

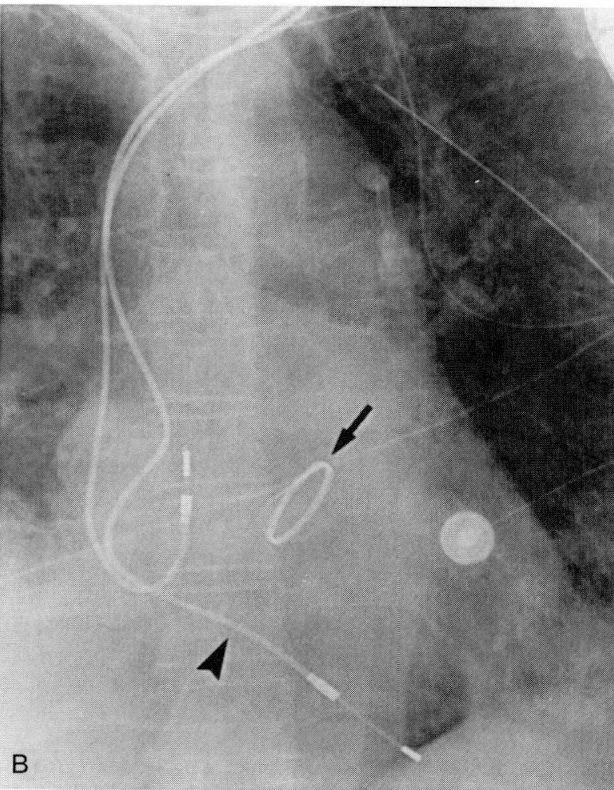

FIGURE 3–9 Cardiac valve sites. **A,** On the lateral CXR, the aortic valve *(arrow)* lies on or above a diagonal line connecting the junction of the sternum and the diaphragm with the carina. **B,** On the frontal (anteroposterior or PA) CXR, the location of the mitral valve is indicated by its prosthesis *(arrow),* and the location of the tricuspid valve is shown by the upward arc *(arrowhead)* in the cable of the right ventricular electrode.

irregular, and most commonly appears in a reversed C or J configuration to the left of the spine and caudal to the auricular appendage on the PA CXR.

Coronary artery calcifications involve the left anterior descending, left circumflex, and right coronary arteries, in order of frequency.[14] Therefore, coronary artery calcification should be sought in anatomically predictable locations on the PA and lateral CXRs. These calcifications are usually subtle and, on the lateral CXR, may be obscured by superimposed pulmonary parenchymal and/or vascular shadows. The plain film signs of cardiomyopathy and of pericardial effusion are so similar as to defy radiographic distinction. Epicardial fat and pericardial cysts alter the cardiac silhouette by obscuring the cardiophrenic angles.

Focal convexity of the left heart border indicates a left ventricular aneurysm. When suspected on the PA CXR, its presence is confirmed on the left posterior oblique radiograph or by fluoroscopy.

Aorta

The location and degree of aortic ectasia and tortuosity and its effect on the trachea, as well as the location and extent of aortic calcification, must be assessed in every patient suspected of cardiovascular disease. *Aortic dissection is not a plain chest film diagnosis.* However, the diagnosis of acute aortic dissection must be considered in every middle-aged or elderly patient with any aortic abnormality, for example ectasia, with or without adjacent tracheal displacement to the right, laminar aortic calcification, and appropriate interscapular pain.[15–17] The diagnosis of aortic dissection can be established or excluded, noninvasively, within 15 minutes by intravenous contrast-enhanced helical (spiral) computed tomography.

Pulmonary Vasculature

Alteration of pulmonary vasculature as recorded on the PA CXR has long been recognized[10, 18] and more recently confirmed[8, 19] as a quantitative reflection of altered pulmonary hemodynamics.

Pulmonary Venous Hypertension

This discussion is limited to the signs of elevated pulmonary venous pressure of cardiac (hydrostatic) etiology. Pulmonary venous pressure greater than 10 to 12 mm Hg results in redistribution ("cephalization") of blood from the lung bases into the upper lobe arteries and veins. Redistribution is manifested on the erect PA CXR by increase in both the number and the caliber of upper lobe vessels, which extend further toward the pleura than normal, and by decrease in caliber of the lower lobe arteries. The upper lobe vascular shadows remain sharply demarcated (Fig. 3–10).

Pulmonary venous pressure between approximately 20 and 30 mm Hg results in interstitial pulmonary edema, which, surrounding the pulmonary vessels, makes their margins indistinct and, surrounding bronchi, results in peribronchial "cuffing" (Fig. 3–11). Accumulation of fluid in interlobular septa is evidenced by Kerley B lines—thin, approximately 1.0-cm linear, pleura-based densities visible along the lateral chest wall on the PA CXR and retrosternally on the lateral radiograph. *Kerley B lines are not a prerequisite for the radiologic diagnosis of pulmonary edema.* Radiographic prominence of the interlobular fissures, usually seen best on the lateral CXR, is caused by edema accumulation in the visceral pleura, subpleural edema, rather than a free effusion in the interlobar pleural space.

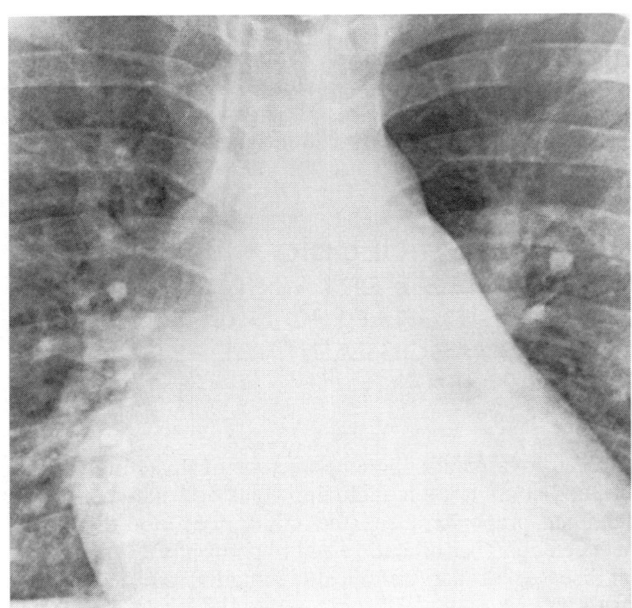

FIGURE 3–10 Elevated pulmonary venous pressure without pulmonary edema. This 18-year-old patient has a ventricular septal defect, as reflected by the cardiac configuration. The intrinsic pulmonary hypervolemia results in increased caliber of the upper lobe vessels, whose margins remain distinct. There is no peribronchial cuffing.

Elevation of pulmonary venous pressure greater than 30 mm Hg results in alveolar pulmonary edema, manifested on PA CXR by bilateral, essentially symmetric confluences of small parenchymal densities ("rosettes") that obscure or obliterate vascular shadows and cause increased peribronchial cuffing (Fig. 3–12). Kerley B and A lines may be visible. Kerley A lines are lymphatic channels that normally carry lymph from the lymphatic channels of the interlobular septa to the hila and are not normally radiographically visible. When visible, the A lines appear as long (2 to 3 cm), irregular linear densities approximately 1 mm in width that course obliquely from the periphery of the lung toward the hilum. *Kerley A lines are not a prerequisite for the radiographic diagnosis of alveolar pulmonary edema.*

Kerley lines are not pathognomic of pulmonary edema, being also found on the CXRs of patients with occupational dust exposure (anthracosis), lymphangitic pulmonary metastasis, and viral pneumonia. Permanent Kerley lines may be found in anthracosis and, owing to deposition of hemosiderin, in chronically elevated pulmonary venous pressure as commonly occurs in mitral stenosis.

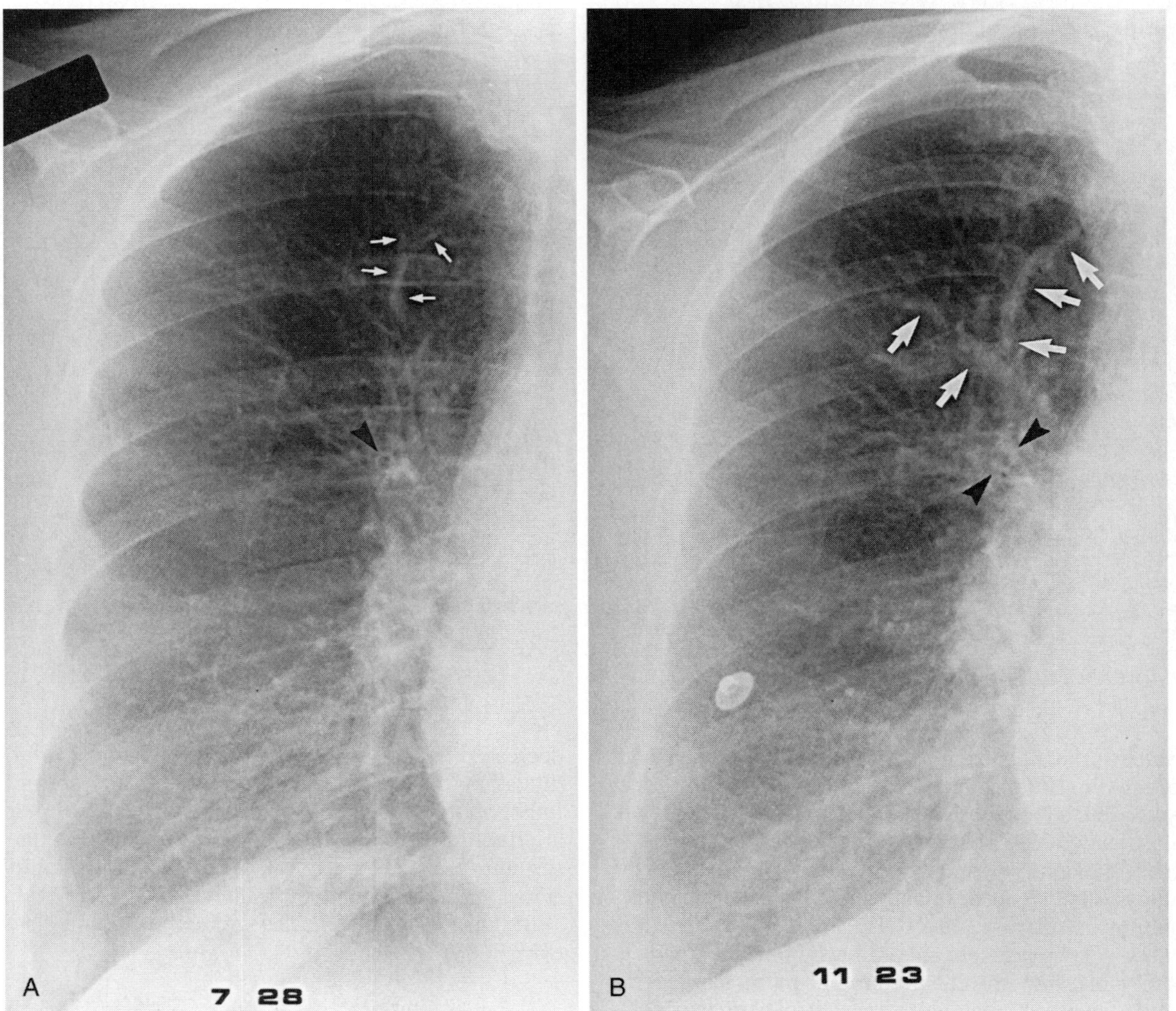

FIGURE 3–11 Interstitial pulmonary edema. **A,** The normal radiographic appearance of this patient's right lung. Note, particularly, the medial right upper lobe artery *(arrows)* and the wall of the bronchus *(arrowhead)*. **B,** Signs of interstitial pulmonary edema include an increase in the number and caliber of right upper lobe vessels whose margins are now indistinct (*arrows,* compare with **A**) and peribronchial "cuffing" *(arrowheads)*, all representative of elevated pulmonary venous pressure with interstitial pulmonary edema.

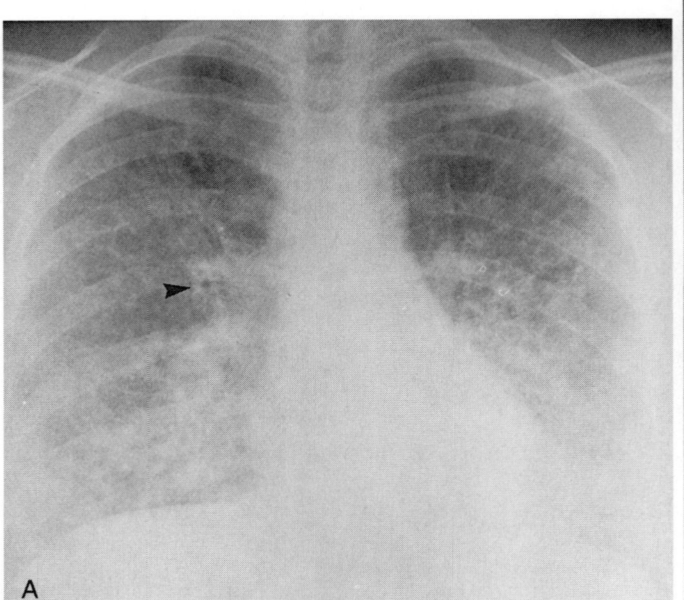

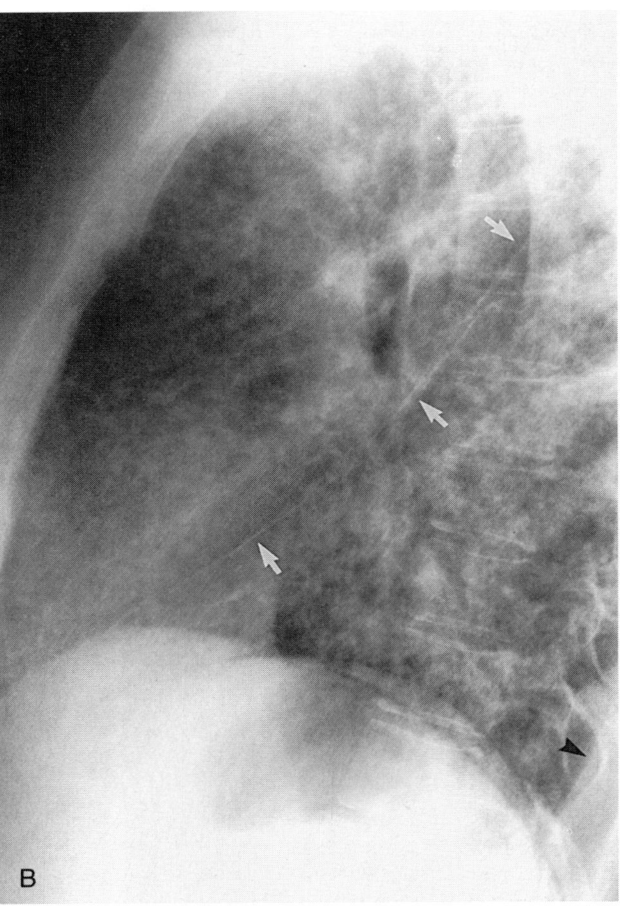

FIGURE 3–12 Alveolar pulmonary edema. **A,** On the PA CXR, pulmonary vasculature is almost completely obscured by the bilateral symmetric alveolar pattern parenchymal densities. Peribronchial "cuffing" *(arrowhead)* is marked. **B,** The lateral CXR shows the "rosette" character of the alveolar fluid, unsharpness of the interlobar fissures *(arrows)* representative of subpleural edema, and a small pleural effusion *(arrowhead).*

Elevated pulmonary venous pressure is associated with cardiomegaly, usually left ventricular preponderance, shaggy cardiac silhouette, and fullness of the azygos vein. Pleural effusions may or may not be present.

Because elevation of pulmonary venous pressure effects both lungs equally, except in patients with chronic obstructive pulmonary disease, the CXR findings of increased pulmonary venous pressure should be symmetric. The central (bat's-wing, butterfly) distribution of pulmonary edema is usually associated with abrupt and severe cardiac decompensation such as in massive myocardial infarction or ruptured valvular leaflets.[8]

Pulmonary Arterial Hypertension

Precapillary hypertension, such as occurs in chronic obstructive pulmonary disease, initially results in spasm of precapillary arterioles. Persistent arterial hypertension causes the spasm to move progressively proximally to involve the small arteries. Persistent spasm results in hypertrophy of the muscular layer (media) of the arteries that, in turn, further elevate pulmonary artery pressure. On the PA CXR, pulmonary arterial hypertension is manifested by decreased caliber of the lower lobe segmental arteries and dilatation of the central, main pulmonary arteries. It is important to be aware of the pathophysiology of pulmonary arterial hypertension in order to understand that the basilar segmental arteries are not "pruned," for example, cut across or amputated, but rather they persist as narrow "stringlike" shadows in their normal anatomic distribution (Fig. 3–13).

Pulmonary Embolism

The most common PA CXR finding in patients with subsegmental pulmonary embolism is a "normal" CXR. Hampton's hump, a pleural-based triangular density, is reserved for pulmonary embolus with infarction. The Westermark sign of proximal pulmonary arterial dilatation and peripheral oligemia has been reported as occurring in 6 to 7 percent of patients with pulmonary embolism.[19]

In patients with clinically suspected pulmonary embolus, ventilation-perfusion scintigraphy or spiral computed tomographic angiography must be considered for definitive evaluation. Recently, the latter has been recommended as the first-line test in patients suspected of pulmonary embolism.

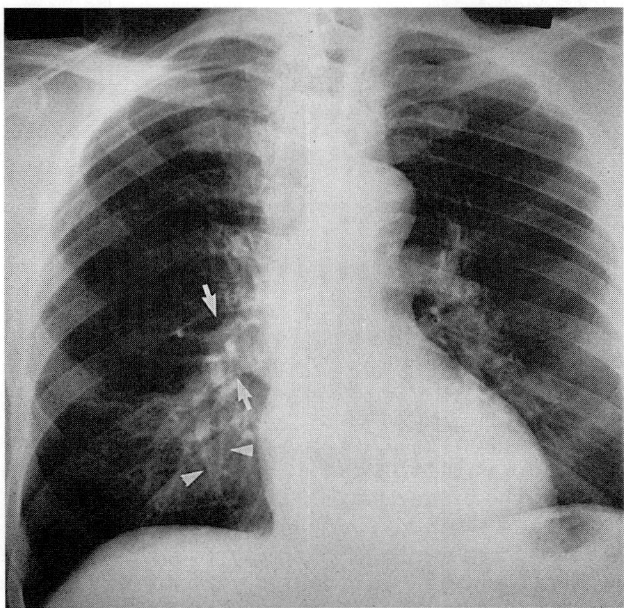

FIGURE 3–13 Pulmonary arterial hypertension, seen in the PA CXR of this patient with chronic obstructive pulmonary disease, is manifest by dilatation of the main pulmonary arteries *(arrows)* and narrowing of the lower lobe segmental arteries *(arrowheads)*. It is important to be aware that the basilar segmental arteries are not "pruned," but rather have a stringlike appearance.

Helical computed tomography is more accurate than scintigraphy in detecting pulmonary embolism and provides for the detection of alternative diagnoses more effectively than ventilation-perfusion scintigraphy.[20–23]

References

1. Curry TS III, Dowdey JE, Murry RC Jr: Christensen's Physics of Diagnostic Radiology. 4th ed. pp. 196–218. Philadelphia: Lea & Febiger, 1990.
2. Hemphill RR, Eisenberg RL: Cardiovascular radiography. Emerg Med Clin North Am 13:855–885, 1995.
3. Tuddenham WJ: Problems of Perception in Chest Roentgenology: Facts and Fallacies. pp. 277–290. Philadelphia: WB Saunders, 1963.
4. Hoffman RB, Rigler LG: Evaluation of left ventricular enlargement in the lateral projection of the chest. Radiology 85:93–100, 1965.
5. Boyden EA: Segmental Anatomy of the Lungs. A Study of the Patterns of the Segmental Bronchi and Related Pulmonary Vessels. New York: McGraw-Hill, 1955.
6. Simon M, Potchen EJ, Le May M: The radiographic assessment of pulmonary hemodynamics. *In* Simon M, Potchen EJ, Le May M (eds): Frontiers of Pulmonary Radiology. pp 189–221. New York: Grune & Stratton, 1969.
7. Harris JH: The pulmonary arteries and veins: their radiographic identification. Med Radiogr Photogr 39:52–53, 1963.
8. Milne ENC, Pistolesi M: Reading the Chest Radiograph. pp. 9–50, 51–79. St. Louis: Mosby–Year Book, 1993.
9. Heitzman ER, Frazier RG, Proto AV, Simon M: American College of Radiology Self-Evaluation Syllabus: Chest Disease III. p. 378. Chicago: Waverly, 1981.
10. Simon M, Potchen EJ, Le May M: The radiographic assessment of pulmonary hemodynamics. *In* Simon M, Potchen EJ, Le May M (eds): Frontiers of Pulmonary Radiology. pp. 205–221. New York: Grune & Stratton, 1969.
11. Danzer CS: The cardio-thoracic ratio: an index of cardiac enlargement. Am J Med Sci 157:513–521, 1919.
12. Miller SW: Cardiac Radiography. The Requisites. p. 6. St. Louis: Mosby, 1996.
13. Miller SW: Cardiac Radiography. The Requisites. p. 16. St. Louis: Mosby, 1996.
14. Miller SW: Cardiac Radiography. The Requisites. p. 21. St. Louis: Mosby, 1996.
15. Razavi M: Acute dissection of the aorta: options for diagnostic imaging. Cleve Clin J Med 62:360–365, 1995.
16. Dowd SB, Wilson BG, Hall JD, et al: Review of techniques used to image aortic dissection. Radiol Technol 67:223–230, 1996.
17. Petasnick JP: Radiologic evaluation of aortic dissection. Radiology 180:297–305, 1991.
18. Healey RF, Dow JW, Sosman MC, Dexter L: The relationships of the roentgenographic appearance of the pulmonary artery to pulmonary hemodynamics. AJR 62:777–787, 1949.
19. Palla A, Petruzzelli S, Donnemaria V, et al: Radiographic assessment of perfusion impairment in pulmonary embolism. Eur J Radiol 5:252–255, 1985.
20. Sheedy PF, Johnson CM, Welch TJ, et al: Fast CT for pulmonary embolus. Semin Ultrasound CT MR 17:324–338, 1996.
21. Russi TJ, Libby DM, Henschke CI: Clinical utility of computed tomography in the diagnosis of pulmonary embolism. Clin Imaging 21:175–182, 1997.
22. Mayo JR, Remy-Jardin M, Muller NL, et al: Pulmonary embolism: prospective comparison of spiral CT with ventilation-perfusion scintigraphy. Radiology 205:447–452, 1997.
23. van Rossum AB, Pattynama PM, Mallens WM, et al: Can helical CT replace scintigraphy in the diagnostic process in suspected pulmonary embolism? Eur Radiol 8:90–96, 1998.

CHAPTER 4

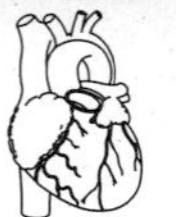

ECHOCARDIOGRAPHY

Eddy Barasch

TECHNIQUES OF EXAMINATION
GENERAL CLINICAL APPLICATIONS OF DOPPLER ECHOCARDIOGRAPHY
Assessment of Left Ventricular Mass, Volume, and Geometry
Left Ventricular Diastolic Function Assessment
Hemodynamics
SPECIFIC CLINICAL APPLICATIONS OF DOPPLER ECHOCARDIOGRAPHY
Valvular Heart Disease
Prosthetic Valves
Infective Endocarditis
Cardiomyopathies
Identification of Intracardiac or Aortic Source of Systemic or Pulmonary Embolism
Coronary Artery Disease
Pericardial Diseases
Congenital Heart Diseases

In 1954, Drs. Edler and Hertz[1] demonstrated that echocardiography can be successfully utilized in the diagnosis of cardiac diseases in humans. For a latent period of about 20 years, only M-mode echocardiography was available, and it was used mainly for evaluation of cardiac anatomy. Thereafter, the rapid development of ultrasound technology allowed the introduction of two-dimensional (2-D) echocardiography followed by the development of spectral and color Doppler. The introduction of transesophageal echocardiography (TEE) into clinical practice made possible the visualization of anatomic structures not seen before, significantly improving the quality of imaging and ultimately enlarging the indications for echocardiography. Since the mid-1980s, three-dimensional (3-D) reconstruction of the cardiac chambers[2]; development of transpulmonary contrast agents with numerous applications[3–7]; automatic assessment of left ventricular volumes[8]; Doppler tissue imaging (DTI)[9–11]; color kinesis[12, 13]; harmonic imaging[14, 15]; power Doppler used with or without contrast medium administration[16, 17]; and currently, the utilization of parallel processing for the beam former, allowing multiple real-time simultaneous-plane display of 2-D images,[18] contribute to a continued refinement of this imaging technique and the development of new and exciting research opportunities and clinical applications. The physical principles of Doppler echocardiography are described elsewhere, and their discussion is beyond the aim of this introductory chapter.

TECHNIQUES OF EXAMINATION

Current display modalities of standard echocardiography are M-mode (*M* stands for motion) and 2-D echocardiography. 3-D echocardiography has passed the stage of feasibility testing and entered clinical development.

In M-mode, a number of cardiac structures aligned along the same interrogation plane are displayed over time at a speed of 1000 frames/s. In contrast, on 2-D display, the moving of the beam sector gives rise to slices of the heart at a frequency of only 30 to 60 frames/s under ideal conditions. This explains the higher accuracy of M-mode echocardiography in identifying the timing of different events occurring during the cardiac cycle.

In 3-D echocardiography utilizing transthoracic or transesophageal windows, data acquisition occurs utilizing different methods in a sequential order along or around an axis or using different reference views. Real-time, 3-D echocardiography allowing continuous scanning at a 65-degree pyramidal volume shows promising results for the assessment of left ventricular volumes.[18] The conventional windows of cardiac investigation are parasternal long-axis view; right ventricular inflow view; parasternal short-axis view; apical four-chamber, five-chamber, and long-axis views; and subcostal and suprasternal views (Fig. 4–1).

TEE utilizing biplane or multiplane probes gives a better definition of cardiac anatomy and enables the visualization of structures, such as atrial appendages, pulmonic veins, and interatrial septum, that are not always possible to visualize or accurately evaluate by transthoracic scanning. In a tomographic manner, in elective cases, the scanning usually starts from the transgastric (deep and mid) views, followed by the visualization of gastroesophageal junction in which coronary sinus can be easily identified. Midesophageal windows display similar views as transthoracic imaging from apical windows in addition to visualization of atrial appendages and pulmonic veins. The bicaval view, in which the anatomy of the interatrial septum can be accurately investigated in addition to the distal segments of the inferior and superior venae cavae, is followed by the imaging of the aortic root in both horizontal and longitudinal planes, which enables the visualization of the proximal and middle segments of all three coronary arteries in many patients.[19] In the upper esophageal view, the main pulmonary artery and its bifurcation into the right and left branches (the right one being better visualized and having under it the short-axis view of the aortic root, superior vena cava, and right upper pulmonic vein) are visualized; and finally, the thoracic descending aorta, aortic arch with

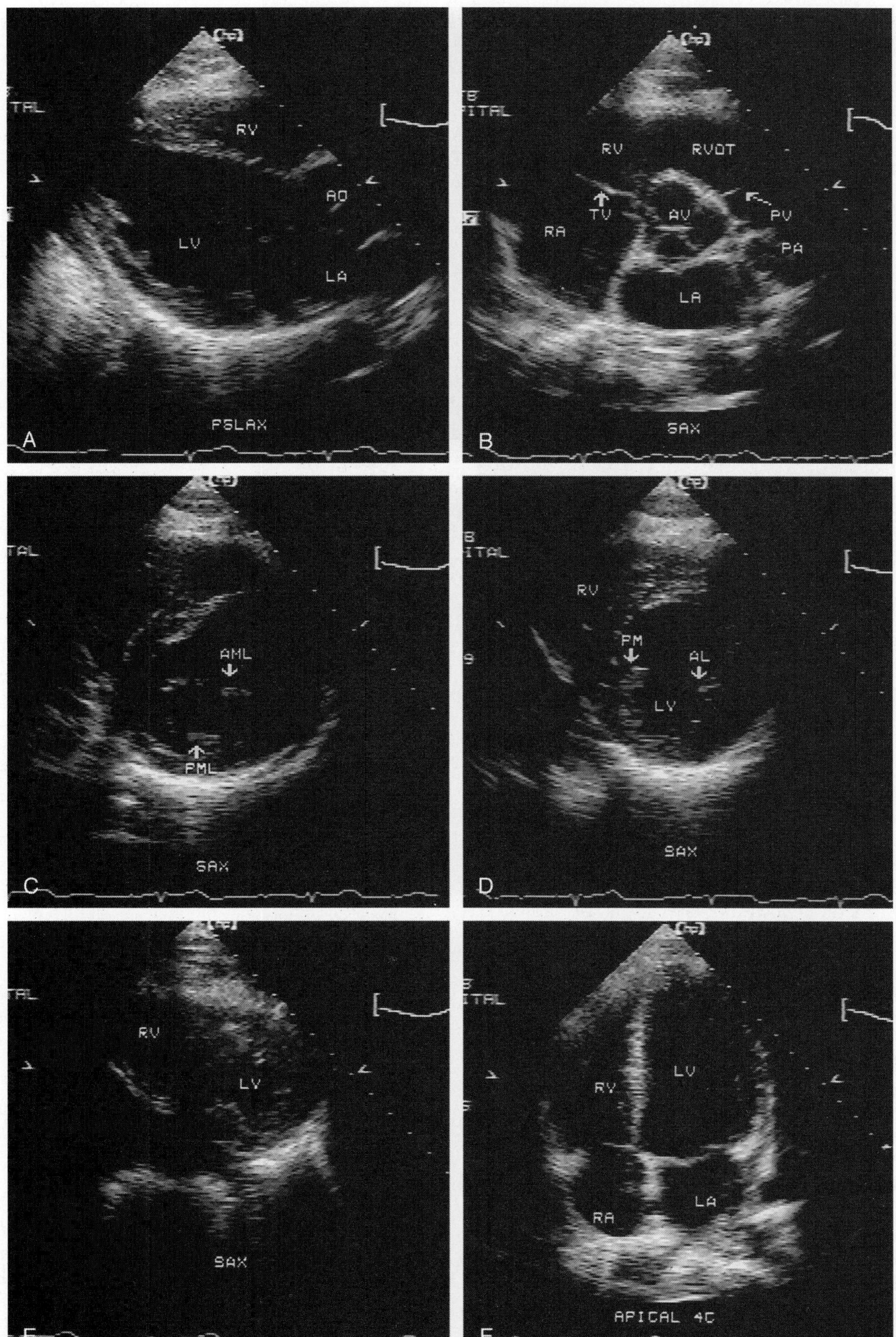

FIGURE 4–1 The normal transthoracic echocardiography (TTE) study shows the usual scanning windows. **A,** Parasternal long-axis (PSLAX) view. AO, aorta; LA, left atrium; LV, left ventricle; RV, right ventricle. **B,** Parasternal short-axis (SAX) view at the level of the aortic valve. AV, aortic valve; PA, pulmonary artery; RA, right atrium; RVOT, right ventricular outflow tract; TV, tricuspid valve. **C,** SAX at the level of the base of the heart (mitral valve). AML, anterior mitral leaflet; PML, posterior mitral leaflet. **D,** SAX at the level of the papillary muscles (midventricular view). AM, anterior mitral (valve); PM, posterior mitral (valve). **E,** SAX at apical level. **F,** Apical four-chamber (4C) view.

Illustration continued on following page

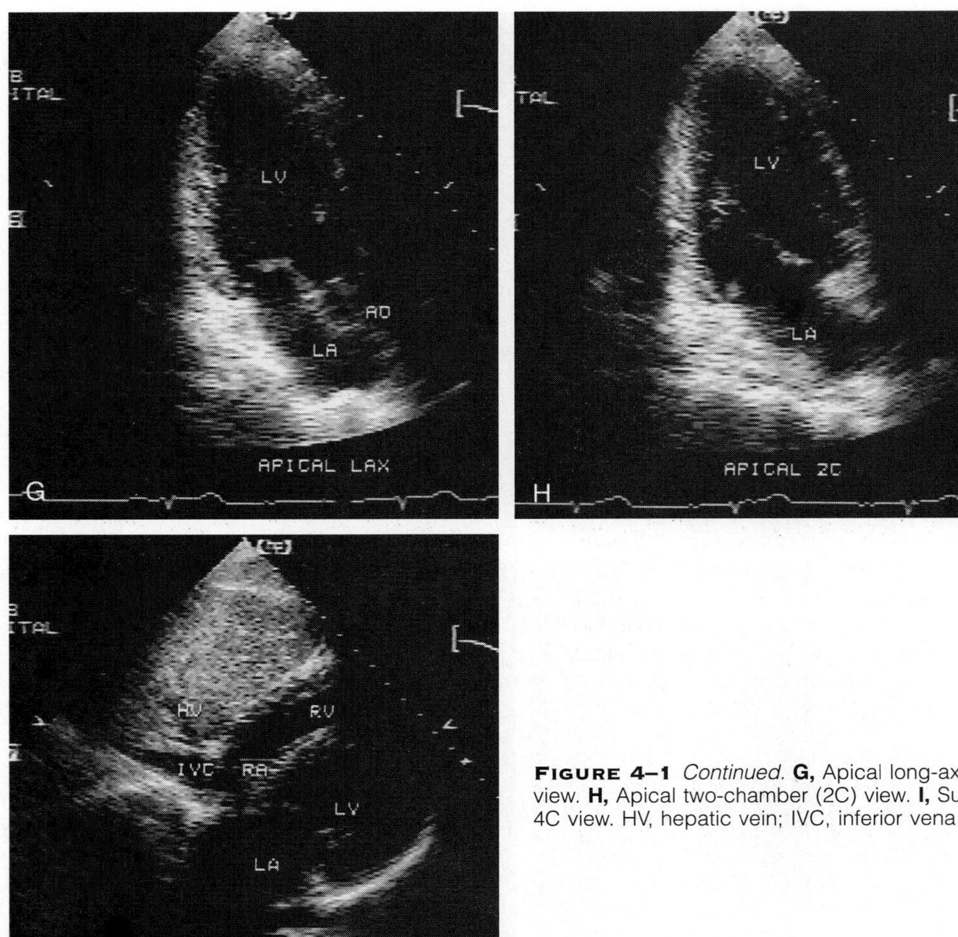

FIGURE 4–1 *Continued.* **G,** Apical long-axis (LAX) view. **H,** Apical two-chamber (2C) view. **I,** Subcostal 4C view. HV, hepatic vein; IVC, inferior vena cava.

its proximal branches, and ascending aorta are the last structures to be identified. The distal third of the ascending aorta and proximal third of the aortic arch cannot always be visualized owing to interposition of the trachea between the probe and the aorta. The good alignment of the Doppler beam with blood-flow direction through the left ventricular outflow tract (LVOT) and aortic root in the deep transgastric view (in horizontal axis) or midtransgastric view (in longitudinal axis) makes calculation of left ventricular stroke volume and aortic valve area possible.

General Clinical Applications of Doppler Echocardiography

Assessment of Left Ventricular Mass, Volume, and Geometry

M-mode, 2-D, and more recently, 3-D echocardiography,[20, 21] can be employed to calculate left ventricular mass.

On M-mode, the Deveroux method assumes that the left ventricle (LV) is a prolate ellipsoid with a ratio of 2:1 between the major and the minor radii.[22–25] Great care has to be taken in order to have a perpendicular alignment of the ultrasound beam on the interventricular septum and posterior wall and to document the absences of regional wall motion abnormalities.

$$\text{Left ventricular mass} = 0.8\{1.04[(\text{IVSd} + \text{LVIDd} + \text{PWd})]^3 - \text{LVIDd}^3]\} + 0.6\ \text{g}$$

where 0.8 = a correction factor for about 20 percent overestimation of left ventricular mass by echocardiography compared with the true anatomic value, IVSd = diastolic interventricular septum thickness, LVIDd = left ventricular diastolic dimension, PWd = posterior wall diastolic dimension, and 1.04 = the specific gravity of the myocardium. In adults, a normal left ventricular mass is 93 ± 22 g/m^2 for men and 76 ± 18 g/m^2 for women.[26] On 2-D, the most utilized methods for calculation of left ventricular mass are the area-length method and the truncated ellipsoid model. For the truncated ellipsoid method, the normal values are 76 ± 13 g/m^2 for men and 66 ± 11 g/m^2 for women.[27] The left ventricular volumes calculated by M-mode are better described by the Teicholtz formula,[28] which takes into consideration the fact that certain diseases may change left ventricular geometry, making it more spherical. Both left ventricular systolic and diastolic volumes can be measured by this formula:

$$Vd = [7/(2.4 + LVIDd)] \times LVIDd^3$$

Utilizing 2-D echocardiography, there are a number of formulas for calculating left ventricular volumes. At present, the one most frequently used is based on the modified Simpson rule stating that the volume of a large geometric figure can be calculated from the sum of a series of smaller similar figures. The normal value of the left ventricular end-diastolic volume (LVEDV) index is 55 ± 10 ml/m^2, and that of the left ventricular end-systolic volume (LVESV) index is 18 ± 6 ml/m^2.[29] On-line assessment of left ventricular volumes is possible utilizing automatic border detection, but the accuracy of the measurements can be confounded by technical problems.[8] Real-time 3-D echocardiography is the newest technology utilized in the assessment of ventricular volumes.[18]

The assessment of global and regional left ventricular systolic function is one of the most frequent indications for performing an echocardiographic study.[30] Global left ventricular ejection fraction (LVEF) is calculated by the formula

$$LVEF = LVEDV - LVESV/LVEDV \times 100$$

Although the ventricular loading conditions and the shortening of the myocardial fibers in the longitudinal plane are disregarded in this method, its general acceptance is based on the simplicity of calculation and on the good correlation between "track-ball" and experienced "eyeball" estimation.[31–33]

The evaluation of the degree of the systolic mitral annulus displacement as a reflection of the contraction of the longitudinal fibers has been strongly correlated with LVEF and can be achieved by 2-D echocardiography,[34] M-mode echocardiography,[35] or more recently, DTI.[36] DTI is able to display tissue motion velocities (low-velocity, high-amplitude Doppler signal) utilizing a signal processing that bypasses the high-pass filter and a lower-gain amplification to eliminate the weaker intensity blood-flow signal.

Using M-mode echocardiography, E point of septal separation—a diastolic event—is a qualitative estimate of the left ventricular systolic dysfunction, the normal value being less than 1 cm.[37] Both by M-mode and on 2-D studies, one may calculate the shortening fraction, the velocity of circumferential fiber shortening, and the left ventricular midwall stress. The generation of pressure-volume loops using 2-D echocardiography and pressure-dimension loops derived from M-mode as a surrogate for volume loops are advances in evaluation of left ventricular function. The first derivative of rise in left ventricular pressure has recently been validated and has good correlation with the invasive method for its measurement.[38] More accurate evaluation of regional myocardial function has been reported with utilization of DTI,[9] color kinesis,[39] and transpulmonary contrast agents.[3–7]

Right ventricular function is more difficult to measure owing to the peculiar geometry of this chamber. 2-D or 3-D echocardiography can be employed for volume calculations.[40–42] Fractional area change and tricuspid annulus systolic displacement are other methods for assessing right ventricular systolic function.[43, 44]

Left Ventricular Diastolic Function Assessment

Since the late 1980s, there has been large body of literature dealing with the assessment of left ventricular diastolic function.[45–51] The three basic abnormalities identified by pulsed-wave interrogation of the mitral inflow—impaired relaxation, pseudonormalization, and restriction—have been of great value in the diagnosis and definition of the most appropriate therapeutic strategy in patients with diastolic heart failure (Plates 4–1 to 4–4). In addition, the deceleration of time of the transmitral E wave predicts an elevated left ventricular end-diastolic pressure (LVEDP)[52] and is an important prognostic variable in patients with congestive heart failure.[53, 54] More recently, the addition of color M-mode propagation across the mitral valve and DTI to the armamentarium of Doppler echocardiography made possible a more accurate evaluation of diastolic function and better differentiation between constriction and restriction physiology.[55, 56] The flow propagation velocity measured with color M-mode Doppler from the mitral leaflets tips to the ventricular apex is negatively correlated with the time constant of relaxation.[57] The time delay between the point of maximal velocity at the tip of the mitral leaflets and at the apex has been prolonged in myocardial ischemia.[58, 59] DTI has been shown to be able to identify regional myocardial dysfunction provoked by ischemia.[40, 41] DTI is utilized for assessing the left ventricular filling pattern,[60] detection of early diastolic changes in patients with secondary left ventricular hypertrophy,[61] differentiation between hypertrophic cardiomyopathy and myocardial hypertrophy in athletes,[62] evaluation of diastolic function in tachycardia,[63] and calculation of right ventricular systolic pressure (RVSP).[64] The reflected left ventricular diastolic filling waves are helpful in assessing myocardial relaxation process.[65]

Hemodynamics

The introduction of Doppler interrogation of the blood-flow direction and velocity facilitated the calculation of pressure gradients, valve area, and shunt volume and the assessment of intracardiac pressures. Numerous validation studies have shown excellent correlation with the data obtained by invasive methods.[66–77] The flow calculation from the product of the cross-sectional area of the orifice and the time velocity integral (TVI) of the particular flow are utilized in the calculation of left ventricular stroke volume and/or shunt volume. The simplified Bernoulli equation, which derives the pressure gradients from the peak velocity of flow, and the continuity equation are the most utilized for assessing the hemodynamics. However, a number of limitations of these equations should be recognized in order to more accurately assess the hemodynamic values; for example, a small error in the measurement of LVOT diameter, when multiplied by itself, can produce significant error in stroke volume calculation. Malalignment of the Doppler beam to the flow direction may produce significant errors in the systolic pulmonary artery pressure (SPAP) estimation or aortic valve area (AVA) calculation. The simplified Bernoulli equation that disregards the velocity proximal to the obstruction should not be used when this velocity is greater than 1 m/s; instead, the expanded equation should be utilized:

$$p1 - p2 = 4(V2^2 - V1^2)$$

where p1 = pressure proximal to an obstruction (e.g., LVOT), p2 = pressure distal to an obstruction (e.g., aortic valve), V1 = velocity proximal to an obstruction, and V2 = velocity distal to an obstruction. The RVSP, which in the absence of right ventricular tract obstruction or pulmonic valve stenosis equals the SPAP, can be derived from the peak velocity of tricuspid regurgitant jet. In the presence of a ventricular septal defect (VSD), RVSP can be calculated from the trans-VSD gradient by subtracting this gradient from the systemic systolic blood pressure. With a patent ductus arteriosus, the same principle can be applied as in VSDs for calculation of RVSP. The mean and diastolic pulmonary artery pressure can be calculated from the early and late peak diastolic gradients to which the right atrial pressure is added.

With valvular heart diseases, the continuity equation is utilized to calculate the functional valve area, whereas the anatomic valve area can be measured by planimetry in short-axis views. In regurgitant lesions, qualitative, semiquantitative, and quantitative methods are used. The calculation of regurgitant volume, regurgitant stroke volume, effective regurgitant orifice area, and regurgitant fraction are quantitative means to estimate the severity of regurgitant lesions and ideally should be applied routinely in clinical practice. New methods were developed for estimation of pulmonary wedge pressure by color M-mode propagation and DTI.[74, 78]

Specific Clinical Applications of Doppler Echocardiography

Valvular Heart Diseases

Mitral Stenosis

Historically, the recognition of mitral stenosis was the first clinical application of echocardiography (Fig. 4–2). The planimetry of mitral valve area in short-axis view from transthoracic or transgastric windows and the pressure half-time method measure the anatomic valve area, whereas other Doppler methods (continuity equation, and proximal isovelocity acceleration [PISA] method) measure the functional valve area. The PISA method is based on the principle of conservation of mass: all the blood flow approaching a regurgitant orifice has to exit through that orifice and in order to cross it has to accelerate to reach a peak velocity

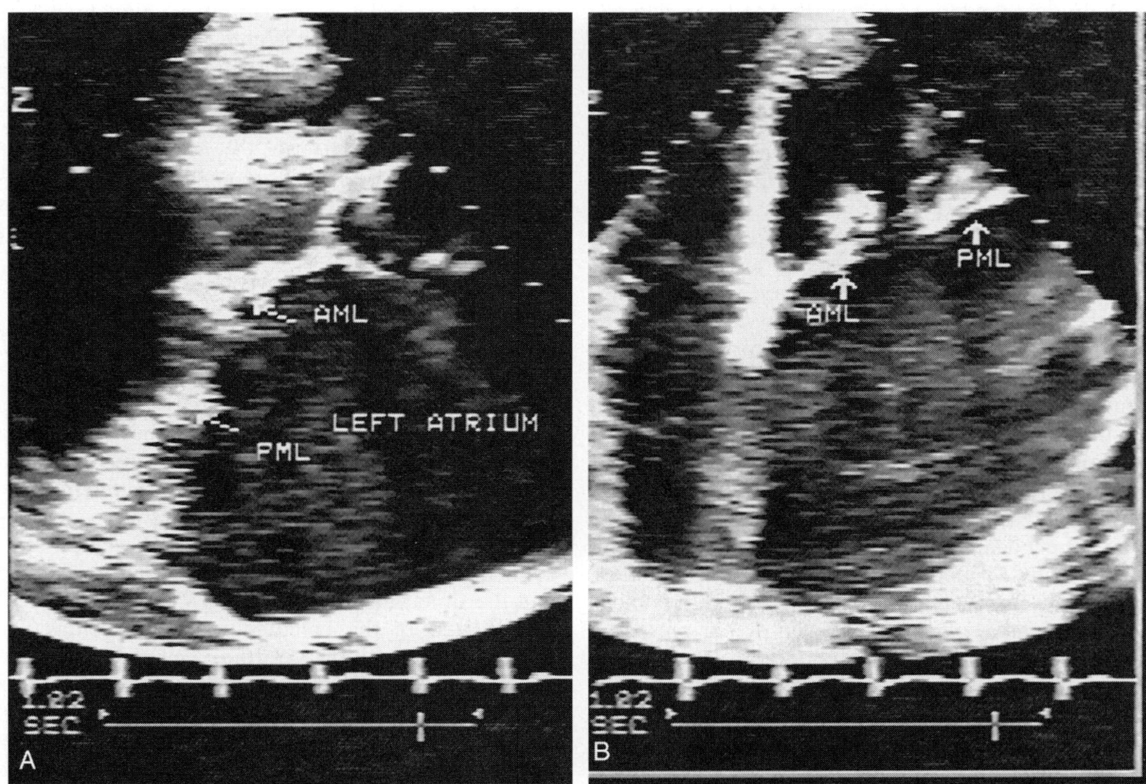

FIGURE 4–2 TTE PSLAX **(A)** and apical four-chamber **(B)** views show a giant left atrium secondary to long-standing mitral stenosis and chronic atrial fibrillation. Spontaneous echo contrast is evident into the left atrium. AML, anterior mitral leaflet; PML, posterior mitral leaflet.

at the orifice. If one knows the radius of the first concentric hemisphere formed proximal to the regurgitant or stenotic orifice and the velocity of blood at that level, a regurgitant volume can be calculated by multiplying cross-sectional area of that hemisphere with the velocity at that point. Effective regurgitant or stenotic orifice can be further determined by dividing instantaneous flow by instantaneous velocity. A factor correcting for the inflow funnel angle formed by the mitral leaflets is used for calculating mitral valve area in mitral stenosis or effective regurgitant area in mitral regurgitation (MR) with an eccentric jet. Besides mitral valve area, the diastolic transmitral gradients at rest and exercise, the degree of left atrial enlargement, the presence of spontaneous echo contrast or thrombus in the left atrium or left atrial appendage, the estimation of SPAP, and the identification of other valvular abnormalities frequently described in rheumatic heart disease complete the echocardiographic evaluation of these patients (Fig. 4–3). Two different echocardiography scores have been proposed for prediction of success of balloon valvuloplasty[79] and the occurrence of postprocedural MR.[80] In most instances, TEE is not required for the evaluation of these patients unless the identification of intra-atrial clots is the clinical question.

Mitral Regurgitation

The echocardiographic examination may reveal the etiology (organic, functional, or ischemic) of mitral regurgitation (MR), evaluate its severity, and determine the optimal timing for surgery. The modern echocardiographic criteria for the diagnosis of mitral valve prolapse (MVP) were described in 1988.[81] Parasternal long-axis and apical long-axis windows are recommended for the diagnosis of MVP. Patients with "classic" MVP (leaflets thickening > 5 mm and upward displacement of the leaflets > 2 mm) have an increased risk of endocarditis and an increased severity of MR requiring surgical therapy (Fig. 4–4),[82] In the absence

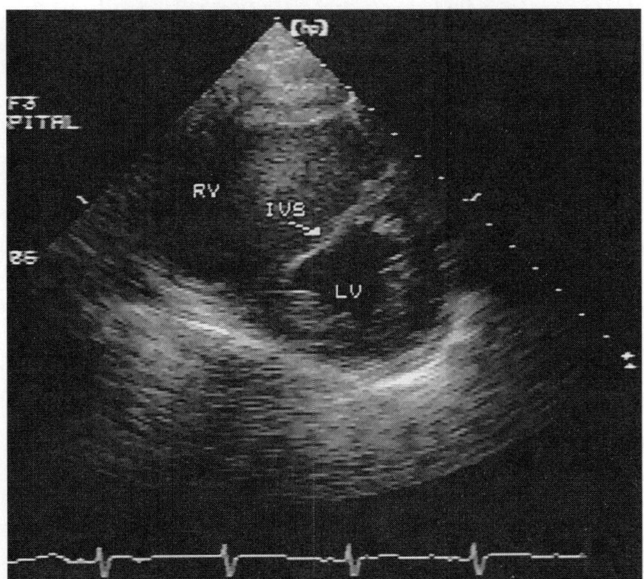

FIGURE 4–3 TTE SAX view shows an enlarged right ventricle (RV) and a D-shaped interventricular septum (IVS), suggesting the presence of pulmonary hypertension. LV, left ventricle.

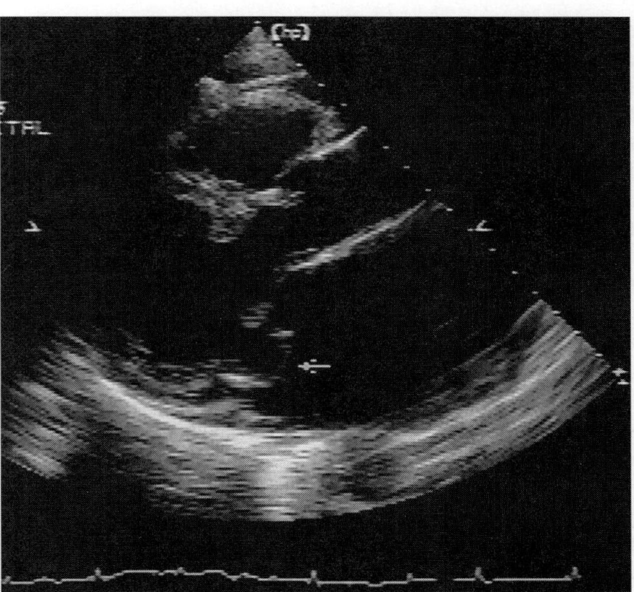

FIGURE 4–4 TTE PSLAX view shows a myxomatous degenerated mitral valve with severe prolapse of the posterior leaflet *(arrow)*.

of MR at rest, patients with MVP who develop MR during exercise have a higher risk of clinical events.[83] Estimates of the severity of MR, left ventricular and right ventricular function, left ventricular systolic and diastolic diameters and volumes, left atrial size, and left ventricular end-systolic wall stress corrected for end-systolic volume index help guide the decision for surgical correction of MR and predict surgical outcome. The evaluation of the severity of MR is done by qualitative and quantitative methods. Although color-flow spatial distribution of MR jet is the most frequent method utilized for the assessment of MR severity in clinical practice, this is not the most accurate one, especially with eccentrically directed jets. The calculation of regurgitant stroke volume and the effective regurgitant orifice area (EOA) by the PISA method[84–87] is very helpful

$$Q = (2\pi r^2)Vr$$

where Vr is the velocity of a hemisphere shell defined by the radius r.

$$EOA = Q/\text{peak velocity of regurgitant jet}$$

The measurement of vena contracta (the narrowest diameter of the color-flow jet just downstream of the regurgitant orifice) correlates well with the severity of MR measured by other methods.[88–90]

Aortic Stenosis

The echocardiogram identifies the location of LVOT obstruction (valvular, subvalvular, or supravalvular), the anatomy of the aortic valve (bicuspid valve being the most frequent etiology of aortic valvular aortic stenosis in individuals < 65 years old), the magnitude of aortic cusps separation (normal > 1.5 cm), the degree of cusp calcification, and the presence of associated lesions (e.g., vegetations). The degree of left ventricular hypertrophy, in the absence of other conditions that increase the left ventricular afterload, usually indicates the severity and duration of LVOT obstruction, and left atrial dilatation may suggest the presence of left ventricular diastolic dysfunction in the absence of mitral valve diseases and/or atrial fibrillation. In patients with bicuspid valves, the descending thoracic aorta should be evaluated for the presence of aortic coarctation. Applying the continuity equation, one may evaluate functional aortic valve area, which is usually smaller than the area calculated at cardiac catheterization, which includes a constant to account for the coefficient of discharge. By continuity equation

$$\text{AVA} = \text{CSA(LVOT)} \times \text{TVI(LVOT)/TVI(AV)}$$

where CSA = cross-sectional area calculated by π multiplied by the square of the LVOT radius. There is a very good correlation between the instantaneous transvalvular gradients measured by continuous-wave Doppler and those measured at cardiac catheterization.[91] The echocardiographic measurement of the anatomic aortic valve area is done by planimetry, and its correlation with the aortic valve area calculated at cardiac catheterization should be excellent when the commissures are well identified. Using TEE, planimetry of AVA has been shown to be a valuable method of measurement of anatomic AVA (Fig. 4–5).[92] If the aortic valve area is not measured, in the presence of preserved left ventricular systolic function, a mean transaortic gradient greater than 50 mm Hg usually signifies severe valvular stenosis (AVA < 1 cm^2), whereas a mean transvalvular gradient less than 20 mm Hg usually indicates mild stenosis (AVA > 1.5 cm^2). A mean transvalvular gradient between 20 and 50 mm Hg defines AVA less accurately, and in such cases, AVA should be calculated.[93] If peak transaortic velocities are considered, a peak velocity greater than or equal to 4 m/s predicts an AVA less than or equal to 0.8 cm^2, whereas a peak transaortic velocity less than or equal to 3 m/s predicts noncritical aortic stenosis. The correlation between transaortic peak velocity and AVA at catheterization was -0.72 in one study.[94] The accurate measurement of the sinotubular junction is required for those patients in whom a stentless prosthetic valve is present. Low-dose dobutamine infusion coupled with echocardiography has been reported to be able to identify those patients with severe aortic stenosis, poor left ventricular systolic function, and low mean transaortic gradients that benefit from surgery. Dobutamine may improve cardiac output and therefore increase AVA with little change in the transvalvular gradient. These patients are unlikely to improve left ventricular systolic function after surgery, in contrast to those patients who exhibit an increase in cardiac output and transvalvular gradients with no change in AVA (fixed aortic stenosis) during dobutamine infusion.[95]

Aortic Regurgitation

In a large number of patients, transthoracic echocardiography (TTE) identifies the mechanism of regurgitation (e.g.,

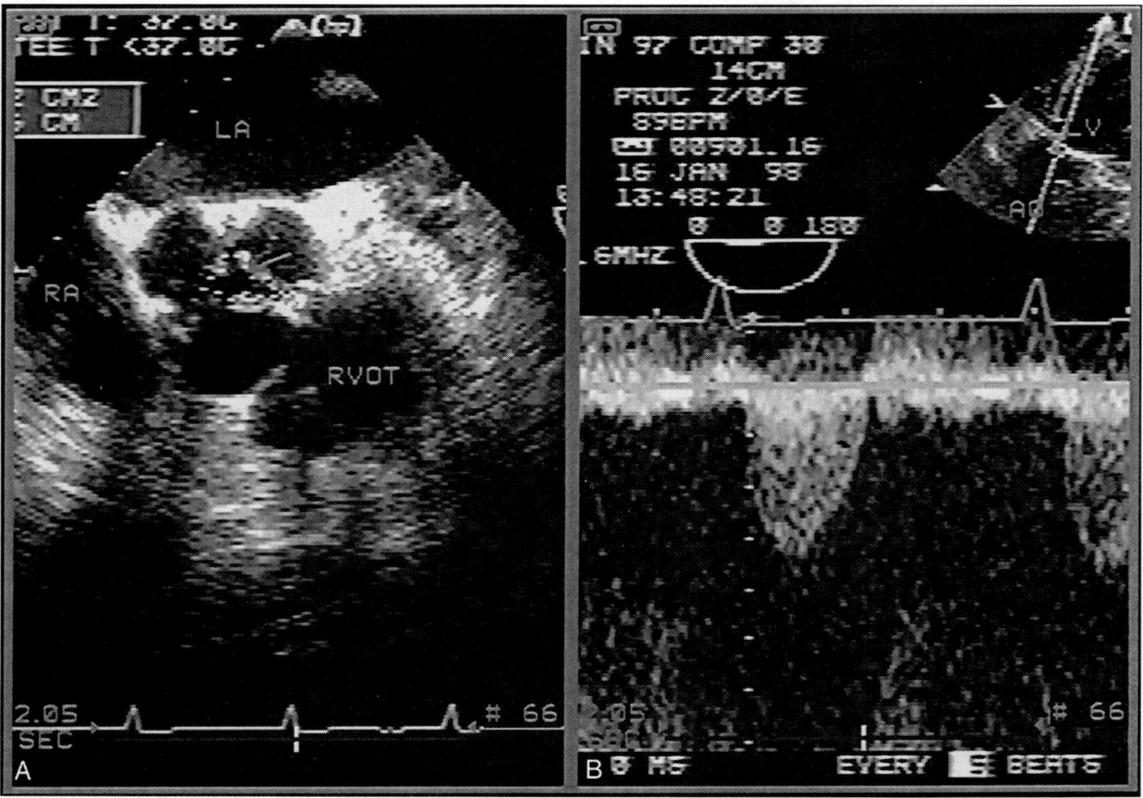

FIGURE 4–5 Transesophageal echocardiography (TEE) horizontal plane view in a patient with moderate calcified valvular aortic stenosis. **A,** Midesophageal view shows the anatomic aortic valve area measured by planimetry (0.9 cm^2). LA, left atrium; RA, right atrium; RVOT, right ventricular outflow tract. **B,** Deep transgastric view, continuous-wave Doppler interrogation of the aortic valve identified a peak gradient of 58 mm Hg and a mean gradient of 31 mm Hg. AO, aorta; LV, left ventricle.

congenital or acquired aortic root dilatation, intimal dissection) and its severity and provides an accurate measurement of aortic annulus, sinotubular junction, aortic arch, and proximal descendent aorta. The geometry of the cusps in systole (triangle sign) has recently been described as a means to identify the aortic root dilatation with practical surgical implications (repair versus replacement).[96] The semiquantification of regurgitation severity is best done by color-flow Doppler in parasternal long-axis view as the ratio between the width of regurgitant jet immediately below the valve and the LVOT.[97] Other semiquantitative methods for evaluation of aortic regurgitation severity are the slope of deceleration of the aortic regurgitation jet interrogated by continuous-wave Doppler (a steeper slope meaning a higher LVEDP and, therefore, a higher degree of severity); identifying holodiastolic reverse flow in the abdominal aorta; and the ratio of diastolic to systolic flow integrals in the ascending or proximal thoracic descending aorta.[98] Aortic regurgitant volume, regurgitant fraction, and EOA can be calculated by Doppler methods or PISA, especially in flat-flow convergence.[99] With acute and severe aortic regurgitation, the rapid and excessive increase in LVEDP will be reflected in premature closure of the mitral valve, diastolic MR, and premature opening of the aortic valve.[100–102] A number of echocardiographic variables have been described to assess the timing for surgery[103] and postoperative outcome.[104–106] In general, it is considered that the optimal timing for aortic valve surgery is before LVEF falls below 55 percent or the end-systolic dimension is larger than 55 mm. When the etiology of aortic regurgitation is suspected to be aortic dissection, a TEE will often define the location and extension of dissection, identify the entry and the exit sites, evaluate involvement of coronary arteries, and detect the presence and severity of aortic regurgitation. TTE from a suprasternal window helps to provide visualization of the distal ascending aorta and proximal aortic arch. We perform annual serial echocardiographic examinations in patients who have repairs of their aortic dissections in order to identify early progression or recurrence of disease (Fig. 4–6).

Prosthetic Valves

Echocardiography has an important role in determining the size of valvular annulus, allowing preoperative consideration of the size of the valve to be placed. Prosthetic valve function can be evaluated by both echocardiography (e.g., mechanical bileaflet prosthetic valves in mitral position will give two parallel linear echo reverberations, reflecting full valve opening in diastole) and Doppler examination (transvalvular gradients). The presence of masses attached to the prosthetic material (thrombus, pannus, or vegetations) may significantly affect the normal valve function, and the dehiscence of the suture lines can generate regurgitant jets, which sometimes may lead to severe hemolysis.[107, 108] TEE has an important role in the evaluation of prosthetic mitral valves and the interannular fibrosa where an abscess can occur (Fig. 4–7 and Plate 4–5).

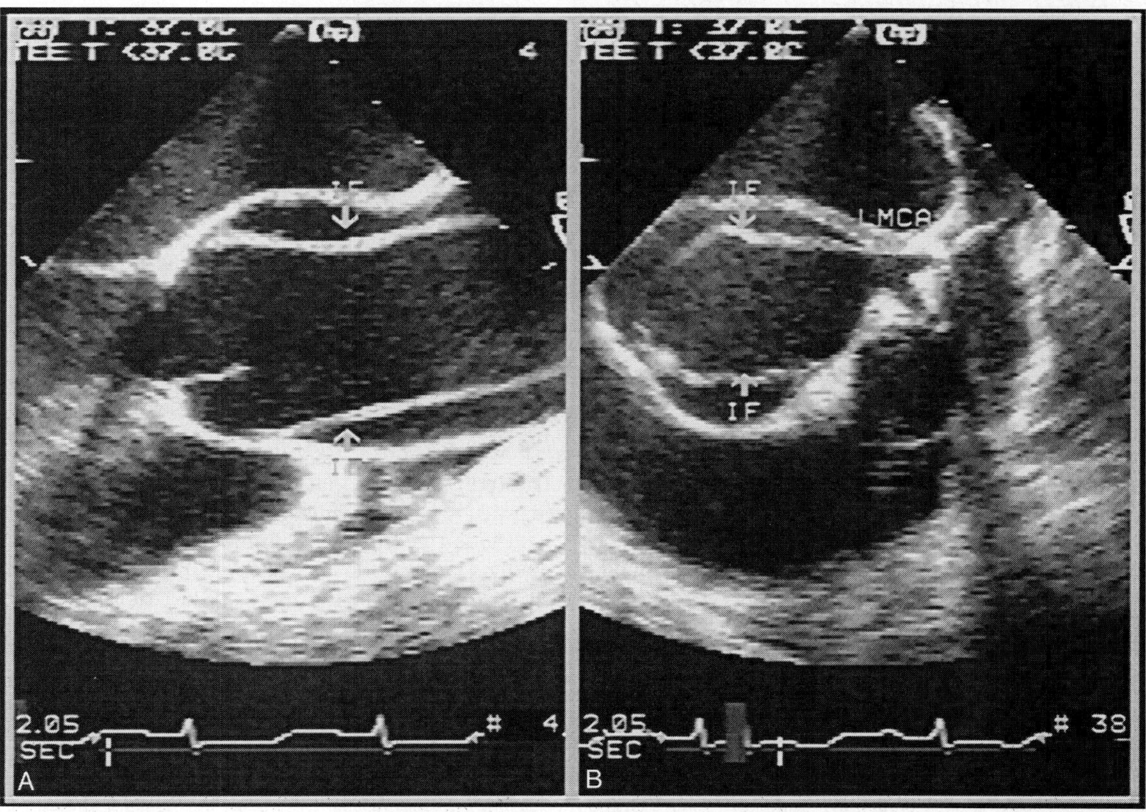

FIGURE 4–6 TEE multiplane probe at 130 degrees **(A)** and 30 degrees **(B)** show a dissecting aneurysm of the ascending aorta. The intimal flap (IF) extends into the ostium of the left main coronary artery (LMCA) **(B)**.

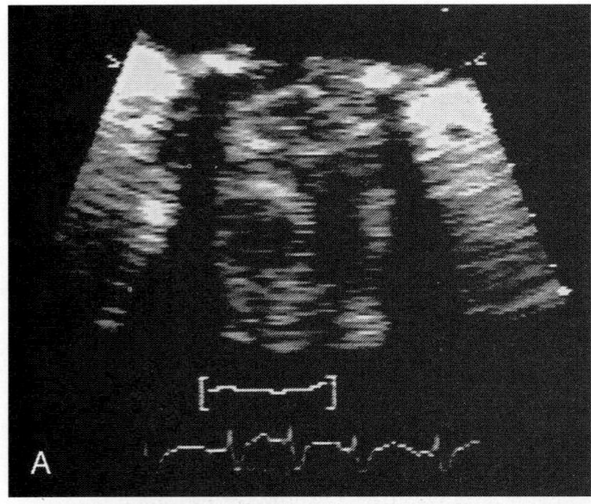

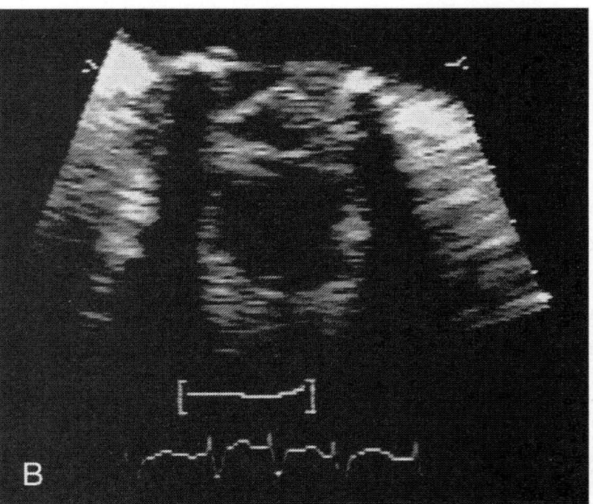

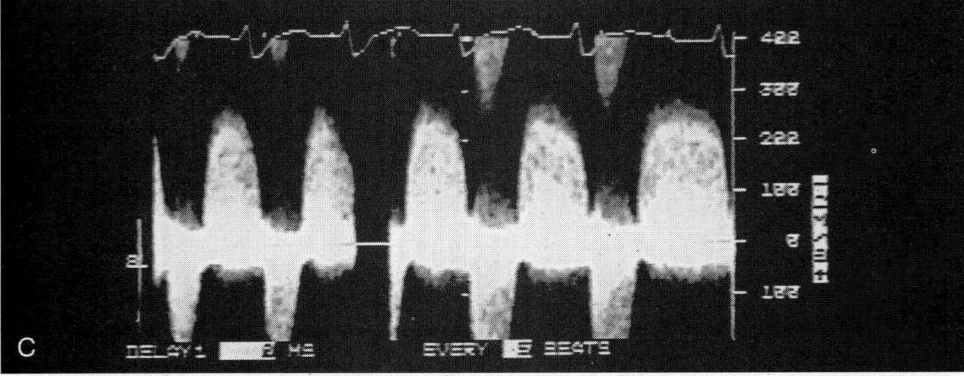

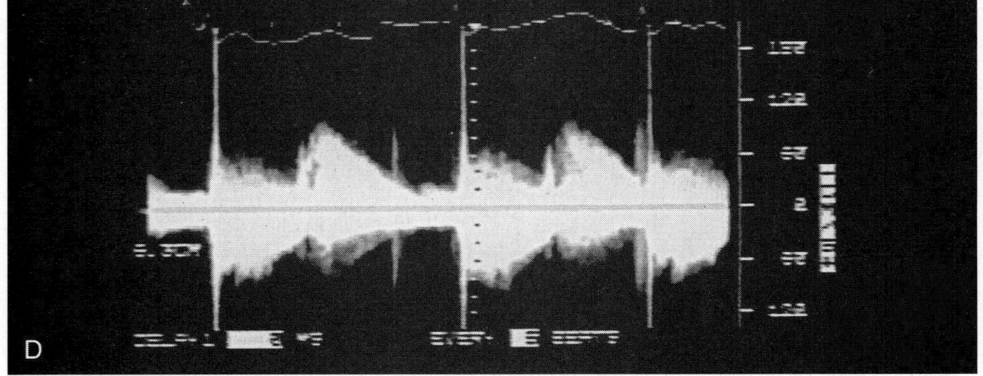

FIGURE 4–7 TEE horizontal plane view shows a thrombosed mechanical bileaflet prosthetic mitral valve with a mean transmitral gradient of 20 mm Hg. **A,** Systolic frame. **B,** Diastolic frame. Note that there is not much movement of the mechanical leaflets between systole and diastole. **C,** Continuous-wave Doppler interrogation of the transmitral flow shows a significant increase in the left atrium–left ventricle gradient. **D,** Continuous-wave Doppler interrogation of the mitral flow after surgery shows the normalization of the transprosthetic gradient (peak gradient = 4 mm Hg).

Infective Endocarditis

Although infective endocarditis is a clinical diagnosis, echocardiography can often identify the presence of vegetations, abscess, dehiscence of prosthetic valves, mycotic aneurysm, or arterial-cameral fistula. Typically, staphylococcal, gram-negative organisms, gonococcal, or fungal vegetations are 2 to 3 cm in diameter or larger. Vegetations larger than 10 mm have a high propensity to embolize.[109] Recently, it has been shown that the diagnostic value of TEE resides mainly in the evaluation of patients who have prosthetic valves and in whom TTE is either technically inadequate or indicates an intermediate probability of endocarditis.[110] In nonbacterial endocarditis, the echocardiographic diagnosis is very helpful because the clinical suspicion is much lower than for infective endocarditis (Fig. 4–8 and Plate 4–6).

Cardiomyopathies

Dilated Cardiomyopathy

Dilated cardiomyopathy has multiple echocardiographic features besides ventricular enlargement: changes in left ventricular geometry (from ellipsoid to spherical), different degrees of systolic dysfunction, different patterns of diastolic filling, and often MR and/or tricuspid regurgitation. The incomplete closure of the mitral valve reflected by an increase in the distance between the mitral annulus and the point of apposition of the mitral leaflets (apical tethering or tenting) (Fig. 4–9)[111] creates functional MR. A thrombus can often be visualized in the cardiac apex in these patients. They frequently have left atrial dilatation and pulmonary hypertension. Although an ischemic etiology of dilated cardiomyopathy can be inferred by the presence of preserved contractility in some left ventricular segments,[112]

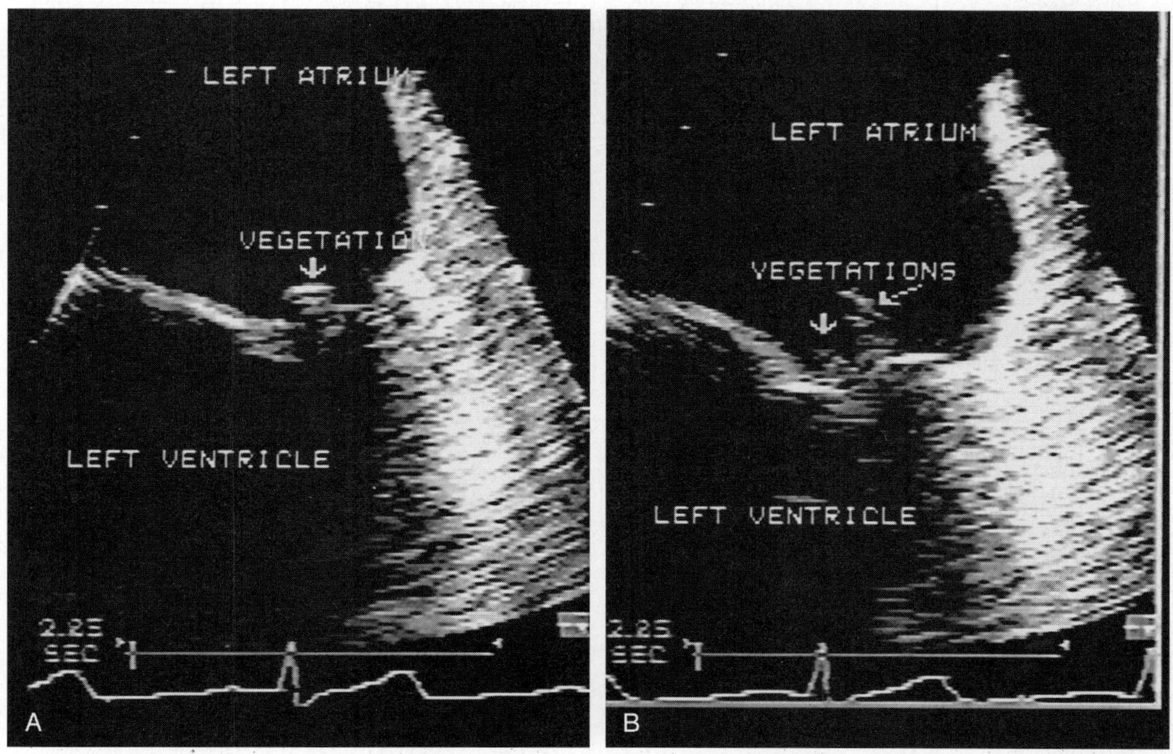

FIGURE 4–8 TEE study shows small, ill-defined masses *(arrows)* attached to the atrial aspect of the mitral valve leaflets, consistent with vegetations in a patient with infective endocarditis.

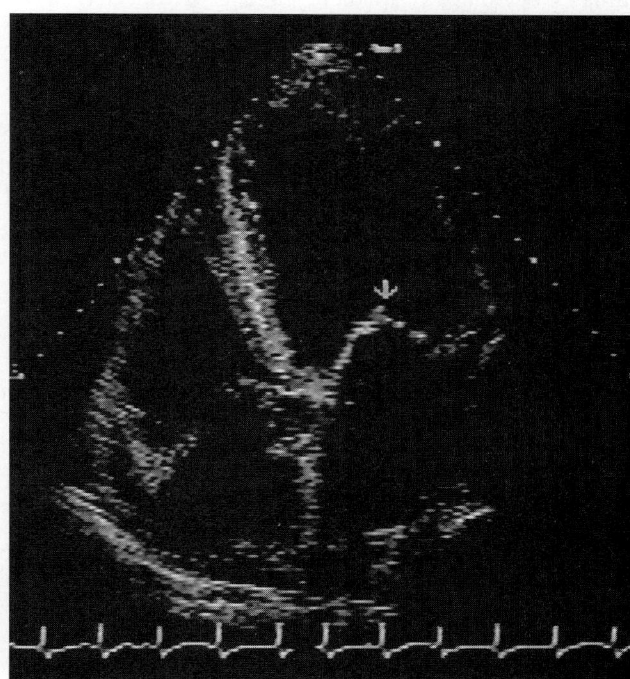

FIGURE 4–9 TTE apical four-chamber view in a patient with dilated cardiomyopathy and spontaneous echo contrast in the left ventricle. In diastole, there is an increase in distance between the mitral annulus plane and the apposition point of the mitral valve leaflets, giving the tenting appearance *(arrow)* of mitral leaflets.

approximately 60 percent of patients with idiopathic dilated cardiomyopathy may also have regional wall motion abnormalities.[113] A restrictive type of left ventricular filling characterized by a transmitral E/A ratio greater than 2, a deceleration time of E wave less than 130 ms, and an isovolumic relaxation time less than 60 ms are predictors of increased mortality in these patients.[53, 54]

Restrictive Cardiomyopathy

Restrictive cardiomyopathy is often characterized by normal-sized ventricles with increased wall thickness, biatrial dilatation, and an increase in diameter of the pulmonic veins signifying high atrial pressures. Small to moderate pericardial effusions have been described in amyloidosis (Fig. 4–10).[114, 115] A speckled or granular sparkling appearance to the LV owing to acoustic mismatch between amyloid fibrils and myocytes[115] occurs in approximately 50 percent of patients, mainly in those with severe disease.[114] Restrictive cardiomyopathy causes left ventricular and/or right ventricular diastolic dysfunction, including an abnormal relaxation pattern, continuing with pseudonormalization, and in advanced stages of the disease, a restrictive pattern is observed.[116]

Hypertrophic Obstructive Cardiomyopathy (Fig. 4–11)

The echocardiogram provides the diagnoses in these patients and will give accurate measurements of the degree of hypertrophy of the left ventricular walls and eventually the right ventricular free wall and will identify unusual forms of hypertrophy (apical, basal, midventricular). Myocardial fiber disarray in these patients is reflected in the "ground-glass" acoustic texture. Left ventricular size may be decreased owing to significant hypertrophy. Systolic anterior motion of the anterior mitral valve leaflet (Plate 4–7) is the hallmark of dynamic obstruction. The left atrium may be dilated. Valsalva maneuver and/or amyl nitrate administration is indicated for detection of latent obstruction; these maneuvers may bring out the systolic anterior motion pattern. In those patients with systolic anterior motion, MR is present (see Plate 4–7). The impact of medication, surgery, or pacemaker therapy on the dynamic gradient across the LVOT is accurately evaluated by Doppler echocardiography. Recent data explain the interindividual differences in MR severity despite similar LVOT gradients by the mismatch of anterior to posterior leaflet length and decreased posterior mitral leaflet mobility.[117]

Identification of Intracardiac or Aortic Source of Systemic or Pulmonary Embolism

The main findings by TTE and/or TEE are infectious or noninfectious vegetations (Fig. 4–12), tumors (Figs. 4–13 and 4–14) or thrombus, interatrial septal abnormalities (atrial septum aneurysm, patent foramen ovale, atrial septal defect), spontaneous echo contrast, and ascending aorta or aortic arch atherosclerotic debris that, when 4 mm or greater, are significant predictors of recurrent cerebral emboli and other vascular events (Fig. 4–15).[118] A vigorous Valsalva maneuver is required to identify a small patent foramen ovale, which may be responsible for a paradoxical embolism. However, in patients with a normal TTE, the TEE has a higher sensitivity for identifying interatrial septum pathology and should be recommended in younger patients (<45 years) with otherwise unexplained events in whom a patent foramen ovale is more prevalent and potentially more important.[119] We recently reported a significant increase in embolic strokes (4.4-fold) in patients with aortic sinotubular debris identified by TTE (Fig. 4–16).[120]

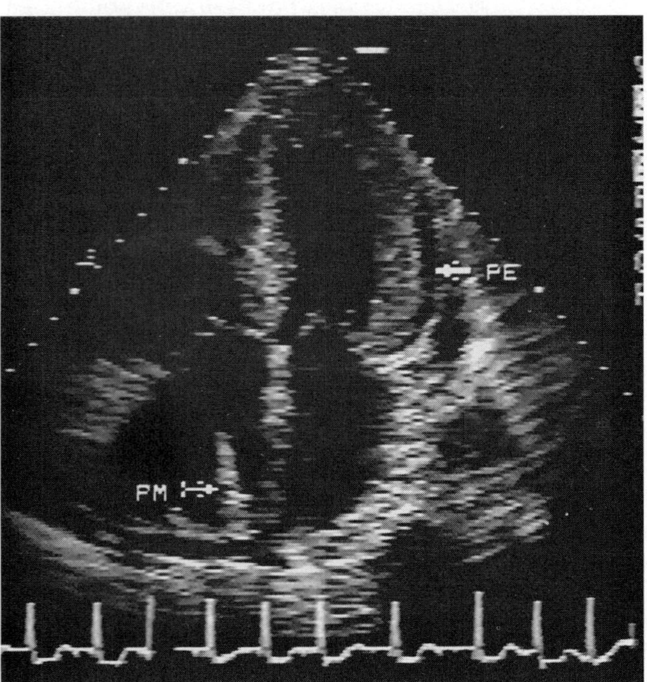

FIGURE 4–10 TTE apical 4-chamber view in a patient with cardiac amyloidosis. The "ground-glass" appearance of the myocardium and the small pericardial effusion (PE; *thick arrow*) are evident. A pacemaker wire (PM; *thin arrow*) is also shown.

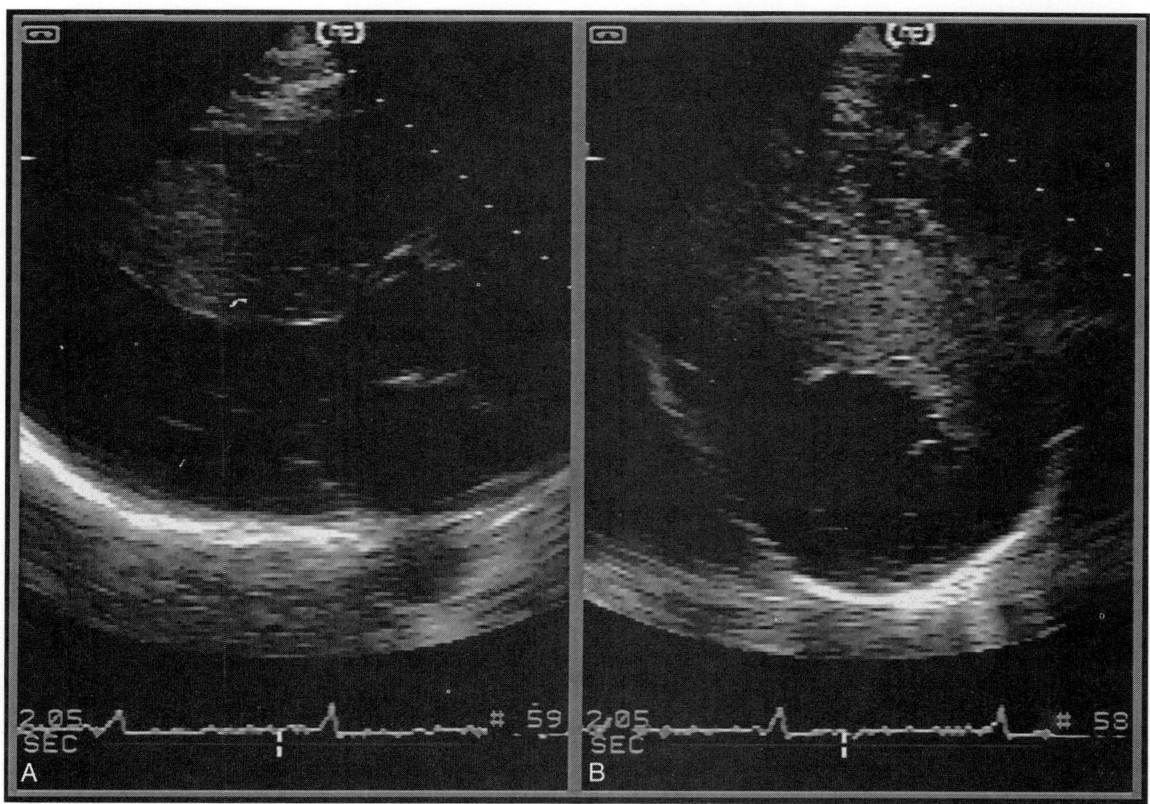

FIGURE 4–11 TTE, PSLAX **(A)** and SAX **(B)** views in a patient with asymmetric septal hypertrophy. The diastolic thickness of the interventricular septum is 3.5 cm.

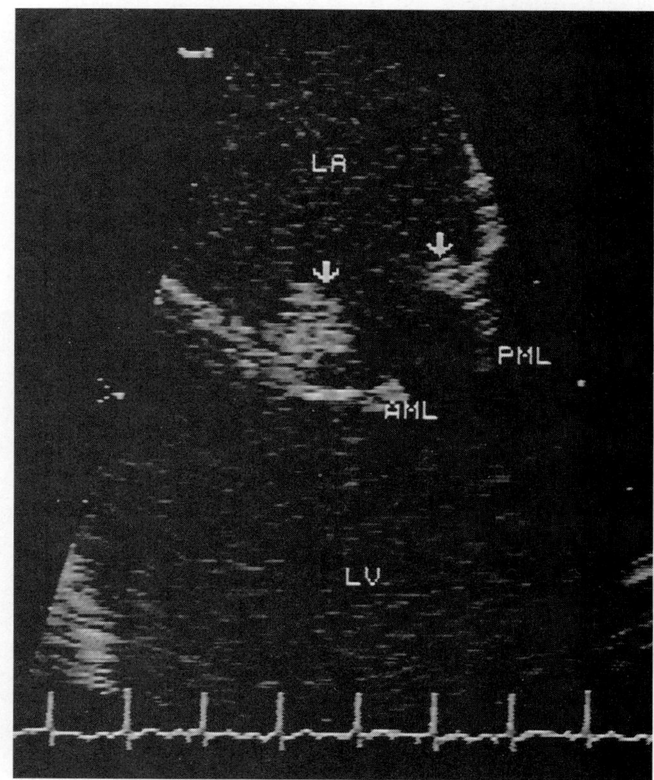

FIGURE 4–12 TEE, horizontal plane, magnified view of the mitral valve shows Libman-Sacks vegetations in a young pregnant woman who presented with a stroke. AML, anterior mitral leaflet; LA, left atrium; LV, left ventricle; PML, posterior mitral leaflet.

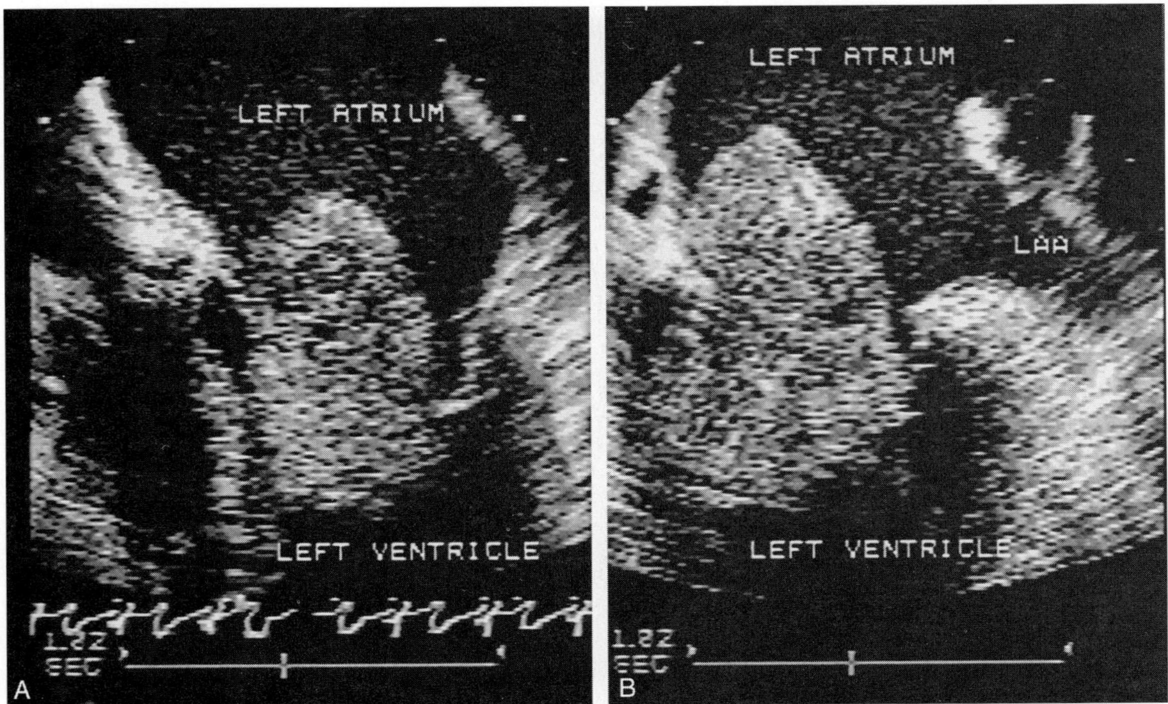

FIGURE 4–13 TEE horizontal **(A)** and longitudinal **(B)** plane views show a large left atrial myxoma prolapsing into the left ventricle in diastole. LAA, left atrial appendage.

Coronary Artery Disease

An abrupt occlusion of a coronary artery will affect both the relaxation and the contraction myocardial properties, the last translating into regional wall motion abnormalities. Patients with acute chest pain of coronary origin can be diagnosed by echocardiography that, from pooled data, has a modest positive predictive value (50 percent) and very high negative predictive value (95 percent) for diagnosing an acute coronary event.[121] In patients with acute myocardial infarction (MI), a rest echocardiogram can identify the location, the extent, and the degree of systolic dysfunction and diastolic impairment. The mechanical complications of an acute MI (Fig. 4–17 and Plate 4–8) (VSD, acute MR, free wall subacute or acute rupture) and recently described LVOT dynamic obstruction in anterior MI when the basal septum is contracting in excess[122, 123] are identifiable by Doppler echocardiography. Contrast echocardiography has proved of great value in determining the success of reperfusion[124–127] and the prognosis after the acute MI.[128] The echocardiographic follow-up of these patients after the acute event is important for evaluation of left ventricular remodeling, thrombus formation, the improvement of regional and global left ventricular function, and the evolution of MR. The risk stratification after an acute MI by stress echocardiography is of considerable value.[129–138] Stress echocardiography has been continuously refined during its more than 20 years of existence,[139] and in competent

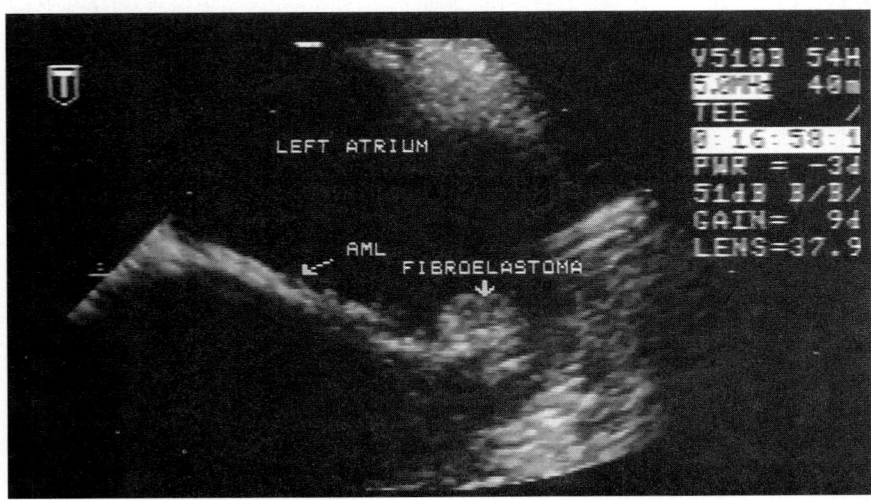

FIGURE 4–14 TEE horizontal plane view shows a well-defined rounded mass attached to the anterior mitral leaflet (AML), suggestive of a fibroelastoma, which was diagnosed at pathology.

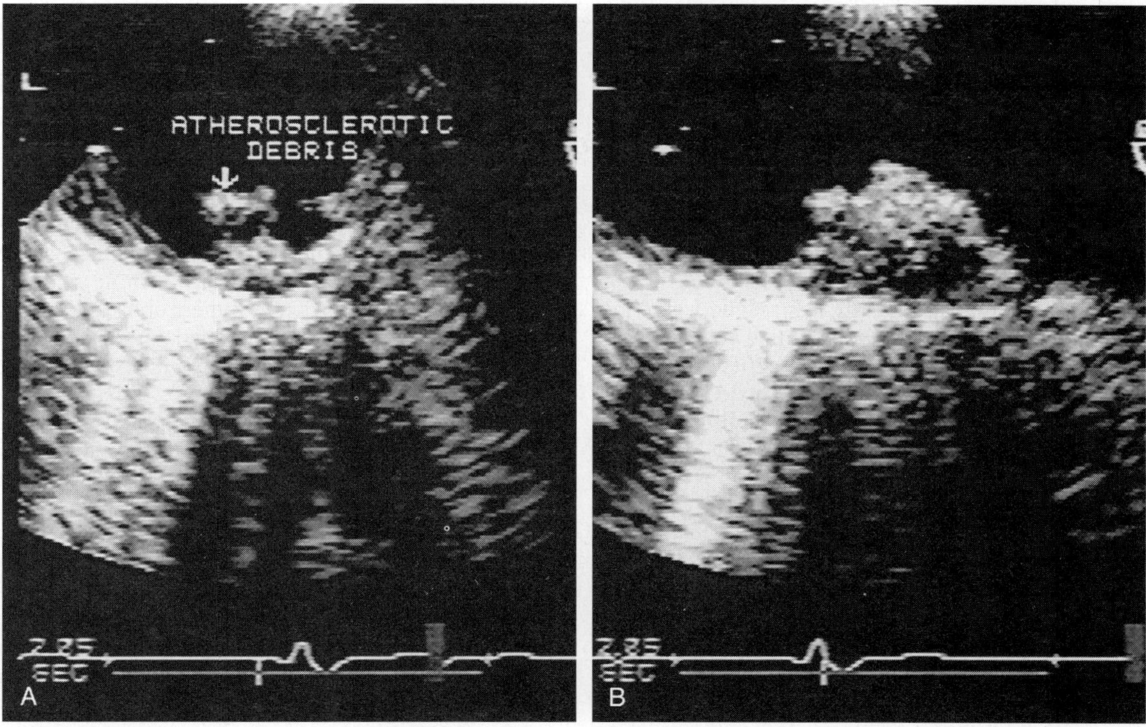

FIGURE 4–15 TEE horizontal **(A)** and longitudinal **(B)** plane views show large atherosclerotic debris in the descending thoracic aorta.

hands, it has sensitivity, specificity, and accuracy similar to those of myocardial nuclear perfusion techniques for the detection and localization of coronary artery disease.[140] Post–treadmill supine bicycle and dobutamine stress echocardiography are the most utilized protocols for exercise and pharmacologic stress, respectively, in the United States today. Identification of viable myocardium by low-dose dobutamine echocardiography in patients with significant left ventricular dysfunction before revascularization procedures (and therefore predicting the postprocedural functional recovery) is another important indication of stress echocardiography.[141–150] In a number of studies comparing

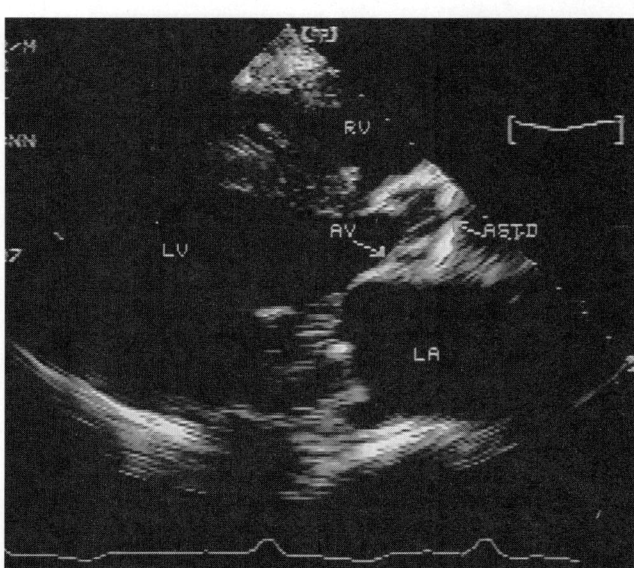

FIGURE 4–16 TTE PSLAX view shows significant aortic sinotubular debris (ASTD; *arrow*). AV, aortic valve; LA, left atrium; LV, left ventricle; RV, right ventricle.

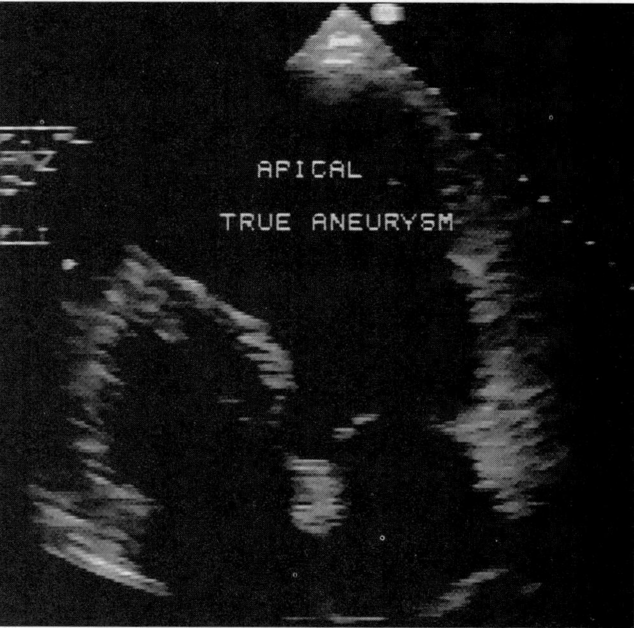

FIGURE 4–17 TTE apical four-chamber view shows a true apical aneurysm in a patient with a large chronic anterior wall myocardial infarction.

dobutamine echocardiography with stress thallium 201 single-photon emission computed tomography (SPECT) for evaluation of viability, dobutamine echocardiography had a higher specificity and a lower sensitivity than that of stress thallium 201 myocardial scintigraphy (90 percent versus 52 percent and 75 percent versus 82 percent).[150, 151] However, the detection of residual viability by thallium 201 does not always correctly predict functional recovery as assessed by the biphasic response during dobutamine echocardiography (improving contractility at low dose and deterioration at high dose). The differences between the evaluation of inotropic reserve by dobutamine echocardiography and the evaluation of myocardial integrity and perfusion by thallium 201 scintigraphy may explain the lower positive predictive value and specificity of thallium.

Pericardial Diseases

The presence, location, semiquantification, and hemodynamic consequences of pericardial effusion can be reliably assessed by Doppler echocardiography. In addition, echocardiography has been shown to be of great value in guiding pericardiocentesis.[152] In small pericardial effusions (<100 ml), the fluid accumulates characteristically around the posterior left ventricular wall. In the absence of a loculated effusion, anterior "echo-free" space represents epicardial fat.[153] Although cardiac tamponade is a clinical diagnosis, a number of echocardiographic findings (right ventricular and right atrial diastolic collapse, inferior vena cava plethora) and Doppler signs (e.g., exacerbation of normal respiratory variation across atrioventricular valves and characteristic hepatic vein flow pattern of significant predominance of systolic flow during the apnea and diminished or reversal diastolic flow velocities on the first beat after the onset of expiration) have been shown to have high accuracy in identifying profound hemodynamic embarrassment that accompanies this condition (Fig. 4–18).[154–159] However, one should be aware of potential confounding factors affecting the interpretation of these highly utilized Doppler echocardiographic variables, including mechanical ventilation, volume status, and the presence of right ventricular hypertrophy and/or pulmonary hypertension. Localized tamponade is usually recognized by TTE, and when clinical suspicion is high (e.g., recent open heart surgery, chest trauma), TEE should be performed.[160]

In patients with a clinical history suggesting constrictive pericarditis (e.g., prior open heart surgery, infectious or connective tissue diseases, trauma) and appropriate symptoms and signs, TEE may allow the best echocardiographic definition of thickened pericardium.[161] The dissociation between intrathoracic and intrapericardial pressures and the strong interventricular coupling existing in constriction explain the Doppler findings in constrictive pericarditis: a significant augmentation of respiratory variation across atrioventricular valves and an expiratory increase flow reversal in hepatic veins.[162, 163] The distinction between constrictive pericarditis and restrictive cardiomyopathy is of considerable importance because the therapeutic options are totally different: surgery for constrictive pericarditis and medical therapy for the patient with restrictive myocardial disease. DTI has been shown to be useful in the differentiation between these two entities. (A peak E′ ve-

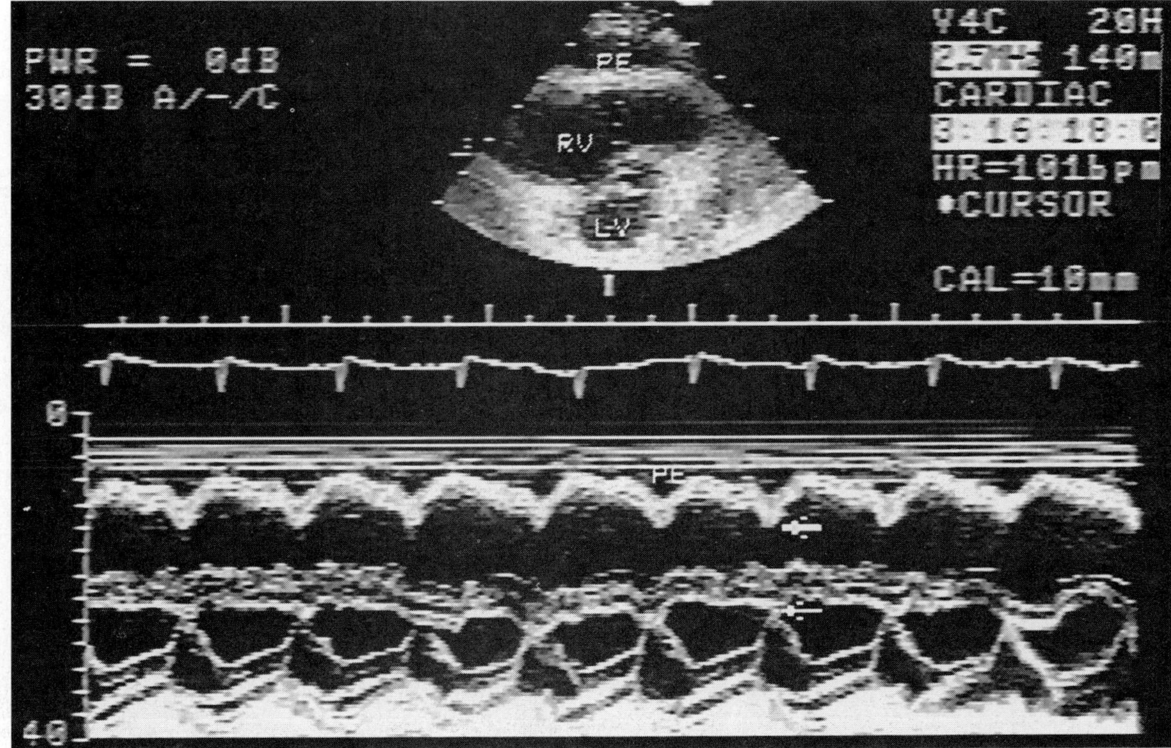

FIGURE 4–18 M-mode echocardiogram parasternal SAX view at the level of the mitral valve shows early diastolic collapse of the right ventricle's (RV) free wall. The nadir of the collapse coincides with the E point of the anterior mitral leaflet. LV, left ventricle; PE, pericardial effusion.

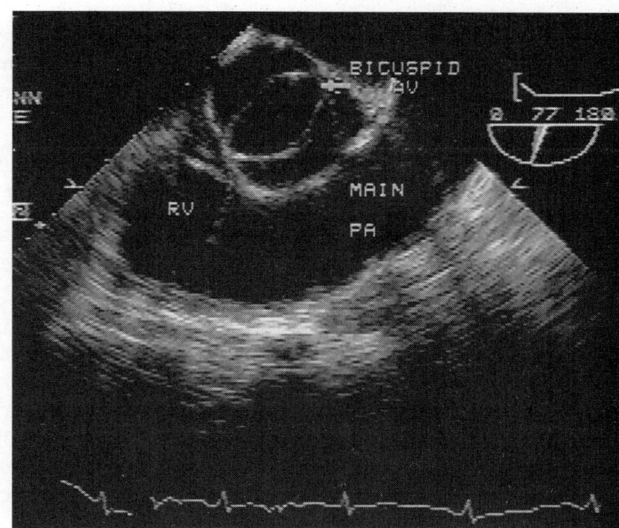

FIGURE 4–19 TEE multiplane probe at 77 degrees shows the characteristic systolic opening of a bicuspid aortic valve (AV). PA, pulmonary artery; RV, right ventricle.

locity < 8 cm/s measured at the lateral mitral annulus or an E′/E index < 0.11 was observed in patients with restrictive cardiomyopathies.[56]) In patients treated with prior radiation therapy, both constriction and restriction physiology can coexist with both pericardial and myocardial fibrosis, making the diagnosis and subsequent treatment more difficult.

Congenital Heart Diseases

For evaluation of complex congenital heart diseases, a segmental analysis is required.[164–166] One should begin with the determination of the atrial situs, continuing with determination of the bulboventricular loops, which describes the location of the ventricles, ventriculoarterial connections (e.g., concordant, discordant, double-outlet), semilunar valves, and finally, the great vessels.

Valvular Abnormalities

Bicuspid aortic valve, the most frequent of congenital heart defects, is usually easily identifiable by TTE finding two instead of three cusps. In cases in which the quality of the TTE study is modest, TEE makes the definitive diagnosis (Fig. 4–19). Progression to stenosis with or without regurgitation is common, and one should search actively for associated lesions like coarctation of the aorta, isolated or in the setting of Shone's complex (supramitral ring, congenital mitral stenosis, discrete subaortic stenosis), and aortic dissection. In Ebstein's anomaly, the septal and posterior leaflets are apically displaced 8 mm/m^2 or more,[167] creating an enlarged right atrium, an atrialized segment of the right ventricle, and a very small right ventricle (Plate 4–9). Severe tricuspid regurgitation and, as associated abnormalities, atrial septal defect or patent foramen ovale are

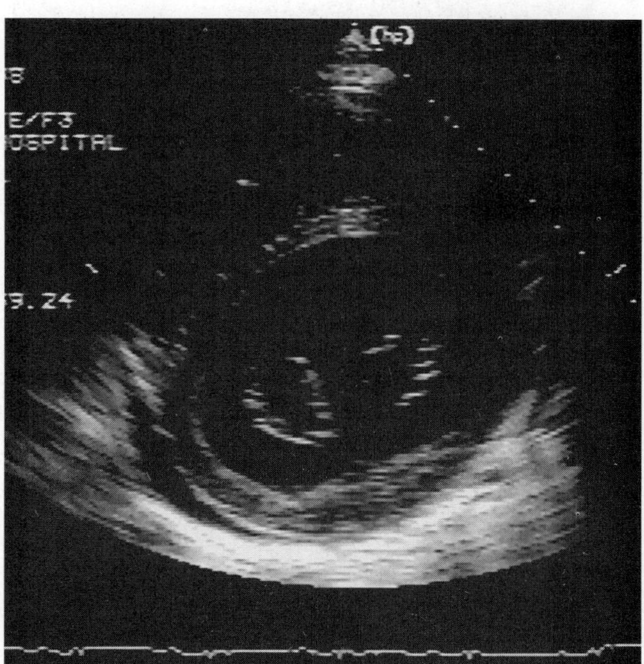

FIGURE 4–20 TTE SAX shows a double-orifice mitral valve. This patient did not have significant mitral regurgitation or mitral stenosis.

usually present.[168] Mitral valve anomalies like parachute valve and double-orifice valve can be identified by transthoracic 2-D echocardiography (Fig. 4–20). Congenital pulmonic valve stenosis can also be diagnosed in adults. A peak transvalvular gradient greater than 50 mm Hg requires balloon valvulotomy or surgical correction.

Cardiac Shunts

VSD, the most common congenital heart disease diagnosed at birth, is found in only about 10 percent of adults (Fig. 4–21).[169] The vast majority of patients have a membranous VSD diagnosed in parasternal views. Supracristal VSD is diagnosed from the parasternal short-axis view at the base of the heart in the vicinity of the pulmonic valve or from the parasternal long-axis view of the right ventricular outflow tract. Aortic insufficiency is more frequently associated with supracristal defects. RVSP and the magnitude of left-to-right shunt can be calculated from transeptal gradient interrogated by continuous-wave Doppler.

In atrial septal defect, the subcostal window usually gives more accurate images. Atrial septum secundum defect is followed by septum primum and sinus venosus defect in decreasing order of frequency. Pulsed-wave, color-flow Doppler and the presence of a "negative" contrast into the right atrium (beware of inferior vena cava or coronary sinus flow, which can also wash out the contrast material from the right atrium) after peripheral injection of 5 to 10 ml of agitated saline solution can identify the defect (Fig. 4–22). MVP (functional or organic) and cleft mitral valve (in septum primum atrial septal defect) can be associated lesions. In the sinus venosus type, one should search for the partial anomalous venous connection. Recently, the value of TEE for diagnosing it has been emphasized.[170, 171] In atrial septal defect, the magnitude of shunt (Qp:Qs) determined by pulmonary (CSA PA $\times$ TVI PA) to systemic (CSA LVOT $\times$ TVI LVOT) flow ratio and pulmonary pressure should be calculated. The degree of right atrial, right ventricular, and main pulmonary artery dilatation should be determined. Patent ductus arteriosus flow is usually visualized by color-flow Doppler from the high left parasternal window at the bifurcation of the main pulmonary artery. Continuous-wave Doppler should be used for estimating pulmonary artery pressure by subtracting the gradient from the systolic systemic arterial pressure.

Complex Congenital Heart Diseases

In tetralogy of Fallot (large VSD, overriding aorta, pulmonary stenosis, and right ventricular hypertrophy), 2-D echocardiography identifies from the parasternal long-axis view the VSD of the anterior malalignment type overriding the dilated aorta (Fig. 4–23). From the parasternal short-axis view, the abnormalities of right ventricular outflow tract, pulmonic valve, and its branches can be determined. In unoperated patients, the shunt across a VSD is small and predominantly right to left (Eisenmenger physiology). Transposition of Fallot with pulmonary atresia has to be differentiated from a truncus arteriosus.

In congenital corrected transposition of the great arteries

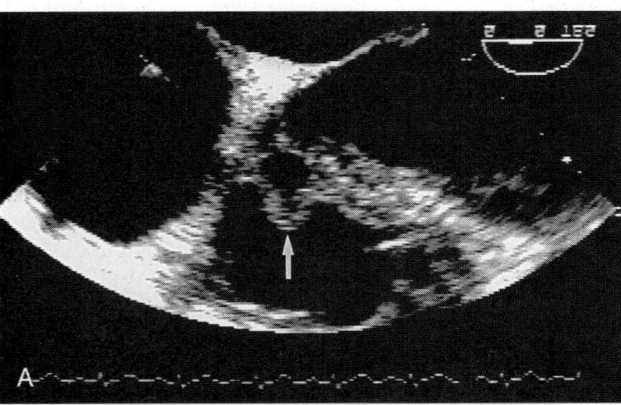

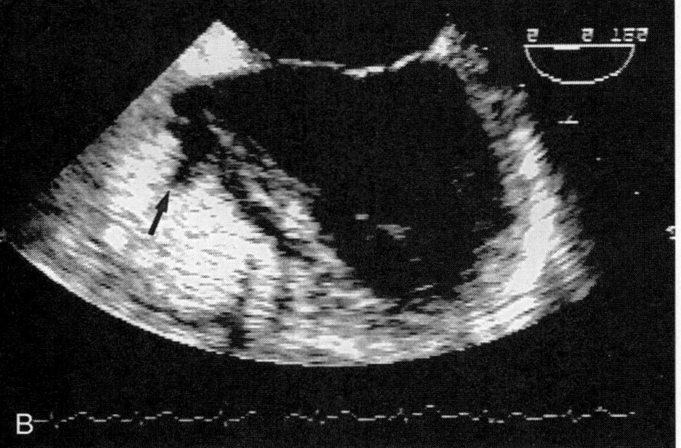

FIGURE 4–21 A, TEE horizontal plane view shows an aneurysm of the membranous interventricular septum *(arrow).* **B,** Contrast study demonstrates a small ventricular septal defect with a left-to-right shunt *(arrow).*

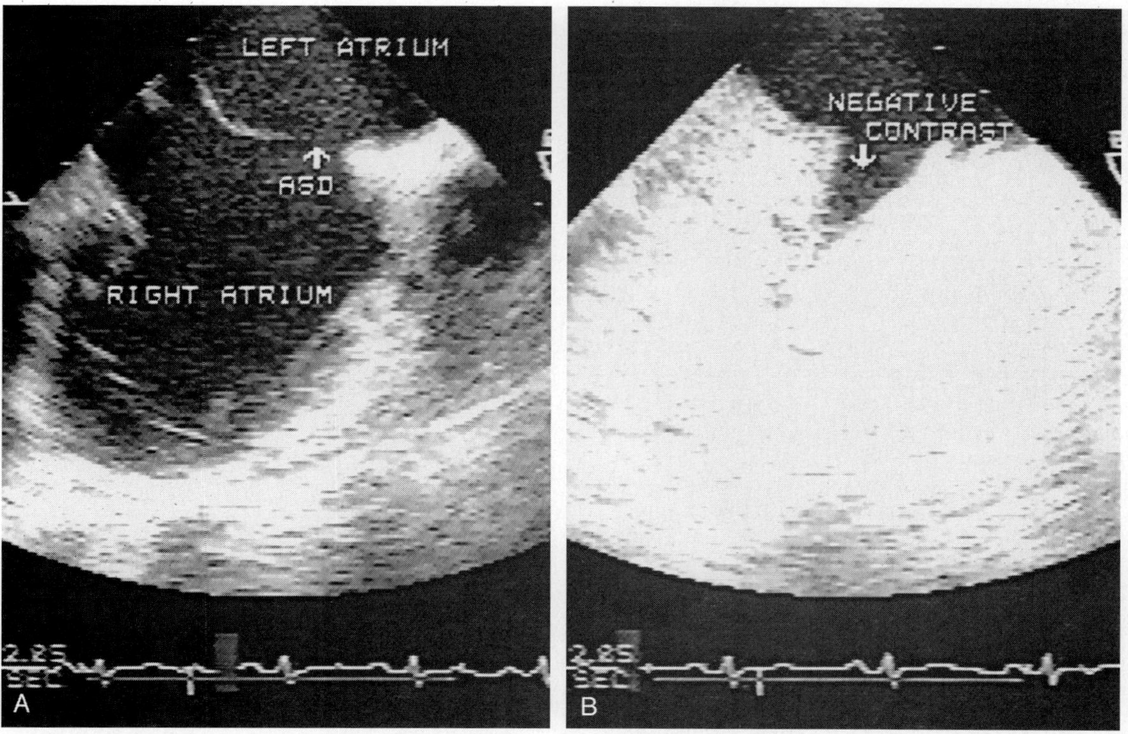

FIGURE 4–22 **A** and **B**, TEE bicaval longitudinal plane views show an atrial septal defect (ASD) secundum type (*arrow* in **A**). The negative contrast in the right atrium (*arrow* in **B**) is explained by the left-to-right shunt washing out the contrast material from the right atrium.

(L-transposition), whereas there is an atrioventricular and a ventricular-arterial discordance, the two arteries run parallel to each other, the aorta being anterior and to the left of the pulmonary artery (Fig. 4–24). Valvular regurgitation is common and associated lesions, including membranous VSD, pulmonary outflow obstruction, and Ebstein anomalies of the tricuspid valve, can be found.

In double-outlet right ventricle in which both arteries emerge from the right ventricle, a VSD is present and the main echocardiographic feature is the lack of continuity between the anterior mitral valve and the most posterior aortic valve cusp.

Because of tremendous progress in pediatric cardiac surgery, the adult cardiologist is required to recognize a number of surgically corrected congenital heart anomalies and to learn their natural history. Patients, with and without

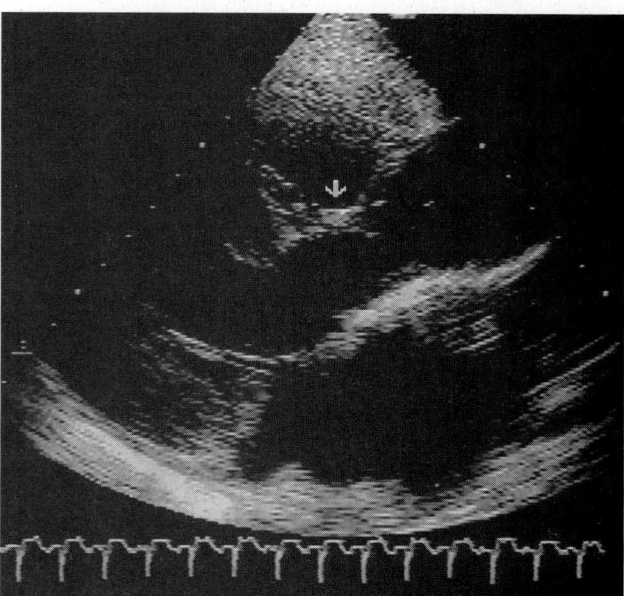

FIGURE 4–23 TTE PSLAX view in an adult patient with tetralogy of Fallot surgically corrected. The aorta overrides the interventricular septum, which has a repaired defect *(arrow)* done in childhood.

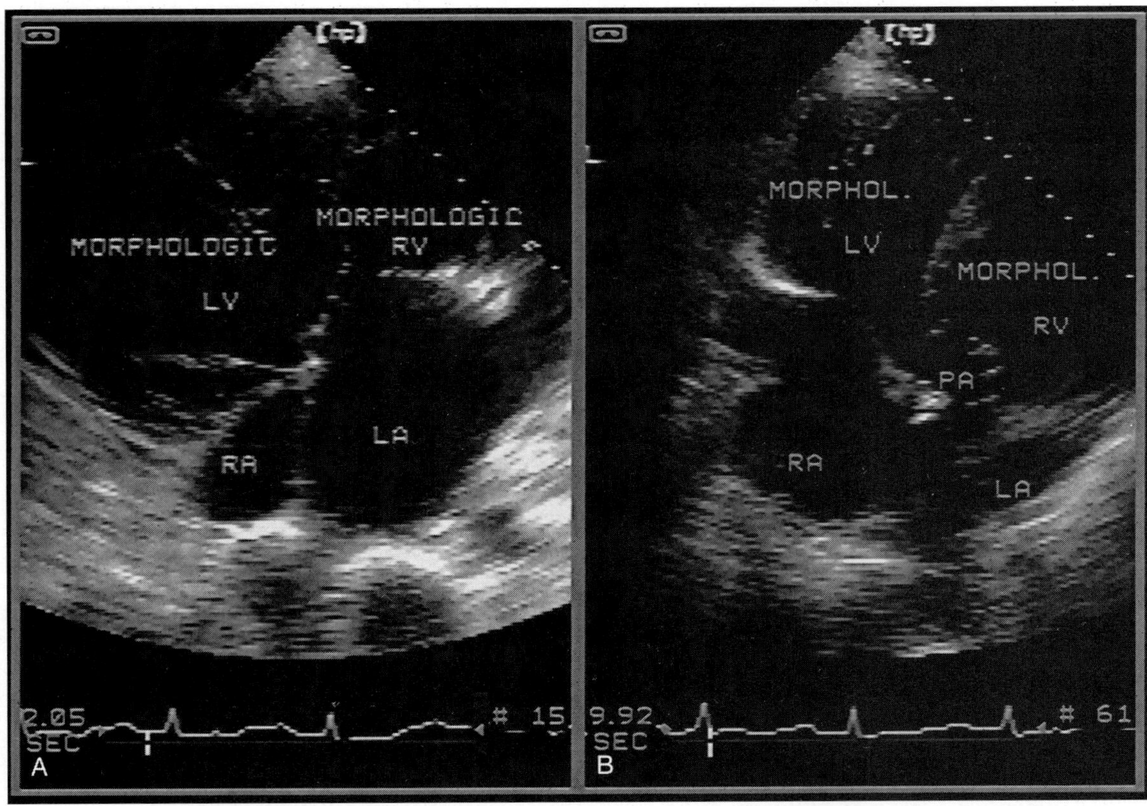

FIGURE 4–24 A and **B,** TTE apical four-chamber views of a congenitally corrected transposition of the great arteries (L-transposition). The morphologic left atrium (LA) is connected with the morphologic right ventricle (RV) from which the aorta emerges. The morphologic right atrium (RA) is connected to the morphologic left ventricle (LV) from which the pulmonary artery (PA) emerges.

surgically corrected congenital heart diseases, should be followed with Doppler echocardiography.

REFERENCES

1. Edler I, Hertz CH: Use of ultrasonic reflectoscope for the continuous recording of movements of heart walls. Kungl Fysiogr Sallsk Lund Forth 24:40, 1954.
2. De Castro S, Yao J, Pandian NG: Three-dimensional echocardiography: clinical relevance and application. Am J Cardiol 81:96G–102G, 1998.
3. Feinstein SB, Ten Cate F, Werner Z, et al: Two-dimensional contrast echocardiography. I. In vitro development and quantitative analysis of echo contrast agents. J Am Coll Cardiol 3:14–20, 1984.
4. Kaul S, Pandian NG, Okada RD, et al: Contrast echocardiography in acute myocardial ischemia: I. In vivo determination of total left ventricular "area at risk." J Am Coll Cardiol 4:1272–1282, 1984.
5. Crouse L, Cheirif J, Hanley D, et al: Opacification and border delineation improvement in patients with suboptimal endocardial border definition in routine echocardiography: results of the phase III Albunex multicenter trial. J Am Coll Cardiol 22:1494–1500, 1993.
6. Villanueva FS, Glasheen WP, Sklenar J, et al: Assessment of risk area during coronary occlusion and infarct size after reperfusion with myocardial contrast echocardiography using left and right atrial injections of contrast. Circulation 88:596–604, 1993.
7. Wei K, Skyba D, Firshke C, et al: Interactions between microbubbles and ultrasound: in vitro and in vivo observations. J Am Coll Cardiol 29:1081–1088, 1997.
8. Morrissey RL, Siu SC, Guerrtro L, et al: Automated assessment of ventricular volume and function by echocardiography: validation of automated border detection. J Am Soc Echocardiogr 7:107–115, 1994.
9. Sutherland GR, Stewart MJ, Groundstroem KWE, et al: Color Doppler myocardial imaging: a new technique for the assessment of myocardial function. J Am Soc Echocardiogr 7:441–458, 1994.
10. Miyatake K, Yamagishi M, Tanaka N, et al: New method for evaluating left ventricular wall motion by color-coded tissue Doppler imaging: in vivo and in vitro studies. J Am Coll Cardiol 25:717–724, 1995.
11. Derumaux G, Ovize M, Loufoua J, et al: Doppler tissue imaging quantitates regional wall motion during myocardial ischemia and reperfusion. Circulation 97:1970–1977, 1998.
12. Lang RM, Vignon P, Weinert L, et al: Echocardiographic quantification of regional left ventricular wall motion with color kinesis. Circulation 93:1877–1885, 1996.
13. Schwarz SL, Cao QL, Vannan MA, et al: Automatic backscatter analysis of regional left ventricular systolic function using color kinesis. Am J Cardiol 77:1345–1350, 1996.
14. Thomas JD, Rubin DN: Tissue harmonic imaging: why does it work? J Am Soc Echocardiogr 11:803–808, 1998.
15. Spencer KT, Bednarz J, Rafter PG, et al: Use of harmonic imaging without echocardiographic contrast to improve two-dimensional image quality. Am J Cardiol 82:794–799, 1998.
16. Tacy TA, Snider R, Vermilion RP: In vitro analysis of regurgitant fraction using Doppler power-weighted sum of velocities. J Am Soc Echocardiogr 11:266–273, 1998.
17. Mor-Avi V, Tan J, Bednarz J, et al: Power mode Doppler imaging with contrast as a basis for automated boundary detection in patients with poor endocardial definition. Circulation 98(17):I-502, 1998.
18. Schmidt MA, Agyeman KO, Laurienzo JM, et al: Left ventricular volume measurements in humans using real-time three-dimensional echocardiography: comparison with magnetic resonance imaging. Circulation 98:I-701, 1998.
19. Tardif JC, Vannan MA, Taylor K, et al: Delineation of extended length of coronary arteries by multiplane transesophageal echocardiography. J Am Coll Cardiol 24:909–919, 1994.
20. Yao J, Cao QL, Masani N, et al: Three-dimensional echocardio-

graphic estimation of infarct mass based on quantification of dysfunctional left ventricular mass. Circulation 96:1660–1666, 1997.

21. Rodevand O, Bjornerheim R, Kolbjornsen O, et al: Left ventricular mass assessed by three-dimensional echocardiography using rotational acquisition. Clin Cardiol 20:957–962, 1997.
22. Devereux R, Reichek N: Echocardiographic determination of left ventricular mass in man. Anatomic validation of the method. Circulation 55:613–618, 1977.
23. Devereux RB, Alonso D, Lutas E, et al: Echocardiographic assessment of left ventricular hypertrophy: comparison to necropsy findings. Am J Cardiol 57:450–458, 1986.
24. Devereux R: Detection of left ventricular hypertrophy by M-mode echocardiography: anatomic validation, standardization and comparison to other methods. Hypertension 9(suppl II):II-19–II-26, 1987.
25. Reichek N: Standardization in the measurement of left ventricular wall mass. Hypertension 9(suppl II):II-27–II-29, 1987.
26. Vuille C, Weyman AE: Left ventricle I: general considerations, assessment of chamber size and function. *In* Weyman AE (ed): Principles and Practice of Echocardiography. 2nd ed. Philadelphia: Lea & Febiger, 1994.
27. Byrd BF 3rd, Wahr D, Wang YS, et al: Left ventricular mass and volume/mass ratio determined by two-dimensional echocardiography in normal adults. J Am Coll Cardiol 6:1021–1025, 1985.
28. Teichholz LE, Kreulen T, Herman MV, et al: Problems in echocardiographic volume determinations: echocardiographic-angiographic correlations in the presence and absence of asynergy. Am J Cardiol 37:7–12, 1976.
29. Wahr DW, Wang YS, Schiller NB: Left ventricular volumes determined by two-dimensional echocardiography in a normal adult population. J Am Coll Cardiol 1:863–868, 1983.
30. Calenda P, Prasoon J, Smith LG: Utilization of echocardiography by internists and cardiologists: a comparative study. Am J Med 101:584–591, 1998.
31. Mueller X, Stauffer JC, Jaussi A, et al: Subjective visual echocardiographic estimate of left ventricular ejection fraction as an alternative to conventional echocardiographic methods: comparison with contrast angiography. Clin Cardiol 14:898–902, 1991.
32. Rich S, Sheikh A, Gallastegui J, et al: Determination of left ventricular ejection fraction by visual estimation during real-time two-dimensional echocardiography. Am Heart J 104:603–606, 1982.
33. Johnson H, Corretti M, Fisher M, et al: Visual estimate of left ventricular ejection fraction (LVEF) by echocardiography: comparison to quantitative echo methods and radionuclide angiography. J Am Soc Echocardiogr 8:384, 1995.
34. Simonson JS, Schiller NB: Descent of the base of the left ventricle: an echocardiographic index of left ventricular function. J Am Soc Echocardiogr 2:25–35, 1989.
35. Keren G, Sonnenblick EH, LeJemtel TH: Mitral annulus motion. Relation to pulmonary venous and transmitral flows in normal subjects and in patients with dilated cardiomyopathy. Circulation 78:621–629, 1988.
36. Gulati VK, Katz WE, Follansbee WP, et al: Mitral annular descent velocity by tissue Doppler echocardiography as an index of global left ventricular function. Am J Cardiol 77:979–984, 1996.
37. Feigenbaum H: Echocardiographic evaluation of cardiac chambers. *In* Feigenbaum H (ed): Echocardiography. 5th ed. pp. 134–180. Baltimore: Williams & Wilkins, 1994.
38. Bargiggia GS, Bertucci C, Recusani F, et al: A new method for estimating left ventricular dP/dt by continuous wave Doppler-echocardiography. Validation studies at cardiac catheterization. Circulation 80:1287–1292, 1989.
39. Lang RM, Vignon P, Weinert L, et al: Echocardiographic quantification of regional ventricular wall motion with color kinesis. Circulation 93:1877–1885, 1996.
40. Levine RA, Gibso TC, Aretz T: Echocardiographic measurements of right ventricular volume. Circulation 69:497–505, 1984.
41. Jiang L, Siu SC, Handschumacher MD: Three-dimensional echocardiography: in vivo validation for right ventricular volume and function. Circulation 89:2342–2350, 1994.
42. Denslow S, Wiles HB: Right ventricular volumes revisited: a simple model and simple formula for echocardiographic determination. J Am Soc Echocardiogr 11:864–873, 1998.
43. Kaul S, Tei C, Hopkins JM, et al: Assessment of right ventricular function using two-dimensional echocardiography. Am Heart J 107:526–531, 1984.
44. Hammarstrom E, Wranne B, Pinto FJ, et al: Tricuspid annular motion. J Am Soc Echocardiogr 4:131–139, 1991.
45. Appleton CP, Hatle L, Popp RL: Relation of transmitral flow velocity patterns to left ventricular diastolic function: new insights from a combined hemodynamic and Doppler echocardiographic study. J Am Coll Cardiol 12:426–440, 1988.
46. Labovitz AJ, Pearson A: Evaluation of left ventricular diastolic function: clinical relevance and recent Doppler echocardiographic insights. Am Heart J 114:836–851, 1987.
47. Nishimura RA, Abel MD, Hatle LK, et al: Assessment of diastolic function of the heart: background and current applications of Doppler echocardiography. Part II: clinical studies. Mayo Clin Proc 64:181–204, 1989.
48. Pinamonti B, Di Lenarda A, Sinagra G, et al: Restrictive left ventricular filling pattern in dilated cardiomyopathy assessed by Doppler echocardiography: clinical, echocardiographic and hemodynamic correlations and prognostic implications. J Am Coll Cardiol 22:808–815, 1993.
49. Thomas JD, Weyman AE: Echo-Doppler evaluation of the left ventricular diastolic function: physics and physiology. Circulation 84:977–999, 1991.
50. Appleton CP, Gonzalez MS, Basnight MA: Relationship of left atrial pressure and pulmonary venous flow velocities: importance of baseline mitral and pulmonary venous flow patterns studied in lightly sedated dogs. J Am Soc Echocardiogr 7:264–275, 1994.
51. Nishimura RA, Tajik AJ: Evaluation of diastolic filling of left ventricle in health and disease: Doppler echocardiography is the clinician's Rosetta stone. J Am Coll Cardiol 30:8–18, 1997.
52. Giannuzzi P, Imparato A, Temporelli PL, et al: Doppler-derived mitral deceleration time of early filling is strong predictor of pulmonary wedge pressure in postinfarction patients with left ventricular systolic dysfunction. J Am Coll Cardiol 23:1630–1637, 1994.
53. Xie G-Y, Berk MR, Smith MD, et al: Prognostic value of Doppler transmitral flow patterns in patients with congestive heart failure. J Am Coll Cardiol 24:132–139, 1994.
54. Pinamonti B, Di Lenarda A, Sinagra G, et al: Restrictive left ventricular filling pattern in dilated cardiomyopathy assessed by Doppler echocardiography: clinical, echocardiographic and hemodynamic correlations and prognostic implications. J Am Coll Cardiol 22:808–815, 1993.
55. Rodriguez L, Ares MA, Vandervoort PM, et al: Does color M-mode flow propagation differentiate between patients with restrictive vs. constructive physiology? J Am Coll Cardiol 27:268A, 1996.
56. Garcia MJ, Rodriguez L, Ares MA, et al: Differentiation of constrictive pericarditis from restrictive cardiomyopathy: assessment of left ventricular diastolic velocities in the longitudinal axis by Doppler tissue imaging. J Am Coll Cardiol 27:108–114, 1996.
57. Brun P, Tribouilloy C, Duval AM, et al: Left ventricular flow propagation during early filling is related to wall relaxation: a color M-mode Doppler analysis. J Am Coll Cardiol 20:420–432, 1992.
58. Stugaard M, Risoe C, Ihlen H, et al: Intracavity filling pattern in the failing left ventricle assessed by color M-mode Doppler echocardiography. J Am Coll Cardiol 24:663–670, 1994.
59. Stugaard M, Smiseth OA, Risoe C, et al: Intraventricular early diastolic filling during acute myocardial ischemia: assessment by multigated color M-mode Doppler echocardiography. Circulation 88:2705–2713, 1993.
60. Sohn DW, Chai IH, Lee DJ: Assessment of mitral annulus velocity by Doppler tissue imaging in the evaluation of left ventricular diastolic function. J Am Coll Cardiol 30:474–480, 1997.
61. Pai RG, Gill KS: Amplitudes, durations, and timings of apically directed left ventricular myocardial velocities II. Systolic and diastolic asynchrony in patients with left ventricular hypertrophy. J Am Soc Echocardiogr 11:112–118, 1998.
62. Palka P, Lange A, Fleming AD, et al: Differences in myocardial velocity gradient measure through cardiac cycle in patients with hypertrophic cardiomyopathy, athletes, and in patients with left ventricular hypertrophy due to hypertension. J Am Coll Cardiol 30:760–768, 1997.
63. Nagueh SF, Mikati I, Kopelen HA, et al: Doppler estimation of left ventricular filling pressure in sinus tachycardia: a new application of tissue Doppler imaging. Circulation 98:1644–1650, 1998.
64. Lim M, Ahn C, Diaz S, et al: The value of tricuspid annular motion (TAM) evaluated by Doppler tissue imaging (DTI) in the diagnosis of pulmonary hypertension (PHT). J Am Soc Echocardiogr 10:408, 1997.

65. Pai RG, Stoletniy L: Clinical and echocardiographic correlates of mitral E-wave transmission inside the left ventricle: potential insights into left ventricular diastolic function. J Am Soc Echocardiogr 10:532–539, 1997.
66. Scalia GM, Greenbert N, McCarthy P, et al: Noninvasive assessment of the ventricular relaxation time constant (*) in humans by Doppler echocardiography. Circulation 95:151–155, 1997.
67. Michalis LK, Thomas MR, Jewitt DE, et al: Echocardiographic assessment of systolic and diastolic left ventricular function using an automatic boundary detection system. Correlation with established invasive and noninvasive parameters. Int J Cardiac Imaging 11:71–80, 1995.
68. Christie J, Sheldahl L, Tristani F, et al: Determination of stroke volume and cardiac output during exercise: comparison of two-dimensional and Doppler echocardiography, Fick oximetry, and thermodilution. Circulation 76:539–547, 1987.
69. Gardin J, Tobis J, Dabestani A, et al: Superiority of two-dimensional measurement of aortic vessel diameter in Doppler echocardiographic estimates of left ventricular stroke volume. J Am Coll Cardiol 6:66–74, 1985.
70. Dittmann H, Jacksch R, Voelker W, et al: Accuracy of Doppler echocardiography in adult patients with atrial septal defect. J Am Coll Cardiol 11:338–342, 1988.
71. Chen C, Rodriguez L, Lethor J-P, et al: Continuous wave Doppler echocardiography of noninvasive assessment of left ventricular dP/dt and relaxation time constant from mitral regurgitant spectra in patients. J Am Coll Cardiol 23:970–975, 1994.
72. Schwammenthal E, Chen C, Giesler M, et al: New method for accurate calculation of regurgitant flow rate based on analysis of Doppler color flow maps of the proximal flow field. Validation in a canine model of mitral regurgitation with initial application in patients. J Am Coll Cardiol 27:161–172, 1996.
73. Foster G, Weissman N, Picard M, et al: Determination of aortic valve area in valvular aortic stenosis by direct measurement using intracardiac echocardiography: a comparison with the Gorlin and continuity equations. J Am Coll Cardiol 27:392–398, 1996.
74. Garcia M, Ares M, Asher C, et al: An index of early left ventricular filling that combined with pulsed Doppler peak E velocity may estimate capillary wedge pressure. J Am Coll Cardiol 29:448–454, 1997.
75. Zamorano J, Wallbridge DR, Ge J, et al: Non-invasive assessment of cardiac physiology by tissue Doppler echocardiography. Eur Heart J 18:330–339, 1997.
76. Conovan KD, Dobb GJ, Newman MA, et al: Comparison of pulsed Doppler and thermodilution methods for measuring cardiac output in critically ill patients. Crit Care Med 15:853–857, 1987.
77. Thys DM, Hillel Z, Goldman ME, et al: A comparison of hemodynamic indices derived by invasive monitoring and two-dimensional echocardiography. Anesthesiology 67:630–634, 1987.
78. Nagueh SF, Middleton KJ, Kopelen HA, et al: Doppler tissue imaging: a noninvasive technique for evaluation of left ventricular relaxation and estimation of filling pressures. J Am Coll Cardiol 30:1527–1533, 1997.
79. Wilkins GT, Weyman AE, Abascal VM, et al: Percutaneous balloon dilatation or the mitral valve: an analysis of echocardiographic variables related to outcome and the mechanism of dilatation. Br Heart J 60:299, 1988.
80. Padial LR, Freitas N, Sagie A, et al: Echocardiography can predict which patients will develop severe mitral regurgitation after percutaneous mitral valvulotomy. J Am Coll Cardiol 27:1225–1231, 1996.
81. Levine RA, Stathogiannis E, Newell JB, et al: Reconsideration of echocardiographic standards for mitral valve prolapse: lack of association between leaflet displacement isolated to the apical four-chamber view and independent echocardiographic evidence of abnormality. J Am Coll Cardiol 11:1013, 1988.
82. Marks AR, Choong CY, Sanfillipo AJ, et al: Identification of high-risk and low-risk subgroups of patients with mitral-valve prolapse. N Engl J Med 320:1031–1036, 1989.
83. Stoddard MF, Prince CR, Dillon S, et al: Exercise-induced mitral regurgitation is a predictor of morbid events in subjects with mitral valve prolapse. J Am Coll Cardiol 25:693–699, 1995.
84. Recusani F, Bargiggia GS, Yoganathan AP, et Al: A new method for quantification of regurgitant flow rate using color Doppler flow imaging of the flow convergence region proximal to a discrete orifice: an in vitro study. Circulation 83:594, 1991.
85. Bargiggia GS, Tronconi L, Sahn DJ, et al: A new method for quantitation of mitral regurgitation based on color flow Doppler imaging of flow convergence proximal to regurgitant orifice. Circulation 84:1481, 1991.
86. Pu M, Vandervoort PM, Griffin BP, et al: Quantification of mitral regurgitation by the proximal convergence method using transesophageal echocardiography: clinical validation of a geometric correction for proximal flow constraint. Circulation 92:2169, 1995.
87. Schwammenthal E, Chen C, Giesler M, et al: New method for accurate calculation of regurgitant flow rate based on analysis of Doppler color flow maps of the proximal flow field. Validation in a canine model of mitral regurgitation with initial application in patients. J Am Coll Cardiol 27:161–172, 1996.
88. Grayburn PA, Fehske W, Omran H, et al: Multiplane transesophageal echocardiographic assessment of mitral regurgitation by Doppler color flow mapping of the vena contracta. Am J Cardiol 74:912–917, 1994.
89. Zhou X, Jones M, Shiota T, et al: Vena contracta imaged by Doppler color flow mapping predicts the severity of eccentric mitral regurgitation better than color jet area: a chronic animal study. J Am Coll Cardiol 30:1393–1398, 1997.
90. Hall SA, Brickner ME, Willett DL, et al: Assessment of mitral regurgitation severity by Doppler color flow mapping of the vena contracta. Circulation 95:636–642, 1997.
91. Currie PJ, Seward JB, Reeder GS, et al: Continuous-wave Doppler echocardiographic assessment of severity of calcific aortic stenosis: a simultaneous Doppler-catheter correlative study in 100 adult patients. Circulation 71:1162, 1985.
92. Hoffmann R, Flachskampf FA, Hanrath P: Planimetry of orifice area in aortic stenosis using multiplane transesophageal echocardiography. J Am Coll Cardiol 22:529, 1993.
93. Oh JK, Taliercio CP, Holmes DR Jr, et al: Prediction of the severity of aortic stenosis by Doppler aortic valve area determination: prospective Doppler-catheterization correlation in 100 patients. J Am Coll Cardiol 11:1227–1234, 1988.
94. Harrison MR, Gurley JC, Smith MD, et al: A practical application of Doppler echocardiography for the assessment of severity of aortic stenosis. Am Heart J 115:622–627, 1988.
95. deFilippi CR, Willett DL, Brickner ME, et al: Usefulness of dobutamine echocardiography in distinguishing severe from nonsevere valvular aortic stenosis in patients with depressed left ventricular function and low transvalvular gradients. Am J Cardiol 75:191–194, 1995.
96. Movsowitz HD, Levine RA, Isselbacher EM: A new echocardiographic sign with mechanistic insight for functional aortic regurgitation due to aortic dilatation. J Am Soc Echocardiogr 11:559, 1998.
97. Perry GJ, Helmcke F, Nanda NC, et al: Evaluation of aortic insufficiency by Doppler color flow mapping. J Am Coll Cardiol 9:952, 1987.
98. Diebold B, Peronneau P, Blanchard D, et al: Non-invasive quantification of aortic regurgitation by Doppler echocardiography. Br Heart J 49:167, 1983.
99. Tribouilloy CM, Enriquez-Sarano M, Fett SL, et al: Application of the proximal flow convergence method to calculate the effective regurgitant orifice area in aortic regurgitation. J Am Coll Cardiol 32:1032–1039, 1998.
100. Ambrose JA, Meller J, Teichholz LE, Herman MP: Premature closure of the mitral valve: echocardiographic clue for diagnosis of aortic dissection. Chest 73:121, 1978.
101. Vandenbossche JL, Englert M: Doppler color flow mapping demonstration of diastolic mitral regurgitation in severe acute aortic regurgitation. Am Heart J 11:889, 1987.
102. Weaver WF, Wilson CS, Rourke T, Caudill CC: Mid-diastolic aortic valve opening in severe acute aortic regurgitation. Circulation 55:145, 1977.
103. Bonow RO, Carabello B, de Leon AC Jr, et al: Guidelines for the management of patients with valvular heart disease. Executive summary: a report of the American College of Cardiology/American Heart Association Task Force on Practice Guidelines (Committee on Management of Patients With Valvular Heart Disease). Circulation 98:1949–1984, 1998.
104. Forman R, Firth BG, Barnard MS: Prognostic significance of preoperative left ventricular ejection fraction and valve lesion in patients with aortic valve replacement. Am J Cardiol 45:1120–1125, 1980.
105. Greves J, Rahimtoola SH, McAnulty JH, et al: Preoperative criteria

predictive of late survival following valve replacement for severe aortic regurgitation. Am Heart J 101:300–308, 1981.
106. Copeland JG, Griepp RB, Stinson EB, et al: Long-term follow-up after isolated aortic valve replacement. J Thorac Cardiovasc Surg 74:875–889, 1977.
107. Maraj R, Jacobs LE, Ioli A, et al: Evaluation of hemolysis in patients with prosthetic heart valves. Clin Cardiol 21:387–392, 1998.
108. Binder T, Baumgartner H, Maurer G: Diagnosis and management of prosthetic valve dysfunction. Curr Opin Cardiol 11:131–138, 1996.
109. Buda AJ, Zotz RJ, Lemire MS, et al: Prognostic significance of vegetations detected by two-dimensional echocardiography in ineffective endocarditis. Am Heart J 112:1291, 1986.
110. Lindner JR, Case RA, Dent JM, et al: Diagnostic value of echocardiography in suspected endocarditis. An evaluation based on the pretest probability of disease. Circulation 93:730–736, 1996.
111. He S, Fontaine AA, Schwammenthal E, et al: Integrated mechanism for functional mitral regurgitation: leaflet restriction versus coapting force: in vitro studies. Circulation 96:1826–1834, 1997.
112. Douglas PS, Morrow R, Ioli A, Reichek N: Left ventricular shape, afterload and survival in idiopathic dilated cardiomyopathy. J Am Coll Cardiol 13:311, 1989.
113. Dec GW, Fuster V: Idiopathic dilated cardiomyopathy. N Engl J Med 331:1564–1575, 1994.
114. Cueto-Garcia L, Tajik AJ, Kyle RA, et al: Serial echocardiographic observations in patients with primary systemic amyloidosis: an introduction to the concept of early (asymptomatic) amyloid infiltration of the heart. Mayo Clin Proc 59:589, 1984.
115. Siqueira-Filho AG, Cunha CL, Tajik AJ, et al: M-mode and two-dimensional echocardiographic features in cardiac amyloidosis. Circulation 63:188, 1981.
116. Klein AL, Hatle LK, Taliercio CP, et al: Serial Doppler-echocardiographic follow-up of left ventricular diastolic function in cardiac amyloidosis. J Am Coll Cardiol 16:1135–1141, 1990.
117. Schwammenthal E, Nakatani S, He S, et al: Mechanism of mitral regurgitation in hypertrophic cardiomyopathy: mismatch of posterior to anterior leaflet length and mobility. Circulation 98:856–865, 1998.
118. The French Study of Aortic Plaques in Stroke Group: Atherosclerotic disease of the aortic arch as a risk factor for recurrent ischemic stroke. N Engl J Med 334:1216–1221, 1996.
119. Leung DY, Black IW, Cranney GB, et al: Selection of patients for transesophageal echocardiography after stroke and systemic embolic events. Role of transthoracic echocardiography. Stroke 26:1820–1824, 1995.
120. Barasch E, Kaushick C, Ahn C: Aortic-sino-tubular atherosclerotic debris associated with cerebral embolic events can be identified by transthoracic echocardiography. Cardiology 90:253–257, 1998.
121. ACC/AHA Guidelines for the Clinical Applications of Echocardiography. A Report of the American College of Cardiology/American Heart Association Task Force on Practice Guidelines (Committee on Clinical Application of Echocardiography). Circulation 95:1686–1744, 1997, and J Am Coll Cardiol 29:862–879, 1997.
122. Armstrong WF, Marcovitz PA: Dynamic left ventricular outflow tract obstruction as a complication of acute myocardial infarction. Am Heart J 131:827–830, 1996.
123. Joffe II, Riley MF, Katz SE, et al: Acquired dynamic left ventricular outflow tract obstruction complicating acute anterior myocardial infarction: serial echocardiographic and clinical evaluation. J Am Soc Echocardiogr 10:717–721, 1997.
124. Lindner JR, Firschke C, Wei K, et al: Myocardial perfusion characteristics and hemodynamic profile of MRX-115, a venous echocardiographic contrast agent, during acute myocardial infarction. J Am Soc Echocardiogr 11:36–46, 1998.
125. Galiuto L, Iliceto S: Myocardial contrast echocardiography in the evaluation of viable myocardium after acute myocardial infarction. Am J Cardiol 81:29G–32G, 1998.
126. Ito H, Iwakura K: Assessing the relation between coronary reflow and myocardial reflow. Am J Cardiol 81:8G–12G, 1998.
127. Grayburn PA: Assessment of myocardial "reperfusion" by contrast echocardiography. Am J Med Sci 315:124–132, 1998.
128. Sakuma T, Hayashi Y, Sumii K, et al: Prediction of short- and intermediate-term prognoses of patients with acute myocardial infarction using myocardial contrast echocardiography one day after recanalization. J Am Coll Cardiol 32:890–897, 1998.
129. Carlos ME, Smart SC, Wynsen JC, et al: Dobutamine stress echocardiography for risk stratification after myocardial infarction. Circulation 95:1402–1410, 1997.
130. Applegate RJ, Dell'Italia LJ, Crawford MH: Usefulness of two-dimensional echocardiography during low-level exercise testing early after uncomplicated myocardial infarction. Am J Cardiol 60:10–14, 1987.
131. Quintana M, Lindvall K, Ryden L, et al: Prognostic value of predischarge exercise stress echocardiography after acute myocardial infarction. Am J Cardiol 76:1115–1121, 1995.
132. Previtali M, Poli A, Lanzarini L, et al: Dobutamine stress echocardiography for assessment of myocardial viability and ischemia in acute myocardial infarction treated with thrombolysis. Am J Cardiol 72:124G–30G, 1993.
133. Smart SC, Sawada S, Ryan T, et al: Low-dose dobutamine echocardiography detects reversible dysfunction after thrombolytic therapy of acute myocardial infarction. Circulation 88:405–415, 1993.
134. Smart SC, Knickelbine T, Stoiber TR, et al: Safety and accuracy of dobutamine-atropine stress echocardiography for the detection of residual stenosis of the infarct-related artery and multivessel disease during the first week after acute myocardial infarction. Circulation 95:1394–1401, 1997.
135. Sicari R, Picano E, Landi P, et al: Prognostic value of dobutamine-atropine echocardiography early after acute myocardial infarction. J Am Coll Cardiol 29:254–260, 1997.
136. Greco CA, Salustri A, Seccareccia F: Prognostic value of dobutamine echocardiography early after uncomplicated acute myocardial infarction: a comparison with exercise electrocardiography. J Am Coll Cardiol 29:261–267, 1997.
137. Picano E, Patrizia L, Bolognese L, et al, for the EPIC Study Group: Prognostic value of dipyridamole echocardiography early after uncomplicated myocardial infarction: a large-scale, multicenter trial. Am J Med 95:608–618, 1993.
138. Camerieri A, Picano E, Landi P, et al: Prognostic value of dipyridamole echocardiography early after myocardial infarction in elderly patients. Echo Persantine Italian Cooperative (EPIC) Study Group. J Am Coll Cardiol 22:1809–1815, 1993.
139. Wann LS, Faris JV, Childress RH, et al: Exercise cross-sectional echo in ischemic heart disease. Circulation 60:1300–1308, 1979.
140. Pellika PA: Stress echocardiography in the evaluation of chest pain and accuracy in the diagnosis of coronary artery disease. Prog Cardiovasc Dis 39:523–532, 1997.
141. Takeuchi M, Araki M, Nakashima Y, et al: The detection of residual ischemia and stenosis in patients with acute myocardial infarction with dobutamine stress echocardiography. J Am Soc Echocardiogr 7:242–252, 1994.
142. Bigi R, Ochi G, Fiorentini C: Dobutamine stress echocardiography for the identification of multivessel coronary artery disease after uncomplicated myocardial infarction: the importance of test end-point. Int J Cardiol 50:51–60, 1995.
143. Elhendy A, van Domburg RT, Roelandt JRTC, et al: Accuracy of dobutamine stress echocardiography for the diagnosis of coronary artery stenosis in patients with myocardial infarction. Heart 76:123–128, 1996.
144. Elhendy A, Geleijnse ML, Roelandt JRTC, et al: Comparison of dobutamine stress echocardiography and 99m-technetium sestamibi SPECT myocardial perfusion scintigraphy for predicting extent of coronary artery disease in patients with healed myocardial infarction. Am J Cardiol 79:7–12, 1997.
145. Smart SC, Knickelbine T, Stoiber TR, et al: Safety and accuracy of dobutamine-atropine stress echocardiography for the detection of residual stenosis of the infarct-related artery and multivessel disease during the first week after acute myocardial infarction. Circulation 95:1394–1401, 1997.
146. Afridi I, Kleiman NS, Raizner AE, et al: Dobutamine echocardiography in myocardial hibernation. Optimal dose and accuracy in predicting recovery of ventricular function after coronary angioplasty. Circulation 91:663–670, 1995.
147. Cigarroa CG, deFilippi CR, Brickner ME, et al: Dobutamine stress echocardiography identified hibernating myocardium and predicts recovery of left ventricular function after coronary revascularization. Circulation 88:430–436, 1993.
148. La Canna G, Alfieri O, Giubbini R, et al: Echocardiography during infusion of dobutamine for identification of reversible dysfunction in patients with chronic coronary artery disease. J Am Coll Cardiol 23:617–623, 1994.
149. Marzullo P, Parodi O, Reisenhofer B, et al: Value of rest thallium-201/technetium-99m sestamibi scans and dobutamine echocardiogra-

phy for detecting myocardial viability. Am J Cardiol 71:166–172, 1993.
150. Arnese M, Cornel JH, Salustri A, et al: Prediction of improvement of regional left ventricular function after surgical revascularization: a comparison of low-dose dobutamine echocardiography with ^{201}Tl single-photon emission computed tomography. Circulation 91:2748–2752, 1995.
151. Vanoverschelde JJ, D'Hondt A, Marwick T: Head-to-head comparison of exercise redistribution-reinjection thallium single-photon emission computed tomography and low dose dobutamine echocardiography for prediction of reversibility of chronic left ventricular ischemic dysfunction. J Am Coll Cardiol 28:432–442, 1996.
152. Tsang TS, Freeman WK, Barnes ME, et al: Rescue echocardiographically guided pericardiocentesis for cardiac perforation complicating catheter-based procedures. The Mayo Clinic experience. J Am Coll Cardiol 32:1345–1350, 1998.
153. Martin RP, Rakowsky H, French JW, et al: Localization of pericardial effusion with wide-angle phased array echocardiography. Am J Cardiol 42:904, 1978.
154. Leimgruber PP, Klopfenstein S, Wann SL, et al: The hemodynamic derangement associated with right ventricular diastolic collapse in cardiac tamponade: an experimental echocardiographic study. Circulation 58:612, 1988.
155. Armstrong WF, Schilt BF, Helper DJ, et al: Diastolic collapse of the right ventricle with cardiac tamponade: an echocardiographic study. Circulation 65:1491, 1982.
156. Singh S, Wann LS, Klopfenstein HS, et al: Usefulness of right ventricular diastolic collapse in diagnosing cardiac tamponade and comparison to pulsus paradoxus. Am J Cardiol 57:652, 1986.
157. Kronzon I, Cohen ML, Winer HE: Diastolic atrial compression: a sensitive echocardiographic sign of cardiac tamponade. J Am Coll Cardiol 4:770, 1983.
158. Himelman RB, Kircher B, Rockey DC, et al: Inferior vena cava plethora with blunted respiratory response: a sensitive echocardiographic sign of cardiac tamponade. J Am Coll Cardiol 12:1420, 1988.
159. Appleton CP, Hatle LK, Popp RL: Cardiac tamponade and pericardial effusion: respiratory variation in transvalvular flow velocities studies by Doppler Echocardiography. J Am Coll Cardiol 11:1020, 1988.
160. Kochar GS, Jacobs LE, Kotler MN: Right atrial compression in postoperative cardiac patients: detection by transesophageal echocardiography. J Am Coll Cardiol 16:511–516, 1990.
161. San Filippo AJ, Weyman AE: Pericardial disease. *In* Weiman AE (ed): Principles and Practice of Echocardiography. 2nd ed. pp. 1102–1134. Philadelphia: Lea & Febiger, 1994.
162. Hatle LK, Appleton CP, Popp RL: Differentiation of constrictive pericarditis and restrictive cardiomyopathy by Doppler echocardiography. Circulation 79:357–370, 1989.
163. Klein AL, Cohen GI, Pietrolungo JF, et al: Differentiation of constrictive pericarditis from restrictive cardiomyopathy by Doppler transesophageal echocardiographic measurements of respiratory variations in pulmonary venous flow. J Am Coll Cardiol 22:1935–1943, 1993.
164. Van Praagh R: The segmental approach to diagnosis in congenital heart disease. *In* Bergsma D (ed): Birth Defects: Original Articles Series. pp. 4–23. Baltimore: Williams & Wilkins, 1972.
165. Shinebourne EA, Macartney FJ, Anderson RH: Sequential chamber localization—logical approach to diagnosis in congenital heart disease. Br Heart J 38:327–340, 1976.
166. Tynan MJ, Becker AE, Macartney FJ, et al: Nomenclature and classification of congenital heart disease. Br Heart J 41:544–553, 1979.
167. Shiina A: Two-dimensional echocardiographic-surgical correlation in Ebstein's anomaly: preoperative determination of patients requiring tricuspid valve plication vs. replacement. Circulation 68:34, 1983.
168. Anderson KR, Zuberbuhler JR, Anderson RH, et al: Morphologic spectrum of Ebstein's anomaly of the heart: a review. Mayo Clin Proc 54:174, 1979.
169. King MEE: Echocardiographic evaluation of the adult and unoperated congenital heart disease. *In* Otto CM (ed): The Practice of Clinical Echocardiography. pp. 697–728. Philadelphia: WB Saunders, 1997.
170. Pascoe RD, Oh JK, Warnes CA, et al: Diagnosis of sinus venosus atrial septal defect with transesophageal echocardiography. Circulation 94:1049–1055, 1996.
171. Ammash NM, Seward JB, Warnes CA, et al: Partial anomalous pulmonary venous connection: diagnosis by transesophageal echocardiography. J Am Coll Cardiol 29:1351–1358, 1997.

CHAPTER 5

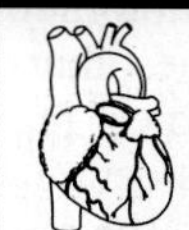

NUCLEAR IMAGING

A. *Iain McGhie*

PHYSICS AND INSTRUMENTATION
Basic Principles
Single-Crystal Gamma Camera
Acquisition Modes
SPECT MYOCARDIAL PERFUSION IMAGING
Physiologic Principles
Choice of Radiopharmaceutical
Choice of Stress
Analysis of Images
Comparison of SPECT and PET Perfusion Imaging
RADIONUCLIDE VENTRICULOGRAPHY
First-Pass Radionuclide Angiocardiography
Gated-Equilibrium Radionuclide Ventriculography
Exercise Radionuclide Ventriculography
Analysis of Radionuclide Ventriculograms
INFARCT IMAGING
Technetium-Labeled Infarct Avid Imaging Agents
Antimyosin Antibody Imaging
Recent Developments in Infarct Imaging
POSITRON EMISSION TOMOGRAPHY
Basic Principles
Coronary Flow Reserve
Positron-Emitting Radiopharmaceuticals in Myocardial Perfusion Imaging
Metabolic Identification of Myocardial Hibernation and Stunning
Myocardial Viability as a State of Reversible Contractile Function at Rest
Identification of Reversibly Dysfunctional Myocardium
Positron-Emitting Radiopharmaceuticals in Assessment of Myocardial Viability
Positron Emission Tomography Approaches for the Identification of Myocardial Viability

PHYSICS AND INSTRUMENTATION

Basic Principles

The use of radionuclides to image the heart depends on the ability to detect emitted electromagnetic radiation from injected radionuclides. The radionuclide is usually taken up by the myocardium, or it remains in the intravascular compartment. The emitted gamma rays are detected by a scintillation counter, where the emitted electromagnetic radiation is converted into electrical energy and transformed into a digital format to produce images of either myocardial activity or the cardiac blood pool.

The *scintillation counter* is usually made of sodium iodide thallium (NaI[Tl])–activated crystal. The purpose of the scintillation crystal is to convert the energy of gamma-radiation into visible light. When a gamma ray interacts with the atom in the crystal, a high-speed electron is produced. This electron in turn disturbs other atoms in its path, creating more high-speed electrons. The number of high-speed electrons generated is in proportion to the gamma-ray's total kinetic energy. These electrons move through the crystal until trapped by an atom of thallium, when their kinetic energy is converted into a photon of light, that is, a scintillation. This whole process occurs within a microsecond of the initial interaction between the high-energy photon and the crystal. Every gamma-ray absorbed by the crystal results in the production of a large number of photons, which is in direct proportion to the energy of the gamma-rays.

Subsequently, a *photomultiplier* converts these photons of light into an electrical signal, which then amplifies the electrical signal. Photons of light are detected by the photomultiplier by use of a thin plate called a *photocathode,* which releases electrons in proportion to the photons striking it. The electrons are then accelerated through a series of usually 10 plates, known as *dynodes,* which multiply the electrons, striking them in proportion to voltage difference between the plates. This results in an amplification factor of approximately 1 million. After this, an anode collects the electrons, and a preamplifier generates an electrical impulse. The energy of the gamma-ray absorbed by the crystal and subsequent light released by the crystal is directly proportional to the height of this electrical pulse, that is, the voltage.

A device, called a *pulse height analyzer,* is used to preselect the range of energies to be counted (energy window) from the distribution of available energies (energy spectrum). Any energies corresponding to gamma-rays out with this predetermined energy window are rejected. Discriminating the energy of the gamma-ray is important because it allows (1) selection of different radionuclides with different energies and (2) the elimination of less energetic gamma-rays scattered by the patient's tissue before detection by the scintillation device. However, pulses generated by the unscattered gamma-rays are not all of exactly the same amplitude, and they are distributed around the exact characteristic energy of the radionuclide (photopeak). The less spread of the radionuclide around the photopeak, the better the energy resolution of the system, and therefore, the better the inherent counting and imaging characteristics of the device.

Single-Crystal Gamma Camera

The single-crystal gamma camera uses a large (300 to 500 mm), thin (75 to 125 mm) NaI(Tl) crystal with an array of photomultiplier tubes covering one side of the crystal. On the other side of the crystal is a lead plate with multiple holes in it called a *collimator* (Fig. 5–1). This causes selective interference by blocking those rays not traveling in the selected direction. In some ways, the collimator is analogous to the lens of a photographic camera, resulting in a preselection of gamma-rays before they strike the crystal. The most commonly used collimator in nuclear cardiology is a parallel-hole collimator. The lead septa between the holes absorb most of the gamma-rays not traveling parallel to the holes. The larger the diameter or shorter the length of the holes, the higher the sensitivity of the collimator, and the smaller the diameter or longer the length of the holes, the higher the spatial resolution of the collimator.

The gamma-rays passing through the holes of the collimator strike the crystal and produce a scintillation. All the photomultiplier tubes detect photons produced by the scintillation; photomultiplier tubes closer to the event gather more light than those further away do. All output from the photomultipliers is relayed into electronic computer circuitry, where it is processed. A *positional analyzer* determines and assigns x and y cartesian coordinates to the point in the crystal where the scintillation occurs. In addition, output of all the photomultipliers is summed, representing the total energy of the gamma-ray that interacted with the crystal, to form an energy, or z, pulse. The z pulse is sent to the pulse height analyzer and it is set to accept a preselected range of energies. If the z pulse is within the predetermined range, it is referred to as either a trigger impulse or a signal pulse. This signals that the scintillation event should be counted. Each time a trigger impulse is received by the cathode ray tube, it allows the emission of electrons from the electron gun. The x and y positional impulses are transmitted to the horizontal and vertical plates, creating a deflection in the path of the electrons that corresponds to the scintillation coordinates. Electrons hit the phosphor screen of the cathode ray tube, creating a small scintillation that can be recorded on photographic film. However, today, computers are used for image display, processing, analysis, and archiving purposes. Therefore, the x, y, and z pulses are also relayed to the computer interface unit. These impulses first must be converted from analog to digital format by use of an *analog-to-digital converter*. The analog-to-digital converter converts the pulse height into discrete numbers. The x and y impulses both have an analog-to-digital converter, whereas the z impulse signals the analog-to-digital converters to convert the analog pulses to digital numbers.

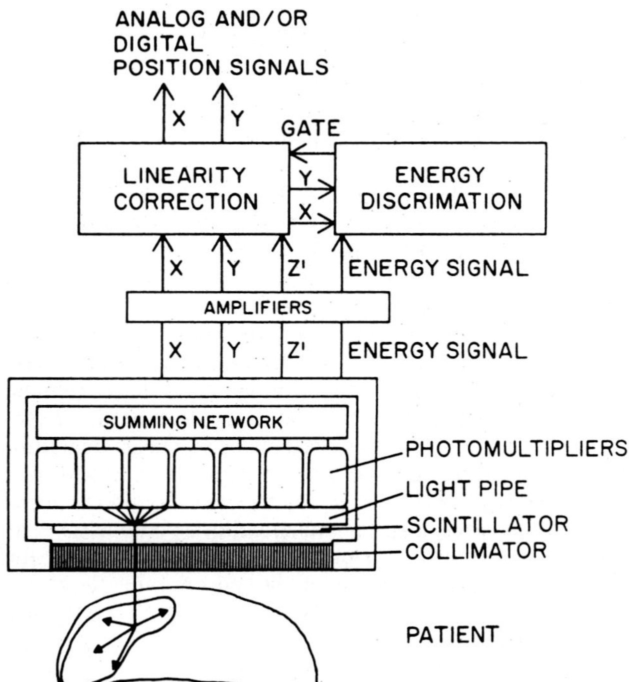

FIGURE 5–1 Schematic diagram of a gamma camera. (From Muehllenher G: The Anger scintillation camera. *In* Gottschalk A, Hoffer PB, Potchon EJ [eds]: Diagnostic Nuclear Medicine. pp. 71–81. Baltimore: Williams & Wilkins, 1988.)

The current generation of gamma cameras performs real-time corrections for (1) tube drift (2) energy variations, and (3) spatial nonlinearity. *Tube drift correction* automatically adjusts the photomultipliers so that each one generates the same pulse voltage when it gathers photons from the same light source. This correction is required because the earth's magnetic field affects the photomultiplier's output as a function of its angle and is particularly important in rotational tomography. The *energy correction factor* compensates for differences in responses of individual photomultiplier tubes, in the crystal, or in regional light gathering properties. Energy-specific field floods need to be acquired periodically to generate the time-dependent energy maps. A correction circuit in real time then applies this predetermined map. This normalizes the relationship of the energy window to the shape of the spectrum and practically abolishes the variations in energy response. *Linearity correction* is required because the gamma camera positioning scheme does not perfectly image straight radioactive line sources. To correct for this, a phantom of straight lines in horizontal and vertical positions is imaged. The displacement is measured and stored, allowing the linearity circuit to correct lines so that they appear perfectly straight in the image.

Acquisition Modes

Planar Acquisition. This the simplest means of acquisition, in which the gamma-camera acquires data in one dimension in multiple projections, usually in three: anterior, left anterior oblique, and left lateral projection. Right anterior and left posterior oblique projections may be obtained, depending on the circumstances. Despite the multiple projections, the spatial resolution is limited. This occurs because of either overlapping activity from noncardiac structures or overlap between normal and abnormal segments within the heart. For example, the presence of adjacent pulmonary activity may overlap the posterolateral wall in the left anterior oblique, making the anteroseptum appear hypoperfused; alternatively, a small perfusion defect may not be detected because of activity in normal myocardium in an adjacent but different plane.

Tomographic Acquisition. Over the past decade, single-photon emission computed tomography (SPECT) has been increasingly used in cardiac imaging. A series of planar images are obtained from a patient around 180 or 360 degrees. Using filtered backprojection, a computer creates a set of transaxial images from these planar images, allowing the radioisotope distribution to be displayed in three dimensions. From these transaxial images, horizontal and vertical long-axis sections and short axis sections are constructed (Plate 5–1). This results in improved contrast and enhanced spatial resolution, which leads to superior accuracy. However, this technique is more exacting in terms of both equipment and acquisition technique, and it requires more rigorous quality control.

SPECT, along with many other tomographic modalities, such as positron emission tomography (PET) and x-ray computed tomography, uses a computer-based algorithm during reconstruction, called *filtered backprojection.* The algorithm is dependent on the fact that each photon, which interacts with the crystal, must pass through the collimator. This defines the path of the photon because the holes in the collimator are parallel. The reconstruction algorithm backprojects or "sends back" the counts from their recorded position on the crystal, along a line perpendicular to the face of the crystal (Fig. 5–2). The back-projected lines cross at the origin of the radiation, and these points are recorded in computer memory from which tomograms are generated. However, the reconstruction algorithm deposits counts in each pixel along the back-projected line, producing a star-shaped artifact and in-plane blurring of the image. In order to reduce these artifacts, the images are modified by a filter, which eliminates unwanted low- and high-frequency statistical noise, hence the term *filtered backprojection.*

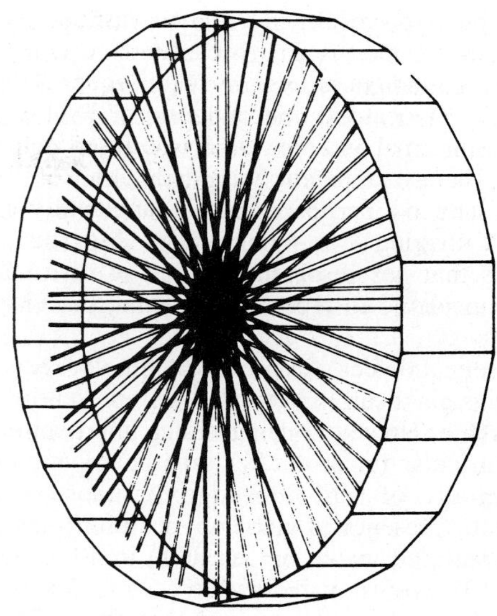

FIGURE 5–2 Schematic representation of the process of backprojection. Multiple planar views are taken around 360 degrees or 180 degrees, with data being backprojected in space to define the origin of the data in space (see text for further details). (Data from Budinger TF, McDonald B: Reconstruction of the Fresnel-coded gamma camera images by digital computer. J Nucl Med 16:309, 1975.)

SPECT Myocardial Perfusion Imaging

Physiologic Principles

Briefly, the underlying physiologic principles of stress-rest perfusion imaging are as follows.[1] At rest, coronary flow is normal even in the presence of a narrowing of up to 85 percent diameter stenosis.[1a, 1b] Stress, usually in the form of dynamic exercise or vasodilatation, results in an increase in coronary flow. In a normal coronary artery, flow increases twofold to 2.5-fold with dynamic exercise or threefold to fourfold with maximal coronary vasodilatation.[2–6] However, the increase in flow in a stenosed coronary is attenuated. Despite an increase in proximal flow, there is an increase in the pressure gradient across the stenosis, resulting in a drop in pressure and flow distal to the stenosis. This causes a heterogeneous distribution of blood flow during stress, with a greater increase in myocardial perfusion in the area subtended by the normal coronary artery relative to the myocardium supplied by the stenotic artery.

In certain circumstances, coronary flow may actually decrease distal to the stenosis, resulting in subendocardial ischemia. This phenomenon of *myocardial steal* may occur in two circumstances. In the presence of a severe coronary stenosis, the coronary pressure distal to the stenosis may decrease enough during stress that it is insufficient to perfuse the endocardium, resulting in subendocardial ischemia despite an increase in total flow in the proximal epicardial artery. This is sometimes referred to as *vertical steal.* Alternatively, in the presence of one or more diseased vessels with collaterals between their distal beds, there may be an unequal fall in the pressure between the two distal perfusion beds. This results in blood being shunted away from the distal bed, with the higher perfusion pressure to the one with the lower perfusion pressure. This is referred to as *horizontal steal* and also can result in the production of subendocardial ischemia in the affected area. The concept of coronary flow reserve is described in detail in the section on positron emission tomography.

Choice of Radiopharmaceutical

Thallium 201. This cation is a potassium analogue and is widely used in the assessment of myocardial perfusion. Myocardium uptake occurs by both active and passive mechanisms involving Na,K-ATPase.[7, 8] Uptake of ^{201}Tl by the myocyte is not affected by either ischemia or hypoxia unless these processes result in cell death.[9–12] There is a linear relationship between ^{201}Tl uptake and coronary blood flow, with a tendency to underestimate and to overestimate at the upper and lower limits of the physiologic range, respectively,[11, 13–15] Thallium washes out of the myocardium by diffusion, with a half-life in the myocardium of 4 to 8 hours. The rate is primarily dependent on the ^{201}Tl concentration gradient between the myocardium and the blood.[16, 17]

In comparison to a normal coronary artery, lower coronary flow rates are achieved in a stenosed artery during stress. As a consequence, there is less ^{201}Tl uptake by the myocardium in this artery's distribution. After stress, coronary flow returns to baseline levels and is the same in both the normal and the stenosed artery. However, because of the unequal distribution of ^{201}Tl in the myocardium during stress, clearance of ^{201}Tl is heterogeneous. The greater concentration gradient between the normal myocardium and the blood results in a higher washout rate of ^{201}Tl than in the hypoperfused myocardium, where the ^{201}Tl concentration gradient is less. As a consequence, there is a trend for the myocardial concentration of ^{201}Tl to equalize with time in normal and abnormally perfused myocardium. Therefore, there is apparent "redistribution" of ^{201}Tl, with the stress-induced perfusion defect apparently reversing during rest imaging 3 to 4 hours later. A perfusion defect after stress that has resolved by time of distribution imaging is considered to represent ischemic but viable myocardium.

Conversely, a defect still present at time of redistribution imaging was classically interpreted as representing nonviable scar tissue. However, using either improvement in regional ventricular function after revascularization or myocardial uptake of ^{18}Fl-fluorodeoxyglucose (FDG) as indicating the presence of viable myocardium, several studies have identified viable myocardium in 40 to 60 percent of fixed ^{201}Tl perfusion defects.[18–20] Several studies from Bonow and associates[21–23] have shown that reinjection of ^{201}Tl in the presence of a persistent perfusion defect at time of redistribution imaging results in reversal of a significant proportion of these "irreversible" defects, and that this correlates with myocardial uptake of FDG. The same workers have also shown that areas with mild or moderate reductions in ^{201}Tl uptake that do not redistribute still contain viable myocardium.[24] However, Kitsiou and associates[25] have shown that although mild-to-moderate perfusion fixed defects contain viable myocardium, these areas are less likely to show functional improvement after revascularization than mild-to-moderate defects that are reversible.

The underlying mechanism by which ^{201}Tl reinjection enhances the detection of viable myocardium is illustrated in Plate 5–2. During stress, there is an unequal distribution of ^{201}Tl because of differences in coronary flow between the normal and the abnormal areas. At rest, coronary flow returns to normal, with a tendency for the ^{201}Tl concentration to equalize between the normal and the abnormal areas as a result of differential washout rates. If there is still heterogeneous distribution of ^{201}Tl after 4 hours, a further dose of ^{201}Tl is reinjected. Because the basal coronary flow rates are normally the same in the normal and the abnormal coronary arteries at this time, the dose of ^{201}Tl should be equally distributed. Therefore, ^{201}Tl concentration increases proportionally more in the previously hypoperfused myocardium. The net result is a decrease in the difference in ^{201}Tl concentration between the abnormal and the normal regions, resulting in reversal of the perfusion defect. However, if flow does not return to normal at rest, differences in myocardial uptake in ^{201}Tl persist. This may explain why some perfusion defects may appear to redistribute, whereas reinjection images may show persistence of the perfusion defect (Plate 5–3). Therefore, it is important to perform both 4-hour redistribution imaging and, if a severe defect is still seen, either reinjection or 24-hour imaging.

^{99m}Technetium–Labeled Perfusion Agents. ^{99m}Tc-labeled radiopharmaceuticals were developed in the early 1980s. Three agents have been approved for clinical use by the United States Food and Drug Administration: sestaMIBI, teboroxime, and tetrofosmin. Compared with ^{201}Tl, the ^{99m}Tc-labeled radiopharmaceuticals offer significant advantages, including (1) a shorter, 6-hour half-life, allowing larger patient doses to be administered, typically 25 to 35 mCi, compared with 3 to 4 mCi of ^{201}Tl, and (2) the higher energy of ^{99m}Tc photons, 140 versus 74 keV, reducing the scatter fraction and resulting in superior energy discrimination. These advantages translate into higher-quality images.[26, 27]

Teboroxime has kinetic properties that are different from those of the other currently available ^{99m}Tc-labeled radiopharmaceuticals. It is extremely lipophilic, and myocardial uptake correlates closely with coronary blood flow over a wide range of flow rates and has very rapid myocardial washout.[28] Unlike ^{201}Tl, teboroxime washout is largely flow dependent, and it appears that the rate of washout from the myocardium may allow differentiation between viable and nonviable tissue.[29–31] However, the short residence time in the myocardium mandates rapid data acquisition. Failure to do so may potentially lead to image artifacts because of the changing myocardial distribution of ^{99m}Tc-teboroxime during acquisition. Despite the clinical utility of ^{99m}Tc-teboroxime,[32] its rapid clearance presented significant constraints on clinical imaging protocols, which resulted in a preference for ^{99m}Tc-labeled radiopharmaceuticals and the subsequent removal of the product from the marketplace by the manufacturer.

In contrast, the kinetics of sestaMIBI are in many ways at the opposite end of the spectrum. It is a lipophilic cation, which accumulates in the myocardium according to blood flow, although at higher coronary flow rates, the relationship becomes nonlinear, resulting in an underestimation of coronary flow. It has a first-pass extraction fraction of 65 percent, which is lower than either ^{201}Tl or teboroxime. However, its net extraction is higher because it is avidly retained by myocytes with little bidirectional exchange of sestaMIBI and minimal redistribution and slow clearance.[33] The volume of distribution for sestaMIBI is so large that saturation of myocardial uptake does not occur. Uptake occurs primarily by diffusion, resulting primarily from negative electrical gradients across sarcolemmal and inner mitochondrial membranes and, to a lesser extent, concentration gradients.[34] Carvalho and associates[35] demonstrated that 90 percent of ^{99m}Tc-MIBI in vivo activity is associated with mitochondria as the original free cationic complex.

Clinical studies indicate that imaging with ^{99m}Tc-sestaMIBI has a similar degree of accuracy for the overall detection of coronary artery disease. In addition, it produces higher-quality images and is more accurate for the detection of individual coronary artery stenoses.[26, 36] Use can be made of ^{99m}Tc-sestaMIBI's long myocardial retention time; it allows patients to be imaged up to 4 to 6 hours after administration of ^{99m}Tc-sestaMIBI. In the setting of acute myocardial infarction, ^{99m}Tc-sestaMIBI can be given at the same time as thrombolytic therapy but allows imaging to be performed later, when the patient is in a more stable condition and environment.[37, 38] The higher count rates and the lack of redistribution also allow gated tomographic acquisitions to be performed (Plate 5–4). This increases the accuracy of the technique and allows the evaluation of endocardial wall motion and myocardial thickening, providing important information on regional and global ventricular function.[39–41]

Tetrofosmin is the most recent ^{99m}Tc-labeled radiopharmaceutical approved for clinical use. Like its predecessor,

^{99m}Tc-sestaMIBI, tetrofosmin is a lipophilic cation, which diffuses across the sarcolemmal and mitochondrial membranes.[42–44] Similar to sestaMIBI, tetrofosmin tends to underestimate flows greater than 2 ml/min/g and to overestimate flows less than 0.2 ml/min/g.[45] Munch and colleagues[46] reported that ^{99m}Tc-tetrofosmin had a shorter myocardial half-life and higher heart-liver ratios than ^{99m}Tc-sestaMIBI. In addition, in a canine model using adenosine, Glover and associates[47] observed that ^{99m}Tc-tetrofosmin uptake underestimated the flow heterogeneity more than ^{201}Tl. A clinical study[48] comparing ^{99m}Tc-tetrofosmin with ^{201}Tl SPECT imaging using dipyridamole stress had findings that tended to support those reported by Glover and associates. In this clinical study, ^{201}Tl imaging identified more reversible defects than ^{99m}Tc-tetrofosmin SPECT imaging, and in addition, they noted that the magnitude of reversible perfusion defects also was more severe in the ^{201}Tl images. Similar findings have also been reported by others.[49, 50] However, in general terms, clinical experience has shown that tetrofosmin is comparable to the other currently available myocardial perfusion agents.[50–53]

Choice of Stress

Exercise

The cardiovascular response to dynamic exercise results in an increase in cardiac output. Peripheral resistance decreases in active muscles and increases in resting tissues; overall, there is a fall in systemic vascular resistance.[54] There is an increase in heart rate in response to exercise that is mediated by alterations in the autonomic nervous system. The increase is linearly related to work load and oxygen uptake. The heart rate response to maximal dynamic exercise is dependent on many factors, especially the individual's age and health. The increases in cardiac output during dynamic exercise increase systolic arterial blood pressure but cause little alteration in diastolic pressure.

Dynamic exercise is the most commonly used means of stress when nuclear techniques are used. The procedure is carried out in a manner almost identical to that of conventional exercise electrocardiography. In addition, the patient should have an intravenous cannula placed in a large vein in the antecubital fossa before stress. This is kept patent with an infusion of saline. At peak exercise, the patient is injected with the radiopharmaceutical and continues exercising for a further 60 seconds. The timing of imaging after exercise is dependent on the particular radiopharmaceutical being used.

Pharmacologic stress is being increasingly used. The main indication for its use is when the patient is unable to exercise adequately. Reasons for this are varied and include concomitant medical conditions (e.g., peripheral vascular disease, morbid obesity, and neurologic disease), poor motivation, and antianginal medications (in particular beta-adrenergic and calcium channel antagonists).

Vasodilators

Dipyridamole is widely used as pharmacologic agent in conjunction with myocardial perfusion imaging agents, and has a diagnostic accuracy similar to that of exercise myocardial perfusion imaging.[55–57] Dipyridamole is a highly basic and hydrophobic pyridimine derivative that induces an increase in endogenous adenosine levels by blocking uptake of adenosine by red cells and endothelium.[58–60] The increased concentrations of adenosine in the interstitial fluid result in relaxation of vascular smooth muscle. This may be mediated by many mechanisms, including (1) an inhibition of slow inward calcium current, resulting in decreased calcium uptake; (2) activation of adenylate cyclase through A_2 receptors in smooth muscle cells; and (3) possible modulation of sympathetic neurotransmission.[61, 62] Dipyridamole may alter systemic hemodynamics, causing a slight fall in blood pressure and slight increases in the heart rate and pressure-rate product. Once adenosine leaves the interstitium, it undergoes rapid intracellular metabolism via adenosine kinase by phosphorylation to adenosine monophosphate or deamination by adenosine deaminase.[63] Dipyridamole undergoes hepatic biotransformation to a monoglucuronide and is excreted in the bile.[64]

Patients should be in a fasting state and should not have taken any xanthine medications (theophylline) in the previous 36 hours and caffeine beverages (including decaffeinated coffee or tea and cola) in the preceding 24 hours. Patients should be in stable condition with no history of recent unstable angina or complicated acute myocardial infarction. It is contraindicated in patients with reversible airways obstruction. The infusion of 0.142 mg/kg/min of dipyridamole is given over 4 minutes, and 3 to 4 mCi of ^{201}Tl is administered 3 to 4 minutes later. Continuous clinical, electrocardiographic, and blood pressure monitoring is performed during the procedure. Imaging is performed in the usual manner, with acquisitions immediately after dipyridamole administration and again 2½ to 4 hours later.

Serious adverse reactions have been reported after intravenous dipyridamole, including fatal and nonfatal myocardial infarction, ventricular fibrillation, symptomatic ventricular tachycardia, transient cerebral ischemia, and bronchospasm.[57] The effects of dipyridamole are usually rapidly reversed by the administration of aminophylline, which antagonizes the effects of adenosine at the A_2 receptor.[65] Side effects are reported in approximately 50 percent of patients after intravenous dipyridamole administration at a dose of 0.568 mg/kg. Chest pain occurs in approximately 15 to 40 percent and ST segment depression in 5 to 20 percent of patients. The presence of either or both does not reliably predict the presence of angiographically significant disease, although it is more common in their presence. Noncardiac symptoms are relatively common and include flushing, nausea, lightheadedness, and mild headaches.

Dipyridamole stress imaging can be supplemented with exercise, usually isometric handgrip, although treadmill exercise can also been used.[66, 67] Dypyridamole and handgrip have been used extensively after evidence of increased coronary flow when used in combination with dipyridamole.[68] More recent data using Doppler-derived indices of flow have produced conflicting evidence.[3] Therefore, it may confer benefit by different mechanisms, such as an increase in afterload or vasoconstriction of small-to-moderate–sized arteries. Exercise may improve image quality by improving target-to-background ratios after dipyridamole administration.[69, 70]

Adenosine, the mediator of dipyridamole's vasodilating action, has also been used as a coronary vasodilator.[71, 72] Maximal coronary vasodilatation is obtained with an intravenous infusion rate of 100 to 140 μg/kg/min. This increases coronary blood flood flow velocity 4.4-fold. The effects are maximal 2 minutes after the onset of the infusion and return to baseline within 2 to 3 minutes of its discontinuation. Adenosine has also been used as an alternative to dipyridamole in conjunction with ^{201}Tl tomography in patients with suspected or known coronary artery disease, and it appears to have comparable diagnostic accuracy.[73–75] Verani and associates[76] reported their experiences with this technique in 607 patients. Small but significant mean increases increases in heart rate and decreases in the systolic and diastolic blood pressures were observed. First- and second-degree atrioventricular block occurred in 10 percent and 4 percent of patients respectively; ischemic ST segment depression was identified in 13 percent of cases. Side effects were frequent but well tolerated; flushing occurred in 35 percent, chest pain in 34 percent, headache in 21 percent, dyspnea in 19 percent of patients. In most patients, the side effects ceased rapidly after the adenosine infusion was stopped. The side effects were severe in only 2 percent of patients and in only 6 of 607 patients was it necessary to discontinue the infusion.

Sympathomimetics

Dobutamine is a potent sympathomimetic agent with stimulatory effects on β_1-, β_2- and α_1-adrenoreceptors with predominantly inotropic and a lesser chronotropic effects.[77, 78] Therefore, dobutamine produces an increase in myocardial oxygen requirement by causing an increase in myocardial contractility and systolic blood pressure and, at higher doses, an increase in heart rate. This is similar to the effects of dynamic exercise, and in the presence of coronary artery disease, myocardial ischemia may be provoked.[78, 79] The dose for dobutamine is usually 5.0 μg/kg/min, increased by increments every 3 to 5 minutes to a maximal infusion rate of 30 to 50 μg/kg/min. Side effects that can occur with this agent include palpitation, headache, paresthesia, nausea, tremor, ventricular arrhythmia, and marked ST-segment depression. Side effects usually resolve rapidly after discontinuation of the infusion. Experimental evidence suggests that dipyridamole produces greater increases in coronary flow rates than dobutamine, making the former the pharmacologic agent of choice in stress myocardial perfusion imaging.[80] However, some studies indicate that the technique has potential clinically; however, larger studies are needed to substantiate these findings.[81, 82] At present, the main role of dobutamine in nuclear cardiology is in patients for whom the use of dipyridamole or adenosine is contraindicated, usually patients with reversible obstructive airways disease.

Analysis of Images

For the most part, tomographic imaging has replaced planar techniques because of enhanced contrast and spatial resolution and consequently improved sensitivity for the identification and localization of coronary artery disease.[83] The myocardial territories subtended by the left anterior descending coronary artery consist of the apical, anterolateral, anterior, and anteroseptal portions of the left ventricle. The left circumflex coronary artery supplies the midportion and posterior portion of the left ventricular wall. The right coronary artery supplies the apical, inferior, and inferoseptal aspects of the left ventricle. Plate 5–5 demonstrates ^{201}Tl tomograms from a patient with disease of the left anterior descending artery. There is a severe perfusion abnormality involving the anterior and septal aspects of the left ventricle. Plate 5–6 are stress and rest ^{201}Tl tomograms from a patient with right coronary artery disease. The reversible perfusion defect can be seen in the inferior and posterior wall of the left ventricle.

Subjective interpretation of ^{201}Tl tomograms is frequently performed. However, gender-related differences in tissue attenuation can make interpretation problematic (Plate 5–7). In males, the anterior and lateral segments normally demonstrate the highest relative activity, and the posterior and septal segments demonstrate lower activity. In contrast, females normally demonstrate somewhat higher activity in the inferoposterior and lateral segments as compared with the anterior and septal segments. These differences relate to the relative anatomic thinness of the ventricular septum and to photon attenuation from intervening body tissue.[84] Quantitative computer techniques for the analysis of ^{201}Tl tomograms, including myocardial uptake and redistribution, when combined with qualitative visual analysis result in improved sensitivity with only marginal effects on specificity.[85–87] The results of these analyses are usually displayed as polar maps or "bull's-eye" displays (Fig. 5–3). The center of the polar map is obtained from an apical short-axis section, with subsequent short-axis sections being obtained from progressively more basal portions of the left ventricle and the most basal short-axis section forming the outer border of the polar map. Polar maps are divided into approximately 100 segments. The profiles from the patient's segments are compared with a data bank of gender-matched normal profiles previously acquired from a group of normal individuals (usually patients with < 5 percent probability of coronary disease). Any of the patient's segments falling 2.5 standard deviations below the normal mean value are plotted (Fig. 5–4).

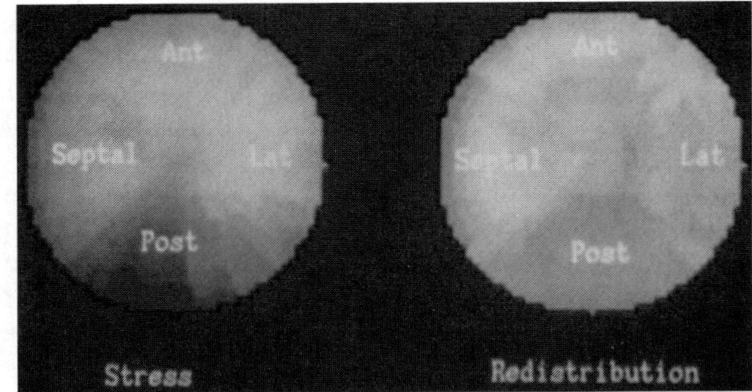

FIGURE 5–3 Polar maps from a patient with right coronary artery disease (see Plate 5–6). There is hypoperfused area involving the inferior and posterolateral aspects of the left ventricle in the stress map. The redistribution map shows that this is almost completely reversible. Ant, anterior; Lat, lateral; Post, posterior.

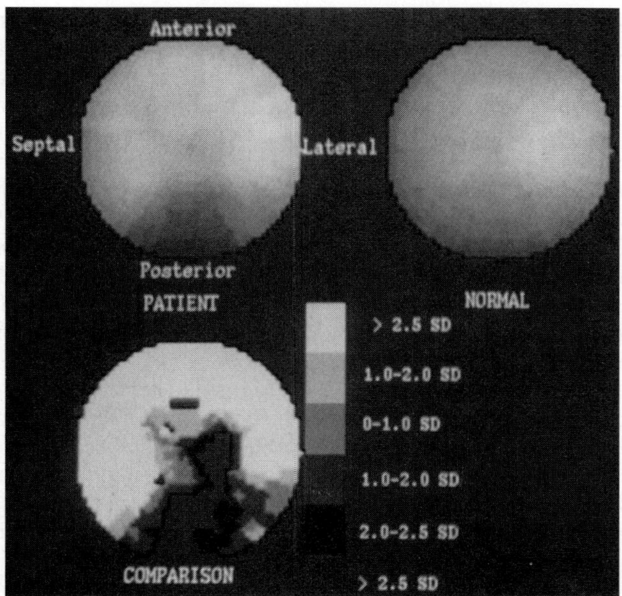

FIGURE 5–4 The patient's polar map *(top left)* is compared with normal polar map *(top right)* obtained from patients with less than a 5 percent likelihood of coronary artery disease. Areas that are outside of 2.5 standard deviations (SDs) of normal are blacked out *(bottom left)*.

Imaging principles and quantitative analytical techniques used to analyze ^{99m}Tc-labeled radiopharmaceuticals are similar to those used for ^{201}Tl tomography.

Recognition of image artifacts is important in the interpretation of SPECT myocardial perfusion images. Many factors have been identified as potentially artifact causes, including patient motion, soft tissue attenuation (breast tissue, lateral chest wall fat, diaphragm), overlying visceral activity, left bundle branch block, left ventricular hypertrophy, reconstruction artifacts, flood field nonuniformity, and center of rotation errors.[88] Breast tissue attenuation is a common occurrence and results in a lower count density in the anterior wall of the left ventricle of women (anterior/inferior count density ratio = 1.0 in women and 1.2 in men). Motion during acquisition is a common cause of image artifacts. This can occur after exercise, resulting in the phenomenon called "upward creep." It is the consequence of changes in depth of respiration from deep to shallower breathing, resulting in the heart "creeping" up in the thorax during the acquisition. Delaying the start of imaging for 10 minutes after cessation of exercise usually eliminates this phenomenon. Patient motion during acquisition may result in the production of factitious perfusion abnormalities and can usually be easily identified by examining a cine display of the planar projection images.[89] The presence of left bundle branch block can result in septal perfusion abnormalities, which may be reversible.[90]

The use of electrocardiographically gated acquisitions (refer to radionuclide ventriculography section for details on electrocardiographically gated acquisitions) during myocardial perfusion imaging provides important incremental data over static imaging.[39, 40, 91–95] It provides important information regarding regional and global ventricular function, including wall thickening, ventricular volumes, and ejection fraction.[91, 95] In addition, the use of gated images appears to improve the specificity of the technique by better identifying perfusion defects that are due to artifacts.[40, 92]

Another important development in SPECT imaging that is under intensive investigation and refinement is the use of attenuation correction.[96–101] With and without attenuation-corrected SPECT, Ficaro and coworkers[98] studied 60 patients with coronary artery disease and 59 patients who had a low likelihood of coronary artery disease. With their method of attenuation correction, the sensitivity and specificity for detection of coronary artery disease increased from 78 and 46 percent to 84 and 82 percent, respectively, with visual analysis and from 84 and 46 percent to 88 and 82 percent, respectively, for quantitative analysis. Many different techniques for correcting for attenuation are under development and evaluation by most of the major gamma camera manufacturers.

Comparison of SPECT and PET Perfusion Imaging

There are several theoretical reasons to believe that PET is more accurate than its single-photon counterpart, ^{201}Tl SPECT. First, the intrinsic resolution of this technology affords higher-resolution images. Second, the ability to correct for attenuation using a transmission scan should also improve the diagnostic accuracy of the technique. There is potential for the production of image artifacts.[102] However, the main disadvantages of the PET technology are its limited availability and significantly higher capital expenditure, running, and maintenance costs.

Several studies of PET in the diagnosis of coronary artery disease have indicated that this technique is accurate for the diagnosis of coronary artery disease.[103–105] Three comparative trials suggest that this technique has diagnostic accuracy superior to that of ^{201}Tl SPECT imaging.[104, 106, 107] However, the evidence is not conclusive; one study did not demonstrate any significant difference; another, which showed significantly higher sensitivity and specificity, has been criticized for its methodology and analysis.[108] Further larger prospective studies are required before it is possible to determine whether the added expense of PET translates into a greater degree of diagnostic accuracy. Having said this, PET imaging is becoming more available, and an increasing number of insurance companies are providing reimbursement for this procedure. In the current climate of containment of health care costs, the future of clinical cardiac PET imaging will depend on the ability to demonstrate convincing evidence of superior diagnostic accuracy.

RADIONUCLIDE VENTRICULOGRAPHY

Radionuclide ventriculography is one of the most widely used techniques for evaluating ventricular function. This essentially noninvasive method of assessing ventricular function can be easily performed and provides a reproducible, accurate evaluation of both right and left ventricular function. There are basically two methods of performing radionuclide ventriculography: first-pass and gated equilibrium radionuclide ventriculography.

First Pass Radionuclide Angiocardiography

This technique involves following the passage of a radioactive tracer through the central circulation. It requires the use of a gamma camera with a high count rate capability, usually 1×10^5 to 5×10^5 counts per second. This high count rate capability is optimally provided by a multicrystal gamma camera, such as Baird-Atomic, which is expensive and can be used solely for first-pass imaging studies. However, the newer digital single crystal Anger gamma cameras have improved count rate capabilities and are reputed to provide satisfactory count statistics.

The radioisotope is administered as a compact bolus, 1 ml plus 20 ml of saline solution flush, through a large vein, usually antecubital or jugular.[109] An anterior or 30-degree right anterior oblique projection is used to optimize separation of the atria from the ventricles. The former is preferred because the position is more reproducible, it enhances resolution by minimizing the distance between the detector and the chest wall, and during exercise studies, motion artifact is minimized by pressing the chest wall firmly against the detector. The right and left ventricles overlap in these projections; however, this does not pose a problem during first pass of the radionuclide bolus. Data are usually acquired in a series of images with high temporal resolution. The optimal framing interval is determined by the sensitivity of the camera and the patient's heart rate. For example, with a multicrystal gamma camera during an exercise study, the framing interval is 25 milliseconds. In a patient with normal hemodynamics, first-pass transit is encompassed by 600 frames. The most commonly used radiopharmaceutical is ^{99m}Tc, complexed either to diethylenetriamine-pentaacetic acid or sulfur colloid. This allows for optimal excretion of the isotope via the kidneys to decrease background accumulation, which is an important consideration if more than one study is being performed.[110] Clinical studies using ^{195}Au have found it to be a suitable alternative to ^{99m}Tc.[111, 112] ^{195}Au has a half-life of only 30.5 seconds, allowing multiple studies to be performed without imposing a prohibitive radiation burden on the patient or increasing the background activity that occurs with ^{99m}Tc.

After acquisition of the data, right and left ventriculograms are constructed from which ejection fractions and ventricular volumes can be calculated.[113] A number of time-activity curves are obtained; the number depends on the time taken for the bolus to traverse the chamber of interest, usually 5 to 10 individual beats in a normal patient. The count rate reaches a maximum at end-diastole, when ventricular volume is largest and falls in proportion to the ventricular volume to reach a minimum at end-systole. Data from individual beats are summed to provide a single curve, which is then corrected, for background. The ejection fraction and ventricular volumes are then calculated from the normalized, background-corrected time-activity curve (Fig. 5–5).

The first-pass technique has the advantage of excellent image contrast and chamber separation because of the absence of background activity from adjacent great vessels and organs, in particular, the lung. In addition, acquisition time is short, usually between 20 and 30 seconds, which is

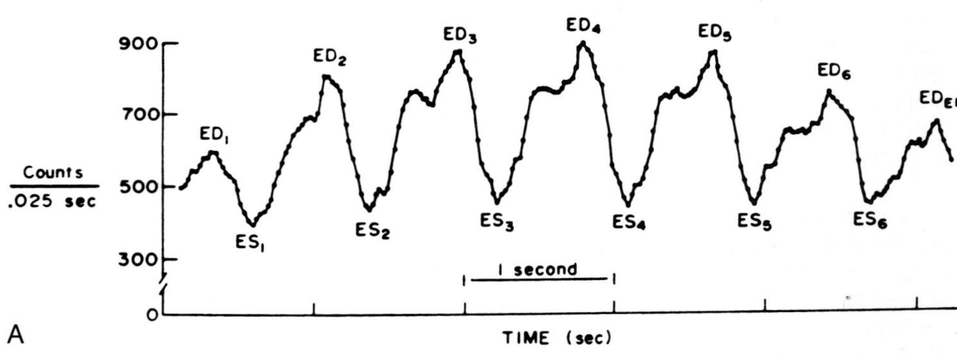

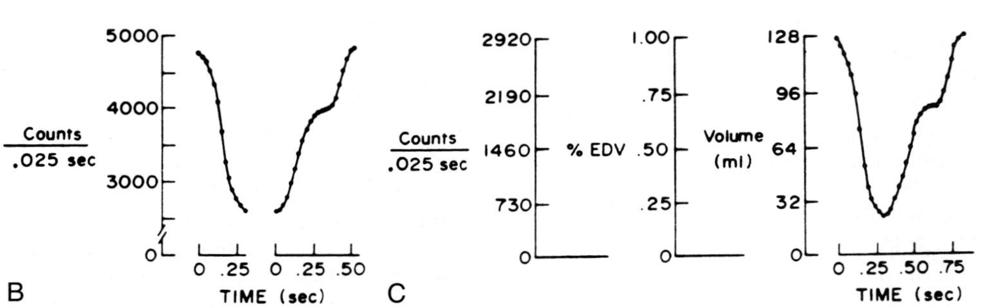

FIGURE 5–5 Calculation of left ventricular ejection fraction and volumes from first-pass radionuclide angiocardiography. **A,** Uncorrected counts measured within the left ventricular region of interest during the levophase. **B,** Summed systolic and diastolic segments. **C,** Final volume curve after normalization and background correction. ED, end-diastole; ES, end-systole; EDV, end-diastolic volume. (**A–C,** From Jones RH: Radionuclide angiography. *In* Marcus ML, Schelbert HR, Skorton DJ, Wolf GL [eds]: Cardiac Imaging: A Companion to Braunwald's Heart Disease. pp. 1006–1026. Philadelphia: WB Saunders, 1991.)

an advantage during exercise studies as acquisition of data occurs only during peak exercise. The first-pass technique also provides a means of detecting and quantifying intracardiac shunts.[114–117] For both right-left and left-right shunts, the time-activity curves that are generated resemble dye-dilution curves and are analyzed by use of a similar methodology. Despite these advantages, it does have significant limitations. First, one is limited to two to three acquisitions per patient study because of the increasing radiation exposure to the patient and the increasing background activity. Second, the technique is more demanding both on personnel and on equipment: (1) it requires a compact bolus injection; (2) any patient motion or ventricular arrhythmia, such as coughing, one ventricular ectopic beat occurring during acquisition, can seriously degrade the radionuclide data; (3) it requires use of a multicrystal gamma camera or a digital Anger camera with high count rate capabilities. Additionally, evaluation of regional wall motion function is poorer than that of the gated equilibrium technique.

Gated-Equilibrium Radionuclide Ventriculography

The most widely used radionuclide technique to assess ventricular function is gated-equilibrium radionuclide ventriculography. In this technique, the patients' red blood cells are labeled with 25 to 35 mCi of ^{99m}Tc-pertechnetate, using either an in vivo or in vitro method. The in vitro or modified in vitro methods result in a consistently higher labeling efficiency. Scintigraphic data are acquired by use of a conventional single crystal Anger gamma camera in multiple planar projections. Usually, an anterior, left anterior oblique, and left lateral or posterior oblique are acquired (Fig. 5–6). The left anterior oblique that best separates the right and left ventricles is chosen, that is, the best septal projection. The detector is also angulated to separate the left atrium from the left ventricle. The anterior projection is usually at 45 degrees less oblique, and the left lateral projection is usually at 45 degrees more oblique than the best septal projection. In addition, the scintigraphic data are acquired gated to the electrocardiogram, with each R-R interval being divided equally into a predetermined number of time bins, usually 16 to 32 time bins (Fig. 5–7). During acquisition, scintigraphic data are stored in memory in one of these time bins, such that at the end of the acquisition, each time bin contains scintigraphic data from several, typically 300, R-R intervals (Fig. 5–8).

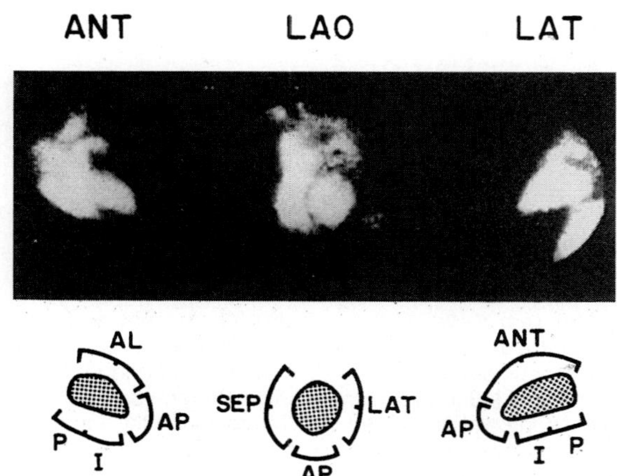

FIGURE 5–6 Assessment of regional left ventricular function from a gated radionuclide ventriculogram. Anterior (ANT), left anterior oblique (LAO), and left lateral (LLAT) projections in end-diastole are shown. Corresponding segmentation is given below. AL, anterolateral; AP, apical; I, inferior; P, posterior; SEP, septal; LAT, lateral. (From Corbett JR, Jansen DE, Willerson JT, et al: Radionuclide ventriculography. II: anatomic and physiologic aspects. Am J Physiol Imag 2:85, 1987.)

Gated-equilibrium radionuclide ventriculography is one of the most accurate means of assessing ventricular function and can be easily performed by use of readily available nuclear imaging systems. It allows acquisition of multiple projections and/or multiple studies up to 6 hours after administration of the isotope. The high count densities achieved, typically 300 counts/cm^2 in the left ventricle, allow superior evaluation of region wall motion to that with the first-pass technique. The technique does have some limitations: (1) overlap between cardiac chambers; however, this can usually be resolved by use of multiple views; (2) limited spatial resolution, when compared with contrast ventriculography or echocardiography; and (3) longer acquisition times are required when compared with first-pass techniques (minimum of 2 minutes), which can pose a problem during exercise studies in patients with limited or unpredictable exercise capabilities.

Many of these problems can be resolved by tomographic gated radionuclide ventriculography by providing an accurate three-dimensional representation of the entire cardiac blood pool.[118–120] With this technique, all chambers are separated in space, and very limited ventricular segments can be assessed without concern about adjacent and potentially superimposed segments (Plate 5–8). This technique allows an accurate means of assessing both global and regional ventricular function with a higher diagnostic accuracy than that of either contrast or planar radionuclide ventriculography.

Exercise Radionuclide Ventriculography

Exercise radionuclide ventriculography is performed by use of either the first-pass or the gated-equilibrium technique. The commonly used gated-equilibrium technique is described here. A resting study is performed in the usual manner, but the left anterior oblique projection is obtained last, with the patient lying supine on a specially designed bicycle table-ergometer, which has adjustable shoulder restraints and handle bars to minimize movement of the patient's torso during exercise. After the resting left anterior oblique projection is obtained, exercise is commenced. The exercise test is performed in exactly the same manner as with other exercise tests, with continual monitoring of the electrocardiogram, heart rate, and blood pressure. Typically, the first stage of exercise is performed at 200 kpm for 3 or 4 minutes and increased by 200-kpm increments (less if the patient has a limited exercise capacity) to a symptom-limited maximum. Scintigraphic data are acquired during the last 2 minutes of each stage of exercise,

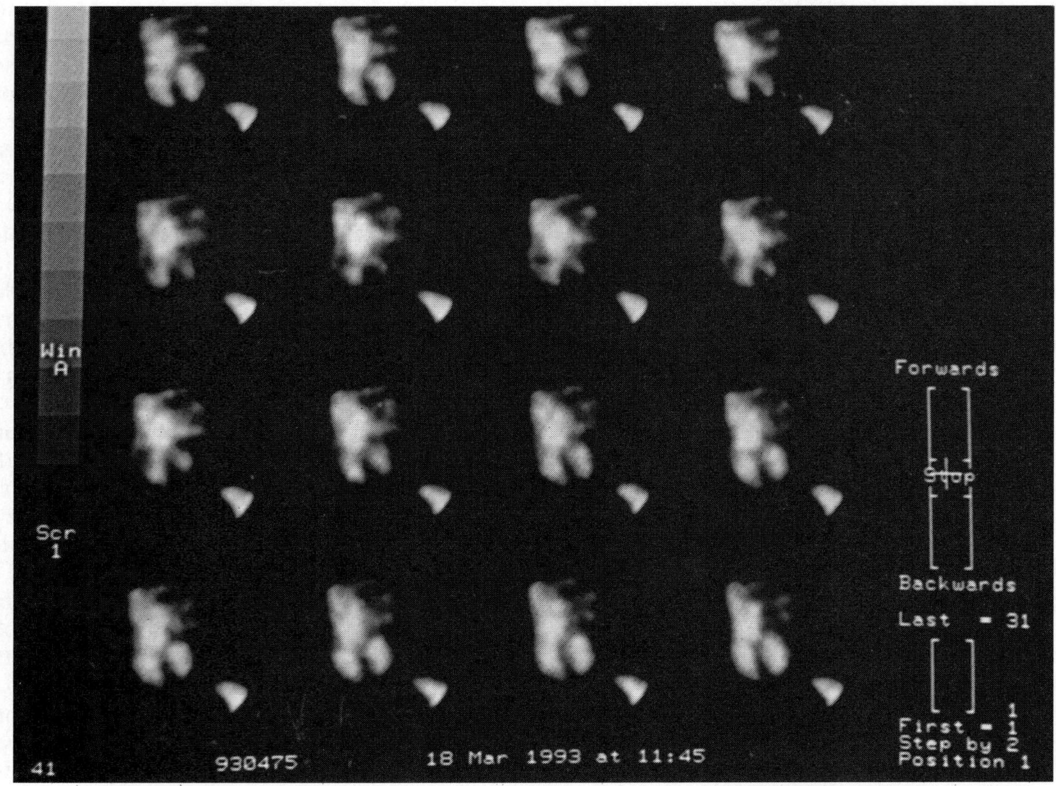

FIGURE 5–7 Sixteen frames from a gated radionuclide ventriculogram in the "best septal" left anterior oblique projection. The end-diastolic frame is the first image, located in the upper left of the figure; the end-systolic frame is the eighth image.

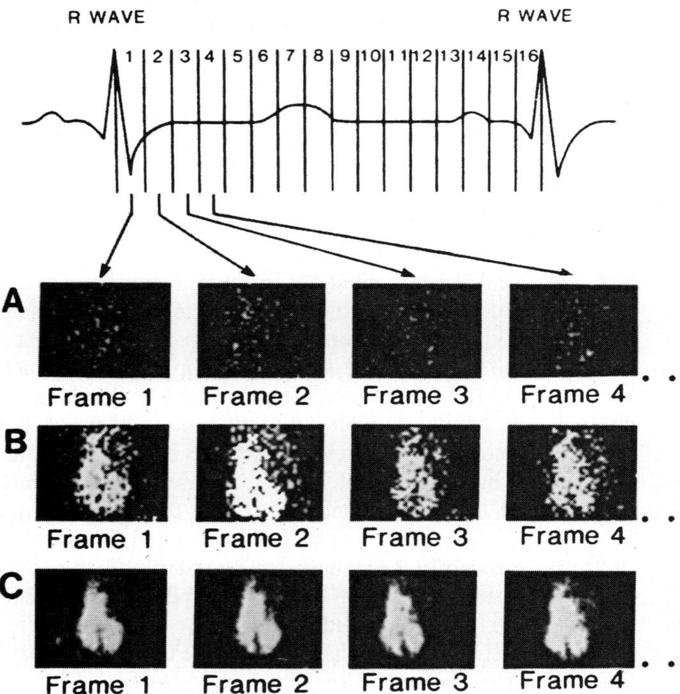

FIGURE 5–8 Schema explaining the principle of electrocardiographic gated acquisition in radionuclide ventriculography. The cardiac cycle is divided into equal intervals (16 in this example). Counts recorded during each interval are stored in different computer frames. After a single cardiac cycle **(row A)**, there are no recognizable images. After 20 cardiac cycles **(row B)**, the images begin to be recognizable. After 400 cardiac cycles (300,000 counts per frame), image quality has improved considerably **(row C)**. (From Parker DA, Karvelis KC, Thrall JH, Froelich JW: Radionuclide ventriculography: methods. *In* Greson C [ed]: Cardiac Nuclear Medicine. pp. 67–84. New York: McGraw-Hill, 1987. Copyright © by McGraw-Hill, Inc. Used by permission of The McGraw-Hill Companies.)

when the hemodynamics have equilibrated. The hemodynamic response is different than with erect exercise.[121, 122] During supine exercise, there is a lesser increase in end-diastolic volume and heart rate, but a greater increase in systolic blood pressure when compared with erect exercise. This does not appear to adversely affect the sensitivity of the technique.[123] There are significant gender-related differences in the left ventricular response to exercise. Women have greater increases in end-diastolic volume and lesser increases in left ventricular ejection fraction than men.[124, 125]

Analysis of Radionuclide Ventriculograms

Data from radionuclide ventriculograms can be used to provide many parameters of ventricular function. The method is relatively independent of geometric assumptions because there is complete mixing of the ^{99m}Tc-labeled red cells in the intravascular compartment, and the activity within the ventricle is proportional to ventricle volume.[126]

Left ventricular ejection fraction (LVEF) is calculated using the left anterior oblique projection by drawing a region of interest (ROI) around the left ventricle in end-diastole and end-systole. After correcting the counts in the ROIs for background activity, the ejection fraction is calculated from the formula

$$LVEF = EDc - ESc/EDc$$

where EDc and ESc are end-diastolic and end-systolic counts corrected for background, respectively.

Ventricular volumes can be calculated by use of a nongeometric count–based technique.[127, 128] This methodology uses measured ventricular activity that is normalized for the acquisition time per frame and the activity in a known volume from a peripheral venous blood sample. Estimation of left ventricular volume is calculated by use of the formula

$$\text{Volume} = K(\text{corrected left ventricular counts})/(\text{no. cardiac cycles})(\text{time/frame})(\text{blood activity})$$

where K is a correction constant to adjust for attenuation, which is usually determined from a regression equation by use of contrast angiography as a reference.

This usually suffices for most individuals who are of normal size and shape, heart size, and so on. However, in some patients, it is necessary to correct for individual variations, which can be successfully done by use of a simple geometric technique.[129, 130] With these data, stroke volume and cardiac output can be calculated by use of radionuclide ventriculography.[131, 132] When the tomographic technique is used, ventricular volume is usually calculated by use of a geometric technique. If the pixel volume is known, the ventricular volume can be calculated by summing the number of pixels in each tomographic section in the left ventricular region of interest. Values obtained with this technique correlate well with other techniques and have the advantage of not requiring any correction for attenuation.[118]

Valvular regurgitation can be evaluated by calculating the ratio of left-to-right ventricular stroke counts.[133, 134] Normally, the right and left ventricular stroke volumes are equal. However, in the presence of valvular regurgitation, the stroke volume is greater in the ventricle with the affected valve. Ventricular stroke counts are obtained by subtracting the end-systolic from the end-diastolic frame, resulting in a stroke volume image. In this image, the activity in the left and right ventricular regions is proportional to their respective stroke volumes. These data can be expressed in terms of either the stroke volume ratio (left ventricular stroke counts/right ventricular stroke counts, normal value < 1.2) or as the regurgitant fraction (left ventricular $-$ right ventricular stroke counts/left ventricular stroke counts $\times$ 100, normal value < 20 percent). The systematic overestimation of this technique results from right atrial/right ventricular overlap. Assessment of valvular regurgitation by use of this technique is somewhat crude. It is not possible to detect mild regurgitation or clearly quantitate the severity of the regurgitation. In addition, the accuracy is increasingly compromised when the left ventricular ejection fraction is 35 percent or less. Valvular regurgitation can also be estimated by use of Fourier amplitude images.[135]

Diastolic function can also be assessed by radionuclide ventriculography.[136, 137] The variables used are the peak filling rate, measured as the slope of a third-order polynomial fit to the rapid filling phase; the time to peak filling rate, measured from end-systole; and rapid diastolic filling and atrial systole, expressed as a percent of stroke volume (Fig. 5–9). However, noninvasive assessment of diastolic function, whether obtained with radionuclide or Doppler echocardiographic techniques, has several limitations. These result from dependence of these variables of diastolic function on other variables, such as heart rate, preload and afterload, and ejection fraction, making their interpretation difficult. Therefore, their clinical utility is limited. However, they may be helpful in patients with clinical features of cardiac failure but a normal ejection fraction.

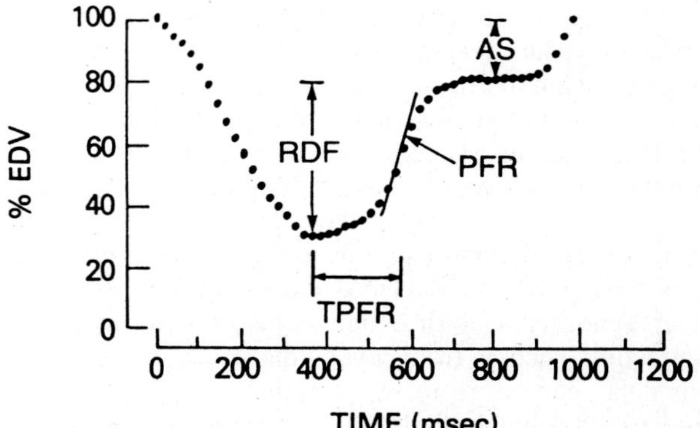

FIGURE 5–9 High temporal resolution time-activity curve obtained from radionuclide ventriculography. Each point represents 20 ms. Variables used to assess left ventricular rapid filling include peak filling rate (PFR), measured as slope of a third-order polynomial fit to the rapid filling phase; time to peak filling rate (TPFR), measured from end-systole; and contributions of rapid diastolic filling (RDF) and atrial systole (AS), expressed as percent of stroke volume. EDV, end-diastolic volume. (From Bonow RO: Left ventricular filling in ischemic and hypertrophic disease. *In* Grossman W, Lorell BH [eds]: Diastolic Relaxation of the Heart. pp. 231–243. New York: Martinus Nijhoff, 1987.)

Regional ventricular function can be assessed either qualitatively or quantitatively by use of radionuclide ventriculography. The former method, using visual analysis of an endless-loop cine display, is the most widely used. There is good correlation between visual assessments of radionuclide and contrast ventriculograms, and reproducibility of the two techniques is comparable.[138, 139] Quantitative techniques have been developed and can be broadly classified into geometric techniques (usually modifications of methods developed for contrast ventriculography) and nongeometric techniques specifically designed for radionuclide ventriculography.

The most commonly used nongeometric techniques use the regional ejection fraction and Fourier transform–derived phase and amplitude images. The regional ejection fraction image is obtained by subtracting the background-corrected end-systolic from the background-corrected end-diastolic frame.[140] The resulting image is normally crescent shaped, delineating the left ventricular borders. If there is an area of regional hypokinesis or akinesis, there is thinning or absence of the crescent in this area. The data can also be presented in actual regional ejection fraction values, with the left ventricle typically being divided into three or five segments.[141]

Fourier phase analysis has been applied to the evaluation of radionuclide ventriculograms.[141a, 142] Each pixel has its own time-activity curve, which is at maximum in end-diastole and at minimum in end-systole, and whose fundamental frequency is determined by the heart rate. The time-activity curve is sinusoidal in shape and can be approximated by use of a single cosine function of the frequency of the time-activity curve. This allows each pixel within the region of the heart to be expressed as a single mathematical value, which can be color coded. The amplitude of this cosine wave, which is equivalent to change in counts during the cardiac cycle, is proportional to the stroke volume of the pixel. Therefore, the amplitude image gives a regional representation of stroke volume. For example, in a region of akinesis, the pixels show time-activity curves of reduced amplitude, resulting in the amplitude image showing absent activity in that region. The phase of the cosine wave can also be expressed in a similar fashion. The R-R interval is considered to represent 360 degrees, with the R wave occurring at zero degrees, which coincides with the peak of the cosine wave. In areas of the ventricle where onset of contraction is delayed, the peak of the cosine wave is also delayed. This may be the result of either abnormal electrical activation or delayed onset of contraction, such as from myocardial ischemia or scarring. This delay can be expressed in terms of "phase delay" or "increased phase angle." For example, an area of dyskinesis results in a phase delay of about 180 degrees. Similarly, pixels in the atria have time-activity curves that are completely out of phase with the ventricles, equivalent to a phase delay of 180 degrees. These data can be expressed in a phase image, in which each pixel is colored coded according to its phase angle. Fourier images are useful in evaluating regional wall motion in patients with coronary artery disease at rest and during exercise.[142–144] These images can also identify conduction abnormalities and have been used to localize the site of arrhythmias and also atrioventricular accessory pathways.[145–147]

INFARCT IMAGING

Technetium-Labeled Infarct Avid Imaging Agents

The recognition of acute myocardial infarction is not always easily accomplished.[148–151] Infarcts are especially difficult to recognize by electrocardiography in individuals who have had previous myocardial infarcts, in those with left bundle branch block, in those who have been cardioverted, and in those who have nontransmural (non–Q wave) myocardial infarcts. Even the most sophisticated enzymatic techniques have certain limitations in identifying the presence or absence of acute myocardial infarction in patients, including the following: (1) there is a temporal dependency in the ability of the enzyme markers to detect severe myocardial injury, and (2) certain clinical circumstances preclude the use of traditional enzyme measurements, including creatine kinase and creatine kinase MB determinations for infarct recognition. Therefore, it is important to have available additional noninvasive means of identifying the presence of myocardial necrosis, which may be used in conjunction with standard techniques for infarct recognition. Additional noninvasive techniques developed should be able to identify the presence or absence of acute myocardial infarction in almost every instance in which it occurs. They should also be relatively noninvasive, as inexpensive as possible, usable in diverse clinical conditions, and subject to repeat measurement with whatever frequency is necessary to evaluate the possibility of extension of myocardial damage or relatively delayed evolution of it.

An infarct avid imaging agent, ^{99m}Tc stannous pyrophosphate (^{99m}Tc-PPi), has been developed for these purposes. This radionuclide myocardial imaging approach has been evaluated in both experimental animals and in patients and its utility in recognizing acute myocardial necrosis has been well established.[152–167] An alternative myocardial scintigraphic method, a monoclonal antibody to cardiac myosin labeled with either iodine, technetium, or indium, has been used for similar purposes.[168–172]

The potential for using ^{99m}Tc-PPi myocardial scintigraphy to recognize myocardial necrosis was first suggested by the observations of Shen and Jennings[173] and D'Agostino,[174] when they demonstrated that calcium is deposited in crystalline and subcrystalline form in irreversibly damaged myocardial cells. These observations led Bonte and associates[156] to question whether ^{99m}Tc-PPi might be able to identify irreversibly damaged myocardial cells on the basis of pyrophosphate complexing with calcium in crystalline or precrystalline form. Subsequently, extensive studies were performed in experimental animals and patients, examining the ability to ^{99m}Tc-PPi to detect irreversibly damaged myocardium and to further elucidate pathophysiologic mechanisms involved in its uptake and concentration in irreversibly damaged myocardium.[157–167] The three most important determinants of ^{99m}Tc-PPi myocardial uptake in the heart

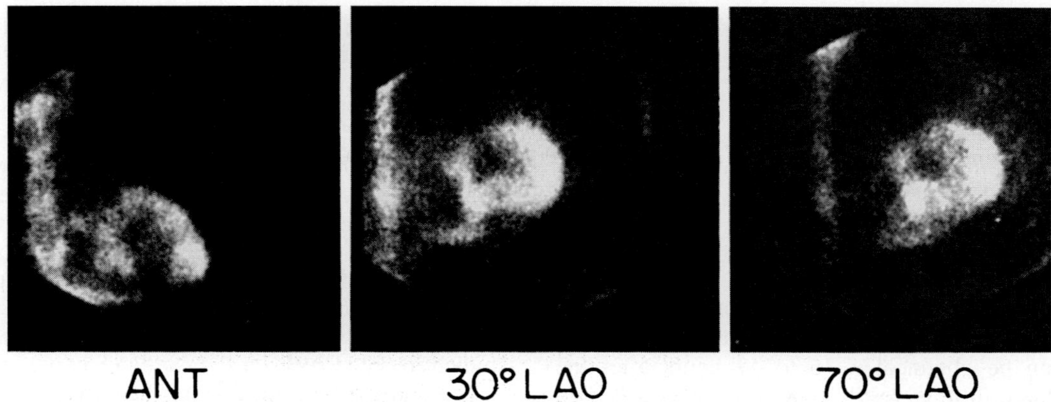

FIGURE 5–10 Anterior (ANT), 30-degree left anterior oblique (LAO), and 70-degree LAO ^{99m}Tc-pyrophosphate scans in a patient with proximal occlusion of the left anterior descending coronary artery with resultant extensive infarction, producing a "doughnut" appearance. (See text for further details.)

are (1) the presence of myocardial necrosis, (2) persistent residual collateral blood flow into the area of irreversible myocardial damage, and (3) time elapsed after the onset of myocardial damage before the ^{99m}Tc-PPi myocardial scintigram is obtained.[157–167, 175–181, 181a] At least 3 g of myocardial necrosis must be present to identify acute myocardial infarcts in experimental animals with fixed coronary occlusion when two-dimensional or planar myocardial imaging is used and ^{99m}Tc-PPi is the imaging agent. However, with SPECT, as little as 1 g of myocardial necrosis may be identified, especially if reperfusion is allowed. Collateral coronary blood flow alterations are also important determinants of ^{99m}Tc-PPi myocardial uptake in irreversibly damaged myocardium. ^{99m}Tc-PPi uptake is greatest is myocardial regions in which coronary blood flow is reduced to levels of 20 to 40 percent of normal with fixed coronary occlusion and experimental myocardial infarction. In experimental animals, if the occlusion is positioned very proximally around the left anterior descending coronary artery, there is initially reduced ^{99m}Tc-PPi uptake in the center of the area of gross necrosis; this scintigraphic pattern has been referred to as the "doughnut" pattern of ^{99m}Tc-PPi uptake.[151, 153, 156, 158] This same phenomenon occurs in patients and is associated with very severe proximal narrowing or complete occlusion of the left anterior descending coronary artery (Figs. 5–10 and 5–11). In experimental animals, when the coronary occlusion is positioned more distally around the left anterior descending coronary artery, or when collateral flow is relatively abundant, the doughnut pattern does not occur. Instead, homogeneous and intense ^{99m}Tc-PPi myocardial uptake is observed when myocardial infarction occurs. The doughnut pattern becomes at least partially filled in during the first few days after myocardial infarction in both animal models and patients; this presumably is the result of collateral blood flow reaching the more central portions of the infarct and reperfusing an area that previously received no flow. These observations emphasize that ^{99m}Tc-PPi uptake is dependent on collateral flow, and three must be some flow reaching the area of damage for increased ^{99m}Tc-PPi myocardial uptake to be detectable. It seems likely that coronary flow–dependent uptake will also be a feature of other "infarct-avid" myocardial imaging agents available or that may be developed to image irreversibly damaged myocardial cells. The need for some collateral flow to the area of injury can be met by serial myocardial imaging over the first 3 to 4 days after myocardial infarction, allowing one to detect infarcts several days later, even if the amount of collateral flow initially is not adequate to do so.

When reperfusion is allowed, ^{99m}Tc-PPi uptake occurs in irreversibly damaged myocardial cells within 2 to 3 hours after the infarct, so virtually immediate scintigraphic detection is possible. Infarcts may be sized accurately when SPECT is used with this technique, especially if a blood pool overlay is allowed and/or one attempts to determine the amount of irreversible damage based on an estimate of the myocardium at risk by use of a concomitant perfusion study, such as with thallium 201 and SPECT imaging with ^{99m}Tc-PPi.[182]

We use a grading scheme (0 to 4+) for the interpretation of ^{99m}Tc-PPi myocardial scintigrams. We regard ^{99m}Tc-PPi myocardial scintigrams that are "2 to 4+" as indicating increased pyrophosphate uptake and the presence of myocardial necrosis. "Two plus" ^{99m}Tc-PPi uptake is the faintest but definitely increased uptake in the region of the heart. "Three-plus" ^{99m}Tc-PPi uptake is uptake equivalent to that noted in bone, and "4+" uptake is greater than the

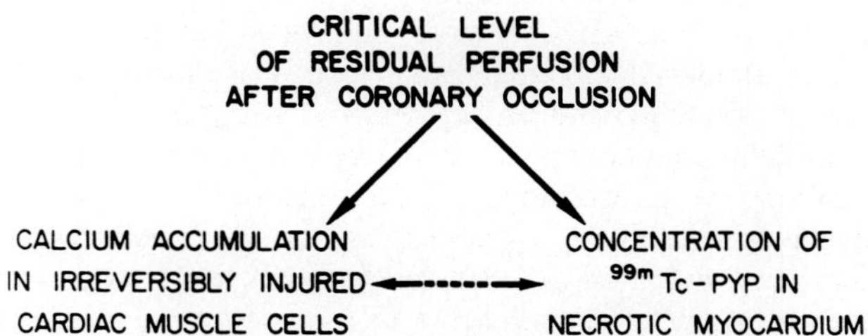

FIGURE 5–11 Relationship between collateral flow blood, pathologic calcification, and concentration of ^{99m}Tc-pyrophosphate (PYP) in necrotic myocardium. (From Willerson JT, McGhie I, Parkey RW, et al: Infarct avid imaging. *In* Marcus ML, Schelbert HR, Skorton DJ, Wolf GL [eds]: Cardiac Imaging: A companion to Braunwald's Heart Disease. pp. 1074–1084. Philadelphia: WB Saunders, 1991.)

surrounding bone. Most Q-wave infarcts evolve to a pattern of being "3 to 4+," but many non–Q wave infarcts demonstrate "2+" and poorly localized ^{99m}Tc-PPi uptake.

Dead and dying cells are the primary cell types that take up increased amounts of ^{99m}Tc-PPi after experimental infarction. This emphasizes that any circumstance in which a significant region of heart muscle is irreversibly injured, including viral myocarditis, cardioversion, trauma to the heart, and metastatic tumor in the heart could result in an abnormal ^{99m}Tc-PPi myocardial scintigram.

In patients, with fixed coronary artery occlusion not receiving thrombolytic therapy, we recommend that the first scintigram be obtained at 36 to 48 hours after the suspected infarct. If this result should be negative, one should repeat the study at 96 hours after the first symptoms that are suggestive of infarction. In patients receiving reperfusion, abnormal ^{99m}Tc-PPi images should be obtained within the first 24 hours after the event.

In some patients, the ^{99m}Tc-PPi myocardial scintigrams remain abnormal for several months after the event, although they ordinarily become negative within 5 days, and even sooner, if reperfusion has been allowed. In patients with persistently positive ^{99m}Tc-PPi myocardial scintigrams after infarction, ongoing myocardial ischemia and progressive cellular injury are responsible for the persistently abnormal result. Coronary artery revascularization interrupts this process, converting the persistently abnormal ^{99m}Tc-PPi scintigram to a negative one. In the patient with a persistently abnormal ^{99m}Tc-PPi myocardial scintigram, it is very difficult to recognize a new infarction.

Antimyosin Antibody Imaging

An alternative to ^{99m}Tc-PPi imaging for infarct detection is the use of an antimyosin antibody labeled with iodine, indium, or technetium.[168, 182–185] With irreversible cellular damage, there are structural defects in the sarcolemmal membrane that allow the penetration of antibodies into the interior of the injured cells. Myosin is degraded slowly after myocardial infarction, and an antibody directed at the heavy chain of myosin complexes with it, and the attached label allows the detection of that region of myocardium as an infarct-avid uptake. The antimyosin antibody has proved to be essentially equally sensitive to ^{99m}Tc-PPi in infarct detection both with and without reperfusion[168, 182–185] (Figs. 5–12 and 5–13). The one major difference between ^{99m}Tc-PPi and antimyosin antibody uptake is that the antimyosin antibody concentrates against a flow gradient so that its uptake is not as dependent on residual collateral blood flow. Nevertheless, the results of antimyosin antibody and ^{99m}Tc-PPi myocardial scintigraphy have been very similar in the relatively small numbers of patients that have been studied to date.[182–185]

The antimyosin antibody has been used to estimate the extent of irreversible damage in experimental animal models and patients; again, the results have been very similar to those with ^{99m}Tc-PPi when SPECT imaging is used.[182–185] Antimyosin antibody uptake also occurs with any condition that causes irreversible cellular injury in the heart, including myocarditis, rejection of the heart after transplantation, and other injury. There are persistently abnormal antimyosin antibody scans just as has been described for ^{99m}Tc-PPi. The absolute significance and total duration of persistently abnormal antimyosin antibody scans remains to be determined, but this does suggest the need for serial imaging in some patients.

Recent Developments in Infarct Imaging

^{99m}Tc-labeled glucarate has been successfully in acute infarct imaging.[186–189] Uptake of ^{99m}Tc-glucarate appears to be very specific for the presence of infarcted myocardium.[189] In a study by Narula and coworkers,[188] ^{99m}Tc-labeled glucarate was rapidly taken up by reperfused and nonreperfused infarcts; reperfused infarcts could be imaged as early as 10 minutes, and nonreperfused infarcts, 30 minutes. A radiopharmaceutical such as glucarate that has a high specificity and has the potential to detect infarction in the very early phase of acute myocardial infarction has obvious attraction because of its application in the clinical arena.

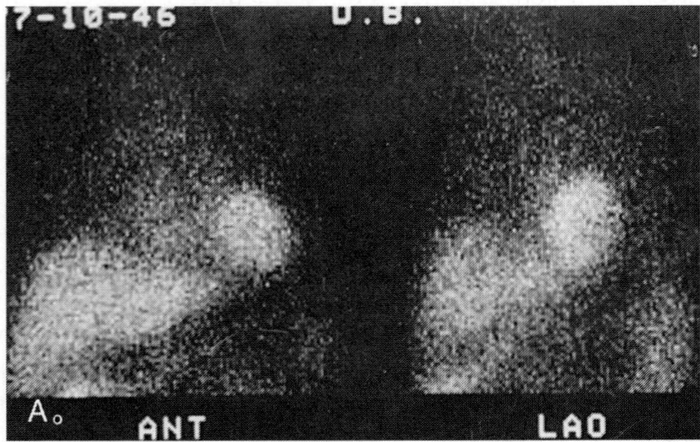

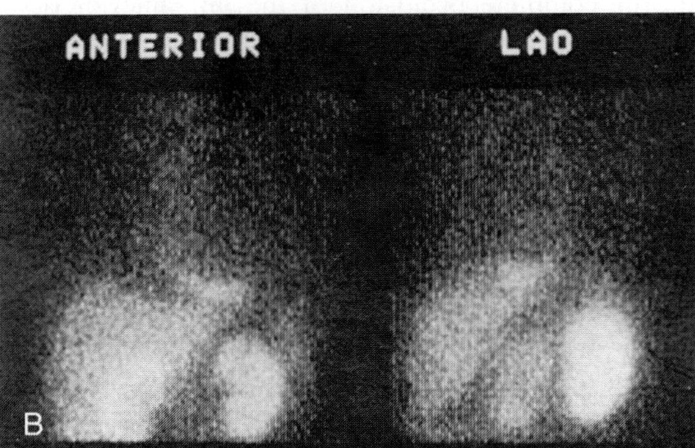

FIGURE 5–12 A, Anterior *(left)* and 45-degree LAO *(right)* indium 111 antimyosin scans, 24 hours after intravenous injection of a patient with acute anterior myocardial infarction and angiographically confirmed, persistently occluded left anterior descending coronary artery. **B,** Anterior *(left)* and 45-degree LAO *(right)* gamma scintigrams 29 hours after injection of a patient with acute inferior myocardial infarction and angiographically confirmed, persistently occluded right coronary artery. (**A** and **B,** From Khaw BA, Yasuda T, Gold HK, et al: Acute myocardial infarct imaging with indium 111-labeled monoclonal antibody Fab. J Nucl Med 8:1671, 1987. Reprinted with permission from the Society of Nuclear Medicine.)

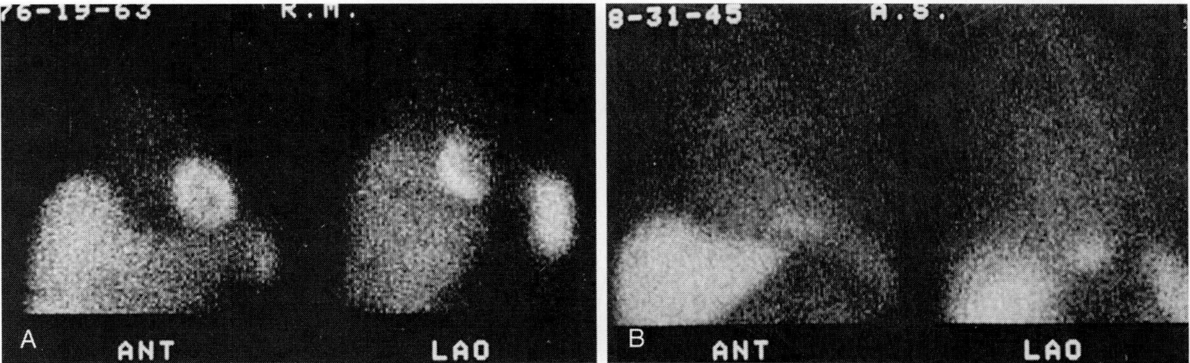

FIGURE 5–13 **A,** Anterior *(left)* and 45-degree LAO *(right)* indium 111 antimyosin scans, 26 hours after intravenous injection of a patient with an acute myocardial infarction and a left anterior descending coronary artery that has been successfully reperfused. **B,** Anterior *(left)* and 45-degree LAO *(right)* gamma scintigrams 25 hours after injection of a patient with an inferior myocardial infarction and right and left circumflex coronary arteries that have been successfully reperfused. (**A** and **B,** From Khaw BA, Yasuda T, Gold HK, et al: Acute myocardial infarct imaging with indium-111-labeled monoclonal antibody Fab. J Nucl Med 28:1671, 1987. Reprinted with permission from the Society of Nuclear Medicine.)

Another class of agents that has shown some promise in this area are the nitroimidazoles.[190–196] These compounds appear to be retained by severely hypoxic tissue. When the pharmaceutical enters a hypoxic cell, it is reduced and, because of the reduced intracellular Po_2, it cannot be reoxidized and is hence trapped within the hypoxic cell. In an experimental setting, several investigators have had varying degrees of success in imaging uptake of this radiopharmaceutical in hypoxic myocardium.[192–194, 196] There may be some potential shortcoming of this class of agents when they are used in patients, in particular, the very high heart-to-liver ratio, which may compromise the imaging quality in clinical studies.[193]

POSITRON EMISSION TOMOGRAPHY

Basic Principles

A positron is a positively charged electron that is emitted by certain unstable atoms in the process of radioactive decay. The positron travels several millimeters in tissue before colliding with an electron. With this interaction, the positron and the electron are annihilated, with conversion of their combined mass into two photons. Each of these two photons has an energy of 511 keV emitted in opposite directions, 180 degrees to each other. This annihilation photon pair can be detected with a pair of radiation detectors connected through an electrical coincidence counting circuit. This circuit is set so that one decay is recorded only if both detectors are activated simultaneously by the photon pair. All other events are rejected. Therefore, radioactive decays occurring outside the sample volume between the detectors are excluded from the count data because an unpaired photon striking only one of the detectors is not counted. Collimation is accomplished electronically with coincidence counting, rather than with lead collimators, as in single-photon imaging. Coincidence counting has several attributes that make positron emission tomography (PET) uniquely quantitative and accurate for clinical imaging, including accurate attenuation correction of emission data, electronic collimation that provides higher efficiency, better count statistics, and better spatial and contrast resolution than single-photon systems.[197]

Generically, PET cameras contain 1000 to 3000 detectors in three to eight banks of rings that are attached to photomultiplier tubes (PMTs) in ratios of 1 to 8 detectors for each PMT. Scintillations from the coincidence detectors are converted to electronic signals from the PMTs, which are subsequently converted to digital information and processed using a computer to reconstruct a tomographic image corrected for attenuation, unlike SPECT imaging, as described earlier. To compensate for the gaps between the detectors to optimize spatial sampling, the banks of detectors are wobbled in an eccentric path, with each coincidence decay assigned a spatial location in the wobble path.

A transmission image for attenuation correction is obtained by placing a ring of activity around the patient to image the target organ before the injection of a radiotracer. The positron radiotracer is then injected intravenously, and an emission image is obtained through back projection techniques. The emission image is corrected for attenuation loss, random coincidences, scattered radiation, deadtime losses, wobble, and variation in detector sensitivity. If performed correctly, a quantitative three-dimensional image of the radiotracer activity can be obtained for the organ imaged.

Coronary Flow Reserve

As discussed earlier, under resting conditions coronary blood flow remains normal during progressive coronary artery narrowing until the coronary arterial lumen is severely reduced, to approximately 85 percent diameter stenosis.[197–202] Consequently, resting coronary flow or myocardial perfusion imaging at rest does not sensitively reflect the presence or severity of coronary artery disease. However, maximum coronary flow, coronary flow reserve, or the capacity to increase flow to high levels in response to exercise stress or pharmacologic coronary arteriolar vasodilators becomes impaired with moderate coronary artery stenosis. Coronary flow reserve, as illustrated in Figure

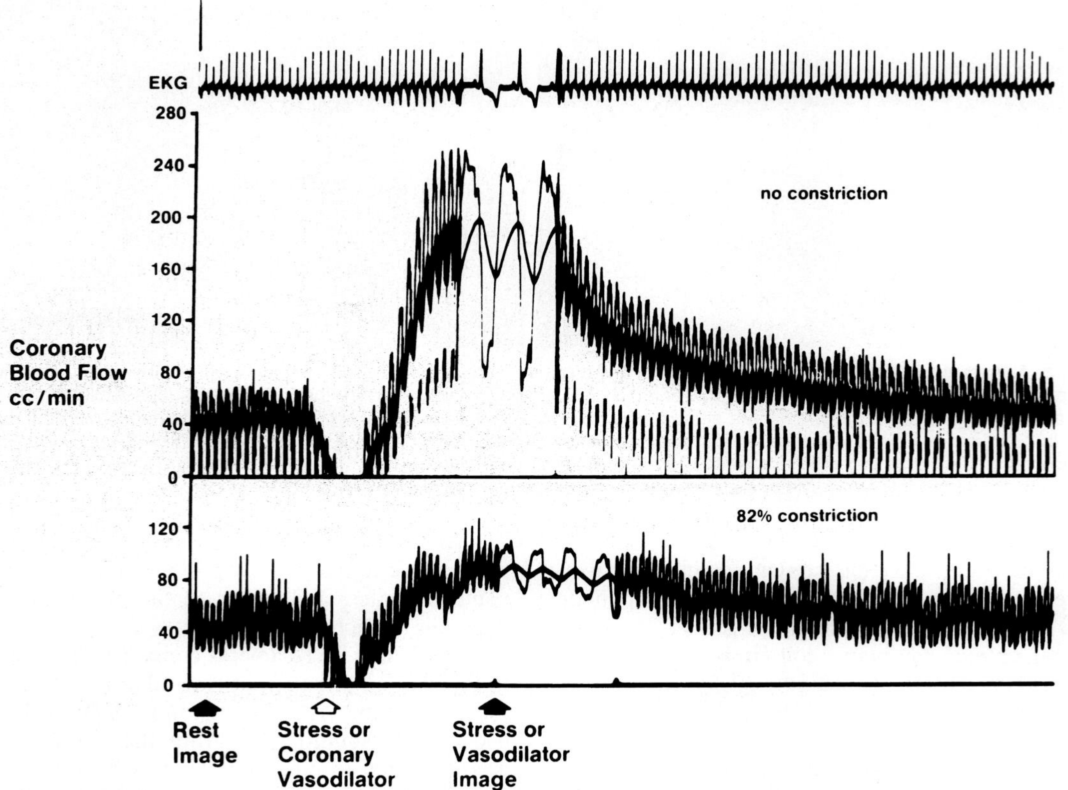

FIGURE 5–14 Top, Coronary blood flow by electromagnetic flowmetry in a normal artery at rest and after a coronary flow stimulus. Flow normally increases four to five times over baseline levels in response to dipyridamole or adenosine, thereby indicating a normal coronary reserve flow of 4 or 5. **Bottom,** The flow response in the presence of an 82 percent diameter constriction of the coronary artery. Resting coronary flow is normal, but the increase in flow is blunted by the coronary artery stenosis, thereby reducing the coronary flow reserve to approximately 2 in this case compared with a normal of 4 or 5. (From Gould KL: Coronary Artery Stenosis. New York: Elsevier, 1990.)

5–14, is defined as the ratio of maximum flow or perfusion during stress or pharmacologic vasodilation to resting flow or perfusion. Figure 5–15 relates stenosis severity (horizontal axis) to coronary flow reserve expressed as the relative increase of flow in multiples times initial baseline resting flow (vertical axis). (The dashed line indicates resting flow and the solid line is flow reserve. The gray zone indicates the range for multiple observations.) With progressive narrowing, baseline flow remains normal until the coronary artery is narrowed by 80 to 85 percent diameter stenosis. However, coronary flow reserve begins to decrease at 40 to 50 percent diameter stenosis for a vasodilatory stimulus increasing flow normally to four times baseline. For a stimulus increasing flow to five or six times baseline levels, coronary flow reserve would be reduced by even milder stenoses of 30 percent diameter stenosis.

For the experimental stenoses on which these figures were based, normal arterial diameter and stenosis length were constant and relatively uniform for each stenosis in a progressive series of experimental coronary artery constrictions. Consequently, percent narrowing related well to flow reserve, with some data scatter (gray area of Fig. 5–15) due to variable physiologic conditions of heart rate and aortic pressure, which may somewhat alter flow reserve.[203] In humans, absolute dimensions and length of stenoses are highly variable, with the consequence that percent diameter stenosis is poorly related to coronary flow reserve.[203–211] However, in both animals and humans, we have shown that directly measured coronary flow reserve is equivalent to, interchangeable with, and predicted by the arteriographic geometry of coronary artery stenoses if all stenosis dimensions are accounted for, including percent stenosis, absolute cross-sectional luminal area, length, and shape.[202, 212–215]

Mechanisms of Coronary Flow Reserve

To explain the maintenance of normal resting coronary flow but reduced coronary flow reserve during progressive coronary constriction, consider the stenotic coronary artery as two resistances in series (i.e., a narrowed tube and a distal coronary vascular bed) as represented schematically in Figure 5–16. Normally, the distal coronary bed resistance at rest is high. In this schema, the driving pressure for flow is the total pressure gradient across the stenosis and distal vascular bed, which is approximately central aortic pressure because venous pressure is relatively small. Therefore, flow is determined approximately by aortic pressure divided by the sum of the resistances of the stenosis (R_s) and of the distal vascular bed (R_b) in series. If the distal bed resistance is large compared with the stenosis resistance, as normally found at rest, large changes in the stenosis resistance will have little effect on flow, which is determined primarily

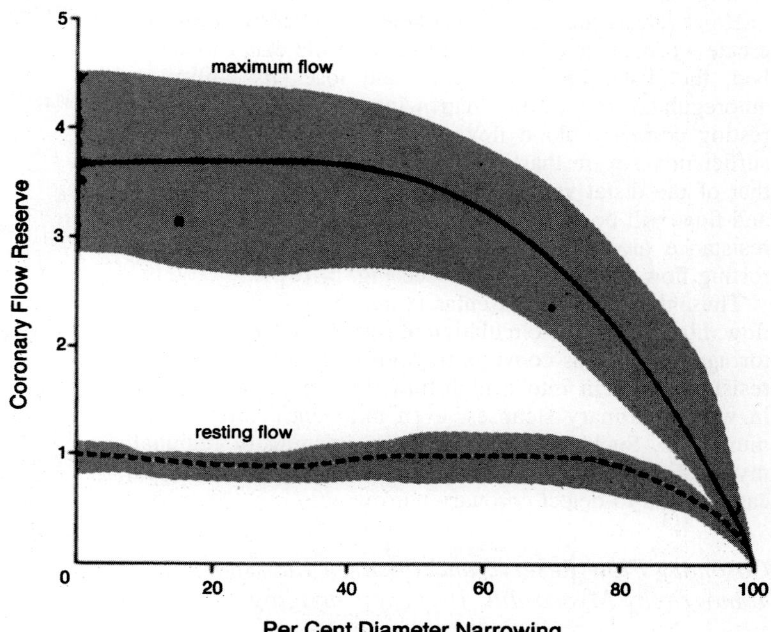

FIGURE 5–15 Coronary flow reserve expressed as a ratio of maximal flow to resting flow is given on the vertical axis, with percent diameter narrowing given on the horizontal axis. With progressive narrowing, resting flow does not change *(dashed lines),* whereas the maximal potential increase in flow or coronary flow reserve begins to fall at approximately 50 percent diameter narrowing. *Shaded areas* represent the limits of variability of data about the mean plotted by the *solid* and *dashed lines.* (From Gould KL: Coronary Artery Stenosis. New York: Elsevier, 1990.)

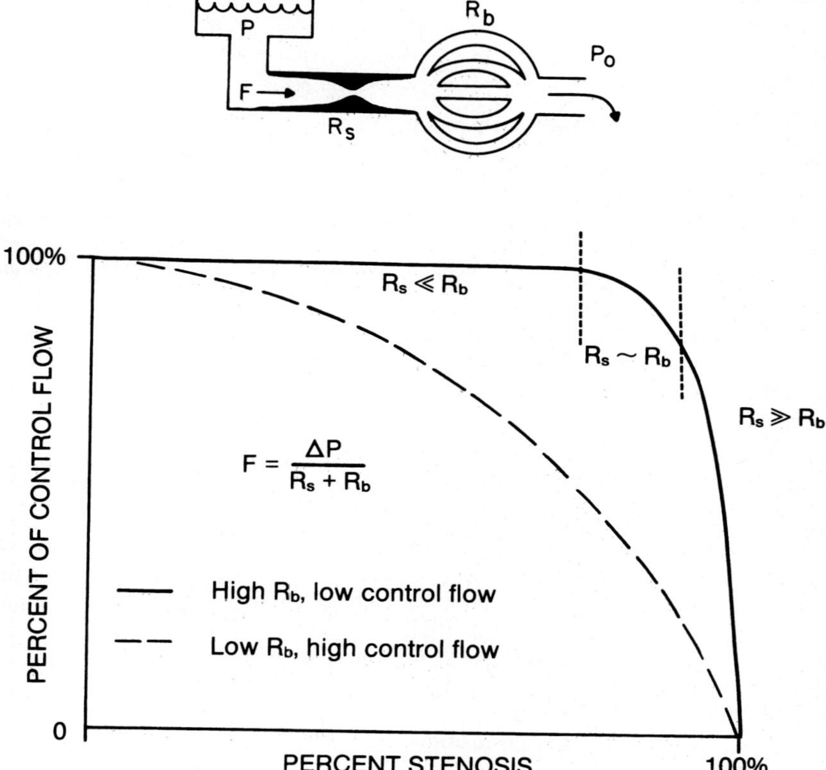

FIGURE 5–16 Diseased coronary circulation as two resistances in series. R_s indicates the resistance of the stenotic artery, and R_b indicates the resistance of the distal vascular bed. The effects of reducing R_b with the use of vasodilators are shown by the *dashed line.* The equation shows the relation between resistance and flow (F) for various segments of the curves. For a given total pressure gradient across the narrowed tube and distal vascular bed, flow is determined primarily by R_b if R_b is large. Changes in the stenotic resistance R_s have little effect until the value of R_s approaches that of R_b. (From Gould KL: Coronary Artery Stenosis. New York: Elsevier, 1990.)

by distal vascular bed resistance. Therefore, a progressive stenosis up to a point will have no hemodynamic effect on resting coronary blood flow.

However, as the stenosis becomes sufficiently severe to create a resistance comparable to that of the distal vascular bed, the distal bed vasodilates and loses its ability to autoregulate, and further narrowing will cause a fall in resting coronary blood flow. When the stenosis becomes sufficiently severe that its resistance is much greater than that of the distal vascular bed, autoregulation will be lost and flow will be determined predominantly by the stenosis resistance alone. Further arterial narrowing then causes resting flow to fall, as shown (see Fig. 5–16).

Thus, the coronary vascular system is normally a low-flow, high-resistance circulation at rest. Coronary vasodilator agents or stress converts this normally low-flow, high-resistance system into a high-flow, low-resistance system in which coronary stenoses, even mild ones, limit maximum flow. Such logic explains why imaging of regional myocardial perfusion at maximum coronary vasodilation can be used to detect coronary narrowing.

Coronary Flow Reserve and Positron Emission Tomography Myocardial Perfusion Imaging

Flow through a moderately severe coronary artery stenosis is normal at rest in the absence of unstable plaque rupture associated with unstable angina. Coronary vasodilators increase flow throughout the heart except in areas of flow-limiting stenoses, thereby causing disparity in regional perfusion relative to areas supplied by normal coronary arteries. This disparity in regional perfusion at high coronary blood flow is imaged as a means of identifying coronary artery disease noninvasively with perfusion tracers.

With marked increases in coronary flow, functionally mild early coronary artery stenoses can be identified. However, with only modest increases in coronary flow as occur during exercise, only more severe coronary stenoses can be identified. An inadequate stimulus for increasing coronary flow or an inadequate perfusion imaging agent or technique will limit the ability to detect or quantify coronary stenoses by perfusion imaging. Based on studies in animals and confirmed in humans,[203, 204, 211–216] there are three essential principles of an imaging method for detecting and assessing the severity of coronary artery disease:

1. A potent stimulus for increasing coronary flow to image the regional disparities in maximum perfusion caused by stenosis
2. A myocardial perfusion imaging agent, which is taken up or deposited in the myocardium in proportion to flow at high coronary blood flow, up to three to four times resting control levels
3. Cross-sectional positron tomography to avoid overlapping structures and to obtain depth-independent resolution for accurate quantitative measurements of coronary flow

Figure 5–17 illustrates these principles as applied to myocardial perfusion imaging. In the top panel, resting coronary flow and distribution are normal despite a severe stenosis.[203] After intravenous dipyridamole, flow increases

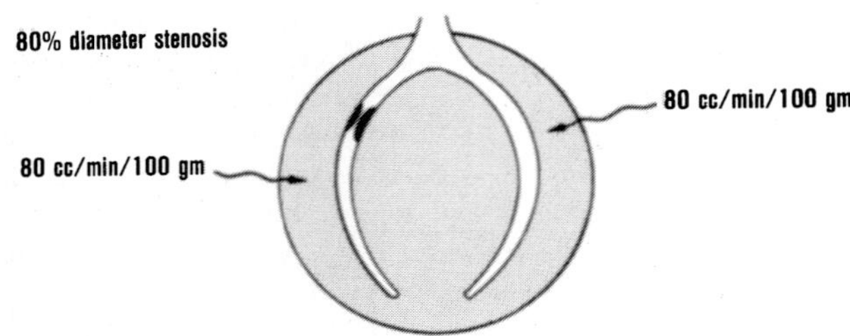

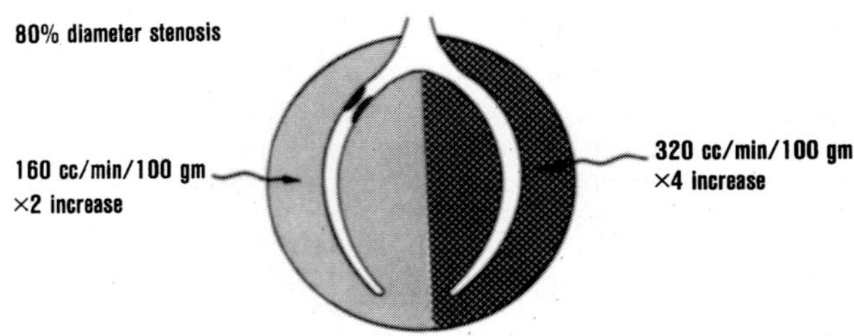

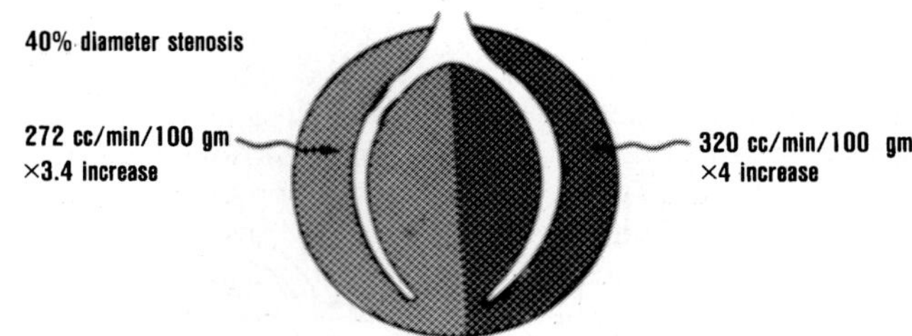

FIGURE 5–17 Principles for the detection of coronary artery disease with perfusion imaging under conditions of maximal coronary vasodilation. With an 80 percent diameter narrowing, coronary flow reserve is limited to an approximately twofold increase over resting levels compared with a fourfold increase in nonstenotic arteries. The abnormal area therefore has 50 percent less activity, reflecting a 50 percent decrease in regional maximal flow compared with the normal maximum. A milder stenosis of approximately 40 percent diameter narrowing will produce a mild relative defect of approximately 15 percent below maximal flow, indicating a mild lesion. (From Gould KL: Coronary Artery Stenosis. New York: Elsevier, 1990.)

to four times baseline level (middle panel) in the normal area but is restricted to a twofold increase in the area supplied by a stenotic artery. An average ratio of 2.5:1, or 150 percent difference, between the normal and affected areas is necessary before being visible as a relative perfusion defect on planar thallium imaging in experimental animals. Using PET, a difference of only 15 percent can be detected (i.e., an abnormal area that is 85 percent of normal maximum), thereby allowing the detection of milder stenoses, which cause less severe abnormalities in maximal perfusion.

Absolute and Relative Coronary Flow Reserve

The concept of coronary flow reserve, defined as maximum flow divided (normalized) by resting control flow, has evolved into an accepted functional measure of stenosis severity since it was first proposed.[202, 211–221] Its validity has been confirmed and applied clinically through noninvasive imaging and invasive methods. These clinical methods measure pharmacologically induced increases in coronary blood flow, with intravenous dipyridamole or adenosine for noninvasive studies and intracoronary adenosine or papaverine for invasive studies. However, changes in aortic pressure and heart rate are known to alter cardiac workload and therefore baseline coronary blood flow, as well as altering maximum coronary flow under conditions of maximal vasodilation.[211] Consequently, absolute coronary flow reserve, as measured by flowmetry, also varies with aortic pressure and heart rate independent of stenosis geometry due to the differential effects of these variables on resting and maximal coronary flow. Under markedly varying physiologic conditions, or from patient to patient, absolute coronary flow reserve may not reliably or specifically reflect the severity of coronary artery narrowing because it may be altered by physiologic factors unrelated to stenosis geometry.

In contrast, relative maximum coronary flow or relative flow reserve is defined as maximum flow in a stenotic artery divided (normalized) by the normal maximum flow in the absence of stenosis. During maximal coronary vasodilation, physiologic variables such as aortic pressure, heart rate, metabolic demand, and vasomotor tone alter distal coronary bed resistance equally for both normal and stenotic arteries. When the maximum flow in the stenotic artery is normalized by normal maximum flow, the effects of pressure, heart rate, or vasomotor tone on flow in the numerator and denominator of this ratio cancel out. Therefore, relative differences in regional maximum flow, or relative flow reserve, are determined primarily by geometric stenosis severity. Relative flow reserve is therefore a measure of stenosis severity relatively independent of physiologic variables.

Rather than considering absolute coronary flow reserve to be competitive or antithetical to relative flow reserve, these measurements are independent variables that provide complementary information. Absolute flow reserve is the flow capacity of the stenotic coronary artery and vascular bed under whatever conditions of pressure, workload, hypertrophy, vasomotor tone, or stenosis are present. It reflects the cumulative summed effects of these various factors without being specific for the mechanism or cause of altered flow reserve. Relative coronary flow reserve reflects more specifically the effects of the stenosis independent of and unaffected by the other physiologic variables if normal maximum flow is sufficiently high. Thus, absolute and relative coronary flow reserves are complementary.

"Balanced" three-vessel coronary artery disease has been viewed as causing a false-negative stress perfusion test depending on the stress stimulus and the imaging technology used. Based on experience with clinical PET, most hearts affected by coronary artery disease have some myocardium supplied by an unaffected artery, even a small one, that serves as a reference area. However, small vessel disease, left ventricular hypertrophy, and theoretically "balanced" three-vessel coronary artery disease are potential causes of diffusely impaired flow reserve that must be accounted for in individual patients. For this purpose, some measure of absolute as well as relative coronary flow reserve may be helpful. Moreover, new concepts in perfusion imaging outlined later have established specific sensitive, abnormal perfusion patterns by PET that characterize diffuse coronary artery disease.

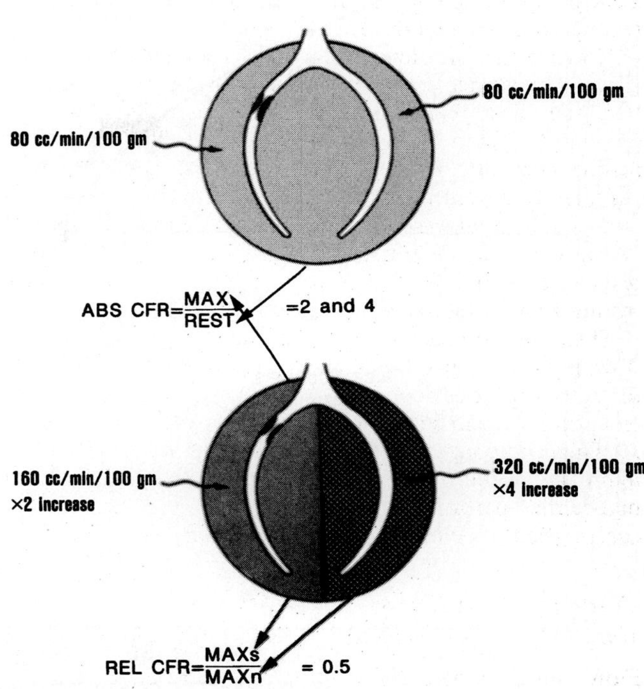

FIGURE 5–18 Concept of absolute coronary flow reserve (ABS CFR) and (REL CFR) relative coronary flow reserve. (Reprinted by permission of the Society of Nuclear Medicine from Gould KL: PET perfusion imaging and nuclear cardiology. J Nucl Med 32:579–606, 1991.)

As shown in Figure 5–18, a stress myocardial perfusion image shows relative maximum perfusion (radiotracer uptake) or relative coronary flow reserve. The ratio of myocardial radionuclide activity on the dipyridamole image to the myocardial activity on the rest image reflects absolute flow reserve. The ratio of activity in a perfusion defect to the normal maximum activity in the distribution of normal coronary arteries on the dipyridamole image alone reflects relative coronary flow reserve. With the quantification of PET perfusion imaging to account for arterial input function and flow-dependent radionuclide extraction, absolute and relative coronary flow reserve may be quantitatively measured by PET.

Relation of Coronary Flow Reserve to Percent Diameter Stenosis in Humans

Coronary flow reserve has been integrated theoretically with and experimentally related to the geometric dimensions of stenoses.[202, 211–221] The commonly used percent diameter stenosis is poorly related to functional severity of human coronary artery narrowing or coronary flow reserve,[217–222] determined by quantitative coronary arteriogra-

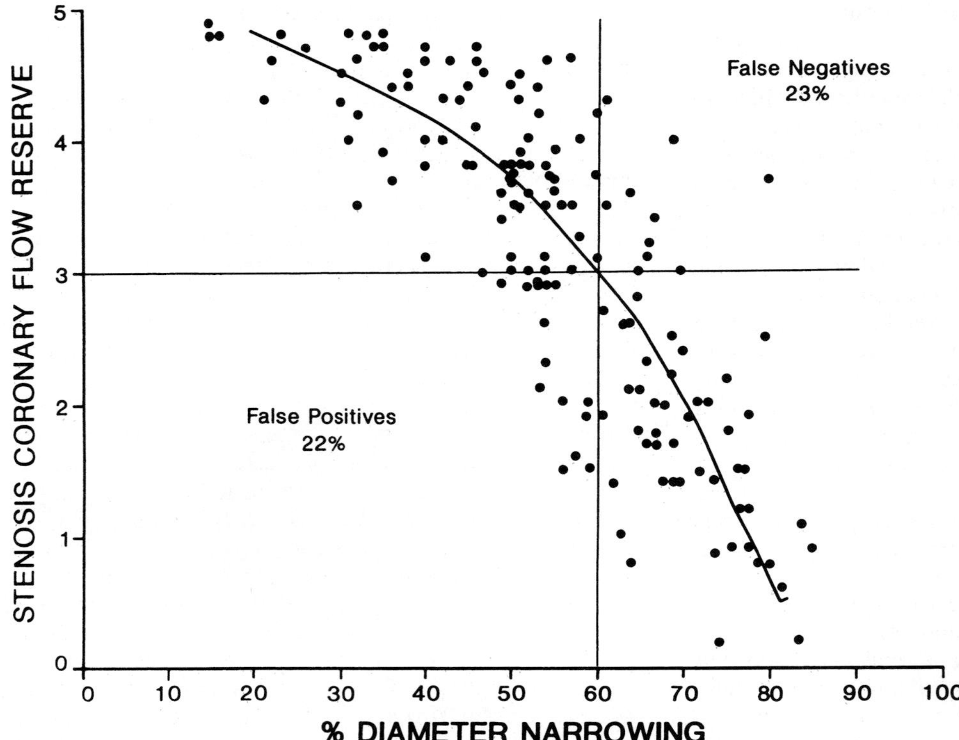

FIGURE 5–19 Relation between stenosis flow reserve and percent diameter narrowing, with both determined from automated quantitative arteriographic measurements of coronary artery stenoses in 100 patients. Because percent diameter narrowing is only one of several factors used to calculate stenosis flow reserve, the scatter in this relation indicates the importance of those factors other than percent stenosis that limit maximal flow capacity through a stenosis. (From Gould KL: PET perfusion imaging and nuclear cardiology. J Nucl Med 32:579–606, 1991; adapted from Demer LL, Gould KL, Goldstein RA, et al: Assessment of coronary artery disease severity by positron emission tomography. Comparison with quantitative arteriography in 193 patients. Circulation 79[4]:825–835, 1989.)

phy as in Figure 5–19 or by directly measured flow reserve using a Doppler catheter.[215, 220] Figure 5–19 also shows why a single threshold percent diameter stenosis is a poor "gold standard" of disease severity for comparison with perfusion imaging. For a hypothetically perfect imaging technique that measured coronary flow reserve exactly as with a flowmeter, false-positive and false-negative tests would be 22 and 23 percent for a threshold of 60 percent diameter stenosis. Thus, perfect physiologic measures of coronary flow reserve would appear diagnostically poor with a sensitivity and specificity of 77 and 78 percent, due to the inadequacy of using a percent stenosis threshold as the gold standard of significant disease.

Positron-Emitting Radiopharmaceuticals in Myocardial Perfusion Imaging

The most commonly used PET perfusion radionuclides for clinical cardiac studies are ^{13}N-ammonia[223–226] and ^{82}Rb.[204, 211–217] From 10 to 20 mCi of ^{13}N-ammonia is injected intravenously for clinical studies. The first-pass extraction fraction of ^{13}N-ammonia at resting conditions is approximately 60 to 70 percent compared with 50 to 60 percent for ^{82}Rb. Rubidium is an alkali metal analogue of potassium with similar chemical and biologic properties. Its first-pass extraction is 50 to 60 percent at resting flow levels, which falls to 25 to 30 percent at high flows, compared with 70 percent at resting conditions and falling to approximately 35 percent at high flows (for ^{13}N-ammonia). ^{82}Rb is eluted from a commercially available ^{82}Sr/^{82}Rb generator (CardioGen-82; Squibb) that provides preset volume, dose, and dose rate of ^{82}Rb to the patient. Typically, with a fresh generator, 30 to 50 mCi is injected intravenously for cardiac PET. Because of its short half-life (75 seconds), ^{82}Rb is excellent for repeated or sequential myocardial imaging, particularly in acute clinical situations in which the patient's condition is changing rapidly or for studies before and after an intervention such as dipyridamole stress.

With appropriately larger doses of rubidium (40 mCi), images are comparable to those of ^{13}N-ammonia (18 mCi), and the diagnostic accuracy is the same for ^{13}N-ammonia and ^{82}Rb. The longer half-life of ^{13}N-ammonia (9.9 minutes) permits injection of the perfusion tracer during treadmill exercise, with subsequent imaging of the ^{13}N-ammonia trapped in the myocardium under conditions of stress imaged later at rest. The shorter half-life of ^{82}Rb does not require the 30-minute decay time between rest and stress images needed for ^{13}N-ammonia. Acquisition time for a cardiac study with ^{82}Rb is 6 minutes compared with 15 to 20 minutes for ^{13}N-ammonia. Therefore, a complete rest-dipyridamole study with ^{82}Rb requires approximately 1 hour, whereas with ^{13}N-ammonia, it requires 2 hours, thereby decreasing patient throughput volume. ^{13}N-ammonia for perfusion imaging requires an on-site cyclotron, whereas ^{82}Rb is generator produced without the high cost of a cyclotron. With the fixed cost of a rubidium generator, the cost per study goes down as patient volume rises. Perfusion imaging with ^{82}Rb therefore is more economically feasible.[227] Although less expensive than a cyclotron, the cost of ^{82}Rb is quite high; however, with the development of more generator-produced positron-emitting radiopharmaceutical agents such as ^{62}Cu-PTSM, these costs are likely to decrease.[228, 229]

Metabolic Identification of Myocardial Hibernation and Stunning

Myocardial ischemia, if sustained, progresses to necrosis and scar tissue formation with an irreversible loss of contractile function. On the other hand, an impairment or a loss of contractile function is not necessarily permanent or irreversible. There are several conditions under which the restoration of adequate tissue perfusion leads to an improvement in or complete recovery of regional myocardial contractile function. The diagnostic challenge to distinguish between an irreversible and a potentially reversible loss of contractile function lies in the fact that both have several features in common. Different from irreversibly injured myocardium, biochemical activity must persist in reversibly dysfunctional myocardium to remain viable. Herein lies the uniqueness of PET as a noninvasive biochemical assay technique. It uncovers the persistence of life-sustaining metabolic processes and thus discriminates between reversibly and irreversibly dysfunctional myocardium. In this chapter, we briefly review the current concepts of reversible dysfunction, describe how PET can identify viable myocardium, and then discuss the value of PET for the assessment of risk and for stratifying patients to the most appropriate therapeutic approach.

Myocardial Viability as a State of Reversible Contractile Dysfunction at Rest

The term *myocardial viability* is frequently used rather indiscriminately. This is particularly true for ^{201}Tl stress-redistribution studies when regional myocardial wall motion is not considered. Determination of regional wall motion that is abnormal only during stress or that is chronically present at rest is critical within the context of assessing myocardial viability. Even if a stress-induced ^{201}Tl defect does not resolve on delayed imaging or after ^{201}Tl reinjection but myocardium contracts normally, then viability is not a question. At issue is a sustained impairment of contractile function at rest. The question is whether such impairment is permanent or whether interventional restoration of coronary blood flow or of tissue perfusion results in a partial or complete recovery of contractile function.

Several conditions of reversibly impaired contractile dysfunction at rest have been described; one is *myocardial hibernation.*[230–232] A chronic reduction in blood flow is matched by a chronic reduction in or down-regulation of contractile function so that according to Rahimtoola,[230, 231] myocardium reduces its energy expenditures as an act of self-preservation. A new balance between reduced supply and reduced demand is attained. A second condition is *myocardial stunning* as a consequence of an acute but only transient ischemic insult.[233–235] Although blood flow has been restored, contractile function remains impaired and recovers only slowly. First observed in animal experiments, it is now known that it also exists in humans. Either transient reductions in blood flow (*low-flow ischemia*) or a transient increase in demand in excess of supply causes stunning.[236–238] The resulting impairment in wall motion would, however, be only transient and recover progressively. A chronically sustained impairment of wall motion due to this condition requires the occurrence of repeated ischemic episodes, or *repetitive stunning,* which precludes the recovery of contractile function and leads to a persistent decrease in wall motion.[239] Observations in patients with collateralized myocardium with near-normal blood flows at rest but a severely limited flow reserve support this possibility.[240]

The distinction between potentially reversible from irreversible states of contractile dysfunction in patients with acute or chronic coronary artery disease can pose considerable diagnostic difficulties; this is because both states of altered contractile function share a number of common features. Although as a general rule parameters of regional contractile dysfunction like diastolic wall thickness, systolic wall motion, or wall thickening are thought to be depressed more severely when contractile function is lost permanently, equally severe depressions may accompany reversible dysfunction.[241] Reductions in blood flow may be equally severe for both conditions.[242] Moreover, electrocardiographic criteria like pathologic Q waves were found to discriminate insufficiently between reversible and irreversible tissue damage.[243] Additional factors further confound the identification of reversibly injured myocardium. Ischemia invariably affects myocardium heterogeneously. Thus, especially in longstanding or end-stage coronary artery disease, reversibly injured myocardium can be interspersed with islands of scar tissue, of normal myocardium, or both. Similarly, stunned myocardium may coexist with *hibernating myocardium.*[244]

Identification of Reversibly Dysfunctional Myocardium

Several clinically relevant questions arise from the complexities of an ischemic injury to human myocardium. First, what is the fraction in a given myocardial segment that is irreversibly injured or replaced by scar tissue? Once this fraction has been determined, then the question becomes what is the fractional distribution between normal and reversibly injured or viable myocardium in the remaining fraction? Furthermore, is the fraction of or the amount of reversibly dysfunctional myocardium sufficiently large to result in an improvement in segmental or, more importantly, global left ventricular contractile function? The answers to these questions should provide criteria that predict whether revascularization will lead to an improvement in regional and, even more significantly, global left ventricular function, physical activity, or congestive heart failure symptoms and in long-term survival rates of patients with end-stage coronary artery disease.

Positron-Emitting Radiopharmaceuticals in Assessment of Myocardial Viability

Together with the availability of numerous tracers of blood flow and substrate metabolism, PET can offer answers to most of these questions. Several positron-emitting tracers are used for the assessment of myocardial viability. Foremost are tracers of blood flow such as ^{15}O-water, ^{82}Rb, and ^{13}N-ammonia for evaluation of the relative distribution of myocardial blood flow and ^{11}C-acetate and ^{18}F-fluorodeoxyglucose (FDG) for the evaluation or quantification of regional myocardial oxidative metabolism and exogenous glucose utilization.[245–255] Additional tracers include ^{15}O-labeled carbon monoxide for labeling red blood cells in carboxyhemoglobin and, thus, for measuring the vascular space of the left ventricular myocardium as well as ^{18}F-misonidazole as a specific marker of hypoxic/ischemic tissue.[256, 257]

The relatively straightforward metabolic rate of acetate affords estimates of substrate fluxes through the tricarboxylic acid (TCA) cycle.[251, 252] Administered intravenously, myocardium avidly extracts the radiotracer from blood and then releases the ^{11}C label at a rate proportional to that of the TCA cycle activity. Because of a close linkage to oxidative phosphorylation, rates of TCA cycle activity provide indirect estimates of regional myocardial oxygen consumption. In contrast, the glucose analogue ^{18}F-FDG traces a key metabolic reaction step in the metabolism of glucose.[255, 258] The agent exchanges across the capillary and sarcolemmal membranes in proportion to glucose, with which it then competes with hexokinase. Unlike glucose-6-phosphate, the phosphorylated glucose analogue is a poor substrate for glycogen synthesis, glycolysis, and the pentose-fructose shunt. Dephosphorylation and, thus, reversed transport of the compound is negligible. Because the phosphorylated FDG is rather impermeable to the sarcolemmal membranes, it becomes virtually trapped in myocardium. Images of the myocardial ^{18}F activity concentrations therefore mirror the relative distribution of regional rates of exogenous glucose utilization. Moreover, quantification of regional rates of exogenous glucose utilization in millimoles of glucose per minute per gram of myocardium is possible.[255, 258] On the other hand, it should be emphasized that the compound traces only the initial uptake of glucose into myocardium and therefore provides only indirect information on the glycolytic rate, and this, again, occurs only under specific conditions.

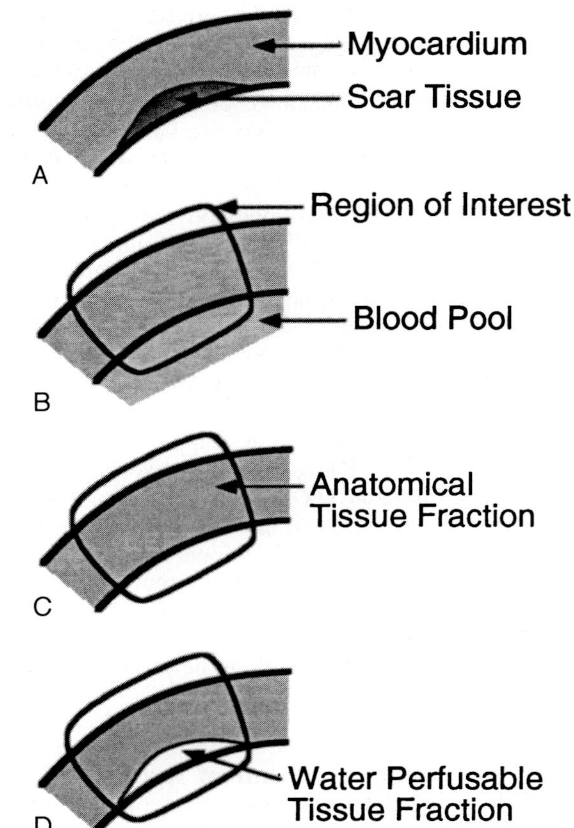

FIGURE 5–20 Water-perfusable tissue index. **A,** A myocardial segment with a subendocardial layer of scar tissue. **B,** The same myocardial segment is shown on a positron emission tomographic transmission image. Because of similar densities, the image does not distinguish between blood flow and myocardium. **C,** The anatomic extravascular tissue fraction contained in the region (or volume) of interest is obtained after subtraction of blood pool activity from the transmission image. **D,** For the same volume of interest, the fraction of the extravascular tissue volume that rapidly exchanges water is then estimated with ^{15}O water (**A–D,** Modified from Yamamoto Y, De Silva R, Rhodes C, et al: A new strategy for the assessment of viable myocardium and regional myocardial blood flow using ^{15}O-water and dynamic positron emission tomography. Circulation 86[1]:167–178, 1992.)

Positron Emission Tomography Approaches for the Identification of Myocardial Viability

Several approaches are available or have been developed to provide answers to the questions stated earlier. These approaches include determination of (1) the water-perfusable tissue index, (2) exogenous glucose utilization relative to blood flow, and (3) persistence of oxidative metabolism in reversibly dysfunctional myocardium.

The Water-Perfusable Tissue Index

Underlying this approach is the assumption that only normal, or viable myocardium, but not necrotic myocardium or scar tissue, rapidly exchanges water.[259, 260] The approach therefore can answer the question of what fraction in a given myocardial segment or the myocardium is injured irreversibly or has been replaced by scar tissue.

Figure 5–20 illustrates the general approach.[260] In PET, transmission images are routinely acquired to correct for photon attenuation. These images are comparable to low spatial resolution computed tomography scans and depict the different tissue densities throughout a cross section of, for example, the chest. Because of similar densities, these images do not discriminate between myocardium and blood pool (see Fig. 5–20B). Therefore, blood pool images obtained after labeling of red blood cells with ^{11}C- or ^{15}O-labeled carbon monoxide are subtracted from the attenuation images, resulting in images of the extravascular myocardial tissue. The extravascular tissue volume in a given region or volume of interest can be obtained by assigning a region of interest to the blood pool corrected transmission image. After the administration of ^{15}O-water, either intravenously or by inhalation of ^{15}O-carbon dioxide, the fraction of this tissue volume that exchanges water is then determined for the same volume of interest.

Preliminary data support the potential value of this approach for quantifying the fraction of irreversibly injured myocardium or, conversely, the fractional amount of myocardium that is either viable or normal. For example, in a group of 11 acute infarct patients with successful thrombolysis or spontaneous coronary recanalization, the perfusable tissue index predicted accurately whether contractile function would or would not improve.[261] In normal myocardium (e.g., in the absence of necrosis or scar tissue), all of the extravascular myocardial space rapidly exchanged water. The perfusable tissue index therefore approached unity. In those clinical "infarct" regions that recovered contractile function when reevaluated with two-dimensional echocardiography 4 months later, the perfusable tissue index ranged from 0.73 to 1.05 and averaged 0.88 ± 0.10. Conversely, the index was significantly lower in segments without an improvement in systolic wall motion. It averaged 0.53 ± 0.11 and ranged from 0.37 to 0.61. The threshold value was a perfusable tissue index of about 0.7. In other words, if more than 30 percent of the extravascular myocardial volume had been injured irreversibly, then contractile function remained permanently impaired. Preliminary observations in 12 patients with chronic coronary artery disease are similarly encouraging.[262] Segments with a perfusable tissue index of less than 0.7 (average, 0.45 ± 0.11) failed to improve segmental wall motion at 3 to 5 months after coronary revascularization compared with an improvement in contractile function in those segments with a perfusable tissue index ranging from 0.67 ± 0.21 to 0.78 ± 0.19. As an additional benefit, estimates of blood flow or of metabolic rates as obtained with PET can be related with this index directly to the amount of viable myocardium. This is in contrast to the more conventional methods in which estimates of such functional processes are related to units of total myocardium and average values are obtained that include both viable and irreversibly injured myocardium. This is exemplified by the data listed in Table 5–1, which indicate that average blood flows were discriminated only poorly between reversible and irreversible impairments of contractile function.

The approach should allow measurements of the fraction of irreversibly injured myocardium as a percentage of the entire left ventricular mass. If, conversely, the remainder of the myocardial mass can be assessed in terms of normal or of stunning or hibernation, it then would be possible to predict the magnitude of improvement in contractile function in a given myocardial segment or of the left ventricle after successful interventional revascularization. In this regard, the high accuracy of the preliminary data described above is somewhat surprising because the perfusable tissue index alone would seem to be unable to distinguish between normal and reversibly injured myocardium. In the early postinfarction patients, the fraction of myocardium that exchanged water can be assumed to have represented mostly stunned myocardium, which then accounts for the improvement in contractile function. The same assumption may, however, not apply to patients with chronic coronary artery disease. Scar tissue in a given myocardial segment may coexist exclusively with normal, contracting myocardium. In such segments, it would therefore be difficult to explain why function improved. It will be important to explore this promising approach in other laboratories and to apply it to patients with poor left ventricular function to substantiate these preliminary observations and to test whether perfusable tissue fractions of 70 percent or greater universally predict an improvement in contractile function.

Oxidative Metabolism as Predictor of Reversibility of Contractile Function

Several reports explored the potential value of estimates of regional oxidative metabolism for distinguishing between a potentially reversible and an irreversible loss of contractile function. Clearance rates of ^{11}C-acetate, derived from the early part of the myocardial time activity curve and defined as k_{mono}, provide, as demonstrated in animal experiments and in human investigations, an index of regional myocardial oxygen consumption.[253, 263, 264] Clearance rates in dysfunctional segments within two standard deviations of clearance rates in normally contracting myocardium were highly accurate in predicting an improvement in contractile function either in early postinfarction patients who had undergone coronary thrombolysis or in patients with chronic coronary artery disease who underwent interventional revascularization.[253, 263–266] Conversely, a reduction in the clearance rate by more than two standard deviations accurately predicted that contractile function would not improve. In a comparative study in patients with chronic coronary artery disease, the authors concluded that the predictive accuracy of the ^{11}C-acetate approach exceeded that of the more traditional blood flow ^{18}F-FDG approach.[267]

The findings made with ^{11}C-acetate are surprising for several reasons; one is the conventional view that oxygen consumption parallels closely myocardial blood flow be-

TABLE 5–1 Water-Perfusable Tissue Index and Contractile Dysfunction

	Normal Myocardium	Dysfunctional Myocardium: Improved	Dysfunctional Myocardium: Unchanged
Acute myocardial infarction and thrombolysis[186]			
PTI	0.98 ± 0.08	0.88 ± 0.10	0.53 ± 0.11
MBF (ml/min/g)	1.00 ± 0.26	0.61 ± 0.33	0.33 ± 0.15
Chronic coronary artery disease and revascularization[185]			
PTI	0.97 ± 0.22	0.67 ± 0.21* (0.78 ± 0.19)†	0.45 ± 0.11
MBF (ml/min/g)	1.10 ± 0.15	0.91 ± 0.09* (1.07 ± 0.12)†	0.62 ± 0.06

Abbreviations: MBF, myocardial blood flow; PTI, water-perfusable tissue index.
*Seven segments that were akinetic.
†Fourteen segments that were hypokinetic but fully recovered contractile function after revascularization.

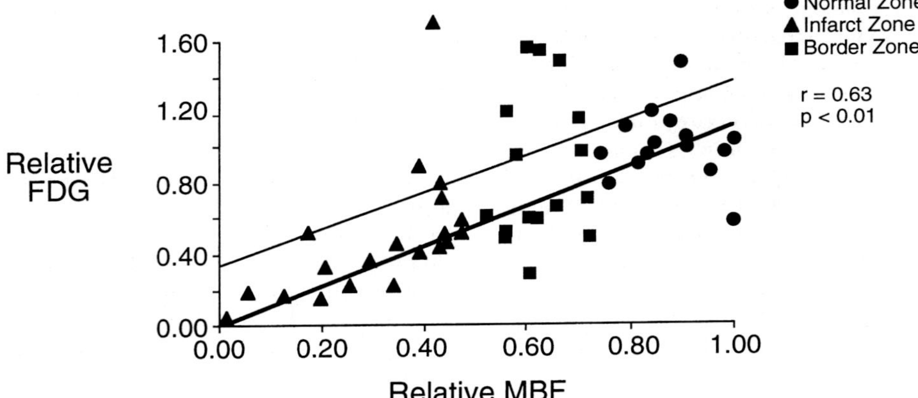

FIGURE 5–21 Regional myocardial blood flow and myocardial viability. Relative reductions in regional myocardial blood flow (MBF) are compared with the relative regional myocardial ^{18}F-deoxyglucose uptake (FDG). The values were obtained from remote (normal zone) and infarct (myocardium) zones and from myocardium bordering the infarct zone. Values for relative glucose uptake on or above the *upper, thin line* indicate "mismatches," whereas values between that line and the *bold line* indicate "matches." Note that mismatches are not observed in regions with severely reduced flows but coexist with matches in regions with intermediate-flow reductions. (From Gewirtz H, Fischman A, Abraham S, et al: Positron emission tomographic measurements of absolute regional myocardial blood flow permits identification of nonviable myocardium in patients with chronic myocardial infarction. Reprinted with permission from the American College of Cardiology [J Am Coll Cardiol, 1994, Vol. 23, pp. 851–859].)

cause the oxygen extraction is high (≈75 percent). This affords little, if any, latitude for modulating the extraction ratio of oxygen so that changes in oxygen demand can be met only by proportionate changes in myocardial blood flow. Consistent with this line of argumentation has been the linear correlation between reductions in blood flow and in oxidative rates and their general correlation with the recoverability of contractile function.[268] For example, modest reductions are more frequently associated with reversibility of contractile function than severe reductions (>50 percent). On the other hand, intermediate flow reductions were found to be associated with both types of functional impairments (Fig. 5–21).[242]

Other studies in experimental animals and in humans have challenged the traditional view of a linear relationship between blood flow and oxygen consumption; rather, these studies demonstrated a piecewise relationship (Fig. 5–22).[269] Flow reductions of 50 percent or less are associated with only modest decrements in oxygen consumption and, thus, in oxygen availability. However, once blood flows decreases below 50 percent of normal, oxygen consumption declines precipitously. A compensatory increase in the oxygen extraction ratio has been invoked as an explanation for this piecewise relationship.[270] Another component of this compensatory increase in oxygen extraction is a decline or even cessation of contractile work as an energy-saving measure. Both increased oxygen extraction and reduced oxygen demand produce a new state of balanced supply and demand and, thus, tissue survival. Measurements of oxygen extractions in patients with a variety of cardiovascular disorders further reveal an average oxygen extraction of only 66 percent (coronary sinus oxygen saturation, 32 ± 2), which also affords a greater latitude for changes in the oxygen extraction ratio compared with the traditional value of about 75 percent or higher[271] and supports the possibility of a compensatory increase in the oxygen extraction ratio.

Despite these observations in early postinfarction patients and the possibility for compensatory increases in the extraction ratio of oxygen, the use of ^{11}C-acetate for the identification of viable myocardium has remained controversial. Clinical studies described a considerable overlap in clearance rates of ^{11}C-acetate between reversibly and irreversibly reduced contractile function in which the magnitude of relative reductions in regional myocardial blood

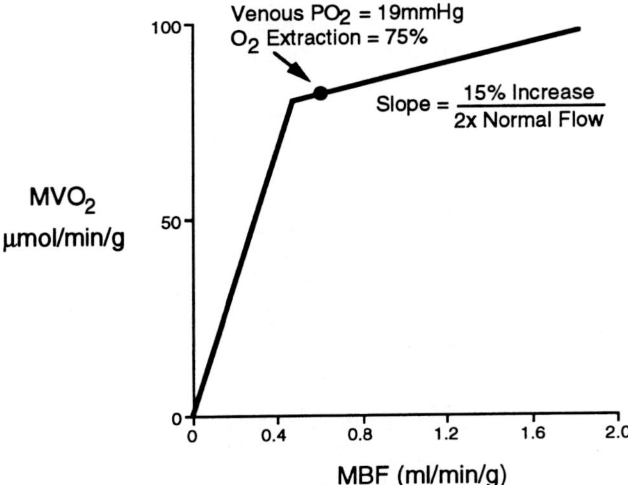

FIGURE 5–22 Relationship between myocardial blood flow and oxygen consumption. Note the piecewise relationship with only modest decreases in oxygen consumption for moderate reductions in blood flow. The solid dot on the line indicates the oxygen consumption for a normal value of blood flow. As indicated, a twofold increase in blood flow is associated with only a 15 percent increase in oxygen consumption. As the figure further indicates, once blood flow declines below values of about 0.5 ml/min/g, oxygen consumption decreases precipitously. (From Feigl E, Neat G, Wuang A: Interrelations between coronary artery pressure, myocardial metabolism, and coronary blood flow. J Mol Cell Cardiol 22:375, 1990.)

flow completely separated the reversibly dysfunctional myocardium from the irreversibly dysfunctional myocardium.[272, 273] In one of these studies, dobutamine infusion raised rates of oxidative metabolism derived from the myocardial clearance rates of ^{11}C-acetate only in reversibly dysfunctional myocardium, so viability could be identified with ^{11}C-acetate only during dobutamine stress.[272, 273] Perhaps these more controversial observations on the use of ^{11}C-acetate prompted more careful conclusions by other investigators, who emphasized the need for the combined evaluation of blood flow and oxidative metabolism.[274] This then would identify compensatory increases in the oxygen extraction ratio as evidence of viable myocardium versus no increases or possibly even reductions in the extraction ratios as indicators of irreversible injury.

Imaging of Blood Flow and Glucose Metabolism

The combined evaluation of regional myocardial blood flow and of exogenous glucose utilization is most widely used for the identification of viable or potentially reversible contractile dysfunction.[275–279] Either ^{82}Rb, ^{15}O-water, or ^{13}N-ammonia can be used to evaluate myocardial blood flow. Exogenous glucose utilization is determined with intravenous ^{18}F-FDG. The approach compares relative reductions in blood flow with relative ^{18}F-FDG concentrations. In effect, the comparison provides an index of the relative regional extraction of glucose in hypoperfused and dysfunctional myocardium.

The well established increase in glycolytic flux during acute myocardial ischemia served as the rationale for the use of this approach.[280–282] Extension of the approach to patients with stable coronary artery disease revealed three different patterns of blood flow and metabolism in dysfunctional myocardial regions (Fig. 5–23).[277] ^{18}F-FDG uptake is reduced in proportion to blood flow (*match*), or in other words, myocardial glucose extraction is constant. A second pattern demonstrates normal blood flow in dysfunctional segments with either normal or elevated ^{18}F-FDG accumulation, whereas a third pattern consists of a segmental reduction in blood flow while ^{18}F-FDG uptake is either elevated, fully preserved, or reduced (also referred to as *mismatch*). Importantly, however, such reductions are disproportionately less than the reductions in blood flow.

Other factors determine the specific pattern observed in a given patient. Foremost is the preferential substrate selection in normal myocardium. If, for example, normal myocardium preferentially utilizes glucose such as after oral glucose loading or during the hyperinsulinemic-euglycemic clamp, then a pattern of normal, slightly elevated, or even reduced glucose utilization is noted in hypoperfused and dysfunctional segments.[254, 283–285] To meet the criterion of a blood flow metabolism mismatch, the difference between segmental ^{18}F-FDG uptake and blood flow must exceed at least two standard deviations of the values established in a normal database. Alternatively, if normal myocardium accumulates little if any ^{18}F-FDG as a consequence of preferential free fatty acid utilization (most frequently induced by at least 4 to 5 hours of fasting but also possibly caused by elevated catecholamine levels), then ^{18}F-FDG uptake is selectively increased in viable but dysfunctional myocardium.[278]

Although it might be argued that the latter approach offers the highest sensitivity in detecting viable myocardium, it has some shortcomings. First, because of low insulin levels, glucose and, consequently, ^{18}F-FDG clear slowly from blood, so the resulting images often exhibit high blood pool activity and low signal-to-noise ratios.[286] Images of suboptimal or poor diagnostic quality result. Second, even if diagnostically adequate images are obtained, the fasted approach may uncover only small islands of reversibly injured myocardium, which are of little, if any, consequence for an improvement in contractile function on restoration of blood flow.[287]

If postrevascularization changes in regional contractile function as assessed also by echocardiography or radionuclide equilibrium ventriculography are used as end points, then maintained blood flow with either normal or increased glucose uptake and the blood flow metabolism mismatch predict an improvement in wall motion with an accuracy ranging from 72 to 95 percent.[273, 277, 279, 288–292] Conversely, a matching reduction in blood flow and glucose metabolism has been found to be from 74 to 100 percent accurate in predicting the absence of such improvement.

A clinically more meaningful end point is the global left ventricular performance after revascularization. Most clinical investigators consistently report an improvement in left ventricular ejection fraction in patients with an extent of viable myocardium that occupies at least 15 to 20

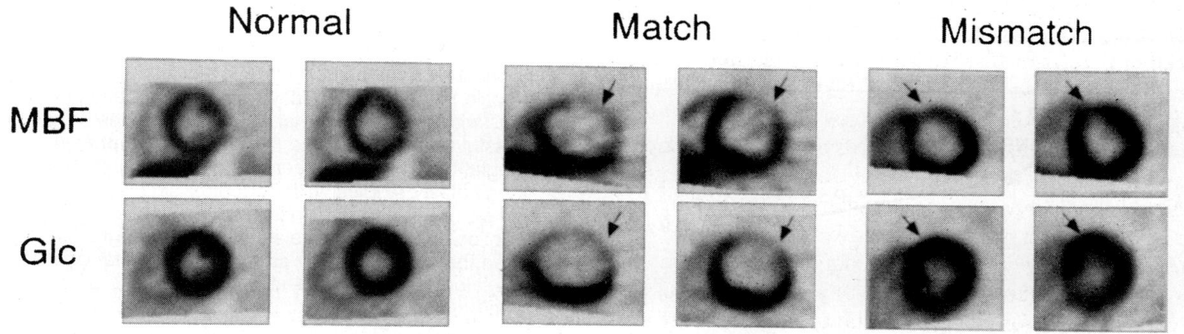

FIGURE 5–23 Patterns of blood flow (MBF) and glucose (Glu) metabolism in ischemic heart disease. Short-axis cross sections through the mid left ventricle are shown in three patients. **Left,** A study with homogeneous blood flow and glucose utilization. **Middle,** Reduced blood flow in the anterior wall associated with a proportionate reduction in ^{18}F-deoxyglucose uptake ("match"). **Right,** Reduced blood flow in the anterior wall but preserved or even modestly elevated glucose utilization ("mismatch").

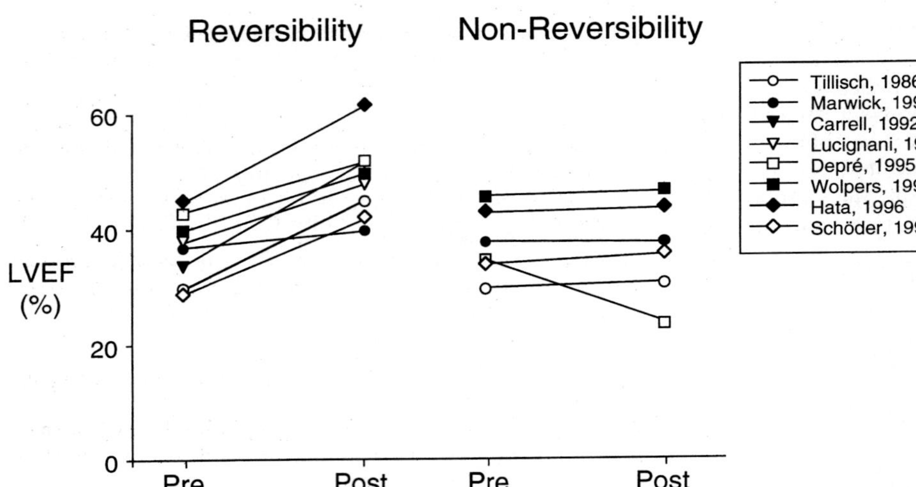

FIGURE 5–24 Comparison of average postrevascularization changes in left ventricular ejection fraction (LVEF) as reported from several studies. **Left,** Changes in patients with blood flow metabolism mismatches. **Right,** Absence of significant changes in patients with only small blood flow metabolism mismatches or without metabolic evidence of myocardial viability.

percent of the left ventricle (Fig. 5–24).[273, 277, 289, 290, 292–297] In fact, more recent, although still preliminary, observations noted a linear correlation between the extent of viable myocardium and the improvement in left ventricular ejection fractions.[298] Conversely, the left ventricular ejection fraction remained unchanged when mismatches were only small (<5 percent of the left ventricular myocardium) or were not present at all.

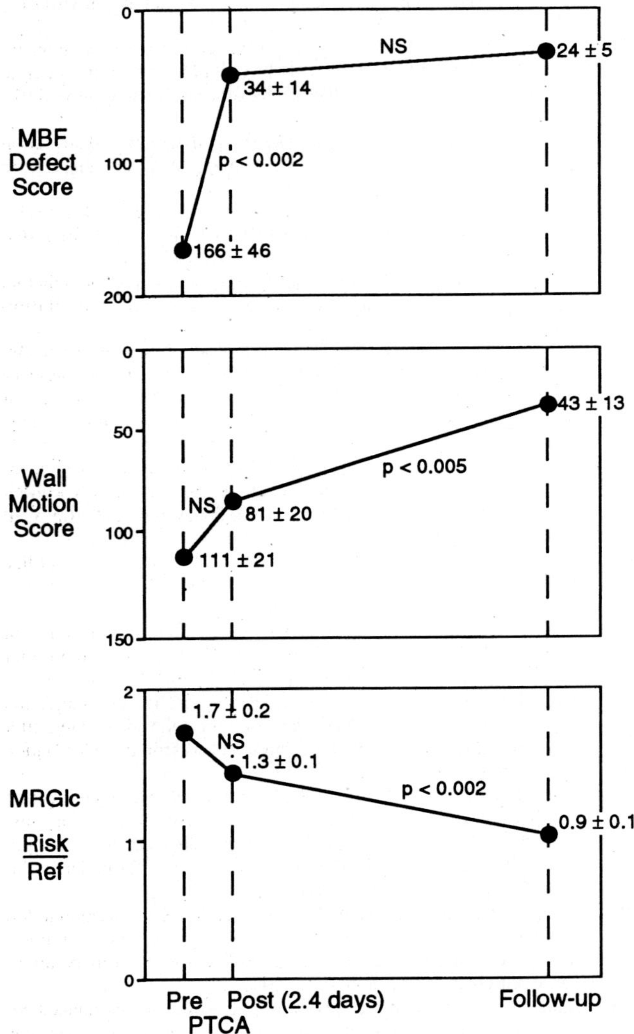

FIGURE 5–25 Sequential changes in blood flow (MBF), contractile function, and relative glucose utilization (MRGlc) in patients with blood flow metabolism mismatches before and after successful angioplasty. Note the significant improvement in segmental blood flow between the preangioplasty and the early postangioplasty studies, with no further significant improvement in late follow-up. In contrast, there was no significant change in the wall motion score and the relative increase in glucose utilization between the preangioplasty and the early postangioplasty studies. However, when reevaluated at the time of late follow-up, both parameters had significantly improved compared with the preangioplasty study. (From Nienaber C, Brunken R, Sherman C, et al: Metabolic and functional recovery of ischemic human myocardium after coronary angioplasty. Reprinted with permission from the American College of Cardiology [J Am Coll Cardiol, 1991, Vol. 18, pp. 966–978].)

Recovery of Contractile Function After Revascularization

Contractile function does not necessarily improve promptly after blood flow to viable myocardium has been restored. Serial studies with PET and two-dimensional echocardiography after percutaneous transluminal coronary angioplasty in 12 patients with metabolic evidence of reversibly dysfunctional myocardium demonstrated improvements in myocardial blood flow 2.4 ± 2.4 days later, whereas systolic wall motion at that time remained unchanged (Fig. 5–25). Reperfused myocardium continued to use more glucose relative to remote or normal myocardium. An average of 67 ± 19 days later, segmental myocardial blood flow had not increased further, but glucose metabolism was now similar to that in normal myocardium. Importantly, segmental wall motion had significantly improved. The postrevascularization delay in recovery of contractile function has been confirmed by more recent, although still preliminary, reports.[299, 300] One study notes a correlation with the severity of the relative flow reduction where segments with more severely reduced blood flow require longer recovery times than in segments with only mildly reduced or even normal flow.[300] The other study reports a slow but gradual improvement in left ventricular dimensions and global left ventricular function paralleled by a gradual gain in contractile function in the mismatch segment.[299] This particular study implicates the severity and extent of histologic and ultrastructural abnormalities determined from intraoperative biopsy samples as one major factor accounting for the delay in functional recovery.[240, 293, 301] Both studies are clinically relevant because they indicate that the success of interventional revascularization cannot necessarily be judged from an early wall motion assessment.

At present, there is uncertainty as to whether the blood flow–glucose metabolism approach discriminates between the dysfunction of *myocardial hibernation* and that of *myocardial stunning.* It is possible, however, that the pattern of normal blood flow associated with normal or elevated ^{18}F-FDG uptake signifies myocardial stunning, whereas reduced blood flow associated with increased glucose extraction reflects hibernating myocardium. On the other hand, accurate identification of the underlying mechanism might be complicated by two factors: the possible coexistence of both patterns in a given anatomical segment and an apparent but artifactual reduction of blood flow in dysfunctional myocardium as a consequence of the partial volume effect.

References

1. Muehllenher G: The Anger scintillation camera. *In* Gottschalk A, Hoffer PB, Potchon EJ (eds): Diagnostic Nuclear Medium. pp. 71–81. Baltimore: Williams Wilkins, 1988.

1a. Budinger TF, McDonald B: Reconstruction of the Fresnet-coded gamma camera images by digital computer J Nucl Med 16:309, 1975.

1b. Gould K, Lipscomb K, Hamilton G. Physiologic basis for assessing critical coronary stenosis: instantaneous flow response and regional distribution during coronary hyperemia as measures of coronary flow reserve. Am J Cardiol 33:87–94, 1974.

2. Holmberg S, Serzysko W, Varnauskas E: Coronary circulation during heavy exercise in control subjects and patients with coronary heart disease. Acta Med Scand 190:465–480, 1971.

3. Rossen JD, Simonetti I, Marcus ML, Winniford MD: Coronary dilation with standard dose dipyridamole and dipyridamole combined with handgrip. Circulation 79:566–572, 1989.

4. Heiss HW, Barmeyer J, Wink K, et al: Studies on the regulation of myocardial bloodflow in man: training effects on bloodflow and metabolism of the healthy heart at rest and during standardized heavy exercise. Basic Res Cardiol 71:658–675, 1976.

5. Ferguson RJ, Cote P, Gauthier P, Bourassa MG: Changes in exercise coronary sinus blood flow with training in patients with angina pectoris. Circulation 58:41–47, 1978.

6. Wilson RF, Laughlin DE, Ackell PH, et al: Transluminal, subselective measurement of coronary artery blood flow velocity and vasodilator reserve in man. Circulation 72:82–92, 1985.

7. McCall D, Zimmer LJ, Katy AM: Kinetics of thallium exchange in cultured rat cells. Circ Res 56:370–376, 1985.

8. Weich HF, Strauss HW, Pitt B: Extraction of thallium-201 by the myocardium. Circulation 56:188–191, 1977.

9. Goldhaber SZ, Newell JB, Alpert NM, et al: Effects of ischemic-like insult on myocardial thallium-201 accumulation. Circulation 67:778–786, 1983.

10. Leppo JA, MacNeil PB, Moring AF, Apstein CS: Separate effects of ischemia, hypoxia and contractility on thallium-201 kinetics in rabbit myocardium. J Nucl Med 27:66–74, 1986.

11. Pohost GM, Alpert NS, Ingwall JS, Strauss HW: Thallium redistribution: mechanisms and clinical utility. Semin Nucl Med 20:70–93, 1980.

12. Leppo JA: Myocardial uptake of thallium and rubidium during alterations in perfusion and oxygenation in isolated rabbit hearts. J Nucl Med 28:878–885, 1987.

13. Strauss HW, Harrison K, Langan VK, et al: Thallium-201 for myocardial imaging: relation of thallium-201 to regional myocardial perfusion. Circulation 51:641–645, 1975.

14. Nielsen AP, Morris KG, Murdock RH, et al: Linear relationship between the distribution of thallium-201 and blood flow in ischemic and nonischemic myocardium during exercise. Circulation 61:797–801, 1980.

15. Pohost GM, Okada RD, O'Keefe DD, et al: Thallium redistribution in dogs with severe coronary artery stenosis of fixed caliper. Circ Res 48:439–446, 1981.

16. Kaul S, Chester DA, Pohost GM, et al: Influence of peak exercise heart rate on normal thallium-201 myocardial clearance. J Nucl Med 27:26–30, 1986.

17. Gewirtz H, O'Keefe DD, Pohost GM, et al: The effect of ischemia on thallium-201 clearance from the myocardium. Circulation 58:216–219, 1978.

18. Brunken R, Tillisch J, Schwaiger M, et al: Regional perfusion, glucose metabolism, and wall motion in patients with chronic electrocardiographic Q wave infarctions: evidence for persistence of viable tissue in infarct regions by positron emission tomography. Circulation 73:951–963, 1986.

19. Brunken R, Schwaiger M, Grover-McKay M, et al: Positron emission tomography detects tissue metabolic activity in myocardial segments with persistent thallium perfusion defects. J Am Coll Cardiol 10:557–567, 1987.

20. Tillisch J, Brunken R, Marshall R, et al: Reversibility of cardiac wall-motion abnormalities predicted by positron emission tomography. N Engl J Med 314:884–888, 1986.

21. Dilsizian V, Rocco TP, Freedman NM, et al: Enhanced detection of ischemic but viable myocardium by the reinjection of thallium after stress-redistribution imaging. N Engl J Med 323:141–146, 1990.

22. Dilsizian V, Smeltzer WR, Freedman NM, et al: Thallium reinjection after stress-reinjection imaging: does 24 hour delayed imaging after reinjection enhance detection of viable myocardium? Circulation 83:1247–1255, 1991.

23. Bonow RO, Dilsizian V, Cuocolo A, Bacharach SL: Identification of viable myocardium in patients with chronic coronary artery disease and left ventricular dysfunction: comparison of thallium scintigraphy with reinjection and PET imaging with 18F-fluorodeoxyglucose. Circulation 83:26–37, 1991.

24. Perrone-Filardi P, Bacharach SL, Dilizian V, et al: Regional left ventricular wall thickening: relation to regional uptake of 18Fluorodeoxyglucose and 201T1 in patients with chronic coronary artery disease. Circulation 86:1125–1137, 1992.

25. Kitsiou AN, Srinivasan G, Quyyumi AA, et al: Stress-induced reversible and mild-to-moderate irreversible thallium defects: are they

equally accurate for predicting recovery of regional left ventricular function after revascularization? Circulation 98:501–508, 1998.
26. Kahn JK, McGhie I, Akers MS, et al: Quantitative rotational tomography with 201T1 and 99mTc 2-methoxy-isobutyl-isonitrile: a direct comparison in normal individuals and patients with coronary artery disease. Circulation 79:1282–1293, 1989.
27. Leppo JA, DePuey EG, Johnson LL: A review of cardiac imaging with sestamibi and teboroxime [see comments]. J Nucl Med 32:2012–2022, 1991.
28. Leppo JA, Meerdink DJ: Comparative myocardial extraction of two technetium-labeled BATO derivatives (SQ30217, SQ32014) and thallium. J Nucl Med 31:67–74, 1990.
29. Gray WA, Gewirtz H: Comparison of 99mTc-Teboroxime with thallium for myocardial imaging in the presence of a coronary stenosis. Circulation 84:1796–1807, 1991.
30. Stewart RE, Heyl B, O'Rourke RA, et al: Demonstration of differential post-stenotic myocardial technetium-99m teboroxime clearance kinetics after experimental ischemia and hyperemic stress. J Nucl Med 32:2000–2008, 1991.
31. Beanlands R, Muzik O, Nguyen N, et al: The relationship of the myocardial retention of technetium-99m teboroxime and myocardial blood flow. J Am Coll Cardiol 20:712–719, 1992.
32. Fleming RM, Kirkeeide RL, Taegtmeyer H, et al: Comparison of technetium-99m teboroxime and thallium-201 tomography with automated coronary arteriography and thallium tomographic imaging. J Am Coll Cardiol 17:1297–1302, 1991.
33. Beller GA, Sinusas AJ: Experimental studies of the physiologic properties of technetium-99m isonitriles. Am J Cardiol 66:5E–8E, 1990.
34. Beanlands RS, Dawood F, Wen WH, et al: Are the kinetics of technetium-99m methoxyisobutyl isonitrile affected by cell metabolism and viability. Circulation 82:1802–1814, 1990.
35. Carvalho PA, Chui ML, Kronauge JF, et al: Subcellular distribution and analysis of technetium-99m-MIBI in isolated perfused rat hearts. J Nucl Med 33:1516–1522, 1992.
36. Kiat H, Maddahi J, Roy L, et al: Comparison of Tc-99m-methoxy-isobutyl isonitrile with T1-201 imaging by planar and SPECT techniques for assessment of coronary disease. Am Heart J 117:1–11, 1989.
37. Verani MS, Jeroudi MO, Mahmarian JJ, et al: Quantification of myocardial infarction during coronary occlusion and myocardial salvage after reperfusion using cardiac imaging with technetium-99m hexakis 2-methoxy isobutyl isonitrile. J Am Coll Cardiol 12:1573–1581, 1988.
38. Sinusas AJ, Trautman KA, Bergin JD, et al: Quantification of area at risk during coronary occlusion and degree of myocardial salvage after reperfusion with technetium-99m methoxyisobutyl isonitrile. Circulation 82:1424–1437, 1990.
39. Germano G, Kiat H, Kavanagh PB, et al: Automatic quantification of ejection fraction from gated myocardial perfusion SPECT. J Nucl Med 36:2138–2147, 1995.
40. DePuey EG, Rozanski A: Using gated technetium-99m-sestamibi SPECT to characterize fixed myocardial defects as infarct or artifact. J Nucl Med 36:952–955, 1995.
41. Berman DS, Kiat HS, Van Train KF, et al: Myocardial perfusion imaging with technetium-99m-sestamibi: comparative analysis of available imaging protocols. J Nucl Med 35:681–688, 1994.
42. Younes A, Songadele JA, Maublant J, et al: Mechanism of uptake of technetium-tetrofosmin. II: uptake into isolated adult rat heart mitochondria [published erratum appears in J Nucl Cardiol 2:560, 1995]. J Nucl Cardiol 2:327–333, 1995.
43. Platts EA, North TL, Pickett RD, Kelly JD: Mechanism of uptake of technetium-tetrofosmin. I: uptake into isolated adult rat ventricular myocytes and subcellular localization [published erratum appears in J Nucl Cardiol 2:560, 1995]. J Nucl Cardiol 2:317–326, 1995.
44. Kelly JD, Forster AM, Higley B, et al: Technetium-99m-tetrofosmin as a new radiopharmaceutical for myocardial perfusion imaging. J Nucl Med 34:222–227, 1993.
45. Sinusas AJ, Shi Q, Saltzberg MT, et al: Technetium-99m-tetrofosmin to assess myocardial blood flow: experimental validation in an intact canine model of ischemia. J Nucl Med 35:664–671, 1994.
46. Munch G, Neverve J, Matsunari I, et al: Myocardial technetium-99m-tetrofosmin and technetium-99m-sestamibi kinetics in normal subjects and patients with coronary artery disease. J Nucl Med 38:428–432, 1997.
47. Glover DK, Ruiz M, Yang JY, et al: Myocardial 99mTc-tetrofosmin uptake during adenosine-induced vasodilatation with either a critical or mild coronary stenosis: comparison with 201T1 and regional myocardial blood flow. Circulation 96:2332–2338, 1997.
48. Shanoudy H, Raggi P, Beller GA, et al: Comparison of technetium-99m tetrofosmin and thallium-201 single-photon emission computed tomographic imaging for detection of myocardial perfusion defects in patients with coronary artery disease. J Am Coll Cardiol 31:331–337, 1998.
49. Matsunari I, Fujino S, Taki J, et al: Comparison of defect size between thallium-201 and technetium-99m tetrofosmin myocardial single-photon emission computed tomography in patients with single-vessel coronary artery disease. Am J Cardiol 77:350–354, 1996.
50. Tamaki N, Takahashi N, Kawamoto M, et al: Myocardial tomography using technetium-99m-tetrofosmin to evaluate coronary artery disease. J Nucl Med 35:594–600, 1994.
51. Rigo P, Leclercq B, Itti R, et al: Technetium-99m-tetrofosmin myocardial imaging: a comparison with thallium-201 and angiography. J Nucl Med 35:587–593, 1994.
52. Zaret BL, Rigo P, Wackers FJ, et al: Myocardial perfusion imaging with 99mTc tetrofosmin: comparison to 201T1 imaging and coronary angiography in a phase III multicenter trial. Tetrofosmin International Trial Study Group [see comments]. Circulation 91:313–319, 1995.
53. Acampa W, Cuocolo A, Sullo P, et al: Direct comparison of technetium 99m-sestamibi and technetium 99m-tetrofosmin cardiac single photon emission computed tomography in patients with coronary artery disease. J Nucl Cardiol 5:265–274, 1998.
54. Higginbotham MB: Cardiac performance during submaximal and maximal exercise in healthy persons. Heart Failure 4:68–76, 1988.
55. Leppo JA: Dipyridamole-thallium imaging: the lazy man's stress test. J Nucl Med 30:281–287, 1989.
56. Beller GA: Pharmacologic stress imaging. JAMA 265:633–638, 1991.
57. Ranhosky A, Kempthorne-Rawson J: The safety of intravenous dipyridamole thallium myocardial perfusion imaging: Intravenous Dipyridamole Thallium Imaging Study Group. Circulation 81:1205–1209, 1990.
58. Miura M, Tominago S, Hashimoto K: Potentiation of reactive hyperemia in the coronary and femoral circulation by the selective use of 2,5-bis-(diethanolamino)-4,8-dipiperidino (5,4-d) pyrimidine. Arzneium Forschrift 17:976–979, 1967.
59. Kubler W, Bretschneider HJ: Competitive inhibition of catalyzed adenosine diffusion as the mechanism of coronary dilating action of a pyrimido-pyrimidine derivative. Pflugers Arch 280:141–157, 1964.
60. Afonso S, O'Brien GS: Mechanism of enhancement of adenosine action by dipyridamole and lidoflazine in dogs. Arch Int Pharmacodyn Ther 194:181–196, 1971.
61. Fenton RA, Bruttig SP, Rubio R, Berne RM: Effect of adenosine on calcium uptake by intact and cultured vascular smooth muscle. Am J Physiol 252:H598–604, 1987.
62. Fredholm BB, Gustafsson LH, Hedqvist P, Sollevi A: Regulatory function of adenosine. *In* Berne RM, Rall TW, Rubio R (eds): Adenosine in the Regulation of Neurotransmitter Release in the Peripheral Nervous System. pp. 479–495. Hague: Martinus Nijhoff, 1983.
63. Rovetto MJ: Myocardial nucleotide transport. Am Rev Physiol 47:605–616, 1985.
64. Hiefsen-Kadsk F, Pedersen AK: Pharmacokinetics of dipyridamole. Acta Pharmacol Toxicol 44:391–399, 1979.
65. Fredholm BB, Persson CG: Xanthine derivatives and adenosine receptor antagonists. Eur J Pharmacol 81:673–676, 1981.
66. Gould KL, Westcott RJ, Albro PC, Hamilton GW: Non-invasive assessment of coronary stenosis by myocardial imaging during pharmacologic coronary vasodilation. II: clinical methodology and feasibility. Am J Cardiol 41:279–287, 1978.
67. Casale PN, Guiney TE, Strauss HW, Boucher CA: Simultaneous low-level treadmill exercise and intravenous dipyridamole stress thallium imaging. Am J Cardiol 62:799–802, 1988.
68. Brown G, Josephesen MA, Petersen RB, et al: Intravenous dipyridamole combined with isometric handgrip for near maximal acute increase in coronary flow in patients with coronary artery disease. Am J Cardiol 48:1077–1085, 1981.
69. Stern S, Greenberg ID, Corne R: Effect of exercise supplementation on dipyridamole thallium-201 image quality. J Nucl Med 32:1559–1564, 1991.

70. De Puey EG: Exercise supplementation of dipyridamole for myocardial perfusion imaging. J Nucl Med 32:1564–1568, 1991.
71. Wilson RF, Wychek K, Christensen BV, et al: Effects of adenosine on human coronary arterial circulation. Circulation 82:1595–1606, 1990.
72. Christensen CW, Rosen LB, Gal RA, et al: Coronary vasodilator reserve: comparison of the effects of papaverine and adenosine on coronary flow, ventricular function, and myocardial metabolism. Circulation 83:294–303, 1991.
73. Nishimura S, Mahmanian JJ, Boyce TM, Verani MS: Quantitative thallium-201 single photon emission computed tomography during maximal pharmacologic coronary vasodilation with adenosine for assessing coronary artery disease. J Am Coll Cardiol 18:736–745, 1991.
74. Verani MS, Mahmarian JJ, Hixson JB, et al: Diagnosis of coronary artery disease by controlled coronary vasodilation with adenosine and thallium-201 scintigraphy in patients unable to exercise. Circulation 82:80–87, 1990.
75. Coyne EP, Belvedere DA, Vande Streek PR, et al: Thallium-201 scintigraphy after intravenous infusion of adenosine compared with exercise thallium testing in the diagnosis of coronary artery disease. J Am Coll Cardiol 17:1289–1294, 1991.
76. Abreu A, Mahmarian JJ, Nishimura S, et al: Tolerance and safety of pharmacologic coronary vasodilation with adenosine in association with thallium-201 scintigraphy in patients with suspected coronary artery disease. J Am Coll Cardiol 18:730–735, 1991.
77. Ruffolo RR: Review: the pharmacology of dobutamine. Am J Med Sci 294:244–248, 1987.
78. Willerson JT, Hutton I, Watson JT, et al: Influence of dobutamine on regional myocardial bloodflow and ventricular performance during acute and chronic myocardial ischemia in dogs. Circulation 53:828–833, 1976.
79. McGillem MJ, Scott BS, DeBoe SF, et al: The effects of dopamine and dobutamine on regional function in the presence of rigid coronary stenoses and subcritical impairments of reactive hyperemia. Am Heart J 115:970–977, 1988.
80. Fung AY, Gallagher KP, Buda AJ: The physiologic basis of dobutamine as compared with dipyridamole stress interventions in the assessment of critical coronary stenosis. Circulation 76:943–951, 1987.
81. Pennell DJ, Underwood SR, Swanton RH, et al: Dobutamine thallium myocardial perfusion tomography. J Am Coll Cardiol 18:1471–1479, 1991.
82. Elliot BM, Robison JG, Zellner JL, Hendrix GH: Dobutamine-201T1 imaging: assessing cardiac risks associated with vascular surgery. Circulation 84(suppl 5):54–60, 1991.
83. Fintel DJ, Links JM, Brinker JA, et al: Improved diagnostic performance of exercise thallium-201 single photon emission computed tomography over planar imaging in the diagnosis of coronary artery disease: a receiver operating characteristic analysis. J Am Coll Cardiol 13:600–612, 1989.
84. Clausen M, Bice AN, Civelek C, et al: Circumferential wall thickness measurements of the human left ventricle: reference data for thallium-201 single photon emission computed tomography. Am J Cardiol 58:827–831, 1986.
85. Maddahi J, Van Train K, Prigent F, et al: Quantitative single photon emission computed thallium-201 tomography for detection and localization of coronary artery disease: optimization and prospective validation of a new technique. J Am Coll Cardiol 14:1689–1699, 1989.
86. Garcia EV, Van Train K, Maddahi J, et al: Quantification of rotational thallium-201 myocardial tomography. J Nucl Med 26:17–26, 1985.
87. DePasquale EE, Nody AC, DePuey EG, et al: Quantitative rotational thallium-201 tomography for identifying and localizing coronary artery disease. Circulation 77:316–327, 1988.
88. DePuey EG, Garcia EV: Optimal specificity of thallium-201 SPECT through the recognition of imaging artifacts. J Nucl Med 30:441–449, 1989.
89. Cooper JA, Neumann PH, McCandless BK: Effect of patient motion on tomographic myocardial perfusion imaging. J Nucl Med 33:1566–1571, 1992.
90. Matzer L, Kiat H, Friedman J, et al: A new approach to the assessment of tomographic thallium-201 scintigraphy in patients with left bundle branch block. J Am Coll Cardiol 17:1309–1317, 1991.
91. Chua T, Kiat H, Germano G, et al: Gated technetium-99m sestamibi for simultaneous assessment of stress myocardial perfusion, postexercise regional ventricular function and myocardial viability: correlation with echocardiography and rest thallium-201 scintigraphy. J Am Coll Card 23:1107–1114, 1994.
92. Taillefer R, DePuey EG, Udelson JE, et al: Comparative diagnostic accuracy of T1-201 and Tc-99m sestamibi SPECT imaging (perfusion and ECG-gated SPECT) in detecting coronary artery disease in women. J Am Coll Cardiol 29:69–77, 1997.
93. Germano G, Erel J, Kiat H, et al: Quantitative LVEF and qualitative regional function from gated thallium-201 perfusion SPECT [see comments]. J Nucl Med 38:749–754, 1997.
94. Germano G, Erel J, Lewin H, et al: Automatic quantitation of regional myocardial wall motion and thickening from gated technetium-99m sestamibi myocardial perfusion single-photon emission computed tomography. J Am Coll Cardiol 30:1360–1367, 1997.
95. Berman DS, Germano G: Evaluation of ventricular ejection fraction, wall motion, wall thickening, and other parameters with gated myocardial perfusion single-photon emission computed tomography. J Nucl Cardiol 4(2 Pt 2):S169–S171, 1997.
96. Matsunari I, Boning G, Ziegler SI, et al: Attenuation-corrected rest thallium-201/stress technetium 99m sestamibi myocardial SPECT in normals. J Nucl Cardiol 5:48–55, 1998.
97. Chouraqui P, Livschitz S, Sharir T, et al: Evaluation of an attenuation correction method for thallium-201 myocardial perfusion tomographic imaging of patients with low likelihood of coronary artery disease. J Nucl Cardiol 5:369–377, 1998.
98. Ficaro EP, Fessler JA, Shreve PD, et al: Simultaneous transmission/emission myocardial perfusion tomography: diagnostic accuracy of attenuation-corrected 99mTc-sestamibi single-photon emission computed tomography. Circulation 93:463–473, 1996.
99. Ficaro EP, Fessler JA, Ackermann RJ, et al: Simultaneous transmission-emission thallium-201 cardiac SPECT: effect of attenuation correction on myocardial tracer distribution [see comments]. J Nucl Med 36:921–931, 1995.
100. Bacharach SL, Buvat I: Attenuation correction in cardiac positron emission tomography and single-photon emission computed tomography. J Nucl Cardiol 2:246–255, 1995.
101. King MA, Tsui BM, Pan TS: Attenuation compensation for cardiac single-photon emission computed tomographic imaging: part 1. Impact of attenuation and methods of estimating attenuation maps. J Nucl Cardiol 2:513–524, 1995.
102. McCord ME, Bacharach SL, Bonow RO, et al: Misalignment between PET transmission and emission scans: its effect on myocardial imaging. J Nucl Med 33:1209–1213, 1992.
103. Schelbert HR, Wisenberg G, Phelps ME, et al: Non-invasive assessment of coronary stenosis by myocardial imaging during pharmacologic coronary vasodilation. VI: detection of coronary artery disease in man with intravenous N-13 ammonia and positron computed tomography. Am J Cardiol 49:1197–1207, 1982.
104. Tamaki N, Yonekura Y, Senda M, et al: Value and limitation of stress 201T1 single photon emission tomography: comparison with nitrogen-13 ammonia positron emission tomography. J Nucl Med 29:1181–1188, 1988.
105. Dehmer LL, Gould KL, Goldstein RA, et al: Assessment of coronary artery disease severity by positron emission tomography: comparison with quantitative coronary arteriography in 193 patients. Circulation 79:825–835, 1989.
106. Go RT, Marwick TH, MacIntyre WJ, et al: A prospective comparison of rubidium-82 PET and thallium-210 SPECT myocardial perfusion imaging utilizing a single dipyridamole stress in the diagnosis of coronary artery disease. J Nucl Med 31:1899–1905, 1990.
107. Stewart RE, Schwaiger M, Molina E, et al: Comparison of rubidium-82 positron emission tomography and thallium-201 SPECT imaging for detection of coronary artery disease. Am J Cardiol 67:1303–1310, 1991.
108. Bonow RO, Berman DS, Gibbons RJ, et al: Cardiac positron emission tomography: a report for health professionals from the Committee on Advanced Cardiac Imaging and Technology on Clinical Cardiology, American Heart Association. Circulation 84:447–454, 1991.
109. Watson DD, Nelson JP, Gottlieb S: Rapid bolus injection of radioisotopes. Radiology 106:347–352, 1973.
110. Berger JH, Mathay RA, Pytlik LM, et al: First-pass radionuclide assessment of right and left ventricular performance in patients with cardiac and pulmonary disease. Semin Nucl Med 9:275–294, 1979.

111. Dymond DS, Elliot AT, Flatman W, et al: The clinical validation of gold-195m: a new short half-life radiopharmaceutical for rapid, sequential, first pass angiocardiography. J Am Coll Cardiol 2:85–92, 1983.
112. Wackers FJ, Stein R, Pytlik L, et al: Gold-195m for serial first pass radionuclide angiocardiography during upright exercise in patients with coronary artery disease. J Am Coll Cardiol 2:497–505, 1983.
113. Jones RH: Radionuclide angiocardiography. *In* Marcus ML, Schelbert HR, Skorton DJ, Wolf GL (eds): Cardiac Imaging: A companion to Braunwald's Heart Disease. pp. 1006–1026. Philadelphia: WB Saunders, 1991.
114. Askenazi J, Amnberg DS, Korngold E, et al: Quantitative radionuclide angiocardiography. Am J Cardiol 97:382–387, 1976.
115. Treves S, Collins-Nakai RL: Radioactive tracers in congenital heart disease. Am J Cardiol 38:711–721, 1976.
116. Gilday DL, DeSouza M: Pediatric nuclear cardiology. *In* Come PC (ed): Diagnostic Cardiology: Noninvasive Imaging Techniques. pp. 159–190. Philadelphia: J B Lippincott, 1985.
117. Peter CA, Armstrong BE, Jones RH: Radionuclide quantitation of right-to-left intracardiac shunts in children. Circulation 64:572–577, 1981.
118. Corbett JR, Jansen DE, Lewis SE, et al: Tomographic gated blood pool radionuclide ventriculography: analysis of wall motion and left ventricular volumes in patients with coronary artery disease. J Am Coll Cardiol 6:349–358, 1985.
118a. Corbett JR, Jansen DE, Willerson JT, et al: Radionuclide ventriculography. II: anatomic and physiologic aspects. Am J Physiol Imag 2:85,1987.
118b. Parker DA, Karvelis CK, Thrall JH, Froelich JW: Radionuclide ventriculography: methods. *In* Greson C (ed): Cardiac Nuclear Medicine. pp. 81–98. New York: McGraw-Hill, 1991.
119. Gill JB, Moore RH, Tamaki N, et al: Multi-gated blood-pool tomography: new method for the assessment of left ventricular function. J Nucl Med 12:1916–1924, 1986.
120. Maublant J, Bailly P, Mestas D, et al: Feasibility of gated single photon transaxial tomography of the cardiac blood pool. Radiology 146:837–839, 1983.
121. Poliner LR, Dehmer GJ, Lewis SE, et al: Left ventricular performance in normal subjects: a comparison of the responses to exercise in the upright and supine position. Circulation 62:528–534, 1980.
122. Manyari DE, Kostuk WJ: Left and right ventricular function at rest and during bicycle exercise in the supine and sitting positions in normal subjects and patients with coronary artery disease. Am J Cardiol 51:36–42, 1983.
123. Freeman MR, Berman DS, Staniloff H, et al: Comparison of upright and supine bicycle exercise in the detection and evaluation of extent of coronary artery disease by equilibrium radionuclide ventriculography. Am Heart J, 102:182–189, 1981.
124. Higgenbotham MB, Morris KG, Coleman E, Cobb FR: Sex-related differences in normal cardiac response to upright exercise. Circulation 70:357–366, 1984.
125. Hanley PJ, Gibbons RJ, Zinsmeister AR, et al: Sex-related differences in cardiac response to supine exercise assessed by radionuclide angiography. J Am Coll Cardiol 13:624–629, 1989.
126. Parker JA, Secker-Walker R, Hill R, et al: A new technique for the calculation of left ventricular ejection fraction. J Nucl Med 13:585–592, 1972.
127. Dehmer GJ, Lewis SE, Hillis LD, et al: Nongeometric determination of left ventricular volumes from equilibrium blood pool scans. Am J Cardiol 45:293–300, 1980.
128. Dehmer GJ, Firth BG, Hillis LD, et al: Nongeometric determinations of right ventricular volumes from equilibrium blood pool scans. Am J Cardiol 49:78–84, 1982.
129. Links JM, Becker LC, Shindledecker JG, et al: Measurement of absolute left ventricular volumes from gated blood pool studies. Circulation 65:82–91, 1982.
130. Starling MR, Dell'Italia LJ, Walsh RA, et al: Accurate estimates of absolute left ventricular volumes from equilibrium radionuclide angiographic count data using a simple geometric attenuation correction. J Am Coll Cardiol 3:789–798, 1984.
131. Dehmer GJ, Firth BG, Lewis SE, et al: Direct measurement of cardiac output by gated equilibrium blood pool scintigraphy: validation of scintigraphic volume measurements by a non-geometric technique. Am J Cardiol 47:1061–1067, 1984.
132. Konstam MA, Wynne J, Holman BL, et al: Use of equilibrium (gated) radionuclide ventriculography to quantitate left ventricular output in patients with and without left-sided valvular regurgitation. Circulation 64:578–585, 1981.
133. Rigo P, Alderson PO, Robertson RM, et al: Measurement of aortic and mitral regurgitation by gated blood pool scans. Circulation 60:306–312, 1979.
134. Nicod P, Corbett JR, Firth BG, et al: Radionuclide techniques for valvular regurgitation index: comparison in patients with normal or depressed ventricular function. J Nucl Med 23:763–769, 1982.
135. Makler PT, McCarthy DM, Velchik MG, et al: Fourier amplitude ratio: a new way to assess valvular regurgitation. J Nucl Med 24:204–207, 1983.
136. Bonow RO: Radionuclide angiographic evaluation of left ventricular diastolic function. Circulation 84(suppl I): I208–I215, 1991.
137. Bonow RO: Left ventricular filling in ischemic and hypertrophic disease. *In* Grossman W, Lorell BH (eds): Diastolic Relaxation of the Heart. pp. 231–243. Boston: Martinus Nijhoff, 1987.
138. Okada RD, Kirshenbaum HD, Kushner FG, et al: Observer variance in the qualitative evaluation of left ventricular wall motion and the quantitation of left ventricular ejection fraction using rest and exercise multigated blood pool imaging. Circulation 61:128–136, 1980.
139. Okada RD, Pohost GM, Nichols AB, et al: Left ventricular regional wall motion assessment by multigated and end-diastolic, end-systolic gated radionuclide left ventriculography. Am J Cardiol 45:1211–1218, 1980.
140. Maddox DE, Holman BL, Wynne J, et al: Ejection fraction image: a non-invasive index of regional left ventricular wall motion. Am J Cardiol 14:1230–1238, 1978.
141. Maddox DE, Wynne J, Uren R, et al: Regional ejection fraction: a quantitative radionuclide index of regional left ventricular performance. Circulation 59:1001–1009, 1979.
141a. Links LM, Douglass KH, Wagner HN: Patterns of ventricular emptying by Fourier analysis of gated blood-pool studies. J Nucl Med 21:978–982, 1980.
142. Ratib O, Henze E, Schon H, Schelbert H: Phase analysis of radionuclide ventriculograms for the detection of coronary artery disease. Am Heart J 104:1–12, 1982.
143. Bacharach SL, Green MV, Bonow RO, et al: A method for objective evaluation of functional images. J Nucl Med 23:285–290, 1982.
144. Walton S, Yiannikas J, Jarritt PH, et al: Phasic abnormalities of left ventricular emptying in coronary artery disease. Br Heart J 46:250–253, 1981.
145. Links JM, Raichlen JS, Wagber HN, Reid PR: Assessment of the site of ventricular activation by Fourier analysis of gated blood pool studies. J Nucl Med 26:27–32, 1985.
146. Botvinick E, Dunn R, Frais M, et al: The phase image: its relationship to patterns of contraction and conduction. Circulation 65:551–560, 1982.
147. Botvinick E, Frais M, O'Connell W, et al: Phase image evaluation of patients with ventricular pre-excitation syndromes. J Am Coll Cardiol 3:799–814, 1984.
148. Roberts WC: The coronary arteries and left ventricle in clinically isolated angina pectoris: a necropsy analysis. Circulation 54:388, 1976.
149. Alison HW, Moraski RE, Mantle JA: Coronary anatomy and arteriography in patients with unstable angina pectoris. Am J Cardiol 35:118, 1975.
150. Eliot RS, Edwards JE: Pathology of coronary atherosclerosis and its complications. In Hurst JW, Logue RB (eds): The Heart. p. 1003. New York: McGraw-Hill, 1974.
151. Poliner LR, Buja LM, Parkey RW, et al: Clinicopathologic correlates of technetium-99m stannous pyrophosphate myocardial scintigraphy in patients. Circulation 54(suppl II): 80, 1975.
152. Parkey RW, Bonte FJ, Meyer SL, et al: A new method for radionuclide imaging of acute myocardial infarction in humans. Circulation 50:540, 1974.
153. Willerson JT, Parkey RW, Bonte FJ, et al: Technetium stannous pyrophosphate myocardial scintigrams in patients with chest pain of varying etiology. Circulation 51:1046, 1975.
154. Willerson JT, Parkey RW, Bonte FJ, et al: Acute subendocardial myocardial infarcts detected by technetium-99m stannous pyrophosphate myocardial scintigrams. Circulation 51:436, 1975.
155. Willerson JT, Parkey RW, Bonte FJ, et al: Technetium-99m stannous pyrophosphate myocardian scintigraphy: a new method of proven value for the diagnosis and localization of acute myocardial infarcts

and for the detection of infarct extension in patients. Tex Med 72:61, 1976.
156. Bonte FJ, Parkey RW, Graham KD, et al: A new method for radionuclide imaging of acute myocardial infarcts. Radiology 110:473, 1974.
157. Buja LM, Parkey RW, Stokely EM, et al: Pathophysiology of technetium-99m stannous pyrophosphate and thallium-201 scintigraphy of acute anterior myocardial infarcts in dogs. J Clin Invest 57:1508, 1976.
158. Buja LM, Parkey RW, Dees JH, et al: Morphologic correlates of technetium-99m stannous pyrophosphate imaging of acute myocardial infarcts in dogs. Circulation 52:596, 1975.
159. Platt MR, Parkey RW, Willerson JT, et al: Technetium-99m stannous pyrophosphate myocardial scintigrams in the recognition of myocardial infarction in patients undergoing coronary artery revascularization. Ann Thorac Surg 21:311, 1976.
160. Platt MR, Mills LJ, Parkey RW, et al: Perioperative myocardial infarction diagnosed by technetium-99m stannous pyrophosphate myocardial scintigrams. Circulation 54(suppl III): 24, 1976.
161. Donsky MS, Curry GC, Parkey RW, et al: Unstable angina pectoris: clinical, angiographic, and myocardial scintigraphic observations. Br Heart J 28:257, 1976.
162. Pugh BR, Buja LM, Parkey RW, et al: Cardioversion and its potential role in the production of "false positive" technetium-99m stannous pyrophosphate myocardial scintigrams. Circulation 54:399, 1976.
163. Stokely EM, Buja LM, Lewis SE, et al: Measurement of acute myocardial infarcts in dogs with technetium-99m stannous pyrophosphate scintigrams: J Nucl Med 17:1, 1976.
164. Willerson JT, Parkey RW, Stokely EM, et al: Infarct sizing with technetium-99m stannous pyrophosphate scintigraphy in dogs and man: the relationship between scintigraphic and precordial mapping estimates of infarct size in patients. Cardiovasc Res 11:291, 1977.
165. Buja LM, Tofe AJ, Kulkarni PV, et al: Site and mechanisms of localization of technetium-99m phosphorus radiopharmaceuticals in acute myocardial infarcts and other tissues. J Clin Invest 60:724, 1977.
166. Parkey RW, Bonte FJ, Stokely EM, et al: Acute myocardial infarction imaged with technetium-99m stannous pyrophosphate and thallium-201: a clinical evaluation. J Nucl Med 17:771, 1976.
167. Lewis M, Buja LM, Saffer S, et al: Experimental infarct sizing utilizing computer processing and a three-dimensional model. Science 1977:167, 197.
168. Beller GA, Khaw BA, Haber E, et al: Localization of radiolabeled cardiac myosin-specific antbody in myocardial infarcts: comparison with technetium-99m stannous pyrophosphate. Circulation 55:74, 1977.
169. Khaw BA, Beller GA, Haber E, Smith TW: Localization of cardiac myosin-specific antibody in myocardial infarction. J Clin Invest 58:439–446, 1976.
170. Khaw BA, Beller GA, Haber E: Experimental myocardial infarct imaging following intravenous administration of iodine-131 labeled antibody $(Fab')_2$ fragments specific for cardiac mysoin. Circulation 57:743–750, 1978.
171. Khaw BA, Fallon JT, Beller GA, Haber E: Specificity of localization of myosin-specific antibody fragments in experimental myocardial infarction: histologic, histochemical, autoradiographic and scintigraphic studies. Circulation 60:1527–1531, 1979.
172. Khaw BA, Gold HK, Yasuda T, et al: Scintigraphic quantification of myocardial necrosis in patients after intravenous injection of myosin-specific antibody. Circulation 74:501–508, 1986.
173. Shen AC, Jennings RB: Myocardial calcium and magnesium in acute ischemic injury. Am J Pathol 67:417, 1972.
174. D'Agostino AN: An electron microscopic study of cardiac necrosis produced by 9α-fluorocortisol and sodium phosphate. Am J Pathol 45:633, 1964.
175. Perez LA: Clinical experience: technetium-99m labeled phosphates in myocardial imaging. Clin Nucl Med 1:2, 1976.
176. Bruno FP, Cobb FR, Rivas F, et al: Evaluation of ^{99m}technetium stannous pyrophosphate as an imaging agent in acute myocardial infarction. Circulation 54:71, 1976.
177. Zaret BL, DiCola VC, Donabedian RK, et al: Dual radionuclide study of myocardial infarction: relationship between myocardial uptake of potassium-43, technetium-99m stannous pyrophosphate, regional myocardial blood flow and creatine phosphokinase depletion. Circulation 53:422, 1976.
178. Poliner LR, Buja LM, Parkey RW, et al: Comparative evaluation of several different noninvasive methods of infarct sizing during experimental myocardial infarction. J Nucl Med 18:517, 1977.
179. Rude R, Parkey RW, Bonte FJ, et al: Clinical implications of the "doughnut" pattern of uptake in myocardial imaging with technetium-99m stannous pyrophosphate. Circulation 56(suppl III): 561, 1977.
180. Buja LM, Poliner L, Parkey RW, et al: Clinicopathologic findings in patients with persistently positive technetium-99m stannous pyrophosphate myocardial scintigrams and myocytolytic degeneration after acute myocardial infarction. Circulation 56:1016, 1977.
181. Stokeley EM, Parkey RW, Bonte FJ, et al: Gated blood pool imaging following technetium-99m phosphate scintigraphy. Radiology 120:433, 1976.
181a. Willerson JT, McGhie I, Parkey RW, et al: Infarct avid imaging. *In* Marcus ML, Schelbert HR, Skorton DJ, Wolf GL (eds): Cardiac Imaging: A Companion to Brawnwald's Heart Disease. pp. 1074–1084. Philadelphia: WB Saunders, 1991.
182. Khaw BA, Haber E: Imaging necrotic myocardium: detection with ^{99m}Tc-pyrophosphate and radiolabeled antimyosin. Cardiol Clin 7:577–588, 1989.
183. Khaw BA, Yasuda T, Gold HK, et al: Acute myocardial infarct imaging with indium-111-labeled monoclonal antimyosin Fab. J Nucl Med 28:1671, 1987.
184. Khaw BA, Strauss HW, Moore R, et al: Myocardial damage delineated by indium-111 antimyosin Fab and technetium-99m pyrophosphate. J Nucl Med 28:76–82, 1987.
185. Takeda K, LaFrance ND, Weissman HF, et al: Comparison of indium-111 antimyosin antibody and technetium-99m pyrophosphate localization in reperfused and nonreperfused myocardial infarction. J Am Coll Cardiol 17:519, 1991.
186. Ohtani H, Callahan RJ, Khaw BA, et al: Comparison of technetium-99m-glucarate and thallium-201 for the identification of acute myocardial infarction in rats. J Nucl Med 33:1988–1993, 1992.
187. Yaoita H, Fischman AJ, Wilkinson R, et al: Distribution of deoxyglucose and technetium-99m-glucarate in the acutely ischemic myocardium. J Nucl Med 34:1303–1308, 1993.
188. Narula J, Petrov A, Pak KY, et al: Very early noninvasive detection of acute experimental nonreperfused myocardial infarction with 99mTc-labeled glucarate. Circulation 95:1577–1584, 1997.
189. Khaw BA, Nakazawa A, O'Donnell SM, et al: Avidity of technetium 99m glucarate for the necrotic myocardium: in vivo and in vitro assessment. J Nucl Cardiol 4:283–290, 1997.
190. Kusuoka H, Hashimoto K, Fukuchi K, Nishimura T: Kinetics of a putative hypoxic tissue marker, technetium-99m-nitroimidazole (BMS181321), in normoxic, hypoxic, ischemic and stunned myocardium. J Nucl Med 35:1371–1376, 1994.
191. Ng CK, Sinusas AJ, Zaret BL, Soufer R: Kinetic analysis of technetium-99m-labeled nitroimidazole (BMS-181321) as a tracer of myocardial hypoxia. Circulation 92:1261–1268, 1995.
192. Rumsey WL, Kuczynski B, Patel B, et al: SPECT imaging of ischemic myocardium using a technetium-99m-nitroimidazole ligand. J Nucl Med 36:1445–1450, 1995.
193. Shi CQ, Sinusas AJ, Dione DP, et al: Technetium-99m-nitroimidazole (BMS181321): a positive imaging agent for detecting myocardial ischemia [see comments]. J Nucl Med 36:1078–1086, 1995.
194. Stone CK, Mulnix T, Nickles RJ, et al: Myocardial kinetics of a putative hypoxic tissue marker, 99mTc-labeled nitroimidazole (BMS-181321), after regional ischemia and reperfusion. Circulation 92:1246–1253, 1995.
195. Fukuchi K, Kusuoka H, Watanabe Y, et al: Ischemic and reperfused myocardium detected with technetium-99m-nitroimidazole. J Nucl Med 37:761–766, 1996.
196. Weinstein H, Reinhardt CP, Leppo JA: Direct detection of regional myocardial ischemia with technetium-99m nitroimidazole in rabbits. J Nucl Med 39:598–607, 1998.
197. Gould KL: Coronary Artery Stenosis and Reversing Heart Disease. 2nd Ed. London: Arnold, 1998, distributed by Oxford University Press.
198. Gould KL: Heal Your Heart: How to Prevent or Reverse Your Heart Disease. Rutgers University Press, 1998.
199. Gould KL, Kirkeeide R, Buchi M: Coronary flow reserve as a physiologic measure of stenosis severity, part I: relative and absolute coronary flow reserve during changing aortic pressure, part II: determination from arteriographic stenosis dimensions under standardized conditions. J Am Coll Cardiol 15:459–474, 1990.

200. Gould KL: Identifying and measuring severity of coronary artery stenosis: quantitative coronary arteriography and positron emission tomography. Circulation 68:237–245, 1988.
201. Kirkeeide RL, Gould KL, Parsel L: Assessment of coronary stenoses by myocardial perfusion imaging during pharmacologic coronary vasodilation, VII: validation of coronary flow reserve as a single integrated functional measure of stenosis severity reflecting all its geometric dimensions. J Am Coll Cardiol 7:103–113, 1986.
202. Gould KL: Coronary Artery Stenosis. New York: Elsevier Scientific, 1990.
203. Gould KL: PET perfusion imaging and nuclear cardiology. J Nucl Med 32:579–606, 1991.
204. Younis LT, Byers S, Shaw L, et al: Prognostic value of intravenous dipyridamole thallium scintigraphy after an acute ischemic event. Am J Cardiol 64:161–166, 1989.
205. Gould KL: Cardiac PET: state of the art. Circulation 84(suppl):1–22, 1991.
206. Gould KL: Percent coronary stenosis: battered gold standard, pernicious relic, or clinical practicality? J Am Coll Cardiol 11:886–888, 1988.
207. Marcus ML, Skorton DJ, Johnson MR, et al: Visual estimates of percent diameter coronary stenosis: "A battered gold standard." J Am Coll Cardiol 41:882–885, 1988.
208. White CW, Wright CB, Doty DB, et al: Does visual interpretation of the coronary arteriogram predict the physiologic importance of a coronary stenosis? N Engl J Med 310:819–824, 1984.
209. Marcus ML, Harrison DG, White CW, et al: Assessing the physiologic significance of coronary obstructions in patients: importance of diffuse undetected atherosclerosis. Prog Cardiol Dis 31:39–56, 1988.
210. Seiler C, Kirkeeide RL, Gould KL: Basic structure-function of the epicardial coronary vascular tree: the basis of quantitative coronary arteriography for diffuse coronary artery disease. J Clin Invest 85:1987–2003, 1992.
211. Gould KL, Kirkeeide R, Buchi M: Coronary flow reserve as a physiologic measure of stenosis severity, part I: relative and absolute coronary flow reserve during changing aortic pressure, part II: determination from arteriographic stenosis dimensions under standardized conditions. J Am Coll Cardiol 15:459, 1990.
212. Gould KL: Identifying and measuring severity of coronary artery stenosis: quantitative coronary arteriography and positron emission tomography. Circulation 68:237, 1988.
213. Gould KL: Quantification of coronary artery stenosis in vivo. Circ Res 57:341, 1985.
214. Kirkeeide RL, Gould KL, Parsel L: Assessment of coronary stenoses by myocardial perfusion imaging during pharmacologic coronary vasodilation, VII: validation of coronary flow reserve as a single integrated functional measure of stenosis severity reflecting all its geometric dimensions. J Am Coll Cardiol 7:103, 1986.
215. Gould KL: PET perfusion imaging and nuclear cardiology. J Nucl Med 32:579, 1991.
216. Gould KL: Cardiac PET: state of the art. Circulation 84(suppl):1–22, 1991.
217. Gould KL: Percent coronary stenosis: battered gold standard, pernicious relic, or clinical practicality? J Am Coll Cardiol 11:886, 1988.
218. Marcus ML, Skorton DJ, Johnson MR, et al: Visual estimates of percent diameter coronary stenosis: "a battered gold standard." J Am Coll Cardiol 41:882, 1988.
219. White CW, Wright CB, Doty DB, et al: Does visual interpretation of the coronary arteriogram predict the physiologic importance of a coronary stenosis? N Engl J Med 310:819, 1984.
220. Marcus ML, Harrison DG, White CW, et al: Assessing the physiologic significance of coronary obstructions in patients: importance of diffuse undetected atherosclerosis. Prog Cardiovasc Dis 31:39, 1988.
221. Seiler C, Kirkeeide RL, Gould KL: Basic structure-function of the epicardial coronary vascular tree: the basis of quantitative coronary arteriography for diffuse coronary artery disease. J Clin Invest 85:1987, 1992.
222. Schelbert HR, Wisenberg G, Phelps ME, et al: Noninvasive assessment of coronary stenosis by myocardial imaging during pharmacologic coronary vasodilation, VI. Detection of coronary artery disease in man with intravenous N-13 ammonia and positron computed tomography. Am J Cardiol 49:1197, 1982.
223. Abraham RD, Freedman SB, Dunn RF, et al: Prediction of multivessel coronary artery disease and prognosis early after acute infarction by exercise electrocardiography and thallium-201 myocardial perfusion scanning. Am J Cardiol 58:423–427, 1986.
224. Schelbert HR, Phelps ME, Huang S, et al: N-13 ammonia as an indicator of myocardial blood flow. Circulation 63:1259–1271, 1981.
225. Nienaber CA, Ratib O, Gambhir S, et al: A quantitative index of regional blood flow in canine myocardium derived noninvasively with N-13 ammonia and dynamic positron emission tomograph. J Am Coll Cardiol 17:260–269, 1991.
226. Schelbert HR, Wisenberg G, Phelps ME, et al: Non-invasive assessment of coronary stenosis by myocardial imaging during pharmacologic coronary vasodilation, VI: detection of coronary artery disease in man with intravenous N-13 ammonia and positron computed tomography. Am J Cardiol 49:1197–1207, 1982.
227. Gould KL, Goldstein RA, Mullani NA: Economic analysis of clinical positron emission tomography of the heart with rubidium-82. J Nucl Med 30:707–717, 1989.
228. Shelton ME, Green MA, Mathias CJ, et al: Kinetics of Copper-PTSM in isolated hearts: a novel tracer for measuring blood flow with positron emission tomography. J Nucl Med 30:1843–1847, 1989.
229. Shelton ME, Green MA, Mathias CJ, et al: Assessment of revional myocardial and renal blood flow with copper PTSM and positron emission tomography. Circulation 82:990–997, 1990.
230. Rahimtoola SH: A perspective on the three large multicenter randomized clinical trials of coronary bypass surgery for chronic stable angina. Circulation 72(suppl V):V123–V135, 1987.
231. Rahimtoola SH: The hibernating myocardium. Am Heart J 117:211–221, 1989.
232. Braunwald E, Rutherford JD: Reversible ischemic left ventricular dysfunction: evidence for "hibernating myocardium." J Am Coll Cardiol 8:1467–1470, 1986.
233. Heyndrickx G, Millard R, McRitchie R, et al: Regional myocardial functional and electrophysiological alterations after brief coronary occlusion in conscious dogs. J Clin Invest, 56:978–985, 1975.
234. Braunwald E, Kloner RA: The stunned myocardium: prolonged, postischemic ventricular dysfunction. Circulation 66:1146–1149, 1982.
235. Vanoverschelde J-L, Wijns W, Borgers M, et al: Chronic myocardial hibernation in humans: from bedside to bench. Circulation 95:1961–1971, 1997.
236. Chatterjee K, Swan H, Parmley W, et al: Influence of direct revascularization on left ventricular asynergy and function in patients with coronary heart disease. Circulation, 47:276–286, 1973.
237. Heyndrickx G, Baig H, Nellens P, et al: Depression of regional blood flow and wall thickening after brief coronary occlusions. Am J Physiol 234:H653–H659, 1978.
238. Kloner R, Allen J, Cox T, et al: Stunned left ventricular myocardium after exercise treadmill testing in coronary artery disease. Am J Cardiol, 68:329–334, 1991.
239. Bolli R: Myocardial "stunning" in man. Circulation 86:1671–1691, 1992.
240. Vanoverschelde J-L, Wijns W, Depré C, et al: Mechanisms of chronic regional postischemic dysfunction in humans: new insights from the study of noninfarcted collateral-dependent myocardium. Circulation 87:1513–1523, 1993.
241. Cabin HS, Clubbs KS, Vita N, Zaret BL: Regional dysfunction by equilibrium radionuclide angiography: a clinicopathologic study evaluating the relation of degree of dysfunction to the presence and extent of myocardial infarction. J Am Coll Cardiol 10:743–747, 1987.
242. Gewirtz H, Fischman A, Abraham S, et al: Positron emission tomographic measurements of absolute regional myocardial blood flow permits identification of nonviable myocardium in patients with chronic myocardial infarction. J Am Coll Cardiol 23:851–859, 1994.
243. Brunken R, Tillisch J, Schwaiger M, et al: Regional perfusion, glucose metabolism and wall motion in chronic electrocardiographic Q-wave infarctions: evidence for persistence of viable tissue in some infarct regions by positron emission tomography. Circulation 73:951–963, 1986.
244. Sun K, Czernin J, Krivokapich J, et al: Effects of dobutamine stimulation on myocardial blood flow, glucose metabolism and wall motion in normal and dysfunctional myocardium. Circulation 94:3146–3154, 1996.
245. Bergmann SR, Herrero P, Markham J, et al: Noninvasive quantitation of myocardial blood flow in human subjects with oxygen-15-labeled water and positron emission tomography. J Am Coll Cardiol 14:639–652, 1989.

246. Araujo L, Lammertsma A, Rhodes C, et al: Noninvasive quantification of regional myocardial blood flow in coronary artery disease with oxygen-15-labeled carbon dioxide inhalation and positron emission tomography. Circulation 83:875–885, 1991.
247. Gould KL, Schelbert HR, Phelps ME, Hoffman EJ: Noninvasive assessment of coronary stenoses with myocardial perfusion imaging during pharmacologic coronary vasodilation, V: detection of 47 percent diameter coronary stenosis with intravenous nitrogen-13 ammonia and emission-computed transaxial tomography in intact dogs. Am J Cardiol 43:200–208, 1979.
248. Gould KL, Goldstein RA, Mullani NA, et al: Noninvasive assessment of coronary stenoses by myocardial perfusion imaging during pharmacologic coronary vasodilation, VIII: clinical feasibility of positron cardiac imaging without a cyclotron using generator-produced rubidium-82. J Am Coll Cardiol 7:775–789, 1986.
249. Kuhle W, Porenta G, Huang S-C, et al: Quantification of regional myocardial blood flow using ^{13}N-ammonia and reoriented dynamic positron emission tomographic imaging. Circulation 86:1004–1017, 1992.
250. Schelbert HR, Phelps ME, Huang SC, et al: N-13 ammonia as an indicator of myocardial blood flow. Circulation 63:1259–1272, 1981.
251. Brown M, Marshall DR, Burton BS, et al: Delineation of myocardial oxygen utilization with carbon-11-labeled acetate. Circulation 76:687–696, 1987.
252. Buxton DB, Schwaiger M, Nguyen A, et al: Radiolabeled acetate as a tracer of myocardial tricarboxylic acid cycle flux. Circ Res 63:628–634, 1988.
253. Armbrecht JJ, Buxton DB, Brunken RC, et al: Regional myocardial oxygen consumption determined noninvasively in humans with [1-^{11}C] acetate and dynamic positron tomography. Circulation 80:863–872, 1989.
254. Phelps ME, Hoffman EJ, Selin CE, et al: Investigation of [^{18}F]2-fluoro-2-deoxyglucose for the measure of myocardial glucose metabolism. J Nucl Med 19:1311–1319, 1978.
255. Ratib O, Phelps ME, Huang SC, et al: Positron tomography with deoxyglucose for estimating local myocardial glucose metabolism. J Nucl Med 23:577–586, 1982.
256. Martin GV, Caldwell JH, Graham MM, et al: Noninvasive detection of hypoxic myocardium using fluorine-18-fluoromisonidazole and positron emission tomography. J Nucl Med 33:2202–2208, 1992.
257. Shelton M, Dence C, Hwang D, et al: In vivo delineation of myocardial hypoxia during coronary occlusion using fluorine-18 fluoromisonidazole and positron emission tomography: a potential approach for identification of jeopardized myocardium. J Am Coll Cardiol 16:477–485, 1990.
258. Gambhir SS, Schwaiger M, Huang SC, et al: Simple noninvasive quantification method for measuring myocardial glucose utilization in humans employing positron emission tomography and fluorine-18 deoxyglucose. J Nucl Med 30:359–366, 1989.
259. Iida H, Kanno I, Takahashi A, et al: Measurement of absolute myocardial blood flow with H_2 ^{15}O and dynamic positron-emission tomography: strategy for quantification in relation to the partial-volume effect. Circulation 78:104–115, 1988.
260. Iida H, Rhodes C, de Silva R, et al: Myocardial tissue fraction—correction for partial volume effects and measure of tissue viability. J Nucl Med 32:2169–2175, 1991.
261. de Silva R, Yamamoto Y, Rhodes CG, et al: Preoperative prediction of the outcome of coronary revascularization using positron emission tomography. Circulation 86:1738–1742, 1992.
262. Yamamoto Y, De Silva R, Rhodes C, et al: A new strategy for the assessment of viable myocardium and regional myocardial blood flow using ^{15}O-water and dynamic positron emission tomography. Circulation 86:167–178, 1992.
263. Henes C, Bergmann S, Walsh M, et al: Noninvasive quantification of myocardial metabolic reserve by positron emission tomography (PET) with C-11 acetate and dobutamine. Circulation 80(suppl II):II-312, 1989.
264. Buxton DB, Nienaber CA, Luxen A, et al: Noninvasive quantitation of regional myocardial oxygen consumption in vivo with [1-^{11}C] acetate and dynamic positron emission tomography. Circulation 79:134–142, 1989.
265. Gropler R, Geltman E, Sampathkumaran K, et al: Functional recovery after coronary revascularization for chronic coronary artery disease is dependent on maintenance of oxidative metabolism. J Am Coll Cardiol 20:569–577, 1992.
266. Gropler R, Siegel B, Sampathkumaran K, et al: Dependence of recovery of contractile function on maintenance of oxidative metabolism after myocardial infarction. J Am Coll Cardiol 19:989–997, 1992.
267. Gropler RJ, Geltman EM, Sampathkumaran K, et al: Comparison of carbon-11-acetate with fluorine-18-fluorodeoxyglucose for delineating viable myocardium by positron emission tomography. J Am Coll Cardiol 22:1587–1597, 1993.
268. Vanoverschelde J, Melin J, Bol A, et al: Regional oxidative metabolism in patients after recovery from reperfused anterior myocardial infarction. Circulation 85:9–21, 1992.
269. Czernin J, Porenta G, Brunken R, et al: Regional blood flow, oxidative metabolism, and glucose utilization in patients with recent myocardial infarction. Circulation 88:884–895, 1993.
270. Feigl E, Neat G, Huang A: Interrelations between coronary artery pressure, myocardial metabolism and coronary blood flow. J Mol Cell Cardiol 22:375–390, 1990.
271. Holmberg S, Serzysko W, Varnauskas E: Coronary circulation during heavy exercise in control subjects and patients with coronary heart disease. Acta Med Scand 190:465–480, 1971.
272. Hata T, Nohara R, Fujita M, et al: Noninvasive assessment of myocardial viability by positron emission tomography with ^{11}C acetate in patients with old myocardial infarction: usefulness of low-dose dobutamine infusion. Circulation 94:1834–1841, 1996.
273. Wolpers H, Burchert W, van den Hoff J, et al: Assessment of myocardial viability by use of ^{11}C-acetate and positron emission tomography. Circulation 95:1417–1424, 1997.
274. Hicks R, Melon P, Kalff V, et al: Metabolic imaging by positron emission tomography early after myocardial infarction as a predictor of recovery of myocardial function after reperfusion. J Nucl Cardiol 1:124–137, 1994.
275. Schelbert HR, Phelps ME, Selin C, et al: Regional myocardial ischemia assessed by ^{18}fluoro-2-deoxyglucose and positron emission computed tomography. *In* Kreuzer H, Parmley WW, Rentrop P, Heiss HW (eds): Quantification of Myocardial Ischemia. pp. 437–447. New York: Gehard Witzstrock Publishing House, 1980.
276. Marshall RC, Tillisch JH, Phelps ME, et al: Identification and differentiation of resting myocardial ischemia and infarction in man with positron computed tomography ^{18}F-labeled fluorodeoxyglucose and N-13 ammonia. Circulation 67:766–778, 1983.
277. Tillisch J, Brunken R, Marshall R, et al: Reversibility of cardiac wall motion abnormalities predicted by positron tomography. N Engl J Med 14:884–888, 1986.
278. Tamaki N, Yonekura Y, Yamashita K, et al: Positron emission tomography using fluorine-18 deoxyglucose in evaluation of coronary artery bypass grafting. Am J Cardiol 64:860–865, 1989.
279. Tamaki N, Kawamoti M, Yonekura Y, et al: Regional metabolic abnormality in relation to perfusion and wall motion in patients with myocardial infarction: assessment with emission tomography using an iodinated branch chain fatty acid analog. J Nucl Med 33:659–667, 1992.
280. Opie LH, Owen P, Riemersma RA: Relative rates of oxidation of glucose and free fatty acids by ischemic and non-ischemic myocardium after coronary artery ligation in the dog. Eur J Clin Invest 3:419–435, 1973.
281. Opie LH: Myocardial ischemia: metabolic pathways and implications of increased glycolysis. Cardio Drugs Ther 4:777–790, 1990.
282. Lopaschuk G, Stanley W: Glucose metabolism in the ischemic heart. Circulation 95:313–315, 1997.
283. Choi Y, Brunken R, Hawkins R, et al: Factors affecting myocardial 2-[F-18]fluoro-2-deoxy-D-glucose uptake in positron emission tomography studies of normal humans. Eur J Nucl Med 20:308–318, 1993.
284. Knuuti MJ, Yki-Jarvinen H, Voipio-Pulkki LM, et al: Enhancement of myocardial [fluorine-18]fluorodeoxyglucose uptake by a nicotinic acid derivative. J Nucl Med 35:989–998, 1994.
285. Maki M, Luotolahti M, Nuutila P, et al: Glucose uptake in the chronically dysfunctional but viable myocardium. Circulation 93:1658–1666, 1996.
286. Berry J, Baker J, Pieper K, et al: The effect of metabolic milieu on cardiac PET imaging using fluorine-18-deoxyglucose and nitrogen-13-ammonia in normal volunteers. J Nucl Med 32:1518–1525, 1991.
287. Chan A, Czernin J, Brunken R, et al: Effects of dietary state on the incidence of myocardial blood flow-metabolism mismatches in patients with chronic coronary artery disease. Circulation 1994.

288. Tamaki N, Yonekura Y, Yamashita K, et al: Value of rest-stress myocardial positron tomography using nitrogen-13 ammonia for the preoperative prediction of reversible asynergy. J Nucl Med 30:1302–1310, 1989.
289. Carrel T, Jenni R, Haubold-Reuter S, et al: Improvement of severely reduced left ventricular function after surgical revascularization in patients with preoperative myocardial infarction. Eur J Cardiothorac Surg 6:479–484, 1992.
290. Lucignani G, Paolini G, Landoni C, et al: Presurgical identification of hibernating myocardium by combined use of technetium-99m hexakis 2-methoxyisobutylisonitrile single photon emission tomography and fluorine-18 fluoro-2-deoxy-D-glucose positron emission tomography in patients with coronary artery disease. Eur J Nucl Med 19:874–881, 1992.
291. vom Dahl J, Altehoefer C, Sheehan F, et al: Recovery of regional left ventricular dysfunction after coronary revascularization: impact of myocardial viability assessed by nuclear imaging and vessel patency at follow-up angiography. J Am Coll Cardiol 28:948–958, 1996.
292. Marwick T, MacIntyre W, Lafont A, et al: Metabolic responses of hibernating and infarcted myocardium to revascularization: a follow-up study of regional perfusion, function, and metabolism. Circulation 85:1347–1353, 1992.
293. Depré C, Vanoverschelde J-LJ, Melin J, et al: Structural and metabolic correlates of the reversibility of chronic left ventricular ischemic dysfunction in humans. Am J Physiol 268:H1265–H1275, 1995.
294. Dreyfus G, Duboc D, Blasco A, et al: Myocardial viability assessment in ischemic cardiomyopathy: benefits of coronary revascularization. Ann Thorac Surg 57:1402–1408, 1994.
295. Maes A, Borgers M, Flameng W, et al: Assessment of myocardial viability in chronic coronary artery disease using technetium-99m sestamibi SPECT. J Am Coll Cardiol 29:62–68, 1997.
296. Schwarz E, Schaper J, vom Dahl J, et al: Myocyte degeneration and cell death in hibernating human myocardium. J Am Coll Cardiol 27:1577–1585, 1996.
297. Schöder H, Campisi R, Ohtake T, et al: Predictive accuracy of PET flow/F-18 FDG mismatch is maintained in type II diabetes mellitus patients. J Nucl Med 38:55P, 1997.
298. Nienaber C, Brunken R, Sherman C, et al: Metabolic and functional recovery of ischemic human myocardium after coronary angioplasty. J Am Coll Cardiol 18:966–978, 1991.
299. Vanoverschelde J, Melin J, Depré C, et al: Time-course of functional recovery of hibernating myocardium after coronary revascularization. Circulation 90(suppl I):I-378, 1994.
300. Haas F, Haebnel N, Augustin N, et al: Prevalence and time-course of functional improvements in stunned and hibernating myocardium in patients with coronary artery disease (CAD) and congestive heart failure (CHF). J Am Coll Cardiol 29:376A, 1997.
301. Maes A, Flameng W, Nuyts J, et al: Histological alterations in chronically hypoperfused myocardium: correlation with PET findings. Circulation 90:735–745, 1994.

CHAPTER 6

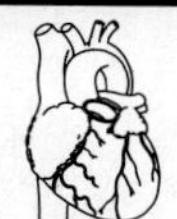

MAGNETIC RESONANCE IMAGING

Warren J. Manning

MRI: TECHNICAL CONSIDERATIONS
SPECIAL CONSIDERATIONS OF MRI IN THE CARDIAC PATIENT
THORACIC AORTA AND GREAT VESSELS
PULMONARY EMBOLISM
CARDIAC TUMORS AND MASSES
PERICARDIUM AND PERICARDIAL EFFUSIONS
CONGENITAL HEART DISEASE
QUANTITATIVE ASSESSMENT OF VENTRICULAR VOLUMES AND MASS
MYOCARDITIS
CARDIOMYOPATHIES
NATIVE VESSEL CORONARY ARTERY DISEASE
CORONARY ARTERY BYPASS GRAFT PATENCY
CARDIAC MRI—FUTURE PERSPECTIVES

More than any other noninvasive imaging technique, the flexibility of cardiac magnetic resonance imaging (MRI) offers the promise of dramatically altering our choice of imaging modalities to evaluate the patient with known or suspected cardiac disease. The combined attributes of superior image quality and flexibility for assessment of cardiac anatomy, ventricular function, great vessel anatomy and blood flow, native coronary artery and coronary artery bypass graft integrity, and myocardial perfusion give MRI tremendous potential for the comprehensive evaluation of the cardiovascular system. Currently accepted clinical applications of cardiac MRI are limited to relatively specific diseases (Table 6–1), but if the pace of technical advances during the 1990s continues, we will soon experience a greatly expanding clinical role for cardiac MRI. Hardware advances now allow for subsecond data acquisitions with "real-time" imaging, whereas software advances and novel contrast agents promise to further exploit MRI's advantages for noninvasive imaging. In all likelihood, the introduction of the comprehensive cardiac MRI examination, in which cardiac anatomy, function, perfusion, and coronary artery assessment is performed during a single session, will lead to decreased utilization for other imaging tests (e.g., echocardiography, radionuclide ventriculography and radionuclide perfusion, diagnostic x-ray coronary angiography). The relative cost advantage/disadvantage of MRI as compared with these other imaging technologies will need to be defined by cost-effectiveness studies.

MRI: TECHNICAL CONSIDERATIONS

A review of MRI physics is beyond the scope of this chapter, and readers are referred elsewhere.[1] It is important to remember that, unlike any other imaging technique, with MRI, blood may appear bright or dark depending on the specific sequence used and whether blood flow is rapid or slow, laminar or turbulent. The most common MRI approaches are the spin-echo and the gradient sequences. With typical spin-echo imaging, rapidly moving blood appears dark because a pair (90 degrees, 180 degrees) of radiofrequency (RF) pulses are used. Rapidly moving blood will flow out of the imaging plane during the time interval between the RF pulses, leading to an absence of signal, or flow void. Stagnant blood, which would be exposed to both RF pulses, will appear bright. Variations may be high-

TABLE 6–1 Current Clinical Applications for Cardiac Magnetic Resonance Imaging

Thoracic Aorta
Aneurysm
Coarctation
Dissection
Hematoma
Congenital Heart Diseases
Spatial relationships of aorta, pulmonary arteries, cardiac chambers, venous system
Identification of anomalous coronary arteries
Quantitation of intracardiac shunt
Quantitation of Left and Right Ventricular Volumes, Ejection Fraction, Mass
Regional and global systolic function
Myocardial infarction
Dobutamine stress magnetic resonance imaging study
Primary or Secondary Cardiac Tumors
Especially those tumors that involve extracardiac structures
Pericardial Diseases
Pericardial thickening (constriction)
Pericardial effusions—quantification, especially loculated effusions
Cardiomyopathies
Hemochromatosis
Hypertrophic cardiomyopathy—distribution of hypertrophy
Myocarditis
Right ventricular dysplasia
Sarcoid cardiomyopathy
Coronary Arteries
Anomalous coronary artery anatomic course
Coronary artery bypass graft patency
Future Research
Native coronary artery integrity
Atherosclerotic plaque characterization
Regional myocardial perfusion

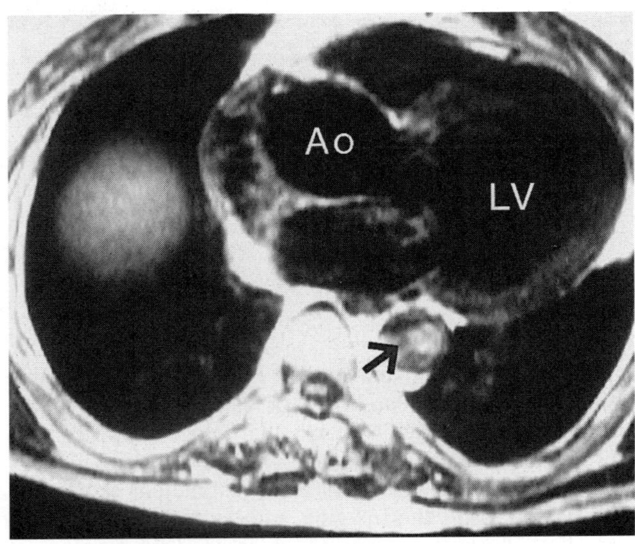

FIGURE 6–1 Electrocardiography-gated spin-echo magnetic resonance imaging (MRI) study acquired in the transverse imaging plane at the base of the heart during early ventricular systole. Note the signal void in the ascending aorta (Ao) due to rapid blood flow, with signal in the descending thoracic aorta *(arrow)* related to stagnant blood flow. LV, left ventricle.

lighted when images obtained during different phases of the cardiac cycle are compared (Fig. 6–1). The flow void can be emphasized using a thin-section or long echo time. Spin-echo imaging is commonly used for assessment of cardiac and great vessel anatomy.

With gradient-echo sequences, only a single RF pulse is applied, with a shorter echo time. Little signal is therefore lost due to washout effects. Instead, stationary tissue (often surrounding blood vessels) become saturated ("dark") because of repeated RF stimulation, whereas regions of rapid blood flow have continuous inflow of unsaturated blood with resultant bright signal. Therefore, on gradient-echo images, rapidly moving blood flow appears bright (Fig. 6–2), and stagnant blood may appear relatively dark. In addition, areas of turbulence (corresponding to stenoses, aortic insufficiency, mitral regurgitation) will appear dark owing to phase dispersion. The relative "size" of these signal voids is dependent on the echo time. Gradient-echo imaging is commonly used for cine MRI of ventricular and valvular function. Exogenous intravenous contrast (typically gadolinium–diethylenetriaminepenta-acetic acid [Gd-DTPA]) may be used in combination with both spin-echo and gradient-echo approaches.

For nearly all cardiac MRI applications, accurate electrocardiographic (ECG) gating for R wave detection is essential. The presence of an irregular rhythm (atrial fibrillation or frequent atrial or premature extrasystoles) often leads to significant image degradation. In limited situations, peripheral pulse gating may be adequate, but we have generally found the resulting image quality to be inferior to ECG gating. Very rapid ("real-time") imaging has recently received increased attention,[2] with the potential for obviating the need for ECG gating. Such an approach may be particularly desirable among patients with irregular rhythms.

Special Considerations of MRI in the Cardiac Patient

In addition to general restrictions regarding MRI (e.g., intracranial clips, transcutaneous electrical nerve stimulation units, intra-auricular implants, shrapnel), there are also special considerations for MRI in the cardiac patient. As mentioned, nearly all current clinical cardiac MRI employs ECG gating to minimize artifacts (blurring) related to bulk cardiac motion. Although the presence of an irregular rhythm (atrial fibrillation, frequent ventricular or atrial ectopic activity) is not in itself a contraindication to MRI, image quality is often suboptimal in these settings and alternative imaging methods (e.g., computed tomography [CT], echocardiography, radionuclide scanning) should be considered.

At current field strengths (1.5 Tesla), MRI is considered safe for both bioprosthetic and mechanical heart valves. There is minimal attractive force (except for preseries 6000 Starr-Edwards prostheses).[3] However, a local image artifact (loss of signal/image distortion) will occur in the region immediately surrounding the valve prosthesis. Similarly, sternotomy wires, thoracic vascular clips, and ostial coronary artery bypass graft markers are not a contraindication to imaging, but localized artifacts are common (Fig. 6–3). The relative size of these artifacts is increased in gradient-echo imaging as compared with spin-echo sequences.

Finally, in general, patients with cardiac pacemakers and automatic implantable cardiodefibrillators should *not* undergo MRI scans, and alternative imaging modalities should be used to obtain the necessary clinical information.

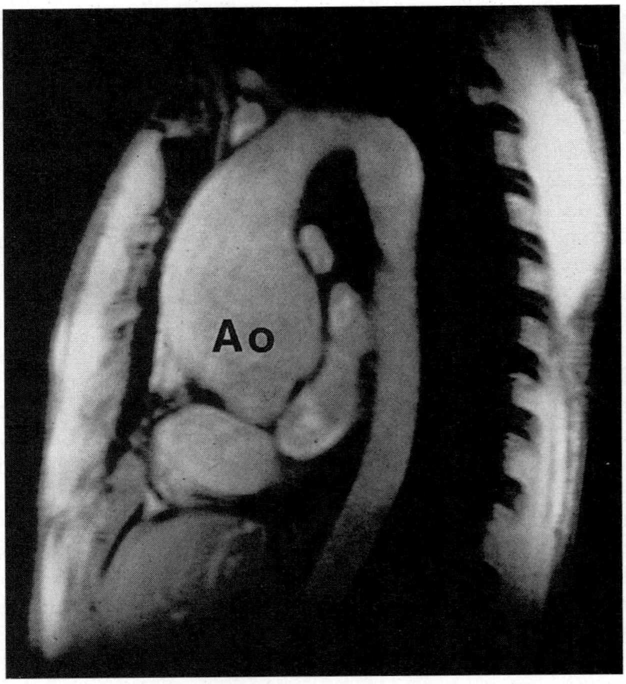

FIGURE 6–2 Ascending aortic aneurysm. No dissection. Sagittal orientation, gradient-echo sequence. Note the markedly dilated ascending aorta (Ao) with normal transverse and descending thoracic aorta.

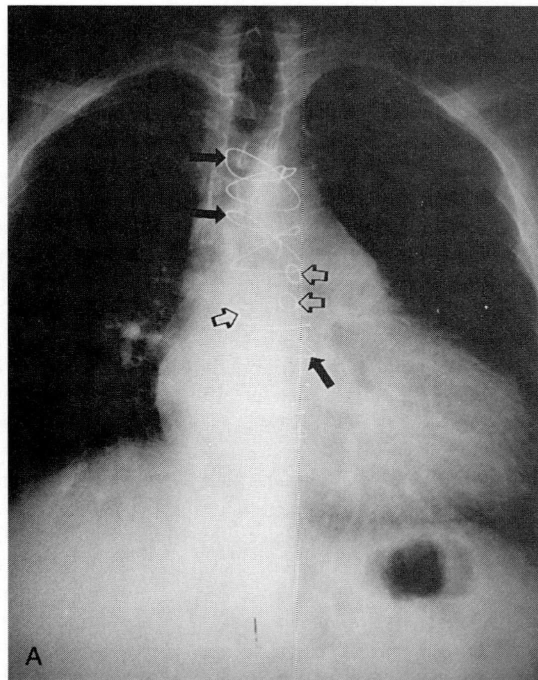

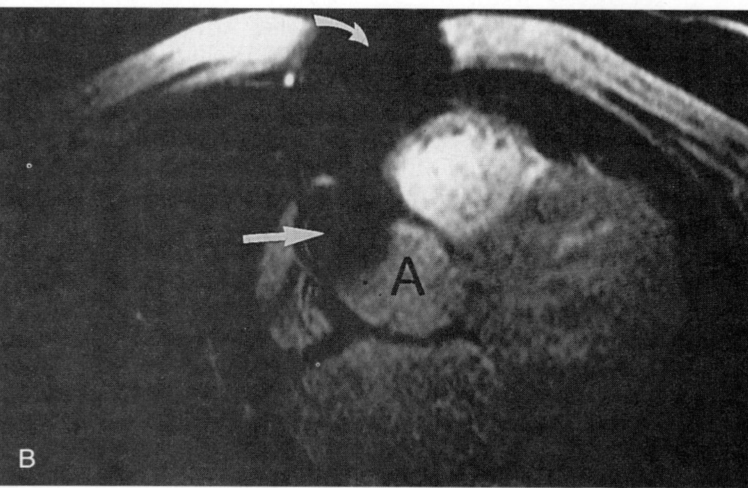

FIGURE 6–3 **A,** Posteroanterior chest x-ray in a patient who had a prior sternotomy and coronary artery bypass. Note the sternal wires *(solid arrows)* and saphenous vein graft markers *(open arrows).* **B,** Gradient-echo MRI study in the transverse plane at the level of the origin of the saphenous vein bypass grafts. Note the artifacts from the saphenous vein markers *(straight arrow)* as well as the sternal wires *(curved arrow).*

This is because of the concern regarding pacemaker reprogramming, direct stimulation of the pacemaker lead/heart during gradient switching, and/or localized heating in the lead system. Similarly, patients with pulmonary artery catheters that include pacing or thermistor wires should also not undergo MRI scans as localized heating has been reported, including melting of the catheter. When MRI is the only imaging modality available, uncomplicated MRI has been performed at low field strengths (0.2 T) using specific protocols[4] and with proper safeguards in place.

THORACIC AORTA AND GREAT VESSELS

Since the late 1980s, cardiac MRI has had its greatest clinical impact on the assessment of the thoracic aorta in the patient with known or suspected thoracic aortic aneurysm (see Fig. 6–2) or aortic dissection (Fig. 6–4). MRI compares favorably to contrast x-ray aortography because MRI has no associated procedural risks or iodinated contrast agent load. Comprehensive data regarding the presence of a dissection, entry and exit points, intraluminal thrombus, involvement of the great vessels, and coexistent aortic insufficiency and a pericardial effusion are also readily obtained. Transverse, coronal, and sagittal images using ECG gating T1-weighted spin-echo techniques are typically acquired for anatomic imaging.[5, 6] The sine qua non of aortic dissection is the identification of an intimal "flap" separating the true and the false lumen. Breath-hold three-dimensional cine gradient-echo imaging[7] with Gd-DTPA contrast (and without ECG gating) is often obtained to further define blood flow in both true and false lumen and flap mobility. In addition to the classic finding of an intimal flap, eccentric aortic wall thickening may also be seen, possibly representing an early dissection or intramural hematoma.[8] In experienced hands, MRI, *helical* CT, and *multiplane* transesophageal echocardiography (TEE)[5, 6, 9] have similarly high sensitivity, specificity, and accuracy for

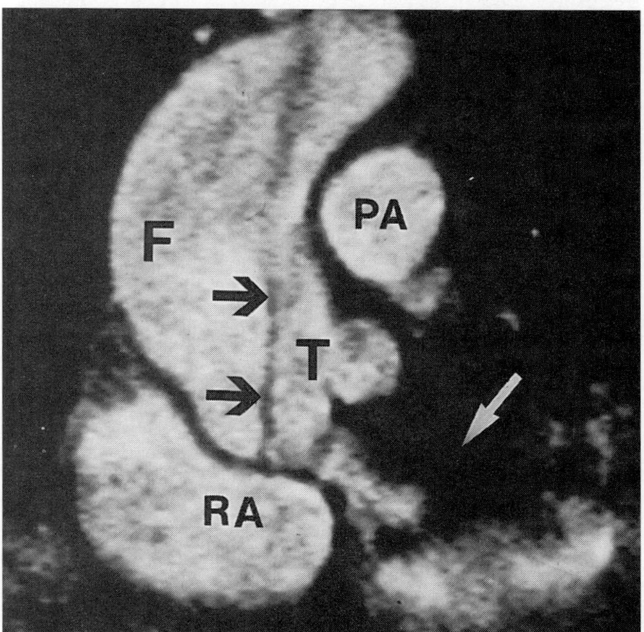

FIGURE 6–4 Ascending aortic dissection. Coronal orientation, gradient-echo sequence. Note that the dissection flap *(black arrows)* begins immediately superior to the aortic valve leaflet. Flow (white signal) is seen in both the true (T) and the false (F) lumen. Signal void *(white arrow)* from local turbulence is seen in the left ventricular cavity immediately below the aortic valve and is due to associated aortic insufficiency. PA, pulmonary artery; RA, right atrium.

identification of thoracic aortic dissection and pericardial effusion. MRI and CT have specific advantages (compared with TEE) for providing information regarding the full extent of the dissection (including involvement of the great vessels, entry and exit sites, and the presence of thrombosed lumen). Both TEE and MRI also permit determination of aortic valve involvement and aortic insufficiency (see Fig. 6–4), although valve morphology and severity of aortic insufficiency are better appreciated by TEE. Both TEE and MRI can often provide information regarding the involvement of the proximal coronary arteries. Using current techniques, the MRI assessment for dissection can generally be completed within 30 minutes. Blood pressure monitoring is strongly recommended during the entire examination. We generally recommend MRI for patients who are hemodynamically stable and for follow-up studies in patients with chronic dissection and refer those with clinical instability, claustrophobia, or pacemakers for multiplane TEE.

In addition to aortic aneurysm and dissection, MRI is also quite useful for the anatomic definition of an aortic coarctation (Fig. 6–5), patent ductus arteriosus, and more complex congenital abnormalities involving the great vessels (also see later). Phase-velocity mapping may be used to quantify velocity gradients.[10] Patients with congenital

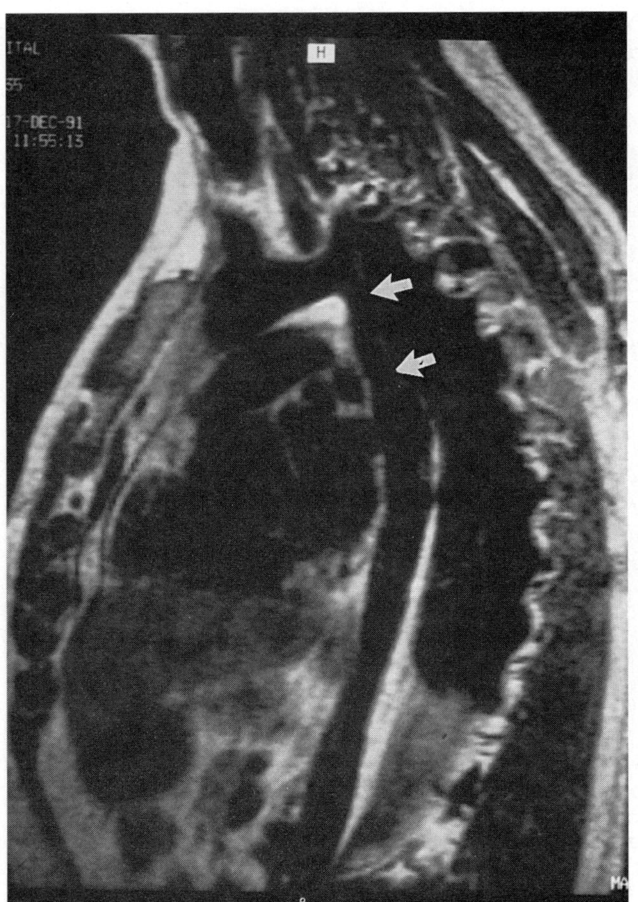

FIGURE 6–5 Spin-echo sagittal oblique image in a patient with aortic coarctation. Note the aortic narrowing *(arrows)*.

lesions are often referred for MRI for confirmation and/or better definition of an abnormality already identified or suspected on a prior imaging (echocardiography, angiography) study.

PULMONARY EMBOLISM

Compared with imaging of the aorta, MRI of the pulmonary artery is more technically demanding owing to artifacts related to motion as the lungs expand and collapse during free breathing. Additionally, pulmonary arteries branch in a complex fashion, with their diameter progressively decreasing at each bifurcation. Finally, susceptibility between blood-tissue interface and air leads to signal loss at the vessel-lung interface. Although spin-echo approaches can be used to define the anatomy of the pulmonary trunk and the proximal portions of the right and left main pulmonary arteries, gradient-echo techniques (often using Gd-DTPA contrast enhancement) are the mainstay of pulmonary magnetic resonance angiography (MRA).

The evaluation and diagnosis of congenital abnormalities of the pulmonary trunk are beyond the scope of this chapter. For adult imaging, the most significant application of pulmonary MRA is for the assessment of suspected acute (and chronic) pulmonary thromboembolism. The clinical "gold standard" for the diagnosis of pulmonary embolism is contrast x-ray pulmonary angiography, a procedure with considerable morbidity and cost. Although radionuclide ventilation-perfusion scans are widely used and offer high sensitivity for the diagnosis of pulmonary embolism, the test specificity is low (~40% indeterminate scans), limiting the diagnostic yield of this test. Contrast-enhanced techniques have been extended to the pulmonary arteries.[11, 12] It is now possible to cover the entire pulmonary tree in a single breath-hold during the injection of Gd-DTPA contrast medium. Pulmonary MRA has been demonstrated to be an excellent noninvasive alternative. Several studies have demonstrated a high sensitivity and specificity. Similar to conventional angiography, pulmonary emboli present as an abrupt discontinuation (signal void) of the arterial lumen (Fig. 6–6).

CARDIAC TUMORS AND MASSES

Although the high spatial resolution of MRI allows for depiction of intracavitary tumors/masses (e.g., myxoma, left ventricular thrombi), these intracavitary "masses" are generally well appreciated and characterized using conventional echocardiography (transthoracic echocardiography and/or TEE). MRI has its greatest value in the situation in which the mass/tumor originates outside of the cardiac chambers and extends into the myocardium and/or neighboring mediastinal structures (e.g., venae cavae, pulmonary veins). The ability of MRI data to be acquired or reconstructed helps to guide the surgical approach in such situations or to determine the surgical approach for advanced lesions.

Although rarely difficult to diagnose from echocardiographic images, benign lipomatous hypertrophy of the in-

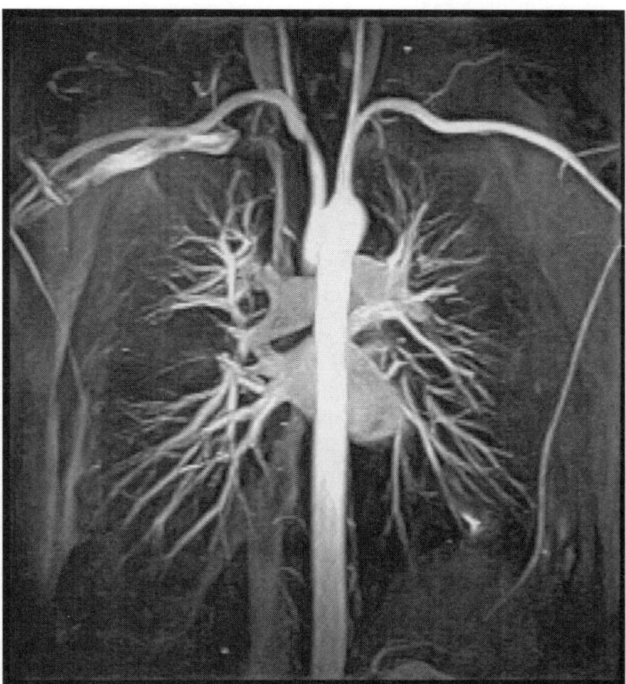

FIGURE 6–6 Three-dimensional gadolinium–diethylenetriaminepenta-acetic acid–enhanced magnetic resonance pulmonary angiogram. (Courtesy of Robert Edelman, M.D.)

teratrial septum as visualized on transthoracic echocardiography or TEE may sometimes lead to the misdiagnosis of an atrial septal "tumor." The characteristic, very intense signal from fatty tissue readily allows for the MRI diagnosis of this benign disorder.[13]

Pericardium and Pericardial Effusions

The normal pericardium is seen as a thin black line between visceral and parietal pericardial fat on spin-echo MRI. Normal pericardial thickness is 3 mm or less.[14] Among patients presenting with constrictive cardiomyopathy, often following recurrent pericarditis or mediastinal radiation, the pericardium is thickened (Fig. 6–7), a finding readily appreciated by spin-echo MRI. Gradient-echo methods are slightly less reliable.[15] CT is also valuable in this situation and is better suited for the specific assessment of pericardial *calcifications* (see Ch. 65, Etiology, Pathophysiology, Clinical Recognition, and Treatment). It should be remembered, however, that although MRI (and CT) will accurately quantify focal pericardial thickening, the presence of thickened pericardium alone is not diagnostic of constrictive physiology. Among patients with constriction, MRI also frequently demonstrates an enlarged inferior vena cava along with right atrial and right ventricular enlargement.[15] MRI is also helpful for delineation of focal pericardial effusions—especially in patients with suboptimal echocardiographic windows. Delineation of hemorrhagic and transudative effusions is another attribute of MRI.

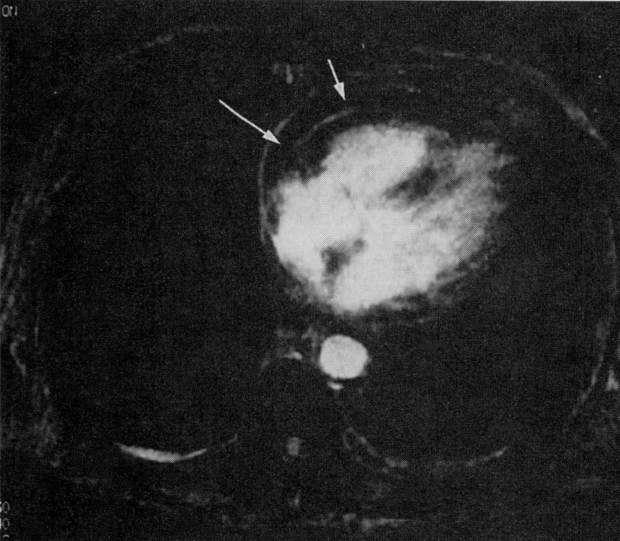

FIGURE 6–7 Constriction. Transverse, spin-echo sequence. Markedly thickened pericardium *(arrows)* around the right atrium as well as the right and left ventricular apex in a patient who is 10 years out from mediastinal radiation for Hodgkin's disease.

Congenital Heart Disease

MRI is quite useful for the assessment of both simple and complex congenital heart disease. Whereas hemodynamically significant atrial septal defects and ventricular septal defects in the adult are usually identifiable by transthoracic echocardiography and/or TEE, phase-contrast MRI can be quite valuable in *quantifying* the pulmonary:systemic flow ratio in patients with known defects.[16] As previously mentioned, MRI is specifically valuable in the characterization of congenital heart disease outside of the cardiac chambers. These include aortic coarctation, anomalous pulmonary venous drainage (Fig. 6–8), and complex congenital heart disease in patients who have undergone corrective or pallia-

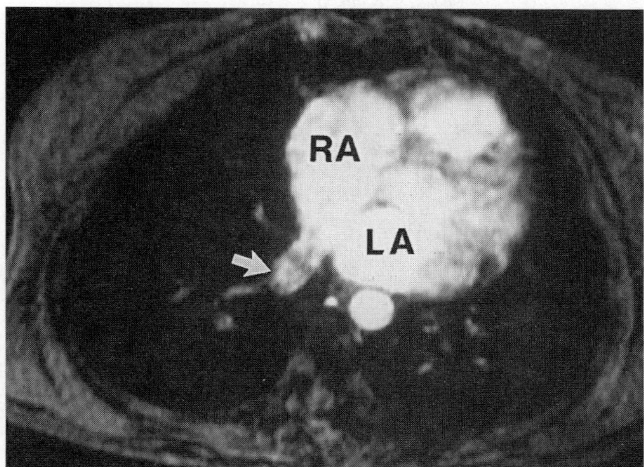

FIGURE 6–8 Anomalous right upper pulmonary vein. Transverse image, gradient-echo sequence. The anomalous pulmonary vein *(arrow)* may be seen entering the right atrium (RA). LA, left atrium.

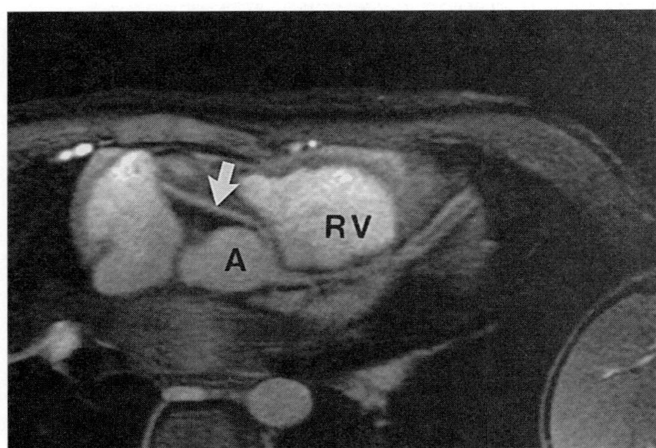

FIGURE 6–9 Anomalous right coronary artery. Transverse image, gradient-echo sequence. The anomalous right coronary artery *(arrow)* may be seen traversing between the aorta (A) and the right ventricular outflow tract (RV).

tive surgery. MRI is particularly useful in the definition of various structural components and their relationships, especially for serial evaluation and planning of subsequent surgical interventions. MRI is also valuable for detection of anomalous pulmonary venous drainage. Spin-echo MRI has been shown to be superior to both echocardiography and conventional angiography.[17] Gradient-echo approaches appear to have an even higher sensitivity in detecting partial anomalous pulmonary venous return.[18]

Although MRI assessment of the native coronary arteries for obstructive disease remains to be defined, the newer breath-hold segmented gradient-echo methods do readily allow for the identification of anomalous coronary arteries. This condition is found in only 1 to 2% of the population and is generally benign. However, there is an increased risk of sudden death and myocardial infarction for the anatomy in which the anomalous vessel courses between the aorta and the pulmonary artery[19] (Fig. 6–9). Even among patients with anomalous coronary arteries identified by invasive x-ray angiography, the anatomic course of the anomalous vessel may be misinterpreted owing to the projection method or operator inexperience, making MRI a preferred technique. Several studies have now reported on the value of MRI in this condition,[20–22] including the finding of initial misinterpretation by conventional x-ray angiography. No data are available on the value of MRI as a "screening" test for anomalous coronary arteries among young adults who present with chest pain.

QUANTITATIVE ASSESSMENT OF VENTRICULAR VOLUMES AND MASS

Although rarely used clinically because of its relative cost disadvantage as compared with echocardiography or radionuclide angiography, MRI is considered the gold standard for the *quantitative* assessment of left and right ventricular volumes, stroke volume, and ejection fraction, as well as regional left ventricular systolic function (Fig. 6–10). Left ventricular aneurysm may be recognized as severe wall thinning (<2 mm) and diastolic bulging of the left ventricular free wall. Left ventricular pseudoaneurysms may also be readily identified using MRI.[23] The false aneurysm is characterized by a relatively narrow neck connecting the left ventricle chamber and body of the aneurysm, with lack of myocardium in the wall of the aneurysm (Fig. 6–11). Left ventricular mural thrombi may be identified on spin-echo images as a density or mass filling the left ventricular apex, especially in an area corresponding to a left ventricular aneurysm.[24] The advantages of MRI include the ability to obtain tomographic data in true short-axis and long-axis orientations, high definition of endocardial borders, and the relative ease of image analysis. As compared with echocardiography, which has suboptimal results in a substantial number of patients, breath-hold cine MRI scans can be readily performed in nearly all patients in less than 10 minutes. Semiautomated methods allow for the delineation of the endocardial and epicardial borders with very high accuracy or reproducibility and determination of ventricular volumes, stroke volume, and ejection fraction in both normal and focally deformed ventricles.[25–27] MRI may be especially valuable for quantitative information

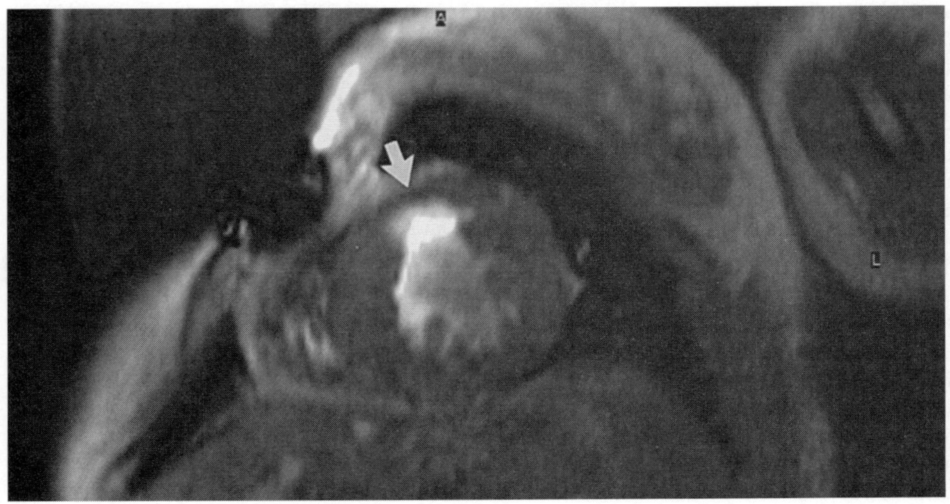

FIGURE 6–10 Gradient-echo MRI study in left ventricular short axis orientation. Note the anterior wall thinning *(arrow)* consistent with chronic anterior infarction.

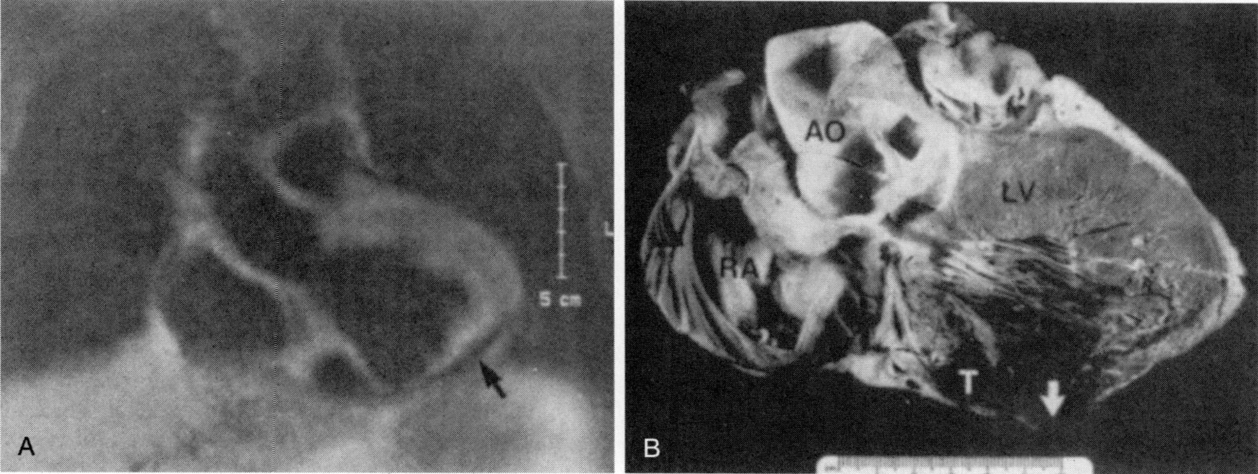

FIGURE 6–11 Correlation of autopsy pathology with cardiac MRI study. **A,** Coronary spin-echo shows inferior left ventricle thinning *(arrow)*. **B,** Coronal section of the heart at autopsy shows a pseudoaneurysm with rupture point *(arrow)* and intramyocardial thrombus (T). AO, aorta; LV, left ventricle; RA, right atrium. (**A** and **B,** From Harrity P, Patel A, Bianco J, Subramanian R: Improved diagnosis and characterization of postinfarction left ventricular pseudoaneurysm by cardiac magnetic resonance imaging. Reprinted from *Clinical Cardiology* [1991, 14:603–606] with permission from Clinical Cardiology Publishing Company, Inc., and/or the Foundation for Advances in Medicine and Science, Inc.)

regarding left ventricular mass and regression of hypertrophy in response to antihypertensive therapy[28] or aortic valve replacement. The accurate quantitative evaluation of *right* ventricular volumes and ejection fraction is also a relatively unique attribute of MRI.[29] For regional assessment of both right and left ventricular systolic function, myocardial tagging techniques have been shown to be more sensitive for quantitation of local dysfunction,[29, 30] although their clinical role remains to be defined.

In combination with dobutamine stress, functional MRI assessment of regional myocardial dysfunction has been shown to be superior to dobutamine stress echocardiography for identification of patients with coronary artery disease.[30a, 30b] A "negative" dobutamine MRI also appears to be predictive for a good prognosis.[30b]

MYOCARDITIS

Viral myocarditis may often present as a nonischemic cardiomyopathy. The diagnosis of acute myocarditis is generally supported by ECG changes or heart block, echocardiographic findings of global ventricular dysfunction, and elevated creatine kinase or troponin T in the absence of epicardial coronary artery disease. Although diagnosis is usually made by endomyocardial biopsy according to the Dallas criteria,[31] inflammation may be focal and the biopsy may be "negative." Recent preliminary data suggest a role for Gd-DTPA–enhanced T1-weighted spin-echo MRI, in which focal enhancement is seen early in the disease with more diffuse or global enhancement seen several weeks after initial presentation.[32]

CARDIOMYOPATHIES

The ability of MRI to acquire images of the entire heart in true tomographic planes makes it ideal for the evaluation of patients with hypertrophic cardiomyopathies, especially patients with focal or asymmetric hypertrophy. Investigative MRI "tagging" methods may also help in the further assessment of patients with hypertrophic cardiomyopathy[33] but remain to be more fully elucidated in larger clinical studies.

In specific conditions, cardiac MRI is also useful in the assessment of patients with a dilated cardiomyopathy. In addition to biventricular volumetric and mass data, MRI may confirm excess iron deposition[34] as the cause of depressed systolic function in a patient with suspected hemochromatosis. With spin-echo imaging, depressed myocardial signal intensity correlates with systolic function as well as severity of iron deposition. In contrast, focal signal enhancement may be found with other diseases such as sarcoidosis or myocarditis.[32] In the absence of clinical suspicion, however, routine MRI in dilated cardiomyopathy is currently not recommended.

MRI is particularly valuable in the evaluation of patients with suspected right ventricular dysplasia, a condition associated with ventricular arrhythmias and sudden death. In this condition, the right ventricular free wall myocardium is often diffusely or focally replaced with fatty or fibrous tissue. Associated focal wall thinning and systolic dysfunction are often present. Spin-echo MRI can be used to identify transmural or focal fatty infiltration in the right ventricular free wall, as well as focal wall thinning (Fig. 6–12).[35, 36]

NATIVE VESSEL CORONARY ARTERY DISEASE

The assessment of native coronary artery integrity using MRI is a field of intense research activity and rapid evolution. Its success will likely lead to an emergence of MRI as the dominant noninvasive imaging technique, since the additional cost of MRI for anatomic and functional data will be minimal. Although current coronary MRA techniques have a relatively limited spatial resolution, which

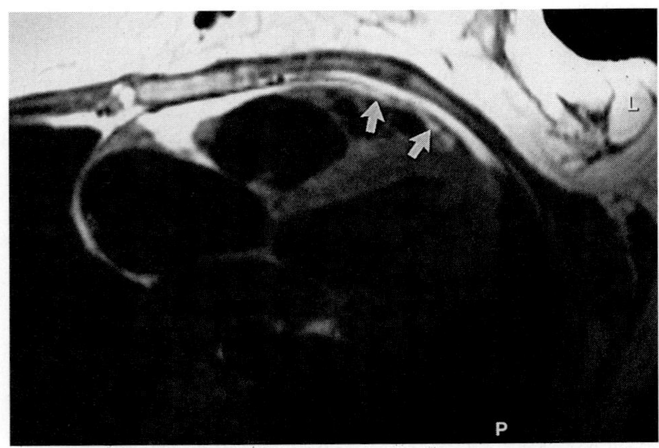

FIGURE 6–12 Right ventricular dysplasia. Transverse orientation, spin-echo sequence. Note the increased signal intensity in the right ventricular free wall *(arrows)* consistent with fatty infiltration/replacement.

precludes *quantitative* coronary MRA, the feasibility of identifying stenoses in the proximal and midcoronary segments has been demonstrated in several clinical series. In most of these, breath-hold segmented k-space gradient-echo techniques are used to image flow within the coronary vessel. With this approach, high signal intensity (bright blood) represents normal, laminar blood flow, with low signal (signal void) at sites of turbulence (stenoses) or absent blood flow. Although initial reports were quite promising in comparison with 50-percent-diameter stenoses on conventional x-ray angiography,[37] subsequent studies[38–42] have had variable success. Differences in patient selection, breath-hold technique, and imaging parameters (including different spatial and temporal resolution) likely account for the wide variability. More recently, coronary MRA was used to evaluate patients who had undergone prior balloon angioplasty and were referred for follow-up angiography because of chest pain. Coronary MRA was found to have high diagnostic yield for assessing restenosis.[42] Non–breath-hold three-dimensional methods, in which MRI navigators are used to gate to the respiratory cycle, have also received considerable attention and appear quite promising (Fig. 6–13).[43, 44]

For patients who have experienced a myocardial infarction, coronary MRA has been shown to accurately evaluate the presence of antegrade flow in the infarct-related artery.[45] The noninvasive determination of patency influences therapy and prognosis in these patients, as it is believed that a patent coronary artery after myocardial infarction leads to more favorable remodeling.

CORONARY ARTERY BYPASS GRAFT PATENCY

In comparison with native vessel coronary MRA, MRI of coronary artery bypass grafts (both saphenous veins and internal mammary arteries) is greatly facilitated by their relatively stationary anterior location, relatively straight and predictable course, and greater lumen diameter. Adequate flow is visualized as a signal void (spin-echo) or as bright signal (gradient-echo) in the anatomic location corresponding to the expected graft position. Identification of flow in at least two contiguous slices, or obtained at different planes perpendicular to the expected bypass graft course, suggests patency (Fig. 6–14). If flow is suggested at only one level, graft patency is considered "indeterminate," and if there is no evidence of flow in any portion of the graft, the graft is considered "occluded." Gd-DTPA–enhanced three-dimensional coronary MRA has been reported to have higher sensitivity (95 to 100 percent) for patency of both saphenous venous and internal mammary grafts. Data from several studies with and without use of MRI contrast,[46–50] comparing MRI data with contrast angiography, are summarized in Table 6–2.

Although the "patency" or "absence of flow" can be determined using MRA, assessment of graft atherosclerotic disease is more challenging. Implanted metallic clips, markers (see Fig. 6–3), or intracoronary stents[51] often create local signal void, precluding assessment in these regions.

CARDIAC MRI—FUTURE PERSPECTIVES

Since the late 1980s, there has been tremendous growth in cardiovascular applications of MRI. The recent introduction of enhanced gradient systems, cardiac-specific receiver coils, intravascular MRI contrast agents, and software advances all continue to provide great promise for cardiac MRI. Already, cardiac MRI laboratories are being developed at many major medical centers, a process that is likely to accelerate and include the general clinical community as well.

TABLE 6–2 Magnetic Resonance Imaging Assessment of Coronary Artery Bypass Graft Patency

Reference	Patients (n)	Grafts (n)	Patent (%)	Sensitivity	Specificity
Spin Echo					
White et al[46]	25	72	69	0.86	0.72
Rubenstein et al[47]	20	47	62	0.90	0.72
Galjee et al[49]	47	84	74	0.98	0.85
Gradient Echo					
Aurigemma et al[48]	45	45	73	0.88	1.00
Galjee et al[49]	47	84	74	0.98	0.88

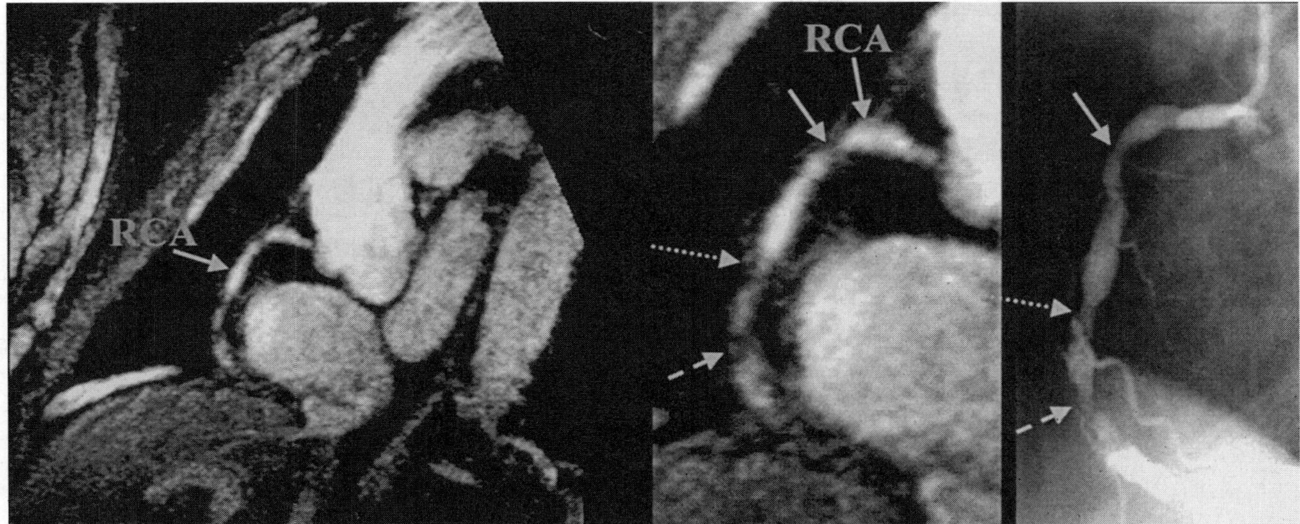

FIGURE 6–13 Three-dimensional coronary magnetic resonance angiogram acquired during free breathing with corresponding x-ray angiogram. Note that the moderate and severe stenoses *(arrows)* seen in the magnetic resonance angiogram correspond to those seen on the x-ray angiogram. RCA, right coronary artery.

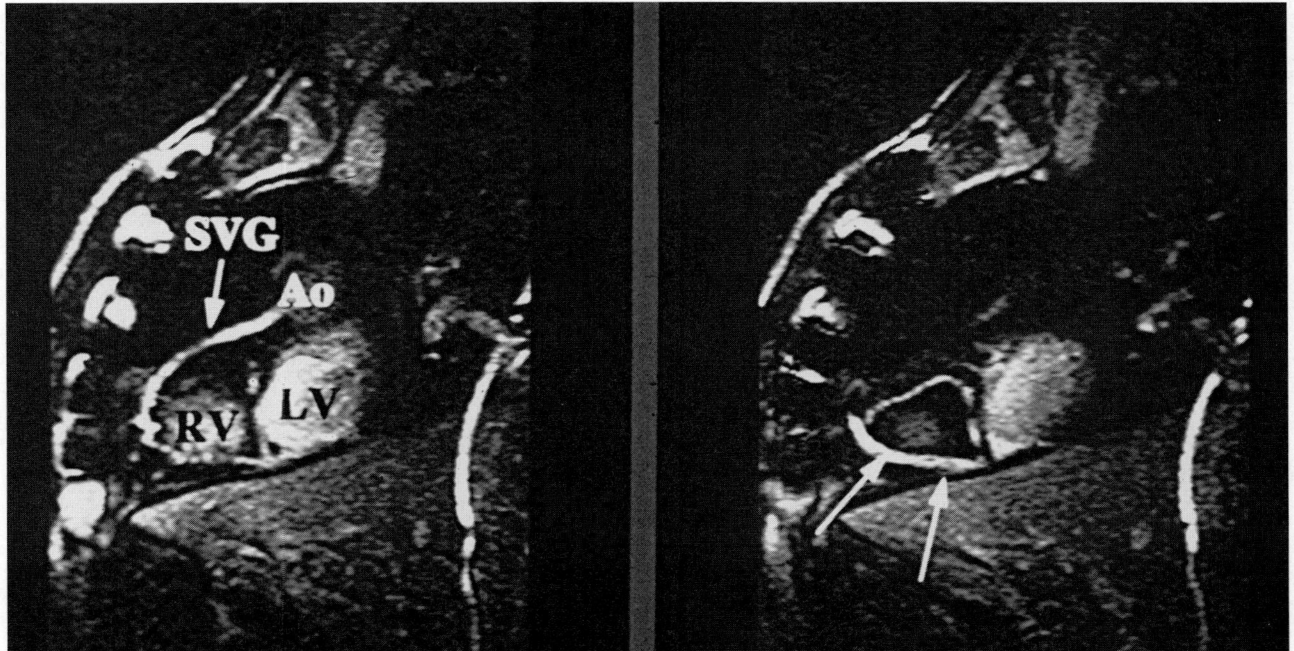

FIGURE 6–14 Breath-hold coronary magnetic resonance angiogram of a normal reverse saphenous vein bypass graft (SVG). Two adjacent images depict the graft *(arrows)* extending from the ascending aorta (Ao) to the posterior descending coronary artery. LV, left ventricle; RV, right ventricle.

REFERENCES

1. Weisskoff RM, Edelman RR: Basic principles of MRI. *In* Edelman RR, Hesselink JR, Zlatkin MB (eds): Clinical Magnetic Resonance Imaging. 2nd ed. pp 3–51. Philadelphia: WB Saunders, 1996.
2. Kerr AB, Pauly JM, Hu BS, et al: Real-time interactive MRI on a conventional scanner. Magn Reson Med 38:355–367, 1997.
3. Shellock FG, Kanal E: Bioeffects and safety of MR procedures. *In* Edelman RR, Hesselink JR, Zlatkin MB (eds): Clinical Magnetic Resonance Imaging. 2nd ed. pp 391–434. Philadelphia: WB Saunders, 1996.
4. Gimbel JR, Johnson D, Levine PA, Wilkoff BL: Safe performance of magnetic resonance imaging on five patients with permanent cardiac pacemakers. Pacing Clin Electrophysiol 19:913–919, 1996.
5. Nienaber CA, von Kodolitsch Y, Nicolas V, et al: The diagnosis of thoracic aortic dissection by noninvasive imaging procedures. N Engl J Med 328:1–9, 1993.
6. Laissy JP, Blanc F, Soyer P, et al: Thoracic aortic dissection: diagnosis with transesophageal echocardiography versus MR imaging. Radiology 194:331–336, 1995.
7. Prince MR, Narasimham DL, Jacoby WT, et al: Three-dimensional gadolinium-enhanced MR angiography of the thoracic aorta. AJR 166:1387–1397, 1996.
8. Murray JG, Manisali M, Flamm SD, et al: Intramural hematoma of the thoracic aorta: MR image findings and their prognostic implications. Radiology 204:349–355, 1997.
9. Keren A, Kim CB, Hu BS, et al: Accuracy of biplane and multiplane transesophageal echocardiography in diagnosis of typical acute aortic dissection and intramural hematoma. J Am Coll Cardiol 28:627–636, 1996.
10. Oshinski JN, Parks WJ, Markou CP, et al: Improved measurement of pressure gradients in aortic coarctation by magnetic resonance imaging. J Am Coll Cardiol 28:1818–1826, 1996.
11. Hatabu H, Gaa J, Kim D, et al: Pulmonary perfusion and angiography: evaluation with breath-hold enhanced three-dimensional fast imaging steady-state precession MR imaging with short TR and TE. AJR 167:653–655, 1996.
12. Meaney JF, Weg JG, Chenevert TL, et al: Diagnosis of pulmonary embolism with magnetic resonance angiography. N Engl J Med 336:1422–1427, 1997.
13. Levine RA, Weyman AE, Dinsmore RE, et al: Noninvasive tissue characterization: diagnosis of lipomatous hypertrophy of the atrial septum by nuclear magnetic resonance imaging. J Am Coll Cardiol 7:688–692, 1986.
14. Sechtem U, Tscholakoff D, Higgins CB: MRI of the normal pericardium. AJR 147:239–244, 1986.
15. Masui T, Finck S, Higgins CB: Constrictive pericarditis and restrictive cardiomyopathy: evaluation with MR imaging. Radiology 182:369–373, 1992.
16. Hundley WG, Li HF, Lange RA, et al: Assessment of left-to-right intracardiac shunting by velocity-encoded, phase-difference magnetic resonance imaging. A comparison with oximetric and indicator dilution techniques. Circulation 91:2955–2960, 1995.
17. Masui T, Seelos KC, Kersting-Sommerhoff BA, Higgins CB: Abnormalities of the pulmonary veins: evaluation with MR imaging and comparison with cardiac angiography and echocardiography. Radiology 181:645–649, 1991.
18. White CS, Baffa JM, Haney PJ, et al: Anomalies of pulmonary veins: usefulness of spin-echo and gradient-echo MR images. AJR 170:1365–1368, 1998.
19. Cheitlin MD, de Casstro DM, McAllister HA: Sudden death as a complication of anomalous left coronary origin from the anterior sinus of Valsalva: a not-so-minor congenital anomaly. Circulation 50:780–787, 1974.
20. McConnell MV, Ganz P, Selwyn AP, et al: Identification of anomalous coronary arteries and their anatomic course by magnetic resonance coronary angiography. Circulation 92:3158–3162, 1995.
21. Post JC, van Rossum AC, Bronzwaer JG, et al: Magnetic resonance angiography of anomalous coronary arteries. A new gold standard for delineating the proximal course? Circulation 92:3163–3171, 1995.
22. Vliegen HW, Doornbos J, de Roos A, et al: Value of fast gradient echo magnetic resonance angiography as an adjunct to coronary arteriography in detecting and confirming the course of clinically significant coronary artery anomalies. Am J Cardiol 79:773–776, 1997.
23. Harrity P, Patel A, Bianco J, Subramanian R: Improved diagnosis and characterization of postinfarction left ventricular pseudoaneurysm by cardiac magnetic resonance imaging. Clin Cardiol 14:603–606, 1991.
24. McNamara MT, Higgins CB: Magnetic resonance imaging of chronic myocardial infarcts in man. AJR 146:315–320, 1986.
25. Cranney GB, Lotan CS, Dean L, et al: Left ventricular volume measurement using cardiac axis nuclear magnetic resonance imaging: validation by calibrated ventricular angiography. Circulation 82:154–163, 1990.
26. Mogelvang J, Stokholm KH, Saunamaki K, et al: Assessment of left ventricular volumes by magnetic resonance in comparison with radionuclide angiography, contrast angiography and echocardiography. Eur Heart J 13:1677–1683, 1992.
27. Sakuma H, Fujita N, Foo TKF, et al: Evaluation of left ventricular volume and mass with breath-hold cine MR imaging. Radiology 188:377–380, 1993.
28. Johnson DB, Foster RE, Barilla F, et al: Angiotensin-converting enzyme inhibitor therapy affects left ventricular mass in patients with ejection fraction >40% after acute myocardial infarction. J Am Coll Cardiol 29:49–54, 1997.
29. Fayad ZA, Ferrari VA, Kraitchman DL, et al: Right ventricular regional function using MR tagging: normals versus chronic pulmonary hypertension. Magn Reson Med 39:116–123, 1998.
30. Kramer CM, Rogers WJ, Theobald TM, et al: Remote noninfarcted region dysfunction soon after first anterior myocardial infarction. A magnetic resonance tagging study. Circulation 94:660–666, 1996.

30a. Nagel E, Lehmkuhl HB, Bocksch W, et al: Noninvasive diagnosis of ischemia-induced wall motion abnormalities with the use of high dose dobutamine stress MRI: comparison with dobutamine echocardiography. Circulation 99:763–770, 1999.

30b. Hundley WG, Hamilton CA, Thomas MS, et al: Utility of fast cine magnetic resonance imaging and display for the detection of myocardial ischemia in patients not well suited for second harmonic stress echocardiography. Circulation 100:1697–1702, 1999.

31. Aretz HT, Billingham ME, Edwards WD, et al: Myocarditis: a histopathologic definition and classification. Am J Cardiovasc Pathol 1:3–14, 1987.
32. Friedrich MG, Strohm O, Schulz-Menger J, et al: Contrast media–enhanced magnetic resonance imaging visualizes myocardial changes in the course of viral myocarditis. Circulation 97:1802–1809, 1998.
33. Kramer CM, Reichek N, Ferrari VA, et al: Regional heterogeneity of function in hypertrophic cardiomyopathy. Circulation 90:186–194, 1994.
34. Johnston DL, Rice L, Vick GW 3rd, et al: Assessment of tissue iron overload by nuclear magnetic resonance imaging. Am J Med 87:40–47, 1989.
35. Carlson MD, White RD, Trohman RG, et al: Right ventricular outflow tract ventricular tachycardia: detection of previously unrecognized anatomic abnormalities using cine magnetic resonance imaging. J Am Coll Cardiol 24:720–727, 1994.
36. Globits S, Kreiner G, Frank H, et al: Significance of morphological abnormalities detected by MRI in patients undergoing successful ablation of right ventricular outflow tract tachycardia. Circulation 96:2633–2640, 1997.
37. Manning WJ, Li W, Edelman RR: A preliminary report comparing magnetic resonance coronary angiography with conventional angiography. N Engl J Med 328:828–832, 1993.
38. Pennell DJ, Bogren HG, Keegan J, et al: Assessment of coronary artery stenosis by magnetic resonance imaging. Heart 75:127–133, 1996.
39. Duerinckx AJ, Urman MK: Two-dimensional coronary MR angiography: analysis of initial clinical results. Radiology 193:731–738, 1994.
40. Post JC, van Rossum AC, Hofman MB, et al: Clinical utility of two-dimensional magnetic resonance angiography in detecting coronary artery disease. Eur Heart J 18:426–433, 1997.
41. Yoshino H, Nitatori T, Kachi E, et al: Directed proximal magnetic resonance coronary angiography compared with conventional contrast coronary angiography. Am J Cardiol 80:514–518, 1997.
42. Muller MF, Fleisch M, Kroeker R, et al: Proximal coronary artery stenosis: three-dimensional MRI with fat saturation and navigator echo. J Magn Reson Imaging 7:644–651, 1997.
43. Woodard PK, Li D, Haacke EM, et al: Detection of coronary stenoses on source and projection images using three-dimensional MR angiography with retrospective respiratory gating: preliminary experience. AJR 170:883–888, 1998.

44. Botnar RM, Stuber M, Danias PG, et al: Improved coronary artery definition with T2-weighted, free-breathing three-dimensional coronary MRA. Circulation 99:3139–3148, 1999.
45. Hundley WG, Clarke GD, Landau C, et al: Noninvasive determination of infarct artery patency by cine magnetic resonance angiography. Circulation 91:1347–1353, 1995.
46. White RD, Caputo GR, Mark AS, et al: Coronary artery bypass graft patency: noninvasive evaluation with MR imaging. Radiology 164:681–686, 1987.
47. Rubinstein RI, Askenase AD, Thickman D, et al: Magnetic resonance imaging to evaluate patency of aortocoronary bypass grafts. Circulation 76:786–791, 1987.
48. Aurigemma GP, Reichek N, Axel L, et al: Noninvasive determination of coronary artery bypass graft patency by cine magnetic resonance imaging. Circulation 80:1595–1602, 1989.
49. Galjee MA, van Rossum AC, Doesburg T, et al: Value of magnetic resonance imaging in assessing patency and function of coronary artery bypass grafts. An angiographically controlled study. Circulation 93:660–666, 1996.
50. Vrachliotis TG, Bis KG, Aliabadi D, et al: Contrast-enhanced breath-hold MR angiography for evaluating patency of coronary artery bypass grafts. AJR 168:1073–1080, 1997.
51. Duerinckx AJ, Atkinson D, Hurwitz R, et al: Coronary MR angiography after coronary stent placement. AJR 165:662–664, 1995.

SECTION II

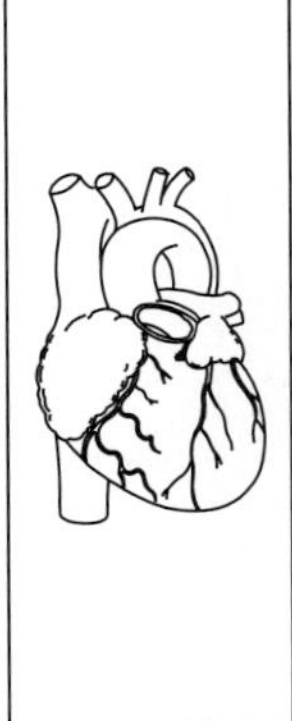

CONGENITAL HEART DISEASE IN THE ADULT

Anatomic Abnormalities

Pathophysiology, Clinical Recognition, and Treatment

Echocardiography

Interventional Therapy

Surgical Treatment

CHAPTER 7

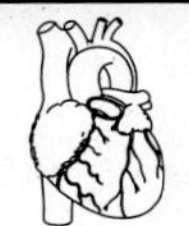

Anatomic Abnormalities

Jack L. Titus and Jesse E. Edwards

NORMAL ANATOMY
ANATOMIC ABNORMALITIES
Obstruction
Valvular Regurgitation
Abnormal Communication Between the Chambers and/or the Great Arteries
Abnormal Connections
Combinations of Anomalies
Abnormal Aortic and Arterial Branching
Syndromes With Heart Disease

Normal Anatomy

Before considering the various anatomic abnormalities of the heart, we review the highlights of the anatomy of the normal heart. These are considered according to the various chambers and the coronary vessels.

The right atrium (RA) (Fig. 7–1) lies to the right and somewhat inferior and anterior to the left atrium (LA)—separated by the atrial septum. The appendage of the RA has a broad base and is positioned on the right of the ascending aorta. Prominent parallel muscle bundles, the pectinate muscles, line the wall of the RA.

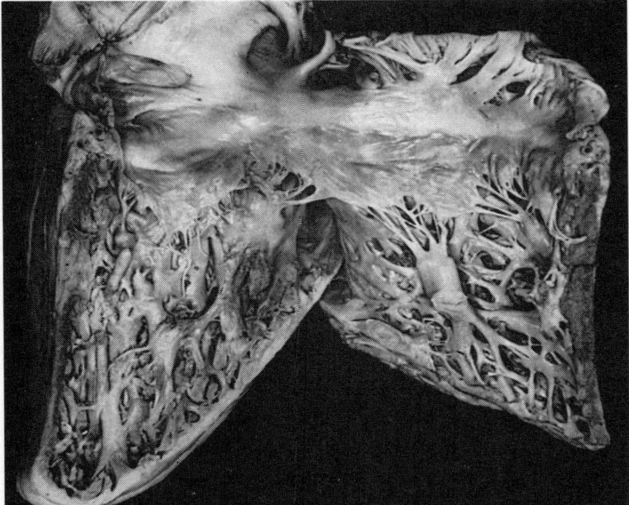

FIGURE 7–1 The right atrium (above), tricuspid valve, and inferior portion of the right ventricle (below) have been opened by an incision along their posterior (inferior) walls to display the atrial and ventricular septa. Toward the left, in the approximate center of the atrial septum, is the fossa ovalis. The interior of the right atrial appendage with prominent pectinate bundles is on the right. The tricuspid valve has three leaflets—septal (on the ventricular septum), anterior, and posterior (inferior).

Entering the superior part of the RA is the superior vena cava (SVC). Between the atrial ostium of the SVC and the base of the atrial appendage is a muscle bundle, the crista terminalis, which is situated in the superior aspect of the RA. The sinoatrial (sinus) node is situated in the anterosuperior part of the crista terminalis at the junction of the SVC with the RA.

The inferior vena cava (IVC) joins the posteroinferior part of the RA near the atrial septum. Its orifice may be guarded by a flaplike valve, the eustachian valve. Inferior to the ostium of the IVC (i.e., toward the tricuspid valve) is the orifice of the coronary sinus. The coronary sinus itself lies in the epicardium of the posterior atrioventricular (AV) sulcus between the LA and the left ventricle (LV).

In the center of the right side of the atrial septum is the fossa ovalis (Fig. 7–2A), which has a raised edge about its superior, anterior, and inferior margins, termed the *limbus fossa ovalis,* with superior and inferior limbi. Normally, a thin membrane lies over the left side of the fossa ovalis, which is the floor of the fossa ovalis, and also the "valve" of the foramen ovale, described later.

In the fetus, a channel in the anterior aspect of the fossa ovalis passes through the atrial septum into the LA; this opening is the foramen ovale (see Fig. 7–2B). In about one third of adults, this channel persists as a valvular competent patent foramen ovale (see Fig. 7–2A). Potential effects of such patency are discussed in the section on Atrial Septal Defects.

The AV valve in the orifice between the RA and the right ventricle (RV) is the tricuspid valve. This valve has three leaflets, each supported by chordae and papillary muscles of the RV.

The RV has inflow and outflow portions. The inflow portion lies posteriorly (inferiorly) (Fig. 7–3), and the outflow portion lies anteriorly (superiorly).

The septal wall of the RV has generally well-defined structures. Beneath the septal leaflet of the tricuspid valve, often at the commissure between septal and anterior leaflets, is the membranous part of the ventricular septum. In part, this structure separates the two ventricles, and in part, the membranous septum separates the RA from the LV.

Superior to the membranous septum is the papillary muscle of the conus (medial papillary muscle, muscle of Luschka, muscle of Lancisi). This receives chordae from the adjacent portions of the septal and anterior tricuspid leaflets (see Fig. 7–3). More superiorly, on the septal wall of the RV, are two muscle bundles having the shape of an

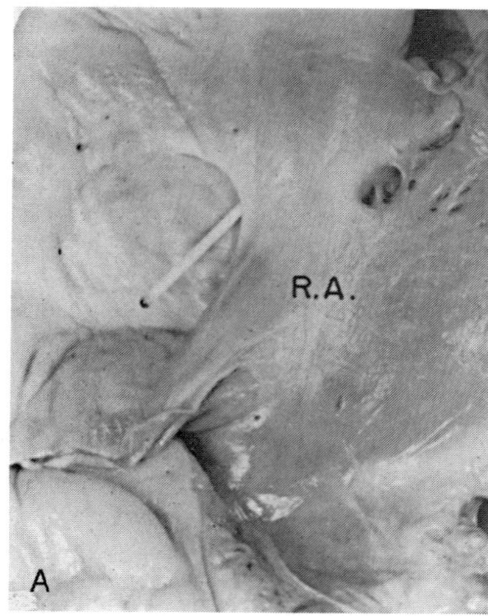

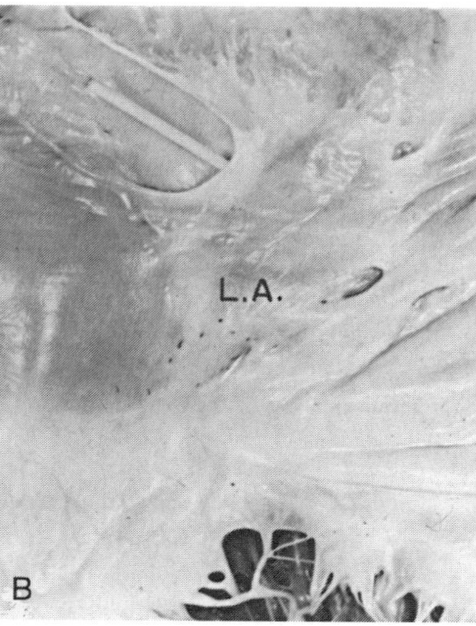

FIGURE 7–2 Valvular competent patent foramen ovale in an adult. **A,** Right atrial (R.A.) aspect. The fossa ovalis appears as a circle; the probe placed in the foramen ovale disappears between the edge of the foramen and the floor of the fossa ovalis or valve of foramen. **B,** Left atrial (L.A.) aspect of the same case demonstrates the probe placed in the foramen ovale at left, appearing in the left atrial cavity between the edge of the foramen ovale and the valve of the fossa ovalis. The valve mechanism is such that left atrial pressure in excess of right atrial pressure tends to close the potential opening. (**A** and **B,** From Schroeckenstein RF, Wasenda GJ, Edwards JE: Valvular competent patent foramen ovale in adults. Minn Med 55:11, 1972.)

inverted U, forming the crista supraventricularis, with the apex of the U-shaped structure located just under the pulmonary valve. The more anterior of the two limbs of the crista is the septal band, and the more lateral limb is the parietal limb.

The right ventricular infundibular outflow tract is a cylindrical, muscular tube, lying between the level of the membranous septum below and the pulmonary valve above. Thus, muscle separates the tricuspid and the pulmonary valves (see Fig. 7–3).

The pulmonary valve is in the most anterosuperior part of the heart. The pulmonary trunk is a relatively short vessel that bifurcates into the left and right pulmonary arteries. The ductus arteriosus of fetal life and early infancy, which becomes the ligamentum arteriosum, connects the superior aspect of the near-origin of the left pulmonary artery and the lower (inferior) part of the aorta at the junction of its distal arch and descending portions.

The LA (Fig. 7–4) lies to the left posterior and somewhat superior to the RA. It receives the pulmonary veins in its upper half. The veins enter somewhat posteriorly in the LA. Classically, pulmonary veins at their junction with the LA are defined as right and left superior and inferior pulmonary veins, although anatomic variations in the number are common.

The left atrial appendage joins the LA anteriorly and inferiorly to the entrance of the left inferior pulmonary vein. The left atrial appendage is more narrow than the right atrial appendage and has an angulated shape. The appendage lies toward the left side of the aorta and pulmonary trunk.

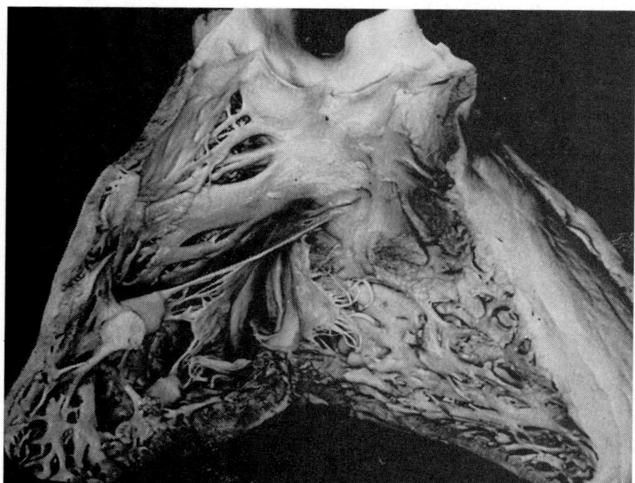

FIGURE 7–3 Right ventricle and pulmonary valve. The outflow portion of the right ventricle is formed by the infundibulum, a muscular tube that separates the tricuspid (below, leftward) and pulmonary (above, center) valves.

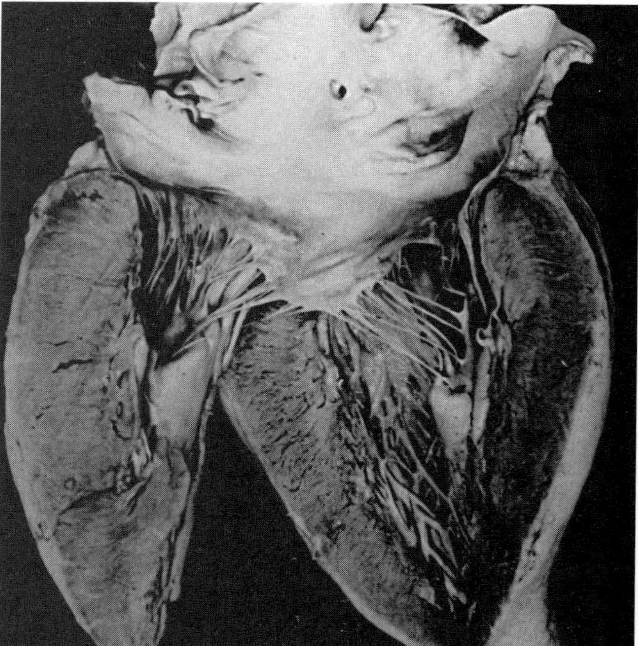

FIGURE 7–4 Left atrium, mitral valve, and left ventricle. The pulmonary venous orifices as they enter the left atrium have been opened. The mitral valve has two leaflets and two sets of papillary muscles—joined by corresponding sets of chordae. Note that each leaflet has a chordal attachment to each papillary muscle. The interior of the left atrium is smooth walled.

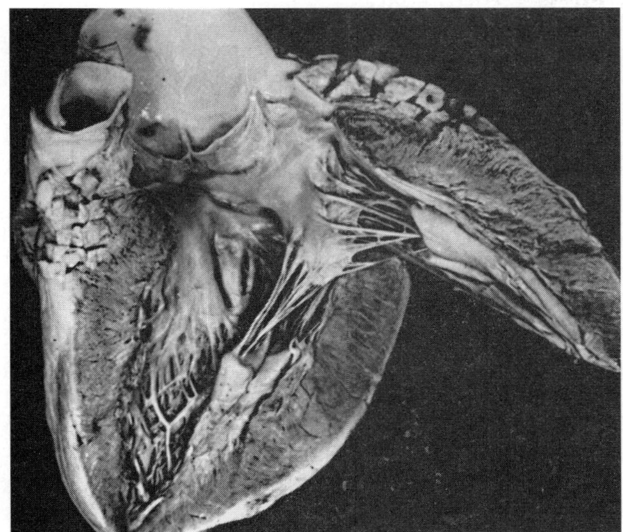

FIGURE 7–5 The outflow tract of the left ventricle and the aortic valve have been opened. The outflow tract is walled, in part, by the ventricular septum and, in part, by the anteromedial leaflet of the mitral valve (right).

The left AV valve (see Fig. 7–4), the mitral valve, has two leaflets, each supported by chordae tendineae attached to the two papillary muscles, the anterolateral and posteromedial of the LV. Each mitral leaflet has chordal connections with each papillary muscle. The LV is somewhat conical, its apex forming the apex of the cone.

The left ventricular outflow tract to the aorta (Fig. 7–5) lies behind the right ventricular infundibulum. The outflow tract is walled by the ventricular septum and the anterior mitral leaflet (see Fig. 7–5). Changes in position of the anterior mitral leaflet with the cardiac cycle change the caliber of the outflow tract. The aortic valve connects with the ventricular septum and anterior wall of the LV, anteriorly and medially, whereas posteriorly and laterally the aortic origin connects with the base of the anterior mitral leaflet (Fig. 7–6A), the connecting unit being the aortomitral intervalvular fibrosa.

The base of the posterior mitral leaflet connects with the LA and LV at a common junction that is often termed the *mitral annulus* or *ring* (see Fig. 7–6B), although it is not a complete ring.

The aortic valve has three semilunar cusps—left, right, and posterior (noncoronary). Each cusp, along with the aortic wall, forms a sinus (aortic sinus, sinus of Valsalva). Each sinus is named according to the corresponding cusp.

The left and right coronary arteries originate from the left and the right aortic sinuses, respectively. The main left coronary artery is short before its division into the anterior descending and left circumflex coronary arteries. A third branch, sometimes called the intermediate coronary artery, may be present at the end of the main left coronary artery. The anterior descending artery passes in the anterior interventricular sulcus toward the cardiac apex. The left circum-

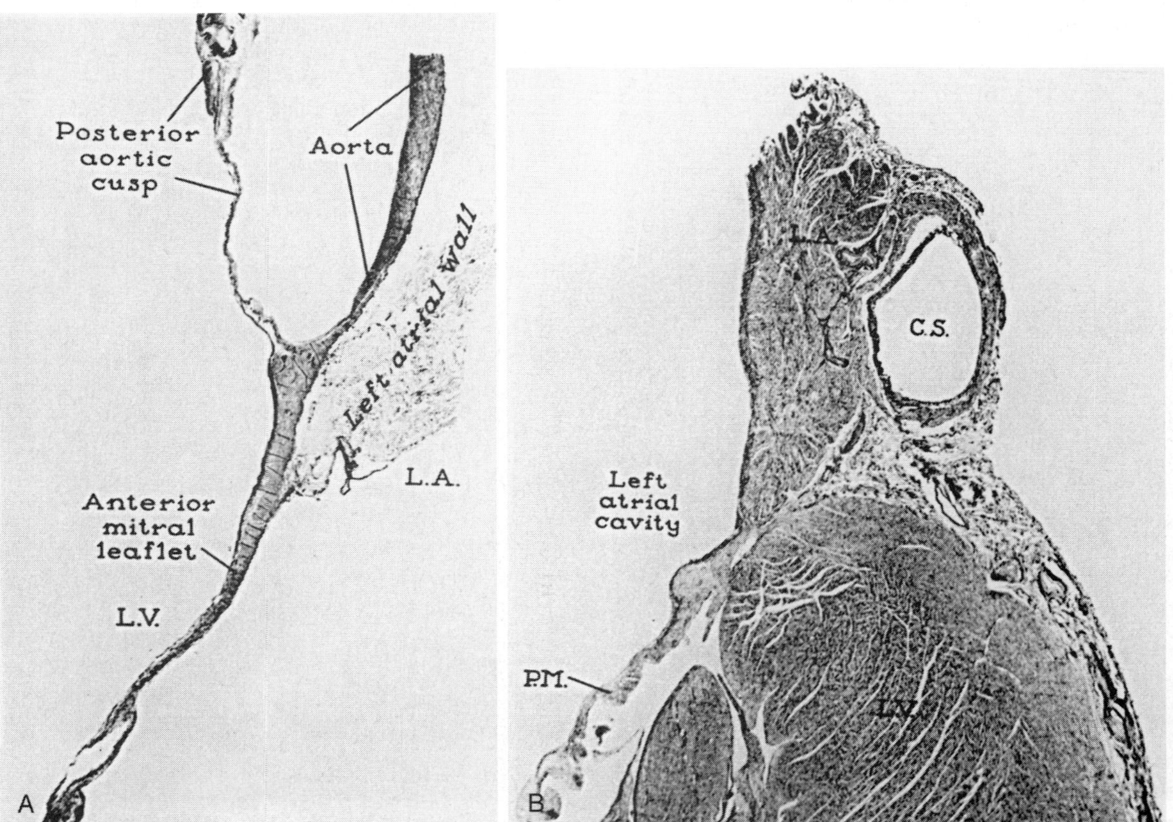

FIGURE 7–6 A, Low-power view of the posterior aortic cusp and anterior mitral leaflet shows fibrous continuity between the two structures. L.A., left atrium; L.V., left ventricle. **B,** Low-power view of the left atrium (L.A.), left ventricle (L.V.), and the posterior mitral leaflet (P.M.). The latter joins a common fibrous meeting place with the atrium and ventricle. The coronary sinus (C.S.) runs in the epicardium of the left atrioventricular sulcus.

flex artery passes in the left AV sulcus. The right coronary artery runs in the right AV sulcus toward the posterior aspect of the heart. Most often, it turns abruptly downward in the posterior interventricular sulcus of the heart as the posterior descending coronary artery. This pattern of the coronary arteries is termed *right dominance*. In the less common *left dominant pattern,* the left circumflex artery continues in the left AV sulcus to give the posterior descending coronary artery.

The coronary veins run in the epicardium, either over the ventricles or in the different cardiac sulci, to terminate in the coronary sinus. The latter lies against the posterior wall of the lower part of the LA (see Fig. 7–6B). Some small coronary veins may join the RA directly, usually as thebesian veins, some of which also may join the LA.

ANATOMIC ABNORMALITIES

This section covers obstruction, valvular regurgitation, abnormal communication between the chambers and/or the great arteries, abnormal connections, combinations of anomalies, abnormal aortic and arterial branching, and syndromes with heart disease.

Obstruction

Congenital obstructions in the cardiovascular system that are seen in the adult include valvular, paravalvular, and vascular conditions.

Valvular and Paravalvular Obstructions

Congenital valvular obstruction may affect any valve, but most commonly, the aortic valve is involved.

States related functionally to aortic valvular stenosis include obstruction in the subaortic region (subaortic stenosis) or in the ascending aorta (supravalvular stenosis). Atresia of any valve may occur. Those involving the left-sided valves tend to be lethal in early life, whereas atresia of the tricuspid and particularly of the pulmonary valve may be tolerated, allowing some patients to survive to adulthood.

AORTIC STENOSIS

The major cause of obstruction at the aortic valve in the adult is the congenital bicuspid aortic valve. Although this condition may be intrinsically obstructive, this is not usually the case in individuals who reach adulthood with a congenital bicuspid aortic valve. However, the congenital bicuspid aortic valve has a strong tendency over time to become calcified and stenotic. It is probable that a congenital bicuspid aortic valve is present in about 1 to 2 percent of the adult populations.[1] Most but not all of these valves become calcified with time, leading to rigidity that causes aortic stenosis.[2, 3] This type of aortic stenosis in the adult accounts for approximately 50 percent of prosthetic valve replacements.[4, 5]

The calcified stenotic bicuspid aortic valve has two cusps, the conjoined cusp and a "single" cusp. A ridge or raphe extends from the aorta onto the center of the aortic aspect of the conjoined cusp (Fig. 7–7). The conjoined cusp usually lies anteriorly. In this situation, both coronary arteries arise from its sinus. Less commonly, the cusps lie in a lateral orientation (right or left cusps). In this state, one coronary artery arises from each of the two aortic sinuses.

Another anomaly of the aortic valve is the unicuspid, unicommissural state in which the valve has the shape of a modified dome.[6] This valve is intrinsically stenotic, the degree of obstruction varying from case to case. This type of valve is the usual cause of aortic stenosis in infants and children. Occasionally, a lesser degree of stenosis can be tolerated for years, even into adulthood. Eventually, calci-

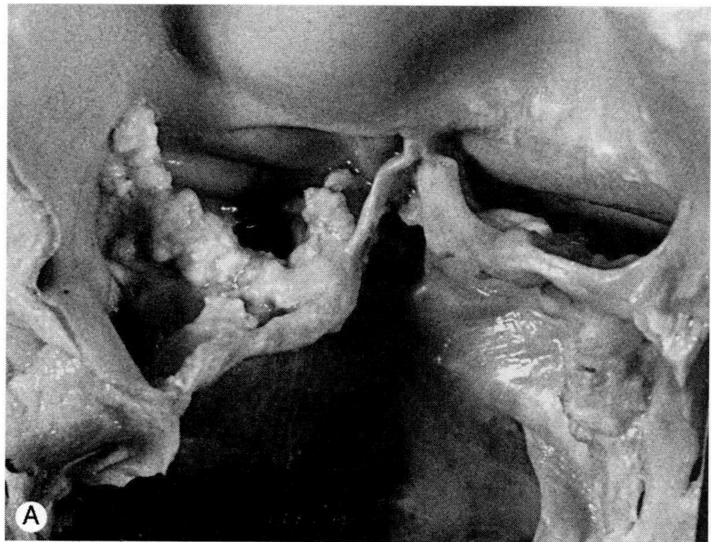

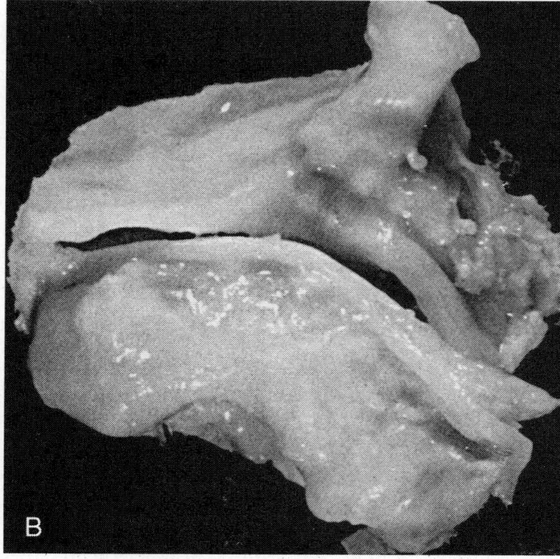

FIGURE 7–7 Congenital bicuspid aortic valve with calcific aortic stenosis. **A,** Autopsy specimen in which the valve has been opened. The conjoined cusp and its calcified raphe lie to the left. Thickening of tissue is caused by heavy calcification of the conjoined cusp and its raphe. **B,** A valve removed at operation. The conjoined cusp lies above, as does its raphe. Calcific thickening of cusps and raphe is the basis for aortic stenosis.

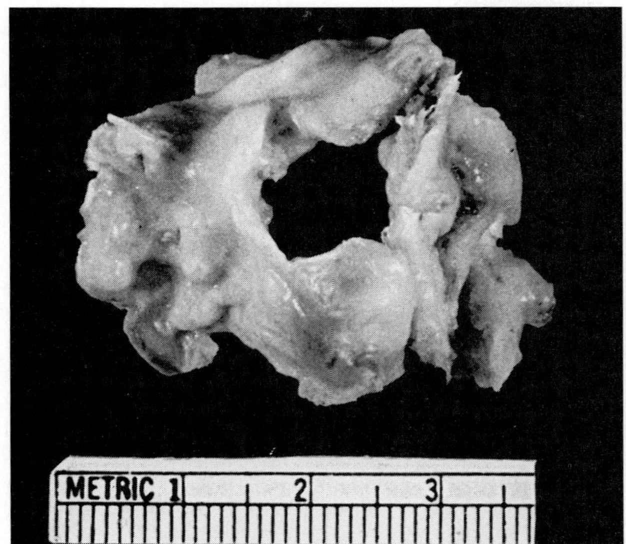

FIGURE 7–8 Congenital unicuspid aortic stenosis in a surgically excised valve from an adult patient. The single commissure is seen at upper right. The valve orifice is fixed, and the funnel-like valve is calcified.

fication may develop, and the aortic stenosis becomes symptomatic. The delay in the appearance of symptoms can be explained as follows. In the natural, noncalcified state, the valve is a flexible dome. During diastole, the fibrotic, noncalcified dome may act as a flutter valve, preventing regurgitation. Later, when calcification has become established, the flutter action is lost, allowing regurgitation to occur (Fig. 7–8). This, in turn, causes an increased volume of blood to be expelled through the aortic valve during the period of contraction, and aortic stenosis therefore becomes apparent. The calcification does not change the caliber of the intrinsically stenotic valve. However, because it allows regurgitation, the increased flow through the orifice is responsible for the transformation from asymptomatic to symptomatic disease.[7]

SUBAORTIC STENOSIS

Adults exhibit two principal types of subaortic stenosis, the muscular type and the membranous type. In addition, an uncommon third type, tunnel subaortic stenosis, has been described.

Muscular Subaortic Stenosis. Henry and associates[8] listed the various names used to describe this condition, including idiopathic hypertrophic subaortic stenosis, muscular subaortic stenosis, asymmetric septal hypertrophy, and obstructive cardiomyopathy, or hypertrophic obstructive cardiomyopathy.

Asymmetrical septal hypertrophy is characterized by asymmetrical hypertrophy of the muscular ventricular septum associated with histologic features of myocardial disarray. The degree of this change varies qualitatively and quantitatively, as does its specific location.

Henry and associates[8] concluded that asymmetric septal hypertrophy is a genetically transmitted condition characterized by a clinically continuous spectrum that includes asymptomatic individuals, symptomatic patients without outflow obstruction, and symptomatic patients with typical left ventricular outflow obstructions. These authors noted that ultrastructural observations suggest a fundamental cardiac defect involving abnormal muscle hypertrophy with or without altered cellular morphogenesis. They were of the opinion that "asymmetric septal hypertrophy" is the best description for this disease, not only providing a concise name but also describing an anatomic abnormality that can be detected noninvasively. This feature distinguishes patients with a disease different from those with other forms of ventricular hypertrophy and dilatation. It also provides a terminology independent of outflow obstruction.

When left ventricular outflow obstruction occurs, it is caused by systolic anterior motion of the anterior leaflet of the mitral valve. As the anterior leaflet impinges against the ventricular septum, outflow obstruction of the LV results, as well as mechanical irritation of the affected mural endocardium. The latter leads to a patch of fibrous deposition over the prominence of the ventricular septum (Fig. 7–9).

Frank and Braunwald[9] reviewed the manifestations and course in 126 patients with idiopathic hypertrophic subaortic stenosis followed for up to 12 years. They divided these patients into two etiologic groups—the familial type (32 percent) and the sporadic type (68 percent)—by studying families of patients. These authors recognized that some cases actually of the familial type were incorrectly assigned to the sporadic type because inadequate numbers of family members had been studied. Among patients with asymmetric septal hypertrophy, obstruction to right ventricular outflow also may be present. In 2 of the patients studied, left ventricular outflow obstruction was absent. Sudden death was a relatively common cause of mortality, occurring in 6 of 10 fatal cases.

Infectious endocarditis was observed in 3 patients. Death did not appear related to the degree of left ventricular outflow obstruction. There was no significant difference in ages between the patients who died suddenly and those whose course was characterized by progressive deterioration. Among the patients who died, the average age of the familial cases (18.8 years) was less than that of the sporadic cases (40.4 years).

Membranous Subaortic Stenosis. Membranous, discrete, or fixed subaortic stenosis is characterized by encirclement of the left ventricular outflow tract with dense fibrous tissue.[10] Because of the anatomic structure of the area involved, the fibrous tissue is attached to the endocardium over the ventricular septum and the anterior wall of the LV and also involves the ventricular aspect of the anterior mitral leaflet. The fibrous tissue causes narrowing of the left ventricular outflow tract and may also extend to and attach irregularly to the aortic cusps (Fig. 7–10).[11] Contracture of this fibrous tissue may lead to aortic regurgitation.

The degree of obstruction may increase with age[12, 13] as the result of contracture of the fibrous tissue. In addition, turbulence of the blood flowing through the narrow channel may lead to an increase in deposition of fibrous tissue. It is probable that the caliber of the outflow tract at the site of the lesion does not increase with age. Therefore, the increase in cardiac output with body growth while the

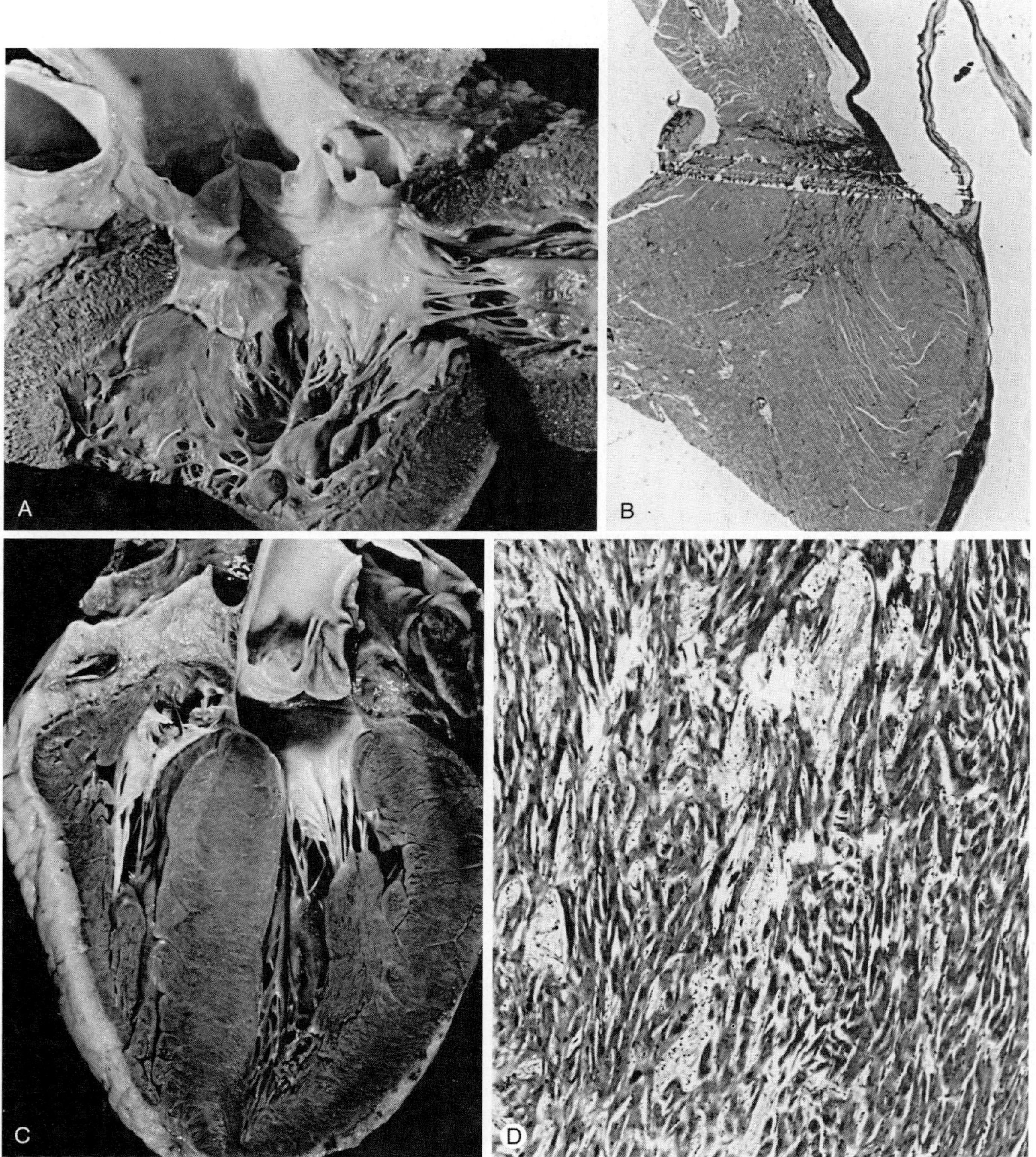

FIGURE 7–9 Hypertrophic cardiomyopathy (asymmetric septal hypertrophy, idiopathic hypertrophic muscular subaortic stenosis) from a 67-year-old man (**A** and **B**) and a 39-year-old man (**C** and **D**). **A,** The left ventricle and aorta have been opened. On the subaortic portion of the ventricular septum, immediately subjacent to the aortic valve, is an endocardial patch characteristic of this condition. **B,** Low-power photomicrograph of the right aortic cusp and the ventricular septum shows the fibrous thickening of the mural endocardium corresponding to the endocardial patch seen in **A**. The muscle is hypertrophied. Elastic tissue stain, ×5. **C,** Frontal section of the ventricular portion of the heart and the aorta shows massive hypertrophy of the myocardium. The anterior mitral leaflet lies against the focus of endocardial thickening of the subaortic portion of the ventricular septum. **D,** Photomicrograph of the ventricular septum shows the characteristic disarray of the myocardial fibers. H&E, ×100.

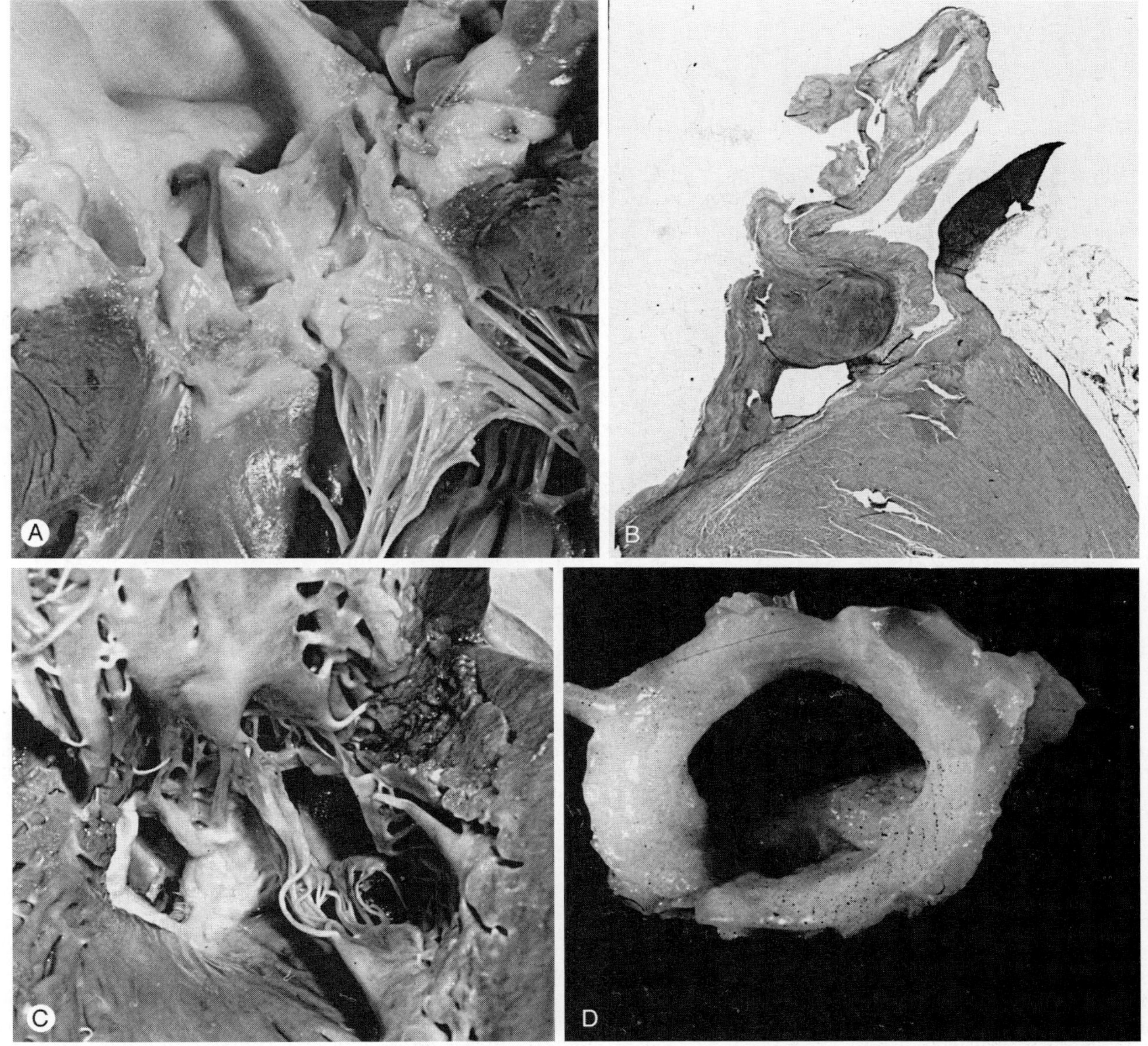

FIGURE 7–10 Membranous subaortic stenosis. **A** and **B,** From an 11-year-old boy. **A,** The opened subaortic area of the left ventricle, the aortic valve, and the ascending aorta. Encirclement of the outflow tract of the left ventricle by fibrous tissue extends onto the anterior mitral leaflet and the aortic cusps. **B,** Low-power photomicrograph of section through the aorta, the aortic valve, and the ventricular septum. Fibrous tissue involves the endocardium of the ventricular septum and extends upward to adhere to aortic valvular tissue. Elastic tissue stain, ×5. **C,** Autopsy specimen from a 62-year-old man. Opened left ventricle. To the left of the anterior mitral leaflet is encirclement of the outflow tract of the ventricle by a fibrous lesion, characteristic of membranous subaortic stenosis. **D,** Surgically excised lesion of membranous subaortic stenosis from a 15-year-old girl.

width of the obstructive channel remains relatively stable causes an additional effective increase in obstruction.

Among the significant complications of membranous subaortic stenosis are major left ventricular hypertrophy and sudden death. Infective endocarditis is a complication seen in the adult,[13, 14] and it is more common in membranous subaortic stenosis than in muscular subaortic stenosis.

Tunnel Subaortic Stenosis. Tunnel subaortic stenosis, characterized by a narrowing of the lumen in the subaortic portion, was described by Maron and colleagues in 1976.[15] The aortic annulus was relatively narrow, and the aortic valvular leaflets exhibited fibrous thickening. Left ventricular hypertrophy was marked. In 2 of 11 patients, there was associated asymmetric septal hypertrophy. The patients ranged in age from 5 to 34 years.

SUPRAVALVULAR AORTIC STENOSIS

The least common form of congenital left ventricular outflow obstruction is supravalvular aortic stenosis. Two major types occur—the hypoplastic type and the hourglass type (Fig. 7–11). The hypoplastic type is a major anomaly and frequently involves the pulmonary trunk as well. It is doubtful that survival to adulthood occurs with this type. In contrast, some patients with the hourglass type do survive to adulthood.[16] This condition may be associated with

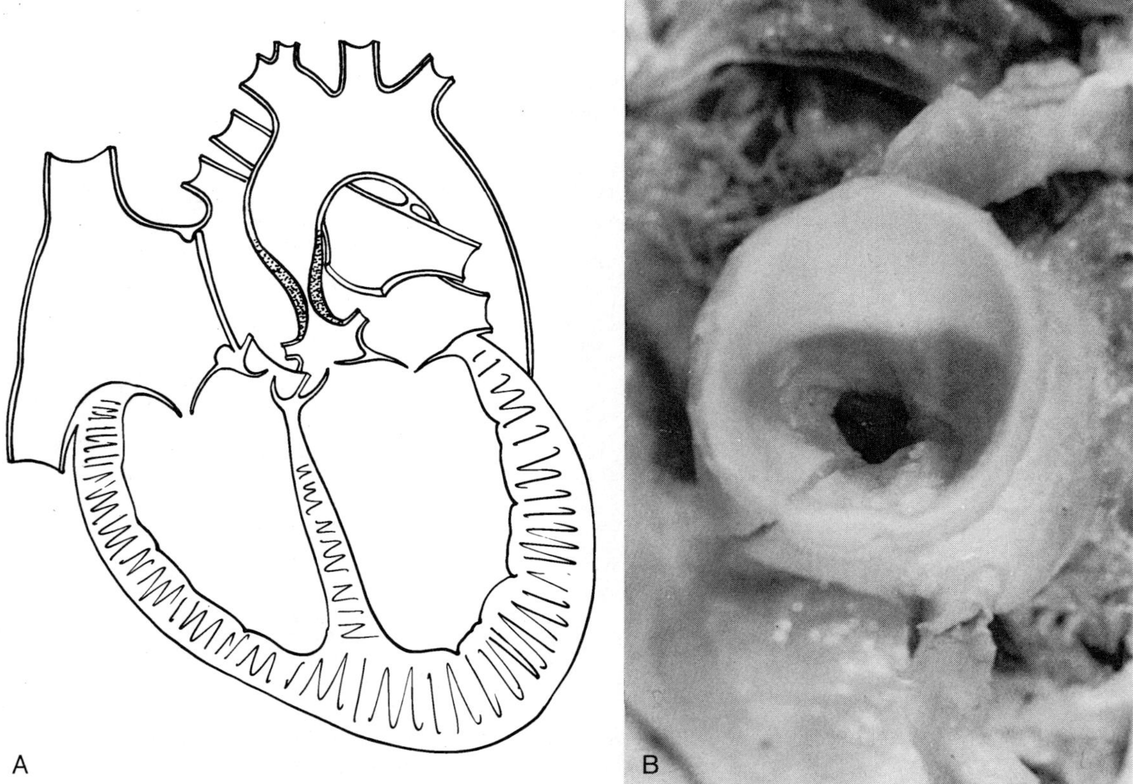

FIGURE 7–11 Hourglass-type of supravalvular aortic stenosis. **A,** Diagrammatic portrayal of the lesion involving the ascending aorta, characterized by thickening of the aortic media and pronounced narrowing of the lumen. **B,** Autopsy specimen from a 50-year-old man. The ascending aorta has been transected, and the view is toward the aortic valve. The obstruction by the narrowed lumen is evident (black).

obstruction of branches of the aortic arch and of the pulmonary artery. Experience with children and adolescents has shown that in untreated patients, the degree of left ventricular outflow obstruction increases with age, whereas the associated pulmonary arterial stenosis may become less severe.[17, 18]

One of the significant problems with supravalvular stenosis is that the coronary arterial lumens lie within the hypertensive compartment during both systole and diastole. This condition is associated with premature coronary atherosclerosis, with the potential for early manifestations of coronary arterial obstruction. The intimal aspect of the aortic lesion may encroach on the ostia of the coronary arteries. In an exceptional case, the free edge of an aortic cusp may be attached along its full length to the lesion in the aorta (Fig. 7–12), resulting in exteriorization of the involved aortic sinus and coronary artery from the aortic lumen and leading to hypoplasia of the involved coronary artery.[16]

Infective endocarditis at the aortic lesion is another potential complication in the hourglass type.

PULMONARY STENOSIS

Individuals with isolated, so-called dome-shaped pulmonary stenosis, even untreated, may survive to adulthood. By definition, the ventricular septum is intact. Major right ventricular hypertrophy exists. Acquired subpulmonary stenosis secondary to myocardial hypertrophy may occur. With few exceptions, the valve takes the shape of a truncated cone. No commissures are present, but three equidistant raphes are characteristic (Fig. 7–13). Exceptions include more than three raphes or a single commissure. Poststenotic dilatation of the pulmonary trunk is common, extending more into the left than into the right pulmonary artery.[19]

In pulmonary stenosis with intact ventricular septum and a patent foramen ovale, a right-to-left shunt may be present at the atrial level. Even though the right-to-left shunt is minor, such patients may develop cerebral abscess.[20] This infectious process is a recognized complication in instances of chronic right-to-left shunts without a focus of infection within the heart. In other instances, infectious endocarditis may develop on the valve or infectious pulmonary arteritis may occur at the area where the jetlike stream has an impact at and near the pulmonary arterial bifurcation.

In patients treated by adequate pulmonary valvotomy, right ventricular hypertrophy may remain for years. Sudden death has occurred in such cases, perhaps as a consequence of residual myocardial hypertrophy.

MITRAL STENOSIS

In most cases of mitral valve stenosis, the condition is considered to be acquired and of rheumatic origin.

The parachute mitral valve is among the causes of con-

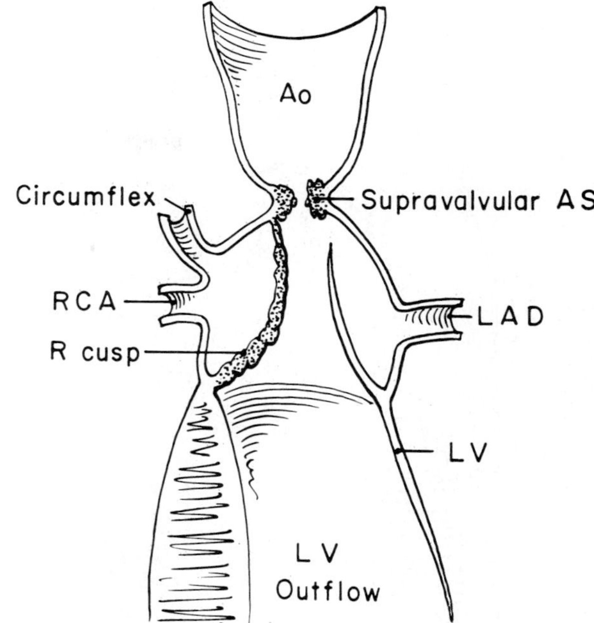

FIGURE 7–12 Hourglass-type of supravalvular aortic stenosis (AS) shows adhesion of the right aortic cusp (R cusp) to the lesion of the aortic wall. The result is exteriorization of the right aortic sinus from the aortic lumen. In this particular patient, a 50-year-old man, both the right coronary artery (RCA) and the left circumflex artery arose from the right aortic sinus. Gross specimen of aorta (Ao) is shown in Fig. 7–11B. LAD, left anterior descending coronary artery; LV, left ventricle; LV Outflow, left ventricular outflow tract.

genital mitral stenosis observed in adults. This condition is characterized by a solitary papillary muscle, into which the chordae of both leaflets converge and insert. This condition may be associated with three other obstructive anomalies in the left side of the heart, together forming the so-called Shone syndrome.[21] The other obstructive anomalies are coarctation of the aorta, subaortic stenosis, and supravalvular ring of the LA (Fig. 7–14). Most patients with the Shone syndrome do not survive to adulthood. In the original article on this subject by Shone and coworkers,[21] one 23-year-old patient was represented.

A report by da Silva and Edwards[22] described a 59-year-old man who died of mitral stenosis, which was considered to be congenital. In this patient, the majority of the mitral chordae inserted into a major papillary muscle, and the remaining chordae inserted into the other papillary muscle,

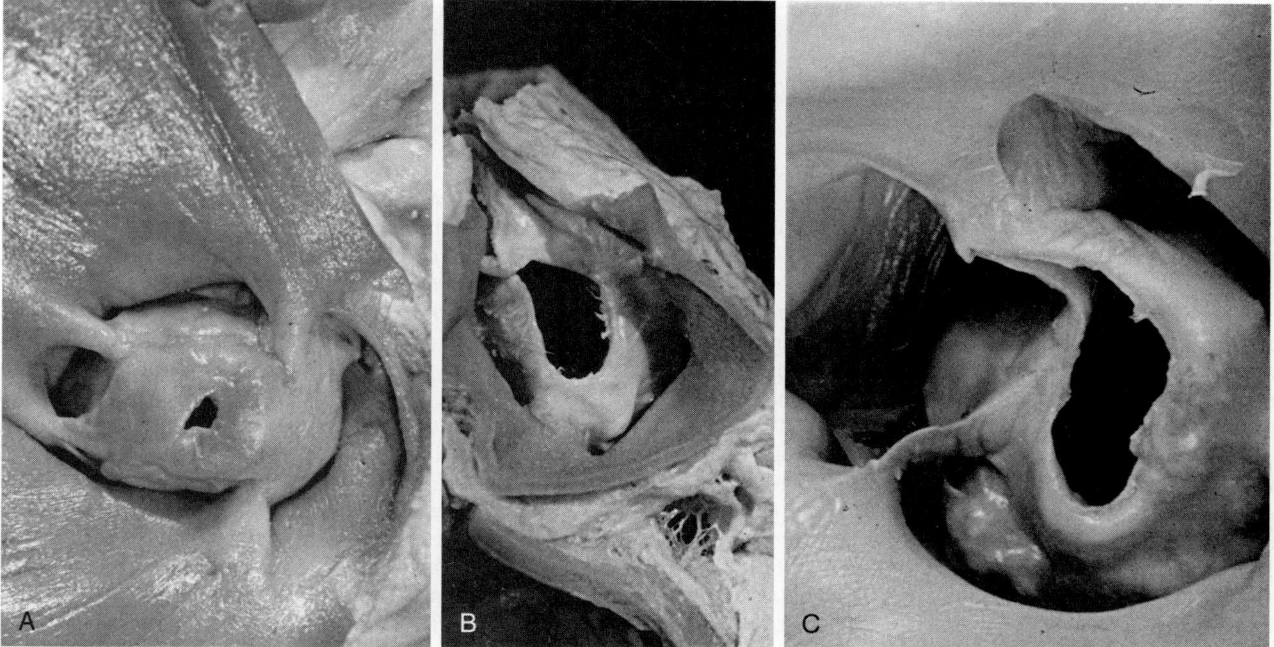

FIGURE 7–13 Autopsy specimens of congenitally stenotic pulmonary valves, each associated with intact ventricular septum. The valves are unopened and are viewed from above. **A,** From a 21-year-old woman. The valve is dome-shaped, with major obstruction. Four raphes are present. **B,** From a 61-year-old woman. There is classical dome-shaped stenosis without commissures, but the obstruction is less than that in **A**. **C,** From a 39-year-old man. A unicommissural valve is present. The commissure is above, and portions of the raphes are at lower left and lower right.

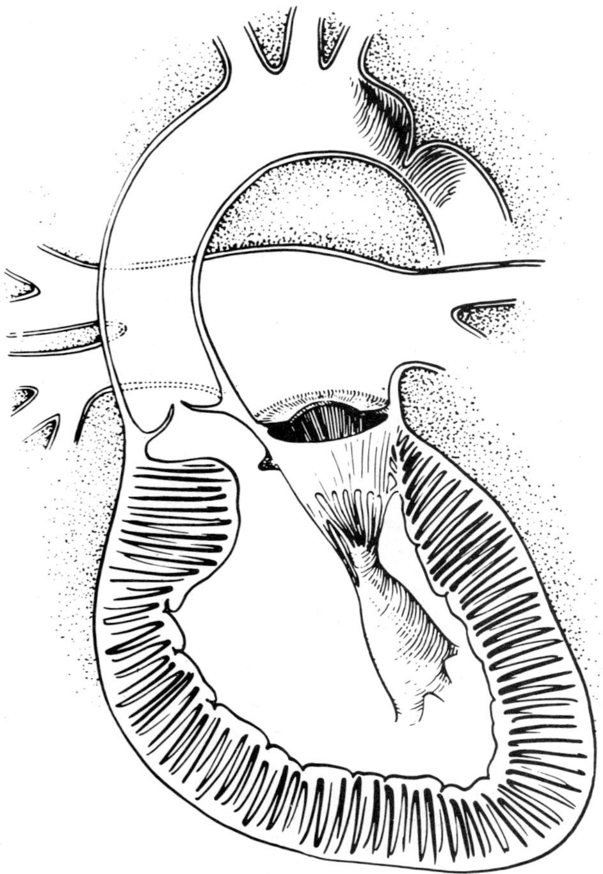

FIGURE 7–14 The Shone syndrome has four congenital obstructions in the left heart and aorta: a supravalvular ring in the left atrium, a parachute mitral valve, subaortic stenosis, and aortic coarctation. (From Shone JD, Sellers RD, Anderson RC et al: The developmental complex of "parachute mitral valve," supravalvular ring of left atrium, subaortic stenosis, and coarctation of aorta. Reprinted with permission from the American College of Cardiology [*Journal of the American College of Cardiology,* 1963, Vol. 11, p. 714].)

which was smaller. This deformity was considered to represent a variant of the parachute mitral valve.

TRICUSPID STENOSIS

Patients with Ebstein's malformation of the tricuspid valve commonly reach adulthood. Only rarely is tricuspid stenosis associated, however. Stenosis or regurgitation may be observed with this malformation, the latter being more common. Ebstein's anomaly is considered in greater detail later.

Tricuspid atresia is a relatively common condition in the young, but it is rare in adults. In an exceptional case, tricuspid atresia in a 56-year-old woman was reported by Hedinger in 1915.[23] This patient had an associated single ventricle and malposition of the great arteries. Incorrect reference to this report as an example of complete transposition of the great arteries has been made in many published reports through the years.

Aortic Coarctation

Among the various arterial obstructive anomalies that allow patients to survive into adulthood, coarctation of the aorta is the most common. The usual site of coarctation is in the general position of the union of the ductus with the aorta. In patients with coarctation who reach adulthood, the obstruction tends to lie distal to the ductal insertion (usually represented by the ligamentum arteriosum) with the aorta.

Externally, at the site of the obstruction, there is an indentation of the superior wall of the aorta. Internally, this site corresponds to a curtain-like protrusion of the aortic media toward the lumen. The curtain extends from the anterior, superior, and posterior walls of the aorta but not from the inferior aspect, the latter being the site into which the ductus inserts. The position of the medial curtain causes the narrowed aortic lumen to lie eccentrically near the inferior wall (Fig. 7–15).[24]

Beyond the obstruction, there is dilatation of the aorta (poststenotic dilatation). The subclavian arteries are wide, as these represent the major channels carrying blood from the proximal to the distal compartments of the aorta.[25] Dilatation and tortuosity of the internal mammary arteries represent part of the subclavian source of blood to the lower extremities. The ostia of the intercostal and lumbar arteries are wider than normal, and the LV is hypertrophied. A congenital bicuspid aortic valve is common, being present in at least 50 percent of cases.[26]

The source of collateral circulation depends principally on the subclavian arteries (Fig. 7–16).[25] These arteries supply two main systems, the anterior and the posterior. The anterior system mainly supplies the lower extremities via the internal mammary and superior and inferior epigastric arteries. The posterior system supplies blood to the thoracic aorta for ultimate supply to the abdominal viscera. The posterior system makes use of parascapular branches of the subclavian arteries. From parascapular arteries, the posterior segments of the intercostal arteries carry blood to the aorta for distribution to the abdominal viscera.

The anterior spinal artery may contribute to the collateral circulation. In coarctation, this vessel is enlarged and tortuous. It connects with arteries at levels both above and below the coarctation, including branches of the vertebral, intercostal, and lumbar arteries.

The potential complications of coarctation are numerous. These include changes in the commonly occurring congenital bicuspid aortic valve, such as calcific aortic stenosis, primary aortic valvular regurgitation, and infectious endocarditis.[3]

Various aortic complications include saccular aneurysm and aortic dissection.[27] The latter condition is confined to the compartment in which it begins. Usually, this is the proximal compartment, leading to the potential for obstruction of coronary arteries and of arteries arising from the aortic arch. External rupture leading to fatal hemopericardium is usual when a dissecting aneurysm originates in the proximal compartment.

In the aorta distal to the coarctation, infection may arise at the site of jet impact of the blood passing through the narrow segment. The infection may lead to a localized mycotic aneurysm. Rupture of the latter may cause hemorrhage into the left lung or left pleural space and, uncommonly, into the right pleural cavity.

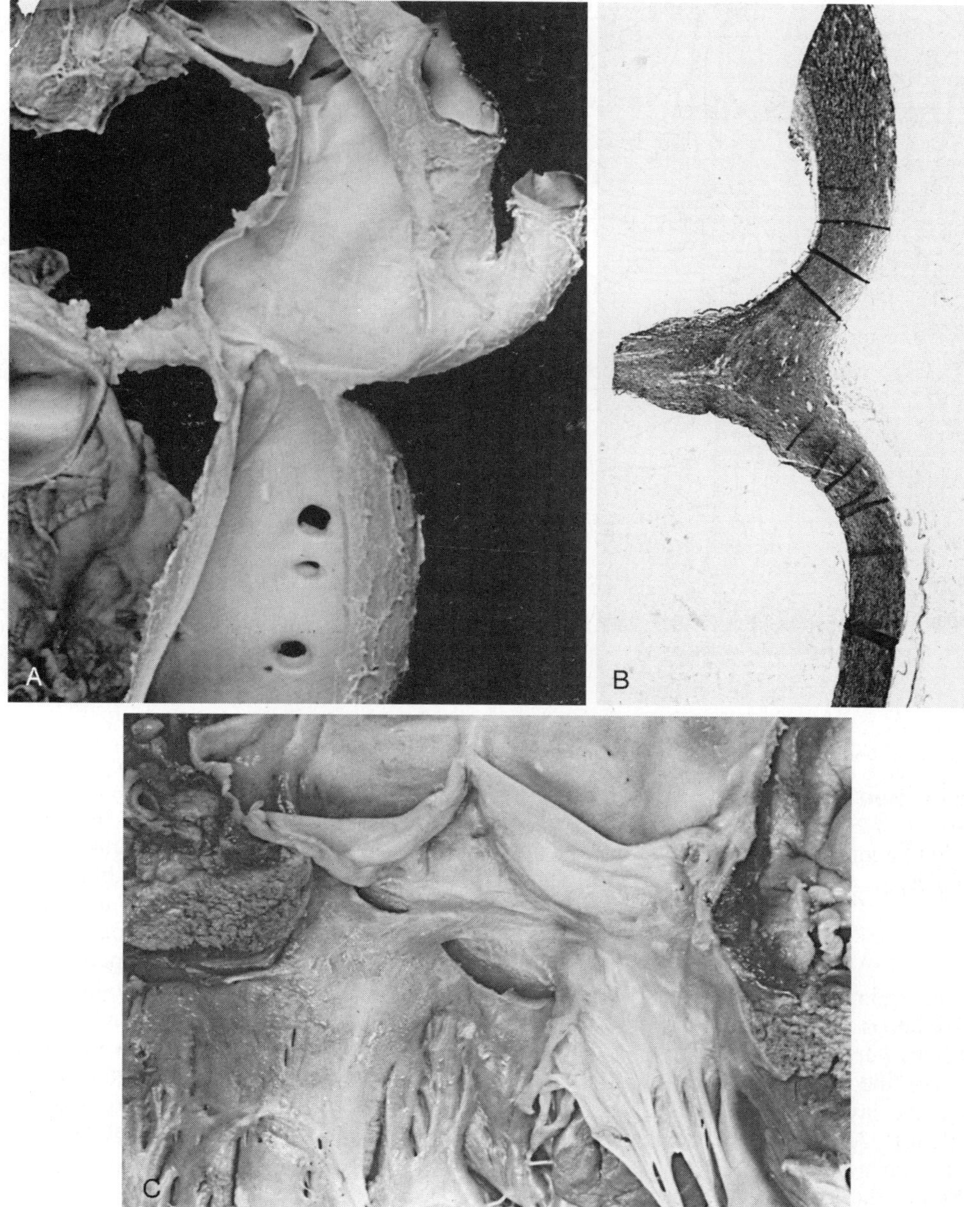

FIGURE 7–15 Coarctation of the aorta in a 20-year-old man who sustained fatal dissection of the ascending aorta, leading to hemopericardium. **A,** The junction of the aortic arch and upper descending aorta. At left is the site of the ligamentum arteriosum and left pulmonary artery. Opposite this, the exterior wall of the aorta shows a major indentation, which corresponds to protrusion of the wall into the lumen, causing the lumen to be eccentric and narrow. Poststenotic dilatation of the upper descending aorta is associated with dilated ostia of intercostal arteries. **B,** Low-power photomicrograph of the indentation and protrusion of the aortic wall characteristic of coarctation. Elastic tissue stain, ×5. **C,** The aortic valve is congenitally bicuspid. The incisions in the subjacent ventricular septum are artifacts.

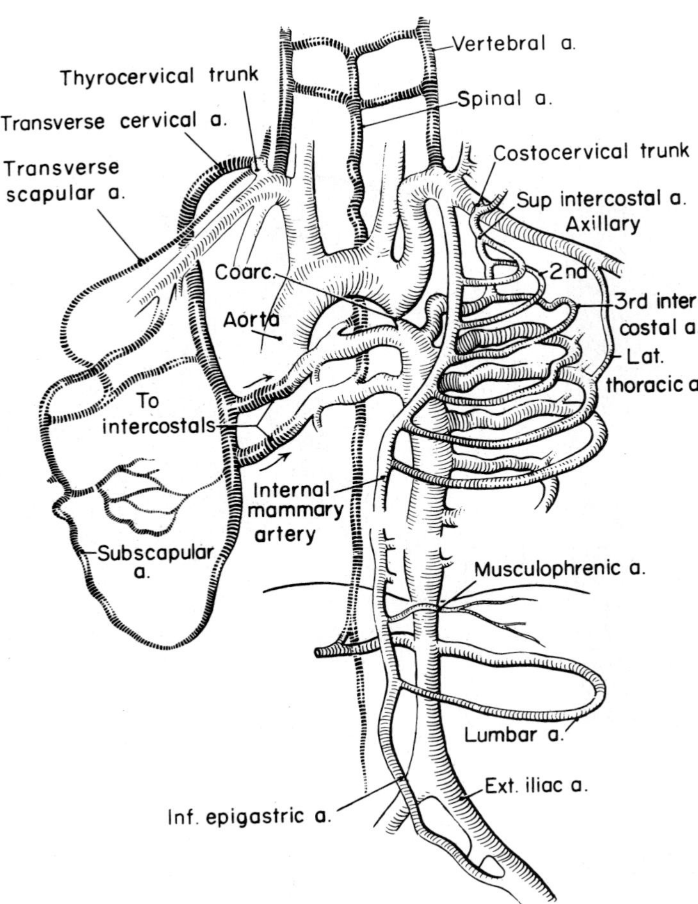

FIGURE 7–16 The collateral circulation in coarctation of the aorta. There are two major routes, the anterior and the posterior, each arising from the subclavian arteries. The anterior system is shown at right and the posterior system at left. The anterior system makes use of the internal mammary artery and the epigastric arteries, leading to flow to the external iliac artery for supply to the lower extremity. The posterior system is derived from collaterals in relation to subclavian branches lying in parascapular positions. These connect with posterior segments of the intercostal arteries for principal supply to the aorta. The anterior spinal artery extends across the level of the coarctation to connect the upper and lower compartments, and so to participate in collateral circulation. (Modified from Edwards JE, Clagett OT, Drake RL, et al: The collateral circulation in coarctation of the aorta. Proc Mayo Clin 23:333, 1948.)

Valvular Regurgitation

A variety of valvular anomalies may be associated with valvular incompetence.

Mitral Valve

Congenital mitral regurgitation in adults is most commonly caused by a myxomatous or prolapsed mitral valve.[28, 29] This condition is characterized by an increase in the midsubstance of the valve, the spongiosa. Excessive spongiosa invades the fibrosa, the layer that is most responsible for the strength of the leaflet. As the leaflets become weakened, interchordal prolapse occurs (Fig. 7–17), characterized by interchordal hooding of the leaflets.[29a] This feature may be responsible for mitral insufficiency. In the myxomatous mitral valve, other features causing regurgitation include an increase in the width of the orifice. Increase in length of the chordae may favor prolapse. A major cause for appearance or accentuation of mitral regurgitation is rupture of chordae. Although this may involve chordae attaching to either leaflet, the most common site involves chordae attaching to the central scallop of the posterior mitral leaflet. In this situation, the systolic regurgitant stream strikes the atrial septum at the same horizontal level as the aortic valve (Fig. 7–18).

It has been shown in mitral valve prolapse that friction between chordae of the posterior mitral leaflet may occur against the related mural endocardium of the LV.[30] The secondary effect is appearance of multiple fibrous thickenings of the mural endocardium. In some cases, the fibrous lesions may coalesce and bind to the chordae, shortening the chordae and leading to mitral regurgitation by restraining the upward excursion of the leaflets. Patients with mitral valve prolapse experience transient cerebral ischemic attacks, probably caused by emboli related to the valvular disease. One potential source is thrombosis on the contact surface of the leaflets. A second site is in the angle between the left atrial endocardium and the base of the atrial surface of the leaflets. Grossly, this yields a line of thrombosis (Fig. 7–19). In mitral valve prolapse associated with calcification of the mitral annulus, the latter process may be accentuated.

Mitral valve prolapse is associated with a tendency toward development of chronic obstructive pulmonary disease. Other sites of potential disease include the aortic and pulmonary valvular cusps and the aortic media. The latter may show cystic medial necrosis, a condition associated with widening of the thoracic aorta.

When mitral valve prolapse and changes in the aorta and aortic valves coexist, one of these is usually dominant and claims the primary diagnosis. Thus, one may observe primary mitral valve prolapse and associated (secondary) aortic and aortic valvular changes. Conversely, the aortic and aortic valvular changes may be primary, whereas the mitral valve prolapse occupies a secondary position.

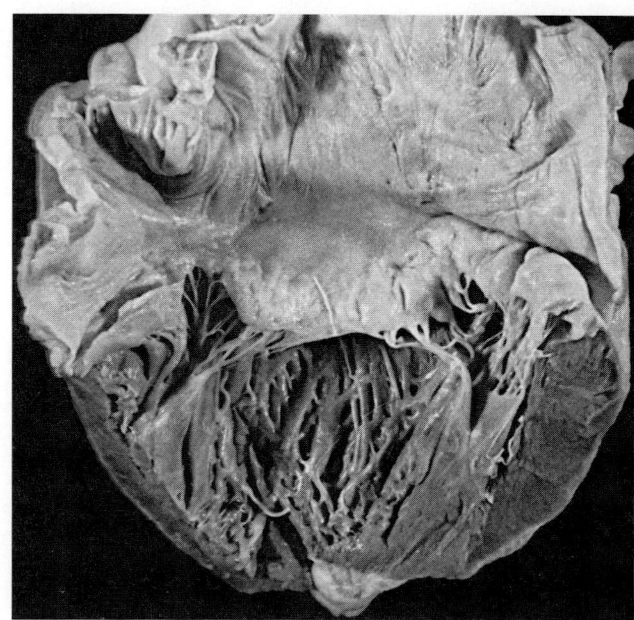

FIGURE 7–17 Mitral valve prolapse in the opened left side of the heart. At right, elements of the posterior mitral leaflet have prolapsed markedly toward the left atrium.

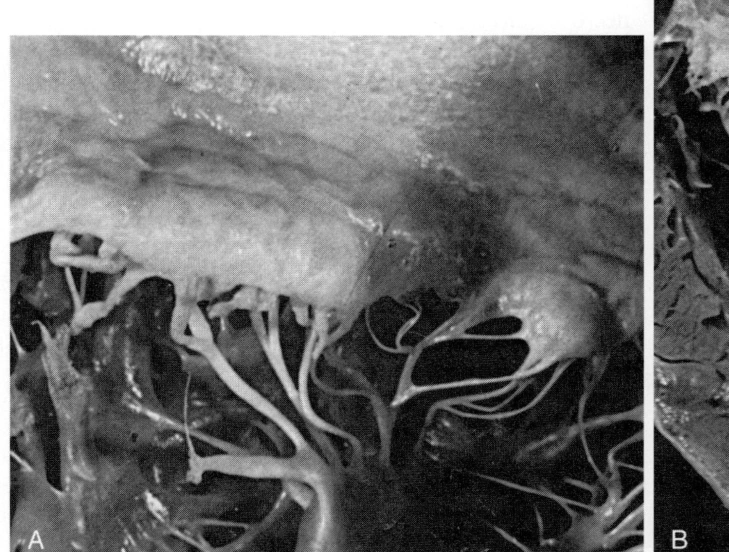

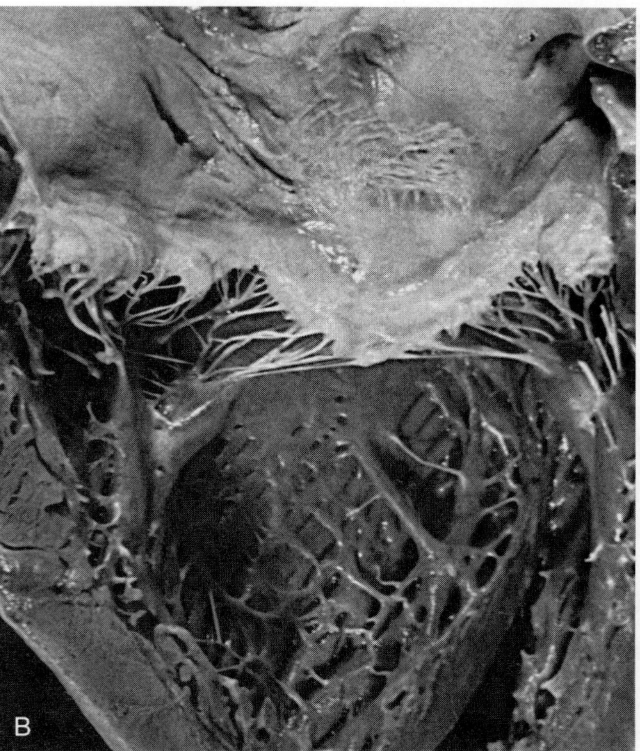

FIGURE 7–18 Mitral valve prolapse with ruptured chordae tendineae. **A,** Parts of the posterior mitral leaflet are shown. The larger of the two leaflets is the central scallop of the posterior leaflet with attached stumps of ruptured chordae. There is an upward deformity of the leaflet. **B,** Left atrium and left ventricle. In the septal wall of the left atrium are many curved endocardial elevations representing jet lesions caused by impact of the regurgitant stream, the latter resulting from the ruptured chordae shown in **A**. The aortic valve (not shown) lies on the opposite side of the atrial septum at the level of the jet lesions.

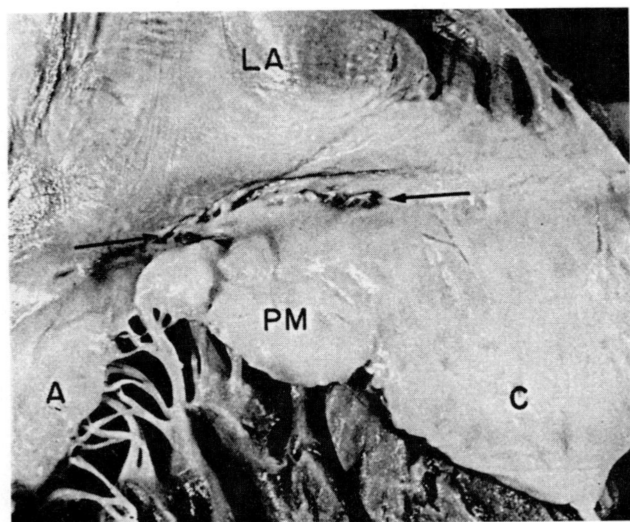

FIGURE 7–19 Left atrium (LA) and left ventricle from an adult with mitral valve prolapse. In the angle between the LA and the base of the posterior mitral leaflet (PM) is a linear deposit of thrombotic material (*arrows*). This is a so-called atrial valvular angle lesion from which the thrombotic material may serve as an embolic source for transient ischemic attacks. A, part of the anterior mitral leaflet; C, central scallop of the PM. (From Titus JL, Edwards JE: Mitral insufficiency other than rheumatic, ischemic, or infective; emphasis on mitral valve prolapse. Semin Thorac Cardiovasc Surg 1:118, 1989.)

Tricuspid Valve

The tricuspid valve may exhibit prolapse (Fig. 7–20). Usually, but not always, the process in the mitral valve is dominant. When chronic obstructive pulmonary disease is associated with tricuspid prolapse, the latter process may be more fully developed than when pulmonary disease is absent. The challenge of right ventricular hypertension tends to expose the valvular abnormalities when the potential for valvular prolapse exists.

Ebstein's malformation is characterized by downward displacement of elements of the valve (Fig. 7–21) (i.e., basal insertion of elements of the valve at a level below that of the annulus). The septal and posterior leaflets are most commonly involved. The abnormality causes some of the RV to be "atrialized." The functional disturbance is reduction in the effective volume of the cavity of the RV.[31] The anterior leaflet usually attaches normally and is large. During systole, the anterior leaflet prolapses toward the atrium, acting in a sense like an aneurysm and compounding the inefficiency of a basically small RV. Minor degrees of tricuspid regurgitation may contribute to the inefficiency of the RV. In the majority of cases, there is an interatrial communication, either an atrial septal defect (ASD) or a valvular competent patent foramen ovale, and therefore some right-to-left shunting. In patients who reach adulthood, a cerebral abscess may complicate the right-to-left shunt. Ebstein's malformation is commonly accompanied by accessory AV myocardial tracts.

Aortic Valve

Congenital aortic regurgitation may result from intrinsic disease of the aortic valve (primary regurgitation) or from disease of the ascending aorta with secondary changes in the aortic valve. Aortic regurgitation may also be associated with a ventricular septal defect (VSD).

Primary aortic valvular regurgitation is usually caused by a congenital bicuspid aortic valve. In this condition, the conjoined cusp is wider than the opposite single cusp. In some cases, however, the conjoined cusp is excessively wide and, during ventricular diastole, prolapses beyond the single cusp. The inappropriate contact allows regurgitation to occur (Fig. 7–22A).[3] Uncommonly, the characteristic raphe of the congenital bicuspid aortic valve is represented by a strand whose rupture may cause loss of support of the conjoined cusp and either establishment or accentuation of aortic regurgitation (see Fig. 7–22B).

The congenital bicuspid valve is subject to infectious endocarditis, which may be an indirect cause of valvular regurgitation through destruction of cuspid tissue (see Fig. 7–22C).

Abnormal width of the aorta caused by cystic medial necrosis, either idiopathic[32] or associated with arachnodactyly (Marfan syndrome),[33] may be a primary basis for aortic regurgitation. In many such cases, the aorta has an intimal-medial tear in its ascending portion. Such a tear may be stable and without extension, but it can also progress to the beginning of an intramural tract of aortic dissection. Aortic valvular regurgitation caused by aortic laceration results from loss of support of aortic cuspid tissue in relation to one or more valvular commissures. Commissural prolapse is an important mechanism that underlies aortic regurgitation.

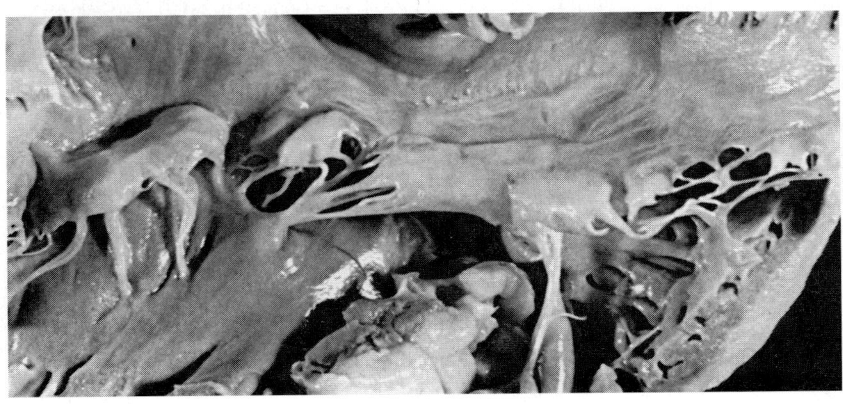

FIGURE 7–20 Tricuspid valve. Several units of the septal and anterior leaflets show interchordal hooding, characteristic of tricuspid valve prolapse.

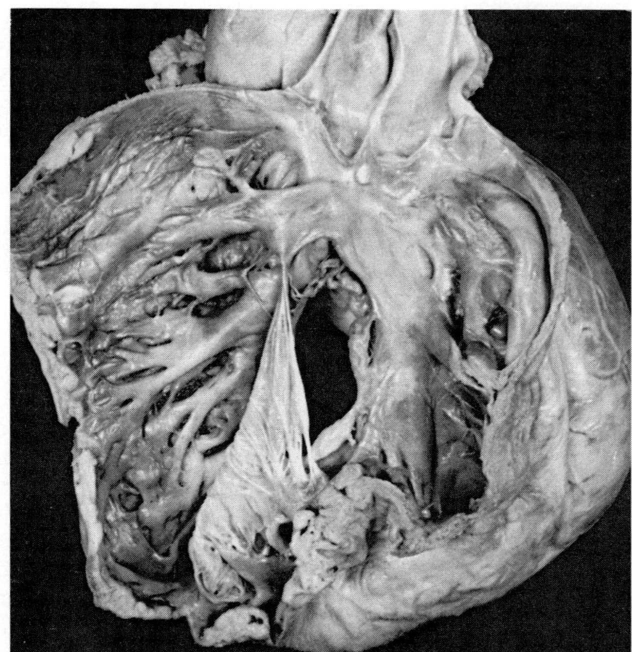

FIGURE 7–21 Ebstein's malformation of the tricuspid valve is shown in this view of the opened right ventricle, pulmonary valve, and pulmonary artery. The right ventricular wall is thin. The large leaflet represents the anterior leaflet, characteristic of this condition. The downward displacement of the septal and posterior leaflets is not seen in this perspective.

Aortic regurgitation may be associated with a VSD (Fig. 7–23). The most common defect is of the supracristal type, lying beneath the left and right aortic cusps.[34] Less commonly, the VSD is of the infracristal type. The basic reason for the aortic regurgitation is that the portion of the aortic root related to the VSD is unsupported. This allows the involved part of the aorta to move out of line from its normal position, causing a "tipping" of the related cusp or cusps. The consequence of the tipping is malalignment of the cusps, resulting in incompetence of the valve.

Pulmonary Valve

Congenital pulmonary valvular regurgitation is usually associated with so-called absence of the pulmonary valve: the pulmonary valve either is truly absent or is represented by hypoplastic units of valvular tissue. In some instances, there are no other associated anomalies. In a rare case reported by Pouget and associates[35] in a 73-year-old patient with an intact ventricular septum, absence of the pulmonary valve was a surprising finding. Most cases exhibit features of tetralogy of Fallot with mild infundibular stenosis. Untreated congenital pulmonary valvular insufficiency usually does not allow survival to adulthood.

In cases of pulmonary stenosis, atresia with intact ventricular septum, or tetralogy of Fallot surgically treated to overcome obstruction, the consequence is an incompetent pulmonary valve. This does not usually constitute a problem, as the right ventricular hypertrophy resulting from the underlying condition serves to prevent significant regurgitation.

In congenital conditions, such as ASD, that result in major dilatation of the pulmonary artery and valve, the pulmonary artery tends to remain dilated and is a potential basis for pulmonary valvular regurgitation similar to that caused by major dilatation of the aorta. However, this potential is usually obviated by correction of the underlying condition.

Abnormal Communication Between the Chambers and/or the Great Arteries

Two categories of conditions fall under this heading, those in which the communication begins proximal to the AV valves and those in which it begins distal to these valves.

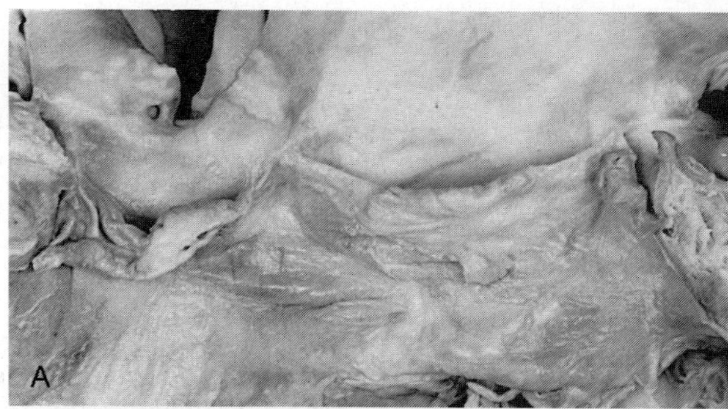

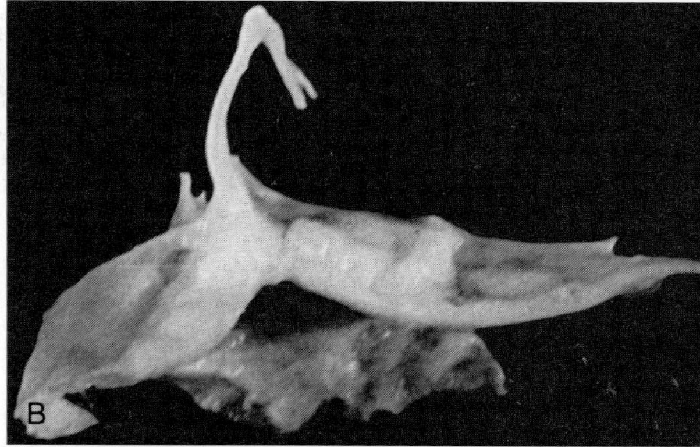

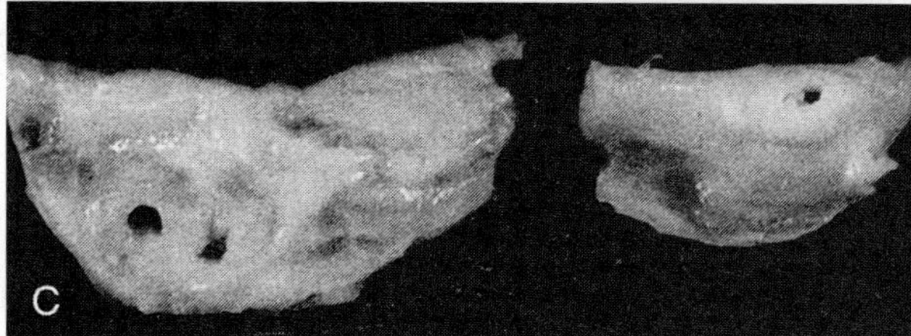

FIGURE 7–22 Congenital bicuspid aortic valve with aortic regurgitation. **A,** Autopsy specimen shows bicuspid aortic valve. The conjoined cusp has been incised. It lies in the right and left portions of the illustration. In the left portion, the raphe of the conjoined cusp is evident, as well as prolapse of that cusp. **B,** From a specimen removed at operation. A bicuspid aortic valve with a strandlike raphe is shown in the upper portion of the illustration. Rupture of this strand resulted in loss of support of the conjoined cusp, leading to aortic regurgitation. **C,** From a specimen removed at operation. Congenital bicuspid aortic valve is shown with perforations of now-healed infectious endocarditis.

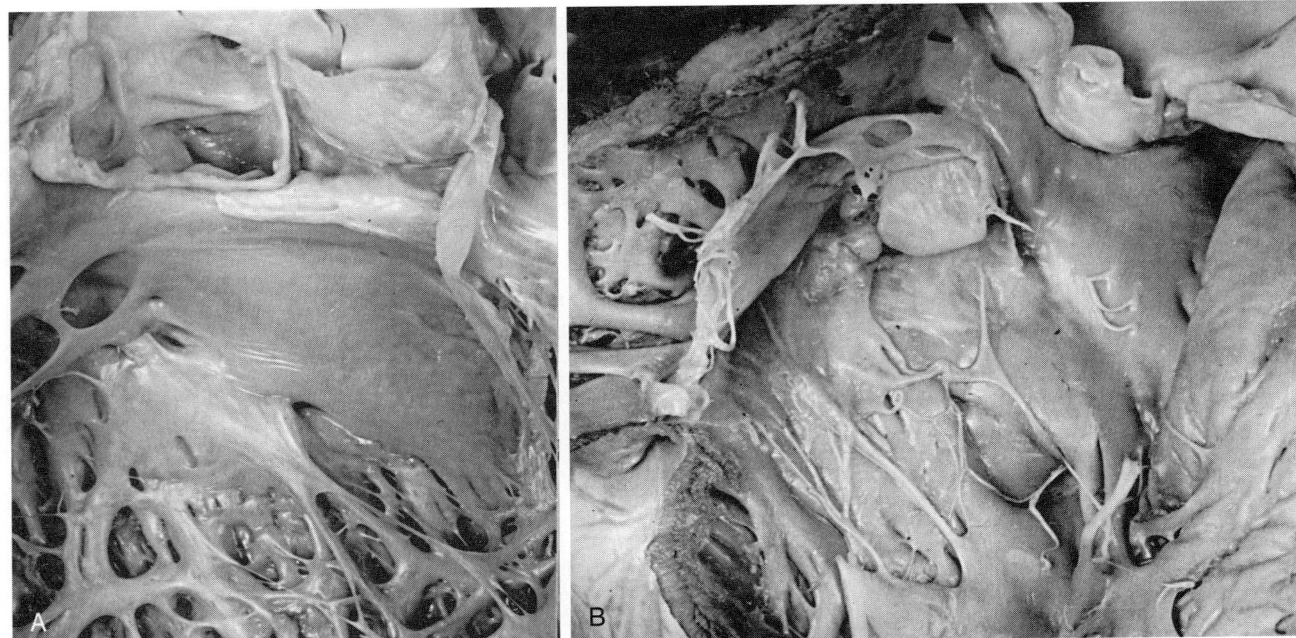

FIGURE 7–23 Ventricular septal defect and aortic insufficiency. **A,** The opened left ventricle reveals an opened bicuspid aortic valve. The conjoined cusp has prolapsed into a ventricular septal defect; the valve obscures the defect. **B,** Right ventricle and pulmonary valve. Under the septal leaflet of the tricuspid valve is a dome representing the fundus of the protruded conjoined cusp of the bicuspid aortic valve seen in **A**.

Proximal to Atrioventricular Valves

Of the communications that begin proximal to the AV valves, the most common is ASD. Less common are various types of anomalous pulmonary venous connections. Although anomalous pulmonary venous connections resemble ASDs in many respects, they are considered in a separate section.

ATRIAL SEPTAL DEFECTS

Different types of ASDs that allow patients to reach adulthood have been described. Included in these are the common defect at the fossa ovalis (so-called secundum type) and the less common sinus venosus type. The latter defect lies near the entrance of the SVC and is associated with anomalous pulmonary venous connection from the right lung.

Defects in the lowermost part of the atrial septum are of the ostium primum type. These are classically associated with either a cleft in the mitral valve or a common AV valve as examples of persistent common AV canal malformations.

In ASD, there is a tendency for large pulmonary flow to be associated with normal pulmonary arterial pressure for many years. In some patients, obstructive pulmonary vascular disease may develop, followed by pulmonary hypertension and right ventricular hypertrophy. The resulting right ventricular hypertrophy is responsible for a difference in the filling characteristics of the ventricles, leading to a basis for right-to-left shunting through the ASD. This complication tends to occur relatively early in adulthood, but usually not before the mid-30s.

The histologic features of the pulmonary vascular bed vary. In the stage of high flow–low pressure, the vascular bed is dilated. Early changes leading to obstructive disease are represented by intimal fibrous proliferation of the pulmonary arterioles. Medial hypertrophy of the muscular arteries follows. Ultimately, nonspecific fibrous proliferation and a plexiform lesion may develop. At this stage, right ventricular hypertrophy has become established. The resulting right-to-left shunt may be manifested by delayed cyanosis. Cerebral abscess, in concert with other states in which a chronic right-to-left shunt is associated, may complicate the course.

In cases of ASD with pulmonary hypertension, the wide right and left pulmonary arteries may become aneurysmal. At aneurysmal sites, laminated thrombi have a tendency to occur (Fig. 7–24).

In a study by Craig and Selzer[36] of patients ranging in age from 18 to over 60 years, the percentages of anatomic types of 112 ASDs were secundum type of defect, 85 percent; sinus venosus, 8 percent; and ostium primum, 6 percent. In one case, the atrial septum was absent. Significant pulmonary hypertension was noted in 22 percent of cases. This complication of ASD had a poor prognosis.

In 1970, Campbell[37] reported on the natural history of ASD. The intent was to work with patients having the fossa ovalis type of defect. Nevertheless, the author recognized that other types of ASD or partial anomalous pulmonary venous connection might have been included. The study showed that of the patients studied, about one fourth had died before 27 years, over half by 36 years, three fourths by 50 years, and 90 percent by 60 years of age. The mean age of death for all patients with ASD was 37.5 ± 4.5 years.

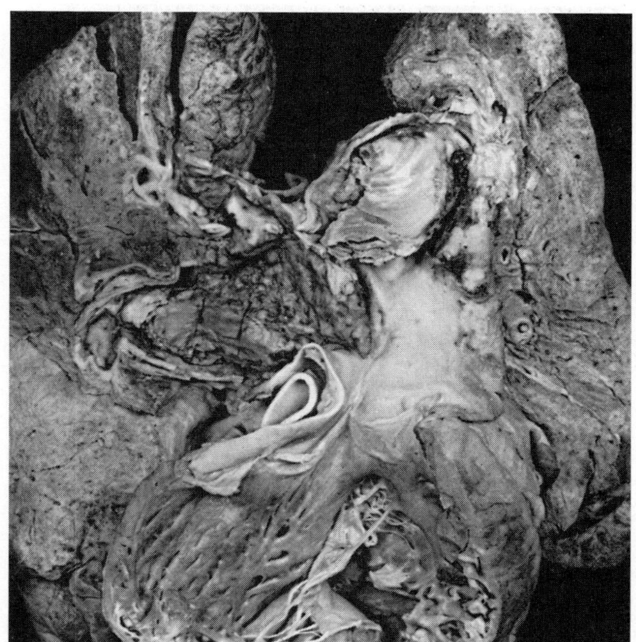

FIGURE 7–24 Right ventricle and major pulmonary arteries in atrial septal defect with pulmonary hypertension. There is aneurysmal dilatation of the pulmonary arteries, which now contain laminated thrombi.

Persistent patency with a competent valve of the foramen ovale throughout life may have functional consequences in certain circumstances. As indicated previously, about one third of the population will have a patent, competent foramen ovale. In such circumstances, the "valve," which is a derivative of septum primum of the developing heart and forms the floor of the fossa ovalis, is normally competent to functionally close the patent foramen ovale as long as postnatal interatrial pressure relationships are normal (i.e., left atrial pressure exceeds right atrial pressure). The potential exists for a right-to-left interatrial shunt through the patent foramen ovale if for any reason during the cardiac cycle, right atrial intracavitary pressure exceeds left atrial pressure and thus opens the "valve" of the foramen ovale. In addition, with anatomic patency of the foramen ovale, the valve may enlarge or appear to enlarge, creating an aneurysm of the fossa ovalis. With an aneurysm of the fossa ovalis related to a patent foramen ovale, the aneurysmal bulge may project toward the right or left atrial cavity with variations in interatrial pressures such as occur with normal respiration. In this situation, the interatrial shunt could be either left to right or right to left. If the shunt is from RA to LA, embolic material from systemic venous sources may cross the foramen ovale into the LA and thereby be distributed to the systemic arterial circulation as a paradoxical embolus. Such an event is recognized to be a cause of so-called cryptogenic ischemic stroke.[38–42, 42a]

Distal to Atrioventricular Valves

Among the abnormal communications beginning distal to the AV valves are VSD, patent ductus arteriosus, aorticopulmonary septal defect, persistent truncus arteriosus, double-outlet RV (origin of both great arteries from the RV), and single ventricle.

In these conditions, there are two principal groups. In one, the communication between the ventricles or the great arteries is narrow; in the other, the communication is wide or nonobstructive. The former category includes primarily the small VSD or the classic patent ductus arteriosus. When no obstruction is present between the two chambers or the arteries, the conditions include large VSD or wide ductus arteriosus, as well as the other conditions listed.

In cases of small VSD or classic patent ductus arteriosus, survival to adulthood is usual. The ventricular systolic pressures are different, and the left and right ventricular pressures are near normal, as is the volume of pulmonary flow. The pulmonary arterial pressure is not elevated. A jetlike stream occurs through a small VSD or classic patent ductus arteriosus. Infection may take place at the sites of impact of the jetlike stream, in the RV in VSD, and in the pulmonary artery in patent ductus arteriosus. The pulmonary vascular bed is within normal limits.

When there is a large VSD, a wide patent ductus arteriosus, or any of the other conditions with unobstructed communication between the ventricles and/or the great arteries, the pulmonary arterial pressure is elevated. The pulmonary and systemic systolic arterial pressures are equal. The pulmonary vascular bed is prone to a variety of obstructive lesions. Ultimately, grade IV of the Heath-Edwards classification may develop, establishing a basis for a right-to-left shunt (Fig. 7–25). In the group of anomalies under consideration, there is considerable variation among individuals. Therefore, although the majority of patients develop major obstructive pulmonary vascular lesions by adulthood, occasional adult patients do not have significant pulmonary vascular lesions and may exhibit different degrees, sometimes large, of left-to-right shunting.

A special condition to be considered is the complete variety of persistent common AV canal. In uncomplicated cases, survival beyond infancy or childhood is highly unusual. However, when this condition is associated with the tetralogy of Fallot, survival to adulthood is common because the tetralogy element introduces a factor of "natural pulmonary arterial banding." In this way, the element of unobstructed interventricular communication is overcome.[43]

The so-called congenital aortic sinus (sinus of Valsalva) aneurysm usually involves either the right or the posterior aortic sinus. The term *congenital,* as applied here, indicates that there may be a congenital weakness in the attachment between the aortic media and the cardiac skeleton. This allows slippage or avulsion of the aortic media from the cardiac skeleton.[44] The result is support of the aorta only by the wall of the RA or RV. An aneurysm then develops and may rupture, leading to a shunt from the aorta to either the RA or the RV (Fig. 7–26A and B). In the so-called congenital right aortic sinus aneurysm, a subvalvular VSD is commonly associated (see Fig. 7–26C and D).

Abnormal Connections

Another group of anomalies is characterized by arteries or veins abnormally joining certain vessels or chambers.

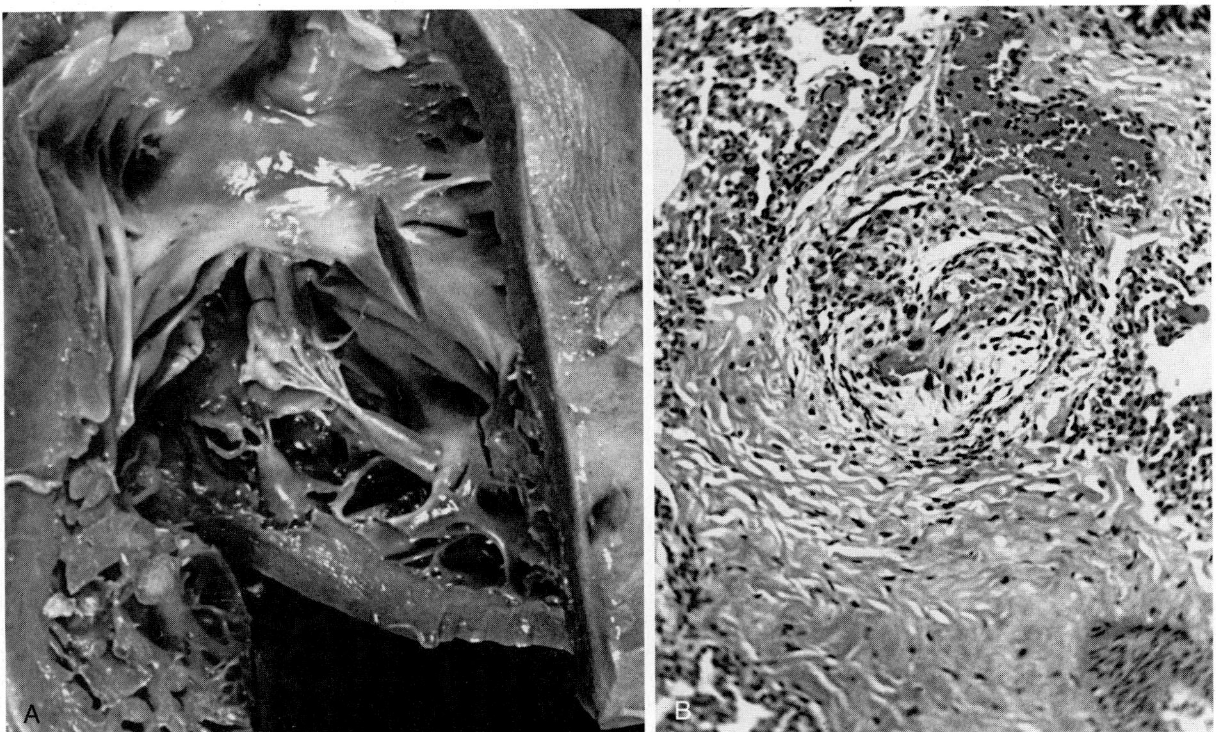

FIGURE 7–25 Previously closed ventricular septal defect in an adult. **A,** Right ventricle. The site of the previous closure is seen at center. **B,** Pulmonary artery shows a plexiform lesion of grade IV hypertensive (obstructive) pulmonary vascular disease.

Communication of a Coronary Artery With a Cardiac Chamber or a Major Thoracic Vessel

Communication of a coronary artery with a cardiac chamber or a major thoracic vessel not infrequently presents in adult life. Reviews by Sakakibara and colleagues[45] and by McNamara and Gross[46] showed that such fistulas beginning with the right coronary artery are more common than those beginning with the left coronary artery (Fig. 7–27).

In about 90 percent of cases, the anomalous termination is to the lesser circulation, usually the RV.[47] The artery proximal to the fistulous connection is wide. Distal to the fistula, the artery narrows precipitously. Localized aneurysm may involve the artery proximal to the fistula. Infectious endocarditis may complicate fistulas beginning with a coronary artery and has been observed in about 10 percent of patients with anomalous termination of a coronary artery.

Transposition or Malposition of the Great Arteries

The condition in which the great arteries join the "incorrect" ventricular chamber is termed *transposition.* Strictly speaking, this definition requires that there be two ventricles, with the aorta joining the anatomic RV and the pulmonary trunk joining the anatomic LV. The transposed aorta usually lies at an anterior level compared with the position of the pulmonary trunk. When there is a single ventricle or when the abnormally positioned great arteries join or arise from only one of two ventricles, the term *malposition of the great arteries* is sometimes used to avoid violation of the strict definition of transposition.

In single ventricle or so-called double-outlet RV, the great vessels are frequently malpositioned. Pulmonary stenosis may be present or absent. In either case, survival to adulthood is possible.

Complete Transposition

In classic complete transposition, the venous connections to the heart are normal. The great arteries are transposed so that the aorta arises from the RV and the pulmonary trunk from the LV. Left untreated, this common condition tends to cause death in early life. In rare cases, survival is longer. Today, cases have been reported in which one of several possible surgical procedures has enabled the patient to survive to adulthood.

Adult patients may have undergone an atrial "switch" operation, such as the Senning or Mustard procedure. Some of these patients may develop obstruction of the SVC or the channel of pulmonary venous flow into the heart. In addition, these operations are frequently followed by scarring of the RA wall and the sinoatrial node, of which the function may be altered.

Corrected Transposition

Corrected transposition is characterized by normal delivery of blood to the atria. The ventricles, however, are inverted, and the great arteries are transposed. *Ventricular inversion* is a condition in which the morphologic LV and RV are on the "wrong sides" of the heart, whereas the atria are normally positioned.

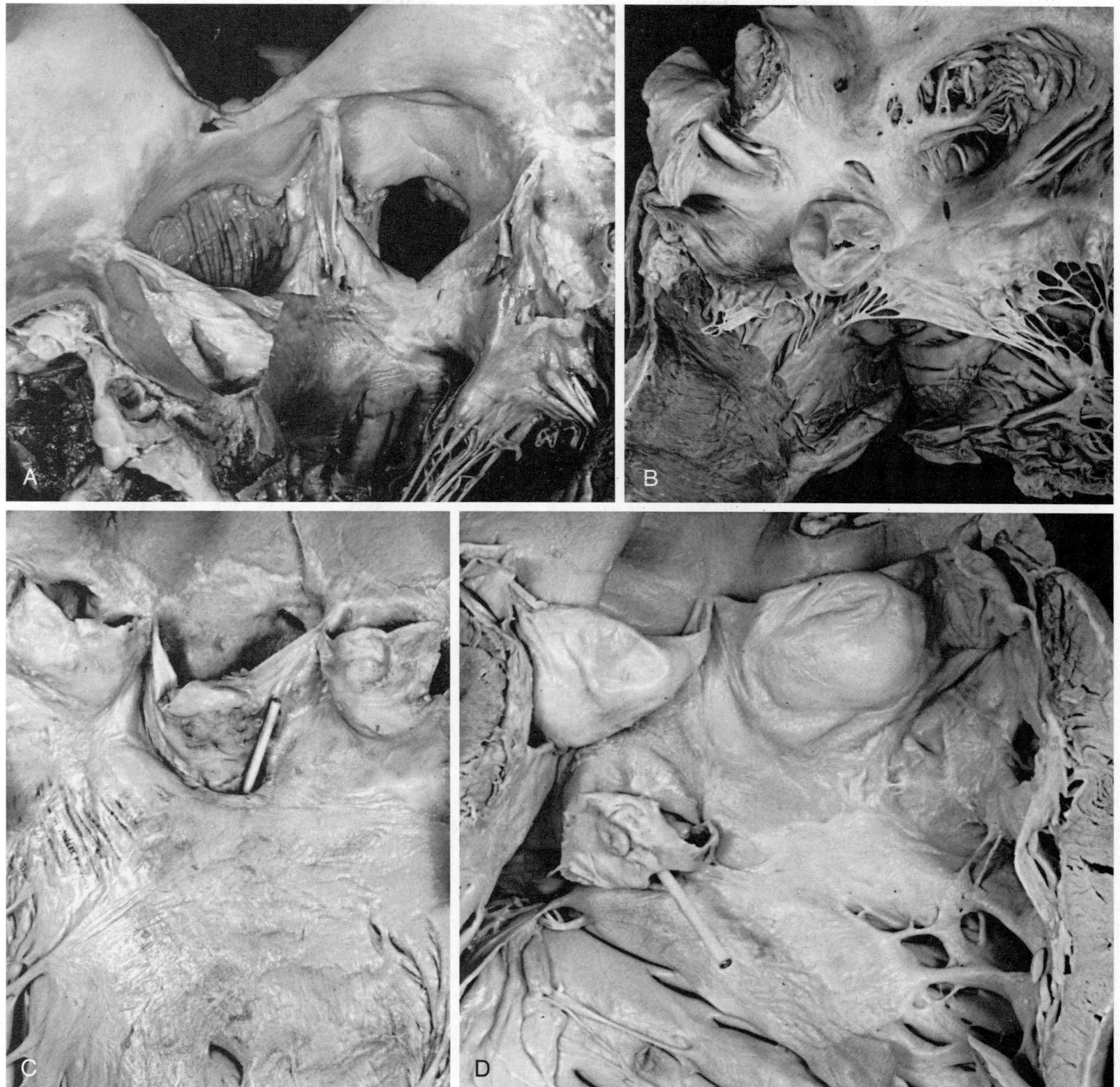

FIGURE 7–26 Congenital aortic sinus aneurysms. **A** and **B,** Aneurysm of the posterior aortic sinus. **A,** Mouth of the aneurysm of the posterior aortic sinus is represented by the dark circular depression at right of center. To the left of this is the right aortic sinus. The myocardium of the infundibular septum is exposed by avulsion of the aortic wall of this sinus, a state that precedes an aneurysm of the posterior aortic sinus. **B,** Right atrium and right ventricle. The domelike sac above the tricuspid valve is the aneurysm of the posterior aortic sinus shown in **A,** which has ruptured. **C** and **D,** Congenital aneurysm of the right aortic sinus. **C,** Left ventricle in a patient with aneurysm of the right aortic sinus and associated ventricular septal defect (probe), as is commonly the case with congenital aneurysm of the right aortic sinus. The aortic ostium of the aneurysm is obscured by the right aortic cusp. **D,** Pulmonary valve and outflow tract of right ventricle. The dome-shaped structure beneath the pulmonary valve represents the aneurysm of the right aortic sinus. One of the perforations of this structure contains a probe. The fundus of the aneurysm obscures the associated ventricular septal defect that lies beneath the pouch of the aneurysm.

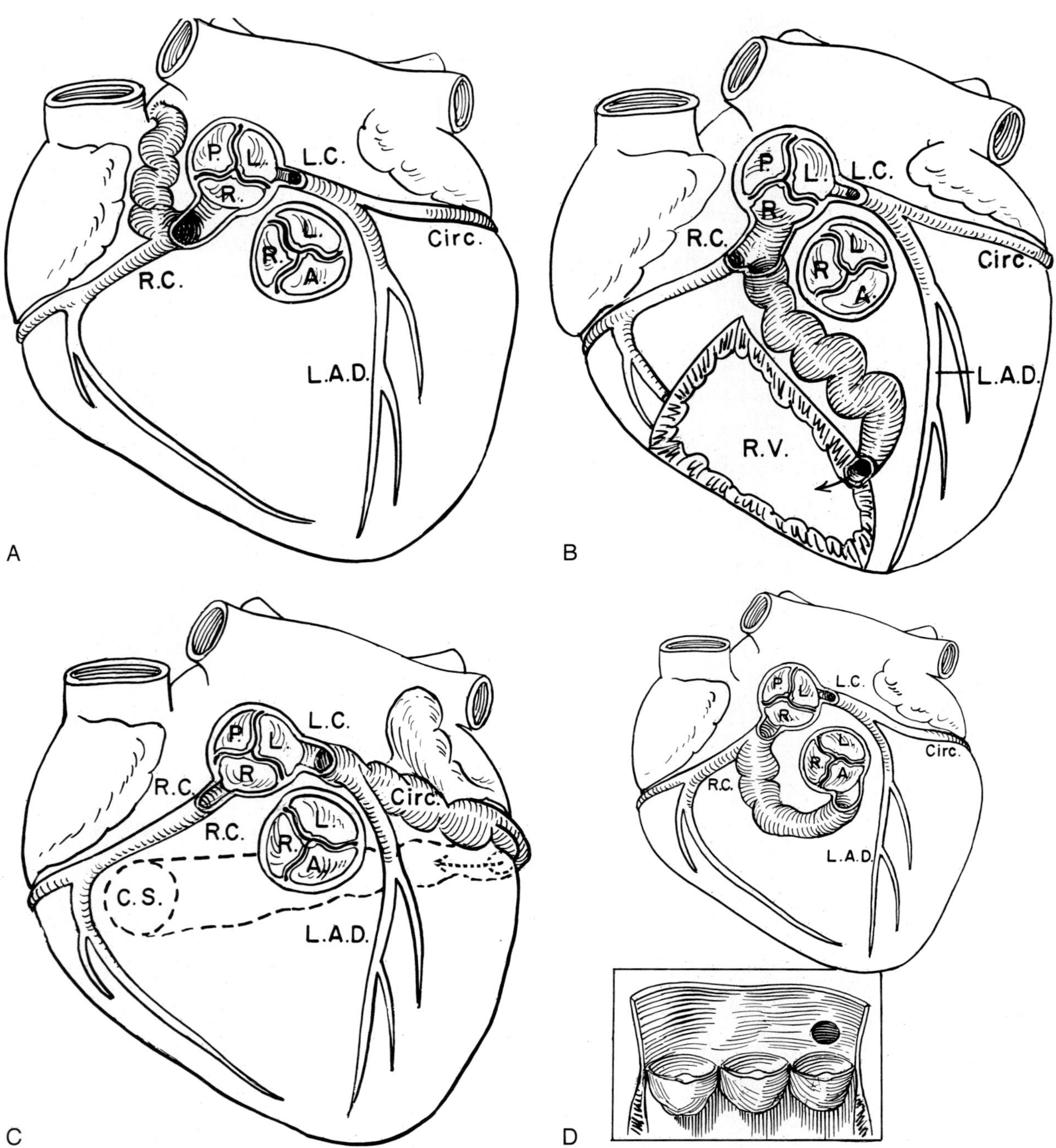

FIGURE 7–27 Examples of coronary arterial fistulas of various chambers or vessels. **A,** Right coronary artery (R.C.) to right atrium. A., anterior; Circ., circumflex coronary artery; L., left; L.A.D., left anterior descending coronary artery; L.C., main left coronary artery; P., posterior; R., right. **B,** Right coronary artery to right ventricle (R.V.). **C,** Left circumflex coronary artery to coronary sinus (C.S.). **D,** Right coronary artery to pulmonary trunk. *Insert* shows position of the ostium in the pulmonary trunk. (**A–D,** From Vlodaver Z, Neufeld HN, Edwards JE: Coronary Arterial Variations in the Normal Heart and in Congenital Heart Disease. New York, Academic, 1975.)

As a result of the two anomalies (ventricular inversion and transposition of the great arteries), the basic connections allow proper delivery of blood. Systemic venous blood is carried to the RA. From this chamber, blood flows into the right-sided, morphologic LV and thence into the transposed pulmonary trunk. Comparable connections on the left side allow pulmonary venous blood to be carried through a morphologic left-sided RV to the transposed aorta.

Without associated anomalies, corrected transposition may allow normal cardiac function.[48] In a case reported by Lieberson and coworkers,[49] the patient lived to the age of 73 years. However, it is rare for corrected transposition to be without associated anomalies.[50] If any are present, they determine the circulatory effect.

In adult patients with corrected transposition, associated conditions include VSD,[51] subpulmonary stenosis, either with intact ventricular septum[52] or with VSD, incompetence of the left-sided AV valve,[53] and congenital complete heart block.[50]

Anomalous Pulmonary Venous Connection

Anomalous pulmonary venous connection may be either total or partial. Total anomalous pulmonary venous connection in the adult is among the types in which the anomalous termination, with one exception, lies above the diaphragm. The common connections are with either the superior vena caval system or the coronary sinus (Fig. 7–28). To our knowledge, total anomalous termination into an infradiaphragmatic vein (usually a part of the portal system) has not been reported in adults.

Partial anomalous pulmonary venous connection may be either a random event or part of a syndrome. Partial anomalous connections do not always introduce a significant cardiovascular problem.

Random connections are exemplified by isolated cases in which a left or a right upper pulmonary vein joins the left innominate vein or the SVC, respectively.[54]

Partial anomalous connection of a right pulmonary vein or veins in association with the sinus venosus type of ASD forms a recognized syndrome. In this condition, anomalous termination of either the right upper or each of the right pulmonary veins occurs in the SVC or in the RA near the superior vena caval termination (Fig. 7–29).[55]

The one exception to cases of infradiaphragmatic connection of pulmonary veins in which patients survive to adulthood is termination of a vein from the right lung in the IVC,[55] either above or below the diaphragm (Fig. 7–30). This venous anomaly may be the sole condition or part of the so-called scimitar syndrome, reviewed by Kiely and associates.[56] In this syndrome, the right lung may lack one or two lobes. Usually, the venous drainage of the upper lobe of the right lung is to the LA. Bronchial anomalies are common, as described by Halasz and colleagues.[57] Anomalous arteries from the descending thoracic or abdominal aorta may supply the lower part of the right lung, but pulmonary sequestration, which commonly is

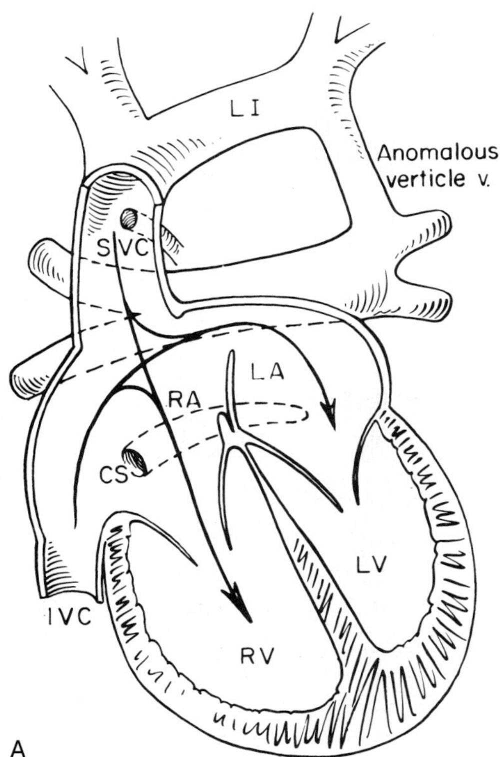

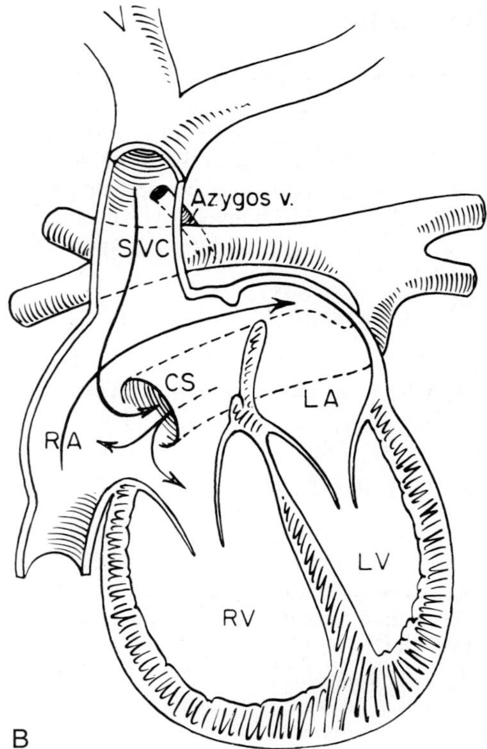

FIGURE 7–28 Total anomalous pulmonary venous connection in an adult. **A,** Termination of the pulmonary venous system in an anomalous vertical vein, which ends at the left innominate vein (LI). An atrial septal defect may be present. CS, coronary sinus; IVC, inferior vena cava; LA, left atrium; LV, left ventricle; RA, right atrium; RV, right ventricle; SVC, superior vena cava. **B,** Total anomalous pulmonary venous connection to the coronary sinus.

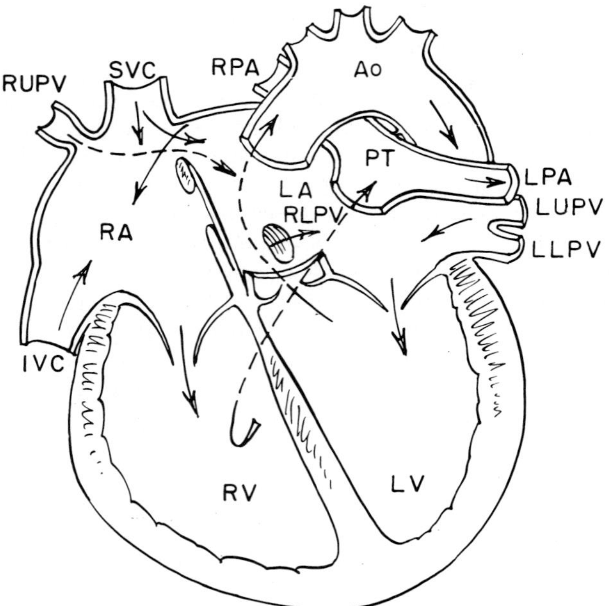

FIGURE 7–29 Sinus venosus type of atrial septal defect. The defect lies in the upper part of the septum and is straddled by the superior vena cava (SVC). Right pulmonary veins (in this instance, the right upper pulmonary vein [RUPV]) join the right atrium (RA) near the atrial septal defect. Ao, aorta; IVC, inferior vena cava; LA, left atrium; LLPV, left lower pulmonary vein; LPA, left pulmonary artery; LUPV, left upper pulmonary vein; LV, left ventricle; PT, pulmonary trunk; RLPV, right lower pulmonary vein; RPA, right pulmonary artery; RV, right ventricle.

associated with the latter arterial variation, is not part of the scimitar syndrome.

The *polysplenic syndrome* is usually characterized by fewer severe cardiovascular anomalies than the *asplenic syndrome,* so that survival to adulthood is more common in the former. Among the anomalies that may occur in the polysplenic syndrome is anomalous connection of pulmonary veins with the RA, which may involve either all of the pulmonary veins or only the right pulmonary veins.[58]

Anomalous Systemic Venous Connection

Major anomalous connections of systemic veins may involve the superior vena caval system, the inferior vena caval system, or both.

INFERIOR VENA CAVAL SYSTEM

Congenital union of the IVC with the LA is rare, although instances of this condition have been described. In a case reported by Gardner and Cole,[59] a cyanotic woman died at the age of 32 years. The atrial septum was intact, and the LA received the IVC. The SVC joined the RA and received a dilated azygos vein. A similar case, involving a 34-year-old cyanotic woman in whom an ASD was also present, was described by Gautam.[60] Black and coworkers[61] described the case of a cyanotic patient with intact atrial septum and termination of the IVC in the LA. Pulmonary arteriovenous fistulas were also present in this patient.

A syndrome is known in which, after repair of the usual type of ASD, the IVC terminates in the LA. This is the result of surgical misinterpretation of the edge of a large valve of the IVC as the posterior edge of an ASD. Sewing this valve to the anterior rim of the ASD not only closes the ASD but also results in the delivery of inferior vena caval blood into the LA.

SUPERIOR VENA CAVAL SYSTEM

Persistent left SVC is a relatively common condition. Classically, in this condition, there are two superior venae cavae. The right SVC joins the RA in the usual position, and the left SVC joins the coronary sinus, through which left superior vena caval blood enters the RA. In cases of this type, a "bridging innominate" vein between the two superior vena cavae is present in about 60 percent of patients.[62]

Among the variations of this condition is that in which the right SVC fails to join the RA. Instead, the right SVC crosses the midline to terminate in a left SVC. The latter then joins the coronary sinus.[63]

A separate condition is that in which the left SVC joins the LA. The site of union is near the base of the left atrial appendage. This condition has been recognized as part of a syndrome[64] in which additional features are the absence of the coronary sinus and the presence of an ASD at the

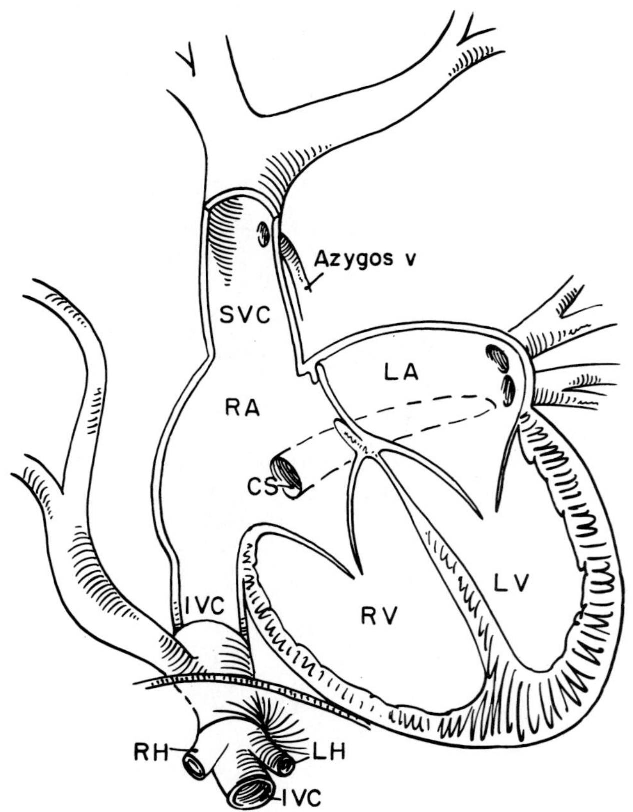

FIGURE 7–30 Anomalous termination of the right lower pulmonary vein in the inferior vena cava (IVC). The termination may be either above, as shown, or below the diaphragm. CS, coronary sinus; LA, left atrium; LH, left hepatic vein; LV, left ventricle; RA, right atrium; RH, right hepatic vein; RV, right ventricle; SVC, superior vena cava.

anticipated location of the coronary sinus ostium. This syndrome may appear as an isolated entity or may be associated with persistent common AV canal (endocardial cushion malformation).

INFERIOR AND SUPERIOR VENAE CAVAE

Interruption of inferior vena cava is a term sometimes used as a synonym for *azygos continuity with inferior vena cava.* In this condition, the IVC just superior to the union of the renal veins deviates toward the right and becomes continuous with the azygos vein. The latter is wide and joins the SVC. The IVC does not have its usual relationship with the liver because the hepatic veins do not join the IVC (Fig. 7–31). Instead, the right and left hepatic veins join to form a common hepatic vein, which passes through the diaphragm at the position of the inferior vena caval ostium and terminates in the RA at the usual site of entrance of the IVC (see Fig. 7–31A).

Continuity of the IVC with the azygos vein is usually, but not always, a part of the polysplenic syndrome. The IVC may be left-sided and join the hemiazygos vein,[65] which leads into a persistent left SVC. The inferior vena caval blood carried into this vessel is delivered to the RA through the coronary sinus (see Fig. 7–31B).

Union of both cavae with the LA is very rare (Fig. 7–32). In a case reported by Gueron and associates[66] involving an extremely cyanotic 15-year-old boy, this condition was associated with an ASD and a hypoplastic RA. Removal of the atrial septum, followed by insertion of an appropriately placed septum of pericardial tissue, resulted in cure.

A case reported by Miller and colleagues[67] was similar to that of Gueron and associates, with the exceptions that the coronary sinus drained into the LA and the left rather than the right SVC drained into the LA. Repair was essentially similar in both cases.

Arteriovenous Fistulas

Congenital arteriovenous fistulas may involve either the systemic or the pulmonary vascular bed.

PULMONARY ARTERIOVENOUS FISTULA

Congenital pulmonary arteriovenous fistulas may be either solitary or multiple. In the latter instance, the condition may involve one or more than one lobe. The individual

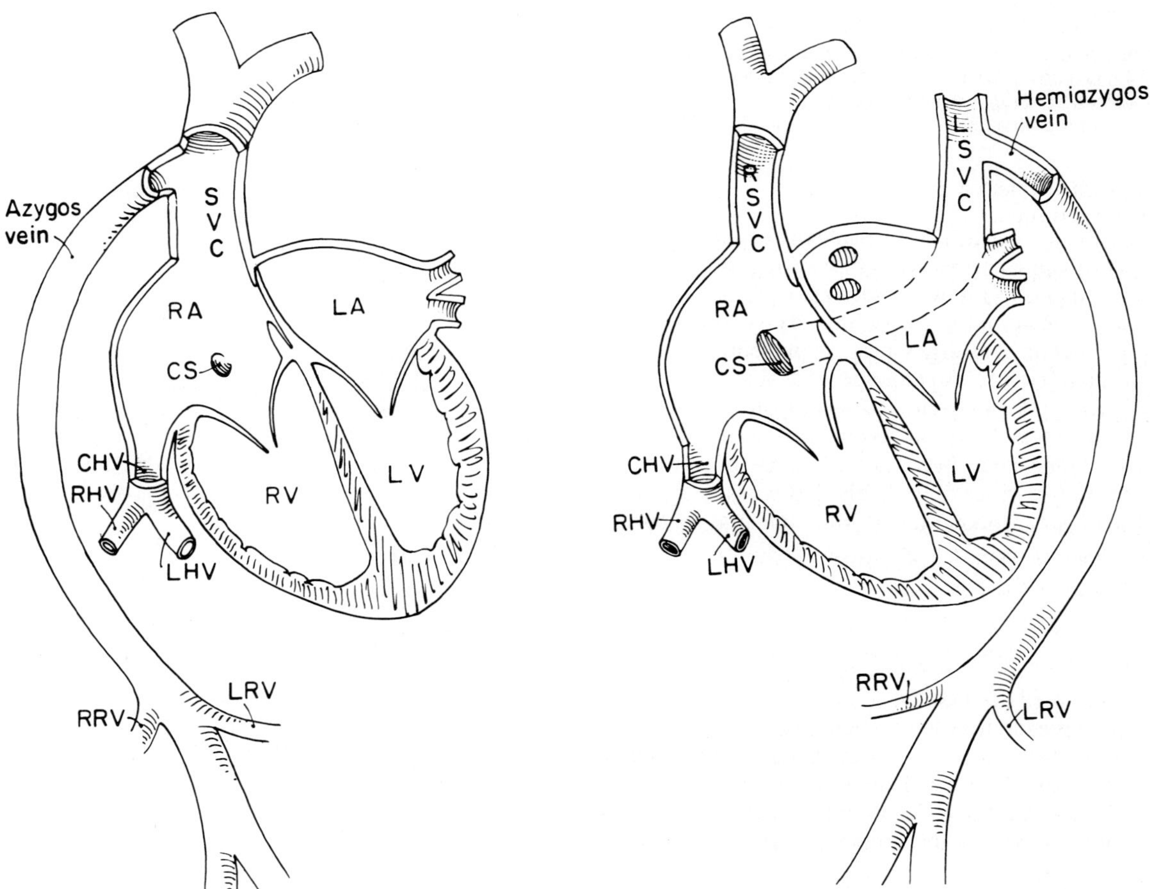

FIGURE 7–31 Azygos continuity of the inferior vena cava with the azygos or hemiazygos systems. **A,** Inferior vena cava to the azygos vein. CHV, common hepatic vein; CS, coronary sinus; LA, left atrium; LHV, left hepatic vein; LRV, left renal vein; LV, left ventricle; RA, right atrium; RHV, right hepatic vein; RRV, right renal vein; RV, right ventricle; SVC, superior vena cava; **B,** Inferior vena cava joins the hemiazygos vein that, in turn, leads into a persistent left superior vena cava (LSVC) for ultimate delivery of blood to the right atrium via the coronary sinus. RSVC, right superior vena cava.

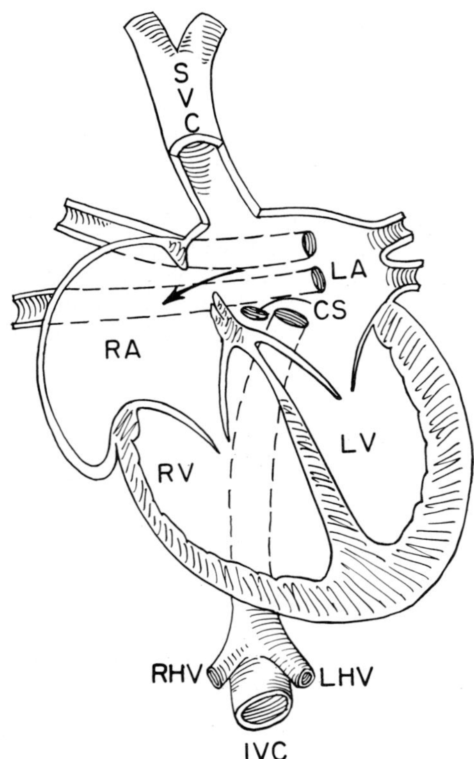

FIGURE 7–32 Termination of the superior (SVC) and inferior (IVC) venae cavae and coronary sinus (CS) in the left atrium (LA), with associated atrial septal defect. LHV, left hepatic vein; LV, left ventricle; RA, right atrium; RHV, right hepatic vein; RV, right ventricle.

lesion is usually characterized by a plexus of intercommunicating arteries and veins within the lung (Fig. 7–33). Because the condition allows desaturated pulmonary arterial blood to be delivered to the pulmonary venous system, cyanosis and clubbing of digits may be evident, depending on the volume of shunt. The condition has a strong hereditary association.[68, 69] The familial Rendu-Osler-Weber syndrome with telangiectasia involving various organs and mucous membranes has been described as occurring in about 35 percent of cases.[70, 71] Cerebral abscess is a potential complication.[72] Uncommonly, infection may occur at the fistula site.[73]

SYSTEMIC ARTERIOVENOUS FISTULA

Congenital arteriovenous fistulas in the coronary system have been discussed previously.

Extracardiac systemic arteriovenous fistulas may occur in any part of the systemic circulation. Those involving the cerebral circulation are usually covered in treatises concerned with intracranial conditions. Other congenital systemic arteriovenous fistulas may involve any part of the body.

A study by Gomes and Bernatz[74] reported on 139 congenital arteriovenous fistulas, excluding those that were intracranially located. In the study were 47 cases of congenital pulmonary arteriovenous fistulas. Among the 92 cases of congenital systemic arteriovenous fistulas, the most common location was in the extremities (80 cases), mainly the lower extremities. The other locations were the face and neck (11 cases) and the pelvis (1 case).

Multiple arteries commonly supply the area of arterial and venous connections. The main arterial trunks are dilated. When an extremity is involved, greater length of that extremity is characteristic. Infectious endophlebitis is a recognized complication.

Combinations of Anomalies

Almost any combination of anomalies is possible. The random association of some anomalies with others has been discussed previously. This section considers primarily the combination of VSD with pulmonary stenosis or atresia. The majority of these conditions are associated with biventricular origin of the aorta and right ventricular hypertrophy, constituting the well-known tetralogy of Fallot. In each case, there is obstruction to pulmonary flow, either atresia or stenosis, at some level or levels between the RV and the pulmonary arterial system. If the pulmonary arteries are identifiable when atresia exists, the condition commonly is called tetralogy of Fallot with atresia or *pseudotruncus arteriosus*. In other instances, the usual major pulmonary arteries either are absent or are represented by atretic cords. Among these, there are major variations in supply of blood to the lung. The cases have variously been classified as pulmonary atresia, solitary aortic trunk, or truncus arteriosus type IV.

Tetralogy of Fallot

In the adult, the tetralogy of Fallot displays the same range of anatomic detail as in the infant or child (Fig. 7–34). The

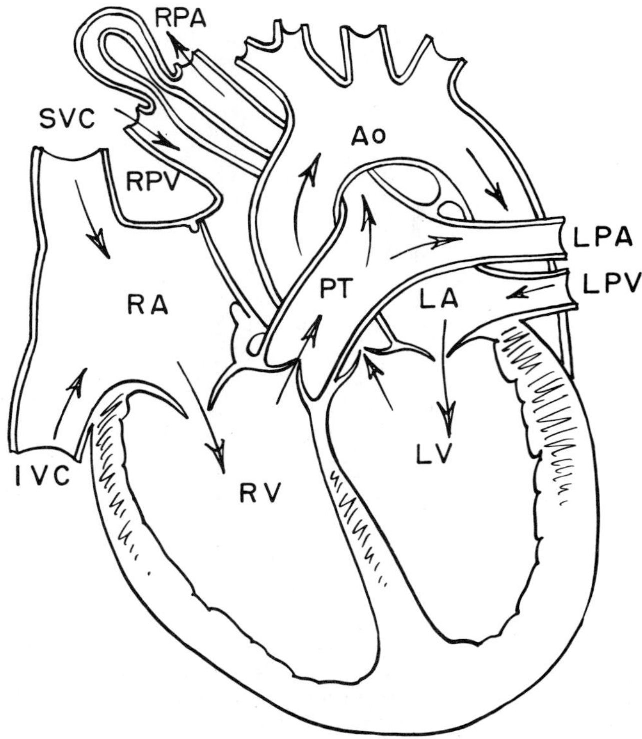

FIGURE 7–33 Pulmonary arteriovenous fistula in the right lung. Abbreviations as in Figs. 7–28 to 7–30.

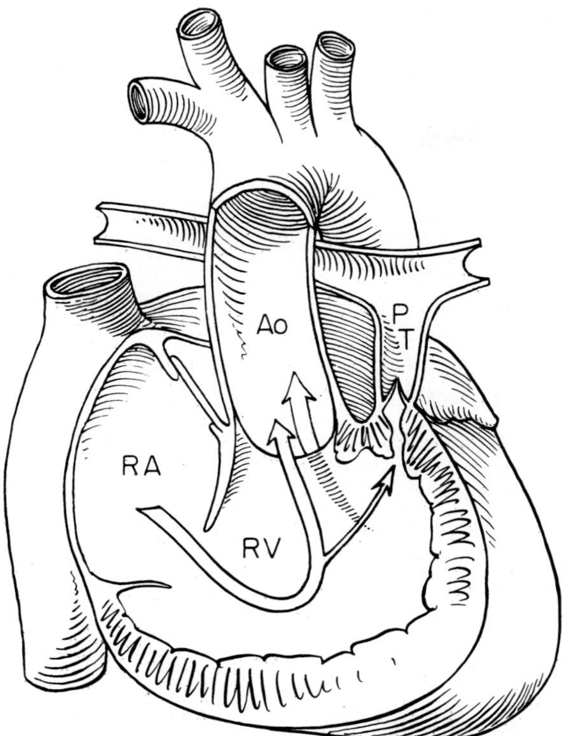

FIGURE 7–34 Classic example of tetralogy of Fallot, exhibiting biventricular origin of the aorta, ventricular septal defect, right ventricular hypertrophy, and obstruction to pulmonary flow. Abbreviations as in Figs. 7–28 to 7–30.

origin of the aorta from the ventricles varies in its degree from each ventricle, and there is also variation in degree of pulmonary stenosis.

When the major part of the aortic origin is primarily from the RV, the condition might be considered as part of double-outlet RV. In our view, however, if there is fibrous continuity of the aortic origin with the mitral valve, we prefer to designate the case as *tetralogy of Fallot with dominant origin of the aorta from the RV* (Fig. 7–35).

The degree of pulmonary stenosis varies, and in some instances, atresia may be present at some level of the pulmonary arterial channel (Fig. 7–36). An interesting point is that patient survival is not directly related to the width of the pulmonary arterial channel. The degree of collateral flow plays a role in determining survival,[75] so that there are instances of major degrees of pulmonary obstruction with long survival.

Solitary Arterial Trunk

An extreme in the level of pulmonary arterial obstruction is that in which the pulmonary trunk is not identifiable. There is a VSD, above which the aorta arises from both ventricles (Fig. 7–37).

Usually, wide collateral channels arise from the aorta, principally the descending aorta, and proceed to the pulmonary hili.[75] This condition has been called *truncus arteriosus type IV.* A source for blood flow to the lungs may also be derived from the descending aorta or arch through so-called distal ductal channels. These represent the peripheral part of ducti. Their site of origin depends on the side of the aortic arch.[76] Distal ductal origin on the side of the aortic arch is represented by a vessel beginning at the anticipated site of ductal origin. From this, the vessel proceeds toward the hilus of the homolateral lung. The distal ductal channel joins a vessel at the pulmonary hilus that is considered to be the true pulmonary artery of that side.

When the distal ductal origin occurs on the side contralateral to the aortic arch, the vessel arises from the base of

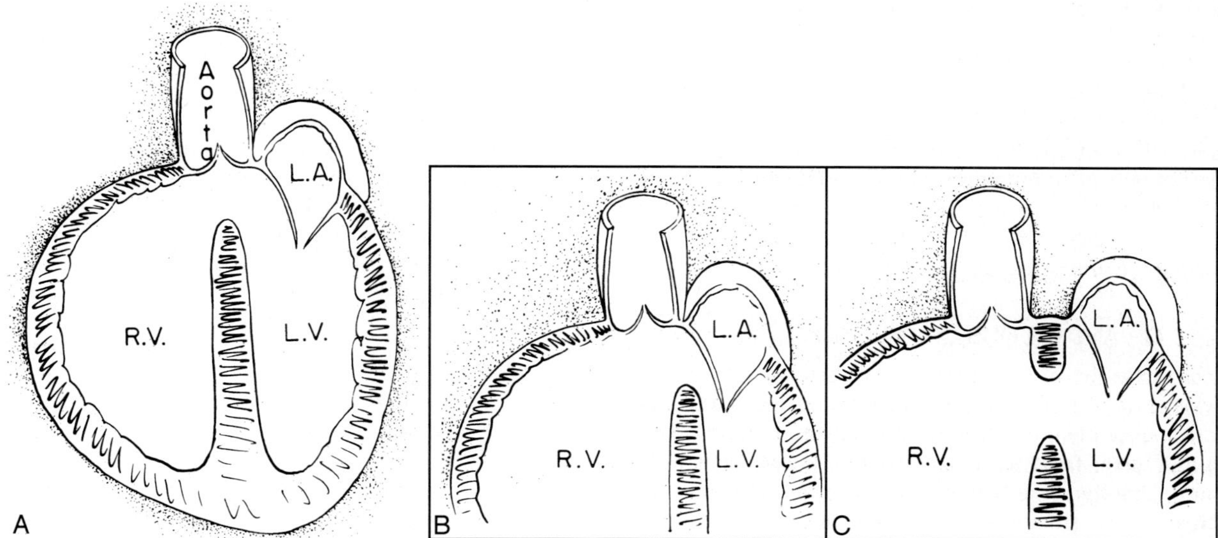

FIGURE 7–35 Variations in relation of the aortic origin to the ventricular septum. **A,** Classic example of biventricular origin of the aorta in tetralogy of Fallot. There is aortic and mitral valve continuity. The aortic origin from each ventricle is about equal. L.A., left atrium; L.V., left ventricle; R.V., right ventricle. **B,** An extreme degree of right-sided position (dextroposition) of the aorta in tetralogy of Fallot. There is maintenance of continuity between the aortic and the mitral valves. **C,** The aorta arises from the right ventricle. There is no continuity between the aorta and the anterior mitral leaflet, yielding double-outlet right ventricle. Similarity of the aortic relationship in the two conditions shown in **B** and **C** is recognized, but they are not identical.

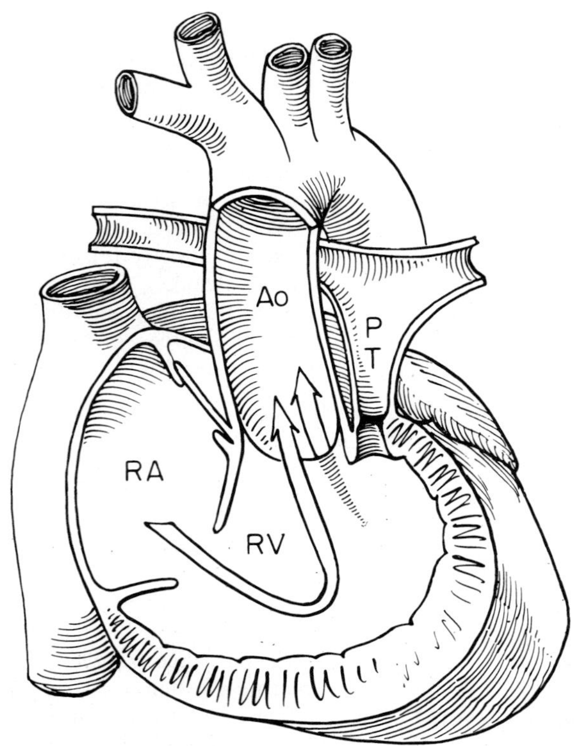

FIGURE 7–36 Tetralogy of Fallot with pulmonary atresia (pseudotruncus arteriosus). Ao, aorta; PT, pulmonary trunk; RA, right atrium; RV, right ventricle.

the homolateral subclavian artery and proceeds to the hilus of the lung on that side.

Abnormal Aortic and Arterial Branching

This section is concerned with variations in branching or origin of major arteries, including the coronary arteries and aorta.

Coronary Arteries

The anomalies of the coronary arteries considered here include ectopic or anomalous origin of a coronary artery from the aorta, coronary arterial dominance, and anomalous origin of a coronary artery from a pulmonary artery, usually the pulmonary trunk.[71a]

ECTOPIC OR ANOMALOUS ORIGIN FROM THE AORTA

In ectopic origin of a coronary artery from the aorta, the artery may arise from a "wrong" sinus of Valsalva (Fig. 7–38), may arise from an unusually high position, or may have an unusually acute angle of origin from the aorta.[77, 78] In each of these situations, the ectopically arising artery makes a flap as it leaves the aorta. This flap (ridge) may obstruct the coronary lumen during diastole. Sudden death, especially during exercise, has occurred in some individuals with ectopic origin of a coronary artery from the aorta. Among such are examples of origin of the right coronary artery from the left aortic sinus or origin of the left coronary artery from the right aortic sinus.

The most common type of ectopic origin is origin of the left circumflex coronary artery either from the proximal segment of the right coronary artery or from the right aortic sinus posterior to the normally situated origin of the right coronary artery. After origin of the left circumflex artery from either location, the artery classically courses along the posterior wall of the aorta. It then turns forward to reach the proximal segment of the left AV sulcus. Claims have been made that sudden death can be caused by this variation.

CORONARY ARTERIAL DOMINANCE

The artery that gives rise to the posterior descending artery is usually designated as the dominant coronary artery. In about 85 percent of the general population, the coronary arterial dominance is right-sided.

When a congenital bicuspid aortic valve is present, the dominance is left-sided in about 30 percent of cases.

ORIGIN OF A CORONARY ARTERY FROM THE PULMONARY ARTERY

Origin of a coronary artery from a pulmonary artery usually involves the left coronary artery. Uncommonly, both coronary arteries arise from the pulmonary trunk, a condition that leads to death in early infancy unless there is an associated condition characterized by pulmonary hypertension.

Usually, the pulmonary arterial segment from which the coronary artery arises is the pulmonary trunk, although rarely a coronary artery may arise from the right pulmonary artery. Origin of the right coronary artery from the pulmonary artery is less common than similar anomalous origin of the left coronary artery. When the right artery is affected, some patients exhibit no evidence of disease.[79] Nevertheless, there are reported cases of middle-aged persons in whom unexpected sudden death was associated with anomalous origin of the right coronary artery from the pulmonary trunk.

Origin of the left coronary artery from the pulmonary trunk is more than five times as common as origin of the right coronary artery from the pulmonary trunk. Untreated, the majority of individuals with anomalous origin of the left coronary artery from the pulmonary trunk die in infancy or childhood. The minority who survive to adulthood manifest major flow from the normally arising right artery through the myocardium and then into the left coronary artery, with the arteriovenous-like flow terminating in the pulmonary artery.[80]

Wesselhoeft and coworkers[81] reviewed 147 cases in which the left coronary artery arose from the pulmonary trunk. Of 11 patients aged 16 to 60 years, 9 died suddenly. The death was unexpected in 8 of these, 5 of whom died after some type of exertion. Wesselhoeft and coworkers[81] divided their cases into four clinical groups: infant syndrome, mitral insufficiency, continuous murmur syndrome, and sudden death in adults.

In the sudden death syndrome, several features were common. These included a large, tortuous right coronary

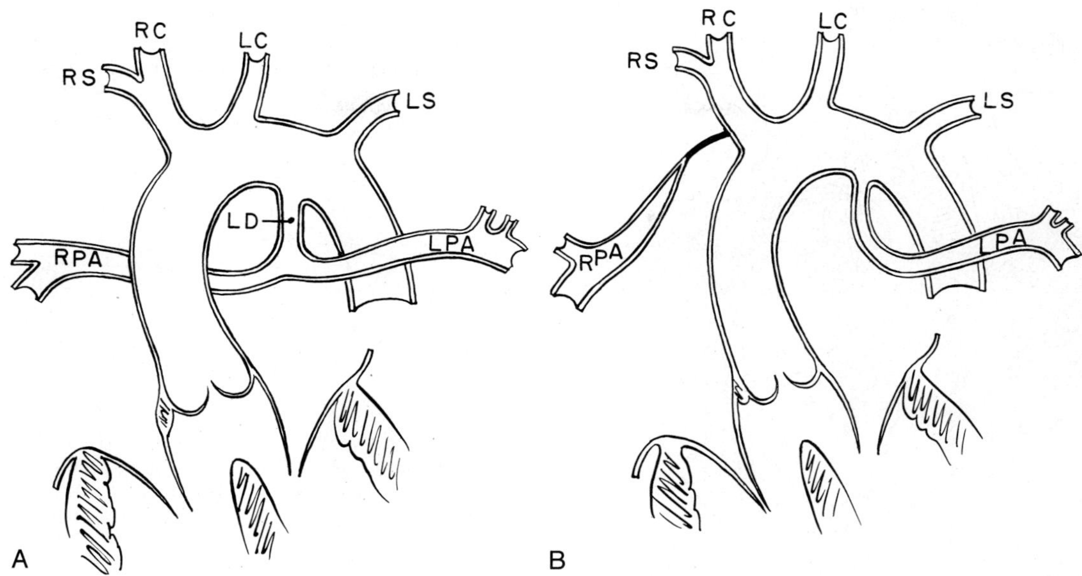

FIGURE 7–37 Variations in origin of pulmonary arteries. **A,** Left aortic arch. The pulmonary trunk and pulmonary valve are absent. The left ductus arteriosus (LD) feeds the confluence of the left and right pulmonary arteries (LPA and RPA). LC, left coronary artery; LS, left subclavian artery; RC, right coronary artery; RS, right subclavian artery. **B,** Left aortic arch with distal ductal origin of each pulmonary artery. The left ductus arises from the aortic arch, and the right ductus (atretic in this case) arises from the base of the innominate artery near the right subclavian artery. (**A** and **B,** From Sotomora RF, Edwards JE: Anatomic identification of so-called absent pulmonary artery. Circulation 57(3):624–633, 1978.)

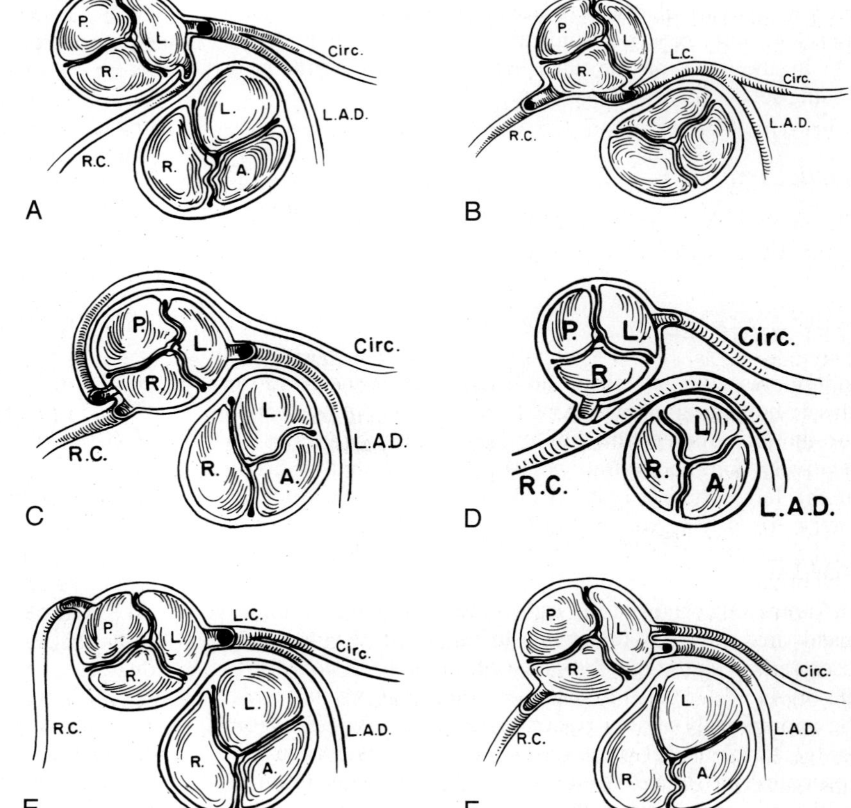

FIGURE 7–38 Ectopic origin of coronary arteries. **A,** Origin of the right coronary artery (R.C.) from the left aortic sinus. A., anterior; Circ., circumflex coronary artery; L., left; L.A.D., left anterior descending coronary artery; P., posterior; R., right. **B,** Origin of the left coronary artery (L.C.) from the right aortic sinus. **C,** Origin of the left circumflex coronary artery from the right aortic sinus. **D,** Origin of the left circumflex coronary artery from the left aortic sinus. A short coronary artery arising from the right aortic sinus bifurcates into the left anterior descending coronary artery and the right coronary artery. **E,** Origin of the right coronary artery from the noncoronary (posterior) aortic sinus. **F,** Independent origins of the left circumflex and anterior descending coronary arteries from the left aortic sinus. There is no true main left coronary artery. (**A–F,** From Mahowald JM, Blieden LC, Coe JI, et al: Ectopic origin of a coronary artery from the aorta. Sudden death in 3 of 23 patients. Chest 89:668, 1986.)

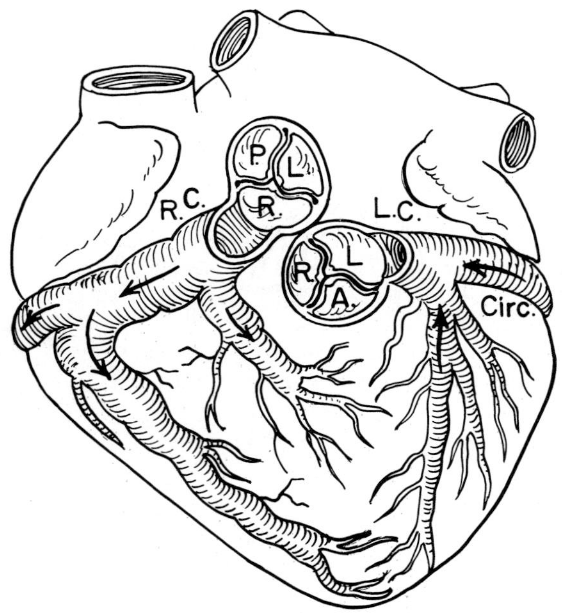

FIGURE 7–39 Origin of the left coronary artery (L.C.) from the pulmonary trunk in an adult. There is major collateral flow from the right coronary (R.C.) to the left, leading to significant widening of the major arterial trunks. A., anterior; Circ., circumflex coronary artery; L., left; P., posterior; R., right.

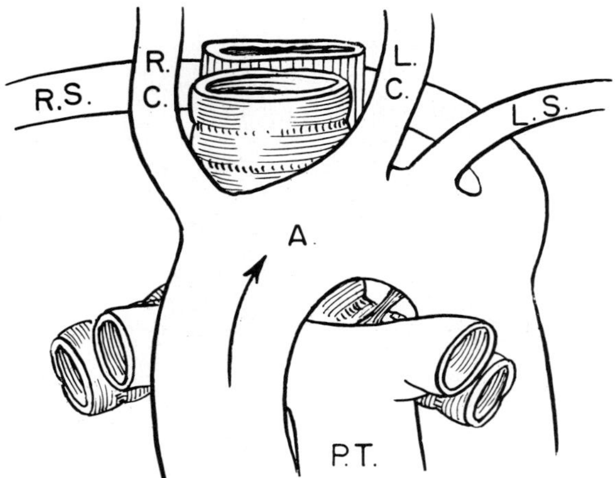

FIGURE 7–40 Anomalous (aberrant) origin of the right subclavian artery (R.S.) from the left aortic arch (A). The anomalously arising artery passes toward the right, closely related to the posterior wall of the esophagus. L.C., left common carotid artery; L.S., left subclavian artery; P.T., pulmonary trunk; R.C., right common carotid artery.

artery; anastomoses between the two coronary systems (although connections were not evident grossly); subendocardial myocardial fibrosis, including fibrosis of papillary muscles; and large sinusoids that communicate with the LV in the area of the distribution of the anomalously arising left coronary artery (Fig. 7–39).

Aortic Arch

The anomalies or variations of the aortic arch system seen in the adult may occur with either a left arch or a right arch.

LEFT AORTIC ARCH

Individuals with left aortic arch have variations from the classic branching pattern. Among these is a common origin for the innominate and left common carotid arteries. A relatively common variation (10 percent) is that of origin of the left vertebral artery from the aortic arch. Such an artery arises just proximal to the origin of the left subclavian artery, and the two arteries commonly share the same adventitia.

Anomalous origin of the right subclavian artery from the distal arch has the following features (Fig. 7–40). The artery arises as the fourth branch of the arch. In contrast to the origin of the usual branches of the arch from its vertex, the anomalously arising right subclavian artery arises from the posterior aspect of the arch. Such a vessel occurs in approximately 1 in 200 individuals (0.5 percent). From its origin, the anomalous right subclavian artery proceeds toward the right axilla, coursing upward and rightward posteriorly to the esophagus.

RIGHT AORTIC ARCH

When a right aortic arch is present, it may be either the only aortic arch or part of a double aortic arch. The double aortic arch is characterized by bifurcation of the ascending aorta into right and left arches (Fig. 7–41). Each arch passes over the homolateral bronchus, joining posteriorly to the esophagus to form the descending aorta. The ligamentum arteriosum joins the junction of the left arch with the descending aorta. The latter lies to the left of the midline.

A right aortic arch may be of two types, either with or without a retroesophageal segment.

Right aortic arch with a retroesophageal segment shows

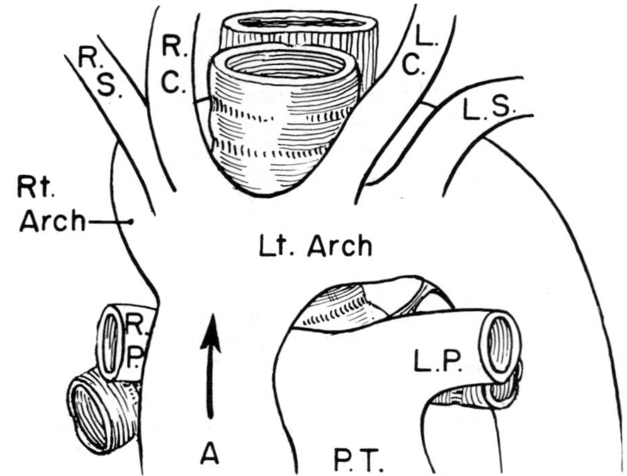

FIGURE 7–41 Double aortic arch. The ascending aorta (A) bifurcates into two arches (Rt. arch; Lt. arch) that join behind the esophagus, thus encircling the trachea and the esophagus. The right aortic arch occupies a retroesophageal position. A left-sided ligamentum arteriosum runs between the left pulmonary artery (L.P.) and the left aortic arch. LC, left common carotid artery; LS, left subclavian artery; PT, pulmonary trunk; RC, right common carotid artery; RS, right subclavian artery.

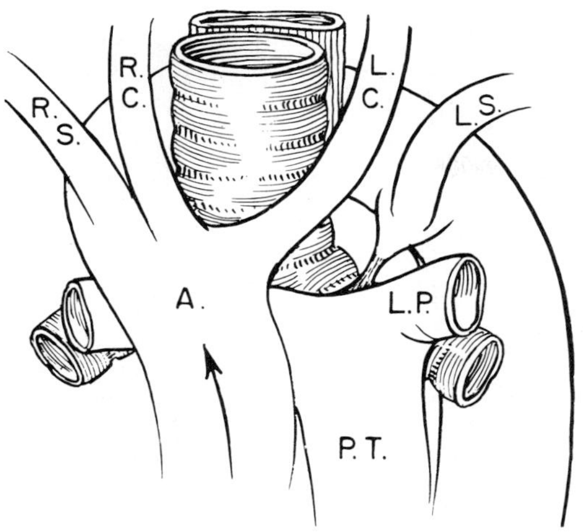

FIGURE 7–42 Right aortic arch with retroesophageal segment. The right aortic arch (A.), after passing over the right bronchus, deviates to the left to join the left-sided descending aorta. The left subclavian artery (L.S.) arises as the fourth branch of the aorta from a diverticulum into which the left ductus arteriosus, or ligamentum arteriosum, inserts. L.C., left common carotid artery; L.P., left pulmonary artery; P.T., pulmonary trunk; R.C., right common carotid artery; R.S., right subclavian artery.

the branches from before, backward, to be the left common carotid, right common carotid, right subclavian, and finally, left subclavian artery (Fig. 7–42). The latter arises from the arch after it has passed in a leftward direction behind the esophagus. The origin of the left subclavian artery is usually from a diverticulum of the arch. The ligamentum arteriosum is left-sided and inserts into the diverticulum. Right aortic arch with a retroesophageal segment is usually not associated with congenital heart disease. Important is the fact that a double aortic arch, as illustrated in Figure 7–41 with an atretic segment between the left common carotid and subclavian arteries, may angiographically resemble the right aortic arch with a retroesophageal segment (Fig. 7–43).

A right aortic arch without a retroesophageal segment is usually associated with congenital heart disease, of which the tetralogy of Fallot is the most common condition. In order of decreasing frequency, the most common patterns of branching are mirror-image branching, aberrant left subclavian artery, and isolation of the left subclavian artery (Fig. 7–44).

Abdominal Aorta

Uncommonly, multiple accessory branches arise from the abdominal aorta or from the nearby lower thoracic aorta and lead to a lung, usually the right. The usual setting is that of pulmonary sequestration. This also may occur in some examples of the scimitar syndrome.

Syndromes With Heart Disease

Congenital cardiovascular disease forms part of many syndromes. Examples of the more common associations are provided in this section.

One recognized association of anomalies is that of aortic coarctation and congenital bicuspid aortic valve, the latter occurring in at least 50 percent of cases with coarctation.

VSD and patent ductus arteriosus have a fairly common association. Elliott and colleagues[82] found that among 154 patients undergoing closure of VSD, 19 (12 percent) had associated patent ductus arteriosus.

The association of persistent common AV canal and tetralogy of Fallot has been recognized as allowing patients to reach adulthood (Fig. 7–45). The complete variety of persistent common AV canal, when untreated, tends to be associated with death in infancy or childhood. The addition of the tetralogy of Fallot introduces an element of "natural banding," leading to survival to adulthood.[43]

Familial Cardiomyopathy

At least two forms of familial myopathy may be manifested in the adult—dilated (congestive) cardiomyopathy and hypertrophic cardiomyopathy.[83] Familial dilated (congestive) cardiomyopathy is structurally similar to apparently acquired congestive cardiomyopathy. The heart is enlarged, with hypertrophied and dilated ventricles. Differing amounts (usually small) of myocardial fibrosis are present, and congestive failure and/or sudden major arrhythmias are common.

Arachnodactyly (Marfan Syndrome)

The connective tissue laxity characteristic of Marfan syndrome commonly affects the cardiovascular system. The elastic arteries show medial foci of mucoid, cystlike deposits (cystic medial necrosis) associated with corresponding interruption and retraction of fibers. In the aorta, the changes are most commonly located in the ascending por-

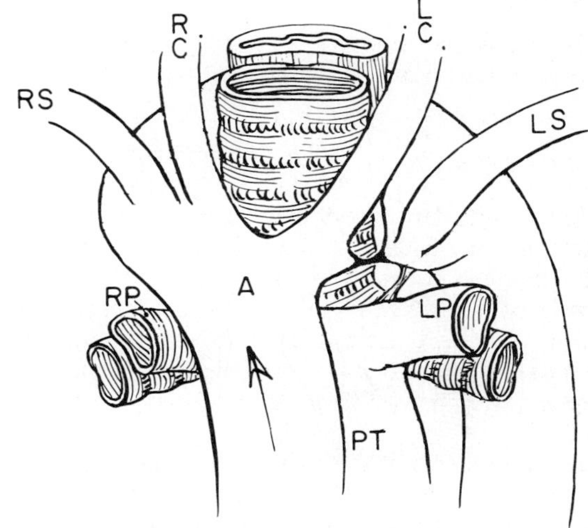

FIGURE 7–43 Double aortic arch with atretic segment (narrow, dark zone) between the left common carotid (LC) and the left subclavian (LS) arteries. Angiographically, this arrangement would give the same picture as that in Fig. 7–42 but is more significant in tracheal and esophageal compression, in that the atretic segment completes a double aortic arch. A, aorta; LP, left pulmonary artery; PT, pulmonary trunk; RC, right common carotid artery; RP, right pulmonary artery; RS, right subclavian artery.

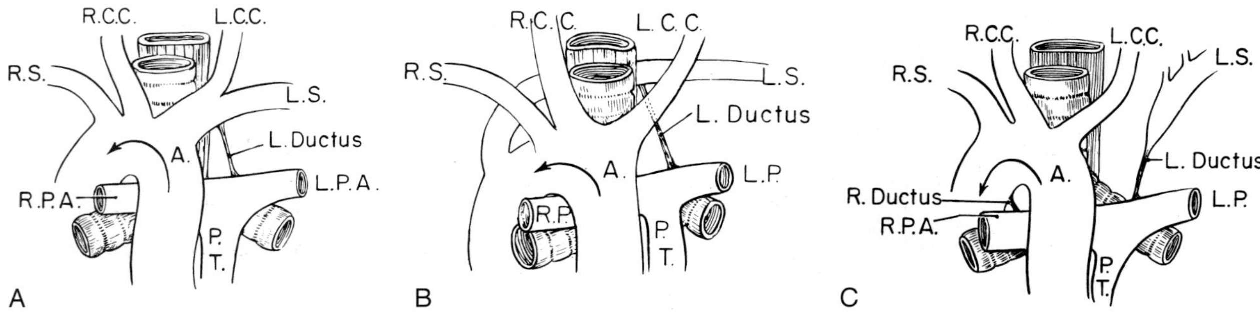

FIGURE 7–44 Right aortic arch without retroesophageal segment. The conditions shown are characteristic of right aortic arch and congenital heart disease, of which the tetralogy of Fallot and truncus arteriosus are most common. **A,** Mirror-image branching of the aorta (A.). L.C.C., left common carotid artery; L. Ductus, left ductus arteriosus; L.P.A., left pulmonary artery; L.S., left subclavian artery; P.T., pulmonary trunk; R.C.C., right common carotid artery; R.P.A., right pulmonary artery; R.S., right subclavian artery. **B,** Aberrant left subclavian artery. L.P., left pulmonary artery; R.P., right pulmonary artery. **C,** Isolation of the left subclavian artery. R. Ductus, right ductus arteriosus.

tion.[84] This leads to dilatation of the ascending aorta in general and of the aortic sinuses as well. Beyond the arch, the process of cystic medial necrosis is less evident than that proximally. Two characteristics of this condition are aortic valvular regurgitation and aortic dissection, each with its classic consequences. Simple aortic regurgitation may result from dilatation of the aorta and coexisting myxomatous changes in the aortic valvular cusps. In the pulmonary trunk, cystic medial necrosis may be present and associated with so-called idiopathic dilatation of the pulmonary artery.[85] The AV valves may exhibit myxomatous change (prolapse) and may be incompetent. Rarely, foci of myxomatous accumulation occur in coronary arterial intimas and may be responsible for significant obstruction.

Holt-Oram Syndrome

The Holt-Oram syndrome is also known as the heart-hand syndrome or the heart–upper limb syndrome. As the synonyms indicate, the condition affects the heart and upper extremities. The usual cardiac anomaly is an ASD at the fossa ovalis. Malformations of the skeleton, particularly of the upper extremities, are characteristic.[86, 87]

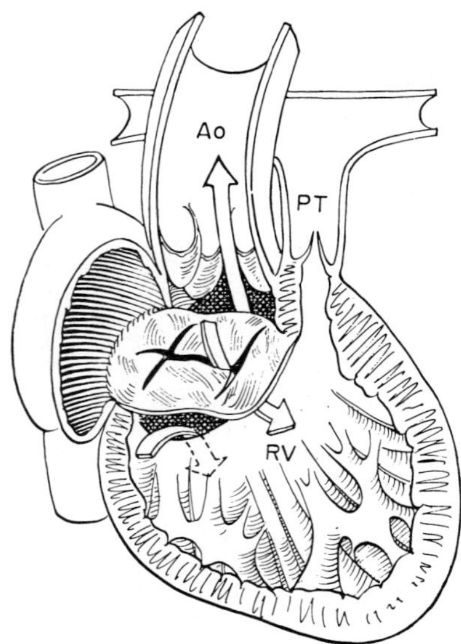

FIGURE 7–45 Tetralogy of Fallot and persistent common atrioventricular canal may coexist. Ao, aorta; PT, pulmonary trunk; RV, right ventricle.

Down Syndrome

Down syndrome is commonly associated with congenital heart disease. About 40 percent of Down syndrome patients have cardiac anomalies. The anomalies are usually derived from the AV endocardial cushions, leading to the endocardial cushion defect (persistent common AV canal). VSD and, rarely, simple cleft of the anterior leaflet of the mitral valve[88] may be expressions of anomalies of the AV cushions.

In a study by Tenckhoff and Stamm[89] of 35 cases of the complete form of persistent common AV canal, 11 patients (31 percent) exhibited Down syndrome.

Turner's Syndrome

Turner's syndrome is commonly associated with coarctation of the aorta.[90] Pulmonary valvular stenosis or VSD occurs less frequently.[91]

REFERENCES

1. Roberts WC: The congenitally bicuspid aortic valve: a study of 85 autopsy cases. Am J Cardiol 26:83, 1970.
2. Bacon APC, Matthews MB: Congenital bicuspid aortic valves and the aetiology of isolated aortic valvular stenosis. Q J Med 28:545, 1959.
3. Edwards JE: The congenital bicuspid aortic valve. Circulation 23:485, 1961.
4. Peterson MD, Roach RM, Edwards JE: Types of aortic stenosis in surgically removed valves. Arch Pathol Lab Med 109:829, 1985.
5. Subramanian R, Olsen LJ, Edwards WD: Surgical pathology of combined aortic stenosis and insufficiency: a study of 213 cases. Mayo Clin Proc 60:247, 1985.
6. Edwards JE: Pathologic aspects of cardiac valvular insufficiencies. Arch Surg 77:634, 1958.
7. Edwards JE: Varieties of valvular heart disease. II. Aortic valvular disease. Pract Cardiol 8:117, 1982.
8. Henry WL, Clark CE, Epstein SE: Asymmetric septal hypertrophy (ASH): the unifying link in the IHSS disease spectrum. Observations regarding its pathogenesis, pathophysiology, and course. Circulation 47:827, 1973.
9. Frank S, Braunwald E: Idiopathic hypertrophic subaortic stenosis.

Clinical analysis of 126 patients with emphasis on the natural history. Circulation 37:759, 1968.
10. Edwards JE: Pathology of left ventricular outflow tract obstruction. Circulation 31:586, 1965.
11. Feigl A, Feigl D, Lucas RV Jr, Edwards JE: Involvement of the aortic valve cusps in discrete subaortic stenosis. Pediatr Cardiol 5:185, 1984.
12. Somerville J, Stone S, Ross D: Fate of patients with fixed subaortic stenosis after surgical removal. Br Heart J 443:629, 1980.
13. Shem-Tov A, Schneeweiss A, Motro M, Neufeld HN: Clinical presentation and natural history of mild discrete subaortic stenosis. Follow-up of 1–17 years. Circulation 66:509, 1982.
14. Morrison RW, Edwards JE: Subaortic stenosis. Report of two cases, one associated with patent ductus arteriosus, the other complicated by bacterial endocarditis. Int Assoc Med Mus Bull 31:73, 1950.
15. Maron BJ, Redwood DR, Roberts WC, et al: Tunnel subaortic stenosis. Left ventricular outflow tract obstruction produced by fibromuscular tubular narrowing. Circulation 54:404, 1976.
16. Peterson TA, Todd DB, Edwards JE: Supravalvular aortic stenosis. J Thorac Cardiovasc Surg 50:734, 1965.
17. Giddins NG, Finley JP, Nanton MA, Roy DL: The natural course of supravalvar aortic stenosis and peripheral pulmonary artery stenosis in Williams's syndrome. Br Heart J 62:315, 1989.
18. Wren C, Oslizlok P, Bull C: Natural history of supravalvular aortic stenosis and pulmonary artery stenosis. J Am Coll Cardiol 15:1625, 1990.
19. D'Cruz IA, Arcilla RA, Agustsson MH: Dilatation of the pulmonary trunk in stenosis of the pulmonary valve and of the pulmonary arteries in children. Am Heart J 68:611, 1964.
20. Parker RL: Pulmonary stenosis: tetralogy of Fallot. Med Clin North Am 32:855, 1948.
21. Shone JD, Sellers RD, Anderson RC, et al: The developmental complex of "parachute mitral valve," supravalvular ring of left atrium, subaortic stenosis, and coarctation of aorta. Am J Cardiol 11:714, 1963.
22. da Silva CL, Edwards JE: Parachute mitral valve in an adult. Arg Bras Cardiol 26:149, 1973.
23. Hedinger E: Transposition der grossen Gefasse dei rudimentarer linker Herzkammer bei einer 56 jahrigen Frau. Zentralbl Allg Pathol 26:529, 1915.
24. Edwards JE, Christensen NA, Clagett OT, McDonald JR: Pathologic considerations in coarctation of the aorta. Proc Mayo Clin 23:324, 1948.
25. Edwards JE, Clagett OT, Drake RL, et al: The collateral circulation in coarctation of the aorta. Proc Mayo Clin 23:333, 1948.
26. Becker AE, Becker MJ, Edwards JE: Anomalies associated with coarctation of aorta. Particular reference to infancy. Circulation 41:1067, 1970.
27. Edwards JE: Aneurysms of the thoracic aorta complicating coarctation. Circulation 48:195, 1973.
28. Edwards JE: Floppy mitral valve syndrome. Cardiovasc Clin 18:249, 1987.
29. Lucas RV Jr, Edwards JE: The floppy mitral valve. Curr Probl Cardiol 7:1, 1982.
29a. Titus JL, Edwards JE: Mitral insufficiency other than rheumatic, ischemic, or infective: emphasis on mitral valve prolapse. Semin Thorac Cardiovasc Surg 1:118, 1989.
30. Salazar AE, Edwards JE: Friction lesions of ventricular endocardium. Relation to chordae tendineae of mitral valve. Arch Pathol Lab Med 90:364, 1970.
31. Shiina A, Seward JB, Edwards WD, et al: Two-dimensional echocardiographic spectrum of Ebstein's anomaly: detailed anatomic assessment. J Am Coll Cardiol 3:356, 1984.
32. Weaver WF, Edwards JE, Brandenburg RO: Idiopathic dilation of the aorta with aortic valvular insufficiency: a possible forme fruste of Marfan's syndrome. Mayo Clin Proc 34:518, 1959.
33. Brown OR, deMots H, Kloster FE, et al: Aortic root dilation and mitral valve prolapse in Marfan's syndrome. An echocardiography study. Circulation 52:651, 1975.
34. Kawashima Y, Danno M, Shimizu Y, et al: Ventricular septal defect associated with aortic insufficiency. Anatomic classification and method of operation. Circulation 47:1057, 1973.
35. Pouget JM, Kelly CE, Pilz CG: Congenital absence of the pulmonic valve. Report of a case in a seventy-three year old man. Am J Cardiol 29:732, 1967.
36. Craig RJ, Selzer A: Natural history and prognosis of atrial septal defect. Circulation 37:805, 1968.
37. Campbell M: Natural history of atrial septal defect. Br Heart J 32:820, 1970.
38. Hagen PT, Scholz DG, Edwards WD: Incidence and size of patent foramen ovale during the first 10 decades of life. Mayo Clin Proc 59:17, 1984.
39. Silver MD, Dorsey JS: Aneurysms of the septum primum in adults. Arch Pathol Lab Med 102:52, 1978.
40. Pearson AC, Nagelhout D, Castello R, et al: Atrial septal aneurysm and stroke. A transesophageal echocardiographic study. J Am Coll Cardiol 18:1233, 1991.
41. Di Tullio M, Sacco RL, Gopal A, et al: Patent foramen ovale as a risk factor for cryptogenic stroke. Ann Intern Med 117:461, 1992.
42. Petty GW, Khandheria BK, Chu CP, et al: Patent foramen ovale in patients with cerebral infarction. A transesophageal echocardiographic study. Arch Neurol 54:819, 1997.
42a. Schroeckenstein RF, Wasenda GJ, Edwards JE: Valvular competent patent foramen ovale in adults. Minn Med 55:11, 1972.
43. Tandon R, Moller JH, Edwards JE: Tetralogy of Fallot associated with persistent common atrioventricular canal (endocardial cushion defect). Br Heart J 36:197, 1974.
44. Edwards JE, Burchell HB, Christensen NA: Specimen exhibiting the essential lesion in aneurysm of the aortic sinus. Proc Mayo Clin 31:407, 464, 1956.
45. Sakakibara A, Yokoyama M, Takao A, et al: Coronary arteriovenous fistula. Nine operated cases. Am Heart J 72:307, 1966.
46. McNamara JJ, Gross RE: Congenital coronary artery fistula. Surgery 65:59, 1969.
47. Cooley DA, Ellis PR Jr: Surgical considerations of coronary arterial fistula. Am J Cardiol 10:467, 1962.
48. Nagle JP, Cheitlin MD, McCarty RJ: Corrected transposition of the great vessels without associated anomalies: report of a case with congestive failure at age 45 years. Chest 60:367, 1971.
49. Lieberson AD, Schumacher RR, Childress RH, Genovese PD: Corrected transposition of the great vessels in a 73-year-old man. Circulation 39:96, 1969.
50. Cumming GR: Congenital corrected transposition of the great vessels without associated intracardiac anomalies. A clinical hemodynamic and angiographic study. Am J Cardiol 10:605, 1962.
51. Bjarke BB, Kidd BSL: Congenitally corrected transposition of the great arteries. A clinical study of 101 cases. Acta Paediatr Scand 65:153, 1976.
52. Levy MJ, Lillehei CW, Elliott LP et al: Accessory valvular tissue causing subpulmonary stenosis in corrected transposition of great vessels. Circulation 27:494, 1963.
53. Edwards JE: Differential diagnosis of mitral stenosis: clinicopathological review of simulating conditions. Lab Invest 3:89, 1954.
54. Hickie JB, Gimlette TMD, Bacon APC: Anomalous pulmonary venous drainage. Br Heart J 18:365, 1956.
55. Hudson R: The normal and abnormal inter-atrial septum. Br Heart J 17:489, 1955.
56. Kiely B, Filler J, Stone S, Doyle EF: Syndrome of anomalous venous drainage of the right lung to the inferior vena cava. A review of 67 reported cases and three new cases in children. Am J Cardiol 20:102, 1967.
57. Halasz NA, Halloran KH, Liebow AA: Bronchial and arterial anomalies with drainage of the right lung into the inferior vena cava. Circulation 14:826, 1956.
58. Peoples WM, Miller JH, Edwards JE: Polysplenia: A review of 146 cases. Pediatr Cardiol 4:129, 1983.
59. Gardner DL, Cole L: Long survival with inferior vena cava draining into left atrium. Br Heart J 17:93, 1955.
60. Gautam P: Left atrial inferior vena cava with atrial septal defect. J Thorac Cardiovasc Surg 55:827, 1968.
61. Black H, Smith GT, Goodale WT: Anomalous inferior vena cava draining into the left atrium associated with intact interatrial septum and multiple pulmonary arteriovenous fistulae. Circulation 29:258, 1964.
62. Winter FS: Persistent left superior vena cava. Survey of world literature and report of thirty additional cases. Angiology 5:90, 1954.
63. Karnegis JN, Wang Y, Winchell P, Edwards JE: Persistent left superior vena cava, fibrous remnant of the right superior vena cava and ventricular septal defect. Am J Cardiol 14:573, 1964.
64. Raghib G, Ruttenberg HD, Anderson RC, et al: Termination of left superior vena cava in left atrium, atrial septal defect, and absence of coronary sinus. A developmental complex. Circulation 31:906, 1965.

65. Moller JH, Nakib A, Anderson RC, Edwards JE: Congenital cardiac disease associated with polysplenia. A developmental complex of bilateral "left-sidedness." Circulation 36:789, 1967.
66. Gueron M, Hirsh M, Borman J: Total anomalous systemic venous drainage into the left atrium. J Thorac Cardiovasc Surg 58:570, 1969.
67. Miller GAH, Ongley PA, Rastelli GC, Kirklin JW: Surgical correction of total anomalous systemic venous connection: report of case. Mayo Clin Proc 40:532, 1965.
68. Goldman A: Arteriovenous fistula of the lung: its hereditary and clinical aspects. Am Rev Tuberc 57:266, 1948.
69. Armentrout HL, Underwood FJ: Familial hemorrhagic telangiectasia with associated pulmonary arteriovenous aneurysm. Am J Med 8:246, 1950.
70. Moyer JH, Glantz G, Brest AN: Pulmonary arteriovenous fistula: physiologic and clinical considerations. Am J Med 32:417, 1962.
71. Dines DE, Arms RA, Bernatz PE, Gomes MR: Pulmonary arteriovenous fistulas. Mayo Clin Proc 49:460, 1974.
71a. Vlodaver Z, Neufeld HN, Edwards JE: Coronary Arterial Variations in the Normal Heart and in Congenital Heart Disease. New York, Academic, 1975.
72. Wodehouse GE: Hemangioma of the lung: a review of four cases, including two not previously reported, one of which was complicated by brain abscess due to *H. influenzae*. J Thorac Surg 17:408, 1948.
73. Maier HC, Himmelstein A, Riley RL, Bunin JJ: Arteriovenous fistula of the lung. J Thorac Surg 17:13, 1948.
74. Gomes MMR, Bernatz PE: Arteriovenous fistulas: a review and ten-year experience at the Mayo Clinic. Mayo Clin Proc 45:81, 1970.
75. Berry BE, McGoon DC, Ritter DG, Davis GD: Absence of anatomic origin from heart of pulmonary arterial supply. Clinical application of classification. J Thorac Cardiovasc Surg 68:119, 1974.
76. Sotomora RF, Edwards JE: Anatomic identification of so-called absent pulmonary artery. Circulation 57:624, 1978.
77. Mahowald JM, Blieden LC, Coe JI, et al: Ectopic origin of a coronary artery from the aorta. Sudden death in 3 of 23 patients. Chest 89:668, 1986.
78. Tuna IC, Bessinger FB, Ophoven JP, Edwards JE: Acute angular origin of left coronary artery from aorta: an unusual cause of left ventricular failure in infancy. Pediatr Cardiol 10:39, 1989.
79. Jordan RA, Dry TJ, Edwards JE: Anomalous origin of the right coronary artery from the pulmonary trunk. Proc Mayo Clin 25:763, 1950.
80. Sabiston DC, Neill CA, Taussig HB: The direction of blood flow in anomalous left coronary artery arising from the pulmonary artery. Circulation 22:591, 1960.
81. Wesselhoeft H, Fawcett JS, Johnson AL: Anomalous origin of the left coronary artery from the pulmonary trunk. Its clinical spectrum, pathology, and pathophysiology, based on a review of 140 cases with seven further cases. Circulation 38:403, 1968.
82. Elliott LP, Ernst RW, Anderson RC, et al: Silent patent ductus arteriosus in association with ventricular septal defect. Clinical, hemodynamic, pathological and surgical observations in forty patients. Am J Cardiol 10:475, 1962.
83. Michels VV, Moll PP, Miller FA, et al: The frequency of familial dilated cardiomyopathy in a series of patients with idiopathic dilated cardiomyopathy. N Engl J Med 326:77, 1992.
84. Wagenvoort CA, Neufeld HN, Edwards JE: Cardiovascular system in Marfan's syndrome and in idiopathic dilatation of the ascending aorta. Am J Cardiol 9:496, 1962.
85. Tung HL, Liebow AA: Marfan's syndrome observation at necropsy: with special reference to medionecrosis of the great vessels. Lab Invest 1:382, 1952.
86. Holt M, Oram S: Familial heart disease with skeletal malformations. Br Heart J 22:236, 1960.
87. Kaufman RL, Rimoin DL, McAlister WH, Hartmann AS: Variable expression of Holt-Oram syndrome. Am J Dis Child 127:21, 1974.
88. Spicer RL: Cardiovascular disease in Down syndrome. Pediatr Clin North Am 31:1331, 1984.
89. Tenckhoff L, Stamm SJ: An analysis of 35 cases of the complete form of persistent common atrioventricular canal. Circulation 48:416, 1973.
90. Palmer CG, Reichmann A: Chromosomal and clinical findings in 100 females with Turner syndrome. Hum Genet 35:35, 1976.
91. Nora JJ, Torres FG, Sinha AK, McNamara DG: Characteristic cardiovascular anomalies of XO Turner syndrome, XX and XY phenotype and XO/XX Turner mosaic. Am J Cardiol 25:639, 1970.

CHAPTER 8

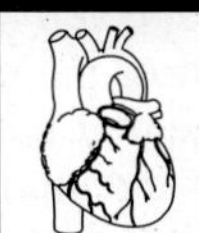

Pathophysiology, Clinical Recognition, and Treatment of Congenital Heart Disease

Yang Wang and Gladwin Das

NATURAL HISTORY
VALVULAR ABNORMALITIES
Aortic Stenosis
Mitral Stenosis
Tricuspid Stenosis and Atresia
Pulmonary Stenosis
Mitral Valve Prolapse
Atrioventricular Valvular Regurgitation
Mitral Valve Regurgitation
Aortic Valve Regurgitation
Pulmonary Valve Regurgitation
Ebstein's Anomaly
OBSTRUCTION OF THE GREAT VESSELS
Coarctation of the Aorta
Pulmonary Artery Stenosis
Superior Vena Caval Obstruction
Inferior Vena Caval Obstruction
ABNORMAL COMMUNICATION BETWEEN CHAMBERS OR GREAT ARTERIES
Interatrial Septal Defect
Atrial Septal Defect, Secundum Type
Septum Primum Defect
Single Atrium
Sinus Venosus Defect
Coronary Sinus Fistula
Partial Anomalous Pulmonary Venous Connection
Ventricular Septal Defects
Patent Ductus Arteriosus
Endocardial Cushion Defects
COMPLEX CONGENITAL HEART DISEASE
Without Cyanosis
With Cyanosis
GREAT VEIN MALPOSITIONS
Partial Anomalous Pulmonary Venous Return (Connection)
Total Anomalous Pulmonary Venous Connection
GENETIC SYNDROMES THAT INCLUDE HEART DISEASE
Osler-Weber-Rendu Syndrome
HYPERTROPHIC CARDIOMYOPATHY (ASYMMETRIC SEPTAL HYPERTROPHY)
RIGHT VENTRICULAR DYSPLASIA
CORONARY ARTERY ANOMALIES
ANEURYSMS OF THE SINUS OF VALSALVA
CONGENITAL ARRHYTHMIAS
Congenital Isolated Complete Atrioventricular Block
PREGNANCY AND CONGENITAL HEART DISEASE

Natural History

Successful open-heart surgery to correct septal defects in humans was ushered in by the pioneering work of C. Walton Lillehei,[1] who closed a ventricular septal defect in a 4-year-old boy, using the boy's father for cross-circulation, on April 20, 1954. The boy is now a middle-aged man. Since that time, because of increasingly sophisticated diagnostic precision, better understanding of the altered hemodynamics, and development of surgical techniques, the natural history of congenital heart disease has changed considerably. In the early days of open-heart surgery, unoperated congenital heart disease among adults was not uncommon, whereas congenital heart disease is now usually corrected by surgery in childhood or adolescence. Therefore, the cardiologist with an interest in congenital heart disease in adults sees mostly patients with congenital heart disease (e.g., Eisenmenger's complex) who are as yet inoperable or those with congenital heart disease that has been surgically corrected and for whom the cardiologist is responsible for the long-term follow-up. Also included in this category are patients who are destined to develop cardiac abnormalities, such as those with Marfan's syndrome, in whom the heart disease may not become overt until adulthood, and those with conditions that easily escape the noncardiologist physician, such as interatrial septal defect and congenital unicuspid or bicuspid aortic valve.

Cardiologists interested in adult congenital heart disease were at one time a rapidly vanishing breed, especially with the burgeoning developments in research, diagnosis, and therapy for coronary artery disease (CAD) and congestive heart failure (CHF). Others have been attracted to the rapidly expanding field of cardiac electrophysiology, which began as a diagnostic field but now includes installation of a bewildering variety of pacemakers, ablation of accessory pathways and arrhythmogenic foci, and evaluation of syncope. However, it has become increasingly apparent that patients who have undergone surgical correction of congenital heart disease frequently have complications later in adulthood. The ligation and division of a patent ductus arteriosus perhaps comes closest to a complete cure. Even patients with closed atrial septal defects are commonly plagued in later life by supraventricular tachyarrhythmias, especially atrial fibrillation and atrial flutter. Therefore, most patients seen by cardiologists interested in adult congenital heart disease are those with previously "corrected" congenital heart disease who have sequelae later in life. However, a significant minority consists of those with hitherto undiagnosed congenital heart disease, inoperable heart disease, or congenital heart disease for which the patient has refused surgery. Significant advances in therapy, including surgery, pacemakers, better treatment modalities for CHF, and improved management of hyperviscosity syndromes, have increased the life expectancy of such patients.

There are many ways to classify congenital heart disease. Perhaps the most "scientific" classification would be in terms of abnormal embryologic development. Unfortunately, such a classification would be of limited clinical usefulness. A reasonable classification would be by clinical categories, such as whether or not there is cyanosis, whether pulmonary hypertension is present, whether cardiac valves are involved, which ventricle is more involved, and whether there are disturbances in heart rhythm. Sophisticated echocardiographic techniques can now delineate the anatomy and often the physiologic disturbance or disturbances, and cardiac catheterization can be used to more precisely quantify the physiologic disturbances and to identify abnormalities that are not easily visualized by echocardiography, such as coronary anomalies, unusual insertions of anomalous pulmonary veins, and pulmonary arteriovenous fistulas. The electrocardiogram (ECG) can be a very useful adjunct in clinical diagnosis because some forms of congenital heart disease, such as atrial septal defect, tricuspid atresia, and the endocardial cushion defects, have electrocardiographic markers.

The cardiologist treating adults should still be able to diagnose congenital heart disease or at least to narrow down the diagnostic possibilities by both clinical and laboratory methods. This is equally true in the long-term follow-up of such patients, especially if they have undergone surgery, because the natural history of the disease will have been altered by the operation itself. This demands a thorough knowledge of the operative techniques used at the time of surgical intervention—many of which have changed considerably.

VALVULAR ABNORMALITIES

The valvular abnormalities include stenosis, regurgitation, and atresia. Mitral and aortic atresia never allow survival into adulthood and are therefore not discussed further.

Aortic Stenosis

Congenital obstruction of the outflow tract of the left ventricle (LV) in the adult is overwhelmingly valvular and commonly results from the development of aortic stenosis because of a congenital bicuspid or unicuspid valve.[2,3] The incidence of aortic valve disease is four to five times higher in males than in females.[4] Idiopathic hypertrophic subaortic stenosis and asymmetric septal hypertrophy are dealt with separately.

Valvular Aortic Stenosis

In nonelderly adults, the overwhelming majority of aortic stenoses develop because of a bicuspid (or unicuspid) aortic valve.[5,6] This is sometimes seen in association with coarctation of the aorta.[7] In general, the valve causes little or no hemodynamic disturbance for the first several decades of life and, in fact, may never cause any hemodynamic disturbance at all. Progressive aortic regurgitation may develop, especially in young adulthood. It appears that most valves with this abnormality develop progressive thickening and fibrosis after the third or fourth decade of life and, as time goes on, increasing calcification and progressively severe aortic stenosis. The presence of mild aortic stenosis may be associated with progressively severe aortic regurgitation when inadequate coaptation outweighs inadequate opening of the valve.[7] The supervention of bacterial endocarditis may also transform the pathophysiologic disturbance from predominant stenosis to predominant regurgitation.

The course of the disease, once stenosis begins, tends to be relentless but has a highly variable timetable. In general, the progression to severe aortic stenosis may take decades, although we have treated two patients who progressed from a zero systolic gradient across the aortic valve to tight aortic stenosis within 5 years. After significant aortic stenosis develops, the natural history is similar to that of aortic stenosis stemming from noncongenital causes. The classic ominous symptoms are syncope, angina, and CHF. Sudden death is a threat once even mild symptoms are noted.[4,8–10] However, evaluation for surgery should be undertaken if there has been any subjective change in exercise tolerance or general sense of well-being. Most patients with predominant aortic stenosis have well-preserved left ventricular function if exertional syncope is the primary manifestation. Although angina may occur in severe aortic stenosis without concomitant CAD, CAD is not uncommon in the presence of aortic stenosis and should always be looked for when surgery on the aortic valve is contemplated.[11–13] The appearance of overt CHF is usually of ominous prognostic import, although some patients may recover virtually normal left ventricular function after successful surgery. Approximately 5 percent of patients with a bicuspid aortic valve have associated cystic medial disease of the aorta, which can become the basis of an aortic dissection. Coarctation of the aorta is sometimes associated with a bicuspid aortic valve (it is far more common for a coarctation of the aorta to be associated with a bicuspid aortic valve, rather than the reverse), which has its own inherent natural history and complications.[14] Before the aortic valve has become heavily calcified, the presence of a bicuspid aortic valve has rather classic physical findings. The most characteristic feature of a bicuspid aortic valve is a loud systolic ejection sound,[15,16] which coincides with the doming of the aortic valve toward the end of isovolumetric contraction of the LV (it can be thought of as a "reversed opening snap"). In the younger age group, this may be the only physical finding, although commonly there is an aortic systolic murmur that starts after the ejection sound. The ejection sound is usually somewhat pronounced, and it is likely that the doming of the aortic valve prolongs the phase of isovolumetric contraction. The aortic systolic murmur, if present, starts with the ejection sound and may be of variable intensity.[17]

The second heart sound characteristically preserves components of A_2 and P_2 until significant aortic stenosis develops, when the second sound becomes single. There may or may not be an early diastolic blowing murmur of aortic regurgitation. The peripheral pulse contour characteristically shows an anacrotic notch. In general, the more severe the stenosis, the more delayed the upstroke and the lower the anacrotic notch on the upstroke.[18] Classically, the heart is not enlarged.[19] If the aortic valve is heavily calcified, it can be visualized, especially in the lateral view of the chest film, and can be readily seen on fluoroscopy. A characteristic finding is dilatation of the ascending aorta (Fig. 8–1).[20, 22] This dilatation is asymmetric, anterior, and to the right and is believed to be due to the direction of the abnormal flow pattern across the bicuspid aortic valve. This "poststenotic dilatation" can be observed even when there is no systolic gradient across the aortic valve. The ECG may be unremarkable throughout the course of the disease up to the time of surgery, although it may demonstrate a characteristic "strain" pattern of left ventricular hypertrophy.

DIAGNOSIS

The clinical diagnosis of aortic valve stenosis is made by auscultating the characteristic ejection systolic murmur, which is harsh and radiates to the neck. This murmur may be mimicked by mitral insufficiency associated with an "overshooting" of the posterior mitral valve leaflet directing the regurgitant jet anteriorly and medially, giving rise to a murmur best heard along the left sternal border and sometimes heard in the neck.[23–25] Valvular pulmonary stenosis may also be heard in the neck. An aortic ejection sound strongly suggests the presence of a bicuspid aortic valve. With time, many or most such aortic valves become more stenotic.[26, 27] The ejection sound may gradually disappear, and its absence is associated with increasing fibrosis and calcification of the valve leaflets.[28, 29] The first heart sound is characteristically soft, and the A_2 component of the second heart sound gradually diminishes as the stenosis becomes progressively more severe. A soft diastolic murmur of aortic insufficiency is not uncommon as the cusps become more rigid. As the stenosis becomes more severe, an S_4 becomes prominent and may sometimes be mistaken for S_1. The peripheral pulses show an anacrotic notch and a somewhat delayed upstroke. In general, the lower the notch, the more severe the stenosis. The heart is usually not grossly enlarged unless there is a significant degree of aortic insufficiency.

The chest x-ray study usually shows the heart to be of normal size unless there is no significant concomitant regurgitation, possibly with some calcification of the aortic valve and "poststenotic" dilatation of the ascending aorta, as previously described (Fig. 8–2). The ECG, even in severe aortic stenosis, may range from normal to that characteristic of left ventricular hypertrophy with a "strain" pattern (Fig. 8–3) and may not be helpful in the clinical evaluation of severity. The echocardiogram shows a thickened aortic valve, which becomes increasingly immobile as it becomes more calcified. The LV exhibits concentric hypertrophy, and the systolic gradient across the aortic valve can be estimated by the velocity of the systolic jet.[30, 31] Similarly, aortic insufficiency can be visualized.

On cardiac catheterization, the LV can be entered either retrograde across the stenotic aortic valve or by trans-septal puncture from the femoral venous approach to the left atrium (LA) and then the LV. Angiography shows the characteristic poststenotic dilatation of the ascending aorta, which does not involve the aortic ring or sinuses. Simultaneous pressures across the aortic valve can be measured, and with simultaneous measurement of cardiac output, the valve area can be calculated from the Gorlin formula,[32]

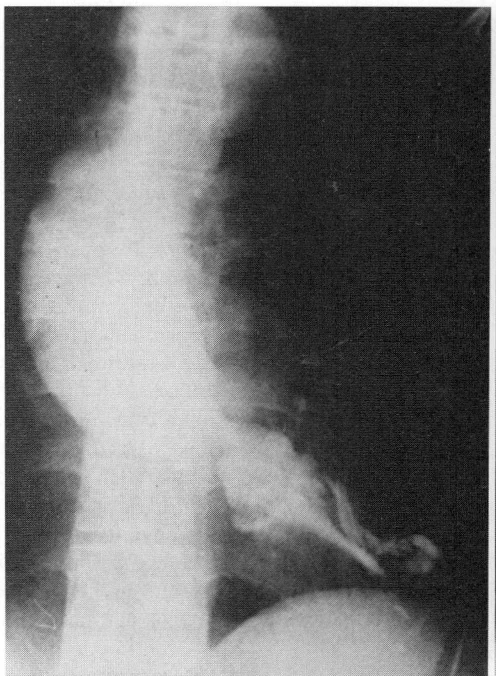

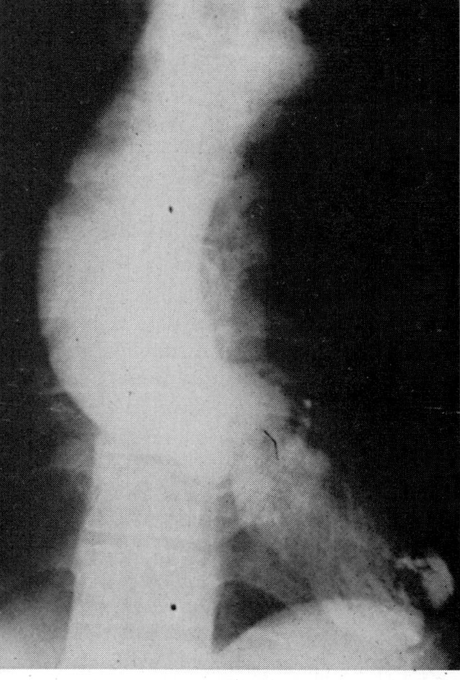

FIGURE 8–1 Aortic stenosis on a congenitally bicuspid aortic valve. Note the eccentric poststenotic dilatation of the ascending aorta, with a normal-sized aortic ring. The ventriculogram illustrates the contraction of the severely hypertrophied left ventricle to a very small end-systolic volume.

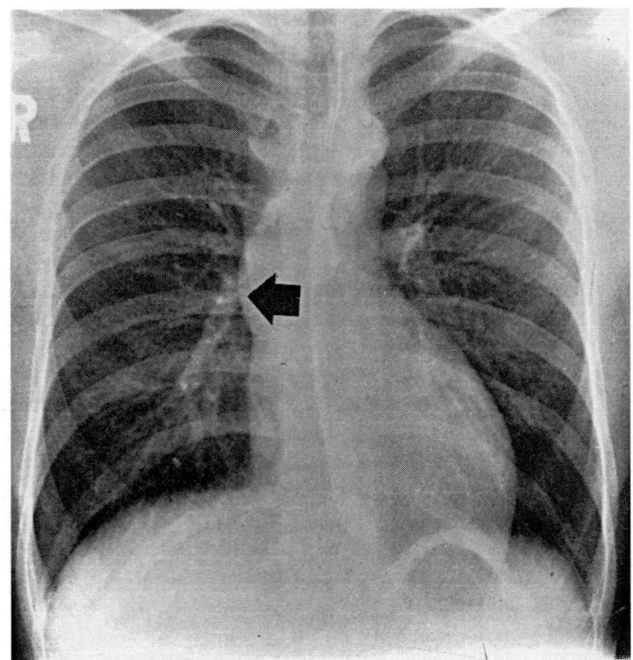

FIGURE 8–2 Posteroanterior (PA) radiograph of a patient with congenital aortic stenosis. The heart is slightly enlarged and has a left ventricular configuration. The pulmonary vasculature is normal. There is striking prominence of the ascending aorta *(arrow)* as a result of poststenotic dilatation. (Courtesy of Kurt Amplatz, M.D.)

assuming inconsequential aortic regurgitation. If the patient has CHF, the clinical picture must be modified to include left ventricular dilatation, decreased contractility, and a ventricular gallop rhythm.

TREATMENT

There is no "magical" aortic valve area that clearly dictates intervention. In general, the patient who is normally active, who has no symptoms, and in whom the clinical signs and the echocardiogram do not suggest severe aortic stenosis can be safely watched. Even when the evidence points to significant aortic stenosis, the total absence of symptoms should outweigh the objective measurements of valve orifice size in continuing careful observation and follow-up.[33] However, with even mild changes in status that can be ascribed to the heart, together with the physical signs of significant aortic stenosis that are confirmed by echocardiography and catheterization, surgical replacement of the aortic valve should be seriously considered. These changes may involve merely a subtle change in well-being or a slight decrease in exercise tolerance.[34] It is advisable to proceed with cardiac catheterization when it is felt that surgery is imminent, both to confirm the clinical and echocardiographic evidence and to visualize the coronary arteries. It is not wise to wait until major symptoms arise, because the incidence of sudden death rises dramatically.[35] In patients with aortic stenosis and angina, there is a significant incidence of coexisting CAD.[11, 12] Treatment involves surgical replacement of the calcified valve[37, 38] by a mechanical or bioprosthesis and coronary artery bypass grafting, if indicated. Even patients older than 80 years benefit from valve replacement; they have an operative mortality of 9.4 percent and a good outcome in 81 percent. Porcine bioprostheses are especially suitable in the elderly, in whom the longevity of such prostheses is better than when they are implanted in younger patients. Balloon valvotomy has been useful in children but disappointing in adults, for whom the benefits are of limited duration, especially with a stiff, calcified valve.[39, 41]

Long-term follow-up on a large cohort of 462 patients with congenital aortic stenosis (mostly children) showed that with gradients of less than 50 mm Hg medical follow-up is appropriate, whereas with gradients of more than 80 mm Hg, intervention is clearly indicated.[38]

Supravalvular Aortic Stenosis

Supravalvular aortic stenosis is a congenital constriction of the ascending aorta just above the superior rim of the sinuses of Valsalva.[42, 43] In children, this is sometimes seen in combination with hypercalcemia and "elfin facies" (Williams' syndrome).[44, 45] We have seen only two adult patients who had supravalvular aortic stenosis alone. A characteristic feature of this anomaly is that the blood pressure in the right arm is hypertensive, whereas that in the left arm is normotensive, with no evidence of stenosis of the left subclavian artery. Although the cardiac findings closely resemble those of valvular aortic stenosis, the striking disparity in the pressure between the two arms should raise the suspicion of supravalvular aortic stenosis, which can be confirmed by the characteristic echocardiographic findings and by those of cardiac catheterization and angiography (Fig. 8–4). The coronary arteries are usually greatly enlarged. Because they are proximal to the stenosis, they may become atherosclerotic and have compromised ostia.[46] Treatment consists of resection of the stenosis.

Subvalvular Aortic Stenosis

Subvalvular aortic stenosis has three types: a subvalvular ring,[47] a fibromuscular tunnel type,[48] and an idiopathic hypertropic subaortic stenosis type. Discrete subaortic stenosis may be familial.[48a]

Subaortic rings are very uncommon in adults. We have seen only two young adults with this condition. Both were symptomatic as young men, presenting with exertional dyspnea with peak systolic gradients of 50 to 60 mm Hg, which were significantly lower than those usually seen in asymptomatic aortic valvular stenosis.[48, 49] An aortic systolic murmur and often an aortic diastolic murmur are present, the latter resulting from aortic valvular regurgitation.[50] This is postulated to be related to impingement of the subvalvular jet on the aortic valve.[51] In patients who have a predominantly muscular ring, a characteristic Brockenbrough's sign may be observed after premature beats (i.e., a fall in the aortic systolic pressure and an increase in the intraventricular pressure after an extrasystole). Treatment of this condition involves resection of the ring. It may be necessary for this resection to be incomplete, lest the anterior leaflet of the mitral valve be damaged.[51, 52]

Idiopathic hypertrophic subaortic stenosis is discussed later.

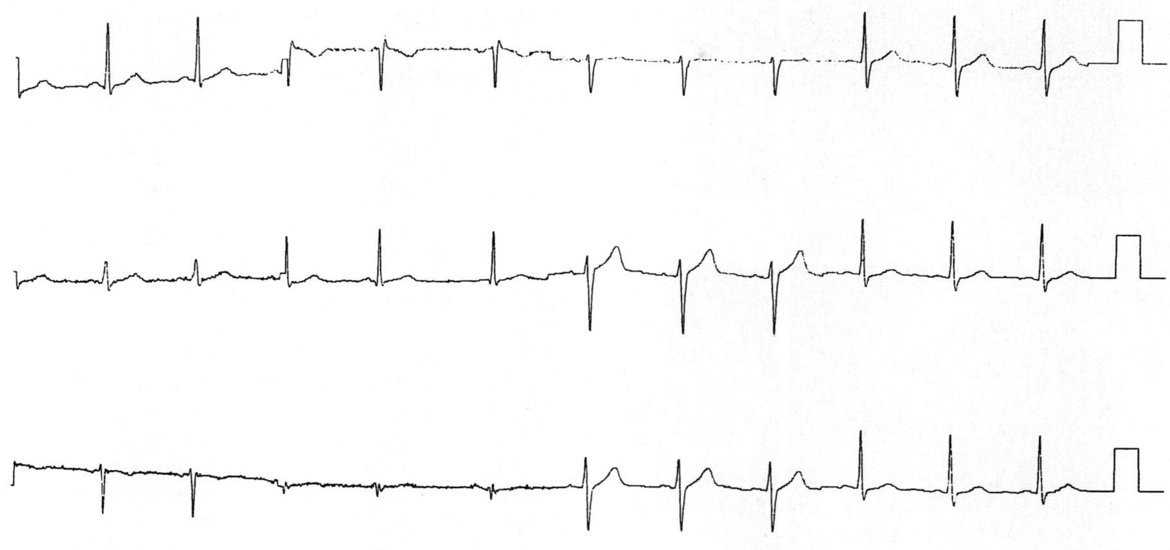

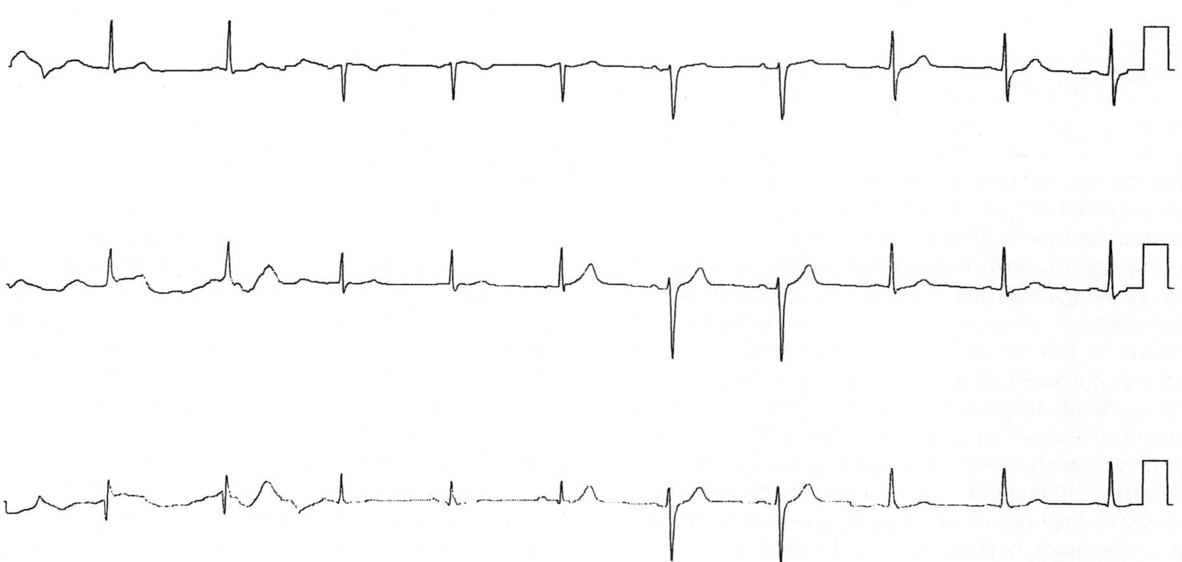

FIGURE 8–3 Electrocardiograms of a patient who developed severe symptomatic aortic stenosis within less than 8 years. Tight stenosis and angina were corrected by valve replacement. Note the absence of significant electrocardiographic changes during this interval.

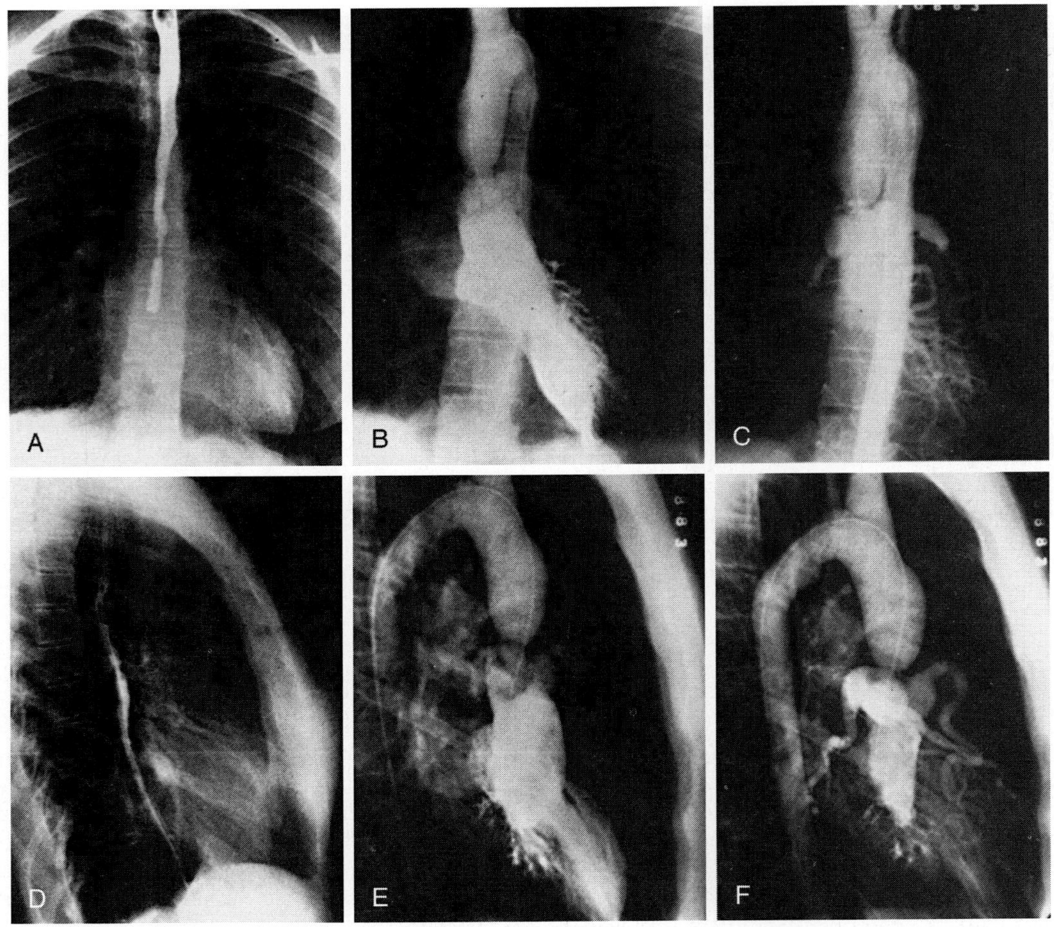

FIGURE 8–4 A–F Supravalvular aortic stenosis in a young woman. **A** and **D,** The plain chest film may be entirely normal. **C** and **F,** Left ventriculogram in diastole and systole, respectively. The severe supravalvular stenosis of the aorta is easily visualized. Note the large coronary arteries associated with high systolic pressures and marked left ventricular hypertrophy.

Mitral Stenosis

Shone's Syndrome

Congenital mitral stenosis in adults is uncommon. We have seen one instance of the Shone syndrome[53, 54] in which supravalvular mitral stenosis was associated with a parachute mitral valve (with only one papillary muscle), but not with subaortic stenosis and coarctation of aorta. The clinical picture resembles that of rheumatic mitral stenosis, in that there is a long and initially asymptomatic history followed by gradually increasing exertional dyspnea and fatigability. Atrial fibrillation may develop secondary to enlargement of the LA as a consequence of the stenosis.

Cardiac examination does not identify the opening snap characteristic of rheumatic mitral stenosis, and a diastolic rumble may or may not be present. However, there may be signs of pulmonary hypertension associated with a loud pulmonary second sound and an active right ventricle (RV). The definitive examination is echocardiography, both transthoracic and transesophageal. However, hemodynamic studies at cardiac catheterization are important for the characterization of pulmonary hemodynamics and for the search for other features of the Shone syndrome.

Treatment consists of excision of the mitral valve with valve replacement, and dilatation of the supravalvular ring if this is significantly stenotic.

Tricuspid Stenosis and Atresia

Congenital Tricuspid Stenosis

Congenital tricuspid stenosis is extremely rare in adults.[55, 56] We have seen one case, in a 26-year-old man who had an atrial septal defect without pulmonary hypertension but with a right-to-left shunt, in the pre-echocardiographic era. This was deduced to be due to congenital tricuspid stenosis. At surgery, tricuspid stenosis was indeed found, as was an atrial septal defect. Most cases of adult tricuspid stenosis are acquired, such as those associated with rheumatic fever, carcinoid syndrome, or right atrial myxoma.

Echocardiography provides a definitive diagnosis by demonstrating a stenotic tricuspid valve with an enlarged right atrium (RA). Cardiac catheterization is usually unnecessary unless the coexistence of other anomalies cannot be entirely excluded by echocardiography.

Ebstein's Anomaly

Ebstein's anomaly is seen in adults, but this is a complex anomaly that is usually associated with tricuspid insufficiency. It is discussed under that category.

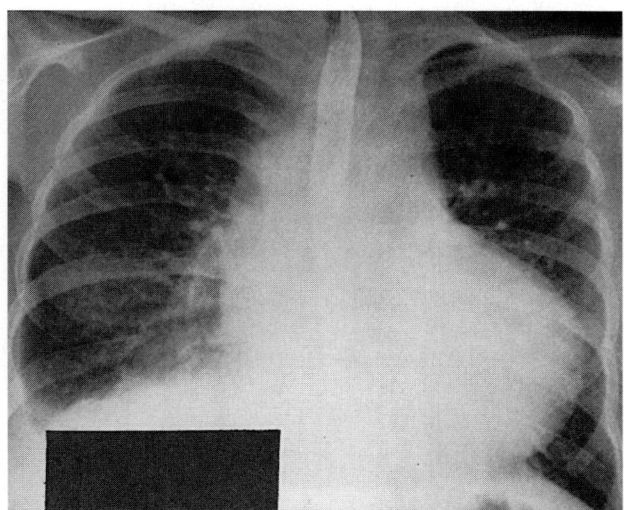

FIGURE 8–5 Tricuspid atresia in a 16-year-old girl. Note that there is unusual cardiomegaly due to the greatly dilated "right atrium," which is actually composed of the true right atrium and the thin-walled, atrialized right ventricle.

Tricuspid Atresia

Tricuspid atresia[57] is unusual but is compatible with survival to adulthood, providing that there is coexisting pulmonary stenosis.[58–60] This anomaly never occurs alone because live birth obligates patency of the foramen ovale or, more commonly, a secundum type of atrial septal defect. In addition, tricuspid atresia is almost always associated with a physiologically common ventricle, the other ventricle being smaller or rudimentary. In patients who survive to adulthood, coexisting pulmonary or subpulmonary stenosis is virtually always present. In approximately one third of the cases, the great arteries exhibit L- or D-transposition. These patients are invariably cyanotic because there is arteriovenous mixing at both the LA and at the common ventricular level. The degree of disability largely depends on the degree of arterial unsaturation. This, in turn, depends on the magnitude of pulmonary flow, which is greatest with mild-to-moderate pulmonary stenosis and with a normal or only mildly elevated vascular resistance. Paradoxically, more severe pulmonary stenosis results in more arterial desaturation but "protects" the pulmonary vasculature.

Clinically, there is always marked cyanosis with clubbing. The characteristic murmur of pulmonary stenosis can be heard. There is some degree of cardiomegaly. On chest x-ray study, the enlarged heart is somewhat bottle shaped, with normal or somewhat decreased pulmonary vasculature (Fig. 8–5). There may be associated skeletal anomalies, such as pectus excavation and kyphoscoliosis.

The ECG shows left axis deviation in patients with normally related great arteries and normal axis with D-transposition. The P waves are often large and bizarre (Figs. 8–6 and 8–7). Atrial arrhythmias are common, especially atrial fibrillation and atrial flutter (Fig. 8–8).

The echocardiogram demonstrates atresia of the tricuspid valve and evidence for an atrial septal defect with right-to-left shunting by the bubble technique, a functionally single ventricle communicating with a rudimentary ventricle via a ventricular septal defect, and often pulmonary stenosis. There may be transposition of the great arteries.

Cardiac catheterization is essential if a Fontan procedure is contemplated.[61] The pulmonary vascular resistance (PVR) must be carefully quantified and adequacy of ventricular function determined. These can be accurately ob-

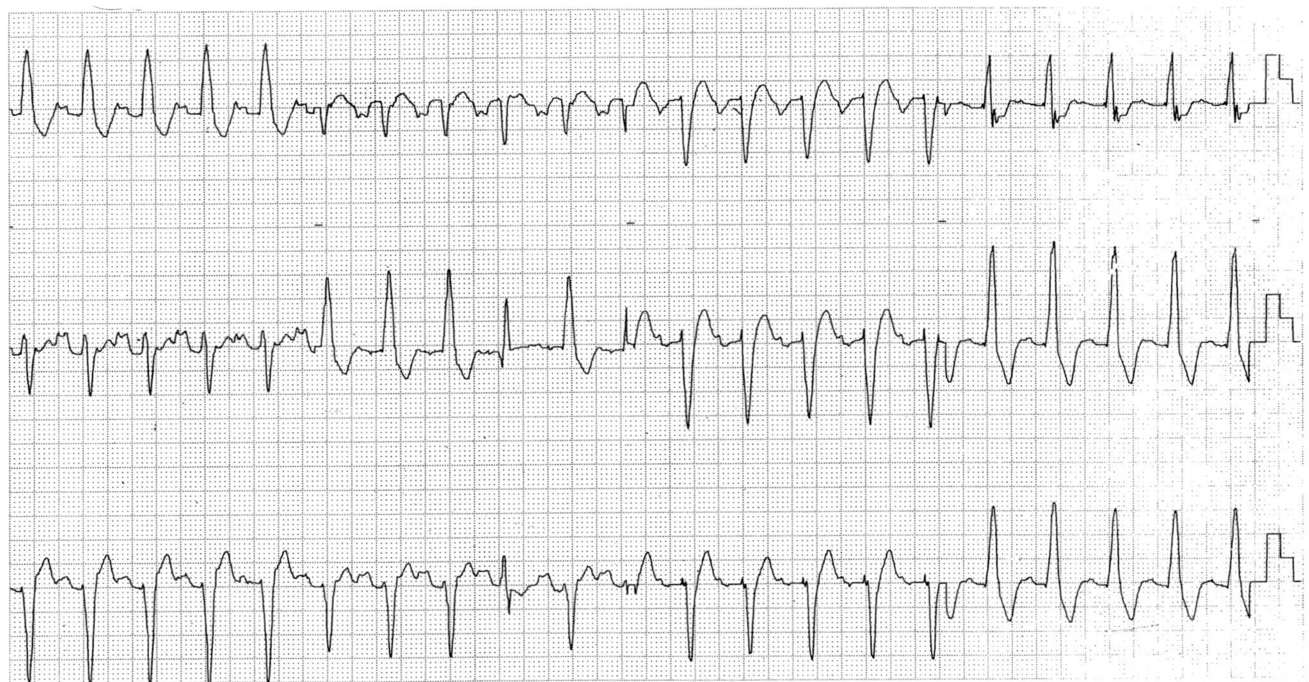

FIGURE 8–6 A 34-year-old man with tricuspid atresia and normally related great vessels. Note the left axis deviation and the unusual P waves.

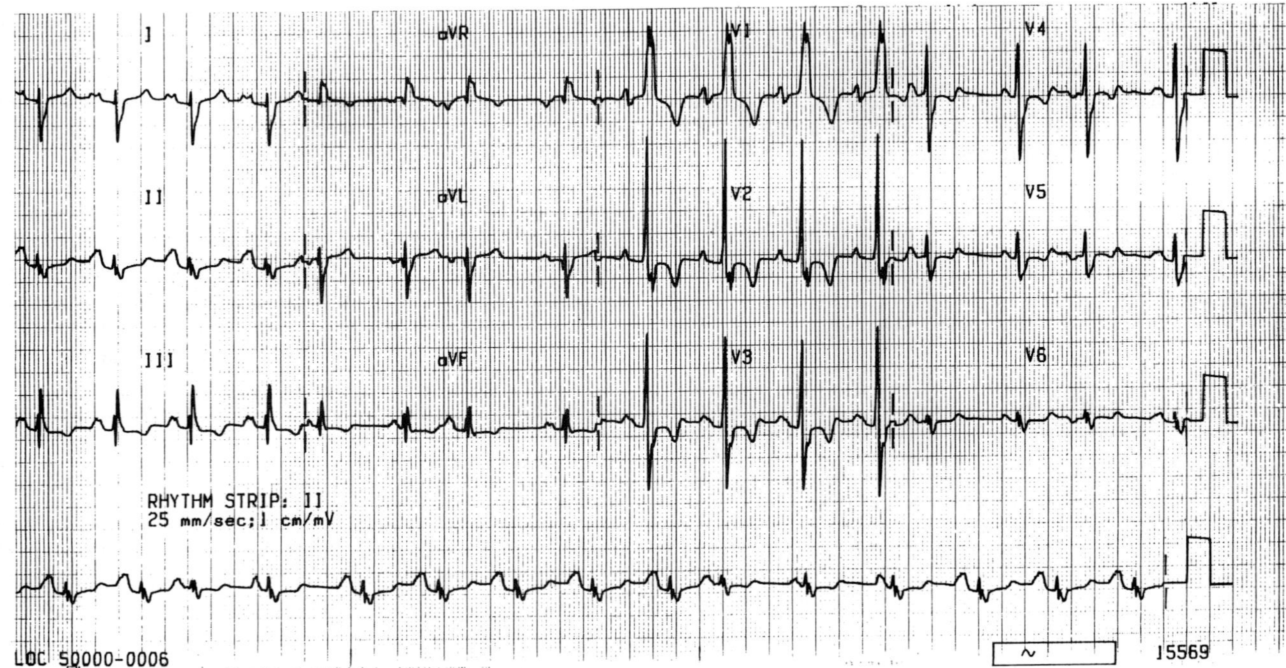

FIGURE 8–7 A 25-year-old man with tricuspid atresia. Note the marked right axis deviation in the frontal plane. This patient had L-transposition of the great arteries.

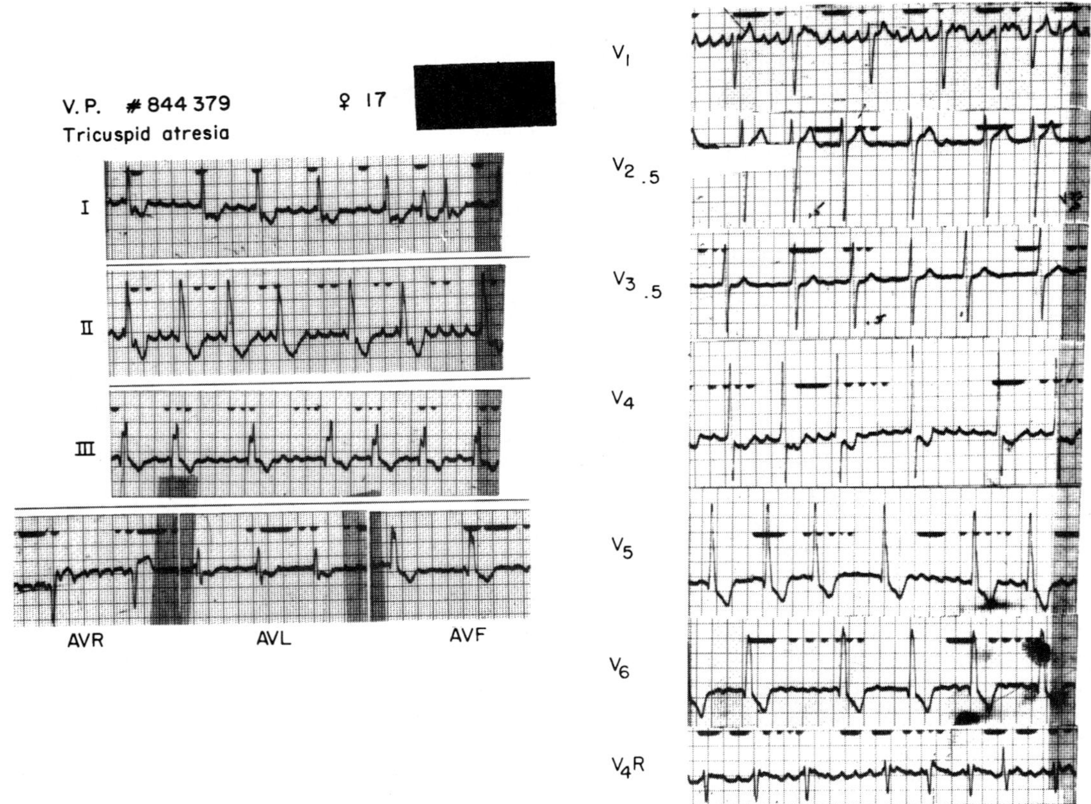

FIGURE 8–8 Electrocardiogram of a young woman with tricuspid atresia and chronic atrial flutter.

tained only with direct measurements of pressures in the pulmonary artery and the two atria and measurement of simultaneous flow by the Fick method. If the pulmonary artery cannot be entered with a catheter, the Radner procedure may be necessary.[61a] Measurement of pulmonary artery pressure is needed to calculate the PVR. Because even a mild elevation of PVR greatly decreases the success of the Fontan procedure, direct measurement is vital.

TREATMENT OF TRICUSPID ATRESIA WITH PULMONARY STENOSIS

Earlier treatment modalities were directed toward increasing pulmonic flow by creating shunts. The earliest treatment was the Blalock-Taussig anastomosis, originally devised for tetralogy of Fallot. The Glenn procedure (anastomosis of the superior vena cava to the right pulmonary artery) was another palliative modality.[62] In the Blalock-Taussig operation, a significant portion of the partially oxygenated arterial blood is recycled into the pulmonary vasculature for more complete oxygenation. In the Glenn procedure, no true shunt is involved, because the operation allows the superior vena cava to bypass the right heart and empty directly into the pulmonary artery. However, blood from the inferior vena cava continues to shunt from right to left, so that although there is some clinical improvement, the increasing desaturation of the inferior vena cava blood associated with work by the lower extremities, such as walking and running, results in shunting of increasingly desaturated blood and therefore a considerable limitation of exercise capacity.

In 1971, Fontan and colleagues[61] devised an ingenious procedure to separate the pulmonary and systemic circulations. The original procedure entailed closing the atrial septal defect, closing the pulmonary stenosis, and anastomosing the RA to the pulmonary artery by means of a conduit. A modification in which the communication between the RA and the pulmonary artery is achieved by anastomosing the right atrial appendage to the pulmonary artery avoids the use of prosthetic material.[63] In this arrangement, flow proceeds from the venous system to the LA entirely by the pressure gradient between the RA and the LA. Two obligatory conditions must be met for this to succeed: a virtually passive pulmonary vascular bed (i.e., an unequivocally normal PVR) and a completely normal left ventricular filling pressure at rest and with exertion.[64] When these conditions are rigidly met, this operation is surprisingly successful and the patients are able to live relatively normal lives with normally saturated arterial blood. Because the right atrial pressure must exceed the left arterial pressure, some of these patients may require diuretics to control edema. However, the cardiac output response to exercise is somewhat limited and, therefore, so is the maximal exercise capacity.[64] The long-term results are uncertain.[65] Palliative shunts should be performed only when the physiologic conditions preclude a Fontan procedure.

This procedure bears out the early observations that the RV can be dispensed within the presence of an otherwise normal circulation. The severe hemodynamic disturbances that may accompany right ventricular infarction are associated with an abnormal LV and its decreased compliance.

Because forward flow depends primarily on the differential atrial pressures, the "pump" function of the RA plays a relatively minor role, and supervention of supraventricular tachyarrhythmias causes symptoms that result from the rapid ventricular rate but not syncope or death.[66–68]

Patients without pulmonary stenosis or in whom the PVR is elevated can be considered for heart transplantation if their physical activity is severely limited. The Fontan procedure has been modified to treat patients with a functionally common ventricle and pulmonary stenosis by surgically closing the tricuspid valve and then proceeding as in the Fontan procedure, providing that the other physiologic criteria are satisfied.[69, 70]

Pulmonary Stenosis

Pulmonary stenosis can be valvular, supravalvular, or subvalvular. Although pulmonary stenosis may occur as an isolated anomaly, it is often associated with an interatrial or interventricular communication or with great artery transposition.

Pulmonary Valvular Stenosis

Pulmonary valvular stenosis is almost always associated with a dome-shaped valve but may be dysplastic.[71, 72] The consequent obstruction to right ventricular outflow results in right ventricular hypertrophy and, when severe, an increase in the right ventricular filling pressure. Patients with isolated mild-to-moderate pulmonary stenosis usually do well,[73, 75] whereas those with severe stenosis (systolic gradient > 80 mm Hg) should be considered for intervention.[76, 77]

Multiple peripheral pulmonary stenoses are rare in the adult (Fig. 8–9).[78–80] These are almost always associated with one of several clinical syndromes, including the following:

1. Williams' syndrome, characterized by elfin facies, unusual dentition, supravalvar aortic stenosis, mental retardation, and sometimes hypercalcemia[44, 45]
2. Noonan's syndrome, characterized by ventricular septal defect and multiple peripheral pulmonary stenoses, mimicking the clinical picture of tetralogy of Fallot[81, 82]
3. Congenital rubella syndrome[83]

In patients who have an associated probe-patent foramen ovale, right-to-left shunting at rest may occur during atrial systole (during which the right atrial pressure exceeds that of the LA) or during exercise or tachycardia, when the pressure in the RA may exceed that of the LA throughout the cardiac cycle, resulting in arterial desaturation. These elevated right atrial pressures result from the decreased compliance of the hypertrophied RV. The Valsalva maneuver at rest may cause a transient increase in the right atrial pressure relative to that of the LA during its release. During all of these conditions, it is possible for paradoxical embolization to occur.

Relatively mild-to-moderate pulmonary stenosis is com-

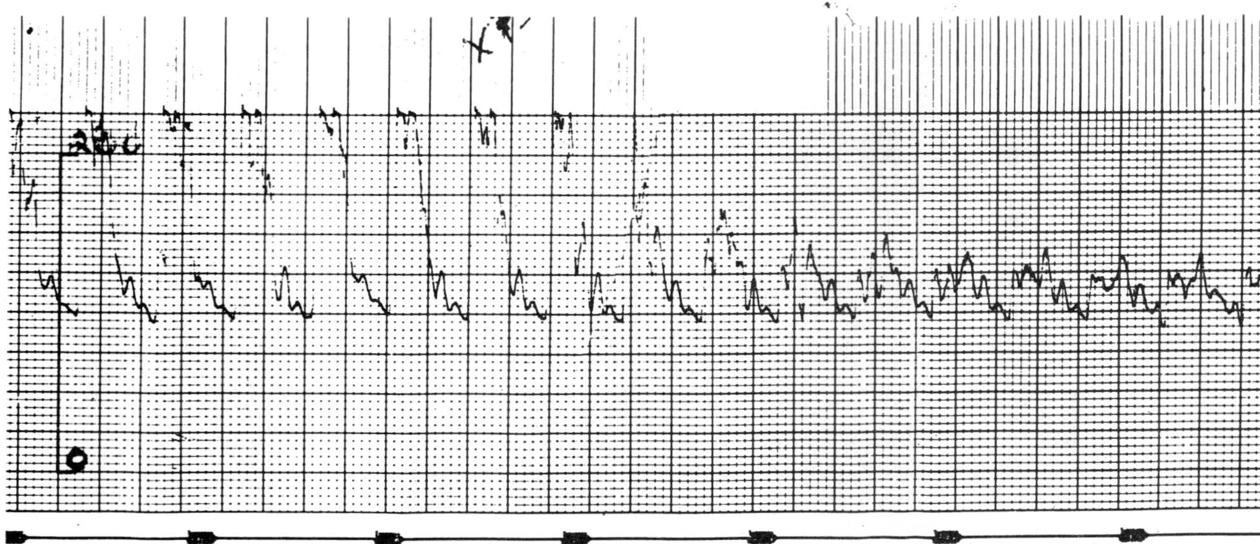

FIGURE 8–9 Tracing of the pulmonary artery pressure as the catheter is being advanced distally. Note the sudden drop in pressure as the catheter advances. This patient had the clinical picture of tetralogy of Fallot with a large ventricular septal defect. The obstruction to pulmonary flow was in the more distal pulmonary arteries rather than at the pulmonary valve.

patible with a normal existence, the chief risk being infective endocarditis.[84] In increasingly severe degrees of pulmonary stenosis, the degree of right ventricular hypertrophy increases and may result in early and significant right-to-left shunting at the atrial level, if there is an interatrial communication with arterial desaturation, and ultimately right ventricular failure. This is now an extremely rare eventuality when adequate medical facilities are available and early intervention can be instituted.

DIAGNOSIS

Pulmonary stenosis is always associated with a pulmonary ejection systolic murmur.[17] On auscultation, it is difficult to distinguish from an aortic systolic murmur because the pulmonic systolic murmur may also be heard in the neck. Two subtle auscultatory features help to confirm the diagnosis of pulmonary versus aortic stenosis. The ejection systolic murmur should be heard throughout the duration of right ventricular systole, and thus beyond A_2 and ending with P_2. Furthermore, the pulmonary systolic murmur is better heard over the left side of the back as opposed to the right. This phenomenon is related to the anatomy of the pulmonary arteries; anatomically, the left pulmonary artery is almost a direct continuation of the main pulmonary artery, whereas the right pulmonary artery comes off at a virtual right angle. There is often a systolic ejection sound (click). The ECG may be normal in mild pulmonary stenosis, but with increasing severity, the ECG demonstrates an increasing right ventricular hypertrophy in the chest leads and a tendency to right axis deviation. The chest x-ray study usually reveals normal heart size with a right ventricular configuration and a left heart border showing prominence of the main and left pulmonary arteries (Figs. 8–10 and 8–11). Calcification of the pulmonary valve is very rare. Patients with only subpulmonary stenosis do not exhibit pulmonary artery dilatation. In patients whose stenosis is far advanced, increasing cardiomegaly is present owing to enlargement of the RV and RA. The skilled observer may suspect "decreased pulmonary blood flow" by the vascular pattern on the chest film. However, this is more reflective of the decreased pulse pressure in the pulmonary arteries than of decreased pulmonary flow because it is the same as the cardiac output. The echocardiogram demonstrates a dome-shaped stenotic pulmonary valve, the severity of which can be gauged by Doppler determination of the pressure gradient and assessment of coexisting infundibular stenosis. The echocardiogram should be accompanied by a bubble study to search for a right-to-left shunt at the atrial level through a probe-patent foramen ovale, using the Valsalva maneuver if necessary.

When the stenosis is mild, the ECG is usually normal.

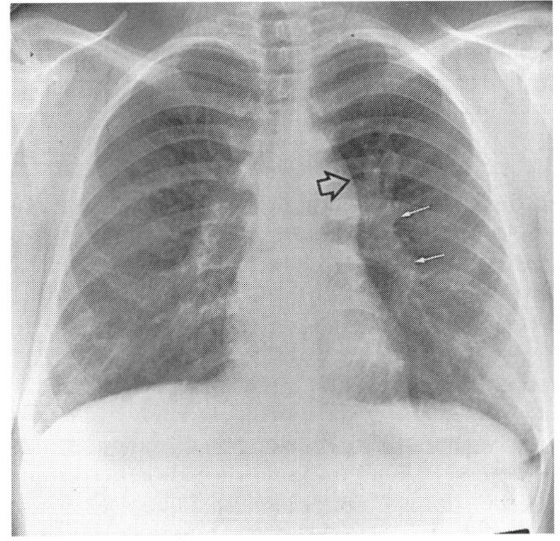

FIGURE 8–10 PA radiograph of a patient with valvular pulmonary stenosis. The heart is normal in size, and there is striking enlargement of the main pulmonary artery *(open arrow)* and the left pulmonary artery *(solid arrow)*. (Courtesy of Kurt Amplatz, M.D.)

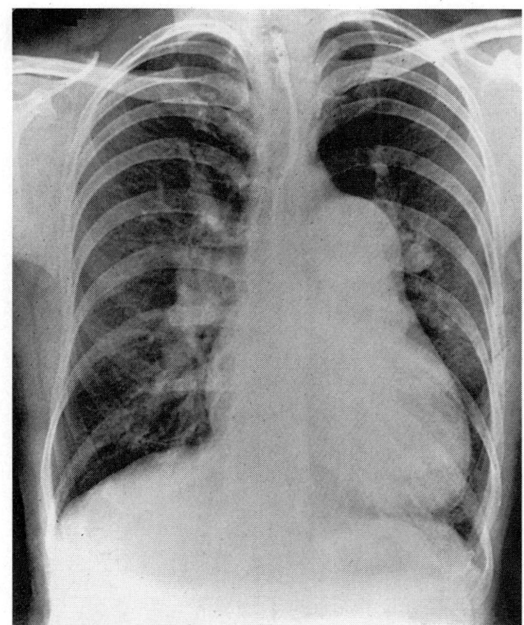

FIGURE 8–11 Pulmonary stenosis with intact ventricular septum in a middle-aged man. The cardiac shadow is unusual in that there is marked poststenotic dilatation of the main pulmonary artery. The cardiomegaly is of right ventricular configuration, typical of long-standing significant pulmonary stenosis in this age group.

With moderate to more severe stenosis (systolic gradient > 50 mm Hg), right ventricular hypertrophy is seen in the chest leads, and "P pulmonale" will be increasingly evident (Fig. 8–12).

Cardiac catheterization for direct measurement of the systolic gradient across the pulmonic valve, combined with simultaneous cardiac output measurements, permits calculation of valve orifice size by the Gorlin formula.[32] The catheter may cross a probe-patent foramen ovale, and, if so, a comparison of the oxygen saturation of the pulmonary vein and that of the systemic artery indicates whether a significant right-to-left shunt is present. Angiography in the RV visualizes the valve and right ventricular outflow tract stenosis.

PROGNOSIS

In the modern era, the prognosis is usually good because the striking murmur demands cardiac evaluation and, when indicated, intervention. However, such patients are always at risk for infective endocarditis.

TREATMENT

Treatment of isolated pulmonary valvular stenosis formerly entailed surgical valvuloplasty, but increasingly, the treatment of choice is percutaneous transvenous balloon valvuloplasty.[85] This is the noninvasive analogue of the older Brock procedure (pulmonary valvotomy)[86] but with more adequate dilatation of the valve. Treatment with balloon valvuloplasty is highly successful and can be repeated if the dilatation is inadequate or restenosis occurs.[87–89] If there is a coexisting probe-patent foramen ovale, consideration should be given to its closure because late paradoxical embolism is possible, but during balloon dilatation, it may be protective.[90] Several devices are involved in trials to close interatrial communications by transcatheter techniques.[91, 92]

Long-term follow-up of patients with pulmonary stenosis shows that the probability of survival is similar to that of the general population after 25 years (95.7 percent) whether medically or, when indicated, surgically treated. Survival is somewhat shorter when associated cardiomegaly is present.[93]

Subpulmonary Stenosis

Subpulmonary stenosis is relatively uncommon as an isolated lesion but is the more common type of pulmonary stenosis associated with a ventricular septal defect (tetralogy of Fallot).[93] Pulmonary stenosis can be either membranous or infundibular and may be clinically indistinguishable from pulmonary valvular stenosis. However, pulmonary valvular stenosis is associated with poststenotic dilatation of the main pulmonary artery, which is readily seen on chest x-ray study, and the echocardiogram is definitive. When the condition is severe, the treatment is surgical, with either resection of the obstruction or roofing of the outflow tract by patching.[94, 95] We have seen one patient in whom the "stenosis" was caused by a tricuspid valve aneurysm during systole.[96]

Mitral Valve Prolapse

Mitral regurgitation is seldom congenital but may occur on a mitral valve that is either congenitally myxomatous or prolapsed.[97, 98] There is thinning and elongation of the chordae tendineae, redundancy of the mitral leaflets, and dilatation of the mitral annulus. In some patients, the mitral leaflets have undergone myxomatous changes. The phenomenon of the valve prolapse is present in up to 10 percent of the population.[99–103] It is usually isolated but may occur in association with conditions such as Marfan's syndrome, atrial or ventricular septal defect, and connective tissue disease.[104]

COURSE

In the overwhelming majority of cases, isolated mitral valve prolapse is completely benign. However, it is the most common cause of isolated mitral regurgitation requiring surgical treatment.[105] Various symptoms have been ascribed to it, including chest pain and palpitations. Because prolapse is so common and chest pain and palpitations are relatively uncommon, there is some question as to whether mitral valve prolapse is causal: some evidence suggests that panic attacks may be responsible for many such symptoms,[106] and autonomic dysfunction has been hypothesized.[107]

Four uncommon but serious complications are chordal rupture with mitral regurgitation,[105, 107] infective endocarditis,[108, 109] stroke, and sudden death.[109, 110] The course of chordal rupture sometimes suggests that the rupture is

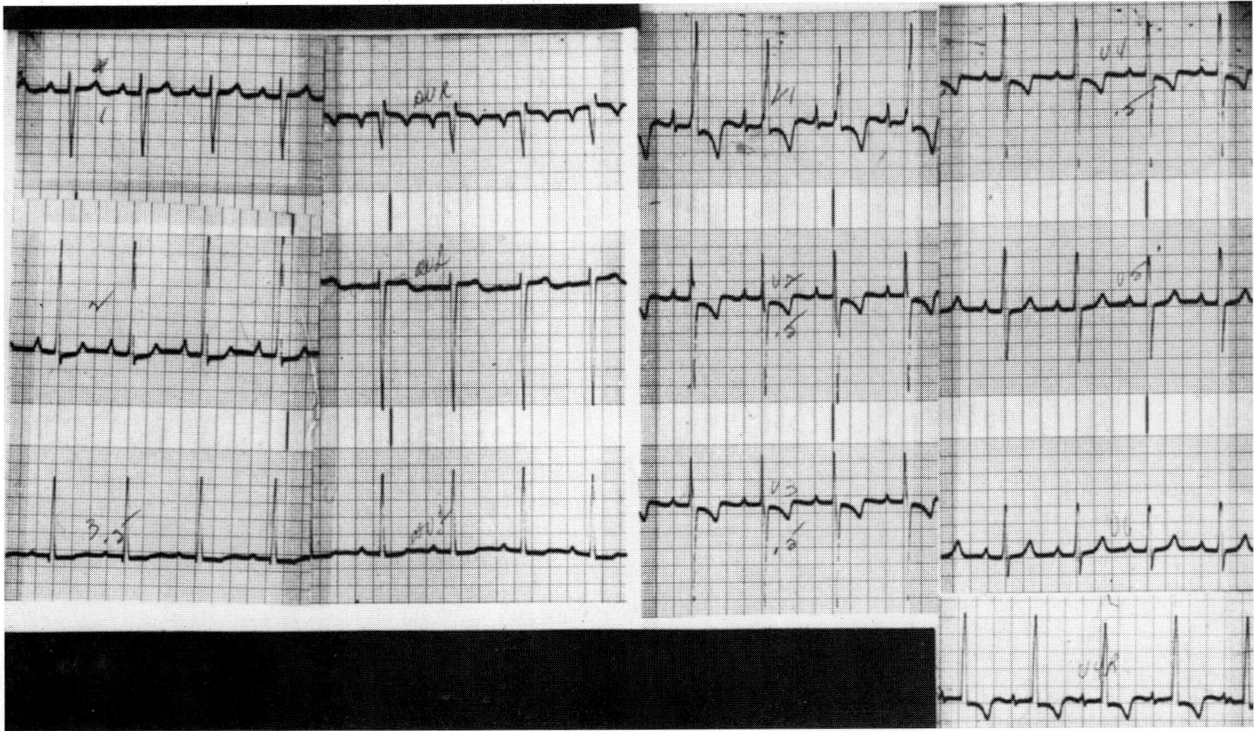

FIGURE 8–12 Electrocardiogram of a patient with severe pulmonary stenosis. Note the right axis deviation and severe right ventricular hypertrophy.

sequential. Initially, a previously asymptomatic patient may experience sudden exertional dyspnea, which rapidly worsens, presumably with rupture of successive chordae. Endocarditis entails some destruction of the valve leaflets, which, to a greater or lesser extent, results in mitral regurgitation. Stroke is a rare complication of mitral valve prolapse. The mechanism is uncertain but is believed to be associated with friction of the chordae against the atrial endocardium.[109] This mildly injured endothelium may then become the site of a thromboembolism.

The vast majority of patients with mitral valve prolapse are asymptomatic. In one series of 1376 autopsies, 7.4 percent had a floppy mitral valve. Of the 102 patients, in only two patients was mitral valve prolapse the cause of death.[111] No patient died suddenly.

DIAGNOSIS

The auscultatory findings of a mid-to-late systolic click at the mitral area and/or a mid-to-late systolic murmur establish the diagnosis. Confirmation of the diagnosis is made by echocardiography, the criterion being that the mitral leaflet or leaflets should prolapse into the LA during systole beyond the level of the mitral ring. In some patients, there is thickening of the mitral leaflets, indicating myxomatous change.[112, 113]

TREATMENT

No treatment is indicated unless the aforementioned complications ensue. If there is severe mitral regurgitation from ruptured chordae creating a flail valve, this should be corrected surgically. Severe mitral regurgitation not only causes hemodynamic disturbances but often is also associated with significant arrhythmias.[114, 115] Whereas previously, such situations always involved replacement of the mitral valve with a valve prosthesis, it is now often possible to repair the valve by reducing redundancy of the leaflets and performing annuloplasty[116] with satisfactory results, obviating anticoagulation and its possible complications. Bacterial endocarditis is a relatively rare complication on a prolapsed mitral valve. There is no general consensus as to when antibiotic prophylaxis against bacterial endocarditis during dental work should be utilized, but it is prudent to do so in the presence of mitral regurgitation.[116, 117] After a stroke, maintenance anticoagulation therapy is advisable. For patients with anxiety attacks or arrhythmias, a beta-adrenergic blocker is sometimes helpful.

Mitral valve prolapse secondary to cardiac or systemic disease has different clinical implications. Mitral valve prolapse occurs frequently in heritable diseases of connective tissue, including Marfan syndrome, pseudoxanthoma elasticum, and Fabry's disease. Although the mitral valve insufficiency under these conditions can be surgically treated, the ultimate prognosis is the prognosis of the primary disease. Surgical treatment should be aimed at repairing the mitral valve (i.e., restoring continuity to the chordae tendineae). If this is not feasible, valve replacement may be necessary.

Atrioventricular Valvular Regurgitation

Atrioventricular (AV) valvular regurgitation, long held to always be pathologic, is now seen as a phenomenon that may at times be "normal" under certain conditions when it is minimal. This has become clear with newer, highly sensitive echocardiographic techniques. Near-instant closure of the AV valves is dependent on normal sinus rhythm, an optimal PR interval, and normal ventricular function. The swiftness of AV valve closure is greatest when there is sinus rhythm with a normal PR interval, resulting in a ventricular contraction that generates the steepest intraventricular pressure rise as a consequence of the presystolic atrial "boost." Therefore, in atrial fibrillation, mild valve regurgitation may occur in the presence of a normal valve. Similarly, in marked first-degree AV block, mild regurgitation may occur because atrial systole is not timely. In AV dissociation or third-degree heart block, mild AV valve regurgitation may be intermittent, depending on the timing of atrial contraction in relation to ventricular systole. Normally, one may see mild tricuspid regurgitation, even with sinus rhythm. Thus, pathologic valvular regurgitation entails more than trivial regurgitation in the presence of sinus rhythm and a normal PR interval.

Mitral Valve Regurgitation

Mitral regurgitation may occur in a mitral valve that is either congenitally redundant or prolapsed, as is discussed later.

Aortic Valve Regurgitation

Primary aortic regurgitation is almost nonexistent in the adult, although it may occur later in life as a result of coalescence of fenestrations. However, it is a frequent complication of the Marfan syndrome.[118–120] In this disease, the fibrillin is defective, resulting in cystic medial changes in the aorta. This may occur in the absence of the Marfan phenotype.[121] If the medial changes are severe, the aorta may gradually undergo dilatation involving the aortic root, with increasingly marked dilatation of the aortic ring, and the sinuses of Valsalva cause the aortic valve to become insufficient. The regurgitation worsens with time, resulting in gradual dilatation of the LV and eventually failure. Frequently, there is mitral valve prolapse, which progresses to severe mitral regurgitation in one fourth of such patients.[122] This course may be interrupted by aortic dissection starting either at the aortic root or at the aortic arch, may involve the great arteries of the aortic arch, or, even more ominously, may dissect down into the pericardium with tamponade, sometimes avulsing the origin of the right coronary artery on the way. This is almost always a lethal sequence of events. The physical findings are those of aortic regurgitation with decreased pulses of the involved arteries. There is characteristically severe chest pain, which is frequently indistinguishable from an acute coronary event, and often severe pain in the upper back, but the event may be silent in Marfan's syndrome. Sometimes, the dissection may spontaneously heal.

The diagnosis is readily made clinically in the presence of the characteristic Marfan's phenotype when aortic and/or mitral regurgitation is present. There is arachnodactyly; long, gangly extremities; dislocated lenses; hyperextensibility of the joints; and often a family history.[123, 124] This is most readily confirmed by echocardiography, which reveals a markedly dilated ascending aorta, including the sinuses of Valsalva, to and including the aortic arch, and mitral valve prolapse.[125, 127] The chest x-ray study may look surprisingly normal in the posteroanterior view, although usually there is unmistakable prominence of the ascending aorta (Fig. 8–13). Much of the dilatation may be camouflaged by the shadow of the heart and great vessels proper, but in the lateral view, the ascending aorta is seen to "hug" the anterior chest wall up to the arch. Transesophageal echocardiography is especially useful in suspected aortic dissection to delineate the extent of the dissection, although it cannot well visualize the aortic arch.[128] The flap separating the true and false lumina of the ascending aorta is readily visualized by echocardiography with or without hemopericardium, and by aortography (Fig. 8–14). Magnetic resonance imaging with contrast gives excellent detail, but echocardiography is much more accessible and rapid.[129]

TREATMENT

Treatment of severe aortic regurgitation and of aortic dissection consists of prompt replacement of the ascending aorta and the entire aortic root and valve with a composite graft and reimplantation of the coronary arteries. Somewhat surprisingly, the operative mortality is low and the results good.[130, 131] This may in part reflect the fact that such patients are usually in the younger adult age group. However, late redissection at the anastomotic sites may occur. In cases in which the dominant lesion is severe mitral insufficiency, mitral valve repair or replacement is feasible.[132] Earlier surgical intervention before serious complica-

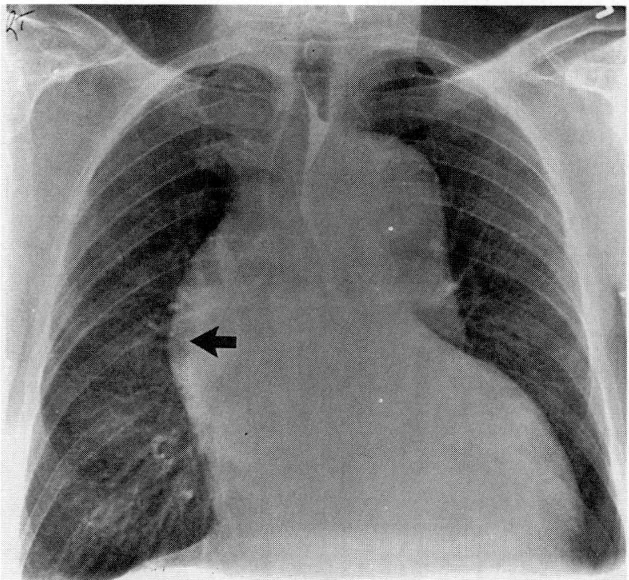

FIGURE 8–13 PA radiograph of a patient with cystic medial necrosis and severe aortic reflux. The heart is massively enlarged because of left ventricular hypertrophy, and the ascending aorta *(arrow)* and the aortic arch are huge. (Courtesy of Kurt Amplatz, M.D.)

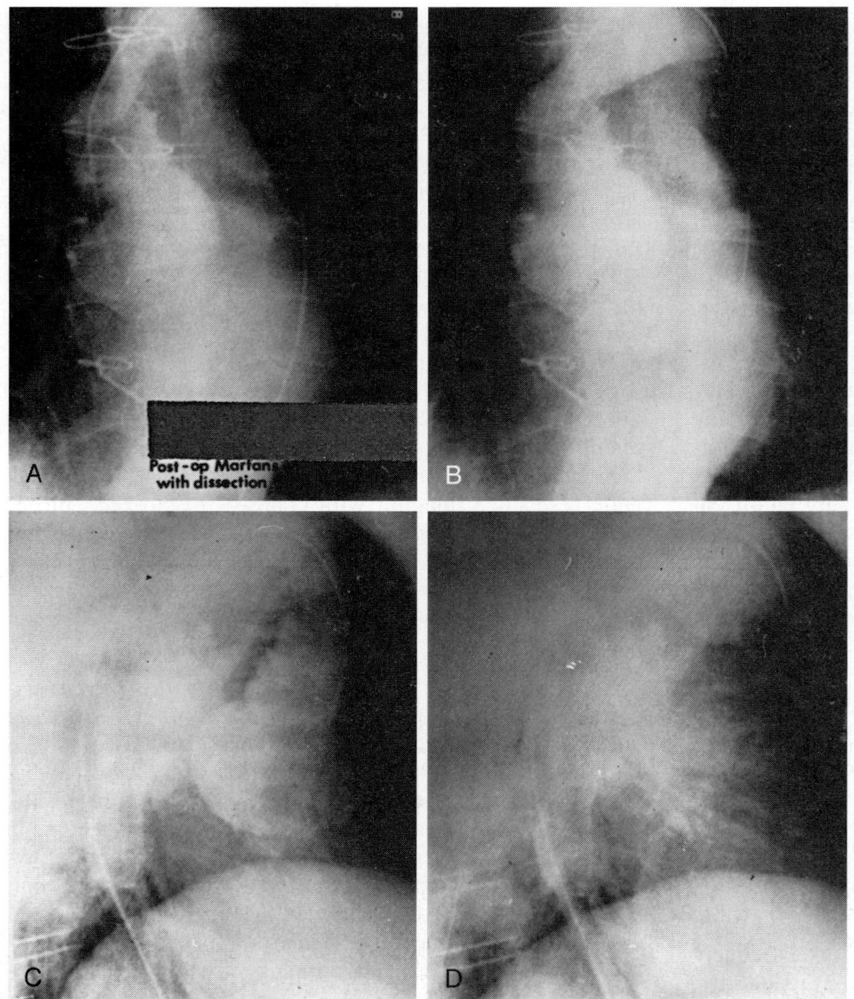

FIGURE 8–14 A–D, Marfan's syndrome with dissection of the ascending aorta and the aortic arch. Note the two channels, which are most evident in the region of the aortic arch, where the true channel is narrow and the false channel large.

tions occur has been suggested when the ascending aorta diameter exceeds 60 mm.[133, 134]

Pulmonary Valve Regurgitation

Congenital absence of the pulmonary valve is rare among adults. We have seen only two such patients. Surprisingly, the isolated condition is well tolerated because there is no pulmonary hypertension and the RV is anatomically adapted for volume load. The physiologic effect of pulmonary regurgitation therefore bears some similarity to the large left-to-right shunts associated with atrial septal defects, which are also well tolerated.

The diagnosis is made clinically by the sound of the early diastolic blowing murmur of semilunar valve regurgitation, which increases with inspiration, and palpation of an right ventricular lift.[135, 136] Echocardiography confirms the diagnosis and excludes aortic insufficiency.

Absence of the pulmonary valve may have serious hemodynamic consequences in infancy. Pulmonary insufficiency in adults is often due to valve dysplasia, and the chief concern would be the possibility of endocarditis. No treatment is usually indicated in adults.

Ebstein's Anomaly

Ebstein's anomaly consists of downward displacement of the tricuspid valve so that the septal and posterior leaflets are adherent to the right ventricular wall, thus to a greater or lesser extent "atrializing" the inflow tract of the RV.[137, 138] The tricuspid valve is deformed and may assume a cribriform appearance, and it is invariably associated with tricuspid regurgitation. Some evidence has linked this anomaly to maternal use of lithium, but this has been disputed.[139]

The physical findings show a characteristic "quadruple cadence" consisting of S_1, a "sail sound" produced by the upward motion of the billowing anterior leaflet, and wide split of S_2 due to the right bundle branch block.

In mild cases of Ebstein's anomaly, there is little or no functional disturbance, and the condition is compatible with a normal life expectancy. We have seen a patient (a surgeon!) admitted for noncardiac reasons who had the classical "sail sound" quadruple cadence who was asymptomatic and proved to have a mild form. Another patient experienced two uneventful pregnancies. When the condition is severe, the entire inflow tract is functionally atrialized, and there is little pump function of the RV. There

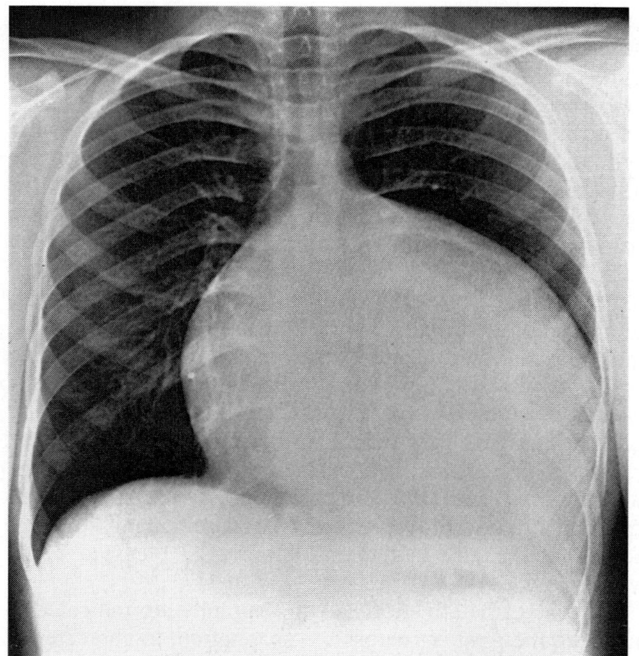

FIGURE 8–15 PA radiograph of a patient with Ebstein's malformation of the tricuspid valve with right-to-left shunt. The cardiac silhouette is huge. There is prominence of the right atrial border. The pulmonary artery segment and aorta are inconspicuous. The pulmonary vasculature is frankly decreased. (Courtesy of Kurt Amplatz, M.D.)

is an associated interatrial communication, with a patent foramen ovale or an atrial septal defect in 50 percent of patients. If right-to-left shunting occurs, cyanosis and fatigability ensue. The large "atrium" also predisposes to atrial fibrillation. The chest x-ray study is characteristic and has been described as a "pumpkin" heart (Fig. 8–15).

The diagnosis is made by echocardiography to delineate the tricuspid valve, assess right ventricular function, and look for right-to-left shunting.[140]

The ECG may show one of two patterns: Wolff-Parkinson-White pattern[141] or an unusual right bundle branch block with a "splintered" QRS complex in V_1 or V_2 (Fig. 8–16). These patients may have an accessory AV pathway that predisposes to supraventricular tachyarrhythmias.

Treatment

No treatment is needed when the condition is mild.[138] If there is considerable atrialization of the RV and some function in the remaining RV, tricuspid valve replacement or reconstruction with closure of the interatrial communication may be indicated. Electrophysiologic studies are appropriate so that an accessory pathway can be interrupted at operation. Severe cases of Ebstein's anomaly, however, do not do well over the long term.

OBSTRUCTION OF THE GREAT VESSELS

Coarctation of the Aorta

By far, the most common congenital aortic obstruction in adults is coarctation of the aorta, which in adults is almost always at or just distal to the ligamentum arteriosum and the take-off of the left subclavian artery. This anomaly is seen in adults who have hypertension in the arms and in whom there is a decrease in the pulse pressure of the femoral arteries. It is twice as common in men and is

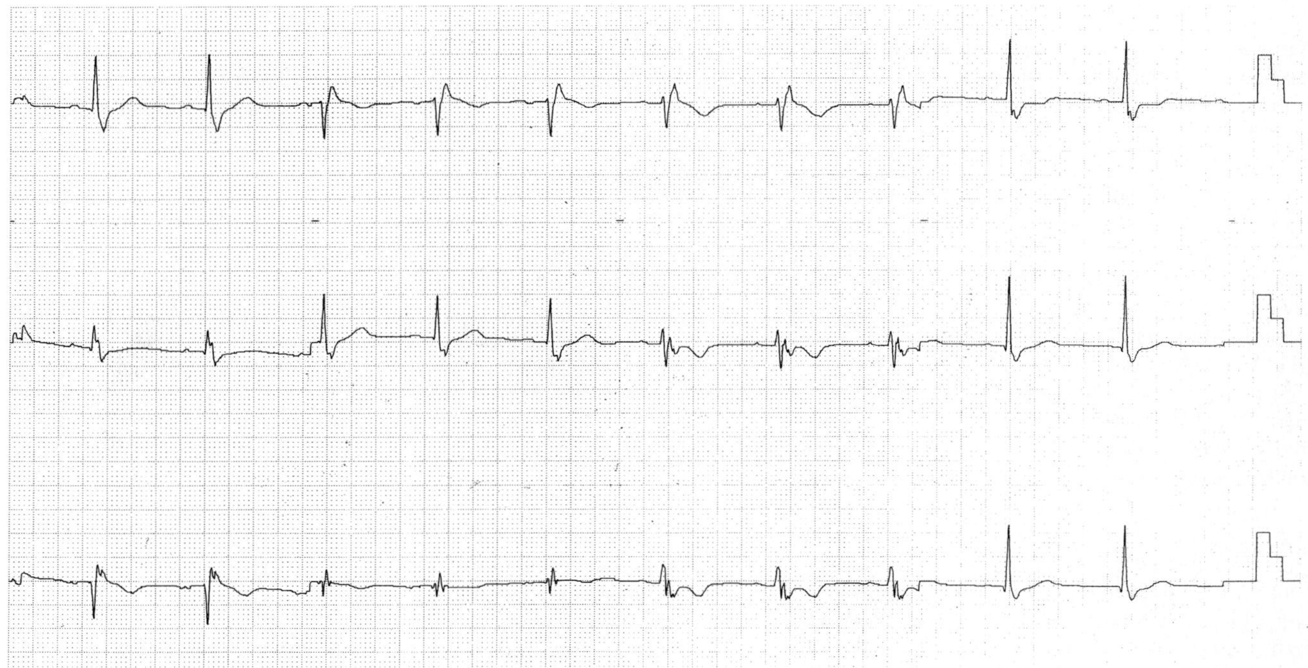

FIGURE 8–16 Electrocardiogram of a 24-year-old man with Ebstein's anomaly. Note the right bundle branch block pattern, with "splintering" of the QRS complex in the V_2 (i.e., R′SS′S).

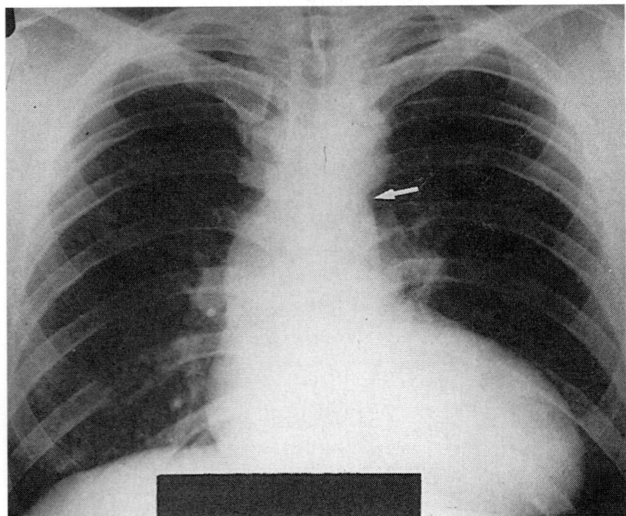

FIGURE 8–17 Coarctation of the aorta in a 24-year-old man. Note the "3" sign just beyond the aortic arch, where the indentation *(arrow)* is the site of the coarctation with a dilated aortic arch proximal to the coarctation because of the hypertension.

sometimes seen in patients with Turner's syndrome.[141a] Sometimes, there is a discrepancy between the blood pressure in the two arms. This may occur either because the coarctation is proximal to the left subclavian artery stenosis or because there is an anomalous origin of the right subclavian artery distal to the coarctation.

Physiologically, there is hypertension of the arterial system proximal to the coarctation and normotension distal to it. The decreased or absent pulses in the distal arteries are due not to low flow but to a narrow pulse pressure. Invariably, the mean pressure in the distal arterial tree is normal.[142] Flow to the distal aorta is by a number of collaterals via arterial anastomoses involving the internal mammary, intercostal, and superior and inferior epigastric arteries. It has been well demonstrated by Shepherd[142] that flow distal to the coarctation is normal at rest and in exercise. This is often not appreciated if it is assumed that impalpable pulses are associated with low flow. The difference in the systolic pressure between the upper and the lower halves of the body is determined by the degree of coarctation and by the caliber and the number of the collateral vessels. The hypertension results primarily from mechanical obstruction, but there is some evidence that damping of pulsatile flow distal to the coarctation may affect the renin-angiotensin system via the juxtaglomerular apparatus.

Mild coarctation may not be associated with significant hypertension, the consequences being those of the associated bicuspid aortic valve. This is the most common congenital cardiovascular disease in Turner's syndrome.[143]

DIAGNOSIS

There are seldom symptoms from hypertension alone. Because blood flow distal to the coarctation is normal, lower body development is normal, and claudication is not part of the clinical picture. In the adult, the clinical picture is asymptomatic until one or more complications develop.[144, 145] The diagnosis is made clinically by the faint or absent pulses in the femoral arteries in the presence of hypertension in the arms. In some instances, the femoral artery pulsations are good, but simultaneous pressure measurements in the arms and legs reveal the systolic pressure in the lower extremities to be somewhat lower than in the arms. A bicuspid aortic valve is present in more than half the cases.[146, 147] Sometimes, the intercostal collaterals are palpable, and murmurs are audible. The chest x-ray study often shows a notch at the site of the coarctation just distal to the aortic arch, the "3" sign (Fig. 8–17), caused by dilatation of the proximal aorta because of the hypertension and poststenotic dilatation distal to the coarctation. There is frequently notching of the posteroinferior border of the ribs after the second rib (Fig. 8–18). These are not directly due to increased flow per se in the intercostal arteries but rather to the tortuosity and resulting "knuckling" of the arteries from increased flow, the notches corresponding to the knuckling. Mild cases of coarctation are sometimes found incidentally in the evaluation of a bicuspid aortic valve (Fig. 8–19).

Cardiac catheterization and angiography are indicated to measure the gradient across the coarctation, to characterize the anatomy (i.e., discrete or tubular), to assess the stenosis or competency of the aortic valve, to study the coronary arteries, and to visualize the adequacy of the collateral circulation. Angiographically, contrast medium injected into the ascending aorta appears to stop at the coarctation, with delayed appearance in the descending aorta via visualizable collateral circulation.

Echocardiography is useful to assess the anatomy and

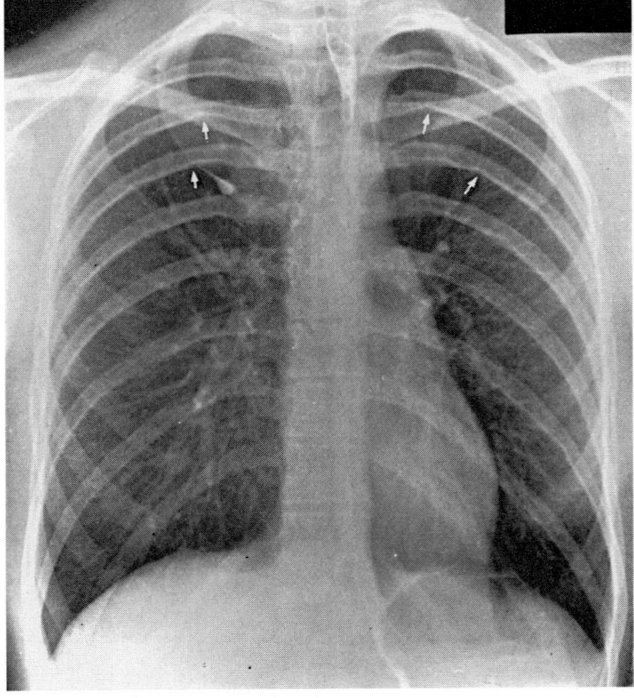

FIGURE 8–18 PA radiograph of a patient with coarctation of the aorta. The heart is not enlarged, and the pulmonary vasculature is normal. The aortic arch is inconspicuous owing to tubular hypoplasia of the distal segment. Rib notching *(arrows)* is demonstrated. (Courtesy of Kurt Amplatz, M.D.)

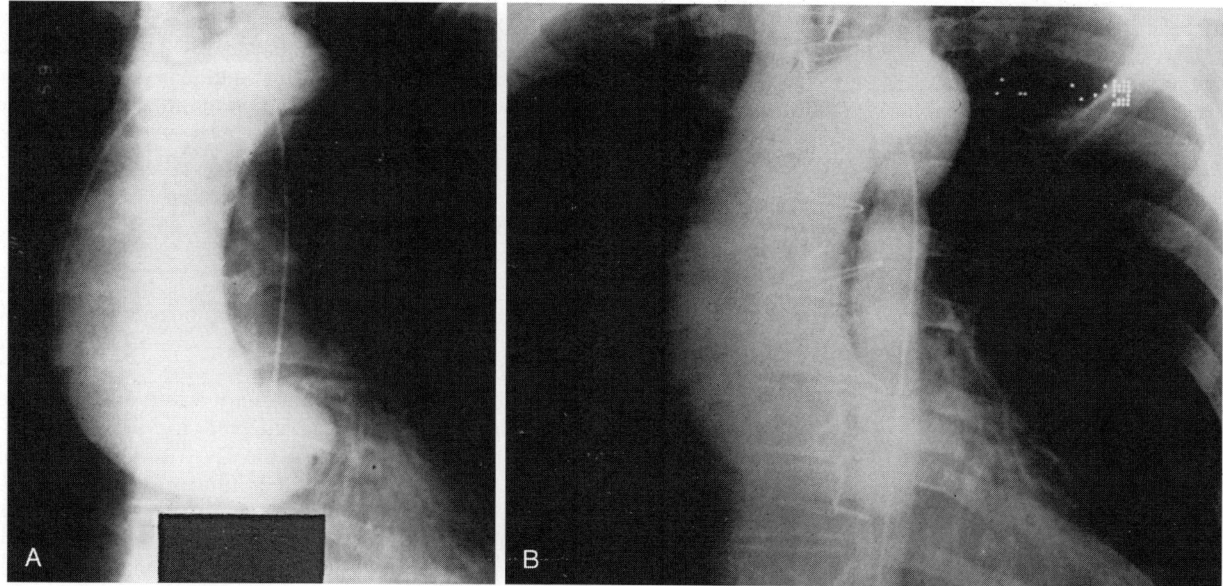

FIGURE 8–19 **A** and **B**, Mild coarctation found incidentally during evaluation of aortic stenosis on a bicuspid aortic valve. Note the characteristic poststenotic dilatation.

function of the aortic valve and the degree of left ventricular hypertrophy and to follow the diameter of the ascending aorta, especially after surgery. Transesophageal echocardiography may or may not visualize the coarctated site well.

PROGNOSIS

The frequently associated congenital bicuspid aortic valve discussed elsewhere influences prognosis separately if it progresses to significant aortic stenosis or reflux. There is an increased incidence of cystic medial changes in the aorta,[148, 149] which may predispose to aortic dissection, the initiation of which may be just above the aortic valve or in the aortic arch.[150] Aortic rupture may occur as an infrequent complication of dissection. Infective endocarditis may occur on the coarctation or, more commonly, on the bicuspid aortic valve. The presence of arterial hypertension from birth predisposes to premature cerebrovascular and CAD if the hypertension persists into adulthood.[151] Cerebral hemorrhage may occur in 20 percent of cases as a result of a frequently associated berry aneurysm of the circle of Willis.[150] In women, pregnancy increases the risk for aortic rupture, CHF due to hypervolemia, and increased hypertension.[152, 153] Most patients who survive childhood reach adulthood asymptomatic but hypertensive until one of the complications supervenes.

TREATMENT

Treatment in adults is surgical and should be undertaken as soon as the diagnosis is made. Balloon dilatation is often performed in the pediatric age group, but recurrence is common.[154] In adults, the most common form of coarctation is a discrete constriction, which is best resected with end-to-end anastomosis.[155] Sometimes, significant restenosis occurs, necessitating re-intervention. Long tubular coarctations are rare in adults. Cross-clamping of the aorta during surgery does not usually cause ischemia of the kidneys or spinal cord, because most of the distal aortic flow is via collaterals. After successful correction in the adult, hypertension often persists but is more readily controlled medically, especially with repair in later adulthood. This persistent hypertension appears to be related to baroceptor resetting and activation of the renin-angiotensin system.[156, 157] Patients must be followed up throughout their lives because of the potential complications associated with hypertension and the frequently associated bicuspid aortic valve.

Pulmonary Artery Stenosis

Peripheral pulmonary artery stenoses, whether occurring in the main branches or distally, are extremely rare in adults, although they may occur as a consequence of surgery for various anomalies, especially tetralogy of Fallot. We have seen one 23-year-old patient with multiple distal pulmonary stenoses associated with the Williams syndrome[44, 45] in the presence of supravalvar aortic stenosis, hypercalcemia, and elfin facies. This is associated with elevation of proximal pulmonary artery pressure, for which there is no satisfactory treatment (see Fig. 8–9). Single-lung transplantation is possible, in theory, but most of these patients have other serious associated anomalies.

Superior Vena Caval Obstruction

Congenital obstruction of the superior vena cava in the adult is virtually nonexistent.

Inferior Vena Caval Obstruction

Interruption of the hepatic portion of the inferior vena cava can be seen in the polysplenic syndromes associated with cyanotic heart disease.[158, 159] This is extremely rare in adults. The inferior caval blood reaches the heart via the hemiazygos-azygos system, draining into the superior vena cava. In fact, it is usually possible with skillful manipulation to pass a catheter from the femoral vein into the right side of the heart via this pathway. There are no consequences of the interruption of the hepatic portion of the inferior vena cava per se, the clinical picture being dominated by the features of the associated heart disease.

Connection of the inferior vena cava to the LA is rare in adults. Treatment requires surgical revision of the atrial septum to divert venous blood to the RA.

ABNORMAL COMMUNICATION BETWEEN CHAMBERS OR GREAT ARTERIES

Abnormal communications between cardiac chambers may be interatrial, interventricular, AV, or aortopulmonary. They may also occur between the aorta and one of the cardiac chambers. Such communications result in shunting of blood, the direction of flow being determined by the pressure gradient and/or the difference in resistance between pulmonic and systemic circulation. Therefore, in these conditions, the shunt may be entirely left to right, entirely right to left with resulting cyanosis, or right to left, occurring only under certain conditions, such as exercise (i.e., tardive cyanosis).

A unique physiologic situation exists if the defect results in formation of a common mixing chamber. For example, a subset of complete AV canal consists of complete absence of the atrial septum (single atrium) and a cleft in the anterior leaflet of the mitral valve, and sometimes in the septal leaflet of the tricuspid valve. In total anomalous pulmonary venous connection, the RA serves as the common mixing chamber. A functionally single or common ventricle in which the other ventricle is rudimentary would constitute a mixing chamber. Finally, the septum between the aorta and the pulmonary artery may be absent (i.e., truncus arteriosus). In all four of these situations, there always is arterial desaturation, regardless of the PVR. Infrequently, one or more pulmonary veins may connect anomalously in the presence of an intact atrial septum and give the clinical picture of an atrial septal defect.

Interatrial Septal Defect

Interatrial communications may be any of the following: an ostium secundum, which represents nonclosure of the foramen ovale; an ostium primum that is a subset of common AV canal and is an endocardial cushion defect; a sinus venosus defect that results from failure of the sinus venosus in the proximal portion of the superior vena cava to be incorporated into the RA; and a coronary sinus defect, in which there is a communication between the coronary sinus and the LA, resulting in flow from the LA to the RA via the coronary sinus.[160] In practice, the overwhelming majority of atrial septal defects are of the secundum type, representing about 70 percent of all interatrial communications, with ostium primum being a poor second. The sinus venosus defect is uncommon, and coronary sinus defect is extremely rare. Patients with uncomplicated interatrial communications frequently arrive at adulthood undiagnosed (Table 8–1).

Atrial Septal Defect, Secundum Type

Atrial septal defect, secundum type, is the most common congenital heart disease in the adult, possibly matched only by the bicuspid aortic valve.[161–163] It is helpful here to review the circulatory physiology in the fetus. During fetal life, the pressures in the pulmonary artery and the aorta are equal; the fetal RV, being adapted for pressure, has the same compliance as that of the LV. Cordal venous blood (arterial blood) flows via the inferior vena cava to the RA and preferentially shunts across the foramen ovale. (Vestigial preferential right-to-left streaming from the inferior vena cava can be demonstrated in adults with atrial septal defects by echocardiography or by indicator dilution techniques; the clinical counterpart is paradoxical embolization.) At birth, with the infant's first breath, there is an immediate drop in PVR, which gradually decreases to normal in the first years of life. At the same time, the RV undergoes regression of myocardial hypertrophy, gradually changing from its cylindrical configuration and thick walls to that characteristic of the adult, in which the cavity is more crescentic and the wall thinner than that of the LV. Therefore, in the fetus, there is virtually no left-to-right shunting across the defect. If the defect persists, as the PVR falls and the compliance of the RV increases, left-to-right shunting results and pulmonary flow may be two to five times the systemic flow. With time, both the RA and the RV enlarge.

Many such patients, although having normal pulmonary artery pressures in childhood and young adulthood, gradually have pulmonary hypertension with increased PVR, but significant pulmonary hypertension seldom occurs before the third or fourth decade.[163–165] The mechanism by which pulmonary hypertension develops is not well understood. It may rarely start in childhood.[166] Although high flow is implicated, it takes many decades for pulmonary hypertension to develop, and not all patients do, in fact, develop

TABLE 8-1 Paradigm for Left-to-Right Shunts at the Atrial Level

	Cyanosis	ECG, Frontal Plane Axis
Atrial septal defect, secundum type	0	Normal
Atrioventricular canal		
Ostium primum	0	Left
Common atrium	+	Left
Complete	+	Left
Anomalous pulmonary venous connection		
Partial	0	Normal
Complete	+	Normal

Abbreviation: ECG, electrocardiogram.

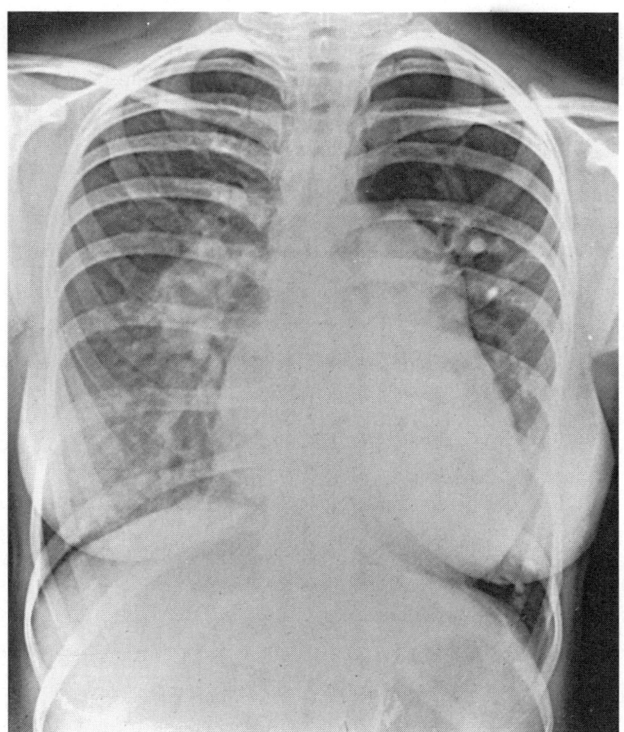

FIGURE 8–20 PA radiograph in a female patient with a large atrial septal defect. The cardiac silhouette is markedly enlarged, the pulmonary vasculature is increased, and the main pulmonary artery is huge. The aorta is inconspicuous, and there is prominence of the right atrial border. (Courtesy of Kurt Amplatz, M.D.)

it.[167] Progressive right ventricular hypertrophy caused by increasing pulmonary hypertension may lead to decreased compliance of the RV compared with that of the LV, and therefore, the exclusive left-to-right shunt also yields some right-to-left shunting. Right-to-left shunting is not a direct effect of the relative pressures of the pulmonary artery and of the aorta, but rather of the compliance of the two ventricles. If left ventricular compliance also decreases, the atrial pressures rise, and classic signs of CHF may be present. The pulmonary artery pressure in atrial septal defects with shunt reversal is almost always significantly lower than the systemic pressure. This contrasts with ventricular septal and aortopulmonary defects, in which shunt reversal and pressure equalization go hand in hand.

Approximately 10 percent of patients with atrial septal defects have one or more anomalously connected pulmonary veins, and mitral insufficiency may coexist in 10 to 20 percent.[168] The insufficiency may be due to prolapse of the posterior leaflet of the mitral valve associated with secundum atrial septal defect.[168a] An interesting syndrome has been described[169–174] in which an atrial septal defect coexists with rheumatic mitral stenosis; patients remain relatively asymptomatic until pulmonary hypertension develops because the atrial septal defect decompresses the LA, and the left atrial pressure is not elevated despite significant mitral valve obstruction (Lutenbacher's syndrome). Patients with secundum-type interatrial septal defects are seldom symptomatic until they begin to experience pulmonary hypertension, usually after the fourth decade, if it occurs. It may not occur, however. Unlike the other interatrial communications, it has a 2:1 female to male preponderance and is sometimes familial.

There is usually a soft systolic flow murmur of markedly increased pulmonary flow. The diagnostic feature, however, is a wide splitting of the second heart sound, which does not noticeably change with the respiratory cycle. This wide, fixed splitting of the second heart sound has been attributed to prolongation of right ventricular systole because of volume overload. However, it is also likely that a conduction abnormality in the RV may contribute to this. The ECG almost always shows an rSR configuration in lead V_1, the R being associated with late activation of the crista supraventricularis. This may explain why, after successful closure of the atrial septal defect, wide splitting of the second heart sound often persists. The development of pulmonary hypertension accentuates P_2, and ultimately cyanosis appears, at least with exercise if not at rest.

LABORATORY FINDINGS

The chest x-ray study (Fig. 8–20) shows an enlarged heart caused by dilatation of the RA and the RV. The central pulmonary arteries are usually enormous, with radiographic evidence of increased pulmonary flow. When significant pulmonary hypertension develops, the radiologic evidence of increased pulmonary flow decreases, and the central pulmonary arteries are often described as a "pruned tree" (Fig. 8–21). The ECG shows an rSR in lead V_1, usually with a normal axis. When pulmonary hypertension develops, electrocardiographic evidence of right ventricular hypertrophy may become manifest in the form of a tall R in lead V_1 and a rightward axis.

The echocardiographic picture of secundum atrial septal

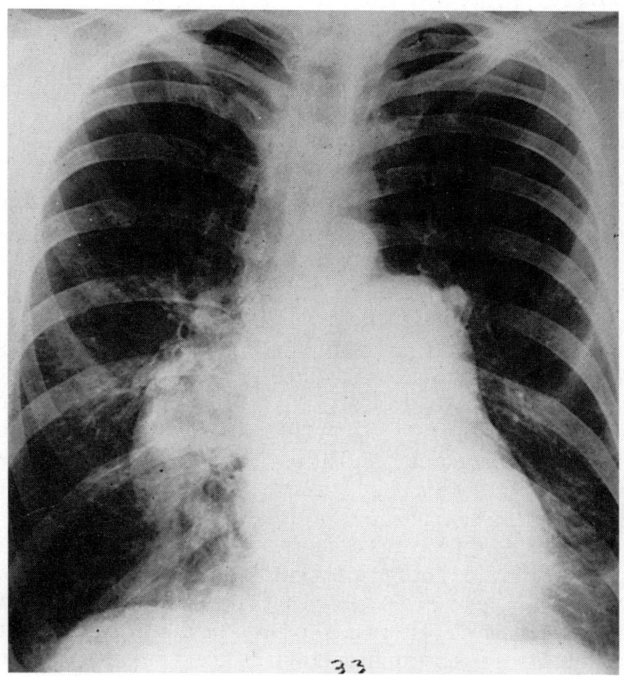

FIGURE 8–21 Interatrial septal defect with severe pulmonary hypertension. Note the increased heart size and the huge central pulmonary arteries with distal "pruning."

defects shows an enlarged RA and RV. The interventricular septum moves paradoxically, as if the septum were coopted by the RV. The interatrial septum can be seen as a "drop-out," especially by transesophageal echocardiography. Shunting is demonstrable by color-flow Doppler, and the pulmonary artery pressure can be estimated.

Cardiac catheterization is no longer indicated to confirm the diagnosis of an atrial septal defect. However, it is appropriate in middle-aged patients to characterize the pulmonary hemodynamics and to evaluate coexisting CAD before surgical correction, and also to rule out anomalous pulmonary veins, if they are not accounted for by echocardiography, for consideration of surgical correction.

PROGNOSIS

Patients with normal or mildly elevated PVR are usually asymptomatic, even with vigorous physical activity. They may have atrial arrhythmias and are at risk for paradoxical embolism. However, the development of significant pulmonary hypertension causes functional impairment, heart failure, and shortened life span, but severe pulmonary hypertension develops only in a minority of patients (<15 percent). However, there is substantial evidence that the persistence of the larger left-to-right shunt in itself shortens life expectancy, with survival beyond age 50 years being less than 50 percent. Factors contributing to this include the development of pulmonary hypertension, which overtaxes the volume-overloaded RV. The decreased diastolic compliance of the aging LV may further increase the left-to-right shunting, and supraventricular tachyarrhythmias and paradoxical embolism further complicate the course.[163–165, 168]

TREATMENT

Because the mortality risk of surgical closure of an uncomplicated secundum atrial septal defect is approximately 1 percent and the adverse consequences (i.e., pulmonary hypertension, paradoxical embolism, and shortened life expectancy) have a higher risk, early closure should be recommended, even when patients are asymptomatic. However, when there is severe pulmonary hypertension, especially with right-to-left shunting, the pulmonary/systemic flow ratio may be closer to 1, and closure would be contraindicated because closure would not be expected to improve pulmonary hypertension. In such cases, lung transplantation with closure of the defect or heart-lung transplantation could be considered. Closure should be recommended, even if patients are asymptomatic. However, should really small atrial septal defects be found in childhood, there is some evidence favoring waiting because about half of such patients have spontaneous closure of the defect (age, 8.4 years).[181a]

Percutaneous Repair

Open-heart surgery for the closure of defects in the atrial septum is currently the "gold standard" for the treatment of such patients. The mortality rate for this procedure is close to zero percent in most contemporary reports.[175–178] However, open-heart surgery is a major procedure, with its attendant morbidity, need for intensive care, and significant hospitalization. The complication rates after surgical closure of atrial septal defects in adult patients can be as high as 13 percent.[179]

The pioneering work of King and Mills[180, 181] resulted in the development of a double-umbrella device and established the feasibility of occluding atrial septal defects with percutaneous devices. The need for a 23 French delivery sheath and the cumbersome procedure led to its abandonment. Many other devices were subsequently developed, including the Rashkind single-disc device,[182–183] the Locke USCI "clamshell" device,[184–188] the "buttoned" device,[189–198] the ASDOS device,[199–202] the Monodisk device,[203] and the Das Angel Wings. All of these devices are essentially umbrella variants. They all have one or more wire struts that go radially from or across the center of the disc or discs to the periphery to support a fabric patch.

In 1993, we were the first to report on the experimental results of a new, self-centering, nitinol-polyester atrial septal defect closure device (Figs. 8–22 and 8–23).[204] A new device made from braided nitinol wire that also self-centers because of a central conjoint ring was later reported on by Sharafudin and coworkers in 1996.[205]

Patients with secundum atrial septal defects that are less than 20 mm in diameter with a distance of at least 4 mm from the AV valves, coronary sinus, and pulmonary veins are candidates for percutaneous closure. On echocardiography, the atrial septal defect has to be central in location. The presence of a deficient anterior rim is not considered to be an indication for exclusion from the procedure because the aortic root behaves as the anterior rim in those with deficient anterior rims. Patients with atrial septal defects also require evidence of right ventricular volume overload on echocardiography. In addition, patients who have a patent foramen ovale with a presumed paradoxical

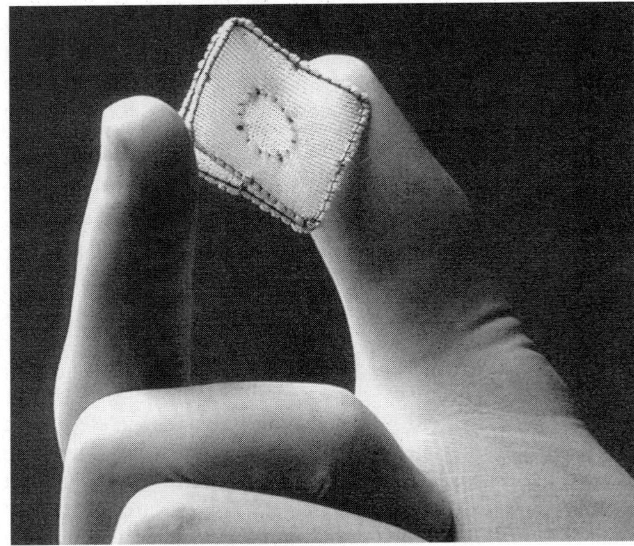

FIGURE 8–22 The Das Angel Wings transcatheter atrial septal defect closure device. This shows the construction of the double-disc device with two square wire frames of "super-elastic" nitinol, which are covered by polyester fabric. The device is photographed from the right atrial disc side, highlighting the prominent conjoint suture ring in the center. Note the corner eyelets, which act as torsion rings.

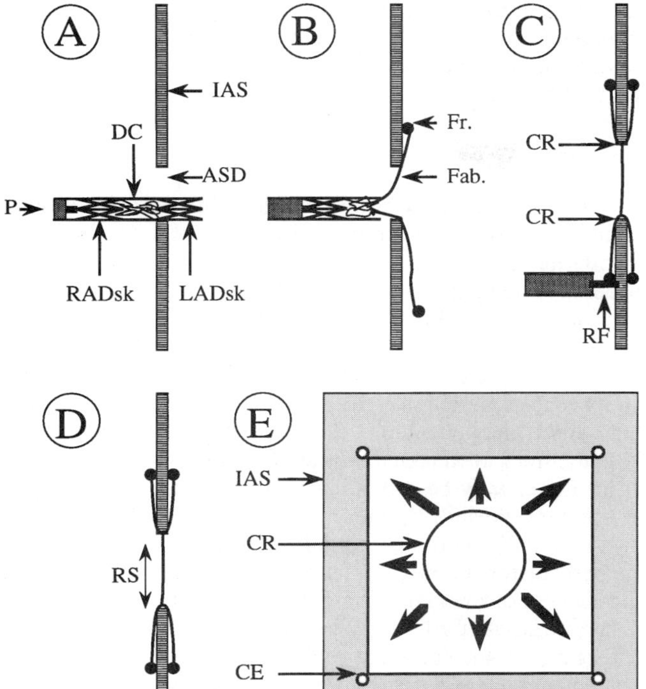

FIGURE 8–23 Schematic illustration of the mechanism of closure. Panels **A** to **D** are sectional views; panel **E** is a frontal view. **A,** The delivery sheath is positioned across the atrial septal defect (ASD). DC indicates delivery catheter; P, pusher. **B,** the left atrial disc (LADsk) has been deployed. Fab. indicates fabric. **C,** The right atrial disc (RADsk) has been deployed with frame (Fr.) attached to the release fixture (RF). **D,** The released implanted device. Note the increase in the diameter of the ASD. RS indicates radial stretch. **E,** The conjoint ring (CR) has been opened. *Radial arrows* illustrate the direction of the radial stretch due to the square super elastic wire frame. CE, corner eyelet; IAS, interatrial septum. (**A–E,** From Das GS, Voss G, Jawis G, et al: Experimental atrial septal defect closure with a new, transcatheter, self-centering device. Circulation 88[4 pt 1]:1754–1764, 1993.)

embolism, patients with significant residual shunts after either surgical or device closure, and patients with a fenestrated Fontan or baffle leak can have percutaneous repair of these defects.

PROSTHESIS

The Das Angel Wings device consists of 2 square frames made of "super-elastic" nitinol wire (0.012-inch diameter) with radiopaque markers of platinum at each corner. Each square frame has four legs that are interconnected by flexible eyelets at the corners.[204] At the midpoint of each leg, there is a flexible eyelet, and these eyelets function as torsion springs that permit the device to be collapsed and loaded into the delivery catheter. The wire frames are covered by polyester fabric, which is sewn onto the wire frames after being stretched taut. A circular hole, whose diameter is approximately half the length of the side of the disc, is punched out from the right atrial disc, and the margin of this orifice is sewn onto the fabric of the left-sided patch to form a conjoint suture ring. The hole is punched out to reduce the bulk of the fabric. The device is available in a range of sizes from 12 to 40 mm. The size of the device refers to the length of each side of the square. The device has a custom-designed delivery system that consists of a control handle connected to either an 11, 12, or 13 French–sized delivery catheter (11 French for the 12-mm device; 12 French for the 18-, 22-, 25-mm devices; and 13 French for the 30-, 35-, and 40-mm devices).

CATHETERIZATION AND DEFECT CLOSURE PROTOCOL

All closures are performed in the cardiac catheterization laboratory using general anesthesia with the patients intubated. Transesophageal echocardiography is used to help guide device deployment. Access is gained percutaneously from both the femoral veins and the left femoral artery for monitoring systemic pressure. After a right heart study, the defect is crossed with an end-hole/NIH angiographic catheter (USCI, Bard, Tewksbury, MA). A left atrial angiogram is performed in the 30-degree left anterior oblique projection with 30-degree cranial angulation and a straight posteroanterior projection. These views are obtained primarily to provide "road maps" for the deployment of the device. The defect is recrossed with an end-hole catheter, and a 0.038-inch, 260-cm-length Amplatz Super Stiff exchange wire (Mansfield Meditech Corp., Watertown, MA) is placed across the defect. A 27- or 33-mm balloon occlusion catheter (Mansfield Meditech) is calibrated outside the body by inflating it with measured volumes of radiographic contrast diluted with saline in a 1:4 dilution. The diameter of the balloon is measured for every 1-ml increase in volume. The balloon catheter is then passed over the wire to the LA. The balloon is inflated to a size larger than the defect, and it is attempted to be pulled through the atrial septal defect using gentle traction. The volume of the balloon is gradually decreased, and the minimum diameter of the balloon that cannot be pulled across the defect is determined. This is referred to as the balloon occlusive diameter.

The device size to balloon occlusive diameter ratio that is selected is approximately 1.5. An appropriate-size device is selected, and a suitable (11/12 or 13 French) Mullins transeptal sheath is passed over the exchange wire until the tip is in the mid-LA. The hub of the Mullins sheath is immersed in a tray with saline to prevent the entry of air. The appropriate-size device in its delivery catheter is then passed through the Mullins sheath and advanced until the tip of the delivery catheter exits the tip of the sheath. The blue actuator ring is torqued clockwise to deploy the left atrial disc. The Mullins sheath and the delivery catheter are then held as a unit, and the left atrial disc is manipulated until it is seated flush against the atrial septum. The right atrial disc is then deployed, and both fluoroscopy and transesophageal echocardiography are used to assess the deployment. If the deployment is satisfactory, the release knob is loosened, and the device is released. After the deployment of the device, right atrial angiography is performed to evaluate the device. No catheters are manipulated into the pulmonary artery to obtain an oximetry run or for angiography because of concern of dislodgment of, or entanglement with, the device. All patients are given broad-spectrum antibiotic prophylaxis for 24 hours. During the procedure, the patients are heparinized to obtain an activated clotting time > 300 seconds. At the completion of the procedure, the effects of heparin are reversed by use of protamine sulfate. The patients are allowed to recover from anesthesia, observed overnight, and discharged from the hospital the next morning. All patients are recommended to take aspirin, 325 mg daily (adult dose), for a period of 6 months. Patients undergo a transesophageal echocardiographic evaluation between 3 and 6 months after the procedure. Echocardiographic residual shunting is graded according to the classification proposed by Boutin and associates.[206]

CURRENT STATUS OF THE DEVICE AND RESULTS

The device is undergoing a United States Food and Drug Administration–approved clinical trial. After successful completion of the phase I trials, the device is in the phase II trials in the United States. At the University of Minnesota, a total of 52 device closures have been performed in adult patients. Procedural success was possible in 51. In a patient with a suboptimal deployment and difficulties in retrieval, surgical retrieval and closure of the atrial septal defect were required. Many retrieval strategies have subsequently been developed, and most of these infrequently encountered suboptimal deployments are likely to be managed per catheter with retrieval of the device and percutaneous closure of the defect. The completion of the United States trials and greater experience with this device in the United States are likely to establish the utility of this device for the percutaneous repair of interatrial communications in adult patients. The manufacturer is also developing a second-generation circular device that is repositionable and retrievable into the delivery catheter. This would make the device more user friendly than at present and obviate surgery for suboptimal deployments.

LATE COMPLICATIONS

A common complication after successful surgical closure is the occurrence of atrial arrhythmias, especially atrial fibrillation or flutter (Fig. 8–24). Atrial flutter in such patients is usually paroxysmal but may be chronic and extraordinarily stable for years, belying the reputation of atrial flutter as an inherently unstable rhythm (Fig. 8–25). The ventricular rate can often be controlled with digitalis, and because the flutter rate may be significantly slower than 300 beats per minute, the electrocardiographic picture is sometimes mistaken for that of digitalis toxicity. Such atrial flutter may be difficult to keep in sinus rhythm after conversion. Atrial fibrillation may likewise be paroxysmal but is usually chronic. Antiarrhythmic drugs sometimes succeed in maintaining sinus rhythm after conversion, but the success of maintaining sinus rhythm in a patient predisposed to atrial fibrillation associated with an enlarged RA and previous atriotomy is problematic.[169] Endocarditis does not occur on the defect but may occur on an insufficient cleft mitral valve.

In patients in whom closure of an atrial septal defect is contraindicated by a low pulmonary/systemic flow ratio, treatment is symptomatic. Adequate control of the ventricular rate, especially with atrial arrhythmias, and judicious use of oxygen are helpful. Anticoagulation with low-dose warfarin (Coumadin) is advisable to minimize paradoxical embolism. Endocarditis does not occur in the secundum type of defect per se, because flow across the large defect

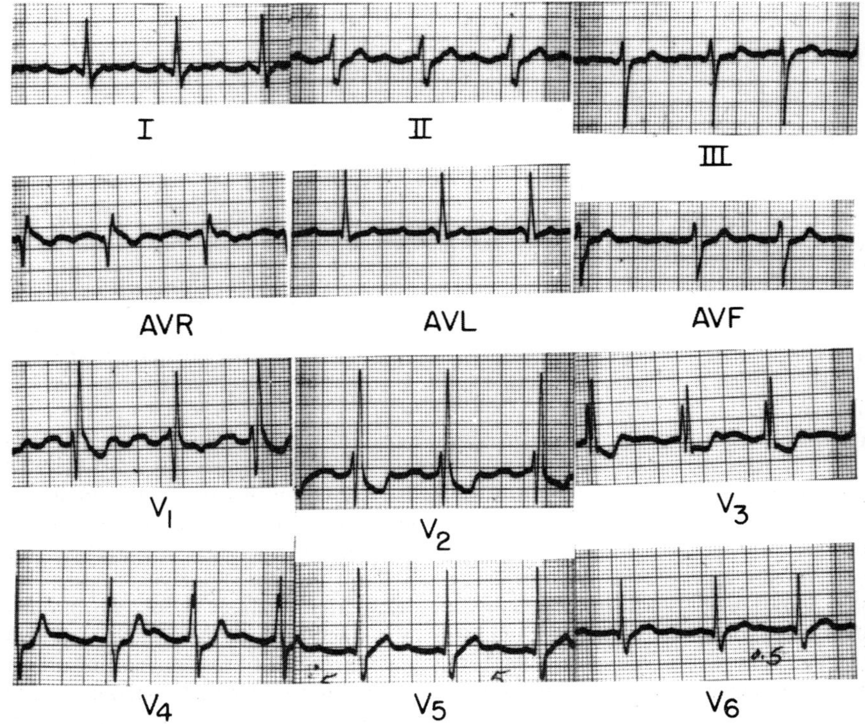

FIGURE 8–24 Electrocardiogram of a patient with an ostium primum defect, severe pulmonary hypertension, and mitral insufficiency through a cleft anterior leaflet. Note the left-axis deviation, right ventricular hypertrophy, and atrial flutter.

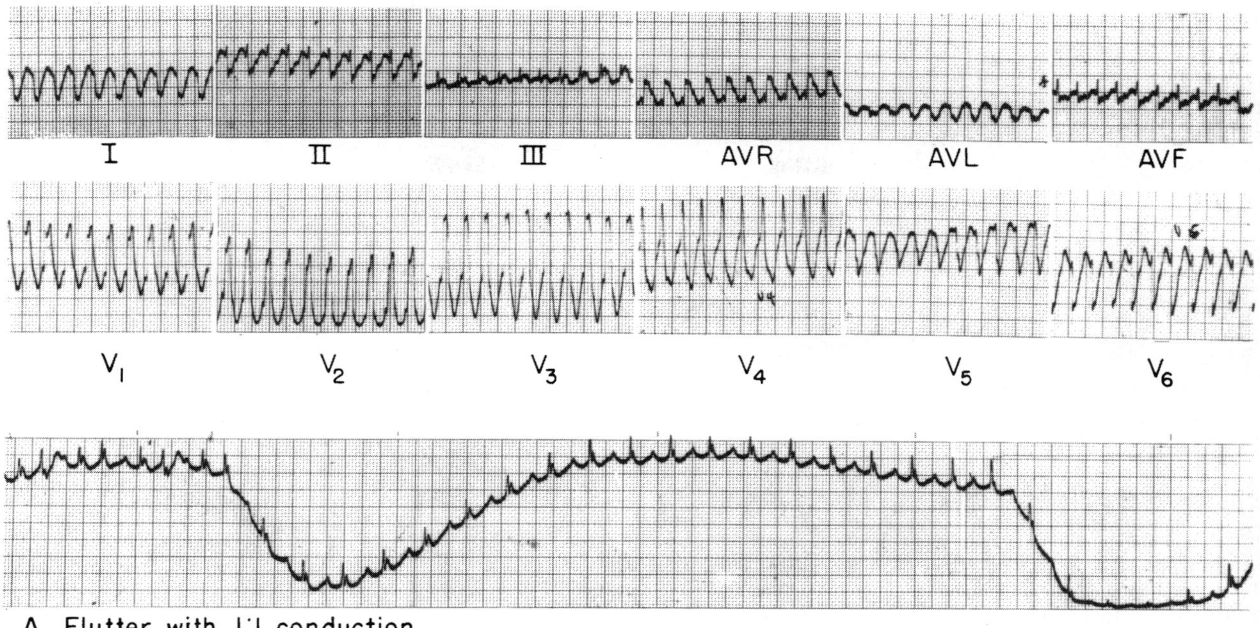

FIGURE 8–25 Rapid atrial flutter with one-to-one conduction in a patient who claimed to "not be feeling well" while walking down the hall. This occurred 1 week after closure of a secundum-type atrial septal defect.

is at a low pressure. However, if mitral valve prolapse coexists, the considerations for infective endocarditis prophylaxis would be those pertaining to isolated mitral valve prolapse. Cardiopulmonary transplantation would be a consideration in patients with advanced disease who are disabled.

Septum Primum Defect

Septum primum defect, commonly termed *ostium primum*, is an endocardial cushion defect in which the septum primum (i.e., the lower portion of the atrial septum) fails to develop, as does the membranous portion of the ventricular septum. In this situation, the anterior leaflet of the mitral valve is attached to the ventricular septum in a somewhat lower position than normal and is therefore no longer in direct continuity with the aortic valve. The anterior leaflet is cleft and, because of its lower position, has characteristic angiographic[171] and echocardiographic[174] features. The mitral valve cleft is associated with various degrees of mitral regurgitation. The considerations governing interatrial shunting and those involved in the development of pulmonary hypertension are similar to those of the secundum type of atrial septal defect. However, if the degree of mitral regurgitation is more than mild, it may cause left ventricular dilatation and both left atrial and right atrial enlargement.

The clinical diagnosis of an ostium primum has many of the features of those associated with a secundum-type atrial septal defect (i.e., hyperactive RV; wide, fixed splitting of the second heart sound; and pulmonary flow murmur). However, there is usually an additional murmur of mitral insufficiency associated with a cleft in the anterior leaflet. This does not necessarily radiate to the axilla, because the regurgitant jet impinges more medially than toward the free wall of the LA. If the mitral regurgitation is severe or if pulmonary hypertension develops, decreased exercise tolerance and exertional dyspnea can be expected. Examination may also show an left ventricular filling sound (the third heart sound of mitral insufficiency) and an S_4. The chest x-ray result is very similar to that of a secundum-type atrial septal defect unless there is severe mitral insufficiency, in which case, there is evidence of left atrial enlargement as well. The ECG has the characteristic rSR in lead V_1, but in addition, the frontal plane axis is always leftward, and there is often first-degree heart block (Fig. 8–26). With pulmonary hypertension, the chest leads show right ventricular hypertrophy (Fig. 8–27).

Until and unless pulmonary hypertension develops, the interatrial shunting is left to right, and there is no cyanosis. When the mitral insufficiency is severe, there may not be a significant elevation of atrial pressures, because the RV is adapted for volume overload and accepts the increased left-to-right shunt. However, with a decrease in compliance of a failing or hypertrophied RV because of pulmonary hypertension, atrial pressures rises, and the pulmonary venous pressure can be estimated from inspection of the neck veins.

The natural history of ostium primum defects differs significantly from that of a secundum-type atrial septal defect. Primum defects are susceptible to infective endocarditis on the cleft mitral valve. If the mitral regurgitation is severe, patients may have dyspnea and left ventricular dysfunction, and if the right ventricular compliance is compromised, there are signs of both right ventricular and left ventricular failure. AV canals as a group are prone to develop increasing degrees of AV block and not infrequently progress from first-degree block to second-degree and then to third-degree block. The last, however, is usually

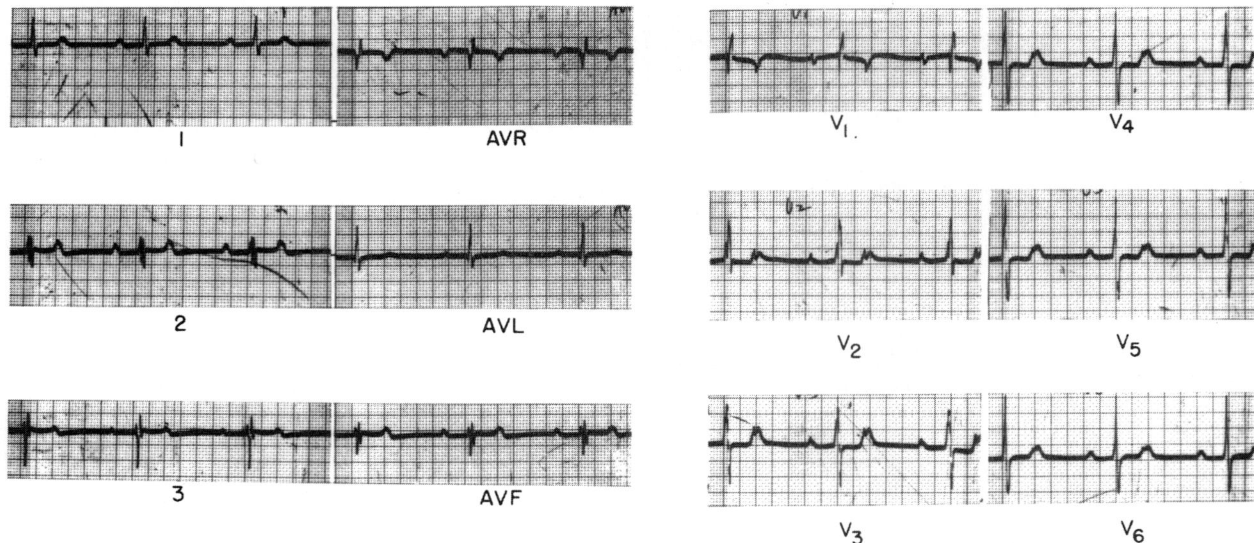

FIGURE 8–26 Electrocardiogram of a patient with an ostium primum. Note the left axis deviation, incomplete right bundle branch block in V_2, and first- and second-degree atrioventricular block.

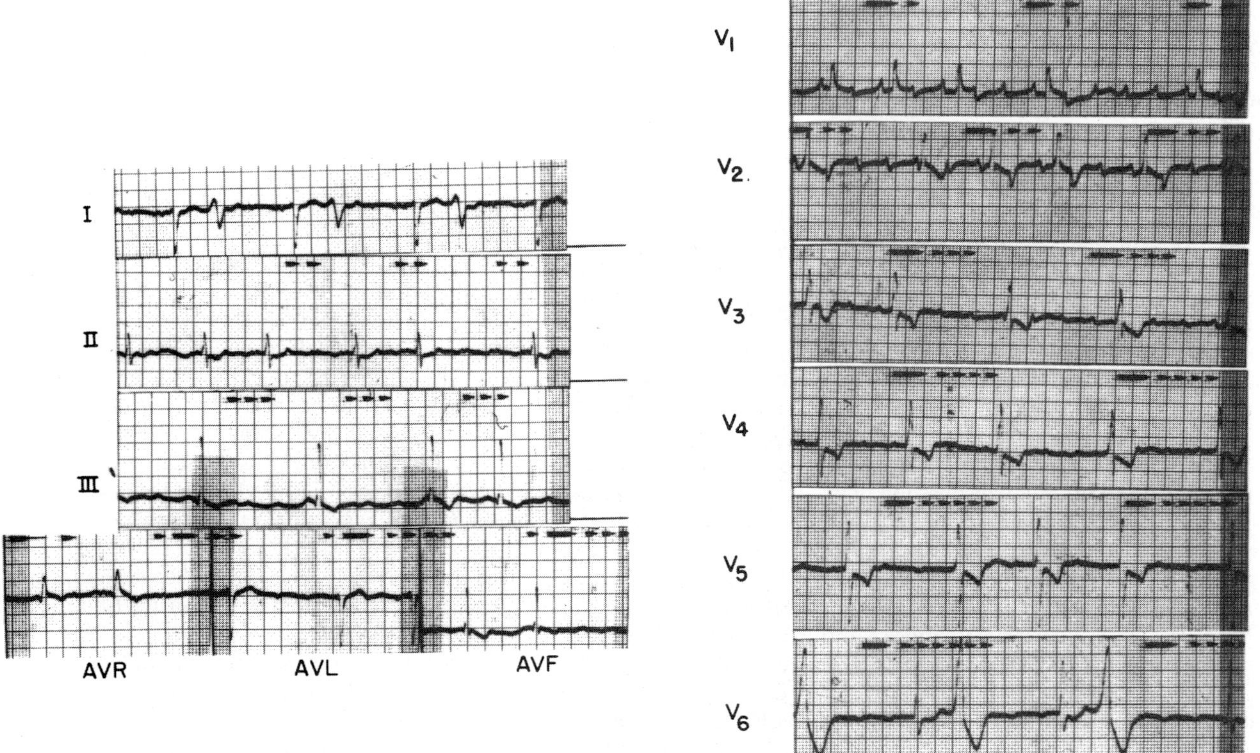

FIGURE 8–27 Electrocardiogram of a patient with an atrial septal defect of secundum type with severe pulmonary hypertension. Note the right-axis deviation and right ventricular hypertrophy. This patient has slow flutter with varying atrioventricular conduction, which resembles "paroxysmal atrial tachycardia with block" and may be mistaken for digitalis intoxication.

associated with a junctional rhythm rather than an idioventricular rhythm.

Patients with complete AV canal seldom survive to late adulthood without cardiac surgery. The ECG shows left-axis, right ventricular hypertrophy, large P waves, and various degrees of AV block (see Fig. 8–26).

LABORATORY STUDIES

The echocardiogram shows a low-lying atrial septal defect with no continuity between the anterior lead of the mitral valve and the aortic valve, and a cleft in the anterior leaflet of the mitral valve.[174] The mitral and tricuspid valves are at the same level. There is mitral insufficiency of varying degree, an enlarged RV, paradoxical septal motion, and enlarged atria. Angiographically, the left ventriculogram reveals a "goose-neck" deformity (Fig. 8–28), related to the unusual attachment of the anterior leaflet of the mitral valve, and some degree of mitral insufficiency.[171]

PROGNOSIS

The large left-to-right shunt may eventually lead to pulmonary hypertension. The cleft mitral leaflet results in increasing mitral regurgitation and left ventricular dysfunction and is susceptible to infective endocarditis. Finally, AV block may develop as part of the natural history of endocardial cushion defects.

TREATMENT

The definitive treatment for an ostium primum defect is early surgical closure.[206a] The condition is not suitable for transcatheter closure, in contrast to the secundum type of septal defect, because the lower border of the defect is in direct continuity with the anterior leaflet of the mitral valve. Precautions during surgical closure include not encroaching on or injuring the AV node and the bundle of His. Therefore, patching rather than direct suturing is required. The treatment of the cleft mitral valve depends on the degree of mitral regurgitation. When there is minimal or mild regurgitation, it is more prudent to leave the mitral valve alone. In more moderate or severe mitral regurgitation, surgical attempts to suture the cleft may aggravate regurgitation because the chordal architecture is quite different from that of a normal valve. However, valvuloplasty is often feasible in skillful hands. Should the patient show evidence of a second- or third-degree heart block, DDD pacing would be advised but only after the atrial septal defect has been closed, because the electrodes are thrombogenic and paradoxical embolization may occur.

PROGNOSIS

The prognosis for ostium premium septal defects that have undergone surgical closure depends on the degree of pulmonary vascular disease, complications associated with mitral valve prostheses, and left ventricular function. If the mitral insufficiency has been relatively severe and longstanding, even mitral valve replacement may provide only a short-term reprieve from eventual failure of the LV.

Single Atrium

Single atrium is a variant of AV canal. It is characterized by a total absence of the interatrial septum and a cleft in

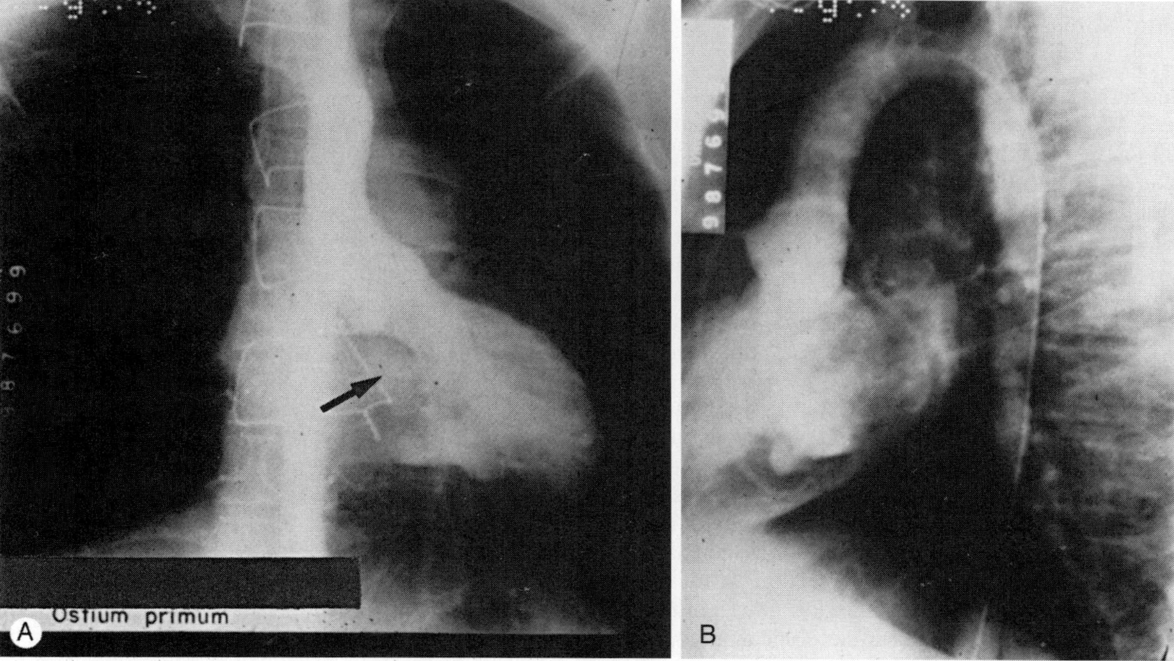

FIGURE 8–28 A and **B,** Left ventriculogram of a 21-year-old woman after surgery for closure of an ostium primum defect. Note the unusual "bite" out of the inferomedial portion of the left ventricle, giving rise to the so-called goose-neck deformity. This is due to the lower attachment of the anterior leaflet of the mitral valve to the ventricular septum so that it is at the same level as the tricuspid valve, whereas normally it is attached more superiorly.

the anterior leaflet of the mitral valve. The clinical profile differs in that these patients invariably have some cyanosis, if not at rest at least with exercise, because the common atrium acts as an incomplete mixing chamber. The ECG is essentially the same as in ostium primum, as is the ventriculogram. The echocardiogram differs in that there is complete absence of the interatrial septum. Because of the arteriovenous mixing, these patients are symptomatic at an earlier age, and surgical creation of an interatrial septum is advisable as soon as the diagnosis is made.

Sinus Venosus Defect

Sinus venosus defect is an atrial septal defect located posteriorly subjacent to the superior vena cava. It is almost always associated with the anomalous insertion of at least one pulmonary vein adjacent to the superior vena cava. Clinically, it is indistinguishable from a secundum type of atrial septal defect. On echocardiography, the defect is seen posteriorly rather than in the area of the foramen ovale, and an anomalous pulmonary vein can be identified. With cardiac catheterization, if the venous catheter enters the heart from the superior vena cava, it very frequently goes out a pulmonary vein when the tip reaches the cavoatrial junction. Successful surgical closure of this defect is more difficult because of the presence of an anomalous pulmonary vein adjacent to the superior vena cava, and some degree of dehiscence of the patch near that area is common. As long as the residual left-to-right shunt is small, it should not cause difficulty.[207, 208]

Coronary Sinus Fistula

A congenital defect may occur between the coronary sinus and the LA, which results in a left-to-right shunt that physiologically resembles an atrial septal defect.[209] This entity can be suspected when echocardiography fails to identify an interatrial septal defect in the presence of clinical and radiographic evidence of a left-to-right shunt. Cardiac catheterization yields an oximetry series that is consistent with a shunt at the atrial level. A useful maneuver is to introduce the catheter into the coronary sinus, which is not difficult in the hands of an experienced operator. The coronary sinus yields a rather high oxygen saturation, in contrast to the normally very low saturation. It may be difficult to distinguish between a coronary sinus fistula and partial anomalous pulmonary venous connection to the coronary sinus. However, the coronary sinus fistula is more proximal, and sampling of the more distal blood in the coronary sinus should yield a low saturation, whereas with an anomalous pulmonary venous connection to the coronary sinus, there is a higher saturation throughout the coronary sinus. This entity is of some clinical importance because the coronary sinus ostium can be rather large, and there have been rare instances in which the coronary sinus ostium has been mistakenly closed for an atrial septal defect.

Partial Anomalous Pulmonary Venous Connection

The connection of one or more pulmonary veins to a structure other than the LA should be considered in patients with clinical or radiographic evidence of left-to-right shunting at the atrial level.[210, 211] Partial anomalous pulmonary venous connection may occur with no interatrial communication.[212–214] It may coexist in approximately 10 percent of secundum-type atrial septal defects. The insertion may be directly into the superior vena cava; into a vertical vein that goes into the innominate vein and then into the superior vena cava; into the RA directly; to the coronary sinus[215]; or, rarely, into the inferior vena cava (scimitar syndrome)[216] (Fig. 8–29). If the cardiologist is alert to the possibility, the echocardiographer who is warned is usually able to identify these. They may also be identified through cardiac catheterization techniques using selective pulmonary arteriography (including the levophase) or by means of selective indicator dilution techniques, as originally pioneered by Wood. It is important to be alert to these veins because the closure of a secundum-type atrial septal defect alone only partially decreases the left-to-right shunt if several anomalous pulmonary veins coexist.

Ventricular Septal Defects

Isolated ventricular septal defects are infrequently seen in adults.[217] About 45 percent of small ventricular septal defects close spontaneously in early childhood, up to the age

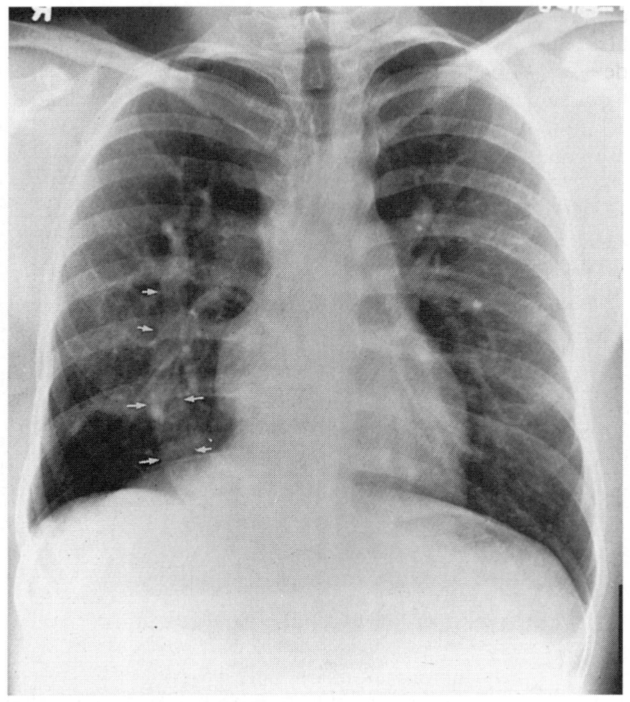

FIGURE 8–29 PA radiograph of patient with partial anomalous venous return to the inferior vena cava (scimitar syndrome). The heart is normal in size, as is the pulmonary vasculature. The anomalous drainage through a large scimitar vein *(arrows)* is well demonstrated. (Courtesy of Kurt Amplatz, M.D.)

of 10 years.[218] When these patients are seen as adults, these defects are associated with little or no hemodynamic disturbance of the LV and result in only a small left-to-right shunt and no pulmonary hypertension. Large defects, defined as exceeding 1 cm^2/m^2, are associated with equalization of pressure in the two ventricles and therefore in the pulmonary artery.[219] The direction and the degree of shunting are determined by the relative resistances of the pulmonary and systemic circuits. The right-to-left and the left-to-right shuntings are more or less balanced if the resistances in the systemic and pulmonary circulations are equal. This is the classic Eisenmenger's complex. Large defects with a low to mildly elevated PVR have large left-to-right shunts and severe volume overload of the LV. These are almost invariably discovered by a pediatric cardiologist, and the defect is closed.[220] Therefore, in adults, the common forms of congenital ventricular septal defect are either large ones of the Eisenmenger physiology or those in association with pulmonary stenosis, in which the pulmonary circulation is "protected," such as in tetralogy of Fallot. Occasionally, one may see patients from Third World countries who have a moderate-size ventricular septal defect (0.5 to 1.0 cm^2/m^2), a large left-to-right shunt, and an enlarged LV and are symptomatic. Unless there are separate, serious comorbid factors, the defect should be closed.

The most common form of congenital isolated ventricular septal defect is of the so-called membranous type, which is posterior and inferior to the crista supraventricularis, involving what would be the membranous septum and some of the adjacent muscular septum.[221] This is situated just under the septal leaflet of the tricuspid valve and is subtended by the aortic valve. The bundle of His courses along the posterior rim of this defect and is therefore not affected, but it is vulnerable during surgical closure of the defect. Multiple muscular septal defects may also occur as isolated congenital lesions.[221] These are present in about 10 percent of the cases of ventricular septal defect. They are generally multiple and small, so that even in the presence of large shunts, there is seldom significant elevation of the right ventricular or pulmonary artery pressure. Although many of these defects close spontaneously, they may persist and are difficult to close completely at the time of surgery because of heavy trabeculation on the right ventricular aspect of the interventricular septum. The seemingly logical left ventricular approach to closure of the lesion would seriously compromise the contractility of the LV.

The predominant type of congenital isolated ventricular septal defect seen in adults is that termed the Eisenmenger complex (i.e., a large ventricular septal defect with severe pulmonary vascular obstruction and bidirectional shunting).[222]

Small Ventricular Septal Defects (Maladie de Roger)

Patients with small ventricular septal defects are totally asymptomatic. The volume overload of the LV is minimal to mild. The heart size remains normal, and pulmonary hypertension does not develop on the basis of this defect alone. The sole risk is that of infective endocarditis.

Rarely, a moderate-size defect may be converted to a smaller defect by adhesion of the septal leaflet of the tricuspid valve, aneurysm formation of the membranous septum, or prolapse of an aortic cusp.[223] This prolapsed cusp may in time become adherent to the ventricular septal defect, partly occluding it functionally. The patient may then present with primarily aortic regurgitation and a small ventricular septal defect.

The diagnosis of a small ventricular septal defect is made clinically by the characteristic holosystolic murmur, starting with the first heart sound. This may be of the so-called diamond shape because of the high-pressure jet through a small orifice. This holosystolic murmur should not be mistaken for mitral insufficiency. It is loudest at the left sternal border but does not radiate to the neck. In mitral regurgitation caused by a redundant anterior leaflet, the murmur is transmitted to the axilla, whereas if it is associated with a redundant posterior leaflet, it radiates medially and often is transmitted to the neck. The chest x-ray study and ECG are normal. The diagnosis is best confirmed echocardiographically with the color-flow Doppler technique.[224, 225] It is also readily visualized on the left ventriculogram (Fig. 8–30). Providing that this is truly a small ventricular septal defect and not one that has been made small by the prolapse of an aortic cusp, surgery is not indicated unless there are other unrelated cardiac defects that require surgical correction. The prognosis is good, and the chief precaution is the need for prophylaxis against infective endocarditis. If a "small" ventricular septal defect is associated with significant aortic regurgitation due to a prolapsed cusp, the major consideration is that of the aortic regurgitation.

Large Ventricular Septal Defect

The rare patient who survives into adulthood with a large ventricular septal defect and a large left-to-right shunt but in whom no Eisenmenger's physiology is yet present may exhibit symptoms similar to those of patients with significant mitral insufficiency, both representing examples of left ventricular volume overload with reflux. The chief manifestation is exertional dyspnea as a consequence of elevated left ventricular filling pressure, and sometimes an angina-like sensation in the presence of marked pulmonary hypertension. Radiographic studies show cardiomegaly, primarily of the LV, and enlarged central pulmonary arteries with radiologic evidence of increased pulmonary flow. The ECG may show tall voltages in the chest leads associated with left ventricular volume overload. Echocardiography is essential not only to confirm the large left-to-right shunt but also to determine the type and the location.[226] Cardiac catheterization is helpful in defining the pulmonary hemodynamics for surgical risk assessment and for ultimate prognosis. Left ventricular angiography in several views is very helpful. Some of these patients may unexpectedly experience a systolic gradient between the RV and the pulmonary artery (Gasul's phenomenon).[227]

Surgical closure of ventricular septal defects is associated with conduction abnormalities in as many as 15 percent of cases, consisting of right bundle branch block and left-axis deviation[228, 229] (Fig. 8–31). There are no extensive data on progression to third-degree heart block, but it

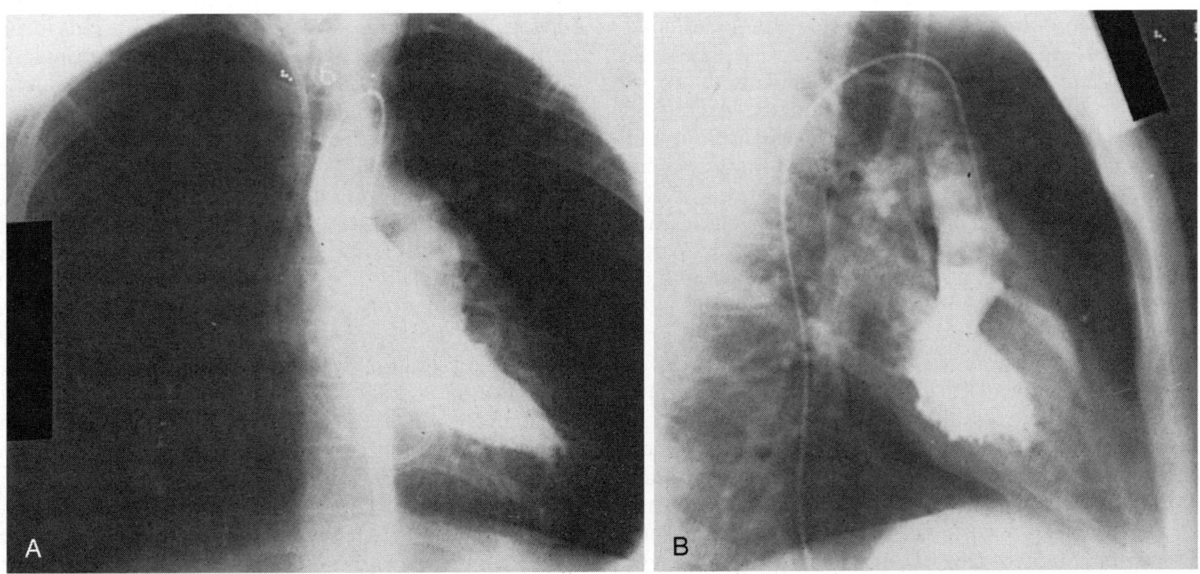

FIGURE 8–30 A and **B,** Left ventriculogram of a small ventricular septal defect, best seen in the lateral view **(B).** Note the normal size of the left ventricle.

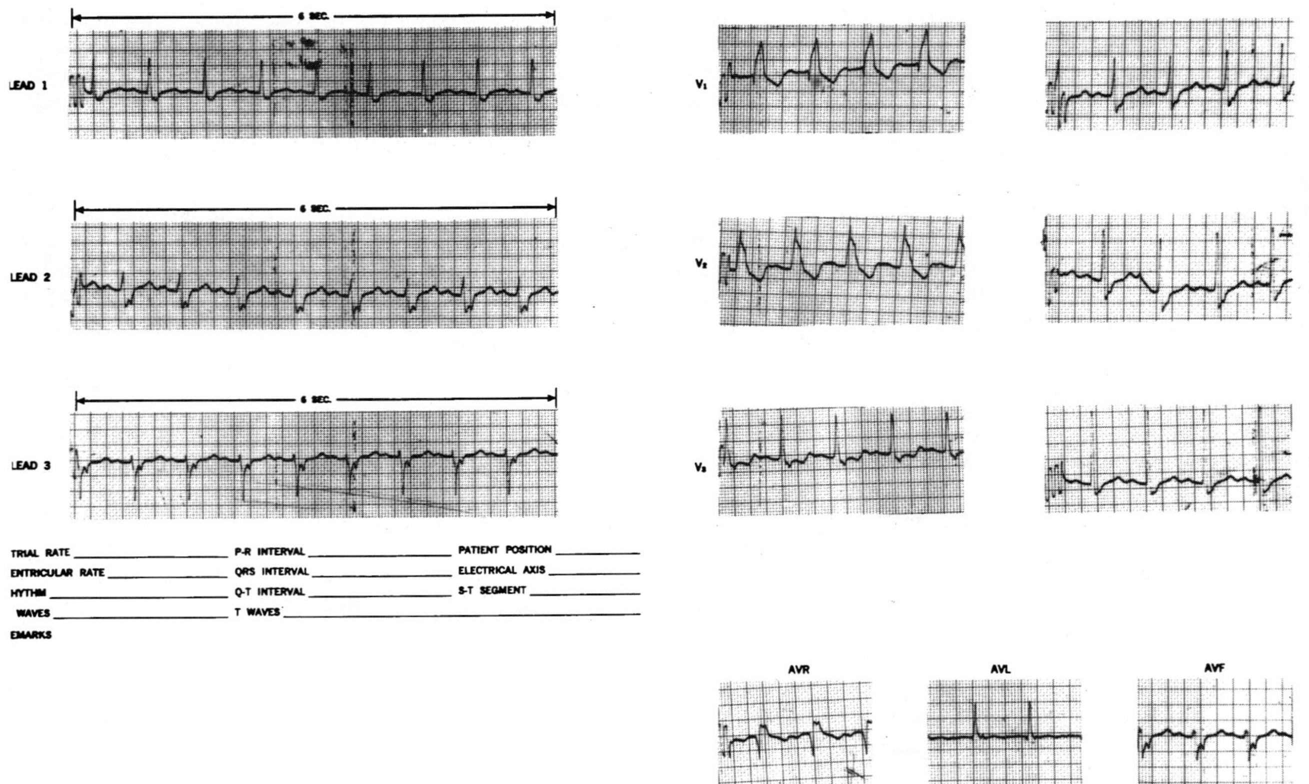

FIGURE 8–31 Electrocardiogram of a patient who underwent closure of a ventricular septal defect. Note the left axis deviation and right bundle branch block, which are commonly seen after ventricular septal defect closure whether as an isolated defect or as part of another entity, such as tetralogy of Fallot. This bifascicular block may uncommonly progress to complete atrioventricular block.

appears to be uncommon, although occasional instances of sudden death have been attributed to it. These conduction abnormalities are related to the close proximity of the bundle of His to the posterior wall of the ventricular septal defect.

Eisenmenger's Complex

Eisenmenger's complex is by far the most common presentation of a large ventricular septal defect in adults.[222] These patients exhibit substantially equal pressures and resistances in the pulmonary and systemic circuits from early childhood onward (see Fig. 8–31). At rest, the patients have a bidirectional shunt. With physical exertion and a decrease in systemic vascular resistance (SVR), the right-to-left shunting increases, resulting in increased arterial desaturation and fatigue. Therefore, these patients are self-restricting and seldom need to have physical restrictions arbitrarily imposed. The longevity of such patients is variable. Causes of death are sudden cardiac death, infective endocarditis, brain abscess, massive hemoptysis, and hyperviscosity. By x-ray study, the heart size is usually normal, the central pulmonary arteries are markedly dilated, and there is no evidence of increased pulmonary flow (Fig. 8–32).

Echocardiography shows the location of a large ventricular septal defect and bidirectional shunting. It can also differentiate between an isolated ventricular septal defect with normally related great vessels from one associated with congenitally corrected transposition or double-outlet RV.

Cardiac catheterization characterizes the hemodynamics (i.e., a large ventricular septal defect through which the venous catheter can be manipulated into both the aorta and the pulmonary artery), severe pulmonary hypertension with markedly elevated PVR, and bidirectional shunting.

Continued survival of such patients requires careful follow-up and management. The erythrocytosis is a consequence of arterial desaturation, and symptoms of hyperviscosity are peculiar to each patient. Most patients have correlating symptoms, such as visual disturbances, lightheadedness, or a "funny feeling," at which time it may be appropriate to phlebotomize them, simultaneously replacing the blood loss with intravenous saline. It is seldom necessary to bring the hemoglobin to much below 20 g. The patients' symptoms are a better guide than arbitrary numeric guides. A word of caution is necessary here. Repeated phlebotomies without iron supplementation result in an iron-deficiency anemia with a disproportion between the hemoglobin and the hematocrit. Because the hematocrit is the main determinant of viscosity, and microcytes may increase viscosity by being more deformable, it is important to reduce the hematocrit while keeping the hemoglobin at a proportionate level. Therefore, iron supplementation may be necessary. Rapid erythrocyte turnover may also lead to folate deficiency, which may require a folic acid supplement. These patients should also be cautioned to maintain adequate fluid intake during hot weather and during exertion.

Patients with Eisenmenger's complex do not progress to CHF unless other factors supervene. Their RVs are adapted to pressure work, and there is no volume overload. However, injudicious and excessive phlebotomies may render the patient relatively anemic, especially if associated with iron deficiency, and CHF may ensue. In some patients, moderate pulmonary insufficiency may develop, creating a volume overload situation that can also lead to CHF. Treatment of the CHF is with inotropes and diuretics; afterload reduction only worsens the right-to-left shunt. If the patient

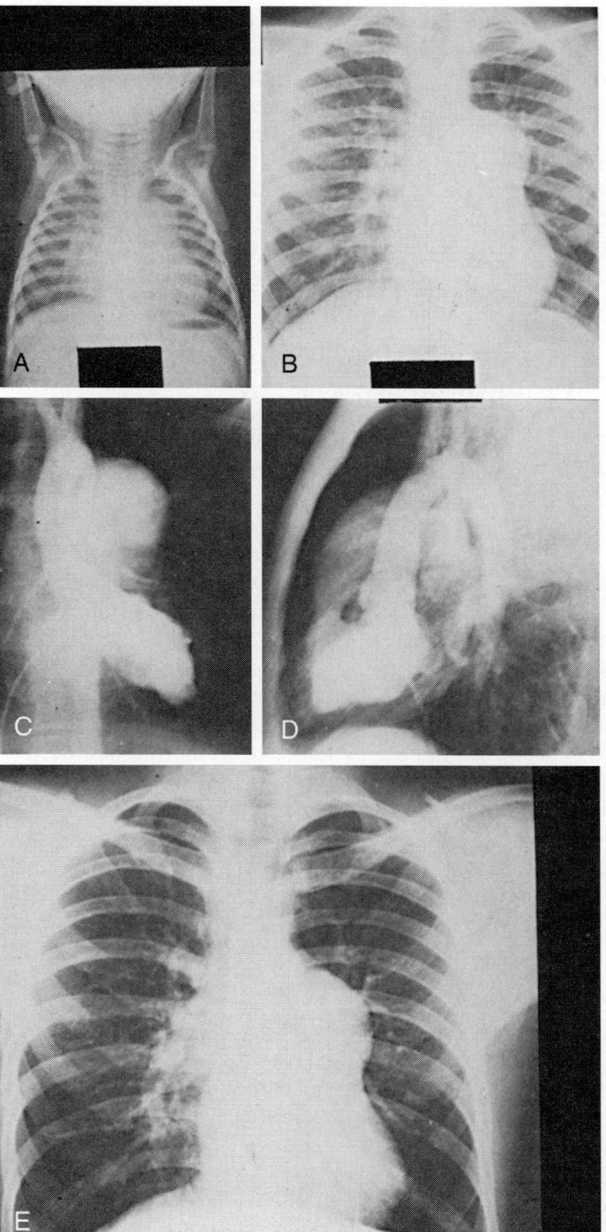

FIGURE 8–32 A–E, Eisenmenger's complex (ventricular septal defect with severe pulmonary hypertension and equal resistances in the pulmonary and systemic circuits). Patient at age 2 **(A)**, at age 10 **(B)**, and at age 20 **(E)**. The left ventriculogram (**C** and **D**) shows the normally related great arteries and markedly dilated pulmonary trunk and left pulmonary artery. Commonly, adults with Eisenmenger's complex have this physiology from early life.

has an iron-deficiency anemia, often owing to repeated phlebotomies, cautious transfusion of packed red cells is sometimes helpful, as is iron replacement.

Many patients with Eisenmenger's complex manage to do reasonably well, holding down full-time jobs and being able to perform many normal activities, although they are not capable of performing strenuous exertion. Ultimately, increasing pulmonary vascular disease with increasing right-to-left shunting and increasing erythrocytosis make existence difficult, and such patients should be considered for heart-lung transplantation.

Patent Ductus Arteriosus

The ductus arteriosus is the main path through which oxygenated cord blood perfuses distal to the aortic arch of the fetus. With delivery and the baby's first breath, there is an immediate drop in PVR, resulting in a reversal of shunt through the ductus arteriosus. Patency normally persists for several days but sometimes for several weeks after delivery until spontaneous closure. The pathophysiologic consequences of persistent patency of the ductus arteriosus depend on the size of the ductus and, to a lesser extent, on the length.[230] There is a continuous left-to-right shunt during systole and diastole through the ductus as long as the PVR is lower than the systemic resistance. When the PVR is equal to or exceeds the SVR, there may be a bidirectional shunt or even an exclusive right-to-left shunt from the pulmonary artery to the descending aorta. Predisposing factors for a patent ductus arteriosus are maternal rubella in the first trimester of pregnancy, prematurity, and high altitude.[230a]

Low-Pressure Patent Ductus Arteriosus

Most patients with a low-pressure patent ductus arteriosus are asymptomatic because the left-to-right shunt is generally mild to moderate. The pathophysiology is similar to that of aortic regurgitation, and there is a rapid run-off with some degree of left ventricular volume overload. The classical physical finding is the machinery murmur of Gibson,[231] heard best in the left subclavicular region and continuous throughout the whole cardiac cycle. This is not to be confused with long murmurs in systole and diastole, such as may occur in combined aortic stenosis and regurgitation, in which the directional shift in flow is marked by a short hiatus between the systolic and the diastolic components. The murmur is identical to that heard in an AV fistula, which it in fact resembles physiologically. The chest x-ray study in patients with a small ductus shows a normal heart size with normal pulmonary vasculature. There is a tendency, however, for the aortic arch to be somewhat wider than usual for the patient's age. With a moderate left-to-right shunt, the heart size may increase somewhat over time, and there may be a suggestion of increased pulmonary flow.

The echocardiogram shows evidence of flow into the left pulmonary artery because the ductus is usually between the distal aortic arch and the left pulmonary artery[232] shortly after its bifurcation. During cardiac catheterization, it is usually possible to manipulate the venous catheter from the proximal left pulmonary artery through the ductus into the descending aorta. The pulmonary artery pressure should be measured simultaneously with the systemic arterial pressure.

PROGNOSIS

The prognosis for a ductus with small-to-moderate left-to-right shunt is excellent,[233, 234] the chief risk being endocarditis. Cardiac catheterization can help to determine the status of the pulmonary vasculature.

Because the ductus is extracardiac, its ligation and division do not require open-heart surgery, making the surgical risk virtually the risk of anesthesia only. At present, however, there are transcatheter techniques for closure of a patent ductus, and these are quite suitable for small to moderate-size ductuses.[235, 236]

Large Patent Ductus

With normal or moderately increased PVR, patients with a large patent ductus have a large continuous left-to-right shunt (Fig. 8–33). They are only rarely seen as adults because the volume overload of the LV and the resultant symptoms betray the diagnosis in childhood, at which time the defect is corrected. A large patent ductus seen in adulthood is almost always one with a PVR slightly less than, equal to, or even greater than the SVR, with either a small bidirectional shunt or an exclusively right-to-left shunt. In many respects, this resembles the Eisenmenger complex associated with a ventricular septal defect (Fig. 8–34).[237–239] These patients experience significant exercise limitations because peripheral vasodilatation serves to in-

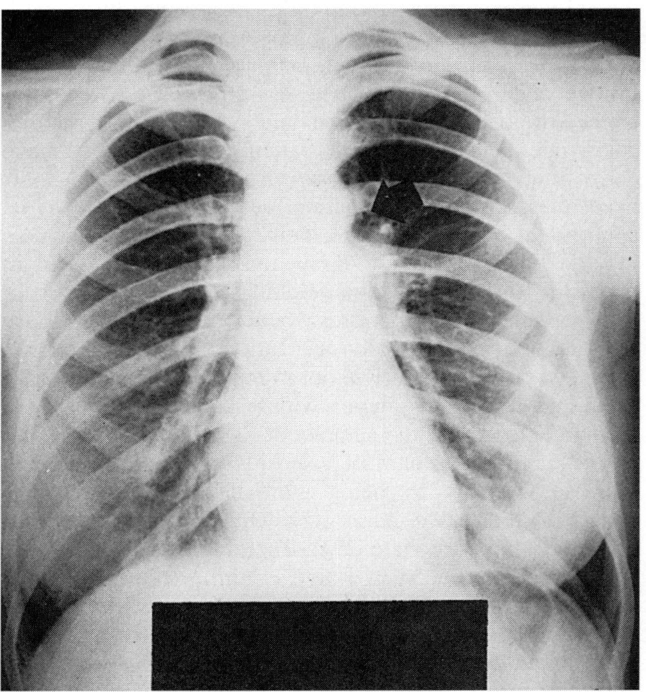

FIGURE 8–33 PA radiograph of a patient with a large patent ductus arteriosus. There is moderate cardiomegaly, with increased pulmonary vasculature and marked enlargement of the main pulmonary artery segment (*arrow* in prominence of the aorta). (Courtesy of Kurt Amplatz, M.D.)

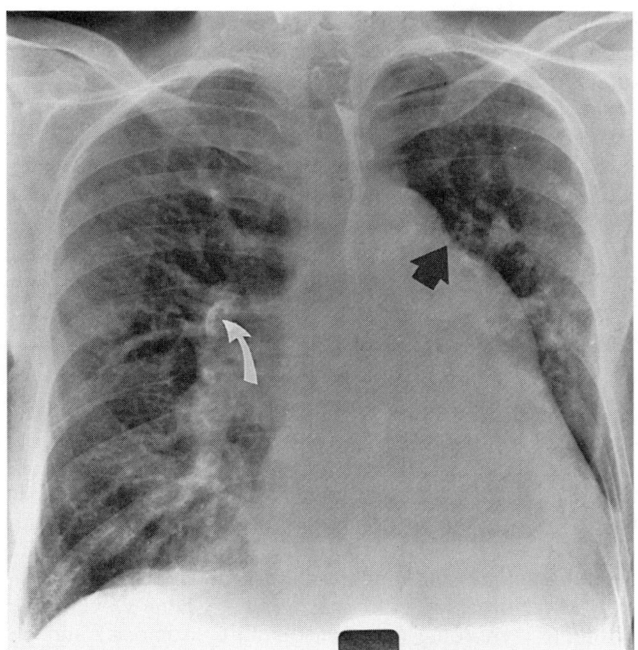

FIGURE 8–34 PA radiograph of a patient with patent ductus arteriosus and severe pulmonary vascular disease, as indicated by calcified plaque in the pulmonary arteries *(curved white arrow).* The ductus arteriosus itself is also calcified *(black arrow).* Pulmonary artery segment and aortic knob are markedly enlarged. (Courtesy of Kurt Amplatz, M.D.)

crease right-to-left shunting and further arterial desaturation. However, unlike the situation in the Eisenmenger complex with a ventricular septal defect, the natural history of a high-pressure, high-resistance ductus may lead to right-sided CHF if the pulmonary artery dilatation results in significant pulmonary insufficiency. The resulting volume overload of the RV with an intact ventricular septum can lead to decompensation.

The clinical history is that of exercise limitation and sometimes angina-like symptoms with exertion. There is definite cyanosis. Classically, the cyanosis should involve the left hand and the feet and not so much the right hand, although this is occasionally seen (Fig. 8–35). Far more common, however, is cyanosis and clubbing of all four extremities, possibly because of backward flow in the ascending aorta during early diastole. Sometimes, there is hoarseness caused by compression of the recurrent laryngeal nerve, especially if the ductus becomes aneurysmal. Hemoptysis may occur, presumably because of the pulmonary hypertension.[240, 241]

LABORATORY STUDIES

The chest x-ray study shows a prominent aortic arch and large central pulmonary arteries. If the PVR is high, the peripheral pulmonary vasculature appears "pruned," as in the Eisenmenger complex. The heart is usually of normal size. Examination of the heart may disclose only a systolic murmur or no murmur, prominent palpable pulsation of the main pulmonary artery, and a loud P_2. By x-ray study, it is possible to see the ductus as a slightly oblique shadow between the distal portion of the aortic arch and the pulmonary artery. This is especially evident when there is calcification of the ductus (see Fig. 8–34).

Echocardiographically, a high-pressure ductus is best seen by the transesophageal technique. Cardiac catheterization is used to define the pulmonary hemodynamics, and the ductus can be visualized angiographically for the surgeon.

PROGNOSIS

In a high-pressure patent ductus in which there is still an appreciable left-to-right shunt and in which the pulmonary/systemic flow ratio is greater than 1.51, the ductus can still be divided and ligated with the anticipation that the pulmonary artery pressure will fall. However, the PVR will still be somewhat elevated. When pulmonary flow and systemic flow are substantially equal, as are their respective resistances, closure of the ductus is contraindicated, and the only treatment would be heart-lung transplantation.[242, 243]

Endocardial Cushion Defects

This is a complex group of anomalies that arise from failure of proper development of the endocardial cushion involving some or all of the following: the lower part of the atrial septum, the upper part of the ventricular septum, and the adjacent leaflets of the two AV valves.[244] The partial AV canal is the ostium primum, in which the lower part of the atrial septum, the upper part of the ventricular septum, and the anterior leaflet of the mitral valve are involved, resulting in an interatrial septal defect and a cleft in the anterior leaflet of the mitral valve. The transitional type is associated with a single atrium with no atrial septum at all but with a cleft leaflet of the mitral valve, resulting in a mixing lesion, as discussed previously. The complete AV canal has all four chambers in communication, there

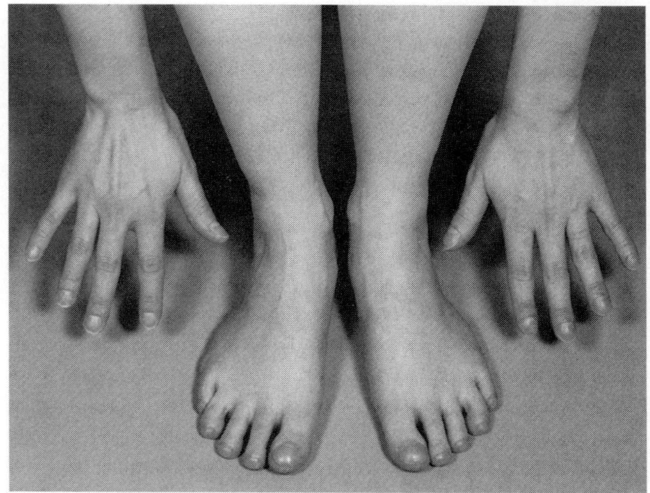

FIGURE 8–35 Differential clubbing in a 23-year-old patient with reversing ductus arteriosus. Note the marked clubbing of the toes and of the fingers of the left hand, with normal nails and fingers of the right hand. Although classic, this is less common than cyanosis and clubbing of all fingers and toes in reversing ductus arteriosus.

being no fusion between the atrial septum, and the ventricular septum and the two AV valves straddle this defect. This common AV valve has four or five leaflets, with an inferior and a superior leaflet straddling the canal and the lateral leaflets attached only to the ipsilateral ventricle. There may be a small fifth leaflet, which is anterior and in the RV.[245, 245a]

Endocardial cushion defects are the most common kind of congenital heart disease associated with Down's syndrome, and patients with Down's syndrome have a high incidence (about 40 percent) of congenital heart disease.[246]

CLINICAL PRESENTATION

The clinical presentation of ostium primum and its close relative, single atrium, was discussed earlier.

Complete AV canal in adults may present in association with either pulmonary stenosis or pulmonary hypertension. In the latter case, it has many of the characteristics of the Eisenmenger syndrome. These patients have a high incidence of mental retardation and cyanosis. The heart is enlarged, there is a loud P_2, there is an absent P_2 in pulmonary stenosis, a loud ejection systolic murmur is heard if pulmonary stenosis is present, and there is evidence of AV valve regurgitation from observation of deep jugular pulses.

LABORATORY STUDIES

The chest x-ray study shows an enlarged heart with a large pulmonary arterial tree and, if there is no pulmonary stenosis, evidence of increased pulmonary flow. Both ventricles and both atria are enlarged. The ECG is the same as that of an ostium primum (i.e., incomplete bundle branch block, left-axis deviation, and often some degree of AV block). Echocardiography visualizes the low-lying atrial septal defect, a corresponding ventricular septal defect, and the characteristic straddling, AV valve.[174] If there is pulmonary stenosis, this can be seen with color-flow Doppler techniques, and the degree of stenosis can be estimated. Measurements should be made of the pulmonary hemodynamics with quantification of the left-to-right and the right-to-left shunts and the respective resistances. Because of the cyanosis, there is secondary erythrocytosis, which must be carefully managed as discussed earlier.

PROGNOSIS

Long-term survival in complete AV canal is uncommon, and such patients rarely survive into adulthood. We have had one patient with co-existing pulmonary stenosis who died at the age of 43 years from septic shock rather than from his heart disease.

TREATMENT

The treatment is surgical correction when the PVR is acceptable or there is pulmonary stenosis. Otherwise, heart-lung transplantation is the only option. These considerations must be tempered by the overall status of the patient, who may have Down's syndrome and is able to function satisfactorily, albeit at a low level of activity. However, patients with mild Down's syndrome with an AV canal should not be denied consideration of surgery if they can function at a more active level.

COMPLEX CONGENITAL HEART DISEASE

Complex congenital heart disease is a group of diseases in which more than one cardiac abnormality is present, which may or may not be associated with cyanosis.

Without Cyanosis

Congenital heart diseases without cyanosis have been alluded to in separate categories. Their clinical presentation is a composite of their individual pathophysiology. Such combinations include interatrial septal defects with one or more anomalous pulmonary veins, Shone's syndrome, Williams' syndrome (supravalvar aortic stenosis) and peripheral pulmonary artery stenoses (with characteristic facies), aortic insufficiency and mitral insufficiency with Marfan's syndrome, coarctation of the aorta and/or ventricular septal defect with Turner's syndrome, and various degrees of AV block with endocardial cushion defects, from first- to second- to third-degree AV block.

With Cyanosis

These conditions involve transposition of the great arteries. Three categories of great vessel transposition can be seen in the adult: D-transposition, L-transposition, and double-outlet RV.

D-Transposition (Complete Transposition)

This transposition involves virtually a direct switch between the two great arteries so that the aorta arises anteriorly from the RV and the pulmonary artery arises posteriorly from the LV (Figs. 8–36 and 8–37). It is evident that without intercommunication, these would be two closed circuits that are incompatible with life. Therefore, there must be a shunt at the atrial level (most common) or at the ventricular level, or else a large patent ductus.[247–249] In patients with atrial or ventricular septal defects, pulmonary stenosis may be present, which "protects" the pulmonary vasculature. Uncorrected D-transposition is compatible with survival into adulthood, but patients are invariably cyanotic. Because the disability is obvious in childhood, these patients now undergo surgery before they reach adulthood. Echocardiography[250] is the diagnostic modality of choice. Cardiac catheterization is essential to characterize the pulmonary vasculature for any consideration of surgery. Surgical treatment for this condition has undergone considerable evolution, from "atrial switching" (actually re-routing of venous blood to the appropriate ventricle) to present-day methods, including arterial switching.[251, 252]

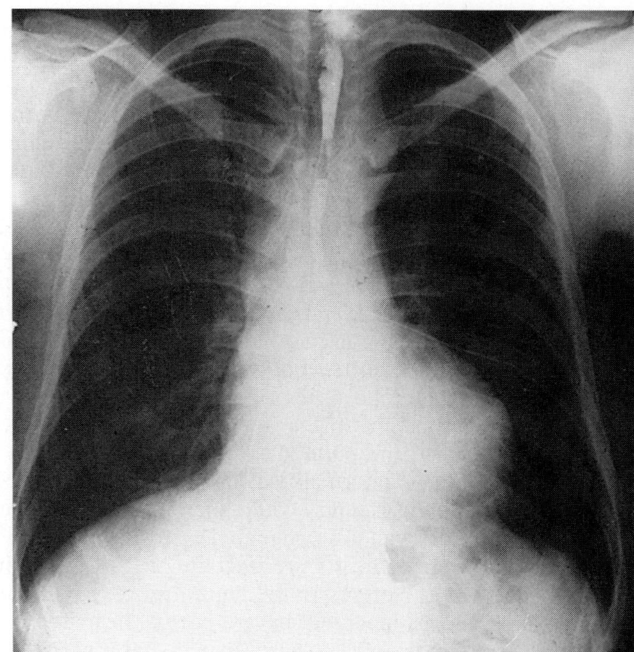

FIGURE 8–36 PA radiograph of a patient with transposition of the great vessels, ventricular septal defect, and pulmonary stenosis. The heart size is at the upper limits of normal, and the pulmonary vasculature is slightly accentuated. The main pulmonary artery segment is absent. (Courtesy of Kurt Amplatz, M.D.)

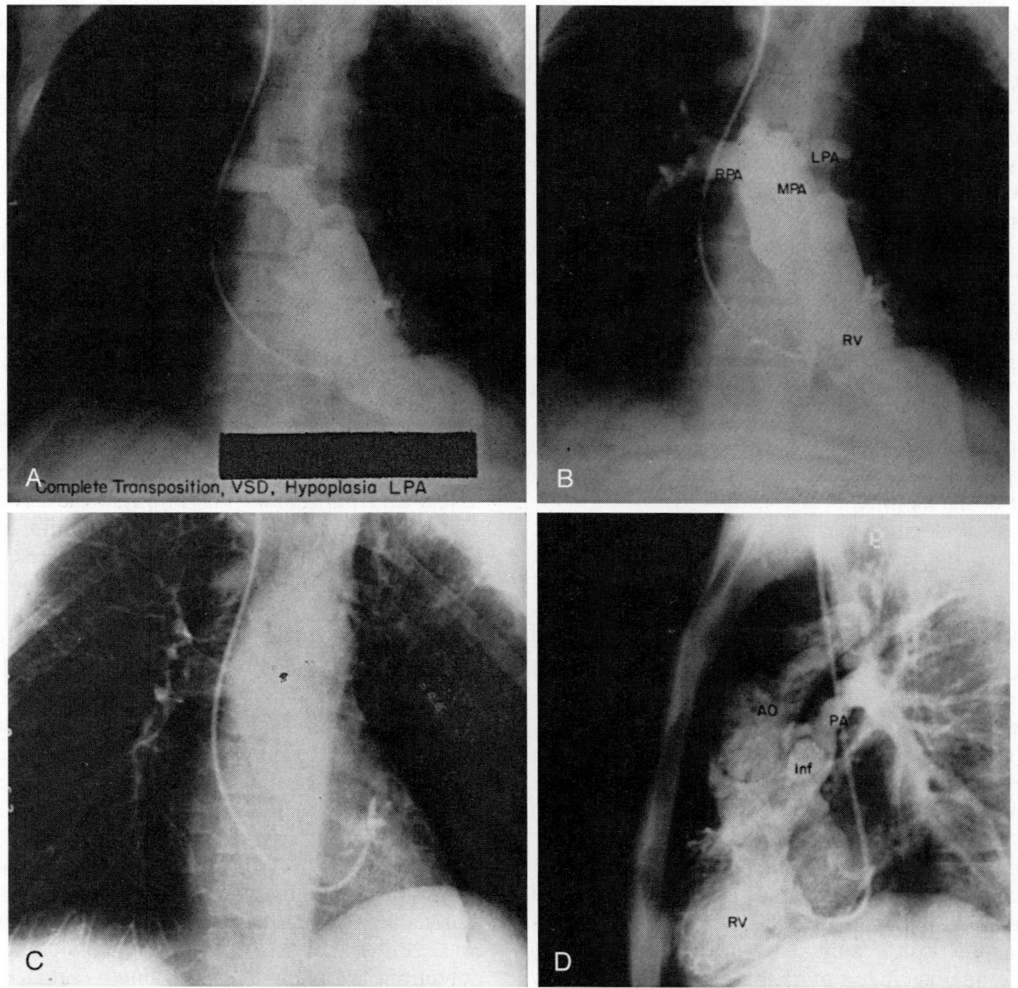

FIGURE 8–37 A–D, D-Transposition in a 28-year-old man. **D,** The completely switched position of the pulmonary artery and the aorta is evident, with the aortic valve anterior to the pulmonary trunk and the pulmonary valve.

L-Transposition (Congenitally Corrected Transposition)

L-Transposition is best described as ventricular inversion. This inversion involves both the AV valves and the semilunar valves, so that the venous ventricle is the anatomic LV, the arterial ventricle is the anatomic RV, and the crista supraventricularis is on the left, as is the tricuspid valve, whereas the mitral valve is the right AV valve. The AV conduction system goes down the left side of the heart. The atria are not involved, and therefore, the venous return to both atria and the coronary sinus is in the normal position. However, the aortic root and the pulmonary trunk do not have an anteroposterior relationship but rather a side-by-side relationship, so that the aortic root forms the left heart border and the pulmonary trunk arises medially. Were there no other abnormalities, this would be a functionally "normal" heart and would therefore not belong under the rubric of cyanotic congenital heart disease.[253–255] However, such normal hearts are uncommon, and in such cases, two common features in the natural history make it unlikely that these patients will have a normal heart for the rest of their natural lives. These patients are prone to develop AV block, which may progress to third-degree block with a narrow QRS.[256] Although they may have Adams-Stokes attacks, this is a less common manifestation, but exercise tolerance may become limited because of the inadequate chronotropic response to exercise. Furthermore, the left-sided AV valve (i.e., the tricuspid valve) is prone to dysplasia or to Ebstein's anomaly.[257] If the patient survives into adulthood, this Ebstein's anomaly is not apt to be severe, but the valve becomes insufficient because of systemic pressure in the arterial ventricle. This may therefore necessitate subsequent valve replacement.[258, 259]

In the vast majority of patients who reach adulthood, there is communication at the ventricular level associated with pulmonary stenosis. A ventricular septal defect or sometimes even a functionally common ventricle may be present. Such patients are always cyanotic but have a pulmonary vasculature that is "protected" against the development of pulmonary hypertension.

The physical findings are those of severe pulmonary stenosis, together with cyanosis and clubbing. The chest x-ray study shows a normal heart size, very often with a straight left heart border, this being the ascending aorta (Figs. 8–38 and 8–39). The heart may have an unusual contour if the inverted RV is prominent (Fig. 8–40). The ECG shows evidence of right ventricular hypertrophy and first-, second-, or third-degree AV block (Figs. 8–41 and 8–42).

The echocardiogram is characteristic.[260] The inversion of the ventricles can be identified by the presence of the crista supraventricularis in the arterial ventricle, the clearly switched AV valves, and the unusual position of the two semilunar valves. Because the aorta and the tricuspid valve are now on the same side, the aortic valve and the left-sided (tricuspid) AV valve are not in continuity, as would be the relationship between the aortic and the mitral valves in the normal heart. Ebstein's anomaly of the left-sided AV valve can also be visualized if present. The ventricular septal defect and the pulmonary stenosis can be further identified. For purposes of possible surgical treatment, one needs to know whether the interventricular communication is a functionally common ventricle or a large ventricular septal defect.

Cardiac catheterization is important for characterizing the hemodynamics, including ventricular function; the degree of pulmonary stenosis; and the PVR. These data are especially important in patients who have a common ventricle, with the possibility of a modified Fontan procedure as a therapeutic option. Angiography can quantify the degree of left AV valve insufficiency and the respective positions of the two great arteries. The pulmonary stenosis can be confirmed as being either valvular or subvalvular. Angiography also helps to detail the anatomy of the coronary arteries. These undergo a curious "rotation," which is described in the pathophysiology section.[254]

Patients who start out in life with a "normal" heart usually have trouble eventually with the supervention of various degrees of heart block and with insufficiency of the left-sided AV valve. The prognosis for patients who have interventricular septal defect with pulmonary stenosis has improved considerably with modern surgical therapy. However, these patients are still susceptible to infective endocarditis. Even with correction of the left-sided AV valve insufficiency, the anatomic RV may not perform optimally over the years,[261] although we have one 65-year-old patient with a normal heart who has third-degree heart block, for which she has a DDD pacemaker, and whose insufficient left-sided AV valve has been replaced with a valve prosthesis. The arterial ventricle, although exhibiting some global hypokinesia, is still performing reasonably well, and the patient is a functional class I.

TREATMENT

The treatment is surgical. Because the clinical profile of such patients closely resembles the tetralogy of Fallot, many of them have undergone a Blalock-Taussig anastomosis with marked improvement in functional capacity and arrive at adulthood only mildly cyanotic. Although they may not be functional class I, they may still be quite functional but receptive to future surgical procedures.

For patients who have an interventricular septal defect and pulmonary stenosis, closure of the ventricular septal defect and pulmonary valvotomy would seem reasonable. The approach to the defect from the right side in congenitally corrected transposition of great vessels is, however, technically difficult. Patients with a common ventricle and pulmonary stenosis may be eligible for a modified Fontan procedure,[61, 63] provided that the PVR and ventricular filling pressure are normal. This can be accomplished by converting the heart into one with tricuspid atresia by closing the tricuspid valve and placing a conduit between the RA and the pulmonary artery.

Double-Outlet Right Ventricle

A double-outlet RV is rarely seen in the adult. Both the aorta and the pulmonary artery arise from the RV (Figs. 8–43 and 8–44). The relationship of the great arteries is more or less usual. There is an obligatory ventricular septal defect.[262, 263] When the ventricular septal defect is under the aortic valve (the Taussig-Bing anomaly), cyanosis is minimal or mild, with left ventricular blood flowing preferentially into the aorta and pulmonary flow coming chiefly

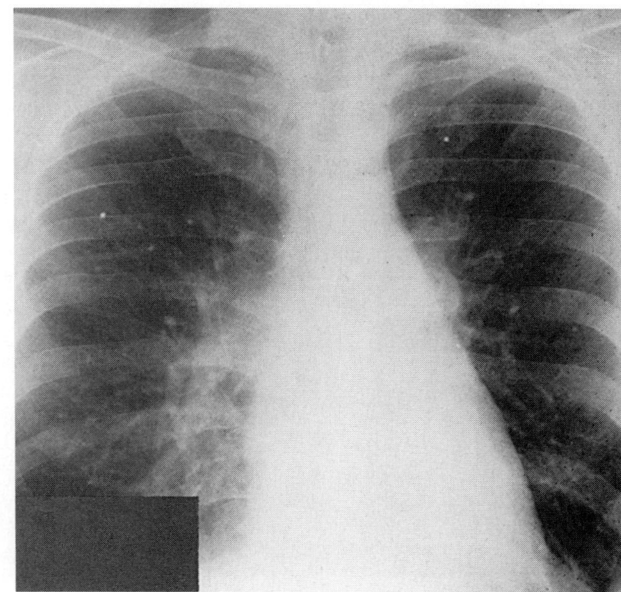

FIGURE 8–38 Congenitally corrected transposition in a 35-year-old man with ventricular septal defect and no pulmonary stenosis. Note the straight left-sided heart border, which is formed by the L-transposed ascending aorta and the inverted right ventricle.

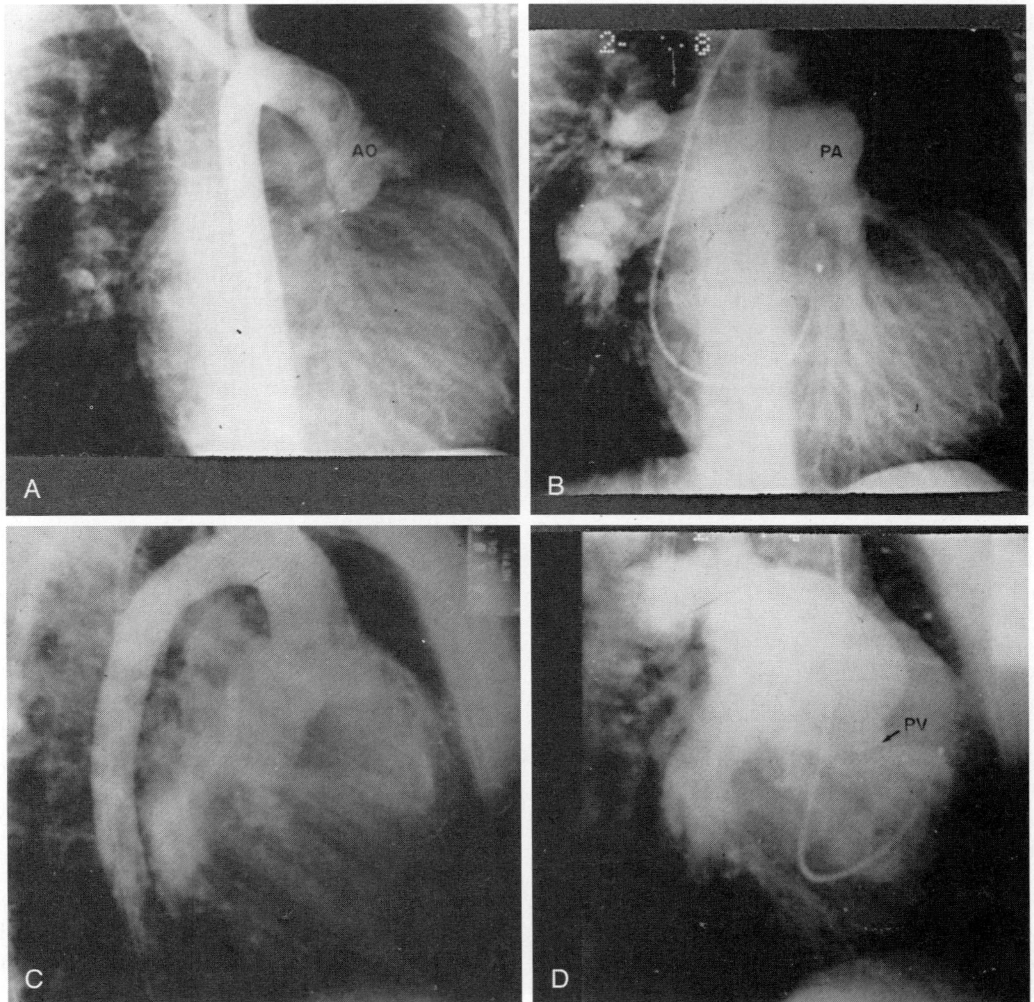

FIGURE 8–39 A–D, An 18-year-old woman with congenitally corrected transposition of the great vessels and a common ventricle. **A** and **B,** The anteroposterior views show that the ascending aorta forms the left-sided heart border and the pulmonary trunk arises more medially. **C** and **D,** The lateral views show that the semilunar valves are more side to side than anteroposterior to each other.

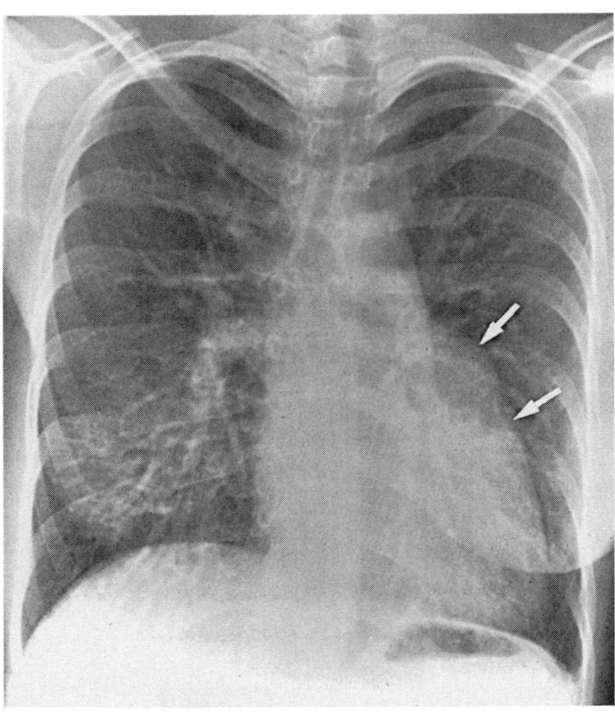

FIGURE 8–40 PA radiograph of a patient with corrected transposition, ventricular septal defect, and pulmonary stenosis. The heart is slightly enlarged, and the pulmonary vasculature is within normal limits. There is a prominent bulge at the left heart contour *(arrows),* representing the inverted right ventricle. The pulmonary segment is absent because the main pulmonary artery lies centrally within the mediastinum and is no longer border forming.

from the RV. Right ventricular flow goes to both great vessels but primarily to the pulmonary artery. When the ventricular septal defect is subjacent to the pulmonary valve, the situation physiologically resembles that of D-transposition of the great vessels with ventricular septal defect. Figure 8–44 shows the chest film and angiogram of such a patient, aged 22 years. He survived to age 35 and was a poor surgical risk because of severe chronic obstructive lung disease caused by smoking. Diagnostic confirmation is by echocardiography[264] and by cardiac catheterization and angiography[265] for consideration of surgical correction.[266, 267]

Tetralogy of Fallot

Tetralogy of Fallot consists of a large ventricular septal defect in the usual position, together with pulmonary stenosis, either valvular or infundibular, or both.[268] The large ventricular septal defect results in equal pressure in the two ventricles. The two other features constituting the tetralogy are right ventricular hypertrophy and overriding of the interventricular septum by the dilated aorta. This malformation is compatible with surviving into adulthood.[269, 270] The more severe the pulmonary stenosis, the greater the degree of right-to-left shunting at the ventricular level. The more complete the arterial unsaturation, the greater the disability. Such patients not only are prone to the usual complications of cyanotic heart disease (i.e., endocarditis, brain abscess, and complications of marked erythrocytosis) but may also experience sudden death, which has been attributed to spasm of the infundibulum.[271] Lesser degrees of pulmonary stenosis result in a lesser degree of right-to-left shunting, with a modestly decreased exercise capacity but with the ability to perform most normal activities. In some patients, the degree of pulmonary stenosis is such that the patient is not visibly cyanotic at rest but only with exercise; such patients are said to have tardive cyanosis.

The usual clinical findings are cyanosis and clubbing and a loud, harsh pulmonary ejection murmur with spilling over A to a very soft P, or P may even be absent. This murmur is often well heard in the neck, and such radiation should not mislead one into thinking that this is of aortic origin. Frequently, there is a systolic ejection sound that arises in the dilated ascending aorta. A faint blowing diastolic murmur of pulmonary insufficiency is sometimes heard either starting with P or, when P is inaudible, starting after a gap from A.

The chest x-ray study (Fig. 8–45) shows a somewhat globular heart of normal size, and on the lateral view, a prominent RV can be seen "hugging" the sternum. There may be a right-sided aortic arch, which deviates the esophagus and the sternum slightly to the left. If the pulmonary stenosis is purely valvular and tricuspid, as occurs in about 20 percent of these cases, poststenotic dilatation of the pulmonary trunk and left pulmonary artery occurs. With the much more common infundibular stenosis, the left heart border is concave because the pulmonary trunk is relatively small. This stenosis usually creates a "third chamber" just subjacent to the pulmonary valve.[272, 273] The ECG shows right ventricular hypertrophy, often with a right bundle branch block pattern. Echocardiography shows the large ventricular septal defect, the overriding large aorta, and the pulmonary valvular or infundibular stenosis and the systolic gradient by Doppler. Cardiac catheterization can quantify the pulmonary artery pressure and the PVR and can measure the systolic gradient between the pulmonary artery and the RV. By careful catheter withdrawal, it is possible to quantify the systolic gradient across the valve and also across the infundibulum, if both co-exist. Right ventriculography can indicate the size and the location of the ventricular septal defect, and biplanar angiography demon-

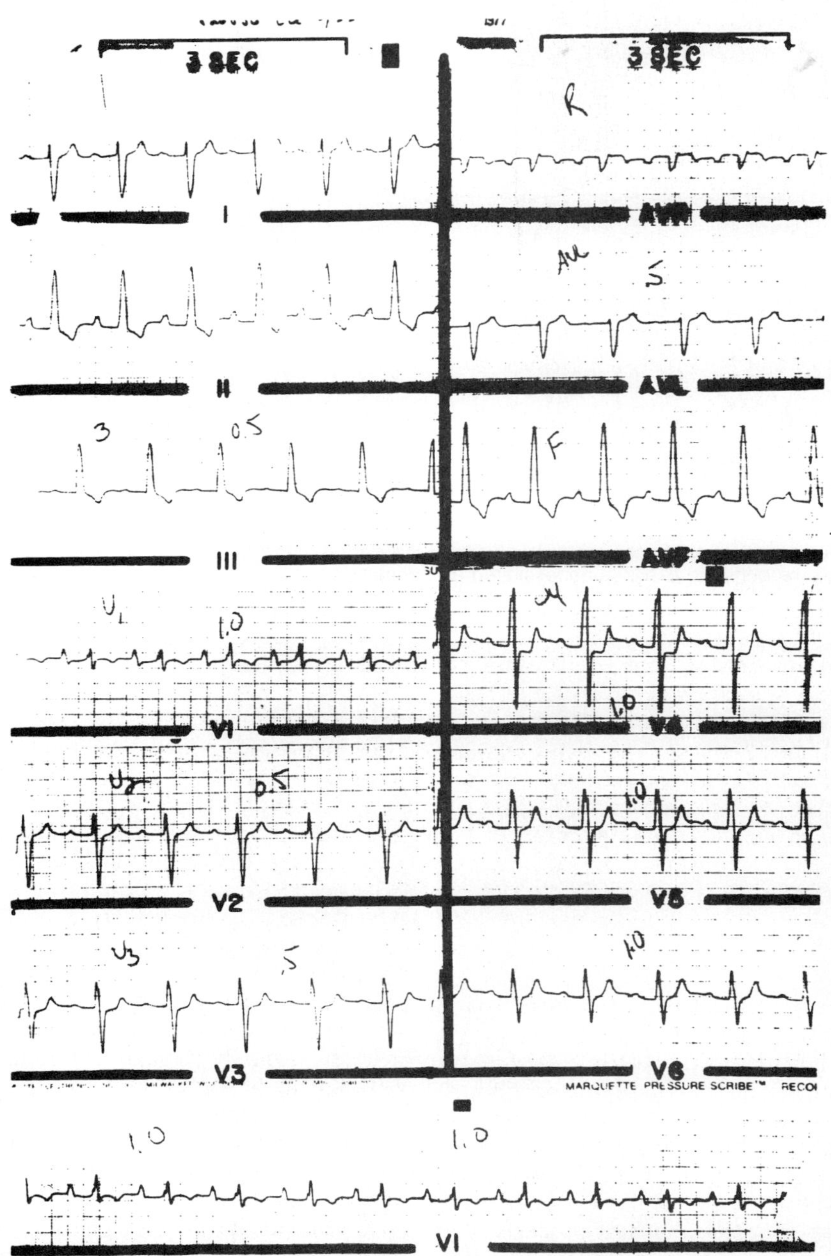

FIGURE 8–41 Electrocardiogram of a 43-year-old patient with congenitally corrected transposition with pulmonary stenosis and ventricular septal defect. Note the absence of a Q wave in the lateral chest leads. This is because of the ventricular inversion, with the septum depolarizing from right to left rather than from left to right.

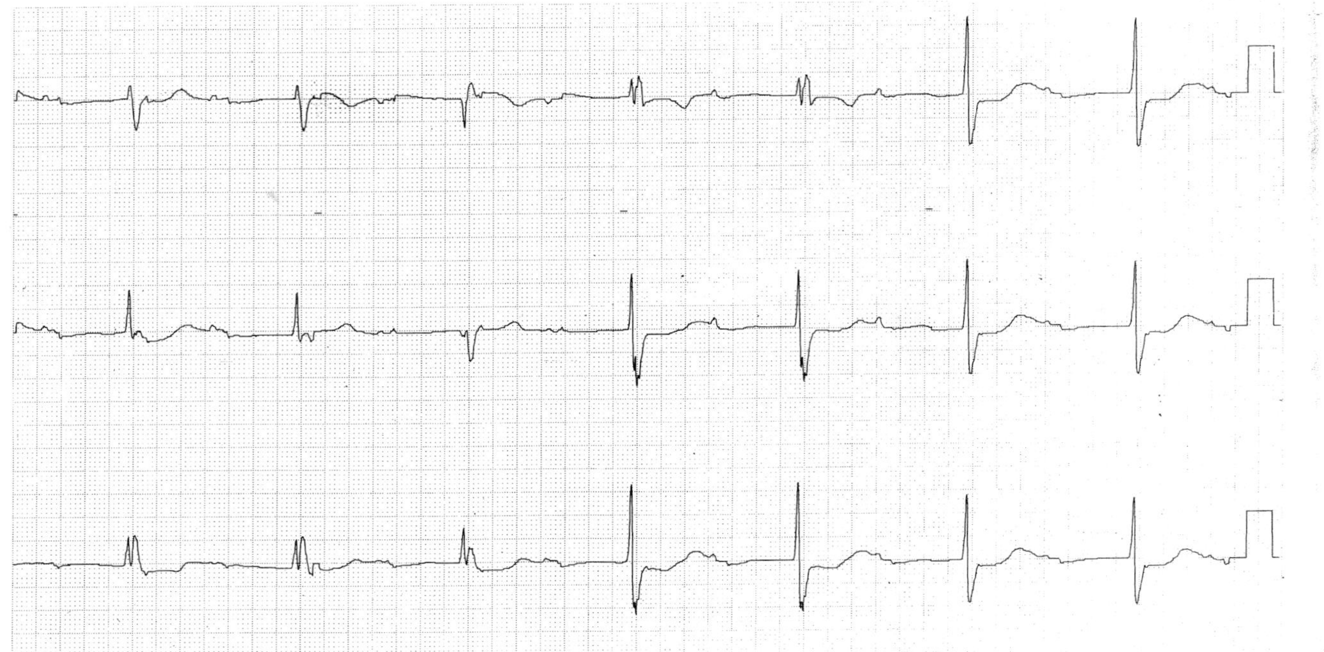

FIGURE 8–42 Electrocardiogram of a 54-year-old woman with a third-degree heart block. She did well over the years, but eventually, the inadequate chronotropic response to exercise necessitated a pacemaker.

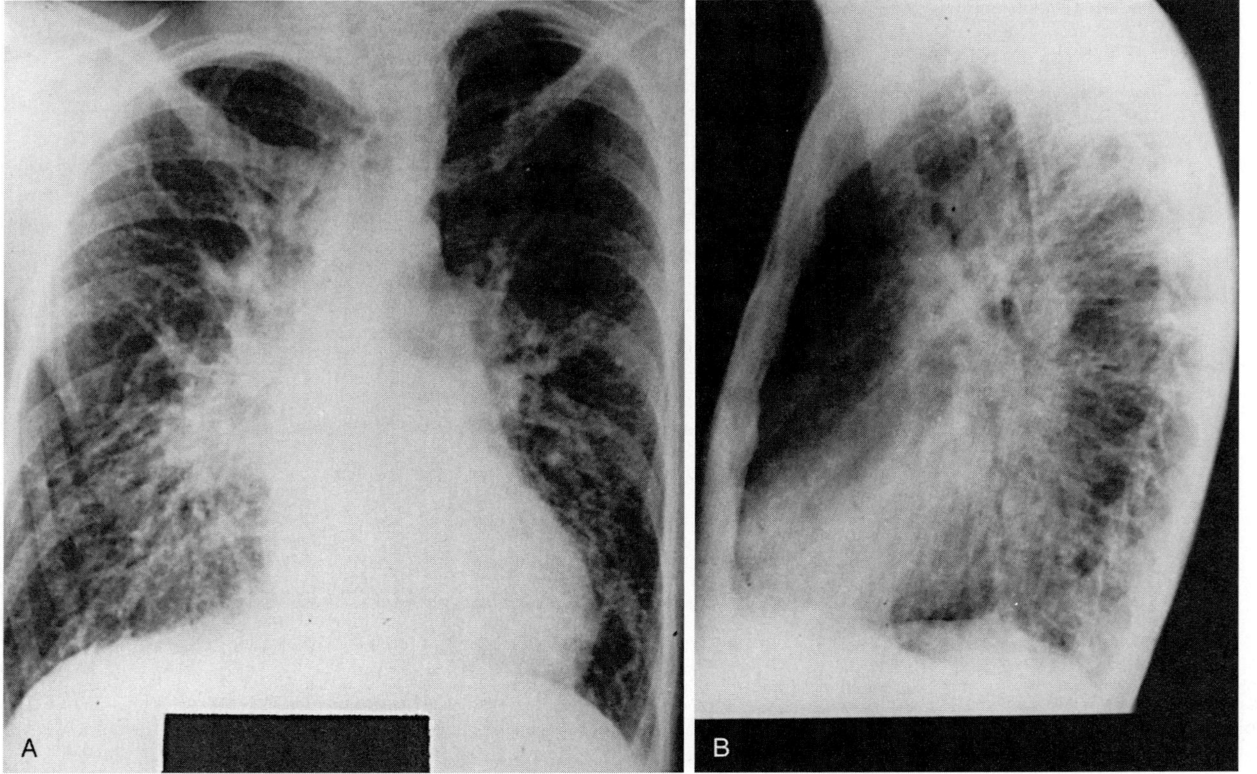

FIGURE 8–43 A and **B,** Double-outlet right ventricle in a 25-year-old man with a supracristal ventricular septal defect with significant left-to-right shunting. Note the kyphoscoliosis, which is not uncommon in cyanotic congenital heart disease.

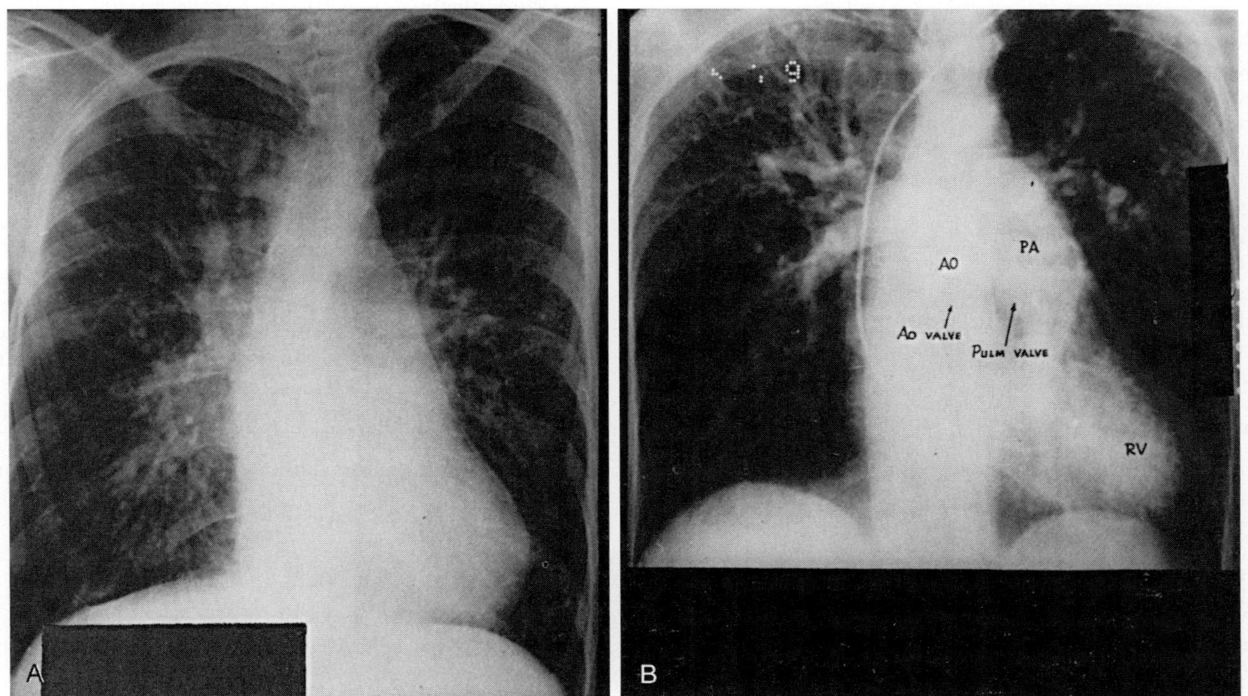

FIGURE 8–44 This 22-year-old man had origin of both great vessels from the right ventricle with the ventricular septal defect under the pulmonary valve. **A,** In the chest film on the left, note the unusual left-sided heart border caused by the markedly dilated pulmonary artery. **B,** The right ventriculogram shows both great vessels arising from the right ventricle. This patient had an Eisenmenger physiology.

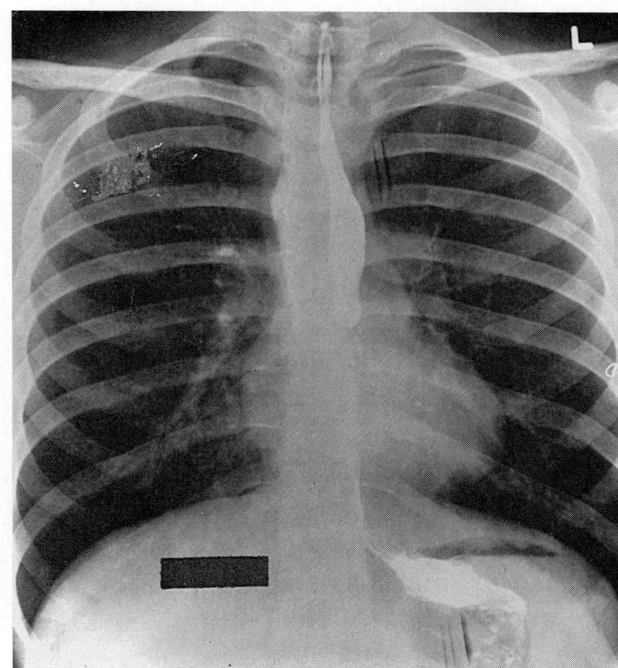

FIGURE 8–45 PA radiograph of a patient with tetralogy of Fallot. The heart is normal in size and boot shaped in configuration. The pulmonary vasculature is decreased. The esophagus is displaced toward the left by a right-sided aortic arch. (Courtesy of Kurt Amplatz, M.D.)

strates the extent of the infundibular stenosis, if present (Fig. 8–46). Sometimes, unusual moderator bands can mimic classic infundibular stenosis.

PROGNOSIS

Patients who reach adulthood with uncorrected tetralogy of Fallot used to be common, but now, the vast majority of such patients are diagnosed in childhood and undergo surgery. However, we have had two women patients who had each borne two children before they were willing to undergo surgical correction. Patients who have had a Potts or a Waterston anastomosis may experience significant rise in PVR, unlike those who have undergone the single Blalock-Taussig anastomosis,[273a] in which pulmonary vascular changes are exceedingly rare. However, a double Blalock-Taussig anastomosis may result in volume overload of the LV (Fig. 8–47).

TREATMENT

The first palliative operation for cyanotic congenital heart disease with pulmonic stenosis was the Blalock-Taussig anastomosis, anastomosing the subclavian artery to the pulmonary artery, resulting in significant functional improvement, with many patients reaching adulthood. Surgical correction now consists of closure of the ventricular septal defect and relief of the pulmonary stenosis. If the pulmonary stenosis is valvular, the entire procedure can be transatrial for both the closure of the ventricular septal defect and the pulmonary valvotomy. In patients in whom the pulmonary stenosis is largely infundibular, it may be necessary to expand and roof the outflow tract and the pulmonary trunk by incision and patching. In general, the postoperative results of such surgery have been extremely gratifying, with restoration of full functional capacity.[274–276] However, late sequelae may include recurrent supraventricular tachyarrhythmias related to the atriotomy, ventricular tachycardias related to ventriculotomy, and mild right-sided CHF resulting from ventriculotomy and pulmonary regurgitation.[277] Such CHF is uncommon, but when it exists, it occurs mostly in patients who have undergone ventriculotomy, either to close the septal defect or to open up the infundibular stenosis rather than using the transatrial approach.

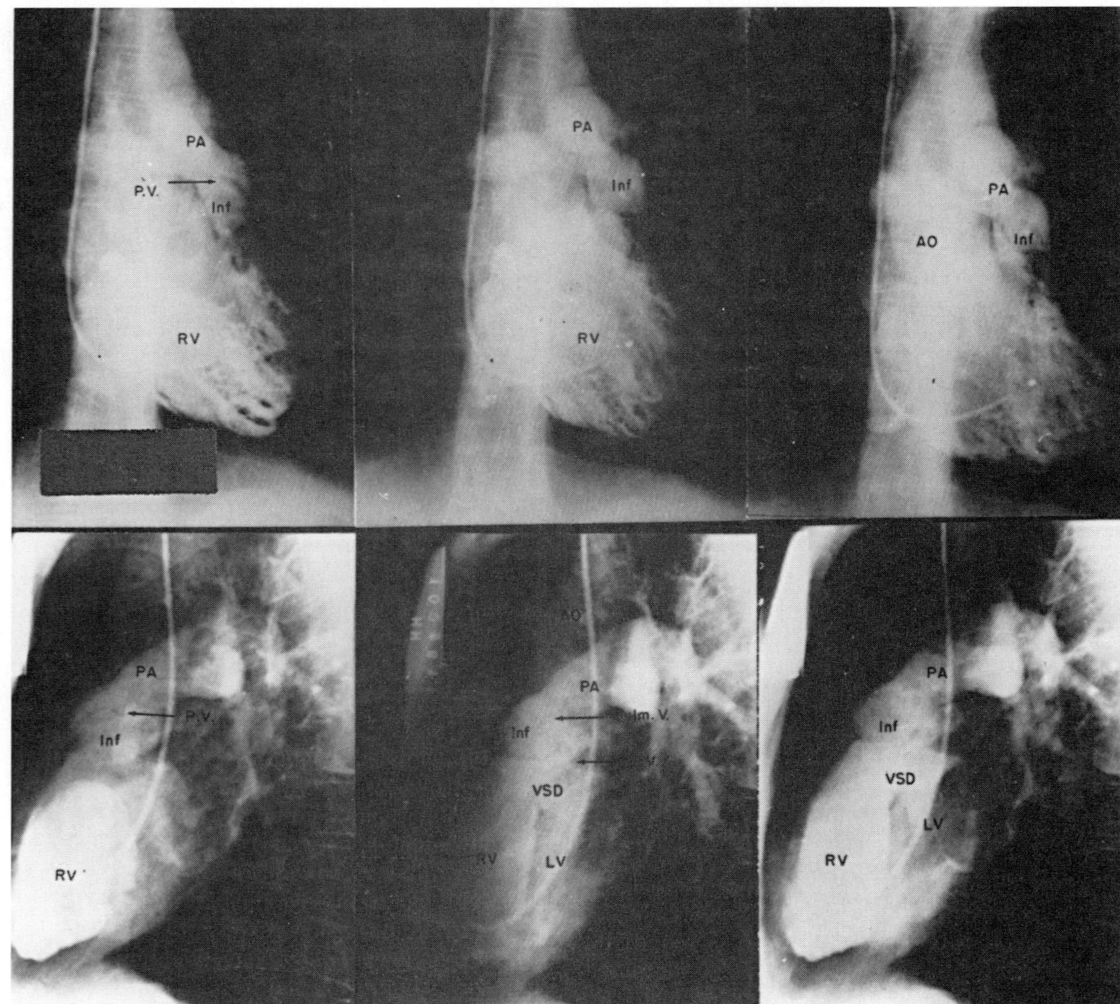

FIGURE 8–46 Right ventriculogram of a 40-year-old patient with tetralogy of Fallot. In the **upper panels** are anteroposterior views showing the normal relationship of the pulmonary trunk and the ascending aorta (AO). The **lower panels** show an infundibular chamber just under the pulmonary valve (Pulm. V.) and also show contrast from the right ventricle (RV) passing through a high ventricular septal defect (VSD) into the left ventricle (LV). The ventricular septum can be clearly seen.

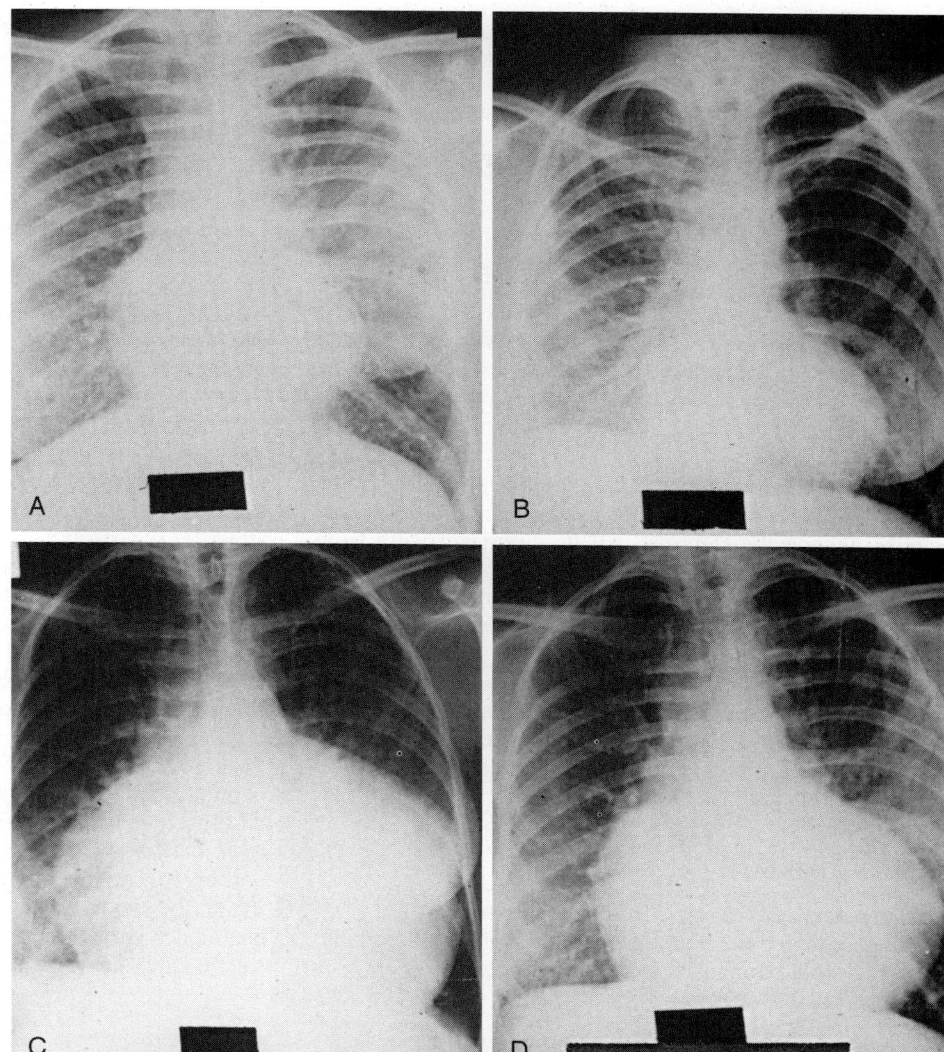

FIGURE 8–47 Tetralogy of Fallot in a 20-year-old woman. **A,** A globular and bulky heart with somewhat increased pulmonary vasculature after a Blalock-Taussig anastomosis. **B,** Some decrease in pulmonary flow is due to decreasing shunt through the anastomosis. **C,** Striking cardiomegaly after a left-sided Blalock-Taussig anastomosis, demonstrating the adverse effect of marked volume overload on the heart. **D,** Decreased heart size after spontaneous closure of the first anastomosis.

Many patients with tetralogy of Fallot have a mild degree of aortic insufficiency, which is related more to the dilatation of aortic root than to intrinsic valvular disease. This is almost never of clinical significance. Over the long term, many problems remain in patients who have undergone "total correction"—impaired right heart function, decreased exercise tolerance, and especially rhythm disorders.[278, 279]

Pulmonary Atresia With Ventricular Septal Defect (Pseudotruncus Arteriosus)

Pulmonary atresia may be associated with a large ventricular septal defect and is sometimes considered the extreme version of the tetralogy of Fallot. A more uncommon situation exists when the pulmonary atresia is seen with an intact ventricular septum and a small RV that is drained by large coronary sinusoids. The latter is almost never seen by cardiologists treating adults.

Pulmonary atresia associated with a ventricular septal defect is more usefully thought of clinically as an entity apart from the tetralogy of Fallot. The clinical manifestations and the surgical considerations are quite different. The pulmonary circulation is derived entirely from large anomalous arteries that arise from the descending aorta, often called *bronchial arteries*[280] (Fig. 8–48). At the junction of these arteries with the pulmonary arteries, it is common to observe significant stenosis, so that the distal pulmonary arteries may be of relatively normal pressure. Pulmonary atresia can range from mere atresia of the pulmonary valve, which is uncommon, to atresia of the pulmonary trunk and often atresia of the proximal left and right arteries. These patients are markedly cyanotic. A characteristic feature on clinical examination is the presence of a continuous murmur throughout the chest, arising from the stenoses of the bronchopulmonary anastomoses. The chest x-ray study shows a large ascending aorta and aortic arch, and absence of the pulmonary trunk and the left and right pulmonary arteries (Fig. 8–49). There are bronchial arteries coming off the descending aorta. Echocardiography can identify the absence of a pulmonary artery in the presence of a large ventricular septal defect. Cardiac catheterization is essential for the measurement of pressures in the distal pulmonary arteries. This is a very difficult procedure, which

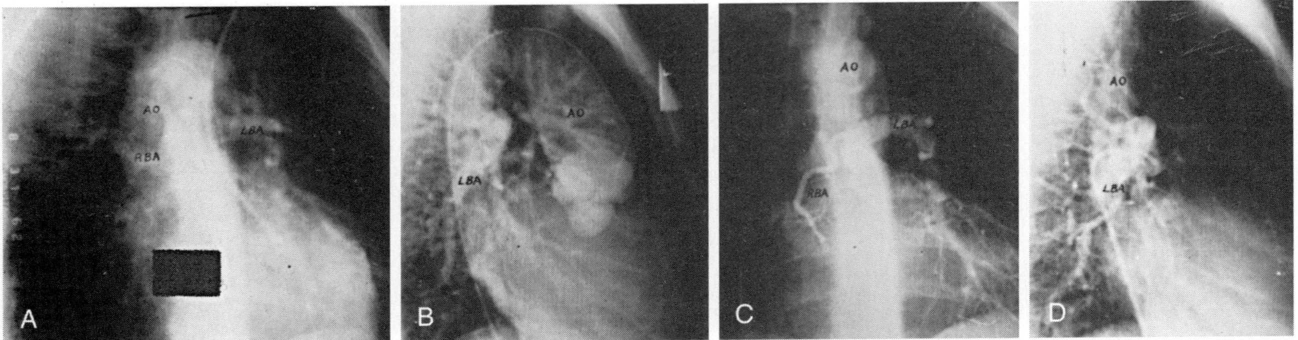

FIGURE 8–48 A–D, Angiogram of a 30-year-old man with pseudotruncus arteriosus. There is a rather dilated ascending aorta, no pulmonary trunk is seen, and the pulmonary vasculature fills from "bronchial" arteries that arise from the descending aorta.

involves cannulating the bronchial arteries arising from the descending aorta and threading the catheter into the distal arteries beyond the stenoses. All the arteries arising from the descending aorta that are supplying the pulmonary vasculature should be thus cannulated.

Arteriography of each of these vessels is also important to define the anatomy. If the anatomy is suitable and the PVR acceptable, some of these patients can be considered for staged open-heart surgery to establish continuity between the RV and the pulmonary arteries. This can be performed only in highly selected individuals and carries a significant surgical risk.[281–283]

Truncus Arteriosus

Truncus arteriosus is an incomplete septation of the ascending aorta and the pulmonary trunk.[284, 285] The semilunar valve is a single truncus valve, which in most cases consists of three cusps but may be either quadricuspid or bicuspid. It is commonly insufficient, sometimes markedly so, and straddles a ventricular septal defect.[286, 287] Truncus defects are divided into three types. Type I has a common trunk, but this gives rise distally to recognizably separate ascending aorta and pulmonary trunk (Fig. 8–50). In type II, the truncus extends up to the right and left pulmonary artery bifurcations, there being no separate pulmonary trunk (Fig. 8–51). In type III, the left and right pulmonary arteries come off either side of the truncus. In adults, the most common type is a type I truncus. Such patients have a regurgitant truncus valve, a common mixing chamber, and Eisenmenger's physiology. In the very young, the PVR may be somewhat less than the SVR, so that surgical correction can be attempted. By adulthood, the PVR is markedly elevated, and few if any of these patients are candidates for corrective surgery. The remaining possible treatment is heart-lung transplantation. When patients are

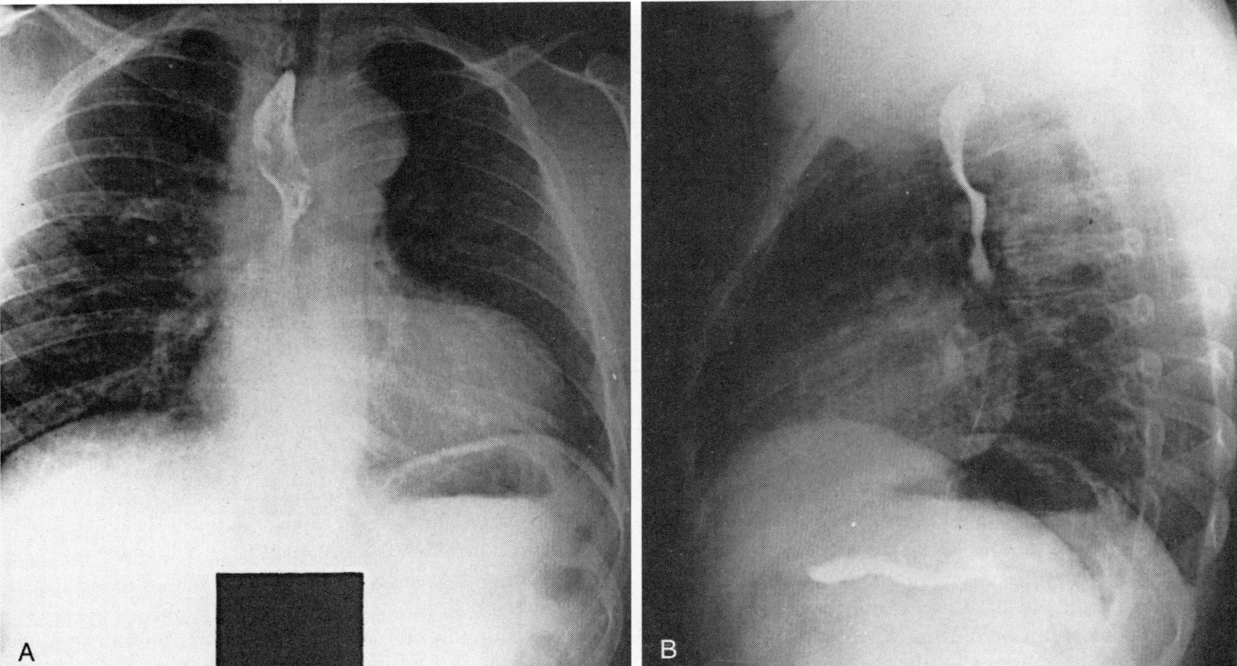

FIGURE 8–49 Pseudotruncus arteriosus in a 24-year-old man. Note the large ascending aorta and aortic arch and marked concavity of the left heart border owing to the absence of the central pulmonary arteries.

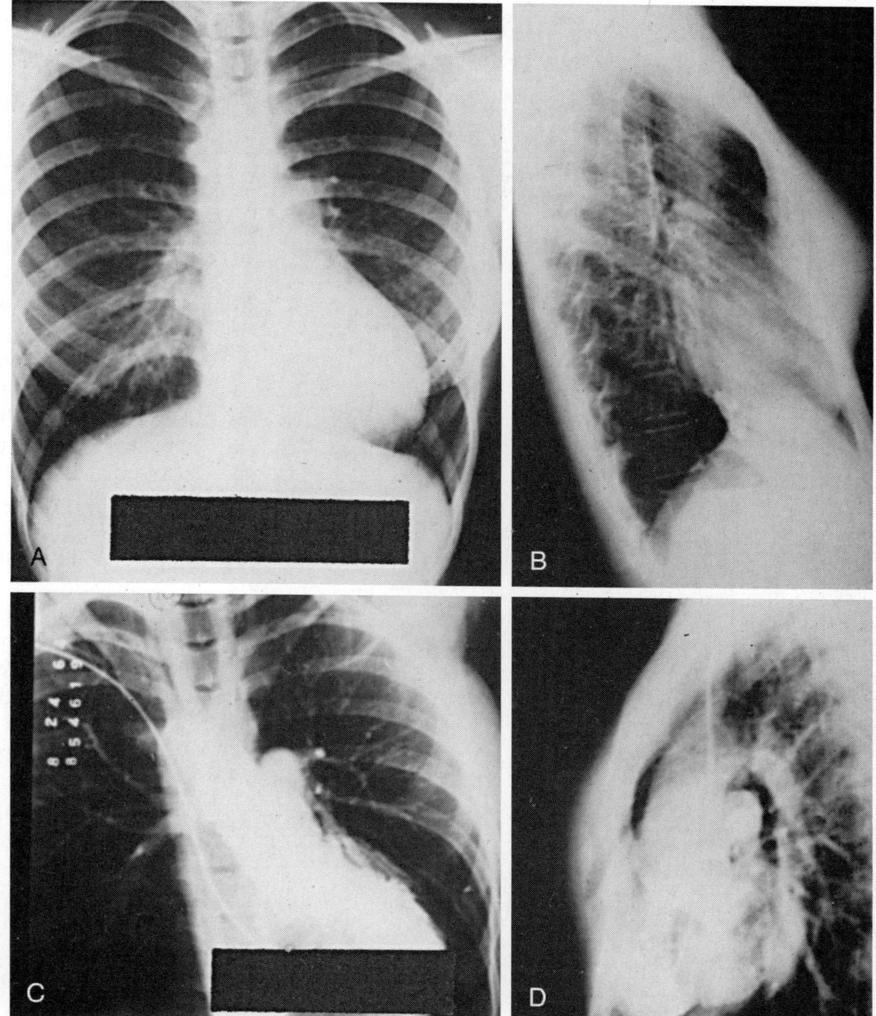

FIGURE 8–50 Truncus arteriosus in an adolescent. **A** and **B,** Note the rather characteristic wide waist of a heart with a somewhat unusual shape but not enlarged. The shape is in part influenced by the presence of pectus excavatum, which is not infrequently seen in patients with congenital heart disease. **C** and **D,** The heart and great vessels, with injection into the right ventricle. The truncus artery is clearly seen in both anteroposterior and lateral views, with the truncus dividing into a separate aorta and pulmonary artery. The ventricular septal defect can be seen in **D,** where the anterior right ventricle and the posterior left ventricle are separated by the ventricular septum.

operated on in childhood, the results are promising for survival to adulthood.[288]

The clinical examination shows the patient to be cyanotic and the digits clubbed. There is usually no systolic murmur, but occasionally, one may be heard. The early diastolic blowing murmur of truncus valve insufficiency is characteristic. Depending on the degree of truncus valve insufficiency, the heart may or may not be enlarged. The chest x-ray study shows the cardiac shadow to have a wide waist, which is the markedly dilated truncus arteriosus. The pulmonary vasculature is similar to that in Eisenmenger's complex (i.e., large central pulmonary arteries and no evidence of increased pulmonary flow). Echocardiography readily visualizes the truncus arteriosus and the truncus valve and can distinguish the type of truncus. Cardiac catheterization is important in characterizing the pulmonary vasculature, especially if there is any consideration of repair, because the PVR should be significantly less than the SVR.

Note should be made of a commonly used term, *pseudotruncus arteriosus*, which is really pulmonary atresia with ventricular septal defect. Despite the single arterial outflow from the two ventricles, this is really not a variant of truncus arteriosus, because the single outflow is the ascending aorta and not a truncus, and the valve is a competent tricuspid aortic valve rather than a truncus valve. Pulmonary flow is via bronchopulmonary anastomoses, as described earlier.

Aorticopulmonary window is a separate entity and is not related to truncus arteriosus.[289] In this condition, there is a window in the septum between the aorta and the pulmonary trunk. The aorta and the pulmonary trunk have separate semilunar valves, and the window does not go down to and involve the semilunar valves. If the window is large, the adult patient presents with Eisenmenger's syndrome (Fig. 8–52). Smaller windows may protect the pulmonary vasculature and allow closure of the defect.

GREAT VEIN MALPOSITIONS

Partial Anomalous Pulmonary Venous Return (Connection)

Partial anomalous pulmonary venous return has been discussed previously and is physiologically similar to left-to-right shunting at the atrial level. There may be one, two, or three pulmonary veins, which are anomalously con-

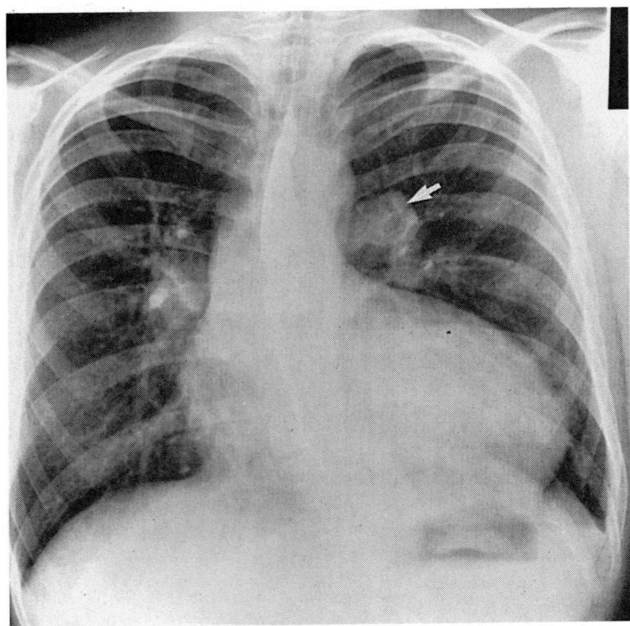

FIGURE 8–51 PA radiograph of a patient with truncus arteriosus type II. The heart is markedly enlarged, and no main pulmonary artery segment is demonstrated. The right and left pulmonary arteries are prominent, as is the aorta. The left pulmonary artery is in an abnormally high position *(arrow).* (Courtesy of Kurt Amplatz, M.D.)

nected, and they may drain together or separately into the innominate–superior vena cava system, coronary sinus, RA, and/or inferior vena cava. These constitute pure left-to-right shunts. When all four pulmonary veins connect anomalously and drain eventually into the RA, there is an obligatory atrial septal defect, the RA becoming a mixing chamber, with right-to-left shunting at the atrial level.

Total Anomalous Pulmonary Venous Connection

Total anomalous pulmonary venous connection is uncommon in the adult.[290–292] The most common form is type I, in which the pulmonary veins drain via a large ascending vertical vein into the left innominate vein and then to the superior vena cava. Less common is type II, in which the veins drain into a left "superior vena cava" and then into the coronary sinus. In type III, the pulmonary veins join to form a long anomalous vein into the inferior vena cava or even into the portal vein. Type III is not seen in adults and, if not corrected during the first few weeks of life, is usually fatal. One may also see a combination of connections, with the veins draining separately but ultimately into the RA.[293, 294]

In all these situations, the oxygen saturation in all four chambers should in theory be identical, but in fact, this is not necessarily so. Drainage into the inferior vena caval system causes the relatively more oxygenated blood to stream preferentially through the atrial septal defect so that the left heart chambers are somewhat more saturated than the right heart chambers. When the connections are by the superior vena caval system, there is apt to be more nearly equal saturation in all four chambers. If all four veins drain to the coronary sinus, the right ventricle and the pulmonary artery may have a higher oxygen content than the left side of the heart.

There are cyanosis and clubbing, but the cardiac findings are similar to those of the secundum type of atrial septal defect, with a wide, fixed splitting of the second heart sound and a hyperactive LV. The ECG is also similar, with incomplete right bundle branch block with rSR in lead V_1 and a normal frontal plane axis. The chest x-ray study is most striking if all four pulmonary veins drain into a venous sinus, then into a common vertical vein and into the innominate vein, and then to the superior vena cava. The marked dilatation of this system gives rise to the so-called snowman or figure-eight configuration of the heart and great vessels (Fig. 8–53). The echocardiogram can identify the drainage site of most or all of the pulmonary veins if the echocardiographer is alerted beforehand to the diagnosis. Sometimes, a transesophageal echocardiogram may be required. Cardiac catheterization is helpful in obtaining the oxygen saturation in all the cardiac chambers and in the pulmonary artery and aorta to give one a clue as to the likely connections. The anomalous connections can be individually cannulated, and angiograms of these anomalous veins and the exact anatomy are extremely helpful to the surgeon, especially if they drain to different sites (Fig. 8–54). It may be necessary to explore the superior vena cava and innominate vein, the coronary sinus, and the inferior vena cava. Selective indicator dilution

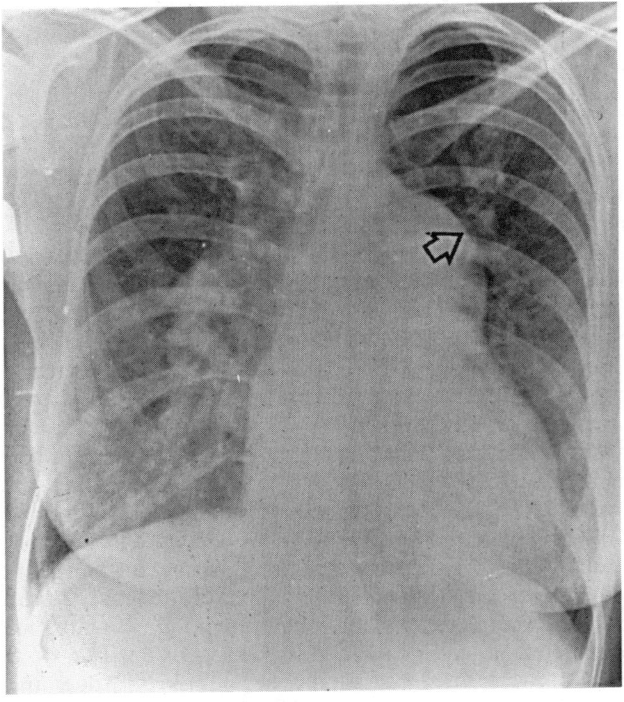

FIGURE 8–52 PA radiograph of a patient with ventricular septal defect and severe pulmonary vascular disease (Eisenmenger's syndrome). The heart is moderately enlarged, and the central pulmonary artery is distinctly enlarged, whereas the peripheral pulmonary vasculature is normal. The main pulmonary artery is huge *(arrow)* as a result of long-standing pulmonary hypertension. (Courtesy of Kurt Amplatz, M.D.)

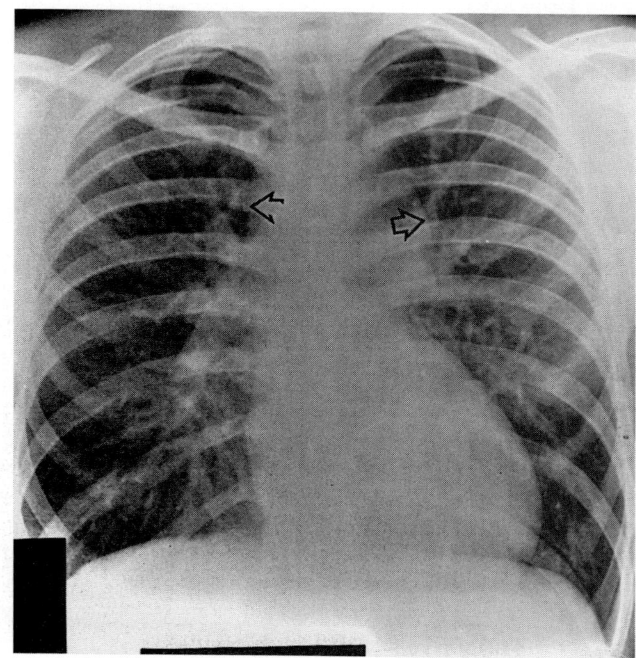

FIGURE 8–53 PA radiograph of a patient with total anomalous venous return to the left superior vena cava. The heart is mildly enlarged, the pulmonary vasculature is increased, and the dilated left and right portions of the superior vena cava are clearly demonstrated *(arrows)*; snowman heart. (Courtesy of Kurt Amplatz, M.D.)

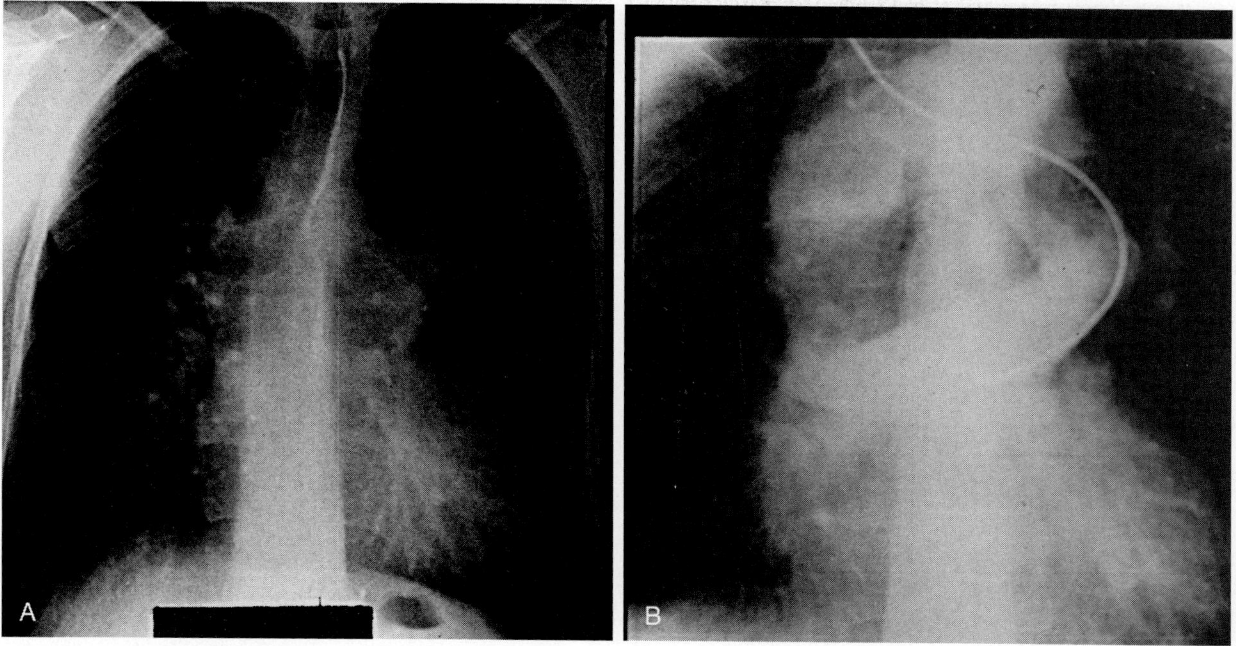

FIGURE 8–54 This 35-year-old patient had total anomalous pulmonary venous connection via a large vertical vein to the superior vena cava. **A,** Chest x-ray shows the characteristic "snowman" or figure-eight configuration. **B,** Angiogram shows the large horizontal vein, being the confluence of the pulmonary veins, which drains by a vertical vein into the innominate vein and thence into a greatly dilated superior vena cava.

curves in the four pulmonary arteries or selective angiography of these vessels can help identify the connections if the anomalous veins are not draining together.

TREATMENT

The treatment is surgical. The type of connection that is most readily amenable to surgery is anomalous pulmonary venous connection of the snowman type, by a side-to-side anastomosis of the common venous sinus to the LA and ligation of the vertical vein.

GENETIC SYNDROMES THAT INCLUDE HEART DISEASE

In adults, the most common genetic syndromes are maternal rubella–caused patent ductus arteriosus; Marfan's syndrome (mitral insufficiency, aortic insufficiency, aortic dissection); Fabry's disease[300] (cardiomyopathy and mitral insufficiency); pseudoxanthoma elasticum[296] (endocardial thickening and mitral insufficiency); well-defined neurologic syndromes, such as Friedreich's ataxia (progress is being made in elucidating the genetics of this condition),[297, 297a] myotonic dystrophy,[298, 299] and others that lead to death from cardiomyopathy; Turner's syndrome (coarctation of the aorta); Noonan's syndrome[240] (pulmonary valve dysplasia or stenosis, atrial septal defect, and sometimes hypertrophic cardiomyopathy); Down's syndrome (usually AV canal, sometimes ventricular septal defect); Carney's syndrome[301, 302] (Cushing's syndrome due to multinodular adrenal hyperplasia or a pigmented carcinoma of the adrenal cortex associated with spotty skin pigmentation and atrial myxomas; these may occur sequentially—this is the only known familial association with atrial myxoma); Goldenhar's syndrome[303] (ventricular septal defect); Osler-Weber-Rendu syndrome[304, 305] (pulmonary arteriovenous fistulas); Ehlers-Danlos syndrome[306] (mitral insufficiency); Duchenne's muscular dystrophy[307]; mucopolysaccharide storage disease,[308] and the Swyer-James syndrome (hyperlucent lung due to a small pulmonary artery and its branches).[308a] Many syndromes associated with congenital heart disease are seen almost exclusively in children and are never seen by cardiologists who work exclusively with adults.

Osler-Weber-Rendu Syndrome

Osler-Weber-Rendu syndrome is diagnosed by the cutaneous phenotype and gastrointestinal bleeding. Patients with this syndrome are often cyanotic because of right-to-left shunting through pulmonary arteriovenous fistulas. If the fistulas are few, the treatment of choice is selective embolization.

HYPERTROPHIC CARDIOMYOPATHY (ASYMMETRIC SEPTAL HYPERTROPHY)

Patients with hypertrophic cardiomyopathy have marked hypertrophy of the interventricular septum, which histologically consists of muscle fibers in disarray.[309] The rest of the left ventricular wall undergoes hypertrophy of the usual kind. During systole, the anterior leaflet of the mitral valve may move anteriorly toward the ventricular septum rather than superiorly to coapt with the posterior leaflet. This results in some degree of mitral regurgitation (Fig. 8–55), but more seriously, it may create hemodynamic obstruction to left ventricular outflow. This entity is also known as idiopathic hypertrophic subaortic stenosis.[310] The genetics of this condition have not been completely elucidated, but there is frequently a familial distribution.

In patients who have normal mitral valve motion, there is nonobstructive hypertrophic cardiomyopathy. Echocardiography has proved to be the definitive diagnostic tool,[311, 312] especially in patients who do not have systolic anterior motion of the anterior mitral valve leaflet. This condition is clinically silent, but affected patients have a predisposition to sudden death, averaging around 3 percent per year.[313] In such patients, the condition is often discovered during the course of cardiac screening of the family of a patient with obstructive hypertrophic cardiomyopathy. There is at present no proven method for decreasing this propensity for sudden death, but the avoidance of strenuous or severe isometric exertion is advisable. This condition, together with concentric myocardial hypertrophy, is the most common cause of unexpected death in young athletes.[314] No definite predictive indices of proneness to sudden death have emerged,[314] except that some families seem to be more prone to sudden death. However, Holter monitoring data suggest that patients who exhibit ventricular instability or ventricular tachycardias are more likely to die suddenly.[315, 316]

In subaortic obstructive hypertrophic cardiomyopathy, the clinical findings are characteristic. The pulse contour may be of the bisferious configuration, the second peak occurring with transiently more flow across the obstructed outflow tract as ventricular relaxation begins and before the aortic valve closes. There is a systolic murmur at the left sternal border of left ventricular outflow obstruction. The Valsalva maneuver causes the intensity of the murmur to increase owing to the fall in aortic pressure and the transient decrease in preload and left ventricular cavity size. Again, echocardiography is the most powerful tool for the diagnosis of this condition and for monitoring the effect of therapy. The echocardiogram can quantify the systolic gradient from the LV to the aorta caused by the systolic anterior motion of the mitral valve, and the Valsalva maneuver during echocardiography increases the systolic gradient.[317, 318]

Cardiac catheterization can also document the systolic gradient from the body of the LV and the aorta. The emptying of the LV is so complete that the apex is virtually obliterated. The ECG sometimes may show a Wolff-Parkinson-White configuration or may be mistaken for an old inferior infarct (Fig. 8–56). The gradient is extremely labile from day to day, or even during the procedure. Of interest is the phenomenon following an extrasystole. Normally, the systolic arterial pressure after a compensated pause is distinctly elevated, and this phenomenon occurs similarly in valvar aortic stenosis. In obstructive hypertrophic cardiomyopathy, after a compensated pause, the intraventricular pressure increases but the aortic pressure decreases, pre-

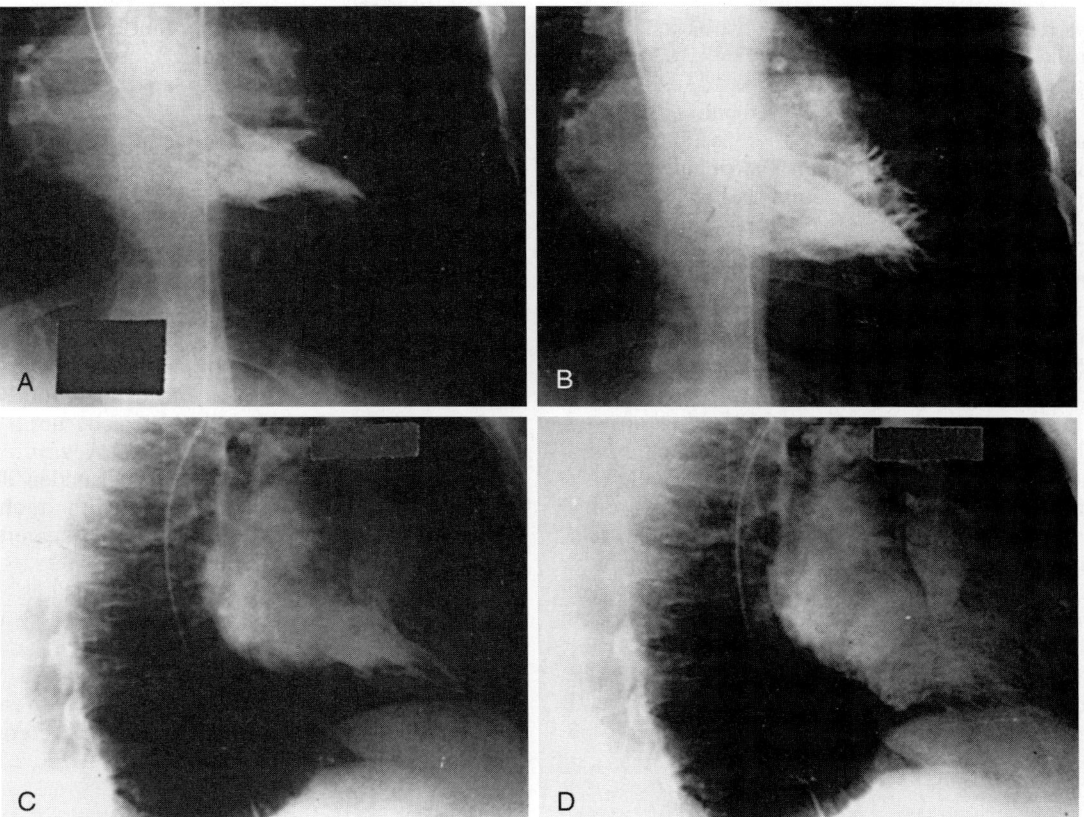

FIGURE 8–55 A–D, Idiopathic hypertrophic subaortic stenosis (obstructive hypertrophic cardiomyopathy) with mitral insufficiency in a 28-year-old man with exertional dyspnea and lightheadedness. Note the significant mitral insufficiency, with a markedly enlarged left atrium, and the hypertrophied left ventricle with a small end-systolic volume.

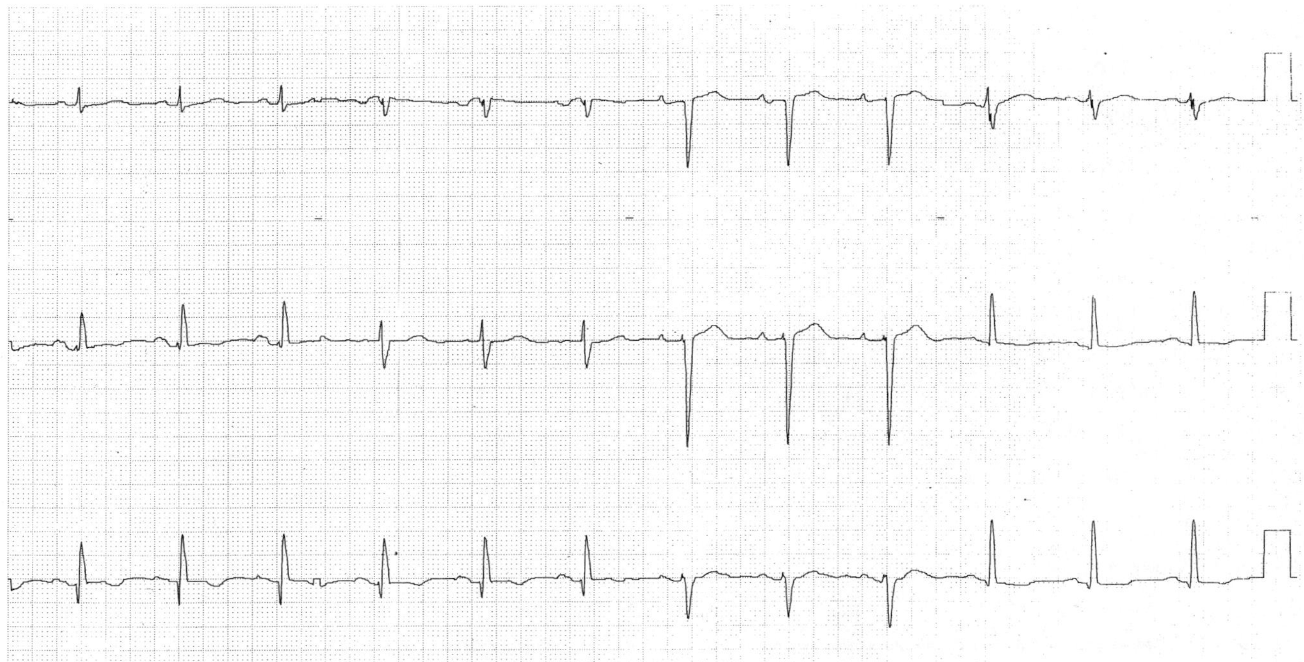

FIGURE 8–56 Electrocardiogram (ECG) of a 49-year-old woman with hypertrophic subaortic stenosis. In this condition, the ECG sometimes can be misread as an old inferior myocardial infarction, the diagnosis that had been made by ECG in this patient on more than one occasion. She had normal coronary arteries.

sumably as a result of increased outflow obstruction related to extrasystolic potentiation[319] (Fig. 8–57).

These patients are usually asymptomatic, especially when they are discovered by family screening, but they may die suddenly and unexpectedly.[320, 321] Symptoms may include exertional dyspnea due to left ventricular diastolic dysfunction,[322, 323] angina,[324] presyncope, and syncope.

Most patients with obstructive hypertrophic cardiomyopathy can be treated medically with negative inotropic agents, such as β-blockers, calcium channel blockers (especially verapamil),[321] and disopyramide, to improve ventricular compliance. These medications, especially β-blockers and verapamil, may significantly improve exercise tolerance and abolish exercise-induced syncope. In the minority of patients in whom these are ineffective, septal myectomy may be helpful.[322] When all other measures fail, replacement of the mitral valve has been reported to alleviate symptoms because the anterior leaflet of the mitral valve no longer obstructs ventricular outflow.[325] It is not clear whether any of these measures prolong life expectancy, because the natural history of the disease has been altered, but such patients can be made much more functional. Successes have been reported with use of dual-chamber pacing, reduction of the outflow tract gradient, and abolition of syncope and improvement of angina.[326] Several reports have reported hemodynamic improvement with the injection of alcohol into the first septal branch of the left anterior descending artery, thereby creating a small, controlled infarct that appears to improve or relieve the obstruction.

Right Ventricular Dysplasia

Right ventricular dysplasia appears to be an abnormality of development and may present as gross cardiomegaly and congestive failure. When it is paper thin, it has been called *Uhl's anomaly.*[326a]

The condition is usually of lesser degree, and there may be no significant right ventricular dysfunction. However, it may be associated with ventricular tachycardia, and this is then termed *arrhythmogenic right ventricular dysplasia.*[326b]

The proneness of such patients to sudden death is believed to be somewhat associated with a characteristic electrocardiographic pattern.[326c] Cardiac surgery has been performed to lessen arrhythmogenesis.[326d]

Coronary Artery Anomalies

Coronary artery anomalies can be divided into four types.[327] The first is anomalous origin of the right coronary artery

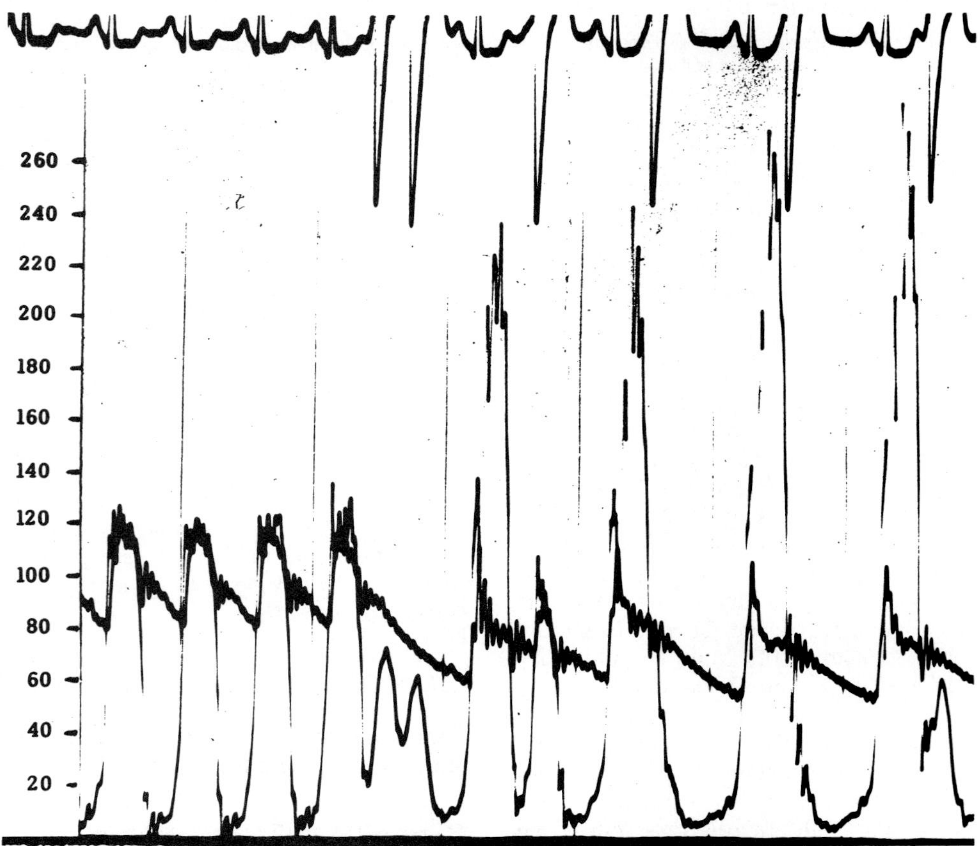

FIGURE 8–57 Obstructive hypertrophic cardiomyopathy: simultaneous tracings in the ascending aorta and the distal left ventricle. The initial four beats show no significant systolic gradient, whereas the supervention of bigeminy markedly increases the intraventricular pressure while decreasing aortic systolic pressure, the Brockenbrough phenomenon. Also note the bifid arterial pulse contour in complexes on the right.

from the left coronary artery, or a branch of the left coronary artery from the right coronary artery, or if the left anterior descending coronary artery and the circumflex artery have separate ostia. These patients are asymptomatic and do well unless they acquire coronary atherosclerosis.

A second type is an ectopic course of the left coronary artery, so that instead of coursing anterior to the pulmonary artery, it goes between the aorta and the pulmonary artery.[328] Sudden deaths have been reported with this anomaly. It is likely that the pathophysiology is not compression of the coronary artery between the aorta and the pulmonary artery, as has been suggested, because the pulmonary artery is essentially a low-pressure vessel. Rather, the course of the coronary artery shortly after its origin from the aorta is at a somewhat acute angle, which during vigorous exercise may become more acute, with resultant myocardial ischemia. The other anomaly in this group is myocardial bridging, in which the epicardial coronary artery dives under the myocardium and then re-emerges. During systole, the vessel undergoes compression. Most such cases are asymptomatic, but an occasional patient has angina and a positive stress test result that is relieved when the bridging is unroofed.[329]

A third anomaly involves fistulas between the coronary arteries and the ventricular cavity.[330] A coronary artery may empty distally directly into a cardiac chamber. This more commonly involves the right coronary artery, which drains into the RV. More often, the coronary artery drains into a telangiectatic structure, which then empties into the RV. Clinically, such patients are usually asymptomatic, but the physical examination may reveal a soft, continuous murmur over the precordium, more commonly near the left sternal border if the right coronary artery is involved. If the shunt is large, there may be a "steal" phenomenon, which may rarely cause angina. The treatment may be either surgical or selective embolization of the distal telangiectatic lesion. Angiographically, this lesion is seen at the terminus of a greatly enlarged coronary artery as a "puddle" from which contrast enters the RV. Fistulas of small coronary arterial branches are sometimes seen in routine angiograms and are of no hemodynamic significance.

If coronary artery fistulas are asymptomatic, it seems that they can be safely watched. Although the details of the lifelong mortality risk of such an anomaly are not entirely known, the evidence that exists suggests that the mortality risk of such fistulas is extremely small and would not necessarily warrant surgical intervention.[330a]

Finally, there may be an anomalous origin of a coronary artery from a pulmonary artery.[331] In this situation, the effect is that of a large coronary artery steal because the pulmonary artery is under low pressure. Therefore, anomalous origin of the left coronary artery from the pulmonary artery is seen less commonly in adults because it is usually fatal in childhood unless it is treated. Formerly, the recommended treatment was ligation of the anomalous artery, but current treatment involves both ligation of the anomalous coronary artery at its take-off from the pulmonary artery and bypass grafting. In the adult, anomalous origin of the right coronary artery from the pulmonary artery is somewhat more common and is usually asymptomatic, although it has been implicated in sudden death.

We have described an unusual situation in which two coronary arteries come off the aorta and a coronary artery also arises from the pulmonary trunk.[332] Myocardial bridging, in which the coronary artery dives under the myocardium before emerging on the surface again, is an uncommon anomaly that generally has been believed to be benign. However, occasional cases of angina have been reported, and even myocardial infarction has been documented at least once.[332a]

Aneurysms of the Sinus of Valsalva

Congenital aneurysm of the sinus of Valsalva is caused by a weakness at the junction of the aortic media and the annulus fibrosus of the aortic valve.[333] By far the most commonly involved sinus is the right aortic sinus. The aneurysm usually protrudes into the outflow tract of the RV or, less commonly, into the RA. Aneurysm of the posterior sinus is much less common, and that of the left coronary sinus is extremely rare. An aneurysm of the sinus of Valsalva is asymptomatic until it ruptures, at which time a sudden large left-to-right shunt develops into the RV or RA, with dyspnea due to pulmonary congestion and even pulmonary edema.[334] The physical findings are those of an arteriovenous fistula (i.e., a loud, continuous murmur over the precordium). The diagnosis is made clinically by the history and physical findings and is corroborated by echocardiography, which can locate the fistula and visualize the shunt. This can also be accomplished by aortic root angiography. The treatment is surgical.

The sinus of Valsalva aneurysm itself is a potential site for infective endocarditis and occasionally is the cause of rupture. The cause of this is unclear developmentally, but there seems to be an association between maternal systemic lupus erythematosus[334a] and anti-Ro (SSA) maternal antibodies.[334b]

Congenital AV block does not include the forms of congenital heart disease in which AV block may be a complication, namely, variants of AV canal and corrected transposition of the great vessels. The prognosis of those who survive into adulthood is not entirely clear because of relatively small numbers. However, in some, complete AV block may improve to the extent that it may go to second-degree or even first-degree AV block.[334c]

The temptation would be to pace all patients with congenital AV block, but it is not clear whether totally asymptomatic patients have a better prognosis with pacing. If there is exercise intolerance, escape arrhythmias, or left ventricular dysfunction, the general consensus is that pacing is indicated.[334d]

Congenital Arrhythmias

Congenital arrhythmias include congenital isolated complete AV block and the Wolff-Parkinson-White syndrome.

Congenital Isolated Complete Atrioventricular Block

The pathology of this condition has been well studied by Lev.[334e]

Pregnancy and Congenital Heart Disease

During pregnancy, there is an increase in intravascular volume starting in the second trimester, reaching a peak at 32 weeks, and declining slightly thereafter until term.[335] There is a corresponding rise in cardiac output owing to the increased volume and the vascularity of the gravid uterus.[336] During the first stage of labor, the hemodynamic alterations are intermittent and transient. The pulmonary artery wedge pressure may rise with each uterine contraction and fall promptly with relaxation, the rise in pulmonary wedge pressure being due to a sudden increase in intravascular volume by up to 500 mm Hg, caused by the contracting uterus. During the second stage of labor, however, vigorous bearing down constitutes a series of giant, prolonged Valsalva maneuvers. During the third stage, there is a loss of blood of about 500 ml and a transient rise in cardiac output without a significant change in arterial blood pressure, which translates into a lower SVR.[337, 338]

Patients with noncyanotic heart disease with left-to-right shunting and normal to moderately elevated PVRs usually tolerate pregnancy well.[339, 340] Examples would be atrial septal defects, patent ductus arteriosus, and small-to-moderate ventricular septal defects. Patients with mild-to-moderate valvular stenosis or insufficiency can also be safely carried through pregnancy. Coarctation of the aorta carries a higher risk during pregnancy because of possible aortic dissection, aortic rupture, or subarachnoid hemorrhage from a berry aneurysm, which is sometimes associated with coarctation of the aorta.[153] In all of these situations, salt restriction to prevent a disproportionate rise in the intravascular volume is of great importance. It is especially important in coarctation of the aorta, in which management of the intravascular volume should coincide with control of hypertension, if present. Salt restriction may also help to control hypertension. However, if drug therapy becomes necessary, the inevitable question of fetal toxicity arises. Verapamil has been used during pregnancy to treat fetal tachycardias without documented fetal toxicity. However, nifedipine has been associated with a high rate of cesarean section and low-birth-weight infants. The β-blockers propranolol and atenolol have been associated with low birth weight, tachycardia, and hypoglycemia. Metoprolol has been well tolerated, as apparently has labetalol. There have been rare reports of adverse effects on the fetus with angiotensin-converting enzyme inhibitors. Diuretics have not been shown to be directly deleterious to the fetus, although they may decrease placental perfusion. The combination of thiazide diuretics and methyldopa has apparently been shown to be safe and effective. There have been reports, however, that thiazides, which cross the placental barrier, are associated with neonatal thrombocytopenia and hyponatremia. Thus, drugs should be reserved for pregnant women who have clear-cut hypertension that cannot be controlled with salt restriction alone.[340]

In patients who have mechanical cardiac prostheses[339] or who might have thromboembolic phenomena caused by secondary erythrocytosis in cyanotic heart disease, use of warfarin should be avoided because of its substantial teratogenicity and fetal wastage. Heparin does not cross the placental barrier because of its molecular size and is the drug of choice for anticoagulation.[341] In the presence of erythrocytosis, self-administration of subcutaneous heparin is practical.[342] For mechanical prostheses, however, more careful monitoring of the activated partial thromboplastin time is necessary, and intravenous administration of heparin via a heparin lock may be necessary. It is precisely these considerations that may make it advisable for women of child-bearing age who have severe congenital valve disease necessitating valve replacement to opt for a bioprosthesis, if they wish to bear children, with the full understanding that a second operation will in all likelihood be necessary some years later, after childbearing has been completed.

For cardiac arrhythmias, digoxin has a long history of safety in pregnancy. Although by itself, it may not be especially effective, in combination with other drugs, it can be useful.[343] In general, quinidine has had a reasonable record of safety, although rarely, it causes damage to the eight cranial nerve of the fetus. Disopyramide, verapamil, metoprolol, and labetalol have a reasonable safety record.[344, 345] The conduct of labor in patients with serious valve disease and cyanotic heart disease optimally should include Swan-Ganz catheterization for monitoring of the pulmonary artery wedge and right atrial pressures, constant blood pressure monitoring, and oximetry.[346] Vaginal delivery, with shortening of the second stage of labor by forceps delivery, if necessary, is feasible in most such patients. However, intractable and serious elevation of the pulmonary artery wedge pressure, significant fall in arterial oxygen saturation, or intractable hypertension or hypotension or fetal distress should raise a serious consideration of cesarean section.

The first stage of labor usually does not cause serious hemodynamic disturbances, except transiently during contractions. However, the second stage should be shortened by forceps if safely feasible, and anesthesia, which minimizes vasodilatation, should be given. The third stage may be dangerous in cyanotic patients, in whom the fall in SVR after delivery, combined with blood loss, may suddenly increase right-to-left shunting. The fall in blood pressure and arterial desaturation may cause progressive deterioration, with a fatal outcome. Therefore, every effort should be made to replenish lost intravascular volume and to maintain blood pressure and adequate oxygenation. Such patients should have been typed and cross-matched, with blood available and arterial vasoconstrictors on hand to maintain the blood pressure and thus increase the SVR if necessary if sudden hypotension occurs. Cesarean section itself is not without risk. There is the risk posed by general anesthesia, the greater blood loss, and the supine hypotension phenomenon of pregnancy (postulated to be due to compression of the inferior vena cava by the gravid uterus). Therefore, cesarean section is an option only when it appears that vaginal delivery is posing an unacceptable risk.[347]

Eisenmenger's syndrome carries a high risk, as high as 38 percent, and causes considerable fetal wastage.[340]

Intrapartum open-heart surgery is almost never necessary with careful medical management and is associated with a high incidence of fetal wastage. Patients with tight aortic or pulmonic valve stenosis may be considered for balloon dilatation, preferably well after the first trimester but before the intravascular volume has peaked.[348]

In general, with careful medical management, most women with congenital heart disease can carry a pregnancy safely to term, with the risk being somewhat higher in cyanotic congenital heart disease. The risk is not only to the mother but also to the fetus, because fetal wastage is higher in cyanotic conditions. The causes are not entirely clear but are probably multifactorial because fetal hemoglobin saturates at relatively low oxygen tensions. The placental circulation is probably adversely affected by low oxygen tension and erythrocytosis.[349]

References

1. Lillehei CW, Cohen M, Warden HE, et al: The results of direct vision closure of ventricular septal defects in 8 patients by means of controlled cross circulation. Surg Gynecol Obstet 101:446, 1955.
2. Fenoglio JJ, McAllister HA Jr, deCastro MC, et al: Congenital bicuspid aortic valve after age 20. Am J Cardiol 39:164, 1977.
3. Edwards JE: Calcific aortic stenosis: pathologic features. Proc Mayo Clinic 36:444, 1961.
4. Friedman WF: Congenital aortic stenosis. *In* Adams FH, Emmanouilides GC (eds): Moss' Heart Disease in Infants: Children and Adolescents. 4th ed. Baltimore: Williams & Wilkins, 1989.
5. Roberts WC: The congenitally bicuspid aortic valve: a study of 85 autopsy cases. Am J Cardiol 26:72, 1970.
6. Storstein O: Etiology of aortic valvular disease. Acta Med Scand 185:17, 1969.
7. Edwards JE: Pathologic aspects of cardiac valvular insufficiencies. Arch Surg 77:634, 1958.
8. Downing DF: Congenital aortic stenosis: clinical aspects and surgical treatment. Circulation 14:188, 1956.
9. Peckham GB, Keith JD, Evans JR: Congenital aortic stenosis: some observations in the natural history and clinical assessment. Can Med Assoc J 91:639, 1964.
10. Johnson AM: Aortic stenosis, sudden death and left ventricular baroreceptors [editorial]. Br Heart J 33:1, 1971.
11. Paquay PA, Anderson G, Diefenthal H, et al: Chest pain as a predictor of coronary artery disease in patients with obstructive aortic valve disease. Am J Cardiol 38:863, 1976.
12. Berndt TB, Hancock EW, Shumway NE, et al: Aortic valve replacement with and without coronary artery bypass surgery. Circulation 50:967, 1974.
13. Linhart JW, de la Torre A, Ramsey HW, Wheat MW: The significance of coronary artery disease in aortic valve replacement. J Thorac Cardiovasc Surg 55:811, 1968.
14. Campbell M: Natural history of coarctation in the aorta. Br Heart J 32:633, 1970.
15. Hancock EW: The ejection sound in aortic stenosis. Am J Med 40:569, 1966.
16. Glancy DL, Epstein SE: Differential diagnosis of type and severity of obstruction of left ventricular outflow. Prog Cardiovasc Dis 14:153, 1971.
17. Leatham A: Systolic murmurs. Circulation 17:601, 1958.
18. Wood P: Aortic stenosis. Am J Cardiol 1:553, 1958.
19. Rodan BA, Chen JTT, Halber MD, et al: Chest roentgenographic evaluation of the severity of aortic stenosis. Invest Radiol 17:453, 1982.
20. Klatte EC, Tampas JP, Campbell JA, Lurie PR: The roentgenographic manifestations of aortic stenosis in aortic valvular insufficiency. Am J Roentgenol Radium Ther Nucl Med 88:57, 1962.
21. Rockoff SD, Levine ND, Austen WG: Roentgenographic clues to the cardiac hemodynamics of aortic stenosis. Radiology 83:58, 1964.
22. Myler RK, Sanders CA: Aortic valve disease and atrial fibrillation: report of 122 patients with electrocardiographic, radiographic, and hemodynamic observations. Arch Intern Med 121:530, 1968.
23. Merendino KA, Hessel EA: The murmur on top of the head in acquired mitral insufficiency. JAMA 199:392, 1967.
24. Caves PK, Sutton GC, Paneth M: Nonrheumatic subvalvular mitral regurgitation: etiology and clinical aspects. Circulation 47:1242, 1973.
25. Ronan JA Jr, Steelman RB, DeLeon AC Jr, et al: The clinical diagnosis of acute severe mitral insufficiency. Am J Cardiol 27:284, 1971.
26. Edwards JE: The congenital bicuspid aortic valve. Circulation 23:485, 1961.
27. Roberts WC: Anatomically isolated aortic valvular disease: the case against its being of rheumatic etiology. Am J Med 49:151, 1970.
28. Stein TD, Sabbah HN, Pitha JV: Continuing disease process of calcific aortic stenosis: role of microthrombi and turbulent flow. Am J Cardiol 39:159, 1977.
29. Stewart JR, Paton BC, Blount SG Jr, Swan H: Congenital aortic stenosis 10 to 20 years after valvulotomy. Arch Surg 113:1248, 1978.
30. Young JB, Quinones MA, Waggoner AD, Miller RR: Diagnosis and quantification of aortic stenosis with pulsed Doppler echocardiography. Am J Cardiol 45:987, 1980.
31. Berger M, Bergdoff RL, Gallerstein PE, Goldberg E: Evaluation of aortic stenosis by continuous wave Doppler ultrasound. J Am Coll Cardiol 3:150, 1984.
32. Gorlin R, Gorlin SG: Hydraulic formula for calculation of area of stenotic mitral valves, other cardiac valves and central circulatory shunts. Am Heart J 41:1, 1951.
33. Roberts WC: Natural history of the adult with aortic stenosis. *In* Roberts WC (ed): Adult Congenital Heart Disease. pp 363–368. Philadelphia: FA Davis, 1987.
34. Cheitlin M, Gertz E, Brundage B, et al: The rate of progression of aortic stenosis in the adult. Am Heart J 98:689, 1979.
35. Ross J Jr, Braunwald E: Aortic stenosis. Circulation 61(suppl V):37, 1968.
36. Frank S, Johnson A, Ross J Jr: Natural history of valvular aortic stenosis. Br Heart J 35:41, 1973.
37. Harris CN, Kaplan MA, Parker BP, et al: Aortic stenosis, angina and coronary artery disease. Br Heart J 37:656, 1975.
38. Keane JF, Driscoll DJ, Gersony WM, et al: Second natural history study of congenital heart defects: results of treatment of patients with aortic valvar stenosis. Circulation 87(suppl II):I-16, 1993.
39. Kuntz RE, Tosteson AN, Berman AD, et al: Predictors of event free survival after balloon aortic valvuloplasty. N Engl J Med 325:17, 1991.
40. O'Keefe JH Jr, Vliestra RE, Bailey KR, et al: Natural history of candidates for balloon aortic valvuloplasty. Mayo Clin Proc 62:986, 1987.
41. Litvack F, Jakubowski AT, Buchbinder NA, et al: Lack of sustained clinical improvement in an elderly population after percutaneous aortic valvuloplasty. Am J Cardiol 62:270, 1988.
42. Peterson TA, Todd DB, Edwards JE: Supravalvar aortic stenosis. J Thorac Cardiovasc Surg 50:734, 1965.
43. Perou ML: Congenital supravalvular aortic stenosis. A morphological study with attempt at classification. Arch Pathol Lab Med 71:453, 1961.
44. Williams JCP, Barratt-Boyes BG, Lowe JB: Supravalvar aortic stenosis. Circulation 24:1311, 1961.
45. Beuren AJ, Schulze C, Eberle P, et al: The syndrome of supravalvular aortic stenosis, peripheral pulmonary stenosis, mental retardation and similar facial appearance. Am J Cardiol 13:471, 1964.
46. Kreel I, Reiss R, Strauss L, et al: Supravalvular stenosis of the aorta. Ann Surg 149:519, 1959.
47. Roberts WC: Valvular, subvalvular and supravalvular aortic stenosis: morphologic features. Cardiovasc Clin 5:97, 1973.
48. Greenspan AM, Morganroth J, Perloff JK: Discrete fibromembranous subaortic stenosis in middle age. Cardiology 64:206, 1979.

48a. Petsas AA, Anastassiades LC, Constantinou EC, et al: Familial discrete subaortic stenosis. Clin Cardiol 21:63,1998.

49. Maron BJ, Redwood DR, Roberts WC: Tunnel subaortic stenosis: left ventricular outflow tract obstruction produced by fibromuscular, tubular narrowing. Circulation 54:404, 1976.
50. Wright GB, Keane JF, Nadas AS, et al: Fixed subaortic stenosis in the young: medical and surgical course in 83 patients. Am J Cardiol 52:830, 1983.
51. Morrow AG, Fort L III, Roberts WC, Braunwald E: Discrete subaortic stenosis complicated by aortic valvular regurgitation: clinical, hemodynamic and pathologic studies and the results of operative treatment. Circulation 31:163, 1965.
52. Reiss RL, Peterson LM, Mason DT, et al: Congenital, fixed subvalvular aortic stenosis: an anatomic classification and correlations with operative results. Circulation 43(suppl I):11, 1971.

53. Shone JD, Sellers RD, Anderson RC, et al: The developmental complex of "parachute mitral valve," supravalvular ring of the left atrium, subaortic stenosis and coarctation of aorta. Am J Cardiol 11:714, 1963.
54. DaSilva CL, Edwards JE: Parachute mitral valve in an adult. Arg Bras Cardiol 26:149, 1973.
55. Keefe JF, Wolk MJ, Levine HJ: Isolated tricuspid valvular stenosis. Am J Cardiol 25:252, 1970.
56. Geron M, Hirsch M, Borman J, Appelbaum A: Isolated tricuspid valvular stenosis: the pathology and merits of surgical treatment. J Thorac Cardiovasc Surg 63:760, 1972.
57. Edwards JE, Burchell HB: Congenital tricuspid atresia: classification. Med Clin North Am 33:1179, 1949.
58. Patterson W, Baxley WA, Karp RB, et al: Tricuspid atresia in adults. Am J Cardiol 49:141, 1982.
59. Patel MM, Overy BC, Kazonis NC, Hadley-Folkes LL: Long-term survival in tricuspid atresia. J Am Coll Cardiol 9:338, 1987.
60. Jordan AC, Sanders CA: Tricuspid atresia with prolonged survival. Am J Cardiol 18:112, 1966.
61. Fontan F, Mounicot FB, Baudet E: Correction de l'atresie tricuspidienne: rapport de deux cas "corrigés par utilization technique chirugicale nouvelle." Ann Chir Thorac Cardiovasc 20:39, 1971.
61a. Radner S: Extended suprasternal puncture technique. Acta Med Scand 107:466, 1954.
62. DeLeon SY, Idriss FS, Ilbawi MN, et al: The role of the Glenn shunt in patients undergoing the Fontan operation. J Thorac Cardiovasc Surg 85:669, 1983.
63. Molina JE, Wang Y, Lucas RV, Moller JH: The technique of the Fontan procedure with posterior right atrium pulmonary connection. Ann Thorac Surg 39:371, 1984.
64. Benshachar G, Fuhrman BP, Wang Y, et al: Rest, exercise and hemodynamics after the Fontan procedure. Circulation 65:1043, 1982.
65. Miller RA, Serratto M: Long-term evaluation of the Fontan operation for tricuspid atresia. *In* Rao RS (ed): Tricuspid Atresia. New York: Futura, 1982.
66. Ward KE, Moak JP, Garson A: Appearance and disappearance of arrhythmias after the Fontan operation. J Am Coll Cardiol 5:427, 1985.
67. Alborais ET, Porter CB, Danielson GK, et al: The results of the modified Fontan operation for congenital heart lesions in patients without preoperative sinus rhythm. J Am Coll Cardiol 6:228, 1985.
68. Weber HS, Hellenbrand WE, Kleinman CS, et al: Predictors of rhythm disturbances and subsequent morbidity after the Fontan operation. Am J Coll Cardiol 64:762, 1989.
69. Danielson GK: Univentricular heart. *In* Stark J, deEval M (eds): Surgery for Congenital Heart Defects. pp. 427–438. London: Grune & Stratton, 1983.
70. Matsuda H, Kawashima Y, Kishimoto H, et al: Problems in the modified Fontan operation for univentricular heart of the right ventricular type. Circulation 76:III-45, 1987.
71. Dow JW, Levine HD, Elkin M, et al: Studies of congenital heart disease. IV: uncomplicated pulmonic stenosis. Circulation 1:267, 1950.
72. Koretzky EM, Moeller JH, Korns ME, et al: Congenital pulmonary stenosis resulting from dysplasia of valve. Circulation 40:43, 1969.
73. Engle MA, Tomiko I, Goldberg HP: The fate of the patient with pulmonic stenosis. Circulation 30:554, 1964.
74. Snellen HA, Hartman H, Bois-Liem TN, et al: Pulmonary stenosis. Circulation 37, 38(suppl V):93, 1968.
75. Nugent EW, Freedom RM, Nora JJ, et al: Clinical course in pulmonary stenosis. Circulation 56(suppl I):38, 1977.
76. Franch RH, Gay BB Jr: Congenital stenosis of the pulmonary artery branches. Am J Med 35:512, 1963.
77. Johnson LW, Grossman W, Dalen J, Dexter L: Pulmonic stenosis in the adult: long-term follow-up study. N Engl J Med 287:1159, 1972.
78. Pexieder T: Teratogens. *In* Pierpont MEM, Moller JH (eds): The Genetics of Cardiovascular Disease. Boston: Martinus Nijhoff, 1987.
79. Delanet TB, Nadas AS: Peripheral pulmonary stenosis. Am J Cardiol 13:451, 1964.
80. Kaplan S, Adolph RJ: Pulmonic valve stenosis in adults. Cardiovasc Clin 10:328, 1979.
81. Peral W: Cardiovascular anomalies in Noonan's syndrome. Chest 71:677, 1977.
82. Mendez HMM, Opitz JM: Noonan's syndrome: a review. Am J Med Genet 21:493, 1985.
83. Nora JJ, Nora AH: Genetics and Counseling in Cardiovascular Diseases. Springfield, IL: Charles C Thomas, 1978.
84. Krabill KA, Wang Y, Einzig S, Moller JH: Rest and exercise hemodynamics in pulmonary stenosis: comparison of children and adults. Am J Cardiol 56:360, 1985.
85. Kan JS, White RI, Mitchell SE, Gardner TJ: Percutaneous balloon valvuloplasty: a new method for pulmonary valve stenosis. N Engl J Med 307:540, 1982.
86. Brockman RC: Pulmonary valvulotomy for relief of congenital pulmonary stenosis: report of three cases. BMJ 1:1121, 1948.
87. Peppine CJ, Gessner IH, Feldman RL: Percutaneous balloon valvuloplasty for a pulmonic valve stenosis in the adult. Am J Cardiol 50:1442, 1982.
88. Fawzy ME, Mercer EN, Dunn B: Late results of pulmonary balloon valvuloplasty using double balloon technique. Int J Cardiol 1:35, 1988.
89. Shrivastara S, Shyam-Sundara, Mukhopadhyaya S, Rajani M: Percutaneous transluminal balloon pulmonary valvuloplasty: long-term results. Int J Cardiol 17:304, 1987.
90. Shuck JW, McCormick DJ, Cohen IS, et al: Percutaneous balloon valvuloplasty of the pulmonary valve: role of right-to-left shunting through a patent foramen ovale. J Am Coll Cardiol 4:132, 1984.
91. Bridges ND, Hellenbrand W, Latson L, et al: Transcatheter closure of patent foramen ovale after presumed paradoxical embolism. Circulation 86:1902, 1992.
92. Das, GS, Voss G, Jarvis G, et al: Experimental atrial septal defect with a new transcatheter self-centering device. Circulation 88:1754, 1993.
93. Edwards JE: Classification. *In* Roberts WC (ed): Adult Congenital Heart Disease. p. 23. Philadelphia: FA Davis, 1987.
94. Bove EL, Byrum CJ, Thomas FD, et al: The influence of pulmonary insufficiency on ventricular function following repair of tetralogy of Fallot. J Thorac Cardiovasc Surg 85:691, 1983.
95. Garson A Jr, Nihill MR, McNamara DG, Cooley DA: Status of the adult and adolescent after the repair of tetralogy of Fallot. Circulation 59:1232, 1979.
96. Cosio FG, Wang Y, Nicoloff DM: Membranous right ventricular outflow obstruction. Am J Cardiol 32:1000, 1973.
97. Davies MJ, Moore VP, Baimbridge MV: The floppy mitral valve: the study of incidence, pathology and complications in surgical necropsy and forensic material. Br Heart J 40:468, 1978.
98. Rippe J, Fishbein MC, Carabello B, et al: Primary myxoma degeneration of cardiac valves: clinical, pathologic, haemodynamic and echocardiographic profile. Br Heart J 44:621, 1980.
99. Pocock WA: Mitral leaflet billowing and prolapse. *In* Barlow JB (ed): Perspectives on the Mitral Valve. pp. 45–112. Philadelphia: FA Davis, 1987.
100. Savage DD, Garrison RJ, Devereux RB, et al: Mitral valve prolapse in the general population. I: epidemiological features: a Framingham Study. Am Heart J 106:571, 1983.
101. Procacci PM, Savran SV, Scheiter SL, Bryson AL: Prevalence of clinical mitral valve prolapse in 1,169 young women. N Engl J Med 294:1086, 1976.
102. Levine RA, Handschumacher MD, San Filippo AJ, et al: Three-dimensional echocardiographic reconstruction of the mitral valve with implications for the diagnosis of mitral valve prolapse. Circulation 80:589, 1989.
103. Wann LS, Grove JR, Schess TR, et al: Prevalence of mitral valve prolapse by two-dimensional echocardiography in healthy young women. Br Heart J 49:334, 1983.
104. Perloff JK, Child JS, Edwards JE: New guidelines for the clinical diagnosis of mitral valve prolapse. Am J Cardiol 57:1124, 1986.
105. Guy FC, MacDonald RPR, Fraser DB, Smith ER: Mitral valve prolapse as a cause of hemodynamically important mitral regurgitation. Can J Surg 23:166, 1980.
106. Devereux RB, Kramer-Fox R, Brown WT, et al: Relation of clinical features of the mitral valve prolapse and echocardiographically documented mitral valve prolapse. J Am Coll Cardiol 8:763, 1986.
107. Weissman NJ, Shear MK, Kramer-Fox R, Devereux RB: Contrasting patterns of autonomic dysfunction in patients with mitral valve prolapse and panic attacks. Am J Med 82:880, 1987.
108. Wilcken DE, Hickey AJ: Lifetime risk for patients with mitral valve prolapse of development of severe valve regurgitation requiring surgery. Circulation 78:10, 1988.
109. MacMahon SW, Roberts JK, Kramer-Fox R, et al: Mitral valve prolapse and infective endocarditis. Am Heart J 113:1291, 1987.

110. Chesler E, King RA, Edwards JE: Myxomatous mitral valve and sudden death. Circulation 67:632, 1983.
111. Lucas RV Jr, Edwards JE: The floppy mitral valve. Curr Probl Cardiol 7:1, 1982.
112. Markiewicz W, Stoner J, London E, et al: Mitral valve prolapse in presumably healthy young females. Circulation 53:464, 1976.
113. Weiss AN, Mimbs JW, Ludbrook PA, Sobel BE: Echocardiographic detection of mitral valve prolapse: exclusion of false-positive diagnosis and determination of inheritance. Circulation 52:1091, 1975.
114. Kligfield P, Hochreitter C, Kramer H, et al: Complex arrhythmias in mitral regurgitation with and without mitral valve prolapse: contrast to arrhythmias in mitral valve prolapse without mitral regurgitation. Am J Cardiol 55:1545, 1985.
115. Kligfield P, Levy D, Devereux RB, et al: Arrhythmias and sudden death in mitral valve prolapse. Am Heart J 113:1298, 1987.
116. Cohn LH, DiSesa VJ, Couper GS, et al: Mitral valve repair for myxomatous degeneration and prolapse of the mitral valve. J Thorac Cardiovasc Surg 98:987, 1989.
116a. Edwards DS, Edwards JE: Aortic coarctation in adult congenital heart disease. *In* Roberts WC (ed): Adult Congenital Heart Disease. Philadelphia: FA Davis, 1987.
117. MacMahon SW, Hickey AJ, Wilcken DEL, et al: Risk and effect of endocarditis in mitral valve prolapse with and without systolic murmurs. Am J Cardiol 59:105, 1987.
118. McKusick EA: The cardiovascular aspects of Marfan's syndrome: a heritable disorder of connective tissue. Circulation 11:321, 1955.
119. Roberts WC, Honig HS: The spectrum of cardiovascular disease in the Marfan's syndrome: a clinicomorphologic study of 18 necropsy patients in comparison with 151 previously reported necropsy patients. Am Heart J 104:115, 1982.
120. Marsalese DO, Moodie DS, Vacante M, et al: Marfan's syndrome: natural history and long-term follow-up of cardiovascular involvement. J Am Coll Cardiol 14:422, 1989.
121. Loeppky CB, Alper KMA, Hamel PC, et al: Extensive aortic dissection from combined-type cystic medial necrosis in a young man without previous predisposing factors. Chest 79:116, 1981.
122. Childs JS, Perloff JK, Kaplan S: The heart of the matter: cardiovascular involvement in Marfan's syndrome. J Am Coll Cardiol 14:429, 1989.
123. Pyeritz RE, Wappel MA: Mitral valve dysfunction in the Marfan's syndrome. Am J Med 74:797, 1983.
124. Beighton P, dePaepe A, Danks D, et al: International Nosology of Heritable Disorders of Connective Tissue, Berlin, 1986. Am J Med Genet 29:581, 1988.
125. Granato JE, Dee T, Gibson RS: Utility of two-dimensional echocardiography in suspected ascending aortic dissection. Am J Cardiol 56:123, 1985.
126. Iliceto S, Nanda NC, Rizzon P, et al: Color Doppler evaluation of aortic dissection. Circulation 75:748, 1987.
127. Layman TE, Wang Y: Idiopathic cystic medionecrosis and aneurysm of dilatation of the ascending aorta. Med Clin North Am 52:1145, 1968.
128. Adachi H, Kyo S, Takamoto S, et al: Early diagnosis of surgical intervention of acute aortic dissection by trans-esophageal color flow mapping. Circulation 82(suppl IV):IV-19, 1990.
129. Schaefer S, Peshock RM, Malloy CR: Nuclear magnetic resonance imaging in Marfan's syndrome. J Am Coll Cardiol 9:70, 1987.
130. Mayer JA, Jr, Lindsay WG, Wang Y, et al: Composite replacement of aortic valve and ascending aorta. J Thorac Cardiovasc Surg 76:816, 1978.
131. Crawford CS, Crawford JL, Stowe CO, et al: Total aortic replacement for chronic aortic dissection occurring in patients with and without Marfan's syndrome. Ann Surg 199:358, 1984.
132. Dietzman RH, Peter ET, Wang Y, Lillehei RC: Mitral insufficiency in Marfan's syndrome: a case report of surgical correction. Chest 51:650, 1967.
133. Crawford ES: Marfan's syndrome: broad spectral surgical treatment cardiovascular manifestations. Ann Surg 198:487, 1983.
134. deSanctis R, Doroghazi RN, Austin WG, et al: Aortic dissection. N Engl J Med 317:1060, 1987.
135. Criscitiello MG, Harvey WP: Clinical recognition of congenital pulmonary valve insufficiency. Am J Cardiol 20:765, 1967.
136. Schloff LD, Wang Y: Congenital isolated pulmonic regurgitation. Chest 55:254, 1969.
137. Ebstein W: A rare case of insufficiency of the tricuspid valve caused by a severe malformation of the same [translated by Schiebler GS, et al]. Am J Cardiol 22:867, 1968.
138. Giuliani ER, Fuster V, Brandenberg RO, Mair DD: Ebstein's anomaly: the clinical features and natural history of the tricuspid valve. Mayo Clin Proc 54:163, 1979.
139. Zalzstein E, Koran G, Einerson T, Freedom RN: A case-controlled study on the association of first trimester exposure to lithium in Ebstein's anomaly. Am J Cardiol 65:817, 1990.
140. Gussenhoven WJ, Spitaels SEC, Bom N, Becker AE: Echocardiographic criteria of Ebstein's anomaly of tricuspid valve. Br Heart J 43:31, 1980.
141. Kastor JA, Goldreier BN, Josephson ME, et al: Electrophysiologic characteristics of Ebstein's anomaly of the tricuspid valve. Circulation 52:987, 1975.
141a. Beekman RH, Robinow M: Coarctation of the aorta as an autosomal dominant trait. Am J Cardiol 56:818, 1985.
142. Shepherd JT: Coarctation of the aorta. *In* Shepherd JT (ed): Physiology of the Circulation in Human Limbs in Health and Disease. Philadelphia: WB Saunders, 1963.
143. Lacro RV, Lyons-Jones K, Benirschki K: Coarctation of the aorta in Turner's syndrome: a pathologic study of fetuses with nuchal cystic hygromas, hydrops fetalis and female genitalia. Pediatrics 81:445, 1988.
144. Campbell M: Natural history of coarctation of the aorta. Br Heart J 32:633, 1970.
145. Liberthson RR, Pennington DG, Jacobs ML, Daggett WM: Coarctation of aorta: review of 234 patients and clarification of management problems. Am J Cardiol 43:835, 1979.
146. Reisenstein G, Levin S, Gross R: Coarctation of the aorta: review of 104 autopsy cases of the "adult type" two years of age or older. Am Heart J 33:146, 1947.
147. Becker AE, Becker MJ, Edwards JE: Anomalies associated with coarctation of aorta: particular reference to infancy. Circulation 41:1067, 1970.
148. Edwards JE: Aneurysms of the thoracic aorta complicating coarctation. Circulation 48:195, 1973.
149. Hirst AE Jr, Johns BJ Jr, Kine SW Jr: Dissecting aneurysm of the aorta: review of 505 cases. Medicine (Baltimore) 37:217, 1958.
150. Hodes HL, Steinfeld L, Blumenthal S: Congenital cerebral aneurysms and coarctation of the aorta. Arch Pediatr 76:28, 1959.
151. Vladover Z, Newfeld HN: Coronary arteries and coarctation of the aorta. Circulation 37:449, 1968.
152. Wittemore R, Hobbins JC, Engle MA: Pregnancy and its outcome in women with and without surgical treatment of congenital heart disease. Am J Cardiol 50:641, 1982.
153. Wachtel HL, Czarnecki SW: Coarctation of the aorta and pregnancy. Am Heart J 72:251, 1966.
154. Tynan M, Finley JT, Fontes V, et al: Balloon angioplasty for the treatment of native coarctation: results of valvuloplasty and angioplasty of congenital anomalies registry. Am J Cardiol 65:790, 1990.
155. Cohen M, Fuster V, Steele PM, et al: Coarctation of the aorta: long-term follow-up and prediction of outcome after surgical correction. Circulation 80:840, 1989.
156. Choy M, Rocchini AT, Beekman RH, et al: Paradoxical hypertension after repair of the coarctation of the aorta in children: balloon angioplasty vs. surgical repair. Circulation 75:1186, 1987.
157. Igler FO, Boerboom LE, Warner PH, et al: Coarctation of the aorta and baroreceptor resetting. Circ Res 48:365, 1981.
158. Anderson C, Devine WA, Anderson RH, et al: Abnormalities of the spleen in relation to congenital malformation of the heart: survey of necropsy findings in children. Br Heart J 63:122, 1990.
159. Peoples WM, Moller JH, Edwards JE: Polysplenia: a review of 146 cases. Pediatr Cardiol 4:129, 1983.
160. Bedford DE: The anatomical types of atrial septal defect: their incidence and clinical diagnosis. Am J Cardiol 6:568, 1960.
161. Craig RJ, Selzer A: Natural history and prognosis of atrial septal defect. Circulation 37:805, 1968.
162. Mattila S, Merikallio E, Talla T: ASD in patients over 40 years of age. Scand J Thorac Cardiovasc Surg 13:21, 1979.
163. Gault JH, Morrow AAG, Gay WA, Ross J: Atrial septal defect in patients over the age of 40 years: hemodynamic studies and the effects of operation. Circulation 37:261, 1968.
164. Steele PM, Fuster V, Cohen M, et al: Isolated atrioseptal defect with pulmonary vascular obstructive disease: long-term follow-up and prediction of outcome after surgical correction. Circulation 76:1037, 1987.

165. Markman PG, Horvitt EG, Wade EG: Atrial septal defect in the middle-aged and elderly. Q J Med 34:409, 1965.
166. Baksmann G, Rey C, Mycinski C, Dupuis C: Communication interauriculaire avec hypertension arterielle pulmonaire severe chez l'enfant: a propos de 9 observations. Arch Mal Coeur 80:455, 1987.
167. Sutton MGS, Tajaik A, McGoon DC: Atrial septal defects in patients ages 60 years or older. Circulation 64:402, 1982.
168. Leachman RD, Cokkinos DV, Cooley DA: Association of ostium secundum atrial septal defects with mitral valve prolapse. Am J Cardiol 38:167, 1976.
168a. Am J Cardiol 35:363, 1975.
169. Bink-Boelkens MTE, Meuzellar KJ, Eygelaar A: Arrhythmias after repair of secundum atrial septal defect: influence of surgical modification. Am Heart J 115:629, 1988.
170. Lutembacher R: De la stenose mitrale avec communication interauriculaire. Arch Mal Coeur 9:237, 1916.
171. Girod D, Raghib G, Wang Y, Amplatz K: Angiographic characteristics of persistent common atrioventricular canal. Radiology 85:442, 1965.
172. McGinn S, White PD: Interauricular septal defect associated with mitral stenosis. Am Heart J 9:1, 1933.
173. Goldfarb B, Wang Y: Mitral stenosis and left-to-right shunt at the atrial level: a broad concept of the Lutembacher syndrome. Am J Cardiol 17:3, 1966.
174. Smallhorn JF, Tommasini G, Anderson RH: Assessment of atrioventricular septal defects by two-dimensional echocardiography. Br Heart J 47:109, 1982.
175. Meijboom F, Hess J, Szatmari A, et al: Long-term follow-up (9 to 20 years) after surgical closure of atrial septal defect at a young age. Am J Cardiol 72:1431–1434, 1993.
176. Pastorek JS, Allen HD, Davis JT: Current outcomes of surgical closure of secundum atrial septal defect. Am J Cardiol 74:75–77, 1994.
177. Nasrallah AT, Hall RJ, Garcia E, et al: Surgical repair of atrial septal defect in patients over 60 years of age: long term results. Circulation 53:329–331, 1976.
178. Konstantinides S, Geibel A, Olschewski M, et al: A comparison of surgical and medical therapy for atrial septal defect in adults. N Engl J Med 333:469–473, 1995.
179. Horvath KA, Burke RP, Collins JJ Jr, Cohn LH: Surgical treatment of adult atrial septal defect: Early and long-term results. J Am Coll Cardiol 20:1156–1159, 1992.
180. King TD, Mills NL: Nonoperative closure of atrial septal defects. Surgery 3:383–388, 1974.
181. King TD, Mills NL: Secundum atrial septal defects: nonoperative closure during cardiac catheterization. JAMA 235:2506–2509, 1976.
181a. Brassard M, Fouron JC, van Doesburg NH, et al: Outcome of children with atrial septal defect considered too small for surgical closure. Am J Cardiol 83:1552, 1999.
182. Rashkind WJ: Interventional cardiac catheterization in congenital heart disease. Int J Cardiol 7:1–11, 1985.
183. Lock JE, Cockerham JT, Keane JF, et al: Transcatheter umbrella closure of congenital heart defects. Circulation 75:593–599, 1987.
184. Lock JE, Rome JJ, Davis R, et al: Transcatheter closure of atrial septal defects. Circulation 79:1091–1099, 1989.
185. Rome JJ, Keane JF, Perry SB, et al: Double umbrella closure of atrial septal defects: initial clinical applications. Circulation 82:751–758, 1990.
186. Perry SB, van der Velde ME, Bridges ND, et al: Transcatheter closure of atrial and ventricular septal defects. Herz 18:135–142, 1993.
187. O'Laughlin MP, Bricker JT, Mullins CE, et al: Transcatheter closure of residual atrial septal defect following cardiac transplantation. Cathet Cardiovasc Diagn 28:162–163, 1993.
188. Ruiz CE, Gamra H, Mahrer P, et al: Percutaneous closure of a secundum atrial septal defect and double balloon valvotomies of a severe mitral and aortic valve stenosis in a patient with Lutembacher's syndrome and severe pulmonary hypertension. Cathet Cardiovasc Diag 25:309–312, 1992.
189. Sideris EB, Sideris SE, Thampoulos BD, et al: Transvenous atrial septal defect occlusion by the buttoned device. Am J Cardiol 66:1524–1526, 1990.
190. Rao PS, Sideris EB, Chopra PS: Catheter closure of atrial septal defects: successful use in a 3.6 kg infant. Am Heart J 121:1826–1829, 1991.
191. Rao PS, Langhough R: Relationship of echocardiographic, shunt flow, and angiographic size to the stretched diameter of the atrial septal defect. Am Heart J 122:505–508, 1991.
192. Rao PS, Wilson AD, Chopra PS: Transcatheter closure of atrial septal defect by "buttoned" devices. Am J Cardiol 69:1056–1061, 1992.
193. Rao PS, Wilson AD, Levy JM, et al: Role of "buttoned" double-disc device in the management of atrial septal defects. Am Heart J 123:191–200, 1992.
194. Rao PS, Sideris EB, Hausdorf G, et al: International experience with secundum atrial septal defect occlusion by the buttoned device. Am Heart J 128:1022–1035, 1994.
195. Lloyd TR, Rao PS, Beekman RH III, et al: Atrial septal defect occlusion with the buttoned device (a multi-institutional U.S. trial). Am J Cardiol 73:286–291, 1994.
196. Arabia FA, Rosado LJ, Lloyd TR, Sethi GK: Management of complications of Sideris transcatheter devices for atrial septal defect closure. J Thorac Cardiovasc Surg 106:886–888, 1993.
197. Zamora R, Lax D, Donnerstein RL, Lloyd TR: Transcatheter closure of residual atrial septal defect following implantation of buttoned device. Cathet Cardiovasc Diagn 36:242–246, 1995.
198. Zamora RP, Lloyd TR, Beekman RH, Sideris EB: Follow-up results of the multi-institutional phase I FDA supervised clinical trials of transcatheter occlusion of atrial septal defects with buttoned device. J Am Coll Cardiol 29:143A, 1997.
199. Babic UU, Grujicic S, Djurisic Z, Vucinic M: Transcatheter closure of atrial septal defects. Lancet 336:566–567, 1990.
200. Sievert H, Babic UU, Ensslen R, et al: Transcatheter closure of large atrial septal defects with the Babic system. Cathet Cardiovasc Diagn 36:232–240, 1995.
201. Hausdorf G, Schneider M, Franzbach B, et al: Transcatheter closure of secundum atrial septal defects with the atrial septal defect occlusion system (ASDOS): initial experience in children. Heart 75:83–88, 1996.
202. Sievert H, Dirks J, Rux S, et al: ASD and PFO closure in adults with the second generation ASDOS device. J Am Coll Cardiol 29:143A, 1997.
203. Pavcnik D, Wright KC, Wallace S: Monodisk: device for percutaneous transcatheter closure of cardiac septal defects. Cardiovasc Intervent Radiol 16:308–312, 1993.
204. Das GS, Voss G, Jarvis G, et al: Experimental atrial septal defect closure with a new, transcatheter, self-centering device. Circulation 88:1754–1764, 1993.
205. Sharafudin MJ, Gu X, Titus JL, Amplatz K: Secundum–ASD closure with a new self-expanding prosthesis in swine. Circulation 94:I-57, 1996.
206. Boutin C, Musewe NN, Smallhorn JF, et al: Echocardiographic follow-up of atrial septal defect after catheter closure by double-umbrella device. Circulation 88:621–627, 1993.
206a. McGrath LB, Gonzalez-Lavin L: Actuarial survival, freedom from reoperation, and other events after repair of atrioventricular septal defects. J Thorac Cardiovasc Surg 94:582, 1987.
207. Kyger ER, Frazier OH, Cooley DA, et al: Sinus venosus atrial septal defect: early and late results following closure in 109 patients. Ann Thorac Surg 25:44, 1978.
208. Trusler GA, Kazenleson G, Freedom RM, et al: Late results following repair of partial anomalous pulmonary venous connection with sinus venosus atrial septal defect. J Thorac Cardiovasc Surg 79:776, 1980.
209. Craig JD: Communications between the left atrium and the coronary sinus. Thesis, University of Minnesota, 1952.
210. McGaughey MD, Trail TA, Brinker JA: Partial left anomalous pulmonary venous return: a diagnostic dilemma. Cathet Cardiovasc Diagn 12:110, 1986.
211. Snellen HA, van Ingen HC, Hoefsmit E: Patterns of anomalous pulmonary venous drainage. Circulation 38:45, 1968.
212. Frye RL, Krebs M, Rahimtoola SH, et al: Partial anomalous pulmonary venous connection without atrial septal defect. Am J Cardiol 22:242, 1968.
213. Zelis R, Fisher RD, Cohen LS, et al: Anomalous pulmonary venous drainage from the entire left lung without cardiac malformations. Arch Intern Med 124:91, 1969.
214. Stewart JR, Schaff HV, Fortunin NJ, Brawley RK: Partial anomalous pulmonary venous return with intact atrial septum: report of four cases. Thorax 38:859, 1983.

215. Lucas RV Jr: Anomalous venous connection, pulmonary and systemic. *In* Adams FH, Emmanoulides GC (eds): Moss' Heart Disease in Infants, Children and Adolescents. 4th ed. p. 580. Baltimore: Williams & Wilkins, 1989.
216. Gikonyo DK, Tandon R, Lucas RV Jr, Edwards JE: Scimitar syndrome in neonates: report of four cases and review of the literature. Pediatr Cardiol 6:193, 1986.
217. Hagler DJ, Edwards WD, Seward DJV, Tajik A: Standardized nomenclature of the ventricular septum and ventricular septal defects with applications for two-dimensional echocardiography. Mayo Clin Proc 60:741, 1985.
218. Weidman WH, Blount SG Jr, DuShane JW, et al: Clinical course in ventricular septal defect: natural history study. Circulation 56 (suppl):I56, 1977.
219. Savard M, Swan HJC, Kirklin JW, Wood EH: Hemodynamic alterations associated with ventricular septal defect. *In* Bass AD, Moe GK (eds): Congenital Heart Disease. p. 141. Washington, DC: American Association for the Advancement of Science, 1960.
220. Dickinson DF, Arnold R, Wilkenson JL: Ventricular septal defects in children born in Liverpool: evaluation of natural course and surgical implications in an unselected population. Br Heart J 46:47, 1981.
221. van Praagh R, Gava T, Kreutzer J: Ventricular septal defects: how should we describe, name and classify them? J Am Coll Cardiol 14:1298, 1989.
222. Eisenmenger V: Ursprung der Aorta aus beiden Ventrikeln beim Defect der Septum ventriculoren. Wien Klin Wochenschr 11:26, 1898.
223. Evans JR, Rowe RD, Keith JD: Spontaneous closure of ventricular septal defects. Circulation 22:1044, 1960.
224. Helmcke F, Souza A, Nanda NC, et al: Two-dimensional color Doppler assessment of ventricular septal defect of congenital origin. Am J Cardiol 63:1112, 1989.
225. Sharif DS, Huhta JC, Marantz P, et al: Two-dimensional echocardiographic determination of ventricular septal defect size: correlation of autopsy. Am Heart J 117:1333, 1989.
226. Kurokawa S, Takahashi M, Kato HY, et al: Noninvasive evaluation of the ratio of pulmonary to systemic flow in ventricular septal defect by means of Doppler two-dimensional echocardiography. Am Heart J 116:1033, 1988.
227. Gasul BM, Dillon RF, Vrla V, Hait G: Ventricular septal defects: their natural transformation into those with infundibular stenosis or into the cyanotic or noncyanotic type of tetralogy of Fallot. JAMA 164:847, 1957.
228. Godman MJ, Roberts NK, Izukawa T: Late post operative conduction disturbances after repair of ventricular septal defect in tetralogy of Fallot. Circulation 49:214, 1974.
229. Okarama EO, Guller B, Molony JD, Weidman WH: Etiology of right bundle branch block pattern after surgical closure of ventricular septal defects. Am Heart J 90:14, 1975.
230. Campbell M: Natural history of persistent ductus arteriosus. Br Heart J 30:4, 1968.
230a. Campbell M: Natural history of persistent ductus arteriosus. Br Heart J 30:4, 1968.
231. Gibson GA: Diseases of the Heart and Aorta. London: Young J Pentland, 1898.
232. Liao PK, Su WJ, Hung JS: Doppler echocardiographic flow characteristics of isolated patent ductus arteriosus: better delineation by Doppler color-flow mapping. J Am Coll Cardiol 12:1285, 1988.
233. Bain CWC: Longevity in patent ductus arteriosus. Br Heart J 19:574, 1957.
234. Marquis RM, Miller HC, McCormack RJM, et al: Persistent ductus arteriosus with left-to-right shunt in the older patient. Br Heart J 48:469, 1982.
235. Allikhan MA, Mullins CE, Nihill MR, et al: Percutaneous catheter closure of the ductus arteriosus in children and young adults. Am J Cardiol 64:218, 1989.
236. Hellenbrand WE, Mullins CE: Catheter closure of congenital cardiac defects. Cardiol Clin 7:351, 1989.
237. Kosh JA: Patent ductus arteriosus: a follow-up study of 73 cases. Br Heart J 19:13, 1957.
238. Smith G: Patent ductus arteriosus of pulmonary hypertension and reversed shunt. Br Heart J 16:233, 1954.
239. McManus BM, Hahn PF, Smith JA, et al: Eisenmenger type patent ductus arteriosus with prolonged survival. Am J Cardiol 54:462, 1984.
240. Ng AS, Liestra RE, Smith HC, et al: Patent ductus arteriosus in patients over 50 years. J Am Coll Cardiol 3:599, 1984.
241. Campbell M: Patent ductus arteriosus: some notes on prognosis and pulmonary hypertension. Br Heart J 17:511, 1955.
242. Whitaker W, Heath D, Brown JW: Patent ductus arteriosus of pulmonary hypertension. Br Heart J 17:121, 1955.
243. Bessenger FB Jr, Blieden LC, Edwards JE: Hypertensive pulmonary vascular disease associated with patent ductus arteriosus. Circulation 52:157, 1975.
244. Tandon R, Moller JH, Edwards JE: Unusual longevity and persistent atrioventricular canal. Circulation 50:619, 1974.
245. Friedman WF: Atrioventricular septal defect. *In* Braunwald E (ed): Heart Disease. 4th ed. p. 908. Philadelphia: WB Saunders, 1992.
245a. Dittrich S, Vogel M, Duhnert I, et al: Surgical repair of tetralogy of Fallot in adults today. Clin Cardiol 22:460, 1999.
246. Clapp S, Perry BL, Farooki ZQ, et al: Down's syndrome: complete atrioventricular canal and pulmonary vascular obstructive disease. J Thorac Cardiovasc Surg 100:115, 1990.
247. Paul MH: D-Transposition of great arteries. *In* Adams FH, Emmanouilides GC (eds): Moss' Heart Disease in Infants, Children and Adolescents. 4th ed. p. 371. Baltimore: Williams & Wilkins, 1989.
248. Anderson RH, Henry GW, Becker AE: Morphologic aspects of complete transposition. Cardiol Young 1:41, 1991.
249. Waldeman JD, Paul MH, Newfeld EA, et al: Transposition of the great arteries with intact ventricular septum and patent ductus arteriosus. Am J Cardiol 39:232, 1977.
250. Rigby ML, Chan KY: The diagnostic evaluation of patients with complete transposition. Cardiol Young 1:26, 1991.
251. Kirklin JW, Colvin EV, McConnell ME, Bargeron LM: Complete transposition of the great arteries: treatment in the current era. Pediatr Clin North Am 37:174, 1990.
252. Kirklin JW: The surgical repair for complete transposition. Cardiol Young 1:13, 1991.
253. Schiebler GL, Edwards JE, Burchell HB, et al: Congenital corrected transposition of great vessels. Pediatrics 27:851, 1961.
254. Cumming GR: Congenital corrective transposition of the great vessels without associated intracardiac anomalies: a clinical, hemodynamic, angiographic study. Am J Cardiol 10:605, 162.
255. Rotem CE, Holtgren HN: Corrective transposition of the great vessels without associated defects. Am Heart J 70:305, 1965.
256. Waldo AL, Pacifico AD, Bargeron LM Jr, et al: Electrophysiologic delineation of specialized AV conduction system in patients with corrected transposition of the great vessels and ventricular septal defect. Circulation 52:435, 1975.
257. Bjarke BB, Kidd BSL: Congenitally corrected transposition of the great arteries: a clinical study of 101 cases. Acta Pediatr Scand 65:153, 1976.
258. Berry WB, Roberts WC, Morrow AG, Braunwald E: Corrected transposition of the aorta and pulmonary trunk: clinical, hemodynamic, and pathologic findings. Am J Med 36:35, 1964.
259. Freedberg DC, Nadas AS: Clinical profile of patients with congenital corrected transposition of the great arteries. N Engl J Med 282:1053, 1970.
260. Meisner MD, Panidis IP, Eshaghpour E, et al: Corrected transposition of the great arteries: evaluation by two-dimensional and Doppler echocardiography. Am Heart J 111:599, 1986.
261. Dimas AP, Moodie DS, Strba R, Gill CC: Long-term function of the morphologic right ventricle in adult patients with corrected transposition of the great arteries. Am Heart J 118:526, 1989.
262. Hagler DJ, Ritter DG, Puga FJ: double-outlet right ventricle. *In* Adams FH, Emmanoulides JC (eds): Moss' Heart Disease in Infants, Children and Adolescents. 4th ed. p. 442. Baltimore: Williams & Wilkins, 1989.
263. Sodheimer HM, Freedom RM, Olley PM: Double-outlet right ventricle: clinical spectrum and prognosis. Am J Cardiol 39:709, 1977.
264. Macartney FJ, Rigby ML, Anderson RH, et al: Double-outlet right ventricle: cross-sectional echocardiographic findings, their anatomic explanation and surgical relevance. Br Heart J 52:164, 1984.
265. Sridaromont S, Ritter DG, Feldt RH, et al: Double-outlet right ventricle: anatomic and angiocardiographic correlation. Mayo Clin Proc 53:55, 1978.
266. Kirklin JW, Pacifico AD, Blackstone EH, et al: Current risk and protocols for surgery for double-outlet right ventricle: derivation of an 18 year experience. J Thorac Cardiovasc Surg 92:913, 1986.
267. Kanter K, Anderson R, Lincoln C, et al: Anatomic correction of

double-outlet right ventricle and subpulmonary ventricular septal defect (the Taussig-Bing anomaly). Ann Thorac Surg 41:287, 1986.
268. Fallot A: Contribution a l'anatomie pathologique de la maladie bleue (cyanose cardiaque). Marseille Med 25:418, 1888.
269. Abraham KA, Cherian G, Rao BD, et al: Tetralogy of Fallot in adults: a report on 147 patients. Am J Med 66:811, 1979.
270. Bertranou EG, Blackstone EH, Hazelrig JB, et al: Life expectance without surgery in tetralogy of Fallot. Am J Cardiol 42:458, 1978.
271. McGrath LB, et al: Determination of infundibular innervation in end amine receptor content in cyanotic and acyanotic myocardium: relation to clinical events in tetralogy of Fallot. Pediatr Cardiol 12:155, 1991.
272. Baffes TG, Johnson FR, Potts WJ, Gibson S: Anatomic variations in tetralogy of Fallot. Am Heart J 46:657, 1953.
273. Brinton WD, Campbell M: Necropsy in some congenital diseases of the heart, mainly Fallot's tetralogy. Br Heart J 15:335, 1953.
273a. Blalock A, Taussig HB: The surgical treatment of malformations of the heart. JAMA 128:189, 1995.
274. Hu DCK, Seward JB, Puga FJ, et al: Total correction of tetralogy of Fallot at age 40 years or older: long-term follow-up. J Am Coll Cardiol 5:40, 1985.
275. Hughes CF, Lim YC, Cartmill TB, et al: Total intracardiac repair of tetralogy of Fallot in adults. Ann Thorac Surg 43:634, 1987.
276. Zhao H, Miller DC, Reitz BA, Shumway NE: Surgical repair of tetralogy of Fallot: long-term follow-up with particular emphasis on late death and reoperation. J Thorac Cardiovasc Surg 89:204, 1985.
277. Carvalho JS, et al: Exercise capacity after complete repair of tetralogy of Fallot: deleterious effects of residual pulmonary regurgitation. Br Heart J 67:470, 1992.
278. Rosenthal A: Adults with tetralogy of Fallot: repaired yes; cured, no [editorial]. N Engl J Med 329:655, 1993.
279. Murphy JG, Gersh BJ, Mair DD, et al: Long-term outcome in patients undergoing surgical repair of tetralogy of Fallot. N Engl J Med 329:593, 1993.
280. Jefferson K, Simon R, Somerville J: Systemic arterial supply to the lungs and pulmonary atresia and its relation to pulmonary artery development. Br Heart J 34:418, 1972.
281. Benson LN, Laks H, Lois J, et al: Surgical correction of pulmonary atresia and ventricular septal defect with large systemic pulmonary collaterals. Ann Thorac Surg 38:522, 1984.
282. Millikan JS, Puga FJ, Danielson GK, et al: Stage survival repair of pulmonary atresia with ventricular septal defect and hypoplastic confluent pulmonary artery. J Thorac Cardiovasc Surg 91:818, 1986.
283. Kirklin JW, Blackstone EH, Shimazaki Y, et al: Survival, functional status and reoperations after repair of tetralogy of Fallot with pulmonary atresia. J Thorac Cardiovasc Surg 96:102, 1988.
284. Marcelletti C, McGoon DC, Mair DD: The natural history of truncus arteriosus. Circulation 54:108, 1976.
285. Collett RW, Edwards JE: Persistent truncus arteriosus: classification according to anatomic types. Surg Clin North Am 29:1245, 1949.
286. Becker AE, Becker MJ, Edwards JE: Pathology of the semilunar valve and persistent truncus arteriosus. J Thorac Cardiovasc Surg 62:16, 1971.
287. Fuglestad SJ, Danielson GK, Puga FJ, Edwards WD: Surgical pathology of the truncal valve: the study of twelve cases. Am J Cardiovasc Pathol 2:39, 1988.
288. DiDonato RM, Fyfe DA, Puga FJ, et al: 15 year experience with surgical repair of truncus arteriosus. J Thorac Cardiovasc Surg 89:414, 1985.
289. Newfeld HN, Lester RG, Adams P Jr, et al: Aorticopulmonary septal defect. Am J Cardiol 9:12, 1962.
290. Gensen JB, Blount SG: Anomalous pulmonary venous return. Am Heart J 82:387, 1971.
291. Miller G, Pollack BE: Total anomalous pulmonary venous drainage. Am Heart J 49:127, 1955.
292. Child JS, Perloff JK: Natural survival patterns. *In* Perloff JK, Child JS: Congenital Heart Disease in Adults. pp 21–59. Philadelphia: WB Saunders, 1991.
293. Burroughs JT, Edwards JE: Total anomalous pulmonary venous connection. Am Heart J 59:913, 1960.
294. Nakib A, Moller JH, Kanjuh BI, Edwards JE: Anomalies of the pulmonary veins. Am J Cardiol 20:77, 1967.
295. Desnick RJ, Blieden LC, Sharpe HL: Cardiac valvular anomalies in Fabry disease: clinical, morphologic and biochemical studies. Circulation 54:818, 1976.
296. Huang S, Kumar G, Steele HD, Parker JO: Cardiac involvement in pseudoxanthoma elasticum: report of a case. Am Heart J 74:680, 1967.
297. Boyer SH, IV, Chisholm AW, McKusick VA: Cardiac aspect of Friedreich's ataxia. Circulation 25:493, 1962.
297a. Isnard R, Kalotka H, Durr A, et al: Correlation between left ventricular hypertrophy and GAA trinucleotide repeat length in Friedreich's ataxia. Circulation 95:2247, 1997.
298. Church SC: The heart and myotonia atrophica. Arch Intern Med 119:176, 1967.
299. Petkovich NJ, Dunn N, Reed W: Myotonic dystrophy. Myotonia dystrophica with AV dissociation and Stokes-Adams attacks: a case report and review of the literature. Am Heart J 68:391, 1964.
300. Phornphutkul C, Rosenthal A, Nadas AS: Cardiomyopathy in Noonan's syndrome: report of three cases. Br Heart J 35:99, 1973.
301. Carney JA, Gordan H, Carpenter PC: The complex of myxomas, spotty pigmentation and endocrine overactivity. Medicine 4:270, 1985.
302. Bain J: Carney's complex. Mayo Clin Proc 61:508, 1986.
303. Pierpont MEM, Moller JH, Gorlin RJ, Edwards JE: Congenital cardiac pulmonary and vascular malformations in oculoauriculovertebral dysplasia. Pediatr Cardiol 2:297, 1982.
304. Terry PB, White JI Jr, Barth KH, et al: Pulmonary arteriovenous malformations: physiologic observations and results of balloon embolization. N Engl J Med 308:119, 1983.
305. Perry WH: Clinical spectrum of hereditary hemorrhagic telangiectasia (Osler-Weber-Rendu disease). Am J Med 82:989, 1987.
306. Leier CV, Call TD, Fulkerson PK, et al: The spectrum of cardiac defects in the Ehlers-Danlos syndrome types I and III. Ann Intern Med 92:171, 1980.
307. Perloff JK, deLeon AC, O'Doherty D: The cardiomyopathy of progressive muscular dystrophy. Circulation 33:625, 1966.
308. Gross DM, Williams JC, Caprioli IC, et al: Echocardiographic abnormalities in mucopolysaccharide storage diseases. Am J Cardiol 61:117, 1988.
308a. Piovan M, Vallis G, Sanson A, Milani L: Echocardiographic findings in one case of Swyer-James syndrome. Clin Cardiol 14:352, 1991.
309. Teare D: Asymmetrical hypertrophy of the heart in young adults. Br Heart J 20:1, 1958.
310. Maron BJ, Epstein SE: Hypertrophic cardiomyopathy. Recent observations regarding the specificity of three hallmarks of the disease: asymmetric septal hypertrophy, septal disorganization, and systolic anterior motion of the anterior mitral leaflet. Am J Cardiol 45:141, 1980.
311. Abbasi AS, MacAlpin RN, Eber LM, Pearce ML: Echocardiographic diagnosis of idiopathic hypertrophic cardiomyopathy without outflow obstruction. Circulation 46:897, 1972.
312. Henry WL, Clark CE, Epstein SE: Asymmetric septal hypertrophy (ASH): echocardiographic identification of the pathognomonic anatomic abnormality of IHSS. Circulation 47:225, 1973.
313. Shah PM, Adelman AG, Weigel ED, et al: The natural (and unnatural) course of hypertrophic obstructive cardiomyopathy: a multicenter study. Circ Res 34, 35 (suppl II):II179, 1973.
314. Maron BJ, Roberts WC, McAllister HA, et al: Sudden death in young athletes. Circulation 62:218, 1980.
315. McKenna WJ, England D, Doi YL, et al: Arrhythmia in hypertrophic cardiomyopathy. I: influence on prognosis. Br Heart J 46:168, 1981.
316. Maron BJ, Savage DD, Wolfson JK, Epstein SE: Prognostic significance of 24 hour ambulatory electrocardiographic monitoring in patients with hypertrophic cardiomyopathy: a prospective study. Am J Cardiol 48:252, 1981.
317. Madeira HC: The mitral valve in hypertrophic cardiomyopathy: an echocardiographic approach. Postgrad Med J 62:563, 1986.
318. Gardin JM, Dabestani A, Glasgow GA, et al: Echocardiographic and Doppler flow observations in obstructed and unobstructed hypertrophic cardiomyopathy. Am J Cardiol 56:614, 1985.
319. Braunwald E, Lambrew CT, Rockoff SD, et al: Idiopathic hypertrophic subaortic stenosis: description of the disease based upon the analysis of 64 patients. Circulation 29(suppl IV):1, 1964.
320. Brigden W: Hypertrophic cardiomyopathy. Br Heart J 58:299, 1987.
321. Hopf R, Kaltenbach M: 10-year results and survival of patients with hypertrophic cardiomyopathy treated with calcium antagonists. Z Kardiol 76:137, 1987.
322. Mohr R, Shaff HB, Danielson GK, et al: The outcome of surgical

treatment of hypertrophic obstructive cardiomyopathy: experience over 15 years. J Thorac Cardiovasc Surg 97:666, 1989.
323. Spirito T, Chiarella F, Carratino L, et al: Clinical course and prognosis of hypertrophic cardiomyopathy in an outpatient population. N Engl J Med 320:749, 1989.
324. Cannon RO, Shenke WH, Maron BJ, et al: Differences in coronary flow and myocardial metabolism at rest and during pacing between patients with obstructive and nonobstructive hypertrophic cardiomyopathy. J Am Coll Cardiol 10:53, 1987.
325. Leachman RD, Krajcer Z, Azic T, Cooley DA: Mitral valve replacement in hypertrophic cardiomyopathy: 10-year follow-up of 54 patients. Am J Cardiol 60:1416, 1987.
326. Jean Renaud X, Goy JJ, Kappenberger L: The effects of dual-chamber pacing in hypertrophic obstructive cardiomyopathy. Lancet 339:1318, 1992.
326a. Uhl HS: A previously undescribed congenital malformation of the heart: almost total absence of the myocardium of the right ventricle. Bull Johns Hopkins Hosp 91:197, 1972.
326b. Marcus FI: Right ventricular dysplasia: a report of 24 adult cases. Circulation 65:384, 1982.
326c. Tada H, Aihara N, Ohe T, et al: Arrhythmogenic right ventricular cardiomyopathy underlies the syndrome of right bundle branch block, ST-segment elevation and sudden death. Am J Cardiol 81:519, 1998.
326d. Guiraudon GM, Klein GJ, Gulamhusein SS, et al: Total disconnection of the right ventricular free wall: surgical treatment of right ventricular tachycardia associated with right ventricular dysplasia. Circulation 67:463, 1983.
327. Roberts WC: Major anomalies of coronary artery origin seen in adulthood. Am Heart J 111:941, 1986.
328. Kragel AH, Roberts WC: Anomalous origin of either the right or left main coronary artery from the aorta. The subsequent coursing between aorta and pulmonary trunk. Analysis of 32 necropsy cases. Am J Cardiol 62:771, 1988.
329. Faruqui AMA, Malloy WC, Felner JM, et al: Symptomatic myocardial bridging of coronary artery. Am J Cardiol 41:1305, 1978.
330. Levin DC, Fellows KE, Abrams HL: Hemodynamically significant primary anomalies of the coronary arteries: angiographic aspects. Circulation 58:25, 1978.
330a. Sherwood MC, Rockenmacher S, Colan SD, Geva T: Prognostic significance of clinically silent coronary artery fistulas: Am J Cardiol 83:407, 1999.
331. Wilson CL, Dlabal PW, Holeyfield RW, et al: anomalous origin of left coronary artery from pulmonary artery: case reports and review of literature concerning teenagers and adults. J Thorac Cardiovasc Surg 73:887, 1977.
332. Gobel FL, Anderson DF, Baltaxe HA, et al: Shunts between the coronary and pulmonary arteries with normal origin of the coronary arteries. Am J Cardiol 25:655, 1970.
332a. Agirbasli M, Martin GS, Stout JB, et al: Myocardial bridge as a cause of thrombus formation and myocardial infarction in a young athlete. Clin Cardiol 20:1032,1997.
333. Botefeu JM, Moret PR, Hahn C, Hauf E: Aneurysms of the sinus of Valsalva: report of 7 cases and review of the literature. Am J Med 65:18, 1983.
334. Mayer ED, Ruffman K, Saggau W, et al: Ruptured aneurysms of the sinus of Valsalva. Ann Thorac Surg 42:81, 1986.
334a. McCue CM, Mantakas ME, Tingelstad JB, Ruddy S: Congenital heart block in newborns of mothers with connective tissue disease. Circulation 56:82, 1977.
334b. Ramsey-Goldman R, Horn D, Deng JS, et al: Anti-SS-A antibodies and fetal outcome in maternal systemic lupus erythematosus. Arthritis Rheum 29:1269, 1986.
334c. Michaëlsson M, Jonzon A, Riesenfeld T: Isolated congenital complete atrioventricular block in adult life: a prospective study. Circulation 92:442, 1995.
334d. Kertesz NJ, Fenrich AL, Friedman RA: Congenital complete atrioventricular block. Tex Heart Inst J 24:301, 1997.
334e. Lev M: Pathogenesis of congenital atrioventricular block. Prog Cardiovasc Dis 15:145, 1972.
335. Ueland K: Maternal cardiovascular dynamics. VII: intrapartum blood volume changes. Am J Obstet Gynecol 126:171, 1976.
336. Robson SC, Hunter S, Boys RJ, et al: Serial study of factors influencing changes in cardiac output during pregnancy. Am J Physiol 256:H1060, 1989.
337. Kjelbsen J: Hemodynamic investigations during labor and delivery. Acta Obstet Gynecol Scand Suppl 89:20, 1979.
338. Ueland K, Hansen JM: Maternal cardiovascular dynamics. III: labor and delivery under local caudal analgesia. Am J Obstet Gynecol 103:8, 1969.
339. Whittemore R, Hobbins JC, Engle MA: Pregnancy and its outcome in women with and without surgical treatment of congenital heart disease. Am J Cardiol 50:641, 1982.
340. Elkayam U, Cobb T, Gleicher N: Congenital heart disease in pregnancy. *In* Elkayam U, Gleicher N (eds): Cardiac Problems in Pregnancy. 2nd ed. New York: Alan R Liss, 1990.
341. Sareli P, England MJ, Berk HR, et al: Maternal and fetal sequelae of anticoagulation during pregnancy in patients with mechanical heart valve prosthesis. Am J Cardiol 63:1462, 1989.
342. Wang RYC, Li PK, Chow JSF, et al: Efficacy of low-dose subcutaneously administered heparin in the treatment of pregnant women with artificial heart valves. Med J Aust 2:126, 1983.
343. Mitani GM, Harrison EC, Steinberg I, et al: Digitalis, glycosides in pregnancy. *In* Elkayam U, Gleicher N (eds): Cardiac Problems in Pregnancy. 2nd ed. pp. 417–646. New York: Alan R Liss, 1990.
344. Ellsworth AJ, Horn JR, Raisys VA, et al: Disopyramide and *N*-monodesalkyodisopyramide in serum and breast milk. Drug Intell Clin Pharm 23:56, 1989.
345. Dicke JM: Cardiovascular drugs in pregnancy. *In* Gleicher N, Elkayam U, Galbraith RM, et al (eds): Principles of Medical Therapy in Pregnancy. p. 646. New York: Plenum, 1985.
346. Lee W, Shah PK, Amin DK, et al: Hemodynamic monitoring of cardiac patients during pregnancy. *In* Elkayam U, Gleicher N (eds): Cardiac Problems in Pregnancy: Diagnosis and Management of Maternal and Fetal Disease. 2nd ed. p. 47. New York: Alan R Liss, 1990.
347. Rosenberg B, Simonberg K, Peretz BA, et al: Eisenmenger's syndrome in pregnancy: controlled segmental epidural block for cesarean section. Reg Anaesth 7:131, 1984.
348. Angel JL, Chapman C, Knappeo RA, et al: Percutaneous balloon aortic valvuloplasty in pregnancy. Obstet Gynecol 72:438, 1988.
349. Gleicher N, Midwall J, Hochberger B, et al: Eisenmenger's syndrome in pregnancy. Obstet Gynecol Surv 34:721, 1979.

CHAPTER 9

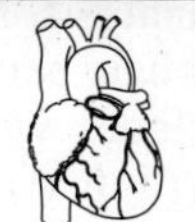

ECHOCARDIOGRAPHY

David S. Bach

ANOMALIES OF VENOUS RETURN
ABNORMALITIES OF THE ATRIAL SEPTUM
Atrial Septal Defect
Flow and Shunt Quantitation
Patent Foramen Ovale
ABNORMALITIES OF VENTRICULAR INFLOW
Cor Triatriatum
Mitral Stenosis
Ebstein's Anomaly
DEFECTS OF THE VENTRICULAR SEPTUM
Ventricular Septal Defect
Tetralogy of Fallot
Endocardial Cushion Defect
OBSTRUCTION OF LEFT VENTRICULAR OUTFLOW
Subvalvular and Supravalvular Aortic Stenosis
Bicuspid Aortic Valve and Valvular Aortic Stenosis
Coarctation of the Aorta
OBSTRUCTION OF RIGHT VENTRICULAR OUTFLOW
ABNORMALITIES OF THE GREAT ARTERIES
Transposition and Corrected Transposition of the Great Arteries
Patent Ductus Arteriosus
ABNORMALITIES OF THE PROXIMAL AORTA
Anomalous Coronary Arteries
Sinus of Valsalva Aneurysm
INTRAUTERINE ECHOCARDIOGRAPHY
GENERAL ECHOCARDIOGRAPHIC APPROACH TO COMPLEX CONGENITAL HEART DISEASE

Two-dimensional (2-D) echocardiographic imaging with accompanying Doppler evaluation has led to dramatic changes in the diagnosis and management of congenital heart disease. The adult cardiologist encounters four categories of patients with congenital heart disease. First is the patient with known congenital heart disease that has not been previously corrected because the abnormality has only minor hemodynamic consequences and is without significant symptoms. A second group consists of patients with congenital heart disease that is known but inoperable at the time of presentation. A third category includes patients with known congenital heart disease who have previously undergone either a corrective or a palliative surgical procedure. With the advances made in cardiac surgical therapy, more patients in this category survive to adulthood. A fourth group includes adults first presenting with congenital heart disease.

The spectrum of congenital heart disease that is first diagnosed in the adult population differs significantly from that in the pediatric population. Because these patients have survived to adulthood without diagnosis, their congenital defects are necessarily less hemodynamically overwhelming and the physical findings are less prominent. Lesions such as ventricular septal defect (VSD), which are usually recognized in the pediatric population, have prominent associated physical findings and are readily diagnosed long before a patient reaches adulthood. In contradistinction, atrial septal defects (ASDs), which are hemodynamically well tolerated and have associated subtle and nonspecific physical findings, are commonly not diagnosed until adulthood. Adult patients first presenting with congenital heart disease may exhibit symptoms of congestive heart failure or signs of progressive cyanosis. Initial presentation may be with a complication secondary to the congenital defect, such as stroke or peripheral embolic event due to paradoxical embolization in the setting of an underlying anatomic abnormality. Finally, a congenital abnormality may be diagnosed as a purely incidental finding during cardiac evaluation for unrelated purposes.

2-D echocardiography, because of its excellent spatial resolution, definition of cardiac anatomy and function, widespread availability, and noninvasive nature, has gained a pivotal role in the diagnosis, follow-up, and management of patients with congenital heart disease. Although of historical interest, M-mode echocardiography plays a very limited role at present in the detection and management of congenital heart disease. The use of transesophageal echocardiography (TEE) adds an additional level of accuracy to echocardiographic imaging in congenital heart disease. By eliminating constraints in imaging windows and limitations in ultrasound penetration and image resolution, TEE allows direct visualization of abnormalities that are less reliably detected on transthoracic imaging. Doppler analysis with spectral and color-flow imaging allows functional assessment of anatomic defects, including the ability to quantify the severity of obstructing lesions, valvular regurgitation, and shunts. In addition, echocardiography has become an integral part of the intraoperative assessment of surgical repair, reconstruction, and conduit placement, and it provides a noninvasive means of following patients who have undergone surgical procedures for congenital heart disease.

This section discusses congenital cardiac lesions encountered in the adult, with emphasis given to those that are more commonly seen in this population. Abnormalities are described from proximal to distal cardiac anatomy, beginning with venous return to the heart, through the atria and ventricles, to ventricular outflow and the great arteries. The discussion concentrates on current echocardiographic modalities for detection and management of congenital heart disease, emphasizing 2-D transthoracic and transesophageal imaging and spectral and color-flow Doppler analysis. M-mode echocardiographic findings are presented when pertinent or of historical interest. The section concludes with a brief discussion of the general echocardiographic approach to patients with complex congenital heart disease.

ANOMALIES OF VENOUS RETURN

Two anomalies of systemic venous return may be encountered in the adult population. Most common is persistence of the left superior vena cava. The left superior vena cava is a venous structure that drains blood from the left upper extremity, most often in a persistent connection to the coronary sinus, and subsequently to the right atrium (RA). Flow through the coronary sinus is increased and the coronary sinus is markedly dilated, which is readily detectable on echocardiographic imaging. Because there is no admixture of venous and arterial circulations, patients remain asymptomatic with this condition. Persistence of a left superior vena cava is usually detected as an incidental finding on echocardiography.

The coronary sinus, located within the atrioventricular (AV) groove, may be directly visualized on transesophageal imaging as it enters the RA near the inferior aspect of the tricuspid annulus. On transthoracic imaging, the coronary sinus is visualized in the parasternal long-axis view and is often detected only when it is enlarged. In this view, the coronary sinus is seen as a clear space located posterior to the mitral valve and within the AV groove. When enlarged, it appears as a distinct circular structure on 2-D scanning. It may be pulsatile and appears to share a thin, common wall with the posterior left atrium (LA). Although echocardiographically detected enlargement of the coronary sinus has been associated with persistence of the left superior vena cava,[1, 2] peripheral venous contrast echocardiographic techniques are invaluable for definitive diagnosis.[3, 4] After injection of peripheral venous contrast material, the normal pattern of echocardiographic contrast enhancement is appearance of contrast medium first in the RA, followed by the right ventricle (RV), and then the pulmonary artery. This pattern is preserved in patients with persistence of the left superior vena cava after venous contrast medium injections from the right arm. However, contrast medium injections from the left arm result in initial opacification of the dilated coronary sinus, followed by appearance of contrast in the RA and RV. An example of this is seen in Figure 9–1. In Figure 9–1A, the dilated coronary sinus is seen immediately posterior to the posterior mitral annulus in this parasternal long-axis view. Figure 9–1B shows the same parasternal long-axis view after peripheral venous injection of agitated saline solution via the left arm. Contrast material is visualized within the dilated coronary sinus. A persistent left-sided superior vena cava has also been described draining to the LA,[4] with an accompanying right-to-left shunt and hypoxia.

A second and rare anomaly of systemic venous return is drainage of the right superior vena cava to the LA.[5, 6] This anomaly is associated with hypoxia secondary to admixture of systemic and pulmonary venous blood at the level of the LA. Again, a diagnosis can be made with contrast echocardiography. Venous injections of contrast medium from either upper extremity result in opacification of the LA followed by the left ventricle (LV), with no contrast medium appearing in the right-sided chambers. Lower extremity venous contrast medium injections, or injections into the inferior vena cava at catheterization, result in opacification of the RA and RV, with no contrast medium seen in the left-sided chambers.

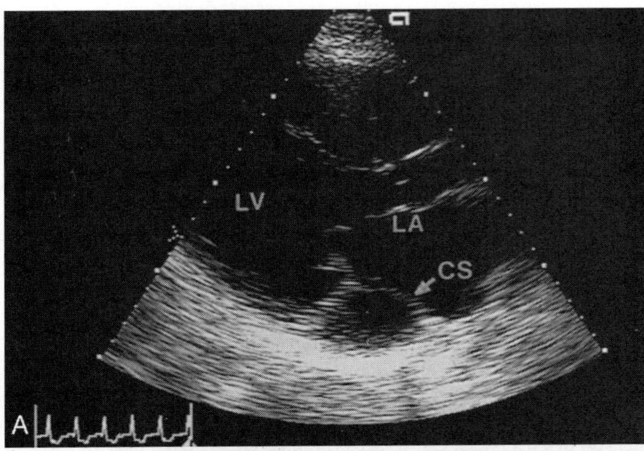

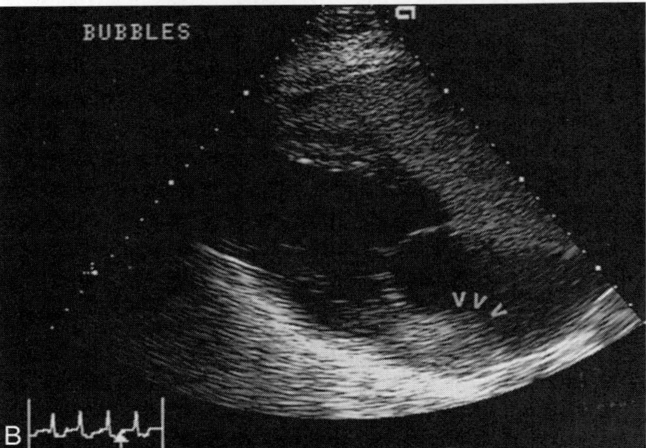

FIGURE 9–1 Parasternal long-axis echocardiograms in persistent left superior vena cava. **A,** A markedly dilated coronary sinus (CS) is demonstrated, located in the posterior atrioventricular groove between the left atrium (LA) and the left ventricle (LV). **B,** Peripheral venous contrast medium injection from the left arm results in opacification of the coronary sinus *(arrowheads).*

Anomalies of pulmonary venous return may be complete or partial. Total anomalous pulmonary venous return is always associated with an ASD, which provides a conduit for blood flow to the systemic arterial circulation and presents during the neonatal period. Partial anomalous venous return may present in the adult patient, usually in conjunction with a sinus venosus–type ASD. Partial anomalous venous return is not reliably visualized directly on transthoracic echocardiographic studies, but detection with transthoracic echocardiography after contrast medium injections in the pulmonary veins or LA at cardiac catheterization has been described.[7] Of note, direct imaging of the four pulmonary veins and their respective atrial connections can be reliably performed using TEE. Direct visualization of the pulmonary veins using TEE makes this the diagnostic method of choice among patients in whom there is suspicion of anomalous pulmonary venous return.

Abnormalities of the Atrial Septum

Atrial Septal Defect

After bicuspid aortic valve, ASD is the second most common congenital abnormality in the adult population. With relatively nonspecific physical findings and hemodynamics that are well tolerated, ASD is the only congenital heart defect with an associated shunt for which diagnosis is routinely made in an adult population. Described by anatomic location, the most common type is the secundum defect, making up approximately 70 percent of ASDs. This defect involves communication of the LA and RA through the foramen ovale and is due to the absence or incomplete formation of the membranous portion of the interatrial septum. Sinus venosus defects involving the basal portion of the interatrial septum account for approximately 15 percent of ASDs. The remaining 15 percent involve the primum portion of the septum, located near the AV junction and the fibrous skeleton of the heart. Primum-type ASDs may be associated with other abnormalities of the midline AV junction, including VSD and cleft anterior mitral valve leaflet, which may be seen together in an endocardial cushion defect.

The identification of echoes attributable to the interatrial septum on early M-mode echocardiography was followed by recognition of the absence of these echoes in patients with ASD and the ability to diagnose ASDs using echocardiography. To a great extent, however, the early echocardiographic diagnosis of ASD relied on the detection of an enlarged RV and accompanying abnormalities in interventricular septal motion.[8–11] On M-mode echocardiography, brisk anterior motion of the interventricular septum is noted at the onset of systole, followed by normal systolic thickening. Exaggeration of the early diastolic posterior ventricular septal motion is also noted and has been correlated with the magnitude of the interatrial shunt.[11] 2-D echocardiographic imaging in the parasternal short-axis view subsequently revealed a diastolic flattening of the interventricular septum in the presence of ASD, with restoration of the normal curvature concave to the LV during systole.[12] This pattern of right ventricular volume overload is not specific to ASD, as it can also be seen in the setting of anomalous pulmonary venous return to the RA or with significant tricuspid regurgitation. The pattern reflects diastolic flattening of the interventricular septum due to increased right ventricular volumes and elevation of the right relative to the left ventricular diastolic pressures. In systole, when the left ventricular pressure again exceeds that of the RV, there is restoration of the normal curvature of the interventricular septum. An example of a right ventricular volume overload pattern in diastole and systole is shown in Figure 9–2.

The pattern of right ventricular volume overload can be differentiated from that of right ventricular pressure overload.[13] In pulmonary hypertension, the interventricular septum assumes a flattened contour in both diastole and systole. The magnitude of perturbation of septal geometry in systole, from a diminished degree of septal concavity toward the LV, to septal flattening, and finally, to assumption of a convex geometry in systole, has been correlated with the magnitude of right ventricular systolic pressures and the severity of pulmonary hypertension.[13–15]

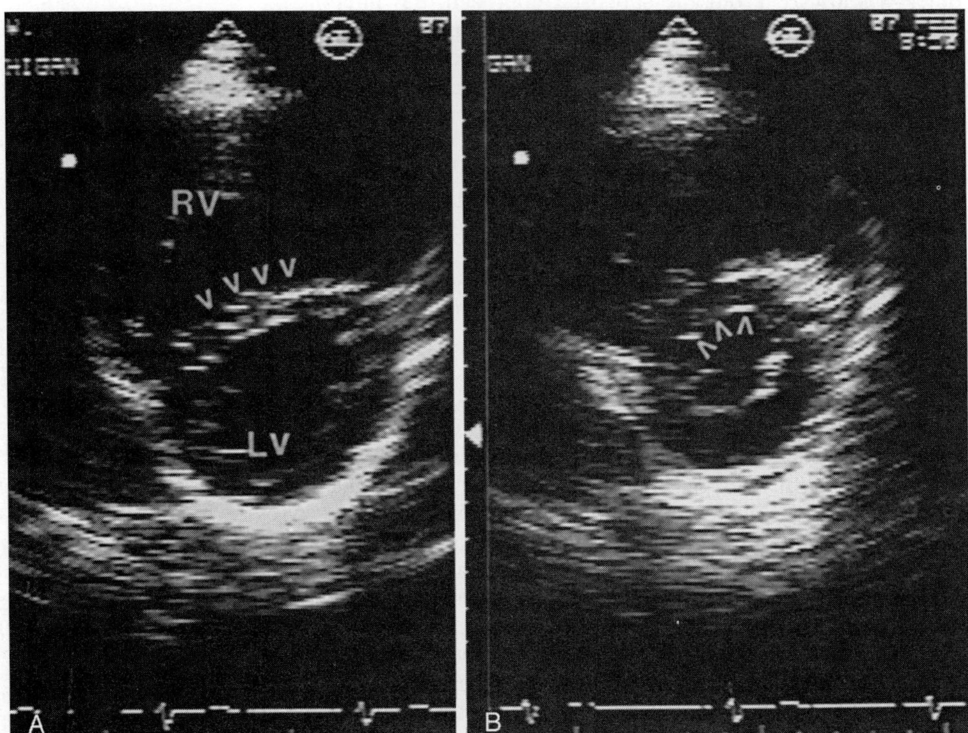

Figure 9–2 Right ventricular volume overload pattern is demonstrated in a parasternal short-axis echocardiogram. **A,** In diastole, the right ventricle (RV) is dilated and there is flattening of the interventricular septum *(arrowheads)*. LV, left ventricle. **B,** In systole, the normal curvature of the interventricular septum *(arrowheads)* is restored.

2-D cross-sectional echocardiography makes direct visualization of the interatrial septum more reliable and therefore adds to the diagnostic capability of echocardiography for ASD. The normal interatrial septum is visualized as a linear echo density extending posteromedially from the aortic root, and a dropout of echoes within this region is associated with an ASD. The use of echo dropout as a diagnostic criterion for ASD is complicated by the normal loss in intensity of the reflected ultrasound signal over distance, the posterior location of the interatrial septum, and in the case of secundum-type defects, the normally thin and difficult to visualize membrane forming the interatrial septum in this location. Whereas dropout of echoes within the primum portion of the interatrial septum has excellent specificity for the presence of an ASD, echo dropout within the secundum portion is less powerful in its ability to differentiate from normal.[16] The pattern of echo dropout is useful in the differentiation of secundum-type ASD from normal. From the apical transducer position, the normal pattern of echo dropout is a direct function of signal attenuation with increasing distance. An apparent tapering and disappearance of echoes within the secundum portion of the interatrial septum is common and is not specific for an ASD. In contrast, an abrupt dropout of echoes with accompanying bright side-lobe artifacts at the level of echo dropout, referred to as a *T sign* for its appearance similar to an inverted letter T, is more specific for ASD.

Albeit with less accuracy, venosus-type ASDs can be detected with transthoracic echocardiography.[17–19] Because of the posterior location of the venosus portion of the interatrial septum and its distance from the transducer, the same phenomenon of distance-related signal attenuation makes detection of this type of ASD less reliable than other forms.[17, 18] For detection of all types of ASDs, a subcostal transducer position appears to be superior to other windows.[17] From the subcostal approach, the interatrial septum can be interrogated with the ultrasound beam perpendicular to the length of the septum, which resolves the distance-related phenomenon of signal attenuation with artifactual echo dropout. An example of a secundum-type ASD visualized from the subcostal approach is shown in Plate 9–1.

Given the technical limitations in direct visualization of defects of the interatrial septum, other modalities have been employed in conjunction with echocardiography to increase diagnostic accuracy. Peripheral venous injections of echocardiographic contrast agents have been utilized extensively for detection of intracardiac shunts.[20–22] The first descriptions of contrast medium injections for detection of ASDs relied exclusively on the detection of right-to-left shunts, with appearance of contrast material within the left-sided cardiac chambers after peripheral venous injections.[22–25] Even in the presence of normal pulmonary arterial pressures and a predominant left-to-right shunt on oximetry, right-to-left crossover of contrast material is detected echocardiographically in a majority of patients.[25] The use of the Valsalva maneuver during contrast medium injections, with a transient rise in right-sided intracardiac pressures, further increases sensitivity. In addition, the detection of contrast medium in the inferior vena cava after upper extremity peripheral venous injections has been reported to be sensitive and specific for the detection of ASDs in patients with a predominant left-to-right shunt.[26] The presence of a left-to-right shunt through an ASD can also be detected by a pattern of "negative contrast" in the RA during peripheral venous contrast medium injections.[27] This pattern indicates an echo-free area within the RA, adjacent to the interatrial septum, where unopacified blood crosses from the LA and displaces opacified blood within the RA.

Of note is that the finding of a right-to-left shunt on intravenous contrast medium injection is not specific for the presence of ASD. Small degrees of right-to-left shunting may persist after surgical repair of an ASD.[28] In addition, the incidence of right-to-left shunting demonstrated by intravenous contrast medium injections during the Valsalva maneuver in a normal population has been estimated at approximately 18 percent.[29] The mechanism for this is presumably a functionally patent foramen ovale, which will be addressed later.

The greatest technical limitations to direct echocardiographic visualization of ASDs are related to the posterior location of the interatrial septum, the distance of the septum from extrathoracic echocardiographic windows, and the distance-associated attenuation of the ultrasound beam. Without exception, these technical limitations can be overcome by the use of transesophageal imaging. Because of the juxtaposition of the esophagus to the LA, interrogation of the interatrial septum and direct visualization of ASDs is routinely feasible using TEE.[30–33] For direct visualization of the interatrial septum, TEE is superior to transthoracic echocardiography.[31–33] Direct visualization provides important information regarding location of a defect within the interatrial septum, size of the defect, and any associated cardiac abnormalities. The diagnostic superiority of TEE is most pronounced for sinus venosus–type defects, which are

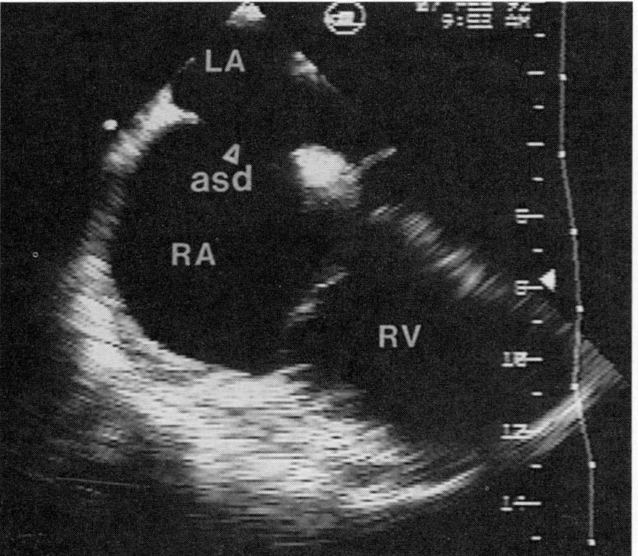

FIGURE 9–3 Transesophageal echocardiogram of secundum-type atrial septal defect (asd). The atrial septal defect is clearly visualized within the membranous portion of the interatrial septum, with drop-out of echoes between the left atrium (LA) and the right atrium (RA). Transesophageal echocardiography is superior to transthoracic imaging for direct visualization of atrial septal defects. RV, right ventricle.

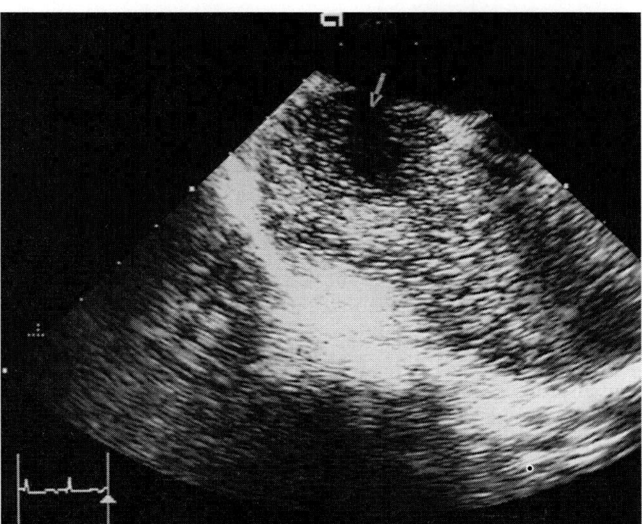

FIGURE 9–4 Transesophageal echocardiogram of atrial septal defect after peripheral venous contrast medium injection. The right atrium and right ventricle are opacified, with an area of "negative contrast" *(arrow)* in the right atrium. The negative contrast is caused by unopacified blood entering the right atrium across the atrial septal defect and is indicative of a left-to-right shunt.

very difficult to visualize via a transthoracic approach. In addition, small defects and multiple defects are more reliably visualized with TEE, as are anomalous pulmonary venous connections in sinus venosus–type defects. Although transthoracic echocardiography is helpful as a screening tool for ASD, transesophageal imaging should be considered in adults with suspected ASD in order to further characterize defect size and location, as well as in patients with clinical suspicion of ASD and a nondiagnostic transthoracic echocardiogram. Figure 9–3 depicts a large secundum-type ASD from the transesophageal approach. Imaging after peripheral venous contrast medium injection, depicted in Figure 9–4, demonstrates complete opacification of the RA with a negative contrast jet detected adjacent to the interatrial septum, consistent with a predominant left-to-right shunt.

Spectral pulsed-wave and color-flow Doppler imaging can be used in conjunction with echocardiographic imaging for detection of ASDs, for assessment of the predominant direction of shunt flow, and for quantification of shunt flow. Color-flow Doppler imaging of secundum-type ASDs is shown in Plate 9–1 from a transthoracic subcostal view and in Plate 9–2 with transesophageal imaging. In both cases, color-flow Doppler demonstrates a predominant left-to-right shunt.

Flow and Shunt Quantitation

Quantification of flow with echo Doppler is based on the principle that flow (Q) can be estimated as a product of area, flow velocity, and heart rate (HR), with flow velocity defined as either the velocity-time integral (VTI) or the product of mean velocity of flow and the duration of flow:

$$Q\ [\text{cm}^3/\text{min}] = \text{area}\ [\text{cm}^2] \times \text{mean velocity}\ [\text{cm/s}] \times \text{flow duration}\ [\text{s}] \times \text{HR}\ [\text{min}^{-1}]$$

or

$$Q\ [\text{cm}^3/\text{min}] = \text{area}\ [\text{cm}^2] \times \text{VTI}\ [\text{cm}] \times \text{HR}\ [\text{min}^{-1}]$$

Noninvasive quantification of right-sided (Q_P) and left-sided (Q_S) cardiac output, indirectly reflecting the magnitude of shunt flow, has been estimated using echo Doppler techniques, with good correlation with invasive methods. For estimation of cardiac output, area is calculated from echocardiographic measurements of diameter and is used in conjunction with Doppler measurements of flow in either the right ventricular outflow tract (RVOT) and the left ventricular outflow tract (LVOT)[34, 35] or in the proximal pulmonary artery and aorta.[36] Shunt flow can then be calculated from the difference between right-sided and left-sided cardiac outputs. Alternatively, shunt flow across an ASD can be directly estimated using the same principles. The diameter of an ASD can be measured by direct echocardiographic visualization,[33] or color-flow Doppler can be used to estimate the effective orifice diameter by measuring the maximal width of the color jet crossing the septum.[18, 31] Estimation of absolute shunt flow can then be made based on the defect diameter, Doppler-derived velocity at the defect, and heart rate.

An alternative technique for noninvasive estimation of shunt flow utilizes the principles of flow quantitation based on radius and velocity at a color Doppler flow convergent zone proximal to the ASD.[37] The principles of a color Doppler proximal isovelocity flow convergence zone take advantage of the aliasing of color Doppler signals as blood accelerates to pass through a restrictive orifice. With the known Nyquist limit of the color spectrum and the measured distance from the restrictive orifice to the zone of color aliasing, shunt volume can be estimated directly by making assumptions with respect to the three-dimensional shape of the flow convergence zone.

The accurate detection of ASDs with echocardiography has been established, and routine cardiac catheterization need not precede surgical repair, in uncomplicated cases.[38, 39] The most reliable method for echocardiographic diagnosis of ASD is by direct visualization utilizing TEE. Without direct visualization of a defect, demonstration of a significant shunt at the atrial level either by peripheral venous contrast medium injection or with Doppler, accompanied by demonstration of right ventricular enlargement and a right ventricular volume overload pattern of interventricular septal motion, is also reliable. Innovative methods for percutaneous closure of ASDs have made direct visualization of even greater importance. Echocardiographic imaging is ideal for the evaluation of defects before attempted percutaneous closure[40] and to help position the percutaneously delivered occluder device. In the assessment of the suitability of ASDs for percutaneous closure, the integrity of surrounding septal tissue must be considered, as well as the size and location of the defect.

Patent Foramen Ovale

In the fetal circulation, right-to-left shunting of blood occurs through the foramen ovale, permitting oxygenated blood to reach the systemic circulation. After birth, the foramen ovale is normally closed by a membrane that constitutes the secundum portion of the interatrial septum. Failure of the membranous division of the LA and RA results in a secundum-type ASD, as discussed previously. A patent foramen ovale results when a small communication remains between the atria owing to incomplete fusion of the membrane to the surrounding muscular interatrial septum. A patent foramen ovale need not have an associated shunt, as the pressure difference between atria usually serves to complete the functional division of the atria. With left atrial pressures normally greater than those in the RA, the membrane is forced against the muscular interatrial septum and right-to-left flow through the foramen ovale is prevented. Increases in right heart pressures resulting from right heart pathology, or transient increases associated with the Valsalva maneuver, may result in right-to-left shunting through a patent foramen ovale. From a clinical standpoint, a patent foramen ovale is of importance only as a potential conduit for paradoxical embolization or for its differentiation from a true ASD with shunt.

Because of its small size, a patent foramen ovale cannot usually be diagnosed echocardiographically by direct visualization, although an abnormal motion of the valve of the foramen ovale has been described on both M-mode and 2-D imaging.[41] Instead, detection of a patent foramen ovale relies on the demonstration of a small magnitude shunt at the atrial level, either at rest or provocable with respiratory maneuvers. As previously noted, a right-to-left shunt on contrast echocardiography has been described in a healthy population[29] as well as in patients with surgically proven absence of ASD.[42] Such small magnitude shunts are usually due to a functionally patent foramen ovale, which is most reliably detected with echocardiography in conjunction with peripheral venous contrast medium injections. Transient increases in right-sided intracardiac pressures using the Valsalva maneuver during contrast medium injection further increase the diagnostic sensitivity for the detection of patent foramen ovale.[29, 43] Conversely, any left-sided heart disease resulting in elevation of left atrial pressure will lessen shunting and may be associated with diminished sensitivity for the detection of patent foramen ovale.[44] It should be noted that the presence of pulmonary arterial-venous malformations permit the appearance of intravenous contrast medium in the LA in the absence of an atrial level shunt. A delay of at least five cardiac cycles between initial contrast opacification of the RA and subsequent appearance of contrast material in the LA should suggest the presence of an extracardiac shunt such as a pulmonary arterial-venous malformation.

Because of the proximity of the transducer position to the LA, TEE with peripheral venous contrast medium injection is highly sensitive for the detection of patent foramen ovale.[45–47] However, the use of intravenous contrast material and transesophageal imaging may result in the detection of extremely small right-to-left shunts that are of unclear clinical significance. The presence of a patent foramen ovale has been implicated as a potentially important risk factor for cerebroembolic events, presumably mediated by paradoxical embolization. This is supported by a greater incidence of echocardiographically detected patent foramen ovale in patients who have suffered a cerebrovascular event than in control subjects.[48] TEE has a sensitivity for detection of the patent foramen ovale superior to that of transthoracic 2-D echocardiography in patients undergoing evaluation for a possible cardiac etiology of embolic stroke,[49–51] in whom the incidence of echocardiographically detected patent foramen ovale has been estimated to be as high as 40 percent.[48] However, although the finding of a probe-patent foramen ovale on surgical or necropsy inspection requires a communication of at least 1 to 2 mm, the size of agitated microbubbles may range as small as 10 μm. Because transesophageal imaging may allow detection of a single microbubble crossing the interatrial septum, caution should be used in the extrapolation of clinical significance for any detectable shunt.[52]

Abnormalities of Ventricular Inflow

Congenital abnormalities of ventricular inflow include defects that cause obstruction of venous return and abnormalities of the AV valves. Obstruction of ventricular inflow may be present at the level of venous return to the atria, within the body of the atria, or at the level of the AV valves. Valvular abnormalities include stenosis of the mitral valve, hypoplasia or atresia of the mitral valve, and Ebstein's anomaly of the tricuspid valve.

Obstruction of venous return to the atria is uncommon. It presents during the neonatal period with signs of peripheral or pulmonary venous congestion. Obstruction of flow within the body of the LA or RA may be due to cor triatriatum or to the presence of a supravalvular membrane, and is discussed later. Valvular obstruction may be due to valvular mitral stenosis, also discussed later, or to the presence of a subvalvular ring. Atresia of the mitral or tricuspid valve is associated with an obligatory ASD that provides an egress for blood from the affected atrium. Similarly, hypoplasia of the mitral valve is associated with other significant cardiac defects, usually as part of the hypoplastic left heart syndrome. All of these abnormalities usually present during the neonatal period and are extremely uncommon in the adult population. Because of its ability to reliably define the anatomy of the atria and AV valves, echocardiography is probably the imaging modality of choice for diagnosis of abnormalities of ventricular inflow and is particularly useful to define the level of obstruction.

Cor Triatriatum

Cor triatriatum is a rare congenital abnormality that causes obstruction of left ventricular filling by a membrane dividing the LA into two chambers. In cor triatriatum sinistrum, a restrictive membrane in the LA impairs filling of the LV. Although usually presenting early in life, cor triatriatum sinistrum may first present in adulthood.[53–55] On echocardiographic imaging, the membrane can usually be seen coursing inferoposteriorly from the posterior aortic root to the posterior wall of the LA. The LA is divided such that the pulmonary veins are in the proximal chamber and the mitral valve and atrial appendage are included in the distal chamber. The proximal and distal chambers communicate through an incomplete portion of the membrane, usually located in the posterior portion of the membrane.

In patients with cor triatriatum, M-mode echocardiography may be able to demonstrate the presence of an intra-atrial membrane, differentiating this cause of ventricular inflow obstruction from valvular obstruction.[56, 57] However, detection of an intra-atrial membrane with M-mode imaging may be unreliable, and 2-D echocardiography is far more reliable.[58] With 2-D imaging, the membrane of cor triatriatum appears in the parasternal long-axis view as an echo-dense structure within the LA, inserting anteriorly at the level of the posterior portion of the aortic root and extending to the posterior portion of the LA wall.[57, 59] In apical views, the membrane is usually parallel to the plane of the mitral annulus. The incomplete portion of the membrane that allows passage of blood between the proximal and the distal atrial chambers is usually located inferoposteriorly and may be visualized. Although the membrane may have several smaller fenestrations within its body, direct visualization of these is usually not possible with standard echocardiographic imaging. Differentiation of the membrane of cor triatriatum from a supravalvular ring is less reliably accomplished with 2-D echocardiography,[58] although a supravalvular ring can be distinguished by its insertion closer to the mitral annulus than the membrane of cor triatriatum.

Because of the proximity of the transducer to the LA, TEE has significant advantages over transthoracic imaging for direct visualization of the membrane of cor triatriatum.[54, 60] On TEE imaging, a membrane within the LA is clearly visualized, with its insertion on the interatrial septum at the level of the fossa ovalis. On the lateral wall of the LA, the membrane inserts such that the atrial appendage is included in the low-pressure chamber distal to the pulmonary veins, thus allowing differentiation from a supravalvular ring.

Doppler analysis provides localization of the level of obstruction within the LA. Turbulence of flow may be seen on color-flow Doppler,[60] and pulsed-wave and continuous-wave Doppler are useful for localization and quantification of the severity of obstruction to ventricular inflow.[61]

Obstruction of flow within the RA has been described on 2-D echocardiography[62, 63] and is termed *cor triatriatum dexter.* Usually not a true membrane, the obstruction to filling in cor triatriatum dexter results from a failure of normal regression of the eustachian valve.

Mitral Stenosis

The echocardiographic differentiation of congenital mitral stenosis from cor triatriatum and supravalvular ring relies on the abnormal valve motion in mitral stenosis and the absence of additional intra-atrial echoes that are associated with a membrane or ring.[58, 64] On M-mode echocardiography, the features of congenital mitral stenosis are similar to those seen in acquired valvular stenosis of the mitral valve. This includes a reduction in the mitral E-to-F slope, diastolic flutter of the mitral leaflets, and a paradoxical anterior motion of the posterior mitral valve leaflet during diastole.[64, 65] On 2-D echocardiography, there is doming of the mitral leaflets in diastole, with restricted motion of the leaflet tips.[66, 67] Differentiation of congenital mitral stenosis from rheumatic disease in an adult relies on visualization of chordal insertions into abnormal papillary muscles, with one of two anatomic types of papillary muscle deformity associated with congenital mitral stenosis. In the "parachute" variety, all of the chordae insert into a single large papillary muscle, whereas in the "arcade" type, the chordae insert into multiple small papillary muscles.

Ebstein's Anomaly

Ebstein's anomaly is an abnormality of the tricuspid valve with the hallmark of apical displacement of the septal tricuspid leaflet. The anterior tricuspid leaflet is elongated and to a variable degree is tethered along its length by chordae inserting into the right ventricular wall. Apical displacement of tricuspid leaflet coaptation results in atrialization of part of the anatomic RV. The right-sided chambers are therefore divided into an anatomic RA, an atrialized portion of the RV, and an abnormally small but functional RV. The functional abnormalities associated with Ebstein's anomaly include the presence of tricuspid regurgitation and a decrease in the functional capacity of the RV. Although presentation may occur later in life, Ebstein's anomaly usually presents in infancy or childhood, and prognosis is related to the size of the functional RV. Because the course of the disease may be benign, many patients survive to adulthood with this abnormality.

M-mode echocardiography in Ebstein's anomaly reveals simultaneous visualization of the mitral and tricuspid leaflets from a single parasternal transducer position.[68–70] In addition, there is a delay of variable degree in the closure of the tricuspid compared with the mitral valve.[71] However, delayed tricuspid closure is not specific for Ebstein's anomaly and may be found in other diseases associated with right heart volume overload, including ASD or severe tricuspid regurgitation. Although a delay in excess of 65 ms has been used as a threshold for the diagnosis of Ebstein's anomaly, the precise delay between mitral and tricuspid valve closure exhibits significant individual variability as a result of differences in transducer position and normal changes with respiration.[72]

The anatomic abnormalities associated with Ebstein's anomaly can be directly visualized on 2-D echocardiography.[73–75] In addition, the degree of apical displacement of the septal tricuspid leaflet, the morphology and degree of tethering of the elongated anterior leaflet, and the size of the functional RV can be quantified.[76–78] Figure 9–5 shows an apical four-chamber view of a patient with Ebstein's anomaly. The septal tricuspid valve leaflet is apically displaced and coapts with an elongated anterior leaflet within the body of the anatomic RV. Plate 9–3 shows tricuspid regurgitation on color-flow Doppler. Note the origin of the regurgitant jet well within the body of the anatomic RV, correlating with the apical displacement of the septal tricuspid leaflet.

The tricuspid valve normally inserts slightly more apically than the mitral valve, and some degree of apical displacement of the tricuspid valve may occur in any form of right heart disease associated with right atrial enlarge-

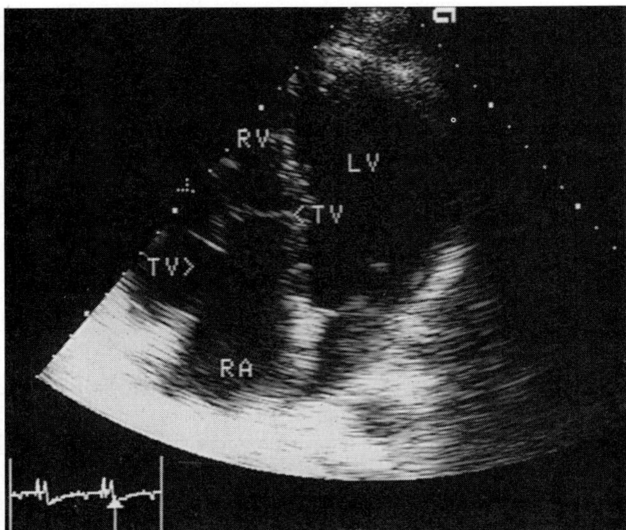

FIGURE 9–5 Apical four-chamber echocardiogram in Ebstein's anomaly of the tricuspid valve. There is apical displacement of the septal leaflet of the tricuspid valve (TV). The right-sided chambers are divided into anatomic right atrium (RA), functional right ventricle (RV), and atrialized right ventricle, which is located between the tricuspid valve leaflets and the tricuspid annulus. LV, left ventricle.

ment. Therefore, attempts have been made to quantify the degree of apical displacement of the tricuspid valve necessary for the diagnosis of Ebstein's anomaly. An absolute tricuspid valve displacement of 20 mm from the mitral insertion can be used for the diagnosis of Ebstein's anomaly in adults.[76] Alternatively, the distance from the mitral valve insertion can be measured and normalized for body surface area, with a value of 8 mm/m^2 accurate for the diagnosis of Ebstein's anomaly.[76] Echocardiographic quantification of the size of the functional RV is an important predictor of prognosis, with a ratio of functional to anatomic RV of less than 35 percent associated with the need for surgical intervention.[78]

Echocardiography is useful for preoperative and intraoperative assessment in the surgical treatment of Ebstein's anomaly. The morphology of the anterior tricuspid leaflet predicts the likelihood of successful valvular reconstruction, with a heavily tethered, restricted anterior leaflet less amenable to reconstruction and more likely to require replacement of the tricuspid valve.[78] Intraoperative TEE has also been used to assess the adequacy of valve reconstruction.[79]

DEFECTS OF THE VENTRICULAR SEPTUM

Ventricular Septal Defect

Defects of the ventricular septum represent the most common form of congenital heart defect in the pediatric population. The prominent associated murmur usually leads to recognition and treatment of VSDs early in infancy and childhood. Adult patients with VSD usually present either with a known restrictive defect that is small and not of hemodynamic importance or having undergone previous surgical repair.

The classification of VSDs is based on the anatomic location of the defect within the ventricular septum. The anatomy of the ventricular septum is usually described as viewed from the right ventricular aspect, owing to the presence of identifying landmarks. The membranous portion of the septum is a small area located at the base of the septum, in continuity with the fibrous support of the aortic valve. Most defects that occur in this area of the septum extend to some degree to involve a portion of the adjacent muscular septum, and therefore are more correctly termed perimembranous than membranous defects. The muscular portion of the interventricular septum is divided into inlet, trabecular, and outlet regions. The inlet region is located in proximity to the right ventricular inflow tract and the tricuspid valve, the outlet portion is in proximity to the RVOT, and the trabecular portion of the muscular septum is between these other two areas. The supracristal region is the most superior portion of the muscular septum, located above the crista supraventricularis. Defects of the muscular portion of the septum are therefore categorized as inlet, trabecular, outlet, or supracristal subarterial or doubly committed defects. The term *Swiss-cheese defect* refers to multiple small defects in the muscular septum.

Both M-mode and 2-D echocardiography have been used for detection and localization of VSDs. Because of its excellent spatial resolution, 2-D imaging is far superior for direct visualization of VSDs.[80–84] As in the detection of ASDs, the finding of dropout of echoes within the septum may not be specific for the presence of a VSD unless the dropout is detected in more than one plane. Views useful for the detection of VSDs include parasternal long-axis and short-axis, apical four-chamber, and subcostal. As in the case of ASDs, the subcostal view is useful for its ability to interrogate a large portion of the septum utilizing the axial resolution of the ultrasound beam.[85] For perimembranous defects, the parasternal views similarly image the affected portion of the septum from a perpendicular axis. From the apical view, the presence of a T sign, as with ASDs, adds specificity to the findings of echo dropout. Factors that limit the direct visualization of VSDs are related to the size and the location of the defect.[86] Perimembranous defects are more reliably visualized than are defects within the muscular septum, and defects within the trabecular portion of the muscular septum are detected less reliably than inlet-type and outlet-type defects. Defects smaller than approximately 2 mm are unreliably visualized directly on echocardiographic imaging.

Doppler interrogation of the RV and ventricular septum adds significant sensitivity to the detection of VSDs.[87–91] Small defects are difficult to visualize echocardiographically but are associated with high-velocity, turbulent left-to-right shunt flow, which is readily detected with color-flow Doppler imaging. Small, restrictive defects are therefore best identified using color-flow Doppler of the RV or RVOT, with the finding of turbulent systolic flow that can be traced back to the interventricular septum. Although pulsed-wave Doppler is sensitive for the detection of VSDs, the ability to detect and localize multiple defects is less reliable than with color-flow Doppler imaging. The presence of pulmonary hypertension may reduce the sensitivity for the detection of VSDs by Doppler analysis.[87] As the systolic pressure gradient between the LV and the RV decreases, shunt through a defect is diminished and turbulent flow is less prominent. In the setting of right ventricular pressures that equal or exceed systemic pressures, such as in Eisenmenger physiology, Doppler sampling of the RV may fail to detect shunt flow through a VSD.

Before the availability of color-flow Doppler imaging, intravenous contrast medium injection was used in conjunction with echocardiographic imaging for detection of shunt flow across a VSD.[20–22, 81, 92] Elevated right ventricular systolic pressure in relationship to left ventricular pressure is associated with a right-to-left shunt detectable on contrast echocardiography, whereas a high pulmonary-to-systemic flow ratio is associated with a "negative contrast" effect in the RV.[81] In addition, various patterns of contrast appearance in the LV have been correlated with defect size and pulmonary resistance.[92] However, peripheral contrast medium injection has a more limited sensitivity for detection of shunt flow at the ventricular than at the atrial level and has effectively been supplanted by the introduction and widespread availability of color-flow Doppler imaging. Plate 9–4 shows a shunt detected with color-flow Doppler through a small muscular VSD. The defect is poorly visualized on routine echocardiographic imaging, but flow is demonstrated within the right ventricular cavity and through the muscular portion of the ventricular septum.

The normal apical displacement of the tricuspid valve relative to the mitral valve is associated with a limited area in which the ventricular septum isolates the LV from the RA. In addition to defects of the ventricular septum with communication between the LV and the RV, defects may occur in this area of the septum and can result in shunting from the LV to the RA. These AV defects tend to be small and are not usually visualized directly by 2-D echocardiography. A low-frequency, high-amplitude systolic flutter of the tricuspid valve can be noted on M-mode and potentially on 2-D echocardiography.[93] Color-flow Doppler imaging demonstrates the high-velocity turbulent flow in the RA. Peripheral venous contrast medium injections may be helpful in this setting with the appearance of contrast material in the LV but not in the LA.[94, 95]

In addition to detection and localization of VSDs, Doppler analysis is useful for quantitation of the pressure gradient between the LV and the RV, thereby differentiating restrictive from nonrestrictive defects.[96–98] Continuous-wave Doppler can be used to quantify the peak velocity of the jet through a VSD, with the gradient derived in the usual manner using the modified Bernoulli equation. Restrictive VSDs are associated with a high jet velocity and nonrestrictive defects with a low jet velocity. In addition, Doppler analysis can be used to provide a noninvasive estimate of the right ventricular systolic pressure by subtracting the peak interventricular pressure gradient from the systolic component of systemic blood pressure. The right ventricular systolic pressure can also be estimated from the peak velocity of tricuspid regurgitation, and the end-diastolic velocity of pulmonic insufficiency can be used to estimate the right ventricular end-diastolic pressure.[84] In the absence of right ventricular outflow obstruction, these estimates of right ventricular systolic pressure correlate well with the pulmonary arterial systolic pressure. A parasternal long-axis view of a perimembranous VSD is shown in Plate 9–5. In this patient, prominent flow is detected in the RV on color-flow Doppler imaging. The restrictive nature of the defect is demonstrated by the high velocity of the left-to-right shunt on continuous-wave Doppler, shown in Figure 9–6. In this example, a peak velocity of approximately 5 m/s predicts a peak interven-

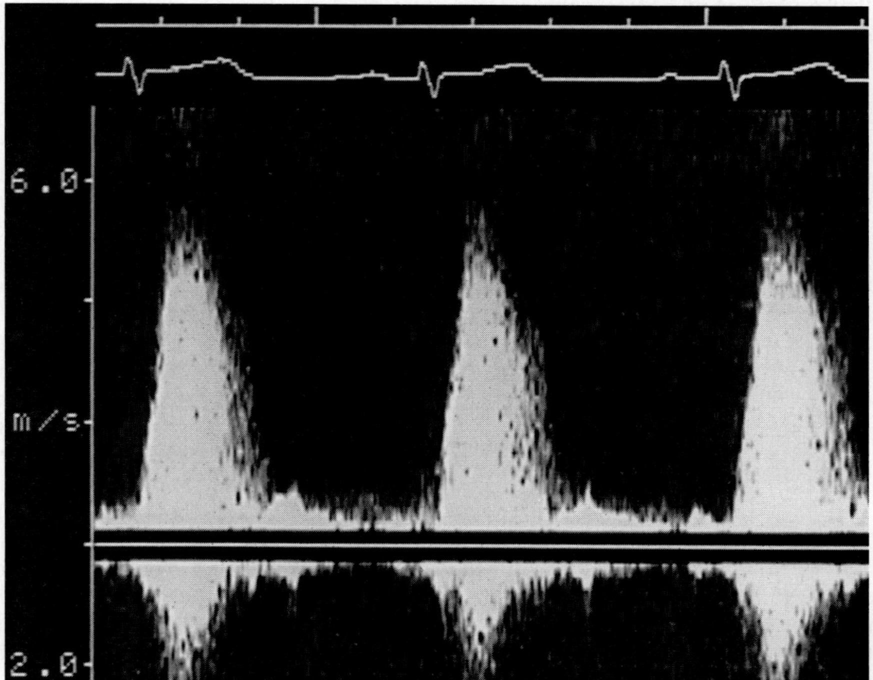

FIGURE 9–6 Continuous-wave Doppler image of flow through the perimembranous ventricular septal defect shown in Plate 1–5. The peak velocity of flow from the left to the right ventricle is approximately 5 m/s, predicting a peak interventricular pressure gradient of approximately 100 mm Hg. The restrictive nature of the ventricular septal defect is demonstrated by the high velocity of flow through the defect.

tricular gradient of approximately 100 mm Hg. A larger perimembranous defect with more prominent shunt flow on color-flow Doppler is shown in Plate 9–6.

As in ASDs, echocardiography and Doppler have been used in VSDs for estimation of shunt flow and of relative flows in the pulmonary and systemic circulations. With M-mode echocardiography, the magnitude of shunt through an isolated VSD has been estimated as a function of the ratio of the size of the LA to that of the aortic root,[99, 100] although correlation with invasively derived measurements of Q_P/Q_S has been poor. As discussed previously for ASDs, estimates of pulmonary and systemic flows can be calculated from the product of mean flows derived by pulsed-wave Doppler and the cross-sectional areas of the aorta and pulmonary artery. Color-flow Doppler imaging has also been used in this situation for noninvasive quantitation of shunt volume across a VSD, utilizing the principles of a proximal flow convergence zone.[101]

Aneurysms of the interventricular septum may develop after spontaneous closure or partial closure of VSDs. Ventricular septal aneurysms are reliably visualized on 2-D echocardiographic imaging from a parasternal window as a mobile echo-dense membrane at the junction of the interventricular septum and the anterior aortic root.[102, 103] In the absence of pulmonary hypertension, the aneurysm bulges into the RVOT during systole. A ventricular septal aneurysm is shown in Plate 9–7. In Plate 9–7A, a small aneurysm is visualized anterior to the membranous portion of the interventricular septum in a parasternal long-axis view. Plate 9–7B demonstrates left-to-right flow on color-flow Doppler through the residual defect.

Echocardiography and Doppler imaging are useful for assessing patients after surgical closure of a VSD. From a functional standpoint, a decrease in left ventricular volume, stroke volume, and mass can be seen postoperatively and ventricular systolic function can be followed.[104] The prosthetic patch can usually be visualized directly as a bright line of echoes along the ventricular septum.[105] A residual shunt may be detected postoperatively,[105] and dehiscence of the patch can be detected as a mobile echo-dense flap moving into the RV during systole.[106] In addition, echocardiography is useful for detection of complications of VSDs. Pulmonary hypertension can be detected and quantified noninvasively with 2-D imaging and Doppler analysis. As a result of compromise of supporting structures associated with a supracristal VSD, prolapse of an aortic valve leaflet may occur and can be visualized echocardiographically.[107, 108] The accompanying aortic insufficiency can be detected and quantified in the usual manner. When infectious endocarditis complicates a VSD, echocardiography is useful for visualization of vegetations involving the right-sided valves or the right ventricular endocardium.[109]

Tetralogy of Fallot

The full cardiac manifestations of tetralogy of Fallot include perimembranous VSD, malposition of the aorta such that it overrides the VSD, a variable degree of obstruction to right ventricular outflow at the valvular or infundibular levels, and right ventricular hypertrophy. Although initial diagnosis is exclusively in infancy, there are an increasing number of patients with tetralogy of Fallot reaching adulthood after palliative or corrective surgery.

The diagnosis of tetralogy of Fallot by M-mode echocardiography relied on the demonstration of an abrupt termination of echoes representing the interventricular septum, with discontinuity of the ventricular septal and anterior aortic root echoes corresponding to the overriding aorta.[110, 111] 2-D echocardiography allows direct visualization of the cardiac defects associated with tetralogy of Fallot and permits assessment of the degree of aortic overriding, RVOT narrowing, and pulmonary stenosis.[112–115] 2-D echocardiography has been shown to have excellent sensitivity for detection of VSDs and for direct visualization of the pulmonary valve and overriding aorta in patients with tetralogy of Fallot.[114] In addition, the severity of infundibular narrowing assessed by 2-D echocardiography has good correlation with angiographic findings. The parasternal long-axis view allows visualization of the size of the VSD. Short-axis views with successive superior angulation allow visualization of the RVOT, pulmonary valve, and main pulmonary artery. Tetralogy of Fallot can be differentiated echocardiographically from other forms of congenital heart disease that involve malposition of the great vessels by the demonstration of preserved continuity between the anterior mitral valve annulus and the posterior aortic root.[112, 113, 115] 2-D echocardiographic imaging also provides a sensitive means for detection of associated abnormalities in patients with tetralogy of Fallot, including congenital absence of the pulmonary valve[116] and abnormalities of the proximal coronary arteries.[117]

Echocardiography and Doppler imaging are useful in the postoperative management of patients after palliative or corrective surgery. Before surgical intervention, flow in the pulmonary circulation in tetralogy of Fallot is diminished by right ventricular outflow obstruction. Echocardiographically, the diminished pulmonary flow is reflected by a small LA, with a ratio of aortic root to left atrial size significantly lower than normal. After palliative surgery for tetralogy of Fallot with a Blalock-Taussig shunt, the increased flow in the pulmonary circulation is reflected by an increase in the ratio of left atrial to aortic root dimensions.[118] The patency of a Blalock-Taussig shunt can be directly assessed by pulsed-wave Doppler,[119] with shunt patency reflected by continuous turbulent flow in the pulmonary artery. In the setting of a patent Blalock-Taussig shunt, flow can be traced back to the shunt, differentiating this from the flow associated with a patent ductus arteriosus.

After corrective surgery for tetralogy of Fallot, the prosthetic patch can be directly visualized and dehiscence detected as in isolated VSD. During the weeks after surgery, the diastolic dimension of the RV decreases and the dimension of the LV increases with maintenance of normal left ventricular systolic function.[120] The abnormal septal motion visualized preoperatively owing to combined volume and pressure overload of the RV is corrected in approximately half of patients after surgery. Echocardiographic assessment of relative right and left ventricular sizes 1 year postoperatively can be used to reflect right ventricular pressures and the degree of residual shunt.[121]

Echocardiographic imaging in adults late after corrective surgery reveals the prosthetic patch closing the VSD and some degree of anterior displacement of the aortic root reflecting its position overriding the interventricular septum. The RVOT can be interrogated for evidence of residual right ventricular outflow obstruction and for pulmonic insufficiency. Right ventricular outflow obstruction may reflect valvular, subvalvular, or supravalvular stenosis. 2-D imaging with pulsed-wave Doppler can usually localize the site of obstruction, and transesophageal imaging may provide additional anatomic information.

Endocardial Cushion Defect

Also termed AV canal defects, endocardial cushion defects are complex congenital abnormalities that involve the midline structures of the AV junction. Cardiac abnormalities include primum-type ASD, perimembranous VSD, cleft anterior mitral valve leaflet, and abnormalities of the septal tricuspid leaflet. The diagnosis of endocardial cushion defect on M-mode echocardiography relies on the detection of discontinuity between the anterior mitral valve leaflet and the interatrial septum,[122] but demonstration of the full spectrum of the defect with M-mode echocardiography is unusual. 2-D echocardiographic imaging provides a reliable means for direct visualization of the cardiac abnormalities present. Atrial and VSDs can be directly visualized, as can the mitral and tricuspid valve abnormalities.[123] In addition, the relative sizes of the RV and the LV can be assessed. An example of the AV defect present in a patient with an endocardial cushion defect is shown in Figure 9–7. In this apical four-chamber view, communication between the left-sided and the right-sided chambers can be seen at both the atrial and the ventricular levels. The accompanying cleft anterior leaflet of the mitral valve is best appreciated in the parasternal short-axis view.

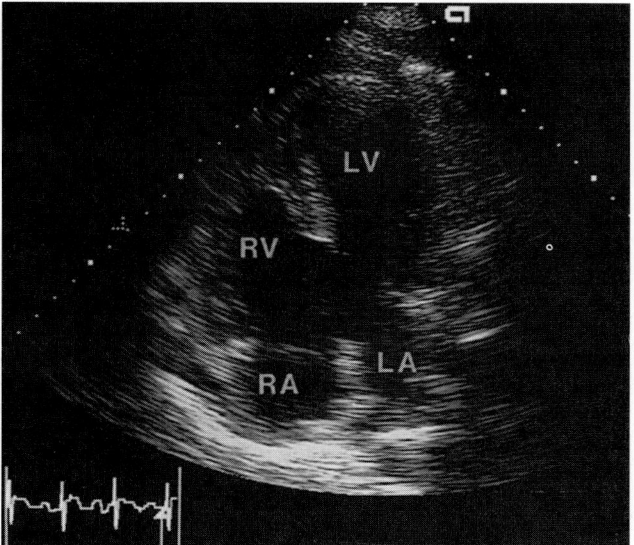

FIGURE 9–7 Apical four-chamber echocardiogram of endocardial cushion defect. Communication between the left and the right chambers is demonstrated at both the atrial and the ventricular levels, with primum-type atrial septal defect and perimembranous ventricular septal defect. LA, left atrium; LV, left ventricle; RA, right atrium; RV, right ventricle.

Obstruction of Left Ventricular Outflow

Obstruction of left ventricular outflow can occur at several anatomic levels, involving abnormalities below, at, or above the level of the aortic valve. Subvalvular aortic stenosis can be caused by the presence of a discrete membrane or fibromuscular ridge in the LVOT or by a longer area of outflow tract narrowing in tunnel subaortic stenosis. When hemodynamically significant, discrete subaortic stenosis is diagnosed in infancy by the presence of a prominent accompanying murmur. Obstruction at the level of the aortic valve may occur in association with a unicuspid or bicuspid valve. Bicuspid aortic valve is the single most common congenital heart abnormality observed in the adult population. A congenitally abnormal aortic valve may not be hemodynamically significant in childhood. However, because the severity of obstruction or insufficiency tends to increase over time owing to progressive valvular sclerosis, calcification, or infection, an initial diagnosis in adulthood is not uncommon. Supravalvular aortic stenosis is a less common congenital cause of left ventricular outflow obstruction and is characterized by an hourglass-shaped narrowing of the ascending aorta, usually in association with other developmental abnormalities including mental retardation and characteristic "elfin" facies. 2-D echocardiographic imaging[124, 125] and pulsed-wave Doppler[126] are highly sensitive for localization of the level of left ventricular outflow obstruction. The severity of outflow obstruction can be estimated with continuous-wave Doppler.[126–128]

Subvalvular and Supravalvular Aortic Stenosis

Discrete subaortic stenosis has been described on M-mode echocardiography and can be differentiated from valvular aortic stenosis by visualization of LVOT narrowing and characteristic coarse flutter of the aortic valve.[129] 2-D echocardiography allows direct visualization of subvalvular anatomy and the extent of outflow tract narrowing.[130–134] Use of multiple imaging planes allows direct visualization and characterization of membranous, fibromuscular, and tunnel obstruction of the outflow tract. Although echocardiographic imaging does not afford reliable quantification of the severity of obstruction,[134] accurate estimation of pressure gradients is possible with Doppler analysis.[126, 127] The impact of the turbulent jet on the aortic valve leads to a high incidence of significant aortic regurgitation among patients with untreated subvalvular obstruction. Patients having undergone percutaneous[135] or surgical intervention[130, 136] are subject to restenosis and aortic insufficiency, which can be evaluated with echocardiographic imaging.

In supravalvular aortic stenosis, direct visualization at the level of stenosis is usually possible with 2-D echocardiographic imaging.[137] In addition to anatomic location, the diameter of obstruction and the extent of the lesion can be assessed.

Bicuspid Aortic Valve and Valvular Aortic Stenosis

The M-mode echocardiographic diagnosis of bicuspid aortic valve and congenital aortic stenosis relied on the demonstration of abnormal leaflet thickness, multiple diastolic cusp lines, and eccentric leaflet closure.[138] These findings, however, are neither sensitive nor specific for the detection of congenital aortic stenosis,[139] with abnormal leaflet eccentricity seen in only 29 percent of patients with aortic stenosis and in up to 20 percent of normal patients. 2-D echocardiographic imaging is superior for detection of bicuspid aortic valve.[140] In the parasternal long-axis view, bicuspid aortic valve can be distinguished from a normal valve by restricted leaflet mobility during systole and from calcific aortic stenosis by the characteristic pattern of leaflet doming. Figure 9–8 shows a parasternal long-axis view of a bicuspid aortic valve, with restricted leaflet excursion and systolic doming. In the short axis, the presence of a bicuspid valve can be confirmed by direct visualization of leaflet anatomy. Leaflet orientation, usually either anterior-posterior with a horizontal commissure or left-right with a vertical commissure, can also be established. Adequate visualization of valve anatomy for the diagnosis of bicuspid aortic valve is possible in a majority of adults,[141] although it is more difficult in smokers.[142] A short-axis view of a bicuspid aortic valve is shown in Figure 9–9. This example from a transesophageal window demonstrates asymmetry of the valve cusps with a discrete area of focal thickening.

As in other forms of aortic stenosis,[128] Doppler analysis allows noninvasive quantification of transvalvular gradients in congenital aortic stenosis.[126, 127] In addition, aortic valve area can be accurately estimated.[143] Echocardiography with Doppler provides an accurate noninvasive means of following patients with congenital aortic stenosis and bicuspid aortic valve both before and after surgical intervention.[144, 145]

Coarctation of the Aorta

Coarctation of the aorta involves a discrete shelflike narrowing of the descending thoracic aorta immediately distal to the left subclavian artery. 2-D echocardiography allows direct visualization of aortic coarctation in almost all pediatric patients,[146–148] although complete visualization of the aorta in adults may be more difficult because of limitations in imaging from the suprasternal window. The severity of obstruction can be estimated by the orifice diameter if visualized, although quantitation of obstruction is more accurately estimated by continuous-wave Doppler from the suprasternal notch. The descending thoracic aorta and aortic coarctation can be reliably visualized on transesophageal imaging.

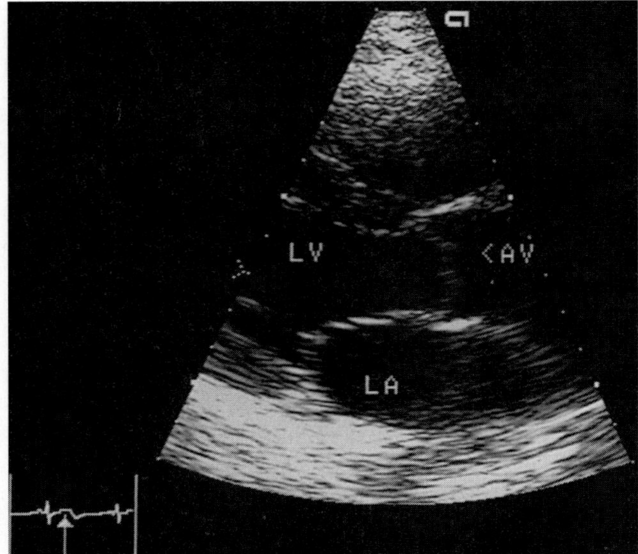

FIGURE 9–8 Parasternal long-axis echocardiogram of bicuspid aortic valve. Characteristic systolic doming of the aortic valve (AV) is noted, caused by restricted excursion of the cusps. LA, left atrium; LV, left ventricle.

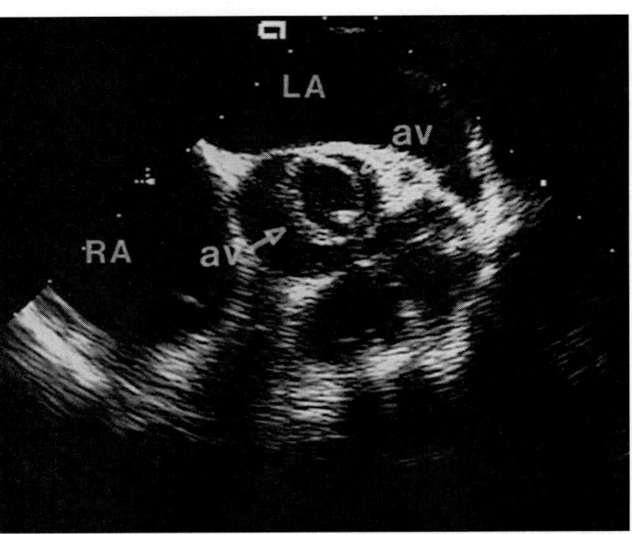

FIGURE 9–9 Transesophageal short-axis view of bicuspid aortic valve. Two discrete aortic valve cusps (av) are identified. There is asymmetry of the cusp sizes and an area of focal thickening involving one cusp. LA, left atrium; RA, right atrium.

OBSTRUCTION OF RIGHT VENTRICULAR OUTFLOW

As in left ventricular outflow obstruction, obstruction of right ventricular outflow may occur below, at, or above the level of the valve. In the subvalvular form, obstruction is caused by infundibular narrowing as the result of hypertrophy of right ventricular muscle bundles. The diagnosis of obstruction within the RVOT by M-mode echocardiography is unreliable, although findings may include coarse systolic flutter and midsystolic closure of the pulmonary valve.[149] 2-D echocardiographic imaging provides a reliable means for direct visualization of the narrowed outflow tract.[150, 151]

Valvular pulmonary stenosis can be reliably detected with 2-D echocardiographic imaging. As in congenital stenosis of the aortic valve, stenosis of the pulmonary valve is distinguished echocardiographically by thickening of the leaflets and by the characteristic pattern of systolic doming.[152] M-mode echocardiography in moderate or severe pulmonary stenosis reveals an increase in depth of the A wave,[153] possibly the result of increased right ventricular end-diastolic pressure and transmission of the force of right atrial contraction. Although the depth of the A wave correlates with the transvalvular pressure gradient, excessive overlap of A wave depth in normal and diseased valves precludes its use in quantification of pulmonary stenosis.[154] The third form of obstruction of right ventricular outflow involves stenosis of the main pulmonary artery or its branches. Echocardiographic imaging usually allows direct visualization of the site of stenosis in the proximal pulmonary artery,[155] but multiple branch stenoses may not be visualized directly.

Quantitation of right ventricular outflow obstruction can be performed with continuous-wave Doppler. Doppler estimates of transvalvular pulmonary flow velocities are easily established owing to the proximity of the RVOT to the parasternal imaging window and because the anterior-posterior orientation of flow allows parallel alignment of the Doppler signal. Using the modified Bernoulli equation for estimation of gradients from peak flow velocities, there is an excellent correlation with invasive techniques of Doppler-derived estimates of both transvalvular gradients[156] and pulmonary valve area.[143] Doppler assessment of the acceleration time of flow through the pulmonary valve may be useful in pulmonary stenosis because it is inversely proportional to the pulmonary artery pressure and allows detection of superimposed pulmonary hypertension.

Continuous-wave Doppler can also be used for quantification of obstruction in infundibular stenosis.[157, 158] By mapping the RVOT, pulsed-wave Doppler is useful in determination of the anatomic level of outflow obstruction. Finally, echocardiographic imaging with accompanying Doppler analysis is useful for determination of right ventricular size and function and of outflow hemodynamics over time in patients treated medically or surgically for obstruction of right ventricular outflow.[159]

Abnormalities of the Great Arteries

Transposition and Corrected Transposition of the Great Arteries

The normal relationship of ventriculoarterial connections is a result of spiral septation. Complete transposition of the great arteries, also referred to as *d*-transposition or dextroloop of the great arteries, reflects ventriculoarterial discordance with reversal of the ventricular origins of the great arteries caused by straight rather than spiral infundibulotruncal septation. In transposition of the great arteries, the origin of the aorta is from the morphologic RV, which receives venous return from the systemic circulation, and the pulmonary artery originates from the morphologic LV, which receives venous return from the pulmonary circulation. Two parallel circuits exist that, without the presence of a concomitant defect permitting shunting of blood between the two circulations, are incompatible with life. The presence of a persistent patent ductus arteriosus, VSD, or ASD is therefore required to sustain life. Corrected transposition or *l*-transposition of the great arteries describes ventriculoarterial discordance in conjunction with AV discordance and malposition of the ventricles. The combination of AV and ventriculoarterial discordance results in normal physiologic blood flow, with the morphologic RV serving in the systemic circulation and the morphologic LV serving in the pulmonary circulation. In the setting of either complete transposition or corrected transposition of the great arteries, the aorta arises from the RV anterior and to the right of the pulmonary artery, rather than in its usual posterior location.

The echocardiographic diagnosis of transposition of the great arteries relies on identification of the morphologic LV and RV and establishment of the identity of the great vessel arising from each. Features useful for identification of the morphologic RV include the coarse trabeculation of the ventricle and its association with a tricommissural AV valve in a relatively apical location, which inserts into multiple irregular papillary muscles.[160] In distinction, the morphologic LV has a fine trabecular pattern and is associated with a bicommissural mitral valve inserting into two discrete papillary muscles. In addition, the mitral valve demonstrates direct fibrous continuity with an associated semilunar valve.

The orientation of the proximal aorta and main pulmonary artery in the normal heart places the aorta posterior and to the right of the main pulmonary artery. Because the great vessels arise from their respective ventricles in a spiral geometry, the long axes of their proximal portions are not in the same plane. Imaging in the parasternal short axis, the proximal ascending aorta is visualized echocardiographically as a circle, with the main pulmonary artery visualized anterior, rightward, and in an oblique long axis. In transposition of the great arteries, the proximal vessels arise with their long axes parallel and located in the same plane. Both arteries are visualized echocardiographically as circular structures when imaged in the parasternal short-axis, located either anterior-posterior or side by side.[161] The great vessels are most reliably distinguished echocardiographically by direct visualization of the proximal bifurcation of the pulmonary artery.[161–163] In transposition of the great arteries, the pulmonary artery arises posterior to the aorta.[112, 113, 161–163]

In the past, the most widely used procedure for surgical treatment of complete transposition of the great arteries was the Mustard operation. In this procedure, the interatrial septum is removed and an intra-atrial baffle is created. The baffle directs blood from the pulmonary veins across the ASD to the morphologic RV and the systemic arterial circulation, and similarly from the systemic venous return to the morphologic LV and the pulmonary arterial circulation. In the first days of life, palliative percutaneous atrial septostomy is performed to allow admixture of blood from the systemic and pulmonary circulations. Echocardiographic imaging is useful for direct visualization of the intra-atrial baffle,[164] for long-term assessment of right ventricular size and function,[165] and for assessment for complications of the Mustard procedure, including superior vena caval obstruction,[164, 166] tricuspid regurgitation, and obstruction within the pulmonary venous atrium.[164] In addition, echocardiographic imaging can be used to assist balloon placement in palliative percutaneous atrial septostomy.[167, 168]

At present, the surgical procedure of choice for treatment of transposition of the great arteries is an anatomically corrective arterial switch operation. Echocardiographic imaging after arterial switch surgery allows direct visualization of the site of the arterial switch and assessment of left and right ventricular function and patency of the coronary ostia.[169] Echocardiographic imaging with Doppler is also useful for long-term assessment of ventricular function and of development of obstruction of ventricular outflow or regurgitant valvular lesions.[170]

Patent Ductus Arteriosus

The ductus arteriosus normally connects the fetal pulmonary and systemic arterial circulations, providing an outlet for oxygenated pulmonary arterial blood to the systemic arterial circulation. The ductus arteriosus is a vascular channel located between the left pulmonary artery immediately after the main pulmonary artery bifurcation and the descending thoracic aorta immediately distal to the left subclavian artery. Normally closing within hours of birth, patency of the ductus arteriosus may persist either as an isolated abnormality or in conjunction with other congenital heart lesions. In neonates, infants, and children, a patent ductus arteriosus can be reliably visualized by 2-D echocardiographic imaging.[171, 172] From the parasternal window, a patent ductus arteriosus is visualized as a continuation of the pulmonary artery to the descending aorta. From the suprasternal window, the ductus arteriosus is demonstrated by a dropout of echoes in the descending aorta, with a short channel to the pulmonary artery. Echocardiographic detection of a patent ductus arteriosus is feasible in adults,[173] although its sensitivity and specificity for detection is not known.

Imaging constraints in adults may preclude direct visualization of a patent ductus arteriosus, and the diagnosis may rest on the demonstration of shunt flow with pulsed-wave and/or color-flow Doppler.[172, 174–176] In an isolated patent ductus arteriosus there is a continuous shunt, with flow directed from the descending aorta to the pulmonary artery. Pulsed-wave Doppler findings in patent ductus arteriosus therefore include disturbance of flow in the pulmonary artery and retrograde diastolic flow in the descending aorta. Aortic and pulmonary insufficiency may also cause disturbances in diastolic flow patterns in the aorta and pulmonary artery, respectively. Doppler criteria for the detection of patent ductus arteriosus are therefore based on detection of diastolic retrograde flow in the descending aorta in the absence of aortic insufficiency, accompanied by diastolic turbulence in the pulmonary artery in the absence of pulmonary insufficiency. The pattern of flow in the pulmonary artery is further influenced by elevations of pulmonary arterial pressures, with abbreviated diastolic flow implying significant pulmonary hypertension. Finally, echocardiography with Doppler is also useful in assessment of percutaneous techniques for closure of patent ductus arteriosus.[177]

ABNORMALITIES OF THE PROXIMAL AORTA

Anomalous Coronary Arteries

Congenital abnormalities of the coronary arteries include anomalous origin or course of one or more coronary arteries and coronary AV fistulas. Either the left or the right coronary artery may originate from the pulmonary artery. Patients with anomalous pulmonary origin of a coronary artery usually present in infancy or childhood with left ventricular dysfunction and congestive heart failure. In such a population, 2-D echocardiographic imaging can reliably demonstrate the anomalous coronary origin by direct visualization both before[178–181] and after[178–182] surgical reimplantation. Pulsed-wave and color-flow Doppler imaging are also useful for detection of anomalous pulmonary origins of either the left or the right coronary artery.[180, 181, 183, 184]

The coronary arteries may originate from an anomalous location in the systemic arterial circulation, including origination from an anomalous sinus of Valsalva or as an abnormal coronary arterial trunk. Because the coronary arteries supply oxygenated blood to the myocardium despite the abnormal origin, such anomalous coronary origins may be clinically unimportant. However, they may present with myocardial ischemia, infarction, or sudden death in the adult population. In an adult population with limitations in imaging of the proximal aortic root, transthoracic 2-D echocardiographic imaging may be useful for detection of anomalous coronary artery origins,[185] although TEE affords significantly greater imaging definition and improved diagnosis.[186–188]

Coronary arterial fistulas have been described using transthoracic[189–191] and transesophageal imaging.[192, 193] Venous connections of coronary arterial fistulas have been described echocardiographically in the RA, LA, coronary sinus, and pulmonary artery.

Sinus of Valsalva Aneurysm

Congenital aneurysms of the sinuses of Valsalva occur as a result of localized weakening of the aortic media. The right coronary sinus is affected most commonly, followed by the noncoronary sinus and, very rarely, the left coronary sinus. Direct visualization of sinus of Valsalva aneurysm by 2-D echocardiographic imaging is possible in a majority of patients. On echocardiographic imaging, the aneurysm appears as a thin-walled structure, usually protruding into the right heart cavities.[194, 195]

Complications resulting from sinus of Valsalva aneurysm are readily detected echocardiographically. Progressive enlargement of an aneurysm may lead to obstruction of the RVOT.[195] Sinus of Valsalva aneurysms originating in the right coronary sinus have been found on echocardiography to dissect into the muscular interventricular septum.[196–198] Aneurysms may rupture, with those originating in the right sinus of Valsalva rupturing into the RV and those originating in the noncoronary sinus into the RA.[194] Rupture of a sinus of Valsalva aneurysm is associated with enlargement of the right heart chambers on echocardiography, diastolic flutter of the tricuspid valve, and premature opening of the pulmonic valve. Peripheral injection of intravenous contrast medium results in a "negative jet" on echocardiographic imaging,[194] as unopacified blood from the proximal aorta enters the contrast-opacified right heart chambers through the ruptured aneurysm. Color-flow Doppler imaging demonstrates turbulent, high-velocity flow detectable in the RA or RV throughout the cardiac cycle and usually allows localization of the jet origin.[199–201] TEE provides additional anatomic information among patients with sinus of Valsalva aneurysm that is not identified on transthoracic imaging[202] and among patients with associated complex cardiac anatomy.[203]

Intrauterine Echocardiography

As the imaging capabilities of ultrasound have improved with advances in technology, 2-D echocardiographic imaging has become an important tool in the cardiac evaluation of the fetus, permitting antenatal diagnosis of congenital diseases. Although satisfactory echocardiographic images of the fetus can be obtained as early as 14 weeks' gestation, diagnostic accuracy is improved with imaging after 18 weeks.[204] The use of pulsed-wave Doppler[205] and color-flow Doppler imaging[206] further add to the utility of fetal cardiac imaging and the detection of cardiac disease in utero.

Fetal echocardiography is useful for detection of cardiac abnormalities in the setting of hydrops fetalis, allowing the diagnosis of hypoplastic left heart syndrome,[204, 207, 208] AV canal, tetralogy of Fallot, pulmonary atresia, intracardiac tumor,[209] and cardiomyopathy.[204] Other congenital cardiac abnormalities diagnosed with intrauterine echocardiography and Doppler include ASD,[206, 210] VSD,[204, 206] coarctation of the aorta,[210] right ventricular hypoplasia,[205] double-outlet RV,[205, 211] Ebstein's anomaly,[204, 212] and endocardial fibroelastosis.[206]

General Echocardiographic Approach to Complex Congenital Heart Disease

The approach to the echocardiographic evaluation of patients with congenital heart disease can differ from that used among most adult patients referred for echocardiography. Most echocardiographic examinations in the adult without congenital heart disease proceed through a set of standard imaging planes that display the cardiac structures for assessment of anatomy and function. Adult patients with isolated congenital heart disease such as ASD or VSD or bicuspid aortic valve can be imaged successfully using standard echocardiographic views. However, among patients with complex congenital heart disease, the cardiac structures used to align the standard imaging planes may be distorted or displaced from their normal positions and relationships. Therefore, among patients with complex congenital heart disease, the identity of cardiac chambers cannot be assumed by their position, and imaging planes must be adapted to existing anatomy.

The echocardiographic examination among patients with complex congenital heart disease requires the identification of cardiac structures and their relationships in addition to the interrogation of their anatomy and function. To accomplish this goal, a systematic approach should be employed. Although the order and details of the examination can vary, it should in general establish the following seven features[213]:

1. Atrial location or situs
2. The number, size, orientation, and identity of ventricles
3. AV connection
4. Great vessel orientation and identity
5. Ventricular connections to the great vessels
6. Presence and direction of intracardiac shunts
7. Presence, location, and severity of outflow obstruction

If the patient has undergone prior palliative surgery, the examination should establish the presence and patency of surgical shunts.

Atrial identity can be established based on the insertion of the inferior vena cava, which almost exclusively returns to the morphologic RA. Ventricular number is determined by the presence or absence of an interventricular septum. Ventricular identity can be established based on either morphologic features of the ventricles or the identity of the associated AV valves. The RV is distinguished by coarse trabeculation and the presence of a muscular moderator band. The tricuspid valve, associated with the morphologic RV, can be distinguished by three leaflets and commissures rather than two associated with the mitral valve, by its insertion apical to that of the mitral valve, and by its association with three rather than two papillary muscles. AV connections are considered *concordant* when the morphologic RA connects to the morphologic RV and the morphologic LA connects to the morphologic LV, and *discordant* when the converse is true.

Identification of the great vessels can be based on their pattern of branching; the pulmonary artery bifurcates, and the aorta forms an arch with multiple branches. However, it is usually possible to assume great vessel identity based on orientation. Normally oriented great vessels cross obliquely as they course away from the LV and RV, and the two vessels are not both seen in the same axis at their origins. In contrast, the great vessels maintain a parallel course at their origins when transposed, and both can be simultaneously imaged in the same axis. When the great vessels cross at their origins, the anterior vessel is always the pulmonary artery and the posterior vessel the aorta. When the great vessels are transposed and one is anterior to the other, the anterior vessel is almost always the aorta and the posterior vessel the pulmonary artery. The relationship of the ventricles to the great vessels can be directly visualized and is defined relative to the plane of the interventricular septum.

Intracardiac shunts, including defects in the interatrial and interventricular septa, have been described previously. Obstruction of left ventricular and right ventricular outflow are quantified in the usual fashion and similarly have been described previously.

References

1. Snider AR, Ports TA, Silverman NH: Venous anomalies of the coronary sinus: detection by M-mode, two-dimensional and contrast echocardiography. Circulation 60:721, 1979.
2. Stewart JA, Fraker TD, Slosky DA, et al: Detection of persistent left superior vena cava by two-dimensional contrast echocardiography. J Clin Ultrasound 7:357, 1979.

3. Hibi N, Fukui Y, Nishimura K, et al: Cross-sectional echocardiographic study of persistent left superior vena cava. Am Heart J 100:69, 1980.
4. Foale R, Bourdillon PD, Somerville J, Rickards A: Anomalous systemic venous return: recognition by two-dimensional echocardiography. Eur Heart J 4:186, 1983.
5. Park HM, Summerer MH, Preuss K, et al: Anomalous drainage of the right superior vena cava into the left atrium. J Am Coll Cardiol 2:358, 1983.
6. King RE, Plotnick GD: Isolated right superior vena cava into the left atrium detected by contrast echocardiography. Am Heart J 122:583, 1991.
7. Danilowicz D, Kronzon I: Use of contrast echocardiography in the diagnosis of partial anomalous pulmonary venous connection. Am J Cardiol 43:248, 1979.
8. Diamond MA, Dillon JC, Haine CL, et al: Echocardiographic features of atrial septal defect. Circulation 153:129, 1971.
9. Meyer RA, Schwartz DC, Benzing G III, Kaplan S: Ventricular septum in right ventricular volume overload. Am J Cardiol 30:349, 1972.
10. Radtke WE, Tajik AJ, Gau GT, et al: Atrial septal defect: echocardiographic observations. Ann Intern Med 84:246, 1976.
11. Chazal RA, Armstrong WF, Dillon JC, Feigenbaum H: Diastolic ventricular septal motion in atrial septal defect: analysis of M-mode echocardiograms in 31 patients. Am J Cardiol 52:1088, 1983.
12. Weyman AE, Wann S, Feigenbaum H, Dillon JC: Mechanism of abnormal septal motion in patients with right ventricular volume overload. A cross-sectional echocardiographic study. Circulation 54:180, 1976.
13. Ryan T, Petrovic O, Dillon JC, et al: An echocardiographic index for separation of right ventricular volume and pressure overload. J Am Coll Cardiol 5:918, 1985.
14. King ME, Braun H, Goldblatt A, et al: Interventricular septal configuration as a predictor of right ventricular systolic hypertension in children: a cross-sectional echocardiographic study. Circulation 68:68, 1983.
15. Shimada R, Takeshita A, Nakamura M: Noninvasive assessment of right ventricular systolic pressure in atrial septal defect: analysis of the end-systolic configuration of the ventricular septum by two-dimensional echocardiography. Am J Cardiol 53:1117, 1984.
16. Dillon JC, Weyman AE, Feigenbaum H, et al: Cross-sectional echocardiographic examination of the interatrial septum. Circulation 55:115, 1977.
17. Shub C, Dimopoulos IN, Seward JB, et al: Sensitivity of two-dimensional echocardiography in the direct visualization of atrial septal defect utilizing the subcostal approach: experience with 154 patients. J Am Coll Cardiol 2:127, 1983.
18. Mehta RH, Helmcke F, Nanda NC, et al: Uses and limitations of transthoracic echocardiography in the assessment of atrial septal defect in the adult. Am J Cardiol 67:288, 1991.
19. Nasser FN, Tajik AJ, Seward JB, Hagler DJ: Diagnosis of sinus venosus atrial septal defect by two-dimensional echocardiography. Mayo Clin Proc 56:568, 1981.
20. Valdes-Cruz LM, Pieroni DR, Roland JMA, Varghese PJ: Echocardiographic detection of intracardiac right-to-left shunts following peripheral vein injections. Circulation 54:558, 1976.
21. Seward JB, Tajik AJ, Hagler DJ, Ritter DG: Peripheral venous contrast echocardiography. Am J Cardiol 39:202, 1977.
22. Serruys PW, Van den Brand M, Hugenholtz PG, Roelandt J: Intracardiac right-to-left shunts demonstrated by two-dimensional echocardiography after peripheral vein injection. Br Heart J 42:429, 1979.
23. Kronik G, Slany J, Moesslacher H: Contrast M-mode echocardiography in diagnosis of atrial septal defect in acyanotic patients. Circulation 59:372, 1979.
24. Fraker TD, Harris PJ, Behar VS, Kisslo JA: Detection and exclusion of interatrial shunts by two-dimensional echocardiography and peripheral venous injection. Circulation 59:379, 1979.
25. Bourdillon PDV, Foale RA, Rickards AF: Identification of atrial septal defects by cross-sectional contrast echocardiography. Br Heart J 44:401, 1980.
26. Gullace G, Savoia MT, Ravizza P, et al: Detection of atrial septal defect with left-to-right shunt by inferior vena cava contrast echocardiography. Br Heart J 47:445, 1982.
27. Weyman AE, Wann LS, Caldwell RL, et al: Negative contrast echocardiography: a new method for detecting left-to-right shunts. Circulation 59:498, 1979.
28. Santoso T, Meltzer RS, Castellanos S, et al: Contrast echocardiographic shunts may persist after atrial septal defect repair. Am Heart J 4:129, 1983.
29. Lynch JJ, Schuchard GH, Gross CM, Wann LS: Prevalence of right to left atrial shunting in a healthy population: detection by Valsalva maneuver contrast echocardiography. Am J Cardiol 53:1478, 1984.
30. Hanrath P, Schluter M, Langenstein BA, et al: Detection of ostium secundum atrial septal defects by transoesophageal cross-sectional echocardiography. Br Heart J 49:350, 1983.
31. Mehta RH, Helmcke F, Nanda NC, et al: Transesophageal Doppler color flow mapping assessment of atrial septal defect. J Am Coll Cardiol 16:1010, 1990.
32. Kronzon I, Tunick PA, Freedberg RS, et al: Transesophageal echocardiography is superior to transthoracic echocardiography in the diagnosis of sinus venosus atrial septal defect. J Am Coll Cardiol 17:537, 1991.
33. Ishii M, Kato H, Inoue O, et al: Biplane transesophageal echo-Doppler studies of atrial septal defects: quantitative evaluation and monitoring for transcatheter closure. Am Heart J 125:1363, 1993.
34. Kitabatake A, Inoue M, Asao M, et al: Noninvasive evaluation of the ratio of pulmonary to systemic flow in atrial septal defect by duplex Doppler echocardiography. Circulation 69:73, 1984.
35. Dittman H, Jacksch R, Voelker W, et al: Accuracy of Doppler echocardiography in quantification of left to right shunts in adult patients with atrial septal defect. J Am Coll Cardiol 2:338, 1988.
36. Valdes-Cruz LM, Horowitz S, Mesel E, et al: A pulsed Doppler echocardiographic method for calculating pulmonary and systemic blood flow in atrial level shunts: validation studies in animals and initial human experience. Circulation 69:80, 1984.
37. Rittoo D, Sutherland GR, Shaw TRD: Quantification of left-to-right atrial shunting and defect size after balloon mitral commissurotomy using biplane transesophageal echocardiography, color flow Doppler mapping, and the principle of proximal flow convergence. Circulation 87:1591, 1993.
38. Shub C, Tajik AJ, Seward JB, et al: Surgical repair of uncomplicated atrial septal defect without "routine" preoperative cardiac catheterization. J Am Coll Cardiol 6:49, 1985.
39. Lipshultz SE, Sanders SP, Mayer JE, et al: Are routine preoperative cardiac catheterization and angiography necessary before repair of ostium primum atrial septal defect? J Am Coll Cardiol 2:373, 1988.
40. Rao PS, Langhough R, Beekman RH, et al: Echocardiographic estimation of balloon-stretched diameter of secundum atrial septal defect for transcatheter occlusion. Am Heart J 124:172, 1992.
41. Kupferschmid C, Lang D: The valve of the foramen ovale in interatrial right-to-left shunt: echocardiographic cineangiocardiographic and hemodynamic observations. Am J Cardiol 51:1489, 1983.
42. Lunde P, Abrahamsen AM: Contrast shunting through a patent foramen ovale in a patient with pulmonary stenosis. Eur J Cardiol 12:129, 1980.
43. Kronik G, Mosslacher H: Positive contrast echocardiography in patients with patent foramen ovale and normal right heart hemodynamics. Am J Cardiol 49:1806, 1982.
44. Siostrzonek P, Lang W, Zangeneh M, et al: Significance of left-sided heart disease for the detection of patent foramen ovale by transesophageal contrast echocardiography. J Am Coll Cardiol 19:1192, 1992.
45. Hausmann D, Mugge A, Becht I, Daniel WG: Diagnosis of patent foramen ovale by transesophageal echocardiography and association with cerebral and peripheral embolic events. Am J Cardiol 70:668, 1992.
46. de Belder MA, Tourikis L, Griffith M, et al: Transesophageal contrast echocardiography and color flow mapping: methods of choice for the detection of shunts at the atrial level? Am Heart J 124:1545, 1992.
47. Stollberger C, Schneider B, Abzieher F, et al: Diagnosis of patent foramen ovale by transesophageal contrast echocardiography. Am J Cardiol 71:604, 1993.
48. Lechat PH, Mas JL, Lascault G, et al: Prevalence of patent foramen ovale in patients with stroke. N Engl J Med 318:1148, 1988.
49. Pearson AC, Labovitz AJ, Tatineni S, Gomez CR: Superiority of transesophageal echocardiography in detecting cardiac source of embolism in patients with cerebral ischemia of uncertain etiology. J Am Coll Cardiol 17:66, 1991.
50. Lee RJ, Bartzokis T, Yeoh TK, et al: Enhanced detection of intracardiac sources of cerebral emboli by transesophageal echocardiography. Stroke 22:734, 1991.

51. Siostrzonek P, Zangeneh M, Gossinger H, et al: Comparison of transesophageal and transthoracic contrast echocardiography for detection of a patent foramen ovale. Am J Cardiol 68:1247, 1991.
52. Homma S, Di Tullio MR, Sacco RL, et al: Characteristics of patent foramen ovale associated with cryptogenic stroke: a biplane transesophageal echocardiographic study. Stroke 25:582, 1994.
53. Lengyl M, Arvay A, Biro V: Two-dimensional echocardiographic diagnosis of cor triatriatum. Am J Cardiol 59:484, 1987.
54. Schlüter M, Langenstein BA, Thier W, et al: Transesophageal two-dimensional echocardiography in the diagnosis of cor triatriatum in the adult. J Am Coll Cardiol 2:1011, 1983.
55. Feld H, Shani J, Rudansky HW, et al: Initial presentation of cor triatriatum in a 55-year-old woman. Am Heart J 124:788, 1992.
56. Canedo MI, Stefadouros MA, Frank MJ, et al: Echocardiographic features of cor triatriatum. Am J Cardiol 40:615, 1977.
57. Östman-Smith I, Silverman NH, Oldershaw P, et al: Cor triatriatum sinistrum. Diagnostic features on cross-sectional echocardiography. Br Heart J 51:211, 1984.
58. Snider RA, Roge CL, Schiller NB, Silverman NH: Congenital left ventricular inflow obstruction evaluated by two-dimensional echocardiography. Circulation 61:848, 1980.
59. Weindorf S, Goldberg H, Goldman M, Reitman M: Diagnosis of cor triatriatum by two-dimensional echocardiography. J Clin Ultrasound 9:97, 1981.
60. Vuocolo LM, Stoddard MF, Longaker RA: Transesophageal two-dimensional and Doppler echocardiographic diagnosis of cor triatriatum in the adult. Am Heart J 124:791, 1992.
61. Radhakrishnan S, Shrivastava S: Doppler echocardiography in the diagnosis of divided left atrium (cor triatriatum sinister). Int J Cardiol 21:180, 1988.
62. Alboliras ET, Edwards WD, Driscoll DJ, Seward JB: Cor triatriatum dexter: two-dimensional echocardiographic diagnosis. J Am Coll Cardiol 9:334, 1987.
63. Burton DA, Chin A, Weinberg PM, Pigott JD: Identification of cor triatriatum dexter by two-dimensional echocardiography. Am J Cardiol 60:409, 1987.
64. Lacorte M, Harada K, Williams RG: Echocardiographic features of congenital left ventricular inflow obstruction. Circulation 54:562, 1976.
65. Driscoll DJ, Gutgesell HP, McNamara DG: Echocardiographic features of congenital mitral stenosis. Am J Cardiol 42:259, 1978.
66. Smallhorn J, Tommasini G, Deanfield J, et al: Congenital mitral stenosis. Anatomical and functional assessment by echocardiography. Br Heart J 45:527, 1981.
67. Grenadier E, Sahn DJ, Valdes-Cruz LM, et al: Two-dimensional echo Doppler study of congenital disorders of the mitral valve. Am Heart J 107:319, 1984.
68. Farooki ZQ, Henry JG, Green EW: Echocardiographic spectrum of Ebstein's anomaly of the tricuspid valve. Circulation 53:63, 1976.
69. Giuliani ER, Fuster V, Brandenburg RO, Mair DD: Ebstein's anomaly. The clinical features and natural history of Ebstein's anomaly of the tricuspid valve. Mayo Clin Proc 54:163, 1979.
70. Daniel W, Rathsack P, Walpurger G, et al: Value of M-mode echocardiography for non-invasive diagnosis of Ebstein's anomaly. Br Heart J 43:38, 1980.
71. Gussenhoven WJ, Spitaels SEC, Bom N, AE Becker: Echocardiographic criteria for Ebstein's anomaly of tricuspid valve. Br Heart J 43:31, 1980.
72. Gussenhoven WJ, Jansen JRC, Bom N, Ligtvoet CM: Variability in the time interval between tricuspid and mitral valve closure in Ebstein's anomaly. J Clin Ultrasound 12:267, 1984.
73. Matsumoto M, Matsuo H, Nagata S, et al: Visualization of Ebstein's anomaly of the tricuspid valve by two-dimensional and standard echocardiography. Circulation 53:69, 1976.
74. Hirschklau MJ, Sahn DJ, Hagan AD, et al: Cross-sectional echocardiographic features of Ebstein's anomaly of the tricuspid valve. Am J Cardiol 40:400, 1977.
75. Kambe I, Ichmiya S, Toguchi M, et al: Cross-sectional echocardiographic study of Ebstein's anomaly using electronic sector scan. J Cardiogr 9:269, 1979.
76. Gussenhoven EJ, Stewart PA, Becker AE, et al: "Offsetting" of the septal tricuspid leaflet in normal hearts and in hearts with Ebstein's anomaly. Am J Cardiol 53:172, 1984.
77. Shiina A, Seward JB, Edwards WD, et al: Two-dimensional echocardiographic spectrum of Ebstein's anomaly: detailed anatomic assessment. J Am Coll Cardiol 3:356, 1984.
78. Shiina A, Seward JB, Tajik A, et al: Two-dimensional echocardiographic-surgical correlation in Ebstein's anomaly: preoperative determination of patients requiring tricuspid valve plication vs replacement. Circulation 68:534, 1983.
79. Quaegebeur JM, Sreeram N, Fraser AG, et al: Surgery for Ebstein's anomaly: the clinical and echocardiographic evaluation of a new technique. J Am Coll Cardiol 17:722, 1991.
80. Meltzer RS, Schwartz J, French J, Popp RL: Ventricular septal defect noted by two-dimensional echocardiography. Chest 76:455, 1979.
81. Funabashi T, Yoshida H, Nakaya S, et al: Echocardiographic visualization of ventricular septal defect in infants and assessment of hemodynamic status using a contrast technique. Comparison of M-mode and two-dimensional imaging. Circulation 64:1025, 1981.
82. Sutherland GR, Godman MJ, Smallhorn JF, et al: Ventricular septal defects. Two dimensional echocardiographic and morphological correlations. Br Heart J 47:316, 1982.
83. Capelli H, Andrade JL, Somerville J: Classification of the site of ventricular septal defect by 2-dimensional echocardiography. Am J Cardiol 51:1474, 1983.
84. Pieroni DR, Nishimura RA, Bierman FZ, et al: Second natural history study of congenital heart defects. Ventricular septal defect: echocardiography. Circulation 87(suppl I):I-80, 1993.
85. Bierman FZ, Fellows K, Williams RG: Prospective identification of ventricular septal defects in infancy using subxiphoid two-dimensional echocardiography. Circulation 62:807, 1980.
86. Canale JM, Sahn DJ, Allen HD, et al: Factors affecting real-time, cross-sectional echocardiographic imaging of perimembranous ventricular septal defects. Circulation 63:689, 1981.
87. Stevenson JG, Kawabori I, Dooley T, Guntheroth WG: Diagnosis of ventricular septal defect by pulsed Doppler echocardiography. Sensitivity, specificity and limitations. Circulation 58:322, 1978.
88. Magherini A, Azzolina G, Wiechmann V, Fantini F: Pulsed Doppler echocardiography for diagnosis of ventricular septal defects. Br Heart J 43:143, 1980.
89. Yokoi K, Kambe T, Ichimiya S, et al: Pulsed Doppler echocardiographic evaluation of the shunt flow in ventricular septal defect. Jpn Heart J 24:175, 1983.
90. Ludomirsky A, Huhta JC, Vick W III, et al: Color Doppler detection of multiple ventricular septal defects. Circulation 74:1317, 1986.
91. Lin SL, Hwang B, Hsieh KS, et al: Efficacy of Doppler color flow mapping in assessing the severity of shunting ventricular septal defect. Am J Card Imaging 2:316, 1988.
92. Serwer GA, Armstrong BE, Anderson PAW, et al: Use of contrast echocardiography for evaluation of right ventricular hemodynamics in the presence of ventricular septal defects. Circulation 58:327, 1978.
93. Grenadier E, Shem-Tov A, Motro M, Palant A: Echocardiographic diagnosis of left ventricular–right atrial communication. Am Heart J 106:407, 1983.
94. Grenadier E, Keidar S, Palant A: Contrast echocardiographic right-to-left flow in left ventricular–to–right atrial shunt. Am Heart J 106:1157, 1983.
95. Shanes JG, Levitsky S, Seyal MS, et al: Diagnosis of left ventricular to right atrial shunt utilizing contrast echocardiography. Am J Cardiol 52:650, 1983.
96. Murphy DJ, Ludomirsky A, Huhta JC: Continuous-wave Doppler in children with ventricular septal defect: noninvasive estimation of interventricular pressure gradient. Am J Cardiol 57:428, 1986.
97. Ge Z, Zhang Y, Kang W, et al: Noninvasive evaluation of interventricular pressure gradient across ventricular septal defect: a simultaneous study of Doppler echocardiography and cardiac catheterization. Am Heart J 124:176, 1992.
98. Ge Z, Zhang Y, Kang W, et al: Noninvasive evaluation of right ventricular and pulmonary artery systolic pressures in patients with ventricular septal defects: simultaneous study of Doppler and catheterization data. Am Heart J 125:1073, 1993.
99. Ahmad M, Hallidie-Smith KA: Assessment of left-to-right shunt and left ventricular function in isolated ventricular septal defect. Echocardiographic study. Br Heart J 41:147, 1979.
100. Fuhrman BP, Epstein ML, Bass JL, Moller JH: Predictive value of the echocardiographic left atrial dimension in isolated ventricular septal defect. J Clin Ultrasound 8:347, 1980.
101. Moises VA, Maciel BC, Hornberger LK, et al: A new method for noninvasive estimation of ventricular septal defect shunt flow by Doppler color flow mapping: imaging of the laminar flow conver-

gence region on the left septal surface. J Am Coll Cardiol 18:824, 1991.
102. Gussenhoven WJ, te Riele JAM, Scherpenzeel W, Roelandt J: Echocardiographic pattern in an aneurysm of the membranous interventricular septum. Chest 77:541, 1980.
103. Canale JM, Sahn DJ, Valdes-Cruz LM, et al: Accuracy of two-dimensional echocardiography in the detection of aneurysms of the ventricular septum. Am Heart J 101:255, 1991.
104. Cordell D, Graham TP, Atwood GF, et al: Left heart volume characteristics following ventricular septal defect closure in infancy. Circulation 54:294, 1976.
105. Andrade JL, Serino W, de Leval M, Somerville J: Two-dimensional echocardiographic assessment of surgically closed ventricular septal defect. Am J Cardiol 52:325, 1983.
106. Mostow N, Riggs T, Borkat G: Echocardiographic features of ventricular septal defect patch dehiscence. Am Heart J 102:941, 1981.
107. Mehta J, Wang Y, Lawrence C, Cohn JN: Aortic regurgitation associated with ventricular septal defect. Echocardiographic and hemodynamic observations. Chest 71:784, 1977.
108. Aziz KU, Cole RB, Paul MH: Echocardiographic features of supracristal ventricular septal defect with prolapsed aortic valve leaflet. Am J Cardiol 43:854, 1979.
109. Agathangelou NE, Dos Santos LA, Lewis BS: Real-time 2-dimensional echocardiographic imaging of right-sided cardiac vegetations in ventricular septal defect. Am J Cardiol 52:420, 1983.
110. Morris DC, Felner JM, Schlant RC, Franch RH: Echocardiographic diagnosis of tetralogy of Fallot. Am J Cardiol 36:908, 1975.
111. Assad-Morell JL, Seward JB, Tajik AJ, et al: Echo-phonocardiographic and contrast studies in conditions associated with systemic arterial trunk overriding the ventricular septum. Truncus arteriosus, tetralogy of Fallot, and pulmonary atresia with ventricular septal defect. Circulation 53:663, 1976.
112. Sahn DJ, Terry R, O'Rourke R, et al: Multiple crystal cross-sectional echocardiography in the diagnosis of cyanotic congenital heart disease. Circulation 50:230, 1974.
113. Henry WL, Maron BJ, Griffith JM: Cross-sectional echocardiography in the diagnosis of congenital heart disease. Identification of the relation of the ventricles and great arteries. Circulation 56:267, 1977.
114. Caldwell RL, Weyman AE, Hurwitz RA, et al: Right ventricular outflow tract assessment by cross-sectional echocardiography in tetralogy of Fallot. Circulation 59:395, 1979.
115. Sanders SP, Bierman FZ, Williams RG: Conotruncal malformations: diagnosis in infancy using subxiphoid 2-dimensional echocardiography. Am J Cardiol 58:1361, 1982.
116. Segni ED, Einzig S, Bass JL, Edwards JE: Congenital absence of pulmonary valve associated with tetralogy of Fallot: diagnosis by 2-dimensional echocardiography. Am J Cardiol 51:1798, 1983.
117. Jureidini SB, Appleton RS, Nouri S: Detection of coronary artery abnormalities in tetralogy of Fallot by two-dimensional echocardiography. J Am Coll Cardiol 14:960, 1989.
118. Reitman M, Goldberg H, Boris G, et al: Echocardiographic assessment of a Blalock-Taussig shunt. J Clin Ultrasound 6:55, 1978.
119. Stevenson JG, Kawabori I, Bailey WW: Noninvasive evaluation of Blalock-Taussig shunts: determination of patency and differentiation from patient ductus arteriosus by Doppler echocardiography. Am Heart J 106:1121, 1983.
120. Oberhänsli I, Friedli B: Echocardiographic study of right and left ventricular dimension and left ventricular function in patients with tetralogy of Fallot before and after surgery. Br Heart J 41:40, 1979.
121. Vick GW III, Serwer GA: Echocardiographic evaluation of the postoperative tetralogy of Fallot patient. Circulation 58:842, 1978.
122. Beppu S, Nimura Y, Nagata S, et al: Diagnosis of endocardial cushion defect with cross-sectional and M-mode scanning echocardiography. Differentiation from secundum atrial septal defect. Br Heart J 38:911, 1976.
123. Hagler DJ, Tajik AJ, Seward JB, et al: Real-time wide-angle sector echocardiography: atrioventricular canal defects. Circulation 59:140, 1979.
124. Weyman AE, Feigenbaum H, Hurwitz RA, et al: Localization of left ventricular outflow obstruction by cross-sectional echocardiography. Am J Med 60:33, 1978.
125. Williams DE, Sahn DJ, Friedman WF: Cross-sectional echocardiographic localization of sites of left ventricular outflow tract obstruction. Am J Cardiol 37:250, 1976.
126. Hatle L: Noninvasive assessment and differentiation of left ventricular outflow obstruction with Doppler ultrasound. Circulation 64:381, 1981.
127. Lima CO, Sahn DJ, Valdes-Cruz LM, et al: Prediction of the severity of left ventricular outflow tract obstruction by quantitative two-dimensional echocardiographic Doppler studies. Circulation 68:348, 1983.
128. Hatle L, Anglelsen BA, Tromsdal A: Non-invasive assessment of aortic stenosis by Doppler ultrasound. Br Heart J 43:284, 1980.
129. Krueger SK, French JW, Forker AD, et al: Echocardiography in discrete subaortic stenosis. Circulation; 59:506, 1979.
130. Weyman AE, Feigenbaum H, Hurwitz RA, et al: Cross-sectional echocardiography in evaluating patients with discrete subaortic stenosis. Am J Cardiol 37:358, 1976.
131. Ten Cate FJ, Van Dorp WG, Hugenholtz PG, Roelandt J: Fixed subaortic stenosis. Value of echocardiography for diagnosis and differentiation between various types. Br Heart J 41:159, 1979.
132. Wilcox WD, Seward JB, Hagler DJ, et al: Discrete subaortic stenosis. Two-dimensional echocardiographic features with angiographic and surgical correlation. Mayo Clin Proc 55:425, 1980.
133. DiSessa TG, Hagan AD, Isabel-Jones JB, et al: Two-dimensional echocardiographic evaluation of discrete subaortic stenosis from the apical long axis view. Am Heart J 101:774, 1981.
134. Motro M, Schneeweiss A, Shem-Tov A, et al: Two-dimensional echocardiography in discrete subaortic stenosis. Am J Cardiol 53:896, 1984.
135. Shrivastava S, Dev V, Bahl VK, Saxena A: Echocardiographic determinants of outcome after percutaneous transluminal balloon dilatation of discrete subaortic stenosis. Am Heart J 122:1323, 1991.
136. Frommelt MA, Snider AR, Bove EL, Lupinetti FM: Echocardiographic assessment of subvalvular aortic stenosis before and after operation. J Am Coll Cardiol 19:1018, 1992.
137. Weyman AE, Caldwell RL, Hurwitz RA, et al: Cross-sectional echocardiographic characterization of aortic obstruction. 1. Supravalvular stenosis and aortic hypoplasia. Circulation 57:491, 1978.
138. Radford DJ, Bloom KR, Izukawa T, et al: Echocardiographic assessment of bicuspid aortic valves: angiographic and pathological correlates. Circulation 53:80, 1976.
139. Kececioglu-Draelos Z, Goldberg SJ: Role of M-mode echocardiography in congenital aortic stenosis. Am J Cardiol 47:1267, 1981.
140. Raizada V, Roth R, Abrams J, Schroeder K: Superiority of two-dimensional echocardiography in the diagnosis of congenitally bicuspid aortic valve. Jpn Heart J 23:305, 1982.
141. Brandenburg RO, Tajik AJ, Edwards WD, et al: Accuracy of 2-dimensional echocardiographic diagnosis of congenitally bicuspid aortic valve: echocardiographic-anatomic correlation in 115 patients. Am J Cardiol 51:1469, 1983.
142. Zema J, Caccavano M: Two dimensional echocardiographic assessment of aortic valve morphology: feasibility of bicuspid valve detection. Prospective study of 100 adult patients. Br Heart J 48:428, 1982.
143. Kosturakis D, Allen HD, Goldberg SJ, et al: Noninvasive quantification of stenotic semilunar valve areas by Doppler echocardiography. J Am Coll Cardiol 3:1256, 1984.
144. Beppu S, Suzuki S, Matsuda H, et al: Rapidity of progression of aortic stenosis in patients with congenital bicuspid aortic valves. Am J Cardiol 71:322, 1993.
145. Nishimura RA, Pieroni DR, Bierman FZ, et al: Second natural history study of congenital heart defects. Aortic stenosis: echocardiography. Circulation 87(suppl I):I-66, 1993.
146. Weyman AE, Caldwell RL, Hurwitz RA, et al: Cross-sectional echocardiographic detection of aortic obstruction. 2. Coarctation of the aorta. Circulation 57:498, 1978.
147. Smallhorn JF, Huhta JC, Adams PA, et al: Cross-sectional echocardiographic assessment of coarctation in the sick neonate and infant. Br Heart J 50:349, 1983.
148. Huhta JC, Gutgesell HP, Latson LA, Huffines FD: Two-dimensional echocardiographic assessment of the aorta in infants and children with congenital heart disease. Circulation 70:417, 1984.
149. Mills P, Wolfe C, Redwood D, et al: Non-invasive diagnosis of subpulmonary outflow tract obstruction. Br Heart J 43:276, 1980.
150. VonDoenhoff LJ, Nanda NC: Obstruction within the right ventricular body: two-dimensional echocardiographic features. Am J Cardiol 51:1498, 1983.
151. Silove ED, deGiovanni JV, Shiu MF, Yi MM: Diagnosis of right ventricular outflow obstruction in infants by cross sectional echocardiography. Br Heart J 50:416, 1983.

152. Weyman AE, Hurwitz RA, Girod DA, et al: Cross-sectional echocardiographic visualization of the stenotic pulmonary valve. Circulation 56:769, 1977.
153. Weyman AE, Dillon JC, Feigenbaum H, Chang S: Echocardiographic patterns of pulmonary valve motion in valvular pulmonary stenosis. Am J Cardiol 34:644, 1974.
154. LeBlanc MH, Paquet M: Echocardiographic assessment of valvular pulmonary stenosis in children. Br Heart J 46:363, 1981.
155. Tinker DD, Nanda NC, Harris JP, Manning JA: Two-dimensional echocardiographic identification of pulmonary artery branch stenosis. Am J Cardiol 50:814, 1982.
156. Lima CO, Sahn DJ, Valdes-Cruz LM, et al: Noninvasive prediction of transvalvular pressure gradient in patients with pulmonary stenosis by quantitative two-dimensional echocardiographic Doppler studies. Circulation 67:866, 1983.
157. Johnson GL, Kwan OL, Handshoe S, et al: Accuracy of combined two-dimensional echocardiography and continuous wave Doppler recordings in the estimation of pressure gradient in right ventricular outlet obstruction. J Am Coll Cardiol 3:1013, 1984.
158. Houston AB, Simpson IA, Sheldon CD, et al: Doppler ultrasound in the estimation of the severity of pulmonary infundibular stenosis in infants and children. Br Heart J 55:381, 1986.
159. Nishimura RA, Pieroni DR, Bierman FZ, et al: Second natural history study of congenital heart defects. Pulmonary stenosis: echocardiography. Circulation; 87(suppl I):I-73, 1993.
160. Hagler DJ, Tajik AJ, Seward JB, et al: Atrioventricular and ventriculoarterial discordance (corrected transposition of the great arteries). Wide-angle two-dimensional echocardiographic assessment of ventricular morphology. Mayo Clin Proc 56:591, 1981.
161. Daskalopoulos DA, Edwards WD, Driscoll DJ, et al: Correlation of two-dimensional echocardiographic and autopsy findings in complete transposition of the great arteries. J Am Coll Cardiol 2:1151, 1983.
162. Houston AB, Gregory NL, Coleman EN: Echocardiographic identification of aorta and main pulmonary artery in complete transposition. Br Heart J 40:377, 1978.
163. Bierman FZ, Williams RG: Prospective diagnosis of *d*-transposition of the great arteries in neonates by subxiphoid, two-dimensional echocardiography. Circulation 60:1496, 1979.
164. Aziz KU, Paul MH, Bharati S, et al: Two dimensional echocardiographic evaluation of Mustard operation for *d*-transposition of the great arteries. Am J Cardiol 47:654, 1981.
165. Ninomiya K, Duncan WJ, Cook DH, et al: Right ventricular ejection fraction and volumes after Mustard repair: correlation of two-dimensional echocardiograms and cineangiograms. Am J Cardiol 48:317, 1981.
166. Silverman NH, Snider AR, Colo J, et al: Superior vena caval obstruction after Mustard's operation: detection by two-dimensional contrast echocardiography. Circulation 64:392, 1981.
167. Allan LD, Leanage R, Wainwright R, et al: Balloon atrial septostomy under two dimensional echocardiographic control. Br Heart J 47:41, 1982.
168. Perry LW, Ruckman RN, Galioto FM Jr, et al: Echocardiographically assisted balloon atrial septostomy. Pediatrics 70:403, 1982.
169. Duncan WJ, Freedom RM, Rowe RD, et al: Echocardiographic features before and after the Jatene procedure (anatomical correction) for transposition of the great vessels. Am Heart J 102:227, 1981.
170. Serraf A, Lacour-Gayet F, Bruniaux J, et al: Anatomic correction of transposition of the great arteries in neonates. J Am Coll Cardiol 22:193, 1993.
171. Sahn DJ, Allen HD: Real-time cross-sectional echocardiographic imaging and measurement of the patent ductus arteriosus in infants and children. Circulation 58:343, 1978.
172. Vick GW III, Huhta JC, Gutgesell HP: Assessment of the ductus arteriosus in preterm infants utilizing suprasternal two-dimensional/Doppler echocardiography. J Am Coll Cardiol 5:973, 1985.
173. Perez JE, Nordlicht SC, Geltman EM: Patent ductus arteriosus in adults: diagnosis by suprasternal and parasternal pulsed Doppler echocardiography. Am J Cardiol 53:1473, 1984.
174. Stevenson JG, Kawabori I, Guntheroth WG: Pulsed Doppler echocardiographic diagnosis of patent ductus arteriosus: sensitivity, specificity, limitations and technical features. Cathet Cardiovasc Diagn 6:255, 1980.
175. Cloez JL, Isaaz K, Pernot C: Pulsed Doppler flow characteristics of ductus arteriosus in infants with associated congenital anomalies of the heart or great arteries. Am J Cardiol 56:845, 1986.
176. Swensson RE, Valdes-Cruz LM, Sahn DJ, et al: Real-time Doppler color flow mapping for detection of patent ductus arteriosus. J Am Coll Cardiol 8:1105, 1986.
177. Bridges ND, Perry SB, Parness I, et al: Transcatheter closure of a large patent ductus arteriosus with the clamshell septal umbrella. J Am Coll Cardiol 18:1297, 1991.
178. Fisher EA, Sepehri B, Lendrum B, et al: Two-dimensional echocardiographic visualization of the left coronary artery in anomalous origin of the left coronary artery from the pulmonary artery. Pre- and postoperative studies. Circulation 63:698, 1981.
179. Worsham C, Sanders SP, Burger BM: Origin of the right coronary artery from the pulmonary trunk: diagnosis by two-dimensional echocardiography. Am J Cardiol 55:232, 1985.
180. Schmidt KG, Cooper MJ, Silverman NH, Stanger P: Pulmonary artery origin of the left coronary artery: diagnosis by two-dimensional echocardiography, pulsed Doppler ultrasound and color flow mapping. J Am Coll Cardiol 11:396, 1988.
181. Jureidini SB, Nouri S, Crawford CJ, et al: Reliability of echocardiography in the diagnosis of anomalous origin of the left coronary artery from the pulmonary trunk. Am Heart J 122:61, 1991.
182. Jureidini SB, Nouri S, Pennington DG: Anomalous origin of the left coronary artery from the pulmonary trunk: repair after diagnostic cross sectional echocardiography. Br Heart J 58:173, 1987.
183. Shah RM, Nanda NC, Hsiung MC, et al: Identification of anomalous origin of the right coronary artery from pulmonary trunk by Doppler color flow mapping. Am J Cardiol 57:366, 1988.
184. Maire R, Gallino A, Jenni R: Initial detection in a teenager of anomalous left coronary artery from the pulmonary artery by color Doppler echocardiography. Am Heart J 125:1802, 1993.
185. Kessler KM, Feldman T, Harding L, et al: Anomalous origin of the right coronary artery from the left sinus of Valsalva: echocardiographic-angiographic correlations. Am Heart J 115:470, 1988.
186. Gaither NS, Rogan KM, Stajduhar K, et al: Anomalous origin and course of coronary arteries in adults: identification and improved imaging utilizing transesophageal echocardiography. Am Heart J 122:69, 1991.
187. Smolin MR, Gorman PD, Gaither NS, Wortham DC: Origin of the right coronary artery from the left main coronary artery identified by transesophageal echocardiography. Am Heart J 123:1062, 1992.
188. Samdarshi TE, Hill DL, Nanda NC: Transesophageal color Doppler diagnosis of anomalous origin of left circumflex coronary artery. Am Heart J 122:571, 1991.
189. Oliver JM, Lopez de Sa E, Dominguez F, et al: Congenital right coronary artery–to–left atrium fistula detected by two-dimensional and Doppler echocardiography. Am Heart J 114:165, 1987.
190. Velvis H, Schmidt KG, Silverman NH, Turley K: Diagnosis of coronary artery fistula by two-dimensional echocardiography, pulsed Doppler ultrasound and color flow imaging. J Am Coll Cardiol 14:968, 1989.
191. Nishiguchi T, Matsuoka Y, Sennari E, et al: Congenital coronary artery fistula: diagnosis by two-dimensional Doppler echocardiography. Am Heart J 120:1244, 1990.
192. Samdarshi TE, Mahan EF III, Nanda NC, Sanyal RS: Transesophageal echocardiographic assessment of congenital coronary artery to coronary sinus fistulas in adults. Am J Cardiol 68:263, 1991.
193. Sunaga Y, Taniichi Y, Okubo N, et al: Biplane transesophageal echocardiographic study of left coronary artery to right atrium fistula. Am Heart J 123:1058, 1992.
194. Terdjman M, Bourdarias JP, Farcot JC, et al: Aneurysms of sinus of Valsalva: two-dimensional echocardiographic diagnosis and recognition of rupture into the right heart cavities. J Am Coll Cardiol 3:1227, 1984.
195. Kiefaber RW, Tabakin BS, Coffin LH, Gibson TC: Unruptured sinus of Valsalva aneurysm with right ventricular outflow obstruction diagnosed by two-dimensional and Doppler echocardiography. J Am Coll Cardiol 7:438, 1986.
196. Engel PJ, Held JS, Van Der Bel-Kahn J, Spitz H: Echocardiographic diagnosis of congenital sinus of Valsalva aneurysm with dissection of the interventricular septum. Circulation 63:705, 1981.
197. Chen WW, Tai YT: Dissection of interventricular septum by aneurysm of sinus of Valsalva. A rare complication diagnosed by echocardiography. Br Heart J 50:293, 1983.
198. Hands ME, Lloyd BL, Hung J: Cross-sectional echocardiographic

diagnosis of unruptured right sinus of Valsalva aneurysm dissecting into the interventricular septum. Int J Cardiol 9:380, 1985.
199. Chow LC, Dittrich HC, Dembitsky WP, Nicod PH: Accurate localization of ruptured sinus of Valsalva aneurysm by real-time two-dimensional Doppler-flow imaging. Chest 94:462, 1988.
200. Chia BI, Ee BK, Choo MH, Yan PC: Ruptured aneurysm of sinus of Valsalva: recognition of Doppler color-flow mapping. Am Heart J 115:686, 1988.
201. Goudevenos J, Kouvaras G, Chronopoulos DG, et al: Color Doppler echocardiography in the diagnosis of ruptured aneurysm of sinus of Valsalva. Eur Heart J 11:666, 1990.
202. Rubin DC, Carliner NH, Salter DR, et al: Unruptured sinus of Valsalva aneurysm diagnosed by transesophageal echocardiography. Am Heart J 124:225, 1992.
203. Flynn MS, Castello R, McBride LW, Labovitz AJ: Ruptured congenital aneurysm of the sinus of Valsalva with persistent left superior vena cava imaged by intraoperative transesophageal echocardiography. Am Heart J 125:1185, 1993.
204. Silverman NH, Golbus MS: Echocardiographic techniques for assessing normal and abnormal fetal cardiac anatomy. J Am Coll Cardiol 5:205, 1985.
205. Shenker L, Reed KL, Marx GR, et al: Fetal cardiac Doppler flow studies in prenatal diagnosis of heart disease. Am J Obstet Gynecol 158:1267, 1988.
206. DeVore GR, Horenstein J, Siassi B, Platt LD: Fetal echocardiography. VII. Doppler color flow mapping: a new technique for the diagnosis of congenital heart disease. Am J Obstet Gynecol 156:1054, 1987.
207. Sahn DJ, Shenker L, Reed KL, et al: Prenatal ultrasound diagnosis of hypoplastic left heart syndrome in utero associated with hydrops fetalis. Am Heart J 104:1368, 1982.
208. Silverman NH, Enderlein MA, Golbus MS: Ultrasonic recognition of aortic valve atresia in utero. Am J Cardiol 53:391, 1984.
209. Kleinman CS, Donnerstein RL, DeVore GR, et al: Fetal echocardiography for evaluation of in utero congestive heart failure. N Engl J Med 306:568, 1982.
210. Allan LD, Tynan M, Campbell S, Anderson RH: Identification of congenital cardiac malformations by echocardiography in midtrimester fetus. Br Heart J 46:358, 1981.
211. Stewart PA, Wladimiroff W, Becker AE: Early prenatal detection of double outlet right ventricle by echocardiography. Br Heart J 54:340, 1985.
212. Roberson DA, Silverman NH: Ebstein's anomaly: echocardiographic and clinical features in the fetus and neonate. J Am Coll Cardiol 14:1300, 1989.
213. Weyman AE: Complex congenital heart disease I: a diagnostic approach. *In* Weyman AE (ed): Principles and Practice of Echocardiography. 2nd ed. p. 979. Philadelphia: Lea & Febiger, 1994.

CHAPTER **10**

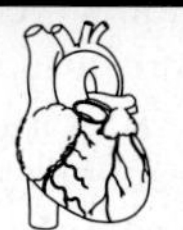

INTERVENTIONAL THERAPY

Sandra K. Clapp and Charles E. Mullins

HISTORY AND GENERAL CONSIDERATIONS
VALVULAR STENOSES
Pulmonary Stenosis
Aortic Stenosis
Mitral Stenosis
Tricuspid Stenosis
OBSTRUCTIONS OF THE GREAT VESSELS
Angioplasty and Stent Placement
Pulmonary Artery Stenosis
Coarctation of the Aorta
Systemic Veins
Pulmonary Veins
PATENT DUCTUS ARTERIOSUS
Rashkind Patent Ductus Arteriosus Occluding Device
Patent Ductus Arteriosus Gianturco Coil Occlusion Device
Gianturco-Grifka Vascular Occlusion Device
Other Devices for Patent Ductus Arteriosus Occlusion
CLOSURE OF ABNORMAL VASCULAR COMMUNICATIONS
ATRIAL SEPTAL DEFECT OCCLUSIONS
Background and General Considerations
General Procedure for Atrial Septal Defect Closure
CardioSEAL Device
Angel Wings Device
Sideris Button Device
Atrial Septal Defect Occluding System
Amplatzer Atrial Septal Defect Occlusion Device
VENTRICULAR SEPTAL DEFECT AND OTHER ABNORMAL COMMUNICATION OCCLUSION
Umbrella Device Occlusion of Other Intravascular Communications
MISCELLANEOUS THERAPEUTIC CATHETER PROCEDURES
Balloon Atrial Septostomy
Blade Atrial Septostomy
Angioplasty Balloon Dilatation of an Atrial Defect
CATHETER REMOVAL OF FOREIGN BODIES
Snare Techniques
Basket Device
Bioptome
Vascular Retrieval Forceps
Cook Deflector Wire
COLLABORATIVE THERAPEUTIC CATHETERIZATION AND SURGICAL PROCEDURES
CONCLUSIONS

HISTORY AND GENERAL CONSIDERATIONS

The development of surgical interventions for patients with congenital heart disease in the 1950s stimulated an increased interest in diagnostic cardiac catheterization and angiography in these patients. As cardiovascular surgeons have become more technically adept at operating on congenital heart disease in smaller, sicker, and bluer patients, they have expected and required better diagnostic information. To accomplish these goals, pediatric cardiologists have been at the forefront of development of new catheterization techniques, better imaging systems, and more recently, an explosion of new therapeutic catheters, devices, and procedures for use in the growing population of surviving patients with congenital heart disease.

Historically, pediatric cardiac catheterization began moving from a strictly diagnostic procedure to a therapeutic procedure in 1966 when Rashkind and Miller introduced balloon atrial septostomy for babies with transposition of the great arteries.[1] This procedure was lifesaving in a limited number of patients. Of equal importance, it demonstrated that transcatheter intracardiac procedures could be performed safely in small babies with good long-term results.

During the same period, the development of diagnostic cardiac catheterization was advanced by the introduction of transseptal left heart catheterization by Cope,[2] Ross and coworkers,[3] and Roveti and colleagues.[4] This procedure became widely used in pediatric cardiology when Duff and Mullins[5] introduced the long transseptal sheath in 1978. The long transseptal sheath encouraged the development of the Park blade septostomy procedure, permitting the septostomy concept to be applied to the older patient with complex lesions.[6]

The most recent and dramatic advances in interventional cardiology began in 1975 when Gruentzig demonstrated that fixed-diameter cylindrical balloons could be positioned within a vessel stenosis and inflated at high pressure to improve the stenosis.[7] In 1982, Kan and associates[8] applied this technique, using larger balloons, to children with pulmonary valvular stenosis. The results were excellent and were enthusiastically accepted by pediatric cardiologists, with rapid extension of the technique to the other cardiac valves and to vascular obstructions. Balloon valvuloplasty and balloon angioplasty have now been effectively applied to all four valves and all major blood vessels in patients of all ages. In the short time since its inception, balloon valvuloplasty has led to a tremendous increase in technology, including the development and use of balloon-expandable stents together with the dilatation of vessels. During this same time, there were dramatic, separate developments in transcatheter devices and techniques for closing abnormal or persistent intracardiac and vascular communications. These included devices for the occlusion of aortopulmonary collateral vessels, patent ductus arteriosus (PDA), and intracardiac septal defects.

As patients with operated congenital heart disease have reached adulthood, it has become clear that many have residual cardiovascular problems that are difficult to approach surgically. Interventional cardiac catheterization procedures in many instances now offer alternatives to surgery for these patients. This chapter discusses therapeutic interventional catheterization techniques that should be considered when evaluating the adult with congenital heart disease. A technical description of each procedure is included. These procedures require special skills and technical training in the individual catheter manipulations and in the use of the specialized equipment. Each procedure also requires a large inventory of specialized expendable equipment. In addition to the procedural and equipment training, the cardiologist performing these procedures must have training and experience in when to use the various techniques or devices and must know the contraindications for each device. For these reasons, not every center should plan to perform every type of therapeutic catheterization procedure. However, cardiologists caring for these patients must be aware that these procedures are available in order to most appropriately advise their patients of their therapeutic options.

Valvular Stenoses

Since Kan first introduced the concept of balloon valvuloplasty for the pulmonary valve in 1982, techniques have developed rapidly for the aortic, mitral, and tricuspid valves and have been perfected for the pulmonary valve in children and young adults. Early in the experience with these techniques, the voluntary Valvuloplasty and Angioplasty of Congenital Anomalies (VACA) Registry was established, initially including 28 centers in which these procedures were performed. This registry was intended to record the results and complications of dilatation procedures. The Registry rapidly accumulated information on a large number of patients with all types of lesions undergoing dilatation procedures by pediatric cardiologists. Now there are many reports documenting results of these procedures in adult patients with congenital and acquired heart disease, which are discussed in this chapter. There is a place for balloon dilatation of stenosis of each of the four cardiac valves. These procedures have special applications in selected adult patients, especially women during later stages of pregnancy and the elderly.

A complete diagnostic cardiac catheterization should be performed to document the anatomy and hemodynamics of the lesion and exclude additional congenital or acquired heart disease before the valvuloplasty procedure is performed. Angiography is performed to exactly delineate the valve anatomy and measure the valve annulus. Additional angiography may be necessary to evaluate valvular insufficiency before balloon valvuloplasty, particularly for the left-sided valves. One should use a calibrated catheter, grid, or sphere of known size as a reference measurement. The reference catheter or object must be recorded in the exact plane of the valve to be dilated so that accurate measurements can be made.

Pulmonary Stenosis

With the current safety of this procedure in experienced hands, indications for transcatheter intervention for pulmonary valvular stenosis are less stringent than for surgical valvulotomy. The indications for treatment of pulmonary stenosis include significant right ventricular outflow tract obstruction, any evidence for right ventricular hypertrophy, or any evidence for right ventricular fibrosis or dysfunction.[9, 10] Severity of pulmonary valvular stenosis correlates quite well with the echo peak instantaneous gradient, but it is determined definitively in the presence of normal cardiac output by the peak systolic gradient across the valve at catheterization. Less than a 10 mm Hg gradient is considered trivial, less than 30 mm Hg is considered a mild gradient, 30 to 60 mm Hg is a moderate obstruction, and greater than 60 mm Hg represents severe stenosis. Natural history studies have documented that moderate and severe pulmonary valve stenoses tend to develop more obstruction with time, whereas mild pulmonary valve stenosis usually does not progress.[11, 12] At the time of catheterization, a patient with a peak systolic gradient of 30 mm Hg or more across the pulmonary valve, when associated with clinical evidence of right ventricular hypertrophy and a favorable valve with fused commissures, should undergo catheter intervention.

A variety of balloons are in use for pulmonary valvuloplasty. These are cylindrical polyethylene balloons that are noncompliant and have a fixed, predetermined diameter and parallel walls at the maximal inflation pressure. The balloons are available in a wide range of diameters from 2 mm to as large as 25 mm. When inflated to their maximal recommended pressure of between 2.5 and 12 atm, they reach their advertised fixed diameter and become rigid.[13] The balloon is prepared by purging it of air with repeated flushing and low-pressure inflations with a solution of contrast medium diluted with saline (1:5 dilution). The same contrast solution will be used to inflate the balloon during the valvuloplasty.

To perform the valvuloplasty, the pulmonary valve, valve annulus, right ventricular outflow tract, and main and branch pulmonary arteries are imaged with a right ventricular angiocardiogram in the posteroanterior (or cranially angulated posteroanterior) and lateral views.[13] Measurements of the valve annulus diameter are obtained using an accurately calibrated reference. When a single balloon is to be used to dilate the pulmonary valve, the balloon diameter should be 1.2 to 1.3 times the diameter of the valve annulus.[10, 13] The length of the balloon is chosen according to the patient's size. In general, much longer balloons (6 to 8 cm) are used in the adult patient.

An end-hole diagnostic catheter is advanced through the right heart and into the distal left pulmonary artery. It is important that this catheter passes through the center of the tricuspid valve and not between or through the chordal attachments. A stiff exchange guide wire is passed through this catheter and into a large distal left pulmonary artery. With the wire carefully fixed in place, the catheter is withdrawn and replaced with the previously prepared balloon catheter. The balloon catheter is advanced over the wire until it lies centered across the annulus. Exact centering is important so that the balloon is not squeezed forward or backward out of the valve during inflation. The balloon is inflated to its designated maximal pressure using an inflation device with a pressure gauge, observing first for the development of a "waist" or circumferential indentation in the balloon, followed by disappearance of this waist. The balloon is then rapidly deflated, with the entire inflation-deflation cycle taking place over less than 10 to 15 seconds. This process should be repeated several times with repositioning of the balloon so that it remains centered over the valve.[13]

Not uncommonly, the valve annulus is too large (>18 mm in diameter) for the single-balloon technique, or the use of a single large balloon would require the introduction of a large and traumatic balloon into the vein. Under these circumstances, the double-balloon technique is used.[14] The balloon diameters are chosen so that the sum of the inflated balloon diameters is 1.5 to 1.6 times the diameter of the pulmonary valve annulus.[14] For this technique, a second exchange wire is introduced from the opposite femoral vein and positioned next to the first wire in the distal left pulmonary artery. The second balloon catheter is advanced over this wire and placed side by side with the first balloon catheter across the valve annulus. The two balloons are then inflated and deflated simultaneously. Because of space between the two inflated balloons, there is generally less detrimental effect on systemic arterial blood pressure during inflation. The double-balloon technique allows the use of smaller profile balloon catheters with less individual vessel trauma for introduction of the balloons. For these reasons, the double-balloon technique is preferentially employed, even when a single larger balloon may be available.[10, 13, 14] Figure 10–1 demonstrates a pulmonary valvuloplasty that required three angioplasty balloons owing to the patient's size.

As the first valve to be successfully dilated and with the relatively easy approach to this valve, data accumulated rapidly. The voluntary VACA Registry reported in 1990 on the results of 784 pulmonary valvuloplasties, including 33 neonates, 716 children, and 35 adults.[15] For the whole group of patients, the gradient across the pulmonary valve decreased from 71 ± 33 mm Hg to 28 ± 21 mm Hg with only a 1.3 percent incidence of complications. In the VACA Registry, there was no difference in success of the procedure with age, but only 9 adults between 21 and 79 years were included. In 196 of the VACA patients, the residual gradient was subdivided into infundibular (18 ± 24 mm Hg) and transvalvular (16 ± 15 mm Hg).[15] Unsuccessful procedures were associated with dysplastic valves and with inability to cross the valve. Pulmonary balloon valvuloplasty is now considered the procedure of choice for children and adults with pulmonary valvular stenosis.

The experience at Texas Children's Hospital has been positive and similar to those mentioned in the VACA report. Pulmonary valvuloplasty was performed in 102 patients, including 3 patients who were 51, 71, and 76 years of age.[13, 16] The mean gradient was reduced by 69 percent for the whole group, which included the early experience before 1988. After the procedure, the valve was shown angiographically to open more widely than before valvuloplasty, with an associated reactive infundibular narrowing that often actually increased temporarily. This residual infundibular obstruction is dynamic and tends to decrease with time.[13]

There is less information available for adult patients with

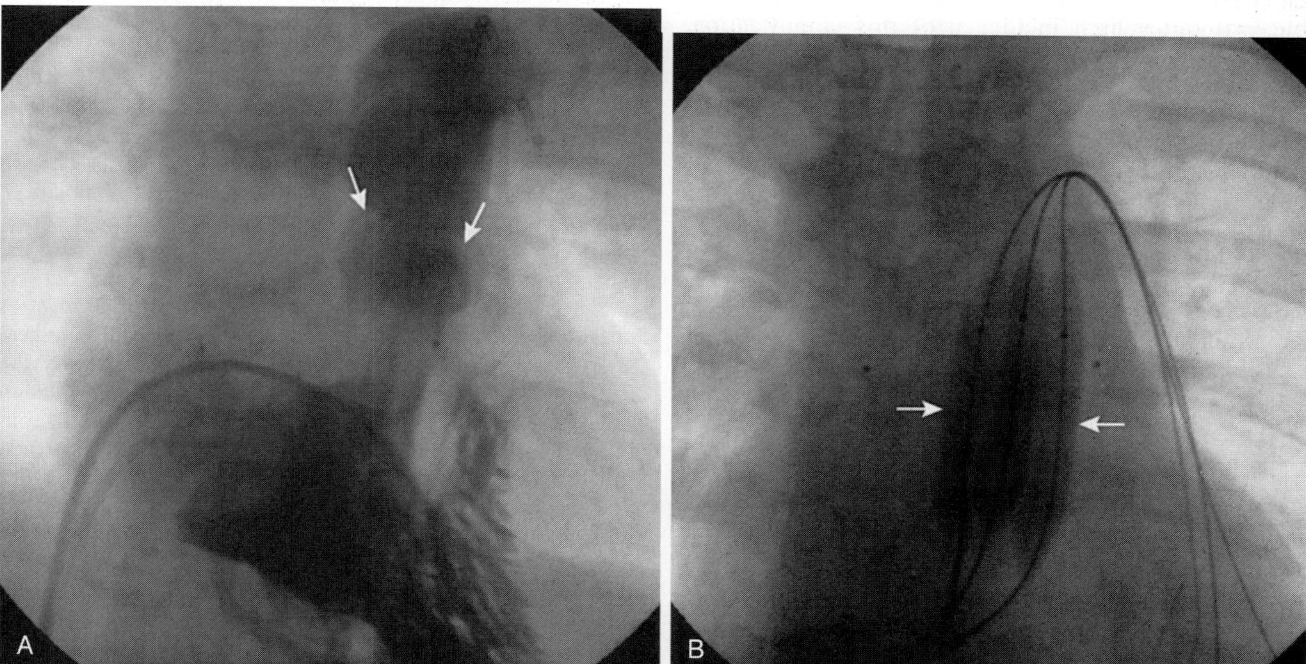

FIGURE 10–1 Pulmonary balloon valvuloplasty. **A,** Right ventricular angiocardiogram in the anteroposterior view. *Arrows* mark the thickened, doming pulmonary valve leaflets. **B,** Three balloon angioplasty catheters are positioned across the pulmonary valve with the balloons simultaneously inflated. *Arrows* demarcate the level of the pulmonary valve, with a slight "waist" present in the middle balloon. Superstiff guide wires for the angioplasty catheters can be identified in position in the distal left pulmonary artery.

pulmonary valvular stenosis because it is relatively rare for a patient with this lesion to reach adulthood without diagnosis and treatment. Chen and colleagues[17] reported their experience in 53 adolescent and adult patients 13 to 55 years of age. With pulmonary balloon valvuloplasty, the systolic pressure gradient across the pulmonary outflow tract decreased from 91 ± 46 mm Hg to 38 ± 32 mm Hg in their patients. There was a further decrease in gradient at follow-up catheterization in 9 patients who were restudied.[17] Teupe and coworkers[18] reported a similar experience in 24 adult patients who were 19 to 65 years of age, 14 of whom had late follow-up at 5 to 9 years. In those 14 patients, the mean peak systolic gradient before valvuloplasty was 82 ± 29 mm Hg. Immediately after intervention, the gradient fell to 37 ± 14 mm Hg, and it was 31 ± 7 mm Hg at a mean follow-up of 6.5 years. Three patients in this study had a peak systolic gradient before valvuloplasty of greater than 100 mm Hg. All 3 had high residual gradients immediately after the procedure that were shown to be muscular and dynamic in nature. In these 3 patients, the subvalvular hypertrophy resolved by 3 months after the procedure, and they had a permanently lower gradient at late follow-up.[18] Both groups of investigators thought that balloon valvuloplasty for pulmonary valvular stenosis in the adult is highly effective and associated with an excellent long-term outcome.[17, 18]

Aortic Stenosis

Aortic valve dilatation was first reported by Labadidi and colleagues in 1984.[19] This technique was slower to gain acceptance than pulmonary valvuloplasty because of concerns regarding the potential development of aortic regurgitation. The early and subsequent experience has been favorable, without a high incidence of this complication. Surgical valvotomy is not without this complication, and valve replacement in children is best delayed, if possible, because of size issues and difficulties with anticoagulation. Children with congenital aortic valve stenosis now routinely undergo balloon valvuloplasty. Indications for balloon valvuloplasty of the aortic valve are the same as those for surgical intervention for aortic stenosis. Although no single set of diagnostic criteria is universally accepted for determining the severity of aortic stenosis, most pediatric cardiologists would agree that in the presence of normal cardiac output, a systolic gradient of 70 mm Hg or greater at rest or a peak gradient of 50 to 70 mm Hg with ischemia or other symptoms indicates the need for some form of intervention.[20, 21] A major contraindication to performing aortic balloon valvuloplasty is the presence of more than mild aortic regurgitation, as 25 to 30 percent of patients develop some increase in degree of regurgitation with this procedure.[22]

The balloon catheters are similar to those used for the pulmonary valve procedure with the exception that longer, 6- to 8-cm balloons are used for the aortic valve. The longer balloons are less likely to be ejected with inflation during systole. In addition to the longer balloons, the use of "superstiff" wires has helped to stabilize the balloons in the aortic orifice. Although a single-balloon technique was originally described,[19] many centers have moved to a double-balloon technique.[13, 14, 20] This technique allows the insertion of a smaller profile balloon catheter in each femoral artery rather than a single, larger profile balloon catheter in the one femoral artery. In addition, with the "lumen" between the two side-by-side balloons across the valve, there is less reduction in systemic cardiac output during balloon inflation. When the double-balloon technique is used, the combined diameter of the two balloons should be 1.1 to 1.2 times the measured diameter of the aortic valve annulus.[13, 14, 20, 22] If only one balloon catheter is used, the diameter of the single balloon should be approximately the same as the diameter of the aortic annulus.[20, 22]

The procedure requires a full cardiac catheterization with complete hemodynamic measurements and assessment of cardiac output. This includes simultaneous measurements of left ventricular and ascending aorta pressures. The transseptal approach allows the transseptal sheath to be positioned in the left ventricle. With a floating balloon catheter 1 French size smaller advanced through this sheath, and from there into the ascending aorta, simultaneous left ventricular and ascending aorta pressure measurements can be obtained before, during, and after aortic valve dilatation without any additional arterial catheterization. Cineangiograms should be obtained in the left ventricle and ascending aorta with careful measurement of the aortic valve annulus diameter using a calibrated reference grid or catheter. The presence and amount of aortic regurgitation must be evaluated initially to assess appropriateness of valvuloplasty.

Once the catheters are introduced for the valvuloplasty, heparin, 50 to 100 units/kg in children or 3000 to 5000 units in adults, is administered intravenously. The appropriate-size balloons are chosen and prepared using a dilute solution of contrast material and saline (1:5). Two end-hole catheters are introduced into the two femoral arteries, and each is advanced retrograde across the aortic valve into the left ventricular apex. A 180-degree curve is preformed at the transition area between the stiff and the floppy portions of the distal ends of two stiff exchange wires. One by one, the wires are positioned through the end-hole catheters into the left ventricular apex with the floppy tip curled toward the outflow tract. With the wires securely fixed in position, the end-hole catheters are withdrawn. The two balloon catheters are advanced retrograde into position across the aortic valve annulus. The balloons are centered side by side across the valve and rapidly inflated until the waist of circumferential narrowing disappears. It is important to keep the balloons stable within the valve annulus by the use of stiff wires and proper positioning of the wires in order to prevent "shear" trauma against the leaflets from the balloons moving in and out of the valve. The total inflation-deflation cycle should be completed within 10 to 15 seconds. Balloon inflations are repeated as many as four to eight times with the balloon catheters repositioned as necessary across the valve. After the procedure is completed, gradient measurements and aortic root angiography are repeated. The balloons are withdrawn, and hemostasis is achieved by careful pressure to the femoral puncture sites.

It is better to delay valve replacement to adulthood and through childbearing years, if possible. Since we realize that both surgical valvotomy and balloon dilatation are palliative, at our institution children and young adults with aortic stenosis severe enough to warrant intervention are offered the alternative of balloon valvuloplasty. Although long-term outcome studies of aortic balloon valvuloplasty are just now appearing, it appears that this procedure is as good as surgical valvotomy for the short-term and mid-term relief of aortic stenosis. This is supported by reports by Justo and associates[23] and by the VACA Registry.[24] Justo and associates compared 110 patients with balloon valvuloplasty with 103 patients after surgical valvotomy and demonstrated that the left ventricle to aorta pressure gradient is reduced equally well in both, with the procedures having a similar likelihood of recurrence of the aortic stenosis with time.[23] Additionally, their study demonstrated an equal but unpredictable risk of creating aortic valve regurgitation with either surgical valvotomy or balloon valvuloplasty.[23] The VACA Registry report, which examined results in 606 patients from 23 participating institutions, also demonstrated a comparable relief of obstruction and development of aortic insufficiency.[24] In this report, the left ventricle to aorta systolic gradient was reduced by a mean of 60 ± 23 percent, with 7.3 percent (n = 46) developing either severe aortic insufficiency or an increase in insufficiency of two or more grades. Independent predictors of development of more severe aortic regurgitation included increased balloon/annulus ratio, larger valves, and the presence of preexisting aortic regurgitation (mild or more severe), all presumed to signify valves with morphologic abnormalities exacerbated by valvuloplasty.[24] Procedure-related mortality for this large cohort of patients was 1.9 percent. The procedure could not be performed or completed in 4.7 percent, with a suboptimal result in 17 percent. Both suboptimal outcome and mortality were highly correlated with young age (<3 months). Midterm follow-up studies continue to suggest that aortic balloon valvuloplasty is an effective and relatively safe palliation for children and adolescents with valvular aortic stenosis.[25, 26]

Balloon valvuloplasty has been demonstrated to have similar outcome for *young* adults with bicuspid aortic valve to that in children.[27] Balloon valvuloplasty should be attempted in active young adults with severe stenosis, particularly those who are at risk from difficulties with anticoagulation due to lifestyle or employment demands, or women interested in becoming pregnant without the known teratogenic effects of warfarin anticoagulation. Aortic balloon valvuloplasty is unlikely to be beneficial in older adults when the valve has undergone calcific degenerative changes.[28, 29] Lieberman and coworkers[28] evaluated the results in 165 symptomatic adult patients who underwent balloon aortic valvuloplasty and found that event-free and actuarial survival after this procedure resembles the natural history of untreated symptomatic aortic stenosis, and it is dismal for patients who are not candidates for aortic valve replacement. Although it has been suggested that balloon valvuloplasty might improve symptoms in the very elderly or alleviate need for surgery, this has not been shown to be the case.[28, 29] Balloon aortic valvuloplasty in the elderly is followed by, at best, only a short period of symptomatic relief, and better overall survival is obtained with direct valve replacement.[29]

Mitral Stenosis

Children and young adults may have either congenital or rheumatic mitral stenosis. Congenital mitral stenosis is a rare form of congenital heart disease that is actually a spectrum of abnormalities. The obstruction may occur in the supravalve area, the annulus, the leaflets, the chordae tendineae, the papillary muscle level, or any combination of these. The most typical form of congenital mitral stenosis consists of thickened leaflets, shortened chordae tendineae, and decreased interchordal spaces.[30, 31] Other typical forms include supravalve mitral membrane and parachute mitral valve.[30, 31] The diagnosis of mitral stenosis may be delayed or masked in these patients owing to associated lesions, most commonly other obstructions to left heart inflow or outflow.[32, 33]

Intervention is indicated for severe mitral stenosis, particularly when it leads to pulmonary hypertension. Symptoms of severe stenosis include shortness of breath and marked exercise limitation. The symptoms are confirmed by echocardiographic evidence of significant mitral gradient and prolonged pressure half-time of 220 ms or greater. The severity of the mitral stenosis is confirmed definitively at catheterization by findings of left atrial hypertension, pulmonary hypertension, and a calculated mitral valve area of 0.5 cm^2/m^2 or less.[30–35]

Surgical mitral valvuloplasty in the congenital lesions is associated with significant morbidity and mortality. Patients with congenital mitral stenosis frequently have a small mitral annulus, and this may also occur with rheumatic mitral stenosis in young adults. Insertion of a prosthetic mitral valve prohibits any further growth of the annulus. In an effort to provide symptomatic relief and allow growth of the mitral annulus and other left heart structures, balloon valvuloplasty has been attempted for severe congenital mitral stenosis in a limited number of children and young adults.[34–37]

The preferred technique for mitral valve dilatation at Texas Children's Hospital is the double-transseptal, double-balloon technique.[13, 37] This technique is applicable to patients of all sizes. After appropriate hemodynamic measurements, including the simultaneous measurement of left atrial and left ventricular pressures, angiography is performed in the left atrium and left ventricle in views appropriate for measurement of the mitral valve annulus. The diameter of the annulus is compared with a calibrated catheter or other measurement device. The two balloons are then selected and prepared in the usual fashion using dilute contrast medium solution. The combined diameter of the two balloons should be approximately equal to the annulus diameter.[37] Relatively long balloons (5 to 6 cm for larger patients) are selected.

Two separate transseptal punctures are performed for this procedure, preferably from opposite legs. If a 12 or 14 French Mullins transseptal set is employed, no further septal dilatation should be necessary to deliver the balloon catheters to the left atrium. The patient is given heparin, 50 to 100 units/kg in children or 3000 to 5000 units in adults, as soon as the transseptal procedures are completed. Curved-tipped or even pigtail end-hole catheters are passed through the transseptal sheaths and through the mitral valve to the left ventricle. Curves are formed on the transition portion of appropriate-size superstiff wires, so that the curve will fit in the apex of the left ventricle and the tip of the wire will curve back on itself in the left ventricle toward the left ventricular outflow tract. The wires are positioned in the left ventricle, and the end-hole catheters are removed. Each of the balloon catheters is then advanced over its wire through the transseptal sheath to the left atrium. Alternately, the sheath may be withdrawn and each balloon catheter passed over its wire into the left atrium through the hole created by the transseptal sheath. The balloons are subsequently manipulated into position, centered side by side across the mitral annulus, and inflated to their maximal advertised pressures. The inflation-deflation cycle is performed as rapidly as possible while the positions of the balloons are carefully controlled, particularly so that they do not move forward into the left ventricular apex or backward toward the atrial septum. The inflation-deflation cycles are repeated with repositioning of the balloons for centering until the circumferential waist disappears in the balloons. If no waist appears and no significant mitral regurgitation has been created, larger balloons may be selected and the procedure repeated. At the end of the procedure, hemodynamic measurements and angiography are repeated.[13, 37]

Other methods are available for delivery of balloon catheters to the mitral valve. One technique employs a single transseptal puncture and special double-lumen Block catheter through which two wires can be delivered to the left ventricle and aorta.[38] This technique requires that both balloon catheters be delivered, side by side, through the same femoral venous and atrial septal puncture sites. The Inoue balloon and technique, which is in wide use for rheumatic mitral stenosis, may be more satisfactory for the adolescent and adult congenital mitral stenosis and should be considered in centers familiar with this technique.[39]

The long-term benefit of mitral valvuloplasty for severe congenital mitral stenosis is unknown. It is likely that all of these patients will eventually need mitral valve replacement. By delaying operative intervention, this procedure will delay the need for chronic anticoagulation therapy and may allow growth of the annulus, permitting the insertion of a larger prosthetic valve when valve replacement is necessary.[34–37] In adults with rheumatic mitral stenosis, balloon valvuloplasty has been proved to be beneficial with longer follow-up.[40–44] Although balloon mitral valvuloplasty has had limited use in congenital mitral stenosis, this should be the initial procedure attempted in selected children, adolescents, and young adults with severe congenital mitral stenosis.

Tricuspid Stenosis

Tricuspid stenosis is very rare in childhood and in adults. The cause can be congenital, rheumatic, or acquired with other illnesses such as carcinoid. When tricuspid stenosis is present in children, it is often associated with a hypoplastic annulus and right ventricle, so that it is rarely amenable to surgical or balloon valvuloplasty. The early and limited experience with tricuspid valvuloplasty in children and young adults for either congenital or acquired tricuspid stenosis has demonstrated that it is possible to achieve satisfactory dilatations in these patients. One of the authors also has had the experience of managing a patient with Ebstein's malformation who had required tricuspid valve replacement. This patient then developed stenosis of the porcine xenograft, which was amenable to balloon valvuloplasty with good short-term relief of symptoms. Symptoms of severe tricuspid stenosis include tiring and peripheral and central edema. These symptoms can be correlated with gradients by echocardiography and catheterization, although the right atrium is extremely compliant, so that the gradient may be lower than expected. The lesion is usually well demonstrated by angiography when obtained in appropriate views.

The procedure for tricuspid stenosis is similar to that described for mitral stenosis, although it appears safer and easier. Owing to the large size of the tricuspid annulus, a double-balloon technique is necessary. The sum of the diameters of the two balloons should match the diameter of the valve annulus, and longer 5.5- or 8-cm balloons should be used. The superstiff wires can be curled in the right ventricular apex, or they can be stabilized in the left pulmonary artery. If there is no waist in the balloons with the inflation-deflation cycle, larger balloons may be necessary.

Case reports of successful tricuspid valvuloplasty are available for adult patients with rheumatic tricuspid stenosis, often accompanying mitral stenosis.[44, 45] This valve has also been successfully dilated during pregnancy to allow completion to term.[46] The procedure should be attempted for any patient with tricuspid stenosis in whom surgery is being considered.

Obstructions of the Great Vessels

Angioplasty and Stent Placement

After the original description of balloon angioplasty for coronary arteries,[7] the procedure was soon extended by pediatric cardiologists to other blood vessels.[47, 48] The techniques for relieving congenital or surgically acquired vascular lesions by balloon angioplasty have now become fairly routine and are employed with variable success for stenoses anywhere within the great vessels.[13, 49–51] The technique is the same for systemic arterial, pulmonary arterial, and systemic venous obstructions. The most common lesions to be dilated are pulmonary branch stenoses and coarctation of the aorta. The vessel to be dilated is identified and measured angiographically, being careful to also film a calibrated measuring device in the same planes at the same time. Discrete stenoses or longer segment lesions can be dilated, and more than one site can be dilated in the same patient during one catheterization. The congenitally stenotic lesions within the pulmonary bed usually require dilatation with a balloon that is at least 50 percent larger than the adjacent normal vessel or three to four times the diameter of the stenosis, whereas systemic artery lesions are dilated with balloons approximating the diameter of the adjacent normal vessel.[13, 48]

The stenotic area is crossed with an end-hole catheter. An exchange-length stiff or superstiff wire is positioned across and distal to the site of stenosis. The diagnostic catheter is removed, and the balloon catheter is advanced over the wire to the area of stenosis. After careful positioning, the balloon is inflated to its maximal advertised pressure for several seconds, while observing for any residual waist or deformity in the balloon. After the balloon is repositioned across the stenotic area, the dilatation can be repeated to achieve maximal effect. After the angioplasty procedure is completed, pressure measurements and angiography are repeated to assess improvement in vessel diameter and identify any irregularities in the vessel wall.

Balloon angioplasty enlarges stenotic vessels by causing a tear in the vessel intima and/or stretching or tearing the scar. This is reasonably safe in stenotic areas due to previous surgical manipulations, as the vessel is supported and surrounded by additional scar tissue that will prevent more extensive tearing or rupture. Care must be taken not to excessively overdilate unoperated vessels, particularly systemic arteries, because this may extend the vessel tear into the media, with potential aneurysm formation or vessel rupture. Care is also advisable in passing wires, catheters, or balloons across freshly angioplastied vessels, as this may create or extend aneurysms. Other concerns related to specific lesions are discussed with each defect.

Balloon angioplasty has variable success, depending on the *criteria for success,* occasionally producing "satisfactory" results but usually leaving the vessel with residual obstruction. Even though the vessel stenosis is dilated to three or four times the size of the original narrowing during balloon angioplasty, it is not uncommon for the postdilatation angiogram to be indistinguishable from the preintervention study because of elastic recoil of the vessel wall or scar tissue being dilated.[52] For these reasons, there was particular interest in the experimental successes of Palmaz and Schatz and colleagues[53,54] when they reported their work with intravascular stents implanted into rabbit aortas and dog coronary arteries in the mid-1980s. These investigators designed a stainless steel mesh stent that could be delivered through the vascular system over an angioplasty balloon and expanded by that balloon to permanently hold the vessel open.[53, 54] Following these reports, Mullins and associates, in 1988,[55] reported an animal study in which the feasibility of stent implantation in the pulmonary arteries and systemic veins was investigated and then began a collaborative investigation of potential pediatric cardiology uses of the device.[55] Others reported laboratory successes with encouraging results,[56, 57] and these excellent results led to the use of stents in children with both native and postoperative pulmonary artery stenoses.[52, 58–60]

The Palmaz balloon expandable stent (Johnson & Johnson Interventional Systems, Warren, NJ) is the most commonly employed and the only stent investigated for the types of vascular stenoses found in growing patients with congenital heart disease. The stent is a stainless steel tube with staggered slots cut along its length that form diamond-shaped spaces during balloon expansion. These "diamonds" are resistant to collapse and, in turn, to the elastic recoil of the dilated vessel. The "iliac" stents most commonly used are 30- or 18-mm lengths with an unexpanded 3.4-mm external diameter. These stents are expanded with angioplasty balloons to a minimal diameter of 6 mm and a maximal diameter of 18 mm. With full expansion, the stents shorten by 35 percent. The smaller diameter "renal" stents with the usual lengths of 20 or 10 mm and an external diameter of 2.4 mm are used in the smaller peripheral vessels. The renal stents have a minimal expanded diameter of 4 mm and a maximal diameter of 10 to 11 mm, and also shorten with full expansion by 35 to 40 percent. The final expanded stent diameter is determined by the diameter of the angioplasty balloon selected to deploy the stent. This stent does not continue to expand after the balloon is removed.[59, 60] Stents can be initially implanted over a smaller angioplasty balloon and can be further expanded with a larger balloon at the same catheterization or at a later time.[61, 62]

When stent implantation is considered, gradient measurements and angiography are first performed in the area of stenosis. The diameter of the stenotic area is carefully measured, along with the diameters of the normal vessel proximal and distal to the site of stenosis and the length of the vessel in the area where the stent is to be placed. The stent and angioplasty balloon are selected using these measurements, so that the expanded stent size will be the same as the diameter of the contiguous normal vessel. The balloon length should approximate the unexpanded length of the stent. If the balloon is too long, the ends of the balloon will inflate first with a "dumbbell" appearance, and this may lead to uneven expansion of the stent, displacement of the stent during inflation, or perforation of the balloon by the stent.

Two or more simultaneous catheters are utilized for the stent procedure, one or more for the delivery of the stents, and an additional catheter for angiography during positioning.[52] The delivery of the Palmaz stent is best accomplished by insertion of a Mullins transseptal or other long sheath beyond the site of stenosis. The sheath diameter required for the combined angioplasty balloon and stent is at least two sheath sizes larger than for the angioplasty balloon catheter itself. This results in a minimum of an 8 French but more commonly a 9 to 12 French diameter sheath.

To position the sheath, a superstiff wire is first introduced beyond the site of stenosis using an end-hole diagnostic catheter, as described for balloon angioplasty. It is important to anchor the superstiff wire as far distally as possible beyond the stenosis so that it will be less likely to be dislodged during the sheath and subsequent stent delivery. The diagnostic catheter is removed, leaving the superstiff wire in place. The long sheath and dilator are advanced over the wire to a site distal to the stenosis. Occasionally, the stenosis must be predilated with a smaller balloon before the sheath and dilator can be introduced.

After the sheath is in place and its dilator removed, the stent is mounted on an angioplasty balloon by carefully crimping the stent circumferentially on the balloon between thumb and forefinger throughout its length. The stent, mounted on its balloon, is advanced over the wire through the sheath to the desired location, and the sheath is withdrawn. Repeat angiography is performed to confirm proper stent position across the site of stenosis. The balloon is expanded to its maximal recommended pressure, which expands the stent and the stenotic area. Inflations can be repeated with repositioning of the balloon within the implanted stent to ensure full expansion of the stent. The angioplasty balloon catheter is withdrawn into the sheath and angiography is repeated. If necessary, the stent can be dilated with a higher pressure or a larger angioplasty balloon, or the proximal and distal ends of the stent can be flared. For long-segment stenoses, overlapping stents can be placed sequentially using the same wire and sheath.

Other types of stents are being tested, including self-expanding nitinol stents,[63] which do not require implantation using a balloon angioplasty catheter. These stents may have some theoretical advantages, including smaller sheath size, but much less information is currently available on their use, and some long-term adverse sequelae have been reported in the congenital locations. Indications and special considerations for Palmaz stent implant are discussed subsequently with individual lesions.

Pulmonary Artery Stenosis

Branch pulmonary artery stenosis occurs frequently in patients with congenital heart disease. This may be seen as an isolated lesion but, more commonly, is part of a congenital heart defect in which there has been reduced intrauterine pulmonary blood flow, as in tetralogy of Fallot or pulmonary atresia. Branch stenoses are also a significant part of the heart disease accompanying rubella syndrome, Williams' syndrome, and Alagille's syndrome. Additionally, branch stenosis frequently occurs after any surgical procedure involving the pulmonary arteries, including systemic to pulmonary artery shunt procedures, previous pulmonary artery banding, the arterial switch procedure, and right ventricle to pulmonary artery conduit repairs for severe forms of tetralogy of Fallot or truncus arteriosus. Whether congenital or after operative intervention, pulmonary artery branch stenosis is a difficult problem for the cardiovascular surgeon because the sites of stenosis are frequently deep within the lungs, distal to the hilus in the lung parenchyma, or embedded in scar tissue.[55] These stenoses can occasionally be improved slightly by balloon angioplasty, but they can usually be corrected with intravascular stent procedures. The only patients unlikely to achieve marked benefit from the pulmonary artery stents are those with generalized hypoplasia or multiple stenoses throughout the pulmonary vascular bed. Indications for intervention include significant right ventricular hypertension, right ventricular failure, unbalanced pulmonary blood flow by perfusion scan, and excessive pulmonary regurgitation.[55, 64] Any visible discrete pulmonary artery obstruction warrants intervention when associated with cavopulmonary anastomosis or other modifications of the Fontan procedure.

The balloon angioplasty procedure is described previously. It is indicated primarily for those patients in whom stent delivery and implant are not possible. The balloon selected for angioplasty should be 3 to 4 times the diameter of the stenosed area, but no more than 1.5 times the diameter of the normal vessel on either side of the stenosis.[13, 48] If there are multiple stenoses in separate vessels, the most severe obstruction should be dilated first. In general, it is better to perform angioplasty on more distal lesions before proximal ones in the same vessel, so that freshly dilated areas are not repeatedly reentered. The success rate of balloon angioplasty of pulmonary branch stenoses varies from 20 to 70 percent, depending on the criteria used for "success."[49, 55–57] Success has been defined as a greater than 50 percent increase in diameter of the lumen, or as little as a 10 mm Hg or greater *drop* in pressure gradient across the stenosed area.[56] This success frequently leaves something to be desired. Although long-term follow-up is not available, persistent or restenosis has been reported in as much as 70 percent of the original successes, with a *serious* complication rate of greater than 5 percent.[56]

Stent implant should be considered in any patient with important pulmonary branch stenoses who is large enough to accommodate the delivery of the larger stents. The procedure itself has been described previously. Patients who are of adolescent or adult size are the most appropriate for stent implant, as they can tolerate placement of the large sheaths required and their stents can be fully expanded to 15 to 18 mm at the time of initial implantation.[52, 64, 65] The experience at Texas Children's Hospital and by others confirms such excellent success and low risk of stent implant in patients with native or postsurgical pulmonary branch stenosis that we no longer attempt angioplasty before stent implant in these patients.[60, 64, 65] The occurrence of significant restenosis after stent implant is extremely low, and residual or restenoses because of vessel growth can be redilated or restented.[66] For some patients with multiple lesions, a combination of balloon angioplasty and stent implantation is best. For example, angioplasty alone may be performed at more distal branch points, particularly if bifurcation or trifurcation vessels are stenotic, and if stenting of one or even two would lead to occlusion of another major branch. In the same patient, one or a series of stents could also be implanted in more proximal and larger vessel stenoses. When two important nearby branches are stenotic or when stent placement will likely block access to a significant neighboring branch, parallel or bifurcating stents will be indicated.[67] For this, two wires and two long sheaths are placed, one across each vessel, and the two stents are implanted simultaneously.[52, 67] Similar considerations must be made when placing a stent in the orifice of the proximal right or left pulmonary artery, as this may partially occlude or "jail" the contralateral pulmonary artery and, at the very least, make it difficult or impossible to reenter the vessel. Figure 10–2 demonstrates simultaneous proximal right and left pulmonary artery stent implants in a patient with bilateral proximal pulmonary artery stenoses.

Stents are relatively contraindicated in proximal conduits because repetitive compression from the beating heart will likely lead to stent fracture.[52] Stents should also not be implanted in a conduit if the diameter of the stenosis is close to the maximal stent diameter, as this may lead to stent embolization.[52] If right ventricular dilatation and failure are already present, care must be taken that stent implantation will not impinge on the pulmonary or homograft valve and cause increased pulmonary regurgitation. On the other hand, *crossing stent* placement in proximal branch stenoses at the obstructed distal end of a conduit or homograft has been very satisfactory at totally relieving obstruction and avoiding further surgery. Whenever large sheaths and stiff wires are placed across a prosthetic conduit, an intimal peel may be lifted and become obstructive.[52, 64] It is important to repeat pressure measurements and angiographic assessment at the end of the procedure to document the final results.

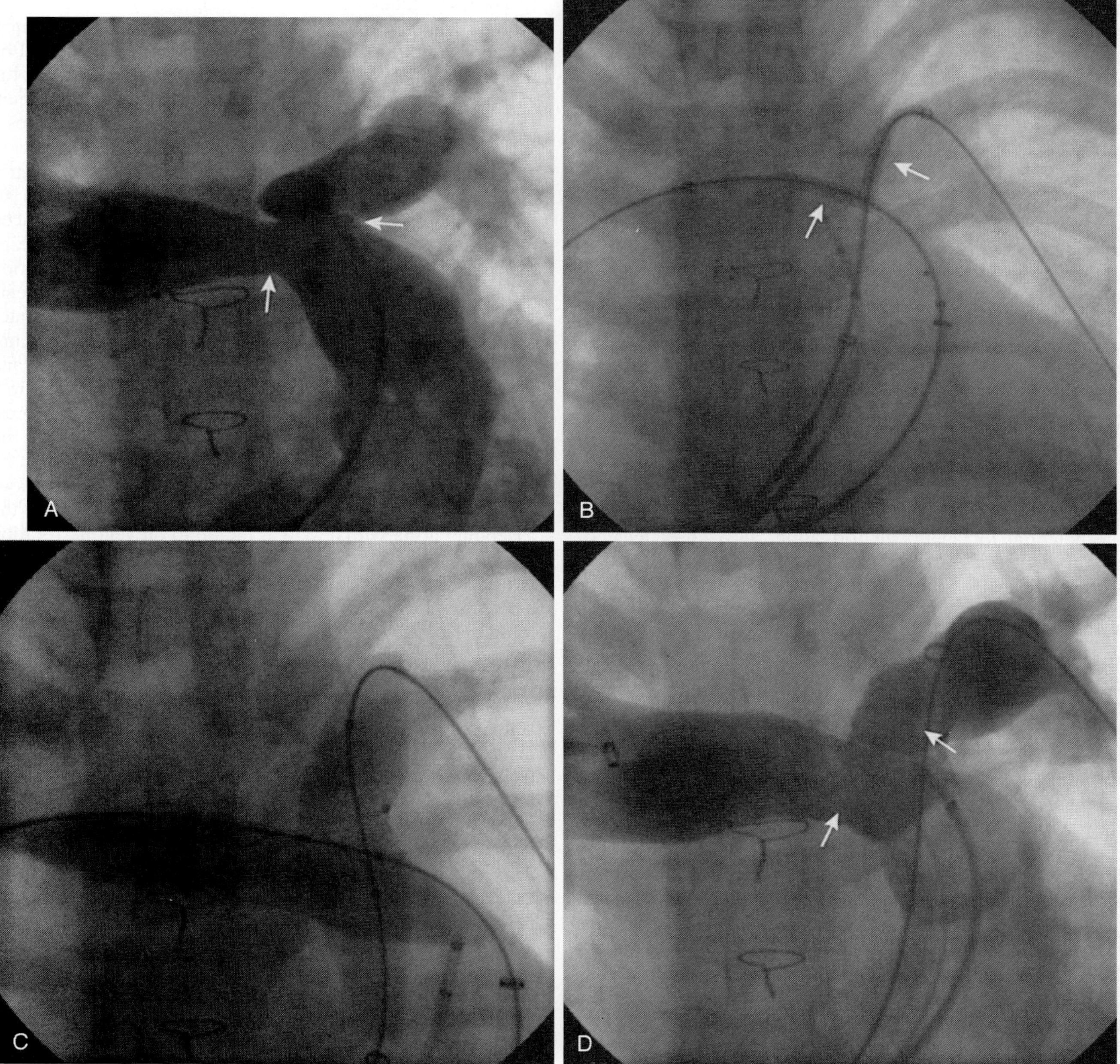

FIGURE 10–2 Stent implant for bilateral proximal pulmonary artery stenoses. **A,** Main pulmonary artery angiogram discloses the right and left proximal pulmonary artery stenoses *(arrows).* There is reflux of contrast material into the right ventricular outflow tract. **B,** Anteroposterior view of the positions of the right and left pulmonary artery stents *(arrows)* before expansion with the angioplasty balloons. The superstiff guide wires are identified in the distal right and left pulmonary arteries. The tips of the long sheaths have been withdrawn into the right ventricular outflow tract *(small circles).* **C,** The angioplasty balloons have been inflated simultaneously, expanding the right and left pulmonary artery stents. **D,** Main pulmonary artery angiogram confirms stent expansion *(arrows)* and improved caliber of the proximal right and left pulmonary arteries.

Coarctation of the Aorta

Coarctation of the aorta is a relatively common form of congenital heart disease with which there is a long surgical experience. The late results of surgical repair of coarctation of the aorta are not always completely satisfactory, particularly when the patient was initially operated in early infancy. A significant number of these patients will have persistent or recurrent obstruction at the aortic isthmus due to isthmic hypoplasia or at the site of previous coarctation repair.[68–70] When at the site of previous coarctation repair, the obstruction may be a persistence of the original membrane or it may be the suture line itself, either of which can be successfully treated by balloon angioplasty. Dilatation of recurrent coarctation of the aorta was one of the first lesions approached with balloon angioplasty.[71] This lesion was thought to be ideal for this procedure because the extensive surrounding scar tissue would provide extravascular support and some safety against bleeding and extension of wall tears.[13] The VACA Registry originally reported on the multicenter experience with dilation in 200 patients with residual or recurrent coarctation of the aorta in 1990.[51] In these patients, the peak systolic pressure difference across the aortic obstruction was decreased from 41.9 ± 19 mm Hg to 13.3 ± 12.1 mm Hg and the diameter of the recurrent coarctation site was increased from 5.2 ± 2.9 mm Hg to 8.9 ± 3.4 mm Hg. A good or excellent result was found in 78.4 percent (residual gradient < 20 mm Hg). Five patients (2.5 percent) died of complications related to the procedure, which included aortic rupture (n = 1), sudden death at 6 and 14 hours after the procedure with probable exaggerated vagal reactions (n = 2), cerebral vascular accident owing to carotid occlusion (n = 1), and persistent congestive heart failure unimproved by angioplasty (n = 1). The angioplasty success rate for recurrent coarctation of the aorta and low mortality compare well with surgical results for reoperation of recurrent coarctation of the aorta.[51]

Balloon angioplasty for native coarctation of the aorta remains more controversial because of concern regarding the potential for aneurysm formation, and subsequent potential difficulties in repairing these aneurysms. Histologic studies of excised human coarctation specimens from surgical repairs of native coarctation have demonstrated cystic medial necrosis of varying degrees in virtually all of the specimens, with severe changes in 67 percent.[72] There is extension of the necrosis into the aorta proximal or distal to the coarctation in 80 percent. This has been proposed as a part of the mechanism of late aneurysm formation after balloon dilatation. In 1981, Lock and coworkers[73] performed balloon angioplasty in seven explanted coarctation segments using a balloon approximately twice the size of the stenotic diameter and were able to increase the vessel diameter by 85 percent. However, four of the specimens had tears extending into the media, and three had complete transmedial tears. In vivo studies on an animal model with surgically created coarctation found less extensive tears of the media after angioplasty and some healing with time.[74] Balloon angioplasty was subsequently performed in children and young adults with native coarctation with variable results, including a continued incidence of aneurysm formation.[50, 75] The original VACA Registry report included the multicenter combined early experience with native coarctation in 140 patients, finding significant complications in 17 percent with 2 early and 6 late aneurysms.[50] The more recent experience at Texas Children's Hospital includes 102 patients with a median 36-month follow-up.[76] The success rate at time of catheterization in this group was 91.2 percent and intermediate-term success rate 77.2 percent (gradient < 20 mm Hg). These data included newborns, who have been shown to have a less successful long-term outcome due to persistence of reactive ductal tissue surrounding the coarctation and to transverse arch and isthmic hypoplasia.[76] There were only 2 aneurysms in the 102 patients at midterm follow-up.[76] This experience suggests improvement in native coarctation angioplasty outcomes, which may reflect improvement in techniques and equipment. Further long-term follow-up is necessary to know whether this procedure can match the low complication rate of operative intervention.

The technique for balloon angioplasty is the same for both native and recurrent coarctation. A complete catheterization including careful gradient measurements should be performed. Ideally, a catheter is positioned prograde in the ascending aorta via transseptal technique for both gradient measurements and angiography. This avoids repeated crossing of the coarctation site during and after angioplasty. A calibrated catheter or grid is filmed at the time of angiography for accurate vessel measurements. When a PDA or large collateral vessels are present, less emphasis is placed on gradient and more on the angiographic appearance of the coarctation itself. The discrete, shelflike coarctation represents the best lesion for successful dilatation. Patients with a long tubular coarctation probably are not candidates for balloon dilatation alone.[76] The narrowest adjacent diameter, regardless of location, is the limiting diameter and determines the diameter of the balloon used for dilatation. The aorta proximal to the coarctation is usually the most narrow site. The angioplasty balloon is selected to be no more than 1 to 2 mm greater than this measurement.

The patient should be anticoagulated using intravenous heparin. A stiff or superstiff wire is positioned in the ascending aorta with a loop at the tip to prevent perforation of the aorta or valve cusps or entrance into the coronary arteries as the procedure is performed. The angioplasty balloon is introduced through a sheath to minimize vessel trauma and advanced retrograde and centered over the coarctation shelf. The balloon is inflated for 5 to 10 seconds to its maximal recommended pressure while observing for a waist or circumferential narrowing from the coarctation. Inflations can be repeated after repositioning until the waist disappears with full inflation. The balloon should be carefully withdrawn from the angioplasty site in order not to increase trauma to the freshly dilated area. An end-hole diagnostic catheter is reintroduced over the curved superstiff wire, and the wire is withdrawn through it so that the wire itself does not tear the angioplasty site. The gradient is measured by either direct withdrawal or simultaneously, with the ascending aorta prograde catheter and the retrograde catheter. Angiography is repeated to visualize the result and to ensure that no dissection or aortic aneurysm has occurred. The patient should be kept well hydrated overnight to minimize the effects of hypovolemia, and persistent discomfort of any type should be considered seriously. Patient follow-up is mandatory and should include magnetic resonance imaging or catheterization with angiography within 1 to 2 years after angioplasty.

Until recently, there has not been much enthusiasm for stent implant as a therapy for coarctation of the aorta. Concerns have included the lack of stents large enough to be dilated to a normal or larger than normal adult aortic diameter and the large size arterial sheath (10 to 12 French) required for implant of large stents. It was obvious that the implant of a smaller stent that could not be dilated to an adult diameter would be creating a lesion worse than the original. To assess the possibility of stent implant for aortic coarctation, Morrow and colleagues implanted stents in the normal aortas of juvenile animals and then reexpanded the stents after vessel growth.[62] They then surgically created coarctation of the aorta in juvenile swine, performed angioplasty with stent implant, and successfully re-expanded the stents in these animals after growth.[77] Histopathologic specimens from the aortas did not suggest significant intimal or medial injury from the initial implantation or subsequent re-expansion of the stents. Diethrich and associates[78] subsequently implanted Palmaz iliac stents in two adult patents with coarctation, and Ebeid and coworkers[79] implanted the same stents in nine older children and adults, all with good short-term success. Palmaz stents that are larger and sturdier than the iliac stents have been developed and are now available in the United States. The relief of obstruction with these stents has been very good, but aneurysms with the stent implant have been reported in several cases. A larger experience, more information about the cause of these aneurysms, and longer follow-up will determine whether stent implant will be a good alternative for treatment of coarctation of the aorta.

Systemic Veins

Obstructions to systemic veins in patients with congenital heart disease are usually due to previous surgical intervention, indwelling intravenous lines, or cardiac catheterization. The most common venous obstruction occurs in the upper limb of the baffle created for superior vena caval flow after either the Mustard or the Senning atrial switch operation for transposition of the great vessels. The inferior vena caval limb of the baffle may also become obstructed, although this is much less common. These operations have now been replaced by the arterial switch procedure at most institutions. However, many patients who had one of the atrial switch operations are now adults. If superior vena cava obstruction occurs, symptoms and findings may include upper trunk and head and neck venous distention, headache, and communicating hydrocephalus. Patients may be asymptomatic with severe upper limb baffle obstruction, but they need this channel for transvenous pacemaker implantation because of arrhythmias common to atrial switch patients. Obstruction to inferior vena caval flow may cause abdominal ascites or peripheral edema. Any of these symptoms or signs in a patient who has had a "venous switch" repair should be investigated with a detailed cardiac catheterization. The surgical approach to these problems requires complete revision of the baffle, frequently with less than satisfactory results owing to dense adhesions and scarring. For these reasons, interventional pediatric cardiologists have been aggressive with procedures to dilate and stent systemic venous inflow problems. Reports of balloon angioplasty for superior vena cava obstruction following Mustard or Senning operation indicated some improvement in vessel diameter after this procedure, but the improvement was frequently only temporary.[80, 81] The use of intravascular stents in systemic venous and systemic venous baffle obstructions has now become the treatment of choice.[55, 82, 83] Indications for stent implant have been expanded to include patients of all ages with superior vena cava syndrome due to malignancy, and this has been very successful.[84]

For stent implant in systemic veins, the diameters of the stenosed segment and the normal vessel proximal and distal to the obstruction are measured by angiography. The obstruction is then crossed with an end-hole catheter. In cases of complete occlusion, the area can be crossed by advancing the end of a glide wire out of an end-hole catheter or a long dilator and through the occluded area. A transseptal needle can be used if more direction and force are needed to penetrate the obstruction.[85] To help in directing the wire or transseptal needle, angiography must be obtained both above and below the obstruction. It is also helpful to leave a catheter in the most distal reachable part of the vessel on the opposite side of the obstruction so that the wire or needle can be aimed at it from the puncturing side. Once a wire has been introduced across the obstructed area, predilatation with a smaller angioplasty balloon will frequently be necessary so that a long transseptal sheath can be introduced across the obstruction for stent implant.[83] The patient should receive heparin before stent implant. The angioplasty balloon selected for stent procedure should be approximately the size of the vessel proximal or distal to the obstruction, whichever is *smaller*.[83] The stent is mounted on the angioplasty balloon and delivered in the usual fashion (discussed previously). After stent implant in systemic veins, the patient should remain on aspirin for at least 6 months. Although extreme long-term follow-up is not yet available for stents placed in systemic veins, lack of symptoms and continued patency of these vessels by echocardiography and early recatheterization for as long as 8 years suggest that there will be good long-term results.[83]

Pulmonary Veins

Pulmonary vein stenosis is very rare and commonly occurs with other congenital heart disease.[86, 87] This lesion has been the most discouraging of all of the stenotic lesions for the cardiovascular surgeon and for the interventional pediatric cardiologist. Balloon dilatation has been attempted in many cases with some immediate success but recurrence of the stenosis within weeks or months.[13, 87] Stent implant has been similarly unsuccessful in the limited number of pediatric patients in whom it has been tried.[88] This is partially due to technical reasons related to the small size of the vessels and difficulty of approach. Progression of underlying sclerotic disease of the affected veins deep within the parenchyma has also been implicated in the failure of all treatments attempted with this disease. Pulmonary venous channel obstruction after Mustard surgery has been successfully treated with stent implant, and this should be considered as the treatment of choice when this problem occurs in adult patients after either of the atrial switch operations.[89]

PATENT DUCTUS ARTERIOSUS

PDA is very common. Occasionally, a PDA can be large in childhood and result in congestive heart failure or pulmonary hypertension. More commonly, PDAs are small or moderate in size, and their main implications for the patient are those of endocarditis and lifelong left ventricular volume overload. Although risk of operative intervention for PDA is generally "low," it does involve the pain and morbidity of surgery; and the risk is higher in the adult patient who has developed heart failure or pulmonary hypertension or has additional coronary artery disease. Surgery is further complicated by calcification of the PDA in older adults.

Interventional cardiologists have been interested in occluding PDAs nonsurgically for a long time. Porstmann and collegues[90] first introduced a catheterization technique for closure of the ductus arteriosus in 1967. The procedure was complicated and required a very large arterial sheath, which limited its usefulness to teenage and adult patients. Rashkind, who developed the atrial septostomy balloon, also developed a device for closure of the PDA.[91] This device was a small umbrella that attached to the ductus by tiny hooks at the ends of the umbrella arms. The first successful use of this early device was published in 1979.[91]

Rashkind Patent Ductus Arteriosus Occluding Device

The Rashkind PDA occluding device was changed to a double umbrella that began clinical trials in 1981. The double-umbrella device implants itself in the ductus by a spring mechanism of the arms that causes them to expand against the vessel wall at each end of the ductus. This device comes in two sizes, which have either opposing 12- or 17-mm-diameter polyurethane foam discs mounted on spring-loaded stainless steel frames. The umbrellas are collapsed away from each other into a specialized loader for folding and loading and then withdrawn into a delivery catheter for delivery. The smaller occluder and delivery system requires an 8 French and the larger an 11 French sheath. The device may be delivered from either the arterial or the venous system, although the venous approach is preferred. An end-hole catheter is first advanced from the femoral vein through the right heart, through the PDA, and into the descending aorta. The catheter in the descending aorta is replaced with a superstiff wire. The end-hole catheter is removed. The appropriate long sheath and dilator are inserted over the wire and placed across the PDA into the upper descending aorta. The occluding device is delivered through the ductus within the long sheath. The distal umbrella is opened on the aortic end of the ductus, the entire system is withdrawn until this umbrella "seats" against the aortic end of the ductus, and the other disc is opened on the pulmonary side of the narrowest portion of the PDA. The tension of the opposing spring mechanisms of the two umbrellas at each end of the ductus fixes the device in position. Once secure in the ductus arteriosus, the device is released from the delivery catheter. Complete closure of the ductus arteriosus is accomplished by thrombus and tissue growth into the fabric of the device.

Of all the therapeutic catheterization procedures and devices for congenital heart lesions, the Rashkind PDA occluding device has had the most extensive and thorough clinical investigation. A collaborative study, which eventually included 12 participating centers, was performed to evaluate this device, and these investigators reported on over 700 PDA occlusion procedures in the United States.[92] Experience at Texas Children's Hospital since the last major modification of the Rashkind occluding device and delivery technique includes 200 procedures with an implant rate of 98 percent and a *total* occlusion of 88 percent.[93] The delivery of the device was improved and now is accomplished in virtually all patients over 6 or 7 kg. Most of the residual leaks after successful implant are tiny, not audible, and detectable only by aortic angiography or by high-quality echocardiographic Doppler studies. It is quite possible that "coil" embolization can supplement the Rashkind device for complete occlusion in those few patients with a small residual PDA. Embolization was the major complication in the early use of the device, and this problem had been virtually eliminated. There were rare cases of hemolysis and one case of endocarditis after implantation of the device. These problems occurred only in patients with major leaks after the implant. In spite of the large and positive experience with the Rashkind device for PDA occlusion, the U.S. Food and Drug Administration (FDA) did not approve it for clinical use in the United States; it has subsequently been abandoned for introduction or possible use in the United States where it was conceived and developed. It is available in most major centers outside of the United States and continues to be widely used for the large, short PDA.

Patent Ductus Arteriosus Gianturco Coil Occlusion Device

The success of the Rashkind device and particularly its subsequent removal from availability in the United States stimulated an intense interest in alternate techniques and devices for nonsurgical correction of the PDA. The most successful of the devices and techniques to come from that interest has been the Gianturco coil, which was already FDA-approved for other uses.[94] Moore and Cambier and associates first described the use of the Gianturco coil experimentally and then clinically for the PDA.[95] The use of the Gianturco coil with various techniques for PDA occlusion has proliferated over a short period, and this method has now been accepted as the standard therapy for small and moderate PDAs in this country and abroad.[96, 97] This procedure is most applicable when the PDA is "conical," with a discrete narrowing toward the pulmonary end, and is less likely to be successful with either short or large tubular PDAs. Fortunately, most PDAs are small to moderate with some discrete stenosis. This technique offers the advantages of easy availability of the coils in a variety of sizes and low cost of the coils. The standard Gianturco coil is usually delivered from the arterial approach for PDA occlusion with low-profile catheters that allow delivery of 0.038-inch caliber coils but can be inserted through a 4 or 5 French arterial sheath.

The technique for coil occlusion of a PDA requires careful angiography of the ductus arteriosus and measurement of the narrowest diameter. A coil is selected that is greater than twice the diameter of the narrowest part of the PDA.[97] This is followed by retrograde crossing of the PDA with an appropriate end-hole catheter for coil delivery. The coil is advanced until one or more loops of the coil are extruded into the pulmonary artery side of the ductus. The catheter is then withdrawn into the aortic ampulla while simultaneously extruding the coil from the delivery catheter so that the remaining two to four loops are delivered into the aortic ampulla of the ductus. The closure rate with this technique is up to 97 percent in some series.[96, 97] Occasionally, there is still some residual ductus shunt after placement of the first coil, which may necessitate placement of additional coils. The procedure for the additional coils is the same, but particular care must be taken not to dislodge the first coil during catheter manipulations. A disadvantage of this technique is the lack of control of withdrawal of the coil once extrusion is started, which may lead to occasional coil embolization. Usually, the coil can be retrieved from the pulmonary circulation if coil embolization occurs.[97]

Modifications of the coil delivery technique have included methods of attaching the delivery wire to the coil to enhance delivery with potential for retraction of the coil if delivery is not optimum.[98] Outside of the United States, these are standard, approved systems with specifically designed, effective screw attachment and release mechanisms that have simplified the technique and made it safer and more effective. Unfortunately, these systems are not approved for clinical use in the United States. A different attach-release mechanism for the coils has been introduced in the United States. However, the coil wires for this system are smaller in diameter and there are fewer "fibers" on each coil. As a consequence, these coils are less robust and less occlusive and have not been very popular. In order to increase the occlusion and stability of these coils, they have been used with the simultaneous delivery of two (or more) coils at the same time through separate catheters. The separate catheters can be from the same vessel approach or one catheter can be inserted from the artery and one catheter from the vein.

In this country, the snare technique for delivering the coil(s) has become more popular. Figure 10–3 demonstrates PDA occlusion using the snare technique. For this modification, the 5 French coil delivery catheter is passed retrograde through the ductus arteriosus into the main pulmonary artery. A snare catheter is advanced from the femoral vein and used to snare the end of the retrograde catheter in the main pulmonary artery. The coil is then advanced through the retrograde catheter until the tip of the coil is extruded 1 to 2 mm out of the tip of the delivery catheter into the main pulmonary artery. The snare is allowed to slip to the tip of the retrograde catheter in order to snare the exposed end of the coil just at the point of extrusion from the tip of the catheter in the main pulmonary artery. The coil and its exact positioning can then be totally controlled by advancing the snare catheter and simultaneously withdrawing the retrograde delivery catheter. A half-loop of coil is held by the snare in the main pulmonary artery, and the rest of the coil is delivered into the arterial side of the ductus ampulla. Even after the coil is fully extruded, it can be pulled farther into the ductus or removed using the venous snare if positioning is not ideal. Angiography is performed while the coil is still held by the snare catheter. If delivery of a second coil is necessary, the retrograde catheter can be repositioned in the main pulmonary artery while still having snare control of the first coil, which avoids the risk of embolization of the first coil. Although a little more complex and time consuming and having the additional expense of the snare catheter, this technique does allow better control of the procedure at all stages.

Gianturco-Grifka Vascular Occlusion Device

The Gianturco-Grifka vascular occlusion device (GGVOD) was developed as a modification of the coil procedure. The GGVOD is applicable for the occlusion of larger, tubular, and higher velocity communications.[99] It has been approved in the United States and is in limited use for PDAs and other abnormal tubular vascular structures. The GGVODs are nylon sacks of varying sizes that are filled (packed) during the procedure with specific lengths of spring guide wire to form tightly packed, occlusive masses within the tubular vessel. For ductus occlusion using the GGVOD, angiography is performed to carefully measure the PDA length as well as the diameter. To use the GGVOD, the vessel to be occluded must be 0.5 mm narrower and 1.5 times the length of the "sack" to be used. All sizes of the GGVOD are delivered through an 8 French system. The 8 French long sheath is introduced antegrade in the usual fashion, and the tip of the sheath is positioned through the ductus into the descending aorta. The empty sack is advanced through the sheath to the aortic ampulla and is partially filled with coil. The sheath and sack are then withdrawn into the tubular portion of the ductus toward the pulmonary end, where the sack is completely filled with coil. Once one is satisfied with the sack position as well as its stability and occlusion of the PDA, the sack is released from the delivery catheter. The sack is totally removable until it is released. It has proved very effective for the moderate-size and large tubular PDAs.

Other Devices for Patent Ductus Arteriosus Occlusion

In addition to the Rashkind device, the various modifications of the coil, and the GGVOD, there are other devices in the rest of the world specifically developed for PDA occlusion.[100] One of these is the Redel Duct-Occlud Device, which has had favorable results outside of the United States and is beginning trials in the United States at this time. The Duct-Occlud Device is a stiff, preformed, tight double coil that comes in various sizes to fit various sizes and shapes of PDAs. It also comes with a very elaborate attach-release-delivery mechanism that gives total control over the delivery of the device until release. There are also a number of atrial septal defect (ASD) occlusion devices in various clinical trials that have been adapted for the closure of the large PDA. These are discussed under the ASD devices.

Closure of Abnormal Vascular Communications

Embolization of abnormal or persistent arterial or arteriovenous structures has been performed since the late 1960s.[93] These embolization techniques were originally developed and perfected by the vascular radiologists to treat abnormal bleeding related to the gastrointestinal tract and central nervous system, particularly in "end artery" vessels. Many materials and devices have been used for these peripheral

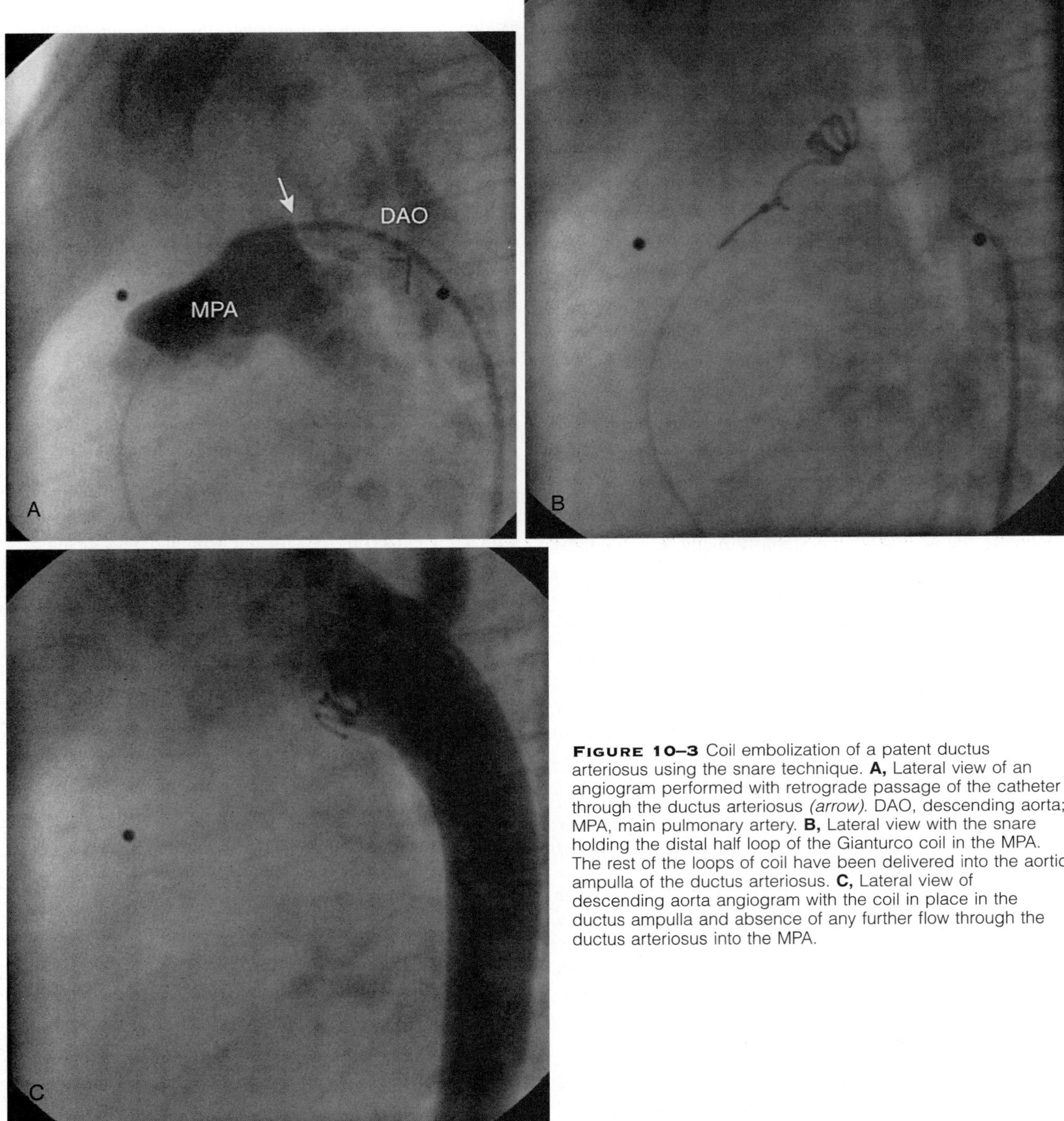

FIGURE 10–3 Coil embolization of a patent ductus arteriosus using the snare technique. **A,** Lateral view of an angiogram performed with retrograde passage of the catheter through the ductus arteriosus *(arrow).* DAO, descending aorta; MPA, main pulmonary artery. **B,** Lateral view with the snare holding the distal half loop of the Gianturco coil in the MPA. The rest of the loops of coil have been delivered into the aortic ampulla of the ductus arteriosus. **C,** Lateral view of descending aorta angiogram with the coil in place in the ductus ampulla and absence of any further flow through the ductus arteriosus into the MPA.

occlusions, including the patient's own clotted blood, Gelfoam, colloidal plugs, "glues," detachable balloons, and coil occlusion devices. In patients with congenital heart disease, there are frequently abnormal aorta to pulmonary collateral vessels or persistent, surgically created systemic to pulmonary artery shunts associated with complex cyanotic lesions. It is appropriate to occlude these vessels when there is competitive flow between the collateral and the normal pulmonary blood flow, particularly when the major defect has been, or is to be, corrected. These communications historically required surgical division during the corrective procedure or as a separate procedure. When surgically managed along with intracardiac repair, the closure of these defects may significantly prolong the surgery and recovery. Occasionally, teenagers and adults with congenital heart disease will develop hemoptysis from spontaneous bleeding of these abnormal collaterals and will require urgent intervention.

Gianturco coils are most commonly used for occlusion of aorta to pulmonary collateral vessels in patients with congenital cardiac defects.[94] These coils are available in a wide variety of sizes. Coils have a wire dimension similar to that of spring guide wires (0.025 to 0.052 inch), a length (2.5 to 15 cm) that ultimately determines the number of loops formed on release, and a loop dimension, which is the predetermined diameter (2 to 15 mm) of the loops formed when the coil is released. For occlusion of abnormal tubular vascular communications, the coil to be used should have a loop diameter approximately 1.5 to 2 times the size of the vessel to be occluded. The delivered coil wire should elongate *slightly* and form an irregular strand, not a "doughnut" circle, in the vessel to be occluded. To deliver the coil, an end-hole catheter with adequate internal diameter for coil delivery is positioned within the vessel as near as possible to the site to be embolized. The coil is packaged as a straight length of wire in a straight metal "loader," used to introduce it into the delivery catheter.

The straightened coil is advanced through the catheter by pushing it with a spring guide wire of the same diameter as the coil wire. When the coil is extruded out of the end of the catheter, it coils like a small pigtail, usually forming three to five circular loops. Once any part of the coil has been advanced past the tip of the catheter, there is no way of withdrawing it back into the delivery catheter. The Gianturco coil occludes the vessel by creating a mass of wire and attached strands of fabric that stimulate thrombus formation. Ideal vessels for Gianturco coil occlusion have a discrete narrowing where the coil can be fixed in place. Without a discrete stenosis, the coils have a potential to migrate farther through the vessel, so that care must be taken in vessel measurement. Without a distal narrowing, coils can be used only in vessels which are up to 7 to 8 mm in diameter when distended. It is often necessary to place several coils in a larger vessel to achieve complete occlusion.[100] For vessels greater than 7 to 8 mm in diameter, coils should be used only in conjunction with other intravascular occlusion devices, especially if there is no discrete stenosis.

Most abnormal aorta to pulmonary communications can now be occluded with Gianturco coils. Other lesions in which Gianturco coils may be useful are arteriovenous fistulas, including systemic coronary-cameral communications and pulmonary arteriovenous fistulas. In both of these lesions, it is critical to advance the delivery catheter as distally as possible beyond more proximal significant normal or vital branches of the vessel before considering coil delivery. It is again important to deliver the coil at a stenotic site or end vessel to reduce the danger of coil embolization through the fistula to a vital systemic structure.

Occasionally, other devices have been used to occlude abnormal vascular channels in patients with congenital heart disease. In 1987, Lock and coworkers[101] described the use of the Rashkind PDA occluder for the closure of a variety of persistent, abnormal vascular communications in very complex congenital heart lesions. These defects included persistent left superior vena cava to the left atrium; persistent systemic to pulmonary artery shunts in patients who had undergone tetralogy of Fallot or pulmonary atresia repair; recurrent systemic venous to right atrium or inferior vena cava channels in postoperative Glenn patients; persistent systemic venous to pulmonary venous communications in patients who had Fontan operations; and persistent atrial communications in patients with right-to-left shunt after repair of complex defects. All of these patients had symptoms from their abnormal communications and were at significantly greater risk for any further surgical intervention. In any defect of this type, the nonsurgical transcatheter approach should be considered. Thoughtful and innovative interventions in these types of patients can significantly improve their quality and length of life.

ATRIAL SEPTAL DEFECT OCCLUSIONS

Background and General Considerations

An ASD usually does not cause problems in childhood, but it may have more serious implications in adult patients. These include the development of congestive heart failure, arrhythmia, paradoxical embolism, or rarely, pulmonary vascular disease. The diagnosis of ASD can be missed in early childhood because of the low-intensity murmur and lack of symptoms, only to have the patient present in adolescence or later with a murmur, symptoms, or abnormal studies. Owing to its significant late complications and, at the same time, relative ease of catheter approach, ASD was the first septal defect to be considered for an occlusion device. King and Mills[102] developed an effective double-umbrella device in 1974 and used it in several patients. Their ASD occlusion device never gained wide acceptance because it required a large delivery system and was rather rigid, limiting its use to adult-sized patients. The few patients treated with this device are still doing well and provide a perspective about the long-term follow-up of catheter-occluded ASDs.

The next major development in catheter closure of ASDs began in 1977 at the same time as the collaborative study on PDAs. At that time, Rashkind and Cuaso[103] employed a device that was a hooked, single umbrella delivered through a smaller catheter system. This device was implanted in humans with ASD for a short time under an investigational protocol. Its use was discontinued because the tiny hooks would often become attached prematurely to structures within the left atrium before the septum could be engaged, which led to erroneous placement in some cases. Although abandoned even for clinical trials, this device stimulated additional development in the area of ASD closure.

Lock and colleagues[104] used experience from the already developed PDA devices to create the next ASD occlusion device. They first used a larger version of the Rashkind PDA double umbrella that did not "clamp" on the septum sufficiently. Their next device added "hinges" or joints to each of the umbrella arms and employed woven Dacron as the umbrella fabric instead of the earlier polyurethane foam. This ASD device had the appearance of a "clamshell" when viewed on edge and was marketed as the *clamshell device*. With this device, an effective delivery system and technique were developed that are still employed with some of the current ASD occlusion devices.

The Bard Clamshell Septal Occluder underwent an FDA Investigational Device Exemption (IDE) protocol clinical trial in five centers and was implanted in 545 patients with 97 percent success.

The occlusion umbrellas were available in 17-, 23-, 28-, 33-, and 40-mm sizes. These measurements represented the maximal transverse diameter of the umbrella occluder device. Because the clamshell umbrella had no centering mechanism, it could position itself entirely to one side of the center of the ASD. For this reason, it was recommended that the clamshell device be at least twice the stretched diameter of the ASD, so the radius of the device by itself would not pull through the defect but could occlude the defect. These ASD devices were delivered with an 11 French delivery catheter through an 11 French long delivery sheath. At follow-up, 64 percent of implanted patients had complete closure of the ASD, and 34 percent had only a very small residual shunt.[105] Unfortunately, on follow-up x-rays, fractures of device legs were identified in some of these patients. The fractures had no clinical consequences on long-term follow-up. Four asymptomatic patients with protrusion of a fractured leg against an adjacent wall developed a mass on the wall by echocardiography. This led to surgery for the four patients. Although the masses turned out to be benign, fibrous, "callous-like" structures, this finding plus the "unknowns" of the fractures led to the withdrawal of the device in the original study. Even though it was removed from clinical trials, the success of the clamshell device demonstrated unequivocally that selected ASDs could be safely and effectively closed nonsurgically. This stimulated a proliferation of new ideas and designs for devices for ASD closure, many of which are employed in Europe and are in trials in the United States now.

General Procedure for Atrial Septal Defect Closure

The suitability of an ASD for closure must be determined during cardiac catheterization with very accurate sizing of the defect. The standard transthoracic echocardiogram is useful in screening patients to confirm the diagnosis and location of the defect and to exclude other intracardiac defects. It is also useful to rule out sinus venosus, ostium primum, and very large ASDs that would be unsuitable for transcatheter closure. The transthoracic echocardiogram *cannot* unequivocally determine the size or suitability of the ASD for transcatheter closure. The transesophageal echocardiogram (TEE) is more accurate for sizing and localizing the ASD, but even it does not correlate accurately enough in borderline cases with the size found at catheterization to make an absolute noninvasive determination of appropriateness for transcatheter closure.

The catheterization procedure is similar for all of the ASD devices currently in trials in the United States. If a patient is considered a possible candidate for ASD occlusion, strict "operating room" sterile precautions should be observed in the catheterization laboratory. Sheaths should be placed in each femoral vein and a needle or dilator in the femoral artery for monitoring. A detailed right heart catheterization is performed to document the presence of the ASD and determine the magnitude of the shunt flow. An angiocardiographic catheter is introduced and advanced to the mouth of the right upper pulmonary vein for angiography. A good angulation for this angiogram is a shallow four-chamber view, with either camera at approximately 30 to 45 degrees left anterior oblique and 25 to 45 degrees cranial angulation. This should produce a good on-edge view of the atrial septum and visualization of the size of the ASD. If the septum is not precisely cut on edge by the first angiogram, it is repeated with different x-ray tube angulation until the septal defect is clearly demonstrated. An appropriate grid or sizing device should also be filmed for defect measurement.

The TEE probe should be introduced by this time and satisfactory imaging obtained to assist with defect measurement and later visualization during implant. If the ASD is suitable for catheter closure, heparin, 50 to 100 units/kg in children or 3000 to 5000 units in adults, is administered to prevent thrombus formation on the wire or delivery catheter or within the large delivery sheath. The right venous sheath is replaced with a 10 or 11 French short sheath with a side port and backbleed valve. An end-hole catheter is introduced through this sheath and advanced through the right heart, through the ASD, and out into the left pulmonary vein. With extreme care to avoid the introduction of air, an exchange length 0.038-inch guide wire is advanced through this catheter into the distal pulmonary vein and the catheter is withdrawn. *Accurate balloon sizing* is next performed to determine the "stretched" size of the ASD. A 33-mm sizing-balloon catheter (Meditech occlusion balloon catheter) is calibrated outside the body by inflation with 1-ml increments of up to 6 ml of diluted contrast material while measuring the exact balloon diameter with each increment of fluid. After calibration, the deflated sizing-balloon catheter is advanced over the exchange wire into the left atrium. The balloon is positioned in the left atrium and inflated with dilute contrast material to reach a size expected to just occlude the ASD. The balloon catheter is gently withdrawn toward the right atrium while the wire is held in place. During this careful withdrawal, the balloon is observed on the fluoroscopy screen for distortion or indentation by the edges of the ASD. If the balloon pulls through the ASD, the deflated balloon is readvanced into the left atrium, an additional milliliter of dilute fluid is used to fill the balloon, and the sizing procedure is repeated. If the balloon is not deformed by the septum when inflated to a 20-mm diameter, then the ASD is too large for safe transcatheter closure. The TEE is particularly helpful for identifying the catheters and sizing balloons within the atria as they are being positioned.

After sizing of the ASD, the inflated sizing balloon is used to occlude the ASD; and the atrial septum is again inspected by TEE to verify that there is occlusion, that there is an adequate rim of septum both above and below the ASD for the device to deploy, that there is enough room to accommodate the length of the device frame in all directions after deployment, and that there are no additional ASDs. A right upper pulmonary vein angiogram can be performed with the sizing balloon in place. This angiogram will demonstrate the adequacy of the balloon sizing and, of more importance, confirm the presence of additional small ASDs or suggest a peculiar shape of the ASD that could prohibit closure with a "square" device.

The sizing catheter is next withdrawn over the wire, and the long 11 French delivery sheath is advanced over the wire into the left atrium. The sheath is then very meticulously cleared of any air or clots. To verify the exact position of the tip of the sheath in the left atrium and confirm that it is not entrapped in the atrial appendage or a pulmonary vein, a slow hand injection of contrast medium can be performed through the sheath. The position of the sheath passing through the septum should also be clearly identified by TEE. It is advisable not to open the ASD occlusion device or the delivery catheter until all the preceding steps have been completed. All ASD devices are expensive and should not remain in the collapsed or folded configuration any longer than absolutely necessary to prevent loss of spring. Figure 10–4 depicts the ASD closure procedure using a CardioSEAL device.

CardioSEAL Device

The CardioSEAL device (Nitinol Medical Technologies) is a totally new version of the original clamshell device (Fig. 10–5). It is produced by a new manufacturer and has a new design, and the arms are manufactured with new MP35n metal alloy that is more flexible and corrosion resistant. Although the device is totally new, it is delivered with the same technique established with the clamshell device. In in vitro studies and animal trials, the new material and design have eliminated the clinical problem of strut fractures. The CardioSEAL device itself consists of opposing umbrellas made of woven Dacron. The two umbrellas are attached at their centers. Each umbrella has four metal arms of MP35n alloy, and each arm has *two* joints along its length in addition to the central hinge point. The two umbrellas are attached in their open positions with the concavity of each facing the other. The two umbrellas fold away from each other for delivery. The CardioSEAL devices are available in 17-, 23-, 28-, 33-, and 40-mm diameters. All sizes are delivered through an 11 French long Mullins sheath.

The CardioSEAL device is supplied in the open position and must be loaded into the delivery catheter. The tips of the distal arms are attached to a pair of sutures that, in turn, pass through a loading device. As with the original clamshell device, the size chosen needs to be at least twice the diameter of the ASD, but it cannot exceed the diameter of the septum itself. The device is attached to the delivery wire/catheter at the center of the proximal umbrella. The CardioSEAL device is folded for delivery by drawing it into the loading device using the sutures attached to the distal arms. It then is loaded by withdrawing it from the loading device into the delivery pod. The long Mullins sheath is positioned in the *left atrium* with the tip between the left pulmonary veins and the left atrial appendage. The delivery catheter with its pod is then introduced into the long sheath and advanced until the pod is in the area of the *right* atrium. With the distal end of the *sheath* fixed in the left atrium and the distal end of the delivery catheter and pod fixed in the right atrium, the delivery wire is advanced, which advances the device into the sheath. This and subsequent maneuvers are observed very closely with both fluoroscopy and TEE. The sheath now functions like a curved extension of the pod and delivery catheter. As the device is slowly advanced beyond the end of the sheath, the distal umbrella will spring open in the left atrium. When all of the distal legs are confirmed to be open and not entangled in the left atrium by both fluoroscopy and TEE, the entire system is withdrawn as a single unit toward the right atrium. Because of the usual and significant "malalignment" of the long axis of the delivery sheath to the perpendicular axis of the septum, the surface of the distal umbrella usually will not align even close to parallel to the septal surface. The more cephalic arms will touch the septum well before the caudal arms and can be visualized against the septum by echocardiography. No attempt should be made to have the more caudal arms approximate the septum because this will cause one or more of the cephalic arms to pull through the septum.

Once the left atrial side of the device is in satisfactory position with the initial legs against the septum, the delivery wire and delivery catheter are fixed in place. The sheath alone is withdrawn, allowing the proximal legs to spring open on the right atrial side of the defect. The device usually aligns itself better on the septum and in a relatively secure position once both umbrellas have been opened. However, while the device is still attached to the delivery wire, all of the legs usually will not come in contact with the septum. When assured by TEE and fluoroscopy of a correct position of all of the legs on the appropriate sides of the septum, the release mechanism is activated. This allows the delivery catheter to pull away from the device. The device usually will spring away and "align" with the septum as it is released. The proper position of the device on the septum and the degree of closure are confirmed by TEE. A right atrial angiocardiogram is obtained with the heart in a four-chamber view to image the right atrial surface of the device as well as the left atrial side during the recirculation phase of the contrast medium through the left heart. Manipulation of the angiocatheter into the pulmonary artery for angiography after the implant is unnecessary and potentially dangerous because of the possibility of dislodging the newly implanted device.

Angel Wings Device

The DAS Angel Wings device (Microvena Corp.) (Fig. 10–6) has undergone a successful FDA clinical pilot trial in the United States. It is in the process of FDA IDE trials in the United States, and it has completed trials and is commercially available in Europe. Not too much information is available except to the investigators about the characteristics of the device in a clinical situation. The device is a square double umbrella with two opposing occluding surfaces of woven Dacron. Both umbrellas have a fairly rigid *square* frame of nitinol wire that does not require support arms from the center. The Dacron umbrellas are connected at their centers by a circular suture line that joins the two fabric squares together. This circular suture line creates a central ring that varies in size according to the size of the ASD and tends to fill the defect and center the device within it. The two umbrellas or discs, once deployed, act to hold the device in place by their contact

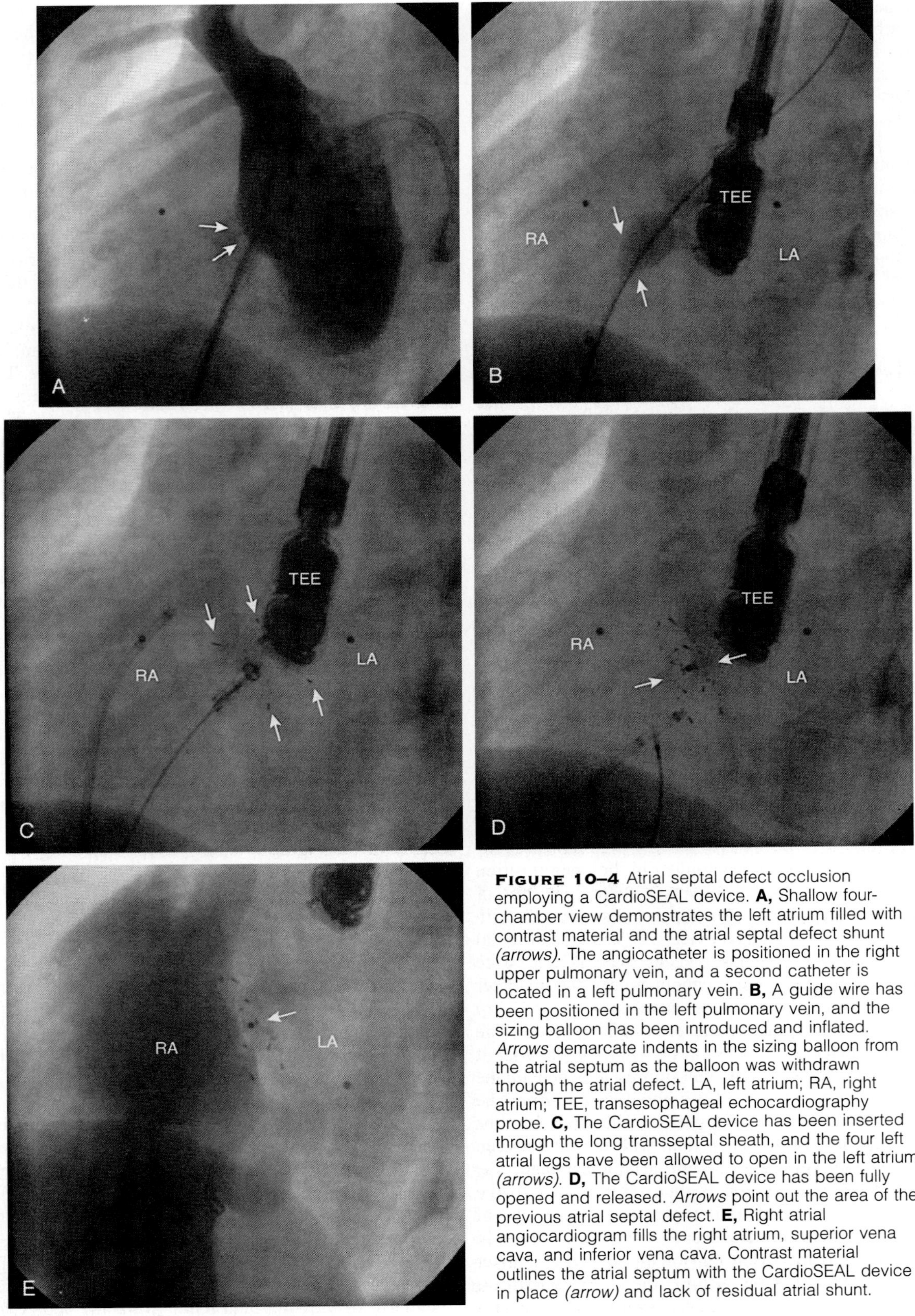

FIGURE 10–4 Atrial septal defect occlusion employing a CardioSEAL device. **A,** Shallow four-chamber view demonstrates the left atrium filled with contrast material and the atrial septal defect shunt *(arrows)*. The angiocatheter is positioned in the right upper pulmonary vein, and a second catheter is located in a left pulmonary vein. **B,** A guide wire has been positioned in the left pulmonary vein, and the sizing balloon has been introduced and inflated. *Arrows* demarcate indents in the sizing balloon from the atrial septum as the balloon was withdrawn through the atrial defect. LA, left atrium; RA, right atrium; TEE, transesophageal echocardiography probe. **C,** The CardioSEAL device has been inserted through the long transseptal sheath, and the four left atrial legs have been allowed to open in the left atrium *(arrows)*. **D,** The CardioSEAL device has been fully opened and released. *Arrows* point out the area of the previous atrial septal defect. **E,** Right atrial angiocardiogram fills the right atrium, superior vena cava, and inferior vena cava. Contrast material outlines the atrial septum with the CardioSEAL device in place *(arrow)* and lack of residual atrial shunt.

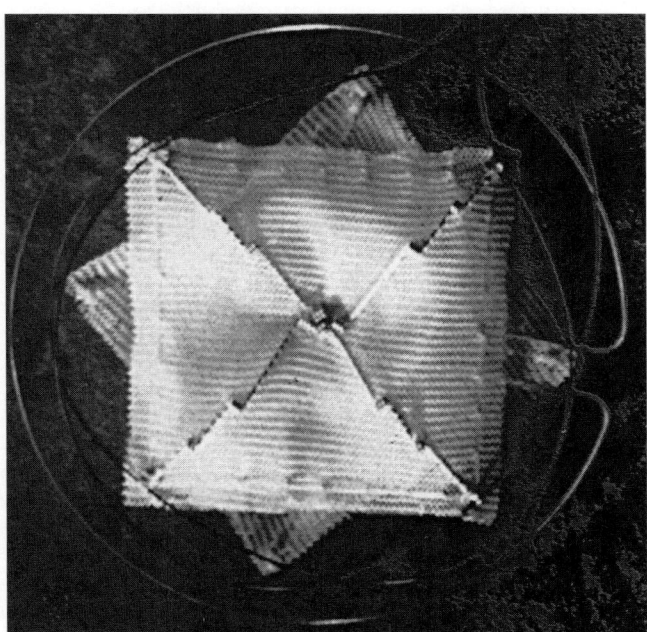

FIGURE 10–5 CardioSEAL device.

on the opposite surfaces of the atrial septum. These devices come in a variety of sizes up to 40 mm in diameter.

The technique of sizing the defect and delivery through a long sheath are similar to those of the CardioSEAL device. The Angel Wings device also requires a 2:1 ratio of device to defect size. An 11 or 12 French delivery sheath is used for deployment. The delivery catheter for the Angel Wings is more complex, and the rigid design of the device frame requires a fair amount of mechanical force to deliver the two umbrellas. The attachment mechanism of the device to the delivery catheter is at one corner of the right atrial umbrella. As a consequence, the device tends to spring out eccentrically when it is advanced out of the delivery catheter. Once the first umbrella is opened, neither of the umbrellas can be withdrawn back into the delivery catheter, and the operator is committed to the delivery of that particular device. A proposed approach for removal of a deployed but misplaced Angel Wings device by a transcatheter technique requires the introduction of an additional large sheath from the internal jugular approach. A retrieval apparatus capable of grasping the Angle Wings device exactly at a *corner* of the device is introduced. If the device has not been released from the delivery system, the corner of the device opposite from the attached corner is grasped with the retrieval device. Traction on these opposite corners allows the square device to be stretched longitudinally into an elongated rhomboid that can be withdrawn into the jugular sheath. If the device has been fully deployed and released, it must be re-caught by one *corner,* and then the opposite *corner* must be grasped with a separate grabbing device. Again, traction is applied in the opposite directions to stretch the square from the opposite corners into a rhomboid that can be pulled into one of the two sheaths. If catching the two opposite corners cannot be accomplished, the patient will have to undergo surgery for device removal. This retrieval mechanism is still untested, and reports of erosion and perforation of adjacent structures by the rigid frame have placed this device on a temporary hold for design changes.

Sideris Button Device

Another device that has undergone at least one FDA clinical pilot study in the United States is the Sideris Button Device (Custom Medical Devices, Athens, Greece). This device has been available longer than many of the other current ASD devices and has had extensive use in numerous centers around the world. It has undergone many modifications to correct deficiencies in earlier designs. The button device began as a single square umbrella of polyurethane foam sheet on a frame of two crossed pieces of spring guide wire that made up the occlusion part of the device. It was held against the septum by a "counteroccluder." The counteroccluder consisted of a single piece of guide wire, the center of which buttoned against the center of the umbrella on the opposite side of the septal defect by a unique latex buttoning mechanism. The umbrella and the counteroccluder were delivered separately through a long sheath and over a long looped control suture. Once these were buttoned together, the delivery catheter was released from the occluder by withdrawing the long retaining suture from the device mechanism. The delivery sheath was then withdrawn. The early generations of this device were very flexible and the polyurethane foam was very compressible, so the device could be folded to a small diameter and delivered through a much smaller sheath than any of the other devices. The newer-generation devices are still square umbrellas of polyurethane, but with a thicker counteroccluder, which is not as compressible. They now reportedly require 10 to 12 French sheaths for delivery. Defect sizing, the ratio of device to defect size, and the delivery through a long sheath are similar to the other devices. The button device is available in very small sizes suitable for the small

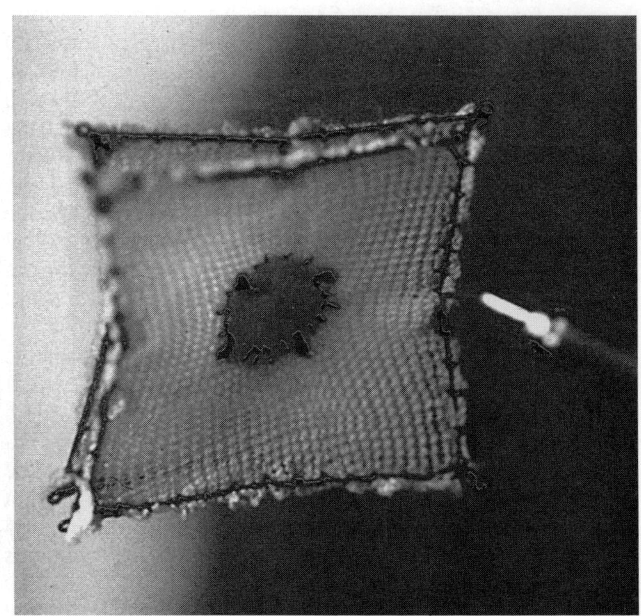

FIGURE 10–6 Angel Wings device.

defects and also in sizes up to 60 mm in diameter for very large ASDs. Because of the attachment with a suture during delivery, the device remains flexible in its seating on the septum. Owing to its flexibility, it is retrievable until, and actually after, it is released.

The earlier generations of button devices had a high incidence of residual and recurrent leaks. There were also reports of embolization from poor fixation or unbuttoning. In view of these problems, the device underwent several significant changes and now it is in its fifth generation since the initial FDA pilot study. Although the button device has been used in many centers throughout the world, there have not been large enough numbers with the same generation of device in any individual center for data analysis. The current generation button device has not undergone an FDA IDE clinical trial but is available for commercial use in many countries outside of the United States.

Atrial Septal Defect Occluding System

The Atrial Septal Defect Occluding System (ASDOS; Salzer Osypka, Rheinfelden, Germany) is still awaiting clinical trials in the United States. This device has undergone an investigational clinical trial in Europe, which was successful. The ASDOS is commercially available in Europe. The ASDOS device is a double umbrella employing a polyurethane membrane for the umbrella material. Each umbrella consists of the membrane supported by five narrow hooplike arms of fine nitinol wire. The umbrella arms have a spring attachment to the central hub of their umbrella that allows them to fold. The central hubs of the two opposing umbrellas then screw together by a very refined and complex mechanism. The ASDOS device comes in sizes up to 60 mm in diameter.

The delivery system of the ASDOS device is the most complex of all of the ASD devices. It is unique in that it requires a guide wire or "rail" system that is through and through for delivery and fixation. An end-hole balloon catheter is advanced from the right heart through the ASD into the left atrium and left ventricle and on into the aorta. A long exchange delivery wire is then advanced through this catheter and out the catheter tip into the aorta. This exchange wire is snared with a small retrograde catheter and withdrawn through the femoral artery puncture site. This produces the rail from the femoral vein through the heart chambers, into the aorta, and out through the femoral artery. A small retrograde catheter is left in place over the wire retrograde to the left atrium to protect the left heart structures from the edge of the wire.

The delivery catheter is next advanced over the exchange wire rail from the venous side into the left atrium. The left and right atrial umbrellas are delivered separately, both from the *venous end* of the rail wire. The left atrial umbrella is opened and positioned on the left atrial side of the septum. The right atrial umbrella is opened in the right atrium and advanced to the right atrial side of the septum over the rail wire, employing a centering tool that appears similar to a transseptal needle without the point on it. The two umbrellas are adjusted together on the septum with the centering tool. After positioning, the two opposing umbrellas are screwed together. When the operator is satisfied with the position, the device is released from the delivery catheter but still has the rail wire passing through it. When the operator is satisfied with the position *and the fixation* of the ASDOS device on the septum, the rail wire is carefully withdrawn through the two catheters and out of the device, leaving the device attached on the septum.

The rail wire provides the unique advantage of allowing the ASDOS device to be retrievable at any time during delivery, deployment, and fixation on the septum, even after the release of the device from the delivery catheter. The device has another advantage of an extensive range of sizes. The capability of adjusting the centering of the device should make it uniquely useful for some of the larger and not ideally centered defects. Disadvantages include the complexity of the delivery, early reports of erosion of tissues from the rigid arms, and tight compression of the arms against the atrial septum. These concerns have so far delayed the further development of this device and its introduction into the United States.

Amplatzer Atrial Septal Defect Occlusion Device

The last occlusion device to be discussed is the Amplatzer Septal Occluder (AGA Medical Corp., Golden Valley, MN). This device has undergone European clinical trials and FDA pilot trials in the United States. It is commercially available in most of the world except the United States and is beginning FDA IDE trials. This device has two retaining discs or "bodies" that are fixed on the opposite sides of the defect, but the concept of this device is different from that of all of the previously described devices. The entire device is a unique and complex "weave" of fine nitinol metal wires that retain their shape from the memory of the nitinol. In its released state, the wire mesh forms a double circular pair of "mushrooms" with the two mushrooms of the device being relatively flat, large-diameter, round discs. The two discs hold the device against the septum over the ASD. The discs are connected with a broad circular central hub or stalk of the same material. The "left" atrial disc is 14 mm larger, and the right atrial disc only 12 mm larger in diameter than the central hub. The central hub is designed to precisely fill the defect and is the occluding portion of the device. The size of the device is determined by the diameter of the hub, which should correspond exactly to the stretched diameter of the ASD. These devices come in variable hub sizes up to 27 mm for occlusion of a 27-mm ASD. There are polyester fibrous strands intertwined in the nitinol mesh of both the hub and the discs to promote thrombosis and occlusion.

In spite of its considerably different design, the Amplatzer device is delivered in a fashion similar to that for the other ASD devices under combined fluoroscopic and TEE guidance. The smaller devices will pass through a 7 French sheath, whereas the larger devices require up to a 9 French sheath. For delivery, the device is attached to a delivery pusher wire by a very fine screw mechanism. It is then stretched into a long thin "braid" of the material for delivery. The stretched device is advanced to the ASD through the long sheath previously positioned across the atrial septum with the tip within the body of the left atrium. As the device reaches the tip of the sheath, it is extruded out the end of the sheath by carefully withdrawing the sheath back toward the right atrium while leaving the device in place within the body of the left atrium. When the left atrial disc is fully extruded and expanded, the sheath together with the remainder of the device is withdrawn until the left atrial disc rests against the septum. The position of the distal disc is confirmed by TEE and fluoroscopy. The sheath alone is withdrawn, allowing first the central hub and then the proximal right atrial disc to expand. With the circular configuration of the central occluding portion, there should be a tight fit within the defect. To check the security of its fixation, the device is test "wiggled." If the device is malpositioned or pulls through the defect *at any stage* of the delivery, it can be withdrawn back into the delivery sheath and repositioned, reimplanted, or removed and a different size device inserted. Once the operator is confident of the fixation, the device is unscrewed from the delivery wire for release.

All of these ASD devices have at one time or another been used to close a patent foramen ovale (PFO) after a documented right-to-left central nervous system embolic event through the PFO. The apparent potential for this use appears staggering. However, the true risk of a PFO for embolism has not been documented to really justify this use very often. At least in the United States, where all of the devices are still in ASD clinical trials, this use of any of the ASD occluding devices for PFOs is not approved as part of any of the ASD trials. Several of the devices are beginning separate randomized, controlled trials for PFO in patients with proven embolic strokes. The PFO equipment and technique are the same as those for ASD closure. Because the defects are small, the smallest ASD devices can be used and the procedure is more straightforward. The exception is the PFO that is on a redundant, "aneurysmal" septum that is, in turn, mobile and has poor "edges." These particular lesions often require the largest umbrellas to cover the entire aneurysm. At the same time, the devices with the smallest hubs are much more of a challenge to implant. The next few years will probably shed more light on this indication for ASD device implant.

The ASD occluding devices discussed in this section are those already developed and clinically available outside of the United States in 1998. Most of these devices are well into clinical trials in the United States and, if the FDA permits, should be near premarket approval submissions within a year or two. More effective and even safer transcatheter ASD occlusion devices may be in investigational trials when this text is published.

Ventricular Septal Defect and Other Abnormal Communication Occlusion

Transcatheter closure of muscular ventricular septal defects (VSDs) was first performed on a compassionate basis using the Rashkind PDA occluding device.[106] The defects chosen were patch leaks after prior surgery, acquired VSDs due to myocardial infarction, and some unoperated congenital apical and midmuscular defects. The Rashkind device frequently was too small, leaving significant residual shunting or causing embolization of the device. The Rashkind device was abandoned during trials of the clamshell ASD device, when the clamshell used for closure of certain VSDs became available under a separate high-risk protocol.[107] The defects chosen for occlusion were in the mid or apical muscular interventricular septum, away from the semilunar and atrioventricular valves. These particular defects are the most difficult for the surgeons to repair and frequently have unsatisfactory surgical results.

The procedure for device closure of these lesions not only is difficult for the surgeon but also is far more complicated and technically difficult for the interventional cardiologist as well. The defects are hard to approach and cross with a catheter from the right side owing to their apical location and the heavy right ventricular trabeculations in the area. The acute angle from the tricuspid valve to the apex makes catheter approach from the femoral vein very difficult, particularly for device delivery. The jugular venous approach with a through and through or rail wire system extending through the left heart has been utilized to overcome some of these problems.

The procedure for VSD closure involves crossing the defect from the left ventricle to the right ventricle with an end-hole catheter. The left ventricle can be entered by either a transseptal or a retrograde approach. A second angiographic catheter is placed in the left ventricle that allows repeated left ventricular angiocardiograms during positioning and delivery of the initial end-hole catheter and eventually the device. The x-ray tubes are positioned to cut the VSD exactly on edge. A left ventricular angiocardiogram is recorded to serve as a road map for the procedure. The x-ray tubes are then kept at the same angles for the remainder of the procedure. Often, the left ventricular side of the muscular VSD will be broad, and the VSD will taper into a relatively narrow interventricular communication as it approaches the right ventricular side.

Entry into the left ventricular side of the VSD can be quite difficult and may require a combination of mechanical tip deflector wires, torqueable catheters, and a floating balloon end-hole catheter. The use of a balloon end-hole catheter for this catheter passage will help ensure passage through the largest opening through the VSD from the left ventricle to the right ventricle. Torqueable guide wires may facilitate catheter guidance to the vicinity of, and through, the defect once the left ventricular "entrance" of the defect has been engaged. After the catheter has been advanced through the ventricular septum into the right ventricle, the wire and catheter are maneuvered retrograde across the tricuspid valve into the right atrium.

A separate venous sheath is introduced into the right jugular vein through which a snare catheter is passed into the right atrium. The free end of the wire that has been passed through the VSD is grasped with the snare. Occasionally, the snare catheter may have to be advanced through the tricuspid valve to snare the tip of the wire or catheter in the right ventricle. Once the wire or catheter has been snared, the wire is externalized through the sheath in the right jugular vein. The catheter through which the wire was introduced is withdrawn into the left ventricle to protect the left heart chambers, valves, and vessels from the cutting effects of the bare wire passing through these structures. A through-and-through or rail wire is thus created with the wire passing from the femoral vein, through the atrial septum to the left atrium, through the mitral valve to the left ventricle, through the VSD to the right ventricle, through the tricuspid valve to the right atrium, and out through the jugular vein.

An alternative approach is to enter the left ventricle in a retrograde fashion to create this rail from the femoral artery to left ventricle, to right ventricle, right atrium, and out through the jugular vein. The jugular venous end of the rail is then utilized to advance the delivery sheath, catheter, and occlusion device through the right ventricle, through the VSD, and into the left ventricle. Traction to the opposite end of the rail wire is frequently needed during the passage of the sheath and dilator combination through the septum and during the advancement of the sheath over the dilator into the left ventricle.

The dilator is slowly and carefully removed over the wire from the sheath. After removal of the dilator, the position of the sheath tip is verified within the left ventricular cavity by a left ventricular angiocardiogram. If the sheath is not exactly in position and needs to be advanced to a more secure position, the dilator should be reintroduced because advancement of the sheath alone is likely to kink the sheath in the right ventricle. Since any movement of the patient or the slightest traction on the sheath can displace the sheath back to the right ventricular side of the septum, the wire should not be removed until the device is loaded and ready for introduction. When the device is ready for delivery and the position of the sheath within the left ventricular cavity is satisfactory, the through and through rail wire is withdrawn from the system. As the wire is removed, the sheath is held firmly in place and, if necessary, *very gently* adjusted forward to keep the sheath tip well within the left ventricle.

Changes in sheath and wire positions should be verified by small left ventricular angiocardiograms. The delivery catheter with the loaded device is introduced into the sheath, and the delivery pod with the device is advanced to the center of the right *atrium*. From there, the device is advanced carefully out of the delivery pod and into the sheath. The sheath must be allowed to advance or move slightly to keep its tip well within the left ventricle because advancement of the device may straighten the sheath and, in turn, pull it back into the VSD or right ventricle. No attempt should be made to deliver the device unless the sheath tip is well through the defect and free within the left ventricle. If delivery is attempted with the sheath in the defect, the device will end up entirely on the right side of the defect because the distal legs may open rapidly and on a very acute angle out of the tip of the sheath.

When the device has been advanced to the tip of the sheath in the left ventricle or against the free wall of the left ventricle, the device is advanced very slightly while withdrawing the sheath the same distance. This is repeated until the distal legs of the device spring open in the left ventricular cavity. Once the left side has opened completely, the entire system is slowly withdrawn into the defect. There is usually a conical folding of the distal left ventricular arms into the left ventricular side of the defect. Angiocardiography should be repeated to verify proper positioning. In spite of what appears to be perfect folding into the defect, the device may still be on the left ventricular rim of the defect and the center of the device may still be within the left ventricle. This would lead to embolization in the left ventricle. With predominantly angiographic and limited TEE guidance, the device is withdrawn well into the defect to ensure that all of the proximal legs open on the right side of the VSD. The sheath is withdrawn farther to allow the proximal, right-sided arms to spring completely open. The right-sided arms are usually entangled in the right ventricular trabeculae and do not open completely or symmetrically. However, they fix very well in the right ventricle. After angiographic confirmation of the positioning and closure of the defect, the device is released and the delivery catheter and sheath are removed. Because of the complexity of this procedure, transcatheter closure of muscular VSDs will certainly be limited to a few centers very active in interventional catheterization.[107]

Umbrella Device Occlusion of Other Intravascular Communications

In addition to the previously discussed ASDs and VSDs, many other, often unique intravascular communications have been closed with the various umbrella occlusion devices. The most notable of this type of use is the closure of the purposely left atrial communication in the so-called fenestrated Fontan procedure. In these patients, a small 3- to 5-mm opening is purposely left in the atrial baffle of a total cavopulmonary anastomosis for single ventricle to allow a small right-to-left shunt during the recovery period. This defect and shunt serve the purpose of shunting a finite amount of systemic venous blood away from the pulmonary circuit and, at the same time, increasing systemic cardiac output by this amount. The shunt does leave the patient cyanotic and with a potential for right-to-left embolization, so that once its usefulness is finished, it is desirable to close it. This has been accomplished similarly but more easily than with the closure of an ASD. Because of the small size and usually rigid baffle material, the umbrella devices seat very simply and securely in these defects. At the moment, these defects are not in the "device protocols" in the United States, so these patients must live with their fenestrations until the FDA "liberates" one or more of these devices from the protocols.

Similarly, the umbrellas have been used in extenuating circumstances for closure of other nonpurposeful residual postoperative leaks, including patch leaks and even a few perivalvular leaks. The applications in these lesions are so rare and so heterogeneous that each is usually a "new" and unique procedure that must be utilized at the discretion of a physician skilled and experienced in the use of the particular device and after an informed discussion and disclosure with the patient. As these unusual and rare uses occur, they will become "accepted" and more of these patients will be spared reoperation.

MISCELLANEOUS THERAPEUTIC CATHETER PROCEDURES

Balloon Atrial Septostomy

The first intracardiac therapeutic catheterization device and procedure specifically for patients with congenital heart disease were the septostomy balloon and the balloon atrial septostomy procedure, created by Rashkind in 1966.[1] This procedure involved *creating an ASD* for babies with transposition of the great arteries. This was not only the first intracardiac therapeutic procedure to be performed in the catheterization laboratory but also the first catheterization procedure that effectively replaced a surgical procedure, the Blalock-Hanlon septectomy. Rashkind convinced United States Catheter Incorporated (USCI) to build a catheter with a lumen through the catheter communicating with a relatively tough, spherical, latex balloon attached at the distal end. He then proceeded to perform balloon atrial septostomy in newborn patients with transposition of the great arteries. This procedure involved positioning the catheter with the balloon in the left atrium, inflating the balloon to its maximal recommended volume, and withdrawing it rapidly with force into the right atrium. This created a tear in the thin, flaplike newborn foramen ovale. The ASD that was created during this procedure allowed mixing of the blood between the two parallel circuits in infants with transposition of the great arteries. The procedure proved to be very successful and has remained essentially unchanged since its inception.

Although the original septostomy procedure has not changed, the balloons have been improved. Shortly after the procedure was introduced, the Edwards Company produced an improved septostomy balloon. This was a larger latex balloon on a smaller, single-lumen shaft. This became the standard balloon employed in this procedure for more than two decades. The balloon could be inflated with up to 6 ml of fluid, which produced a firm, tough sphere almost 2 cm in diameter. The disadvantages of this balloon included (1) the need for a 7 French introducer sheath, (2) the balloon was moderately compliant at less than 6 ml inflation, and (3) there was a possibility of rupture of the balloon with distant embolization of latex. The Nu-Med Company now produces a septostomy balloon made of polyethylene material that has received FDA approval. This balloon has the advantage of achieving a hard, noncompliant sphere with only 2 ml of fluid, and yet it produces the nearly the same tearing effect as the larger, more compliant balloon and can be introduced through a smaller sheath. It also has less chance of rupture, and there is no loss of pieces of the balloon if rupture does occur.

Balloon atrial septostomy is still an essential procedure in every pediatric catheterization laboratory. The use of balloon atrial septostomy has been extended to other lesions in which mixing is needed through the atrial septum to sustain life. Such lesions include tricuspid and pulmonary atresia, in which all of the systemic venous blood must pass through the ASD; mitral atresia, in which all of the pulmonary venous blood must pass through the ASD; and total anomalous pulmonary venous connection, in which all of the combined mixed systemic and pulmonary venous blood that sustains systemic output must cross the ASD. In the newborn, balloon atrial septostomy proved very effective and, in many cases, has served to palliate these infants indefinitely. In the later newborn period, even as young as 6 weeks, the atrial septum becomes much tougher, and balloon atrial septostomy is less effective. Balloon septostomy at this age and older may only temporarily stretch the atrial septum with transient relief of symptoms.

Blade Atrial Septostomy

The inability to create an adequate atrial communication with balloon septostomy in children beyond the newborn period led to the development of the Park blade septostomy catheter and the blade septostomy procedure. Indications for this procedure are similar to those for balloon septostomy and have been further expanded to include teenagers and adults with persistent complex lesions or pulmonary vascular disease, who may benefit from an atrial "pop-off" to improve cardiac output and decrease pulmonary congestion or right heart failure.[108] The Park blade septostomy catheter (Cook Inc., Bloomington, IN) was designed to initiate a cut in a thicker or tougher atrial septum.[6] This incision is then extended with a balloon septostomy or dilatation procedure. The original Park blade septostomy catheter was a 6 French catheter with a 1.0-cm knife blade recessed in a slot in the distal end of the catheter. The blade was controlled by a sliding wire that ran from the proximal end of the catheter to the blade located distally. When the control wire was advanced, the blade would extend out of the slot on the catheter and form a triangle, with the apex of the triangle away from the catheter. When the blade was open, the cutting edge faced the proximal end of the catheter. The Park blade septostomy catheter underwent a small, nonrandomized collaborative trial and received FDA approval for use in 1979.[109] Shortly after its approval, two larger blades were built and approved. These blades were 1.34 and 2.0 cm long. The 1.34-cm blade was similar to the original 1.0-cm blade and was mounted on a 6 French catheter, whereas the 2.0-cm blade was much sturdier and was mounted on an 8 French catheter.

Indications for blade septostomy in the adult are in patients with inoperable complex congenital lesions with inadequate "venting" of either atrium and in patients with cor pulmonale secondary to pulmonary vascular disease.[108] In the presence of the muscular atrial septum found in the adult, it is better to start with the *blade* septostomy procedure even if a small ASD is present. If a balloon septostomy alone is attempted first, it will only stretch the restrictive atrial communication. Stretching of the defect will cause the blade to pull through the stretched orifice while *not* producing the desired initial cut.

The Park blade septostomy catheter is introduced through a long Mullins sheath that has been passed either through an existing atrial communication or, preferably, via a separate transseptal puncture adjacent to the existing atrial communication into the left atrium. The blade location in the left atrium is verified on biplane fluoroscopy. The sheath is withdrawn from the blade well into the right atrium or the inferior vena cava. With the blade apparatus positioned well into the left atrium, the catheter is rotated until the blade points toward the patient's anterior chest wall and to the patient's right or left. The blade is carefully opened to approximately 45 degrees while its position is checked to be sure it is not in the left atrial appendage or in a pulmonary vein. The blade is locked in the open position, and the blade catheter is slowly withdrawn to the atrial septum. Resistance will be felt at the septum, and the blade may tend to rotate as it engages the septum. A continued firm, *slow,* and *controlled* withdrawal of the catheter and blade is performed until the blade snaps through the septum. Often, the entire septum will be displaced caudally almost into the inferior vena cava before the blade pulls through the septum. When the blade pulls through the septum, it is important that the open blade is *not* withdrawn down into the inferior vena cava after the cut is made.

After the successful cut, the blade is closed and the blade apparatus is withdrawn back into the catheter shaft. The blade catheter is reinserted into the left atrium, and the blade pull-through is repeated three to five times. Each time, the angle of the blade is changed until no more resistance is felt as the blade is withdrawn through the septum. After the blade withdrawals are completed, the blade catheter is replaced with a balloon septostomy catheter. A balloon atrial septostomy procedure is performed to enlarge the opening created with the blade. The balloon atrial septostomy remains the most hazardous part of the procedure.

Angioplasty Balloon Dilatation of an Atrial Defect

Angioplasty balloon dilatation of the atrial defect may be necessary in conjunction with blade atrial septostomy or as a primary procedure in the adult patient with a tough atrial septum. It is also indicated when there is compromised access from the inferior vena cava or in a very tall patient in whom the standard balloon septostomy catheter is not long enough to be advanced to the left atrium. Balloon dilatation of the atrial septum is usually more effective after an initial blade septostomy, because even a tiny initial incision will initiate a *tear* that can be extended with the dilatation. To perform a balloon dilatation of the atrial septum, a transseptal procedure is performed followed by blade septostomy.

An end-hole catheter is then used to introduce a stiff exchange wire through the atrial septum and out into a pulmonary vein. An angioplasty balloon is chosen with a diameter at least twice the size of the atrial defect. With the wire stabilized in this position, the appropriate angioplasty dilatation catheter is introduced over the wire and advanced into the atrial septum. The angioplasty balloon is partially inflated to visualize the indentation on the balloon made by the restrictive septum. Once the balloon is centered precisely within the septum, the dilatation balloon is inflated to its maximal recommended pressure, followed by rapid deflation. The balloon should be closely observed on fluoroscopy during the inflation to be sure that it is not displaced out of the septum during full inflation. The procedure should be repeated several times to ensure the dilatation has achieved maximal tearing of the septum. During the repeat inflations, there should be no waist or indentation of the balloon even initially as the balloon is inflated. In large adult patients, a single angioplasty balloon may not achieve an adequate ASD owing to balloon size and pressure limitations. In these patients, venous access can be obtained from both groin areas, and two sheaths can be placed. Two stiff wires are introduced to the pulmonary veins for simultaneous balloon inflations of two angioplasty balloons in the atrial septum. Once the procedure is completed, the balloon angioplasty catheters are removed and the hemodynamics are repeated to be sure an adequate septal opening has been achieved.

In most of the patients with complex lesions and restrictive "mixing" or inadequate "venting," the largest ASD possible is created using the large blade and double balloons. This may occasionally require making multiple punctures, blade septostomy cuts, and balloonings. The pulmonary vascular disease patient is the other extreme, requiring only a *very* small defect (4 to 6 mm) initially, enlarged in 1-mm increments until a balance is reached between improvement in right heart failure and development of systemic desaturation.

CATHETER REMOVAL OF FOREIGN BODIES

Transcatheter removal of foreign bodies has become an important part of the armamentarium of the interventional cardiologist. This is due to the general increase in the use of indwelling catheters and the increased number of therapeutic devices implanted in the catheterization laboratory. Most, if not all, of the foreign bodies within the vascular system are iatrogenic. In the past, the majority of these foreign bodies were pieces of indwelling chronic intravenous tubing from chemotherapy, hyperalimentation, and neurosurgical shunts that were broken during removal, leaving pieces floating in the circulation. Now, many of the foreign bodies are a consequence of interventional procedures, including occlusion coils that have migrated or embolized, tips of catheters or wires, pieces of balloon dilatation catheters, umbrella occlusion devices, and even intravascular stents. Virtually all intravascular foreign bodies can and should be removed in the cardiac catheterization laboratory. The biplane congenital catheterization laboratory is particularly well suited for these retrievals. The key to the successful removal of foreign bodies is the three-dimensional localization of the foreign body within the vascular system with *biplane* fluoroscopy. Without the use of both fluoroscopic views, the retrieval becomes a random "fishing expedition."

A variety of catheter devices are available for the removal of foreign bodies. These devices are commonly inserted through a long sheath, which should be of sufficient diameter to allow the *grasped foreign body* to be withdrawn into the sheath before withdrawal from the body. This occasionally will require a 14 or 16 French long sheath. An end-hole catheter is first advanced to a location distal to the foreign body. A stiff or superstiff wire is advanced and fixed distal to the foreign body so that the long sheath and dilator can be maneuvered over the wire to a location *immediately adjacent* to the foreign body. The retrieval device is passed through the long sheath and out of its tip so that the foreign body can be grasped and withdrawn into the sheath for removal.

Snare Techniques

The most frequently used retrieval device is the snare catheter. Several snare catheters are available, including "homemade" snares using a loop of standard spring guide wire inserted through an end-hole catheter. The most sophisticated and now "standard" snare system is made of nitinol wire by Microvena. These nitinol snares have several advantages over previous snares. The snare catheter is a 4 or 5 French end-hole catheter that can be inserted through a short sheath, a long sheath, or a 7 French end-hole catheter that has been positioned near the foreign body. The snare itself is a wire with a fixed-diameter loop at its distal tip that, when advanced out of the distal end of the snare catheter, aligns perpendicular to the shaft of the catheter. The proximal end of the snare wire extends out of the proximal end of the catheter. The loop of the snare is advanced from the tip of the catheter and manipulated to encircle the foreign body. The snare loop is made smaller by advancing the catheter forward over the proximal loop while holding the back end of the wire, which tightens the loop at its distal end around the object.

The Microvena snare loop has virtually infinite memory, so that no matter how many times the loop is advanced to open or is withdrawn back into the catheter, it resumes its original shape and orientation. Another advantage is that the snare loop is 90 degrees offset from the shaft of the catheter. The loop catheter angle has the same memory as the loop, which places it perpendicular to the catheter shaft at all times. This allows the loop to pass around the object as the snare catheter is advanced, rather than requiring advancement past the object and trying to "catch" it from the side as the snare is withdrawn. For this technique to work, there must be a free end or piece of the foreign body extending into the circulation that the loop of the snare can encircle. This snare is most useful for the retrieval of pieces of indwelling lines or pieces of catheters.

Basket Device

Another frequently used retrieval device is the "basket" device. This is a catheter and core wire system that has a helix or basket of three or four strands of wire at the distal end. The basket opens as it is extruded from the catheter. Several different designs of the helix are available in various sizes. When extruded from the catheter, the basket opens. It is rotated as it expands, which encircles or entangles the foreign body. The basket wires must be able to encircle at least part of the foreign body to trap it. When the basket is withdrawn into its catheter, it compresses, and in this way, grasps the foreign body securely. The basket device can be used for the retrieval of pieces of catheter or other foreign bodies that have a free end. The basket will also work if a separate wire can encircle or pass through the foreign body and the combination can then be entrapped by the basket. This technique is essential in the retrieval and extraction of fractured pieces of embedded transvenous pacing leads. The basket is also useful for embolized occlusion devices including coils, umbrellas, and even stents.

Bioptome

A cardiac bioptome with serrated jaws can be used as an alternative to grasp foreign objects in some circumstances. The advantage of a bioptome is that it can be used to grasp a free *side* as well as the ends of a small object. A limitation of the bioptome is that it must be manipulated so that its jaws open perpendicular to the object to be grabbed. The bioptome jaws may also not open widely enough to accommodate larger foreign bodies and, once the object is grabbed, may not be strong enough to hold and withdraw the object. Another disadvantage of the bioptome is the difficulty and patience (and fluoroscopy) it takes to grab a small, moving object with such a small jaw. A common use of the bioptome would be to grasp the center of a piece of catheter or wire that extends across the main pulmonary artery when no free end is accessible. Although retrieval may not be accomplished with the bioptome, at least one end can be pulled free to allow it to be grasped by one of the stronger devices.

Vascular Retrieval Forceps

Another retrieval device, the vascular retrieval forceps (Cook, Inc.) has a very tiny, angled, serrated jaw that extends from one side near the distal end of a very small 3 French catheter. It is operated much as for the jaw operation on the Cook bioptome catheter. This tiny device can be passed *into or through* a mass of foreign body wedged distally in a vessel. The grasping jaw can then be opened and closed within the mass to catch part of the object and pull it proximally, if not out of the vascular system. The tiny tip and catheter can also be passed under the middle of a catheter or wire that is against a vessel or chamber wall and used to pull the foreign material away from the wall. This device is useful both for small foreign objects and to initially dislodge or move larger objects into more favorable positions for grasping with sturdier retrieval systems.

Cook Deflector Wire

The Cook deflector wire can be used in a manner similar to that for the small jaws device to encircle and dislodge foreign bodies that have no free ends. The straight wire is passed between the foreign body and the vascular wall, the deflector system is activated, and the foreign material will be encircled by the 360-degree loop of the deflected tip of the wire.

The type and size of the foreign body, the location of the foreign body, the length of time that the foreign body has been in place, and the adequacy of access vessels all will determine the success of foreign body retrieval. The larger foreign bodies certainly can be grasped within the vascular system, but they may be too large to be withdrawn into a sheath or otherwise completely out of the vascular system. If a large, jagged foreign body, such as an open occlusion device, cannot be withdrawn into the large sheath enough to cover sharp parts of the device, it should *not* be withdrawn through the cardiac structures. If the foreign body can be drawn into a peripheral vessel, it can usually be removed by a small cut-down over the peripheral vessel using local anesthesia, rather than requiring a thoracotomy. If a large foreign body within the lung can be grasped and freed from its distal site, but cannot be withdrawn sufficiently into the sheath, it can still be held in the main or proximal branch pulmonary arteries so that the surgeon has easier access to it. All of these things should be considered in preparation for foreign body removal.

Collaborative Therapeutic Catheterization and Surgical Procedures

An added bonus to the new therapeutic catheterization procedures has been an increased collaboration between the pediatric cardiologists and the pediatric cardiac surgeons in staged repairs of complex defects.[110] One of the earliest examples of this preplanned cooperation was in the use of the fenestrated Fontan procedure, for which the immediate surgical morbidity is reduced by leaving a residual ASD that can be closed in the catheterization laboratory once the patient is recovered from the surgery. The most notable example of this type of multistaged collaboration is in patients with pulmonary artery atresia and VSD, where the surgical creation of a right ventricle to pulmonary artery connection early in the course of management provides the interventional cardiologist access to the pulmonary vessels for dilatation and intrapulmonary stent implant in preparation for the eventual more definitive repair. This type of cooperation and its complementary beneficial results for the patient contribute to a far better outcome for many of the extremely complex lesions.

Conclusions

The therapeutic cardiac catheterization procedures discussed in this chapter represent some of the greatest advances in the care of patients with heart disease since the advent of the first surgical corrections. The procedures are performed with less immediate risk and certainly far less acute trauma to the patient than repeated surgical intervention. Even with the additional expense of the specialized catheters and devices and of the more extensive catheterization procedure, the direct costs of the therapeutic catheterization procedure are significantly less than for the comparable surgical procedure. The indirect expense savings for a patient and the family may be even greater than the savings in direct expense. The patient and family are away from home and work for only 1 or 2 days, compared with 1 or 2 weeks for the surgical procedure. After the catheterization procedure, the patient is able to go home and immediately return to full activity of either school or work. This compares with a minimum of 4 to 8 weeks of convalescence after a surgical procedure. With these multiple advantages to the therapeutic catheterization procedures, many such procedures have already replaced the surgical alternatives. With further developments and improvements in the catheter techniques, many more nonsurgical corrections should be included in this "standard" category of treatment within the next several years.

References

1. Rashkind WJ, Miller WW: Creation of an atrial septal defect without thoracotomy: palliative approach to complete transposition of the great arteries. JAMA 196:991, 1966.
2. Cope C: Technique for transseptal catheterization of the left atrium: preliminary report. J Thorac Surg 37:482–486, 1959.
3. Ross JJ, Braunwald E, Morrow AG: Transseptal left atrial puncture: new technique for the measurement of left atrial pressure in man. Am J Cardiol 3:353–365, 1959.
4. Roveti GC, Ross RS, Bahmson HT: Transseptal left heart catheterization in the pediatric age group. J Pediatr 61:855–858, 1962.
5. Duff DF, Mullins CE: Transseptal left heart catheterization in infants and children. Cathet Cardiovasc Diagn 4:213–223, 1978.
6. Park SC, Zuberbuler JR, Neches WH, et al: A new atrial septostomy technique. Cathet Cardiovasc Diagn 1:195, 1975.
7. Gruentzig AR: Transluminal dilation of coronary artery stenosis. Lancet 1:263, 1975.
8. Kan JS, White RI Jr, Mitchell SE, et al: Percutaneous balloon valvuloplasty: a new method for treating congenital pulmonary valve stenosis. N Engl J Med 370:540–542, 1982.
9. Beekman RH, Rocchini AP, Rosenthal A: Therapeutic cardiac catheterization for pulmonary valve and pulmonary artery stenosis. Cardiol Clin 7:331–340, 1989.
10. Fedderly RT, Beekman RH: Balloon valvuloplasty for pulmonary valve stenosis. J Interven Cardiol 8:451–461, 1995.
11. Johnson LW, Grossman W, Dallen JE, et al: Pulmonic stenosis in the adult: long-term follow-up results. N Engl J Med 287:1159–1163, 1972.
12. Mody MR: The natural history of uncomplicated valvular pulmonic stenosis. Am Heart J 90:317–321, 1975.
13. Mullins CE: Therapeutic cardiac catheterization. *In* Garson A Jr, Bricker JT, McNamara DG (eds): The Science and Practice of Pediatric Cardiology. pp. 2183–2209. Philadelphia: Lea & Febiger, 1990.
14. Mullins CE, Nihill MR, Judd VE, et al: Double balloon technique for dilation of valvular or vessel stenosis in congenital and acquired heart disease. J Am Coll Cardiol 10:107–114, 1987.
15. Stanger P, Cassidy SC, Girod DA, et al: Balloon pulmonary valvuloplasty: results of Valvuloplasty and Angioplasty of Congenital Anomalies Registry. Am J Cardiol 65:775–783, 1990.
16. Nihill MR, Mullins CE: Balloon valvuloplasty of congenital lesions. *In* Vogel JHK, King SB (eds): Interventional Cardiology: Future Directions. St. Louis: CV Mosby, 1989.
17. Chen CR, Cheng TO, Huang T, et al: Percutaneous balloon valvuloplasty for pulmonic stenosis in adolescents and adults. N Engl J Med 35:21–25, 1996.
18. Teupe CHJ, Berger W, Schrader R, Zeiher AM: Late (five to nine years) follow-up after balloon dilation of valvular pulmonary stenosis in adults. Am J Cardiol 80:240–242, 1997.
19. Labadidi Z, Wu RJ, Walls TJ: Percutaneous balloon aortic valvuloplasty: results in 23 patients. Am J Cardiol 53:194–197, 1984.
20. Beekman RH, Rocchini AP, Crawley DC, et al: Comparison of single and double balloon valvuloplasty in children with aortic stenosis. J Am Coll Cardiol 12:480–485, 1988.
21. Grifka RG, Mullins CE: Therapeutic cardiac catheterization for congenital heart disease. Cardiac Chron 6:1–11, 1992.
22. O'Laughlin MP, Khan MA, Al-Yousef S, et al: Pediatric therapeutic cardiac catheterization: update 1992. J Saudi Heart Assoc 5:65–72, 1993.
23. Justo RN, McCrindle BW, Benson LN, et al: Aortic valve regurgitation after surgical versus percutaneous balloon valvotomy for congenital aortic valve stenosis. Am J Cardiol 77:1332–1338, 1996.
24. McCrindle BW, for the Valvuloplasty and Angioplasty of Congenital Anomalies (VACA) Registry investigators: Independent predictors of immediate results of percutaneous balloon aortic valvotomy in childhood. Am J Cardiol 77:286–293, 1996.
25. O'Connor BK, Beekman RH, Rocchini AP, et al: Intermediate-term effectiveness of balloon valvuloplasty for congenital aortic stenosis: A prospective follow-up study. Circulation 84:732–738, 1991.
26. Moore P, Egito E, Mowrey H, et al: Midterm results of balloon dilation of congenital aortic stenosis: predictors of success. J Am Coll Cardiol 27:1257–1263, 1996.
27. Sandhu SK, Lloyd TR, Crawley DC, et al: Effectiveness of balloon valvuloplasty in the young adult with congenital aortic stenosis. Cathet Cardiovasc Diagn 36:122–127, 1995.

28. Lieberman EB, Bashore TM, Hermiller JB, et al: Balloon aortic valvuloplasty in adults: failure of procedure to improve long-term survival. J Am Coll Cardiol 26:1522–1528, 1995.
29. Kvidal PD, Stahle E, Nygren A, et al: Long-term follow up study on 64 elderly patients after balloon aortic valvuloplasty. J Heart Valve Dis 6:480–486, 1997.
30. Ruckman R, Van Praagh R: Anatomic types of congenital mitral stenosis: report of 49 autopsy cases with consideration of diagnosis and surgical implications. Am J Cardiol 42:592–601, 1978.
31. Strasburger J: Congenital mitral valve disease. *In* Garson A Jr, Bricker JT, McNamara DG (eds): The Science and Practice of Pediatric Cardiology. pp. 1308–1315. Philadelphia, Lea & Febiger, 1990.
32. Shone J, Sellers R, Anderson R, et al: The developmental complex of "parachute mitral valve": supravalvular ring of left atrium, subaortic stenosis, and coarctation of the aorta. Am J Cardiol 11:714–725, 1963.
33. Daoud G, Kaplan S, Perrin EV, et al: Congenital mitral stenosis. Circulation 27:185–196, 1963.
34. Kveselis D, Rocchini A, Beekman R, et al: Balloon angioplasty for congenital and rheumatic mitral stenosis. Am J Cardiol 57:348–350, 1986.
35. Alday L, Juaneda E: Percutaneous balloon dilation in congenital mitral stenosis. Br Heart J 57:479–482, 1987.
36. Spevak P, Bass J, Ben-Shachar G, et al: Balloon angioplasty for congenital mitral stenosis. Am J Cardiol 66:472–476, 1989.
37. Grifka RG, O'Laughlin MP, Nihill MR, Mullins CE: Double-transseptal, double-balloon valvuloplasty for congenital mitral stenosis. Circulation 85:123–129, 1992.
38. Palacios IF, Block PC, Brandi S, et al: Percutaneous balloon valvuloplasty for patients with severe mitral stenosis. Circulation 75:778–784, 1987.
39. Babic UU, Pejcic P, Vucinic M, et al: Percutaneous transarterial balloon valvuloplasty for mitral valve stenosis. Am J Cardiol 57:1101–1104, 1986.
40. Turi ZG, Reyes VP, Raju S, et al: Percutaneous balloon versus surgical closed commissurotomy for mitral stenosis: a prospective randomized trial. Circulation 83:1179–1185, 1991.
41. Arora R, Nair M, Kalra GS, et al: Immediate and long-term results of balloon and surgical closed mitral valvotomy: a randomized comparative study. Am Heart J 125:1091–1094, 1993.
42. Reyes VP, Raju S, Wynne J, et al: Percutaneous balloon valvuloplasty compared with open surgical commissurotomy for mitral stenosis. N Engl J Med 331:961–967, 1994.
43. Orrange SE, Kawanishi DT, Lopez BM, et al: Actuarial outcome after catheter balloon commissurotomy in patients with mitral stenosis. Circulation 95:382–389, 1997.
44. Robalino BB, Whitlaw PL, Marwick T, et al: Percutaneous balloon valvuloplasty for the treatment of isolated tricuspid stenosis. Chest 100:867–869, 1991.
45. Patel TM, Dani SI, Shah SC, Patel TK: Tricuspid balloon valvuloplasty: a more simplified approach using Inoue balloon. Cathet Cardiovasc Diagn 37:86–88, 1996.
46. Gamra H, Betbout F, Ayari M, et al: Recurrent miscarriages as an indication for percutaneous tricuspid valvuloplasty during pregnancy. Cathet Cardiovasc Diagn 40:283–286, 1997.
47. Sos T, Sniderman KW, Rettek-Sos B, et al: Percutaneous transluminal dilatation of coarctation of the thoracic aorta post mortem. Lancet 2:970–971, 1979.
48. Lock JE, Nierni T, Amplatz K, et al: Transvenous angioplasty of experimental branch pulmonary artery stenosis in newborn lambs. Circulation 64:886–893, 1981.
49. Rothman A, Perry SB, Keane JF, et al: Early results and follow-up of balloon angioplasty for branch pulmonary artery stenosis. J Am Coll Cardiol 15:1109–1117, 1990.
50. Tynan M, Finley JP, Fontes V, et al: Balloon angioplasty for the treatment of native coarctation: results of Valvuloplasty and Angioplasty of Congenital Anomalies Registry. Am J Cardiol 65:790–792, 1990.
51. Hellenbrand WP, Allen H, Golinko R, et al: Balloon angioplasty for aortic recoarctation: results of Valvuloplasty and Angioplasty of Congenital Anomalies Registry. Am J Cardiol 65:793–779, 1990.
52. O'Laughlin MP: Balloon-expandable stenting in pediatric cardiology. J Interven Cardiol 8:463–475, 1995.
53. Palmaz JC, Windeler SA, Garcia F, et al: Atherosclerotic rabbit aortas: expandable intraluminal grafting. Radiology 160:723–726, 1986.
54. Schatz RA, Palmaz JC, Tio FO, et al: Balloon expandable intracoronary stents in the adult dog. Circulation 76:450–457, 1987.
55. Mullins CE, O'Laughlin MP, Vick GW III, et al: Implantation of balloon-expandable intravascular grafts by catheterization in pulmonary arteries and systemic veins. Circulation 77:188–199, 1988.
56. Benson LN, Hamilton F, Dasmahapatra H, et al: Percutaneous implantation of a balloon-expandable endoprosthesis for pulmonary artery stenosis: an experimental study. J Am Coll Cardiol 18:1303–1308, 1991.
57. Rocchini AP, Meliones JN, Beekman RH, et al: Use of balloon-expandable stents to treat experimental peripheral pulmonary artery and superior vena caval stenosis: preliminary experience. Pediatr Cardiol 13:92–96, 1992.
58. O'Laughlin MP, Mullins CE: Balloon dilation and stenting of hypoplastic pulmonary arteries: a new area of cooperation between interventional pediatric cardiologists and cardiac surgeons. Tex Heart Inst J 19:185–189, 1992.
59. Rothman A, Perry SB, Keane JF, et al: Early results and follow-up of balloon angioplasty for branch pulmonary artery stenosis. J Am Coll Cardiol 15:1109–1117, 1990.
60. Perry SB, O'Laughlin MP, Mullins CE, Lock JE: Endovascular stents in congenital heart disease. Prog Pediatr Cardiol 1:35–43, 1992.
61. Grifka RG, Vick GW III, O'Laughlin MP, et al: Balloon expandable intravascular stents: aortic implantation and late further dilation in growing minipigs. Am Heart J 126:979–984, 1993.
62. Morrow WR, Palmaz JC, Tio FO, et al: Re-expansion of balloon-expandable stents after growth. J Am Coll Cardiol 22:2007–2013, 1993.
63. Dotter CT, Buschmann RW, McKinney MK, et al: Transluminal expandable nitinol coil stent grafting: preliminary report. Radiology 147:259–260, 1983.
64. O'Laughlin MP, Perry SB, Lock JE, Mullins CE: Use of endovascular stents in congenital heart disease. Circulation 83:1923–1939, 1991.
65. Shaffer KM, Mullins CE, Grifka RG, et al: Intravascular stents in congenital heart disease: short- and long-term results from a large single-center experience. J Am Coll Cardiol 31:661–667, 1998.
66. Ing FF, Grifka RG, Nihill MR, Mullins CE: Repeat dilation of intravascular stents in congenital heart defects. Circulation 92:893–897, 1995.
67. O'Laughlin MP, Slack MC, Grifka RG, et al: Implantation and intermediate-term follow-up of stents in congenital heart disease. Circulation 88:605–614, 1993.
68. Beerman L, Neches W, Patnode R, et al: Coarctation of the aorta in children. Late results after surgery. Am J Dis Child 134:464–466, 1980.
69. Kopf G, Hellenbrand W, Kleinman C, et al: Repair of aortic coarctation in the first three months of life: immediate and long-term results. Ann Thorac Surg 41:425–430, 1986.
70. Beekman R, Rocchini A, Brehrendt D, et al: Long-term outcome after repair of coarctation in infancy: subclavian flap angioplasty does not reduce the need for reoperation. J Am Coll Cardiol 8:1406–1411, 1986.
71. Kan J, White R, Mitchell S, et al: Treatment of coarctation by percutaneous transluminal angioplasty. Circulation 68:1087–1094, 1983.
72. Isner JM, Donaldson RF, Fulton D, et al: Cystic medial necrosis in coarctation of the aorta: a potential factor contributing to adverse consequences observed after percutaneous balloon angioplasty of coarctation sites. Circulation 75:689–695, 1992.
73. Lock JE, Castaneda-Zuniga WR, Bass JL, et al: Balloon dilation of excised aortic coarctations. Radiology 143:689–691, 1982.
74. Lock JE, Nierni T, Burke BA, et al: Transcutaneous angioplasty for experimental aortic coarctation. Circulation 66:1280–1286, 1982.
75. Cooper RS, Ritter SB, Rothe WB, et al: Angioplasty for coarctation of the aorta: long-term results. Circulation 75:600–604, 1987.
76. Fletcher SE, Nihill MR, Grifka RG, et al: Balloon angioplasty of native coarctation of the aorta: midterm follow-up and prognostic factors. J Am Coll Cardiol 25:730–734, 1995.
77. Morrow RW, Smith VC, Mullins CE, et al: Balloon angioplasty with stent implantation in experimental coarctation of the aorta. Circulation 89:2677–2683, 1994.

78. Diethrich EB, Heuser RR, Cardenas JR, et al: Endovascular techniques in adult aortic coarctation: the use of stents for native and recurrent coarctation repair. J Endovasc Surg 2:183–188, 1995.
79. Ebeid MR, Prieto LR, Latson LA: Use of balloon-expandable stents for coarctation of the aorta: initial results and intermediate-term follow-up. J Am Coll Cardiol 30:1847–1852, 1997.
80. Wisselink W, Money SR, Becker MO, et al: Comparison of operative reconstruction and percutaneous dilatation for central venous obstruction. Am J Surg 166:200–205, 1993.
81. Chatelain P, Meier B, Friedli B: Stenting of superior vena cava and inferior vena cava for symptomatic narrowing after repeated atrial surgery for D-transposition of the great arteries. Br Heart J 66:466–468, 1991.
82. Rosenthal E, Qureshi SA, Tynan M, Bucknall CA: Percutaneous pacemaker lead extraction and stent implantation for superior vena cava occlusion due to pacemaker leads. Am J Cardiol 77:670–672, 1996.
83. Ward CJB, Mullins CE, Nihill MR, et al: Use of intravascular stents in systemic venous and systemic venous baffle obstructions: short-term follow-up results. Circulation 91:2948–2954, 1995.
84. Gross CM, Kramer J, Waigand J, et al: Stent implantation in patients with superior vena cava syndrome. AJR 169:429–432, 1997.
85. Abdulhamed JM, Alyousef SA, Kahn MAA, Mullins CE: Balloon dilatation of complete obstruction of the superior vena cava after Mustard operation for transposition of the great arteries. Br Heart J 72:482–485, 1994.
86. Sade RM, Freed MD, Matthews EC, Castaneda AR: Stenosis of individual pulmonary veins. Review of the literature and report of a surgical case. J Thorac Cardiovasc Surg 67:953–957, 1974.
87. Driscoll DJ, Hesslein PS, Mullins CE: Congenital stenosis of individual pulmonary veins: clinical spectrum and unsuccessful treatment by transvenous balloon dilation. Am J Cardiol 49:1767–1771, 1982.
88. Mendelshon AM, Bove EL, Lupinetti FM, et al: Intraoperative and percutaneous stenting of congenital pulmonary artery and vein stenosis. Circulation 88:210–217, 1993.
89. Abdulhamed JM, Alyousef SA, Mullins CE: Endovascular stent placement for pulmonary venous obstruction after Mustard operation for transposition of the great arteries. Heart 75:210–212, 1996.
90. Porstmann W, Wierny L, Warnke H: Der Verschluss des Ductus arteriosus persistens. Ohne Thorakotomie (1 Mitteilung). Thoraxchirurgie 15:199–203, 1967.
91. Rashkind WJ, Cuaso CC: Transcatheter closure of patent ductus arteriosus: successful use in a 3.5 kilogram infant. Pediatr Cardiol 1:3–7, 1979.
92. Rashkind WJ, Mullins CE, Hellenbrand WE, et al: Nonsurgical closure of patent ductus arteriosus: clinical application of the Rashkind PDA Occluder System. Circulation 75:583–592, 1987.
93. O'Laughlin MP, Nihill MR, Mullins CE: Patent ductus arteriosus occlusion: results in 205 patients [abstract]. Circulation 82(suppl III):582, 1990.
94. Gianturco C, Anderson JH, Wallace S: Mechanical devices for arterial occlusion. AJR 124:428–435, 1975.
95. Cambier PA, Kirby WC, Moore JW, et al: Percutaneous closure of the small (<2.5 mm) patent ductus arteriosus using coil embolization. Am J Cardiol 69:815–816, 1992.
96. Lloyd TR, Fedderly R, Beekman RH, et al: Transcatheter occlusion of patent ductus arteriosus with Gianturco coils. Circulation 88:1412–1420, 1993.
97. Moore JW, Cambier PA: Transcatheter occlusion of patent ductus arteriosus. J Interven Cardiol 8:517–531, 1995.
98. Neuss MB, Le TP, Coe JE, et al: Retrievable coils for interventional treatment of persistent ductus arteriosus: first clinical results. J Am Coll Cardiol 23:390A, 1994.
99. Grifka RG, Mullins CE, Gianturco C, et al: New Gianturco-Grifka vascular occlusion device: initial studies in a canine model. Circulation 91:1840–1846, 1995.
100. Lock JE, Keane JF, Fellows KE: Diagnostic and Interventional Catheterization in Congenital Heart Disease. pp. 126–135. Boston: Martinus Nijhoff, 1987.
101. Lock JE, Cockerham JT, Keane JF, et al: Transcatheter umbrella closure of congenital cardiac defects. Circulation 73:593–599, 1987.
102. King TD, Mills NL: Nonoperative closure of atrial septal defects. Surgery 75:383–388, 1974.
103. Rashkind WJ, Cuaso CC: Transcatheter closure of atrial septal defects in children. Proc Assoc Eur Pediatr Cardiol 13:49, 1977.
104. Lock JE, Rome JJ, David F, et al: Transcatheter closure of atrial septal defects: experimental studies. Circulation 79:1091–1099, 1989.
105. Latson LA, Benson LN, Hellenbrand WE, et al: Transcatheter closure of ASD: early results of multicenter trial of the Bard Clamshell Septal Occluder. Circulation 84(suppl II):544, 1991.
106. Lock JE, Block PC, McKay RG, et al: Transcatheter closure of ventricular septal defects. Circulation 78:361–368, 1988.
107. Bridges ND, Lock JE: Transcatheter closure of ventricular septal defects. Prog Pediatr Cardiol 1:72–77, 1992.
108. Nihill MR, O'Laughlin MP, Mullins CE: Effects of atrial septostomy in patients with terminal cor pulmonale due to pulmonary vascular disease. Cathet Cardiovasc Diagn 24:166–172, 1991.
109. Park SC, Neches WH, Mullins CE, et al: Blade atrial septostomy: collaborative study. Circulation 66:258–266, 1982.
110. Bridges ND, Lock JE, Castaneda AR: Collaborative transcatheter and surgical treatment of complex congenital heart disease. Prog Pediatr Cardiol 1:78–84, 1992.

CHAPTER 11

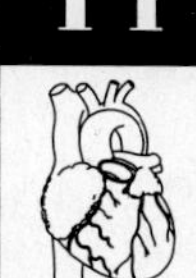

SURGICAL TREATMENT

Magdi Yacoub, Michael Gatzoulis, Sara Thorne, and Rosemary Radley-Smith

GENERAL CONSIDERATIONS
SPECIFIC CONGENITAL DEFECTS IN THE ADULT
Aortic Stenosis
Aortic Regurgitation
Mitral Valve Disease
Tricuspid Valvular Disease
Pulmonary Valve
Ventricular Outflow Tract Obstruction
Coarctation of the Aorta
Septal Defects and Anomalous Pulmonary Veins
Patent Arterial Ducts
Coronary Artery Anomalies
Cyanotic Heart Disease
Transposition of the Great Arteries
Tricuspid Atresia and Double-Inlet Ventricle
Heart-Lung Transplantation for Congenital Heart Disease
CONCLUSIONS

During the 1980s and 1990s, there was a determined effort to "correct" congenital heart disease during infancy, usually within the first few days or weeks of life,[1–5] in an attempt to prevent secondary functional and anatomic changes in the heart and other organs and to avoid the stress of repeated hospitalization and surgery in older children and adults. Despite this, a significant proportion of patients with uncorrected congenital heart disease grow to adulthood because of the relatively "benign" nature of the condition or because they were not offered or they refused surgical treatment. In addition, a number of patients who have undergone palliative or supposedly corrective surgery require further surgical treatment in adulthood. The increasing number and the specific nature of these operations have created a new subspecialty of surgery for congenital heart disease.[6, 7] This section considers some of the general features and specific conditions of congenital heart surgery in the adult.

GENERAL CONSIDERATIONS

Congenital heart defects produce progressive changes in cardiac form and function, as well as secondary effects resulting from chronic systolic or diastolic overload[8] that can involve myocardial cells,[9] the connective tissue framework of the heart,[10–12] or the microvasculature and endocardium.[13] These abnormalities are qualitatively different for systolic and diastolic overload. Although many of these changes initially have the potential to be reversed, they may become irreversible if left uncorrected. Other cardiac effects may involve progression or development of new obstructive lesions, such as that observed in tetralogy of Fallot,[14] ventricular septal defect (VSD), or aortic outflow obstruction in double-inlet ventricle with malposition of the great arteries.[15, 16] Continued blood turbulence may affect the structure and function of the atrioventricular (AV) or semilunar valves, with thickening or calcification of the cusps or dilatation of the annulus. Poststenotic changes in the great arteries can lead to either dilatation or arterial wall changes as the result of turbulence or failure of development and growth due to chronic reduction in flow. The pulmonary vascular changes caused by an increase in flow and pressure include medial hypertrophy and reactivity of smooth muscle cells, functional and structural intimal changes,[17] and eventual development of irreversible plexogenic lesions.[18, 19] The rate at which such changes occur varies among different conditions and among individual patients. Other changes that may occur are the direct result of previous surgery, which can produce distortion of vessels on intracardiac shunting. Cerebral, hepatic, and renal function may be affected by hypoperfusion, cyanosis, or embolism. Accurate characterization of the extent and reversibility of secondary changes is of special importance in planning the time and type of surgical intervention in adults with congenital heart disease.

SPECIFIC CONGENITAL DEFECTS IN THE ADULT

Aortic Stenosis

Congenital bicuspid aortic valve commonly results in progressive stenosis due to thickening and calcification of the cusps (Fig. 11–1). Valve-conserving surgery is rarely possible in adults, and therefore valve replacement is the most commonly performed surgical procedure. Advances in myocardial protection and other intraoperative techniques have led to a reduction in the perioperative mortality rates for both initial and successive surgery to approximately 1 to 3 percent.[20] The most important issue is the choice of a valve substitute, which should match the characteristics of the valve to the requirements of the patient.

Although a considerable amount of information is available about the performance and suitability of the different valve substitutes, this information is often incomplete, and other factors, such as the experience, predictions, and bias of the surgical team, cardiologist, and patient, can influence the choice. The available substitutes include prosthetic valves and stented or unstented xenografts.

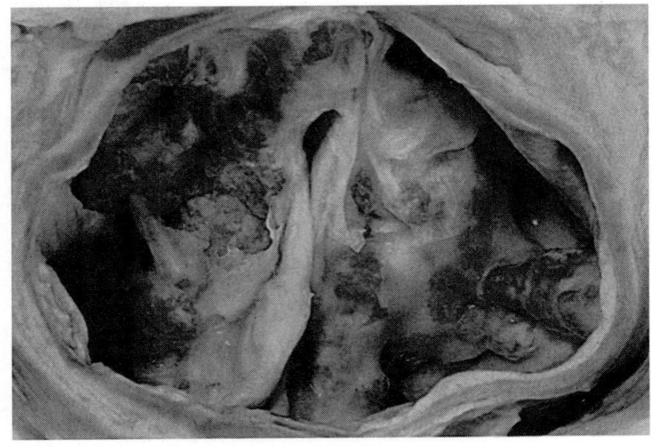

FIGURE 11–1 Severe aortic stenosis of a congenitally bicuspid valve. (From Becker AE, Anderson RH: Cardiac Pathology. New York: Churchill Livingstone, 1983.)

Homografts and Pulmonary Autografts

Prosthetic valves are the most commonly used valve substitutes and have the advantages of ease of insertion and superior durability. However, the need for continuous postoperative anticoagulation can lead to a small but significant morbidity and mortality incidence,[21] particularly in women during the childbearing years.[22] Stented xenografts offer the advantage of predictability, ease of insertion, and low incidence of thromboembolic complications. However, their durability is limited, particularly in patients younger than 35 years. In addition, the stent can become obstructive (Fig. 11–2), which has negative implications for hemodynamic performance and possibly for long-term left ventricular (LV) function. Homograft valves are inserted in the subcoronary position either via a two-suture-line technique[23, 24] (Fig. 11–3) or as a root replacement (Fig. 11–4) with reimplantation of the coronary arteries (see Fig. 11–4).[25, 26] These valves have excellent hemodynamic performance (Fig. 11–5), are free of thromboembolic complications, and have greater durability than xenografts, particularly in children. However, their insertion is somewhat technically demanding, they are less readily available, and they must be replaced after a period of time.[27] Pulmonary autografts make use of the patient's pulmonary valve to replace the aortic valve, with insertion of a pulmonary or aortic allograft in the pulmonary position (Fig. 11–6).[28–30] The autograft is inserted in the aortic position using a two-suture-line technique or as a root replacement. The latter technique is more predictable with regard to achieving immediate competence, but there is some concern about the late dilatation of the autograft root. The pulmonary autograft is the only valve substitute capable of continued growth, and it shares most of the advantages of the allograft but with greater durability. The main disadvantages include the extensive surgery required, the risk to the first septal artery, and the involvement of two valves with the need for further surgery, at least for the right ventricular (RV) outflow valve. This operation, however, has an important role, particularly in young patients. There is an increasing realization that reparative procedures or valve substitutes that preserve or reproduce the dynamic nature of valve function may produce superior results in terms of both cardiac function and possibly survival.[31]

Aortic Regurgitation

Severe aortic regurgitation in adults may be secondary to congenital abnormalities of the aortic sinuses, sinotubular

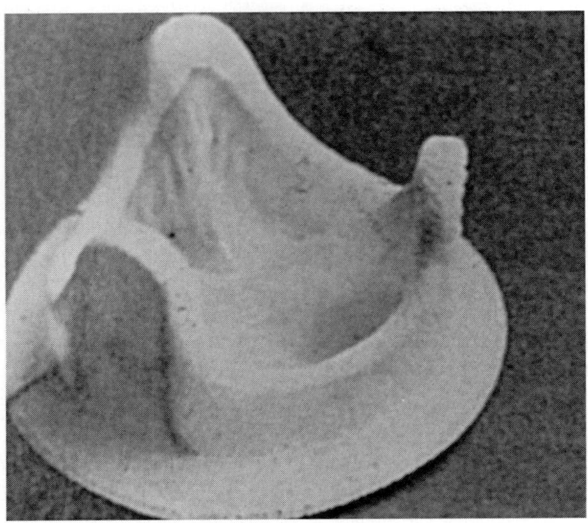

FIGURE 11–2 A stented xenograft valve; porcine bioprosthesis. (From Bauer G, Geha AS, Hammond GL, et al [eds]: Glenn's Thoracic and Cardiovascular Injury. 5th ed. New York: Prentice-Hall International, 1991. With permission of The McGraw-Hill Companies.)

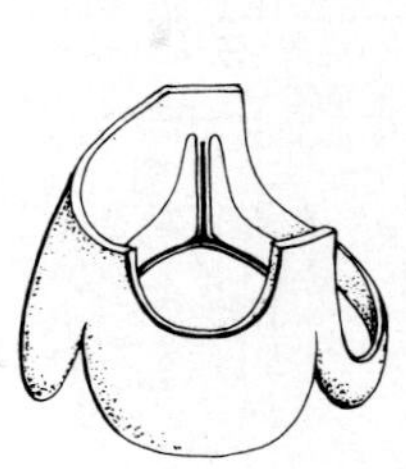

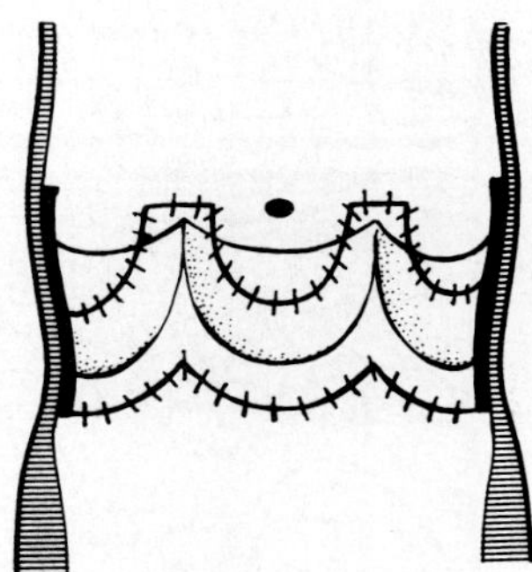

FIGURE 11–3 Homograft aortic valve replacement; the two-suture-line technique.

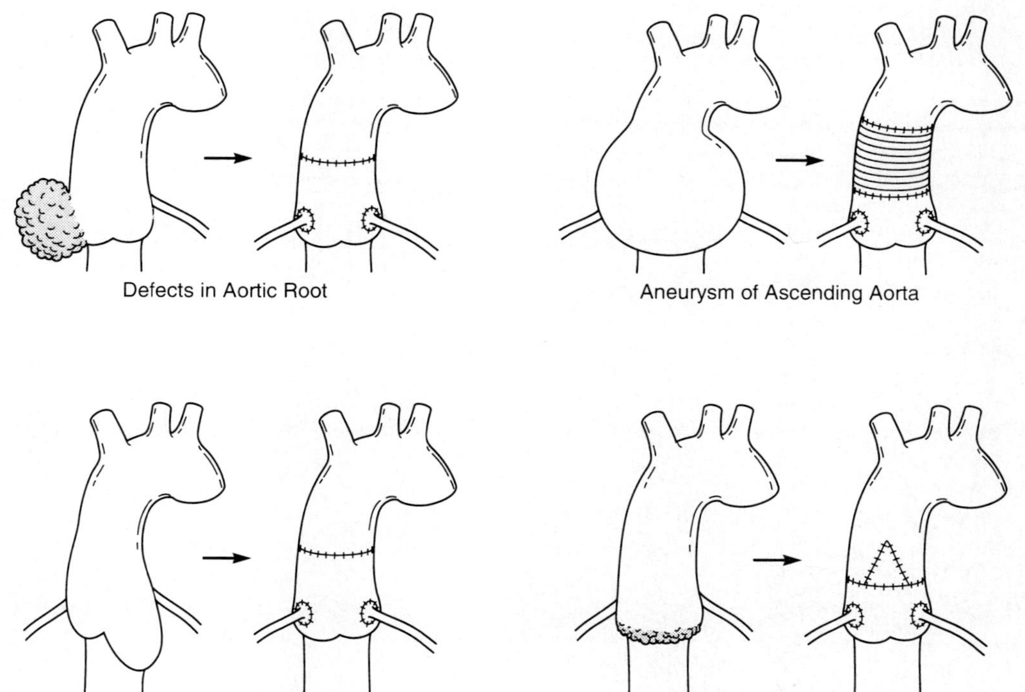

FIGURE 11–4 Homograft aortic root replacement with reimplantation of the coronary ostia. (From Dhella et al: In Bodner F, Yacoub MH [eds]: Biologic and Bioprosthetic valves. 1st ed. London: Yorke Medical Books, 1986.)

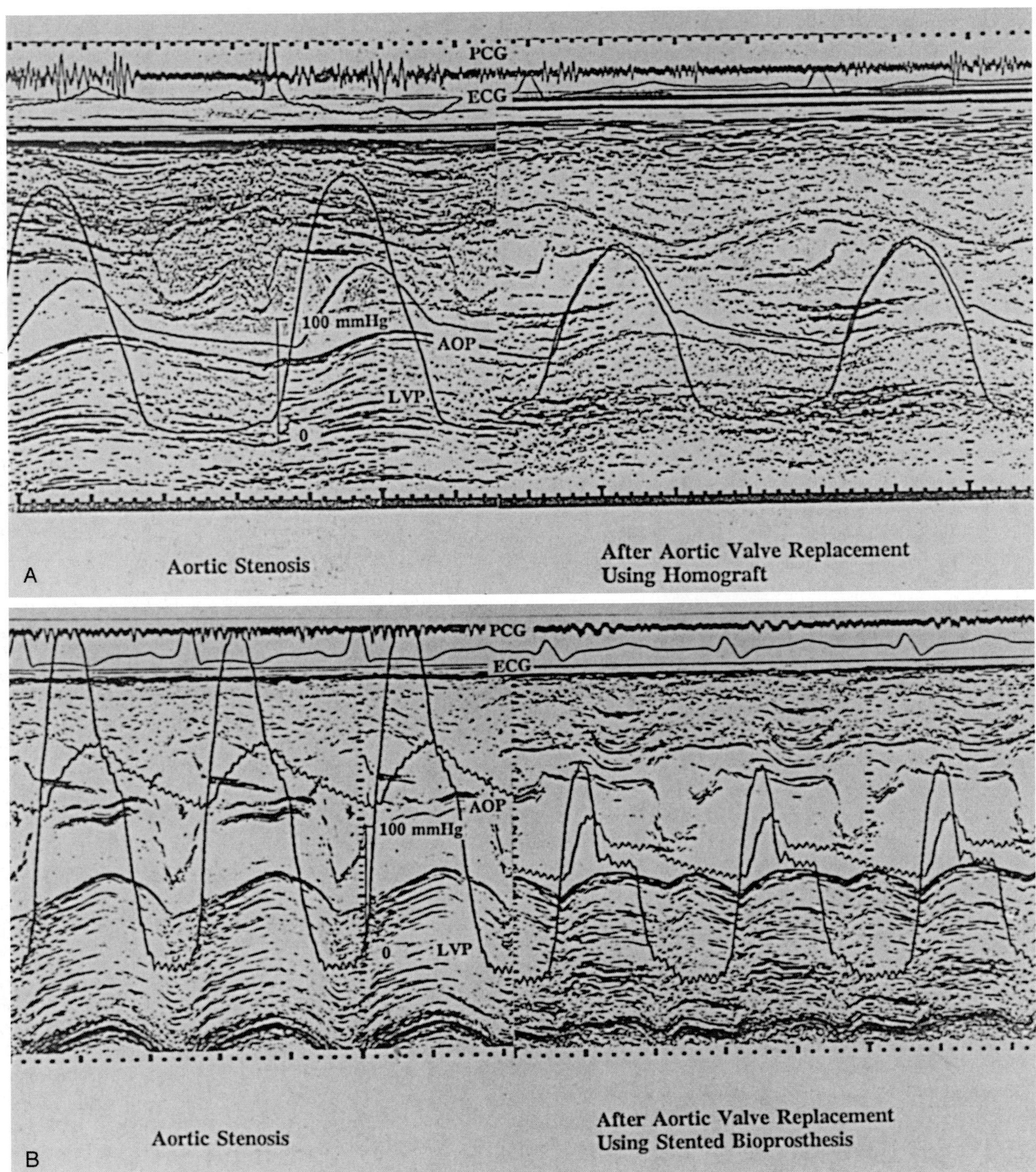

FIGURE 11–5 Simultaneous left ventricular pressure (LVP) (solid-state catheter) and M-mode echocardiogram show left ventricular wall movement and transventricular peak systolic gradient immediately after aortic valve replacement with homograft **(A)** and stented xenograft **(B)**. AOP, aortic pressure; ECG, electrocardiogram; PCG, phonocardiogram.

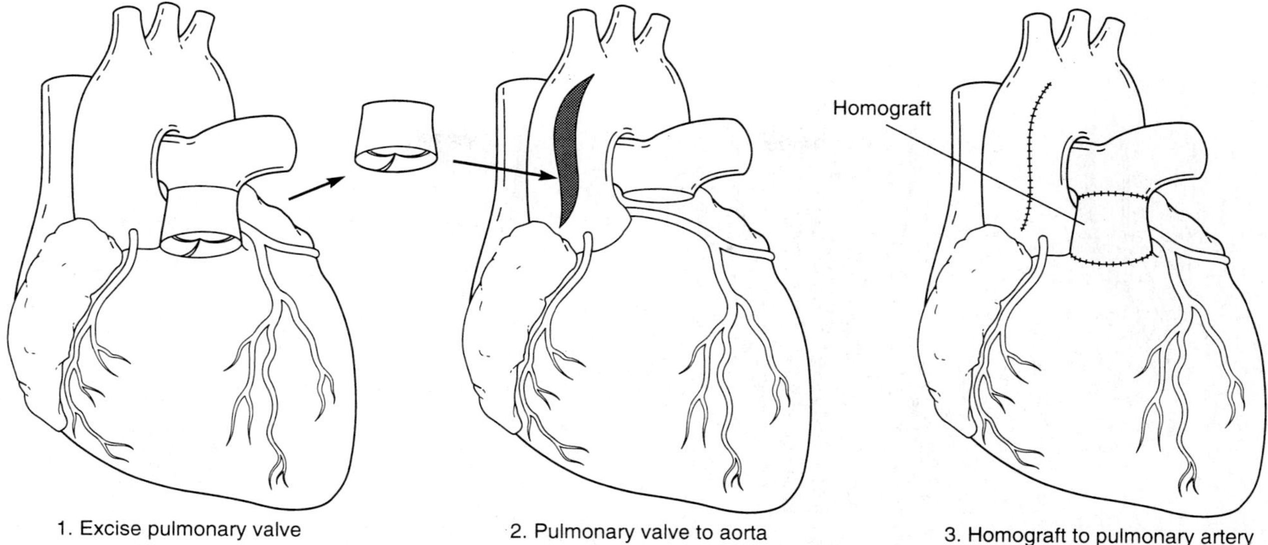

FIGURE 11–6 Pulmonary autograft replacement in the aortic position; two-suture-line technique. Pulmonary autograft as a root replacement (see Fig. 11–4). (From Ross DN: Evolution of the biological concept in cardiac surgery: a pilgrim's progress. *In* Yankah AC, Hetzer R, et al [eds]: Cardiac Valve Allografts 1962–1987. New York: Springer-Verlag, 1988.)

junction, or cusps and may be associated with VSD. Valve-preserving reparative procedures are possible in a high proportion of these patients[32–36] and depend on a thorough understanding of the anatomic and functional components of the particular condition, factors that influence progression and evolution of safe, predictable methods of surgical repair. These principles are exemplified in repair of the syndrome of dilatation of the right coronary sinus, VSD, and aortic regurgitation[32] (Figs. 11–7 and 11–8), as well as aortic regurgitation due to dilatation of the aortic sinus or sinotubular junction in patients with connective tissue disorders, such as Marfan's syndrome[37–40] (Fig. 11–9), or after the correction of certain congenital malformations, such as truncus arteriosus.[41]

Cusp extension with the use of fresh autologous or glutaraldehyde-treated or homologous pericardium dura mater has been used with good initial results (Fig. 11–10).[42–44] Although this technique can be used to tide patients for a period of time, relatively fast degeneration of the cusp extension, especially in young individuals, limits its wider use. The development of more durable materials, possibly through tissue engineering, is needed for this method to reach its potential.

Mitral Valve Disease

Congenital abnormalities of the mitral valve can present in adulthood with severe regurgitation secondary to a cleft in the anterior cusp or to cusp prolapse (Fig. 11–11) caused by myxomatous degeneration.[45–50] Valve repair is the procedure of choice for these lesions and is appropriate for the majority of patients. Accurate characterization of the anatomic lesion is usually achieved with intraoperative echocardiography (Fig. 11–12). Intraoperative testing of the mitral valve, using a technique that subjects the valve to physiologic pressures with a beating heart, allows selective repair of the responsible lesion (Fig. 11–13).

Congenital mitral stenosis secondary to a parachute valve almost always presents in infancy or childhood. A supravalvular membrane attached to the upper surface of the mitral valve can present in late childhood or early adulthood (Fig. 11–14).[51] We have observed the progression of supravalvular membranes in adulthood. Although the membrane is commonly fused to the atrial surface of the mitral valve cusps, it is usually possible to excise it with preservation of the valve. The left AV valve in ventriculoarterial discordance is usually abnormal, with resulting progressive regurgitation in adult life.[52, 53] These valves usually require replacement and are very rarely suitable for repair. Furthermore, after surgery, the regurgitation is usually associated with varying degrees of dysfunction of the systemic morphologic right ventricle.

Tricuspid Valvular Disease

The most common congenital defects of the tricuspid valve presenting in adulthood are the less severe forms of Ebstein's anomaly, with displacement of attachment of the posterior and septal leaflets into the right ventricle, resulting in varying degrees of tricuspid regurgitation, as well as RV and LV dysfunction. Repair is possible in approximately two thirds of the patients, with a variety of techniques (Fig. 11–15).[54, 55] In patients with advanced RV dysfunction in the presence of severe LV dysfunction, total cavopulmonary shunt can be considered. In patients with advanced RV and LV dysfunction, cardiac transplantation is indicated.

Pulmonary Valve

Isolated pulmonary valvular stenosis occasionally presents for the first time in adult life. Although the valve is thicker and may be calcified, open valvotomy is usually possible.

Text continued on page 295

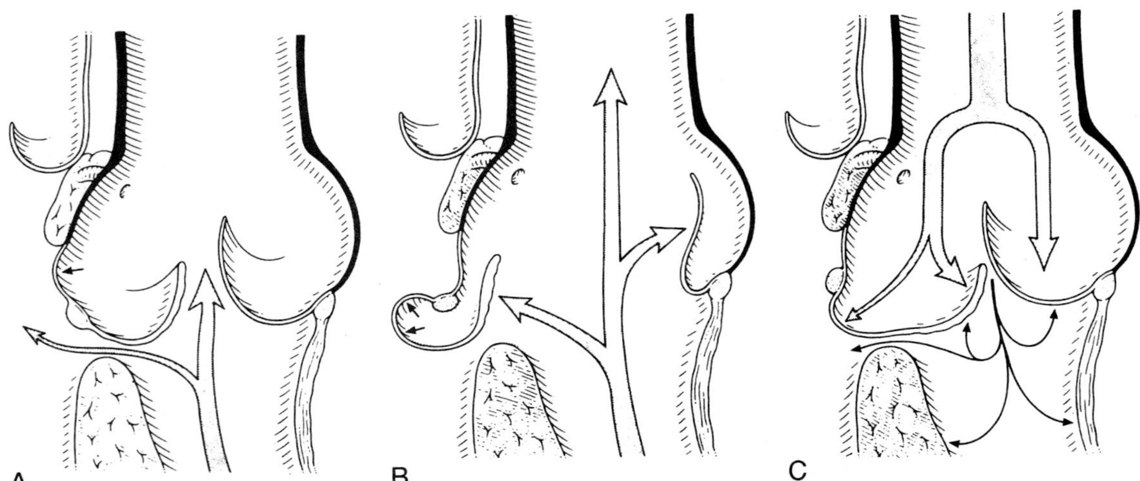

FIGURE 11–7 Hemodynamic forces that influence progression of the syndrome during early systole **(A)**, late systole **(B)**, and diastole **(C)**. (**A–C,** From Yacoub M, Khan H, Stavri G, et al: Anatomic correction of the syndrome of prolapsing right coronary aortic cusp, dilatation of the sinus of Valsalva and ventricular septal defect. J Thorac Cardiovasc Surg 113:253–261, 1997.)

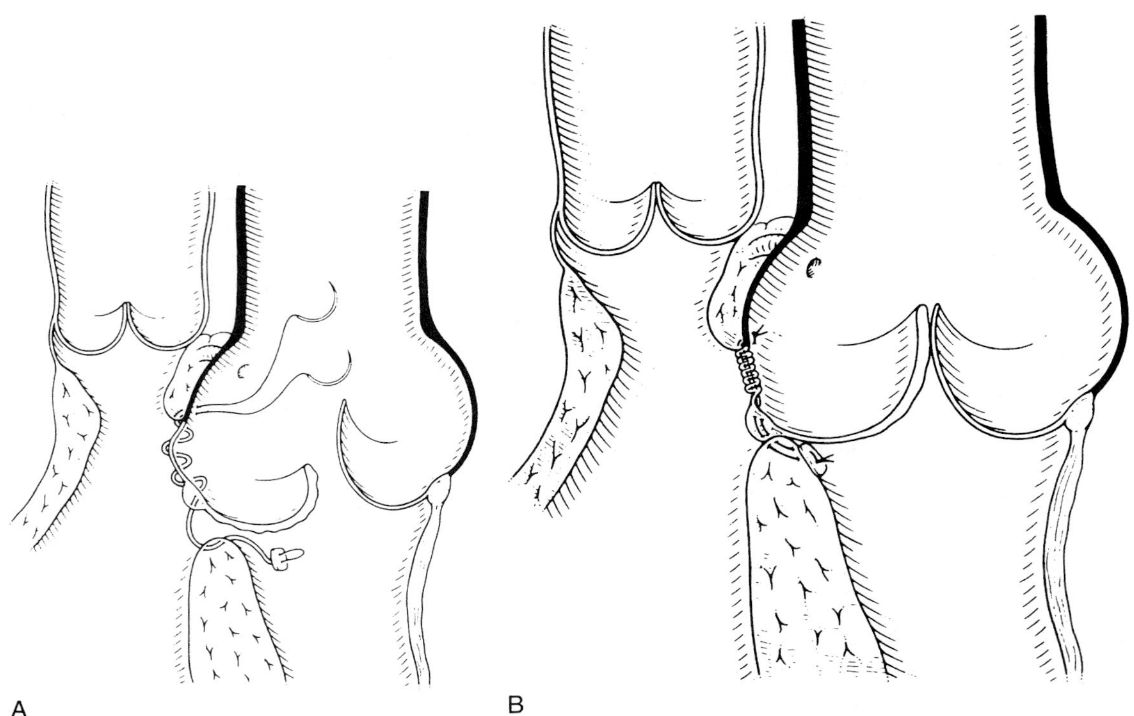

FIGURE 11–8 **A** and **B,** Section in the aortic root illustrates the plicating sutures used to close the ventricular septal defect, elevate the annulus, reduce the size of the sinus, and restore competence of the aortic valve. (**A** and **B,** From Yacoub M, Khan H, Stavri G, et al: Anatomic correction of the syndrome of prolapsing right coronary aortic cusp, dilatation of the sinus of Valsalva and ventricular septal defect. J Thorac Cardiovasc Surg 113:253–261, 1997.)

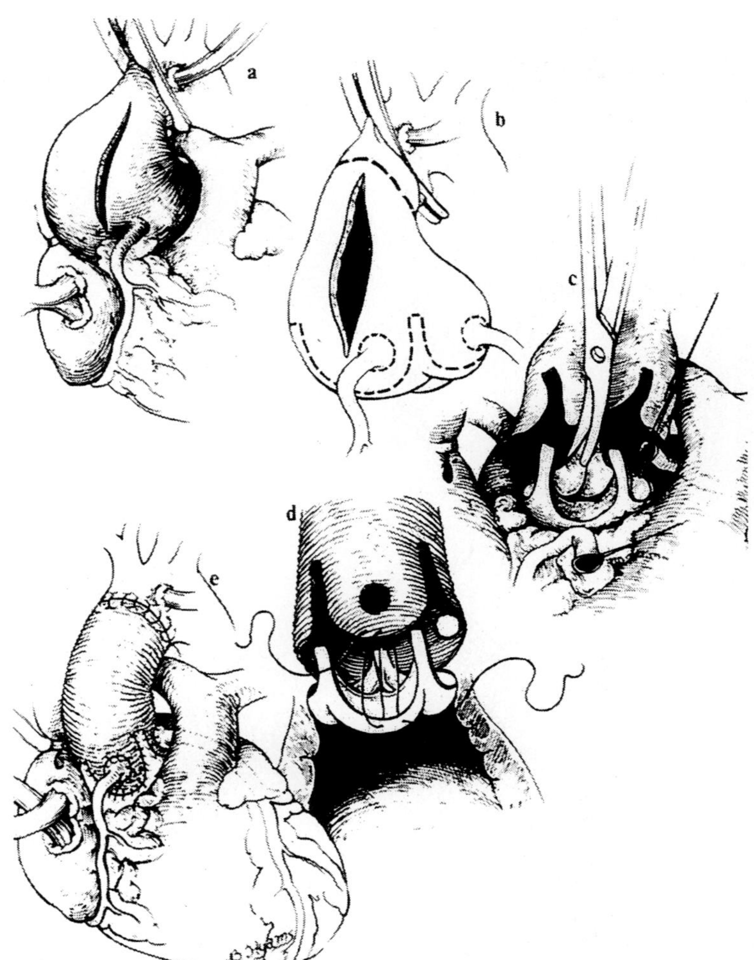

FIGURE 11–9 a–e, Operative technique of the valve-sparing operation used in this series (see the text). (**a–e,** From Yacoub MH, Gehle P, Chandrasekaram V, et al: Late results of a valve preserving operation in patients with aneurysms of the ascending aorta and root. J Thorac Cardiovasc Surg 115:1080–1090, 1998.)

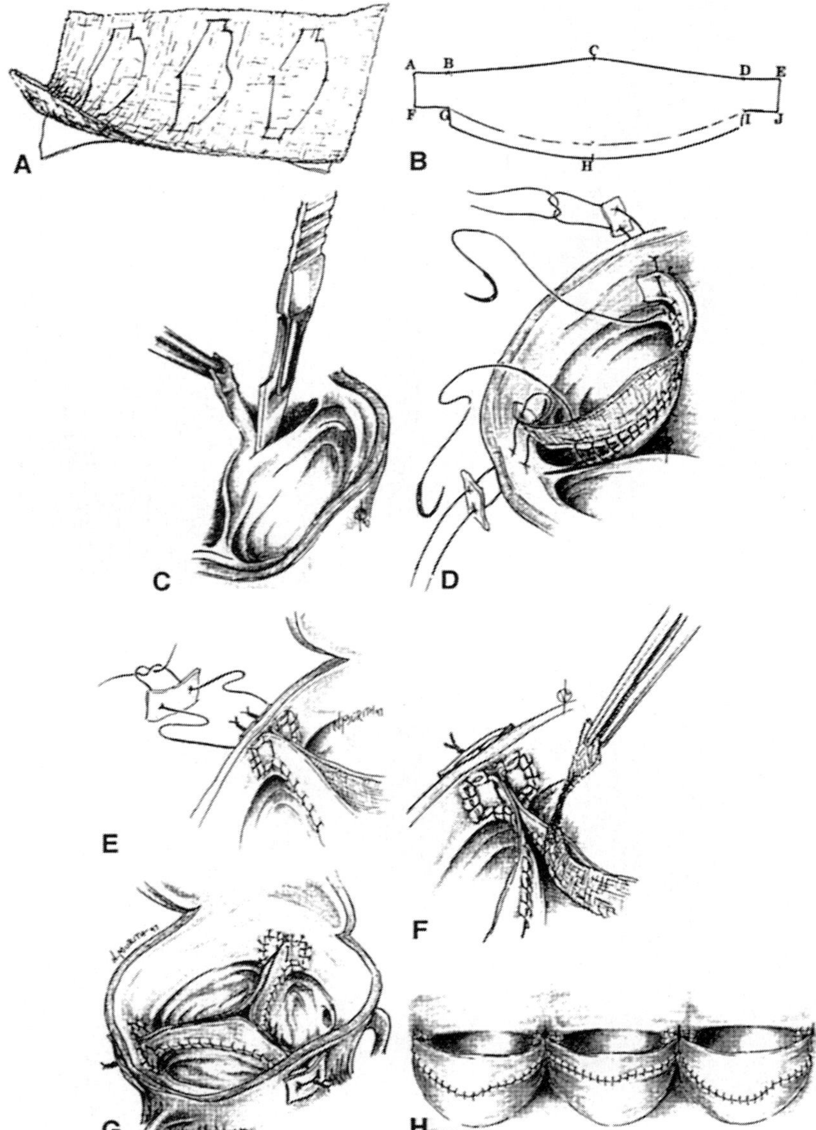

FIGURE 11–10 A–H, Surgical technique of aortic cusp extension with fresh autologous pericardium. (**A–H,** From Kalangos A, Beghetti M, Baldovinos A, et al: Aortic valve repair by cusp extension with the use of fresh autologous pericardium in children with rheumatic aortic insufficiency. J Thorac Cardiovasc Surg 118:225–236, 1999.)

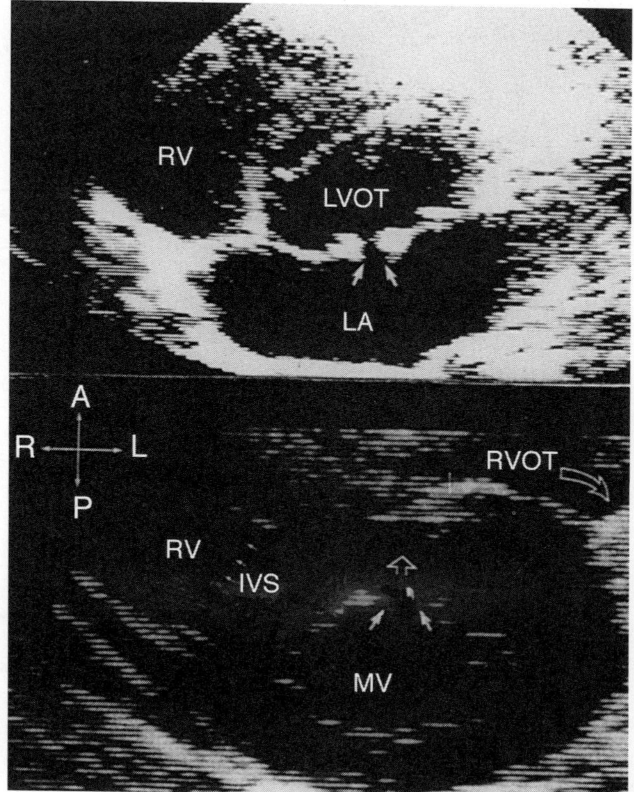

FIGURE 11–11 Top, Short-axis cut at the level of the left ventricular outflow tract (LVOT) in a patient with an isolated cleft in the anterior mitral leaflet. Note the cleft, indicated by the *two arrows* pointing toward the outflow tract, and not the right ventricle (RV). LA, left atrium. **Bottom,** Short-axis cut at the level of the mitral valve (MV). Note again the cleft indicated by the *arrows,* pointing toward the outlet of the heart and not the right ventricle. IVS, interventricular septum; MV, mitral valve. (From Smallhorn JF, de Leval M, Stark J, et al: Isolated anterior mitral cleft two dimensional echocardiography assessment. Br Heart J 48:109–116, 1982.)

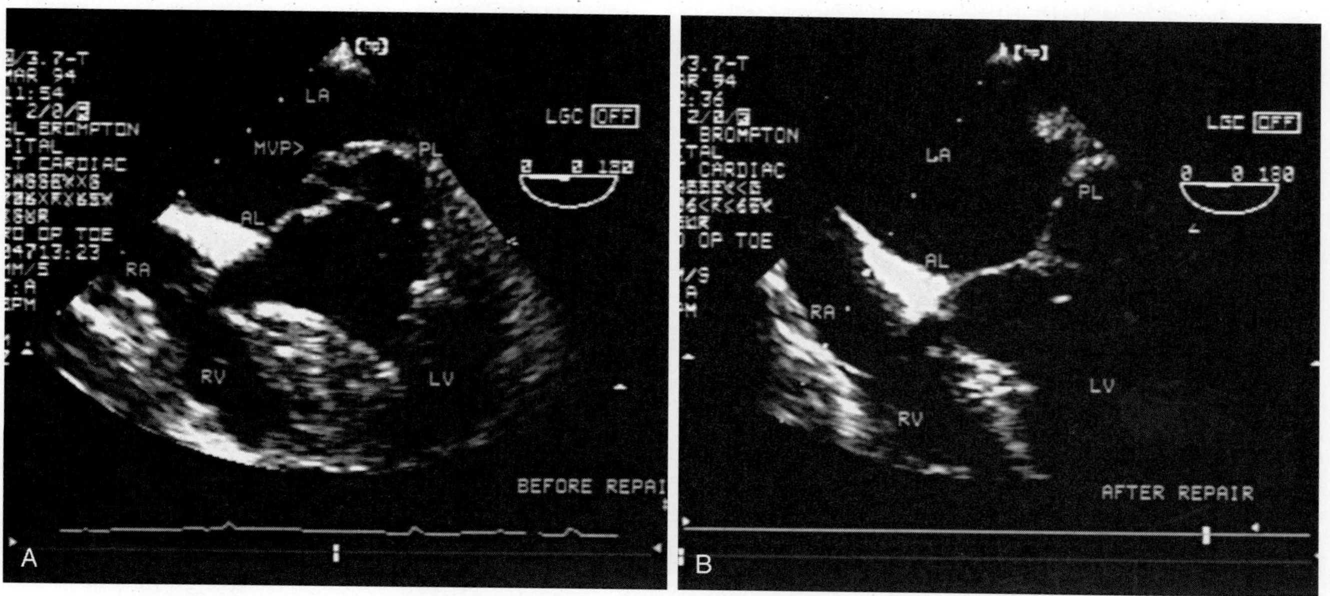

FIGURE 11–12 A and **B,** Typical features of mitral valve prolapse (MVP) as shown by intraoperative transesophageal echocardiography. AL, anterior leaflet; LA, left atrium; LV, left ventricle; RA, right atrium; RV, right ventricle.

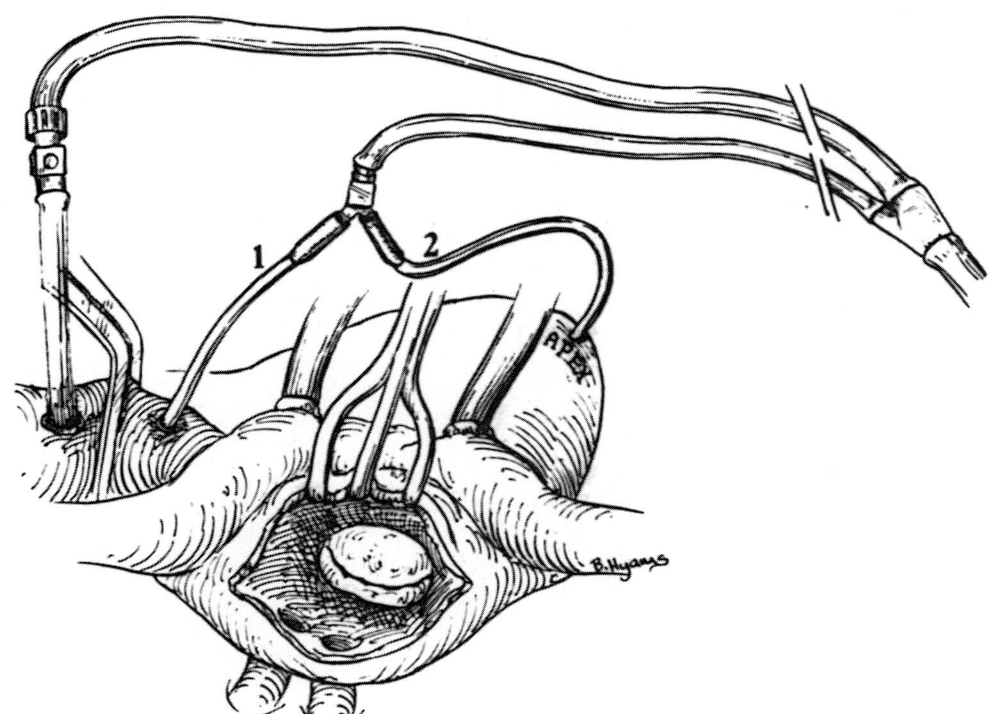

FIGURE 11–13 Intraoperative testing of mitral valve repair. Note use of a bifurcated coronary line directing blood into the left ventricle via the apex and into the aortic root proximal to the cross-clamp. The mitral valve can be safely inspected in the beating heart.

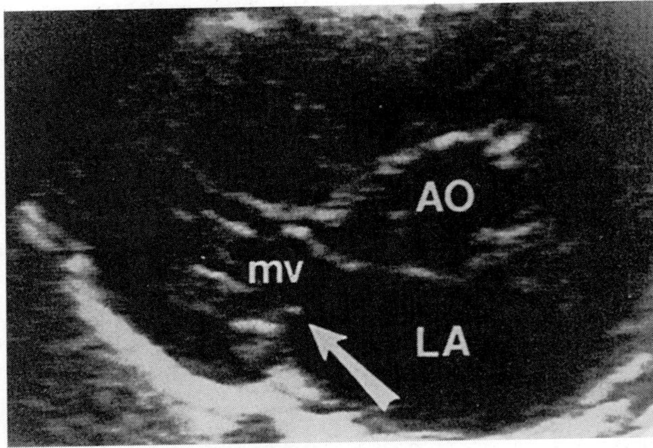

FIGURE 11–14 Congenital stenosing supravalvular membrane attached to the atrial side of the mitral valve (mv). Note that in contrast to the situation in cor triatriatum, the pulmonary veins and left atrial appendage enter the left atrium (LA) proximal to or above the supravalvular membrane. AO, aorta. (From Hurst JW: Atlas of the Heart. New York: Gower Medical, 1988.)

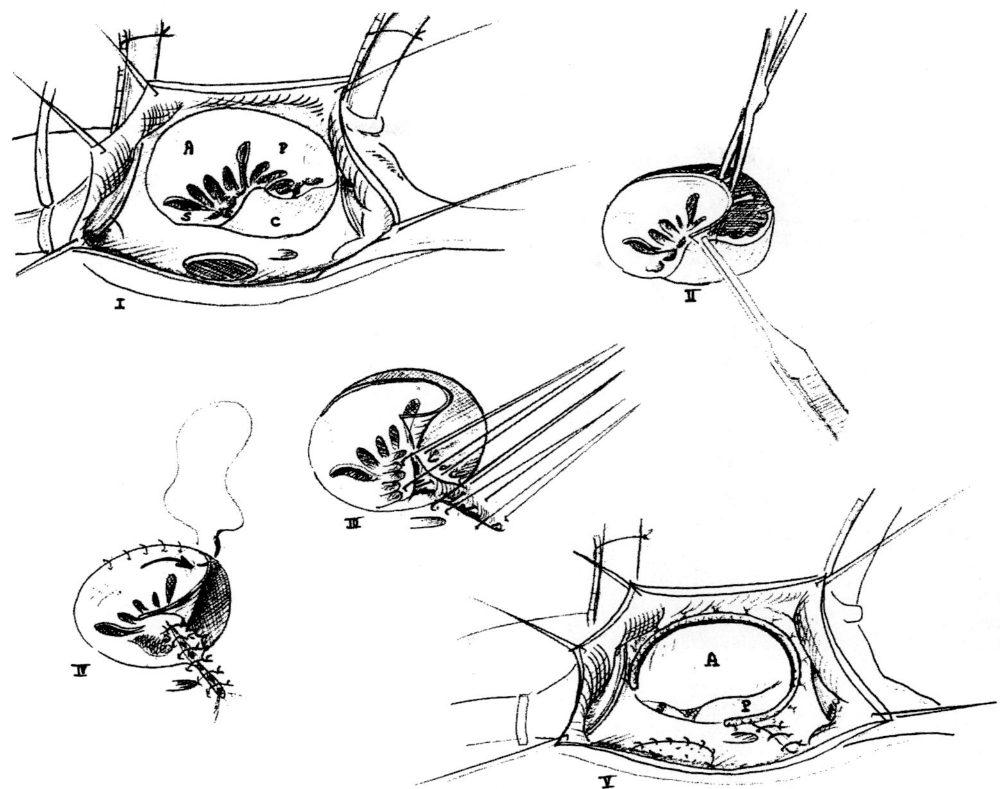

FIGURE 11–15 Surgical technique. **I,** Operative view. A, Anterior leaflet; C, atrialized chamber; P, posterior leaflet; S, septal leaflet. **II,** Anterior leaflet and adjacent portion of posterior leaflet are detached from the annulus. Leaflet tissue is mobilized by cutting fibrous bands attached to the ventricular wall. Interchordal spaces are fenestrated if obliterated. **III,** Longitudinal plication of right ventricle by simple sutures passed through the septal and posterior leaflet remnants. Tricuspid annulus and right atrium are plicated. **IV,** Anterior and posterior leaflets are sutured to the tricuspid annulus after clockwise rotation (*arrow*) to cover the entire orifice area. **V,** Prosthetic ring is inserted to remodel the orifice and to reinforce repair. Atrial septal defect is closed. (From Carpentier A, Chauraud S, Mace L: A new reconstructive operation for Ebstein's anomaly of the tricuspid valve. J Thorac Cardiovasc Surg 96:92–101, 1988.)

Pulmonary valve replacement is rarely necessary. Recurrent or residual pulmonary valvular dysfunction after previous repair or angioplasty is uncommon except in patients with tetralogy of Fallot who have received transannular patches or previous insertion of a valve conduit for correction of a variety of complex congenital anomalies.[56] In these patients, the calcified conduit could be adherent to the sternum and therefore at risk of being injured during sternotomy. To avoid this, profound hypothermia with femorofemoral cannulation may be used. The preferred valve at both the first and second operation is a pulmonary homograft, although both aortic homografts and xenografts have been used with varying degrees of success.

Ventricular Outflow Tract Obstruction

Outflow tract obstruction due to causes other than valvular disease may occur at the subvalvular and supravalvular levels. On the left side, subaortic obstruction may be caused by muscular or fibromuscular tissue, which may be mild at birth but can progress during adulthood (Figs. 11–16 and 11–17).[57–60] Adequate relief of obstruction can be achieved in almost all cases with transaortic excision of the obstructing tissue, starting from a point below the midportion of the right coronary cusp and extending laterally toward the left fibrous trigone, clearing the angle between the muscular septum and the anterolateral attachment of the anterior mitral leaflet with mobilization of both fibrous trigones (Fig. 11–18) and thus restoring the dynamic nature of the subaortic region (Fig. 11–19).[60] Subaortic obstruction due to hypertrophic obstructive cardiomyopathy can be relieved with transaortic wide excision of the obstructive muscle. Mobilization of the fibrous trigones may be necessary in some of these patients.[60] A very small minority of patients with tunnel-type obstruction requires more radical procedures.[61–63]

Supravalvular aortic stenosis is usually associated with hypoplasia of the ascending aorta. This condition can be adequately treated by the insertion of a bifid (Fig. 11–20)[64] and trifoliate (Fig. 11–21)[65] patch of autogenous pericardium or Dacron.

On the right side, isolated infundibular stenosis can usually be relieved through the pulmonary valve or through a transverse ventriculotomy.

Coarctation of the Aorta

Uncorrected and recurrent coarctation[66, 67] or complications related to previous repair,[68] such as false aneurysms or hypertension, can present in adult life. In these patients, an

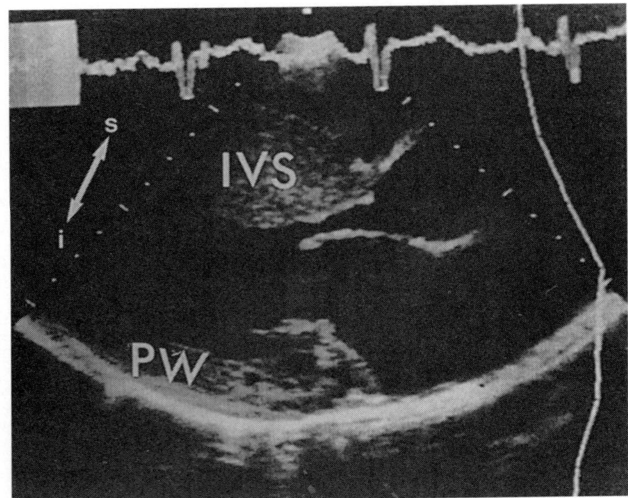

FIGURE 11–16 Left ventricular outflow tract obstruction due to subvalvular muscular hypertrophy. IVS, interventricular septum; PW, posterior wall. (From Nitkoyannopoulos P [ed]: Cardiac Ultrasound Cardiomyopathy. New York: Churchill Livingstone, 1993.)

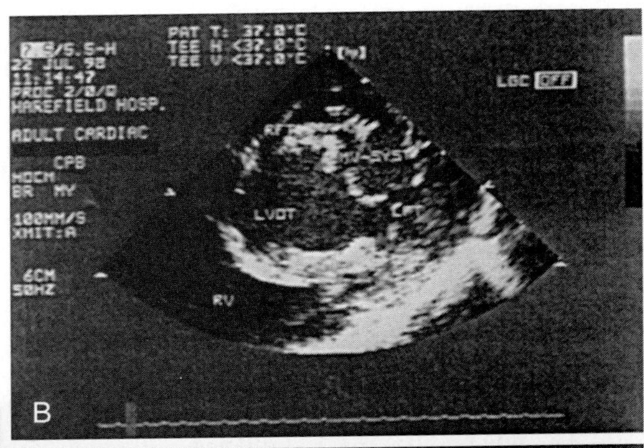

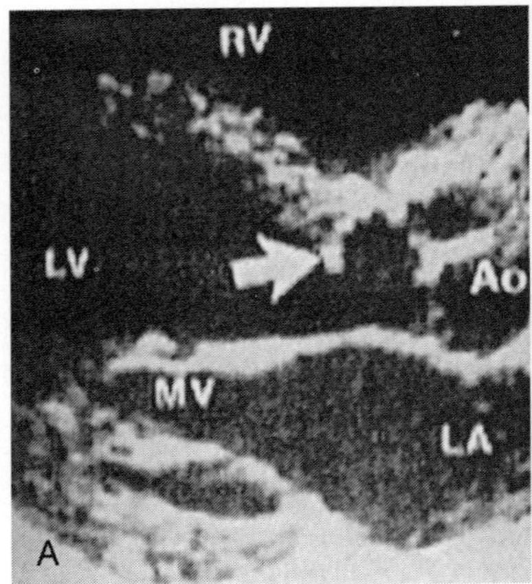

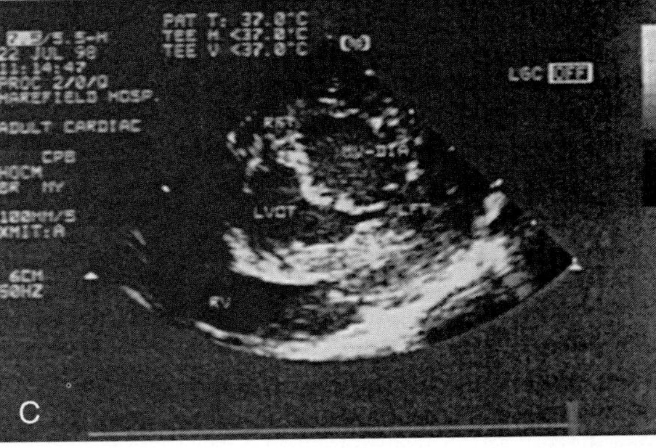

FIGURE 11–17 Echocardiogram shows the anterior component of the subaortic stenosis **(A)**, postoperative transesophageal echocardiogram of the left ventricular outflow tract (LVOT) during systole and diastole **(B)**, and the mobilized hinge mechanism of the right and left fibrous trigones **(C)**. Ao, aorta; LA, left atrium; LV, left ventricle; MV, mitral valve; RV, right ventricle. (**A–C,** From Yacoub M, Onuzo O, Riedel B, Radley-Smith R: Mobilization of the left and right fibrous trigones for relief of severe left ventricular outflow obstruction. J Thorac Cardiovasc Surg 117:126–133, 1999.)

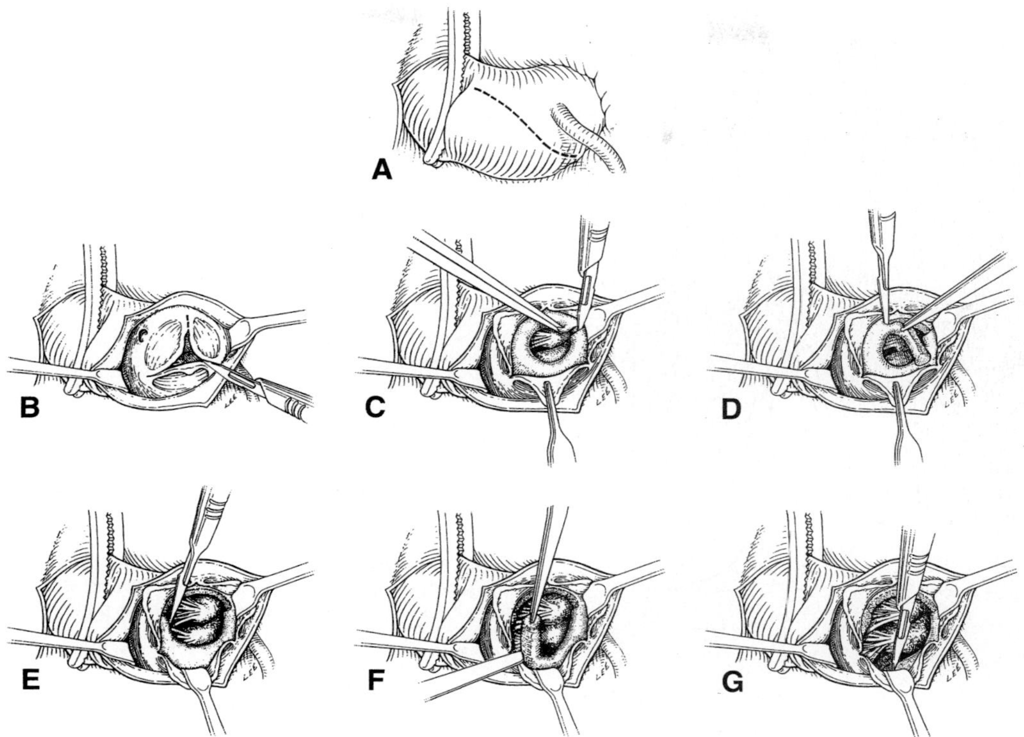

FIGURE 11–18 A–G, Diagrams show the different steps of surgical relief of fixed subaortic stenosis with mobilization of the fibrous trigones (see the text for details). (**A–G,** From Yacoub M, Onuzo O, Riedel B, Radley-Smith R: Mobilization of the left and right fibrous trigones for relief of severe left ventricular outflow obstruction. J Thorac Cardiovasc Surg 117:126–133, 1999.)

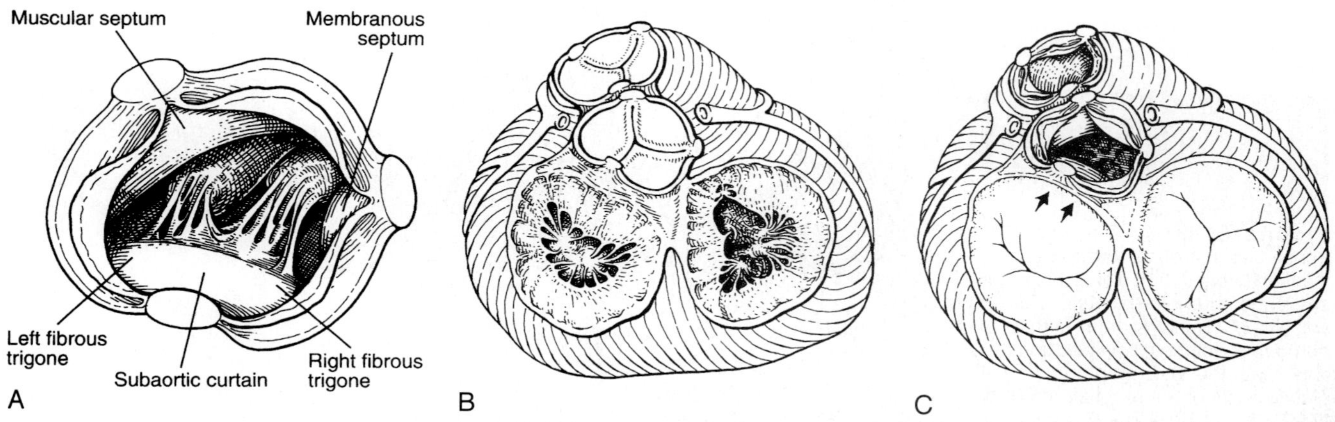

FIGURE 11–19 Diagrams show the interaction between the mitral and the aortic orifices **(B** and **C)**, with the two fibrous trigones acting as a hinge mechanism for the movement of the subaortic curtain and anterior leaflet of the mitral valve during different phases of the cardiac cycle and the structures surrounding the left ventricular outflow tract **(A)**. (**A–C,** From Yacoub M, Onuzo O, Riedel B, Radley-Smith R: Mobilization of the left and right fibrous trigones for relief of severe left ventricular outflow obstruction. J Thorac Cardiovasc Surg 117:126–133, 1999.)

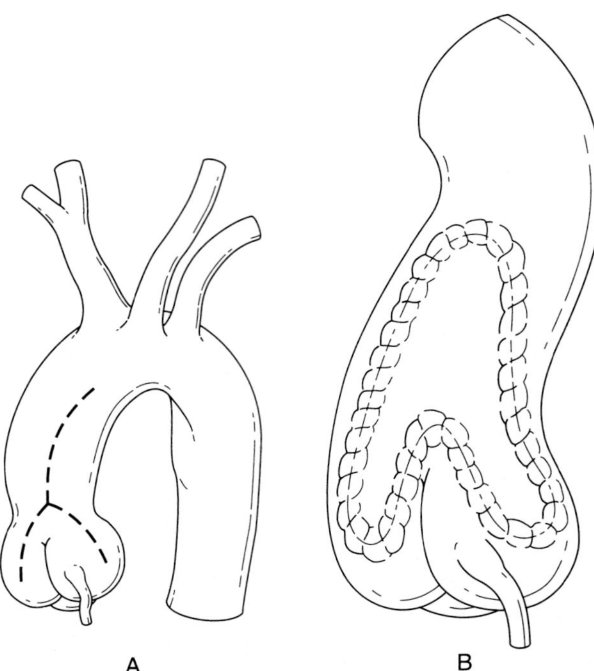

FIGURE 11–20 A and **B,** Repair of supravalvular aortic stenosis with a patch of autologous pericardium. (**A** and **B,** From Van Son JAM, Danielson GK, Puga FJ, et al: Supravalvular aortic stenosis. J Thorac Cardiovasc Surg 107:103–115, 1994.)

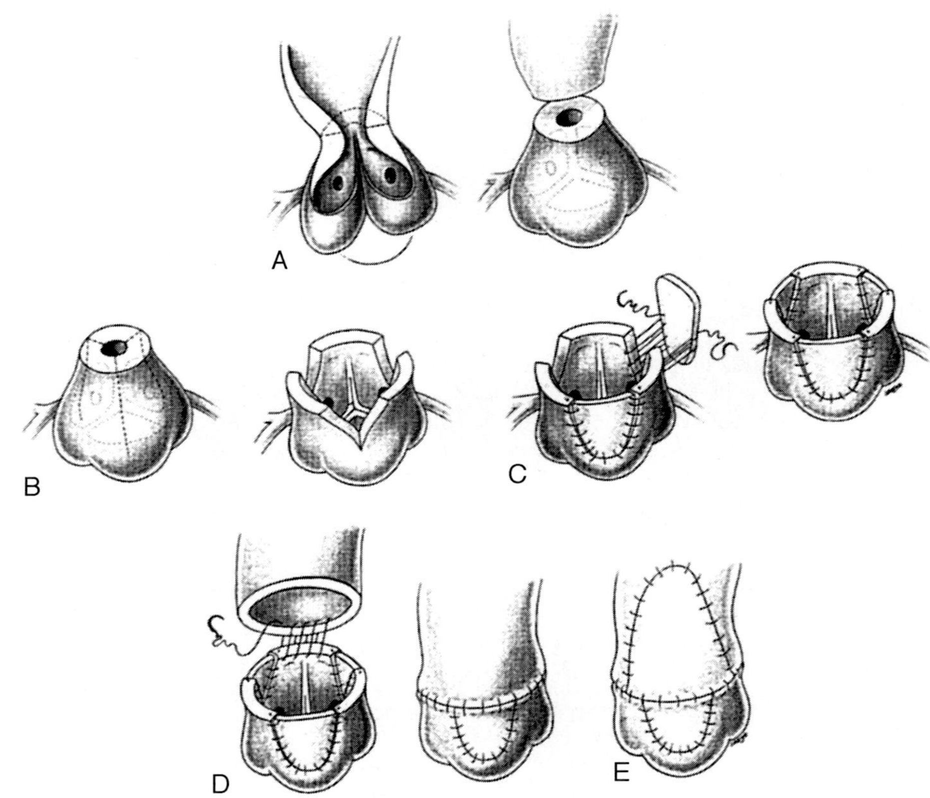

FIGURE 11–21 A, The aorta is transected just distal to the area of maximal stenosis. **B,** Three incisions are made, one into each sinus of Valsalva. **C,** Restoration of normal aortic root geometry by insertion of three patches. **D,** End-to-end anastomosis of the reconstructed root to the ascending aorta. **E,** Enlargement of the ascending aorta by an additional patch. (**A–E,** From HazeKamp MG, Kappeteia AP, Schoof PF, et al: Brom's three-patch technique for repair of supravalvular aortic stenosis. J Thorac Cardiovasc Surg 118:252–258, 1999.)

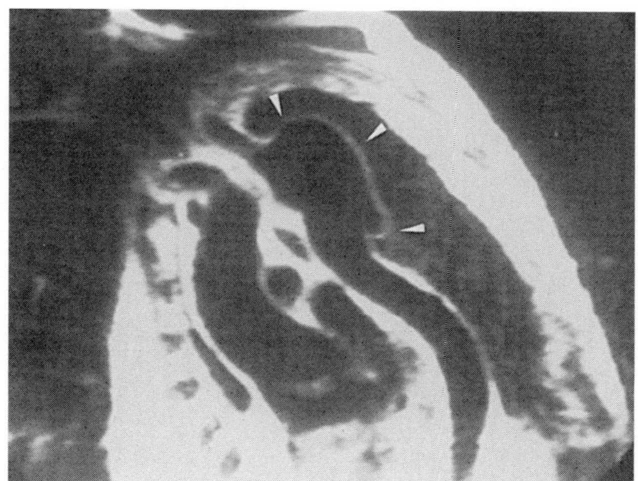

FIGURE 11–22 Dacron patch aneurysm *(arrowheads)* shown by spin-echo magnetic resonance imaging in the region of the previous Dacron patch repair.

accurate diagnosis of the exact anatomic lesion with the use of magnetic resonance imaging[69] (Fig. 11–22), computed tomography scanning, or angiography is necessary. The use of patch angioplasty has resulted in a high incidence of late false aneurysms. The operation of choice is excision of the lesion with direct end-to-end anastomosis; in some patients, however, interposition of a Dacron graft or the use of a bypass graft from the proximal to the distal segment may be necessary, and possibly safer. The use of balloon dilatation should be considered in these patients.[70]

Septal Defects and Anomalous Pulmonary Veins

Secundum Atrioseptal Defect

Secundum atrioseptal defect (ASD) can present in adulthood and may be associated with atrial fibrillation, marked enlargement of the right ventricle and pulmonary arteries (Fig. 11–23), and occasionally, mitral valve prolapse. Varying degrees of pulmonary vascular disease may occur later in life. Large defects should be closed with a pericardial or Dacron patch to avoid tension on the slightly rigid tissues. The sudden postoperative drop in flow through the markedly enlarged pulmonary arteries may lead to intravascular thrombosis, which may be prevented by postoperative anticoagulation for a period of 1 month to 1 year, depending on the size of the pulmonary arteries. Defects with echocardiographic evidence of right heart dilatation, a pulmonary/systemic flow ratio of more than 1.5, or both, should be closed electively to prevent long-term complications. Older patients with nonrestrictive ASDs and established atrial flutter or fibrillation, paroxysmal or chronic, may still benefit from elective ASD closure. However, these patients remain at the risk of persistent postoperative arrhythmia (Fig. 11–24), and for this reason, additional procedures targeting the arrhythmia (maze procedure) should be considered at the time of surgical closure of the defect.[71–73] Numerous transcatheter devices are under evaluation by different investigators for nonsurgical closure of ASDs. However, most of these devices are not suitable for large ASDs, and their use is restricted to a limited number of centers.

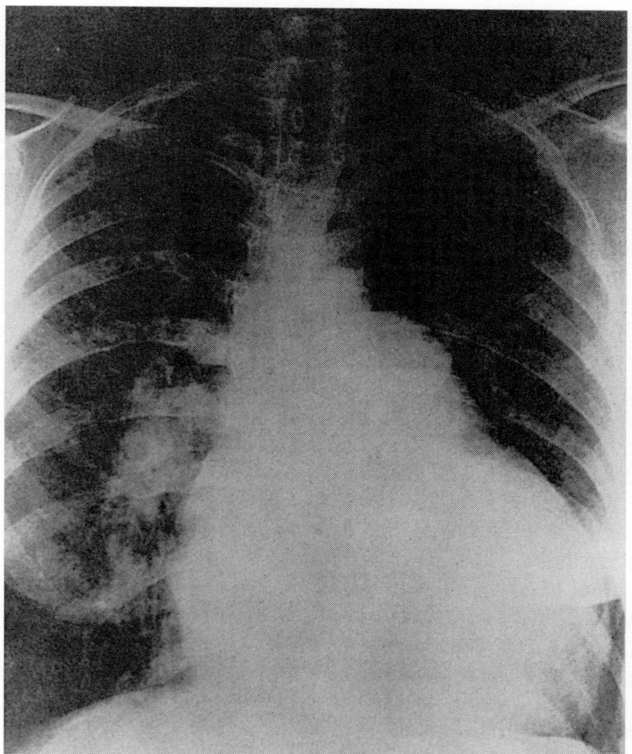

FIGURE 11–23 Right ventricular enlargement associated with a secundum atrial septal defect presenting in adult life. (From Shapiro LM, Fox KM [eds]: A Colour Atlas of Adult Congenital Heart Disease. London: Wolfe Medical, 1990.)

Atrioventricular Septal Defect

Patients with partial atrioventricular septal defects (AVSDs) share the same hemodynamic burden of chronic right heart

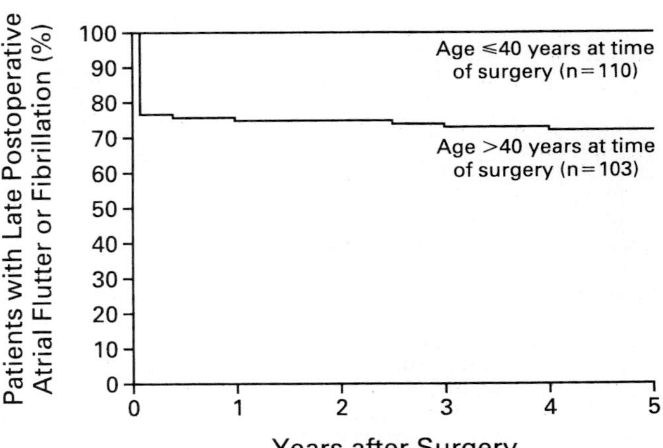

FIGURE 11–24 Kaplan-Meier estimates of late postoperative atrial flutter or fibrillation. (From Gatzoolis MA, Freeman MA, Sui SC, et al: Atrial arrhythmia after surgical closure of atrial septal defects in adults. N Engl J Med 340:839–846, 1999. Copyright 1999 Massachusetts Medical Society. All rights reserved.)

volume overload with secundum ASDs, with the additional hazard of left AV valve regurgitation. Patients with more severe forms of left AV valve regurgitation tend to present earlier. Repair of partial AVSD in adulthood, combined with elective left AV valvuloplasty, carries a low operative risk with an excellent long-term outcome and may reduce the need for reoperation on the left AV valve.[74]

Patients with complete AVSDs, in contrast, develop early pulmonary vascular disease, and although they may still survive to adulthood without an operation, they develop the Eisenmenger complex. Occasionally, the pulmonary circulation in the older patient with complete AVSD is protected by natural pulmonary stenosis or the early insertion of pulmonary artery banding. Ideally, complete AVSD should be corrected during the first year of life, including those with tetralogy of Fallot, unless there are specific contraindications.[75]

After repair of the AVSD, a significant number of patients develop progressive left AV valve regurgitation. This is usually secondary to separation of the two repaired components of the reconstructed septal leaflet of the new left AV valve and can be repaired by inserting extra sutures (Fig. 11–25). Occasionally, valvular tissue is deficient, necessitating valve replacement with a low-profile valve to prevent LV outflow obstruction by the prosthetic valve. Subaortic stenosis can develop late after repair of AVSD. This is usually due to turbulence produced by the abnormal attachment of the left AV valve, resulting in the development of a discrete fibrous shelf. Radical excision of the fibrous tissue is usually sufficient to relieve the obstruction (see discussion on subaortic stenosis). Occasionally, more complex forms of reconstruction are required.

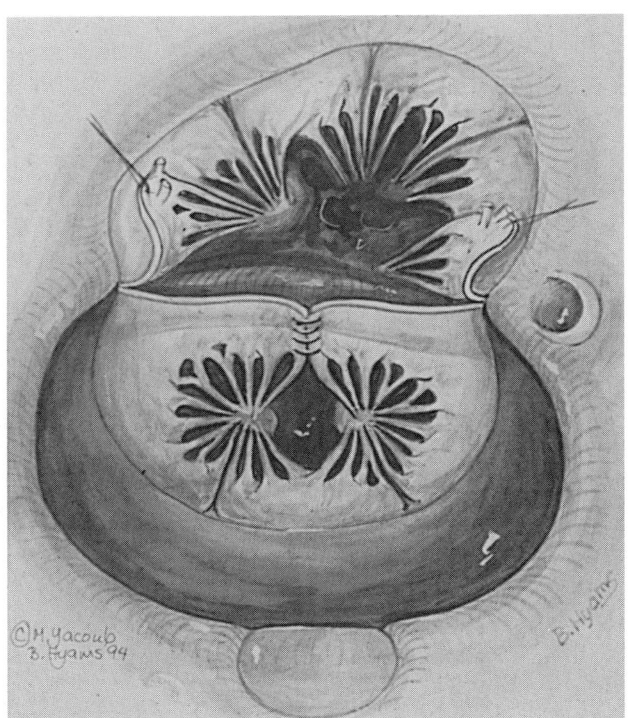

FIGURE 11–25 Reattachment of the two components of the reconstructed septal leaflet of the left atrioventricular valve.

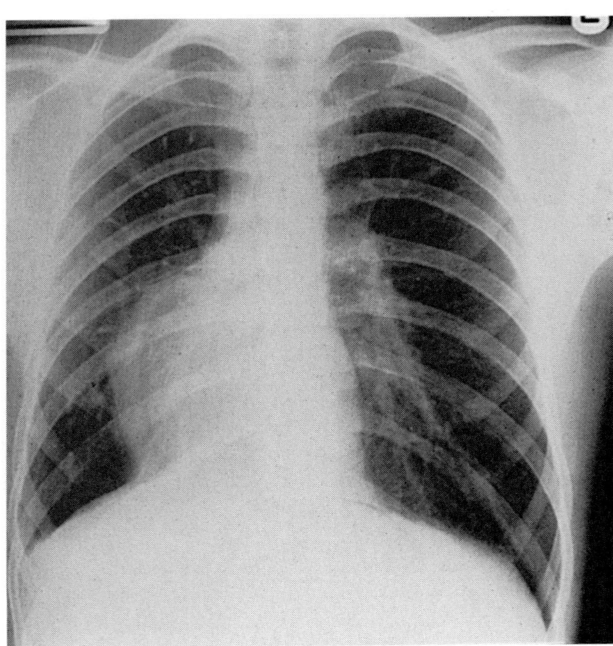

FIGURE 11–26 Hemianomalous pulmonary venous drainage in association with right lung hypoplasia (scimitar syndrome).

Anomalous Pulmonary Veins

Anomalous drainage of one or more pulmonary veins is occasionally encountered in adult life. This may be isolated or associated with a small ASD or specific syndrome of right pulmonary hypoplasia (*scimitar syndrome*) (Fig. 11–26). As in isolated ASD, the need for correction depends on the size of the left-to-right shunt.

Ventricular Septal Defect

Small VSDs may be diagnosed in adulthood during routine medical examination or during repeated episodes of infectious endocarditis involving the tricuspid valve on the RV wall. The defect may be closed after adequate treatment of the endocarditis with intravenous antibiotics. Emergency excision of the infected tissue and repair of the VSD during the acute stage are indicated in patients with uncontrolled infection or uncontrolled heart failure. There still is no agreement about the management of small defects diagnosed during routine medical examination. The risk for death or major complications (i.e., endocarditis) is very small and probably equal to the risk of surgical correction. Occasionally, small defects present with RV outflow obstruction or aortic cusp prolapse and aortic regurgitation. Resuspension of the right coronary or noncoronary cusp often reveals a larger VSD—partially occluded by the cusp—and may preserve the aortic valve.[32] Patients with large unoperated defects present with advanced pulmonary vascular disease and are considered for heart-lung transplantation or double-lung transplantation, and repair of the defect (see later).

Patent Arterial Ducts

Small patent ductus arteriosus diagnosed in adulthood carries a relatively high risk for endarteritis (about 1 to 2 percent) because of the turbulence created, which may produce endothelial damage and infection; therefore, these defects should be electively closed. In middle-aged patients, calcification and aneurysmal dilatation around the area of the duct may necessitate the use of cardiopulmonary bypass to handle the additional lesion. The presence of a large patent ductus arteriosus in adults is usually associated with severe pulmonary vascular disease, which may require heart-lung or double-lung transplantation.

Coronary Artery Anomalies

Anomalies of the mode of origin or course of the proximal coronary arteries can have a profound effect on myocardial blood flow and can lead to severe ischemia or sudden death. Although these anomalies are uncommon, familiarity with the different anatomic types and with the exact mechanisms involved in ischemia is essential if the treating clinician is to recognize and effectively treat these potentially correctable conditions before they produce irreversible damage.

In addition, recognition of benign coronary anomalies and aberrant vessels is important in planning surgical repair of congenital heart disease. Anomalies occur in 10 to 30 percent of cases of tetralogy of Fallot—most commonly, a prominent conus artery arising from the right coronary artery or the left anterior descending coronary or circumflex artery arising from the right aortic sinus or right coronary artery. If the aberrant vessel crosses the RV outflow tract, it may be jeopardized at the time of surgical repair. There are several surgically important variations of coronary anatomy in transposition of the great arteries (AV concordance, VA discordance) to be considered when performing the arterial switch operation in an infant.[76]

Anomalous Origin of the Coronary Arteries From an Inappropriate Aortic Sinus

Origin of the left coronary artery from the right coronary sinus and, less commonly, the right coronary artery from the left coronary sinus[77] is known to produce sudden death or episodic ischemia. The exact mechanism responsible has been debated and was originally thought to be compression of the proximal coronary artery by the pulmonary artery. However, the most probable cause is compression of the intramural segment of the anomalous coronary artery that runs inside the aortic wall superficial to the intercoronary commissure of the aortic valve. Clinical diagnosis of the anomaly may be difficult, because objective evidence of ischemia may be lacking unless the patient undergoes repeated stress exercise testing to reproduce the exact conditions necessary to produce ischemia. Surgical treatment involves removal of the intramural course of the artery by laying it open into the lumen of the aorta, with careful reattachment of the intima.[77] This technique is effective, but there is a risk of damaging the aortic valve or producing coronary dissection or obstruction by the intimal flaps. Alternatively, the coronary artery can be bypassed, preferably using an arterial graft.

Anomalous Origin of the Left Coronary Artery From the Pulmonary Artery

This rare condition usually presents in infancy when pulmonary vascular resistance decreases, with myocardial ischemia and LV failure. However, 10 to 15 percent of patients survive into adulthood because an adequate circulation is established between the right and left coronary arteries via intercoronary collateral vessels.[78–80] Adults may be asymptomatic or present with myocardial ischemia or mitral regurgitation due to papillary muscle dysfunction. Even if there is no resting myocardial ischemia and ventricular function is normal, repair is warranted because such patients remain at risk of ischemia, syncope, and sudden death. Although several surgical strategies for treating this condition have been described,[81–85] the operation of choice is to create a two-coronary artery system by transplanting the anomalously arising vessel from the pulmonary artery. A reliable technique of anatomic correction of this anomaly with aortic transfer of the coronary ostium to the middle of the left coronary aortic sinus has been developed.[86, 87] The exact location of the coronary ostium in the sinus could have important implications to coronary flow.[88] The technique consists of limited mobilization of the pulmonary artery button bearing the coronary orifice, followed by threading it through the transverse sinus into the lumen of the aorta after making a circular hole in the aortic sinus. The anastomosis is performed from inside the aorta (Fig. 11–27). Mitral valve repair may also be required. Survival after surgical repair depends on the amount of ischemic myocardial damage and degree of mitral regurgitation.

Coronary Artery Fistulas

Coronary artery fistulas consist of a heterogeneous group of anomalies characterized by the presence of a fistulous tract between part of the coronary artery tree and a low-pressure chamber such as the right ventricle (40 percent of cases), the right atrium (25 percent), the pulmonary artery (15 percent), and rarely, the left atrium, pulmonary veins, or superior vena cava. In almost all of these conditions, survival to adulthood is usual, but longevity could be reduced. The evolution of the anomaly and its clinical importance depend on several factors, including the initial size and the exact location. Small fistulous communications between the proximal left anterior descending or right coronary artery on one side and the pulmonary artery on the other side usually cause trivial shunts and no significant coronary steal and appear to remain very small and therefore require no treatment. In contrast, large fistulous tracts between one of the aortic sinuses near the coronary orifice or from one of the large coronary arteries usually continue to grow in size and length, becoming progressively more tortuous.

The relationship between the fistulous tract and the coronary artery system can be complex in that the portion of the coronary artery proximal to the origin of the fistula can markedly enlarge and appear to be part of the fistulous tract but can be distinguished by the fact that it gives origin to coronary artery branches and, to some extent, by its location, which follows the normal course of the particular artery affected. Definition of the exact location of the

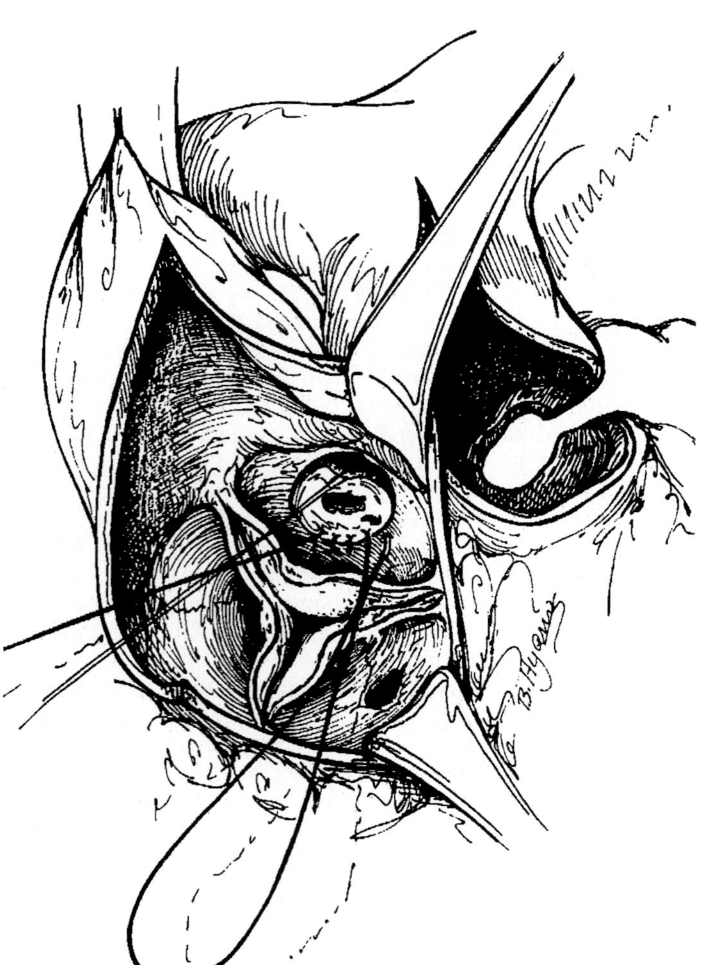

FIGURE 11–27 Technique of anatomic correction of an anomalous left coronary artery with transfer of the coronary ostium to the middle of the left coronary aortic sinus.

coronary arteries to the fistulous tract is essential in planning the appropriate corrective procedure. The objective is to remove the fistulous tract in its entirety while preserving coronary artery supply without ectatic segments. Attempts at defining the exact cause of the fistulous tract and the associated coronary orifice in relation to the fistulous tract can be determined at the time of operation after opening the fistulous tract. Restoration of near-normal coronary anatomy (after excision of the fistulous tract) can be accomplished via various reconstructive procedures involving anastomosing a flap or a button carrying the main coronary artery back to the aorta, occasionally combined with arterial grafts to the distal coronary branches. Distal interruption of the fistulas is inadequate because it could result in recurrence through rupture of the blind end into the same or another chamber or progressive thrombosis involving some of the coronary artery branches. Similarly, transcatheter closure may be accompanied by such complications.[89]

Cyanotic Heart Disease

Tetralogy of Fallot

Uncorrected tetralogy of Fallot encountered in adulthood is usually associated with many secondary changes, including various degrees of RV fibrosis, acquired calcification and/or atresia of the pulmonary valve, aortic valvular abnormalities (regurgitation or annular calcification), and occasionally, dilatation of the ascending aorta. In addition, the possibility of coronary artery disease should be excluded by angiography. Late repair is usually feasible but carries a slightly higher risk.[90–92] Such patients do not tolerate well free pulmonary regurgitation, and the use of a valve in the pulmonary position under these circumstances is advisable. Previous palliative procedures, such as shunts, must be taken down, with repair of any distortion or narrowing of the pulmonary arterial tree produced by the shunt. The shunts of Waterston and Pott require separation of the aorta from the pulmonary artery, with reconstruction of both vessels, which may be extensive in some patients. The use of extracardiac conduits to relieve the RV outflow obstruction is required more often than in the pediatric age group. Pulmonary or aortic homografts[93,94] are the preferred types of conduits because of their superior hemodynamic performance and durability compared with other types of conduits, such as stented porcine xenografts,[95,96] pericardial valve conduits, or prosthetic valves.

Residual or recurrent hemodynamic lesions leading to RV dilatation are not uncommon in the adult patient with previous repair of tetralogy of Fallot. These lesions should be corrected before they produce irreversible changes. Pulmonary regurgitation secondary to transannular patches, malfunctioning monocusp, or complete conduit is well tolerated. Pulmonary regurgitation, however, in the long term may lead to reduced exercise capacity, RV dysfunction, arrhythmia, and possibly sudden death.[97] QRS duration from the surface electrocardiogram relates to RV size; when it exceeds 180 milliseconds, it becomes a sensitive and specific marker of sustained ventricular tachycardia and sudden death late after repair of tetralogy of Fallot.

Restoration of RV outflow competence with pulmonary valve implantation, therefore, should be considered when progressive RV dilatation and early dysfunction occur or the patient becomes symptomatic.[98]

Tetralogy of Fallot With Pulmonary Atresia

A significant number of patients with tetralogy of Fallot with pulmonary atresia survive into adulthood when there is pulmonary blood supply through a set of true pulmonary arteries supplied by a patent ductus arteriosus, a previously constructed shunt, or multiple aortopulmonary collateral arteries (MAPCAs). The intracardiac anatomy is usually identical to that found in tetralogy of Fallot with atresia or absence of the RV outflow tract. Aortic root dilatation is often marked in these patients and may predispose to aortic root rupture and sudden death.

Management of this condition depends largely on the anatomy of the pulmonary circulation. The blood supply to the different segments may be absent or may be taken by a transpulmonary artery (connected to a central pulmonary artery derived from the sixth arch), by an MAPCA, or by a combination (dual blood supply).[99] Accurate definition of all the branches supplying the lung (Fig. 11–28) is essential to the formulation of a plan for surgical treatment, consisting of one or, usually, more multiple stages of unifocalization[100–102] of the pulmonary arteries by direct anastomosis of the different branches or interposition of segments of azygos vein or Gore-Tex shunt combined with ligation of MAPCAs supplying segments with dual blood supply. Total correction is performed by closing the VSD and inserting a homograft conduit from the right ventricle and the reconstructed pulmonary artery tree (Fig. 11–29). In some patients with absent central pulmonary arteries, unifocalization is not a real option; for these patients, lung or heart-lung transplantation may be the only recourse.

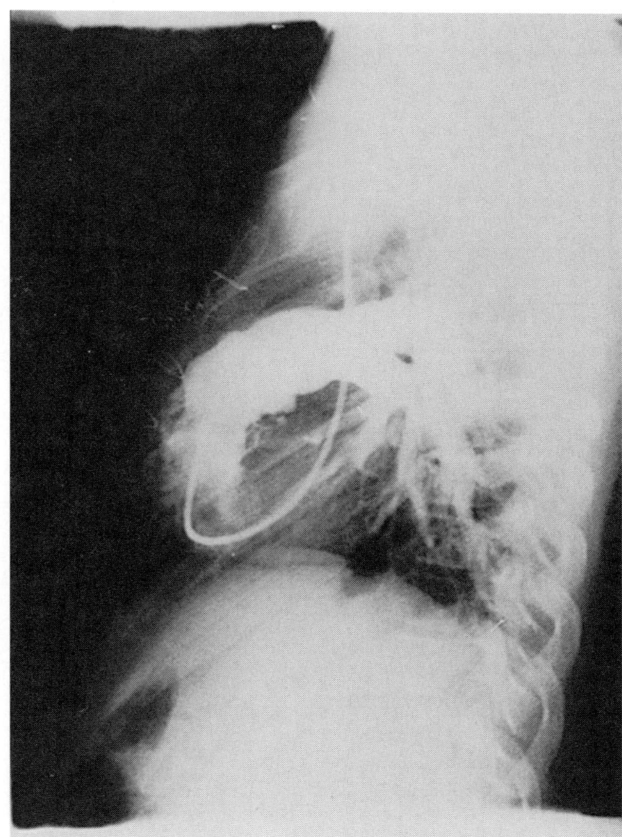

FIGURE 11–29 Repair of pulmonary atresia with homograft conduit from the right ventricle to the central pulmonary artery.

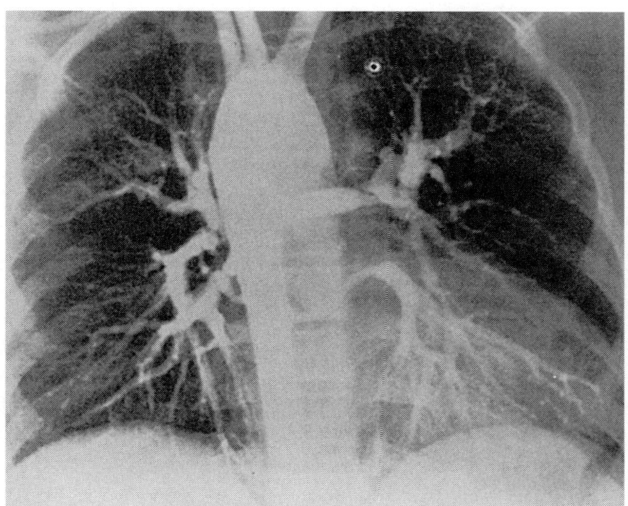

FIGURE 11–28 Aortopulmonary collateral arteries in a patient with tetralogy of Fallot and pulmonary atresia. (From Mair DD, Julsrud PR: Diagnostic evaluation of PA and VSD. Prog Pediatr Cardiol 1:23–36, 1992.)

Transposition of the Great Arteries

Uncorrected transposition is incompatible with survival into adulthood unless there are additional lesions that ensure adequate mixing of blood and possible protection against pulmonary vascular disease. The most common such additional abnormalities are large VSDs with or without pulmonary stenosis. Patients with transposition and large VSDs develop severe pulmonary vascular disease at an earlier age than those without transposition.[103] In severely symptomatic patients, heart-lung transplantation is the only treatment option.[104, 105] The combination of transposition of the great arteries, VSD, and pulmonary stenosis can be treated with the Rastelli operation,[106] which consists of redirection of blood through the VSD to the RV outflow tract into the aorta and insertion of an extracardiac conduit from the right ventricle to the transected pulmonary artery (Fig. 11–30). The Le Compte operation (*redirection entre ventriculaire*, or the REV operation) constitutes an alternative approach (Fig. 11–31).[107] Incomplete or L-transposition of the great arteries is usually associated with AV and

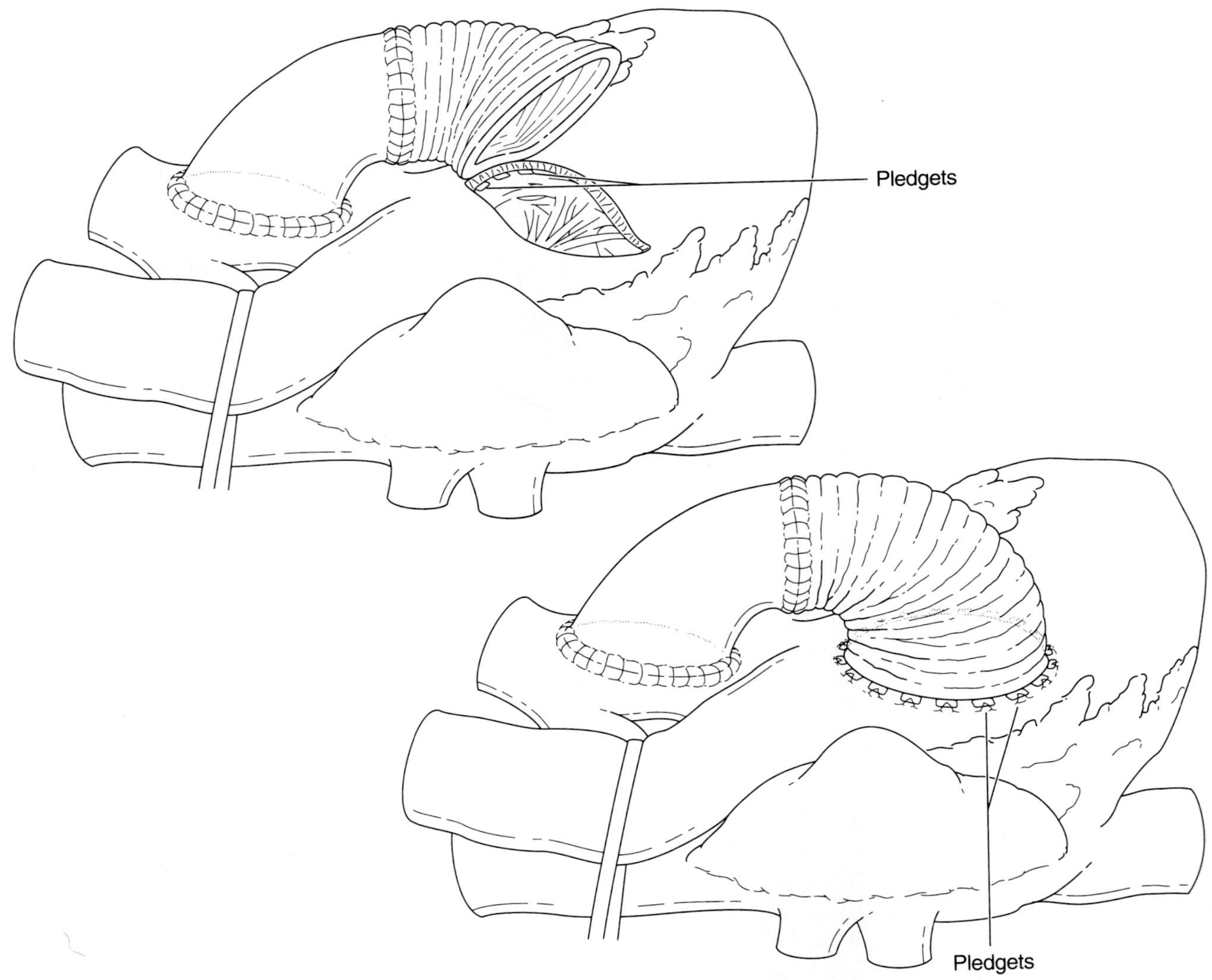

FIGURE 11–30 Use of a right ventricle–to–pulmonary artery conduit in the Rastelli operation. (From Kirklin JW, Barratt-Boyes BG: Complete transposition of the great arteries. *In* Kirklin JW, Barratt-Boyes BG [eds]: Cardiac Surgery. 2nd ed. pp. 1383–1467. New York: Churchill Livingstone, 1993.)

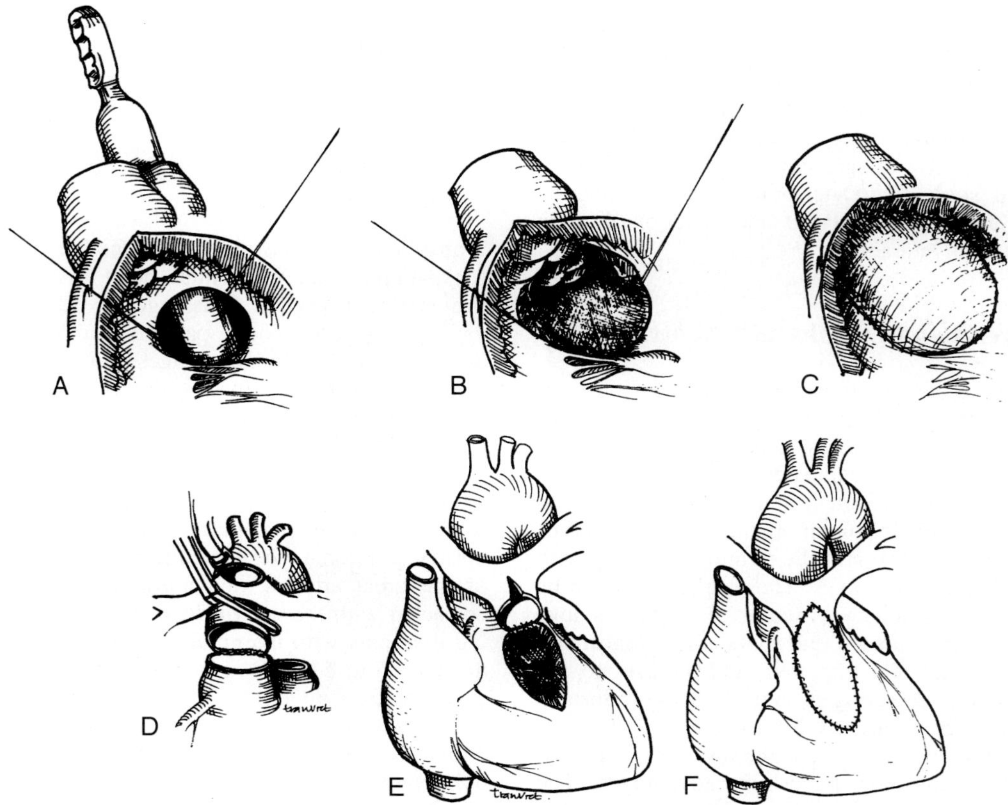

FIGURE 11–31 Correction of transposition of the great arteries with ventricular septal defect and pulmonary stenosis **A,** View from right ventricular infundibulotomy of the ventricular septal defect and the portion of the interventricular septum to be excised. **B,** The infundibular septum has been resected. **C,** The intraventricular baffle has been sutured into place. **D,** The pulmonary bifurcation is passed anterior to the ascending aorta. **E,** The posterior rim of the distal pulmonary trunk is sutured to the top of the infundibulotomy. **F,** An anterior patch is sewn over the pulmonary outflow tract. (**A–F,** From Lecompte Y, Neveux JY, Leca F, et al: Reconstruction of the pulmonary outflow tract without prosthetic conduit. J Thorac Cardiovasc Surg 84:727–733, 1982.)

ventriculoarterial discordance (corrected transposition). In these patients, surgical treatment is commonly required for left AV valve regurgitation and associated anomalies such as VSD and pulmonary outflow obstruction.

Adults with transposition of great arteries who have undergone a previous atrial switch procedure (Mustard or Senning) may present with arrhythmia or symptoms due to stenosis of the systemic or pulmonary venous pathways or RV dysfunction. Relief of baffle obstruction can be achieved with baffle revision, enlargement of the pulmonary venous atrium, or both. Anatomic correction (takedown of the Mustard or Senning procedure combined with an arterial switch) after pulmonary artery banding (to retrain the left ventricle for the systemic circulation) has been considered a "conventional" option for patients with failing systemic right ventricles.[108] However, there are very limited data on the use of this approach in this group of patients. The future application of this strategy will depend on the timing of the operations and possibly on the use of strategies to induce physiologic hypertrophy as suggested by experimental studies.[109] Deterioration in RV function can ultimately affect LV structure and function through ventriculoventricular interaction.[110]

Tricuspid Atresia and Double-Inlet Ventricle

The conditions of tricuspid atresia and double-inlet ventricle are characterized by severe hypoplasia or absence of one of the ventricular chambers, rendering biventricular repair impossible or impractical. These patients are considered for operations that direct systemic venous return to the lung.[111–113] The original Fontan operation[111] consisted of anastomosing the right atrium to the pulmonary artery with interposition of homograft valves. These operations can be considered only if pulmonary vascular resistance is low, the pulmonary arteries are of adequate size, ventricular function is not significantly impaired, and there is no AV valvular dysfunction. Directing systemic venous return to the lung can also be achieved by total cavopulmonary shunt,[114, 115] which avoids the use of the atrium as a pumping chamber. This approach has many advantages. The extracardiac Fontan modification has been used by some groups; this procedure consists of a combination of the bidirectional Glenn procedure with an extracardiac lateral tunnel connecting the inferior vena cava with the pulmonary artery.[116]

In patients with marginally elevated pulmonary vascular resistance, the addition of a fenestration of about 2 cm in diameter between the systemic venous channel and the atrium has added substantially to the safety of the operation.[117] The fenestration can then be closed by transcatheter insertion of an umbrella device, providing balloon occlusion of the orifice does not cause excessive rise in systemic venous pressure (>15 mm Hg). We have used another technique of fenestration that does not require closure; this consists of making a cusp-shaped incision in the baffle. In addition, protagonists of the extracardiac Fontan operation have advocated that the need for fenestration be assessed after cardiopulmonary bypass is discontinued, when hemodynamics can be accurately evaluated.[118] Another approach that we have used is the creation of a temporary "fenestration" by a cruciate incision in the baffle that closes spontaneously after a period of several weeks or months.

The judicious use of the Fontan operation has provided good palliation for a large number of patients. There are still concerns, however, regarding the very long-term results of this procedure. Some patients can be adequately palliated by systemic-to-pulmonary artery shunts, a Glenn anastomosis, or both as a long-term solution.[119] Survival rates for such selected patients with definitive non-Fontan palliations may compare favorably with those from published Fontan series. Arrhythmia is a major cause of morbidity for these patients and relates to both ventricular dysfunction and death. Another serious complication of a Fontan-type operation is *protein losing enteropathy.*[120] This condition may respond to conversion of the Fontan operation to total cardiopulmonary correction or could necessitate heart transplantation.[121]

Heart-Lung Transplantation for Congenital Heart Disease

Transplantation constitutes an effective form of treatment for patients with congenital heart disease who develop irreversible myocardial damage or advanced pulmonary vascular disease. These patients can experience specific anatomic and functional changes related to congenital heart disease or secondary to complex or less complex surgical treatment. This point must be addressed if transplantation is to be successfully accomplished.

Abnormalities of situs, such as situs inversus or situs ambiguus, can be treated through technical modifications of the transplant procedure (Fig. 11–32).[122] Similarly, abnormal pulmonary or systemic venous return, malposition of the great arteries, and aortic artery anomalies can be corrected with the use of donor tissue.

In patients with marginally elevated pulmonary vascular disease (3 to 5 units), cardiac transplantation can lead to severe and acute failure of the thin-walled normal donor right ventricle. In patients with potentially reversible pulmonary vascular disease, such as those with long-standing pulmonary venous hypertension due to chronic heart failure, tests of reversibility, using pulmonary vasodilators[123] such as prostacyclin or inhaled nitric oxide, can be of value in deciding whether orthotopic heart transplantation should be considered. In these patients, a large heart or a heart from a domino procedure for a patient who requires heart-lung transplantation for a condition causing some degree of pulmonary hypertension can be valuable. Alternatively, heterotopic heart transplantation can be considered if the recipient heart has a relatively healthy pulmonary ventricle capable of supporting the pulmonary circulation.[124–126]

Heart-lung transplantation is the procedure of choice for patients in whom both the heart and lungs are badly and irreversibly damaged or malformed. In patients with severe pulmonary hypertension, heart-lung or double-lung transplantation is the procedure of choice. Although single-lung transplantation with repair of the intracardiac lesion has been successfully used in some patients,[127] this approach has the disadvantage of potentially dangerous ventilation perfusion imbalance during bouts of acute rejection or infection of the transplanted lung as the entire cardiac

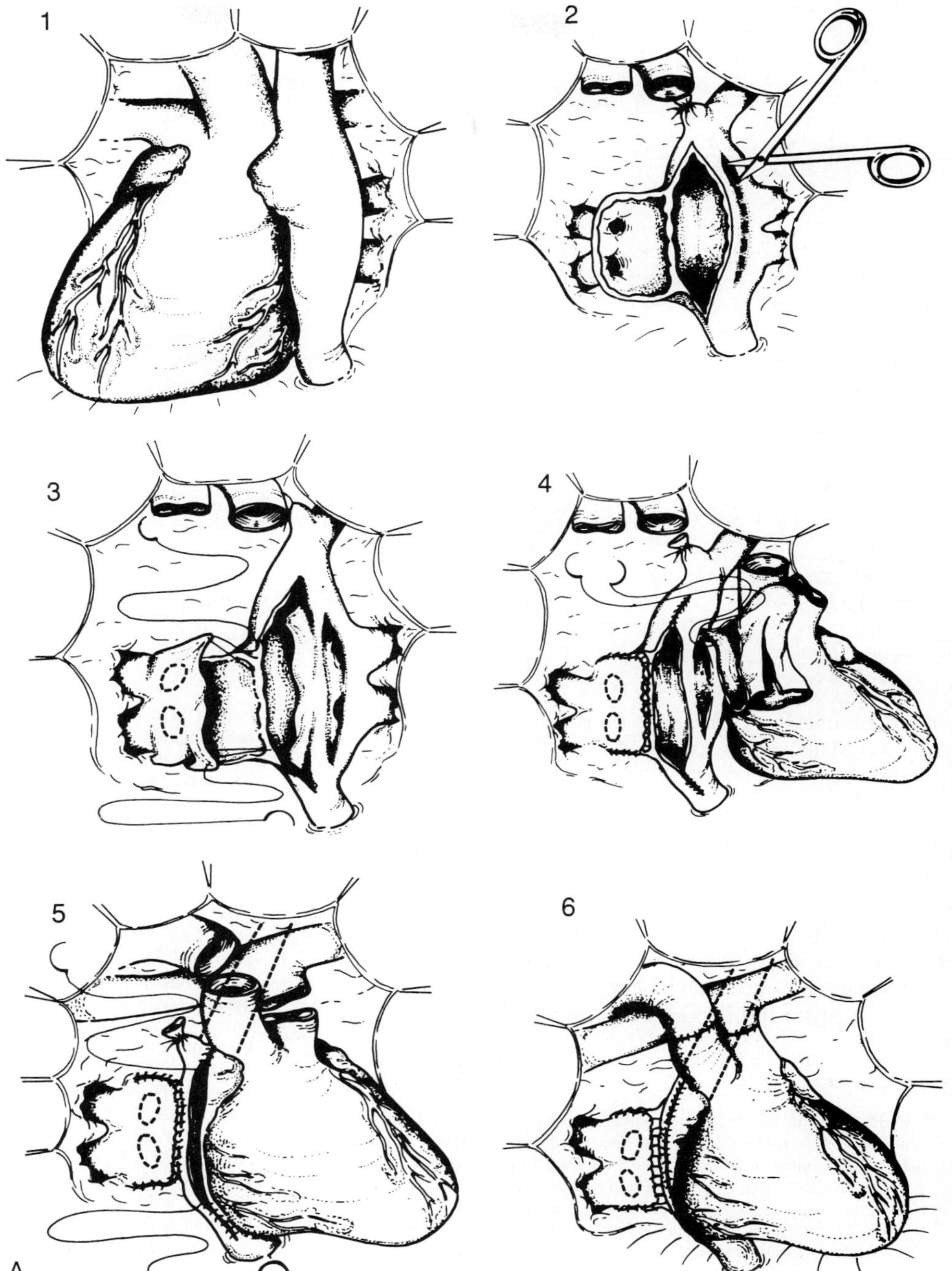

FIGURE 11–32 Technique of heart implantation in recipients with abnormalities of situs inversus **(A)** and situs ambiguus **(B)**. (**A** and **B,** From Yacoub M, Mankad P, Ledingham S: Donor procurement and surgical techniques for cardiac transplantation. Semin Thorac Cardiovasc Surg 2:153–161, 1990.)

Illustration continued on following page

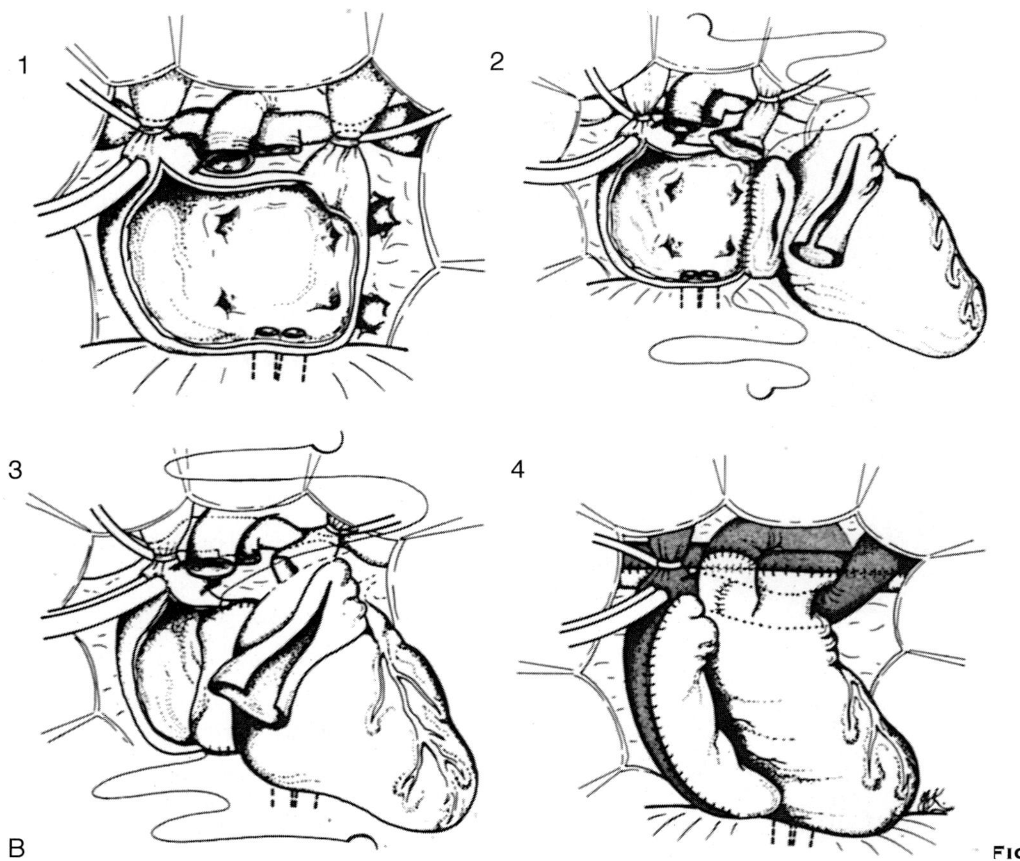

FIGURE 11–32 *Continued*

output continues to perfuse the transplanted lung, which is badly ventilated due to reduced compliance during these episodes.

CONCLUSIONS

Successful surgical treatment of congenital heart disease in adults depends on a thorough understanding of the specific anatomic and physiologic changes in that age group. Although many advances have been made, there is still room for improvement through specialization and research.

REFERENCES

1. Reddy VM, McElhinney DB, Sagrado T, et al: Results of 102 cases of complete repair of congenital heart disease in patients weighing 700–2500 grams. J Thorac Cardiovasc Surg 117:324–331, 1999.
2. Weintraub RG, Brawn WJ, Venables AW, Mee RBB: Two-patch repair of complete atrioventricular septal defect in the first year of life. J Thorac Cardiovasc Surg 90:320–326, 1990.
3. Reddy VM, Liddicoat JR, McElhinney DB, et al: Routine primary repair of tetralogy of Fallot in neonates and infants less than 3 months of age. Ann Thorac Surg 60:592–596, 1995.
4. Bartmus DA, Driscoll DJ, Offord KP, et al: The modified Fontan operation for children less than 4 years old. J Am Coll Cardiol 15:429–435, 1990.
5. Rajasinghe HA, McElhinney DB, Reddy VM, et al: Long term follow-up of truncus arteriosus repaired in infancy. J Thorac Cardiovasc Surg 113:869–879, 1997.
6. Dorc A, Glacy DL, Stone S, et al: Cardiac surgery for grown up congenital heart patients: survey of 307 consecutive operations from 1991 to 1994. Am J Cardiol 80:906–913, 1997.
7. Perloff JK: Congenital heart disease in adults: a new cardiovascular subspecialty. Circulation 84:1881–1890, 1991.
8. Swynghedauw B: Remodeling of the heart in response to chronic mechanical overload. Eur Heart J 10:935–943, 1989.
9. Wong K, Boheler KR, Petrou M, Yacoub MH: Pharmacological modulation of pressure overload cardiac hypertrophy. Circulation 96:2239–2246, 1997.
10. Holubarsh C, Holubarsh T, Jacob R, et al: Passive elastic properties of myocardium in different models and stages of hypertrophy. *In* Alpert NR (ed): Myocardial Hypertrophy and Failure. pp. 323–336. New York: Raven, 1983.
11. Doering CW, Jalil JE, Janiki JS, et al: Collagen network remodelling and diastolic stiffness of the rat left ventricle with pressure overload hypertrophy. Cardiovasc Res 22:686–695, 1988.
12. Weber KT, Brilla CG: Pathological hypertrophy and cardiac interstitium: fibrosis and renin-angiotensin aldosterone system. Circulation 83:1849–1865, 1991.
13. Lewis MJH, Shah AM, Smith JA, Henderson AH: Does endocardium modulate myocardial contractile performance? Cardio Sci 1:83–87, 1990.
14. Norwood WI, Rosenthal A, Castaneda AR: Tetralogy of Fallot with acquired pulmonary atresia and hypoplasia of pulmonary arteries. J Thorac Cardiovasc Surg 72:454–457, 1976.
15. Matitiau A, Geva T, Colan SD, et al: Bulboventricular foramen size in infants with double-inlet left ventricle or tricuspid atresia with transposed great arteries: influence on initial palliative operation and rate of growth. J Am Coll Cardiol 19:142–148, 1992.
16. Somerville J, Becu L, Ross D: Common ventricle with acquired subaortic obstruction. Am J Cardiol 34:206–214, 1974.
17. Hoffman JIE, Rudolph AM, Heyman MA: Pulmonary vascular disease with congenital heart lesions: pathologic features and causes. Circulation 64:873–877, 1981.
18. Wagenvoort CA. Wagenvoort N: Primary pulmonary hypertension: a pathologic study of the lung vessels in 156 clinically diagnosed cases. Circulation 42:1163–1184, 1970.
19. Tuder RM, Groves BM, Badesch DB, Voelkel NF: Exuberant endo-

thelial cell growth and elements of inflammation are present in plexiform lesions of pulmonary hypertension. Am J Pathol 144:275–285, 1994.
20. Blackstone EH, Kirklin JW: Death and other time related events after valve replacement. Circulation 72:753–767, 1985.
21. Cannegieter SC, Rosendaal FR, Briet E: Thromboembolic and bleeding complications in patients with mechanical heart prostheses. Circulation 89:635–641, 1994.
22. Oakley CM: Pregnancy and valve replacement. *In* Yacoub MH, Carpentier AF (eds): Tenth Annual of Cardiac Surgery 89–94. London: Rapid Science, 1997.
23. Ross DN, Yacoub MH: Homograft replacement of the aortic valve. Prog Cardiovasc Dis 11:275–293, 1969.
24. Yacoub M, Rasmi NR, Sundt TM, et al: Fourteen year experience with homovital homografts for aortic valve replacement. J Thorac Cardiovasc Surg 110:186–193, 1995.
25. Gula G, Ahmed M, Thompson R, et al: Combined homograft replacement of the aortic valve and aortic root with reimplantation of the coronary arteries. Circulation 54(suppl II):II-150, 1976.
26. Yacoub MH: Allograft aortic root replacement. *In* Yankah AC, Metzer R, Miller DC, et al (eds): Cardiac Valve Allografts, 1962–1987. p. 149. New York: Springer-Verlag, 1988.
27. Lund O, Chandrasekaran V, Grocott-Mason R, et al: Primary aortic valve replacement with allografts over 25 years: valve-related and procedure-related determinants of outcome. J Thorac Cardiovasc Surg 117:77–91, 1999.
28. Ross DN: Replacement of the aortic and mitral valves with a pulmonary autograft. Lancet 2:956–958, 1967.
29. Kouchoukos NT, Davila-Roman VG, Spray TL, et al: Replacement of the aortic root with a pulmonary autograft in children and young adults with aortic valve disease. N Engl J Med 330:1–6, 1994.
30. Santini F, Dyke C, Edwards S, et al: Pulmonary autograft versus homograft replacement of the aortic valve: a prospective randomized trial. J Thorac Cardiovac Surg 113:894–899, 1997.
31. Yacoub M, Kilner PJ, Birks E, Misfeld M: The aortic outflow and root: a tale of dynamism and crosstalk. Ann Thorac Surg 68:S38–S45, 1999.
32. Yacoub M, Khan H, Stavri G, et al: Anatomic correction of the syndrome of prolapsing right coronary aortic cusp, dilatation of the sinus of Valsalva and ventricular septal defect. J Thorac Cardiovasc Surg 113:253–261, 1997.
33. Lambry CP: Trante des Maladies Congitales du Coeur. Paris: JB Bailliere, 1921.
34. Trusler GA, Williams WG, Smallhorn JF, Freedom RM: Late results after repair of aortic insufficiency associated with ventricular septal defect. J Thorac Cardiovasc Surg 103:276–281, 1992.
35. Kawashima Y, Danno M, Shimuzu Y, et al: Ventricular septal defect associated with aortic insufficiency and anatomic classification and method of operation. Circulation 47:1057–1064, 1973.
36. Garamella JJ, Cruz AB, Heupel WH, et al: Ventricular septal defect with aortic insufficiency: successful surgical correction of both defects by the transaortic approach. Am J Cardiol 5:266–272, 1960.
37. Yacoub M, Fagan A, Stassano P, Radley-Smith R: Results of valve conserving operations for aortic regurgitation. Circulation 68:311–321, 1983.
38. Yacoub M, Sundt TM, Rasmi N: Management of aortic valve incompetence in patients with Marfan's syndrome. *In* Hetzer R, Gehle P, Ennker J (eds): Cardiovascular Aspects of Marfan's Syndrome. pp. 71–81. Darmstadt: Steinkopf, 1995.
39. Birks EJ, Webb C, Child A, et al: Early and long-term results of a valve sparing operation for Marfan syndrome. Circulation 1999.
40. David TE, Feindel CM, Bos RN: Repair of the aortic valve in patients with aortic insufficiency and aortic root aneurysm. J Thorac Cardiovasc Surg 109:345–352, 1995.
41. Black MD, Adatia I, Freedom RM: Truncal valve repair: initial experience in neonates. Ann Thorac Surg 65:1737–1740, 1998.
42. Duran CMG, Alonso J, Gaite L, et al: Long term results of conservative repair of the rheumatic aortic valve insufficiency. Eur J Cardiothorac Surg 2:217–223, 1988.
43. Yacoub MH, Gehle P, Chandrasekaram V, et al: Late results of a valve preserving operation in patients with aneurysms of the ascending aorta and root. J Thorac Cardiovasc Surg 115:1080–1090, 1998.
44. Kalangos A, Beghetti M, Baldovinos A, et al: Aortic valve repair by cusp extension with the use of fresh autologous pericardium in children with rheumatic aortic insufficiency. J Thorac Cardiovasc Surg 118:225–236, 1999.
45. Barlow JB, Bosman CK, Pocock WA, Marchand P: Late systolic murmurs and non-ejection ("mid-late") systolic clicks: an analysis of 90 patients. Br Heart J 30:203–218, 1968.
46. Jeresaty RM, Edwards JE, Chawla SK: Mitral valve prolapse and ruptured chordae tendineae. Am J Cardiol 55:138–142, 1985.
47. McKay R, Yacoub M: Clinical and pathological findings in patients with "floppy" valves treated surgically. Circulation 38(suppl III):III-63–III-73, 1973.
48. Yacoub M, Halim M, Radley-Smith R, et al: Surgical treatment of mitral regurgitation caused by floppy valves: repair versus replacement. Circulation 64(suppl II):II-210–II-216, 1981.
49. Enriquez-Sarano M, Schaff JV, Orszulak TA, et al: Valve repair improves the outcome of surgery for mitral regurgitation. Circulation 91:1022–1028, 1995.
50. Reul RM, Cohn LH: Mitral valve reconstruction for mitral valve insufficiency. Prog Cardiovasc Dis 39:567–599, 1997.
51. Anabtawi IN, Ellison RG: Congenital stenosing ring of the left atrioventricular canal (supravalvular mitral stenosis). J Thorac Cardiovasc Surg 49:944–1005, 1965.
52. Williams WG, Suri R, Shindo G, et al: Repair of major intracardiac anomalies associated with atrioventricular discordance. Ann Thorac Surg 31:527–531, 1981.
53. Horvath P, Szufladowicz M, de Leval MR, et al: Tricuspid valve abnormalities in patients with atrioventricular discordance: surgical implications. Ann Thorac Surg 57:941–945, 1994.
54. Danielson GK, Fuster V: Surgical repair of Ebstein's anomaly. Ann Surg 196:499–504, 1982.
55. Carpentier A, Chauraud S, Mace L, et al: A new reconstructive operation for Ebstein's anomaly of the tricuspid valve. J Thorac Cardiovasc Surg 96:92–101, 1988.
56. Sano S, Karl TR, Mee RBB: Extracardiac valved conduits in the pulmonary circuit. Ann Thorac Surg 52:285–290, 1991.
57. Somerville J, Stone S, Ross D: Fate of patients with fixed subaortic stenosis after surgical removal. Br Heart J 43:629–647, 1980.
58. Gewillig M, Daenen W, Dumoulin M, Van der Hawaert L: Rheologic genesis of discrete subvalvular stenosis: a Doppler echocardiographic study. J Am Coll Cardiol 19:818–824, 1992.
59. Coleman DH, Smallhorn JF, McCrundle BW, et al: Postoperative follow up of fibromuscular subaortic stenosis. J Am Coll Cardiol 24:1558–1564, 1994.
60. Yacoub M, Onuzo O, Riedel B, Radley-Smith R: Mobilization of the left and right fibrous trigones for relief of severe left ventricular outflow obstruction. J Thorac Cardiovasc Surg 117:126–133, 1999.
61. Konno S, Imai Y, Lida Y, et al: A new method for prosthetic valve replacement in congenital aortic stenosis associated with hypoplasia of the aortic ring. J Thorac Cardiovasc Surg 70:909–917, 1975.
62. Vouhe PR, Poulain H, Bloch G, et al: Aortoseptal approach for optimal resection of diffuse subvalvular aortic stenosis. J Thorac Cardiovasc Surg 87:887–893, 1984.
63. Vouhe PR, Neveux JY: Surgical management of diffuse subaortic stenosis: an integrated approach. Ann Thorac Surg 52:654–661, 1991.
64. van Son JAM, Danielson GK, Puga FJ, et al: Supravalvular aortic stenosis. J Thorac Cardiovasc Surg 107:103–115, 1994.
65. Hazekamp MG, Kappeteiu AP, Schoof PF, et al: Brom's three patch techniques for repair of supravalvar aortic stenosis. J Thorac Cardiovasc Surg 118:252–258, 1999.
66. Wells WJ, Prendergast TW, Berdjis F, et al: Repair of coarctation of the aorta in adults: the fate of systolic hypertension. Ann Thorac Surg 61:1168–171, 1996.
67. Sakopoulos AG, Hahn TL, Turrentino M, Brown JW: Recurrent aortic coarctation: is surgical repair still the gold standard? J Thorac Cardiovasc Surg 116:560–565, 1998.
68. Mendolsohn AM, Crowley DC, Lindauer A, Beekman RH: Rapid progression of aortic aneurysm after patch aortoplasty repair of coarctation of the aorta. J Am Coll Cardiol 20:381–385, 1992.
69. Greenberg SB, Marks LA, Eshaghpour EE: Evaluation of magnetic resonance imaging in coarctation of the aorta: the importance of multiple imaging planes. Pediatr Cardiol 18:287–349, 1997.
70. Fawzy ME, Swanandam V, Galal O, et al: 1–10 year follow-up results of balloon angioplasty of native coarctation. J Am Coll Cardiol 30:1542–1546, 1997.
71. Gatzoulis MA, Freeman MA, Sui SC, et al: Atrial arrhythmia after

surgical closure of atrial septal defects in adults. N Engl J Med 340:839–846, 1999.
72. Kobayashi J, Yamamoto F, Nakano K, et al: Maze procedure for atrial fibrillation associated with atrial septal defect. Circulation 98:(suppl II):II-399–II-402, 1998.
73. Cox JL, Jaquiss RDB, Schuessler RB, Boineau JP: Modification of the Maze procedure for atrial flutter and fibrillation. II: surgical technique of the Maze III procedure. J Thorac Cardiovasc Surg 110:485–495, 1995.
74. Gatzoulis MA, Hechter S, Webb GD, Williams WG: Surgery for partial atrioventricular septal defect in adults. Ann Thorac Surg 67:504–510, 1999.
75. Gatzoulis MA, Shore D, Yacoub M, Shinebourne EA: Complete atrioventricular septal defect with tetralogy of Fallot: diagnosis and management. Br Heart J 71:579–583, 1994.
76. Yacoub M, Radley-Smith R: Anatomy of the coronary arteries in transposition of the great arteries and methods for their transfer in anatomical correction. Thorax 33:418–424, 1978.
77. Mustapha I, Gula G, Radley-Smith R, et al: Anomalous origin of the left coronary artery from the anterior aortic sinus: a potential cause of sudden death. J Thorac Cardiovasc Surg 82:297–300, 1981.
78. Keith JD: The anomalous origin of the left coronary artery from the pulmonary artery. Br Heart J 21:149–161, 1959.
79. Edwards JE: The direction of blood flow in coronary arteries arising from the pulmonary trunk. Circulation 29:163–166, 1964.
80. Wesselhoeft H, Fawcett JS, Johnson AL: Anomalous origin of the left coronary artery from the pulmonary trunk. Circulation 38:403–425, 1968.
81. Cooley DA, Hallman GL, Bloodwell RD: Definitive surgical treatment of anomalous origin of left coronary artery from pulmonary artery: indications and results. J Thorac Cardiovasc Surg 52:798–808, 1966.
82. Bunton R, Jonas R, Lang P, et al: Anomalous origin of left coronary artery from pulmonary artery: ligation versus establishment of two coronary artery system. J Thorac Cardiovasc Surg 93:103–108, 1987.
83. Neches WH, Mathews RA, Park SC, et al: Anomalous origin of the left coronary artery from the pulmonary artery. Circulation 50:582–587, 1974.
84. Takeuchi S, Imamura H, Katsumoto K, et al: New surgical method for repair of anomalous left coronary artery. J Thorac Cardiovasc Surg 78:7–11, 1979.
85. Cochrane AD, Coleman DM, Davis AM, et al: Excellent long-term functional outcome after an operation for anomalous left coronary artery from the pulmonary artery. J Thorac Cardiovasc Surg 117:332–342, 1999.
86. Mustafa I, Gula G, Coe Y, et al: Anomalous origin of the coronary arteries: clinical significance and surgical treatment. p. 335. Abstracts of the World Congress on Paediatric Cardiology, London, June 2–6, 1980.
87. Laks H, Ardehali A, Grant PW, Allada V: Aortic implantation of anomalous left coronary artery. J Thorac Cardiovasc Surg 109:519–523, 1995.
88. Bellhouse BJ, Bellhouse FH: Fluid mechanics of the aortic root with application to coronary flow. Nature 219:1059–1061, 1968.
89. Reidy F, Anjos RI, Qureshi SA, et al: Transcatheter embolisation in the treatment of coronary artery fistulas. J Am Coll Cardiol 18:187–192, 1991.
90. Rosenthal A: Adults with tetralogy of Fallot: repaired, yes. Cured, no. N Engl J Med 329:655–656, 1993.
91. Hu DC, Seward JB, Puga FJ, et al: Total correction of tetralogy of Fallot at age 40 years and older: long term follow-up. J Am Coll Cardiol 5:40–44, 1985.
92. Dittrich S, Vogel M, Dahnert I, et al: Surgical repair of tetralogy of Fallot in adults today. Clin Cardiol 22:460–464, 1999.
93. Ross DN, Somerville J: Correction of pulmonary atresia with a homograft aortic valve. Lancet 2:1446–1447, 1966.
94. Radley-Smith R, Ahmed M, Yacoub M: Late results of aortic homograft reconstruction of the right ventricular outflow tract in infants and children. Thoraxchirurgie 23:455–459, 1975.
95. Bisset GS, Schartz DC, Benzing G, et al: Late results of reconstruction of right ventricular outflow tract with porcine xenografts in children. Ann Thorac Surg 31:437–443, 1981.
96. Jonas RA, Freed MD, Mayer JE, Castanada AR: Long term following of patients with synthetic right heart conduits. Circulation 72(suppl XII):XII-77–XII-83, 1985.
97. Gatzoulis MA, Till JA, Somerville J, Redington AN: Mechanoelectrical interaction in tetralogy of Fallot: QRS prolongation relates to right ventricular size and predicts malignant ventricular arrhythmias and sudden death. Circulation 92:231–237, 1995.
98. Bove EL, Byrum CJ, Sondheimer MH, et al: Improved right ventricular function following late pulmonary valve replacement for residual pulmonary insufficiency or stenosis. J Thorac Cardiovasc Surg 90:50–55, 1985.
99. Anderson RH, Seo JW, Ho SY: The pulmonary arterial supply in tetralogy of Fallot with pulmonary atresia. *In* Yacoub M, Pepper J (eds): Annual of Cardiac Surgery 1990–91. pp. 77–83. London: Current Science.
100. Haworth SG, Rees PG, Taylor JFN, et al: Pulmonary atresia with ventricular septal defect and major aortopulmonary collateral arteries: effect of systemic pulmonary anastomosis. Br Heart J 45:133–141, 1981.
101. Castenada AR, Mayer JE, Lock JE: Tetralogy of Fallot, pulmonary atresia, and diminutive pulmonary arteries. Prog Pediatr Cardiol 1:50–60, 1992.
102. Shanley CJ, Lupinetti FM, Shah ML, et al: Primary unifocalisation for the absence of intrapericardial pulmonary arteries in the neonate. J Thorac Cardiovasc Surg 106:237–247, 1993.
103. Newfeld EA, Paul MH, Muster AJ, Idriss FS: Pulmonary vascular disease in complete transposition of the great arteries: a study of 200 patients. Am J Cardiol 34:75, 1974.
104. Reitz BA, Wallwork JL, Hunt SA, et al: Heart-lung transplantation: successful therapy for patients with pulmonary vascular disease. N Engl J Med 306:557–564, 1982.
105. Yacoub MH, Banner NR: Recent developments in heart and lung transplantation. *In* Morris P, Tilney NL (eds): Transplantation Reviews, Vol. 3. pp. 1–29. Philadelphia: WB Saunders, 1989.
106. Rastelli GC, McGoon DC, Wallace RB: Anatomic correction of transposition of the great arteries with ventricular septal defect and pulmonary stenosis. J Thorac Cardiovasc Surg 58:545–552, 1969.
107. Lecompte Y, Neveux JY, Leca F, et al: Reconstruction of the pulmonary outflow tract without prosthetic conduit. J Thorac Cardiovasc Surg 84:727–733, 1982.
108. Cochrane AD, Karl TR, Mee RBB: Staged conversion to arterial switch for late failure of the systemic right ventricle. Ann Thorac Surg 56:854–862, 1993.
109. Wong K, Boheler KR, Bishop J, et al: Clenbuterol induces cardiac hypertrophy with normal functional morphological and molecular features. Cardiovasc Res 37:115–122, 1998:
110. Yacoub MH: Two hearts that beat as one. Circulation 92:156–157, 1995.
111. Fontan F, Baudet E: Surgical repair of tricuspid atresia. Thorax 26:240–248, 1971.
112. Yacoub MH, Radley-Smith R: Use of a valved conduit from right atrium to pulmonary artery for correction of single ventricle. Circulation 54(suppl III):III-63–III-70, 1976.
113. Danielson GK: Surgical management of double inlet ventricle. *In* Anderson RH, Crupi G, Parenzan L (eds): Double Inlet Ventricle. pp. 174–182. Tunbridge Wells, UK: Castle House, 1987.
114. Kawashima Y, Kitamura S, Matsuda H, et al: Total cavopulmonary shunt operation in complex cardiac anomalies. J Thorac Cardiovasc Surg 87:74–81, 1984.
115. de Leval MR, Kilner P, Gewllig M, Bull C: Total cavopulmonary connection: a logical alternative to atriopulmonary connection for complex Fontan operations: experimental studies and early clinical experience. J Thorac Cardiovasc Surg 96:682–695, 1988.
116. Laschinger JC, Ringer RE, Brenner JI, McLaughlin JS: The extracardiac total cavopulmonary connection for definitive conversion to the Fontan circulation. J Card Surg 8:524–533, 1993.
117. Bridges ND, Meyer JEJ, Lock JE, et al: Effect of baffle fenestration on outcome of the modified Fontan operation. Circulation 86:1762–1769, 1992.
118. LeNardo DT, Petrossian E, McElhinney DB, et al: Is it necessary to routinely fenestrate an extracardiac Fontan? J Am Coll Cardiol 34:539–544, 1991.
119. Gatzoulis MA, Munk M-D, Williams WG, Webb DG: Definitive palliation with cavopulmonary or aortopulmonary shunts for adults with single ventricle physiology. Heart 82, 1999.
120. Feldt RH, Driscoll DJ, Offord KP, et al: Protein losing enteropathy after Fontan operation. J Thorac Cardiovasc Surg 112:672–680, 1996.

121. Mertens L, Hagler DJ, Sauer U, et al: Protein losing enteropathy after the Fontan operation: an international multicentre study. J Thorac Cardiovasc Surg 115:1063–1073, 1998.
122. Yacoub M, Mankad P, Ledingham S: Donor procurement and surgical techniques for cardiac transplantation. Semin Thorac Cardiovasc Surg 2:153–161, 1990.
123. Addonizio LJ, Gersony WM, Robbins RC, et al: Elevated pulmonary vascular resistance and cardiac transplantation. Circulation 76(suppl V):V-52–V-55, 1987.
124. Yacoub MH: Haemodynamics of "domino" heart transplantation. G Ital Cardiol 27:540–543, 1997.
125. Galbraith HT, Yacoub M: Heterotropic heart transplantation: operative technique and results. *In* Myerowitz PD (ed): Heart Transplantation. pp. 155–162. Mt. Kisco, NY: Futura, 1987.
126. Cochrane AD, Adams DR, Radley-Smith R, et al: Heterotopic heart transplantation for elevated pulmonary vascular resistance in pediatric patients. J Heart Lung Transplant 14:296–301, 1995.
127. Pasque MK, Trulock EP, Kaiser LR, Cooper JD: Single lung transplantation for pulmonary hypertension: three month hemodynamic follow-up. Circulation 84:2275, 1991.
128. Becker AE, Anderson RH: Cardiac Pathology. New York: Churchill Livingstone, 1983.
129. Whittlesey D, Geha AS: Selection and complications of cardiac valvular prostheses. *In* Bauer G, Geha AS, Hammond GL, et al (eds): Glenn's Thoracic and Cardiovascular Surgery. 5th ed. New York: Prentice Hall International, 1991.
130. Dhalla N, Khaghani A, Radley-Smith R, Yacoub M: Early and longterm performance of aortic homograft root replacement. *In* Bodner F, Yacoub MH (eds): Biologic and Bioprosthetic Valves. 1st ed. London: Yorke Medical Books, 1986.
131. Ross DN: Evolution of the biological concept in cardiac surgery: a pilgrim's progress. *In* Yankah AC, Hetzer R, Yacoub MH (eds): Cardiac Valve Allografts 1962–1987. New York: Springer-Verlag, 1988.
132. Smallhorn JF, de Leval M, Stark J, et al: Isolated anterior mitral cleft two dimensional echocardiographic assessment. Br Heart J 48:109–116, 1982.
133. Hurst JW: Atlas of the Heart. New York: Gower Medical, 1988.
134. Nitkoyannopoulos P (ed): Cardiac Ultrasound Cardiomyopathy. New York: Churchill Livingstone, 1993.
135. Shapiro LM, Fox KM (eds): A Colour Atlas of Adult CUD. London: Wolfe Medical Publications, 1990.
136. Mair DD, Julsrud PR: Diagnostic evaluation of pulmonary atresia and VSD. Prog Pediatr Cardiol 1:23, 1992.
137. Kirklin JW, Barratt-Boyes BG: Complete transposition of the great arteries. *In* Cardiac Surgery. 2nd ed. pp. 1383–1467. New York: Churchill Livingstone, 1993.

SECTION III

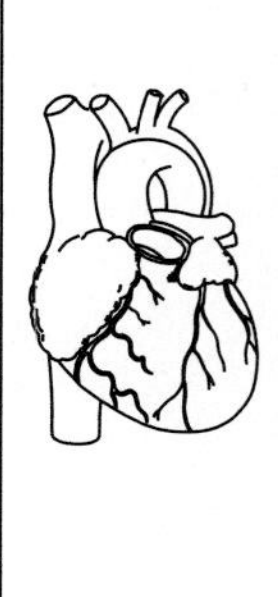

VALVULAR HEART DISEASE

Anatomic Abnormalities

Aortic Valve Disease

Pulmonary and Tricuspid Valve Disease

Mitral Valve Disease

Mitral Valve Prolapse (Myxomatous Mitral Valve)

Acute Rheumatic Fever

Infective Endocarditis

Cardiac Catheterization

Echocardiography and Doppler Evaluation

Radionuclide Techniques of Evaluation

Balloon Dilatation of the Cardiac Valves

Surgical Treatment

CHAPTER 12

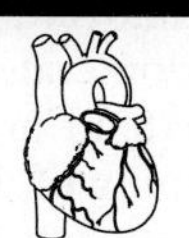

ANATOMIC ABNORMALITIES

Hugh A. McAllister, Jr., L. Maximilian Buja, and Victor J. Ferrans

CONGENITAL VALVULAR HEART DISEASE
COLLAGEN VASCULAR DISEASES
Rheumatic Valvulitis
Rheumatoid Valvulitis
Lupus Erythematosus Valvulitis
Other Collagen Vascular and Related Diseases
Lesions Resembling Collagen Vascular Disease Valvulitis
ENDOCRINE AND METABOLIC DISEASES
FLOPPY VALVE (MYXOMATOUS DEGENERATION) AND CONNECTIVE TISSUE DYSCRASIAS
INFECTIVE ENDOCARDITIS
PROSTHETIC HEART VALVES
Types
Complications

CONGENITAL VALVULAR HEART DISEASE

The most common congenital malformation of heart valves is the *bicuspid aortic valve*. Unless it is the site of associated dysplasia, this valve is not inherently stenotic, although it frequently becomes stenotic in later life. Stenosis is secondary to fibrosis and calcification of the cusps and usually not to fusion of the commissures, as is seen in rheumatic aortic stenosis.[1] Classically, the calcific deposits form nodules at the base of the cusps in the sinuses of Valsalva and extend to, but frequently do not involve, the free edge of the valve cusps (Plate 12–1). In addition, there are foci of calcification and extensive fibrosis within the substance of the cusps. Commissural fusion is usually minimal, involves only one commissure, and is only rarely extensive.[2] Another common reason for surgical excision of a bicuspid aortic valve is infective endocarditis. The extremely high incidence of infective endocarditis in patients with bicuspid aortic valves is well known. Therefore, each of these valves must be examined closely by the surgical pathologist for superimposed infective endocarditis, and if suspicious lesions are noted, sections must be taken for microbiologic culture before fixation.

The *quadricuspid aortic valve* is far less common than the bicuspid valve. The most frequent indication for surgical excision of these valves is aortic insufficiency. Most commonly, one of the cusps is rudimentary; however, the gross and microscopic appearance of the valves is usually otherwise normal. *Quadricuspid pulmonary valves* rarely cause cardiac dysfunction unless there is associated dysplasia of the valve or a coexisting congenital cardiac defect. As in quadricuspid aortic valves, the fourth cusp is usually small and rudimentary, with the remaining cusps appearing morphologically normal.[3]

Valve dysplasia may affect any of the cardiac valves, most frequently the aortic valve; however, 25 percent of patients have multiple valve involvement.[4] The dysplastic changes may be severe and extensive, so that the entire valve is distorted, or mild and focal, so that valve function is not impaired. A dysplastic stenotic pulmonary valve is frequently present in patients with Noonan's syndrome. The dysplastic semilunar valve may be unicuspid, bicuspid, or tricuspid; failure of development of the commissures also may occur, resulting in a dome-shaped valve. Stenosis is secondary to the marked thickening of the individual valve cusps. The spongiosa of the dysplastic valve is quite cellular and composed primarily of small spindle cells resembling fibroblasts, set in an acid mucopolysaccharide matrix and haphazardly arranged bundles of collagen.[5] This loose connective tissue encroaches on and often replaces the ventricularis and fibrosa of the valve cusps. The majority of involved cusps consist entirely of this loose connective tissue; however, remnants of the ventricularis and fibrosa, interrupted by accumulations of abnormal loose connective tissue, are often found at the base of the cusps. Inflammation and calcification are not features of the dysplastic valve. The abnormal valve tissue of the dysplastic or incompletely differentiated valve resembles the embryonic connective tissue of the cardiac valves in 8- to 12-week-old fetuses.[4]

COLLAGEN VASCULAR DISEASES

Rheumatic Valvulitis

Acute rheumatic fever produces a pancarditis; however, valvular involvement is responsible for the most important long-term consequences. In the *acute phase* of rheumatic valvulitis, the most conspicuous lesions are minute, translucent nodules (verrucae) along the lines of closure (Plate 12–2). These are most frequently observed in the mitral and aortic valves, less often in the tricuspid, and rarely in the pulmonary valve. They vary in diameter from less than 1 mm to 3 mm and are located on the atrial surface of the atrioventricular valves and on the ventricular surface of the semilunar valves.[6] Occasionally, a few verrucae may be distributed elsewhere over the cusps. They are also characteristically present on the chordae tendineae, especially those of the mitral valve; and not infrequently, they extend over the posterior leaflet of the mitral valve onto the endocardium of the left atrium. The verrucae tend to conglomerate on the corpora arantii of the aortic valve and extend in a row along the semilunar cusps. Diffuse thickening of the valves, except the pulmonary, is a less conspicuous but frequent gross alteration.

Microscopically, the verrucae may have the appearance of either thrombi, formed by the deposition of platelets and fibrin on the surface of the valve, or extruded collagen that has undergone fibrinoid degeneration. The region immediately adjacent to the vegetation shows marked proliferation of fibroblasts, as well as edema and numerous lymphocytes (Fig. 12–1).[6] The inflammatory process is observed most frequently in the auricularis layer of the atrioventricular valves and the ventricularis layer of the semilunar valves. A nonspecific inflammatory process, which may involve the entire valve and ring, consists of edema, increased numbers of capillaries, and a variety of inflammatory cells (mainly lymphocytes; occasionally polymorphonuclear leukocytes predominate). Plasma cells, fibroblasts, and other mononuclear cells are often present in variable numbers. Usually the valve also contains Anitschkow and Aschoff cells, which may be arranged in nodules or in rows and often surround foci of eosinophilic fragmented collagen, fibrinoid, or both. Aschoff cells may be multinucleated.[7]

Gross alterations of the cardiac valves become more pronounced as a result of *recurrent* rheumatic valvulitis. Thickening, irregularity of the surfaces, and gross vascularization are usually present. This thickening is usually most pronounced in the distal third of the valve leaflets.[6] The chordae tendineae become thicker and shorter, with especially prominent thickening at their insertions into the valve leaflets. Verrucae in various stages of activity and healing may be observed. In addition to being thickened, the aortic cusps may be considerably shortened, with their free margins rolled and inverted toward the sinus pocket. Fibrous adhesions are commonly present at the commissures, and verrucae in various stages of activity may extend across the commissures of aortic cusps. In recurrent valvulitis, there is a higher incidence of verrucae on the valves of the right side of the heart, and microscopic observation reveals considerable fibrosis, an apparent increase in elastic tissue, and inflammatory changes in various stages of activity.[6, 8] The fibrosis and inflammation involve the rings as well as the leaflets. This histologic pattern differs from that of acute valvulitis, in which the thickening of the valves is the result only of edema and inflammation. Also in contrast to the appearance of acute valvulitis are numerous arteries with thick muscular walls in the ring and proximal portion of the valve.

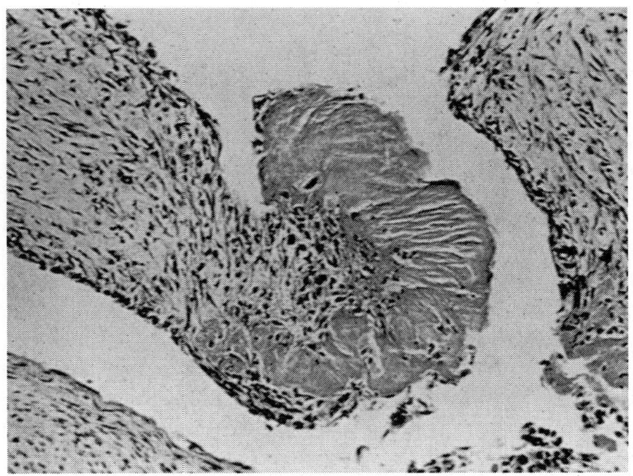

FIGURE 12–1 Acute rheumatic valvulitis, mitral valve. Fibrinoid necrosis of the valve collagen with extrusion through the surface. The region adjacent to the vegetation contains marked proliferation of fibroblasts, as well as edema and scattered lymphocytes (H&E, ×200).

In *chronic* rheumatic valvulitis, the alterations described in recurrent valvulitis are more advanced. Usually, the diffuse thickening and fibrosis of the valves have resulted in loss of elasticity and in narrowing of the orifice (Plate 12–3). Thickening, fusion, and shortening of the chordae tendineae of the mitral valve are usually pronounced (Plate 12–4). In addition, focal deposits of calcium salts may be present. These deposits may be extensive and may project to the atrial and ventricular surfaces, causing further distortion. Ossification, complete with hematopoiesis, may occur, causing further distortion.[8] Verrucae are less frequent in chronic valvulitis than in recurrent valvulitis and are broad and flat. Active inflammation is less pronounced in chronic than in recurrent valvulitis and usually consists of scattered foci of perivascular cuffing with lymphocytes. The grossly apparent thickening is due to an increase in fibrous and elastic tissue throughout the entire leaflet, including the rings and the tips of the valves. The fibrous connective tissue is usually homogeneous and hyaline. These valves are vascularized by capillaries and thick-walled vessels, which are most numerous in the superficial layers. The verrucae no longer consist of material showing fibrinoid necrosis, but are organized and contain fibroblasts and collagen fibers. As chronicity progresses, the number of fibroblasts decreases, and the verrucae become dense, hyalinized scars.

Rheumatoid Valvulitis

Rheumatoid granulomas may occur in any of the cardiac valves but are most common in the mitral and aortic valves.[9] Involvement may be focal or diffuse and is usually most prominent in the midportion or base of the valve (Fig. 12–2). The chordae tendineae are usually uninvolved, but occasionally, they may be fibrotic and shortened. Commissural fusion is rare. Rheumatoid nodules are most commonly located within the valve leaflets and are enclosed by fibrous tissue; rarely, a rheumatoid nodule may erode the surface of the valve, so that the necrotic center of the nodule communicates with a cardiac cavity (Plate 12–5). In these unusual occurrences, there may be superimposed thrombus or infective endocarditis. Verrucae of fibrinoid necrosis, common in rheumatic valvulitis and systemic lupus erythematosus, are not a feature of pure rheumatoid valvulitis.

Lupus Erythematosus Valvulitis

Lupus erythematosus valvulitis (atypical verrucous endocarditis of Libman and Sacks) is recognized as a specific

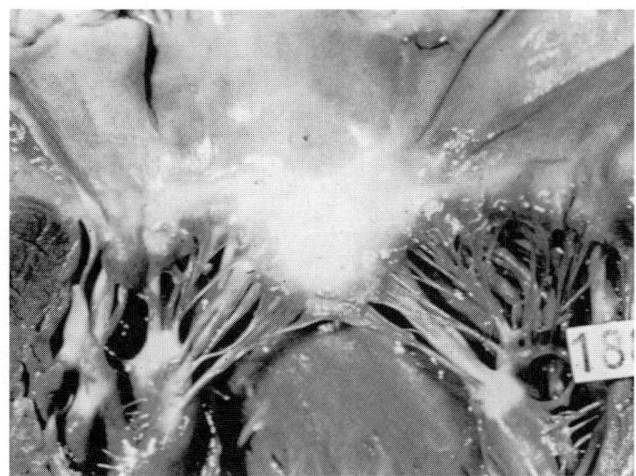

FIGURE 12–2 Rheumatoid valve disease, mitral valve. Involvement may be focal or diffuse, as in this case, and is usually most prominent in the midportion or base of the valve. The chordae tendineae are usually uninvolved, and commissural fusion is rare.

valvular abnormality occurring in systemic lupus erythematosus. Any valve may be involved, but the mitral and tricuspid valves are most often affected (Plate 12–6). The verrucae may be located on either side of a valve cusp but most frequently are present on the ventricular surface of the posterior mitral leaflet or in the valve ring; involvement of the anterior mitral leaflet is infrequent. They have no special tendency to occur along the free edge of the valves and may be scattered on the chordae tendineae and atrial or ventricular mural endocardium. The lesions are small, usually ranging in size from 1 to 4 mm in diameter but, rarely, may reach a diameter of 8 to 10 mm. They are sterile, dry, granular pink vegetations that may be single or multiple in conglomerates.[6] Histologically, the verrucae consist of a finely granular, eosinophilic, fibrinoid material, which may contain hematoxylin bodies. In a general sense, these hematoxylin bodies are the tissue equivalent of the lupus erythematosus cell of the blood and bone marrow.[6] The verrucous endocardial lesions result from degenerative and inflammatory processes of the endocardium and deeper layers of the valves. An intense valvulitis is present, which is characterized by fibrinoid necrosis of the valve substance and is often contiguous with the vegetations. Exudative and proliferative cellular reactions are present in the deeper layers of the valve. Healing of these lesions may produce foci of granulation tissue, which develop into focal fibrous thickening in the valves or in the mural endocardium. Rarely, bacterial endocarditis may be superimposed on the Libman-Sacks lesions.[9]

Other Collagen Vascular and Related Diseases

Valvular lesions in scleroderma are distinctly rare; the most common lesion is nonbacterial thrombotic endocarditis. In patients with *thrombotic thrombocytopenic purpura*, nonbacterial thrombotic endocarditis frequently is present. In both diseases, the cardiac valves most commonly involved are the mitral and the aortic.[9] Valvulitis is most unusual in *Wegener's granulomatosis*. The mitral valve is most commonly involved by the inflammatory process, which may result in subsequent fibrosis with commissural fusion resembling rheumatic mitral stenosis.[10] Primary valvulitis is not a feature of *dermatomyositis*. Diseases that may result in valvulitis but are manifested most commonly by *aortitis* include syphilis, ankylosing spondylitis, psoriatic arthritis, Reiter's syndrome, and granulomatous aortitis.

Lesions Resembling Collagen Vascular Disease Valvulitis

Although not collagen vascular diseases, three entities that may result in fibrous thickening of the cardiac valves and thickening and fusion of chordae tendineae are Whipple's disease, endomyocardial fibrosis with eosinophilia, and radiation-induced disease. In *Whipple's disease*, the valve most commonly involved is the mitral, then the tricuspid and the aortic valves. The gross deformity closely resembles that seen in chronic rheumatic heart disease, with diffuse thickening and fibrosis of the valve leaflets and chordae tendineae and rolling of the free edges of the leaflets (Fig. 12–3). Microscopically, the valve substance contains large macrophages filled with granules that are positive for the periodic acid–Schiff reaction; these granules are identical to those found in the epithelial cells of the small intestine in patients with this disease. Proliferating fibrous tissue and chronic inflammatory cells are commonly associated with the periodic acid–Schiff–positive macrophages. Scattered rod-shaped bodies, measuring 1.5 to 2.0 μm in length and 0.2 to 0.4 μm in diameter, are present intracellularly and extracellularly. These bodies, as well as membrane-bound masses of fibrillar material within the macrophages, are identical to those described in jejunal biopsies of patients with Whipple's disease[11] and are thought to represent bacteria *(Tropheryma whippelii)*, which are known to be associated with this disease.[12]

In *endomyocardial fibrosis with eosinophilia*, the valves most commonly involved are the mitral and the tricuspid,

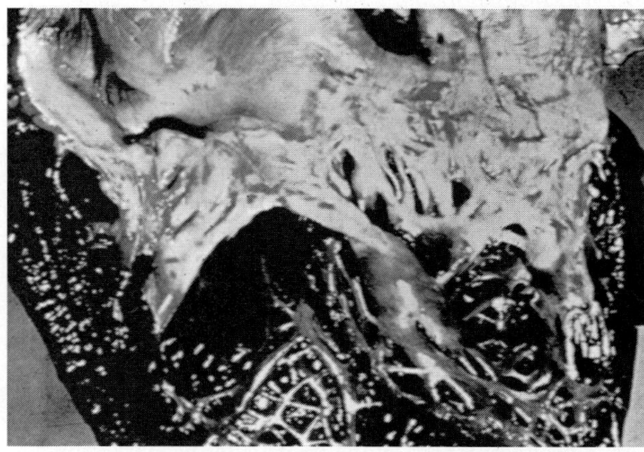

FIGURE 12–3 Whipple's disease, mitral valve. The gross deformity closely resembles that seen in chronic rheumatic valve disease, with diffuse thickening and fibrosis of the valve leaflets and chordae tendineae and rolling of the free edges of the leaflets.

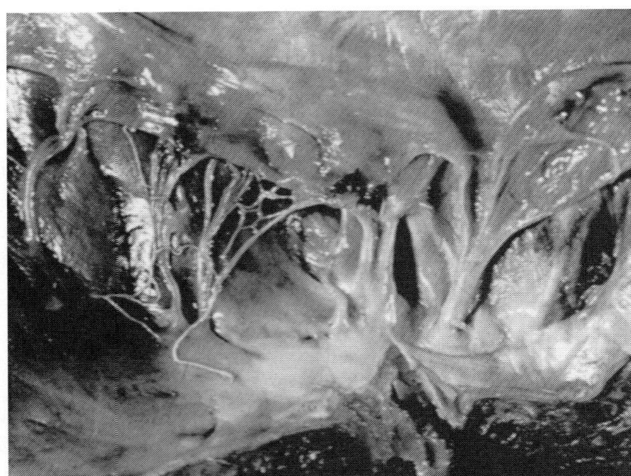

FIGURE 12–4 Endomyocardial fibrosis with eosinophilia. The posterior and septal leaflets of the tricuspid valve are tethered to the subvalvular endocardium by organizing thrombus, resulting in valvular insufficiency.

with a lesser incidence of aortic valve involvement. There is fibrous thickening of endocardium, with superimposed fibrin thrombus beneath either the posterior mitral leaflet or the posterior or septal tricuspid leaflet (Plate 12–7). These leaflets become adherent to the underlying mural endocardium, which results in regurgitation (Fig. 12–4).[13] The aortic valve cusps are occasionally thickened by vascularized fibrous tissue, which is superimposed on the ventricular aspects of the cusps. The commissures of the aortic valve may become fused by fibrous tissue with superimposed fibrin thrombus. Eosinophilic leukocytes in varying numbers are usually present at the periphery of the fibrous lesions.

Rarely, patients receiving *mediastinal irradiation* may develop lesions of the cardiac valves.[14, 15] The valves most commonly involved are the tricuspid and the mitral, followed by the aortic and the pulmonary. The fibrous valvular thickenings are focal, and the anterior tricuspid leaflet and the anterior mitral leaflet are usually more markedly involved than are the posterior leaflets. The chordae tendineae also may be focally thickened by fibrous tissue.

ENDOCRINE AND METABOLIC DISEASES

In *carcinoid heart disease*, there is either focal or diffuse plaquelike thickening of valvular and mural endocardium and, occasionally, of the intima of the great veins, coronary sinus, pulmonary trunk, and main pulmonary arteries. The fibrous tissue is atypical and limited in the majority of instances to the right side of the heart. When the pulmonary valve is involved, deposition is almost exclusively on the arterial aspect of the valve cusps (Plate 12–8). When the tricuspid valve is involved, however, the fibrous tissue is located predominantly on the ventricular aspect, often causing the leaflets to adhere to the adjacent ventricular wall.[6] Similar lesions may be observed in the mitral and aortic valves in patients with a patent foramen ovale or a functioning bronchial carcinoid tumor.[16] In some patients with predominant right-sided carcinoid heart disease, the mitral and aortic valves also may be involved to a lesser degree. Microscopically, these lesions contain fibroblasts, myofibroblasts, and smooth muscle cells embedded in a distinctive stroma, which is rich in collagen and proteoglycans but lacking in elastic fibers. Blood vessels, often thick-walled, may be immediately adjacent to the valve leaflets. Lymphocytes and plasma cells are frequently located adjacent to these blood vessels.

Histologically, similar valvular and endocardial lesions have been described in patients taking methysergide[17] and ergot[18]; however, the mitral and aortic valves are most commonly involved in these cases. Recently, similar valvular lesions have been described in patients taking fenfluramine phentermine for appetite suppression.[19]

The heart valves are involved in 50 percent of patients with cardiac *amyloidosis*. Valvular involvement is usually minimal, but discrete nodules measuring from 1 to 4 mm in diameter are occasionally present on the valves, either in the cusps or in the annulus.[20] Rarely, valvular involvement is diffuse, resulting in thick, rigid cusps and stenotic or regurgitant orifices (Plate 12–9). The four cardiac valves are affected with almost equal frequency.

All heart valves and valvular annuli, especially the mitral and aortic valves, are sites of heavy pigment deposition in patients with *ochronosis* (Plate 12–10).[20] Although the pigment deposition is most prominent at the bases of the mitral and aortic valves and annulus fibrosus, the edges of the cusps may be roughened and fused for 1 to 2 mm at their bases; the cusps may be focally calcified. The ochronotic pigment appears blue-black on gross examination and yellow-tan in histologic sections. Infective endocarditis may occasionally be superimposed, especially when the valves are heavily calcified.

The cardiac valves may be involved in any of the *mucopolysaccharidoses*, most frequently in Hurler's syndrome (mucopolysaccharidosis I).[20] The valves are considerably thickened, particularly the mitral valve; right-sided cardiac valves are less severely affected than those in the left side of the heart (Fig. 12–5). The valvular thickening is most

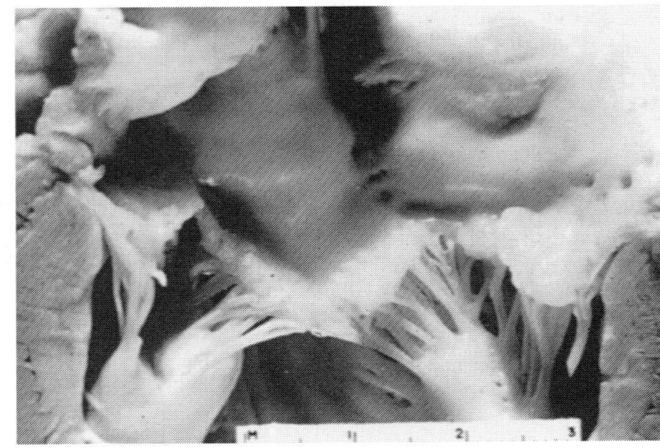

FIGURE 12–5 Hurler's syndrome, mitral valve. The valvular thickening is most pronounced at the free margins, which have an irregular, nodular appearance. The commissures are not fused. The chordae tendineae are moderately shortened and thickened.

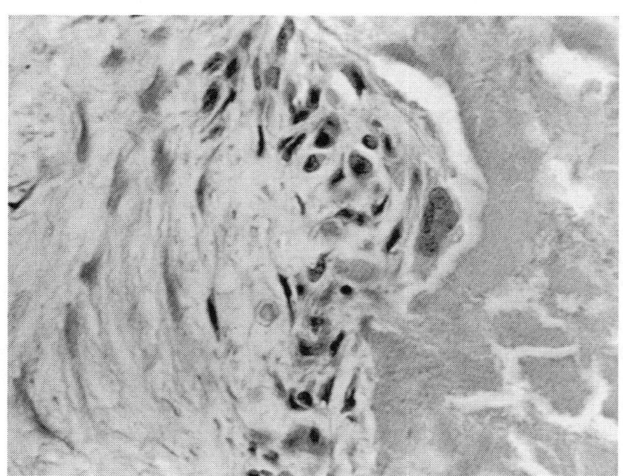

FIGURE 12–6 Gout, tophus involving the mitral valve. Multinucleated giant cells and dense fibrous tissue adjacent to accumulated uric acid (H&E, ×300).

pronounced at the free margins, which have an irregular, nodular appearance. The commissures are not fused. The chordae tendineae of the atrioventricular valves are moderately shortened and thickened. Calcific deposits occur in the angle just beneath the basal attachment of the posterior mitral leaflet (mitral annular calcification), in the mitral leaflets, and in the aortic aspect of the aortic valve cusps. The valves contain large, oval or rounded connective tissue cells (Hurler cells) filled with numerous clear vacuoles, which are the sites of deposition of acid mucopolysaccharide.[20] This material is extremely soluble and difficult to preserve. In addition, small granular cells are present, which contain membrane-limited electron-dense material associated with fragments of collagen fibrils. The valve thickening is due to the presence of these cells and to an increase in the amount of fibrous connective tissue.

In *Fabry's disease*, the glycosphingolipid is deposited within the cardiac valves, occasionally resulting in valvular dysfunction.[20] The mitral and aortic valves are the two valves that most commonly present clinical problems. There may be thickening of the valves with interchordal hooding, or there may be attenuation of the chordae with thickening and ballooning of the mitral valve. Commissural fusion is not a feature of Fabry's disease.

Type II hyperlipoproteinemia (familial hypercholesterolemia) exists in homozygous and heterozygous forms, which differ in the severity and age of onset of clinical symptoms. Aortic valvular disease is frequent in homozygous patients but does not usually occur in heterozygous patients. The aortic valve may be markedly stenosed by fibrous tissue, deposits of foam cells, and cholesterol crystals in the cusps. Thickening of the mitral valve, which results in both stenosis and regurgitation, and thickening of the pulmonary valve and endocardium by foam cells also occur.[20]

Patients with *gout* most commonly develop dysfunction due to hypertension secondary to renal damage; however, tophi occasionally may be present in the heart, most commonly in the mitral valve (Fig. 12–6) and the endocardium of the left ventricle and, less frequently, in the mitral annulus and aortic and tricuspid valve leaflets.[20, 21] To establish the diagnosis histologically, appreciable amounts of uric acid must be identified in the tophi to distinguish them from small amounts of uric acid that may be deposited on previously existing fibrocalcific lesions. Urate deposits are histochemically identifiable by fixation in absolute ethanol, followed by staining by the De Galantha method.

Floppy Valve (Myxomatous Degeneration) and Connective Tissue Dyscrasias

Although myxomatous degeneration has been described in tricuspid aortic and pulmonary valves, the mitral valve is most commonly involved, and the posterior leaflet is affected more often and more severely than is the anterior leaflet. Grossly, the most outstanding feature is a marked increase in surface area of the affected leaflet (Fig. 12–7), which are voluminous, hooded, and white; however, they transilluminate with ease, especially before fixation. On sectioning, the myxomatous consistency of the center of the cuspid is often apparent on gross examination. Small foci of ulceration with occasional superimposed thrombi may be noted on the atrial surface of the affected mitral leaflet.[5] The chordae tendineae often are elongated and thin; however, some localized thickening may be present at their insertions into the valve leaflets (Fig. 12–8). Rupture of the chordae tendineae is common in myxomatous degeneration of the mitral valve; less frequently, myxomatous degeneration may result in aneurysmal dilatation and rupture of a mitral leaflet. Commissural fusion is not a feature of the floppy valve. Because these valves are predisposed to infective endocarditis, gross evidence of this complication must be sought by the surgical pathologist, so that appropriate sections can be obtained for culture before fixation of the valve.

Microscopically, the spongiosa contains stellate cells embedded in a matrix rich in proteoglycans. Characteristically,

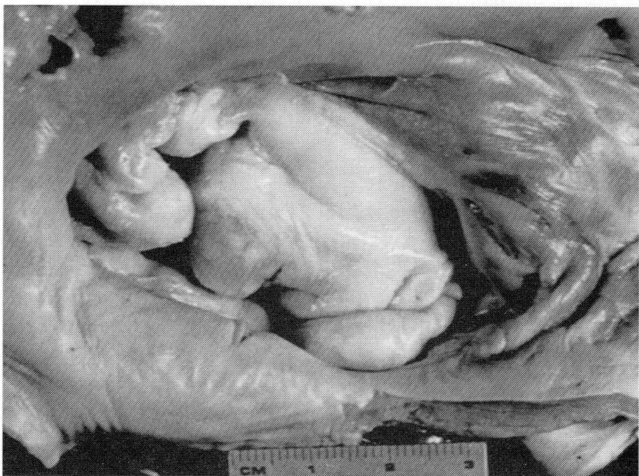

FIGURE 12–7 Floppy mitral valve. The most outstanding feature is a marked increase in the surface area of the leaflets. They are voluminous, hooded, and white; however, they transilluminate with ease. Commissural fusion is not a feature of the floppy valve.

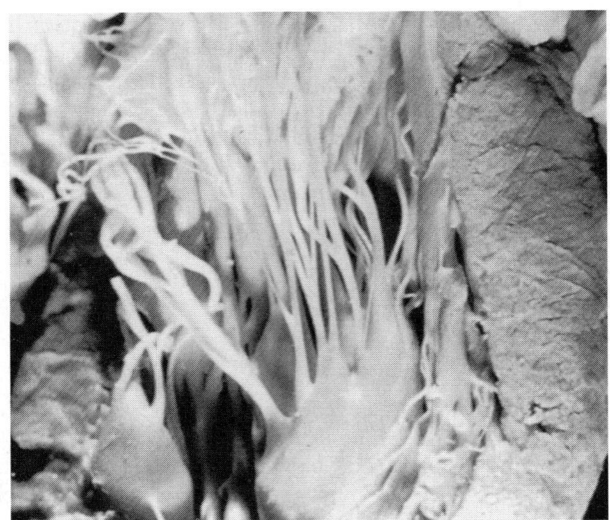

FIGURE 12–8 Floppy mitral valve. The chordae tendineae are often elongated and thin; however, some localized thickening may be present at their insertion into the valve leaflets.

there is focal to extensive replacement of the normal dense, homogeneous collagen of the fibrosa by this myxomatous tissue. This histologic pattern is in contrast to that seen in most valvular heart diseases, in which the spongiosa of the leaflets is partially or completely replaced by dense fibrous tissue. The collagen in the chordae tendineae may show changes similar to those in the fibrosa. The atrialis of the leaflet generally contains a variable degree of fibroelastic proliferation, and superficial ulceration with microscopic fibrin deposition is not uncommon. Unless there is superimposed infective endocarditis, there is no evidence of inflammation or vascularization. Ultrastructurally, there is focal loss of the normal orderly cross-banding of collagen fibers. Microscopically, small areas of myxomatous degeneration may be found near the free edges of normal or diseased valves and should not be confused with the diffuse findings in floppy valves.

Myxomatous degeneration of the cardiac valves, with resulting insufficiency, often occurs in connective tissue dyscrasias such as Marfan's syndrome, osteogenesis imperfecta, cutis laxa, and relapsing polychondritis. This group of diseases may also be associated with cystic medial degeneration of the aorta. Adults with *Marfan's syndrome* most commonly have myxomatous degeneration of the aortic valve; in children, however, the mitral valve is more commonly involved.[20] The affected mitral and aortic leaflets contain an accumulation of myxoid material, mainly in the spongiosa. Recent studies have shown the importance of matrix metalloproteinases in the pathogenesis of these lesions in the Marfan syndrome.[22] The *Ehlers-Danlos syndrome* is a heterogeneous group of several genetically distinct disorders of connective tissue synthesis, which differ in major clinical features, inheritance patterns, and biochemical defects. Cardiovascular lesions have been described in types I to IV; however, myxomatous degeneration and prolapse of the mitral valve appear to be more common in type III, the benign hypermobile form.[20] The most common valvular lesion in *osteogenesis imperfecta* is aortic regurgitation; mitral regurgitation and combined aortic and mitral regurgitation are less common. The aortic regurgitation results from dilatation of the aortic root and deformity of the valvular leaflets, which become abnormally translucent, weak, and elongated. Aneurysms of the sinuses of Valsalva also occur. The mitral annulus is dilated, the mitral leaflets are attenuated and redundant and tend to prolapse, and the chordae tendineae may rupture.[20] In *cutis laxa*, the most common cardiac lesions involve the aorta, pulmonary artery, and pulmonary veins; less commonly, there may be myxomatous degeneration of the aortic or mitral valves.[20] The aortic and mitral valves are the cardiac valves most commonly involved in *relapsing polychondritis*. Lesions may be microscopically identical to those in the other connective tissue dyscrasias.[5]

INFECTIVE ENDOCARDITIS

The relative frequency of involvement of the cardiac valves is similar for infective endocarditis and rheumatic heart disease: mitral, aortic, aortic and mitral combined, tricuspid, and pulmonary valves, in decreasing order of frequency. The tricuspid and pulmonary valves are not commonly involved, with the notable exception of intravenous drug abusers. In many cases of combined aortic and mitral involvement, the anterior leaflet of the mitral valve appears to be infected by regurgitation-induced deposition of organisms from the aortic vegetation. Lesions usually originate on the atrial surface of the atrioventricular valves and the ventricular surface of the semilunar valves and vary from tiny granular or flat vegetations to large polypoid masses. They may be single or multiple and may be firm or soft, but are usually friable. Grossly, they may appear yellow-white to red or brown.[23] The affected valve exhibits destruction and loss of tissue. Valvular ulceration, perforation, or formation of aneurysm of the valve may occur. Rupture of chordae tendineae is common. Infection may spread into the contiguous structures, resulting in annular or myocardial abscesses or aneurysms of the sinuses of Valsalva. Microscopically, the vegetations are composed of masses of necrotic tissue, fibrin, platelets, erythrocytes, leukocytes, and organisms. Classically, there is a superficial zone of fibrin, organisms, and leukocytes; an intermediate zone of amorphous necrotic material; and a basal zone of granulation tissue extending from the substance of the valve. Small foci of calcification are common.

Bicuspid aortic valves or valves with acquired deformities are most frequently involved in infective endocarditis; however, the disease may develop in previously normal valves, including the pulmonary and tricuspid valves, especially in patients over 60 years of age. In previously normal valves, the lesions tend to be larger, and tissue destruction is more extensive. Staphylococci and Gram-negative organisms are more likely to be the etiologic agents than in the case of infection of deformed valves, in which *Streptococcus viridans* is the most common organism encountered. Infected but previously normal valves often show marked necrosis and inflammation, which are less common findings in infected, previously scarred valves.

Although streptococci and staphylococci are the most common microorganisms responsible for infection, a wide variety of bacteria and fungi have been recovered from patients with infective endocarditis. *Candida* species in particular are recovered from addicts and patients with prosthetic heart valves. Gram-negative bacilli account for only a small percentage of infections, despite the relative frequency of Gram-negative bacteremia, and are more likely to be encountered in addicts or in patients with prosthetic heart valves. Rarely, infections are due to other organisms, such as meningococci, pneumococci, gonococci, *Brucella, Haemophilus, Corynebacterium*, mycobacteria, rickettsiae, and *Aspergillus* and other fungal species.[24] Fungal vegetations, in particular, tend to be large and friable, with a tendency to produce embolization (Plate 12–11). Because fungal endocarditis is frequently indolent clinically, it is important for the surgical pathologist to obtain appropriate special stains on any thromboembolus removed from a systemic artery. Any valve removed surgically that has gross lesions suggestive of infective endocarditis should have sections taken for microbiologic culture before fixation. Merely taking a swab of the surface of the valve for culture is not adequate. Indeed, even if the valve appears grossly normal, patients in whom the clinical history or physical findings suggest the possibility of infective endocarditis should have sections of the valve taken for culture.

Healing of vegetations may occur as a result of therapy or spontaneously, without antimicrobial therapy.[23] These healed vegetations often result in multiple, calcified, polypoid lesions on the surface of the valve. Contracture of scar tissue may further reduce the surface area of the valve. The healed vegetations in the heart valves or chordae tendineae are similar in gross appearance to those with active infection.[23] Occasionally, well-circumscribed defects with smooth edges remain in the heart valve after the healing of perforations that resulted from infective endocarditis. Usually, the etiology of these morphologic abnormalities cannot be identified, especially if there is no known antecedent infection. Histologic study rarely helps to resolve these issues because the alterations resulting from the healing of the inflammatory process tend to be similar in their end-stage appearance.[23]

PROSTHETIC HEART VALVES

Types

Prosthetic heart valves in current use can be classified into two major groups: rigid-framed (mechanical) valves and tissue valves (bioprosthesis). Rigid-framed valves are of three types: (1) valves with a centrally placed occluder (ball or disc), which moves up and down in a metal cage and allows only lateral blood flow, (2) valves with a tilting disc, which permits semicentral flow, and (3) valves with two hinged, semicircular plates (St. Jude type), which allow central flow. Tissue valves include (1) fresh and variously treated homografts, (2) human dura mater or fascia lata valves, (3) bovine pericardial valves, and (4) porcine aortic valves. The metal and plastic mounting frames and the preimplantation chemical treatments vary from one type of tissue valve to another. Tissue valves without supporting frames (unstented porcine valves) are beginning to be used clinically. Knowledge of the frames and treatments is necessary to interpret morphologic findings in tissue valves. Radiographs may be useful in the identification and evaluation of explanted valves.[25, 26] Essential for the evaluation of any prosthetic valve is knowledge of the length of time the valve was in place and the specific reason for its removal.

Complications

Certain complications are common to all types of prosthetic heart valves. Among these are thrombosis, embolization, infection, dehiscence of the valvular ring, paravalvular leak, disproportion, turbulent flow, and hemolysis. Complications limited to rigid-framed prostheses[27, 28] are related to wear and fracture of mechanical components, resulting in interference with proper motion of the occluder (and sometimes also in embolic phenomena), whereas complications peculiar to tissue valves[27, 28] are related to calcification or breakdown of the prosthetic tissue leaflets.

Complications Common to All Types of Prosthetic Valves

Thrombus formation in mechanical prostheses is most common at the base of the struts forming the cage. From this area, thrombi can spread and interfere with motion of the occluder, with seating of the occluder on the orifice, or with blood flow (Fig. 12–9). These thrombi can undergo organization, become infected, or be sources of emboli. Ball valves with cloth-covered cage struts are less likely to form thrombi than are those with uncovered struts. Tissue valves are least likely to form large thrombi, although aggregates of platelets do develop on their surfaces. Thrombi can splint the cusps of bioprostheses and render them stenotic.[29, 30] Thrombi removed from prosthetic heart valves must be examined (by histology and by culture) for evidence of infection.[8] *Dehiscence of a valvular ring* must be regarded as due to infection until proved otherwise. *Paravalvular leaks* most frequently result from a prosthesis having been sutured to a ring that is heavily calcified or weakened (as occurs in patients with Marfan's syndrome

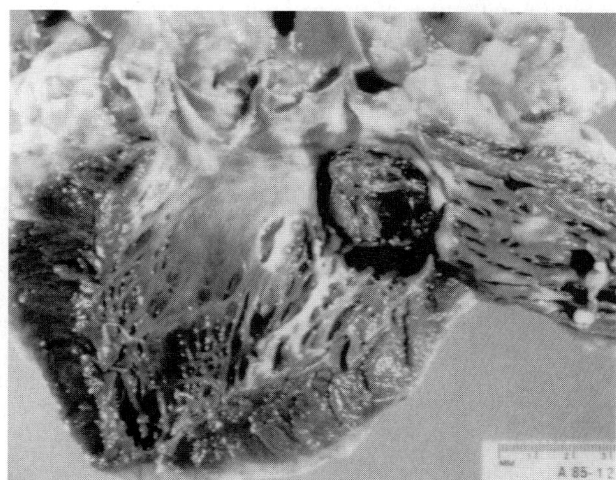

FIGURE 12–9 Mechanical prosthesis, mitral valve. Thrombus formation in mechanical prostheses is most common at the base of the struts forming the cage, as illustrated in this heart.

or other connective tissue disorders). Anemia and renal hemosiderosis are typical findings in *hemolysis* produced by prosthetic heart valves.

Disproportion is caused by prosthetic heart valves that are too large for the chamber in which they are placed. This can result in interference with movement of the poppet, as in the case of large ball valves placed in a small ascending aorta (particularly in patients with combined mitral and aortic valve disease in whom the aortic root is usually not dilated) or in a small left ventricle (as in patients with combined mitral and aortic stenosis in whom the left ventricle is hypertrophied but not dilated). If a porcine bioprosthesis is improperly placed in the mitral orifice, one of its struts may obstruct the left ventricular outflow tract. In the case of double valve replacement, the prosthetic mitral valve may be inadvertently placed in such a way as to interfere with proper seating of the poppet of the prosthetic aortic valve. Disproportion also may result from normal growth of the heart of a child in whom a small prosthetic valve was implanted at an early age.

Complications Limited to Rigid-Framed (Mechanical) Prosthetic Valves

Turbulent blood flow produced by caged-ball prostheses may lead to *diffuse endocardial fibroelastotic thickening* and to intimal proliferation in the ascending aorta, sometimes with extension of the thickening into the coronary arterial ostia. Degeneration (variance) of the silicone rubber poppet was common in the caged-ball prostheses implanted before 1967. This complication, which resulted from surface abrasion and lipid infiltration, has not been reported in the metallic hollow poppet. Wear of a caged disc, causing "grooving" and disc cocking, has been described in most caged-disc prostheses. Disc cocking remains a potential problem with all caged-disc valves, and it may be totally unrecognized as a cause of fatalities. Wear of the cloth covering on the struts and the orifice occurred in some of the older models of completely cloth-covered caged-ball prostheses, but strut cloth wear has not been reported in the newer Starr-Edwards models with metal tracks. Dislodgment of caged discs and poppets has been reported in association with wear of these components or with fracture of struts.

Complications Limited to Bioprosthetic (Tissue) Valves

The various types of bioprosthetic heart valves developed since the late 1970s have the following characteristics in common: collagen is their major structural component; they are mounted (except for some of the homografts) on metal and plastic stents; the incidence of clinical episodes of thromboembolism is lower with these valves than with rigid-framed valves; and they have problems of long-term durability because they can become stenotic as a result of calcification or regurgitant due to alterations in collagen.[31]

PORCINE AORTIC VALVES

Porcine aortic valves treated with a low (<1 percent) concentration of glutaraldehyde (to crosslink tissue proteins, to sterilize the tissue, and to eliminate problems of antigenicity) and mounted on flexible stents have become the most widely used type of valvular bioprosthesis. During the first 5 years after implantation, these valves usually have excellent function, although they can develop extensive anatomic changes. After the first 5 years, appreciable incidences of calcification and cuspal damage become evident (Fig. 12–10). Calcific deposits develop more frequently and earlier in children and young adults than in older individuals and also are more frequent in patients with chronic renal disease. Cuspal perforations have no relation to patient age.

A bioprosthetic heart valve removed because of dysfunction should first be examined for evidence of infection, perforation, or calcification, and cultures should be taken as indicated by clinical or anatomic findings; then it should be radiographed and photographed before the cusps are detached from the frame for histologic sectioning. These valves are fragile and should be handled only by the mounting frame to avoid producing artifactual damage to the cusps. Connective tissue stains and stains for calcium are useful in evaluating these valves. Transmission electron microscopy provides the best method for studying the collagen, and scanning electron microscopy is the method of choice for examining the surfaces.

Histologically, porcine aortic valves are composed of the following three layers, which also are recognizable in the bioprosthesis even after having been in place for long periods of time: (1) the ventricularis, which faces the ventricular cavity when the valve is in its anatomic position and which contains collagen and abundant elastic fibers, (2) the spongiosa, which is the proteoglycan-rich middle

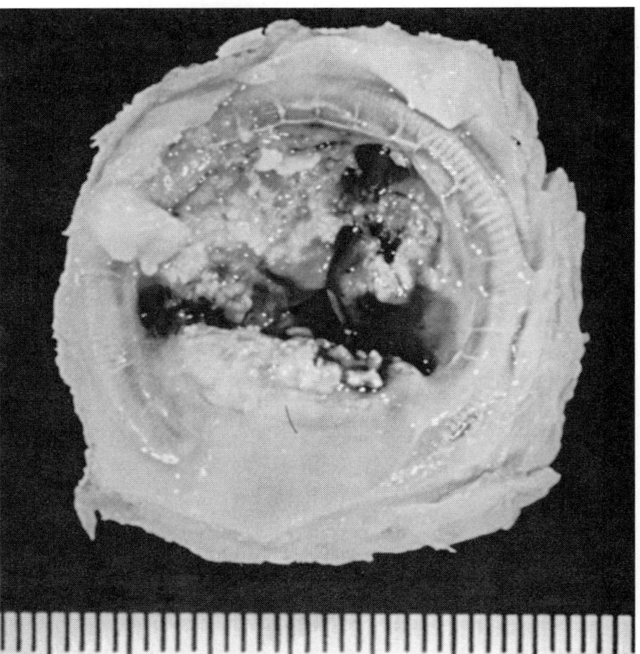

FIGURE 12–10 Porcine aortic valve prosthesis. After years of implantation, appreciable incidences of calcification and cuspal damage become evident. Calcific deposits develop more frequently and earlier in children and young adults and are more frequent in patients with chronic renal disease.

layer, and (3) the fibrosa, which contains densely packed collagen but only small, scanty elastic fibers and which faces the aortic wall. Proteoglycans are lost from the spongiosa during commercial processing and soon after implantation of the bioprosthesis, leaving empty spaces that gradually are filled with deposits of plasma proteins. The surfaces of porcine valvular bioprostheses usually do not become endothelialized, although they may be covered by macrophages, multinucleated giant cells, platelet aggregates, and small fibrin deposits. Polymorphonuclear leukocytes are very scanty or absent unless infection is present. Macrophages show little tendency to invade the bioprosthetic tissue, and there is no evidence that immunologic rejection plays a role in its deterioration.

Calcific deposits usually develop in association with collagen in foci of loss of proteoglycans and with surface thrombi, especially in regions near the commissures; they form yellow, plaquelike or raised lesions.[32] Calcific deposits also develop in the aortic wall just adjacent to the cusps and in cardiac muscle cells in a muscular shelf extending from the ventricular septum into the base of the right coronary cusp of the porcine aortic valve. This cusp is larger than the others, and its base is less translucent. Calcific deposits can also be associated with perforations, perhaps because collagen adjacent to these deposits undergoes severe mechanical stresses.[32] The collagen in bioprostheses undergoes a time-dependent process of degeneration, which may be related to material fatigue and may result in perforation of the cusps. Perforations in porcine valves occur most frequently near the basal attachment of the cusps. In pericardial valves, particularly those implanted in the mitral position, cuspal tears are likely to involve the free edge near the attachment to the post. It has been suggested that such tears begin at the attachment suture. Infection of porcine valvular bioprostheses differs from that of rigid-framed valves: it is likely to involve the cusps (rather than the sewing ring), is less likely to result in formation of a ring abscess, and usually extends into the collagen in the cusps.[31] The incidence of infection in the two types of valves appears to be similar.

OTHER BIOPROSTHETIC VALVES

Fresh, antibiotic-sterilized, freeze-dried, and chemically treated aortic valve homografts (allografts) have been used infrequently in the United States. However, cryopreserved aortic valve allografts have been used more extensively in recent years. In contrast to glutaraldehyde-treated bioprostheses, allografts tend to become covered with a fibrous sheath of host origin. These valves become completely acellular, and apoptosis has recently been shown to play an important role in the loss of the valvular cells.[33] Complications of allograft valves include calcification, cuspal rupture, and fibrous retraction of the edges of the cusps. *Autologous fascia lata valves* implanted without any chemical treatment have had a very poor record of durability and a high incidence of degeneration, thrombosis, calcification, and fibrous contraction of the cusps. Their use has been completely discontinued. *Human dura mater valves* preserved by glycerol treatment have been used extensively in Latin America. Bioprostheses made of *glutaraldehyde-treated bovine pericardium* have also been used as substitute cardiac valves. Both dura mater and pericardium consist of dense collagenous sheets with sparse elastic fibers. Their layered structure is easily distinguishable histologically from that of porcine aortic valves. Complications of pericardial and dura mater valves are similar to those of porcine valves, consisting mainly of calcification and cuspal dehiscence.[27]

CONDUITS

Conduits composed of various synthetic materials have been used to correct hypoplasia or atresia of the pulmonary artery. Valveless conduits were first used; subsequently, conduits containing mechanical (Björk-Shiley) valves were employed but were found to be prone to valvular thrombosis. More recently, extensive use has been made of pulmonic conduits with bioprosthetic (porcine or pericardial) valves; in addition, left ventricular apical-aortic conduits have had limited use for correction of tunnel aortic stenosis.[27] The most frequent complication of conduits is obstruction, which can result from one or more of the following causes: (1) muscular compression of the proximal end of the conduit during ventricular systole, (2) accumulation of thrombotic or fibrous material (fibrous peel) in the wall of the conduit, (3) compression of the conduit by the sternum, (4) calcific or thrombotic stenosis of the bioprosthesis, and (5) stenosis at the distal end (the most common cause of obstruction) because of the small size of the artery at the anastomotic site.

REFERENCES

1. Cheitlin MD, Fenogho JJ, McAllister HA Jr, et al: Congenital aortic stenosis secondary to dysplasia of congenital bicuspid aortic valves without commissural fusion. Am J Cardiol 42:102, 1978.
2. Fenogho JJ, McAllister HA Jr, DeCastro CM, et al: Congenital bicuspid aortic valve after age 20. Am J Cardiol 39:164, 1977.
3. Davia JE, Fenogho JJ, DeCastro CM, et al: Quadricuspid semilunar valves. Chest 72:186, 1977.
4. Hyams VJ, Manion WC: Incomplete differentiation of the cardiac valves. A report of 197 cases. Am Heart J 76:173, 1968.
5. Pomerance A, Davies MJ: The Pathology of the Heart Oxford, Blackwell Scientific, 1975.
6. Baggenstoss AH, Titus JL: Rheumatic and collagen disorders of the heart. *In* Gould SE (ed): Pathology of the Heart and Blood Vessels. p. 701. Springfield, IL, Charles C Thomas, 1968.
7. Ferrans VJ, Butany JW: Ultrastructural pathology of the heart. *In* Trump BF, Jones RT (eds): Diagnostic Electron Microscopy. Vol. 4. p. 319. New York: Churchill Livingstone, 1983.
8. McAllister HA Jr, Ferrans VJ: The heart and blood vessels. *In* Silverberg SJ (ed): Principles and Practice of Surgical Pathology. p. 787. New York: Churchill Livingstone, 1991.
9. McAllister HA Jr: Collagen diseases and the cardiovascular system. *In* Silver MD (ed): Cardiovascular Pathology. p. 1151. New York: Churchill Livingstone, 1991.
10. Fauci AS, Wolff SM: Wegener's granulomatosis and related diseases. Dis Mon 23(7):1, 1977.
11. McAllister HA Jr, Fenogho JJ: Cardiac involvement in Whipple's disease. Circulation 52:152, 1975.
12. Eck M, Muller-Hermelink HK, Harmsen D, Kreipe H: Invasion and destruction of mucosal plasma cells by *Tropheryma whippelii*. Hum Pathol 28:1424–1428, 1997.
13. Olsen EGJ, Spry CJF: The pathogenesis of Loffler's endomyocardial disease, and its relationship to endomyocardial fibrosis. Prog Cardiol 8:281, 1979.
14. Roberts WC, Dangel JC, Bulkley BH: Nonrheumatic valvular cardiac disease: a clinicopathologic survey of 27 different conditions causing valvular dysfunction. Cardiovasc Clin 5:333, 1973.

15. McAllister HA Jr, Hall RJ: Iatrogenic heart disease. *In* Cheng TO (ed): The International Textbook of Cardiology. p. 871. New York: Pergamon, 1986.
16. McAllister HA Jr: Pathology of the heart in endocrine disorders. *In* Silver MD (ed): Cardiovascular Pathology. p. 1181. New York: Churchill Livingstone, 1991.
17. Redfield MM: Ergot alkaloid heart disease. *In* Hurst JW (ed): New Types of Cardiovascular Diseases: Topics in Clinical Cardiology. pp. 63–76. New York: Igaku-Shoin Medical, 1994.
18. Redfield MM, Nicholson WJ, Edwards WD, Tajik AJ: Valve disease associated with ergot alkaloid use: echocardiographic and pathologic correlations. Ann Intern Med 117:50–52, 1992.
19. Connolly HM, Cresy JL, McGoon MD, et al: Valvular heart disease associated with fenfluramine-phentermine. N Engl J Med 337:581–588, 1997.
20. Ferrans VJ: Metabolic and familial diseases. *In* Silver MD (ed): Cardiovascular Pathology. p. 1973. New York: Churchill Livingstone, 1991.
21. McAllister HA Jr: Pathology of the cardiovascular system in chronic renal failure. *In* Lowenthal DT, Pennock RL, Likoff W et al (eds): Management of Cardiovascular Disease in Renal Failure. p. 1. Philadelphia: FA Davis, 1981.
22. Segura AM, Luna RE, Horiba K, et al: Immunohistochemistry of matrix metalloproteinases and their inhibitors in thoracic aortic aneurysms and aortic valves of patients with the Marfan's syndrome. Circulation 98:II331–II337, 1998.
23. Titus JL: Infective endocarditis, active and healed. *In* Edwards JE, Lev M, Abell MR (eds): The Heart. p. 176. Baltimore: Williams & Wilkins, 1974.
24. Freedman LR: Endocarditis updated. Dis Mon 26(3):1, 1979.
25. Silver MD, Datta BN, Bowes VF: A key to identify heart valve prostheses. Arch Pathol 99:132, 1975.
26. Steiner RM, Flicker S: The radiology of prosthetic heart valves. *In* D Morse, RM Steiner, J Fernandez (eds): Guide to Prosthetic Cardiac Valves. p. 53. New York: Springer-Verlag, 1985.
27. Lefrak EA, Starr A: Cardiac Valve Prostheses. East Norwalk, CT: Appleton & Lange, 1979.
28. Zeien LB, Klatt EC: Cardiac valve prostheses at autopsy. Arch Pathol Lab Med 144:933, 1990.
29. Platt MR, Mills LJ, Estrera AS, et al: Marked thrombosis and calcification of porcine heterograft valves. Circulation 62:862, 1980.
30. Croft CH, Buja LM, Floresca MZ, et al: Late thrombotic obstruction of aortic porcine bioprosthesis. Am J Cardiol 57:355, 1986.
31. Ferrans VJ, Tomita Y, Hilbert SL, et al: Evaluation of operatively excised prosthetic tissue valves. *In* Waller BF (ed): Pathology of the Heart and Great Vessels. p. 311. New York: Churchill Livingstone, 1988.
32. Hilbert SL, Ferrans VJ, McAllister HA Jr, Cooley DA: Ionescu-Shiley bovine pericardial bioprosthesis: histologic and ultrastructural studies. Am J Pathol 140:1195, 1992.
33. Hilbert SL, Luna RE, Zhang J, et al: Allograft heart valves: the role of apoptosis-mediated cell loss. J Thorac Cardiovasc Surg 117:454–462, 1999.

CHAPTER 13

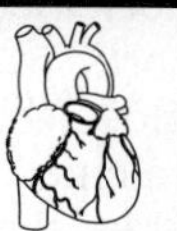

Aortic Valve Disease

Otto M. Hess, Urs Scherrer, Blase A. Carabello, Pascal Nicod, and Robert L. Frye

AORTIC STENOSIS
Pathophysiology
Physical Examination
Doppler Echocardiography Examination of Aortic Stenosis
Natural History
Medical Treatment
DIFFERENTIATION OF REVERSIBLE FROM IRREVERSIBLE LEFT VENTRICULAR SYSTOLIC DYSFUNCTION IN PATIENTS WITH AORTIC STENOSIS
Blase A. Carabello
Consequences of Hypertrophy
Clinical Implications of Left Ventricular Dysfunction in Aortic Stenosis
Summary
AORTIC REGURGITATION
Pathophysiology
Physical Examination
Natural History
Medical Treatment

Aortic Stenosis

Pathophysiology

Obstruction to left ventricular outflow is localized most commonly at the aortic valve, but it may also occur above *(supravalvular)* or below *(subvalvular)* the valve. This chapter focuses on valvular aortic stenosis alone. A reduction of the aortic valve area to 1 cm^2 is usually associated with a systolic pressure gradient that, in turn, results in an increase in the load on the left ventricle and in the left ventricular (LV) muscle mass. LV hypertrophy can usually maintain LV function for many years without a reduction in cardiac output or development of cardiac symptoms. In general, aortic stenosis is considered to be severe when the mean pressure gradient exceeds 50 mm Hg in the presence of a normal cardiac output, or when the aortic valve orifice area is less than 0.80 cm^2 (i.e., less than one fourth that of the normal valve orifice).[1,2] Severe aortic stenosis is usually accompanied by typical symptoms, such as angina pectoris, dizziness, syncope during exertion, or dyspnea. Angina pectoris is a manifestation of myocardial ischemia caused by a mismatch between oxygen supply and demand. Oxygen demand is heightened because of the increase in muscle mass, and supply is decreased because of low perfusion pressure, increased end-diastolic filling pressure, shortened diastolic perfusion interval, and increase in the oxygen diffusion distance owing to muscle fiber hypertrophy.[3] As a result of these "pressure overload" demands on the myocardium, patients with severe aortic stenosis may develop congestive heart failure as an additional mode of clinical presentation. In addition, coronary artery vasodilatation is attenuated by severe ventricular hypertrophy.[3] In patients with severe aortic stenosis, coronary blood flow/100 g muscle mass can be reduced not only during exercise but also under resting conditions.[4] Associated coronary artery disease may further compromise myocardial oxygen supply/demand imbalances and aggravate the hemodynamic burden on the heart. Sudden strenuous exercise leading to a decrease in peripheral vascular resistance may provoke a drop in systolic blood pressure and cause syncope. Normally, the decline in peripheral vascular resistance during exercise is compensated for by an increase in cardiac output, thus maintaining arterial pressure and cerebral perfusion at normal levels. However, in severe aortic stenosis, reflex vasodilatation may be triggered by stimulation of inhibitory ventricular baroreceptors as the result of high intraventricular pressure, leading to withdrawal of sympathetic drive and syncope.[5] Dysfunction of ventricular baroreceptors has been thought to be responsible for the arterial hypertension sometimes observed in patients after surgical correction of aortic stenosis, despite adequate relief of the pressure burden. Other causes of syncope in valvular aortic stenosis include ventricular tachyarrhythmias, intermittent atrioventricular (AV) block, and atrial fibrillation with loss of the "atrial kick."

Long-standing LV hypertrophy is associated with changes in the collagen structure of the left ventricle (structural remodeling), which may impair systolic and diastolic function.[6] Severe concentric hypertrophy may be associated with increased myocardial stiffness and LV end-diastolic pressure at a time when LV systolic function is still normal. Indeed, approximately 50 percent of patients with normal LV systolic function exhibit evidence of diastolic dysfunction.[7] Such diastolic dysfunction may itself lead to an increase in mean left atrial (LA) pressure, pulmonary congestion, and secondary pulmonary hypertension.

In rare cases, severe septal hypertrophy of the left ventricle bulges into the right ventricular (RV) outflow tract and causes an RV systolic pressure gradient (Bernheim effect). Dilatation of the left ventricle may occur late in the course of patients with severe aortic stenosis and is associated with a large increase in LV end-diastolic pressure and a decrease in cardiac output. At this stage, mitral regurgitation may develop as a result of mitral annular dilatation.

The pathologic basis for valvular aortic stenosis has changed over the past several decades. The relative frequency of postinflammatory disease of the aortic valve has decreased.[8] In patients less than 70 years of age undergoing aortic valve replacement for isolated aortic stenosis, the most common finding in aortic valves replaced was a calcified bicuspid valve in 50 percent of patients; in those older than 70 years, degenerative (senile) calcification of tricuspid aortic valves was the most common finding.[9] More recent studies have challenged the concept of a passive degenerative process with evidence of an active inflammatory process in aortic valves obtained at autopsy,[10] and others have suggested a possible role for infection of the aortic valve in the pathogenesis of aortic stenosis.[11] An additional potential mechanism for the pathogenesis of aortic stenosis is the process of atherosclerosis with deposition of apolipoproteins in the early lesions.[12] Consistent with such a mechanism is the occurrence of calcific aortic stenosis in patients with familial hypercholesterolemia.[13] An important pathologic finding of clinical importance relates to those extensively calcified aortic valves in which the calcification may impinge on the conduction system sufficiently to cause complete heart block, and in certain patients after aortic valve replacement, permanent pacemakers may be required as a result of such changes.

Physical Examination

Clinical recognition of valvular aortic stenosis is most commonly based on the presence of a systolic ejection murmur with radiation to the neck. Other forms of LV outflow tract obstruction may be suspected at the bedside, but objective imaging studies are usually required for definitive classification. Features that suggest severe obstruction include a long systolic murmur with a delay in the peak intensity of the murmur[14] associated with characteristic changes in the carotid pulse of a slow upstroke (pulsus lentus), delayed peaking (pulsus tardus), and decreased amplitude (pulsus parvus) (Fig. 13–1).

Estimates of severity of aortic stenosis at the bedside based on analysis of the carotid pulse are open to considerable error, particularly in the elderly as a result of changes in arterial compliance. Intensity of the murmur of aortic stenosis is also a poor predictor of severity of obstruction. Of critical clinical importance is the recognition that in the presence of low cardiac output and depressed LV function, the classic findings of severe aortic stenosis may be absent. As a result, in the setting of congestive heart failure, systolic ejection murmurs that seem clinically insignificant may be associated with critical aortic stenosis.

Simulation of aortic stenosis by prolapse of the posterior leaflet of the mitral valve with a large regurgitant jet directed anteriorly along the atrial septum to the base of the heart is well recognized. Distinguishing the murmur of aortic stenosis from that of mitral regurgitation may be accomplished at the bedside by noting the increase in the murmur of aortic stenosis after the pause of a premature contraction or longer cycle length in the setting of atrial fibrillation. In contrast, the murmur of mitral regurgitation remains the same or decreases in intensity. In addition, there is a decrease in the murmur during a Valsalva maneuver in patients with aortic stenosis as a result of decrease in the stroke volume.

Other ancillary findings in the setting of valvular aortic stenosis may be noted at the bedside, including an aortic ejection click suggesting a bicuspid aortic valve,[15] paradoxical splitting of the second heart sound,[16] a prominent S_4,[17] and a high-pitched musical murmur at the apex.[18]

Careful attention to the details of the entire clinical picture of the patient at the bedside is essential to making the appropriate decisions to establish an accurate anatomic and physiologic diagnosis in a cost-effective manner. This is best accomplished with Doppler echocardiographic studies performed with careful attention for accurate assessment of valvular hemodynamics. High-quality Doppler echocardiographic analysis of patients with aortic stenosis allows clinical decision making without requiring left heart catheterization except in unusual circumstances.[19]

Doppler Echocardiographic Examination of Aortic Stenosis

The Doppler echocardiographic examination of the aortic valve and aortic hemodynamics has radically changed the

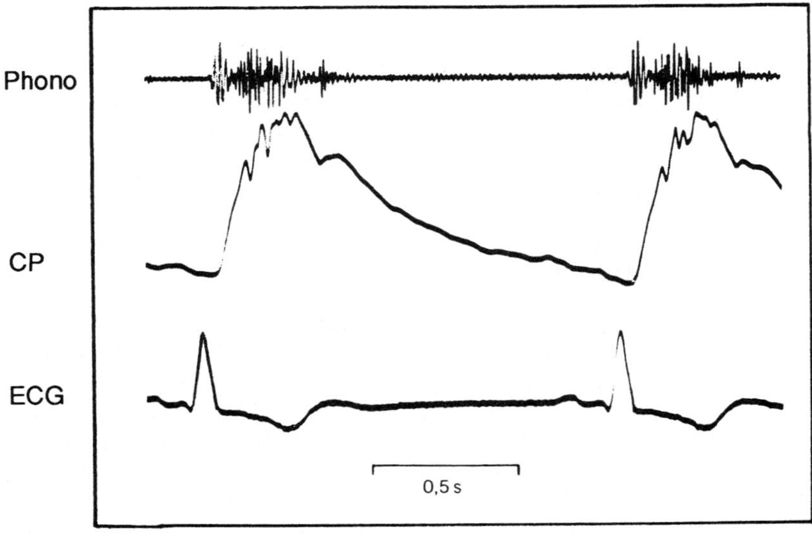

FIGURE 13–1 Carotid pulse contour (CP) in a 56-year-old patient with aortic stenosis. The pulse upstroke is slow (pulsus lentus) and displays shuddering. On the phonocardiogram (Phono), the peak intensity of the murmur is delayed toward midsystole. The electrocardiogram (ECG) shows typical ST-segment changes (strain).

approach to aortic stenosis.[20–22] It allows the indirect visualization of the valve with its morphologic abnormalities and the assessment of transvalvular hemodynamics and LV function.

Morphologic Assessment

The two-dimensional echocardiographic examination allows determination of the presence of calcification,[23] the number of aortic cusps, and in particular, the presence of bicuspid aortic valve. This determination may be difficult if the valve is heavily calcified or if the fusion of a commissure mimics a bicuspid valve. Aortic stenosis due to rheumatic disease is characterized by fusion of the commissures, whereas "degenerative" aortic stenosis is due to limitation of movement of the cusps owing to the deposition of calcium and perhaps other substances within the body of the cusps. The distinction of these two mechanisms of obstruction is possible using two-dimensional or even three-dimensional echocardiography at an early stage of the disease, but this is often not possible when the cusps are massively calcified.[24]

The amplitude of separation of the cusps is inversely proportional to the degree of stenosis. The separation of cusps measured by M-mode echocardiography has been widely used when no other direct method of measurement of the degree of stenosis was available. However, the limitations of the M-mode method have been recognized, and it has been replaced by the direct planimetry of the orifice using the high-resolution imaging of transesophageal echocardiography.[25] This method has provided important insight into the pathophysiology of aortic stenosis[26] but remains disputed with regard to its reliability and accuracy,[27] especially in heavily calcified valves.[28] Furthermore, it is also limited by the fact that in patients with reduced LV function, the movement of the cusps may be limited owing to low cardiac output despite modest degrees of stenosis.

The morphologic assessment also involves the measurement of the LV outflow tract, which may be used for sizing of certain valve substitutes. Usually, the proximal ascending aorta is dilated (poststenotic dilatation) but not aneurysmal. The LV size is usually normal in pure aortic stenosis, but it may be increased in patients with reduced LV function and in those with associated aortic regurgitation of significant degree. LV hypertrophy, present in patients with moderate or severe stenosis, can sometimes be absent despite severe stenosis.[29] The end-systolic wall stress is normalized by the compensatory hypertrophy, but the causal role of insufficient hypertrophy in the development of excess afterload with high wall stress and secondary reduction of LV function is unclear.[30]

Color-Flow Imaging

Color-flow imaging shows the acceleration of the flow at the level of the leaflets with mosaic pattern, but its most conspicuous utility is in the assessment of the degree of associated regurgitation. The qualitative assessment using the size of the jet of aortic regurgitation is the most utilized method, but in cases with more significant degree of regurgitation, a quantitative assessment is possible.

Hemodynamic Assessment

A profound change in management of patients with aortic stenosis occurred with the availability of continuous-wave Doppler.[20] With the advent of continuous-wave Doppler and its ability to detect high blood velocity, the transvalvular aortic gradient has become measurable noninvasively. The simplified Bernoulli equation neglects the prestenotic velocity and the viscous and convective components of the equation. It is applicable under most circumstances to assess obstruction to the aortic flow.[31] Simultaneous catheter and Doppler studies have shown that the Doppler assessment is highly accurate.[32] The major pitfall of Doppler is the possible angle between the beam of ultrasound and the aortic flow that, if superior to 30 degrees, may lead to notable underestimation of gradient. The only approach to avoid this potential underestimation is a multiwindow, comprehensive examination, aiming at recording the maximal aortic velocity. The confrontation of invasive and Doppler data has led to the recognition of semantic differences leading to potential misunderstandings. The invasive peak-to-peak gradient—the difference between the peaks of the LV and the aortic pressures—is not a simultaneous gradient and has no corresponding Doppler measure and should not be used. The peak gradient usually occurs before the peak ventricular or aortic pressures and is easily measured using the Doppler peak velocity. The mean gradient obtained by planimetry of the pressure or Doppler signals is the best measure of the integrated obstruction to flow. A possible cause of higher gradients by Doppler than by catheterization is the pressure-recovery phenomenon,[33] characterized by a progressive increase in pressure distal to the aortic orifice with deceleration of blood.[34, 35] This difference is usually small but may be notable in patients with moderate stenosis and a small aorta.[35]

Another major advance has been the measurement of the aortic valve area (AVA),[36] using the combination of the peak transvalvular velocity (PVel) and the subvalvular (left ventricular outflow tract [LVOT]) velocity (Vel) and area as:

$$\text{AVA} = (\text{LVOT area}) \cdot (\text{LVOT Vel})/\text{PVel}$$

The velocity can also be replaced by the time-velocity integral of the Doppler signals of the jet and LVOT to calculate the mean AVA. This measurement is accurate and reproducible,[37, 38] if adequate precautions are taken to record the peak transvalvular velocity. This measure of the lesion severity in aortic stenosis has long been considered as the absolute reference standard, but several points deserve emphasis. First, the threshold for defining severe aortic stenosis has not been based on outcome data and has varied between 0.75 and 1.0 cm^2. We use thresholds of 0.75, 1.0, 1.5 to define aortic stenosis of severe, moderately severe, and moderate degrees, respectively, but outcome studies are needed to provide evidence regarding the risk associated with specific AVAs. Second, the AVA is not a fixed measure[39] for several reasons.[40] With very low flow, the profile of velocity at the vena contracta (smallest area of transvalvular flow) tends to become less flat, suggesting that through the same effective orifice less flow may pass, resulting in a decreased calculated effective AVA.[41] Also the orifice of the aortic valve in aortic stenosis is limited more by the inertia of the calcified leaflets than by a commissural fusion and, therefore, may vary[42] with the driving force of flow, that is, the quality of ventricular contraction. The concept of the variable aortic orifice has been disputed and requires additional investigation.[43]

Special Problems

Aortic Stenosis in Atrial Fibrillation. In atrial fibrillation, a marked beat-to-beat variability of transvalvular flow and gradient is observed, and the values reported should be the average of large numbers of beats, at least 6 to 10. The AVA is particularly difficult to calculate[44] and requires the use of matching cycle lengths for the jet and LVOT measurements and averaging. However, with these precautions adequate measures can be obtained.

Aortic Stenosis With Reduced Left Ventricular Function and Low Gradient. Concerns in such patients are of two types. If the AVA is in the range of moderate stenosis, the concern is usually that Doppler may have underestimated the gradient and degree of stenosis. In this context, the observation of only mild or absent calcification or of a wide opening of leaflet is of great value. If the AVA is consistent with severe stenosis, the concern is that the reduced valve area may be due to the low flow state[45] secondary to an unrelated cause of LV dysfunction and not to primary severe aortic stenosis. In this context, two approaches have been recommended. The calculation of aortic valve resistance has been touted as less sensitive to flow than that of valve area,[45, 46] but the usefulness of that index[46, 47] has not been fully confirmed in large clinical series.[48] A low-dose dobutamine stress test is useful[49, 50] to discriminate the truly severe aortic stenosis in which the gradient increases with dobutamine from the mild stenosis in which the gradient increases mildly and the valve area increases markedly.

Aortic Stenosis With Subaortic Stenosis. In some patients, the LV hypertrophy of aortic stenosis predominates at the base of the septum and is associated with a systolic anterior motion of the mitral valve, leading to LVOT obstruction. This combination has important consequences. First, with these combined successive obstructions, the assumptions of the continuity equation are not respected and the valve area cannot be calculated accurately. Second, the subaortic obstruction may increase postoperatively, and it is important that the surgeon be aware of the situation in order to consider a myectomy in association with the aortic valve replacement.

Combined Aortic Stenosis and Regurgitation. Aortic regurgitation associated with stenosis is usually mild, but moderate or more severe regurgitation, if present, modifies the hemodynamic profile and results in a higher mean gradient than would be justified by the stenosis alone, owing to the increased transvalvular flow. Therefore, mixed aortic valve disease with both moderate stenosis (AVA $>$ 0.75 cm^2) and regurgitation ($<$4+) may result in a severe lesion that can be diagnosed on the basis of a high gradient.

Natural History

Patients with aortic stenosis may remain asymptomatic for many years despite the presence of moderate to severe valve obstruction. However, 3 to 5 percent of these patients may die suddenly without exhibiting cardiac symptoms.[1, 2] More recent studies have challenged the risk of sudden death in asymptomatic patients with moderate to severe aortic stenosis, and management of these patients is controversial. In the prospective study of patients with asymptomatic aortic stenosis by Otto and associates,[51] the likelihood of being alive without aortic valve replacement at 2 years after entry was a mean of 21 percent for patients with a jet velocity of greater than 4.0 m/s (Fig. 13–2). Such event rates in this prospective study are higher than previously reported in observational studies.[52] The rate of progression of aortic valve stenosis in asymptomatic patients may vary considerably, but on average, aortic jet velocity increased by 0.70 $\pm$ 0.58 m/s, mean transaortic gradient by 14 $\pm$ 13 mm Hg, and valve area decreased -0.25 ± 0.28 cm^2.[51] Progression of valvular obstruction and the short duration between onset of symptoms and sudden death in some patients require careful follow-up of asymptomatic patients with moderate to severe aortic stenosis, and in those with the most severe degrees of obstruction, aortic valve replacement may be justified in those centers with operative mortality rates of 1 to 2 percent for elective aortic valve replacement.[52] Other clinical features that may justify consideration of aortic valve replacement in the setting of severe aortic stenosis and an asymptomatic patient include LV systolic dysfunction, abnormal response to exercise (hypotension), marked or excessive LV hypertrophy ($\geq$15 mm), and/or aortic valve area less than 0.6 cm^2.[53]

The natural history is much worse in patients with symptomatic aortic stenosis. In Rapaport's series,[54] 40 percent of symptomatic patients with severe aortic stenosis survived for 5 years and 20 percent for 10 years (Fig. 13–3). Other studies reported 5-year survival rates ranging between 52 and 76 percent in moderately symptomatic patients and between 17 and 22 percent in severely symptomatic patients.[55–59] Among those who died, more than half died suddenly. When patients with aortic stenosis become symptomatic, the average survival time is approximately 5 years in patients with angina, 3 years in those with syncope, and 1.5 years in those who develop heart failure[60] (Fig. 13–4). The occurrence of any of these symptoms usually indicates that aortic stenosis is severe and that aortic valve replacement is indicated. The importance of associated coronary artery disease in the adult patient with aortic stenosis needs emphasis. Documentation of the presence of significant coronary disease requiring combined coronary bypass surgery with aortic valve replacement compromises long-term survival rates compared with those in patients having aortic valve replacement with normal coronary arteries.[61]

Those patients with severe aortic stenosis who present with congestive heart failure and impaired LV systolic function deserve special emphasis. Clinical recognition of the importance of aortic stenosis in the etiology of heart failure may be difficult, but this is essential because these patients may benefit dramatically from successful aortic valve replacement in spite of severe symptoms and depression of the LV function, although operative mortality rates are higher than in patients with normal ventricles.[62] These patients may have gradients across the aortic valve

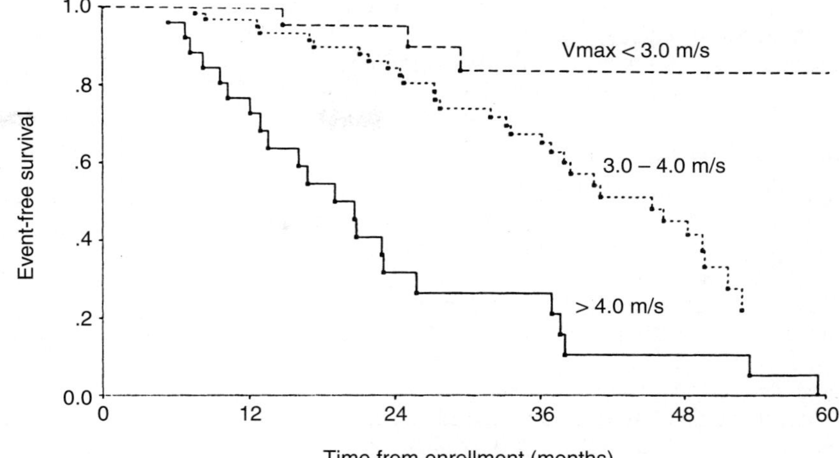

FIGURE 13–2 Cox regression analysis shows event-free survival in groups defined by aortic jet velocity at entry ($P < .0001$ by log-rank test). (From Otto CM, Burwash IG, Legget ME, et al: Prospective study of asymptomatic valvular aortic stenosis: clinical, echocardiographic, and exercise predictors of outcome. Circulation 95:2262, 1997.)

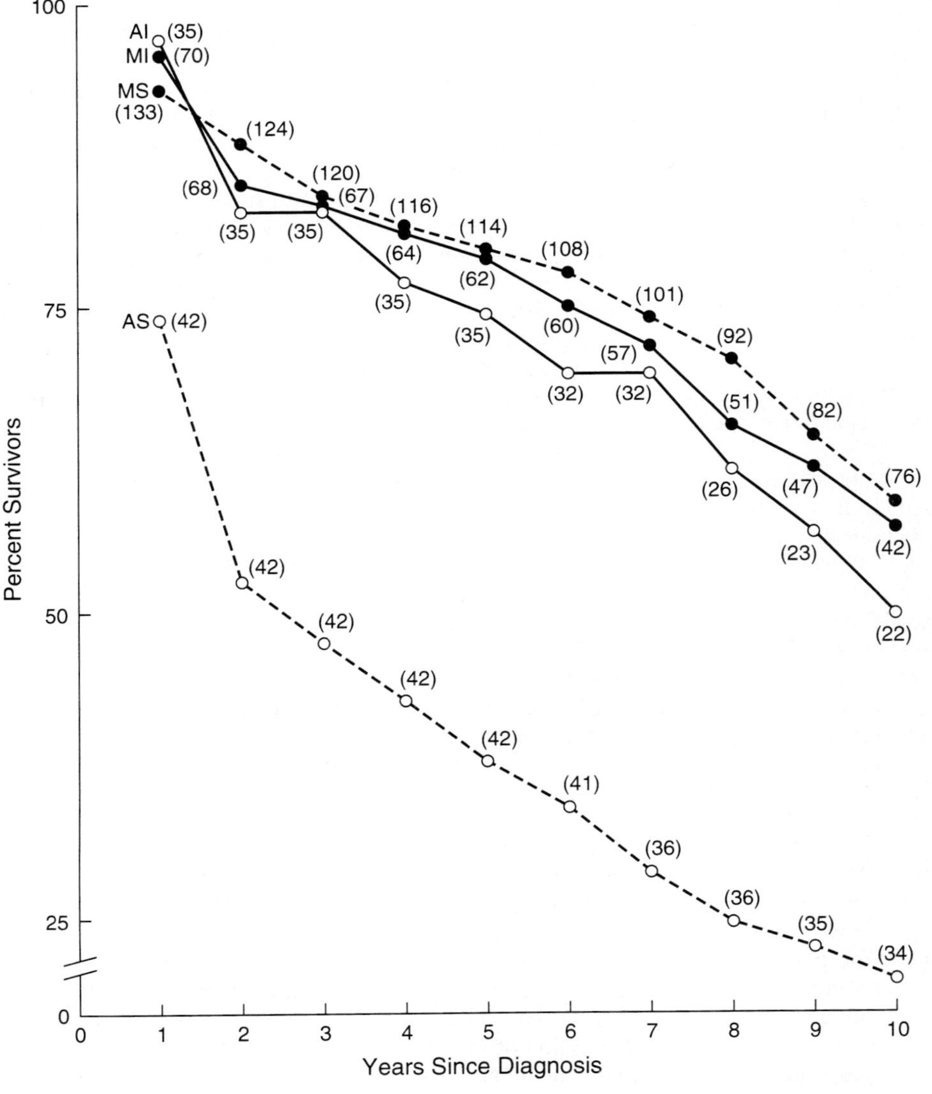

FIGURE 13–3 Survival rates in 42 patients with aortic stenosis (AS, *open circles with dotted line*), 35 with aortic regurgitation (AI, *open circles with solid line*), and 133 with mitral regurgitation (MI, *closed circles with solid line*). Clinical course in aortic regurgitation, mitral stenosis (MS, *closed circles with dotted line*), and mitral regurgitation is similar, with a 5-year survival rate of approximately 80 percent and a 10-year survival rate of 60 percent. Patients with aortic stenosis have a worse prognosis with 5- and 10-year survival rates of approximately 40 percent and 20 percent, respectively. (Reprinted from Rapaport E: Natural history of aortic and mitral valve disease. Am J Cardiol 35:221, 1975, with permission from Excerpta Medica Inc.)

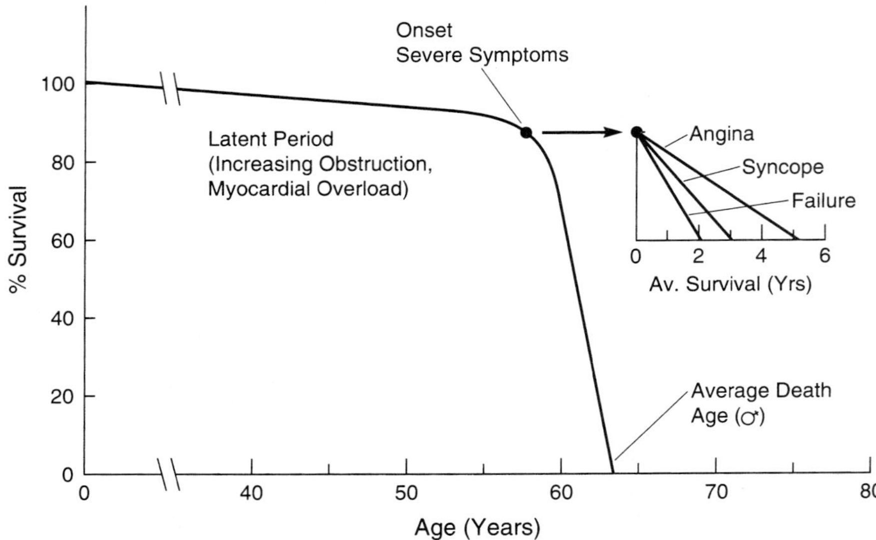

FIGURE 13–4 Natural history in patients with aortic stenosis. After an asymptomatic period of several decades, survival is approximately 5 years with the occurrence of angina pectoris, 3 years with syncope, and 2 years with the development of heart failure. (From Ross J Jr, Braunwald E: Aortic stenosis. Circulation 38[suppl V]:V61, 1968.)

that appear to be insignificant, even less than 30 mm Hg. In such patients with "low gradient, low-cardiac output" aortic stenosis, further assessment of the degree of aortic valve stenosis during dobutamine stress may provide critical information.

An additional subgroup of patients that demand special consideration are those with mild to moderate aortic stenosis in need of coronary artery bypass surgery. A dilemma exists in the management of the aortic valve disease in such patients because of a relatively high operative mortality rate in those patients who subsequently require aortic valve replacement after coronary artery bypass surgery.[63] Thus, patients with mean gradients of 25 to 30 mm Hg across the aortic valve, with a normal cardiac output, may be considered for elective replacement of the aortic valve as a combined procedure for those patients in whom coronary artery bypass grafting is the primary reason for surgery, although this remains controversial.

In summary, the natural history of aortic stenosis confirms the need for aortic valve replacement in symptomatic patients with significant obstruction without undue delay.[53] In asymptomatic patients, careful annual follow-up of those with moderate obstruction is essential, whereas selected patients with severe asymptomatic aortic stenosis may be candidates for aortic valve replacement in selected centers with excellent surgical results. Patients who present with congestive heart failure, depressed LV function, and low cardiac output must be carefully evaluated at the bedside and with echocardiographic stress studies to accurately diagnose severe aortic stenosis, a diagnosis that might otherwise be missed.

Medical Treatment

There is no specific medical treatment for patients with severe aortic stenosis other than to treat symptomatically those with active symptoms until aortic valve surgery can be performed. In the setting of congestive heart failure and depressed LV function, use of diuretics and digitalis may be necessary until surgery is performed. However, in such patients, surgery should not be delayed because all efforts with medical therapy only will ultimately fail, and delays in performing surgery should be avoided, depending on other significant comorbidities. Although there may be debate regarding the occurence of sudden death in asymptomatic patients with aortic stenosis, it is clear that patients with severe aortic stenosis, once symptoms begin, may die suddenly.

For those patients with mild to moderate aortic stenosis who are being managed medically, several clinical recommendations are generally accepted. Strenuous exercise should be avoided in the presence of significant aortic stenosis because of the risk for sudden death. This does not apply to patients with mild aortic stenosis, who should be followed clinically on an annual basis and with appropriate use of noninvasive testing. The importance of bacterial endocarditis prophylaxis with annual follow-up examinations cannot be overemphasized.

Differentiation of Reversible From Irreversible Left Ventricular Systolic Dysfunction in Patients With Aortic Stenosis

Blase A. Carabello

Aortic stenosis places a pressure overload on the left ventricle that is compensated by the development of concentric hypertrophy. The law of Laplace calculates the stress on a given portion of the myocardium as stress = pressure × radius ÷ 2 × thickness. Grossman and colleagues[64] hypothesized that when aortic stenosis causes an increase in LV pressure in the LaPlace numerator, it sets in motion the metabolic machinery that increases thickness in the denominator (concentric hypertrophy) and stress is normal-

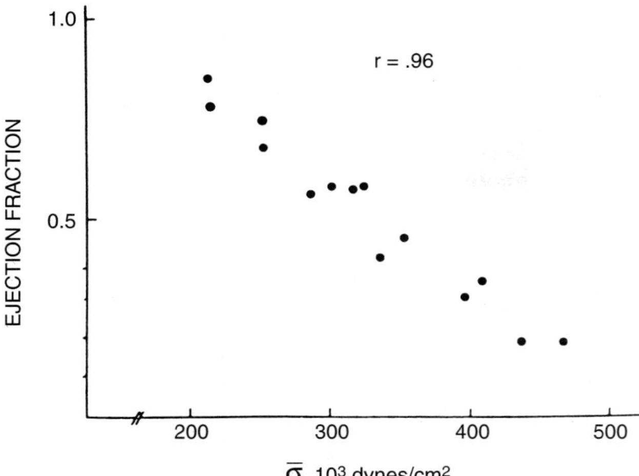

FIGURE 13–5 The relation of afterload (stress, σ) and ejection fraction is shown for aortic stenosis patients. As afterload increases, ejection fraction decreases. (From Gunther S, Grossman W: Determinants of ventricular function in pressure-overload hypertrophy in man. Circulation 59[4]:679–688, 1979.)

ized. Because the three major determinants of LV ejection performance are preload, afterload, and contractility and because, as shown in Figure 13–5, an increase in afterload causes ejection fraction to fall in a predictable manner, normalization of afterload by the development of concentric hypertrophy is clearly compensatory.[65, 66] However, in many cases as aortic stenosis progresses, the compensatory nature of the hypertrophy may vanish, the hypertrophy becomes pathologic, and there is a transition to heart failure that worsens prognosis.[67]

As shown in Figure 13–4, prognosis in aortic stenosis is nearly normal with only a 1 to 2 percent risk of sudden death per year until the development of symptoms, at which time there is a precipitous decline in survival. After the development of angina, only 50 percent of the patients with aortic stenosis can be expected to live for 5 years unless aortic valve replacement is performed. After syncope develops, only 50 percent live for 3 years, and after the development of heart failure, only a 2-year 50 percent survivorship is expected. Two of these three cardinal symptoms, angina and heart failure, are based on the development of LV hypertrophy.

Consequences of Hypertrophy

Angina

Angina, in the broad sense, occurs when myocardial nutrient demand exceeds its supply. It is well established that coronary blood flow reserve (supply) is diminished in aortic stenosis.[68] Mechanisms for this finding include insufficient capillary ingrowth and increased LV diastolic pressure.[69, 70] As hypertrophy develops, the ratio of capillaries to mass diminishes, potentially limiting the increase in coronary blood flow per gram of tissue that can occur during stress. Alternatively or in concert, diastolic filling pressure that is elevated in aortic stenosis (see later) compresses the endocardium during diastole (when coronary blood flow occurs) and diminishes coronary blood flow by vascular compression.

Heart Failure in Aortic Stenosis

DIASTOLIC DYSFUNCTION

Diastole is conventionally separated into two components, active relaxation followed by passive filling, both of which are usually abnormal in aortic stenosis. The time constant of isovolumic decline in LV pressure fall (tau) represents active relaxation and is the time it takes LV pressure to reach half of its nadir. It is prolonged when concentric LV hypertrophy is present.[71] This finding presumably reflects a decline in the rate at which cross-bridge cycling diminishes in diastole, suggesting a delay in calcium reuptake by the sarcoplasmic reticulum. The effect of delayed relaxation on ventricular filling is that diastole begins later and at a higher pressure, in turn imputing the consequences of elevated diastolic filling pressure and LA hypertension on the lungs.

LV stiffness describes passive filling of the ventricle and is the change in pressure divided by change in volume ($\Delta P \div \Delta V$) (Fig. 13–6).[72, 73] In stiffer ventricles, any increase in volume is accompanied by a progressively larger change in pressure, so that increased ventricular stiffness causes an increase in filling pressure and its consequences. Stiffness is increased in aortic stenosis for at least two reasons. First, the development of ventricular hypertrophy that helps compensate systolic function must by itself worsen diastolic function because it is intrinsically harder to fill a thicker chamber than a thinner one.[74] In addition to myocyte hypertrophy, the collagen weave that supports the myocardium and transduces movements generated by myocyte contraction into overall shortening of the ventricle increases in extent and thickness, causing ventricular stiffening.[75, 76]

SYSTOLIC DYSFUNCTION

Afterload Mismatch. The two major determinants of systolic ejection performance are afterload and contractil-

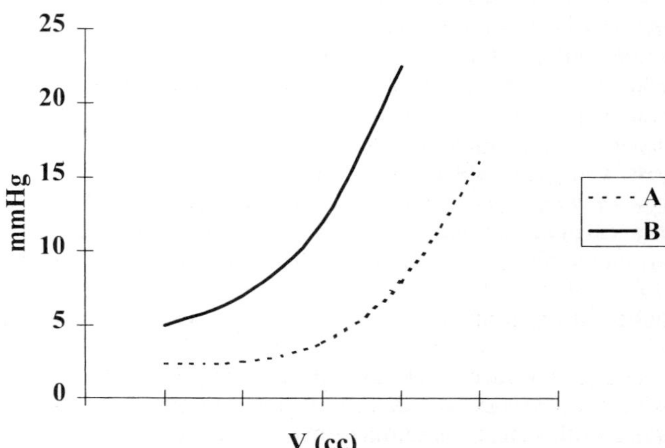

FIGURE 13–6 The pressure-volume relationships of a normal **(A)** versus a hypertrophied ventricle **(B)** are shown. For ventricle B, any filling volume is associated with a higher filling pressure.

ity, both of which may be altered in aortic stenosis. As noted previously, the development of concentric hypertrophy helps to normalize afterload. In many cases, this compensation is well matched to the pressure overload present. However, in other cases there may be too little an increase in wall thickness (inadequate hypertrophy) or, conversely, "excessive" hypertrophy.[66, 77–79] As shown in Figure 13–5, the result from inadequate hypertrophy is a rise in afterload and a fall in ejection fraction. Thus, in many cases of aortic stenosis, there may be a severe reduction in ejection performance predicated primarily on afterload mismatch.[77, 80] In fact, afterload mismatch explains all or part of diminished LV performance in about 75 percent of aortic stenosis patients.[78] In other patients, especially elderly women, there may be a greater thickness than is required to normalize stress, so stress declines and ejection performance becomes supernormal.[79] Whereas this setting does not contribute to systolic dysfunction, it invariably leads to a stiffer ventricle and diastolic dysfunction.

Why some patients have adequate hypertrophy while others have inadequate hypertrophy or excessive hypertrophy is unclear. In Grossman and colleagues[64] feedback loop concept of the Laplace relationship, just enough increase in wall thickness should occur to normalize stress and turn off the hypertrophy process. By definition, the adequacy of this feedback system fails when there is either excessive or inadequate hypertrophy. This variation in response to pressure overload may be controlled genetically. They noted that normal dogs have a wide differential in the amount of muscle mass present for a given stress.[81] When an identical pressure overload is placed on dogs with this varying background, those with less mass for a given stress at baseline never develop enough mass to normalize stress and hypertrophy is predictably inadequate. Other dogs that demonstrate larger mass at a given stress at baseline develop more exuberant hypertrophy when a pressure overload is placed on the myocardium and stress remains normal. Thus, some of the differences in hypertrophic compensation in patients with aortic stenosis are probably not predicated on differences in the disease process itself, but rather reflect inherited differences in a "set-point" for the myocardium's response to pressure overload.

Contractile Dysfunction. Whereas some patients have systolic dysfunction based on afterload excess as noted previously, in others, there is a deficit in force generation (contractility) in addition to or in isolation from afterload excess.[77, 78] The mechanisms by which LV contractile dysfunction develops remain unclear, but theories center around myocardial ischemia, calcium handling, myocyte loss, and cytoskeletal abnormalities.

Ischemia. It is known that coronary blood flow to the concentrically hypertrophied myocardium is abnormal.[68] In normal subjects, the ratio of endocardial to epicardial blood flow is about 1.2:1, appropriately meeting the greater metabolic demands of the endocardium. With hypertrophy, this ratio is reversed, and during stress, the subendocardium becomes underperfused and dysfunctional.[82–84] However, whereas repeated episodes of ischemia might lead to damage and fibrosis, it is unlikely that chronic ischemia causes chronic LV dysfunction. Even in severe hypertrophy, coronary flow reserve is not exhausted at rest.[82] In view of the exquisite autoregulatory nature of the coronary bed, it is implausible that ischemia is chronically present, yet existing reserve is not used to offset the demands for flow. Thus, ischemia is probably involved in the LV dysfunction of aortic stenosis, primarily during exercise when demand outstrips supply.

Calcium Handling. Although much is known about calcium handling in cardiomyopathic states, less is known in concentric hypertrophy. However, a variety of abnormalities have been described. The sarcoplasmic reticulum becomes distorted,[85] abnormalities in calcium flux and excitation-contraction coupling develop,[86, 87] and ryanodine receptors are diminished.

Gross and Ultrastructural Abnormalities. As hypertrophy progresses, there is myocyte dropout with replacement fibrosis.[88, 89] In addition, Cooper and coworkers[90] found that when concentric hypertrophy is inadequate to normalize wall stress, there is a densification of cytoskeletal microtubules that act as an internal viscous load on the myocyte, inhibiting shortening. When the tubules are dissolved with physical or chemical measures, contractile function is restored.

It is unlikely that any one of the pathophysiologic problems associated with hypertrophy noted previously is exclusively responsible for the transition to failure. Rather, they probably act in concert, with one mechanism being more prominent than another in a given pathophysiologic situation.

Clinical Implications of Left Ventricular Dysfunction in Aortic Stenosis

Low Ejection Fraction, High Gradient

As noted previously, untreated heart failure owing to aortic stenosis has a grave prognosis, with most patients succumbing in 2 to 3 years. It seems clear that there is no medical therapy for this mechanical obstruction to outflow. Rather, effective therapy can only be provided by mechanical relief of outflow obstruction (aortic valve replacement). In many patients with severely reduced ejection fraction, the postoperative outcome is amazingly favorable[77, 91]; ejection fraction increases dramatically, survivorship is prolonged, and the symptoms of heart failure abate. Improvement after surgery is based on an initial decrease in afterload as the outflow obstruction is relieved, followed by an improvement in contractile performance, presumably due to some form of "healing" of the myocardium. Figure 13–7 demonstrates the dramatic improvement in ejection fraction that can occur after valve replacement for aortic stenosis.[91] Thus, whereas reduced ejection fraction denotes a high operative risk in many other forms of valvular and nonvalvular heart disease, low ejection fraction in aortic stenosis should not be viewed as a contraindication to aortic valve replacement in most cases because low ejection fraction is due in part to excess afterload, which can be surgically relieved.

The Patient With Low Ejection Fraction, Low Cardiac Output, and Low Transvalvular Gradient

An exception to the favorable outcome for low-ejection-fraction aortic stenosis patients noted previously is the

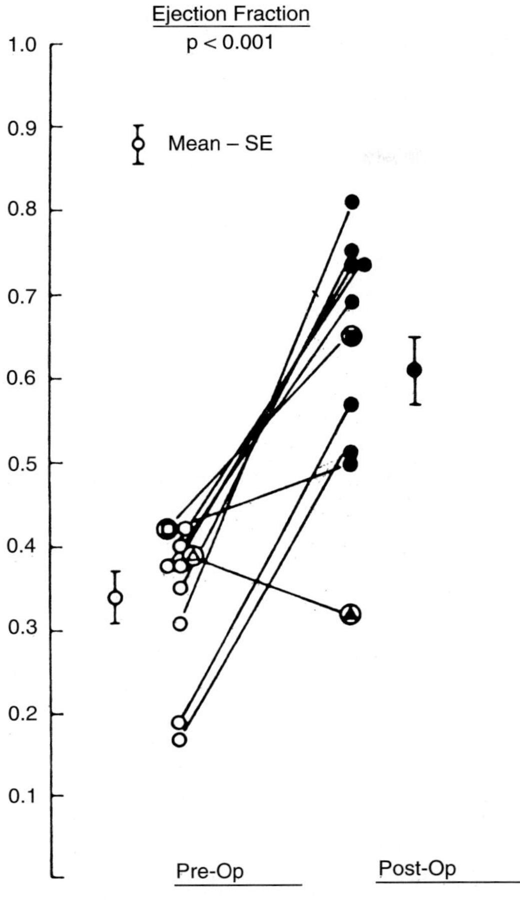

FIGURE 13–7 Ejection fraction is shown preoperatively and postoperatively for a group of patients with preoperative left ventricular dysfunction. In almost all cases, ejection fraction improved dramatically after obstruction to flow was reduced. CHB, complete heart block; MI, myocardial infarction. (From Smith N, McAnulty JH, Rahimtoola SH: Severe aortic stenosis with impaired left ventricular function and clinical heart failure: results of valve replacement. Circulation 58(2):255–264, 1978.)

patient with a low gradient, low cardiac output, and low ejection fraction. In 1980, it was noted that patients with a low transvalvular gradient and low ejection fraction had a poor prognosis after aortic valve replacement.[77] This concept has been amplified in subsequent studies and is true whether or not coronary artery disease is present.[92, 93] Poor outcome in such patients is based on advanced LV dysfunction out of proportion to afterload mismatch; thus, even after the surgeon relieves the outflow obstruction, the degree of afterload reduction that occurs is small, depriving the patient of the robust improvement in ejection performance that usually occurs when the afterload reduction is more prominent.

However, even in this poor-prognosis group of patients with reduced ejection fraction and low gradient, some patients improve after surgery (Fig. 13–8).[93] It appears that approximately half of such patients improve, while the other half either die perioperatively or fail to improve. The clinical issue is obvious: which of the low-ejection-fraction, low-gradient patients might improve with surgery and thus should not be denied it, and which patients are likely to die perioperatively and might therefore have a better prognosis treated medically? Although yet unproved, it is likely that the answer to the question resides in the degree of perioperative valvular obstruction and its relationship to ventricular contractile dysfunction. Those patients who have truly severe aortic stenosis in whom the severity of valvular heart disease has led to ventricular dysfunction are probably the patients likely to benefit from the relief of obstruction. In this case, valve disease has caused ventricular dysfunction, giving rise to the hope that relief of the primary problem would lead to secondary improvement in the ventricle. On the other hand, there appears to be patients with primary LV dysfunction and concomitant mild-to-moderate aortic valve disease in whom a primarily weakened ventricle cannot open a mildly diseased valve. In this group of patients, it is unlikely that aortic valve replacement will be beneficial because the valve lesion is not at the apex of the problem. How are these two entities distinguished? Traditionally, the severity of obstruction has been identified by the aortic valve area.[94] The presumption was that the stenotic aortic valve was a fixed rigid orifice, with smaller valve areas correlating with worse stenosis. It is now clear that this approach often fails in this group of patients with low gradient and low output because calculated valve area, whether by the Gorlin formula or by the continuity equation, is flow dependent, especially at low flows (Fig. 13–9).[95–97] Since calculated valve area increases with flow, it is often not possible to use a single valve area to determine the true severity of obstruction when output is low. In Table 13–1, the patient shown initially would have been thought to have severe aortic stenosis because the calculated valve area was 0.6 cm^2. However, when flow was increased, valve area increased in parallel fashion into the

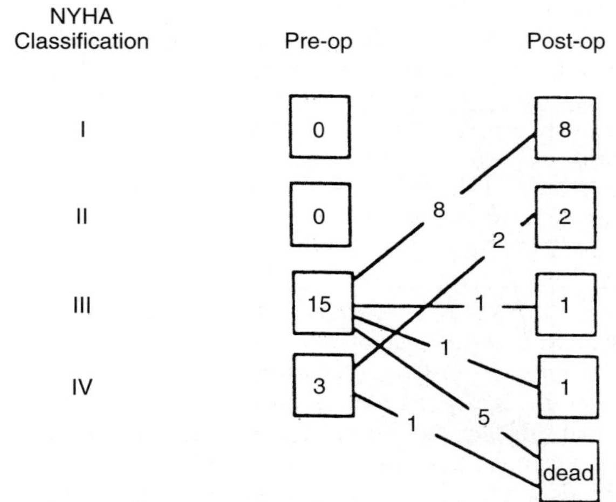

FIGURE 13–8 Symptomatic status for patients with aortic stenosis and low transvalvular gradient is shown before and after surgery. Ten patients improved. NYHA, New York Heart Association. (From Brogan WC III, Grayburn PA, Lange RA, et al: Prognosis after valve replacement in patients with severe aortic stenosis and a low transvalvular pressure gradient. Reprinted with permission from the American College of Cardiology [J Am Coll Cardiol, 1993, Vol. 21, pp. 1657–1660].)

TABLE 13-1 **Effect of Cardiac Output on Valve Area**

	Rest	Dopamine 7.5 μg/kg/min
CO	3.0 L/min	5.0 L/min
Gradient	24 mm Hg	25 mm Hg
AVA	0.6 cm²	1.0 cm²

Abbreviations: AVA, aortic valve area; CO, cardiac output.

moderate range, no longer indicating surgery. How are these data reconciled? It is likely that at low flows, a physiologically smaller orifice is calculated because the valve is in fact less widely opened than when higher flows open the sclerotic but not stenotic valve to a greater extent. Alternatively, problems with the formulas themselves may be involved. The commonly used Gorlin formula, which calculates valve area from cardiac output and gradient, involves the use of discharge coefficients that were never calculated for the aortic valve, but have erroneously been assumed to be 1.0.[94] In any case, valve areas obtained at higher flows (>4.5 L/min) appear to better predict actual stenosis severity.

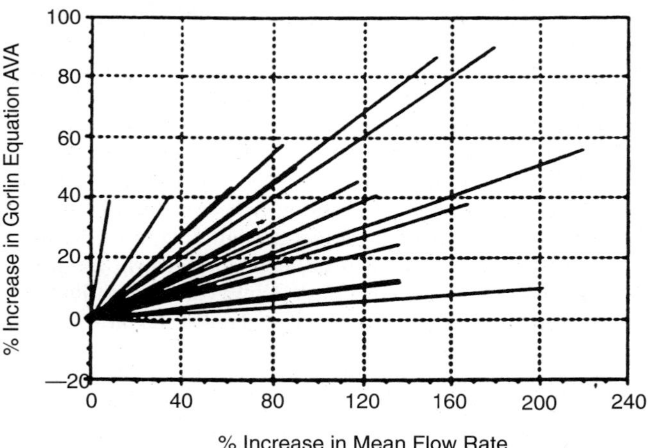

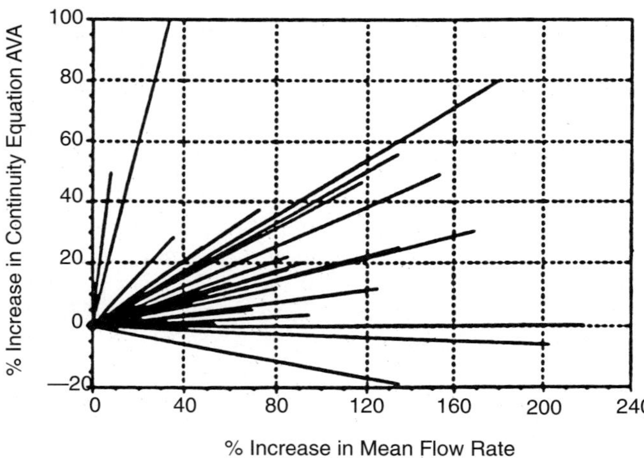

FIGURE 13–9 Changes in calculated valve area are plotted against increases in flow. As flow increases, calculated area increases. AVA, aortic valve area. (From Burwash IG, Thomas DD, Sadahiro M, et al: Dependence of Gorlin formula and continuity equation valve areas on transvalvular volume flow rate in valvular aortic stenosis. Circulation 89[2]:827–835, 1994.)

Low-Gradient, Low-Ejection-Fraction, Low-Output Aortic Stenosis: Who Benefits From Surgery?

As noted previously, this is a very high-risk group of patients in whom only about half could expect benefit. The most reasonable approach is to separate those patients with mild aortic stenosis and severe primary LV dysfunction from those patients in whom severe aortic stenosis has caused LV dysfunction. The best approach (as yet examined in only a small number of patients) is to raise cardiac output and recalculate the valve area. Since flow dependence of calculated area plateaus around 4.5 L/min[97] it seems advisable to use pharmacologic intervention to increase flow to this level of output and then recalculate valve area. In most instances, dobutamine has been infused to increase cardiac output. Three responses have been noted.[98–100] The first is that typified by Table 13–1, in which there is large increase in cardiac output associated with only a small or no increase in transvalvular gradient, resulting in a large increase in AVA. This type of patient almost certainly does not have true aortic stenosis and should be treated medically. In a second group of patients, the increase in output is met with a concomitant increase in gradient, and valve area increases only slightly and remains within the critical range. It is likely that it is this group of patients who really have severe valvular obstruction and might benefit from surgery. Apart from anecdotal experience, proof of this concept is currently lacking. In the third group of patients, dobutamine infusion has no effect, presumably owing to severe beta-receptor downregulation and the lack of inotropic reserve. What the fate of this group of patients would be, if operated, is unknown.

As noted previously, dobutamine has usually been used to increase output. However, the author has frequently used infusion of nitroprusside instead. Although nitroprusside carries with it the risk of hypotension in those patients with true aortic stenosis, it has the benefit of demonstrating the therapeutic value of vasodilators in those patients in whom the obstruction to outflow is only mild. If nitroprusside is used it is done so with great caution, gradually increasing the infusion by 0.25 μg/kg/min every 2 or 3 minutes.

Because of the difficulties in calculating valve area and because the discharge coefficients for the Gorlin formula were never developed, valve resistance has been examined as another tool for determining stenosis severity.[96, 101] Resistance is simply gradient divided by flow:

$$\text{Resistance} = \frac{G \times HR \times SEP \times 1.33}{CO}$$

where G = mean gradient, HR = heart rate, SEP = systolic ejection period (in seconds), CO = cardiac output in liters per minute, and 1.33 is a factor that converts to dynes-sec-cm^{-5} and involves no discharge coefficient. It seems to be less flow-dependent than valve area.[96] An aortic valve resistance of greater than 250 dynes-sec-cm^{-5} appears coincident with severe aortic stenosis.[96] Whether or not this measure will add to the output augmentation technique noted previously is unclear at this time.

Summary

When the symptoms of congestive heart failure develop in the patient with aortic stenosis, prognosis dramatically worsens, such that only 50 percent of such patients will be alive without operative therapy 2 years later. Heart failure ensues from diastolic dysfunction owing to abnormalities in both active relaxation and passive filling, and from systolic dysfunction, which is due to both afterload mismatch and contractile dysfunction. When afterload mismatch is the major cause of the systolic dysfunction, an excellent postoperative prognosis can be expected, even when ejection fraction is severely reduced, because afterload reduction leads to improved postoperative function and a decrease in symptoms. However, when diminished contractility is the primary cause of the LV dysfunction, postoperative outcome is much less certain. Whereas all patients with low output, low ejection fraction, and low gradient remain at high risk, some patients do improve after surgery. It is probably those patients, with true obstruction to aortic outflow in whom aortic stenosis was the primary cause of the LV dysfunction, who are likely to benefit from surgery. Conversely, those patients in whom primary LV dysfunction causes low output and low force generation (incapable of opening a mildly but not severely stenotic valve) have a primary cardiomyopathy and will not benefit from aortic valve replacement. These patients are more likely to benefit from vasodilator therapy. At the current time, the best method for distinguishing these two groups is recalculation of AVA at a pharmacologically induced higher output, greater than 4.5 L/min. In those patients in whom gradient increases concomitantly with output, severe aortic stenosis is probably present, and it is these patients who are most likely to benefit from aortic valve replacement.

Aortic Regurgitation

Pathophysiology

Chronic Form

In developed countries, aortic regurgitation is most often caused by dilatation of the ascending aorta (aortic root disease or aortoannular ectasia) secondary to a variety of disorders or by incomplete closure and/or prolapse of a congenitally bicuspid valve. Rheumatic valvular disease of the aortic valve, on the other hand, has become relatively rare. A newly reported potential etiologic basis for valvular regurgitation in general, which includes the aortic valve, is the use of anorectic drugs such as the combination of fenfluramine and phentermine.[102] Diastolic reflux through the aortic valve leads to an LV volume overload. The severity of aortic regurgitation is dependent on the diastolic valve area, the diastolic pressure gradient between the aorta and the left ventricle, and the duration of diastole.[103] An increase in heart rate and a decrease in peripheral resistance diminish regurgitation, and dynamic exercise may therefore be associated with a reduction in aortic regurgitation. Such a reduction of regurgitant flow during exercise causes an increase in forward flow and a decrease in filling pressure, which may explain why patients with severe aortic regurgitation are often asymptomatic and have normal physical working capacity.

The increase in systolic stroke volume, together with the low diastolic aortic pressure, produces the increased pulse pressure typically seen in aortic regurgitation. The low diastolic aortic pressure may have an adverse effect on coronary perfusion, which occurs mainly during diastole and is dependent on the pressure gradient between the aorta and the left ventricle. In patients with severe aortic valve lesions, this decrease in coronary perfusion in the face of an increase in oxygen requirement caused by the augmentation of LV muscle mass and wall stress may result in a potentially critical imbalance between oxygen supply and demand.

Diastolic backflow from the aorta into the left ventricle leads to an enlargement of the ventricular cavity and an increase in LV filling pressure. LV muscle mass is increased (eccentric hypertrophy), presumably by serial replication of sarcomeres. In animal studies, evidence of an increase in protein turnover has been demonstrated, including the specific myosin heavy chain and actin protein.[104] The increasing hypertrophy may explain why LV end-diastolic pressure is normal or only slightly elevated despite massive enlargement of the ventricular chamber. Diastolic chamber stiffness is decreased, and patients may therefore have no clinical symptoms until late in the disease (Fig. 13–10). Myocardial stiffness, which is calculated from the diastolic stress-strain relations, is often increased, suggesting that structural alterations have occurred. Approximately 90 percent of all patients with aortic regurgitation and normal systolic function already have abnormal diastolic function.[7] Therefore, either diastolic dysfunction precedes systolic dysfunction or diastolic function variables may be more sensitive indicators of altered ventricular function than systolic ones. After long-standing severe aortic regurgitation, reduced systolic ejection may occur, associated with increased cardiovascular mortality and an increased risk for persistent postoperative LV dysfunction. Exploration of the influence of the proto-oncogene *c-myc* has been reported in human patients with severe aortic regurgitation with evidence to suggest a role for gene mediated myocardial remodeling in the adaptation of the ventricle to the stress of large regurgitant volume.[105]

Alterations of the collagen network have been described in patients with aortic regurgitation: increased amounts of total collagen, subendocardial fibrosis, and enhanced cross-hatching of the collagen fibers have been reported in preoperative patients.[106] Although the consequences of such alterations in the collagen network are not clear, they may contribute to the observed changes in diastolic and systolic function.[107]

Acute Form

The most common causes of acute severe aortic regurgitation include bacterial endocarditis, dissection of the ascending aorta, and an abrupt structural collapse of a congenitally anomalous valve, including a ruptured aneurysm of a sinus of Valsalva.

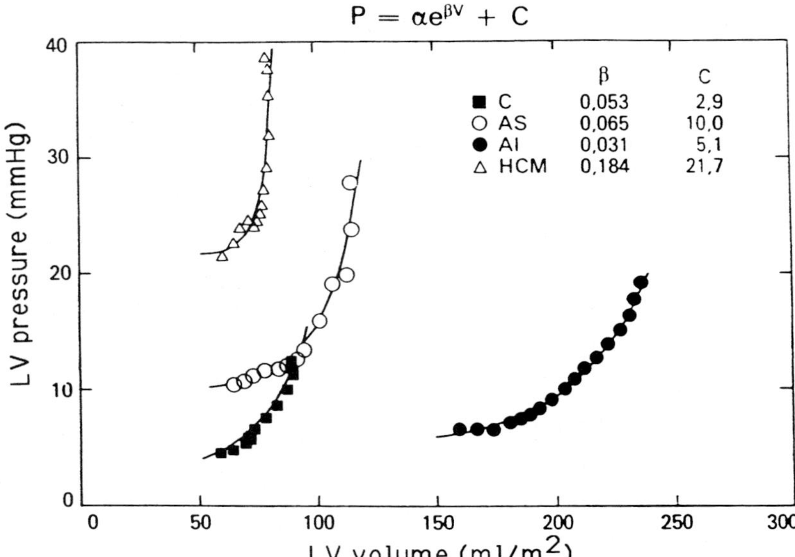

FIGURE 13–10 Left ventricular (LV) pressure-volume relationship in a control patient (C), a patient with aortic stenosis (AS), a patient with aortic regurgitation (AI), and a patient with hypertrophic cardiomyopathy (HCM). Chronic volume overload in aortic regurgitation is associated with a rightward shift of the pressure-volume curve (decrease in chamber stiffness), whereas chronic pressure overload in patients with aortic stenosis is accompanied by an upward shift (increase in chamber stiffness). The decrease in chamber stiffness explains why patients with volume overload often remain asymptomatic for many years, because the increase in stroke volume (forward volume + regurgitant volume) can be achieved with a small increase in end-diastolic pressure. β is equal to the coefficient of chamber stiffness (ml^{-1}) or represents the slope of the pressure-volume curve, and C is equal to the pressure asymptote (mm Hg). (From Hess OM, Krayenbuehl HP: Diastolische Function des linken Ventrikels. Schweiz Med Praxis 77:685, 1988.)

In contrast to chronic regurgitation, the sudden increase in regurgitant volume in acute aortic regurgitation is associated with a rapid increase in LV diastolic filling pressure because the left ventricle cannot accommodate the combined regurgitant volume and the inflow from the left atrium (Fig. 13–11). Therefore, forward stroke volume declines and the rapid rise in LV diastolic pressure leads to premature closure of the mitral valve.

LV end-diastolic pressure is often higher than mean LA pressure. Therefore, closure of the mitral valve protects the pulmonary venous bed from backward transmission of the markedly elevated end-diastolic pressure. Premature closure of the mitral valve, together with tachycardia, reduces the diastolic filling time interval during which the mitral valve is open (see Fig. 13–11). Since aortic diastolic pressure cannot decline below the elevated end-diastolic pressure, the arterial pulse pressure increases only slightly.

Physical Examination

Clinical signs of aortic regurgitation are caused by the forward and backward flow of blood across the aortic valve, leading to increased stroke volume and hyperdynamic cardiac and vascular motion. The degree of regurgitation is determined not only by the extent of valvular incompetence but also by LV compliance and end-diastolic volume, which may be significantly increased only in chronic aortic insufficiency. Clinical signs are therefore prominent in severe chronic aortic regurgitation but are

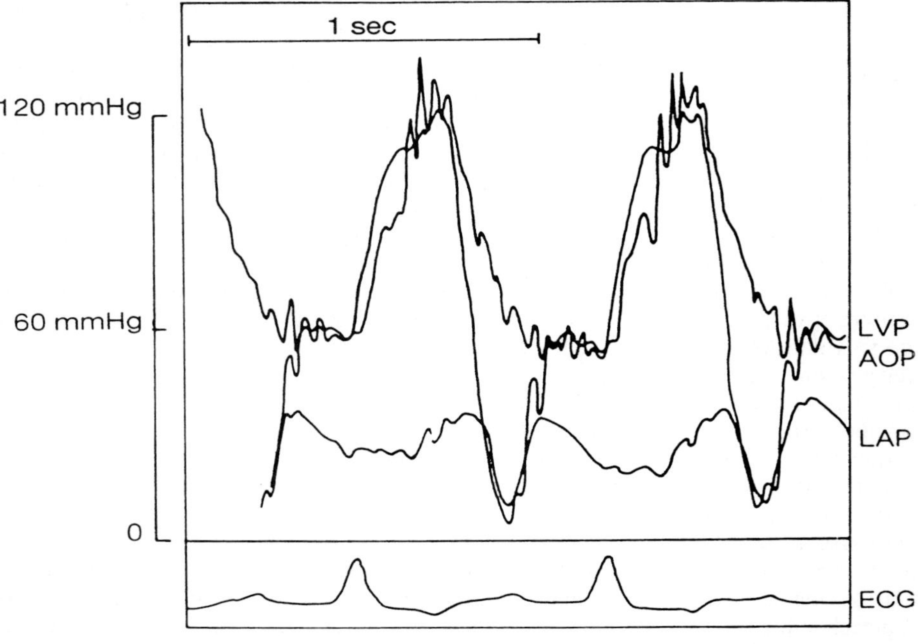

FIGURE 13–11 Pressure recording in a patient with acute aortic regurgitation after bacterial endocarditis. Aortic (AOP) and left ventricular pressure (LVP) are equalized during mid-diastole. Left ventricular pressure exceeds left atrial pressure (LAP) during early diastolic filling and causes premature mitral valve closure. Early valve closure prevents the transmission of the high late diastolic filling pressure to the pulmonary vascular bed. ECG, electrocardiogram. (From Krayenbuehl HP, Hess OM: Chronic valvular insufficiency. *In* Parmley WW, Chatterjee K [eds]: Cardiology. pp. 1–28. Philadelphia: JB Lippincott, 1991.)

more subtle in mild chronic aortic regurgitation or in acute aortic regurgitation, where both the small LV cavity and elevation of end-diastolic pressure limit the regurgitant volume.

In patients presenting with unexplained heart failure, or other cardiac symptoms such as dyspnea, recognition that bedside clinical assessment may underestimate the severity of aortic regurgitation is important to avoid overlooking highly treatable valvular heart disease that may be the basis for the patient's disability.

Chronic Aortic Regurgitation

Pulse pressures exceed 100 mm Hg in severe cases. Diastolic pressures are low, with Korotkoff sounds persisting sometimes to 0 mm Hg, owing to emptying of the aorta both backward and forward during diastole. Systolic pressures are usually increased except in young patients and may be substantially higher in popliteal arteries than in brachial arteries (Hill sign).[108] Diastolic pressures above 70 mm Hg can be seen in acute aortic regurgitation, in mild chronic aortic regurgitation, and in the presence of LV failure.

In patients with significant chronic aortic regurgitation, the pulse may be bounding, with a quick upstroke and rapid collapse (Corrigan pulse), leading to bobbing of the head (Musset sign).[109, 110] A bisferiens pulse may be present, which is best palpated on carotid, brachial, or femoral arteries. There may be visible capillary pulsations of the nail beds (Quincke sign) and pulsations of the uvula (Müller sign). Loud systolic sounds may be heard over the femoral arteries (Traube sign), and compression of these arteries with the stethoscope may produce a systolic-diastolic murmur (Duroziez sign) proximal to the compression.[111]

Jugular vein distention may occur if RV failure develops secondary to postcapillary pulmonary hypertension. Palpation of the precordium reveals a hyperdynamic apical impulse, which is enlarged and is displaced laterally and inferiorly.[112] An early diastolic filling impulse may occasionally be felt, which correlates with the presence of an S_3.[113] A systolic thrill may be felt at the base and sometimes in the carotids, even in the absence of significant stenosis.[114] A diastolic thrill is rare and a sign of severe regurgitation. All these signs may be attenuated or absent when only mild aortic regurgitation is present.

On auscultation, the intensity of S_1 is usually normal but may be decreased when partial closure of the mitral valve occurs,[115] secondary to severe aortic regurgitation, prolongation of the PR interval, or sinus bradycardia.[116] S_1 may also be decreased in the presence of associated myocardial dysfunction. An ejection click may be heard, caused by rapid distention of the aorta during early systole. S_2 may be normal or decreased in severe aortic regurgitation because of poor leaflet coaptation, or when P_2 is buried in the early component of the diastolic murmur. S_2 may be single or paradoxically split owing to a prolongation of the LV ejection time.[117] In LV failure, the intensity of P_2 may be increased because of associated pulmonary hypertension. An S_3 is commonly heard as the result of rapid early diastolic filling, but this is more common in the setting of ventricular dysfunction. Only rarely can the mid-diastolic closure of the mitral valve be heard (Fig. 13–12).

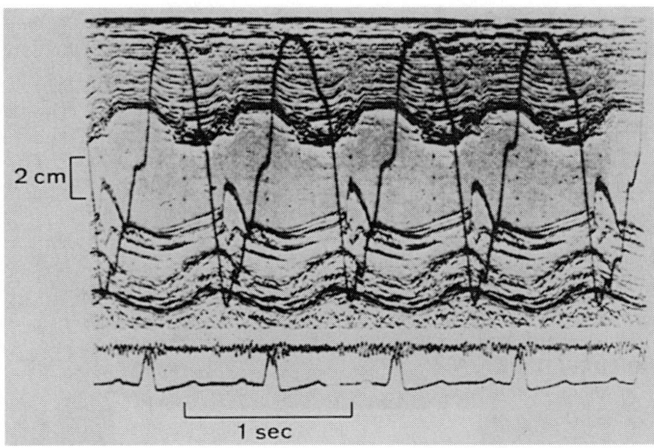

FIGURE 13–12 Echocardiogram of a 17-year-old patient with severe chronic aortic regurgitation shows premature closure of the mitral valve. The superimposed apexcardiogram shows a prominent rapid filling wave, mimicking an A wave. However, the left atrial contraction cannot contribute to left ventricular filling because the mitral valve is closed at mid-diastole. On the phonocardiogram at the bottom of the figure, a sound can be seen corresponding to the mid-diastolic closure of the mitral valve.

A decrescendo diastolic murmur is best heard while the patient is leaning forward on deep expiration. It is located at the mid left sternal border but may well radiate to the apex and the upper right sternal border. When the murmur is predominant at the right sternal border, aortic dilatation or dissection must be considered.[118] The severity of aortic regurgitation is more closely related to the length of the murmur during diastole than to its intensity. The murmur is usually high pitched and blowing. It may become musical or "cooing" in the presence of fenestration, laceration, or eversion of the valves.[119, 120] An apical diastolic rumble (Austin Flint murmur) may be heard in mid or late diastole in the absence of mitral stenosis.[121, 122] This murmur is due to the early partial closure of the mitral valve and the production of a functional mitral stenosis. It correlates with diastolic fluttering of the anterior leaflet of the mitral valve on echocardiography, and it is a bedside finding indicative of severe aortic insufficiency. It can be differentiated from the murmur of mitral stenosis by the absence of a loud S_1 and an opening snap. A systolic murmur may be heard at the base of the heart, radiating to the carotids and the apex. It is sometimes as loud as in aortic stenosis and may be accompanied by a thrill, but it takes place during early systole.

The diastolic murmur increases with all maneuvers that increase blood pressure, such as squatting, infusion of pressor agents, or isometric exercise. It is attenuated by vasodilators or the Valsalva maneuver. The murmur must be differentiated from that of pulmonic insufficiency, which occurs later in diastole, after P_2, and is not accompanied by a widened systemic pressure.

Acute Aortic Regurgitation

Clinical signs of acute aortic regurgitation differ from those of chronic regurgitation because the regurgitant volume is limited by a relatively small, noncompliant left ventricle. Pulse pressure is often not significantly widened.[123, 124] Hyperdynamic pulses and the apical impulse are less prominent than in chronic aortic insufficiency. S_1 may be muffled because of early closure of the mitral valve during diastole,[125, 126] which may be heard as a mid-diastolic sound. The diastolic decrescendo murmur may be soft and shortened by a rapidly rising LV end-diastolic pressure. The Austin Flint rumble may be limited to early diastole.[127] Signs of LV failure, such as S_3 and pulmonary rales, are prominent and may overshadow the subtle auscultatory findings of acute aortic regurgitation.

Natural History

Chronic Form

Chronic aortic regurgitation has a protracted course and may cause little disability for many years. In patients with chronic aortic regurgitation (see Fig. 13–3), approximately 75 percent are alive after 5 years and 50 percent after 10 years.[54] In patients with mild to moderate regurgitation, 10-year survival rates may be as high as 85 to 95 percent.[128, 129] However, when the patient becomes symptomatic, deterioration is usually rapid and surgery should be considered without undue delay. Spagnuolo and associates[130] reported that 87 percent of patients with severe cardiomegaly, electrocardiographic evidence of LV hypertrophy, and a diastolic pressure of 40 mm Hg or greater developed congestive heart failure or died within 6 years. After the onset of congestive heart failure, most patients die within 2 years, whereas after the onset of angina pectoris, the average survival rate is approximately 5 years.[54] Two- and 5-year survival rates from several clinical studies are summarized in Table 13–2. Most studies reported 5-year survival rates of between 66 and 73 percent in mildly symptomatic (New York Heart Association [NYHA] class I to II) and between 29 and 38 percent in severely symptomatic patients (NYHA class III to IV). Even during the asymptomatic period, gradual deterioration of LV function, with a decrease in ejection fraction and an increase in end-systolic volume, may occur. Therefore, it is important to intervene surgically before these changes become irreversible.[131] The conclusion that patients with severe aortic regurgitation and mild symptoms should be considered for earlier intervention is also supported by analysis of surgical results. Klodas and colleagues[132] reported higher operative mortality rates in patients with class III or IV symptoms (7.8 percent) compared with those in class I or II (1.2 percent) (Fig. 13–13).

TABLE 13–2 Survival Rates in Aortic Regurgitation

First Author	Yr	n	NYHA	2-Yr (%)	5-Yr (%)
Rapaport[54]	1955–1975	35	Various	82	75
Haerten[59]	1967–1976	30	III–IV	54	37
Horstkotte[58]	1968–1981	25	III–IV	51	38
Schwarz[57]	1975–1985	40	I–II	92	66
Turina[2]	1963–1983	80	I–II	93	73
			III–IV	57	29
Mean	Total 210			72	53
±1 SD				20	21

Abbreviation: NYHA, New York Heart Association.

From Turina J, Hess O, Sepulcri F, Krayenbuehl HP: Spontaneous course of aortic valve disease, Eur Heart J 8:471, 1987.

Long-term survival is also significantly compromised for those with class III or IV symptoms at the time of surgery for aortic valve replacement (45 percent) compared with those in class I or II at the time of aortic valve replacement (78 percent). Although patients with severe LV dilatation (diastolic dimension $\geq$ 80 mm) associated with severe aortic regurgitation remain candidates for surgery, operative mortality is higher and there may be some compromise in long-term results, depending on the degree of impairment in systolic function preoperatively.[133] Furthermore, it is clear that persistent LV systolic dysfunction after successful aortic valve replacement relates to the duration of profound LV dilatation.[134] Thus, patients should not be advised to delay surgery in the presence of severe LV dilatation unless comorbidities or other considerations make surgery an unreasonable option.

Acute Form

Although mild acute aortic regurgitation is well tolerated, the prognosis is poor in severe forms despite intensive medical therapy. Even a normal left ventricle cannot sustain the burden of acute severe volume overload for a long time because the regurgitant volume has to be ejected in a high-impedance system. Because early death due to LV failure is common, prompt surgical intervention is necessary. Outcomes in surgical treatment of patients with severe acute aortic regurgitation is heavily dependent on the anatomic basis for the disruption of aortic valve competence. In patients with acute aortic valve endocarditis 75 percent survival rates at 10 years have been reported after aortic valve replacement, with 91 percent free of recurrent endocarditis at 10 years.[135]

Medical Treatment

Patients with mild aortic regurgitation can be followed clinically by noninvasive methods and can lead a normal life. An increasingly frequent clinical finding is mild degrees of aortic regurgitation in the elderly population. These patients may have only mild degenerative changes in the aortic valve combined with some dilatation of the root of the aorta, and most will not progress to more severe degrees of insufficiency requiring surgical intervention.

Identifying those patients with moderate to severe aortic regurgitation and mild symptoms who may deteriorate early has been facilitated by noninvasive testing. Load-adjusted variables of LV function including size, ejection fraction, and end-systolic wall stress measured with radionuclide ventriculography predict progression, indications for aortic valve replacement as well as sudden death.

Patients with moderate to severe chronic aortic regurgitation who are asymptomatic with normal LV systolic function should be considered for a trial of medical therapy with emphasis on afterload reduction and careful attention to monitoring indices of LV function to determine therapeutic response. A variety of vasodilators have been studied to determine whether afterload reduction may delay or prevent the deterioration in LV function and need for aortic valve replacement with viable results.[136–138] Angiotensin-converting enzyme inhibitors have been demonstrated to reduce LV mean wall stress, and achieve a significant

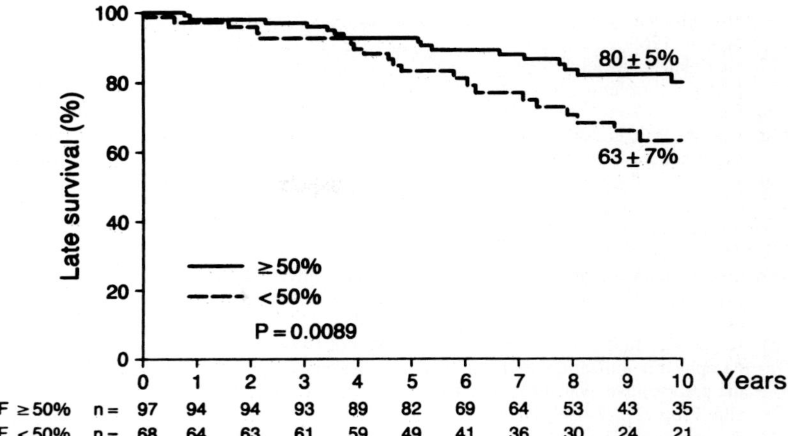

FIGURE 13–13 Late survival in male patients stratified according to preoperative ejection fraction (EF). Late survival was worse in all patients with an abnormal preoperative ejection fraction. (From Klodas E, Enriquez-Sarano M, Tajik AJ, et al: Aortic regurgitation complicated by extreme left ventricular dilation; long-term outcome after surgical correction. Reprinted with permission from the American College of Cardiology [J Am Coll Cardiol, 1996, Vol. 27, pp. 670–677].)

regression in LV mass, end-diastolic and end-systolic volume indices.[139, 140] Hypertension should be treated because it can increase the regurgitant volume and consequently worsen congestive heart failure. Arrhythmias should be promptly treated. In particular, bradycardia should be avoided because it may increase the diastolic regurgitant time and lead to congestive heart failure. If a program of afterload reduction is instituted, LV function should be followed serially and surgical treatment should be advised if LV dilatation or dysfunction progresses in spite of afterload reduction and control of hypertension. A consensus panel provides specific recommendations for surgical intervention in patients with moderate to severe valve incompetence.[141] With highly experienced surgeons providing low operative mortality rates and improved prosthetic valves combined with advances in managing chronic anticoagulant therapy, it is important to avoid delay of aortic valve replacement until severe symptoms or deterioration in left ventricular function occur that may seriously compromise long-term results.[141]

Acute severe aortic regurgitation is poorly tolerated, and urgent surgical repair or replacement of the aortic valve is usually required. Patients can be stabilized by the use of inotropic agents and vasodilators if blood pressure is adequate. The use of an intra-aortic counterpulsation balloon is contraindicated in this setting because it would increase aortic root diastolic pressure and the severity of the aortic insufficiency. Valve replacement should not be delayed in patients who have persistent congestive heart failure despite medical therapy.[141] In patients with infectious endocarditis who are stable on medical therapy, 7 to 10 days of antibiotics can usually be given before surgery, with the antibiotics continued a full 4- to 6-week course after aortic valve replacement or repair. In patients with severe acute aortic insufficiency from bacterial endocarditis with staphylococci, gram-negative organisms, gonococcus, and fungi, emergent aortic valve replacement with continuing intravenous antibiotics is indicated with the earliest signs of congestive heart failure.

The reader is referred to the websites of the American College of Cardiology (www.acc.org) and the American Heart Association (www.americanheart.org) for the ACC/AHA Guidelines for the Management of Patients with Acute Myocardial Infarction.

REFERENCES

AORTIC STENOSIS

1. Chizner MA, Pearle DL, DeLeon AC Jr: The natural history of aortic stenosis in adults. Am Heart J 99:419, 1980.
2. Turina J, Hess O, Sepulcri F, Krayenbuehl HP: Spontaneous course of aortic valve disease. Eur Heart J 8:471, 1987.
3. Marcus ML, Dotv DB, Hiratzka LF, et al: Decreased coronary reserve: a mechanism for angina pectoris in patients with aortic stenosis and normal coronary arteries. N Engl J Med 307:1362, 1982.
4. Eberli FR, Ritter M, Schwitter J, et al: Coronary reserve in patients with aortic valve disease before and after successful aortic valve replacement. Eur Heart J 12:127, 1991.
5. Mark AL, Kioschos JM, Abboud FM, et al: Abnormal vascular responses to exercise in patients with aortic stenosis. J Clin Invest 52:1138, 1973.
6. Weber KT, Brilla CG, Janicki JS: Structural remodeling of myocardial collagen in systemic hypertension: functional consequences and potential therapy. Heart Failure 4:129, 1990.
7. Villari B, Hess OM, Kaufmann PH, et al: Effect of aortic valve stenosis (pressure overload) and regurgitation (volume overload) on left ventricular systolic and diastolic function. Am J Cardiol 69:927, 1992.
8. Selzer A: Changing aspects of the natural history of valvular aortic stenosis. N Engl J Med 317:91, 1987.
9. Passik CS, Ackerman DM, Pluth JR, et al: Temporal changes in the causes of aortic stenosis: a surgical pathologic study of 646 cases. Mayo Clin Proc 62:119, 1987.
10. Otto CM, Kuusisto J, Reichenbach DD, et al: Characterization of the early lesion of "degenerative" valvular aortic stenosis. Histological and immunohistochemical studies. Circulation 90:844, 1994.
11. Juvenon J, Laurila A, Juvonen T, et al: Detection of *Chlamydia* pneumonia in human nonrheumatic stenotic aortic valves. J Am Coll Cardiol 29:1054, 1997.
12. O'Brien KD, Reichenbach DD, Marcovina SM, et al: Apolipoproteins B, (a), and E accumulate in the morphologically early lesion of "degenerative" valvular aortic stenosis. Arterioscler Thromb Vasc Biol 16:523, 1996.
13. Allen JM, Thompson GR, Myant NB, et al: Cardiovascular complications of homozygous familial hypercholesterolemia. Br Heart J 44:361, 1980.
14. Oakley CM, Hallidie-Smith KA: Assessment of site and severity in congenital aortic stenosis. Br Heart J 29:367, 1967.
15. Perloff JK: Clinical recognition of aortic stenosis. The physical signs and differential diagnosis of the various forms of obstruction to left ventricular outflow. Prog Cardiovasc Dis 10:323, 1968.
16. Braunwald E, Roberts WC, Goldblatt A, et al: Aortic stenosis:

physiological, pathological, and clinical concepts. Ann Intern Med 58:494, 1963.
17. Goldblatt A, Aygen MM, Braunwald E: Hemodynamic-phonocardiographic correlations of the fourth heart sound in aortic stenosis. Circulation 26:92, 1962.
18. Roberts WC, Perloff JK, Costantino T: Severe valvular aortic stenosis in patients over 65 years of age. Am J Cardiol 27:497, 1971.
19. Roger VL, Tajik AJ, Reeder GS, et al: Effect of Doppler echocardiography on utilization of hemodynamic cardiac catheterization in the preoperative evaluation of aortic stenosis. Mayo Clin Proc 71:141–149, 1996.
20. Otto CM, Pearlman AS: Doppler echocardiography in adults with symptomatic aortic stenosis. Diagnostic utility and cost-effectiveness. Arch Intern Med 148:2553–2560, 1988.
21. Roger VL, Tajik AJ, Reeder GS, et al: Effect of Doppler echocardiography on utilization of hemodynamic cardiac catheterization in the preoperative evaluation of aortic stenosis [see comments]. Mayo Clin Proc 71:141–149, 1996.
22. Popovic AD, Thomas JD, Neskovic AN, et al: Time-related trends in the preoperative evaluation of patients with valvular stenosis. Am J Cardiol 80:1464–1468, 1997.
23. Lindroos M, Kupari M, Heikkila J, Tilvis R: Prevalence of aortic valve abnormalities in the elderly: an echocardiographic study of a random population sample. J Am Coll Cardiol 21:1220–1225, 1993.
24. Wong M, Tei C, Sadler N, et al: Echocardiographic observations of calcium in operatively excised stenotic aortic valves. Am J Cardiol 59:324–329, 1987.
25. Hofmann T, Kasper W, Meinertz T, et al: Determination of aortic valve orifice area in aortic valve stenosis by two-dimensional transesophageal echocardiography. Am J Cardiol 59:330–335, 1987.
26. Tardif JC, Miller DS, Pandian NG, et al: Effects of variations in flow on aortic valve area in aortic stenosis based on in vivo planimetry of aortic valve area by multiplane transesophageal echocardiography. Am J Cardiol 76:193–198, 1995.
27. Bernard Y, Meneveau N, Vuillemenot A, et al: Planimetry of aortic valve area using multiplane transoesophageal echocardiography is not a reliable method for assessing severity of aortic stenosis. Heart 78:68–73, 1997.
28. Cormier B, Iung B, Porte JM, et al: Value of multiplane transesophageal echocardiography in determining aortic valve area in aortic stenosis. Am J Cardiol 77:882–885, 1996.
29. Seiler C, Jenni R: Severe aortic stenosis without left ventricular hypertrophy: prevalence, predictors, and short-term follow up after aortic valve replacement. Heart 76:250–255, 1996.
30. Rohde LE, Zhi G, Aranki SF, et al: Gender-associated differences in left ventricular geometry in patients with aortic valve disease and effect of distinct overload subsets. Am J Cardiol 80:475–480, 1997.
31. Hatle L, Angelsen BA, Tromsdal A: Non-invasive assessment of aortic stenosis by Doppler ultrasound. Br Heart J 43:284–292, 1980.
32. Currie PJ, Seward JB, Reeder GS, et al: Continuous-wave Doppler echocardiographic assessment of severity of calcific aortic stenosis: a simultaneous Doppler-catheter correlative study in 100 adult patients. Circulation 71:1162–1169, 1985.
33. Cape EG, Jones M, Yamada I, et al: Turbulent/viscous interactions control Doppler/catheter pressure discrepancies in aortic stenosis. The role of the Reynolds number. Circulation 94:2975–2981, 1996.
34. Laskey WK, Kussmaul WG: Pressure recovery in aortic valve stenosis. Circulation 89:116–121, 1994.
35. Niederberger J, Schima H, Maurer G, Baumgartner H: Importance of pressure recovery for the assessment of aortic stenosis by Doppler ultrasound. Role of aortic size, aortic valve area, and direction of the stenotic jet in vitro. Circulation 94:1934–1940, 1996.
36. Skjaerpe T, Hegrenaes L, Hatle L: Noninvasive estimation of valve area in patients with aortic stenosis by Doppler ultrasound and two-dimensional echocardiography. Circulation 72:810–818, 1985.
37. Zoghbi WA, Farmer KL, Soto JG, et al: Accurate noninvasive quantification of stenotic aortic valve area by Doppler echocardiography. Circulation 73:452–459, 1986.
38. Oh JK, Taliercio CP, Holmes DR Jr, et al: Prediction of the severity of aortic stenosis by Doppler aortic valve area determination: prospective Doppler-catheterization correlation in 100 patients. J Am Coll Cardiol 11:1227–1234, 1988.
39. Badano L, Cassottano P, Bertoli D, et al: Changes in effective aortic valve area during ejection in adults with aortic stenosis. Am J Cardiol 78:1023–1028, 1996.
40. Burwash IG, Thomas DD, Sadahiro M, et al: Dependence of Gorlin formula and continuity equation valve areas on transvalvular volume flow rate in valvular aortic stenosis. Circulation 89:827–835, 1994.
41. DeGroff CG, Shandas R, Valdes-Cruz L: Analysis of the effect of flow rate on the Doppler continuity equation for stenotic orifice area calculations: a numerical study. Circulation 97:1597–1605, 1998.
42. Burwash IG, Pearlman AS, Kraft CD, et al: Flow dependence of measures of aortic stenosis severity during exercise. J Am Coll Cardiol 24:1342–1350, 1994.
43. Tardif JC, Rodrigues AG, Hardy JF, et al: Simultaneous determination of aortic valve area by the Gorlin formula and by transesophageal echocardiography under different transvalvular flow conditions. Evidence that anatomic aortic valve area does not change with variations in flow in aortic stenosis. J Am Coll Cardiol 29:1296–1302, 1997.
44. Panidis IP, Mintz GS, Ross J: Value and limitations of Doppler ultrasound in the evaluation of aortic stenosis: a statistical analysis of 70 consecutive patients. Am Heart J 112:150–158, 1986.
45. Bermejo J, Garcia-Fernandez MA, Torrecilla EG, et al: Effects of dobutamine on Doppler echocardiographic indexes of aortic stenosis. J Am Coll Cardiol 28:1206–1213, 1996.
46. Cannon JD Jr, Zile MR, Crawford FA Jr, Carabello BA: Aortic valve resistance as an adjunct to the Gorlin formula in assessing the severity of aortic stenosis in symptomatic patients. J Am Coll Cardiol 20:1517–1523, 1992.
47. Isaaz K, Munoz L, Ports T, Schiller NB: Demonstration of postvalvuloplasty hemodynamic improvement in aortic stenosis based on Doppler measurement of valvular resistance. J Am Coll Cardiol 18:1661–1670, 1991.
48. Roger VL, Seward JB, Bailey KR, et al: Aortic valve resistance in aortic stenosis: Doppler echocardiographic study and surgical correlation. Am Heart J 134:924–929, 1997.
49. deFilippi CR, Willett DL, Brickner ME, et al: Usefulness of dobutamine echocardiography in distinguishing severe from nonsevere valvular aortic stenosis in patients with depressed left ventricular function and low transvalvular gradients. Am J Cardiol 75:191–194, 1995.
50. Shively BK, Charlton GA, Crawford MH, Chaney RK: Flow dependence of valve area in aortic stenosis: relation to valve morphology. J Am Coll Cardiol 31:654–660, 1998.
51. Otto CM, Burwash IG, Legget ME, et al: Prospective study of asymptomatic valvular aortic stenosis: clinical, echocardiographic, and exercise predictors of outcome. Circulation 95:2262, 1997.
52. Pellikka PA, Nishimura RA, Bailey KR, et al: The natural history of adults with asymptomatic hemodynamically significant aortic stenosis. J Am Coll Cardiol 15:1012, 1990.
53. Guidelines for the Management of Patients with Valvular Heart Disease ACC/AHA Practice Guidelines. Executive Summary. Circulation 98:1949, 1998.
54. Rapaport E: Natural history of aortic and mitral valve disease. Am J Cardiol 35:221, 1975.
55. Frank S, Johnson A, Ross J: Natural history of valvular aortic stenosis. Br Heart J 35:41, 1973.
56. Wagner HR, Ellison RC, Keane JF, et al: Clinical course in aortic stenosis. Circulation 56(suppl I):I47, 1977.
57. Schwarz F, Ehrmann J, Olschewski M, et al: Langzeitprognose medikamentös und chirurgisch behandelter Patienten mit erworbenen Aortenklappenfehlern: Ueberlebensstatisk und multivariate Cox-Regressionanalyse. Z Kardiol 74:598, 1985.
58. Horstkotte D, Loogen F, Kelikamp G, et al: Der Einfluss des prosthetischen Herzklappenersatzes auf den natürlichen Verlauf von isolierten Mitral- und Aortenklappenfehlern sowie Mehrklappenerkrankungen. Klinische Ergebnisse bei 783 Patienten bis zu 8 Jahre nach Implantation von Björk-Shiley-Kippscheibenprothesen. Z Kardiol 72:494, 1983.
59. Haerten K, Dohn G, Dohn V, et al: Natürlicher Verlauf operationswürdiger Aortenklappenvitien bei konservativer Therapie. Z Kardiol 69:757, 1980.
60. Ross J Jr, Braunwald E: Aortic stenosis. Circulation 38 (suppl V):V61, 1968.
61. Mullany CS, Elvebach LR, Frye RL, et al: Coronary artery disease and its management: influence on survival in patients undergoing aortic valve replacement. J Am Coll Cardiol 10:66–72, 1987.
62. Lund O: Preoperative risk evaluation and stratification of long-term survival after valve replacement for aortic stenosis. Circulation 82:124, 1990.

63. Connolly HM, Oh JK, Orszulak TA, et al: Aortic valve replacement for aortic stenosis with severe left ventricular dysfunction—prognostic indicators. Circulation 95:2395–2400, 1997.

Differentiation of Reversible From Irreversible Left Ventricular Systolic Dysfunction in Patients With Aortic Stenosis

64. Grossman W, Jones D, McLaurin LP: Wall stress and patterns of hypertrophy in the human left ventricle. J Clin Invest 56:56–64, 1975.
65. Grossman W: Cardiac hypertrophy: useful adaptation or pathologic process? Am J Med 69:576–584, 1980.
66. Gunther S, Grossman W: Determinants of ventricular function in pressure-overload hypertrophy in man. Circulation 59:679–688, 1979.
67. Ross J Jr, Braunwald E: Aortic stenosis. Circulation 38(suppl V):V61–V67, 1968.
68. Marcus ML, Doty DB, Hiratzka LF, et al: Decreased coronary reserve: a mechanism for angina pectoris in patients with aortic stenosis and normal coronary arteries. N Engl J Med 307:1362–1367, 1982.
69. Breish EA, Houser SR, Carey RA, et al: Myocardial blood flow and capillary density in chronic pressure overload of the feline left ventricle. Cardiovasc Res 14:469–475, 1980.
70. Dunn RB, Griggs DM: Ventricular filling pressure as a determinant of coronary blood flow during ischemia. Am J Physiol 244:H429–H436, 1983.
71. Gwathmey JK, Morgan JP: Altered calcium handling in experimental pressure-overload hypertrophy in the ferret. Circ Res 57:836, 1985.
72. Zile MR: Diastolic dysfunction: detection, consequences, and treatment. Part 2: diagnosis and treatment of diastolic dysfunction. Mod Conc Cardiovasc Dis 59:1–6, 1990.
73. Grossman W: Diastolic dysfunction and congestive heart failure. Circulation 81(suppl III):III-1–III-7, 1990.
74. Lorell BH, Grossman W: Cardiac hypertrophy: the consequences for diastole. J Am Coll Cardiol 9:1189–1193, 1987.
75. Weber KT, Janicki JS, Shroff SG, et al: Collagen remodeling of the pressure overloaded, hypertrophied nonhuman primate myocardium. Circ Res 62:757–765, 1988.
76. Weber KT: Cardiac interstitium in health and disease: the fibrillar collagen network. J Am Coll Cardiol 13:1637–1652, 1989.
77. Carabello BA, Green LH, Grossman W, et al: Hemodynamic determinants of prognosis of aortic valve replacement in critical aortic stenosis and advanced congestive heart failure. Circulation 62:42–48, 1980.
78. Huber D, Grimm J, Koch R, Krayenbuhl HP: Determinants of ejection performance in aortic stenosis. Circulation 64:126–134, 1981.
79. Carroll JD, Carroll EP, Feldman T, et al: Sex-associated differences in left ventricular function in aortic stenosis of the elderly. Circulation 86:1099–1107, 1992.
80. Ross J Jr: Afterload mismatch and preload reserve: a framework for the analysis of ventricular function. Prog Dis 18:255, 1976.
81. Koide M, Nagatsu M, Zile MR, et al: Premorbid determinants of left ventricular dysfunction in a novel model of gradually induced pressure overload in the adult canine. Circulation 95:1601–1610, 1997.
82. Rembert JC, Kleinman LH, Fedor JM, et al: Myocardial blood flow distribution in concentric left ventricular hypertrophy. J Clin Invest 62:379–386, 1978.
83. Nakano K, Corin WJ, Spann JF Jr, et al: Abnormal subendocardial blood flow in pressure overload hypertrophy is associated with pacing-induced subendocardial dysfunction. Circ Res 65:1555–1564, 1989.
84. Fujii AM, Gelpi RJ, Mirsky I, Vatner SF: Systolic and diastolic dysfunction during atrial pacing in conscious dogs with left ventricular hypertrophy. Circ Res 62:462–470, 1988.
85. Dalen H, Saetersdal T, Odegarden S: Some ultrastructural features of the myocardial cells in the hypertrophied human papillary muscle. Virchows Arch A 410:281, 1987.
86. Maier LS, Brandes R, Pieske B, Bers DM: Effects of left ventricular hypertrophy on force and Ca^{2+} handling in isolated rat myocardium. Am J Physiol 274:H1361–H1370, 1998.
87. McCall E, Ginsburg KS, Bassani RA, et al: Ca flux, contractility, and excitation-contraction coupling in hypertrophic rat ventricular myocytes. Am J Physiol 274:H1348–H1360, 1998.
88. Meerson FZ: The myocardium in hyperfunctional, hypertrophied heart failure. Circ Res 25(suppl 2):1, 1969.
89. Ferrans VJ: Morphology of the heart in hypertrophy. Heart J 18:67, 1983.
90. Tsutsui H, Ishihara K, Cooper G: Cytoskeletal role in the contractile dysfunction of hypertrophied myocardium. Science 260:682–687, 1993.
91. Smith N, McAnulty JH, Rahimtoola SH: Severe aortic stenosis with impaired left ventricular function and clinical heart failure: results of valve replacement. Circulation 58:255–264, 1978.
92. Lund O: Preoperative risk evaluation and stratification of long-term survival after valve replacement for aortic stenosis. Reasons for earlier operative intervention. Circulation 82:124–139, 1990.
93. Brogan WC III, Grayburn PA, Lange RA, et al: Prognosis after valve replacement in patients with severe aortic stenosis and a low transvalvular pressure gradient. J Am Coll Cardiol 21:1657–1660, 1993.
94. Gorlin R, Gorlin G: Hydraulic formula for calculation of area of stenotic mitral valve, other cardiac values and central circulatory shunts. Am Heart J 41:1, 1951.
95. Burwash IG, Thomas DD, Sadahiro M, et al: Dependence of Gorlin formula and continuity equation valve areas on transvalvular volume flow rate in valvular aortic stenosis. Circulation 89:827–835, 1994.
96. Cannon JD Jr, Zile MR, Crawford FA Jr, et al: Aortic valve resistance as an adjunct to the Gorlin formula in assessing the severity of aortic stenosis in symptomatic patients. J Am Coll Cardiol 20:1517–1523, 1992.
97. Marcus R, Bednarz J, Abruzzo J, et al: Mechanism underlying flow-dependency of valve orifice area determined by the Gorlin formula in patients with aortic valve obstruction [abstract]. Circulation 88(suppl I):I-103, 1993.
98. De Filippi CR, Willett DL, Brickner E, et al: Usefulness of dobutamine echocardiography in distinguishing severe from nonsevere valvular aortic stenosis in patients with depressed left ventricular function and low transvalvular gradients. Am J Cardiol 75:191–194, 1995.
99. Casale PN, Palacios IF, Abascal VM, et al: Effect of dobutamine on Gorlin and continuity equation valve areas and valve resistance in valvular aortic stenosis. Am J Cardiol 70:1175–1179, 1992.
100. Lin S, Roger V, Pellikka P: Dobutamine stress echocardiography in aortic stenosis: use and surgical correlations. Circulation 94(suppl I):I-31, 1996.
101. Ford LE, Feldman T, Chiu CY, Carroll JD: Hemodynamic resistance as a measure of functional impairment in aortic valvular stenosis. Circ Res 66:1–7, 1990.

Aortic Regurgitation

102. Connolly HM, Crary JL, McGoon MD, et al: Valvular heart disease associated with fenfluramine-phentermine. N Engl J Med 337:581–588, 1997.
103. Krayenbuehl HP, Hess OM: Chronic valvular insufficiency. *In* Parmley WW, Chatterjee K (eds): Cardiology. pp. 1–28. Philadelphia: JB Lippincott, 1991.
104. King RK, Magid NM, Opio G, Borer JS: Protein turnover in compensated chronic aortic regurgitation. Cardiology 88:518–525, 1997.
105. Taketani S, Sawa Y, Taniguchi K, et al: *C-Myc* expression and its role in patients with chronic aortic regurgitation. Circulation 96(suppl):II-83–II-87, 1997.
106. Villari B, Campbell SE, Hess OM, et al: Influence of collagen network on left ventricular systolic and diastolic function in aortic valve disease. J Am Coll Cardiol 22:1477, 1993.
107. Weber KT: Cardiac interstitium in health and disease: the fibrillar collagen network. J Am Coll Cardiol 13:1637, 1989.
108. Hill L, Rowlands RA: Systolic blood pressure: (1) in change of posture. (2) in cases of aortic regurgitation. Heart 3:219, 1911.
109. Constant J: Arterial and venous pulsations in cardiovascular diagnosis. J Cardiovasc Med 5:973, 1980.
110. Corrigan DJ: Permanent patency of the mouth of the aortic valves. Edinb Med Surg J 37:225, 1832.
111. Braunwald E, Morrow AG: A method for the detection and estimation of aortic regurgitant flow in man. Circulation 17:505, 1958.
112. Conn RD, Cole JS: The cardiac apex impulse: clinical and angiographic correlations. Ann Intern Med 75:185, 1971.

113. Abdulla AM, Frank MJ, Erdin RA Jr, Canedo MI: Clinical significance and hemodynamic correlates of the third heart sound gallop in aortic regurgitation. Circulation 64:464, 1981.
114. Alpert JS, Veiweg WVR, Hagan AD: Incidence and morphology of carotid shudders in aortic valve disease. Am Heart J 92:435, 1976.
115. Meadows WR, Van Pragh S, Indreika M, Sharp JT: Premature mitral valve closure. A hemodynamic explanation for absence of the first sound in aortic insufficiency. Circulation 28:251, 1963.
116. Segal J, Harvey WP, Hufnagel CL: A clinical study of one hundred cases of severe aortic insufficiency. Am J Med 21:200, 1956.
117. Sabbah HN, Khaja F, Anbe DT, Stein PD: The aortic closure sound in pure aortic stenosis. Circulation 56:859, 1977.
118. Harvey WP, Corrado MA, Perloff JK: "Right-sided" murmurs of aortic insufficiency (diastolic murmurs better heard to the right of the sternum than to the left). Am J Med Sci 245:533, 1963.
119. Bellet S, Gouley B, Nichols CF, McMillian TM: Loud, musical diastolic murmurs of aortic insufficiency. Am Heart J 18:483, 1939.
120. Groom D, Boone JA: The "dove-coo" murmur and murmurs heard at a distance from the chest wall. Ann Intern Med 42:1214, 1955.
121. Flint A: On cardiac murmurs. Am J Med Sci 44:29, 1862.
122. Reddy PS, Curtiss EI, Salerni R, et al: Sound pressure correlates of the Austin Flint murmur: an intracardiac sound of study. Circulation 53:210, 1976.
123. Welch GH, Braunwald E, Sarnoff SJ: Hemodynamic effects of quantitatively varied experimental aortic regurgitation. Circ Res 5:546, 1957.
124. Perloff JK: Acute severe aortic regurgitation: recognition and management. J Cardiovasc Med 8:209, 1983.
125. Spring DA, Folts JD, Young WP, Rowe GG: Premature closure of the mitral and tricuspid valves. Circulation 45:663, 1972.
126. Botvinick EH, Schiller NB, Wickramasekaran R, et al: Echocardiographic demonstration of early mitral valve closure in severe aortic insufficiency. Circulation 51:836, 1975.
127. Mann T, McLaurin L, Grossman W, Craige E: Assessing the hemodynamic severity of acute aortic regurgitation due to infective endocarditis. Lancet 2:115, 1971.
128. Hegglin R, Scheu H, Rothlin M: Aortic insufficiency. Circulation 37 (suppl V):V77, 1968.
129. Goldschlager N, Pfeifer J, Cohn K, et al: The natural history of aortic regurgitation. Am J Med 54:577, 1973.
130. Spagnuolo M, Kloth H, Taranta A, et al: Natural history of rheumatic aortic regurgitation. Criteria predictive of death, congestive heart failure and angina in young patients. Circulation 44:368, 1971.
131. Bonow RO, Rosing DR, McIntosh CL, et al: The natural history of asymptomatic patients with aortic regurgitation and normal left ventricular function. Circulation 68:509, 1983.
132. Klodas E, Enriquez-Sarano M, Tajik AJ, et al: Optimizing timing of surgical correction in patients with severe aortic regurgitation. Role of symptoms. J Am Coll Cardiol 30:746–752, 1997.
133. Klodas E, Enriquez-Sarano M, Tajik AJ, et al: Aortic regurgitation complicated by extreme left ventricular dilation: long-term outcome after surgical correction. J Am Coll Cardiol 27:670–677, 1996.
134. Bonow RO, Rosing DR, Maron BJ, et al: Reversal of left ventricular dysfunction after aortic valve replacement for chronic aortic regurgitation: influence of duration of preoperative left ventricular dysfunction. Circulation 70:570–579, 1984.
135. Pompilio G, Brockman C, Bruneau M, et al: Long term survival after aortic valve replacement for native aortic valve endocarditis. Cardiovasc Surg 6:126–132, 1998.
136. Greenberg BH, DeMots H, Murphy E, Rahimtoola SH: Mechanisms for improved cardiac performance with arteriolar dilators in aortic insufficiency. Circulation 63:263, 1981.
137. Greenberg B, Massie B, Bristow JD, et al: Long-term vasodilator therapy of chronic aortic insufficiency. Circulation 78:92, 1988.
138. Scognamiglio R, Fasoli G, Ponshia A, Dalla-Volta S: Long-term nifedipine unloading therapy in asymptomatic patients with chronic severe aortic regurgitation. J Am Coll Cardiol 16:424, 1990.
139. Levine HJ, Gaasch WH: Vasoactive drugs in chronic regurgitant lesions of the mitral and aortic valves. J Am Coll Cardiol 28:1083–1091, 1996.
140. Schön HR, Dorn R, Fischer M, Blömer H: ACE-Hemmer verzögern den Zeitpunkt des Aortenklappenersatzes bei Patienten mit schwerer asymptomatischer chronischer Aorteninsuffizienz [abstract]. Z Kardiol 1992, p. 128.
141. ACC/AHA guidelines for the management of patients with valvular heart disease. A Report of the American College of Cardiology/American Heart Association Task Force on Practice Guidelines (Committee on Management of Patients With Valvular Heart Disease). J Am Coll Cardiol 32:1486–1588, 1998.

CHAPTER 14

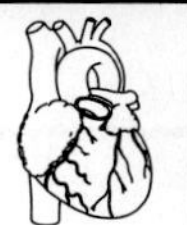

Pulmonary and Tricuspid Valve Disease

Otto M. Hess, Urs Scherrer, and Pascal Nicod

PATHOPHYSIOLOGY
PHYSICAL EXAMINATION
Pulmonary Valve Disease
Tricuspid Valve Disease
NATURAL HISTORY
MEDICAL/SURGICAL TREATMENT

Pathophysiology

Acquired pulmonary valve disease is extremely rare. Occasionally, rheumatic inflammation may be seen, but this rarely leads to serious deformity. Infective endocarditis and leaflet destruction of the pulmonic valve may be observed in drug addicts. Thickening or retraction of the pulmonary valve leaflets has also been described in patients with carcinoid syndrome.[1] Finally, *low-pressure pulmonary regurgitation* may be observed in patients with dilatation of the valvular ring, as in idiopathic dilatation of the pulmonary artery, in connective tissue disorders, or after valvotomy for pulmonary stenosis.

By far the most common disorder is pulmonary regurgitation secondary to dilatation of the valvular ring in patients with pulmonary hypertension or severe mitral valve disease. This disorder, called *high-pressure pulmonary regurgitation,* is usually overshadowed by the underlying disease and is characterized by a high-pitched diastolic murmur (Graham Steell's murmur).

Tricuspid stenosis is almost always rheumatic in origin and is typically accompanied by mitral stenosis. A reduction in tricuspid valve area to less than 1.5 cm^2 is usually associated with an increase in right atrial pressure. Severe tricuspid stenosis is present if valve area is less than 1 cm^2. Under these circumstances, right atrial pressure increases to 10 mm Hg or greater, and venous congestion with peripheral edema and ascites occurs.

Tricuspid regurgitation can be relative or organic. By far, the most common cause is relative tricuspid regurgitation secondary to dilatation of the right ventricle (RV) and the tricuspid annulus, often associated with pressure overload of the RV. Organic tricuspid regurgitation is usually more severe and may be caused by right atrial myxoma, endocarditis, carcinoid syndrome, Ebstein's anomaly, or myxomatous degeneration of the tricuspid valve leaflets and supporting structures, that is, tricuspid valve prolapse.

Physiologic pulmonary or tricuspid regurgitation in normal individuals is common and can be found in 80 (pulmonary) to 95 percent (tricuspid valve) of all subjects.

Physical Examination

Pulmonary Valve Disease

Physical findings of pulmonary regurgitation vary according to the presence or absence of pulmonary hypertension. The carotid pulse is usually normal unless cardiac output is decreased. Jugular venous pressure may be normal or increased when tricuspid valve disease or RV failure is present. A prominent A wave can be seen with pulmonary hypertension. A parasternal RV impulse may be present, and a pulsatile pulmonary artery may be felt in the second left intercostal space. On auscultation, the pulmonary component of S_2 is usually normal and delayed, causing variable wide splitting of S_2. If significant pulmonary hypertension is present, P_2 becomes louder with narrow splitting of S_2. An ejection click and an S_3 may be heard. The regurgitant murmur, in the absence of pulmonary hypertension, follows S_2 in a crescendo-decrescendo pattern with a medium pitch and is best heard in the third and fourth left intercostal spaces.[2, 3] When pulmonary hypertension is present, the murmur becomes decrescendo and has a higher pitch, similar to that of aortic insufficiency.

When pulmonary stenosis is associated with pulmonary regurgitation, a thrill may be felt in the second left intercostal space. An ejection click is usually not heard in acquired mixed pulmonary stenosis and regurgitation. A systolic crescendo-decrescendo murmur is found in the second left parasternal intercostal space, with delayed peaking. Typically, murmurs of pulmonary valve disease increase with inspiration or with inhalation of amyl nitrite.

Tricuspid Valve Disease

Tricuspid Stenosis

The physical findings of tricuspid stenosis are often obscured by the concomitant presence of stenosis or regurgitation of other valves. The most prominent finding is the presence of a large A wave in the jugular veins of patients who are in sinus rhythm (Fig. 14–1).[4] The distinction from pulsating carotid arteries can be made by concomitant palpation of the upstroke of the carotid pulse, which fol-

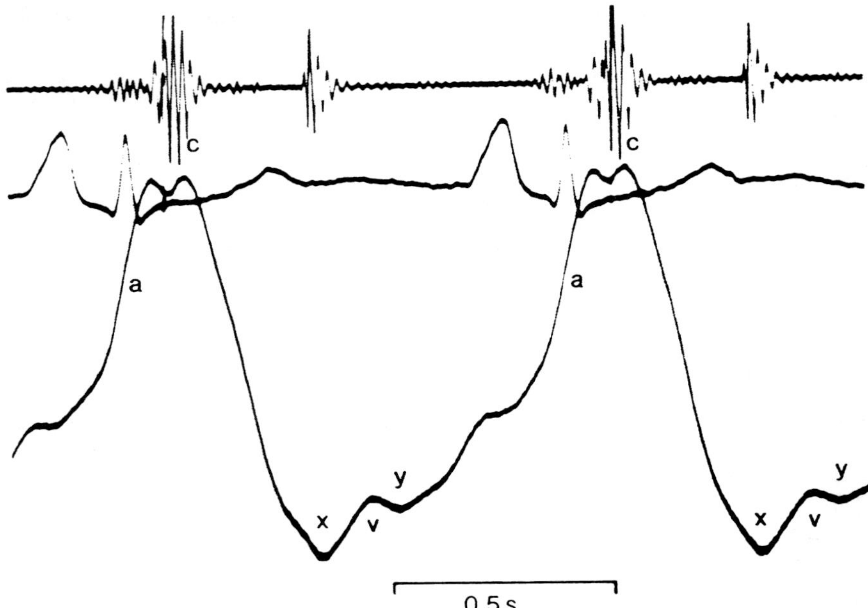

FIGURE 14–1 Right-sided venous pulse pressure in a 39-year-old patient with tricuspid stenosis. The A wave is predominant, and the *y* descent is decreased. On the phonocardiogram, a diamond-shaped presystolic rumble can be appreciated. P waves on the electrocardiogram are suggestive of right atrial enlargement.

lows the jugular A wave. In patients with atrial fibrillation, jugular turgescence may be accompanied by a slow *y* descent, owing to an impairment of RV filling in early diastole.[5]

Palpation is usually normal unless associated valvular disease is present. Occasionally, a thrill may be felt over the left lower sternal border, and pulsation of the right atrium may be detected in the right parasternal area.

S_2 may be narrowly split, with little respiratory variation as a result of impaired RV filling. An opening snap is often difficult to differentiate from that of mitral stenosis but may occur later in diastole. The diastolic murmur after the opening snap is usually of low frequency, or on occasion, of higher frequency and decrescendo. It is maximal over the lower left sternal border. In patients with sinus rhythm, a presystolic murmur may be heard and can be differentiated from that of mitral stenosis by an earlier appearance, a crescendo-decrescendo pattern, and termination before S_1.[4]

The murmur of tricuspid stenosis and the opening snap typically increase in intensity with deep inspiration (Carvallo sign). All other maneuvers that cause an increase in cardiac output, such as leg raising, exercise, and inhalation of amyl nitrite, also increase the intensity of the murmur and the opening snap, whereas the Valsalva maneuver and sudden standing position decrease their intensity.

Tricuspid Regurgitation

Tricuspid regurgitation is often associated with pulmonary hypertension or other valvular lesions. Prominent jugular V waves may be seen in the neck (Fig. 14–2).[5–7] They should be differentiated from the A wave of tricuspid stenosis by their slower upstroke and their appearance after the carotid pulse and in association with the second heart sound. They may be accompanied by a pulsatile liver and signs of RV failure. The *y* descent is also present. The RV impulse may be prominent and hyperdynamic. A systolic right atrial impulse may rarely be felt in the right parasternal area. On auscultation, P_2 may be increased in presence of pulmonary hypertension. A prominent S_3 that increases with inspiration may be heard. The murmur is usually holosystolic and located in the lower left parasternal area but may be heard over the lower sternum and the subxyphoid area. Occasionally, it may be early systolic, particularly in the presence of acute tricuspid regurgitation, or limited to midsystole or even late systole. Sometimes, a diastolic flow rumble may be heard, as a result of increased diastolic flow across the tricuspid valve.

The murmur typically increases with deep inspiration (Carvallo sign) as a result of increased venous return (Fig. 14–3) and decreases with the Valsalva maneuver. However, this inspiratory increase in the intensity of the murmur may be lacking in the presence of markedly elevated venous pressure.

NATURAL HISTORY

The natural history of pulmonary and tricuspid valve disease is dependent on the underlying disorder. Acquired pulmonary valve disease is extremely rare. Pulmonary or tricuspid regurgitation due to infective endocarditis may be seen in drug addicts or after surgical interventions. In the absence of pulmonary hypertension, tricuspid regurgitation is usually well tolerated for many years. However, when pulmonary hypertension and tricuspid regurgitation coexist, right-sided congestive heart failure with reduced cardiac output and painful congestive hepatomegaly may occur.[8] In patients with combined tricuspid regurgitation and mitral valve disease, the natural history is usually determined by the latter.

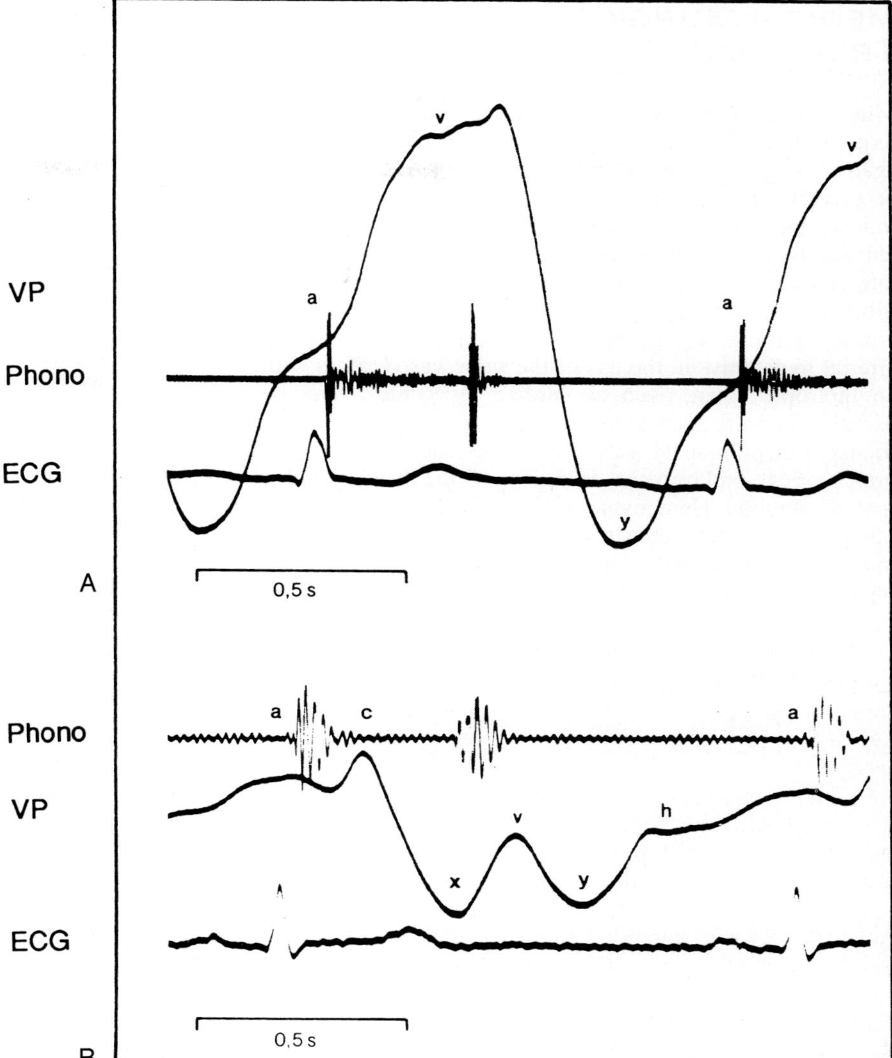

FIGURE 14–2 A, Right-sided venous pulse pressure (VP) in a 39-year-old patient with tricuspid regurgitation. There is a prominent V wave, followed by a rapid *y* descent. A phonocardiogram (Phono) reveals a holosystolic murmur. **B,** Right-sided venous pressure in a 26-year-old patient without heart disease. The A wave is typically taller than the V wave. Both the *x* and the *y* descents can be seen. ECG, electrocardiogram.

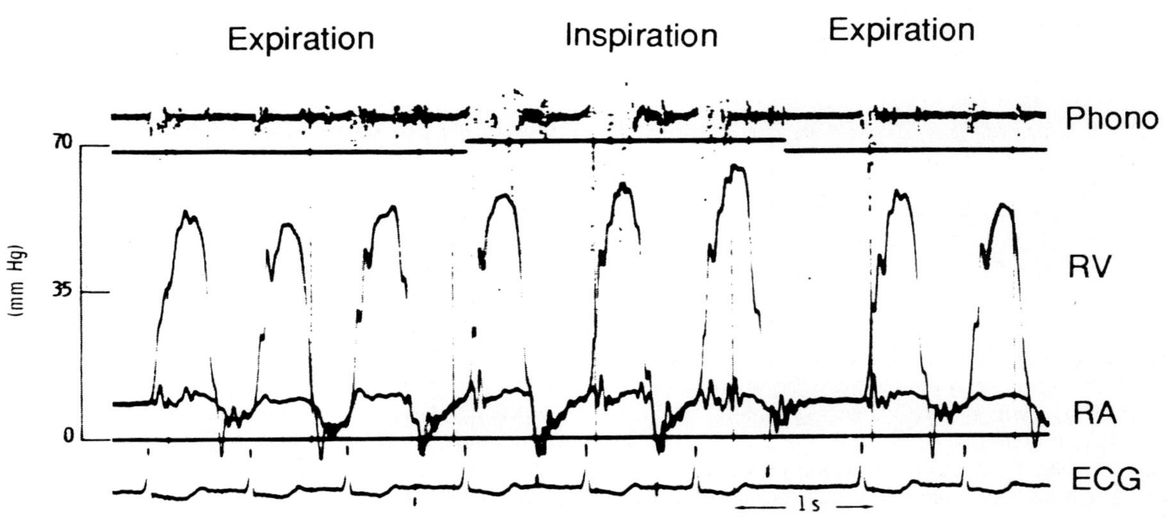

FIGURE 14–3 Phonocardiographic recording (Phono) in a patient with tricuspid regurgitation. There is a marked inspiratory increase of the intensity of the murmur (Carvallo sign), followed by a third heart sound. The right atrial (RA) pressure recording shows no inspiratory fall in pressure, whereas right ventricular (RV) systolic pressure increases during inspiration. ECG, electrocardiogram.

MEDICAL/SURGICAL TREATMENT

Mild tricuspid or pulmonary valvular insufficiency does not require specific therapy other than antibiotic prophylaxis against subacute bacterial endocarditis before dental work or surgery. Hemodynamically significant tricuspid or pulmonary insufficiency in the presence of pulmonary hypertension is best treated with vasodilators and unloading interventions, such as angiotensin-converting enzyme inhibitors, nifedipine, hydralazine, and prazosin, with or without nitrates. In the absence of important pulmonary arterial hypertension, the use of the same vasodilators with an inotropic agent, such as cardiac glycosides, may be useful, especially if atrial fibrillation is present. With severe tricuspid or pulmonary valvular insufficiency and RV failure, surgical replacement or repair of the leaking valve may be required. Hemodynamically important valvular pulmonic or tricuspid stenosis with associated limiting symptoms is treated by valvuloplasty or sometimes by surgical replacement or repair of the valve.

The reader is referred to the websites of the American College of Cardiology (www.acc.org) and the American Heart Association (www.americanheart.org) for the ACC/AHA Guidelines for the Management of Patients with Acute Myocardial Infarction.

REFERENCES

1. Hedinger Ch, Isler P: Metastasierendes Dünndarmkarzinoid mit schweren, vorwiegend das rechte Herz betreffenden Klappenfehlern und Pulmonalstenose: ein eigenartiger Symptomenkomplex? Schweiz Med Wochenschr 83:4, 1953.
2. Nemickas R, Roberts J, Gunnar RM, Tobin JR: Isolated congenital pulmonic insufficiency: differentiation of mild from severe regurgitation. Am J Cardiol 14:456, 1964.
3. Bousvaros GA, Deuchar DC: The murmur of pulmonary regurgitation which is not associated with pulmonary hypertension. Lancet 2:962, 1961.
4. Perloff JK, Harvey WP: Clinical recognition of tricuspid stenosis. Circulation 22:346, 1960.
5. Messer AL, Hurst JW, Rappaport MB, et al: A study of the venous pulse in tricuspid valve disease. Circulation 1:388, 1950.
6. Schilder DP, Harvey WP: Confusion of tricuspid incompetence with mitral insufficiency: a pitfall in the selection of patients for mitral surgery. Am Heart J 54:352, 1957.
7. Amidi M, Irwin JM, Salerni R, et al: Venous systolic thrill and murmur in the neck: a consequence of severe tricuspid insufficiency. J Am Coll Cardiol 7:942, 1986.
8. Braunwald E: Heart Disease. 5th Ed. Philadelphia: WB Saunders, 1997.

CHAPTER 15

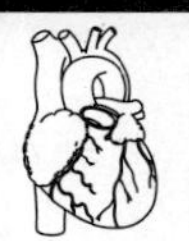

MITRAL VALVE DISEASE

Otto M. Hess, Urs Scherrer, Pascal Nicod, Elliot Chesler, Robert L. Frye, and Maurice Enriquez-Sarano

MITRAL STENOSIS
Pathophysiology
Physical Examination
Natural History
Medical Treatment
MITRAL REGURGITATION
Pathophysiology
Physical Examination
Natural History
Medical Treatment
ASSESSMENT OF SEVERITY OF MITRAL REGURGITATION AND ITS TREATMENT
Robert L. Frye and Maurice Enriquez-Sarano
Doppler Echocardiographic Semiquantitative Methods
Doppler Echocardiographic Quantitative Methods
Cardiac Catheterization
Strategy of Laboratory Testing
MITRAL PROLAPSE (MYXOMATOUS MITRAL VALVE)
Elliot Chesler
History
Nomenclature
Pathology
Genetics
Epidemiology
Associated Abnormalities
Clinical Findings
Electrocardiography
Echocardiography
Cardiac Catheterization and Angiocardiography
Complications
Prognosis
Management

MITRAL STENOSIS

Pathophysiology

The predominant cause of mitral stenosis is rheumatic heart disease. The end products of the rheumatic process are shrinkage of the valvular apparatus and contraction and fusion of the chordae tendineae. When the valvular orifice is reduced to 2 cm^2 (normal valve area, 4 to 6 cm^2), blood flow through the stenotic valve is still normal under resting conditions, but during exercise, left atrial (LA) pressure and mean pulmonary artery pressure increase abnormally.[1] When the mitral valve orifice is reduced to 1 cm^2, which is considered to represent severe mitral stenosis, LA pressure is augmented at rest, and atrioventricular (AV) pressure gradients of more than 10 mm Hg can be observed (Fig. 15–1). Such patients have a reduced cardiac output and have dyspnea during mild exercise or even at rest. The AV pressure gradient is directly dependent on transvalvular flow rate and heart rate (Fig. 15–2). Tachycardia augments the transmitral diastolic flow rate and pressure gradient by decreasing diastolic time and, therefore, elevating LA pressure. This explains why previously asymptomatic patients who develop atrial fibrillation suddenly become symptomatic. Furthermore, a small increase in blood flow is associated with a large increase in the pressure gradient because the pressure gradient is a square function of flow rate; thus, doubling the flow rate quadruples the pressure gradient.[2]

LA function plays an important hemodynamic role in mitral stenosis. Chronic elevation of LA pressure is associated with dilatation of the atrial chamber. LA contraction

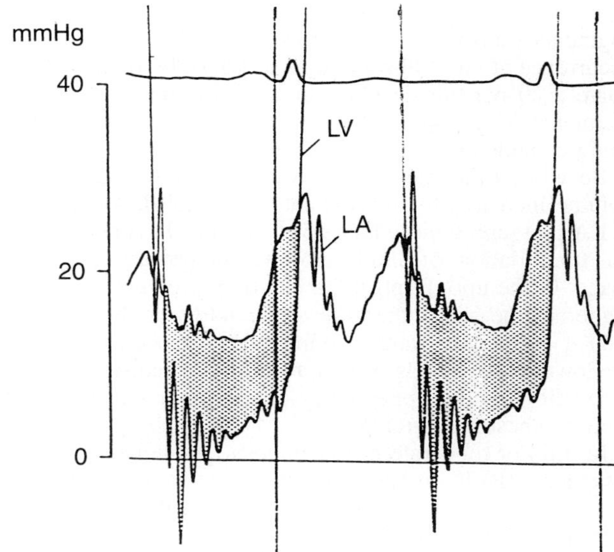

FIGURE 15–1 Pressure recordings in a young patient with rheumatic mitral stenosis. Left ventricular (LV) and left atrial (LA) pressure show the typical pressure gradient, with presystolic accentuation during atrial contraction. Note that early diastolic pressures can become negative due to diastolic suction caused by rapid relaxation and elastic recoil in patients with mitral stenosis. MVA, mitral valve area; ΔP, mean diastolic pressure gradient.

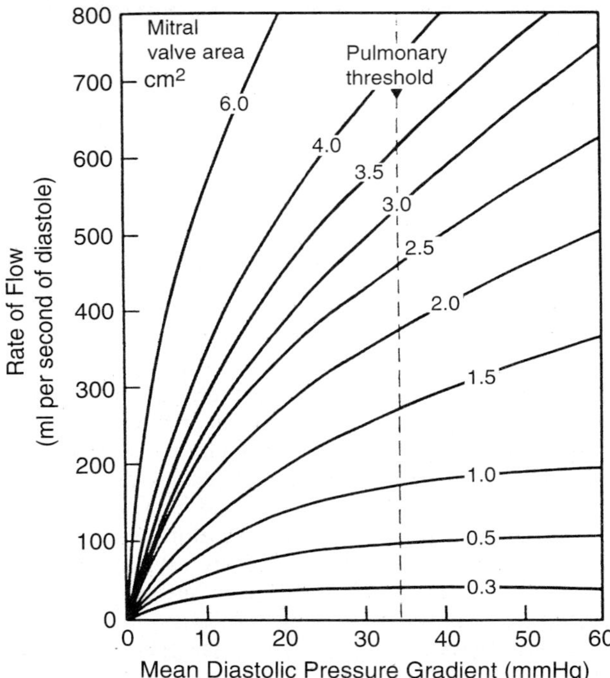

FIGURE 15–2 Relation between mean diastolic pressure gradient and diastolic flow rate across the mitral valve as predicted by the Gorlin formula. A small increase in flow rate in patients with severe mitral stenosis (mitral valve area ≤ 1 cm²) causes a large increase in diastolic pressure gradient. (From Wallace AG: Pathophysiology of cardiovascular disease. *In* Smith LH Jr, Thier SO [eds]: International Textbook of Medicine. Vol. 1. Philadelphia: WB Saunders, 1981.)

augments transmitral blood flow (see Fig. 15–1), and the occurrence of atrial fibrillation is responsible for an approximately 20 percent decrease in cardiac output. Therefore, maintenance of sinus rhythm is important for the well-being of patients with mitral stenosis.

Because of the increase in LA pressure, pulmonary blood volume increases by approximately one third. An increase in LA pressure to more than 25 to 30 mm Hg is responsible for transudation of fluid into the pulmonary interstitial space. In the upright position, capillary pressure is slightly higher in the lower than the upper lobes of the lung. To reduce pulmonary transudation, reflex vasoconstriction of the lower lobe vessels occurs, resulting in redistribution of blood flow to the upper lobes of the lung, which can be seen on chest radiography.

In mild or moderate mitral stenosis, pulmonary vascular resistance (PVR) remains normal, but it increases with more severe stenosis when transudation of fluid occurs into the interstitium. Reflex vasoconstriction due to pulmonary hypoxemia may contribute to secondary pulmonary hypertension. PVR can reach values of 1000 dynes·sec·cm^{-5} or more. This increase has been attributed mainly to pulmonary vasoconstriction, because PVR falls and may even normalize after successful valvuloplasty or surgery, although structural alterations of the pulmonary vessels have been described.[3]

Physical Examination

The general appearance of patients with mitral stenosis is normal except in patients with tight stenosis, in whom a low cardiac output may produce peripheral and malar cyanosis ("facies mitralis"). Pulse pressure is usually normal but may be reduced if stroke volume is decreased due to severe stenosis or atrial fibrillation. The jugular veins may be normal in mild stenosis. Prominent A waves are seen in patients with secondary pulmonary hypertension who remain in sinus rhythm. Jugular vein distention, peripheral edema, and liver enlargement appear in patients with right ventricular (RV) failure. Prominent V waves suggest the presence of associated tricuspid regurgitation.

Palpation of the precordium may reveal an RV impulse in patients with secondary pulmonary hypertension.[4] The pulmonary component of S_2 may be felt in the left upper sternal border. The apical impulse is usually normal but may be displaced laterally in the presence of an enlarged right ventricle or associated mitral regurgitation (MR). Closure of S_1 may be felt at the apex, and a diastolic thrill can sometimes be found while the patient lies on the left side ("frennissment mitrale").

S_1 is characteristically accentuated in mitral stenosis (Fig. 15–3). The mitral valve is held open longer because of increased LA pressure. Mitral closure occurs later, as measured by an increased qS_1 interval, at a time when dP/dt of the ventricle is steeper and causes forceful closure of the valve and increased S_1 intensity.[5, 6] With decreased leaflet mobility, S_1 may become softer and the opening snap may disappear.[7] S_2 may be normal in mild mitral stenosis. With the appearance of progressive pulmonary hypertension, the pulmonary component of S_2 becomes louder and the splitting of S_2 may progressively disappear, due to earlier closure of the pulmonary valve. Right-sided S_4 or S_3 may be present, becoming louder during inspiration. A pulmonary ejection click may be heard in the presence of pulmonary hypertension and may be slightly softer during inspiration but often does not change in intensity.

An opening snap follows aortic closure by 0.03 to 0.13 second, and it is best heard at the apex as a high-pitched sound (see Fig. 15–3).[6, 8–10] The opening snap may be attenuated when valve excursion is limited by thickening or calcification. The presence of mitral regurgitation or aortic valve disease may also attenuate the intensity of the opening snap. The time interval between A_2 and the opening snap is an indicator of the severity of mitral stenosis. An interval of less than 0.06 second is suggestive of severe mitral stenosis, and an interval of more than 0.08 second indicates a milder degree of stenosis, although such an interval can be seen in the presence of severe stenosis when valve excursion is impaired by *thickening and calcification*. The A_2-opening snap interval is influenced by changes in LA pressure or cardiac output, being shortened during exercise or rapid atrial fibrillation and lengthened in the standing position or when cardiac failure develops. Associated MR, aortic valve disease, and systemic hypertension may also influence the A_2-opening snap interval.

A diastolic rumble can be best heard by placing the bell of the stethoscope over the apical impulse while the patient lies on the left side. There is a correlation between the severity of the stenosis and the duration of the diastolic murmur but not with its intensity.[9] Although the presence of a holodiastolic rumble suggests severe stenosis, it may be present even in mild mitral stenosis when heart rate is accelerated. In rapid atrial fibrillation, the presence of a

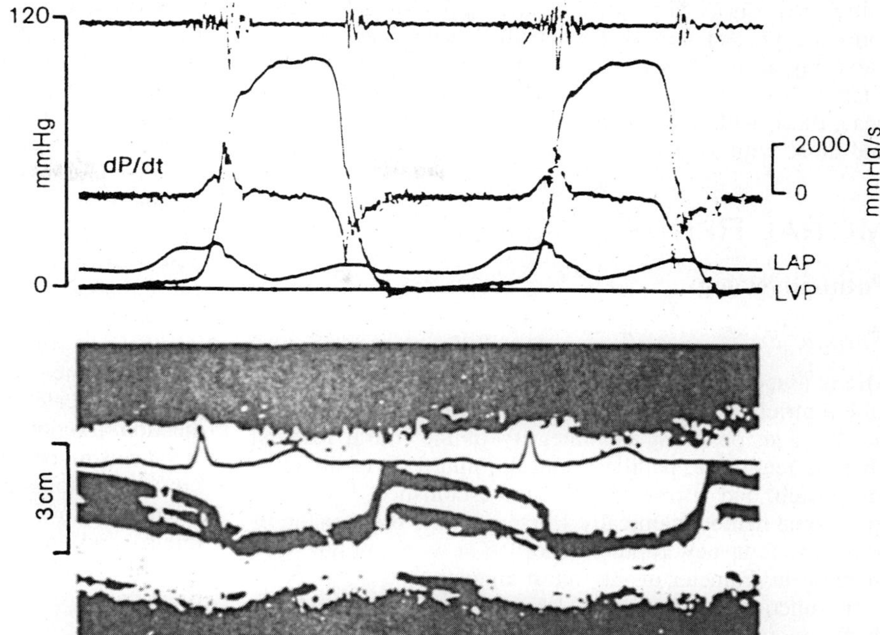

FIGURE 15–3 Echocardiogram of a 49-year-old patient with mitral stenosis. The thickened mitral leaflets can be clearly seen with diastolic anterior motion of the posterior leaflet. Simultaneous left ventricular (LVP) and left atrial (LAP) pressures reveal the presence of a holodiastolic pressure gradient. **Top,** On the phonocardiogram, an opening snap and a presystolic accentuation of the murmur can be seen. S_1 is increased in intensity because closure of the mitral valve is delayed and occurs at a time when dP/dt of the left ventricle is increased.

holodiastolic rumble should be sought during long RR intervals. Presystolic accentuation of the murmur is typical in sinus rhythm (see Fig. 15–3) but has been occasionally described in atrial fibrillation.[11] The diastolic rumble may be difficult to hear in the presence of obesity or emphysema. In severe mitral stenosis, a low cardiac output, resulting in increased turbulence across the valve, and the displacement of the left ventricular (LV) apex by an enlarged right ventricle may render the mitral stenosis "silent."[12]

A murmur of tricuspid insufficiency may be heard in the left lower parasternal area and can be due to the presence of pulmonary hypertension, associated tricuspid valve disease, or both. In pulmonary hypertension, a pulmonary insufficiency murmur may be also heard along the left parasternal area (Graham Steell's murmur) and should be differentiated from aortic insufficiency by the absence of peripheral signs, such as bounding pulses.[13]

The diastolic rumble may be increased and the A_2-opening snap interval reduced by maneuvers that cause increased cardiac output, such as exercise, squatting, leg raising, or inhalation of amyl nitrite. Conversely, the Valsalva maneuver or standing may decrease the intensity of the rumble and widen the A_2-opening snap interval.

Natural History

In temperate climates, most patients with mitral stenosis after acute rheumatic fever remain asymptomatic for a decade or longer. In tropical regions or underdeveloped areas, the disease may progress more rapidly, and severe mitral stenosis may already be present in early adolescence. Although the reason for this difference in the progression of the disease is not clear, it may be related to differences in socioeconomic conditions, virulence of bacterial strains, or genetic factors. Once mitral stenosis has become symptomatic, it takes approximately 5 to 7 years for most patients to progress from mild to severe disability. However, medical treatment that emphasizes heart rate control with digoxin or beta-blockers and treatment with diuretics and oral anticoagulation may improve the clinical course and allow the postponement of interventions with valvuloplasty, valvulotomy, or mitral valve replacement. In the presurgical era,[14] 5- and 10-year survival rates in mildly symptomatic patients were 62 and 38 percent, respectively, whereas severely symptomatic patients had a 5-year survival rate of only 15 percent and no survival after 8 years.

Medical Treatment

Clinical conditions such as anemia, fever, pregnancy, or heavy exercise, which are associated with a significant increase in cardiac output, should be avoided in patients with severe mitral stenosis. Diuretics and low doses of nitrates may be used to treat symptoms of pulmonary congestion. Digitalis, β-blockers, and selected calcium antagonists are useful in patients with atrial fibrillation to slow the ventricular response rate and increase the diastolic filling time. The use of β-blockers in patients with sinus rhythm may prevent exercise-induced tachycardia and improve exercise tolerance.[15]

Anticoagulants should be administered to patients with atrial fibrillation and those who have had previous episodes of peripheral emboli. There is, however, no clear-cut evidence that anticoagulants are beneficial in patients in sinus rhythm, although they are advised for patients with moderate to severe mitral stenosis in sinus rhythm.

Percutaneous mitral valvuloplasty is recommended when

mitral stenosis is hemodynamically important and symptoms are present at a well controlled heart rate. Surgical valve replacement is indicated only in calcified, severely altered valves with thickened and shortened chordae tendineae, those with associated significant mitral insufficiency, and those with associated LA thrombi.

MITRAL REGURGITATION

Pathophysiology

Chronic Form

MR is associated with volume overload of the left atrium and ventricle. Proper function of the mitral valve depends on the size, position, and integrity of the mitral leaflets, chordae tendineae, papillary muscle, mitral valve annulus, left atrium, and left ventricle. Once established, MR tends to become hemodynamically worse with the progression of lesions such as new ruptured chordae or with a progressive increase in diameter of the mitral annulus.

In functional MR due to localized or generalized LV dysfunction, the increase in LV cavity size displaces the papillary muscle laterally and downward, resulting in abnormal systolic traction on the chordae tendineae that prevents coaptation of the mitral leaflets.[16–18]

MR leads to an increase in LA V-wave pressure (Fig. 15–4) that is dependent on the severity of regurgitation, the distensibility of the left atrium, and the loading conditions.[19, 20] In patients with chronic MR and a large left atrium (low LA chamber stiffness), the V-wave pressure is usually small despite severe regurgitation because the pressure is absorbed in the large atrium and is not transmitted to the pulmonary veins. However, in acute MR, V-wave pressure is large because the left atrium is small (high LA chamber stiffness) and is not prepared to accommodate a large regurgitant volume. The V-wave pressure may be transmitted backward into the pulmonary arterial bed and lead to the occurrence of a "pulmonary artery V wave." Acute changes in preload and afterload are associated with changes in the severity of MR. For example, a large increase in V-wave pressure can be observed when MR is acutely increased during isometric (handgrip) exercise (see Fig. 15–4).[21]

Patients with severe regurgitation and chronically augmented LA pressure develop secondary pulmonary hypertension and RV hypertrophy. LV afterload, as assessed on the basis of mean systolic and end-systolic wall stress, is usually normal but if elevated is inversely related to systolic ejection performance.[22] LV pump function, however, remains preserved for a long time because the ventricle empties against a low-impedance system. Therefore, in the compensated state, LV ejection phase indices such as ejection fraction, systolic axis shortening, and velocity of circumferential fiber shortening are slightly elevated. "Normalization" of ejection fraction may actually reflect impaired myocardial function, whereas moderately decreased values (e.g., ejection fractions of 0.40 to 0.50) usually indicate severely impaired contractile function. An ejection fraction of less than 0.40 is usually a sign of advanced myocardial dysfunction. Such patients may improve symptomatically after mitral surgery but often, with progression of LV dysfunction, present with recurrent heart failure and incur a high mortality rate.[23] Patients with ischemic MR who frequently present with reduced LV function are also at an increased operative risk.[24, 25]

Acute Form

If MR develops suddenly with disruption of the mitral valve apparatus, the left atrium is unprepared and the rapid rise in LA pressure leads to dilatation of the left atrium, intimal proliferation with media hypertrophy of the pulmonary vessels, and hypertrophy of the right ventricle.[3] The low-impedance leak into the left atrium allows the left ventricle to maintain both ejection fraction and cardiac output at normal levels. However, when regurgitation is severe, stroke volume cannot be maintained and cardiac output falls. Acute severe MR, such as that seen in patients with mitral valve prolapse and ruptured chordae tendineae, or with perforation of leaflets, is often associated with acute pulmonary edema. The progression of these patients from the acute to the chronic stage is characterized by the enlargement of the left atrium and ventricle, which allows normalization of filling pressures and symptomatic improvement. Another important basis for acute severe MR is rupture of a papillary muscle in the setting of acute inferior wall myocardial infarction. Most commonly, this

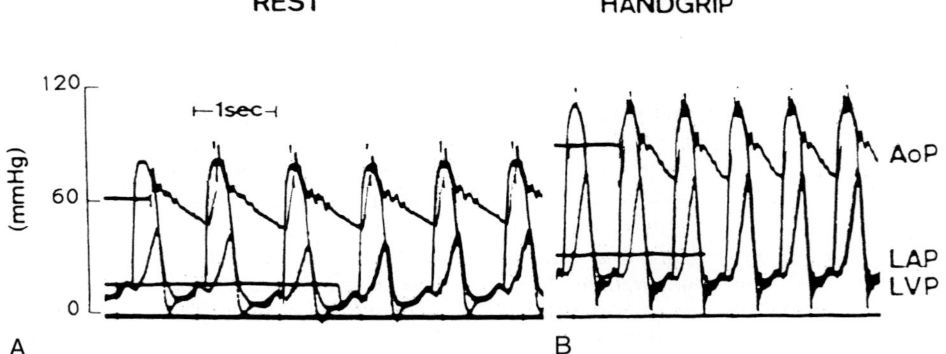

FIGURE 15–4 Pressure recording in a patient with severe mitral regurgitation at rest **(A)** and during maximal handgrip exercise for 2 minutes **(B)**. Aortic (AoP), left ventricular (LVP), and left atrial (LAP) pressures are shown, with the large V wave as an expression of mitral regurgitation. With isometric exercise, mean diastolic pressure *(solid line)* is doubled and V-wave pressure increases to 60 mm Hg.

occurs 2 to 3 days after the infarction and usually presents abruptly with shock and pulmonary edema. Prompt recognition of papillary muscle rupture in the setting of an inferior wall myocardial infarction is critical because surgery is lifesaving and must not be delayed.[26, 27]

Physical Examination

In chronic MR, a portion of the clinical findings result from a progressive enlargement of the LV and LA chambers to accommodate the regurgitant volume. The upstroke of the pulse pressure may be brisk, but because the left ventricle is unable to sustain forward ejection during the entire systole in the presence of severe regurgitation, the amplitude is normal or decreased, which allows differentiation from aortic regurgitation.[28] Jugular vein distention can occur in the presence of RV failure. Prominent A waves may accompany pulmonary hypertension, whereas large V waves may be seen with associated tricuspid regurgitation.

The apical impulse can be enlarged, displaced laterally and downward, and hyperdynamic in severe chronic MR. An early diastolic wave may be felt, which corresponds to the rapid filling phase and the presence of an S_3. A left parasternal RV lift may be felt in the presence of pulmonary hypertension and is difficult to differentiate from systolic expansion due to filling of the left atrium, which occurs later during systole.[29, 30]

S_1 is usually of normal or decreased intensity and is sometimes buried in a loud early holosystolic murmur. S_1 may be increased in intensity with associated mitral stenosis or when late systolic murmurs are present.

S_2 may be normal. The P_2 component may be prominent when pulmonary hypertension is present. A wide splitting of S_2 is sometimes present because of early closure of the aortic valve due to shortened LV ejection. A third heart sound may be heard even in the absence of LV failure when the regurgitation is significant. This sound must be distinguished from an opening snap, which occurs earlier in diastole, has a higher pitch, and is well heard with the diaphragm of the stethoscope.

The characteristic auscultatory finding of MR is a holosystolic murmur that begins with the first heart sound and extends beyond the closure of the aortic valve. The murmur is of blowing quality and high pitched, and typically radiates toward the axilla and the left infrascapular area. The radiation may be directed toward the left parasternal area when MR is due to an abnormal or a failing posterior leaflet, because the turbulent regurgitant jet is directed anteriorly.[31] In the presence of a failing anterior leaflet, the radiation may be posterior, to the back, and over the spine and may rarely be transmitted to the skull.[32, 33] The intensity of murmur is grossly correlated to the degree of regurgitation, although grade 3/6 murmurs observed in a large number of patients are of indeterminate significance.[34] Factors such as obesity, chest deformity, and ventricular dilatation may obscure the murmur. The severity of regurgitation can be better appreciated by the presence of LV enlargement, signs of hyperdynamism, S_3, and a diastolic flow murmur; the latter can be found in the absence of mitral stenosis and is caused by increased diastolic flow across the mitral valve.[35]

In mitral valve prolapse, a systolic click may be heard 0.14 second or longer (occasionally earlier with ejection timing) after S_1.[36–38] It may be followed, but rarely preceded, by a systolic murmur and is best heard with the diaphragm along the left sternal border. The click and the murmur may vary in intensity, and their delay after S_1 may vary with LV filling.[39] An early diastolic click or murmur may also be heard on the return of the prolapsing valve in the ventricle.[40] The severity of regurgitation tends to correlate with the length of the murmur during systole but not with the intensity of the murmur.

Late systolic murmurs may also be heard with papillary muscle dysfunction. They characteristically vary in intensity, being loud and sometimes holosystolic during ischemia and disappearing when ischemia is relieved.[41]

Unlike the murmur of aortic stenosis, the intensity of the murmur of mitral regurgitation varies little with changes in the cardiac cycle length. There also is little respiratory variation of the murmur. On the other hand, maneuvers that increase aortic pressure, such as squatting, isometric exercise, or infusion of pressor agents, increase the murmur, whereas sudden standing, the Valsalva maneuver, and inhalation of amyl nitrite diminish it.

The click and murmur of mitral valve prolapse are displaced toward S_1 by any maneuver that decreases LV volume, such as the Valsalva maneuver, inhalation of amyl nitrite, inspiration, or standing, because the prolapse tends to occur earlier. Conversely, maneuvers such as leg raising, squatting, and isometric exercise tend to increase LV size and delay the onset of the click and murmur.

In acute MR, the left ventricle and atrium are only slightly enlarged. A marked increase in LA pressure is seen, caused by a lack of adaptation and poor atrial compliance. Physical signs often include pulmonary congestion or edema, particularly when MR is associated with LV infarction. The LV impulse is not enlarged or displaced, but it may be hyperdynamic. A thrill is unusual. S_2 may be prominent, with associated pulmonary hypertension, and it may rarely be paradoxically split due to an early closure of the pulmonary valve caused by a large retrograde V wave. A prominent S_3 is heard when the mitral insufficiency is moderately severe or worse. The systolic murmur is often low pitched and decrescendo and may finish before A_2, when a marked increase in LA pressure limits the regurgitant flow. The radiation of the murmur depends on the cause of regurgitation, but often it is directed toward the base of the heart or to the back, as described earlier. In many patients, the murmur of MR associated with papillary muscle rupture in the setting of acute myocardial infarction may be absent or unimpressive. Prompt echocardiographic studies at the bedside or proceeding directly to cardiac catheterization is essential to establish the diagnosis and thus provide the opportunity for lifesaving surgical intervention.

Natural History

The clinical course in MR is a function of the severity of regurgitation. Patients with mild regurgitation may remain asymptomatic for their entire lives, whereas patients with mild to moderate regurgitation may show slow progression, with the appearance of symptoms in the fifth or sixth decade.[19, 21] With severe MR, progression is usually more rapid, but patients may remain asymptomatic until serious and irreversible ventricular dysfunction has occurred. This course contrasts with the progression of patients with mitral stenosis, who often already have symptoms at an early stage of the disease.[21] The development of atrial fibrillation may adversely affect the clinical course but not as dramatically as in mitral stenosis. Nevertheless, the natural history is often variable and depends on the severity of regurgitation, the state of the myocardium, and the underlying disease. Regurgitation tends to progress more rapidly in patients with connective tissue disorders than in those with rheumatic valve disease. Acute severe regurgitation may occur in patients with infective endocarditis, in those with myxomatous mitral valves when chordae tendineae rupture acutely, or secondary to papillary muscle rupture after myocardial infarction.

In an unselected group of patients with MR,[1] approximately 80 percent of patients survived after 5 years and 60 percent survived after 10 years (see Fig. 13–3).[19, 21] In patients with flail mitral leaflet, which exemplifies severe mitral MR, an excess mortality rate is observed in comparison with expected survival rates and is directly related to the valve regurgitation.[42] In these patients, a high morbidity rate also occurs; at 10 years after the diagnosis, 60 percent of patients have incurred heart failure, 30 percent have atrial fibrillation, and 90 percent of patients have undergone surgery or died.[42] In such patients, early operation immediately after diagnosis appears to improve prognosis.[43]

For patients with combined mitral stenosis and regurgitation, the prognosis is worse than that for those with pure MR. The survival rate is approximately 70 percent after 5 years and 30 percent after 10 years.

Fortunately, the refinement of surgical technique to repair valves with severe prolapse combined with intraoperative transesophageal echocardiography has led to earlier intervention in patients with severe MR. The rationale for early intervention in such patients is based on studies that demonstrate the advantage of repair versus replacement of the mitral valve[44] and the penalty associated with a delay in surgery until LV function is depressed.[45] Preoperative LV ejection fraction is the most powerful predictor of survival in patients with severe MR, and postoperative depression of LV function may persist even with preoperative LV ejection fractions between 0.50 and 0.60, particularly if end-systolic dimensions of the left ventricle exceed 40 mm[46] (Fig. 15–5). Furthermore, a delay in the repair of severe MR until patients have class 3/4 congestive heart failure is associated with a compromise in long-term survival.[47] Furthermore, as might be expected, patients with a compromise in preoperative LV function as assessed by estimates of LV ejection fraction have a greater likelihood of compromise in quality of life, with higher rates of congestive heart failure in long-term follow-up. A somewhat surprising rate of cardiac mortality and other events has been reported in patients with mitral flail leaflet and severe MR[48] (Fig. 15–6). Although these observational studies may be used to support early surgical intervention in patients with severe MR with mild or no symptoms, it is important to note that there are no randomized trials of early surgical intervention compared with pharmacologic treatment. Any recommendation for early mitral valve repair must be based on clear documentation of severe MR by quantitative echo-Doppler studies (or contrast ventriculography), lack of major comorbidities, and documented surgical expertise in the successful repair of mitral valves.

Medical Treatment

Digitalis and diuretics may relieve the symptoms of cardiac failure and are effective even in patients with normal sinus rhythm. For patients with atrial fibrillation, digitalis or β-blockers may also improve hemodynamics and symptoms by slowing the ventricular response rate. However, patients with severe MR should ideally have relief of their LV volume overload before progression to severe symptoms or deterioration of LV function.

Acute MR may respond dramatically to the use of vasodilators, such as nitroprusside. This major beneficial effect is due to the decrease in LA pressure, but the decrease in the degree of regurgitation achieved has not been documented.[49] Intra-aortic balloon counterpulsation may be lifesaving in patients with severe regurgitation and marked

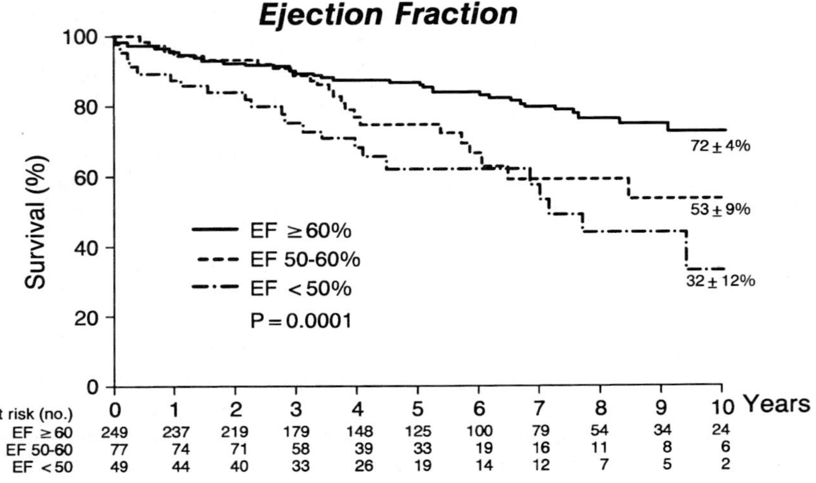

FIGURE 15–5 Postoperative survival according to preoperative ejection fraction (EF) in patients with chronic organic mitral regurgitation. Note the significant and major differences among the three subsets. (Reproduced with authorization from the American Heart Association.)

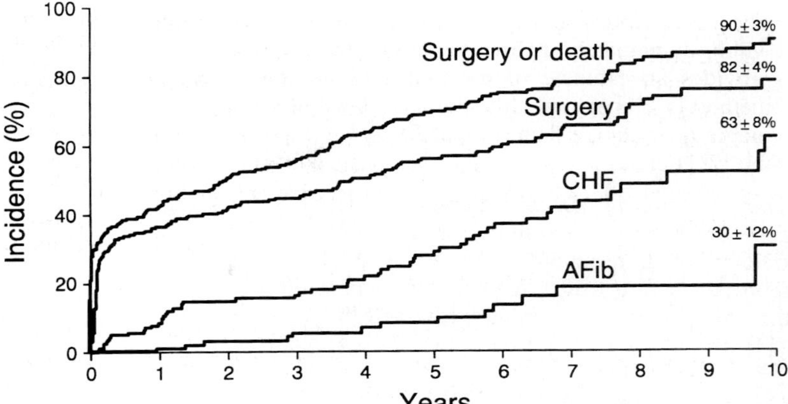

FIGURE 15–6 Cardiovascular events occurring after the diagnosis of mitral regurgitation owing to flail leaflets. Note the high morbidity rates. At 10 years, 90 percent of patients either died or were operated on, showing that surgery is almost unavoidable in these patients. AFib, atrial fibrillation; CHF, congestive heart failure. (Reproduced with authorization of the Massachusetts Medical Society.)

cardiac failure or shock while they are being prepared for surgery.

Vasodilators, especially angiotensin-converting enzyme inhibitors, have been shown to reduce regurgitant volume and to decrease LV size and mitral orifice area, both acutely and chronically.[50–52] In other studies, no significant decrease in the degree of MR could be observed with the use of these medications.[53] Similarly, a beneficial effect of angiotensin-converting enzyme inhibitors on LV remodeling in patients with MR due to organic valve disease is uncertain.[54–56]

Assessment of Severity of Mitral Regurgitation and Its Treatment

Robert L. Frye and Maurice Enriquez-Sarano

Doppler Echocardiographic Semiquantitative Methods

Color flow imaging of the jet demonstrates the origin and direction of the jet. The jet length, the ratio of the jet area to the left atrial area,[57] and the jet area[58] have been suggested as good indices of the severity of regurgitation. Small jets, such as those seen in normal subjects, consistently correspond to mild regurgitation[59]; however, color flow imaging has significant limitations that are technical, but also, more importantly, intrinsically related to the nature of regurgitant jets. The extent of a jet is determined by its momentum and thus as much as by regurgitant velocity as by regurgitant flow. In addition, jets are constrained by the left atrium and expand more in large atria.[57, 59] The eccentric jets of valve prolapse[60] impinge on the LA wall[61] and tend to underestimate the MR.[59, 62] The central jets of ischemic or functional MR expand markedly in the enlarged left atrium and tend to overestimate the MR.[59] Transesophageal echocardiography usually shows larger jets but does not suppress these limitations of color flow imaging.

The density of the *continuous-wave Doppler* signal[63] reflects grossly the degree of MR in that it is determined by the number of moving red blood cells within the beam of ultrasound. However, eccentric jets are often captured on a short length and are often of low density.

Pulmonary venous velocity profile is useful to assess the degree of MR.[64, 65] Systolic reversal of flow in the pulmonary veins is a strong argument for severe regurgitation. Unfortunately, there is an important interaction among MR severity, direction of the jet, LA pressure, and the occurrence of pulmonary venous flow reversal.[66] This sign may be absent or asymmetric in severe MR.[66] It is not specific of severe regurgitation and may be observed in patients with elevated LA pressure or a markedly enlarged left atrium.

Doppler Echocardiographic Quantitative Methods

The *goal of quantitative methods* is to assess the volume overload expressed as the regurgitant volume per beat or the regurgitant fraction, which is the proportion of the LV ejection volume regurgitated in the left atrium. The regurgitant lesion can be expressed as the effective regurgitant orifice (ERO) area.[67, 68]

The *methods used* for the quantification of MR are as follows:

- *Quantitative Doppler* is based on the calculation of the mitral and aortic stroke volumes with the use of pulsed-wave Doppler.[69, 70] The principle is simple and applicable in most cases, but the measurement of the mitral stroke volume is technically demanding, with a significant learning phase.[69]
- *Quantitative two-dimensional echocardiography* is of a similar principle but is based on the measurement of LV volumes for total stroke volume calculation.[71]
- Conversely, the *proximal isovelocity surface area* method directly measures the regurgitant flow by analyzing the flow convergence region proximal to the regurgitant orifice; the method is based on the principle of conservation of mass.[72] Because color flow mapping allows the precise determination of the velocity in the flow convergence region, the regurgitant flow can be calculated.[73] With knowledge of the regurgitant flow and the regurgitant velocities, the ERO and the regurgitant volume can be calculated.[68, 74] This method is simple and accurate if the assumptions are respected.[75]

- The *vena contracta* method measures the smallest jet width immediately below the regurgitant orifice[76] and provides an estimate of the radius of the ERO.[77] This method is simple, and although it does not provide physiologic quantitative data, it appears to correlate well with the ERO area.[78]

The *gradation of MR* with these quantitative indices suggests that regurgitant volumes of at least 60 ml, regurgitant fraction of at least 50%, and ERO of at least 40 mm^2 represent severe MR.[79] A vena contracta width of at least 0.5 cm appears to represent severe MR.[80]

Cardiac Catheterization

The major hemodynamic consequences of MR are a reduced cardiac output and an elevated LA pressure; however, the LA pressure may be normal because of the compensatory effect of LA enlargement.[81] Similarly, a large V wave is less frequent in chronic than in acute MR and is not specific for MR.[82]

The degree of MR can be assessed with LV selective angiography and can be qualitatively graded in three or four grades on the basis of the degree and persistence of opacification of the left atrium.[83] This classic method has limitations similar to those of all qualitative methods.[84]

The quantification of MR can be obtained by comparing the angiographic stroke volume with the forward stroke volume as calculated by the Fick or by the thermodilution method[85] to calculate the regurgitant volume and fraction. The angiographic stroke volume usually overestimates the true stroke volume, and correction factors have been used to minimize the overestimation of the regurgitant volume. Angiographic quantification of MR is difficult and has a potentially high range of error,[86] which cannot be verified by the use of combined methods or by repeating the measurements.

Strategy of Laboratory Testing

It is not necessary to perform all of the tests in all patients with MR.

Transthoracic Doppler echocardiography is used to confirm the diagnosis of MR, demonstrate associated valvular disease, and assess the morphologic lesions of the mitral valve and is performed in most cases for the initial diagnosis, for follow-up, and for presurgical assessment. Transesophageal echocardiography provides high-resolution imaging, but its incremental value has not been fully documented.[87] In our practice, it is reserved preoperatively for patients in whom the presence of lesions (especially if endocarditis is suspected) or the severity of MR is uncertain, but it is used on a large scale intraoperatively to monitor the results of valve repair.[88, 90]

LV angiography is not mandatory unless there is concern regarding the validity of echocardiographic studies.[91] Although discrepancies between color flow Doppler and angiography may be observed,[92] the understanding of the pitfalls of color Doppler[59] and the introduction of quantitative methods have reduced the need for redundant tests.

Coronary angiography is indicated as a presurgical procedure depending on age. Coronary stenoses may be present even in the absence of angina,[93, 94] and coronary angiography is ordinarily performed in patients older than 40 to 50 years.[95]

These general guidelines should be individualized in clinical practice. In our practice, the use of tests is performed stepwise and based on the patient's characteristics and the results of noninvasive studies.

MITRAL PROLAPSE (MYXOMATOUS MITRAL VALVE)

Elliot Chesler

History

Interest in the mid ejection or nonejection systolic click has fascinated clinicians for a long time and was seminal in development of the knowledge of *mitral valve prolapse.* In 1913, Gallavardin[96] thought the click was of extracardiac origin, but in 1961, Reid[97] recorded a midsystolic click followed by a late systolic murmur and correctly reasoned that both probably arose from one of the atrioventricular valves. The relationship among the late systolic murmur, nonejection click, prolapse of the mitral leaflets, and MR was firmly established by Barlow and Pocock[98] in 1963 with cine-angiography. These authors credited the assistance of Criley and associates,[99] who interpreted their angiograms and subsequently introduced the term *prolapse* to describe the appearance produced by protrusion of the posterior mitral leaflet into the left atrium.

There followed the rapid recognition of various clinical and electrocardiographic abnormalities. Complications such as infective endocarditis, rupture of the chordae tendineae, systemic embolism, dysrhythmias, sudden death, and neuroendocrine and psychiatric abnormalities were described in rapid succession.[100–112] The advent of M-mode echocardiography helped clarify the effects of posture and other maneuvers that affect the click and murmur and was widely used for population surveys. The interest of echocardiographers was further boosted by the two-dimensional technique, which greatly facilitated the detection of abnormal leaflets and rupture of chordae tendineae.[100, 102–104]

Importantly, pathologists precisely defined the gross and microscopic abnormalities of the mitral valve by showing that *myxomatous degeneration* was the crucial alteration in the leaflets that predisposed them to redundancy, prolapse, and sometimes rupture of chordae tendineae. In addition, genetic studies identified that the myxomatous mitral valve is transmissible as an autosomal dominant associated with other heritable abnormalities of connective tissue, typically Marfan's syndrome.[105–108]

In the 1990s alone, more than 1500 articles relating to mitral valve prolapse (MVP) were published in peer-reviewed journals.[109, 110] Other articles in daily tabloids may have contributed to the establishment of centers for treatment and support groups for "victims" of MVP. Although this may have surrounded the condition with some atmosphere of pantomime, there should be no illusion about its importance; it affects approximately 4 percent of the population and after the decline in the incidence of rheumatic fever has become the leading cause of MR in the United States.

Nomenclature

The surfeit of names given to this condition indicates the confusion and disagreement among physicians. Apart from eponyms such as "Barlow's syndrome," other terminology refers to some anatomic or functional abnormality: "myxomatous," "floppy," "hooded," "billowing," "prolapsing" mitral valve, the "systolic click-murmur syndrome," "anatomic MVP," "MVP syndrome," and "billowing mitral leaflet syndrome," among others.

This semantic confusion has been aggravated by echocardiographers attempting to measure and define what constitutes "normal" superior systolic displacement as distinct from "abnormal prolapse" of mitral valve leaflets.[111, 112] Prolapse detected with echocardiography does not necessarily imply that the valve is abnormal. In atrial septal defect and hypertrophic obstructive cardiomyopathy, the prolapse of normal leaflets may occur due to a disproportionate relation between the volume of the left ventricle and the size of the mitral annulus ("secondary MVP").[113, 114] This may also occur in inferior myocardial infarction and other myocardial diseases such as myocarditis and cardiomyopathy due to the failure of chordal systolic tension. Under these circumstances, the clinical picture is usually dominated by the underlying disease, and prolapse is a secondary finding. The prolapse of normal leaflets has also been reported in trained athletes and nonathletic young women.[115, 116] In all of these instances, the leaflets appear thin and do not have the thickness and redundancy of a myxomatous mitral valve or its associated pathologic features such as LV endocardial friction lesions and LA angle lesions, which are recognizable by two-dimensional echocardiography.

Definition

Because the term *mitral valve prolapse* is widely accepted, it seems reasonable to restrict its use to that condition in which the observed clinical and echocardiographic features are compatible with those of a myxomatous mitral valve. Prolapse of normal leaflets (secondary MVP) observed as an incidental complication of diseases of the left ventricle should not enter into this consideration.

Pathology

Normal Mitral Valve

GROSS ANATOMY

The mitral valve has two leaflets attached at their bases to the annulus fibrosis and by their free edges to their chordae tendineae[105, 107, 108] (Fig. 15–7). Each leaflet has a rough zone toward the free edge and a central clear zone toward the base. The anterior leaflet forms one third and the posterior leaflet forms two thirds of the annulus. The anterior leaflet is approximately triangular in shape, and its base is attached by a fibrous connection to the root of the aorta. The posterior leaflet is narrower than the anterior leaflet and is a continuation of the LA endocardium across the AV ring.

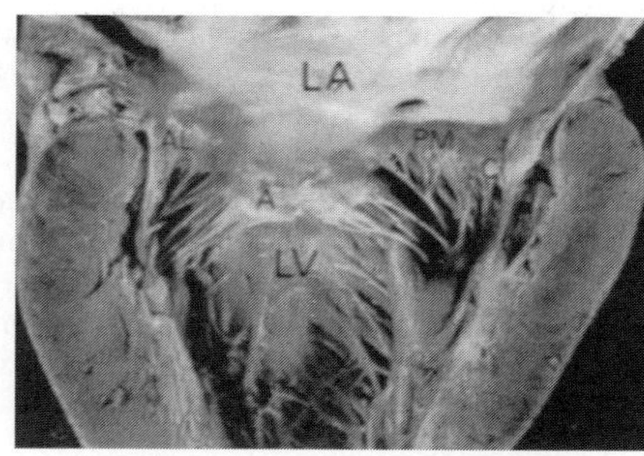

FIGURE 15–7 Normal mitral valve. The anterior leaflet (A) is large and triangular. The posterior leaflet has three scallops: anterolateral (AL), posteromedial (PM), and central (C). Mild interchordal hooding is present at the edge of the leaflet. LA, left atrium. LV, left ventricle. (From Lucas R, Edwards JE: The floppy mitral valve. Curr Probl Cardiol 7:5, 1982.)

Although the leaflets are of different shapes, their surface areas are approximately the same. In most patients, the posterior leaflet is composed of three scallops, named according to their position in relation to the commissures of the mitral valve: *posteromedial, central,* and *anterolateral.* In the normal mitral valve, there also are interchordal convexities protruding toward the left atrium that vary considerably in height. Because the leaflets are thin and pliable, LV pressure causes a certain amount of "hooding" of interchordal tissue, even in the normal valve.

MICROSCOPIC ANATOMY

The leaflets are composed of four layers: auricularis, fibrosa, ventricularis, and spongiosa.

The *auricularis* is composed of collagen and elastic tissue that forms the contact or atrial aspect of the leaflet (Fig. 15–8). This layer is continuous with the endocardium of the left atrium.

The *fibrosa* constitutes the basic support for the leaflet and is composed of thick collagen. This layer is continuous

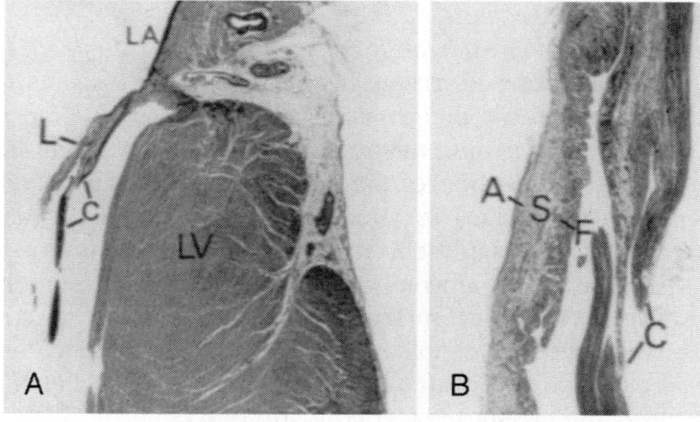

FIGURE 15–8 Photomicrographs of normal mitral valve **(A)** and components of the leaflet **(B)**. A, auricularis; C, chordae; F, fibrosa; L, leaflets; LA, left atrium; LV, left ventricle; S, spongiosa. (**A** and **B,** From Guthrie RB, Edwards JE: Pathology of the myxomatous mitral valve. Minn Med 59:637, 1976.)

at its base with either the fibrous tissue of the annulus, as in the case of the posterior leaflet, or the aortic root, as in the case of the anterior leaflet. Its free edge is continuous with the chordae tendineae.

The *ventricularis* is a thin layer of collagen and elastic tissue that covers the ventricular aspect of the fibrosa and is continuous in the case of the posterior leaflet with LV endocardium; it is considered to be part of the fibrosa.

The *spongiosa* or fourth layer is situated between the auricularis and fibrosa layers and is formed by delicate myxomatous connective tissue.

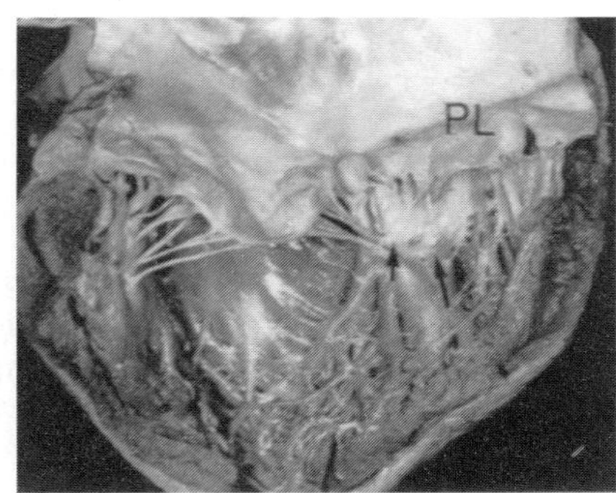

FIGURE 15–9 Myxomatous mitral valve shows redundancy of anterior and posterior mitral leaflets with obvious prolapse. Note extensive endocardial fibrosis below the posterior mitral leaflet (PL). (From The Jesse E. Edwards Registry of Cardiovascular Diseases.)

Myxomatous Mitral Valve

GROSS ANATOMY

The criteria for making a gross diagnosis of myxomatous mitral valve have been well summarized (Fig. 15–9)[117]:

1. Interchordal hooding involving both rough and clear zones of the involved leaflet or leaflets
2. Height of interchordal hooding exceeding 4 mm
3. Interchordal hooding involving at least half of the anterior leaflet or two thirds of the posterior leaflet

Typically, the posterior leaflet is involved either alone or more prominently than the anterior leaflet. The leaflet tissue, which is abnormally hooded, is also translucent or opaque. The degree of interchordal hooding is variable, so there is an intermediate zone between the obviously abnormal and the clearly normal that even experienced pathologists may find difficult to evaluate without histologic confirmation. The condition of the chordae tendineae is variable: some are elongated, thickened, and even fused, and this may be confused with rheumatic disease. However, commissural fusion is absent, and this makes the distinction possible.

SECONDARY EFFECTS

1. *Fibrosis of the free aspect of the leaflet.* Fibrosis at the summit of the atrial aspect of prolapsing portions of the leaflet is believed to be a response to injury when the leaflet makes contact with an opposite element or adjacent segment of the valve. The fibrosis involves the auricularis layer.
2. *Fibrous deposits on the LV surface of the leaflets.* Fibrous deposits occur in the noncontact aspects of the leaflets in the concavity of prolapsed segments and are a response to stretching and tension that occur when that portion of the leaflet prolapses. Occasionally, this fibrous reaction between inserting chordae extends to related chordae, but the basic anatomy of the leaflets remains normal. This is important in making the distinction from chronic rheumatic mitral valve disease: a myxomatous mitral valve may become fibrotic, but not all layers of the leaflet are affected as in chronic rheumatic mitral valve disease. In addition, like marked secondary leaflet fibrosis, commissural fusion is characteristically absent.
3. *LV endocardial friction lesions.* A secondary effect produced by the myxomatous mitral valve involves the mural endocardium of the left ventricle in relation to the insertion of chordae into the posterior mitral valve leaflet (Fig. 15–10). Initially, the chordae tendineae are long and thin, but eventually they may become thickened by aggregation of fibrous tissue on their surfaces. When the posterior mitral leaflet protrudes into the left atrium, the chordae make contact with the related LV mural endocardium, causing a fibrous reaction. These lesions initially are discrete linear thickenings of the endocardium but subsequently may coalesce so that considerable portions of the base of the left ventricle become thickened and even calcified. Because the chordae adhere to the mural endocardium, they may become shortened and incorporated into the fibrous tissue. This may yield a complex picture that can easily be misinterpreted as the end result of infective endocarditis or rheumatic fever.

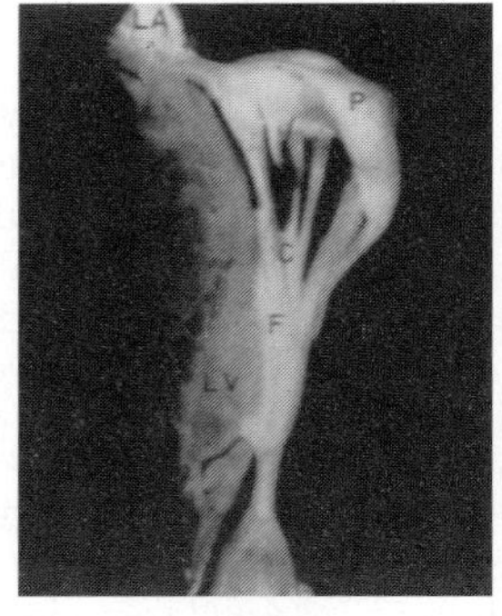

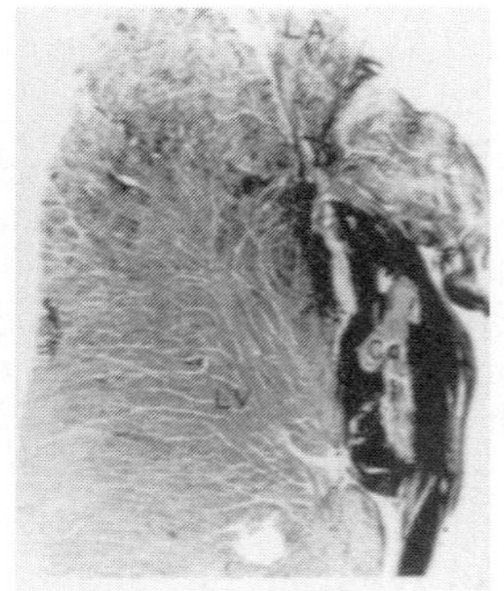

FIGURE 15–10 A, Cross section of myxomatous posterior mitral leaflet, chordae, adjacent left ventricle, and left atrium. Mural endocardium of the left ventricle is markedly thickened, and lower portions of the chordae are incorporated into this fibrous tissue. **B,** Photomicrograph of region illustrated in **A** shows myxomatous posterior mitral leaflet above an extensive, calcified endocardial friction lesion. C, chordae; CA, calcification; F, mural left ventricle endocardium; LA, left atrium; LV, left ventricle; P, posterior mitral leaflet. (**A** and **B,** Reprinted from Am J Cardiol, Vol. 60, Chesler E, Gomick C, Edwards J, Calcification of the mural endocardium of the left ventricle complicating the myxomatous mitral valve, p. 1197, Copyright 1987, with permission from Elsevier Science.)

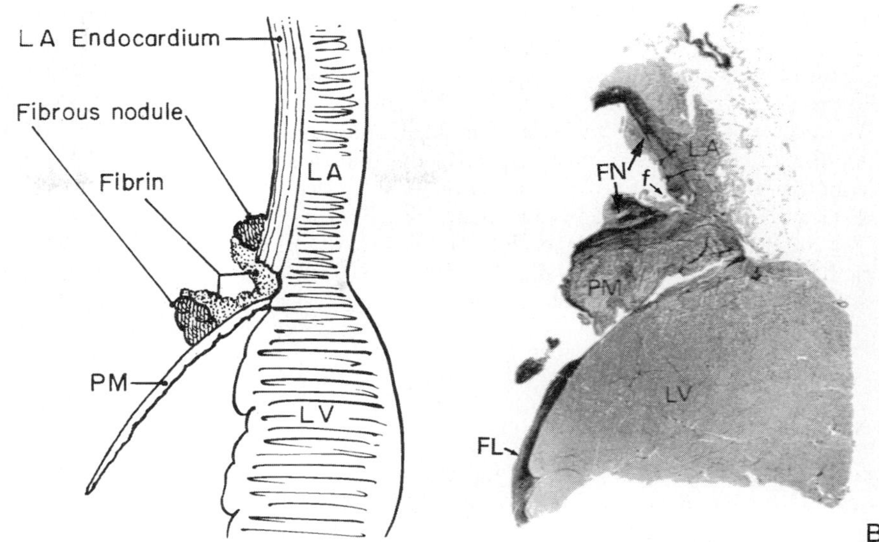

FIGURE 15–11 Diagram **(A)** and photomicrograph **(B)** of the junction of the left atrium (LA) and the posterior mitral leaflet (PM) and related left ventricular wall (LV). There is deposition of fibrin (f) in the angle between the posterior mitral leaflet and the left atrial (LA) endocardium. Fibrous nodules (FN) are present both above the angle, involving the left atrial wall, and below the angle, involving the superior surface of the posterior mitral leaflet. A friction lesion (FL) of the left ventricular endocardium is present in **B**. (Elastic tissue stain, magnification 40×.) (**A** and **B,** From Chesler E, King R, Edwards J: The myxomatous mitral valve and sudden death. Circulation 67:632, 1983.)

4. *LA angle lesion.* The LA angle lesion is situated in the angle between the posterior mitral leaflet and the LA wall; it also consists of an aggregation of platelets and thrombus that may eventually calcify (Fig. 15–11). The lesion occurs as a result of friction between the posterior leaflet and the LA wall.[118]
5. *Contact thrombosis.* Contact thrombosis may be found on the atrial aspect of prolapsed units. It consists of an aggregation of platelets and thrombi. Contact thrombosis on either the leaflets or the LA angle lesion is considered a source of systemic embolism.

MICROSCOPIC ANATOMY

The primary abnormality occurs in the spongiosa layer, which is characteristically thickened by the deposition of acid mucopolysaccharides (Fig. 15–12). This layer encroaches on and invades the other layers, particularly the fibrosa. Because the fibrosa represents the chief support for the leaflets, focal interruption by myxomatous infiltration weakens the leaflet, and "hooding" into the left atrium results from the force of LV systole in stretching the interchordal tissue.

Genetics

Most studies strongly favor that the myxomatous mitral valve is inherited. Family studies indicate that expression of the genes for the myxomatous valve is affected by both age and sex. In the first 93 families studied by Devereux and associates,[119] the proportion of affected first-degree relatives was approximately 50 percent among adult, female first-degree relatives younger than 50 years, which is compatible with a fully expressed autosomal dominant disorder. Lower prevalence rates were found among adult men, older women, and children.

Epidemiology

Most studies of the prevalence of MVP have been based on findings derived from echocardiography. These studies have inherent disadvantages, not only because the criteria for diagnosis of degrees of prolapse are extremely variable among the study groups but also because of considerable variation in interobserver and intraobserver interpretation. Other studies have been biased because subjects volunteered in response to advertisement, making it difficult to exclude the possibility that the "volunteers" knew they had some form of heart disease.[116] As indicated earlier, some interchordal hooding is present even in the normal mitral valve; therefore, the findings from large-scale echocardiographic epidemiologic studies should be interpreted with caution. The hazard of attempting to identify minor degrees of prolapse is that it artificially increases the "background prevalence" of the condition and increases the chances of finding a coincidental association with some other disease or symptom.

Most studies indicate that the myxomatous mitral valve is identified in approximately 4 percent of the population.[112] The prevalence rate is lower in childhood and adolescence but increases with advancing years. Clinical observations indicate a higher frequency in older age groups, particularly men, who also tend to have more severe valve and LV dysfunction.[120] The prevalence rate in women, but not in men, decreases with age.

Associated Abnormalities

Skeletal

Pectus excavatum, straight back, scoliosis, and high-arched palate are associated with MVP. When these thoracic deformities are present, a diligent search should be made for the presence of a myxomatous mitral valve.[121, 122]

Inherited Disorders of Connective Tissue

An association with Marfan's and Ehlers-Danlos syndromes is well established. These findings suggest that there is a reasonable possibility of finding a myxomatous mitral valve in patients with other generalized disorders of connective tissue, such as pseudoxanthoma elasticum.[122]

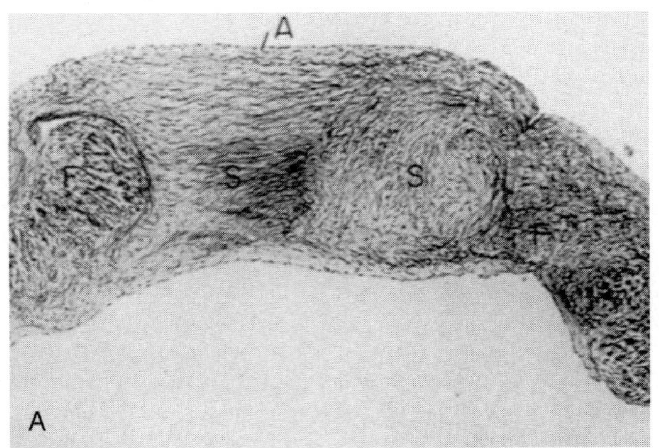

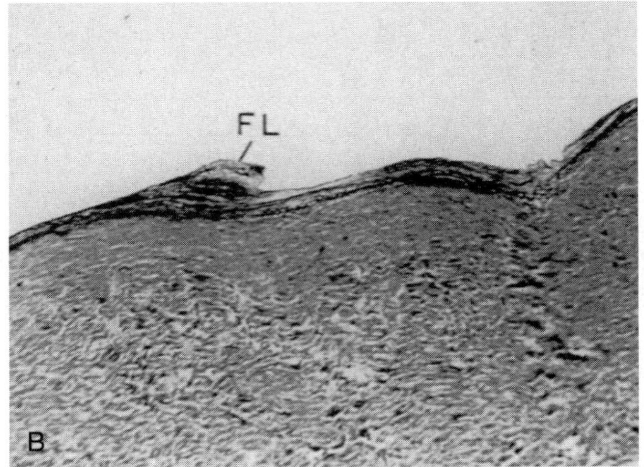

FIGURE 15–12 Photomicrographs of posterior mitral leaflet **(A)** and related left ventricular endocardium **(B)**. Spongiosa layer (S) in the leaflet is increased and encroaches on the atrialis (A) and fibrosa (F) layers. **B,** A fibrous friction lesion (FL) of endocardium adjacent to chordae of the posterior leaflets. (**A** and **B,** From Chesler E, King R, Edwards J: The myxomatous mitral valve and sudden death. Circulation 67[3]:632–639, 1983.)

Other Conditions

MVP has been described in association with a host of other disorders, such as rheumatic endocarditis, coronary artery disease, congestive and hypertrophic cardiomyopathy, myocarditis, trauma, LA myxoma, systemic lupus erythematosus, LV aneurysm, migraine, hypomagnesemia, and congenital heart disease (including atrial and ventricular septal defects, patent ductus arteriosus, absence of the pericardium, membranous subaortic stenosis, and others).[123] However, it was pointed out earlier that many of these associations relate to "secondary MVP," in which LV-LA disproportion produces minor bulging of normal leaflets into the left atrium.

Obviously, there must be a fortuitous concurrence of a myxomatous valve with other abnormalities. Because MVP is identified in approximately 4 percent of the population, coincidental association will be most likely when some other condition, whether cardiac or noncardiac (e.g., migraine[124] or mitral annular calcification), also occurs with some frequency in the general population. For example, it is not surprising that MVP has been described in association with mitral annular calcification in women in their 70s because approximately three fourths of such individuals are found to have some degree of calcification at autopsy.[125] Similarly, a pathologic study found a high incidence (18 percent) of myxomatous valves among patients with ventricular septal defect, but a careful comparison with other information in that report suggested that they were unrelated occurrences.[125]

The effect of *patient selection* and *ascertainment bias* is illustrated by the purported association between MVP and hyperthyroidism. By studying the prevalence of all types of thyroid disorders among family members with and without MVP, Zullo and colleagues[126] were unable to demonstrate a valid statistical link between hyperthyroidism and symptomatic subjects with MVP. Such noncausal associations are likely to be identified in populations that share multiple symptoms: in MVP and hyperthyroidism, the common symptom is palpitation, and this leads to ascertainment bias.[127]

Clinical Findings

Symptoms

It is virtually certain that the majority of subjects with myxomatous mitral valve and varying degrees of MVP are asymptomatic and never seek medical attention. However, there is a group of patients purported to have an "MVP syndrome" who present with a variety of symptoms that have attracted considerable attention. These nonspecific symptoms include palpitation, fatigue, left inframammary pain, dizziness, syncope, or presyncope. The difficulty in reconciling the ocurrence of similar auscultatory, echocardiographic, and electrocardiographic features among patients with and without the above symptoms was clearly recognized by Barlow and Pocock,[123] who emphasized that patients with marked prolapse are not necessarily symptomatic, yet some with mild prolapse may have numerous symptoms.[123]

The symptoms described in association with MVP are indistinguishable from those occurring in DaCosta's syndrome, neurocirculatory asthenia, and "Soldier's heart" and were considered by Paul Wood to be a psychiatric disorder (anxiety state).[128] In modern terminology, these symptoms are classified as "panic disorder with somatization"[129] and affect 2 to 5 percent of the general population, 10 to 14 percent of patients in cardiologic practice, and 6 to 10 percent of patients attending primary care clinics.[130, 131] In a review of 55 patients with panic disorder, Katon[129] noted that such patients often focus on one or two somatic symptoms of the disorder for which they seek medical help; primary among the somatic presentations are cardiac symptoms.[129]

Some authors have claimed an association among anxiety state, panic disorder, agoraphobia, and MVP, but others have denied this relationship. Leatham and Brigden[132] believed that "isolated disease of the mitral valve causing mild or moderate reflux seldom causes symptoms other than those of iatrogenic anxiety." Hickey and associates[133] studied 103 patients with echocardiographically proved MVP and found that the scores for neuroticism and neurotic symptoms did not differ from those in patients with other cardiac diseases or from patients presenting to primary care physicians. Uretsky[134] studied 927 patients in an adult general medical population and found that the incidence of atypical chest pain (17.4 versus 17.2 percent) and chronic anxiety (7.1 versus 10.7 percent) was not significantly different for patients with MVP compared with healthy subjects. A study of 42 young soldiers with neurocirculatory asthenia found that the prevalence of MVP was similar to that in the general population.[135] In our study of 10 patients, the results of the Minnesota Multiphasic Personality Inventory, State Trait Anxiety Score, and Psychological Present State Examination showed no difference between patients with MVP and control subjects.[136] In an extensive review, Margraf and colleagues[137] concluded that there was no functional relationship between MVP and panic disorders and that *comorbidity* in highly symptomatic individuals was the likely explanation. Thus, it is highly likely that there is no causal relationship between psychiatric disorder and the myxomatous mitral valve and that the symptoms are probably a result of superimposed or iatrogenic-induced anxiety in a select group of individuals who have been subjected to excessive medical attention.

Physical Examination

GENERAL FINDINGS

Occasionally, there are some features of Marfan's syndrome or formes frustes (i.e., high arched palate or chest wall deformity such as pectus excavatum or scoliosis).

PRECORDIAL PALPATION

This is normal unless there is significant MR associated with severe prolapse or rupture of the chordae. Under these circumstances, palpation may detect evidence of hyperdynamic LV enlargement and, occasionally, a late systolic "LA lift" produced by severe MR.

AUSCULTATION

The Click. This is a high-pitched sound occurring in midsystole that has therefore been termed "nonejection." It is frequently the feature that attracts medical attention. It is heard in the region between the apex and the left sternal border. Careful timing in the use of M-mode echocardiography has shown that the click coincides with the position of maximal excursion of the posterior leaflet in midsystole, when there is likely to be the most tension on the chordal-leaflet structures. Occasionally, a diastolic sound may be recorded when a voluminous posterior leaflet slaps against the anterior leaflet in early diastole[100] (Fig. 15–13).

Depending on volume changes in the left ventricle, the click may occur quite early in systole (Fig. 15–14). However, it can be differentiated from an aortic ejection click because it occurs after the beginning of the upstroke of the carotid pulse. Not infrequently, there are multiple systolic

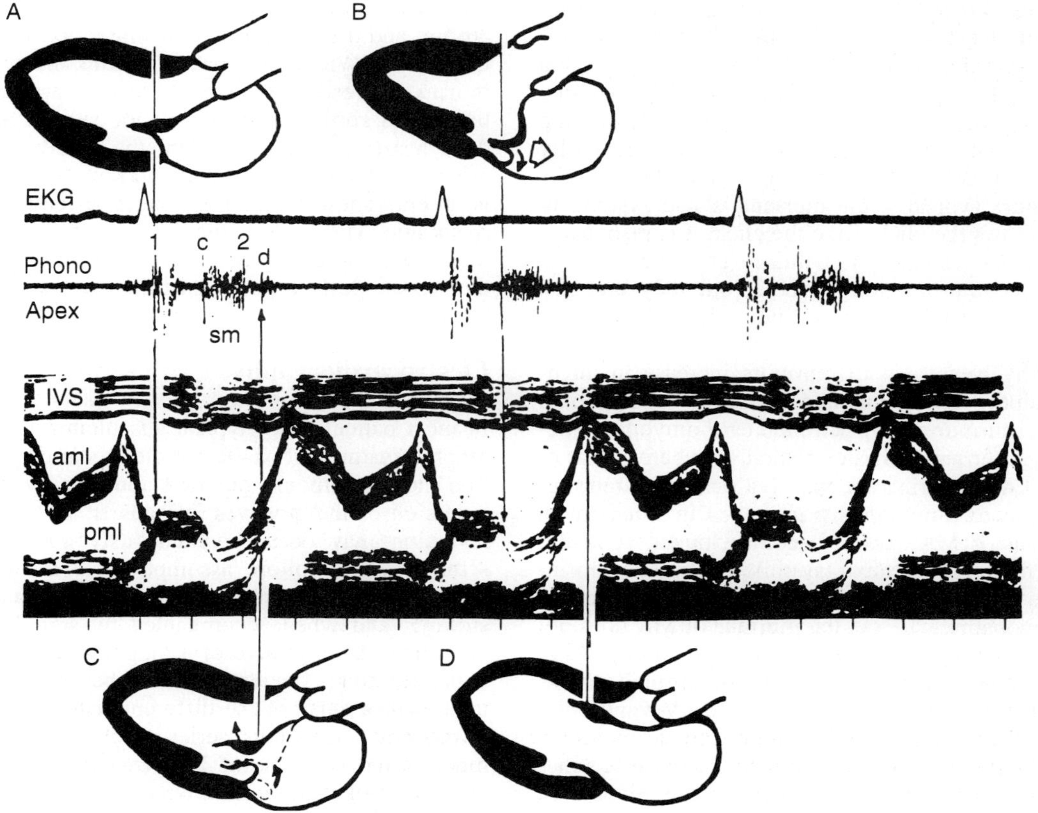

FIGURE 15–13 Simultaneous electrocardiogram (EKG), phonocardiogram (Phono), and M-mode echocardiogram in mitral valve prolapse. Ventricular angiography is depicted in **A–D**. The phonocardiogram demonstrates a midsystolic click (c), late systolic murmur (M), and an opening sound early in diastole (D). First heart sound occurs at the onset of ventricular systole **(A)**; in midsystole **(B)**, there is a click and late systolic murmur as the mitral valve leaflets bulge into the left atrium. In early diastole **(C)**, the leaflets swing open, resulting in a diastolic opening sound (d); in **D**, the leaflets reach their maximal diastolic excursion as the anterior mitral leaflet (aml) echo strikes the ventricular septum. IVS, interventricular septum; pml, posterior mitral leaflet. (**A–D,** From Criley JM, Siegel RJ: Functional anatomy and pathophysiology of mitral valve prolapse. *In* Mitral Valve Prolapse and the Mitral Valve Prolapse Syndrome. Mount Kisco, NY: Futura, 1988.)

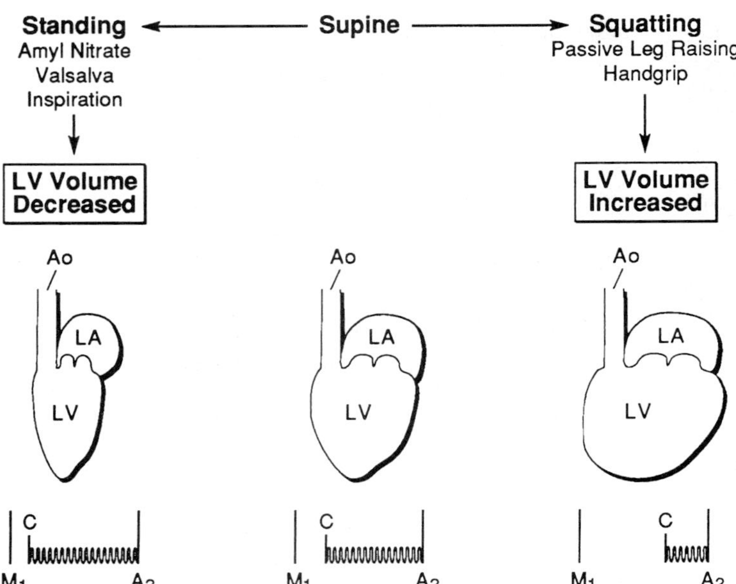

FIGURE 15–14 Diagram illustrates the effect of volume changes on portions of click and murmur. (See text for details.)

clicks. The clue to the proper identification of nonejection systolic clicks is the dynamic demonstration of their mobility induced by changes in LV volume. Maneuvers that increase ventricular volume, such as squatting, phenylephrine administration, and passive leg raising, shift the click later in systole, whereas maneuvers that decrease LV volume, such as standing, amyl nitrate inhalation, or Valsalva maneuver, shift the click earlier in systole. These volume changes within the left ventricle are responsible for the characteristic day-to-day and often hour-to-hour variability that occurs in the detection and timing of the click.

The Murmur. Typically, the murmur is late systolic in timing and follows the click. Like the click, it is responsive to maneuvers that change LV volume. The intensity and character of the murmur are variable, but they are best heard at the apex or left midprecordium when MR is mild. The murmur may be confused with that of hypertrophic cardiomyopathy because both murmurs increase in intensity and duration with standing and decrease with squatting. However, the murmur of hypertrophic cardiomyopathy becomes louder after amyl nitrate inhalation, whereas that of MR does not. Also, during the Valsalva strain, the murmur of hypertrophic cardiomyopathy increases in intensity in contrast to that of MR, which becomes longer. A useful auscultatory finding is postextrasystolic potentiation in intensity of the murmur, which is quite marked in hypertrophic cardiomyopathy, whereas the murmur of MR does not usually change or may actually decrease in intensity. In any event, the other typical features of hypertrophic cardiomyopathy, such as jerky pulses and severe LV ventricular hypertrophy detected clinically with electrocardiography and echocardiography, usually suffice to make the distinction.

When the myxomatous change in the leaflets is severe, and particularly when the chordae rupture, the murmur of MR is holosystolic and may have a loud vibratory "honking" quality. The clinical picture produced by rupture of chordae tendineae to the *posterior leaflet* is quite characteristic. Because the regurgitant jet is often directed anteriorly, striking the atrial septum adjacent to the aortic root, the systolic murmur is most prominent in the aortic area and may therefore be confused with the murmur of aortic stenosis. When chordae to the *anterior leaflet* rupture, the regurgitant jet is directed to the posterior wall of the left atrium, and the murmur is transmitted to the spine, or even the occiput. With both types of rupture, the systolic murmur is usually crescendo-decrescendo in shape and terminates before the aortic component of the second heart sound. A third heart sound is common, the first heart sound is of normal or increased intensity, and a mid-diastolic murmur is absent. These findings are quite different from those of rheumatic MR, where the first heart sound is soft, the holosystolic murmur ends after the second heart sound, and there is a significant mid-diastolic murmur.

Electrocardiography

In most patients with typical auscultatory and echocardiographic features of MVP, the electrocardiogram is normal. The most commonly reported abnormality is flattening or inversion of the T waves in leads II, III and aVF. T-wave inversion may occur spontaneously and independent of effort or may follow assumption of the erect position. Occasionally, these inferior repolarization changes are quite striking, and when accompanied by significant Q waves, they may be suggestive of a diagnosis of inferior myocardial infarction. The exact prevalence of these findings is unknown because of the different criteria for the selection of patients in various series. McLaren and associates[138] reported an incidence of 7 percent in a survey of asymptomatic black school children with MVP in Johannesburg. On the other hand, the Framingham Heart Study of the general population showed that persons with and without echocardiographically proved MVP were equally likely to have repolarization abnormalities.[139] Furthermore, studies that compared unaffected relatives and spouses of relatives in the families of affected patients with MVP showed no

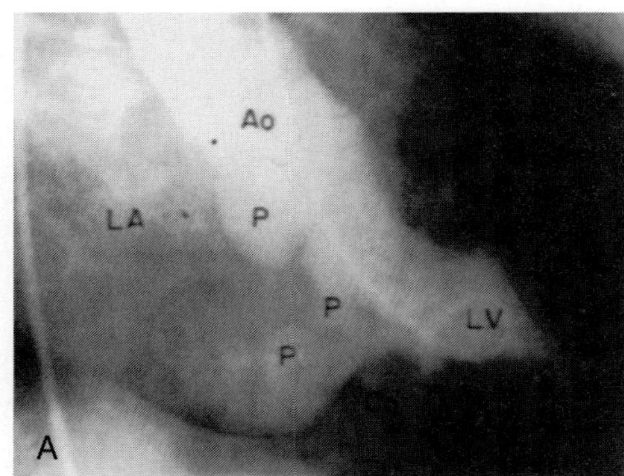

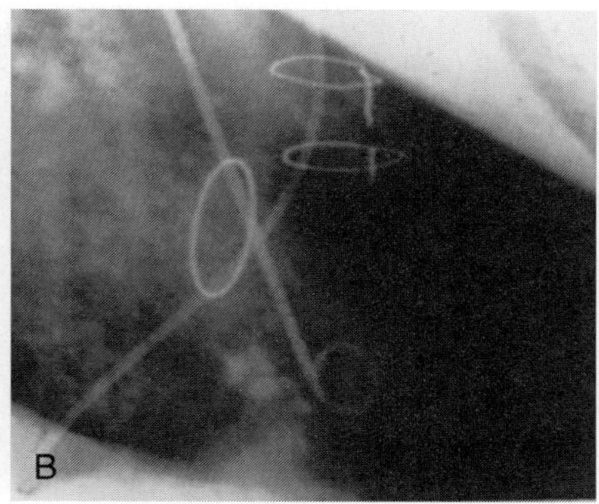

FIGURE 15–15 **A,** Left ventricular cineangiogram in the right anterior oblique projection. Severe mitral regurgitation and prolapsing mitral leaflets with subannular mural calcification of the endocardium are present. **B,** Postoperatively, the calcification is demonstrated below the mitral annulus. Ao, aorta; Ca, calcification; LA, left atrium; LV, left ventricle; P, prolapsing mitral leaflets. (**A** and **B,** Reprinted from Am J Cardiol, Vol. 60, Chesler E, Gomick C, Edwards J, Calcification of the mural endocardium of the left ventricle complicating the myxomatous mitral valve, p. 1196, Copyright, 1987, with permission from Elsevier Science.)

difference in the incidence of electrocardiographic repolarization abnormalities compared with control subjects. Such studies among relatives of patients with MVP have the advantage of being free of the selection bias that affects the referral of patients to specialized centers.[140]

The pathogenesis of these electrocardiographic abnormalities is unknown, but it is tempting to speculate that they may be related to endocardial friction lesions. It is not generally appreciated that fibrosis involving the endocardium of the left ventricle beneath the posterior leaflet of the mitral valve may be so extensive, confluent, and calcified that it can be detected with angiography and echocardiography and distinguished from mitral annular calcification[141] (Figs. 15–15 and 15–16). Perhaps repolarization changes that are transient result from varying degrees of chordal-endocardial friction induced by changes in LV volume before permanent endocardial scarring ensues.

Echocardiography

Both M-mode and two-dimensional techniques play a pivotal role in the diagnosis and assessment of patients with MVP.[100, 102–104, 111, 142] Paradoxically, the advent of echocardiography contributed to the current "epidemic" of MVP because the diagnosis was based on findings that were, in fact, variants of the normal. Epidemiologic studies based on loose echocardiographic criteria have reported the incidence of MVP in 5 to 21 percent of the healthy population. Such fallacies may be avoided by using at least two criteria for diagnosis: (1) clear echocardiographic evidence of leaflet redundancy and thickening with chordal lengthening compatible with myxomatous degeneration of the valve and (2) the presence of some degree of MR detectable *clinically* and not merely with color-flow Doppler, which is overly sensitive.

M-Mode Echocardiography

This technique has the limitation that the ultrasonic beam is narrow and provides a restricted window ("ice-pick" view). However, there are findings that supplement the two-dimensional technique:

Mid or Late Systolic Buckling. This sudden posterior displacement of the leaflets is quite characteristic of MVP and is extremely useful in timing the onset of the click and

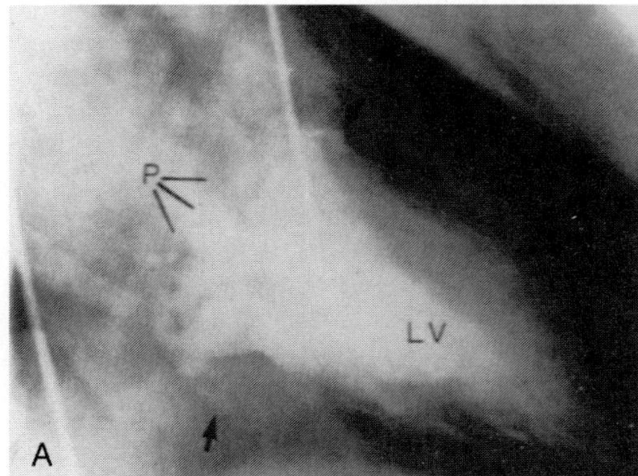

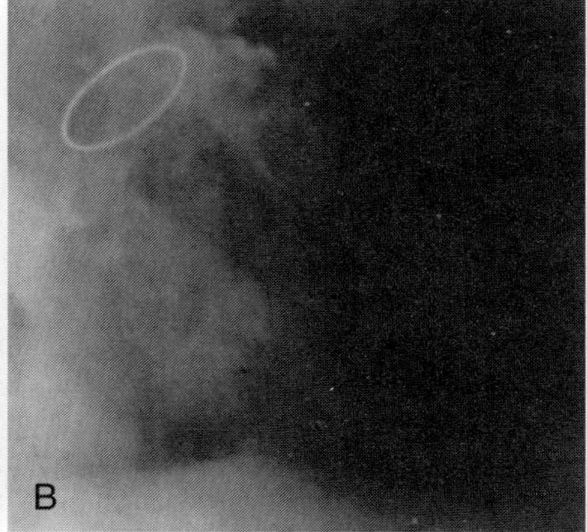

FIGURE 15–16 Left ventricular cineangiogram in the right anterior oblique view. **A,** Calcified mitral annulus *(arrows),* prolapsed mitral leaflets, and severe mitral regurgitation. **B,** Postoperatively, the sewing ring of the porcine prosthesis clearly locates the calcification in the mitral annulus. LV, left ventricle; P, prolapsed mitral leaflets. (**A** and **B,** From Chesler E, Gomick C, Edwards J: Calcification of the mural endocardium of the left ventricle complicating the myxomatous mitral valve. Am J Cardiol 60:1196, 1987.)

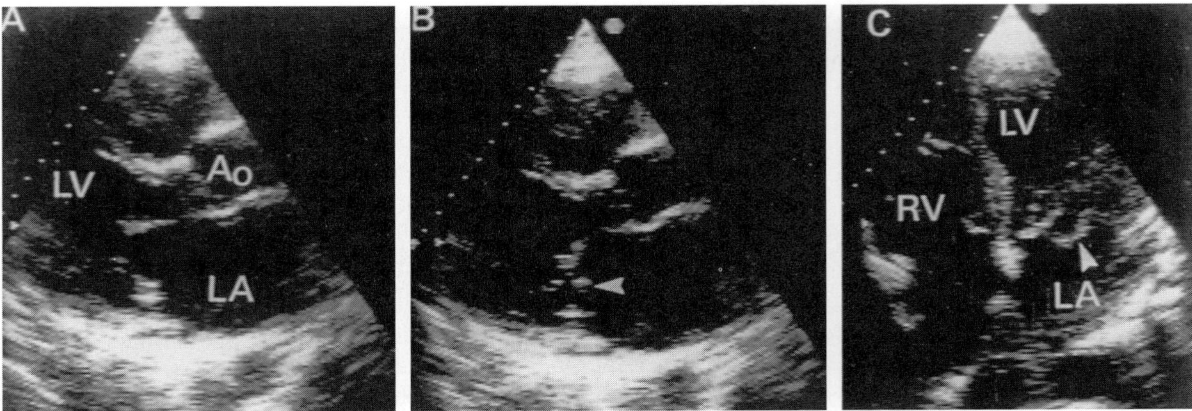

FIGURE 15–17 Two-dimensional echocardiogram in mitral valve prolapse. **A,** Thickened anterior and posterior mitral leaflets open in diastole. **B,** Prolapse of the posterior leaflet *(arrowhead).* **C,** Four-chamber view shows prolapse of the posterior leaflet into the left atrium (LA). Ao, aorta; LV, left ventricle; RV, right ventricle.

murmur (see Fig. 15–13). This finding is very reliable, and there are few false-positives. Posterior prolapse of one or both leaflets is the opposite movement as SAM (systolic anterior motion) encountered in hypertrophic obstructive cardiomyopathy, where the anterior mitral leaflet moves *anteriorly* toward the ventricular septum in midsystole.

Holosystolic "Hammocking." Holosystolic posterior displacement is not absolutely specific for MVP. False-positive results may occur when there is excessive cardiac movement in systole (e.g., pericardial effusion). Because a small amount of posterior movement of the normal mitral valve occurs during systole, it has been suggested that the diagnosis be made only when this exceeds 2 mm. However, such arbitrary values increase the number of false-positives and the likelihood of misleading epidemiologic data. Reliance should instead be placed on the two-dimensional technique.

Two-Dimensional Echocardiography

This technique provides much better spatial visualization of the leaflets, chordae, and papillary muscle and is particularly useful in the diagnosis of ruptured chordae. The important changes are as follows:

Thickening of the Leaflets and Chordae With Superior Systolic Displacement of Segments of the Valve Into the Left Atrium Above the Plane of the Mitral Annulus. Using multiple views, it is possible to detect which portions of the leaflets are redundant and prolapsing (Fig. 15–17). The rupture of chordae is readily diagnosed by echocardiography, which is also helpful in excluding infective endocarditis as the cause. The following findings are readily elicited with good technique: (1) failure of leaflet coaptation with the edges frequently observed in several views and (2) a whipping motion of the leaflet and attached chordae seen when a sizeable portion of a leaflet is detached. (3) In addition, color-flow Doppler is useful but not essential in the diagnosis and clearly demonstrates the eccentricity and direction of the jet depending on which chordae have ruptured.

The Presence of Calcified LA Angle Lesion *Above* and LV Endocardial Friction Lesions *Below* the Mitral Annulus. The *transesophageal* technique is particularly useful in defining the anatomy more precisely and readily recognizes failure of leaflet coaptation and lengthening and rupture of the chordae tendineae (Fig. 15–18).

Cardiac Catheterization and Angiocardiography

Invasive procedures are rarely indicated because clinical and echocardiographic findings are so accurate. The hemodynamics are normal unless there is severe MR. Although

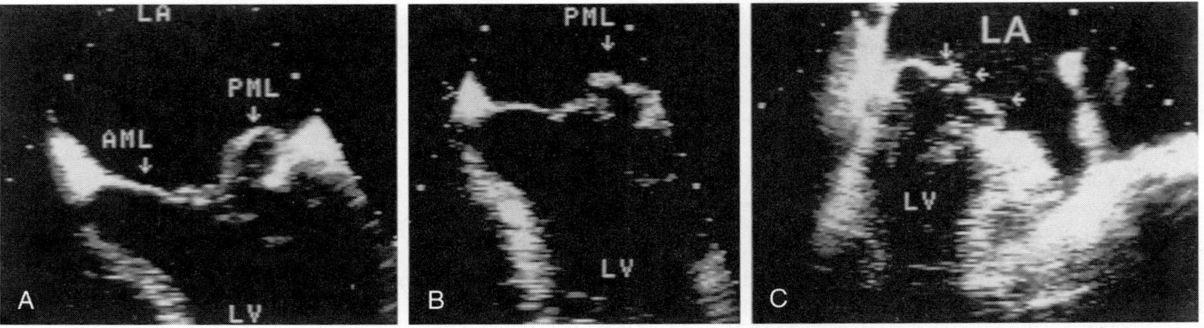

FIGURE 15–18 Transesophageal echocardiograms in mitral valve prolapse show fine detail of leaflet anatomy. **A,** Prolapse of the posterior mitral leaflet (PML). **B** and **C,** Scallops *(arrows).* AML, anterior mitral leaflet; LA, left atrium; LV, left ventricle.

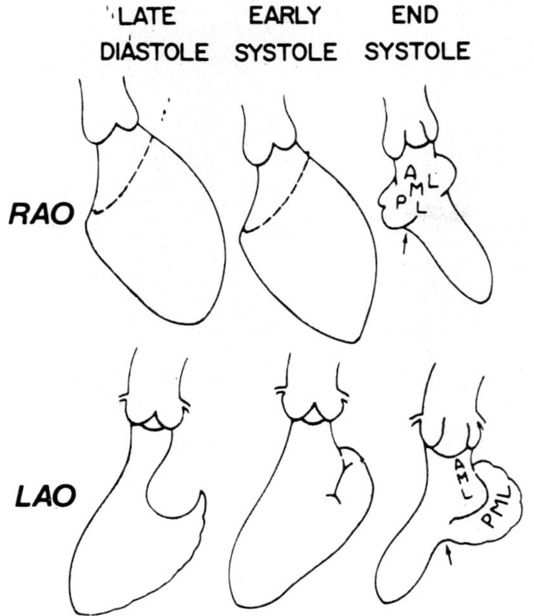

FIGURE 15–19 Diagrammatic representation of angiographic anatomy in mitral valve prolapse, in the 45-degree right anterior oblique (RAO) and 60-degree left anterior oblique (LAO) projections. **Top right,** "Anterior hump," RAO projection represents anterior commissural scallop of the posterior leaflet. **Bottom right,** "Ballerina foot" deformity is illustrated in the LAO projection. (From Hager J, Criley JM: Prolapse mitral leaflet syndrome. Cardiovasc Clin 10:1, 213, 1979.)

earlier reports incriminated a myocardial factor,[143] there is no consistent abnormality other than the "ballerina foot" deformity of the LV contour in systole found when there is marked prolapse (Fig. 15–19). This deformity of the inferior LV wall is a frequent finding and is a result of traction on the papillary muscles by the leaflet that is prolapsing. Traction on the LV wall may also be demonstrated with apex cardiography (Fig. 15–20). The "ballerina foot" disappears after mitral valve replacement.

In a typical case of MVP, angiography demonstrates protrusion of the mitral leaflet beyond the plane of the annulus. Much like echocardiography, there has been considerable disagreement as to what constitutes an abnormal protrusion of the various scallops beyond the annulus. The posterior leaflet is best evaluated in the right anterior oblique position. It should be noted that there is a normal protrusion below the valve attachment in the "fornix," or subannular pouch, that may be confused with prolapse of the posterior leaflet if it is not appreciated that the fornix is inferior to the annulus (Fig. 15–21). The posteromedial, middle, and anterolateral scallops of the posterior leaflet are readily identifiable with high-quality cineangiography.[99] The anterior commissural scallop of the posterior mitral leaflet is frequently confused with the anterior mitral leaflet as it forms a bump anterior to and beneath the aortic valve in the right oblique projection. Prolapse of the anterior leaflet is usually better visualized in the 60-degree left anterior oblique view, where it can be followed from its attachment to the aortic root to its position in systole where it coapts with the posterior leaflet. When the anterior leaflet prolapses, it extends posterior to the shadow of the annulus into the left atrium, inferior and posterior to the aortic root (see Fig. 15–19).

Complications

Mitral Regurgitation

The myxomatous valve is a leading cause of MR in patients in the United States because of a decline in the incidence of rheumatic fever and a greater awareness of the condition by clinicians and pathologists. Some instances of "rheumatic" MR were in fact myxomatous valves associated with secondary fibrosis erroneously diagnosed as healed rheumatic or infective endocarditis. Signs of severe MR and heart failure supervene in a small proportion of patients with MVP; men older than 45 years are particularly prone to this complication[140, 144] The mechanisms for increasing MR include (1) increasing prolapse when progressive myxomatous degeneration weakens the leaflets, (2) dilatation of the annulus, which goes along with, and may aggravate, increasing degrees of regurgitation, and (3) rupture of the chordae tendineae.

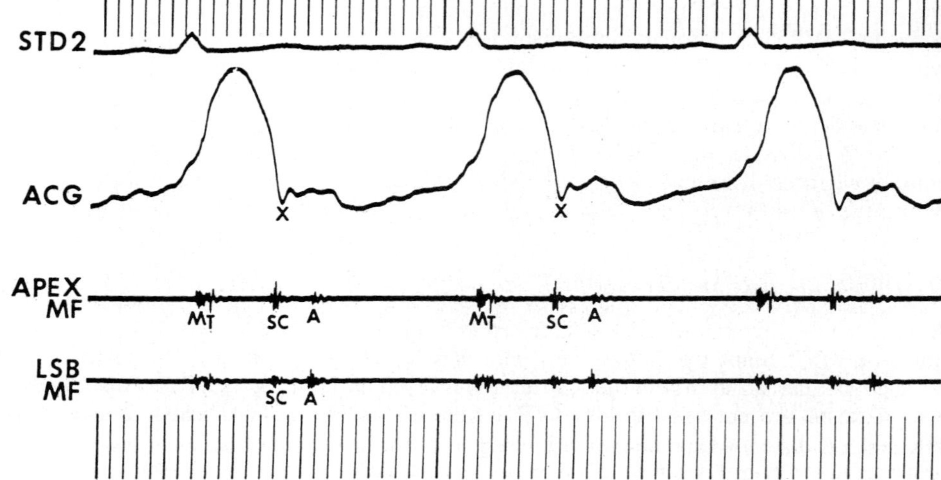

FIGURE 15–20 Simultaneous electrocardiogram (standard lead II [STD2]), apex cardiogram (ACG), and phonocardiogram at apex and left sternal border (medium frequency [MF]) demonstrate a midsystolic click (SC) and retraction of the apex "X." (From Barlow JB, Pocock W: Perspectives on the Mitral Valve. Philadelphia: FA Davis, 1987.)

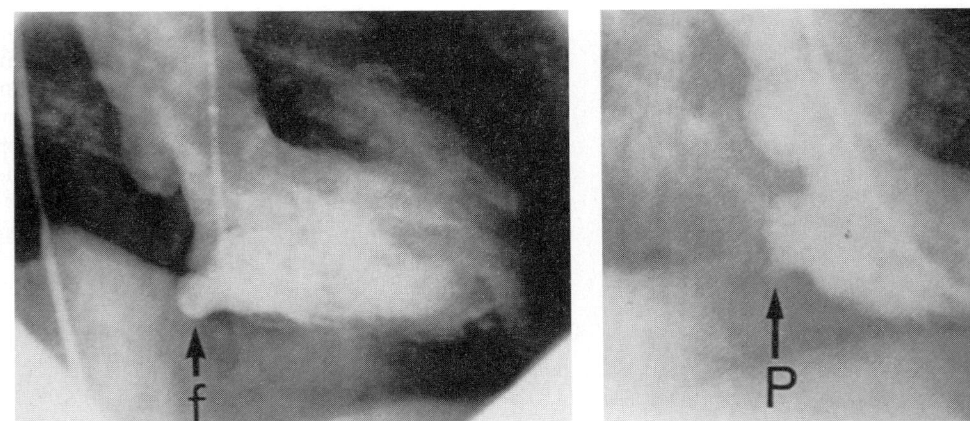

FIGURE 15–21 A, Cineangiogram in the right anterior oblique position demonstrates the fornix (f) or subannular pouch *(arrow)* in the normal mitral valve. Note that the leaflets are not displaced beyond the annulus. **B,** Prolapse (P) of the posterior mitral leaflet.

Infective Endocarditis

Patients with MVP and a late systolic murmur are at an increased risk of infective endocarditis.[145–148] Most clinicians agree that such patients should receive antibiotic prophylaxis before any procedure that places them at risk.[133] This does not completely solve the problem, however, because patients with MVP who have systolic murmurs intermittently may also be at an increased risk. Certainly, antibiotic prophylaxis is strongly indicated when additional factors such as thickened redundant leaflets are identified with echocardiography and when there is a predisposition to frequent bacteremia due to drug addiction immunosuppression.

Systemic Embolism

Several studies have reported an increased risk for stroke among subjects with MVP. Barnett and associates[149, 150] found a much higher incidence of systemic embolism in younger patients with MVP than in control subjects. However, a population-based study in Olmsted County, Minnesota, found that the age at first stroke among individuals with MVP was similar to that in an unselected population: in the absence of ischemic heart disease, congestive heart failure, diabetes mellitus, and MVP, their risk for stroke was not increased.[151] There also is a possible association between MVP and coronary embolism in young people who have had myocardial infarction with angiographically normal coronary arteries.[152] Although the exact mechanism for systemic embolism has not been documented, there are at least two sources for platelet, fibrin, and even calcific emboli: surfaces of redundant leaflets and the angle lesion within the left atrium.

Dysrhythmias and Sudden Death

A wide range of dysrhythmias has been reported in association with MVP. Some dysrhythmias, such as supraventricular tachycardia, atrial fibrillation, atrial flutter, and atrial ectopic beats, are not specific for MVP but are a result of MR and LA distention, and they complicate significant MR of any cause. Other dysrhythmias, such as those complicating the Wolff-Parkinson-White syndrome, are a result of concurrence of two common conditions.

It is the ventricular dysrhythmias, particularly high-grade ventricular ectopy and ventricular tachycardia, that have attracted so much attention and have been correlated with the risk of sudden death. However, it should be strongly emphasized that sudden unexpected death resulting from dysrhythmia among young people with MVP is rare.[118, 153–157] Not only are adequate clinical details and electrocardiographic recordings of the final event poorly documented, but detailed pathologic findings are also usually absent. In 1983, we reviewed 39 reported cases of sudden death attributed to the myxomatous mitral valve and found that autopsies had been performed in only 19 patients; in most, the information was so sparse that other diseases could not be definitely excluded.[118] Many cases of sudden death attributed to MVP were, in fact, the result of drug toxicity, electrolyte imbalance, or other unrecognized and unrelated cardiac pathology, such as cardiomyopathy.

In their meticulous follow-up of patients with MVP, Pocock and associates[153] encountered only one patient who died suddenly. This young woman had been treated for multifocal ventricular extrasystoles, and a myxomatous mitral valve was the chief finding at autopsy; ventricular fibrillation was the presumed cause of death. Nishimura and colleagues[104] reported six cases of sudden death among 237 asymptomatic or mildly symptomatic patients with MVP whom they had followed for a mean of 6.2 years. In addition, Duren and associates[144] encountered three cases of sudden death in a prospective follow-up of 300 patients (mean follow-up, 6.1 years). In neither series were autopsies available, and Duren and associates pointed out that their data may have been biased because their patients had been referred to a cardiac center for evaluation, so their findings did not necessarily apply to the natural history in the general population.

These findings in so few cases must be reconciled with other evidence and considered against the background prevalence of dysrhythmias and risk of sudden death in the general population. Frequent atrial and ventricular premature beats are unusual in a young population, but one study of 50 male medical students without apparent heart disease showed that one subject had a short run of ventricular tachycardia and three other subjects with ventricular ectopy manifested the R-on-T phenomenon.[158] In the Framingham Heart Study, dysrhythmias were detected with similar frequency on resting 12-lead, exercise, and 1-hour ambulatory electrocardiography in subjects with and without MVP.[159] This study was population based and avoided the selection bias evident in other studies from tertiary referral centers that reported life-threatening cardiac dysrhythmias. Kramer and colleagues[160] clearly demonstrated the effect of selection bias when they compared patients with MVP with similarly symptomatic controls: patients with MVP did not have an excessive prevalence of dysrhythmias.

MECHANISM OF DYSRHYTHMIAS

In our report of 14 patients with sudden death, it was documented that the myxomatous valve was the only pathologic finding.[118] We noted that 3 of the 14 patients showed only mild grades of prolapse. In one of these patients (a 14-year-old girl), a family pedigree was available. The girl's mother died suddenly at age 36, and two of the girl's siblings died suddenly at ages 11 and 12, respectively. All had mild grades of prolapse and no history of dysrhythmias. There was no recording of the final dysrhythmia in five patients, but because premature ventricular systoles had been documented at some time, the final event was assumed to be ventricular dysrhythmia. It was postulated that the mechanism for dysrhythmia might be mechanical stimulation of the endocardium by chordae of the posterior mitral leaflet, a notion supported by experiments showing that traction on papillary muscles may produce ventricular ectopy.[161] These observations may be in concert with those rare patients with hemodynamically mild MR and repeated ventricular tachycardia in whom valvuloplasty of the voluminous leaflets abolished the dysrhythmia.[162]

Electrophysiologic studies have not contributed to definition of the role of ventricular ectopy. Some patients with mild MVP and high-grade ventricular ectopy have demonstrated normal intracardiac conduction and refractoriness.[163] Other authors have pointed out that programmed ventricular stimulation, which induced polymorphic ventricular tachycardia among patients with MVP, could simply be a nonspecific response to an aggressive stimulation protocol.[164]

Episodes of sudden death among the general population are not usually recorded with ambulatory electrocardiography.[157, 165] Usually, ventricular tachycardia and fibrillation are responsible and complicate cases of ischemic heart disease. It is interesting to note that in pathology and forensic literature, there also are cases of sudden death in young people that have not been associated with any demonstrable cardiac abnormality and the conduction system has been normal.[154, 166] Perhaps such cases are related to the phenomenon of asystolic cardiac arrest that has been documented in young people. Milstein and associates[167] reported the findings in six survivors of cardiac asystole, none of whom had clinically detectable heart disease. A hypotensive-bradycardic response with syncope was reproduced by passive orthostatic tilt and thought to be neurally mediated by mechanoreceptors in the left ventricle. This raises the possibility that some cases of sudden death may have been erroneously attributed to a myxomatous mitral valve when the actual cause was neurally mediated hypotension and cardiac asystole. This association has, in fact, been documented by Leichtman and colleagues,[168] who described 11 members of a family with a high prevalence of MVP and syncope: orthostatic tilt induced hypotension, bradycardia, and syncope. Santos and associates[169] reported similar findings in 12 of 86 patients with MVP, but unfortunately there were no controls in their study, so the association could be a result of selection bias.

Thus, the causal relationship between MVP and sudden death remains unclear. What is clear is that in the absence of severe MR and LV dysfunction,[170] the risk of sudden death in young people who do not have ventricular dysrhythmia, syncope, or presyncope is so remote that they should not be informed of this possibility.

Autonomic Dysfunction

The term *billowing mitral leaflet syndrome* was introduced by Barlow and Pocock[171] for symptoms such as anxiety, fatigue, weakness, and palpitation associated with MVP. The term *mitral valve prolapse syndrome* was coined by Boudoulas and associates[121] to categorize symptomatic patients whom they believe to have neuroendocrine or autonomic dysfunction and a "hyperadrenergic" state. These authors proposed that MVP may be a marker for autonomic dysfunction.[172]

Several reports have pointed to autonomic dysfunction among patients with MVP. Pasternac and colleagues[173] studied 15 symptomatic patients and measured plasma norepinephrine levels, heart rate, and supine and standing systolic and diastolic blood pressures. Total plasma catecholamine and norepinephrine levels were significantly increased in patients in both positions, and heart rate was lower than normal in patients in the supine position but returned to normal in the upright position. These investigators believe that this hyperadrenergic and vagotonic state could explain many of the findings and manifestations of the MVP syndrome. These observations were confirmed by Coghlan and associates[174] but somewhat at variance with those of Gaffney and associates,[175] who found diminished vagal response to the diving reflex and phenylephrine infusion. Boudoulas and colleagues[176] found increased 24-hour urinary norepinephrine and epinephrine excretion in symptomatic patients with MVP. In addition, isoproterenol infusion produced a dose-related increase in heart rate in MVP patients in excess of that of control subjects. These authors believe that MVP may be a specific marker in certain people "for the constitutional, neuroendocrine-cardiovascular process that is currently designated as the MVP syndrome."[177] However, other studies reported decreased epinephrine excretion and increased vagal tone in patients with MVP.[178] Chesler and associates[136] showed that among 11 consecutive patients with MVP encountered in hospital practice who were evenly matched with control subjects for age and sex, there was no significant difference between norepinephrine levels, heart rates, and blood pressures in response to orthostatic tilt. Similarly, Lenders and colleagues[179] found no differences in neurohumoral responses to orthostatic tilt in a comparison of symptomatic and asymptomatic patients with MVP. Mantysaari[180] compared patients with neurocirculatory asthenia and normal control subjects and reported no significant difference in response to hyperventilation, orthostatic tilt, Valsalva maneuver, cold pressor test, or isometric hand grip.

These conflicting findings are likely a result of several factors[173, 175, 176, 178]:

1. Many study populations have been small and composed mostly of highly symptomatic young women.
2. Not all control populations have been clearly defined.
3. MVP has not always been excluded with echocardiography in control groups.
4. Some studies have drawn conclusions from the measurements of catecholamine levels at rest or during passive standing rather than during orthostatic stress and isometric exercise, which is the preferred method. Anxiety may induce a hyperadrenergic state. For example, plasma norepinephrine levels have been shown to increase by more than 50 percent and epinephrine levels to more than double during public speaking by young physicians at conferences.[181, 182]

Taylor and associates[183] studied normal control subjects, asymptomatic MVP patients, and patients with MVP who had symptoms suggestive of autonomic dysfunction. Responses to ice water immersion and the administration of isoprotenolol, epinephrine, and tyramine were the same in patients with similar symptoms and did not distinguish between those with and those without MVP. These authors emphasized that autonomic responses to physiologic maneuvers and agonist drugs in control subjects and in patients with MVP are heterogeneous, and this may be partially responsible for the divergent findings reported in the literature; bias in patient selection and small sample size could favor one abnormality over another. One may conclude, therefore, that definite proof of a connection between autonomic dysfunction and MVP is lacking.

Prognosis

Although it is difficult to precisely define the natural history of such a common disorder, there can be little doubt that the outlook for patients with MVP is excellent, with the majority of subjects remaining asymptomatic for their lifetimes without any complications. Pathologic studies comparing the age at death of patients with myxomatous valves with control autopsy material showed that patients with myxomatous valves in fact lived longer.[108] The incidence of infective endocarditis and systemic embolism is low, and the risk of sudden death is minuscule. Progressive MR may occur, particularly in older men among whom sudden deterioration is frequently a result of ruptured chordae or infective endocarditis.

Management

The majority of patients with MVP are asymptomatic and should be reassured that their condition is benign. When a nonejection click is followed by a late systolic murmur, there is a risk of infective endocarditis, and patients should be advised of the necessary prophylactic measures.

Patients who have significant MR should be examined at regular intervals of approximately 1 year, particularly in the case of elderly men with a holosystolic murmur and echocardiographic evidence of leaflet redundancy and chordal lengthening; LV function should be carefully assessed at each visit. LV dysfunction is a major hazard for patients with significant regurgitation. When the preoperative ejection fraction is less than 50 percent, there is considerable risk of postoperative LV dysfunction and eventual heart failure. Among patients with preserved LV function and without coronary artery disease, conservative repair of the mitral valve may be accomplished with low mortality rates and excellent functional result.[184] At centers in which surgeons have considerable experience with valvuloplasty, correction should be seriously considered even in asymptomatic patients when the ejection fraction is more than 0.60 and the LV end-systolic dimension is 45 mm or less. The variety of techniques include annuloplasty, leaflet plication, leaflet resection, and chordal transposition. Transesophageal Doppler echocardiography is extremely useful in assessing whether the valve is suitable for repair and is of great value in the operating room to assess the efficacy of repair. In cases in which the anatomy is unsuitable for repair, valve replacement should be accomplished with a metallic prosthesis or porcine heterograft.

The small group of patients who complain of dizziness, presyncope, or syncope and have ventricular arrhythmias demonstrated by 24-hour electrocardiographic monitoring or treadmill exercise testing should be treated aggressively: if necessary, provocative electrophysiologic testing should be used to select the most efficacious drug.

The reader is referred to the websites of the American College of Cardiology (www.acc.org) and the American Heart Association (www.americanheart.org) for the ACC/AHA Guidelines for the Management of Patients with Acute Myocardial Infarction.

References

Mitral Stenosis

1. Rapaport E: Natural history of aortic and mitral valve disease. Am J Cardiol 35:221–227, 1975.
2. Wallace AG: Pathophysiology of cardiovascular disease. *In* Smith LH Jr, Thier SO (eds): International Textbook of Medicine. Vol. 1. Philadelphia: WB Saunders, 1981.
3. Harris P, Heath D: The Human Pulmonary Circulation. Edinburgh: Churchill Livingstone, 1977.
4. Mounsey JPD: Inspection and palpation of the cardiac impulse. Prog Cardiovasc Dis 10:187–206, 1967.
5. Wooley CF, Klassen KP, Leighton RF, et al: Left atrial and left ventricular sound and pressure in mitral stenosis. Circulation 38:295–307, 1968.
6. Barrington WW, Boudoulas H, Bashore T, et al: Mitral dome excursion and M1 and the mitral opening snap—the concept of reciprocal heart sounds. Am Heart J 115:1280–1290, 1988.
7. Dack S, Bleifer S, Grishman A, Donoso E: Mitral stenosis: auscultatory and phonocardiographic findings. Am J Cardiol 5:815, 1960.
8. Ebringer R, Pitt A, Anderson ST: Haemodynamic factors influencing opening snap interval in mitral stenosis. Br Heart J 32:350–354, 1970.
9. Craige E: Phonocardiographic studies in mitral stenosis. N Engl J Med 257:650, 1957.
10. Legler JF, Benchimol A, Dimond EG: The apex cardiogram in the study of the 2-OS interval. Br Heart J 25:246, 1963.
11. Bonner AJ Jr, Stewart J, Travel ME: "Presystolic" augmentation of diastolic heart sounds in atrial fibrillation. Am J Cardiol 37:427–431, 1976.
12. Harvey WP: Silent valvular heart disease. Cardiovasc Clin 2:77–95, 1973.
13. McArthur JD, Sukumar IP, Munsi SC, et al: Reassessment of Graham Steell murmur using platinum electrode technique. Br Heart J 36:1023–1027, 1974.

14. Olesen KH: The natural history of 271 patients with mitral stenosis under medical treatment. Br Heart J 24:349, 1962.
15. Jose AD, Taylor RR, Bernstein L: The influence of arterial pressure on mitral incompetence in man. J Clin Invest 43:2094, 1964.

MITRAL REGURGITATION

16. Boltwood C, Tei C, Wong M, Shah P: Quantitative echocardiography of the mitral complex in dilated cardiomyopathy: the mechanism of functional mitral regurgitation. Circulation 68:498–508, 1983.
17. He S, Fontaine A, Schwammenthal E, et al: Integrated mechanism for functional mitral regurgitation. Circulation 96:1826–1834, 1997.
18. Otsuji Y, Handschumacher M, Schwammenthal E, et al: Insights from three dimensional echocardiography into the mechanism of functional mitral regurgitation. Circulation 96:1999–2008, 1997.
19. Braunwald E (ed): Heart Disease. 5th ed. Philadelphia: WB Saunders, 1997.
20. Grossman W, Baim DS: Cardiac Catheterization, Angiography, and Intervention. Philadelphia: Lea & Febiger, 1991.
21. Krayenbuehl HP, Hess OM: Chronic valvular insufficiency. *In* Parmley WW, Chatterjee K (eds): Cardiology. Philadelphia: JB Lippincott, 1991.
22. Corin WJ, Monrad ES, Murakami T, et al: The relationship of afterload to ejection performance in chronic mitral regurgitation. Circulation 76:59, 1987.
23. Enriquez-Sarano M, Schaff H, Orszulak T, et al: Congestive heart failure after surgical correction of mitral regurgitation: a long-term study. Circulation 92:2496–2503, 1995.
24. Zile MR, Gaasch WH, Carroll JD, Levine HJ: Chronic mitral regurgitation: predictive value of preoperative echocardiographic indexes of left ventricular function and wall stress. J Am Coll Cardiol 48:467, 1981.
25. Philips HR, Levine FH, Carter JE, et al: Mitral valve replacement for isolated mitral regurgitation: analysis of clinical course and later postoperative left ventricular ejection fraction. Am J Cardiol 48:647, 1981.
26. Nishimura, RA, Schaff HV, Shub C, et al: Papillary muscle rupture complicating acute myocardial infarction; analysis of 17 cases. Am J Cardiol 51:373–377, 1983.
27. Calvo CE, Figueras J, Cortadellas J, et al: Severe mitral regurgitation complicating acute myocardial infarction: clinical and angiographic differences between patients with and without papillary muscle rupture. Eur Heart J 18:606–610, 1997.
28. Elkins RC, Morrow AG, Vasko JS, Braunwald E: The effects of mitral regurgitation on the pattern of instantaneous aortic blood flow: clinical and experimental observations. Circulation 36:45–53, 1967.
29. Basta LL, Wolfson P, Eckberg DL, Abboud FM: The value of left parasternal impulse recordings in the assessment of mitral regurgitation. Circulation 48:1055, 1973.
30. Armstrong TG, Meeran MK, Gotsman MS: The left atrial lift. Am Heart J 82:764–769, 1971.
31. Antman EM, Angoff GH, Sloss LJ: Demonstration of the mechanism by which mitral regurgitation mimics aortic stenosis. Am J Cardiol 42:1044–1048, 1978.
32. Giuliani ER: Mitral valve incompetence due to flail anterior leaflet: a new physical sign. Am J Cardiol 20:784–788, 1967.
33. Merendino KA, Hessl EA II: The "murmur on top of the head" in acquired mitral insufficiency: pathological and clinical significance. JAMA 199:892–896, 1967.
34. Desjardins V, Enriquez-Sarano M, Tajik A, et al: Intensity of murmurs correlates with severity of valvular regurgitation. Am J Med 100:149–156, 1996.
35. Bleifer S, Dack S, Grishman A, Donoso E: The auscultatory and phonocardiographic findings in mitral regurgitation. Circulation 5:836, 1960.
36. Perloff JK, Child JS, Edwards JE: New guidelines for the clinical diagnosis of mitral valve prolapse. Am J Cardiol 57:1124–1129, 1986.
37. Devereux RB, Perloff JK, Reichek N, Josephson ME: Mitral valve prolapse. Circulation 54:3–4, 1976.
38. Epstein EJ, Coulshed N: Phonocardiogram and apex cardiogram in systolic click–late systolic murmur syndrome. Br Heart J 35:260–275, 1973.
39. Fontana ME, Wooley CG, Leighton RF, Lewis RP: Postural changes in left ventricular and mitral valvular dynamics in the systolic click–late systolic murmur syndrome. Circulation 51:165–213, 1975.
40. Wei J, Fortuin NJ: Diastolic sounds and murmurs associated with mitral valve prolapse. Circulation 63:559–564, 1981.
41. Shelburne JC, Rubenstein D, Gorlin R: A reappraisal of papillary muscle dysfunction. Am J Med 46:862–871, 1969.
42. Ling H, Enriquez-Sarano M, Seward J, et al: Clinical outcome of mitral regurgitation due to flail leaflets. N Engl J Med 335:1417–1423, 1996.
43. Ling L, Enriquez-Sarano M, Seward J, et al: Early surgery in patients with mitral regurgitation due to partial flail leaflet: a long-term outcome study. Circulation 96:1819–1825, 1997.
44. Enriquez-Sarano M, Schaff HV, Orszulak TA, et al: Valve repair improves the outcome of surgery for mitral regurgitation: a multivariate analysis. Circulation 91:1022–1028, 1995.
45. Enriquez-Sarano M, Tajik AJ, Schaff HV, et al: Echocardiographic prediction of survival after successful correction of organic mitral regurgitation. Circulation 90:830–837, 1994.
46. Enriquez-Sarano M, Tajik AJ, Schaff HV, et al: Echocardiographic prediction of left ventricular function after correction of mitral regurgitation: results and clinical implications. J Am Coll Cardiol 24:1536–1543, 1994.
47. Enriquez-Sarano M, Schaff HV, Orszulak TA, et al: Congestive heart failure after surgical correction of mitral regurgitation: a long term study. Circulation 92:2496–2503, 1995.
48. Ling H, Enriquez-Sarano M, Seward J, et al: Clinical outcome of mitral regurgitation due to flail leaflets. N Engl J Med 335:1417–1423, 1996.
49. Kizilbash A, Willett D, Brickner M, et al: Effects of afterload reduction on vena contracta width in mitral regurgitation. J Am Coll Cardiol 32:427–431, 1998.
50. Klein HO, Sareli P, Schamroth CL, et al: Effects of atenolol on exercise capacity in patients with mitral stenosis with sinus rhythm. Am J Cardiol 56:598–601, 1985.
51. Greenberg BH, Massie MB, Brundage BH, et al: Beneficial effects of hydralazine in severe mitral regurgitation. Circulation 58:273–279, 1978.
52. Goodman DJ, Rossen RM, Holloway EL, et al: Effect of nitroprusside on left ventricular dynamics in mitral regurgitation. Circulation 50:1025–1032, 1974.
53. Rothlisberger C, Sareli P, Wisenbaugh T: Comparison of single dose nifedipine and captopril for chronic severe mitral regurgitation. Am J Cardiol 73:978–981, 1994.
54. Tishler M, Rowan M, LeWinter M: Effect of Enalapril on left ventricular mass and volumes in asymptomatic chronic, severe mitral regurgitation secondary to mitral valve prolapse. Am J Cardiol 82:242–245, 1998.
55. Marcotte F, Honos G, Walling A, et al: Effect of angiotensin converting enzyme inhibitor therapy in mitral regurgitation with normal left ventricular function. Can J Cardiol 13:479–485, 1997.
56. Wisenbaugh T, Sinovich V, Dullbh A, Sareli P: Six month pilot study of captopril for mildly symptomatic, severe isolated mitral and isolated aortic regurgitation. J Heart Valve Dis 3:197–204, 1994.

ASSESSMENT OF SEVERITY OF MITRAL REGURGITATION

57. Helmcke F, Nanda N, Hsiung M, et al: Color Doppler assessment of mitral regurgitation with orthogonal planes. Circulation 75:175–183, 1987.
58. Spain M, Smith M, Grayburn P, et al: Quantitative assessment of mitral regurgitation by Doppler color flow imaging: angiographic and hemodynamic correlations. J Am Coll Cardiol 13:585–590, 1989.
59. Enriquez-Sarano M, Tajik A, Bailey K, Seward J: Color flow imaging compared with quantitative Doppler assessment of severity of mitral regurgitation: influence of eccentricity of jet and mechanism of regurgitation. J Am Coll Cardiol 21:1211–1219, 1993.
60. Pearson A, St. Vrain J, Mrosek D, Labovitz A: Color Doppler echocardiographic evaluation of patients with a flail mitral leaflet. J Am Coll Cardiol 16:232–239, 1990.
61. Cape E, Yoganathan A, Weyman A, Levine R: Adjacent solid boundaries alter the size of regurgitant jets on Doppler color flow maps. J Am Coll Cardiol 17:1094–1102, 1991.
62. Chen C, Thomas J, Anconina J, Harrigan P, et al: Impact of impinging wall jet on color Doppler quantification of mitral regurgitation. Circulation 84:712–720, 1991.
63. Utsunomiya T, Patel D, Doshi R, et al: Can signal intensity of the

continuous wave Doppler regurgitant jet estimate severity of mitral regurgitation? Am Heart J 123:166–171, 1992.

64. Castello R, Pearson A, Lenzen P, Labovitz A: Effect of mitral regurgitation on pulmonary venous velocities derived from transesophageal echocardiography color-guided pulsed Doppler imaging. Am Coll Cardiol 17:1499–1506, 1991.
65. Klein A, Obarski T, Stewart W, et al: Transesophageal Doppler echocardiography of pulmonary venous flow: a new marker of mitral regurgitation severity. J Am Coll Cardiol 18:518–526, 1991.
66. Enriquez-Sarano M, Dujardin K, Tribouilloy C, et al: Determinants of pulmonary venous flow reversal in mitral regurgitation and its usefulness in determining the severity of the mitral regurgitation. Am J Cardiol (in press).
67. Enriquez-Sarano M, Seward J, Bailey K, Tajik A: Effective regurgitant orifice area: a noninvasive Doppler development of an old hemodynamic concept. J Am Coll Cardiol 23:443–451, 1994.
68. Vandervoort P, Rivera J, Mele D, et al: Application of color Doppler flow mapping to calculate effective regurgitant orifice area: an in vitro study and initial clinical observations. Circulation 88:1150–1156, 1993.
69. Enriquez-Sarano M, Bailey K, Seward J, et al: Quantitative Doppler assessment of valvular regurgitation. Circulation 87:841–848, 1993.
70. Rokey R, Sterling L, Zoghbi W, et al: Determination of regurgitant fraction in isolated mitral or aortic regurgitation by pulsed Doppler two-dimensional echocardiography. J Am Coll Cardiol 7:1273–1278, 1986.
71. Blumlein S, Bouchard A, Schiller N, et al: Quantitation of mitral regurgitation by Doppler echocardiography. Circulation 74:306–314, 1986.
72. Bargiggia G, Tronconi L, Sahn D, et al: A new method for quantitation of mitral regurgitation based on color flow Doppler imaging of flow convergence proximal to regurgitant orifice. Circulation 84:1481–1489, 1991.
73. Chen C, Koschyk D, Brockhoff C, et al: Noninvasive estimation of regurgitant flow rate and volume in patients with mitral regurgitation by Doppler color mapping of accelerating flow field. J Am Coll Cardiol 21:374–383, 1993.
74. Enriquez-Sarano M, Miller FJ, Hayes S, et al: Effective mitral regurgitant orifice area: clinical use and pitfalls of the proximal isovelocity surface area method. J Am Coll Cardiol 25:703–709, 1995.
75. Nozaki S, Shandas R, DeMaria N: Requirement for accurate measurement of regurgitant stroke volume by the combined continuous-wave Doppler and color Doppler flow convergence method. Am Heart J 133:19–28, 1997.
76. Tribouilloy C, Shen W, Quere J, et al: Assessment of severity of mitral regurgitation by measuring regurgitant jet width at its origin with transesophageal Doppler color flow imaging. Circulation 85:1248–1253, 1992.
77. Mele D, Vandervoort P, Palacios I, et al: Proximal jet size by Doppler color flow mapping predicts severity of mitral regurgitation. Circulation 91:746–754, 1995.
78. Hall S, Brickner M, Willett D, et al: Assessment of mitral regurgitation by Doppler color flow mapping of the vena contracta. Circulation 95:636–642, 1997.
79. Dujardin K, Enriquez-Sarano M, Bailey K, et al: Grading of mitral regurgitation by quantitative Doppler echocardiography: calibration by left ventricular angiography in routine clinical practice. Circulation 96:3409–3415, 1997.
80. Heinle S, Hall S, Brickner E, et al: Comparison of vena contracta width by multiplane transesophageal echocardiography with quantitative Doppler assessment of mitral regurgitation. Am J Cardiol 81:175–179, 1998.
81. Braunwald E, Awe W: The syndrome of severe mitral regurgitation with normal left atrial pressure. Circulation 27:29–35, 1963.
82. Fuchs R, Heuser R, Yin F, Brinker J: Limitations of pulmonary wedge V waves in diagnosing mitral regurgitation. Am J Cardiol 49:849–854, 1982.
83. Sellers R: Left retrograde cardioangiography in acquired heart disease: technic, indications and interpretations in 700 cases. Am J Cardiol 14:437–447, 1964.
84. Croft C, Lipscomb K, Mathis K, et al: Limitations of qualitative angiographic grading in aortic or mitral regurgitation. Am J Cardiol 53:1593–1598, 1984.
85. Sandler H, Dodge H, Hay R, Rackley C: Quantitation of valvular insufficiency in man by angiocardiography. Am Heart J 65:501–513, 1963.
86. Lopez J, Hanson S, Orchard R, Tan L: Quantification of mitral valvular incompetence. Cathet Cardiovasc Diag 11:139–152, 1985.
87. Hozumi T, Yoshikawa J, Yoshida K, et al: Direct visualization of ruptured chordae tendineae by transesophageal two-dimensional echocardiography. J Am Coll Cardiol 16:1315–1319, 1990.
88. Reichert S, Visser C, Moulijn A, et al: Intraoperative transesophageal color-coded Doppler echocardiography for evaluation of residual regurgitation after mitral valve repair. J Thorac Cardiovasc Surg 100:756–761, 1990.
89. Sheikh K, Bengtson J, Rankin J, et al: Intraoperative transesophageal Doppler color flow imaging used to guide patient selection and operative treatment of ischemic mitral regurgitation. Circulation 84:594–604, 1991.
90. Freeman W, Schaff H, Khanderia B, et al: Intraoperative evaluation of mitral valve regurgitation and repair by transesophageal echocardiography: incidence and significance of systolic anterior motion. J Am Coll Cardiol 20:599–609, 1992.
91. Leitch J, Mitchell A, Harris P, et al: The effect of cardiac catheterization upon management of advanced aortic and mitral regurgitation. Eur Heart J 12:602–607, 1991.
92. Slater J, Gindea A, Freedberg R, et al: Comparison of cardiac catheterization and Doppler echocardiography in the decision to operate in aortic and mitral valve disease. J Am Coll Cardiol 17:1026–1036, 1991.
93. Ramsdale D, Bennett D, Bray C, et al: Angina, coronary risk factors and coronary artery disease in patients with valvular disease: a prospective study. Eur Heart J 5:716–726, 1984.
94. Enriquez-Sarano M, Klodas E, Garratt KN, et al: Secular trends in coronary atherosclerosis: analysis in patients with valvular regurgitation. N Engl J Med 335:316–322, 1996.
95. Ramsdale D, Bray C, Bennett D, et al: Routine coronary angiography is unnecessary in all patients with valvular heart disease. Z Kardiol 75:61–67, 1986.

Mitral Prolapse

96. Gallavardin L: Pseudo dedoublement du deuxieme bruit de du coueur simultant le dedoublement mitral par bruit extracardiac telesystolique surajoute. Lyon Med J 121:409, 1913.
97. Reid J: Mid-systolic clicks. S Afr Med J 35:353, 1961.
98. Barlow J, Pocock W: The significance of late systolic murmurs and mid-late systolic clicks. Maryland State Med J 12:76, 1963.
99. Criley J, Lewis K, Humphries J, Ross R: Prolapse of the mitral valve: clinical and cine-angiographic findings. Br Heart J 28:488, 1966.
100. Criley J, Heger J: Prolapsed mitral leaflet syndrome. Cardiovasc Clin 10:213, 1979.
101. Barlow J, Pocock W, Marchand P, Denny M: The significance of late systolic murmurs. Br Heart J 66:443, 1968.
102. Abbasi A, DeCristofaro D, Anabtawi J, Irwin L: Mitral valve prolapse: comparative value of M-mode, two-dimensional and Doppler echocardiography. J Am Coll Cardiol 2:1219, 1983.
103. Popp RL, Brown OR, Silverman JF, Harrison DC: Echocardiographic abnormalities in the mitral valve prolapse syndrome. Circulation 49:428, 1974.
104. Nishimura R, McGoon M, Shub C, et al: Echocardiographically documented mitral valve prolapse: long-term follow-up of 237 patients. N Engl J Med 313:1305, 1985.
105. Pomerance A: Ballooning deformity (mucoid degeneration) of atrioventricular valves. Br Heart J 31:343, 1969.
106. Ranganathan N, Lam J, Wigle E, Silver M: Morphology of the human mitral valve, II: the valve leaflets. Circulation 41:459, 1970.
107. Salazar A, Edwards J: Friction lesions of ventricular endocardium: relation to chordae tendineae of mitral valve. Arch Pathol Lab Med 90:364, 1970.
108. Lucas RJ, Edwards J: The floppy mitral valve. Curr Probl Cardiol 7:1, 1982.
109. Cheitlin M: Mitral valve prolapse. Circulation 59:610, 1979.
110. Chesler E, Gornick C: Maladies attributed to myxomatous mitral valve. Circulation 82:328, 1991.
111. Warth D, King ME, Cohen JM, et al: Prevalence of mitral valve prolapse in normal children. J Am Coll Cardiol 5:1173, 1985.
112. Perloff JC, Edwards JE: New guidelines for the clinical diagnosis of mitral valve prolapse. Am J Cardiol 57:1124, 1986.

113. Schreiber T, Feigenbaum H, Weyman A: Effect of atrial septal defect repair on left ventricular geometry and degree of mitral valve prolapse. Circulation 61:888, 1980.
114. Barlow J, Pocock W: The mitral valve prolapse enigma: two decades later. Mod Concepts Cardiovasc Dis 53:13, 1984.
115. Lewis J, Maron B, Diggs J, et al: Preparticipation echocardiographic screening for cardiovascular disease in a large, predominantly black population of collegiate athletes. Am J Cardiol 64:1029, 1989.
116. Markiewicz W, Stoner J, London E, et al: Mitral valve prolapse in one hundred presumably healthy young females. Circulation 53:464, 1976.
117. Edwards J: Floppy mitral valve syndrome. Cardiovasc Clin 18:249, 1987.
118. Chesler E, King R, Edwards J: The myxomatous mitral valve and sudden death. Circulation 67:632, 1983.
119. Devereaux R, Brown W, Kramer-Fox R, Sachs I: Inheritance of mitral valve prolapse: effect of age and sex on gene expression. Ann Intern Med 97:826, 1982.
120. Devereaux R, Hawkins I, Kramer-Fox R, et al: Complications of mitral valve prolapse: disproportionate occurrence in men and older patients. Am J Med 81:751, 1986.
121. Boudoulas H, Kolibach A, Baker P, et al: Mitral valve prolapse and the mitral valve prolapse syndrome: a diagnostic classification and pathogenesis of symptoms. Am Heart J 118:797, 1989.
122. Leier C, Call T, Fulkerson P, Wooley C: The spectrum of cardiac defects in the Ehlers-Danlos syndrome, types I and III. Ann Intern Med 92:171, 1980.
123. Barlow J, Pocock W: Mitral valve prolapse, the specific billowing mitral leaflet syndrome, or an insignificant non-ejection systolic click. Am Heart J 97:277, 1979.
124. Amat G, Louis P, Loisy C, et al: Migraine and mitral valve prolapse syndrome. Adv Neurol 33:27, 1982.
125. Lucas R, Edwards J: Floppy mitral valve and ventricular septal defect: an anatomic study. J Am Coll Cardiol 15:1337, 1983.
126. Zullo M, Devereaux R, Kramer-Fox R, et al: Mitral valve prolapse and hyperthyroidism: effect of patient selection. Am Heart J 110:977, 1985.
127. Motulsky A: Biased ascertainment and the natural history of disease. N Engl J Med 298:1196, 1978.
128. Wood P: Diseases of the Heart and Circulation. 3rd ed. p. 937. London: Eyre & Spottiswoode, 1962.
129. Katon W: Panic disorder and somatization. Am J Med 77:101, 1984.
130. Cohen M, Bodal D, Kilpatrick A, et al: The high familial prevalence of neurocirculatory asthenia. Am J Hum Genet 3:126, 1951.
131. Rice R: Symptom patterns of the hyperventilation syndrome. Am J Med Sci 8:691, 1951.
132. Leatham A, Brigden W: Mild mitral regurgitation and the mitral prolapse fiasco. Am Heart J 99:659, 1980.
133. Hickey A, MacMahon S, Wilcken D: Mitral valve prolapse and bacterial endocarditis: when is antibiotic prophylaxis necessary? Am Heart J 109:431, 1985.
134. Uretsky B: Does mitral valve prolapse cause nonspecific symptoms? Int J Cardiol 1:435, 1982.
135. Leor R, Markiewicz W: Neurocirculatory asthenia and mitral valve prolapse: two unrelated entities? Isr J Med Sci 17:1137, 1981.
136. Chesler E, Weir E, Braatz G, Francis G: Normal catecholamine and hemodynamic responses to orthostatic tilt in subjects with mitral valve prolapse. Am J Med 78:754, 1985.
137. Margraf J, Ehlers A, Roth W: Mitral valve prolapse and panic disorder: a review of their relationship. Psychosom Med 50:93, 1988.
138. McLaren MJ, Hawkins DM, Lachman AS, et al: Non-ejection clicks and late systolic murmurs in black school children of Soweto Johannesburg. Br Heart J 38:718, 1976.
139. Savage D, Devereaux R, Garrison R, et al: Mitral valve prolapse in the general population; 2: clinical features: the Framingham Study. Am Heart J 106:577, 1983.
140. Devereaux R, Kramer-Fox R, Kligfield P: Mitral valve prolapse: causes, clinical manifestations, and management. Ann Intern Med 111:305, 1989.
141. Chesler E, Gornick C, Edwards J: Calcification of the mural endocardium of the left ventricle complicating the myxomatous mitral valve. Am J Cardiol 60:1196, 1987.
142. Dillon JC, Chang CS: Use of echocardiography in patients with prolapsed mitral valve. Circulation 43:503, 1971.
143. Tresh D, Soin J, Siegel R, et al: Mitral valve prolapse: evidence for a myocardial perfusion abnormality. Am J Cardiol 41:441, 1978.
144. Duren D, Becker A, Dunning A: Long-term follow-up of idiopathic mitral valve prolapse in 300 patients: a prospective study. J Am Coll Cardiol 11:42, 1988.
145. Lachman A, Bramwell-Jones D, Lakier J, et al: Infective endocarditis in the billowing leaflet syndrome. Br Heart J 37:326, 1975.
146. MacMahon S, Hickey A, Wilcken D, et al: Risk of infective endocarditis in mitral valve prolapse with and without precordial systolic murmurs. Am J Cardiol 59:105, 1987.
147. MacMahon S, Roberts J, Kramer-Fox R, et al: Mitral valve prolapse and infective endocarditis. Am Heart J 113:1291, 1987.
148. Danchin N, Briancon S, Mathieu P, et al: Mitral valve prolapse as a risk factor for infective endocarditis. Lancet 1:743, 1989.
149. Barnett H, Jones M, Boughner D, Kostuk W: Cerebral ischemic events associated with prolapsing mitral valve. Arch Neurol 33:777, 1976.
150. Barnett H, Boughner D, Taylor D, et al: Further evidence relating mitral valve prolapse to cerebral ischemic events. N Engl J Med 302:129, 1980.
151. Orencia AJ, Petty GW, Khandheria BK, et al: Risk of stroke with mitral valve prolapse in population based cohort study. Stroke 26:7, 1995.
152. Chesler E, Matisonn R, Lakier J, et al: Acute myocardial infarction with normal coronary arteries: a possible manifestation of the billowing mitral leaflet syndrome. Circulation 54:203, 1976.
153. Pocock W, Bosman C, Chesler E, et al: Sudden death in primary mitral valve prolapse. Am Heart J 107:378, 1984.
154. Topaz O, Edwards J: Pathologic features of sudden death in children, adolescents, and young children. Chest 87:476, 1985.
155. Kligfield P, Devereux R: Is the mitral valve prolapse patient at high risk of sudden death identifiable? Cardiovasc Clin 21:143, 1990.
156. Jeresaty R: Sudden death in the mitral valve prolapse–click syndrome. Am J Cardiol 37:317, 1976.
157. Dollar A, Roberts W: Morphologic comparison of patients with mitral valve prolapse who died suddenly with patients who died from severe valvular dysfunction or other conditions. J Am Coll Cardiol 17:921, 1991.
158. Brodsky M, Wu D, Denes P, et al: Arrhythmias documented by 24 hour continuous electrocardiographic monitoring in 50 male medical students without apparent heart disease. Am J Cardiol 39:390, 1977.
159. Savage H, Kissane J, Becher E, et al: Analysis of ambulatory electrocardiograms in 14 patients who experienced sudden cardiac death during monitoring. Clin Cardiol 10:621, 1987.
160. Kramer H, Kligfield P, Devereaux R, et al: Arrhythmias in mitral valve prolapse. Arch Intern Med 144:2360, 1984.
161. Gornick C, Tobler H, Pritzker M, et al: Electrophysiologic effects of papillary muscle traction in the intact heart. Circulation 73:1013, 1986.
162. Kay J, Krohn B, Zubiate P, Hoffman R: Surgical correction of severe mitral prolapse without mitral insufficiency but with pronounced cardiac arrhythmias. J Thorac Cardiovasc Surg 78:259, 1979.
163. Senges J, Zebe H, Pelzer J, et al: Nitrates and ectopic ventricular activity in mitral valve prolapse: clinical and experimental data. Z Kardiol 68:26, 1979.
164. Morady F, Shen E, Bhandari A, et al: Programmed ventricular stimulation in mitral valve prolapse: analysis of 36 patients. Am J Cardiol 53:134, 1984.
165. Hohnloser S, Weiss M, Zeiher A, et al: Sudden cardiac death recorded during ambulatory electrocardiographic monitoring. Clin Cardiol 7:517, 1984.
166. Davis M, Popple A: Sudden unexpected cardiac death: a practical approach to the forensic problem. Histopathology 3:255, 1979.
167. Milstein S, Buetikofer J, Lesser J, et al: Cardiac asystole: a manifestation of neurally-mediated hypotension-bradycardia. J Am Coll Cardiol 14:1626, 1989.
168. Leichtman D, Nelson R, Gobel F, et al: Bradycardia with mitral valve prolapse. Ann Intern Med 85:453, 1976.
169. Santos A, Mathew P, Hilal A, Wallace W: Orthostatic hypotension: a commonly unrecognized cause of symptoms in mitral valve prolapse. Am J Med 11:746, 1977.
170. Holmes J, Kubo S, Cody R, Klingfield P: Arrhythmias in ischemic and nonischemic dilated cardiomyopathy: prediction of mortality by ambulatory electrocardiography. Am J Cardiol 55:146, 1985.

171. Barlow J, Pocock W: Perspectives on the Mitral Valve. p. 45. Philadelphia: FA Davis, 1987.
172. Boudoulas H, King B, Wooley C: Mitral valve prolapse: a marker for anxiety or overlapping phenomenon. Psychopathology 17:98, 1984.
173. Pasternac A, Tabau J, Puddu P, et al: Increased plasma catecholamine levels in patients with symptomatic mitral valve prolapse. Am J Med 73:783, 1982.
174. Coghlan H, Phares P, Cowley M, et al: Dysautonomia in mitral valve prolapse. Am J Med 67:236, 1979.
175. Gaffney H, Karlsson E, Campbell W, et al: Autonomic dysfunction in women with mitral valve prolapse syndrome. Circulation 59:894, 1979.
176. Boudoulas H, Reynolds J, Mazzaferri E, Wooley C: Metabolic studies in mitral valve prolapse syndrome: a neuroendocrine-cardiovascular process. Circulation 61:1200, 1980.
177. Boudoulas H, Reynolds J, Mazzaferri E, Wooley C: Mitral valve prolapse syndrome: the effect of adrenergic stimulation. J Am Coll Cardiol 2:638, 1983.
178. Weisman N, Shear K, Kramer-Fox R, Devereaux R: Contrasting patterns of autonomic dysfunction in mitral valve prolapse and panic attacks. Am J Med 82:880, 1987.
179. Lenders J, Fast J, Blankers J, et al: Normal sympathetic neural activity in patients with mitral valve prolapse. Clin Cardiol 9:177, 1986.
180. Mantysaari M: Hemodynamic reactions to circulatory stress tests in patients with neurocirculatory dystonia. Scand J Clin Lab Invest 44:1, 1984.
181. Dimsdale JE, Moss J: Plasma catecholamines in stress and exercise. JAMA 243:340, 1980.
182. Taggart P, Carruthers M, Somerville W: Electrocardiogram, plasma catecholamines and lipids, and their modification by oxpreolol when speaking before an audience. Lancet 2:341, 1973.
183. Taylor A, Davis A, Mares A, et al: Spectrum of dysautonomia in mitral valvular prolapse. Am J Med 86:267, 1989.
184. Spencer FC, Galloway AC, Grossi EA, et al: Recent developments and evolving techniques of mitral valve reconstruction. Ann Thorac Surg 65:307, 1998.

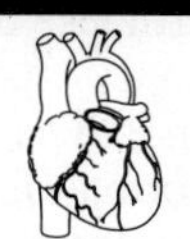

CHAPTER 16

MITRAL VALVE PROLAPSE (MYXOMATOUS MITRAL VALVE)

Elliot Chesler

HISTORY
NOMENCLATURE
DEFINITION
PATHOLOGY
Normal Mitral Valve
Myxomatous Mitral Valve
GENETICS
EPIDEMIOLOGY
ASSOCIATED ABNORMALITIES
Skeletal Disorders
Inherited Disorders of Connective Tissue
Other Conditions
CLINICAL FINDINGS
Symptoms
Physical Examination
ELECTROCARDIOGRAPHY
ECHOCARDIOGRAPHY
M-Mode Echocardiography
Two-Dimensional Echocardiography
CARDIAC CATHETERIZATION AND
ANGIOCARDIOGRAPHY
COMPLICATIONS
Mitral Regurgitation
Infective Endocarditis
Systemic Embolism
Dysrhythmias and Sudden Death
Autonomic Dysfunction
PROGNOSIS
MANAGEMENT

HISTORY

Interest in the midejection or nonejection systolic click has fascinated clinicians for a long time and was seminal in the development of our knowledge of *mitral valve prolapse* (MVP). In 1913, Gallavardin[1] thought the click was of extracardiac origin, but it was not until 1961 that Reid[2] recorded a midsystolic click followed by a late-systolic murmur and correctly reasoned that both probably arose from one of the atrioventricular valves. The relationship among the late-systolic murmur, nonejection click, prolapse of the mitral leaflets, and mitral regurgitation was firmly established by Barlow and Pocock in 1963[3] using cineangiography. These authors credited the assistance of Criley, who interpreted their angiograms and subsequently introduced the term *prolapse* to describe the appearance produced by protrusion of the posterior mitral leaflet into the left atrium.[4]

After this came rapid recognition of various clinical and electrocardiographic abnormalities. Complications such as infective endocarditis, rupture of the chordae tendineae, systemic embolism, dysrhythmias, sudden death, and neuroendocrine and psychiatric abnormalities were described in rapid succession.[5–17] The advent of M-mode echocardiography helped clarify the effects of posture and other maneuvers affecting the click and murmur, and this technique was widely used for population surveys. The interest of echocardiographers was further boosted by the two-dimensional technique that greatly facilitated detection of abnormal leaflets and rupture of chordae tendineae.[5–9]

Importantly, pathologists precisely defined the gross and microscopic abnormalities of the mitral valve by showing that *myxomatous degeneration* was the crucial alteration in the leaflets that predisposed to their redundancy and prolapse and, sometimes, rupture of chordae tendineae. Also, genetic studies identified that the myxomatous mitral valve is transmissible as an autosomal dominant trait associated with other heritable abnormalities of connective tissue, typically Marfan's syndrome.[10–13]

Since the late 1980s alone, more than 1500 articles relating to MVP were published in peer-reviewed journals.[14, 15] Other articles published in daily tabloids may have contributed to establishing centers for treatment and support groups for "victims" of MVP. Although this may have surrounded the condition with some atmosphere of pantomime, there should be no illusion about its importance—it affects approximately 4% of the population and, following the decline in incidence of rheumatic fever, has become the leading cause of mitral regurgitation in the United States.

NOMENCLATURE

The surfeit of names given to this condition indicates the confusion and disagreement among physicians. Apart from eponyms such as *Barlow's syndrome,* other terms refer to some anatomic or functional abnormality. Thus, we have, among others, *myxomatous, floppy, hooded, billowing,* and *prolapsing* mitral valve, the *systolic click-murmur syndrome, anatomic MVP, MVP syndrome,* and *billowing mitral leaflet syndrome.*

This semantic confusion has been aggravated by echocardiographers who attempt to measure and define what constitutes "normal" superior systolic displacement as distinct from abnormal "prolapse" of mitral valve leaflets.[16, 17]

Prolapse detected by echocardiography does not necessarily imply that the valve is abnormal. In atrial septal defect and hypertrophic obstructive cardiomyopathy, prolapse of normal leaflets may occur because of disproportion between the volume of the left ventricle and the size of the mitral annulus (secondary MVP).[18, 19] This may also occur in inferior myocardial infarction and other myocardial diseases, such as myocarditis and cardiomyopathy, because of failure of chordal systolic tension. Under these circumstances, the clinical picture is usually dominated by the underlying disease and prolapse is a secondary finding. Prolapse of normal leaflets has also been reported in trained athletes and nonathletic young women.[20, 21] In all these instances, the leaflets appear thin and they do not have the thickness and redundancy of a myxomatous mitral valve nor its associated pathologic features, such as left ventricular endocardial friction lesions and left atrial angle lesions, which are recognizable by two-dimensional (2-D) echocardiography.

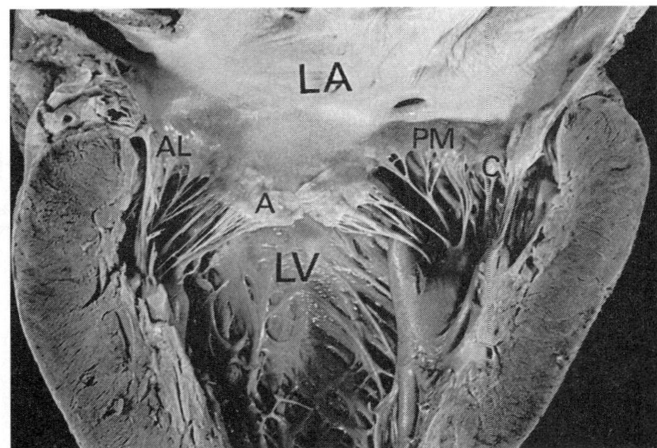

FIGURE 16–1 Normal mitral valve. The anterior leaflet (A) is large and triangular. The posterior leaflet has three scallops: anterolateral (AL), posteromedial (PM), and central (C). Mild interchordal hooding is present at the edge of the leaflet. LA, left atrium; LV, left ventricle. (From Lucas R, Edwards JE: The floppy mitral valve. Curr Probl Cardiol 7:5, 1982.)

DEFINITION

Since the term *mitral valve prolapse* is now widely accepted, it seems reasonable to restrict its use to that condition in which the observed clinical and echocardiographic features are compatible with those of a myxomatous mitral valve. Prolapse of normal leaflets (secondary MVP) observed as an incidental complication of diseases of the left ventricle should not enter into this consideration.

PATHOLOGY

Normal Mitral Valve

Gross Anatomy[10, 12, 13]

The mitral valve has two leaflets attached at their bases to the annulus fibrosis and by their free edges to their chordae tendineae (Fig. 16–1). Each leaflet has a rough zone toward the free edge and a central clear zone toward the base. The anterior leaflet forms one third and the posterior leaflet two thirds of the annulus. The anterior leaflet is approximately triangular, and its base is attached by fibrous connection to the root of the aorta. The posterior leaflet is narrower than the anterior and is actually a continuation of left atrial endocardium across the atrioventricular ring.

Although the leaflets are of different shapes their surface area is approximately the same. In most patients, the posterior leaflet is composed of three scallops, named according to their position in relation to the commissures of the mitral valve—*posteromedial, central,* and *anterolateral.* In the normal mitral valve, there are also interchordal convexities protruding toward the left atrium that vary considerably in height. Since the leaflets are thin and pliable, left ventricular pressure causes a certain amount of "hooding" of interchordal tissue, even in the normal valve.

Microscopic Anatomy

The leaflets are composed of four layers: auricularis, fibrosa, ventricularis, and spongiosa (Fig. 16–2).

The *auricularis* is composed of collagen and elastic tissue, which form the contact or atrial aspect of the leaflet. This layer is continuous with the endocardium of the left atrium.

The *fibrosa* constitutes the basic support for the leaflet and is composed of thick collagen. This layer is continuous at its base with either the fibrous tissue of the annulus, in the case of the posterior leaflet, or the aortic root, in the case of the anterior leaflet. Its free edge is continuous with the chordae tendineae.

The *ventricularis* is a thin layer of collagen and elastic tissue that covers the ventricular aspect of the fibrosa and is continuous in the case of the posterior leaflet with left ventricular endocardium. It is considered to be part of the fibrosa.

The *spongiosa* or fourth layer is situated between the auricularis and the fibrosa layers and is formed of delicate myxomatous connective tissue.

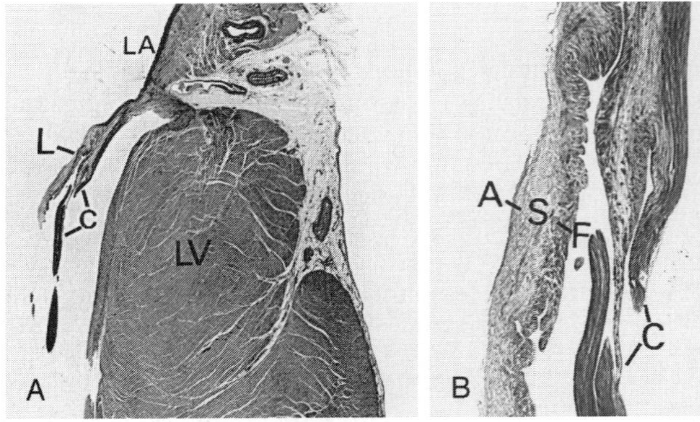

FIGURE 16–2 Photomicrographs of the normal mitral valve **(A)** and components of the leaflet (L) **(B)**. LA, left atrium; LV, left ventricle; A, auricularis; C, chordae; F, fibrosa; S, spongiosa. (**A** and **B,** From Guthrie RB, Edwards JE: Pathology of the myxomatous mitral valve. Minn Med 59:637, 1976.)

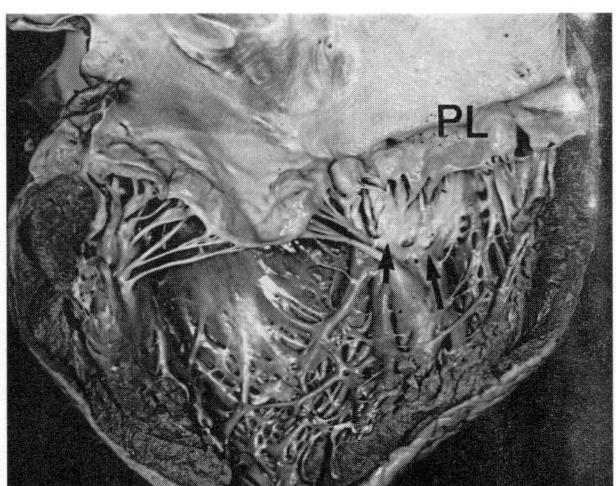

FIGURE 16–3 Myxomatous mitral valve shows redundancy of the anterior and posterior mitral leaflets with obvious prolapse. Note extensive endocardial fibrosis *(arrows)* below the posterior mitral leaflet (PL). (Courtesy of The Jesse E. Edwards Registry of Cardiovascular Diseases.)

Myxomatous Mitral Valve

Gross Anatomy

The criteria for making a gross diagnosis of myxomatous mitral valve have been well summarized by Edwards[22] (Fig. 16–3):

1. Interchordal hooding involving both rough and clear zones of the involved leaflet or leaflets
2. Height of interchordal hooding exceeding 4 mm
3. Interchordal hooding involving at least half of the anterior leaflet or two thirds of the posterior leaflet

Typically, the posterior leaflet is involved either alone or more prominently than the anterior leaflet. The leaflet tissue, which is abnormally hooded, is also translucent or opaque. The degree of interchordal hooding is variable, so that there is an intermediate zone between the obviously abnormal and the clearly normal that even experienced pathologists may find difficult to evaluate without histologic confirmation. The condition of the chordae tendineae is variable: some are elongated, thickened, and even fused, and this may be confused with rheumatic disease. However, commissural fusion is absent, and this makes the distinction possible.

Secondary Effects

Fibrosis of the Free Aspect of the Leaflet. Fibrosis at the summit of the atrial aspect of prolapsing portions of the leaflet is believed to be a response to injury when the leaflet makes contact with an opposite element or adjacent segment of the valve. The fibrosis involves the auricularis layer.

Fibrosis Deposits on the Left Ventricular Surface of the Leaflets. Fibrous deposits occur in the noncontact aspects of the leaflets in the concavity of prolapsed segments and are a response to stretching and tension that occurs when that portion of the leaflet prolapses. Occasionally, this fibrous reaction between inserting chordae may extend to related chordae, but the basic anatomy of the leaflets remains normal. This is important in making the distinction from chronic rheumatic mitral valve disease: a myxomatous mitral valve may become fibrotic but not all layers of the leaflet are affected, as in chronic rheumatic mitral valve disease. Also, like marked secondary leaflet fibrosis, commissural fusion is characteristically absent.

Left Ventricular Endocardial Friction Lesions. A secondary effect produced by the myxomatous mitral valve involves the mural endocardium of the left ventricle in relation to chordae inserting into the posterior mitral valve leaflet. Initially, the chordae tendineae are long and thin but, eventually, may become thickened by aggregation of fibrous tissue on their surfaces. When the posterior mitral leaflet protrudes into the left atrium, the chordae make contact with the related left ventricular mural endocardium, causing a fibrous reaction (Fig. 16–4). These lesions are initially discrete linear thickenings of the endocardium, but subsequently, they may coalesce, so that considerable portions of the base of the left ventricle become thickened and even calcified. Because the chordae adhere to the mural endocardium, they may become shortened and incorporated into the fibrous tissue. This may yield a complex picture

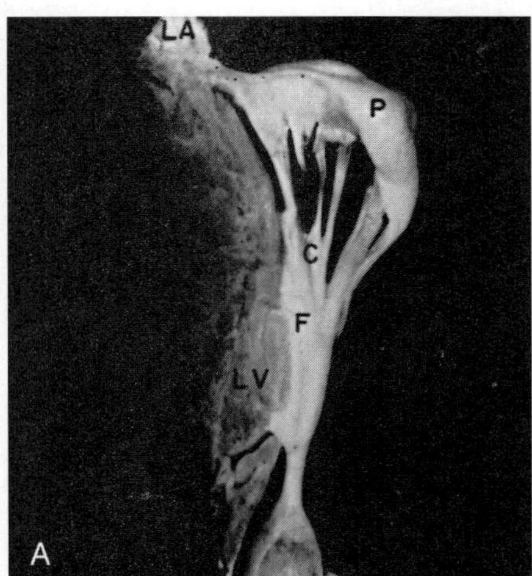

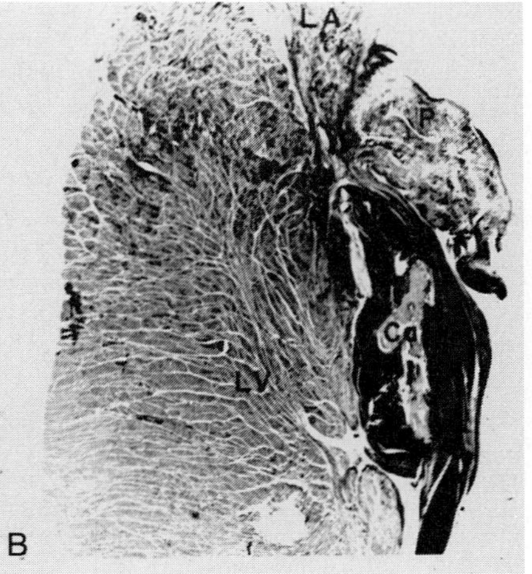

FIGURE 16–4 A, Cross section of the myxomatous posterior mitral leaflet (P) chordae, adjacent left ventricle (LV) and left atrium (LA). The mural endocardium of the left ventricle (F) is markedly thickened and lower portions of the chordae (C) are incorporated into this fibrous tissue. **B,** Photomicrograph of region illustrated in **A** shows the myxomatous posterior mitral leaflet above an extensive, calcified endocardial friction lesion (Ca). (**A** and **B,** Reprinted from Am J Cardiol, Vol. 60, Chesler E, Gornick C, Edwards J, Calcification of the mural endocardium of the left ventricle complicating the myxomatous mitral valve, p. 1197, Copyright 1987, with permission from Excerpta Medica Inc.)

that may easily be misinterpreted as the end result of infective endocarditis or rheumatic fever.

Left Atrial Angle Lesion. The left atrial angle lesion (Fig. 16–5) is situated in the angle between the posterior mitral leaflet and the left atrial wall and also consists of an aggregation of platelets and thrombus that may eventually calcify. The lesion occurs as a result of friction between the posterior leaflet and the left atrial wall.[23]

Contact Thrombosis. Contact thrombosis may be found on the atrial aspect of prolapsed units. It consists of an aggregation of platelets and thrombi.

Both contact thrombosis on the leaflets and the left atrial angle lesion are considered to be sources for systemic embolism.

Microscopic Anatomy

The primary abnormality occurs in the spongiosa layer, which is characteristically thickened by deposition of acid mucopolysaccharides (Fig. 16–6). This layer encroaches on and invades the other layers, particularly the fibrosa. Because the fibrosa represents the chief support for the leaflets, focal interruption by myxomatous infiltration weakens the leaflet, and "hooding" into the left atrium results from the force of left ventricular systole stretching the interchordal tissue.

GENETICS

Most studies strongly favor that the myxomatous mitral valve is inherited. Family studies indicate that expression of the genes for the myxomatous valve is affected by both age and gender. In the first 93 families studied by Devereux and colleagues,[24] the proportion of affected first-degree relatives was approximately 50 percent among adult, female first-degree relatives under the age of 50 years, which is compatible with a fully expressed autosomal dominant disorder. Lower prevalences were found among adult men, older women, and children.

EPIDEMIOLOGY

Most studies of the prevalence of MVP have been based on findings derived from echocardiography. These studies have inherent disadvantages, not only because the criteria for diagnosis of degrees of prolapse is extremely variable among the authors but also because there is considerable variation in interobserver and intraobserver interpretation. Other studies have been biased because subjects volunteered in response to an advertisement, making it difficult to exclude the possibility that the "volunteers" knew they had some form of heart disease.[21] As indicated previously, some interchordal hooding is present even in the normal mitral valve. Therefore, the findings from large-scale echocardiographic epidemiologic studies should be interpreted with caution. The hazard of attempting to identify minor degrees of prolapse is that it artificially increases the "background prevalence" of the condition and increases the chances of finding a coincidental association with some other disease or symptom.

Most studies indicate that the myxomatous mitral valve is identified in approximately 4 percent of the population.[17] The prevalence is lower in childhood and adolescence but increases with advancing years. Clinical observations

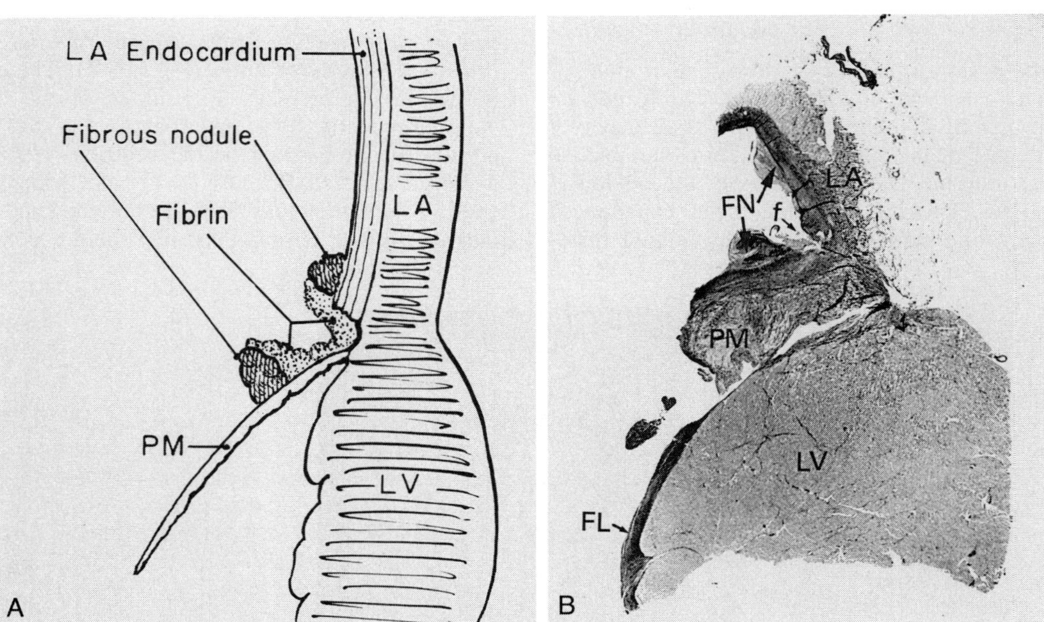

FIGURE 16–5 Diagram **(A)** and photomicrograph **(B)** of the junction of the left atrium (LA), and the posterior mitral leaflet (PM) and the related left ventricular wall (LV). There is deposition of fibrin (f) in the angle between the posterior mitral leaflet and the left atrial endocardium. Fibrous nodules (FN) are present both above the angle, involving the left atrial wall, and below, involving the superior surface of the posterior mitral leaflet. A friction lesion (FL) of the left ventricular endocardium is present in **B**. (Elastic tissue stain, magnification × 40.) (**A** and **B**, From Chesler E, King R, Edwards J: The myxomatous mitral valve and sudden death. Circulation 67:632, 1983.)

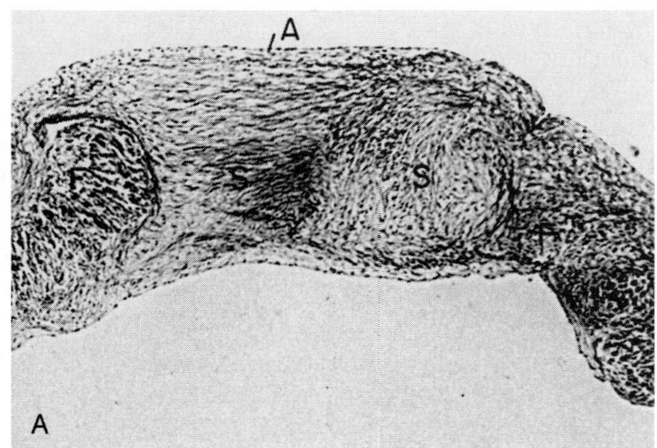

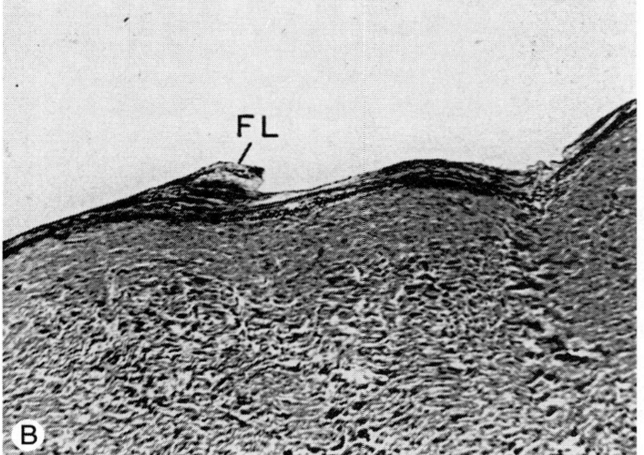

FIGURE 16–6 Photomicrographs of posterior mitral leaflet **(A)** and related left ventricular endocardium **(B)**. The spongiosa layer (S) in the leaflet is increased and encroaches on the atrialis (A) and fibrosa (F) layers. **B,** Fibrous friction lesion (FL) of endocardium is adjacent to the chordae of the posterior leaflets. (**A** and **B,** From Chesler E, King R, Edwards J. et al: The myxomatous mitral valve and sudden death. Circulation 67:632, 1983.)

indicate a higher frequency in older age groups, particularly males, who also tend to have more severe valve and left ventricular dysfunction.[25] The prevalence in women, but not in men, decreases with age.

ASSOCIATED ABNORMALITIES

Skeletal Disorders

Pectus excavatum, straight back, scoliosis, and high-arched palate are associated with MVP. When these thoracic deformities are present, a diligent search should be made for the presence of a myxomatous mitral valve.[26, 27]

Inherited Disorders of Connective Tissue

An association with Marfan's and Ehlers-Danlos syndromes is well established. These findings suggest that there is a reasonable possibility of finding a myxomatous mitral valve in patients with other generalized disorders of connective tissue, such as pseudoxanthoma elasticum.[27]

Other Conditions

MVP has been described in association with a host of other disorders, such as rheumatic endocarditis, coronary artery disease, congestive and hypertrophic cardiomyopathy, myocarditis, trauma, left atrial myxoma, systemic lupus erythematosus, left ventricular aneurysm, migraine, hypomagnesemia, and congenital heart disease (including atrial and ventricular septal defects, patent ductus arteriosus, absence of the pericardium, and membranous subaortic stenosis).[28] However, it has been pointed out earlier that many of these associations relate to so-called secondary MVP, in which left ventricular–left atrial disproportion produces minor bulging of normal leaflets into the left atrium.

Obviously, there must be a fortuitous concurrence of a myxomatous valve with other abnormalities. Since MVP is identified in approximately 4 percent of the population, coincidental association will be most probable when some other condition, whether cardiac or noncardiac (e.g., migraine[29] or mitral annular calcification), also occurs with some frequency in the general population. For example, it is not surprising that MVP has been described in association with mitral annular calcification in women in their 70s because approximately three quarters of such individuals are found to have some degree of calcification at autopsy (J. E. Edwards, M.D., personal communication, 1991) Similarly, a pathologic study found a high incidence (18 percent) of myxomatous valves among patients with ventricular septal defect, but careful comparison with other information in that report suggested that they were unrelated occurrences.[30]

The effect of *patient selection* and *ascertainment bias* is illustrated by the purported association between MVP and hyperthyroidism. By studying the prevalence of all types of thyroid disorders among family members with and without MVP, Zullo and coworkers[31] were unable to demonstrate a valid statistical link between hyperthyroidism and symptomatic subjects with MVP. Such noncausal associations are likely to be identified in populations that share multiple symptoms: in MVP and hyperthyroidism, the common symptom is palpitation, and this leads to ascertainment bias.[32]

CLINICAL FINDINGS

Symptoms

It is virtually certain that the majority of subjects with myxomatous mitral valve and varying degrees of MVP are asymptomatic and never seek medical attention. However, there is a group of patients purported to have an *MVP syndrome* who present with a variety of symptoms that have attracted considerable attention. These nonspecific symptoms include palpitation, fatigue, left inframammary pain, dizziness, syncope, or presyncope. The difficulty in reconciling the occurrence of similar auscultatory, echocardiographic, and electrocardiographic features among patients with and without these symptoms was clearly recognized by Barlow and Pocock,[28] who emphasized that patients with marked prolapse are not necessarily symptomatic, yet some with mild prolapse may have numerous symptoms.

The symptoms described in association with MVP are indistinguishable from those occurring in D'Acosta's syndrome, neurocirculatory asthenia, and "soldier's heart," and were considered by Wood[33] to be a psychiatric disorder (anxiety state). In modern terminology, these symptoms are classified as "panic disorder with somatization"[34] affecting 2 to 5 percent of the general population, 10 to 14 percent of patients seen in cardiologic practice, and 6 to 10 percent of patients attending primary care clinics.[35, 36] In a review of 55 patients with panic disorder, Katon[34] noted that such patients often focus on one or two somatic symptoms of the disorder for which they seek medical help. Primary among the somatic presentations are cardiac symptoms.

Some authors have claimed an association between anxiety state, panic disorder, agoraphobia, and MVP, but others have denied this relationship. Leatham and Brigden[37] believed that "isolated disease of the mitral valve causing mild or moderate reflux seldom causes symptoms other than those of iatrogenic anxiety." Hickey and associates[38] studied 103 patients with echocardiographically proved MVP and found that the scores for neuroticism and neurotic symptoms did not differ from those in patients with other cardiac diseases or from those patients presenting to primary care departments. Uretsky[39] studied 927 patients in an adult general medical population and found that the incidence of atypical chest pain (17.4 versus 17.2 percent) and chronic anxiety (7.1 versus 10.7 percent) was not significantly different for patients with MVP compared with healthy subjects. A study of 42 young soldiers with neurocirculatory asthenia found that the prevalence of MVP was similar to that in the general population.[40] In our study of 10 patients, the Minnesota Multiphasic Personality Inventory, State Trait Anxiety Score, and Psychological Present State Examination showed no difference between patients with MVP and control subjects.[41] In an extensive review, Margraf and colleagues[42] concluded that there was no functional relationship between MVP and panic disorders and that *comorbidity* in highly symptomatic individuals was the probable explanation. Thus, it is highly likely that there is no causal relationship between psychiatric disorder and the myxomatous mitral valve and that the symptoms are probably a result of superimposed or iatrogenic-induced anxiety in a select group of individuals who have been subjected to excessive medical attention.

Physical Examination

General Findings

Occasionally, there are some features of Marfan's syndrome or formes frustes thereof, that is, high-arched palate or chest wall deformity, such as pectus excavatum or scoliosis.

Precordial Palpation

Precordial palpation is normal unless there is significant mitral regurgitation associated with severe prolapse or rupture of the chordae. Under these circumstances, palpation may detect evidence of hyperdynamic left ventricular enlargement and, occasionally, a late-systolic left atrial lift produced by severe mitral regurgitation.

Auscultation

THE CLICK

The click is a high-pitched sound occurring in midsystole, and it has therefore been termed *nonejection.* It is frequently the feature that attracts medical attention. It is high pitched and heard in the region between the apex and the left sternal border. Careful timing by M-mode echocardiography has shown that the click coincides with the position of maximal excursion of the posterior leaflet in midsystole when there is probably the most tension on the chordal leaflet structures. Occasionally, a diastolic sound may be recorded when a voluminous posterior leaflet slaps against the anterior leaflet in early diastole[5] (Fig. 16–7).

Depending on volume changes in the left ventricle, the click may occur quite early in systole (Fig. 16–8). However, it can be differentiated from an aortic ejection click because it occurs after the beginning of the upstroke of the carotid pulse. Not infrequently, there are multiple systolic clicks. The clue to proper identification of nonejection systolic clicks is the dynamic demonstration of their mobility induced by changes in left ventricular volume. Maneuvers that increase ventricular volume, such as squatting, phenylephrine administration, and passive leg raising, shift the click later in systole, whereas maneuvers that decrease left ventricular volume, such as standing, amyl nitrate inhalation, or Valsalva maneuver, shift the click earlier in systole. These volume changes within the left ventricle are responsible for the characteristic day-to-day and often hour-to-hour variability in detection and timing of the click.

THE MURMUR

Typically, the murmur is late systolic in timing and follows the click. Like the click, it is responsive to maneuvers that change left ventricular volume. The intensity and character of the murmur are variable but are best heard at the apex or left midprecordium when mitral regurgitation is mild. The murmur may be confused with that of hypertrophic cardiomyopathy because both murmurs increase in intensity and duration with standing and decrease with squatting. However, the murmur of hypertrophic cardiomyopathy becomes louder after amyl nitrate inhalation whereas that of mitral regurgitation does not. Also, during the Valsalva strain, the murmur of hypertrophic cardiomyopathy increases in intensity in contrast to that of mitral regurgitation, which becomes longer. A useful auscultatory finding is postextrasystolic potentiation in intensity of the murmur that is quite marked in hypertrophic cardiomyopathy, whereas the murmur of mitral regurgitation does not usually change or may actually decrease in intensity. In any event, the other typical features of hypertrophic cardiomyopathy, such as jerky pulses, and severe left ventricular hypertrophy detected clinically by electrocardiogram and echocardiogram usually suffice to make the distinction.

When myxomatous change in the leaflets is severe, and particularly when the chordae rupture, the murmur of mitral

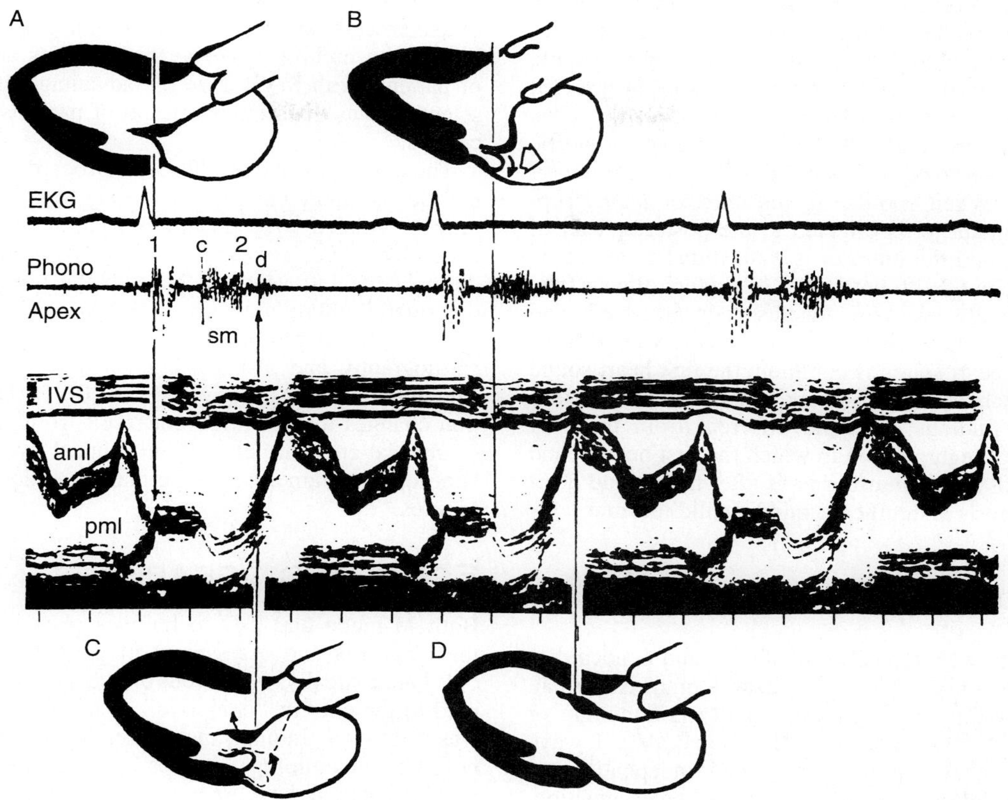

FIGURE 16–7 Simultaneous electrocardiogram (EKG), phonocardiogram (Phono), and M-mode echocardiogram in mitral valve prolapse. **A–D,** Ventricular angiography is depicted. The phonocardiogram demonstrates a midsystolic click (c), a late systolic murmur (sM), and a opening sound early in diastole (d). **A,** The first heart sound occurs at the onset of ventricular systole. **B,** In midsystole, there is a click and a late-systolic murmur as the mitral valve leaflets bulge into the left atrium. **C,** In early diastole, the leaflets swing open, resulting in a diastolic opening sound (d). **D,** The leaflets reach their maximal diastolic excursion as the anterior mitral leaflet (aml) echo strikes the ventricular septum. IVS, interventricular septum; pml, posterior mitral leaflet. (**A–D,** From Criley JM, Siegel RJ: Functional anatomy and pathophysiology of mitral valve prolapse. In Boudoulas H, Wooley CF [eds]: Mitral Valve Prolapse and the Mitral Valve Prolapse Syndrome. Mount Kisco, NY: Futura, 1988.)

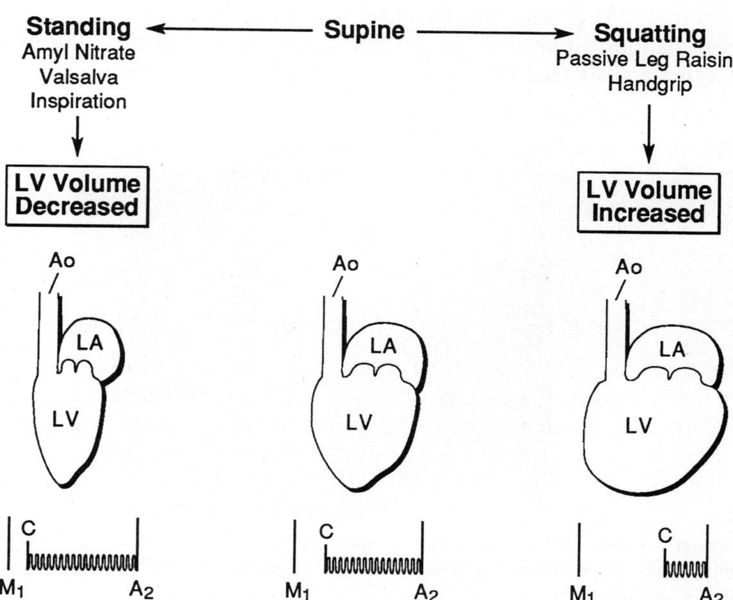

FIGURE 16–8 Diagram illustrates the effect of volume changes on portions of click and murmur (see text). A_2, second heart sound; Ao, aorta; C, click; LA, left atrium; LV, left ventricle; M_1, mitral first heart sound.

regurgitation is holosystolic and may have a loud vibratory "honking" quality. The clinical picture produced by rupture of chordae tendineae to the *posterior leaflet* is quite characteristic. Because the regurgitant jet is often directed anteriorly, striking the atrial septum adjacent to the aortic root, the systolic murmur is most prominent in the aortic area and may therefore be confused with the murmur of aortic stenosis. When chordae to the *anterior leaflet* rupture, the regurgitant jet is directed to the posterior wall of the left atrium, and the murmur is transmitted to the spine or even the occiput. With both types of rupture, the systolic murmur is usually crescendo-decrescendo in shape and terminates before the aortic component of the second heart sound. A third heart sound is common, the first heart sound of normal or increased intensity and a middiastolic murmur absent. These findings are quite different from those of rheumatic mitral regurgitation in which the first heart sound is soft, the holosystolic murmur ends after the second heart sound, and there is a significant middiastolic murmur.

ELECTROCARDIOGRAPHY

In most patients with typical auscultatory and echocardiographic features of MVP, the electrocardiogram is normal. The most commonly reported abnormality is flattening or inversion of the T waves in leads II, III, and aVF. T wave inversion may occur spontaneously and independent of effort or may follow assumption of the erect position. Occasionally, these inferior repolarization changes are quite striking and, when accompanied by significant Q waves, may be suggestive of a diagnosis of inferior myocardial infarction. The exact prevalence of these findings is unknown because of different criteria of selection of patients in various series. McLaren and coworkers[43] reported an incidence of 7 percent in a survey of asymptomatic black school children with MVP in Johannesburg, South Africa. On the other hand, the Framingham study of the general population showed that persons with and without echocardiographic MVP were equally likely to have repolarization abnormalities.[44] Furthermore, studies comparing unaffected relatives and spouses of relatives in the families of affected patients with MVP showed no difference in the incidence of electrocardiographic repolarization abnormalities compared with control subjects. Such studies among relatives of patients with MVP have the advantage of being free of selection bias that affects referral of patients to specialized centers.[45]

The pathogenesis of these electrocardiographic abnormalities is unknown, but is tempting to speculate that they may be related to endocardial friction lesions. It is not generally appreciated that fibrosis involving the endocardium of the left ventricle beneath the posterior leaflet of the mitral valve may be so extensive, confluent, and calcified that it can be detected by angiography and echocardiography and also distinguished from mitral annular calcification[46] (Figs. 16–9 and 16–10). Perhaps repolarization changes that are transient result from varying degrees of chordal-endocardial friction induced by changes in left ventricular volume, before permanent endocardial scarring ensures.

ECHOCARDIOGRAPHY

Both M-mode and 2-D techniques play a pivotal role in the diagnosis and assessment of patients with MVP.[5, 7–9, 16, 47] Paradoxically, the advent of echocardiography contributed to the current "epidemic" of MVP because diagnosis was based on findings that were, in fact, variants of the normal. Epidemiologic studies based on loose echocardiographic criteria have reported the incidence of MVP at anywhere between 5 and 21 percent of the healthy population. Such fallacies may be avoided by using at least two criteria for diagnosis: (1) clear echocardiographic evidence of leaflet redundancy and thickening with chordal lengthening compatible with myxomatous degeneration of the valve; and (2) the presence of some degree of mitral regurgitation detectable *clinically* and not merely by color-flow Doppler, which is overly sensitive.

M-Mode Echocardiography

This technique suffers from the limitation that the ultrasonic beam is narrow and provides a restricted window

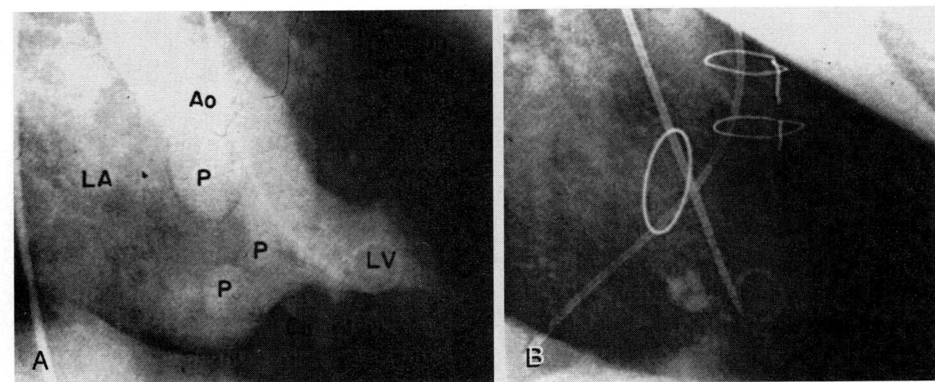

FIGURE 16–9 A, Left ventricular cineangiogram, right anterior oblique projection. Severe mitral regurgitation and prolapsing mitral leaflets (P) with subannular mural calcification (Ca) of the endocardium are present. Ao, aorta; LA, left atrium; LV, left ventricle. **B,** Postoperatively, the calcification is demonstrated below the mitral annulus. (**A** and **B,** Reprinted from Am J Cardiol, Vol. 60, Chesler E, Gornick C, Edwards J, Calcification of the mural endocardium of the left ventricle complicating the myxomatous mitral valve, p. 1196, Copyright 1987, with permission from Excerpta Medica Inc.)

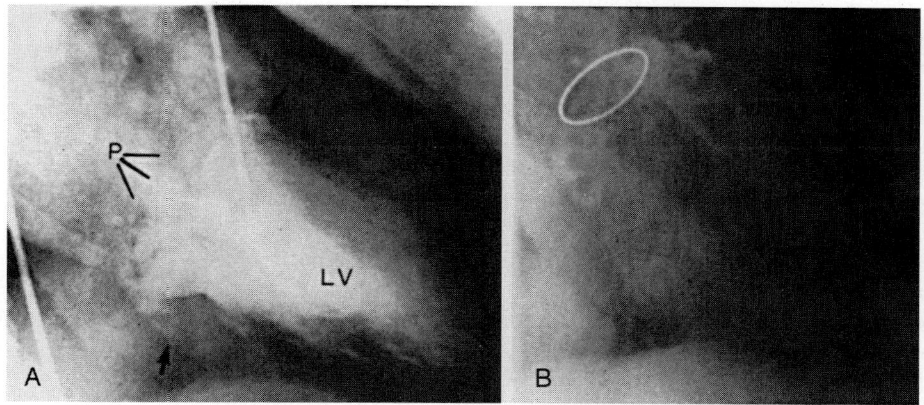

FIGURE 16–10 Left ventricular cineangiogram, right anterior oblique view. **A,** Calcified mitral annulus (*arrows*), prolapsed mitral leaflets (P), and severe mitral regurgitation. LV, left ventricle. **B,** Postoperatively, the sewing ring of the porcine prosthesis clearly locates the calcification in the mitral annulus. (**A** and **B** Reprinted from Am J Cardiol, Vol. 60, Chesler E, Gornick C, Edwards J, Calcification of the mural endocardium of the left ventricle complicating the myxomatous mitral valve, p. 1196, Copyright 1987, with permission from Excerpta Medica Inc.)

(so-called ice-pick view). However, there are findings that supplement the 2-D technique.

1. *Midsystolic or late-systolic buckling:* This sudden posterior displacement of the leaflets is quite characteristic of MVP and is extremely useful in timing the onset of the click and murmur (see Fig. 16–7). This finding is very reliable, and there are few false-positive results. Posterior prolapse of one or both leaflets is the opposite movement to systolic anterior motion encountered in hypertrophic obstructive cardiomyopathy in which the anterior mitral leaflet moves *anteriorly* toward the ventricular septum in midsystole.
2. *Holosystolic "hammocking":* Holosystolic posterior displacement is not absolutely specific for MVP. False-positive results may occur when there is excessive cardiac movement in systole (e.g., pericardial effusion). Since a small amount of posterior movement of the normal mitral valve occurs during systole, it has been suggested that the diagnosis be made only when this exceeds 2 mm. However, such arbitrary numbers increase the number of false-positive results and the likelihood of misleading epidemiologic data. Reliance should rather be placed with the 2-D technique.

Two-Dimensional Echocardiography

Two-dimensional echocardiography provides much better spatial visualization of the leaflets, chordae, and papillary muscle and is particularly useful in the diagnosis of ruptured chordae. The important changes are

1. Thickening of the leaflets and chordae with superior systolic displacement of segments of the valve into the left atrium above the plane of the mitral annulus. Using multiple views, it is possible to detect which portions of the leaflets are redundant and prolapsing (Fig. 16–11). Rupture of chordae is readily diagnosed by echocardiography, which is also helpful in excluding infective endocarditis as the cause. The following findings are readily elicited with good technique: (1) failure of leaflet coaptation with the edges frequently observed in several views; (2) a whipping motion of the leaflet and attached chordae seen when a sizable

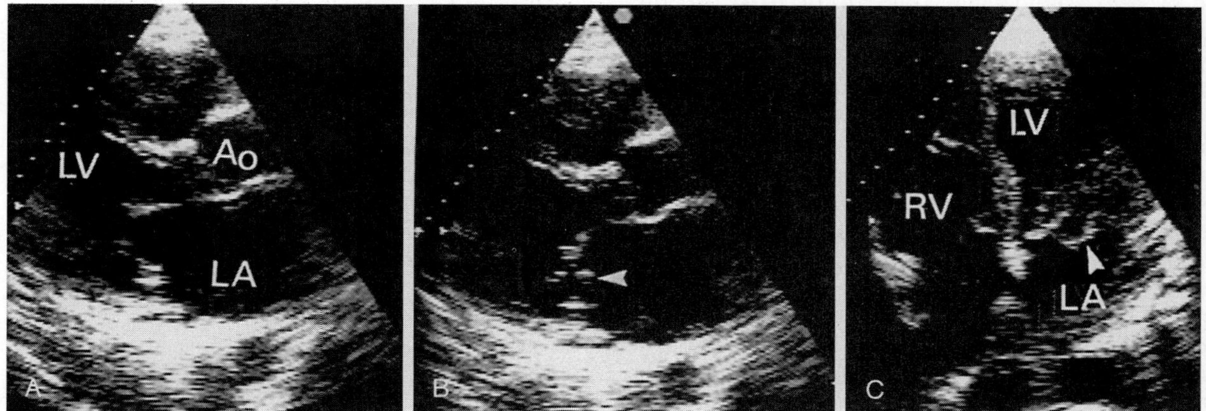

FIGURE 16–11 Two-dimensional echocardiogram in mitral valve prolapse. **A,** Thickened anterior and posterior mitral leaflets are open in diastole. Ao, aorta; LA, left atrium; LV, left ventricle. **B,** Prolapse of the posterior leaflet (*arrowhead*) is shown. **C,** Four-chamber view shows prolapse of the posterior leaflet (*arrowhead*) into the left atrium. RV, right ventricle.

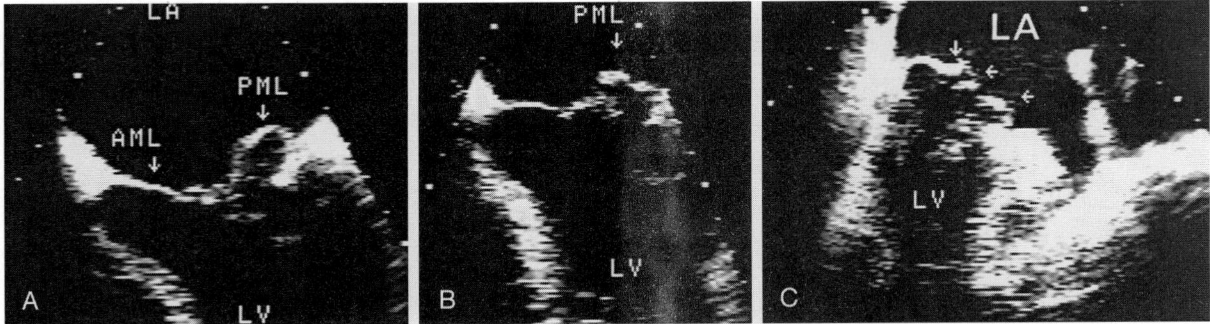

FIGURE 16–12 Transesophageal echocardiograms in mitral valve prolapse show how the technique demonstrates the fine detail of leaflet anatomy. **A,** Prolapse of the posterior mitral leaflet (PML). AML, anterior mitral leaflet; LA, left atrium; LV, left ventricle. **B** and **C,** The scallops (*arrows*).

portion of a leaflet is detached; (3) Color-flow Doppler is useful, but not essential, in diagnosis and clearly demonstrates the eccentricity and direction of the jet, depending on which chordae have ruptured.

2. The presence of calcified left atrial angle lesion *above* and left ventricular endocardial friction lesions *below* the mitral annulus.

The *transesophageal* technique is particularly useful in defining the anatomy more precisely and readily recognizes the failure of leaflet coaptation and lengthening and rupture of the chordae tendineae (Fig. 16–12).

CARDIAC CATHETERIZATION AND ANGIOCARDIOGRAPHY

Invasive procedures are rarely indicated nowadays because clinical and echocardiographic findings are so accurate. The hemodynamics are normal unless there is severe mitral regurgitation. Although earlier reports incriminated a myocardial factor,[48] there is no consistent abnormality other than the so-called ballerina-foot deformity of the left ventricular contour in systole, found when there is marked prolapse (Fig. 16–13). This deformity of the inferior left ventricular wall is a frequent finding and a result of traction on the papillary muscles by the leaflet that is prolapsing. Traction on the left ventricular wall may also be demonstrated by apex cardiography (Fig. 16–14). The ballerina foot disappears after mitral valve replacement.

Angiography in a typical case of MVP demonstrates protrusion of the mitral leaflet beyond the plane of the annulus. Much like echocardiography, there has been considerable disagreement as to what constitutes an abnormal protrusion of the various scallops beyond the annulus. The posterior leaflet is best evaluated in the right anterior oblique position. It should be noted that there is a normal protrusion below the valve attachment in the so-called fornix or subannular pouch that may be confused with prolapse of the posterior leaflet if it is not appreciated that the fornix is inferior to the annulus (Fig. 16–15). The posteromedial, middle, and anterolateral scallops of the posterior leaflet are readily identifiable by high-quality cineangiography.[4] The anterior commissural scallop of the posterior mitral leaflet is frequently confused with the anterior mitral leaflet as it forms a bump anterior to and beneath the aortic valve in the right oblique projection. Prolapse of the anterior leaflet is usually better visualized in the 60-degree left anterior oblique view, where it can be followed from its attachment to the aortic root to its position in systole where it coapts with the posterior leaflet. When the anterior leaflet prolapses, it extends posterior to the shadow of the annulus into the left atrium, inferior and posterior to the aortic root (see Fig. 16–13).

COMPLICATIONS

Mitral Regurgitation

The myxomatous valve is now a leading cause of mitral regurgitation in the United States. This is because of a

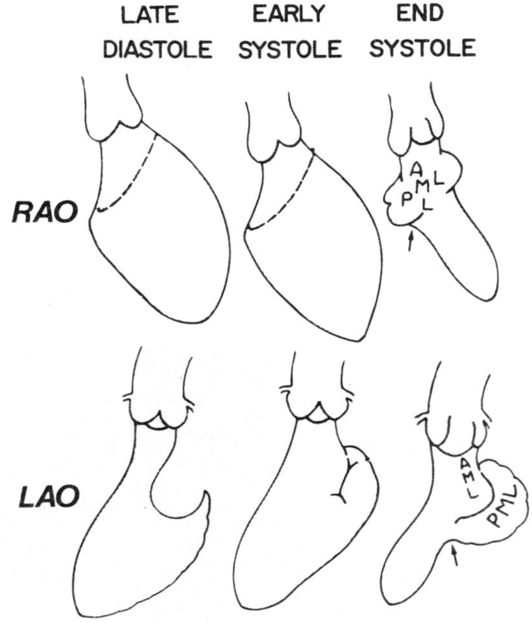

FIGURE 16–13 Diagrammatic representation of angiographic anatomy in mitral valve prolapse. In the 45-degree right anterior oblique (RAO) and the 60-degree left anterior oblique (LAO) projections. The "anterior hump" right upper figure, RAO projection, represents an anterior commissural scallop of the posterior mitral leaflet (PML). "Ballerina-foot" deformity is illustrated in the LAO projection, lower right panel. AML, anterior mitral leaflet. (From Hager J, Criley JM: Prolapse mitral leaflet syndrome. Cardiovasc Clin 10:1, 213, 1979.)

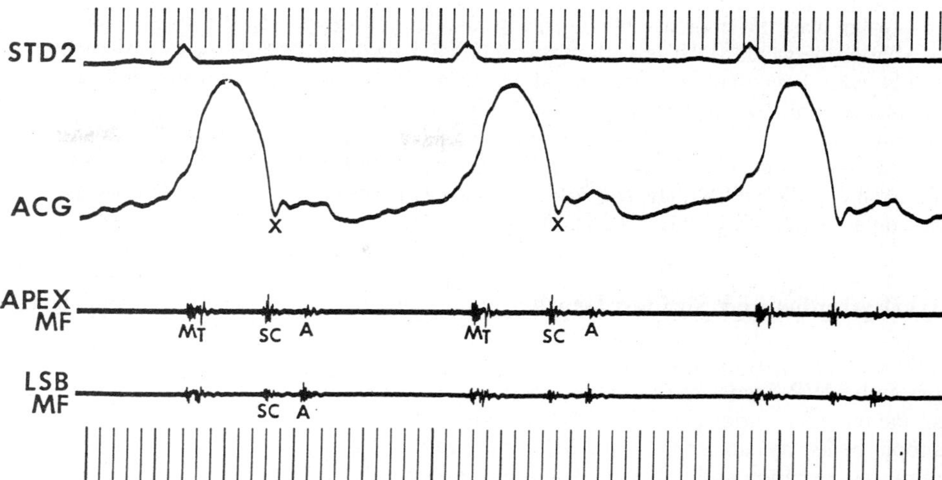

FIGURE 16–14 Simultaneous electrocardiogram (standard lead II [STD2]), apex cardiogram (ACG), phonocardiograms at the apex and the left sternal border (LSB) (medium frequency [MF]) demonstrating a midsystolic click (SC) and retraction of the apex (X). A, aortic valve closure; M, mitral valve closure; T, tricuspid valve closure. (From Barlow JB: Perspectives on the Mitral Valve. Philadelphia: FA Davis, 1987.)

decline in the incidence of rheumatic fever and a greater awareness of the condition by clinicians and pathologists. Some instances of "rheumatic" mitral regurgitation were in fact myxomatous valves associated with secondary fibrosis erroneously diagnosed as healed rheumatic or infective endocarditis. Signs of severe mitral regurgitation and heart failure supervene in a small proportion of patients with MVP, and men above the age of 45 years are particularly prone to this complication.[45, 49] The mechanisms for increasing mitral regurgitation include: (1) increasing prolapse when progressive myxomatous degeneration weakens the leaflets; (2) dilatation of the annulus that goes along with, and may aggravate, in a vicious circle, increasing degrees of regurgitation; and (3) rupture of the chordae tendineae.

Infective Endocarditis

Patients with MVP and a late systolic murmur are at increased risk for infective endocarditis.[50–53] Most clinicians agree that such patients should receive antibiotic prophylaxis before any procedure that places them at risk.[38] This does not completely solve the problem, however, because those patients with MVP who have systolic murmurs intermittently may also be at increased risk. Certainly, antibiotic prophylaxis is strongly indicated when additional factors, such as thickened redundant leaflets, are identified by echocardiography and when there is a predisposition to frequent bacteremia because of drug addition or immunosuppression.

Systemic Embolism

Several studies have reported an increased risk for stroke among subjects with MVP. Barnett and associates[54, 55] found a much higher incidence of systemic embolism in younger patients with MVP than in control subjects. However, a population-based study in Olmsted County, Minnesota, found the age at first stroke among individuals with MVP was similar to that in an unselected population: in the absence of ischemic heart disease, congestive heart failure, diabetes mellitus, and mitral valve replacement, the risk

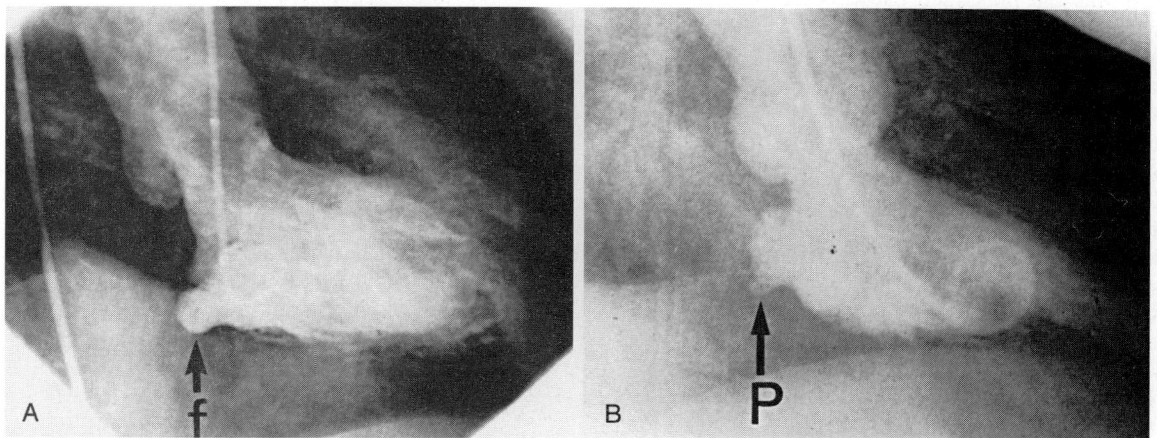

FIGURE 16–15 A, Cineangiogram, right anterior oblique position, demonstrates the formix (F), or subannular pouch (*arrow*), in the normal mitral valve. Note that the leaflets are not displaced beyond the annulus. **B,** Prolapse (P) of the posterior mitral leaflet is also shown.

for stroke was not increased.[56] There is also a possible association between MVP and coronary embolism in young people who have had myocardial infarction with angiographically normal coronary arteries.[57] Although the exact mechanism for systemic embolism has not been documented, there are at least two sources for platelet, fibrin, and even calcific emboli: surfaces of redundant leaflets and the angle lesion within the left atrium.

Dysrhythmias and Sudden Death

A wide range of dysrhythmias has been reported in association with MVP. Some dysrhythmias, such as supraventricular tachycardia, atrial fibrillation, atrial flutter, and atrial ectopic beats, are not specific for MVP but are a result of mitral regurgitation and left atrial distention and complicate significant mitral regurgitation of any cause. Other dysrhythmias, such as those complicating the Wolff-Parkinson-White syndrome, are a result of concurrence of two common conditions.

The ventricular dysrhythmias, particularly high-grade ventricular ectopy and ventricular tachycardia, have attracted attention and have been correlated with the risk of sudden death. However, it should be strongly emphasized that sudden unexpected death resulting from dysrhythmia among young people with MVP is rare.[23, 58–62] Not only are adequate clinical details and electrocardiographic recordings of the final event poorly documented, but detailed pathologic findings are also usually absent. In 1983, we reviewed 39 reported cases of sudden death attributed to the myxomatous mitral valve and found that autopsies had been performed in only 19, and in most, the information was so sparse that other diseases could not be definitely excluded.[23] Many cases of sudden death attributed to MVP were in fact, the result of drug toxicity, electrolyte imbalance, or other unrecognized and unrelated cardiac pathology, such as cardiomyopathy.

In their meticulous follow-up of patients with MVP, Pocock and colleagues[58] encountered only one patient who died suddenly. This young woman had been treated for multifocal ventricular extrasystoles, and a myxomatous mitral valve was the chief finding at autopsy. Ventricular fibrillation was the presumed cause of death.[58] Nishimura and coworkers[9] reported 6 cases of sudden death among 237 asymptomatic or mildly symptomatic patients with MVP whom they had followed for a mean of 6.2 years. Also, Duren and associates,[49] in a prospective follow-up of 300 patients (mean follow-up, 6.1 years), encountered 3 cases of sudden death. In neither series were autopsies available, and Duren and associates[49] pointed out that their data may have been biased because their patients had been referred to a cardiac center for evaluation, so that their findings did not necessarily apply to the natural history in the general population.

These findings in so few cases must be reconciled with other evidence and considered against the background prevalence of dysrhythmias and risk of sudden death in the general population. Frequent atrial and ventricular premature beats are unusual in a young population, but one study of 50 male medical students without apparent heart disease showed that 1 subject had a short run of ventricular tachycardia and 3 others with ventricular ectopy manifested the R-on-T phenomenon.[63] In the Framingham study, dysrhythmias were detected with similar frequency by resting 12-lead, exercise, and 1-hour ambulatory electrocardiography in subjects with and without MVP.[64] This study was population-based and avoided the selection bias evident in other studies from tertiary referral centers that reported life-threatening cardiac dysrhythmias. Kramer and colleagues[65] clearly demonstrated the effect of selection bias when they compared patients with MVP with similarly symptomatic controls: patients with MVP did not have an excessive prevalence of dysrhythmias.

Mechanism for Dysrhythmias

In our report of 14 patients with sudden death, it was documented that the myxomatous valve was the only pathologic finding.[23] We noted that 3 of the 14 patients showed only mild grades of prolapse. A family pedigree was available in 1 of these cases (a girl age 14 years). The girl's mother died suddenly at age 36 years, and two of the girl's siblings died suddenly at ages 11 and 12 years. All had mild grades of prolapse and no history of dysrhythmias. There was no recording of the final dysrhythmia in 5 patients, but because premature ventricular systoles had been documented at some time, the final event was assumed to be ventricular dysrhythmia. It was postulated that the mechanism for dysrhythmia might be mechanical stimulation of the endocardium by chordae of the posterior mitral leaflet, a notion supported by experiments showing that traction on papillary muscles may produce ventricular ectopy.[66] These observations may be in concert with those rare patients with hemodynamically mild mitral regurgitation and repeated ventricular tachycardia in whom valvuloplasty of the voluminous leaflets abolished the dysrhythmia.[67]

Electrophysiologic studies have not contributed to defining the role of ventricular ectopy. Some patients with mild MVP and high-grade ventricular ectopy have demonstrated normal intracardiac conduction and refractoriness.[68] Other authors have pointed out that programmed ventricular stimulation, which induced polymorphic ventricular tachycardia among patients with MVP, could be simply a nonspecific response to an aggressive stimulation protocol.[69]

Episodes of sudden death among the general population are not usually recorded by ambulatory electrocardiography.[64, 70] Usually, ventricular tachycardia and fibrillation are responsible and complicate cases of ischemic heart disease. In pathology and forensic literature, there are also cases of sudden death in young people that have not been associated with any demonstrable cardiac abnormality, and the conduction system has been normal.[59, 71] Perhaps such cases are related to the phenomenon of asystolic cardiac arrest recently documented in young people. Milstein and coworkers[72] reported the findings in six survivors of cardiac asystole, none whom had clinically detectable heart disease. A hypotensive-bradycardic response with syncope was reproduced by passive orthostatic tilt and thought to be neurally mediated by mechanoreceptors in the left ventricle. This raises the possibility that some cases of sudden death may have been erroneously attributed to a myxomatous mitral valve when the actual cause was neurally mediated hypotension and cardiac asystole. This association has, in fact, been documented by Leichtman and associates,[73] who described 11 members of a family with a high prevalence of MVP and syncope: orthostatic tilt-induced hypotension, bradycardia, and syncope. Santos and colleagues[74] reported similar findings in 12 of 86 patients with MVP, but unfortunately, there were no controls in their study, so the association could be a result of selection bias.

Thus, the causal relationship between MVP and sudden death remains unclear. What is clear is that in the absence of severe mitral regurgitation and left ventricular dysfunction,[75] the risk of sudden death in young people who do not have ventricular dysrhythmia, syncope, or presyncope is so remote, they should not be informed of this possibility.

Autonomic Dysfunction

The term *billowing mitral leaflet syndrome* was introduced by Barlow and Pocock[76] to apply when symptoms such as anxiety, fatigue, weakness, and palpitation are associated with MVP. More recently, the term *mitral valve prolapse syndrome* was coined by Boudoulas and coworkers[26] to categorize symptomatic patients whom they believe to have neuroendocrine or autonomic dysfunction and a "hyperadrenergic" state. Boudelas and colleagues[26, 77] proposed that MVP may be a marker for autonomic dysfunction.

Several reports have pointed to autonomic dysfunction among patients with MVP. Pasternac and coworkers[78] studied 15 symptomatic patients and measured plasma norepinephrine levels, heart rate, and supine and standing systolic and diastolic blood pressures. Total plasma catecholamine and norepinephrine levels were significantly increased in patients in both positions, and heart rate was lower than normal in patients in the supine position but returned to normal in the upright position. These investigators believe that this hyperadrenergic and vagotonic state could explain many of the findings and manifestations of the MVP syndrome.

These observations were confirmed by Coghlan and associates,[79] but were somewhat at variance with those of Gaffney and colleagues,[80] who found diminished vagal response to the diving reflex and phenylephrine infusion. Boudoulas and coworkers[81] found increased 24-hour urinary norepinephrine and epinephrine excretion in symptomatic patients with MVP. Additionally, isoproterenol infusion produced a dose-related increase in heart rate in MVP patients in excess of that of controls. These authors believe that MVP may be a specific marker in certain people "for the constitutional, neuroendocrine-cardiovascular process that is currently designated as the MVP syndrome."[82] However, other studies reported decreased epinephrine excretion and increased vagal tone in patients with MVP.[83] Chesler and associates[41] showed that among 11 consecutive patients with MVP encountered in hospital practice evenly matched in control for age and gender, there was not a significant difference between norepinephrine levels, heart rates, and blood pressure in response to orthostatic tilt. Similarly, Lenders and colleagues[84] found no differences in neurohumoral responses to orthostatic tilt comparing symptomatic and asymptomatic patients with MVP. Mantysaari[85] compared patients with neurocirculatory asthenia and normal controls and reported no significant difference in response to hyperventilation, orthostatic tilt, Valsalva maneuver, cold pressor test, or isometric hand grip.

These conflicting findings are likely a result of several factors:

1. Many study populations have been small in size and composed mostly of highly symptomatic young women.
2. Not all control populations have been clearly defined.
3. MVP has not always been excluded by echocardiography in control groups.
4. Some studies have drawn conclusions from measuring catecholamines at rest or during passive standing rather than during orthostatic stress and isometric exercise, which is the preferred method.[78, 80, 81, 83] Anxiety may induce a hyperadrenergic state. For example, plasma norepinephrine levels have been shown to increase by more than 50 percent and epinephrine levels to more than double during public speaking by young physicians at conferences.[86, 87]

Taylor and coworkers[88] studied normal controls, asymptomatic MVP patients, and patients with MVP who had symptoms suggestive of autonomic dysfunction. Responses to ice-water immersion and administration of isoproterenol, epinephrine, and tyramine were the same in patients with similar symptoms and did not distinguish between those with and those without MVP. These authors emphasized that autonomic responses to physiologic maneuvers and agonist drugs in controls and in patients with MVP are heterogenous, and this may be partially responsible for the divergent findings reported in the literature. Bias in patient selection and small sample size could favor one abnormality over another. One may conclude, therefore, that definite proof of a connection between autonomic dysfunction and MVP is lacking.

Prognosis

Although it is difficult to precisely define the natural history of such a common disorder, there can be little doubt that the outlook for patients with MVP is excellent, the majority of subjects remaining asymptomatic for their lifetimes without any complications. Pathologic studies comparing the age at death of patients with myxomatous valves with control autopsy material showed that patients with myxomatous valves in fact, lived longer.[13] The incidence of infective endocarditis and systemic embolism is low, and the risk of sudden death is minuscule. Progressive mitral regurgitation may occur, particularly in older men among whom sudden deterioration is frequently a result of ruptured chordae or infective endocarditis.

Management

The majority of patients with MVP are asymptomatic and should be reassured that their condition is benign. When a nonejection click is followed by a late-systolic murmur, there is a risk of infective endocarditis, and patients should be advised of the necessary prophylactic measures.

Patients who have significant mitral regurgitation should be examined at regular intervals of approximately 1 year, particularly in the case of elderly men with a holosystolic murmur and echocardiographic evidence of leaflet redundancy and chordal lengthening. Left ventricular function should be carefully assessed at each visit. Left ventricular dysfunction is a major hazard for patients with significant regurgitation. When the preoperative ejection fraction is less than 50 percent, there is considerable risk for postoperative left ventricular dysfunction and eventual heart failure. Among patients with preserved left ventricular function and without coronary artery disease, conservative repair of the mitral valve may be accomplished with low mortality and excellent functional result.[89] In centers where surgeons have considerable experience with valvuloplasty, correction should be seriously considered, even in asymptomatic patients when the ejection fraction is more than 60 percent and the left ventricular end-systolic dimension is 45 mm or less. Techniques include annuloplasty, leaflet plication, leaflet resection, and chordal transposition. Transesophageal Doppler echocardiography is extremely useful in assessing whether the valve is suitable for repair and is also of great value in the operating room to assess the efficacy of repair. In those cases in which anatomy is unsuitable for repair, valve replacement should be with a metallic prosthesis or porcine heterograft.

The small group of patients who complain of dizziness, presyncope, or syncope who have ventricular arrhythmias demonstrated by 24-hour electrocardiographic monitoring or treadmill exercise testing should be treated aggressively. If necessary, provocative electrophysiologic testing should be employed to select the most efficacious drug.

REFERENCES

1. Gallavardin L: Pseudo dedoublement du deuxieme bruit du coeur simultant le dedoublement mitral par bruit extracardiac telesystolique surajoute. Lyon Med J 121:409, 1913.
2. Reid J: Mid-systolic clicks. S Afr Med J 35:353, 1961.
3. Barlow J, Pocock W: The significance of late systolic murmurs and mid-late systolic clicks. Md State Med J 12:76, 1963.
4. Criley J, Lewis K, Humphries J, Ross R: Prolapse of the mitral valve: Clinical and cine-angiographic findings. Br Heart J 28:488, 1966.
5. Criley JM, Heger J: Prolapsed mitral leaflet syndrome. Cardiovasc Clin 10:213, 1979.
6. Barlow J, Pocock W, Marchand P, Denny M: The significance of late systolic murmurs. Br Heart J 66:443, 1968.
7. Abbasi AS, DeCristofaro D, Anabtawi J, Irwin L: Mitral valve prolapse: comparative value of M-mode, two-dimensional and Doppler echocardiography. J Am Coll Cardiol 2:1219, 1983.
8. Popp RL, Brown O, Silverman JF, Harrison DC: Echocardiographic abnormalities in the mitral valve prolapse syndrome. Circulation 49:428, 1974.
9. Nishimura R, McGoon M, Shub C, et al: Echocardiographically documented mitral valve prolapse: long-term follow-up of 237 patients. N Engl J Med 313:1305, 1985.
10. Pomerance A: Ballooning deformity (mucoid degeneration) of atrioventricular valves. Br Heart J 31:343, 1969.
11. Ranganathan N, Lam J, Wigle E, Silver M: Morphology of the human mitral valve: II. The valve leaflets. Circulation 41:459, 1970.
12. Salazar A, Edwards J: Friction lesions of ventricular endocardium: relation to chordae tendineae of mitral valve. Arch Pathol Lab Med 90:364, 1970.
13. Lucas RJ, Edwards J: The floppy mitral valve. Curr Probl Cardiol 7:1, 1982.
14. Cheitlin M: Mitral valve prolapse. Circulation 59:610, 1979.
15. Chesler E, Gornick C: Maladies attributed to myxomatous mitral valve. Circulation 82:328, 1991.
16. Warth D, King ME, Cohen JM, et al: Prevalence of mitral valve prolapse in normal children. J Am Coll Cardiol 5:1173, 1985.
17. Perloff JC, Edwards JE: New guidelines for the clinical diagnosis of mitral valve prolapse. Am J Cardiol 57:1124, 1986.
18. Schreiber T, Feigenbaum H, Weyman A: Effect of atrial septal defect repair on left ventricular geometry and degree of mitral valve prolapse. Circulation 61:888, 1980.
19. Barlow J, Pocock W: The mitral valve prolapse enigma—two decades later. Mod Concepts Cardiovasc Dis 53:13, 1984.
20. Lewis J, Maron B, Diggs J, et al: Preparticipation echocardiographic screening for cardiovascular disease in a large, predominantly black population of collegiate athletes. Am J Cardiol 64:1029, 1989.
21. Markiewicz W, Stoner J, London E, et al: Mitral valve prolapse in one hundred presumably healthy young females. Circulation 53:464, 1976.
22. Edwards J: Floppy mitral valve syndrome. Cardiovasc Clin 18:249, 1987.
23. Chesler E, King R, Edwards J: The myxomatous mitral valve and sudden death. Circulation 67:632, 1983.
24. Devereaux R, Brown W, Kramer-Fox R, Sachs I: Inheritance of mitral valve prolapse: effect of age and sex on gene expression. Ann Intern Med 97:826, 1982.
25. Devereaux R, Hawkins I, Kramer-Fox R, et al: Complications of mitral valve prolapse: disproportionate occurrence in men and older patients. Am J Med 81:751, 1986.
26. Boudoulas H, Kolibach A, Baker P, et al: Mitral valve prolapse and the mitral valve prolapse syndrome: a diagnostic classification and pathogenesis of symptoms. Am Heart J 118:797, 1989.
27. Leier C, Call T, Fulkerson P, Wooley C: The spectrum of cardiac defects in the Ehlers-Danlos syndrome, types I and III. Ann Intern Med 92:171, 1980.
28. Barlow J, Pocock W: Mitral valve prolapse, the specific billowing mitral leaflet syndrome, or an insignificant non-ejection systolic click. Am Heart J 97:277, 1979.
29. Amat G, Louis P, Loisy C, et al: Migraine and mitral valve prolapse syndrome. Adv Neurol 33:27, 1982.
30. Lucas R, Edwards J: Floppy mitral valve and ventricular septal defect: an anatomic study. J Am Coll Cardiol 15:1337, 1983.
31. Zullo M, Devereaux R, Kramer-Fox R, et al: Mitral valve prolapse and hyperthyroidism: effect of patient selection. Am Heart J 110:977, 1985.
32. Motulsky A: Biased ascertainment and the natural history of disease. N Engl J Med 298:1196, 1978.
33. Wood P: Diseases of the Heart and Circulation. 3rd ed. p. 937. London: Eyre and Spottiswoode, 1962.
34. Katon W: Panic disorder and somatization. Am J Med 77:101, 1984.
35. Cohen M, Bodal D, Kilpatrick A, et al: The high familial prevalence of neurocirculatory asthenia. Am J Hum Genet 3:126, 1951.
36. Rice R: Symptom patterns of the hyperventilation syndrome. Am J Med Sci 8:691, 1951.
37. Leatham A, Brigden W: Mild mitral regurgitation and the mitral prolapse fiasco. Am Heart J 99:659, 1980.
38. Hickey A, MacMahon S, Wilcken D: Mitral valve prolapse and bacterial endocarditis: when is antibiotic prophylaxis necessary? Am Heart J 109:431, 1985.
39. Uretsky B: Does mitral valve prolapse cause nonspecific symptoms? Int J Cardiol 1:435, 1982.
40. Leor R, Markiewicz W: Neurocirculatory asthenia and mitral valve prolapse—two unrelated entities? Isr J Med Sci 17:1137, 1981.
41. Chesler E, Weir E, Braatz G, Francis G: Normal catecholamine and hemodynamic responses to orthostatic tilt in subjects with mitral valve prolapse. Am J Med 78:754, 1985.
42. Margraf J, Ehlers A, Roth W: Mitral valve prolapse and panic disorder: a review of their relationship. Psychosom Med 50:93, 1988.
43. McLaren MJ, Hawkins DM, Lachman AS, et al: Non-ejection clicks and late systolic murmurs in black school children of Soweto, Johannesburg. Br Heart J 38:718, 1976.
44. Savage D, Devereaux R, Garrison R, et al: Mitral valve prolapse in the general population: 2. Clinical features: the Framingham Study. Am Heart J 106:577, 1983.
45. Devereaux R, Kramer-Fox R, Kligfield P: Mitral valve prolapse: causes, clinical manifestations, and management. Ann Intern Med 111:305, 1989.

46. Chesler E, Gornick C, Edwards J: Calcification of the mural endocardium of the left ventricle complicating the myxomatous mitral valve. Am J Cardiol 60:1196, 1987.
47. Dillon JC, Chang CS: Use of echocardiography in patients with prolapsed mitral valve. Circulation 43:503, 1971.
48. Tresh D, Soin J, Siegel R, et al: Mitral valve prolapse—evidence for a myocardial perfusion abnormality. Am J Cardiol 41:441, 1978.
49. Duren D, Becker A, Dunning A: Long-term follow-up of idiopathic mitral valve prolapse in 300 patients: a prospective study. J Am Coll Cardiol 11:42, 1988.
50. Lachman A, Bramwell-Jones D, Lakier J, et al: Infective endocarditis in the billowing leaflet syndrome. Br Heart J 37:326, 1975.
51. MacMahon S, Hickey A, Wilcken D, et al: Risk of infective endocarditis in mitral valve prolapse with and without precordial systolic murmurs. Am J Cardiol 59:105, 1987.
52. MacMahon S, Roberts J, Kramer-Fox R, et al: Mitral valve prolapse and infective endocarditis. Am Heart J 113:1291, 1987.
53. Danchin N, Briancon S, Mathieu P, et al: Mitral valve prolapse as a risk factor for infective endocarditis. Lancet 1:743, 1989.
54. Barnett H, Jones M, Boughner D, Kostuk W: Cerebral ischemic events associated with prolapsing mitral valve. Arch Neurol 33:777, 1976.
55. Barnett H, Boughner D, Taylor D, et al: Further evidence relating mitral valve prolapse to cerebral ischemic events. N Engl J Med 302:129, 1980.
56. Orencia AJ, Petty GW, Khandheria BK, et al: Risk of stroke with mitral valve prolapse in population based cohort study. Stroke 26:7, 1995.
57. Chesler E, Matisonn R, Lakier J, et al: Acute myocardial infarction with normal coronary arteries: a possible manifestation of the billowing mitral leaflet syndrome. Circulation 54:203, 1976.
58. Pocock W, Bosman C, Chesler E, et al: Sudden death in primary mitral valve prolapse. Am Heart J 107:378, 1984.
59. Topaz O, Edwards J: Pathologic features of sudden death in children, adolescents, and young children. Chest 87:476, 1985.
60. Kligfield P, Devereux R: Is the mitral valve prolapse patient at high risk of sudden death identifiable? Cardiovasc Clin 21:143, 1990.
61. Jeresaty R: Sudden death in the mitral valve prolapse–click syndrome. Am J Cardiol 37:317, 1976.
62. Dollar A, Roberts W: Morphologic comparison of patients with mitral valve prolapse who died suddenly with patients who died from severe valvular dysfunction or other conditions. J Am Coll Cardiol 17:921, 1991.
63. Brodsky M, Wu D, Denes P, et al: Arrythmias documented by 24 hour continuous electrocardiographic monitoring in 50 male medical students without apparent heart disease. Am J Cardiol 39:390, 1977.
64. Savage H, Kissane J, Becher E, et al: Analysis of ambulatory electrocardiograms in 14 patients who experienced sudden cardiac death during monitoring. Clin Cardiol 10:621, 1987.
65. Kramer H, Kligfield P, Devereaux R, et al: Arrhythmias in mitral valve prolapse. Arch Intern Med 144:2360, 1984.
66. Gornick C, Tobler H, Pritzker M, et al: Electrophysiologic effects of papillary muscle traction in the intact heart. Circulation 73:1013, 1986.
67. Kay JH, Krohn BG, Zubiate P, Hoffman RL: Surgical correction of severe mitral prolapse without mitral insufficiency but with pronounced cardiac arrhythmias. J Thorac Cardiovasc Surg 78:259, 1979.
68. Senges J, Zebe H, Pelzer J, et al: Nitrates and ectopic ventricular activity in mitral valve prolapse: clinical and experimental data. Z Kardiol 68:26, 1979.
69. Morady F, Shen E, Bhandari A, et al: Programmed ventricular stimulation in mitral valve prolapse: analysis of 36 patients. Am J Cardiol 53:134, 1984.
70. Hohnloser S, Weiss M, Zeiher A, et al: Sudden cardiac death recorded during ambulatory electrocardiographic monitoring. Clin Cardiol 7:517, 1984.
71. Davis M, Popple A: Sudden unexpected cardiac death—a practical approach to the forensic problem. Histopathology 3:255, 1979.
72. Milstein S, Buetikofer J, Lesser J, et al: Cardiac asystole: a manifestation of neurally-mediated hypotension-bradycardia. J Am Coll Cardiol 14:1626, 1989.
73. Leichtman D, Nelson R, Gobel F, et al: Bradycardia with mitral valve prolapse. Ann Intern Med 85:453, 1976.
74. Santos A, Mathew P, Hilal A, Wallace W: Orthostatic hypotension: a commonly unrecognized cause of symptoms in mitral valve prolapse. Am J Med 11:746, 1977.
75. Holmes J, Kubo S, Cody R, Klingfield P: Arrhythmias in ischemic and nonischemic dilated cardiomyopathy: prediction of mortality by ambulatory electrocardiography. Am J Cardiol 55:146, 1985.
76. Barlow J, Pocock W: Perspectives on the Mitral Valve. p. 45. Philadelphia: FA Davis, 1987.
77. Boudoulas H, King B, Wooley C: Mitral valve prolapse: a marker for anxiety or overlapping phenomenon. Psychopathology 17:98, 1984.
78. Pasternac A, Tabau J, Puddu P, et al: Increased plasma catecholamine levels in patients with symptomatic mitral valve prolapse. Am J Med 73:783, 1982.
79. Coghlan H, Phares P, Cowley M, et al: Dysautonomia in mitral valve prolapse. Am J Med 67:236, 1979.
80. Gaffney H, Karlsson E, Campbell W, et al: Autonomic dysfunction in women with mitral valve prolapse syndrome. Circulation 59:894, 1979.
81. Boudoulas H, Reynolds J, Mazzaferri E, Wooley C: Metabolic studies in mitral valve prolapse syndrome: a neuroendocrine-cardiovascular process. Circulation 61:1200, 1980.
82. Boudoulas H, Reynolds J, Mazzaferri E, Wooley C: Mitral valve prolapse syndrome: the effect of adrenergic stimulation. J Am Coll Cardiol 2:638, 1983.
83. Weisman N, Shear K, Kramer-Fox R, Devereaux R: Contrasting patterns of autonomic dysfunction in mitral valve prolapse and panic attacks. Am J Med 82:880, 1987.
84. Lenders J, Fast J, Blankers J, et al: Normal sympathetic neural activity in patients with mitral valve prolapse. Clin Cardiol 9:177, 1986.
85. Mantysaari M: Hemodynamic reactions to circulatory stress tests in patients with neurocirculatory dystonia. Scand J Clin Lab Invest 44:1, 1984.
86. Dimsdale JE, Moss J: Plasma catecholamines in stress and exercise. JAMA 243:340, 1980.
87. Taggart P, Carruthers M, Somerville W: Electrocardiogram, plasma catecholamines and lipids, and their modification by oxpreolol when speaking before an audience. Lancet 2:341, 1973.
88. Taylor A, Davis A, Mares A, et al: Spectrum of dysautonomia in mitral valvular prolapse. Am J Med 86:267, 1989.
89. Spencer FC, Galloway AC, Grossi EA, et al: Recent developments and evolving techniques of mitral valve reconstruction. Ann Thorac Surg 65:307, 1998.

CHAPTER 17

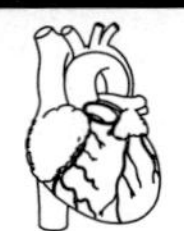

Rheumatic Fever

Robert D. Leachman, D. Richard Leachman, and Jagat Narula

HISTORY
ETIOPATHOGENESIS
EPIDEMIOLOGY
PATHOLOGY
CLINICAL FEATURES
Joint Symptoms
Cardiac Involvement
Sydenham's Chorea
Skin Manifestations
LABORATORY INVESTIGATIONS
NATURAL HISTORY
TREATMENT
STREPTOCOCCAL VACCINE

Rheumatic fever (RF) is a febrile inflammatory illness that affects multiple organ systems. It may affect the skin, brain, cardiovascular system, and the serous membranes of the pericardium, as well as the joints and the abdominal and pleural cavities. In the cardiovascular system, RF causes inflammatory changes, particularly involving the myocardium and the valves. Although the arthritis induced by an acute attack of RF will resolve, leaving no sequelae, the carditis frequently damages the cardiac valves. It has been said that "rheumatic fever licks the joints, but bites the heart."[1]

History

Thomas Sydenham gave the earliest clinical description of acute rheumatism in 1676; it is most common during the autumn, it usually occurs in young, healthy individuals, and after 1 or 2 days, it attacks the joints, sometimes migrating from joint to joint.[2, 3] In his writing, Sydenham distinguished RF from other rheumatic diseases but did not appreciate its effect on the heart. David Pitcairn was the first to note the association of the two in 1788, and Edward Jenner noted this in 1789.[4] Although C. Parry, another early clinician, identified disorders of the heart and blood vessels that appeared to be related to acute rheumatism,[5] it was J. Corvisart (the physician to Napoleon), however, who first used the term *carditis.* He also described the physical finding of the thrill produced in diastole by mitral stenosis.[6] Subsequently, Jean Baptiste Bouillaud drew attention to the relationship between rheumatism and the heart through his descriptions of rheumatic pericarditis and valve lesions. In France and in some parts of South America, acute rheumatism is still known by the eponym *Bouillaud's disease.*[7] In 1840, Bouillaud[8] defined the law of coincidence, which stated that "in the great majority of cases of diffuse acute articular rheumatism with fever, there exists in a variable degree a rheumatism of the serofibrous tissue of the heart. The coincidence is the rule, and the noncoincidence the exception."

In 1904, Aschoff[9] gave the first clear description of the specific rheumatic myocardial lesions seen microscopically, which have since been termed *Aschoff bodies.* In 1948, White[10] translated Aschoff's description of the lesions, noting that the histologic characteristics of the myocardial reaction to the rheumatic infection had been established by finding "these peculiar nodules which appear to be specific." According to the description, the nodules were regularly found near small and medium-sized blood vessels.

The connection between the previous history of a sore throat and RF was suggested by Schlesinger in 1930[11] and later established in 1931 by the bacteriologic and epidemiologic studies of Collis in England[12] and Colburn in the United States.[13] After this, immunologic studies further confirmed the close relationship between group A streptococcal pharyngitis and RF.

Etiopathogenesis

The clinical features of RF tend to develop 10 to 20 days after group A beta-hemolytic streptococcal upper respiratory tract infection. Among the various serotypes of group A streptococci, some appear more likely to be epidemiologically related to acute RF, whereas other strains are more likely to result in postacute streptococcal glomerulonephritis. The exact mechanism by which group A β-hemolytic streptococci initiate RF is unclear, and it is also not known why throat infections and not other streptococcal infections lead to RF.

RF was earlier believed to be the result of direct injury mediated by streptococci[14] or its toxins,[15] but subsequent investigations have suggested that RF is an immune-mediated injury.[16–18] It is believed that rheumatogenic streptococci contain multiple antigenic determinants[19–21] that partially mimic normal human tissue antigens.[22, 23] These antigens, which are recognized as foreign by the susceptible host, induce a hyperactive humoral and cellular immune response. The *N*-acetyl glucosamine moiety of group A polysaccharide cross-reacts with antibodies to the heart valve tissue,[24] which are abundantly observed in patients with rheumatic heart valve disease.[18, 21] On the other hand, the streptococcal M proteins demonstrate homology with contractile (e.g., myosin and tropomyosin) and interstitial (e.g., keratin, laminin, and vimentin) proteins. The M protein epitopes not only can trigger heart cross-reactive antibodies[25, 26] but also can act as superantigens to result in a more widespread immune response by overriding the histocompatibility barrier.[27] It is not yet clear how the cross-reactive antibodies react with contractile protein antigens sequestered intracellularly by sarcolemma. Furthermore, the humoral theory of the genesis of rheumatic carditis through damage to the myocardium does not appear attractive because myocyte necrosis is not a prominent characteristic of myocarditis[28] and cross-reactive antibodies have also been seen in patients without evidence of carditis.[29] The interstitial reaction of anti–M protein antibody may offer an explanation for the induction of myocarditis, whereas the cellular immunity to shared antigenic determinants may contribute to the pathogenesis of valvulitis. A significant T-cell infiltration is observed in the valvular tissue, and the cells isolated from valvular tissue of patients with rheumatic heart disease (RHD) respond to streptococcal M5 protein sequence stretches and cross-react with cardiac myosin.[30] In fact, both humoral[21] and cellular[31] immune responses are more vigorous in patients than in normal subjects. This has been partly attributed to superantigenic property of streptococcal M protein.[27] The superantigen does not bind to antigen-binding cleft in T or B cells but amplifies the immune response through clonal expansion of T and B cells, release of cytokines, and upregulation of adhesion molecules.

Although there is overwhelming evidence that a relationship exists between group A streptococci and RF, the majority of individuals with streptococcal group A infections do not develop RF. There is no satisfactory explanation for this. Studies have shown that a familial or genetic susceptibility to RF exists apart from the environmental risk of exposure to streptococcal infection.[32–34] There is some evidence that the human leukocyte antigens (HLA) may account for individual susceptibility to rheumatic fever and may explain unusual patterns of infection. The HLA types are genetically determined and are not the same in all individuals of a family cohort, although they are the same in monozygotic twins. This may explain why within a family in whom all individuals have been infected with *Streptococcus,* only a few develop RF, and why the incidence is three times higher in monozygotic than in dizygotic twins. Studies have shown a statistically significant association between specific HLA class II antigens and RF. The risk has been associated with the increased prevalence of HLA DR4 in the United States[35, 36] and Saudi Arabia[37] and with the increased prevalence of DR3 and DQw2 in India.[38] Some other markers, such as B-cell alloantigen D8/17, have shown a strong association with susceptibility to RF.[38, 39]

EPIDEMIOLOGY

RF has largely disappeared as a major cause of illness in the United States in the past 30 years.[40–42] According to a summary of notifiable disease in the United States published by the Department of Health and Human Services in 1990,[43] there were approximately 6000 to 9000 cases of acute RF per year up to 1960, when the incidence of acute RF began to decline (Fig. 17–1). By 1970, the incidence had dropped to about 30 percent of the number reported in 1961, and by 1980, the number had declined further to approximately 5 percent. The decline in the incidence of

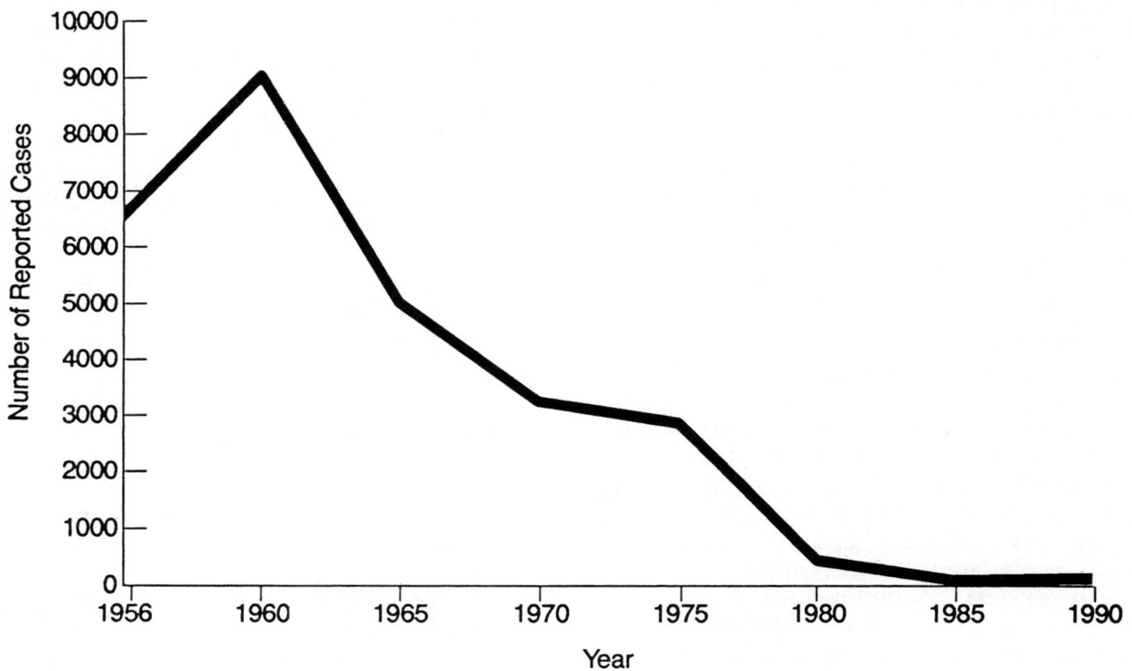

FIGURE 17–1 Summary of reported cases of rheumatic fever in the United States for 1956 to 1990. Note: Before 1956, rheumatic fever was not notifiable nationally. Numbers are given here after 1956 in 5-year increments. The number of reported cases actually peaked in 1961 at 10,470. (Adapted from U.S. Department of Health and Human Services: Summary of Notifiable Disease, United States, 1990. Vol. 39, No. 53, 1990.)

RF may be partially attributed to the introduction of antibiotics to prevent streptococcal pharyngitis and hence recurrences of the disease, although the decline actually began before the antibiotic era (Fig. 17–2).[44] However, a return of RF in sporadic increases was noted in various sections of economically developed countries in the 1980s.[45] The World Health Organization[46] reported an incidence in acute RF of fewer than 5 cases per 100,000 population per year in the industrialized world, which was believed to increase to 100 cases per 100,000 population in some areas of the eastern Mediterranean and the western Pacific. Similarly, several outbreaks had occurred in the United States in portions of Utah and Ohio and at U.S. Naval Training Centers.[45] The return was speculated to be due to the resurgence of more virulent strains of group A *Streptococcus*.

It has long been known that RF tends to occur in socioeconomic groups who are poor, live in crowded conditions, and have inadequate nutrition. This concept has been supported by the frequency of RF outbreaks during World War II, which tended to occur among people concentrated in barracks. The idea that crowded conditions contribute to the distribution of the disease is also supported by the increased incidence among families. It should be obvious that any environmental situation that tends to increase the possibility of dissemination of streptococcal infection will be associated with an increase in RF. Failure to sterilize food utensils and common drinking cups in schools could easily lead to additional transmission. Accordingly, RHD continues to be the most common cause of cardiovascular complications and death in young persons in the developing countries.[46–48] It accounts for more than one third of cardiovascular admissions to hospitals in these countries and constitutes a major indication for cardiac surgery.[48, 49] RF and RHD impose a significant economic burden on the total health budget in developing countries.

PATHOLOGY

The noncardiac inflammatory process produced by RF in the skin, joints, and brain tends to regress spontaneously without any residual effects. There is swelling with serous effusion in the joints, and inflammatory infiltration and edema are evident in the synovial membranes. A fibrinoid exudate frequently lines the membranes. The blood vessels in the articular and periarticular areas are often inflamed and show infiltration with lymphocytes and polymorphonuclear leukocytes. On the other hand, the subcutaneous nodules have a center of fibrinoid necrosis with peripheral inflammatory reaction of lymphocytes and occasional polymorphonuclear leukocytes.

Cardiac involvement in RF affects all three layers: pericardium, myocardium, and endocardium. The pericarditis is typically fibrinous (Fig. 17–3). The histopathologic findings in myocardium include the "pathognomonic" Aschoff

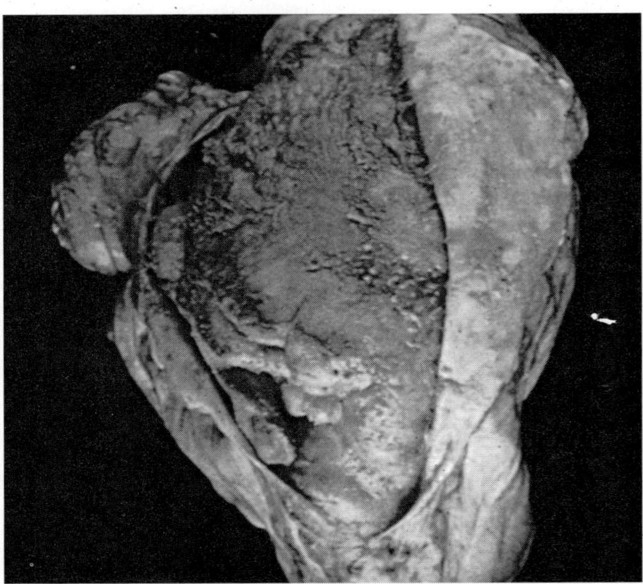

FIGURE 17–3 Pericarditis. Gross pathologic specimen obtained from a patient who died of rheumatic fever. The outer, or parietal, layer of the pericardium has been partially reflected away, revealing the epicardium, which is covered with shaggy fibrinous exudates as if a buttered sandwich had been pulled apart—hence the term *bread-and-butter pericarditis*. (Modified from Massell BF, Narula J: Rheumatic fever and carditis. *In* Braunwald E [ed]: The Atlas of Heart Diseases. pp. 10.1–10.20. Philadelphia: Current Medicine, 1994.)

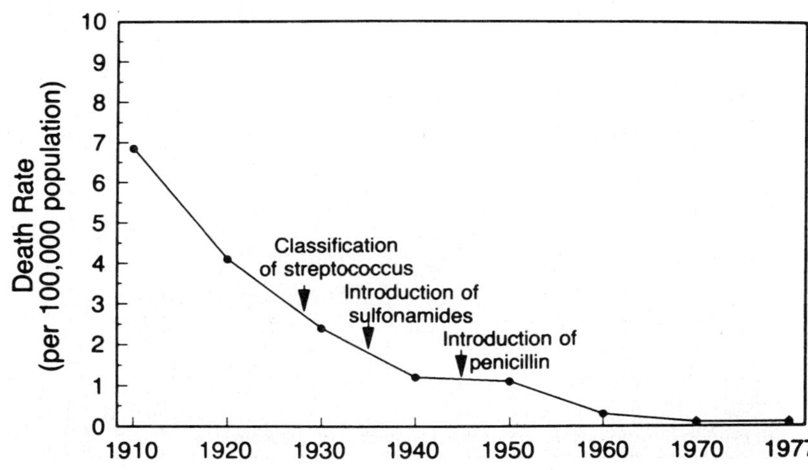

FIGURE 17–2 Unadjusted rates of death due to rheumatic fever in the United States for 1910 to 1977. (From Gordis L: The virtual disappearance of rheumatic fever in the United States: lessons in the rise and fall of the disease: T. Duckett Jones Memorial Lecture. Circulation 72:1155, 1985.)

nodule (Fig. 17–4).[9, 50] The Aschoff granuloma consists of a central area of fibrinoid necrosis surrounded by cells of histiocytic-macrophage origin (Anitschkow cells) which show a typical owl eye–shaped nucleus. These cells are usually found in the subendocardial or perivascular regions in the myocardium. There is surprisingly little histopathologic damage to the myocardium, even in patients with florid clinical carditis and heart failure.[28, 51, 52] Myocyte necrosis is uncommon, and the cellular infiltrate is confined to the interstitium.[53] The conduction system also shows little pathology even in the presence of clinical conduction defects.[54]

The valves bear the brunt of pathologic damage.[42] The valves are inflamed and thickened during the acute stage of the rheumatic activity. The surface of the valves develops small vegetations or verrucae, particularly along the edges of the leaflets (Fig. 17–5). These vegetations are sterile because bacterial colonization does not occur. These vegetations almost never result in thromboembolic sequelae. A mild degree of inflammation leads to fusion of the cusps; further inflammatory reaction involves the chordae tendineae and papillary muscle and results in significant distortion of the valve, which affects the subvalvular apparatus as well. Mitral stenosis never develops in acute stages; it usually requires at least 2 to 8 years, and the obstruction is slow and progressive. Mitral regurgitation, however, occurs very promptly, partly in response to the inflammatory reaction in the valve but also in relation to the dilatation of the left ventricle or mitral annulus. Similarly, tricuspid regurgitation may occur acutely with active rheumatic carditis and dilatation of the annulus. Aortic incompetence also occurs as a consequence of thickening and distortion of the valve leaflets. The scarring process may be gradual, and patients with acute RF may be seen without evidence of aortic valve affliction only to develop aortic regurgitation at a later date. Aortic stenosis also requires a long latent period before becoming evident. There is fusion of the edges of the cusps with fibrinoid inflammatory reaction, followed by fibrosis and obstruction.

The endocardium of the left ventricle and atrium often shows inflammation, including Aschoff bodies. A scar in

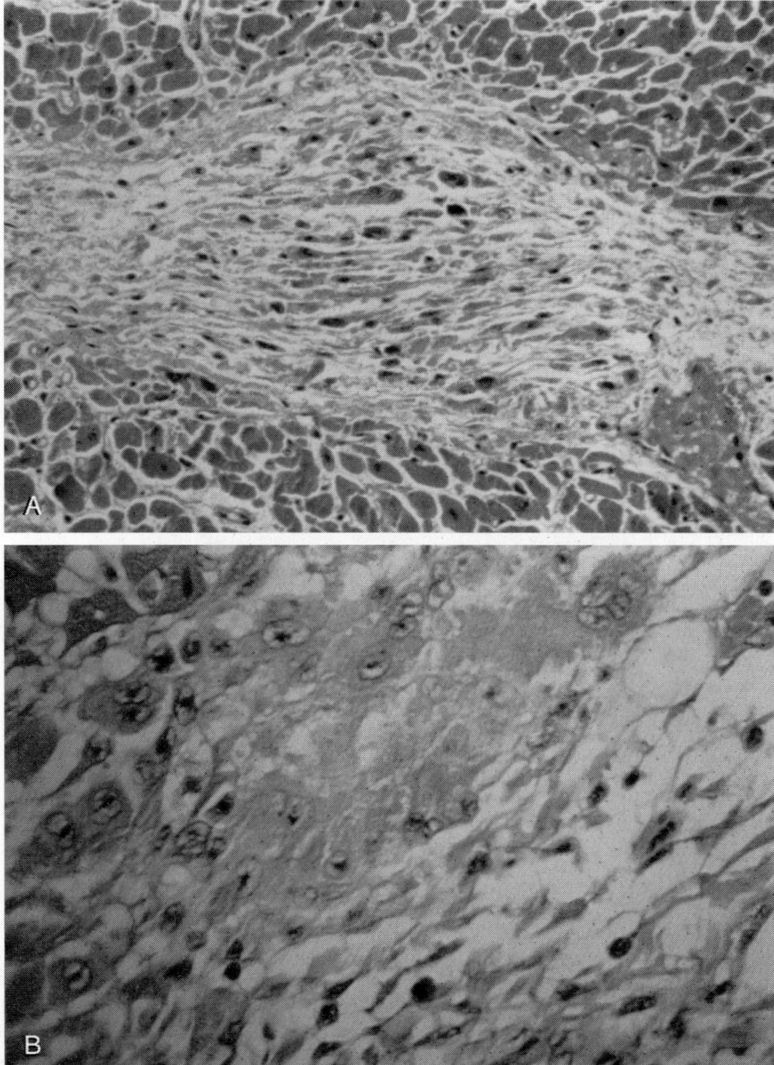

FIGURE 17–4 A, Low-power microscopic intramyocardial view shows Aschoff bodies. Note the nodular aggregate of Aschoff cells immediately adjacent to a coronary arteriole (H&E; magnification, 120×). **B,** High-power microscopic view of an Aschoff body illustrates the characteristic "owl-and-caterpillar" nuclei (H&E; magnification 250×). (**A** and **B,** Courtesy of Hugh A. McAllister, Jr., M.D., Texas Heart Institute at St. Luke's Episcopal Hospital, Houston, Texas.)

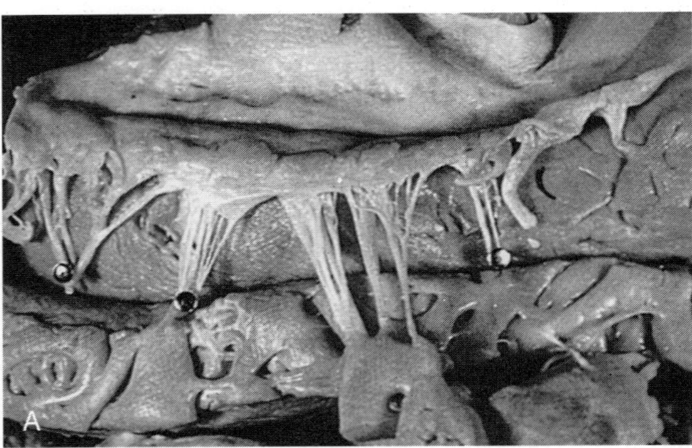

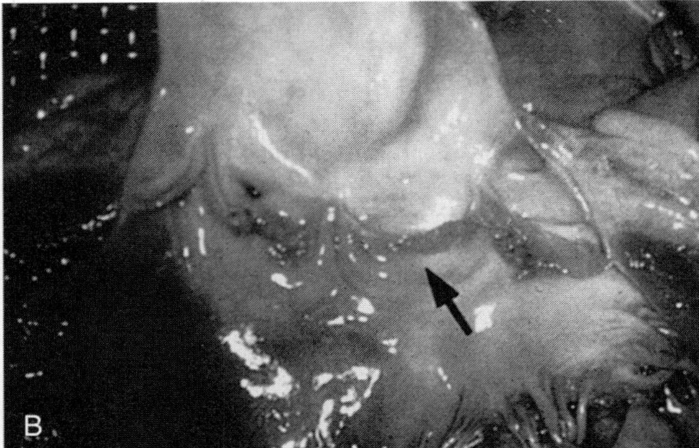

FIGURE 17–5 Valvulitis. **A,** Gross appearance of the mitral valve shows characteristic tiny, wartlike verrucae or vegetations on its inflow side (atrial surface). **B,** Similar verrucae on the ventricular surface of the aortic valve *(arrow).* The verrucae are sterile and small and only rarely result in embolization (unlike vegetations of bacterial endocarditis). (**A** and **B,** Modified from Massell BF, Narula J: Rheumatic fever and carditis. *In* Braunwald E [ed]: The Atlas of Heart Diseases. pp. 10.1–10.20. Philadelphia: Current Medicine, 1994.)

the left atrium, *McCallum's patch,* probably represents a site of impact of mitral regurgitant jet rather than rheumatic inflammation. Older literature has also described vasculitis with areas of fibrinoid necrosis in the aorta and in muscular myocardial vessels.

CLINICAL FEATURES

There is no single diagnostic test or pathognomonic sign that allows an absolute diagnosis of RF. In 1944, Jones[55] described the clinical manifestations of RF and divided them into major and minor manifestations. Since that time, the Jones criteria have been modified several times under the auspices of the American Heart Association[56–59] (Table 17–1). The major manifestations include the presence of carditis, chorea, subcutaneous nodules, migratory arthritis involving large joints, and the skin rash known as erythema marginatum. The minor manifestations include fever, prolonged joint pains, prolonged electrocardiographic PR interval, laboratory indicators of inflammation, and acute phase reactants. An elevated ASO titer or other evidence of preceding streptococcal infection is considered a prerequisite.

TABLE 17-1 Jones Criteria for Diagnosis of Acute Fever*

Major Criteria	Minor Criteria
Carditis	Arthralgia
Polyarthritis	Fever
Chorea	Elevated erythrocyte sedimentation rate
Subcutaneous nodules	Positive C-reactive protein
Erythema marginatum	Leukocytosis
	Prolonged PR interval

*Two major criteria or one major plus two minor criteria are required for the diagnosis of rheumatic fever. Supportive evidence of recent streptococcal infection is also required for all diagnoses. Chorea, indolent carditis, and poststreptococcal arthritis may not fulfill Jones criteria at the time of diagnosis.[59]

Joint Symptoms

Arthritis is the earliest manifestation of RF and frequently brings the patient to clinical attention.[42] Arthritis occurs in at least two thirds of patients,[60, 61] more commonly in older patients with RF. Although larger joints of the extremities are commonly involved, the occasional involvement of smaller joints in the hand and feet may be seen; hips, spine, or axial joints are rarely affected. The joints are swollen, hot, red, and tender.[42] The joints are inflamed at different times and for various intervals to impart a migratory character to joint pains. Monoarticular arthritis is not common.[62] Arthritis usually resolves in 3 to 4 weeks, responds instantly to aspirin treatment, and does not lead to permanent damage. Arthralgia without objective signs of inflammation is common in younger patients, in the presence of carditis, particularly in rheumatic recurrences,[42, 63] and in RHD patients in the developing countries.[64, 65]

Some forms of polyarthritis after streptococcal pharyngitis may represent a reactive phenomenon. Poststreptococcal arthropathy is characterized by recurrent, severe, prolonged polyarthritis in adults that is not very responsive to nonsteroidal anti-inflammatory agents. Although other manifestations of RF are not associated with arthropathy, some patients end up with residual heart disease.[66, 67] Prophylaxis in reactive arthropathy remains similar to that for patients with RF, but very little data are available to provide definite recommendations.

Cardiac Involvement

Carditis is the only manifestation of RF that results in permanent deformity.[68] The cardiac involvement in RF has been reported to occur in nearly one third of to almost all cases in various studies and in up to one half of cases in a prospective series.[68] Clinical carditis was seen in 72 percent of patients in the recent resurgence of RF in Salt Lake City,[69] which is similar to the prevalence in the early part of the century in the United States,[70] possibly due to more virulent strains of streptococci. Evidence of valvular regurgitation was seen in 19 percent of additional cases with the use of echocardiography. Active rheumatic carditis can present in a number of ways, including subclinical cardiac involvement, acute or even fulminant congestive heart failure, and, occasionally, chronic ongoing carditis. Younger patients often present with carditis, whereas joint involvement is more common in older patients.[42] The introduction of penicillin and a change in rheumatogenicity of *Streptococcus* have rendered the carditis milder. Although episodes of carditis occur less frequently in older patients, they present more often with unexplained worsening of congestive heart failure. The clinical findings may be suggestive of pericarditis, myocarditis, and valvulitis, and the guidelines for the diagnosis of rheumatic carditis are summarized in Table 17–2.

Endocarditis. Endocardial inflammation most commonly affects the mitral and aortic valves, and the clinical diagnosis of rheumatic endocarditis is based on the demonstration of mitral or aortic regurgitation murmurs, or both. Mitral valve disease is seen in approximately 70 percent of patients; mitral and aortic valve disease occurs in an additional 25 percent, and isolated aortic valve disease occurs in 5 to 8 percent. Clinical tricuspid or pulmonary valve involvement is rare (in the first attack) of RH.[71] The use of echocardiography has clarified the mechanism of valve regurgitation in RF.[53] Although mild-to-moderate mitral regurgitation is due to left ventricular dilatation with mild or no annular dilatation, more severe degrees of mitral regurgitation are associated with marked annular dilatation, chordal elongation, and anterior mitral leaflet prolapse.[72] Rarely, chordae may rupture to result in flail leaflets and severe regurgitation. Because mitral regurgitation frequently disappears on follow-up,[73, 74] it is likely that a functional mechanism rather than structural alteration in the valve or annulus underlies the development of mitral regurgitation. On the other hand, inflammatory changes in the aortic valves and the aortic ring result in aortic regurgitation; aortic valve prolapse may contribute occasionally.

Myocarditis. Myocardial involvement is generally associated with new-onset cardiomegaly, an interval increase in cardiac size, or the development of congestive heart failure.[51, 75] The left ventricular systolic function and myocardial contractility indexes are normal in patients with rheumatic carditis, and only minimal myocyte damage is pathologically seen in rheumatic carditis.[28] It has been thought that hemodynamically significant valvular lesions lead to the development of congestive heart failure.[75]

Pericarditis. Clinical rheumatic pericarditis occurs in up to 15 percent of patients during the acute stage of RF, and the presence of an evanescent pericardial friction rub in this setting is evidence of rheumatic carditis. Rheumatic pericarditis is almost always associated with findings of valvular involvement. A pericardial rub can sometimes mask the underlying valvular murmurs, but after the resolution of pericarditis, if no valvulitis-related murmur is audible, then the pericarditis can be assumed to be nonrheumatic.[68] Rheumatic pericarditis is often associated with a mild-to-moderate serosanguineous effusion, and the development of pericardial tamponade[76] or pericardial constriction[77] is rare. The presence of pericarditis usually indicates severe carditis.[42]

TABLE 17-2 Simplified Schema for the Diagnosis of Acute Rheumatic Carditis*

Criteria	First Attacks	Recurrences
Valvulitis	New onset apical systolic murmur or aortic regurgitation murmur	Change in murmur
		New-onset murmur
	Carey-Coombs murmur	
Myocarditis	Unexplained cardiomegaly	Worsening cardiomegaly
	Unexplained congestive heart failure/ gallop sounds	Worsening congestive heart failure
Pericarditis	Pericardial rub	Pericardial rub
	Pericardial effusion	Pericardial effusion
Miscellaneous	Conduction disturbances or unexplained tachycardia†	
	Echocardiographic imaging‡	
	Nuclear imaging‡	
	Morphologic evidence at surgery	
	Histologic evidence at biopsy or pathology	

*Supportive evidence is required for the presence of acute rheumatic fever according to the Jones criteria. In patients with known rheumatic heart disease, acute rheumatic fever can be diagnosed with minor criteria *along with* evidence of antecedent streptococcal infection.

†These would be considered soft criteria.

‡The significance of these methods is controversial.

Modified from Narula J, Chopra P, Talwar KK, et al: Does endomyocardial biopsy aid in the diagnosis of active rheumatic carditis? Circulation 88:2198–2205, 1993.

Sydenham's Chorea

Chorea is a late manifestation of RF that is characterized by a series of involuntary movements that commonly involve the face and extremities associated with emotional lability (Fig. 17–6).[42] It commonly affects children between the ages of 7 and 14 years, and occurs more frequently in females; it is rarely seen in adults.[42] Chorea is often associated with carditis and subcutaneous nodules, but it appears several weeks after an acute attack of RF and when these manifestations have disappeared. The patients do not fulfill the Jones criteria at this time. The course of chorea is rather gradual as the patient appears increasingly nervous, becomes dysarthric, makes grimacing gestures, develops difficulty in writing, and shows characteristic purposeless movements of the arms and legs, which may be associated with muscular weakness. The chronic movements are exaggerated in effort or excitement but subside during sleep. Chorea is usually a self-limited condition and resolves without residual damage.

Skin Manifestations

Subcutaneous nodules and erythema marginatum are two important skin manifestations of RF (Fig. 17–7).[42] Subcutaneous nodules occur late in the course of rheumatic fever. They are observed in up to 20 percent of patients, and their presence is usually associated with carditis. Subcutaneous nodules occur on bony prominences, vertebral spinous processes, or extensor tendons and are painless. They usually appear in crops, are variable in size, and disappear within 2 to 3 months. On the other hand, erythema marginatum can be an early or a late manifestation. It occurs

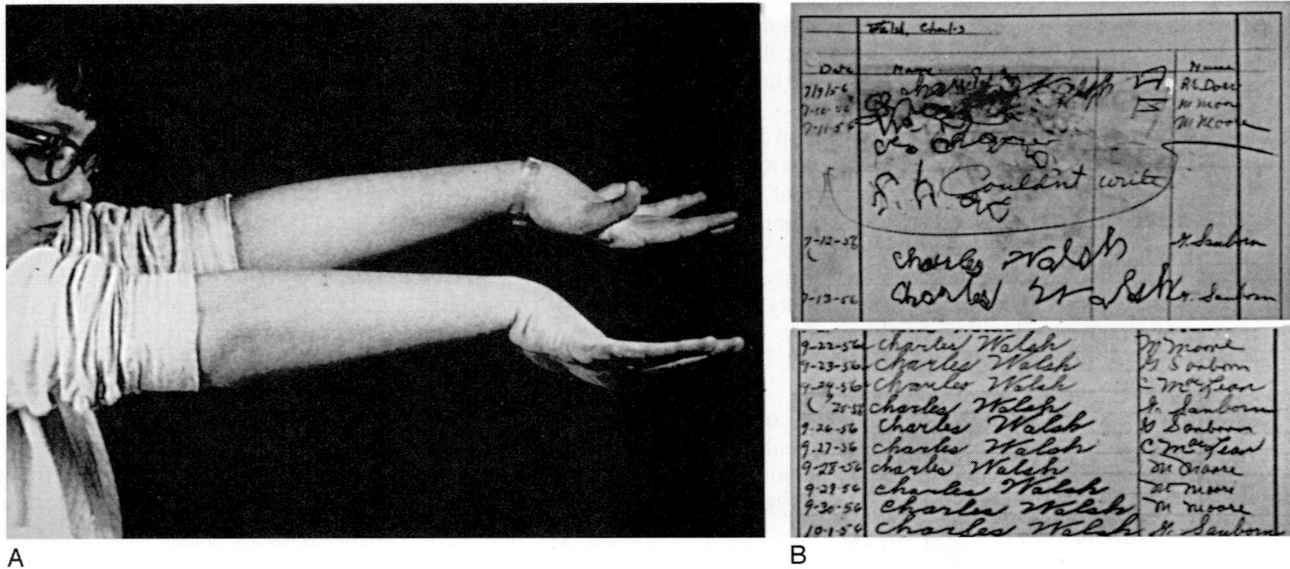

FIGURE 17–6 A, Chorea, a neurologic manifestation of rheumatic fever, is characterized by purposeless, jerky, involuntary movements. The posture of the outstretched hands in chorea often shows a typical "silver-fork" appearance (sometimes called "spooning"). **B,** Handwriting is shown by a patient with severe chorea and after the recovery. Keeping a record of handwriting is a good objective way to follow the progress of patients with chorea. (**A** and **B,** Modified from Massell BF, Narula J: Rheumatic fever and carditis. *In* Braunwald E [ed]: The Atlas of Heart Diseases. pp. 10.1–10.20. Philadelphia: Current Medicine, 1994.)

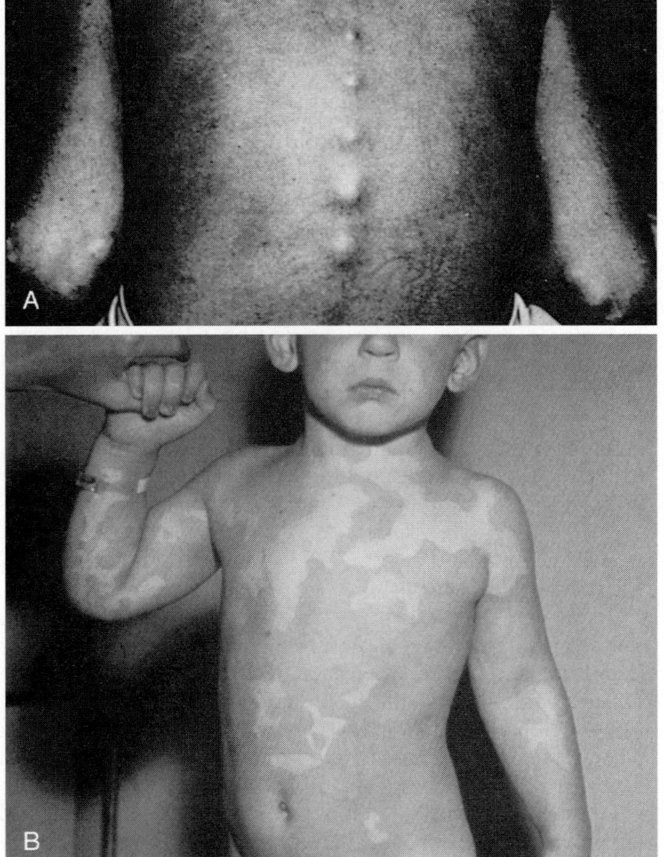

FIGURE 17–7 Skin manifestations of rheumatic fever. **A,** Subcutaneous nodules of the spine. **B,** Skin rash (erythema marginatum) in a child with acute rheumatic fever.

in fewer than 15 percent of patients and is present on the trunk and proximal extremities as a serpiginous, macular, nonpruritic, and evanescent rash.

Although Jones criteria provide an excellent set of guidelines for the diagnosis of RF, such manifestations may be present in varying degrees in other systemic illnesses, leading to the potential for misdiagnosis. For example, streptococcal infection is relatively common, and an elevated antistreptolysin O (ASO) titer indicates only previous infection. Similarly, arthralgia is prevalent in association with several viral syndromes, and carditis may occur as a consequence of coxsackie B virus, Lyme disease, or Kawasaki's infection. The early manifestations of other collagen diseases, such as systemic lupus erythematosus, may also lead to confusion in diagnosis when they are associated with inflammatory abnormalities of the heart valves, particularly the mitral valve. Although rheumatoid arthritis usually does not involve the heart, it may produce aortic regurgitation. A similar inflammatory reaction within the pericardium or conduction system may result in pericarditis or heart block. There may be an erythema multiforme type of rash and laboratory evidence of an elevated erythrocyte sedimentation rate (ESR), anemia, and marked leukocytosis. For these reasons, rheumatoid arthritis is easily confused with RF. In a patient who has streptococcal infection and carditis, particularly with evidence of migratory polyarthritism, the diagnosis of RF should be assumed until proved otherwise.

Laboratory Investigations

Evidence of preceding streptococcal infection is a prerequisite for the diagnosis of RF. Because RF is a postinfectious immunologic complication, microbiological evidence is limited, and the evidence for recent streptococcal infection is usually obtained with the antistreptococcal antibody tests. The most commonly used antibody assays include ASO and antideoxyribonuclease B (anti–DNase B), and other antibody tests such as hyaluronidase, streptokinase, and nicotinamide adenine dinucleotidase are occasionally used.[78] The antibody response to various streptococcal antigens develops within the first month and remains detectable up to 3 to 6 months after the infection.[79] ASO titers are determined by an agglutination test or a hemolytic inhibition test, and in healthy adults, the titers are usually less than 85 Todd Units/ml, whereas school-age children can have ASO titers up to 170 U. Generally, an ASO level of more than 240 U in adults or more than 330 U in children is used for diagnosis,[78] but a better diagnostic specificity is obtained by the demonstration of an interval increase in ASO in two serial samples.[57] Because ASO titers rise and fall more rapidly, the anti–DNase B test can be performed if ASO is nondiagnostic. A rapid slide agglutination test that looks at antibodies against several (five) streptococcal antigens, the Streptozyme test, has been proposed to improve the detection of streptococcal infection.[58]

The electrocardiogram may be normal in a patient with acute rheumatic fever. In patients who have cardiac involvement, ST-segment change may signal pericarditis, and repolarization abnormalities, including QT prolongation and T inversion, may occur in myocarditis. In addition, there may be associated arrhythmias with extrasystoles, supraventricular tachycardia, and atrioventricular blocks. First-degree atrioventricular block is commonly seen in patients with RF but is equally common in patients with or without carditis.[42] The chest radiograph has been traditionally used to evaluate cardiomegaly and is an inexpensive way to study the evolution of the patient under treatment.

Echocardiography has become the tool of choice in diagnosis and monitoring the evolution of chronic rheumatic valvular disease. Current echocardiography-Doppler techniques were not available at the time of major RF epidemics, and one way to optimize their role in RF is to include this modality in the Jones criteria with multiple caveats (Fig. 17–8). Echocardiography will have a useful role in countries with widespread access to health care and with low RF burden (e.g., the United States), where patients are more likely to be seen during the first attack of RF and the additional cost and workload imposed by routine echocardiography is small.[80] Echocardiographic documentation of a normal heart or unrelated causes of cardiac murmurs in this population will have obvious prognostic implications. An echocardiogram will also quickly resolve whether a clinically undetectable murmur is truly absent and will protect patients with clinical carditis from being grouped with noncarditic patients, who have a more benign prognosis and require shorter secondary prophylaxis regimen. There is, however, a lot of concern that echocardiography may lead to the overdiagnosis of rheumatic carditis if strict criteria are not applied for the exclusion of physiologic valvular regurgitation. Even if echocardiography inappropriately overdetected subclinical carditis, serial echocardiographic studies will resolve the significance of such valve dysfunction and an abbreviated prophylaxis regimen can be prescribed. Therefore, the detection of subclinical carditis and even mislabeling a minority of patients with RF as having carditis for a short period of time until their clinical situation is resolved should not adversely affect the overall management strategy. On the other hand, the clinical situation is quite different in the developing world,[80] where the incidence of RF and the prevalence of RHD are very high and access to medical care is limited. First attacks are rarely witnessed, and patients present with recurrences and usually with established heart disease. Physical examination is the most commonly used method to detect patients with and without cardiac involvement. Echocardiography in advanced disease does not demonstrate any incremental diagnostic benefit.[53] Furthermore, echocardiographic facilities are not widely available, and the cost and additional workload imposed with the universal use of echocardiography in RF episodes are likely to be enormous. Therefore, the detection of subclinical carditis in this population not only is very costly but also probably will not change the management strategy very much because the initial period of prophylaxis is no different in patients without and with mild carditis.[80] In this population, the presence of RHD is a reason for life-long prophylaxis, and echocardiography should be performed at the time of discontinuation of prophylaxis. The absence of heart disease at this time should allow the withdrawal of prophylaxis, whereas the presence of valvular disease should prompt life-long pro-

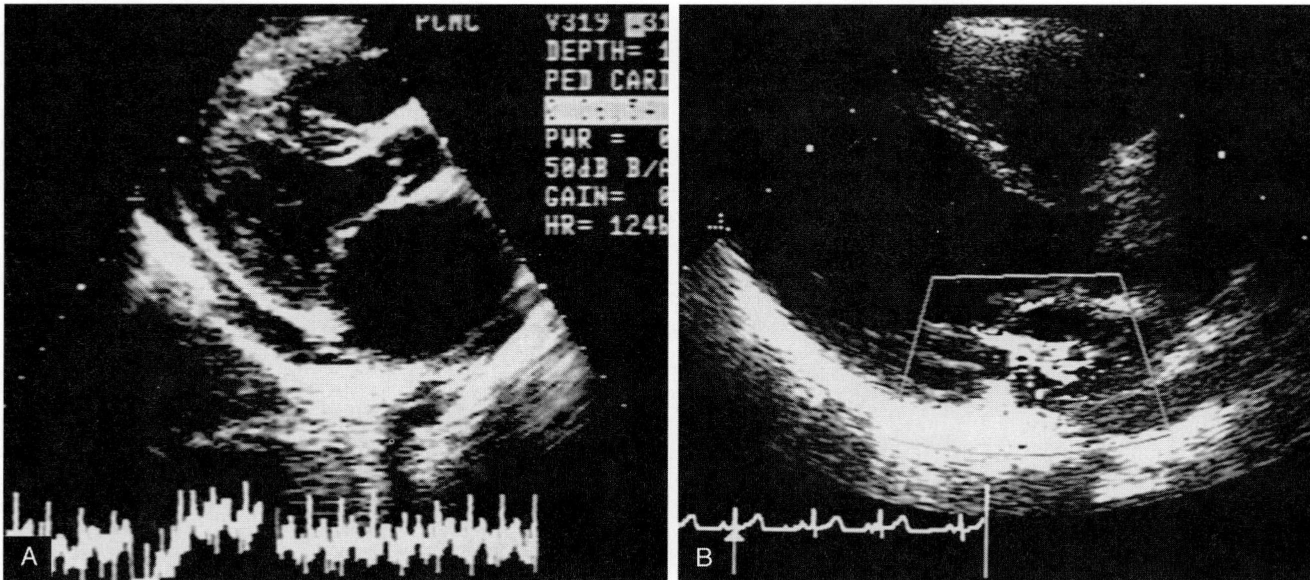

FIGURE 17–8 Echocardiography in rheumatic fever. **A,** Pericarditis. Two-dimensional echocardiogram (freeze-frame of the parasternal long-axis view) obtained in a 10-year-old boy with acute rheumatic fever. Note the echo-free space posterior to the left ventricle due to a small pericardial effusion. The left atrium is dilated. **B,** Endocarditis. Significant murmurs are the most common and the earliest clinical signs of carditis in acute rheumatic fever, and early endocarditis may also be detected with echocardiography and Doppler studies. Two-dimensional echocardiogram with Doppler color-flow imaging (parasternal long-axis view) obtained in a 12-year-old girl with acute rheumatic fever. Note that there is a high-velocity systolic turbulence in the left atrium due to a jet of mitral regurgitation, which is central and extends backup to half of the left atrium. (**A** and **B,** Courtesy of L. George Veasy, Primary Children's Medical Center, University of Utah School of Medicine, Salt Lake City.)

phylaxis. Therefore, echocardiography cannot be recommended as a prerequisite for the investigation of RF in these countries.[80] Of course, the role of echocardiography in the detection and management of established RHD is unquestioned in any population.

Computed tomography or magnetic resonance imaging[81] may also be useful in distinguishing between myocardial dilatation and pericardial effusion, which may not be detected by simple radiography. These techniques may be especially useful in evaluating the results of treatment. Endomyocardial biopsies have been performed in persons with acute rheumatic carditis. Aschoff nodules, which are pathognomonic features of rheumatic carditis, are observed in 40 percent of subjects, thereby offering a test of limited sensitivity.[28] However, because the biopsy results are always normal in patients with chronic RHD or noncarditic manifestations of RF, the specificity of the test is very high. In addition, various radionuclide imaging approaches have been evaluated in rheumatic carditis with variable success[82, 83]; these include imaging with ^{111}In-labeled antimyosin antibodies, radiolabeled leukocytes, and ^{67}Ga scintigraphy.

NATURAL HISTORY

The best evaluation of the natural course of RF comes from observations made during the 1940s. Before that time, there were no adequate anti-inflammatory treatments or prophylactic measures against repeated and recurrent infections. One of the difficulties in treating RF is in determining when the disease has ceased to progress. One can assume that the disease has become quiescent when the patient has had no fever for several weeks, the ESR has become normal, and there are no signs of inflammation of the pericardium, pleura, or articular areas. In addition, heart size is important in patients who have active RF. A dilated heart in a patient with acute RF is often a manifestation of continued rheumatic activity and may be an indication for additional treatment.

First attacks of RF in children characteristically occur between the ages of 5 and 15 years. RF rarely occurs in children younger than 2 years, and first attacks after the age of 30 years are also less common. Individuals who have RF are susceptible to recurrences of the disease. RF can recur with various manifestations at intervals of weeks, months, or years, with apparent inactivity between these episodes (Fig. 17–9). In the past, it was customary to recommend bed rest and relative inactivity for children with RF as long as they had persistent symptoms. Once the symptoms disappeared and the ESR and heart size return to normal (by radiographic examination), the patient was allowed to gradually resume normal activities. Frequent evaluations were made at 2- to 3-week intervals to check the ESR, chest radiographs, and electrocardiograms to determine the status of carditis and the inflammatory state within the body. An increase in heart size or ESR was presumptive of reaction. At present, echographic and Doppler analyses greatly improve the precise evaluation of heart contractility and valve function.

A 1948 report[84] revealed that more children died within the first year after acute RF than in any subsequent year. However, long-term survival was shown in several studies in patients who had no evident heart disease with the onset

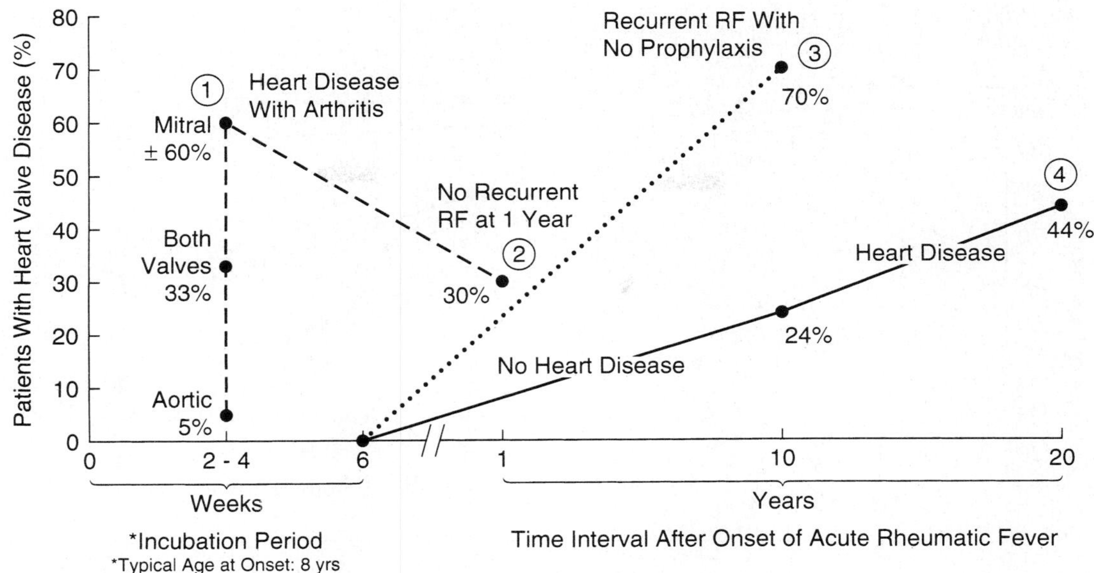

FIGURE 17–9 Frequency of valvular heart disease in different clinical presentations of acute rheumatic fever (RF). 1, The frequency of heart valve involvement in rheumatic heart disease. Mitral valve disease will occur at a greater frequency (~70 percent) than aortic valve disease (5 percent). Both valves will be involved in 33 percent of patients. (Data from White PD: Changes in relative prevalence of various types of heart disease in New England. JAMA 152:303, 1953.) 2, Course of rheumatic heart disease. In 30 percent of patients with signs of rheumatic heart disease, signs will disappear immediately or within 1 year after the onset of rheumatic fever. Note: This differs from the studies of Bland and Jones,[86] in whose patients with rheumatic heart disease signs disappear in 11 percent after 10 years and in 16 percent after 20 years. 3, Recurrence rate of rheumatic activity during a 10-year period with prophylaxis is 70 percent. 4, No heart disease with the first attack of rheumatic fever. Of patients with no obvious signs of heart disease after the onset of rheumatic fever, 25 percent will have heart disease after 10 years, and the number affected will increase to 44 percent at 20 years. Note: One study[115] has shown the following percentages of recurrent activity of rheumatic fever at different ages (usual onset is 8 years of age, as shown earlier): 25 percent at 10 years of age, 8.6 percent at 15 years, and 5 percent at 20 years. (1 and 2, Data from Cooperative Rheumatic Fever Study: The treatment of acute rheumatic fever in children: a cooperative clinical trial of ACTH, cortisone, and aspirin. Circulation 11:343, 1955. 3 and 4, Data from Bland EF, Jones TD: Observation of 10 years of rheumatic infection in children. Am Heart J 36:89, 1948.)

of RF (Fig. 17–10). In one study by Keith and coworkers,[85] the survival rate was 95 percent at 20 years in patients with no evident heart disease. A long-term follow-up report by Bland and Jones[86] of 1000 patients with acute RF revealed that of 347 patients who did not initially have evidence of heart disease, none had died of heart disease at the end of 20 years. The cause of death in most acute rheumatic cases was congestive heart failure with gross cardiomegaly. In fact, the worst prognostic indicator may be the failure of cardiomegaly and congestive cardiac failure to improve with treatment. Within 10 years after the initial attack, 70 to 80 percent of the patients with carditis in these reported series had died. The patients with the initial syndrome of Sydenham's chorea had lower mortality and morbidity rates than did those with arthritis. In this preantibiotic era, death was the result of subacute bacterial endocarditis in 10 percent of the fatal cases. Recurrence of active RF increases heart damage. Recurrence is less common with progressing age and occurred in 20 percent of the patients during the first 5 years, in 10 percent during the second 5 years, in 5 percent in the third 5 years, and in only 1.4 percent 15 to 20 years after the original attack. The severity of RF is evidenced by the fact that before effective treatments were available, 59 percent of the patients who survived their first attacks and had heart disease were dead 20 years later. Most of the deaths occurred within 5 years after the initial attack.

As indicated in the previously mentioned studies, the long-term course in the absence of treatment is quite gloomy. The symptoms of acute RF are obviously related to the degree to which multiple systems of the body are involved, but most of these changes disappear. The prognosis depends principally on the degree of heart involvement (Fig. 17–11). Inflammation of the pericardium rarely, if ever, develops into chronic constrictive pericarditis. The cardiac symptoms are those secondary to inflammatory reaction of the valvular apparatus, and hemodynamic alterations produced by acute mitral or aortic valve regurgitation represent a significant factor in both the short- and long-term prognosis. It is well known that the failure of improvement in heart failure in RF is associated with a high mortality rate. It has been postulated that severe mechanical dysfunction of the aortic or mitral valve with active rheumatic carditis tends to prohibit or retard recovery from active interstitial myocarditis. Surgical treatment of valvular disease during the acute rheumatic process seems to improve the chance of survival in these patients, and in some patients, it is life saving.

In patients who have no major valvular damage, the prevention of recurrent attacks leads to a significantly better prognosis with regard to overall survival and freedom from heart disease. If there is valvular involvement, the scarring process may lead to long-term impairment of valve function. Mitral, aortic, and tricuspid regurgitations are frequently seen during acute RF. The inflammatory reaction of the valves leads to an insidious, slow scarring process

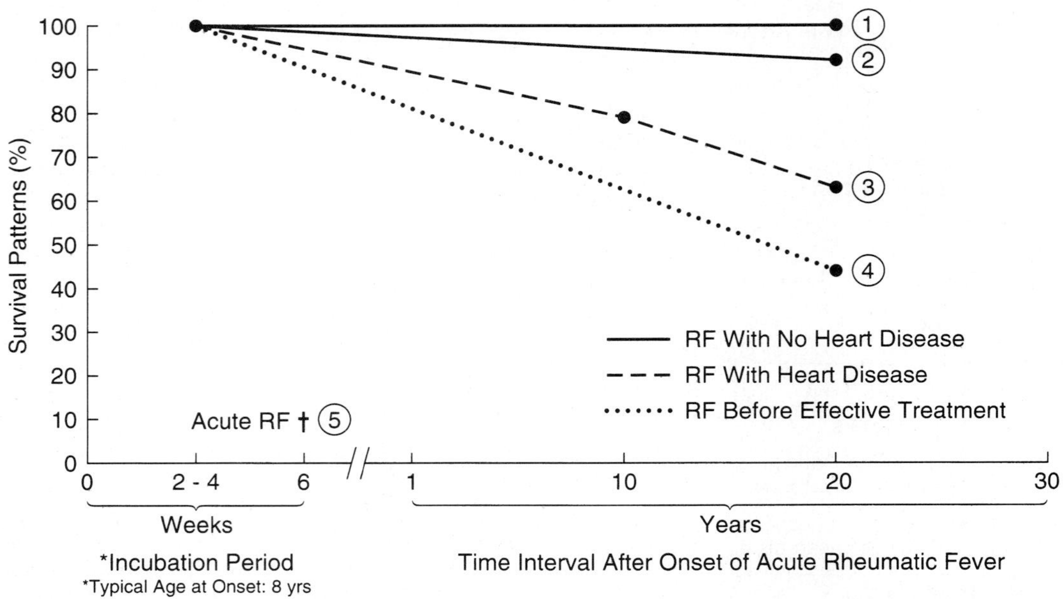

FIGURE 17–10 Survival patterns in acute rheumatic fever (RF). 1, Survival after the initial attack of rheumatic fever with no evidence of heart disease: 100 percent at 20 years. 2, Survival after the initial attack of rheumatic fever with no heart disease: 95 percent at 20 years. 3, Survival after rheumatic heart disease at 10 years (73 percent) and at 20 years (60 percent). 4, Survival after onset of rheumatic fever with heart disease before effective antibiotic treatment: 50 percent at 20 years. 5, Death caused by severe congestive heart failure in cases of acute rheumatic fever (3 percent). (1 and 4, Data from Bland EF, Jones TD: Observation of 10 years of rheumatic infection in children. Am Heart J 36:89, 1948. 2 and 3, Data from Keith JD, Rowe RD, Vlad P: Heart Disease in Infancy and Childhood. 2nd ed. New York: Macmillan, 1967. 5, Data from Bland EF, Jones TD: Rheumatic fever and rheumatic heart disease: a 20-year report on 1000 patients followed since childhood. Circulation 4:836–843, 1951.)

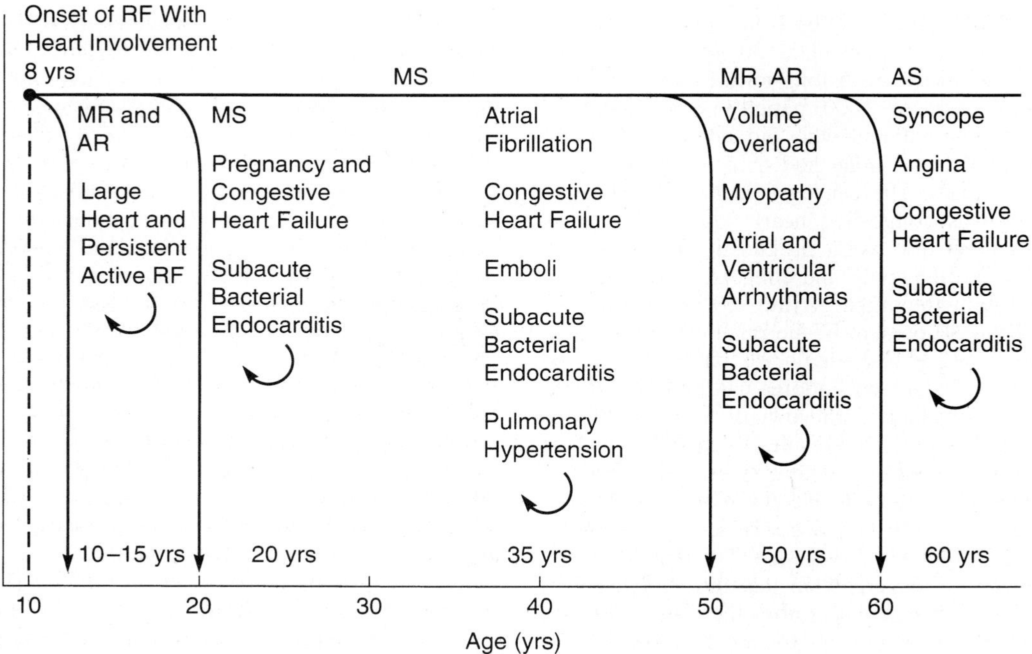

FIGURE 17–11 Simplified chart of the natural history of rheumatic heart disease. AR, aortic regurgitation; AS, aortic stenosis; MR, mitral regurgitation; MS, mitral stenosis.

that progresses over 10 to 30 years, with various combinations of stenosis and regurgitation. Perhaps the most insidious of these is mitral stenosis, which may develop very late—as long as 20 years after the onset of the acute infection—often with no symptoms until the onset of atrial fibrillation.[87] This arrhythmia may be related to rheumatic scarring within the atrium, hydromechanical overload, or both. The onset of arrhythmia usually results in the congestive syndrome and is the beginning of rather rapid deterioration and death from heart failure or thrombotic complications. In association with atrial fibrillation, the formation of free-floating intra-atrial thrombi may acutely obstruct the valve.[88, 89] Thrombi may also form in the atrial appendage and fragment, resulting in systemic embolization and its consequences.[90]

Delayed obstruction may occur in the aortic and tricuspid valves, similar to that which occurs in the mitral valve. It may take as long as 10 or 20 years for valvular obstruction to develop after RF with carditis. The onset of symptoms heralds a rapid progression to death. Even with minimal functional abnormality, these diseased valves are susceptible to infection. Therefore, patients who have recovered from RF are at risk for subacute bacterial endocarditis later in life, even though the mechanical function of the heart is normal. They should therefore receive prophylactic antibiotics during periods when they are at risk for infection (e.g., dental work or gastrointestinal or genitourinary interventions).

Treatment

The primary objective in the treatment of the patient with acute RF is the elimination of offending streptococci with appropriate antibiotic therapy; penicillin remains the agent of choice. The second objective of treatment of acute RF is to eliminate the inflammatory state, particularly that involving vital organs such as the heart. Salicylates, predominantly aspirin, have been used for many years as anti-inflammatory agents in RF.[91] The discovery of adrenocorticotropic hormone and the cortisone derivatives first reported by Hench and associates[92, 93] in 1949 led quickly to their trial in the treatment of RF. At present, corticosteroids are used in patients with severe carditis and heart failure. In the absence of rheumatic carditis or valvulitis, salicylates alone or other nonsteroidal anti-inflammatory drugs may be sufficient to control the arthritic symptoms.

The diagnosis of RF is suspected if high-dose salicylates do not significantly resolve joint pain and inflammation within 48 hours. Relatively high doses are needed: up to 8 to 10 g/da (100 mg/kg/da) for a period of 3 to 4 weeks. Owing to the possibility of clinical rebound after the discontinuation of salicylates, a gradual taper is recommended. There are no data to suggest that salicylates alter the natural history of the disease. On the other hand, because RF is considered a hyperactive immune response to streptococcal moieties, the immunosuppressive effects of steroids are likely to be of benefit. Steroids rapidly suppress the toxic state, subside inflammation, help prevent the appearance of new murmurs, help murmurs disappear faster, allow faster resolution of pericardial effusions, and may be life saving in critical illness.[74, 94–96] One hundred thirty-five studies, which included 11 randomized trials, evaluated the role of steroids and compared them with salicylates, but their meta-analysis could not distinctly demonstrate the superiority of steroids in reducing residual heart disease as assessed by the prevalence of mitral murmurs 1 year after RF.[97] Because these studies are very old, have used varying methodologies and entry criteria, allowed a significant crossover of patients to the steroid group, and did not have sufficient power in some cases, the question of the efficacy of steroids is still not clear. In clinical practice, however, a short course of steroids is commonly used in patients with severe carditis. Prednisone at 1 to 2 mg/kg/da is used for a period of 3 weeks with a tapering schedule once the acute symptoms resolve. There are no definitive end points for discontinuing anti-inflammatory therapy in RF. General measures include the absence of clinical symptoms and signs of rheumatic activity, in addition to normalization of acute-phase reactants, usually ESR. Too rapid reduction can be accompanied by a rebound. The steroid taper is occasionally covered with salicylates to prevent a relapse. If heart failure continues to persist despite steroid therapy, surgical repair of mechanical lesions should be considered instead of prolonged trials with high-dose steroids.

It has long been believed that surgery should not be undertaken during an acute inflammatory state, because earlier studies had showed increased surgical mortality rates in patients with acute RF.[98, 99] However, a recent study by Essop and associates[75] reported no deaths among patients with mitral or mitral and aortic valve replacement during active carditis, and surgery was associated with rapid and remarkable improvement, including a reduction in left ventricular dimensions. A subsequent series with a much longer follow-up period has shown that surgery during acute rheumatic carditis may be associated with less favorable outcome of mitral valve repair, and surgical option during the acute episode should be reserved for subjects who are refractory to medical therapy.[100] In this study of Skoularigis and colleagues,[100] there was a relatively higher incidence of valve failure (27 percent), and the presence of acute carditis was the strongest predictor of reoperation.

The third important objective in the treatment of RF is to prevent recurrences of rheumatic activity.[101] The secondary prophylaxis program should begin during the acute episode of RF and is essentially based on the ability to prevent streptococcal pharyngitis. RF is a recurrent disease, and patients with carditis in previous attacks have a higher recurrence rate per streptococcal infection than those without previous carditis. The likelihood of risk of recurrence per streptococcal infection may range up to 40 to 60 percent in young patients with established RHL,[102, 103] and every recurrence further damages the heart. RF recurrences can be prevented by chemoprophylaxis of streptococcal infections, which results in an eventual reduction in the prevalence of residual heart disease[103–109] and a subsequent reduction in mortality rates due to RHD. The duration of prophylaxis is dependent on the anticipated risk of a recurrence of RF with each throat infection with *Streptococcus* and is determined by the presence of carditis in the index RF episodes and the likelihood of acquiring streptococcal infection. The recurrence of RF is likely to be higher in

TABLE 17-3 Secondary Prevention of Rheumatic Fever

Agent	Dose	Mode	Duration
Benzathine penicillin G*	1.2 million U	IM	Every 4 wk†
Penicillin V‡	250 mg bid	PO	Daily
Sulfadiazine§		PO	Daily
<27 kg (60 lb)	500 mg		
>27 kg (60 lb)	1000 mg		
With penicillin and sulfa allergy			
Erythromycin	250 mg bid	PO	Daily

*Use drug at room temperature and with procaine penicillin to reduce pain.
†Consider three times weekly in high-risk situations, including in Third World countries.
‡May interfere with oral contraception.
§Avoid use in pregnancy. More effective than oral penicillin.
Based on recommendations from Dajani A, Taubert K, Ferrieri P, et al: Treatment of acute streptococcal pharyngitis and prevention of rheumatic fever: a statement for health professionals. Pediatrics 96:758–764, 1995.

patients with carditis or residual heart disease, multiple previous attacks, and younger age, whereas the risk decreases with the interval after the last attack. Streptococcal infections are more common in school children, their parents, teachers or health personnel in contact with children, and persons living in closed quarters or in crowded housing. The recommendations for the choice of antibiotics and duration of prophylaxis are listed in Tables 17–3 and 17–4.[101] The need for prophylaxis should be reassessed periodically. In all situations, the decision to discontinue prophylaxis should be made after discussing the potential risks and benefits with the patient.

STREPTOCOCCAL VACCINE

The most effective way to reduce the global burden of RHD would be the development of an antistreptococcal vaccine.[110] The streptococcal M protein, which is the most important determinant of streptococcal virulence, is type specific for each strain, and the development of antibodies to a particular M protein confers immunity only to that strain. The N-terminal sequence (which is devoid of possible homology with human myocardial tissue) from all putative strains that could cause RF in a community are lined in tandem for a multivalent streptococcal vaccine. One of the current vaccines includes an octavalent antigenic peptide,[111] and the other contains recombinant M protein fragments linked to *Escherichia coli*–labile toxin.[112] Yet another type of streptococcal vaccine has used the C-terminal sequence of M protein.[113] The advantage of this approach is that the C-terminal region is relatively conserved[114] through streptococcal strains, and the development of opsonizing antibodies to it would be useful against multiple streptococcal strains. An effective streptococcal vaccine is likely to be available soon.[115]

TABLE 17-4 Duration of Secondary Rheumatic Fever Prophylaxis*

		Risk of Recurrent Streptococcal Infections†	
		High	*Not High*
Category	**Duration**	<40 yr	>40 yr‡
RHD	Lifelong	Until 40 yr‡	None‡
History of carditis and no RHD§	Until 40 yr of age‡	Until 21 yr of age‡ or 10 yr since last attack¶	None‖
RF and no carditis	Until 21 yr of age‡ or 10 yr from last attack¶	Until 21 yr of age‖ or 5 yr since last attack¶	None‖

Abbreviations: RF, rheumatic fever; RHD, residual rheumatic heart disease of any severity.
Patients from developing countries, with large RF burden, should be considered at high risk for recurrent infections.
*Each case is judged individually after considering the clinical situation and patient wishes.
†Modify prophylaxis in epidemic situations, especially if virulent streptococci reemerge.
‡Should be at least 10 yr since last attack and should not have history of multiple attacks.
§Use echocardiography if possible to prove or disprove RHD.
‖Should be at least 5 yr since last attack and should not have history of multiple attacks.
¶Whichever is longer in duration.

REFERENCES

1. Contreras R: Lesiones de la fiebre rheumatica. *In* Mongografia Sobre Fiebre Rheumatica. pp. 17–37. Madrid: 1970.
2. Sydenham T: The Works of Thomas Sydenham. Vol. 1. London: Sydenham Society, 1848.
3. Parkinson J: Rheumatic fever and heart disease: the Harveian oration. Lancet 2:657, 1945.
4. Cosh JA, Lever JV: Rheumatic fever. *In* Rheumatic Diseases and the Heart. pp. 1–21. Heidelberg: Springer-Verlag, 1988.
5. Parry CH: An inquiry into the symptoms and cause of the syncope anginosa commonly called angina pectoris. London: 1799.
6. Corvisart JN: Essai sur les Maladies et le Lesions Organiques du Coeur et des Gros Vaisseau. Paris: Imprimerie de Migneret, 1806. (A Treatise on the Diseases and Organic Lesions of the Heart and Great Vessels. English translation by C. H. Hebb, London, 1813.)
7. Rolleston JD: Jean Baptiste Bouillaud: a pioneer in cardiology and neurology. Proc R Soc Med 24: 1253, 1931.
8. Bouillaud JB: Traite clinique de rhumatisme articulaire. Paris: JB Bailliere, 1840.
9. Aschoff L: Zur Myocarditis frag. Berhandl Deutsch Pathol Ges 8:46, 1904.
10. White P: Rheumatic heart disease: acute and chronic. *In* Heart Disease. 2nd ed. pp. 324–350. New York: Macmillan, 1944.
11. Schlesinger B: The relationship of throat infection to acute rheumatism in childhood. Arch Dis Child 5:411, 1930.
12. Collis WRF: Acute rheumatism and hemolytic streptococci. Lancet 1:1341, 1931.
13. Coburn AF: Relationships of the rheumatic process to the development of alterations in the tissues. Am J Dis Child 45:933, 1933.
14. Thompson S, Innes J: Hemolytic streptococci in the cardiac lesions of acute rheumatism. BMJ, 2:733–736, 1940.
15. Hirschhorn K, Schreibman RR, Verbo S, Grushkin RH: The action of streptolysin S on peripheral leukocytes of normal subjects and patients with acute rheumatic fever. Proc Natl Acad Sci U S A 52:1151–1157, 1964.
16. Kaplan MH, Meyeserian M, Kushner I: Immunologic cross reaction between group A streptococcal cells and human heart tissue. Lancet 1:706–710, 1962.
17. Kaplan MH, Suchy ML: Immunologic relation of streptococcal and tissue antigens, II: cross reaction of antisera to mammalian heart tissue to the cell wall constituents of certain strains of group A streptococci. J Exp Med 119:643–650, 1964.
18. Dudding BA, Ayoub EM: Persistance of streptococcal group A antibody in patients with rheumatic valvular disease. J Exp Med 128:1081–1098, 1968.
19. Dale JB, Beachey EH: Epitopes of streptococcal M protein shared with cardiac myosin. J Exp Med 162:583–591, 1985.
20. Bessen D, Jones KF, Fischetti VA: Evidence for two distinct classes of streptococcal M protein and their relationship to rheumatic fever. J Exp Med 169:269–283, 1989.
21. Ayoub EM, Dudding BA: Streptococcal group A carbohydrate antibody in rheumatic and non rheumatic bacterial endocarditis. J Lab Clin Med 76:322–332, 1970.

22. Stollerman GH: Rheumatogenic streptococci and autoimmunity. Clin Immunol Immunopathol 61:131–142, 1991.
23. Zabriskie JB: Mimetic relationships between group A streptococci and mammalian tissues. Adv Immunol 7:147–188, 1967.
24. Goldstein I, Halpern B, Robert L: Immunological relationship between streptococcus A polysaccharide and the structural glucoproteins of heart valve. Nature 213:44–47, 1967.
25. Cunningham MW, McCormack JM, Fenderson PG, et al: Human and murine antibodies cross reactive with streptococcal M protein and myosin recognise the sequence GLN-LYS-SER-LYS-GLN in M protein. J Immunol 143:2677–2683, 1989.
26. Manjula BN, Trus BL, Fischetti VA: Presence of two distinct regions in the coiled coil structure of the streptococcal Pep M5 protein: relationship to mammalian coiled coil proteins and implications to its biological properties. Proc Natl Acad Sci U S A 82:1064–1068, 1985.
27. Tomai MA, Kotb M, Majumdar G, Beachey EH: Superantigenicity of streptococcal M protein. J Exp Med 172:359–362, 1990.
28. Narula J, Chopra P, Talwar KK, et al: Does endomyocardial biopsy aid in the diagnosis of active rheumatic carditis? Circulation 88:2198–2205, 1993.
29. Zabriskie JB, Hsu KC, Seegal BC: Heart reactive antibody associated with rheumatic fever: characterisation and diagnostic significance. Clin Exp Immunol 7:147–159, 1970.
30. Guilherme L, Cuhna-Neto E, Coehlo V, et al: Human heart infiltrating T cell clones from rheumatic heart disease recognize both streptococcal and cardiac proteins. Circulation 92:415–420, 1995.
31. Read SE, Reid HF, Fischetti V, et al: Serial studies on the cellular immune response to streptococcal antigens in acute and convalescent rheumatic fever patients in Trinidad. J Clin Immunol 6:433–441, 1986.
32. Hafez M, el Battoty MF, Hawas S, et al: Evidence of inherited susceptibility of increased streptococcal adherence to pharyngeal cells of children with rheumatic fever. Br J Rheumatol 38:304, 1989.
33. Khanna AK, Buskirk DR, Williams RC Jr, et al: Presence of a non-HLA B cell antigen in rheumatic fever patients and their families as defined by a monoclonal antibody. J Clin Invest 83:1710, 1989.
34. Taranta A: Rheumatic fever made difficult: a critical review of pathogenetic theories. Paediatrician 5:74, 1976.
35. Ayoub EM: The search for host determinants of susceptibility to rheumatic fever: the missing link. Circulation 69:197–201, 1984.
36. Anastasiou-Nana MI, Anderson HL, Carlquist ZL, Nanas HN: HLA-DR typing and lymphocyte subset evaluation in rheumatic heart disease: a search for immune response factors. Am Heart J 112:992–997, 1986.
37. Rajapakse CN, Halim K, Al-Orainay I, et al: A genetic marker for rheumatic heart disease. Br Heart J 58:659–662, 1987.
38. Taneja V, Mehra NK, Reddy KS, et al: HLA-DR/DQ and reactivity to B cell alloantigen D8/17 in Indian patients with rheumatic heart disease. Circulation 80:335–340, 1989.
39. Patarroyo ME, Winchester RJ, Vejerano A, et al: Association of a B cell alloantigen with susceptibility to rheumatic fever. Nature (Lond) 278:173–174, 1979.
40. Land MA, Bisno AL: Acute rheumatic fever: a vanishing disease in suburbia. JAMA 249:895, 1983.
41. Gordis L: The virtual disappearance of rheumatic fever in the United States: lessons in the rise and fall of the disease. T. Duckett Jones Memorial Lecture. Circulation 72:1155, 1985.
42. Massell BF, Narula J: Rheumatic fever and carditis. *In* Braunwald E (ed): The Atlas of Heart Diseases. pp. 10.1–10.20. Philadelphia: Current Medicine, 1994.
43. U.S. Department of Health and Human Services: Summary of notifiable disease, United States, 1990. Vol 39, No. 53, 1990.
44. Bisno AL: Group A streptococcal infections and acute rheumatic fever. N Engl J Med 325:783, 1991.
45. Kaplan EL: Report on return of rheumatic fever. J Pediatr 111:224, 1987.
46. World Health Organization: Rheumatic fever and rheumatic heart disease: report of a WHO Study Group. WHO Tech Rep Ser 764, 1988.
47. Markowitz M: Observations on the epidemiology and preventability of rheumatic fever in developing countries. Clin Ther 4:240–251, 1981.
48. Vijaykumar M, Narula J, Reddy KS, Kaplan EL: Incidence of rheumatic fever and prevalence of rheumatic heart disease in India. Int J Cardiol 43:221–228, 1994.
49. Krishnaswami S, Joseph G, Richard J: Demands on tertiary care for cardiovascular diseases in India: analysis of data for 1960–89. Bull WHO 69:325–330, 1991.
50. Virmani R, Roberts WC: Aschoff bodies in operatively excised atrial appendages and in papillary muscles: frequency and clinical significance. Circulation 55:559–563, 1977.
51. Veasy GL: Myocardial dysfunction in active rheumatic carditis. J Am Coll Cardiol 24:578, 1994.
52. Klibanoff E, Frieden J, Spagnuolo M, Feinstein AR: Rheumatic activity: a clinicopathologic correlation. JAMA 195:895–900, 1966.
53. Vasan R, Shrivastava S, Vijaya Kumar K, et al: Echocardiographic evaluation of patients with acute rheumatic fever and rheumatic carditis. Circulation 94:73–82, 1996.
54. Gross G, Fried BM: Lesions in the atrioventricular conduction system occurring in rheumatic fever. Am J Pathol 12:31–43, 1936.
55. Jones TD: The diagnosis of rheumatic fever. JAMA 126:281, 1944.
56. Committee on Standards and Criteria for Programs of Care of the American Heart Association: Jones criteria (modified) for guidance in the diagnosis of rheumatic fever. Circulation 13:617, 1956.
57. American Heart Association: Jones criteria (revised) for guidance in the diagnosis of rheumatic fever. Circulation 32:664, 1965.
58. Committee on the Prevention of Rheumatic Fever and Bacterial Endocarditis of the American Heart Association: The Jones criteria (revised) (Abstract). Circulation 70:893A, 1984.
59. Special Writing Group of the Committee on Rheumatic Fever, Endocarditis, and Kawaski Disease of the Council of Cardiovascular Disease in the Young of the American Heart Association: Guidelines for the diagnosis of rheumatic fever: Jones criteria, 1992 update. JAMA 268:2069, 1992.
60. Feinstein AR, Spagnuolo M: The clinical pattern of acute rheumatic fever: a reappraisal. Medicine 41:279–305, 1962.
61. Sanyal SK, Thapar MK, Ahmed AH, et al: The initial attack of rheumatic fever during childhood in North India: a prospective study of the clinical profile. Circulation 49:7–12, 1974.
62. Amigo MC, Martinez-Levin M, Reyes PA: Acute rheumatic fever. Rheum Clin North Am 19:333–350, 1993.
63. Markowitz M: Evolution and critique of changes in the Jones criteria for the diagnosis of rheumatic fever. N Z Med J 101:392–394, 1988.
64. Battacharya S, Tandon R: The diagnosis of rheumatic fever: evaluation of Jones criteria. Int J Cardiol 12:285–294, 1986.
65. Pamavati S, Gupta V: Reappraisal of Jones criteria: the Indian experience. N Z Med J 101:391–392, 1988.
66. Fink CW: The role of the streptococcus in post-streptococcal reactive arthritis and childhood polyarteritis nodosa. J Rheumatol 29:14–20, 1991.
67. Deighton C: Beta hemolytic streptococci and reactive arthritis in adults. Ann Rheum Dis 52:475–482, 1993.
68. Kothari SS, Chandrashekhar Y, Tandon RK: Rheumatic Carditis. *In* Narula J, Tandon R, Reddy KS, Virmani R (eds): Rheumatic Fever. Washington, DC: AFIP Press, 1998.
69. Veasy LG, Wiedmeier SE, Orsmond GS, et al: Resurgence of acute rheumatic fever in the intermountain area of the United States. N Engl J Med 316:421–427, 1987.
70. Bland EF, Jones TD: Rheumatic fever and rheumatic heart disease: a 20-year report on 1,000 patients followed since childhood. Circulation 4:836–843, 1951.
71. Kinare SG: Chronic valvular heart disease. Ann Indian Acad Med Sci 8:48–51, 1972.
72. Marcus RH, Sareli P, Pocock WA, et al: Functional anatomy of severe mitral regurgitation in active rheumatic carditis. Am J Cardiol 63:577–584, 1989.
73. Stollerman GH: Rheumatic carditis. Lancet 346:390–391, 1995.
74. Massell BF, Fyler DC, Roy SB: The clinical picture of rheumatic fever: diagnosis, immediate prognosis, course and therapeutic implications. Am J Cardiol 1:436–449, 1958.
75. Essop MR, Wisenbaugh T, Sareli P: Evidence against a myocardial factor as the cause of left ventricular dilation in active rheumatic carditis. J Am Coll Cardiol 22:826–829, 1993.
76. Tan AT, Mah PK, Chia BL: Cardiac tamponade in acute rheumatic carditis. Ann Rheum Dis 42:699–701, 1983.
77. Przybojewski JZ: Rheumatic constrictive pericarditis: a case report and review of the literature. S Afr Med J 59:682–686, 1981.
78. Burdash NM, Teti G, Hund P: Streptococcal antibody tests in rheumatic fever. Ann Clin Lab Sci 16:163–170, 1986.
79. Ayoub EM, Wannamaker LW: Evaluation of the streptococcal DNase

B and DNase antibody tests in acute rheumatic fever and glomerulonephritis. Pediatrics 29:527–538, 1962.

80. Narula J, Chandrashekhar Y, Rahimtoola SH: Diagnosis of active rheumatic carditis: the echoes of change. Circulation 100:1576–1581, 1999.
81. Gagliardi MG, Bevilacqua M, DiRenzi P, et al: Usefulness of magnetic resonance imaging for diagnosis of acute myocarditis in infants and children, and comparison with endomyocardial biopsy. Am J Cardiol 69:1089, 1991.
82. Narula J, Malhotra A, Yasuda T, et al: Usefulness of antimyosin imaging for the detection of active rheumatic carditis. Am J Cardiol 84:946–950, 1999.
83. Bhatnagar A, Calegaro JUM, Narula J: Radionuclide imaging in rheumatic fever. *In* Narula J, Virmani R, Reddy KS, Tandon R (eds): Rheumatic Fever. Washington, DC: American Registry of Pathology, 1999, pp 329–338.
84. Bland EF, Jones TD: Observation of 10 years of rheumatic infection in children. Am Heart J 36:89, 1948.
85. Keith JD, Rowe RD, Vlad P: Heart Disease in Infancy and Childhood. 2nd ed. New York, Macmillan, 1967.
86. Bland EF, Jones TD: Rheumatic fever and rheumatic heart disease: a 20 year report on 1000 patients followed since childhood. Circulation 4:836, 1951.
87. Wood P: An appreciation of mitral stenosis. BMJ 1:1051–1113, 1954.
88. Levine SA: Intracardiac thrombi. Am J Med Sci 1939.
89. Sellers TH, Bedford DE, Somerville W: Valvotomy in the treatment of mitral stenosis. BMJ 2:1059, 1953.
90. Wallach JB, Lukash L, Angrist AA: An interpretation of the incidence of mural thrombi in the left auricle and appendage with particular reference to mitral commissurotomy. Am Heart J 45:252, 1953.
91. Coburn AF: Salicylate therapy in rheumatic fever: rational technic. Bull Johns Hopkins Hosp 73:435, 1943.
92. Hench PS, Slocumb CH, Barnes AR et al: The effects of the adrenal cortical hormone 17-hydroxy-11-dehydrocorticorticosterone (compound E) on the acute phase of rheumatic fever: preliminary report. Proc Staff Meet Mayo Clin 25:277, 1949.
93. Hench PS, Kendall EC, Slocumb CH, Polley HF: Effects of cortisone acetate and pituitary ACTH on rheumatoid arthritis, rheumatic fever and certain other conditions: a study in clinical physiology. Arch Intern Med 85:545, 1950.
94. Rothman PE: Treatment of rheumatic carditis: a critical review. Clin Pediatr 4:619–625, 1965.
95. Markowitz M, Kuttner AG: Treatment of acute rheumatic fever. Am J Dis Child 104:137–144, 1962.
96. Czoniczer G, Amezcua F, Pelagronio S, Massell BF: Therapy of severe rheumatic carditis: comparison of adrenocortical steroids and aspirin. Circulation 29:813–819, 1964.
97. Albert DA, Harel L, Karrison T: The treatment of rheumatic carditis: a review and meta analysis. Medicine 74:1–12, 1995.
98. Duran CMG, Gometza B, De Vol EB: Valve repair in rheumatic mitral disease. Circulation 84(suppl III)III-125–III-132, 1991.
99. Lewis BS, Geft IL, Milo S, Gotsman MS: Echocardiography and valve replacement in the critically ill patients with acute rheumatic carditis. Ann Thorac Surg 27:529–55, 1978.
100. Skoularigis J, Sinovich V, Joubert G, Sareli P: Evaluation of the long-term results of mitral valve repair in 254 young patients with rheumatic mitral regurgitation. Circulation 90(Suppl II):II-167–II-174, 1994.
101. Chandrashekhar Y: Secondary prevention: theory, practice and analysis of available trials. *In* Narula J, Tandon R, Reddy KS, Virmani R (eds): Rheumatic Fever. Washington, DC: AFIP Press, 1999, pp 399–442.
102. Taranta A, Kleinberg E, Feinstein AR, et al: Rheumatic fever in children and adolescents: a long-term epidemiologic study of subsequent prophylaxis, streptococcal infections, and clinical sequelae. V. Relation of the rheumatic fever recurrence rate per streptococcal infection to preexisting clinical features of the patients. Ann Intern Med 60(suppl 5):58–67, 1964.
103. Massell BF: Factors in the pathogenesis of rheumatic fever recurrences. A study of streptococcal infections and rheumatic fever. J Maine Med Assoc 53:88–93, 1962.
104. United Kingdom and United States Joint Report on Rheumatic Heart Disease: The natural history of rheumatic fever and rheumatic heart disease: ten-year report of a cooperative clinical trial of ACTH, cortisone, and aspirin. Circulation 32:457–476, 1965.
105. Sanyal SL, Berry AM, Duggal S, et al: Sequelae of the initial attack of acute rheumatic fever in children from North India: a prospective 5-year follow-up study. Circulation 65:375–379, 1982.
106. Majeed HA, Bhatnagar S, Yousof AM, et al: Acute rheumatic fever and the evolution of rheumatic heart disease: a prospective 12-year follow-up report. J Clin Epidemiol 45:871–875, 1992.
107. Tompkins DG, Boxerbaum B, Liebman J: Long-term prognosis of rheumatic fever patients receiving regular intramuscular benzathine penicillin. Circulation 45:543–551, 1972.
108. Majeed HA, Yousof AM, Khuffash FA, et al: The natural history of acute rheumatic fever in Kuwait: a prospective six year follow-up report. J Chron Dis 39:361–369, 1986.
109. Taranta A: Should adults with rheumatic heart disease be kept on continuous prophylaxis? Am J Cardiol 18;627–629, 1966.
110. Stollerman GH: Changing streptococci and prospects for global eradication of rheumatic fever. Perspec Biol Med 40:165–189, 1997.
111. Dale JB, Simmons M, Chiang EC, Chiang EY: Recombitant octavalent group A streptococcal vaccine. Vaccine 14:944–948, 1996.
112. Dale JB, Chiang EC: Intranasal immunization with recombinant group A streptococcal M protein fragment fused to the B subunit of *E coli* labile toxin protects mice against systemic challenge infections. J Infect Dis 171:1038–1041, 1995.
113. White PD: Changes in relative prevalence of various types of heart disease in New England. JAMA 152:L303, 1953.
114. Cooperative Rheumatic Fever Study: The treatment of acute rheumatic fever in children: a cooperative clinical trial of ACTH, cortisone, and aspirin. Circulation 11:343, 1955.
115. Wilson MG, Lubschez R: Recurrence rates in rheumatic fever: the evaluation of etiologic concepts and consequent preventive therapy. JAMA 126:447, 1944.

CHAPTER 18

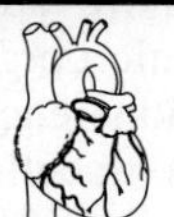

INFECTIVE ENDOCARDITIS*

Walter R. Wilson and Eddy Barasch

INCIDENCE, ANATOMIC CONSIDERATIONS, AND PATHOPHYSIOLOGY
CLINICAL RECOGNITION
Physical Examination
Laboratory Examination
MICROBIOLOGIC ETIOLOGY
MEDICAL TREATMENT
Penicillin-Susceptible Streptococci
Enterococci
Staphylococci
TREATMENT OF COMPLICATIONS
Cardiac Complications
Extracardiac Complications
PREVENTION OF ENDOCARDITIS

The term *infective endocarditis* (IE) describes infection of the endocardium caused by a microorganism. Endocarditis most often involves the heart valves but may involve septal defects, mural endocardium, atriovenous shunts, or a patent ductus arteriosus. The terms *acute* and *subacute* were used previously to classify patients with IE. These terms were based on the progression of untreated patients and are primarily of historic interest. Most authorities now use the term *infective endocarditis* rather than *subacute* or *acute bacterial endocarditis* to describe endocardial infection.

In the preantibiotic era, the fact that patients recovered from serious bacterial infections is testimony to the major role played by host defense mechanisms in controlling or eradicating bacterial infection. This is not the case with IE; host defense mechanisms play little role in the control of IE, and the mortality rate among untreated patients is virtually 100 percent. In no other infectious diseases is cure so dependent on the administration of appropriate bactericidal antimicrobial agents. The successful management of patients with IE is based on (1) recognition of the syndrome consistent with IE, (2) recovery of microorganisms from blood or cardiac valve vegetation cultures, (3) administration of appropriate antimicrobial agents, (4) management of complications, and (5) adequate prophylactic measures.

INCIDENCE, ANATOMIC CONSIDERATIONS, AND PATHOPHYSIOLOGY

A population-based study in Olmsted County, Minnesota, showed the estimated age- and sex-adjusted incidence of IE to be 4.9 per 100,000 person years.[1] Males (rate ratio 2.51) and advanced age (rate ratio 8.81 for age $\geq$ 65 years compared with $<$ 65 years) were associated with higher rates of endocarditis. In another study, endocarditis accounted for approximately 1 case per 1000 hospital admissions.[2] The cardiac valve involved with endocarditis varies among reported series. The rate of infection of the mitral valve alone ranged from 24 to 45 percent; for the aortic valve alone, the rate was 5 to 36 percent; and for the aortic and mitral valves combined, the rate was 0 to 35 percent.[3–6] The aortic valve is more commonly involved among male patients, and mitral valve infections dominate in female patients. Tricuspid valve involvement ranged from 0 to 6 percent, and pulmonary valve involvement was less than 1 percent. Tricuspid valve endocarditis has increased in incidence since about 1980 because of the large number of addicts who abuse intravenous drugs. In the United States, mitral valve prolapse (MVP) with regurgitation is the most common underlying cardiac defect predisposing to IE; previously, rheumatic valvular heart disease was the most common predisposing condition. Underlying congenital heart disease has been reported in 6 to 24 percent of patients with IE. However, as many as 40 percent of patients develop IE with no demonstrable underlying valvular heart disease.[5] Presumably, these patients are at risk because of calcified mitral or aortic valves or other degenerative cardiac diseases or because of infection with virulent microorganisms that infect previously normal cardiac valves.

Pathophysiologic events that result in IE involving a normal cardiac valve differ from those affecting a previously abnormal valve. Endocarditis affecting a previously abnormal cardiac valve results from a series of factors or events. Valvular insufficiency, congenital cardiac lesions such as septal defects, or other valvular abnormalities produce turbulent blood flow and a jet effect that traumatizes the endothelial surface and results in deposition of a fibrin–platelet matrix called *nonbacterial thrombotic endocarditis*.[8] Transient bacteremias occur frequently, often in association with procedures such as dental extraction, tooth brushing, or chewing or as a result of manipulations of the urogenital system, gastrointestinal tract, or oral respiratory tract. Colonization of nonbacterial thrombotic lesions during transient bacteremia results in IE. Once colonization occurs, vegetations enlarge through further deposition of fibrin, platelets, and bacteria. The dense fibrin–platelet matrix provides a sanctuary for bacteria against host defenses and impairs penetration of antibiotics into the vegetation. Certain microorganisms, such as viridans streptococci, enterococci, staphylococci, and *Pseudomonas aeruginosa,* are

*Prosthetic valve endocarditis and its treatment are discussed in the Appendix.

more adherent to cardiac valve endothelium than other microorganisms not commonly associated with IE.[9] The adherence of streptococci may be in part related to the extracellular production of a polysaccharide called *dextran.*[10] Platelets may also play a role in the pathophysiology of IE. Staphylococci and streptococci stimulate platelet aggregation, and these aggregates may have an increased affinity for nonbacterial thrombotic lesions.[11]

Nonbacterial thrombotic endocarditis probably does not play a major role, if any, in the pathophysiology of IE involving normal cardiac valves. The organisms responsible for IE involving previously normal cardiac valves, such as *Staphylococcus aureus, Streptococcus pneumoniae, Neisseria gonorrhoeae,* and *Streptococcus pyogenes,* differ from those that usually infect an abnormal cardiac valve. IE in the former patients is usually caused by bacteremia originating from the focus of infection, such as the skin, musculoskeletal system, or genitourinary tract. Although the pathophysiology of IE in these patients is poorly understood, it may be related to the high magnitude of bacteremia, virulence of the microorganisms, and possibly binding to specific receptors on the surface of endothelial cells.

CLINICAL RECOGNITION

Physical Examination

The clinical manifestations of IE may involve any organ system and are largely dependent on the infecting microorganism. Patients with acute fulminant IE caused by *S. aureus, S. pneumoniae,* or *N. gonorrhoeae* usually present with fever, metastatic abscesses, rapid valvular destruction, and the sudden onset of severe congestive heart failure (CHF) and have a high mortality rate. More commonly, patients present with a subacute or chronic form of IE that is usually caused by viridans streptococci, enterococci, or fastidious gram-negative bacilli of the HACEK group (*Haemophilus* species, *Actinobacillus actinomycetemcomitans, Cardiobacterium hominis, Eikenella* species, and *Kingella kingae*). The history of a preceding dental procedure, genitourinary tract manipulation, or urinary tract infection is present in 20 to 30 percent of patients with viridans streptococcal or enterococcal endocarditis.[5] Initial symptoms are nonspecific and include anorexia, weight loss, fatigue, fever, headaches, myalgias, and arthralgias. This condition may be confused with a number of other chronic febrile illnesses, such as lymphoma, other malignancies, other chronic infectious diseases, and collagen vascular disorders. The duration of symptoms in the subacute or chronic form ranges from 1 to 2 weeks to more than 1 year.

Although fever is present in virtually all patients with IE, it may be absent in patients who have received antimicrobial therapy. A cardiac murmur is present in at least 85 percent of patients but may be absent in patients with right-sided endocarditis. A change in a preexisting murmur or the development of a new regurgitant murmur is an important finding. Peripheral embolic or hypersensitivity phenomena occur in at least 60 percent of patients with the subacute or chronic form of IE.[5] *Osler nodes* occur in 10 to 25 percent of patients and are characterized by small, tender, slightly nodular lesions usually located on the palms of the hands and soles of the feet. Osler nodes are thought to occur as a result of the deposition of circulating immune complexes or, possibly, microemboli of vegetations that contain bacteria. *Roth spots* occur in about 10 percent of patients with IE and are characteristically present in the conjunctiva or retina. Approximately 10 percent of patients develop macular, nontender, erythematous lesions on the palms and soles, known as *Janeway lesions.* Splenomegaly occurs in 25 to 60 percent of patients with IE, and myalgias and arthralgias occur in at least 40 percent. Large systemic emboli have been observed in 10 to 30 percent of patients and are more often associated with infection caused by nutritionally variant viridans streptococci, members of the HACEK group, group B streptococci, and fungal endocarditis. Headaches have been reported in up to 60 to 80 percent of patients with IE.[12, 13] Approximately 20 to 40 percent of patients develop neurologic manifestations, including ataxia, aphasia, alterations in mental status, or other changes resulting from cerebral emboli or hypersensitivity phenomena.[13] Intracranial mycotic aneurysms are documented in approximately 1 percent of patients with IE; they may be asymptomatic or present with catastrophic complications resulting from rupture and hemorrhage.[12]

Laboratory Examination

Because patients with IE may present with a chronic, nonspecific febrile illness that may mimic a wide variety of other diseases, clinicians must be alert to the possibility of IE. This is especially true for patients who have received partial treatment with antibiotics that has rendered blood cultures negative and temporarily eliminated the fever. It may therefore be necessary in these patients to observe them after the withdrawal of antibiotic therapy and to periodically obtain blood cultures.

The diagnosis of IE depends on recognition of the clinical syndrome and the recovery of bacteria or fungi from two or more cultures of blood obtained at intervals during a 48-hour period. In most cases, bacteremia associated with IE is continuous, and if any blood culture is positive, most of the other specimens cultured will also be positive. Therefore, it is usually unnecessary to obtain more than three sets of blood cultures within a 24-hour period on 2 consecutive days. Collection of blood for culture during temperature elevations does not increase the likelihood of a positive blood culture. However, cases of IE caused by nutritionally variant viridans streptococci or members of the HACEK group may have intermittently positive blood cultures. The recovery of these microorganisms from more than one blood culture has such a high association with IE that this diagnosis must be considered even in the absence of physical findings suggestive of IE.

Durack and colleagues[14] (from Duke University [Duke criteria]) proposed a new diagnostic strategy to define cases of IE. The Duke criteria combine important traditional diagnostic parameters, such as persistent bacteremia, newly developed valvular insufficiency, and peripheral manifestations, with echocardiographic findings. According to the Duke criteria, patients suspected of having IE may be classified into one of three categories: definite, possible, or

TABLE 18–7 **Standard Therapy for Endocarditis Due to Enterococci***

Antibiotic	Dosage and Route	Duration (wk)	Comments
Aqueous crystalline penicillin G sodium	18–30 million U/24 h IV either continuously or in 6 equally divided doses	4–6	4-wk therapy recommended for patients with symptoms < 3 mo in duration; 6-wk therapy recommended for patients with symptoms > 3 mo in duration
With gentamicin sulfate†	1 mg/kg IM or IV every 8 h	4–6	
Ampicillin sodium	12 g/24 h IV either continuously or in 6 equally divided doses	4–6	
With gentamicin sulfate†	1 mg/kg IM or IV every 8 h	4–6	
Vancomycin hydrochloride†‡	30 mg/kg per 24 h IV in 2 equally divided doses, not to exceed 2 g/24 h unless serum levels are monitored	4–6	Vancomycin therapy is recommended for patients allergic to β-lactams; cephalosporins are not acceptable alternatives for patients allergic to penicillin
With gentamicin sulfate†	1 mg/kg IM or IV every 8 h	4–6	

*All enterococci causing endocarditis must be tested for antimicrobial susceptibility to select optimal therapy (see text). This table is for endocarditis due to gentamicin- or vancomycin-susceptible enterococci, viridans streptococci with a minimum inhibitory concentration of > 0.5 µg/ml, nutritionally variant viridans streptococci, or prosthetic valve endocarditis caused by viridans streptococci or *Streptococcus bovis*. Antibiotic dosages are for patients with normal renal function.

†For specific dosing adjustment and issues concerning gentamicin (obese patients, relative contraindications), see Table 18–5 footnotes.

‡For specific dosing adjustment and issues concerning vancomycin (obese patients, length of infusion), see Table 18–5 footnotes.

From Wilson WR, Karchmer AW, Dajani AS, et al: Antibiotic treatment of adults with infective endocarditis due to streptococci, enterococci, staphylococci, and HACEK microorganisms. JAMA 274:1706–1713, 1995. Copyrighted 1995, American Medical Association.

with a combination of penicillin and low-dose gentamicin (see Table 18–7).[17]

Patients with pneumococcal IE often present with an acute fulminant course. These patients should receive therapy with penicillin G, a cephalosporin, or vancomycin administered for 4 weeks. Few data are available concerning the optimal therapy for IE caused by group B streptococci. Most authorities recommend 4-week therapy with penicillin, a cephalosporin, or vancomycin, combined with low-dose gentamicin for the first 2 weeks of treatment.

Enterococci

Enterococci (*S. faecalis, S. faecium, S. durans*) are inhibited but not killed in vitro by penicillin or vancomycin alone. Successful therapy of enterococcal endocarditis requires the administration of penicillin, ampicillin, or vancomycin together with an aminoglycoside, usually gentamicin. The most important factor in the outcome of patients with enterococcal endocarditis is the duration of symptoms before the initiation of effective antimicrobial therapy. Patients with symptoms of infection for more than 3 months have significantly higher relapse and mortality rates than do those with a shorter duration of illness.[18] Patients with symptoms for less than 3 months can be treated successfully for 4 weeks with penicillin or ampicillin, together with gentamicin (see Table 18–7).[17] Patients ill for more than 3 months and those with PVE should receive 6 weeks of therapy. Concentrations of gentamicin in serum should be monitored closely to ensure that the 1-hour concentration is 3 g/ml and the trough concentration is 1 g/ml. The administration of higher dosages of gentamicin does not improve efficacy or enhance synergy with penicillin. However, it does significantly increase the risk for nephrotoxicity.

The treatment of enterococcal endocarditis is becoming increasingly complicated because of the development of resistance of enterococci to multiple antimicrobial agents. Enterococci are uniformly resistant to the cephalosporins. Since the late 1980s, strains of enterococci have been recovered with high-level resistance in vitro to gentamicin, streptomycin, and other aminoglycosides; penicillin and ampicillin; and vancomycin. Enterococci that are highly resistant to an aminoglycoside are not killed synergistically by combinations of either penicillin or vancomycin together with that aminoglycoside. Moreover, vancomycin-resistant strains of enterococci frequently exhibit high-level resistance to aminoglycosides and often to penicillins. Currently, no bactericidal regimen is available for the treatment of patients with enterococcal IE caused by these multiply resistant microorganisms. A small number of patients with multiply resistant enterococcal IE have been treated successfully with a combination of imipenem and ampicillin. Quinupristin-dalfopristin (Synercid) has been effective treatment in some patients with IE caused by vancomycin-resistant strains of *Streptococcus faecium.* The treatment of patients with infections caused by strains of multiply resistant enterococci should be performed in collaboration with an infectious disease specialist and a cardiothoracic surgeon.[17] Cardiac valve replacement may offer these patients the only hope of survival.

Staphylococci

S. aureus *(Methicillin Susceptible)*

Patients with *S. aureus* native valve left-sided endocarditis or PVE should receive 6 weeks of therapy with nafcillin, oxacillin, a first-generation cephalosporin (e.g., cefazolin), or vancomycin (Table 18–8).[17] In in vitro and in animal model studies of experimental endocarditis, the combination of nafcillin and gentamicin was more effective than either drug alone.[20, 21] The administration of nafcillin for 6 weeks combined with gentamicin for the first 2 weeks of therapy did not improve survival rates or reduce complications compared with patients treated with nafcillin alone.[22] However, the combination of nafcillin and gentamicin did significantly shorten the duration of *S. aureus* bacteremia compared with patients who received therapy with nafcillin

TABLE 18–8 **Therapy for Endocarditis Due to Staphylococcus in the Absence of Prosthetic Material***

Antibiotic	Dosage and Route	Duration	Comments
Methicillin-Susceptible Staphylococci			
Regimens for non–β-lactam–allergic patients			
Nafcillin sodium or oxacillin sodium	2 g IV every 4 h	4–6 wk	Benefit of additional aminoglycosides has not been established
With optional addition of gentamicin sulfate†	1 mg/kg IM or IV every 8 h	3–5 da	
Regimens for β-lactam–allergic patients			
Cefazolin (or other first-generation cephalosporins in equivalent dosages)	2 g IV every 8 h	4–6 wk	Cephalosporins should be avoided in patients with immediate-type hypersensitivity to penicillin
With optional addition of gentamicin†	1 mg/kg IM or IV every 8 h	3–5 da	
Vancomycin hydrochloride‡	30 mg/kg per 24 h IV in 2 equally divided doses, not to exceed 2 g/24 h unless serum levels are monitored	4–6 wk	Recommended for patients allergic to penicillin
Methicillin-Resistant Staphylococci			
Vancomycin hydrochloride‡	30 mg/kg per 24 h IV in 2 equally divided doses, not to exceed 2 g/24 h unless serum levels are monitored	4–6 wk	

*For treatment of endocarditis due to penicillin-susceptible staphylococci (minimum inhibitory concentration ≤ 0.1 μg/ml), aqueous crystalline penicillin G sodium (Table 18–5, first regimen) can be used for 4 to 6 wk instead of nafcillin or oxacillin. Shorter antibiotic courses have been effective in some drug addicts with right-sided endocarditis due to *Staphylococcus aureus* (see text). See text for comments on use of rifampin.

†For specific dosing adjustment and issues concerning gentamicin (obese patients, relative contraindications), see Table 18–5 footnotes.

‡For specific dosing adjustment and issues concerning vancomycin (obese patients, length of infusion), see Table 18–5 footnotes.

From Wilson WR, Karchmer AW, Dajani AS, et al: Antibiotic treatment of adults with infective endocarditis due to streptococci, enterococci, staphylococci, and HACEK microorganisms. JAMA 274:1706–1713, 1995. Copyrighted 1995, American Medical Association.

alone. If clinicians prefer to use the combination of nafcillin and gentamicin, the dosage of gentamicin could be the same as that for patients with viridans streptococcal endocarditis and the duration of gentamicin therapy should not exceed the initial 3 to 5 days of treatment. Antimicrobial therapy for *S. aureus* PVE is shown in Table 18–9.[17] Intravenous drug abusers with right-sided methicillin-susceptible *S. aureus* IE who do not have extrapulmonary or extracardiac foci of infection can be treated successfully with a combination of nafcillin and low-dose tobramycin or gentamicin for 2 weeks.[23] Addicts who do not qualify for the 2-week regimen should receive therapy for 4 to 6 weeks.

S. aureus *(Methicillin Resistant)*

Patients with methicillin-resistant IE should be treated for 6 weeks with vancomycin (see Table 18–8).[17] The only effective alternative is cotrimoxazole therapy (trimethoprim/sulfamethoxazole).

Coagulase-Negative Staphylococci (S. epidermidis)

Native valve IE caused by coagulase-negative staphylococci is relatively uncommon, and most strains are susceptible to nafcillin. These patients should be treated with the same therapy used to treat methicillin-susceptible left-sided *S. aureus* endocarditis. Patients with infective endocarditis caused by methicillin-resistant strains should receive vancomycin therapy for 6 weeks. Coagulase-negative staphylococci are the most common cause of early-onset PVE.[24, 25] Most of these strains are resistant to nafcillin or cefazolin. The most effective therapy for patients with coagulase-negative staphylococcal PVE is a combination of vancomycin and rifampin administered for 6 weeks with low-dose gentamicin therapy for the first 2 weeks of treatment (see Table 18–9).[17]

HACEK Group

Endocarditis caused by the HACEK group of microorganisms accounts for about 5 percent of non–addict-associated cases. Previous studies have shown that these patients can be treated successfully with 3 weeks of intravenous ampicillin therapy.[26] However, occasional strains of *H. parainfluenzae* produce beta-lactamase. Susceptibility tests are difficult to perform on the HACEK group of microorganisms. Therefore, they should be considered to be β-lactamase producers until shown otherwise. Ceftriaxone administered in a single dose of 2 g/d for 3 weeks is effective treatment for IE caused by this group of microorganisms (Table 18–10).[17]

Other Gram-Negative Bacillary Microorganisms

Non–addict-associated native valve IE caused by gram-negative bacilli other than the HACEK group is rare. Most cases of native valve gram-negative bacillary endocarditis occur in addicts and are most often caused by *P. aeruginosa, Serratia,* and *Klebsiella.* The choice of effective antimicrobial therapy should be based on in vitro susceptibility tests, and the selection of a specific antimicrobial agent should be the least toxic, most active agent in vitro. In general, therapy should be administered for 4 to 6 weeks.

TABLE 18–9 **Treatment of Staphylococcal Endocarditis in the Presence of a Prosthetic Valve or Other Prosthetic Material***

Antibiotic	Dosage and Route	Duration (wk)	Comments
Regimen for Methicillin-Resistant Staphylococci			
Vancomycin hydrochloride†	30 mg/kg per 24 h IV in 2 or 4 equally divided doses, not to exceed 2 g/24 h unless serum levels are monitored	≥6	
With rifampin‡	300 mg PO every 8 h	≥6	Rifampin increases the amount of warfarin sodium required for antithrombotic therapy
And with gentamicin sulfate§‖	1.0 mg/kg IM or IV every 8 h	2	
Regimen for Methicillin-Susceptible Staphylococci			
Nafcillin sodium or oxacillin sodium	2 g IV every 4 h	≥6	First-generation cephalosporins or vancomycin should be used in patients allergic to β-lactam; cephalosporins should be avoided in patients with immediate-type hypersensitivity to penicillin or with methicillin-resistant staphylococci
With rifampin‡	300 mg PO every 8 h	≥6	
And with gentamicin sulfate§‖	1.0 mg/kg IM or IV every 8 h	2	

*Dosages recommended are for patients with normal renal function.
†For specific dosing adjustment and issues concerning vancomycin (obese patients, length of infusion), see Table 18–5 footnotes.
‡Rifampin plays a unique role in the eradication of staphylococcal infection involving prosthetic material (see text); combination therapy is essential to prevent emergence of rifampin resistance.
§For specific dosing adjustment and issues concerning gentamicin (obese patients, relative contraindications), see Table 18–5 footnotes.
‖Use during initial 2 wk.
From Wilson WR, Karchmer AW, Dajani AS, et al: Antibiotic treatment of adults with infective endocarditis due to streptococci, enterococci, staphylococci, and HACEK microorganisms. JAMA 274:1706–1713, 1995. Copyrighted 1995, American Medical Association.

Gram-negative bacilli are the second most common cause of early-onset PVE. The same principles of therapy for the selection of an antimicrobial agent or a combination of agents used for addict-associated IE should be applied to patients with gram-negative bacillary PVE. The duration of therapy should be 4 to 6 weeks.

Fungal Endocarditis

Endocarditis caused by *Candida* should be treated with amphotericin B or, if susceptible, with fluconazole. After 7 to 10 days of therapy, the infected cardiac valve should be excised. There are few documented cases of cure of fungal endocarditis with medical therapy alone. *Aspergillus* endocarditis most often occurs in association with cardiac valve replacement surgery. Aspergilli are relatively resistant to amphotericin B and other antifungal agents. Therapy should be initiated with amphotericin B, followed by early surgical intervention. Fungal endocarditis is associated with the formation of large cardiac valve vegetations, and embolization to systemic vessels is common. The mortality rate associated with fungal endocarditis, especially that with prosthetic valve infection, is high.

Culture-Negative Endocarditis

Culture-negative endocarditis most often occurs in patients who have received recent antimicrobial therapy. Unless the need for antimicrobial therapy is urgent, it is preferable to withhold therapy for a few days until positive blood cultures establish the microbiologic diagnosis. For patients with acute fulminating IE or those in whom blood cultures remain negative, therapy should be started with a combination of vancomycin and low-dose gentamicin. As described

TABLE 18–10 **Therapy for Endocarditis Due to HACEK Microorganisms***

Antibiotic	Dosage and Route	Duration (wk)	Comments
Ceftriaxone sodium†	2 g once daily IV or IM†	4	Cefotaxime sodium or other third-generation cephalosporins may be substituted
Ampicillin sodium‡	12 g/24 h IV either continuously or in 6 equally divided doses	4	
With gentamicin sulfate§	1 mg/kg IM or IV every 8 h	4	

Abbreviation: HACEK, *Haemophilus* species, *Actinobacillus actinomycetemcomitans, Cardiobacterium hominis, Eikenella* species, and *Kingella kingae.*
*Antibiotic dosages are for patients with normal renal function.
†Patients should be informed that IM injection of ceftriaxone is painful. For patients unable to tolerate β-lactam therapy, consult text.
‡Ampicillin should not be used if laboratory tests show β-lactamase production.
§For specific dosing adjustment and issues concerning gentamicin (obese patients, relative contraindications), see Table 18–5 footnotes.
From Wilson WR, Karchmer AW, Dajani AS, et al: Antibiotic treatment of adults with infective endocarditis due to streptococci, enterococci, staphylococci, and HACEK microorganisms. JAMA 274:1706–1713, 1995. Copyrighted 1995, American Medical Association.

earlier, patients with culture-negative endocarditis should be evaluated for Q fever, chlamydia, mycoplasma, or fungal endocarditis. Patients with nutritionally variant viridans streptococcal IE and those with HACEK endocarditis may have intermittently positive blood cultures, and prolonged incubation may be required before results are positive.

TREATMENT OF COMPLICATIONS

The complications of IE will be considered as those that involve the heart and adjacent structures or those that are extracardiac. Complications chosen for discussion here are those that occur most commonly and are accessible to diagnosis and treatment.

Cardiac Complications

Heart Failure

Heart failure caused by valvular insufficiency is the most common serious complication of IE and is the leading cause of death. Patients with moderate to severe CHF caused by IE who are unresponsive to medical therapy alone have a higher mortality than do patients with CHF who are treated with a medical regimen and cardiac valve replacement.[27–31] Aortic valve IE is associated with a higher mortality rate than is mitral valve infection.[28] Our approach to the management of patients with CHF caused by IE is shown in Figure 18–2.[30] The most important factor in the decision to proceed with cardiac valve replacement and the timing of surgical intervention is the hemodynamic status of the patient. Among patients with severe CHF who fail to respond to medical therapy after 24 to 48 hours, consideration should be given to prompt surgical intervention regardless of the duration of preoperative antimicrobial therapy. In these patients, procrastination in cardiac valve replacement in an attempt to complete the course of antimicrobial therapy preoperatively usually results in death from CHF. The operative mortality rate of patients who undergo cardiac valve replacement owing to CHF caused by IE is directly related to the degree of CHF present at the time of surgery. In a 13-year study done at the Mayo Clinic, the operative mortality rate was highest in patients with class IV disability preoperatively, and the operative mortality rate in patients with or without IE was remarkably similar when the degree of heart failure was the same as that at the time of operation.[31]

Echocardiography is useful in the management of patients with IE and heart failure. Assessment of valvular dysfunction and hemodynamic status by echocardiography is important in decision-making concerning the necessity and timing of surgical intervention.[5, 32–35]

Echocardiography is used to define ventricular function, size, and wall motion, and valvular insufficiency may be quantified. Progressive increase in ventricular size, elevation of pulmonary artery pressure, and wall motion abnormalities on serial echocardiography suggest the onset or worsening of heart failure and suggest the need for surgical intervention (Table 18–11).[15]

Reportedly, there is a higher frequency of complications, including CHF and need for cardiac valve replacement, myocardial abscess, and death, among patients with IE in whom vegetations were detected on echocardiography compared with patients without echocardiographic evidence of vegetation. Patients with larger vegetations (Fig. 18–3) were also reportedly at high risk for complication in some studies[33, 36, 37] but not in others.[32, 38] On the basis of

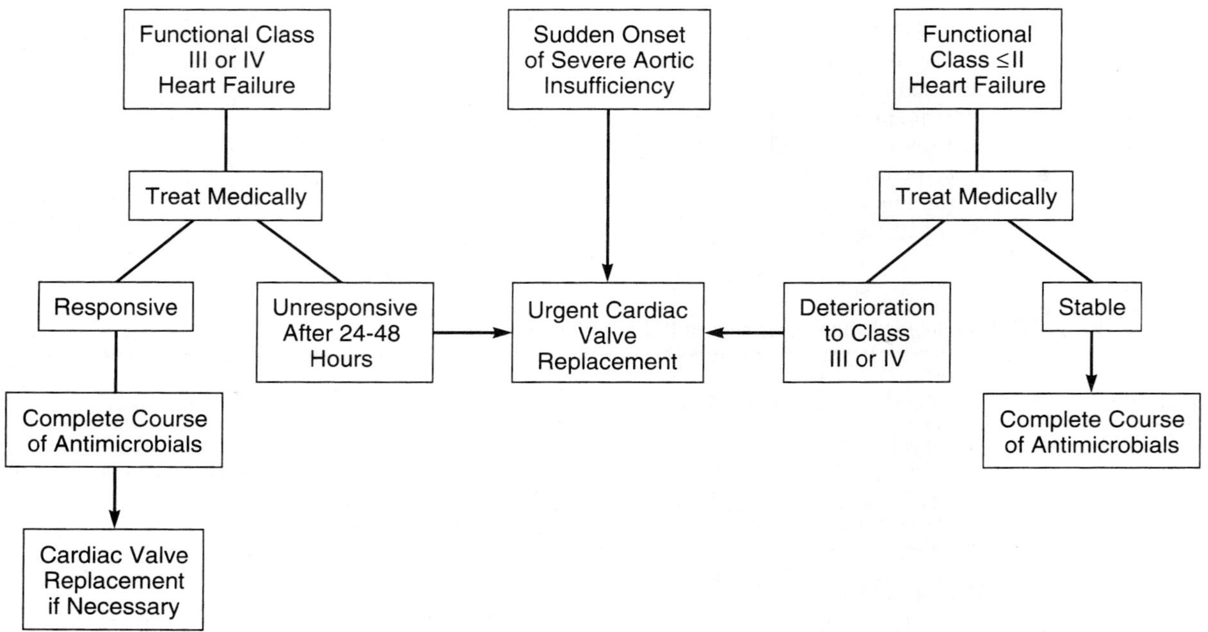

FIGURE 18–2 Diagram of our approach to the management of patients with infective endocarditis and heart failure. Class II, III, or IV indicates New York Heart Association functional classification. (From Wilson WR, Giuliani ER, Danielson GK, Geraci JE: Management of complications of infective endocarditis. Mayo Clin Proc 57:152, 1982.)

TABLE 18-11 Echocardiographic Features Suggesting Potential Need for Surgical Intervention*

Vegetation

Persistent vegetation after systemic embolization
- Anterior mitral leaflet vegetation, particularly with size > 10 mm†
- One or more embolic events during first 2 wk of antimicrobial therapy†
- Two or more embolic events during or after antimicrobial therapy†

Increase in vegetation size after 4 wk of antimicrobial therapy†‡

Valvular Dysfunction

Acute aortic or mitral insufficiency with signs of ventricular failure‡
Heart failure unresponsive to medical therapy‡
Valve perforation or rupture‡

Perivalvular Extension

Valvular dehiscence, rupture, or fistula‡
New heart block‡
Large abscess, or extension of abscess despite appropriate antimicrobial therapy‡

*See text for more complete discussion of indications for surgery based on vegetation characterizations.
†Surgery may be required because of risk of embolization.
‡Surgery may be required because of heart failure or failure of medical therapy.
From Bayer AS, Bolger AF, Taubert KA, et al: Diagnosis and management of infective endocarditis and its complications. Circulation 98:2936, 1998.

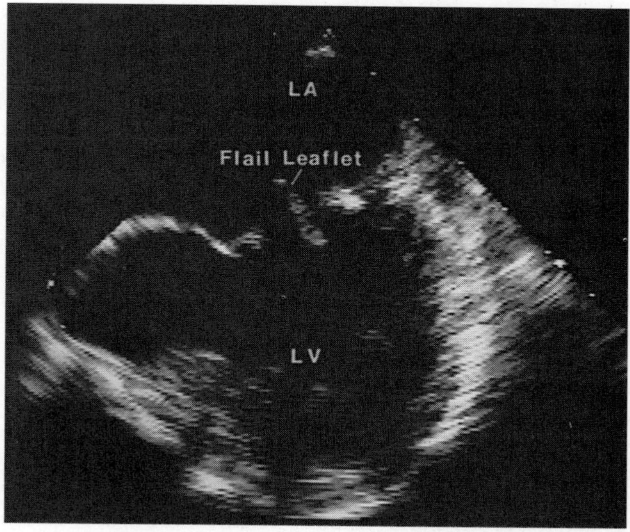

FIGURE 18–4 Transesophageal imaging of the left atrium (LA) and left ventricle (LV) shows a flail posterior leaflet of the mitral valve resulting from ruptured chordae.

these observations, some authorities have recommended early surgical intervention if valvular vegetations are detected by echocardiography.[39–42]

Although these studies reported a high incidence of CHF in patients with echocardiographic detection of vegetations compared with those without vegetations, Lutas and associates[38] reported that the presence or size of vegetations on echocardiography did not significantly increase the incidence of CHF or the need for cardiac valve replacement. O'Brien and Geiser[43] reported that 50 percent of patients without vegetations on echocardiogram developed heart failure. Patients whose echocardiograms demonstrated fluttering of the anterior mitral valve leaflets, premature closure of the mitral valve, chordal (Fig. 18–4) or cusp rupture, or Doppler ultrasound evidence of moderate to severe valvular regurgitation were at higher risk for the development of CHF and the need for cardiac valve replacement.[41–45]

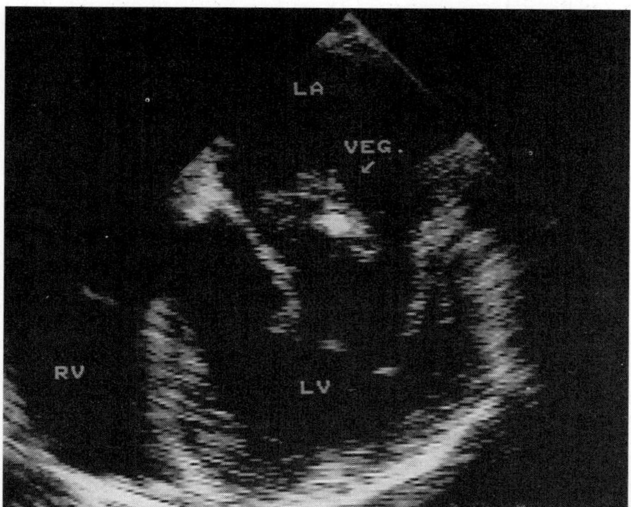

FIGURE 18–3 Transesophageal echocardiographic imaging of the right ventricle (RV), left atrium (LA), and left ventricle (LV) shows a large vegetation (VEG) that involves the atrial surface of the mitral valve.

Echocardiographic imaging is operator dependent and is influenced by such factors as obesity, chest wall deformity, trauma, recent thoracic surgery, and the use of ventilating equipment. Not surprisingly, considerable variability is reported for the incidence of complications and the need for cardiac valve replacement associated with the presence of vegetations detected on echocardiography. Medical regimens and indications for cardiac valve replacement differ among institutions, and the detection of vegetations by echocardiography may have in itself influenced the decision to intervene surgically.

In summary, we do not believe that patients should be subjected to cardiac valve replacement only on the basis of echocardiographic detection of cardiac valve vegetations. The mere presence, location, size, or persistence of vegetations visualized by echocardiography do not necessarily imply that all of these patients will develop CHF. The hemodynamic status of the patient and the response to medical therapy are the most important factors in the decision for surgical intervention. Echocardiography is useful as a means to closely monitor patients with endocarditis during and after the completion of antimicrobial therapy. Patients with torn aortic cusps that produce severe aortic regurgitation and premature closure of mitral valve or ruptured mitral valve chordae that produce severe mitral regurgitation are at higher risk for CHF and should be followed closely for early detection of left ventricular dysfunction and CHF so that prompt surgical intervention can be performed.

Cardiac valve replacement can be performed successfully in patients who have active IE and severe heart failure.[46–49] Previously, we described 11 patients with active IE who underwent urgent cardiac valve replacement; 8 of these patients had positive blood cultures within 48 hours preoperatively.[49] Three of the 11 patients died: 2 of complications of sudden-onset severe aortic regurgitation and 1 of coagulase-negative staphylococcal PVE. The risk of valve dehiscence in PVE may be higher in patients with active IE at the time of operation than in those who have completed a course of antimicrobial therapy preoperatively, but this risk is justified by the excessively high mortality rate in patients with severe CHF who do not undergo early cardiac valve replacement. For patients with sudden-onset severe aortic insufficiency, urgent cardiac valve replacement offers the only hope for survival.

Relapse

In a series of 629 consecutive cases of endocarditis in patients seen at the Mayo Clinic, relapse occurred in 4 percent.[1] All patients with IE should be evaluated carefully to determine the portal of entry of infection. If a source of infection is identified, it should be eliminated while the patient is receiving antimicrobial therapy for IE. Because the oral cavity and urinary tract are the most frequently identified portals of entry, urine culture, urologic evaluation if necessary, and assessment of dentition and any necessary dental procedures should be performed. Metastatic infection is most likely to occur in patients with *S. aureus* IE, and a diligent search for possible metastatic foci of infection, especially located intra-abdominally, using imaging techniques should be conducted.

Our approach to the management of patients with relapse of IE is shown in Figure 18–5.[30] We believe that in all patients with bacterial IE who are stable hemodynamically and who have not had recurrent multiple large emboli, at least one attempt should be made to sterilize the infected valve by antimicrobial therapy before cardiac valve replacement is considered. Patients with *S. aureus* IE who experience a relapse despite adequate antimicrobial therapy should be considered for cardiac valve replacement, espe-

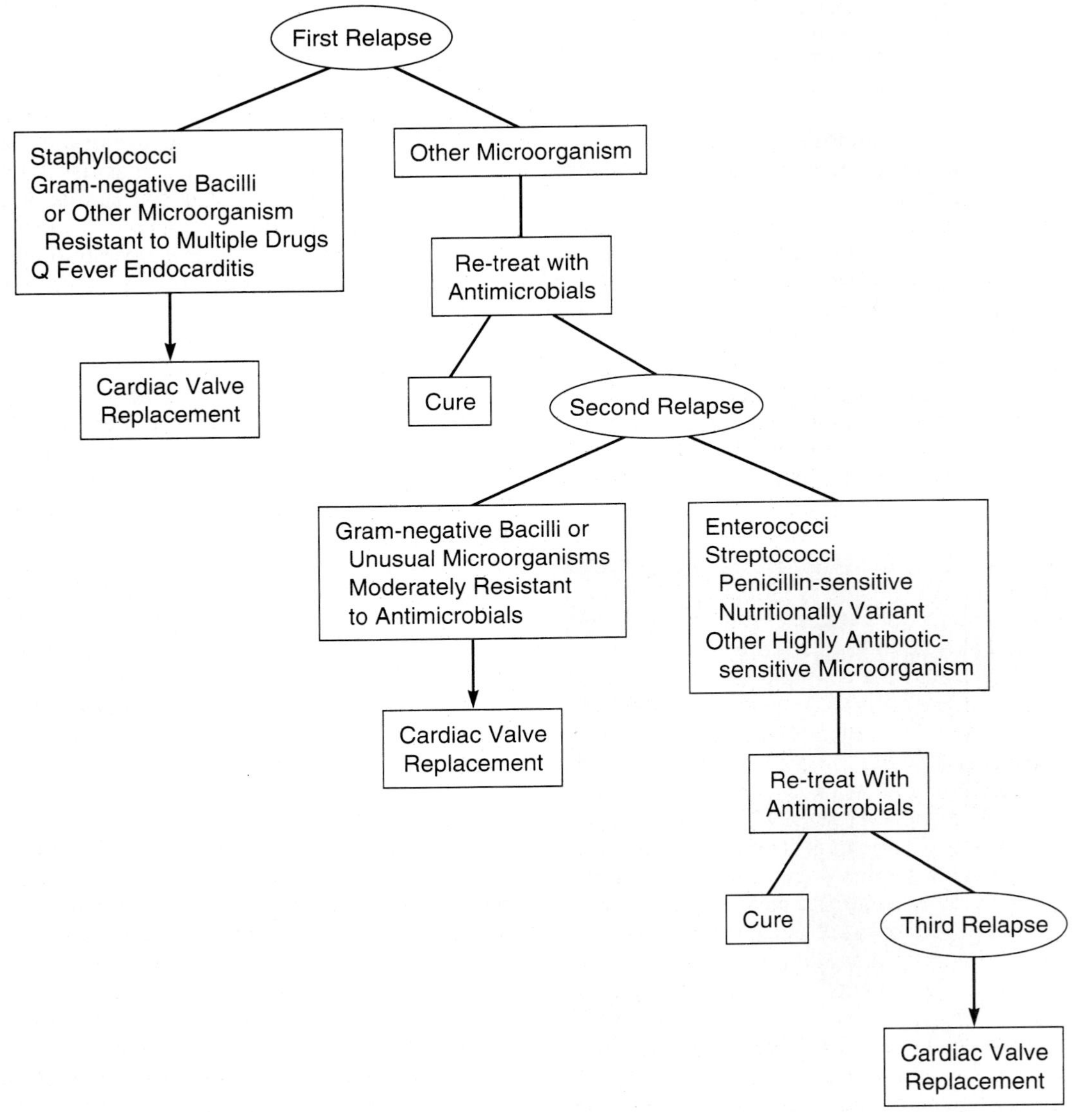

FIGURE 18–5 Diagram of our approach to management of patients with relapse of infective endocarditis. (Modified from Wilson WR, Giuliani ER, Danielson GK, Geraci JE: Management of complications of infective endocarditis. Mayo Clin Proc 57:152, 1982.)

cially if a second relapse occurs and if no metastatic focus of infection to account for the relapse is identified.

Patients with penicillin-susceptible streptococcal IE or enterococcal IE are usually responsive to antimicrobial therapy, and relapses, when they occur, are usually cured by a second course of antimicrobial therapy.

Perivalvular Extension of Infection, Myocardial Abscess, Myocardial Conduction Defects, Infarction, and Pericarditis

The extension of infection involving cardiac valves beyond the valve annulus may result in conduction defects, myocardial abscess, increased risk of valve dehiscence, and the development of heart failure and is associated with a higher mortality rate and need for cardiac surgery. In aortic valve IE, infection may extend from the annulus into the membranous septum and involve the atrioventricular node, resulting in myocardial abscess or heart block. Perivalvular extension of infection is more likely to occur in aortic valve IE than in mitral or tricuspid valve IE. PVE is especially susceptible to perivalvular extension of infection and valvular dehiscence. Persistent bacteremia despite appropriate antimicrobial therapy, recurrent emboli, or the development of heart block or worsening valvular insufficiency or dehiscence suggests perivalvular extension of IE. The use of TEE is more sensitive and specific than TTE for the detection of perivalvular extension of infection.[50] Moreover, TEE combined with spectral and color Doppler echocardiography may demonstrate fistulas, pseudoaneurysms, or myocardial abscess associated with perivalvular extension of infection. Accordingly, TEE is the procedure of choice for the diagnosis of perivalvular extension of infection in patients with IE.

Some patients with perivalvular extension of infection may be successfully treated without surgical intervention; these patients include those without heart block, echocardiographically demonstrated progression of abscess during appropriate antimicrobial therapy, or valvular dehiscence. These patients should be monitored closely with serial echocardiography during and after the completion of antimicrobial therapy.

At the Mayo Clinic, we have observed patients with presumed myocardial abscess diagnosed by echocardiography in whom antimicrobial therapy alone resulted in disappearance of the abscess. In addition, autopsies performed on patients with previously healed endocarditis may demonstrate healed abscess cavities after medical therapy alone. Therefore, the detection of an abscess by echocardiography is not an absolute indication for surgical intervention.

Daniel and colleagues[50] reported their experience in patients with myocardial abscesses documented at surgery or autopsy. TEE in these patients detected abscesses in 87 percent of cases, whereas only 28 percent were identified by two-dimensional echocardiography ($P < .001$). In this study, patients with PVE had a higher percent of abscesses than did those with native valve IE. In patients with IE, we believe that two-dimensional echocardiography should be performed initially, followed by TEE if necessary. The two procedures complement each other and are not mutually exclusive. Patients with myocardial abscesses diagnosed by echocardiography should be followed closely for signs of extension of the abscess, valve dehiscence, development of heart block on electrocardiography, CHF, or persistence of infection despite adequate medical therapy. Patients who exhibit one or more of these complications of myocardial abscess should receive prompt surgical intervention.

Cardiac rhythm disturbances or heart block may result from involvement of the cardiac conduction system by extension of IE. Patients with conduction defects should be monitored closely and may require the insertion of a transvenous pacemaker or other surgical intervention. The goal of surgical intervention in patients with perivalvular extension of IE is eradication of infection, correction of hemodynamic abnormalities including cardiac valve replacement, drainage of abscess, and debridement and closure of fistulous tracts. In patients with perivalvular infection who require cardiac valve replacement, the use of aortic hemographs may be associated with a lower risk of persistence of infection than the use of an artificial prosthesis.

Myocardial infarction results from vegetations that dislodge and embolize to the coronary arteries. In our experience, the frequency of myocardial infarction associated with IE is 3 percent. Patients with myocardial infarction associated with IE should be treated similarly to those with infarction associated with atherosclerosis. Pericarditis is most often associated with *S. aureus* IE. Echocardiography is useful in the detection of pericardial fluid, but the diagnosis of purulent pericarditis must be established by pericardiocentesis. Purulent pericarditis should be treated with prompt surgical drainage and antimicrobial therapy.

Extracardiac Complications

Emboli

The frequency of clinically apparent emboli in patients with IE has been reported to be from 22 to 50 percent.[32, 51] The highest percentage of patients with major embolic events occurs in association with *S. aureus* or those infections that produce large bulky vegetations, such as those caused by the HACEK group of microorganisms, nutritionally variant viridans streptococci, group B streptococci, or fungi (especially *Aspergillus*).[52, 53] Because embolic events may result in irreversible organ dysfunction or death, prevention is a desirable goal. Elective cardiac valve replacement has been recommended for patients who have recurrent emboli or who are at high risk for additional emboli.[40, 54]

The relationship between echocardiographically visualized cardiac valve vegetations, systemic embolization, and the need for cardiac valve replacement is controversial. Valvular vegetations have been detected by echocardiography in 13 to more than 78 percent of patients with endocarditis,[32–34] and their presence has been reported to increase the risk of embolization in some studies[33, 40, 42–44, 55] but not in others.[32, 56–59] Large, mobile vegetations detected by echocardiography, especially those in excess of 10 mm in diameter, have also been reported to increase the risk of embolization in some reports[33, 42, 60] but not in others.[32, 38, 44, 58, 59, 61] The results of these studies led to the controversial

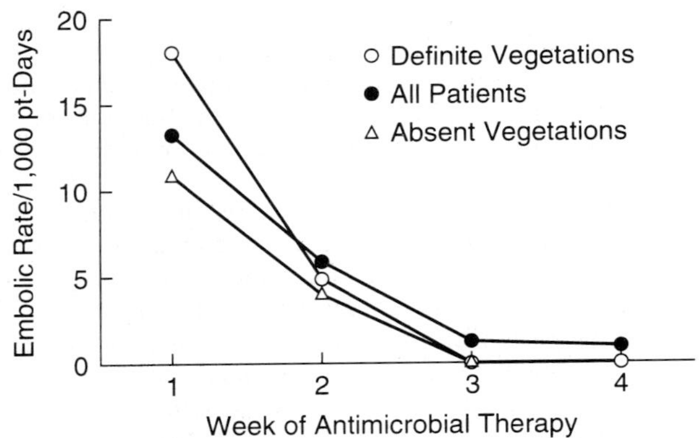

FIGURE 18–6 Incidence of embolic events in patients (pt) with infective endocarditis. (From Steckelberg JM, Murphy JG, Ballard D, et al: Emboli in infective endocarditis: the prognostic value of echocardiography. Ann Intern Med 114:635, 1991.)

recommendation that elective cardiac valve replacement be considered in patients with vegetations detected by echocardiography on the presumption that the presence of vegetations is predictive of future embolic events.

We reported the incidence of first embolic event after the onset of effective antimicrobial therapy in more than 200 patients with left-sided native valve IE.[32] Vegetations were detected by echocardiography in 38 percent of patients and were absent in 40 percent. In the remaining patients, vegetation status was indeterminate. We observed no statistically significant difference in the incidence rate of embolic events among patients with definite valve vegetations compared with those with absent or indeterminate vegetation. Moreover, no increased rate of embolization was noted with increasing vegetation size from 3 to 30 mm in diameter, nor was there a statistically significant difference in the rate of emboli among patients with vegetations greater than 10 mm in diameter compared with those with smaller vegetations. There was no significant effect of vegetation size on the rate of embolization in subsets of patients with aortic or mitral valve involvement except in patients with streptococcal IE who had a higher rate of embolization. The incidence rate of emboli decreased over time during antimicrobial therapy ($P < .001$). The incidence of embolic events among all patients fell from 13 per 1000 patient days during week 1 of antimicrobial therapy to fewer than 1.2 per 1000 patient days after week 2 of therapy (Fig. 18–6).

TABLE 18–12 Dental Procedures and Endocarditis Prophylaxis

*Endocarditis Prophylaxis Recommended**

Dental extractions
Periodontal procedures including surgery, scaling and root planing, probing, and recall maintenance
Dental implant placement and reimplantation of avulsed teeth
Endodontic (root canal) instrumentation or surgery only beyond the apex
Subgingival placement of antibiotic fibers or strips
Initial placement of orthodontic bands but not brackets
Intraligamentary local anesthetic injections
Prophylactic cleaning of teeth or implants where bleeding is anticipated

Endocarditis Prophylaxis Not Recommended

Restorative dentistry† (operative and prosthodontic) with or without retraction cord‡
Local anesthetic injections (nonintraligamentary)
Intracanal endodontic treatment; postplacement and buildup
Placement of rubber dams
Postoperative suture removal
Placement of removable prosthodontic or orthodontic appliances
Taking of oral impressions
Fluoride treatments
Taking of oral radiographs
Orthodontic appliance adjustment
Shedding of primary teeth

*Prophylaxis is recommended for patients with high- and moderate-risk cardiac conditions.
†This includes restoration of decayed teeth (filling cavities) and replacement of missing teeth.
‡Clinical judgment may indicate antibiotic use in selected circumstances that may create significant bleeding.
From Dajani AS, Taubert KA, Wilson WR, et al: Prevention of bacterial endocarditis: recommendations of the American Heart Association. JAMA 277:1794, 1977.

TABLE 18–13 Other Procedures and Endocarditis Prophylaxis

Endocarditis Prophylaxis Recommended

Respiratory tract
- Tonsillectomy and/or adenoidectomy
- Surgical operations that involve respiratory mucosa
- Bronchoscopy with a rigid bronchoscope

Gastrointestinal tract*
- Sclerotherapy for esophageal varices
- Esophageal stricture dilatation
- Endoscopic retrograde cholangiography with biliary obstruction
- Biliary tract surgery
- Surgical operations that involve intestinal mucosa

Genitourinary tract
- Prostatic surgery
- Cystoscopy
- Urethral dilation

Endocarditis Prophylaxis Not Recommended

Respiratory tract
- Endotracheal intubation
- Bronchoscopy with a flexible bronchoscope, with or without biopsy†
- Tympanostomy tube insertion

Gastrointestinal tract
- Transesophageal echocardiography†
- Endoscopy with or without gastrointestinal biopsy†

Genitourinary tract
- Vaginal hysterectomy†
- Vaginal delivery†
- Cesarean section
- In uninfected tissue
  - Urethral catheterization
  - Uterine dilatation and curettage
  - Therapeutic abortion
  - Sterilization procedures
  - Insertion or removal of intrauterine devices
- Other
  - Cardiac catheterization, including balloon angioplasty
  - Implanted cardiac pacemakers, implanted defibrillators, and coronary stents
  - Incision or biopsy of surgically scrubbed skin
  - Circumcision

*Prophylaxis is recommended for high-risk patients; it is optional for medium-risk patients.
†Prophylaxis is optional for high-risk patients.
From Dajani AS, Taubert KA, Wilson WR, et al: Prevention of bacterial endocarditis: recommendations of the American Heart Association. JAMA 277:1794, 1977.

Many studies, including ours cited earlier,[32] have attempted to identify patients with IE who are at high risk of emboli who might benefit from surgical intervention to avoid embolization. Mitral valve vegetations reportedly are more likely to result in peripheral embolization (25 percent) than in aortic valve vegetations (10 percent). The highest rate of embolization (37 percent) was observed when the vegetations were located on the anterior leaflet rather than the posterior leaflet of the mitral valve.[62, 63] This higher rate may be related to the mechanical effects of the abrupt excursion of the anterior mitral valve during the cardiac cycle which subject vegetations located on the anterior leaflet to fragmentation and embolization. The risk of emboli is greater when associated with an increase in vegetation size demonstrable by TEE during 4 to 8 weeks of antimicrobial therapy. The risk of emboli in these patients was twice that of patients in whom vegetations remained unchanged or decreased in size during therapy.

The American Heart Association published guidelines suggesting the potential need for surgical intervention in patients with valvular vegetations demonstrable by echocardiography (see Table 18–11).[15] Antimicrobial therapy reduces the risk of embolization during the first 2 weeks of therapy. Accordingly, benefit from surgery to prevent embolic events is highest early in the course of antimicrobial therapy. In selected patients, surgical intervention may prevent a primary or recurrent serious embolic event. The decision for surgical intervention to prevent embolization should be individualized in each patient. Surgery should be considered when large vegetations are detected on the mitral valve, especially the anterior leaflet, and in patients whose vegetation increases in size after 4 weeks of antimicrobial therapy or in patients who have one or more embolic events during the first 2 weeks of antimicrobial therapy or two or more embolic events during or after antimicrobial therapy.

Mycotic Aneurysm

Mycotic aneurysm is a rare complication of IE. During a 16-year period at the Mayo Clinic, we were able to identify only 32 patients with mycotic aneurysm among 628 patients with IE (5 percent).[12] Intercranial mycotic aneurysms are associated with higher morbidity and mortality rates than mycotic aneurysms located elsewhere. Patients with intracranial mycotic aneurysms may be asymptomatic, and the diagnosis is usually made after a sudden massive, often fatal subarachnoid or intracerebral hemorrhage. Our experience suggests, however, that the diagnosis of intracranial mycotic aneurysm can be made early before massive hemorrhage occurs. A severe unremitting localized headache or a homonymous hemianopsia is a finding that is highly suggestive of intracranial mycotic aneurysm. Contrast-enhanced computed tomography scanning may detect an intracerebral bleed in 90 to 95 percent of instances and may indirectly suggest the locations of a mycotic aneurysm.[15] Magnetic resonance angiography may be useful for the diagnosis of intracranial mycotic aneurysm, but its sensitivity for the detection of an aneurysm of less than 5 mm is less than that of cerebral angiography. Accordingly, cerebral angiography remains the diagnostic procedure of choice. Cerebral angiography should be performed in these patients.

Although many authorities believe that most intracranial mycotic aneurysms will rupture if untreated, Bingham[64] reported that the outcome of patients with intracranial mycotic aneurysm is similar in those administered adequate antimicrobial therapy compared with those treated with both antibiotics and surgical excision of the aneurysm.

Some patients with mycotic aneurysm require both cardiac valve replacement surgery and ligation of an intracranial mycotic aneurysm. The more life-threatening problem dictates the surgical procedure to be performed first. The use of a bioprosthetic cardiac valve that does not require the administration of anticoagulant therapy may be preferable to mechanical valve prosthesis in these patients.

Most, if not all, intrathoracic and intra-abdominal mycotic aneurysms will rupture if not excised. Peripheral mycotic aneurysms are most accessible to early diagnosis and are associated with the best prognosis. The risk of rupture of an untreated peripheral mycotic aneurysm is high, and prompt surgical intervention is imperative. Most

TABLE 18–14 Prophylactic Regimens for Dental, Oral, Respiratory Tract, or Esophageal Procedures

Situation	Agent	Regimen
Standard general prophylaxis	Amoxicillin	Adults: 2.0 g; children: 50 mg/kg PO 1 h before procedure
Unable to take oral medications	Ampicillin	Adults: 2.0 g IM or IV; children: 50 mg/kg IM or IV within 30 min before procedure
Allergic to penicillin	Clindamycin or	Adults: 600 mg; children: 20 mg/kg PO 1 h before procedure
	Cephalexin† or cefadroxil† or	Adults: 2.0 g; children: 50 mg/kg PO 1 h before procedure
	Azithromycin or clarithromycin	Adults: 500 mg; children: 15 mg/kg PO 1 h before procedure
Allergic to penicillin and unable to take oral medications	Clindamycin or	Adults: 600 mg; children: 20 mg/kg IV within 30 min before procedure
	Cefazolin†	Adults: 1.0 g; children: 25 mg/kg IM or IV within 30 min before procedure

*Total children's dose should not exceed adult dose.
†Cephalosporins should not be used in individuals with immediate-type hypersensitivity reaction (urticaria, angioedema, or anaphylaxis) to penicillins.
From Dajani AS, Taubert KA, Wilson WR, et al: Prevention of bacterial endocarditis: recommendations of the American Heart Association. JAMA 277:1794, 1977.

TABLE 18-15 **Prophylactic Regimens for Genitourinary/Gastrointestinal (Excluding Esophageal) Procedures**

Situation	Agents*	Regimen†
High-risk patients	Ampicillin plus gentamicin	Adults: ampicillin 2.0 g IM or IV plus gentamicin 1.5 mg/kg (not to exceed 120 mg) within 30 min of starting procedure: 6 h later, ampicillin 1 g IM/IV or amoxicillin 1 g PO Children: ampicillin 50 mg/kg IM or IV (not to exceed 2.0 g) plus gentamicin 1.5 mg/kg within 30 min of starting the procedure; 6 h later, ampicillin 25 mg/kg IM/IV or amoxicillin 25 mg/kg orally
High-risk patients allergic to ampicillin/amoxicillin	Vancomycin plus gentamicin	Adults: vancomycin 1.0 g IV over 1–2 h plus gentamicin 1.5 mg/kg IV/IM (not to exceed 120 mg): complete injection/infusion within 30 min of starting procedure Children: vancomycin 20 mg/kg IV over 1–2 h plus gentamicin 1.5 mg/kg IV/IM; complete injection/infusion within 30 min of starting procedure
Moderate-risk patients	Amoxicillin or ampicillin	Adults: amoxicillin 2.0 g PO 1 h before procedure, or ampicillin 2.0 g IM/IV within 30 min of starting procedure
Moderate-risk patients allergic to ampicillin/amoxicillin	Vancomycin	Adults: vancomycin 1.0 g IV over 1–2 h; complete infusion within 30 min of starting procedure Children: vancomycin 20 mg/kg IV over 1–2; complete infusion within 30 min of starting procedure

*Total children's dose should not exceed adult dose.
†No second dose of vancomycin or gentamicin is recommended.
From Dajani AS, Taubert KA, Wilson WR, et al: Prevention of bacterial endocarditis: recommendations of the American Heart Association. JAMA 277:1794, 1977.

authorities believe that the treatment of choice for patients with peripheral mycotic aneurysm is ligation and excision and that it is preferable to sacrifice the limb, if necessary, rather than the life of the patient.

Splenic Abscess

Splenic infarction is a common complication of left-sided IE (approximately 40 percent of cases); however, only about 5 percent of patients with splenic infarction develop splenic abscess.[15] Viridans streptococci or *S. aureus* is the most common cause of splenic abscess. Patients with persistent left upper quadrant pain and those with persistent or recurrent bacteremia or fever despite appropriate antimicrobial therapy should be suspected of having splenic abscess. Abdominal computed tomography or magnetic resonance imaging is the most sensitive test for the diagnosis of splenic abscess. Differentiation of splenic abscess from infarction may be difficult with these imaging tests. Persistent sepsis, positive blood cultures, or enlargement of the splenic defect on computed tomography or magnetic resonance imaging suggests an abscess rather than an infarction. Percutaneous drainage of splenic abscess has been performed successfully[15] and, in experienced hands, has replaced splenectomy as the treatment of choice. In patients with splenic abscess who require cardiac valve replacement surgery, splenectomy should be performed before valve replacement surgery because of the risk of bacteremia and infection of the valve prosthesis.

Metastatic Infection

Patients with metastatic infection are at risk for relapse of IE, which most often occurs in patients with staphylococcal endocarditis. Imaging techniques such as computed tomography, magnetic resonance imaging, and radioisotope scanning may be helpful in localizing occult metastatic foci of infection. The persistence of fever, localized pain or tenderness, persistently abnormal liver function tests, and breakthrough bacteremia suggest the diagnosis of metastatic abscess.

Central Nervous System Abnormalities

Central nervous system abnormalities have been reported to occur in 9 to 80 percent of patients with IE; these include headache, confusion, stroke, meningoencephalitis, brain abscess, and mycotic aneurysm.[12, 13] The management of patients with mycotic aneurysms or embolic events was discussed earlier. Most patients with central nervous system abnormalities show improvement with supportive care and appropriate antimicrobial therapy. Patients with a large solitary brain abscess may require stereotactic or open surgical drainage, but most patients with small abscesses do not require neurosurgical intervention. In patients with brain abscess, the duration of antimicrobial therapy should often be extended beyond that usually required for the treatment of uncomplicated IE.

PREVENTION OF ENDOCARDITIS

The American Heart Association published recommendations for prophylaxis of IE for patients with cardiac valve abnormalities, congenital heart disease, intercardiac prostheses, or other cardiac abnormalities (Tables 18–12 to 18–15).[65] It is important for clinicians to be aware of the indications for prophylaxis and the recommendations for the use of specific antimicrobial prophylactic regimens. Patients should be provided with the card that is published and distributed through the American Heart Association.

References

1. Steckelberg JM, Melton LJ III, Ilstrup DM, et al: Influence of referral bias on the apparent clinical spectrum of infective endocarditis. Am J Med 88:582, 1990.
2. Von Reyn CR, Levy BS, Arbeit RD, et al: Infective endocarditis: an analysis based on strict case definitions. Ann Intern Med 94:505, 1981.
3. Garvey GJ, Neu HC: Infective endocarditis—an evolving disease. Medicine 57:105, 1978.
4. Come PC: Infective endocarditis: current perspectives. Compr Ther 8:57, 1982.
5. Scheld WM, Sande MA: Endocarditis and intravascular infections. *In* Mandell GL, Douglas RG Jr, Bennett JE (eds): Principles and Practice of Infectious Diseases. 3rd ed. p. 670. New York: John Wiley & Sons, 1990.
6. Pelletier LL Jr, Petersdorf RG: Infective endocarditis: a review of 125 cases from the University of Washington Hospitals, 1963–1972. Medicine 56:287, 1977.
7. Kaye D: Definitions and demographic characteristics. *In* Kaye D (ed): Infective Endocarditis. p. 1. Baltimore: University Park Press, 1976.
8. Angrist AA, Oka M, Nakao K, et al: Experimental endocarditis. *In* Kaye D (ed): Infective Endocarditis. p. 11. Baltimore: University Park Press, 1976.
9. Gould K, Ramirez-Ronda CH, Holmes RK, et al: Adherence of bacteria to heart valves in vitro. J Clin Invest 56:1364, 1976.
10. Scheld WM, Valone JA, Sande MA: Bacterial adherence in the pathogenesis of endocarditis: interaction of bacterial dextran, platelets, and fibrin. J Clin Invest 61:1394, 1978.
11. Clawson CC, Rao GHR, White JG: Platelet interaction with bacteria. IV. Stimulation of the release reaction. Am J Pathol 81:411, 1975.
12. Wilson WR, Lie JT, Houser OW, et al: The management of patients with mycotic aneurysm. Curr Clin Top Infect Dis 2:151, 1981.
13. Jones HR Jr, Siekert RG, Geraci JE: Neurologic manifestations of bacterial endocarditis. Ann Intern Med 71:21, 1969.
14. Durack DT, Lukes AS, Bright DK, et al: New criteria for diagnosis of infective endocarditis: utilization of specific echocardiographic findings. Am J Med 96:200, 1994.
15. Bayer AS, Bolger AF, Taubert KA, et al: Diagnosis and management of infective endocarditis and its complications. Circulation 98:2936, 1998.
16. Fowler VG Jr, Li J, Corey GR, et al: Role of echocardiography in evaluation of patients with *Staphylococcus aureus* bacteremia: experience in 103 patients. J Am Coll Cardiol 30:1072–1078, 1997.
17. Wilson WR, Karchmer AW, Dijani AS, et al: Antibiotic treatment of adults with infective endocarditis due to streptococci, enterococci, staphylococci, and HACEK microorganisms. JAMA 274:1706, 1995.
18. Wilson WR, Wilkowske CJ, Wright AJ, et al: Treatment of streptomycin-susceptible and streptomycin-resistant enterococcal endocarditis. Ann Intern Med 100:816, 1984.
19. Francioli P, Etienne J, Hoigne R, et al: Treatment of streptococcal endocarditis with a single daily dose of ceftriaxone sodium for 4 weeks: efficacy and outpatient treatment feasibility. JAMA 267:264, 1992.
20. Sande MA, Courtney KB: Nafcillin-gentamicin synergism in experimental staphylococcal endocarditis. J Lab Clin Med 88:118, 1976.
21. Steigbigel RT, Greenman RL, Remington JS: Antibiotic combinations in the treatment of experimental *Staphylococcus aureus* infection. J Infect Dis 131:245, 1975.
22. Korzeniowski O, Sande MA, and the National Collaborative Endocarditis Study Group: Combination antimicrobial therapy for *Staphylococcus aureus* endocarditis in patients addicted to parenteral drugs and in nonaddicts: a prospective study. Ann Intern Med 97:496, 1982.
23. Chambers HF, Miller RT, Newman MD: Right-sided *Staphylococcus aureus* endocarditis in intravenous drug abusers: two-week combination therapy. Ann Intern Med 109:619, 1988.
24. Dismukes WE, Karchmer AW, Buckley MJ, et al: Prosthetic valve endocarditis: analysis of 38 cases. Circulation 48:365, 1973.
25. Wilson WR, Danielson GK, Giuliani ER, et al: Prosthetic valve endocarditis. Mayo Clin Proc 57:75, 1982.
26. Geraci JE, Wilson WR: Endocarditis due to gram-negative bacteria: report of 56 cases. Mayo Clin Proc 57:145, 1982.
27. Mills J, Utley J, Abbott J: Heart failure in infective endocarditis: predisposing factors, course, and treatment. Chest 66:151, 1974.
28. Griffin FM Jr, Jones G, Cobbs CG: Aortic insufficiency in bacterial endocarditis. Ann Intern Med 76:23, 1972.
29. Neville WE, Magno M, Foxworthy DT, Moffat JE: Emergency aortic valve replacement in bacterial endocarditis. J Thorac Cardiovasc Surg 61:916, 1971.
30. Wilson WR, Giuliani ER, Danielson GK, Geraci JE: Management of complications of infective endocarditis. Mayo Clin Proc 57:152, 1982.
31. Wilson WR, Danielson GK, Giuliani ER, et al: Cardiac valve replacement in congestive heart failure due to infective endocarditis. Mayo Clin Proc 54:223, 1979.
32. Steckelberg JM, Murphy JG, Ballard D, et al: Emboli in infective endocarditis: the prognostic value of echocardiography. Ann Intern Med 114:635, 1991.
33. Mugge A, Daniel WG, Frank G, Lichtlen PR: Echocardiography in infective endocarditis: reassessment of prognostic implications of vegetation size determined by the transthoracic and the transesophageal approach. J Am Coll Cardiol 14:631, 1989.
34. Erbel R, Rohmann S, Drexler M, et al: Improved diagnostic value of echocardiography in patients with infective endocarditis by transesophageal approach: a prospective study. Eur Heart J 1:43, 1988.
35. Martin RP: The diagnostic and prognostic role of cardiovascular ultrasound in endocarditis: bigger is not better. J Am Coll Cardiol 15:1234, 1990.
36. Bardy G, Talano JV, Reisberg B, Lesch M: Sensitivity and specificity of echocardiography in a high-risk population of patients for infective endocarditis: significance of vegetation size. J Cardiovasc Ultrasonogr 2:23, 1983.
37. Strom J, Frishman WH, Klein N, et al: Effect of vegetation size on the outcome of patients with infective endocarditis. Circulation 66(suppl II):II-103, 1979.
38. Lutas EM, Roberts RB, Devereux RB, Prieto LM: Relation between the presence of echocardiographic vegetations and the complication rate in infective endocarditis. Am Heart J 112:107, 1986.
39. Wann LS, Dillon JC, Weyman AE, Feigenbaum H: Echocardiography in bacterial endocarditis. N Engl J Med 295:P135, 1976.
40. Pratt C, Whitcomb C, Neumann BS, et al: Relationship of vegetations on echo to the clinical course and systemic emboli in bacterial endocarditis. Am J Cardiol 41:384, 1978.
41. Wong D, Chandraratna PAN, Wishnow RM, et al: Clinical implications of large vegetations in infective endocarditis. Arch Intern Med 143:1874, 1983.
42. Egeblad H, Wennevold A, Bernning J, Lauridsen P: Mitral valve replacement in infective endocarditis as prophylaxis against embolism. Identification of patients at risk by 2-dimensional echocardiography. Eur J Cardiol 10:369, 1979.
43. O'Brien JT, Geiser EA: Infective endocarditis and echocardiography. Am Heart J 108:386, 1984.
44. Jaffe WM, Morgan DE, Pearlman AS, Otto CM: Infective endocarditis. 1983–1988: echocardiographic findings and factors influencing morbidity and mortality. J Am Coll Cardiol 15:1227, 1990.
45. Roy P, Tajik AJ, Giuliani ER, et al: Spectrum of echocardiographic findings in bacterial endocarditis. Circulation 53:474, 1976.
46. Mintz GS, Kotler MN, Segal BL, Parry WR: Survival of patients with aortic valve endocarditis: the prognostic implications of the echocardiogram. Arch Intern Med 139:862, 1979.
47. Wilson LC, Wilcox BR, Sugg WL, Peters RM: Valvular regurgitation in acute infective endocarditis: early replacement. Arch Surg 101:756, 1970.
48. Manhas DR, Mohri H, Hessel EA II, Merendino KA: Experience with surgical management of primary infective endocarditis: a collected review of 139 patients. Am Heart J 84:738, 1972.
49. Wilson WR, Danielson GK, Giuliani ER, et al: Valve replacement in patients with active infective endocarditis. Circulation 58:585, 1978.
50. Daniel WG, Mugge A, Martin RP, et al: Improvement in the diagnosis of abscesses associated with endocarditis by transesophageal echocardiography. N Engl J Med 324:795, 1991.
51. Weinstein L, Schlesinger JJ: Pathoanatomic, pathophysiologic and clinical correlations in endocarditis. N Engl J Med 291:832, 1974.
52. Geraci JE, Wilkowske CJ, Wilson WR, Washington JA II: *Haemophilus* endocarditis: report of 14 patients. Mayo Clin Proc 52:209, 1977.
53. Merchant RK, Louria DB, Geisler PH, et al: Fungal endocarditis: review of the literature and report of three cases. Ann Intern Med 48:242, 1958.
54. Strom J, Becker R, Davis R, et al: Echocardiographic and surgical

correlations in bacterial endocarditis. Circulation 62(suppl I):I-164, 1980.
55. Stulz P, Pfisterer M, Jenzer HR, et al: Emergency valve replacement for active infective endocarditis. J Cardiovasc Surg (Torino) 30:20, 1989.
56. Come PC, Isaacs RE, Riley MF: Diagnostic accuracy of M-mode echocardiography in active infective endocarditis and prognostic implications of ultrasound detectable vegetations. Am Heart J 103:839, 1982.
57. Young JB, Wilton D, Quinones MA, et al: Prognostic significance of valvular vegetations identified by M-mode cardiography in infective endocarditis. Circulation 58(suppl II):II-41, 1978.
58. Martin RP, Meltzer RS, Chia BL, et al: Clinical utility of two dimensional echocardiography in infective endocarditis. Am J Cardiol 46:379, 1980.
59. Manolis AS, Meltia H: Echocardiographic and clinical correlates in drug addicts with infective endocarditis: implications of vegetation size. Arch Intern Med 148:2461, 1988.
60. Sheikh MV, Covarrubias EA, Ali N, et al: M-mode echocardiographic observations during and after healing of active bacterial endocarditis limited to the mitral valve. Am Heart J 101:37, 1981.
61. Buda AJ, Zotz RJ, Lemire MS, Bach DS: Prognostic significance of vegetations detected by two-dimensional echocardiography in infective endocarditis. Am Heart J 112:1291, 1986.
62. Rohmann S, Erbel R, Darius H, et al: Prediction of rapid versus prolonged healing of infective endocarditis by monitoring vegetation size. J Am Soc Echocardiogr 4:465–474, 1991.
63. Rohmann S, Erbel R, Gorge G, et al: Clinical relevance of vegetation localisation by transoesophageal echocardiography in infective endocarditis. Eur Heart J 13:446–452, 1992.
64. Bingham WF: Treatment of mycotic intracranial aneurysms. J Neurosurg 46:428, 1977.
65. Dajani AS, Taubert KA, Wilson WR, et al: Prevention of bacterial endocarditis: recommendations of the American Heart Association. JAMA 277:1794, 1997.

CHAPTER 19

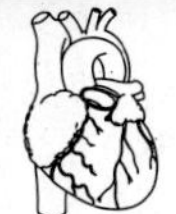

Cardiac Catheterization

Yang Wang and Gladwin Das

ADVANCES IN RADIOGRAPHIC CONTRAST MEDIA
MITRAL VALVE DISEASE
Mitral Stenosis
Mitral Regurgitation
Mixed Mitral Stenosis and Regurgitation
AORTIC VALVE DISEASE
Aortic Stenosis
Aortic Regurgitation
Mixed Aortic Stenosis and Regurgitation
PULMONARY VALVE DISEASE
TRICUSPID VALVE DISEASE
VALVE PROSTHESES
THERAPEUTIC CARDIAC CATHETERIZATION FOR VALVULAR HEART DISEASE
MITRAL VALVULOPLASTY
BALLOON AORTIC VALVULOPLASTY
PULMONARY VALVULOPLASTY

The basic radiograph in the diagnosis of valvular heart disease is the posteroanterior (PA) and lateral chest film; a simultaneous barium swallow is often helpful. The barium highlights the indentation of the esophagus by a large left atrium, and an enlarged left ventricle extends posterior to the esophagus. Right ventricular (RV) enlargement is best seen in the lateral view and poststenotic dilatation of the aorta is seen in both PA and lateral views.

Cardiac catheterization and echocardiography are the tools for quantifying the degree of stenosis or regurgitation of a given heart valve. Modern sophisticated techniques for hemodynamic and angiographic studies of the heart originated in a brash self-experiment by Forssmann[1] in 1929, when he catheterized his own right atrium from an arm vein. No further human studies were performed until 1941, when Cournand and colleagues[2] laid the foundations for hemodynamic studies of the heart. In 1946, Dexter and colleagues[3] showed that the pulmonary artery wedge pressure was a close approximation of the left atrial (LA) pressure.[4] This was followed by left-sided heart catheterizations,[5, 6] the simplification of arterial access by Seldinger in 1953 and transseptal catheterization of the left side of the heart by Ross,[7] modified by Brockenbrough and Braunwald in 1960. Sones and Shirey[8] performed coronary angiography in 1959 and the flow-directed right heart balloon-tipped catheter was developed in 1970.[9] Rapid advances in radiographic equipment with improved image intensification, a 35-mm cine camera, and the capability to image from any angle desired have paralleled these technical developments.

Advances in Radiographic Contrast Media

All standard contrast media are iodinated derivations of benzoic acid, but they vary in viscosity, osmolality, and ion concentration.[9–11] Anionic contrast media have been developed that are reported to be less arrhythmogenic and nephrotoxic.[12] An undoubted virtue is the mitigation of severe discomfort when a large bolus must be injected during a ventriculogram or a peripheral arteriogram. We now use only anionic contrast media in our practice. There has been a substantial reduction in costs.

The technical expertise of the laboratory should allow entry into all heart chambers and major blood vessels for the purposes of hemodynamic measurements and angiographic studies. These should include the retrograde crossing of a tightly stenotic aortic valve, transseptal puncture for access into the left atrium and left ventricle and direct left ventricular (LV) puncture. The most common access sites are the femoral artery and vein, using the Seldinger technique to introduce an appropriately sized thin-walled sheath into each vessel, through which catheters can be introduced and exchanged. Technical considerations may sometimes necessitate the use of the brachial artery approach (which is less satisfactory because of limitations of catheter size) in circumstances such as peripheral vascular disease (stenoses or extreme tortuosity), occlusion of the abdominal aorta, and morbid obesity. In general, the left brachial artery is preferred because most preformed coronary artery catheters are easier to manipulate into the desired vessels from this side.

Hemodynamic evaluations of heart valves demand simultaneous measurement of pressures on both sides of the valve and measurement of the cardiac output. The "pullback" technique can be used but is less satisfactory, especially where access is difficult, such as in aortic valve stenosis. Cardiac output can be determined by any of the standard techniques, including the Fick principle, the thermodilution technique, and the cardio green dye indicator–dilution method, but each technique has limitations. Valve regurgitation is best assessed angiographically.

Mitral Valve Disease

Mitral Stenosis

Acquired mitral stenosis is almost always of rheumatic origin.[13–15] The carcinoid syndrome[16] may cause mitral ste-

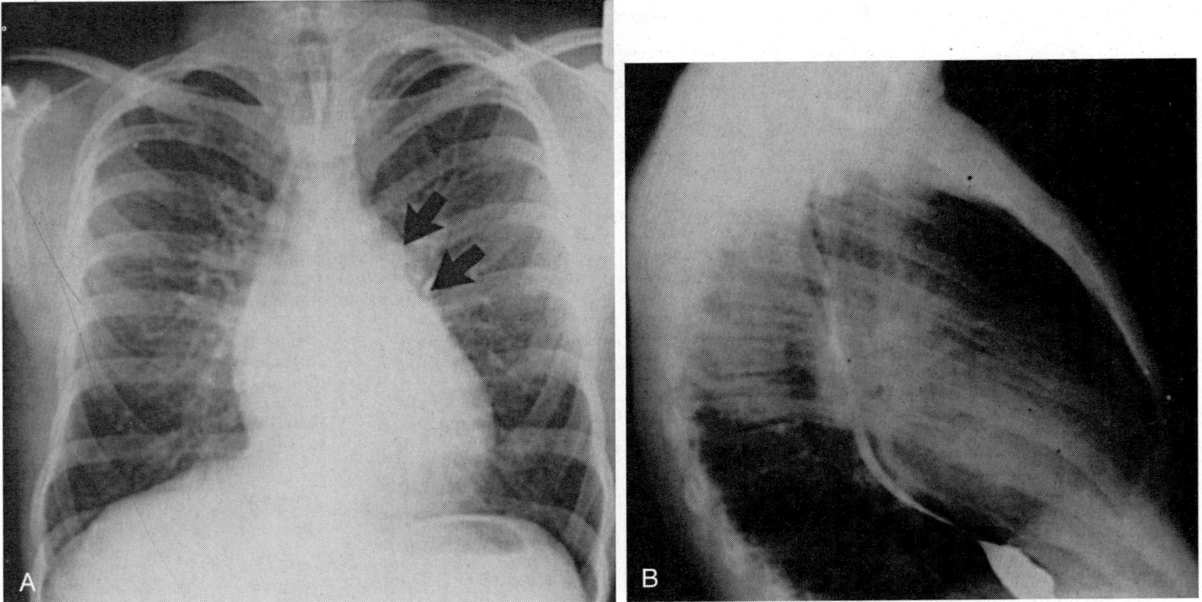

FIGURE 19–1 A and **B,** A 33-year-old man with mitral stenosis. Note the straight left heart border formed by the main pulmonary artery enlarged by pulmonary hypertension, and the enlarged left atrial appendage *(arrows).* The overall heart size is not enlarged. On the lateral view, the barium swallow shows a characteristic indentation caused by an enlarged left atrium.

nosis if an atrial septal defect is present, and rarely, stenosis may be caused by rheumatoid arthritis.[17] The characteristic PA chest film in clinically significant mitral stenosis shows the heart size to be either normal or enlarged, the latter caused by enlargement of the two atria and the right ventricle (Fig. 19–1). The left heart border shows a "straightening" caused by an enlarged main pulmonary artery (Fig. 19–2) and the prominent left atrial appendage (Fig. 19–3A). There may be pulmonary vascular congestion and even Kerley B lines. The latter are horizontal lines at the lung bases, which are present with marked pulmonary venous congestion. On the lateral view, especially with a barium swallow, there is a characteristic smooth indentation of the esophagus posteriorly by the enlarged left atrium, which is the only posterior heart structure directly adjacent to the esophagus (see Fig. 19–1).[18–20]

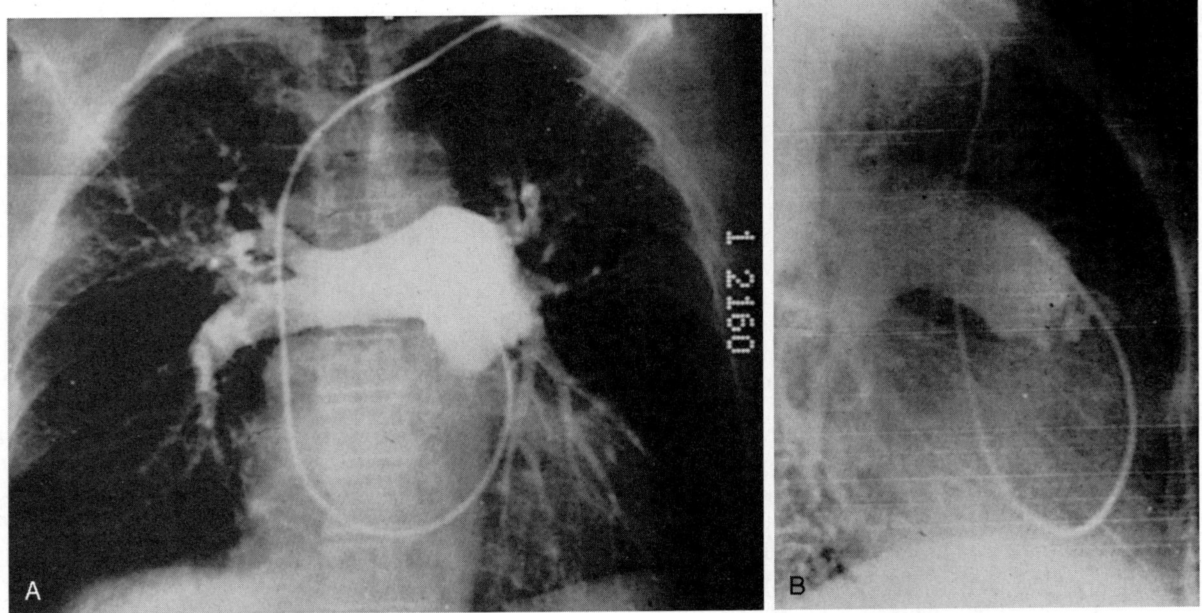

FIGURE 19–2 A and **B,** Pulmonary angiogram in a patient with mitral stenosis. Note the enlargement of the pulmonary arteries associated with pulmonary hypertension.

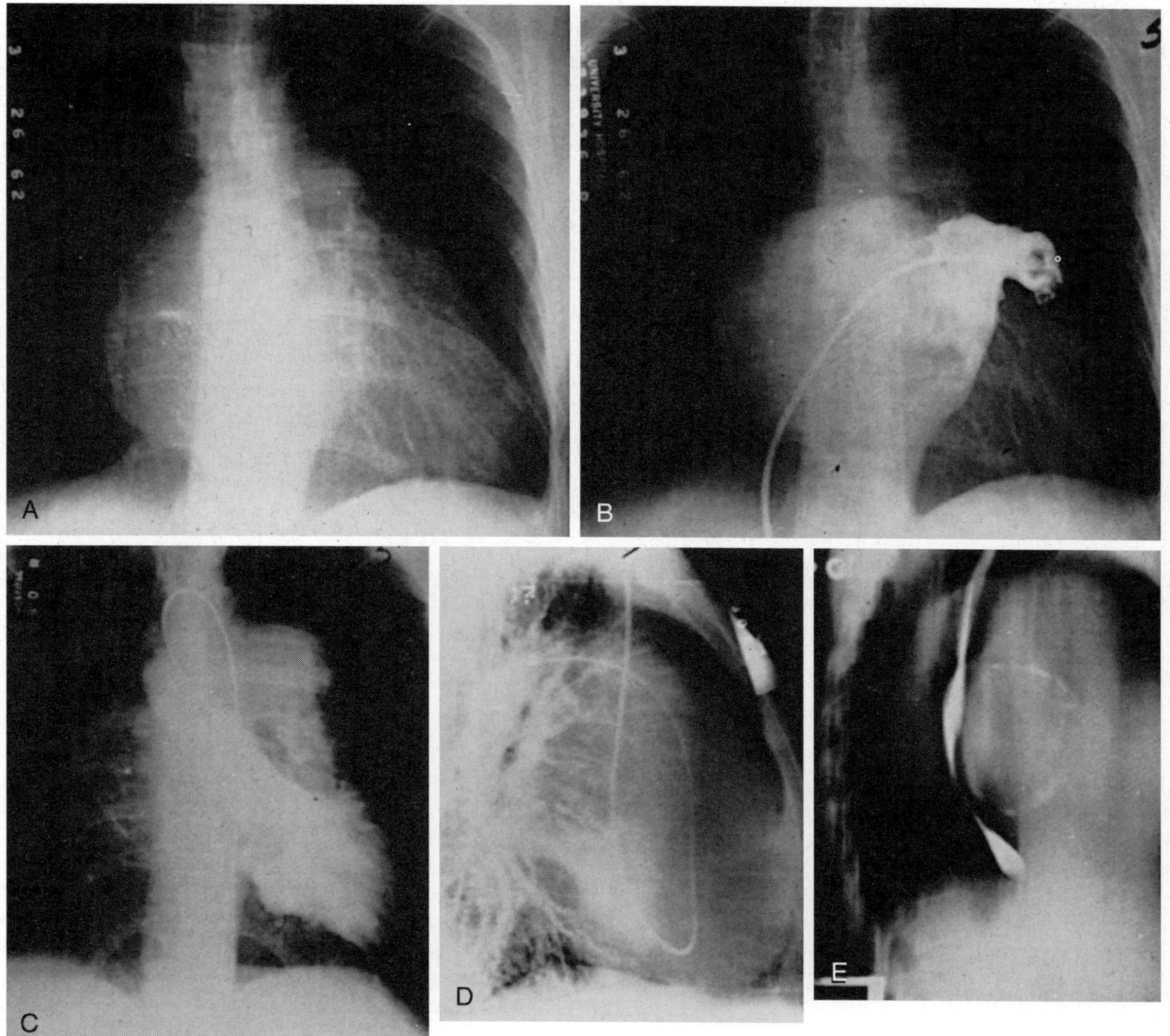

FIGURE 19–3 A, Prominent left atrial appendage on the radiograph. **B,** Left atriogram by transseptal technique shows a markedly enlarged left atrium and the prominent left atrial appendage. **C,** Normal-sized left ventricle. **D,** Opacified left ventricle markedly displaced posteriorly by an enlarged right ventricle (the angiographic catheter was withdrawn quickly before the end of the ventriculogram because of ventricular irritability). **E,** Calcification of the left atrial wall.

A heavily calcified mitral valve is now seldom seen in industrialized countries, but it is still seen in patients from Third World countries, in whom mitral stenosis may be symptomatic for decades before treatment is sought. There may be calcification in the left atrial (LA) wall as a result of calcification of a long-standing laminated clot (Fig. 19–3E).

The key measurements are simultaneous pressures in the left atrium (or the pulmonary artery wedge pressure) together with the simultaneous cardiac output, and a long pressure tracing to determine the diastolic filling period (Fig. 19–4). This is especially the case if the patient is in atrial fibrillation with widely varying diastolic filling periods. The pulmonary artery wedge pressure closely approximates the LA pressure,[3, 4, 6, 21] but this requires that great care be taken to ensure that the pulmonary artery wedge pressure is indeed a true wedge pressure: there should be a significant abrupt change in pressure compared with the pulmonary artery, and the pressure contour should be of venous configuration with a large A wave if the patient is in sinus rhythm, but with atrial fibrillation, it may be fairly nondescript.[21, 22] Ideally, a blood sample drawn from the wedge position should be fully saturated; some desaturation does not necessarily indicate that the catheter is not wedged, because alveolar ventilation at rest is not uniform. As an added precaution when the balloon-tipped flow-directed catheter is used, it may be wise to advance the deflated tip as far as it can go into the distal pulmonary artery and then gently inflate until the wedge pressure appears. Sometimes, advancing distally yields the characteristic pattern without inflation. If there is uncertainty about the validity of the wedge pressure after these precautions are observed and wedging occurs at several sites, direct measurement of LA pressure may be necessary.[21, 23] This technique is described further.[7] The pulmonary artery wedge pressure contour shows a prominent A wave of atrial systole and a leisurely *y* descent resulting from delayed emptying of the left atrium with mitral obstruction. With atrial fibrillation, there will be no A wave (see Fig.

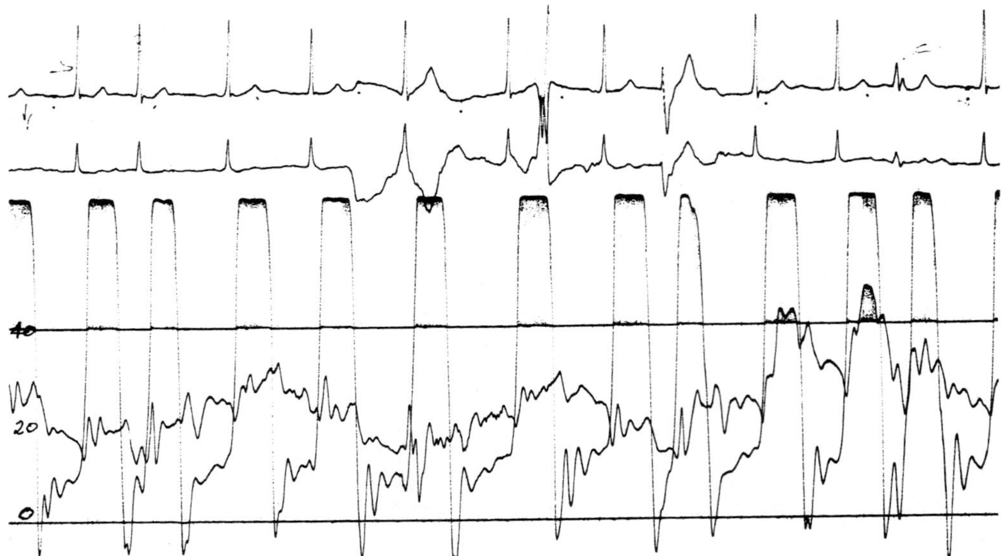

FIGURE 19–4 Simultaneous pressure recordings in the pulmonary artery wedge and in the left ventricle in a patient with mitral stenosis. There is atrial fibrillation and therefore no A wave. The features of the pulmonary artery wedge tracing are fairly nondescript, without a prominent CV wave to suggest the possibility of mitral regurgitation. As the tracing proceeds, the catheter is no longer in a wedge position and "snaps" into the pulmonary artery proper. The mean pressure in the left atrium is 24 mm Hg, and the end-diastolic pressure in the left ventricle is 12 mm Hg. Both the mean diastolic gradient and the end-diastolic pressure gradient are increased.

19–4). The A wave in the left ventricle is either absent or markedly attenuated in mitral stenosis.

Gorlin's original formulation for calculating valve areas[23–26] was derived from two hydraulic equations. In the first (Bernoulli):

$$Q = A \cdot V \cdot K_1$$

where Q is flow, A is valve area, V is velocity, and K_1 is an empirical constant. In the second (Torricelli):

$$V^2 = K_2 \sqrt{2}\, gh$$

where g is the acceleration factor, h is the fall in pressure, and K_2 is an empirical constant for the mitral valve, there is a correction factor of 0.85; thus:

$$MVA = \frac{Q_d}{37.7 \sqrt{\Delta p}}$$

where Qd is the cardiac output/diastolic filling period in s/min and p is the mean diastolic gradient corresponding to "h."

The validity of this calculation depends on the identity of pulmonary artery wedge pressure and LA pressure.[6, 7, 22, 26–29] If there is reasonable doubt, the direct LA pressure should be used, and the constant is 39.9.[29] Here, Q_d is the flow across the mitral valve per minute of diastole. The diastolic filling period is measured from the simultaneous wedge and LV diastolic tracings, but in practice, it can be taken from an ascending aortic tracing. This diastolic filling period is multiplied by the heart rate and is divided into the cardiac output to give the cardiac output per minute or second of diastole. p is the mean diastolic gradient measured as the difference in pressure between the LA (pulmonary wedge) pressure and the LV pressure over time and is best measured planimetrically. The normal cross-sectional area of the mitral valve is greater than 4 cm.^{2} Between 1.5 and 2 cm^2 is considered to reflect mild mitral stenosis and less than 1 cm^2 is considered to reflect critical mitral stenosis. The relationship of mean diastolic gradient to diastolic flow in mitral stenosis is an exponential rather than a linear one (Fig. 19–5). It is evident that the pressure gradient across the valve is a function of heart rate as well as of flow because diastole is proportionately shortened more than systole during tachycardia (Fig. 19–6) and increases the pressure gradient. Therefore, both exercise and uncontrolled tachycardia, such as atrial fibrillation, raise the diastolic gradient; the more severe the stenosis, the

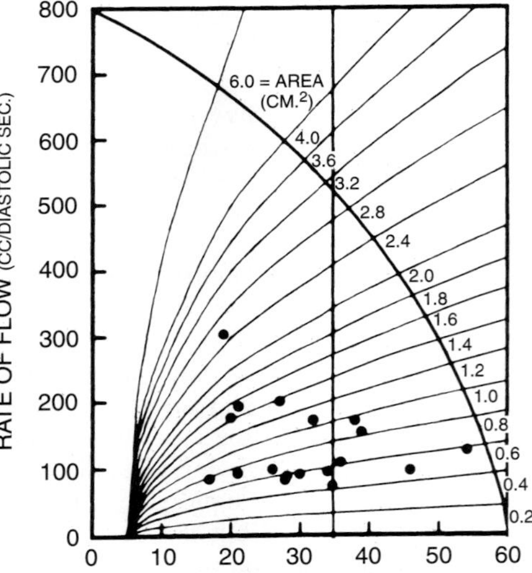

FIGURE 19–5 Diagramatic representation of the Gorlin formula relates pulmonary artery wedge pressure and diastolic flow to mitral valve area.

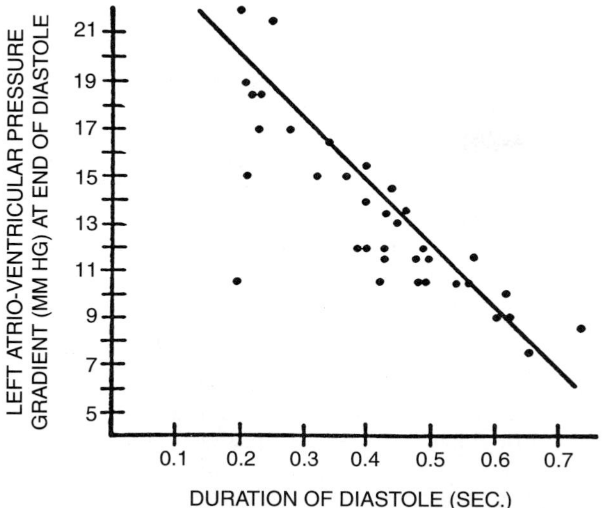

FIGURE 19–6 Relationship between mean diastolic gradient and the pressure gradient across the stenotic mitral valve and the duration of diastole.

greater the rise. Pulmonary vascular congestion occurs with rises in the LA pressure. Because the oncotic pressure of plasma is 30 to 35 mm Hg, as LA mean pressures approach these levels, the pulmonary vascular congestion is increased, and pulmonary edema eventually occurs.[3]

An increase in cardiac output, given a constant mitral valve area, causes an increase in the pressure gradient. In advanced mitral stenosis, cardiac output rises with exertion to a relatively limited degree, but the rise in heart rate in the presence of either sinus rhythm or atrial fibrillation raises the LA pressure and causes dyspnea (see Fig. 19–6). A subgroup of patients with only moderate mitral stenosis is capable of normal increases in cardiac output with exercise. This significantly elevates the LA pressure, despite moderate mitral stenosis. These patients should not be denied treatment simply because their valve stenoses have not reached a "critical" value.

The calculated mitral valve area is subject to many possible errors (Table 19–1).[21, 30] Pulmonary artery wedge pressure is used for LA pressure, the "constant" may be variable,[23–25] and significant mitral regurgitation may coexist. Cardiac output measurements also have a margin of error. Therefore, the calculated valve areas obtained from the Gorlin formula should be used by the cardiologist together with all ancillary clinical and laboratory data in arriving at a judgment of the degree to which valve stenosis is responsible for the patient's clinical disability.

TABLE 19–1 Hemodynamic Data of a Subject at Rest and During Exercise Demonstrating the Difficulty of Measuring Mitral Valve Stenosis*

Measurement	Rest	Exercise
PAWP	15	35
PA pressure	35/15	62/30
Brachial artery pressure	105/58	110/60
Mitral valve end-diastolic gradient	15	—
Cardiac output	5.7	7.0
Oxygen consumption (cm²/min)	263	564
Systemic resistance	1120	940
PAR	98	114

Abbreviations: PA, pulmonary artery; PAR, pulmonary arterial resistance.

* Subject is a 27-year-old man whose resting measurements are misleadingly near normal. With moderate exercise, his cardiac output rises (as does his heart rate). His pulmonary artery wedge pressure (PAWP) doubles. This illustrates the importance of planning cardiac catheterization around the clinical picture.

Pulmonary hypertension in mitral stenosis may result from passive rise caused by an elevated pulmonary artery wedge pressure, by pulmonary arteriolar vasoconstriction, and sometimes by tissue changes associated with long-standing pulmonary hypertension.[31] The pulmonary vascular resistance is estimated by the formula

$$PVR = \frac{\overline{PAP} - \overline{PAW}}{Q_p}$$

where $\overline{PAP}$ is the mean pulmonary artery pressure; $\overline{PAW}$ is the pulmonary artery wedge pressure, and Qp is pulmonary flow.

The simple ratio is known as a *Wood unit,* which is dimensionless. A dimensional value is obtained by multiplying this value by 80 to yield dyne·sec·cm^{-5}. The formula is a recasting of the Poiseuille equation and is not strictly applicable to pulsatile flow. In significant mitral stenosis, there is pulmonary hypertension, and the pulmonary vascular resistance is elevated. It decreases and may even normalize with corrective valve surgery.[32, 33]

The decreased cardiac output response in mitral stenosis is in part a function of the increased pulmonary vascular resistance and, in long-standing cases, due to RV dysfunction, associated tricuspid regurgitation.

Each method of measuring cardiac output has limitations. In the thermodilution method,[34–37] a bolus of saline is injected into the right atrium and is sensed by a thermistor in the pulmonary artery. The results may be invalid in the presence of severe tricuspid regurgitation and/or RV dilatation and dysfunction. Indicator dilution curves[38, 39] obtained by injecting into the pulmonary artery and sampling in the ascending aorta may be invalid in the presence of a huge left atrium and low flow. Under these circumstances, one may need to resort to the Fick principle,[40, 41] which has its own inherent problems.[42, 43] A longer period of steady state is needed to allow the time to collect the expired air, and respirations must be regular and uniform (the most extreme example in which the Fick principle cannot be applied is Cheyne-Stokes respiration). However, the Fick principle has the virtue of being usable in severe RV or LV failure, severe valve regurgitation, and intracardiac shunts. It is usually difficult and unwise to enter the left ventricle retrograde across a mechanical aortic valve prosthesis because the catheter itself markedly alters the hemodynamics. Often it is impossible to cross a tightly stenotic aortic valve. Here, the transseptal technique is useful (see Fig. 19–3A). The technique has been described in extenso elsewhere.[7, 44] Briefly, a venous catheter with a preshaped distal curve and tapered tip is introduced over a guide wire via the right femoral vein to the superior vena cava. With an aortic prothesis or aortic valve calcification, the level of the aortic valve is readily identified. Otherwise, a pigtail catheter should be advanced into the aortic cusps to mark the level of the valve. A Brockenbrough needle with a curved tip and an arrow at its hilt to indicate the direction of the curve at the tip is advanced through the catheter to within 1 cm of the catheter tip. The entire assembly is gently pulled down until the tip of the catheter is in the upper right atrium. At this juncture, it is important to make sure that the tip of the catheter is pointing posteromedially to avoid the aorta. We prefer to turn the entire assembly counterclockwise until the tip just points medially, thus ensuring that it is posterior. Clockwise rotation may be associated with a catching of the tip, resulting in a possible torque so that the tip may be still be anterior. The lumen of the needle is then connected to pressure, and the assembly is slowly drawn down until the tip "gives." If this is at the level of the aortic valve, this usually represents the upper limbus of the fossa ovalis. The needle is then extended through the catheter so that approximately 1 cm of the needle is exposed. The patient is then instructed to report any chest or throat pain. The operator then gently pushes the needle posteromedially until it gives easily, the sensation being somewhat similar to that of a successful lumbar puncture. If the patient has pain in the chest or throat, the needle is not in the fossa but rather in the muscular part of the septum and must be repositioned. When the needle enters the left atrium, a pressure change is obvious. The chamber can further be confirmed by a blood sample, which should be fully saturated. The catheter then can be smoothly extended over the needle into the left atrium and the needle withdrawn (see Fig. 19–3). The tip can then be maneuvered into the left ventricle. I prefer to maneuver a J-tipped 35 guide wire with graduated stiffness (floppy wire) into the left ventricle and then to pass the catheter over the wire.

In terms of technical considerations, there are at least three contraindications to transseptal puncture: left atrial myxoma (which is commonly attached to the atrial septum at the rim of the fossa ovalis), cystic medial disease with massive dilatation of the aorta, and significant thrombi in the left atrium, especially in the presence of long-standing atrial fibrillation. Significant thrombi can be excluded with reasonable confidence by transesophageal echocardiography. The transseptal technique is also useful in that it is the route used for balloon dilatation of mitral stenosis. When it is performed correctly, complications should be very infrequent. Perforation of the atrial free wall may occur and may lead to tamponade, although in patients with previous open-heart surgery, this is not as much of a concern. If the needle is pointing anteriorly, the aorta may be entered. If the needle is too low, one may mistake the coronary sinus for the fossa ovalis, but this is largely obviated by noting the level of the aortic valve. Because of the possibility of perforation of the atrial free wall, the patient should not be heparinized until after completion of the transseptal puncture and when there have not been several unsuccessful passes. Transseptal puncture is sometimes performed with echocardiography, which has much to commend it. However, experience and meticulous care and attention to contraindications are essential to a low complication rate. The patient should be periodically questioned about possible pericardial pain for up to half an hour after transseptal puncture. RA and intra-arterial pressure should be monitored, and a pericardiocentesis set should be available. Echocardiographic assessment for pericardial fluid should be performed immediately if there is any doubt.

Left ventriculography should be performed in the right and left anterior oblique views. Pure or predominant mitral stenosis should show little or no mitral regurgitation (see Fig. 19–3B). An enlarged right ventricle displaces the left ventricle posteriorly (Fig. 19–3D). The left ventricle is usually of normal size. Sometimes, mitral stenosis is associated with LV dysfunction in the absence of mitral regurgitation or aortic valve disease.[45–47] Therefore, the left ventricle must be evaluated for dilatation, ejection fraction, and regional wall motion abnormalities. Although the angiography may yield important information concerning the pliability of the valve and the subvalvar mitral apparatus, these are better evaluated by echocardiography.

Left atriography can be accomplished via the transseptal catheter. Because this is an end-hole catheter, the use of a tip occluder, consisting of a wire with a beaded tip, adds a margin of safety. Alternatively, injection of a large amount of contrast material into the pulmonary artery may enable good visualization of the left atrium during the levophase. LA angiography has been largely superseded by echocardiography for assessment of valve mobility and the presence of thrombi.

Mitral Regurgitation

Acquired mitral regurgitation may be due to chronic rheumatic heart disease,[48] dilated mitral annulus due to dilatation of the left ventricle,[49] ruptured chordae tendineae,[50] or ischemic heart disease,[50–54] among other causes. The chest film in mitral regurgitation is dependent on the acuteness, severity, and duration of mitral insufficiency. In relatively mild mitral insufficiency, the chest x-ray is usually unremarkable. With significant mitral insufficiency of some duration, the left atrium is usually markedly enlarged and in extreme cases may be almost as large as the rest of the heart itself. This is evidenced by a large atrial appendage, the elevation of the left mainstem bronchus, the "double density" through the cardiac shadow, and the right heart border formed by the left atrium rather than the right atrium (Fig. 19–7). With time, volume overload of the left ventricle causes LV dilatation, which can be seen as leftward extension of the cardiac apex and, on the lateral view, posterior extension of a large LV shadow. If the film is taken with a barium swallow, there will be LA indentation of the enlarged left atrium, but the left ventricle extends posterior to the esophagus without displacing it.[52, 53] Depending on the LA pressure, there may or may not be pulmonary congestion. In chronic severe mitral insufficiency with an enlarged dysfunctional left ventricle, elevation of the LV filling pressure, and therefore the LA pressure, manifests itself by pulmonary venous congestion and even Kerley B lines, as in mitral stenosis.[52] Acute mitral insufficiency, such as by papillary muscular rupture secondary to an acute myocardial infarction,[54] spontaneous chordal rupture,[50, 54–56] or infective endocarditis, is associated with prominent pulmonary vasculature and may even be associated with pulmonary edema, with a rather unremarkable cardiac contour.

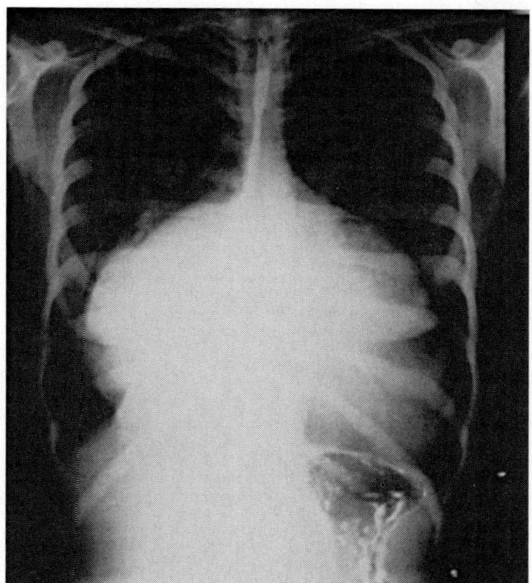

FIGURE 19–7 A markedly enlarged left atrium in the presence of severe mitral insufficiency. In the posteroanterior view, both the right heart border and the upper left heart border are formed by the left atrium.

Evaluation of mitral insufficiency by cardiac catheterization involves both hemodynamic measurements and angiography. As discussed earlier, the right-sided heart catheter should be advanced to the pulmonary artery wedge position and the arterial catheter into the left ventricle. The wedge tracing classically shows a steep rise in a CV wave, with a rapid *y* descent as the unobstructed valve opens (Fig. 19–8). In pure mitral insufficiency, there should be little or no end-diastolic gradient across the mitral valve. The magnitude of the CV wave is dependent on both the magnitude of regurgitant flow and the compliance of the left atrium.[57] CV waves are therefore impressively tall in acute mitral regurgitation, where there is large regurgitant volume and a relatively noncompliant left atrium. In chronic mitral regurgitation, a large CV wave may or may not be present because progressive dilatation of the left atrium may be associated with markedly increased compliance, so that even a large regurgitant volume may not elicit characteristic pressure contour changes in the left atrium. Quantification of regurgitation flow is not entirely satisfactory. Left ventriculography, using the right and left anterior oblique views, is commonly used to assess the magnitude of regurgitant flow. A commonly used grading is from I to IV, I being trivial-to-mild insufficiency and IV being massive regurgitation into the left atrium, where opacification of the left atrium lingers. Grades II and III are in between, II being mild to moderate and III being moderately severe (Fig. 19–9). The ejection fraction and size of the left ventricle can be measured by standard techniques. Hemodynamically, the volume regurgitation may be approximated; thus, the forward stroke volume is calculated from hemodynamic studies (i.e., cardiac output divided by heart rate); the volume ejected can be calculated as the difference

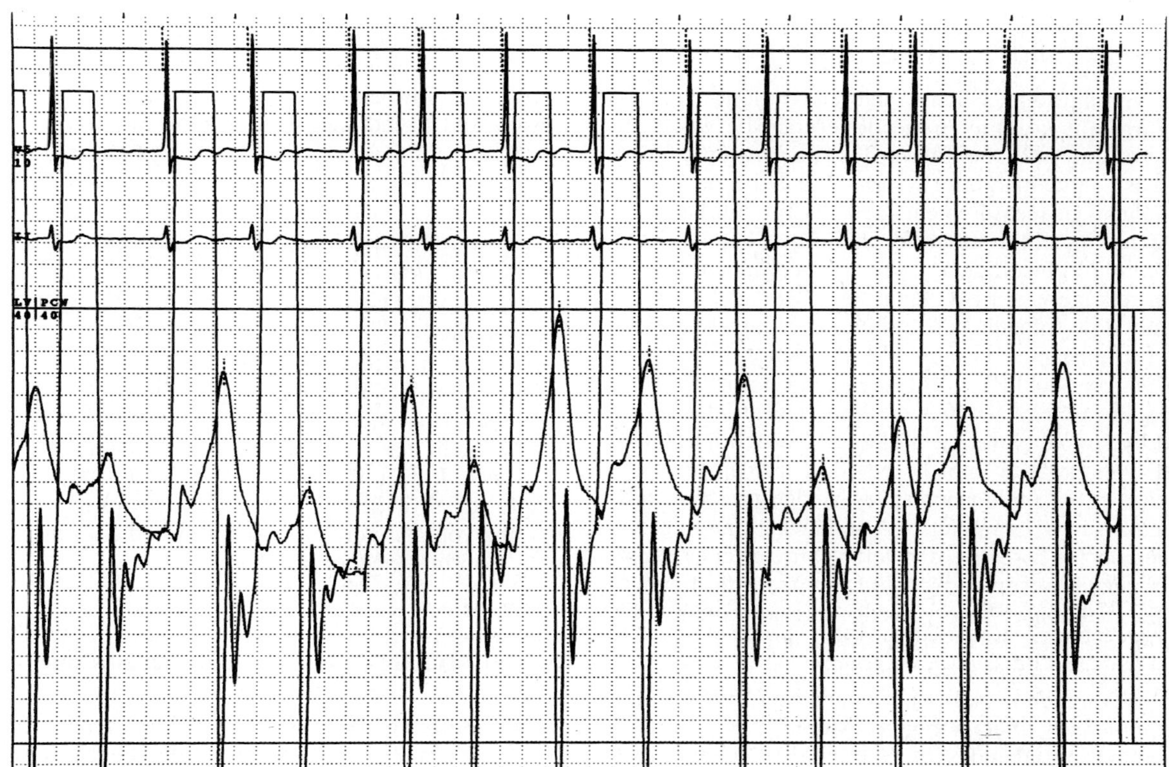

FIGURE 19–8 Simultaneous recording of pulmonary artery wedge pressure and left ventricular diastolic pressure in a patient with predominant mitral insufficiency. Note the large CV wave with slurring of the C wave into the V wave, with a rapid *y* descent. The peak of the CV wave is at the intersection of the wedge tracing and the fall in pressure of the left ventricle. There is a small end-diastolic gradient, indicating that this is mixed mitral disease with predominant mitral regurgitation.

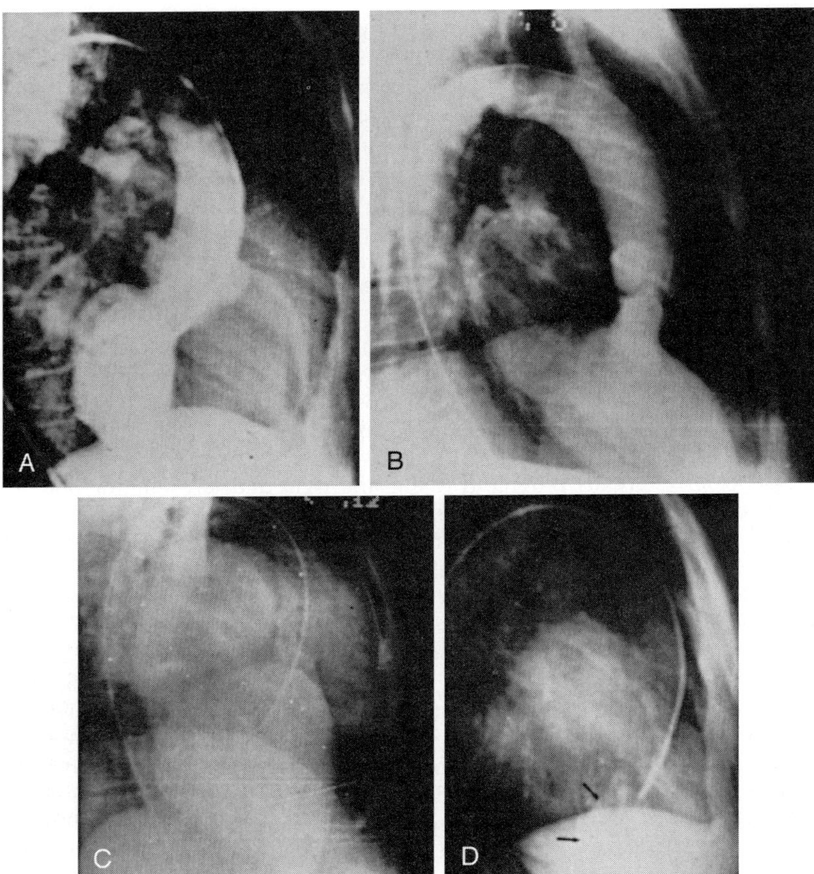

FIGURE 19–9 The four panels are illustrative of angiographic estimation of degrees of mitral regurgitation. All are left ventriculograms taken in the lateral view. **A,** A small puff of mitral regurgitation posteriorly. **B,** General outlining of the left atrium but with the predominant opacification being in the left ventricle. **C,** Equal opacification of the left atrium and the left ventricle. **D,** More opacification of the left atrium than of the left ventricle. These would be grades I, II, III, and IV, respectively.

between end-diastolic volume and end-systolic volume. The regurgitant volume is the difference between the ejected volume and the forward stroke volume. This method has a large margin of error and must be carried out with simultaneous measurements to be useful. Furthermore, it is probably invalid in atrial fibrillation.

In acute mitral insufficiency, the ventriculogram demonstrates a relatively normal ventricular size and massive regurgitant flow into the left atrium. In symptomatic patients, what appears to be normal LV function by ejection fraction at rest should be further assessed. Some idea of the compliance characteristics of the left ventricle can be obtained by simple elevation of the legs, which introduces a sudden volume load into the heart. A sudden and prolonged rise in the pulmonary artery wedge pressure indicates decreased LV compliance. A somewhat more quantitative method for assessing the left ventricle under stress can be obtained by supine bicycle exercise, with monitoring of the pulmonary artery wedge pressure with each increase in the level of exercise. Although this does not duplicate normal physiologic activities, it is helpful in evaluating LV function and in correlating dyspnea with the level of pulmonary artery wedge pressure.

A commonly used index of ventricular function is the ejection fraction. Although it is a relatively gross measure, it is useful for longitudinal comparisons. The ejection fraction of the left ventricle can be obtained from the 30-degree right anterior oblique plane by the area-length method of Dodge and coworkers.[58, 59] Measurement of volume at end-systole and at end-diastole yields the following:

$$\text{Ejection fraction} = \frac{\text{EDV} - \text{ESV}}{\text{EDV}} = \frac{\text{SV}}{\text{EDV}}$$

where EDV is end-diastolic volume, ESV is end-systolic volume, and SV is stroke volume. This normally should be 0.67 ± 0.80. Mitral regurgitation may be misleading, in that the marked LV systolic unloading into the left atrium may mask impaired ventricular systolic function. Therefore, ejection fraction values approaching 50 percent should be regarded as indicative of possible myocardial dysfunction, which may not be overt until the regurgitation is abolished. In fact, the end-systolic volume may be the most helpful of all indices of LV function, with increasing end-systolic volume indicating compromised LV function, even with a normal ejection fraction.[60]

Mixed Mitral Stenosis and Regurgitation

Mixed mitral stenosis and regurgitation occur when there is a significantly elevated diastolic gradient across the mitral valve as well as angiographically significant regurgitation of contrast into the left atrium. Here, the level of the left atrium (or pulmonary artery wedge) pressure, regurgitant volume, and LV function are collectively the determining factors for decisions regarding valve dilatation or replacement.

Aortic Valve Disease

Aortic Stenosis

Aortic stenosis in the adult is most commonly based on a congenital unicuspid or bicuspid aortic valve. The valve may not be truly stenotic in the young, but with age, degenerative changes and ultimately calcification render the valve increasingly stenotic.[61–63] This is by far the most common cause of aortic stenosis in the adult. The most common type of bicuspid aortic valve has two separate cusps, one of which is a conjoint cusp containing a raphe. Although there initially is no stenosis in the sense of a measurable pressure gradient across the valve, "poststenotic" dilatation is seen very early. This dilatation is eccentric, involving the anterolateral aspect of the ascending aorta, presumably as a result of the direction of the aortic flow jet through the eccentric orifice. The characteristic chest x-ray study in the patient with a congenital bicuspid valve shows anterolateral dilatation of the ascending aorta in both the PA and the lateral views (Fig. 19–10). Calcific aortic stenosis of the degenerative type is common in the elderly and is often related to atherosclerosis and hypercholesterolemia.[64] Because this form of aortic stenosis is acquired late in life, the configuration of the ascending aorta does not resemble that of the bicuspid valve (Fig. 19–11). Rheumatic aortic stenosis is rare in the absence of mitral valve involvement and has become uncommon in industrialized countries. Calcification of the aortic valve is common in long-standing aortic stenosis and is usually best seen in the lateral view of the chest film.

Cardiac catheterization in the patient with significant aortic valve disease is essential to evaluate the coronary status in patients who are middle aged or older. Cardiac catheterization should include both right- and left-sided heart catheterization, preferably with two arterial catheters for gradient measurement. The most important hemodynamic measurements are simultaneous pressures in the ascending aorta and the left ventricle and a simultaneous cardiac output (Fig. 19–12). Again, using the formula of Gorlin,[23, 24, 26]

$$\text{AVA (cm}^2\text{)} = \frac{\text{cardiac output/systolic filling period}}{44.3\sqrt{\Delta p}}$$

where AVA is aortic valve area and p is mean systolic gradient (Fig. 19–13). This should be obtained planimetrically. The peak-to-peak systolic pressure gradient is often used, and the resulting valve area agrees well with the planimetric method when the stenosis is significant. However, strictly speaking, there is no peak-to-peak gradient, because the peak pressures in the left ventricle and aorta are not simultaneous, occurring later in the aorta.[65]

In aortic stenosis, the assumption is that all flow across the valve occurs during systole; therefore, cardiac output is divided by the systolic ejection period times the heart rate to obtain systolic flow per minute. The cardiac output may be obtained by the Fick principle, thermodilution, or dye dilution techniques, simultaneously with measurement of the pressure gradient. Care must be taken in measurements of the pressure gradient. Damping underestimates the peak systolic pressure; conversely, if overshoots are not recognized, the peak pressure may be overestimated. Optimally, the aortic pressure should be measured in the ascending aorta because the systolic pressure in the femoral artery is frequently higher and peaks later than the pressure in the ascending aorta.[65, 66] Only if the pressures obtained from the ascending aorta and the femoral artery are identical should the femoral artery pressure be used. The signifi-

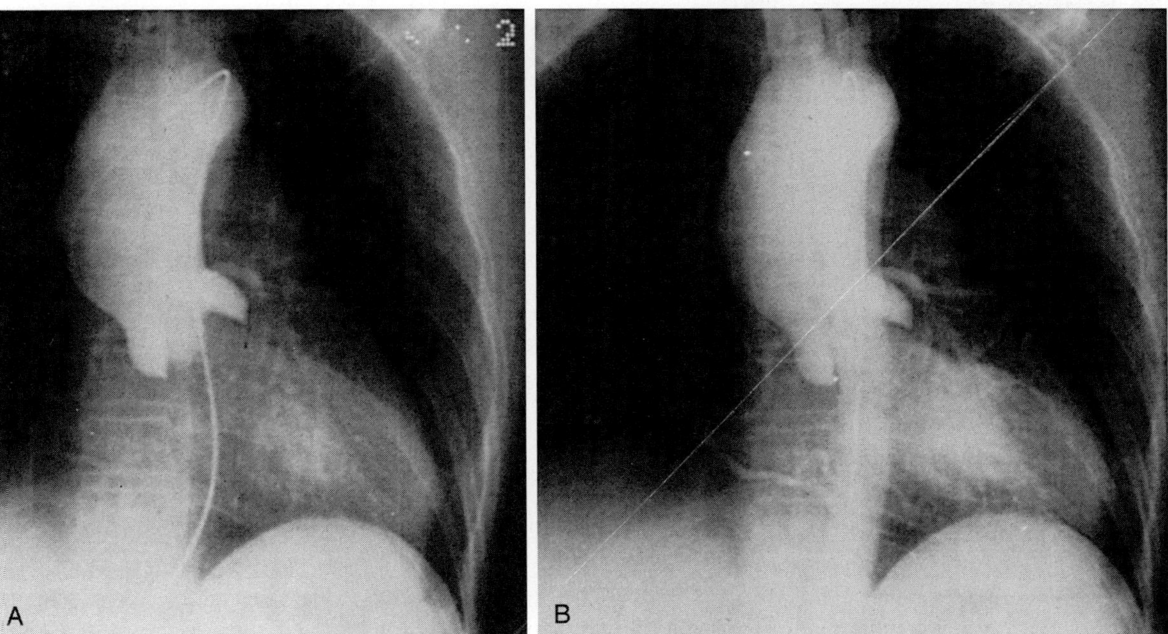

FIGURE 19–10 A and **B,** This aortogram in a patient with aortic stenosis on the basis of bicuspid valve shows the anterolateral dilatation of the ascending aorta, which is also recognizable in the posteroanterior chest film.

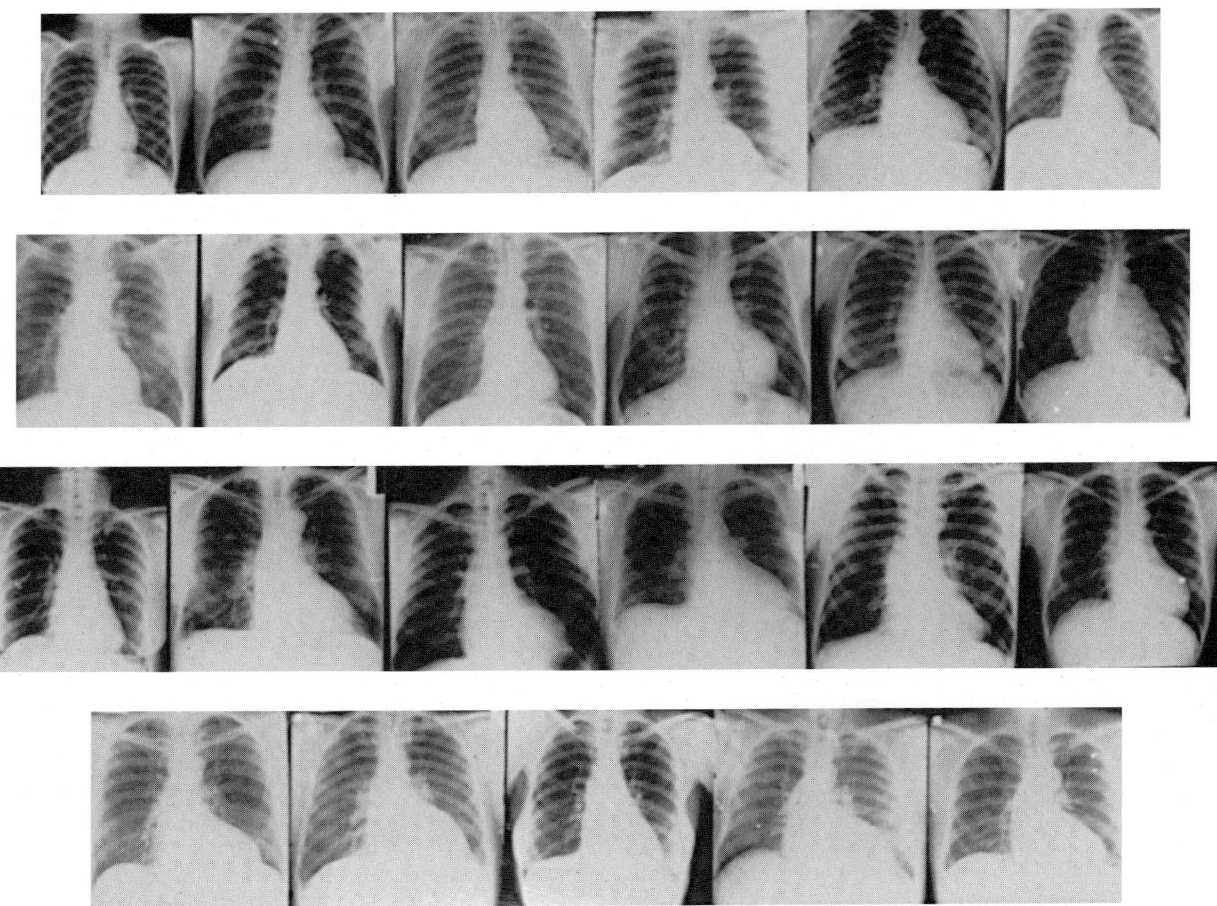

FIGURE 19–11 Posteroanterior chest films of 23 adult patients with predominant aortic stenosis. There is no consistent characteristic pattern, but in some, the anterolateral dilatation of the ascending aorta can be seen.

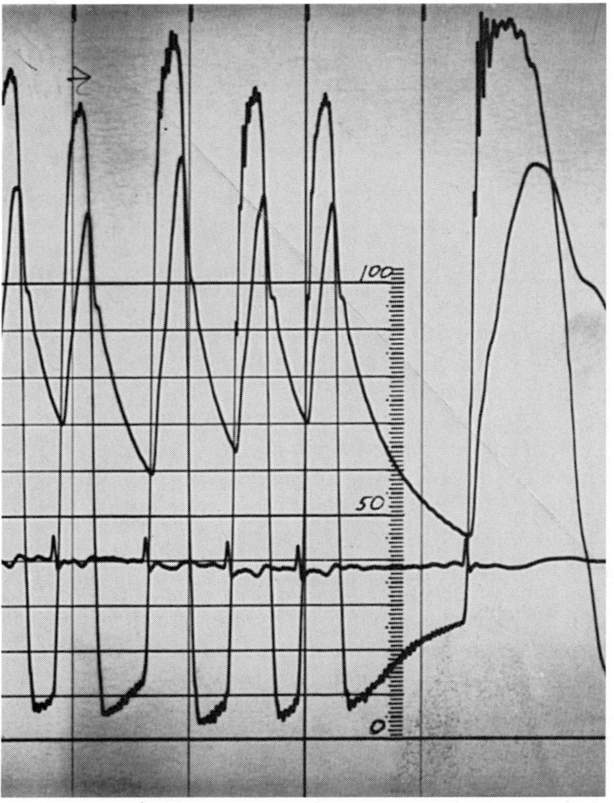

FIGURE 19–12 Simultaneous pressure tracings of the left ventricle and ascending aorta. The anacrotic notch in the ascending aortic tracing is about halfway up the upstroke. The upstroke is delayed and reaches its peak during early diastole. Therefore, the peak-to-peak pressure is not a true peak systolic gradient.

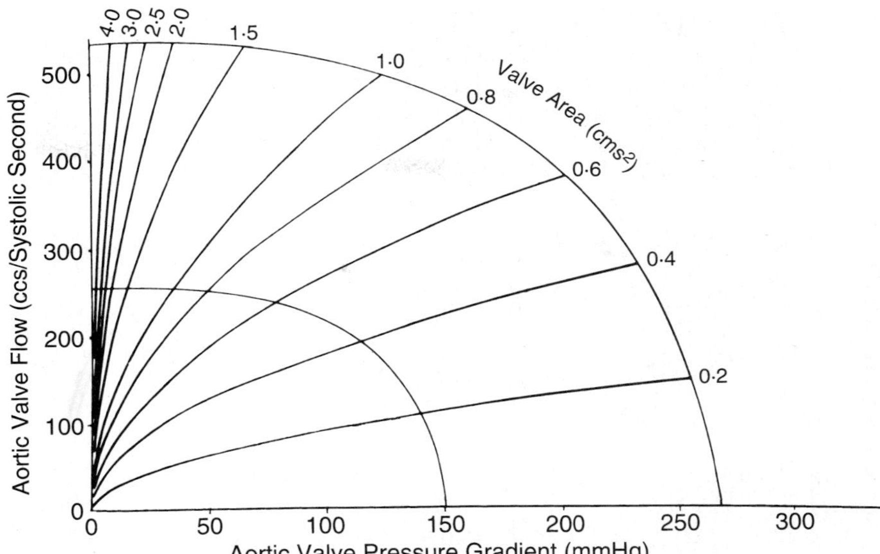

FIGURE 19–13 The relation between the aortic valve systolic gradient and the valve area is seen to be exponential.

cantly stenotic aortic valve is usually calcified and distorted.

Manipulation of the pigtail angiographic catheter through the stenotic valve into the left ventricle requires considerable skill. This is related in part to the small and distorted orifice and in part to the somewhat downward and leftward displacement of the valve itself by the poststenotic dilatation of the ascending aorta. A straight-tipped guide wire should be used to straighten out the pigtail curvature, and a systematic probing of the aortic valve is undertaken, making use of the curvature in the catheter itself to alter the angle of the probing wire. Should the pigtail catheter be unsuccessful in entering the LV, one is often successful with use of the Judkins right coronary catheter with a guidewire. Then, by use of an exchange wire, the Judkins catheter can be exchanged for a pigtail catheter. Once the catheter is successfully introduced into the left ventricle, it should not be withdrawn until all of the desired studies have been completed, including ventriculography to evaluate ventricular function and regional wall motion abnormalities. Therefore, a second arterial catheter is useful. I have made use of a thin-walled No. 5 radiopaque catheter introduced by the Seldinger technique just adjacent to the original entry site of the femoral arterial sheath. This enables simultaneous measurement of pressures in the ascending aorta and left ventricle and accurate measurement of the mean systolic gradient across the aortic valve. Rarely, it is impossible to cross the aortic valve retrogradely, and one must resort to transseptal puncture to gain access to the LV, as described earlier. The aortic pressure contour shows a characteristic delay and an anacrotic notch (see Fig. 19–12) in the upstroke.

It is uncommon for an aortic valve of more than 1 cm^2 to be the cause of cardiac symptoms on the basis of valve stenosis alone, although in conjunction with significant coronary artery disease, the high intraventricular pressure may be an important factor in causing ischemia and angina. Therefore, it is routine practice to perform coronary angiography in older patients with significant aortic stenosis. It is difficult to say precisely what aortic valve area is critical in the absence of coexisting pathology such as coronary artery disease. However, aortic valve areas less than 0.8 cm^2 are generally considered to represent severe valvular aortic stenosis. In the presence of good LV function, the resting systolic pressure gradient may exceed 100 mm Hg without symptoms at rest or with exercise. It has also been shown that with normal LV function, increases in cardiac output with exercise may be normal in severe aortic stenosis, owing to a disproportionately prolonged ejection period and, in part, perhaps to a "stretching" of the valve at higher systolic pressures (Fig. 19–14).[67] The pressure gradient across the valve is a function of heart rate and flow, and systolic gradient alone may therefore be misleading because a relatively modest systolic gradient may be associated with severe aortic stenosis in the presence of a low cardiac output and LV dysfunction. Again, the calculated valve area is to be used together with the clinical evaluation in judging its contribution to the degree of disability or symptoms.

Aortic Regurgitation

The chest film in aortic regurgitation depends on the degree of regurgitation, its duration, and its cause. Aortic regurgitation caused by a bicuspid aortic valve shows the characteristic anterolateral poststenotic dilatation of the ascending aorta as in aortic stenosis of a bicuspid valve (see Fig. 19–10). Aortic regurgitation caused by cystic medial disease, especially in Marfan's syndrome, shows balloon-like dilatation of the ascending aorta involving the entire aortic root. This may be more evident in the lateral (Fig. 19–15) view. Surprisingly, generalized dilatation of the ascending aorta may be missed on the chest film.

LV size is increased in moderate-to-severe regurgitation and with time may reach immense proportions with enlargement of the heart to the left on PA view and posteriorly on the lateral view in the absence of symptoms. Acute aortic regurgitation (in the absence of cystic medial disease), such as from trauma or from perforation in acute

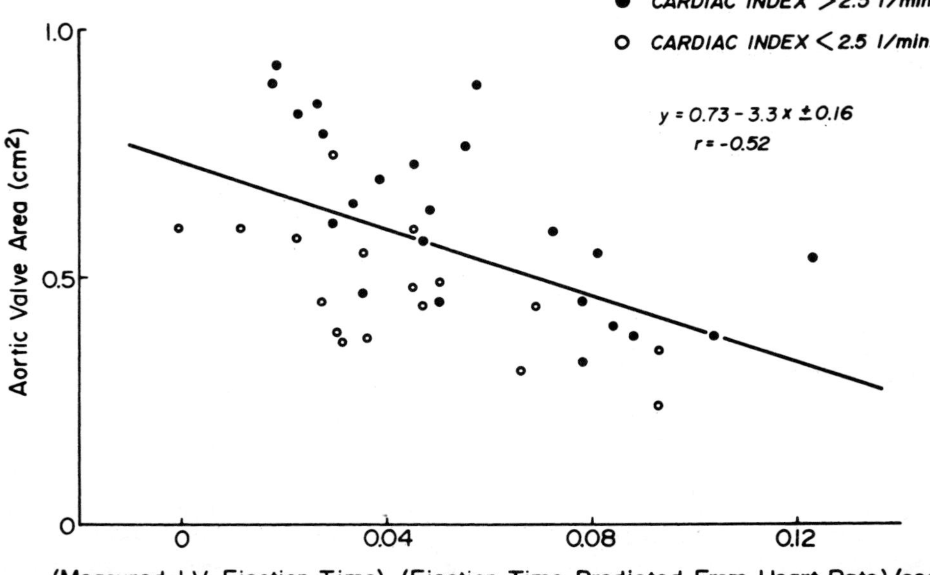

FIGURE 19–14 Prolongation of ejection time as a function of heart rate with critical aortic stenosis. This was true irrespective of adequate or decreased cardiac output. LV, left ventricular. (Modified from Bache RJ, Wang Y, Greenfield JC Jr: Left ventricular ejection time in valvular aortic stenosis. Circulation 47:527, 1973. By permission of the American Heart Association, Inc.)

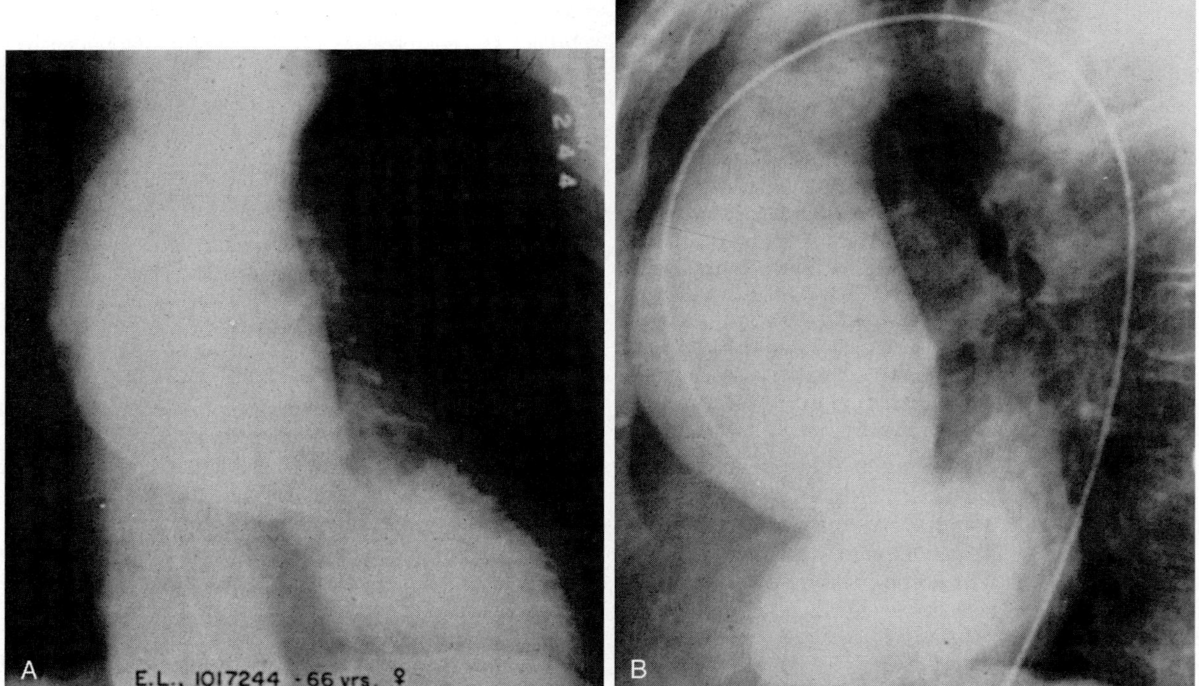

FIGURE 19–15 A and **B,** Angiogram in a patient with cystic medial disease of the aorta and severe aortic regurgitation. Note the balloon-shaped dilatation of the ascending aorta involving the aortic root, including the sinus of Valsalva.

infective endocarditis, shows pulmonary vascular congestion in the presence of a normal-sized heart. Right-sided heart catheterization is performed to measure the LA (wedge) pressure. Ascending aortography is used to obtain an estimate of the degree of regurgitation (Fig. 19–16). The morphology of the ascending aorta helps to distinguish aortic regurgitation caused by a tricuspid aortic valve from cystic medial disease. Injection of contrast into the aortic root and at the aortic arch is indicated in the evaluation for possible aortic dissection, to locate the origin of the dissection and the site of re-entry.

The arterial pulse contour in severe and pure aortic regurgitation shows a steep rise and fall that corresponds to the water-hammer pulse. Left ventriculography in the right anterior oblique plane measures LV volume, ejection fraction, and end-systolic volume. A less than normal ejection fraction and a large end-systolic volume are unfavorable.[68, 69]

Mixed Aortic Stenosis and Regurgitation

Calculation of valve area is not possible with more than mild aortic regurgitation. Judgment of the severity of the aortic valve disease must rely on the systolic gradient, regurgitant volume, and LV function.

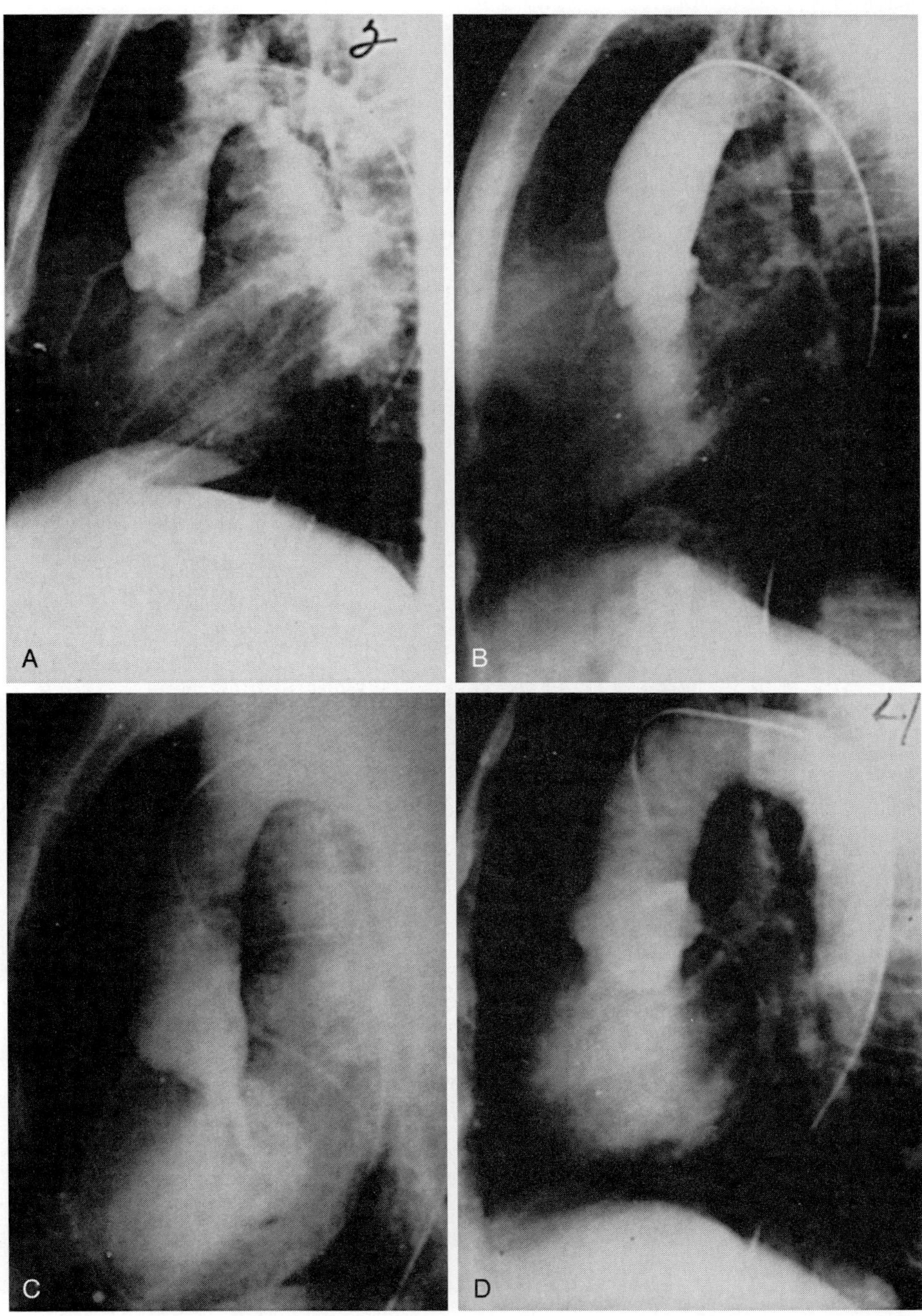

FIGURE 19–16 Estimation of degree of aortic insufficiency by ascending aortography. **A,** Mild aortic regurgitation. **B,** Mild-to-moderate regurgitation. **C,** Moderately severe regurgitation with a jet still evident. **D,** Severe aortic regurgitation with a broad regurgitant "band."

PULMONARY VALVE DISEASE

Acquired pulmonary valve stenosis is uncommon. It may occur in the carcinoid syndrome.[70] This is always valvar and never infundibular. Rheumatic involvement is extremely rare.[71] The chest x-ray study shows no remarkable characteristics, unlike congenital pulmonary valve stenosis, in which there is poststenotic dilatation of the main and left pulmonary arteries. During cardiac catheterization, pressures should be obtained in the pulmonary artery and in the right ventricle with simultaneous cardiac output. The pressures can be taken simultaneously or by withdrawal (Fig. 19–17). The pulmonary valve area can be calculated by the Gorlin formula[23, 24] by use of the mean systolic gradient. In practice, the severity of the stenosis is judged by the RV pressure. In acquired pulmonary stenosis, the stenosis is seldom of sufficient severity to require intervention.

The pulmonary regurgitation associated with severe mitral stenosis, which is heard as a Graham Steell murmur, is a consequence of pulmonary hypertension and pulmonary artery dilatation. Pulmonary regurgitation may also be acquired in congenital heart disease from long-standing severe pulmonary hypertension. Pulmonary angiography with severe pulmonary hypertension carries an increased risk and is seldom performed for this indication when the diagnosis is clinically evident and any uncertainty can be resolved echocardiographically.

TRICUSPID VALVE DISEASE

Acquired tricuspid stenosis is uncommon but may be of rheumatic origin[72, 73] or may be associated with the carcinoid syndrome,[74, 75] but it is often found as part of mixed tricuspid disease, with regurgitation as well. Hemodynamic evaluation of tricuspid stenosis includes simultaneous pressure recordings in the right atrium and the right ventricle and simultaneous measurement of cardiac output and heart rate and determination of the diastolic filling period. The valve area can then be calculated in accordance with the Gorlin formula,[23, 24] providing that the regurgitation is mild.

The right atrial tracing in tricuspid stenosis will show sustained elevation of the right atrial pressure (Fig. 19–18). In both severe tricuspid stenosis and tricuspid insufficiency, the usual rhythm is atrial fibrillation, and an A wave is seldom seen. Practically speaking, the presence of a consistent end-diastolic gradient establishes the diagnosis because functional tricuspid regurgitation alone should not be associated with an end-diastolic gradient.

Tricuspid insufficiency is a diagnosis best made by a skilled clinician. The hallmark of tricuspid insufficiency is large CV waves in the right atrial pressure tracing that give rise to deep jugular pulsations readily apparent on inspection of the neck veins. RV angiography adds little to the physical examination because some tricuspid regurgitation is often seen on color Doppler in normals.

VALVE PROSTHESES

Valve prostheses are either bioprosthetic or mechanical. Bioprosthetic valves may deteriorate with time but are often used in elderly patients to avoid anticoagulation and its complications.

Mechanical prostheses are of three types: ball-in-cage

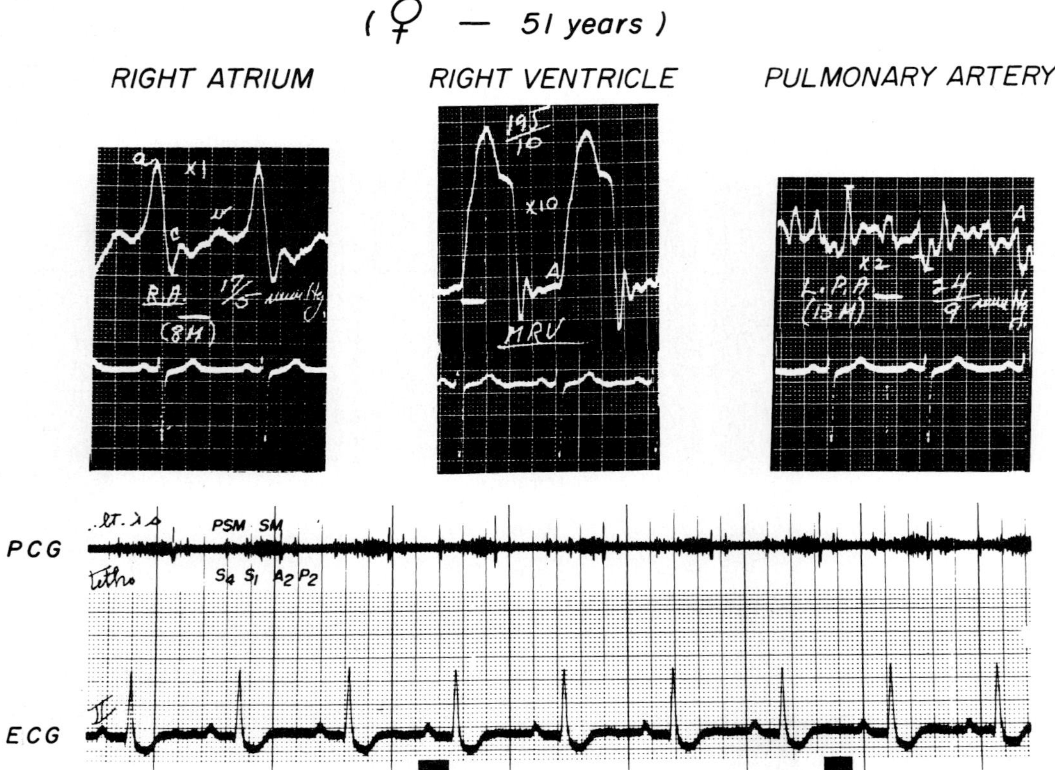

FIGURE 19–17 Pressure measurements obtained during cardiac catheterization.

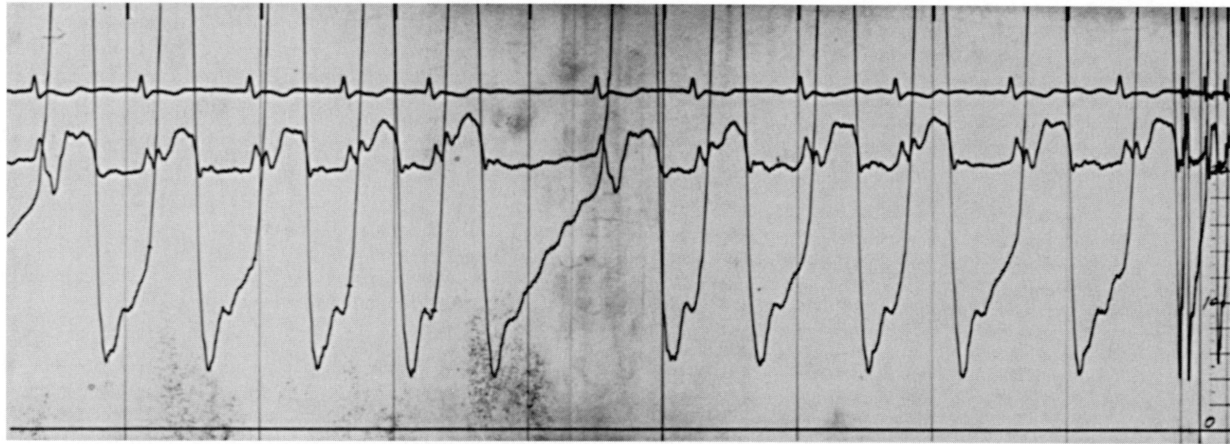

FIGURE 19–18 Simultaneous right atrial and right ventricular tracings in a patient with rheumatic tricuspid stenosis. Note the persistent elevation of the right atrial pressure and the large mean-diastolic gradient.

(Starr-Edwards),[76, 77] tilting disc,[78] and bileaflet (St. Jude).[79, 80] At present, the St. Jude prosthesis and its variants are regarded as having the least stenosis or abnormal pressure gradient across the valve (Table 19–2).

Valve prostheses are evaluated hemodynamically by methods identical to those for native valves. However, unlike native valves, mechanical prostheses cannot be crossed with a catheter without producing acute regurgitation, thereby invalidating any measurement. A mitral prosthesis can be evaluated with the pulmonary artery wedge (Fig. 19–19) and LV pressures. A prominent V wave is commonly seen in the wedge pressure in the presence of a mitral prosthesis without regurgitation, but the C wave is preserved and not slurred into a CV wave. The prominent V wave may be due to decreased atrial compliance in the presence of the prosthesis. With a mechanical aortic prosthesis, transseptal access to the LV is necessary.[79] In situations in which both the aortic and the mitral valves have been replaced with mechanical prostheses, access to the left ventricle can only be by LV puncture. This involves locating the cardiac apex and ascertaining that the apex is left ventricular. If this is uncertain and if the RV is large, the needle puncturing the apex may enter the left anterior descending artery. This uncertainty can be resolved by echocardiographic guidance. A sheathed LV puncture needle is then introduced transthoracically under local anesthesia and with either echocardiographic or fluoroscopic guidance into the apex, aiming toward the right shoulder and slightly posteriorly, advancing until a sudden "give" is felt. The needle is then withdrawn, leaving the sheath in situ, and entry into the LV cavity is confirmed by pulsatile flow and high saturation. To advance the sheath, a J-tipped guide wire is introduced through the sheath, and the sheath is further advanced into the LV cavity over the guide wire. Although these patients are receiving warfarin anticoagulation, complications are minimal because the pericardial cavity has usually been obliterated by previous open-heart surgery. Furthermore, the puncture is through the LV wall,

TABLE 19–2 Comparative Results of Transvalvular Pressure Gradient and Effective Valve Area*

	St. Jude Medical		Lillehei-Kaster		Starr-Edwards	
Tissue Annulus Diameter (mm)	***Gradient (mm Hg)***	***Valve Area (cm^2)***	***Gradient (mm Hg)***	***Valve Area (cm^2)***	***Gradient (mm Hg)***	***Valve Area (cm^2)***
21	0 (1)†	—‡	45 (9) (R 27–70)	0.8 (9) (R 0.5–1.1)	29 (5) (R 13–54)	1.0 (5) (R 0.7–1.4)
23	4 ± 0 (2)	2.5 ± 0 (2)	28 (12) (R 5–57)	1.1 (12) (R 0.9–1.3)	18 (7) (R 1–32)	1.1 (7) (R 0.8–1.5)
25	2.2 ± 1 (12) (R 0–9)	2.1 ± 0.2 (4)‡ (R 1.6–2.4)	22 (15) (R 10–42)	1.3 (15) (R 0.9–1.8)	13 (7) (R 6–22)	1.3 (7) (R 0.9–1.7)
26	3 ± 3 (2) (R 0–6)	2.4 (1)‡	—	—	21 (6) (R 16–26)	1.3 (6) (R 1.1–1.5)
27	0 (1)	—‡				
27.5			15 (4) (R 13–20)	1.9 (4) (R 1.7–2.3)	13 (1)	1.8 (1)

Abbreviation: R, range.
* Data on Lillehei-Kaster and Starr-Edwards prostheses from Pyle et al.[84]
† Indicates number of patients.
‡ Patients with 0 mm Hg transvalvular gradient not included.
From Pyle RB, Mayer JE Jr, Lindsay WG, et al: Hemodynamic evaluation of Lillehei-Kaiser and Starr-Edwards prosthesis. Ann Thorac Surg 26:336–343, 1978. Reprinted with permission from the Society of Thoracic Surgeons.

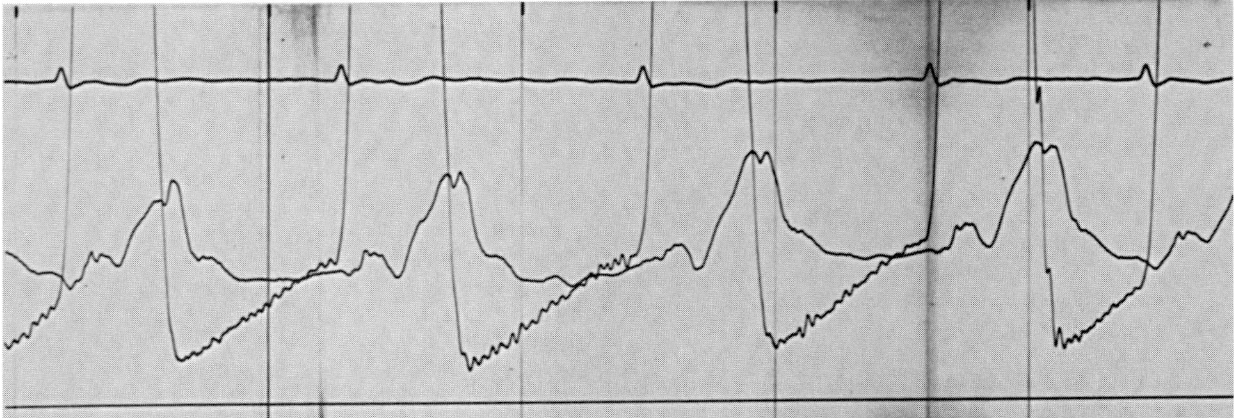

FIGURE 19–19 Simultaneous pulmonary artery wedge and left ventricular diastolic pressure in a patient with a St. Jude mitral prosthesis. The C and V waves are distinct, and there is no end-diastolic gradient. The prominent V wave is commonly seen with well-functioning mitral prostheses.

which is not easily lacerated, and the tract after withdrawal of the sheath does not give rise to significant bleeding problems because it is occluded with each ventricular systole. Nevertheless, it is prudent to discontinue warfarin for 1 or more days before the procedure.

Mechanical valve areas can be calculated as for native valves.[64, 65] This calculated area does not correspond to any structural area, but rather is a number that is useful for functional comparison with the native valve. We have often used the term *effective valve area.* The significance of the calculated area would be an index of the degree of obstruction to flow. Estimation of valve gradients and valve areas by echocardiography and by cardiac catheterization of native valves is usually in agreement. Sometimes, the estimations are divergent, the valve gradients being somewhat higher in mechanical prostheses with echocardiography. It seems that whereas the hemodynamic measurement measures the overall pressures, the continuous-wave Doppler measures velocity, and for a mechanical prosthesis such as the bileaflet St. Jude valve, the highest velocity and therefore the highest gradient may be between the two leaflets. Therefore, whereas hemodynamic measurements often yield no flow gradient across the St. Jude prosthesis, echocardiography usually yields a small-to-modest systolic gradient, and allowances should be made accordingly in data interpretation.[81]

Bioprostheses pose no technical difficulties for cardiac catheterization. They can be crossed readily without significantly altering hemodynamics. Tricuspid valve prostheses are commonly bioprosthetic, but tilting disc valves can be cautiously traversed in this low-pressure system. Even patients with triple valve prostheses can be evaluated hemodynamically by use of the aortic pressure, the LV pressure by direct LV puncture,[82, 83] and, with a right catheter, the pulmonary artery and pulmonary artery wedge pressures and RA pressure (Table 19–3).

Therapeutic Cardiac Catheterization for Valvular Heart Disease

Balloon valvuloplasty for stenotic valves, including mitral, aortic, pulmonary and tricuspid, have been reported by numerous groups from countries across the world[85–148] and it has become the standard of care for certain well-defined subsets of patients. Although rheumatic heart disease has been on the decline in the United States, it still is seen in a large number of patients in the Far and Middle East, and many groups have reported extensively on the results with mitral valvuloplasty.[85–126]

Mitral Valvuloplasty

Inoue and coworkers[85] were among the initial workers to report on the utility of balloon valvuloplasty with a spe-

TABLE 19-3 Hemodynamic Data on a Rheumatic Fever Patient Who Underwent Valve Replacement (2-Year Follow-Up)*

Measurement	Preoperative Data	2-Year Follow-Up Data
PAWP	M 35, A 36, V42	M 13, A 14, V 18
LV	170/4–8	128/0–8
AO	120/65	128/78
PA	80/35	34/16
RV	80/5–8	34/2–8
RA	M 12, A 15, V 13	M 7, A 8, V 8
MVEDG	20 (0.5 cm²)	0
TVEDG	4–6	0
AVPSG	50	0
MI	<1+	
AI	2+	
CO	2.54 L/min	4.8
CI	1.59 L/min/m²	3.7
HR	70	81
SV	36 ml	59 ml
HgB	13.2%	9.7 (retics. 9%)

Abbreviations: A, a wave; AI, aortic incompetence; AO, aorta; AVPSG, aortic valve peak systolic gradient; CI, cardiac index; CO, cardiac output; HgB, hemoglobin; HR, heart rate; LV, left ventricle; M, mean pressure; MVEDG, mitral valve end-diastolic gradient; PA, pulmonary artery; PAWP; pulmonary artery wedge pressure; RA, right atrium; RV, right ventricle; SV, stroke volume; TVEDG, tricuspid valve end-diastolic gradient; V, v wave.

*This patient with rheumatic heart disease initially had an aortic valve replaced by a Starr-Edwards prosthesis; in 1970, Lillehei-Kaster prostheses were used for the mitral valve for mitral stenosis and for the tricuspid valve for severe mixed tricuspid disease. Two years after the last operation, she had no abnormal gradients across her valves. She died in 1981.

cially developed balloon catheter for mitral stenosis. After this there was a tremendous amount of interest in the utility of balloon techniques for the percutaneous valvuloplasty of stenotic mitral valves, especially in centers in the Far East, including Asia, where "closed" surgical commissurotomy was the standard of care for patients with mitral stenosis with flexible valves and commissural fusion. This has been largely replaced with balloon valvuloplasty, which produces similar results.[110–112]

Percutaneous valvuloplasty of the mitral valve in adults is generally performed with sedation without general anesthesia. Transseptal catheterization is performed via the right femoral vein by use of standard techniques. The valvuloplasty itself can be performed with either a single-balloon or a double-balloon technique. The mitral valve is crossed by use of a balloon catheter, and one or two exchange wires are placed across it. The atrial septum is dilated with an 8- or 6-mm balloon. A single- or double-balloon valvuloplasty is performed. This is determined by the height and weight or the body surface area of the patient. With the Inoue technique, the Inoue guide wire is introduced in the left atrium, and the femoral entry site and atrial septal puncture site are dilated with a rigid 14 French dilator. The balloon is introduced into the left atrium, and the balloon size is chosen in accordance with the patient's height: 24 mm in patients shorter than 1.47 m, 26 mm in patients 1.47 to 1.6 m, 28 mm in patients 1.6 m to 1.8 m, and 30 mm in patients taller than 1.8 m.[86] The distal portion of the balloon is inflated with 1 to 2 ml of diluted contrast medium. The balloon is then pulled back into the mitral valve orifice, and then the proximal part of the balloon is inflated with disappearance of the central waist. It is recommended that the balloon be deflated and returned back into the left atrium after every increment in diameter and the severity of the mitral regurgitation assessed by color Doppler, as also measurements of the pressure gradient across the valve. The end point is the achievement of good immediate results, which are usually defined as mitral valve area larger than 1.5 cm^2, without mitral regurgitation greater than II/IV. The technical details of performance of the procedure have been well documented by numerous authors.[85, 88, 90, 92, 96–98] The mechanism of benefit has been clearly established because of commissural splitting of the valve, which is akin to surgical commissurotomy. Many groups have reported on the comparable results between percutaneous mitral commissurotomy and surgical commissurotomy.[111, 112] The ideal patients are young adults with pliable mitral valves as a result of commissural fusion with only moderate subvalvular disease (echo score < 8). Although such patients are more commonly seen in Eastern countries, the typical patients seen in the United States are older and often have an unfavorable anatomy and significant fibrosis, with calcification and subvalvular deformity. In patients with echo scores of 8 to 12 with extensive subvalvular disease or mitral valve calcification, we usually recommend proceeding to mitral valve replacement rather than balloon mitral valvuloplasty. In countries where large populations of patients have mitral stenosis, the cost of balloon valvuloplasty is considerably higher than that of closed surgical commissurotomy, and, hence, there is a definite financial burden on these patients. Attempts have been made to develop a percutaneous valvulotomy device that features a metallic valvulotome instead of the balloon.[149] This is an ingenious new device that is similar to the surgical dilators used by surgeons for closed-chest commissurotomy. The device is delivered percutaneously through the mitral valve, and the valve is dilated by activation of a handheld pliers. The results of the initial experience would suggest that this technique is comparable to balloon valvuloplasty, and it might soon find wider acceptance. The reusable nature of the device is an attractive option for indigent patients.

Balloon Aortic Valvuloplasty

The technique of percutaneous balloon valvuloplasty was described in the late 1980s by Cribier and colleagues[127] and McKay and associates.[128] There was a great deal of interest in investigating this technique for patients with calcific aortic stenosis who are poor risks for surgery. Over the past 13 years, the results of balloon valvuloplasty, high restenosis rates, the ability of cardiac surgeons to effectively operate on fairly old patients with calcified aortic valves, and the use of porcine heart valves rather than mechanical valves have markedly reduced the enthusiasm for this particular procedure. The procedure is performed percutaneously. The aortic valve is crossed with any standard end-hole catheter, and a stiff guide wire is positioned across the aortic valve. We recommend using 14 French arterial sheaths, rather than passing the balloon percutaneously. The aortic valve is then dilated sequentially with a 15-mm balloon catheter, which is approximately 5 cm in length. We then progress to a 20-mm balloon and, if required, a 23-mm balloon. Oversized balloons have been reported to be associated with severe aortic regurgitation or aortic annular rupture, and hence, in our practice, most of these patients are dilated with either a single 15-mm or 20-mm balloon. The balloons are dilated with hand injection and are deflated immediately when the balloon has dilated. We perform three inflations for every balloon size, and the aortic gradient, valve area, and severity of aortic regurgitation should be assessed with each balloon catheter size. The aim is to achieve a mean gradient of less than 30 mm Hg and/or a greater than 100 percent increase in valve area. The mechanism of balloon aortic valvuloplasty has been previously described and is related to fracture of calcium deposits and separation of the commissures.[128] We believe that in adult patients with calcific aortic stenosis, this should be reserved primarily as a means of palliation for elderly, frail patients with severe congestive heart failure who are not candidates for open-heart surgery.

Pulmonary Valvuloplasty

Valvar pulmonary stenosis is infrequently seen in adults. However, since the early descriptions of pulmonary valvuloplasty[136, 138, 139] and the substantial experience of pediatric cardiologists, the technique has been fairly well standardized. This procedure is easy to perform and has a fairly low complication rate and practically no mortality. Most patients have a domed, pliable, pulmonic valve, which is seen in a right ventricular angiogram, especially in the lateral view. In adults, there may be some amount of calcification, which may restrict mobility as well. The procedure is relatively straightforward. It is performed in adult patients under local anesthesia without the need for any general anesthesia. The right femoral vein is accessed. An angiographic catheter is passed into the right ventricle, and an angiogram is performed in the anteroposterior and lateral projection. The pulmonary annulus diameter is measured from the lateral view. Then an end-hole catheter is passed from the right femoral vein across the pulmonic valve, and the pressure gradient across the valve is measured. For pulmonary annulus diameters of less than 20 mm, we tend to perform single-balloon valvuloplasty. If the annulus diameter is larger than 20 mm, we tend to perform a double-balloon valvuloplasty. For double-balloon valvuloplasty, a second guide wire is passed through an end-hole catheter from the left femoral vein, and both of these 0.035-inch stiff guide wires are placed in the left pulmonary artery. Balloon catheters are chosen so that the combined diameter is approximately 130 percent of the pulmonary annulus diameter. These are passed over the wire and positioned at the pulmonic valve. We use 4- to 5-cm-long balloons to prevent inflation of longer balloons within the right ventricular cavity. Once the balloons are positioned, the balloons are partially inflated in order to center the balloons, and then by hand injection, the balloons are inflated until the waist disappears. We deflate the balloons immediately and typically perform three inflations for every size of balloon or balloons. One of the balloons then is withdrawn, and the pressure gradient is measured across the pulmonary valve. We attempt to reduce the systolic gradient to less than 30 mm Hg. At the conclusion of the procedure, a right ventricular angiogram is again performed. Balloon valvuloplasty for pulmonic stenosis can be performed quite safely in adults, with practically no mortality and infrequent complications of arrhythmias or heart block. Several groups have reported on the results of pulmonary valvuloplasty in adult patients, with substantial reduction of the systolic gradients and with persistent relief on follow-up for as long as 5 years.[140, 143–147]

References

1. Forssmann W: Die Sondierung des rechten Herzens. Klin Wochenschr 8:2085, 1929.
2. Cournand AF, Riley RL, Breed ESD, et al: Measurement of cardiac output in man using the technique of catheterization of the right auricle. J Clin Invest 24:106, 1945.
3. Dexter L, Burwell CS, Haynes FW, et al: Oxygen content of the pulmonary "capillary" blood in unanesthetized human beings. J Clin Invest 25:913, 1946.
4. Dexter L, Haynes FW, Burwell SC, et al: Studies of congenital heart disease. II: the pressure and oxygen content of blood in the right auricle, ventricle and pulmonary artery in control patients with observations on the oxygen saturation of pulmonary "capillary" blood. J Clin Invest 26:544, 1947.
5. Zimmerman HA, Scott RW, Becker B, Becker ND: Catheterization of the left side of the heart in man. Circulation 1:357, 1950.
6. Bjork VO, Malmstrom G: Left heart catheterization. Circ Res 2:424, 1954.
7. Ross J Jr: Transseptal left heart catheterization: a new method of left atrial puncture. Ann Surg 149:295, 1959.
8. Sones FM Jr, Shirey EK: Cine coronary arteriography. Mod Concepts Cardiovasc Dis 31:735, 1962.
9. Swan HJC, Ganz W, Forrester JL, et al: Catheterization of the heart in man with use of a flow-directed balloon-tipped catheter. N Engl J Med 283:447, 1970.
10. Benotti J: Comparative effects of ionic versus nonionic agents in cardiac catheterization. Invest Radiol 23(suppl 2):S-366, 1988.
11. Bettmann MA, Bourdillon PD, Barry WH, et al: Contrast agents for cardiac angiography: effect of a nonionic agent vs a standard ionic. Radiology 153:583, 1984.
12. Missri J, Jeresaty RM: Ventricular fibrillation during coronary angiography: reduced incidence with nonionic contrast media. Cathet Cardiovasc Diagn 19:4, 1990.
13. Wood P: An appreciation of mitral stenosis. BMJ 1:1051, 1113, 1954.
14. Olson LJ, Subramanian R, Ackermann DM: Surgical pathology of the mitral valve: a study of 712 cases spanning 21 years. Mayo Clin Proc 62:22, 1987.
15. Selzer A, Cohn KE: Natural history of mitral stenosis: a review. Circulation 45:878, 1972.
16. Millward MJ, Blake MP, Byrne MJ, et al: Left heart involvement with cardiac shunt complicating carcinoid heart disease. Aust N Z J Med 19:716, 1989.
17. Bortolotti U, Valente M, Agozzino L, et al: Rheumatoid mitral stenosis requiring valve replacement. Am Heart J 107:1049, 1984.
18. Amplatz K: The roentgenographic diagnosis of mitral and aortic valvular disease. Am Heart J 64:556, 1962.
19. Melhem RE, Dunbar JE, Booth RW: "B" lines of Kerley. Left atrial size and mitral valve disease: their correlation with mean atrial pressure as measured by left atrial puncture. Radiology 76:65, 1961.
20. Chen JTT, Behar VS, Morris JJ Jr, et al: Correlation of roentgen findings with hemodynamic data in pure mitral stenosis. Am J Roentgenol Radium Ther Radium Ther Nucl Med 102:280, 1968.
21. Werko L, Varnauskas H, Eliasch H, et al: Further evidence that the pulmonary capillary venous pressure pulse in man reflects cyclic pressure changes in the left atrium. Circ Res 1:337, 1953.
22. Lange RA, Moore DM Jr, Cigarros RG, Hillis LD: Use of pulmonary capillary wedge pressure to assess severity of mitral stenosis: is true left atrial pressure needed in this condition? J Am Coll Cardiol 13:825, 1989.
23. Gorlin R, Gorlin SG: Hydraulic formula for calculation of the area of the stenotic valve, other cardiac valves, and central circulatory shunts. Am Heart J 41:1, 1951.
24. Gorlin R: Calculation of orifice areas within the cardiovascular system. Methods Med Res 7:102, 1958.
25. Cohen MV, Gorlin R: Modified orifice equation with a calculation of mitral valve area. Am Heart J 84:839, 1972.
26. Gorlin R: Calculations of cardiac valve stenosis: restoring an old concept for advanced applications. J Am Coll Cardiol 10:920, 1987.
27. Walston A, Kendall ME: Comparison of pulmonary wedge and left atrial pressure in man. Am Heart J 86:159, 1973.
28. Connolly DC, Tompkins RG, Lev R, et al: Pulmonary artery wedge pressures in mitral valve disease, relationship to left atrial pressure. Proc Staff Meet Mayo Clin 28:72, 1953.
29. Chambers JB, Cochrane T, Black MM, et al: The Gorlin formula validated against directly observed orifice area in porcine mitral bioprostheses. J Am Coll Cardiol 13:348, 1989.
30. Hammermeister JE, Murray JA, Blackmon JR: Revision of Gorlin constant for calculation of mitral valve area from left heart pressures. Br Heart J 35:392, 1973.
31. Smith RC, Burchell HB, Edwards JE: Pathology of the pulmonary vasculature. IV: structural changes in the pulmonary vessels in chronic left ventricular failure. Circulation 10:801, 1954.
32. Dalen JE, Matloff JM, Evans GL, et al: Early reduction of pulmonary vascular resistance after mitral valve replacement. N Engl J Med 277:387, 1967.
33. Braunwald E, Braunwald NS, Ross J Jr: Effects of mitral valve replacement on cardiovascular dynamics of patients with pulmonary hypertension. N Engl J Med 273:509, 1965.
34. Fegler G: Measurement of cardiac output in anesthetized animals by a thermodilution method. Q J Exp Physiol 39:153, 1954.
35. Stetz CW, Miller RG, Kelly GE, et al: Reliability of the thermodilution method in the determination of cardiac output in clinical practice. Annu Rev Respir Dis 126:1001, 1982.
36. Fromer A, Ganz I: Measurement of flow in single blood vessels including cardiac output by local thermodilution. Circ Res 8:175, 1960.
37. Ganz W, Donoso R, Marcus HS, et al: A new technique for measure-

ment of cardiac output by thermodilution in man. Am J Cardiol 27:394, 1971.
38. Hamilton WF, Riley RL, Attyah AM, et al: Comparison of Fick and dye injection methods of measuring cardiac output in man. Am J Physiol 153:309, 1948.
39. Fox IJ, Wood EH: Circulatory system methods indicator dilution techniques in study of normal and abnormal circulation. *In* Glasser O (ed): Medical Physics. Vol. 3. pp. 163–168. Chicago: Chicago Yearbook, 1960.
40. Fick A: Ueber die Messung des Blutquantums in den Herzventrikel. Sitzungsb Phys Med Ges Wurzburg 36, 1870.
41. Richards DW Jr: Cardiac output by catheterization in various clinical conditions. Fed Proc 4:215, 1945.
42. Stow RW: Systematic errors in flow determination by the Fick method. Minn Med 37:30, 1954.
43. Visscher MB, Johnson JA: The Fick principle: analysis of potential errors in the conventional application. J Appl Physiol 5:635, 1953.
44. Brockenbrough EC, Braunwald E: A new technique for cardioangiography and transseptal left heart catheterization. Am J Cardiol 6:1062, 1960.
45. Bolen JL, Lopes MG, Harrison DC, et al: Analysis of left ventricular function in response to afterload changes in patients with mitral stenosis. Circulation 52:894, 1975.
46. Hildner FJ, Javier RP, Cohen LS, et al: Myocardial dysfunction associated with valvular heart disease. Am J Cardiol 30:319, 1972.
47. Selzer A, Cohn K: The "myocardial factor" in valvular heart disease. Cardiovasc Clin 5:177, 1973.
48. Davis MJ: Aetiology and pathology of the diseases mitral valve. *In* Ionescu MI, Cohn LH (eds): Mitral Valve Disease: Diagnosis and Treatment. pp. 27–42. London: Butterworth, 1985.
49. Keren G, Sonnenblick EH, Lejemtel TH: Mitral annulus motion: relation to pulmonary venous transmitral flows in normal subjects and in patients with dilated cardiomyopathy. Circulation 78:621, 1988.
50. Oliveira DBG, Dawkins DK, Kay PH, et al: Chordal rupture I: aetiology and natural history. Br Heart J 50:312, 1983.
51. Burch GE, DePasquale NP, Phillips JH: The syndrome of papillary muscle dysfunction. Am Heart J 75:339, 1968.
52. Priest EA, Finlayson JK, Shou DS: The x-ray manifestations in the heart and lungs of mitral regurgitations. Prog Cardiovasc Dis 5:291, 1962.
53. Selzer A, Katayama F: Mitral regurgitation: clinical patterns, pathophysiology, and natural history. Medicine (Baltimore) 51:337, 1972.
54. Sanders RJ, Naubuerger KT, Ravin A: Rupture of papillary muscles: occurrence of rupture of the posterior muscle in posterior myocardial infarction. Dis Chest 31:316, 1957.
55. Sanders CA, Armstrong PW, Willerson JT, et al: Etiology and differential diagnosis of acute mitral regurgitation. Prog Cardiovasc Dis 14:129, 1971.
56. Selzer A, Kelly JJ Jr, Vannitamby M, et al: The syndrome of mitral insufficiency due to isolated rupture of chordae tendineae. Am J Med 43:822, 1967.
57. Kihara Y, Sasayama S, Miyazaki S, et al: Role of the left atrium in adaptation of the heart to chronic mitral regurgitation in conscious dogs. Circ Res 62:543, 1988.
58. Dodge HT, Sheehan H: Quantitative contrast angiography for assessment of ventricular performance in heart disease. J Am Coll Cardiol 1:73, 1983.
59. Dodge HT, Baxley WA: Left ventricular volume and mass and their significance in heart disease. Am J Cardiol 23:528, 1969.
60. Schuler G, Peterson KL, Johnson A, et al: Temporal response of left ventricular performance to mitral valve surgery. Circulation 59:1218, 1979.
61. Ellis HF Jr, Kirklin JW: Congenital valvular aortic stenosis: anatomic findings and surgical technique. J Thorac Cardiovasc Surg 43:199, 1962.
62. Passick CS, Ackermann DM, Pluth JR, Edwards ND: Temporal changes in the causes of aortic stenosis: a surgical pathologic study of 646 cases. Mayo Clin Proc 52:119, 1987.
63. Edwards JE: Calcific aortic stenosis: pathologic features. Mayo Clin Proc 36:444, 1961.
64. Pomerance A: Pathogenesis of aortic stenosis and its relation to age. Br Heart J 34:569, 1972.
65. Folland ED, Parisi AF, Carbone C: Is peripheral arterial pressure a satisfactory substitute for ascending aortic pressure when measuring aortic valve gradients? J Am Coll Cardiol 4:1207, 1984.
66. Raber G, Goldberg H: Left ventricular, central aortic, and peripheral pressure pulses in aortic stenosis. Am J Cardiol 1:572, 1958.
67. Bache RJ, Wang Y, Greenfield JC Jr: Left ventricular ejection time in valvular aortic stenosis. Circulation 47:527, 1973.
68. Ramanthan KP, Knowles J, Connor MJ, et al: Natural history of chronic aortic insufficiency: relation of peak systolic pressure/end-systolic volume ratio to morbidity and mortality. J Am Coll Cardiol 3:1412, 1984.
69. Borow K, Green LH, Mann T, et al: End-systolic volume as a predictor of postoperative left ventricular performance in volume overload from valvular regurgitation. Am J Med 68:655, 1980.
70. Ross EM, Roberts WC: The carcinoid syndrome: comparison of 21 necropsy subjects with carcinoid heart disease to 15 necropsy subjects without carcinoid heart disease. Am J Med 79:339, 1985.
71. Altrichter PM, Olson LJ, Edwards WD, et al: Surgical pathology of the pulmonary valve: a study of 116 cases spanning 15 years. Mayo Clin Proc 64:1352, 1989.
72. McCord MC, Swan H, Blonut SG Jr: Tricuspid stenosis: clinical and physiological evaluation. Am Heart J 48:405, 1954.
73. Hauck AJ, Freeman DP, Ackermann DM, et al: Surgical pathology of the tricuspid valve: a study of 363 cases spanning 25 years. Mayo Clin Proc 68:851, 1988.
74. Graham-Smith DG: The carcinoid syndrome. Am J Cardiol 21:376, 1968.
75. Carpena C, Kay JH, Mendez AM, et al: Carcinoid heart disease: surgery for tricuspid and pulmonary valve lesions. Am J Cardiol 32:229, 1973.
76. Starr A, Edwards, ML: Mitral replacement: clinical experience with a ball valve prosthesis. Ann Surg 154:726, 1961.
77. Grunkemeier GS, Starr A: Twenty five year experience with Starr-Edwards heart valves: follow-up methods and results. Can J Cardiol 4:381, 1988.
78. Austin EH III: Other mechanical prosthesis. *In* Crawford FA (ed): Cardiac Surgery: Current Heart Valve Prostheses. Vol. 1. p. 237. Philadelphia: Hanley & Belfus, 1987.
79. Emery RW, Anderson RW, Lindsay WG, et al: Clinical and hemodynamic results with a St. Jude Medical aortic valve prosthesis. Surg Forum 30:235, 1979.
80. Emery RW, Anderson RW, Lindsay WG, et al: Clinical and hemodynamic results with the St. Jude Medical aortic valve prosthesis, a 3 year experience. Surg Forum 30:235, 1979.
81. Baumgartner H, Kahn S, DeRobertis M, et al: Effect of a prosthetic valve design on Doppler-catheter gradient correlation: an in-vitro study of normal, St. Jude, Medtronic-Hall, Starr-Edwards and Hancock valves. J Am Coll Cardiol 19:324, 1992.
82. Lehman JS, Musser BG, Lyken HD: Cardiac ventriculography: direct transthoracic needle puncture opacification of the left (or right) ventricle. AJR 77:207, 1957.
83. Levy MJ, Lillehei CW: Percutaneous direct cardiac catheterization: a new method with results in 122 patients. N Engl J Med 271:273, 1964.
84. Pyle RB, Mayer JE Jr, Lindsay WG, et al: Hemodynamic evaluation of Lillehei-Kaiser and Starr-Edwards prosthesis. Ann Thorac Surg 26:336, 1978.
85. Inoue K, Owaki T, Nakamura T, et al: Clinical application of transvenous mitral commissurotomy by a new balloon catheter. J Thorac Cardiovasc Surg 87:394, 1984.
86. Iung B, Cormier B, Ducimetiere P, et al: Immediate results of percutaneous mitral commissurotomy. Circulation 94:2124, 1996.
87. Vahanian A, Michel PL, Cormier B, et al: Results of percutaneous mitral commissurotomy in 200 patients. Am J Cardiol 63:847, 1989.
88. Vahanian A, Cormier B, Iung B: Percutaneous transvenous mitral commissurotomy using the Inoue balloon: international experience. Cathet Cardiovasc Diagn 2:8, 1994.
89. Iung B, Cormier B, Ducimetiere P, et al: Functional results 5 years after successful percutaneous mitral commissurotomy in a series of 528 patients and analysis of predictive factors. J Am Coll Cardiol 27:407, 1996.
90. McKay RG, Lock JE, Safian RD, et al: Balloon dilatation of mitral stenosis in adult patients: postmortem and percutaneous mitral valvuloplasty studies. J Am Coll Cardiol 9:723, 1987.
91. Kaplan JD, Isner JM, Karas RH, et al: In vitro analysis of mechanisms of balloon valvuloplasty of stenotic mitral valves. Am J Cardiol 59:318, 1987.
92. Zaibag M, Al Kasab S, Ribeiro PA, et al: Percutaneous double-

balloon mitral valvotomy for rheumatic mitral valve stenosis. Lancet 1:757, 1986.
93. Palacios IF, Block PC, Brandi S, et al: Percutaneous balloon valvotomy for patients with severe mitral stenosis. Circulation 75:778, 1987.
94. McKay CR, Kawanishi DT, Rahimtoola SH: Catheter balloon valvuloplasty of the mitral valve in adults using a double-balloon technique: early hemodynamic results. JAMA 257:1753, 1987.
95. Nobuyoshi M, Hamasaki N, Kimura T, et al: Indications, complications, and short-term clinical outcome of percutaneous transvenous mitral commissurotomy. Circulation 80:782, 1989.
96. Bassand JP, Schiele F, Bernard Y, et al: The double-balloon and Inoue techniques in percutaneous mitral valvuloplasty: comparative results in a series of 232 cases. J Am Coll Cardiol 18:982, 1991.
97. Ribeiro PA, Fawzy ME, Arafat MA, et al: Comparison of mitral valve area results of balloon mitral valvotomy using the Inoue and double-balloon techniques. Am J Cardiol 68:687, 1991.
98. Ruiz CE, Zhang HP, Macaya C, et al: Comparison of Inoue single-balloon versus double-balloon technique for percutaneous mitral valvotomy. Am Heart J 123:942, 1992.
99. Patel J, Vythilingum S, Mitha AS: Balloon dilatation of the mitral valve by a single bifoil (2 × 19 mm) or trefoil (3 × 15 mm) catheter. Br Heart J 64:342, 1990.
100. Bonhoeffer P, Piechaud JF, Sidi D, et al: Mitral dilatation with the multi-track system: an alternative approach. Cathet Cardiovasc Diagn 36:189, 1995.
101. Roth BR, Block PC, Palacios IF: Predictors of increased mitral regurgitation after percutaneous mitral balloon valvotomy. Cathet Cardiovasc Diagn 20:17, 1990.
102. Tuzcu EM, Block PC, Palacious IF: Comparison of early versus late experience with percutaneous mitral balloon valvuloplasty. J Am Coll Cardiol 17:1121, 1991.
103. Arora R, Singh Kalra G, Ramachandra Murty GS, et al: Percutaneous transatrial mitral commissurotomy: immediate and intermediate results. J Am Coll Cardiol 23:1327, 1994.
104. Chen CR, Cheng TO: Percutaneous balloon mitral valvuloplasty by the Inoue technique: a multicenter study of 4832 patients in China. Am Heart J 129:1197, 1995.
105. Lock JE, Khalilullah M, Shrivastava S, et al: Percutaneous catheter commissurotomy in rheumatic mitral stenosis. N Engl J Med 313:1515, 1985.
106. The National Heart, Lung, and Blood Institute Balloon Valvuloplasty Registry Participants: Multicenter experience with balloon mitral commissurotomy: NHLBI Balloon Valvuloplasty Registry report on immediate and 30-day follow-up results. Circulation 85:448, 1992.
107. The National Heart, Lung, and Blood Institute Balloon Valvuloplasty Registry: Complications and mortality of percutaneous balloon mitral commissurotomy. Circulation 85:2014, 1992.
108. Lefevre T, Bonan R, Serra A, et al: Percutaneous mitral valvuloplasty in surgical high-risk patient. J Am Coll Cardiol 17:348, 1991.
109. Levine MJ, Weinstein JS, Diver DJ, et al: Progressive improvement in pulmonary vascular resistance after percutaneous mitral valvuloplasty. Circulation 79:1061, 1989.
110. Turi ZG, Reyes VP, Soma Raju B, et al: Percutaneous balloon versus surgical closed commissurotomy for mitral stenosis. Circulation 83:1179, 1991.
111. Patel JJ, Shama D, Mitha AS, et al: Balloon valvuloplasty versus closed commissurotomy for pliable mitral stenosis: a prospective hemodynamic study. J Am Coll Cardiol 18:1318, 1991.
112. Reyes VP, Raju BS, Wynne J, et al: Percutaneous balloon valvuloplasty compared with open surgical commissurotomy for mitral stenosis. N Engl J Med 331:961, 1994.
113. Harrison KJ, Wilson JS, Hearne SE, et al: Complications related to percutaneous transvenous mitral commissurotomy. Cathet Cardiovasc Diagn 2:52, 1994.
114. Drobinski G, Montalescot G, Evans J, et al: Systemic embolism as a complication of percutaneous mitral valvuloplasty. Cathet Cardiovasc Diagn 25:327, 1992.
115. Essop MR, Wisenbaugh T, Skoularigis J, et al: Mitral regurgitation following mitral balloon valvotomy: differing mechanisms for severe versus mild-to-moderate lesions. Circulation 84:1669, 1991.
116. Herrmann HS, Lima JAC, Feldman T, et al: Mechanisms and outcome of severe mitral regurgitation after Inoue balloon valvuloplasty. J Am Coll Cardiol 27:783, 1993.
117. Hernandez R, Macaya C, Benuelos C, et al: Predictors, mechanisms and outcome of severe mitral regurgitation complicating percutaneous mitral valvotomy with the Inoue balloon. Am J Cardiol 70:1169, 1993.
118. Padial LR, Freitas N, Sagie A, et al: Echocardiography can predict which patients will develop severe mitral regurgitation after percutaneous mitral valvulotomy. J Am Coll Cardiol 27:1225, 1996.
119. Fields CD, Slovenkai GA, Isner JM: Atrial septal defect resulting from mitral balloon valvuloplasty: relation of defect morphology to trans-septal balloon catheter delivery. Am Heart J 119:568, 1990.
120. Wilkins GT, Gillam LD, Weyman AE, et al: Percutaneous balloon dilatation of the mitral valve: an analysis of echocardiographic variables related to outcome and the mechanism of dilatation. Br Heart J 60:299, 1988.
121. Herrmann HC, Ramaswamy K, Isner JM, et al: Factors influencing immediate results, complications and short-term follow-up status after Inoue balloon mitral valvotomy: a North-American multicenter study. Am Heart J 124:160, 1992.
122. Palacios IF, Block PC, Wilkins GT, et al: Follow-up of patients undergoing percutaneous mitral balloon valvotomy. Circulation 79:573, 1989.
123. Cohen DJ, Kuntz RE, Gordon SPF, et al: Predictors of long-term outcome after percutaneous balloon mitral valvuloplasty. N Engl J Med 327:1329, 1992.
124. Reid CL, Kawanishi DT, Stellar W, et al: Long-term incidence of atrial septal defects after catheter balloon commissurotomy for mitral stenosis [abstract]. J Am Coll Cardiol 17(suppl A):339A, 1991.
125. Rediker DE, Block PC, Abascal VM, et al: Mitral balloon valvuloplasty for mitral restenosis after surgical commissurotomy. J Am Coll Cardiol 11:252, 1988.
126. Cheng TO: Percutaneous balloon mitral valvuloplasty: are Chinese and western experiences comparable? Cathet Cardiovasc Diagn 31:23, 1994.
127. Cribier A, Savin T, Saoudi N, et al: Percutaneous transluminal valvuloplasty of acquired aortic stenosis in elderly patients: an alternative to valve replacement: Lancet 1:63, 1986.
128. McKay RG, Safian RD, Lock JE, et al: Balloon dilatation of calcific aortic stenosis in elderly patients: postmortem, intra-operative, and percutaneous valvuloplasty studies. Circulation 74:119, 1986.
129. Cribier A, Savin T, Berland J, et al: Percutaneous transluminal balloon valvuloplasty of adult aortic stenosis: report on 92 cases. Am J Cardiol 9:381, 1987.
130. Litvack F, Jakubowski AT, Burchbinder NA, Eigler N: Lack of sustained clinical improvement in an elderly population after percutaneous aortic valvuloplasty. Am J Cardiol 62:270, 1988.
131. Lembo NJ, King SB, Roubin GS, et al: Fatal aortic rupture during percutaneous balloon valvuloplasty for valvular aortic stenosis. Am J Cardiol 60:733, 1987.
132. Holmes DR Jr, Nishimura RA, Reeder GS: In-hospital mortality after balloon aortic valvuloplasty: frequency and associated factors. J Am Coll Cardiol 17:187, 1991.
133. Berland J, Cribier A, Savin T, et al: Percutaneous balloon valvuloplasty in patients with severe aortic stenosis and low ejection fraction: immediate results and 1-year follow-up. Circulation 79:1189, 1989.
134. McKay RG, Safian RD, Lock JF, et al: Assessment of left ventricular and aortic valve function after balloon aortic valvuloplasty in adult patients with critical aortic stenosis. Circulation 75:192, 1987.
135. Cribier A, Remadi F, Koning R, et al: Emergency balloon valvuloplasty as initial treatment of patients with aortic stenosis and cardiogenic shock. N Engl J Med 323:646, 1992.
136. Kan JS, White RI, Mitchell SE, Gardner TJ: Percutaneous balloon valvuloplasty: a new method for treatment of congenital pulmonary-valve stenosis. N Engl J Med 307:540, 1982.
137. Lababidi Z, Wu JR: Percutaneous balloon pulmonary valvuloplasty. Am J Cardiol 52:560, 1983.
138. Stanger P, Cassidy SC, Girod DA, et al: Balloon pulmonary valvuloplasty: results of the Valvuloplasty and Angioplasty of Congenital Anomalies Registry. Am J Cardiol 65:775, 1990.
139. Pepine CJ, Gessner IH, Feldman RL: Percutaneous balloon valvuloplasty for pulmonary valve stenosis in the adult. Am J Cardiol 50:1442, 1982.
140. Al Kasab S, Ribeiro PA, al Raibag M, et al: Percutaneous double balloon pulmonary valvotomy in adults. Am J Cardiol 62:822, 1988.

141. Rao PS, Thapar MK, Kutayli F: Causes of restenosis after balloon valvuloplasty for valvular pulmonary stenosis. Am J Cardiol 62:979, 1988.
142. Rao PS: Influence of balloon size on short-term and long-term results of balloon pulmonary valvuloplasty. Tex Heart Inst J 14:57, 1987.
143. Tentolouris CA, Kyriakidis MK, Gaualiatsis IP, et al: Percutaneous pulmonary valvuloplasty in an octogenarian with calcific pulmonary stenosis. Chest 101:1456, 1992.
144. Herrmann HC, Hill JA, Krol J, et al: Effectiveness of percutaneous balloon valvuloplasty in adults with pulmonic valve stenosis. Am J Cardiol 68:1111, 1991.
145. Sherman W, Hershman R, Alexopoulos D, et al: Pulmonic balloon valvuloplasty in adults. Am Heart J 119:186, 1990.
146. Fawzy ME, Mercer EN, Dunn B: Late results of pulmonary balloon valvuloplasty in adults using double balloon technique. J Intervent Cardiol 1:35, 1988.
147. Chen CR, Cheng TO, Huang T, et al: Percutaneous balloon valvuloplasty for pulmonary stenosis in adolescents and adults. N Engl J Med 335:21, 1996.
148. McCrindle BW, Kan JS: Long-term results after balloon pulmonary valvuloplasty. Circulation 83:1915, 1991.
149. Cribier A, Rath PC, Letac B: Percutaneous mitral valvotomy with a metal dilatator. Lancet 349:1667, 1997.

C H A P T E R **20**

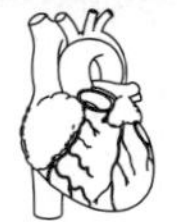

ECHOCARDIOGRAPHY AND DOPPLER EVALUATION

William F. Armstrong and Peter G. Hagan

PRINCIPLES OF EVALUATION
Ultrasound Techniques
AORTIC VALVE DISEASE
Evaluation of Aortic Stenosis
Doppler Evaluation of Aortic Stenosis
Concurrent Valvular Lesions
Other Anatomic Features
Aortic Insufficiency
Determination of Regurgitation Severity
Assessment of Ventricular Function
MITRAL VALVE DISEASE
Normal Anatomy
Mitral Stenosis
Mitral Regurgitation
Mitral Valve Repair
Mitral Valve Prolapse
TRICUSPID AND PULMONARY VALVE DISEASE
Tricuspid Stenosis
Tricuspid Regurgitation
Pulmonary Hypertension
Pulmonary Stenosis
Prosthetic Heart Valves
MISCELLANEOUS VALVULAR CONDITIONS
Valvulopathy Associated With Anorectic Agents
Marfan's Syndrome
Aortic Dissection
Echocardiographic Findings in Endocarditis

Valvular heart disease, although less common in adult patients than ischemic heart disease, remains a challenging diagnostic and therapeutic dilemma of substantial proportion. Patients with valvular heart disease may come to medical attention with a broad range of clinical presentations including syncope, congestive heart failure, chest pain, fatigue, and arrhythmias. The presentation can be acute, chronic, or subacute. In addition, valvular heart disease can coexist with other forms of organic heart disease. Because therapy of these entities is distinct for each, accurate identification of the component of valvular heart disease is essential for appropriate management.

Modern cardiac ultrasound techniques afford a widely disseminated, easily performed, low-risk, and relatively low-cost means of evaluating all forms of valvular heart disease. This chapter reviews the principles of ultrasound evaluation of valvular heart disease and its application to specific lesions.

PRINCIPLES OF EVALUATION

Cardiac ultrasound techniques, because they afford excellent visualization of all four cardiac chambers, all four valves, and the great vessels, are an ideal tool for assessing valvular disease. The two-dimensional echocardiogram is an excellent tool for determining left ventricular (LV) function, which is a critical factor in management of patients with valvular lesions. By combining Doppler techniques, an accurate assessment of the severity of most valvular lesions, whether regurgitant or stenotic, is also easily obtained. An appropriate assessment of the underlying anatomy and subsequent physiologic effects is essential for planning appropriate therapy, decision-making regarding timing of intervention, and the appropriateness of medical therapy. The extensive role of echocardiography in the evaluation of patients with valvular heart disease has been outlined in the American Heart Association/American College of Cardiology documents on the management of patients with valvular heart disease and guidelines on utilization of echocardiography.[1, 2]

Ultrasound Techniques

Modern cardiac ultrasound machines support a wide variety of transducers and imaging approaches. Transthoracic imaging involves placing a transducer on the surface of the chest or, alternately, in the subxiphoid or suprasternal area.[3, 4] The ultrasound beam is then directed as a fan-shaped array into the mediastinum, where tomographic imaging planes of the heart are recorded. Transesophageal echocardiography (TEE) involves inserting a modified gastroscope into the esophagus. Modern probes provide imaging in multiple planes and support M-mode and all Doppler modalities and three-dimensional image reconstruction.[5, 6]

The complete cardiac ultrasound examination is multimodal. The basic screening tool is the two-dimensional (2-D) echocardiogram, which records a high-resolution view of all four cardiac chambers and all four valves (Figs. 20–1 to 20–3). Chamber sizes and systolic function can be easily assessed. The anatomic characteristics of valvular lesions are also accurately determined. The accuracy and resolution of the technique are such that linear dimensions are accurate within a 3- to 4-mm range of error and volumetric measurements within a 5 to 10 percent range of error in experienced laboratories.[7–11]

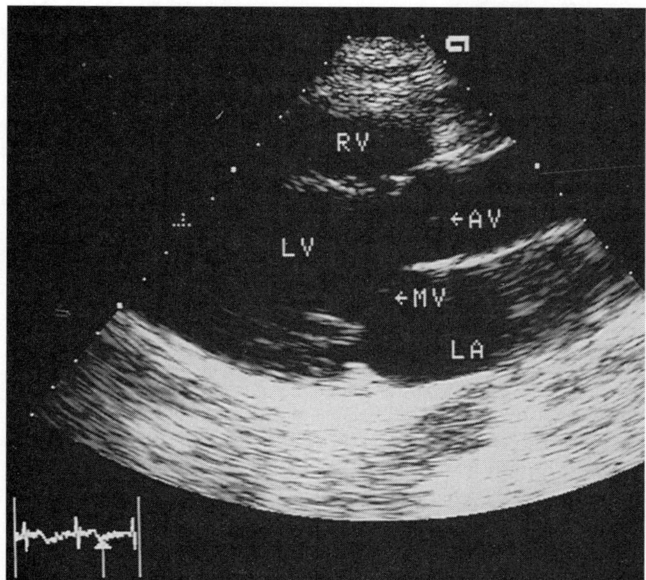

FIGURE 20–1 Parasternal long-axis two-dimensional echocardiogram in a normal patient. The proximal aorta and the aortic (AV) and mitral (MV) valves are visible, as are the ventricular septum, left ventricular cavity, and posterior left ventricular wall. LA, left atrium; LV, left ventricle; RV, right ventricle.

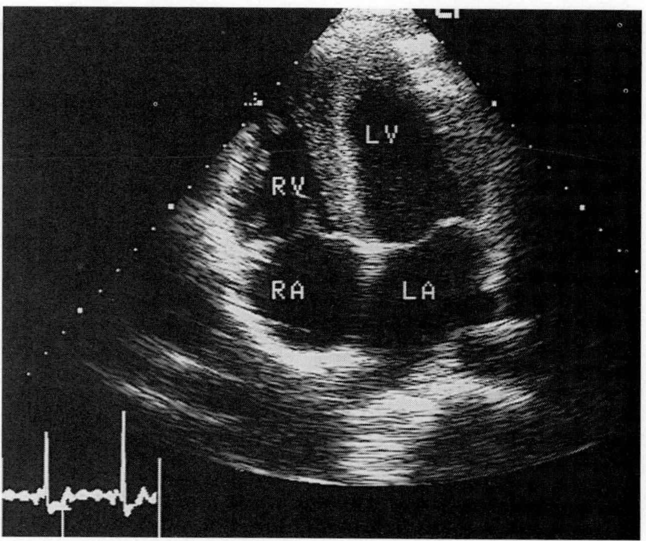

FIGURE 20–3 Four-chamber view of the left (LV) and right (RV) ventricles recorded from the apical transducer position. All four cardiac chambers as well as the ventricular septum and interatrial septum are visible. The mitral and tricuspid valves are likewise seen. LA, left atrium; RA, right atrium.

The *Doppler phenomenon* refers to the change in frequency in ultrasound as it is reflected from a moving target (red blood cells).[12, 13] This change in frequency (the Doppler shift) can then be used to calculate the velocity of the moving red blood cells. From the velocity, the pressure gradient between two chambers can be determined.

Spectral Doppler, from which these measurements are made, can be recorded in two different formats. The first is pulsed-wave Doppler, in which a small, user-selectable area of interrogation is defined and superimposed on the cardiac image. The interrogation of the Doppler shift occurs only at this location. The advantage of pulsed-wave Doppler is that the operator can precisely localize an area within the heart and determine flow velocity and direction exclusively at that point. Its disadvantage is the limited maximal velocity that can be detected. As typically employed, the maximal velocity that can be accurately recorded with pulsed-wave Doppler is approximately 2 m/s. However, many pathologic states have velocities greater than 2 m/s.

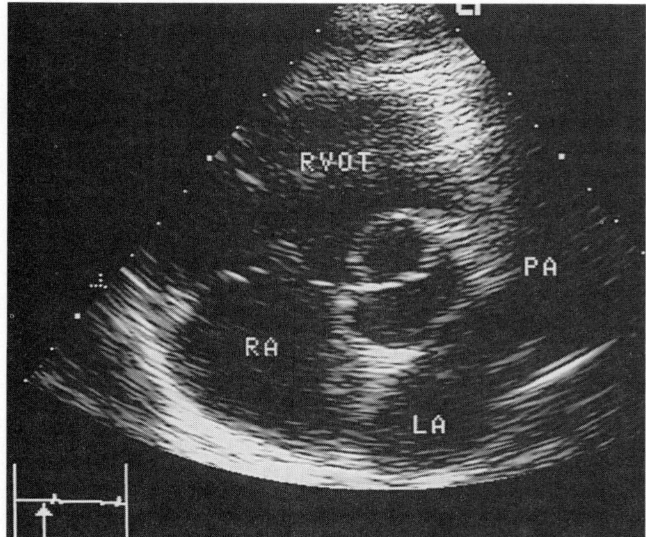

FIGURE 20–2 Short-axis view of the left ventricle at the base of the heart recorded from the parasternal position. The tricuspid valve, right ventricular outflow tract (RVOT), pulmonary artery (PA), aorta, and left (LA) and right (RA) atria are all visualized.

The second format available for processing of spectral signals is continuous-wave Doppler. With continuous-wave Doppler, there is constant transmission and reception of the Doppler beam. This affords an unlimited range of spectral shifts and velocities that can be recorded accurately but results in "range ambiguity." Although the line of interrogation can be user-selected, the location along the line of interrogation at which the maximal velocity occurs is unknown. Because maximal velocity occurs at the area of greatest stenosis, the location of the gradient can often be surmised from the anatomic information available from the 2-D image.

Calculation of transvalvular gradients relies on utilization of the Bernoulli equation.[12, 13] This well-validated equation stipulates that the difference in pressure (P) between two chambers can be related to the velocity of flow (V) between the two chambers, convective acceleration, viscous friction, and mass of the fluid in motion. In most biologic systems, and within the limits of most disease processes encountered, viscous friction and convective acceleration are not pertinent. Therefore, the Bernoulli equation can be simplified to the form

$$P = 4V^2$$

This simplified form assumes that the velocity on the proximal side of the stenotic orifice is trivial in magnitude compared with that distal to the stenosis. This may not be applicable in all patients. Exceptions, such as serial stenoses (hypertrophic myopathy in combination with aortic stenosis is a classic example) or severe aortic insufficiency combined with aortic stenosis, are occasionally encountered, in which case the proximal velocity must also be considered.

The modified Bernoulli equation allows calculation of a pressure gradient at any instant in time. By integrating the instantaneous pressure gradient at multiple time points, the mean pressure gradient can be accurately calculated.

Information content from the spectral signals is not limited to peak velocity and pressure alone. The timing, duration, and intensity of spectral signal provide information regarding the nature and severity of the lesion. The contour of the spectral signal can be analyzed for information regarding both the relaxation properties of the ventricle in diastole and the contractile properties of the ventricle in systole.[14–18]

The third major Doppler recording mode is color-flow imaging.[19–21] Color-flow imaging involves the simultaneous recording of multiple pulsed-wave interrogation sites. These multiple sites are superimposed on the anatomic image and updated at variable intervals. The direction and velocity of flow at each of the individual interrogation points are color encoded. The color-encoding scheme most commonly employed uses various shades of red to indicate flow toward the transducer and various shades of blue to indicate flow away from the transducer. Superimposed on this red-blue scheme is a variance map that color-encodes in green those areas that represent turbulent or high-velocity flow beyond the limits for accurate representation in red or blue. Color-flow imaging provides a means for simultaneously interrogating large areas of the cardiac chambers for both normal and abnormal flow. It allows the dimension and orientation of regurgitant jets to be assessed within chambers. By interrogating from multiple views, the three-dimensional size of regurgitant jets can be surmised. The clinical utility of this observation is discussed later. The subsequent portions of this chapter deal with the applicability of cardiac ultrasound to specific valvular lesions.

Aortic Valve Disease

Disease of the aortic valve in adults occurs in several forms (Table 20–1). Each can result in either stenosis or regurgitation. Classically, however, one or the other predominates. Anatomic assessment of the aortic valve is performed with 2-D echocardiographic imaging from both transthoracic and transesophageal approaches. Features to be noted from an anatomic standpoint include the number, size, shape, thickness, mobility, and degree of calcification of leaflets.[22–25] Congenital lesions, such as unicuspid, bicuspid, and quadricuspid valves, are usually readily apparent (Fig. 20–4). With modern techniques, experienced laboratories can identify the number of leaflets in the aortic valve in the majority of patients.[26] Ancillary anatomic features to be noted at the time of the examination include the size and shape of the aortic root, specifically the annular dimension, presence and absence of dilatation of the sinuses of Val-

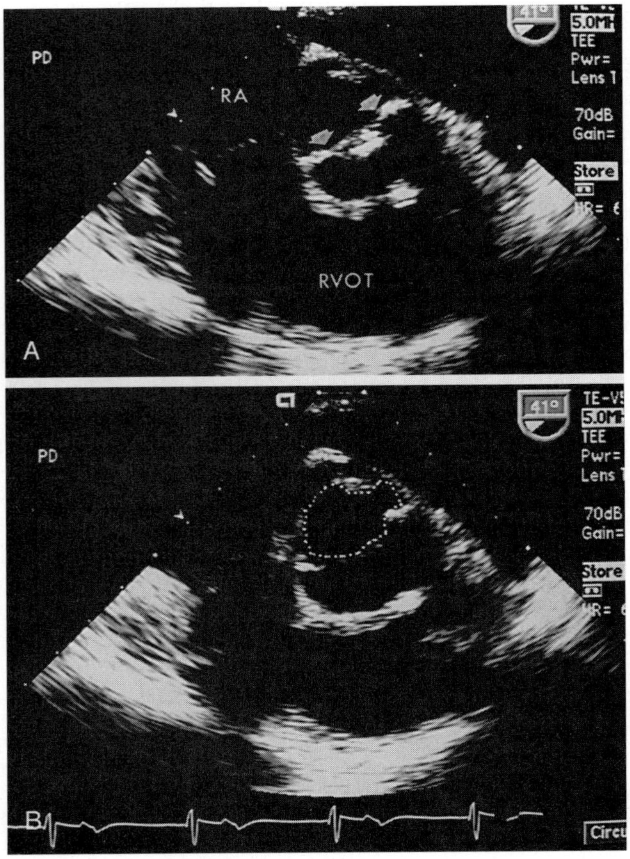

Figure 20–4 Transesophageal echocardiogram (TEE) recorded in a patient with a bicuspid aortic valve. This view is recorded in both diastole **(A)** and systole **(B)**. In this view, the aorta is seen in its cross section as a circular structure surrounded by the right atrium (RA) and right ventricular outflow tract (RVOT). In diastole, the closure line of the bicuspid valve can be seen (*arrows*). **B** was recorded in systole, and the eccentric, nearly circular opening of the bicuspid aortic valve is outlined by the *dotted line*.

salva, and the size, shape, and configuration of the tubular aorta. TEE can accurately estimate the aortic annulus size usually to within 1 mm.

The type of aortic dilatation can give valuable clues to the etiology of aortic valve disease. A classic example is that of Marfan's syndrome, in which predominantly dilatation of the sinuses occurs, with secondary involvement of the aortic annulus or the valve itself.[27, 28]

Once the number of leaflets has been established, attention should be turned to the leaflet characteristics. The normal aortic valve has three almost equally sized leaflets that are thin and highly mobile (see Fig. 20–1). They are free of calcification, and the mobility of all three leaflets is equivalent. The mobility is such that the leaflets typically lie against the wall of the aorta during systole and close in a midline fashion. The degree of thickening can range from mild, without associated calcification, to heavily calcified, almost immobile leaflets, as seen in calcific aortic stenosis (Figs. 20–5 and 20–6).

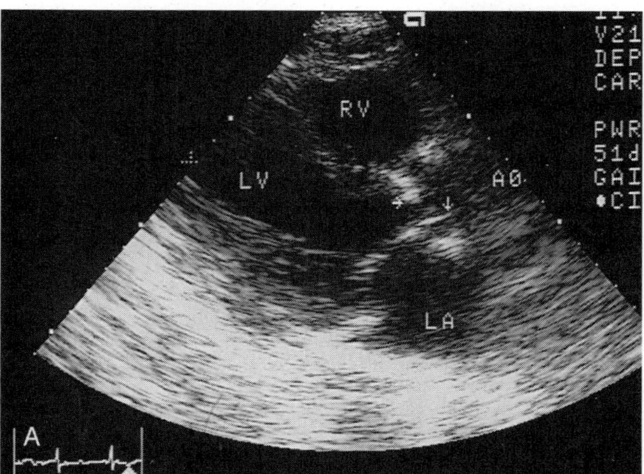

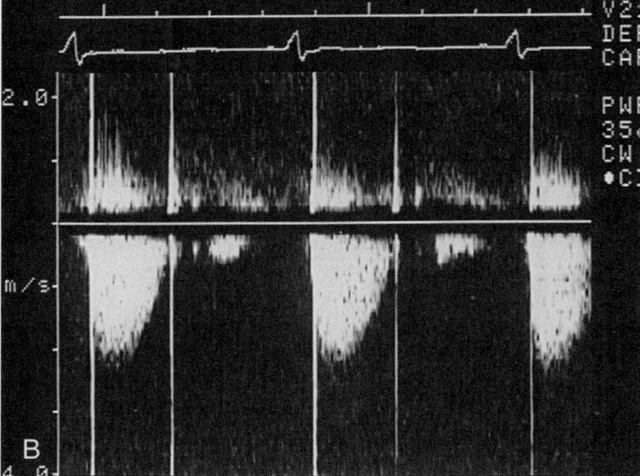

FIGURE 20–5 Two-dimensional echocardiogram and continuous-wave Doppler recorded in a patient with mild aortic stenosis. **A,** Systole. Note the fixed, anteriorly located leaflet of the right coronary cusp in the aorta (AO) and the freely mobile noncoronary cusp (*vertical arrow*). LA, left atrium; LV, left ventricle; RV, right ventricle. **B,** Note the continuous-wave Doppler recorded from the apical transducer position. The peak velocity is 2.2 ms, which corresponds to a peak instantaneous gradient of 19 mm Hg across the aortic valve.

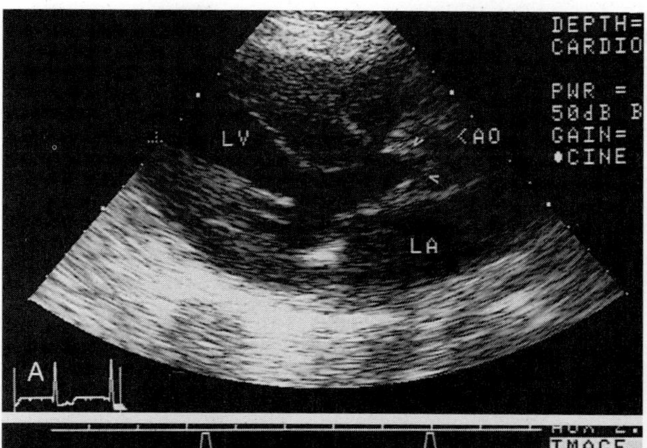

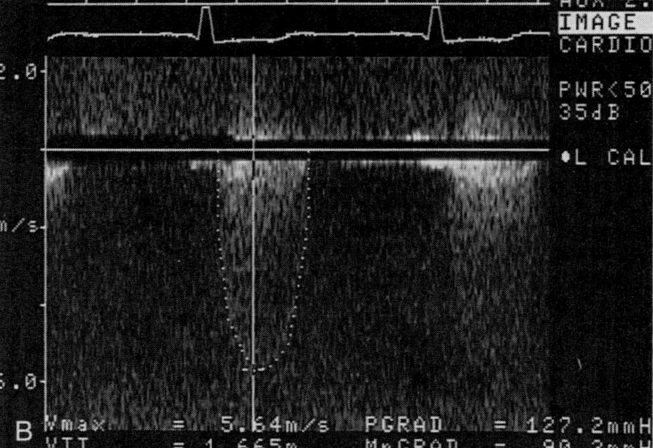

FIGURE 20–6 A, Parasternal long-axis view recorded in systole in a patient with severe aortic stenosis. Note the marked left ventricular hypertrophy with thickening of the septum and posterior wall. The aortic valve is dense and immobile (*arrowheads*). AO, aortic valve; LA, left atrium; LV, left ventricle. **B,** Continuous-wave Doppler from the apex. The peak instantaneous gradient is 127 mm Hg and the mean gradient is 90 mm Hg.

Increased leaflet mobility is less frequently seen, but some degree may occur in bicuspid (Fig. 20–7) and unicuspid valves, which may appear to prolapse below the level of the aortic valve annulus. The aortic valve can also be

TABLE 20–1 Aortic Valve Disease

Congenital	
Bicuspid	*(S > R)*
Unicuspid	*(S > R)*
Quadricuspid	*(R > S)*
Acquired	
Rheumatic	R = S
Degenerative	S > R
Senile	S > R
Connective tissue disease–related	R > S
Endocarditis	R >> S
Related to aortic pathology	R
Miscellaneous	
Cystic medial necrosis	R
Myxomatous disease	R

Abbreviations: S, stenotic physiology predominates; R, regurgitant physiology predominates.

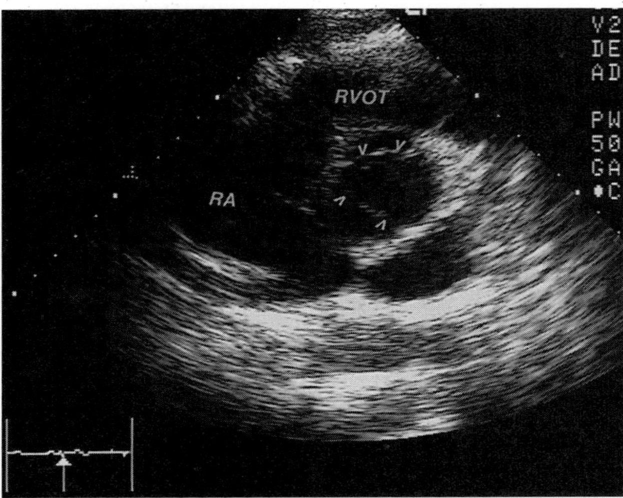

FIGURE 20–7 Parasternal short-axis view in a patient with a bicuspid aortic valve. In this systolic frame, note the two leaflets with commissures running horizontally (*arrowheads*). RA, right atrium; RVOT, right ventricular outflow tract.

involved in myxomatous valve degeneration, at which point associated sinus dilatation and diffuse thickening of the aortic valve leaflets are often seen. Secondary causes of aortic valve disease, such as aortic dissection, can also be detected with cardiac ultrasound techniques.[29, 30]

Other types of aortic valve disease include infective endocarditis. With high-frequency transducers, vegetations as small as 3 mm can be readily identified. Identification and characterization of vegetations with regard to their diffuse or focal nature, size, and mobility can also be performed and may provide prognostic information concerning the likelihood of complications.[31–35]

Once the anatomic type of aortic valve disease has been established, its functional consequences must be determined, including both the severity of stenosis or regurgitation and any subsequent effects on ventricular size and function.

Evaluation of Aortic Stenosis

The evaluation of aortic stenosis is both anatomic and functional, and most of the information can be gained from a good-quality transthoracic study (Table 20–2). An echocardiogram is indicated to diagnose and assess severity of stenosis, to assess LV size and function, and to re-evaluate specific patients with known aortic stenosis.[2]

While TEE may provide clearer structural details, Doppler pressure assessment of the aortic valve is better performed from a surface echocardiogram. The normal adult aortic valve orifice is 3 to 4 cm^2. An aortic valve area greater than 1.5 cm^2 is considered mild, and less than 1.0 cm^2 is considered severe aortic stenosis. Obviously, the clinical significance of a given valve area will vary according to patient characteristics such as body size, age, gender, and cardiac work.[22–25] The echocardiographic evaluation of aortic stenosis begins with assessment of anatomy, leaflet thickening, calcification, and mobility. LV size, function, hypertrophy, and associated lesions can be evaluated, and the underlying pathophysiologic process can frequently be determined.

Doppler Evaluation of Aortic Stenosis

The key to evaluating the severity of aortic stenosis is to determine the transvalvular gradient. This can be accomplished in the majority of patients with aortic stenosis by aligning a continuous-wave Doppler beam parallel to flow through the stenotic orifice and determining flow velocity. Care must be taken not to contaminate the signal with mitral regurgitation and to look for nonvalvular causes of a pressure gradient, such as dynamic subaortic muscular obstruction, which is typically seen in elderly patients. Using modifications of the Bernoulli equation, both the instantaneous and the mean transvalvular gradients can be obtained. When compared with directly measured pressure gradients in the catheterization laboratory, there is excellent correlation for both instantaneous peak and mean pressure gradients (Fig. 20–8; see also Figs. 20–6 and 20–7).[36–44] Nonsimultaneous measurements, as are typically acquired, often result in underestimation of transvalvular gradients by Doppler ultrasound techniques.[37] The most common reason for this is that in the catheterization laboratory, patients are studied in an excited state during which cardiac output and stroke volume are increased compared with that seen during the resting state in the echocardiography laboratory. Because the transvalvular pressure gradient is directly related to stroke volume, the lower cardiac output in a calm patient results in a lower valvular gradient determined in the echocardiography laboratory.

A mean pressure gradient of greater than 50 mm Hg typically correlates with severe stenosis. In patients with decreased cardiac output, calculated valve area may reflect decreased valve opening and overestimate the severity of stenosis. In addition to determination of peak and mean gradients, aortic valve areas can be calculated by the continuity equation.[45–50] The continuity equation is based on the assumption that all flow at the left ventricular outflow tract (LVOT) subsequently moves through the stenotic aortic valve. As volumetric flow can be calculated as the product

TABLE 20–2 Echocardiographic Assessment of the Aortic Valve

Aortic Stenosis

Anatomic features: etiology, calcification, leaflet number, mobility
Continuous-wave Doppler: mean and peak pressure gradient
Valve area calculation: continuity equation, planimetry
Dobutamine echo in low-gradient LV dysfunction
Secondary/associated abnormalities: LVH, LV dysfunction, poststenotic dilatation, mitral regurgitation

Aortic Regurgitation

Anatomic features: etiology, bicuspid valve, dilated annulus
Color-flow Doppler: jet width, jet area, PISA
Spectral Doppler
Continuous-wave: pressure half-time, intensity
Pulsed-wave: diastolic flow reversal in aorta, LVOT velocity, regurgitant fraction, flow reversal in descending aorta

Abbreviations: LV, left ventricular; LVH, left ventricular hypertrophy; LVOT, left ventricular outflow tract; PISA, proximal isovelocity surface area.

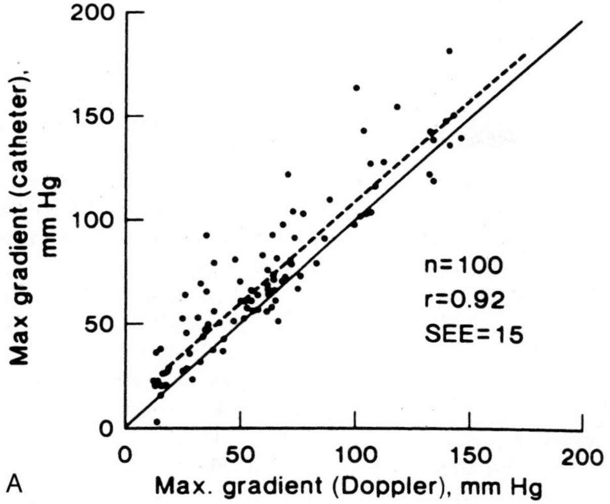

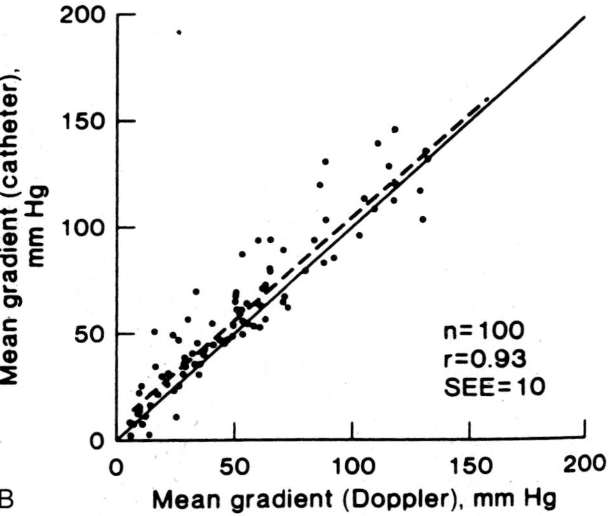

FIGURE 20–8 Graphic comparison of Doppler-derived and simultaneous catheterization-derived aortic valve gradients in 100 patients. **A,** Maximal gradient by Doppler and catheterization. **B,** Mean gradients. Note the superb correlation between the two techniques over a broad range of pressure gradients. (**A** and **B** from Currie PJ, Seward JB, Reeder GS, et al: Continuous-wave Doppler echocardiographic assessment of severity of calcific aortic stenosis: a simultaneous Doppler-catheter correlative study in 100 adult patients. Circulation 71[6]:1162–1169, 1985.)

of cross-sectional area (volume thickness index [VTI]) and mean velocity, the simple equation

$$\text{Aortic valve area} = \frac{\text{Area(LVOT)} \times \text{VTI(LVOT)}}{\text{VTI (valve)}}$$

can then be solved. In high-quality studies, where the LVOT dimension can be reliably determined, this method for calculating the aortic orifice compares very favorably with that determined invasively from the Gorlin formula.[10] The major limitation of this calculation is accurate determination of LVOT size. In suboptimal studies, substantial inaccuracy can occur. Although the continuity equation allows calculation of an aortic valve area independent of both LV function and the presence of aortic insufficiency, valve area itself can vary with changes in transaortic volume flow rate.

Clinically, one is frequently faced with the dilemma of a relatively low transvalvular aortic valve gradient in the presence of critical aortic stenosis as seen in patients with significant LV dysfunction.[44] If uncertainty regarding clinical decision-making remains, evaluation of transvalvular gradients can be achieved at two different flow rates by performing studies at rest and after dobutamine infusion.[51]

Aortic valve area may be directly measured by planimetry either from a transthoracic study or more readily by TEE (see Fig. 20–4).

Concurrent Valvular Lesions

It is important to note the presence or absence of concurrent valvular lesions in patients with aortic stenosis. Aortic insufficiency ranging from mild to severe can coexist with stenosis and complicates the calculation of valve area from the Gorlin formula. As noted previously, the continuity equation is not dependent on the presence of isolated aortic stenosis and remains an accurate means of determining aortic valve area when concurrent insufficiency is present. The presence or absence of concurrent mitral valve disease can also be assessed. Up to two thirds of patients with aortic stenosis will have concomitant mitral regurgitation, and it appears that reduction in mitral regurgitation postoperatively appears to be related to decreased LV pressure and changes in morphology.[52]

Other Anatomic Features

In addition to evaluation of valve anatomy and severity of stenosis, an assessment of LV size, function, hypertrophy, and degree of poststenotic dilatation of the aorta can be obtained from the ultrasound examination.[18, 44, 53–56] As a general rule, LV systolic dysfunction is not considered a contraindication to aortic valve replacement in the presence of critical aortic stenosis. It is important, however, to determine aortic valve area to ensure that the degree of dysfunction is compatible with the degree of stenosis. Similarly, valve area should be consistent with the observed pressure gradient.

The average rate of progression of aortic stenosis has been estimated at 0.12 cm^2, although the rate of progression in a given valve cannot be predicted.[57]

According to recently published guidelines, echocardiography should be performed at least annually in patients with severe stenosis, biannually in patients with moderate stenosis, and every 5 years for mild stenosis.[1]

Aortic Insufficiency

Aortic insufficiency has many etiologies that may overlap with aortic stenosis. These are listed in Table 20–1 and include the sequelae of rheumatic heart disease; degenerative disease; endocarditis; congenital anomalies, such as the bicuspid valve; and developmental anomalies, such as those associated with myxomatous valvular disease,

Marfan's syndrome, or aortic insufficiency acquired as a result of dissecting aortic aneurysms. The management approach is heavily dependent on the anatomy of the aortic valve and of the aorta itself. Echocardiography can serve as the sole diagnostic technique for identifying the underlying anatomic defect and planning appropriate surgical procedures in many instances. Doppler echocardiography is a sensitive technique for the determination of regurgitation, and a mild degree of regurgitation is often seen in normal adults.[58]

Multiple methods should be combined to obtain a semiquantitative assessment (see Table 20–2). The degree of regurgitation at a given time may vary significantly depending on factors that affect pressure gradients and flow across the valve, such as blood pressure, heart rate, and myocardial loading conditions. Also, because measurements are subjective and no "gold standard" is available, precise assessment is often difficult.[1]

As noted for stenosis of this valve, the anatomy can be defined as either a two-leaflet or a three-leaflet valve, and nonvalvular primary pathology involving the aortic root. TEE may be necessary for accurate description of pathology involving the aorta predominantly, but the valve itself can often be completely characterized from the transthoracic approach.

Determination of Regurgitation Severity

A number of algorithms have been proposed for determining the severity of aortic insufficiency, including depth of penetration and overall size of the aortic insufficiency jet (Plate 20–1).[56, 60–62] Unlike mitral regurgitation, these algorithms are less accurate in aortic insufficiency. Refinements on color-flow Doppler quantitation of aortic insufficiency have included determining the diameter of the regurgitant jet at its orifice.[59, 60] By doing so, a fairly accurate estimate of the severity of aortic regurgitation, compared with quantitative or qualitative catheterization determinations, can be derived. The effective regurgitant orifice of the aortic regurgitation jet can be calculated by dividing the aortic regurgitant volume by the TVI of the regurgitant jet. This measurement is less affected by heart rate and loading conditions than other techniques.[63, 64]

Aortic regurgitation is considered severe if greater than 50 percent of the LVOT is filled by the regurgitant jet at its origin and mild if the jet occupies less than 20 percent of the LVOT. Evaluation of eccentric jets is more challenging, and severity is often underestimated. Calculating regurgitant volume from the proximal isovelocity surface area is based on the principle that blood accelerates in a laminar fashion toward a regurgitant orifice, forming multiple hemispheres of isovelocity. The flow rate through any given hemisphere will equal the regurgitant flow rate. Color-flow Doppler can be used to determine the flow rate, which in turn, is used to calculate regurgitant volume.

An additional method for determining the severity of aortic insufficiency is examination of the spectral profile of the insufficiency jet.[13] The velocity of the insufficiency jet can be related to the instantaneous pressure gradient between the aorta and the left ventricle.[61, 62, 65] The rate at which these two pressures equilibrate in diastole is directly related to the severity of the regurgitant lesion. Severe aortic regurgitation allows rapid equilibration of diastolic aortic and LV pressures, and therefore, the deceleration of the aortic insufficiency jet is rapid. Mild degrees of aortic insufficiency do not cause equilibration of pressure, and therefore, the deceleration of the jet velocity is substantially longer. The half-time of deceleration can be quantified and appears to relate directly to the severity of aortic insufficiency. A pressure half-time of less than 300 ms is consistent with severe aortic regurgitation. As with mitral pressure half-time, this assessment is dependent on the presence of isolated aortic insufficiency and no other significant derangement of ventricular performance. Similarly, in severe aortic regurgitation, mitral inflow velocity reflects elevated LV pressure with a rapid deceleration time and an increased E/A ratio.

Other features on Doppler assessment that suggest severe aortic regurgitation are holodiastolic reversal of flow in the descending aorta and LVOT velocity greater than 1.8 m/s.

Assessment of Ventricular Function

Many decisions to proceed to surgical replacement of the aortic valve for aortic regurgitation are based as much on the degree of subsequent LV dilatation and systolic dysfunction as they are on the severity of the regurgitation itself. Long-term follow-up studies in patients with chronic aortic insufficiency suggest that serial echocardiographic measurements of LV size and systolic performance are valuable tools for following patients with aortic insufficiency.[1, 66–70] Patients with substantial LV dilatation, baseline reduction in systolic function, or substantial serial increases in size or decreases in ventricular function are appropriate candidates for aortic valve replacement. If undertaken before the occurrence of severe LV dysfunction, aortic valve replacement is highly successful in relieving symptoms and preventing long-term LV dysfunction.[71–74] Conversely, patients with marked LV dilatation and poor systolic function are less likely to have recovery of function after aortic valve replacement and less likely to experience symptomatic relief.

MITRAL VALVE DISEASE

Because the appropriate decision for operative versus nonoperative intervention and the nature of an intervention are heavily dependent on the valvular anatomy in mitral valve disease, it is on lesions of this valve that echocardiography often has the greatest impact. This is true for both stenotic and regurgitant lesions. Multiple etiologies exist for regurgitant and stenotic lesions of the mitral valve (Table 20–3).

Normal Anatomy

The normal mitral valve is a bileaflet structure, typically with the anterior leaflet being longer and having a greater surface area than the posterior leaflet (see Fig. 20–1). The leaflet inserts in the fibrous skeleton of the heart. The mitral annulus represents a geometric figure equivalent to

TABLE 20-3 Mitral Valve Disease

Congenital	
Parachute deformity	S >> R
Other stenosis	S > R
Cleft valve	R
Acquired	
Rheumatic	S > R
Endocarditis	R >> S
Ischemic-functional	R
Ruptured papillary muscle	R
Annular degeneration	R >> S
Ruptured chordae/flail leaflet	R
Miscellaneous	
Myxomatous with prolapse	R
Nonmyxomatous prolapse	R

Abbreviations: S, stenotic physiology predominates; R, regurgitant physiology predominates.

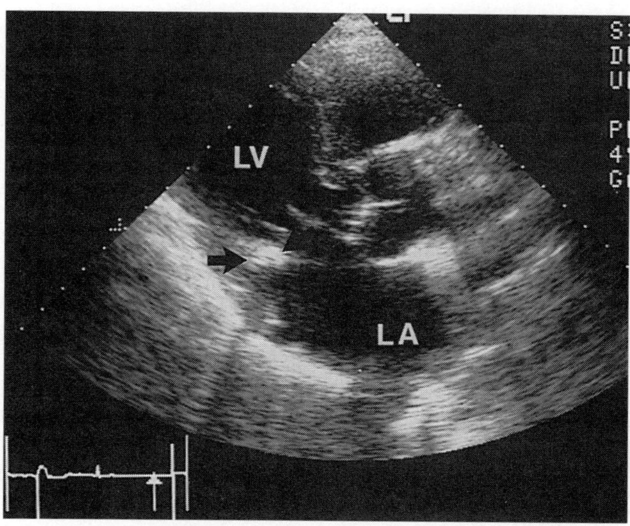

FIGURE 20–10 Parasternal long-axis view of a patient with a calcified mitral valve annulus. Note the dilated left atrium (LA) and the echo-dense mass of tissue in the posterior mitral annulus (*arrows*). LV, left ventricle.

a hyperbolic parabaloid.[75] From an anatomic standpoint, the mitral valve should be considered as consisting of several structures including the annulus, the leaflets, the chordae tendineae, and the papillary muscles. Any or all of the components of the mitral valve apparatus can be involved in pathologic processes. Certain pathophysiologic states affect one area of the mitral apparatus more than another. Examples are rheumatic valvular disease, which classically affects the mitral valve tips and chordae (Fig. 20–9); degenerative disease, which classically affects the mitral annulus (Fig. 20–10); and mitral valve prolapse (MVP) with myxomatous changes, which affects the body of the leaflet and the chordae (Fig. 20–11). Once the anatomic description of mitral valve pathology has been determined, assessments of its long-term behavior can be made and therapy decisions often can be made on the basis of the echocardiogram alone.

Depending on the nature of the anatomic defect, either stenosis or regurgitation can be present and, in many instances, can coexist. An assessment of the severity of either lesion is readily available from modern Doppler ultrasound techniques. Assessment of ventricular function can be made from the 2-D echocardiogram. Specific considerations for distinct mitral valve pathology follow.

Mitral Stenosis

In adults, mitral stenosis is almost exclusively due to the sequelae of rheumatic heart disease. Rare patients with congenital mitral stenosis may escape detection until adulthood, and a small percentage of patients with severe, ag-

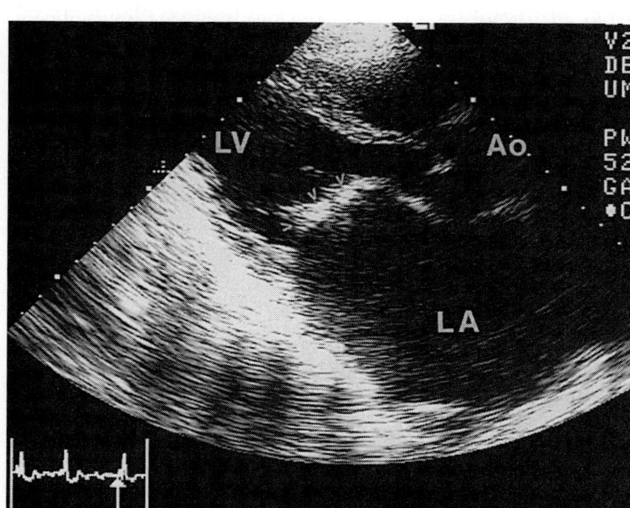

FIGURE 20–9 Parasternal long-axis echocardiogram in a patient with mitral stenosis. Note the dilated left atrium (LA) and the fibrotic, partially calcified mitral valve, which "domes" in diastole. AO, aorta; LV, left ventricle.

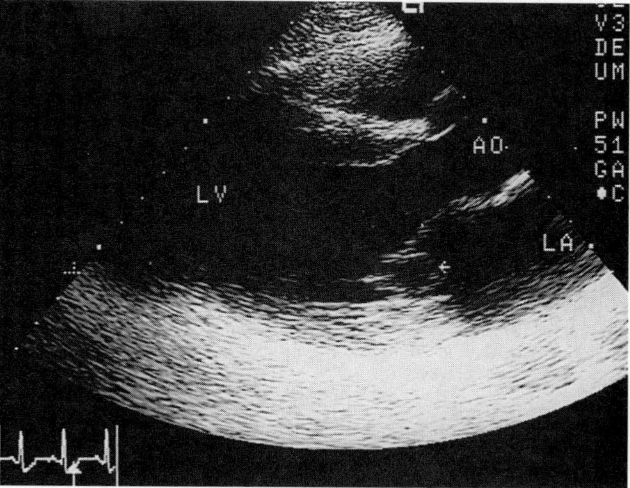

FIGURE 20–11 Parasternal long-axis echocardiogram in a patient with mitral valve prolapse with myxomatous changes. Note the redundant, thickened mitral valve leaflets and the buckling of the mitral valve into the left atrium (LA) in systole (*arrow*). AO, aorta; LV, left ventricle.

gressive mitral annular calcification can develop functional stenosis. These subsets of obstruction to the mitral orifice are relatively rare and can be readily identified by 2-D echocardiography. The hallmark of rheumatic mitral stenosis on 2-D echocardiography is fibrosis and thickening at the level of the mitral valve tips and proximal chordae. This causes fusion along the commissures and a reduction in the opening at the tips of the leaflet. The relatively cylindrical mitral valve channel then becomes more funnel-shaped, with its restrictive orifice at the level of the tips (see Fig. 20–9). Early in the disease process, the belly of the leaflet may remain uninvolved, causing a characteristic "doming" of the belly of the leaflet. With progression of the disease, fibrosis of the belly of the leaflet occurs and subsequent calcification can also be seen. Involvement of the submitral apparatus may also occur.

The hemodynamic effect of the restrictive orifice is to restrict the flow from the left atrium to the left ventricle, and a pressure gradient therefore occurs. The magnitude of this pressure gradient is directly proportional to the severity of the stenosis and the volumetric flow. The subsequent elevation in left atrial (LA) pressure, which is present throughout the cardiac cycle, results in progressive dilatation of the left atrium with attendant complications of atrial fibrillation, stasis of blood, and thrombus formation in the left atrium. The chronically elevated LA and pulmonary venous pressures can eventually lead to pulmonary hypertension. In its fully developed form, critical mitral stenosis can be associated with a massively dilated and fibrillating atrium with pulmonary hypertension, subsequent right ventricular (RV) failure, and tricuspid regurgitation. Milder forms may exist for several decades in an isolated form, resulting in only mild to moderate pressure gradients between the left atrium and the left ventricle.

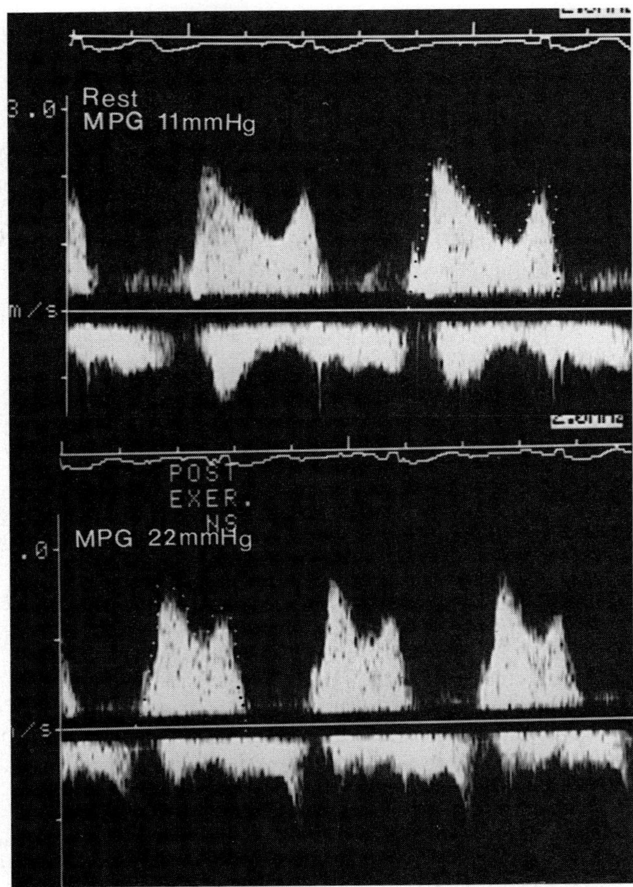

FIGURE 20–12 Continuous-wave Doppler recorded from the apex of the left ventricle in a patient with mitral stenosis. **A,** The characteristic mitral stenosis spectral flow profile was recorded at rest. A mean pressure gradient of 11 mm Hg is noted. **B,** after 60 seconds of leg lifts, the mean pressure gradient has doubled to 22 mm Hg.

Assessment of Severity

Assessment of the severity of mitral stenosis involves the determination not only of its anatomic severity but also its physiologic importance (Table 20–4). Anatomically, the degree of fibrosis and calcification should be noted from the echocardiogram. By careful scanning in the short-axis plane, images can be recorded through the actual restrictive orifice of the mitral valve, which can then be planimetered. This orifice area compares favorably with the hemodynamically determined mitral valve areas from the Gorlin equation.[76, 77]

In addition to this direct assessment of mitral valve area, pressure gradients can be measured with Doppler techniques.[36] With the transducer placed at the apex of the left ventricle, using either pulsed-wave or continuous-wave Doppler recordings, the spectral display of the LA to LV blood flow can be recorded (Fig. 20–12). From this, the mean pressure gradient can be accurately calculated. This calculated transvalvular gradient compares favorably with that determined at the time of simultaneous cardiac catheterization. In addition, gradients can be determined after exercise.[78] In patients with mitral stenosis, the simple maneuver of 60 seconds of leg lifts is often sufficient to demonstrate unequivocal increases in the mitral valve pressure gradients. Demonstration of dramatic increases in mitral transvalvular pressures often provides the clinical explanation for symptoms in patients who otherwise appear to have only modest degrees of obstruction at rest (see Fig. 20–12).

TABLE 20–4 Echocardiographic Assessment of the Mitral Valve

Mitral Stenosis
Anatomic features: etiology, diastolic doming, leaflet thickening, degree of calcification
Continuous-wave Doppler: mean and peak pressure gradient at rest and exercise, pressure half-time
Valve area calculation: planimetry
Valve area calculation: continuity equation
Color-flow Doppler: PISA
Mitral Regurgitation
Anatomic features: etiology, annular dilatation, prolapse, flail leaflet
Color-flow Doppler: jet area, jet width, PISA
Spectral Doppler
Continuous-wave: intensity, peak velocity
Pulsed-wave: pulmonary vein systolic flow reversal, regurgitant fraction

Abbreviation: PISA, proximal isovelocity surface area.

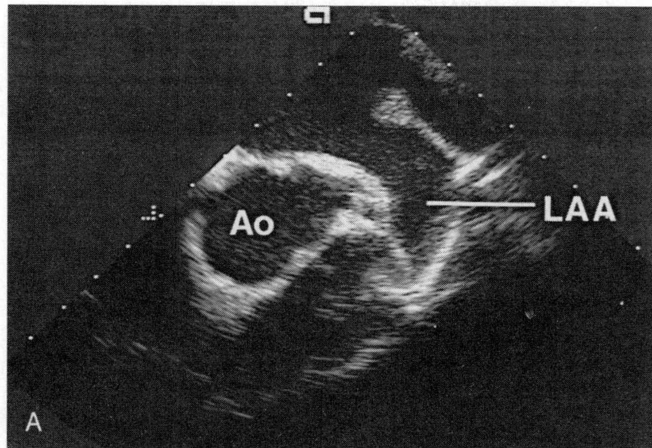

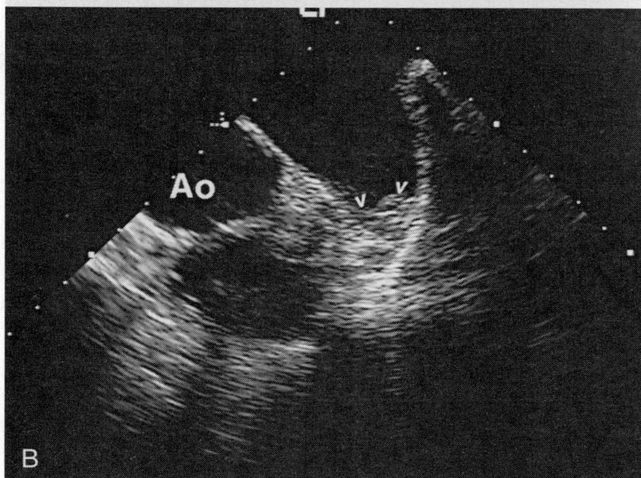

FIGURE 20–13 TEEs recorded in two patients. **A,** Note the normal left atrial appendage (LAA), which is free of spontaneous contrast or thrombus. AO, aorta. **B,** TEE recorded in a patient with mitral stenosis and a left atrial appendage thrombus (*arrowheads*).

A final method for determining the severity of mitral stenosis is from the mitral pressure gradient half-time of decay.[79–82] This concept, initially developed from hemodynamic data in the cardiac catheterization laboratory, appears applicable to patients in sinus rhythm with isolated mitral stenosis and without other major abnormalities of intracardiac physiology. The mechanism for determining mitral stenosis severity from the pressure half-time is recognition that an empirical constant (220 milliseconds) can be related to mitral valve area. The pressure half-time is the time (in milliseconds) required for the initial peak instantaneous transmitral gradient to decay to half its highest value. The equation is

$$\text{Mitral valve area} = 220 \div P\tfrac{1}{2}T$$

This calculation may not be valid in patients with concurrent mitral regurgitation, aortic insufficiency, or severe ventricular hypertrophy.[80–82] It does appear to be accurate in patients with isolated mitral stenosis. It should be relied on with extreme caution otherwise.

Decisions Regarding Intervention

Once mitral stenosis is recognized in a symptomatic patient, a decision for operative or nonoperative intervention is often made. Accurate definition of the anatomic details of the lesion is critical for this assessment. The three interventional options available are replacement with a prosthetic valve, open commissurotomy and reconstruction, and mitral balloon valvotomy. When properly selected, patients will benefit from each of these interventions. However, mitral valvotomy and mitral valve reconstruction may be of limited practicality in patients with certain anatomic features.

It appears that increasing degrees of calcification, especially involving the commissures, substantial involvement of the submitral apparatus, and severe diffuse mitral fibrosis and immobility all militate against successful balloon valvotomy, and probably against open repair as well.[83–85]

When patients with these features are recognized, mitral valve replacement with a prosthetic valve is in order rather than attempting balloon valvotomy. Other features that have an impact on the decision to proceed with balloon valvotomy versus open repair include the presence of coexisting mitral regurgitation, which is a relative contraindication to balloon valvotomy.

TEE should be employed for a more refined assessment of mitral valve anatomy and to evaluate for the presence or absence of LA thrombus, which has been considered a contraindication to attempted balloon valvotomy (Figs. 20–13 and 20–14).[86] In patients with atrial fibrillation and/or embolic events, TEE plays a critical role in screening for potential cardiac sources of emboli, such as LA thrombus and stagnant blood. Decisions regarding the use of anticoagulants can be made on the basis of these findings.

After a mitral valve intervention (either operative or catheter-based), the 2-D echocardiogram and Doppler can be used to evaluate the success of these procedures.[83, 84, 87–89] The anatomic changes in the valve are often more

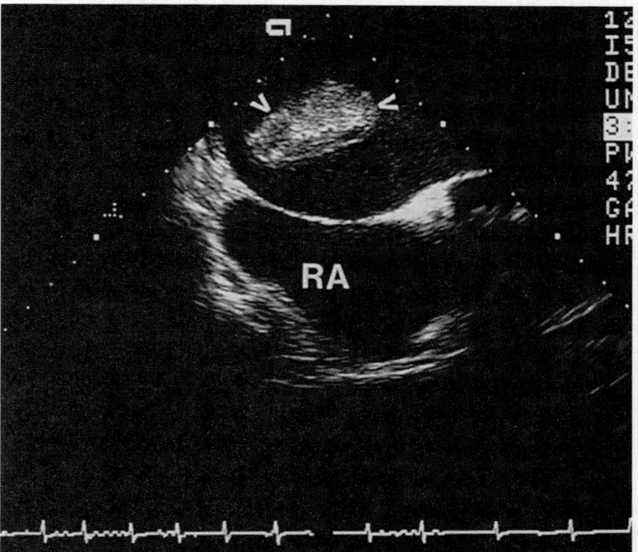

FIGURE 20–14 TEE from a patient with severe mitral stenosis and a massively dilated left atrium. Note the 2 × 4-cm thrombus in the body of the left atrium (*arrowheads*). RA, right atrium.

difficult to elucidate than the beneficial effect on transvalvular pressure gradients. Once instrumented, the mitral valve orifice frequently becomes irregular and direct quantitation becomes difficult. The transvalvular mitral gradient, however, remains accurate and can be determined both at rest and with exercise. The pressure half-time measurement is not accurate for determination for mitral valve area shortly after mitral valvotomy.[89] In addition to relief of obstruction, documentation of the subsequent degree of mitral regurgitation can be made.

Mitral Regurgitation

The severity and the mechanism of mitral regurgitation can be accurately determined from 2-D echocardiography and Doppler recordings (see Table 20–4). The potential mechanisms of mitral regurgitation are listed in Table 20–3, the majority of which are accurately identified from 2-D imaging. It is imperative to determine the mechanism of mitral regurgitation, as important therapeutic considerations will hinge on this. Some forms of mitral regurgitation (e.g., flail posterior leaflet) are readily approached surgically with a high degree of success in skilled hands.[90–92] Other forms are less likely to be repairable, and mitral valve replacement may be necessary.

One specific form of mitral regurgitation requiring comment is the flail mitral valve leaflet.[93, 94] The etiology of the flail leaflet can often be determined from the echocardiogram. Various etiologies include myxomatous change with ruptured chordae, vegetations with subsequent destruction of the chordal supporting apparatus, ischemic events with rupture of a papillary muscle head, trauma, and a certain subset that remains undefined. The hallmark of a flail leaflet is abnormal coaptation of the leaflet tips, so that one leaflet tip coapts behind the other (Fig. 20–15 and Plate 20–2). In addition, the leaflet tip may point backward into the left atrium and often has excessive random motion. Careful scanning in multiple planes, including TEE, enables the diagnosis of a flail leaflet to be made in the majority of cases. In addition to the direct visualization of an anatomic flail leaflet, color-flow Doppler imaging can provide valuable clues to the presence of a flail leaflet and can assist in determining which leaflet is flail.[90] The mechanism of regurgitation in a flail leaflet is that a jet forms along the LV boundary of the flail leaflet and is directed along the opposing leaflet. Therefore, an anterior flail leaflet results in a posterolaterally directed jet and a posterior flail leaflet in an anteriorly or septally directed jet (Plate 20–3). The jet direction, even when the flail leaflet is not seen, is highly accurate in determining which leaflet is flail.

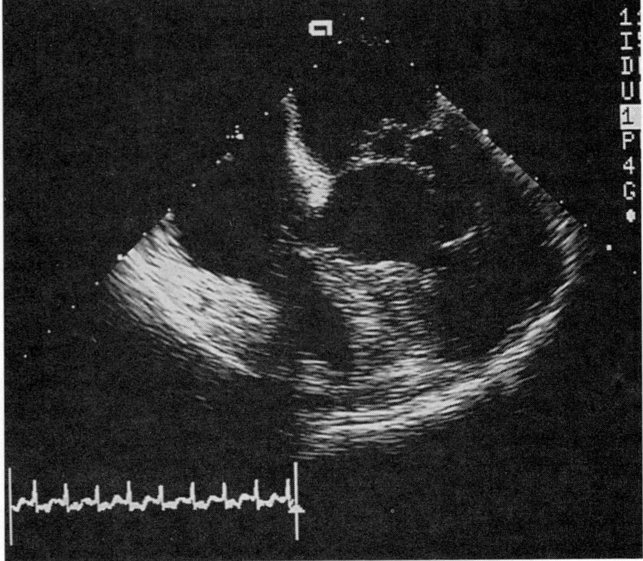

FIGURE 20–15 TEE in a patient with a flail posterior mitral valve leaflet. Note the redundant posterior leaflet, which coapts behind the anterior leaflet.

Determination of Regurgitation Severity

Determination of the severity of mitral regurgitation hinges on detecting the anatomic extent of the regurgitant jet. This is most efficiently done by color-flow Doppler imaging, from either the transthoracic or the transesophageal route. Many algorithms have been developed for assessing the severity of mitral regurgitation. These include determination of the depth of penetration into the left atrium, determination of the width of the jet, determination of the area of the jet and the jet area indexed to the LA size, and calculation of the proximal isovelocity surface area.[95–100]

A central jet area less than 20 percent is consistent with mild regurgitation and greater than 60 percent is consistent with severe regurgitation. As with aortic regurgitation, the effective regurgitant orifice of mitral regurgitation can be calculated. In general, severe mitral regurgitation is associated with an effective regurgitant orifice greater than 35 mm^2. Also, an intense signal on continuous-wave Doppler results from a large number of red blood cells in the jet. Other features of continuous-wave Doppler that suggest severe mitral regurgitation are peak velocity of less than 4 m/s (secondary to increased LA pressure) and an E velocity of greater than 2.2 m/s. Reversal of systolic flow in the pulmonary vein by pulsed-wave Doppler is suggestive of severe mitral regurgitation.[101] Doppler-determined grades of mitral regurgitation correlate favorably with those determined invasively in the cardiac catheterization laboratory.[99]

Several pitfalls can occur in making this assessment. These include dependency of the severity of mitral regurgitation on the driving pressure on the left ventricle. It is important to note the systolic blood pressure at the time of assessment of mitral regurgitation. Second, the pressure generating the regurgitant volume will not be directly and linearly related to the area of the jet. The perceived area of a regurgitation jet includes not only the regurgitant blood flow but also the blood already present in the left atrium, which has been forced into motion by the regurgitant jet. At higher driving pressures, the amount of "recruitment" is greater and therefore the jet area is greater.

A second well-described pitfall arises because of the Coanda effect.[102–104] This phenomenon refers to the apparent decrease in absolute jet volume when a regurgitant jet is adjacent to a solid boundary. A centrally located jet of any given size will assume a greater absolute and relative area than a regurgitant jet of identical volume that is eccentric and adjacent to the wall of the receiving chamber. Therefore, the absolute size of an eccentric jet will consistently underestimate (by as much as 40 percent) the amount of regurgitation that would be found if it had been centrally located. Recognition of these factors is essential to avoid inaccurate determination of mitral regurgitation severity. TEE is often helpful in determining anatomy and degree of severity of mitral regurgitation, particularly in the presence of an eccentric jet.

It is also critical to assess ventricular size and function in mitral regurgitation. Patients with a dilated left ventricle and markedly reduced systolic function are frequently poor candidates for mitral valve repair and are less likely to experience recovery of function and abolition of symptoms after valve replacement.

Mitral Valve Repair

Contemporary surgical techniques in mitral valve disease include an increasing reliance on repair rather than replacement of the mitral valve.[90–92] A variety of surgical techniques exist for repair of regurgitant mitral valves, including leaflet resection, chordal shortening, leaflet transplantation, and annular rings. It is important to appropriately select patients for mitral valve repair rather than replacement. The advantages of mitral valve repair are that it preserves LV function, obviates the need for long-term anticoagulation, and appears to have an excellent long-term follow-up. Complications of repair can include iatrogenic mitral stenosis and various degrees of residual mitral regurgitation.

Echocardiographic and Doppler techniques can play a critical role in selecting patients for mitral valve repair. The classic posterior flail leaflet can be readily identified as a lesion highly likely to be amenable to repair in skilled hands and to result in a successful repair. More complex forms of valvular disease, such as anterior flail leaflets or papillary muscle rupture, are less likely to result in a good repair and a gratifying clinical response. Therefore, the 2-D echocardiogram (transthoracic and transesophageal) can play a critical role in selection of patients for attempted repair rather than valve replacement.

TEE is used in virtually all high-volume surgical centers at the time of mitral valve repair to monitor the success of this procedure on-line.[90–92] After repair, the severity of residual regurgitation can be readily assessed by TEE and the complications of iatrogenic stenosis screened for (Plate 20–4). A decision to revise the operation can then be made before fully removing the patient from cardiopulmonary bypass. It is estimated that TEE will lead to a change in the planned surgical procedure in 15 to 30 percent of cases and can obviate the need for a second surgery.[90]

Mitral Valve Prolapse

The diagnosis of MVP is made on the basis of a combination of clinical and echocardiographic features. MVP is at present considered to exist in two basic forms[105–108]: (1) prolapse of a thin, otherwise anatomically normal, leaflet, and (2) myxomatous degeneration with chordal involvement and mitral prolapse. The thin leaflet with only mild degrees of prolapse may be within the range of normal anatomic variation and appears to confer a relatively benign prognosis. Conversely, substantial leaflet thickening has been associated with complications arising from MVP, such as an increased risk for endocarditis and the risk of developing progressive mitral regurgitation that would necessitate valve replacement. The diagnosis of MVP is made on the basis of several features detectable with echocardiography, including the degree of displacement of the belly of the mitral valve beyond the plane of the mitral annulus. The specificity of this finding is least in the apical four-chamber view and greatest in the apical two-chamber and parasternal long-axis views. The nonplanar shape of the mitral annulus must be appreciated because its complex geometric configuration will result in apparent displacement of the belly of the mitral leaflet behind the mitral annulus in one or more views.[109] This does not necessarily represent pathologic MVP. The degree of thickening, if any, has been alluded to previously and should be noted from the echocardiogram as an integral aspect of the assessment of MVP. In addition to the anatomic description and identification of prolapse, determination of the severity of mitral regurgitation, if any, can also be made. Routine repeated studies should not be performed, and an echocardiogram is not indicated for MVP in the absence of physical evidence of structural heart disease or a family history of myxomatous disease.

TRICUSPID AND PULMONARY VALVE DISEASE

Tricuspid Stenosis

Isolated tricuspid stenosis is an exceptionally rare entity. Tricuspid stenosis can occur as a result of rheumatic heart disease, in which case there will almost always be concurrent mitral stenosis and usually aortic valve involvement as well. Rheumatic tricuspid stenosis has many of the hallmarks of rheumatic mitral valve disease, and similarly results in fusion of the tips of the leaflets along the commissures, with reduction in the tricuspid orifice and subsequent elevation in right atrial (RA) and systemic venous pressures. The anatomic features of tricuspid stenosis can be readily appreciated and, as with the mitral valve, gradients accurately determined by Doppler techniques.

A fairly classic form of tricuspid stenosis can be seen in carcinoid heart disease. In this disease, the tricuspid leaflets become progressively fibrotic, beginning at their more distal tips, and the leaflets subsequently become shrunken and nearly immobile. This results in a fairly characteristic echocardiographic appearance associated with various degrees of tricuspid stenosis and regurgitation. The pulmonary valve is frequently involved in a similar process in patients with carcinoid heart disease.

Tricuspid Regurgitation

Isolated tricuspid regurgitation has only a limited number of etiologies and is infrequently encountered in adult populations. It can occur in an isolated, primary form due to congenital anomalies of the tricuspid valve, such as Ebstein's anomaly, or can be due to tricuspid valve prolapse or endocarditis. More commonly, tricuspid regurgitation is encountered secondary to other forms of organic heart disease that predominate in the left ventricle. These include valvular, ischemic, and myopathic disease, which may result in pulmonary hypertension and various degrees of RV dilatation and dysfunction, or primary pulmonary vascular events, which have also resulted in pulmonary hypertension. The normal tricuspid valve frequently has small physiologic degrees of regurgitation, which may be encountered in up to 75 percent of overtly normal individuals.[110] More severe forms of regurgitation are seen in patients with either primary tricuspid valve disease or tricuspid regurgitation secondary to left-sided heart disease or pulmonary hypertension.

Appreciation of the mechanism of tricuspid regurgitation is crucial to decision-making. In many instances, tricuspid regurgitation does not require a specific therapeutic approach. Instead, an approach to the primary LV pathology is in order.

The tricuspid regurgitant jet can be utilized to calculate RV systolic pressure.[111, 112] By employing the Bernoulli equation, the tricuspid valve gradient (right ventricle to right atrium) can be reliably determined. By then adding the measured or estimated RA pressure to this gradient, an estimated RV systolic pressure can be determined (Fig. 20–16). Several schemes for taking into account RA pressure have been proposed, including clinical estimation of jugular venous pressure, measurement of RA pressure by comparison with inspiratory pressures, and addition of sliding scale constants or a fixed constant. It appears that all of these algorithms are equally successful at predicting RV systolic pressure. The addition of an empirical constant, which obviously is the simplest scheme, appears to accurately predict RV systolic pressure in the majority of patients, with a degree of precision sufficient for clinical decision-making. Assessment of severity of tricuspid regurgitation and estimation of RV systolic pressure are pertinent in patients with valvular and nonvalvular heart disease. They are an integral part of assessing the severity of mitral stenosis or regurgitation.

Pulmonary Hypertension

Other mechanisms for assessing the severity of pulmonary hypertension include evaluation of the pulmonary valve motion with M-mode echocardiography and assessment of the pulmonary artery Doppler flow profile. With substantial degrees of pulmonary hypertension (typically $>$ 50 mm Hg systolic), the normal presystolic opening of this valve (the A wave) is lost and notching occurs during midsystole in the valve.[109, 110] This assessment is fairly specific for the presence of clinically important pulmonary hypertension

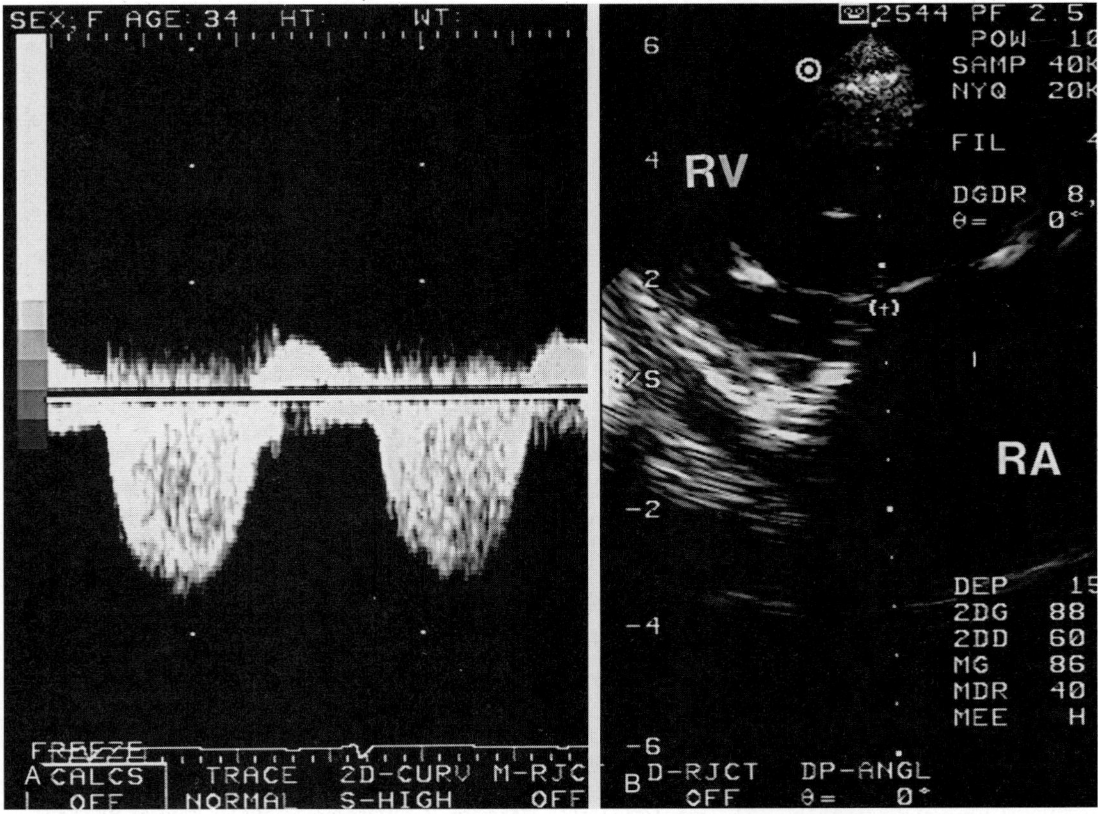

FIGURE 20–16 Parasternal right ventricular inflow tract view recorded in a patient with pulmonary hypertension and tricuspid regurgitation. **A,** The continuous-wave Doppler sample can be appreciated. **B,** Note the tricuspid regurgitation jet with a peak velocity of 3 m/s. This corresponds to a right ventricular to right atrial gradient of 36 mm Hg, from which the right ventricular systolic pressure can be estimated to be 50 mm Hg. RA, right atrium; RV, right ventricle.

but does not allow estimation of actual pulmonary artery pressures.

Examination of the spectral profile of the pulmonary artery flow can give more quantitative clues to the severity of pulmonary hypertension.[115] The normal pulmonary outflow velocity profile consists of a smooth, relatively gradual acceleration to peak velocity. In normal individuals, the time of onset of flow to peak velocity is typically greater than 140 milliseconds. With progressive degrees of pulmonary artery systolic hypertension, this acceleration time progressively shortens. Although a definite linear relationship exists between the pulmonary artery pressure and the acceleration time, the scatter in this observation is substantial and does not allow accurate prediction of pulmonary artery pressures, which is better accomplished using the tricuspid regurgitation jet.

Pulmonary Stenosis

Pulmonary stenosis is rarely encountered in adult populations as a previously unrecognized entity. It is far more common in childhood. The pulmonary valve is readily interrogated with both 2-D imaging and Doppler techniques. Because flow from the RV outflow tract into the main pulmonary artery across the pulmonary valve is directed almost precisely posteriorly, little difficulty is encountered in aligning a Doppler beam parallel to the flow. Therefore, an accurate assessment of transvalvular gradients in pulmonary stenosis is available in the majority of patients. The same techniques regarding peak and mean pressure determination and calculation of stenotic valve areas that were discussed for aortic stenosis can be employed for determining the severity of pulmonary stenosis.[116]

In addition to accurately determining the severity of pulmonary stenosis, other features that can be detected and should always be investigated include the degree of any dynamic infundibular stenosis, which occurs as a secondary phenomenon in patients with pulmonary stenosis, and the presence or absence of pulmonary insufficiency. In addition, the degree of RV hypertrophy, dilatation, and systolic dysfunction can be assessed.

Prosthetic Heart Valves

Echocardiography can be used to assist in determining the size of the prosthetic valve that will be required at surgery in any given patient.[27] Prosthetic heart valves may be classified as *tissue* (biologic) or *nontissue* (mechanical), and all prosthetic valves produce some degree of obstruction that is valve dependent. Prosthetic heart valves are prone to complications, including infection, obstruction, and dehiscence or structural deterioration (Plate 20–5). Although echocardiography usually allows adequate evaluation of prosthetic valve function, acoustic shadowing and reverberation from the prosthetic material, especially in metal valves, often limit the assessment. The principles of evaluation are the same as for native valves. Pitfalls in the Doppler evaluation of prosthetic heart valves include falsely low velocities due to eccentric jets or the central occluder of ball-type valves and falsely elevated velocity secondary to the phenomenon of pressure recovery.

Effective orifice area may be calculated from the continuity equation. Continuous-wave Doppler determination of transvalvular pressure gradients generally correlates well with invasive measurements. Since velocity across a valve may be increased without stenosis, as in high-output state or severe regurgitation, upstream velocity must be factored into the Bernoulli equation. It is useful to have early postoperative assessment of prosthetic valves by echocardiogram with gradients in order to have reference values at follow-up. Normal echocardiography-derived hemodynamic measurements and effective orifice areas for various prostheses have been published.[117]

As with native valve assessment, gradients should be reassessed after exercise whenever the resting gradient appears incongruous with the clinical scenario. TEE is often needed in combination with transthoracic echocardiography to fully assess prosthetic valve function, especially for prosthetic valves in the mitral position, and contrast medium infusion may enhance spectral signals.[118]

A small amount of regurgitation is typical in many valves, and normal characteristic patterns are seen in bileaflet and tilting disc prostheses.

MISCELLANEOUS VALVULAR CONDITIONS

Several forms of valvular heart disease require specific comment.

Valvulopathy Associated With Anorectic Agents

Fenfluramine and phentermine were commonly prescribed anorectic agents with over 18 million prescriptions written in the United States in 1996. Concern about associated valvular heart disease subsequently led to the withdrawal of these agents. Echocardiography revealed unusual valve morphology associated with regurgitation. Pulmonary hypertension was a common associated feature. Both right-sided and left-sided heart valves were involved, although a left-sided valve was involved in all cases.[119–121]

In patients requiring surgery, affected valves had a glistening white appearance. Histopathologic features were similar to those seen in carcinoid or ergotamine-induced valvular disease. The relationship and mechanism of valvulopathy in these patients have yet to be determined.

Marfan's Syndrome

The Marfan syndrome typifies the heritable disorders of connective tissue in which vascular structures are prominently involved.[28, 122] The classic cardiac abnormality in Marfan's syndrome is cystic medial necrosis of the proximal aorta, resulting in various degrees of aortic root dilatation. This entity is not infrequently associated with MVP with myxomatous thickening.

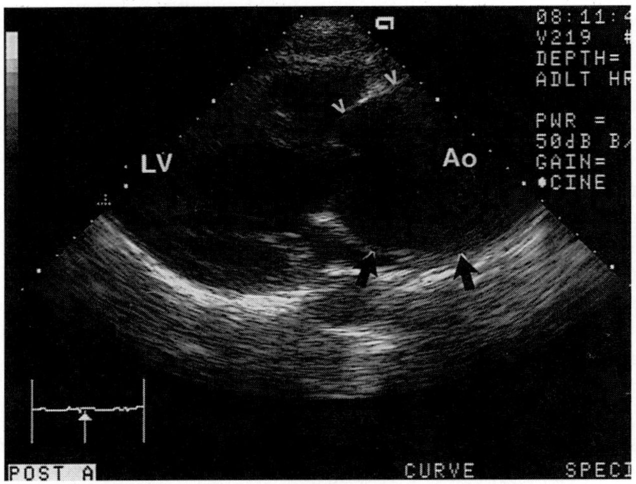

FIGURE 20–17 Parasternal long-axis echocardiogram recorded in a patient with Marfan's syndrome. Note the massively dilated proximal aortic root, which measures 7 cm in diameter (*arrowheads*). AO, aorta; LV, left ventricle.

The classic echocardiographic abnormality in Marfan's syndrome is dilatation of the aortic root at the level of the sinuses of Valsalva (Fig. 20–17). The aortic annular dimension may remain near normal early in the course of this process, and dilatation is seen exclusively at the level of the sinuses. With more severe degrees of involvement, there can be massive sinus dilatation and subsequent dilatation of the aortic annulus itself. With marked secondary annular dilatation, aortic insufficiency ensues and can vary in severity from trivial to severe. Occult dissection is frequently seen in the more advanced cases, and obviously, clinically recognized dissection or rupture represents a major cause of death in these patients.

From an echocardiographic standpoint, these patients can be serially followed and managed with transthoracic ultrasound techniques alone in many instances. Echocardiographic studies should be tailored to high-quality examinations of the proximal aorta, from which annular, sinus, and tubular aortic dimensions can be determined and followed serially. Long-term clinical studies suggest that with diameters greater than 55 mm, the risk of dissection or rupture of the aortic root is sufficiently high to warrant prophylactic surgical intervention.[123]

Aortic Dissection

Dissection of the proximal aorta often causes disruption of the integrity of the aortic valve and various degrees of aortic insufficiency. Typically, this an acute cardiovascular event requiring urgent surgical intervention. TEE is highly accurate and reliable for detecting aortic dissection and determining its extent.[124, 125]

Echocardiographic Findings in Endocarditis

The pathologic findings in valvular endocarditis include direct invasive destruction of valve structures as well as superimposed thrombus formation and deposition of inflammatory tissue, all of which may be either actively infected or resolving. Independent of the valve involved, from both a pathologic and an echocardiographic standpoint, a mass distorting the normal architecture of the valve develops and leads to disruption of normal valvular function. Echocardiographic features form an integral part of the Duke clinical criteria for the diagnosis of infective endocarditis.[126] Vegetations are typically discrete, located on the low-pressure aspect of the valve, in the path of turbulent flow, and along the sewing ring of prosthetic valves; excessive mobility of the valve may be noted (Fig. 20–18).[32–35] Differential diagnosis of infective vegetations include benign fibrotic lesions of the valve, thrombus, ruptured chordae, and valve excrescences.

Different schemes for stratifying the embolic potential or risk of other complications of vegetations have been proposed. Although controversial, mobility, size, extent, and texture of vegetation by echocardiography may be predictive of embolic events.[33–35] In addition to the presence or absence of a vegetation, other indirect evidence regarding a destructive infectious process should be investigated. These include evidence of an abscess of either the aortic or the mitral annulus and spread of infection to a contiguous valve. The classic example of the latter is involvement of the anterior mitral valve leaflet in aortic insufficiency due to endocarditis. Although transthoracic echocardiography may detect vegetations in up to 80 percent of patients, TEE is more sensitive, especially in prosthetic valves and in diagnosing complications such as perivalvular extension of infection.[127] However, when the valvular structure or pathology is well visualized by transthoracic echocardiography, there is no indication to perform TEE.[2]

In conclusion, modern cardiac ultrasound techniques include an anatomic assessment with 2-D echocardiography and a physiologic assessment with Doppler modalities. They allow an almost complete evaluation of patients with virtually any form of valvular heart disease. The accuracy

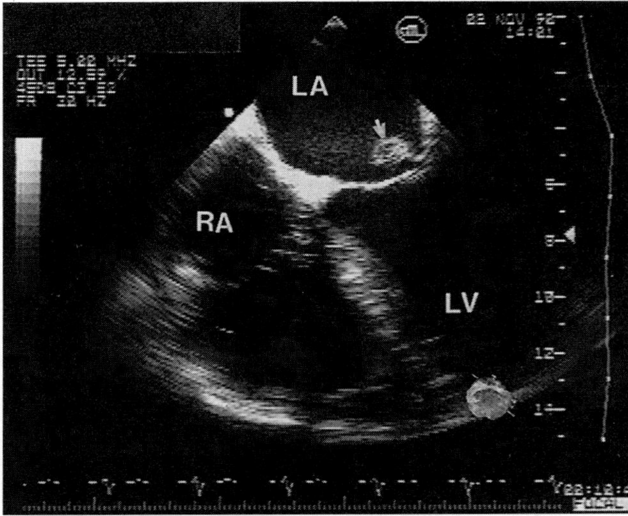

FIGURE 20–18 TEE recorded in a patient with endocarditis and a vegetation on the posterior leaflet of the mitral valve. Note the 1-cm mass attached to the mitral valve leaflet (*arrow*). LA, left atrium; LV, left ventricle; RA, right atrium.

of the technique is sufficiently high to supplant cardiac catheterization as a necessary diagnostic tool before proceeding to surgical intervention. In addition, the success of more recently developed invasive procedures for valve reconstruction can frequently be predicted on the basis of the echocardiographic findings.

REFERENCES

1. Bonow RO, Carabello B, de Leon AC Jr, et al: Guidelines for the management of patients with valvular heart disease: executive summary. A report of the American College of Cardiology/American Heart Association Task Force on Practice Guidelines (Committee on Management of Patients with Valvular Heart Disease). Circulation 98:1949, 1998.
2. Cheitlin MD, Alpert JS, Armstrong WF, et al: ACC/AHA guidelines for the clinical application of echocardiography: a report of the American College of Cardiology/American Heart Association Task Force on Practice Guidelines (Committee on Clinical Application of Echocardiography), developed in collaboration with the American Society of Echocardiography. Circulation 95:1686, 1997.
3. Feigenbaum H: Echocardiography. 4th ed. Philadelphia: Lea & Febiger, 1986.
4. Henry WL, DeMaria A, Gramiak R, et al: Report of the American Society of Echocardiography Committee on Nomenclature and Standards in Two-Dimensional Echocardiography. pp. 1–10. Raleigh, NC: American Society of Echocardiography.
5. Tardif JC, Schwartz SL, Vannan MA, et al: Clinical usefulness of multiple plane transesophageal echocardiography: comparison to biplanar imaging. Am Heart J 128:156, 1994.
6. Warner JG Jr, Nomier AM, Salim M, Kitzman DW: A prospective, randomized, blinded comparison of multiple and biplane transesophageal echocardiographic techniques. J Am Soc Echocardiogr 9:865, 1996.
7. Schiller NB, Shah PM, Crawford M, et al: Recommendations for quantitation of the left ventricle by two-dimensional echocardiography. J Am Soc Echocardiogr 2:358, 1989.
8. Starling MR, Crawford MH, Sorensen SG, et al: Comparative accuracy of apical biplane cross-sectional echocardiography and gated equilibrium radionuclide angiography for estimating left ventricular size and performance. Circulation 63:1075, 1981.
9. Petrovic O, Feigenbaum H, Armstrong WF, et al: Digital averaging to facilitate two-dimensional echocardiographic measurements. J Clin Ultrasound 14:367, 1986.
10. Zoghbi WA, Buckey JC, Massey MA, et al: Determination of left ventricular volumes with use of a new nongeometric echocardiographic method: clinical validation and potential application. J Am Coll Cardiol 15:610, 1990.
11. Schiller NB, Acquatella H, Ports TA, et al: Left ventricular volume from paired biplane two-dimensional echocardiography. Circulation 60:547, 1979.
12. Feigenbaum H: *In* Meltzer RS, Vered Z, Neufeld HN (eds): Noninvasive Cardiac Imaging: Recent Developments. Mount Kisco, NY: Futura, 1988.
13. Handshoe R, Demaria AN: Doppler assessment of intracardiac pressures. Echocardiography 2:127, 1985.
14. Bargiggia GS, Bertucci C, Recusani F, et al: A new method for estimating left ventricular dP/dt by continuous wave Doppler-echocardiography. Circulation 80:1287, 1989.
15. Chen C, Rodriquez L, Guerrero JL, et al: Noninvasive estimation of the instantaneous first derivative of left ventricular pressure using continuous-wave Doppler echocardiography. Circulation 83:2101, 1991.
16. Thomas JD, Weyman AE: Echocardiographic Doppler evaluation of left ventricular diastolic function. Circulation 84:977, 1991.
17. Nishimura RA, Abel MD, Hatle LK, Tajik AJ: Assessment of diastolic function of the heart: background and current applications of Doppler echocardiography. Part II. Clinical studies. Mayo Clin Proc 64:181, 1989.
18. Nishimura RA, Tajik AJ: Evaluation of diastolic filling of left ventricle in health and disease: Doppler echocardiography in the clinician's Rosetta Stone. J Am Coll Cardiol 30:8, 1997.
19. Omoto R, Kasai C: Physics and instrumentation of Doppler color flow mapping. Echocardiography 4:467, 1987.
20. Demaria AN, Smith M, Branco M, et al: Normal and abnormal blood flow patterns by color Doppler flow imaging. Echocardiography 3:475, 1986.
21. Pandian NG, Kusay BS, Caldeira M, et al: Color Doppler flow imaging in cardiac diagnosis. Echocardiography 6:99, 1989.
22. Weyman AE, Feigenbaum H, Hurwitz RA, et al: Cross-sectional echocardiographic assessment of the severity of aortic stenosis in children. Circulation 55:773, 1977.
23. Huhta JC, Latson LA, Gutgesell HP, et al: Echocardiography in the diagnosis and management of symptomatic aortic valve stenosis in infants. Circulation 70:438, 1984.
24. Godley RW, Green D, Dillon JC, et al: Reliability of two-dimensional echocardiography in assessing the severity of valvular aortic stenosis. Chest 79:657, 1981.
25. DeMaria AN, Bommer W, Joye J, et al: Value and limitations of cross-sectional echocardiography of the aortic valve in the diagnosis and quantification of valvular aortic stenosis. Circulation 62:304, 1980.
26. Brandenburg RO, Tajik AJ, Edwards WD, et al: Accuracy of 2-dimensional echocardiographic diagnosis of congenitally bicuspid aortic valve: echocardiographic-anatomic correlation in 115 patients. Am J Cardiol 51:1469, 1983.
27. Harpaz D, Shah P, Bezante G, et al: Transthoracic and transesophageal echocardiographic sizing of the aortic annulus to determine prosthesis size. Am J Cardiol 72:1411, 1993.
28. Come PC, Fortuin NJ, White RI, McKusick VA: Echocardiographic assessment of cardiovascular abnormalities in the Marfan syndrome. Am J Med 74:465, 1983.
29. Nienaber CA, Spielmann RP, von Kodolitsch Y, et al: Diagnosis of thoracic aortic dissection. Circulation 85:434, 1992.
30. Ballal RS, Nanda NC, Gatewood R, et al: Usefulness of transesophageal echocardiography in assessment of aortic dissection. Circulation 84:1903, 1991.
31. Hecht SR, Berger M: Right-sided endocarditis in intravenous drug users. Prognostic features in 102 episodes. Ann Intern Med 117:560, 1992.
32. Smith MD, Kwan OL, DeMaria AN: The role of echocardiography in the diagnosis and management of infective endocarditis. Pract Cardiol 10:78, 1984.
33. Mugge A, Daniel WG, Frank G, Lichtlen PR: Echocardiography in infective endocarditis: reassessment of prognostic implications of vegetation size determined by the transthoracic and the transesophageal approach. J Am Coll Cardiol 14:631, 1989.
34. Lindner JR, Case RA, Dent JM, et al: Diagnostic value of echocardiography in suspected endocarditis. An evaluation based on the pretest probability of disease. Circulation 93:730, 1996.
35. Sanfilippo AJ, Picard MH, Newell JB, et al: Echocardiographic assessment of patients with infectious endocarditis: prediction of risk for complications. J Am Coll Cardiol 18:1191, 1991.
36. Stamm RB, Martin RP: Quantification of pressure gradients across stenotic valves by Doppler ultrasound. J Am Coll Cardiol 2:707, 1983.
37. Currie PJ, Hagler DJ, Seward JB, et al: Instantaneous pressure gradient: a simultaneous Doppler and dual catheter correlative study. J Am Coll Cardiol 7:800, 1986.
38. Currie PJ, Seward JB, Reeder GS, et al: Continuous-wave Doppler echocardiographic assessment of severity of calcific aortic stenosis: a simultaneous Doppler-catheter correlative study in 100 adult patients. Circulation 71:1162, 1985.
39. Smith MD, Dawson PL, Elion JL, et al: Systematic correlation of continuous-wave Doppler and hemodynamic measurements in patients with aortic stenosis. Am Heart J 111:245, 1986.
40. Otto CM, Pearlman AS: Doppler echocardiography in adults with symptomatic aortic stenosis. Arch Intern Med 148:2553, 1988.
41. Otto CM, Pearlman AS, Gardner CL: Hemodynamic progression of aortic stenosis in adults assessed by Doppler echocardiography. J Am Coll Cardiol 13:545, 1989.
42. Geibel A, Gornandt L, Kasper W, et al: Reproducibility of Doppler echocardiographic quantification of aortic and mitral valve stenoses: comparison between two echocardiography centers. Am J Cardiol 67:1013, 1991.
43. Bengur AR, Snider AR, Serwer GA, et al: Usefulness of the Doppler mean gradient in evaluation of children with aortic valve stenosis and comparison to gradient at catheterization. Am J Cardiol 64:756, 1989.

44. Otto CM, Nishimura RA, Davis KB, et al: Doppler echocardiographic findings in adults with severe symptomatic valvular aortic stenosis. Am J Cardiol 68:1477, 1991.
45. Teirstein P, Yeager M, Yock PG, et al: Doppler echocardiographic measurement of aortic valve area in aortic stenosis: a noninvasive application of the Gorlin formula. J Am Coll Cardiol 8:1059, 1986.
46. Skjaerpe T, Hegrenaes L, Hatle L: Noninvasive estimation of valve area in patients with aortic stenosis by Doppler ultrasound and two-dimensional echocardiography. Circulation 72:810, 1985.
47. Otto CM, Pearlman AS, Comess KA, et al: Determination of the stenotic aortic valve area in adults using Doppler echocardiography. J Am Coll Cardiol 7:509, 1986.
48. Zoghbi WA, Farmer KL, Soto JG, et al: Accurate noninvasive quantification of stenotic aortic valve area by Doppler echocardiography. Circulation 73:452, 1986.
49. Bengur AR, Snider AR, Meliones JN, et al: Doppler evaluation of aortic valve area in children with aortic stenosis. J Am Coll Cardiol 18:1499, 1991.
50. Myreng Y, Molstad P, Endresen K, et al: Reproducibility of echocardiographic estimates of the area of stenosed aortic valves using the continuity equation. Int J Cardiol 26:349, 1990.
51. deFilippi CR, Willet DL, Brickner ME, et al: Usefulness of dobutamine echocardiography in distinguishing severe from nonsevere valvular aortic stenosis in patients with depressed left ventricular function and low transvalvular gradients. Am J Cardiol 75:191, 1995.
52. Harris KM, Malenka DJ, Haney MF, et al: Improvement in mitral regurgitation after aortic valve replacement. Am J Cardiol 80:741, 1997.
53. Otto CM, Pearlman AS, Amsler LC: Doppler echocardiographic evaluation of left ventricular diastolic filling in isolated valvular aortic stenosis. Am J Cardiol 63:313, 1989.
54. Aziz KU, van Grondelle A, Paul MH, et al: Echocardiographic assessment of the relation between left ventricular wall and cavity dimensions and peak systolic pressure in children with aortic stenosis. Am J Cardiol 40:775, 1977.
55. Carabello BA, Green LH, Grossman W, et al: Hemodynamic determinants of prognosis of aortic valve replacement in critical aortic stenosis and advanced congestive heart failure. Circulation 62:42, 1980.
56. Bouchard A, Yock P, Schiller NB, et al: Value of color Doppler estimation of regurgitant volume in patients with chronic aortic insufficiency. Am Heart J 117:1099, 1989.
57. Otto CM, Burwash IG, Legget ME, et al: Prospective study of asymptomatic valvular aortic stenosis: clinical, echocardiographic, and exercise predictors of outcome. Circulation 95:2262, 1997.
58. Sahn DJ, Maciel BC: Physiological valvular regurgitation. Doppler echocardiography and the potential for iatrogenic heart disease. Circulation 78:1075, 1998.
59. Tribouilloy C, Shen WF, Slama M, et al: Assessment of severity of aortic regurgitation by M-mode colour Doppler flow imaging. Eur Heart J 12:352, 1991.
60. Perry GJ, Helmcke F, Nanda NC, et al: Evaluation of aortic insufficiency by Doppler color flow mapping. J Am Coll Cardiol 9:952, 1987.
61. Pye M, Rae AP, Hutton I, et al: Quantification of aortic regurgitation using continuous and pulsed wave Doppler echocardiography. Int J Cardiol 27:101, 1990.
62. Teague SM, Heinsimer JA, Anderson JL, et al: Quantification of aortic regurgitation utilizing continuous wave Doppler ultrasound. J Am Coll Cardiol 8:592, 1986.
63. Wilkenshoff UM, Kruck I, Gast D, Schroder R: Validity of continuous wave Doppler and colour Doppler in the assessment of aortic regurgitation. Eur Heart J 15:1227, 1994.
64. Enriquez-Sarano M, Seward JB, Bailey KR, Tajik AJ: Effective regurgitant orifice area: a noninvasive Doppler development of an old hemodynamic concept. J Am Coll Cardiol 23:443, 1994.
65. Samstad SO, Hegrenaes AL, Skjaerpe T, et al: Half time of the diastolic aortoventricular pressure difference by continuous wave Doppler ultrasound: a measure of the severity of aortic regurgitation? Br Heart J 61:336, 1988.
66. Henry WL, Bonow RO, Borer JS, et al: Observations on the optimum time for operative intervention for aortic regurgitation. Circulation 61:471, 1980.
67. Henry WL, Bonow RO, Rosing DR, Epstein SE: Observations on the optimum time for operative intervention for aortic regurgitation. Circulation 61:484, 1980.
68. Borow KM, Green LH, Mann T, et al: End-systolic volume as a predictor of postoperative left ventricular performance in volume overload from valvular regurgitation. Am J Med 68:655, 1980.
69. Bonow RO, Rosing DR, McIntosh CL, et al: The natural history of asymptomatic patients with aortic regurgitation and normal left ventricular function. Circulation 68:509, 1983.
70. Bonow RO, Lakatos E, Maron BJ, et al: Serial long-term assessment of the natural history of asymptomatic patients with chronic aortic regurgitation and normal left ventricular systolic function. Circulation 84:1625, 1991.
71. Bonow RO, Picone AL, McIntosh CL, et al: Survival and functional results after valve replacement for aortic regurgitation from 1976 to 1983: impact of preoperative left ventricular function. Circulation 72:1244, 1985.
72. Bonow RO, Dodd JT, Maron BJ, et al: Long-term serial changes in left ventricular function and reversal of ventricular dilatation after valve replacement for chronic aortic regurgitation. Circulation 78:1108, 1988.
73. Kumpuris AG, Quinones MA, Waggoner AD: Importance of preoperative hypertrophy, wall stress and end-systolic dimension as echocardiographic predictors of normalization of left ventricular dilatation after valve replacement in chronic aortic insufficiency. Am J Cardiol 49:1091, 1982.
74. Gaasch WH, Andrias CW, Levine HJ: Chronic aortic regurgitation: the effect of aortic valve replacement on left ventricular volume, mass and function. Circulation 58:825, 1978.
75. Levine RA, Handschumacher MD, Sanfilippo AJ, et al: Three-dimensional echocardiographic reconstruction of the mitral valve, with implications for the diagnosis of mitral valve prolapse. Circulation 80:589, 1989.
76. Martin RP, Rakowski H, Kleiman JH, et al: Reliability and reproducibility of two dimensional echocardiographic measurement of the stenotic mitral valve orifice area. Am J Cardiol 43:560, 1979.
77. Heger JJ, Wann LS, Weyman AE, et al: Long-term changes in mitral valve area after successful mitral commissurotomy. Circulation 59:443, 1979.
78. Voelker W, Jackson R, Dittmann H, et al: Validation of continuous-wave Doppler measurements of mitral valve gradients during exercise—a simultaneous Doppler-catheter study. Eur Heart J 10:737, 1989.
79. Hatle L, Angelsen B, Techn DR, et al: Noninvasive assessment of atrioventricular pressure half-time by Doppler ultrasound. Circulation 60:1096, 1979.
80. Karp K, Teien D, Bjerle P: Reassessment of valve area determinations in mitral stenosis by the pressure half-time method: impact of left ventricular stiffness and peak diastolic pressure difference. J Am Coll Cardiol 13:594, 1989.
81. Flachskampf FA, Weyman AE, Gillam L, et al: Aortic regurgitation shortens Doppler pressure half-time in mitral stenosis: clinical evidence, in vitro simulation and theoretic analysis. J Am Coll Cardiol 16:396, 1990.
82. Smith MD, Wisenbaugh T, Grayburn PA, et al: Value and limitations of Doppler pressure half-time in quantifying mitral stenosis: a comparison with micromanometer catheter recordings. Am Heart J 121:480, 1991.
83. Abascal VM, Wilkins GT, O'Shea JP, et al: Prediction of successful outcome in 130 patients undergoing percutaneous balloon mitral valvotomy. Circulation 82:448, 1990.
84. Nobuyoshi M, Hamasaki N, Kimura T, et al: Indications, complications, and short-term clinical outcome of percutaneous transvenous mitral commissurotomy. Circulation 80:782, 1989.
85. Cannan CR, Nishimura RA, Reeder GS, et al: Echocardiographic assessment of commissural calcium: a simple predictor of outcome after percutaneous mitral balloon valvotomy. J Am Coll Cardiol 29:175, 1997.
86. Aschenberg W, Schluter M, Kremer P, et al: Transesophageal two-dimensional echocardiography for the detection of left atrial appendage thrombus. J Am Coll Cardiol 7:163, 1986.
87. Pan J, Lin S, Go JU, et al: Frequency and severity of mitral regurgitation one year after balloon mitral valvuloplasty. Am J Cardiol 67:264, 1991.
88. Abascal VM, Wilkins GT, Choong CY, et al: Mitral regurgitation after percutaneous balloon mitral valvuloplasty in adults: evaluation

by pulsed Doppler echocardiography. J Am Coll Cardiol 11:257, 1988.
89. Thomas JD, Wilkins GT, Choong CYP, et al: Inaccuracy of mitral pressure half-time immediately after percutaneous mitral valvotomy. Circulation 78:980, 1988.
90. Stewart WJ, Currie PJ, Salcedo EE, et al: Intraoperative Doppler color flow mapping for decision-making in valve repair for mitral regurgitation. Circulation 81:556, 1990.
91. Currie PJ, Stewart WJ: Intraoperative echocardiography in mitral valve repair for mitral regurgitation. Am J Card Imaging 4:192, 1990.
92. Reichert SLA, Visser CA, Moulijn AC, et al: Intraoperative transesophageal color-coded Doppler echocardiography for evaluation of residual regurgitation after mitral valve repair. J Thorac Cardiovasc Surg 100:756, 1990.
93. Himelman RB, Kusumoto F, Oken K, et al: The flail mitral valve: echocardiographic findings by precordial and transesophageal imaging and Doppler color flow mapping. J Am Coll Cardiol 17:272, 1991.
94. Pearson AC, St Vrain J, Mrosek D, et al: Color Doppler echocardiographic evaluation of patients with a flail mitral leaflet. J Am Coll Cardiol 16:232, 1990.
95. Blumlein S, Bouchard A, Schiller NB, et al: Quantitation of mitral regurgitation by Doppler echocardiography. Circulation 1:40, 1987.
96. Spain MG, Smith MD, Grayburn PA, et al: Quantitative assessment of mitral regurgitation by Doppler color flow imaging: angiographic and hemodynamic correlations. J Am Coll Cardiol 13:585, 1989.
97. Ascah KJ, Stewart WJ, Jiang L, et al: A Doppler-two-dimensional echocardiographic method for quantitation of mitral regurgitation. Circulation 72:377, 1985.
98. Helmcke F, Nanda NC, Hsiung MC, et al: Color Doppler assessment of mitral regurgitation with orthogonal planes. Circulation 75:175, 1987.
99. Yoshida K, Yoshikawa J, Yamaura Y, et al: Assessment of mitral regurgitation by biplane transesophageal color Doppler flow mapping. Circulation 82:1121, 1990.
100. Chen C, Koschyk D, Brockhoff C, et al: Noninvasive estimation of regurgitant flow rate and volume in patients with mitral regurgitation by Doppler color mapping of accelerating flow field. J Am Coll Cardiol 21:374, 1993.
101. Klein AL, Obarski TP, Stewart WJ, et al: Transesophageal Doppler echocardiography of pulmonary venous flow: a new marker of mitral regurgitation severity. J Am Coll Cardiol 18:518, 1991.
102. Cape EG, Yoganathan AP, Weyman AE, et al: Adjacent solid boundaries alter the size of regurgitant jets on Doppler color flow maps. J Am Coll Cardiol 17:1094, 1991.
103. Chao K, Moises VA, Shandas R, et al: Influence of the Coanda effect on color Doppler jet area and color encoding. Circulation 85:333, 1992.
104. Chen C, Thomas JD, Anconina J, et al: Impact of impinging wall jet on color Doppler quantification of mitral regurgitation. Circulation 84:712, 1991.
105. Devereux RB, Kramer-Fox R, Kligfield P: Mitral valve prolapse: causes, clinical manifestations, and management. Ann Intern Med 111:305, 1989.
106. Levine RA, Stathogiannis E, Newell JB, et al: Reconsideration of echocardiographic standards for mitral valve prolapse: lack of association between leaflet displacement isolated to the apical four chamber view and independent echocardiographic evidence of abnormality. J Am Coll Cardiol 11:1010, 1988.
107. Marks AR, Choong CY, Sanfilippo AJ, et al: Identification of high-risk and low-risk subgroups of patients with mitral-valve prolapse. N Engl J Med 320:1031, 1989.
108. Chandraratna PAN, Nimalasuriya A, Kawanishi D, et al: Identification of the increased frequency of cardiovascular abnormalities associated with mitral valve prolapse by two-dimensional echocardiography. Am J Cardiol 54:1283, 1984.
109. Levine RA, Triulzi MO, Harrigan P, et al: The relationship of mitral annular shape to the diagnosis of mitral valve prolapse. Circulation 75:756, 1987.
110. Yoshida K, Yoshikawa J, Shakudo M, et al: Color Doppler evaluation of valvular regurgitation in normal subjects. Circulation 78:840, 1988.
111. Chan K, Currie PJ, Seward JB, et al: Comparison of three Doppler ultrasound methods in the prediction of pulmonary artery pressure. J Am Coll Cardiol 9:549, 1987.
112. Berger M, Haimowitz A, van Tosh A, et al: Quantitative assessment of pulmonary hypertension in patients with tricuspid regurgitation using continuous wave Doppler ultrasound. J Am Coll Cardiol 6:359, 1985.
113. Heger JJ, Weyman AE: A review of M-mode and cross-sectional echocardiographic findings of the pulmonary valve. J Clin Ultrasound 7:98, 1979.
114. Weyman AE: Pulmonary valve echo motion in clinical practice. Am J Med 62:843, 1977.
115. Mallery JA, Gardin JM, King SW, et al: Effects of heart rate and pulmonary artery pressure on Doppler pulmonary artery acceleration time in experimental acute pulmonary hypertension. Chest 100:470, 1991.
116. Johnson GL, Kwan OL, Handshoe S, et al: Accuracy of combined two-dimensional echocardiography and continuous wave Doppler recordings in the estimation of pressure gradient in right ventricular outlet obstruction. J Am Coll Cardiol 3:1013, 1984.
117. Reisner SA, Meltzer RS: Normal values of prosthetic valve Doppler echocardiographic parameters: a review. J Am Soc Echocardiogr 1:201, 1998.
118. Terasawa A, Miyatake K, Nakatani S, et al: Enhancement of Doppler flow signals in the left heart chambers by intravenous injection of sonicated albumin. J Am Coll Cardiol 21:737, 1993.
119. Connolly HM, Crary JL, McGoon MD, et al: Valvular heart disease associated with fenfluramine-phentermine. N Engl J Med 337:581, 1997.
120. Weissman NJ, Tighe JF Jr, Gottdiener JS, Gwynne JT: An assessment of heart valve abnormalities in obese patients taking dexfenfluramine, sustained-release dexfenfluramine, or placebo. N Engl J Med 339:725, 1998.
121. Khan MA, Herzog CA, St Peter JV, et al: The prevalence of cardiac valvular insufficiency assessed by transthoracic echocardiography in obese patients treated with appetite-suppressant drugs. N Engl J Med 339:713, 1998.
122. Murdoch JL, Walker BA, Halpern BL, et al: Life expectancy and causes of death in the Marfan syndrome. N Engl J Med 286:804, 1972.
123. McDonald GR, Schaff HV, Pyeritz RE, et al: Surgical management of patients with the Marfan syndrome and dilatation of the ascending aorta. J Thorac Cardiovasc Surg 81:180, 1981.
124. Erbel R, Borner N, Steller D, et al: Detection of aortic dissection by transesophageal echocardiography. Br Heart J 58:45, 1987.
125. Hashimoto S, Kumada T, Osakada G, et al: Assessment of transesophageal Doppler echography in dissecting aortic aneurysm. J Am Coll Cardiol 14:1253, 1989.
126. Durack DT, Lukes AS, Bright DK, for the Duke Endocarditis Service: New criteria for diagnosis of infective endocarditis: utilization of specific echocardiographic findings. Am J Med 96:200, 1994.
127. Shapiro SM, Young E, De Guzman S, et al: Transesophageal echocardiography in diagnosis of infective endocarditis. Chest 105:377, 1994.

CHAPTER 21

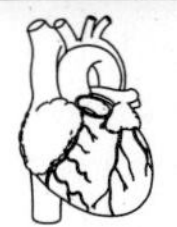

RADIONUCLIDE TECHNIQUES OF EVALUATION

A. Iain McGhie

REGURGITANT VALVULAR LESIONS
Aortic Regurgitation
Mitral Regurgitation
CONGENITAL HEART DISEASE: QUANTIFICATION OF SHUNTS

Nuclear imaging techniques are primarily used in the diagnosis and management of patients with known or suspected coronary heart disease. However, radionuclide techniques can play an important role in patients with valvular heart disease, especially aortic regurgitation, and they also provide a means for quantification of cardiac shunts in patients with congenital heart disease.

REGURGITANT VALVULAR LESIONS

Regurgitant valvular lesions result in ventricular volume overload that may be either acute or chronic. If the onset is acute, there is inadequate time for the cardiovascular system to adapt to the hemodynamic consequences, and patients often develop fulminant heart failure or circulatory collapse. Radionuclide techniques have a limited role in the management of such patients; therefore, only chronic valvular regurgitation is discussed.

Radionuclide ventriculography can be used to estimate the degree of regurgitation by calculating either the difference between left and right ventricular stroke volumes or both the absolute and the forward stroke volumes. The former technique is easily performed using the "best septal" projection from a gated-equilibrium radionuclide ventriculogram. Using either a stroke volume or a Fourier-transform amplitude image, the relative stroke counts (volume) of the right and left ventricles are estimated.[1–3] This technique works on the premise that right and left ventricular volumes are equal under normal physiologic conditions. In the presence of mitral or aortic regurgitation, left ventricular stroke counts will be greater than right ventricular stroke counts. Results are expressed either as a stroke volume ratio (left ventricular stroke counts/right ventricular stroke counts) or as a regurgitant fraction (left − right ventricular stroke counts/left ventricular stroke counts). However, this technique has some significant limitations. First, one has to assume there is no concomitant right-sided valvular regurgitation (e.g., tricuspid regurgitation) or the presence of an intracardiac shunt. Second, the inevitable right atrial and right ventricular overlap that occurs in the left anterior oblique projection results in systematic overestimation of the right ventricular stroke volume. Some workers have suggested a method for correcting for the contribution of right atrial counts.[4] Left atrial enlargement resulting from mitral regurgitation may also produce overlap between the left-sided chambers. However, this can be minimized using craniocaudal angulation of the gamma camera. Another additional limitation is the restricted accuracy of this estimate in the presence of moderate to severe left ventricular dysfunction.[3]

Alternatively, the regurgitant volume can be determined using a combination of first-pass and gated-equilibrium radionuclide ventriculography.[5, 6] Using the cardiac output calculated from the first-pass data curve, the forward stroke volume (cardiac output divided by heart rate) is measured. The left ventricular ejection fraction and end-diastolic volume are measured using a gated-equilibrium acquisition, allowing the absolute stroke volume to be calculated. The regurgitant fraction is obtained by subtracting the forward from the absolute stroke volume. The advantage of this technique is that no assumptions regarding competency of the right-sided valves are required. Other workers have also reported success in calculating regurgitant fractions using deconvoluted lung and left ventricular time-activity curves obtained by factor analysis from first-pass radionuclide angiograms.[7]

Aortic Regurgitation

Aortic regurgitation results from disease of the aortic valve, the aortic root, or both. Increased end-diastolic volume is the main hemodynamic compensatory mechanism in chronic aortic regurgitation. This results in increased end-diastolic wall stress, which is associated with development of eccentric hypertrophy, replication of sarcomeres in series, and elongation of myocardial fibers. These adaptive processes increase left ventricular wall thickness, returning end-diastolic wall stress to normal.

Overall, the natural history of patients with chronic aortic regurgitation is relatively good, even in those with moderate to severe regurgitation. However, after symptoms develop, the prognosis is poor without surgical intervention.[8] The main preoperative predictors of outcome after valve replacement for aortic regurgitation include left ventricular function, duration of left ventricular dysfunction, and the patient's symptomatic status.[9] In asymptomatic patients, the status of left ventricular function is important to determining both the natural history and the outcome of valve replacement.[10] Asymptomatic patients with normal resting left ventricular systolic function have a benign prognosis with an annual mortality rate less than 0.5 percent.[11] In contrast, the majority of asymptomatic patients with left ventricular dysfunction will develop symptoms and require surgical intervention within 2 to 3 years.[12, 13] The timing of surgical intervention is critical. Delay may result in irreversible changes in ventricular function associated with increased postoperative mortality and morbidity. Conversely, intervening too early exposes the patients to unnecessary risks associated with a prosthetic valve and the additional risks of anticoagulation in the case of mechanical prostheses. Bonow and associates[14] demonstrated that serial radionuclide ventriculography is very useful in managing asymptomatic patients with aortic regurgitation (Fig. 21–1). Asymptomatic patients can be followed carefully with serial evaluation of left ventricular function, undergoing valve replacement only after the onset of symptoms or the development of left ventricular dysfunction, as evidenced by an increase in left ventricular end-systolic volume greater than 2 standard deviations from normal or a decreased left ventricular ejection fraction (0.45 was used by Bonow and associates in their studies, which is the lower limit of normal for their laboratory). It should be noted that although exercise tolerance of patients is a determinant of outcome after valve replacement, the left ventricular ejection fraction response to exercise is of limited value.[15] This most likely relates to the fact that the change in the left ventricular ejection fraction from rest to peak exercise in these patients is principally determined by the peripheral vascular response.[16]

Mitral Regurgitation

Mitral regurgitation can result from lesions involving the mitral valve annulus, leaflets, chordae, papillary muscles, or a combination of these structures. The regurgitant volume is ejected from the left ventricle during early systole (50 percent before aortic valve opening) into the low-impedance left atrium.[17] The decreased left ventricular afterload results in an elevated left ventricular ejection fraction in patients with severe mitral regurgitation. Patients with cardiac failure resulting from mitral regurgitation often have left ventricular ejection fractions within the normal range. By the time the ejection fraction has fallen below 40 percent, there is already advanced myocardial dysfunction.[8]

End-systolic volume has been found to be a better predictor of outcome than ejection fraction or end-diastolic volume in these patients. Patients with an end-systolic volume index less than 30 ml/m^2 have preserved left ventricular function postoperatively; in contrast, an end-systolic index of 90 ml/m^2 preoperatively is associated with increased perioperative mortality and left ventricular dysfunction postoperatively. In comparison with aortic regurgitation, patients with mitral regurgitation with the same end-systolic volume usually have more severe left ventricular function.[18] This has led to the recommendations that, in general terms, patients with mitral regurgitation should

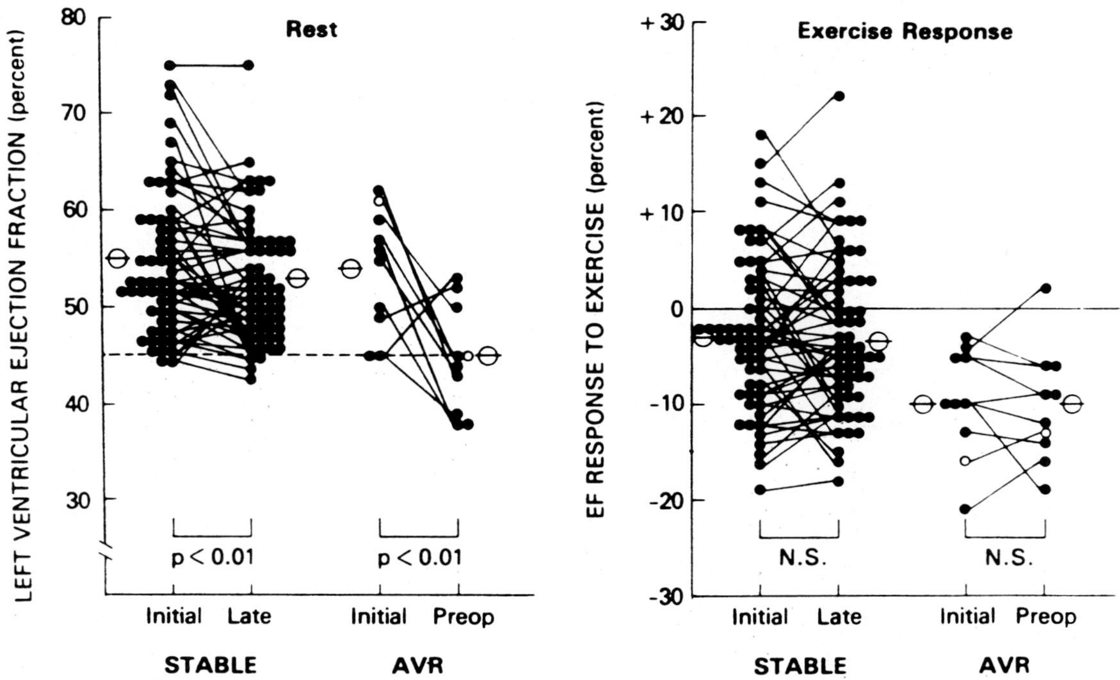

FIGURE 21–1 Change in radionuclide angiographic data during follow-up studies (6 to 8 months) in patients who remained asymptomatic with normal left ventricular function (Stable) and those who subsequently underwent aortic valve replacement (AVR). *Dashed line,* lower limit of normal ejection fraction (EF) at rest (45 percent); *slashed circles,* mean values. (Adapted from Bonow RO, Rosing DR, McIntosh CL, et al: The natural history of asymptomatic patients with aortic regurgitation and normal left ventricular function. Circulation 68:509–517, 1983. By permission of The American Heart Association, Inc.)

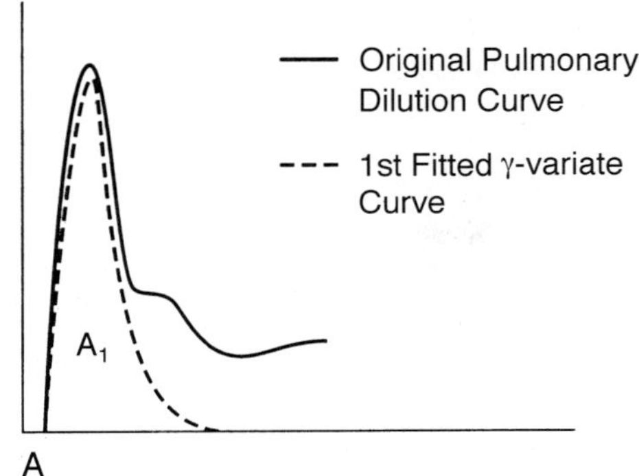

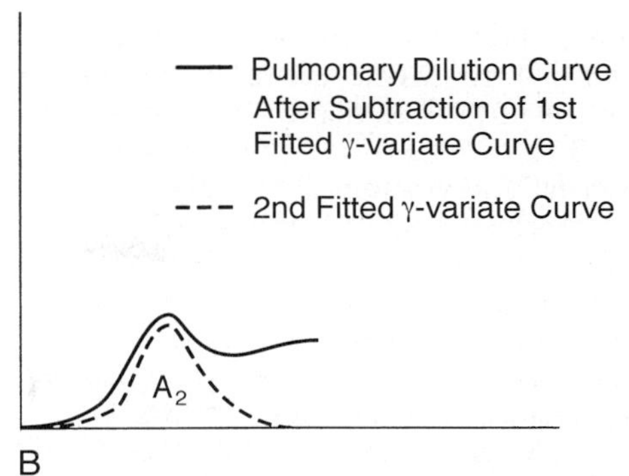

FIGURE 21–2 A, Gamma-variate curve fitted to pulmonary dilution curve. The area under curve A_1 is calculated, representing Q_p, the quantity of blood flowing through the lungs. **B,** Each point on the gamma-variate curve in **A** is subtracted from the corresponding point in the original dilution curve. The resultant curve is shown, representing the recirculation of activity through the lungs. Using this portion of this curve from the beginning of its upslope until immediately after its peak, a second gamma-variate curve is fitted. The area under this second gamma-variate curve (A_2) represents pulmonary flow minus systemic flow ($Q_p - Q_s$). The ratio $A_1/(A_1 - A_2)$ is equal to Q_p/Q_s. (**A** and **B,** Adapted from Gelfand MJ, Hannon DW: Pediatric cardiology. *In* Greson MC [ed]: Cardiac Nuclear Medicine. pp. 432–474. New York, McGraw-Hill, 1987.)

undergo surgical intervention before the ejection fraction falls below 55 to 60 percent and before the end-systolic volume index increases above 55 ml/m^2.[19]

Right ventricular function also appears important in patients with mitral regurgitation. Using radionuclide ventriculography, Hochreiter and colleagues[20] studied 53 patients with chronic mitral regurgitation and found that the patients' symptomatic status and exercise tolerance correlated with their right ventricular ejection fractions. In a subgroup of patients who underwent cardiac catheterization, the pulmonary arterial systolic and capillary wedge pressures correlated with the right ventricular ejection fraction. In 35 patients managed medically, the presence of a depressed right and/or left ventricular function was associated with a poor prognosis. However, Cox model analysis of survival identified no covariable that added significantly to the resting right ventricular ejection fraction as a prognostic factor related to survival.

Congenital Heart Disease: Quantification of Shunts

The role of nuclear cardiology is limited in congenital heart disease, with two-dimensional and Doppler echocardiography and magnetic resonance imaging being the most useful noninvasive techniques in this setting. However, first-pass radionuclide angiography is useful in detecting and quantitating intracardiac shunts.

Radionuclide data are obtained using a gamma camera with first-pass capabilities, and acquired data are analyzed using a dedicated computer. Pulmonary time-activity curves are obtained by placing a region of interest over the right lung that is not contaminated by activity from the heart or great vessels. A normal pulmonary time-activity curve typically rapidly reaches a peak that then decreases exponentially. However, in the presence of a left-to-right shunt, there is early recirculation of the tracer, altering the rapid exponential decline of the time activity. If the shunt is large enough, it may result in the appearance of a second peak. The time-activity curve is usually analyzed by using curve fitting by a gamma-variate method (Fig. 21–2). A curve with an exponential decay is fitted corresponding to the rapid upstroke of the pulmonary time-activity curve. The area under this curve (A_1) is directly proportional to pulmonary flow (Q_p). This curve is subtracted from the original time-activity curve, and another curve is fitted to the remaining data. The area under this second curve (A_2) is directly proportional to flow through the shunt; therefore, $A_1 - A_2$ is equal to systemic flow (Q_s). This allows quantification of the shunt as a ratio of pulmonary/systemic flow (Q_p/Q_s). Close correlation between results obtained from this method and those calculated with Fick oximetry have been reported.[21, 22] Experimental and clinical data suggest that radionuclide technique may be more accurate than Fick oximetry, particularly in patients with atrial septal defects when it can be difficult to obtain an accurate mixed venous O_2 saturation.[23, 24]

Right-to-left shunts have also been quantified using first-pass radionuclide angiography.[25] Peter and coworkers[25] acquired time-activity curves over the carotid artery, avoiding contamination from heart and lung activity in 20 children with congenital heart disease. The presence of a right-to-left shunt was indicated by the early appearance of activity in the systemic circulation. Carotid time-activity curves were analyzed with techniques analogous to those used for quantitating left-to-right shunts. The results correlated well with Fick oximetry. Despite these encouraging preliminary results, the technique has not found wide application, possibly because of low count rates obtained over the peripheral artery. Radiolabeled macroaggregates of albumin have also been used to quantitate right-to-left cardiac shunts.[26] Normally, in the absence of right-to-left shunting, all the labeled macroaggregates become lodged in the pulmonary capillaries after intravenous administration. However, in the presence of right-to-left shunting, some of the macroaggregates enter the systemic circulation and become trapped in systemic capillaries. By whole body counting, it is possible to derive the size of the shunt by comparing the systemic and pulmonary counts. Careful attention to particle size is required to prevent clinically significant embolization.

Radionuclide ventriculography can also be of value in assessing resting left and right ventricular function and in evaluating ventricular function during exercise to determine cardiac reserve in patients with congenital heart disease. The role of perfusion imaging is poorly defined, but this technique may be of value in assessing patients with congenital abnormalities of the coronary artery circulation.

REFERENCES

1. Rigo P, Alderson PO, Robertson RM, et al: Measurement of aortic and mitral regurgitation. Circulation 60;306–312, 1979.
2. Nicod P, Corbett JR, Firth BG, et al: Radionuclide techniques for valvular regurgitant index: comparison in patients with normal and depressed ventricular function. J Nucl Med 23:763–769, 1982.
3. Makler PT, McCarthy DM, Velchik MG, et al: Fourier amplitude ratio: a new way to assess valvular regurgitation: J Nucl Med 24:204–207, 1983.
4. Dae M, Botvinick EH, O'Connell WO, et al: Increased accuracy of scintigraphic quantitation of valvular regurgitation using atrial corrected-Fourier amplitude ratios. Am J Noninvas Cardiol 1:155–162, 1987.
5. Kelbaek H, Hartling OJ, Skagen K, et al: First-pass radionuclide determination of cardiac output: an improved gamma camera method. J Nucl Med 28:1330–1334, 1987.
6. Kelbaek H, Aldershville J, Svendsen JH, et al: Combined first pass and equilibrium radionuclide cardiographic determination of stroke volume for quantitation of valvular regurgitation. J Am Coll Cardiol 11:769–773, 1988.
7. Philippe L, Mena I, Darcourt J, French WJ: Evaluation of valvular regurgitation by factor analysis of first-pass angiography. J Nucl Med 29:159–167, 1988.
8. Braunwald E: Valvular heart disease. *In* Braunwald (ed): Heart Disease. A Textbook of Cardiovascular Disease. Philadelphia: WB Saunders, 1992.
9. Bonow RO, Dodd JT, Maron BJ, et al: Long-term serial changes in left ventricular function and reversal of ventricular dilatation after valve replacement for chronic aortic regurgitation. Circulation 78:1108–1120, 1988.
10. Bonow RO: Radionuclide angiography in management of asymptomatic aortic regurgitation. Circulation 84 (suppl I):296–302, 1991.
11. Seimienczuk D, Greenberg B, Morris C, et al: Chronic aortic insufficiency: factors associated with progression to aortic valve replacement. Ann Intern Med 110:587–592, 1989.
12. Henry WL, Bonow RO, Rosing DR, Epstein SE: Observations on the optimum time for operative intervention for aortic regurgitation: II. Serial echocardiographic evaluation of asymptomatic patients. Circulation 61:484–492, 1980.
13. McDonald IG, Jelinek VM: Serial M-mode echocardiography in severe chronic aortic regurgitation. Circulation 62:1291–1296, 1980.
14. Bonow RO, Rosing DR, McIntosh CL, et al: The natural history of asymptomatic patients with aortic regurgitation and normal left ventricular function. Circulation 68:509–517, 1983.
15. Kawanishi DT, McKay CR, Chandraratna AN, et al: Cardiovascular response to dynamic exercise in patients with chronic symptomatic mild-to-moderate and severe aortic regurgitation. Circulation 73:62–72, 1986.
16. Stewart RE, Gross MD, Starling MR: Mechanisms for an abnormal radionuclide left ventricular ejection fraction to exercise in patients with chronic, severe aortic regurgitation. Am Heart J 123:453–461, 1992.
17. Eckberg DL, Gault FH, Bouchard R, et al: Mechanics of left ventricular contraction in chronic severe mitral regurgitation. Circulation 47:1252–1259, 1973.
18. Wisenbaugh T, Spann JF, Carabello BA: Differences in myocardial performance and load between patients with similar amounts of chronic aortic versus chronic mitral regurgitation. J Am Coll Cardiol 3:916–923, 1984.
19. Bonow RO, Carabello B, de Leon AC Jr et al: Guidelines for the management of patients with valvular heart disease: executive summary. A report of the American College of Cardiology/American Heart Association Task Force on Practice Guidelines (Committee on Management of Patients with Valvular Heart Disease). Circulation 18:1949–1984, 1998.
20. Hochreiter C, Niles N, Devereux RB, et al: Mitral regurgitation: relationship of noninvasive descriptors of right and left ventricular performance to clinical and hemodynamic findings and to prognosis in medically and surgically treated patients. Circulation 73:900–912, 1986.
21. Alderson PO, Jost RG, Strauss AW, et al: Radionuclide angiocardiography. Improved diagnosis and quantitation of left-to-right shunts using area ratio techniques in children. Circulation 51:1136–1143, 1975.
22. Askenazi J, Ahnberg DS, Korngold E, et al: Quantitative radionuclide angiocardiography: detection and quantitation of left to right shunts. Am J Cardiol 37:382–387, 1976.
23. Alderson PO, Gaudiani VA, Watson DC, et al: Quantitative radionuclide angiocardiography in animals with experimental atrial septal defects. J Nucl Med 19:364–369, 1978.
24. Baker EJ, Ellam SV, Lorber A, et al: Superiority of radionuclide over oximetric measurements of left to right shunts. Br Heart J 53:535–540, 1985.
25. Peter CA, Armstrong BE, Jones RH: Radionuclide quantitation of right-to-left intracardiac shunts in children. Circulation 64:572–577, 1981.
26. Gates GF, Orme HW, Dore EK: Measurement of cardiac shunting with technetium labeled albumin aggregates. J Nucl Med 12:746–749, 1971.
27. Gelfand MJ, Hannon DW: Pediatric cardiology. *In* Greson MC (ed): Cardiac Nuclear Medicine. pp. 432–474. New York, McGraw-Hill, 1987.

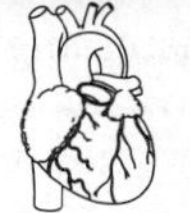

CHAPTER 22

BALLOON DILATATION OF THE CARDIAC VALVES

Igor F. Palacios

PERCUTANEOUS PULMONIC VALVULOPLASTY
PERCUTANEOUS MITRAL BALLOON VALVOTOMY FOR PATIENTS WITH RHEUMATIC MITRAL STENOSIS
Patient Selection
Technique
Mechanism
Immediate Outcome
Predictors of an Increase in Mitral Valve Area and Procedural Success With PMV
Complications
Clinical Follow-Up
PERCUTANEOUS AORTIC BALLOON VALVULOPLASTY
Procedure
Mechanism
Immediate Results
Complications
Long-Term Follow-Up After PAV
PAV as a Bridge to Aortic Valve Replacement
PAV for Patients in Cardiogenic Shock
PAV for Patients With Congenital Aortic Stenosis
PERCUTANEOUS TRICUSPID BALLOON VALVULOPLASTY

Before 1982, cardiac surgery was the conventional form of treatment for symptomatic stenotic valvular heart lesions. Today, percutaneous balloon dilatation of stenotic cardiac valves is being used in many centers for the treatment of patients with pulmonic, mitral, aortic, and tricuspid stenosis.

PERCUTANEOUS PULMONIC VALVULOPLASTY

Since its introduction by Kan and associates in 1982, percutaneous balloon pulmonary valvuloplasty (PPV) has become the treatment of choice for patients with isolated pulmonic valvular stenosis.[1–3] In both children and adults with valvular pulmonic stenosis, balloon valvuloplasty produces excellent immediate and long-term results. Patients with isolated pulmonic stenosis and a transvalvular gradient greater than 40 mm Hg are candidates for this technique.[3–8]

The technique of PPV is relatively simple—it is performed under sedation and local anesthesia. Before PPV, accurate measurement of the pulmonary annulus by two-dimensional (2-D) echocardiography and angiography is fundamental in the appropriate selection of balloon size. Complete right and left catheterization and right ventricular cineangiography in both the anteroposterior and the lateral projections are performed before PPV to document the severity of the stenosis and the presence of associated lesions.

The stenotic pulmonic valve is crossed with an end-hole balloon wedge catheter, and the catheter is placed in the left pulmonary artery. A 0.035- or 0.038-inch exchange guidewire is advanced in the distal left pulmonary artery, and the catheter and venous introducer are removed. When using the double-balloon technique, a second guide wire could be placed parallel to the first guide wire with the help of a double-lumen catheter. In smaller children, double-balloon PPV can be performed by introducing a dilating balloon through each of the femoral veins. The balloon or balloons dilating catheters are then advanced and placed straddling the pulmonic valve. A balloon combination that provides a diameter 20 to 30 percent greater than the pulmonary annulus is used to provide adequate relief of the stenosis. The valvuloplasty balloons are then inflated by hand until the waist produced by the stenotic pulmonic valve disappears. Two to four brief inflations are performed to minimize the period of hypotension. The inflation/deflation process takes between 15 and 20 seconds.

Double-balloon PPV is tolerated better than single-balloon PPV, resulting in less hypotension and bradycardia during balloon inflations. After the dilatations are completed, the deflated catheters are removed and hemodynamics and right ventricular cineangiography are repeated. At the end of the procedure, the catheters are removed and hemosthesis is achieved by local pressure. In most adults, two balloons are required. Patients are observed after the procedure in a general medical ward and discharged the following day.

PPV produces a significant decrease in pulmonic gradient. In general, pulmonic gradient decreases by 50 to 80 percent. The results of PPV from different centers are shown in Table 22–1. Patients with severe pulmonary dysplasia with hypoplasia of the pulmonic annulus are unlikely to have improvement after PPV. In some patients, a significant gradient could develop across the infundibulum after relief of the valvular pulmonic stenosis and may be reduced by the use of beta-blockers or calcium channel blockers. This infundibular gradient has no clinical importance and disappears or markedly decreases at follow-up cardiac catheterization or Doppler echocardiography.

Complications of PPV are rare. They are more frequent in neonates. Perforation of the right ventricular outflow

TABLE 22-1 Immediate Results of Percutaneous Pulmonic Valvuloplasty

Author	Patients (n)	Pulmonary Gradient (mm Hg)	
		Pre-PPV	*Post-PPV*
Khan et al	20	68	23
Rao et al	71	91 ± 41	26 ± 19
VACA registry*	784	71 ± 33	28 ± 21
Beekman et al	90	70 ± 24	30 ± 17
Ali Khan et al	257	97 ± 30	22 ± 20
Schmaltz et al*	305	72 ± 32	32 ± 25
MGH†	39	69 ± 26	17 ± 11

Abbreviations: MGH, Massachusetts General Hospital; PPV, percutaneous pulmonic valvuloplasty.
*Multicenter study.
†Adults.

tract has been reported to occur in neonates when attempts have been made to cross the pulmonary valve. Similarly, vessel trauma is more frequent in neonates and infants and can be diminished by using the double-balloon technique. Mild pulmonary insufficiency occurs frequently but does not have significant clinical or hemodynamic consequences.

Follow-up studies have shown that restenosis is uncommon. Follow-up cardiac catheterization and Doppler echocardiography studies have demonstrated that significant restenosis appears to be uncommon. Recurrent stenosis is much less likely if the final gradient after PPV is less than 30 mm Hg. The residual gradient measured 6 months after PPV has been significantly smaller than the one measured immediately after the procedure. This finding is probably related to improvement in the infundibulum stenosis, which frequently occurs immediately after PPV.

Percutaneous Mitral Balloon Valvotomy for Patients With Rheumatic Mitral Stenosis

Since its introduction in 1984 by Inoue and colleagues,[9] percutaneous mitral balloon valvotomy (PMV) has been used successfully as an alternative to open or closed surgical mitral commissurotomy in the treatment of patients with symptomatic rheumatic mitral stenosis.[10–26] PMV produces good immediate hemodynamic outcome, a low complication rate, and sustained clinical improvement in the majority of patients with mitral stenosis.[10–26] PMV is safe and effective. The immediate and long-term results appear to be similar to those of surgical mitral commissurotomy.[10–26] Today, PMV is the preferred form of therapy for relief of mitral stenosis for a selected group of patients with symptomatic mitral stenosis.

Patient Selection

Selection of patients for PMV should be based on symptoms, physical examination, and 2-D and Doppler echocardiographic findings. PMV is usually performed electively. However, emergency PMV can be performed as a lifesaving procedure in patients with mitral stenosis and severe pulmonary edema refractory to medical therapy and/or cardiogenic shock. Patients considered for PMV should be symptomatic (New York Heart Association [NYHA] ≥ II), have no recent thromboembolic events, have less than two grades of mitral regurgitation by contrast ventriculography (using the Seller classification), and have no evidence of left atrial thrombus on 2-D and transesophageal echocardiography. Transthoracic and transesophageal echocardiography should routinely be performed before PMV. Patients in atrial fibrillation and those with previous embolic episodes should be anticoagulated with warfarin with a therapeutic prothrombin time for at least 3 months before PMV. Patients with left atrium thrombus on 2-D echocardiography should be excluded. However, PMV could be performed in these patients if left atrium thrombus resolves after warfarin therapy.

Technique

PMV is performed with the patient in the fasting state under mild sedation. Antibiotics (dicloxacillin 500 mg PO q/6 hours for 4 doses started before the procedure, or cefazolin 1 g IV at the time of the procedure) are used. Patients allergic to penicillin should receive vancomycin 1 g IV at the time of the procedure.

All patients carefully chosen as candidates for PMV should undergo diagnostic right and left and transseptal left heart catheterization. After transseptal left heart catheterization, systemic anticoagulation is achieved by the intravenous administration of 100 U/kg of heparin. In patients older than 40 years, coronary arteriography should also be performed.

Hemodynamic measurements, cardiac output, and left ventricular cineangiography are performed before and after PMV. Cardiac output is measured by thermodilution and Fick method techniques. Mitral valve calcification and angiographic severity of mitral regurgitation (Seller classification) are graded qualitatively from grade 0 to 4 as previously described.[11] An oxygen diagnostic run is performed before and after PMV to determine the presence of left-to-right shunt across the atrial septum after PMV.

There is no single unique technique of PMV. Most of the techniques of PMV require transseptal left heart catheterization and use of the antegrade approach. Antegrade PMV can be accomplished using a single-[10–11, 14] or a double-balloon technique.[11–13, 15] In the latter approach, the two balloons could be placed through a single femoral vein and single transseptal punctures[11–13, 15] or through two femoral veins and two separate atrial septal punctures.[12] In the retrograde technique of PMV, the balloons' dilating catheters are advanced percutaneously through the right and left femoral arteries over guide wires that have been snared from the descending aorta.[27] These guide wires have been advanced transseptally from the right femoral vein into the left atrium, the left ventricle, and the ascending aorta. A retrograde nontransseptal technique of PMV has also been described.[28] A technique of PMV using a newly designed metallic valvulotome was recently introduced.[29] The device consists of a detachable metallic cylinder with two articulated bars screwed onto the distal end of a disposable catheter whose proximal end is connected to an activating pliers. Squeezing the pliers opens the bars up to a maximum of 40 mm. The results with this device are at least comparable to those of the other balloon techniques of PMV. However, multiple uses after sterilization should markedly decrease procedural costs.

Antegrade Double-Balloon Technique

In performing PMV using the antegrade double-balloon technique (Fig. 22–1), two 0.0038-inch, 260-cm-long Teflon-coated exchange wires are placed across the mitral valve into the left ventricle, through the aortic valve into the ascending and then the descending aorta.[30] Care should be taken to maintain large and smooth loops of the guide wires in the left ventricular cavity to allow appropriate placement of the dilating balloons. If a second guide wire cannot be placed into the ascending and descending aorta, a 0.038-inch Amplatz-type transfer guide wire with a preformed curlew at its tip can be placed at the left ventricular apex. In patients with an aortic valve prosthesis, both guide wires with preformed curlew tips should be placed at the left ventricular apex. When one or both guide wires are placed in the left ventricular apex, the balloons should be inflated sequentially. Care should be taken to avoid forward movement of the balloons and guide wires to prevent left ventricular perforation. Two balloon dilating catheters, chosen according to the patient's body surface area, are then advanced over each one of the guide wires and positioned across the mitral valve parallel to the longitudinal axis of the left ventricle. The balloon valvotomy catheters are then inflated by hand until the indentation produced by the stenotic mitral valve is no longer seen. Generally one but occasionally two or three inflations are performed. After complete deflation, the balloons are removed sequentially.

Inoue Technique

PMV can also be performed using the Inoue technique (Fig. 22–2).[9, 23–25] The Inoue balloon is a 12 French shaft, coaxial, double-lumen catheter. The balloon is made of a double layer of rubber tubing with a layer of synthetic micromesh in between. After transseptal catheterization, a stainless steel guide wire is advanced through the transseptal catheter and placed with its tip coiled into the left atrium and the transseptal catheter is removed. A 14 French dilator is advanced over the guide wire and used to dilate the femoral vein and the atrial septum. A balloon catheter chosen according to the patient's height is advanced over the guide wire into the left atrium. The distal part of the balloon is inflated and advanced into the left ventricle with the help of the spring wire stylet, which has been inserted through the inner lumen of the catheter. Once the catheter is in the left ventricle, the partially inflated balloon is moved back and forth inside the left ventricle to assure that it is free of the chordae tendinae. The catheter is then gently pulled against the mitral plane until resistance is felt. The balloon is then rapidly inflated to its full capacity and deflated quickly. During inflation of the balloon, an indentation should be seen in its midportion. The catheter is withdrawn into the left atrium, and the mitral gradient and cardiac output are measured. If further dilatations are required, the stylet is introduced again and the steps are repeated at a larger balloon volume. After each dilatation, the effect should be assessed by pressure measurement, auscultation and 2-D echocardiography. If mitral regurgitation occurs, further dilatation of the valve should not be performed.

Mechanism

The mechanism of successful PMV is splitting of the fused commissures toward the mitral annulus, resulting in commissural widening. This mechanism has been demonstrated by pathologic,[14–31] surgical,[31] and echocardiographic

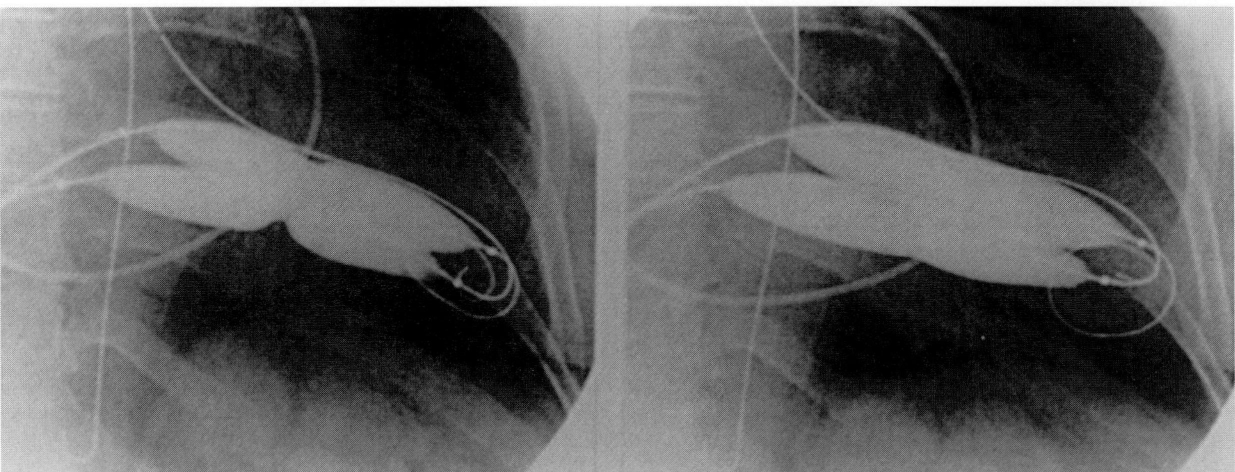

FIGURE 22–1 Double-balloon percutaneous mitral balloon valvotomy (PMV). Two guide wires are advanced into the ascending and descending aorta, with the tip at the level of diaphragm. Two balloon catheters are placed straddling the stenotic mitral valve; markers identifying the proximal end of the balloons are inflated by hand until the waist produced by the stenotic valve disappears.

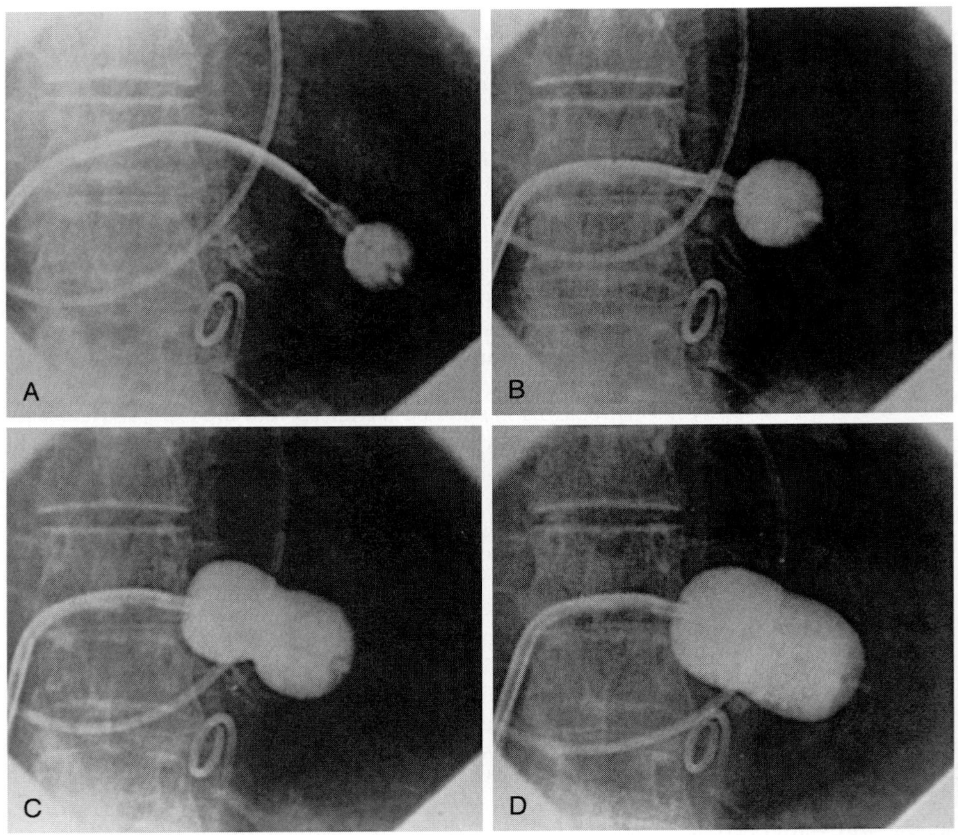

FIGURE 22–2 The Inoue technique of PMV. **A,** A partially inflated Inoue balloon catheter is placed into the left ventricle. **B,** It is gently pulled against the mitral plane until resistance is felt. The balloon is therewith rapidly inflated by hand. **C,** An indentation is seen in the balloon's mid portion straddling the stenotic mitral valve. **D,** The balloon inflated until the waist produced by the stenotic valve disappears.

studies.[32] In addition, in patients with calcific mitral stenosis, the balloons could increase mitral valve flexibility by the fracture of the calcified deposits in the mitral valve leaflets.[14] Although rare, undesirable complications such as leaflet tears, left ventricular perforation, tear of the atrial septum, and rupture of chordae, mitral annulus, and papillary muscle could also occur.

Immediate Outcome

Figure 22–3 shows the hemodynamic changes produced by PMV in one patient. PMV resulted in a significant decrease in mitral gradient, mean left atrial pressure, and mean pulmonary artery pressure, and an increase in cardiac output and mitral valve area. Table 22–2 shows the changes in mitral valve area reported by several investigators using different techniques of PMV. In most series, PMV is reported to increase mitral valve area from less than 1.0 cm^2 to 2.0 cm^2 or greater.[10–30, 32–34]

Eight hundred and sixty consecutive patients with mitral stenosis have undergone PMV at the Massachusetts General Hospital between July 1986 and July 1999. As shown in Figure 22–4, in this group of patients PMV resulted in a significant decrease in mitral gradient from 15 ± 1 mm Hg to 5 ± 1 mm Hg. The mean cardiac output increased from 3.9 ± 0.1 L/min to 4.5 L/min, and the calculated mitral valve area increased from 0.9 ± 0.1 cm^2 to 2.0 ± 0.1 cm^2. In addition, mean pulmonary artery pressure decreased from 37 ± 1 mm Hg to 28 ± 1 mm Hg (P <

TABLE 22–2 **Changes in Mitral Valve Area**

Author	Institution	Patients (n)	Age (yr)	Pre-PMV	Post-PMV
Palacios	MGH	860	57 ± 12	0.9 ± 0.3	2.0 ± 0.2
Vahanian	Tenon	1514	45 ± 15	1.0 ± 0.2	1.9 ± 0.3
Stefanadis	Athens University	438	44 ± 11	1.0 ± 0.3	2.1 ± 0.5
Chen	Guangzhou	4832	37 ± 12	1.1 ± 0.3	2.1 ± 0.2
NHLBI	Multicenter	738	54 ± 12	1.0 ± 0.4	2.0 ± 0.2
Inoue	Takeda	527	50 ± 10	1.1 ± 0.1	2.0 ± 0.1
Inoue registry	Multicenter	1251	53 ± 15	1.0 ± 0.3	1.8 ± 0.6
Farhat	Fattouma	463	33 ± 12	1.0 ± 0.2	2.2 ± 0.4
Arora	G.B. Pan	600	27 ± 8	0.8 ± 0.2	2.2 ± 0.4
Cribier	Ruen	153	36 ± 15	1.0 ± 0.2	2.2 ± 0.4

Abbreviations: MGH, Massachusetts General Hospital; NHLBI, National Heart, Lung, and Blood Institute; PMV, percutaneous mitral balloon valvotomy.

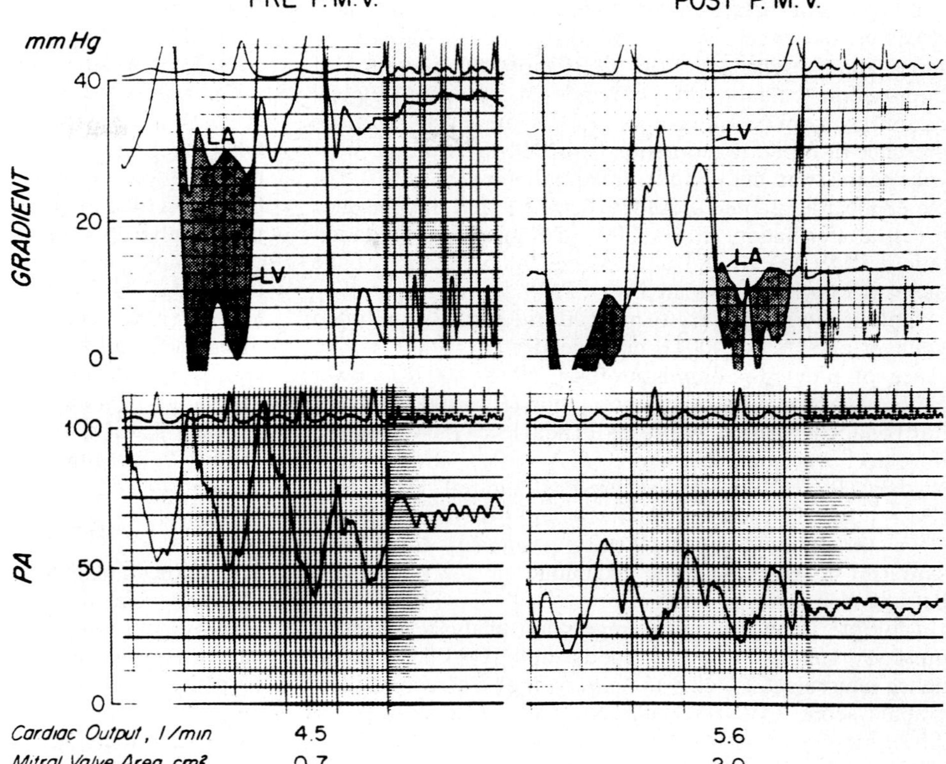

FIGURE 22–3 Hemodynamic changes produced by a successful PMV in one patient with severe mitral stenosis. **Top,** Simultaneous left atrium and left ventricular pressures before **(right)** and after **(left)** PMV. **Bottom,** The phasic and mean pulmonary artery pressures before **(right)** and after **(left)** PMV. The corresponding cardiac outputs and calculated mitral valve areas are also displayed. LA, left atrium; LV, left ventricle; PA, pulmonary artery pressure; PMV, percutaneous mitral balloon valvuloplasty.

.0001). The mean left atrial pressure decreased from 25 ± 1 mm Hg to 16 ± 1 mm Hg ($P < .0001$) and the calculated pulmonary vascular resistances decreased significantly after PMV.

A successful hemodynamic outcome (defined as a post-PMV mitral valve area ≥ 1.5 cm², ≤ 2-grade increase in mitral regurgitation by angiography, and a QP/QS < 1.5/1) was obtained in 79 percent of the patients. Although a suboptimal result occurred in 21 percent of the patients, a post-PMV mitral valve area 1.0 cm² or less (critical mitral valve area) was present in only 7 percent of these patients.

Predictors of an Increase in Mitral Valve Area and Procedural Success With PMV

Univariate analysis demonstrated that the increase in mitral valve area with PMV is directly related to the balloon size

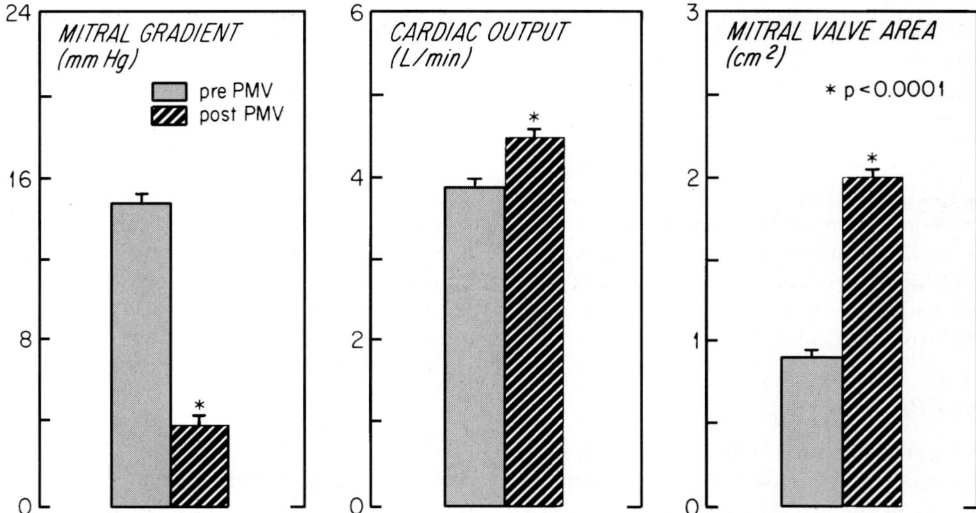

FIGURE 22–4 Mean changes in mitral gradient, cardiac output, and mitral valve area produced by percutaneous mitral balloon valvotomy (PMV) in 732 consecutive patients undergoing PMV at the Massachusetts General Hospital.

employed as it reflects in the effective balloon dilating area (EBDA) and inversely related to the echocardiographic score, the presence of atrial fibrillation, the presence of fluoroscopic calcium, the presence of previous surgical commissurotomy, older age, NYHA pre-PMV, and the presence of mitral regurgitation before PMV. Multiple stepwise regression analysis identified balloon size ($P < .02$), the echocardiographic score ($P < .0001$), and the presence of atrial fibrillation ($P < .009$) and mitral regurgitation before PMV ($P < .03$) as independent predictors of the increase in mitral valve area with PMV.

Univariate predictors of procedural success included younger age ($P = .0001$), male gender ($P = .0003$), absence of previous commissurotomy ($P = .0078$), lower NYHA functional status at presentation ($P = .0001$), lower fluoroscopic mitral valve calcification ($P = .0001$), lower echocardiographic score ($P = .0001$), normal sinus rhythm ($P = .0001$), larger pre-PMV mitral valve area ($P = .0001$), lower pre-PMV mitral regurgitation ($P = .0001$), lower pre-PMV mean pulmonary artery pressure ($P = .001$), and the technique of PMV (double-balloon technique, $P = .05$).

Multiple stepwise logistic regression analysis identified pre-PMV mitral valve area (odds ratio [OR] 138, confidence intervals (CIs) 43.8 to 46.6, $P < .0001$), echocardiographic score 8 or less (OR 1.92, CI 1.26 to 2.94, $P = .002$), male gender (OR 2.32, CI 1.37 to 4.16, $P = .002$) absence of previous surgical commissurotomy (OR 1.79, CI 1.09 to 2.94, $P = .01$), and younger age (OR 6.25, CI 2.5 to 16.6, $P = .0002$) as independent predictors of procedural success.

Echocardiographic Score

The echocardiographic score is the more important predictor of the immediate and long-term outcome of PMV. In this morphologic score, leaflet rigidity, leaflet thickening, valvular calcification, and subvalvular disease are each scored from 0 to 4.[32, 35] A higher score would represent a heavily calcified, thickened, and immobile valve with extensive thickening and calcification of the subvalvular apparatus. Among the four components of the echocardiographic score, valve leaflet thickening and subvalvular disease correlate best with the increase in mitral valve area produced by PMV. The increase in mitral valve area with PMV is inversely related to the echocardiographic score. The best outcomes with PMV occur in those patients with echocardiographic scores of 8 or less. The increase in mitral valve area is significantly greater in patients with echocardiographic scores of 8 or less than in those with echocardiographic scores greater than 8. Suboptimal results with PMV are more likely to occur in patients with valves that are more rigid and more thickened and in those with more subvalvular fibrosis and calcification.

Balloon Size and EBDA

The increase in mitral valve area with PMV is directly related to balloon size. This effect was first demonstrated in the subgroup of patients treated with repeat PMV.[17] They initially underwent PMV with a single balloon, resulting in a mean mitral valve area of 1.2 ± 0.2 cm^2. The repeat PMV used the double-balloon technique, which increased the EBDA normalized by body surface area (EBDA/BSA) from 3.41 ± 0.2 cm^2/m^2 to 4.51 ± 0.2 cm^2/m^2. The mean mitral valve area in this group after repeat PMV was 1.8 ± 0.2 cm^2. The increase in mitral valve area in patients who underwent PMV at the Massachusetts General Hospital using the double-balloon technique (EBDA 6.4 ± 0.03 cm^2) was significantly greater than the increase in mitral valve area achieved in patients who underwent PMV using the single-balloon technique (EBDA 4.3 ± 0.02 cm^2). The mean mitral valve areas were 2.0 ± 0.1 cm^2 and 1.4 ± 0.1 cm^2 for patients who underwent PMV with the double-balloon and the single-balloon techniques, respectively. However, care should be taken in the selection of dilating balloon catheters in order to obtain an adequate final mitral valve area and no change or a minimal increase in mitral regurgitation.

Mitral Valve Calcification

The immediate outcome of patients undergoing PMV is inversely related to the severity of valvular calcification seen by fluoroscopy. Patients without fluoroscopic calcium have a greater increase in mitral valve area after PMV than do patients with calcified valves. Patients with either no or 1+ fluoroscopic calcium have a greater increase in mitral valve area after PMV (2.1 ± 0.1 cm^2 and 1.9 ± 0.1 cm^2, respectively) than those patients with 2, 3, or 4+ of calcium (1.7 ± 0.1 cm^2, 1.5 ± 0.1 cm^2, and 1.4 ± 0.1 cm^2, respectively).

Previous Surgical Commissurotomy

Although the increase in mitral valve area with PMV is inversely related to the presence of previous surgical mitral commissurotomy, PMV can produce a good outcome in this group of patients. The mean mitral valve area in 102 patients with previous surgical commissurotomy was 1.7 ± 0.1 cm^2 compared with a valve area of 2.0 ± 0.1 cm^2 in patients without previous surgical commissurotomy. In this group of patients, an echocardiographic score of 8 or less was again the most important predictor of a successful immediate hemodynamic outcome.

Age

The immediate outcome of PMV is directly related to the age of the patient. The percentage of patients obtaining a good result with this technique decreases as age increases. A successful hemodynamic outcome from PMV was obtained in less than 50 percent of patients 65 years old or older.[22] This inverse relationship between age and the immediate outcome from PMV is due to the higher frequency of atrial fibrillation and calcified valves and the higher echocardiographic scores in elderly patients.

Atrial Fibrillation

The increase in mitral valve area with PMV is inversely related to the presence of atrial fibrillation; the post-PMV mitral valve area of patients in normal sinus rhythm was 2.1 ± 0.1 cm^2 compared with a valve area of 1.7 ±

TABLE 22-3 Complications

Author	Patients (n)	Mortality (%)	Tamponade (%)	Severe MR (%)	Embolism (%)
Palacios	860	0.3	0.6	3.3	1.0
Vahanian	1514	0.4	0.3	3.4	0.3
Stefanadis	438	0.2	0.0	3.4	0.0
Chen	4832	0.1	0.8	1.4	0.5
NHLBI	738	3.0	4.0	3.0	3.0
Inoue	527	0.0	1.6	1.9	0.6
Inoue registry	1251	0.6	1.4	3.8	0.9
Farhat	463	0.4	0.7	4.6	2.0
Arora	600	1.0	1.3	1.0	0.5
Cribier	153	0.0	0.7	1.4	0.7

Abbreviations: MR, mitral regurgitation; NHLBI, National Heart, Lung, and Blood Institute.

0.1 cm^2 of those patients in atrial fibrillation. The inferior immediate outcome of PMV in patients with mitral stenosis who are in atrial fibrillation is more likely related to the presence of clinical and morphologic characteristics associated with inferior results after PMV. Patients in atrial fibrillation are older and present more frequently with echocardiographic scores of 8 or greater, NYHA functional class IV, calcified mitral valves under fluoroscopy, and a previous history of surgical mitral commissurotomy.

Mitral Regurgitation Before PMV

The presence and severity of mitral regurgitation before PMV is an independent predictor of unfavorable outcome of PMV. The increase in mitral valve area after PMV is inversely related to the severity of mitral regurgitation determined by angiography before the procedure. This inverse relationship between the presence of mitral regurgitation and the immediate outcome of PMV is in part due to the higher frequency of atrial fibrillation, higher echocardiographic scores, calcified mitral valves under fluoroscopy, and older age in patients with mitral regurgitation before PMV.

Complications

Table 22–3 shows the complications reported by several investigators using the double-balloon and the Inoue techniques of PMV.[9–28, 32–35] Mortality and morbidity with PMV are low and similar to those of surgical commissurotomy. There is a less than 1 percent mortality. Severe mitral regurgitation (4 grades by angiography) has been reported in 1 to 5.2 percent of the patients. Some of these patients required in-hospital mitral valve replacement. Thromboembolic episodes and stroke have been reported in 0 to 3.1 percent and pericardial tamponade in 0.2 to 4.1 percent of cases in these series. Pericardial tamponade can occur from transseptal catheterization and, more rarely, from ventricular perforation. PMV is associated with a 3 to 16 percent incidence of left-to-right shunt immediately after the procedure. However, the pulmonary-to-systemic flow ratio is 2:1 or greater in only a minimal number of patients.

We have demonstrated that severe mitral regurgitation (4 grades by angiography) occurs in about 2 percent of patients undergoing PMV.[35–37] An undesirable increase in mitral regurgitation ($\geq$2 grades by angiography) occurred in 12.5 percent of patients.[35–37] This undesirable increase in mitral regurgitation is well tolerated in most patients. Furthermore, more than half of them have less mitral regurgitation at follow-up cardiac catheterization. We have demonstrated that the ratio of the EBDA/BSA is the only predictor of increased mitral regurgitation after PMV. The EBDA is calculated using standard geometric formulas. The incidence of mitral regurgitation is lower if balloon sizes are chosen so that the EBDA/BSA is 4.0 cm^2/m^2 or less. The single-balloon technique results in a lower incidence of mitral regurgitation but provides less relief of mitral stenosis than the double-balloon technique. Thus, there is an optimal EBDA between 3.1 and 4.0 cm^2/m^2 that achieves a maximal mitral valve area with a minimal increase in mitral regurgitation.[37] An echocardiographic score for the mitral valve that can predict the development of severe mitral regurgitation after PMV has been reported by Padial and coworkers.[38, 39] This score takes into account the distribution (even or uneven) of leaflet thickening and calcification, the degree and symmetry of commissural disease, and the severity of subvalvular disease (Table 22–4).

TABLE 22-4 Echocardiographic Score for Severe Mitral Regurgitation After Percutaneous Mitral Balloon Valvotomy

I–II: Leaflets Thickening (score each leaflet separately)
1. Leaflet near normal (4–5 mm) or with only one thick segment
2. Leaflet fibrotic and/or calcified evenly; no thin areas
3. Leaflet fibrotic and/or calcified with uneven distribution; the thinner segments are mildly thickened (5–8 mm)
4. Leaflet fibrotic and/or calcified with uneven distribution; the thinner segments are near normal (4–5 mm)

III: Commissure Calcification
1. Fibrosis and/or calcium in only one commissure
2. Both commissures mildly affected
3. Calcium in both commissures; one markedly affected
4. Calcium in both commissures; both markedly affected

IV: Subvalvular Disease
1. Minimal thickening of chordal structure just below the valve
2. Thickening of chordae extending up to one third of chordal length
3. Thickening to distal third of the chordae
4. Extensive thickening and shortening of all chordae extending down to the papillary muscle

Total score is the sum of each of these echocardiographic features (maximum, 16)

Left-to-right shunt through the created atrial communication occurred in 3 to 16 percent of the patients undergoing PMV. The size of the defect is small, as reflected in the pulmonary-to-systemic flow ratio of 2:1 or less in the majority of patients. Older age, fluoroscopic evidence of mitral valve calcification, higher echocardiographic score, pre-PMV lower cardiac output, and higher pre-PMV NYHA functional class are the factors that predispose patients to develop left-to-right shunt post-PMV.[39] Clinical, echocardiographic, surgical, and hemodynamic follow-up of patients with post-PMV left-to-right shunt demonstrated that the defect closed in 59 percent. Persistent left-to-right shunt at follow-up is small (QP/QS < 2:1) and clinically well tolerated. In the series from the Massachusetts General Hospital, there is one patient in whom the atrial shunt remained hemodynamically significant at follow-up. This patient underwent percutaneous transcatheter closure of her atrial defect with a clamshell device.[40]

Desideri and associates[41] reported atrial shunting determined by color-flow transthoracic echocardiography in 61 percent of 57 patients immediately after PMV. The shunt persisted in 30 percent of patients at 19 ± 6 (range 9 to 33) months follow-up.[41] They identified the magnitude of the post-PMV atrial shunt (QP/QS > 1.5:1), use of the Bifoil balloon (two balloons on one shaft), and smaller post-PMV mitral valve area as independent predictors of the persistence of atrial shunt at long-term follow-up.[41]

Clinical Follow-Up

Follow-up studies after PMV are encouraging.[19, 22–25, 34, 40–45] After PMV, the majority of patients have marked clinical improvement and become NYHA class I or II. The symptomatic, echocardiographic, and hemodynamic improvement produced by PMV persists in intermediate and long-term follow-up. The best long-term results are seen in patients with echocardiographic scores of 8 or less. When PMV produces a good immediate outcome in this group of patients, restenosis is unlikely to occur at follow-up.[19, 22–25, 34, 40–45] Although PMV can result in a good outcome in patients with echocardiographic scores of 8 or greater, hemodynamic and echocardiographic restenosis is frequently demonstrated at follow-up despite ongoing clinical improvement.[19, 22–25, 34, 40–45] Table 22–5 shows long-term follow-up results of patients undergoing PMV at different institutes. We reported an estimated 10-year survival rate of 79 percent in a cohort of 734 patients undergoing PMV at the Massachusetts General Hospital (Fig. 22–5). Death at follow-up was directly related to age, post-PMV pulmonary artery pressure, pre-PMV NYHA functional class, and echocardiographic score. In the same group of patients, the 10-year event-free survival (freedom from mitral valve replacement or mitral valve repair or redo-PMV) was 36 percent. Cox regression analysis identified post-PMV mitral regurgitation of 3+ or greater (risk ratio [RR] 2.88,

TABLE 22–5 **Clinical Follow-Up After Percutaneous Mitral Balloon Valvotomy**

Author	Patients (n)	Age (yr)	Time of Follow-Up (mo)	Survival (%)	Event-Free Survival (%)
Palacios	698	57	61	89	60
Vahanian	606	46	60	94	66
Farhat	430	33	36		95
NHLBI	736	54	48	84	60
Pan	350	46	60	94	85
Orrange	132	44	84	83	65
Cohen	146	59	36	76	51

Abbreviation: NHLBI, National Heart, Lung, and Blood Institute.

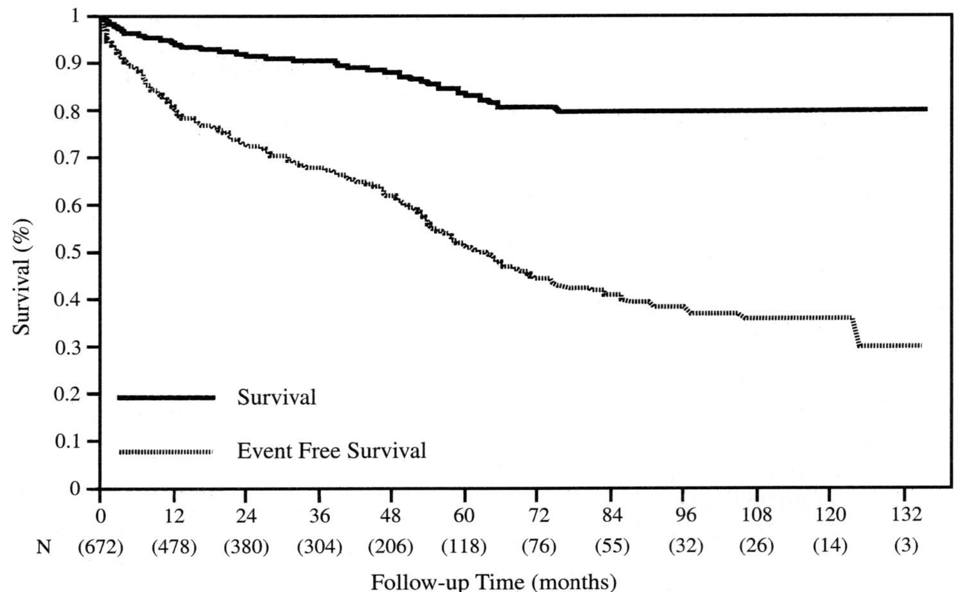

FIGURE 22–5 Eleven-year actuarial survival and event-free survival of 732 patients undergoing PMV at the Massachusetts General Hospital.

CI 2.05 to 3.97, $P < .0001$), echocardiographic score of 8 or greater (RR 1.48, CI 1.12 to 1.97, $P = .005$), age (RR 1.02, CI 1.01 to 1.03, $P < .0001$), post-PMV mitral valve area (RR 0.78, CI 0.63 to 0.93, $P = .01$), and post-PMV mean pulmonary artery pressure (RR 1.02, CI 1.01 to 1.03, $P = .0001$) as independent predictors of combined events at long-term follow-up.

Patients with echocardiographic scores of 8 or less have a significantly greater survival, survival with freedom from mitral valve surgery, and event-free survival (death, mitral valve surgery and NYHA class ≥ III) than those patients with echocardiographic scores of 8 or greater (Fig. 22–6). Patients with echocardiographic scores of 8 or less have an 86 percent survival and a 41 percent event-free survival at 10-year follow-up. In contrast, patients with echocardiographic scores of 8 or greater have a 55 percent survival and a 21 percent event-free survival at the same follow-up time. Similar follow-up studies have been reported in other series with the double-balloon technique and with the Inoue technique of PMV.[19, 22–25, 34, 40–45] With the Inoue technique of PMV at intermediate long-term follow-up of 51 months, young patients with pliable valves, in sinus rhythm, and with no evidence of calcium under fluoroscopy were free of cardiovascular events. In contrast, 84 percent of patients with calcified valves and/or severe subvalvular disease were free of cardiovascular events at 48 months' follow-up.[23–25] Cohen and colleagues[26] reported the clinical follow-up of 146 patients undergoing PMV. The overall survival rate was 88 percent at 2 years and 76 percent at 5 years. Event-free survival was 74 percent at 2 years and 51 percent at 5 years. Ninety-six percent of patients alive at follow-up were NYHA class I or II. These authors identi-

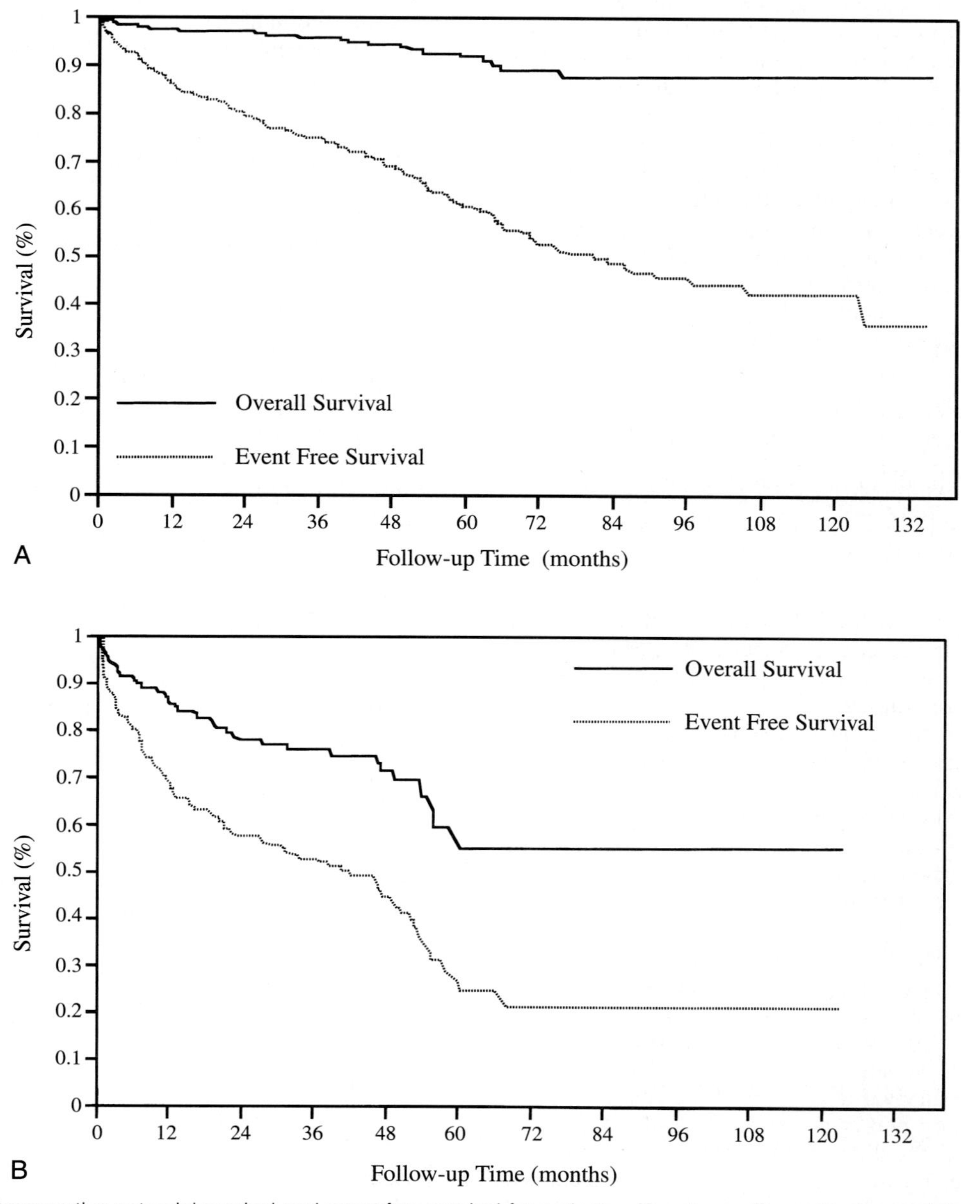

FIGURE 22–6 Comparative actuarial survival and event-free survival for patients with echocardiographic score of 8 or less **(A)** and greater than **(B)** undergoing PMV at the Massachusetts General Hospital.

fied a lower echocardiographic score, lower left ventricular end-diastolic pressure, and final mitral valve area post-PMV as independent predictors of longer event-free survival. The lower 5-year event-free survival can be explained by a larger number of patients with higher echocardiographic scores and mitral valve calcification. Furthermore, in that study, 39 percent of the patients were considered to be high surgical risk candidates owing to the presence of important coexisting conditions or advanced age.

Follow-Up in the Elderly

Tuzcu and coworkers[22] reported the outcome of PMV in 99 elderly patients (≥65 yr). A successful outcome (valve area ≥ 1.5 cm^2, without ≥ 2+ increase in mitral regurgitation, and without left-to-right shunt of ≥ 1.5:1) was achieved in 46 patients. The best multivariate predictor of success was the combination of echocardiographic score, NYHA functional class, and inverse of mitral valve area. Patients who had an unsuccessful outcome from PMV were in a higher NYHA functional class and had higher echocardiographic scores and smaller mitral valve areas pre-PMV compared with those patients who had a successful outcome. Actuarial survival and combined event-free survival at 3 years were significantly better in the successful group. Mean follow-up was 16 ± 1 months. Actuarial survival (79 ± 7 percent versus 62 ± 10 percent, P = .04), survival without mitral valve replacement (71 ± 8 percent versus 41 ± 8 percent, P = .002); and event-free survival (54 ± 12 percent versus 38 ± 8 percent, P = .01) at 3 years were significantly better in the successful group of 46 patients than the unsuccessful group of 53 patients. Low echocardiographic score was the independent predictor of survival, and lack of mitral valve calcification was the strongest predictor of event-free survival.

Follow-Up of Patients With Calcified Mitral Valves

The presence of fluoroscopically visible calcification on the mitral valve influences the success of PMV. Patients with heavily (≥3 grades) calcified valves under fluoroscopy have a poorer immediate outcome as reflected in a smaller post-PMV mitral valve area and greater post-PMV mitral valve gradient. Immediate outcome is progressively worse as the calcification becomes more severe. The long-term results of PMV are significantly different in calcified and uncalcified groups and in subgroups of the calcified group.[46] The estimated 2-year survival is significantly lower for patients with calcified mitral valves than for those with uncalcified valves (80 percent versus 99 percent). The survival curve becomes worse as the severity of valvular calcification becomes more severe. Freedom from mitral valve replacement at 2 years was significantly lower for patients with calcified valves than for those with uncalcified valves (67 percent versus 93 percent). Similarly, the estimated event-free survival at 2 years in the calcified group became significantly poorer as the severity of calcification increased. The estimated event-free survival at 2 years was significantly lower for the calcified than for the uncalcified group (63 percent versus 88 percent). The actuarial survival curves with freedom from combined events at 2 years in the calcified group became significantly poorer as the severity of calcification increased.[46] These findings are in agreement with several follow-up studies of surgical commissurotomy that demonstrate that patients with calcified mitral valves had a poorer survival compared with those patients with uncalcified valves.[47–49]

Follow-Up of Patients With Previous Surgical Commissurotomy

PMV has also been shown to be a safe procedure in patients with previous surgical mitral commissurotomy.[18, 50–52] Although a good immediate outcome is frequently achieved in these patients, follow-up results are not as favorable as those obtained in patients without previous surgical commissurotomy.[50–52] Although there is no difference in mortality between patients with and those without a history of previous surgical commissurotomy at 4-year follow-up, the number of patients who required mitral valve replacement (26 percent versus 8 percent) and/or were in NYHA class III or IV (35 percent versus 13 percent) was significantly higher among those patients with previous commissurotomy. However, when the patients are carefully selected according to the echocardiographic score (≤8), the immediate outcome and the 4-year follow-up results are excellent and similar to those seen in patients without previous surgical commissurotomy.[18, 50–52]

Follow-Up of Patients With Atrial Fibrillation

We recently reported that the presence of atrial fibrillation is associated with inferior immediate and long-term outcome after PMV, as reflected in a smaller post-PMV mitral valve area and a lower event-free survival (freedom from death, redo-PMV, and mitral valve surgery) at a median follow-up time of 61 months (32 percent versus 61 percent, $P < .0001$).[53] Analysis of preprocedural and procedural characteristics revealed that this association is most likely explained by the presence of multiple factors in the atrial fibrillation group that adversely affect the immediate and long-term outcome of PMV. Patients in atrial fibrillation are older and presented more frequently with NYHA class IV, echocardiographic score greater than 8, calcified valves under fluoroscopy, and a history of previous surgical commissurotomy. In the group of patients in atrial fibrillation, Leon and associates[53] identified severe post-PMV mitral regurgitation (≥3+) (P = .0001), echocardiographic score greater than 8 (P = .004) and pre-PMV NYHA class IV (P = .046) as independent predictors of combined events at follow-up.[53] The presence of atrial fibrillation per se should not be the only determinant in the decision process regarding treatment options in a patient with rheumatic mitral stenosis. The presence of an echocardiographic score of 8 or less primarily identifies a subgroup of patients in atrial fibrillation in whom PMV is very likely to be successful and to provide good long-term results. Therefore, in this group of patients, PMV should be the procedure of choice.

Follow-Up of Patients With Pulmonary Artery Hypertension

The degree of pulmonary artery hypertension before PMV is inversely related to the immediate and long-term outcome of PMV. Chen and colleagues[54] divided 564 patients undergoing PMV at the Massachusetts General Hospital into three groups on the basis of the pulmonary vascular resistance (PVR) obtained at cardiac catheterization immediately before PMV: group I with a PVR of 250 dynes-sec/cm^{-5} or lower (normal/mildly elevated resistance) comprised 332 patients (59 percent); group II with a PVR between 251 and 400-dynes-sec/cm^{-5} (moderately elevated resistance) comprised 110 patients (19.5 percent); group III with a PVR of 400 dynes-sec/cm^{-5} or greater comprised 122 patients (21.5 percent). Patients in groups I and II were younger and had less severe heart failure symptoms measured by NYHA class and a lower incidence of echocardiographic scores greater than 8, atrial fibrillation, and calcium noted on fluoroscopy than patients in group III. Before and after PMV, patients with higher PVR had a smaller mitral valve area, lower cardiac output, and higher mean pulmonary artery pressure. For groups I, II, and III patients, the immediate success rates for PMV were 68 percent, 56 percent, and 45 percent, respectively. Therefore, patients in the group with severely elevated pulmonary artery resistance before the procedure had lower immediate success rates of PMV. At long-term follow-up, patients with severely elevated PVRs had a significant lower survival and event-free survival (survival with freedom from mitral valve surgery or NYHA class III or IV heart failure).

Follow-Up of Patients With Tricuspid Regurgitation

The degree of tricuspid regurgitation before PMV is inversely related to the immediate and long-term outcome of PMV. Sagie and coworkers[55] divided patients undergoing PMV at the Massachusetts General Hospital into three groups on the basis of the degree of tricuspid regurgitation determined by 2-D and color-flow Doppler echocardiography before PMV. Patients with severe tricuspid regurgitation before PMV were older and had more severe heart failure symptoms measured by NYHA class and a higher incidence of echocardiographic scores greater than 8, atrial fibrillation, and calcified mitral valves on fluoroscopy than patients with mild or moderate tricuspid regurgitation. Patients with severe tricuspid regurgitation had a smaller mitral valve area before and after PMV than the patients with mild or moderate tricuspid regurgitation. At long-term follow-up, patients with severe tricuspid regurgitation had a significantly lower survival and event-free survival (survival with freedom from mitral valve surgery or NYHA class III or IV heart failure).

Follow-Up of the Best Patients for PMV

In patients identified as optimal candidates for PMV, this technique results in excellent immediate and long-term outcome. Optimal candidates for PMV are those patients meeting these characteristics: (1) age less than 65 years, (2) normal sinus rhythm, (3) echocardiographic score of 8 or less, (4) no fluoroscopic mitral valve calcification, and (5) pre-PMV mitral regurgitation of 1+ or lower Seller grade. From 780 consecutive patients undergoing PMV, we identified 202 patients with optimal preprocedure characteristics. In these patients, PMV results in an 81 percent success rate and a 3.4 percent incidence of major in-hospital combined events (death and/or mitral valve regurgitation). In these patients, PMV results in a 97 percent survival and a 76 percent event-free survival rate at a median follow-up of 61 months[56] (Fig. 22–7).

The Double-Balloon Versus the Inoue Techniques of PMV

Today, the Inoue and the double-balloon techniques of PMV are more widely used. However, there is controversy

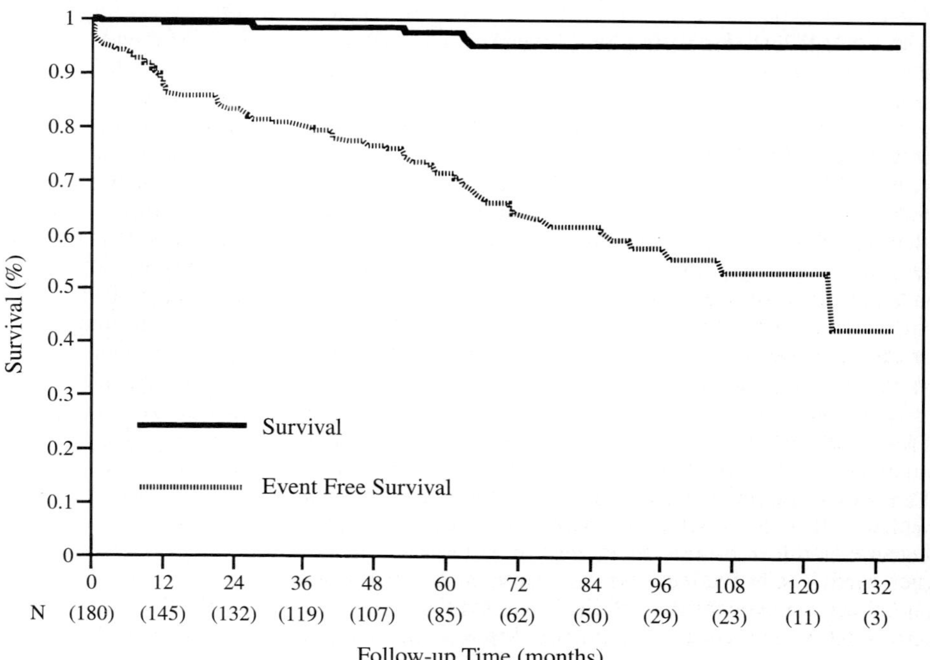

FIGURE 22–7 Actuarial survival and event-free survival for optimal patients for PMV undergoing PMV at the Massachusetts General Hospital.

as to which technique provides superior immediate and long-term results. We compared the immediate procedural and the long-term clinical outcomes after PMV using the double-balloon (n = 621) and the Inoue (n = 113) techniques.[34] There were no statistically significant differences in baseline clinical and morphologic characteristics between the double-balloon and the Inoue patients. The double-balloon technique resulted in superior immediate outcome, as reflected in a larger post-PMV mitral valve area (1.9 ± 0.7 cm^2 versus 1.7 ± 0.6 cm^2, P = .005) and a lower incidence of 3+ mitral regurgitation post-PMV (5.4 percent versus 10.6 percent, P = .05). The superior immediate outcome of the double-balloon technique was observed only in the group of patients with echocardiographic score of 8 or less (post-PMV mitral valve areas 2.1 ± 0.7 cm^2 versus 1.8 ± 0.6 cm^2, P = .004). Despite the difference in immediate outcome, there were no significant differences between the two techniques in event-free survival at long-term follow-up.[34]

Echocardiographic and Hemodynamic Follow-Up

Follow-up studies have shown that the incidence of hemodynamic and echocardiographic restenosis is low 2 years after PMV.[19, 21, 23–25, 40] A study of a group of patients undergoing simultaneous clinical evaluation, 2-D Doppler echocardiography and transseptal catheterization 2 years after PMV reported 90 percent of patients in NYHA classes I and II and 10 percent of patients in NYHA class ≥III or higher.[21] In this study, hemodynamic determination of mitral valve area using the Gorlin equation showed a significant decrease in mitral valve area from 2.0 cm^2 immediately after PMV to 1.6 cm^2 at follow-up. However, there was no significant difference between the echocardiographic mitral valve areas immediately after PMV and at follow-up (1.8 cm^2 and 1.6 cm^2, respectively, P = NS). Although there was a significant difference in the mitral valve area after PMV determined by the Gorlin equation and by 2-D echocardiography (2.0 cm^2 versus 1.8 cm^2), there was no significant difference between the mitral valve area determined by the Gorlin equation and the echocardiographic calculated mitral valve area (1.6 cm^2 for both) at follow-up. The discrepancy between the 2-D echocardiographic and the Gorlin equation determined post-PMV mitral valve areas is due to the contribution of left-to-right shunting (undetected by oximetry) across the created interatrial communication, which results in both an erroneously high cardiac output and an overestimation of the mitral valve area by the Gorlin equation.[57] Desideri and associates[41] showed no significant differences in mitral valve area (measured by Doppler echocardiography) at 19 ± 6 (range 9 to 33) months follow-up between the post-PMV and the follow-up mitral valve areas. Mitral valve areas were 2.2 ± 0.5 cm^2 and 1.9 ± 0.5 cm^2, respectively. Echocardiographic restenosis (mitral valve area ≤ 1.5 cm^2 with > 50 percent reduction of the gain) was seen in 21 percent of the patients.[43] Predictors of restenosis included age, smaller post-PMV mitral valve area, and higher echocardiographic score.[40] With the Inoue technique, Chen and coworkers[24] showed no significant differences in mitral valve area determined by 2-D Doppler echocardiography in 85 patients at a mean follow-up of 5 ± 1 years (range 43 to 79 months). Post-PMV and follow-up mitral valve areas were 2.0 ± 0.4 cm^2 and 1.8 ± 0.5 cm^2, respectively (P = NS).

PMV Versus Surgical Mitral Commissurotomy

Results of surgical closed mitral commissurotomy have demonstrated favorable long-term hemodynamic and symptomatic improvement. A restenosis rate of 4.2 to 11.4 per 1000 patients per year was reported by John and associates[58] in 3724 patients who underwent surgical closed mitral commissurotomy. Survival after PMV is similar to that reported after surgical mitral commissurotomy. Although freedom from mitral valve replacement (87 percent versus 92 percent) and freedom from all events (67 percent versus 80 percent) after PMV are lower than those reported after surgical commissurotomy, freedom from both mitral valve replacement and all events in patients with echocardiographic scores of 8 or less are similar to those reported after surgical mitral commissurotomy.[34, 40, 48, 49, 58–64]

Restenosis after both closed and open surgical mitral commissurotomy has been well documented.[58–66] Although surgical closed mitral commissurotomy is uncommonly performed in the United States, it is still used frequently in other countries. Long-term follow-up of 267 patients who underwent surgical transventricular mitral commissurotomy at the Mayo Clinic showed 79 percent, 67 percent, and 55 percent survival at 10, 15, and 20 years, respectively. Survival with freedom from mitral valve replacement was 57 percent, 36 percent, and 24 percent, respectively.[67] In this study, age, atrial fibrillation, and male gender were independent predictors of death, and mitral valve calcification, cardiomegaly, and mitral regurgitation were independent predictors of repeat mitral valve surgery.[67] Because of similar patient selection and mechanism of mitral valve dilatation, similar long-term results should be expected after PMV. Indeed, prospective, randomized trials comparing PMV and surgical closed mitral commissurotomy have shown no differences in immediate and 3-year follow-up results between both groups of patients.[68, 69] Furthermore, restenosis at 3-year follow-up occurred in 10 percent and 13 percent of the patients treated with PMV and surgical commissurotomy, respectively.[69] Results of randomized clinical trials comparing PMV and surgical open commissurotomy show similar results.

Interpretation of long-term clinical follow-up of patients undergoing PMV as well as their comparison with surgical commissurotomy series are confounded by heterogeneity in patient populations. Most surgical series have involved a younger population with optimal mitral valve morphology: pliable with no calcification and no evidence of subvalvular disease. Differences in age and valve morphology may account for the lower survival and event-free survival of PMV series from United States and Europe. For example, in the series from the Massachusetts General Hospital, 497 patients with echocardiographic scores of 8 or less and a mean age of 51 ± 14 years have an 85 percent survival and a 45 percent event-free survival at 8-year follow-up. In contrast, 237 patients with echocardiographic scores greater than 8 and a mean age of 63 ± 14 years have a

55 percent 8-year survival, and only 20 percent of them were free of combined events at 8-year follow-up.

A larger number of patients with higher echocardiographic scores and mitral valve calcification may account for the 5-year 76 percent survival and a 51 percent combined event-free survival reported by Cohen and colleagues[26] in a group of 146 patients undergoing PMV. Furthermore, 39 percent of the patients in Cohen and colleagues'[26] series were considered to be high-surgical-risk candidates owing to the presence of important coexisting conditions or advanced age.

Conversely, survival and event-free survival rates after PMV in optimal patients for this technique appear to be similar to those reported after surgical mitral commissurotomy. In the series from the Massachusetts General Hospital, 202 optimal candidates—defined as patients less than 65 years old, in normal sinus rhythm, with echocardiographic scores of 8 or less, without mitral valve calcification, and with pre-PMV mitral regurgitation of 1 grade or less—had an excellent immediate and long-term outcome, as reflected in a 97 percent survival and a 76 percent event-free survival at a median follow-up of 61 months[56] (see Fig. 22–7). In patients with optimal mitral valve morphology, surgical mitral commissurotomy has favorable long-term hemodynamic and symptomatic improvement. Similar to PMV, patients with advanced age, calcified mitral valves, and with atrial fibrillation had a poorer survival and event-free survival.

Several studies have compared the immediate and early follow-up results of PMV with closed surgical commissurotomy in optimal patients for these techniques. The results of these studies have been controversial, showing either superior outcome from PMV or no significant differences between the techniques.[70–72] Patel and colleagues[70] randomized 45 patients with mitral stenosis and optimal mitral valve morphology to closed surgical commissurotomy and to PMV. These authors demonstrated a larger increase in mitral valve area with PMV (2.1 ± 0.7 cm^2 versus 1.3 ± 0.3 cm^2). Shrivastava and associates[71] compared the results of single-balloon PMV, double-balloon PMV, and closed surgical commissurotomy in three groups of 20 patients each. The mitral valve area postintervention was larger for the double-balloon technique of PMV. Postintervention valve areas were 1.9 ± 0.8 cm^2, 1.5 ± 0.4 cm^2, and 1.5 ± 0.5 cm^2 for the double-balloon, the single-balloon, and the closed surgical commissurotomy techniques, respectively. Conversely, Arora and coworkers[72] randomized 200 patients with a mean age of 19 ± 7 years and mitral stenosis with optimal mitral valve morphology to PMV and to closed mitral commissurotomy. Both procedures resulted in similar postintervention mitral valve areas (2.39 ± 0.9 cm^2 versus 2.2 ± 0.9 cm^2 for the PMV and the mitral commissurotomy groups, respectively) and no significant differences in event-free survival at a mean follow-up period of 22 ± 6 months. Restenosis documented by echocardiography was low in both groups, 5 percent in the PMV group and 4 percent in the closed commissurotomy group. Turi and associates[68] randomized 40 patients with severe mitral stenosis to PMV and to closed surgical commissurotomy. The postintervention mitral valve area at 1 week (1.6 ± 0.6 cm^2 versus 1.6 ± 0.7 cm^2) and 8 months (1.6 ± 0.6 cm^2 versus 1.8 ± 0.6 cm^2) after the procedures were similar in both groups.[68] Reyes and colleagues[69] randomized 60 patients with severe mitral stenosis and favorable valvular anatomy to PMV and to surgical commissurotomy. They reported no significant differences in immediate outcome, complications, and 3.5-year follow-up between both groups of patients. Improvement was maintained in both groups, but mitral valve areas at follow-up were larger in the PMV group (2.4 ± 0.6 cm^2 versus 1.8 ± 0.4 cm^2).

Farhat and coworkers[73] reported the results of a randomized trial designed to compare the immediate and long-term results of double-balloon PMV with those of open and closed surgical mitral commissurotomy in a cohort of patients with severe rheumatic mitral stenosis. This group of patients were from the clinical and morphologic point of view optimal candidates for both PMV and surgical commissurotomy (closed or open) procedures. They had a mean age of less than 30 years, absence of mitral valve calcification on fluoroscopy and 2-D echocardiography, and an echocardiographic score of 8 or less in all patients. The results demonstrate that the immediate and long-term results of PMV are comparable with those of open mitral commissurotomy and superior to those of closed commissurotomy. The hemodynamic improvement, in-hospital complications, and long-term restenosis rate and need for reintervention were superior for the patients treated with either PMV or open commissurotomy than for those treated with closed commissurotomy. The postintervention mitral valve areas achieved with PMV were similar to the one obtained after open surgical commissurotomy (1.5 ± 0.5 cm^2 versus 2.2 ± 0.4 cm^2) but larger than those obtained after closed commissurotomy. These initial changes resulted in an excellent long-term follow-up in the group of patients treated with PMV that was comparable with the open commissurotomy group and superior to the closed commissurotomy group. The inferior results of closed mitral commissurotomy presented by Farhat and coworkers[73] are in disagreement with previous studies showing no significant differences in immediate and follow-up results between PMV and closed surgical mitral commissurotomy.[70–72] However, the increase in mitral valve area after closed commissurotomy is not uniform and is often unsatisfactory. Since open commissurotomy is associated with a thoracotomy, need for cardiopulmonary bypass, higher cost, longer length of hospital stay, and longer period of convalescence, PMV should be the procedure of choice for the treatment of patients with rheumatic mitral stenosis who are from the clinical and morphologic point of view optimal candidates for PMV.[73, 74]

PMV in Pregnant Women

Surgical mitral commissurotomy has been performed in pregnant women with severe mitral stenosis. Since the risk of anesthesia and surgery for the mother and the fetus are increased, this operation is reserved for those patients with incapacitating symptoms refractory to medical therapy.[75, 76] Under these conditions, PMV can be performed safely after the 20th week of pregnancy with minimal radiation to the fetus.[77, 78]

Conclusions

PMV produces a good immediate outcome and good clinical long-term follow-up results in a high percentage of patients with mitral stenosis. Patients with echocardiographic scores of 8 or less have the best results, particularly if they are young, are in sinus rhythm, and have no evidence of calcification of the mitral valve under fluoroscopy. The immediate and long-term results of PMV in this group of patients are similar to those reported after surgical mitral commissurotomy. Patients with echocardiographic scores greater than 8 have only a 50 percent chance of obtaining a successful hemodynamic result with PMV, and long-term follow-up results are less good than those from patients with echocardiographic scores of 8 or less. In patients with echocardiographic scores of 12 or greater, it is unlikely that PMV could produce good immediate or long-term results. These patients should preferably undergo open-heart surgery. However, PMV could be performed in these patients if they are non–high-risk surgical candidates.

Surgical therapy for mitral stenosis should be reserved for patients who have 2 or more grades of Seller mitral regurgitation by angiography that can be better treated by mitral valve repair and for those patients with severe mitral valve thickening and calcification or with significant subvalvular scarring to warrant valve replacement.

PERCUTANEOUS AORTIC BALLOON VALVULOPLASTY

Aortic valve replacement is the treatment of choice for symptomatic, severe aortic stenosis in the elderly.[79–82] However, associated major medical comorbid conditions increase perioperative complications significantly, and in some cases the risk is so high that surgeons classify these patients as nonsurgical candidates. Previous bypass surgery, severe congestive heart failure, low left ventricular ejection fraction, recent myocardial infarction, diabetes mellitus, renal failure, and most of all, emergent operation are independent predictors for operative death in elderly patients undergoing aortic valve replacement.[83–86] Furthermore, 54 percent of octogenarians require concomitant surgical procedures including coronary artery bypass surgery and/or mitral valve replacement.[82, 87] Elective perioperative mortality for octogenarians undergoing aortic valve replacement and coronary artery bypass graft is 24 percent.[87] Emergent perioperative mortality increases to 37 percent in patients with severe congestive heart failure requiring pressors[88] and can be as high as 50 percent in patients with cardiogenic shock.[89] Finally, a complicated postoperative course including encephalopathy with discharge to a rehabilitation facility is present in 38 percent of the patients.[90]

Since the initial report by Cribier and coworkers in 1986,[91] percutaneous aortic balloon valvuloplasty (PAV) has been considered as a palliative form of treatment for elderly patients with calcific aortic stenosis. PAV is associated with significant immediate clinical and hemodynamic improvement.[92, 93] However, the risk of major complications and the high restenosis rate during the first year are major limitations of this technique.[94, 95] In fact, because PAV does not change the natural history of severe aortic stenosis,[96–99] its use in some institutions has been abandoned.[100] Therefore, elderly patients with profound hemodynamic instability due to severe aortic stenosis present a challenging dilemma in critical care medicine. If surgery is not an option, PAV can be effectively used as a lifesaving procedure for immediate relief of the transaortic valve gradient with subsequent hemodynamic stabilization and further consideration for elective bridge to aortic valve replacement.

Procedure

The technique of PAV is not complex and can be performed using either the retrograde or the antegrade technique.[93]

Retrograde Technique

After crossing the aortic valve and determining resting hemodynamics, a 0.038-inch Amplatz-type heavy exchange wire is advanced through the retrograde catheter and placed into the left ventricular cavity. The retrograde catheter is then removed, leaving the guide wire across the stenotic aortic valve coiled in the left ventricular apex. A dilating balloon catheter chosen according to the size of the aortic annulus is then advanced over the guide wire, placed across the aortic valve, and inflated by hand (Fig. 22–8).

Antegrade Technique

The left atrium is entered using transseptal catheterization with a modified Brockenbrough needle and a Mullin sheath. A balloon wedge catheter is advanced through the Mullin sheath and passed into the left ventricle and then antegrade through the stenotic aortic valve. A soft 0.038-inch exchange wire is advanced through the catheter into the ascending and descending aorta, and the catheter and Mullin sheath are removed. A chosen dilating balloon catheter is then advanced antegrade across the mitral valve, placed across the aortic valve, and inflated.

With both techniques, multiple balloon inflations are performed to relieve the stenosis. To monitor systemic blood pressure during and immediately after balloon inflations, a radial arterial line should be in place before the inflations. In two thirds of the patients, inflations are well tolerated and longer balloon inflations (>30 seconds) can be performed. In the other third of the patients, only short balloon inflations (15 to 30 seconds) can be performed because of significant hypotension during balloon inflation. Short balloon inflations and a longer period between inflations are used in patients with severe depression of left ventricular ejection fraction as well as in those with severe coronary artery disease or carotid disease. The size of the dilating balloon catheter (18 to 25 mm in diameter) is chosen according to the size of the aortic annulus (not greater than 100 percent of annulus) determined by 2-D echocardiography or angiography.

Hemodynamic measurement and cardiac output using the thermodilution method are determined before and after completion of the procedure. For patients with significant tricuspid regurgitation and/or left-to-right shunting, cardiac output is determined using the Fick method. The aortic

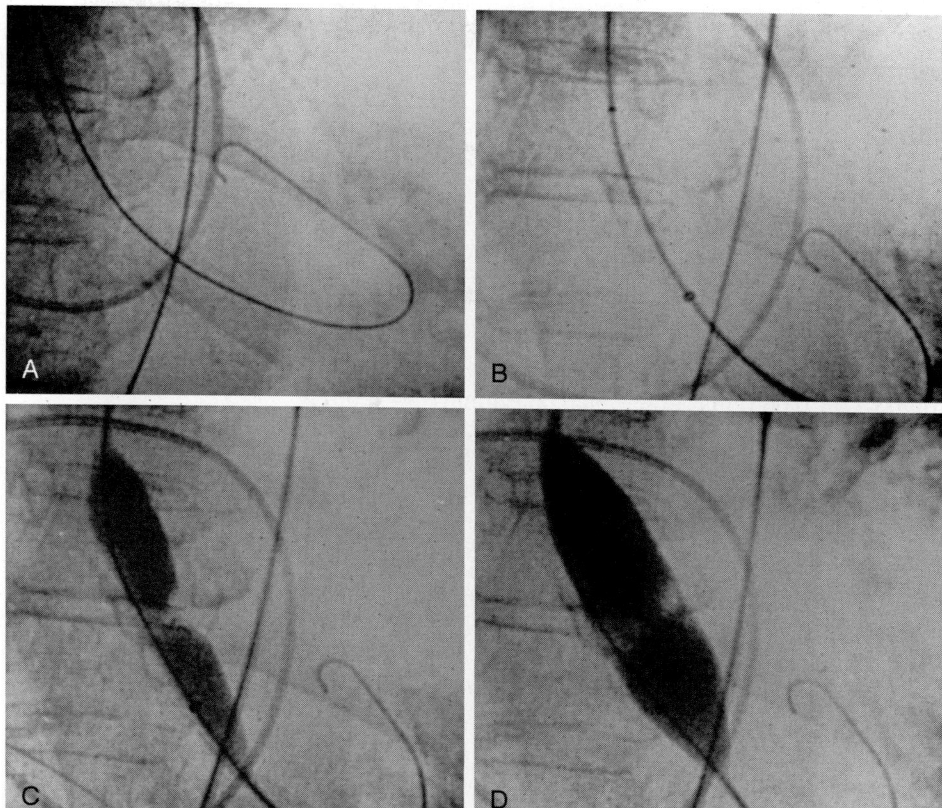

FIGURE 22–8 Cineangiographic frames of retrograde percutaneous aortic balloon valvuloplasty (PAV) **A,** The guide wire is in place across the aortic valve, with a loop into the left ventricle. **B,** The dilating balloon catheter is placed across the aortic valve. **C,** The dilating balloon catheter is partially inflated across the stenotic aortic valve. Note the indentation in the balloon caused by the stenotic aortic valve. **D,** Full inflation of the dilating balloon across the aortic valve is achieved.

valve area is calculated using the Gorlin equation.[101] Aortic valve resistance, proposed as a better indicator of the hemodynamic significance of aortic stenosis before and after PAV, can be calculated as previously described.[102] Left ventricular ejection fraction is calculated by contrast ventriculography and/or 2-D echocardiography.

Mechanism

The final aortic valve area obtained with PAV is most likely related to the underlying valve pathology.[103, 104] Fresh postmortem studies of patients with degenerative calcific aortic stenosis in whom commissural fusion is minimal have shown that the increase in aortic valve area in these patients occurs as result of the fracture of calcium deposits in the aortic leaflets.[104] In patients with commissural fusion such as rheumatic aortic stenosis and some patients with noncalcific bicuspid valve stenosis, PAV produces commissural splitting with or without cuspal crack. In addition, PAV produces stretching of the aortic wall at nonfused commissural sites. Stretching is probably transient and is responsible for the cases of early restenosis seen in some patients. Although opening of fused commissures is probably the most effective mechanism of PAV, commissure fusion seldom occurs in the elderly with calcific aortic stenosis.[105]

Immediate Results

Between February 1986 and February 1993, 394 PAVs were performed at the Massachusetts General Hospital in 310 symptomatic patients with severe, calcific, aortic stenosis.[97] The patients were considered non–high-risk or very-high-risk surgical candidates at the time of presentation because of associated major comorbid conditions. In addition, PAV was performed in patients with severe aortic stenosis, discovered at the time of evaluation for major noncardiac surgery, in 65 patients who presented with symptomatic aortic valve restenosis after a previous successful procedure (redo-PAV) and in 21 patients who presented in cardiogenic shock owing to critical aortic stenosis. There were 180 females and 130 males with a mean plus or minus standard error of the mean age of 79 $\pm$ 1 (range 35 to 96) years. Mean left ventricular ejection fraction was 48 $\pm$ 15 (range 10 to 81) percent. Ninety percent of the patients were in NYHA functional classes III to IV. All patients had more than one major comorbid condition (average 1.3/patient) at the time of presentation, including chronic renal failure, previous stroke, severe chronic obstructive pulmonary disease, liver failure, hip fracture, pulmonary hemorrhage, pulmonary embolism, Alzheimer's disease, sepsis, diabetes with multiple organ complications, thyroid disease, bleeding disorders, incapacitating arthritis, multiple myeloma, and AIDS. Major comorbid conditions are shown in Table 22–6.

PAV results in a decrease in aortic gradient and a modest increase in aortic valve area in the great majority of patients with degenerative calcific aortic stenosis. The hemodynamic changes produced by PAV are shown in Table 22–7. PAV resulted in a significant decrease in mean systolic aortic gradient from 56 $\pm$ 1 mm Hg to 25 $\pm$ 1 mm Hg ($P = .0001$) and a significant increase in both cardiac output

TABLE 22-6 **Associated Comorbid Conditions**

Condition	Patients
Chronic obstructive pulmonary disease	64 (21%)
Chronic renal failure	64 (21%)
Peripheral vascular disease	54 (17%)
Cancer	48 (15%)
Cerebrovascular disease	48 (15%)
Other*	112 (38%)

*Liver failure, hip fracture, gastrointestinal bleeding, complicated diabetes, Alzheimer's disease, sepsis, thyroid disease, AIDS.

TABLE 22-7 **Hemodynamic Parameters Before and After Percutaneous Aortic Balloon Valvuloplasty***

Variables	Pre-PAV	Post-PAV	*P* Value
Mean aortic gradient (mm Hg)	56 ± 1	25 ± 1	.0001
Cardiac output (L/min)	3.7 ± 0.1	3.9 ± 0.1	.0001
Aortic valve area (cm²)	0.49 ± 0.01	0.87 ± 0.02	.0001
Systolic aortic pressure (mm Hg)	129 ± 2	144 ± 2	.0001
Systolic pulmonary artery pressure (mm Hg)	49 ± 1	45 ± 2	.03

Abbreviation: PAV, percutaneous aortic balloon valvuloplasty.
*Values are expressed in mean ± SEM.

from 3.7 ± 0.06 L/min to 3.9 ± 0.06 L/min (*P* = .0001) and aortic valve area from 0.5 ± 0.01 cm² to 0.9 ± 0.02 cm² (*P* = .0001). Failure of PAV (no change in aortic valve area) occurs in only 3 percent of the patients. An aortic valve area of 0.7 cm² or less is obtained in about 38 percent of the patients. An aortic valve area greater than 0.7 cm² is obtained in 59 percent of the patients, including 27 percent of patients in whom PAV results in an aortic valve area of 1.0 cm² or greater. The increase in aortic valve area with PAV is inversely related to the NYHA functional class before PAV and to the severity of aortic stenosis as reflected in a higher aortic gradient and a smaller aortic valve area before PAV.

Complications

Procedural mortality (death in the catheterization laboratory) occurred in 12 patients (3 percent); in-hospital (30-day) mortality occurred in 34 patients (8.6 percent); local vascular complications in 49 patients (12 percent), including a need for vascular surgery in 38 patients (9.6 percent), 2 of whom required leg amputation (0.5 percent). Cerebrovascular accident occurred in 5 patients (1.2 percent); severe aortic regurgitation in 6 patients (1.5 percent); acute renal failure in 7 patients (1.7 percent); significant atrial septal defect in 2 patients (0.5 percent) who had antegrade PAV; cholesterol emboli in 3 patients (0.8 percent); nonfatal ventricular fibrillation in 7 patients (1.7 percent); myocardial infarction in 6 patients (1.5 percent); and left ventricular perforation in 1 patient (0.2 percent).

Long-Term Follow-Up After PAV

Although PAV results in immediate hemodynamic and symptomatic improvement in the great majority of patients, the long-term results of PAV show that clinical restenosis occurs frequently 6 to 12 months after PAV.[92, 94] Estimated actuarial survival rates at 1, 3, and 5 years follow-up of the Massachusetts General Hospital series were 55 ± 3 percent, 25 ± 3 percent, and 22 ± 3 percent (Fig. 22–9). The corresponding estimated actuarial event-free survival rates were 33 ± 2 percent, 13 ± 2 percent, and 2 ± 1 percent, respectively (see Fig. 22–9). Clinical follow-up of the patients who have undergone PAV has demonstrated

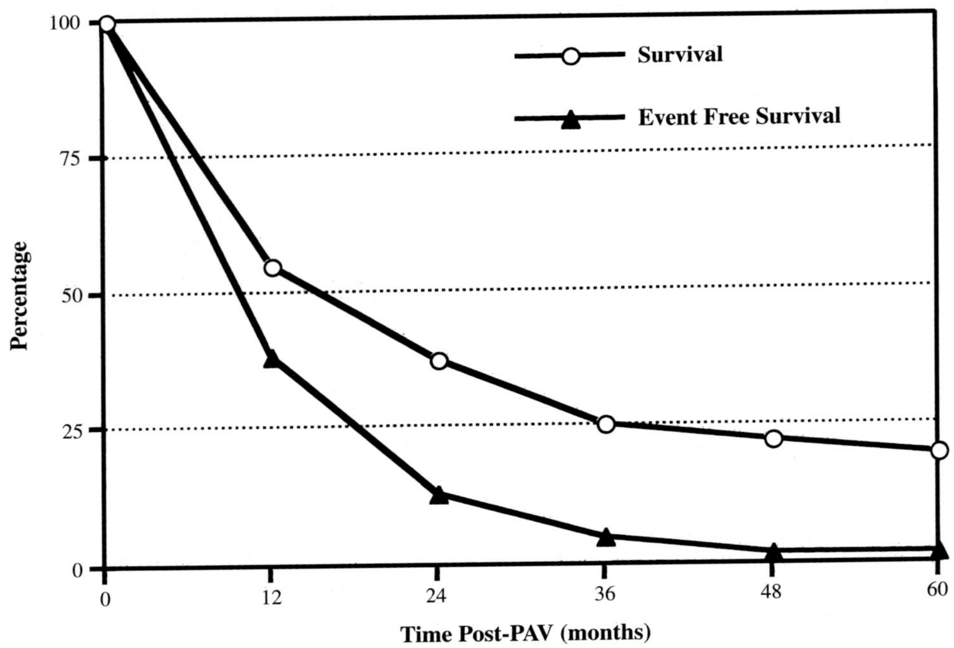

FIGURE 22–9 Actuarial survival and event-free survival curves for patients with severe aortic stenosis treated with percutaneous aortic balloon valvuloplasty (PAV) at the Massachusetts General Hospital.

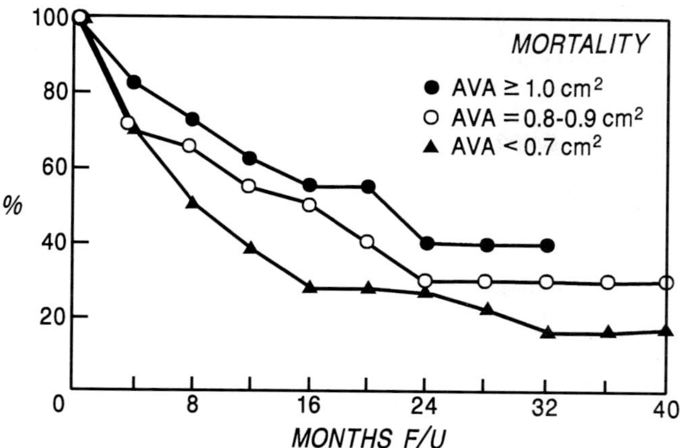

FIGURE 22–10 Actuarial survival curves for patients with severe aortic stenosis treated with PAV at the Massachusetts General Hospital. Curves for three different post-PAV aortic valve areas (AVA) achieved with the procedure are shown.

that cardiac mortality and clinical restenosis (defined as cardiac mortality plus patients returning to the pre-PAV NYHA functional class) after balloon valvuloplasty is very high.

Although mortality is greater in those patients in whom PAV resulted in an aortic valve area less than 0.7 cm² than in those with post-PAV valve areas greater than 0.7 cm² (Fig. 22–10), the survival curve of the natural history of patients with severe aortic stenosis treated medically is unaffected by balloon valvuloplasty (Fig. 22–11). The presence of left ventricular dysfunction and the presence of coronary artery disease adversely affect the prognosis of patients undergoing PAV. The decrease in aortic valve area at follow-up is inversely related to the post-PAV aortic valve area. One-year clinical restenosis is greater in patients in whom post-PAV aortic valve area was 0.7 cm² or less than in those in whom post-PAV aortic valve area was greater than 0.7 cm². A high restenosis rate (>50 percent) was also present in patients who had a second or third PAV with larger balloon sizes.

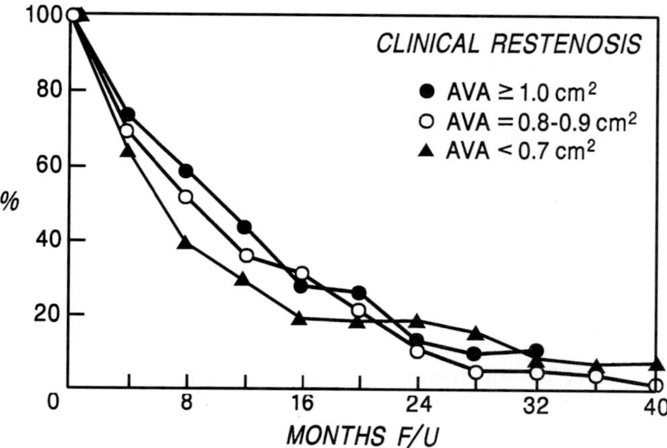

FIGURE 22–11 Curves for clinical restenosis after PAV for patients with severe aortic stenosis treated with PAV at the Massachusetts General Hospital. Curves for three different post-PAV aortic valve areas (AVA) achieved with the procedure are shown.

A high incidence of restenosis after PAV in elderly patients with calcific aortic stenosis is not unexpected. Previous attempts at surgical aortic valvuloplasty using a wide variety of instruments were accompanied by a high rate of restenosis. Healing of the fractured calcium nodules could be expected to occur early after PAV, resulting in the high incidence of restenosis. However, it is possible that if commissure splitting had occurred at the time of PAV, restenosis might not be as rapid. Although only speculative, this mechanism may account in part for those patients with superior long-term results.

PAV as a Bridge to Aortic Valve Replacement

From our cohort of 310 patients who underwent PAV at the Massachusetts General Hospital, there were 40 patients (14 percent), 21 males and 19 females, mean age of 75 ± 2 years, who underwent aortic valve replacement 6 ± 1 months after PAV. When compared with the group that did not undergo aortic valve replacement after PAV (n = 270), the group of patients bridged to surgery were younger (*P* = .003), had a higher cardiac output (*P* < .003), higher aortic valve area (*P* = .006), and higher left ventricular end-diastolic pressure (*P* < .034) before PAV (Table 22–8). Left ventricular ejection fraction was similar in both groups. With PAV, the mean aortic gradient decreased from 57 ± 3 mm Hg to 26 ± 2 mm Hg (*P* < .001), the cardiac output increased from 4.2 ± 1 L/min to 45 ± 1 L/min (*P* = .11) and the aortic valve area increased from 0.6 ± 0.04 cm² to 1.0 ± 0.07 cm² (*P* < .001).

Patients who underwent aortic valve replacement had both higher cardiac output (*P* < .001) and larger aortic valve area (*P* = .03) after PAV than the group of patients who did not undergo surgery. In-hospital surgical mortality was 10 percent. There were 7 deaths occurring at 18 ± 6 months after PAV. There was a significant improvement in symptoms after aortic valve replacement. At a mean follow-up of 35 ± 3 months, 87 percent of the patients bridged to aortic valve replacement after PAV were in NYHA classes I and II and 13 percent were in classes III

TABLE 22–8 Percutaneous Aortic Balloon Valvuloplasty as a Bridge to Aortic Valve Replacement

	AVR	Control	*P* Value
Patients (n)	40	270	
Age (yr)	75 ± 280 ± 1	0.003	
Ejection fraction (pre-PAV)	0.47 ± 0.15	0.49 ± 16	NS
Mean aortic gradient (mm Hg)			
Pre-PAV	57 ± 3	56 ± 1	NS
Post-PAV	26 ± 225 ± 1	NS	
Cardiac output (L/min)			
Pre-PAV	4.2 ± 0.2	3.6 ± 0.2	.003
Post-PAV	4.5 ± 0.2	3.8 ± 0.2	.001
Aortic valve area (cm²)			
Pre-PAV	0.6 ± 0.04	0.5 ± 0.01	.006
Post-PAV	1.0 ± 0.07	0.9 ± 0.02	.03

Abbreviations: AVR, aortic valve replacement; NS, not significant; PAV, percutaneous aortic balloon valvuloplasty.

and IV. As shown in Figure 22–12, estimated actuarial survival curves at 1, 3, and 5 years were significantly better for the group of patients bridged to aortic valve replacement after PAV.

PAV for Patients in Cardiogenic Shock

PAV can be performed successfully in patients with cardiogenic shock owing to severe aortic stenosis.[106] PAV resulted in a significant decrease in aortic gradient and a significant increase in aortic valve area and systolic arterial pressure in 90 percent of these moribund patients. From our cohort of 310 patients who underwent PAV at the Massachusetts General Hospital, there were 21 patients, 10 males and 11 females, mean age of 74 ± 3 (range 35 to 90) years, mean left ventricular ejection fraction of 29 ± 3 percent (range 15 to 61 percent) who underwent PAV for cardiogenic shock. All patients met the following criteria of cardiogenic shock: (1) sustained arterial hypotension with systolic blood pressure less than 90 mm Hg despite maximal inotropic and pressor pharmacologic support, (2) cardiac index less than 2.2 L/min/m², (3) mean pulmonary capillary wedge pressure and/or left ventricular end-diastolic pressure greater than 20 mm Hg, (4) urinary output less than 0.5 ml/kg/h; and (5) clinical evidence of decreased tissue perfusion.

The hemodynamic characteristics of patients with and without cardiogenic shock are shown in Table 22–9. Before PAV, patients with cardiogenic shock exhibit a lower left ventricular ejection fraction ($P = .001$), and lower cardiac index ($P < .0003$), than the group of patients without cardiogenic shock. PAV resulted in a significant reduction in mean aortic gradient from 49 ± 4 mm Hg to 21 ± 3 mm Hg ($P = .0001$), a borderline improvement in cardiac index from 1.8 ± 0.1 L/min/m² to 2.2 ± 0.1 L/min/m² ($P = .06$), and a significant improvement in aortic valve area from 0.5 ± 0.04 cm² to 0.8 ± 0.06 cm² ($P = .0001$) in the group of patients presenting in cardiogenic shock (see Table 22–9). Sixteen of these patients were

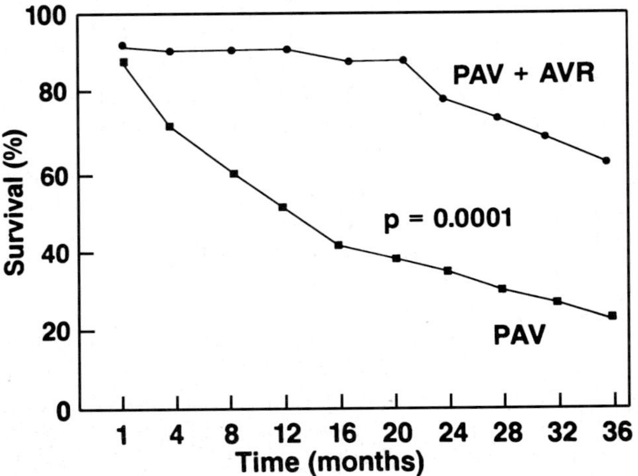

FIGURE 22–12 Comparative actuarial survival for patients undergoing percutaneous aortic balloon valvuloplasty (PAV) at the Massachusetts General Hospital as a bridge to aortic valve replacement (AVR) with those who did not undergo AVR.

TABLE 22–9 Percutaneous Aortic Balloon Valvuloplasty for Cardiogenic Shock due to Aortic Stenosis

	Cardiogenic Shock	Control	*P* Value
Patients (n)	21	289	
Age (yr)	74 ± 3	79 ± 2	.001
NYHA	4 ± 0	3.4 ± 0.04	.0001
LVEF (pre-PAV)	29 ± 3	49 ± 1	.0001
Mean aortic gradient (mm Hg)			
Pre-PAV	49 ± 4	57 ± 1	.05
Post-PAV	21 ± 3	25 ± 1	NS
Cardiac index (L/min/m²)			
Pre-PAV	1.8 ± 0.1	2.2 ± 0.03	.003
Post-PAV	2.2 ± 0.1	2.4 ± 0.04	NS
Aortic valve area (cm²)			
Pre-PAV	0.5 ± 0.04	0.5 ± 0.01	NS
Post-PAV	0.8 ± 0.06	0.9 ± 0.02	NS

Abbreviations: LVEF, Left ventricular ejection fraction; NS, not significant; NYHA, New York Heart Association; PAV, percutaneous aortic balloon valvuloplasty.

successfully weaned from the inotropic support in the first 24 hours after the valvuloplasty procedure. Complications in this cohort of patients included procedural mortality in 2 patients (9.5 percent), total in-hospital (30-day) mortality in 9 patients (43 percent), local vascular complications in 5 patients (24 percent), local vascular surgery in 3 patients (14 percent), cerebrovascular accident in 1 patient (5 percent), severe aortic regurgitation in 1 patient (5 percent), and cholesterol embolization in 1 patient (5 percent). The major cause of in-hospital mortality was multiorgan failure despite successful PAV.[106]

Actuarial survival was 38 ± 11 percent at 27 months' follow-up. Cox regression analysis identified post-PAV cardiac index as the only predictor for longer survival ($P = .02$). Although high, the procedure-related mortality after PAV in this group of patients with cardiogenic shock compares favorably with the extremely high mortality rate reported in previous surgical studies in patients with cardiogenic shock and severe aortic stenosis.[88, 89] Even though surgical correction with aortic valve replacement is the only therapy that will alter the natural history of severe, symptomatic aortic stenosis in the elderly, important guidelines have to be kept in mind when managing elderly patients with cardiogenic shock owing to critical aortic stenosis:

1. Sustained hypotension-associated severe congestive heart failure constitutes a medical emergency, and pharmacologic therapy and bedside hemodynamic monitoring should be started immediately.
2. There is no time for procrastination, and emergent interventional therapy (PAV valvuloplasty or aortic valve replacement) should be done as soon as possible.
3. PAV should be considered as a bridge to aortic valve replacement, and aortic valve replacement with myocardial revascularization, if needed, should be performed early after PAV.[106]

PAV is a palliative treatment for adult patients with aortic stenosis who are not candidates for aortic valve replacement.[91–100, 107] PAV provides immediate hemodynamic and clinical improvement with low incidence of life-threatening complications. However, the major limitation of PAV is the high incidence of restenosis within 1 year after the procedure. Although PAV results in immediate hemodynamic and symptomatic improvement in the great majority of patients, the long-term results of PAV show that clinical restenosis occurs frequently 6 to 12 months after PAV. It is well known that the onset of symptoms in patients with severe aortic stenosis begins after a latent period of several years, during which increasing left ventricular obstruction and myocardial overload occur. After the onset of symptoms, the prognosis of patients with aortic stenosis without aortic valve replacement is very poor. The 5-year survival is less than 50 percent when congestive heart failure, syncope, or angina develops in patients treated medically. Congestive heart failure carries the worst prognosis; the 50 percent survival of these patients is 2 years if surgery is not performed. Thus, once symptoms develop, medical therapy has a limited role in the treatment of patients with aortic stenosis. Aortic valve replacement is the treatment of choice for these patients. This technique has been clearly demonstrated to change the natural history of patients with severe aortic stenosis. Aortic valve replacement can be performed with low operative mortality and morbidity. Follow-up studies of these patients demonstrated significant improvement in symptoms and excellent long-term survival. Although aortic valve replacement in elderly patients, particularly octogenarians, with severe aortic stenosis is associated with a greater morbidity and mortality, it can be performed safely with low mortality in a selected group of these patients. Furthermore, after surgery, the survival of these patients is no different than the survival of other octogenarians with no cardiac diseases.[90]

Although the hemodynamic and clinical improvement produced by PAV in patients with degenerative calcific aortic stenosis is short-lived, it provides a window of opportunity, making this technique an attractive alternative for a selected group of patients with symptomatic calcific aortic stenosis. Today, PAV indications for patients with severe degenerative aortic stenosis include:

1. Patients who are not-high-risk or very-high-risk surgical candidates and are incapacitated by symptoms of aortic stenosis. Consultation with a cardiac surgeon is recommended to identify patients who are truly not candidates for cardiac surgery. Elderly patients with aortic stenosis should not be denied the opportunity for aortic valve replacement solely on the basis of age.
2. As a bridge to aortic valve replacement in patients with calcific aortic stenosis who require urgent major noncardiac surgical intervention for other organ dysfunction. These patients may have PAV to transiently improve their hemodynamics and therefore the safety of their urgent major surgical procedure. After recovery from this surgery, the decision to replace the aortic valve should be made.
3. As a bridge to aortic valve replacement in patients with severe heart failure or cardiogenic shock owing to aortic stenosis.
4. In patients with "the Gorlin conundrum" characterized by poor left ventricular function, low cardiac output, and small transaortic gradient whose calculated aortic valve areas by the Gorlin formula are small. In these patients, the low left ventricular ejection fraction could be secondary to a myopathic left ventricle with an aortic valve that is not stenotic but with a low flow state that results in a falsely low calculated aortic valve area or secondary to afterload mismatch owing to a severely stenotic aortic valve. In the former, surgery will not be of benefit and the surgical risk is very high; in the latter, aortic valve replacement should be performed. PAV can be used to solve this dilemma. Improvement of left ventricular ejection fraction after a successful PAV indicates that aortic stenosis was present and the patient should undergo aortic valve replacement. On the contrary, lack of improvement in left ventricular ejection fraction after a successful PAV indicates that aortic stenosis was never present and the patient was suffering from a cardiomyopathy. Under these latter conditions, aortic valve replacement should not be performed.

PAV for Patients With Congenital Aortic Stenosis

Lababidi and associates[108] introduced PAV for congenital valvular aortic stenosis in 1982. The aortic valve in patients with congenital aortic stenosis is most commonly bicuspid with two commissures, less frequently is unicommissural or noncommissural, and rarely the valve is tricuspid with fusion of one or more of the three commissures. PAV in this patient population provides effective gradient relief with minimal restenosis at follow-up.[103, 108] In this patient cohort, PAV is a good alternative to surgical valvuloplasty, and this latter technique should be reserved for those patients with congenital aortic stenosis in whom PAV is unsuccessful or impossible. Complications are rare, and most of them are transient. Arterial access problems owing to the large balloon size are the most common complications. The incidence and degree of aortic regurgitation post-PAV are comparable with that associated with surgical open valvuloplasty. Appropriate balloon sizing (a balloon diameter equal to or less than the aortic annulus measured by echocardiography and/or cineangiography) is essential to decrease the incidence of severe aortic regurgitation and/or disruption of the aortic annulus after PAV.[103, 108]

Percutaneous Tricuspid Balloon Valvuloplasty

Tricuspid stenosis is rare and is associated with mitral stenosis. Percutaneous tricuspid balloon valvuloplasty (PTV) has been performed in few isolated cases with good outcome.[109, 110] Because of the large tricuspid annulus, it is necessary to employ the double-balloon technique. Results from PTV have been similar to those reported for surgery. PTV results in a dramatic clinical and hemodynamic improvement in patients with tricuspid stenosis. With PTV, there is a decrease in tricuspid gradient and an increase in cardiac output. Significant tricuspid regurgitation rarely occurs, and restenosis at follow-up is infrequent. Patients with associated moderate or severe tricuspid regurgitation are not candidates for PTV.

REFERENCES

1. Kan JS, White RI, Mitchell SE, Gardner TJ: Percutaneous balloon valvuloplasty: a new method for treating congenital pulmonary-valve stenosis. N Engl J Med 307:540–542, 1982.
2. Lababidi Z, Wu JR: Percutaneous balloon pulmonary valvuloplasty. Am J Cardiol 52:560–562, 1983.
3. Kan JS, White RI Jr, Mitchell E, et al: Percutaneous transluminal balloon valvuloplasty for pulmonary valve stenosis. Circulation 69:554–560, 1984.
4. Radtke W, Keane JF, Fellows KE, et al: Percutaneous balloon valvotomy of congenital pulmonary stenosis using oversized balloons. J Am Coll Cardiol 8:909–915, 1986.
5. Rocchini AP, Kveselis DA, Crowley D, et al: Percutaneous balloon valvuloplasty for treatment of congenital pulmonary valvular stenosis in children. J Am Coll Cardiol 3:1005–1012, 1984.
6. Pepine CJ, Gessner IH, Feldman RL: Percutaneous balloon valvuloplasty for pulmonary valve stenosis in the adult. Am J Cardiol 50:1442–1445, 1982.
7. Rao PS, Mardini MK: Pulmonary valvotomy without thoracotomy: the experience with percutaneous balloon valvuloplasty. Ann Saudi Med 5:149, 1985.
8. Rao PS: Influence of balloon size on short-term and long-term results of balloon pulmonary valvuloplasty. Tex Heart Inst J 14:57, 1987.
9. Inoue K, Owaki T, Nakamura T, et al: Clinical application of transvenous mitral commissurotomy by a new balloon catheter. J Thorac Cardiovasc Surg 87:394–402, 1984.
10. Lock JE, Kalilullah M, Shrivastava S, et al: Percutaneous catheter commissurotomy in rheumatic mitral stenosis. N Engl J Med 313:1515–1518, 1985.
11. Palacios I, Block PC, Brandi S, et al: Percutaneous balloon valvotomy for patients with severe mitral stenosis. Circulation 75:778–784, 1987.
12. Al Zaibag M, Ribeiro PA, Al Kassab SA, Al Fagig MR: Percutaneous double balloon mitral valvotomy for rheumatic mitral stenosis. Lancet 1:757–761, 1986.
13. Vahanian A, Michel PL, Cormier B, et al: Results of percutaneous mitral commissurotomy in 200 patients. Am J Cardiol 63:847–852, 1989.
14. McKay RG, Lock JE, Safian RD, et al: Balloon dilatation of mitral stenosis in adult patients: postmortem and percutaneous mitral valvuloplasty studies. J Am Coll Cardiol 9:723–731, 1987.
15. McKay CR, Kawanishi DT, Rahimtoola SH: Catheter balloon valvuloplasty of the mitral valve in adults using a double balloon technique. Early hemodynamic results. JAMA 257:1753–1761, 1987.
16. Abascal VM, O'Shea JP, Wilkins GT, et al: Prediction of successful outcome in 130 patients undergoing percutaneous balloon mitral valvotomy. Circulation 82:448–456, 1990.
17. Herrman HC, Wilkins GT, Abascal VM, et al: Percutaneous balloon mitral valvotomy for patients with mitral stenosis: analysis of factors influencing early results. J Thorac Cardiovasc Surg 96:33–38, 1988.
18. Rediker DE, Block PC, Abascal VM, Palacios IF: Mitral balloon valvuloplasty for mitral restenosis after surgical commissurotomy. J Am Coll Cardiol 2:252–256, 1988.
19. Palacios IF, Block PC, Wilkins GT, Weyman AE: Follow-up of patients undergoing percutaneous mitral balloon valvotomy: analysis of factors determining restenosis. Circulation 79:573–579, 1989.
20. Abascal VM, Wilkins GT, Choong CY, et al: Echocardiographic evaluation of mitral valve structure and function in patients followed for at least 6 months after percutaneous balloon mitral valvuloplasty. J Am Coll Cardiol 12:606–615, 1988.
21. Block PC, Palacios IF, Block EH, et al: Late (two year) follow-up after percutaneous mitral balloon valvotomy. Am J Cardiol 69:537–541, 1992.
22. Tuzcu EM, Block PC, Griffin BP, et al: Immediate and long term outcome of percutaneous mitral valvotomy in patients 65 years and older. Circulation 85:963–971, 1992.
23. Nobuyoshi M, Hamasaki N, Kimura T, et al: Indications, complications, and short term clinical outcome of percutaneous transvenous mitral commissurotomy. Circulation 80:782–792, 1989.
24. Chen CR, Cheng TO, Chen JY, et al: Percutaneous mitral valvuloplasty with the Inoue balloon catheter. Am J Cardiol 70:1455–1458, 1992.
25. Hung JS, Chern MS, Wu JJ, et al: Short and long term results of catheter balloon percutaneous transvenous mitral commissurotomy. Am J Cardiol 67:854–862, 1991.
26. Cohen DJ, Kuntz RE, Gordon SPF, et al: Predictors of long-term outcome after percutaneous mitral valvuloplasty. N Engl J Med 327:1329–1335, 1991.
27. Babic UU, Pejcic P, Djurisic Z, et al: Percutaneous transarterial balloon valvuloplasty for mitral valve stenosis. Am J Cardiol 57:1101–1104, 1986.
28. Stefanides C, Stratos C, Pitsavos C, et al: Retrograde nontransseptal balloon mitral valvuloplasty. Immediate results and long term follow-up. Circulation 85:1760–1767, 1992.
29. Cribier A, Eltchaninoff H, Koning R, et al: Percutaneous mechanical mitral commissurotomy with a newly designed metallic valvulotome. Circulation 99:793–799, 1999.
30. Palacios IF, Lock JE, Keane JF, Block PC: Percutaneous transvenous balloon valvotomy in a patient with severe calcific mitral stenosis. J Am Coll Cardiol 7:1416–1419, 1986.
31. Block PC, Palacios IF, Jacobs M, et al: The mechanism of percutaneous mitral valvotomy. Am J Cardiol 59:178–179, 1987.
32. Wilkins GT, Weyman AE, Abascal VM, et al: Percutaneous mitral valvotomy: an analysis of echocardiographic variables related to outcome and the mechanism of dilatation. Br Heart J 60:299–308, 1988.
33. Ruiz CE, Zhang HP, Macaya C, et al: Comparison of Inoue single balloon versus double balloon techniques for percutaneous mitral valvotomy. Am Heart J 123:942–947, 1992.
34. Leon MN, Harrell LC, Simosa HF, et al: Comparison of immediate and long-term results of mitral balloon valvotomy with the double balloon versus Inoue techniques. Am J Cardiol 83:1356–1363, 1999.
35. Abascal VM, Wilkins GT, Choong CY, et al: Mitral regurgitation after percutaneous mitral valvuloplasty in adults: evaluation by pulsed Doppler echocardiography. J Am Coll Cardiol 2:257–263, 1988.
36. The National Heart, Lung, and Blood Institute Balloon Valvuloplasty Registry: Complications and mortality of percutaneous balloon mitral commissurotomy. Circulation 85:2014–2024, 1992.
37. Roth RB, Block PC, Palacios IF: Predictors of increased mitral regurgitation after percutaneous mitral balloon valvotomy. Cathet Cardiovasc Diagn 20:17–21, 1990.
38. Padial LR, Freitas N, Sagie A, et al: Echocardiography can predict which patients will develop severe mitral regurgitation following percutaneous mitral valvulotomy. J Am Coll Cardiol. 27:1225–1231, 1996.
39. Padial LR, Abascal VM, Moreno PR, et al: Echocardiography can predict the development of severe mitral regurgitation after percutaneous mitral valvuloplasty by the Inoue technique. Am J Cardiol 83:1210–1213, 1999.
40. Casale P, Block PC, O'Shea JP, Palacios IF: Atrial septal defect after percutaneous mitral balloon valvuloplasty: immediate results and follow-up. J Am Coll Cardiol 15:1300–1304, 1990.
41. Desideri A, Vanderperren O, Serra A, et al: Long term (9 to 33 months) echocardiographic follow-up after successful percutaneous mitral commissurotomy. Am J Cardiol 69:1602–1606, 1992.
42. Babic UU, Grujicic S, Popovic Z, et al: Percutaneous transarterial balloon dilatation of the mitral valve. Five year experience. Br Heart J 67:185–189, 1992.
43. The National Heart, Lung, and Blood Institute Balloon Valvuloplasty Registry Participants: Multicenter experience with balloon mitral commissurotomy. NHLBI balloon valvuloplasty registry report on immediate and 30 day follow-up results. Circulation 85:448–461, 1992.
44. Pan M, Medina A, de Lezo JS, et al: Factors determining late success after mitral balloon valvotomy. Am J Cardiol 71:1181–1185, 1993.
45. Herrmann HC, Kleaveland P, Hill JA, et al: The M-Heart percutaneous balloon mitral Valvuloplasty Registry: initial results and early follow-up. J Am Coll Cardiol 15:1221–1226, 1990.
46. Tuzcu EM, Block PC, Griffin B, et al: Percutaneous mitral balloon valvotomy in patients with calcific mitral stenosis: immediate and long term outcome. J Am Coll Cardiol 23:1604–1609, 1994.
47. Harken DE, Ellis LB, Ware PF: The surgical treatment of mitral stenosis. I. Valvuloplasty. N Engl J Med 239:801, 1948.

48. Williams JA, Littmann D, Warren R: Experience with the surgical treatment of mitral stenosis. N Engl J Med 258:623–630, 1958.
49. Scannell JG, Burke JF, Saidi F, Turner JD: Five-year follow-up study of closed mitral valvotomy. J Thorac Cardiovasc Surg 40:723–730, 1960.
50. Medina A, Delezo JS, Hernandez E, et al: Balloon valvuloplasty for mitral restenosis after previous surgery. A comparative study. Am Heart J 120:568–571, 1990.
51. Davidson CJ, Bashore TM, Mickel M, et al: Balloon mitral commissurotomy after previous surgical commissurotomy. Circulation 86:91–99, 1992.
52. Jang IK, Block PC, Newell JB, et al: Percutaneous mitral balloon valvotomy for recurrent mitral stenosis after surgical commissurotomy. Am J Cardiol 75:601–605, 1995.
53. Leon M, Harrell L, Mahdi N, et al: Immediate and long term outcome of percutaneous mitral balloon valvotomy in patients with mitral stenosis and atrial fibrillation. J Am Coll Cardiol (in press).
54. Chen MH, Semigran M, Schwammenthal E, et al: Impact of pulmonary resistance on short and long term outcome after percutaneous mitral valvuloplasty. Circulation (suppl I):1825, 1993.
55. Sagie A, Schwammenthal E, Newell JB, et al: Significant tricuspid regurgitation is a marker for adverse outcome in patients undergoing mitral balloon valvotomy. J Am Coll Cardiol 24:696–702, 1994.
56. Lopez-Cuellar JC, Leon MN, Pathan A, et al: Ten year follow-up of optimal candidates for percutaneous mitral balloon valvuloplasty. Circulation 96(suppl I): 2225, 1997.
57. Petrossian GA, Tuzcu EM, Ziskind AA, et al: Atrial septal occlusion improves the accuracy of mitral valve area determination following percutaneous mitral balloon valvotomy. Cathet Cardiovasc Diagn 22:21–24, 1991.
58. John S, Bashi VV, Jairaj PS, et al: Closed mitral valvotomy: early results and long term follow up of 3724 patients. Circulation 68:891–896, 1983.
59. Ellis LR, Harken DE, Black H: A clinical study of 1,000 consecutive cases of mitral stenosis two to nine years after mitral valvuloplasty. Circulation 19:803, 1959.
60. Elis FH, Kirklin JW, Parker RL, et al: Mitral commissurotomy: an overall appraisal of clinical and hemodynamic results. Arch Intern Med 94:774, 1954.
61. Hoeksema TD, Wallace RB, Kirklin JW: Closed mitral commissurotomy. Am J Cardiol 17:825–828, 1966.
62. Kirklin JW: Percutaneous balloon versus surgical closed commissurotomy for mitral stenosis. Circulation 83:1450–1451, 1991.
63. Higgs LM, Glancy DL, O'Brien KP, et al: Mitral restenosis: an uncommon cause of recurrent symptoms following mitral commissurotomy. Am J Cardiol 26:34–37, 1970.
64. Glover RP, Davila JC, O'Neil TJE, Janton OH: Does mitral stenosis recur after commissurotomy? Circulation 11:14–28, 1955.
65. Hickey MSJ, Blackstone EH, Kirklin JW, Dean LS: Outcome probabilities and life history after surgical mitral commissurotomy: implications for balloon commissurotomy. J Am Coll Cardiol 17:29–42, 1991.
66. Scalia D, Rizzoli G, Campanile F, et al: Long-term results of mitral commissurotomy. J Thorac Cardiovasc Surg 105:633–642, 1993.
67. Rihal CS, Schaff HV, Frye RL, et al: Long-term follow-up of patients undergoing closed transventricular mitral commissurotomy: a useful surrogate for percutaneous balloon mitral valvuloplasty. J Am Coll Cardiol 20:781–786, 1992.
68. Turi ZG, Reyes VP, Raju BS, et al: Percutaneous balloon versus surgical closed commissurotomy for mitral stenosis: a prospective, randomized trial. Circulation 83:1179–1185, 1991.
69. Reyes VP, Raju BS, Wynne J, et al: Percutaneous balloon valvuloplasty compared with open surgical commissurotomy for mitral stenosis. N Engl J Med 331:961–967, 1994.
70. Patel JJ, Sharma D, Mitha AS, et al: Balloon valvuloplasty versus closed commissurotomy for pliable mitral stenosis: a prospective hemodynamic study. J Am Coll Cardiol 18:1318–1322, 1991.
71. Shrivastava S, Mathur A, Dev V, et al: Comparison of immediate hemodynamic response of closed mitral commissurotomy, single-balloon, and double-balloon mitral valvuloplasty in rheumatic mitral stenosis. J Thorac Cardiovasc Surg 104:1264–1267, 1992.
72. Arora R, Nair M, Kalra GS, et al: Immediate and long-term results of balloon and surgical closed mitral valvotomy: a randomized comparative study. Am Heart J 125:1091–1094, 1993.
73. Farhat MB, Ayari M, Maatouk F, et al: Percutaneous balloon versus surgical closed and open mitral commissurotomy: seven year follow-up results of a randomized trial. Circulation 97:245–250, 1998.
74. Palacios IF: Farewell to surgical mitral commissurotomy for many patients. Circulation 97:223–226, 1998.
75. Bernal Y, Miralles: Cardiac surgery with cardiopulmonary bypass during pregnancy. Obstet Gynecol Surg 41:1, 1998.
76. Vosloo S, Reichart B: The feasibility of closed mitral valvotomy in pregnancy. J Thorac Cardiovasc Surg 93:675–679, 1987.
77. Palacios IF, Block PC, Wilkins GT, et al: Percutaneous mitral balloon valvotomy during pregnancy in patients with severe mitral stenosis. Cathet Cardiovasc Diagn 15:109–111, 1988.
78. Mangione JA, Zuliani MF, Del Castillo JM, et al: Percutaneous double balloon mitral valvuloplasty in pregnant women. Am J Cardiol 64:99–102, 1989.
79. Straumann E, Kiowski W, Langer I, et al: Aortic valve replacement in elderly patients with aortic stenosis. Br Heart J 71:449–453, 1994.
80. Pupello DF, Bessone LN, Hiro SP, et al: Aortic valve replacement: procedure of choice in elderly patients with aortic stenosis. J Card Surg 9(2 suppl):148–153, 1994.
81. Ruygrot PN, Barratt-Boyes BG, Agnew TM, et al: Aortic valve replacement in the elderly. Heart Valve Dis 2:550–557, 1993.
82. Aranki SF, Rizzo RJ, Couper GS, et al: Aortic valve replacement in the elderly. Effect of gender and coronary artery disease on operative mortality. Circulation 88:II-17–II-23, 1993.
83. Fighali AU, Sayid F, Avendano A, et al: Early and late mortality of patients undergoing aortic valve replacement after previous coronary artery bypass graft surgery. Circulation 92:II-163–II-168, 1995.
84. Fremes SE, Goldman BS, Ivanov J, et al: Valvular surgery in the elderly. Circulation 80:I-77–I-90, 1989.
85. Smith N, McAnulty JH, Rahimtoola SH: Severe aortic stenosis with impaired left ventricular function and clinical heart failure: results of aortic valve replacement. Circulation 58:255–264, 1978.
86. Carabello BA, Green LH, Grossman W, et al: Hemodynamic determinants of prognosis of aortic valve replacement in critical aortic stenosis and advanced congestive heart failure. Circulation 62:42–48, 1980.
87. Elayda MA, Hall RJ, Reul RM, et al: Aortic valve replacement in patients 80 years and older. Operative risks and long-term results. Circulation 88:II-11–II-16, 1993.
88. Hutter A Jr, De Sanctis R, Nathan M, et al: Aortic valve surgery as an emergent procedure. Circulation 51:623–627, 1970.
89. Kirklin JW: Aortic valve disease. *In* Kirklin JW, Barrat-Boyes B (eds): Cardiac Surgery: Morphology, Diagnostic Criteria, Natural History, Techniques and Indications. p. 528. New York: Churchill Livingstone, 1993.
90. Levinson JR, Akins CW, Buckley MJ, et al: Octogenarians with aortic stenosis. Outcome after aortic valve replacement. Circulation 80:I-49–I-56, 1989.
91. Cribier A, Savin T, Saoudi N, et al: Percutaneous transluminal valvuloplasty of acquired aortic stenosis in elderly patients: an alternative to valve replacement? Lancet 63–67, 1986.
92. Block PC, Palacios IF: Aortic and mitral balloon valvuloplasty: the United States experience. *In* Topol EJ (ed): Textbook of Interventional Cardiology. 2nd ed. pp. 1189–1205. WB Saunders, Philadelphia: 1994.
93. Block PC, Palacios IF: Comparison of hemodynamic results of anterograde versus retrograde percutaneous balloon valvuloplasty. Am J Cardiol 60:659–662, 1987.
94. McKay RG, for the Mansfield Scientific Aortic Valvuloplasty Registry: Balloon aortic valvuloplasty in 285 patients: initial results and complications. Circulation 78:II–594, 1988.
95. Block PC, Palacios IF: Clinical and hemodynamic follow-up after percutaneous aortic valvuloplasty in the elderly. Am J Cardiol 62:760–763, 1988.
96. Palacios IF: Percutaneous aortic balloon valvuloplasty. *In* Robicseck F (ed): Cardiac Surgery: State of the Art Reviews. Vol. 5, No. 2. pp. 267–272. Philadelphia: Hanley & Belfus, 1991.
97. Moreno PR, Jang I-K, Newell JB, et al: Percutaneous aortic balloon valvuloplasty in the elderly: the Massachusetts General Hospital experience. Circulation 88:I-340, 1993.
98. Otto CM, Mickel MC, Kennedy JW, et al: Three year outcome after balloon aortic valvuloplasty. Insights into prognosis of valvular aortic stenosis. Circulation 89:642–650, 1994.
99. O'Keefe JH Jr, Vlietstra RE, Bailey KR, Holmes DR Jr: Natural history of candidates for balloon aortic valvuloplasty. Mayo Clin Proc 62:986–991, 1987.

100. Bernard Y, Etivent J, Mourand JL, et al: Long-term results of percutaneous aortic valvuloplasty compared with aortic valve replacement in patient more that 75 years old. J Am Coll Cardiol 20:796–801, 1992.
101. Gorlin R, Gorlin G: Hydraulic formula for calculation of area of stenotic mitral valve, other cardiac valves and central circulatory shunts. Am Heart J 41:1, 1951.
102. Ford L, Felman T, Chiu C, et al: Hemodynamic resistance as a measurement of functional impairment in aortic valve stenosis. Circ Res 66:1–7, 1990.
103. Sholler GF, Keane JF, Perry SB, et al: Balloon dilation of congenital aortic valve stenosis. Results and influence of technical and morphological features on outcome. Circulation 78:351–360, 1988.
104. Safian RD, Mandell VS, Thurer RE, et al: Postmortem and intraoperative balloon valvuloplasty of calcific aortic stenosis in elderly patients: mechanisms of successful dilatation. J Am Coll Cardiol 9:655–660, 1987.
105. Roberts WD, Perloff JK, Constantino T: Severe valvular aortic stenosis in patients over 65 years of age. A clinico-pathologic study. Am J Cardiol 27:497–506, 1971.
106. Moreno PR, Jang IK, Newell JB, et al: The role of percutaneous aortic valvuloplasty in patients with cardiogenic shock due to severe aortic stenosis. J Am Coll Cardiol 23:1071–1075, 1994.
107. Rahimtoola SH: Catheter balloon valvuloplasty for severe calcific aortic stenosis: a limited role. J Am Coll Cardiol 23:1076–1078, 1994.
108. Lababidi Z, Wu J, Walls JT: Percutaneous balloon aortic valvuloplasty: results in 23 patients. Am J Cardiol 53:194–197, 1984.
109. Al Zaibag M, Ribeiro PA, Al Kasab S: Percutaneous balloon valvotomy in tricuspid stenosis. Br Heart J 57:51–53, 1987.
110. Ribeiro PA, Al Zaibag MA, Al Kasab SA, et al: Percutaneous double balloon valvotomy for rheumatic tricuspid stenosis. Am J Cardiol 61:660–662, 1988.

CHAPTER 23

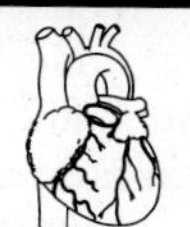

Surgical Treatment

Denton A. Cooley, O. H. Frazier, and Michael S. Sweeney

GENERAL CONSIDERATIONS
Traditional Versus Minimally Invasive Valve Surgery
Valve Repair Versus Replacement
INITIATION OF CARDIOPULMONARY BYPASS
MITRAL VALVE PROCEDURES
Mitral Stenosis
Mitral Insufficiency
AORTIC VALVE PROCEDURES
TRICUSPID VALVE PROCEDURES
Primary Lesions
Secondary Lesions
FINAL STEPS IN VALVE SURGERY
POSTOPERATIVE CARE
CONCLUSION

Although the first direct attack on valvular heart disease occurred in the 1920s, cardiac valve surgery was not taken seriously by most surgeons until World War II, when Harken[1] successfully removed bullets and other foreign bodies from the heart. Once surgeons realized that the heart could be operated on successfully, attention turned toward correcting congenital defects, including valvular stenosis and insufficiency, and modern valvular surgery began its evolution. In the late 1940s, Harken and associates,[2] Bailey,[3] and Brock and coworkers[4] reported successful repair of mitral valve disease. Not until the development of cardiopulmonary bypass and open heart surgery in the 1950s, however, were surgeons able to attack acquired valvular disease. The past few decades have seen continual advancement in valvular prostheses and repair techniques. Moreover, cardiopulmonary bypass has been simplified and improved by the practice of hemodilution and by the use of cell-saver techniques.

Of the 2500 open heart operations performed each year at the Texas Heart Institute in Houston, about 20 percent involve valve replacement or repair. Surgery for these valvular lesions can be done successfully today with low operative risk. This chapter describes our standard surgical techniques for treating acquired valvular heart disease.[5–12]

General Considerations

In adults, cardiac valve lesions are usually caused by rheumatic heart disease, which produces stenosis, incompetence, or both of these disorders. Whereas the aortic and mitral valves may be affected either alone or in combination, the tricuspid valve is rarely subject to isolated disease. The indications for operation should be based on symptoms as well as on physiologic and pathologic findings, and the risk-benefit ratio should be carefully examined in each case. Generally, surgery should be considered for patients who remain in New York Heart Association functional class III despite optimal medical management.

The best surgical approach depends on the degree of physiologic disturbance, the extent and nature of the pathologic changes, and the expertise of the surgeon. Whichever approach is used, intraoperative echocardiography is valuable for monitoring the operation.[13–15]

Traditional Versus Minimally Invasive Valve Surgery

During the past few years, minimally invasive techniques have been extended to heart valve surgery, and a number of approaches have been described for performing valve replacement or repair through so-called keyhole incisions. Because we seldom perform minimally invasive valve surgery, these techniques are not described here. Interested surgeons may consult the numerous articles on this subject that have been published recently in the literature.[16–22]

We prefer the traditional approach for the following reasons.[23] Traditional valve surgery is extremely safe and effective, and it allows direct access to the heart if a complication arises. We do not believe that a smaller incision is necessarily preferable. Moreover, minimally invasive procedures entail significantly longer (40 percent or more) cardiopulmonary bypass, myocardial ischemia, and overall operative times, which not only increase patient risk but also may increase the cost of the procedure. Postoperatively, the reduction in the hospital stay is minimal, and the patient does not always experience less pain. Therefore, we believe that further prospective studies are needed to clarify the role of minimally invasive valve surgery. Meanwhile, surgeons must use discretion and sound judgment in choosing the optimal approach for each specific case.

Valve Repair Versus Replacement

Whenever possible, we perform valve repair rather than replacement.[24–26] Repair has a number of advantages, eliminating not only the need for lifelong anticoagulation but also the threat of mechanical dysfunction and paravalvular leakage.[27–29]

When valve replacement is unavoidable, we prefer the St. Jude Medical bileaflet valve (St. Jude Medical, Inc., St. Paul, MN) or the CarboMedics bileaflet valve (Sulzer CarboMedics, Inc., Austin, TX). Both of these valves have two pyrolytic carbon tilting discs, an extremely low profile, excellent hemodynamic characteristics, and a low rate of complications, including thromboembolism. Our experience with bioprostheses has primarily been with the Ionescu-Shiley bovine pericardial valve, which is no longer being used. In comparison, the St. Jude and CarboMedics valves are less susceptible to infection, freer from complications, and associated with a lower overall mortality.[25, 30–36] We currently use bioprostheses only in older patients, women of childbearing age, and those for whom anticoagulants are contraindicated. We seldom use homografts, but elsewhere interest in these valves is growing because of improved tissue preservation and surgical techniques.[37, 38]

Having tried various methods of suturing valvular prostheses, we reverted to using a continuous monofilament polypropylene suture in most cases.[11] This simple technique expedites implantation in any valve position and provides even more security than individual mattress sutures. The technique also eliminates the need for porous felt pledgets, which can become a source of infection.

To prevent infective endocarditis, we routinely administer bactericidal antibiotics to all patients undergoing prosthetic valve replacement. Antibiotics are given before surgery and continued until all catheters are removed.

Initiation of Cardiopulmonary Bypass

The valve is approached through a standard median sternotomy. To prevent costal and brachial plexus trauma, the sternum must not be opened too widely nor the shoulders hyperextended.

After heparin (3 mg/kg) has been administered, access to the systemic arterial system is gained by cannulating the ascending aorta through a pursestring suture. To prevent rupture of the aortic lumen, the suture should be carefully placed into the adventitia of the aortic wall. Cannulation for venous outflow depends on which valve is involved. For aortic valve procedures, we use a single, large-bore (52 French) right atrial cannula with numerous perforations. We position the tip of the device in the orifice of the inferior vena cava so that some of the perforations are in the right atrium. For single or combined procedures involving the mitral valve, the venae cavae are cannulated separately because traction on the atrium could cause a single cannula to become occluded.

In patients undergoing valve replacement, we routinely use moderate systemic hypothermia and cardiac hypothermia as well as a membrane oxygenator. Our cardiopulmonary bypass time rarely exceeds 1 hour.

Once cardiopulmonary bypass has been initiated and hemodilution established, the ascending aorta is cross-clamped. Hypothermic cardiac arrest is induced by injecting the ascending aorta with 500 to 700 ml of cold, lactated Ringer's solution (with 5 percent dextrose) containing 2 mEq/ml of potassium chloride. We insert a sump drain into the left atrium by making an incision dorsal to the right interatrial groove, near the orifice of the right superior pulmonary vein.

Patients with severe left ventricular hypertrophy may benefit from the addition of propranolol to the cardioplegic solution (approximately 1 mg for a normal adult). In such patients, retrograde coronary sinus blood cardioplegia may also be considered useful for myocardial protection. For more complex cardiac procedures, retrograde myocardial perfusion through the coronary sinus is used.

In combined mitral and aortic procedures, the mitral valve is treated first. Traditionally, double-valve replacement necessitates two separate incisions to visualize the valve apparatus. When this approach is impractical, as in patients who have undergone a previous median sternotomy, the mitral valve can be replaced through the aortic root after the aortic valve has been excised (Fig. 23–1).[6]

Mitral Valve Procedures

Surgical treatment of mitral valve lesions depends on the operative findings. Many mitral lesions can be repaired by means of a commissurotomy or an annuloplasty. When deterioration is advanced, however, valve replacement is unavoidable.

Mitral Stenosis

The time-honored method for alleviating "pure" mitral stenosis with minimal or no calcification is a commissurotomy with subvalvular dissection of fibrosed chordae tendineae and papillary muscles. Usually, the valve is fused at both commissures and has a slitlike opening. Freeing the fused commissures produces a functional, near-normal valve. The distended left atrium is incised parallel and posterior to the interatrial groove (Fig. 23–2A). An atrial retractor is inserted, and the valve is exposed (see Fig. 23–2B). The valve is then examined and débrided of calcium and fibrinous deposits. The commissures and line of leaflet fusion should serve as anatomic landmarks for separation of the leaflets. We routinely use scissors to incise the fused anterolateral commissure (see Fig. 23–2C) and a scalpel to divide the posteromedial commissure (see Fig. 23–2D). After these structures have been freed (see Fig. 23–2E and F), leaflet mobility can be increased by subvalvular dissection and mobilization. If fibrosis extends into the chordae tendineae and papillary muscles, subvalvular dissection is also necessary. The fibrotic and fused chordae are separated, and the papillary muscles are divided longitudinally. At the end of the procedure, the atriotomy is repaired with continuous sutures (see Fig. 23–2G).

Although a closed commissurotomy is possible with the aid of a transventricular dilator, we almost routinely perform an open procedure with cardiopulmonary bypass support. This approach enables us not only to assess the extent of disease and determine the best operative strategy but also to perform an anatomic repair. Moreover, the open approach facilitates accurate division of the commissure and allows left atrial thrombi to be extracted.

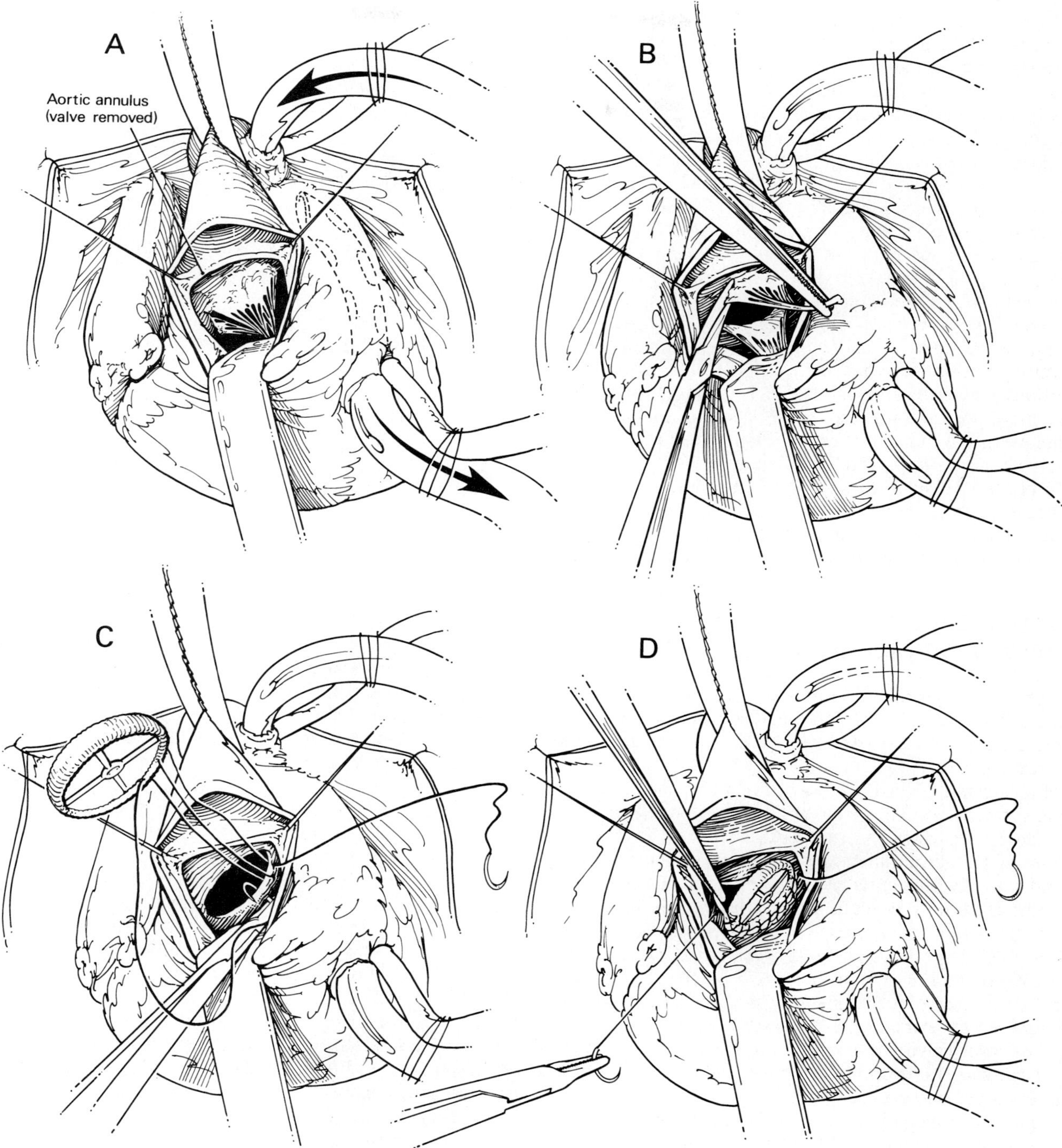

FIGURE 23–1 Single transverse aortotomy for combined valve replacement. **A,** Once the aortic valve has been excised, the mitral valve is exposed through the aortic root. **B,** The mitral valve is removed. **C** and **D,** The mitral prosthesis is inserted through the aortic root and secured with a continuous suture (alternatively, interrupted sutures could be used). (**A–D,** From Carmichael MJ, Cooley DA, Favor AS: Aortic and mitral valve replacement through a single transverse aortotomy: a useful approach in difficult mitral valve exposure. Tex Heart Inst J 10:415, 1983.)

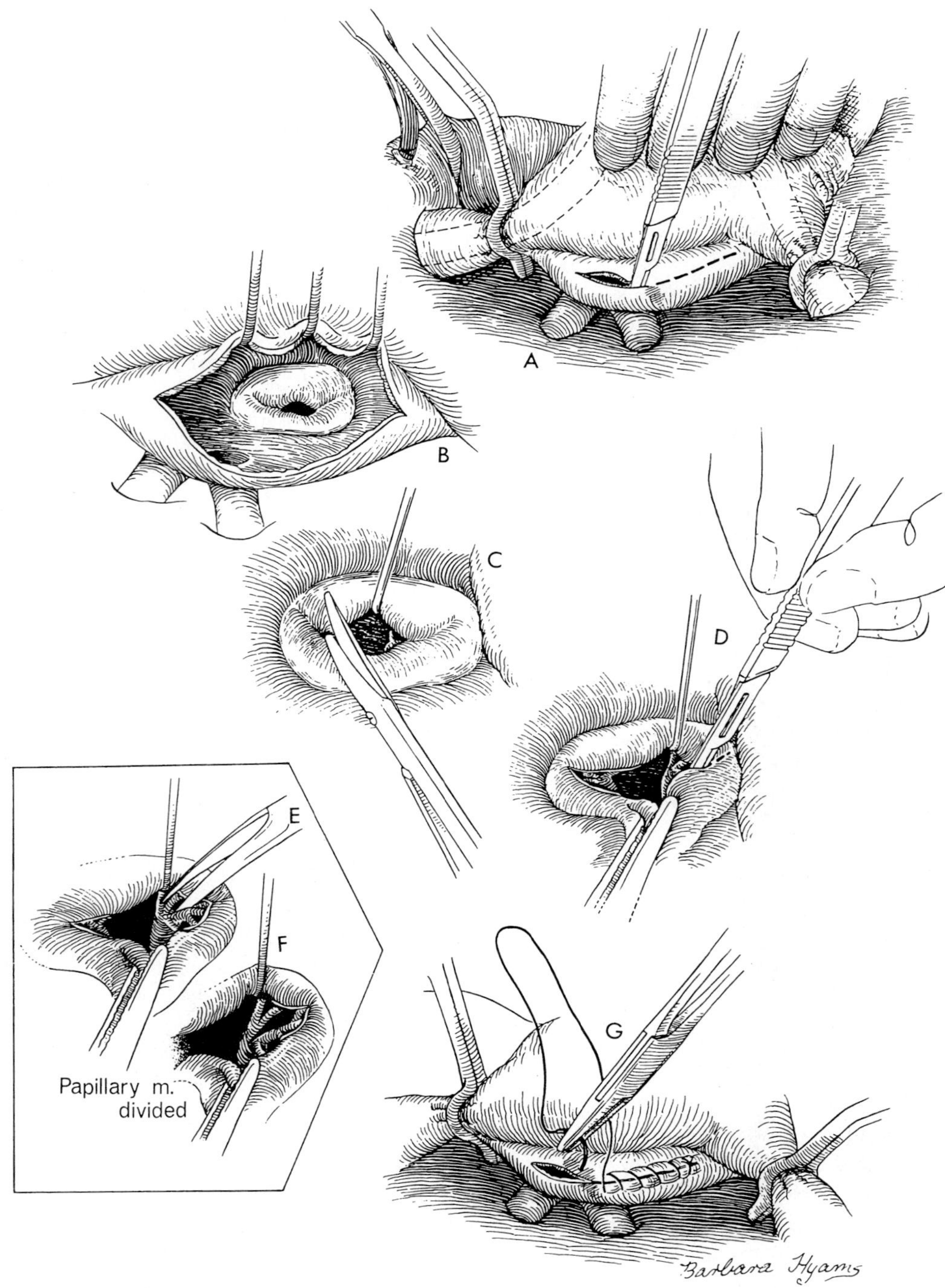

FIGURE 23–2 A–G, Open mitral commissurotomy (see text). (**A–G,** From Cooley DA: Techniques in Cardiac Surgery. 2nd ed. pp. 201–214. Philadelphia: WB Saunders, 1984.)

For patients with extensive calcification or severe fibrotic distortion, especially in the subvalvular area, valve replacement is the only option.

Mitral Insufficiency

Repair Techniques

In more than 90 percent of the cases, repair is appropriate for incompetent nonrheumatic mitral valves.[28] As long as the anterior leaflet is functional, there are no absolute contraindications to reconstruction. Compared with valve replacement, repair is associated with improved left ventricular function and better long-term survival. A variety of reconstructive techniques have been described.[27–29] Although we still occasionally perform annuloplasty by means of commissural plication, we prefer to insert an annuloplasty ring. Both of these methods reduce the annular circumference without necessitating the placement of restrictive sutures in either the anterior leaflet or the anterior portion of the annulus.

We also use an annuloplasty ring to treat mitral incompetence secondary to valve prolapse. Depending on the surgeon's preference, a Carpentier, Cooley, Duran, Puig-Massana-Shiley, or Cosgrove-Edwards ring can be used.[10, 39, 40] The device reduces the overall circumference of the annulus, thereby eliminating prolapse of the posterior leaflet. We generally use a cut section of a 22-mm Dacron graft. This ring is simple and inexpensive to produce.

After the valve is exposed, it is examined visually and a nerve hook is used to inspect the leaflets and chordae. If the posterior leaflet is partially ruptured, we remove the flail scallop (Fig. 23–3A[a]) and repair the remaining por-

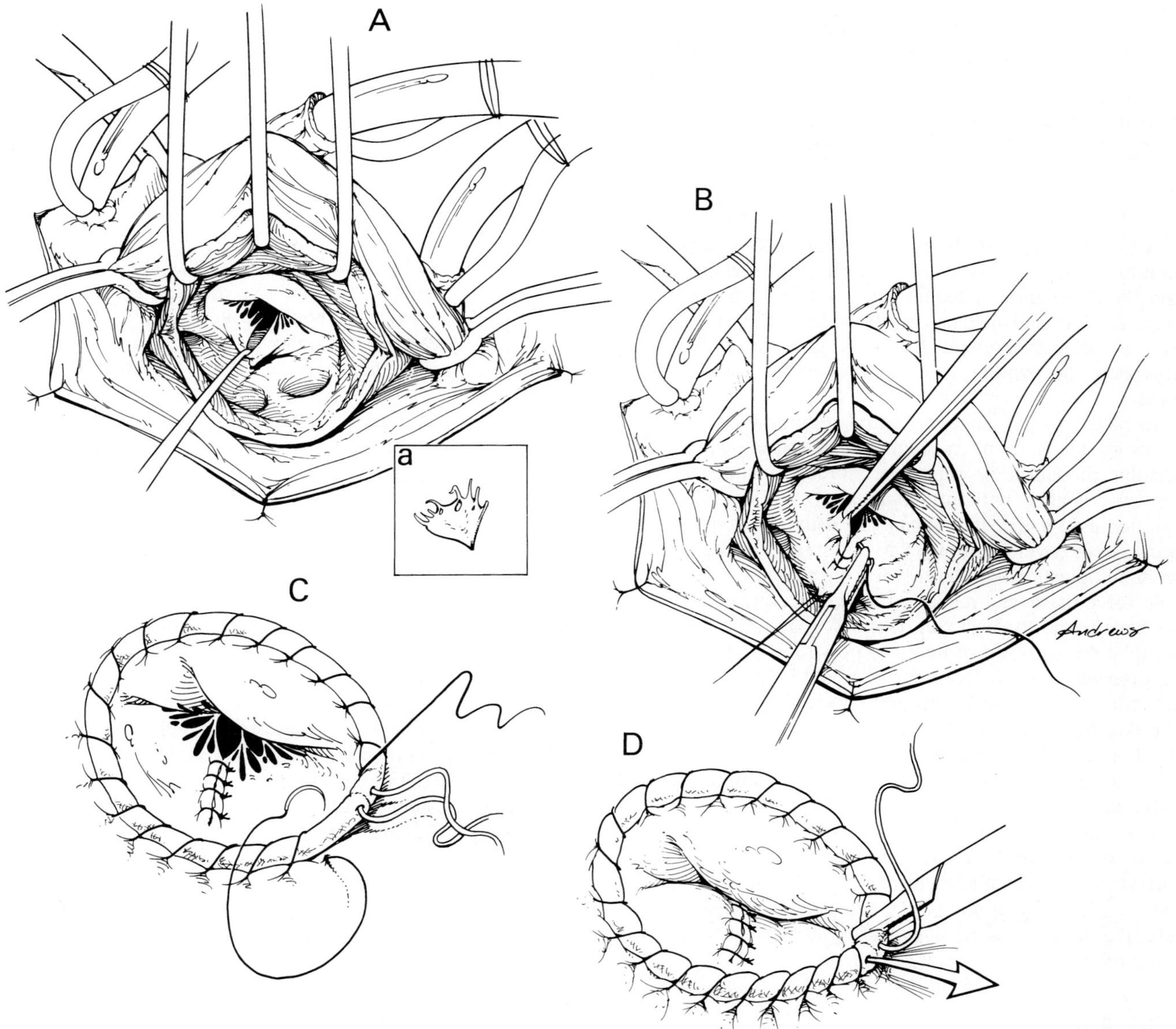

FIGURE 23–3 A–D, Annuloplasty using a circumferential fabric ring to reduce and support the annulus (see text). (**A–D,** From Murphy JP Jr, Sweeney MS, Cooley DA: The Puig-Massana-Shiley annuloplasty ring for mitral valve repair: experience in 126 patients. Reprinted with permission from the Society of Thoracic Surgeons [The Annals of Thoracic Surgery, 1987, Vol. 43, p. 52].)

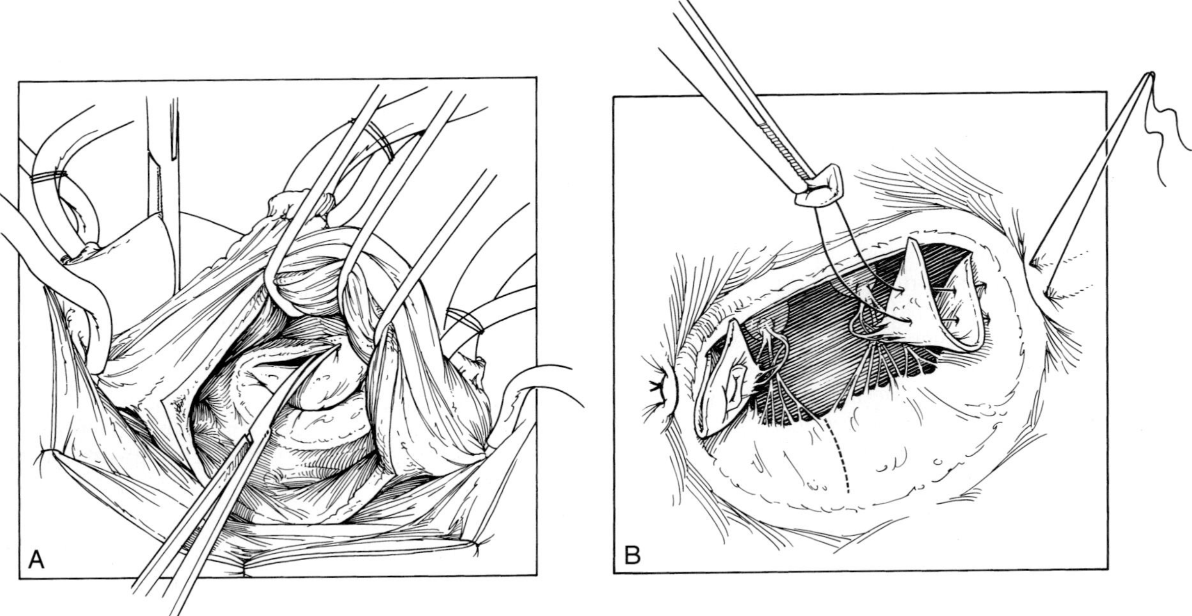

FIGURE 23–4 If the anterior mitral leaflet interferes with flow, it is incised **(A)** and fastened to the side of the annulus **(B)**. (**A** and **B**, From Frazier OH, Sweeney MS, Cooley DA: Valvular heart disease. *In* Willerson JT [ed]: Treatment of Cardiovascular Disease. pp. 6.13–6.43. New York, Gower Medical, 1993.)

tion (see Fig. 23–3B) before reducing and supporting the annulus with a circumferential fabric ring (see Fig. 23–3C and D). If the anterior leaflet hinders flow, it can be incised (Fig. 23–4A) and fastened to the side of the annulus (see Fig. 23–4B), after which the valve is replaced. With this approach, the papillary muscle is conserved and strengthened.

In patients with ischemic mitral regurgitation, the valve structure tends to be normal. When these patients have annular dilatation or ruptured chordae tendineae on the posterior leaflet without calcification or leaflet fibrosis, annuloplasty and leaflet repair are usually satisfactory. To decrease the overall annular circumference, we again insert an annuloplasty ring, thereby making the best use of available valve tissue and rendering the valve competent. Again, we have found the best annuloplasty rings to be the supple, complete rings made of nylon or polyester. These rings can be inserted quickly. Even for combined coronary-valvular procedures, our mean ischemic time is 55 minutes. If chordae tendineae are ruptured, they should be removed; the leaflet is then either excised or imbricated. When chordal or papillary rupture affects the anterior leaflet, valve replacement is necessary.

For mitral incompetence associated with a ventricular aneurysm, we perform an endoaneurysmorrhaphy[9] by inserting an oval patch graft inside the left ventricle to restore the ventricular anatomy. Once the papillary muscles have returned to their normal position, mitral dysfunction is often relieved.

Valve Replacement

In advanced rheumatic heart disease with foreshortening and thickening of the mitral leaflets and in instances of subacute bacterial endocarditis (Fig. 23–5), valve replacement is the only available option. To ensure maximal postoperative ventricular function, the chordal attachments to the papillary muscles should be preserved.[41–44] Therefore, insofar as possible, we remove only the anterior mitral leaflet, sparing the posterior leaflet and the chordal attachments.

In excising the mitral valve, the surgeon must take care not to damage the posterior annulus. This structure can rupture if an oversized valve is inserted or excessive tissue is removed. Furthermore, the nearby circumflex coronary artery may be injured if sutures are placed too deeply during valve replacement or annuloplasty.

The valve is usually approached through a standard left atrial incision. If the case is complex, however, or if the patient has undergone previous mitral surgery, a transseptal route may be more appropriate. For combined mitral-aortic procedures, a single transverse aortotomy can be used, as described previously. The valve is exposed with a handheld retractor. Once the anterior leaflet has been excised, an appropriately sized prosthesis is lowered into the annulus and continuous sutures are implanted with a 60-inch-long segment of 2-0 monofilament polypropylene and a noncutting needle (Davis & Geck, Danbury, CT). The posterior suture line is begun at the point farthest to the surgeon's left and is advanced toward the surgeon (Fig. 23–6A). It is tightened with a right-angle hook (see Fig. 23–6B) (8.5-inch right-angle suture hook [R7025]; Royal Surgical Instrument Company, Lewistown, IL), and the valve holder is removed. A similar technique is used to complete the anterior suture line (see Fig. 23–6C), and multiple throws are used to secure the continuous suture. Alternatively, two long sutures can be used to implant the valve by means of a curved-hook technique, as in aortic

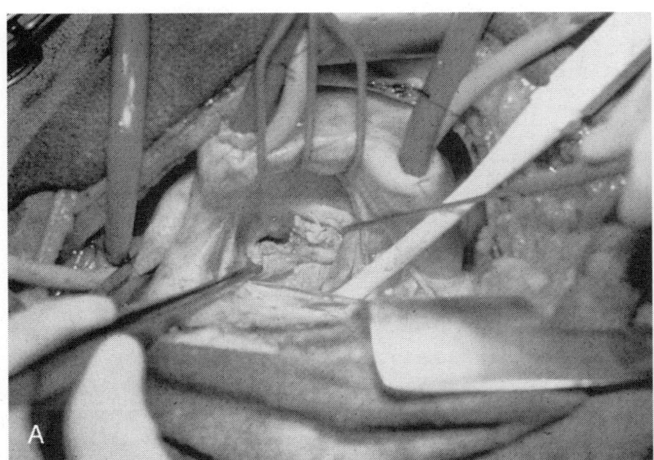

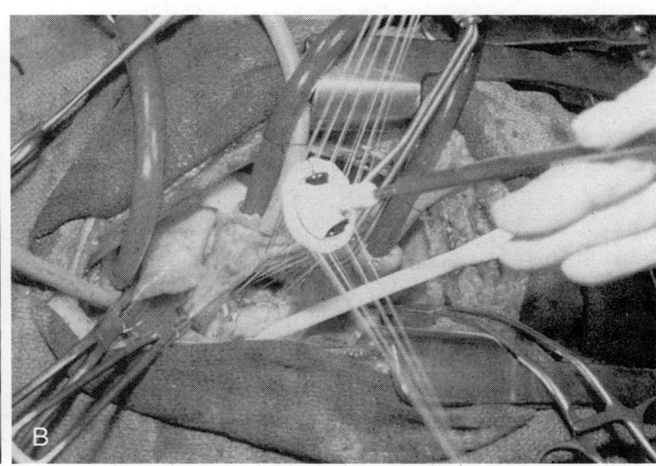

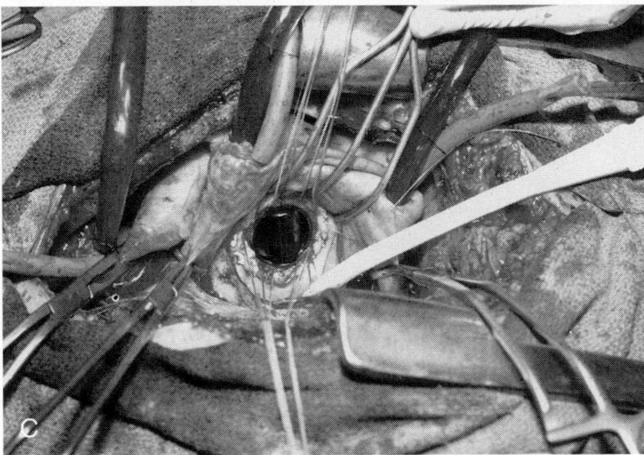

FIGURE 23–5 Mitral valve replacement in a patient with subacute bacterial endocarditis and severe mitral regurgitation. **A,** On examination, the valve was found to have a flail posterior leaflet, and both leaflets had vegetations that were causing chordal disruption. **B** and **C,** The valve was removed and replaced with a 29-mm St. Jude mechanical valve. To secure the sewing ring to the annulus, we now frequently use continuous sutures rather than interrupted mattress sutures, as shown here.

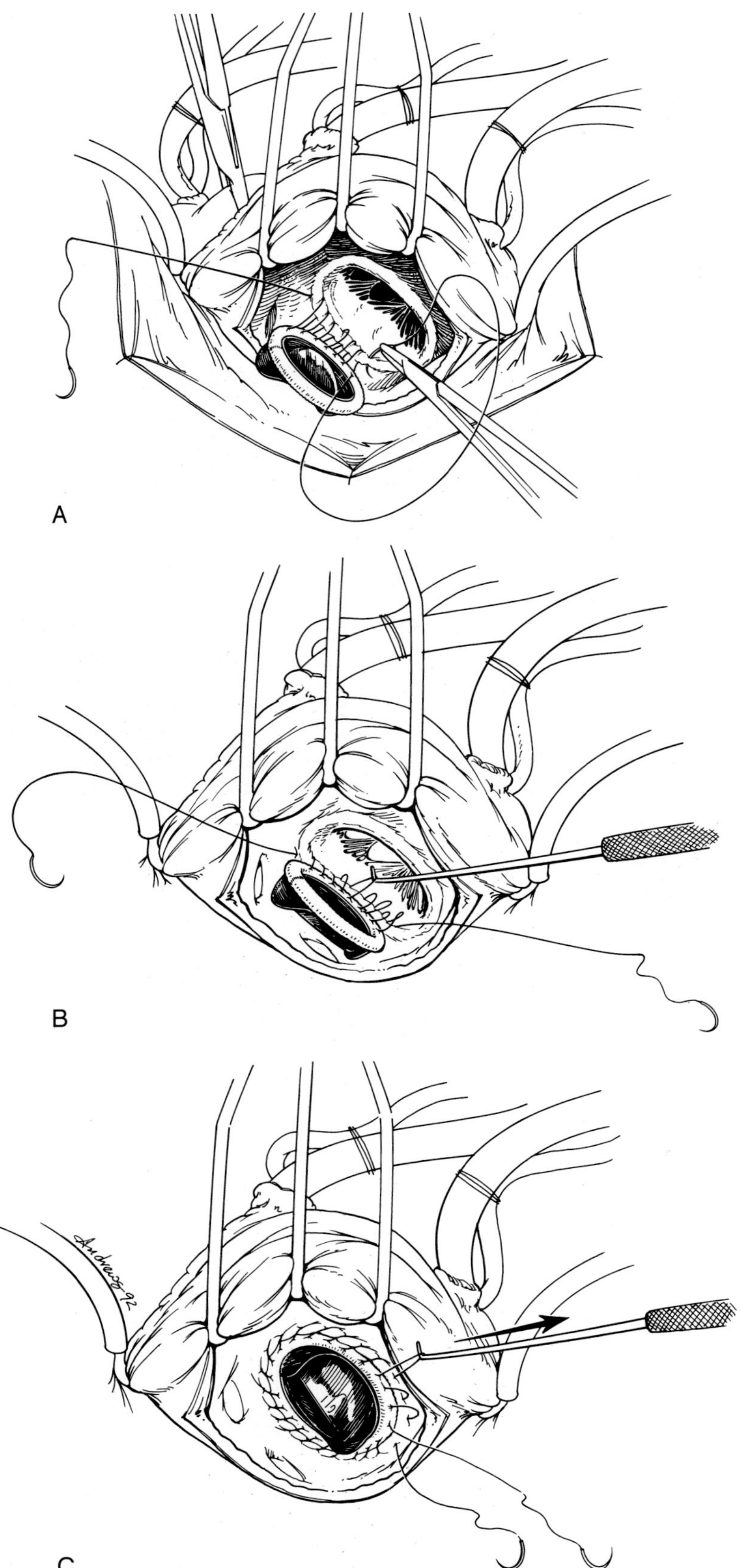

FIGURE 23–6 A–C, Mitral valve replacement with a continuous suture technique (see text). (**A–C,** From Cooley DA: Simplified techniques of valve replacement. J Cardiac Surg 7:357, 1992.)

valve replacement (see later). Because the annular tissue may be extremely fragile, the surgeon should take adequate tissue bites and avoid excessive suture tension. Once the valve has been secured in place, the atriotomy is repaired with a continuous 3-0 polypropylene suture.

Intravalvular Implantation

In patients with sound, flexible mitral leaflets and supple chordae, we sometimes use a technique known as in situ intravalvular implantation, particularly if the annular tissue is of poor quality.[8] To prevent obstruction of the valve prosthesis, we divide the anterior leaflet and insert it into the annulus. We then implant a low-profile prosthesis, affixing it to the valve leaflet and annulus with continuous sutures. In this manner, we are able to spare both the anterior and the posterior chordal and papillary mechanisms.

Aortic Valve Procedures

Although congenital aortic valve disease in children is often amenable to repair, the same cannot be said for acquired aortic valve disease. Therefore, in adults, operations for incompetent or stenotic aortic valves almost always entail valve replacement.

Once cardiac arrest has been instituted and most of the blood has been drained from the left side of the heart, the valve is exposed through an aortotomy. After assessing the extent of disease and determining the best operative strategy, the surgeon places a traction suture at each of the three commissural points to maximize exposure of the annulus (Figs. 23–7A and 23–8). The valve leaflets are removed, and the annulus is débrided. The surgeon should be particularly cautious in excising the leaflets of a calcified valve. If too much tissue is removed at the first cut, the annulus and sinus of Valsalva may be disrupted, resulting in uncontrollable hemorrhage and making valve implantation quite difficult. Before the residual calcium is débrided, a sponge is inserted into the left ventricle to trap any calcium fragments.

The valve is secured with a 60-inch-long 2-0 polypropylene monofilament suture. Usually, two thirds of the suture length is needed to fasten the sewing ring to the left and noncoronary cusps. When suturing the latter structure, the surgeon should be careful not to damage the bundle of His. The posterior suture line is completed first, beginning at the point farthest to the surgeon's left and advancing toward the surgeon. The anterior sutures are placed in a similar manner (see Fig. 23–7B). The sutures are then gathered onto three curved suture hooks (8.5-inch blunt curved suture hook [R7025]; Royal Surgical Instrument, Lewistown, IL), which are applied with their tips extending outward (see Fig. 23–7C). The prosthesis is eased into the annulus with the valve holder, which is then withdrawn.

The sutures are removed from the curved hooks one by one and are tightened sequentially (see Fig. 23–7D). When implantation is completed, the suture is tied at the commissure between the right and the noncoronary cusps (see Fig. 23–7E). The leaflets are opened to confirm proper valve placement and to detect any obstruction. The aortotomy is then closed with continuous 4-0 or 3-0 polypropylene sutures.

Tricuspid Valve Procedures

Acquired lesions of the tricuspid valve may be either primary or secondary. In managing tricuspid disease, the surgeon must weigh each case carefully and select the treatment plan that offers the best chance of long-term success. Functional tricuspid insufficiency, which sometimes accompanies mitral stenosis, usually resolves after correction of the mitral condition.

Primary Lesions

Primary tricuspid lesions include rheumatic valvulitis, bacterial endocarditis, and traumatic rupture. Stenosis or regurgitation caused by rheumatic valvulitis can be alleviated by an annuloplasty, a valvotomy, or a combination of these procedures. Alternatively, valve replacement can be performed.

When bacterial endocarditis results in advanced tricuspid valve destruction, as it frequently does in drug addicts, the surgeon is advised to perform a total valvectomy rather than to implant a foreign body or an artificial valve.[45] If the patient survives, she or he may then undergo elective valve replacement once the infectious process has resolved.

Traumatic disruption of the tricuspid valve can result from a closed, crushing chest injury. We have treated several automobile accident victims with papillary muscle disruption. Such cases always necessitate valve replacement or repair.[46]

Secondary Lesions

Secondary tricuspid lesions tend to be more common than primary ones. Secondary lesions arise when rheumatic valvulitis in the mitral (and perhaps also the aortic) position results in pulmonary hypertension and increased pulmonary vascular resistance, thereby straining the right ventricle and causing pulmonary and tricuspid valve insufficiency by secondary annular dilatation. Treatment of secondary lesions requires sound surgical judgment and expertise. If the leaflets are relatively normal, repair can be achieved by decreasing the overall circumference of the tricuspid annulus. However, if the leaflets are calcified or eroded because of infection or ruptured chordae tendineae, valve replacement may be necessary.

Final Steps in Valve Surgery

Once valve surgery is completed, the anesthesiologist exerts pressure on the lungs to eliminate most of the air from the left atrium and the pulmonary vein. Air in the ascending aorta is removed by suction, and a 19-gauge needle is used to aspirate air from the ventricular apex.

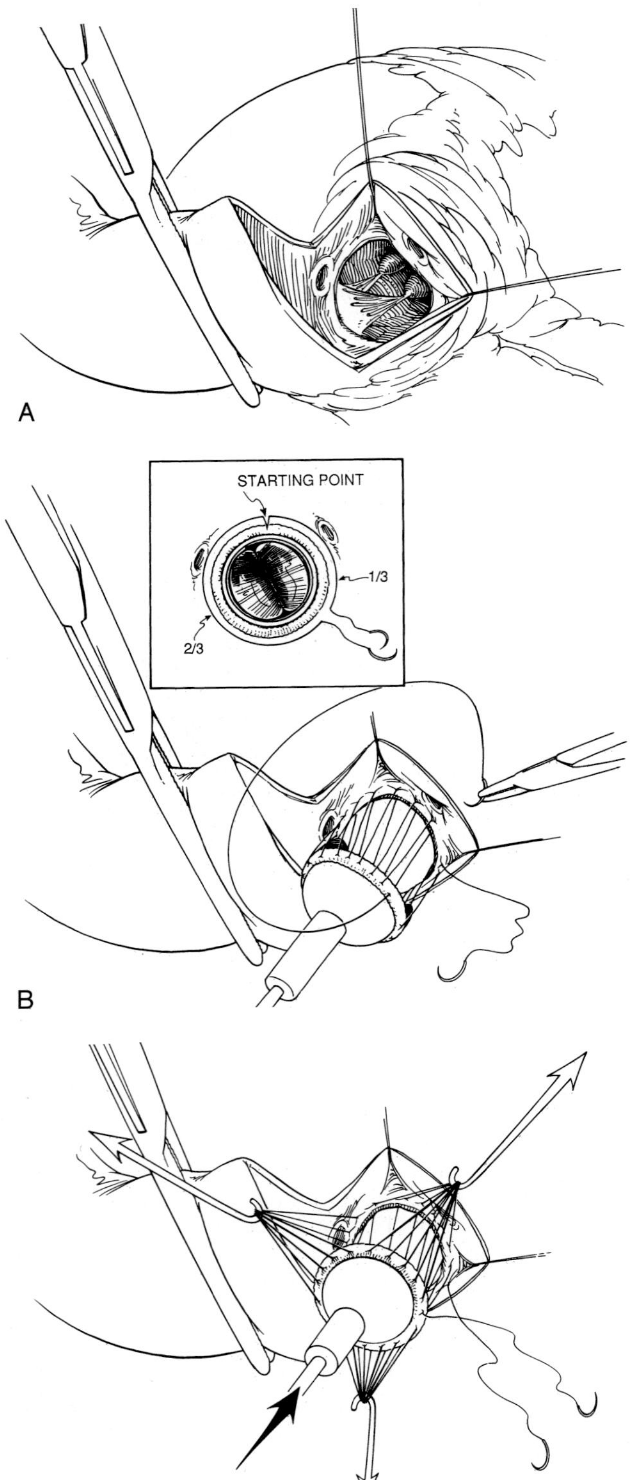

FIGURE 23–7 A–C, Aortic valve replacement with a continuous suture technique (see text). (**A–E,** From Cooley DA: Simplified techniques of valve replacement. J Cardiac Surg 7:357, 1992.)

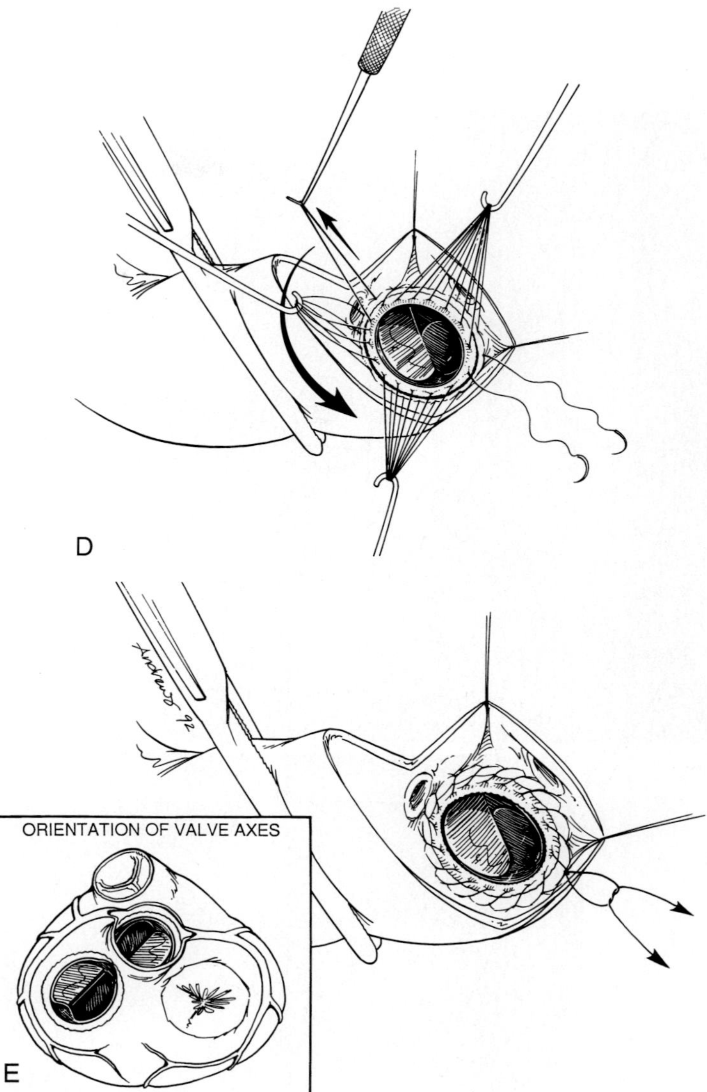

FIGURE 23–7D–E *Continued*

When the patient has been weaned from cardiopulmonary bypass, the aspirating needle is removed from the ascending aorta. The adventitia is carefully sutured so as not to penetrate the aortic lumen. The left atrial sump is withdrawn and the aortic cannula is removed. The cannulation site is reinforced with a pursestring suture, again only in the adventitia. The effect of heparin is reversed with protamine sulfate (in a 1:1 ratio), and the suture lines are carefully inspected for bleeding.

To decrease the need for transfusion, venous line blood remaining in the pump is returned to the patient before she or he leaves the operating room. Any additional blood is saved for retransfusion by means of cell-saver techniques.

If atrial fibrillation occurs, normal rhythm can be reinstituted with countershock. Most patients who undergo valve replacement receive temporary pacing electrodes to prevent heart block or other arrhythmias during the early postoperative period. The pacing wires are usually removed after 4 or 5 days. A mediastinal chest tube is inserted and left in place for 48 hours. Extrapericardial mediastinal tissue is placed over the aorta to prevent dense adhesions, which would make a future sternotomy difficult. The sternum is closed with evenly twisted heavy-gauge wires. Finally, nonabsorbable sutures are used to close the subcutaneous tissue in a single layer, with care not to entrap the sternal wires.

Postoperative Care

Optimal postoperative care depends on familiarity with the potential complications of valve surgery. The most feared threat is thromboembolism, which is mainly associated with mechanical prostheses. Patients with such devices in the mitral position should routinely take an anticoagulant such as sodium warfarin (Coumadin). Those with aortic prostheses should also undergo anticoagulation on a long-term basis. However, patients with low-profile valves such as the St. Jude or CarboMedics models can be kept at lower levels of anticoagulation, particularly if the valve is

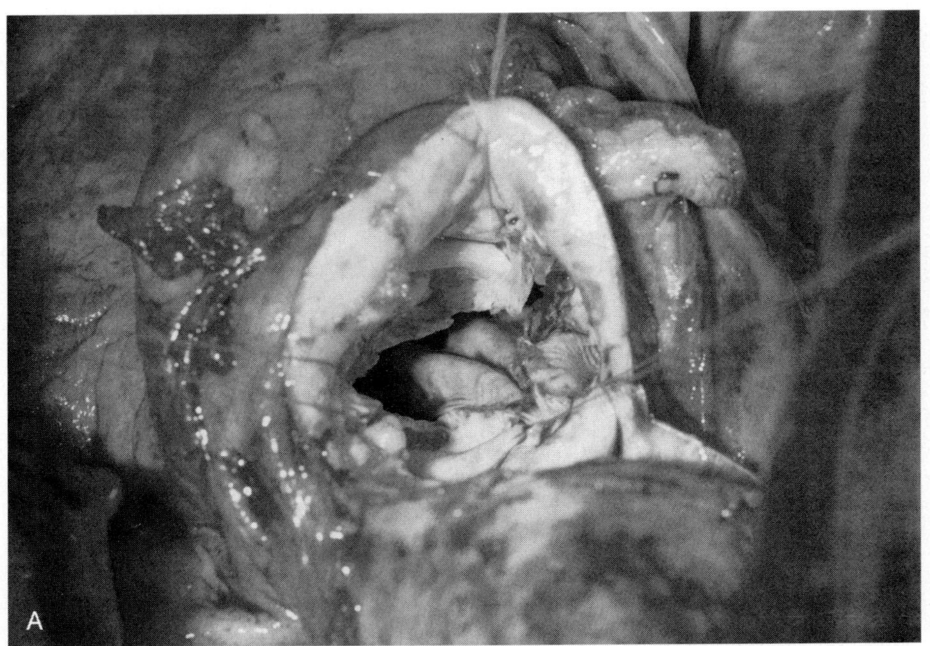

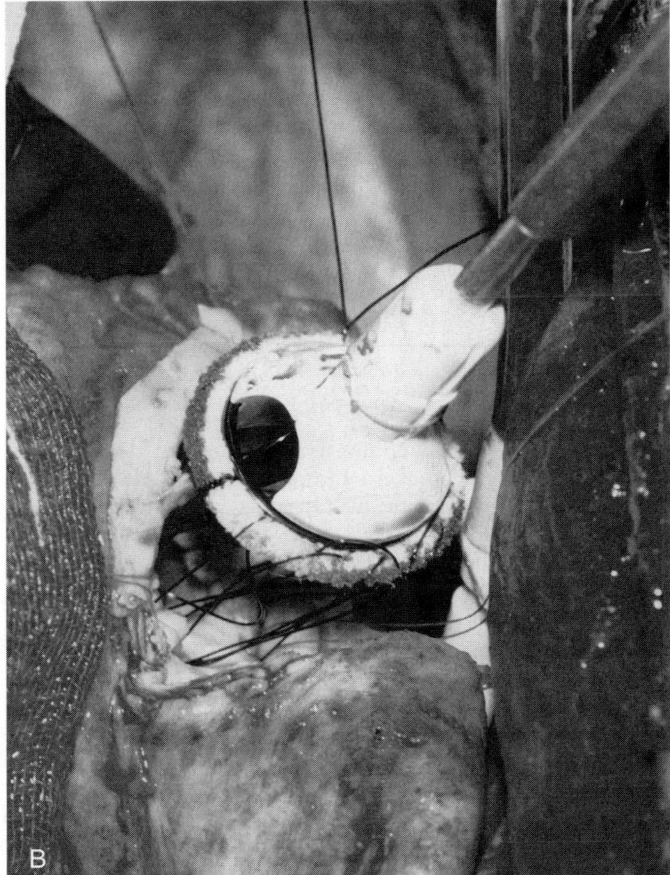

FIGURE 23–8 Aortic valve replacement in an 82-year-old man with aortic stenosis and coronary insufficiency. Exploration revealed an aortic valve with fused commissures and calcification in the aortic root. Some calcification was also noted in the ascending aorta. **A,** Traction sutures were placed at the commissures, and excision of the valve leaflets was begun. Care was taken to débride all loose calcium from the valve annulus as well as from the adjacent aorta. **B,** A 23-mm St. Jude mechanical prosthesis was sewn into the annulus with a single continuous 2-0 suture.

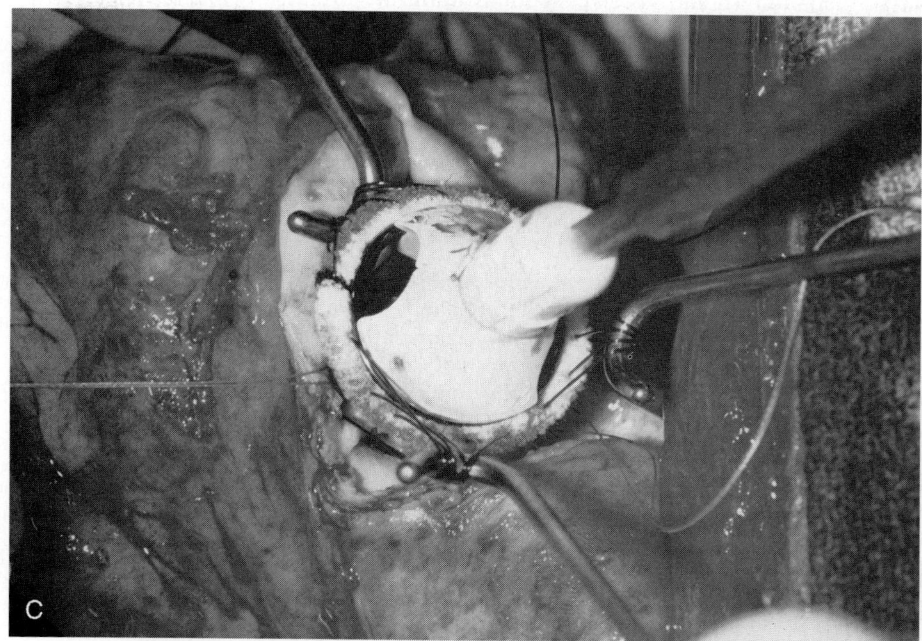

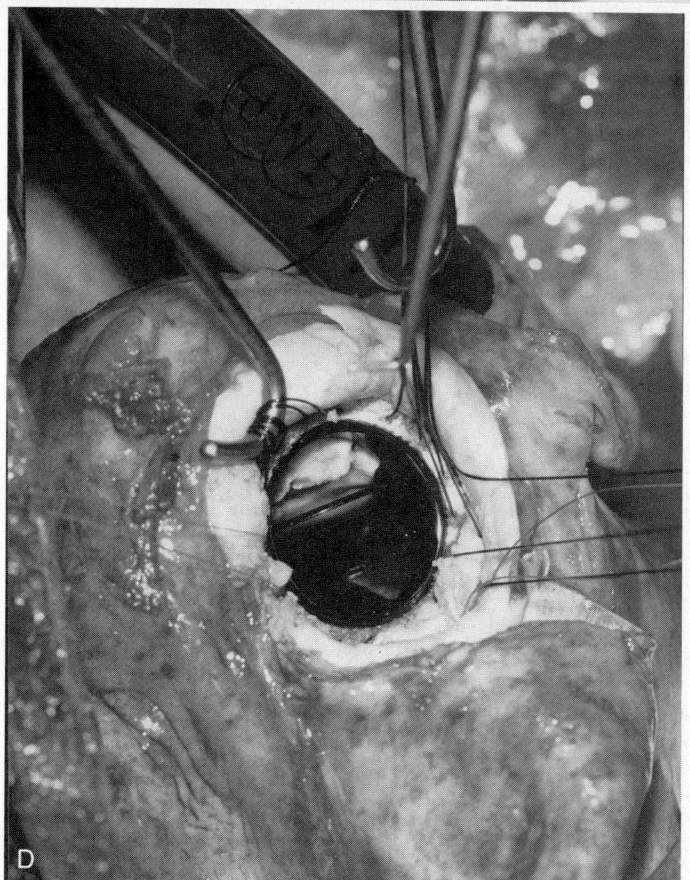

FIGURE 23–8C–D *Continued.* Once the continuous suture was in place **(C)**, it was tightened sequentially with three separate curved suture hooks and then tied **(D)**. The valve was noted to open fully and easily. After the aortotomy was repaired, a triple coronary artery bypass procedure was performed.

implanted in the aortic position. Although anticoagulants are not always prescribed for patients with bioprostheses, patients with chronic atrial fibrillation or extensive left atrial dilatation should receive sodium warfarin for an indefinite period.

Infection is a relatively rare complication of prosthetic valve implantation. In patients with valve prostheses, we routinely continue postoperative bactericidal antibiotic therapy until all invasive catheters have been removed. Subsequently, these patients should receive prophylactic antibiotics whenever they undergo dental procedures or operations on the lower genitourinary or gastrointestinal tract.

When bacterial endocarditis is diagnosed, a second operation may be necessary to replace the prosthetic valve. In such cases, we begin antibiotic therapy preoperatively to sterilize the blood stream, but we do not delay valve replacement, since we have found this operation to be successful even in the presence of active infection. Moreover, delay can be dangerous if it results in irreversible hemodynamic deterioration.

Valve dehiscence may occasionally result from infection, technical errors, or tissue failure. This complication can be alleviated by a repeat open cardiac procedure in which additional sutures are inserted to secure the valve.

Today's mechanical prostheses are extremely durable, and valve fracture or failure is quite uncommon. When such problems do arise, however, a repeat operation is mandatory.

CONCLUSION

Valve operations account for a large proportion of the caseload at most cardiac centers. Thanks to ongoing advances in prosthetic design and surgical technique, patients with valvular heart disease have an excellent chance to overcome their disability and enjoy a normal life. The foregoing guidelines will facilitate the management of these patients.

REFERENCES

1. Harken DE: Management of retained foreign bodies in the heart and great vessels, European Theater of Operations. pp. 393–395. *In* Surgery in World War II. Vol. 2. Thoracic Surgery. Washington, DC: Office of the Surgeon General, Department of the Army, 1965.
2. Harken DE, Ellis LB, Ware PF, Norman LR: The surgical treatment of mitral stenosis (mitral commissurotomy). Dis Chest 15:377, 1949.
3. Bailey CP: The surgical treatment of mitral stenosis. N Engl J Med 239:801, 1948.
4. Baker C, Brock RC, Campbell M: Valvulotomy for mitral stenosis: report of six successful cases. BMJ 1:1283, 1950.
5. Cooley DA: Current status of surgical treatment of acquired valvular heart disease. Tex Med 79:41, 1983.
6. Carmichael MJ, Cooley DA, Favor AS: Aortic and mitral valve replacement through a single transverse aortotomy: a useful approach in difficult mitral valve exposure. Tex Heart Inst J 10:415, 1983.
7. Cooley DA: Techniques in Cardiac Surgery. 2nd ed. pp. 201–214. Philadelphia: WB Saunders, 1984.
8. Cooley DA, Ingram MT: Intravalvular implantation of mitral valve prostheses. Tex Heart Inst J 14:188, 1987.
9. Cooley DA: Ventricular endoaneurysmorrhaphy: results of an improved method of repair. Tex Heart Inst J 16:72, 1989.
10. Murphy JP Jr, Sweeney MS, Cooley DA: The Puig-Massana-Shiley annuloplasty ring for mitral valve repair: experience in 126 patients. Ann Thorac Surg 43:52, 1987.
11. Cooley DA: Simplified techniques of valve replacement. J Cardiac Surg 7:357, 1992.
12. Frazier OH, Sweeney MS, Cooley DA: Valvular heart disease. *In* Willerson JT (ed): Treatment of Cardiovascular Disease. pp. 6.13–6.43. New York, Gower Medical, 1993.
13. Armstrong WF: Echocardiographic evaluation of valvular heart disease. ACC Curr J Rev 7:69, 1998.
14. Grimm RA, Stewart WJ: The role of intraoperative echocardiography in valve surgery. Cardiol Clin 16:477, 1998.
15. Falk V, Walther T, Diegeler A, et al: Echocardiographic monitoring of minimally invasive mitral valve surgery using an endoaortic clamp. J Heart Valve Dis 5:630, 1996.
16. Cohn LH, Adams DH, Couper GS, et al: Minimally invasive cardiac valve surgery improves patient satisfaction while reducing costs of cardiac valve replacement and repair. Ann Surg 226:421, 1997.
17. Svensson LG, D'Agostino RS: Minimal-access aortic and valvular operations, including the "J/j" incision. Ann Thorac Surg 66:431, 1998.
18. Cosgrove DM, Sabik JF: Minimally invasive approach for aortic operations. Ann Thorac Surg 62:596, 1996.
19. Aklog L, Adams DH, Couper GS, et al: Techniques and results of direct-access minimally invasive mitral valve surgery: a paradigm for the future. J Thorac Cardiovasc Surg 116:705, 1998.
20. Weinschelbaum E, Stutzbach P, Machain A, et al: Valve operations through a minimally invasive approach. Ann Thorac Surg 66:1106, 1998.
21. Letsou GV, Reardon MJ: Minimally invasive valve surgery. Curr Opin Cardiol 13:105, 1998.
22. Loulmet DF, Carpentier A, Cho PW, et al: Less invasive techniques for mitral valve surgery. J Thorac Cardiovasc Surg 115:772, 1998.
23. Cooley DA: Minimally invasive valve surgery versus the conventional approach. Ann Thorac Surg 66:1101, 1998.
24. Hammond GL, Franco KL: Mitral, tricuspid, and aortic valve repair or reconstruction. Curr Opin Cardiol 12:100, 1997.
25. Grossi EA, Galloway AC, Miller JS, et al: Valve repair versus replacement for mitral insufficiency: when is a mechanical valve still indicated? J Thorac Cardiovasc Surg 115:389, 1998.
26. Lawrie GM: Mitral valve repair vs replacement. Current recommendations and long-term results. Cardiol Clin 16:437, 1998.
27. Espada R, Westaby S: New developments in mitral valve repair. Curr Opin Cardiol 13:80, 1998.
28. Spencer FC, Galloway AC, Grossi EA, et al: Recent developments and evolving techniques of mitral valve reconstruction. Ann Thorac Surg 65:307, 1998.
29. Cooper HA, Gersh BJ: Treatment of chronic mitral regurgitation. Am Heart J 135:925, 1998.
30. Sweeney MS, Reul GJ, Cooley DA, et al: Comparison of bioprosthetic and mechanical valve replacement for active endocarditis. J Thorac Cardiovasc Surg 90:676, 1985.
31. Duncan JM, Cooley DA, Reul GJ, et al: Experience with the St. Jude Medical valve and the Ionescu-Shiley bovine pericardial valve at the Texas Heart Institute. pp. 233–245. *In* Matloff JM (ed): Cardiac Valve Replacement: Current Status. Boston, Martinus Nijhoff, 1985.
32. Remadi JP, Bizouarn P, Baron O, et al: Mitral valve replacement with the St. Jude Medical prosthesis: a 15-year follow-up. Ann Thorac Surg 66:762, 1998.
33. Stahlberg K, Mattila I, Heikkila L, et al: St. Jude versus CarboMedics: follow-up after prosthetic valve replacement. J Cardiovasc Surg 38:577, 1997.
34. Copeland JG: The CarboMedics prosthetic heart valve in the mitral position: results of the multicenter international trial. J Card Surg 12:205, 1997.
35. Bernal JM, Rabasa JM, Gutierrez-Garcia F, et al: The CarboMedics valve: experience with 1,049 implants. Ann Thorac Surg 65:137, 1998.
36. Jamieson WR, Munro AI, Miyagishima RT, et al: Multiple mechanical valve replacement surgery comparison of St. Jude Medical and CarboMedics prostheses. Eur J Cardiothorac Surg 13:151, 1998.
37. Doty DB, Acar C: Mitral valve replacement with homograft. Ann Thorac Surg 66:2127, 1998.
38. Staab ME, Nishimura RA, Dearani JA, Orszulak TA: Aortic valve homografts in adults: a clinical perspective. Mayo Clin Proc 73:231, 1998.

39. Dall'Agata A, Taams MA, Fioretti PM, et al: Cosgrove-Edwards mitral ring dynamics measured with transesophageal three-dimensional echocardiography. Ann Thorac Surg 65:485, 1998.
40. Cosgrove DM 3rd, Arcidi JM, Rodriguez L, et al: Initial experience with the Cosgrove-Edwards annuloplasty system. Ann Thorac Surg 60:499, 1995.
41. Hansen DE, Cahill PD, Derby GC, Miller DC: Relative contributions of the anterior and posterior mitral chordae tendineae to canine global left ventricular systolic function. J Thorac Cardiovasc Surg 93:45, 1987.
42. Westaby S: Preservation of left ventricular function in mitral valve surgery. Heart 75:326, 1996.
43. Aagaard J, Andersen UL, Lerbjerg G, et al: Mitral valve replacement with total preservation of native valve and subvalvular apparatus. J Heart Valve Dis 6:274, 1997.
44. Fontaine AA, He S, Stadter R, et al: In vitro assessment of prosthetic valve function in mitral valve replacement with chordal preservation techniques. J Heart Valve Dis 5:186, 1996.
45. Sethia B, Williams BT: Tricuspid valve excision without replacement in a case of endocarditis secondary to drug abuse. Br Heart J 40:579, 1978.
46. Sugita T, Watarida S, Katsuyama K, et al: Valve repair with chordal replacement for traumatic tricuspid regurgitation. J Heart Valve Dis 6:651, 1997.

SECTION IV

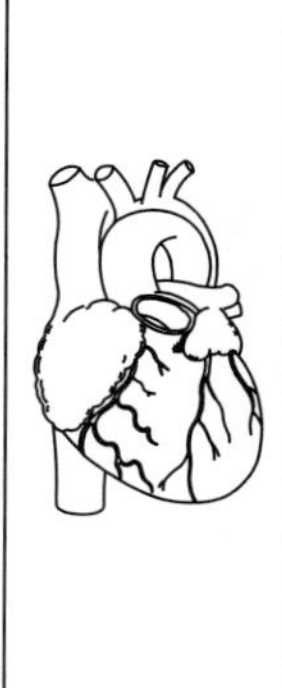

CORONARY ARTERY DISEASE

Anatomic Abnormalities and Pathogenesis

Regulation of Coronary Blood Flow

Pathophysiology and Clinical Recognition of Coronary Artery Disease Syndromes

Silent Ischemia

Coronary Artery Disease in Women

Exercise Testing

Coronary Angiography

Echocardiography

Nuclear Imaging in Coronary Artery Disease

Natural History

Medical Treatment of Stable Angina

Medical Treatment of Unstable Angina and Non–Q Wave Myocardial Infarction

Medical Treatment of Acute Q Wave Myocardial Infarction

Percutaneous Coronary Interventions for Stable Angina Pectoris

Percutaneous Coronary Intervention for Unstable Coronary Artery Disease

Percutaneous Coronary Intervention for Acute Myocardial Infarction

Radiation Therapy

Surgical Treatment

Coronary Artery Bypass Graft Surgery and Percutaneous Coronary Intervention: Impact on Morbidity and Mortality in Patients With Coronary Artery Disease

Cardiac Rehabilitation

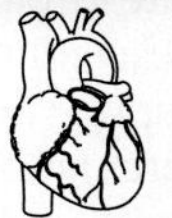

CHAPTER 24

Anatomic Abnormalities and Pathogenesis

L. Maximilian Buja and Hugh A. McAllister, Jr.

THE CORONARY CIRCULATION
CORONARY ATHEROSCLEROSIS
CORONARY THROMBOSIS AND OTHER ACUTE CORONARY LESIONS
NONATHEROSCLEROTIC CORONARY VASCULAR DISEASES
PATHOLOGY OF ANGINA PECTORIS AND SUDDEN CARDIAC DEATH
PATHOLOGY OF ACUTE MYOCARDIAL INFARCTION
BASIC BIOLOGY OF MYOCARDIAL ISCHEMIC INJURY
DETERMINANTS OF INFARCT DEVELOPMENT AND SIZE
REPERFUSION, PRECONDITIONING, STUNNING, AND HIBERNATION
PATHOLOGY OF INTERVENTIONALLY TREATED CORONARY ARTERY DISEASE
NEW APPROACHES TO MYOCARDIAL MODULATION

The clinical manifestations of coronary artery disease (CAD), also known as ischemic heart disease, are diverse, with a spectrum that encompasses various forms of angina pectoris, myocardial infarction (MI), sudden cardiac death, and chronic CAD. These syndromes result from complex interactions between the coronary circulation and the myocardium, usually with coronary atherosclerosis as a major factor.[1–3]

The Coronary Circulation

Blood is normally supplied to the heart via the left and right coronary arteries, which originate via their ostia from the left and right aortic sinuses of Valsalva, located just distal to the aortic valve (Fig. 24–1).[1–3] The short left coronary artery divides into left anterior descending and left circumflex branches and, occasionally, a left marginal branch. The anterior portion of the left ventricle (LV) and the interventricular septum are supplied by the left anterior descending coronary artery and its left diagonal and septal branches. The lateral LV is supplied by the left circumflex coronary artery and its circumflex marginal branches. The right coronary artery supplies the right ventricle (RV), and in about 90 percent of hearts, it extends posteriorly to give rise to the posterior-descending coronary artery.

There is considerable variation in the anatomic distribution of the coronary arterial branches. However, in most hearts, branches of the left circumflex and right coronary arteries contribute to the blood supply of the posterior LV, creating a "balanced circulation." In about 10 percent of hearts, the right coronary artery is diminutive, and the

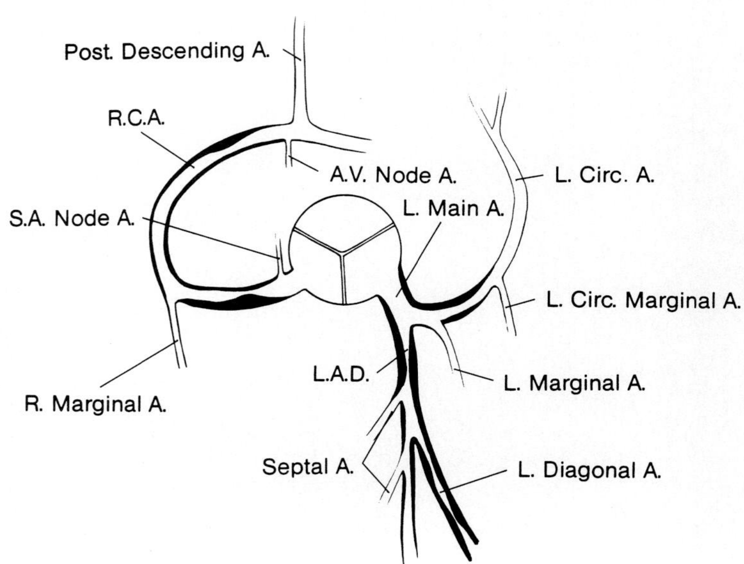

FIGURE 24–1 Diagram of the usual anatomic distribution of the coronary arteries, shows a typical distribution of atherosclerotic plaque (dark areas). A., artery; Circ., circumflex; Post. posterior; S.A., sinoatrial; R., right; L., left; A.V. atrioventricular; L.A.D., left anterior descending coronary artery; R.C.A., right coronary artery. (From Willerson JT, Hillis LD, Buja LM: Ischemic Heart Disease: Clinical and Pathophysiological Aspects. New York: Raven, 1982.)

left circumflex coronary artery gives rise to the posterior descending coronary artery and provides the sole blood supply for the posterior LV, creating a "left dominant circulation." Rarely, the converse "right dominant circulation" is formed when the left circumflex artery is diminutive and the posterior LV is supplied primarily via left ventricular branches of the right coronary artery.

With regard to the conduction system, the artery to the sinoatrial node arises from the proximal right coronary artery in about 60 percent of hearts and from the left circumflex coronary artery in about 40 percent of hearts. The major atrioventricular nodal artery takes origin from the coronary artery that gives rise to the posterior descending branch and therefore originates from the right coronary artery in about 90 percent of hearts and from the left circumflex coronary artery in about 10 percent of hearts.

The epicardial coronary arteries deliver oxygenated blood to the myocardial arteries, arterioles, and capillaries. After oxygen and substrate extraction in the myocardium, a small amount of unoxygenated blood flows directly into the ventricular cavities via the thebesian veins. Most blood, however, returns via myocardial venules and veins into the epicardial veins, which drain into the coronary sinus located in the inferoposterior region of the right atrium.

Normal embryologic development of the coronary circulation includes the formation of collateral vessels, which connect different components of the coronary arterial circulation.[1, 2] The coronary collateral system is composed of four types of vessels: intramural branches of the same coronary artery (homocoronary collateral vessels), intramural branches of two or more coronary arteries (intercoronary collateral vessels), atrial branches that connect with the vasa vasorum of the aorta and other vessels (extracardiac collateral vessels), and intramural branches that communicate with the cardiac cavities (arterioluminal vessels).[3] In the normal adult heart, the collateral vessels are small, thin-walled channels, usually less than 50 μm in diameter, that contribute little to total coronary blood flow. In response to coronary arterial narrowing and myocardial ischemia, myocardial collateral vessels can increase in diameter to 200 to 600 μm or greater, develop muscular media, and transport a significant proportion of blood flow.[4] In addition to the collateral vessels described previously, collateral channels develop between segments of a coronary artery proximal and distal to a stenosis.[3, 4]

CORONARY ATHEROSCLEROSIS

The major cause of CAD is coronary atherosclerosis (arteriosclerosis), a process that develops as a response of the vessel wall to chronic, multifactorial injury and leads to the formation of atherosclerotic plaques (fibrous plaques, atheromas).[5–7] These plaques are regions of thickened intima that are composed of varying mixtures of fibrous tissue, cells, and lipid (Fig. 24–2).[8–10]

Initially, atherosclerosis is a focal disease. There is a predilection for the formation of atherosclerotic plaques adjacent to branch points in areas of low-velocity flow and low shear stress adjacent to areas of high shear stress.[11, 12] It is postulated that the flow patterns in such regions promote endothelial dysfunction and increased contact of endothelium with monocytes and platelets. Areas of predilection for severe atherosclerosis in the coronary system include the proximal left anterior descending coronary artery and the proximal and distal right coronary arteries (see Fig. 24–1). Established atherosclerosis involves all three layers of the arterial wall such that in addition to intimal thickening, diseased areas exhibit medial degeneration and weakening and intimal fibrosis, with lymphocytic inflammatory infiltrates.

Atherosclerotic disease leads to extensive remodeling of

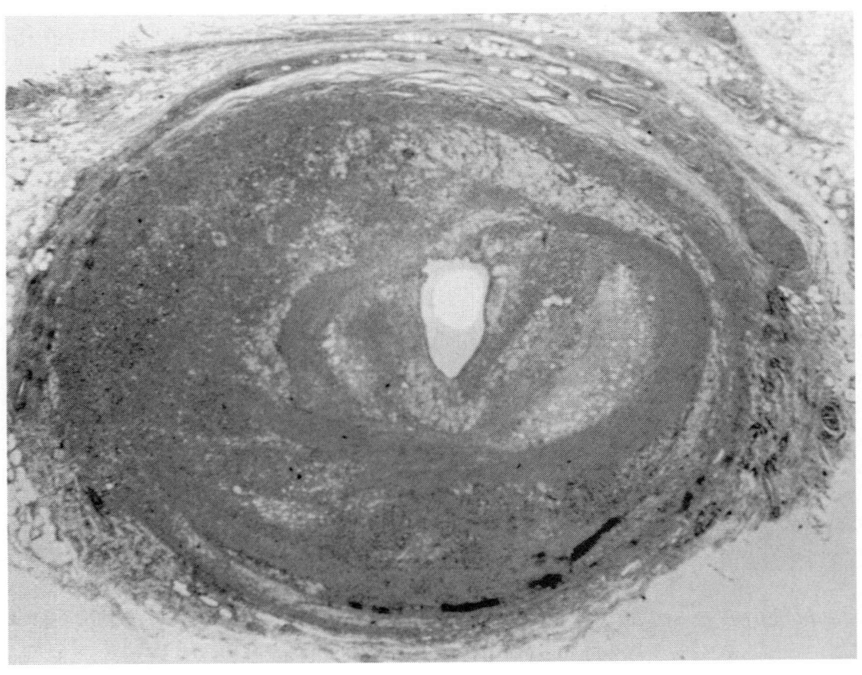

FIGURE 24–2 Left main coronary artery from a 6-year-old girl with homozygous familial hypercholesterolemia. The artery is severely involved with atherosclerotic plaque. The plaque is composed of fibrous tissue (dark areas) and foam cells and lipid (light areas). (H&E, ×16.) (From Buja LM, Clubb FJ Jr, Bilheimer DW, et al: Pathobiology of human familial hypercholesterolemia and a related animal model, the Watanabe heritable hyperlipidaemic model. Eur Heart J 11[suppl E]:41–52, 1990.)

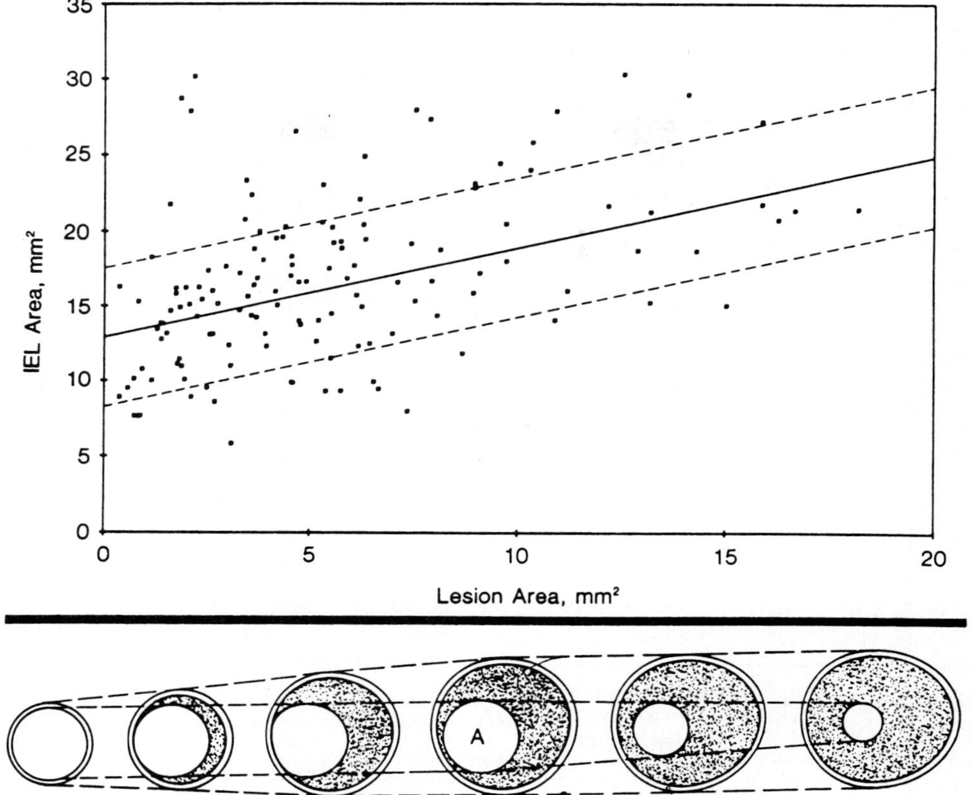

FIGURE 24–3 Compensatory enlargement of human coronary arteries in relation to plaque formation. In graph, the area encompassed by internal elastic lamina (IEL Area) is plotted against lesion area for sections of the left main coronary artery from 136 adult hearts obtained postmortem. The IEL area is potential luminal area if no plaque is present. The IEL area progressively increases as lesion area increases in a linear manner ($r = .44$; $P < .001$; standard error of 4.8 mm² indicated by the *dotted lines* above and below regression line). Below the graph is a diagrammatic representation of the sequence of changes in atherosclerotic arteries, which may eventually lead to luminal narrowing. Arteries initially enlarge, preserving nearly normal luminal cross section, but it appears that normal luminal area may not be maintained once the lesion occupies more than 40 percent of the IEL area (A). (From Glagov S, Zarins C, Giddens DP, et al: Hemodynamics and atherosclerosis: insights and perspectives gained from studies of human arteries. Arch Pathol Lab Med 112:1018–1031, 1988. Copyright 1988, American Medical Association).

the vessel wall. Dilatation of the vessel occurs in such a way that the lumen is maintained despite the presence of intimal plaque, which may develop in an eccentric or a concentric pattern (Fig. 24–3).[11, 12] Luminal narrowing occurs only when atherosclerotic disease is advanced. Approximately 50 percent narrowing of luminal diameter (75 percent luminal area) must occur before blood flow is affected. Areas of severe narrowing often develop in the setting of multifocal disease. All of these changes can lead to an underestimation of the extent and severity of coronary atherosclerosis on visual inspection of coronary arteriograms (*luminograms*) (Fig. 24–4).[13] Quantitative coronary arteriography can provide more objective measurements of absolute coronary dimensions and flow.

Coronary Thrombosis and Other Acute Coronary Lesions

Acute CAD is often initiated by acute changes superimposed on atherosclerotic plaques (Fig. 24–5).[14–16] The spectrum of thrombotic lesions includes platelet aggregates, mural (nonocclusive) thrombi, and occlusive thrombi (Plates 24–1 and 24–2).[17–26] Major thrombi are frequently associated with significant disruptions in the plaque surface, which may appear as fissures, erosion, ulceration, or rupture (Figs. 24–6 to 24–8; Plate 24–3). Coronary lesions that are particularly susceptible to such changes are atheromatous plaques with thin fibrous capsules and large cores of lipid-rich debris. Factors that probably contribute to endothelial injury and disruption of the plaque surface include hemodynamic trauma, local attachment and activation of platelets and blood cells, inflammatory processes in the plaques, and cytotoxic effects of plaque contents, possibly including enzyme release from mononuclear cells that often are present at the sites of plaque rupture.[14–26] The likely pathogenetic sequence of plaque rupture is endothelial injury, influx of blood components, increase in intraplaque pressure, and outward rupture of the fibrous capsule (see Figs. 24–6 and 24–7).[19, 23] Plaque fissuring is a more discrete process (see Fig. 24–8).[23, 24] There is evidence of a higher incidence of plaque rupture in men dying suddenly during exertion than in men dying suddenly at rest.[26] Furthermore, plaque rupture with exertion is characterized by a relatively thin fibrous capsule, relatively nu-

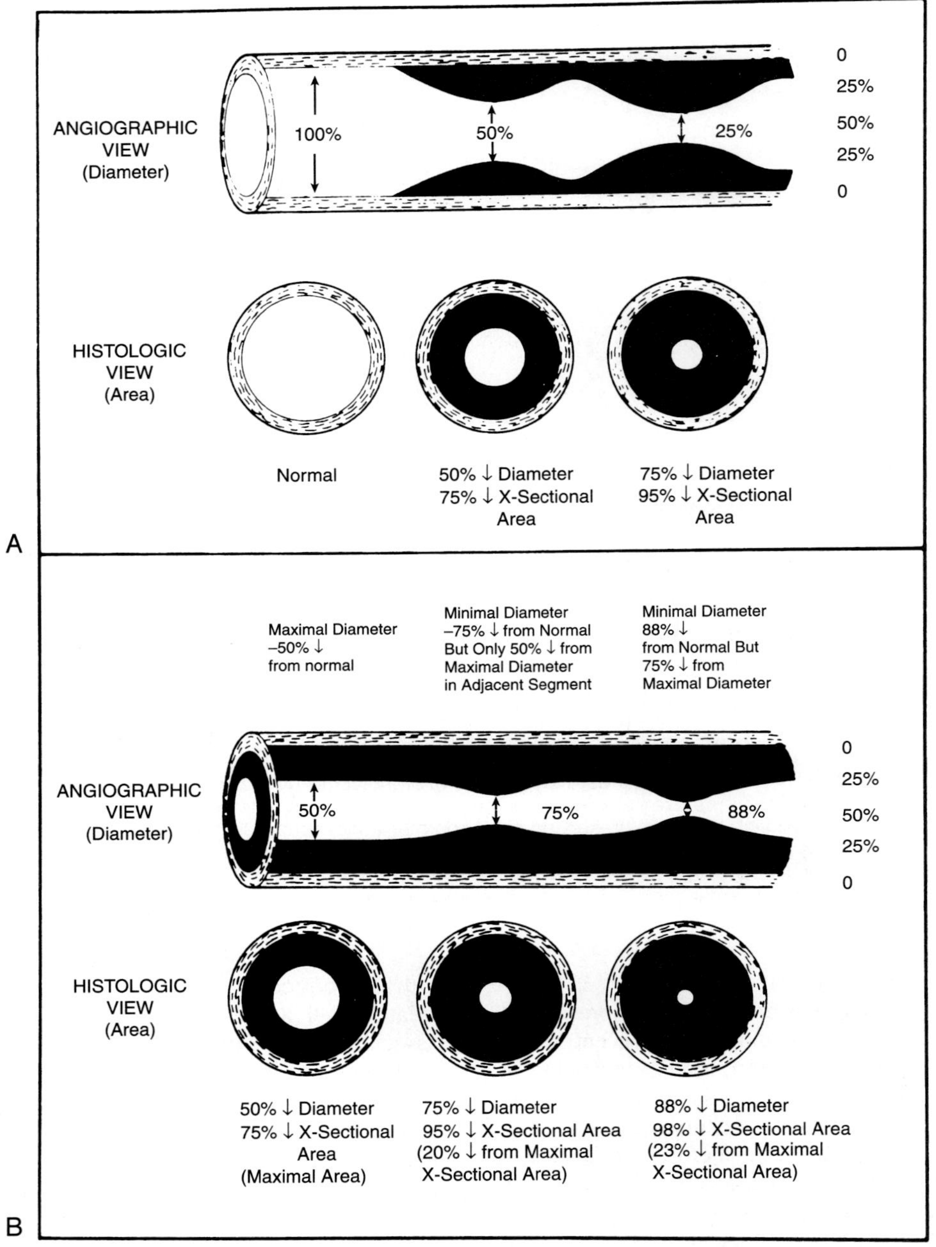

FIGURE 24–4 Relationship between reduction in diameter (as seen with selective coronary arteriography) and cross-sectional area (as seen with histologic examination). **A,** A coronary artery with a 50 percent reduction in diameter narrowing has a 75 percent diminution in cross-sectional area, and a coronary artery with a 75 percent reduction in diameter narrowing has a 95 percent reduction in cross-sectional area. **B,** In many patients who undergo coronary arteriography, stenosed segments are not compared with totally normal segments but rather with segments of the coronary artery that are somewhat narrowed diffusely. Thus, if the least-narrowed segment actually is 50 percent narrowed, what appears to be a 50 percent diameter narrowing in an adjacent segment is in fact a 75 percent diameter narrowing and therefore a 95 percent cross-sectional area reduction. Similarly, what appears to be a 75 percent diameter narrowing is in fact an 88 percent diameter narrowing, which in turn is a 98 percent cross-sectional diameter narrowing. Because many patients with coronary artery disease have diffuse luminal narrowings in addition to discrete stenoses, **B** more accurately reflects the true clinical situation in such cases. (**A** and **B,** From Arnett EN, Isner JM, Redwood DR, et al: Coronary artery narrowing in coronary heart disease: comparison of cineangiographic and necropsy findings. Ann Intern Med 91:350–356, 1979.)

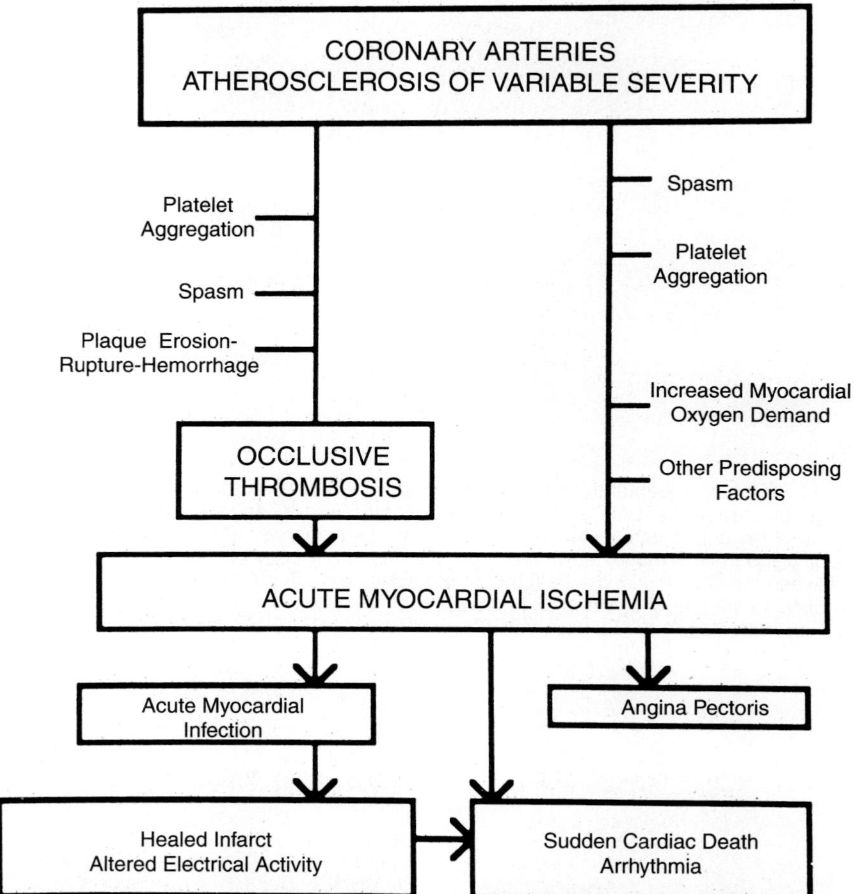

FIGURE 24–5 Pathogenetic mechanisms of acute ischemic heart disease and potential clinical outcomes. (Adapted from Buja LM, Hillis LD, Petty CS, et al: The role of coronary arterial spasm in ischemic heart disease. Arch Pathol Lab Med 105:221–226, 1981. Copyright 1981, American Medical Association.)

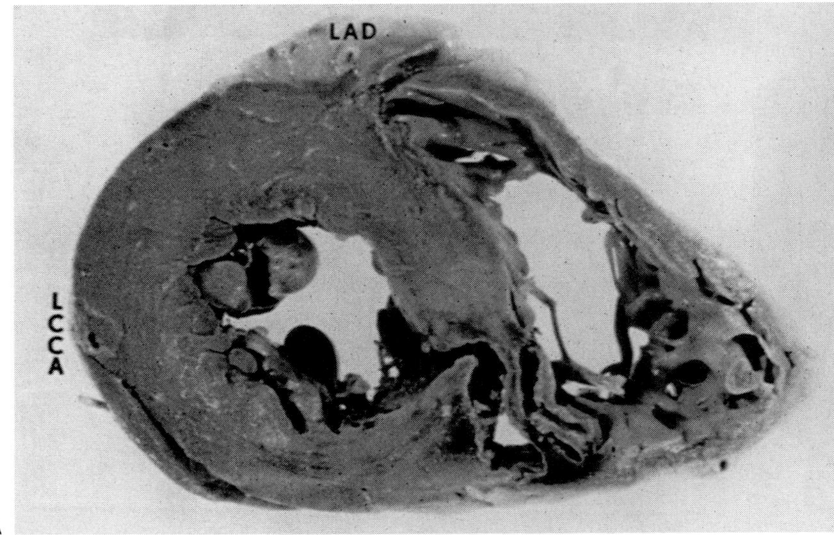

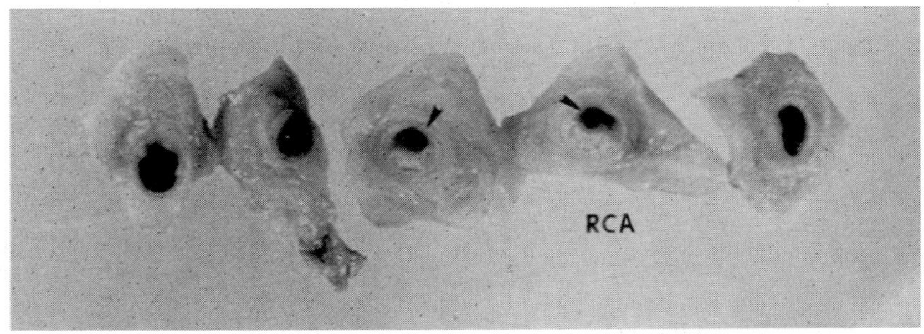

FIGURE 24–6 Two-day-old inferoposteroseptal transmural myocardial infarct with ventricular septal rupture in a 51-year-old woman. **A,** The left anterior descending coronary artery (LAD) shows moderate atherosclerosis, and the left circumflex coronary artery (LCCA) is free of disease. **B,** At the site of the only severely stenotic plaque in the right coronary artery (RCA), there is an occlusive thrombus adjacent to an area of major plaque hemorrhage. *Arrows* indicate a plane of demarcation formed by a thin strand of attenuated and eroded plaque capsule between the centrally located thrombus and the peripheral plaque hemorrhage. Thrombus is also located immediately proximal and distal to the plaque. (**A** and **B,** From Buja LM, Willerson JT: Clinicopathological correlates of acute ischemic heart disease syndromes. Reprinted from Am J Cardiol, Vol. 47, pp. 343–356, Copyright 1981, with permission from Excerpta Medica Inc.)

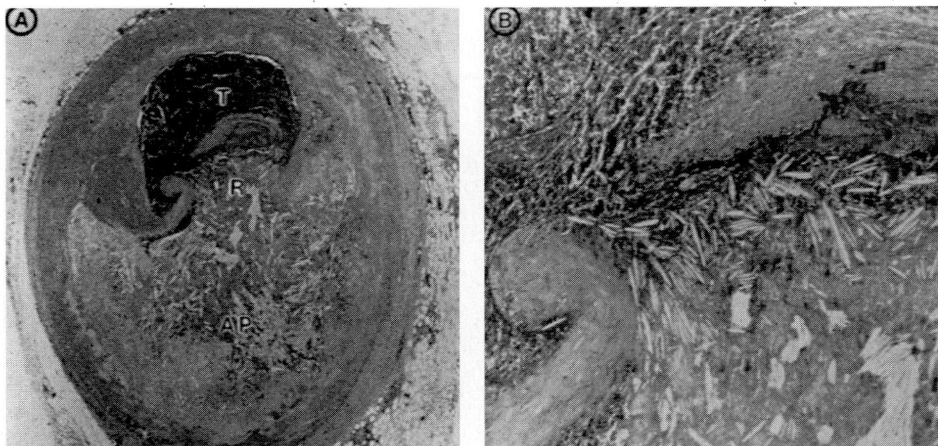

FIGURE 24–7 Histopathologic features of a coronary occlusion with plaque rupture, hemorrhage, and thrombosis. **A,** The atherosclerotic plaque (AP) shows rupture of the capsule (R), outward displacement of plaque contents across the rupture site, and communication with the overlying thrombus (T). (H&E, ×13.5.) **B,** Higher magnification of the site of plaque rupture shows continuity between thrombus and atheromatous material of the plaque core. Note the abundant cholesterol crystals in the atheromatous material. (H&E, ×57.) (**A** and **B,** From Buja LM, Willerson JT: Clinicopathologic correlates of acute ischemic heart disease syndromes. Reprinted from Am J Cardiol, Vol. 47, pp. 343–356, Copyright 1981, with permission from Excerpta Medica Inc.)

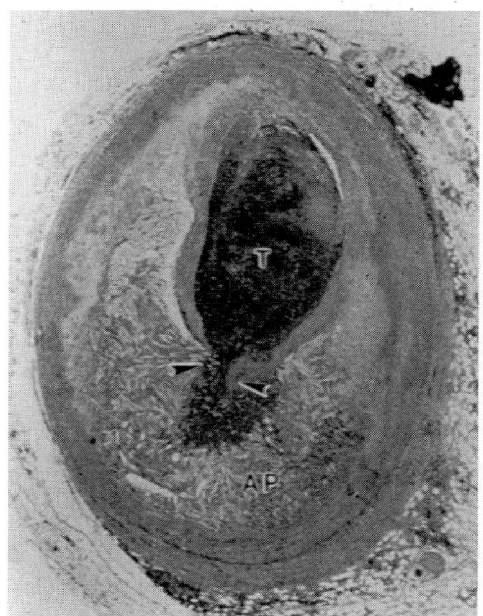

FIGURE 24–8 Coronary artery from a patient with an acute myocardial infarct is occluded by a thrombus (T) superimposed on an atherosclerotic plaque (AP), which exhibits a fissure in the capsule (*arrowheads*) and hemorrhage (dark material) at the fissure site. (H&E ×10.) (From Buja LM, Willerson JT, Murphree SS: Pathobiology of arterial wall injury, atherosclerosis, and coronary angioplasty. *In* Black AJR, Anderson HV, Ellis SG [eds]: Complications of Coronary Angioplasty. New York: Marcel Dekker, 1991, by courtesy of Marcel Dekker, Inc.)

merous vasa vasorum, and rupture in the midcap, whereas plaque rupture at rest tends to occur at the shoulder region of the fibrous cap.[26] Disruption of the plaque surface via any mechanism predisposes to the formation of intraluminal and intramural (intraplaque) thrombi. Plaque hemorrhage may occur with or without thrombus. Two mechanisms of intraplaque hemorrhage are influx of blood across the damaged endothelial surface of the plaque and influx of blood from small intraplaque vessels derived from the vasa vasorum.

Little information is available regarding the anatomic correlates of coronary spasm.[14] Spasm is usually associated with atherosclerotic lesions but, in some cases, occurs without angiographically evident disease.[27, 28] In isolated cases, transverse ridges in the coronary artery[29] and increased numbers of adventitial mast cells have been reported in association with coronary spasm.[30] Prominent adventitial inflammation has been found to be more prevalent in coronary arteries of patients with a recent history of unstable angina pectoris at rest than in control subjects, further suggesting a role for inflammatory mediators in the pathophysiology of coronary spasm.[31]

NONATHEROSCLEROTIC CORONARY VASCULAR DISEASES

In a small number of cases of CAD, the coronary arteries are free of atherosclerosis and the clinical disease is related to some other condition. There is an interesting spectrum of nonatherosclerotic causes of CAD, including congenital anomalies, dissection (Fig. 24–9; Plates 24–4 and 24–5), emboli, vasculitis (Figs. 24–10 and 24–11), and other conditions of the coronary arteries (Table 24–1).[32, 33] Cocaine use can precipitate acute myocardial ischemia and MI as a result of coronary spasm, thrombosis, or both.[34, 35]

PATHOLOGY OF ANGINA PECTORIS AND SUDDEN CARDIAC DEATH

The usual pathologic correlate of angina pectoris is coronary atherosclerosis with significant luminal narrowing of one or more of the major coronary arteries.[1, 14–16, 22] However, there is considerable variation in the anatomic extent of large vessel CAD associated with the development of symptomatic CAD. The variability is influenced by a number of interrelated factors, including the rate of progression of large vessel disease and the development of the coronary collateral circulation. Depending on the extent of coronary collateral blood flow, coronary occlusion may lead to major MI or to little or no myocardial damage.

Unstable angina pectoris and related syndromes (prein-

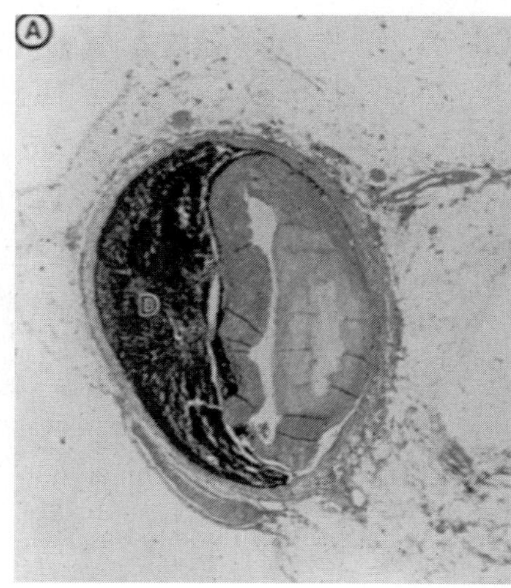

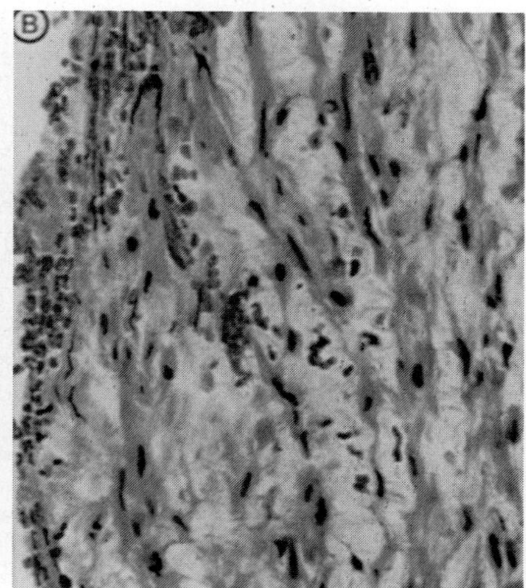

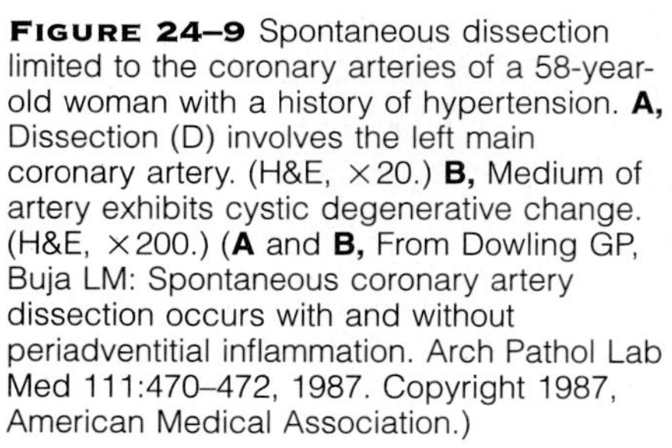
FIGURE 24–9 Spontaneous dissection limited to the coronary arteries of a 58-year-old woman with a history of hypertension. **A,** Dissection (D) involves the left main coronary artery. (H&E, ×20.) **B,** Medium of artery exhibits cystic degenerative change. (H&E, ×200.) (**A** and **B,** From Dowling GP, Buja LM: Spontaneous coronary artery dissection occurs with and without periadventitial inflammation. Arch Pathol Lab Med 111:470–472, 1987. Copyright 1987, American Medical Association.)

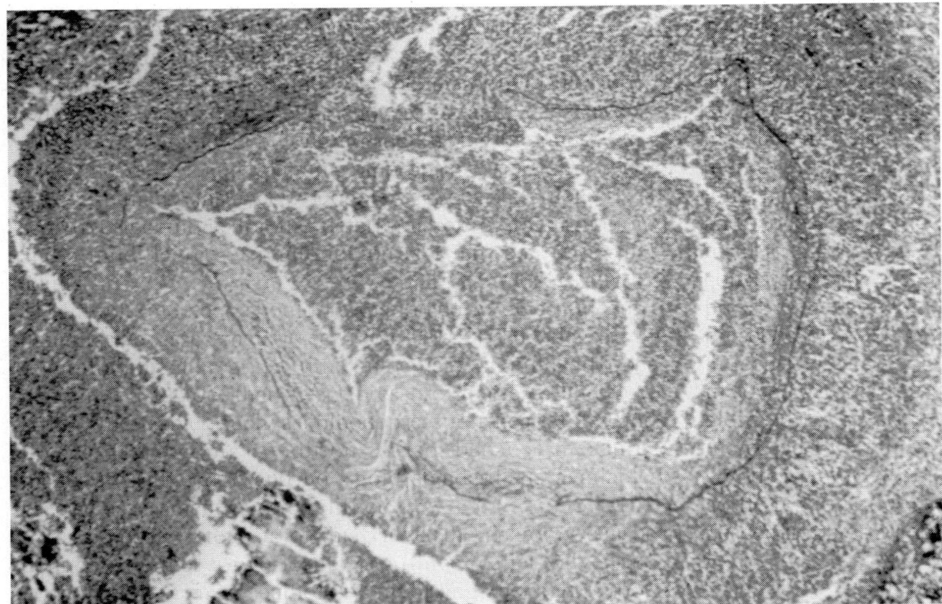

FIGURE 24–10 Mycotic aneurysm of the coronary artery in a patient with infective endocarditis of the aortic valve. Septic embolus has lodged in the coronary artery and led to necrotizing vasculitis with massive accumulation of neutrophils and destruction of the arterial wall. (Trichrome stain, ×60.)

farction angina, coronary insufficiency) are associated with a high incidence of acute alterations of plaques (*unstable plaques*) with superimposed thrombotic lesions, usually platelet aggregates or nonocclusive thrombi, as well as platelet aggregates in the microcirculation of the myocardium.[1, 14–16, 22, 36, 37] The accumulation of mononuclear cells at sites of unstable plaques, suggesting an inflammatory component to these vascular lesions, has also been demonstrated.[25]

Coronary atherosclerosis is the most frequent anatomic substrate of sudden cardiac death.[38, 39] In large series, approximately 90 percent of patients exhibit significant atherosclerotic narrowing of at least one coronary artery.[40–43] Many of the patients also show evidence of previous myocardial injury, manifest as multifocal myocardial scarring, healed infarction, or both. Most cases do not exhibit an anatomically demonstrable acute MI. There is considerable variability in the reported incidence of acute plaque alterations and thrombotic lesions[39–45]; however, evidence of coronary plaque disruption and thrombosis has been documented in a significant subset of patients, particularly those with a prior history of unstable angina pectoris.[42–45] Such patients also frequently show evidence of platelet aggregation in the coronary microcirculation.[36, 37]

Women and men exhibit differences regarding sudden cardiac death.[26, 44–47] Sudden cardiac death occurs more frequently in men than in women. Differences in coronary lesions have been observed, with superficial plaque erosion

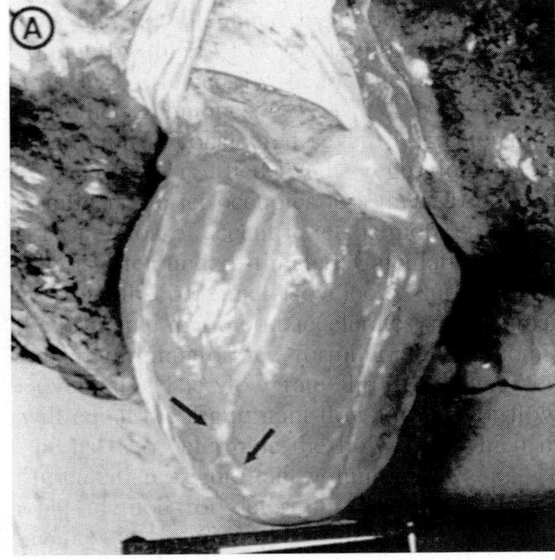

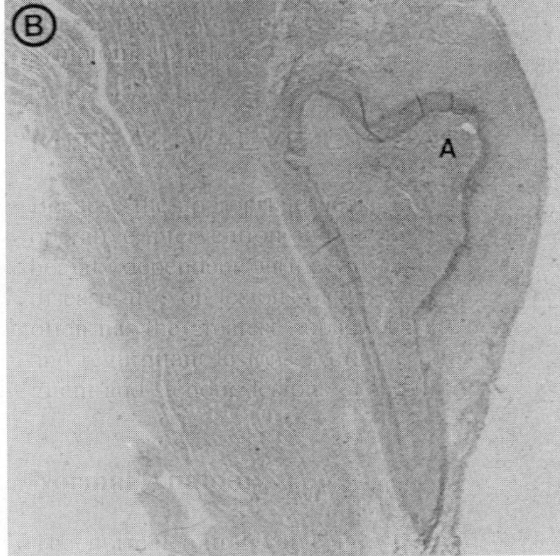

FIGURE 24–11 Polyarteritis nodosa involving the coronary arteries. **A,** Posterior view of the heart reveals numerous nodular (nodose) lesions (*arrows*) of the coronary arteries. **B,** The nodose lesions correspond to microaneurysms (A) of the coronary arteries, which result from inflammatory destruction of the arterial wall. (H&E, low magnification.)

TABLE 24–1 Causes of Myocardial Ischemia and Infarction Without Coronary Atherosclerosis

Coronary Artery Disease Other Than Atherosclerosis

Arteritis
- Luetic
- Granulomatous (Takayasu's disease)
- Polyarteritis nodosa
- Mucocutaneous lymph node (Kawasaki's) syndrome
- Disseminated lupus erythematosus
- Rheumatoid arthritis
- Ankylosing spondylitis

Trauma to coronary arteries
- Laceration
- Thrombosis
- Iatrogenic

Coronary mural thickening with metabolic diseases or intimal proliferative disease
- Mucopolysaccharidoses (Hurler's disease)
- Homocystinuria
- Fabry's disease
- Amyloidosis
- Juvenile intimal sclerosis (idiopathic arterial calcification of infancy)
- Intimal hyperplasia associated with contraceptive steroids or with the postpartum period
- Pseudoxanthoma elasticum
- Coronary fibrosis caused by radiation therapy

Luminal narrowing by other mechanisms
- Spasm of coronary arteries (Prinzmetal's angina with normal coronary arteries)
- Spasm after nitroglycerin withdrawal
- Dissection of the aorta
- Dissection of the coronary artery

Emboli to Coronary Arteries

Infective endocarditis
Prolapse of mitral valve
Mural thrombus from left atrium, left ventricle
Prosthetic valve emboli
Cardiac myxoma
Associated with cardiopulmonary bypass surgery and coronary arteriography
- Paradoxic emboli
- Papillary fibroelastoma of the aortic valve ("fixed embolus")

Congenital Coronary Artery Anomalies

Anomalous origin of left coronary from pulmonary artery
Left coronary artery from anterior sinus of Valsalva
Coronary arteriovenous and arteriocameral fistulas
Coronary artery aneurysms

Myocardial Oxygen Demand-Supply Disproportion

Aortic stenosis, all forms
Incomplete differentiation of the aortic valve
Aortic insufficiency
Carbon monoxide poisoning
Thyrotoxicosis
Prolonged hypotension

Hematologic (In Situ Thrombosis)

Polycythemia vera
Thrombocytosis
Disseminated intravascular coagulation
Hypercoagulability
Hypercoagulability, thrombosis, thrombocytopenic purpura

Miscellaneous

Myocardial contusion
Myocardial infarction with normal coronary arteries

Modified from Cheitlin M, McAllister HA, de Castro CM: Myocardial infarction without atherosclerosis. JAMA 231:951, 1975. Copyright 1975, American Medical Association.

rather than plaque rupture occurring more frequently in younger individuals and in women.[45] In summary, clinicopathologic studies support the concept of three major mechanisms of sudden cardiac death: ischemia-induced ventricular arrhythmia without acute MI, acute MI with ventricular arrhythmia, and primary ventricular arrhythmia associated with old myocardial damage and altered electrical conduction (see Fig. 24–5).[35]

Pathology of Acute Myocardial Infarction

MI is defined as the death of heart muscle resulting from severe, prolonged ischemia. MIs usually involve the LV.[1, 48] The relatively unusual right ventricular infarcts occur in association with left ventricular infarcts, particularly posterior transmural left ventricular infarcts, or as isolated entities, usually in association with pulmonary hypertension. Most MIs are confined to the distribution of a single coronary artery and are designated as anterior, anteroseptal, lateral, and posteroinferior (Plate 24–6). Multiregional MIs also occur. MIs are designated as subendocardial (non–Q wave) when the necrosis is limited to the inner half of the ventricular wall (Plate 24–7) or transmural (Q wave) when the necrosis involves not only the inner half but also significant amounts of the outer half of the ventricular wall. The electrocardiographic correlates are ST-segment elevation with Q wave pattern for transmural infarcts and ST-segment depression without Q wave pattern for subendocardial infarcts.

The overall incidence of occlusive coronary thrombosis and associated plaque fissure or rupture is high (>75 percent) for acute MI.[14–24] The thrombus typically involves the major coronary artery in the distribution of the infarcted myocardium. However, there is a significant difference in the incidence of thrombosis according to the type of infarct. In autopsy studies, occlusive coronary thrombi are found in more than 90 percent of cases of transmural (non–Q wave) MI but in only about one third of cases of subendocardial (Q wave) MI. Subendocardial MI without occlusive thrombosis is related to the influence of other factors, such as more subtle coronary lesions (e.g., platelet aggregation, nonocclusive thrombi) or factors that increase myocardial oxygen demand (e.g., aortic stenosis, systemic hypertension, cardiac hypertrophy, excessive stress, or exertion) (see Fig. 24–5). The occurrence of subendocardial MI without occlusive thrombosis highlights the increased susceptibility of the human subendocardium to ischemic injury. This susceptibility is caused by a more tenuous oxygen supply-demand balance in this region versus the subepicardium. This in turn is related to the pattern of distribution of the collateral circulation and to local metabolic differences in subendocardial versus subepicardial myocytes.

The major complications of acute MI are infarct expansion (shape change leading to stretching and thinning of the ventricular wall), infarct extension (additional necrosis), ventricular aneurysm (Plate 24–8), cardiogenic shock or recurrent ventricular arrhythmias related to large infarct size (generally > 33 to 40 percent of left ventricular mass), papillary muscle dysfunction, papillary muscle rupture

(Plate 24–9), external cardiac rupture (Plates 24–10 and 24–11), ventricular pseudoaneurysm (due to sealing off of a relatively slowly evolving rupture), ventricular septal rupture (Plate 24–12; see also Fig. 24–6), pericarditis (nonspecific and autoimmune, such as Dressler's syndrome), systemic embolization from a left ventricular mural thrombus, and pulmonary thromboembolism.[49]

The risk for infarct rupture is significant during the first week of MI before significant organization of the necrotic tissue.[48, 49] Healing of MI involves neutrophil infiltration, followed by formation of granulation tissue. Granulation tissue is grossly visible at approximately 10 days and completely replaces the necrotic tissue by 2 to 3 weeks; thereafter, the granulation tissue is converted to a dense scar; this process is completed in 2 to 3 months.

Basic Biology of Myocardial Ischemic Injury

The pathogenesis of ischemic myocardial cell injury and necrosis involves complex metabolic and structural alterations induced by severely reduced blood flow (Fig. 24–12).[50–58] As a result of oxygen deprivation, mitochondrial oxidative phosphorylation rapidly ceases, with a resultant loss of the major source of adenosine triphosphate (ATP) synthesis. Initially, there is a compensatory increase in anaerobic glycolysis, but this process leads to an accumulation of hydrogen ions and lactate, with a resultant intracellular acidosis and inhibition of glycolysis, as well as mitochondrial fatty acid and energy metabolism.[50]

The metabolic alterations are associated with inhibition of contraction (excitation-contraction uncoupling) and associated alterations in ionic transport systems located in the sarcolemma and organellar membranes.[50] The initial alteration is loss of intracellular K^+ due to increased efflux of the ion.[58] Although the mechanism is unclear, it may involve the activation of ATP-dependent K^+ channels due to a change in the ratio of ATP to adenosine diphosphate (ADP). Another early change is an increase in free Mg^{2+}, followed by a decrease in total Mg^{2+}. Once ATP decreases substantially, Na^+,K^+-ATPase is inhibited, resulting in a further loss of K^+ and an increase in Na^+. The accompanying influx of extracellular fluid leads to cell swelling. An

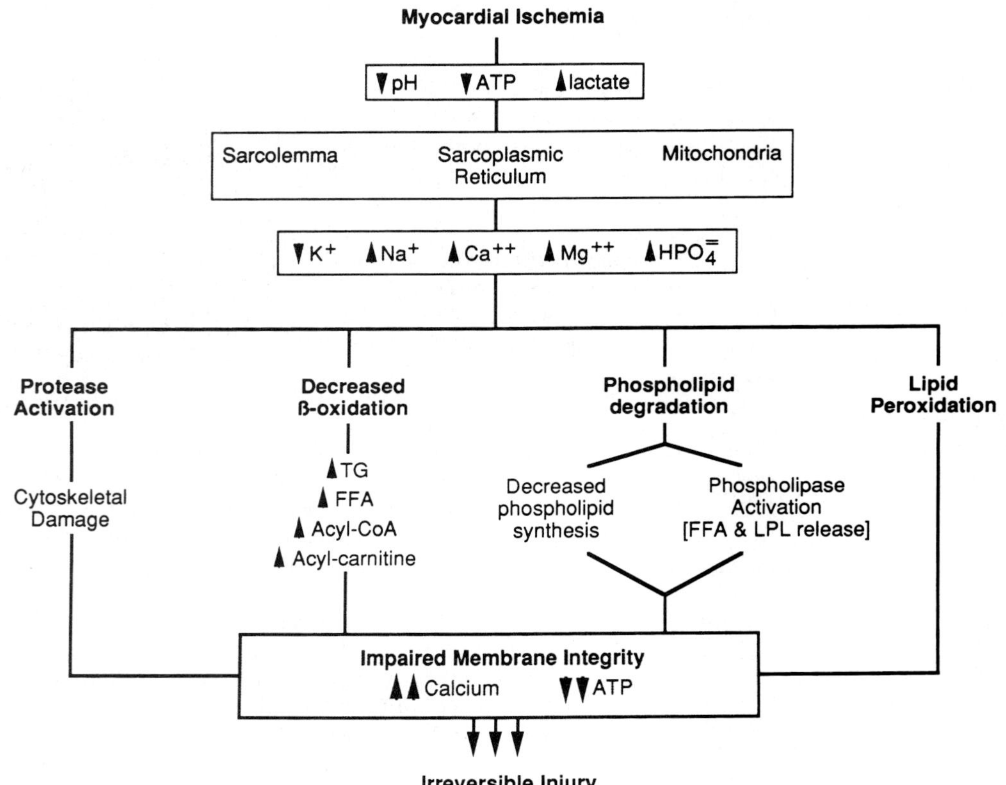

FIGURE 24–12 Postulated sequence of alterations involved in the pathogenesis of irreversible myocardial ischemic injury. Oxygen deficiency induces metabolic changes, including decreased adenosine triphosphate (ATP), decreased pH, and lactate accumulation, in ischemic myocytes. The altered metabolic milieu leads to impaired membrane transport with resultant derangements in intracellular electrolytes. An increase in cytosolic Ca^{2+} may trigger the activation of proteases and phospholipases with resultant cytoskeletal damage and impaired membrane phospholipid balance. Lipid alterations include increased phospholipid degradation with release of free fatty acids (FFA) and lysophospholipids (LPL) and decreased phospholipid synthesis. Lipid peroxidation occurs as a result of attack by free radicals produced at least in part by the generation of excess electrons in oxygen-deprived mitochondria. Free radicals also may be derived from metabolism of arachidonic acid and catecholamines, metabolism of adenine nucleotides by xanthine oxidase in endothelium (species dependent), and activation of neutrophils and macrophages. The irreversible phase of injury appears to be mediated by severe membrane damage produced by phospholipid loss, lipid peroxidation, and cytoskeletal damage. Acyl-CoA, acyl coenzyme A; TG, triglycerides. (Reprinted from Trends Cardiovasc Med, Vol. 1, Buja LM, Lipid abnormalities in myocardial cell injury, pp. 40–45, Copyright 1991, with permission from Elsevier Science.)

early increase in cytosolic Ca^{2+} also occurs as the result of multifactorial changes in transport systems of the sarcolemma and sarcoplasmic reticulum.[54–58]

Advanced ischemic myocardial cell injury is mediated by progressive membrane damage involving several contributory factors (see Fig. 24–12).[52, 56] Calcium accumulation or other metabolic changes lead to phospholipase activation and resultant phospholipid degradation and the release of lysophospholipids and free fatty acids. Impaired mitochondrial fatty acid metabolism leads to the accumulation of various lipid species, including long-chain acyl coenzyme A (acyl CoA) and acyl carnitine, which together with products of phospholipid degradation can incorporate into membranes and impair their function. Free radicals, including toxic oxygen species, are generated from ischemic myocytes, ischemic endothelium, and activated leukocytes. These toxic chemicals induce peroxidative damage to fatty acids of membrane phospholipids. Probably as a result of protease activation, cytoskeletal filaments, which normally anchor the sarcolemma to adjacent myofibrils, become damaged, and their anchoring and stabilizing effect on the sarcolemma is lost. All of these changes lead to a progressive increase in membrane permeability, further derangements in the intracellular ionic milieu, and ATP exhaustion. The terminal event in initiation of irreversible myocyte injury appears to be physical disruption of the sarcolemma of the swollen myocyte.[52, 56]

The sequence of abnormalities described previously constitutes the well-documented pathophysiologic basis of cell injury that leads to cell death in cardiac myocytes subjected to a major ischemic or hypoxic insult. Several discoveries have raised the possibility that other pathophysiologic mechanisms may contribute to myocardial cell injury and death. After the recognition of apoptosis as a major and distinctive mode of cell death, reports have been published that implicate apoptosis in MI, reperfusion injury, and other forms of cardiovascular pathology.[59–61] Apoptosis is characterized by a series of molecular and biochemical events, including (1) gene activation (programmed cell death), (2) perturbations of mitochondria, including membrane permeability transition and cytochrome *c* release, (3) activation of a cascade of cytosolic aspartate–specific cysteine proteases (caspases), (4) endonuclease activation leading to double-stranded DNA fragmentation, and (5) altered phospholipid distribution of cell membranes and other surface properties with preservation of selective membrane permeability.

Apoptosis is also characterized by distinctive morphologic alterations featuring cell and nuclear shrinkage and fragmentation. In contrast, numerous studies have reported ischemic myocardial damage to be characterized by cell swelling with altered cellular ionic composition due to altered membrane permeability. This pattern of cell injury and death with cell swelling has been designated as *oncosis.* Although some reports have proposed a major role for apoptosis in myocardial ischemic injury and infarction, such a role for apoptosis may be overstated because of overinterpretation of evidence of DNA fragmentation, which is not specific for apoptosis.[60, 61] Although certain assays have been proposed to be more reliable for the detection of patterns of DNA fragmentation characteristic of apoptosis, the overall sensitivity and specificity of these assays require confirmation.[60, 61] Nevertheless, research with caspase inhibitors suggests that both apoptosis and oncosis may contribute to the overall magnitude of ischemic necrosis.[60, 61]

The rate and magnitude of ATP reduction may be critical determinants of whether an injured myocyte progresses to death via apoptosis or oncosis because an ATP analog, dATP, is a key component of a molecular complex that mediates cytochrome *c* release with activation of the caspase cascade and apoptotic death.[60, 61] It is likely, then, that severely ischemic myocytes progress rapidly to cell death with swelling (oncosis), whereas less severely ischemic myocytes may develop apoptosis.

Determinants of Infarct Development and Size

After coronary artery occlusion, the myocardium can withstand up to about 20 minutes of severe ischemia without developing irreversible injury; after about 20 to 30 minutes of severe ischemia, irreversible myocardial injury begins.[52, 53] The subsequent degradative changes give rise to recognizable myocardial necrosis. In the human and dog, myocardial necrosis first appears in the ischemic subendocardium because this area usually has a more severe reduction in perfusion than the subepicardium. During the ensuing 3 to 6 hours, irreversible myocardial injury progresses in a wavefront pattern from the subendocardium into the subepicardium (Fig. 24–13).[51] In the experimental animal and probably also in humans, most MIs are completed within approximately 6 hours after the onset of coronary occlusion. However, a slower pattern of evolution of MI can occur when the coronary collateral perfusion is abundant or when the stimulus for myocardial ischemia is intermittent (e.g., in the case of episodes of intermittent platelet aggregation before occlusive thrombosis).

Established MIs have distinct central and peripheral regions (Fig. 24–14).[52–55] In the central zone of severe ischemia, the necrotic myocytes exhibit clear sarcoplasm with separation of organelles (evidence of edema): clumped nuclear chromatin, stretched myofibrils with widened I bands, swollen mitochondria containing amorphous matrix (flocculent) densities composed of denatured lipid and protein and linear densities representing fused cristae, and defects (holes) in the sarcolemma. In the peripheral region of an infarct, which has some degree of collateral perfusion, many necrotic myocytes exhibit edematous sarcoplasm: disruption of the myofibrils with the formation of dense transverse (contraction) bands, swollen mitochondria containing calcium phosphate deposits as well as amorphous matrix densities, varying amounts of lipid droplets, and clumped nuclear chromatin. A third population of cells at the outermost periphery of infarcts contains excess numbers of lipid droplets but does not exhibit the features of irreversible injury just described. The pattern of injury seen in the infarcted periphery is also characteristic of myocardial injury produced by temporary coronary occlusion followed by reperfusion. In general, the most reliable ultrastructural features of irreversible injury are the amorphous matrix densities in the mitochondria and the sarcolemmal defects.

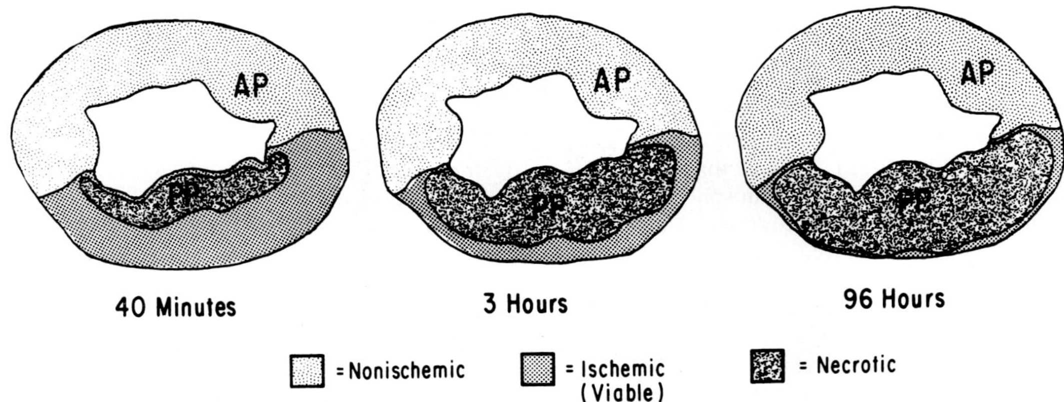

FIGURE 24–13 Progression of cell death versus time after circumflex coronary occlusion in dogs. Necrosis occurs first in the subendocardial myocardium. With longer occlusions, a wavefront of cell death moves from the subendocardial zone across the wall to involve progressively more of the transmural thickness of the ischemic zone. In contrast, the lateral margins in the subendocardial region of the infarct are established as early as 40 minutes after occlusion and are sharply defined by the anatomic boundaries of the ischemic bed. AP, anterior papillary muscle; PP, posterior papillary muscle. (From Reimer KA, Jennings RB: The "wavefront" phenomenon of myocardial ischemic cell death: II. Transmural progression of necrosis within the framework of ischemic bed size [myocardium at risk] and collateral flow. Lab Invest 40[6]:633–644, 1979.)

The myocardial *bed at risk,* or *risk zone,* refers to the mass of myocardium that receives its blood supply from a major coronary artery that develops occlusion (see Fig. 24–13).[51] After occlusion, the severity of the ischemia is determined on the basis of the amount of preexisting collateral circulation into the myocardial bed at risk. The collateral blood flow is derived from collateral channels connecting the occluded and nonoccluded coronary systems. With time, there is a progressive increase in coronary collateral blood flow, but much of this increase in flow may occur too late to salvage significant amounts of myocardium.

The size of the MI is determined on the basis of the mass of necrotic myocardium within the bed at risk (see Figs. 24–13 and 24–14). The bed at risk will also contain viable but injured myocardium. The border zone refers to the non-necrotic but dysfunctional myocardium within the ischemic bed at risk. The size of the border zone varies inversely with the relative amount of necrotic myocardium, which increases with time as the wavefront of necrosis progresses. The border zone exists primarily in the subepicardial half of the bed at risk and has a very small lateral dimension, due to a sharp demarcation between vascular beds supplied by the occluded and the patent major coronary arteries.

The major determinants of ultimate infarct size, therefore, are the duration and severity of ischemia, the size of the myocardial bed at risk, and the amount of collateral blood flow available shortly after coronary occlusion. Infarct size can also be influenced by the major determinants of myocardial metabolic demand: heart rate, wall tension (determined by blood pressure), and myocardial contractility.

REPERFUSION, PRECONDITIONING, STUNNING, AND HIBERNATION

A number of factors can significantly modulate the myocardial response and subsequent outcome of an ischemic episode.[61] The progression of myocardial ischemia can be profoundly influenced by *reperfusion,* but the effects of reperfusion are complex.[62–64] Reperfusion clearly can limit the extent of myocardial necrosis if instituted early enough after the onset of coronary occlusion. However, reperfusion also changes the pattern of myocardial injury by causing hemorrhage within the severely damaged myocardium and by producing a pattern of myocardial injury characterized by contraction bands and calcification. Reperfusion also accelerates the release of intracellular enzymes from damaged myocardium. This may lead to a marked elevation in serum levels of these enzymes without necessarily implying further myocardial necrosis. The timing of reperfusion is critical to the outcome, with the potential for myocardial salvage being greater with earlier intervention. Although reperfusion can clearly salvage myocardium, it may also induce additional injury. The concept of reperfusion injury implies the development of further damage, as a result of the reperfusion, to myocytes that were injured but remained viable during a previous ischemic episode. Such injury may involve functional impairment, arrhythmia, or progression to cell death.[61–64]

The rate of progression of myocardial necrosis can be influenced by prior short intervals of coronary occlusion and reperfusion. Specifically, experimental evidence indicates that the extent of myocardial necrosis after 60 to 90 minutes of coronary occlusion is significantly less in animals that had been pretreated with one or more 5-minute intervals of coronary occlusion before the induction of permanent occlusion.[61, 65, 66] However, after 120 minutes of coronary occlusion, the effect on infarct size is lost. This phenomenon is known as *preconditioning.*[61, 65, 66] Evidence has indicated that a reduced rate of ATP depletion correlates with the beneficial effects of preconditioning.[65, 66] Further studies have suggested that the activation of adenosine receptors and ATP-dependent potassium channels may mediate the process of preconditioning.[61, 67, 68] After a refractory period, a second late phase of myocardial protection during a subsequent ischemic event develops.[69] This phenomenon, known as the *second window of protection,* is related to ischemia-induced gene activation with the

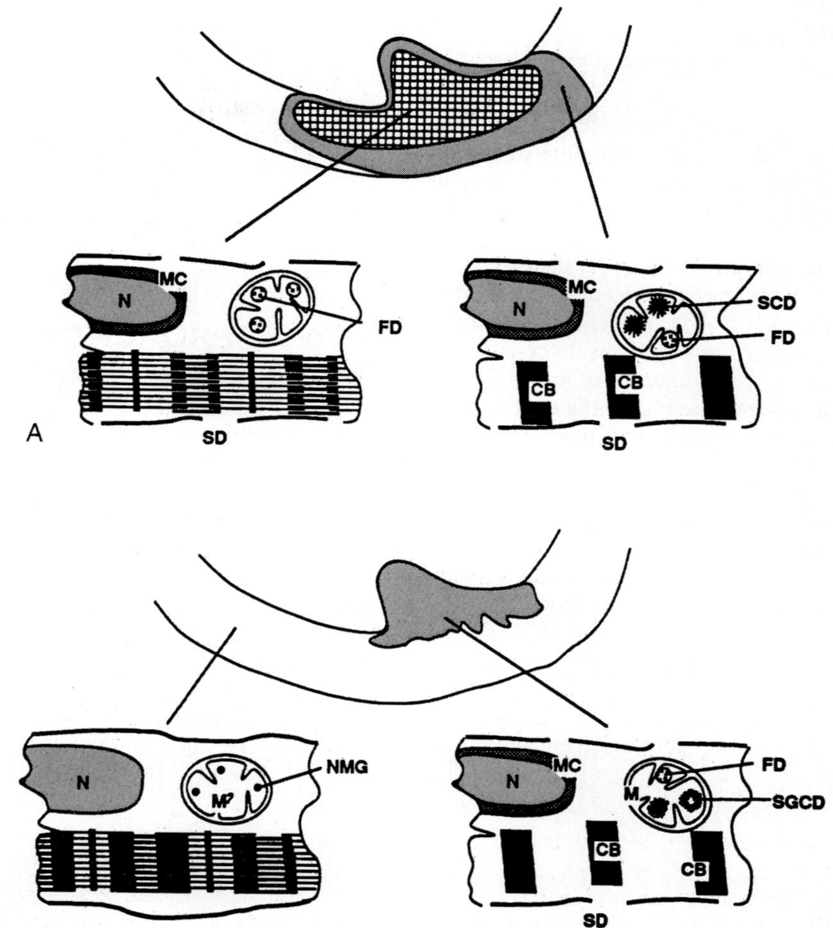

FIGURE 24–14 Schematic diagram of the morphologic features of myocardial cell injury present in different regions of transmural infarcts produced by permanent coronary occlusion **(A)** and subendocardial infarcts produced by temporary ischemia followed by reperfusion **(B)**. With prolonged coronary occlusion, myocardial necrosis is established in the subendocardium within 40 to 60 minutes, progresses in a wavefront pattern into the subepicardium of the region at risk (risk zone), and is completed by 3 to 6 hours. With prolonged coronary occlusion, the myofibrils of myocytes in the central infarct region are hyperrelaxed compared with those in the normal tissue depicted in **B**, and the mitochondria contain flocculent densities (FD) composed of denatured lipid and protein. The myofibrils of myocytes in the peripheral infarct region are formed into contraction bands (CB), and the mitochondria show calcium deposits as well as flocculent densities. With temporary ischemia and reperfusion, injury is limited to the subendocardium and is characterized by myofibrillar contraction bands and early mitochondrial calcification. MC, marginated chromatin; N, nucleus; NMG, normal matrix granule; SCD, large spicular calcium deposit; SD, sarcolemmal defect; SGCD, small granular calcium deposit. (**A** and **B**, From Hagler HK, Buja LM: Subcellular calcium shifts in ischemia and reperfusion. *In* Piper HM [ed]: Pathophysiology of Severe Ischemic Myocardial Injury. pp. 283–296. Dordrecht: Kluwer Academic, 1990, with kind permission from Kluwer Academic Publishers.)

production of various gene products, including stress (heat shock) proteins and nitric oxide synthase.[61, 69]

Prolonged functional depression, requiring as much as 24 hours or longer for recovery, develops on reperfusion even after relatively brief periods of coronary occlusion, such as 15 minutes, which is insufficient to cause myocardial necrosis. This phenomenon has been referred to as *myocardial stunning.*[61] A related condition, termed *hibernation,* refers to chronic depression of myocardial function due to a chronic moderate reduction in perfusion.[61] Preconditioning and stunning are independent phenomena; the preconditioning effect is short term, transient, and not mediated through stunning. Free radical effects and calcium loading have been implicated in the pathogenesis of stunning, as well as other components of reperfusion injury.[61, 70, 71] After longer intervals of coronary occlusion, on the order of 2 to 4 hours, necrosis of the subendocardium develops and even more severe and persistent functional depression occurs.[72] In experimental studies, after 2 hours of coronary occlusion, left ventricular regional sites of moderate dysfunction during ischemia recovered to normal or near-normal regional contractile function after 1 to 4 weeks of reperfusion, whereas after 4 hours of coronary occlusion, contractile dysfunction persisted after 4 weeks of reperfusion.[72]

Depending on the interval of coronary occlusion before reperfusion, varying degrees of contractile dysfunction, necrosis, or both, are seen with reperfusion. These observations emphasize the need for early intervention to salvage myocardium.[61, 73] On balance, early reperfusion results in a major net positive effect, making early reperfusion an important goal in the treatment of acute CAD.[74, 75]

Pathology of Interventionally Treated Coronary Artery Disease

The use of percutaneous transluminal coronary angioplasty can produce a variety of acute effects, including dilatation of the vessel caused by stretching of the intima and media, damage to the endothelial surface, multiple fissures in the plaque, and dissection of the media (Plate 24–13).[7, 76] The acute injury initiates a reparative response that leads to intimal proliferation.[7, 77] Similar effects occur after atherectomy and laser angioplasty.[78, 79] The resultant fibrocellular tissue is composed of modified smooth muscle cells (*myofibroblasts*) and connective tissue matrix without lipid deposits. A similar lesion is seen in animal models of arterial injury (Fig. 24–15).[77] Experimental evidence supports a role for platelet activation in the pathogenesis of the lesion.[77] This process of intimal proliferation leads to restenosis of lesions in 30 to 40 percent of cases within 6 months. The use of vascular stents in conjunction with angioplasty has significantly improved the long-term patency rates, although the stents invoke some intimal reaction.[80, 81]

Saphenous vein–coronary artery bypass grafts develop diffuse fibrocellular intimal thickening, medial degeneration and atrophy, and vascular dilatation within several months after implantation (Fig. 24–16).[82–84] Subsequently, the grafts are prone to the development of eccentric intimal plaques with lipid deposition (atherosclerosis). Plaque fissuring and thrombosis also may develop (Fig. 24–17). Therefore, all of the changes seen in naturally occurring atherosclerosis may also develop in the saphenous veins, thereby creating a finite limit to the beneficial effects of these grafts. With improvements in surgical technique, the use of internal mammary arteries for coronary bypass has taken on more widespread application. The internal mammary arteries are more resistant to the intimal injury and intimal proliferation observed in saphenous veins, and therefore, the arterial bypass grafts have prolonged potency.[85, 86]

New Approaches to Myocardial Modulation

A new era is developing in therapy regarding the pathogenesis of CAD. Ongoing testing is being conducted to successfully achieve genetic manipulation (gene therapy) of the processes responsible for the response of the arterial wall to injury, with the goals of retarding or preventing intimal proliferation and thrombosis at sites of coronary injury.[87–89] New pharmacologic interventions are being tested based on the possible contributions of both apoptosis and oncosis to MI.[61, 62] The debate regarding whether cardiac myocytes are terminally differentiated has been revived.[90, 91] Molecular mechanisms responsible for the mitotic block of mature myocytes are under investigation with the potential for genetic manipulation of myocyte proliferation.[90, 91] Other approaches are being explored, in-

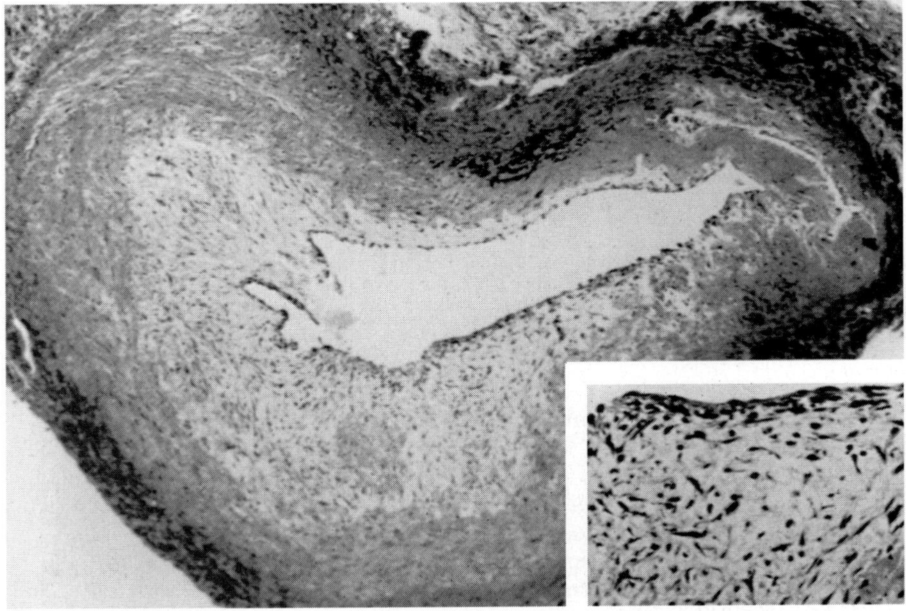

FIGURE 24–15 Histologic section of a coronary artery from a dog with endothelial injury and coronary artery stenosis of the proximal left anterior descending coronary artery; the dog had frequent cyclic coronary blood flow variations during the first week after instrumentation and endothelial injury. The constrictor site shows extensive intimal proliferation. (Trichrome stain, ×62.) *Inset,* At higher magnification, the area of intimal profileration is composed of loose connective tissue containing numerous elongated cells shown to have features of modified smooth muscle cells by electron microscopy. There are also round monocytes adjacent to the luminal surface. (Trichrome stain, ×150.) Similar lesions occur in approximately 30 to 40 percent of patients after percutaneous transluminal coronary angioplasty. (From Willerson JT, Yao S-K, McNatt J, et al: Frequency and severity of cyclic flow alteration and platelet aggregation predict the severity of neointimal proliferation following experimental coronary stenosis and endothelial injury. Proc Natl Acad Sci USA 88:10624–10628, 1991.)

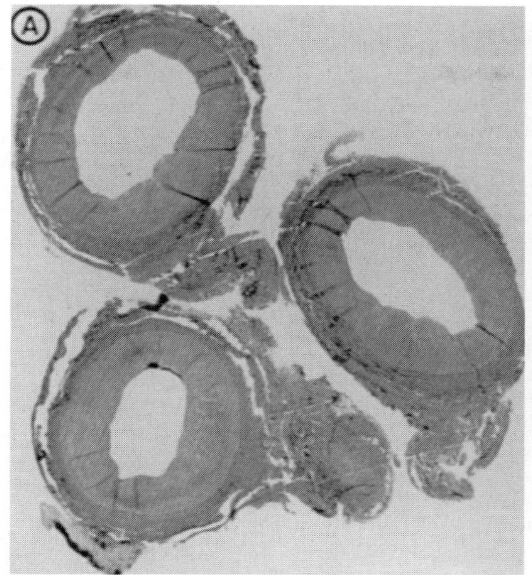

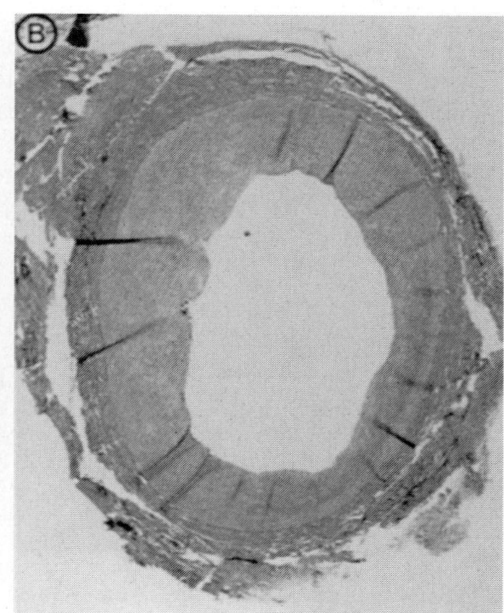

FIGURE 24–16 Saphenous vein–coronary artery bypass graft implanted for several months. **A,** The vein graft shows diffuse concentric fibromuscular intimal thickening. (H&E, ×5.6.) **B,** Higher magnification view of one segment of vessel. (H&E, ×12.) (**A** and **B,** From Willerson JT, Hillis LD, Buja LM: Ischemic Heart Disease: Clinical and Pathophysiological Aspects. New York: Raven, 1982.)

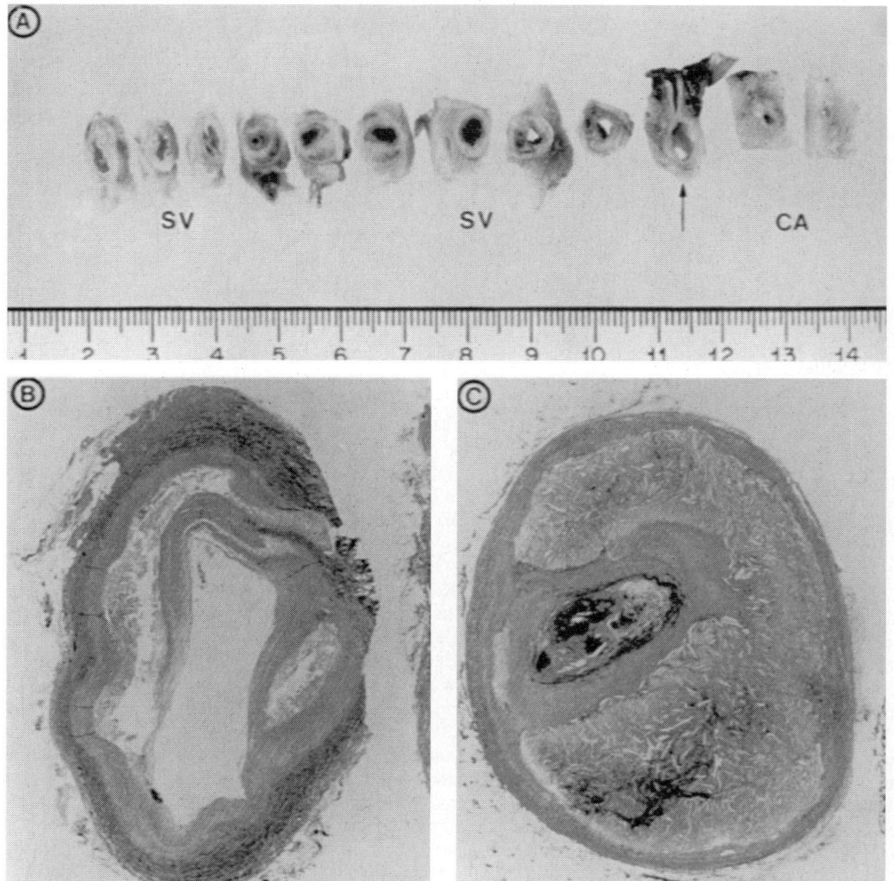

FIGURE 24–17 Severe atherosclerosis in a saphenous vein graft in place for 7 years. **A,** Multiple cross sections through the saphenous vein (SV), distal anastomosis (*arrow*), and distal coronary artery (CA). The saphenous vein shows marked atherosclerosis and acute occlusive thrombosis with plaque hemorrhage. The distal coronary artery has focal plaque, but a residual lumen is present. There was a massive acute myocardial infarct in the distribution of the occluded vein graft. **B,** Histological section of a segment of the vein graft shows foci of lipid in the diffusely thickened intima. (Trichrome stain, ×7.5.) **C,** This segment of vein graft is involved by a large atheroma with a lipid-laden core and thin fibrous capsule. Hemorrhage is present in the plaque core. The lumen is occluded by recent thrombus. (H&E, ×7.5.) (**A–C,** From Willerson JT, Hillis LD, Buja LM: Ischemic Heart Disease: Clinical and Pathophysiological Aspects. New York: Raven, 1982.)

cluding microinjection of genetically engineered myocytes for repopulation of damaged myocardium.[92, 93] Alternative approaches are being explored for the treatment of intractable angina pectoris[94, 95]; one surgical approach is the use of transmyocardial laser treatment to create new myocardial microvasculature.[95–98] An alternate approach is the intravascular delivery of genetically engineered growth factors, including vascular endothelial growth factor and fibroblast growth factor.[99–102] These approaches have considerable promise for the treatment of CAD.

REFERENCES

1. Willerson JT, Hillis LD, Buja LM: Ischemic Heart Disease: Clinical and Pathophysiological Aspects. New York: Raven, 1982.
2. James TN: The coronary circulation and conduction system in acute myocardial infarction. Prog Cardiovasc Dis 10:410–446, 1968.
3. Baroldi G: Diseases of extramural coronary arteries. *In* Silver MD (ed): Cardiovascular Pathology. 2nd ed. pp. 487–563. New York: Churchill Livingstone, 1991.
4. Gregg DE, Patterson RE: Functional importance of coronary collaterals. N Engl J Med 303:1404–1406, 1980.
5. Ross R: The pathogenesis of atherosclerosis—an update. N Engl J Med 314:488–500, 1986.
6. Munro JM, Cotran RS: The pathogenesis of atherosclerosis: atherogenesis and inflammation. Lab Invest 58:249–261, 1988.
7. Buja LM, Willerson JT, Murphree SS: Pathobiology of arterial wall injury, atherosclerosis, and coronary angioplasty. *In* Black AJR, Anderson HV, Ellis SG (eds): Complications of Coronary Angioplasty. pp. 11–33. New York: Marcel Dekker, 1991.
8. Schwartz CJ, Mitchell JRA: The morphology, terminology and pathogenesis of arterial plaques. Postgrad Med J 38:25–34, 1962.
9. Pearson TA, Kramer EC, Solez K, Heptinstall RH: The human atherosclerotic plaque. Am J Pathol 86:657–664, 1977.
10. Buja LM, Clubb FJ Jr, Bilheimer DW, Willerson JT: Pathobiology of human familial hypercholesterolemia and a related animal model, the Watanabe heritable hyperlipidaemic rabbit. Eur Heart J 11(suppl E):41–52, 1990.
11. Glagov S, Zarins C, Giddens DP, Nu DN: Hemodynamics and atherosclerosis: insights and perspectives gained from studies of human arteries. Arch Pathol Lab Med 112:1018–1031, 1988.
12. Glagov S, Weisenberg E, Zarins CK, et al: Compensatory enlargement of human atherosclerotic coronary arteries. N Engl J Med 316:1371–1375, 1987.
13. Arnett EN, Isner JM, Redwood DR, et al: Coronary artery narrowing in coronary heart disease: comparison of cineangiographic and necropsy findings. Ann Intern Med 91:350–356, 1979.
14. Buja LM, Hillis LD, Petty CS, Willerson JT: The role of coronary arterial spasm in ischemic heart disease. Arch Pathol Lab Med 105:221–226, 1981.
15. Buja LM, Willerson JT: The role of coronary artery lesions in ischemic heart disease: insights from recent clinicopathologic, coronary arteriographic, and experimental studies. Hum Pathol 18:451–461, 1987.
16. Fuster V, Badimon L, Badimon JJ, Chesebro JH: The pathogenesis of coronary artery disease and the acute coronary syndromes. N Engl J Med 326:242–250, 310–318, 1992.
17. Davies MJ, Woolf N, Robertson WB: Pathology of acute myocardial infarction with particular reference to occlusive coronary thrombi. Br Heart J 38:659–664, 1976.
18. Ridolfi RL, Hutchins GM: The relationship between coronary artery lesions and myocardial infarcts: ulceration of atherosclerotic plaques precipitating coronary thrombosis. Am Heart J 93:468–486, 1977.
19. Horie T, Sekiguchi M, Hirosawa K: Coronary thrombosis in pathogenesis of acute myocardial infarction: histopathological study of coronary arteries in 108 necropsied cases using serial section. Br Heart J 40:153–161, 1978.
20. Davies MJ, Fulton WFM, Robertson WB: The relation of coronary thrombosis to ischemic myocardial necrosis. J Pathol 172:99–110, 1979.
21. Silver MD, Baroldi G, Mariani F: The relationship between acute occlusive coronary thrombi and myocardial infarction studied in 100 consecutive patients. Circulation 61:219–227, 1980.
22. Buja LM, Willerson JT: Clinicopathologic correlates of acute ischemic heart disease syndromes. Am J Cardiol 47:343–356, 1981.
23. Falk E: Plaque rupture with severe preexisting stenosis precipitating coronary thrombosis: characteristics of coronary atherosclerotic plaques underlying fatal occlusive thrombi. Br Heart J 50:127–134, 1983.
24. Davies MJ, Thomas AEC: Plaque fissuring—the cause of acute myocardial infarction, sudden ischemic death, and crescendo angina. Br Heart J 53:363–373, 1985.
25. Casscells W, Hathorn B, David M. et al: Thermal detection of cellular infiltrates in living atherosclerotic plaques: possible implications for plaque rupture and thrombosis. Lancet 347:1447–1451, 1996.
26. Burke AP, Farb A, Malcom GT, et al: Plaque rupture and sudden death related to exertion in men with coronary artery disease. JAMA 281:921–926, 1999.
27. Roberts WC, Curry RC Jr, Isner JM, et al: Sudden death in Prinzmetal's angina with coronary spasm documented by angiography: analysis of three necropsy patients. Am J Cardiol 50:203–210, 1982.
28. MacAlpin RN: Relation of coronary arterial spasm to sites of organic stenosis. Am J Cardiol 46:143–153, 1980.
29. El-Maraghi NRH, Sealey BJ: Recurrent myocardial infarction in a young man due to coronary arterial spasm demonstrated at autopsy. Circulation 61:199–207, 1980.
30. Forman MB, Oates JA, Robertson D, et al: Increased adventitial mast cells in a patient with coronary spasm. N Engl J Med 313:1138–1141, 1985.
31. Kohchi K, Takebayashi S, Hiroki T, Nobuyoshi M: Significance of adventitial inflammation of the coronary artery in patients with unstable angina: results at autopsy. Circulation 71:709–716, 1985.
32. Cheitlin MD, McAllister HA, de Castro CM: Myocardial infarction without atherosclerosis. JAMA 231:951–959, 1975.
33. Dowling GP, Buja LM: Spontaneous coronary artery dissection occurs with and without periadventitial inflammation. Arch Pathol Lab Med 111:470–472, 1987.
34. Stenberg RG, Winniford MD, Hillis LD, et al: Simultaneous acute thrombosis of two major coronary arteries following intravenous cocaine use. Arch Pathol Lab Med 113:521–524, 1989.
35. Kloner RA, Hale S, Alker K, Rezkalla S: The effects of acute and chronic cocaine use on the heart. Circulation 85:407–419, 1992.
36. El-Maraghi N, Genton E: The relevance of platelet and fibrin thromboembolism of the coronary microcirculation with special reference to sudden cardiac death. Circulation 62:936–944, 1980.
37. Davies MJ, Thomas AC, Knapman PA, Hangartner JR: Intramyocardial platelet aggregation in patients with unstable angina pectoris suffering sudden ischemic cardiac death. Circulation 73:418–427, 1986.
38. Zipes DP, Wellens HJJ: Sudden cardiac death. Circulation 98:2334–2351, 1998.
39. Buja LM, Willerson JT: Relationship of ischemic heart disease to sudden cardiac death. J Forens Sci 36:25–33, 1991.
40. Reichenbach DD, Moss NS, Meyer E: Pathology of the heart in sudden cardiac death. Am J Cardiol 39:865–872, 1977.
41. Baroldi G, Falzi G, Mariani F: Sudden coronary death: a postmortem study in 208 selected cases compared to 97 "control" subjects. Am Heart J 98:20–31, 1979.
42. Warnes CA, Roberts WC: Sudden coronary death: comparison of patients with to those without coronary thrombus at necropsy. Am J Cardiol 54:1206–1211, 1984.
43. Davies MJ, Thomas A: Thrombosis and acute coronary-artery lesions in sudden cardiac ischemic death. N Engl J Med 310:1137–1140, 1984.
44. Farb A, Tang AL, Burke AP, et al: Sudden coronary death: frequency of active lesions, inactive coronary lesions, and myocardial infarction. Circulation 92:1701–1709, 1995.
45. Farb A, Burke AP, Tang AL, et al: Coronary plaque erosion without rupture into a lipid core: a frequent cause of coronary thrombosis in sudden coronary death. Circulation 93:1354–1363, 1996.
46. Burke AP, Farb A, Malcom GT, et al: Coronary risk factors and plaque morphology in men with coronary disease who die suddenly. N Engl J Med 336:1276–1282, 1997.
47. Burke AP, Farb A, Malcom GT, et al: Effect of risk factors on the

CHAPTER 25

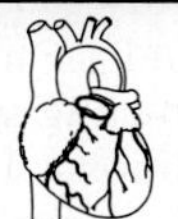

Regulation of Coronary Blood Flow

Robert J. Bache

DETERMINANTS OF MYOCARDIAL OXYGEN CONSUMPTION
Systolic Wall Tension
Contractility
Heart Rate
Rate-Pressure Product
EPICARDIAL CORONARY ARTERIES
CORONARY RESISTANCE VESSELS
Coronary Arterioles
Myogenic Mechanisms
Resistance Arteries
ENDOTHELIUM-DEPENDENT VASODILATATION
Nitric Oxide
Prostacyclin
Hyperpolarizing Factor
TRANSMURAL DISTRIBUTION OF MYOCARDIAL BLOOD FLOW
CORONARY COLLATERAL CIRCULATION
CORONARY STEAL
LEFT VENTRICULAR HYPERTROPHY

Over a wide range of activity, coronary blood flow is closely regulated to maintain a high level of oxygen extraction from the blood perfusing the myocardial capillaries. During resting conditions, 70 to 80 percent of the oxygen perfusing the coronary capillaries is extracted by the myocardium, so there is little ability to increase oxygen uptake during exercise by means of increasing oxygen extraction.[1] For this reason, increases of oxygen demands must be met by proportionate increases in coronary flow. Close coupling of coronary blood flow to cardiac work is further mandated by the strongly oxidative nature of energy production by the heart. More than 95 percent of the adenosine triphosphate (ATP) produced by the myocardium is generated through oxidative phosphorylation, which requires a continuous supply of oxygen to the mitochondria.[2] Since the ATP pool of the heart turns over four to five times per minute, failure of ATP production to equal ATP consumption results in loss of contractile function within a few seconds. Reductions of coronary blood flow by as little as 10 to 20 percent result in contractile dysfunction and depletion of high-energy phosphates.[3, 4] These considerations suggest that the myocardium functions at the brink of ischemia and emphasizes the importance of the control mechanisms by which coronary vasomotor tone is adjusted in response to beat-to-beat changes of myocardial energy demands. Despite the seemingly precarious relationship between coronary blood flow and myocardial energy demands, there is no evidence that increased cardiac work can result in ischemic dysfunction in the normal heart, except possibly in the presence of severe anemia or hypoxia. Ischemia occurs when diseased coronary vessels are unable to deliver sufficient arterial inflow to meet myocardial metabolic demands. When coronary flow is limited by an arterial stenosis, myocardial oxygen demands play a decisive role in setting the threshold for ischemia.

Determinants of Myocardial Oxygen Consumption

Approximately 85 percent of the ATP produced in the heart is utilized to support contractile activity, so that indices that measure cardiac pump function can be used to estimate myocardial oxygen demands. Consequently, therapies that decrease the response of contractile work during exercise or other stress can prevent the development of ischemia in myocardial regions in which flow reserve is limited by a coronary stenosis. The hemodynamic variables that determine contractile energy consumption are discussed later.

Systolic Wall Tension

Force produced by the contracting myocardium to generate pressure is expressed in terms of wall tension. Systolic wall tension is directly proportional to left ventricular intracavitary systolic pressure. Since wall tension is expressed as force per unit of cross-sectional area, it is directly proportional to left ventricular cavity diameter and inversely proportional to wall thickness. Since wall tension cannot be directly measured, systolic arterial pressure is commonly used as a surrogate for systolic wall tension. Because the effects of left ventricular cavity diameter and wall thickness are neglected, the relationship between systolic arterial pressure and absolute myocardial oxygen consumption is imprecise. However, changes in systolic pressure are directly proportional to changes in systolic wall stress, so that such changes during exercise or other stress are predictive of changes in oxygen consumption.

Contractility

Myocardial contractility describes the rate of tension development during cardiac contraction. An increase in contractility causes an increase in the rate of pressure development and an increase in the velocity of shortening of the contracting myocardium, which is independent of loading conditions. The first time derivative of left ventricular pressure during isovolumic contraction (dP/dt_{max}) is commonly used to estimate myocardial contractility. This variable changes in parallel with contractility but is influenced by both left ventricular preload (end-diastolic pressure) and afterload (systolic pressure). Because determination of this index of contractility requires high-fidelity measurements of left ventricular systolic pressure, it can be obtained only in the catheterization laboratory.

Heart Rate

Heart rate is a summing factor for the energy cost of cardiac contraction. Since systolic wall tension and contractility are computed on a per-beat basis, changes in heart rate bear a strong relationship to changes in myocardial oxygen uptake. Furthermore, heart rate directly influences contractility, so that increases of heart rate during exercise or other stress result in increased contractility.

Rate-Pressure Product

The product of heart rate and systolic arterial pressure (rate-pressure product) is a convenient index for estimating changes in myocardial oxygen demands. Proportional changes in heart rate or systolic pressure have equal effects on myocardial oxygen consumption.[5] The rate-pressure product is especially useful for estimating the degree of cardiac stress during exercise testing. It should be noted that the rate-pressure product reflects changes in global left ventricular oxygen consumption. In regions in which a coronary stenosis prevents an adequate increase in blood flow, the insufficient oxygen availability will result in failure of contractile function.

Epicardial Coronary Arteries

The epicardial arteries form a network of vessels that arborize over the surface of the heart and give off perpendicular branches that penetrate into the myocardium. Normal epicardial arteries are true conduit vessels that do not contribute significantly to total coronary vascular resistance. The epicardial arteries are richly innervated with sympathetic nerve fibers, and coronary artery smooth muscle cells contain both alpha adrenoceptors, which mediate vasoconstriction, and beta receptors, which cause vasodilatation.[6] In the normal heart, exercise results in endothelium-dependent vasodilatation of the epicardial arteries which is mediated by nitric oxide (NO), so that blockade of NO production prevents normal coronary artery vasodilatation during exercise.[7, 8] Furthermore, endothelial dysfunction resulting from hyperlipidemia, hypertension, or atherosclerosis blunts or abolishes the normal epicardial artery dilatation during exercise.[9]

Autopsy studies of patients with atherosclerotic disease have demonstrated that approximately 75 percent of coronary atheromas are eccentric in location, leaving part of the vessel wall uninvolved. The finding of a relatively uninvolved segment explains the observation that coronary stenoses often do not cause fixed narrowings, but have some degree of compliance and are able to undergo active vasomotion.[10] The intra-arterial pressure within a stenosis opposes the vasomotor tone and elasticity of the arterial wall, which act to constrict the vessel. Compliant stenoses can interact with the distal resistance vessels as the result of hydrodynamic changes that occur at the stenotic segment. Thus, when exercise results in vasodilatation of the distal resistance vessels, the increased blood velocity (kinetic energy) within the stenotic segment causes a proportionate decrease in pressure (potential energy) acting to distend the stenosis. As the distending pressure in the stenosis decreases with increasing flow, the arterial wall elasticity and vasoconstrictor tone act to collapse the stenosis and increase stenosis severity.[11] This effect is augmented by endothelial dysfunction in the atherosclerotic coronary circulation, since the normal flow-mediated vasodilator response is absent.[12]

When a stenosis is severe, the effects of increasing blood velocity within the stenosis can be sufficient to cause a paradoxical decrease in blood flow in response to resistance vessel dilators such as adenosine or dipyridamole. Furthermore, an uninvolved segment of arterial wall at the site of a stenosis can undergo vasoconstriction in response to sympathetic nervous system activation or agonists such as ergonovine, serotonin, or thromboxane. Sympathetic vasoconstriction is augmented in the atherosclerotic coronary circulation because adrenergic stimulation causes endothelial release of NO, which opposes vasoconstriction in normal coronary vessels but is lost in atherosclerotic vessels.[13] Isometric exercise causes greater activation of the sympathetic nervous system than does dynamic exercise. Consequently, the tendency toward constriction of stenotic coronary artery segments is more prominent with isometric than with dynamic exercise.[10]

Coronary Resistance Vessels

The principal resistance to blood flow resides in coronary microvessels smaller than 400 μm in diameter. These vessels are responsible for autoregulation, by which blood flow is maintained constant over a range of perfusion pressures, as well as metabolic vasoregulation, by which blood flow is adjusted to myocardial demands in response to changes in cardiac workload. The resistance vessels can be divided functionally into two separate segments. Metabolic vasoregulation and autoregulation occur in arterioles smaller than 100 μm in diameter, whereas as much as 40 percent of total coronary resistance resides in the small arteries 100 to 300 μm in diameter. Because of important differences in the responses of the coronary arterioles and the resistance arteries, these vascular segments are discussed separately.

Coronary Arterioles

Regulation of coronary blood flow in response to changing myocardial needs occurs at the level of the coronary arterioles. The principal mechanism for coupling arteriolar vasomotor tone to myocardial metabolic demands involves ATP-sensitive potassium channels (K^+_{ATP}) in coronary vascular smooth muscle cells.[14–17] Opening of K^+_{ATP} channels results in outward flux of potassium from the cell that increases the sarcolemmal membrane potential. This hyperpolarization causes voltage-dependent calcium channels to close; the resultant decreased influx of calcium causes relaxation of the vascular smooth muscle and vasodilatation.[14] Inhibition of K^+_{ATP} channel opening with glibenclamide has been demonstrated to impair coronary autoregulation, metabolic vasoregulation, and ischemic vasodilatation.[15, 16] Thus, decreases of coronary perfusion pressure result in vasodilatation of the coronary arterioles, which is abolished by inhibition of K^+_{ATP} opening.[15] In contrast, reductions of coronary perfusion pressure cause a decrease in the diameter of the resistance arteries, indicating passive collapse of these vessels with no response to the metabolic state of the myocardium. In addition, blockade of K^+_{ATP} channels causes a decrease of coronary blood flow that results in impaired contractile performance and metabolic evidence of ischemia.[16, 17] These findings demonstrate that K^+_{ATP} channel activity is essential for coupling of coronary blood flow to myocardial metabolic demands. The mechanism responsible for regulation of K^+_{ATP} channel activity during physiologic conditions is unclear. These channels open in response to marked decreases of intracellular ATP, increases of adenosine diphosphate (ADP), or both. Such marked alterations of high-energy phosphates can occur during ischemia, but they cannot account for coronary vasodilatation that occurs during physiologic increases of myocardial oxygen demands during exercise or other stress.

Adenosine has been suggested as a mediator of metabolic coronary vasodilatation.[18] When cardiac work is increased, the rate of ATP utilization by the contractile apparatus transiently exceeds the rate of resynthesis of ATP through oxidative phosphorylation, resulting in an increase of free ADP. Adenylate kinase can then act on two molecules of ADP to form one molecule each of ATP and adenosine monophosphate (AMP). AMP released by this reaction can be catabolized to adenosine, which can be transported out of the cell into the interstitial fluid. Adenosine in the interstitial fluid can engage specific receptors on the coronary smooth muscle cell membrane to cause vasodilatation.[18] Adenosine can be reassimilated by the myocardial myocytes for reincorporation into the adenine nucleotide pool or can be deaminated to inosine, which has little vasodilator activity. These reactions occur very quickly, so that the half-life of adenosine is only a few seconds. The vasodilator effects of adenosine can be inhibited by methyl xanthines such as theophylline that act as adenosine receptor blockers.

Adenosine exerts its vasodilator effect, at least in part, by causing opening of ATP-sensitive potassium channels.[19] However, adenosine receptor blockade does not interfere with the normal increase in myocardial blood flow during exercise or other increases of oxygen demands, suggesting that adenosine is not a principal mediator of metabolic vasoregulation.[20] However, adenosine production increases markedly during ischemia and contributes to vasodilatation of the coronary resistance vessels in ischemic myocardial regions. Other perturbations that occur during ischemia, including accumulation of hydrogen ion and lactate, can also cause coronary vasodilatation, but these changes are not likely to contribute to regulation of arteriolar tone during physiologic conditions. Decreases of arterial oxygen tension and increases of carbon dioxide tension exert vasodilator effects on coronary resistance vessels, with evidence for a synergistic interaction between these variables.[21] Oxygen diffusion out of the coronary microvessels occurs so rapidly that oxygen tensions in arterioles and even small arteries are lower than in coronary artery blood, suggesting a direct role for oxygen in the local regulation of blood flow.[22]

Myogenic Mechanisms

Myogenic automaticity refers to the intrinsic property of smooth muscle to respond to stretch with a counteracting increase in contractile force. Thus, an increase in intraluminal distending pressure causes the vascular smooth muscle to contract, whereas a decrease in pressure results in vasodilatation. Myogenic activity is an intrinsic property of coronary arterioles less than 125 μm in diameter and is not altered by endothelial denudation.[23] Myogenic responses to changes of intraluminal pressure are more prominent in arterioles from the subepicardium than from the subendocardium of the left ventricle, suggesting that intrinsic differences in responsiveness could contribute to the lesser ability to autoregulate in the subendocardium.[24] Although myogenic activity can be demonstrated in isolated coronary arterioles, the contribution of myogenic mechanisms to regulation of blood flow in the intact heart is probably of less importance than metabolic or endothelium-mediated responses.

Resistance Arteries

The small arteries (100 to 300 μm in diameter) contribute up to 40 percent of total coronary resistance, but unlike the arterioles, these vessels are not responsive to the metabolic state of the myocardium.[25] However, when increased cardiac activity results in metabolic vasodilatation of the coronary arterioles, the resultant increase of blood flow causes shear-mediated endothelium-dependent dilatation of the resistance arteries. However, in patients in whom hyperlipidemia, atherosclerosis, or hypertension has resulted in endothelial dysfunction, it is probable that flow-mediated dilatation of the resistance arteries is impaired. Loss of flow-mediated vasodilatation of the resistance arteries could impair vasodilator reserve even in the absence of occlusive coronary artery disease. This is supported by the finding that vasodilator reserve measured with positron emission tomography is impaired in patients with hyperlipidemia but with angiographically normal coronary arteries and that this abnormality can be corrected by lipid-lowering therapy.[26]

The penetrating arteries are a distinct group of arterial

vessels that deliver blood from the epicardial arteries to the subendocardial microvasculature. Estes and coworkers[27] divided the intramyocardial arteries into two classes. *Class A arteries* arborize soon after entering the myocardium and supply principally the outer two thirds of the left ventricular wall, whereas *class B arteries* penetrate deep into the myocardium before arborizing to supply blood to the subendocardium. The class B vessels are also called *penetrating arteries*. The potential influence of the penetrating arteries on blood flow is documented by the finding that pressure in arterioles in the subendocardium is less than in subepicardial arterioles, indicating that a significant pressure loss occurs across the penetrating arteries.[28] Furthermore, vasomotor activity of the penetrating arteries can selectively influence blood flow to the subendocardium. Although the small arteries that supply the subepicardium could also influence blood flow, their contribution to subepicardial resistance is less than the contribution of the penetrating arteries to subendocardial resistance. Vasodilatation of the penetrating arteries appears to be a mechanism by which nitroglycerin can selectively augment blood flow to the subendocardium in ischemic myocardial regions.[29]

ENDOTHELIUM-DEPENDENT VASODILATATION

Nitric Oxide

The importance of the vascular endothelium in mediating vasodilator responses was first demonstrated by Furchgott and Zawadski,[30] who observed that acetylcholine caused relaxation of isolated coronary artery rings when the endothelium was intact but produced contraction when the endothelium was removed. Subsequent studies demonstrated that a number of agonists, including acetylcholine, bradykinin, histamine, and thrombin, cause coronary vasodilatation indirectly by engaging specific receptors on the endothelium that trigger the release of one or more endothelium-derived relaxing factors.[21] The principal mediator of this vasodilatation is NO, which is produced when the constitutive endothelial cell enzyme nitric oxide synthase (eNOS) acts on arginine to produce citrulline with liberation of NO.[31] eNOS is a calcium-calmodulin–dependent cytochrome P-450 enzyme. Agonists that produce endothelium-dependent NO-mediated vasodilatation act by causing increases of intracellular calcium to activate the enzyme.[31] NO produced by eNOS can diffuse into the vascular smooth muscle, where it results in activation of guanylate cyclase. The resultant increase in cyclic guanosine monophosphate causes relaxation of the vascular smooth muscle.[32] The shearing force of blood flow can also activate eNOS, providing a physiologic mechanism by which coronary arteries undergo vasodilatation in response to increased blood flow during exercise or other stress.[31] Coronary NO production has been shown to increase during exercise, and direct measurements of epicardial coronary artery diameter have demonstrated that normal coronary arteries undergo vasodilatation during exercise.[7] This response is mediated by NO, since blockade of NO production with N^G-nitro-L-arginine, a competitive blocker of NO production, prevented coronary artery dilatation during exercise.[33] eNOS is distinct from inducible nitric oxide synthase, which can be induced in many cells by cytokines and which is not regulated by the intracellular calcium content.

Endothelium-dependent NO-mediated coronary vasodilatation is impaired in the setting of hyperlipidemia or atherosclerosis. Impairment of NO-dependent vasodilatation appears to result from increased oxygen free radical production in the atherosclerotic vessel, which quenches NO, thereby attenuating its biologic actions.[32] There is some evidence that arginine administration can improve endothelium-dependent vasodilator mechanisms.[34] Since intracellular arginine is present in excess for eNOS activity, arginine deficiency is unlikely to directly limit NO production. However, circulating arginine analogues, such as asymmetric dimethylarginine, have been identified that can act as competitive inhibitors of arginine.[35] Arginine administration could potentially exert a beneficial effect by competition with these endogenous inhibitors of NO synthase.

Prostacyclin

Prostacyclin is a coronary vasodilator and potent inhibitor of platelet aggregation that is produced from arachidonic acid by vascular endothelial cells. Prostacyclin is synthesized by the enzyme cyclooxygenase, so that nonsteroidal anti-inflammatory agents that inhibit cyclooxygenase decrease prostacyclin production.[36] The rate-limiting step for prostacyclin synthesis appears to be the availability of arachidonic acid mobilized from membrane phospholipids by phospholipase A_2. Basal prostacyclin production in the coronary circulation is insufficient to be detected using current technology.[36] Prostacyclin is released in response to agonists that interact with specific endothelial cell surface receptors, including bradykinin, histamine, and thrombin, as well as by increased endothelial shear forces that cause release of calcium from intracellular stores, thereby activating phospholipase A_2.[37] Production of prostacyclin in response to these stimuli is transient even when the agonist is continuously present. Most evidence suggests that the principal role of prostacyclin is as an antiplatelet and antithrombotic molecule with only a modest influence on coronary vasomotor activity in the normal heart.

Hyperpolarizing Factor

Studies in isolated coronary vessels have demonstrated that the vasodilator effects of acetylcholine and certain other agonists that are dependent on intact endothelium cannot be fully accounted for by NO or prostacyclin. These agents cause hyperpolarization of the vascular smooth muscle cell membrane by opening of calcium activated potassium channels. Membrane hyperpolarization decreases calcium influx, thereby resulting in vasodilatation.[38] The mediators of this effect have been termed *endothelium-dependent hyperpolarizing factors*; current evidence suggests that they are cytochrome P-450–dependent metabolites of arachidonic acid. The extent to which endothelium-dependent hyperpolarizing factors contribute to regulation of coronary blood flow during physiologic conditions is unknown.

Transmural Distribution of Myocardial Blood Flow

In the normal heart, blood flow to the subendocardium is maintained 20 to 40 percent higher than flow to the subepicardium, reflecting greater systolic tension development and greater oxygen utilization in the subendocardium.[39] Maintenance of this perfusion gradient favoring the subendocardium requires active vasomotion of the coronary resistance vessels. During systole, the contracting myocardium compresses the thin-walled microvessels within the wall of the left ventricle. The interaction between the extravascular forces acting to collapse the vessels and the intravascular distending pressure, which resists collapse of the vessels, is termed the *vascular waterfall*.[40] Since the extravascular compressive forces increase from epicardium to endocardium, impedance to blood flow is greatest in the subendocardium. To compensate for underperfusion of the subendocardium during systole, during diastole vasomotor tone of the resistance vessels is maintained lower in the subendocardium than in the subepicardium. As a result, vasodilator reserve is lower in the subendocardium than in the subepicardium.[41]

In response to an arterial stenosis, the coronary resistance vessels undergo vasodilatation to compensate for the additional resistance caused by the stenosis. The need for vasodilatation to maintain blood flow during basal conditions compromises the ability for further vasodilatation to increase blood flow in response to exercise or other stress. A stenosis that is sufficiently severe to elicit maximal vasodilatation of the resistance vessels is termed a *critical stenosis,* inasmuch as an increase in myocardial metabolic demand cannot be met by an increase in blood flow, so that ischemia results. When a coronary stenosis limits blood flow below the metabolic demands of the myocardium, the limited arterial inflow is redistributed toward the subepicardium, so that hypoperfusion and ischemia are most severe in the subendocardium. This redistribution of blood flow away from the subendocardium initially occurs because vasodilator reserve is lowest in the subendocardium. In addition, ischemic vasodilatation of the coronary resistance vessels can result in a marked pressure drop across a stenosis. As distal coronary artery pressure falls, intramyocardial tissue pressure acts to compress the microvessels. Since intramyocardial pressure is highest in the subendocardium, impedance to blood flow is greatest in this region. Increases of left ventricular diastolic intracavitary pressure augment subendocardial compressive forces and amplify the redistribution of blood flow away from the subendocardium caused by a coronary stenosis.

Coronary Collateral Circulation

Normal human hearts possess a rudimentary network of intercoronary collateral anastomoses 20 to 300 μm in diameter.[42] These intrinsic collateral vessels, which are insufficient to limit myocardial injury during acute coronary occlusion, form a scaffold for the development of an effective collateral circulation in response to occlusive coronary artery disease.[42] Collateral vessel development is stimulated by hemodynamically significant coronary artery stenoses. If a coronary occlusion occurs gradually, sufficient time for collateral vessel development can prevent myocardial infarction, despite total coronary occlusion. High-grade coronary stenotic lesions are required to stimulate growth of well-developed collateral vessels. A stenosis causing less than 80 percent luminal narrowing is rarely associated with well-developed collaterals, whereas stenoses causing 95 percent narrowing are almost always associated with good collateral filling.[43] The rate of collateral development has been studied in patients hospitalized for acute myocardial infarction. Sequential coronary angiograms demonstrated that approximately half of patients developed an effective collateral circulation within 2 weeks and approximately two thirds by 2 months after acute coronary occlusion.[44] It is unclear whether collateral vessel growth proceeds at a similar rate in patients with high-grade coronary stenotic lesions and recurrent ischemia but without tissue necrosis.

Development of collateral vessels can proceed by sprouting of new vessels (angiogenesis) or by growth and remodeling of the rudimentary intercoronary anastomoses that exist in normal hearts (arteriogenesis).[45] Angiogenesis predominates in regions adjacent to infarcted myocardium, probably as the result of growth factors released from necrotic myocytes and recruited inflammatory cells. In contrast, collateral vessel growth in response to a coronary stenosis in the absence of infarct occurs principally through arteriogenesis.[46] It is probable that endothelial shearing forces trigger collateral vessel growth in response to a coronary stenosis. In the normal heart, there is little flow in the rudimentary collateral vessels, since blood pressure in adjacent coronary arteries is essentially equal. However, when a pressure drop occurs across a coronary stenosis, blood flow from the adjacent arteries flows through the rudimentary collateral vessels into the low-pressure vessel. The resultant endothelial shear causes expression of adhesion molecules that attract monocytes.[46] Activated monocytes can release growth factors that exert mitogenic effects on endothelial and smooth muscle cells, as well as proteases that break down extracellular matrix to provide space for the enlarging collateral vessels. Administration of recombinant basic fibroblast growth factor has been shown to accelerate collateral vessel growth in dogs subjected to coronary occlusion.[47] Vascular endothelial growth factor is an endothelial cell mitogen found in regions of collateral vessel growth; it has also been discovered to accelerate collateral vessel growth in animal models of coronary artery occlusion.[48]

Although marked collateral vessel growth can occur in response to coronary artery occlusion, vasodilator reserve is not normal in regions perfused by collateral vessels. Thus, developed collateral vessels can provide adequate arterial inflow to meet myocardial needs during resting conditions, but the ability to augment flow in response to exercise or other stress may be limited.[49] Furthermore, occlusive disease in the donor arteries from which collateral vessels originate can impair the ability to increase blood flow. Well-developed collateral vessels have a well-organized muscular media and are responsive to vasodilator and vasoconstrictor stimuli; as a result, collateral vessels do not behave as fixed conduits but can undergo vasomotor activity. Vasoconstriction of collateral vessels can worsen hypoperfusion of a collateral-dependent region of myocardium and lower the threshold for ischemia during exercise.[50, 51] In experimental animals, well-developed collateral vessels have intact endothelium-dependent vasodilator mechanisms, so that the increase in blood flow during exercise would be expected to cause flow-mediated collateral vessel dilatation.[52] However, if hyperlipidemia or hypertension has resulted in endothelial dysfunction, vasodilatation of the collateral vessels in response to increases of endothelial shear would be absent. Nitroglycerin is a potent collateral vessel dilator that has been demonstrated to improve exercise tolerance in patients with single-vessel coronary occlusion and a region of viable collateral-dependent myocardium.[51]

Coronary Steal

Coronary steal describes the situation in which resistance vessel dilatation causes an increase of coronary blood flow in one myocardial region but a paradoxical decrease in flow in an adjacent region. This phenomenon most commonly occurs when adjacent collateral-dependent and normally perfused myocardial regions derive their arterial blood supply from a common stenotic coronary artery. During basal conditions, the arterioles in the collateralized region must maintain sufficient vasodilatation to compensate for the resistance of the collateral vessels. As a result, the capacity for further vasodilatation is limited. In response to a stimulus for vasodilatation such as exercise, the arterioles in the collateralized region will achieve maximal vasodilatation at a time when the vessels in the normal region still have capacity for further vasodilatation. Because the resistance vessels in the normally perfused zone have a greater capacity for vasodilatation, flow will be preferentially shunted toward the normal region at the expense of the collateral-dependent region.[53] Any stimulus that causes resistance vessel dilatation, such as exercise or pharmacologic dilators such as adenosine or dipyridamole, can cause coronary steal.[54] Agents such as nitroglycerin that act to dilate the collateral vessels and proximal coronary arteries oppose the development of steal.

Left Ventricular Hypertrophy

Left ventricular hypertrophy is associated with structural and functional abnormalities of the coronary circulation. Myocardial hypertrophy is associated with increased vulnerability to ischemia during exercise or other stress. In patients with hypertension, left ventricular hypertrophy confers an increased risk for development of angina pectoris, congestive heart failure, and sudden death.[55] Furthermore, a coronary stenosis that limits arterial inflow during exercise causes more severe subendocardial hypoperfusion in animals with left ventricular hypertrophy than in normal animals.[56] Acute coronary occlusion results in infarction of a greater fraction of the myocardial region at risk and a higher incidence of sudden death in animals with left ventricular hypertrophy than in normal animals.[57] Epicardial coronary artery lumen diameter is increased in left ventricular hypertrophy, but this is less than expected for the increase in myocardial mass.[58] Maximal coronary flow rates per gram of myocardium are impaired in the hypertrophied heart. This impairment of maximal coronary flow results both from failure of the coronary vessels to grow in proportion to the increased myocardial mass and because of increased extravascular forces that act to compress the intramural coronary microvasculature.[59] The effects of the increased extravascular forces in the hypertrophied heart are most prominent in the subendocardium, so that exercise can result in transmural redistribution of blood flow away from the subendocardium even in the absence of atherosclerotic coronary artery disease. In patients with severe pressure overload hypertrophy, especially that resulting from aortic stenosis, the abnormalities of coronary perfusion can be sufficient to result in exertional angina pectoris even in the absence of occlusive coronary artery disease.

References

1. von Restorff W, Holtz J, Bassenge E: Exercise induced augmentation of myocardial oxygen extraction in spite of normal coronary dilatory capacity in dogs. Pflugers Arch 372:181–185, 1977.
2. Taegtmeyer H: Energy metabolism of the heart: from basic concepts to clinical applications. Curr Probl Cardiol 19:59–113, 1994.
3. Vatner W: Correlation between acute reductions in myocardial blood flow and function in conscious dogs. Circ Res 47:201–207, 1980.
4. Path G, Robitaille P-M, Merkle H, et al: Correlation between transmural high energy phosphate levels and myocardial blood flow in the presence of graded coronary stenosis. Circ Res 67:660–673, 1990.
5. Rooke GA, Feigl EO: Work as a correlate of canine left ventricular oxygen consumption, and the problem of catecholamine wasting. Circ Res 50:273–286, 1982.
6. Feigl EO: Coronary physiology. Physiol Rev 63:1–205, 1983.
7. Schwartz JS, Baran KW, Bache RJ: Effect of a stenosis on exercise-induced dilation of large coronary arteries. Am Heart J 119:520–524, 1990.
8. Wang J, Wolin MS, Hintze TH: Chronic exercise enhances endothelium-mediated dilation of epicardial coronary artery in conscious dogs. Circ Res 73:829–838, 1993.
9. Gordon JB, Ganz P, Nabel EG, et al: Atherosclerosis influences the vasomotor response of epicardial coronary arteries to exercise. J Clin Invest 83:1946–1952, 1989.
10. Brown BG, Bolson EL, Dodge HT: Dynamic mechanisms in human coronary stenosis. Circulation 70:917–922, 1984.
11. Schwartz JS, Bache RJ: Effect of arteriolar dilation on coronary artery diameter distal to coronary stenoses. Am J Physiol 249:H981–H988, 1985.
12. Gage JE, Hess OM, Murakami T, et al: Vasoconstriction of stenotic coronary arteries during dynamic exercise in patients with classic angina pectoris: reversibility by nitroglycerin. Circulation 73:865–876, 1986.
13. Jones CJH, DeFily DV, Patterson JL, Chilian WM: Endothelium-dependent relaxation competes with α_1- and α_2-adrenergic constriction in the canine epicardial coronary microcirculation. Circulation 87:1264–1274, 1993.
14. Standen NB, Quayle JM, Davies NW, et al: Hyperpolarizing vasodilators activate ATP-sensitive K^+ channels in arterial smooth muscle. Science 245:177–180, 1989.
15. Komaru T, Lamping KG, Eastham CL, Dellsperger KC: Role of ATP-sensitive potassium channels in coronary microvascular autoregulatory responses. Circ Res 69:1146–1151, 1991.
16. Duncker DJ, van Zon NS, Altman JD, et al: Role of K^+_{ATP} channels in coronary vasodilation during exercise. Circulation 88:1245–1253, 1993.
17. Samaha FF, Heineman FW, Ince C, et al: ATP-sensitive potassium channel is essential to maintain basal coronary vascular tone in vivo. Am J Physiol 262:C1220–C1227, 1992.

18. Berne RM, Rubio R: Regulation of coronary blood flow. Adv Cardiol 12:303–317, 1974.
19. Duncker DJ, van Zon NS, Pavek T, et al: Endogenous adenosine opposes hypoperfusion and loss of wall motion during exercise produced by K^+_{ATP} channel-blockade. J Clin Invest 95:285–295, 1995.
20. Bache RJ, Dai X-Z, Schwartz JS, Homans DC: Role of adenosine in coronary vasodilation during exercise. Circ Res 62:846–853, 1988.
21. Broten TP, Feigl EO: Role of myocardial oxygen and carbon dioxide in coronary autoregulation. Am J Physiol 262:H1231–H1237, 1992.
22. Duling BR, Berne RM: Longitudinal gradients in periarteriolar oxygen tension. A possible role for the participation of oxygen in local regulation of blood flow. Circ Res 28:669–678, 1970.
23. Muller JM, Davis MJ, Chilian WM: Integrated regulation of pressure and flow in the coronary microcirculation. Cardiovasc Res 32:668–678, 1996.
24. Kuo L, Davis MJ, Chilian WM: Myogenic activity in isolated subepicardial and subendocardial coronary arterioles. Am J Physiol 255:H1558–H1562, 1988.
25. Chilian WM, Eastham CL, Marcus ML: Microvascular distribution of coronary vascular resistance in beating left ventricle. Am J Physiol 251:H779–H788, 1986.
26. Czernin J, Barnard RJ, Sun KT, et al: Effect of short-term cardiovascular conditioning and low-fat diet on myocardial blood flow and flow reserve. Circulation 92:197–204, 1995.
27. Estes EH, Entman ML, Dixon HB, Hackel DB: The vascular supply of the left ventricular wall: Anatomic observations, plus a hypothesis regarding acute events in coronary artery disease. Am Heart J 171:58–67, 1966.
28. Chilian WM: Microvascular pressures and resistances in the left ventricular subepicardium and subendocardium. Circ Res 69:561–570, 1991.
29. Ishibashi Y, Mizrahi J, Duncker DJ, Bache RJ: The nitric oxide donor ITF 1129 augments subendocardial blood flow during exercise-induced myocardial ischemia. J Cardiovasc Pharmacol 30:374–382, 1997.
30. Furchgott RF, Zawadski JV: The obligatory role of endothelial cells in the relaxation of arterial smooth muscle by acetylcholine. Nature 288:373–376, 1980.
31. Bassenge E: Coronary vasomotor responses: role of endothelium and nitrovasodilators. Cardiovasc Drugs Ther 8:601–610, 1994.
32. Harrison DG, Venema RC, Arnal JF, et al: The endothelial cell nitric oxide synthase: is it really constitutively expressed? Agents Actions Suppl 45:107–117, 1995.
33. Bernstein RD, Ochoa Y, Xu X, et al: Function and production of nitric oxide in the coronary circulation of the conscious dog during exercise. Circ Res 79:840–848, 1996.
34. Creager MA, Gallagher SJ, Girerd XJ, et al: L-Arginine improves endothelium-dependent vasodilatation in hypercholesterolemic humans. J Clin Invest 90:1248–1253, 1992.
35. MacAllister RJ, Parry H, Kimoto M, et al: Regulation of nitric oxide synthesis by dimethylarginine dimethylaminohydrolase. Br J Pharmacol 119:1533–1540, 1996.
36. Carter TD, Pearson JD: Regulation of prostacyclin synthesis in endothelial cells. News Physiol Sci 7:64–69, 1992.
37. Allan TJ, Pearson JD, Needham L: Thrombin-stimulated elevation of endothelial cell cytoplasmic free calcium concentration causes prostacyclin production. Biochem J 257:243–249, 1988.
38. Quilley J, Fulton D, McGiff JC: Hyperpolarizing factors. Biochem Pharmacol 54:1059–1070, 1997.
39. Weiss HH, Neubauer JD, Lipp JD, Sinha AK: Quantitative determination of regional oxygen consumption in the dog heart. Circ Res 42:394–401, 1978.
40. Farhi ER, Klocke FJ, Mates RE, et al: Tone-dependent waterfall behavior during venous pressure elevation in isolated canine hearts. Circ Res 68:392–401, 1991.
41. Hoffman JIE: Determinants and prediction of transmural myocardial perfusion. Circulation 58:381–391, 1978.
42. Baroldi G, Scomazzoni G: Coronary Circulation in the Normal and Pathologic Heart. Washington DC: Armed Forces Institute of Pathology, 1967.
43. Cohen M, Sherman W, Rentrop KP, Gorlin R: Determinants of collateral filling observed during sudden controlled coronary artery occlusion in human subjects. J Am Coll Cardiol 13:297–303, 1989.
44. Schwartz H, Leiboff RH, Bren GB, et al: Temporal evolution of the human coronary collateral circulation after myocardial infarction. J Am Coll Cardiol 4:1088–1093, 1984.
45. Schaper W, Schaper J (eds): Collateral Circulation. Norwell, MA: Kluwer Academic, 1993.
46. Schaper W, Ito WD: Molecular mechanisms of coronary collateral vessel growth. Circ Res 79:911–919, 1996.
47. Lazarous DF, Shou M, Scheinowitz M, et al: Comparative effects of basic fibroblast growth factor and vascular endothelial growth factor on coronary collateral development and the arterial response to injury. Circulation 94:1074–1082, 1996.
48. Banai S, Jaklitsch MT, Shou M, et al: Angiogenic-induced enhancement of collateral blood flow to ischemic myocardium by vascular endothelial growth factor in dogs. Circulation 89:2183–2189, 1994.
49. Bache RJ, Schwartz JS: Myocardial blood flow during exercise after gradual coronary occlusion in the dog. Am J Physiol 245:131–138, 1983.
50. Foreman BW, Dai XZ, Bache RJ: Vasoconstriction of canine coronary collateral vessels with vasopressin limits blood flow to collateral-dependent myocardium during exercise. Circ Res 69:657–664, 1991.
51. Pupita G, Maseri A, Kaski JC, et al: Myocardial ischemia caused by distal coronary-artery constriction in stable angina pectoris. N Engl J Med 323:514–520, 1990.
52. Altman J, Dulas D, Pavek T, et al: Endothelial function in well developed canine coronary collateral vessels. Am J Physiol 264:H567–H572, 1993.
53. Bache RJ, Duncker DJ: Coronary Steal. ACC Curr J Rev 3:9–12, 1994.
54. Bache RJ: Effect of exercise and pharmacologic interventions on coronary collateral blood flow. *In* Schaper W, Schaper J (eds): Collateral Circulation. pp. 173–194. Norwell, MA: Kluwer Academic, 1993.
55. Koren MJ, Devereaux RB, Casale PN, et al: Relation of left ventricular mass of geometry to morbidity and mortality in uncomplicated essential hypertension. Ann Intern Med 114:345–352, 1991.
56. Bache RJ, Wright L, Laxson DL, Dai X: Effect of a coronary stenosis on myocardial blood flow during exercise in the chronically pressure overloaded hypertrophied left ventricle. Circulation 81:1967–1973, 1990.
57. Mueller TM, Tomanek RJ, Kerber RE, Marcus ML: Myocardial infarction in dogs with chronic hypertension and left ventricular hypertrophy. Am J Physiol 239:H731–H735, 1980.
58. Imball BP, LiPreti V, Bui S, Wigle EG: Comparison of proximal left anterior descending and circumflex coronary artery dimensions in aortic valve stenosis and hypertrophic cardiomyopathy. Am J Cardiol 65:767–771, 1990.
59. Duncker DJ, Zhang J, Pavek TJ, et al: Effect of exercise on the coronary pressure-flow relationship in the hypertrophied left ventricle. Am J Physiol 269:H271–H281, 1995.

CHAPTER 26

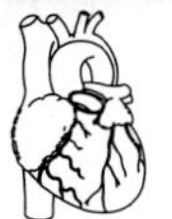

Pathophysiology and Clinical Recognition of Coronary Artery Disease Syndromes

James T. Willerson and Attilio Maseri

STABLE ANGINA
Pathophysiology
Physical Examination/Bedside Findings
UNSTABLE ANGINA
Pathophysiology
Physical Examination/Bedside Findings
VARIANT ANGINA ("PRINZMETAL'S ANGINA")
ACUTE MYOCARDIAL INFARCTION
UNSTABLE ATHEROSCLEROTIC PLAQUE
Pathophysiology
Clinical Recognition of Myocardial Infarction
Differential Diagnosis
Estimation of Infarct Size
Evaluation of Ventricular Function
Prognosis

Stable Angina

Pathophysiology

The coronary heart disease syndromes are listed in Table 26–1. *Angina pectoris* is the clinical term used to describe chest pain resulting from a relative oxygen deficiency in heart muscle. Heberden[1] named this entity when he identified a "disorder of the breast marked with strong and peculiar symptoms and considerable for the kind of danger belonging to it" associated with a "strangling and anxiety," which he suggested should be called "angina pectoris." This description was enlarged on by Herrick in 1912.[2] Angina is usually described by the patient as a left precordial tightness or ache provoked by exercise or emotion and relieved by rest. Angina occurs when oxygen demand exceeds supply.[3–7] Most individuals with angina have underlying atherosclerotic coronary artery disease (CAD) (Figs. 26–1 and 26–2). However, angina may also develop in some patients with ventricular hypertrophy, left ventricular (LV) outflow obstruction, severe aortic valvular regurgitation or stenosis, cardiomyopathy, or dilated ventricle(s) in whom coronary artery stenoses are not present. The explanation for the occurrence of angina when CAD is not present is that even normal coronary arteries may not adequately supply hypertrophied, dilated, or failing heart muscle with oxygen. On occasion, a limited coronary vasodilator reserve may explain angina, especially in some patients with ventricular hypertrophy associated with LV outflow obstruction, including valvular aortic stenosis and hypertrophic obstructive cardiomyopathy, and in patients with poorly controlled systemic arterial hypertension.[8, 9] Coronary artery vasoconstriction occurring with exercise or stress may also be a contributing factor.[10, 11] Most humans without coronary heart disease or ventricular hypertrophy do not develop angina, probably because the heart is protected from an important imbalance between oxygen supply and demand by other factors that limit physical activity, such as dyspnea and fatigue.

The predisposing pathologic alteration in coronary arteries responsible for angina is atherosclerosis, atherothrombosclerosis, and neointimal fibrous proliferation (Fig. 26–3; see also Figs. 26–1 and 26–2). These terms describe the relative importance of each of the components of atherothrombosclerosis, including atherothrombosis and fibroproliferation, in the development of the process that has long been called *atherosclerosis* but, in fact, very often includes evidence of thrombosis in the progressive atherosclerotic plaque. Embolic atherosclerotic debris and platelet aggregates almost certainly play a role in more distal coronary artery occlusion and limitation of coronary flow reserve (see Fig. 26–3). Severe narrowing of the lumen of the coronary artery results in a decreased ability to deliver oxygen, especially when oxygen demand in the heart is increased, as with increases in heart rate, contractile state, or myocardial wall tension, or a combination of these.[3–7] Therefore, angina may develop during exercise, cold exposure, or emotional stress or after eating a large meal. Angina may also occur because of extracardiac influences.

TABLE 26–1 **Coronary Heart Disease Syndromes**

Stable angina pectoris
Unstable angina pectoris
Variant angina ("Prinzmetal's angina")
Acute myocardial infarction
"Non–Q wave" (usually nontransmural infarcts)
"Q wave" (usually transmural myocardial infarcts)

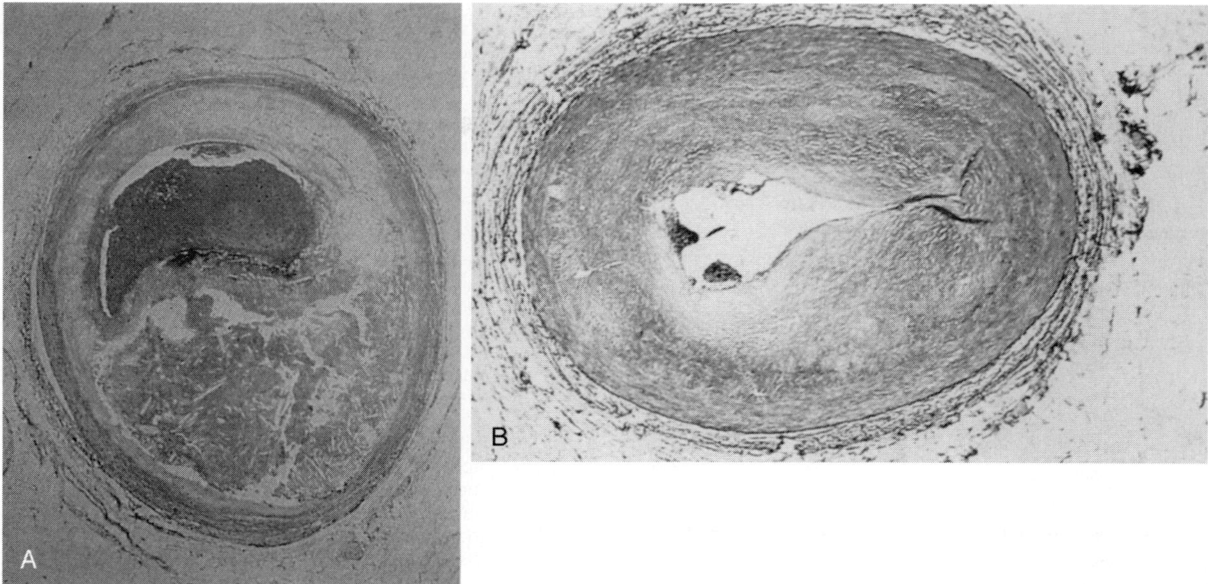

FIGURE 26–1 **A,** A typical atherosclerotic plaque in which plaque has ruptured, leading to the development of coronary artery thrombosis. Such a patient may or may not have had angina at effort before the plaque rupture and thrombosis, and may have abruptly developed severe chest pain and a myocardial infarction (MI) with plaque rupture and coronary artery thrombosis. **B,** The neointimal proliferation occurring with restenosis after coronary artery angioplasty, leading to coronary artery luminal diameter narrowing and the need for some additional revascularization procedure is shown. Patients who develop coronary heart disease after cardiac transplantation also demonstrate this same alteration in their coronary arteries (i.e., neointimal proliferation). Native atheromas have substantial fibroproliferative alterations as well. (**A,** From Becker AE, Anderson RH: Cardiac Pathology. London: Gower Medical, 1988. **B,** From Hurst JW, Anderson RH, Becker AE, et al: Atlas of the Heart. p. 63. New York: Gower Medical, 1988.)

In particular, severe anemia or carbon monoxide exposure limits the capacity of the blood to carry or release oxygen and may result in angina under conditions that would otherwise be well tolerated. Increases in systemic arterial pressure and consequent dilatation of the heart may result in angina. Increases in heart rate or contractile state, as with hyperthyroidism, pheochromocytoma, and exogenous administration or release of catecholamines, may also lead to angina. Cold exposure decreases oxygen delivery by causing coronary artery vasoconstriction and increases systemic blood pressure, ventricular wall tension, and oxygen demand.

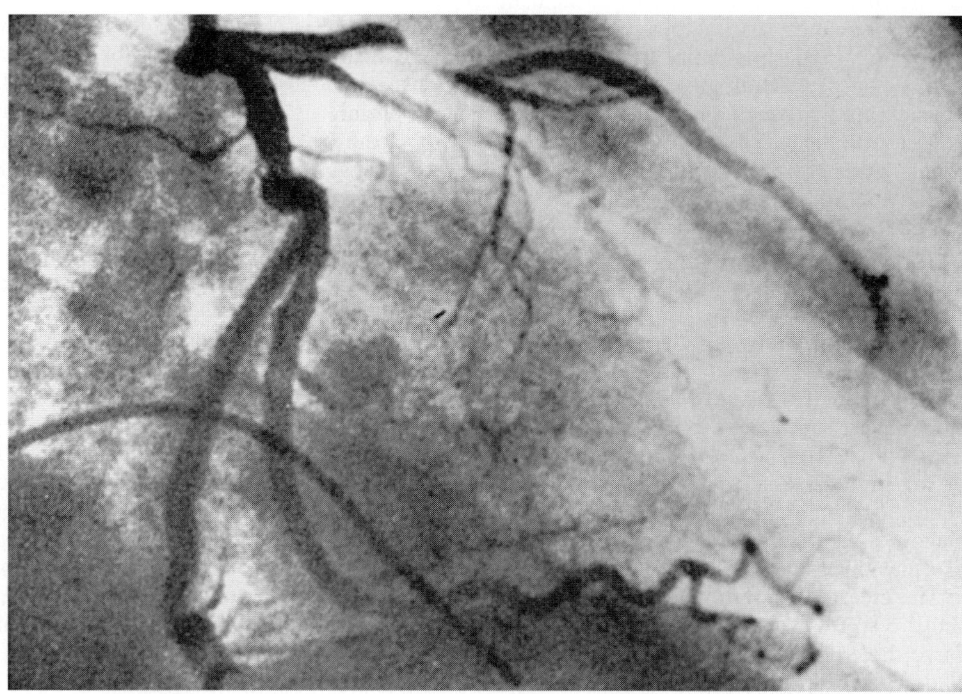

FIGURE 26–2 Typical narrowing and occlusion of the coronary artery by atherosclerosis in patients with unstable angina and MI. In many other patients, the severity of the left anterior descending coronary artery stenosis is less than that demonstrated in this right anterior oblique projection of the left coronary artery by coronary arteriography. (From Willerson JT: Treatment of Heart Disease. New York: Gower Medical, 1992.)

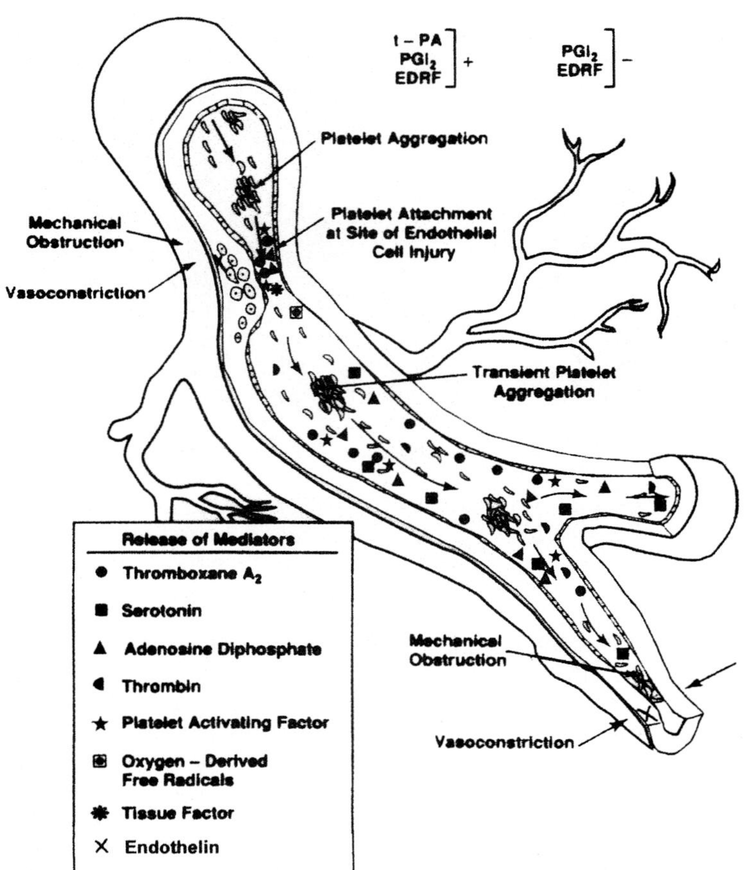

FIGURE 26–3 Schematic diagram suggests probable mechanisms responsible for the conversion from chronic coronary heart disease to acute coronary artery disease syndromes. In this scheme, endothelial injury, generally at sites of atherosclerotic plaques and usually plaque ulceration or fissuring, is associated with platelet adhesion and aggregation and the release and activation of selected mediators, including thromboxane A_2, serotonin, adenosine diphosphate, platelet-activating factor, thrombin, oxygen-derived free radicals, and endothelin. Local accumulation of thromboxane A_2, serotonin, platelet-activating factor, thrombin, adenosine diphosphate, and tissue factor promotes platelet aggregation. Thromboxane A_2, serotonin, thrombin, and platelet activating factor are vasoconstrictors at sites of endothelial injury. Therefore, the conversion from chronic stable to acute unstable coronary heart disease syndromes is usually associated with endothelial injury, platelet aggregation, accumulation of platelet and other cell-derived mediators, further platelet aggregation, and vasoconstriction, with consequent dynamic narrowing of the coronary artery lumen. In addition to atherosclerotic plaque fissuring or ulceration, other reasons for endothelial injury include flow shear stress, hypertension, immune complex deposition and complement activation, infection, and mechanical injury to the endothelium as it occurs with coronary artery angioplasty and after heart transplantation. EDRF, endothelium-derived relaxing factor, PGI_2, prostaglandin I_2; t-PA, tissue-type plasminogen activator. (From Willerson JT: Treatment of Heart Disease. New York: Gower Medical, 1992; modified from Willerson JT, Golino P, Eidt JF, et al: Specific platelet mediators and unstable coronary artery lesions. Experimental evidence and potential clinical implications. Circulation 80:198, 1989.)

Physical Examination/Bedside Findings

The findings on physical examination in the patient with stable angina pectoris are highly variable. Sometimes, there are no localizing or suggestive physical findings. Alternatively, associated risk factors such as systemic arterial hypertension, hyperlipidemia, valvular heart disease, heart failure, or peripheral atherosclerosis result in a specific physical finding, such as elevated blood pressure, a prominent fourth heart sound (S_4), accentuated aortic closure sound, a paradoxically split second heart sound (S_2) (systemic arterial hypertension during an episode of angina or reflecting left bundle branch block [LBBB]), reduced peripheral pulse (i.e., carotid, femoral, or lower extremity pulse with or without bruit over the artery [atherosclerosis]), murmur of aortic stenosis or mitral insufficiency (the most commonly associated valvular heart disease with CAD), or a third heart sound (S_3) with heart failure or rapid filling of the ventricle, such as occurs with moderately severe and severe mitral insufficiency. Thus, the patient with coronary heart disease and stable angina may or may not have an enlarged heart, frequent or complex ventricular premature beats, S_4, murmur of mitral insufficiency, S_3 and moist rales, and/or evidence of peripheral vascular disease.

The electrocardiogram (ECG) may be normal, or it may show ST-T wave changes, usually ST depression and T wave flattening or inversion. When the ECG demonstrates changes, it often varies on different ECGs, with intermittent normalization and return to the abnormal pattern. On occasion, the ST-T wave depression or inverted T waves persist for weeks or longer, presumably reflecting chronic ischemia. The ECG may also demonstrate ventricular ectopic beats or evidence of a prior Q wave myocardial infarction (MI). An echocardiogram may be normal at rest or may show regional or global wall motion abnormalities, including reduced left ventricular ejection fraction or increased LV dimensions, consistent with myocardial ischemia or infarction, or mitral insufficiency. Chest x-ray may show a normal-sized or enlarged heart with or without heart failure. On occasion, one sees coronary artery calcification on the chest x-ray.

Rapid-speed computed tomography (CT) (or electron beam [EB] CT) identifies coronary artery calcification. Several studies[12–16] have shown that coronary calcium assessment using fluoroscopy or EB CT imaging has a sensitivity for significant angiographic stenoses comparable with that of exercise tests when used with symptomatic patients, but the specificity is lower. Symptomatic patients with coronary calcium have at least a fourfold increased risk of death or infarction when compared with those with less or no calcification. The fluoroscopic finding of at least one calcified coronary artery or the EB CT identification of a coronary calcium score exceeding 100 has been shown to be predictive of the presence of advanced coronary plaque and stenosis. This may be useful in making subsequent decisions about the need for invasive studies. In general, greater degrees of calcification in coronary arteries are consistent with greater amounts of atherosclerotic plaque and more advanced coronary luminal diameter narrowing. An advantage of an assessment of coronary artery calcium is that it can be done irrespective of the patient's ability to exercise to a maximal level and regardless of the presence or absence of resting electrocardiographic abnormalities. However, the most valuable finding in the symptomatic patient is a negative EB CT study for coronary calcium. The negative predictive value of such a calcium scan for significant stenosis of a major coronary artery is greater than 90 percent. Thus, EB CT scanning might be an appropriate first test in individuals with atypical cardiac symptoms in whom the likelihood for ischemic disease is considered to be small by the responsible physician. Patients with a zero or very low calcium score (i.e., <10) may be reassured and further testing directed at noncardiac etiologies of chest pain. On the other hand, if the calcium score is consistent with moderate or severe atherosclerotic plaque development, additional cardiac evaluation, including stress testing with or without perfusion or functional evaluation, may be indicated.

Asymptomatic individuals differ from symptomatic patients in that the risk of subsequent morbid events is relatively small. Data available at this time are not yet conclusive regarding the ability of coronary calcification in asymptomatic individuals to predict short-term coronary artery risks.[12] Figure 26–4 demonstrates, however, that prevalence-risk relationships decrease with age. Although serious overprediction may occur in the young, overprediction is only moderate in the elderly.

Hemodynamic monitoring typically shows increases in mean pulmonary capillary wedge pressure during angina pectoris. With the onset of myocardial ischemia, the initial hemodynamic change in the left ventricle is a decrease in myocardial compliance and an increase in stiffness. This results in a sharp increase in mean pulmonary capillary wedge pressure during angina, with a return to baseline as the angina resolves. The change in compliance is followed by ST-T wave changes on the ECG, a decline in regional systolic wall thickening, and finally, the development of chest pain, with this entire sequence occurring within a few seconds.

Unstable Angina

Pathophysiology

Angina occurring in a crescendo pattern, with limited physical activity or at rest, is known as *unstable angina*. The chest discomfort is typically milder than that occurring with acute MI, being described as recurrent chest or epigastric "tightness" or "pressure" and as usually "not severe" in character. Typically, the episodes of angina last less than 30 minutes; they may or may not be associated with nausea. On occasion, however, unstable angina is associated with more severe and prolonged chest pain or nausea, making its differentiation from acute MI at the bedside difficult. In these situations, serial ECGs and measurement of serum creatine kinase (CK) and its relatively specific cardiac isoenzyme, CK-MB, and of troponin I are needed to distinguish unstable angina from acute MI.

Unstable angina is usually caused by a primary decrease in coronary blood flow and myocardial oxygen delivery that occurs as a consequence of atherosclerotic plaque fissuring or ulceration (or other injury).[17–20] The atherosclerotic plaque fissuring or ulceration is followed by platelet adhesion and aggregation at the site of plaque disruption and transient thrombosis and dynamic vasoconstriction. Platelet adhesion occurs by platelet attachment to exposed collagen and to von Willebrand binding sites largely through platelet glycoprotein Ib receptors. Thrombosis and vasoconstriction are promoted by the local accumulation of powerful promoters of platelet aggregation and vasoconstriction at these same sites, including thromboxane A_2, serotonin, adenosine diphosphate, selected leukotrienes, platelet-activating factor, thrombin, oxygen-derived free radicals, and endothelin (see Fig. 26–3).[17–38] Unstable angina may also occur in the individual with a severe coronary artery stenosis or partially occluded coronary artery

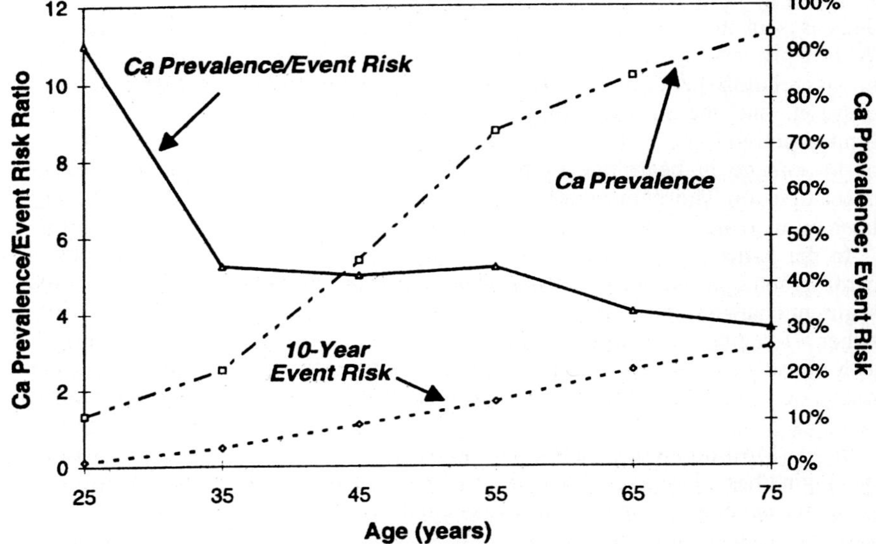

FIGURE 26–4 Coronary artery calcium prevalence, 10-year event risk, and prevalence/risk ratio in asymptomatic men. Event risk and calcium prevalence are plotted against the right axis, and prevalence/risk ratio is plotted against the left axis. Prevalence/risk curve decreases with age, demonstrating serious overprediction in the young and moderate overprediction in the elderly. (From Wexler L, Brundage B, Crouse J, et al: Coronary artery calcification: pathophysiology, epidemiology, imaging methods, and clinical implications. Circulation 94[5]:1175–1192, 1996.)

when myocardial oxygen demand is increased by intense emotion, tachycardia, or systemic hypertension. Alternatively, unstable angina may occur as a result of reduction in myocardial blood flow associated with severe and progressive coronary artery atherosclerosis or dynamic coronary artery constriction associated with coronary artery spasm.[39, 40]

Physical Examination/Bedside Findings

The patient with unstable angina and angina at rest typically appears concerned. Findings on physical examination are similar to those in the patient with stable angina. There may be no localizing finding or the patient may have an audible S_4, cardiac enlargement, congestive heart failure (CHF), mitral insufficiency, or evidence of peripheral vascular disease.

The resting ECG between episodes of unstable angina may be normal or may show the same ST-T wave changes or prior MI found in the patient with stable angina. However, typically the ECG demonstrates ST-T wave changes during rest angina, usually ST depression or T wave flattening or inversion in the electrocardiographic leads, reflecting myocardial perfusion of the "culprit" artery. These same electrocardiographic changes are usually found in the patient with non–Q wave MI, thereby making it impossible to distinguish unstable angina and non–Q wave MI electrocardiographically. On occasion, episodes of unstable angina are not associated with recognizable ST-T wave changes on the ECG, but this is very unusual.

Echocardiographic findings are as highly variable as in the patient with stable angina, but they may include reversible or fixed reductions in regional wall motion or global LV functional abnormalities. In some patients, reductions in regional wall motion occur with episodes of rest angina and resolve as the angina resolves.

The chest x-ray also shows great variability in findings from a normal-sized heart to cardiomegaly with CHF, just as is true in the patient with stable angina. Hemodynamic findings are similar to those during angina in the patient with stable angina.

Coronary artery spasm leads to abrupt and dynamic decreases in myocardial oxygen delivery (Fig. 26–5).[39, 40] With a primary decrease in coronary blood flow, there is no association between the development of angina and exertion, and the majority of anginal episodes occur at limited activity and rest. These patients usually have little or no change in heart rate or blood pressure before the onset of pain. The pain occurs first and may be followed later by increased blood pressure or heart rate.

In the patient with unstable angina, continuous electrocardiographic monitoring often documents transient ST-segment change immediately before the onset of chest pain, either ST-segment elevation indicating transmural ischemia as a consequence of spasm in a major epicardial coronary artery or platelet-initiated transient coronary artery thrombosis (see Figs. 26–3 and 26–5) or ST-segment depression.[41, 42] Most commonly, however, the patient with unstable angina has ST-segment depression when subendocardial ischemia develops as a result of transient thrombosis and vasoconstriction-induced narrowing of a coronary artery with flow distribution to the subendocardial region of the heart. In some individuals, ST-segment alterations occur in the absence of chest pain; this is referred to as *silent ischemia*. Silent ischemia has the same prognosis as painful episodes of ischemia.[41–43]

VARIANT ANGINA ("PRINZMETAL'S ANGINA")

Patients with variant angina pectoris ("Prinzmetal's angina") have angina at rest, often in the early morning hours, associated with ST-segment elevation on the ECG and the presence of coronary artery spasm, that is, focal obliteration of a coronary artery lumen (see Fig. 26–5).[39, 40]

In the early descriptions of typical angina, Latham[44] and Osler[45] suggested that this entity was due to periodic spasm of a large coronary artery. Subsequently, however, clinical studies with anatomic correlations suggested that fixed atherosclerotic CAD was responsible for typical angina and MI. In 1959, Prinzmetal and coworkers[46] revived interest in coronary arterial spasm when they described a group of individuals with "variant angina." The clinical features of this syndrome are distinctly different from those of typical angina.[39, 46–57] First, the patients described by Prinzmetal and coworkers[46] usually had chest pain at rest rather than with physical exertion or emotional stimulation. Second, the episodes of pain tended to recur at roughly the same time every day, often during the early morning hours, awakening the patient from sleep. Third, the patient with variant angina usually had ST-segment elevation on the ECG recorded during chest pain (see Fig. 26–5). Fourth, the episodes of chest pain were sometimes accompanied by atrioventricular block or ventricular ectopic activity, and occasionally, the patients had transient ventricular tachycardia. Finally, the chest discomfort of variant angina was quickly relieved by nitroglycerin, after which the ST-segment elevation resolved. Prinzmetal's patients did not undergo selective coronary arteriography, but Prinzmetal and coworkers[46] hypothesized that patients with variant angina had severe proximal stenoses of one or more large coronary arteries in which spasm occurred periodically. Since the original description of variant angina by Prinzmetal and coworkers, many observers[46–57] have confirmed the existence of this syndrome and have shown the presence of coronary artery spasm at sites of fixed coronary artery stenosis and in regions of the coronary vasculature where no obvious stenosis exists. In patients with clinically active coronary artery spasm, variant angina can often be induced by ergonovine maleate.[58–68] Other maneuvers that have been used to produce coronary artery spasm in susceptible patients include hyperventilation with the administration of an alkaline buffer, cold pressor testing, and the administration of methacholine, a parasympathomimetic agent, acetylcholine, or serotonin.[63, 66–73] We have speculated that endothelial or adventitial injury, often in association with coronary artery stenosis, leads to the accumulation of platelets and white blood cells, mononuclear cells, including mast cells, and T cells, and the release of humoral mediators, including serotonin, thromboxane A_2, prostaglandin D_2, thrombin, leukotrienes, platelet-activating factor, endothelin, or histamine, which singly or in combina-

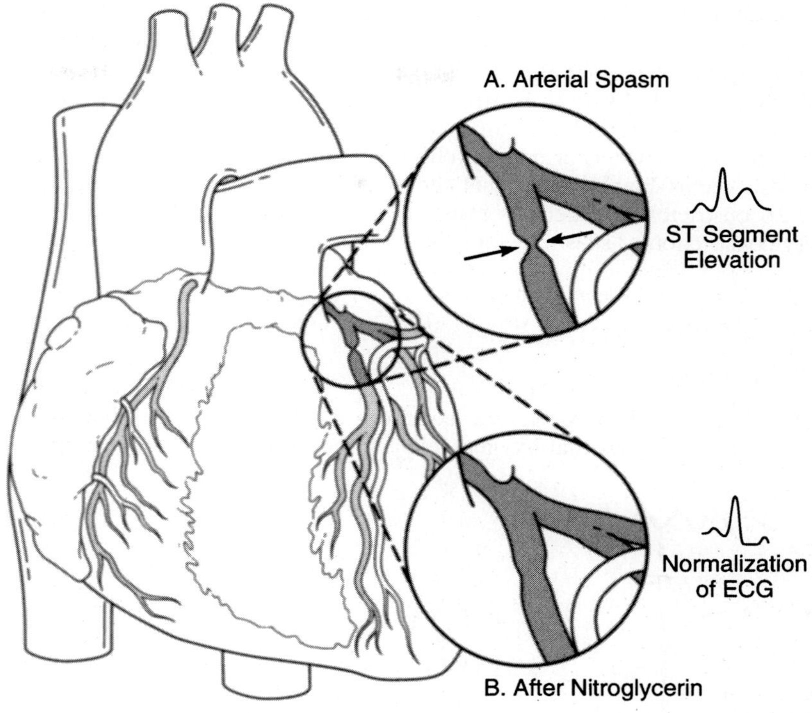

Channel 1

Channel 2

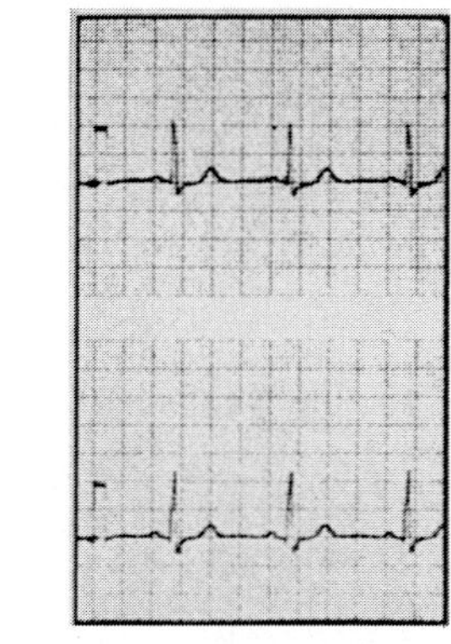

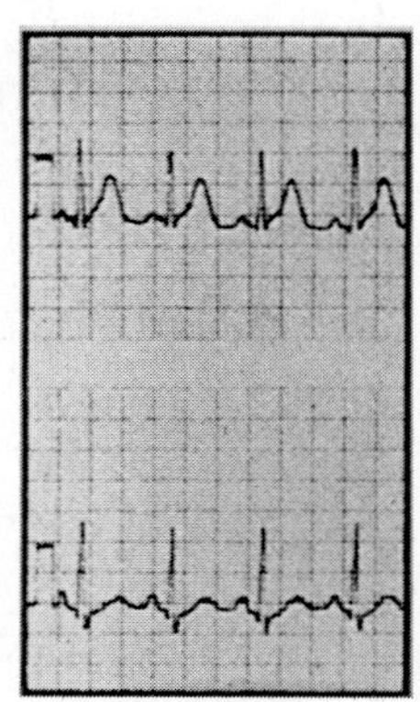

Channel 1

Channel 2

C

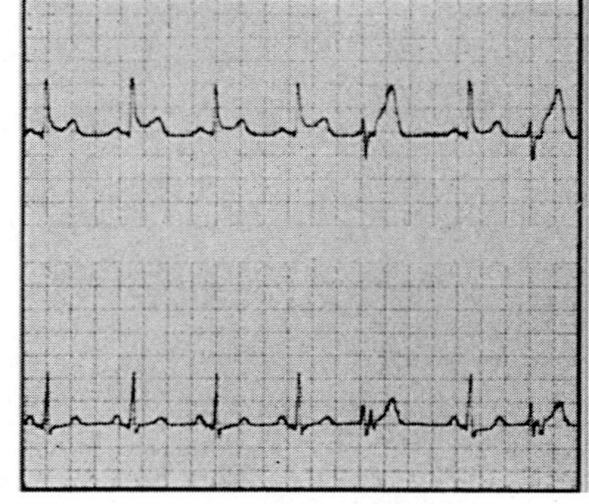

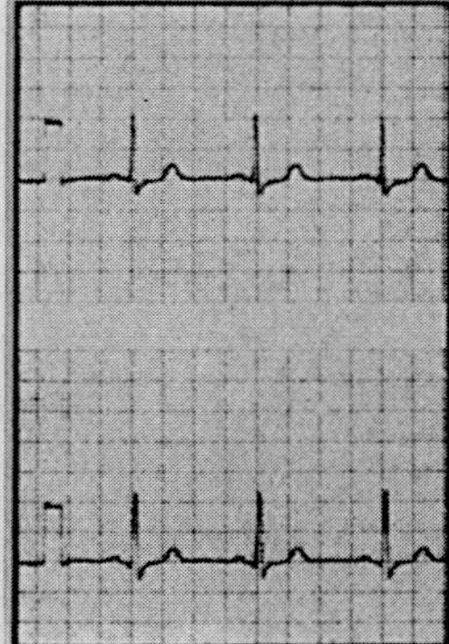

FIGURE 26–5 **A,** Focal obliteration of the coronary artery lumen caused by coronary artery spasm at a spot marked by the *arrows. Inset,* The associated ST-segment elevation that occurs with coronary artery spasm. **B,** Resolution of the coronary artery spasm after administration of nitroglycerin. *Inset,* Normalization of the electrocardiogram (ECG). **C,** Continuous 24-hour Holter recording in a patient with coronary artery spasm before chest pain *(top two panels),* as chest pain begins *(top right panel),* during chest pain *(bottom left panel),* and with pain relief *(bottom right panel).* The T wave prominence and ST-segment elevation that occur with coronary artery spasm are demonstrated. (**A–C,** From Willerson JT: Treatment of Heart Disease. New York: Gower Medical, 1992.)

tion may cause coronary artery spasm (see Figs. 26–3 and 26–5).[31–35] Exposure of tissue factor[74] and accumulation of local inhibitors of thrombolysis, such as the endogenous inhibitor of tissue plasminogen activator,[75] and activation of procoagulant factors, such as factors X and Xa (Fig. 26–6),[76] may also contribute to the development of thrombosis. This is especially likely to be true when endothelial injury decreases vascular concentrations of nitric oxide, tissue plasminogen activator, or prostacyclin (see Fig. 26–3).[32–35] It also seems highly likely that the endothelium-derived vasoconstrictor endothelin is responsible for coronary artery constriction or spasm in some patients (see Fig. 26–3).[32–35]

ACUTE MYOCARDIAL INFARCTION

Acute MI occurs when there are severe reductions in coronary blood flow and myocardial oxygen delivery for more than 20 minutes. The infarct begins on the inner wall or subendocardium of the heart and is confined there in the first 20 minutes to 1 hour (Figs. 26–7 and 26–8) (non–Q wave or ST depression infarcts, generally subendocardial infarcts). If the coronary artery thrombosis is transient or does not cause complete coronary artery occlusion, the infarct usually remains confined to the subendocardium and a *non–Q wave* MI develops. If the coronary artery occlusion is sustained, the myocardial necrosis progresses vertically outward toward the epicardium in the next 2 to 3 hours (Q wave, ST elevation, or transmural MI). Herrick[2] described acute MI caused by coronary artery thrombosis in 1912. Subsequently, the role of coronary artery thrombosis in causing MI was debated[77] until studies by DeWood and colleagues[78] demonstrated by coronary arteriography that coronary artery thrombosis is virtually always the cause of acute Q wave MIs. Buja and Willerson[79] confirmed the association between thrombosis of the infarct-related coronary artery and the development of acute Q wave

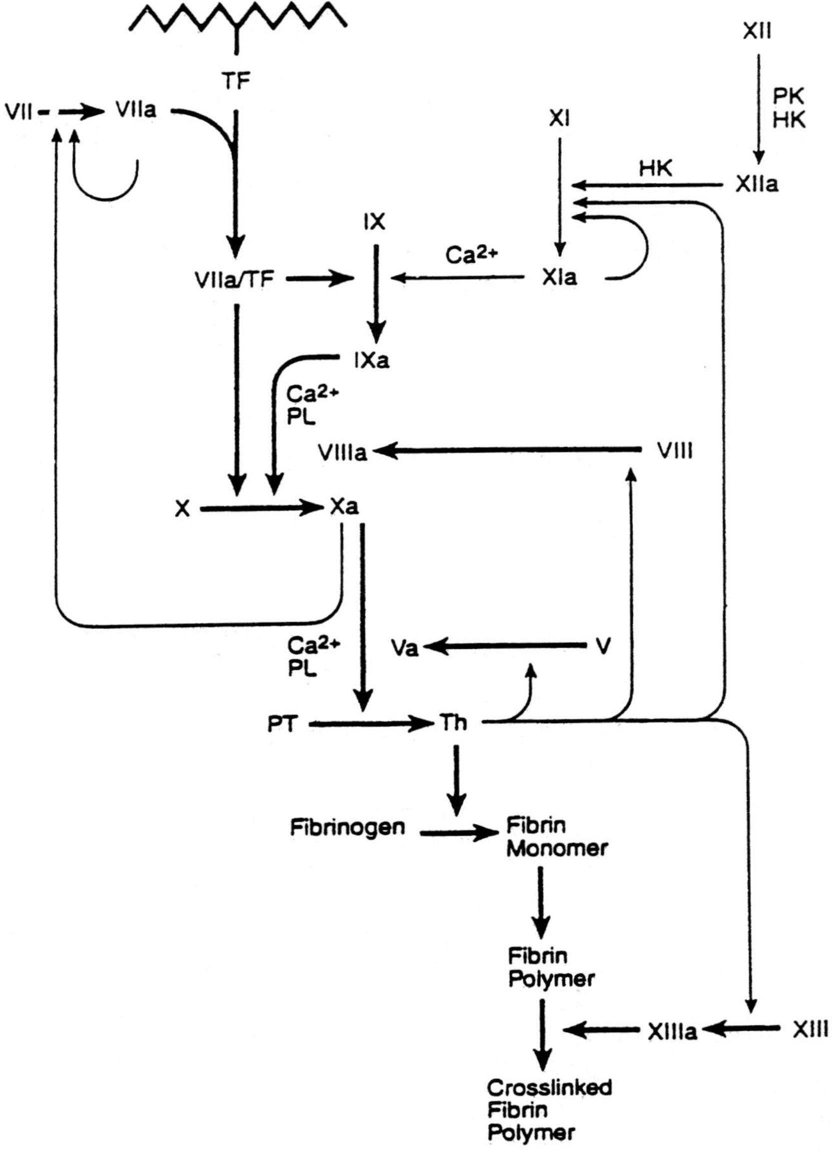

FIGURE 26–6 Schematic representation of the role of tissue factor (TF), factors IX, X, XI, XII, and VIII in the formation of thrombin (Th) and the subsequent role of thrombin in the formation of fibrin. HK, high-molecular-weight; PK, prekallikrein; PL, phospholipid; PT, prothrombin. (From Schafer AI: Coagulation cascade: an overview. *In* Loscalzo J, Schafer A [eds]: Thrombosis and Hemorrhage. p. 7. Boston: Blackwell Scientific, 1994.)

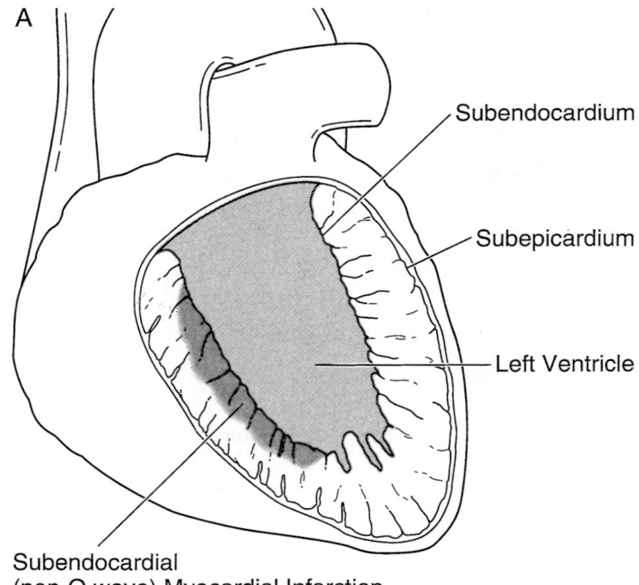

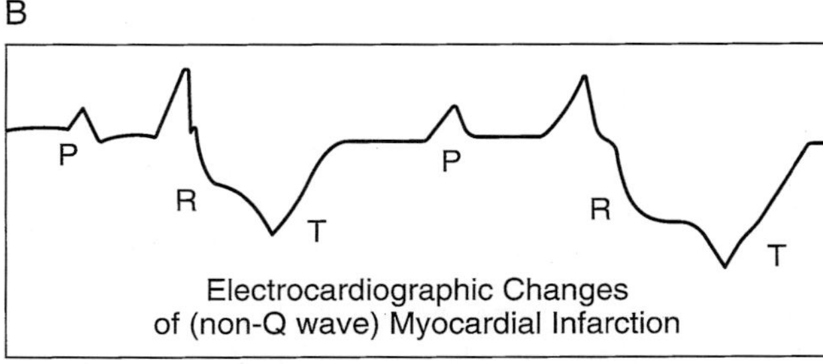

FIGURE 26–7 A, Schematic diagram shows the location of myocardial necrosis with subendocardial or non–Q wave myocardial infarcts and a representation of the typical electrocardiographic changes. **B,** Typical electrocardiogram (ECG) in a patient with acute non–Q wave MI. With these infarcts, the ECG is unable to provide specific evidence of the presence of the infarct but ST-segment depression of varying magnitude and T wave abnormalities, usually T wave flattening or inversion, often develop. The only evolution of the electrocardiographic abnormalities is a return to the normal pattern. (**A** and **B,** From Willerson JT: Treatment of Heart Disease. New York: Gower Medical, 1992.)

(transmural) MI by detailed clinicopathologic correlations. Ninety percent or more of acute Q wave MIs (usually transmural MIs) have persistent and occlusive coronary artery thrombosis in the infarct-related coronary artery.[78, 79]

Acute Q wave MI is usually caused by persistent thrombotic occlusion of a coronary artery resulting in sustained reductions in coronary blood flow and myocardial oxygen availability. Occasionally, increases in myocardial oxygen demand above the ability of a stenotic coronary artery to deliver oxygen cause MI, often non–Q wave MI. Such increases in oxygen demand occur in some patients with CAD who have severe systemic arterial hypertension, sustained tachycardia, or both. Alternatively, sustained reductions in myocardial oxygen delivery associated with severe systemic arterial hypotension may lead to MI, often non–Q wave MI. Approximately 30 percent of patients with non–Q wave MIs have an occlusive thrombus in the infarct-related artery.[79–81] In most patients with non–Q wave MI, transient coronary artery occlusion—initiated by platelet aggregation and with associated vasoconstriction lasting more than 30 minutes and less than 2 hours—is present (see Figs. 26–3 and 26–7).

When critical reductions in myocardial blood flow persist for more than 2 hours, the resultant infarct is usually a transmural or Q wave MI (see Fig. 26–8). The local accumulation of thromboxane A_2, serotonin, platelet-activating factor, adenosine diphosphate, oxygen-derived free radicals, and thrombin activation at sites of endothelial

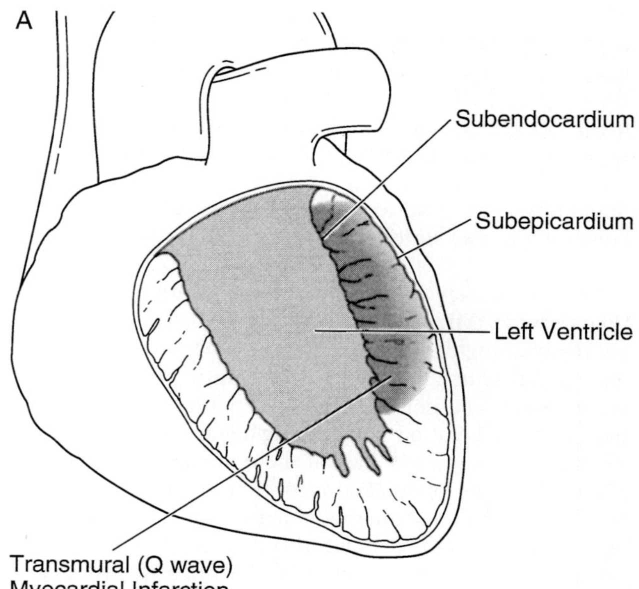

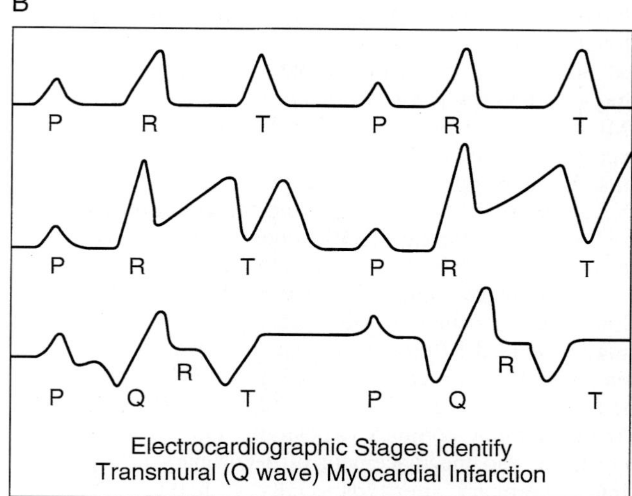

FIGURE 26–8 A, Schematic diagram of the topographic location of myocardial necrosis with transmural or Q wave MI and the associated electrocardiographic changes. **B,** The sequential electrocardiographic alterations that document the development of a new Q wave infarct, beginning with T wave prominence *(top),* followed by hyperacute ST-segment elevation *(middle),* T wave inversion and the development of a significant Q wave (0.04 s in duration) *(bottom).* (**A** and **B,** From Willerson JT: Treatment of Heart Disease. New York: Gower Medical, 1992.)

injury contributes to vasoconstriction, platelet aggregation, and thrombosis (see Fig. 26–3).[33–36] Increases in systemic and local catecholamine concentrations associated with the development of unstable angina and MI increase platelet aggregation and may contribute to coronary vasoconstriction. Local accumulation of endothelin causes marked vasoconstriction; serotonin, adenosine diphosphate, thrombin, and endothelin are mitogens, and they are very likely to contribute to subsequent local fibroproliferation with increases in the neointima, further narrowing the lumen of the endothelium-injured coronary artery.[82] In 30 percent (or more) of patients with unstable angina and non–Q wave MIs, there is a rapid anatomic progression in the severity of the coronary luminal diameter narrowing, most likely associated with the inclusion of organized thrombus within the plaque and the fibroproliferation that follows plaque fissuring and ulceration.[82] Reductions in fibrinolytic capability at sites of vascular endothelial injury associated with decreases in vascular tissue concentrations of prostacyclin, tissue plasminogen activating factor, and nitric oxide undoubtedly contribute to coronary artery thrombosis, vasoconstriction, and fibroproliferation at these same sites (see Fig. 26–3).[33–35]

We and others have suggested that unstable angina, non–Q wave MI, and Q wave MI represent a continuum pathophysiologically.[33–35] The process begins with coronary endothelial injury, usually atherosclerotic plaque ulceration or fissuring. The degree of coronary artery stenosis where the plaque ulceration or fissuring occurs may be mild or severe. Approximately half of the coronary stenoses where plaque fissuring or ulceration occurs are sites of less than 50 per cent luminal diameter narrowing.[83] We have suggested that when the platelet-fibrin thrombus and associated severe vasoconstriction persist for periods of less than 20 minutes and often recur, the syndrome of unstable angina develops.[33–35] However, when the reduction in coronary blood flow and oxygen delivery to the heart is more prolonged, lasting 30 minutes to 1 to 2 hours, a non–Q wave MI occurs.[33–35] When the period of inadequate myocardial oxygen delivery persists for more than 2 hours, a Q wave MI results (see Fig. 26–3).[33–35] When unstable angina and acute MI are viewed in this manner, it is easy to appreciate that patients with unstable angina and non–Q wave MI have "aborted" Q wave MIs, and therefore, they remain at risk for new infarction and its consequences in the ensuing 6 weeks.[79, 80, 84–87] The authors believe that the risk for renewed unstable angina and MI persists until the endothelial injury is repaired. Other causes of endothelial injury may also lead to this same sequence of events, including endothelial injury associated with systemic arterial hypertension, flow shear stress, smoking, diabetes, infection, aging, immune complex deposition, substance abuse (e.g., cocaine), and the placement of a coronary artery catheter into a coronary artery, especially with the interventional procedures of percutaneous transluminal coronary angioplasty (PTCA) and stent placement.[33–35]

Fissuring and ulceration of the plaque most commonly occur in the asymmetric portion or "shoulder region" with a thin fibrous cap that is lipid laden. Inflammation at sites of thin fibrous plaques with adjacent lipid cores best predicts the "unstable" atherosclerotic plaque and one likely to fissure or ulcerate.[17–26] Inflammation is characterized in the unstable plaque by the accumulation of monocyte-derived macrophages, activated T cells, and mast cells. Most likely, proteases released from the infiltrating mononuclear cells contribute to thinning of the fibrous cap through their degradation of collagen and subsequent atherosclerotic plaque fissuring and ulceration (Fig. 26–9).[26, 33–35, 82–101]

UNSTABLE ATHEROSCLEROTIC PLAQUE

Pathophysiology

Figure 26–9 demonstrates the characteristics of the unstable atherosclerotic plaque herein defined as one likely to ulcerate or fissure or otherwise promote platelet adherence and aggregation and vasoactive mediator accumulation, leading to the development of thrombosis, dynamic vasoconstriction, and fibroproliferation. The morphologic characteristics of the unstable plaque include a thin fibrous cap, the presence of numerous inflammatory cells on or beneath the atherosclerotic plaque surface, and an adjacent lipid core. Casscells, Willerson, and associates have shown that such plaques in the human carotid artery have temperature heterogeneity with temperatures varying by 0.8° to 4°C in that part of the plaque where the inflammation exists (Fig. 26–10).[102] More recently, others have confirmed these observations and shown the same temperature heterogeneity in vivo in human coronary arteries in patients with unstable angina and acute MI (Fig. 26–11).[103]

Several studies have shown that patients with unstable angina and non–Q wave MIs with elevated serum C-reactive protein or fibrinogen at hospital discharge, elevations in serum troponin I or T at hospital admission, and/or increases in serum interleukin-6 concentrations during their hospital admission have an increased risk of future coronary events, presumably reflecting the importance of inflammation in the instability of their unstable atherosclerotic plaques.[104–114] The increases in troponin I and T identify myocardial necrosis and possibly more extensive plaque instability, longer duration of platelet-derived thrombosis and vasoconstriction and, possibly, of platelet emboli and occlusive disease of distal arterial networks (Figs. 26–12 to 26–15).[106–114]

Berk and coworkers[109] were among the first to demonstrate an increase in C-reactive protein in patients with acute coronary heart disease syndromes. Subsequently, several studies, including those by Maseri and colleagues, demonstrated a poorer prognosis in patients with severe unstable angina who also have increases in their serum C-reactive protein and serum amyloid-A protein.[110] Ridker and associates[113] and Koenig and coworkers[108] demonstrated that increases in serum C-reactive protein predict the development of future coronary events, even in otherwise apparently healthy individuals. Figure 26–12 demonstrates that for patients with unstable angina and non–Q wave MIs with C-reactive protein values 0.3 mg/dl or higher, there is an increased risk of future coronary events, including urgent coronary artery bypass surgery or angioplasty, cardiac death, or MI. Similar data have been pro-

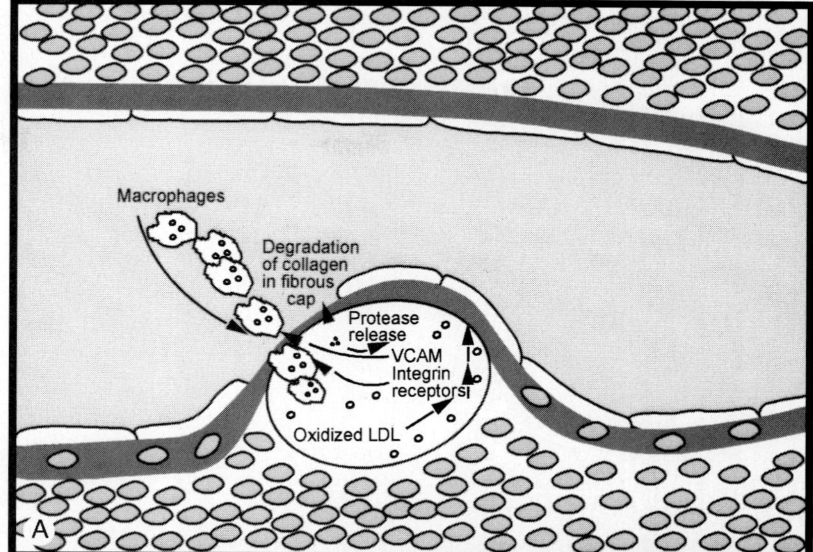

Anatomy of 30% of Fatal Myocardial Infarctions: Erosion

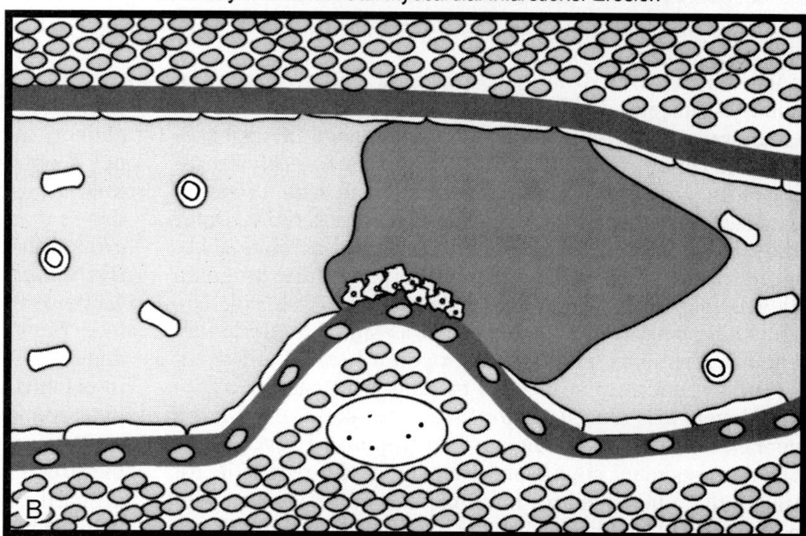

Anatomy of 60% of Fatal Myocardial Infarctions: Rupture

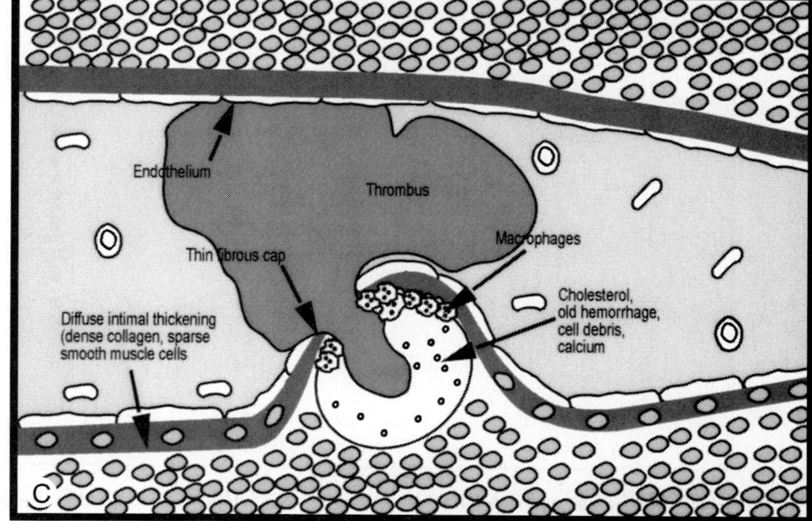

FIGURE 26–9 A, Potential mechanisms responsible for atherosclerotic plaque fissuring and ulceration. Oxidized low-density lipoprotein (LDL) within the atherosclerotic plaque promotes the upregulation of vascular cell adhesion molecule (VCAM) and other integrins, resulting in the recruitment of inflammatory cells, primarily monocyte-derived macrophages but including activated T cells and mast cells; subsequent protease release from the mononuclear cells; and degradation of collagen in the fibrous cap, leading to its fissuring and ulceration. **B,** Atherosclerotic plaque fissuring, leading to platelet adhesion and aggregation and thrombosis. **C,** Atherosclerotic plaque ulceration and thrombosis. (**B** and **C,** Drawn with the assistance of Dr. Ward Casscells.)

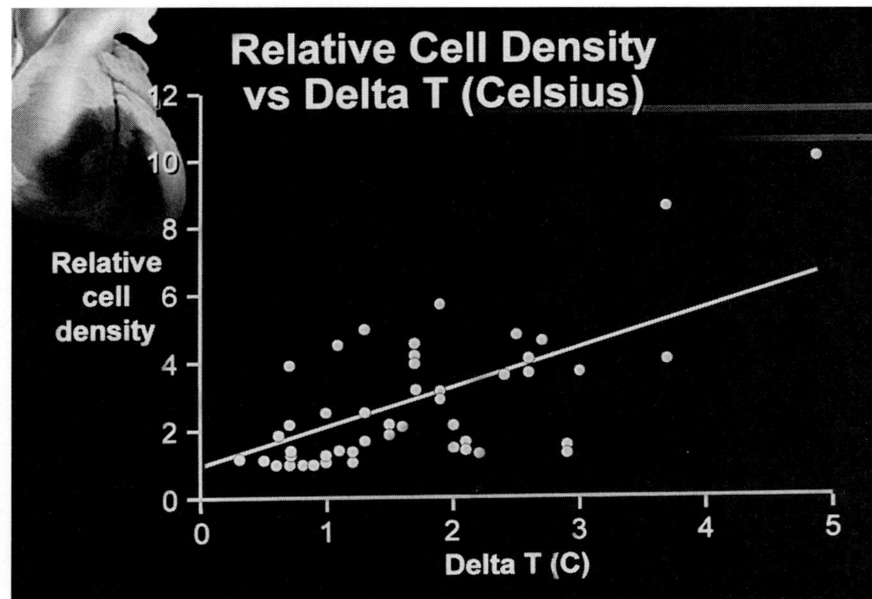

FIGURE 26–10 Relationship between temperature heterogeneity and inflammatory cell presence in human carotid plaques removed at carotid endarterectomy. (From Casscells W, Hathorn B, David M, et al: Thermal detection of cellular infiltrates in living atherosclerotic plaques: possible implications for plaque rupture and thrombosis. Lancet 347:1447, 1996. © by The Lancet Ltd 1996.)

vided for patients who have elevated serum fibrinogen values at hospital discharge.[111]

Several groups have shown the importance of increases in serum levels of troponin I as prognostic factors indicative of increased future risk for patients with acute coronary syndromes. Antman and colleagues,[106] in a multicenter study of 1404 symptomatic patients, found a relation between mortality at 42 days and the serum cardiac troponin I levels at patient admission to the hospital (see Fig. 26–15). The mortality rate at 42 days was significantly higher in the 573 patients with cardiac troponin I levels of 0.4 ng/ml and greater than in the 831 patients with cardiac troponin I levels less than 0.4 ng/ml (see Fig. 26–15). For each increase of 1 ng/ml in the cardiac troponin I level, there was an associated significant increase in the risk ratio for death, after adjustment for baseline characteristics that were independently predictive of mortality, including ST-segment depression and age 65 years or older. Similar data have been provided for serum values for troponin T in patients with unstable coronary heart disease. Lindahl and associates[105] found that the risk of cardiac events in these patients increased with increasing maximal levels of troponin T obtained in the initial 24 hours after admission. The lowest quartile (<0.06 μg/L) constitutes a low-risk group, the second quartile (0.06 to 0.18 μg/L) an intermediate group, and the three highest quartiles (≥0.18 μg/L) relatively high-risk groups with 4.3 percent, 10.5 percent, and 16 percent risk of either MI or cardiac death, respectively (see Fig. 26–13).[105] Recently, Biasucci and coworkers[114] demonstrated an increased risk for future coronary events in patients whose serum interleukin-6 increases during hospital admission.

Stability of an atherosclerotic plaque depends largely on the structural integrity of its fibrous cap, which is composed primarily of extracellular matrix components rich in collagen. Evidence supports a role for the release of matrix-degrading enzymes called *matrix metalloproteinases* (MMPs) in the catabolism of the structural macromolecules

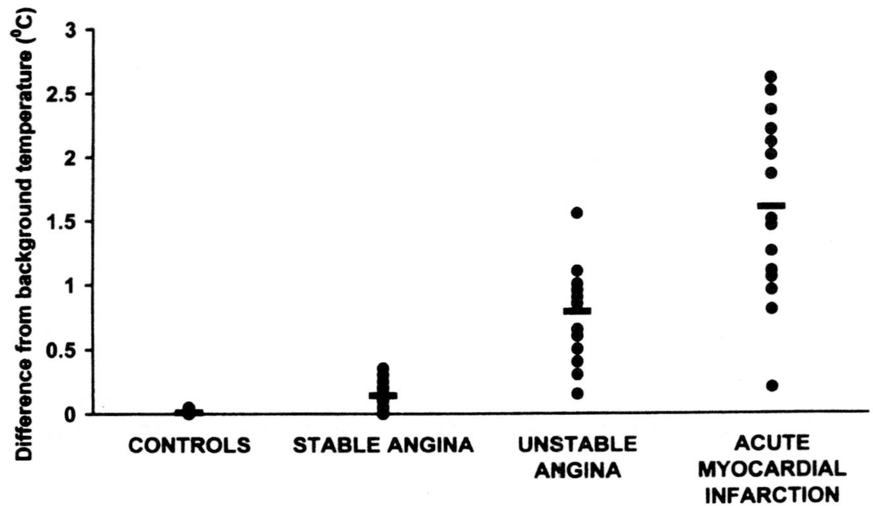

FIGURE 26–11 Increased temperature of infarct-related plaques in patients with unstable angina and with acute MI compared with controls and with patients with stable angina. (From Stefanadis C, Diamantopoulos L, Vlachopoulos C, et al: Thermal heterogeneity within human atherosclerotic coronary arteries detected in vivo. A new method of detection by application of a special thermography catheter. Circulation 99[15]:1965–1971, 1999.)

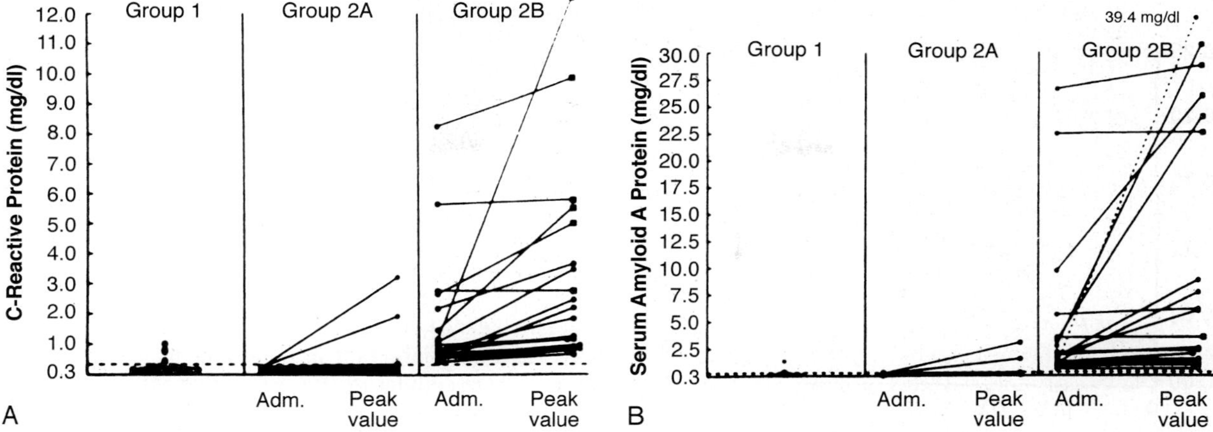

FIGURE 26–12 Plasma levels of C-reactive protein **(A)** and serum amyloid A protein **(B)** in patients with stable angina (group 1), in patients with unstable angina and levels of C-reactive protein < 0.3 mg/dl on admission (Adm.) (group 2A), and in patients with unstable angina and levels of C-reactive protein ≥ 0.3 mg/dl on admission (group 2B). *Circles,* urgent coronary artery bypass or angioplasty; *squares,* cardiac death or MI. In one patient, the peak value for serum amyloid A protein, which exceeded the values on the scale, is shown numerically and joined by a *dashed line* to the corresponding value on admission. The level of C-reactive protein is < 0.3 mg/dl (*dashed horizontal line* in **A**) in 90 percent of normal subjects. The median normal level of serum amyloid A protein is 0.3 mg/dl (*dashed horizontal line* in **B**); 96 percent of normal subjects have levels of serum amyloid A protein < 1.0 mg/dl. (**A** and **B,** From Liuzzo G, Biasucci LM, Gallimore JR, et al: The prognostic value of C-reactive protein in severe angina. N Engl J Med 331:407, 1994. Copyright © 1994, Massachusetts Medical Society. All rights reserved.)

causing a dissolution of the fibrous cap of the plaque.[95–101] Table 26–2 provides a classification of the MMPs.

The MMP family includes at least 19 structurally related, zinc-dependent enzymes that function at physiologic pH in the extracellular space. In addition, membrane-type (MT) metalloproteinases have been identified that have the designations MT1-MMP through MT4-MMP (see Table 26–2).

MMPs have been broadly classified into three main groups on the basis of substrate specificity. They include the collagenases (MMP-1, -8, and -13) that degrade intact fibrillar collagens. The gelatinases (MMP-2 and -9) hydrolyze the denatured collagen fibril and basement membrane collagen type IV. The stromelysins (MMP-3, -7, -10, and -11) have broad substrate specificity (see Table 26–2). For some of the remaining MMPs, substrate specificity has not yet been identified.

The MMPs share a similar five-domain structure. The leader sequence targets the enzyme for secretion and is cleaved during secretion from the cells. The N-terminal domain contains a highly conserved PRCGVPD sequence that maintains latency of the proenzyme through interaction with its unpaired cysteine residue and the active site zinc in the catalytic domain.

Regulation of MMPs occurs at three levels including: (1) control of the rate of gene transcription; (2) conversion of the inactive translational product, and inactive zymogen precursor, to the active form; and (3) inactivation by a family of endogenous inhibitors known as *tissue inhibitors of metalloproteinases* (TIMPs) (Table 26–3).

Human peripheral blood monocytes produce little MMP, but differentiation into macrophages yields higher levels of MMP-9.[95–101] Secretion of MMP-9 from macrophages can

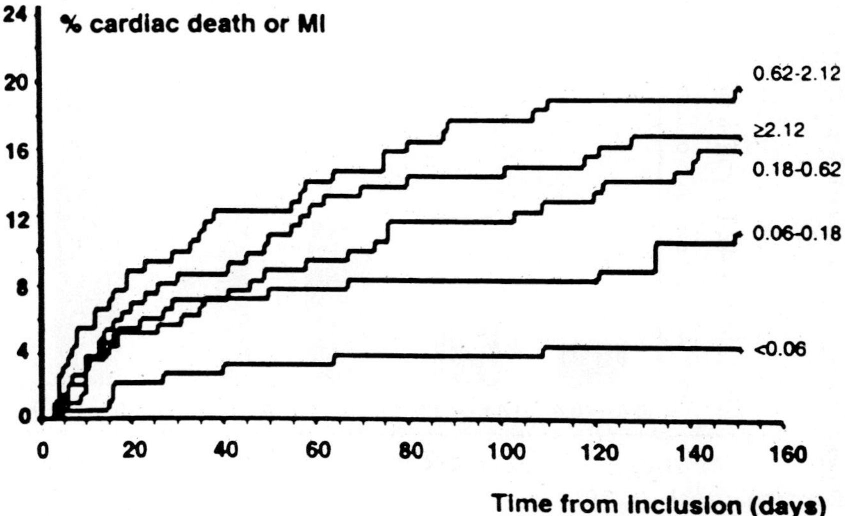

FIGURE 26–13 Cumulative risk and time of occurrence of cardiac death or MI in patients with unstable coronary heart disease grouped on the basis of increase in quintiles of maximal serum troponin T levels (micrograms per liter). The numbers of patients in each group (lowest through highest) were 187, 201, 190, 191, and 194, respectively. Pooled log rank $P < .0001$. (From Lindahl B, Venge P, Wallentin L, for the FRISC Study Group: Relation between troponin T and the risk of subsequent cardiac events in unstable coronary artery disease. Circulation 93[9]:1651–1657, 1996.)

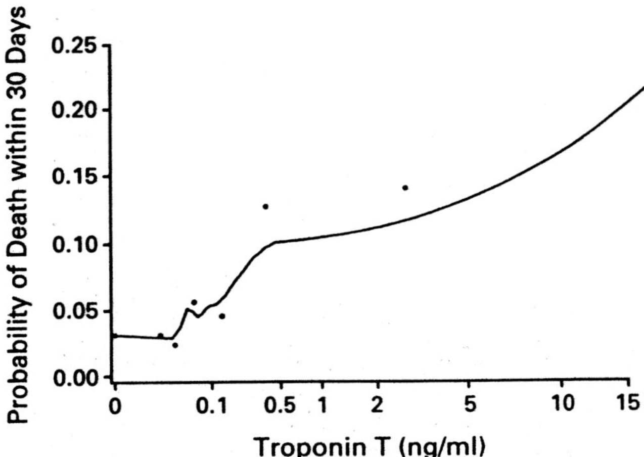

FIGURE 26–14 Probability of death within 30 days according to the serum troponin T level at hospital admission. *Dots* represent simple estimates of mortality derived from ranges of the troponin T level that contained at least 70 patients. (From Ohman EM, Armstrong PW, Christenson RH, et al, for the GUSTO-IIa Investigators: Cardiac troponin T levels for risk stratification in acute myocardial ischemia. N Engl J Med 335:1337, 1996.)

be induced by tumor necrosis factor-alpha, interleukin-1-beta, and CD40. Expression of collagenase (MMP-1) and stromelysin (MMP-3) in macrophages is regulated by certain bacterial products, including lipopolysaccharide (endotoxin) and yeast zymosan. Activated T lymphocytes may cause collagenase and stromelysin expression in the human monocyte-derived macrophages.

MMPs are secreted from cells as inactive zymogens and require activation in the extracellular milieu before they are capable of degrading extracellular matrix molecules. Macrophage-derived reactive oxygen species activate MMP-2 and MMP-9 and thrombin activates MMP-2. MMPs themselves, once processed from the zymogen to active form, can trigger activation of other members of the MMP family. Mast cells within atheroma may release serine proteinases that activate MMPs.

The endogenous inhibitors known as TIMPs help regulate MMP activity under normal circumstances (see Table 26–3). Four TIMPs have been described thus far. They exhibit sequence homology and share domains of identical protein structures that consist of highly conserved N-terminal regions believed to be critical for inhibition of the enzyme.

The balance between MMP activities and their inhibition by TIMPs is important in the maintenance of homeostasis for the extracellular matrix. Excessive MMP activity occurs in a number of disease states, including metastatic cancer, rheumatoid arthritis, and glomerulosclerosis. There is evidence that MMPs play a role in accelerated connective tissue turnover associated with degenerative diseases of vessels, including aortic aneurysms and vein graft stenoses, as well as migration of smooth muscle cells from the media to the intima after arterial injury.

Several of the MMPs and TIMPs have been found in atherosclerotic plaques,[95–101] including MMP-1 (collagenase), MMP-9 (gelatinase B), and stromelysin-1 (MMP-3). Each of these has been found in the fibrous cap, the atherosclerotic lesions' shoulders, and the base of the lipid core. MMP-7 (matrilysin) is found primarily in macrophages overlying the lipid core. A high expression of MMPs has also been detected in lipid-laden macrophages in experimental animal lesions.

Similarly, constitutive expression of TIMP-1 and -2 has been described in both normal and diseased arteries and TIMP-3 has been found in atheromas. Thus, the spatial distribution of selected TIMPs within atheroma correlates with that described for MMP expression. Most of the MMPs and TIMPs in atheromas are in macrophages, thereby identifying the macrophage as probably a key participant in the regulation of the balance between synthesis

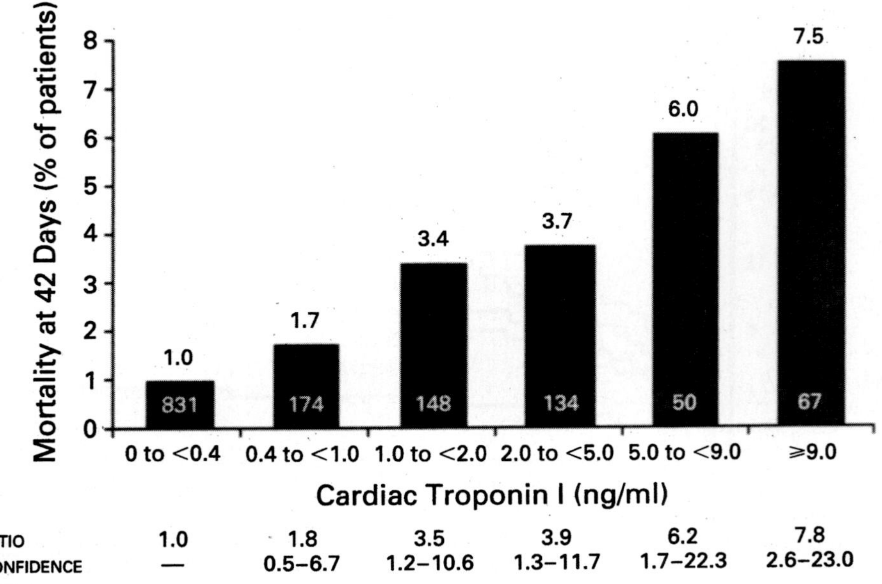

FIGURE 26–15 The mortality incidence at 42 days in patients admitted to the hospital with unstable angina or non–Q wave MI based on their initial cardiac troponin serum levels (nanograms per milligram). The number of patients in each category is shown within each *black bar.* (From Antman EM, Tanasijevic MJ, Thompson B, et al: Cardiac-specific troponin I levels to predict the risk of mortality in patients with acute coronary syndromes. N Engl J Med 335:1342–1349, 1996.)

TABLE 26–2 **Classification of Matrix Metalloproteinases**

Enzyme Names	MMP	Size (kD)	ECM Substrates
Collagenase, interstitial (fibroblast-type)	MMP-1	55	Collagens I, II, III, VII, VIII, X; gelatin: PG core protein
PMN collagenase (neutrophil)	MMP-8	75	Same as above
Collagenase-3	MMP-13	54	Collagen II, aggrecan
Stromelysin-1 Transin-1	MMP-3	57	PG core protein; fibronectin; laminin; collagen IV, V, IX, X; elastin'oCL
Stromelysin-2 Transin-2	MMP-10	57	Same as above
Stromelysin-3	MMP-11		Fibronectin, laminin, gelatin, PG
Putative metalloproteinase-1 (PUMP-1), matrilysin	MMP-7	28	Fibronectin, laminin, collagen IV, gelatin, procollagenase, PG core protein
Gelatinase, 72 kD (A) Type IV collagenase	MMP-2	72	Gelatin; collagens IV, V, VII, X, XI; elastin; fibronectin; PG core protein, laminin
Gelatinase, 92 kD (B) Type IV collagenase	MMP-9	92	Gelatin; collagens IV, V; glastin; PG core protein
Macrophage metalloelastase	MMP-12	53	Elastin
MT1-MMP	MMP-14	66	Interstitial collagens, gelatin, cartilage PG, fibronectin, vitronectin, laminin
MT2-MMP	MMP-15	66	n.d.
MT3-MMP	MMP-16	69	Gelatin, casein
MT4-MMP	MMP-17	57	n.d.
	MMP-18		n.d.
	MMP-19	56	n.d.

Abbreviations: ECM, extracellular material; MMP, matrix metalloproteinase; MT, membrane-type; n.d., not determined; PG, prostaglandin; PMN, polymorphonuclear neutrophil.
Modified from Birkedal-Hansen H: Matrix metalloproteinases: a review. Crit Rev Oral Biol Med 4:197–250, 1993.

and degradation of extracellular matrix macromolecules in the atherosclerotic plaque.

Current evidence suggests a probable role for metalloproteinase release in excess of TIMP presence leading to degradation of collagen in the fibrous cap and the subsequent fissuring and ulceration that predisposes to unstable angina and acute MI (see Fig. 26–9). The proposed scheme includes the oxidation of low-density lipoprotein (LDL) within the plaque and the chemoattractant influence of oxidized LDL and other oxidation products to promote the expression of selected adhesion molecules, including vascular cell adhesion molecule and intracellular adhesion molecule, and the subsequent recruitment of monocyte-derived macrophages, activated T lymphocytes, and mast cells within the plaque, with subsequent release of selected MMPs in excess of their TIMP concentration locally. The excess MMPs degrade plaque collagen within the fibrous cap and lead to consequent fissuring and ulceration of the atherosclerotic plaque. One anticipates future clinical trials with inhibitors of selected MMPs, but the redundancy within the system—that is, the number of MMPs and other proteases within plaques that are nonmetalloenzymes, may make effective inhibition of these plaque-degrading enzymes difficult. Other approaches to inhibiting inflammation and the recruitment of monocyte-derived macrophages that may be protective of atherosclerotic plaques include inhibiting macrophage homing to unstable atherosclerotic plaques using inhibitors of vascular cell adhesion molecule and intracellular adhesion molecule[115] or of cyclooxygenase-2; the use of antioxidants, inhibitors of selected cytokines, especially tumor necrosis factor-α, nitric oxide donors, inhibitors of NF-κB; and marked lipid lowering with the use of medications capable of providing marked reductions in serum cholesterol and LDL.

At least three major clinical studies (the Scandinavian Simvastatin Survival Study [4S], the West of Scotland trial, and the Cholesterol and Recurrent Events [CARE] trial) have shown a decreased frequency of future acute coronary events in patients in the 1 to 2 years after they receive a 3-hydroxy-3-methylglutaryl coenzyme A reductase inhibitor with subsequent marked lowering of serum cholesterol and LDL (Fig. 26–16).[116–118] Recent data from the CARE trial suggest that marked serum cholesterol and LDL lowering reduces C-reactive protein values, thereby indicating a close association between serum (and presumably intraplaque)

TABLE 26–3 **Tissue Inhibitors of Matrix Metalloproteinases**

Designation	Enzyme Preference	Type
TIMP-1	proMMP-9	Soluble
TIMP-2	proMMP-2	Soluble
TIMP-3	All	Matrix bound
TIMP-4	n.d.	Soluble

Abbreviations: MMP, matrix metalloproteinase; n.d., not determined; TIMP, tissue inhibitor of matrix metalloproteinases.

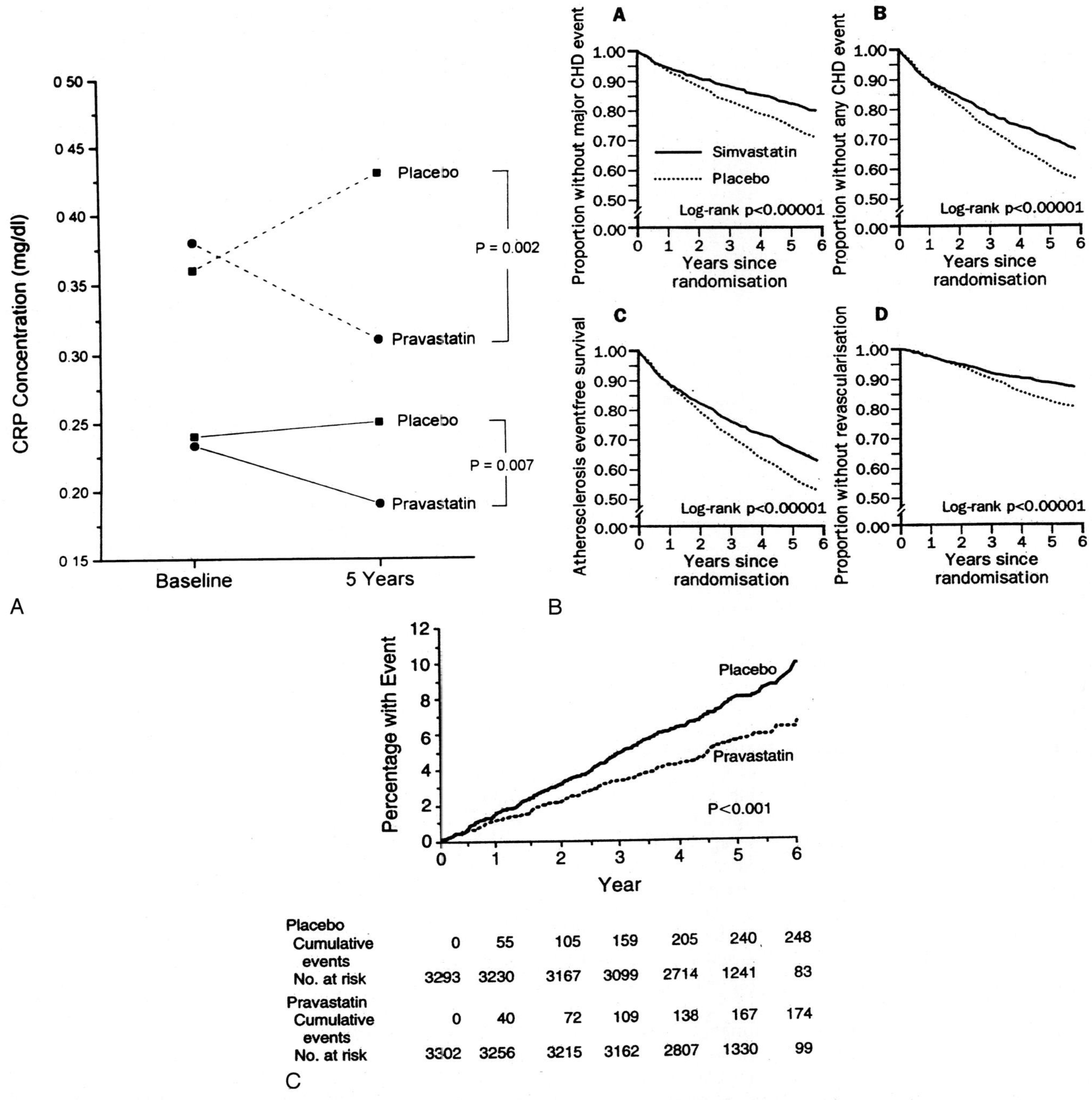

FIGURE 26–16 **A,** These data are obtained from analyses of patients treated in the Cholesterol and Recurrent Events (CARE) trial. With lowering of serum cholesterol and low-density lipoprotein (LDL) values by the 3-hydroxy-3-methylglutaryl coenzyme A (HMG CoA) reductase inhibitor pravastatin, there is a reduction in C-reactive protein (CRP) concentration in the serum in association with the lowering of total serum cholesterol and LDL values. This implies a reduction in inflammation in these patients in association with reducing their serum cholesterol and LDL values. **B,** The insert panels show data from the Scandinavian Simvastatin Survival Study and the reduction in major coronary heart disease (CHD) events (*A* and *B*); survival without an atherosclerosis event *(C)*; and the reduction in the need for future revascularizations *(D)* associated with simvastatin therapy and a reduction in serum cholesterol and LDL values. **C,** Kaplan-Meier analysis of the time to a definite nonfatal MI or death from coronary heart disease, according to treatment group. (**A,** From Ridker CM, Rifai N, Pfeffer MA, et al: Long-term effects of pravastatin on plasma concentration of C-reactive protein. Circulation 100[2]:230–235, 1999. **B,** From Scandinavian Simvastatin Survival Study Group: Randomized trial of cholesterol lowering in 4444 patients with coronary heart disease: the Scandinavian Simvastatin Survival Study [4S]. Lancet 344:1383, 1994. **C,** From Shepherd J, Cobbe SM, Ford I, et al, for the West of Scotland Coronary Prevention Study Group: Prevention of coronary heart disease with pravastatin in men with hypercholesterolemia. N Engl J Med 333:1301–1307, 1995.)

cholesterol and LDL values and the presence of inflammation (see Fig. 26–16).[119]

Clinical Recognition of Myocardial Infarction

History

The history is of the utmost importance in the recognition of acute MI.[1, 2, 120] Typically, the patient complains of very severe chest or epigastric pain that lasts until analgesic medication is administered, usually 30 minutes or longer. The pain is often described as being retrosternal or left precordial, as a "heaviness," "tightness," or "like a weight on my chest," and is usually associated with nausea and diaphoresis. It may radiate to the back, neck, jaw, or left arm, particularly down its ulnar aspect. Occasionally, the pain exists only in the back, jaw, left arm, or neck. It usually lasts longer than 30 minutes. The pain is usually described as the most severe the individual has ever experienced. It gradually builds in severity, reaches a peak, and then recedes. Many patients with acute MI have unstable angina pectoris for hours to days before their infarct. It should be emphasized, however, that 10 to 20 percent of patients with diabetes mellitus who have MIs have "silent" (i.e., painless) acute MIs.[121–123] Silent MIs also occur in patients who develop CAD (transplant vasculopathy) after cardiac transplantation, occasionally in other individuals with neuromyopathic abnormalities, and in some seemingly otherwise normal subjects. One should have a high index of suspicion for the patient who presents with new CHF, ventricular arrhythmias, hypotension, heart murmur of mitral insufficiency, or systemic embolic events, or is resuscitated from sudden death, especially in the diabetic patient. Serial serum measurements of CK, CK-MB, and troponin I and serial ECGs should be obtained in such patients.

Physical Examination

Patients with small MIs, particularly non–Q wave infarcts, may not have any detectable abnormality on physical examination. At the other extreme, patients with extensive damage to the left ventricle (≥40 percent of the LV mass) often develop "power-failure" complications of their infarct, including development of cardiogenic shock, severe LV failure, or medically refractory arrhythmias (Fig. 26–17).[124–128]

Inspection and Palpation

The findings on physical examination in patients with acute MI depend primarily on the extent of the myocardial damage. Most patients are in obvious discomfort and diaphoretic. Those with extensive myocardial damage develop a reduction in systemic arterial blood pressure, ranging from mild to severe, including the development of cardiogenic shock. *Cardiogenic shock* is defined as hypotension resulting from extensive myocardial damage coexisting with evidence that the reduced blood pressure is inadequate for normal systemic perfusion, so that cool skin, mental confusion, and oliguria are usually present. Patients with extensive LV myocardial necrosis may also have an alternating pulse force (pulsus alternans) (Fig. 26–18) and frequent premature ventricular beats. If second- or third-degree (complete) atrioventricular block with sinus rhythm is present, the patient will have intermittent "cannon" A waves in the jugular venous pulse (Fig. 26–19). Patients with atrial fibrillation do not have an A wave in the jugular venous pulse but instead have an irregularly irregular pulse. Those with important tricuspid insufficiency have prominent V waves in their jugular venous pulse (Fig. 26–20). Patients with right ventricular (RV) failure have an increased jugular venous pressure, and they may have hepatomegaly, right upper quadrant tenderness when acute hepatic congestion develops, ascites if the RV failure is severe, and peripheral or sacral edema.

With acute Q wave MI, a precordial "ectopic impulse" may sometimes be palpated over the left precordium, typically along the lower left sternal border or between the left sternal border and the apex. This impulse is caused by an increase in regional LV compliance within the area of injury, with a resultant systolic distention or bulging (dyskinesia) of the injured tissue. Over hours to a few days after MI, the compliance of this region decreases (stiffness increases) and the systolic bulging is replaced by reduced (hypokinetic) or absent (akinetic) regional wall motion. If the systolic bulging persists, a ventricular aneurysm may be present.

Auscultation

S_4 is heard in most patients with acute and chronic CAD (Fig. 26–21) and is often soft and best heard with light application of the bell of the stethoscope over the middle and lower left precordium. S_4 is caused by a more forceful atrial contraction against a ventricle whose compliance is reduced as a consequence of increased ventricular stiffness (reduced compliance) caused by the physiologic effects of CAD.

When the mitral valve apparatus is damaged, a murmur of mitral insufficiency may be audible. These murmurs have variable auscultatory characteristics; they may be ejection in quality, peaking in intensity in mid to late systole, or they may be holosystolic (Fig. 26–22). Intermittent myocardial ischemia with transient dysfunction of the posterior papillary muscle of the mitral valve leads to a murmur of papillary muscle dysfunction typically associated with mild to moderate mitral insufficiency. The murmur of papillary muscle dysfunction usually begins after the first heart sound (S_1), peaks in mid to late systole, and extends up to S_2. It is heard at the cardiac apex and may radiate toward the left sternal border or into the axilla. If caused by intermittent myocardial ischemia, the murmur is transient. If caused by infarction of the papillary muscle, the murmur is usually permanent. Rupture of a papillary muscle with acute MI causes severe mitral insufficiency and often a soft apical holosystolic murmur. However, sometimes no audible murmur occurs with a ruptured papillary muscle, even though severe mitral insufficiency develops. Acute mitral insufficiency occurs most commonly in patients with Q wave inferior or lateral MI and in those with non–Q wave MI.[129–135] Similarly, those with inferior

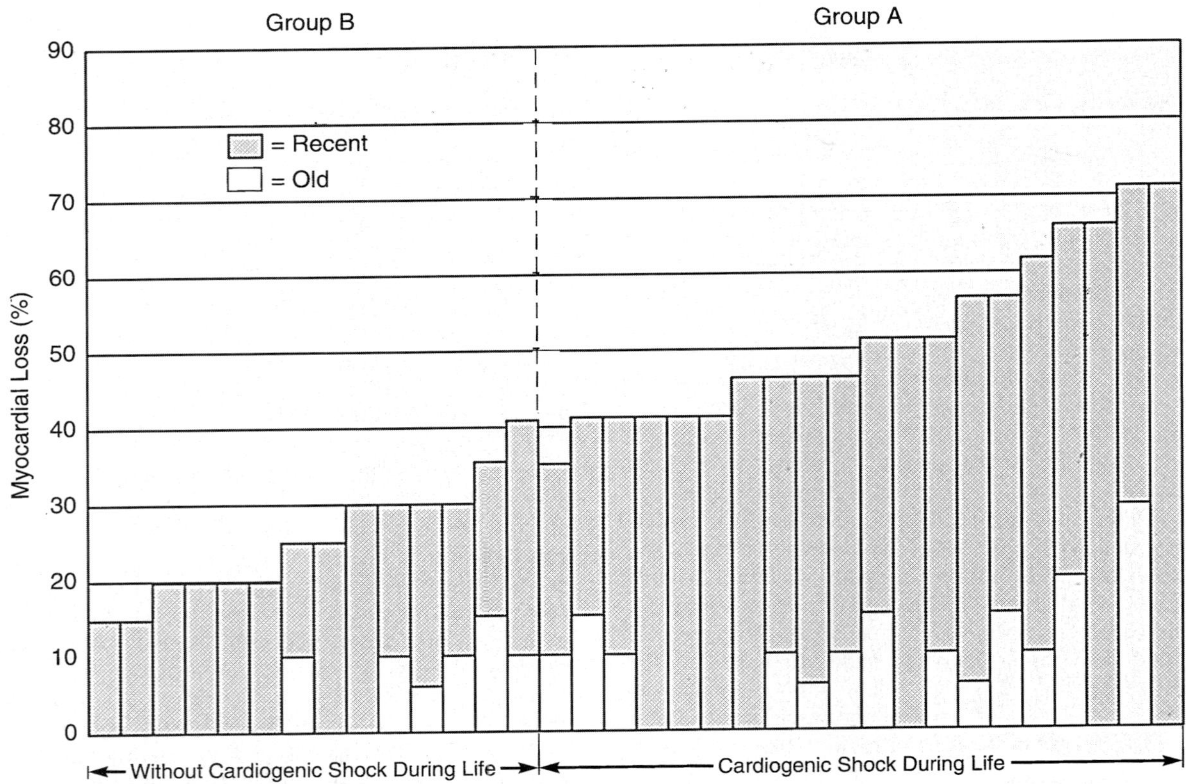

FIGURE 26–17 Development of "power failure" complications of MI, including cardiogenic shock, occurs in patients with the most extensive myocardial necrosis from their infarcts. (From Page DL, Caulfield JB, Kastor JA, et al: Myocardial changes associated with cardiogenic shock. N Engl J Med 285:133, 1971.)

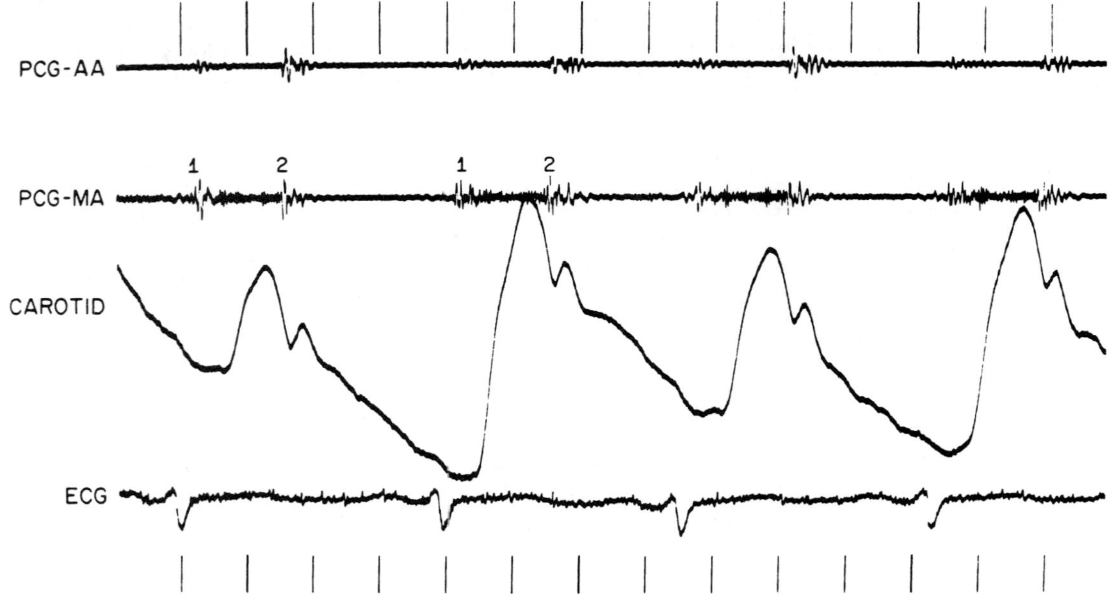

FIGURE 26–18 Heart sounds *(top)*, carotid pulse tracing *(middle)*, and electrocardiogram (ECG) *(bottom)*. Pulsus alternans is shown as the alternating height in the pulse wave tracing in a woman with a dilated cardiomyopathy. AA, aortic area; MA, mitral area; PCG, phonocardiogram. (From Willerson JT, Sanders CA: Clinical Cardiology. New York: Grune & Stratton, 1977.)

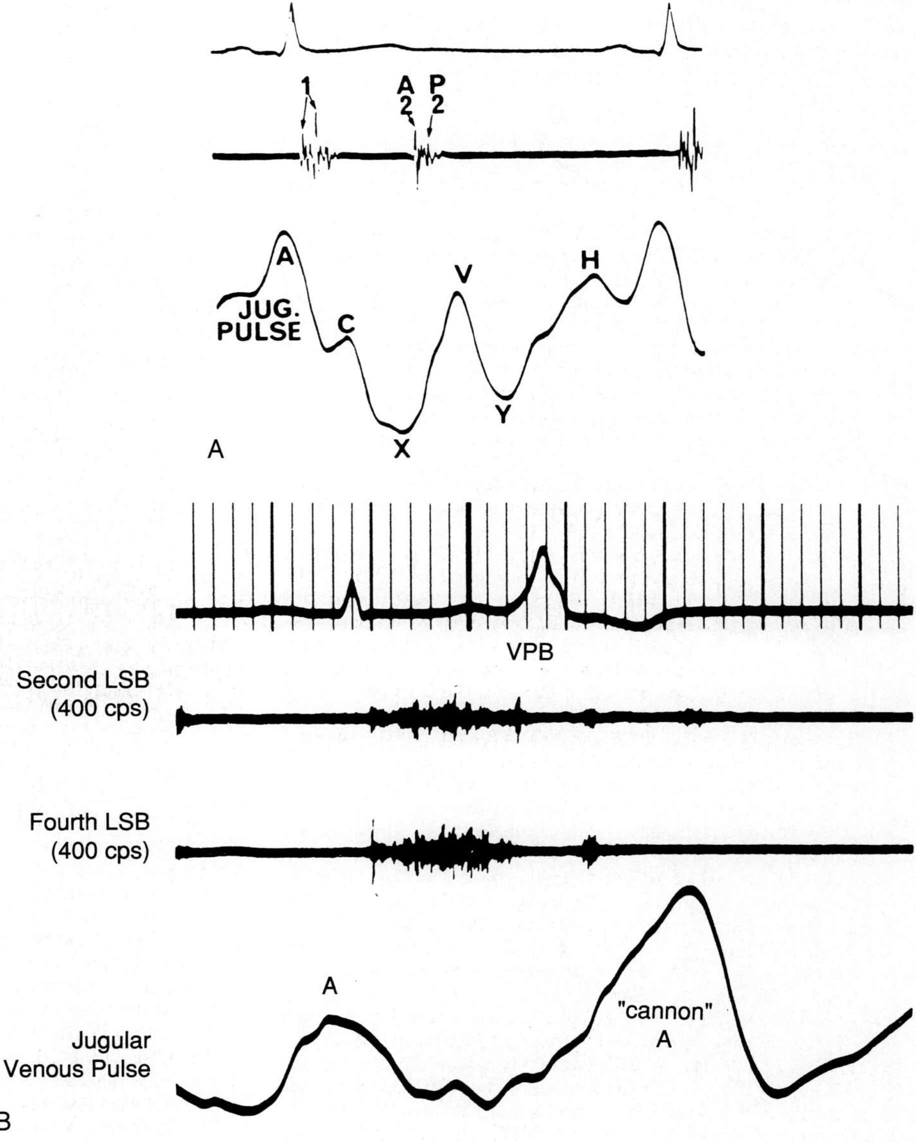

FIGURE 26–19 A, Normal jugular (jug.) venous pulse configuration. Note the prominence of the A wave and that the X trough is deeper than the Y trough. Heart sounds and the ECG are shown *(top)*. **B,** A "cannon" A wave in the jugular venous pulse. Heart sounds are shown along with the ECG *(top)*. LSB, left sternal border; VPB, ventricular premature beat.

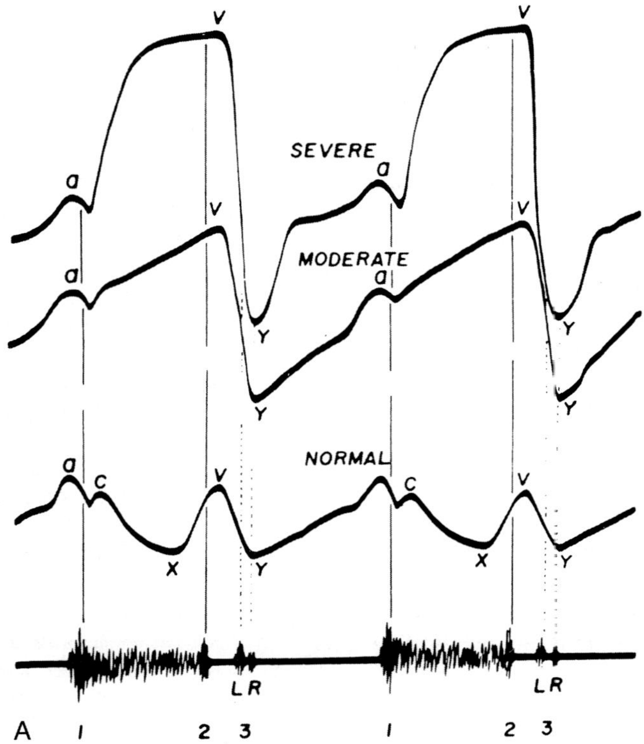

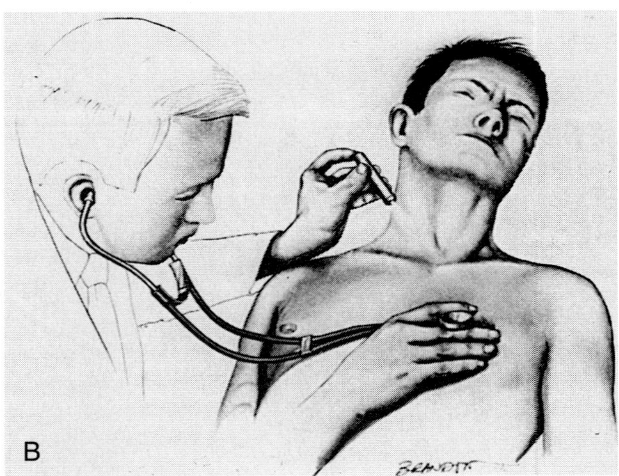

FIGURE 26–20 A, The jugular venous pulse normally *(bottom)* and with moderate *(middle)* and severe tricuspid insufficiency *(top)*. Note the marked prominence of the V wave with moderate and severe tricuspid insufficiency. The V wave correlates with the second heart sound (*bottom,* 2). The holosystolic murmur of tricuspid insufficiency is also shown *(bottom)*. Typically, it becomes louder along the lower left sternal border with inspiration. L and R, timing of left and right ventricular third heart sounds (3). Third heart sounds occur with moderately severe and severe valvular regurgitation, and those emanating from the right heart become louder with inspiration. **B,** A preferred way to evaluate the jugular venous pulse waveform is to examine the right external jugular vein as shown and simultaneously listen to the heart sounds, timing the A wave with the first heart sound and the V wave with the second heart sound. (**A** and **B,** From Willerson JT, Sanders CA: Clinical Cardiology. New York: Grune & Stratton, 1977; adapted from Hurst JW: The Heart. 5th ed. pp 158–159. New York: McGraw-Hill, 1990.)

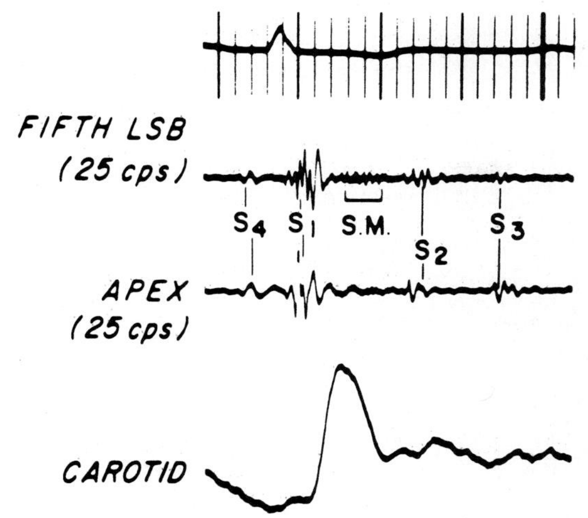

FIGURE 26–21 Fourth heart sound (S_4), third heart sound (S_3), and a systolic ejection murmur (SM), representing mitral insufficiency. LSB, left sternal border; S_1, first heart sound; S_2, second heart sound. (From Willerson JT, Hillis LD, Buja LM: Ischemic Heart Disease: Clinical and Pathophysiological Aspects. New York: Raven, 1982.)

infarcts and structural damage to the tricuspid valve may develop tricuspid insufficiency.

Rupture of the interventricular septum occurs most commonly in patients with acute anterior infarction, although it may also occur in the patient with an inferior MI (Fig. 26–23).[136–145] The murmur caused by a ventricular septal defect (VSD) is located along the lower left sternal border, is holosystolic, and is often associated with a left sternal border systolic thrill. As pulmonary artery pressure and vascular resistance increase, the systolic murmur of a VSD becomes shorter, ultimately disappearing altogether with the development of severe pulmonary hypertension (see Fig. 26–23). Functionally large acute VSDs (pulmonary to systemic blood flows of 1.5 to 1 or greater) should be closed by surgical intervention when CHF develops in the patient with MI; otherwise, rapidly progressive CHF and death may ensue. We recommend prompt coronary arteriography and surgical repair of a VSD with the development of CHF.

A murmur of relative mitral or tricuspid insufficiency occurs in patients with LV or RV failure, respectively; it is the result of a spatial abnormality in the orientation of the papillary muscles of the mitral and tricuspid valves caused by marked dilatation of the left or right ventricle. The mitral and tricuspid insufficiency with these entities is usually mild or moderate and diminishes in severity with diuresis.

S_3 occurs in patients with acute MIs who have ventricular filling pressures (LV end-diastolic pressures) of 15 mm Hg or greater and in those with moderately severe or severe mitral, aortic, or tricuspid valvular insufficiency (Fig. 26–24). S_3 is heard in patients with CHF and in those with rapid filling of the ventricles as a consequence of moderate or severe mitral, tricuspid, or aortic valve incompetence. S_3 may be heard normally in some young individuals (i.e., those under 30 years of age) as a result of rapid filling of the ventricle.

S_2 normally splits into two components with inspiration, the earlier aortic and the later pulmonary valve closure sound, because inspiration increases venous return to the right heart and delays pulmonary valve closure (Fig. 26–25). However, this second sound may be paradoxically split (i.e., wider splitting of the second sound during expiration) in the patient with angina pectoris, as well as in the patient with severe LV failure, systemic arterial hypertension, left bundle branch block (LBBB) or pacing from the right ventricle, and with the various forms of LV outflow obstruction, including valvular, supravalvular, and subval-

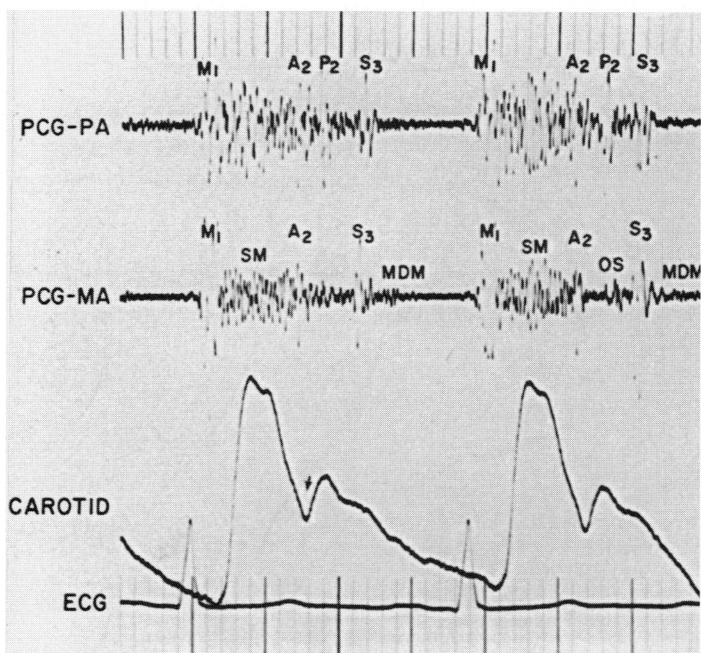

FIGURE 26–22 Use of two simultaneous phonocardiograms (PCGs) to identify heart sounds in the patient with mitral regurgitation. A loud holosystolic murmur (SM) is noted at both the pulmonary area (PCG-PA) and the mitral area (PCG-MA). The aortic component of the second heart sound (A_2) is masked by the latter part of the murmur, but it can be identified as the widely transmitted sound immediately preceding the incisura of the carotid pulse tracing *(arrow)*. In this patient, mixed mitral regurgitation and stenosis coexist and a mitral valve opening snap (os) can be seen occurring slightly later than the second pulmonic heart sound (P_2) in the cardiac cycle. A prominent third sound (S_3) is seen in both PCG channels, and a mid-diastolic murmur (MDM) is present at the mitral area.

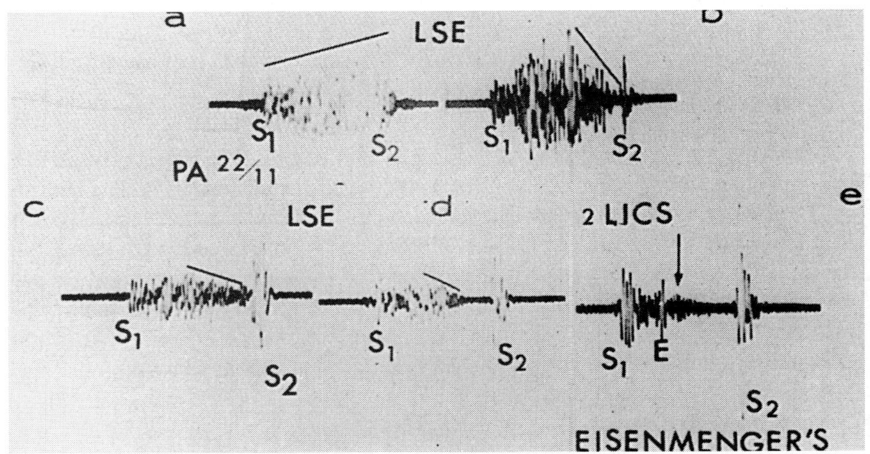

FIGURE 26–23 The typical holosystolic murmur of a ventricular septal defect (VSD) and the influence of increasing pulmonary artery (PA) pressure on the murmur. *a,* Murmur of a VSD with normal PA pressure. *b–e,* The influence of increasing PA pressure on the murmur of a VSD shows that with the development of severe pulmonary hypertension, the murmur becomes shorter and ejection in timing. With severe pulmonary hypertension, the systolic murmur of a VSD disappears. E, ejection click; LICS, second left intercostal spaces; LSE, lower sternal edge. (From Perloff JK: The Clinical Recognition of Congenital Heart Disease, p. 321. Philadelphia: WB Saunders, 1970.)

vular aortic stenosis (see Fig. 26–25). The pulmonary closure sound is increased in intensity in the patient with pulmonary hypertension resulting from LV failure.

A pericardial friction rub is detected in less than 10 percent of patients with acute Q wave MIs. Patients with audible pericardial friction rubs are usually those with the largest transmural MIs and a relatively poorer prognosis. If a large pericardial effusion develops, the heart sounds may be distant and the jugular venous pressure elevated. Cardiac tamponade results in the development of hypotension, pulsus paradoxus (reduction in systolic blood pressure during inspiration of more than 10 mm Hg), distant heart sounds, and an elevated jugular venous pressure.

Bibasilar or more extensive moist rales develop in patients with LV failure. Pulmonary edema occurs with extensive MI, in those with myocardial ischemia superimposed on extensive previous MI, and in some who develop mechanical complications (acute VSDs, acute mitral insufficiency, or large ventricular aneurysms) as a complication of acute MI.

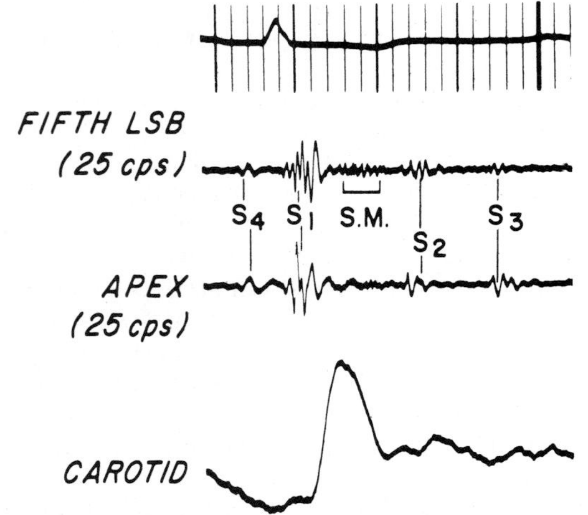

FIGURE 26–24 A fourth (S_4) and a third heart sound (S_3). Both the S_3 and the S_4 are relatively low-frequency sounds and were recorded well at 25 cps. Note that the S_4 is presystolic and the S_3 mid-diastolic in timing. This record was obtained from a patient with idiopathic hypertrophic subaortic stenosis. A systolic murmur (S.M.) and rapid carotid upstroke were also demonstrated. LSB, left sternal border.

Myocardial Stunning and Hibernation

Transient myocardial ischemia followed by reperfusion may lead to protracted recovery of segmental ventricular function, known as *myocardial stunning*. This is probably caused by cellular calcium overload and free radical generation.[146–153] Stunned myocardial segments may contribute to the development of CHF when the area of ischemia or infarction is large. Alternatively, persistent ischemia can lead to chronic depression of segmental ventricular function, known as *myocardial hibernation,*[149–153] which may also contribute to CHF and can be reversed, thereby correcting severe CHF, in selected patients who undergo coronary artery revascularization.

Electrocardiographic Diagnosis

The ECG provides an excellent means for recognizing acute Q wave MI (Figs. 26–26 to 26–28). The characteristic sequence of electrocardiographic alterations with Q wave MI includes (1) the initial development of prominent, peaked T waves in the electrocardiographic leads, representing sites of epicardial injury; (2) the development of hyperacute ST-segment elevation; and (3) the development of Q waves, 0.04 second in duration, or 40 percent or greater loss of R wave amplitude. The rapidity with which these electrocardiographic changes develop is variable. They can occur within minutes or may be delayed for several hours after symptom onset. Some patients with acute MIs have relatively normal ECGs during the first few hours.

In addition to the sometimes variable time-related evolution of the ECG when an acute Q wave MI occurs, there are other potential problems in using the ECG to identify acute MI. First, with LBBB, acute anterior MI is not recognizable from the ECG, since the LBBB pattern simulates that of an anterior MI in the left precordial leads. However, if the LBBB pattern is otherwise altered by the presence of diminutive R wave voltage, S waves, or initial Q waves in leads I, AVL, and/or V_5 and V_6, the patient may have had prior anterior and lateral MI. Inferior Q wave MIs can be recognized in the patient with LBBB because the evolution of the inferior Q wave MI is not altered by LBBB. Abnormal T wave vectors reversed from the normal pattern—that is, inverted T waves in V_1 to V_3

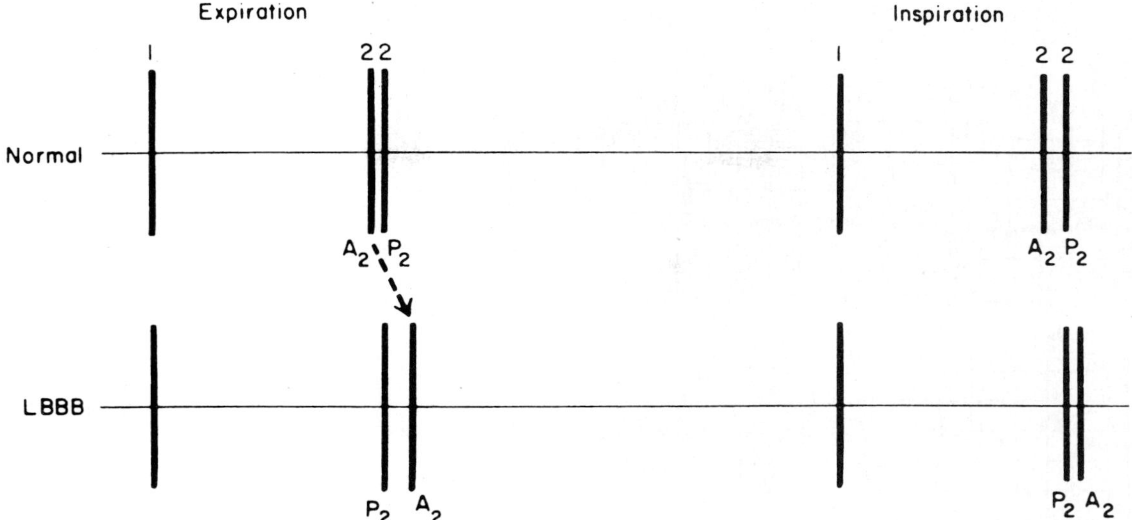

FIGURE 26–25 Normal and paradoxical splitting of the second heart sound are shown at *top* and *bottom,* respectively. The influence of left bundle branch block (LBBB) to produce paradoxical splitting of the second heart sound is shown (*bottom*). (From Willerson JT, Hillis LD, Buja LM: Ischemic Heart Disease: Clinical and Pathophysiological Aspects. New York: Raven, 1982.)

and/or upright T waves in leads V_4 to V_6—may indicate anterior or lateral ischemia or infarction. Second, with previous Q wave MI, recognition of new injury in the same general regions of the left ventricle is more difficult. Finally, with rapid electrocardiographic evolution of the MI, it may not be possible to differentiate old from new MI from the ECG alone. ST-segment elevation may also occur under other circumstances: (1) with normal early repolarization (Fig. 26–29); (2) with transient myocardial ischemia, as in Prinzmetal's angina, or with ischemia in an area of previous MI; (3) in some individuals with chronic ventricular aneurysms (Fig. 26–30); (4) transiently after electrical cardioversion; (5) in the anterior precordial electrocardiographic leads in patients with LBBB; (6) in the anterior precordial leads in some patients with LV hypertrophy; and (7) in an occasional patient with hyperkalemia.

Although the ECG is useful in the recognition of acute Q wave MI, it does not enable one to recognize acute non–Q wave MI with certainty. In these patients, the ECG usually demonstrates ST depression and T wave inversion, and the only evolution is a return to baseline (Fig. 26–31; see also Fig. 26–7). Unfortunately, subendocardial ischemia, ventricular hypertrophy, tachycardia, severe emotion, electrolyte alterations (especially hypokalemia, hypomagnesemia, hypocalcemia), and the use of certain medications (including cardiac glycosides) may produce similar electrocardiographic changes. Indeed, bizarre and deeply inverted T wave alterations occur in some patients with acute intracerebral hemorrhage. The only useful rule in the electrocardiographic recognition of non–Q wave MI is that the deeper the ST-segment depression and the longer it lasts, the more likely is an acute non–Q wave MI.

Serum Enzyme and Cardiac Intracellular Substance Changes

The relationship of changes in cardiac enzyme concentrations and other intracellular myocardial substances to the development of acute MI is shown in Figure 26–32. A previously preferred enzymatic technique was the measurement of CK and, in particular, the myocardium-specific CK-MB isoenzyme, measured either by spectrophotometry, fluorometry, or radioimmunoassay.[154–169] CK-MB increases in the sera of patients approximately 2 to 3 hours after the onset of acute MI, reaches a peak at 10 to 12 hours, and returns to normal within 24 hours after the event in patients with small infarcts and in those who have reperfusion after thrombolytic therapy or with endogenous thrombolysis. In patients with large infarcts, those not receiving thrombolytic therapy, and those who fail to experience reperfusion after thrombolytic therapy, CK and CK-MB often peak later (e.g., 18 to 24 hours after infarction) and return to normal 30 to 40 hours after the event. *Stuttering infarcts,* defined as repeated episodes of infarction with recurrent chest pain over hours to days, result in repeated elevations of serum CK and CK-MB.

Radioimmunoassay measurement of alterations in serum myoglobin concentration allows a slightly earlier recognition of acute MI, but there is no means to distinguish myoglobin release from the heart and skeletal muscle when skeletal muscle injury occurs. Therefore, in the patient with skeletal muscle damage from trauma, intramuscular injection, recent surgery, cardioversion, heat exposure, consumption of alcohol in excess, or primary skeletal muscle disorders, determining the presence of MI is not possible by measurement of serum myoglobin levels. However, in the patient without skeletal muscle injury, measurement of serum myoglobin by radioimmunoassay provides a sensitive and relatively rapid means to detect MI within 1 to 2 hours of the event. Myoglobin is released from injured myocardial cells within 1 to 2 hours of the event, peaks within 4 to 6 hours, and returns to normal values within 10 to 12 hours.

Radioimmunoassay measurement of alterations in the serum concentration of the light chain of myosin may also allow a relatively early and precise recognition of acute

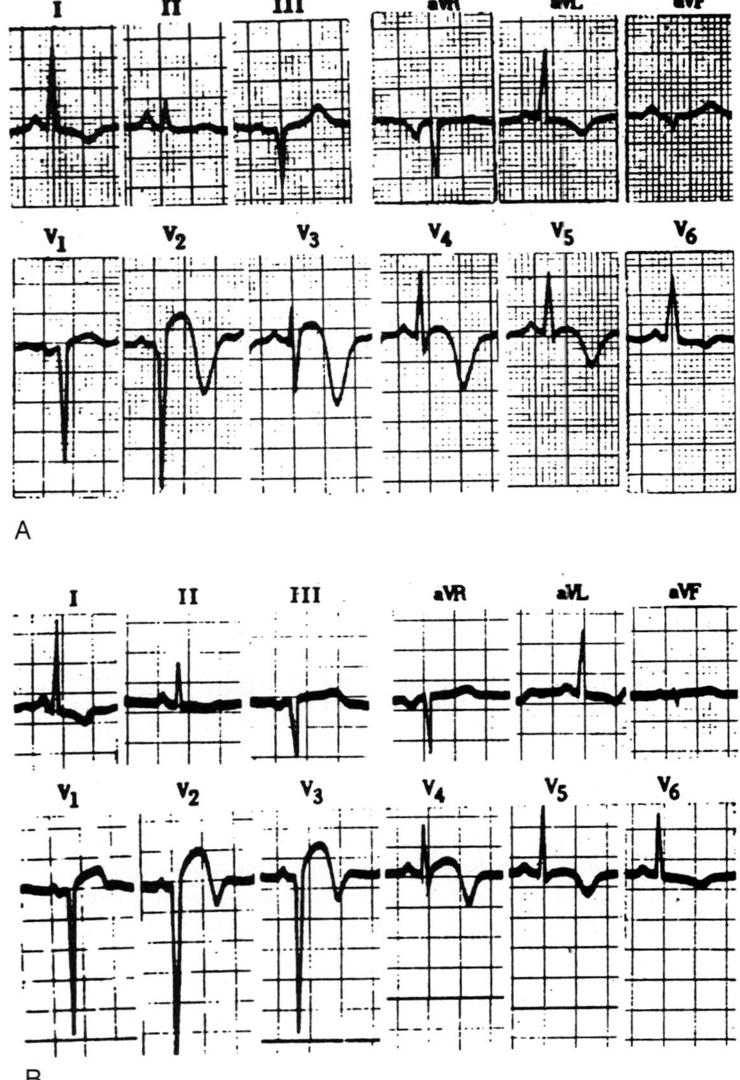

FIGURE 26–26 An evolving Q wave anterolateral MI **(A)** and the completed evolution of this infarct **(B)**. (**A** and **B,** From Willerson JT, Hillis LD, Buja LM: Ischemic Heart Disease: Clinical and Pathophysiological Aspects. New York: Raven, 1982.)

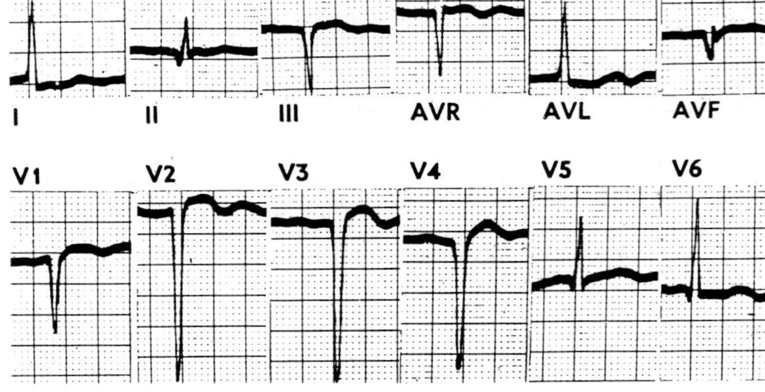

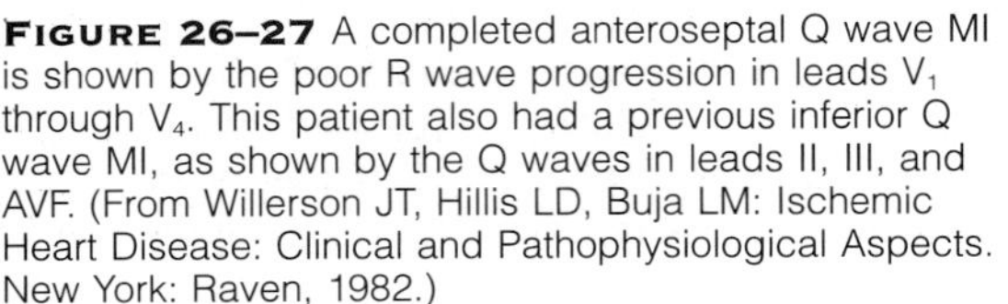

FIGURE 26–27 A completed anteroseptal Q wave MI is shown by the poor R wave progression in leads V_1 through V_4. This patient also had a previous inferior Q wave MI, as shown by the Q waves in leads II, III, and AVF. (From Willerson JT, Hillis LD, Buja LM: Ischemic Heart Disease: Clinical and Pathophysiological Aspects. New York: Raven, 1982.)

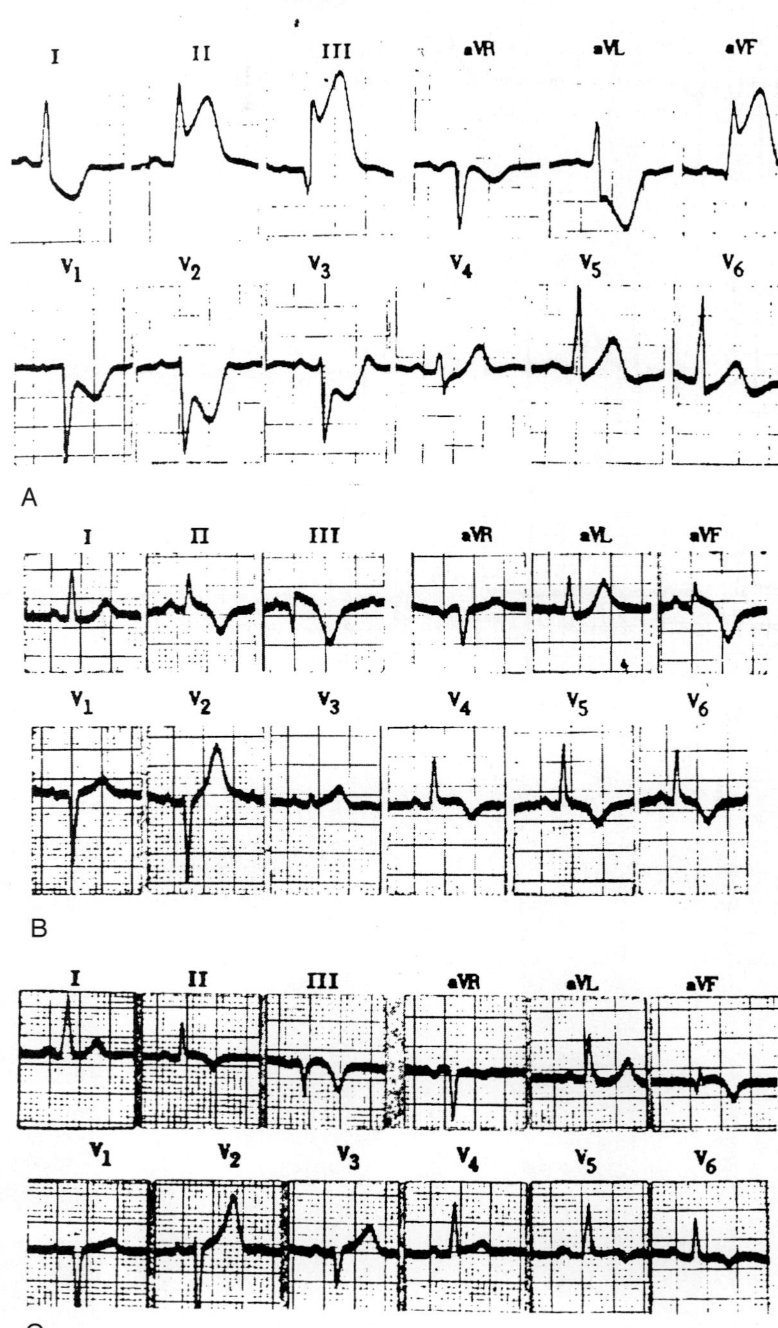

FIGURE 26–28 Evolution of a Q wave inferior MI. **A,** Note the hyperacute ST-segment elevation in leads II, II, and aVF and the reciprocal changes in leads V_1 through V_4. **B,** Further evolution of the infarct patterns. **C,** Completed evolution of the infarct. (**A–C,** From Willerson JT, Hillis LD, Buja LM: Ischemic Heart Disease: Clinical and Pathophysiological Aspects. New York: Raven, 1982.)

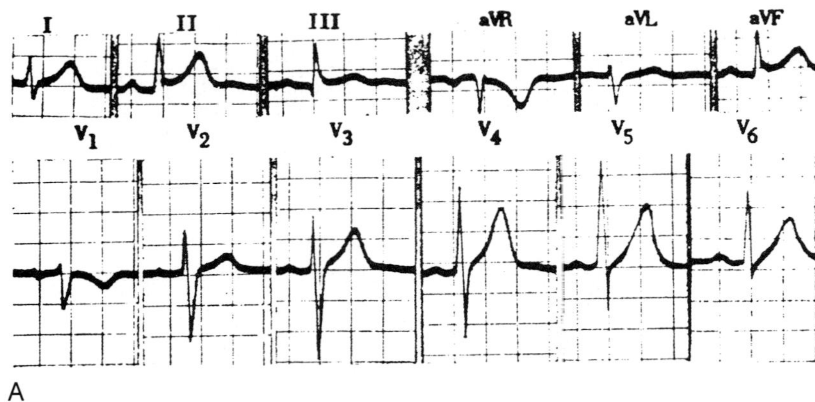

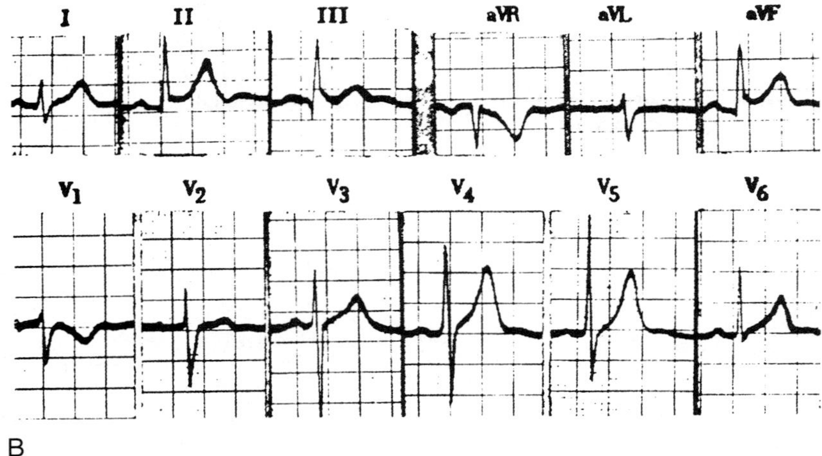

FIGURE 26–29 A and **B,** Normal early repolarization, in which upward sloping ST-segment elevation is seen in leads II, III, and aVF. The ECG is stable over time. On occasion, the elevated ST segment diminishes slightly during exercise. (**A** and **B,** From Willerson JT, Hillis LD, Buja LM: Ischemic Heart Disease: Clinical and Pathophysiological Aspects. New York: Raven, 1982.)

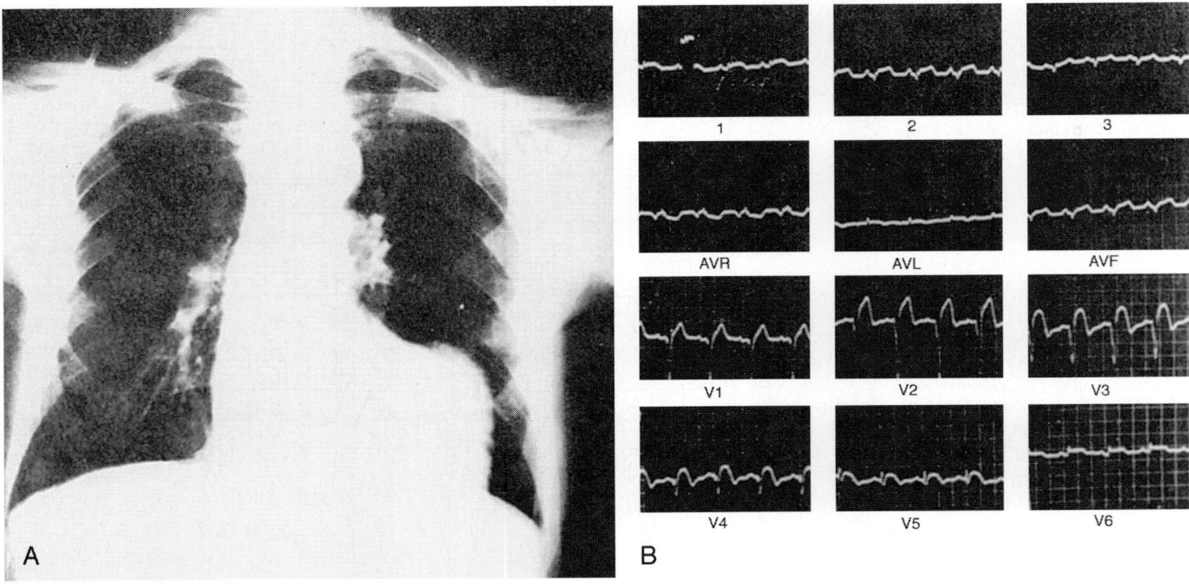

FIGURE 26–30 Chest radiograph **(A)** and corresponding ECG **(B)** reflect a ventricular aneurysm. Note the high lateral bulge in the left ventricular silhouette in the chest x-ray and the persistent ST-segment elevation across the pretorium (leads V_1 through V_6). (**A** and **B,** From Weisfeldt ML, Flaherty JR: Myocardial infarction. *In* Willerson JT, Sanders CA [eds]: Clinical Cardiology. pp. 346–369. New York: Grune & Stratton, 1977.)

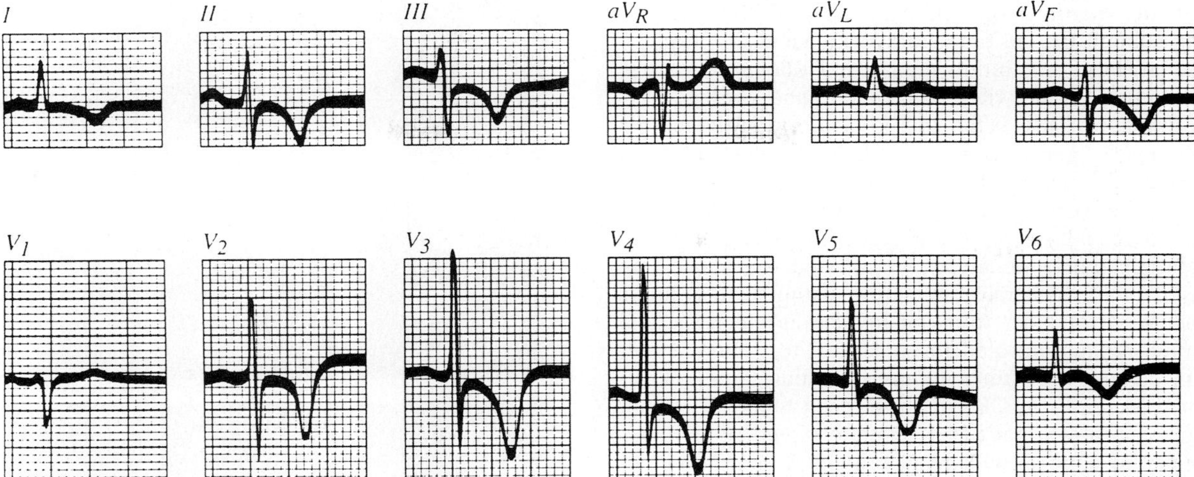

FIGURE 26–31 Electrocardiographic patterns seen with an acute non–Q wave MI. The T wave inversion in leads II, III, and AVF and the ST-segment depression and T wave inversion in the lateral precordial leads (leads V_4 through V_6) suggest the presence of subendocardial infarction. (From Willerson JT, Hillis LD, Buja LM: Ischemic Heart Disease: Clinical and Pathophysiological Aspects. New York: Raven, 1982.)

MI.[160, 161] Measurements of serum transaminase values were made in the past, but these are nonspecific and they are not relied on at present for MI detection. Serial serum measurements of lactic dehydrogenase (LDH) and LDH isoenzymes have also been used to recognize acute MI. There are five LDH isoenzymes, and increases in LDH isoenzymes 1 and 2 are consistent with MI, such that when LDH-1 and/or -2 elevations represent more than 50 percent of the total, they are often indicative of an acute MI. Increases in LDH occur 18 to 30 hours after MI and usually return to normal within 48 to 72 hours. Therefore, LDH measurements allow the detection of some patients with MI who delay their hospital admission in whom it is not possible to rely on changes in CK and CK-MB for infarct detection. More recent studies have indicated that damaged heart muscle releases the proteins troponin I and T, which increase in the circulation within 6 to 8 hours after the onset of chest pain and remain elevated for 2 or 3 days (see later).

Measurements of CK isoforms, as well as myoglobin, have proved useful in detecting reperfusion after thrombolytic therapy or release of an experimental coronary artery occlusion.[163–167] The conversion of CK isoform from CKMM-1 to CKMM-2 in the peripheral circulation appears to correlate with successful reperfusion therapy. Staccato increases in serum myoglobin in the first 4 to 6 hours after MI are indicative of reperfusion; rapid peaking of increases in serum CK and CK-MB (within 10 to 12 hours from symptom onset) are also often indicative of reperfusion of the MI.

Three troponin subunits regulate muscle contraction by modulating the calcium-dependent interaction of actin and

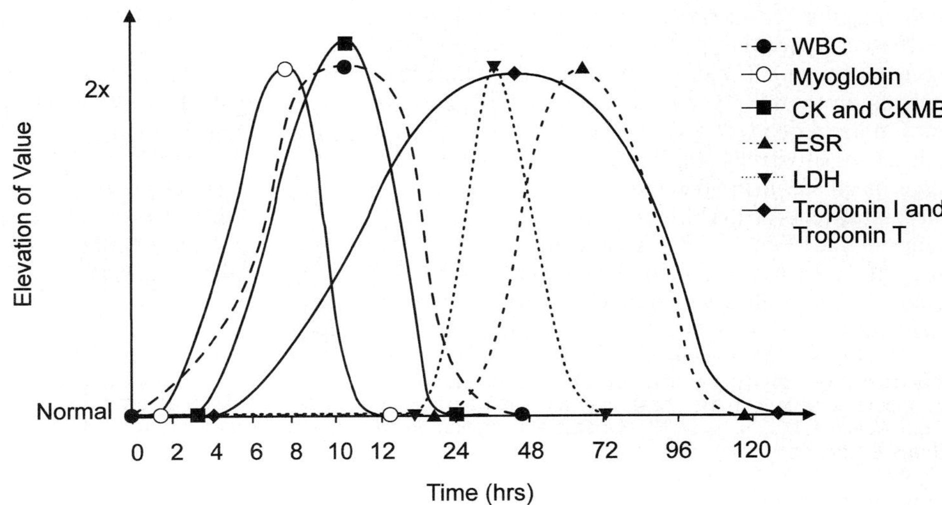

FIGURE 26–32 Typical changes in several enzymes measured in a patient with an evolving acute MI. Increases in serum myoglobin concentration are the earliest change indicative of MI. Note that the white blood cell count (WBC) rises early after infarction and that the serum creatine kinase (CK) and MB isoenzyme of CK (CKMB) rise before the serum troponin I and T. The erythrocyte sedimentation rate (ESR) and lactic dehydrogenase (LDH) rise relatively late after acute MI. (Modified from Willerson JT, Hillis LD, Buja LM: Ischemic Heart Disease: Clinical and Pathophysiological Aspects. New York: Raven, 1982.)

myosin: the tropomyosin-binding subunit T, the calcium-binding subunit C, and the actomyosin–adenosine triphosphatase [ATPase]–inhibiting subunit I. Troponin I exists in three isoforms: slow-twitch, fast-twitch, and cardiac. Cardiac troponin I (cTn-I) is the 26.5-kD isoform of the muscle subunit and is genetically and structurally distinct from that produced in extracardiac muscle.

Previous studies have shown that cTn-I and cardiac troponin T (cTn-T) correlate with acute myocardial necrosis in the general population.[162, 168, 169] Both substances are increased in the systemic circulation within 6 to 8 hours after acute MI or other forms of myocardial necrosis, and they often remain elevated for at least 2 to 3 days. However, in patients with renal failure, spurious cTn-T elevations and increases in CK-MB have been found.[107] Recent studies have shown that cTn-I accurately predicts myocardial injury in patients with renal failure. A study done by Martin and coworkers[107] evaluated 56 patients with acute or chronic renal failure or end-stage renal disease, assessing the sensitivity and specificity of cTn-I for detecting myocardial injury in these patients. During a 6-month period, patients admitted with suspected MI were evaluated. These patients had end-stage renal disease, chronic or acute renal failure, and a mean age of 62 years. There were an equal number of males and females. Further cardiac testing, including echocardiography, stress testing, or arteriography, was performed at the discretion of the primary physician. Positive cTn-I levels were associated with increased in-hospital mortality. The sensitivity and specificity for CK-MB were 44 percent and 56 percent, respectively, whereas they were 94 percent and 100 percent for cTn-I. In this study, elevated cTn-I levels were associated with increased short-term mortality and an ability to risk-stratify patients with severe renal failure and true myocardial injury. Troponin T values were slightly elevated in patients with renal disease, although not necessarily outside of the normal range. Troponin I values appeared to be more reliable in infarct detection in these patients.[107]

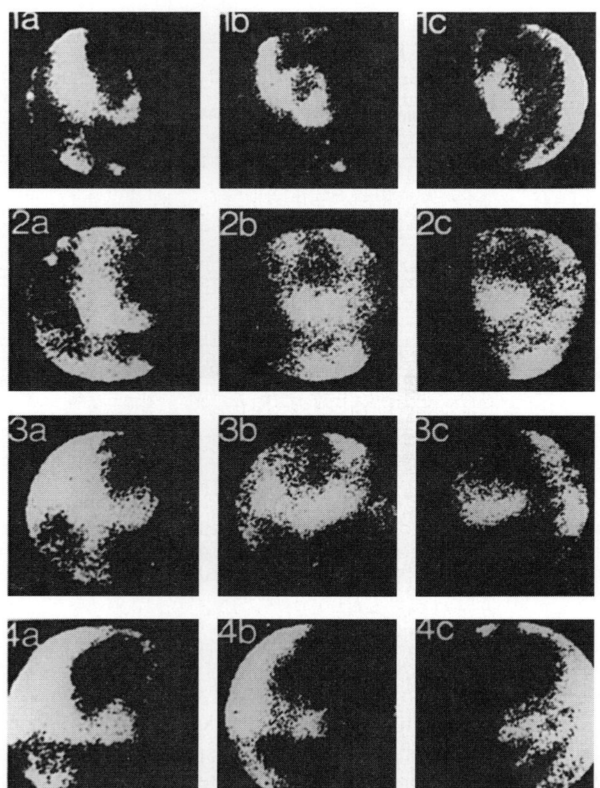

FIGURE 26–33 Various transmural MIs as evidenced by technetium 99m stannous pyrophosphate myocardial scintigraphy in the anterior, left anterior oblique, and left lateral imaging views. **1a–1c,** Large "doughnut" anterolateral MI. **2a–2c,** Inferior MI. **3a–3c,** Inferolateral MI. **4a–4c,** True posterior MI. (From Willerson JT, Hillis LD, Buja LM: Ischemic Heart Disease: Clinical and Pathophysiological Aspects. New York: Raven, 1982.)

Myocardial Scintigraphy

Radionuclide myocardial scintigraphy techniques for identification of acute MI can be useful.[170–182] These techniques enable one to visualize the region(s) of acute MI (*infarct-avid* imaging technique) or to identify areas of severely decreased myocardial perfusion (*myocardial perfusion* imaging technique). The prototype infarct-avid imaging agent, technetium 99m (^{99m}Tc) stannous pyrophosphate, accumulates in irreversibly damaged myocardium 1 to 5 days after MI; its sensitivity in the detection of acute MIs of 3 g or larger is greater than 90 percent (Fig. 26–33).[172, 173, 182] With successful reperfusion, MI may be detected within 2 to 3 hours of the event.[177, 178] An alternative to pyrophosphate imaging is the use of an antimyosin antibody labeled with technetium or iodine, which binds to myosin with myocyte membrane injury and MI.[179–181] It has the same sensitivity in MI detection as pyrophosphate, but it does not accumulate in bone. Thallium 201 (^{201}Tl) and Tc-sestamibi are myocardial perfusion imaging agents that accumulate in the myocardium in direct proportion to blood flow (Fig. 26–34).[175, 176] When used within 24 hours after acute MI, their sensitivities for infarct detection are approximately 90 percent. The size of the initial ^{201}Tl or ^{99m}Tc-sestamibi defect after acute MI appears to have prognostic significance, as do persistently abnormal pyrophosphate scintigrams,[182] that is, ones that remain abnormal for 3 months or longer after MI. Large MIs, as detected by extensive perfusion defect or by pyrophosphate or antimyosin uptake, and persistently abnormal pyrophosphate scintigrams, are associated with an increased risk for future coronary events and heart failure. ^{99m}Tc sestamibi provides information similar to that of ^{201}Tl, but it also allows an evaluation of regional systolic function, including systolic wall thickening.

In addition to these imaging techniques, the cardiovascular blood pool can be identified with technetium-labeled erythrocytes to characterize the impact of acute MI on regional and global ventricular function by dynamic myocardial scintigraphy.[183–186] This latter technique allows measurement of ventricular ejection fraction, ventricular volumes, regional wall motion, left-to-right shunts (i.e., VSDs), and valvular insufficiency, including mitral or tricuspid regurgitation and the identification of ventricular aneurysms.

Two-dimensional (or three-dimensional) echocardiographic measurements can also be used to detect intramyocardial masses and to evaluate global and segmental ven-

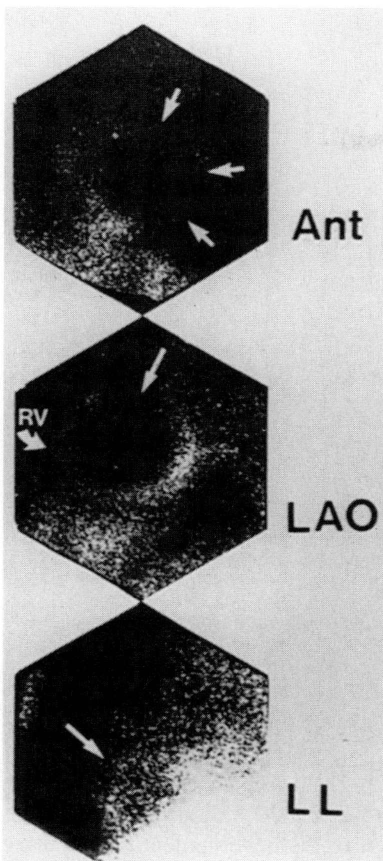

FIGURE 26–34 A thallium 201 myocardial scintigram from a patient with an acute MI in the anterior (Ant), left anterior oblique (LAO), and left lateral (LL) views. Only a portion of the interior and posterior wall of the heart are normally perfused. The anteroseptal and anterolateral aspects of the heart have marked decrease in thallium 201 perfusion, as shown by the *straight arrows.* RV, right ventricle *(curved arrow).*

tricular functional alterations in patients with acute MI.[187–191] Transthoracic and transesophageal two-dimensional echocardiography can also be used for detection of LV thrombi complicating acute MIs (Fig. 26–35).[189–191] Patients with acute anterior Q wave MIs more frequently develop LV mural thrombi acutely (10 to 40 percent of such individuals). These patients have an increased risk for systemic embolic events, requiring that they receive anticoagulants unless there is some exceptional contraindication. Echocardiography with Doppler, transthoracic and transesophageal, enables one to detect and estimate the severity of mitral insufficiency and VSDs, to identify ventricular aneurysms and pseudoaneurysms, and to assess the extent of wall motion abnormality in patients with infarction (Figs. 26–36 to 26–38).[192–209] Detection of these abnormalities is often important, especially in the patients with a low-output state, hypotension, or heart failure, since proper medical management or surgical repair may save the patient's life.

Pseudoaneurysms (false aneurysms) developing after MI represent partial tears in the left ventricle and a risk for complete rupture. They are distinguished from true aneurysms by demonstration—on two-dimensional echocardiogram, angiography, radionuclide ventriculography, or magnetic resonance imaging—of communication with the true left ventricle by a narrow channel or neck (Fig. 26–39). True LV aneurysms communicate with the LV cavity by an imperceptible pathway. False LV aneurysms rupture spontaneously and should be surgically corrected as soon as they are identified. Patients at greatest risk for heart

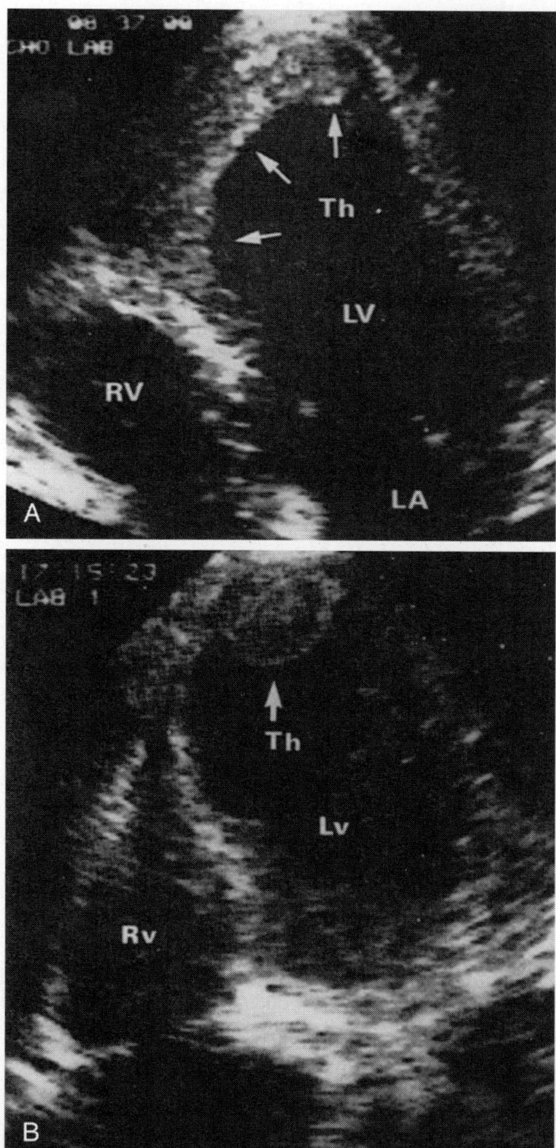

FIGURE 26–35 **A,** Apical four-chamber view demonstrates a large apical aneurysm in a patient status post-MI with a large layered thrombus (Th) in the apex of the left ventricle (LV). LA, left atrium; RV, right ventricle. **B,** Apical four-chamber view of a patient with an anterior MI demonstrates a mobile echolucent thrombus *(arrow)* in the apex. Note how an unconventional scan plane optimized visualization of the thrombus with the transducer tilted more inferiorly than for a standard apical four-chamber view. Lv, left ventricle; Rv, right ventricle; Th, thrombus. (**A** and **B,** From Schnittger I: Cardiac and extracardiac masses: echocardiographic evaluation. *In* Marcus ML, Schelbert HR, Skorton DJ, et al [eds]: Cardiac Imaging: A Companion to Braunwald's Heart Disease. pp. 511–537. Philadelphia: WB Saunders, 1991.)

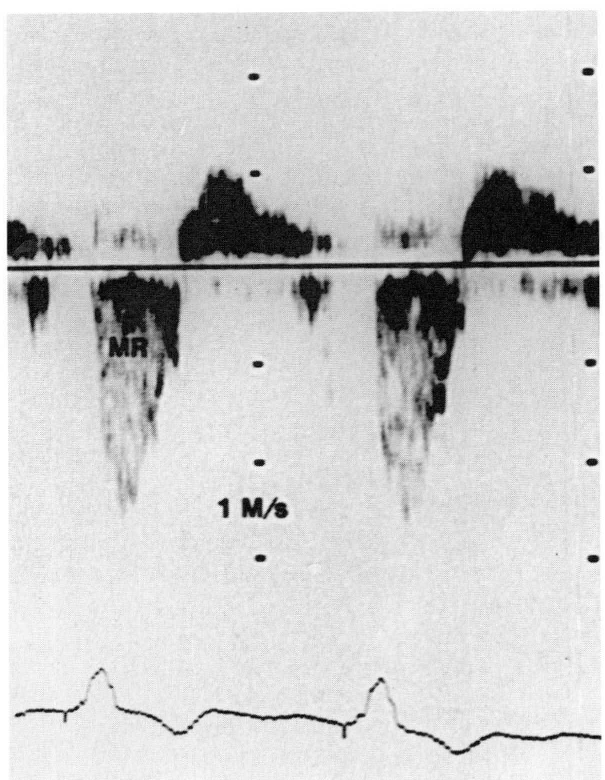

FIGURE 26–36 Continuous-wave Doppler in a patient with acute mitral regurgitation (MR). The maximal velocity peaks early in systole and then decreases abruptly. This occurs presumably on the basis of a large V wave with rapid reduction of the pressure difference between the left atrium and the left ventricle in mid to late systole. (From Kotler MN, et al: *In* Kerber RE [ed]: Echocardiography in Coronary Artery Disease. p. 17. Mt. Kisco, NY: Futura, 1988.)

rupture after MI are those who have systemic arterial hypertension and are experiencing their first MI and elderly patients. Blood pressure elevations should be prevented in patients with MI to minimize this risk. When myocardial rupture occurs after MI, most patients die suddenly of exsanguination or cardiac tamponade. A few develop tamponade with a sealing of the tear by a blood clot in the pericardial space. Although blood does not usually clot in the pericardial space, in the patient with extensive MI, it may clot as a consequence of the loss of segmental wall motion in the infarcted segment. Thus, continued bleeding is prevented, providing the observant physician an opportunity to recognize the development of an enlarging pericardial effusion with early tamponade and to intervene surgically to correct the tamponade and repair the myocardial rupture. In these patients, it appears best to place them on cardiopulmonary bypass and evacuate the pericardial fluid/thrombosis while on bypass rather than attempting to treat the pericardial tamponade by pericardiocentesis before placing the patient on bypass. The classic finding in the patient with sudden myocardial rupture is the development of electromechanical dissociation (EMD), in which the patient loses blood pressure and becomes unresponsive but has continuing electrical activity on the ECG for the

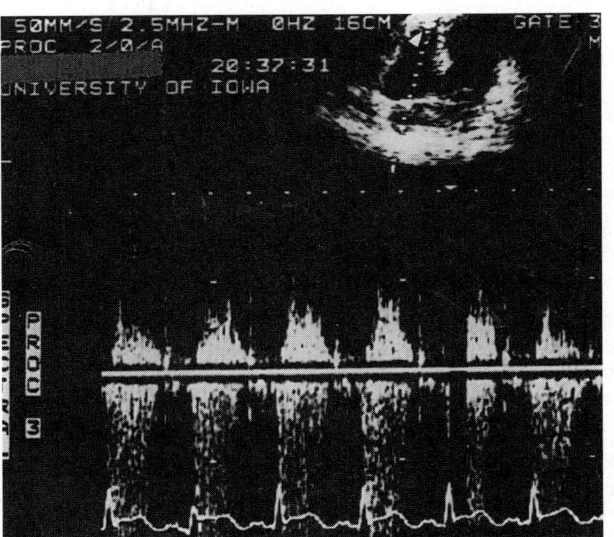

FIGURE 26–37 A pulsed-wave Doppler recording in a patient with a postinfarction ventricular septal defect. **Top,** The sample gate *(arrowhead)* is in the right ventricle adjacent to the septum. **Bottom,** There is an abnormal flow pattern in systole away from the transducer at the sampling point in the right ventricle, indicating left ventricular to right ventricular flow across a septal defect. (From Kerber RE: Echocardiography in coronary artery disease: myocardial ischemia and infarction. *In* Marcus ML, Schelbert HR, Skorton DJ, et al [eds]: Cardiac Imaging: A Companion to Braunwald's Heart Disease. pp. 594–603. Philadelphia: WB Saunders, 1991.)

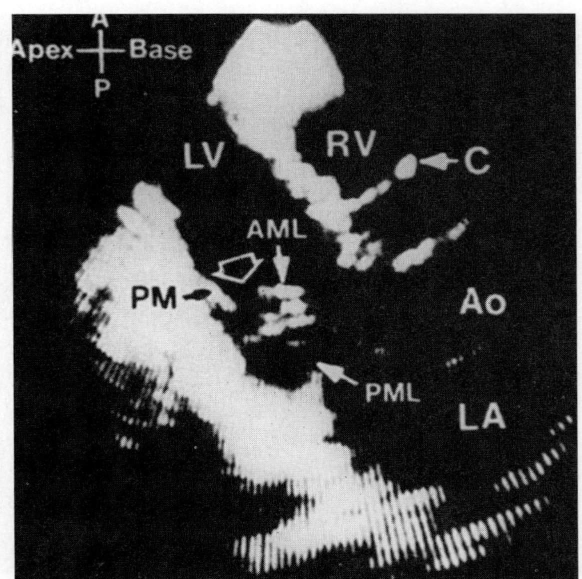

FIGURE 26–38 Parasternal long-axis view. The head of a ruptured papillary muscle (PM) is attached to the anterior mitral leaflet (AML). Ao, aorta; C, catheter; LA, left atrium; LV, left ventricle; PML, posterior mitral leaflet; RV, right ventricle. (From Mintz GS, Victor MF, Kotler MN, et al: Two-dimensional echocardiographic identification of surgically correctable complications of acute myocardial infarction. Circulation 64:91, 1981.)

subsequent few seconds to minutes. Electromechanical dissociation is not specific for myocardial rupture because it may also occur with a large anteroseptal infarct, pericardial tamponade of any etiology, and severe systemic hypoxemia or acidosis.

Differential Diagnosis

In theory, the differential diagnosis of acute MI includes any cause of chest pain, cardiac arrhythmias, new systolic murmur of mitral insufficiency or VSD, heart failure, and sudden death. Important diagnostic considerations include (1) unstable angina, (2) Prinzmetal's angina, (3) pericarditis, and (4) dissecting aortic aneurysm. Other diagnostic considerations, although less commonly presenting with pain classical for MI, include (1) peptic ulcer disease, (2) pancreatitis, (3) cholecystitis, (4) pulmonary embolic disease, (5) spontaneous pneumothorax, and (6) pneumonitis. Careful attention to history, physical examination, relevant blood tests, ECGs, and noninvasive or invasive imaging test results usually enables one to make the correct diagnosis.

Estimation of Infarct Size

Accurate measurements of the extent of reversible and irreversible cell damage can be useful in predicting prognosis and selecting the optimal future therapy for patients. Ideally, such measurements should be relatively noninvasive, applicable early in the patient's clinical course, capable of being repeated with reasonable frequency, able to provide quantitation of the extent of damage with various types of infarcts, and generally available. No perfect measurement of infarct size or of the extent of ischemic damage exists at present, although several methods have been used: (1) enzymatic indices of infarct size, most importantly, measurement of CK-MB enzyme release from the heart[210]; (2) scintigraphic measurements of infarct size, including infarct-avid scintigraphic techniques (with ^{99m}Tc stannous pyrophosphate or antimyosin antibody)[211–213] and myocardial perfusion techniques (^{201}Tl or ^{99m}Tc-sestamibi and other technetium-based perfusion markers); (3) two-dimensional transthoracic or transesophageal echocardiography; and (4) dynamic myocardial scintigraphy to estimate abnormalities of global and segmental ventricular function, using either first-pass or equilibrium techniques. One anticipates that evaluation of global LV function with magnetic resonance imaging will allow estimation of infarct size in the future. Each of these techniques has its limitations, but each also provides important information concerning the location or relative size of an infarction.

Three-dimensional estimates of the extent of myocardial damage are needed for accurate scintigraphic measurements (single-photon emission computed tomography) and with other imaging techniques, including three-dimensional echocardiography and magnetic resonance imaging. Distinction of reversibly ("viable" myocardium) and irreversibly injured myocardium can be made in patients by positron emission tomography evaluation that combines estimates of myocardial perfusion (rubidium or other positron emission tomography perfusion marker) and fluorodeoxyglucose studies to identify reversibly injured myocardium as regions with persistent metabolic activity. Persistent metabolic activity is indicated by uptake and utilization of fluorodeoxyglucose (indicative of reversible injury to the myocardium) even when perfusion is markedly reduced or absent. One may also demonstrate reversible wall motion abnormalities by echocardiography, radionuclide ventriculography, or magnetic resonance imaging when potent inotropic stimuli, such as dobutamine, dopamine, or paired electrical stimulations, are used, or during low-level exercise 5 to 7 days after MI.[214–223]

Evaluation of Ventricular Function

Invasive and noninvasive techniques can be used to allow more precise characterization of ventricular function in

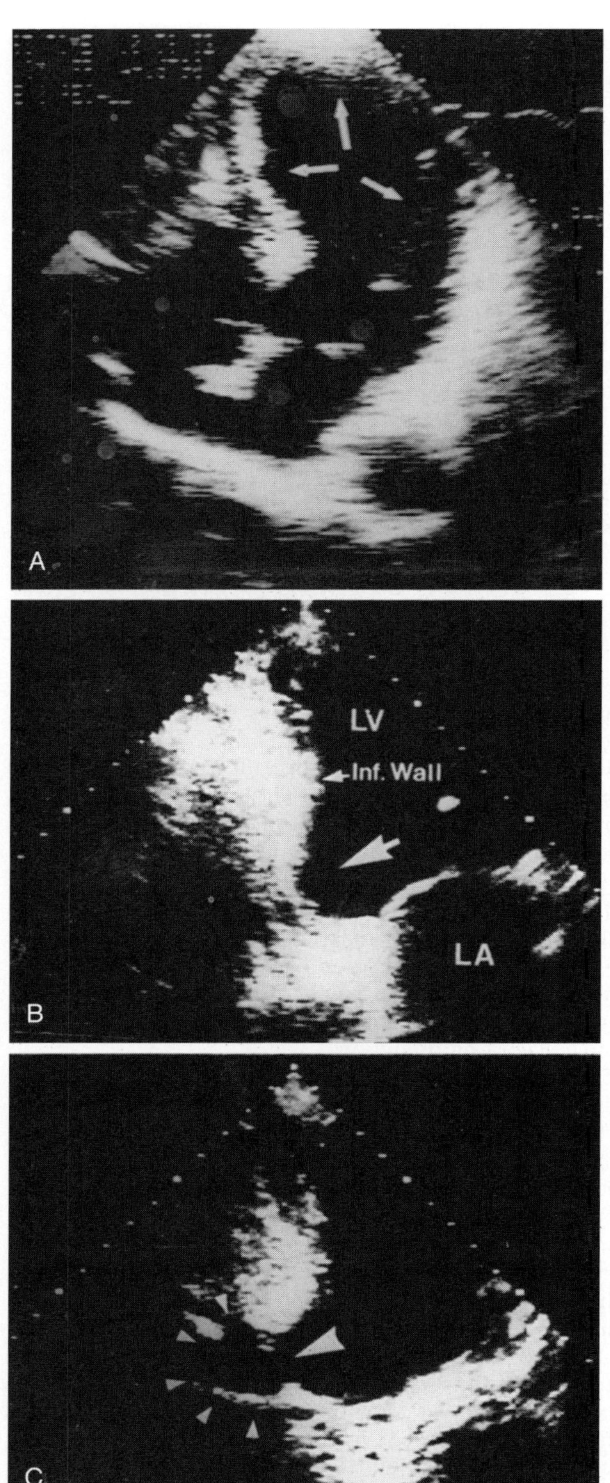

FIGURE 26–39 A, Apical four-chamber view demonstrates an apical left ventricular aneurysm *(arrows)*. **B,** Apical two-chamber view in a patient with a large inferior wall infarction *(large arrow)*. LA, left atrium; LV, left ventricle. **C,** Off-axis view reveals a narrow communications orifice *(large arrow)*. The pseudoaneurysm is outlined by the *small arrows*. (**A–C,** From Kotler MN, et al: *In* Kerber RE [ed]: Echocardiography in Coronary Artery Disease. p. 17. Mt. Kisco, NY: Futura, 1988.)

patients with reduced systemic arterial blood pressure and uncertain LV functional status. Flow-directed catheters, such as the Swan-Ganz catheter, allow measurement of LV filling pressure without entering a systemic artery or the left ventricle (Fig. 26–40).[224] This balloon-tipped, flow-directed catheter can be placed in the pulmonary artery from a systemic vein. The Swan-Ganz catheter is positioned in the pulmonary artery either with the aid of fluoroscopy or with continuous pressure monitoring to identify the characteristic right atrial, RV, and pulmonary artery pressures. Once the catheter is in the pulmonary artery, the balloon is inflated, allowing the measurement of pulmonary capillary wedge pressure. In the absence of mitral valve disease, the mean pulmonary capillary wedge pressure is

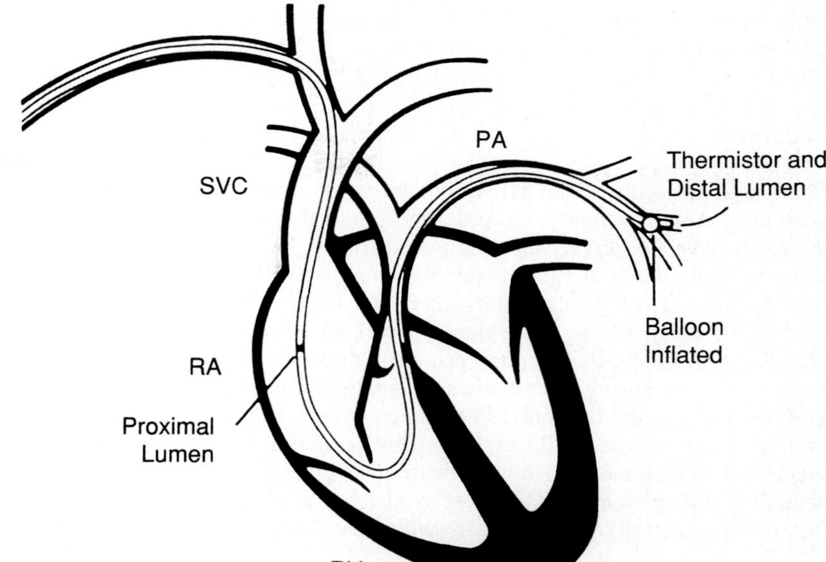

FIGURE 26–40 Path taken by a Swan-Ganz catheter. The catheter is inserted into a systemic vein, threaded into the right heart, and positioned in the pulmonary artery (PA). In this location, pulmonary artery and pulmonary capillary wedge pressures and cardiac output may be measured. RA, right atrium; RV, right ventricle; SVC, superior vena cava. (From Willerson JT, Hillis LD, Buja LM: Ischemic Heart Disease: Clinical and Pathophysiological Aspects. NY: Raven, 1982.)

similar to the LV end-diastolic or filling pressure (Fig. 26–41).

Measurement of LV filling pressure with the Swan-Ganz catheter enables one to differentiate hypotension caused by hypovolemia from cardiogenic shock and LV failure. Mean pulmonary capillary wedge pressures less than 12 mm Hg with hypotension occur with hypovolemia and those 15 mm Hg or higher are usually associated with cardiogenic shock and LV failure. In addition, cardiac output may be measured with the same catheter. The patient with an acute MI and shock should also have an indwelling arterial cannula placed to allow accurate measurement of and to detect moment-to-moment changes in systemic arterial pressure. The flow-directed pulmonary arterial catheter may also be utilized to help idealize mean pulmonary capillary wedge pressure at values of 15 to 18 mm Hg in the hypotensive patient.

LV and RV function after acute MI can be assessed noninvasively with either dynamic myocardial scintigraphy, echocardiography (Fig. 26–42), or with magnetic resonance imaging. These methodologies allow measurement of ventricular ejection fraction, ventricular dimensions or volumes, and segmental wall motion. Two-dimensional echocardiography and transesophageal echocardiography with Doppler assessment allow the detection of LV thrombi, VSDs, and mitral insufficiency, as well as an estimation of their severity. Transesophageal echocardiography allows a more precise detection of intracardiac thrombi than does transthoracic echocardiography. Three-dimensional echocardiography is being developed at present, and it may

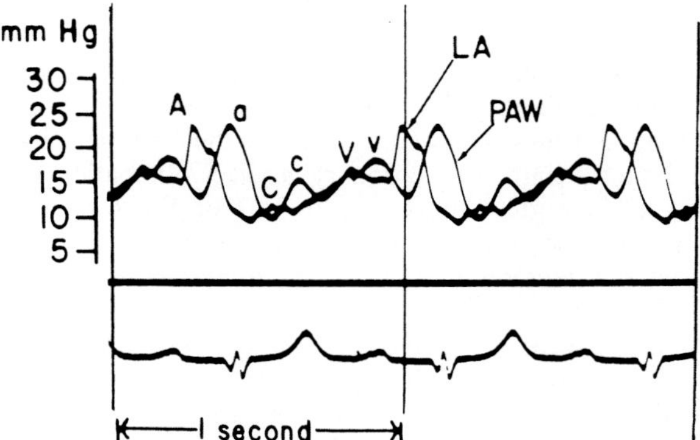

FIGURE 26–41 Simultaneous recordings of the left atrial (LA) and pulmonary capillary wedge (PAW) pressures. These pressures should be equal in the absence of important mitral valve disease. (From Willerson JT, Hillis LD, Buja LM: Ischemic Heart Disease: Clinical and Pathophysiological Aspects. New York: Raven, 1982.)

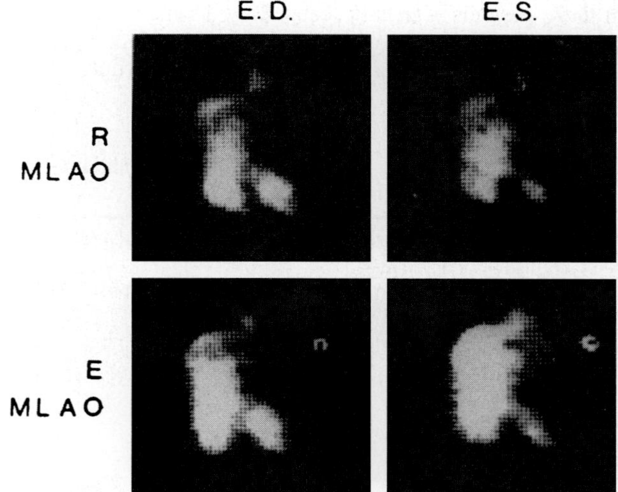

FIGURE 26–42 Gated dynamic myocardial scintigrams obtained by in vivo labeling of red blood cells in the end-diastolic (E.D.) and end-systolic (E.S.) silhouettes. Rest (R) and exercise (E) images are shown in a modified left anterior oblique (MLAO) imaging projection that separates the right and the left ventricles. (From Willerson JT, Hillis LD, Buja LM: Ischemic Heart Disease: Clinical and Pathophysiological Aspects. New York: Raven, 1982.)

allow even more accurate characterization of systolic function and detection of thrombi in the future.

Prognosis

Most patients with acute MI who survive to reach the hospital and subsequently receive appropriate therapy for their MIs have a relatively uncomplicated course. However, some patients develop life-threatening complications during the first 1 to 2 weeks, and others die (Table 26–4). During the early 1970s, more than 50 percent of patients died before reaching the hospital, primarily due to ventricular arrhythmias during the seconds or minutes after onset of chest pain. Since the late 1980s, emergency ambulance systems have achieved a 25 to 30 percent reduction in the incidence of death before hospitalization in patients with acute MI and sudden cardiac arrest syndromes.[225–227] Early thrombolytic therapy or angioplasty within the first 3 hours after MI, especially within the first hour, has reduced mortality to less than 6 percent.

Overall mortality in patients with acute MI who reach the hospital ranges from 3 to 30 percent, depending on the population studied and the promptness and success of the therapy given in opening the infarct-related artery. However, with very rapid administration of thrombolytic therapy or angioplasty followed by reperfusion within the first 1 to 2 hours after MI, mortality rates have decreased to 5 to 6 percent or less. In general, patients with anterior MIs have a higher mortality than those with inferior MIs, probably because of a greater loss of LV muscle.

Patients can be categorized into groups with differing prognoses on the basis of their initial hemodynamic measurements. Patients without LV failure and with a mean systolic arterial pressure of greater than 110 mm Hg, an average cardiac index greater than 2.5 L/min/m^2, and a normal pulmonary capillary wedge pressure (or pulmonary artery diastolic pressure) have low mortality rates. Death in these patients is usually caused by a ventricular arrhythmia, later infarct extension, or a mechanical complication (e.g., myocardial, septal, or papillary muscle rupture).

TABLE 26–4 Life-Threatening Complications of Acute Myocardial Infarction

- Ventricular arrhythmias (ventricular tachycardia, ventricular fibrillation or asystole)
- Extremely rapid atrial arrhythmias in association with extensive MI (atrial flutter or atrial fibrillation)
- Heart block (second-degree [Mobitz II] or third-degree)
- Marked bradycardia
- Infarction $\geq$ 40% of left ventricle
- Extensive RV infarction
- Acute ventricular septal defects
- Acute and severe mitral regurgitation
- Severe pulmonary edema
- Rupture of the heart
- Systemic and/or pulmonary emboli
- Extension of the MI
- Markedly increased LV end-systolic volume after MI
- Occluded proximal LAD after anterior MI

Abbreviations: LAD, left anterior descending coronary artery; LV, left ventricular; MI, myocardial infarction; RV, right ventricular.

A ruptured papillary muscle of the mitral valve leads to fulminant left heart failure with pulmonary edema and often hypotension, and the patient is typically unresponsive to diuretics and unloading interventions. This catastrophic event should be suspected when a patient with an inferior, lateral, or non–Q wave MI abruptly develops fulminant left heart failure with a new apical murmur, often soft, of mitral insufficiency. On occasion, however, the severity of the LV failure is such that no murmur is generated. Prominent V waves are usually found in the pulmonary capillary wedge tracing by flow-directed catheter. An echocardiogram and Doppler evaluation demonstrate severe mitral regurgitation and sometimes a flail mitral leaflet. Ordinarily, the only chance for survival is immediate surgical repair or replacement of the mitral valve.

Papillary muscle dysfunction, mediated by ischemia with a transient apical systolic murmur or by infarction with a permanent apical systolic murmur, usually causes less severe mitral regurgitation, and the patient can generally be stabilized by unloading therapy with a diuretic and nitroprusside or, if needed, temporary intra-aortic balloon support.

Chordae tendineae rupture is not usually caused by MI, but instead may lead to acute mitral regurgitation as a consequence of spontaneous rupture, as in the Marfan patient or the woman with mitral valve prolapse, with chest wall trauma, or secondary to the trauma on the mitral valve apparatus of significant valvular aortic insufficiency, with endocarditis, or as a consequence of acute rheumatic fever.

Acute VSDs occur primarily in the muscular septum and develop within 1 day to 2 weeks after MI, resulting in a new holosystolic murmur along the lower left sternal border, often associated with a systolic thrill in the same location and a significant oxygen step-up between the right atrium and the right ventricle. The VSD places a pressure and volume load on the left and right ventricles and may result in sudden, or gradual, hemodynamic decompensation, with severe CHF, hypotension, and relentless hemodynamic deterioration. We believe that immediate surgical correction of a large VSD is indicated with the development of the earliest signs of hemodynamic deterioration (e.g., increased respiratory rate, tachycardia, hypotension). In the future, it may be possible to do this in the cardiac catheterization laboratory with a device, such as a "clam shell" occluder. Such patients are often placed on an intra-aortic balloon and other unloading therapy and are usually taken to the cardiac catheterization suite for coronary arteriography and then to surgery to repair the VSD and bypass significantly narrowed coronary arteries. In patients with large left-to-right shunts, 1.5 to 2.0 or greater, surgical closure of the VSD becomes mandatory to prevent the subsequent development of severe pulmonary artery hypertension. However, in the hemodynamically stable patient, VSD closure can be delayed for 4 to 6 weeks with resultant lowering of operative risk. Antibiotic prophylaxis against infective endocarditis with dental or surgical work is necessary in these patients, even after VSD closure.

Patients with cardiogenic shock and systolic arterial pressures of 80 mm Hg or less, decreased peripheral perfusion without a reversible cause, reduced mean cardiac index (<2 L/min/m^2), and an increased pulmonary capillary wedge or pulmonary artery diastolic pressure (>25 mm

Hg) have an increased mortality, usually greater than 50 percent, unless the infarct-related artery can be opened by PTCA or thrombolytic therapy within the first 1 to 2 hours after the event. PTCA is capable of more rapid reperfusion in the desperately ill patient with MI and cardiogenic shock and, if the cardiac catheterization facility is available and an experienced team on site or very close by, is the preferred means for providing rapid and potentially lifesaving reperfusion in these patients.[228] Those with clinical evidence of LV failure and a normal or elevated systemic arterial pressure have an expected mortality of 5 to 30 percent. Very early reperfusion in these patients with cardiogenic shock or severe heart failure by PTCA or thrombolytic therapy with successful reperfusion may save the lives of more than half of them.[228]

Longer-term mortality after recovery from an initial MI is related to the presence of ventricular arrhythmias, the extent of myocardial damage, the age of the patient, and the LV end-systolic volume (Fig. 26–43). Persistent occlusion of the infarct-related artery, most especially the proximal left anterior descending coronary artery, is also associated with a reduced long-term survival (Fig. 26–44). In general, if the patient is less than 50 years of age at the time of the initial MI, the annual mortality rate is approximately 5 percent or less. If the patient is over 50 years of age, the mortality rate is approximately doubled. If a patient survives for 1 year after MI, there is a 75 percent chance of 5-year survival. If a patient survives for 5 years after MI, there is an approximately 50 percent or greater chance of 15-year survival. These numbers will improve in the coming years with extensive efforts at prevention of future coronary events, utilizing potent lipid-lowering, antioxidant, and antithrombotic therapies.

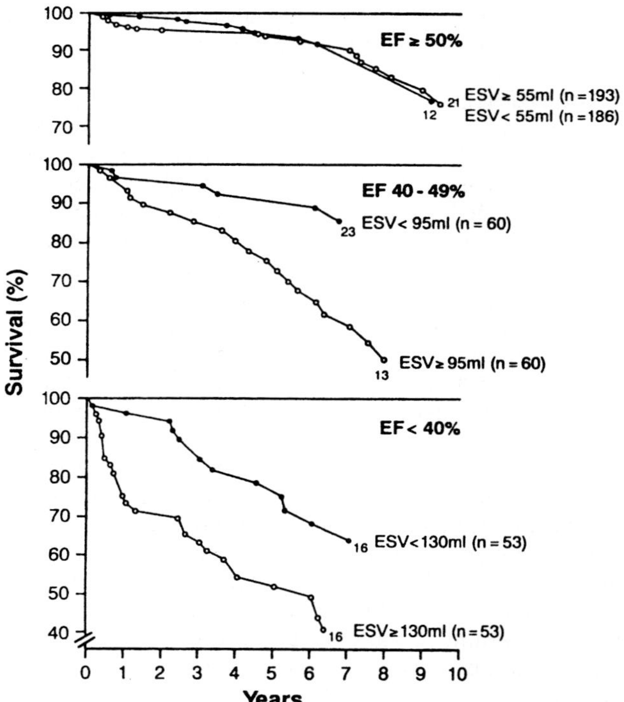

FIGURE 26–43 Actuarial survival curves for patients with low–end-systolic volume (ESV) versus high-ESV at various ejection fractions (EFs) after MI. In patients with left ventricular EFs < 50 percent, ESV plays a greater role in predicting survival than does left ventricular EF. (From White HD, Norris RM, Brown MA, et al: Left ventricular end-systolic volume as the major determinant of survival after recovery from myocardial infarction. Circulation 76[1]:44–51, 1987.)

In-hospital and immediate post-hospital complications are related directly to infarct size. When more than 40 percent of the LV muscle mass is irreversibly damaged and reperfusion is not accomplished by angioplasty, thrombolytic therapy, or surgical revascularization within the first 1 to 2 hours, one can expect power-failure complications, including cardiogenic shock, CHF, and medically refractory ventricular arrhythmias. Patients with small MIs (irrespective of the location) are less likely to experience such complications. However, a strategically located small MI may cause heart block, acute development of a VSD, or papillary muscle dysfunction or rupture resulting in acute mitral insufficiency. In addition, patients with multiple small MIs may ultimately develop cardiogenic shock, medically refractory CHF, or medically refractory arrhythmias as a consequence of the cumulative muscle loss. Even a small MI may be associated with ventricular arrhythmias; therefore, continuous electrocardiographic monitoring is necessary for at least 2 to 3 days after MI, irrespective of infarct size or clinical complications.

Accurate predictors of longer-term prognosis in patients with acute MI are needed. Serum CK measurements are important prognostically, as patients with the largest MIs are most likely to experience cardiogenic shock, refractory CHF, or refractory ventricular arrhythmias; however, several hours to a few days are required to complete such measurements. Myocardial perfusion imaging, ^{201}Tl or ^{99m}Tc-sestamibi myocardial scintigraphy may be used at hospital admission to estimate the extent of the myocardial perfusion defect. Patients with the largest perfusion defects have a poorer prognosis during hospitalization and a higher mortality in the short-term follow-up. Similarly, patients with the most extensive ventricular functional abnormalities (as detected by radionuclide ventriculography, echocardiography, magnetic resonance ventriculography, or angiography) and those with large anterior MIs may develop "pump failure" and important ventricular arrhythmias. Patients with anterior Q wave MI who extend their infarction in hospital have increased morbidity and mortality.[229–231]

Patients with ventricular ejection fractions below 40 percent and those with similar ventricular dysfunction and complex ventricular ectopy (frequent ventricular premature beats, coupled ventricular premature beats, or short bursts of ventricular tachycardia) at the time of hospital discharge, and those with severe global and segmental ventricular dysfunction or a reversible perfusion or function defect on low-level exercise or stress testing at the time of hospital discharge, have a relatively poor prognosis when they have not been treated with thrombolytic agents or angioplasty.[232–237] Whether the same is true for patients who receive thrombolytic therapy or angioplasty and are reperfused after MI is at present unclear. Finally, persistently abnormal ^{99m}Tc-stannous pyrophosphate myocardial scintigrams several months after MI indicate chronic ischemic injury and the risk for progressive decline in ventricular function. Whether this is also true for persistently abnormal antimyosin antibody scans is unknown at present.

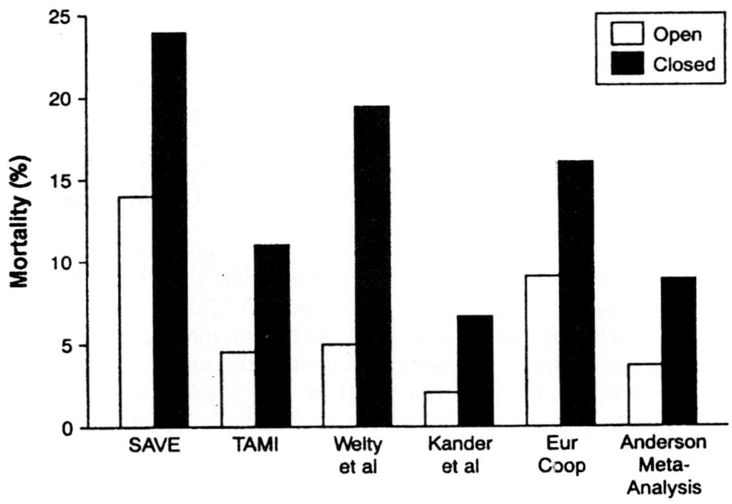

FIGURE 26–44 Mortality in patients with an open versus a closed infarct-related artery after MI. The presence of an open artery at discharge confers a significant survival benefit in the first year after acute MI. (From Topol EJ: Textbook of Cardiovascular Medicine. p. 485. Philadelphia: Lippincott, 1997.)

Remodeling of the Left Ventricle ("Infarct Expansion")

Infarct expansion or *remodeling* of the infarct and peri-infarct regions refers to shape alterations in the infarct and peri-infarct areas that result from stress and strain alterations in the infarct and adjacent areas. Most likely, metalloproteinase release and alterations in myocardial wall stress related to the local influence of angiotensin and endothelin play a role in the remodeling process. The remodeling phenomenon causes changes in contractile patterns in the infarct and peri-infarct regions and dilatation of the heart over time.[238–244] Infarct expansion or remodeling occurs primarily in patients with anterior Q wave MIs, in those with larger MIs, in those with systemic arterial hypertension, in those with occluded infarct-related arteries, and in older individuals. Infarct remodeling leads to increases in LV end-diastolic and end-systolic volumes and dimensions and decline in LV function with a fall in LV ejection fraction in the several weeks to years after the infarct. Previous studies have demonstrated that angiotensin-converting enzyme inhibitors reduce the magnitude of the remodeling phenomenon and preserve LV function when administration is begun several hours to days after MI, especially in patients with anterior Q wave MIs.[241–249] The same is likely to be true for the angiotensin receptor antagonists and the combination of angiotensin-converting enzyme inhibitors and angiotensin receptor antagonists in the future. Revascularization with a subsequent patency of the infarct-related artery also reduces the magnitude of post-MI remodeling.

Infarct Extension

Infarct extension is the result of new MI hours to a few days after the original event, often associated with reocclusion of the infarct-related artery after thrombolytic therapy or angioplasty or as a consequence of increases in myocardial oxygen demand or relative decreases in LV regional oxygen availability, such as occur with tachycardia, severe systemic arterial hypertension, hypotension, and/or worsening CHF. Reductions in myocardial oxygen delivery associated with hypotension or decreased substrate availability as with hypoglycemia may extend MIs. Every effort should be made to prevent increases in myocardial oxygen demand and decreases in oxygen delivery in patients with CAD, especially those with MIs. Infarct extension is poorly tolerated hemodynamically in those with anterior and previous MIs and seems to occur most commonly in those with non–Q wave and possibly those with anterior MIs who are not treated with thrombolytic therapy or angioplasty. Predictors of patients whose infarct-related artery is most likely to close after it has been opened by thrombolytic therapy are not yet agreed on, but every effort is made to keep such arteries patent by using antithrombin interventions (heparin at present, but perhaps more direct inhibitors of thrombin in the future) for 24 to 36 hours after thrombolytic therapy. Antiplatelet agents, aspirin at present as 1 aspirin (325 mg) tablet daily, but potentially even more potent antiplatelet therapies in the future, including the adenosine diphosphate antagonist clopidogrel, low-molecular-weight heparin for several weeks after hospital discharge, or orally available inhibitors of platelet glycoprotein IIb/IIIa receptors, if such agents can be shown in the future to be safe and effective.

Van Belle and colleagues,[250] using coronary angioscopic techniques in patients with MIs, have recently shown that healing of the infarct-related coronary artery lesion requires more than 1 month and that an unstable yellow plaque with adherent thrombus is commonly present during that period. These findings may help explain the risk for some patients with unstable angina and acute MI to reocclude the culprit artery in this time period and the need to provide effective antithrombotic therapy for at least several weeks after the event. Reclosure of the infarct-related artery is associated with a poor prognosis.

REFERENCES

1. Heberden W: Some account of a disorder of the breast. Med Trans R Coll Phys II London, 1786, p. 59.
2. Herrick JB: Clinical features of sudden obstruction of the coronary arteries. JAMA 59:2015, 1912.
3. Sarnoff SJ, Braunwald E, Welch GHJ: Hemodynamic determinants

of oxygen consumption of the heart with special reference to the tension-time index. Am J Physiol 192:148, 1958.
4. Rude RE, Izquierdo C, Buja LM, Willerson JT: Effects of inotropic and chronotropic stimuli on acute myocardial ischemic injury. I. Studies with dobutamine in the barbiturate-anesthetized dog. Circulation 65:1321, 1982.
5. Rude RE, Izquierdo C, Bush LR: Effects of inotropic and chronotropic stimuli on acute myocardial ischemic injury. II. Studies with dopamine and ouabain in the barbiturate-anesthetized dog. J Cardiovasc Pharmacol 5:717, 1983.
6. Rude RE, Bush LR, Izquierdo C, et al: Effects of inotropic and chronotropic stimuli on acute myocardial ischemic injury. III. Influences of basal heart rate. Am J Cardiol 53:1688, 1984.
7. Sonnenblick EH, Ross JJ, Braunwald E: Oxygen consumption of the heart: newer concepts of its multifactorial determination. Am J Cardiol 22:328, 1969.
8. Marcus ML, Doty DB, Hiratzka LF: Decreased coronary reserve—a mechanism for angina pectoris in patients with aortic stenosis and normal coronary arteries. N Engl J Med 307:1362, 1982.
9. Marcus ML, Mueller TM, Eastham CL: Effects of short- and long-term left ventricular hypertrophy on coronary circulation. Am J Physiol 24:H358, 1981.
10. Berkenboom GM, Abramowicz M, Vandermoten P, Degre SG: Role of alpha-adrenergic coronary tone in exercise-induced angina pectoris. Am J Cardiol 57:195, 1986.
11. Gage JE, Hess OM, Murakami T, et al: Vasoconstriction of stenotic coronary arteries during dynamic exercise in patients with classic angina pectoris: reversibility by nitroglycerin. Circulation 73:865, 1986.
12. Wexler L, Brundage B, Crouse J, et al: Coronary artery calcification: pathophysiology, epidemiology, imaging methods, and clinical implications. Circulation 94:1175, 1996.
13. Agatson AS, Janowitz WR, Hildner FJ, et al: Quantification of coronary artery calcium using ultrafast computed tomography. J Am Coll Cardiol 15:872, 1990.
14. Detrano R, Hsiai T, Wang S, et al: Prognostic value of coronary calcification and angiographic stenoses in patients undergoing coronary angiography. J Am Coll Cardiol 27:285, 1996.
15. Secci A, Wong N, Tang W, et al: Electron beam computed tomographic coronary calcium as a predictor of coronary events: comparison of two protocols. Circulation 96:1122, 1997.
16. Arad Y, Spadaro LA, Goodman K, et al: Predictive value of electron beam computed tomography of the coronary arteries. Circulation 93:1951, 1996.
17. Constantinides P: Plaque fissuring in human coronary thrombosis. J Atheroscler Res 6:1, 1966.
18. Davies MJ, Thomas AEC: Plaque fissuring—the cause of acute myocardial infarction, sudden ischemic death, and crescendo angina. Br Heart J 53:363, 1985.
19. Falk E: Plaque rupture with severe preexisting stenosis precipitating coronary thrombosis: characteristics of coronary atherosclerotic plaques underlying fatal occlusive thrombi. Br Heart J 50:127, 1983.
20. Buja LM, Willerson JT: Clinicopathologic correlates of acute ischemic heart disease syndromes. Am J Cardiol 47:343, 1981.
21. Davies MJ, Fulton WFM, Robertson WB: The relation of coronary thrombosis to ischemic myocardial necrosis. J Pathol 172:99, 1979.
22. Buja LM, Willerson JT: The role of coronary artery lesions in ischemic heart disease: insights from recent clinicopathologic, coronary arteriographic, and experimental studies. Hum Pathol 18:451, 1987.
23. Buja LM, Tofe AJ, Kulkarni PV, et al: Sites and mechanisms of localization of technetium-99m phosphorus radiopharmaceuticals in acute myocardial infarcts and other tissues. J Clin Invest 60:7245, 1977.
24. Davies JM, Thomas AC, Knapman PA, Hangartner JR: Intramyocardial platelet aggregation in patients with unstable angina pectoris suffering sudden ischemic cardiac death. Circulation 73:418, 1986.
25. Willerson JT, Hillis LD, Buja LM: Ischemic Heart Disease: Clinical and Pathophysiological Aspects. New York: Raven, 1982.
26. Fuster V, Badimon L, Badimon JJ, Chesebro JH: The pathogenesis of coronary artery disease and the acute coronary syndromes. N Engl J Med 326:242, 310, 1992.
27. Fuster V, Lewis A: Mechanisms leading to myocardial infarction: insights from studies of vascular biology. Connor Memorial Lecture. Circulation 91:256, 1995.
28. Libby P: Molecular bases of the acute coronary syndromes. Circulation 91:2844, 1995.
29. Bush L, Campbell WB, Tilton GD, et al: Effects of the selectin thromboxane synthase inhibitor, dazoxiben, on cyclic flow variations in stenosed canine arteries. Trans Assoc Am Physicians 96:103, 1983.
30. Ashton JH, Ogletree ML, Michel IM, et al: Serotonin and thromboxane A_2/prostaglandin H_2 receptor activation cooperatively mediate cyclic flow variations in dogs with severe coronary artery stenoses. Circulation 76:952, 1987.
31. Golino P, Ashton JH, Buja LM, et al: Local platelet activation causes vasoconstriction of large epicardial canine coronary arteries in vivo: thromboxane A_2 and serotonin are possible mediators. Circulation 79:154, 1989.
32. Bush LR, Campbell WB, Kern K, et al: The effects of alpha-adrenergic and serotonergic receptor antagonists on cyclic blood flow alterations in stenosed canine coronary arteries. Circ Res 55:642, 1984.
33. Willerson JT, Hillis LD, Winniford MD, Buja LM: Speculation regarding mechanisms responsible for acute ischemic heart disease syndromes. J Am Coll Cardiol 8:245, 1986.
34. Willerson JT, Campbell WB, Winniford MD, et al: Conversion from chronic to acute coronary artery disease: speculation regarding mechanisms. Am J Cardiol 54:1349, 1984.
35. Willerson JT, Golino P, Eidt JF, et al: Specific platelet mediators and unstable coronary artery lesions. Experimental evidence and potential clinical implications. Circulation 80:198, 1989.
36. Hirsh PD, Hillis LD, Campbell WB, et al: Release of prostaglandins and thromboxane into the coronary circulation in patients with ischemic heart disease. N Engl J Med 304:685, 1981.
37. Eidt JF, Allison P, Noble S, et al: Thrombin is an important mediator of platelet aggregation in stenosed and endothelially-injured canine coronary arteries. J Clin Invest 84:18, 1989.
38. van den Berg EK, Schmitz JM, Benedict CR, et al: Transcardiac serotonin concentration is increased in selected patients with limiting angina and complex coronary lesion morphology. Circulation 49:116, 1989.
39. Maseri A, Severi S, De Nes M: "Variant" angina: one aspect of a continuous spectrum of vasospastic myocardial ischemia; pathogenic mechanisms, estimated incidence and clinical and coronary arteriographic findings in 138 patients. Am J Cardiol 42:1019, 1978.
40. Dalen JE, Ockene IS, Alpert JS: Coronary spasm, coronary thrombosis and myocardial infarction. Am Heart J 104:1119, 1982.
41. Gottlieb SO, Weisfeldt ML, Ouyang P, et al: Silent ischemia as a marker for early unfavorable outcomes in patients with unstable angina. N Engl J Med 314:1214, 1986.
42. Fleg JL, Gerstenblith G, Zonderman AB: Prevalence and prognostic significance of exercise-induced silent myocardial ischemia detected by thallium scintigraphy and electrocardiography in asymptomatic volunteers. Circulation 81:428, 1990.
43. Weiner DA, Ryan TJ, McCabe CH: Significance of silent myocardial ischemia during exercise testing in patients with coronary artery disease. Am J Cardiol 59:725, 1987.
44. Latham P: Collected Works. Vol. 1. London: New Sydenham Society, 1876.
45. Osler W: The Lumleian lectures on angina pectoris. Lancet 1:697, 1910.
46. Prinzmetal M, Kennamer R, Merliss R: Angina pectoris. I. A variant form of angina pectoris. Am J Med 27:375, 1959.
47. Hillis LD, Braunwald E: Coronary artery spasm. N Engl J Med 299:695, 1978.
48. Silverman ME, Flamm MDJ: Variant angina pectoris: anatomic findings and prognostic implications. Ann Intern Med 75:339, 1971.
49. Cheng TO, Bashour R, Kelser GA: Variant angina of Prinzmetal with normal coronary arteriograms a variant of the variant. Circulation 47:476, 1973.
50. Wiener L, Kasparian H, Duca PR: Spectrum of coronary arterial spasm: clinical, angiographic, and myocardial metabolic experience in 29 cases. Am J Cardiol 38:945, 1976.
51. Dhurandhar RW, Watt DL, Silver MD: Prinzmetal's variant form of angina with arteriographic evidence of coronary arterial spasm. Am J Cardiol 30:902, 1972.
52. Oliva PB, Potts DE, Pluss RG: Coronary arterial spasm in Prinzmetal angina: documentation by coronary arteriography. N Engl J Med 288:745, 1973.

53. Maseri A, Mimmo R, Chierchia S: Coronary artery spasm as a cause of acute myocardial ischemia in man. Chest 68:625, 1975.
54. Higgins CB, Wexler L, Silverman JF: Clinical and arteriographic features of Prinzmetal's variant angina: documentation of etiologic factors. Am J Cardiol 37:831, 1976.
55. Maseri A, Parodi O, Severi S: Transient transmural reduction of myocardial blood flow, demonstrated by thallium-201 scintigraphy, as a cause of variant angina. Circulation 54:280, 1976.
56. McLaughlin PR, Doherty PW, Martin RP: Myocardial imaging in a patient with reproducible variant angina. Am J Cardiol 39:126, 1977.
57. Berman ND, McLaughlin PR, Huckell VF: Prinzmetal's angina with coronary artery spasm: angiographic, pharmacologic, metabolic, and radionuclide perfusion studies. Am J Med 60:727, 1976.
58. Ricci DR, Orlick AE, Doherty PW: Reduction of coronary blood flow during coronary artery spasm occurring spontaneously and after provocation by ergonovine maleate. Circulation 57:392, 1978.
59. Nelson C, Nowak B, Childs H: Provocative testing for coronary arterial spasm: rationale, risk, and clinical illustrations. Am J Cardiol 40:624, 1977.
60. Schroeder JS, Bolen JL, Quint RA: Provocation of coronary spasm with ergonovine maleate: new test with result in 57 patients undergoing coronary arteriography. Am J Cardiol 40:487, 1977.
61. Curry RC Jr, Pepine CJ, Sabom MB, et al: Effects of ergonovine in patients with and without coronary artery disease. Circulation 56:803, 1977.
62. Heupler FA, Proudfit WL, Razavi M, et al: Ergonovine maleate provocative test for coronary arterial spasm. Am J Cardiol 41:631, 1978.
63. Helfant R: Coronary arterial spasm and provocative testing in ischemic heart disease. Am J Cardiol 41:787, 1978.
64. Buxton A, Goldberg S, Hirshfeld JW, et al: Refractory ergonovine-induced coronary vasospasm: importance of intracoronary nitroglycerin. Am J Cardiol 46:329, 1980.
65. Scherf D, Perlman A, Schlachman M: Effect of dihydroergonovine on the heart. Proc Soc Exp Biol Med 71:420, 1949.
66. Heupler FA Jr: Provocative testing for coronary arterial spasm: risk, method, and rationale. Am J Cardiol 46:335, 1980.
67. Fester A: Provocative testing for coronary arterial spasm with ergonovine maleate. Am J Cardiol 46:338, 1980.
68. Cipriano PR, Guthaner DF, Orlick AE, et al: The effects of ergonovine maleate on coronary arterial size. Circulation 59:82, 1979.
69. Endo M, Hirosawa K, Kaneko N, et al: Prinzmetal's variant angina: coronary arteriogram and left ventriculogram during angina attack induced by methacholine. N Engl J Med 294:252, 1976.
70. Yasue H, Horio Y, Imoto N, et al: Induction of coronary artery spasm by acetylcholine in patients with variant angina: possible role of the parasympathetic nervous system in the pathogenesis of coronary artery spasm. Circulation 74:955, 1986.
71. Raizner AE, Chahine RA, Ishimori T, et al: Provocation of coronary artery spasm by the cold pressor test: hemodynamic, arteriographic, and quantitative angiographic observations. Circulation 62:925, 1980.
72. Mudge GH Jr, Grossman W, Mills RM Jr, et al: Reflex increase in coronary vascular resistance in patients with ischemic heart disease. N Engl J Med 295:1333, 1976.
73. Hasue H, Nagao M, Omote S, et al: Coronary arterial spasm and Prinzmetal's variant form of angina induced by hyperventilation and tris-buffer infusion. Circulation 58:56, 1978.
74. Nemerson Y: The phospholipid requirement of tissue factor in blood coagulation. J Clin Invest 47:72, 1968.
75. Hamsten A, Wiman B, Faire U, Blomback M: Increased plasma levels or rapid inhibition of tissue plasminogen activator in young survivors of myocardial infarction. N Engl J Med 313:1557, 1985.
76. Schafer AI: Coagulation cascade: an overview. *In* Loscalzo J, Schafer A (eds): Thrombosis and Hemorrhage. p. 3. Boston: Blackwell Scientific, 1993.
77. Chandler AB, Chapman I, Erhardt LR, et al: Coronary thrombosis in myocardial infarction. Report of a workshop on the role of coronary thrombosis in the pathogenesis of acute myocardial infarction. Am J Cardiol 34:823, 1974.
78. DeWood MA, Spores J, Notshe R, et al: Prevalence of total coronary occlusion during the early hours of transmural myocardial infarction. N Engl J Med 303:897, 1980.
79. Buja LM, Willerson JT: Clinicopathologic findings in 100 episodes of acute ischemic heart disease (acute myocardial infarction or coronary insufficiency) in 83 patients. Am J Cardiol 47:343, 1981.
80. Gibson RS, Beller GA, Gheroghiade M, et al: The prevalence and clinical significance of residual myocardial ischemia 2 weeks after uncomplicated non–Q wave infarction: a prospective natural history study. Circulation 73:1186, 1986.
81. Falk E: Unstable angina with fatal outcome: dynamic coronary thrombosis leading to infarction and/or sudden death. Circulation 71:699, 1985.
82. Haft JI, Haik BJ, Goldstein JE, Brodyn NE: Development of significant coronary artery lesions in areas of minimal disease. A common mechanism for coronary disease progression. Chest 94:731, 1988.
83. Little WC, Constantinescu M, Applegate RJ, et al: Can coronary angiography predict the site of a subsequent myocardial infarction in patients with mild-to-moderate coronary artery disease? Circulation 78:1157, 1988.
84. The RISC Group: Risk of myocardial infarction and death during treatment with low dose aspirin and intravenous heparin in men with unstable coronary artery disease. Lancet 336:827, 1990.
85. Lewis HD, David JW, Archibald DG, et al: Protective effects of aspirin against acute myocardial infarction and death in men with unstable angina. N Engl J Med 209:396, 1983.
86. Freeman MR, Williams AE, Chisholm RJ, Armstrong PW: Intracoronary thrombus and complex morphology in unstable angina. Relation to timing of angiography and in-hospital cardiac events. Circulation 80:17, 1989.
87. Sherman CT, Litvak F, Grundfest W, et al: Coronary angioscopy in patients with unstable angina pectoris. N Engl J Med 315:913, 1986.
88. Libby P, Hansson GK: Involvement of the immune system in human atherogenesis: current knowledge and unanswered questions. Lab Invest 64:5, 1991.
89. Hansson GK, Jonasson L, Seifert PS, Stemme S: Immune mechanisms in atherosclerosis. Arteriosclerosis 9:567, 1989.
90. Gerrity RG: The role of the monocyte in atherogenesis. I. Transition of blood-borne monocytes into foam cells in fatty lesions. Am J Pathol 103:181, 1981.
91. Jonasson L, Holm J, Skalli O, et al: Regional accumulation of T cells, macrophages and smooth muscle cells in the human atherosclerotic plaque. Arteriosclerosis 6:131, 1986.
92. Parthasarathy S, Printz DJ, Boyd D, et al: Macrophage oxidation of low-density lipoprotein generates a modified form recognized by the scavenger receptor. Arteriosclerosis 6:505, 1986.
93. Forman MB, Oates JA, Robertson D, et al: Increased adventitial mast cells in a patient with coronary spasm. N Engl J Med 313:1138, 1985.
94. Carry M, Korley V, Willerson JT, et al: Increased urinary leukotriene excretion in patients with cardiac ischemia: in vivo evidence for 5-lipoxygenase activation. Circulation 85:230, 1992.
95. Henney AM, Wakeley PR, Davies MJ, et al: Localization of stromelysin gene expression in atherosclerotic plaques by in situ hybridization. Proc Natl Acad Sci U S A 88:8154, 1991.
96. Nikkari ST, O'Brien KD, Ferguson M, et al: Interstitial collagenase (MMP-1) expression in human carotid atherosclerosis. Circulation 92:1393, 1995.
97. Sukhova G, Schönbeck U, Rabkin E, et al: Evidence for increased collagenolysis by interstitial collagenases-1 and -3 in vulnerable human atheromatous plaques. Circulation 99:2503, 1999.
98. Galis ZS, Sukhova GK, Lark MW, Libby P: Increased expression of vascular matrix metalloproteinases induced in vitro by cytokines and in regions of human atherosclerotic lesions. Ann N Y Acad Sci 748:501, 1995.
99. Moreno PR, Falk E, Palacios IF, et al: Macrophage infiltration in acute coronary syndromes. Implications for plaque rupture. Circulation 90:775, 1994.
100. Henney AM, Wakeley PR, Davies MJ, et al: Localization of stromelysin gene expression in atherosclerotic plaques by in situ hybridization. Proc Natl Acad Sci U S A 88:8154, 1991.
101. Rajavashisth TB, Xiao-Ping X, Jovinge S, et al: Membrane type I matrix metalloproteinase expression in human atherosclerotic plaques. Evidence for activation by proinflammatory mediators. Circulation 99:3103, 1999.
102. Casscells W, Hathorn B, David M, et al: Thermal detection of cellular infiltrates in living atherosclerotic plaques: possible implications for plaque rupture and thrombosis. Lancet 347:1447, 1996.
103. Stefanadis C, Diamantopoulos L, Vlachopoulos C, et al: Thermal heterogeneity within human atherosclerotic coronary arteries detected in vivo. A new method of detection by application of a special thermography catheter. Circulation 99:1965, 1999.

104. Ohman EM, Armstrong PW, Christenson RH, et al: Cardiac troponin T levels for risk stratification in acute myocardial ischemia. N Engl J Med 335:1333, 1996.
105. Lindahl B, Venge P, Wallentin L, for the FRISC Study Group: Relation between troponin T and the risk of subsequent cardiac events in unstable coronary artery disease. Circulation 93:1651, 1996.
106. Antman EM, Tanasijevic MJ, Thompson B, et al: Cardiac-specific troponin I levels to predict the risk of mortality in patients with acute coronary syndromes. N Engl J Med 335:1342, 1996.
107. Martin GS, Becker B, Schulman G: Cardiac troponin-I accurately predicts myocardial injury in renal failure. Nephrol Dial Transplant 13:1709, 1998.
108. Koenig W, Sund M, Frölich M, et al: C-reactive protein, a sensitive marker of inflammation, predicts future risk of coronary heart disease in initially healthy middle-aged men. Circulation 99:237, 1999.
109. Berk BC, Weintraub WS, Alexander RW: Elevation of C-reactive protein in "active" coronary artery disease. Am J Cardiol 65:168, 1990.
110. Liuzzo G, Biasucci LM, Gallimore JR, et al: The prognostic value of C-reactive protein in severe angina. N Engl J Med 331:407, 1994.
111. Kruskal JB, Commerford PJ, Franks JJ, Kirsch RE: Fibrin and fibrinogen related antigens in patients with stable and unstable coronary artery disease. N Engl J Med 317:1361, 1987.
112. Haverkate F, Thompson SG, Pyke SDM, et al, for the European Concerted Action on Thrombosis and Disabilities Angina Pectoris Study Group: Production of C-reactive protein and risk of coronary events in stable and unstable angina. Lancet 349:462, 1997.
113. Ridker PM, Cushman M, Stampfer MJ, et al: Inflammation, aspirin, and the risk of cardiovascular disease in apparently healthy men. N Engl J Med 336:973, 1997.
114. Biasucci LM, Liuzzo G, Fantuzzi G, et al: Increasing levels of interleukin (IL)-1Ra and IL-6 during the first 2 days of hospitalization in unstable angina are associated with increased risk of in-hospital coronary events. Circulation 99:2079, 1999.
115. Patel SS, Willerson JT, Yeh ETH: Inhibition of macrophages homing to the atherosclerotic plaques in the ApoE deficient mice by anti-α_4 antibody. Circulation 97:25–81, 1998.
116. Shepherd J, Cobbe SM, Ford I, et al, for the West of Scotland Coronary Prevention Study Group: Prevention of coronary heart disease with pravastatin in men with hypercholesterolemia. N Engl J Med 333:1301–1307, 1995.
117. Scandinavian Simvastatin Survival Study Group: Randomised trial of cholesterol lowering in 4444 patients with coronary heart disease: the Scandinavian Simvastatin Survival Study (4S). Lancet 344:1383, 1994.
118. Sacks FJ, Pfeffer MA, Moye LA, et al, for the Cholesterol and Recurrent Events Trial Investigators: The effect of pravastatin on coronary events after myocardial infarction in patients with average cholesterol levels. N Engl J Med 335:1001, 1996.
119. Ridker RP, Rifai N, Pfeffer MA, et al: Long term effects of pravastatin on plasma concentration in C reactive protein. Circulation 100:230, 1999.
120. Weisfeldt ML, Flaherty JR: Myocardial infarction. *In* Willerson JT, Sanders CA (eds): Clinical Cardiology. pp. 346–369. New York: Grune & Stratton, 1977.
121. Kannel WB, Abbott RD: Incidence and prognosis of unrecognized myocardial infarction. N Engl J Med 311:1144, 1984.
122. Younis LT, Byers S, Shaw L, et al: Prognostic importance of silent myocardial ischemia detected by intravenous dipyridamole thallium myocardial imaging in asymptomatic patients with coronary artery disease. J Am Coll Cardiol 14:1635, 1989.
123. Weiner DA, Ryan TJ, McCabe C, et al: Risk of developing an acute myocardial infarction or sudden coronary death in patients with exercise-induced silent myocardial ischemia. A report from the Coronary Artery Surgery Study (CASS) registry. Am J Cardiol 62:1155, 1988.
124. Page DL, Caulfield JB, Kastor JA, et al: Myocardial changes associated with cardiogenic shock. N Engl J Med 285:133, 1971.
125. Alonso DR, Scheidt S, Post M, Killip T: Pathophysiology of cardiogenic shock: quantification of myocardial necrosis, clinical, pathologic, and electrocardiographic correlation. Circulation 48:588, 1973.
126. Willerson JT, Curry GC, Watson JT, et al: Intraaortic balloon counterpulsation in patients in cardiogenic shock, medically refractory left ventricular failure, and/or recurrent ventricular tachycardia. Am J Med 58:183, 1975.
127. Platt MR, Willerson JT, Watson JT, et al: The use of AVCO intraaortic balloon circulatory assistance for patients with cardiogenic shock, severe left ventricular failure and refractory, recurrent ventricular tachycardia. *In* Norman JC (ed): Coronary Artery Medicine and Surgery: Concepts & Controversies. pp. 401–409. New York: Appleton-Century-Crofts, 1975.
128. Sehapayak G, Watson JT, Curry GC, et al: The late development of intractable ventricular tachycardia following acute myocardial infarction. J Thorac Cardiovasc Surg 67:818, 1974.
129. Austen WG, Sanders CA, Aberill JH, et al: Ruptured papillary muscle: report of a case with successful mitral valve replacement. Circulation 32:597, 1965.
130. Nishimura RA, Schaff HV, Shub C, et al: Papillary muscle rupture complicating acute myocardial infarction: analysis of 17 patients. Am J Cardiol 51:373, 1983.
131. Ballester M, Tasca R, Marin L: Different mechanisms of mitral regurgitation in acute and chronic forms of coronary heart disease. Eur Heart J 4:557, 1983.
132. Barbour DJ, Roberts WC: Rupture of a left ventricular papillary muscle during acute myocardial infarction: analysis of 22 necropsy patients. J Am Coll Cardiol 8:588, 1986.
133. Meister SG, Helfant RH: Rapid bedside differentiation of ruptured interventricular septum from acute mitral insufficiency. N Engl J Med 287:1024, 1972.
134. Coma-Canella I, Gamallo C, Onsurbe PM, Jadraque LM: Anatomic findings in acute papillary muscle necrosis. Am Heart J 118:1188, 1989.
135. Come PC, Riley MF, Weintraub R, et al: Echocardiographic detection of complete and partial papillary muscle rupture during acute myocardial infarction. Am J Cardiol 56:787, 1985.
136. Radford MJ, Johnson RA, Daggett WM, et al: Ventricular septal rupture: a review of clinical and physiologic features and an analysis of survival. Circulation 64:454, 1981.
137. Moore CA, Nygaard TW, Kaiser DL, et al: Post infarction ventricular septal rupture: the importance of location of infarction and right ventricular function in determining survival. Circulation 74:45, 1986.
138. Bansal RC, Eng AK, Shakudo M: Role of two-dimensional echocardiography, pulsed, continuous wave and color flow Doppler techniques in the assessment of ventricular septal rupture after myocardial infarction. Am J Cardiol 65:852, 1990.
139. Cummings RG, Reimer KA, Califf R, et al: Quantitative analysis of right and left ventricular infarction in the presence of postinfarction ventricular septal defect. Circulation 77:33, 1988.
140. Mann JM, Roberts WC: Acquired ventricular septal defect during acute myocardial infarction: analysis of 38 unoperated necropsy patients and comparison with 50 unoperated necropsy patients without rupture. Am J Cardiol 62:8, 1988.
141. Edwards BS, Edwards WD, Edwards JE: Ventricular septal rupture complicating acute myocardial infarction: identification of simple and complex types in 53 autopsied hearts. Am J Cardiol 54:1201, 1984.
142. Jones MT, Schofield PM, Dark JF, et al: Surgical repair of acquired ventricular septal defects: determinants of early and late outcome. J Thorac Cardiovasc Surg 93:680, 1987.
143. Norell MS, Gershlick AH, Pillai R, et al: Ventricular septal rupture complicating myocardial infarction: is earlier surgery justified? Eur Heart J 8:1281, 1987.
144. Miller DC, Stinson EB: Surgical management of acute mechanical defects secondary to myocardial infarction. Am J Surg 141:677, 1981.
145. Lader E, Colvin S, Tunick P: Myocardial infarction complicated by rupture of both ventricular septum and right ventricular papillary muscle. Am J Cardiol 52:424, 1983.
146. Heyndrickx GR, Millard RW, McRitchie RJ, et al: Regional myocardial functional and electrophysiological alterations after brief coronary occlusion in conscious dog. J Clin Invest 56:978, 1975.
147. Bush LR, Buja LM, Tilton GD, et al: Effects of propranolol and diltiazem alone and in combination on the recovery of left ventricular segmental function after long-term reperfusion following temporary coronary occlusion in conscious dogs. Circulation 72:413, 1985.
148. Ellis SG, Henschke CI, Sandor T, et al: Time course of functional and biochemical recovery of myocardium salvaged by reperfusion. J Am Coll Cardiol 1:1047, 1983.

149. Braunwald E, Kloner RA: The stunned myocardium: prolonged, postischemic ventricular dysfunction. Circulation 66:1146, 1982.
150. Rahimtoola SH: The hibernating myocardium. Am Heart J 117:211, 1989.
151. Fedele FA, Gerwitz H, Capone RJ: Metabolic response to prolonged reduction of myocardial blood flow distal to a severe coronary artery stenosis. Circulation 78:729, 1988.
152. Marban E: Myocardial stunning and hibernation: the physiology behind the colloquialisms. Circulation 83:681, 1991.
153. Schaefer S, Schwartz GG, Gober JR, et al: Relationship between myocardial metabolites and contractile abnormalities during graded regional ischemia: phosphorus-31 nuclear magnetic resonance studies of porcine myocardium in vivo. J Clin Invest 85:706, 1990.
154. Roberts R, Sobel BE, Parker CW: Radioimmunoassay of creatine kinase isoenzymes. Science 194:855, 1976.
155. Roberts R, Sobel BE: Isoenzymes of creatine phosphokinase and diagnosis of myocardial infarction. Ann Intern Med 79:741, 1973.
156. Willerson JT, Stone MJ, Ting R, et al: Radioimmunoassay of creatine kinase-B isoenzyme in human sera: results in patients with acute myocardial infarction. Proc Natl Acad Sci U S A 74:1711, 1977.
157. Stone MJ, Willerson JT, Gomez-Sanchez CE, Waterman M: Radioimmunoassay of myoglobin in human serum: results in patients with acute myocardial infarction. J Clin Invest 56:1334, 1975.
158. Stone MJ, Waterman MR, Murray G, et al: The serum myoglobin level as a diagnostic test in patients with acute myocardial infarction. Br Heart J 38:375, 1977.
159. Gilkeson G, Stone MJ, Waterman M, et al: Detection of myoglobin by radioimmunoassay in human sera: its usefulness and limitations as an emergency room screening test for acute myocardial infarction. Am Heart J 95:70, 1978.
160. Trahern CA, Gere JB, Krauth GH, et al: Clinical assessment of serum myosin light chains in the diagnosis of acute myocardial infarction. Am J Cardiol 41:641, 1978.
161. Khaw BA, Gold H, Fallon J, et al: Detection of serum cardiac myosin light chains in acute experimental myocardial infarction: radioimmunoassay of cardiac myosin light chains. Circulation 58:1130, 1978.
162. Katus HA, Remppis A, Newmann FJ, et al: Diagnostic efficiency of troponin T measurements in acute myocardial infarction. Circulation 83:902, 1991.
163. Stone MJ, Waterman MR, Poliner LR, et al: Myoglobinemia is an early and quantitative index of acute myocardial infarction. Angiology 29:386, 1978.
164. Ellis AK, Little T, Mausud ARZ, et al: Early noninvasive detection of successful reperfusion in patients with acute myocardial infarction. Circulation 78:1352, 1988.
165. Puleo PR, Perryman B, Bressner MA, et al: Creatine kinase isoforms analysis in the detection and assessment of thrombolysis in man. Circulation 75:1162, 1987.
166. Abendschein D, Seacord LM, Nohara R, et al: Prompt detection of myocardial injury by assay of creatine kinase isoforms in initial plasma samples. Clin Cardiol 11:661, 1988.
167. Mair J, Morandell D, Genser N, et al: Equivalent early sensitivities of myoglobin, creatine kinase MB mass, creatine kinase isoform ratios, and cardiac troponins I and T for acute myocardial infarction. Clin Chem 41:1266, 1995.
168. Adams JE III, Bodor GS, Davila-Roman VG, et al: Cardiac troponin I: a marker with high specificity for cardiac injury. Circulation 88:101, 1993.
169. Cummins B, Auckland MI, Cummins P: Cardiac-specific troponin I radioimmunoassay in the diagnosis of acute myocardial infarction. Am Heart J 113:1333, 1987.
170. Bonte FJ, Parkey RW, Graham KD, et al: A new method for radionuclide imaging of myocardial infarcts. Radiology 110:473, 1974.
171. Willerson JT, Parkey RW, Stokely EM, et al: Infarct sizing with technetium-99m stannous pyrophosphate scintigraphy in dogs and man: the relationship between scintigraphic and precordial mapping estimates of infarct size in patients. Cardiovasc Res 11:291, 1977.
172. Parkey RW, Bonte FJ, Meyer SL, et al: A new method for radionuclide imaging of acute myocardial infarction in humans. Circulation 50:540, 1974.
173. Willerson JT, Parkey RW, Bonte FJ, et al: Technetium stannous pyrophosphate myocardial scintigrams in patients with chest pain of varying etiology. Circulation 51:1046, 1975.
174. Wackers FJ III, Schoot JB, Sokole EB, et al: Noninvasive visualization of acute myocardial infarction in man with thallium-201. Br Heart J 37:741, 1975.
175. Wackers FJ, Busemann S, Samson G, et al: Value and limitations of thallium-201 scintigraphy in the acute phase of myocardial infarction. N Engl J Med 295:1, 1975.
176. Silverman KJ, Becker LC, Bulkley BC, et al: Value of early thallium-201 scintigraphy for predicting mortality in patients with acute myocardial infarction. Circulation 61:996, 1980.
177. Wheelan K, Wolfe C, Corbett J, et al: Early positive technetium-99m stannous pyrophosphate images as a marker of reperfusion in patients receiving thrombolytic therapy for acute myocardial infarction. Am J Cardiol 56:252, 1985.
178. Parkey RW, Kulkarni PV, Lewis S, et al: Effect of coronary blood flow and site of injection on Tc-99m-PPi detection of early canine myocardial infarcts. J Nucl Med 22:133, 1981.
179. Dec GW, Palacios I, Yasuda T, et al: Antimyosin antibody cardiac imaging: its role in the diagnosis of myocarditis. J Am Coll Cardiol 16:97, 1990.
180. Johnson LL, Seldin DW, Becker LC, et al: Antimyosin imaging in acute transmural myocardial infarctions: results of a multicenter clinical trial. J Am Coll Cardiol 13:27, 1989.
181. Carrio I, Bernia L, Ballester M, et al: Indium-111 antimyosin scintigraphy to assess myocardial damage in patients with suspected myocarditis and cardiac rejection. J Nucl Med 29:1900, 1988.
182. Buja LM, Poliner LR, Parkey RW, et al: Clinicopathologic study of persistently positive technetium-99m stannous pyrophosphate myocardial scintigrams and myocytologic degeneration after acute myocardial infarction. Circulation 56:1016, 1977.
183. Sanford CF, Corbett J, Curry GL, et al: Value of radionuclide ventriculography in the immediate characterization of patients with acute myocardial infarction. Am J Cardiol 49:637, 1982.
184. Stokely EM, Parkey RW, Bonte FJ, et al: Gated blood pool imaging following technetium-99m phosphate scintigraphy. Radiology 120:433, 1976.
185. Strauss HW, Zaret BL, Hurley PJ, et al: A scintigraphic method for measuring left ventricular ejection fraction in man without cardiac catheterization. Am J Cardiol 28:575, 1970.
186. Schelbert HR, Verba JW, Johnson AD, et al: Nontraumatic determination of left ventricular ejection fraction by radionuclide angiography. Circulation 51:902, 1975.
187. Nixon JW, Narahara K, Smitherman TC: Estimation of myocardial involvement in patients with acute myocardial infarction by two-dimensional echocardiography. Circulation 62:1248, 1980.
188. Sheiban I, Casarotto D, Trevi G, et al: Two-dimensional echocardiography in the diagnosis of intracardiac masses: a prospective study with anatomic validation. Cardiovasc Intervent Radiol 10:157, 1987.
189. Stratton JR, Resnick AD: Increased embolic risk in patients with left ventricular thrombi. Circulation 75:1004, 1987.
190. Spirito P, Bellotti P, Chiarella F, et al: Prognostic significance and natural history of left ventricular thrombi in patients with acute anterior myocardial infarction: a two-dimensional echocardiographic study. Circulation 72:774, 1985.
191. Schnittger I: Cardiac and extracardiac masses: echocardiographic evaluation. *In* Marcus ML, Schelbert HR, Skorton DJ, et al (eds): Cardiac Imaging: A Companion to Braunwald's Heart Disease. pp. 511–537. Philadelphia: WB Saunders, 1991.
192. Peralman AS, Otto CM: Quantification of valvular regurgitation. Echocardiography 4:271, 1987.
193. Pearson AC, Labovitz AJ, Mrosek D, et al: Assessment of diastolic function in normal and hypertrophied hearts: comparison of Doppler echocardiography and M-mode echocardiography. Am Heart J 113:1417, 1987.
194. Stein PD, Sabbah HN, Albert DE, Snyder JE: Continuous wave Doppler for the noninvasive evaluation of aortic blood velocity and rate of change of velocity: evaluation in dogs. Med Instrum 21:177, 1987.
195. Rokey R, Kuo LC, Zoghbi WA, et al: Determination of parameters of left ventricular diastolic filling by pulsed Doppler echocardiography: comparison with cineangiography. Circulation 71:543, 1985.
196. Loeppky JA, Greene ER, Hoekenga ED, et al: Beat-by-beat stroke volume assessment by pulsed Doppler in upright and supine exercise. J Appl Physiol 50:1173, 1981.
197. Aschenberg W, Schluter M, Kremer P, et al: Transesophageal two-dimensional echocardiography for detection of left atrial appendage thrombus. J Am Coll Cardiol 7:163, 1986.

198. Nellessen U, Daniel WG, Matheis G, et al: Impending paradoxical embolism from atrial thrombus: correct diagnosis by transesophageal echocardiography and prevention by surgery. J Am Coll Cardiol 5:1002, 1985.
199. Lee W, Schiller NB: Transesophageal echocardiography in clinical cardiology. *In* Marcus ML, Schelbert HR, Skorton DJ, et al (eds): Cardiac Imaging: A Companion to Braunwald's Heart Disease. pp. 605–616. Philadelphia: WB Saunders, 1991.
200. Nordrehaug JE, Johannessen KA, von der Lippe G: Usefulness of high-dose anticoagulants in preventing left ventricular thrombus in acute myocardial infarction. Am J Cardiol 55:1941, 1985.
201. Halperin JL, Fuster V: Left ventricular thrombus and stroke after myocardial infarction: toward prevention or perplexity? J Am Coll Cardiol 14:912, 1989.
202. Weintraub WS, Ba'albaki HA: Decision analysis concerning the application of echocardiography to the diagnosis and treatment of mural thrombi after anterior wall acute myocardial infarction. Am J Cardiol 64:708, 1989.
203. Ascah KJ, Stewart WJ, Kiang L, et al: Doppler-two-dimensional echocardiographic method for quantitation of mitral regurgitation. Circulation 72:377, 1985.
204. Mintz GS, Kotler MN, Segal BL, Parry WR: Two-dimensional echocardiographic recognition of ruptured chordae tendineae. Circulation 57:244, 1978.
205. Spain MG, Smith MD, Grayburn PA, et al: Quantitative assessment of mitral regurgitation by Doppler color flow imaging: angiographic and hemodynamic correlations. J Am Coll Cardiol 13:585, 1989.
206. Gillam LD, Hogan RD, Foale A, et al: A comparison of quantitative echocardiographic methods for delineating infarct-induced abnormal wall motion. Circulation 70:113, 1984.
207. Guyer DE, Foale RA, Gillam LD, et al: An echocardiographic technique for quantifying and displaying the extent of regional left ventricular dysynergy. J Am Coll Cardiol 8:830, 1986.
208. Gatewood RP, Nanda N: Differentiation of left ventricular pseudoaneurysm from true aneurysm with two-dimensional echocardiography. Am J Cardiol 46:869, 1980.
209. Kerber RE: Echocardiography in coronary artery disease: myocardial ischemia and infarction. *In* Marcus ML, Schelbert HR, Skorton DJ, et al (eds): Cardiac Imaging: A Companion to Braunwald's Heart Disease. pp. 594–603. Philadelphia: WB Saunders, 1991.
210. Sobel BE, Bresnahan GF, Shell WE, et al: Estimation of infarct size in man and its relation to prognosis. Circulation 46:640, 1972.
211. Jansen DE, Corbett JR, Lewis SE, et al: Quantification of myocardial infarction: a comparison of single photon emission computed tomography with pyrophosphate to serial plasma MB-CK measurements. Circulation 72:327, 1985.
212. Wolfe CL, Lewis SE, Corbett JR, et al: Measurement of infarction fraction using single photon emission computed tomography. J Am Coll Cardiol 6:145, 1985.
213. Corbett JR, Lewis SE, Wolfe CL, et al: Measurement of myocardial infarct size in patients by technetium pyrophosphate single photon tomography. Am J Cardiol 54:1231, 1984.
214. Corbett JR, Nicod PH, Huxley RL, et al: Left ventricular functional alterations at rest and during submaximal exercise in patients with acute myocardial infarction. Am J Med 74:577, 1983.
215. Corbett JR, Nicod P, Lewis SE, et al: Prognostic value of submaximal exercise radionuclide ventriculography following acute transmural and nontransmural myocardial infarction. Am J Cardiol 52:82A, 1983.
216. Dehmer GJ, Lewis SE, Hillis LD, et al: Exercise induced alterations in left ventricular volumes in man: usefulness in predicting the relative extent of coronary artery disease. Circulation 63:1008, 1981.
217. Corbett J, Dehmer GJ, Lewis SE, et al: The prognostic value of submaximal exercise testing with radionuclide ventriculography prior to hospital discharge in patients with recent myocardial infarction. Circulation 64:535, 1981.
218. Pulido J, Doss J, Twieg D, et al: Submaximal exercise testing in patients following acute myocardial infarction: myocardial scintigraphic and electrocardiographic observations. Am J Cardiol 42:19, 1978.
219. Gibson RS, Watson DD, Taylor GJ, et al: Prospective assessment of regional myocardial perfusion before and after coronary revascularization surgery by quantitative thallium-201 scintigraphy. J Am Coll Cardiol 1:804, 1983.
220. Melin JA, Wijns W, Keyeux A, et al: Assessment of thallium-201 redistribution versus glucose uptake as predictors of viability after coronary occlusion and reperfusion. Circulation 77:927, 1988.
221. Armstrong WF, O'Donnell J, Ryan T, Feigenbaum H: Effect of prior myocardial infarction and extent and location of coronary disease on accuracy of exercise echocardiography. J Am Coll Cardiol 10:531, 1987.
222. Applegate RJ, Dell'Italia LJ, Crawford MH: Usefulness of two-dimensional echocardiography during low-level exercise testing early after uncomplicated acute myocardial infarction. Am J Cardiol 60:10, 1987.
223. Crawford MH, Petru MA, Amon KW, et al: Comparative value of 2-dimensional echocardiography and radionuclide angiography for quantitating changes in left ventricular performance during exercise limited by angina pectoris. Am J Cardiol 53:42, 1984.
224. Swan HJC, Ganz W, Forrester J, et al: Catheterization of the heart in men with the use of a flow-directed balloon-tipped catheter. N Engl J Med 280:447, 1970.
225. Cobb LA, Baum RS, Alvarez H III, et al: Resuscitation from out-of-hospital ventricular fibrillation: 4 year follow-up. Circulation 52(suppl III):223, 1975.
226. Liberthson RR, Nagel EL, Hirschmann JC, Nussenfeld SR: Prehospital ventricular defibrillation: prognosis and follow-up course. N Engl J Med 291:317, 1974.
227. Liberthson RR, Nagel EL, Hirschmann JC, et al: Pathophysiologic observations in prehospital ventricular fibrillation and sudden cardiac death. Circulation 49:790, 1974.
228. Lee L, Bates ER, Pitt B, et al: Percutaneous transluminal coronary angioplasty improves survival in acute myocardial infarction complicated by cardiogenic shock. Circulation 78:1345, 1988.
229. Rothkopf M, Boerner J, Stone MJ, et al: Detection of myocardial infarct extension by CK-B radioimmunoassay. Circulation 59:268, 1979.
230. Muller JE, Rude RE, Braunwald E, et al: Myocardial infarct extension: incidence, outcome, and risk factors in the MILIS study. Ann Intern Med 108:1, 1988.
231. Marmor A, Sobel BE, Roberts R: Factors presaging early recurrent myocardial infarction ("extension"). Am J Cardiol 48:603, 1981.
232. Schulze RA, Strauss HW, Pitt B: Sudden death in the year following myocardial infarction: relations to late hospital VPC's and left ventricular ejection fraction. Am J Med 62:192, 1977.
233. Rapaport E, Remedios P: The high-risk patient after recovery from myocardial infarction: recognition and management. J Am Coll Cardiol 1:391, 1983.
234. Moss AJ, Bigger JT, Odoroff CL: Post infarction risk stratification. Prog Cardiovasc Dis 29:389, 1987.
235. Norris RM, Barnaby PF, Brandt PWT, et al: Prognosis after recovery from first acute myocardial infarction: determinants of reinfarction and sudden death. Am J Cardiol 53:408, 1984.
236. Mukharji J, Rude RE, Poole WK, et al, for the MILIS Study Group: Risk factors for sudden death after acute myocardial infarction: two-year follow-up. Am J Cardiol 54:31, 1984.
237. Hung J, Goris M, Nash E, et al: Comparative value of maximal treadmill testing, exercise thallium myocardial perfusion scintigraphy and exercise radionuclide ventriculography for distinguishing high- and low-risk patients soon after acute myocardial infarction. Am J Cardiol 53:1221, 1984.
238. Hammerman H, Schoen FJ, Braunwald E, et al: Drug-induced expansion of infarct: morphologic and functional correlations. Circulation 69:611, 1984.
239. Eaton LW, Weiss JL, Bulkley BH, et al: Regional cardiac dilatation after acute myocardial infarction. Recognition by two-dimensional echocardiography. N Engl J Med 300:57, 1979.
240. McKay RG, Pfeffer MA, Pasternak RC, et al: Left ventricular remodeling after myocardial infarction. A corollary to infarct expansion. Circulation 74:693, 1986.
241. Pfeffer MA, Lamas GA, Vaughan DE, et al: Effect of captopril on progressive ventricular dilatation. N Engl J Med 319:80, 1988.
242. The SOLVD Investigators: Effect of enalapril on mortality and the development of heart failure in asymptomatic patients with reduced left ventricular ejection fractions. N Engl J Med 327:685, 1992.
243. The CONSENSUS Trial Study Group: Effects of enalapril on mortality in severe congestive heart failure: results of the Cooperative North Scandinavian Enalapril Survival Study (CONSENSUS). N Engl J Med 316:1429, 1987.

244. Hutchins GM, Bulkley BH: Infarct expansion versus extension: two different complications of acute myocardial infarction. Am J Cardiol 41:227, 1978.
245. The Acute Infarction Ramipril Efficacy (AIRE) Study Investigators: Effect of ramipril on mortality and morbidity of survivors of acute myocardial infarction with clinical evidence of heart failure. Lancet 342:821, 1993.
246. ISIS-4: A randomized factorial trial assessing early oral captopril, oral mononitrate, and intravenous magnesium sulfate in 58,050 patients with suspected acute myocardial infarction. Lancet 345:669, 1995.
247. Gruppo Italiano Per Lo Studio Della Streptochinasi Well' Inforto Miocardico Investigators: Six month effects of early treatment lisinopril and transdermal glyceryl trinitrate singly and together withdrawn 6 weeks after acute myocardial infarction. GISSI 3 Trial. J Am Coll Cardiol 22:337, 1996.
248. Kober L, Torp-Pedersen C, Carlsen JE, et al: A clinical trial of the angiotensin-convertin-enzyme inhibitor trandolapril in patients with left ventricular dysfunction after myocardial infarction. Trandolapril Cardiac Evaluation (TRACE) Study Group. N Engl J Med 333:1670, 1995.
249. Lindpaintner K, Ganten D: The cardiac renin-angiotensin system. Circ Res 68:905, 1991.
250. Van Belle E, Lablanche JM, Bauters C, et al: Coronary angioscopic findings in the infarct-related vessel within 1 month of acute myocardial infarction. Circulation 97:26, 1998.

CHAPTER 27

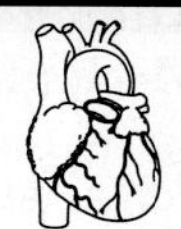

Silent Ischemia

Wojciech Mazur, Grzegorz Kaluza, and Neal S. Kleiman

MECHANISMS OF ALTERED PAIN PERCEPTION DURING MYOCARDIAL ISCHEMIA
Altered Central Nervous System Processing Mechanism
CENTRAL NERVOUS SYSTEM PROCESSING: EVALUATION OF PAIN THRESHOLD
PSYCHOLOGICAL ASPECTS IN SILENT ISCHEMIA
SIZE OF THE ISCHEMIC AREA ("ISCHEMIC BURDEN") AND ANGINA
HEMODYNAMICS AND LEFT VENTRICULAR FUNCTION
SILENT ISCHEMIA IN PATIENTS WITH DIABETES MELLITUS
Mechanism of Silent Ischemia in Diabetes
DETECTION AND DOCUMENTATION OF SILENT ISCHEMIA
Exercise Stress Testing
Ambulatory Electrocardiographic Monitoring
Limitations of Ambulatory Electrocardiographic Monitoring
Relation Between Ambulatory Electrocardiographic Monitoring and Exercise Stress Testing
Nuclear Scintigraphy
Relation Between Ambulatory Electrocardiographic Monitoring and Myocardial Perfusion Imaging
Exercise and Dobutamine Stress Electrocardiography
Prognosis in Silent Ischemia
RESULTS OF SUPPRESSION OF ISCHEMIA

Since the original description by Heberden in 1772[1] of an exertional "disorder of the breast" and the subsequent recognition that angina pectoris was associated with obstructive narrowing of the coronary arteries, clinicians caring for patients with coronary artery disease (CAD) have regarded angina as the benchmark by which to measure the prognosis and gauge the treatment of patients with coronary arterial atherosclerosis. However, reports of coronary atherosclerosis, occasionally severe, in asymptomatic young soldiers killed in World War I and the Korean War[1, 2] and in pilots,[3] coupled with the increasing recognition that the electrocardiographic (ECG) changes in infarction were often present in individuals with no history of chest pain,[4–6] led to the uneasy acceptance that the interruption of blood supply to the myocardium was not necessarily heralded by angina pectoris. As the ability to recognize myocardial ischemia increased, so did the awareness that objective measures of detection were necessary in patients either who were asymptomatic or whose symptoms were not typical. It is well accepted that a large proportion of patients have evidence of remote myocardial infarction (MI) but no clinical history suggesting such an event. The development and acceptance of Masters' two-step test from the 1920s through the 1950s, and later of the exercise treadmill test, led to the recognition that as in many other disease processes, not only MI and sudden death but also myocardial ischemia could occur in the absence of symptoms.

The results of an early study by Twiss and Sokolow,[7] in which 21 of 66 patients with exertional angina pectoris underwent two-step exercise testing without developing chest discomfort, led the authors to declare, "the electrocardiographic changes after exercise are not dependent on the reproduction of pain while allowing that the percentage of positive results is much greater if pain is induced." Eventually, the use of more mechanistically based, and hence more sensitive and specific, nuclear and echocardiographic imaging adjuncts to stress testing reinforced the prognostic significance of decreased blood flow to viable areas of myocardium both in the presence and in the absence of symptoms. Similarly, the development of drugs that could delay the development of ischemia and of successful revascularization techniques that could prevent the development of previously demonstrable ischemia led to increased interest in the study of and characterization of asymptomatic, or "silent," ischemia. This effort was followed by attempts to determine whether the treatment of silent ischemia would improve the outcome of patients in whom it was present. It was no longer clear whether adequate control of symptoms constituted optimal treatment for all patients with ischemic heart disease.

Mechanisms of Altered Pain Perception During Myocardial Ischemia

It is likely that a multitude of mechanisms are responsible for the variability in an individual's ability (or willingness) to sense pain as a result of myocardial ischemia. Experimental studies have demonstrated that activation of the baroreceptor reflex arc by pressor agents can induce hypoanalgesia in rats. Accordingly, stimulation of the efferent loop of this arc (cardiopulmonary vagal pathways) may be responsible for the absence of pain in humans.[8] Because increases in blood pressure repeatedly stimulate this pathway, it has been postulated that hypertensive patients have a higher pain threshold than do nonhypertensives. Patients with angiographically documented CAD and hypertension, for example, tend to have a higher mean dental pain threshold than do normotensive patients and experience fewer episodes of angina during daily life.[9] Patients with infiltrative autonomic neuropathies, such as that associated with diabetes, may also have diminished afferent loop sensitivity. This group is discussed separately in a later section.

Altered Central Nervous System Processing Mechanism

For a noxious stimulus to be perceived as pain, frontal cortical activation must occur. Cortical activation can be traced physiologically through the detection of increased blood flow with positron emission tomography. A comparison of changes in regional cerebral flow reveals equivalent degrees of thalamic activation in both angina and silent ischemia, but a lesser extent of cortical activation in patients with painless ischemia.[10] This finding suggests differential gating of afferent stimuli at the thalamic level with only some impulses being allowed to pass through to the frontal cortex.

Endorphins and Angina

Beta-endorphins are recognized as modulators of pain; elevated plasma endorphin levels raise an individual's threshold for experiencing pain. In patients with established CAD, β-endorphin levels in patients with silent ischemia have been reported to be almost twice as high as those in asymptomatic individuals.[11] The same finding has been noted in patients undergoing percutaneous transluminal coronary angioplasty (PTCA): plasma levels of β-endorphins are lower in symptomatic patients and decrease significantly during balloon inflation. In patients with silent ischemia, plasma levels of β-endorphins are higher before and remain stable during angioplasty, suggesting that endogenous opiate levels and their variation during ischemia are associated with individual experience.[12] In a recent investigation of PTCA-induced ischemia, Hikita and associates[13] suggested that there may be a threshold beyond which β-endorphins must increase to suppress anginal symptoms in response to ischemic stimuli.

Central Nervous System Processing: Evaluation of Pain Threshold

Silent ischemia is induced daily in many patients undergoing coronary angioplasty of a vessel supplying viable myocardium; however, it has been estimated that 16 to 47 percent of patients do not experience pain during the procedure. Consequently, this procedure may provide a model for the evaluation of silent ischemia. Falcone and colleagues[27] evaluated pain threshold using dental stimulation in patients with and without angina during daily life who were undergoing PTCA. During pulpal stimulation, 66.2 percent of patients reported pain, whereas 33.7 percent remained asymptomatic, even at maximal stimulation. The study cohort was then divided into two groups according to the presence or absence of angina during myocardial ischemia. Although the two groups appeared to be demographically similar, dental pain could be provoked in 81 percent of patients with and 36 percent of patients without symptoms during PTCA. The authors concluded that duration or intensity of ischemia and left ventricular dysfunction were not absolute factors in the determination of the occurrence of angina.[27] However, it is worth noting that the same may not apply to angina during exercise or during daily living, possibly due to the different pathophysiologic mechanisms that are involved.

Psychological Aspects in Silent Ischemia

In CAD as in most other disease states, psychological factors may influence the perception of discomfort as pain. These factors may also affect the response to therapy. The psychological comfort associated with increased medical surveillance, as well as the perception that a medical strategy is being pursued, may result in a significant "placebo effect." For example, Amsterdam and colleagues[14] reported that in patients with silent ischemia, placebo therapy led to a 44 percent reduction in ischemic episodes and a 50 percent reduction in total duration of ST depression.

In an elegant study, Friedman and associates[15] showed a strong relation between silent ischemia and "type A" personality. When 10 patients with this behavioral trait underwent psychological counseling, which resulted in marked decreases in the feeling of "time urgency" and hostility (markers of type A personality), the mean frequency of ischemic episodes declined from an initial 6.6 to 3.1 ischemic episodes per 24 hours. Whether this decrease resulted from a truly altered perception threshold or reduction in endorphin secretion and in rate-pressure product is not known.

Size of the Ischemic Area ("Ischemic Burden") and Angina

The relation between the amount of ischemic myocardium and the presence and severity of symptoms is hotly debated. In a study of 963 patients, Narin and coworkers[16] examined the differences between patients with silent ischemia and those with symptomatic ischemia during exercise testing 1 to 6 months after recovery from a coronary event. Compared with patients with symptomatic ischemia during testing, those with silent ischemia had less extensive reversible defects on stress thallium scintigraphy, less functional impairment during treadmill testing (longer exercise duration and longer time to ST-segment depression), and less frequent ST-segment depression during ambulatory electrocardiographic (AECG) monitoring.[16]

In another study of 300 consecutive patients with documented CAD and reversible hypoperfusion on exercise sestamibi tomography, Marcassa and colleagues[17] compared the degree of hypoperfusion and the presence of symptoms during exercise stress testing. Patients with painful ischemia had lower values for workload, exercise time, and peak rate-pressure product. These patients more frequently had significant ST-segment depression during exercise than did patients with silent ischemia. Patients with symptoms during ischemia had more evidence of reversible hypoperfusion than did patients with silent ischemia (16 ± 10 percent versus 11 ± 7 percent) despite comparable extent of stress hypoperfusion (22 ± 12 percent versus 22

± 13 percent).[17] However, discordant results have been reported in at least 10 studies that used myocardial perfusion scintigraphy to compare the amount of ischemic myocardium in patients with and without chest pain during exercise testing.[18–26] Several potential explanations exist for these discrepant findings. The earlier studies were conducted using widely different patient populations, ranging from clinically asymptomatic patients to only those with evidence of a marked ischemic response to exercise. Multivariable analysis was seldom performed in these studies, and varying definitions of silent ischemia were used.

Hemodynamics and Left Ventricular Function

Similar discrepancies exist in the literature concerning left ventricular performance during exercise testing in patients with silent and symptomatic ischemia. In a study that included 131 patients with angiographically documented CAD, Bonow and associates[28] found that patients with silent ischemia were less likely to develop a decrease in left ventricular ejection fraction during exercise radionuclide ventriculography than were patients who developed angina during testing. A similar observation was made by Matsubara and coworkers[12]: pulmonary artery wedge pressure at peak exercise was significantly lower and cardiac index was significantly higher in patients with silent ischemia than in patients who experienced angina. On the other hand, Cohn and associates[28a] and Vassiliadis and colleagues[28b] found no differences in global ejection fraction or regional wall motion abnormalities during exercise testing in symptomatic and asymptomatic patients. The inclusion of patients with prior MI in the latter two studies may explain the differences from the former study.

Silent Ischemia in Patients With Diabetes Mellitus

Patients with diabetes represent a classic example of patients in whom the afferent loop of the cardiac sensory mechanism is altered. It is well established that CAD is a major complication of diabetes mellitus, representing the ultimate cause of death in more than half of all the patients with this disease.[29] Furthermore, MI in diabetic patients is usually more extensive and more severe than in nondiabetic patients and is associated with a higher mortality rate.[30–33] There are conflicting data regarding the frequency of silent ischemia in patients with diabetes mellitus. The Framingham Heart Study investigators initially reported that in diabetic patients, the incidence of painless MI was higher than that in nondiabetic patients.[34] Several studies suggested that diabetic patients may have a high incidence of transient silent ST changes during Holter monitoring.[35, 36] In a well-controlled patient population, Nesto and coworkers[35, 36] demonstrated that only 28 percent of diabetic patients with thallium scintigraphic indications[37] of ischemia experienced angina pectoris during a treadmill test compared with 68 percent of nondiabetic patients.

Different results were reported by Caracciolo and associates[38] in an analysis of diabetic patients in the Asymptomatic Cardiac Ischemia Pilot Investigators (ACIP) database study. The authors compared 77 diabetic and 481 nondiabetic patients. As expected, multivessel disease was more common in the diabetic group (87 versus 74 percent). However, the percentages of patients without angina during the exercise test were similar in the diabetic and the nondiabetic groups (36 and 39 percent, respectively). The percentage of patients with only asymptomatic ST-segment depression during the 48-hour AECG monitoring were also comparable (94 versus 88 percent, respectively). An even more surprising finding was that despite more extensive and diffuse CAD, diabetic patients tended to have less measurable ischemia during the 48-hour AECG monitoring, perhaps related to lower workloads. Diabetic patients had less total ischemic time per 24 hours, lesser ischemic time per episode, and lesser maximal depth of ST-segment depression compared with nondiabetic individuals.

Several surrogate clinical markers of an increased frequency of silent ischemia in diabetics (as assessed with AECG monitoring) have been identified, such as autonomic neuropathy,[36] the presence of microalbuminuria,[39] and left ventricular hypertrophy.[39a] It is likely that these associations represent longer duration of the disease and possibly a greater propensity to develop end-organ damage.

Mechanism of Silent Ischemia in Diabetes

The mechanism of decreased anginal pain perception in diabetics is likely to be different from that in the nondiabetic population. There is a high prevalence of autonomic neuropathy affecting impulse conduction in patients with longstanding diabetes. Scanning with a synthetic radiolabeled norepinephrine analogue, metaiodobenzylguanidine (MIBG), which shares the same uptake mechanism as norepinephrine, into sympathetic nerve terminals revealed that MIBG uptake is nonhomogeneous in normal control subjects and in diabetic patients, with the lowest uptake in the apex compared with the middle two thirds of the left ventricle. MIBG uptake in diabetic patients is significantly lower than that in normal subjects at all levels of the left ventricular long axis. When MIBG uptake is corrected for perfusion abnormalities, diabetic patients had significantly greater mismatch in MIBG uptake than did nondiabetic subjects.[40]

Detection and Documentation of Silent Ischemia

Exercise Stress Testing

Exercise testing has been the hallmark of the detection of myocardial ischemia since the development of the two-step exercise test by Masters and Geller.[41] Although ST-segment deviation in individuals with previously undetected CAD is a well-accepted phenomenon and is the sine qua non of a "positive" test when used for screening purposes in a large and generally asymptomatic population, and although jeopardized coronary arterial flow can similarly be demonstrated scintigraphically in a few asymptomatic individuals at low risk,[42] most interest in "silent ischemia" has been focused on events in patients who are known to have CAD. In a retrospective analysis of 1698 patients with CAD who underwent exercise treadmill testing, Mark and associates[43] reported that ST-segment deviation occurred in 842 (49 percent). These ECG changes were painless in 242 (14 percent) and were accompanied by angina in 600 (35 percent). In this study (as in a report from the Coronary Artery Surgery Study [CASS] Registry),[44] prior angina and more frequent episodes of angina during daily activity were more common among patients with symptoms during ischemia. Those with exercise-induced angina were more likely to have three-vessel CAD, a shorter peak exercise time, and a lower peak heart rate, although the median degree of ST-segment deviation observed with electrocardiography was not different.

Ambulatory Electrocardiography Monitoring

Much interest has been directed toward the detection of silent ischemia with the use of AECG (Holter) monitoring, perhaps because it has extended the ability to detect ischemia from the clinic to the daily activities of life and because it has demonstrated that "ambulant" ischemia commonly occurs during daily activities even in the absence of angina. Golding and coworkers[45] initially reported that transient elevation of the ST segment occurred in 7 of 174 patients undergoing Holter monitoring for detection of arrhythmias. It is unlikely that all episodes of ST-segment depression (especially in a general population) represent myocardial ischemia. However, even in patients in whom exercise-induced ischemia can be demonstrated, it is rare to detect prolonged ST-segment depression in normal subjects if proper data acquisition techniques are used. Because transient changes in position can produce brief periods of deviation in the ST segment, changes are usually required to last for at least 30 seconds before they are interpreted as representative of possible ischemic events. Studies of individuals with a low likelihood of CAD and without cardiac symptoms have revealed episodes of ST-segment depression exceeding 30 seconds in fewer than 5 percent of subjects.[46]

In patients with CAD, it is considerably more common to find ST-segment deviation on Holter monitoring. Other corroborating evidence of ischemia during daily life can be found during such episodes of asymptomatic ST-segment depression. Experience with a lightweight nonimaging radionuclide gamma camera that can be worn strapped to a patient's chest has demonstrated frequent episodic asymptomatic reductions in left ventricular ejection fraction during daily activity, especially during periods of mental stress.[47] These episodes are often, but not always, accompanied by ST-segment depression.[48] It is therefore likely that many episodes of ST-segment depression that occur in patients with obstructive CAD represent actual ischemic events in the myocardium. Conversely, ST-segment depression without reduction in the left ventricular ejection fraction may represent ischemia that does not involve an amount of myocardium sufficient to cause left ventricular dysfunction or may be nonischemic in origin.

Painless depression of the ST segment on AECG monitoring has been reported in 40 to 85 percent of patients with CAD.[41, 49–58] In patients with unstable rest angina or recent MI, reports from some centers have indicated that as many as 50 percent have evidence of ambulatory ischemia,[54–58] although considerable controversy exists concerning the frequency with which ambulant ischemia can be detected. For example, in the National Heart, Lung, and Blood Institute–sponsored Thrombolysis in Myocardial Ischemia study (TIMI 3) of 1473 patients with unstable angina or non–Q wave MI, ischemia exceeding 20 minutes in duration, observed during 24 hours of Holter monitoring with results interpreted in an experienced core laboratory, was present in fewer than 4 percent of patients.[59] In most cases when ischemia is detected, multiple daily episodes are present with considerable variation in each patient from day to day and week to week.[50] In most such studies, between two thirds and three fourths of such episodes in any given patients are not accompanied by angina.

Limitations of Ambulatory Electrocardiographic Monitoring

Several important limitations of AECG monitoring should be kept in mind. Studies have repeatedly shown that ischemic ST-T changes, even though strictly defined by the Minnesota code, are not specific for CAD and can be seen in healthy individuals or in patients with documented CAD but without provocable ischemia. In addition, changes in left ventricular afterload may produce alterations in left ventricular function, particularly in patients with depressed ejection fractions, which may be mistakenly interpreted as representing ischemia.[11] Among the many causes are T wave inversions recorded in young adults, electrolyte disturbances, valvular heart disease, cardiomyopathy, drugs, intracranial lesions, and recent food ingestion.[60]

In comparison with standard electrocardiograms, AECG monitoring is relatively insensitive for the detection of ischemia, even when identical leads are monitored. Detection of silent ischemia may be significantly enhanced with a 12-lead portable microprocessor-driven real-time ECG monitor. Studies with this device are under way.[61] The use of AECG monitoring as a quantitative technique is also unclear. Neither the total duration of ischemic ST-segment depression nor the total number of ischemic episodes correspond well with the size of scintigraphic perfusion defects[62] or with the anatomic extent of angiographic CAD.[63]

Relation Between Ambulatory Electrocardiographic Monitoring and Exercise Stress Testing

Studies that have focused on the correspondence between painless ST-segment shifts on AECG monitoring and symptomatic status during exercise testing have not necessarily shown concordance between the two. Differences between ischemic responses noted on treadmill testing and on ambulatory monitoring ischemia may be related in part to dissimilarities in the provoking stimuli. Episodes of ambulatory ischemia often occur during sedentary activity and can be provoked by stressors as diverse as mental stress,[52, 64] cold exposure,[53] and cigarette smoking.[65] Psychological stressors, especially situations that trigger emotional distress, cause increases in heart rate and blood pressure and may also trigger coronary vasoconstriction.[66–68] In addition, in patients who have painless ischemic responses on AECG monitoring, ischemia induced during exercise testing may be accompanied by angina. Most patients exhibit a combination of both symptomatic and symptomless ST-segment changes, although the difference between ECG characteristics of silent and symptomatic episodes in a given patient is not well documented. Both the degree of ST-segment deviation and the duration of the episodes appear to be similar. When patients with CAD are subjected to differing exercise protocols, ischemic ST-segment depression usually occurs at similar rate-pressure products. However, the ischemic threshold on AECG monitoring is considerably more variable[67, 69] and usually occurs at a lower rate-pressure product than on treadmill exercise,[50, 51, 69–73] even in circumstances when an increase in rate-pressure product precedes the onset of ischemia.[74]

Deanfield and colleagues[50] reported that among patients with ST-segment depression on exercise testing, the ST-segment changes noted during ambulatory monitoring occurred, on average, at heart rates of 20 beats/min less than the ischemic threshold detected on exercise testing. These episodes also occurred more frequently in the morning hours after rising,[70, 74, 75] following established circadian patterns for physiologic increases in plasma catecholamines[76] and platelet aggregability,[77] as well as in blood pressure,[78] heart rate,[71] and for such clinical events as MI[79–81] and sudden cardiac death.[82]

Assessment of asymptomatic ischemia is often used to assess the adequacy of medical therapy. However, it must be noted that exercise testing and AECG monitoring may detect different effects of antianginal treatments. For example, the Canadian Amlodipine/Atenolol In Silent Ischemia (CASIS) Investigators evaluated the influence of amlodipine and atenolol on myocardial ischemia during exercise stress testing and AECG monitoring. Ischemia during treadmill testing was more effectively suppressed by amlodipine, whereas ischemia during AECG monitoring was more effectively suppressed by atenolol. The combination of both drugs was more effective than either drug alone in either setting.[83]

Nuclear Scintigraphy

The same issues of sensitivity and specificity that led to the introduction of nuclear imaging for detection of CAD also apply to the detection of ischemia (Table 27–1). Tomographic imaging is highly reproducible and has allowed the quantification of the amount of ischemic myocardium. When these studies are interpreted by competent readers, the variation in measuring the size of an ischemia defect is less than 10 percent in 95 percent of patients.[84] As a consequence, exercise single-proton emission computed tomography (SPECT) has become accepted as an accurate technique for the evaluation of ischemia suppression.[85–87] Adenosine SPECT, combined with pharmacologic stressors, can also be used to track changes in myocardial ischemia after medical therapy as well as after mechanical revascularization.[88]

Relation Between Ambulatory Electrocardiographic Monitoring and Myocardial Perfusion Imaging

As mentioned, AECG changes in a patient with CAD may not necessarily represent active ischemia. In the ACIP study, 106 patients with recent coronary angiography underwent both AECG monitoring and stress SPECT within 3 days of one another. Seventy-four percent of patients with significant CAD had SPECT abnormalities, whereas 61 percent had ischemia by AECG monitoring. The most important predictors of SPECT abnormalities were the se-

TABLE 27–1 Thallium 201 Myocardial Perfusion Scintigraphic Studies Comparing the Amount of Ischemic Myocardium in Patients With or Without Chest Pain During Exercise Testing*

Reference	Year	Patients (n)	Method	Selection Criteria	Reversible Defects (% of Patients)
Amount of Ischemia Equal in Patients With or Without Chest Pain					
Hecht et al[19]	1989	112	SPECT	CAD, reversible defects	100
Gasperetti et al[20]	1989	103	Planar	Reversible defects	100
Heller et al[21]	1990	234	Planar	Reversible defects	100
Mahmarian et al[22]	1990	356	SPECT	Unselected	54
Baandu et al[100]	1994	294	SPECT	Unselected	94
Amount of Ischemia Greater in Patients With Than in Those Without Chest Pain					
Kurata et al[23]	1990	471	SPECT	Unselected	37
Galli et al[24]	1990	200	Planar	Old MI, reversible defects	100
Travin et al[25]	1991	268	Planar	Reversible defects	100
Hendler et al[26]	1992	152	SPECT	Ex ECG+	83
Klein et al[18]	1994	117	SPECT	Ex ECG+	80

Abbreviations: CAD, coronary artery disease; Ex ECG+, positive exercise electrocardiogram; MI, myocardial infarction; SPECT, single-photon emission computed tomography.

*In patients with CAD.

verity of coronary stenosis, followed by total exercise duration and patient age. The only predictor of AECG abnormalities was the presence of ST-segment depression on the initial treadmill test. The concordance observed between the SPECT and the AECG results was only 50 percent, and no relation was observed between the frequency or duration of AECG ischemia and the quantified myocardial perfusion defect size as assessed with SPECT. Thus, these techniques may detect different pathophysiologic manifestations of ischemia and may be complementary in more fully defining the functional significance of CAD.[62]

Exercise and Dobutamine Stress Echocardiography

Exercise and pharmacologic stimulation with catecholamine derivatives increase cardiac contractility in normal subjects. Consequently, when normal segments of myocardium are visualized with echocardiography, hyperkinetic wall motion is observed. In patients with obstructive CAD and normal wall motion at baseline, ischemia becomes manifest as an abnormality of local wall contractility. Stress echocardiography has been validated as a sensitive method of ischemia detection; however, the method of evaluating wall motion during a stress test depends on a semiquantitative visual evaluation with a limited scoring scale of different grades of dyssynergy.[89, 90] Despite this limitation, at least one study has shown that stress echocardiography and SPECT have similar sensitivities in the detection of ischemia, ranging from 58 and 61 percent (with echocardiography and SPECT, respectively) for one-vessel disease to 94 percent for three-vessel disease.[91] The infusion of dobutamine during stress echocardiography increases the degree of left ventricular dysfunction patients with functionally significant CAD and thus may be a more sensitive indicator of ischemia.[92] On the other hand, as stressors are compounded, the degree to which this intense combination of tachycardia and increased activity reproduces the stresses experienced by an individual during everyday life becomes questionable. Anginal chest pain is frequently induced in patients with stable CAD during stress testing. However, after MI, pain during stress testing may not be associated as clearly with an increased risk of adverse event compared with patients who did not experience angina despite a similar extent of CAD.[93]

Prognosis in Silent Ischemia

As mentioned in the section on the methods of detection of silent ischemia, different methods tend to select different populations at risk; thus, it is difficult to compare studies in which the burden of ischemia was assessed with AECG monitoring with studies that used strictly nuclear quantitative methods.

Standard 12-Lead Electrocardiography and Prognosis

In the largest report published to date (the Reykjavik study), 9139 randomly selected men were screened with the use of standard resting 12-lead electrocardiography and followed for 4 to 24 years. The prevalence of ST-T changes (classified as ischemic according to the Minnesota code) in the absence of angina among men without overt CAD was strongly influenced by age, increasing from 2 percent at age 40 years to 30 percent at age 80 years. Men with ST-T changes but no symptoms were older and had higher serum triglyceride levels, more frequently were hypertensive, had left ventricular hypertrophy, and took antihypertensive medications, digitalis, or diuretics. The serum cholesterol level did not differ between the two groups. After adjustment for other risk factors, the risk ratio was 2.0 for death from CAD and 1.6 for subsequent MI in men with these ST changes.[94]

Ambulatory Electrocardiographic Monitoring, Exercise Stress Testing, and Prognosis

The prognosis associated with asymptomatic myocardial ischemic detected electrocardiographically appears to be related to the overall clinical risk group from which patients are selected. As mentioned previously, AECG findings in patients hospitalized in a coronary care unit with unstable rest angina are associated with a high likelihood of impending MI. On the other hand, studies in patients with stable manifestations of CAD tend to indicate that the risk associated with silent myocardial ischemia is more questionable. Quyyumi and colleagues[63] studied with CAD categorized as low risk (i.e., excluding patients with left main disease, three-vessel disease with left ventricular dysfunction at rest, three-vessel disease with inducible ischemia, two-vessel disease with impaired left ventricular function, and inducible ischemia). Among these "low-risk" patients, 39 percent had ST-segment depression during AECG monitoring; 82 percent of those episodes were asymptomatic, which however, did not predict higher risk for cardiac events in the future.[63]

In a retrospective analysis of 1402 patients with ECG evidence of ischemia during treadmill testing, Cole and Ellestad[95] found that coronary events (cardiac death, MI, or progression of angina) were twice as frequent in patients with symptomatic ischemia than those with silent ischemia. In a review of the 5-year outcome of 842 consecutive patients in the Duke Cardiovascular Database who had angiographically documented CAD and abnormal exercise test results, Mark and associates[43] found that patients with silent ischemia during exercise testing had significantly better overall survival and infarct-free survival rates than did patients with angina. Similarly, there was a mortality rate difference among 1773 veterans referred for treadmill testing at 2 years based on the development of angina during exercise.[96]

The importance of asymptomatic ischemia on exercise testing after MI is often debated. Villella and coworkers[97] studied 6296 patients undergoing an exercise test an average 28 days after intravenous thrombolytic therapy for an MI. Residual ischemia was detected in 26 percent of patients, of whom 67 percent were asymptomatic. The 6-month mortality rate was 1.7 percent for those with a positive test, 0.9 percent for those who had a negative test, and 1.3 percent for those whose test was not diagnostic. After adjustment for myocardial ischemia accompanied by symptoms of angina, only symptomatic induced ischemia and low-work capacity were associated with an increased risk of death at 6 months, although asymptomatic ischemia was not. Even after analysis of silent ischemia based on the occurrence of ST-segment depression at maximal or submaximal levels of exercise or on the degree of ST-segment depression, exercise-induced asymptomatic myocardial ischemia was not significantly associated with a higher risk of death compared with exercise stress testing with negative results. The ability to exercise for more than 6 minutes was a predictor of good prognosis regardless of the associated ECG changes.[97]

The ACIP Trial contributed significantly to understanding of the importance of silent ischemia. Conti and associates[98] compared the outcome of patients who had angina either within the 6 weeks before enrollment or during the study period. These investigators reported that symptomatic patients in the ACIP Trial had a higher incidence of death, MI, or hospitalization for ischemic events (15.3 percent symptomatic versus 7.8 percent asymptomatic per 12 months). Interestingly, this difference was driven mainly by patients who had angina within 6 weeks preceding the study period. Unlike patients who were symptomatic during the period of recruitment, patients with angina observed that angina occurring only during AECG monitoring or stress testing was not associated with a higher incidence of adverse cardiac events than occurred in asymptomatic patients.[98]

Nuclear Imaging and Prognosis

In recent years, tomographic myocardial scintigraphy has gained acceptance as the most widely used and reliable measure of the quantity of myocardium that was ischemic. Consequently, the relationship between ischemic defect size and prognosis has garnered much attention. Reports from several large nuclear laboratories indicate a largely dichotomous relationship. Defects exceeding 15 to 20 percent of the myocardium are associated with a significantly higher likelihood of catastrophic events at 1 to 2 years than are smaller defects. Although the concept that the quantity of myocardium at risk determines a patient's outcome is not new, it is worth noting that several investigators have established that the size of an ischemic defect is a critical determinant of outcome, independent of symptoms.[99]

To determine whether suppression of asymptomatic myocardial ischemia is beneficial, it is necessary to determine whether asymptomatic ischemia can be suppressed at all. Because the degree of suppression is likely to be continuous and is also likely to be quite variable from patient to patient, information concerning the ability to suppress ischemia is best derived from several large clinical trials.

The ACIP Trial was designed as a pilot study to precisely determine whether suppression of silent ischemia was possible with one of three strategies: angina-guided medical therapy, ischemia-guided medical therapy, or revascularization. Patients selected for this study had evidence of myocardial ischemia on both ambulatory and exercise treadmill testing. Ischemia suppression through medical therapy was performed using one of two regimens: (1) atenolol and nifedipine, or (2) diltiazem and isosorbide dinitrate.

With a regimen of atenolol and nifedipine, ischemic changes on AECG monitoring could be suppressed in 47 percent of patients. In the group treated with diltiazem and isosorbide, ischemia was suppressed in 31 percent of patients after a period of 12 weeks. The degree of ischemia suppression was similar in the ischemia- and angina-guided groups. The revascularization strategy led to suppression of ischemia in 70 percent of the bypass surgery group versus 46 percent of the angioplasty group. It is noteworthy that in the medical therapy group, the average doses (combined ischemia- and angina-guided therapy) of each medication at 12 weeks were as follows: 84 mg of atenolol, 34 mg of nifedipine, 91 mg of diltiazem, and 36 mg of isosorbide dinitrate. Thus, the degree of medical therapy can be described as moderately intense.

The findings of other trials have been similar. In the CASIS, patients were selected according to the presence of ischemia during treadmill testing and ambulatory monitoring and subsequently assigned to receive either atenolol or amlodipine. Each group underwent a counterbalanced, crossover evaluation of single drug and placebo, followed by evaluation of the combination. The suppression of ischemia during exercise testing and ambulatory monitoring was similar in patients with and without exercise-induced angina. Exercise time to angina improved by 29 percent with amlodipine, 16 percent with atenolol, and 39 percent with combination therapy. Similarly, in the American Stop Smoking Intervention Study (ASSIST), after 4 weeks of treatment with atenolol of patients with Canadian Cardiovascular Class I or II angina, the number and duration of ischemic episodes on AECG monitoring decreased significantly compared with placebo.

In a smaller study, Dakik and coworkers[88] compared intensive medical therapy with percutaneous revascularization in minimally symptomatic patients with large (>15 percent of the left ventricle) ischemic defects on thallium scintigraphy in patients after recent MI compared with those in other studies. The medical regimen in this trial was much more intense. The average daily doses of medications were 113 ± 23 mg of isosorbide dinitrate, 131 ± 57 mg of metoprolol, and 272 ± 58 mg of diltiazem, and the extent of ischemia was measured with highly reproducible adenosine ^{201}TI tomography (SPECT). This medical regimen resulted in a 12 ± 10 percent reduction in the ischemic defect size and was equally effective as angioplasty.

Results of Suppression of Ischemia

The relationship between suppression of ischemia and clinical outcome remains uncertain. However, in the ACIP Trial, the mortality rate at 1 year was 4.4 percent in the angina-guided group, 1.6 percent in the ischemia-guided group, and 0 percent in the revascularization group. There was a direct correlation between number of ischemic episodes on AECG monitoring and event rate. However, it must be kept in mind that the latter trial was a pilot study with confidence levels too broad to allow definitive conclusions to be drawn. In ASSIST, there was a nonsignificant trend for fewer serious events (death, resuscitation from ventricular fibrillation/tachycardia, nonfatal MI, or hospitalization for unstable angina) in atenolol-treated patients compared with those assigned to placebo. The most powerful univariate and multivariate correlate of event-free survival was the absence of ischemia on AECG monitoring 4 weeks after the start of therapy. In conclusion, most data available indicate that event-free survival is likely to be related to reduction in the amount of ischemia present regardless of the presence or absence of symptoms and the treatment chosen. Large trials that compare revascularization with maximal medical therapy (COURAGE, SMART) are in the design phase or under way.

REFERENCES

1. Heberden W: Some account of a disorder of the breast. Med Trans Coll Physicians (Lond) 2:59, 1772.
2. Enos WF, Holmes RH, Beyer J: Coronary artery disease among United States soldiers killed in action in Korea: preliminary report. JAMA 152:1090, 1953.
3. Mason JK: Asymptomatic disease of coronary arteries in young men. BMJ 5367:1234, 1963.
4. Matthewson FA, Varnam GS: Abnormal electrocardiograms in apparently healthy people. Circulation 21:204–213, 1960.
5. Margolis JR, Kannel WS, Feinleib M, et al: Clinical features of unrecognized myocardial infarction—silent and symptomatic: eighteen year follow-up: the Framingham study. Am J Cardiol 32:1–7, 1973.
6. Sullivan W, Vlodaver Z, Tuna N, et al: Correlation of electrocardiographic and pathologic findings in healed myocardial infarction. Am J Cardiol 42:724–732, 1978.
7. Twiss A, Sokolow M: Angina pectoris: significant electrocardiographic changes following exercise. Am Heart J 23:498–512, 1942.
8. Randich A, Maixner W: Interactions between cardiovascular and pain regulatory systems. Neurosci Biobehav Rev 8:343–367, 1984.
9. Falcone C, Auguadro C, Sconocchia R, Angoli L: Susceptibility to pain in hypertensive and normotensive patients with coronary artery disease: response to dental pulp stimulation. Hypertension 30:1279–1283, 1997.
10. Rosen SD, Paulesu E, Nihoyannopoulos P, et al: Silent ischemia as a central problem: regional brain activation compared in silent and painful myocardial ischemia. Ann Intern Med 124:939–949, 1996.
11. Falcone C, Sconocchia R, Guasti L, et al: Dental pain threshold and angina pectoris in patients with coronary artery disease. J Am Coll Cardiol 12:348–352, 1988.
12. Matsubara K, Yokota M, Miyahara T, et al: Left ventricular performance during exercise testing in patients with silent and symptomatic myocardial ischemia. Am Heart J 129:459–464, 1995.
13. Hikita H, Etsuda H, Takase B, et al: Extent of ischemic stimulus and plasma beta-endorphin levels in silent myocardial ischemia. Am Heart J 135:813–818, 1998.
14. Amsterdam EA, Wolfson S, Gorlin R: New aspects of the placebo response in angina pectoris. Am J Cardiol 24:305–306, 1969.
15. Friedman M, Breall WS, Goodwin ML, et al: Effect of type A behavioral counseling on frequency of episodes of silent myocardial ischemia in coronary patients. Am Heart J 132:933–937, 1996.
16. Narins CR, Zareba W, Moss AJ, et al: Clinical implications of silent versus symptomatic exercise-induced myocardial ischemia in patients with stable coronary disease. J Am Coll Cardiol 29:756–763, 1997.
17. Marcassa C, Galli M, Baroffio C, et al: Ischemic burden in silent and painful myocardial ischemia: a quantitative exercise sestamibi tomographic study. J Am Coll Cardiol 29:948–954, 1997.
18. Klein J, Chao S, Bermand D, Rozanski A: Is "silent" ischemia really as severe as symptomatic ischemia? The analytical effect of patient selection biases [abstract]. Circulation 89:1958–1966, 1994.
19. Hecht H, Shaw R, Bruce T, Myler R: Silent ischemia: evaluation by exercise and redistribution tomographic thallium-201 imaging [abstract]. J Am Coll Cardiol 14:895–900, 1989.
20. Gasperetti C, Burwell L, Beller G: Prevalence and variables associated with silent myocardial ischemia on exercise thallium-201 stress testing [abstract]. J Am Coll Cardiol 16:115–123, 1990.
21. Heller L, Tresgallo M, Sciacca R, et al: Prognostic significance of silent myocardial ischemia on thallium stress test. Am J Cardiol 65:718–721, 1990.
22. Mahamarian J, Pratt C, Cocanougher M, Verani M: Altered myocardium perfusion in patients with angina pectoris or silent ischemia during exercise as assessed by quantitative thallium-201 single photon emission computed tomography. Circulation 82:1305–1315, 1990.
23. Kurata C, Sajata K, Taguchi T, et al: Exercise-induced silent myocardial ischemia: evaluation by thallium-201 emission computed tomography. Am Heart J 119:557–567, 1990.
24. Galli M, Bosimini E, Giordano A, Tavazzi L: Scintigraphic evidence of silent ischemia in post-MI patients: prognostic implication. Adv Cardiol 37:244–260, 1990.
25. Travin M, Flores A, Boucher C, et al: Silent versus symptomatic ischemia during a thallium-201 exercise test. Am J Cardiol 1991;68:1600–1608, 1991.
26. Hendler A, Greyson N, Robinson M, Freeman M: Patients with symptomatic ischemia have larger thallium perfusion abnormalities and more adverse prognosis than patients with silent ischemia. Can J Cardiol 8:814–818, 1992.
27. Falcone C, Auguadro C, Sconocchia R, et al: Susceptibility to pain during coronary angioplasty: usefulness of pulpal test. J Am Coll Cardiol 28:903–909, 1996.
28. Bonow RO, Bacharach SL, Green MV, et al: Prognostic implications of symptomatic versus asymptomatic (silent) myocardial ischemia induced by exercise in mildly symptomatic and in asymptomatic patients with angiographically documented coronary artery disease. Am J Cardiol 60:778–783, 1987.

28a. Cohn PF, Brown EJ Jr, Wynne J, et al: Global and regional left ventricular ejection fraction abnormalities during exercise in patients with silent myocardial ischemia. J Am Coll Cardiol 1:931–933, 1983.

28b. Vassiliadis IV, Machac J, O'Hara M, et al: Exercise-induced myocardial dysfunction in patients with coronary artery disease with and without angina. Am Heart J 121:1403–1408, 1991.

29. Garcia MJ, McNamara PM, Gordon T, Kannel WB: Morbidity and mortality in diabetics in the Framingham population: sixteen year follow-up study. Diabetes 23:105–111, 1974.
30. Mak KH, Moliterno DJ, Granger CB, et al: Influence of diabetes mellitus on clinical outcome in the thrombolytic era of acute myocardial infarction: GUSTO-I Investigators: Global Utilization of Streptokinase and Tissue Plasminogen Activator for Occluded Coronary Arteries. J Am Coll Cardiol 30:171–179, 1997.
31. Malmberg K, Ryden L: Myocardial infarction in patients with diabetes mellitus. Eur Heart J 9:259–264, 1988.
32. Zuanetti G, Latini R, Maggioni AP, et al: Influence of diabetes on mortality in acute myocardial infarction: data from the GISSI-2 study. J Am Coll Cardiol 22:1788–1794, 1993.
33. Herlitz J, Bang A, Karlson BW: Mortality, place and mode of death and reinfarction during a period of 5 years after acute myocardial infarction in diabetic and non-diabetic patients. Cardiology 87:423–428, 1996.
34. Kannel WB, Abbott RD: Incidence and prognosis of unrecognized myocardial infarction: an update on the Framingham study. N Engl J Med 311:1144–1147, 1984.
35. Chiariello M, Indolfi C, Cotecchia MR, et al: Asymptomatic transient ST changes during ambulatory ECG monitoring in diabetic patients. Am Heart J 110:529–534, 1985.
36. Zarich S, Waxman S, Freeman RT, et al: Effect of autonomic nervous system dysfunction on the circadian pattern of myocardial ischemia in diabetes mellitus. J Am Coll Cardiol 24:956–962, 1994.
37. Nesto RW, Phillips RT, Kett KG, et al: Angina and exertional myocardial ischemia in diabetic and nondiabetic patients: assessment by exercise thallium scintigraphy. Ann Intern Med 108:170–175, 1988. (Published erratum appears in Ann Intern Med 104:646, 1988.)
38. Caracciolo EA, Chaitman BR, Forman SA, et al: Diabetics with coronary disease have a prevalence of asymptomatic ischemia during exercise treadmill testing and ambulatory ischemia monitoring similar to that of nondiabetic patients: an ACIP database study. ACIP Investigators: Asymptomatic Cardiac Ischemia Pilot Investigators. Circulation 93:2097–2105, 1996.

39. Earle KA, Mishra M, Morocutti A, et al: Microalbuminuria as a marker of silent myocardial ischaemia in IDDM patients. Diabetologia 39:854–856, 1996.
39a. Sachs RN, Valensi P, Lormeau B, et al: Determinants of endocardiographically measured left ventricular mass in diabetic patients with or without silent myocardial ischaemia. Diabetes Metab 25:128–136, 1999.
40. Langer A, Freeman MR, Josse RG, Armstrong PW: Metaiodobenzylguanidine imaging in diabetes mellitus: assessment of cardiac sympathetic denervation and its relation to autonomic dysfunction and silent myocardial ischemia. J Am Coll Cardiol 25:610–618, 1995.
41. Masters AM, Geller AJ: Magnitude of silent coronary artery disease. N Y State J Med 64:2865, 1964.
42. Cregler LL, Mark H: Relation of acute myocardial infarction to cocaine abuse. Am J Cardiol 56:794, 1985.
43. Mark DB, Hlatky MA, Califf RM, et al: Painless exercise ST deviation on the treadmill: long-term prognosis. J Am Coll Cardiol 14:885–892, 1989.
44. Weiner DA, Ryan TJ, McCabe CH, et al: Risk of developing an acute myocardial infarction or sudden coronary death in patients with exercise-induced silent myocardial ischemia: a report from the Coronary Artery Surgery Study (CASS) Registry. Am J Cardiol 81:428–436, 1988.
45. Golding B, Wolf E, Tzivoni D, Stern S: Transient S-T elevation detected by 24-hour ECG monitoring during normal daily activity. Am Heart J 86:501–507, 1973.
46. Deanfield JE, Ribiero P, Oakley K, et al: Analysis of ST-segment changes in normal subjects: implications for ambulatory monitoring in angina pectoris. Am J Cardiol 54:1321–1325, 1984.
47. Legault SE, Freeman MR, Langer A, Armstrong PW: Pathophysiology and time course of silent myocardial ischaemia during mental stress: clinical, anatomical, and physiological correlates. Br Heart J 73:242–249, 1995.
48. Taki J, Yasuda T, Tamaki N, et al: Temporal relation between left ventricular dysfunction and chest pain in coronary artery disease during activities of daily living. Am J Cardiol 66:1455–1458, 1990.
49. Deanfield JE, Shea M, Ribiero P, et al: Transient ST-segment depression as a marker of myocardial ischemia during daily life. Am J Cardiol 54:1195–1200, 1984.
50. Deanfield JE, Maseri A, Selwyn AP, et al: Myocardial ischaemia during daily life in patients with stable angina: its relation to symptoms and heart rate changes. Lancet 2:753–758, 1983.
51. Cecchi AC, Dovellini EV, Marchi F, et al: Silent myocardial ischemia during ambulatory electrocardiographic monitoring in patients with effort angina. J Am Coll Cardiol 1983;1:934–939, 1983.
52. Deanfield JE, Shea M, Kensett M, et al: Silent myocardial ischaemia due to mental stress. Lancet 2:1001–1005, 1984.
53. Shea MJ, Deanfield JE, deLandsheere CM, et al: Asymptomatic myocardial ischemia following cold provocation. Am Heart J 114:469–476, 1987.
54. Gottlieb SO, Weisfeldt ML, Ouyang P, et al: Silent ischemia as a marker for early unfavorable outcomes in patients with unstable angina. N Engl J Med 314:1214–1219, 1986.
55. Nademanee K, Intarachot V, Singh PN, et al: Characteristics and clinical significance of silent myocardial ischemia in unstable angina. Am J Cardiol 58:26B–33B, 1986.
56. Nademanee K, Intarachot V, Josephson MA, et al: Prognostic significance of silent myocardial ischemia in patients with unstable angina. J Am Coll Cardiol 10:1–9, 1987.
57. Gerstenblith G: Treatment of unstable angina pectoris. Am J Cardiol 70:32G–37G, 1992.
58. Taylor GJ, Katholi RE, Womack K, et al: Increased incidence of silent ischemia after acute myocardial infarction. JAMA 268:1448–1450, 1992.
59. The TIMI IIIB Investigators: Effects of tissue plasminogen activator and a comparison of early invasive and conservative strategies in unstable angina and non–Q-wave myocardial infarction: results of the TIMI IIIB Trial. Circulation 89:1545–1556, 1994.
60. Ostrander LDJ: The relation of "silent" T wave inversion to cardiovascular disease in an epidemiologic study. Am J Cardiol 25:325–328, 1970.
61. Thompson RC, Mackey DC, Lane GE, et al: mproved detection of silent cardiac ischemia with a 12-lead portable microprocessor-driven real-time electrocardiographic monitor. Mayo Clin Proc 70:434–442, 1995.
62. Mahmarian JJ, Steingart RM, Forman S, et al: Relation between ambulatory electrocardiographic monitoring and myocardial perfusion imaging to detect coronary artery disease and myocardial ischemia: an ACIP ancillary study: the Asymptomatic Cardiac Ischemia Pilot (ACIP) Investigators. J Am Coll Cardiol 29:764–769, 1997.
63. Quyyumi AA, Panza JA, Diodati JG, et al: Prognostic implications of myocardial ischemia during daily life in low risk patients with coronary artery disease. J Am Coll Cardiol 21:700–708, 1993.
64. Rozanski A, Bairey CN, Krantz DS, et al: Mental stress and the induction of silent myocardial ischemia in patients with coronary artery disease. N Engl J Med 318:1005–1012, 1988.
65. Deanfield JE, Shea MJ, Wilson RA, et al: Direct effects of smoking on the heart: silent ischemic disturbances of coronary flow. Am J Cardiol 57:1005–1009, 1986.
66. Campbell S, Barry J, Rocco MB, et al: Features of the exercise test that reflect the activity of ischemic heart disease out of hospital. Circulation 74:72–80, 1986.
67. Benhorin J, Moriel M, Gavish A, et al: Usefulness of severity of myocardial ischemia on exercise testing in predicting the severity of myocardial ischemia during daily activities. Am J Cardiol 68:176–180, 1991.
68. Borzak S, Fenton T, Glasser SP, et al: Discordance between effects of antiischemic therapy on ambulatory ischemia, exercise performance and anginal symptoms in patients with stable angina pectoris: the Angina and Silent Ischemia Study Group (ASIS). J Am Coll Cardiol 21:1605–1611, 1993.
69. Benhorin J, Pinsker G, Moriel M, et al: Ischemic threshold during two exercise testing protocols and during ambulatory electrocardiographic monitoring. J Am Coll Cardiol 22:671–677, 1993.
70. Deedwania PC, Nelson JR: Pathophysiology of silent myocardial ischemia during daily life: hemodynamic evaluation by simultaneous electrocardiographic and blood pressure monitoring. Circulation 82:1296–1304, 1990.
71. Deedwania PC, Carbajal EV: Role of myocardial oxygen demand in the pathogenesis of silent ischemia during daily life. Am J Cardiol 70:19F–24F, 1992.
72. Rocco MB, Barry J, Campbell S, et al: Circadian variation of transient myocardial ischemia in patients with coronary artery disease. Circulation 75:395–400, 1987.
73. Mulcahy D, Keegan J, Cunningham D, et al: Circadian variation of total ischaemic burden and its alteration with anti-anginal agents. Lancet 2:755–759, 1988.
74. Deedwania PC, Carbajal EV: Prevalence and patterns of silent myocardial ischemia during daily life in stable angina patients receiving conventional antianginal drug therapy. Am J Cardiol 65:1090–1096, 1990.
75. Cohn PF, Lawson WE: Characteristics of silent myocardial ischemia during out-of-hospital activities in asymptomatic angiographically documented coronary artery disease. Am J Cardiol 59:746–749, 1987.
76. Brezinski DA, Tofler GH, Muller JE, et al: Morning increase in platelet aggregability: association with assumption of the upright posture. Circulation 78:35–40, 1988.
77. Tofler GH, Brezinski D, Schafer Al, et al: Concurrent morning increase in platelet aggregability and the risk of myocardial infarction and sudden cardiac death. N Engl J Med 316:1514–1518, 1987.
78. Millar-Craig MW, Bishop CN, Raftery EB: Circadian variation of blood-pressure. Lancet 1:795–797, 1978.
79. Muller JE, Stone PH, Turi ZG, et al: Circadian variation in the frequency of onset of acute myocardial infarction. N Engl J Med 313:1315–1322, 1985.
80. Hjalmarson A, Gilpin EA, Nicod P, et al: Differing circadian patterns of symptom onset in subgroups of patients with acute myocardial infarction. Circulation 80:267–275, 1989.
81. Hansen O, Johansson BW, Gullberg B: Circadian distribution of onset of acute myocardial infarction in subgroups from analysis of 10,791 patients treated in a single center. Am J Cardiol 69:1003–1008, 1992.
82. Muller JE, Ludmer PL, Willich SN, et al: Circadian variation in the frequency of sudden cardiac death. Circulation 75:131–138, 1987.
83. Davies RF, Habibi H, Klinke WP, et al: Effect of amlodipine, atenolol and their combination on myocardial ischemia during treadmill exercise and ambulatory monitoring: Canadian Amlodipine/Atenolol In Silent Ischemia Study (CASIS) Investigators. J Am Coll Cardiol 25:619–625, 1995.

84. Mahmarian JJ, Moye LA, Verani MS, et al: High reproducibility of myocardial perfusion defects in patients undergoing serial exercise thallium-201 tomography. Am J Cardiol 75:1116–1119, 1995.
85. Aoki M, Sakai K, Koyanagi S, et al: Effect of nitroglycerin on coronary collateral function during exercise evaluated by quantitative analysis of thallium-201 single photon emission computed tomography. Am Heart J 121:1361–1366, 1991.
86. Mahmarian JJ, Fenimore NL, Marks GF, et al: Transdermal nitroglycerin patch therapy reduces the extent of exercise-induced myocardial ischemia: results of a double-blind, placebo-controlled trial using quantitative thallium-201 tomography. J Am Coll Cardiol 24:25–32, 1994.
87. Mahamarian JJ, Moye LA, Nasser GA, et al: Nicotine patch therapy in smoking cessation reduces the extent of exercise-induced myocardial ischemia. J Am Coll Cardiol 30:125–130, 1997.
88. Dakik HA, Kleiman NS, Farmer JA, et al: Intensive medical therapy versus coronary angioplasty for suppression of myocardial ischemia in survivors of acute myocardial infarction: a prospective, randomized pilot study. Circulation 98:2017–2023, 1998.
89. Sawada SG, Segar DS, Ryan T, et al: Echocardiographic detection of coronary artery disease during dobutamine infusion. Circulation 83:1605–1614, 1991.
90. Salustri A, Fioretti PM, McNeill AJ, et al: Pharmacological stress echocardiography in the diagnosis of coronary artery disease and myocardial ischaemia: a comparison between dobutamine and dipyridamole. Eur Heart J 13:1356–1362, 1992.
91. Quinones MA, Verani MS, Haichin RM, et al: Exercise echocardiography versus ^{201}TI single-photon emission computed tomography in evaluation of coronary artery disease: analysis of 292 patients. Circulation 85:1026–1031, 1992.
92. Elhendy A, Geleijnse ML, Roelandt JR, et al: Stress-induced left ventricular dysfunction in silent and symptomatic myocardial ischemia during dobutamine stress test. Am J Cardiol 75:1112–1115, 1995.
93. Bigi R, Galati A, Curti G, et al: Different clinical and prognostic significance of painful and silent myocardial ischemia detected by exercise electrocardiography and dobutamine stress echocardiography after uncomplicated myocardial infarction. Am J Cardiol 81:75–78, 1998.
94. Sigurdsson E, Sigfusson N, Sigvaldason H, Thorgeirsson G: Silent ST-T changes in an epidemiologic cohort study—a marker of hypertension or coronary heart disease, or both: the Reykjavik study. J Am Coll Cardiol 27:1140–1147, 1996.
95. Cole JP, Ellestad MH: Significance of chest pain during treadmill exercise: correlation with coronary events. Am J Cardiol 41:227–232, 1978.
96. Callaham PR, Froelicher VF, Klein J, et al: Exercise-induced silent ischemia: age, diabetes mellitus, previous myocardial infarction and prognosis. J Am Coll Cardiol 14:1175–1180, 1989.
97. Villella A, Maggioni AP, Villella M, et al: Prognostic significance of maximal exercise testing after myocardial infarction treated with thrombolytic agents: the GISSI-2 data-base: Gruppo Italiano per lo Studio della Sopravvivenza Nell'Infarto. Lancet 346:523–529, 1995.
98. Conti CR, Geller NL, Knatterud GL, et al: Anginal status and prediction of cardiac events in patients enrolled in the Asymptomatic Cardiac Ischemia Pilot (ACIP) study: ACIP investigators. Am J Cardiol 79:889–892, 1997.
99. Pancholy SB, Schalet B, Kuhlmeier V, et al: Prognostic significance of silent ischemia. J Nucl Cardiol 1:434–440, 1994.
100. Bandu I, Friedman H, Raggi P: Symptoms of patients with silent ischemia as detected by thallium stress testing. Chest 105:1009–1012, 1994.

CHAPTER 28

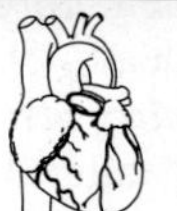

Coronary Artery Disease in Women*

Renu Virmani, Allen P. Burke, Andrew Farb, and Frank D. Kolodgie

EPIDEMIOLOGY OF SUDDEN DEATH IN WOMEN
RISK FACTORS FOR CORONARY HEART DISEASE IN WOMEN
DEFINITION OF PLAQUE RUPTURE AND EROSION
CLINICAL AND MORPHOLOGIC DIFFERENCES OF PLAQUE RUPTURE VERSUS SUPERFICIAL EROSION
INFLUENCE OF RISK FACTORS ON PLAQUE MORPHOLOGY IN WOMEN
DEMOGRAPHICS
RISK FACTOR AND MECHANISM OF DEATH
COMPARISON OF PLAQUE MORPHOLOGY BY AGE IN MEN AND WOMEN
SUMMARY

Sudden cardiac death occurs in more than 300,000 persons annually in the United States and is the most frequent cause of death in the industrialized world. The most frequent cause of sudden death is coronary artery disease, and it is thought to be a male-predominant disease.[1]

Epidemiology of Sudden Death in Women

Data from the Framingham Heart Study show that sudden death in women lags behind that in men by almost 20 years. The annual rate of sudden death in women is approximately half that in men for all ages combined. In the Framingham study, only 94 of 2873 women died suddenly compared with 230 of 2336 men of comparable age.[2] The incidence of sudden death in men and women increased with age, approximately doubling with each decade of life in women. In both sexes, 26 percent of deaths occurred in persons without overt coronary heart disease. In women, 63 percent of deaths occurred in the absence of prior coronary heart disease compared with 44 percent in men. Of the deaths in men and women due to coronary heart disease, 76 percent were sudden deaths. In persons with prior coronary heart disease, 34 percent of deaths in men were sudden compared with 16 percent in women.[2] It appears that sudden coronary death is less frequent in women than in men but is more likely to occur in women without prior coronary disease.

Risk Factors for Coronary Heart Disease in Women

The usual risk factors for coronary heart disease—cigarette smoking, diabetes mellitus, hypertension, dyslipidemia, obesity, sedentary lifestyle, and poor nutrition—are similar in women and in men. More than 50 percent of myocardial infarctions among middle-aged women are attributable to cigarette smoking.[3] It has been reported that the excess risk for coronary heart disease in women from smoking was twofold to fourfold and was similar to that in men.[4] Similarly, epidemiologic studies have documented a strong association between high blood pressure (systolic and diastolic) and the risk of coronary heart disease in men and women. After adjustment for other risk factors, 29 percent of coronary heart disease events in women (≥30 years old) were attributable to blood pressure levels that exceed high normal levels (≥130/85 mm Hg).[5]

Serum cholesterol and low-density lipoprotein levels are established risk factors of coronary heart disease in men and women. In contrast to men, women show only a weak association of total cholesterol and low-density lipoprotein levels with coronary heart disease[6]; however, high-density lipoprotein cholesterol (HDL-C) is closely and inversely associated with coronary heart disease risk in women. Triglycerides are an independent predictor of coronary artery disease in older women but not in men.[4, 6, 7]

Diabetes mellitus is a greater risk factor for the presence and severity of coronary heart disease in women than in men. Diabetes is linked to both hyperlipidemia and obesity in men and women, but especially in women.[8, 9]

Obesity and sedentary lifestyle in the United States have been linked to increased risk of coronary artery disease in men and women. The prevalence of obesity has increased in the 1990s, and it is estimated that at least 30 percent of adult women are obese.[10–12] Dietary habits also influence coronary heart disease risk; diets low in saturated fat and high in fruits, whole grain, and fiber are associated with a reduction in the risk of coronary heart disease.[13, 14]

Definition of Plaque Rupture and Erosion

We reported our findings on the type of atherosclerotic lesion underlying luminal thrombi in individuals with sud-

*The opinions or assertions contained herein are the private views of the authors and are not to be construed as official or reflecting the views of the Department of the Army, the Department of the Air Force, or the Department of Defense.

den coronary death.[15] Of 96 cases of sudden coronary death, 50 (52 percent) had coronary thrombi. *Sudden coronary death* was defined as witnessed sudden unexpected death within 6 hours of the onset of symptoms or death of an individual who had been seen in stable condition less than 24 hours antemortem. To diagnose whether death had been due to coronary disease, at least one major coronary artery had to have at least 75 percent cross-sectional area luminal narrowing or a histologically confirmed acute luminal thrombus.[15]

Coronary artery thrombi were separated into two categories based on the morphology of the underlying plaque. Coronary *plaque rupture* was defined as a luminal thrombus overlying a disrupted fibrous cap; the lipid core was in contact with the thrombus. Conversely, *plaque erosion* (superficial erosion) was characterized as a thrombus with direct contact with the intimal plaque without rupture into a lipid pool. The plaque under the thrombus was rich in smooth muscle cells that lie within a proteoglycan-rich matrix, but macrophages and T cells may be present. The lipid pool either was absent or formed an insignificant part of the plaque and did not communicate with the thrombus on serial sectioning. Based on these definitions, 28 (56 percent) thrombi were secondary to plaque rupture and 22 (44 percent) were secondary to plaque erosion.[15]

Clinical and Morphologic Differences of Plaque Rupture Versus Superficial Erosion

The mean age in cases of coronary thrombosis due to plaque rupture was 53 ± 10 years versus 44 ± 7 years in erosion ($P < .003$). In the plaque rupture group, 5 of 28 (18 percent) patients were women compared with 11 of 22 (50 percent) in the eroded plaque group ($P = .03$). The mean percent cross-sectional area stenosis (excluding the thrombus itself) was greater in plaque ruptures (78 ± 12 percent) than in erosions (70 ± 11 percent, $P < .03$). Plaque calcification was present in 19 ruptures (69 percent) compared with 5 erosions (23 percent, $P = .002$). The thrombus was occlusive in 12 cases of rupture (43 percent) and nonocclusive in 16 (57 percent); only 4 eroded plaques (18 percent) demonstrated complete thrombotic occlusion ($P = .08$ versus rupture into a necrotic core). Thrombi were predominantly composed of platelets in 13 (48 percent) cases of plaque rupture and fibrin in 15 (52 percent). A similar distribution was noted in eroded plaques whereby 14 (52 percent) were predominantly composed of platelets and 8 (35 percent) were mostly fibrin ($P = .26$). Increased fibrin content may represent early organization of the thrombus progressing from initial platelet deposition to infiltration and stabilization by fibrin. Thirteen ruptured arteries were concentric (46 percent) and 15 (54 percent) were eccentric. Only 4 eroded arteries without lipid core rupture were concentric (18 percent), whereas the remaining 18 (82 percent) were eccentric ($P = .07$ versus rupture into a necrotic core). An acute myocardial infarction was present in 10 coronary rupture cases (36 percent) compared with 6 erosion cases (27 percent, $P = .56$). The frequency of healed myocardial infarction was similar in coronary ruptures and erosions (11 [39 percent] ruptures and 7 erosions [32 percent], $P = .77$).[15]

Identification of cell type through immunohistochemical staining demonstrated several differences between ruptures and erosions (Table 28–1 and Plate 28–1). In plaque ruptures, macrophages were typically seen infiltrating the thin fibrous cap at the margins of the rupture site (Fig. 28–1). The foci of KP-1–positive macrophages were present in all 28 plaque ruptures and in only 11 (50 percent) of erosions ($P < .0001$). When present, macrophages in eroded plaques were sparsely distributed in the upper layers of the lesions away from the luminal surface. Conversely, clusters of α-actin–positive smooth muscle cells were seen at the luminal surface adjacent to the thrombus in 21 plaque erosions (95 percent) compared with only 11 (33 percent) cases of rupture ($P < .0001$). In plaque rupture, smooth muscle cells were predominantly seen in the fibrous cap away from the rupture site. T cells were present near the rupture site in 21 (75 percent) cases of rupture compared with 7 (32 percent) cases of eroded arteries ($P < .004$). Cell activation, indicated by anti–human leukocyte antigen (HLA)–DR staining, was identified in both macrophages and T cells in 25 (89 percent) cases of rupture and in macrophages in 8 (36 percent) cases of eroded plaques ($P = .0002$).[15]

Our results are dramatically different from those of van der Wal and colleagues[16] because HLA-DR–positive cells consisted predominantly of macrophages and T cells and, only occasionally, smooth muscle cells. We observed marked difference in plaque erosion and rupture, with a predominance of macrophages and T cells in rupture and fewer of these cells in plaque erosion. Smooth muscle cells were most common in plaque erosions, whereas they were infrequent in ruptures. We quantified the number of macrophages and T cells in rupture and erosion; the number of

TABLE 28–1 Coronary Thrombosis With Rupture Into a Lipid Core (Plaque Rupture) Compared With Thrombosis Associated With Eroded Plaque Without Lipid Pool Rupture (Plaque Erosion)

	Plaque Rupture (n = 28)	Plaque Erosion (n = 22)	P
Male/female	23/5	11/11	.03
Age (yr)	53 ± 10	44 ± 7	<.02
Stenosis (%)	78 ± 12	70 ± 11	<.03
Calcified plaque	19 (69%)	5 (23%)	.002
Occlusive/nonocclusive thrombus	12/16 (43/57%)	4/18 (18/82%)	.08
Concentric/eccentric	13/15 (46/54%)	4/18 (18/82%)	.07
Macrophages*	28 (100%)	11 (50%)	<.0001
T cells*	21 (75%)	7 (32%)	<.004
Smooth muscle cells*	11 (33%)	21 (95%)	<.0001
HLA-DR positive*	25 (89%)	8 (36%)	.0002

*Cellular collections at plaque rupture or erosion sites. Unless otherwise indicated, values are given as n or mean ± SD.

From Farb A, Burke AP, Tang AL, et al: Coronary plaque erosion without rupture into a lipid core: a frequent cause of coronary thrombosis in sudden coronary death. Circulation 93(7):1354–1363, 1996.

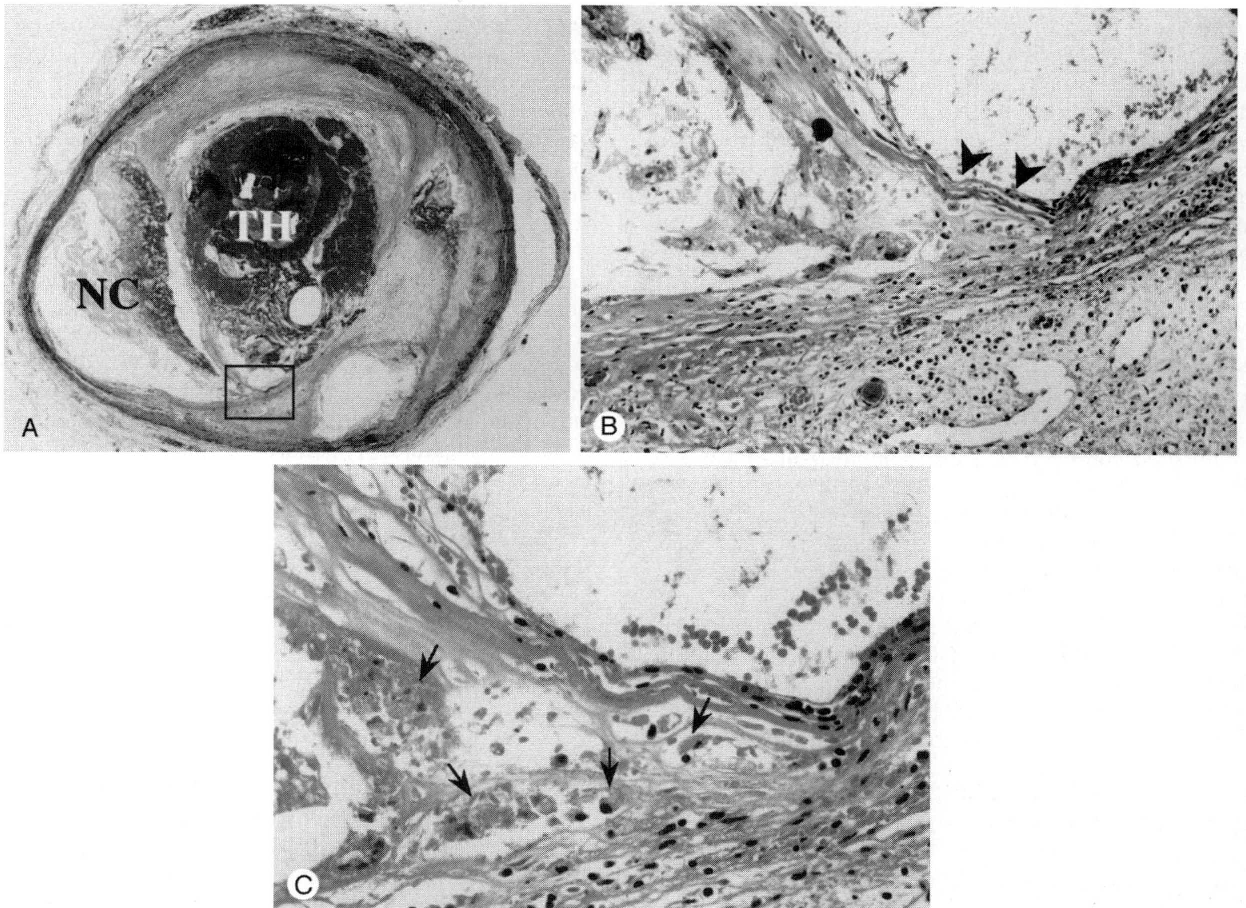

FIGURE 28–1 A 54-year-old woman with no previous medical history had a witnessed cardiac arrest after sudden onset of back pain. The patient's risk factor analysis showed a serum total cholesterol of 256 mg/dl, high-density lipoprotein cholesterol of 35 mg/dl, absence of systemic hypertension, and glucose intolerance. **A,** At autopsy, there was a 70 percent (cross-sectional area luminal narrowing) concentric atherosclerotic plaque in the mid–right coronary artery with a superimposed occlusive thrombus (TH) due to plaque rupture. There was a concentric atherosclerotic plaque at the site of the thrombus with a thin fibrous cap, macrophage infiltration, and an underlying necrotic core (NC). (Movat pentachrome, ×5.) **B,** High-power view of the area in the *boxed area* in **A** near the rupture site; note the thin fibrous cap (*arrowheads*). (Movat pentachrome. ×100.) **C,** High-power micrograph shows a thin fibrous cap infiltrated by macrophages (*arrows*). (H&E, ×200.)

macrophages were significantly greater in ruptures than in erosions (585 ± 219 versus 251 ± 159 mm^{-2}, P = .0007). However, there were no significant differences among the two entities in the number of T cells. For quantification of smooth muscle cells in the fibrous cap, cell counts were performed to a depth of 100 μm. The number of smooth muscle cells were significantly greater in erosion (794 ± 334 mm^{-2}) than in rupture (164 ± 177 mm^{-2}, $P < .0001$). Thus, it appears that what we describe as plaque erosion may be morphologically different from that of van der Wal and colleagues.[16]

The production of extracellular matrix (ECM) by smooth muscle cells contributes to the pathogenesis of atherosclerosis, and the increased expression of ECM proteoglycans is a unique feature of plaque erosion. Although the ECM accounts for the most of the plaque burden, it is also involved in modulation of cell proliferation and is a regulator of growth factor synthesis. The expressions of two proteoglycans in particular—biglycan and decorin—have been shown in atherosclerotic plaques.[17] Evidence further suggests that biglycan, in particular, may contribute to the pathogenesis of atherosclerosis by trapping lipoproteins in the artery wall.[18] In plaque erosion, we found intense expression of biglycan in hypercellular areas, whereas decorin staining was mostly restricted to areas of dense connective tissue (Plate 28–2). In vitro studies in arterial smooth muscle cells have demonstrated up-regulation of biglycan and down-regulation of decorin by transforming growth factor-β (also present in erosion, see Plate 28–2), which may explain the strong expression of biglycan.[19] Clearly, different proteoglycans may play distinct roles during lesion progression and may dictate the cellular composition of erosions.

The mechanisms of thrombosis in plaque erosion are unknown. Furthermore, unlike plaque rupture, in which a precursor plaque can be identified (i.e., *vulnerable plaque*), no such "pre-erosion lesion" has been described. Indeed, the formation of thrombi in plaque erosion most likely involves multiple factors, including fibrinolytic dysfunction or abnormalities to surface endothelium, smooth muscle cells, or both. Fibrinolytic dysfunction—in particular, elevated plasma and tissue levels of tissue factor and plasminogen activator inhibitor-1—may represent a risk factor for coronary thrombosis. Studies have shown alterations in the plasminogen activator system in human coronary plaques.[20] Further studies of eroded coronary plaques in our laboratory have shown this tissue factor expression in both smooth muscle cells and macrophages. Intimal expression of plasminogen activator inhibitor-1 was 75 percent in eroded vessels compared with 20 percent in control nonthrombosed arteries.[21]

Influence of Risk Factors on Plaque Morphology in Women

We compared coronary plaque morphology in 51 cases of sudden coronary deaths in women (mean age, 50 ± 12 years) with that in 15 women (mean age, 50 ± 19 years) who died of trauma. The risk factor analysis was performed in all cases at autopsy. The postmortem serum was evaluated for total cholesterol (TC), HDL-C, and thiocyanate levels. Smokers were identified as those with a thiocyanate level of higher than 90 mg/dl. Glucose intolerance (diabetic screen) was determined on the case of red blood cell glycosylated hemoglobin, and hypertension was assessed through renal vascular morphometric analysis.

Demographics

Of the 51 coronary deaths, 21 occurred in women older than 50 years, and 30 occurred in women younger than 50 years. There were a greater number of younger women because autopsies are performed more frequently in younger individuals. Acute thrombi resulting from plaque erosion were present in 18 hearts (35 percent), plaque rupture in 8 (16 percent), stable plaque with healed myocardial infarction in 18 (35 percent), and stable plaque without myocardial infarction in 7 (14 percent) (Table 28–2). Of the 51 sudden coronary deaths, 36 (71 percent) were witnessed (11 of 18 plaque erosions, 7 of 8 plaque ruptures, 11 of 18 stable plaques with healed myocardial infarction, and 7 of 7 stable plaques without healed myocardial infarction). Of the 36 witnessed coronary death, 22 percent (8 patients) had chest pain. Symptoms other than chest pain were noted in 33 percent (12 patients); these symptoms included back pain (2 patients), dizziness (3 patients), nausea and vomiting (1 patient), fever and chills (1 patient), stomach distention (1 patient), left shoulder tingling (1 patient), shortness of breath (1 patient), malaise (1 patient), and fatigue (1 patient), which occurred immediately before death. No symptoms were described in 45 percent of patients. There was no correlation between category of death and chest pain. A history of heart disease was present in 9 patients (7 of 18 with stable plaque and healed myocardial infarction, 1 of 8 with plaque rupture, and 1 of 8 with stable plaque without healed myocardial infarction). Of the 2 patients with a documented history of previous myocardial infarction, both had healed infarctions at autopsy. Cardiac history pertinent to risk factors included systemic hypertension in 11 patients, insulin-dependent diabetes mellitus in 5 patients, and hypercholesterolemia in 1 patient. One patient, a 46-year-old women with plaque erosion, was receiving estrogen replacement after hysterectomy/oophorectomy. Another patient with erosion had a hysterectomy without an oophorectomy.

TABLE 28–2 Risk Factors and Mechanism of Death for 51 Women With Severe Coronary Atherosclerosis

Risk Factor*	Plaque Rupture (n = 8)	Plaque Erosion (n = 18)	Stable Plaque, Healed MI (n = 18)	Stable Plaque, No MI (n = 7)	*P* (if < .05)
Age (yr)	58 ± 12†	45 ± 8‡	54 ± 13	43 ± 9	†.01 versus erosion; .02 versus stable, no MI; ‡.04 versus stable plaque, healed MI
Age >50 yr	7 (87%)†	3 (17%)	9 (50%)	2 (29%)	†.001 versus plaque erosion; .03 versus stable plaque, no infarct
TC (mg/dl)	270 ± 55†	188 ± 48	203 ± 71	201 ± 57	†.007 versus erosion; .007 versus stable plaque, healed MI; .02 versus stable plaque
HDL-C (mg/dl)	46 ± 12	39 ± 21	40 ± 23	48 ± 32	
TC/HDL-C	6.2 ± 1.8	6.0 ± 3.7	6.6 ± 3.9	5.2 ± 2.7	
BMI (kg/m²)	31 ± 4†	27 ± 4	28 ± 9	30 ± 11	†.02 versus erosion
Glycosylated hemoglobin (%)	8.8 ± 4.4	6.7 ± 0.7	10.2 ± 5.0†	8.0 ± 4.5	†.006 versus erosion
Heart weight (g)	483 ± 108	372 ± 87†	460 ± 105	375 ± 129	†.01 versus rupture and stable plaque, healed MI
Heart weight/BMI	1.6 ± 0.5	1.4 ± 0.4	1.7 ± 0.4†	1.3 ± 0.2	†.02 versus stable plaque; .04 versus erosion
Smokers	4 (50%)	14 (78%)	9 (50%)	2 (29%)	
Hypertension	3 (38%)	4 (22%)	9 (50%)	2 (29%)	

Abbreviations: BMI, body mass index; HDL-C, high-density lipoprotein cholesterol; MI, myocardial infarction; TC, total cholesterol.
*Values are given as n or mean ± SD.
From Burke AP, Farb A, Malcom GT, et al: Effect of risk factors on the mechanism of acute thrombosis and sudden coronary death in women. Circulation 97(21):2110–2116, 1998.

Risk Factor and Mechanism of Death

In the 66 women studied, there were no significant differences between TC in women younger than 50 years (194 ± 63 mg/dl) and those older than 50 years (221 ± 61 mg/dl). HDL-C levels also were similar in the groups (47 ± 18 versus 42 ± 24 mg/dl, respectively), as was the frequency of presumed cigarette smoking (50 versus 58 percent, respectively). The percentage of glycosylated hemoglobin was lower in younger than in older women (7.1 ± 2.4 versus 9.3 ± 5.6 percent, P = .04). Hypertension was more frequent in older (48 percent) than in younger women (20 percent, P = .03). Body mass index and mean heart weight were not significantly different between younger and older women.

Overall, plaque rupture occurred in older women (mean age, 58 ± 12 years) with a high serum TC level (mean, 270 ± 55 mg/dl) and body mass index (31 ± 4 kg/m^2) (see Table 28–2). Eighty-seven percent of women with plaque rupture were older than 50 years. Conversely, plaque erosion was more frequent in younger women (45 ± 8 years), with a significantly lower TC level (188 ± 48 mg/dl), body mass index, and heart weight than women with rupture (see Table 28–2). Women with stable plaque and healed myocardial infarction were older (54 ± 13 years) and had a higher glycohemoglobin (10.2 ± 5.0 percent) than patients with plaque erosion (see Table 28–2).

Compared with control subjects, women with acute rupture had higher serum TC levels and heart weights (Table 28–3). TC/HDL-C ratio was significantly higher in women with stable plaques and healed infarction than in control subjects. The incidence of smoking was greater in women with erosions than in control subjects. Women with stable plaques and healed myocardial infarction were more likely hypertensive and have elevated glycohemoglobin (see Table 28–3). By multivariate analysis, these associations were independent of other risk factors (Table 28–4). Compared with control subjects, the odds ratio of elevated cholesterol (>210 mg/dl) was 7 in women with plaque rupture, and the odds ratio of smoking in women with plaque erosion was 21. The odds ratio of hypertension was 15, and the odds ratio of elevated glycosylated hemoglobin of higher than 10 percent was 41 in women with stable plaque and healed myocardial infarction versus control subjects (see Table 28–4). There was no significant association between risk factors and stable plaques without healed infarctions.

The maximal percent cross-sectional area stenosis was 81 ± 11 percent for plaque rupture and 73 ± 17 percent for erosion. The percent stenosis in women with stable plaque without myocardial infarction was 81 ± 6 percent, and that in women with stable plaque with healed myocardial infarction was 88 ± 10 percent. In women older than 50 years, the maximal percent stenosis was 84 ± 10 percent, and in women younger than 50 years it was 78 ± 16 percent. There were no significant differences noted in these few patients. Coronary thrombi were most common in the proximal segments (62 percent of cases) and mostly associated with the left anterior descending coronary artery.

TABLE 28–3 Risk Factors for 15 Control Women With Comparison to Coronary Deaths by Mechanism (Univariate Analysis)*

Risk Factor†	Trauma Controls (n = 15)	*P* Versus Acute Ruptures (n = 8)	*P* Versus Acute Erosions	*P* Versus Stable Plaque, Healed MI
TC (mg/dl)	194 ± 44	**.002**	.17	.6
Smokers	5 (33%)	.4	**.01**	.3
Glycosylated hemoglobin	6.4 ± 0.4	.1	.8	**.001**
Hypertension	2 (15%)	.2	.2	**.03**
TC/HDL-C	4.3 ± 1.7	**.03**	.2	**.05**
Heart weight (g)	384 ± 86	**.03**	.7	**.03**
Heart weight/BMI (m^2 × 10)	1.3 ± 0.3	.1	.4	**.006**
BMI (kg/m^2)	31 ± 9	.9	.14	.8
Age (yr)	50 ± 16	.3	.2	.5
HDL-C (mg/dl)	50 ± 19	.6	.2	.2

Abbreviations: BMI, body mass index; HDL-C, high-density lipoprotein cholesterol; MI, myocardial infarction; TC, total cholesterol.
*Boldface numbers indicate statistical significance.
†Values are given as n or mean ± SD.
From Burke AP, Farb A, Malcom GT, et al: Effect of risk factors on the mechanism of acute thrombosis and sudden coronary death in women. Circulation 97(21):2110–2116, 1998.

TABLE 28–4 Risk Factors in Women Who Died of Severe Coronary Disease: Multivariate Comparison With Control Subjects by Mechanism of Death*

Mechanism of Death	Risk Factor	*P* Versus Controls	Odds Ratio Versus Controls
Plaque rupture	TC	.02	7†
	Low HDL-C	.14	
	Age	.2	
	Others	>.4	
Plaque erosion	Smoking	.03	21
	Hypertension	.2	
	Low HDL-C	.19	
	Age‡	.17	
	TC‡	.2	
	Others	>.4	
Stable plaque, healed MI	Hypertension	.02	15
	Glycosylated hemoglobin	.03	41§
	TC	.17	
	Heart weight	.2	
	Smoking	.3	
	Others	>.4	

Abbreviations: HDL-C, high-density lipoprotein cholesterol; MI, myocardial infarction; TC, total cholesterol.
*Multivariate analysis using stepwise logistic regression, P = .4 for removing, P = .2 for entering. Odds ratios given only if P < .05.
†Odds ratio calculated if used as dichotomous variable, cut-off 210 mg/dl for TC, 10 percent. Odds ratio as continuous variable, 1.04.
‡Negative association.
§Odds ratio calculated if used as dichotomous variable, cut-off 10 percent glycosylated hemoglobin. Odds ratio as continuous variable, 9.
From Burke AP, Farb A, Malcom GT, et al: Effect of risk factors on the mechanism of acute thrombosis and sudden coronary death in women. Circulation 97(21):2110–2116, 1998.

TABLE 28-5 Mean Vulnerable Plaques in Hearts From 51 Women Who Died Suddenly of Severe Coronary Disease Compared by Presence of Risk Factors

Risk Factor	Mean Vulnerable Plaques Quantified in Each Heart (n ± SD)	*P*
Age ≤ 50 yr	0.2 ± 0.4	<.0001
Age > 50 yr	1.3 ± 0.9	
Normal cholesterol	0.3 ± 0.5	.03
TC > 210 + TC/HDL-C > 5	1.1 ± 1.1	
Normal glycohemoglobin	0.6 ± 0.7	.2
Glycohemoglobin > 10%	1.0 ± 1.2	
Nonsmoker	0.4 ± 0.8	.09
Smoker	0.8 ± 0.1	
Normal weight	0.5 ± 0.9	>.5
BMI > 28 kg/m^2	0.8 ± 0.9	
Normotensive	0.4 ± 0.8	>.5
Hypertensive	0.6 ± 0.8	

Abbreviations: BMI, body mass index; HDL-C, high-density lipoprotein cholesterol; MI, myocardial infarction.

From Burke AP, Farb A, Malcom GT, et al: Effect of risk factors on the mechanism of acute thrombosis and sudden coronary death in women. Circulation 97(21):2110–2116, 1998.

Coronary thrombi were located in the midportion of the arteries in 31 percent, and were rarely found in the distal arteries.

Vulnerable plaques are defined as plaques with a large necrotic core and a thin fibrous cap (<65 μm) infiltrated by macrophages. The mean number of vulnerable plaques was associated with increasing TC (r^2 = 0.3, P = .002), age (r^2 = 0.03, P = .03), and glycohemoglobin (r^2 = 0.2, P = .05). When risk factors of hypercholesterolemia (TC > 210 and HDL-C > 5), diabetes (glycohemoglobin > 10), and age (>50 years) were considered as categorical variables, vulnerable plaques were more numerous in hearts from patients with increasing age (P < .0001) and abnormal TC and TC/HDL-C levels (Table 28–5). By multivariate analysis, age of more than 50 years and TC level were independently associated with number of vulnerable plaques (P = .002 and .007, respectively).

Comparison of Plaque Morphology by Age in Men and Women

Data analysis was performed to better understand the effects of age in men and women older or younger than 50 years. It is well known that the incidence of coronary heart disease in men younger than 60 years is three times that in women. It has been thought that menopausal status negates the beneficial effects of estrogen and leads to accelerated disease in older women. It is reported that it takes 20 years after menopause for the incidence of coronary disease to parallel that of men. In our series of randomly collected cases of sudden coronary death, women represented one third of the patients. Interestingly, women younger than 50 years had a higher incidence of plaque erosion than did women older than 50 years (Table 28–6). Conversely, the overall incidence of plaque erosion in men younger and older than 50 years was not different. The percentage of patients with acute thrombi at autopsy who were younger and older than 50 years was similar in men and women (see Table 28–6). In some instances, thrombosis may arise from de-endothelialization caused by extensive calcification protruding into the lumen; this type of lesion is only seen in men and accounts for only 3 percent of acute thrombi (see Table 28–6).

Summary

Coronary artery thrombi are just as frequent in women as in men who die of sudden coronary death. Women younger than 50 years have thrombi secondary to plaque erosion and tend to be smokers. The percent stenosis is frequently less than 50 percent diameter reduction in women with plaque erosion, and therefore, these lesions may not be detected with angiography. Coronary thrombi in women older than 50 years most often arise from plaque rupture and are associated with hypercholesterolemia (TC > 210 mg/dl and TC/HDL-C > 5). Stable plaque in the presence of a healed myocardial infarction is associated with glucose

TABLE 28-6 Frequency of Different Plaque Morphologies of Culprit Plaques in Men and Women Younger or Older Than 50 Years*

Age and Sex	Acute Thrombus	Plaque Rupture	Plaque Erosion	Calcified Nodule	Organized Thrombus	Stable Plaque
Women						
≤50 yr	16 (59)	1 (4)	15 (55)†	0	4 (15)	7 (25)
>50 yr	10 (47)	7 (53)‡	3 (14)	0	4 (19)	7 (34)
Men						
≤50 yr	38 (59)	25 (38)	13 (19)	1 (2)	13 (19)	15 (22)
>50 yr	22 (47)	15 (28)	7 (13)	3 (6)	4 (7)	25 (46)
Total	86 (51)	48 (29)	38 (23)	4 (3)	25 (15)	54 (32)

*Values are given as n (%).

One hundred sixty-nine patients were studied. Acute thrombi were classified as those arising from plaque rupture, plaque erosion, or superficial calcified nodules breaching the luminal space; the frequency of the latter was relatively low. The incidence of plaque rupture was higher in women older than 50 years than in women younger than 50 (‡P = .0004). No such age-dependent differences were noted for men. Conversely, the occurrence of plaque erosion was higher in women younger than 50 years than in women older than 50 years (†P = .0004). Again, no such differences were noted for men. In comparison among the sexes, plaque rupture in women younger than 50 years was significantly less than in men younger than 50 years (P = .0004). Conversely, plaque erosion in women younger than 50 years was significantly higher than in men younger than 50 years (P = .008).

intolerance and systemic hypertension. Collectively, these data suggest that risk factor modification is different for women with coronary artery disease who are younger or older than 50 years.

References

1. Gillum RF: Sudden coronary death in the United States: 1980–1985. Circulation 79:756–765, 1989.
2. Kannel WB, Wilson PW, D'Agostino RB, Cobb J: Sudden coronary death in women. Am Heart J 136:205–212, 1998.
3. Willett WC, Green A, Stampfer MJ, et al: Relative and absolute excess risks of coronary heart disease among women who smoke cigarettes. N Engl J Med 317:1303–1309, 1987.
4. Rich-Edwards JW, Manson JE, Hennekens CH, Buring JE: The primary prevention of coronary heart disease in women. N Engl J Med 332:1758–1766, 1995.
5. Wilson PW, D'Agostino RB, Levy D, et al: Prediction of coronary heart disease using risk factor categories. Circulation 97:1837–1847, 1998.
6. Miller VT: Lipids, lipoproteins, women and cardiovascular disease. Atherosclerosis 108(suppl):S73–S82, 1994.
7. Criqui MH, Heiss G, Cohn R, et al: Plasma triglyceride level and mortality from coronary heart disease. N Engl J Med 328:1220–1225, 1993.
8. Kannel WB: Range of serum cholesterol values in the population developing coronary artery disease. Am J Cardiol 76:69C–77C, 1995.
9. Kannel WB, D'Agostino RB, Wilson PW, et al: Diabetes, fibrinogen, and risk of cardiovascular disease: the Framingham experience. Am Heart J 120:672–676, 1990.
10. Kuczmarski RJ, Flegal KM, Campbell SM, Johnson CL: Increasing prevalence of overweight among US adults: the National Health and Nutrition Examination Surveys, 1960 to 1991. JAMA 272:205–211, 1994.
11. Manson JE, Colditz GA, Stampfer MJ: Parity, ponderosity, and the paradox of a weight-preoccupied society. JAMA 271:1788–1790, 1994.
12. Manson JE, Colditz GA, Stampfer MJ, et al: A prospective study of obesity and risk of coronary heart disease in women. N Engl J Med 322:882–889, 1990.
13. Willett WC, Lenart EB: Dietary factors. *In* Mason JE, Ridker PM, Gaziano JM, Hennekens CH (eds): Prevention of Myocardial Infarction. pp. 351–383. New York: Oxford, 1996.
14. Willett WC, Manson JE, Stampfer MJ, et al: Weight, weight change, and coronary heart disease in women: risk within the "normal" weight range. JAMA 273:461–465, 1995.
15. Farb A, Burke A, Tang A, et al: Coronary plaque erosion without rupture into a lipid core: a frequent cause of coronary thrombosis in sudden coronary death. Circulation 93:1354–1363, 1996.
16. van der Wal AC, Becker AE, van der Loos CM, Das PK: Site of intimal rupture or erosion of thrombosed coronary atherosclerotic plaques is characterized by an inflammatory process irrespective of the dominant plaque morphology. Circulation 89:36–44, 1994.
17. Evanko SP, Raines EW, Ross R, et al: Proteoglycan distribution in lesions of atherosclerosis depends on lesion severity, structural characteristics, and the proximity of platelet-derived growth factor and transforming growth factor-beta. Am J Pathol 152:533–546, 1998.
18. O'Brien KD, Olin KL, Alpers CE, et al: Comparison of apolipoprotein and proteoglycan deposits in human coronary atherosclerotic plaques: colocalization of biglycan with apolipoproteins. Circulation 98:519–527, 1998.
19. Schonherr E, Jarvelainen HT, Kinsella MG, et al: Platelet-derived growth factor and transforming growth factor-beta 1 differentially affect the synthesis of biglycan and decorin by monkey arterial smooth muscle cells. Arterioscler Thromb 13:1026–1036, 1993.
20. Raghunath PN, Tomaszewski JE, Brady ST, et al: Plasminogen activator system in human coronary atherosclerosis. Arterioscler Thromb Vasc Biol 15:1432–1443, 1995.
21. Farb A, Burke AP, Kolodgie FK, et al: Determinants of coronary thrombosis in sudden cardiac death. Mod Pathol 9:29(A), 1997.

CHAPTER 29

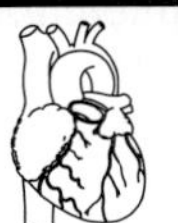

EXERCISE TESTING

A. Iain McGhie and James T. Willerson

INDICATIONS AND CONTRAINDICATIONS
INTERPRETATION
EXERCISE TESTING IN THE DIAGNOSIS OF CORONARY ARTERY DISEASE
PROGNOSTIC USE OF EXERCISE ELECTROCARDIOGRAPHY IN PATIENTS WITH KNOWN OR SUSPECTED CORONARY ARTERY DISEASE
EXERCISE TESTING AFTER MYOCARDIAL INFARCTION
OTHER USES OF EXERCISE TESTING

Exercise testing is a technique widely used primarily for the diagnostic and functional evaluation of patients with known or suspected coronary artery disease (CAD). Exercise testing is often used in conjunction with an imaging procedure, such as myocardial perfusion imaging or echocardiography, to enhance its diagnostic accuracy. In general, exercise testing is a safe procedure; however, approximately 10 myocardial infarctions, deaths, or both, occur per 10,000 tests performed. The risk of an adverse event during an exercise test versus during usual activity is estimated to be 60- to 100-fold greater in patients with CAD.[1] The risk is greater in patients after myocardial infarction and in patients undergoing evaluation for malignant ventricular arrhythmias. Because of the risks, albeit small, exercise testing should be performed only by well-trained technicians and physicians. In addition, these personnel must be trained in cardiopulmonary resuscitation and have immediate access to appropriate equipment and medications to perform cardiopulmonary resuscitation if required.

INDICATIONS AND CONTRAINDICATIONS

Sound clinical judgment is the most important factor in determining the indications and contraindications for exercise testing.[1] The patient should not eat or smoke for 3 to 4 hours before the test and should dress appropriately for exercise. A brief history and physical examination should be performed to rule out contraindications to testing. Patients with a history of increasing or unstable angina should not undergo exercise testing until the condition stabilizes. Patients with poorly controlled blood pressure or heart failure and those with significant valvular or congenital heart disease, particularly severe aortic stenosis, should be identified and usually should not undergo vigorous exercise testing. Table 29–1 summarizes contraindications to exercise testing.

The indication for performing the test in any particular patient should be known; the general indications are summarized in Table 29–2. The procedure and the attendant risks of exercise testing should be explained to the patient, and written consent should be obtained. The Mason-Likar modification of the standard 12-lead electrocardiogram (ECG) is widely used for exercise testing. This modification involves moving the limb electrodes to the torso to minimize motion artifact; however, this modification results in alterations in the voltages in the inferior leads and causes a rightward shift in the axis. A standard resting 12-lead ECG should be obtained before performance of the exercise test.[2] After the limb leads have been moved to the torso, tracings should be recorded with the patient in the supine and erect positions. Table 29–3 summarizes the main indications for termination of an exercise test.

Bicycle Ergometer Protocols. Bicycle ergometers have mechanical or electrical brakes to vary workloads that are

TABLE 29–1 Contraindications to Exercise Testing

Absolute
Acute myocardial infarction (within 2 days)
Unstable angina not previously stabilized with medical therapy*
Uncontrolled cardiac arrhythmias causing symptoms or hemodynamic compromise
Symptomatic severe aortic stenosis
Uncontrolled symptomatic heart failure
Acute pulmonary embolus or pulmonary infarction
Acute myocarditis or pericarditis
Acute aortic dissection
Relative†
Left main coronary stenosis
Moderate or worse aortic valvular stenosis
Electrolyte abnormalities
Severe arterial hypertension‡
Tachyarrhythmias or bradyarrhythmias
Hypertrophic cardiomyopathy and other forms of outflow tract obstruction
Mental or physical impairment leading to inability to exercise adequately
High-degree atrioventricular block

*Appropriate timing of testing depends on level of risk of unstable angina, as defined by the Agency for Health Care Policy and Research Unstable Angina Guidelines.
†Relative contraindications can be superseded if the benefits of exercise outweigh the risks.
‡In the absence of definitive evidence, the committee suggests a systolic blood pressure of > 200 mm Hg and/or diastolic blood pressure of > 110 mm Hg.
Adapted from Fletcher GF, Balady G, Froelicher VF, et al: Exercise standards: a statement for healthcare professionals from the American Heart Association. Special report. Circulation 91(2):580–615, 1995.

TABLE 29-2 Indications for Exercise Testing

Definitely Indicated

Diagnosis of CAD in men with atypical stymptoms
Risk stratification and functional evaluation in patients with known CAD
Patients with recurrent symptomatic exercise-induced arrhythmia

Possibly Indicated

Diagnosis of CAD in women with typical or atypical angina pectoris
Evaluation of functional capacity to monitor cardiovascular therapy in patients with CAD and heart failure
Evaluation of patients with variant angina
Serial evaluation (≥1-year intervals) of patients with known CAD
Evaluation of asymptomatic men older than 40 years
Those with special occupations (pilots, fire fighters, police officers, bus or truck drivers, or railroad engineers)
Those with ≥ 2 atherosclerotic risk factors or
Those planning to enter a vigorous exercise program

Abbreviation: CAD, coronary artery disease.

calibrated in kiloponds (kpm) or watts (W). The initial power output is usually 25 or 50 W depending on the ability of the particular patient, followed by increases of 25 to 50 W every 3 minutes until the end point of the test is reached. Bicycle ergometers are usually less expensive, occupy less space, and make less noise than a treadmill. In addition, upper body motion is usually less than that with a treadmill, making it easier to measure blood pressure, auscultate the chest, and record the ECG. However, a significant proportion of patients experience difficulty in performing optimally on a bicycle compared with a treadmill. In addition, maximal oxygen uptake tends to be 5 to 10 percent lower than with treadmill exercise, and maximal cardiac output and stroke volume are correspondingly reduced. These differences are not usually clinically important.[3]

Treadmill Protocols. There are several different treadmill protocols; it is important to select a protocol that is suited to the patient's physical ability. An optimal protocol should last at least 6 to 12 minutes. The most popular is the Bruce protocol; there is much published data on the diagnostic and prognostic use of exercise testing with this protocol.[4, 5] In patients with limited exercise capacity, the Bruce protocol can be modified by adding an initial zero stage (1.7 mph at 0 percent incline) and one-half stage (1.7 mph at 5 percent incline). The main disadvantages of this protocol are the large increments in work that occur between stages and the additional energy requirements in patients who are required to run rather than walk in the fourth or subsequent stages of the protocol.

Postexercise Period. Although attention is directed to the patient's response to exercise, it is important to be aware that some abnormal responses occur only in recovery after exercise.[6] To achieve maximal sensitivity, patients should be in the supine position during the postexercise period; however, this is not always desirable. In patients who experience severe angina, dyspnea, or ventricular arrhythmias during the exercise test, the lower preload associated with the sitting or erect position is preferable. In other patients, particularly those patients who attain a high workload, it is preferable to have a cool-down period to avoid postexercise hypotension, which occasionally occurs. However, a cool-down period can delay or eliminate the appearance of ST-segment depression. Monitoring should continue for approximately 6 minutes after exercise or until hemodynamic changes stabilize and heart rate and ECG have returned close to baseline.

TABLE 29-3 Indications for Termination of an Exercise Test

Absolute Indications

Progressive fall (>10 mm Hg) or drop in systolic blood pressure persistently below baseline despite an increase in workload
Progressive, increasing anginal chest pain
Central nervous system symptoms (ataxia, dizziness, or near syncope)
Signs of poor peripheral perfusion (cyanosis or pallor)
Serious arrhythmias (e.g., high-grade ventricular arrhythmias)
Technical difficulties monitoring the ECG or systolic blood pressure

Relative Indications

Marked ST or QRS changes
Increasing chest pain
Marked fatigue, dyspnea, wheezing, leg cramps, or intermittent claudication
Less serious arrhythmias (e.g., supraventricular tachycardias)
Development of bundle-branch block when the underlying rhythm cannot be determined

Abbreviation: ECG, electrocardiogram.

INTERPRETATION

Symptoms. Chest pain induced by the exercise test and relieved by rest is strongly predictive of CAD even in the absence of ST-segment depression. It is important to obtain an accurate account of symptoms, in particular, chest pain, that occur during exercise testing.

Physical Signs. Cardiac examination immediately after exercise may reveal a precordial bulge or added heart sounds resulting from left ventricular dysfunction. Papillary muscle dysfunction due to transitory ischemia may result in a mitral regurgitant murmur.

Heart Rate and Blood Pressure Response. Blood pressure is dependent on cardiac output and peripheral resistance. Normally, systolic blood pressure rises to 160 to 220 mm Hg at peak exercise.[4, 5] Diastolic blood pressure does not usually change by more than ±10 mm Hg from the resting value. Systolic blood pressure at maximal exertion or on immediate cessation of exertion is considered a clinically useful first approximation of the heart's inotropic capacity. An inadequate rise (<120 mm Hg) or a progressive fall in systolic blood pressure (>10 mm Hg) during exercise usually is associated with severe CAD and ischemic dysfunction. However, some normal subjects have a transient drop in systolic blood pressure at maximal exercise. An inappropriate increase in the heart rate with exercise may be observed in patients with impaired left ventricular dysfunction. Alternatively, this response may be observed in patients who are physically deconditioned, hypovolemic, or anemic or who have a metabolic disorder.

Electrocardiographic Changes. During exercise, there are changes in virtually all components of the ECG in normal subjects, including progressive shortening of the PR and QT intervals. The amplitude of the P wave increases and the amplitude of the T wave decreases during exercise. There is also a progressive rightward shift in the QRS axis. Changes in the R wave have also been noted to occur during exercise. The usual response of the R wave amplitude in normal subjects is to increase during submaximal exercise and decrease with maximal exercise.

Myocardial ischemia most often manifests itself as ST-segment shifts. As the UP segment disappears during exercise, the ST level is measured relative to the PR segment. ST elevation is measured as the deviation from the baseline ST level. ST-segment depression is measured from the isoelectric PR level because the normal response is a downward shift from early repolarization. If the baseline ST segment is depressed, the deviation from that level to the level during exercise or recovery is considered. The ST level is measured 60 or 80 ms after the J point. ST-segment depression is the most common manifestation of exercise-induced myocardial ischemia. The standard criterion for this abnormal response is horizontal or downsloping ST-segment depression of 0.10 mV or more at 60 to 80 ms after the J point in three consecutive beats (Fig. 29–1). A slow, upward sloping ST-segment depression (>1 mV/s) of 0.15 to 0.20 mV at 60 to 80 ms after the J point in three consecutive beats is also considered by some to be a manifestation of exercise-induced myocardial ischemia (see Fig. 29–1).[7] In the presence of baseline abnormalities, exercise-induced ST-segment depression is less specific for ischemia. Other factors related to the probability and severity of CAD include the type of ST-segment depression (downward more than horizontal), amount, time of appearance, duration, and number of leads with ST-segment depression. In addition, the lower the workload and double product (heart rate multiplied by systolic blood pressure) at which it occurs, the worse the prognosis and the more likely the presence of multivessel disease. The persistence of ST-segment depression in the recovery phase is also related to the severity of CAD.

ST-segment elevation may also be an indicator of myocardial ischemia. ST-segment elevation occurring in a lead without a Q wave is usually indicative of transmural ischemia and is often associated with severe proximal coronary disease or coronary spasm. In this situation, the localization of the ST-segment elevation is relatively specific for the distribution of the coronary artery involved. This is in contrast to ST-segment depression, which results from subendocardial ischemia and has little or no localization value.[8] However, the significance of ST-segment elevation is different in the presence of prior myocardial infarction and Q wave development. In this situation, ST-segment elevation during exercise is often associated with the presence of dyskinetic areas or ventricular aneurysms. Approximately 50 percent of patients with anterior myocardial infarction and 15 percent of patients with inferior myocardial infarction exhibit this finding during exercise. These changes may result in reciprocal ST-segment depression, which may be misinterpreted as indicating ischemia.

Exercise-induced U wave inversion in patients with a normal resting ECG may be a marker of myocardial ischemia in the left anterior descending coronary artery. Pseudonormalization of T waves (i.e., inverted T waves that become upright with exercise) is a nonspecific finding.

Exercise Testing in the Diagnosis of Coronary Artery Disease

In a meta-analysis of 58 published trials of patients undergoing exercise testing and coronary arteriography for the

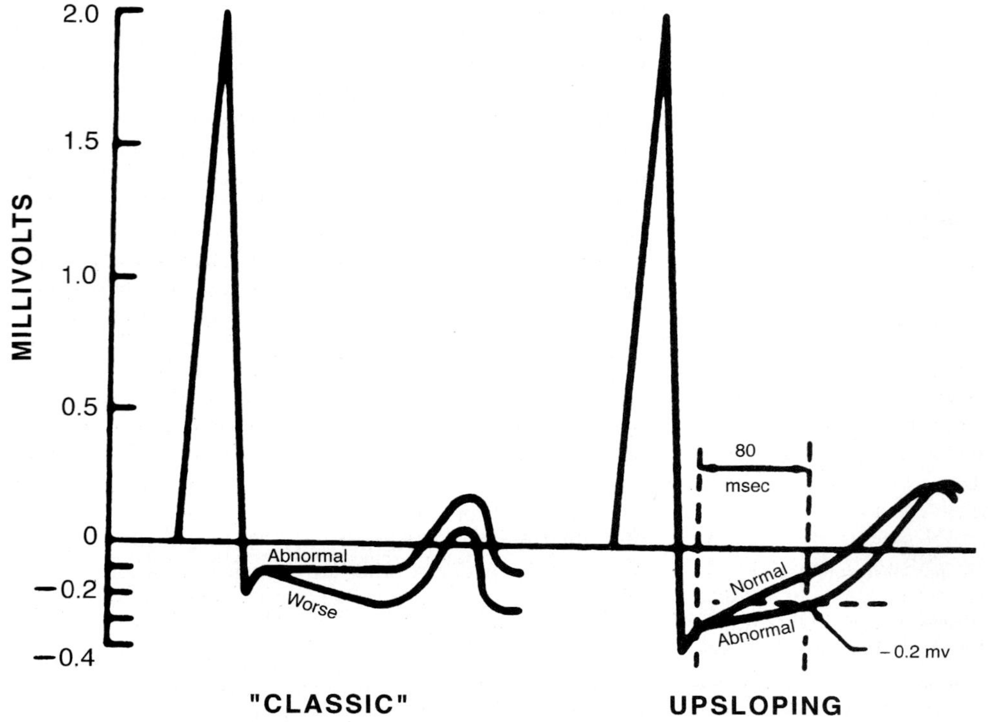

Figure 29–1 Schematic diagram of ST-segment responses. Classic indicates horizontal or downward sloping ST-segment depression. Upsloping indicates normal ST-segment response to exercise; abnormal shows slowly upward ST segment with depression of 0.2 mV at 80 msec after the J point. (Adapted from Pina IL, Madonna DW, Sinnamon EA: Exercise test interpretation. Cardiol Clin 11:215–227, 1993.)

diagnosis of CAD, the mean sensitivity and specificity were 67 and 72 percent, respectively.[9] However, when only studies that avoided workup biases were included in the meta-analysis, the sensitivity and specificity of 1-mm downward or horizontal ST-segment depression was 50 and 90 percent, respectively.[9]

There are several situations in which the electrocardiographic changes are not interpretable with exercise. There are also specific patient populations that are associated with a high incidence of false-positive electrocardiographic responses. Patients with left bundle-branch block, ST-segment depression of at least 1 mm, ventricular paced rhythm, Wolff-Parkinson-White syndrome, or left ventricular hypertrophy have changes with exercise that are uninterpretable; therefore, usually the exercise test is performed in conjunction with an imaging procedure (i.e., nuclear or echocardiographic) to better identify myocardial ischemia. In addition, patients receiving cardiac glycosides usually have abnormal resting ST-T waves, and those with electrocardiographic evidence of left ventricular hypertrophy with or without repolarization abnormalities have a high incidence of "falsely positive" electrocardiographic changes with exercise. Patients with mitral valve prolapse have a very high incidence of typical electrocardiographic changes of ischemia during exercise, even though almost all of them have angiographically normal epicardial coronary arteries. Historically, women have also been thought to have an increased likelihood of having "falsely positive" exercise ECGs; however, this apparently lower specificity is in large part due to a lower prevalence of CAD and the concomitant prevalence of other diseases, such as mitral valve prolapse or ventricular hypertrophy. If the woman has a normal baseline ECG, is not receiving digoxin, does not have mitral valve prolapse or ventricular hypertrophy, and can exercise adequately, the predictive accuracy of the exercise ECG is probably comparable to that of a man.[9–11] The authors have found stress perfusion studies especially useful in women with the above-mentioned problems.

Prognostic Use of Exercise Electrocardiography in Patients with Known or Suspected Coronary Artery Disease

Exercise testing provides important prognostic information in patients with CAD (Table 29–4).

Mark and colleagues[12] devised a treadmill score and applied it to patients who were being evaluated for possible CAD to help determine which patients required coronary angiography and possible revascularization. The treadmill score was calculated on the basis of the duration of exercise, the amount of maximal electrocardiographic depression, and the presence or absence of symptoms occurring during exercise (Fig. 29–2). The authors found that the treadmill score was a better discriminator than clinical assessment and appeared to separate patients who subsequently died from those who lived for 4 years. Approximately two thirds of patients had scores indicating low risk (≤5) and had a 99 percent 4-year survival rate (i.e., annual mortality rate of 0.25 percent). High-risk scores (≥10) occurred in 4 percent of patients; the mortality rate in this group was twenty times greater, with an annual mortality rate of 5 percent (4-year survival rate of 79 percent).

TABLE 29–4 Exercise Test Parameters Associated With Poor Prognosis and/or Increased Severity of Coronary Artery Disease

Duration of symptom-limiting exercise
- Failure to complete stage II of Bruce protocol or equivalent workload (≤6.5 METS*) with other protocols

Exercise HR at onset of limiting symptoms
- Failure to attain HR ≥ 120 beats/min (off beta blockers)

Time of onset, magnitude, morphology, and postexercise duration of abnormal horizontal or downsloping ST-segment depression
- Onset at HR < 120 beats/min or ≤ 6.5 METS
- Magnitude ≥ 2.0 mm
- Postexercise duration ≥ 6 min
- Depression in multiple leads

Systolic BP response during or after progressive exercise
- Sustained decrease of > 10 mm Hg or flat BP response (≤130 mm Hg) during progressive exercise

Other potentially important determinants
- Exercise-induced ST-segment elevation in leads other than aVR
- Angina pectoris during exercise
- Exercise-induced U wave inversion
- Exercise-induced ventricular tachycardia

Abbreviations: BP, blood pressure; HR, heart rate; METS, metabolic equivalents.
*Energy expenditure at rest, equivalent to an oxygen uptake of approximately 3.5 ml O_2/kg body weight/min.
Adapted from Schlant RC, Blomqvist CG, Brandenburg RO, et al: Guidelines for exercise testing: a report of the Joint American College of Cardiology/American Heart Association Task Force on Assessment of Cardiovascular Procedures (Subcommittee on Exercise Testing). Circulation 74(3):653A–667A, 1986.

Exercise Testing After Myocardial Infarction

Exercise electrocardiographic testing after myocardial infarction is widely practiced to risk-stratify patients and evaluate their functional capacity (Fig. 29–3). The latter is useful in providing some indication of the patient's ability to perform daily activities during and after convalescence. Typically, a submaximal exercise test is performed before hospital discharge (days 4 through 7), followed by a maximal test performed either early (14 to 21 days) or late (3 to 6 weeks) after discharge. The value of exercise testing for risk stratification after myocardial infarction has been somewhat controversial, in large part because of the very powerful influence of left ventricular function on prognosis after myocardial infarction.[13] In addition, the introduction of new management strategies for patients with acute myocardial infarction since the mid-1980s, such as reperfusion therapies, antiplatelet agents, beta blockade, and angiotensin-converting enzyme inhibitors, has resulted in a marked

Treadmill score = exercise duration (in min) − [(5× maximum ST-segment depression [in mm] + 4× treadmill angina index)]

Treadmill angina index: 0, no angina; 1, nonlimiting angina; 2, exercise-limiting angina.

FIGURE 29–2 The Duke Treadmill Score. (Data from Mark DB, Shaw L, Harrell FE Jr, et al: Prognostic value of a treadmill exercise score in outpatients with suspected coronary artery disease. N Engl J Med 325:849–853, 1991.)

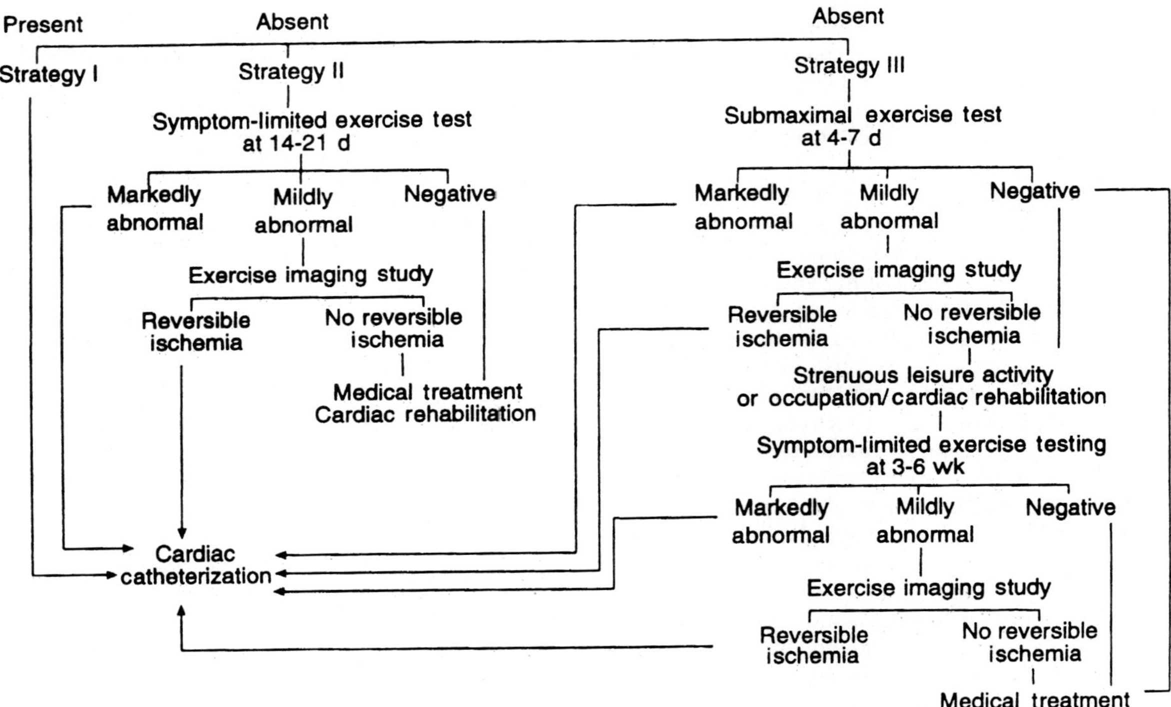

FIGURE 29–3 Clinical indications of high risk at predischarge.

reduction in mortality rates. In particular, patients who have received reperfusion therapy have a very low mortality rate. This has reached such a low level that although the relative mortality rate increases by twofold in a patient with symptomatic ischemic ST-segment depression on exercise testing after a recent myocardial infarction treated with reperfusion therapy, the absolute mortality rate remains very low (1.7 percent after 6 months).[13]

OTHER USES OF EXERCISE TESTING

Revascularization. An exercise ECG may be performed before revascularization to provide objective evidence of myocardial ischemia. However, one must be cognizant that the exercise ECG is not particularly sensitive in demonstrating ischemia in patients with one-vessel coronary disease. In addition, exercise electrocardiographic testing is of little value in demonstrating ischemia in a culprit vessel because of its inability to localize ischemia except in the presence of ST-segment elevation.[8] Therefore, stress testing is usually performed in combination with a nuclear imaging procedure to determine the location and evaluate the extent of disease in these patients.

Valvular Heart Disease. As a general rule, exercise testing should not be performed in patients with significant aortic stenosis. However, in certain circumstances, it may be of value—usually when the clinician is uncertain about the functional capacity of a patient with moderate to severe valvular disease.[14] Objective knowledge of the functional status can provide the clinician with important information to assist in the patient's management. For example, in a patient with severe aortic or mitral stenosis, the main indication for surgery is the presence of symptoms. However, great caution must be used in exercising patients with hemodynamically significant valvular disease, especially patients with aortic stenosis. The testing should be carried out only by a physician who is very familiar with the patient, and the test should be terminated if there is an inappropriate increase or fall in blood pressure or increase in heart rate or the development of arrhythmia or symptoms.

Arrhythmias and Peripheral Arterial Disease. Exercise testing can be of value in the diagnosis of exercise-induced cardiac arrhythmias and in the evaluation of the severity of peripheral arterial disease, as well as in monitoring response to therapy.[15–17]

REFERENCES

1. Fletcher GF, Froelicher VF, Hartley H, et al: AHA Medical/Scientific Statement: special report: exercise standards: a statement for health professionals from the American Heart Association. Circulation 82:2286–2322, 1990.
2. Sevilla DC, Dohrmann ML, Somelofski CA, et al: Invalidation of the resting electrocardiogram obtained via exercise electrode sites as a standard 12-lead recording. Am J Cardiol 63:35–39, 1989.
3. Blomquist GC, Mitchell JH: Heart disease and exercise testing. *In* Willerson JT, Sanders CA (eds): Clinical Cardiology. pp. 213–220. New York: Grune & Stratton, 1977.
4. Froelicher VF: Exercise and the Heart: Clinical Concepts. 2nd ed. Chicago: Year Book Medical, 1987.
5. Ellestad MH: Stress Testing: Principles and Practice. Vol. 3. Philadelphia: FA Davis, 1986.

6. Lachterman B, Lehmann KG, Abrahamson D, et al: "Recovery only" ST-segment depression and the predictive accuracy of the exercise test [published erratum appears in *Ann Intern Med* 113:333–334, 1990]. Ann Intern Med 112:11–16, 1990.
7. Sheffield LT: Upward ST segments: easy to measure, hard to agree upon. Circulation 84:426–428, 1991.
8. Mark DB, Hatky MA, Lee KL, et al: Localizing coronary artery obstructions with the exercise treadmill test. Ann Intern Med 106:53–55, 1987.
9. Gibbons RJ, Balady GJ, Beasley JW, et al: ACC/AHA Guidelines for Exercise Testing: a report of the American College of Cardiology/American Heart Association Task Force on Practice Guidelines (Committee on Exercise Testing). J Am Coll Cardiol 30:260–315, 1997.
10. Barolsky SM, Gilbert CA, Faruqui A, et al: Differences in electrocardiographic response to exercise of women and men: a non-bayesian factor. Circulation 60:1021–1027, 1979.
11. Weiner DA, Ryan TJ, McCabe CH, et al: Correlations among history of angina, ST-segment response and prevalence of coronary-artery disease in the Coronary Artery Surgery Study (CASS). N Engl J Med 301:230–235, 1979.
12. Mark DB, Shaw L, Harrell FE Jr, et al: Prognostic value of a treadmill exercise score in outpatients with suspected coronary artery disease. N Engl J Med 325:849–853, 1991.
13. Ryan TJ, Anderson JL, Antman EM, et al: ACC/AHA guidelines for the management of patients with acute myocardial infarction: a report of the American College of Cardiology/American Heart Association Task Force on Practice Guidelines (Committee on the Management of Acute Myocardial Infarction). Circulation 28:1328–1428, 1996.
14. Bonow RO, Carabello B, de Leon AC, et al: Guidelines for the management of patients with valvular heart disease: executive summary: a report of the American College of Cardiology/American Heart Association Task Force on Practice Guidelines (Committee on Management of Patients with Valvular Heart Disease). Circulation 98:1949–1984, 1998.
15. Hiatt WR, Hirsch AT, Regensteiner JG, et al: Clinical trials for claudication: assessment of exercise performance, functional status, and clinical end points. Circulation 92:614–621, 1995.
16. Hiatt WR, Nawaz D, Regensteiner JG, et al: The evaluation of exercise performance in patients with peripheral vascular disease. J Cardiopulm Rehabil 12:525–532, 1988.
17. Gardner AW, Skinner JS, Cantwell BW, et al: Progressive vs single-stage treadmill tests for evaluation of claudication. Med Sci Sports Exerc 23:402–408, 1991.

CHAPTER 30

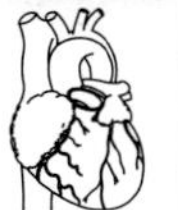

Coronary Angiography

Robert F. Wilson and Carl W. White

TECHNICAL ASPECTS OF CORONARY ANGIOGRAPHY
Facility Requirements
Techniques of Coronary Angiography
COMPLICATIONS OF CORONARY ANGIOGRAPHY
Complications of Arterial Cannulation
Drug Reactions and Toxicity
Arrhythmias
Hemodynamic Deterioration
CORONARY ANATOMY AND RADIOGRAPHIC EVALUATION
Coronary Anatomy
Angiographic Views
Coronary Artery Dimensions
Congenital Coronary Anomalies
CORONARY ATHEROSCLEROSIS
Angiographic Assessment of Stable Coronary Atherosclerosis
Angiographic Findings in Myocardial Infarction and Acute Coronary Syndromes
Coronary Collaterals
NONATHEROSCLEROTIC CORONARY ARTERY DISEASE
Coronary Vasospasm
Spontaneous Coronary Artery Dissection
Myocardial Infarction in Patients With Angiographically Normal Coronary Arteries
Microcirculatory Coronary Disease
Radiation-Induced Coronary Artery Disease
Transplant-Related Arteriopathy
Coronary Abnormalities Associated With Vasculitis
Coronary Artery Aneurysms
Coronary Embolism

The advent of selective coronary angiography over three decades ago revolutionized the clinical practice of cardiology and, since then, has added immeasurably to our understanding of coronary artery disease and its sequelae. Since its inception in the 1950s, coronary angiography has become one of the most common invasive medical procedures. In 1991, coronary angiography was performed in over 1 million patients in more than 1500 catheterization laboratories in the United States and in an estimated 3 million patients worldwide.[1]

Technical Aspects of Coronary Angiography

Facility Requirements

Radiographic Imaging

Radiographic imaging of coronary arteries is demanding because they are small and move quickly with contraction of the heart. A radiographic imaging system can be divided into an x-ray generator, consisting of a high-voltage transformer and x-ray tube, and an imaging chain, which is composed of an image intensifier and display (video or film). The general schematic is shown in Figure 30–1.[2-4]

X-RAY GENERATION

The x-ray photons are generated by a vacuum tube that has a stationary cathode and a rotating anode. A focal spot on the anode is bombarded by electrons from the cathode, exciting the anode to produce high-energy photons with x radiation wavelengths (>1 Å). The energy of the electrons, and hence the *energy* (or wavelength) of the generated photons, is determined by the voltage potential between the cathode and the anode. A high-tension, three-phase transformer is used to generate the voltage potential, which normally ranges between 50 and 100 kV. The number of available electrons accelerated into the anode, and hence the *number* of photons produced, is controlled by the amount of current (measured in milliamperes) passed through a filament in the cathode. In practice, about 350 to 1000 mA of current through the cathode is needed to generate an x-ray beam adequate for cineangiography.

Less than 1 percent of the electron energy delivered to the anode results in x-ray photons that become part of the x-ray beam leaving the tube. A large fraction of the delivered energy is converted into photons, which are reabsorbed within the anode, and heat. Rotation of the anode effectively increases the surface area over which the heat generation can be dispersed. The capacity of the x-ray tube to dissipate heat is of considerable practical importance to angiographic laboratories because tubes with a low heat capacity limit the rate at which angiographic pictures can be taken during the procedure.

The sharpness of the image cast onto the imaging device is affected by the size of the focal spot on the anode (the area of the anode bombarded with electrons). The smaller the focal spot, the crisper the shadow the x-ray beam can cast. Conversely, however, fewer photons can be generated from small focal spots. For thinner adults and shallow radiographic angles, a focal spot of 0.6 to 0.7 mm provides good resolution with an adequate number of photons to create a good image, but focal spots of 1.0 to 1.2 mm may be needed for larger patients and extreme angulation.

All x-ray tube anodes are beveled (see Fig. 30–1). Less acute bevels on the rotating anode reduce the focal spot and beam angle and refine the x-ray beam because more lower-energy photons are absorbed within the anode. As the anode angle is reduced, however, the amount of heat

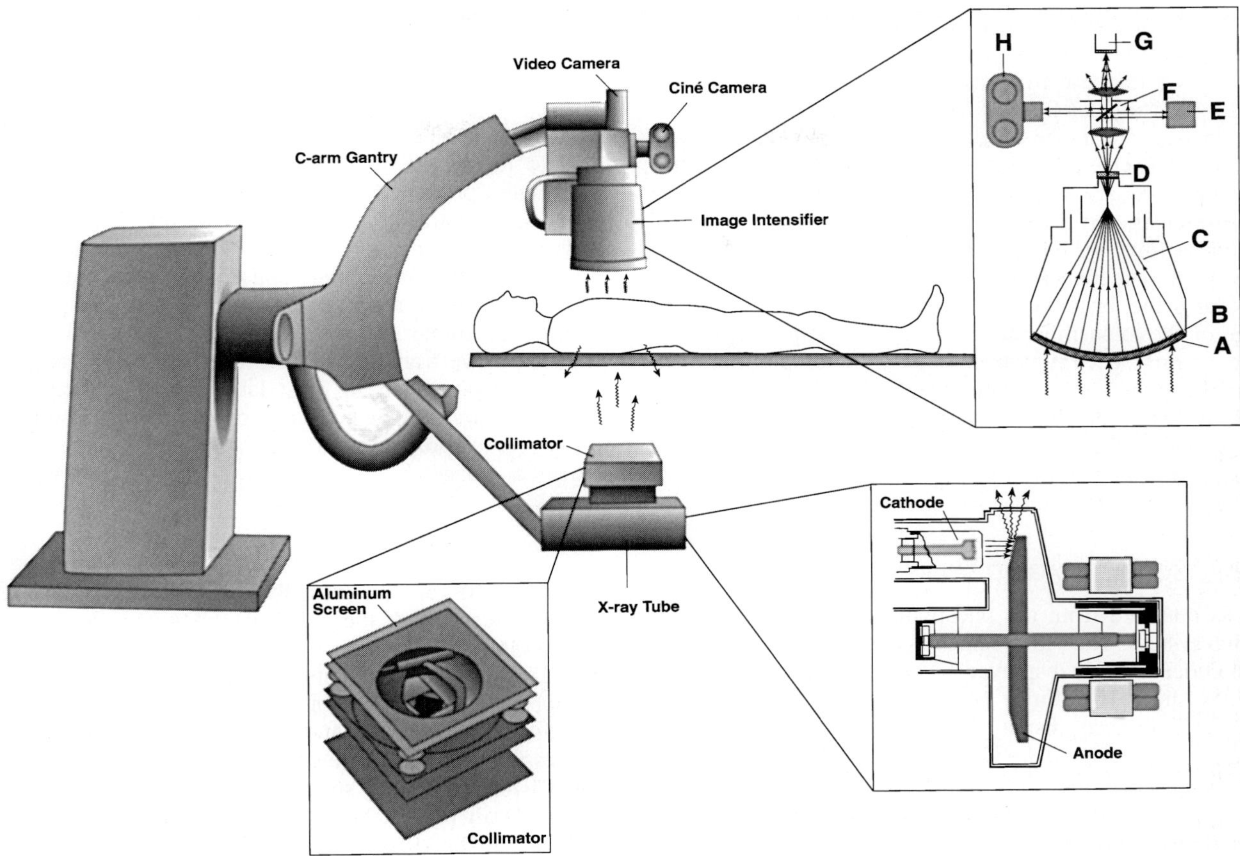

FIGURE 30–1 Schematic of radiographic imaging system for cineangiography. The x-ray beam is generated by an x-ray tube (*lower right box*). The beam passes through a collimator (*lower left box*), where lead apertures form and limit the beam. On intersection with the patient, most of the beam is reflected or absorbed. The remaining photons pass through to the image intensifier (*upper right box*), where they impact on a cesium iodide crystal **(A).** Photons from the crystal cause electron emission from the photocathode **(B).** The electrons are accelerated **(C)** and focused on a phosphor screen **(D).** The image on the screen is split optically **(F)** and imaged with a video pick-up device **(G)** or 35-mm cine film **(H).** A photo detector **(E)** measures the photon output from the central zone of the phosphor image and provides feedback to adjust the x-ray dose and iris settings.

generated increases. In practice, modern x-ray tubes for coronary angiography have an anode angle of 8 to 10 degrees.

Within the emitted x-ray beam, the photons vary from lower-energy "soft" radiation to higher-energy "hard" radiation. By increasing the voltage potential (kilovoltage) between the cathode and the anode, a harder, higher-energy spectrum is produced. This leads to increased radiographic penetration and contrast. Good imaging also requires enough photons, or quantum, to create the image. An insufficient number of photons reaching the imaging device leads to a grainy image appearance (termed *quantum mottling*).

IMAGE DETECTION

After photon emission from the x-ray tube, the beam passes through a filter to eliminate low-energy photons and through a collimator, a series of lead apertures, that form and limit the beam directed at the patient. On interfacing with the patient, some photons are absorbed, some are reflected (scatter radiation), and some pass through entirely, reaching the image intensifier. A grid over the image intensifier helps screen out scatter radiation by passing only photons that are relatively perpendicular to the image intensifier face. On impact with the cesium iodide crystal on the face of the image intensifier, the x-ray photons are absorbed and cause the emission of lower-energy photons. These photons are absorbed by a photocathode coating the inner surface of the crystal and cause electron emission from the photocathode. The electrons are accelerated and focused onto a phosphor screen, where they liberate photons in the visible light range. The light from the phosphor screen of the image intensifier is picked up on a television camera and displayed as a fluoroscopic video image or recorded onto cineangiographic film (usually 35 mm).

The diameter of the image intensifier determines size of the field that can be imaged. Most image intensifiers are bimodal or trimodal. The entire cesium iodide crystal face can be focused onto the phosphor screen, or a smaller portion can be imaged, ignoring photons from the periphery of the crystal. Focusing on a smaller part of the input crystal face increases the magnification of the image on the phosphor screen but decreases the signal intensity (fewer electrons are focused onto the same size phosphor screen). This is compensated for by increasing the x-ray dose, which increases the number of x-ray photons and, hence, the number of electrons emitted per area of the central crystal. The increase in x-ray dose to the patient is mitigated by the smaller field of radiation. Larger field sizes (9 to 11 inches) are needed for ventriculography, and smaller sizes (4 to 5 inches) may be required for pediatric angiography. For coronary angiography, the optimal size of the image intensifier is 5 to 7 inches (13 to 18 cm).

Modern imaging equipment optimizes x-ray generation by way of a feedback loop with the imaging chain. By measuring the brightness of the center of the phosphor image of the intensifier, the amount and energy of photons emitted from the x-ray tube can be varied to obtain optimal image brightness. Automatic brightness control systems adjust for the radiodensity of the patient by varying kilovoltage and milliamperage delivered to the x-ray tube and by adjusting an iris between the phosphor output screen and the imaging system (video or film).

FLUOROSCOPIC IMAGE DISPLAY

Images obtained from the phosphor tube are displayed on a video system. The video image is composed of horizontal lines. Older systems displayed 525 lines per image. Modern displays show 1024 lines per image. Older systems also used an interlaced display mode that was employed in commercial television (NTSC standard). Using the interlaced display method, every other line on the video output is scanned every 1/60th second. By alternating the scans, a complete image is displayed every 1/30th second. This interlacing process eliminates the apparent image flicker that the eye perceives when images are scanned at 30 frames/s. Images of a rapidly moving heart, however, can be blurred because motion has occurred between the first and the second interlacing scans that paint the entire image.

More recent systems use a progressive scan method in which the entire image is displayed line by line every 1/60th second. This process permits better resolution of moving objects. However, it also leads to additional electronic noise and some quantum mottle (see earlier). Most manufacturers have now also employed systems that pulse the x-ray exposure. This "pulse fluoro" approach can further improve image sharpness. Radiation is only modestly reduced (and is even increased in one system), however.

CINEANGIOGRAPHY

For cineangiography, an x-ray beam must be pulsed to provide for adequate stop-motion imaging and to limit x-ray exposure. Thirty to 60 exposures/s are needed to give the appearance of a "live" continuous image. Frame rates greater than 30/s are needed only in patients with rapid heart rates. The exposure duration per frame should not exceed 5 to 8 msec to prevent motion blurring.[5] Exposure time control is achieved by pulsing the current to the x-ray tube. Initially, this was accomplished by pulsing the power to the high-energy transformer (the generator) leading to the x-ray tube. The capacitive effects of the high-voltage side of the transformer and cables, however, led to a slow dissipation of current to the tube and excessive soft radiation emission at the end of each pulse. Modern switching systems pulse the high-voltage side of the transformer output, yielding relatively square pulse waves. Pulsing has now been applied to fluoroscopy with some reduction in radiation exposure as reported by one laboratory.[6]

A 35-mm film camera is used to record the phosphor screen image as cineangiography. The film itself should be able to record all of the image density information (i.e., gray scale) presented by the image phosphor. Each type of film has a characteristic log scale of image density. The 35-mm film frame is rectangular, but the image from the image intensifier is circular. Consequently, the entire circular image can be recorded on film, leaving the periphery of the film frame unexposed, or the image can be "overframed." Overframing cuts off the peripheral display on the image phosphor. In most laboratories, maximal horizontal overframing (which cuts off the top and bottom of the image) is preferred and retains about 84 percent of the phosphor image.

DIGITAL PROCESSING

Nearly all newer radiographic systems incorporate digital image processing of the video pickup signal. For coronary angiography, a pixel matrix of at least 512 × 512 density and 256 gray levels (8 bits) per frame are needed to give acceptable resolution and a 1024 × 1024 matrix is needed for diagnostic quality angiography. A variety of pixel-processing algorithms are employed to enhance image clarity. Display monitors should be able to show all of the image detail presented by the image chain. Monitors display at 525 or 1023 to 1049 lines per screen. The higher line rate provides more resolution but also decreases the signal-to-noise ratio. At present, cine film resolution still exceeds that displayed on a high-resolution video monitor.

Regardless of the display mode, image distortion occurs because

1. Magnification of image is dependent on the distance between the x-ray tube, the patient, and the image intensifier. Objects closer to the tube are more magnified.
2. Images close to the x-ray tube and far from the image intensifier are more blurred.
3. The image intensifier is not entirely flat—it is curved like a pin cushion and increases the apparent size of objects at the periphery. (This is less of a problem with modern intensifiers.)
4. Photon scatter within the image intensifier and subsequent phosphor display pickup (veiling glare) can lead to a loss of contrast.

IMAGE RESOLUTION

The image quality can be defined by several methods. Image resolution is measured as the ability of the eventual image display (film or video) to distinguish closely spaced lead wires. To provide adequate resolution of fine coronary detail, the cineangiographic film resolution should exceed 3.5 to 4.0 line pairs per millimeter for a 6- to 7-inch image intensifier field.[5] Image intensifier veiling glare is tested by filming a circular lead disc. The contrast ratio of the disc to the surrounding area should by 20:1. Film density curves can be obtained by filming a "step-wedge" phantom that has a set of known densities and analyzing the film frame with a densitometer.

Radiation Protection

Radiation protection is an important responsibility for the all-catheterization laboratory personnel.[7–14] To achieve adequate imaging, the newer image intensifiers need to receive 10 to 40 μR/frame (varying inversely with image intensifier field size).[14] For routine fluoroscopy using a 6- to 7-inch field, this amounts to a skin entrance dose of approximately 3 to 10 R/min (increasing with angulation and patient density) because most of the x-ray beam is absorbed or reflected by the patient. Cineangiography increases the skin entrance dose to approximately 20 to 70 mR/frame (0.6 to 2.1 R/s at 30 frames/s, increasing with angulation and patient density). The deep midline tissue dose is approximately one tenth of the skin dose, and it should be kept in mind that the field of radiation is small, so that the average total body dose is substantially smaller than the chest dose. Patient radiation exposure can be minimized primarily by keeping the foot off the x-ray on-off switch, by proper collimation of the x-ray beam to prevent needless exposure of peripheral structures, and by maintaining the radiographic equipment such that a minimal x-ray dose is needed for adequate imaging.

Unless personnel place their hands in the radiation path, they should receive very little direct radiation exposure because by U.S. law all of the direct radiation emitting from the collimator must land on the image intensifier. However, only about 2 percent of the x-ray photons emitted from the x-ray tube ever reach the image intensifier, the rest being absorbed or reflected. Most of the radiation exposure to laboratory personnel results from scatter radiation from the patient (primarily internal reflection). Scatter radiation increases directly with the size of the patient and the number of photons in the x-ray beam and inversely with the energy of the photons (higher kilovolt energy photons are less likely to be reflected).

The radiation exposure for personnel can be reduced by attention to the patient exposure factors described previously, by staying as far away as possible from the x-ray source (the dose falls inversely with distance), and by wearing radiation shielding.[12, 13] Most of the reflected radiation is directed away from the beam direction (i.e., away from the image intensifier). Physician exposure is greatest when the image intensifier is pointed away from the physician (Fig. 30–2).[10, 12] The brachial artery approach to catheter insertion increases physician radiation exposure by nearly 40 percent compared with the femoral approach.[8]

All personnel should wear lead aprons with 0.5-mm lead lining, a thyroid shield, and eye protection.[8] Aprons with 0.5-mm lead shielding absorb 90 percent of the x-ray dose (70 percent for 0.25-mm lead lining), and leaded glasses reduce lens exposure by approximately 40 percent. Leaded surgical gloves, however, absorb only 10 percent of the radiation dose and have minimal efficacy. A table shield is also effective in reducing scatter radiation and should be used in all laboratories.

All personnel should also wear radiation detection badges to quantitate their own exposure and identify faulty equipment. The annual environmental radiation exposure (e.g., from radon, cosmic rays) is about 360 rem/yr in most parts of the United States. Current accepted limits (United States) for radiation exposure for personnel are 30 rem/yr superficial skin dose, 75 rem/yr for the hands and forearms, and 5 rem/yr (and < 3 rem for any 3-mo period) deep dose (under the lead apron) and for the lens.[11] The National Council on Radiation Protection and Measurement has called for an increase in the lens dose limit to 15 rem/yr and a yearly maximal skin dose of 50 rem.[11]

Physical Layout and Physiologic Recording Equipment

A catheterization laboratory should provide at least 600 square feet of laboratory and control room space and adequate facilities for x-ray equipment (e.g., generator) and storage.[2, 5] A physiologic monitor for recording the electrocardiogram (in multiple leads) and intravascular pressures should be located outside the radiation field. It is important that the pressure recording system be calibrated daily and that optimal transducer damping is adjusted. Modern physiologic recorders digitize the pressure waveforms and computer analyze a variety of hemodynamic parameters (e.g., end-diastolic pressures, systolic or diastolic pressure gradients between two transducers, waveform differentiation). It is important to be familiar with the algorithms used to derive these parameters before relying on the computer-derived parameters for clinical decision making.

All catheterization laboratories should be equipped to manage the complications of catheterization. This includes a full stock of catheters and emergency drugs, the capability for rapid defibrillation and right heart pacing, and the immediate availability of an intra-aortic balloon pump.

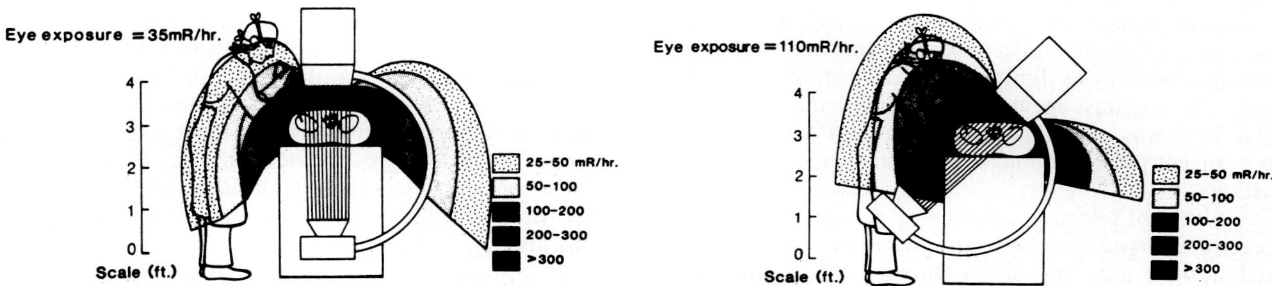

FIGURE 30–2 Radiation exposure to personnel during fluorography. Angulation of the x-ray tube toward personnel increases the exposure. (From Geise RA, Hunter DW: Personnel exposure during fluoroscopy procedures. Postgrad Radiol 8:162–173, 1988.)

Personnel

In addition to the cardiologist performing the procedure, a physiologic recording technician should be monitoring and recording the electrocardiogram and pressure measurements.[5] A circulating nurse should be present during angiography to administer drugs and fluids and to retrieve catheters. A radiologic technician (or equivalent) should be available to assist in operating the radiographic equipment and moving the x-ray table. In many laboratories, a scrub nurse or technician is also available to assist in catheter preparation. Should a complication develop, additional personnel should be immediately available.

For percutaneous procedures that do not involve a cutdown or prolonged catheter placement, the personnel in the room should observe good principles of hygiene. The same intensity of sterile practices performed in an operating room is not supported for percutaneous catheterizations, primarily because the rate of infection for these procedures is extraordinarily low.[15] Personnel at the site of catheter insertion should wash their hands thoroughly and wear gloves. A gown, mask, and protective eyewear should be worn to protect the operator against blood-borne pathogens (e.g., human immunodeficiency virus, hepatitis). If vascular access is accomplished by cutdown, sterile apparel (gown, glove, and mask) and limited room access should be undertaken because the rate of infection is approximately 10-fold that of percutaneous procedures.[15]

Techniques of Coronary Angiography

Technical History of Coronary Angiography

Nonselective angiography of the coronary arteries was accomplished first in the 1920s and 1930s using an aortic injection of radiographic contrast media and cut film imaging.[16] Coronary imaging was limited by the toxicity and limited opacity of the di-iodinated contrast media, the restricted rate of contrast injection through the needle or small-lumen catheters used for intravascular access, and poor radiographic imaging resolution. A variety of methods were subsequently used to enhance coronary filling, including acetylcholine-induced cardiac arrest and occlusion of the distal aorta to limit peripheral arterial runoff.[17] Although normal proximal coronary anatomy could be discerned by these methods, the structure of distal vessels and diseased arteries was poorly defined.

Semiselective coronary angiography was performed later, using a circular catheter with numerous sideholes.[18] When placed in the aorta, some of the sideholes opposed the coronary ostia and contrast medium injection opacified these arteries. Selective injection of contrast media into the coronary arteries was limited by fear that the available radiographic contrast agents would cause ventricular fibrillation. This was quite justified because in an era before direct current cardioversion, fibrillation was a lethal complication.

The advent of selective coronary opacification was introduced by Mason Sones, who inadvertently selectively injected a right coronary artery during an attempted left ventricular angiogram. The patient did not develop ventricular fibrillation, and Sones and Shirey[19] went on to develop a selective coronary catheter that could be deflected off the aortic valve into either coronary ostium, whereupon contrast medium could be injected. Changes in contrast media and improvements in radiographic imaging led to better resolution of the coronary tree with less toxicity and radiation exposure. Improvements in radiographic positioning equipment enabled steep, angulated views of the coronary circulation that are needed to effectively image the proximal left coronary vessels.

With the prior introduction of the Seldinger method of peripheral vascular cannulation, Judkins, Amplatz, Abrams, Schoonmaker, and others invented preformed catheters that could be passed with great ease from the femoral artery to the coronary ostium.[19–24] Since then, an explosion of catheter material and shapes has made possible nearly effortless cannulation of most coronary arteries and bypass grafts. As Judkins is quoted as saying, "The catheter will find the coronary ostium unless impeded by the operator." The technique of coronary cannulation and opacification is important, however, because both the safety and the quality of coronary arteriography can be improved by rigorous attention to certain principles.

Patient Preparation

The evaluation of patients about to undergo coronary angiography should emphasize a detailed history concerning factors that affect the approach and risks of angiography, a physical examination concentrating on the cardiovascular system, and a frank discussion of the procedure and its anticipated risks and benefits.[24a]

The history should include questions about prior experience with angiography and prior or current vascular diseases (e.g., stroke, transient ischemic attack, claudication) and previous vascular procedures (particularly aortic or iliofemoral revascularization). Additionally, the presence of factors increasing sensitivity to drugs used during catheterization should be noted so that appropriate precautions can be taken. This includes sensitivity to radiographic contrast materials (e.g., diabetes, preexisting nephropathy, prior reaction to contrast medium), protamine sulfate (e.g., alpha$_1$-antitrypsin deficiency), narcotics, heparin, and thrombolytic drugs (e.g., gastrointestinal disease).

The physical examination should concentrate on the vascular system and elements that might change the approach for the procedure. The quality of the pulses in both upper (brachial, radial, and ulnar) and lower extremities (femoral, dorsalis pedis, popliteal, and posterior tibial) should be recorded because problems in obtaining vascular access may necessitate a change in cannulation site, and embolic complications can occur in any vascular territory. Particular attention should also be paid to the quality of carotid artery upstroke and the presence of carotid, abdominal (renal), or femoral bruits. Although not always possible, it is better to obtain arterial access in arteries without diminished pulse or bruit. The presence of an abdominal aneurysm should be assessed because aneurysms frequently contain thrombus or other friable material that can be embolized during vascular cannulation.

The physical examination should also concentrate on the cardiovascular illness necessitating angiography. The jugular venous pressure and waveform should be noted to assess right heart filling pressure and possible tricuspid regurgitation. The presence of left heart failure should be assessed, and the ability of the patient to lie flat for prolonged periods should be ascertained (usually by observing the patient supine for 15 to 30 minutes). If possible, patients with severe left heart failure should undergo diuresis before angiography.

After interviewing and examining the patient, the anticipated procedure should be explained in sufficient detail to give the patient an understanding of what will be done, when it will be done, what will occur after the procedure, and what the likely expected findings might be. The main goals of this discussion are to ensure informed consent and to allay anxiety on the day of the procedure. The procedural description can be supplemented with written or video format materials. It can also be quite useful to discuss the implications of certain findings in order to lay the groundwork for future recommendations for treatment. We find it quite useful to involve a responsible family member in the preangiography preparation.

After a discussion of the procedure itself, a frank discussion of the potential risks should occur, and informed consent should be obtained. A description of potential complications should be tailored to the patient's risk factors to provide an estimate that is as accurate as possible (see later). It is to no one's advantage to minimize or exaggerate the risks of angiography.

Before angiography, an electrocardiogram should be obtained. The serum potassium and creatinine concentrations and hemoglobin concentration should be measured to assure that special precautions need not be taken. Generally, measurement of blood clotting time (prothrombin time or partial thromboplastin time) is not required unless there is a clinical suspicion that they might be abnormal (e.g., anticoagulant use, liver disease, severe right heart failure, bleeding history).[25] If the patient has had prior coronary bypass or other heart surgery, the operative report should be read and the position of bypass grafts noted. The patient's report of the operation or the brief notes of other physicians can frequently be incomplete or inaccurate.

On the day of the procedure, the patient should be instructed to withhold oral intake for 6 hours before the procedure. Medications should generally be continued, except for hypoglycemic agents. Oral hypoglycemic agents should be held the day of the procedure. Doses of long-acting insulin should be halved, and regular insulin should be held. If insulin is given, a 5 percent glucose solution should be infused until catheterization and supplemental oral glucose can be given as needed. Metformin, an oral hypoglycemic agent, should be held before and after angiography in patients with increased risk of renal failure. The drug can lead to lactic acidosis in the presence of renal failure.[26]

In all patients, a reliable intravenous access line should be established before angiography. The infusion port should be large enough to permit a rapid infusion of fluid, should the patient develop reduced intravascular pressure (e.g., as a result of increased vagal tone or nitrate-induced venorelaxation). Patients with renal dysfunction, particularly those with diabetes, should be adequately hydrated before angiography. Dehydration increases the risk of contrast-induced renal failure.[26] Many angiographers also administer mannitol to patients with renal dysfunction (particularly those with diabetes) before and during angiography to increase tubular urine flow (see later). Some caution should be used in patients with heart failure because mannitol increases intravascular volume and may transiently increase the pulmonary capillary wedge pressure. There is little evidence to support the use of mannitol or furosemide (Lasix) before angiography to reduce renal dysfunction. A recent study suggests that maintenance of continuous urine flow during and after angiography is the best deterrent to renal failure.[27]

Proper sedation is also an important preparation of the patient. Patients awaiting angiography are anxious. Treatment with anxiolytic drugs can improve their perception of the procedure, although elderly patients may have paradoxical excitation with benzodiazepines and other sedatives. Before coming to the catheterization laboratory, the patient should void urine and take a nonsoporific sedative (e.g., benzodiazepine). If a long procedure is anticipated, insertion of a urinary catheter may be useful in men with prostatism or other patients who have trouble voiding.

Vascular Access

Access to the arterial vasculature can be accomplished by cutdown and direct catheter insertion or by the percutaneous Seldinger technique.[28] For many years, the brachial artery was exposed directly and incised with a blade to insert Sones catheters into the central circulation. After arteriography, the catheter was withdrawn and the artery was sutured closed. The advantages of cutdown cannulation are control of the artery and minimal bleeding after the completion of the repair. The disadvantage is a higher risk of arterial thrombosis or injury (see later), infection, a scar on the arm, and limited reuse of the same access site.

Introduction of a direct percutaneous needle puncture method for angiography made possible the development of femoral approach angiography, the method used overwhelmingly at present.[28] The skin and subcutaneous tissues about the artery are infiltrated with a local anesthetic (e.g., lidocaine or the longer-acting bupivacaine). The common femoral artery is punctured with a thin-walled needle. The site of entry is important because an inferior puncture may enter the smaller superficial femoral artery and a superior puncture may pass through the peritoneal cavity or increase the risk of retroperitoneal bleeding. The common femoral artery can be located by finding the superior, anterior iliac crest and the symphysis pubis (landmarks of the inguinal ligament). The puncture site should be approximately 5 cm inferior to the line at the site of the pulse. Particularly in obese patients, the puncture site may be above the groin crease. Where landmarks are difficult to ascertain, fluoroscopy can be used. In 97 percent of patients, a portion of the common femoral artery overlies the medial femoral head.[29]

Once the artery is punctured, a 0.035- to 0.038-inch (0.88- to 0.95-mm) flexible guide wire with a J tip is passed through the needle into the arterial lumen.[30] Heparin coating on the wire reduces platelet adhesion.[31] Once the guide wire is in place, a dilator is employed to enlarge the tract into the artery, after which a catheter (with a tip tapered down to the wire) or hemostatic sheath (a short tube with a one-way valve) is advanced into the vessel. The angiographic catheters are advanced through a hemostatic valve in the sheath and up to the ascending aorta with the aid of the J-tipped guidewire. If a hemostatic sheath is used, the outer diameter of arteriotomy will be about 0.3 mm larger than the inner diameter of the sheath, enlarging the puncture site by 1 French size.

Although not preferred to a native femoral artery, vascular access can be obtained through prosthetic femoral artery grafts (e.g., Dacron), provided that the grafts have been in place long enough to develop extraluminal fibrosis (i.e., 2 to 4 months). Fears of uncontrollable bleeding, infection, and disruption of the pseudointima within the graft, in general, have not been realized,[32, 33] and catheter insertion into grafts is usually safe. In our experience, however, it may take slightly longer to achieve hemostasis after catheter withdrawal, and dislodgment of the pseudointima within the graft can occur very infrequently. It has been suggested that catheters in vascular grafts be removed after straightening with a guidewire.[34] Brachial artery or radial artery approaches have enjoyed resurgence recently. The available evidence, however, suggests that these sites of cannulation may have a higher risk of vascular complication (e.g., vessel occlusion) and should be reserved for patients with poor femoral arterial access or a diseased descending aorta.

After angiography, the extremity with the arteriotomy site should be extended and held straight. The catheters should be withdrawn from the artery, aspirating during withdrawal to help avoid extrusion of thrombus. Immediately after decannulation, the arterial puncture site should be compressed by hand or, in the case of femoral puncture, with the use of a device (i.e., a C clamp) to apply local pressure. Although some authors suggest that compression devices lead to a higher complication rate, there is little evidence to support this view. However, an unwatched C clamp or other hemostatic device can be dangerous because changes in patient position or muscle tone alter the pressure applied to the artery and may lead to bleeding or total vessel occlusion. The C clamp is meant to save the hands, not time.

Regardless of method used for hemostasis, the distal pulse should be monitored frequently until pressure is withdrawn and for at least several hours thereafter (e.g., every 15 minutes for 1 hour after hemostasis, then every 30 to 60 minutes). The patient should avoid actions that increase arterial pressure (e.g., coughing, straining to urinate, sitting up) for 2 to 6 hours. The precise duration of bed rest needed after arterial puncture is not clear but probably decreases with the size of the catheter used.[27]

Coronary Catheters

The essential features of a coronary angiographic catheter are an adequate lumen area, shape retention, torque control, radiographic opacity, and safety. Catheters used to cannulate the coronary arteries were initially constructed of a woven Dacron or hydrocarbon polymers. Dacron catheters are very durable and can be reused, but they have a relatively thick wall and tend to lose their shape quickly after insertion into the vasculature. Polymers, predominantly polyurethanes and polyethylenes, are advantageous because they can be extruded and easily shaped. Their drawbacks are that they can also soften when inserted into the body and frequently do not transmit torque to the catheter tip. To improve shape retention and torque transmission, most manufacturers use wire braiding within the catheter wall. Improved polymers have allowed a reduction in the thickness of the catheter wall, preserving the caliber of the inner lumen without a significant loss in handling characteristics.

After Sones developed catheters for brachial approach angiography, Judkins and Amplatz and others designed a series of coronary catheters for cannulation from the femoral approach.[19–24] Each design has a primary and a secondary curve and tapers at the tip to hug the guidewire (Figs. 30–3 and 30–4).[19–24]

Catheter caliber is measured in French size (French size equals circumference in millimeters). Seven and 8 French diagnostic coronary catheters, which provide a large inner lumen area and allow rapid contrast medium injections at low injection pressure (<100 psi), were used routinely until recently. Ambulation 6 to 8 hours after 8 French catheter removal is safe.[34] Recently, catheter construction has improved remarkably, allowing the manufacture of 4 to 6 French sizes. The smaller arteriotomy required by 4 to 6 French catheters has reduced the time needed for hemostasis and bed rest after catheter withdrawal and may prevent peripheral vascular complications.[27, 34a, 35] However, smaller catheters (particularly less than 6 French) can have insufficient lumen area to inject contrast medium adequately into the coronary artery (leading to contrast streaming), poor torquing characteristics, and instability within the coronary lumen.[36] Rapid injection through a small catheter end-hole orifice can lead to damage of the coronary wall.[73] The likelihood of coronary injury is directly related to the energy content of the contrast medium jet. A single report also describes an increase in catheter-induced coronary artery dissections associated with 6 French catheter use by less experienced operators.[38] Newer small catheters

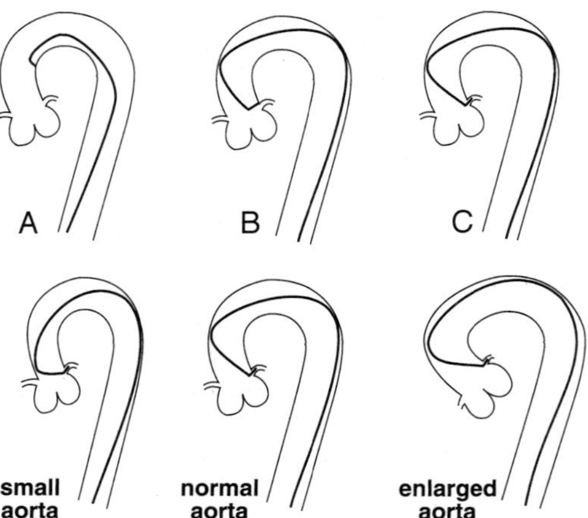

FIGURE 30–3 Cannulation of the left coronary artery using a Judkins curve catheter. **A,** The catheter is passed to the proximal aorta using a guidewire (not shown). **B** and **C,** The catheter is then advanced to the coronary ostium while pressure is monitored from the catheter tip. The tip should be coaxial with the artery. The length of the catheter between the primary and the secondary curves should increase with the diameter of the aorta (*lower panel*). (**A–C,** Adapted from Judkins MP: Selective coronary arteriography: Part I: a percutaneous transfemoral technic. Radiology 89:815–824, 1967.)

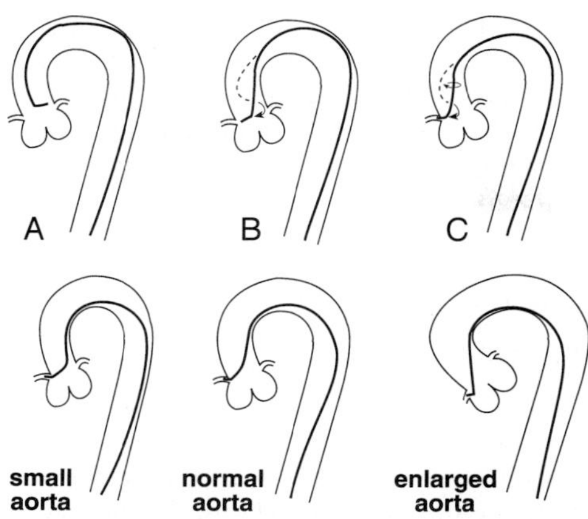

FIGURE 30–4 Cannulation of the right coronary artery using a Judkins curve catheter. **A,** The catheter is passed to the proximal aorta using a guidewire (not shown). **B** and **C,** The catheter is then advanced to the level of the coronary ostium and rotated clockwise while pressure is monitored from the catheter tip. The tip should be coaxial with the artery. The length of the catheter between the primary and the secondary curves and the angle of the primary curve should increase with the size of the aorta (*lower panel*). (**A–C,** Adapted from Judkins MP: Selective coronary arteriography: Part I: a percutaneous transfemoral technic. Radiology 89:815–824, 1967.)

have a remarkably large lumen area and may be safer than earlier versions. In general, however, newer catheters 4 to 6 French in size produce acceptable angiography, particularly when used with a mechanical injector.

Cannulation of the Coronary Ostia

Cannulation of the coronary ostium is the most important step in angiography. Catheters should be advanced to the ascending aortic root with the use of a guide wire. Inserting catheters without a guide wire can lead to retrograde peripheral arterial dissection. After aspirating the catheter to ensure that any debris or air has been removed, the catheter should be filled with contrast medium and connected to the pressure transducer. Left coronary Amplatz and Judkins catheters can be advanced to the coronary ostium directly and usually require little manipulation (see Figs. 30–3 and 30–4).[20, 22] Right coronary Amplatz and Judkins catheters should be advanced to the aortic valve, withdrawn 1 to 1½ cm and rotated clockwise until the ostium is engaged (see Fig. 30–4).

When cannulating a coronary ostium, fluoroscopy in the 40- to 45-degree left anterior oblique (LAO) projection can be useful because the coronary ostia are nearly perpendicular to the view. If the coronary ostium cannot be cannulated, a different catheter shape should be used, keeping in mind the shape of the aorta, the angle of the coronary origin, and the rotation of the heart. If a coronary ostium cannot be found, the possibility of an aberrant origin should be considered (see later).

After cannulation, the pressure at the catheter tip should be observed. Pressure damping implies that the catheter has burrowed into the wall of the artery, that there is catheter-induced vasospasm, or that there is an organic ostial stenosis. If present, injection of contrast medium should be avoided because it could cause a coronary dissection. The catheter should be withdrawn slowly. If the pressure normalizes with the catheter in the orifice, a test injection should be done. Free-flowing contrast medium without staining of the arterial wall should be observed before angiography. Since contrast medium emerges from the catheter as a jet, it is important that the catheter tip is coaxial with the proximal artery to avoid contrast-jet–induced injury to the ostial wall.

Pressure damping from an improper catheter position or vasospasm is common in the right coronary artery, but in the left coronary, it should alert the angiographer to the possibility of stenosis in the left main coronary, a particularly dangerous problem. A test injection below the artery or use of a "cusp" catheter can define the coronary ostium and permit selection of the best catheter shape. Administration of nitroglycerin can reduce the tendency for catheter-induced ostial vasospasm, although it is not always effective.

BYPASS GRAFT ANGIOGRAPHY

Coronary artery bypass graft angiography is usually straightforward if the grafts are in their usual position. The common aortic anastomosis sites of bypass grafts are shown in Figure 30–5. Left coronary vein grafts are usually

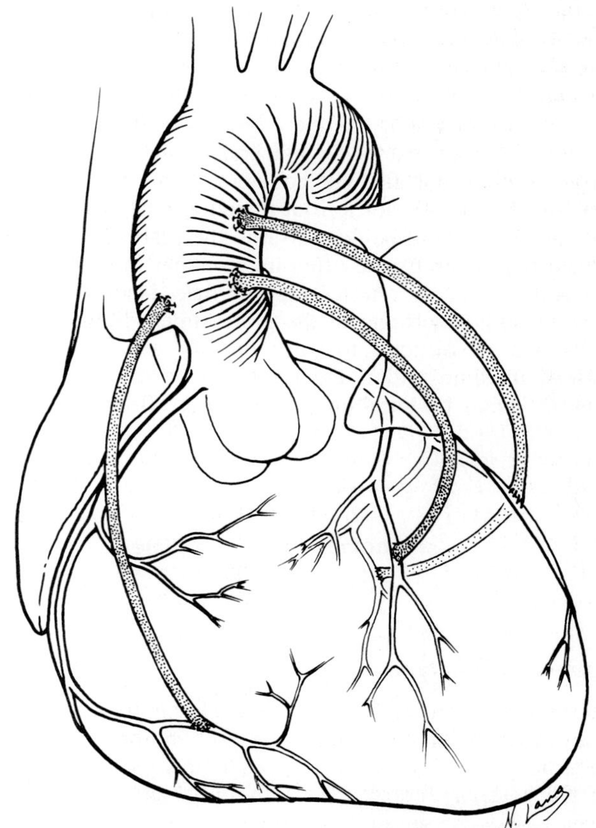

FIGURE 30–5 Typical locations of coronary artery vein bypass grafts. The vein graft to the circumflex marginal branch is usually the most superior and leftward vein-aorta anastomosis. The vein graft to the left anterior descending artery typically arises inferior and anterior to the circumflex graft. The right coronary graft arises lowest on the aorta and in an anterior-rightward position.

located on the anterolateral portion of the aorta and can be cannulated with a left vein bypass curve catheter or with a variety of other coronary catheters (e.g., Judkins right 4 curve, Amplatz right 1 or left 1 curves). A small number of surgeons pass the circumflex vein graft through the transverse sinus and anastomose it to the right-posterior aorta (to minimize graft kinking). If the circumflex graft cannot be found, the posterior aorta should be searched with a left vein bypass graft or Amplatz left catheter.

The right coronary vein grafts usually arise at a very shallow angle from the aorta and can be cannulated easily with a right vein graft curve catheter. Other catheters (e.g., Judkins right 4 curve, Amplatz right 1 or left 1 curves) may also be successful, particularly when the aortic root is enlarged or if the aortic anastomosis is more horizontal.

Internal mammary artery grafts are best cannulated with an internal mammary curve catheter, although a Judkins right 3.5 or 4 curve may suffice. If the internal mammary cannot be engaged selectively, patency can be established with a subclavian artery angiogram performed after inflation of a blood pressure cuff to reduce peripheral runoff into the ipsilateral arm. Injection of contrast material into the internal mammary artery can be painful if the artery still perfuses the chest wall. Low-osmolality contrast material is better tolerated.

The most common problems in bypass graft angiography are failure to determine graft patency, failure to fully opacify the graft and distal coronary, and failure to define a stenosis at the coronary anastomotic site. *It is of paramount importance that the angiographer know the origin and destination of each bypass graft.* The only reliable source for such information is the operative report. If a convincing aortic vein graft stump is not found and the recipient coronary does not fill via collaterals, the vein graft is probably patent. An aortic root injection with dense aortic opacification should be done to find the graft or its stump.

Vein bypass grafts are often much larger in caliber than the native coronary arteries they perfuse, leading to slow velocity within portions of the graft lumen. Large caliber grafts can be difficult to fully opacify and layering of contrast medium within the graft can be mistaken for a stenotic lesion or intraluminal thrombus. Better injection (often using an angioplasty-guiding catheter) will minimize the effects of streaming. The coronary anastomosis may also be difficult to define because of overlapping bypass graft or native arteries. It is important that at least one view be obtained in a radiographic angle that is nearly normal to the anastomosis.

Radiographic Contrast Material

PREPARATIONS

Iodine, an element that absorbs x-ray photons, is the essential constituent of angiographic contrast material. In all biologically compatible angiographic contrast agents, the iodine is organically bound to a benzene carbon ring (Fig. 30–6). The compounds are highly water soluble, stay within the extracellular space, and are excreted primarily by renal glomerular filtration (with minimal biliary, salivary, and small bowel excretion). An iodine concentration of at least 320 mg/ml is required for adequate definition of the coronary arterial tree and higher concentrations (e.g., 350 to 370 mg iodine/ml) are desirable.

In all modern contrast media, three iodine atoms are bound to a benzene ring (see Fig. 30–6). In so-called ionic contrast media, the ring is a benzoic acid derivative, and in solution, it dissociates into two charged particles.[39] Each cationic iodinated benzene ring has a corresponding anion (usually meglumine and sodium in a ratio of 6.6:1). The ionic nature of contrast medium increases its osmolality (osmolality equals number of particles/volume), which can have profound physiologic effects.

Many other constituents of contrast solution are important. In the past, a high or low concentration of sodium cations led to increased ventricular arrhythmias, but now almost all contrast media used for coronary angiography have a sodium concentration between 150 and 190 mmol/L.[40] Ethylenediaminetetraacetic acid (EDTA) is added to nearly all preparations to remove heavy metal contaminants. Additionally, the acidic pH of diatrizoate is neutralized with a variety of bases (e.g., sodium hydroxide, sodium citrate). Citrate and EDTA can bind calcium, reducing the ionized calcium concentration in the blood and intersti-

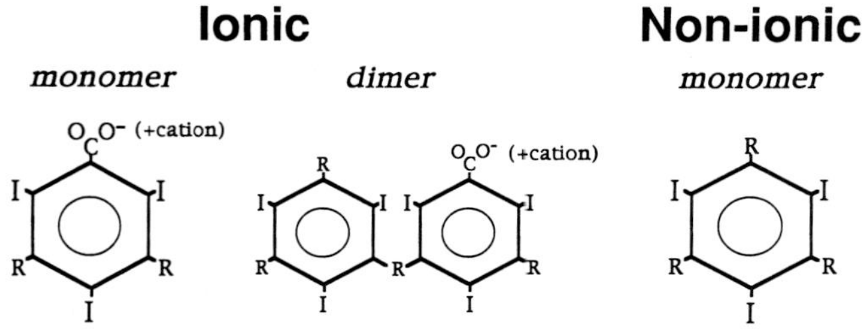

Ionic — *monomer*, *dimer*; **Non-ionic** — *monomer*

	Ionic monomer	Ionic dimer	Non-ionic monomer
Preparations	diatrizoate salt (Hypaque®-76, Renografin®-76)	ioxaglate	iohexol iopamidol iopromide ioversol
Cation	meglumine and sodium	meglumine and sodium	none
Osmolality (osm/kg)	1.57-2.02	.60	.79-.84
Viscosity (cp @37°C)	4.2-8.5	7.5	9.0-10.4
Density (gm/ml)	1.34	1.32	1.33-1.41
LD_{50} (g I/kg)	7.5	15-17	10-24

FIGURE 30–6 Structure and characteristics of radiographic contrast agents.

tial space, which promotes ventricular fibrillation.[41–44] Agents with added calcium (e.g., calcium edetate) and those without citrate cause fewer ventricular arrhythmias and are preferred.[41, 42, 44]

Many of the unwanted effects of contrast material are related to the high osmolality of the contrast solution needed to obtain an adequate iodine concentration. To reduce the osmolality, an ionic dimer (ioxaglate [Hexabrix]) was developed (see Fig. 30–6). This compound has only one cation for each two benzene rings (six iodine atoms/three particles), reducing osmolality by 30 percent over the diatrizoate salts. Ioxaglate is better tolerated than the ionic monomer preparations.[45]

"Nonionic," lower-osmolality solutions have been developed by creating an iodinated benzene ring that does not dissociate, resulting in yet lower osmolality and the absence of toxic effects associated with the cations. Even these solutions, however, still have an osmolality much greater than that of blood and are quite viscous. Although the nonionic, lower-osmolar solutions are substantially more expensive, they confer significant advantages, particularly in patients with severe coronary artery disease, reduced ventricular function, or a history of sensitivity to ionic contrast media.[46–49] Recently, nearly iso-osmotic, nonionic contrast media have been developed. These agents may further reduce the risk of angiography.

PHYSIOLOGIC EFFECTS OF CONTRAST MATERIAL

Injection of contrast material initially causes a brief (<5-second) fall in coronary blood flow caused by passage of the viscous solution through the microcirculation (following Poiseuille's law, Fig. 30–7). Immediately thereafter, blood flow increases by 2.5- to 4.0-fold of basal blood flow and returns to normal within about 15 to 20 seconds.[50, 51] The cause of the hyperemic response appears to be related in part to the high osmolality of contrast media, since a similar response is seen after injection of hyperosmolar dextrose solution.[52, 53] Stimulation of chemoreceptors in the myocardium may contribute to coronary (and peripheral) vasodilatation through the Bezold-Jarisch reflex,[52] and a direct effect on the microcirculation cannot be excluded. The hyperemic response after nonionic contrast medium injection is less than that seen after ionic contrast injection (see Fig. 30–7).[54]

Ventricular dP/dt falls within seconds after contrast medium injection, followed by a reduction in systemic blood pressure.[55, 56] A reflex-mediated rebound increase in blood pressure often occurs 8 to 10 seconds later. Ventricular compliance decreases, causing end-diastolic pressure to rise.[57–59] The negative inotropic response is more pronounced and lasts longer in the presence of coexistent left ventricular dysfunction or myocardial ischemia (up to 20 minutes).[60, 61] Nonionic and low-osmolar contrast media have substantially less deleterious effect on ventricular function and should be used in patients with acute ischemic syndromes, heart failure, severe aortic stenosis, and left main coronary artery disease.[46, 48, 55, 56] In these patients, the additional cost of nonionic media may be offset by the lower incidence of costs related to complications.[62]

Contrast medium significantly reduces the rate of sinoatrial node depolarization and prolongs the action potential and repolarization. Intracoronary contrast medium injection causes an increase in QRS voltage and a lengthening of the QRS and QT intervals, in addition to ST-segment shifts.[55] The effects on the QT interval may be exacerbated by local hypothermia induced by use of room temperature contrast material. These effects are short lasting (<2 minutes).

The bradycardia and reduced atrioventricular node conduction are caused by a direct effect of contrast material on conduction tissue and indirectly by stimulation of afferent chemoreceptors in the ventricle. Chemoreceptor discharge causes a reflex-mediated increase in vagal tone and peripheral sympathetic withdrawal (the Bezold-Jarisch reflex).[52, 53, 63] The vagally mediated bradycardia can be blocked by atropine, although in most patients its brief duration does not merit treatment. Prophylactic pacemaker placement to avoid bradycardia is not recommended because its routine use increases the frequency of ventricular arrhythmias, including fibrillation, without significant benefit.[64, 65]

Contrast media also alter blood coagulation by multiple mechanisms.[66–69] High concentrations of diatrizoate salts reduce activation of platelets and increase the thrombin time, which may prevent clotting within the coronary catheter and thromboembolic complications. Nonionic contrast media have less effect on coagulation. Iopamidol (a non-

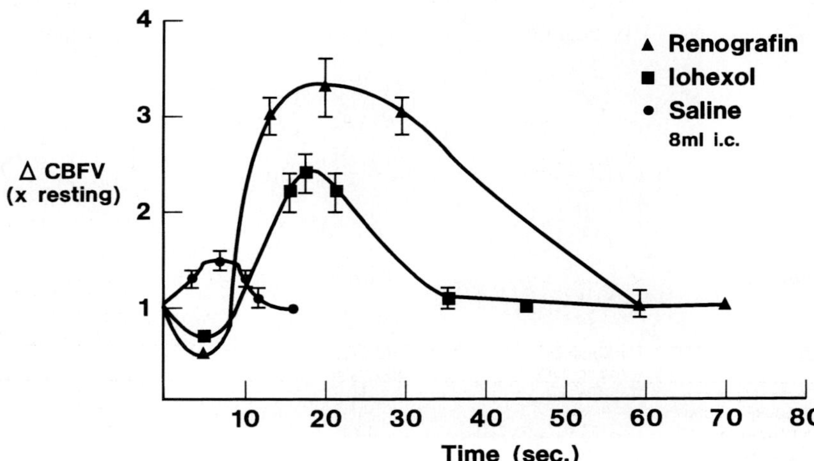

FIGURE 30–7 Changes in coronary blood flow velocity (Δ CBFV) after intracoronary injection of ionic contrast media (Renografin), nonionic contrast media (Iohexol), and saline solution. An initial fall in coronary blood flow velocity after contrast medium injection (but not saline) is followed by a hyperemic response that is more marked after ionic contrast medium injection.

ionic agent) decreases platelet surface charge, which may facilitate platelet aggregation, but it also prevents fibrin monomer assembly and prolongs the thrombin time (although less than ionic salts).[67, 68] The high osmolarity of contrast media also causes transient shrinkage of red blood cells and endothelial cells, increasing vascular permeability.[67] It has been suggested that ionic contrast media (diatrizoate salts) be used in patients with thrombotic coronary syndromes (e.g., infarction or unstable angina), but in clinical studies, the overall incidence of thrombotic complications is very low when nonionic agents are employed.[70]

INJECTION OF CONTRAST MEDIA

Contrast media can be injected into the coronary arteries with the use of a motorized injector or by a hand-held syringe. Hand injection is accomplished with a syringe attached to the coronary catheter via a manifold of stopcocks (Fig. 30–8). The setup varies widely among laboratories, but the essential elements are a clear syringe (to ensure that bubbles can be seen before injection) connected to a stopcock manifold. Using clear tubing, the manifold is connected to a contrast medium container, a pressure transducer (for monitoring pressure at the catheter tip), and a pressurized bag of saline solution to facilitate connecting the coronary catheter to the injection manifold without introducing air. The paramount importance of keeping the entire injection system free of air cannot be overemphasized. This can be accomplished by a thorough purging of the manifold and tubing system with contrast medium or saline solution during the setup and vigilance during the procedure. It should be kept in mind, however, that all liquids contain microbubbles that can cause transient microcirculatory obstruction.[71]

Motorized injectors permit the injection of a specified amount of contrast material at a specified constant injection rate. Typically, the left coronary is injected with 5 to 12 ml of contrast material at 3 to 5 ml/s and the right coronary with 2 to 5 ml at 1 to 4 ml/s. The rate should be adjusted for the size of the perfusion field and the rate of blood flow in the recipient artery or bypass graft. For each contrast injection, most angiographers prefer to progressively increase the initial injection rate by using a ramp (a specified rate of rise in injection speed) to prevent the injection jet from causing the angiographic catheter to "kick" out of the artery. It is important that the ramp not be too slow, because a good initial injection of contrast medium reduces coronary blood flow transiently and enhances the angiographic image (see Fig. 30–7). A slow injection results only in contrast hyperemia, which further dilutes the injected contrast medium. The advantages of motorized injectors are consistency, the ability to deliver large contrast medium volumes at high flow rates (e.g., to hypertrophied hearts), and the ease of injection. The disadvantage is an inability to adjust the flow rate during injection. A semiautomated mechanical injector has been developed for coronary angiography.

Anticoagulation

Catheterization itself is associated with platelet activation and a rise in thromboxane A_2 metabolite excretion.[72] The presence of catheters within the vascular lumen causes endothelial denudation and, combined with the foreign body of the catheter, is a stimulus for intravascular thrombosis. Several, but not all, studies suggest that systemic anticoagulation with heparin reduces the incidence of thrombotic complications of angiography (primarily thrombosis at the site of catheter insertion),[73–75] although heparin has also been reported to cause additional activation of platelets.[76] Anticoagulation is not necessary for patients undergoing routine diagnostic angiography from the femoral approach. There is uniform agreement, however, that heparin (e.g., 2000 U into the artery and 3000 U intravenously) should be given to all patients in whom the brachial or radial approach is used, because of the higher incidence of thrombosis at the catheter insertion site. In patients undergoing femoral approach angiography, the risk of thrombotic complications probably increases with the duration of the procedure, a smaller femoral artery or larger catheter, and the presence of peripheral vascular disease. Patients at higher risk of thrombosis should be anticoagulated (3000 to 5000 U intravenously) unless a contraindication exists.

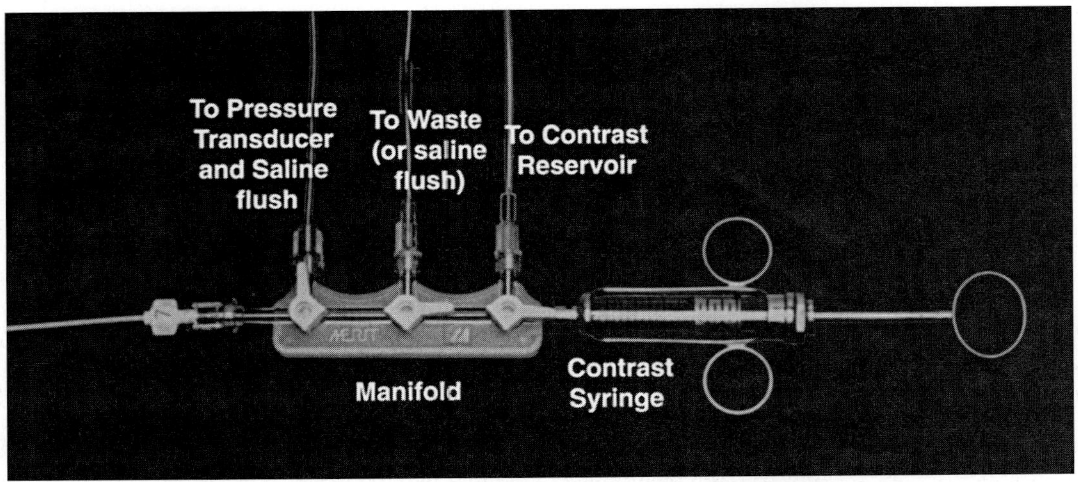

FIGURE 30–8 One variation of the manifold and syringe system used to inject the coronary arteries by hand.

The optimal dose of heparin may vary between patients because plasma antithrombin III and platelet factor IV (which binds heparin) concentrations affect heparin efficacy and availability, respectively.[77] Heparin pharmacokinetics are not affected by the type of contrast medium selected.[78] Aspirin decreases platelet activation caused by angiography, but its efficacy in reducing complications has not been evaluated.[72]

At the end of the procedure, the anticoagulant effects of heparin can be reversed by administering protamine.[79] Protamine is a polycationic compound derived from fish sperm (primarily from salmon and herring) that binds to heparin. One mg of protamine binds approximately 100 U (1 mg) of heparin.[9] Since heparin is essentially eliminated by first-order kinetics, the amount of protamine needed is a function of the initial heparin dose and the time since administration. For a 5000-unit heparin dose, the initial protamine dose should be 50 mg if less than 20 minutes has passed and progressively less thereafter (e.g., 30 mg if 60 minutes has elapsed).[8] If insufficient protamine is given, a phenomenon known as *heparin rebound* can occur.[10] After initial normalization of clotting times from the first protamine dose, protamine degradation by proteinases leads to release of free heparin and a rebound increase in clotting time.[80, 81]

Protamine should be administered cautiously to patients with a prior exposure to the drug (such as NPH insulin or protamine sulfate or chloride) and patients with a "fish allergy" and should not be given to patients with alpha$_1$-antitrypsin deficiency (see later).[82, 83] Very large protamine doses (>4.0:1 protamine:heparin concentration) can have an anticoagulant effect, although it is rarely observed in a clinical setting.[9]

Management of Epicardial Coronary Artery Tone

The lumen caliber of epicardial coronary arteries measured at angiography reflects a variable degree of tone. Both atherosclerotic and normal coronary arteries dilate after nitroglycerin, but proximal vessels exhibit less dilatation than distal epicardial vessels (9 percent versus 34 percent diameter increase).[84] Stenotic lesions also relax after nitroglycerin, although severely narrowed segments usually dilate little.[85] Removal of tone by nitroglycerin permits an assessment of maximal coronary caliber, effectively eliminates vasospastic coronary lesions, and facilitates assessments of stenosis severity.

Nitroglycerin primarily affects the large diameter epicardial portion of the coronary artery, and dilatation in these vessels lasts for 10 to 20 minutes. When administered by the intracoronary route, only small doses of nitroglycerin (100 μg in the right coronary, 150 μg in the left coronary artery) are needed to effect maximal epicardial coronary dilatation, and these doses have a minimal impact on systemic hemodynamics.[84] A 400-μg sublingual dose of nitroglycerin also causes maximal dilatation of the conduit coronary arteries. Nitroglycerin administered into the coronary ostium also has very brief effects on the microcirculation (usually causing a 1.5- to 2.5-fold increase in coronary blood flow lasting less than 2 minutes), but it causes negligible changes in blood flow when given by intravenous infusion or by mouth.[86, 87]

It should be remembered that the nitrate response in the large coronary arteries is not complete for 2 minutes after intracoronary administration and 4 minutes after a sublingual dose. Additionally, patients undergoing angiography are often intravascular volume–depleted because oral intake has been withheld for some time. This can lead to an increased sensitivity to nitrate-induced venodilatation and transient hypotension. Since coronary caliber is dependent on distending pressure, the reproducibility of coronary angiographically defined measurements of coronary diameter over time is dependent on maintenance of arterial pressure.[88] In patients without heart failure, saline solution is often given before nitroglycerin administration to blunt the fall in arterial pressure.

Special Situations

LEFT MAIN CORONARY STENOSIS

Coronary angiography in patients with stenosis of the left main coronary artery is associated with significantly higher incidence of complications.[89, 90] Left main stenosis occurs in 2 to 11 percent of patients undergoing angiography but accounts for a significantly greater fraction of mortality associated with the procedure.[90] A procedural mortality rate of 0.75 percent was found in patients with left main coronary stenosis in the Coronary Artery Surgery Study.[91] Myocardial infarction, persistent angina, profound hypotension, and ventricular fibrillation also can occur during or immediately after angiography in patients with left main coronary stenosis. The likelihood of complications is greater in patients with angina within 24 hours of catheterization and if the stenosis is in the proximal left main coronary (within 6 mm of the angiographic catheter tip).[89]

Complications can be minimized by rapidly identifying the presence of left main stenosis, which occurs more often in patients with widespread, severe atherosclerosis and may be associated with pressure damping on left coronary cannulation. When left main stenosis is suspected, a "cusp" injection about the ostium may identify its presence and morphology. When a significant left main stenosis is present, nonionic contrast medium should be used and the number of angiograms should be limited to only those views required to identify the vessels needing bypass grafts. A catheter tip shape that will not deeply cannulate the ostium should be used. If the pressure at the catheter tip always damps on left main cannulation, the catheter may need to be withdrawn between injections, although repeated cannulation of a stenotic left main may increase the possibility of catheter-induced injury. If adequate filling can be obtained, a nonselective cusp injection should be used. The pulmonary capillary wedge pressure monitoring during angiography can be important in patients with severe stenosis or reduced left ventricular function because contrast material may precipitously reduce left ventricular function. If the wedge pressure rises significantly, angiography should be stopped until hemodynamics are controlled.

Coronary cannulation causes endothelial denudation, which may be responsible in part for the ischemic complications of angiography in this patient group. After angiography, patients with a significant (>50 percent) left main stenosis should be monitored because of the higher frequency of ischemia and hemodynamic deterioration over the following 24 hours. Semiurgent revascularization should be considered after angiography in patients with severe left main stenosis (>90 percent), particularly if the lesion is in the proximal left main.

HEART FAILURE AND ABNORMAL LEFT VENTRICULAR FUNCTION

Coronary angiography always causes a transient reduction in left ventricular function. The decrease in diastolic compliance usually exceeds the effect on systolic contraction. Therefore, it is expected that angiography will increase the ventricular end-diastolic filling pressure in all patients. Those patients with preexisting increases in filling pressures may develop frank pulmonary edema during or shortly after angiography because of the reduction in compliance and the concomitant volume load from hypertonic contrast material and other fluids given during angiography. In patients with marked left heart failure or an inability to lie flat because of high left atrial pressure, diuresis should be accomplished before angiography if possible.

Nonionic, low-osmolar contrast agents have a less pronounced effect on myocardial function and intravascular volume than do ionic agents and should be used in patients with significantly elevated left heart filling pressures. In addition, in patients with poor compensation, the pulmonary artery wedge pressure should be monitored during angiography. If the mean wedge pressure rises above 20 mm Hg, angiography should be stopped and appropriate steps should be taken to reduce the filling pressures (e.g., administration of nitrates or diuretics, afterload reduction, intra-aortic balloon pump). Assiduous attention to the wedge pressure can prevent pulmonary edema and emergency intubation.

SHOCK

Coronary angiography in patients with cardiogenic shock is challenging. In most patients, placement of an intra-aortic balloon pump before angiography is important for stabilization and to prevent hemodynamic collapse during angiography. The balloon pump increases diastolic coronary blood flow in addition to improving systemic blood flow.[92] Nonionic contrast media should be used routinely, and the minimal number of contrast medium injections necessary to plan treatment should be obtained. Special care should be taken in cannulation of the left main coronary artery because of the increased frequency of left main stenosis in patients with cardiogenic shock.

AORTIC DILATATION

Aortic root dilatation, common in patients with aortic valve disease, prolonged hypertension, and Marfan's syndrome, presents a particular challenge for coronary cannulation (Amplatz, Judkins). Large curve left coronary catheters are required (e.g., Judkins left 5 to 7 curve, Amplatz left 3 curve). Right coronary cannulation can be especially problematic because the root is enlarged, elongated, and horizontal. Catheter manipulation can be difficult because of associated tortuosity of the descending aorta and peripheral vessels. Occasionally, an Amplatz left curve or a specially steamed catheter may be needed to cannulate the right coronary. The rapid coronary blood flow associated with hypertrophy from aortic valve disease or hypertension makes it essential to use a catheter of adequate caliber to deliver a rapid injection of contrast material (which should be warmed to 37°C to reduce viscosity and the effects of cold contrast medium–induced hypothermia on the myocardium).

TRANSPLANTATION

After transplantation, the majority of patients undergo annual surveillance angiography to detect transplant-related vasculopathy. Several factors are unique to transplanted hearts.[93] The aortic anastomosis causes a ridge in the ascending aorta, making it important to pass the Judkins left coronary catheter nearly to the sinus of Valsalva to avoid the catheter being hung up on the ridge as it is advanced to the left coronary ostium. The transplanted heart is usually rotated clockwise (from the diaphragmatic perspective), and the left coronary ostium is more posterior and the right ostium more anterior than usual. Additionally, the ascending aorta is often longer and more horizontal in its more proximal segment. Frequently, the right coronary artery is better cannulated from a right anterior oblique (RAO) projection and may require a catheter that can reach more anteriorly, such as a Judkins right 5 curve or Amplatz right 2 or left 1 curve.

Outpatient Angiography

Although once performed exclusively as an inpatient procedure, a large fraction of angiography procedures can now be performed in the outpatient setting.[94–98] This has been made possible by smaller, more well-constructed catheters, better experience by operators, and concerns over the costs of angiography. Outpatient angiography generally has a 25 percent lower hospital cost, but it places some strains on preangiography patient preparation.[94, 98] It also imposes more responsibility on the patient for precatheterization medication and site preparation and postangiography catheter insertion site observation.

Outpatient angiography requires selection of patients who are expected to have a low risk of late complications. Patients with acute ischemic syndromes (unstable angina, infarction) should not go home immediately after angiography because of the risk of recurrent ischemic episodes.[97] Patients with left main or severe three-vessel coronary disease, severe heart failure, bleeding diathesis, and severe aortic valve stenosis should generally be observed longer after contrast medium angiography.[97] About 10 to 12 percent of patients undergoing outpatient angiography are admitted to the hospital after the procedure, 4 to 5 percent for observation after a complication and the remainder for a surgical procedure (e.g., bypass surgery).[94, 95, 98]

Coronary angiography has been performed in mobile truck trailers stationed at smaller hospitals.[99, 100] With the exclusion of higher-risk patients through proper patient selection, the complications of *mobile angiography* appear not to be increased and patient satisfaction may be improved.[100] Several logistical problems remain. Since a significant fraction of patients undergo a revascularization procedure based on the information gained from the angiogram, many (if not the majority) patients will need to travel to a larger hospital anyway, obviating the advantages of mobile angiography. In addition, patients who subsequently have angioplasty may need to have two procedures (at two hospitals) instead of proceeding with angioplasty in the same procedure as the angiogram. More information will be needed to know whether catheterization in mobile structures is cost effective.

COMPLICATIONS OF CORONARY ANGIOGRAPHY

Coronary arteriography is generally a safe procedure, but serious complications can occur. The overall incidence of complications and mortality (Table 30–1) increases directly with the extent of coronary artery disease (particularly left main coronary stenosis), the presence of coexistent significant valvular disease, a reduced ventricular ejection fraction, reduced functional state, and advancing age.[91, 101–104] The complications fall into several groups: those resulting from arterial cannulation, embolization from the aorta, catheter-induced coronary arterial spasm or dissection, arrhythmias, allergic-type reactions from drugs and radiographic contrast material, and angiography-induced deterioration in hemodynamics.

Complications of Arterial Cannulation

Peripheral Vascular Complications

Arterial cannulation performed by the Seldinger method usually causes endothelial denudation at the site of catheter or sheath insertion. During arterial puncture, the needle may also pass into or through the posterior wall of the artery, and advancement of a guide wire into the posterior wall can result in arterial dissection. Fortunately, the arterial flap proceeds against the flow of blood and is usually sealed rather than propelled down the vessel by the arterial pulse. Dissection, along with endothelial injury, may promote local thrombosis and arterial occlusion, however. Perforation of peripheral arteries by a guide wire or catheter is uncommon but probably occurs more frequently in patients with tortuous vessels and when stiff wires or catheters are used.

The development of a hematoma, arterial pseudoaneurysm, or arteriovenous fistula after arterial catheter removal remains an important and probably underreported complication. The importance of immediately obtaining adequate hemostasis cannot be overemphasized. Once a small perivascular hematoma has formed, it becomes more difficult to apply effective pressure to the puncture site because applied force is spread equally throughout the hematoma. Conversely, prolonged overcompression of the site can occlude the vessel, leading to vascular stasis and thrombosis. The affected extremity should be immobilized for at least 4 hours if a catheter of 6 French size is used. Sandbags applied over the arteriotomy site are ineffective in preventing complications. A collagen plug device, implanted into the puncture site above the artery, has been developed and appears to markedly reduce the time needed for hemostasis.[105]

The incidence of arterial cannulation site complications is higher in women, the elderly, in the presence of peripheral vascular disease, when blood flow is reduced (e.g., low cardiac output state or catheter occlusion of the vessel), and with brachial access or a low femoral puncture site, probably related to the smaller size of these vessels.[102, 106–109] Although common sense suggests that arterial complications would be less frequent if smaller catheters were used and arterial access time was minimized, an increase in vascular complications has been shown only for catheters larger than 8 French (>2.5-mm outer diameter).[107] Patients with synthetic (e.g., Dacron) femoral artery grafts may also have a higher incidence of cannulation-related complications, although the reported experience suggests that cannulation of grafts that have been in place for at

TABLE 30–1 Incidence of Complications After Elective Coronary Angiography

	Bourassa and Noble[101] 1970–1974	Davis et al[91] 1975–1976		Kennedy[102] 1979–1980	Noto et al[103] 1990
Route	F	F	B	F or B	F or B
Number of patients	5250	6328	1187	53,581	59,972
Death (%)	0.23	0.15	0.50	0.14	0.11
Myocardial infarction (%)	0.09	0.22	0.42	0.07	0.05
Vascular complication (%)	0.85	0.36	2.8	0.57*	0.43*
Thrombosis (%)	0.68	0.2	1.9	0.23	NS
Dissection/perforation (%)	0.17	0.1	0.9	0.04	NS
Stroke/TIA (%)	0.13	0.02	NS	0.07	0.07
Embolic complication (%)	0.07	0.08	0.17	NS	NS
Arrhythmia (%)	1.23	0.63†	NS	0.56	0.38
Ventricular fibrillation/tachycardia	0.40	NS	NS	0.44	NS
Asystole/severe bradycardia	0.25	NS	NS	0.09	NS
Contrast reaction (%)	NS	NS	NS	NS	0.37
Hemodynamic deterioration	0.1	NS	NS	NS	0.26

Abbreviations: B, brachial artery approach; F, femoral artery approach; NS, not specified; TIA, transient ischemic attack.
*True incidence is probably underestimated because only "in laboratory" complications were reported.
†All patients.

least several months is safe.[32, 33] Heparin anticoagulation during the catheterization reduces the incidence of arterial thrombosis and the need for surgical embolectomy but may increase the incidence of hematoma formation.[74, 75, 107]

Septic complications (access site infection and bacteremia) are very uncommon and associated almost exclusively with prolonged cannulation or repeated instrumentation of the same site within a short time.[15, 110] The most common organism is *Staphylococcus aureus,* although other staphylococcal species, streptococci, gram-negative organisms, and anaerobic species can be involved.[110] The mortality associated with bacteremic episodes can be significant.

The development of Doppler echocardiographic methods for imaging these complications has revealed that small femoral artery pseudoaneurysms are more common after femoral angiography than had been clinically suspected. Additionally, the incidence of pseudoaneurysms and arteriovenous fistulas may have increased with the more frequent use of aspirin, anticoagulants, and thrombolytic drugs. Many close spontaneously within 1 to 2 months.[111] Until recently, all persistent femoral artery pseudoaneurysms were repaired surgically because late enlargement and rupture can occur. It has been shown more recently that prolonged compression (average 30 minutes) during ultrasound imaging can be used to close more than 90 percent of pseudoaneurysms and small arteriovenous fistulas.[112, 113]

EMBOLIZATION

Embolization of arterial circulation can occur from catheter-induced dislodgment of atherosclerotic plaque or vascular thrombus (e.g., clot in an abdominal aneurysm), dislodgment of left ventricular thrombus (e.g., in a ventricular aneurysm or a recently infarcted ventricle), and from debris or clot extruded from an improperly aspirated angiographic catheter. Catheter-induced embolization can lead to a variety of complications, depending on the target organ and makeup of the embolus.[114–121]

Systemic embolization is more likely when the aorta has severe atherosclerosis or mural thrombus, when a large abdominal aortic aneurysm is present (typically containing thrombus), and in elderly patients. A study of patients undergoing cardiopulmonary bypass showed that transesophageal echocardiographic identification of protruding atheroma in the aorta may identify patients at risk for embolic complications and that pedunculated, mobile aortic masses may be a source of catheterization-related embolism.[122, 123] The brachial approach is preferred in patients predisposed to peripheral embolization unless significant disease in the aortic arch or upper extremity vessels is present.

The sequelae of systemic emboli vary widely, from no symptoms to severe tissue necrosis. Thrombotic embolism frequently results in a loss of the peripheral pulse and occlusion of larger branch arteries that can be treated by embolectomy, anticoagulation, and in some cases, thrombolytic drugs. Cholesterol emboli affect 58- to 800-μm-diameter vessels, and the syndrome is characterized by skin changes of livedo reticularis, tissue ischemia with intact peripheral pulses, renal dysfunction, eosinophilia, and an elevated erythrocyte sedimentation rate.[114–121] The renal insufficiency associated with cholesterol embolization can cause immediate anuria but, more frequently, leads to delayed oliguria. It can be differentiated from contrast medium–induced renal failure by its minimal reversibility (contrast medium nephropathy usually is reversible), associated skin findings of embolization, and eosinophilia. Embolization of the splanchnic bed can cause abdominal pain, ileus, or bowel or spleen infarction, usually with onset of symptoms within hours of catheterization. Treatment for cholesterol embolization consists of supportive care. Anticoagulation is ineffective.

Large peripheral air embolization can occur after accidental injection of air or, more commonly, from inspiration of air through a central venous access catheter in the jugular or subclavian venous systems. Venous air embolisms larger than 50 to 100 ml can cause acute pulmonary hypertension and hypoxemia.[124] Arterial air embolism can lead to profound transient tissue ischemia, including stroke, myocardial ischemia, and cardiac arrest.[125] The immediate treatment is to tilt the patient head-down (Trendelenburg position) and on the left side to prevent air from rising to the head or passage from the venous system to the left atrium via a patent foramen ovale. Venous air can pass to the arterial circulation without a clear defect connecting the two circulations, presumably through the pulmonary arteriovenous shunts.[125] Aspiration of air with a catheter in the right atrium or ventricle may be partially effective.[126] Breathing 100 percent oxygen may help treat hypoxemia associated with pulmonary artery flow obstruction. For large emboli, a hyperbaric chamber may be useful if employed promptly.[127]

Neurologic Complications

Neurologic complications of coronary angiography include local brachial nerve injury from brachial artery cannulation, ulnar nerve compression during prolonged procedures, transient central ischemic attacks, and stroke. Significant neurologic events are uncommon, although they are probably underreported (see Table 30–1) because the vast majority resolve within 24 to 72 hours after the procedure.[128–130] Most central ischemic neurologic events occur in the posterior distribution, although any territory can be affected.[128–131] In one careful series, transient visual disturbance occurred in 1 percent of patients.[130] Women and patients with an anginal syndrome and normal coronary angiograms were more commonly affected.[130] The most likely mechanism of central neurologic events is embolism of clot or atheromatous debris from the aorta or cardiac chambers, although vasospasm and transient hypotension during angiography may also be operative in some patients.

Transient cortical blindness can result from contrast administration. This syndrome lasts for 1 to 2 days and resolves spontaneously. Brain imaging (computed tomography or magnetic resonance imaging) is normal.[131a]

Coronary Artery Complications and Myocardial Infarction

Catheter-induced spasm is common in the right coronary artery but uncommon in the left.[132–135] For the most part, the spasm occurs at the catheter tip and may be related to mechanical traction on the artery. Rarely, catheter-induced spasm distal to the catheter tip has been observed. There is no proven significance of catheter-induced spasm, although some have postulated that patients with catheter-induced spasm may be more prone to spontaneous spasm.[132, 135] Catheter-induced spasm can usually be prevented by administration of nitrates and by using an angiographic catheter that does not tent the artery.

Myocardial infarction is usually caused by catheter-induced coronary injury or embolization from the catheter or left ventricular thrombus. Catheter-induced arterial injury is usually caused by the tip of the catheter burrowing into the arterial plaque or media raising an arterial flap that can be extended further by blood flow or by contrast medium injection through the catheter into the arterial wall.[136] The most common and important sites of catheter-induced injury are the coronary arterial ostia, where dissection can lead to thrombosis, spasm, or an extensive spiral dissection down the vessel.[137]

Normal coronary arteries and arteries with ostial lesions or acute angle origins are more likely to suffer catheter-induced injury. The occurrence of catheter injury can be reduced by carefully cannulating the ostia with soft-tipped catheters, monitoring the pressure at the catheter tip (pressure at the catheter tip will be damped if the catheter has burrowed into the wall), and advancing the catheter to the ascending aorta using a flexible guide wire (to prevent the tip from shoveling into the vessel wall). Ostial coronary stenosis is a rare complication of coronary cannulation.[138]

Coronary artery embolization usually results from injection of air or debris from within the catheter. Small air emboli typically cause ischemia for 5 to 10 minutes. On angiography, blood flow to the embolized segment is slow, but the epicardial arteries appear to be intact and no filling defect is seen. Thrombotic emboli, however, almost always lead to occlusion of an artery visible on angiography. Infarction is common, and rapid reperfusion with angioplasty can be effective in limiting injury. Coronary cholesterol embolism can cause a picture similar to either thrombotic or air embolism, but the effects are usually not reversible. In one series, cholesterol emboli were seen at autopsy in 26 percent of patients undergoing coronary angiography, but most emboli were in the myocardium.[120] This underscores the importance of aspirating the coronary catheter and discarding the aspirate before intracoronary injection. Aspiration of shimmering cholesterol crystals is not rare.

Drug Reactions and Toxicity

Radiographic Contrast Material

Although usually well tolerated, iodinated contrast material can have deleterious consequences related to its normal physiologic effects and to allergic-type reactions. The negative inotropic effects on ventricular function and intravascular volume expansion can lead to hemodynamic decompensation, primarily in patients with reduced ventricular reserve (either diastolic or systolic) and ischemic syndromes.[46, 48, 61, 139] The effects on the conduction system can cause transient severe sinus bradycardia or heart block, and the effects on ventricular repolarization can cause ventricular fibrillation (see later).

RENAL DYSFUNCTION

Contrast agents can also cause renal dysfunction, which is usually transient but can be severe. A transient increase in glomerular filtration, an osmotic diuresis, and proteinuria all occur soon after contrast medium administration.[140] Clinically evident renal dysfunction with increased serum creatinine concentration and reduced urine output, however, occurs 48 to 72 hours later. The etiology of contrast medium–induced renal failure is unclear, but transient renal ischemia, physical obstruction of the renal tubules, superoxide radical release, and endothelial injury have been proposed.

Patients with diabetic nephropathy, preexisting renal dysfunction, dehydration, low cardiac output, and, possibly, multiple myeloma are predisposed to develop contrast medium–induced renal failure, which ranges from an asymptomatic increase in serum creatinine concentration to frank anuria.[141–144] The likelihood rises sharply with the amount of contrast medium administered, although renal dysfunction is uncommon in patients with a serum creatinine concentration < 150 μmol/L (<1.7 mg/dl).[142] In diabetics with preexisting renal insufficiency (serum creatinine concentration > 150 μmol/L), Parfrey and associates[142] found that the risk of a 25 percent increase in creatinine concentration was 7.2 percent. In nondiabetic patients with mild renal insufficiency (creatinine 150 to 250 μmol/L), there was no significant reduction in renal function after angiography using small-to-moderate contrast medium volumes (<200 ml). The reported incidence of renal failure after contrast medium exposure varies widely, but nearly all investigators find that the likelihood of a transient increase in creatinine and oliguria rises sharply in patients with a creatinine concentration greater than 250 μmol/L.[141–145]

The primary method for preventing contrast media–induced renal failure is to limit the amount of contrast media used to the minimum required to obtain an adequate study and to avoid administering contrast media to dehydrated patients. Nonionic media probably reduce the risk of contrast nephropathy, but the degree of protection offered is relatively modest.[46, 48, 145, 146] Several studies suggest that administration of mannitol (e.g., 25 g in 250 ml of 155 mM saline solution) to increase urine flow before and during angiography can substantially reduce the risk of renal failure in predisposed patients.[147, 148] Simultaneous administration of the loop diuretic furosemide has been proposed, and one small, preliminary study found a beneficial effect.[149] In general, however, there is no convincing evidence that either mannitol or furosemide reduces the incidence of renal failure after contrast media administration.

ALLERGIC-TYPE REACTIONS

Contrast material can also give rise to allergic-type reactions, but the mechanisms are poorly understood. Nonspecific mast cell degranulation and activation of complement have been implicated, but true immunoglobulin (Ig) E–

related allergy is rare. Contrast medium reactions vary from simple urticaria to nausea to an anaphylactoid reaction characterized by hypotension and bronchospasm. Patients with a prior history of contrast medium reaction or multiple allergies (including seafood) and patients who receive ionic contrast media (especially with a high sodium content) are more likely to have a contrast agent reaction.[47, 150, 151]

Patients with a history of allergic-type reactions should be treated with corticosteroid drugs the day before the procedure.[150] We typically give prednisone (60 mg orally) the night before the procedure, and before angiography, give another dose (30 mg prednisone orally or 250 mg hydrocortisone intravenously) and an antihistamine (e.g., hydroxyzine, 50 mg intravenously). In patients predisposed to a contrast medium reaction, administration of prednisone at least 12 hours before angiography reduces the incidence of mild-to-moderate reactions by half. Treatment on the day of angiography only has no effect.[150] An additional reduction in risk of less severe reactions (e.g., bradycardia, mild hypotension, brief angina) will occur if nonionic contrast medium is utilized.[151] Although H_2-receptor antagonists (e.g., cimetidine) have also been used to prevent reactions, their efficacy is unclear and probably minimal.[152]

Treatment of a reaction is tailored to the symptom. Urticaria is treated with intravenous antihistamines. Nausea, possibly related to intestinal mast cell release, can be lessened with antiemetic compounds. Hypotension is treated with vasopressor drugs, large doses of corticosteroid drugs (e.g., 1 g methylprednisolone), and antihistamines. Bronchospasm is treated with theophylline, inhaled $beta_2$-adrenoreceptor agonists, and corticosteroids.

Anticoagulants

The second most frequent important source of allergic reactions occurs in association with the anticoagulation used during angiography. Protamine sulfate, given to bind heparin and reverse its effects before decannulation, can be associated with several adverse reactions, including urticaria, severe hypotension, bradycardia, bronchospasm, and noncardiogenic pulmonary edema.[153] Severe reactions can require vasopressor drug support for several days. The etiology of protamine reactions may vary among patients. IgE and IgG antibodies, complement activation, direct myocardial depression, increases in endothelial permeability owing to interaction with membrane-bound heparan sulfates, and protamine-stimulated nitric oxide release from the endothelium have been postulated.[82, 154, 155] IgG antibodies are the predominant mechanism in patients without prior protamine exposure.[82] In one series, protamine given after catheterization reduced white blood cell count by an average of 23 ± 4 percent.[156]

Patients with recent protamine exposure or a "fish allergy," diabetic patients exposed to NPH insulin and patients with $alpha_1$-antitrypsin deficiency are particularly sensitive to protamine.[153] Additionally, protamine, when given rapidly to any patient, transiently reduces vascular resistance and can cause hypotension (possibly related to protamine-stimulated nitric oxide release from the endothelium).[155] To minimize complications, a small test dose of protamine can be given into the arterial cannula. If the patient has local erythema or hypotension, the drug should be avoided.

Heparin can result in thrombocytopenia that can be dependent on the type of heparin used (e.g., bovine, porcine).[157] Arterial aggregation and thrombosis can also be caused by heparin, although reactions from brief exposure are rare.[158]

Anesthetics

True allergies to local "-caine-type" anesthetics are *very* rare. Patients sometimes claim to be allergic to "novocaine" as a result of a syncopal episode during a prior procedure (usually neurally mediated syncope) or a complication related to rapid or excessive lidocaine administration (e.g., seizure, dysarthria). These "reactions" are not allergic in nature, and based on the exceptionally low incidence of true lidocaine allergy, we usually continue to administer lidocaine local anesthesia unless the patient gives a clear history consistent with an IgE-mediated reaction. To date, no patient with a "lidocaine allergy" has had an adverse reaction. The maximal subcutaneous dose should not exceed 5 mg/kg, and solutions containing epinephrine should not be used. In patients with a bona fide allergic reaction or local sensitivity to lidocaine, the offending agent is usually the preservative methylparaben. In these patients, lidocaine without the preservative (intravenous-use lidocaine) or procainamide (1 to 2 mg/ml) can be substituted.

Arrhythmias

Arrhythmias during angiography can occur from abrasion of the conduction system by catheters, contrast material–induced changes in repolarization, reflex-mediated changes in cardiac neural traffic to the heart, and transient myocardial ischemia from hemodynamic deterioration. The left bundle branch of the conduction system courses near the surface of the left ventricular septum and can be injured transiently during cannulation of the left ventricle.[159, 160] The right bundle branch is located near the tricuspid annulus and can be rendered dysfunctional by a right heart catheter (particularly if the catheter is rubbed against the superior annulus repeatedly). In a patient with a preexisting contralateral bundle branch block, complete heart block can occur.[159, 160] In these patients, the immediate availability of cardiac pacing (externally or by catheter) should be ascertained before catheterization.

Contrast media can induce sinus bradycardia, sinus node block, and atrioventricular node block by two mechanisms. The hyperosmolar and chemical properties of contrast media cause activation of ventricular afferent chemoreceptors that reflexively trigger a parasympathetic surge, reducing sinus and atrioventricular node repolarization.[52, 53, 63] The reflex is blocked by muscarinic receptor blockade with atropine. Neurally mediated syncope can also complicate angiography, particularly when the patient is dehydrated and experiences pain. Contrast material may also directly depress conduction tissue repolarization and transiently slow heart rate. Vigorous coughing can maintain blood pressure but does not hasten clearance of contrast material from the coronary circulation.[161]

Prolongation of the ventricular refractory period by contrast media can initiate ventricular fibrillation. Fibrillation occurs more commonly after right than left coronary injection, and the incidence is less with "nonionic" contrast material and "ionic" contrast medium that does not contain calcium-binding agents.[41–44, 49] The probability of ventricular fibrillation is also higher if an excessive volume of contrast material is injected in a single dose.

Hemodynamic Deterioration

Although catheterization of the coronary arteries does not by itself change ventricular function (unless the catheters obstruct blood flow in patients with ostial coronary stenosis or vasospasm), injection of contrast medium causes a reduction in diastolic compliance and can reduce systolic function. In patients with normal or near-normal ventricular function, the ventricular effects of contrast medium are not clinically important. Patients with markedly reduced systolic function (ejection fraction < 35 percent) or elevated ventricular filling pressure (regardless of systolic function), however, must be approached with caution, for these are the patients who develop pulmonary edema after contrast medium injection.[46, 48, 61] We routinely ascertain the left ventricular end-diastolic or pulmonary artery wedge pressures before angiography in patients with a prior history of congestive left heart failure, pulmonary edema, or severe left ventricular dysfunction. If the pulmonary wedge pressure is more than 20 mm Hg, it should be reduced before contrast medium injection and the pulmonary wedge or mean pressure should be monitored during the angiogram. If the pressure rises significantly, contrast medium injections should be withheld. It is important to remember that contrast medium can affect ventricular diastolic function for up to 20 minutes. Additionally, intravenous nitroglycerin or nitroprusside infusion during angiography can be used to rapidly reduce filling pressures and facilitate angiography.

Coronary Anatomy and Radiographic Evaluation

Angiographic visualization of the heart, great vessels, and coronary arteries is fundamental to the accurate diagnosis of the wide spectrum of cardiovascular diseases that are characterized by morphologic abnormalities. Whereas the angiographic evaluation of the past several decades was based solely on a visual assessment of the anatomy, today this visual assessment is frequently aided by computer-assisted quantitation of vessel dimensions and physiologic information, allowing assessment of the functional effects of the anatomic abnormalities.

Coronary Anatomy

Coronary Ostia

In humans as well as all birds, reptiles, and mammals, the arterial supply to the heart arises from two ascending aortic branches. The position of these branches that transverse the atrioventricular and interventricular sulci in the shape of a crown led early anatomists to designate the vessels as coronary (or "crown") arteries.[162–163a]

The coronary ostia are normally located in the right and left aortic sinuses of Valsalva. The ostia originate at the center of each sinus, close to the free edge of the aortic cusp and just below or no more than 1 cm above the superior edge of the aortic cusp. Ostia located more than 1 cm above the cusp edge are abnormal, occurring in less than 3 percent of patients.[164] Although two coronary ostia (one in each sinus) are the rule, three or four separate ostia are considered normal variants. In up to 30 percent of cases, the artery to the pulmonary conus (conal artery) originates from a separate ostium rather than its usual position as a branch from the proximal right coronary artery. Absence of a left main coronary trunk resulting in separate aortic origins for the left anterior descending and circumflex arteries occurs in 0.5 to 1 percent of patients.[164] Most commonly, these two ostia are closely juxtaposed with the dual ostia, existing as a "double barrel." Widely separated left anterior descending and circumflex ostia are uncommon.

Orientation of Coronary Trunks

The anatomic configuration of the aortic-coronary junctions has made careful quantitative measurements of the normal coronary-aortic branching angles difficult. Using corrosion casts obtained by injecting casting material through the aorta under physiologic perfusion pressure, Zamir and Sinclair[165] measured coronary-aortic branching angles in both horizontal and vertical planes in normal hearts obtained at autopsy. The mean horizontal branching angle was 25 degrees (range 0 to 55 degrees) for the left main coronary artery and 35 degrees (range 0 to 88 degrees) for the right main coronary artery. The mean vertical branching angle was 102 degrees (range 77 to 145 degrees) for the left main coronary artery and 69 degrees (range 34 to 110 degrees) for the right main coronary artery. These measured branching angles correlate poorly with what would be considered optimal on theoretical grounds. Such data suggest that this geometry reflects more the anatomy of the aortic root rather than the fluid dynamic principles that usually govern arterial branching.

Left Main Coronary Artery

The left main coronary artery has a single initial trunk in 92 to 96 percent of autopsy cases.[162, 163, 166] The length of the left main coronary artery, as derived from pathologic examinations, is 1.0 ± 0.3 cm.[167] Premortem and postmortem angiographic studies have reported that patients with bicuspid aortic valves have a higher incidence of short left main coronary arteries[168] and left coronary dominance,[169, 170] although the findings have been refuted by some[167, 171] and affirmed by others.[172] Although angiographic measurements of coronary diameter are probably more accurate than postmortem pathologic studies (owing to changes inherent in the postmortem state), angiographic measurements of coronary length are probably less accurate owing to underestimation of the effects of rotation, angulation, and foreshortening. Virmani and colleagues[167] found no correlation of left main coronary artery length with age, gender, heart weight, extent of coronary disease, or left ventricular wall thickness.

The left main coronary artery consists of three portions: the ostium or origin from the aorta, the midportion, and the distal portion, which includes the bifurcating segments. Histologically, the left main ostium lacks adventitia and has a larger proportion of elastic tissue than any other area in the coronary tree. These anatomic and histologic features may account for some of the differences in the response of the left main coronary artery to interventional procedures. Since the left main ostium lies within the wall of the aorta, it is vulnerable to diseases primarily affecting the aorta: syphilitic aortitis, rheumatoid arthritis, radiation-induced aortitis, and Takayasu's arteritis.[167a]

Left Anterior Descending Artery

The left anterior descending artery is a direct continuation of the left main coronary artery, with its course along the anterior interventricular sulcus. Several normal variations of the length and distribution of this vessel have been recognized. It is not essential for the anterior descending artery to reach the cardiac apex or to have well-defined septal or diagonal branches to qualify as the anterior descending artery, although both are usually true.[164] The number and prominence of diagonal branches are variable. The diagonal branch in its proximal portion may give rise to septal perforating branches. This is especially likely in cases of chronic ischemic disease with anterior descending occlusion. Hence, the angiographic recognition of a septal branch does not conclusively identify the left anterior descending artery. The cardiac apex is usually perfused by the anterior descending artery but may be supplied by an unusually long diagonal branch or right posterior descending artery.

Left Circumflex Artery

The left circumflex artery is also a continuation of the left main artery. Its initial course is in the left posterior atrioventricular groove, circumscribing the mitral valve. The extent and distribution of the left circumflex artery and right coronary artery are generally reciprocal. If the left circumflex artery is extensive in its supply to the posterior and inferior walls of the heart, the right coronary artery will usually be small, with fewer branches to these regions. The variability of this reciprocal arrangement is great, with some hearts exhibiting a dual vascular supply to the same anatomic regions (e.g., the inferior septum) from both the right coronary and the circumflex arteries.

Ramus Intermedius Branch

In some hearts, the left main coronary artery exhibits a trifurcation at its origin instead of the usual bifurcation. This third artery, termed *ramus intermedius* (or *diagonalis*), acts functionally as a circumflex branch, supplying a portion of the obtuse margin of the heart. In a pathologic study of 150 hearts, Baptista and coworkers[172] found that the left main coronary artery exhibited a bifurcation configuration in 55 percent, trifurcation (with the ramus branch) in 39 percent, and a quadrification (ramus intermedius and a separate diagonal branch) in 7 percent. A trifurcation pattern was most commonly found (60 percent) in the hearts of female nonwhites. The length of the ramus varied from 20 to 50 mm, and its relative length varied from 21 to 50 percent of the length of the left ventricle.

Right Coronary Artery

The right coronary artery runs in the anterior atrioventricular groove and circumscribes the tricuspid valve. The first branch of the right coronary artery is usually to the right ventricular outflow tract (the conal branch), although this artery often arises separately or from a common aortic ostium with the right coronary artery. In midcourse, the right coronary artery normally supplies branches to the right ventricle that usually reach the acute margin of the heart (so-called acute marginal branches). In a small number of cases, the right coronary artery may have an anomalous intra-atrial subendocardial course.[173] This unusual condition has no known adverse clinical outcomes and is generally recognized only at autopsy. The anatomy of the distal right coronary artery, particularly its size and course over the left ventricle, is quite variable. In 50 to 60 percent of patients, the right coronary artery bifurcates at the crux of the atrioventricular groove and the interventricular septum, giving rise to the posterior descending branch (which runs in the posterior interventricular sulcus to meet the anterior descending artery coming from the anterior sulcus) and the posterolateral branch (which perfuses the posterolateral left ventricle). In other cases, however, the posterior descending branch may arise before the crux, either at the acute margin (13 percent) or at an intermediate position (19 percent).[174] In 10 to 20 percent of patients, none of the left ventricular branches arises from the right coronary artery, coming instead from the terminal portion of the circumflex artery (see Coronary Dominance, later).[166, 175]

Sinus Node Artery

In 51 to 70 percent of humans, the sinus node artery arises from the right coronary artery.[174, 175] In contrast, the sinus node artery of swine and dogs almost always (90 to 100 percent) arises from the right coronary artery.[176, 177] The sinus node artery arises from the circumflex artery in the remainder of patients. The sinus node artery is usually the second branch of the right coronary artery (excluding the conal branch) and is generally the first and largest atrial branch. When the sinus node artery does not originate from the right coronary artery, it is usually a branch of the circumflex artery. In an anatomic study of 300 human hearts, Nerantzis and Avgoustakis[177] found that the sinus node artery arose from the circumflex artery in 37 percent of cases. Although this circumflex sinus node artery usually arises near the origin of the circumflex artery, in 21 percent of patients with a circumflex artery origin, the artery is an S-shaped vessel that originates from the posterolateral branch of the circumflex artery. This S-shaped sinus node artery can function as a bridge between the right and the left coronary trunks in the case of proximal coronary occlusions.

Atrioventricular Nodal Artery

The atrioventricular nodal artery in humans arises from the right coronary artery in the area of the crux in nearly 90 percent of patients. In the remainder of cases, this artery is a branch of the circumflex artery. This pattern of vascular supply is similar to that seen in swine, but differs greatly from that in the dog.[176] In canines, because of a small nondominant right coronary artery, the atrioventricular nodal artery arises from the left circumflex artery in almost 100 percent of cases.[176, 177]

Vascular Supply to the Interventricular Septum

In over 99 percent of patients, the blood supply to the anterior interventricular septum is from the left anterior descending coronary artery.[178] In the majority of patients, there is no dominant septal artery; rather, the proximal septal vessels are of equal caliber. In 38 percent, a large dominant septal perforator occurs, and this is usually, but not always, the first septal. Septal perforators may exhibit bifurcation or trifurcation. The branching pattern is unordered (e.g., tertiary branches may arise from the primary vessel).[179]

Septal branches from the posterior descending artery, arising from either the right coronary or the left circumflex artery, are the usual vascular supply to the posterior septum. In rare instances, the posterior descending artery may originate from the first septal branch of the anterior descending artery or from an obtuse marginal branch of the circumflex artery. A more common variant, which occurs to differing degrees, is the "wraparound" left anterior descending artery. In such cases, the posterior septum is supplied by the anterior descending artery. Distal left anterior descending occlusion can result in an inferior wall ischemic pattern on the electrocardiogram.

Coronary Dominance

The term *coronary dominance* was introduced by Schlesinger[180] in 1940. The "dominant" coronary artery is the one that gives rise to the posterior descending artery, traversing the posterior interventricular sulcus and supplying the posterior part of the ventricular septum and often the posterolateral wall of the left ventricle as well.[181] The right coronary artery is dominant in approximately 70 percent of humans.[182] If the circumflex artery terminates in the posterior descending artery, left dominance is present. This is seen in 15 percent. In the remaining 15 percent, the posterior septum is supplied by branches arising from both the right coronary and the left circumflex artery. In this situation, the circulation is said to be "balanced" (or codominant) and the posterior descending artery is either dual or absent,[181] being supplied by a network of small branches. It should be noted that anatomic dominance does not imply physiologic dominance. Although the right coronary artery is usually dominant, the left coronary artery almost always supplies a greater myocardial mass.[183]

Angiographic Views

The importance of obtaining adequate angiographic views of the coronary arteries cannot be overemphasized. Since the orientation between the planes of the major cardiac grooves and septum are different from the standard anteroposterior and lateral projections utilized for chest roentgenology, oblique views must be used to obtain optimal angiographic visualization of the coronary arteries. An understanding of the orientation of these structures and the coronary vessels in the oblique positions can be difficult for the novice, but several teaching models have been developed to facilitate understanding.[184–186]

We have utilized the following schematic diagram. In Figure 30–9, the eyes represent the line of sight of the

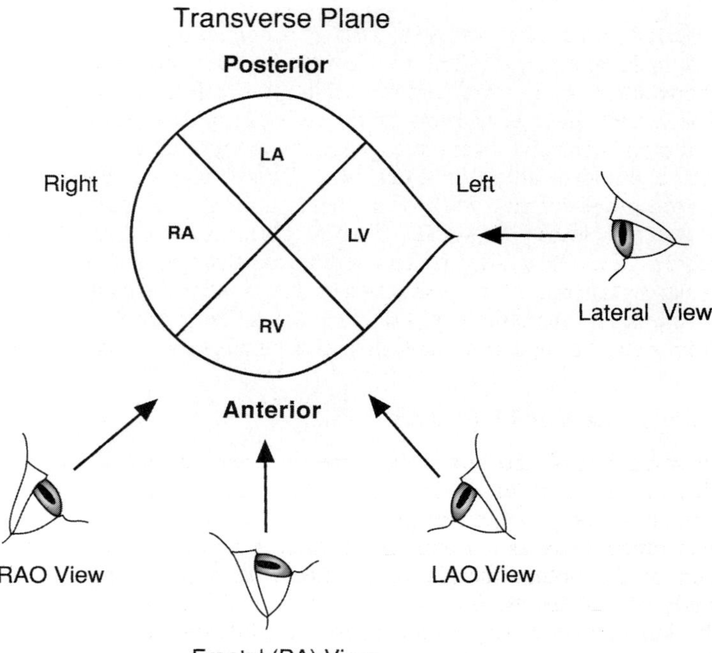

FIGURE 30–9 Schematic diagram depicts cardiac chamber locations as viewed in the four standard radiographic projections: frontal (posteroanterior [PA]), lateral, right anterior oblique (RAO), and left anterior oblique (LAO). The eyes represent the viewer's line of sight. LA, left atrium; LV, left ventricle; RA, right atrium; RV, right ventricle.

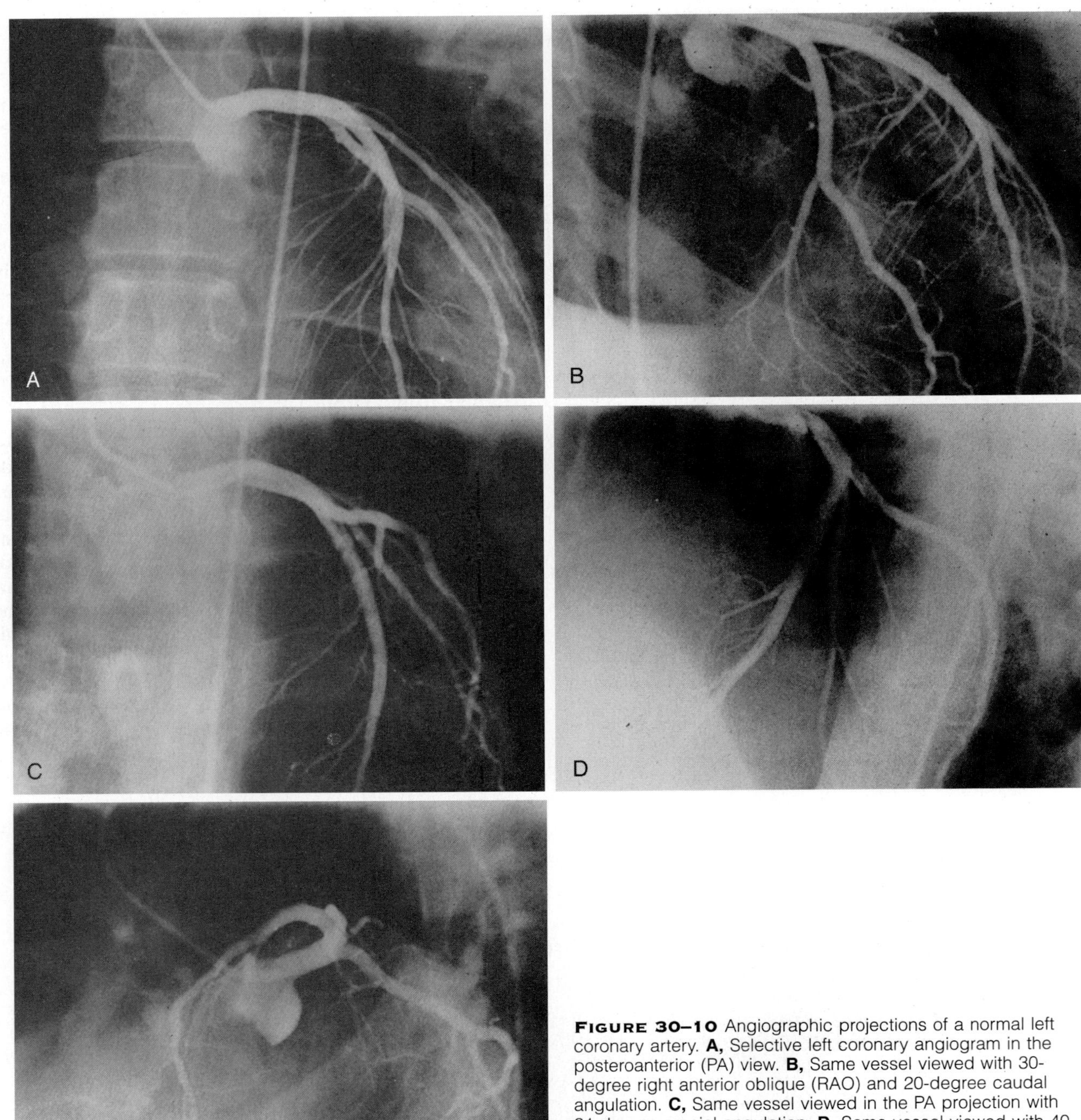

FIGURE 30–10 Angiographic projections of a normal left coronary artery. **A,** Selective left coronary angiogram in the posteroanterior (PA) view. **B,** Same vessel viewed with 30-degree right anterior oblique (RAO) and 20-degree caudal angulation. **C,** Same vessel viewed in the PA projection with 31-degree cranial angulation. **D,** Same vessel viewed with 40-degree left anterior oblique (LAO) and 35-degree cranial angulation. **E,** Same vessel viewed with 30-degree LAO and 30-degree caudal angulation.

viewer. In the LAO projection, the viewer is sighting down the interventricular and interatrial septum. All left-sided cardiac chambers appear to the viewer's right. In the LAO projection, the anterior and posterior descending coronary arteries are seen coursing vertically in the middle of the cardiac silhouette, following the path of the interventricular septum. In the RAO projection, the viewer's line of sight is the atrioventricular groove plane. In this projection, the two atria and the two ventricles are superimposed. The proximal circumflex and proximal right coronary arteries are well visualized as they follow their course in the atrioventricular groove.

The angiographer must evaluate the entire vessel in several different views to avoid the effects of vessel foreshortening that can hide a stenotic lesion and because coronary lesions are frequently eccentric. Although the severity of a coronary stenosis is often reported as the most severe appearance measured in any of the views, physiologic studies show that an integration of lumen stenosis from many views more accurately predicts the degree of blood flow impairment imparted by the lesion.[187] In truth, if the lesion can be well visualized, all views contribute toward assessing stenosis severity. Additionally, when quantitative angiographic methods are employed, coronary lesions are best evaluated in at least two orthogonal projections (e.g., LAO 60 degree and RAO 30 degree) in which the lesion can be seen well in both projections without foreshortening or overlap.[186]

In 1981, Paulin[188] proposed that radiographic projections be named by following the course of the x-ray beam as it passes through the heart. The x-ray gantry can be angled in the horizontal and coronal planes. The position of the imaging device defines the projection. In the LAO projection, the x-ray beam is angled in the horizontal plane such that it is projected from under and to the right of the patient (right posterior) to the image intensifier, which is anterior and to the patient's left. Similarly, the x-ray beam of the RAO view originates in the left posterior aspect and passes to the image tube, which is anterior and rotated to the patient's right. In caudocranial views, the x-ray beam is angled in the coronal (frontal) plane. In the cranial view, the x-ray beam originates caudally and passes through the heart to the image intensifier, which is angled cranially. Conversely, in a caudal projection, the x-ray tube is angled cranially and projects the x-ray beam caudally to the image tube. The use of multiple oblique views in the anterolateral projection in conjunction with angulation in the caudocranial plane has greatly facilitated optimal visualization of coronary lesions and minimized the problem of foreshortening of the coronary arteries.

The use of a "standard set of optimal projections" for coronary angiography is at best only a guide, since variations in normal coronary anatomy are the rule rather than the exception. The following suggestions may be of some help. The left main coronary artery, which under most circumstances should be visualized first and with great care, can be seen best in the posteroanterior (Fig. 30–10) or in a very shallow oblique projection (either RAO or LAO) so that the left main coronary artery is just off the spine. The circumflex artery and its marginal branches can be defined in the RAO projection (20- or 30-degree angulation) with 20 to 30 degrees of caudal angulation (see Fig. 30–10). A second less steep RAO or posteroanterior view coupled with marked cranial angulation (30 degrees) (see Fig. 30–10) may be helpful in delineating the course of the anterior descending artery, avoiding overlap by other branches. A steep LAO view (40 degrees) with severe cranial angulation (40 degrees) (see Fig. 30–10) is essential in viewing the left anterior descending artery and diagonal branch bifurcation. An additional LAO caudal view (LAO 40 degrees, caudal 30 degrees, the so-called spider view) (see Fig. 30–10) may be of use in visualizing the bifurcation of the left main coronary artery, the proximal circumflex and left anterior descending arteries, and at times, the distal left anterior descending artery. The proximal and mid-right coronary artery are usually well seen in a 30 to 45 degree LAO projection. A moderate LAO view with cranial angulation (LAO 20 degrees, cranial 20 degrees) (Fig. 30–11A) may be ideal for viewing the bifurcation of the distal right coronary artery into the posterior descending and posterolateral branches. One view of the right coronary artery in the RAO view is necessary. At times, visualization of the distal right coronary artery is helped by adding

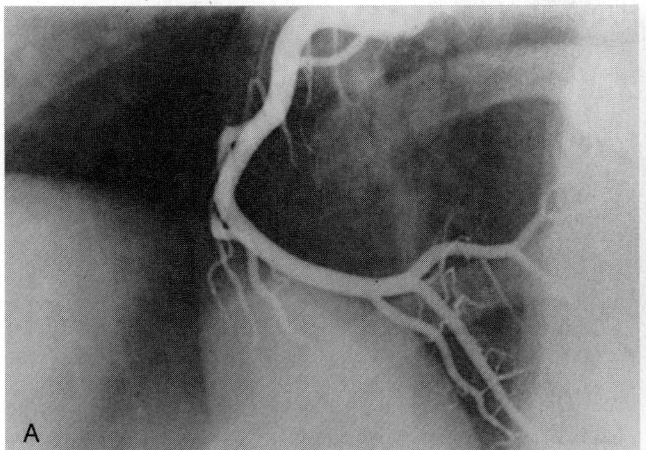

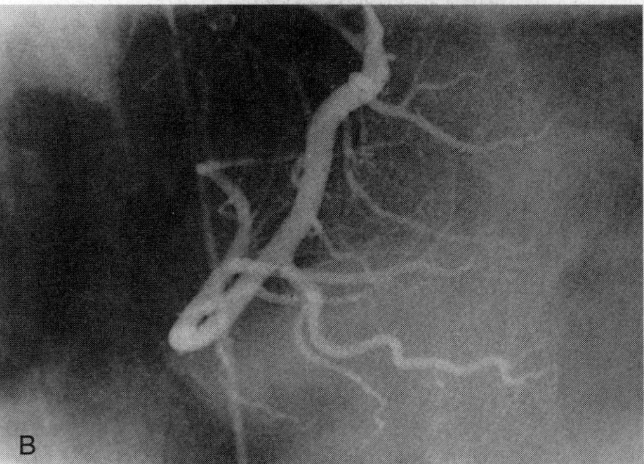

FIGURE 30–11 Angiographic projections of a normal right coronary artery. **A,** Selective right coronary angiogram viewed with 20-degree LAO and 20-degree cranial angulation. **B,** Same vessel viewed with 30-degree RAO and 50-degree cranial angulation.

cranial angulation (sometimes up to 60 degrees) to the RAO view (see Fig. 30–11B).

Coronary Artery Dimensions

Normal Dimensions in Humans

It has become recognized increasingly that measurements of coronary artery dimensions at autopsy do not correlate well with in vivo angiographic measurements of coronary diameter.[189–193] The importance of accurate measurements of normal coronary caliber is underscored by the understanding that coronary atherosclerosis is primarily a diffuse disease process that may be difficult to recognize angiographically.[194] Thus, without knowing the "true" caliber of an artery, it is often difficult to conclude whether a given coronary segment that appears normal angiographically is normal anatomically.[195] The importance of recognizing diffuse coronary narrowing is underscored by studies in patients with advanced atherosclerosis showing that angiographic measurements based on lesion percent stenosis (as a fraction of the diameter of the adjacent "normal segment") correlate poorly with physiologic measurements of the effect of a given focal stenosis on coronary blood flow.[196, 197] The rationale for expressing lesion severity as percent stenosis has been rendered even more tenuous by the findings that in atherosclerosis, compensatory coronary enlargement precedes the process of luminal narrowing and often compensates for any narrowing until this narrowing reaches 40 percent of the intimal lumen (Fig. 30–12).[198]

Dodge and associates[199] used computer-based quantitation of angiograms to measure coronary lumen diameter at 96 points in 32 defined coronary segments or major branches in normal arteriograms carefully selected from over 9000 consecutive studies. In these angiograms, absolutely smooth lumen borders were used to indicate likely freedom from atherosclerotic disease. For these normal arteries, a round cross section was assumed, and the cross-sectional area was estimated to be

$$(\text{coronary diameter})^2 \div (\pi \cdot 4)$$

The summed cross-sectional areas of the main right coronary, the proximal left anterior descending, and the proximal circumflex arteries was called the *total coronary area*. A summary of these results is given in Table 30–2 and Figure 30–13. In men with a large dominant right coronary distribution, the total coronary area was 32.1 ± 7.3 mm^2, with the right coronary artery contributing 38 percent of the total area, the circumflex artery 29 percent, and the left anterior descending artery 33 percent. The *total* coronary area was not statistically different between patients with small right coronary, balanced, and dominant left coronary distributions (33.5 ± 9.3 mm^2, 26.8 ± 5.2 mm^2, and 30.7 ± 5.5 mm^2, respectively).[199] Using these measurements and those of others,[200, 201] it is generally possible to estimate "normal" coronary segment diameter in men and women to within ±25 percent (coefficient of variation). Unfortunately, nitroglycerin was not given in these studies, so the effects of differences in coronary vasomotor tone were not standardized.

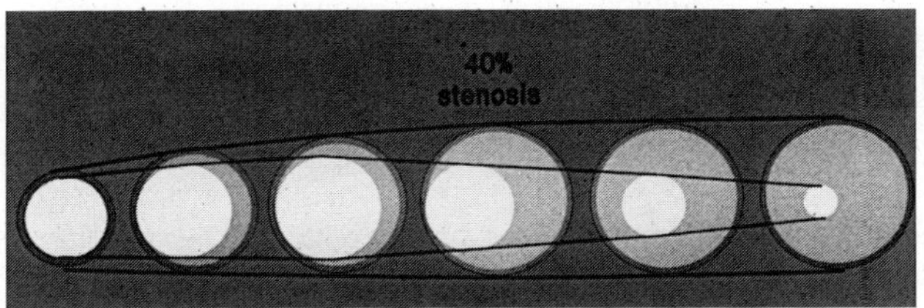

FIGURE 30–12 Concept of compensatory coronary dilatation as initially proposed by Glagov et al. The early atherosclerotic plaque development is associated with a compensatory increase in lumen area. No decrease in lumen caliber is seen until the stenosis reaches nearly 40 percent. (From Glagov S, Weisenberg E, Zarins CK, et al: Compensatory enlargement of human atherosclerotic coronary arteries. N Engl J Med 316:1371–1375, 1987. Copyright 1987 Massachusetts Medical Society. All rights reserved.)

Influence of Coronary Artery Length and Dominance on Coronary Caliber

The normal diameter of a coronary artery is proportionately related to the length of the vessel. Although the diameters of the left main and the left anterior descending segments are unaffected by anatomic perfusion field size, the left circumflex artery or right coronary artery is usually significantly larger when dominant.[199] The diameter of the posterior descending artery, however, is similar regardless of whether it arises from the right or the circumflex arteries.[199]

The epicardial distribution, characterized by the arterial length relative to the distance from its origin to the left ventricular apex, is the principal determinant of branch diameter. There is a close correlation between the lumen area of a coronary artery at each point along its length and the corresponding summed distal branch lengths and regional myocardial mass, in patients both with and without coronary artery disease.[202]

Effects of Other Physiologic and Pathologic Variables on Coronary Caliber

Multiple other physiologic and pathologic processes affect coronary caliber. Acute changes in perfusion pressure

TABLE 30–2 Diameter Measurements of the Main Coronary Arteries in Normal Men*

Location	RCA Dominant	Small Dominant RCA	Balanced	LCA Dominant
LM mid	4.5 ± 0.5	4.6 ± 0.7	4.4 ± 0.4	4.6 ± 0.4
LAD1 mid	3.6 ± 0.5	3.8 ± 0.4	3.6 ± 0.4	3.7 ± 0.2
LAD3 mid	1.7 ± 0.5	1.9 ± 0.5	1.8 ± 0.4	2.0 ± 0.3
LCX1 mid	3.4 ± 0.5	3.5 ± 0.8	3.4 ± 0.5	4.2 ± 0.6‡
LCX3 mid	1.6 ± 0.6	2.2 ± 0.8†	2.5 ± 0.5	3.2 ± 0.5‡
RCA1 mid	3.9 ± 0.6	3.8 ± 0.5	3.0 ± 0.5	2.8 ± 0.5‡
RCA3 mid	3.1 ± 0.5	2.6 ± 0.6†	2.0 ± 0.6	1.1 ± 0.4‡

Abbreviations: LAD, left anterior descending artery; LCA, left coronary artery; LCX, left circumflex artery; LM, left main coronary artery; RCA, right coronary artery.

*Values are mean ± SD.

†$P < .05$, small-RCA, balanced, or LCA-dominant groups compared with RCA-dominant group.

‡$P < .01$, small-RCA, balanced, or LCA-dominant groups compared with RCA-dominant group.

From Dodge JT, Brown BG, Bolson EL, Dodge HT: Lumen diameter of normal human coronary arteries: influence of age, sex, anatomic variation, and left ventricular hypertrophy or dilation. Circulation 86:232–246, 1992.

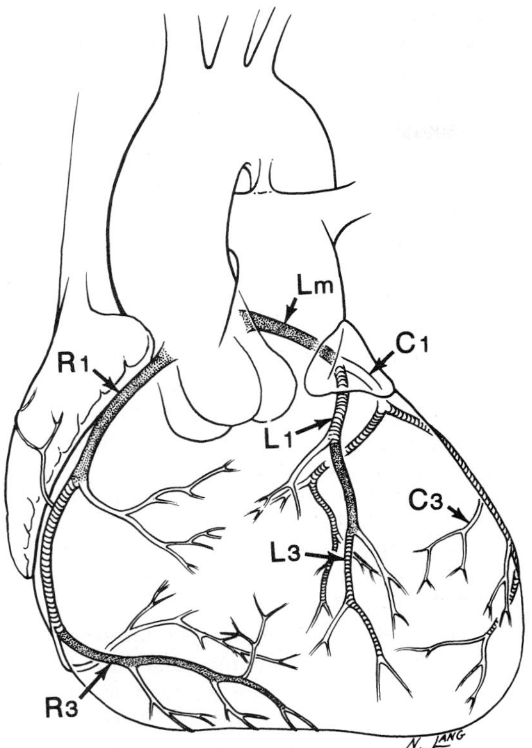

FIGURE 30–13 Diagram of coronary artery segment nomenclature for a right coronary dominant circulation. C1, proximal circumflex; C3, distal circumflex; L1, proximal left anterior descending; L3, distal left anterior descending; Lm, left main; R1, proximal right coronary; R3, distal right coronary (see Table 30–2). (From Dodge JT, Brown BG, Bolson EL, Dodge HT: Lumen diameter of normal human coronary arteries: influence of age, sex, anatomic variation, and left ventricular hypertrophy or dilation. Circulation 86:232–246, 1992.)

markedly alter coronary diameter by changing the distending force.[203] Increased blood flow from heightened myocardial oxygen demand (e.g., increased heart rate) or drug administration leads to coronary relaxation by an endothelium-dependent mechanism that affects coronary smooth muscle vasomotor tone.[204] The effects of endothelium-mediated dilatation on coronary caliber can be altered significantly by vascular pathology.[205, 206]

Other conditions lead to anatomic coronary dilatation via a chronic increase in coronary blood flow. Hypertension and the wide range of conditions resulting in left ventricular hypertrophy[207–209] result in marked increases in epicardial vessel size.[207] When body surface area is used to normalize for differences in body size, men with left ventricular hypertrophy or dilated cardiomyopathy have 37 percent or 31 percent larger coronary segment areas, respectively, than do normal men.[199] Coronary dilatation and increased coronary tone are also seen in long-distance runners.[210] Coronary dilatation can also result from fistulous connections between the artery and a cardiac chamber or vein.

Effects of Gender, Weight, Age, and Tortuosity on Coronary Caliber

Evidence suggests that females have higher morbidity and mortality resulting from attempts at coronary revascularization with either angioplasty[211] or bypass surgery.[212, 213] Speculation as to the reasons for the apparent differences in the results has focused on differences in coronary size between men and women. In one report, the proximal coronary lumen diameter of women with normal arteries and a right dominant coronary circulation was -9 ± 8 percent, less than in similar men.[199] In the same study, women had 15.3 percent smaller main coronary branch areas when normalized for body surface area. In a collaborative study involving multiple institutions in northern New England, O'Connor and colleagues[213] prospectively recorded body weight and the luminal diameter of the mid–left anterior descending artery in 1325 patients undergoing coronary artery bypass surgery. Vessel size was strongly related to both gender and body size (body surface area, mass index, height, and weight). Within each quartile of body size measurements, the mid–left anterior descending artery diameter in men was greater than that in women, with a mean difference range of 0.14 to 0.23 mm. The smaller left anterior descending artery diameter in women was also associated with increased risk of mortality from coronary bypass surgery. Differing results were found when Kornowski and coworkers[214] compared coronary cross-sectional area luminal narrowing, plaque quality, plaque calcium, and lumen location in 549 men and 169 women with chronic stable angina using intravascular ultrasound. These investigators found that when corrected for body surface area, no differences in these parameters of atherosclerosis between men and women could be identified.

Age, if considered separate from an increased possibility of the presence of diffuse atherosclerosis, is thought generally to *increase* coronary caliber.[215] Dodge and associates,[199] however, found no age-related trend toward increased total coronary area in normal men when the coronary diameter was normalized for body surface area. Total coronary area in men with apparently normal coronary arteries was virtually constant at 15.2 ± 3.6 mm²/m². Of note, however, in the left anterior descending artery, a positive correlation was found between age and vessel tortuosity, but not between tortuosity and lumen diameter. In contrast, Leung and associates[215a] found a progressive age-related decrease in the cross-sectional area of each proximal coronary and reduced total coronary cross-sectional area. These authors speculate that such changes may be due to decreased coronary flow requirements, attenuated endothelial vasodilatory responses, or age-related changes in myocardial composition.

Effects of Normal Variations in Coronary Vasomotor Tone on Coronary Caliber

The importance of coronary vasomotor tone on measurements of coronary caliber, although widely acknowledged, is often ignored. Normal proximal epicardial coronary caliber can increase up to 30 percent after administration of nitroglycerin, if coronary perfusion pressure is maintained.[216] Angiographic studies show striking variations in coronary tone depending on time of day[217] and psychological stress.[218] In atherosclerotic monkeys, coronary vasomotor responses can be modulated by estrogen treatment.[219] Despite the acknowledgment of the importance of coronary vasomotor tone, quantitative studies of atherosclerosis progression or regression are too frequently performed with this important variable uncontrolled.

Although vasodilatation in response to nitroglycerin is seen in normal coronary segments of all sizes, the response varies in magnitude.[85] Those epicardial coronary segments with the smallest basal diameter show the greatest relative change in dimension.[85] Since most coronary stenoses have a portion of the vascular circumference that is relatively normal, even severe stenoses may dilate in response to nitroglycerin. However, if stenosis severity is calculated as percent stenosis (comparing lesion diameter to the diameter of the adjacent normal segment), the stenosis may artifactually appear to worsen after nitroglycerin administration because of a comparatively greater dilatory effect on the adjacent "normal segment."[220]

Relationship Between Angiographic Coronary Anatomy and Myocardial Perfusion Field (Risk Region)

There is considerable experimental data relating myocardial infarct size and consequent clinical outcomes to the mass of myocardium perfused by an infarct-related coronary artery.[183, 221–223] Calculation of the infarct/risk area ratio is critical to the assessment of interventions aimed at limiting infarct size. Relating coronary anatomy as viewed from the coronary arteriogram to the myocardial perfusion volume or risk area, however, has proved difficult to accomplish in the clinical setting. Quantitating these relationships in patients with atherosclerosis is difficult because of complexities introduced by the presence of diffuse luminal narrowing and vessel occlusion.

Experimental studies in normal animals have shown that geometric characteristics of the arterial tree relate directly to regional myocardial perfusion volume. Koiwa and colleagues[224] have shown in dogs that the maximally dilated coronary artery luminal cross-sectional area is related linearly to the volume it perfuses. The cumulative length of arterial branches is also related to the myocardial perfusion volume.[224]

In humans, radioisotopic techniques have been used to measure the region at risk. Using a method initially validated in the pig,[225] technetium 99m–radiolabeled albumin microspheres were injected directly into both coronary arteries of patients presenting with acute infarction during the period of total coronary occlusion and again following achievement of lumen patency after intracoronary thrombolysis.[183] Delayed scanning revealed perfusion deficits that could be quantitated as the area at risk and correlated with the exact site of coronary occlusion determined with acute coronary angiography (Fig. 30–14). Data from a limited number of patients studied with these techniques revealed that inferior infarcts secondary to right or circumflex coronary artery occlusions were associated with areas of risk ranging from 10 to 26 percent (mean 18 percent) of left ventricular mass. In contrast, anterior infarctions resulting from left anterior descending artery occlusions had risk areas of 14 to 49 percent (mean 39 percent). Two patients who subsequently expired had risk regions of over 40 percent of the left ventricular mass. Importantly, the area of the region at risk could not be predicted by careful visual assessment of the coronary angiogram.

Intravenous technetium 99m sestamibi has also been used to measure the area at risk in patients with acute infarction.[226, 227] The lack of redistribution with this radiopharmaceutical permits imaging to be done with single-photon emission computed tomography up to 6 hours after injection. Using this technique, quantitative measurements of the infarct risk area in patients with an initial acute infarction correlated poorly with the "best estimate" of two experienced angiographers.[227] This data emphasizes again the variability of risk areas that are not predictable by the anatomic site of coronary occlusion and the inability of angiographers to predict the risk area in individual patients.

Leung and others[215a, 228] developed a semiquantitative method for determining the myocardial territory supplied by a nutrient vessel based on the relative size of the vessel as judged by the summed length of the terminal vessel segment. Although this method is easy to use and has acceptable interobserver variability, it has not been validated in an animal model.

Congenital Coronary Anomalies

Embryology

Although a thorough description of the genesis of the coronary circulation is beyond the scope of this text, a few

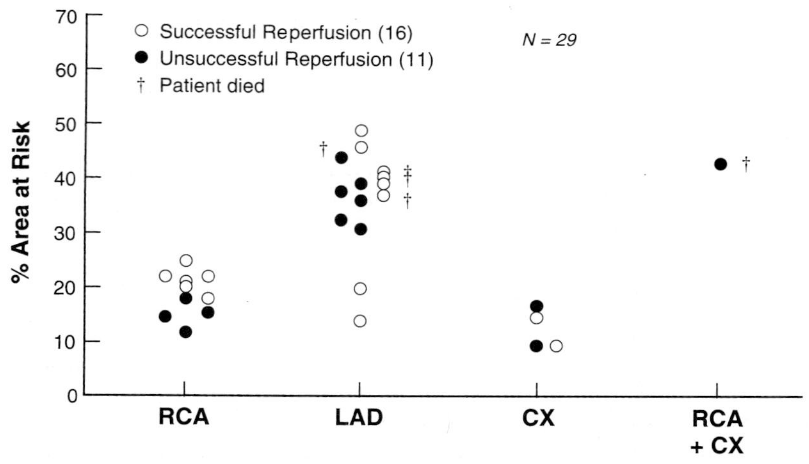

FIGURE 30–14 Relationship between the site of coronary occlusion and the size of the risk area. CX, circumflex coronary artery; LAD, left anterior descending coronary artery; RCA, right coronary artery. (From Feiring AJ, Johnson MR, Kioschos JM, et al: The importance of the determination of the myocardial area at risk in the evaluation of the outcome of acute myocardial infarction in patients. Circulation 75:980–987, 1987.)

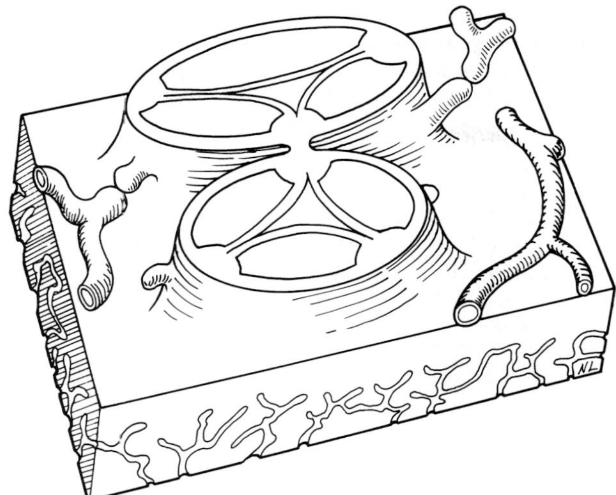

FIGURE 30–15 Schematic illustration of the three major components responsible for the development of the coronary arterial bed: myocardial sinusoids, in situ vascular network, and coronary anlage (buds). (From Angelini P: Normal and anomalous coronary arteries: definitions and classification. Am Heart J 117:418, 1989.)

important considerations are appropriate. There are at least three major anatomic components important in the development of the coronary arterial bed: the myocardial sinusoids, the in situ vascular network, and the coronary anlage (Fig. 30–15).[164] The myocardial sinusoids are an elongation of the trabeculae into the developing myocardium. The sinusoids are the earliest sites of metabolic exchange between the blood contained in the cavities and the cardiac mesenchyme (myocardial jelly). The in situ vascular endothelial network develops separately in the subepicardium 31 days after ovulation. The coronary anlage (buds) sprout from the wall of the aorta–pulmonary trunk as septation is proceeding. After completion of aortopulmonary septation, these latter two components fuse and a normal coronary circulation begins. Although the coronary ostia are formed quite early, the distal coronary branching pattern remains as a variable interbranching network until the cardiac chambers develop.

The size and distribution of the coronary arteries are related to and dependent on subsequent myocardial chamber development. According to Angelini,[164] a true mismatch between the dependent myocardium and its related coronary arteries is embryologically improbable. Therefore, on physiologic grounds, the finding of coronary atresia or hypoplasia is unlikely. Instead, either the dependent myocardium is also hypoplastic or, more commonly, the opposite coronary is relatively oversized. Thus, at birth, the coronary circulation is usually effectively normal in global physiologic terms, and the angiographic finding of a coronary artery that appears hypoplastic is usually only an infrequently occurring coronary arterial pattern. Some coronary anomalies still occur, however, and are well recognized to be associated with major adverse clinical consequences.

Incidence and Classification

Tabulations of coronary angiograms suggest that coronary anomalies occur in the adult population with an incidence ranging from 0.6 to 1.3 percent.[229–230c] Yamanaka and Hobbs[229] reported the Cleveland Clinic experience from 1960 to 1988, reviewing data from 126,595 angiograms. Coronary artery anomalies were found in 1686 patients, an incidence of 1.3 percent. Of the coronary anomalies, 87 percent involved the origin and distribution of the vessel, and 13 percent were coronary artery fistulas. Table 30–3 shows the occurrence rate for various coronary anomalies from the Cleveland Clinic study. Since the angiograms were obtained primarily to assess coronary atherosclerosis in adults, congenital coronary anomalies resulting in early or sudden death are not represented.

A variety of classification schemes for congenital coronary anomalies have been proposed.[230d] Although each has its attributes, the most clinically useful classification divides congenital coronary anomalies into those that are usually associated with a benign outcome and those whose natural history is associated with adverse events. Most adverse outcomes appear to result from decreased myocardial perfusion, although the mechanism of such an ischemia is speculative. Coronary atherosclerosis does not seem to occur with increased incidence in anomalous vessels, nor is the presence of coronary anomalies protective against coronary artery disease.[229]

Congenital Coronary Anomalies, Often Benign

MYOCARDIAL BRIDGES

That portions of the conduit coronary arteries may take a short intramural course and be covered by a muscle "bridge" has been part of the anatomic literature since 1737.[231] However, the clinical significance of such anatomy is more recent in origin. Muscular myocardial bridges are recognized angiographically by the characteristic narrowing of the coronary lumen that is seen during systole and that is absent during diastole. Although most cases of angiographic systolic narrowing correspond with anatomic myocardial bridges, this finding may occasionally be caused by other mechanisms, such as pericardial fibrosis, tumors, or foreign bodies.[232–232b]

Coronary arterial location in mammalian hearts has been classified into three main types: type A (hamster, squirrel, rat, guinea pig, and rabbit), in which the coronary arteries are entirely intramyocardial; type B (goat, sheep, dog, cat, macaque, and human), in which the coronary arteries are predominately epicardial but myocardial bridging is fre-

TABLE 30–3 Incidence of Coronary Artery Anomalies, Detected by Angiography

First Author	Patients (n)	Anomalies (n)	Incidence (%)
Liberthson[250]	Not stated	21	0.6
Engel[230b]	4250	51	1.2
Chaitman[248]	3750	31	0.83
Baltaxe[230c]	1000	9	0.9
Kimbiris[230]	7000	45	0.64
Hobbs[256]	9153	601	1.55
Wilkins[230a]	10,661	83	0.78
Yamanaka[229]	126,595	1686	1.3

TABLE 30–4 Anatomic Incidence of Muscular Bridges*

	Polacek	Chen	Zapedowski		Edwards
Cases (n)	70	100	200		270
Gender	NS	NS	Male	Female	NS
Incidence of MB (%)					
LCA + RCA	85.7	NS	NS	NS	5.4
LCA	77.7	76/2	85.7	38.8	5.1
LAD	60.0	60.0	59.0	30.5	4.7
DIAG	18.5	6.1	50.5	28.4	NS
CX	40.0	NS	42.9	11.6	NS
OM	14.2	19.1	52.4	28.4	0.4
RCA	41.4	NS	NS	NS	0.4

Abbreviations: CX, circumflex artery; DIAG, diagonal branch; LAD, left anterior descending artery; LCA, left coronary artery; MB, muscular bridges; NS, not stated; OM, obtuse marginal branch; RCA, right coronary artery.

*Incidence of muscular bridges. Percentage of patients with muscular bridges in different locations.

From Angelini P, Trivellato M, Donis J, Leachman RD: Myocardial bridges: a review. Progr Cardiovasc Dis 26:75–88, 1983.

quent; and type C (horse, cow, pig), in which the coronary arteries are entirely epicardial and bridging is rarely if ever seen.[233] In humans and other type B mammals, myocardial bridges are found most frequently in the left anterior descending artery. Table 30–4 details the incidence of muscular bridges in the experience of four groups of investigators. When the results of eight separate autopsy studies were pooled, myocardial bridges were found in 449 of 1652 cases (27 percent).[234] This high frequency coupled with the comparative anatomic data suggests that myocardial bridging is often a "normal" finding.

The most frequent site of bridging is the midsegment of the left anterior descending artery (Fig. 30–16). A typical muscular bridge in this artery is 10 to 20 mm long and 2 to 4 mm thick.[232b] Portions of other arteries that are located in the atrioventricular groove (such as the proximal, mid-right, and circumflex arteries) are frequently surrounded by scattered muscular fibers continuous with the atrial myocardium and may also exhibit systolic narrowing. These are referred to as *myocardial loops*. As another variant, arteries such as the obtuse marginal branch and ramus intermedius that are located over the free wall of the left ventricle may plunge into the myocardium at some point in their course. These arteries frequently do not resurface. Anatomic studies suggest that the prevalence of myocardial bridging involving major coronary veins is less than 5 percent.[233]

Angiographic studies of myocardial bridging in humans have shown a much lower prevalence than is seen in autopsy studies, usually ranging from 0.5 to 7.5 percent.[232b, 235, 236] In one series, however, the occurrence was 16 percent.[237] For systolic narrowing to occur, the external muscular compressive force must exceed the arterial pressure and the intrinsic arterial wall stiffness. During angiography, the increased intraluminal pressure resulting from the pressure of contrast medium injection may act to diminish recognition of lesser intramyocardial bridges than might be detected in anatomic studies. In one study, the mean maximal corrected length of artery involved in the muscle bridge was 15 mm (range 9 to 44 mm) and the maximal percent reduction in diameter during systole was 56 percent (range 30 to 100 percent).[235] Long myocardial bridges, often referred to as *tunnels,* have been described.

Although scattered reports have attributed chest pain in patients with normal coronary arteries to the finding of a myocardial bridge, these two conditions are not frequently related causally. Patients with equal degrees of systolic narrowing do not exhibit a similar clinical or pathophysiologic response. Since coronary flow is predominantly diastolic and some animals have wholly intramyocardial arter-

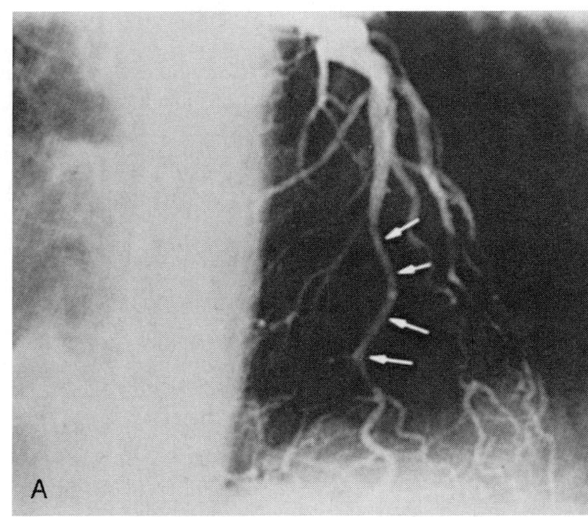

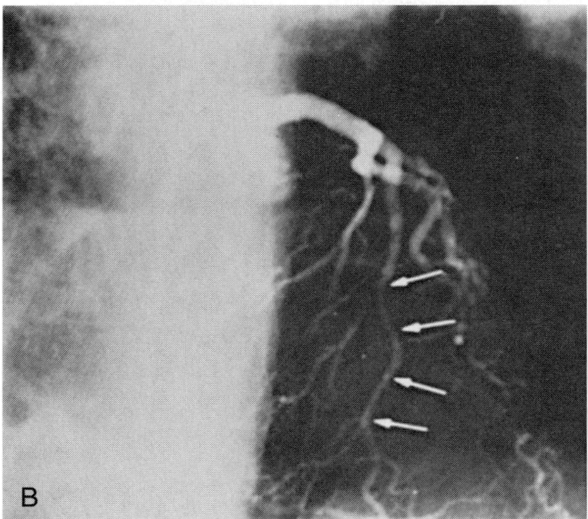

FIGURE 30–16 **A** and **B,** Selective coronary angiogram shows a distinct muscular bridge (*arrows*) in the left anterior descending artery. **A,** Diastolic. **B,** Systolic.

ies, luminal compression during systole is unlikely to play a frequent role in causing myocardial ischemia. Experimental studies in dogs have shown that systolic myocardial contraction does not limit coronary flow at heart rates less than 160 beats/min or unless coronary compression extends into early diastole.[238] Doppler flow studies in one patient with myocardial bridging and normal arteries have confirmed these findings.[107]

Delayed diastolic relaxation in the bridged segment in humans has been reported[239a, 239b] using intravascular ultrasound. Rapid atrial pacing with marked shortening of the coronary diastolic perfusion time, especially if combined with left ventricular hypertrophy, may rarely result in myocardial ischemia in patients with bridging.[240] Thus, it is possible that certain myocardial bridges, especially those of long length that course deeply within the myocardium,[240a] may be responsible for sudden unexpected cardiac death following tachycardia-related ischemia. These occurrences are likely quite rare, although this anomaly has been reported as the sole cardiac anomaly in young patients with sudden unexpected death.[240b]

Several anatomic studies have reported a "protective" effect of myocardial bridging.[232–232b, 240c] In rabbits whose proximal coronary arteries are exclusively intramural, cholesterol-induced atherosclerosis spares these arteries even when "severe lesions" develop in the subendocardial arteries.[232] The mechanism of such a protective effect is unknown but may involve protection from systolic wall stress. In humans, myocardial bridges may slightly increase the chances of proximal coronary atherosclerosis while protecting the bridged segment and the distal artery. Postmortem human morphometric studies have shown that when proximal myocardial bridging is present, intimal thickening and macroscopic raised atherosclerotic lesions are increased just before the bridge. Under the bridge, eccentric plaques and raised lesions are absent, although there is often concentric intimal thickening.[241, 241a] There are isolated case reports of acute myocardial infarction associated with muscle bridges.[242, 243] However, when carefully examined, the overall frequency of myocardial infarction is the same in patients with and without myocardial bridges.

Myocardial bridges have been recognized with increased frequency after cardiac transplantation. Review of the angiograms of 64 cardiac transplant patients revealed a 33 percent incidence of myocardial bridging, an incidence much higher than would be expected in the normal population.[244] Administration of nitroglycerin accentuated the degree of systolic narrowing.[245]

There is a well-described association between left ventricular hypertrophy (as seen in aortic stenosis, hypertrophic cardiomyopathy, and hypertension) and an increased incidence of myocardial bridges.[235, 246] This may relate to a greater contractile force generated by the myocardium. Although angiographically detected systolic compression occurs rarely in normal intramural septal arteries, septal "twinkling" or "squeeze" resulting from prominent widespread systolic septal compression is commonly seen in patients with aortic stenosis (71 percent) and hypertrophic cardiomyopathy (74 percent).[246]

ORIGIN OF THE LEFT CIRCUMFLEX ARTERY FROM THE RIGHT CORONARY SINUS

In the United States, the origin of the left circumflex artery from the right aortic sinus or from the right coronary artery is the most common anomaly of coronary arterial origin.[247, 248] Most patients have no other associated anomalies. The anomalous circumflex artery courses posterior to the aortic root and the noncoronary sinus to enter the left atrioventricular groove and ultimately perfuse its usual territory (Fig. 30–17). The size and variation of the perfusion field is similar to that of the normal circumflex artery.

An anomalous origin of the circumflex artery should be suspected when contrast material injection into the left coronary artery reveals what appears to be an unusually long left main coronary artery or flush occlusion of the circumflex artery (Fig. 30–18).[247] The anomalous circumflex origin is often missed during right coronary angiography because deep seating of the right coronary catheter may prevent sufficient reflux of contrast medium to opacify the aberrant origin (Fig. 30–19). If suspected, the catheter should be withdrawn slowly and repositioned posteriorly in the right sinus of Valsalva and the injection repeated (Fig. 30–20). A right vein bypass curve catheter can be useful in cannulating the circumflex ostium, which is often directed inferiorly.[249]

In this anomaly, the proximal circumflex artery invariably runs a retroaortic course and does not cross between the great vessels. It has no clinical significance unless the angiographer assumes the vessel is occluded or a significant stenosis in the artery is not identified.

SEPARATE ORIGINS OF THE LEFT ANTERIOR DESCENDING AND LEFT CIRCUMFLEX ARTERIES FROM THE LEFT SINUS OF VALSALVA

In this common anomaly, the left anterior descending and circumflex arteries arise from separate but adjacent ostia, and a common left main trunk is absent (Fig. 30–21).[249a] The distribution pattern of both arteries is otherwise normal. The anomaly is associated with aortic valve disease

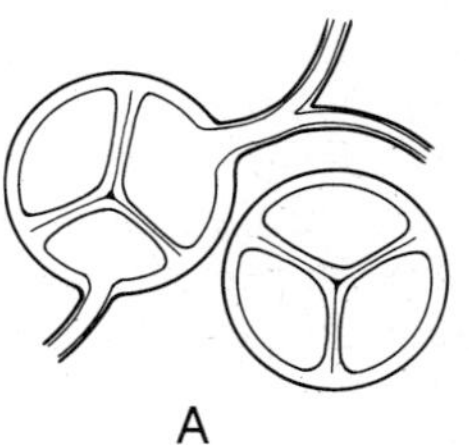

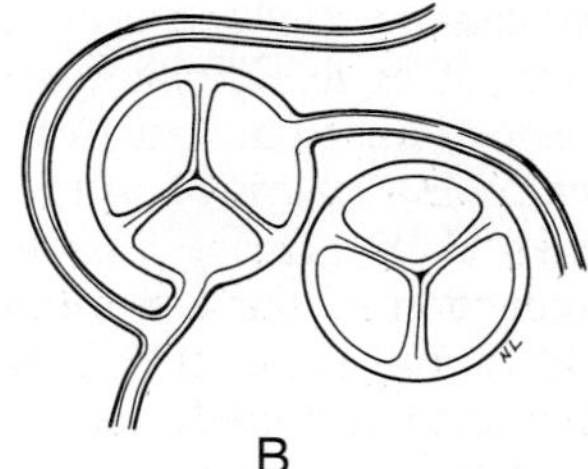

FIGURE 30–17 Views of the aortic and pulmonary valves show the normal origin of the coronary arteries **(A)** and the anomalous origin of the circumflex artery from the right coronary artery and its usual course posterior to the aorta **(B)**.

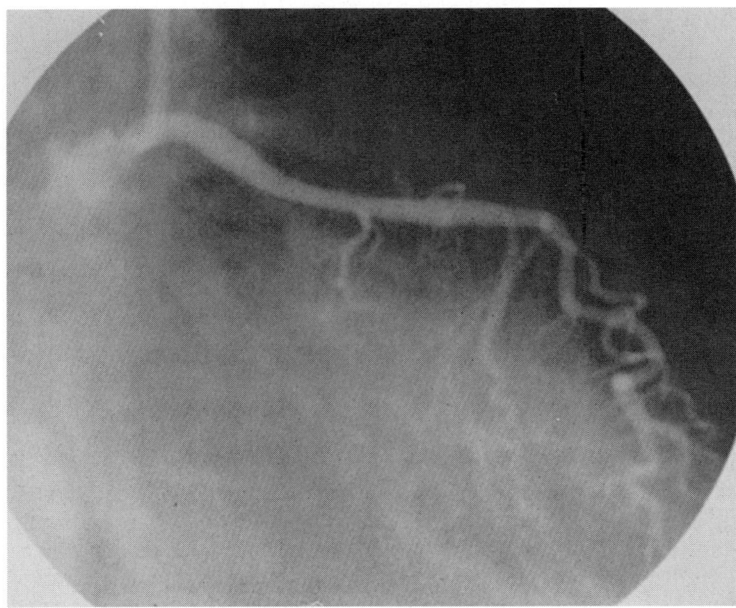

FIGURE 30–18 Selective left coronary artery angiogram in a patient with anomalous origin of the left circumflex from the right coronary artery. Note the apparent very long left main coronary caused by the absence of a circumflex branch.

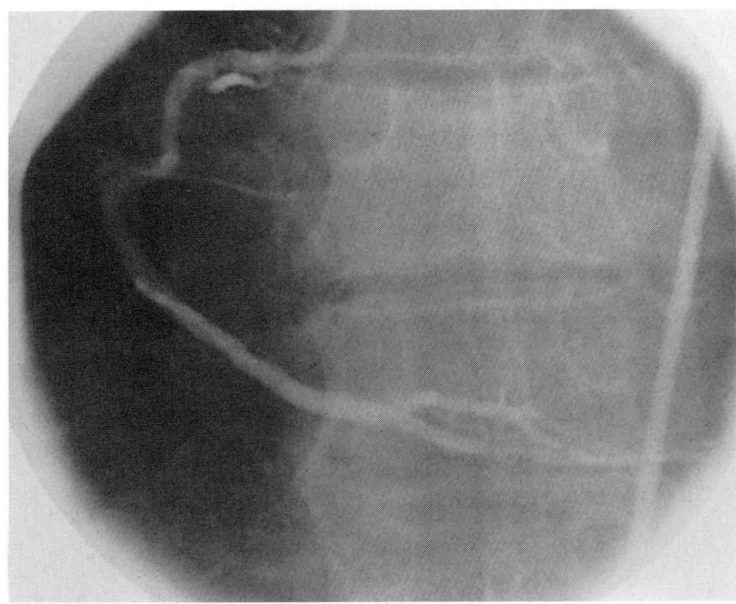

FIGURE 30–19 Selective right coronary angiogram from the same patient as in Figure 30–18. Note that the catheter is positioned deeply into the ostium of the vessel so that no contrast reflux into the sinus is seen. No anomalous circumflex artery is demonstrated.

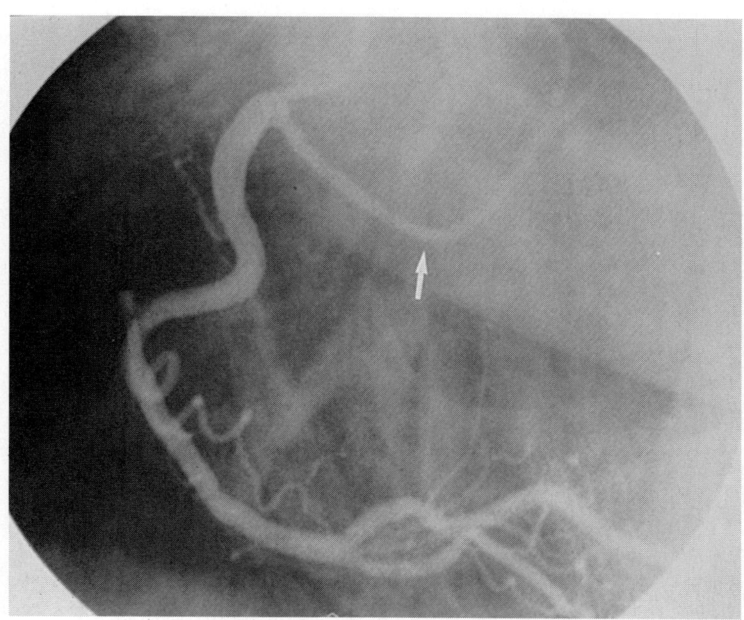

FIGURE 30–20 Repeat selective right coronary angiogram from the same patient as in Figure 30–19. The catheter has been pulled back and the anomalous circumflex (*arrow*) is now apparent.

and left coronary dominance.[250] At angiography, it can be difficult to determine whether the left main coronary artery is truly absent or very short, or if a common ostium is present. Occasionally, different catheter curves are needed to inject contrast medium into the separate left anterior descending and circumflex branches (Fig. 30–22A and B). If unrecognized at catheterization, one of the major left coronary branches may be misinterpreted as being totally occluded.

ANOMALOUS CORONARY ARTERY ORIGIN ABOVE THE SINOTUBULAR RIDGE

In this anomaly, either the right (most frequently) or, occasionally, the left coronary ostium is located 1 to 2 cm above the sinotubular ridge. The distribution of the affected coronary artery is otherwise normal. This common anomaly should be suspected when the angiographer is unable to visualize either coronary ostium using standard angiographic catheters and usual techniques. An aortic root angiogram may be necessary to identify the anomalous origin and facilitate selective catheterization.

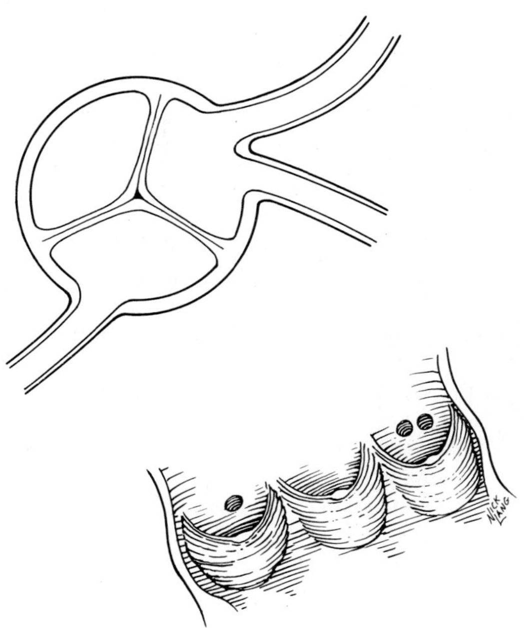

FIGURE 30–21 Separate ostia for the left anterior descending and the left circumflex arteries from the left sinus of Valsalva.

ANOMALOUS CORONARY ARTERY ORIGIN FROM THE POSTERIOR SINUS OF VALSALVA

Either the right coronary artery or the left main coronary artery can take its origin from the posterior sinus of Valsalva (the usual noncoronary sinus). Both of these variants are rare, although an ectopic right coronary origin is more common. Except for the anomalous origin, the anatomic course is normal and no significant clinical complications have been reported.[251]

ABSENT LEFT CIRCUMFLEX

In this rare anomaly, a large "superdominant" right coronary artery crosses the crux of the heart, ascending the atrioventricular groove to perfuse the posterior and lateral wall of the heart. The left anterior descending artery is normal.

Coronary Arterial Anomalies Associated With Adverse Outcomes

ANOMALOUS ORIGIN OF EITHER MAJOR CORONARY ARTERY WITH A PROXIMAL INTERARTERIAL OR SEPTAL COURSE

It is the course of an anomalous coronary artery, rather than the location of the coronary ostium, that is the major determinant of whether the anomaly is benign or associated with clinical consequences (e.g., angina, ventricular arrhythmias, syncope, or sudden death).[229, 250, 251] These adverse outcomes usually occur when the anomalous coronary artery passes between the aorta and the pulmonary artery

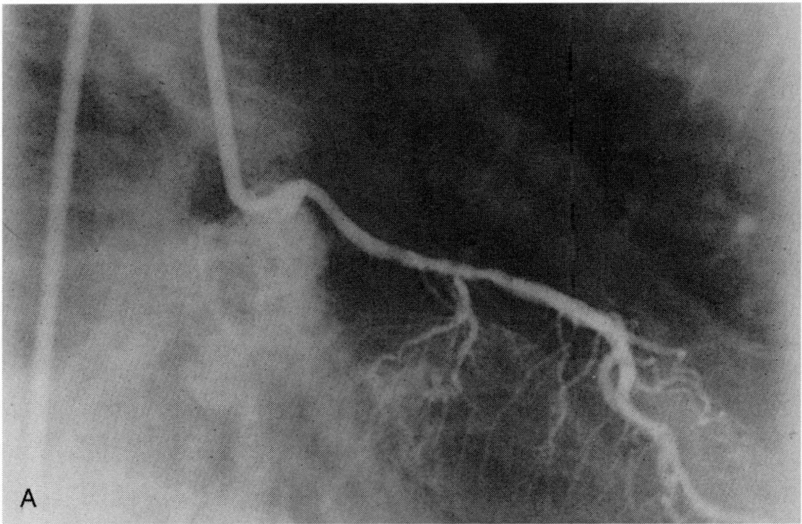

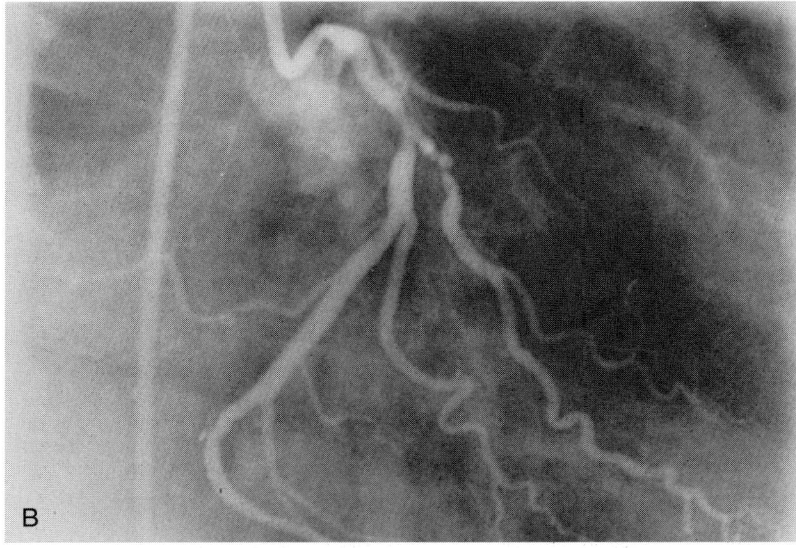

FIGURE 30–22 Selective left coronary angiogram in a patient with separate ostia for the left anterior descending and the left circumflex arteries. **A,** Selective injection reveals only the left anterior descending artery. **B,** Catheter reposition now reveals a large dominant circumflex vessel. The left anterior descending artery is now not seen.

or, less commonly, via a septal pathway. Clinical events, particularly sudden death, are usually seen during exertion in young individuals in the absence of coronary atherosclerosis. It is postulated that exercise results in kinking or in some way causes transient limitation in coronary flow because of the orientation of the vessel at its origin or because it is compressed during its anomalous course.[254]

It is often difficult to delineate angiographically the proximal course of an anomalous vessel. Although some angiographers have suggested that performing coronary angiography in a lateral projection after passing a pulmonary artery catheter localizes the course of the vessel, this technique is of limited value because in the lateral view both a septal and an interarterial course (between the aorta and the pulmonary artery) will appear posterior to the pulmonary artery and anterior to the aorta if the septum is caudal to both great vessels. A ventriculogram or aortic angiogram performed in the RAO projection is needed.[255] Serota and coworkers[255] have developed a clever "dot and eye" recognition pattern technique for localization of the initial pathway that may be helpful. Although coronary angiography, if carefully done, can often define the cause of the anomalous vessel, the concomitant use of magnetic resonance coronary angiography has been shown to be especially helpful owing to the ability of this technique to acquire data noninvasively in double-oblique orientations.[12]

Several coronary variants sharing a common physiology appear at greatest risk:

1. *Origin of the right coronary artery from the left sinus of Valsalva.* When the right coronary artery arises from the left coronary cusp or proximal left main coronary artery, it almost invariably (>99 percent)[229] follows one path. This course runs between the aorta and the pulmonary artery, placing the patient at risk for adverse events (Fig. 30–23).[256] This variant should be suspected when the right coronary ostium is unable to be cannulated in the right coronary sinus or above the sinotubular ridge, yet collateral vessels are absent. This is the most common variant associated with adverse clinical events.
2. *Origin of the left anterior descending coronary artery from the right sinus of Valsalva.* If the right aortic cusp or right sinus gives rise to the left anterior

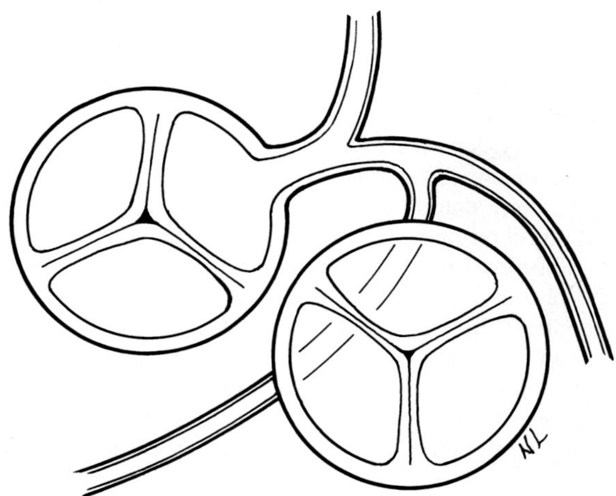

FIGURE 30–23 Schematic diagram illustrates the origin of the right coronary artery from the left sinus of Valsalva. The usual course of this vessel is between the aorta and the pulmonary artery (see text for details).

descending artery, the artery may initially follow a septal or an anterior free wall course. The anterior free wall path is associated with tetralogy of Fallot. If unrecognized, it can lead to catastrophic complications at the time of surgical repair. Although the septal pathway occurs less commonly, only patients with a septal course are at risk for sudden cardiac death.[255]

3. *Origin of the entire left coronary artery from the right sinus of Valsalva, arising separately or sharing a common ostium with the right coronary artery.* In this anomaly, the left main coronary artery may follow one of the four pathways shown in Figure 30–24, the septal pathway being the most frequent. The low incidence of this anomaly makes assessment of the risk difficult. If unrecognized, any of these anomalous courses may be associated with complications at the time of cardiac surgery.[256]
4. *Single coronary artery.* There are multiple patterns of the single coronary artery, although this anomaly is rare in the absence of other abnormalities of the heart and great vessels. The Lipton classification schema as modified by Yamanaka designates the anomalous coronary by the ostium of origin, its anatomic course, and the relationship to the great arteries.[229] In the type I pattern, a single coronary artery from a single ostium perfuses the entire heart. This extremely rare anomaly generally has a benign clinical course. In the type II single coronary pattern, the anomalous coronary arises from the proximal part of the normal coronary. The greatest adverse risk would be expected to occur in those cases in which the anomalous vessel passes between the great vessels.

Although the association between the abnormal intergreat vessel or septal course of the coronary artery and adverse clinical events is well documented in the Western medical literature, an investigation from Japan raises interesting questions. Kaku and associates[256b] reported the clini-

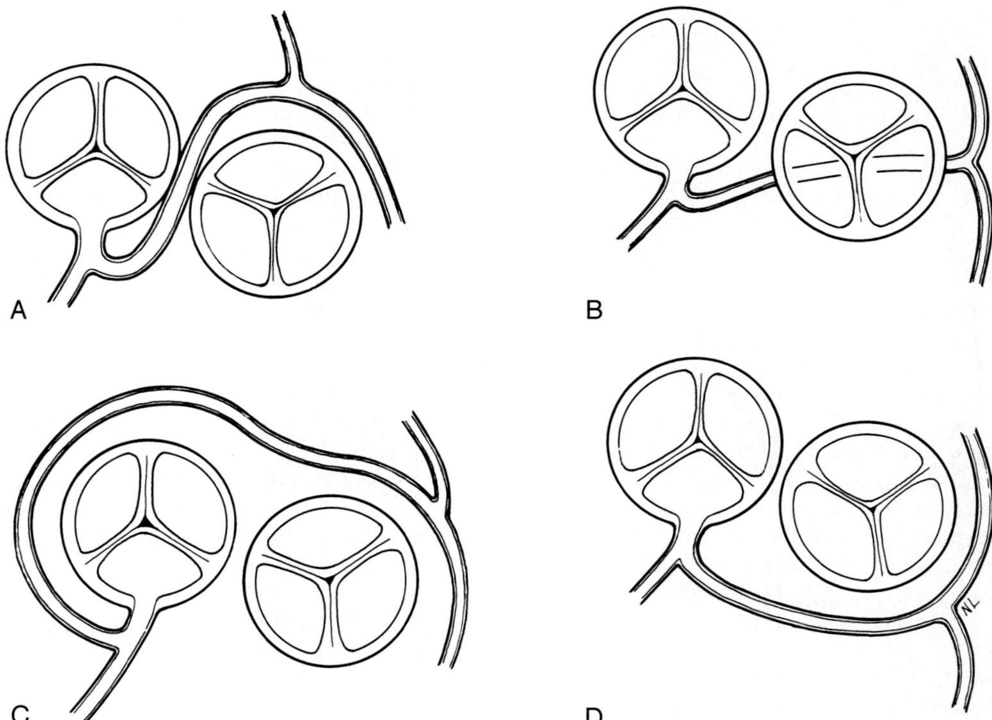

FIGURE 30–24 Variations in the course of the left coronary artery (LCA) when it arises from the right sinus of Valsalva. **A,** Interarterial course of the LCA. **B,** Transseptal course of the LCA. **C,** Course of the LCA posterior to the aorta. **D,** Course of the LCA anterior to the aorta.

cal features of 56 patients (0.32 percent) with anomalous origins of the coronary arteries after review of 17,000 patients with angiograms taken between 1968 and 1994, mean age 56 years. Despite a similar overall incidence of anomalous origin of the coronary artery in Japan and in the United States, the most frequent anomalous coronary course in the Japanese population was the right coronary artery originating from the left sinus of Valsalva and coursing between the great vessels (79 percent). An anomalous posterior course of the left circumflex artery, which occurs most frequently in the United States, was seen in only 11 percent. The left main coronary artery arising from the posterior sinus occurred in 7 percent. During a mean follow-up period of 5.6 ± 4.2 years and despite the lack of surgical treatments, there were no deaths directly related to the anomalous coronary origins. Syncope (14 percent) and aortic regurgitation (21 percent) were the most common adverse events.

ORIGIN OF A CORONARY ARTERY FROM THE PULMONARY ARTERY

Origin of the left coronary artery from the pulmonary artery, sometimes referred to as the *Bland-White-Garland syndrome,*[257] results in perfusion of the left ventricle via collaterals from the right coronary artery and a shunt into the pulmonary artery (Fig. 30–25).[258] It generally results in myocardial ischemia and is characterized clinically by wheezing, tachypnea, failure to thrive, and angina. Ninety percent of these patients die in infancy, and very few survive to adult life.[259]

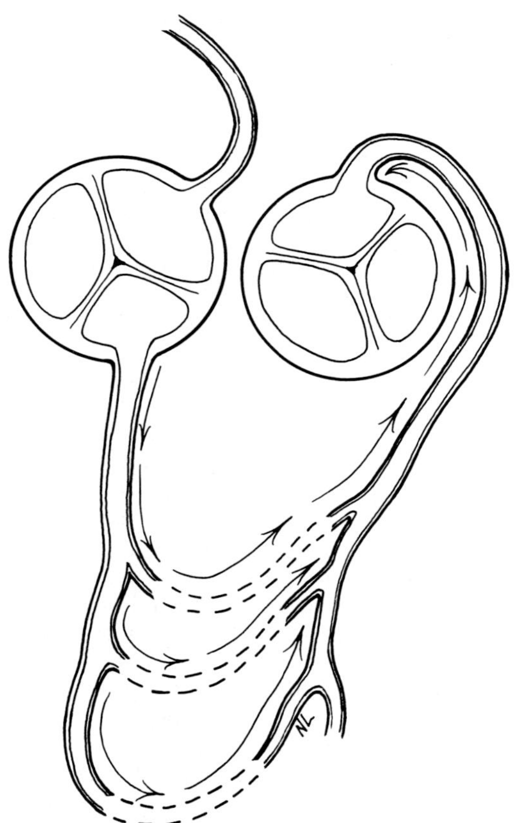

FIGURE 30–25 Origin of the left coronary artery from the pulmonary artery results in a steal phenomenon (aorta left, pulmonary artery right). *Arrows* indicate the direction of coronary blood flow.

Survival is occasionally permitted by the development of intercoronary collaterals, although collateral blood flow from the contralateral artery is drained partially into the low-pressure pulmonary artery via the aberrant coronary artery. This steal phenomenon can permit identification of the aberrant artery when the contralateral vessel is injected with contrast medium. Undiagnosed adults may present with angina, mitral regurgitation, a continuous murmur, heart failure, or sudden death (and are resuscitated). If such patients receive a premortem diagnosis, surgical treatment (coronary reimplantation into the aorta) is advised.[260]

LEFT MAIN CORONARY ATRESIA

Left main coronary atresia is a very rare coronary anomaly in which there is no left coronary atrium. The proximal left main trunk ends blindly, and blood flows via small collaterals into at least one of the left-sided arteries.[260a] Pediatric patients are overtly symptomatic early in life. This condition can occur in the adult population secondary to gradual atherosclerotic obstruction and is occasionally compatible with normal resting global left ventricular function.[260b, 260c] Origin of the right coronary artery from the pulmonary artery is extremely rare.

Coronary Artery Fistula

Although fistulas are relatively common congenital anomalies that have the potential to alter myocardial perfusion, more than half of patients with a fistula are entirely asymptomatic. Small coronary fistulas are quite common and are seen in 0.1 to 0.2 percent of all patients undergoing coronary angiography.[260g] Most arise from a small coronary branch and drain into a single cardiac chamber. The majority of small fistulas originate from the left anterior descending artery and drain into the pulmonary artery.[261] These are angiographically identifiable by contrast medium swirling as "smoke" in the otherwise unopacified pulmonary artery. Most are not associated with detectable intracardiac shunting or with auscultatory abnormalities (e.g., a continuous murmur). The clinical course is usually benign. Patients with small asymptomatic fistulas should be managed medically.

Although the majority of coronary artery fistulas are congenital,[260d, 260e] many are acquired and have been reported secondary to deceleration accidents, coronary angioplasty, repeated endomyocardial biopsies in heart transplant patients, permanent ventricular pacing leads, and cardiac surgery. These acquired forms of coronary fistulas have been increasing in frequency over the last several decades.[260d]

Large congenital fistulas may occasionally persist undetected into adult life. These abnormalities may be asymptomatic, detected only by a continuous murmur, or may present with complications such as endocarditis, heart failure, ischemia, or infarction.[260f] Large fistulas are associated with the development of very tortuous ectatic coronary arteries proximal to the origin of the fistula (Fig. 30–26)

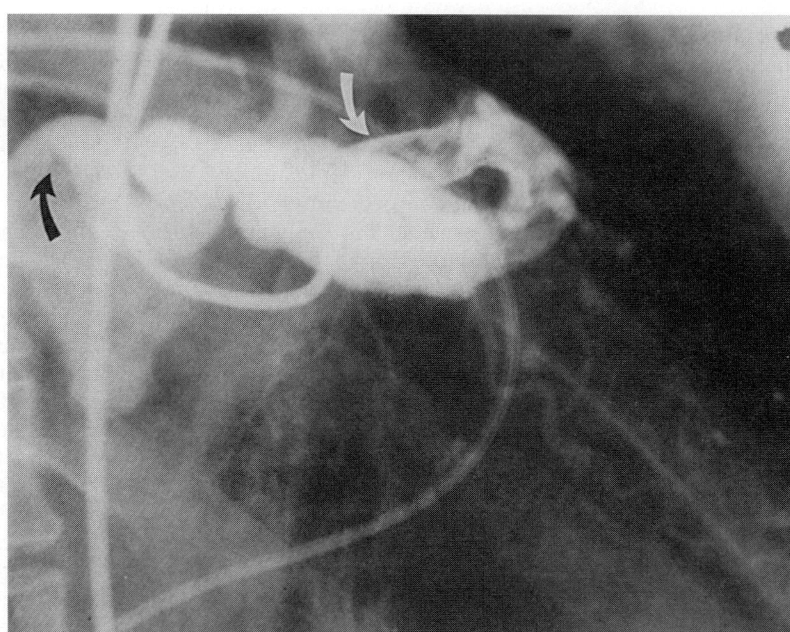

FIGURE 30–26 A large fusiform aneurysm (*arrows*) of the left anterior descending artery in a patient with coronary atherosclerosis.

and may empty into any cardiac chamber. About 50 percent of fistulas arise from the right coronary artery, 42 percent from the left coronary artery, and 5 percent from both.[261] The right atrium, pulmonary artery, or coronary sinus are the most common sites for emptying. The decision as to which fistulas should necessitate therapy is at present difficult.[262] If therapy is undertaken, the treatment should obliterate the fistula yet maintain antegrade coronary flow.[263] In the past, this usually entailed coronary artery bypass grafting with coronary reimplantation. More recently, percutaneous transcatheter embolization techniques have been used. Although these techniques are usually successful and have low morbidity and mortality rates, the obliteration of arterial perfusion to the distal bed makes these techniques not suitable for large congenital fistulas.

Another variant is the occurrence of diffuse coronary-to–ventricular chamber fistulas that resemble an unusually prominent thebesian drainage system.[264, 265, 265] In these patients, coronary injection results in diffuse endocardial opacification and filling of the ventricular cavity. Either or both coronary artery branches can be affected. Symptoms consistent with ischemia and abnormal thallium scintigraphy can occur but are uncommon.[266, 267] Acquired fistulas to the ventricular cavity can also occur at myocardial biopsy sites.[268]

CORONARY ATHEROSCLEROSIS

For over a quarter century, selective coronary angiography has remained the ultimate diagnostic test for assessing the significance of atherosclerotic lesions in the coronary circulation of humans. Despite criticism regarding interpretation and the development of many noninvasive techniques designed to detect myocardial ischemia, the coronary angiogram has maintained a preeminent position for the evaluation of coronary atherosclerosis.

Angiographic Assessment of Stable Coronary Atherosclerosis

Atherosclerosis is a disease of the arterial wall that can encroach on the vessel lumen and limit blood supply to the myocardium. In interpreting coronary angiograms, it is important to understand the nature of the atherosclerotic process as it relates to coronary dimensions and the angiographic appearance of atherosclerosis.

Coronary Changes of Atherosclerosis

COMPENSATORY CORONARY DILATATION

Glagov and colleagues,[198] using pressure-perfused postmortem hearts, demonstrated that early in the atherosclerotic process, coronary arteries undergo a compensatory increase in outer diameter of the artery. Although different segments of the same artery may respond differently, this compensatory dilatation acts to maintain lumen caliber despite thickening of the wall. These investigators found that coronary arterial lumen encroachment does not begin until the atherosclerotic plaque occupies about 40 percent of the original lumen area, as determined by the internal elastic lamina (see Fig. 30–12). Only at this point is angiography able to detect the presence of disease. This is an extremely important observation that may explain the frequent discrepancy between pathologic and angiographic assessments of experimental atherosclerosis.

Clarkson and coworkers[268a] studied the pathology of coronary arteries in monkeys with diet-induced atherosclerosis and in humans (men and women). These investigations found that as plaque intimal area enlarged, so did the artery size as judged in the internal elastic laminar area. However, there was large individual variability. Although the intimal area was significantly associated with lumen area, it was a poor predictor, explaining only 7.5 percent of the variability. In humans, a lack of compensation (decreased lumen size as plaques enlarged) and a history of coronary heart disease were significantly correlated.

CORONARY CALCIFICATION

It has been known for decades that calcification of the atherosclerotic plaque is a common occurrence, is associated with an advanced disease state, and is easily detectable in the coronary arteries by fluoroscopy or angiography. Evidence derived from electron beam computed tomography (EBCT) has challenged the old dogma that coronary plaque calcification is mainly a marker of end-stage plaque degeneration, but instead has demonstrated that intramural calcium can be observed in all degrees of atherosclerotic involvement.[268b] Some investigations have proposed using EBCT as a noninvasive screening test for coronary atherosclerosis. Janowitz and associates[268c] have shown that regardless of gender, the prevalence and extent of coronary calcification increases with age with an epidemiologic pattern similar to that known for coronary atherosclerosis. The total area of coronary calcification detected by EBCT correlates linearly with histologically determined coronary plaque.[268d] However, the total area of coronary plaque calcification significantly underestimates the total associated coronary plaque area. Calcium may be absent or undetectable in small plaques, and the location of coronary calcification may not correlate with the most significant atherosclerotic narrowing. Studies using intravascular ultrasound have confirmed this general premise, showing that coronary calcification correlates with total plaque burden but not with the degree of luminal compromise.[268e]

Absence of detectable coronary artery calcification on EBCT is highly unlikely in the presence of a severe luminal coronary obstruction and has been proposed as a screening tool to identify patients at low risk (80 percent chance of having angiographically normal arteries). Schmermund and colleagues,[268f] using EBCT in patients who had recently diagnosed coronary disease and had undergone angiography, found that quantitation of coronary artery calcification was comparable to coronary angiography in measuring the effect of established cardiovascular risk factor on coronary atherosclerosis.

ANGIOGRAPHICALLY INAPPARENT DIFFUSE ATHEROSCLEROSIS

Pathology studies demonstrate consistently that atherosclerosis is more widespread than angiograms depict.[189, 269] Although early pathology studies were flawed because they measured the size of coronary vessels in an undistended state (leading to overestimation of stenosis), two independent techniques have reconfirmed the essential findings. Using high-frequency epicardial echocardiography, the coronary vessels of living human hearts have been evaluated at the time of cardiac surgery.[195] The ratio of coronary artery lumen diameter to the thickness of the coronary wall was used to quantify the severity of coronary lesions. In patients without atherosclerosis, the mean coronary lumen/wall thickness ratio was 5.9 ± 0.3 (± standard error of the mean). In patients with atherosclerotic disease at the site of examination, the mean ratio was markedly reduced (2.3 ± 0.2), consistent with the marked wall thickening at the site of obstruction. In *angiographically normal* arterial segments of patients with atherosclerosis elsewhere, however, mean ratio (4.1 ± 0.3) was also reduced, suggesting diffuse wall thickening. Thus, in patients with atherosclerosis elsewhere, even normal appearing epicardial segments showed significant unrecognized thickening of the arterial wall.[269]

Intravascular ultrasound techniques have demonstrated similar findings and have confirmed the insensitivity of coronary angiograms for detecting early atheromatous changes.[270, 271] Using intravascular ultrasound, abnormally high intimal/medial thickness measurements have been found in the coronaries of the majority of young donor hearts before cardiac transplantation—all of which appeared angiographically normal.[272] The lack of angiographic sensitivity to early, diffuse vascular disease is also demonstrated compellingly in cardiac transplant recipients.[273] In one study of 60 patients studied 1 year or more after transplantation, all had at least minimal intimal thickening and 63 percent had moderate or severe intimal thickening even though 70 percent of the patients had arteries that appeared normal angiographically. Postmortem examination of one cardiac transplant patient who died of severe left ventricular dysfunction 2 weeks after normal coronary angiography showed severe, diffuse accelerated coronary vasculopathy.[274] These findings of inapparent diffuse disease in angiographically normal coronary arterial segments are an additional reason why conclusions of stenosis severity based on relative measurements of percent luminal narrowing, either area or diameter, are often in error.

DIABETES AND CORONARY ATHEROSCLEROSIS

The problem of coronary atherosclerosis in diabetes mellitus, both types 1 and 2, is especially vexing. Not only is diabetes a highly potent risk factor in the pathogenesis of atherosclerosis and the major cause of death in this population, but also typical symptoms of this condition are atypical and often absent. Angiographically, the widespread presence of often diffuse disease makes calcification of percent stenosis as a marker of disease severity in this patient population most unreliable. "Normal" lumen diameters necessary for a reference segment value in this calculation are often impossible to determine. Diabetics have accelerated progression of disease after diagnosis, a condition also worsened by renal failure and the need for dialysis that may accompany diabetic renal disease.[274a] A decreased ability to exhibit compensatory luminal enlargement has been found in patients with diabetes, which may contribute to the diffuse nature and accelerated course of this condition.[274b] Diabetics also have a lesser degree of coronary collateral circulation associated with severe stenotic lesions.[274c]

Visual Assessment of Coronary Arterial Stenosis

Data obtained from analysis of the coronary arteriogram are traditionally expressed in anatomic terms, describing the vessel narrowing as a percentage reduction of the adjacent, apparently normal lumen caliber. Reams of studies obtained from over 20 years of investigations relate the number, severity, and distribution of coronary obstructive lesions, assessed by visual analysis of the angiogram to a host of clinical outcomes. The effect of a given stenosis in limiting coronary blood flow and thus affecting myocardial ischemia is generally assumed and rarely assessed directly.

The clinical maxim that a coronary stenosis does not become functionally significant until it causes a greater than 50 percent diameter narrowing is an outgrowth of studies in animals by Gould[275] showing that maximally augmented coronary flow is not limited until the stenosis is greater than 50 percent (Fig. 30–27). Although these studies were performed in animals using externally applied constrictors, it was assumed that similar findings would apply to human atherosclerotic lesions.

SOURCES OF ERROR IN VISUAL ASSESSMENTS OF LESION SEVERITY

Although visual assessment of the severity of luminal narrowing remains the standard for patient care today, many investigators since the late 1980s have realized increasingly the inadequacy of this approach.[198, 276–279] Marked intraobserver and interobserver variability in interpretation of lesion severity has been documented repeatedly. Visual intraobserver variability (±1 standard deviation) ranges from 7 to 18 percent, depending on technique.[280–283] The lower value was obtained from analyses of individual cine frames rather than on unselected cine runs. Disagreements of 30 to 35 percent have been reported when maximal stenosis severity has been assessed using either a 50 percent or a 70 percent diameter criterion.[283] Factors increasing observer variability include lesion location (left main[284] or distal lesion[283]), recent angioplasty,[285] and poor-quality angiograms.[283] Variability is lessened by the use of manual or electronic calipers or a calibrated magnifying eyepiece.[286, 287]

It is widely known that visual interpretation usually overestimates the severity of relatively high-grade lesions[288] and underestimates or totally overlooks low-grade lesions. Although visual interpretation has been reported to underestimate lesions greater than 50 percent based on necropsy data, such conclusions may be somewhat inaccurate because pathologic assessment of the coronary stenosis was carried out in "deflated," nonpressure-fixed specimens, exaggerating the degree of luminal compromise.[289] Ex vivo autopsy studies have also shown a high incidence of severely eccentric or slitlike coronary lumens; however, such lumen shapes are rarely seen angiographically.

Although it has been suggested that observer variability improves with angiographic experience, frequency of reading, and the use of consensus panels, the superiority of using a group of experienced angiographers to quantitatively grade angiograms does not withstand careful scrutiny.[280] There is very high agreement (95 percent) regarding lesion severity when determined by panel consensus[290]; however, the standard deviation of these interpretations of percent stenosis was ±14 percent. No improvement in correlation between three individual observers and a three-member consensus panel has been found.[291] Fortunately, quantitative methods for determining stenosis severity (see Quantitative Coronary Angiography) have today gained ascendancy in research investigations, and digital methodologies are frequently used in clinical angiographic evaluations.

Quantitative Coronary Angiography

Since the visual interpretation of coronary angiograms is inherently flawed, numerous computer-assisted systems have been developed to aid in the geometric assessment of epicardial coronary lesions.[292–295] Although quantitation of coronary stenoses is a giant step forward (compared with visual assessment), it must be remembered that quantitative

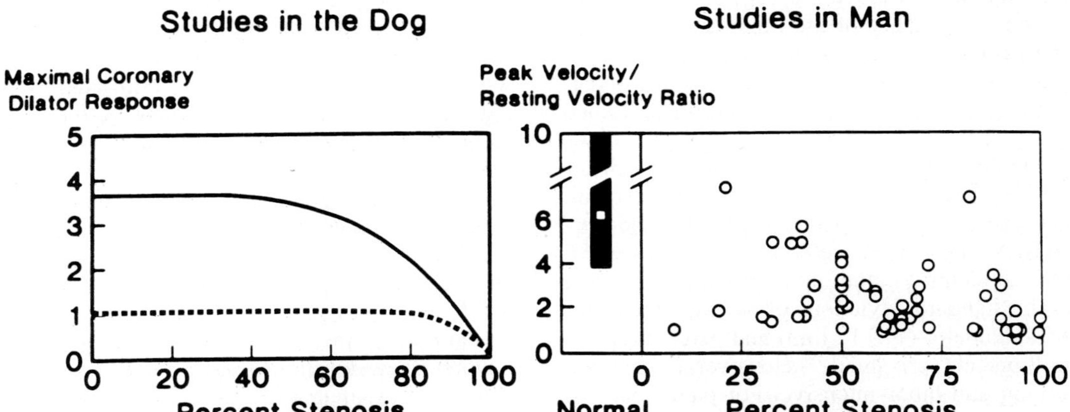

FIGURE 30–27 Relationship between maximal coronary blood flow or blood flow velocity and percent stenosis in an experimental study[275] and a clinical study. **Left,** In the animal experiment, a short concentric stenosis was placed on a normal coronary artery in an awake, chronically instrumented dog. Resting coronary blood flow (*dashed line*) was not significantly decreased until the percent diameter stenosis was greater than 85 percent. In contrast, maximal hyperemic coronary blood flow (*solid line*) was limited when the percent diameter stenosis was in the 50 to 60 percent range. **Right,** In the clinical study, maximal coronary blood flow (expressed as a ratio of peak velocity to resting velocity) was measured after transient ischemia. The range of normal responses in humans is shown by the *black bar* on the right. Each *open circle* represents a study in one patient. In contrast to the close relationship between percent diameter stenosis and maximal coronary blood flow in dogs, angiographically determined percent diameter stenosis was unrelated to hyperemic blood flow impairment in humans with widespread atherosclerosis. (From White CW, Wright CB, Doty DB, et al: Does visual interpretation of the coronary arteriogram predict the physiologic importance of a coronary stenosis? N Engl J Med 310:819–824, 1984.)

angiography is an anatomic but not a physiologic measurement tool. The coronary angiogram is a two-dimensional representation of the lumen of the artery under investigation. Changes in the size or configuration from an assumed normal vessel may not be sufficient to understand the physiology involved or to recognize the anatomic extent of the atherosclerotic process (see Physiologic Assessment of Coronary Arterial Stenoses). Despite these limitations, the development and implementation of quantitative methods for analysis of stenosis severity have improved evaluation of coronary artery lesions.

CALIPER METHOD

In 1979, Gensini and associates[296] described an electronic caliper system in which the borders of the arterial lesion could be manually defined using moving cursors. Errors related to visual parallax, systematic underestimation of severe obstructions (>75 percent diameter stenosis), and overestimation of less severe obstructions make this technique an imprecise substitute for computer-based methods.[292, 297, 298]

BROWN-DODGE METHOD

Development of quantitative coronary angiography by Brown and colleagues[186] at the University of Washington provided the seminal advance in the assessment of coronary angiograms. Images obtained from standard 35-mm cine film are projected at five-power magnification onto a grid. The vessel edges of the lesion and the adjacent proximal and distal "normal" segments are traced manually. The angiographic catheter is used as a scaling device to correct for magnification. The drawn arterial outlines from two orthogonal angiographic views are manually digitized. The outlines are corrected for magnification and distortion using a previously entered record of each angiographic laboratory's x-ray beam divergence and pincushion distortion and using the actual diameter of the angiographic catheter. The outlines are computer-matched at the minimal diameter or another standard point of reference visible in both views. Two orthogonal views are then combined to form a three-dimensional representation, assuming an elliptical lumen contour.

From this composite image, lesion minimal diameter and cross-sectional area are determined in absolute (square millimeter) and relative (lesion percent diameter and percent area stenosis) terms. This method has been used for many research applications and is highly accurate and reproducible. The standard deviations of repeated measurements of arterial diameter (± 0.12 mm) and percent diameter stenosis (± 3 percent) are small.[186] However, the method is time consuming and labor intensive. For these reasons, it has not seen widespread clinical utilization.

AUTOMATED EDGE DETECTION SYSTEMS

Reiber and coworkers[299–301] developed a semiautomated method for detecting the edges of coronary artery segment of interest and of the calibrating catheter (Coronary Artery Analysis System [CAAS]). Similar methods have been developed by others, but all use a digitized image obtained from a cineangiographic film frame or video signal. Nearly all techniques detect the arterial edge by videodensitometric methods, usually employing a weighted average of the first and second derivatives of the density change across the artery to identify the edge.[302]

Unlike the early Brown-Dodge system, these methods do not match orthogonal images and thus give only lumen diameter rather than cross-sectional area measurements. Manual matching of the data obtained from orthogonal views using the Reiber-CAAS system, however, correlates highly with cross-sectional area measured using the Brown-Dodge system.[303]

OTHER METHODS—VIDEODENSITOMETRY

A number of other investigators have developed other systems for computer-assisted quantitative coronary angiography[304, 305] or have made important contributions to the field.[306–313] Although most of these methods assess stenosis severity using geometric methods, considerable research has been directed toward nongeometric methods. Videodensitometry has been most commonly used. This technique is based on the Lambert-Beer law, which states that the logarithmic attenuation of the x-ray beam is proportional to the thickness of column of contrast medium within the vessel. This approach is fundamentally different from others previously described because it requires minimal assumptions regarding the geometry of the lesion being examined. With this approach, the operator performs an analysis at the site of the narrowest portion of the vessel as well as at a smooth proximal "normal" reference segment. The diameter of the adjacent normal segment is determined geometrically using the catheter as a scaling device. The normal lumen is assumed to be circular. Using a previously determined density calibration curve, the gray scale level along the arterial segment is converted to an optical density profile that is corrected for the optical density of a corresponding background point. An integrated optical density across the diameter of each arterial segment is calculated. The minimal integrated optical density of the coronary lesion is divided by the density of the normal segment, and the quotient is multiplied by the normal segment area. The resulting value is the minimal cross-sectional area of the artery.

Under very carefully controlled circumstances and in a small number of patients, one videodensitometric approach appeared to correlate well with minimal luminal area measured using Brown-Dodge quantitative coronary angiography as well as measurements of coronary flow reserve (CFR).[313] However, there are many theoretical and practical limitations to the use of videodensitometric techniques. Theoretically, densitometric techniques are less sensitive to variations in imaging system resolution, quantum noise, and stenosis cross-sectional shape than are edge detection techniques.[314] However, densitometry is also much more sensitive than edge detection to densitometric nonlinearities, overlapping structures (e.g., bone, diaphragm), and a nonperpendicular relationship between the vessel and the x-ray beam. The frequent occurrence of vessel foreshortening in many of the radiographic views results in artifactual increases in density and greatly limits the clinical utility of this technique. At present, the usual error with densitometric angiography appears to be between 5 and 20 percent, but it can approach 50 percent.[314] For these reasons and despite initially promising results, videodensitometric approaches to lesion quantitation have not yet seen widespread application.

PROBLEMS IN QUANTITATIVE ANGIOGRAPHY

Technical Problems. Although under ideal circumstances quantitative angiography can be a reliable and highly accurate measurement technique, many potential pitfalls exist. Blurring of the vessel edges, the penumbra effect, and cardiac motion can lead to a widened vessel edge, making edge detection less accurate.[292] Compared with visual assessment, quantitative angiography requires greater attention to optimal angiographic technique. Vessel overlap and unrecognized lesion foreshortening may produce major errors because single film frames are examined.

Inaccurate calibration from the angiographic catheter can be a major problem for quantitative angiography.[315–317] The use of small catheters (5 or 6 French) as the calibration source can lead to significantly less accuracy in the calculation of absolute diameter measurements.[305] Nylon catheters are also poorly suited for quantitation because they are less radiopaque (some newer nylon catheters are impregnated with radiopaque material). Even catheters of the same size from various manufacturers can vary by as much as 25 percent in diameter.[306] Inaccuracies in angiographic measurement of the true catheter size of up to 35 percent can also occur owing to inaccurate determination of the outer catheter edge (e.g., tracing of the contrast medium–filled inner lumen rather than the outer contour of the catheter).[298] Some authorities suggest that catheter calibration should be based on a catheter empty of contrast medium, before beginning the coronary medium injection, although this is not a widely held view.[319] Reference tables for the true size of a variety of angiographic catheters together with a comparison of their angiographic measurements as calculated by two different algorithms are available.[316]

Variations in Lesion Geometry. Most quantitative angiographic systems calculate only one lumen diameter measurement and assume a cylindrical shape if a lesion area measurement is calculated. The true geometry of a coronary lesion may vary widely. The Brown-Dodge system assumes an elliptical lesion shape and uses integration of two orthogonal views to obtain lumen area. Although major deviations from an elliptical shape occur rarely, the use of orthogonal views and the assumption of an elliptical geometry do not solve all geometric problems. Two acceptable truly orthogonal views are obtainable in only about 50 percent of lesions examined.[294] The maximal error for two arbitrary orthogonal views is small (<25 percent) only for mild degrees of ellipticity (major/minor axis < 2).[315, 320] The error increases as the angle between views becomes less orthogonal and as lesion ellipticity increases.

For angioplasty patient populations, quantitative measurements of vessel diameters taken from only one view in which the lesion appears worst compare quite closely with the average of two diameter measurements from nearly orthogonal views (minimal diameters of the two views within ± 5 percent in 90 percent and within ± 10 percent in all but 2.7 percent).[321] From these data, one could conclude that quantitative measurement of one view is adequate for routine clinical purposes. However, for research purposes, orthogonal views may sometimes be required. *Our experience comparing angiography to Doppler flow reserve measurements has led to the conclusion that integration of lesion diameters as seen in all views appears to relate best to physiologic measures of lesion severity.*

Variations in Vasomotor Tone. Day-to-day changes in coronary smooth muscle motor tone increase the interstudy variability of angiographic measurements and reduce the power of angiographic methods to detect small changes in coronary caliber in sequential studies. Removal of tone by nitroglycerin permits an assessment of maximal coronary caliber during similar conditions between studies.

Physiologic Assessment of Coronary Arterial Stenoses

The inaccuracies inherent in even the most sophisticated methods of anatomic assessment have led to the development of physiologically based methods to assess coronary stenosis severity. In 1939, Katz and Lindner[322] described the coronary reactive hyperemia response that has subsequently become the "gold standard" for the physiologic assessment of stenosis severity. In normal coronary arteries, myocardial blood flow is primarily regulated by the resistance of the arteriolar vessels ($\leq$400 μm diameter); the epicardial coronary arteries provide little resistance to coronary blood flow under physiologic circumstances. As a stenosis progresses in an epicardial vessel, a trans-stenotic pressure gradient develops. The microvessels dilate to compensate for the reduced distal perfusion pressure, thus maintaining normal resting blood flow to the myocardium.

Studies in animals have shown that resting coronary blood flow can be maintained at normal levels until more than 75 percent of the arterial cross-sectional area (50 percent of the diameter if the obstruction is concentric) is obstructed. At this point, the vasodilator reserve of the arterioles is exhausted, and further vasodilatation is impossible.[275] Resting blood flow does not decrease until 90 percent of the lumen is obstructed. Coronary stenoses that limit myocardial blood flow during maximal arteriolar vasodilatation are termed *physiologically significant* (Fig. 30–28).[323] The ratio of maximal hyperemic blood flow (e.g., induced by coronary occlusion or drugs) to resting blood flow is termed *coronary vasodilator reserve* (or *coronary flow reserve*).

The ratio of the intracoronary pressure distal to a stenosis to the proximal coronary or aortic pressure *during conditions of maximal hyperemia* is termed the *fractional flow reserve* (FFR). These two physiologic measurements (CFR and FFR) have provided important clinical techniques to assess limitations in hyperemic blood flow imparted by a stenosis.

CORONARY FLOW RESERVE

Utilization of Doppler methods for measuring blood flow velocity has provided the major principles for clinical investigation of CFR. Initial studies in humans were performed using a Doppler crystal applied at surgery to the epicardial surface of a coronary vessel.[324] These experi-

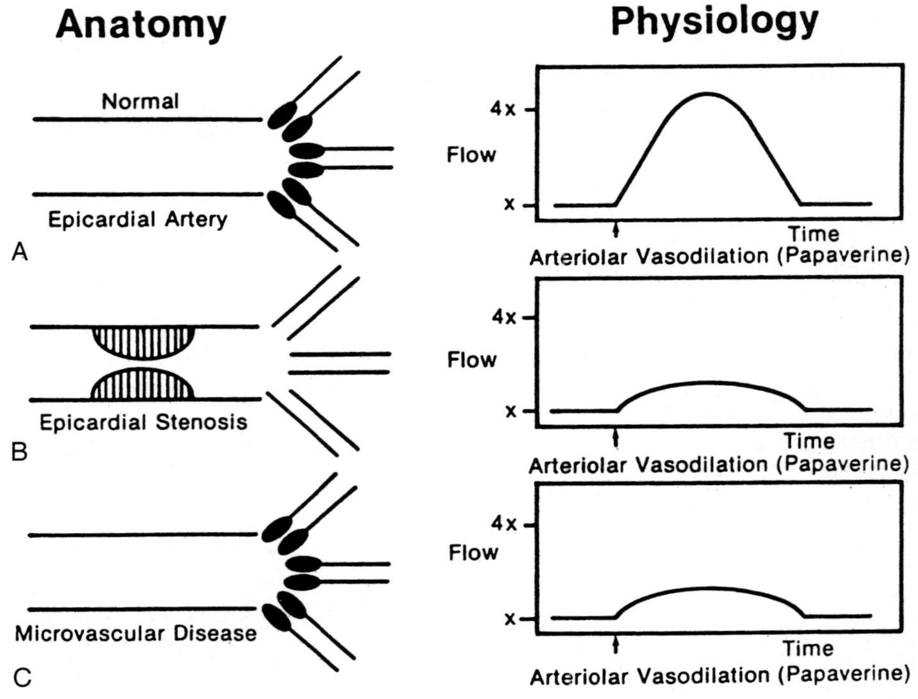

FIGURE 30–28 The effects of an epicardial stenosis on coronary flow reserve. **A,** Dilatation of a normal microvasculature with papaverine causes blood flow to increase fourfold. **B,** An epicardial stenosis causes partial microvascular dilatation, and papaverine has little additional effect. Flow reserve is reduced. **C,** Microvascular disease prevents normal arteriolar dilatation, reducing flow reserve.

ments showed that the reactive hyperemic response in normal human coronary arteries was similar to that obtained in anesthetized animals. However, the experiments failed to confirm in humans the relationship between luminal stenosis and flow impairment previously observed in normal animals (see Fig. 30–27). In patients with multivessel coronary atherosclerosis and isolated discrete coronary lesions varying in severity between 10 and 95 percent stenosis, measurements of the anatomic stenosis severity were not correlated significantly with the reactive hyperemic response ($r = -.25$).[324] Underestimation of lesion severity occurred in 95 percent of vessels with greater than 60 percent diameter stenosis by angiography. Both overestimation and underestimation of lesions with less than 60 percent stenoses were common.

The development and validation of small Doppler catheters[325] and subsequently Doppler guide wires[326] made possible the subselective measurement of coronary blood flow velocity in individual coronary vessels at the time of angiography (Fig. 30–29). Subselective techniques for measuring flow velocity were necessary for clinical usefulness of this methodology because coronary atherosclerosis had a heterogeneous distribution throughout the coronary tree. Since coronary occlusion is not practical during angiography, pharmacologic vasodilators were given to create a maximal hyperemic response. The original studies utilized intracoronary papaverine, which results in maximal increases in coronary flow comparable with those achieved with intravenous transient coronary occlusion or dipyridamole.[327] Although the short half-life coupled with little effect on systemic hemodynamics made papaverine a useful drug for this purpose, occasional QT prolongation and rare but potentially serious transient arrhythmias can occur.[328] For this reason, intracoronary adenosine, which has an even shorter half-life than papaverine, has now generally replaced papaverine as the drug of choice for physiologic studies of the coronary circulation under hyperemic conditions.[329]

In contrast to measurements obtained in patients with severe coronary atherosclerosis studied at cardiac surgery,[324] flow reserve measurements obtained in the catheterization laboratory in patients with only single-vessel disease show a curvilinear relationship between percent stenosis and flow reserve, similar to that found in animals with normal coronary vessels (Fig. 30–30).[187]

Lesions causing less than 70 percent area stenosis did not cause a significant reduction of hyperemic blood flow. The disparate results seen in patients with limited versus those with more widespread coronary atherosclerosis probably relates to the unrecognized presence of diffuse luminal encroachment. Percent stenosis measurements of a focal lesion in an artery with diffuse luminal narrowing lead to underestimation of lesion severity based on an inaccurate determination of the normal adjacent lumen reference segment. Since the coronary angiogram is a "lumenogram," it is impossible to know whether a segment of a vessel appearing angiographically normal has inapparent diffuse disease. As the degree of diffuse narrowing increases, lesser focal stenoses are required to impair maximal hyperemic blood flow.[330] As shown in Figure 30–31, a 50 percent stenosis has greatly different effects on limiting flow, depending on the true area of the normal segment.

Absolute measurements of the coronary caliber can provide important information that is independent of diffuse luminal narrowing. A minimal lesion cross-sectional area of 2.5 mm^2 or more (≥ 3.5 mm^2 in the proximal left anterior descending artery) almost always indicates the absence of flow impairment by the lesion, regardless of the adjacent arterial diameter.

One should not conclude from these studies that moder-

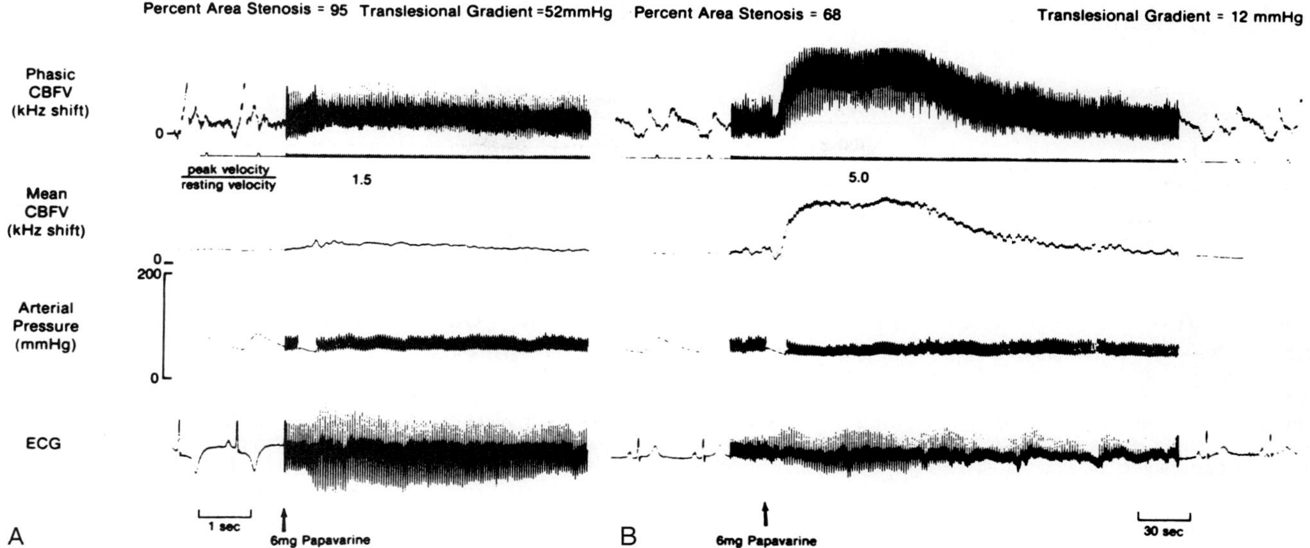

FIGURE 30–29 Record obtained from patient undergoing right coronary artery angioplasty. *Top,* Phasic coronary blood flow velocity (CBFV). *Second from top,* Mean coronary blood flow velocity. *Bottom two panels,* The arterial pressure and electrocardiogram (ECG). **A,** Before angioplasty, the lesion produced 95 percent area stenosis with an associated translesional pressure gradient of 52 mm Hg. Six milligrams of intracoronary papaverine produced only a 1.5-fold increase in blood flow velocity. **B,** After angioplasty, the percent area stenosis was decreased to 68 percent and the translesional pressure gradient was reduced to 12 mm Hg. Six milligrams of intracoronary papaverine resulted in a 5.0-fold increase in blood flow velocity, demonstrating that physiologically significant obstruction to coronary blood flow had been removed.

ate inapparent diffuse coronary atherosclerosis alone impairs the vasodilator reserve.[289]

In a study from our laboratory,[330] hyperemic blood flow was normal in atherosclerotic vessels perfused by bypass grafts as long as the graft perfused a nonstenotic coronary vessel subserving normal myocardium. This occurred despite the fact that cross-sectional area of the bypassed artery is diffusely narrowed (40 percent smaller than a similar site in matched normal vessels).

FRACTIONAL FLOW RESERVE

Intracoronary pressure measurements can also provide important physiologic information regarding the functional significance of coronary stenoses.[330a] Commonly termed the fractional flow reserve, this technique in reality compares the intracoronary pressure measured proximal and distal to a stenosis under conditions of maximal hyperemic flow.[330b] A ratio of proximal/distal intracoronary pressure measured with a fiberoptic pressure-monitoring guide wire during adenosine infusion has been used to assess the physiologic significances of coronary stenoses of moderate severity (40 to 50 percent). In 45 patients an FFR of greater than 0.75 has been shown to correlate highly with noninvasive tests of myocardial ischemia. The overall sensitivity, specificity, positive and negative predictive values, and accuracy were 88 percent, 100 percent, 100 percent, 88 percent, and 93 percent, respectively.[330c]

Such FFR measurements can be used to assess the results of balloon angioplasty.[330d] Using a pressure-monitoring wire to replace a standard angioplasty guide wire, Bech and colleagues[330d] showed that an FFR greater than 0.90 stratified patients into an optimal post–percutaneous transluminal coronary angioplasty result. A small amount of additional stratification value was obtained when a quantitatively determined residual percent diameter stenosis of less than 35 percent was combined with the FFR.

In addition to assessing the efficiency of angioplasty, physiologic measurements evaluating the functional significance of intermediate coronary lesions has been used to

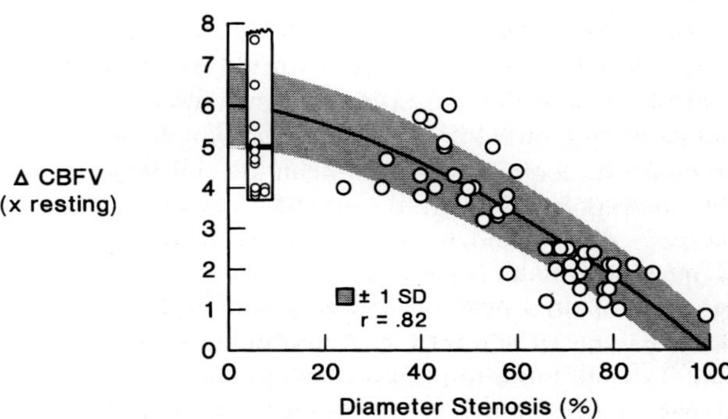

FIGURE 30–30 Relationship between the most severe diameter stenosis measured in the LAO or RAO projection and the coronary flow reserve (Δ CBFV). The *open bar* represents the range of coronary flow reserve measured in 13 patients with normal coronary vessels. The *shaded area* along the regression line represents 1 standard deviation (SD) above and below the mean. (From Wilson RF, Marcus ML, White CW: Prediction of the physiologic significance of coronary arterial lesions by quantitative lesion geometry in patients with limited coronary artery disease. Circulation 75:723–732, 1987.)

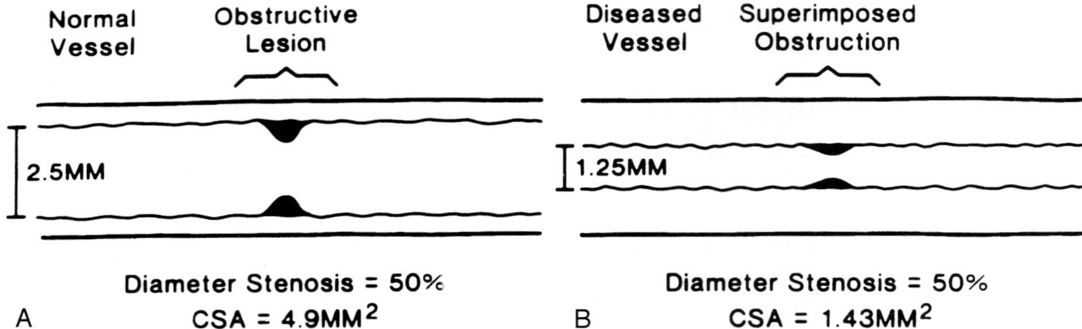

FIGURE 30–31 The effects of a 50 percent diameter stenosis in a normal vessel **(A)** and a diffusely diseased vessel **(B)**. A 50 percent stenosis in a "normal" artery leaves significantly greater residual cross-sectional area (CSA) than does a 50 percent stenosis in an artery that is already diffusely narrowed. Since the amount of diffuse coronary narrowing cannot be well assessed from a visual analysis of a coronary angiogram, a focal 50 percent stenosis on the angiogram may have vastly different effects on coronary blood flow. (**A** and **B,** From Marcus ML, Harrison DG, White CW, et al: Assessing the physiologic significance of coronary obstructions in patients: importance of diffuse undetected atherosclerosis. Prog Cardiovasc Dis 31:39, 1988.)

make a decision NOT to dilate non–flow-limiting lesions.[330e, 330f] These data indicate that deferral of a coronary intervention based on a normal CFR or an FFR of 0.75 or greater is associated with a lower clinical event rate than would be expected if the procedure had been performed as originally planned.

LIMITATIONS IN THE USE OF PHYSIOLOGIC FLOW AND PRESSURE MEASUREMENTS: DUAL ROLES OF THE CORONARY EPICARDIAL AND MICROCIRCULATIONS

Although attractive in concept, there are many limitations in utilizing coronary flow or pressure reserve measurements to define the physiologic significance of a given atherosclerotic lesion. Inherent in understanding these limitations is the fact that the coronary circulation can be regulated by two distinct vascular components connected in series: the epicardial vessels and the microcirculation. Coronary atherosclerosis affects primarily the epicardial vessels, and the microcirculation subserved by any given epicardial artery may be normal or abnormal. A variety of pathophysiologic conditions (e.g., anemia and polycythemia, diabetes, hypertrophy, infarction, vasculitis, wall motion abnormalities, and other conditions involving the coronary microcirculation) can reduce flow reserve in myocardium supplied by anatomically normal epicardial vessel or by one containing atherosclerotic lesions.[333–337] Hence, a reduction in the CFR or in the FFR of a coronary artery with a stenosed vessel cannot be taken as prima facie evidence that blood flow is limited by the stenosis.

The CFR is altered by the hemodynamic conditions existing at the time of study.[338] Increases in heart rate or preload reduce flow reserve because these conditions increase resting blood flow without changing hyperemic flow. In contrast, acute changes in mean arterial pressure within the autoregulatory range do not alter the flow reserve ratio because resting and hyperemic blood flow are increasing proportionately as arterial pressure rises. It has been suggested that flow reserve measurements be obtained during atrial pacing to eliminate the confounding effects of heart rate. Despite these limitations, serial measurements of flow reserve are highly reproducible over time in the absence of conditions known to alter resting or hyperemic coronary blood flow.[339] Repeated measurements of flow reserve separated by 1 year, performed on patients under these conditions, showed a very high degree of correlation ($r = 0.95$).

The FFR has been shown to be independent of loading conditions.[339a] However, this measurement is greatly affected by the ability of the microcirculation to increase flow, and the theoretical and experimental models for normal and abnormal FFR assume a normal microcirculation.[339a] When assessing the effects of a coronary stenotic lesion in patients with small vessel disease, such as diabetes, or after myocardial infarction, the FFR (as well as the CFR) can underestimate the severity of a stenosis because microcirculatory flow may be suboptimally increased. Thus, to assess both epicardial disease and microcirculatory abnormalities, both pressure and flow under hyperemic conditions should be assessed.

LIMITATIONS OF AN OPTIMAL HEMODYNAMIC EVALUATION OF A CORONARY LESION

Despite the importance of determining the hemodynamic impact of individual coronary lesions, the pathophysiologic consequences of non–flow-limiting lesions must not be overlooked. Little and Applegate[340] have shown that lesions of only mild-to-moderate severity are most frequently the source of plaque rupture and progression to acute myocardial infarction. This is perhaps not surprising when one considers the usual frequency of occurrence of mild versus severe atherosclerosis lesions in the coronary tree. For these reasons, one cannot predict the site of the coronary lesion that will likely progress to subtotal occlusion from a retrospective review of angiograms taken shortly before development of the acute event.[340] Thus, it is unlikely that a coronary interventional approach will play a dominant role in preventing acute infarction.

Angiography can also be very important in yielding clues to aid in clarification of clinical syndromes. Unimpressive intraluminal coronary lucencies, both de novo and after angioplasty, may forecast impending total coronary occlusion. Specific morphologic characteristics, such as the ruptured plaque or the lucency of a spontaneous coronary dissection, may serve as important clues in the diagnosis of the cause of chest pain in the absence of alterations in CFR. Similarly physiologic abnormalities in coronary blood flow regulation induced by atherosclerosis (e.g., endothelial dysfunction as assessed by infusions of acetylcholine or substance P) or other abnormalities may potentiate the effects of a focal coronary lesion or lead to ischemia in the absence of a hemodynamically significant stenosis in the epicardial arteries.[344, 345] *Hence, the absence of a flow-limiting stenosis at the time of angiography should not imply the absence of myocardial ischemia or risk of vessel closure.*

Angiographic Findings in Myocardial Infarction and Acute Coronary Syndromes

It has been commonly believed that a severe coronary lesion was the forerunner of acute myocardial infarction and that coronary arteries with less than 50 percent obstructions were relatively free of thrombotic risk.[346] Some studies have convincingly refuted this dogma and given evidence that coronary angiography cannot be used to accurately predict the *site* of a subsequent occlusion that will result in myocardial infarction.[347]

Although retrospective reviews of angiograms performed shortly before the development of acute infarction have identified high-grade coronary stenoses as a risk factor for subsequent total coronary occlusion, studies in patients having angiograms both months to years before and shortly after infarction showed that the infarction-related occlusion frequently occurred in a coronary segment without a severe stenosis on the early angiogram. In only 38 percent of patients was the most severe angiographic stenosis found to be responsible for the subsequent infarction.[348] In 60 percent of patients, the most severe luminal diameter stenosis present in the infarct-related artery before the infarction was less than 50 percent. Similar studies by a number of investigators[349–351] have confirmed these results.

In patients with unstable angina, quantitative angiographic studies show a strikingly different picture. In such patients, angiograms have a high predictive value in determining the culprit lesion. Lesions associated with unstable angina usually have a percent diameter stenosis of greater than 85 percent, a lesion cross-sectional area of less than 0.9 mm^2, and a morphology consistent with an irregular eccentric lesion, occasionally with thrombotic intraluminal filling defects (see later).[352] Hence, such obstructions are usually visually obvious. Patients presenting with symptoms of rest angina who do not have coronary lesions of this severity should be carefully evaluated for the possibility of coronary spasm.

Pathologic-Angiographic Correlates

Coronary angiography performed very soon after the onset of clinical symptoms of myocardial infarction usually demonstrates total occlusion of the coronary artery perfusing the infarct zone. The incidence of total occlusion is nearly 90 percent if angiography is performed as early as 1 hour after symptoms, but drops to about 70 percent if angiography is delayed to 12 to 24 hours.[353] Total occlusion is found less frequently (26 percent) in patients having angiography within 24 hours of symptom onset of a non–Q wave infarction.[354] This reduction in frequency of total coronary occlusion is probably the result of spontaneously occurring thrombolysis.

To understand the angiographic findings of acute coronary syndromes, it is important to consider the underlying events occurring in the artery during acute infarction. Fissuring or rupture of the atherosclerotic plaque appears to be the inciting event in both unstable angina and acute myocardial infarction (Figs. 30–32 and 30–33).[355, 356] Rupture of the fibrous cap also allows blood from the vessel lumen to dissect into the intima and media, thus causing the plaque to expand. Plaque rupture as the nidus for subsequent thrombus formation can be seen only if the entire thrombus is examined by serial histologic sections and is thus often missed on routine autopsy examination.

Pathologic and clinical evidence suggests that coronary thrombosis after plaque rupture is a dynamic process.[355, 356] The occlusive thrombus typically has a multilayered structure, suggesting that it is often formed successively over an extended period of time (days to weeks), rather than occurring as a single, abrupt event.[357] This finding fits with the often stuttering course of ischemic symptoms. In addition, clot fragmentation with distal microembolization has been identified in 73 percent of cases carefully studied and can be seen on the angiogram in a smaller fraction of patients.[357] Although aggregated platelets are the major early component of the thrombus, within 1 or 2 days this platelet thrombus is infiltrated and consolidated, leading to a more distinct angiographic edge.[357]

If the coronary lumen is totally occluded, the blood between the occlusion site and the nearest proximal side branch will stagnate with the production of a stasis thrombus. The volume of stasis clot is usually (but not always) relatively small. A recent total coronary occlusion is characterized angiographically by a small remaining vessel stump that can accumulate contrast material. Injection into

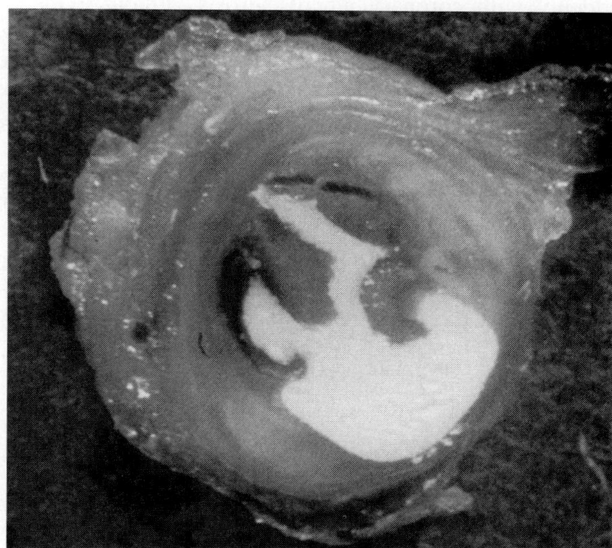

FIGURE 30–32 Section of a coronary arterial cast (the lumen area was filled with barium gel) from a patient with unstable angina. Note the plaque rupture with extension of the lumen into the arterial wall (plaque ulcer). (Courtesy of Erling Falk, M.D.)

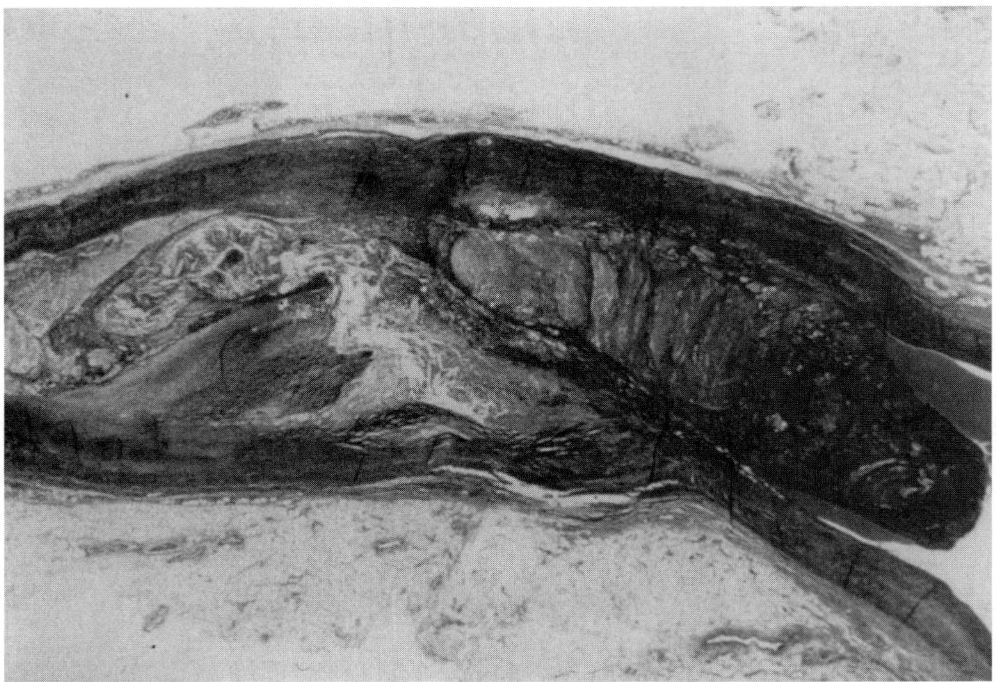

FIGURE 30–33 Longitudinal section of a coronary artery at the site of total thrombotic occlusion resulting from atherosclerotic plaque rupture. Proximal obstruction (*right*) is stasis (red blood cell) clot. Distal obstruction (*left*) is atheromatous debris and primarily platelet clot. (Courtesy of Erling Falk, M.D.)

this stump usually reveals an often "feathered" hangup of contrast medium with indistinct margins and slow washout. The angiographic cut-off of an occluded bypass graft usually occurs at the aortic anastomosis because occlusion within the graft body or at the coronary insertion leads to total graft thrombosis.

Plaque fissuring, a multilayered thrombus, and distal microembolization are also seen at postmortem examination in patients with unstable angina and in humans dying suddenly with coronary atherosclerosis without evidence of myocardial infarction.[356] Clinically and angiographically, despite evidence of plaque rupture, patients with unstable angina have a much smaller burden of clot within the affected arterial segment than do patients with Q or non–Q wave infarction. Coronary angioscopy performed in vivo in patients with unstable angina has shown complex plaques and small intraluminal clots that are sometimes not visible angiographically.[358] Although patients with unstable angina after thrombolytic therapy show small increases in luminal areas assessed using quantitative angiography, such improvements are often not visually apparent nor usually clinically sufficient.[346, 359] A small fraction of patients may have a more dramatic response.

Angiographic Findings

Angiographic features of atherosclerotic plaque disruption have been described qualitatively. Postmortem angiograms in the setting of plaque rupture have a "complicated" appearance characterized by irregular arterial borders and intraluminal filling defects.[360, 361] In vivo angiographic studies of coronary lesions in patients with unstable angina also show eccentric lesion shapes, characterized by a narrow neck and overhanging edges or scalloped borders, a high incidence of stenosis irregularity, and intraluminal filling defects that presumably are clot. After thrombolytic therapy for acute infarction, similar findings are seen with marked stenosis irregularities and an increased incidence of intraluminal filling defects.[361] In addition, an ulcer crater that was obscured by overlying thrombus may become evident after thrombolysis (Fig. 30–34).

Ambrose and associates[362, 363] developed a system for classifying coronary stenosis morphology based on its angiographic appearance (Fig. 30–35). Lesions associated with acute thrombotic syndromes (unstable angina and infarction) were usually of type II eccentric morphology, and in most thrombotic lesions, the edges of the lesion were irregular and scalloped.[362]

Visual interpretation of stenosis morphology is fraught with marked intraobserver and interobserver variability. For these reasons, quantitative indices of lesion irregularity applicable for use with computer-assisted quantitative angiography have been developed.[352] One such quantitative measure, the ulceration index is defined as the diameter of the least severe narrowing within the lesion (the downward lip of the ulcer) divided by the maximal intralesional diameter. This index decreases as the irregularity increases and is independent of stenosis severity (in terms of lumen obstruction). In one study of patients with stable angina, unstable angina, or recent myocardial infarction, the severity of the coronary lesion measured either as percent stenosis or in absolute terms as minimal cross-sectional area was similar in all groups, although lesions causing unstable

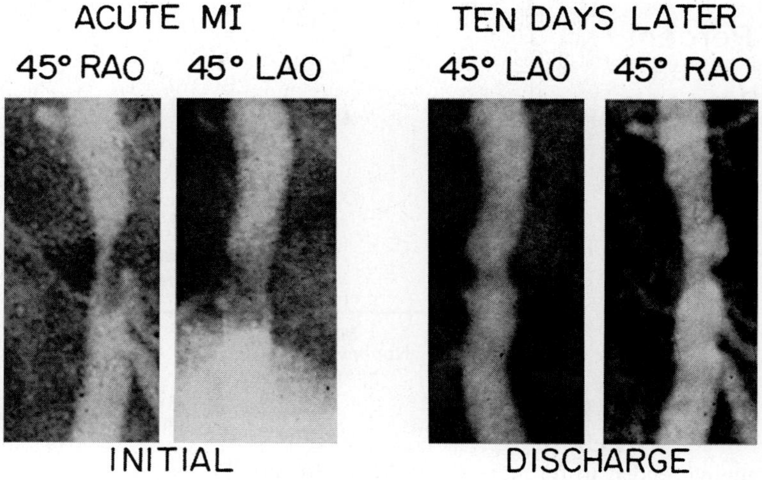

ACUTE MI
45° RAO 45° LAO
INITIAL

TEN DAYS LATER
45° LAO 45° RAO
DISCHARGE

FIGURE 30–34 Angiogram obtained from a patient with acute myocardial infarction demonstrates clot lysis over time. Angiography soon after presentation revealed a large clot adherent to the arterial wall and protruding into the vessel lumen (leftmost panel). Ten days later, angiography showed an "ulcer" at the site of clot attachment (rightmost panel).

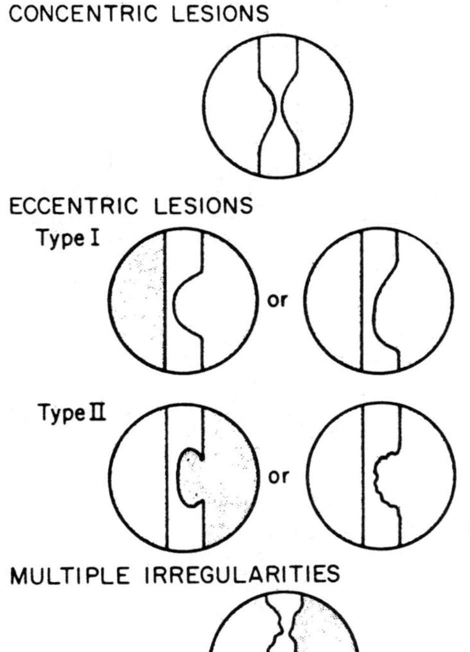

FIGURE 30–35 Angiographic morphology of coronary arterial stenoses. Type A lesions: smooth and concentric. Type B_1 lesions: eccentric with a smooth border. Type B_2 lesions: eccentric with overhanging edges or irregular borders, frequently associated with lesion thrombosis. Type C lesions: multiple irregularities. (From Ambrose JA, Winters SL, Arora RR, et al: Coronary angiographic morphology in myocardial infarction: a link between the pathogenesis of unstable angina and myocardial infarction. Reprinted with permission from the American College of Cardiology [J Am Coll Cardiol 6:1233–1238, 1985].)

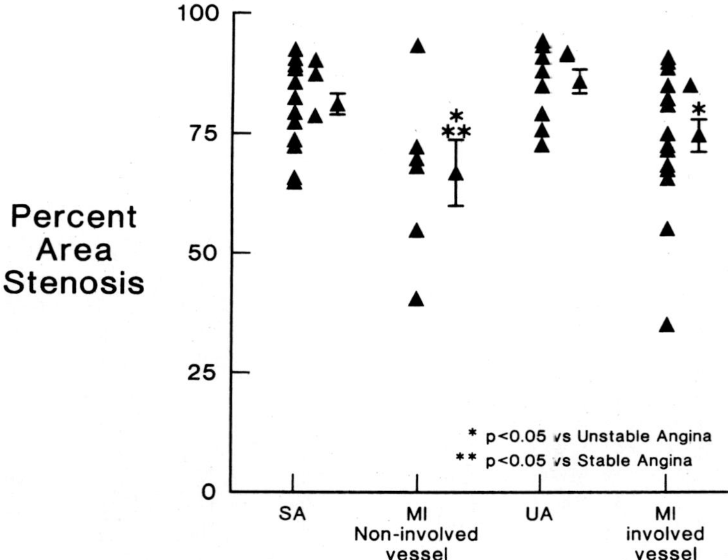

FIGURE 30–36 Percent area stenosis of lesions causing stable angina (SA), myocardial infarction (MI), unstable angina (UA), and non–infarct-related lesions in patients with acute infarction. Although lesions associated with unstable angina tended to be more severe than those associated with infarction or unstable angina, there was significant overlap among groups. (From Wilson RF, Holida MD, White CW: Quantitative angiographic morphology of coronary stenoses leading to myocardial infarction or unstable angina. Circulation 73:286–293, 1986.)

angina tended to be more severe (Fig. 30–36). The ulceration index (Fig. 30–37), however, was significantly lower in lesions causing unstable angina (0.62 ± 0.05) or infarction (0.61 ± 0.03) than in lesions causing stable angina (0.90 ± 0.01).[352] A modified index has also been found useful but is not independent of the stenosis severity.[365]

The angiographic appearance of blood flow in the artery distal to a thrombotic lesion also carries some significance. A system for grading blood flow was developed for the Thrombosis in Myocardial Infarction (TIMI) trial and has been generally used since then.[364] The TIMI flow classification is as follows:

0 No antegrade blood flow
1 Faint antegrade blood flow that does not fill the distal vessel
2 Reduced antegrade blood flow that fills the distal vessel
3 Normal antegrade blood flow

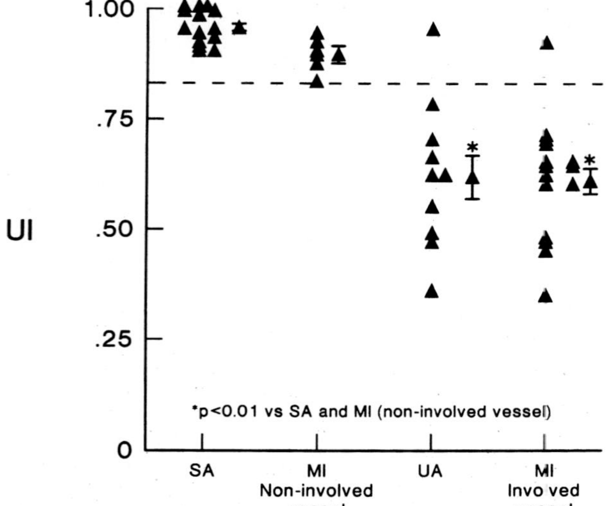

FIGURE 30–37 Calculated ulceration index (UI) of lesions causing stable angina (SA), myocardial infarction (MI), and unstable angina (UA), and non–infarct-related lesions in patients with acute infarction. The ulceration index of lesions involved in myocardial infarction or unstable angina was significantly less than that of lesions uninvolved in infarction or associated with stable angina. (From Wilson RF, Holida MD, White CW: Quantitative angiographic morphology of coronary stenoses leading to myocardial infarction or unstable angina. Circulation 73:286–293, 1986.)

Although visual interpretation of the rapidity and completeness of angiographic coronary flow after myocardial infarction has proved helpful in assessing the efficacy and subsequent clinical outcomes of various therapies, this methodology (TIMI flow assessment) has recently been shown to exhibit considerable variability. This variability can be diminished by counting the angiographic frames from initial vessel opacification until filling of the distal bed.[365]

Although coronary flow in the infarct subserving vessel has been the subject of the greatest study, flow in the angiographically normal noninvolved vessel in acute infarction may not be normal. Using Doppler catheter techniques and acetylcholine infusions, endothelial dysfunction of the noninvolved epicardial resistance vessels was found in 75 percent of patients with acute myocardial infarction.

Coronary Reocclusion and Lesion Remodeling After Myocardial Infarction

Coronary angiography has been helpful in identifying patients at increased risk of recurrent ischemic events after thrombolysis. Typical plaque rupture morphology is often not visible immediately after thrombolysis, presumably because of unlysed but inapparent thrombus laminated along the vessel wall (see Fig. 30–34).[366] The characteristic morphology of the infarct-related lesion after thrombolysis was found in one study,[367] but not in another,[368] to be a marker of subsequent reocclusion.

Quantitative angiographic studies show that clot lysis

continues after thrombolytic therapy for acute infarction and restoration of vessel patency. In our initial studies,[366] the minimal lesion cross-sectional area increased 116 ± 34 percent during the 7 to 10 days after intracoronary thrombolysis and initial lumen patency. In 7 of 17 patients, minimal luminal cross-sectional area more than doubled. Similar data have been obtained by other investigators.[369, 370]

The residual lumen caliber immediately after reperfusion has been used to identify patients at high risk for reclosure within the first 2 weeks after thrombolysis. In quantitative angiographic studies after successful intracoronary thrombolysis with streptokinase, rethrombosis occurred exclusively in vessels with a minimal lesion cross-sectional area of less than 0.4 mm^2.[366, 369, 370] In that group, 54 percent of patients who had initially successful reperfusion with intracoronary streptokinase developed rethrombosis within 2 weeks.[366] Similar conclusions were reached when lesion severity was evaluated by videodensitometry.

Data compiled from trials in which thrombolysis was achieved using recombinant tissue plasminogen activator found that recurrent ischemic events in these patients could not be predicted by any angiographic variable: percent diameter stenosis, absolute lesion diameter, angiographically defined thrombus, or stenosis morphology.[371] Although the incidence of recurrent ischemic events was similar to those reported for streptokinase (about 20 percent), after recombinant tissue plasminogen activator reclosure occurred in 8 percent of patients with a minimal diameter stenosis greater than 0.6 mm (about 0.3 mm^2) and in patients in whom the residual diameter stenosis was as low as 55 percent. These disparate results may be due to fundamental differences in the mechanisms of these agents in creating the thrombolytic state.[372]

Coronary Collaterals

A preexisting network of structural connections between various portions of the coronary arterial supply to the heart (coronary collaterals) has been recognized for centuries.[373] However, the importance of this network in providing a degree of structural protection against the effects of ischemia owing to atherosclerotic coronary obstructions has only recently become clear.

Major species differences exist in the extent and function of coronary collaterals.[374] Rats, pigs, and other species have no native collateral network, and acute coronary occlusion results in rapid myocardial necrosis.[374–376] Conversely, coronary occlusion in guinea pigs causes no infarction at all because they have a well-developed collateral network that maintains normal perfusion in spite of total coronary occlusion.[377]

Where does the human coronary circulation fit in this species listing? Autopsy studies have shown the presence of small coronary anastomoses (native collaterals) 50 to 250 μm in diameter in nearly all normal human hearts.[378, 379] In human coronary disease, this preexisting collateral network is enhanced by the development of an increased plexus of subendocardial collateral vessels that link the perfusion field at risk of infarction with other better-perfused areas.[380] In patients with severe coronary atherosclerosis, a diffuse subendocardial plexus of collateral vessels can be seen angiographically as an outline of the left ventricular cavity.

In the human atherosclerotic state, antemortem or postmortem angiograms also often reveal larger *epicardial* anastomoses (stimulated collaterals). Such connections often connect proximal and distal segments of the same occluded artery, connect adjacent arteries, or may traverse the atrium to connect two arteries with adjacent atrial branches.[381] These connections are more like what is seen in the dog after the placement of ameroid constrictors, which cause the gradual development of coronary obstruction.

Human Coronary Collateral Pathways

The preferred anatomic pathways taken by collateral channels have been described in detail by other authors.[382, 383] Some of the more common anatomic connections are

I. Collateral pathways to the left anterior descending coronary artery
   A. From the posterior descending artery via septal branches or around the apex
   B. From the conal branch of the right coronary artery via the Vieussen ring
   C. From the acute marginal branch of the right coronary artery
   D. From the obtuse marginal branch of the circumflex artery
II. Collateral pathways to the right coronary artery
   A. From the left anterior descending artery via septal branches or around the apex to the posterior descending artery
   B. From the distal circumflex or obtuse marginal branches to the posterolateral branch; at times via the atrioventricular nodal artery
   C. From the conal or right ventricular branch to the more distal right coronary branches
   D. From the left atrial circumflex artery
III. Collateral pathways to the circumflex coronary artery
   A. From a diagonal branch of the left anterior descending artery to a marginal circumflex branch
   B. From a proximal marginal or left atrial circumflex artery to the more distal circumflex marginals
   C. From the distal right coronary artery to the distal circumflex artery
   D. From the posterolateral branch of the right coronary artery to the obtuse marginal branch

Intermittent or gradual coronary occlusion results in the growth of coronary collaterals.[384, 385] This maturation process involves not only an increase in the lumen of the vessel but also the development of new vascular smooth muscle.[381] In the dog, at 6 months after coronary occlusion, a well-developed tunica media is present.[386] Collateral vessels respond to several neurohumoral substances, but the response of mature coronary collaterals differs substantially from that of native coronary arteries and immature collateral vessels.[386] Mature collaterals are also responsive to the vasoconstrictor effects of vasopressin[386] and ergonovine.[387]

Visible and Recruitable Coronary Collaterals

Human coronary collaterals become demonstrable by coronary angiography only when the parent vessel is subtotally or totally occluded. Unfortunately, angiographic grading of coronary collaterals based on collateral caliber is not accurate in predicting the functional ability of the collateral to provide coronary perfusion. There are several reasons for this:

1. Coronary collaterals in the 100-μm range are not angiographically visible.[239]
2. Angiographic techniques in humans for quantitating collateral function are not well validated.[239]
3. In the absence of near-total vessel occlusion, collateral vessels are not visible in the resting state (e.g., during angiography). They can, however, be rendered visible if contrast material is injected into the contralateral artery during coronary spasm[388] or during temporary balloon occlusion of the recipient artery.[389] These collaterals have been termed *recruitable*.[390]

It is likely that these shortcomings in evaluating collateral flow were responsible for much of the controversy over the last several decades regarding the functional importance of coronary collaterals in humans. Until the mid-1960s, the myocardial protective effects of collaterals were widely accepted.[380] In the 1970s, however, these prevailing concepts were called into question[391, 392] with the finding of a higher incidence of wall motion disturbances in patients with versus those without collaterals. Concepts then shifted to reflect the view that collaterals were only a marker of severe disease, which offered no beneficial effects.

At present, the pendulum has returned to the conclusions of the earlier era[393] as a result of several important observations. For any given location of acute coronary occlusion, the degree of deterioration of left ventricular function is inversely related to the presence of angiographically visible coronary collaterals.[394] In addition, the incidence of late aneurysm formation after myocardial infarction is reduced in patients with an angiographically significant collateral circulation, with or without successful reperfusion.[395] The risk of hemodynamically severe consequences from acute infarction is mitigated greatly by the presence of a preexisting severe stenosis and, thus, the protective effect of a developed collateral circulation. Conversely, when acute coronary occlusion occurs in the presence of a mild stenosis and thus poor collateral development, it is likely to have more severe clinical consequences.[396] More recently, it has been shown that the presence of angiographically defined coronary collaterals extends the "window of time" for the beneficial effect of reperfusion therapy of myocardial infarction and results in greater improvement in cardiac function and reduction in infarct size.[397]

Collateral flow can be graded using the following scale devised by Rentrop and colleagues[398]:

Grade 0	No angiographically visible filling of any collateral channels
Grade 1	Collateral filling of the distal branches of the recipient artery, but not the epicardial portion of the artery
Grade 2	Partial collateral filling of the recipient epicardial artery
Grade 3	Complete collateral filling of the recipient epicardial artery

Angiographic methods for assessing collateral blood flow are at best semiquantitative measures. The coronary wedge pressure (e.g., the distal coronary pressure during transient balloon occlusion at the time of angioplasty) has been used to more accurately assess collateral function. Spontaneously visible collaterals are present at angioplasty four times as often as recruitable collaterals. Meier and coworkers[390] found the coronary wedge pressure in patients with collaterals of either type to be 44 ± 12 mm Hg (spontaneously visible collaterals 41 ± 12 mm Hg, recruitable collaterals 36 ± 12 mm Hg). The coronary wedge pressure in patients without collaterals was 18 ± 4 mm Hg. Signs and symptoms during angioplasty balloon occlusion of ischemia occur with a significantly greater frequency in patients with a low coronary wedge pressure.

Many studies in dogs have shown that even well-developed mature collaterals have a minimal vascular resistance that is two to four times greater than normal minimal resistance. Thus, coronary flow during maximal dilatation to areas supplied by angiographically large caliber collaterals is usually significantly reduced when compared with regions supplied by normal coronaries.[399] This may explain the frequent clinical observation that exertional angina is not infrequent when an area of the left ventricle with normal or minimally impaired contraction is supplied by a totally occluded coronary, even when large angiographic collaterals are visible.

NONATHEROSCLEROTIC CORONARY ARTERY DISEASE

Coronary Vasospasm

The diagnosis of coronary vasospasm can be made at the time of angiography by giving drugs that provoke spasm or occasionally by observing spontaneous spasm.[400–407] The most commonly administered agent is an ergot derivative, usually ergonovine maleate or ergometrine, although methacholine was used to induce vasospasm in early pioneering studies in the catheterization laboratory. Ergot derivatives are potent constrictors of vascular smooth muscle. For over 2000 years, ergot drugs have been known to cause gangrene when given in large doses, but the mechanism of action is still not clear. They appear to have alpha-adrenergic and serotonin receptor agonist activity and dopamine antagonist properties and may also inhibit central vasomotor centers.[408]

Before ergonovine administration, an electrocardiogram should be obtained and a coronary arteriogram should show the absence of severe coronary obstruction. When vasospasm is suspected, ergonovine generally is given in incremental intravenous doses, starting at 50 μg and increasing doses until a total dose of 350 to 400 μg is given. Although ergonovine appears safe in doses up to 800 μg, the vast majority of patients with vasospastic angina develop spasm at doses of less than 200 μg.[402–406, 409] In addition, a small fraction of patients with clinical vasospasm (transient electrocardiographic ST-segment elevation during chest pain) do not have vasospasm inducible by ergonovine.

In normal patients, ergonovine causes an increase in systemic arterial pressure (10 to 20 percent) and a small increase in left ventricular end-diastolic pressure (0 to 4 mm Hg) and does not change heart rate or lactate extraction.[405, 407] Normal patients also exhibit mild, diffuse coronary constriction in the epicardial arteries (10 to 20 percent decrease in diameter).[410] The response is more pronounced in the distal vessels.

In patients with vasospastic angina, ergonovine causes focal, usually severe coronary constriction—frequently leading to transient, total coronary occlusion (Fig. 30–38). The peak response occurs 2 to 5 minutes after administration, although onset of spasm 15 to 20 minutes later has been reported. In its classical description, coronary spasm leads to chest pain, ST-segment elevation on the electrocardiogram, increased left ventricular end-diastolic pressure, and myocardial lactate release.[407] In as many as half of patients with vasospastic angina, the response to ergonovine is less intense. ST-segment depression (rather than elevation) is often observed in patients with incomplete coronary occlusion with spasm, in patients with collateral arteries to the ischemic bed, and if spasm occurs in a small vessel.[411–415] Most investigators would consider the test positive if the patient's symptoms are reproduced, if focal spasm greater than 75 percent is demonstrated, and if there are electrocardiographic changes (ST-segment elevation or depression).[402]

Coronary spasm induced by ergonovine is usually easily reversed by nitroglycerin, although intracoronary administration can be required. Vasospasm has been induced while a patient was receiving an intravenous infusion of nitroglycerin and nitrate-resistant induced spasm can occur, but it is rare.[416] It is important to remember that the blood half-life of ergonovine is 30 to 120 minutes, much longer than that of nitroglycerin.[417, 418] Consequently, patients with spasm induced by ergonovine should have nitroglycerin or a calcium channel antagonist administered for at least 6 hours after the procedure.

Ergonovine provocative studies are relatively safe, with complication rates comparable with those of routine angiography. Ventricular tachycardia or fibrillation, the most common complication, occurs in 0.2 to 0.4 percent, myocardial infarction in 0 to 0.03 percent, and significant heart block or severe bradycardia in about 0 to 0.2 percent.[419, 420] We do not recommend prophylactic temporary pacemaker insertion unless the patient has previously developed bradycardia during angina. Platelet activation after induction of vasospasm is reported, but its relationship to the induction of or propensity for spasm is unclear.[421, 422]

Coronary spasm may be slightly more likely in the right coronary, followed by the left anterior descending and circumflex arteries. Vein bypass grafts can also exhibit spasm, but rarely do.[423] Patients with vasospastic angina appear to have more constriction in nonspastic coronary segments, suggesting a generalized coronary abnormality, and may also have enhanced resting tone, as evidenced by a greater degree of relaxation after nitroglycerin administration.[424–427]

Coronary spasm occurs in two broad settings—spasm associated with atherosclerosis or other arterial diseases and spasm that occurs in the absence of identifiable arteriopathy.[402, 404, 420, 428, 429] The former is common, but the latter is not.[402] Bertrand and associates[420] administered ergonovine to 1089 patients undergoing coronary arteriography and found that spasm was more common in patients with recent coronary thrombosis (Fig. 30–39). Vasospasm could be induced in 20 percent of patients with a recent infarction and 38 percent of patients with unstable or rest angina but in only 4.3 percent of patients with stable exertional angina. Equally important, only 1.2 percent of patients with chest pain atypical for angina had inducible spasm, emphasizing that spasm is not a common cause of atypical chest pain.

Patients with inducible vasospasm and a significant (>75 percent) stenotic lesion have a higher incidence of death, infarction, and atherosclerosis progression than patients with isolated stenotic lesions without inducible vasospasm or vasospasm alone.[430–432] Harding and colleagues[419] and others[433] retrospectively analyzed ergonovine provocative studies and found that smoking (odds ratio 4.7 to 7.7:1 compared with nonsmokers) and atherosclerosis were significant risk factors for inducible spasm.

Other agents have also been used to induce spasm at the time of catheterization. Muscarinic receptor agonists (acetylcholine and methacholine) appear to cause vasospasm in a large fraction of patients with ergonovine-induced spasm.[434] The specificity and sensitivity of cholinergic agents is not well described. Induction of vasospasm by muscarinic receptor agonists suggests the possibility that endothelial dysfunction may play a role in coronary spasm.[434] Other agents (cold pressor test, histamines, hyper-

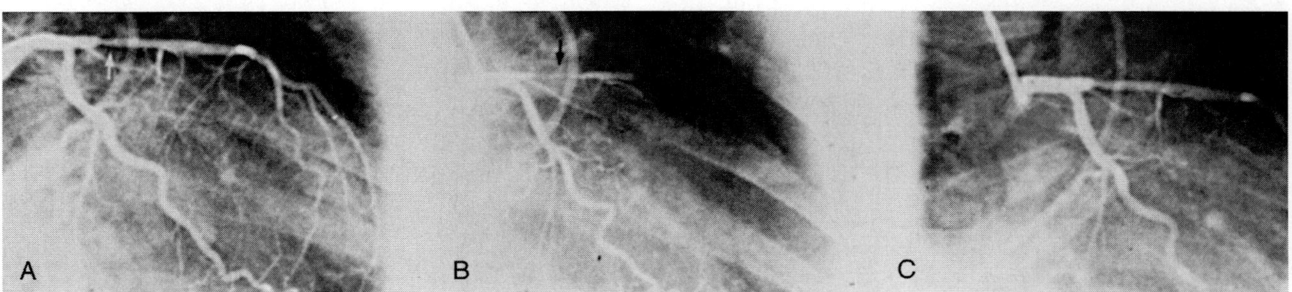

FIGURE 30–38 Angiogram from a patient with vasospasm induced by ergonovine. **A,** Before ergonovine, there is a 50 percent diameter stenosis (*arrow*) in the proximal left anterior descending artery. **B,** After ergonovine (100 μg intravenously), the left anterior descending artery develops spasm at the site of the lesion (*arrow*) and there is minimal antegrade blood flow. **C,** After nitroglycerin (200 μg, intracoronary), the spasm is relieved and blood flow is restored.

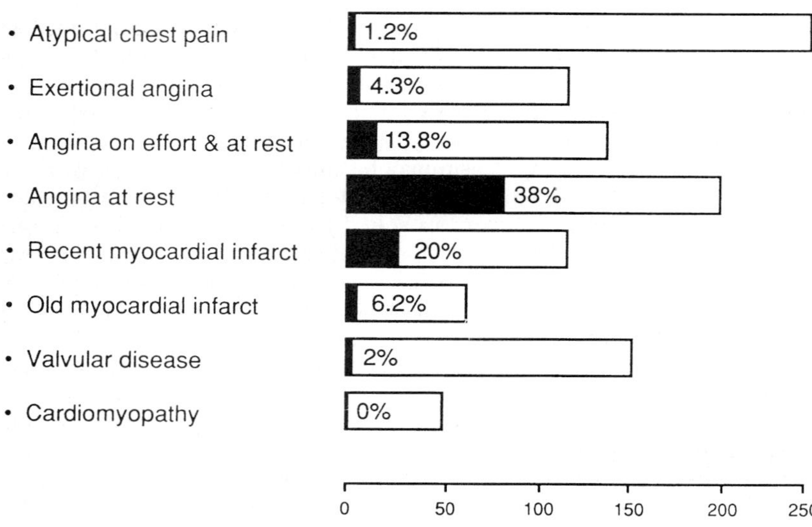

FIGURE 30–39 The frequency of coronary vasospasm induced by ergonovine in 1089 patients undergoing cardiac catheterization. The incidence of provocable spasm was high in patients with angina at rest and recent myocardial infarction, but spasm was uncommon in patients with chest pain atypical for myocardial ischemia. (From Bertrand ME, LaBlanche JM, Tilmant PY, et al: Frequency of provoked coronary arterial spasm in 1089 consecutive patients undergoing coronary arteriography. Circulation 65:1299–1308, 1982.)

ventilation) have also been reported to induce spasm, but not enough information is known to assess the potency and specificity of these agents.[435, 436]

Catheter-Induced Vasospasm

Coronary cannulation can cause vasospasm at the catheter tip, thought usually to result from mechanical traction on the artery. Catheter-induced spasm is much more common in the right than in the left coronary artery and, rarely, may occur distal to the catheter tip or in vein grafts.[132–135] It may occur more frequently in patients with vasospastic disease in other coronary segments, but the association with clinical vasospasm is uncommon.

Spontaneous Coronary Artery Dissection

Naturally occurring coronary artery dissection happens most commonly in conjunction with aortic dissection and involves the right coronary artery more often than the left. Isolated spontaneous coronary artery dissection, however, is a rare event that involves all coronary arteries with approximately equal overall incidence, although in women it may more frequently involve the left coronary artery and in men the right (Fig. 30–40).[437–442] It occurs most frequently in young women, particularly in the peripartum period, but may also be associated with blunt chest trauma, atherosclerosis (possibly related to plaque rupture), obstruction immediately above the aortic valve (e.g., an obstructed prosthetic ball valve), and iatrogenic complications of coronary artery cannulation.[438, 443–446a] Histologic examinations have shown a variety of abnormalities.[438, 440, 441, 445] The most common observation is a hematoma within the arterial media and luminal compression.[438, 441] A rent in the intima leading to the medial hematoma is observed inconsistently, as are changes of cystic medial necrosis.[440] Atherosclerosis with aneurysm or plaque rupture has been reported.[440] Perivascular eosinophilia has also been found late after dissection, but it is not clear whether eosinophils were related to the cause or occurred as a response to the dissection.[447]

At angiography, spontaneous dissection appears as a radiolucent linear filling defect that spirals down the coronary artery.[437, 439, 442, 448, 449, 449a] After intracoronary contrast medium injection, contrast material frequently persists in the false lumen. The dissection may be complicated by total thrombotic coronary occlusion that is amenable to throm-

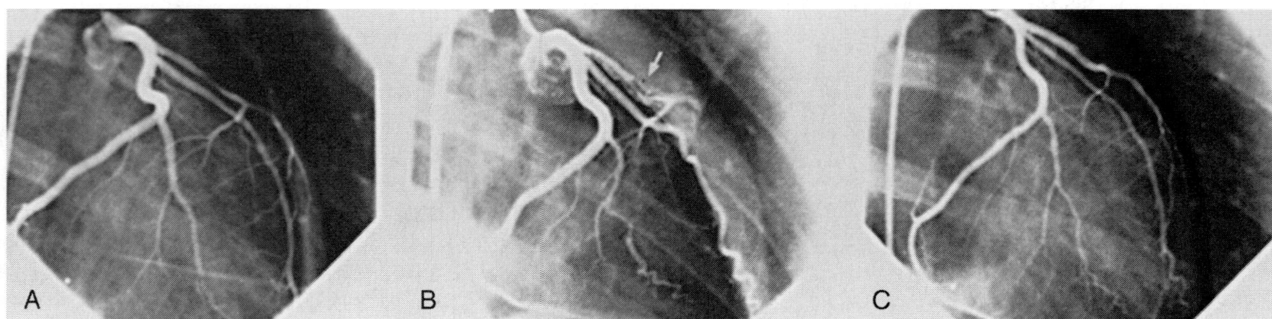

FIGURE 30–40 Serial angiograms obtained from a patient with a spontaneous dissection of the left anterior descending coronary artery. **A,** Angiogram obtained before presentation revealed mild diffuse narrowing of the left anterior descending artery. **B,** After the patient developed signs of acute myocardial infarction, the angiogram revealed subtotal occlusion of the anterior descending coronary artery and a linear intraluminal filling defect along the occlusion (*arrow*). **C,** Angiography months after presentation and treatment with streptokinase showed healing of the dissection and minimal stenosis. (**A–C,** Courtesy of Lyle Swenson, M.D.)

bolytic drug treatment. Distal emboli with abrupt vessel cut-offs are not uncommon.[442] Unless complicated by lumen thrombosis or death, most spontaneous dissections heal, but permanent true and false channel lumens may persist.[437, 448, 449, 449a] A similar dual-lumen vessel can be seen late after angioplasty complicated by a spiral dissection. In one series of patients with spontaneous dissection,[437] the mortality rate was 18 percent. Thrombolytic therapy has been used to successfully treat acute coronary occlusion related to spontaneous dissection,[450] as has stenting.[450a] Recurrent dissection in another artery is uncommon, but it may occur more frequently in women.

Myocardial Infarction in Patients With Angiographically Normal Coronary Arteries

One to 16 percent of patients with documented acute myocardial infarction are found at angiography to have normal or near-normal coronary arteries.[451, 452] Coronary embolism, in situ coronary thrombosis with spontaneous lysis, and vasospasm have been proposed as possible mechanisms.[453–456] Compared with patients with infarction associated with coronary atherosclerosis, those with a normal coronary angiogram after infarction tend to be younger (16 to 22 percent of patients are less than 35 years of age) and have fewer antecedent symptoms of angina and fewer risk factors for atherosclerosis.[457, 458] In contrast to the strong male predominance of atherosclerosis-associated infarction, men and women are approximately equally affected.[455, 458] Associations with tobacco smoking, a prior history of migraine headaches, Raynaud's syndrome, mitral valve prolapse, cocaine abuse, and birth control pill use have been reported.[458–460] Cocaine, sumatriptan, nifedipine, or excessive alcohol use also may precipitate infarction, presumably by causing vasospasm or transient thrombosis.[460a] Coronary spasm induced by ergonovine can be demonstrated in a minority of patients, but no definitive underlying mechanism can be found in most.[455]

Infarctions associated with a normal coronary angiogram tend to be smaller than those associated with atherosclerosis, and the mortality rate may be lower.[458] The long-term prognosis is generally good in terms of mortality, but recurrent infarction and stroke may be more common than in patients with atherosclerosis.[452, 458]

Microcirculatory Coronary Disease

Studies in highly selected patient populations suggest that microvascular coronary dysfunction may be a frequent cause of symptoms in the 10 to 25 percent of patients undergoing coronary angiography for chest pain, but in whom no significant obstruction to blood flow is found in the epicardial vessels.[461–464a] Of patients with angiographically normal coronary arteries, Cannon[465] reported that 71 percent had abnormal microvascular function, and Geltman and colleagues[466] found reduced CFR in 50 percent. It is now accepted that microvascular dysfunction can cause clinically important myocardial ischemia, including anginal syndromes, exertional dyspnea, and left ventricular dysfunction, but the mechanisms and incidence are unclear.[463, 464, 467–469] One investigator[469a] has recently become skeptical of the diagnosis and its clinical importance.

A number of diseases are associated with or cause microvascular dysfunction. These include prolonged hypertension, hypertrophy, cardiomyopathies, collagen vascular diseases, and atherosclerosis,[470–474] diseases associated with endothelial dysfunction. Although common, these specific disease entities are present in less than half of patients found at catheterization to have microvascular disease. Hence, it is likely that other, still uncharacterized, syndromes alter microvascular function in these patients.

The function of the microcirculation can be tested in several ways at the time of angiography, although the clinical significance of abnormalities in function in the absence of symptoms is not yet certain. Maximal coronary conductance can be assessed by measurements of CFR (the ratio of peak hyperemic blood flow/resting flow).[187, 326, 339, 475] In patients with a severe epicardial coronary stenosis (e.g., atherosclerotic stenosis), treadmill exercise performance is reduced proportionately to coronary reserve.[341] Patients with fixed microvascular disease may have similarly reduced coronary reserve, suggesting a fixed reduction in maximal coronary conductance.

Cannon and coworkers[463, 464, 467, 468] identified a subgroup of patients with chest pain and angiographically normal arteries who, after ergonovine administration, failed to normally increase coronary blood flow conductance during atrial pacing. The majority of these patients also had abnormally low maximal coronary conductance after dipyridamole, reduced left ventricular compliance, failure to increase the ventricular ejection fraction with exercise, and abnormally low myocardial lactate uptake (even lactate release) during pacing at a rapid heart rate. Furthermore, many of these patients may also have reduced forearm flow reserve, suggesting a systemic microvascular abnormality.[476] The mechanism of this abnormality is not known.

It has been postulated that endothelial dysfunction may play an important etiologic role in microvascular disease syndromes.[477] The functional integrity of the endothelium can be tested at the time of angiography by measuring the amount of large vessel dilatation and the change in blood flow (i.e., microvascular dilatation) during intracoronary infusion of pharmacologic agents that normally elicit the release of endothelial dilating factors. The responses to two agents have been characterized in humans: acetylcholine and substance P. When normal endothelium is present, acetylcholine causes a dose-dependent epicardial coronary and microvascular dilatation.[345] In the absence of endothelium, acetylcholine causes short-acting constriction. Hence, the response to intracoronary acetylcholine infusion (dilatation or no change/constriction) is one marker of endothelial function that can be tested in humans. The acetylcholine response is abnormal in several diseases with known endothelial dysfunction (atherosclerosis, transplantation).[345, 478] The endothelial response to acetylcholine was also abnormal in both the large conduit coronary arteries and the coronary microcirculation (i.e., constriction or subnormal dilatation) in a series of nine patients with anginal symptoms and normal coronary angiography even though the response to non–endothelium-dependent pharmacologic vasodilators was preserved.[478a, 479] Functional as well as fixed abnormalities in the coronary microcirculation may be causes of ischemia in the absence of epicardial atherosclerosis.

Radiation-Induced Coronary Artery Disease

Chest irradiation can lead to narrowing or occlusion of the epicardial and intramural coronary arteries, typically presenting several months to 12 years after the exposure.[480–487] Radiation-induced injury usually leads to adventitial fibrosis, smooth muscle cell loss in the media, and intimal proliferation.[480, 481] Atherosclerotic changes have also been observed, although lipid deposition is less marked than in patients with typical atherosclerosis. The angiographic findings are similar to those of atherosclerosis.[483] The coronary lumen can be diffusely narrowed or occluded entirely from radiation-induced fibrosis. Acute myocardial infarction has been reported.[485] The proximal vessels are affected more commonly. Generally, a dose of over 3000 R is associated with increased risk of radiation-induced coronary disease. In one series of 16 young patients (<33 years of age) who had received more than 3500 R to the heart, 6 had severe focal epicardial coronary stenoses.[483]

Transplant-Related Arteriopathy

The most persistent problem in patients surviving more than 1 year after transplantation has been the development of coronary arteriopathy characterized by diffuse intimal thickening of the transplanted arterial wall.[488–492] The process extends from the large conduit arteries into smaller branch vessels greater than 400 μm in diameter. Serial angiographic studies demonstrate the development of luminal irregularities or frank stenosis within 3 years of transplantation in 25 to 45 percent of patients.[493–501] Serial angiographic measurements of coronary luminal cross-sectional area using quantitative angiography show that the large conduit arteries decrease in diameter by 6 to 10 percent in the first year after transplantation, but thereafter, the lumen diameter remains fairly stable until more advanced vasculopathy occurs.[497]

The angiographic studies probably underestimate the frequency of arteriopathy because they detect only luminal encroachment but do not reflect wall thickening that may occur in an abluminal manner.[492] Intravascular ultrasound imaging of transplanted coronary arteries generally demonstrates a substantially greater degree of intimal thickening than is observed using angiography.[492a, 492b] The presence of angiographically undetected intimal thickening may predict progression to more severe arteriopathy over time.[492c, 492d] At the present time, many angiographers routinely image the coronary arteries at the time of angiography. Nonetheless, development of angiographically detectable vasculopathy is associated with shortened survival.[501]

In its classical angiographic description, transplant vasculopathy is characterized by diffuse luminal obliteration that is most marked in the smaller branch vessels seen on angiography (Fig. 30–41). In reality, the process affects the entire conduit artery, and focal stenoses in the large epicardial arteries—similar in angiographic morphology to atherosclerotic lesions—are not infrequent (Fig. 30–42). The typical patterns of transplant vasculopathy observed in 81 transplant recipients were described by Gao and associates.[495] Angiographic hallmarks of vasculitis are absent.

Several physiologic abnormalities of coronary vasomotion also have been detected. Endothelial function is frequently abnormal.[478] In many patients, intracoronary acetylcholine administration fails to elicit the expected coronary dilatation and increase in blood flow, suggesting a failure of the endothelium to normally release endothelium-derived relaxing factor. Some transplant recipients have frank vasoconstriction in response to acetylcholine. Whether an abnormal endothelial function presages more severe vasculopathy is unclear, but preliminary studies suggest a link. Endothelial function testing during angiography may have a role in research institutions.[478a]

Epicardial coronary tone is also reduced in the first several months after transplantation.[502] Tone returns to normal by 1 year after transplantation, but the reemergence of normal tone is not related to reinnervation. Spontaneous focal coronary spasm also has been observed during angiography in transplanted hearts.[503] Tone can be misinterpreted as diffuse narrowing. Nitroglycerin should be ad-

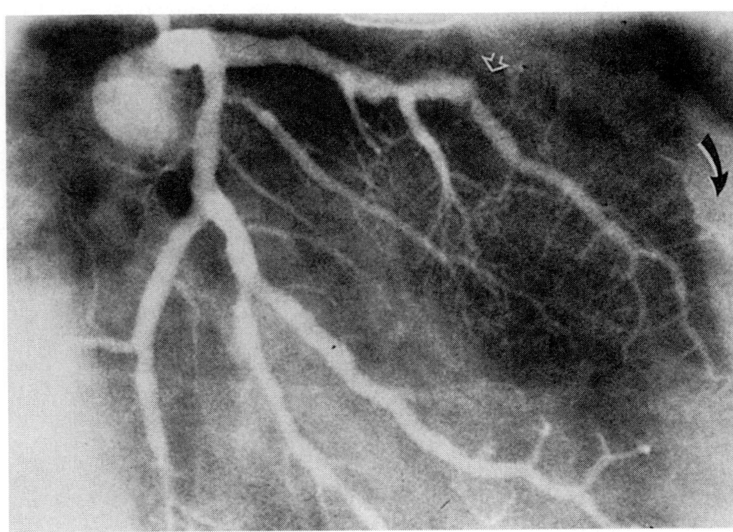

FIGURE 30–41 Angiogram of the left coronary artery of a patient with transplant-related vasculopathy. The left anterior descending artery is occluded (*open arrow*) and fills distally by faint collaterals (*solid arrow*). The remainder of the coronary tree has diffuse irregularities and pruning of the distal branches.

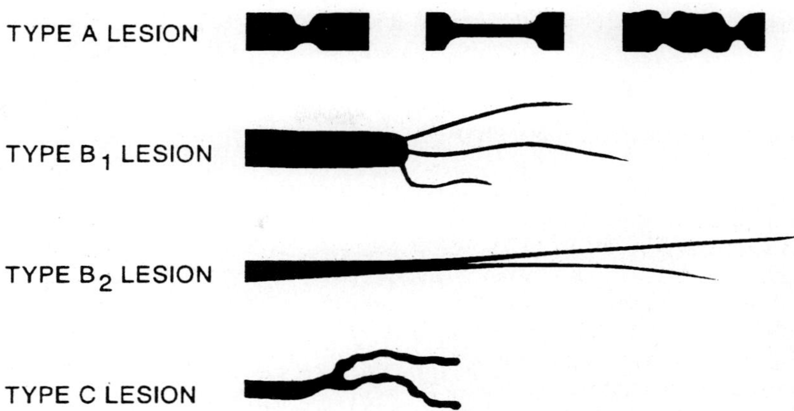

FIGURE 30–42 Angiographic morphologies of coronary lesions associated with transplant vasculopathy. Lesion type A: discrete tubular or multiple stenoses. Lesion type B_1: distal concentric narrowing and obliterated vessels with sparing of proximal vessel. Lesion type B_2: diffuse concentric narrowing. Lesion type C: narrow irregular distal branches with abrupt terminations. (From Gao SZ, Alderman EL, Schroeder JS, et al: Accelerated coronary vascular disease in the heart transplant patient: coronary arteriographic findings. Reprinted with permission from the American College of Cardiology [J Am Coll Cardiol 12:334–340, 1988].)

ministered immediately before angiography to allow a true assessment of the lumen caliber.

Coronary Abnormalities Associated With Vasculitis

Coronary vasculitis can result from vascular infection or collagen vascular diseases and causes four angiographically detectable coronary abnormalities: focal stenotic lesions, diffuse narrowing, thrombosis, and late aneurysmal dilatation.[504, 505] Lesions may be located from the aortic origin of the coronary arteries to the microcirculation. Aortitis associated with syphilis, Takayasu's arteritis, and more rarely, tuberculosis can cause stenosis of the coronary ostia.[506] Involvement of the larger epicardial coronary arteries is reported, but rare.[504, 507]

Of the collagen vascular diseases, systemic lupus erythematosus most commonly involves the angiographically visible epicardial coronary vessels, although large coronary involvement can be seen in polyarteritis nodosa, progressive systemic sclerosis, and more rarely, giant cell arteritis and rheumatoid arthritis.[508–512] The epicardial lesions associated with vasculitis typically resemble atherosclerotic lesions.[505] Diffuse luminal narrowing is less common, and the typical beaded appearance of vasculitis seen in other vascular beds is notably absent, although one case of a huge coronary aneurysm associated with systemic lupus erythematosus is reported.[508, 510, 513] Thrombosis of vasculitic segments can occur, leading to total arterial occlusion or the typical angiographic appearance of a thrombotic lesion.

The incidence of coronary vasculitis is probably underestimated by angiography because the findings are so similar to those of atherosclerosis.[508] In young patients with systemic lupus erythematosus and no important risk factors for atherosclerosis, coronary lesions and myocardial infarction should be assumed to be due to vasculitic involvement of the coronary arteries until shown otherwise, although accelerated atherosclerosis owing to corticosteroid therapy may also account for angiographically detected lesions. Late aneurysmal dilatation of the large coronary arteries, especially in periarteritis nodosa, has been reported to occur in nearly all of the vasculitic syndromes, and rupture of the aneurysm has been reported as a rare consequence.[508, 510, 514]

Microcirculatory vasculitis occurs frequently in patients with systemic lupus erythematosus, scleroderma, and rheumatoid arthritis. In these patients, maximal coronary conductance (e.g., CFR) is usually reduced, and ischemia due to microvascular obstruction or dysfunction has been proposed.[515, 516]

The most common infectious agent to involve the angiographically visible coronary vessels is Kawasaki's disease (mucocutaneous lymph node syndrome). It is characterized by coronary aneurysmal dilatation, stenosis, and thrombosis occurring primarily in the proximal coronary arteries.[517] The aneurysms can be huge. Late after the acute illness, about half of the aneurysms present during the febrile episode resolve.[518, 519] In angiographic studies of 1100 patients at an average of 25 months after disease onset, Suzuki and coworkers[520] found that 36 percent had frank aneurysms, 28 percent had coronary dilatation, 24 percent had localized coronary stenosis, and 8 percent had an occluded coronary. Aneurysmal calcification can occur.[521] Most of the Kawasaki disease–associated aneurysms were in the proximal coronary arteries, but about one in five were in the more distal vessels. Large aneurysms (>9 mm in diameter) were particularly prone to occlude or develop stenotic lesions.[522] Kawasaki's disease should be considered in the differential diagnosis of young adults presenting with coronary artery disease or myocardial infarction.

Coronary Artery Aneurysms

True aneurysms of the coronary arteries are associated with thinning of the tunica media and are very uncommon but, when present, can be over 2 cm in diameter (Fig. 30–43).[523–525] The angiographic morphology of coronary aneurysms can be saccular or fusiform. They frequently contain thrombotic material laminated against the borders of the aneurysm that may not be identifiable on the angiogram. Occasionally, the majority of the aneurysmal cavity can be filled with thrombus, leaving the angiographic appearance of a normal artery. After angioplasty or thrombolytic drug treatment, a portion of the aneurysm cavity can be revealed and at first may resemble a coronary perforation.

Aneurysms can be congenital in origin or occur as a result of atherosclerosis, inherited diseases of connective tissue (e.g., periarteritis nodosa, systemic lupus erythemato-

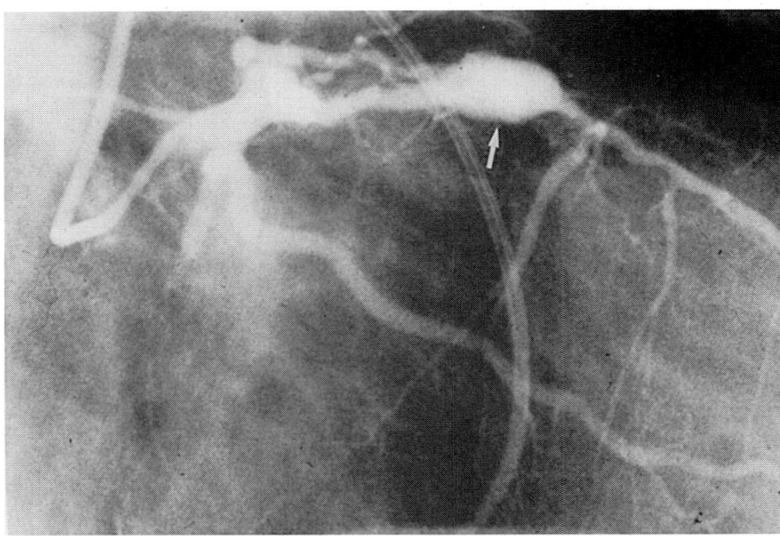

FIGURE 30–43 A large fusiform aneurysm of the left anterior descending coronary artery (*arrow*).

sus), inflammatory arteritis (e.g., Kawasaki's disease), mycotic-embolic events, or coronary trauma (usually iatrogenic). True atherosclerotic coronary aneurysms are very uncommon, occurring in only 0.2 percent of coronary arteriographic studies,[523, 525a] but the overall incidence from all causes ranges from 0.5 percent to 1.1 percent of coronary angiographic studies.[526] When associated with atherosclerosis, there are usually coexistent stenotic lesions in multiple vessels. Atherosclerotic aneurysms almost never rupture, but they may contain thrombotic material and can cause myocardial infarction by in situ thrombosis or embolization. Dissection of atherosclerotic aneurysms has been reported, but is also uncommon.[441]

Congenital disorders of connective tissue are associated with multiple aneurysms, particularly of the proximal arteries. Ehlers-Danlos syndrome type IV is characterized by dilatation of the proximal and mid-coronary artery.[527] One case of rupture and another of thrombosis have been reported. Both angiography-related dissection of the coronary ostium and peripheral vascular pseudoaneurysm have been linked to the syndrome.

True coronary aneurysms can also result from interventional coronary artery procedures including laser angioplasty, atherectomy, stent placement, and balloon dilatation.[528–530] One report suggests that use of corticosteroids around the time of the stent placement may promote aneurysm formation.[530] Aneurysms have also developed at the site of coronary anastomosis of vein bypass grafts.[531] Pseudoaneurysms can occur after coronary rupture from balloon dilatation (Fig. 30–44).[532]

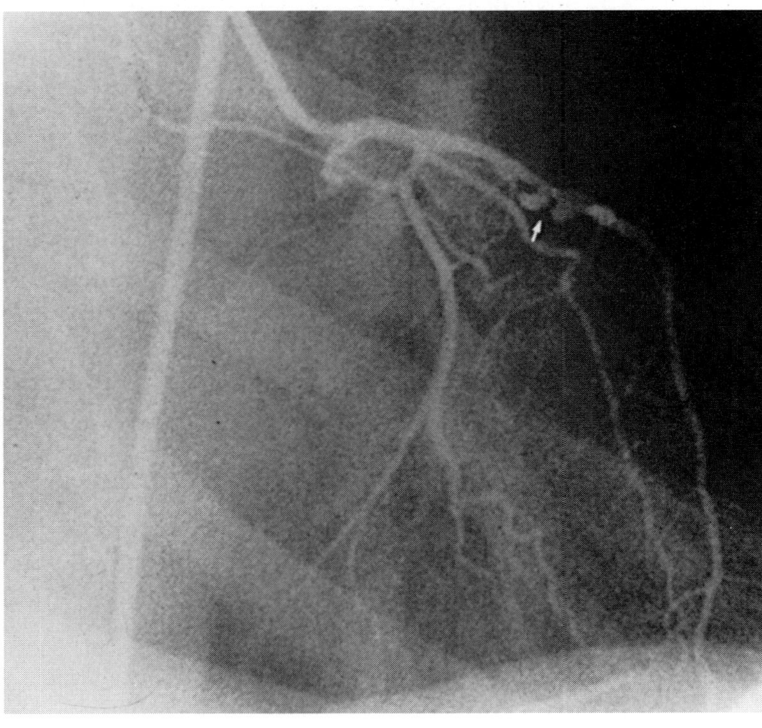

FIGURE 30–44 Angiogram of the left coronary artery of a patient who underwent angioplasty 6 months previously and developed an irregular, saccular pseudoaneurysm at the site of dilatation (*arrow*).

Coronary Embolism

Angiography soon after embolization of the coronary circulation can reveal abrupt occlusion of a coronary artery with persistence of contrast media proximal to the occlusion (usually to the nearest proximal branch) or a filling defect with the coronary lumen. Embolism from an infected mitral or aortic valve can lead to mycotic aneurysm formation and rupture. Embolism should be suspected in patients with an acute ischemic syndrome, otherwise normal coronary arteries with a smooth luminal surface, and a source of emboli (e.g., abnormal native or prosthetic valves with thrombus or infectious vegetation and left atrial or ventricular thrombus).[533, 534]

References

Radiographic Imaging

1. Department of Health and Human Services, National Center for Health Statistics: National Hospital Discharge Survey Annual Summary, 1995. Washington, DC: U.S. Government Printing Office, 1998.
2. Judkins ML: Angiographic equipment: the cardiac catheterization laboratory. *In* Abrams HL (ed): Coronary Arteriography: A Practical Approach. pp. 1–51. Boston: Little, Brown, 1983.
3. Kruger RA: X-ray digital cine angiography. *In* Collins SM, Skorton DJ (eds): Cardiac Imaging and Image Processing. pp. 29–40. New York: McGraw-Hill, 1986.
4. Macorski A: Medical Imaging Systems. pp. 36–62. Englewood Cliffs, NJ: Prentice-Hall, 1983.
5. Pepine CJ, Allen HD, Bashore TM, et al: ACC/AHA guidelines for cardiac catheterization and cardiac catheterization laboratories. Circulation 84:2227–2247, 1991.
6. Holmes DR, Bove AA, Wondrow MA, et al: New technique for decreasing x-ray exposure without decreasing image quality during cardiac catheterization. Mayo Clin Proc 61:321–338, 1986.

Radiation Protection

7. Judkins MP: Guidelines for radiation protection in the cardiac catheterization laboratory. Cathet Cardiovasc Diagn 10:87–92, 1984.
8. Miller SW, Castronovo FP: Radiation exposure and protection in cardiac catheterization laboratories. Am J Cardiol 55:171–176, 1985.
9. Rueter FG: Physician and patient exposure during cardiac catheterization. Circulation 58:135–139, 1978.
10. Geise RA, Hunter DW: Personnel exposure during fluoroscopy procedures. Postgrad Radiol 8:162–173, 1988.
11. National Council on Radiation Protection and Measurements: Recommendations on limits for exposure to ionizing radiation. Report No. 91. Bethesda, MD: NCRP Publications, 1987.
12. Gertz EW, Wisneski JA, Gould RG, Akin JR: Improved radiation protection for physicians performing cardiac catheterization. Am J Cardiol 50:1283–1286, 1982.
13. Judkins MP, for the Laboratory Performance Standards Committee: Guidelines for radiation protection in the cardiac catheterization laboratory. Cathet Cardiovasc Diagn 10:87–92, 1984.
14. National Council on Radiation Protection and Measurements: Quality assurance for diagnostic imaging. Report No. 99. Bethesda, MD: NCRP Publications, 1990.

Personnel

15. Leaman DM, Zelis RF: What is the appropriate "dress code" for the cardiac catheterization laboratory? Cathet Cardiovasc Diagn 9:33–38, 1983.

Technical History of Coronary Angiography

16. Diguglielmo L, Guttaduro M: Roentgenologic study of coronary arteries in living man. Acta Radiol Suppl 97, 1952.
17. Baltaxe HA, Amplatz K, Levin DC: Coronary Angiography. pp. 3–9. Springfield, IL: Charles C Thomas, 1973.
18. Bellman S, Frank HA, Lambert PB, et al: Coronary angiography I. Differential opacification of the aortic stream by catheters of special design—experimental development. N Engl J Med 262:325–329, 1960.
19. Sones FM Jr, Shirey EK: Cine coronary arteriography. Mod Concepts Cardiovasc Dis 31:735–738, 1962.
20. Judkins MP: Selective coronary arteriography: Part I: a percutaneous transfemoral technic. Radiology 89:815–824, 1967.
21. Ricketts HJ, Abrams HL: Percutaneous selective coronary cine arteriography. JAMA 181:620–624, 1962.
22. Amplatz K, Formanek G, Stanger P, Wilson W: Mechanics of selective coronary artery catheterization via femoral approach. Radiology 89:1040–1047, 1967.
23. Schoonmaker FW, King SB: Coronary arteriography by the single catheter percutaneous technique. Circulation 50:735, 1974.
24. Paulin S: Coronary angiography: a technical, anatomic and clinical study. Acta Radiol Suppl 233, 1964.

Patient Preparation

24a. Eisenberg RL, Bank WO, Hedgecock MW: Renal failure after major angiography. Am J Med 68:43–46, 1980.
25. Robbins JA, Rose SP: Partial thromboplastin time as a screening test. Ann Intern Med 90:796–802, 1979.
26. Nawaz S, Cleveland T, Gaines PA, Chan P: Clinical risk associated with contrast angiography in metformin treated patients: a clinical review. Clin Radiol 53:342–344, 1998.
27. Stevens MA, McCullough PA, Tobin KJ, et al: A prospective randomized trial of prevention measures in patients at high risk for contrast nephropathy: results of the P.R.I.N.C.E. Study. Prevention of Radiocontrast Induced Nephropathy Clinical Evaluation. J Am Coll Cardiol 33:403–411, 1999.

Technique

28. Seldinger SI: Catheter replacement of the needle in percutaneous arteriography. Acta Radiol 39:368–376, 1952.
29. Dotter CT, Rosch J, Robinson M: Fluoroscopic guidance in femoral artery puncture. Radiology 127:266–267, 1978.
30. Judkins MP, Kidd HJ, Frische LH, Dotter CT: Lumen-following safety J-guide for catheterization of tortuous vessels. Radiology 88:1127–1130, 1967.
31. Ovitt TW, Durst S, Moore R, Amplatz K: Guide wire thrombogenicity and its reduction. Radiology 111:43–46, 1974.
32. Eisenberg RL, Mani RL, McDonald EJ: The complication rate of catheter angiography by direct puncture through aorto-femoral bypass grafts. AJR 126:814–816, 1976.
33. Giustra PE, Root JA, Killoran PJ: Percutaneous selective visceral catheterization through aortofemoral Dacron prosthesis. Radiology 126:261, 1978.
34. Lau KW, Tan A, Koh TH, et al: Early ambulation following diagnostic 7 French catheter catheterization: a prospective randomized trial. Cathet Cardiovasc Diagn 28:34–38, 1993.
34a. Mani RL, Copstin BS: Catheter angiography through aortofemoral grafts: prevention of catheter separation during withdrawal. AJR 128:328–329, 1977.
35. Hui WKK, Klinke WP, Kubac G, Talibi T: Comparison of 5F and 7/8F catheters for left ventricular and coronary angiography. Cathet Cardiovasc Diagn 19:84–85, 1990.
36. Pande AK, Meier B, Urban P, et al: Coronary angiography with four French catheters. Am J Cardiol 70:1085–1086, 1992.
37. Abbott JA, Lipton MJ, Kosek J, et al: Cardiac trauma from angiographic injections: a quantitative study. Circulation 57:91–98, 1978.
38. Prewitt KC, Zen B, Wortham DC, Pearson C: Increased risk of coronary artery dissection during coronary angiography with 6F catheters. Angiology 44:107–113, 1993.

Contrast Material

39. Dawson P: Conventional angiography. *In* Skucas J (ed): Radiographic Contrast Agents. 2nd ed. p. 152. Rockville, MD: Aspen, 1989.
40. Paulin S, Adams DF: Increased ventricular fibrillation during coro-

nary arteriography with a new contrast medium preparation. Radiology 101:45–50, 1971.

41. Murdock DK, Euler DE, Kozeny G, et al: Ventricular fibrillation during coronary angiography in dogs: the role of calcium-binding additives. Am J Cardiol 54:897–901, 1984.
42. Zukerman LS, Friehling TD, Wolf NM, et al: Effect of calcium-binding additives on ventricular fibrillation and repolarization changes during coronary angiography. J Am Coll Cardiol 10:1249–1253, 1987.
43. Morris TW, Sahler LG, Fischer HW: Calcium binding by radiopaque media. Invest Radiol 17:501–505, 1982.
44. Piao ZE, Murdock DK, Hwang MH, et al: Contrast media–induced ventricular fibrillation: a comparison of Hypaque-76, Hexabrix, and Omnipaque. Invest Radiol 23:466–470, 1988.
45. Fischer HW: Catalog of intravascular contrast media. Radiology 159:561–563, 1986.
46. Ritchie JL, Nissen SE, Douglas JS, et al: Use of nonionic or low osmolar contrast agents in cardiovascular procedures. American College of Cardiology Cardiovascular Imaging Committee. J Am Coll Cardiol 21:269–273, 1993.
47. Gertz EW, Wisneski JA, Miller R, et al: Adverse reactions of low osmolality contrast media during cardiac angiography: a prospective randomized multicenter study. J Am Coll Cardiol 19:899–906, 1992.
48. Barrett BJ, Parfrey PS, Vavasour HM, et al: A comparison of nonionic, low-osmolality radiocontrast agents with ionic, high-osmolality agents during cardiac catheterization. N Engl J Med 326:431–436, 1992.
49. Missri J, Jeresaty RM: Ventricular fibrillation during coronary angiography: reduced incidence with nonionic contrast media. Cathet Cardiovasc Diagn 19:4–7, 1990.
50. Wilson RF, White CW: Intracoronary papaverine: an ideal vasodilator for studies of the coronary circulation. Circulation 73:444–451, 1986.
51. Bookstein JJ, Higgens CB: Comparative efficacy of coronary vasodilatory methods. Invest Radiol 12:121–127, 1977.
52. White CW, Eckberg DL, Inasaka T, Abboud FM: Effects of angiographic contrast media on sino-atrial nodal function. Cardiovasc Res 10:214–223, 1976.
53. Eckberg DL, White CW, Kioschos JM, Abboud FM: Mechanisms mediating bradycardia during coronary arteriography. J Clin Invest 54:1455–1461, 1974.
54. Wilson RF, White CW: Iohexol does not have minimal effects on coronary hemodynamics [abstract]. Circulation 74(suppl II):405, 1986.
55. Bettmann MA, Bourdillon PD, Barry WH, et al: Contrast agents for cardiac angiography: effects of a nonionic agent vs. a standard ionic agent. Radiology 153:583–587, 1984.
56. Mancini GBJ, Bloomquist JN, Bhargava V, et al: Hemodynamic and electrocardiographic effects in man of a new nonionic contrast agent (iohexol): advantages over standard ionic agents. Am J Cardiol 51:1218–1222, 1983.
57. Hirshfeld JW, Laskey W, Martin JL, et al: Hemodynamic changes induced by cardiac angiography with ioxaglate: comparison with diatrizoate. J Am Coll Cardiol 2:954–957, 1983.
58. Thomson KR, Evill CA, Fritzsche J, Beness GT: Comparison of iopamidol, ioxaglate and diatrizoate during coronary arteriography in dogs. Invest Radiol 15:234–241, 1980.
59. Feldman RL, Jalowiec DA, Hill JA, Lambert CR: Contrast media–related complications during cardiac catheterization using Hexabrix or Renografin in high risk patients. Am J Cardiol 61:1334–1337, 1988.
60. Yamazaki H, Banka VS, Bodenheimer MM, et al: Differential effects of Renografin-76 on the ischemic and nonischemic myocardium. Am J Cardiol 47:597–602, 1981.
61. Cohn PF, Horn HR, Teicholz LE, et al: Effects of angiographic contrast medium on left ventricular function in coronary artery disease. Am J Cardiol 32:21–26, 1973.
62. Powe NR, Davidoff AJ, Moore RD, et al: Net costs from three perspectives of using low versus high osmolality contrast medium in diagnostic angiocardiography. J Am Coll Cardiol 21:1701–1709, 1993.
63. Mark AL: The Bezold-Jarisch reflex revisited: clinical implications of inhibitory reflexes originating in the heart. J Am Coll Cardiol 1:90–102, 1983.
64. Palomo AR, Schwartz AM, Trohman RG, et al: Cardiac arrhythmias associated with prophylactic pacing during coronary angiography. Am J Cardiol 58:100–103, 1986.
65. Lehmann MH, Cameron A, Kemp HG: Increased risk of ventricular fibrillation associated with temporary pacemaker use during coronary angiography. Pacing Clin Electrophysiol 6:923–929, 1983.
66. Stormorken H, Skalpe IO, Testart MC: Effect of various contrast media on coagulation, fibrinolysis, and platelet function in in vitro and in vivo study. Invest Radiol 21:348–354, 1986.
67. Dawson P, Hewitt P, Mackie IJ, et al: Contrast, coagulation and fibrinolysis. Invest Radiol 21:248–252, 1986.
68. Gabriel DA, Jones MR, Reece NS, et al: Platelet and fibrin modification by radiographic contrast media. Circ Res 68:881–887, 1991.
69. Greenbaum RA, Barradas MA, Mikhailidis DP, et al: Effect of heparin and contrast medium on platelet function during routine cardiac catheterization. Cardiovasc Res 21:878–885, 1987.
70. Davidson CJ, Mark DB, Pieper KS, et al: Thrombotic and cardiovascular complications related to nonionic contrast media during cardiac catheterization: analysis of 8,517 patients. Am J Cardiol 65:1481–1484, 1990.
71. Markus H, Loh A, Israel D, et al: Microscopic air embolism during cerebral angiography and strategies for its avoidance. Lancet 341:784–787, 1993.
72. Ciabattoni G, Ujang S, Sritara P, et al: Aspirin, but not heparin, suppresses the transient increase in thromboxane biosynthesis associated with cardiac catheterization or coronary angioplasty. J Am Coll Cardiol 21:1377–1381, 1993.
73. Davis K, Kennedy JW, Kemp HG, et al: Complications of coronary arteriography from the Collaborative Study of Coronary Artery Surgery (CASS). Circulation 59:1105–1112, 1979.
74. Eyer KM: Complications of transfemoral coronary arteriography and their prevention using heparin. Am Heart J 86:428–435, 1973.
75. Walker WJ, Mundall SJ, Broderick HG, et al: Systemic heparinization for femoral percutaneous coronary arteriography. N Engl J Med 288:826–830, 1973.
76. Greenbaum RA, Barradas MA, Mikhailidis DP, et al: Effect of heparin and contrast medium on platelet function during routine cardiac catheterization. Cardiovasc Res 21:878–885, 1987.
77. Shanberge JN, Quattrociocchi-Longe TM, Martens MH: Interrelationship of protamine and platelet factor 4 in the neutralization of heparin. Thromb Res 46:89–100, 1987.
78. Becker RC, Clyne C, Weiner BH, et al: Heparin pharmacokinetics and in vitro anticoagulant activity in patients receiving non-ionic contrast media. Cardiology 79:31–38, 1991.
79. Dehmer GJ, Haagen D, Malloy CR, Schmitz JM: Anticoagulation with heparin during cardiac catheterization and its reversal by protamine. Cathet Cardiovasc Diagn 13:16–21, 1987.
80. Shanberge JN, Murato M, Quattrociocchi-Longe T, Van Neste L: Heparin-protamine complexes in the production of heparin rebound and other complications of extracorporeal bypass procedures. Am J Clin Pathol 87:210–217, 1987.
81. Kesteven PJ, Ahmed A, Aps C, et al: Protamine sulphate and heparin rebound following open-heart surgery. J Cardiovasc Thorac Surg 27:600–603, 1986.
82. Weiss ME, Nyhan D, Peng Z, et al: Association of protamine IgE and IgE antibodies with life threatening reactions to intravenous protamine. N Engl J Med 320:886–892, 1989.
83. Harrow JC: Protamine: a review of its toxicity. Anesth Analg 64:348–361, 1985.

Nitroglycerin

84. Feldman RL, Marx JD, Pepine CJ, Conti CR: Analysis of coronary responses to various doses of intracoronary nitroglycerin. Circulation 66:321–327, 1982.
85. Feldman RL, Pepine CJ, Conti CR: Magnitude of dilatation of large and small coronary arteries by nitroglycerin. Circulation 64:324–333, 1981.
86. Macho P, Vatner SF: Effects of nitroglycerin and nitroprusside on large and small coronary vessels in conscious dogs. Circulation 64:1101–1107, 1981.
87. Mehta J, Pepine CJ: Effect of sublingual nitroglycerin on regional flow in patients with and without coronary disease. Circulation 58:803–807, 1978.
88. Dick C, Wyche K, Homans DC, White CW: Effect of distending pressure on intravascular ultrasound measurement of lumen dimensions [abstract]. Circulation 83(suppl III):459, 1990.

LEFT MAIN CORONARY STENOSIS

89. Gordon PR, Abrams C, Gash AK, Carabello BA: Pericatheterization risk factors in left main coronary artery stenosis. Am J Cardiol 59:1080–1083, 1987.
90. Conti CR, Selby JH, Christie LG, et al: Left main coronary artery stenosis: clinical spectrum, pathophysiology, and management. Progr Cardiovasc Dis 22:73–105, 1979.
91. Davis K, Kennedy JW, Kemp HG, et al: Complications of coronary arteriography from the Collaborative Study of Coronary Artery Surgery (CASS). Circulation 59:1105–1112, 1979.
92. Kern MJ, Aguirre F, Bach R, et al: Augmentation of coronary blood flow by intra-aortic balloon pumping in patients after coronary angioplasty. Circulation 87:500–511, 1993.
93. Alderman EL, Wexler L: Angiographic implications of cardiac transplantation. Am J Cardiol 64:16E–21E, 1989.

OUTPATIENT CATHETERIZATION

94. Block PC, Ockene I, Goldberg RJ, et al: A prospective randomized trial of outpatient versus inpatient cardiac catheterization. N Engl J Med 319:1251–1255, 1988.
95. Pink S, Fiutowski L, Gianelly RE: Outpatient cardiac catheterizations: analysis of patients requiring admission. Clin Cardiol 12:375–378, 1989.
96. Clements SD, Gatlin S: Outpatient cardiac catheterization: a report of 3,000 cases. Clin Cardiol 14:477–480, 1991.
97. Clark DA, Moscovich MD, Vetrovec GW, Wexler L: Guidelines for the performance of outpatient catheterization and angiographic procedures. Cathet Cardiovasc Diagn 27:5–7, 1992.
98. Oldroyd KG, Phadke KV, Phillips R, et al: Cardiac catheterization by the Judkins technique as an outpatient procedure. BMJ 298:875–876, 1989.
99. Health and Public Policy Committee: The safety and efficacy of ambulatory cardiac catheterization in the hospital and freestanding setting. Ann Intern Med 103:294–298, 1985.
100. Kahn KL: The efficacy of ambulatory cardiac catheterization in the hospital and free-standing setting. Am Heart J 111:152, 1986.

COMPLICATIONS

101. Bourassa MG, Noble J: Complication rate of coronary arteriography: a review of 5250 cases studied by a percutaneous femoral technique. Circulation 53:106–114, 1976.
102. Kennedy JW: Complications associated with cardiac catheterization and angiography. Registry Committee of the Society for Cardiac Angiography. Cathet Cardiovasc Diagn 8:5–11, 1982.
103. Noto TJ, Johnson L, Krone R, et al: Cardiac catheterization 1990: a report of the Registry of the Society for Cardiac Angiography and Interventions (SCA&I). Cathet Cardiovasc Diagn 24:75–83, 1991.
104. Gersh BJ, Kronmal RA, Frye RL, et al: Coronary arteriography and coronary artery bypass surgery: morbidity and mortality in patients ages 65 years or older. A report from the Coronary Artery Surgery Study. Circulation 67:483–491, 1983.
105. Ernst SMPG, Tjonjoegin RM, Schrader R, et al: Immediate sealing of arterial puncture sites after cardiac catheterization and coronary angioplasty using a biodegradable collagen plug: results of an international registry. J Am Coll Cardiol 21:851–855, 1993.
106. McCann RL, Schwartz LB, Pieper KS: Vascular complications of cardiac catheterization. J Vasc Surg 14:375–381, 1991.
107. Muller DWM, Shamir KJ, Ellis SG, Topol EJ: Peripheral vascular complications after conventional and complex percutaneous coronary interventional procedures. Am J Cardiol 69:63–68, 1992.
108. Altin RS, Flicker S, Naidech HJ: Pseudoaneurysm and arteriovenous fistula after femoral artery catheterization: association with low femoral punctures. AJR 152:629–631, 1989.
109. Khoury M, Batra S, Berg R, et al: Influence of arterial access sites and interventional procedures on vascular complications after cardiac catheterizations. Am J Surg 164:205–209, 1992.
110. McCready RA, Siderys H, Pittman JN, et al: Septic complications after cardiac catheterization and percutaneous transluminal coronary angioplasty. J Vasc Surg 14:170–174, 1991.
111. Kotval PS, Khoury A, Shah PM, Babu SC: Doppler sonographic demonstration of the progressive spontaneous thrombosis of pseudoaneurysms. J Ultrasound Med 9:185–190, 1990.
112. Agrawal SK, Pinheiro L, Roubin GS, et al: Nonsurgical closure of femoral pseudoaneurysms complicating cardiac catheterization and percutaneous transluminal coronary angioplasty. J Am Coll Cardiol 20:610–615, 1992.
113. Fellmeth BD, Baron SB, Brown PR, et al: Repair of postcatheterization femoral pseudoaneurysms by color flow ultrasound-guided compression. Am Heart J 123:547–551, 1992.
114. Colt HG, Begg RJ, Saporito JJ, et al: Cholesterol emboli after cardiac catheterization. Medicine 67:389–400, 1988.
115. Oda H, Miida T, Sato H, Higuma N: Treatment of unstable angina with cholesterol embolization as a complication of left heart catheterization. Jpn Circ J 54:487–492, 1990.
116. Rosman HS, David TP, Reddy D, Goldstein S: Cholesterol embolization: clinical findings and implications. J Am Coll Cardiol 15:1296–1299, 1990.
117. Ong HT, Elmsly WG, Friedlander DH: Cholesterol atheroembolism: an increasingly frequent complication of cardiac catheterization. Med J Aust 154:412–414, 1991.
118. Kalter DC, Rudolph A, McGavran M: Livedo reticularis due to multiple cholesterol emboli. J Am Acad Dermatol 13:235–242, 1985.
119. Gaines PA, Kennedy A, Moorhead P, et al: Cholesterol embolization: a lethal complication of vascular catheterization. Lancet 1(8578):168–170, 1988.
120. Ramirez G, O'Neill WM, Lambert R, Bloomer A: Cholesterol embolization: a complication of angiography. Arch Intern Med 138:1430–1432, 1978.
121. Rose M, Dinour D, Chisin R: Splenic infarction: a complication of cardiac catheterization. Clin Cardiol 15:697–698, 1992.
122. Katz ES, Tunick PA, Rusinek H, et al: Protruding aortic atheromas predict stroke in elderly patients undergoing cardiopulmonary bypass: experience with intraoperative transesophageal echocardiography. J Am Coll Cardiol 20:70–77, 1992.
123. Karalis DG, Chandrasekaran K, Victor MF, et al: Recognition and embolic potential of intraaortic atherosclerotic debris. J Am Coll Cardiol 17:73–78, 1991.
124. O'Quin RJ, Lakshminarayan S: Venous air embolism. Arch Intern Med 142:2173–2176, 1982.
125. Gottdiener JS, Papademetriou V, Notargiacomo A, et al: Incidence and cardiac effects of systemic venous air embolism: echocardiographic evidence of arterial embolization via non-cardiac shunt. Arch Intern Med 148:795–800, 1988.
126. Marco AP, Furman WR: Venous air embolism, airway difficulties, and massive transfusion. Surg Clin North Am 73:213–228, 1993.
127. Calverley RK, Dodds WA, Trapp WG, Jenkins LC: Hyperbaric treatment of cerebral air embolism: a report of a case following cardiac catheterization. Can Anaesth Soc J 18:665–674, 1971.
128. Keilson GR, Schwartz WJ, Recht LD: The preponderance of posterior circulatory events is independent of the route of cardiac catheterization. Stroke 23:1358–1359, 1992.
129. Kosmorsky G, Hanson MR, Tomsak RL: Neuro-ophthalmologic complications of cardiac catheterization. Neurology 38:483–485, 1988.
130. Vik-Mo H, Todnem K, Folling M, Rosland GA: Transient visual disturbance during cardiac catheterization with angiography. Cathet Cardiovasc Diagn 12:1–4, 1986.
131. Dawson DM, Fischer EG: Neurologic complications of cardiac catheterization. Neurology 27:496–497, 1977.
131a. Sticherling C, Berkefeld J, Auch-Schwelk W, Lanfermann H: Transient bilateral cortical blindness after coronary angiography. Lancet 351:570, 1998.
132. Deckelbaum LI, Isner JM, Konstam MA, Salem DN: Catheter-induced versus spontaneous spasm—do these coronary bedfellows deserve to be estranged? Am J Med 79:1–4, 1985.
133. Deligonul U, Kern MJ, Caralis D: Left main and right catheter-induced coronary artery spasm in a patient with vasospastic angina. Cathet Cardiovasc Diagn 17:39–44, 1989.
134. Heijman J, Gamal ME, Michels R: Catheter induced spasm in aortocoronary vein grafts. Br Heart J 49:30–32, 1983.
135. Schwartz RE, Butman S: Catheter-induced nonproximal coronary artery spasm. Am J Cardiol 53:352–354, 1984.
136. Haas JM, Peterson CR, Jones RC: Subintimal dissection of the coronary arteries: a complication of selective coronary arteriography and the transfemoral percutaneous approach. Circulation 38:678–683, 1968.
137. Tortoledo F, Zacca NM, Chahine RA: Coronary artery spasm superimposed on coronary artery dissection. Am J Cardiol 53:363–364, 1984.

138. Wilson VE, Bates ER: Subacute bilateral coronary ostial stenoses following cardiac catheterization and PTCA. Cathet Cardiovasc Diagn 23:114–116, 1991.
139. Hammermeister KE, Warbasse JR: Immediate hemodynamic effects of cardiac angiography in man. Am J Cardiol 31:307–314, 1973.
140. Golman K, Almen T: Contrast media–induced nephrotoxicity: survey and present state. Invest Radiol 20:S92–S96, 1985.
141. D'Elia JA, Gleason RE, Alday M, et al: Nephrotoxicity from angiographic contrast material. Am J Med 72:719–723, 1982.
142. Parfrey PS, Griffiths SM, Barrett BJ, et al: Contrast material–induced renal failure in patients with diabetes mellitus, renal insufficiency, or both. N Engl J Med 320:143–149, 1989.
143. Rich MW, Crecelius CA: Incidence, risk factors, and clinical course of acute renal insufficiency after cardiac catheterization in patients 70 years of age. Arch Intern Med 150:1237–1242, 1990.
144. Talierco CP, Vliestra RE, Fisher LD, Burnett JC: Risks for renal dysfunction with cardiac angiography. Ann Intern Med 104:501–504, 1986.
145. Talierco CP, Vliestra RE, Ilstrup DM: A randomized comparison of nephrotoxicity of iopamidol and diatrizoate in high risk patients undergoing coronary angiography. J Am Coll Cardiol 17:384–390, 1991.
146. Hill JA, Winniford M, VanFossen DB, et al: Nephrotoxicity following cardiac angiography: a randomized double-blind multicenter trial of ionic and nonionic contrast media in 1194 patients [abstract]. Circulation 84:III-333, 1991.
147. Anto HR, Chou SY, Porush JG, Shapiro WB: Infusion intravenous pyelography and renal function. Arch Intern Med 141:1652–1656, 1981.
148. Old CW, Duarte CM, Lehrner LH, et al: A prospective evaluation of mannitol in the prevention of radiocontrast acute renal failure [abstract]. Clin Res 29:472A, 1981.
149. Beroniade VC: Prevention of acute renal failure secondary to radiocontrast agents. Abstracts of the 8th International Congress of Nephrology. p. 380. Athens: University Studio Publishing, 1981.
150. Lasser EC, Berry CC, Talner LB, et al: Pretreatment with corticosteroids to alleviate reactions to intravenous contrast material. N Engl J Med 317:845–849, 1987.
151. Steinberg EP, Moore RD, Powe NR, et al: Safety and cost effectiveness of high-osmolality as compared with low-osmolality contrast material in patients undergoing cardiac angiography. N Engl J Med 326:425–430, 1992.
152. Greenberger PA, Patterson R, Tapio CM: Prophylaxis against repeated radiocontrast media reactions in 857 cases. Arch Intern Med 145:2197–2200, 1985.
153. Horrow JC: Protamine: a review of its toxicity. Anesth Analg 64:348–361, 1985.
154. Hobbhahn J, Conzen PF, Habazettl H, et al: Heparin reversal by protamine in humans—complement, prostaglandins, blood cells, and hemodynamics. J Appl Physiol 71:1415–1421, 1991.
155. Pearson PJ, Evora PRB, Ayrancioglu K, Schaff HV: Protamine releases endothelium-derived relaxing factor from systemic arteries: a possible mechanism of hypotension during heparin neutralization. Circulation 86:289–294, 1992.
156. Friedman HS, Trivelli LA, Nguyen T, et al: Hematologic changes occurring with cardiac catheterization. Cathet Cardiovasc Diagn 15:89–91, 1988.
157. Bell WR, Royall RM: Heparin-associated thrombocytopenia: a comparison of three heparin preparations. N Engl J Med 303:902–907, 1980.
158. Ansell J, Deykin D: Heparin-induced thrombocytopenia and recurrent thromboembolism. Am J Hematol 8:325–332, 1980.
159. Gaglani RD, Turk AA, Mehra MR, Lach RD: Ventricular standstill complicating left heart catheterization in the presence of uncomplicated right bundle branch block. Cathet Cardiovasc Diagn 26:212–214, 1992.
160. Munsif AN, Schechter E: Complete block below the His bundle induced by left-sided cardiac catheterization. Cathet Cardiovasc Diagn 24:189–191, 1991.
161. Little WC, Reeves RC, Coughlan HC, Rogers EW: Effect of cough on coronary perfusion pressure: does coughing help clear the coronary arteries of angiographic contrast medium? Circulation 65:604–610, 1982.

Coronary Anatomy and Dimensions

162. Dryander (1541). Anatomia Mundini. Anatomia Mundini, 30–34. Marburg.
163. Saunders JB, O'Malley CD: The Anatomical Drawings of Andreas Vesalius. New York: Bonanza, 1982.
163a. James TN: Anatomy of the Coronary Arteries. New York: Harper & Row, 1961.
164. Angelini P: Normal and anomalous coronary arteries: definitions and classification. Am Heart J 117:418–434, 1989.
165. Zamir M, Sinclair P: Roots and calibers of the human coronary arteries. Am J Anat 183:226–234, 1988.
166. Baroldi G, Scomazzoni G: Coronary Circulation in the Normal and Pathologic Heart. pp. 5–90. Washington, DC: Department of the Army, United States Government Printing Office, 1967.
167. Virmani R, Chun PKC, Rainowitz M, et al: Lack of correlation to coronary artery dominance and bicuspid aortic valve: an autopsy study of 54 cases. Arch Pathol Lab Med 108:638–641, 1984.
167a. Bergelson BA, Tommaso CL: Left main coronary artery disease: assessment, diagnosis, and therapy. Am Heart J 129:350–359, 1995.
168. Kronzon I, Deutsch P, Glassman E: Length of the left main coronary artery: its relation to the pattern of coronary arterial distribution. Am J Cardiol 34:787–789, 1974.
169. Higgins CB, Wexler L: Reversal of dominance of the coronary arterial system in isolated aortic stenosis and bicuspid aortic valve. Circulation 52:292–296, 1975.
170. Murphy ES, Rosch J, Rahimtoola SH: Frequency and significance of coronary arterial dominance in isolated aortic stenosis. Am J Cardiol 39:505–509, 1977.
171. Green GE, Bernstein S, Reppert EH: The length of the left main coronary artery. Surgery 62:1021–1024, 1967.
172. Baptista CAC, DiDio LJA, Prates JC: Types of division of the left coronary artery and the ramus diagonalis of the human heart. Jpn Heart J 31:323–335, 1991.
173. Kolodziej AW, Lobo FV, Walley VM: Intra-atrial course of the right coronary artery and its branches. Can J Cardiol 10:263–267, 1994.
174. Adams J, Treasure T: Variable anatomy of the right coronary artery supply to the left ventricle. Thorax 40:618–620, 1985.
175. Gregg DE: Coronary Circulation in Health and Disease. Philadelphia: Lea & Febiger, 1950.
176. Weaver ME, Pantely GA, Bristow JD, Ladley HD: A quantitative study of the anatomy and distribution of coronary arteries in swine in comparison with other animals and man. Cardiovasc Res 20:907–917, 1986.
177. Nerantzis C, Avgoustakis D: An S-shaped atrial artery supplying the sinus node area. Chest 78:274–278, 1980.
178. Ilia R, Goldfarb B, Katz A, et al: Variations in blood supply to the anterior interventricular septum: incidence and possible clinical importance. Cathet Cardiovasc Diagn 24:277–282, 1991.
179. Tomanek RJ: Microanatomy of the coronary circulation. *In* Spaan JAE, Bruschke AVG, Gittenberger AC, De Groot DD (eds): Coronary Circulation: From Basic Mechanisms to Clinical Implications. pp. 3–12. Dordrecht, The Netherlands: Martinus Nijhoff, 1987.
180. Schlesinger MJ: Relation of anastomotic pattern to pathologic conditions of the coronary arteries. Arch Pathol 30:403–415, 1940.
181. Allwork SP: Angiographic anatomy. *In* Anderson RH, Becker AE (eds): Cardiac Anatomy. London: Churchill Livingstone, 1980.
182. Allwork SP: The applied anatomy of the arterial blood supply to the heart in man. J Anat 153:1–16, 1987.
183. Feiring AJ, Johnson MR, Kioschos JM, et al: The importance of the determination of the myocardial area at risk in the evaluation of the outcome of acute myocardial infarction in patients. Circulation 75:980–987, 1987.
184. Sos TA, Kligfield PD, Sniderman KW: A method for understanding three-dimensional coronary anatomy. JAMA 243:252–254, 1980.
185. Coleman C, Castaneda-Zuniga WR, Amplatz K: Three-dimensional teaching model for coronary angiography. Cardiovasc Intervent Radiol 5:154–156, 1982.
186. Brown BG, Bolson E, Frimer M, Dodge HT: Quantitative coronary arteriography: estimation of dimensions, hemodynamic resistance, and atheroma mass of coronary artery lesions using the arteriogram and digital computation. Circulation 55:329–337, 1977.
187. Wilson RF, Marcus ML, White CW: Prediction of the physiologic significance of coronary arterial lesions by quantitative lesion geometry in patients with limited coronary artery disease. Circulation 75:723–732, 1987.
188. Paulin S: Terminology for radiographic projections in cardiac angiography [letter]. Cathet Cardiovasc Diagn 7:341, 1981.

189. Arnett EN, Isner JM, Redwood DR, et al: Coronary artery narrowing in coronary heart disease: comparison of cineangiographic and necropsy findings. Ann Intern Med 91:350, 1979.
190. Isner JM, Kishel J, Kent KM, et al: Inaccuracy of angiographic determination of left main coronary arterial narrowing. Circulation 60(suppl II):II–161, 1979.
191. Hutchins GM, Bulkley BH, Ridolfi RL, et al: Correlation of coronary arteriograms and left ventriculograms with postmortem studies. Circulation 56:32, 1977.
192. Grondin CM, Dyrda I, Pasternac A, et al: Discrepancies between cineangiographic and postmortem findings in patients with coronary artery disease and recent myocardial revascularization. Circulation 49:703, 1974.
193. Marcus ML, Armstrong ML, Heistad DD, et al: A comparison of three methods of evaluation of coronary obstructive lesions: postmortem arteriography, pathological examination and measurement of regional myocardial perfusion during maximal vasodilation. Am J Cardiol 49:1699–1706, 1982.
194. Johnson MR: A normal coronary artery: what size is it? Circulation 86:331–333, 1992.
195. McPherson DD, Hiratzka LF, Lamberth WC, et al: Delineation of the extent of coronary atherosclerosis by high-frequency epicardial echocardiography. N Engl J Med 316:304–309, 1987.
196. Langille BI, O'Donnell F: Reductions in arterial diameter produced by chronic decreases in blood flow are endothelium dependent. Science 231:405–407, 1986.
197. Marcus ML, Skorton DJ, Johnson MR, et al: Visual estimates of percent diameter in coronary stenosis: "a battered gold standard." J Am Coll Cardiol 11:882–885, 1988.
198. Glagov S, Weisenberg E, Zarins CK, et al: Compensatory enlargement of human atherosclerotic coronary arteries. N Engl J Med 316:1371–1375, 1987.
199. Dodge JT, Brown BG, Bolson EL, Dodge HT: Lumen diameter of normal human coronary arteries: influence of age, sex, anatomic variation, and left ventricular hypertrophy or dilation. Circulation 86:232–246, 1992.
200. Vieweg WVR, Alpert JS, Hagan AD: Caliber and distribution of normal coronary arterial anatomy. Cathet Cardiovasc Diagn 2:269–280, 1976.
201. MacAlpin RN, Abbasi AS, Grollman JH, Eber L: Human coronary artery size during life. Radiology 108:567–576, 1973.
202. Seiler C, Kirkeeide RL, Gould KL: Basic structure-function relations of the epicardial coronary vascular tree. Basis of quantitative coronary arteriography for diffuse coronary artery disease. Circulation 85:1987–2003, 1992.
203. Dick C, Wyche K, Homans DC, White CW: Effect of distending pressure on intravascular ultrasound measurement of lumen dimensions [abstract]. Circulation 82:III-459, 1990.
204. Drexler H, Zeiher AM, Wollschläger H, et al: Flow-dependent coronary artery dilatation in humans. Circulation 80:466–474, 1989.
205. Cox DA, Vita JA, Treasure CB, et al: Atherosclerosis impairs flow-mediated dilation of coronary arteries in humans. Circulation 80:458–465, 1989.
206. Egashira K, Inou T, Hirooka Y, et al: Impaired coronary blood flow response to acetylcholine in patients with coronary risk factors and proximal atherosclerotic lesions. J Clin Invest 91:29–37, 1993.
207. O'Keefe JH, Owen RM, Bove AA: Influence of left ventricular mass on coronary artery cross-sectional area. Am J Cardiol 59:1395–1397, 1987.
208. Lewis BS, Gotsman MS: Relation between coronary artery size and left ventricular wall mass. Br Heart J 35:1150–1153, 1973.
209. Paulsen S, Vetner M, Hagerup SM: Relationship between heart weight and the cross-sectional area of the coronary ostia. Acta Pathol Microbiol Scand 83:529–532, 1975.
210. Haskell WL, Sims C, Myll J, et al: Coronary artery size and dilating capacity in ultradistance runners. Circulation 87:1076–1082, 1993.
211. Kalin JK, Rutherford BD, McConabay DR, et al: Comparison of procedural results and risks of coronary angioplasty in men and women for conditions other than acute myocardial infarction. Am J Cardiol 69:1241–1242, 1992.
212. Fisher LD, Kennedy JW, Davis KB, et al: Association of sex, physical size and operative mortality after coronary artery bypass in the Coronary Artery Surgery Study (CASS). J Thorac Cardiovasc Surg 84:334–341, 1982.
213. O'Connor NJ, Morton JR, Birkmeyer JD, et al: Effect of coronary artery diameter in patients undergoing coronary bypass surgery. Northern New England Cardiovascular Disease Study Group. Circulation 93:652–655, 1996.
214. Kornowski R, Lansky AJ, Mintz GS, et al: Comparison of men versus women in cross-sectional area luminal narrowing, quantity of plaque, presence of calcium in plaque, and lumen location in coronary arteries by intravascular ultrasound in patients with stable angina pectoris. Am J Cardiol 79:1601–1605, 1997.
215. Neufeld HN, Wagenvoort CA, Edwards JE: Coronary arteries in fetuses, infants, juveniles and young adults. Clin Invest 11:837–844, 1962.
215a. Leung WH, Stadius ML, Alderman EL: Determinants of normal coronary artery dimensions in humans. Circulation 84:2294–2306, 1991.
216. Jost S, Rafflenbeul W, Reil G, et al: Reproducible uniform coronary vasomotor tone with nitrocompounds: prerequisite of quantitative coronary angiographic trials. Cathet Cardiovasc Diagn 20:168–173, 1990.
217. Yasue H, Omati S, Takizawa A, et al: Circadian variation in exercise capacity in patients with Prinzmetal's variant angina: role of exercise induced coronary arterial spasm. Circulation 59:938–948, 1979.
218. Williams JK, Vita JA, Manuck SB, et al: Psychosocial factors impair responses of coronary arteries. Circulation 84:2146–2153, 1991.
219. Williams JK, Adams MR, Klopfenstein HS: Estrogen modulates responses of atherosclerotic coronary arteries. Circulation 81:1680–1687, 1990.
220. Brown BG, Petersen RB, Pierce CD, et al: Dynamics of human coronary stenosis: interaction among stenosis flow, distending pressure and vasomotor tone. *In* Santamore WP, Bove AA (eds): Coronary Artery Disease. p. 199. Baltimore: Urban & Schwarzenberg, 1982.
221. Lee JT, Ideker RE, Reimer KA: Myocardial infarct size and location in relation to the coronary vascular bed at risk in man. Circulation 64:526, 1981.
222. Koyanagi S, Eastham CL, Harrison DG, Marcus ML: Transmural variation in the relationship between myocardial infarct size and risk area. Am J Physiol 242:H867–H874, 1982.
223. Liu YH, Bahn RC, Ritman EL: Myocardial volume perfused by coronary artery branches: a three-dimensional x-ray computed tomographic evaluation in pigs. Invest Radiol 27:302–307, 1992.
224. Koiwa Y, Bahn RC, Ritman EL: Regional myocardial volume perfused by the coronary branch: estimation in vivo. Circulation 74:157–163, 1986.
225. Feiring AJ, Bruch PM, Husayni TS, et al: Premortem assessment of myocardial risk area employing intracoronary technetium macroaggregated albumin and gated nuclear imaging. Circulation 73:551, 1986.
226. Gibbons RJ, Verani MS, Behrenbeck T, et al: Feasibility of tomographic ^{99m}Tc-hexakis-2-methoxy-2-methylprophyl-isonitrile imaging for the assessment of myocardial area at risk and the effect of treatment in acute myocardial infarction. Circulation 80:1277–1286, 1989.
227. Huber KC, Bresnahan JF, Bresnahan DR, et al: Measurement of myocardium at risk by technetium-99m sestamibi: correlation with coronary angiography. J Am Coll Cardiol 19:67–73, 1992.
228. Freiman PC, Cooper SM, Harrison DC: Relationship between angiographic lesion location and left ventricular anatomic risk area [abstract]. Clin Res 35:831A, 1987.

Coronary Anomalies

229. Yamanaka O, Hobbs RE: Coronary artery anomalies in 126,595 patients undergoing coronary arteriography. Cathet Cardiovasc Diagn 21:26–40, 1990.
230. Kimbris D, Iskandrian AS, Segal BL, Bemis CE: Anomalous aortic origin of coronary arteries. Circulation 58:606–615, 1978.
230a. Wilkins CE, Betancourt B, Mathur VS, et al: Coronary artery anomalies: a review of more than 10,000 patients from the Clayton Cardiovascular Laboratories. Tex Heart Inst J15:166–173, 1988.
230b. Engel HJ, Tomes C, Page HL: Major variations in anatomical origin of the coronary arteries: angiographic observations in 4,250 patients without associated congenital heart disease. Cathet Cardiovasc Diagn 1:157–169, 1975.

230c. Baltaxe HA, Wixson D: The incidence of congenital anomalies of the coronary arteries in the adult population. Radiology 122:47–52, 1977.

230d. Becker AE: Congenital coronary arterial anomalies of clinical relevance. Coron Artery Dis 6:187–193, 1995.

231. Reyman HC: Dissertatio de vasis cordis propriis. Haller, Bibioth Anat 2:366, 1737.

232. Angelini P, Trivellato M, Donis J, Leachman RD: Myocardial bridges: a review. Progr Cardiovasc Dis 26:75–88, 1983.

232a. Lee SS, Wu TL: The role of mural coronary artery in prevention of coronary atherosclerosis. Arch Pathol 93:32, 1972.

232b. Stolte M, Weis P, Prestele H: Muscle bridges over the left anterior descending coronary artery: their influence on arterial disease. Virchows Arch Pathol Anat 375:23, 1977.

233. Polacek P, Zechmeister A: The occurrence and significance of myocardial bridges and loops on coronary arteries. Opuscola Cardiologica. Brno, Acta Facultatis Medicae Universitatis Brunensis Brno, 1968.

234. Morales A, Romanelli R, Boucek R: The mural left anterior descending coronary artery, strenuous exercise and sudden death. Circulation 62:230–237, 1980.

235. Channer KS, Bukis E, Hartnell G, Rees JR: Myocardial bridging of the coronary arteries. Clin Radiol 40:355–359, 1989.

236. Irvin RG: The angiographic prevalence of myocardial bridging in man. Chest 81:198–202, 1982.

237. Hashimoto A, Takekoshi N, Murakami E: Clinical significance of myocardial bridging of the coronary artery. Jpn Heart J 25:913–922, 1984.

238. Katz SA, Feigl EO: Systole has little effect on diastolic coronary artery blood flow. Circ Res 62:443–451, 1988.

239. Marcus ML: The Coronary Circulation in Health and Disease. New York: McGraw-Hill, 1983.

239a. Jain SP, White CJ, Ventura HO: De novo appearance of a myocardial bridge in heart transplant: assessment by intravascular ultrasonography, Doppler, and angiography. Am Heart J 126:453–456, 1993.

239b. Ge J, Erbel R, Rupprecht H-S, et al: Comparison of intravascular ultrasound and angiography in the assessment of myocardial bridging. Circulation 89:1725–1732, 1994.

240. Noble J, Bourassa MG, Petitclerc R, Dyrda I: Myocardial bridging and the milking effect of the left anterior descending coronary artery: normal variant or obstruction. Am J Cardiol 37:993–999, 1976.

240a. Ferreira AG, Trotter SE, König B, et al: Myocardial bridges: morphological and functional aspects. Br Heart J 6:364–367, 1991.

240b. Corrado D, Thiene G, Cocco P, Frescura C: Nonatherosclerotic coronary artery disease and sudden death in the young. Br Heart J 68:601–607, 1992.

240c. Ishii T, Asuwa N, Masuda S, Ishikawa Y: The effects of a myocardial bridge on coronary atherosclerosis and ischaemia. J Pathol 185:4–9, 1998.

241. Ishii T, Hosoda Y: The significance of myocardial bridge upon atherosclerosis in the left anterior descending coronary artery. J Pathol 148:279–291, 1986.

241a. Edwards JC, Burnsides CH, Swarm RL, et al: Arteriosclerosis in the intramural and extramural portions of coronary arteries in the human heart. Circulation 13:235, 1956.

242. van Brussel BL, van Tellingen C, Ernst SMPG, Plokker HWM: Myocardial bridging: a cause of myocardial infarction? Int J Cardiol 6:78–82, 1984.

243. Feldman AM, Baugham KL: Myocardial infarction associated with a myocardial bridge. Am Heart J 111:784–787, 1986.

244. Wymore P, Yedlicka JW, Garcia-Medina V, et al: The incidence of myocardial bridges in heart transplants. Cardiovasc Intervent Radiol 12:202–206, 1989.

245. Ischimori T, Raizner AE, Chahine RA, et al: Myocardial bridges in man: clinical correlations and angiographic accentuation with nitroglycerin. Cathet Cardiovasc Diagn 3:59–65, 1977.

246. Kramer JR, Kitazume H, Krauthamer D, et al: The prevalence of myocardial bridging and septal squeeze in patients with significant aortic stenosis. Cleve Clin Q 51:35–38, 1984.

247. Page HL Jr, Engel JH, Campbell WB, Thomas SC: Anomalous origin of the left circumflex coronary artery. Recognition, angiographic demonstration and clinical significance. Circulation 50:768–773, 1974.

248. Chaitman BR, Lesperance J, Saltiel J, Bourassa MG: Clinical, angiographic, and hemodynamic findings in patients with anomalous origin of the coronary arteries. Circulation 53:122, 1975.

249. Topaz O, DiSciascio G, Goudreau E, et al: Coronary angioplasty of anomalous coronary arteries: notes on technical aspects. Cathet Cardiovasc Diagn 21:106–111, 1990.

249a. Dicicco BS, McManus BM, Waller BF, Roberts WC: Separate aortic ostium of the left anterior descending and left circumflex coronary arteries from the left aortic sinus of Valsalva (absent left main coronary artery). Am Heart J 104:53, 1982.

250. Liberthson RR, Dinsmore RE, Bharati S, et al: Aberrant coronary artery origin from the aorta: diagnosis and clinical significance. Circulation 50:774–779, 1974.

251. Roberts WC: Major anomalies of coronary arterial origin seen in adulthood. Am Heart J 111:941–963, 1986.

252. Barth CW III, Roberts WC: Left main coronary artery originating from the right sinus of Valsalva and coursing between the aorta and pulmonary trunk. J Am Coll Cardiol 7:366–373, 1986.

253. Donaldson RM, Raphael M, Rodley-Smith R, et al: Angiographic identification of primary coronary anomalies causing impaired myocardial perfusion. Cathet Cardiovasc Diagn 9:237–249, 1983.

254. Brandt B III, Martins JB, Marcus ML: Anomalous origin of the right coronary artery from the left sinus of Valsalva. N Engl J Med 10:596, 1983.

255. Serota H, Barth CW, Seuc CA, et al: Rapid identification of the course of anomalous coronary arteries in adults: the "dot and eye" method. Am J Cardiol 65:891–898, 1990.

256. Hobbs RE, Millit HD, Raghavan PV, et al: Congenital coronary anomalies: clinical and therapeutic implications. *In* Vidt D (ed): Cardiovascular Therapy. p. 43. Philadelphia: FA Davis, 1982.

256a. Kragel AH, Roberts WC: Anomalous origin of either the right or left main coronary artery from the aorta with subsequent coursing between aorta and pulmonary trunk: analysis of 32 necropsy cases. Am J Cardiol 62:771–777, 1988.

256b. Kaku B, Shimizu M, Yoshio H, et al: Clinical features of prognosis of Japanese patients with anomalous origin of the coronary artery. Jpn Circ J 60:7331–7341, 1996.

257. Bland EF, White PD, Garland J: Congenital anomalies of the coronary arteries: report of an unusual case associated with cardiac hypertrophy. Am Heart J 8:787–801, 1933.

258. Greenberg MA, Fish BG, Spindola-Franco H: Congenital anomalies of the coronary arteries. Radiol Clin North Am 27:1127–1146, 1989.

259. Wesselhoeft H, Fawcett JS, Johnson AL: Anomalous origin of the left coronary artery from the pulmonary trunk: its clinical spectrum, pathology, pathophysiology, based on a review of 140 cases with seven further cases. Circulation 38:403–425, 1968.

260. Guikahue M, Sidi D, Kachaner J, et al: Anomalous left coronary artery arising from the pulmonary artery in infancy: is early operation better? Br Heart J 60:522–526, 1988.

260a. Musiani A, Cernigliaro C, Sansa M, et al: Left main coronary artery atresia: literature review and therapeutical considerations. Eur J Cardiothorac Surg 11:505–514, 1997.

260b. White CW, Chandra MS: Total occlusion of the main left coronary artery: a lethal lesion? Angiology 27:587, 1976.

260c. Vogt PR, Tkebuchava T, Arbenz U, et al: Anomalous origin of the right coronary artery from the pulmonary artery. Thorac Cardiovasc Surg 42:125–127, 1994.

260d. Rittenhouse EA, Doty DB, Ehrenhaft JL: Congenital coronary artery–cardiac chamber fistula. Review of operative management. Ann Thorac Surg 20:468–485, 1975.

260e. Said SA, el Gamal MI, van der Werf T: Coronary arteriovenous fistulas: collective review and management of six new cases—changing etiology, presentation, and treatment strategy. Clin Cardiol 20:748–752, 1997.

260f. Jaffe RB, Glancy DL, Epstein SE, et al: Coronary arterial–right heart fistulae: long-term observations in seven patients. Circulation 48:133–143, 1973.

260g. Gillebert C, Van Hoof R, van de Werf F, et al: Coronary artery fistulas in an adult population. Eur Heart J 7:437–443, 1986.

261. Levin DC, Fellow KE, Abrams HL: Hemodynamically significant primary anomalies of the coronary arteries. Circulation 58:25, 1978.

262. Karagoz HY, Zorlutuna YI, Babacan KM, et al: Congenital coronary artery fistulas: diagnostic and surgical considerations. Jpn Heart J 30:685–694, 1989.

263. Rittenhouse EA, Doty DB, Ehrenhaft JL: Congenital coronary artery–cardiac chamber fistula. Review of operative management. Ann Thorac Surg 20:468–485, 1975.

264. Chia BL, Chan ALK, Tan LKA, Ng RAL: Coronary artery–left ventricular fistula. Cardiology 68:167–179, 1981.
265. Martens J, Haseldoncks C, van de Werf F, de Geest H: Silent left and right coronary artery–left ventricular fistulas: an unusual prominent thebesian system. Acta Cardiol 38:139–142, 1983.
265a. Coussement P, de Geest H: Multiple coronary artery–left ventricular communications: an unusual prominent thebesian system. A report of four cases and review of the literature. Acta Cardiol 49:165–173, 1994.
266. Ahmed SS, Haider B, Regen TJ: Silent left coronary artery–cameral fistula: probable cause of myocardial ischemia. Am Heart J 102:869–870, 1982.
267. Cheng TO: Left coronary artery to left ventricular fistula: demonstration of coronary steal phenomenon. Am Heart J 102:870–871, 1982.
268. Henzlova MJ, Nath H, Bucy RP, et al: Coronary artery to right ventricle fistula in heart transplant recipients: a complication of endomyocardial biopsy. J Am Coll Cardiol 14:258–261, 1989.

Coronary Atherosclerosis

268a. Clarkson TB, Prichard RW, Morgan TM, et al: Remodeling of coronary arteries in human and non-human primates. JAMA 271:289–294, 1994.
268b. Rumberger JA, Sheedy PF II, Breen JF, Schwartz RS: Coronary calcium, as determined by electron beam computed tomography, and coronary disease on arteriogram: effect of patient's sex on diagnosis. Circulation 91:1363–1367, 1995.
268c. Janowitz WR, Agatston AS, Kaplan G, Viamonte M Jr: Differences in prevalence and extent of coronary artery calcium detected by ultrafast computed tomography in asymptomatic men and women. Am J Cardiol 72:247–254, 1994.
268d. Rumberger JA, Simons DB, Fitzpatrick LA, et al: Coronary artery calcium area by electron-beam computed tomography and coronary atherosclerotic plaque area: a histopathologic correlative study. Circulation 92:2157–2162, 1995.
268e. Mintz GS, Pichard AD, Popma JJ, et al: Determinants and correlates of target lesion calcium in coronary artery disease: a clinical, angiographic and intravascular ultrasound study. J Am Coll Cardiol 29:268–274, 1997.
268f. Schmermund A, Baumgart D, Gorge G, et al: Measuring the effect of risk factors on coronary atherosclerosis: coronary calcium score versus angiographic disease severity. J Am Coll Cardiol 31:1267–1273, 1998.
269. Vlodaver Z, Kahn HA, Neufeld HN: The coronary arteries in early life in three different ethnic groups. Circulation 39:541–550, 1969.
270. Waller BF, Pinkerton CA, Slack JD: Intravascular ultrasound: a histological study of vessels during life. Circulation 85:2305–2310, 1992.
271. Mintz GS, Painter JA, Pichard AD, et al: Atherosclerosis in angiographically "normal" coronary artery reference segments: an intravascular ultrasound study with clinical correlations. J Am Coll Cardiol 25:1479–1485, 1995.
272. St. Goar FG, Pinto FJ, Alderman EL, et al: Detection of coronary atherosclerosis in young adult hearts using intravascular ultrasound. Circulation 86:756–763, 1992.
273. St. Goar FG, Pinto FJ, Alderman EL, et al: Intracoronary ultrasound in cardiac transplant recipients. Circulation 85:979–987, 1992.
274. Johnson TH, McDonald K, Nakhleh R, et al: Allograft vasculopathy and death in a cardiac transplant patient with angiographically normal coronary arteries. Cathet Cardiovasc Diagn 24:37–40, 1991.
274a. Herzog CA, Ma JZ, Collins AJ: Poor long-term survival after acute myocardial infarction among patients on long-term dialysis. N Engl J Med 339:799–805, 1998.
274b. Vavuranakis M, Stefanadis C, Toutouzas K, et al: Impaired compensatory coronary artery enlargement in atherosclerosis contributes to the development of coronary artery stenosis in diabetic patients. An in vivo intravascular ultrasound study. Eur Heart J 18:1090–1094, 1997.
274c. Schaper W, Buschmann I: Collateral circulation and diabetes. Circulation 99:2224–2226, 1999.
275. Gould KL: Quantification of coronary artery stenosis in vivo. Circ Res 47:341, 1985.
276. Marcus ML, Harrison DG, White CW, et al: Assessing the physiologic significance of coronary obstructions in patients: importance of diffuse undetected atherosclerosis. Prog Cardiovasc Dis 31:39, 1988.
277. White CW: Physiologic assessment of coronary artery stenosis severity. Trends Cardiovasc Med 1:70–75, 1991.
278. Gould KL: Percent coronary stenosis: battered gold standard, pernicious relic or clinical practicality? J Am Coll Cardiol 11:8868, 1988.
279. Raphael MJ, Donaldson RM: A "significant" stenosis: thirty years on. Lancet 1:207, 1989.
280. Beauman GJ, Vogel RA: Accuracy of individual and panel visual interpretations of coronary arteriograms: implications for clinical decisions. J Am Coll Cardiol 16:108–113, 1990.
281. Detre KM, Wright E, Murphy ML, Takaro T: Observer agreement in evaluating coronary angiograms. Circulation 52:979–986, 1975.
282. Zir LM, Miller SW, Dinsmore RE, et al: Interobserver variability in coronary arteriography. Circulation 53:627–632, 1976.
283. DeRouen TA, Murphy JA, Owen W: Variability in the analysis of coronary arteriograms. Circulation 55:324–328, 1977.
284. Fisher LD, Judkins MP, Lesperance J, et al: Reproducibility of coronary arteriographic reading in the Coronary Artery Surgery Study (CASS). Cathet Cardiovasc Diagn 8:565–575, 1982.
285. Serruys PW, Reiber JHC, Wijns W, et al: Assessment of percutaneous transluminal angioplasty by quantitative angiography: diameter versus densitometric area measurements. Am J Cardiol 54:482–488, 1984.
286. Meier B, Gruentzig AR, Goebel N, et al: Assessment of stenoses in coronary angioplasty: inter- and intraobserver variability. Int J Cardiol 3:159–169, 1983.
287. Scoblionko DP, Brown BG, Mitten S, et al: A new digital electronic caliper for measurement of coronary artery stenosis: comparison with visual estimates and computer-assisted measurements. Am J Cardiol 53:689–693, 1984.
288. Eusterman JH, Achor RWP, Kincaid OW, Brown AL Jr: Atherosclerotic disease of the coronary arteries. A pathologic-radiologic correlative study. Circulation 26:1288, 1962.
289. Marcus ML, Harrison DG, White CW, et al: Assessing the physiologic significance of coronary obstructions in patients: importance of diffuse undetected atherosclerosis. Prog Cardiovasc Dis 31:39–56, 1988.
290. Sanmarco ME, Brooks SH, Blankenhorn DH: Reproducibility of a consensus panel in the interpretation of coronary angiograms. Am Heart J 96:430–437, 1978.
291. Galbraith JE, Murphy ML, de Soyza N: Coronary angiogram interpretation. JAMA 240:2053–2056, 1978.
292. Hermiller JB, Cusma JT, Spero LA, et al: Quantitative and qualitative coronary angiographic analysis: review of methods, utility and limitations. Cathet Cardiovasc Diagn 25:110–131, 1992.
293. Mancini JGB: Quantitative coronary arteriography: development of methods, limitations and clinical applications. Am J Card Imaging 2:98–109, 1988.
294. Brown BG, Bolston EL, Dodge HT: Quantitative computer techniques for analyzing coronary arteriograms. Prog Cardiovasc Dis 18:403–418, 1986.
295. Reiber JHC: Morphologic and densitometric quantitation of coronary stenoses: an overview of existing quantitation techniques. *In* Reiber JHC, Serruys PW (eds): New Developments in Quantitative Coronary Arteriography. p. 34. Dordrecht, The Netherlands: Martinus Nijhoff, 1988.
296. Gensini GG, Kelly AE, DaCosta BCB, Huntington PP: Quantitative angiography: the measurement of coronary vasomobility in the intact animal and man. Chest 60:522–530, 1971.
297. Kalbfleisch SJ, McGillem MJ, Pinto IMF, et al: Comparison of automated quantitative coronary angiography with caliper measurements of percent diameter stenosis. Am J Cardiol 65:1181–1184, 1990.
298. Scoblionko DP, Brown BG, Mitten S, et al: A new digital electronic caliper for measurement of coronary arterial stenosis: comparison with visual estimates and computer-assisted measurements. Am J Cardiol 53:689–693, 1984.
299. Reiber JHC, Kooijman CJ, Slager CG, et al: Coronary artery dimension from cineangiograms: methodology and validation of a computer assisted analysis procedure. IEEE Trans Med Imaging MI-3:131–141, 1984.
300. Reiber JHC, Serruys PW, Kooijman CJ, et al: Approaches to standardization in acquisition and quantitation of arterial dimensions from cineangiograms. *In* Reiber JHL, Serruys PW (eds): State of the Art in Quantitative Coronary Arteriography. p. 145. Dordrecht, The Netherlands: Martinus Nijhoff, 1986.

301. Reiber JHC: Morphologic and densitometric analysis of coronary arteries. *In* Heintzen PH, Bursch JH (eds): Progress in Digital Angiocardiography. p. 137. London: Kluwer Academic, 1988.
302. Reiber JHC, Serruys PW, Kooijman CJ, et al: Assessment of short-, medium-, and long-term variations in arterial dimensions from computer-assisted quantitation of coronary cineangiograms. Circulation 71:280–288, 1985.
303. Langer A, Wilson RF: Comparison of manual versus automated edge detection for determining degrees of luminal narrowing by quantitative coronary angiography. Am J Cardiol 67:885–889, 1991.
304. Mancini GBJ, Simon SB, McGillem MJ, et al: Automated quantitative coronary arteriography: morphologic and physiologic validation in vivo of a rapid digital angiographic method. Circulation 75:452–460, 1987.
305. Cusma JT, Spero LA, Hanemann JD, et al: A multiuser environment for the display and processing of digital cardiac angiographic images. Proc SPIE 1233:310–320, 1990.
306. Spears JR, Sandor T: Quantitation of coronary artery stenosis severity: limitations of angiography and computerized information extraction. *In* Reiber JHC, Serruys PW (eds): State of the Art in Quantitative Coronary Arteriography. p. 103. Dordrecht, The Netherlands: Martinus Nijhoff, 1986.
307. Sanders WJ, Alderman EL, Harrison DC: Coronary artery quantitation using digital image processing. Comput Cardiol 15, 1979.
308. Kirkeeide RL, Smalling RW, Gould KL: Automated measurements of artery diameter from arteriograms [abstract]. Circulation 66:II-325, 1982.
309. Doiot PA: On the accuracy of densitometric measurements of coronary artery stenosis based on Lambert-Beer's absorption law. *In* Reiber JHC, Serruys PW (eds): New Developments in Quantitative Coronary Arteriography. p. 115. Dordrecht, The Netherlands: Martinus Nijhoff, 1988.
310. Parker DL, Pope DL, Petersen JC, et al: Quantitation in cardiac video-densitometry. Comput Cardiol 119, 1984.
311. Nichols AB, Gabrieli CFO, Fenoglio JJ Jr, Esser PD: Quantification of relative coronary arterial stenosis by cinevideodensitometric analysis of coronary arteriograms. Circulation 69:512, 1984.
312. LeFree MT, Simon SB, Lewis RJ, et al: Digital radiographic coronary artery quantification. Comput Cardiol 99, 1985.
313. Johnson MR, Skorton DJ, Ericksen EE, et al: Videodensitometric analysis of coronary stenoses. In vivo geometric and physiologic validation in humans. Invest Radiol 23:891–898, 1988.
314. Whiting JS, Pfaff JM, Eigler NL: Advantages and limitations of videodensitometry in quantitative coronary angiography. *In* Reiber JHC, Serruys PW (eds): Quantitative Coronary Arteriography. p. 43. Dordrecht, The Netherlands: Kluwer Academic, 1991.
315. Spears JR, Sandor T, Als AV, et al: Computerized image analysis for quantitative measurement of vessel diameter from cineangiograms. Circulation 68:453–461, 1983.
316. Leung WH, Demopulos PA, Alderman EL, et al: Evaluation of catheters and metallic catheter markers as calibration standard for measurement of coronary dimension. Cathet Cardiovasc Diagn 21:148–153, 1990.
317. Reiber JHC, Kooijman CJH, den Boer A, Serruys PW: Assessment of dimensions and image quality of coronary contrast catheters from cineangiograms. Cathet Cardiovasc Diagn 11:521–531, 1985.
318. Ellis SG, Pinto IMF, McGillem MJ, et al: Accuracy and reproducibility of quantitative coronary arteriography using 6 and 8 French catheters with cineangiographic acquisition. Cathet Cardiovasc Diagn 22:52–55, 1991.
319. DiMario C, Hermans WRM, Rensing BJ, Serruys PW: Calibration using angiographic catheters as scaling devices—importance of filming the catheters not filled with contrast medium. Am J Cardiol 69:1377–1378, 1992.
320. Fortin DF, Spero LA, Cusma JT, et al: Pitfalls in the determination of absolute dimensions using angiographic catheters as calibration devices in quantitative angiography. Am J Cardiol 68:1176–1182, 1991.
321. Lesperance J, Hudon G, White CW, et al: Comparison by quantitative angiographic assessment of coronary stenoses of one view showing the severest narrowing to two orthogonal views. Am J Cardiol 64:462–465, 1989.
322. Katz LN, Lindner E: Quantitative relation between reactive hyperemia and the myocardial ischemia which it follows. Am J Physiol 126:283, 1939.
323. Click RL, Holmes DR, Vliestra RE, et al: Anomalous coronary arteries: location, degree of atherosclerosis and effect on survival—a report from the Coronary Artery Surgery Study. J Am Coll Cardiol 13:531–537, 1989.
324. White CW, Wright CB, Doty DB, et al: Does visual interpretation of the coronary arteriogram predict the physiologic importance of a coronary stenosis? N Engl J Med 310:819–824, 1984.
325. Wilson RF, Laughlin DE, Holida MD, et al: Transluminal subselective measurement of coronary blood flow velocity and vasodilator reserve in man. Circulation 72:82–92, 1985.
326. Wilson RF, Laughlin DE, Ackell PH, et al: Transluminal, subselective measurement of coronary artery blood flow velocity and vasodilator reserve in man. Circulation 72:82, 1985.
327. Wilson RF, White CW: Intracoronary papaverine: an ideal coronary vasodilator for studies of the coronary circulation in conscious humans. Circulation 73:444, 1986.
328. Wilson RF, White CW: Serious ventricular dysrhythmias after intracoronary papaverine. Am J Cardiol 62:1301–1302, 1988.
329. Wilson RF, Wyche K, Christensen BV, et al: Effects of adenosine on human coronary arterial circulation. Circulation 82:1595–1606, 1990.
330. Wilson RF, White CW: Does coronary bypass surgery restore normal coronary flow reserve? The effect of diffuse atherosclerosis and focal obstructive lesions. Circulation 76:563–571, 1987.
330a. Wilson RF: Assessing the severity of coronary artery stenoses. N Engl J Med 1735–1737, 1996.
330b. Pijls NHJ, Van Gelder B, Van der Voort P, et al: Fractional flow reserve. A useful index to evaluate the influence of an epicardial coronary stenosis on myocardial blood flow. Circulation 92:3183–3193, 1995.
330c. Pijls NHJ, De Bruyne B, Peels K, et al: Measurement of fractional flow reserve to assess the functional severity of coronary-artery stenoses. N Engl J Med 334:1703–1708, 1996.
330d. Bech GJW, Pijls NHJ, De Bruyne B, et al: Usefulness of fractional flow reserve to predict clinical outcome after balloon angioplasty. Circulation 99:883–888, 1999.
330e. Bech GJWS, De Bruyne B, Bonnier HJRM, et al: Long-term follow-up after deferral of percutaneous transluminal coronary angioplasty of intermediate stenosis on the basis of coronary pressure measurement. J Am Coll Cardiol 31:841–847, 1998.
330f. Lesser JR, Wilson RF, White CW: Physiologic assessment of coronary stenoses of intermediate severity can facilitate patient selection for coronary angioplasty. Coron Artery Dis 1:697–705, 1990.
331. Doucette JW, Corl D, Payne H, et al: Validation of a Doppler guide wire for intravascular measurement of coronary artery flow velocity. Circulation 85:1899–1911, 1992.
332. Vanyi J, Bowers T, Jarvis G, White CW: Can an intracoronary Doppler wire accurately measure changes in coronary blood flow velocity? Cathet Cardiovasc Diagn 29:240–246, 1993.
333. von Restorff W, Hofling B, Holtz J, Bassenge E: Effect of increased blood fluidity through homodilution on coronary circulation at rest and during exercise in dogs. Pflugers Arch 357:15–24, 1975.
334. Marcus ML, Doty DB, Hiratzka LF, et al: Decreased coronary reserve: a mechanism for angina pectoris in patients with aortic stenosis and normal coronary arteries. N Engl J Med 307:1362–1366, 1982.
335. Olinger GN, Mulder DG, Maloney JV Jr, Buckberg GD: Phasic coronary flow: intraoperative evaluation of flow distribution, myocardial function, and reactive hyperemic response. Ann Thorac Surg 21:397–404, 1976.
336. White CW: Clinical applications of Doppler coronary flow reserve measurements. Am J Cardiol 71:10D–16D, 1993.
337. Ophertz D, Zebe H, Weihe E, et al: Reduced coronary dilator capacity and ultrastructural changes in patients with angina pectoris but normal coronary arteriograms. Circulation 63:817–825, 1981.
338. Klocke FJ: Measurements of coronary flow reserve: defining pathophysiology versus making decisions about patient care. Circulation 76:1183, 1987.
339. McGinn AL, White CW, Wilson RF: Interstudy variability of coronary flow reserve: influence of heart rate, arterial pressure, and ventricular preload. Circulation 81:1319–1328, 1990.
339a. Pijls NHJ, Van Son JAM, Kirkeeide RL, et al: Experimental basis of determining maximum coronary, myocardial and collateral blood flow by pressure measurements for assessing functional stenosis

severity before and after percutaneous transluminal coronary angioplasty. Circulation 87:1354–1367, 1993.
340. Little WC, Applegate RJ: Role of plaque size and degree of stenosis in acute myocardial infarction. Cardiol Clin 14:221–228, 1996.
341. Wilson RF, Marcus ML, Christensen BV, et al: The accuracy of exercise electrocardiography in predicting the physiologic significance of coronary arterial stenoses. Circulation 83:412–421, 1991.
342. Wijns TL, Serruys PW, Reiber JH, et al: Quantitative angiography of the left anterior descending coronary artery: correlations with pressure gradient and results of exercise thallium scintigraphy. Circulation 71:273–279, 1985.
343. Lesser JR, Wilson RF, White CW: Physiologic assessment of coronary stenoses of intermediate severity can facilitate patient selection for coronary angioplasty. Coron Artery Dis 1:697–705, 1990.
344. Crossman DC, Larkin SW, Fuller RW, et al: Substance P dilates epicardial coronary arteries and increases coronary blood flow in humans. Circulation 80:475–484, 1989.
345. Ludmer PL, Selwyn AP, Shook TL, et al: Paradoxical vasoconstriction induced by acetylcholine in atherosclerotic coronary arteries. N Engl J Med 315:1046–1051, 1986.

Angiographic Findings in Myocardial Infarction and Acute Coronary Syndromes

346. Wilson RF, Ackell PH, Wysham DG, et al: Effect of tissue plasminogen activator (rt-PA) on coronary luminal dimensions in patients with abrupt onset of unstable angina [abstract]. Clin Res 34:905A, 1986.
347. Little WC, Constantinescu M, Applegate RJ, et al: Can coronary angiography predict the site of a subsequent myocardial infarction in patients with mild to moderate coronary artery disease? Circulation 78:1157–1166, 1988.
348. Little WC: Angiographic assessment of the culprit coronary artery lesion before acute myocardial infarction. Am J Cardiol 66:44G–47G, 1990.
349. Ambrose JA, Tannenbaum MA, Alexopoulos D, et al: Angiographic progression of coronary artery disease and the development of myocardial infarction J Am Coll Cardiol 12:56–62, 1988.
350. Hacket D, Verwilghen J, Davies G, Maseri A: Coronary stenoses before and after acute myocardial infarction. Am J Cardiol 63:1517–1518, 1989.
351. Webster MWI, Chesebro JH, Smith HC, et al: Myocardial infarction and coronary artery occlusion: a prospective 5 yr angiographic study. J Am Coll Cardiol 15:218A, 1990.
352. Wilson RF, Holida MD, White CW: Quantitative angiographic morphology of coronary stenoses leading to myocardial infarction or unstable angina. Circulation 73:286–293, 1986.
353. DeWood MA, Spores J, Notske RN, et al: Incidence of total coronary occlusion and thrombosis in the early phase of acute transmural myocardial infarction. Clin Res 27:162, 1979.
354. DeWood MA, Stifter WF, Simpson CS, et al: Coronary arteriographic findings soon after non–Q-wave myocardial infarction. N Engl J Med 315:417–423, 1986.
355. Falk E: Thrombosis in unstable angina: pathologic aspects. Cardiovasc Clin 18:137–149, 1987.
356. Davies MJ, Thomas AC: Plaque fissuring—the cause of acute myocardial infarction, sudden ischaemic death, and crescendo angina. Br Heart J 53:363–373, 1985.
357. Falk E: Coronary thrombosis: pathogenesis and clinical manifestations. Am J Cardiol 68:288–358, 1991.
358. Sherman CT, Litvack F, Grundfest W, et al: Coronary angioscopy in patients with unstable angina pectoris. N Engl J Med 315:913–919, 1986.
359. Ambrose JA, Hjemdahl-Monsen C, Borrico S, et al: Quantitative and qualitative effects of intracoronary streptokinase in unstable angina and non–Q wave infarction. J Am Coll Cardiol 9:1156–1165, 1987.
360. Levin DC, Fallon JT: Significance of the angiographic morphology of localized coronary stenosis: histopathologic correlations. Circulation 66:316, 1982.
361. Davies SW, Marchant B, Lyons JP, et al: Coronary lesion morphology in acute myocardial infarction: demonstration of early remodeling after streptokinase treatment. J Am Coll Cardiol 16:1079–1086, 1990.
362. Ambrose JA, Winters SL, Arora RR, et al: Angiographic evolution of coronary artery morphology in unstable angina. J Am Coll Cardiol 7:472–478, 1986.
363. Ambrose JA, Winters SL, Arora RR, et al: Coronary angiographic morphology in myocardial infarction: a link between the pathogenesis of unstable angina and myocardial infarction. J Am Coll Cardiol 6:1233–1238, 1985.
364. TIMI Research Group: Immediate vs delayed catheterization and angioplasty following thrombolytic therapy for acute myocardial infarction: TIMI IIA results. JAMA 260:2849–2858, 1988.
365. Gibson CM, Murphy SA, Rizzo MJ, et al: Relationship between TIMI frame count and clinical outcomes after thrombolytic administration. Thrombolysis in Myocardial Infarction (TIMI) Study Group. Circulation 99:1945–1950, 1999.
366. Harrison DG, Ferguson DW, Collins SM, et al: Rethrombosis after reperfusion with streptokinase: importance of geometry of residual lesions. Circulation 69:991–999, 1984.
367. Davies SW, Marchant B, Lyons JP, et al: Irregular lesion morphology after thrombolysis predicts early clinical instability. J Am Coll Cardiol 18:669–674, 1991.
368. Freeman MR, Langer A, Wilson RF, et al: Thrombolysis in unstable angina: randomized double blind trial of tPA and placebo. Circulation 85:150–157, 1992.
369. Brown BG, Gallery CA, Badger RS, et al: Incomplete lysis of thrombus in the moderate underlying atherosclerotic lesion during intracoronary infusion of streptokinase for acute myocardial infarction: quantitative angiographic observations. Circulation 73:653–661, 1986.
370. Satler LF, Pallas RS, Bond OB, et al: Assessment of residual coronary arterial stenosis after thrombolytic therapy during acute myocardial infarction. Am J Cardiol 59:1231–1233, 1987.
371. Ellis SG, Topol EJ, George BS, et al: Recurrent ischemia without warning—analysis of risk factors for in-hospital ischemic events following successful thrombolysis with intravenous tissue plasminogen activator. Circulation 80:1159–1165, 1989.
372. White CW: Recurrent ischemic events after successful thrombolysis in acute myocardial infarction: the Achilles' heel of thrombolytic therapy. Circulation 80:1482–1485, 1989.
373. Lower R: Tractus de Corde. Amsterdam: Elsevier, 1669.
374. Schaper W, Gorge G, Winkler B, Schaper J: The collateral circulation of the heart. Prog Cardiovasc Dis 31:57–77, 1988.
375. Winkler B, Sass S, Binz K, et al: Myocardial blood flow and myocardial infarction in rats, guinea pigs, and rabbits [abstract]. J Mol Cell Cardiol 16:48, 1984.
376. Schaper W: Experimental infarcts and the microcirculation. *In* Hearse DJ, Yellon DM (eds): Therapeutic Approaches to Myocardial Infarct Size Limitations. p. 79. New York: Raven, 1984.
377. Roesen R, Marsen A, Klaus W: Local myocardial perfusion and epicardial NADH-fluorescence after coronary artery ligation in the isolated guinea pig heart. Basic Res Cardiol 79:59–67, 1984.
378. Baroldi G, Mantero O, Scomazzoni G: The collaterals of the coronary arteries in normal and pathologic hearts. Circ Res 4:223–229, 1956.
379. Fulton WFM: Arterial anastomoses in the coronary circulation. II. Distribution, enumeration and measurement of coronary arterial anastomoses in health and disease. Scott Med J 8:466–474, 1963.
380. Fulton WF: The Coronary Arteries. Springfield, IL: Charles C Thomas, 1965.
381. Schaper W, Sharma HS, Quinkler W, et al: Molecular biologic concepts of coronary anastomoses. J Am Coll Cardiol 15:513–518, 1990.
382. Assessment of coronary artery disease. *In* Yang SS, Bentivoglio LG, Maranhao V, Goldberg H (eds): From Cardiac Catheterization Data to Hemodynamic Parameters. 3rd ed. p. 256. Philadelphia: FA Davis, 1988.
383. Levin DC: Pathways and functional significance of the coronary collateral circulation. Circulation 50:831, 1974.
384. Franklin D, McKnown D, McKnown M, et al: Development and regression of coronary collaterals induced by repeated, reversible ischemia in dogs [abstract]. Fed Proc 40:339, 1981.
385. Yamamoto H, Tomoike H, Shimokawa H, et al: Development of collateral function with repetitive coronary occlusion in a canine model reduces myocardial reactive hyperemia in the absence of significant coronary stenosis. Circ Res 55:623–632, 1984.
386. Harrison DG, Sellke FW, Quillen JE: Neurohumoral regulation of

coronary collateral vasomotor tone. Basic Res Cardiol 85(suppl l):21–129, 1990.

387. Bache RJ, Foreman B, Hautamaa PV: Response of canine coronary collateral vessels to ergonovine and alpha-adrenergic stimulation. Am J Physiol 261:H1019–H1025, 1991.
388. Takeshita A, Koiwaya Y, Nakamura M, et al: Immediate appearance of coronary collaterals during ergonovine-induced arterial spasm. Chest 82:319, 1982.
389. Rentrop KP, Cohen M, Blanke H, Phillips RA: Changes in collateral channel filling immediately after controlled coronary artery occlusion by angioplasty balloon in human subjects. J Am Coll Cardiol 5:587, 1985.
390. Meier B, Luethy P, Finci L, et al: Coronary wedge pressure in relation to spontaneously visible and recruitable collaterals Circulation 75:906–913, 1987.
391. Helfant RH, Vokonas PS, Gorlin R: Functional importance of the human coronary collateral circulation. N Engl J Med 284:1277–1281, 1971.
392. Gorlin R: Coronary collaterals. *In* Smith LH (ed): Coronary Artery Disease. Philadelphia: WB Saunders, 1976.
393. Sasayama S, Fujita M: Recent insights into coronary collateral circulation. Circulation 85:1197–1204, 1992.
394. Rentrop KP, Thorton JC, Feit F, Buskirk MV: Determinants and protective potential as assessed by an angioplasty model of coronary arterial collaterals. Am J Cardiol 61:677–684, 1988.
395. Hirai T, Fujita M, Nakajima H, et al: Importance of collateral circulation for prevention of left ventricular aneurysm formation in acute myocardial infarction. Circulation 79:791–796, 1989
396. Epstein SE: Influence of stenosis severity on coronary collateral development and importance of collaterals in maintaining left ventricular function during acute coronary occlusion. Am J Cardiol 61:866–868, 1988.
397. Topol EJ, Ellis SG: Coronary collaterals revisited: accessory pathway to myocardial preservation during infarction. Circulation 83:1084–1086, 1991.
398. Rentrop KP, Cohen M, Blanke H, Phillips RA: Changes in collateral channel filling immediately after controlled coronary occlusion by an angioplasty balloon in human subjects. J Am Coll Cardiol 5:587–592, 1985.
399. Schaper W: Residual Perfusion of Acutely Ischemic Heart Muscle. p. 345. Amsterdam: Elsevier Biomedical, 1979.

Coronary Vasospasm

400. Ginsburg R, Schroeder JS: Coronary spasm producing coronary thrombosis. N Engl J Med 309:648, 1983.
401. Oliva PB, Potts DE, Pluss RG: Coronary arterial spasm in Prinzmetal angina. N Engl J Med 288:745–751, 1973.
402. Maseri A, Chierchia S: Coronary artery spasm: demonstration, definition, diagnosis, and consequences. Prog Cardiovasc Dis 25:169–192, 1982.
403. Schroeder JS, Bolen JL, Quint RA, et al: Provocation of coronary spasm with ergonovine maleate. Am J Cardiol 40:487–491, 1977.
404. Heupler FA, Proudfit WL, Razavi M, et al: Ergonovine maleate provocative test for coronary arterial spasm. Am J Cardiol 41:631–640, 1978.
405. Curry RC, Pepine CJ, Sabom MB, et al: Effects of ergonovine in patients with and without coronary artery disease. Circulation 56:804–809, 1977.
406. Chahine RA, Raizner AE, Ishimori T, et al: The incidence and clinical implications of coronary artery spasm. Circulation 52:972–978, 1975.
407. Curry RC, Pepine CJ, Sabom MB, et al: Hemodynamic and myocardial metabolic effects of ergonovine in patients with chest pain. Circulation 58:648–654, 1978.
408. Rall TW: Oxytocin, prostaglandins, ergot alkaloids, and other drugs: tocolytic agents. *In* Gilman G, Goodman LS, Rall TW, Murad F (eds): The Pharmacological Basis of Therapeutics. pp. 936–940. New York: Macmillan, 1985.
409. Feldman RL, Curry RC, Pepine CJ, et al: Regional coronary hemodynamic effects of ergonovine in patients with and without variant angina. Circulation 62:149–159, 1980.
410. Cipriano PR, Guthaner DF, Orlick AE, et al: The effects of ergonovine maleate on coronary arterial size. Circulation 59:82–89, 1979.
411. Magder SA, Johnstone DE, Huckell VF, Adelman AG: Experience with ergonovine provocative testing for coronary arterial spasm. Chest 79:638–646, 1981.
412. Kodama K, Yamagishi M, Nanto S, et al: Comparison of coronary hemodynamic and cardiac metabolic alterations during coronary artery spasm associated with ST segment elevation or depression. Jpn Circ 49:422–431, 1985.
413. Whittle JL, Feldman RL, Pepine CJ, et al: Variability of electrocardiographic responses to repeated ergonovine provocation in variant angina patients with coronary artery spasm. Am Heart J 103:161–167, 1982.
414. Matsuda Y, Ogawa H, Moritani K, et al: Transient appearance of collaterals during vasospastic occlusion in patients without obstructive coronary atherosclerosis. Am Heart J 109:759–763, 1985.
415. Takeshita A, Koiwaya Y, Nakamura M, et al: Immediate appearance of coronary collaterals during ergonovine-induced arterial spasm. Chest 82:319–322, 1982.
416. Hom GA, Brent BN: Coronary artery vasospasm during treatment with intravenous nitroglycerin. Cathet Cardiovasc Diagn 11:423–426, 1985.
417. Kurnik PB, Spadaro JJ, Nordlicht SM, et al: Prolonged coronary vasoconstrictor effect of ergonovine maleate. Cathet Cardiovasc Diagn 10:353–361, 1984.
418. Mantyla R, Kanto J: Clinical pharmacokinetics of methylergometrine (methylergonovine). Int J Clin Pharmacol Ther Toxicol 19:386–391, 1981.
419. Harding MB, Leithe ME, Mark DB, et al: Ergonovine maleate testing during cardiac catheterization: a 10-year perspective in 3,447 patients without significant coronary artery disease or Prinzmetal's variant angina. J Am Coll Cardiol 20:107–111, 1992.
420. Bertrand ME, LaBlanche JM, Tilmant PY, et al: Frequency of provoked coronary arterial spasm in 1089 consecutive patients undergoing coronary arteriography. Circulation 65:1299–1308, 1982.
421. Ogasawara K, Aizawa T, Nishimura K, et al: Beta-thromboglobulin release within coronary circulation—a potential role of platelets in ergonovine-induced coronary vasospasm. Int J Cardiol 10:15–22, 1986.
422. Yui Y, Hattori R, Takatsu Y, Kawai C: Selective thromboxane A_2 synthetase inhibition in vasospastic angina pectoris. J Am Coll Cardiol 7:25–29, 1986.
423. Maleki M, Manley JC: Venospastic phenomena of saphenous vein bypass grafts: possible causes for unexplained postoperative recurrence of angina or early or late occlusion of vein bypass grafts. Br Heart J 62:57–60, 1989.
424. Hosio A, Kotake H, Mashiba H: Significance of coronary artery tone in patients with vasospastic angina. J Am Coll Cardiol 14:604–609, 1989.
425. Hill JA, Feldman RL, Pepine CJ, Conti CR: Regional coronary artery dilation response in variant angina. Am Heart J 104:226–233, 1982.
426. Kaski JC, Maseri A, Vejar M, et al: Spontaneous coronary artery spasm in variant angina is caused by a local hyperreactivity to a generalized constrictor stimulus. J Am Coll Cardiol 14:1456–1463, 1989.
427. Feldman RL, Pepine CJ, Whittle JL, et al: Coronary hemodynamic findings during spontaneous angina in patients with variant angina. Circulation 64:76–83, 1981.
428. Bentivoglio LG, Leo LR, Wolf NM, Meister SG: Frequency and importance of unprovoked coronary spasm in patients with angina pectoris undergoing percutaneous transluminal coronary angioplasty. Am J Cardiol 51:1067–1071, 1983.
429. Bott-Silverman C, Heupler FA, Yiannikas J: Variant angina: comparison of patients with and without fixed severe coronary artery disease. Am J Cardiol 54:1173–1175, 1984.
430. Mark DB, Califf RM, Morris KG, et al: Clinical characteristics and long-term survival of patients with variant angina. Circulation 69:880–888, 1984.
431. Egashira K, Kikuchi Y, Sagara T, et al: Long-term prognosis of vasospastic angina without significant atherosclerotic coronary artery disease. Jpn Heart J 28:841–849, 1987.
432. Nobuyoshi M, Tanaka M, Nosaka H, et al: Progression of coronary atherosclerosis: is coronary spasm related to progression? J Am Coll Cardiol 18:904–910, 1991.
433. Caralis DG, Deligonul U, Kern MJ, Cohen JD: Smoking is a risk factor for coronary spasm in young women. Circulation 85:905–909, 1992.

434. Suzuki Y, Tokunaga S, Ikeguchi S, et al: Induction of coronary artery spasm by intracoronary acetylcholine: comparison with intracoronary ergonovine. Am Heart J 124:39–47, 1992.
435. Wright CM, Engler R, Maisel A: Coronary thrombosis precipitated by hyperventilation-induced vasospasm. Am Heart J 116:867–869, 1988.
436. Ginsburg R, Bristow MR, Kantrowitz N, et al: Histamine provocation of clinical coronary artery spasm: implications concerning pathogenesis of variant angina pectoris. Am Heart J 102:819–822, 1981.

Spontaneous Coronary Artery Dissection

437. DeMaio S, Kinsella SH, Silverman ME: Clinical course and long-term prognosis of spontaneous coronary artery dissection. Am J Cardiol 64:471–474, 1989.
438. Bulkley BH, Roberts WC: Dissecting aneurysm (hematoma) limited to coronary artery. Am J Med 55:747–756, 1973.
439. Mathieu D, Larde D, Vasile N: Primary dissecting aneurysms of the coronary arteries: case report and literature review. Cardiovasc Intervent Radiol 7:71–74, 1984.
440. Claudon DG, Claudon DB, Edwards JE: Primary dissecting aneurysm of coronary artery. Circulation 45:259–266, 1972.
441. Brody GL, Burton JF, Zawadzki ES, French AJ: Dissecting aneurysms of the coronary artery. N Engl J Med 273:1–5, 1965.
442. Yeoh J, Choo H, Soo C, et al: Spontaneous coronary artery dissection in a young man with anterior myocardial infarction. Cathet Cardiovasc Diagn 24:186–188, 1991.
443. Heilbrunn A, Zimmerman JM: Coronary artery dissection: a complication of cannulation. J Thorac Cardiovasc Surg 49:767, 1965.
444. Roy P, Finci L, Bopp P, Meier B: Emergency balloon angioplasty and digital subtraction angiography in the management of an acute iatrogenic occlusive dissection of a saphenous vein graft. Cathet Cardiovasc Diagn 16:176–179, 1989.
445. Thayer JO, Healy RW, Maggs PR: Spontaneous coronary artery dissection. Ann Thorac Surg 44:97–102, 1987.
446. Orbe LC, Gallego FG, Sobrino N, et al: Acute myocardial infarction after blunt chest trauma in young people. Cathet Cardiovasc Diagn 24:182–185, 1991.
446a. Lee FH, Yeung AC, Fowler MB, Fitzgerald PJ: Spontaneous postpartum dissection. Circulation 99:721, 1999.
447. Robinowitz M, Virmani R, McAllister H: Spontaneous coronary artery dissection and eosinophilic inflammation: a cause and effect relationship? Am J Med 72:923–927, 1982.
448. Nishikawa H, Nakanishi S, Nishiyama S, et al: Primary coronary artery dissection observed at coronary angiography. Am J Cardiol 61:645–648, 1988.
449. Alvarez J, Deal CW: Spontaneous dissection of the left main coronary artery: case report and review of the literature. Aust N Z J Med 21:891–892, 1991.
449a. Himbert D, Makowski S, Laperche T, et al: Left main coronary spontaneous dissection: progressive angiographic healing without coronary surgery. Am Heart J 22:747–756, 1991.
450. Behnam R, Tillinghast S: Thrombolytic therapy in spontaneous coronary artery dissection. Clin Cardiol 14:611–614, 1991.
450a. Vale PR, Baron DW: Coronary stenting for spontaneous coronary dissection: a case report and review of the literature. Cathet Cardiovasc Diagn 45:280–286, 1998.

Myocardial Infarction With Angiographically Normal Coronary Arteries

451. Betriu A, Pare JC, Sanz GA, et al: Myocardial infarction with normal coronary arteries: a prospective clinical-angiographic study. Am J Cardiol 48:28–32, 1981.
452. Thompson SI, Vieweg WVR, Alpert JS, Hagan AD: Incidence and age distribution of patients with myocardial infarction and normal coronary arteriograms. Cathet Cardiovasc Diagn 3:1–9, 1977.
453. Cipriano PR, Koch FH, Rosenthal SJ, et al: Myocardial infarction in patients with coronary artery spasm demonstrated by angiography. Am Heart J 105:542–547, 1983.
454. Gersh BJ, Chesebro JH, Bove AA: Myocardial infarction with angiographically "normal" coronary arteries: is this rapid progression of early coronary artery disease? Chest 84:654–656, 1984.
455. Legrand V, Deliege M, Henrard L, et al: Patients with myocardial infarction and normal coronary arteriogram. Chest 82:678–685, 1982.
456. Lindsay J, Pichard A: Acute myocardial infarction with normal coronary arteries. Am J Cardiol 54:902–904, 1984.
457. Rosenblatt A, Selzer A: The nature and clinical features of myocardial infarction with normal coronary arteriogram. Circulation 55:578–580, 1977.
458. Ciraulo DA, Bresnahan GF, Frankel PS, et al: Transmural myocardial infarction with normal coronary angiograms and with single vessel coronary obstruction. Chest 83:196–202, 1983.
459. Glover MU, Kuber MT, Warren SE, Vieweg WVR: Myocardial infarction before age 36: risk factor and arteriographic analysis. Am J Cardiol 49:1600–1603, 1982.
460. Smith HWB, Liberman HA, Brody SL, et al: Acute myocardial infarction temporally related to cocaine use: clinical, angiographic and pathophysiologic observations. Ann Intern Med 107:13–18, 1987.
460a. Ottervanger JP, Wilson JH, Stricker BH: Drug-induced chest pain and myocardial infarction. Reports to a national centre and review of the literature. Eur J Clin Pharmacol 53:105–110, 1997.

Microcirculatory Angina

461. Likoff W, Segal BL, Kasparian H: Paradox of normal selective coronary arteriograms in patients considered to have unmistakable coronary heart disease. N Engl J Med 276:1063, 1967.
462. Kemp HG: Left ventricular function in patients with the anginal syndrome and normal coronary arteriograms. Am J Cardiol 32:375, 1973.
463. Cannon RO, Schenke WH, Leon MB, et al: Limited coronary flow reserve after dipyridamole in patients with ergonovine-induced coronary vasoconstriction. Circulation 75:163, 1987.
464. Cannon RO, Bonow RO, Bacharach SL, et al: Left ventricular dysfunction in patients with angina pectoris, normal epicardial coronary arteries, and abnormal vasodilator reserve. Circulation 7:218, 1985.
464a. Hasdai D, Holmes DR Jr, Higano ST, et al: Prevalence of coronary blood flow reserve abnormalities among patients with nonobstructive coronary artery disease and chest pain. Mayo Clin Proc 73:1133–1140, 1998.
465. Cannon RO: Microvascular angina: pathophysiology, diagnostic techniques and interventions. *In* Braunwald E (ed): Heart Disease: A Textbook of Cardiovascular Medicine. 3rd ed. Update 15. pp. 343–350. New York: WB Saunders, 1991.
466. Geltman EM, Henes CG, Senneff MJ, et al: Increased myocardial perfusion at rest and diminished perfusion reserve in patients with angina and angiographically normal coronary arteries. J Am Coll Cardiol 16:586–595, 1990.
467. Cannon RO, Epstein SE: "Microvascular angina" as a cause of chest pain with angiographically normal coronary arteries. Am J Cardiol 61:1338, 1988.
468. Cannon RO 3rd, Watson RM, Rosing DR, et al: Angina caused by reduced vasodilator reserve of the small coronary arteries. J Am Coll Cardiol 1:1359–1373, 1983.
469. Opherk D, Zebe H, Weihe E, et al: Reduced coronary dilatory capacity and ultrastructural changes of the myocardium in patients with angina pectoris but normal coronary arteriograms. Circulation 63:817 ,1981.
469a. Cannon RO III: Cardiovascular syndrome X: is it real? Contemp Intern Med 10:7–16, 1998.
470. Marcus ML, Mueller TM, Gascho JA, Kerber KE: Effects of cardiac hypertrophy secondary to hypertension on the coronary circulation. Am J Cardiol 44:747–753, 1979.
471. Opherk D, Schwartz F, Mall G, et al: Coronary dilatory capacity in idiopathic dilated cardiomyopathy: analysis of 16 patients. Am J Cardiol 51:1657–1662, 1983.
472. Brush JE, Cannon RO, Schenke WH, et al: Angina due to coronary microvascular disease in hypertensive patients without left ventricular hypertrophy. N Engl J Med 319:1302–1307, 1988.
473. Ryan TJ, Treasure CB, Yeung AC, et al: Impaired endothelium-dependent dilation of the coronary microvasculature in patients with atherosclerosis [abstract]. Circulation 84:II-624, 1991.
474. Selke FW, Armstrong ML, Harrison DG: Endothelium-dependent vascular relaxation is abnormal in the coronary microcirculation of atherosclerotic primates. Circulation 81:1586, 1990.
475. Wilson RF, Christensen BV, Zimmer S, Laxson D: The effects of adenosine on human coronary circulation. Circulation 82:1595–1606, 1990.

476. Sax FL, Cannon RO, Hanson C, Epstein SE: Impaired forearm vasodilator reserve in patients with microvascular angina. N Engl J Med 317:1366–1370, 1987.
477. Egashira K, Inou T, Hirooka Y, et al: Evidence of impaired endothelium dependent coronary vasodilation in patients with angina pectoris and normal coronary angiograms. N Engl J Med 328:1659–1664, 1993.
478. Fish RP, Nabel EG, Selwyn AP, et al: Responses of coronary arteries of cardiac transplant patients to acetylcholine. J Clin Invest 81:21–31, 1988.
478a. Davis SF, Yeung AC, Meredith IT, et al: Early endothelial dysfunction predicts the development of transplant coronary artery disease at 1 year posttransplant. Circulation 93:457–462, 1996.
479. Vogt M, Rabenau O, Motz W, Strauer BE: Evidence of endothelial dysfunction in patients with angina pectoris and angiographically normal coronary arteries [abstract]. Circulation 80:II-436, 1989.

RADIATION-INDUCED CORONARY ARTERY DISEASE

480. McReynolds RA, Gold GL, Roberts WC: Coronary heart disease after mediastinal irradiation for Hodgkin's disease. Am J Med 60:39–45, 1976.
481. Steward JR, Cohn KE, Fajardo LF, et al: Radiation-induced heart disease. Radiology 89:302–310, 1967.
482. Pohjola-Sintonen S, Totterman KJ, Almo M, Siltanen P: Late cardiac effects of mediastinal radiotherapy in patients with Hodgkin's disease. Cancer 60:31–37, 1987.
483. Brosius FC, Waller BF, Roberts WC: Radiation heart disease: analysis of 16 young (aged 15–33 years) necropsy patients who received over 3,500 rads to the heart. Am J Med 70:519–530, 1981.
484. Tracy GP, Brown DE, Johnson LW, Gottlieb AJ: Radiation-induced coronary artery disease. JAMA 228:1660–1662, 1974.
485. Prentice RTW: Myocardial infarction following radiation. Lancet 2:388, 1965.
486. Stewart RJ, Cohn K, Hancock EW, et al: Radiation induced heart disease. Radiology 89:302–310, 1967.
487. Carmel RJ, Kaplan HS: Mantle irradiation in Hodgkin's disease: an analysis of technique, tumor eradication and complications. Cancer 37:2813–2825, 1976.

TRANSPLANT-RELATED ARTERIOPATHY

488. Oguma S, Okazaki H, Jimbo M, et al: Vascular rejection and arteriosclerosis. Transplant Proc 19:63–70, 1987.
489. Lurie KG, Billingham ME, Jamieson SW, et al: Pathogenesis and prevention of graft arteriosclerosis in an experimental heart transplant model. Transplantation 31:41–47, 1981.
490. Pucci AM, Forbes RDC, Billingham ME: Pathologic features in long-term cardiac allografts. J Heart Transplant 9:339–345, 1990.
491. Johnson DE, Gao SZ, Schroeder JS, et al: The spectrum of coronary artery pathologic findings in heart cardiac allografts. J Heart Transplant 8:349–359, 1989.
492. Libby P, Salomon RN, Payne DD, et al: Functions of vascular wall cells related to development of transplantation-associated coronary arteriosclerosis. Transplant Proc 21:3677–3684, 1989.
492a. Kapadia SR, Nissen SE, Tuzcu EM: Impact of intravascular ultrasound in understanding transplant coronary artery disease. Curr Opin Cardiol 14:140–150, 1999.
492b. Kapadia SR, Nissen SE, Ziada KM, et al: Development of transplantation vasculopathy and progression of donor-transmitted atherosclerosis: comparison by serial intravascular ultrasound imaging. Circulation 98:2672–2678, 1998.
492c. Liang DH, Gao SZ, Botas J, et al: Prediction of angiographic disease by intracoronary ultrasonographic findings in heart transplant recipients. J Heart Lung Transplant 15:980–987, 1996.
492d. Gao HZ, Hunt SA, Alderman EL, et al: Relation of donor age and preexisting coronary artery disease on angiography and intracoronary ultrasound to later development of accelerated allograft coronary artery disease. J Am Coll Cardiol 29:623–629, 1997.
493. Uretsky BF, Murali S, Reddy PS, et al: Development of coronary artery disease in cardiac transplant patients. Circulation 76:827–834, 1987.
494. Gao SZ, Schroeder JS, Alderman EL, et al: Prevalence of accelerated coronary artery disease in heart transplant survivors. Circulation 80(suppl III):III-100–III-105, 1989.
495. Gao SZ, Alderman EL, Schroeder JS, et al: Accelerated coronary vascular disease in the heart transplant patient: coronary arteriographic findings. J Am Coll Cardiol 12:334–340, 1988.
496. Olivari MT, Homans DC, Wilson RF, et al: Coronary artery disease in cardiac transplant patients receiving triple-drug immunosuppressive therapy. Circulation 80(suppl III):III-111–III-115, 1989.
497. Gao SZ, Alderman EL, Schroeder JS, et al: Progressive coronary luminal narrowing after cardiac transplantation. Circulation 82(suppl IV):IV-269–IV-275, 1990.
498. Nitkin RS, Hunt SA, Schroeder JS: Accelerated atherosclerosis in a cardiac transplant patient. J Am Coll Cardiol 6:243–245, 1985.
499. Mulvagh SL, Thornton B, Frazier OH, et al: The older cardiac transplant donor: relation to graft function and recipient survival longer than 6 years. Circulation 80(suppl III):III-126–III-132, 1989.
500. O'Neill B, Pflugfelder PW, Singh NR, et al: Frequency of angiographic detection and quantitative assessment of coronary arterial disease one and three years after cardiac transplantation. Am J Cardiol 63:1221–1226, 1989.
501. Sharples LD, Mullin PA, Cary NRB, et al: A method of analyzing the onset and progression of coronary occlusive disease after transplantation and its effect on patient survival. Transplantation 12:381–387, 1993.
502. McGinn AL, Christensen BV, Meyer S, et al: Early impairment of nitroglycerine-induced coronary dilation after human cardiac transplantation [abstract]. J Am Coll Cardiol 17:309A, 1991.
503. Goldenberg IF, Levine TB: Coronary artery spasm in a denervated orthotopic transplanted human heart. Cathet Cardiovasc Diagn 12:44–47, 1986.

VASCULITIS

504. Lie JT: Coronary vasculitis: a review in the current scheme of classification of vasculitis. Arch Pathol Lab Med 111:224–233, 1987.
505. Kawai S, Fukuda Y, Okada R: Atherosclerosis of the coronary arteries in collagen disease and allied disorders, with special reference to vasculitis as a preceding lesion of coronary atherosclerosis. Jpn Circ J 46:1208–1221, 1982.
506. Tanaka M, Abe T, Takeuchi E, et al: Revascularization for coronary ostial stenosis in Takayasu's disease with calcified aorta. Ann Thorac Surg 53:894–895, 1992.
507. Ishikawa K: Diagnostic approach and proposed criteria for the clinical diagnosis of Takayasu's arteriopathy. J Am Coll Cardiol 12:964–972, 1988.
508. Cassling RS, Lortz JB, Olson DR, et al: Fatal vasculitis (periarteritis nodosa) of the coronary arteries: angiographic ambiguities and absence of aneurysms at autopsy. J Am Coll Cardiol 6:707–714, 1985.
509. Rallings P, Exner T, Abraham R: Coronary artery vasculitis and myocardial infarction associated with antiphospholipid antibodies in a pregnant woman. Aust N Z J Med 19:347–350, 1989.
510. Wilson VE, Eck SL, Bates ER: Evaluation and treatment of acute myocardial infarction complicating systemic lupus erythematosus. Chest 101:420–424, 1992.
511. Bulkley BH, Roberts WC: The heart in systemic lupus erythematosus and changes induced in it by corticosteroid therapy. Am J Med 58:243–263, 1975.
512. Haider YS, Roberts WC: Coronary arterial disease in systemic lupus erythematosus: quantification of degrees of narrowing in 22 necropsy patients (21 women) aged 16–37. Am J Med 70:775–778, 1981.
513. Vasquez JJ, San Martin P, Barbado FJ, et al: Angiographic findings in systemic vasculitis. Angiology 11:773–779, 1981.
514. Diaz-Rivera RS, Miller AJ: Periarteritis nodosa: a clinicopathological analysis of seven cases. Ann Intern Med 24:420–443, 1946.
515. Strauer BE: The significance of coronary reserve in clinical heart disease. J Am Coll Cardiol 15:775–783, 1990.
516. Nitenberg A, Foult JM, Kahan A, et al: Reduced coronary flow and resistance reserve in primary scleroderma myocardial disease. Am Heart J 112:309–315, 1986.
517. Suzuki A, Kamiya T, Ono Y, et al: Clinical significance of morphologic classification of coronary arterial segmental stenosis due to Kawasaki disease. Am J Cardiol 71:1169–1173, 1993.
518. Kato H, Ichinose E, Yoshioka F, et al: Fate of coronary aneurysms in Kawasaki disease: serial coronary angiography and long-term follow-up study. Am J Cardiol 49:1758–1766, 1982.
519. Takahashi M, Mason W, Lewis AB: Regression of coronary aneurysms in patients with Kawasaki syndrome. Circulation 75:387–394, 1987.

520. Suzuki A, Kamiya T, Kuwahara N, et al: Coronary arterial lesions of Kawasaki disease: cardiac catheterization findings of 1100 cases. Pediatr Cardiol 7:3–9, 1986.
521. Kato H, Inoue O, Kawasaki T, et al: Adult coronary artery disease probably due to childhood Kawasaki disease. Lancet 340:1127–1129, 1992.
522. Kuribayashi S, Ootaki M, Tsuji M, et al: Coronary angiographic abnormalities in mucocutaneous lymph node syndrome: acute findings and long-term follow-up. Radiology 172:629–633, 1989.

CORONARY ANEURYSM

523. Tunick PA, Slater J, Kronzon I, Glassman E: Discrete atherosclerotic coronary artery aneurysms: a study of 20 patients. J Am Coll Cardiol 15:279–282, 1990.
524. Myler RK, Schechtmann NS, Rosenblum J, et al: Multiple coronary artery aneurysms in an adult associated with extensive thrombus formation resulting in acute myocardial infarction: successful treatment with intracoronary urokinase, intravenous heparin, and oral anticoagulation. Cathet Cardiovasc Diagn 24:51–54, 1991.
525. Rath S, Har-Zahav Y, Battler A, et al: Fate of nonobstructive aneurysmatic coronary artery disease: angiographic and clinical follow-up report. Am Heart J 109:785–791, 1985.
525a. Koh HK, Yoo DH, Yoo TS, et al: Coexistence of coronary aneurysm and total occlusion of the coronary arteries in systemic lupus erythematosus. Clin Exp Rheumatol 16:739–742, 1998.
526. Lipton MJ, Pfeifer JF, Lopes MG, Hultgren HN: Aneurysms of the coronary arteries in the adult: clinical and angiographic features. Radiology 117:11–18, 1975.
527. Eriksen UH, Aunsholt NA, Nielsen TT: Enormous right coronary arterial aneurysm in a patient with type IV Ehlers-Danlos syndrome. Int J Cardiol 35:259–261, 1992.
528. Cohen AJ, Banks A, Cambier P, Edwards FH: Post-atherectomy coronary artery aneurysm. Ann Thorac Surg 54:1216–1218, 1992.
529. Nakamura F, Kvasnicka J, Decoster HL, Geschwind HJ: Aneurysmal formation after successful pulsed laser coronary angioplasty. Cathet Cardiovasc Diagn 27:125–129, 1992.
530. Rab ST, King SB III, Roubin GS, et al: Coronary aneurysms after stent placement: a suggestion of altered vessel wall healing in the presence of anti-inflammatory agents. J Am Coll Cardiol 18:1524–1528, 1991.
531. deHaan HPJ, Huysmans HA, Weeda HWH, et al: Anastomotic pseudoaneurysm after aorto-coronary bypass grafting. Thorac Cardiovasc Surg 33:55–56, 1985.
532. Saito S, Arai H, Kim K, Aoki N: Pseudoaneurysm of coronary artery following rupture of coronary artery during coronary angioplasty. Cathet Cardiovasc Diagn 26:304–307, 1992.

EMBOLIZATION

533. Walley VM, Giannoccaro P, Beanlands DS, Keon WJ: Death at cardiac catheterization: coronary artery embolization of calcium debris from Ionescu-Shiley bioprosthesis. Cathet Cardiovasc Diagn 21:92–94, 1990.
534. Johnson D, Gonzalez-Lavin L: Myocardial infarction secondary to calcific embolization: an unusual complication of bioprosthetic valve degeneration. Ann Thorac Surg 42:102–103, 1986.

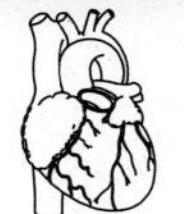

CHAPTER 31

ECHOCARDIOGRAPHY*

Francis T. Thandroyen and Eddy Barasch

REGIONAL WALL MOTION ABNORMALITIES
DETECTION OF ACUTE MYOCARDIAL ISCHEMIA
DETECTION OF ACUTE MYOCARDIAL INFARCTION
PROGNOSTIC INFORMATION IN ACUTE MYOCARDIAL INFARCTION
DETECTION OF COMPLICATIONS OF ACUTE MYOCARDIAL INFARCTION
Pericardial Effusion
Ventricular Aneurysm
Infarct Expansion
Mural Thrombus
Papillary Muscle Rupture Producing Mitral Regurgitation
Cardiac Rupture
Ventricular Septal Defect
Ventricular Pseudoaneurysm
DETECTION OF VIABLE MYOCARDIUM ON REVASCULARIZATION AFTER ACUTE MYOCARDIAL INFARCTION
INFARCT-RELATED ARTERY PATENCY AND DOBUTAMINE STRESS ECHOCARDIOGRAPHY
STRESS ECHOCARDIOGRAPHY FOR DETECTION OF ACUTE MYOCARDIAL ISCHEMIA
Exercise Stress
Pharmacologic Stress
INTRAOPERATIVE ECHOCARDIOGRAPHY FOR DETECTION OF ACUTE MYOCARDIAL ISCHEMIA OR INFARCTION
IDENTIFICATION OF CORONARY ARTERY STENOSIS
INTRAVASCULAR IMAGING OF CORONARY ARTERIES

The use of echocardiography in the diagnosis of coronary artery disease (CAD) is based on the concept that acute myocardial ischemia or infarction (MI) produces impairment in regional left ventricular (LV) mechanical function that can be detected with the use of echocardiography. Reduction in coronary blood flow secondary to intracoronary thrombus produces acute regional myocardial ischemia, which may progress to acute MI if the obstruction is not relieved. Experimental evidence indicates that the fall in adenosine triphosphate (ATP) content in ischemic muscle decreases the transsarcolemmal inward calcium current, whereas the accumulation of hydrogen ions in ischemic muscle results in ionic competition with calcium for binding sites on troponin C, thereby impairing actin-myosin coupling. The initial clinical manifestation of acute myocardial ischemia therefore is a decline in LV pressure development, characterized echocardiographically as a regional wall motion abnormality. The reduction in ATP and the accumulation of hydrogen ions in ischemic heart muscle also inhibit calcium uptake by the sarcoplasmic reticulum, thereby impairing ventricular relaxation, which manifests clinically as an increase in the LV end-diastolic pressure.

REGIONAL WALL MOTION ABNORMALITIES

Regional wall motion abnormalities are characterized by abnormal endocardial motion, the failure of ischemic muscle to thicken during systolic contraction, or even segmental bulging during systole.[1–4] The absence of wall thickening during systole is more suggestive of ischemia than are endocardial wall motion alterations,[5–8] because the latter alteration may be affected by cardiac rotation and translation during contraction, cardiac motion during respiration, and changes in ventricular preload or afterload. The American Association of Echocardiography has recommended standardization of the various wall segments of the left ventricle.[8] The relationship between the various wall segments of the left ventricle and the coronary artery circulation is illustrated in Figure 31–1. A revised grading system classifies formations as grades 1 to 5, with normal represented by 1; hypokinesis, 2; akinesis, 3; dyskinesis, 4; and aneurysm, 5. This system is used to characterize wall motion in each segment. The composite score divided by the number of segments provides a semiquantitative evaluation of wall motion abnormalities. The sensitivity of echocardiography in the detection of alterations in regional wall motion is dependent on two factors: a reduction in resting coronary blood flow of at least 50 percent[9, 10] and the involvement of transmural myocardial ischemia or MI in at least 20 percent of the LV wall.[6, 11] Regional wall motion abnormalities are not diagnostic of acute myocardial ischemia because they also occur with chronic myocardial ischemia or cardiomyopathies. Alterations in regional wall motion must be evaluated in the context of the clinical setting—specifically, their relationship to chest pain and electrocardiographic (ECG) alterations in ST-T wave segments, the development of Q waves, or both. In one study, the addition of measured cardiac troponin T levels to the echocardiographic examination of patients presenting with chest pain gave a positive predictive value of 84 percent and a negative predictive value of 90 percent for adverse cardiac events at 1-year follow-up.[12]

*Current principles applicable to and methods used in echocardiography are described in some detail in Chapters 4 and 20. These details are not repeated here, but the interested reader is referred to those discussions.

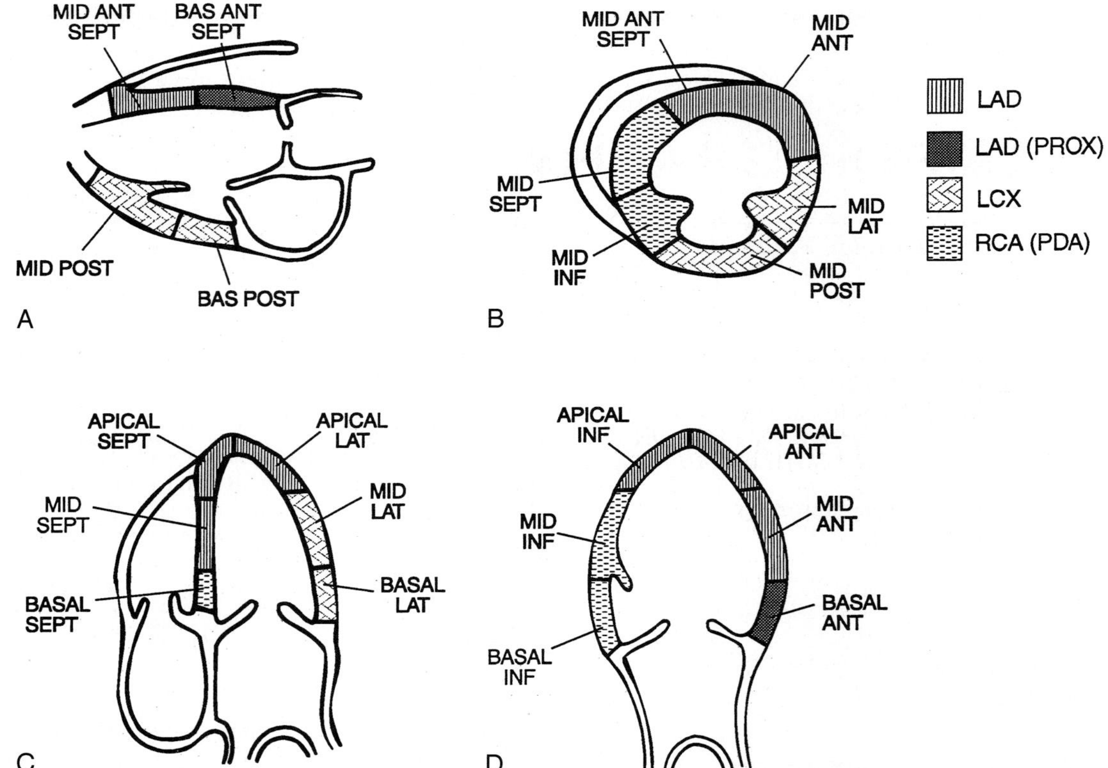

FIGURE 31–1 Transthoracic two-dimensional imaging of the heart illustrates parasternal long-axis view **(A),** parasternal short-axis view **(B),** apical four-chamber view **(C),** and apical two-chamber view **(D).** The left ventricle is divided into multiple segments, thereby allowing visual evaluation of regional wall motion. The relationship between the various wall segments of the left ventricle and the normal coronary artery circulation is depicted. ANT, anterior; BAS, basal; INF, inferior; LAD, left anterior descending coronary artery; LAT, lateral; LCX, left circumflex artery; MID, middle; POST, posterior; PROX, proximal; RCA (PDA), right coronary artery (posterior descending artery); SEPT, septa.

DETECTION OF ACUTE MYOCARDIAL ISCHEMIA

The use of two-dimensional echocardiography during an episode of acute chest pain that is typical of angina may demonstrate regional wall motion abnormalities. In contrast, the use of two-dimensional echocardiography during the pain-free period will reveal normal regional wall motion in the previously abnormal muscle segment, unless the duration of ischemic insult was sufficiently long to induce myocardial stunning, thereby characterizing the reversible nature of the wall motion abnormality. The transient nature of the wall motion abnormality differentiates a brief episode of acute myocardial ischemia from acute MI. In patients who present with atypical chest pain, echocardiographic detection of wall motion abnormalities is especially helpful because it provides a diagnosis of acute myocardial ischemia. In patients with unstable angina who are responding to medical treatment, transient regional wall motion abnormalities are associated with a favorable prognosis.[4] In contrast, the persistence or progression of regional wall motion abnormalities in patients with unstable angina often correlates with an adverse clinical prognosis at 3 months after hospital discharge.[4] In patients with LV dysfunction associated with normal or dilated left ventricles,[13] regional wall motion abnormalities are highly sensitive in the detection of significant CAD. In one study, the sensitivity, specificity, and predictive values of regional wall motion abnormalities in the detection of significant CAD in patients with LV dysfunction and normal-sized ventricles were 95, 100, and 95 percent, respectively.[13]

DETECTION OF ACUTE MYOCARDIAL INFARCTION

In patients who present to the emergency department with acute, prolonged chest pain, two-dimensional echocardiography is highly sensitive and more efficacious than electrocardiography for the initial diagnosis of acute myocardial ischemia or MI.[14] Validation studies with ^{201}TP scintigraphy, pyrophosphate (^{99m}Tc-PYP) scintigraphy, serum creatine kinase–MB levels, and coronary arteriography demonstrate that two-dimensional echocardiography accurately detects and identifies the anatomic location of MI.[3, 15–17] The location of regional wall motion abnormalities correlates with the distribution of the occluded coronary artery, especially if the obstruction involves left anterior descending or posterior descending coronary arteries.[18] Two-dimensional echocardiography has been used to quantify MI size; in animals, a good correlation was found with infarct size through the use of ^{99m}Tc stannous pyrophosphate (^{99m}Tc-PPI).[3] However, in humans, there are some limitations resulting from inadequate sensitivity to differentiate old from new infarction and overestimation of anatomic infarct size[16] due to quantification of infarcted and ischemic myocardium and the adjacent border zone, which may have normal perfusion but impaired contractile function. Two-dimensional echocardiography can be used to characterize segmental ventricular function of the uninvolved myocardium. With acute MI, the uninvolved myocardium shows a compensatory hyperdynamic contractile response, the absence of which indicates multivessel disease and an increased risk for the development of angina pectoris, acute MI, and death.[19] Two-dimensional echocardiography is less sensitive (60 to 75 percent) in the detection of nontransmural MI, presumably because the extent of transmural muscle loss is less than 20 percent and the preservation of contractility of subepicardial myocardial layers can mask subendocardial dysfunction.[20]

Two-dimensional echocardiography may also be used to detect right ventricular (RV) MI, which may manifest as abnormal wall motion and RV enlargement.[21–24] None of these alterations are specific. A prerequisite for the diagnosis of RV MI is the presence of an inferior wall MI. RV MI is an important diagnosis because it represents a potentially reversible cause of cardiogenic shock, the clinical picture may simulate that in patients with cardiac tamponade, and the therapeutic strategy is different from that for LV MI.

Prognostic Information in Acute Myocardial Infarction

Two-dimensional echocardiography can be used to detect patients with acute MI who are at high risk for short-term complications in the hospital and for long-term complications after discharge from the hospital.[25–28] Patients with extensive regional wall motion abnormalities are especially prone to develop congestive heart failure (CHF), hypotension, and sudden death. Horowitz and Morganroth[25] found that echocardiography had a sensitivity of 83 percent and a specificity of 85 percent in the detection of patients with in-hospital complications. In contrast, the Killip classification was found to be relatively insensitive in the detection of in-hospital complications during MI.[26, 27] Nishimura and colleagues[27] found that predischarge echocardiography showing extensive wall motion abnormalities predicted a higher incidence of long-term out-of-hospital complications. In addition, two-dimensional echocardiography allows an estimation of both RV and LV ejection fractions and, therefore, global RV and LV function, which is of prognostic importance in patients with MI. Dobutamine stress echocardiography has been successfully used for risk stratification of patients after an acute MI.[29–31] In addition, contrast echocardiography performed with the intracoronary or intravenous administration of a myocardial contrast agent can differentiate between vessel recanalization and myocardial reperfusion.[32–34]

Detection of Complications of Acute Myocardial Infarction

LV pump failure usually accounts for hemodynamic deterioration. However, in a small number of patients, the cause may be a complication of MI, such as rupture of the ventricular septum, free wall, or a papillary muscle; pericardial effusion; LV pseudoaneurysm; or the development of a ventricular aneurysm. These complications of MI should be actively sought in the patient with hypotension, tachycardia, a new systolic murmur, CHF, or a systemic embolus. Two-dimensional echocardiography, pulsed-wave, and color-flow Doppler imaging provide a comprehensive assessment of anatomic and hemodynamic status at the bedside and therefore are very useful in patients with hemodynamic deterioration.

Pericardial Effusion

Pericardial effusion may result from pericarditis, rupture of a pseudoaneurysm, or heparin therapy, especially in the patient with pericarditis. Two-dimensional echocardiography (Fig. 31–2) and M-mode echocardiography (Fig. 31–3) demonstrate pericardial effusion as an echo-free space located anteriorly or posteriorly to the heart. In addition to therapeutic implications, the presence of pericardial effusion has been shown to have prognostic value. In patients undergoing primary percutaneous transluminal coronary angioplasty (PTCA) for the first Q wave acute MI, the finding of pericardial effusion and a pericardial rub increases by sixfold the risk of death compared with patients without pericardial effusion (19 versus 3 percent; P = .02).[35] The presence of right atrial (RA) diastolic collapse and RV diastolic collapse (see Figs. 31–2 and 31–3) provides early evidence of cardiac tamponade. Pulsed-wave Doppler interrogation of transmitral and transtricuspid diastolic flow profiles may provide identification of cardiac tamponade. Specifically, the evidence consists of an increase in the transtricuspid early filling wave and a de-

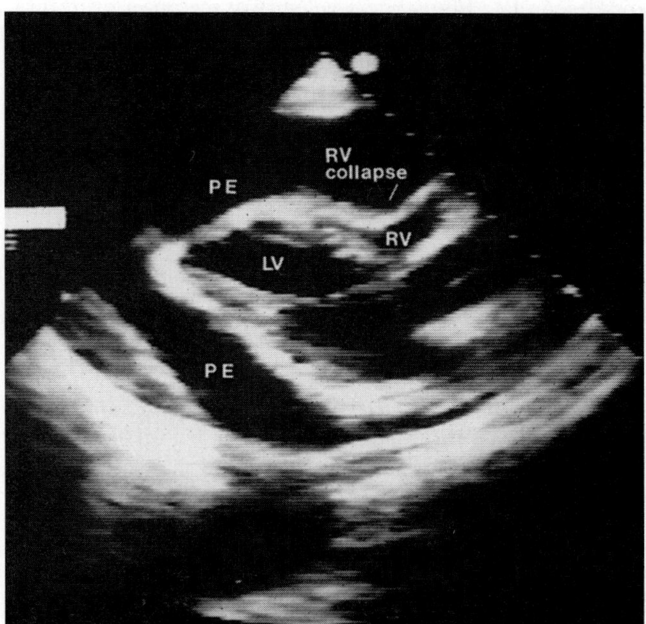

Figure 31–2 Transthoracic parasternal long-axis view of the heart illustrates large pericardial effusion (PE) located anterior and posterior to the left ventricle (LV). In addition, there is right ventricular (RV) collapse.

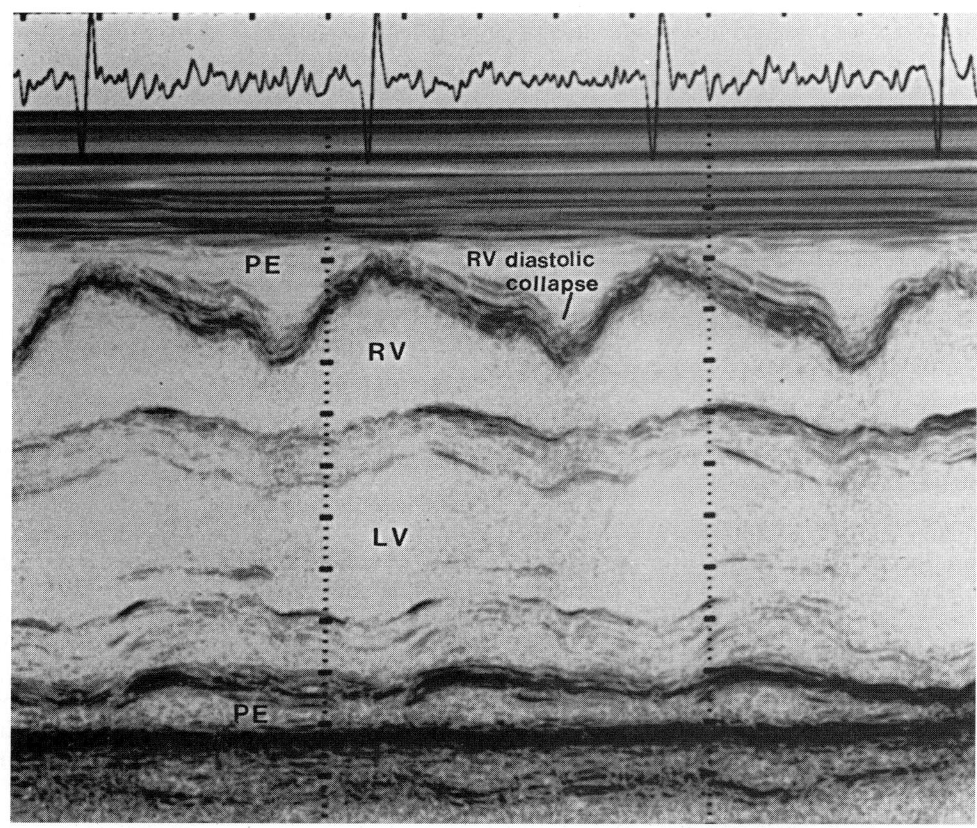

FIGURE 31–3 Transthoracic M-mode imaging of the heart illustrates pericardial effusion (PE) anterior to the right ventricle (RV) and posterior to the left ventricle (LV). In addition, there is right ventricular (RV) diastolic collapse.

crease in late filling wave velocity at the onset of inspiration and reversal of these changes during expiration and of a decrease in the transmitral early filling wave and an increase in late filling wave velocity at the onset of inspiration and reversal of these changes during expiration.[28]

Ventricular Aneurysm

A true ventricular aneurysm develops in approximately 20 to 40 percent of patients with acute MI,[36–38] and it is often located at the cardiac apex and the anterolateral wall (see Fig. 4–17). A true ventricular aneurysm is diagnosed echocardiographically when there is an alteration in the LV geometry. The characteristic findings are the presence of a wide neck and a thin wall that fails to thicken during systolic contraction, producing the appearance of a "bulge" during systole and diastole.[36, 39] In contrast to pseudoaneurysm, true aneurysms do not have the propensity to rupture due to an abundance of fibrotic tissue in the wall of the aneurysm. Doppler echocardiography can be used to detect a low-velocity flow profile with "swirling" motion in the aneurysm. Two-dimensional echocardiography has a sensitivity of 93 percent and a specificity of 94 percent in the detection of LV aneurysm. Serial echocardiography after acute MI demonstrates that aneurysm formation may occur within 5 days of the onset of infarction; early aneurysm formation is associated with high mortality rates (80 percent) within 1 year.[37] The usual time course of aneurysm formation is within 3 months of the onset of MI. LV aneurysm development may be complicated by CHF, ventricular arrhythmias, and thrombus formation. The rupture of a true aneurysm is highly unlikely due to the increased amount of fibrotic tissue in its walls. Two-dimensional echocardiography has been used to evaluate the efficacy of aneurysmectomy in patients with ventricular aneurysm. Ryan and colleagues[38] found that a fractional shortening of more than 17 percent in the uninvolved myocardium (measured at the base of the heart) was associated with improved surgical outcome, whereas patients with a fractional shortening of less than 17 percent were without subsequent clinical or surgical improvement. The finding of an elevated C-reactive protein level (>20 mg/dl) was reported to have a risk ratio of 2.1 (P = .03) for aneurysm formation in patients with the first Q wave acute MI.[40]

Infarct Expansion

In postmortem studies, approximately 70 percent of patients who died within 1 month of acute MI were found to have thinning and dilatation of the infarcted segment of myocardium. Two-dimensional echocardiographic findings of infarct expansion, thinning of the infarcted wall, and ventricular dilatation were associated with a higher mortality rate.[41–43] Furthermore, severe regional wall motion abnormalities distant from the infarcted segment were associ-

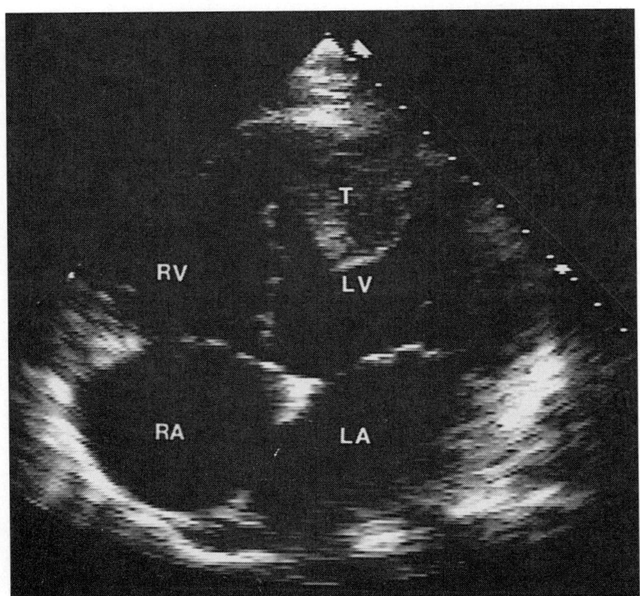

FIGURE 31–4 Transthoracic apical view shows the left ventricle (LV), left atrium (LA), right ventricle (RV), and right atrium (RA). There is a large thrombus (T) in the apex of the LV.

ated with a higher incidence of angina pectoris and reinfarction and were predictive of subsequent hemodynamic deterioration. Echocardiographic evidence of infarct expansion provides important information for the management and risk stratification of patients after an MI.

Mural Thrombus

Mural thrombus is a common complication of acute MI, with an incidence of up to 40 percent in patients with anterior and apical infarction in the prethrombolytic era and a prognosis for higher mortality rates. Thrombus is observed at the site of abnormal wall motion or within an aneurysm and appears as a mobile or an immobile opaque intracavity mass (Fig. 31–4) that may be laminar or pedunculated or may protrude into the ventricular cavity.[44–46] Thrombi are usually located at the apex and, less frequently, along the septum and the inferior regions of the heart.[44] Transthoracic two-dimensional echocardiography has a sensitivity of 75 percent, a specificity of 87 percent, and a predictive value of 84 percent in the detection of LV thrombus.[45, 46] Inadequate visualization of the apex and of thrombi of smaller than 6 mm are causes for failure of echocardiography to detect them. Thrombus forms within 2 weeks of acute MI and is located adjacent to the infarcted area; it is especially common in patients with anterior Q wave MIs. Spontaneous resolution of thrombi has been reported to occur. Two-dimensional echocardiography is the method of choice for the detection of intracardiac thrombi. Thrombi that are pedunculated and mobile within the ventricular cavity are more likely to embolize to the peripheral vasculature; the highest incidence occurs within 3 months after acute MI. In the Gruppo Italiano per lo Studio della Sopravvivenza nell'Infarto miocardio III (GISSI-3) study, LV thrombus was found in 5.1 percent of patients undergoing a predischarge echocardiogram. Patients with an anterior MI had a fivefold higher prevalence of thrombus formation than did patients with other infarct locations (11.5 versus 2.3 percent, respectively[47]).

Papillary Muscle Rupture Producing Mitral Regurgitation

Severe mitral regurgitation resulting from papillary muscle rupture is a common cause of sudden clinical and hemodynamic deterioration in a patient with MI, including the fulminant onset of acute left heart failure. The acute development of a holosystolic murmur at the apex occurs with this lesion and usually requires immediate diagnostic and interventional management. The median duration of survival is 3 days.[48] It is important to recognize that severe mitral regurgitation may occur in the absence of a cardiac murmur or in the presence of a very soft murmur with complete rupture of the papillary muscle; therefore, this diagnosis must be considered with a high index of suspicion in the appropriate clinical setting. Transesophageal echocardiographic imaging from basal short-axis and four-chamber views can detect the origin of the regurgitant jet (Plate 31–1) and the anatomic profile of the mitral and submitral valvular apparatus (Fig. 31–5).[49] Complete rupture of the papillary muscle may present with echocardiographic features of abnormal cut-off of the papillary muscle, a mobile mass attached to the mitral valve, or a flail mitral leaflet.[50] Transesophageal echocardiography has become an invaluable technique for the diagnosis of acute mitral regurgitation complicating MI, especially in the hemodynamically compromised patient in the intensive care unit.

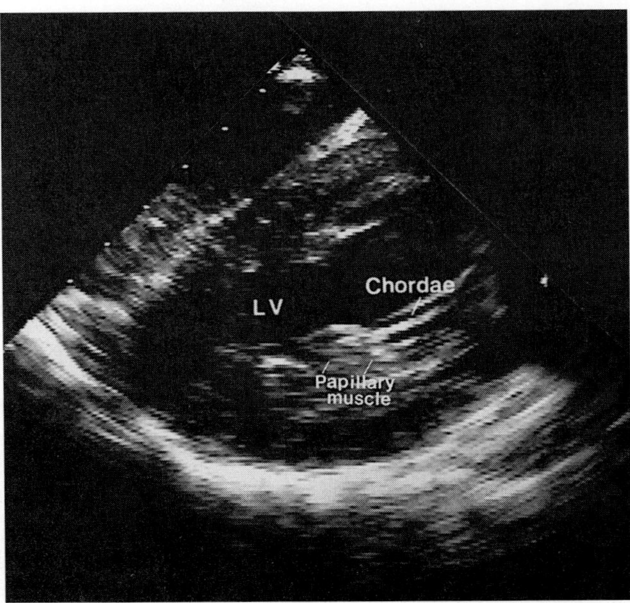

FIGURE 31–5 Transesophageal long-axis view of the left ventricle (LV) and left atrium precisely delineates chordae attached to the papillary muscle.

Cardiac Rupture

Rupture of the free wall of the left or right ventricle occurs in as many as 1 percent of patients with MI and has a mortality rate of 65 percent within 2 weeks.[50] Rupture of the ventricular wall may complicate inferior MI. Acute rupture, which usually results in electromechanical dissociation[51] and death, may be detected echocardiographically by the acute development of pericardial effusion in a patient with MI and the recurrence of chest pain. If rupture is more gradual, intramural dissection occurs and produces the characteristic echocardiographic findings of translucency within ventricular muscle and dyskinesis of the wall.[50–53] The most common site of rupture is posteriorly. The defect may be direct or irregular and serpiginious with inferior basal infarction.[52] Delayed hospital admission or undue in-hospital physical activity was reported to increase the risk of rupture in patients with a first transmural acute MI, the absence of overt heart failure, and advanced age.[54] LV wall subacute rupture is an important clinical entity identified through echocardiography; once recognized, it requires serial studies to assess the increase in pericardial effusion if surgery is not undertaken immediately on its diagnosis.

Ventricular Septal Defect

Two-dimensional echocardiography may demonstrate echo dropout in the interventricular septum in the region of abnormal wall motion. Color-flow Doppler imaging may define the site of septal rupture (Plate 31–2) and may show the presence of single or multiple rupture sites.[52, 53] Pulsed-wave Doppler imaging undertaken on the right side of the interventricular septum (at the site of the defect) usually characterizes a high-velocity jet directed from the left ventricle to the right ventricle. A semiquantitative estimate of the size of the left-to-right shunt can be obtained through measurement of the volumetric flow across the pulmonary valve and the LV outflow tract, provided there is no valvular regurgitation. RV systolic pressure can be estimated by subtracting the peak gradient obtained across the interventricular septum from the systolic (systemic) blood pressure, provided there is no aortic stenosis. Contrast two-dimensional echocardiography can also be used to identify a ventricular septal defect. Thus, two-dimensional echocardiography and color-flow Doppler imaging can rapidly and reliably provide both anatomic diagnosis and estimation of hemodynamic status at the bedside. Because the prognosis is dependent on early surgical intervention, echocardiography has become invaluable for the rapid evaluation of this complication.

Ventricular Pseudoaneurysm

LV pseudoaneurysm, or false aneurysm, results from a localized rupture of the ventricular free wall, producing a localized hemopericardium that is limited by parietal pericardium and blood clot. There is an absence of heart muscle in the wall of a false aneurysm. Two-dimensional echocardiography can be used to detect discontinuity of the ventricular free wall and a narrow neck communicating with the aneurysm and to identify the presence or absence of pericardial tamponade.[55] The false aneurysm is usually pulsatile and may contain thrombus. Color-flow Doppler imaging shows the characteristic bidirectional flow in both systole and diastole, resulting from communication between the false aneurysm and the ventricular cavity (Plate 31–3).[56] The detection of a pseudoaneurysm is important because a rupture is common and death frequently ensues. Two-dimensional echocardiography and color-flow Doppler imaging provide the most sensitive methods for the detection of pseudoaneurysms. These aneurysms should be surgically corrected as soon as possible. Dynamic LV outflow tract obstruction has been reported to constitute a correctable cause of hypotension in patients with an anteroapical MI. The altered septal geometry and hypercontractility of the basal septal segments create conditions for systolic anterior motion of the mitral valve and the generation of a dynamic LV outflow tract obstruction. The withdrawal of inotropic therapy and avoidance of ventricular unloading are essential therapeutic measures for correction of this condition.[57]

Detection of Viable Myocardium on Revascularization After Acute Myocardial Infarction

In experimental animals, coronary artery occlusions of 15- to 60-minute duration followed by reperfusion are associated with reversible ischemia but with regional wall motion abnormalities that may persist for 15 minutes to several days to weeks.[58, 59] This phenomenon of myocardial "stunning" does not appear to be caused by impairment of energy metabolism but instead is considered to result from abnormal regulation of intracellular calcium, possibly through oxidation byproducts. The recovery of regional LV function is related to early reperfusion (i.e., a short time interval between the onset of chest pain and the initiation of thrombolysis and the ability of thrombolysis to open the infarct-related vessel). In patients subjected to reperfusion before the development of Q waves on electrocardiography, the recovery of wall motion abnormalities was nearly complete. In contrast, in patients with Q wave abnormalities, the recovery of wall motion abnormalities was not present in the majority of cases. The value of dobutamine stress echocardiography (DSE) in the identification of myocardial viability and, therefore, in the selection of patients who may benefit from the revascularization procedure is well established. Coronary revascularization performed in patients with significant global LV dysfunction but little viable myocardium does not improve global systolic function.[60, 61] In a number of studies in which postrevascularization echocardiography has been used to assess the LV functional recovery after catheter-based or surgical revascularization,[62–68] the average sensitivity of DSE to predict recovery was 84 percent, specificity was 81 percent, positive predictive value was 81 percent, and negative predictive value was 87 percent. It appears that DSE has a higher specificity and a lower sensitivity than ^{201}Tl myocardial scintigraphy for the identification of functional recovery after the revascularization of dysfunctional myocardial segments.[69] The detection of residual viability by ^{201}Tl does not always correlate with the functional recovery predicted by the biphasic response of DSE. The differences between the evaluation of inotropic reserve with DSE and myocardial integrity and perfusion with ^{201}Tl scintigraphy may account for the lower positive predictive value and specificity of thallium. When transthoracic DSE was compared with transesophageal DSE for the detection of myocardial viability and ^{18}F-fluorodeoxyglucose positron emission tomography as taken as the "gold standard," the agreement between transthoracic and transesophageal DSE was close to 90 percent, suggesting the lack of an incremental value of transesophageal echocardiography if optimal images can be acquired from transthoracic windows.[70–73] Contrast echocardiography has been shown to be a promising tool for the assessment of myocardial capillary blood volume and, therefore, the presence of viable myocardium.

Infarct-Related Artery Patency and Dobutamine Stress Echocardiography

DSE was used in a number of studies to evaluate the prediction of infarct-related artery (IRA) patency.[74–77] In those studies, in which the DSE protocol did not include the biphasic response (improvement of contractility at low dose and worsening at high dose), the sensitivity, specificity, and predictive values for the detection of IRA patency were 56 to 93, 82 to 91, and 63 to 93 percent, respectively. In contrast, in one study in which the biphasic response was used, the sensitivity, specificity, and predictive values for the detection of IRA patency were 82, 80, and 82 percent, respectively.[78] PTCA and coronary artery bypass graft surgery improve myocardial perfusion in the distribution of the previously narrowed coronary artery.[79–81] Two-dimensional echocardiography detects recovery of hypokinetic and akinetic segments and ventricular systolic and diastolic function after PTCA and characterizes the resolution of regional wall motion abnormalities after coronary artery bypass graft surgery.

Stress Echocardiography for Detection of Acute Myocardial Ischemia

Exercise Stress

Patients with CAD may have a normal echocardiogram at rest but may have regional wall motion abnormalities during acute myocardial ischemia evoked with treadmill exercise or bicycle ergonometry.[82, 83] Regional wall motion abnormalities usually recover within 2 to 3 minutes after the completion of exercise and by 5 minutes may show a hyperdynamic response, thereby obviating the requirement for echocardiographic imaging during the exercise procedure and allowing measurement immediately on completion of the exercise test. Both the pretest and the post-test exercise echocardiograms can be performed with the patient in the identical supine position used for imaging analysis. Reportable studies have been detected in 90 to 92 percent of patients undergoing exercise echocardiography. The following aspects have enhanced the diagnostic accuracy of stress echocardiography:

1. The ability to sequentially image the segment
2. The introduction of continuous cine-loop analysis with digital echocardiography, requiring single cardiac cycle analysis displayed on a quadratic screen
3. The concomitant decrease in ejection fraction and development of regional wall motion abnormalities

Ryan and colleagues[84] reported that stress echocardiography has a sensitivity and specificity of 78 and 100 percent, respectively, in the detection of patients with CAD; the values are 60 and 50 percent for treadmill exercise tests. Exercise echocardiography was more sensitive than treadmill exercise for the noninvasive recognition of one-vessel disease. Overall, the reported sensitivity and specificity values for post–treadmill echocardiography are 88 and 82 percent, respectively,[85] when significant CAD is defined as a luminal diameter stenosis of 50 percent or more. The reported sensitivity and specificity values for bicycle echocardiography are 91 and 85 percent, respectively.[86–89] The average sensitivity of exercise echocardiography for the detection of individual CAD[87, 90–93] was 77 percent for left anterior descending coronary artery (LAD), 75 percent for right coronary artery (RCA), and 49 percent for circumflex artery. Regarding the number of diseased vessels, in a study of 104 patients (mean age, 58 ± 8 years; 13 women), the sensitivity was 76 percent for the detection of one-vessel disease, 95 percent for two-vessel disease, and 100 percent for three-vessel disease.[94]

The American College of Cardiology reported that stress echocardiography is a useful adjunct to the standard exercise test and provides a more sensitive and specific form of testing to detect myocardial ischemia; the diagnostic accuracy is similar to that of nuclear technologies, but stress echocardiography can be performed at a considerably lower cost. The situations listed in Table 31–1 have been

TABLE 31-1 Indications for Stress Echocardiography

Patients with a previous nondiagnostic routine treadmill stress test
Patients who are likely to have a high false-positive stress rate for ECG changes with stress tests, such as women and patients undergoing drug therapy that alters the ECG response
Patients with conduction or repolarization abnormalities in whom the ECG diagnosis of stress-induced myocardial ischemia may be difficult
Patients with a high pretest likelihood of a positive test in whom the echocardiogram is performed to provide additional information about the extent and location of ischemic regional wall motion abnormalities
Patients who have had or are going to have acute invasive interventions in whom the exercise echocardiogram is performed to observe the physiologic significance of a lesion and/or to follow the changes after vascular intervention
Patients in whom prognostic information is needed after myocardial infarction

Abbreviation: ECG, electrocardiographic.

reported to be appropriate indications for the use of stress echocardiography.

Pharmacologic Stress

Nonexercise stress or pharmacologic stress (dobutamine, dipyridamole, and adenosine) induces and detects acute myocardial ischemia in patients with CAD.[96–103]

Dobutamine stimulates the beta-adrenergic receptors, thereby increasing myocardial oxygen consumption (increased heart rate and contractility) and exceeding myocardial oxygen supply in the setting of a fixed reduction in coronary flow reserve due to CAD. Dobutamine may also increase or decrease myocardial blood flow to the ischemic region and cause redistribution of flow from subendocardial to subepicardial regions, thereby producing ischemia.

Dipyridamole inhibits the cellular uptake of adenosine, thereby leading to an accumulation of high levels of this nucleoside. In the presence of fixed coronary flow reserve due to CAD, *adenosine* accumulation may cause a decrease in the coronary perfusion pressure and also may induce redistribution of blood flow from the ischemic region to normally perfused myocardial regions, thereby decreasing oxygen supply and inducing acute myocardial ischemia.

DSE data analyzed from 17 studies from single centers (total of 1454 patients) showed overall (weighted mean) sensitivity, specificity, and predictive values of 81 percent (95 percent confidence interval [CI], 79 to 84 percent), 85 percent (95 percent CI, 82 to 87 percent), and 82 percent (95 percent, CI 80 to 85 percent), respectively. The overall abnormality rate was 92 percent.[104] In a meta-analysis of 15 studies, the sensitivity for one-, two-, and three-vessel disease was 74, 86, and 92 percent, respectively. The individual detection of CAD showed the highest sensitivity in LAD territory (72 percent) followed by circumflex (55 percent) and RCA (76 percent). The highest specificity was in the circumflex territory (93 percent), followed by RCA (89 percent) and LAD (88 percent).[104] Some investigators[105, 106] reported more false-positive results in the posterior wall than in the anterior wall, especially in patients with resting wall motion asynergy. This might be explained by the overlap in the perfusion area between the RCA and the circumflex artery,[107] observer error due to suboptimal visualization, or wall motion abnormalities associated with unidentified nonischemic mechanisms. When DSE was compared with dipyridamole echocardiography (DET), pooled data from six studies[108–113] (422 patients) showed that DET had a significantly lower sensitivity than DSE (65 versus 73 percent) due to a higher sensitivity of DSE in patients with one-vessel disease. The specificity and predictive values of these two tests were similar (89 versus 82 percent and 72 versus 76 percent, respectively).

Safety of DSE. In a retrospective analysis of 3020 DSE studies from a single institution,[114] DSE was terminated prematurely due to side effects in 7% of patients: ventricular tachycardia (VT) occurred in 0.8 percent, and supraventricular tachycardia occurred in 0.5 percent. Sustained VT occurred in five patients, and an acute MI occurred in one patient. Women, diabetics, and patients receiving β-blockers, calcium channel blockers, or both, were more likely to have suboptimal stress. Overall, major side effects occurred in 0.2 percent of patients. In an analysis of 1118 DSE studies performed at another institution, Mertes and coworkers[115] reported that patients with a recent MI more frequently had dobutamine-induced angina than did patients without a recent MI, but there were no significant differences in the incidence of arrhythmias between the two groups. No deaths, acute MIs, or sustained VTs occurred. Overall, the frequency of noncardiac side effects (nausea, anxiety, headache, tremor, urgency) was 26 percent, but the major side effects occurred in only 3 percent of the patients. The most frequent side effects were arrhythmia, hypotension, nausea, and dyspnea. Of 1000 DSE studies reported from the Mayo Clinic,[116] 12 percent of patients reported palpitations, 7 percent developed supraventricular tachycardia, 6 percent developed nonsustained VT, and one patient had an acute MI. The occurrence of acute MI during DSE, although extremely rare, has been attributed to platelet activation secondary to dobutamine administration.[117] In another study reported by European investigators of 2949 patients who received atropine in addition to dobutamine, 12 percent of tests were interrupted due to complex ventricular arrhythmia.[118]

Intraoperative Echocardiography for Detection of Acute Myocardial Ischemia or Infarction

Intraoperative echocardiography is increasingly used for the assessment of LV function in patients who are at an increased cardiac risk due to CAD, impaired LV function, or peripheral vascular disease. Intraoperative echocardiography permits the detection of intraoperative myocardial ischemia and alteration in LV function due to changes in loading conditions.[119–124] In transesophageal echocardiography, a transgastric transverse short-axis view is used to monitor LV size and function, as determined by changes in end-diastolic and end-systolic short-axis dimensions. In this view, all three major coronary arteries supply blood flow to the myocardium. The intraoperative development of regional wall motion abnormalities has been shown to occur earlier and to be a more sensitive indicator of myocardial ischemia than ECG evidence of ST-segment changes. Certain reservations should be noted. First, monitoring of wall motion abnormalities at the level of the papillary muscles precludes assessment of ischemia at the apex of the left ventricle and the right ventricle. Second, bundle-branch block development and ventricular pacing during surgery each may induce regional wall motion abnormalities. Intraoperative cross-sectional area measurement at the level of the papillary muscle provides an accurate index of ejection fraction but does not provide a reasonable estimate of changes in LV end-diastolic volume, probably because information is obtained from only one anatomic plane.

Identification of Coronary Artery Stenosis

The use of high-frequency transducers (5.0 to 7.5 MHz), the availability of transducers with biplanar analysis, and

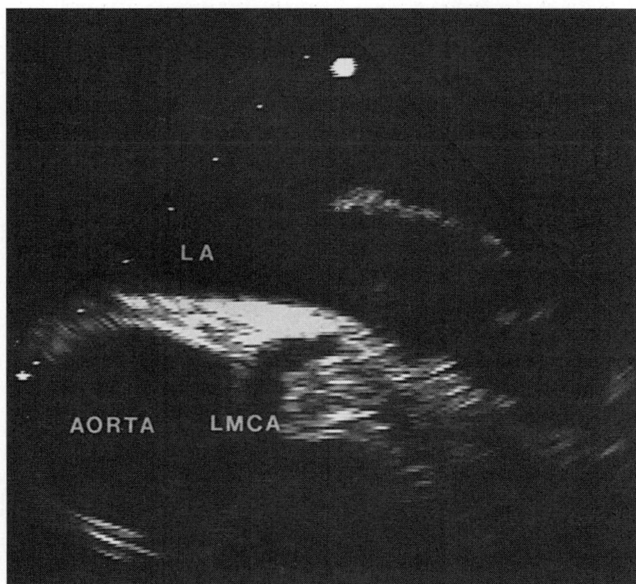

FIGURE 31–6 Transesophageal view of the aortic root defines the origin of the left main coronary artery (LMCA). LA, left atrium.

the direct and unobstructed imaging window from the esophagus have enabled imaging of the left main coronary artery. Transesophageal color-flow Doppler imaging provides adequate visualization of the entire length of the left main coronary artery (Fig. 31–6)[121, 122] reportedly in approximately 90 percent (10 of 11) of patients,[125, 126] as well as visualization of the origin of the right main coronary artery (Fig. 31–7). Transesophageal echocardiography appears to be a potentially valuable technique in the precatheterization diagnosis of left main coronary artery stenosis, especially as this condition is associated with an increased incidence of complications and sudden death during coronary arteriography. With the use of multiplane transesophageal echocardiography, Tardif and colleagues[127] reported values of 100% for sensitivity and specificity in the detection of left main coronary artery stenosis and 80 percent for the sensitivity in the detection of coronary stenosis in the proximal segments of the LAD, circumflex artery, and RCA, with a specificity of 100 percent in the same arteries. The proximal segment of the LAD was visualized in 69 percent of patients, whereas the proximal segment of the circumflex artery and RCA was visualized in 80 percent of patients. Recently, the use of adenosine in a dosage of 140 μg/kg/min in conjunction with transesophageal echocardiography for the assessment of coronary flow reserve was reported.[128] Coronary flow reserve is defined as the ratio between maximal flow and resting flow. After visualization of the LAD, the pulsed-wave Doppler image is aligned with the coronary flow, which is recorded at rest and during the administration of adenosine. A flow ratio of more than 2.1 has a sensitivity of 86 percent, a specificity of 79 percent, a positive predictive value of 46 percent, and a negative predictive value of 96 percent for the detection of critical LAD stenosis. When dipyridamole was used in conjunction with transesophageal echocardiography in a group of 47 patients,[129] the authors found that a coronary flow reserve of less than 2.3 was more sensitive for the detection of CAD than were wall motion abnormalities. The combination of coronary flow reserve of less than 2.3 and wall motion monitoring was more sensitive than was index alone: 94 percent at both 0.56 and 0.84 mg/kg.

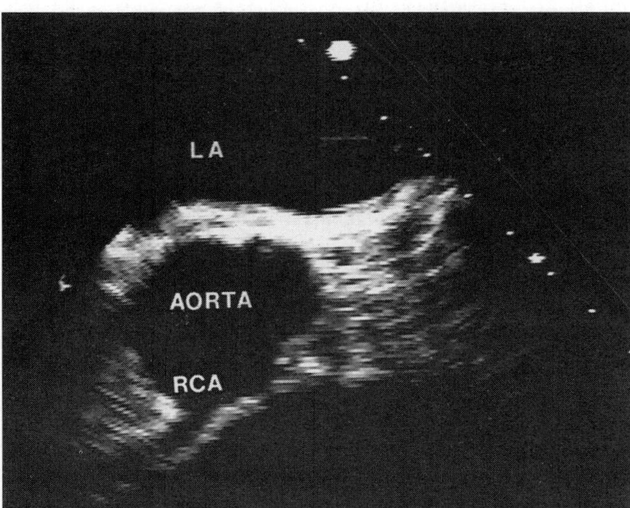

FIGURE 31–7 Transesophageal view of the aortic root defines the origin of the right coronary artery (RCA). LA, left atrium.

Intravascular Imaging of Coronary Arteries

Recent advances have allowed the use of two-dimensional intravascular echocardiography in the cardiac catheterization laboratory for identification of the presence and composition of atherosclerotic plaques. The intracoronary placement of a catheter housing a miniature high-frequency (20 to 30 mHz) transducer allows tomographic imaging of the cross-sectional area of a coronary artery and characterization of the morphology of the intima, media, and adventitia of the coronary artery wall.[130, 131] Three-dimensional reconstruction of coronary arteries with intravascular ultrasound generates a spatial visualization of vascular pathology and longitudinal and volumetric measurement of luminal and plaque dimensions.[132] Intracoronary ultrasound provides valuable information regarding the (1) identification and characterization of the atherosclerotic plaque, (2) degree of luminal cross-sectional area reduction in the coronary artery, (3) efficacy of angioplasty and the placement of intracoronary stents in patients undergoing atherectomy, and (4) coronary vasculopathy in cardiac transplant patients.[133]

References

1. Feigenbaum H, Corya BC, Dillon JC, et al: Role of echocardiography in patients with coronary artery disease. Am J Cardiol 37:775, 1976.
2. Kisslo JA, Robertson D, Gilbert VW, et al: A comparison of real time, two dimensional echocardiography and cineangiography in detecting left ventricular asynergy. Circulation 55:134, 1977.
3. Heger JJ, Weyman AE, Wann LS, et al: Cross sectional echocardiography in acute myocardial infarction: detection and localization of regional left ventricular asynergy. Circulation 60:531, 1979.

4. Nixon JV, Narahara K, Smitherman TC: Estimation of myocardial involvement in patients with acute myocardial infarction by two-dimensional echocardiography. Circulation 62:1248, 1980.
5. Gallagher KP, Kumada T, Kozioli MD, et al: Significance of regional wall thickening abnormalities relative to transmural myocardial perfusion in anesthetized dogs. Circulation 62:1266, 1980.
6. Lieberman AN, Weiss JI, Jugdutt BI, et al: Two-dimensional echocardiography and infarct size: relationship of regional wall motion and thickening to the extent of myocardial infarction in the dog. Circulation 63:739, 1981.
7. Ren JF, Kotler MN, Hakki AH, et al: Quantitation of regional left ventricular function by two-dimensional echocardiography in normals and in patients with coronary artery disease. Am Heart J 110:552, 1985.
8. Schiller NB, Shah PM, Crawford M, et al: Recommendation for quantitation of the left ventricle by two-dimensional echocardiography. J Am Soc Echocardiogr 2:358, 1989.
9. Wyatt HL, Forrester JS, Tyberg JV, et al: Effect of graded reductions in regional coronary perfusion on regional and total cardiac function. Am J Cardiol 36:185, 1975.
10. Kerber RE, Marcus ML, Ehrhardt J: Correlation between echocardiographically demonstrated segmental dyskinesis and regional myocardial perfusion. Circulation 52:1097, 1975.
11. Ellis SG, Henschke CI, Sandor T: Relation between transmural extent of acute myocardial infarction and associated myocardial contractility two weeks after infarction. Am J Cardiol 55:1412, 1985.
12. Mohler ER 3rd, Ryan T, Segar DS, et al: Clinical utility of troponin T levels and echocardiography in the emergency department. Am Heart J 135:253, 1998.
13. Medina R, Panidis IP, Morganroth J, et al: The value of echocardiographic regional wall motion abnormalities in detecting coronary artery disease in patients with or without a dilated left ventricle. Am Heart J 109:799, 1985.
14. Kaul S: Echocardiography in coronary artery disease. Curr Probl Cardiol 15:239, 1990.
15. Pierard LA, Sprynger M, Carlier J: Echocardiographic prediction of the site of coronary artery obstruction in acute myocardial infarction. Eur Heart J 8:116, 1985.
16. Nixon JV, Brown CN, Smitherman TC: Identification of transient and persistent segmental: wall motion abnormalities in patients with unstable angina pectoris by two-dimensional echocardiography. Circulation 65:1497, 1985.
17. Heger JJ, Weyman AE, Wann LS, et al: Cross sectional echocardiographic analyses of the extent of left ventricular asynergy in acute myocardial infarction. Circulation 61:1113, 1980.
18. Gibson RS, Bishop HL, Stamm RB, et al: Value of two dimensional echocardiography in patients with acute myocardial infarction. Am J Cardiol 49:1110, 1982.
19. Parisi AF, Moynihan PF, Folland ED, et al: Echocardiography in acute and remote myocardial infarction. Am J Cardiol 46:1205, 1980.
20. Arvan S, Varat MA: Two-dimensional echocardiography versus surface electrocardiography for the diagnosis of non-Q wave myocardial infarction. Am Heart J 110:44, 1985.
21. Armstrong WF: Echocardiography in coronary artery disease. Prog Cardiovasc Dis 4:267, 1988.
22. Lopez-Sendon J, Garcia-Fernandez MA, Coma-Canella I, et al: Segmental right ventricular function after acute myocardial infarction: two-dimensional echocardiographic study in 63 patients. Am J Cardiol 51:390, 1983.
23. D'arcy B, Nanda NC: Two dimensional echocardiographic features of right ventricular infarction. Circulation 65:167, 1982.
24. Shah PK, Maddhavi J, Berman DS, et al: Scintigraphically detected predominantly right ventricular dysfunction in acute myocardial infarction: clinical and hemodynamic correlates and implications for therapy and prognosis. J Am Coll Cardiol 6:1264, 1985.
25. Horowitz RS, Morganroth J: Immediate detection of early high-risk patients with acute myocardial infarction using two-dimensional echocardiographic evaluation of left ventricular regional wall motion abnormalities. Am Heart J 103:814, 1982.
26. Nishimura RA, Tajik AJ, Shub C: Role of two-dimensional echocardiography in the prediction of in hospital complications after acute myocardial infarction. J Am Coll Cardiol 4:1080, 1984.
27. Nishimura RA, Reeder GS, Miller FA: Prognostic value of predischarge 2-dimensional echocardiogram after acute myocardial infarction. Am J Cardiol 53:429, 1984.
28. Appleton CP, Hatle LK, Popp RL: Cardiac tamponade and pericardial effusion: respiratory evaluation in transvalvular flow velocities studied by Doppler echocardiography. J Am Coll Cardiol 11:1020, 1988.
29. Carlos ME, Smart SC, Wynsen JC, Sagar KB: Dobutamine stress echocardiography for risk stratification after myocardial infarction. Circulation 95:1402, 1997.
30. Quintana M, Lindvall K, Ryden L, Brolund F: Prognostic value of predischarge exercise stress echocardiography after acute myocardial infarction. Am J Cardiol 76:1115, 1995.
31. Smart SC, Knickelbine T, Stoiber TR, et al: Safety and accuracy of dobutamine-atropine stress echocardiography for the detection of residual stenosis of the infarct-related artery and multivessel disease during the first week after acute myocardial infarction. Circulation 95:1394, 1997.
32. Brochet E, Czitrom D, Karila-Cohen D, et al: Early changes in myocardial perfusion patterns after myocardial infarction: relation with contractile reserve and functional recovery. J Am Coll Cardiol 32:2011, 1998.
33. Sakuma T, Hayashi Y, Sumii K, et al: Prediction of short- and intermediate-term prognoses of patients with acute myocardial infarction using myocardial contrast echocardiography one day after recanalization or intravenous administration, of a myocardial contrast agent. J Am Coll Cardiol 32:890, 1998.
34. Porter TR, Li S, Oster R, Deligonul U: The clinical implications of no reflow demonstrated with intravenous pefluorocarbon containing microbubbles following restoration of Thrombolysis in Myocardial Infarction (TIMI) 3 flow in patients with acute myocardial infarction. Am J Cardiol 82:1173, 1998.
35. Sugiura T, Tekehana K, Hatada K, et al: Pericardial effusion after primary percutaneous transluminal angioplasty in first Q-wave acute myocardial infarction. Am J Cardiol 81:1090, 1998.
36. Schlichter J, Hellerstein HK, Katz LN: Aneurysm of the heart: a correlative study of one hundred and two proved cases. Medicine 33:43, 1954.
37. Visser CA, Kan G, Meltzer RS: Incidence, timing and prognostic value of left ventricular aneurysm formation after myocardial infarction: a prospective, serial echocardiographic study of 158 patients. Am J Cardiol 57:729, 1986.
38. Ryan T, Petrovic O, Armstrong WF: Quantitative two dimensional echocardiographic assessment of patients undergoing left ventricular aneurysmectomy. Am Heart J 111:714, 1986.
39. Abrams DL, Edelist A, Luria MH, Miller AJ: Ventricular aneurysm, a reappraisal based on a study of sixty-five consecutive autopsied cases. Circulation 27:164, 1963.
40. Anzai T, Yoshikawa T, Shiraki H, et al: C-reactive protein as a predictor of infarct expansion and cardiac rupture after a first Q-wave acute myocardial infarction. Circulation 96:778, 1997.
41. Hutchins GM, Bulkley BH: Infarct expansion versus extension: two different complications of acute myocardial infarction. Am J Cardiol 41:1127, 1978.
42. Schuster EH, Bulkley BH: Expansion of transmural myocardial infarction: a pathophysiologic factor in cardiac rupture. Circulation 60:1532, 1979.
43. Erlebacher JA, Weiss JL, Weisfeldt ML, Bulkley BH: Early dilatation of the infarcted segment in acute transmural infarction: role of infarct expansion in acute left ventricular enlargement. J Am Coll Cardiol 4:201, 1984.
44. Come PC, Markis JE, Vine HS, et al: Echocardiographic diagnosis of left ventricular thrombi. Am Heart J 100:524, 1980.
45. Nixon J: Left ventricular mural thrombus. Arch Intern Med 143:1567, 1983.
46. Visser CA, Kan G, Meltzer RS, et al: Embolic potential of left ventricular thrombus after myocardial infarction: a two dimensional echocardiographic study in 119 patients. J Am Coll Cardiol 5:1276, 1985.
47. Chiarella F, Santoro E, Domeniocucci S, et al: Predischarge two-dimensional echocardiographic evaluation of left ventricular thrombosis after acute myocardial infarction in the GISSI-3 study. Am J Cardiol 81:822, 1998.
48. Lechman KG, Francis CK, Dodge HT: Mitral regurgitation in early myocardial infarction is the strongest predictor of mortality. Circulation 74(suppl II):II-304, 1986.
49. Come PC, Riley MF, Weintraub R: Echocardiographic detection of complete and partial papillary muscle rupture during acute myocardial infarction. Am J Cardiol 56:787, 1985.

50. Vlodover Z, Edwards JE: Rupture of the ventricular septum or papillary muscle complicating myocardial infarction. Circulation 55:815, 1977.
51. Figueras J, Curos A, Cortadellas J, Soler-Soler J: Reliability of electromechanical dissociation in the diagnosis of left ventricular free wall rupture in acute myocardial infarction. Am Heart J 131:861, 1996.
52. Freeman WK, Miller FA, Oh JK, et al: Postinfarct ventricular septal rupture: diagnosis and management facilitated by two-dimensional and Doppler echocardiography. Echocardiography 4:75, 1987.
53. Miyatake K, Okamoto M, Kinoshita N, et al: Doppler echocardiographic features of ventricular septal rupture in myocardial infarction. J Am Coll Cardiol 5:182, 1985.
54. Figueras J, Cortadellas J, Calvo F, Soler-Soler J: Relevance of delayed hospital admission on development of cardiac rupture during acute myocardial infarction: study in 225 patients with free wall, septal or papillary muscle rupture. J Am Coll Cardiol 32:135, 1998.
55. Katz RJ, Simpson A, Di Bianco R, et al: Non-invasive diagnosis of left ventricular pseudoaneurysm. Am J Cardiol 44:372, 1979.
56. Gatewood RP, Nanda NC: Differentiation of left ventricular pseudoaneurysm from true aneurysm with two dimensional echocardiography. Am J Cardiol 46:869, 1980.
57. Armstrong WF, Marcovitz PA: Dynamic left ventricular outflow tract obstruction as a complication of acute myocardial infarction. Am Heart J 131:827, 1996.
58. Heyndrickx GR, Millard RW, McRitchie RS, et al: Regional myocardial function and electrophysiological alterations after brief coronary artery occlusion in conscious dogs. J Clin Invest 75:978, 1975.
59. Bush LR, Buja LM, Tilton G, et al: Effects of propranolol and diltiazem alone and in combination on the recovery of left ventricular segmental function after temporary coronary occlusion and long term reperfusion in conscious dogs. Circulation 72:413, 1985.
60. Gropler JR, Bergmann SR: Flow and metabolic determinants of myocardial viability assessed by positron-emission tomography. Cor Art Dis 4:495, 1993.
61. Sawada SG, Allman KC, Muzik O: Positron emission tomography detects evidence of viability in rest technetium-99m sestamibi defects. J Am Coll Cardiol 23:92, 1994.
62. Afridi I, Kleiman NS, Raizner AE, Zoghbi WA: Dobutamine echocardiography in myocardial hibernation: optimal dose and accuracy in predicting recovery of ventricular function after coronary angioplasty. Circulation 91:663, 1995.
63. La Canna G, Alfieri O, Giubbini R, et al: Echocardiography during infusion of dobutamine for identification of reversible dysfunction in patients with chronic coronary artery disease. J Am Coll Cardiol 23:617, 1994.
64. Arnese M, Cornel JH, Salustri A: Prediction of improvement of regional left ventricular function after surgical revascularization: a comparison of low-dose dobutamine echocardiography with ^{201}Tl single-photon emission computed tomography. Circulation 91:2748, 1995.
65. Charney R, Schwinger ME, Ryan T: Dobutamine echocardiography and rest redistribution thallium-201 scintigraphy predicts recovery of hibernating myocardium after coronary revascularization. Am Heart J 128:864, 1994.
66. Perrone-Filardi P, Pace L, Prastaro M: Dobutamine echocardiography predicts improvement of dysfunctional myocardium after revascularization in patients with coronary artery disease. Circulation 91:2556, 1995.
67. Vanoverschelde JJ, D'Hondt A, Marwick T: Head-to-head comparison of exercise redistribution-reinjection thallium single-photon emission computed tomography and low dose dobutamine echocardiography for prediction of reversibility of chronic left ventricular ischemic dysfunction. J Am Coll Cardiol 28:432, 1996.
68. De Fillipi CR, Willett DL, Irani WN: Comparison of myocardial contrast echocardiography and low-dose dobutamine stress echocardiography in predicting recovery of left ventricular function after coronary revascularization in chronic ischemic heart disease. Circulation 92:2863, 1995.
69. Bax JJ, Wijns W, Cornel JH, et al: Accuracy of currently available techniques for prediction of functional recovery after revascularization in patients with left ventricular dysfunction due to chronic coronary artery disease: comparison of pool data. J Am Coll Cardiol 30:1451, 1997.
70. Baer FM, Voth E, Deutsch HJ, et al: Assessment of viable myocardium by dobutamine transesophageal echocardiography and comparison with fluorine-18 fluorodeoxyglucose positron emission tomography. J Am Coll Cardiol 24:342, 1994.
71. Gerber B, Vanoverschelde JI, Robert A: Dobutamine echocardiography, 201 thallium scintigraphy, and positron emission tomography: which test for the prediction of myocardial viability? Circulation 90(suppl I):I-314, 1994.
72. Hepner AM, Bach DS, Bolling SF: Positive dobutamine stress echocardiography predicts viable myocardium in ischemic cardiomyopathy: a comparison with positron emission tomography. Circulation 90(suppl I):I-117, 1994.
73. Baer FM, Voth E, Deutsch HJ, et al: Dobutamine-transesophageal echocardiography versus ^{18}F-fluorodeoxyglucose positron emission tomography: predictive value for the improvement of akinetic myocardium after revascularization. Circulation 92(suppl I):I-778, 1995.
74. Takeuchi M, Araki M, Nakashima Y, Kuroiwa A: The detection of residual ischemia and stenosis in patients with acute myocardial infarction with dobutamine stress echocardiography. J Am Soc Echocardiogr 7:242, 1994.
75. Bigi R, Ochi G, Fiorentini C: Dobutamine stress echocardiography for the identification of multivessel coronary artery disease after uncomplicated myocardial infarction: the importance of test endpoint. Int J Cardiol 50:51, 1995.
76. Elhendy A, Van Domburg RT, Roelandt JRTC: Accuracy of dobutamine stress echocardiography for the diagnosis of coronary stenosis in patients with myocardial infarction. Heart 76:123, 1996.
77. Elhendy A, Geleijnse ML, Roelandt JRTC: Comparison of dobutamine stress echocardiography and 99m-technetium sestamibi SPECT myocardial perfusion scintigraphy for predicting extent of coronary artery disease in patients with healed myocardial infarction. Am J Cardiol 79:7, 1997.
78. Smart SC, Knickelbine T, Stoiber TR, et al: Safety and accuracy of dobutamine-atropine stress echocardiography for the detection of residual stenosis of the infarct-related artery and multivessel disease during the first week after acute myocardial infarction. Circulation 95:1394, 1997.
79. Hirzel HO, Nuesch K, Gruentzig A, Luetolf UM: Short and long term changes in myocardial perfusion after percutaneous transluminal coronary angioplasty assessed by thallium-201 exercise scintigraphy. Circulation 63:1001, 1981.
80. Topol EJ, Weiss JL, Guzman PA, et al: Immediate improvement of dysfunctional myocardial segments after coronary revascularization: detection by intraoperative transesophageal echocardiography. J Am Coll Cardiol 4:1123, 1984.
81. Van Den Berg EK, Popma JJ, Dehmer GJ, et al: Reversible segmental left ventricular dysfunction after coronary angioplasty. Circulation 81:1210, 1990.
82. Armstrong WF, O'Donnell J, Dillion JC, et al: Complementary value of two dimensional exercise echocardiography to routine exercise treadmill testing. Ann Intern Med 105:829, 1986.
83. Robertson WS, Feigenbaum H, Armstrong WF, et al: Exercise echocardiography: a clinically practical addition in the evaluation of coronary artery disease. J Am Coll Cardiol 2:1085, 1983.
84. Ryan T, Vasey CG, Prsti CF, et al: Exercise echocardiography: detection of coronary artery disease in patients with normal left ventricular function. J Am Coll Cardiol 11:993, 1988.
85. Pellika AP: Stress echocardiography in the evaluation of chest pain and accuracy in the diagnosis of coronary artery disease. Prog Cardiovasc Dis 39:523, 1997.
86. Galanti G, Sciagria R, Comeglio M: Diagnostic accuracy of peak exercise echocardiography in coronary artery disease: comparison with thallium-201 myocardial scintigraphy. Am Heart J 122:1609, 1991.
87. Ryan T, Segar DS, Sawada SG: Detection of coronary artery disease with upright bicycle exercise echocardiography. J Am Soc Echocardiogr 6:186, 1993.
88. Hecht HS, DeBord L, Shaw R: Digital supine bicycle stress echocardiography: a new technique for evaluating coronary artery disease. J Am Coll Cardiol 21:950, 1993.
89. Dagianti A, Penco M, Agati L: Stress echocardiography: comparison of exercise, dipyridamole and dobutamine in detecting and predicting the extent of coronary artery disease. J Am Coll Cardiol 26:18, 1995.
90. Armstrong WF: Stress echocardiography: introduction, history and methods. Prog Cardiovasc Dis 39:499, 1997.

91. Armstrong WF, O'Donell J, Ryan T: Effect of prior myocardial infarction and extent and location of coronary disease on accuracy of exercise echocardiography. J Am Coll Cardiol 10:531, 1987.
92. Marwick TH, Nemec JJ, Pashkow FJ: Accuracy and limitations of exercise echocardiography in a routine clinical setting. J Am Coll Cardiol 19:74, 1992.
93. Pozzoli MM, Fioretti PM, Salustri A: Exercise echocardiography and technetium-99m MIBI single-photon emission computed tomography in the detection of coronary artery disease. Am J Cardiol 67:350, 1991.
94. Marangelli V, Iliceto S, Piccinni G, et al: Detection of CAD by stress echocardiography: comparison of exercise, transesophageal atrial pacing and dipyridamole echocardiography. J Am Coll Cardiol 24:117, 1994.
95. Stress Echocardiography Task Force of the Nomenclature and Standard Committee of the American Society of Echocardiography: Stress echocardiography: recommendations for performance and interpretation of stress echocardiography. J Am Soc Echocardiogr 11:97, 1998.
96. Willerson JT, Hutton I, Watson JT, et al: Influence of dobutamine on regional myocardial blood flow and ventricular performance during acute and chronic myocardial ischemia in dogs. Circulation 53:828, 1976.
97. Meyer SL, Curry GC, Donsky MS, et al: Influence of dobutamine on hemodynamics and coronary blood flow in patients with and without coronary artery disease. Am J Cardiol 38:103, 1976.
98. Mannering D, Cripps T, Leech G, et al: The dobutamine stress test as an alternative to exercise testing after acute myocardial infarction. Br Heart J 59:521, 1988.
99. Cohen JL, Greene TO, Alston JR, et al: Usefulness of oral dipyridamole digital echocardiography for detecting coronary artery disease. Am J Cardiol 64:385, 1989.
100. Jain S, Suarez J, Mahmarian JJ, et al: Functional significance of myocardial perfusion defects induced by dipyridamole using thallium-201 single photon emission computed tomography and two-dimensional echocardiography. Am J Cardiol 66:802, 1990.
101. Sawada SG, Segar DS, Ryan T, et al: Dobutamine stress echocardiography: assessment of prognosis after myocardial infarction [Abstract]. Circulation 82:75, 1990.
102. Cohen JL, Greene TO, Ottenweller J, et al: Dobutamine digital echocardiography for detecting coronary artery disease. Am J Cardiol 67:131, 1991.
103. Cheirif J, Zoghbi WA: Adenosine echocardiography: a new pharmacologic stress test in coronary artery disease. Eur Heart J 5:564, 1991.
104. Geleijnse ML, Fioretti PM, Roelandt JRTC: Methodology, feasibility, safety and diagnostic accuracy of dobutamine stress echocardiography. J Am Coll Cardiol 30:595, 1997.
105. Mazeika PK, Nadazdin A, Oakley CM: Dobutamine stress echocardiography for detection and assessment of coronary artery disease. J Am Coll Cardiol 19:1203, 1992.
106. Bach DS, Hepner A, Marcovitz PA, Armstrong WF: Dobutamine stress echocardiography: prevalence of nonischemic response in a low-risk population. Am Heart J 125:1257, 1993.
107. Segar DS, Brown SE, Sawada SG, et al: Dobutamine stress echocardiography: correlation with coronary lesion severity as determined by quantitative angiography. J Am Coll Cardiol 19:1197, 1992.
108. Ostojic D, Picano E, Beleslin B, et al: Dipyridamole-dobutamine echocardiography: a novel test for the detection of milder forms of coronary artery disease. J Am Coll Cardiol 23:1115, 1994.
109. Previtali M, Lanzarini L, Fetiveau R: Comparison of dobutamine stress echocardiography, dipyridamole stress echocardiography and exercise stress testing for diagnosis of coronary artery disease. Am J Cardiol 72:865, 1993.
110. Dagianti A, Penco M, Agati L: Stress echocardiography: comparison of exercise, dipyridamole and dobutamine in predicting the extent of coronary artery disease. J Am Coll Cardiol 26:18, 1995.
111. Martin TW, Seaworth JF, Johns JP: Comparison of adenosine, dipyridamole, and dobutamine in stress echocardiography. Ann Intern Med 116:190, 1992.
112. Salustri A, Fioretti PM, El-Said EM, et al: Pharmacological stress echocardiography in the diagnosis of coronary artery disease and myocardial ischemia; a comparison between dobutamine and dipyridamole. Eur Heart J 13:1356, 1992.
113. Sochowski RA, Yvorchuk KJ, Yang YY, et al: Dobutamine and dipyridamole stress echocardiography in patients with a low incidence for severe coronary artery disease. J Am Soc Echocardiogr 8:482, 1995.
114. Secknus MA, Marwick TH: Safety and efficacy of dobutamine-atropine stress: prediction of submaximal stress in 3020 patients studied at a single center. Circulation 94(suppl I):I-383, 1996.
115. Mertes H, Sawada SG, Ryan T, et al: Symptoms, adverse effects, and complications associated with dobutamine stress echocardiography: experience of 1118 patients. Circulation 88:15, 1993.
116. Pellika PA, Roger VL, Oh JK, et al: Stress echocardiography, part II: dobutamine stress echocardiography: techniques, implementation, clinical applications, and correlations. Mayo Clin Proc 70:16, 1995.
117. Arena FJ, Paglioroni T, Wun T, et al: Platelet activation during dobutamine stress echocardiography. Circulation 92(suppl I):I-70, 1995.
118. Picano E, Mathis W Jr, Pingitore A, et al: Safety and tolerability of dobutamine-atropine stress echocardiography: a prospective, multicenter study: Echo Dobutamine International Cooperative Study group. Lancet 344:1190, 1994.
119. Smith JS, Cahalan MK, Benefiel DJ, et al: Intraoperative detection of myocardial ischemia in high-risk patients: electrocardiography versus two-dimensional transesophageal echocardiography. Circulation 72:1015, 1985.
120. Beaupre PN, Kremer PF, Cahalan MK: Intraoperative detection changes in left ventricular segmental wall motion by transesophageal two dimensional echocardiography. Am Heart J 107:1021, 1984.
121. Roizen MF, Beaupre PN, Alpert RA: Monitoring with two dimensional transesophageal echocardiography: comparison of myocardial function in patients undergoing supraceliac, suprarenal-infraceliac, or infrarenal-aortic occlusion. J Vasc Surg 1:1300, 1984.
122. Urbanopwicz JH, Shaaban MJ, Cohen NH, et al: A comparison of transesophageal echocardiographic and scintigraphic estimates of left ventricular end diastolic volume index and ejection fraction in patients following coronary artery bypass grafting. Anesthesiology 72:607, 1990.
123. Leung JM, Okelly JMB, Browner WS: Prognostic importance of postbypass regional wall motion abnormalities in patients undergoing coronary artery bypass surgery. Anesthesiology 71:16, 1989.
124. Kuecherer HK: Estimation of mean left atrial pressure from transesophageal pulse wave Doppler echocardiography of pulmonary venous flow. Circulation 82:1127, 1990.
125. Taams MA, Gussenhoven EJ, Cornel JH, et al: Detection of left coronary artery stenosis by transesophageal echocardiography. Eur Heart J 9:1162, 1988.
126. Yoshida K, Yoshikawa J, Hozumai J, et al: Detection of left main coronary artery stenosis by transesophageal color Doppler and two-dimensional echocardiography. Circulation 81:127, 1990.
127. Tardif JC, Vannan MA, Taylor K, et al: Delineation of extended length of coronary arteries by multiplane transesophageal echocardiography. J Am Coll Cardiol 24:909, 1994.
128. Redberg RF, Sobol Y, Chou TM, et al: Adenosine-induced coronary vasodilatation during transesophageal, Doppler echocardiography: rapid and safe measurement of coronary flow reserve ratio can predict significant left anterior descending coronary stenosis. Circulation 92:190, 1995.
129. Hutchinson SJ, Shen A, Soldo S, et al: Transesophageal assessment of coronary flow velocity reserve during "regular" and "high"-dose dipyridamole stress testing. Am J Cardiol 77:1164, 1996.
130. Waller BF, Pinkerton CA, Slack JD: Intravascular ultrasound: a histological study of ischemia during life. Circulation 85:2305, 1992.
131. Gura GM: Video Atlas of Color Flow Doppler Echocardiography. Boston: Little, Brown, 1990.
132. von Birgelen C, Erbel R, Di Mario C, et al: Three-dimensional reconstruction of coronary arteries with intravascular ultrasound. Herz 20:277, 1995.
133. Kapadia SR, Nissen SE, Ziada KM, et al: Development of transplantation vasculopathy and progression of donor-transmitted atherosclerosis: comparison of serial intravascular ultrasound imaging. Circulation 98:2672, 1998.

CHAPTER 32

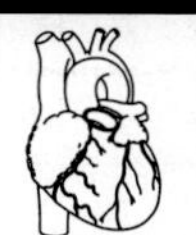

NUCLEAR IMAGING IN CORONARY ARTERY DISEASE

A. Iain McGhie, K. Lance Gould, Heinrich R. Schelbert, and James T. Willerson

SINGLE-PHOTON EMISSION COMPUTED TOMOGRAPHY: CLINICAL APPLICATIONS
Diagnosis of Coronary Artery Disease
Prognosis of Patients With Known or Suspected Coronary Artery Disease
Evaluation of Patients After Myocardial Infarction
Preoperative Assessment
Assessment of Revascularization Procedures
RADIONUCLIDE VENTRICULOGRAPHY: CLINICAL APPLICATIONS
Diagnosis of Coronary Artery Disease
Evaluation of Patients With Known or Suspected Coronary Artery Disease
Evaluation of Patients After Myocardial Infarction
Assessment of Right Ventricular Function
Other Uses of Radionuclide Ventriculography
POSITRON EMISSION TOMOGRAPHY
Myocardial Perfusion Imaging
Assessment of Myocardial Viability
Coronary Flow Reserve

SINGLE-PHOTON EMISSION COMPUTED TOMOGRAPHY: CLINICAL APPLICATIONS

Diagnosis of Coronary Artery Disease

Single-photon emission computed tomography (SPECT) ^{201}Tl imaging is widely used both in the diagnosis of coronary artery disease and in the functional assessment of patients with known coronary artery disease. In the former role, the concept of Bayes' theorem is of paramount importance; this relates the predictive value of any test to the underlying probability of the disease being present in any individual patient, which determines the clinical value of the test being used.[1, 2]

Determining the diagnostic accuracy of ^{201}Tl imaging in patients with chest pain is a complex issue that is fraught with problems. Despite the limitations of sensitivity and specificity, they are the most widely used variables to evaluate the accuracy of medical tests.[3, 4] Several factors may influence the accuracy of the technique:

- *Referral bias* resulting from preferential selection of patients based on the results of ^{201}Tl imaging for verification by coronary arteriography; this causes an increase in sensitivity and a decrease in specificity.
- The study of *skewed patient populations* that are not representative of the population in whom the test is used clinically (e.g., inclusion of a high proportion of patients with previous myocardial infarction and the use of "normal volunteers" for a normal reference group) will artificially increase the sensitivity and specificity of the test.[5]
- The effect of achieving *inadequate levels of exercise* (e.g., concomitant antianginal medications) will have an adverse effect on sensitivity.
- The *form of stress used* (i.e., exercise, dipyridamole, dobutamine) will influence the accuracy.
- The *method of data acquisition* is important. As mentioned earlier, the spatial localization and accuracy of SPECT is superior to those of planar acquisition. Another potential factor is inadequate quality assurance, which can adversely affect sensitivity and specificity; this can be a factor particularly when using the technically more demanding SPECT technology.
- The *method of analysis* used is important. Compared with qualitative analysis, quantitative analysis of ^{201}Tl distribution and washout generally improves sensitivity, but it is usually at the expense of some loss in specificity.

In an analysis of 122 studies in which stress ^{201}Tl myocardial perfusion imaging was used in patients with suspected or known coronary artery disease, the mean sensitivity and specificity for planar exercise ^{201}Tl imaging were 84 percent (1775 of 2118) and 87 percent (990 of 1140), respectively.[6] SPECT ^{201}Tl imaging is widely used; a review of 13 studies in which this technology was used in patients with suspected or known coronary disease reveals a mean sensitivity and specificity of 88 and 87 percent, respectively (Table 32–1). However, as discussed, these sensitivities and specificities may not truly reflect the accuracy of the technique in routine clinical practice.

The pretest likelihood of a patient with a particular disease having coronary disease is important in determining the clinical usefulness of that particular test. Diamond and Forrester[17] analyzed data from several clinical studies and postmortem data that represented 4952 patients. Patients were classified according to age, sex, character of chest pain, and calculated probability of coronary artery disease (Table 32–2).

With the pretest likelihood of coronary artery disease and the sensitivity and specificity of the technique used, the post-test likelihood can be calculated. The following three hypothetical cases illustrate the importance of these concepts in the clinical management of patients.

TABLE 32–1 **Sensitivity and Specificity of ^{201}Tl Single-Photon Emission Computed Tomography Imaging**

Investigator	Sensitivity	Specificity*	Form of Stress
Tamaki et al[7]	98 (80/82)	91 (20/22)	Exercise
Garcia et al[8]	89 (25/28)	92 (23/25)*	Exercise
Van Train et al[9]	94 (184/196)	82 (62/76)	Exercise
DePasquale et al[10]	95 (170/179)	74 (21/31)*	Exercise
Iskandrian et al[11]	82 (23/28)	82 (9/11)	Exercise
Maddahi et al[12]	95 (87/92)	86 (24/28)*	Exercise
Iskandrian et al[11]	84 (224/268)	93 (123/131)*	Exercise
Mahmarian et al[12a]	87 (190/219)	88 (64/73)	Exercise
Nguyen et al[13]	92 (49/53)	100 (7/7)	Adenosine
Nishimura et al[14]	87 (61/170)	90 (28/31)	Adenosine
Gupta et al[15]	82 (49/60)	80 (32/40)	Exercise
	83 (50/60)	87 (35/40)	Adenosine
Quinones et al[16]	76 (65/86)	81 (21/26)	Exercise
Total	88 (1257/1421)	87 (469/541)	

*Denotes specificity estimated using patients with < 5% pretest likelihood of coronary artery disease.

CASE 1

A 39-year-old asymptomatic woman who is an accountant in an investment bank is referred for an "executive health screen." She is a life-long nonsmoker, and her physical examination and electrocardiogram are normal.

The pretest probability of coronary artery disease is 0.8 percent. Stress myocardial perfusion imaging, with a sensitivity of 90 percent and a specificity of 80 percent, is performed. If 1000 such women are evaluated with the use of this test, the following 2 × 2 table can be constructed.

	Abnormal Test	Normal Test	Total
CAD present	9	1	10
CAD absent	198	792	990
Total	207	793	1000

If the test is abnormal, the post-test probability of coronary artery disease (CAD) remains low at 4 percent (9 of 207). If the study is negative, the post-test probability is 0.1 percent. Therefore, the test result has little relevance to the management of this patient.

This case demonstrates the limited value of performing these tests in asymptomatic individuals who have a very low probability of coronary artery disease. In addition, even a technique that is 100 percent accurate for detecting myocardial ischemia has significant limitations when used to screen asymptomatic populations. This in part relates to the nonlinear course of the atherosclerotic plaque.[18]

CASE 2

A 60-year-old man presents with a 6-month history of substernal exertional chest pain that relieved with rest or sublingual nitroglycerin. The physical examination and electrocardiogram are normal.

The pretest probability of coronary artery disease in this patient is 95 percent. The same stress myocardial perfusion procedure is performed as was performed for the patient in case 1.

	Abnormal Test	Normal Test	Total
CAD present	904	46	950
CAD absent	10	40	50
Total	914	86	1000

If the study is positive, the post-test probability of coronary artery disease (CAD) has increased by only 4 percent to 99 percent (904 of 914). If a negative result is obtained, the post-test probability of coronary artery disease is still 53 percent (46 of 86). Therefore, regardless of the result, the study does not contribute to the diagnosis of coronary artery disease.

TABLE 32–2 **Probability of Coronary Artery Disease in Symptomatic Patients According to Age and Gender**

	Nonanginal Chest Pain*		Atypical Chest Pain†		Typical Chest Pain‡	
Age (yr)	Men	Women	Men	Women	Men	Women
30–39	5.2 ± 0.8	0.8 ± 0.3	21.8 ± 2.4	4.2 ± 1.3	69.7 ± 3.2	25.8 ± 6.6
40–49	14.1 ± 1.3	2.8 ± 0.7	46.1 ± 1.8	13.3 ± 2.9	87.3 ± 1.0	55.2 ± 6.5
50–59	21.5 ± 1.7	8.4 ± 1.2	58.9 ± 1.5	32.4 ± 3.0	92.0 ± 0.6	79.4 ± 2.4
60–69	28.1 ± 1.9	18.6 ± 1.9	67.1 ± 1.3	54.4 ± 2.4	94.3 ± 0.4	90.6 ± 1.0

Chest pain characteristics are substernal location, relief within 10 minutes with rest or nitroglycerin, and precipitation by exertion.
*Nonanginal pain: fewer than two characteristics.
†Atypical angina: two of three characteristics.
‡Typical angina: all three characteristics.
Adapted from Diamond GA, Forrester JS: Analysis of probability as an aid in the clinical diagnosis of coronary-artery disease. N Engl J Med 300:1350–1358, 1979.

CASE 3

A 49-year-old man is referred for evaluation. He has a 3-month history of intermittent, sharp, anterior chest pains that last for 1 to 15 minutes. These episodes do not usually occur with exertion but have occurred on occasions while walking. The physical examination and electrocardiogram are normal.

The pretest probability of coronary artery disease in this patient is 46 percent. The same stress myocardial perfusion procedure is performed.

	Abnormal Test	Normal Test	Total
CAD present	405	45	450
CAD absent	110	440	550
Total	515	485	1000

If the test is abnormal, the post-test probability of coronary artery disease (CAD) has increased to 79 percent (405 of 515) from 46 percent. If the study is negative, the post-test probability has decreased to only 9 percent (45 of 485). Therefore, the test result makes a significant contribution to the management of such a patient.

Even a test with a very high sensitivity and specificity contributes little to the diagnosis in patients with either a low pretest likelihood or a high likelihood of coronary artery disease. However, in the case of the patient with a very high likelihood of coronary disease, it would still be useful to perform stress ^{201}Tl imaging to evaluate the functional and prognostic significance of the coronary disease.

Prognosis of Patients With Known or Suspected Coronary Artery Disease

^{201}Tl imaging is increasingly being used to assess the functional significance of documented coronary disease, such as in patients with arteriographically defined disease, after myocardial infarction, and before or after revascularization. The most important role for myocardial perfusion imaging probably in the prediction of the prognosis of patients with suspected or known coronary artery disease. The goal of such a strategy is to stratify these patients into low- and high-risk groups. The hypothesis is that patients at a low risk may be managed with medical therapy, whereas those with a higher risk may be candidates for a revascularization procedure and therefore require coronary arteriography.

There is much in the literature regarding this role of ^{201}Tl imaging.[19] Brown and associates[20] reported on a series of 100 patients without prior myocardial infarction who presented with chest pain. The results of ^{201}Tl imaging were found to have more predictive value than clinical, electrocardiographic, or angiographic data. The number of reversible perfusion defects was the best predictor of future cardiac events (e.g., myocardial infarction, cardiac death). A subsequent study by Landenheim and colleagues[21] of 1689 patients with suspected coronary artery disease confirmed the independent prognostic value of the extent and severity of myocardial hypoperfusion. Another study of 299 patients who were followed for a mean of 4.6 years reported the number of diseased vessels at time of coronary arteriography to be the most powerful prognostic variable, with the number of reversible hypoperfused segments on ^{201}Tl imaging being the next most important prognostic factor.[22] When all of the data from the exercise ^{201}Tl stress test are considered (i.e., heart response, ST-segment change, ventricular premature beats on exercise), it had the same prognostic value as coronary arteriography. The combination of the results from coronary arteriography and exercise ^{201}Tl imaging complemented each other, being superior to either alone. In a similar study, Kaul and associates[23] found that the quantitative lung/heart ratio of ^{201}Tl activity was the most important prognostic predictor, followed by the number of diseased vessels, patient gender, and change in heart rate.

Patients presenting with chest pain who have normal ^{201}Tl images have a good prognosis, regardless of whether they have coronary artery disease. An analysis of 16 studies of patients with known or suspected coronary artery disease who had normal planar ^{201}Tl imaging revealed a low cardiac event rate (mean of 0.9 percent per annum). Machecourt and associates[24] reported similar findings with SPECT ^{201}Tl imaging and observed an annual event rate of less than 0.42 percent compared with 2.1 percent in individuals with abnormal ^{201}Tl images ($P < .0001$). Other similar studies with ^{99m}Tc-labeled sestamibi have also shown a very low event rate in patients with normal SPECT images.[25, 26] For example, in a cohort of patients with stable chest pain syndromes, Stratmann and colleagues[25] reported an event rate of 0.4 percent per annum in patients with normal ^{99m}Tc sestamibi SPECT images compared with an event rate of 7 percent in patients with abnormal ^{99m}Tc sestamibi SPECT images. Berman and associates have also reported extensively on the prognostic power of SPECT perfusion imaging in the management of patients with known or suspected coronary artery disease.[27–31] This group has consistently shown that results from nuclear imaging provide additional powerful and independent prognostic information in all subgroups of patients who have already been risk stratified through the use of clinical and exercise testing data. Their data also suggest that nuclear testing is most cost effective in patient groups who have an intermediate-to-high likelihood of having underlying coronary artery disease.[27] Stress ^{201}Tl imaging also has a role to play in the evaluation of patients with unstable angina. The presence of reversible ^{201}Tl perfusion defects is an important independent predictor of future adverse cardiac events in patients with unstable angina who have been stabilized with medical therapy.[32, 33]

Evaluation of Patients After Myocardial Infarction

Many clinical and laboratory variables have been used to identify the survivors of myocardial infarction who are at a high risk of future cardiac events, including recurrent angina, clinical left heart failure, depressed left ventricular ejection fraction, and complex ventricular arrhythmia.[34–36] The rationale for the use of noninvasive tests after myocardial infarction is to stratify patients into high- and low-risk groups. Exercise electrocardiography can provide important prognostic information after an acute myocardial infarction.[37, 38] However, stress myocardial perfusion imaging offers several advantages, including a higher sensitivity and specificity for the detection of multivessel disease in infarct survivors, the ability to localize ischemia to particular coronary distributions, and the ability to detect ischemia in the infarct zone as well as the noninfarct zone.

Gibson and associates[39] compared the use of predischarge submaximal ^{201}Tl imaging with clinical, exercise electrocardiographic, and angiographic data in patients with acute myocardial infarction. Perfusion defects that redistributed, defects that involved multiple vascular territories, and increased ^{201}Tl lung uptake were important prognostically. The authors also showed that stratification of patients into low- and high-risk groups on the basis of the ^{201}Tl findings had greater discrimination than either exercise electrocardiographic or angiographic data (Fig. 32–1). Subsequent work has confirmed the predictive value of submaximal ^{201}Tl imaging,[40] although not all researchers have found ^{201}Tl results to have an independent predictive value.[41, 42]

Dipyridamole/adenosine stress has theoretical advantages over exercise in some patients after a recent acute myocardial infarction. Dipyridamole/adenosine produces greater increases in coronary flow than submaximal exercise and should be more sensitive in detecting ischemic myocardium. In addition to providing maximal stress, dipyridamole/adenosine results in only a minor increase in myocardial O_2 requirements, and its effects can be rapidly reversed with intravenous aminophylline or by discontinuing the adenosine infusion. Therefore, it allows maximal stress to be performed relatively safely in the setting of a recent uncomplicated acute myocardial infarction. Several workers have found ^{201}Tl imaging with vasodilator stress to be of value in this setting.[43–45] It has also been used early (1 to 4 days) after infarction, with no adverse events being experienced. In a group of 50 patients, a multivariate analysis of several clinical, electrocardiographic, angio-

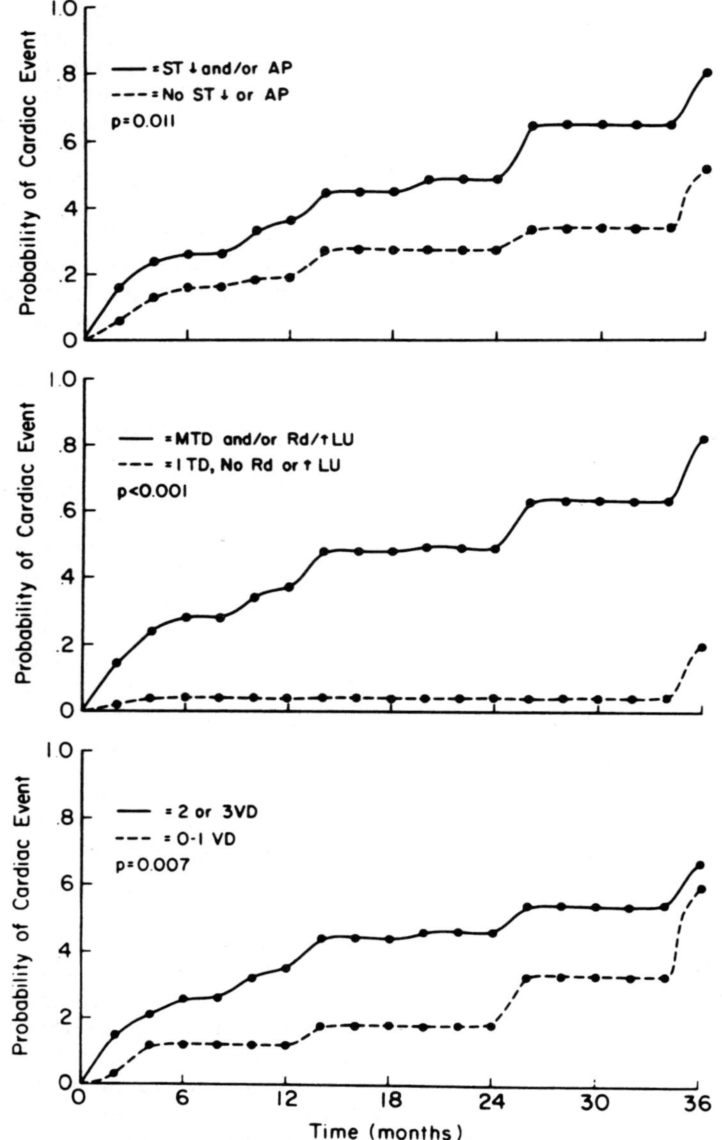

FIGURE 32–1 Cumulative probability of a cardiac event in the 36 months after myocardial infarction. Patients are categorized into high- and low-risk groups according to the results of submaximal exercise test (SMXT) **(top)**, ^{201}Tl scintigraphy **(middle)**, and coronary arteriography **(bottom)**. AP, angina pectoris; LU, lung uptake of ^{201}Tl; MTD, multiple transient defects; RD, redistribution; ST, ST segment; VD, vessel disease. (From Gibson RS, Watson DD, Craddock GB, et al: Prediction of cardiac events after uncomplicated myocardial infarction: a prospective study comparing predischarge exercise thallium-201 scintigraphy and coronary angiography. Circulation 68[2]:321–336, 1983.)

graphic, and ^{201}Tl data was performed.[46] The presence of ^{201}Tl redistribution in the infarct zone (present in 45 percent of patients) was the only predictor of in-hospital events (P = .001). None of the angiographic variables were significant predictors of cardiac events.

However, many of these studies were performed in the 1980s, before implementation of the remarkable changes that have occurred in the management of patients with acute myocardial infarction. The use of reperfusion therapy (thrombolytic agents or primary angioplasty), aspirin, beta-adrenergic receptor blockers, and angiotensin-converting enzyme inhibitors has become widespread and accepted as the standard of care. In addition, the use of coronary arteriography and revascularization, especially coronary angioplasty, has become much more widely practiced. These changes in the management of acute myocardial infarction have resulted in dramatic reductions in in-hospital and 1-year mortality rates, particularly in patients treated with reperfusion and revascularization therapy. Patients who have received reperfusion therapy tend to be younger, less likely to have multivessel disease, and to have smaller infarcts with less left ventricular dysfunction.

The consequence of this very low cardiac event rate has been the lowering of the positive predictive value of risk stratification strategies. Initially, the results of some studies performed in the "reperfusion era" have suggested that the predictive value of stress perfusion imaging is significantly reduced[47–49]; however, other studies have tended to contradict this suggestion.[50, 51] Dakik and associates[50] studied 71 patients with acute myocardial infarction who were treated with thrombolytic therapy over 26 months and found, with the use of multivariate analysis, that the significant predictors of risk were ejection fraction ($P < .0005$) and size of the ischemic perfusion defect (P = .005). In addition, they found that the combination of ejection fraction and SPECT ^{201}Tl results added significant incremental prognostic information to the clinical data, whereas the use of angiography did not further improve a model that included clinical, ejection fraction, and SPECT ^{201}Tl variables. Similar findings have been published with the use of adenosine ^{201}Tl SPECT imaging in patients with acute myocardial infarction who were managed in the "thrombolytic era."[51] In this study, the risk of subsequent events after acute myocardial infarction was best predicted by the combination of the extent of ischemia detected with adenosine ^{201}Tl SPECT and left ventricular ejection fraction.

In conclusion, predischarge stress myocardial perfusion imaging is an effective means of risk stratifying survivors of acute myocardial infarction, allowing the identification of patients with multivessel coronary disease and ventricular dysfunction who are at a high risk of having future cardiac events. The presence of extensive or reversible perfusion defects, perfusion defects in a multivessel distribution, increased lung uptake, transient ischemic dilatation of the left ventricle, and depressed left ventricular function are all important predictors of a poor outcome after myocardial infarction.

Preoperative Assessment

The preoperative assessment of patients undergoing elective vascular surgery poses unique problems. These patients have a high probability of concomitant coronary artery disease[52–54] but often are unable to exercise sufficiently during conventional testing. Dipyridamole or adenosine myocardial perfusion imaging has obvious attractions in this situation. Several studies have confirmed the usefulness of this technique in the preoperative assessment of patients with and without known coronary artery disease who are undergoing reconstructive vascular surgery,[55–58] although some studies have contradicted these findings.[59, 60] Patients with a normal or mildly abnormal or fixed perfusion defect have a low perioperative event rate, whereas those with a large or multiple perfusion defect have a higher perioperative event rate. A review of the literature indicates the positive predictive value can range from 4 to 20 percent. However, when clinical markers of increased cardiac risk are taken into account, the diagnostic accuracy of the technique can be substantially improved. Eagle and colleagues[61] showed that the presence of Q waves, ventricular ectopy, diabetes mellitus, advanced age, and angina were all associated with an increased risk. Patients with three or more of these risk factors had a cardiac event rate of 50 percent. Patients with one or two clinical markers were of intermediate risk and could be risk stratified with dipyridamole ^{201}Tl imaging. In patients with no risk factors, there was no observed benefit of dipyridamole ^{201}Tl imaging. The use of dipyridamole^{201}Tl imaging in the preoperative assessment of patients undergoing nonvascular surgery is less compelling, but data are limited.[62, 63] The usefulness of stress perfusion imaging in this situation probably depends both on the nature of the surgical procedure being performed and on whether coronary artery disease is present in the patient being evaluated. Guidelines for the perioperative evaluation of patients undergoing noncardiac surgery have been published.[64]

Assessment of Revascularization Procedures

Stress myocardial perfusion imaging is of value in evaluating patients before revascularization procedures, in particular, coronary angioplasty. It can be used to demonstrate the presence a stress-induced perfusion defect associated with a particular coronary artery stenosis, allowing targeting of the appropriate "culprit lesion." After angioplasty, myocardial perfusion has been used to evaluate the adequacy of revascularization and to predict restenosis. However, there is a poor correlation between angiographic results and the results of perfusion imaging performed early after angioplasty, with the presence of areas of hypoperfusion despite good angiographic results.[65, 66] These perfusion abnormalities are transient, usually resolving within 3 months of an angiographically successful dilatation. Similarly, Doppler-derived measurements of coronary flow have demonstrated transient abnormalities in coronary flow reserve after angiographically successful procedures. This transient phenomenon probably results from abnormal flow reserve due to endothelial injury occurring at the time of angioplasty. However, if myocardial perfusion imaging is delayed for 4 to 6 weeks after angioplasty, the predictive value is much improved. When myocardial perfusion imaging is performed at this time, patients with normal myocardial perfusion imaging have a very low restenosis rate, whereas patients with abnormal perfusion studies have an 85 and 96 percent restenosis rate after 6 and 12 months, respectively.[67] Interestingly, the use of oral dipyridamole and ^{201}Tl imaging approximately 3 days after coronary angioplasty was a relatively accurate means of predicting restenosis.[68] Ten of 14 (71 percent) patients with reversible defects developed restenosis, whereas only 3 of 27 (11.5 percent) patients without reversible defects developed restenosis.

Myocardial perfusion imaging is also of value in evaluating patients after coronary artery bypass graft surgery and is generally superior to exercise electrocardiography in determining the status of graft patency.[69–71] Gibson and associates[72] prospectively evaluated 47 patients before and after coronary artery bypass graft surgery with ^{201}Tl imaging. In this study, the presence of normal perfusion after grafting in segments that previously showed evidence of reversible or partially reversible hypoperfusion was associated with graft patency and improved left ventricular function.

Radionuclide Ventriculography: Clinical Applications

Diagnosis of Coronary Artery Disease

Exercise radionuclide ventriculography can be used to detect coronary artery disease by inducing myocardial ischemia in the distribution of a stenosed coronary artery that results in regional and global ventricular dysfunction. The normal response to the left ventricle to exercise is characterized by an increase in ejection fraction by at least 5 units, a decrease in end-systolic volume index, an increase in systolic pressure/volume index, and more vigorous segmental contraction. However, the same caveats about pretest probability apply to exercise radionuclide ventriculography as they do to any noninvasive technique used for the diagnosis of coronary artery disease. The reported sensitivity and specificity of exercise radionuclide ventriculography for detecting coronary artery disease have been inconsistent. In the first large series, Borer and associates[73] reported a sensitivity of 95 percent and a specificity of 100 percent for the detection of coronary artery disease. These values were probably artificially high and reflected the patient population studied. The study group included a normal database acquired using "normal volunteers," which may have artificially increased the specificity of the procedure. A later study reported a similar sensitivity (90 percent) but a much lower specificity (58 percent).[74] There probably are several reasons for the lower specificity, including postreferral bias (i.e., only patients with an abnormal response would undergo coronary arteriography, resulting in the inclusion of patients with noncoronary causes of abnormal left ventricular function either at rest or during exercise, such as cardiomyopathy, hypertension, and valvular heart disease).[75] In general, the current practice is to perform stress myocardial perfusion imaging in preference to exercise radionuclide ventriculography in patients with suspected coronary artery disease.

Evaluation of Patients With Known or Suspected Coronary Artery Disease

The noninvasive assessment of ventricular function at rest and exercise has widespread application in the assessment of patients with known coronary artery disease. Both coronary anatomy and resting left ventricular function are important prognostic indicators in patients with chronic stable coronary artery disease.[76, 77] Data from the Coronary Artery Surgery Study (CASS) registry also revealed that resting ventricular dysfunction was associated with a higher mortality rate, which was independent of coronary anatomy. In a group of medically treated patients, the 4-year mortality rate was 8 percent in patients with an ejection fraction of more than 0.50, 17 percent in patients with an ejection fraction of 0.35 to 0.49, and 43 percent in patients with an ejection fraction of less than 0.35.[78]

As with stress ^{201}Tl imaging, exercise radionuclide ventriculography has been used to stratify patients into low- and high-risk groups. The rationale is that the latter group of patients requires more aggressive investigation and management, possibly benefiting from revascularization. Jones and associates[79] reported a 20 percent higher mortality rate after 3 years in patients with an abnormal exercise ejection fraction compared with patients with a normal response, despite no significant differences in the resting ejection fraction. Bonow and colleagues[80] followed for 4 years a group of minimally symptomatic patients with three-vessel coronary disease who had normal or near-normal left ventricular function. The 18-month survival rate was less than 80 percent in patients with severe exercise-induced ischemia as demonstrated by a fall in the ejection fraction, ST-segment depression, and a limited exercise capacity. In comparison, all other patients had an excellent prognosis (Fig. 32–2). Another study of patients with one- and two-vessel disease and a resting ejection fraction of less than

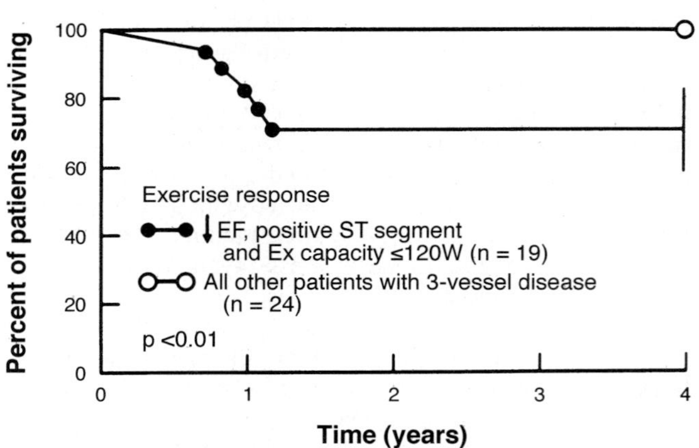

FIGURE 32–2 Prognostic value of exercise radionuclide ventriculography in 43 patients with three-vessel coronary disease and a resting left ventricular ejection fraction (EF) of 0.40. Patients with a fall in the EF during exercise, a positive (abnormal) ST-segment response, and reduced exercise (Ex) capacity had a significantly poorer prognosis than other patients when treated with medication. (From Bonow RO, Kent KM, Rosing DR, et al: Exercise-induced ischemia in mildly symptomatic patients with coronary artery disease and preserved left ventricular function: identification of subgroups at risk of death during medical therapy. N Engl J Med 311:1339–1345, 1984.)

0.50 produced similar results. Patients with a fall in the exercise ejection fraction, at least 1.0-mm ST-segment depression, and a peak workload of 600 kg/m/min or less had a significantly higher event rate after 1 year than did those who did not (33 versus 2 percent).[81]

These results suggest that rest and exercise radionuclide ventriculography is an important prognostic tool in patients with coronary artery disease. It provides data regarding both resting ventricular function and the physiologic importance of coronary disease, complementing anatomic information obtained from arteriography.

Evaluation of Patients After Myocardial Infarction

The prognosis after acute myocardial infarction is determined primarily by the functional state of the left ventricle and the extent to which myocardium is jeopardized by additional obstructed coronary arteries.[35, 82–84] Therefore, rest and exercise radionuclide ventriculography are well suited for the noninvasive assessment of the impact of myocardial infarction on ventricular function and for identification of the physiologic importance of coronary stenoses outside the infarct distribution. Left ventricular ejection fraction and other indices of ventricular performance, such as end-systolic volume and end-systolic pressure/volume ratio, are useful for stratification of patients after acute myocardial infarction and can be calculated using radionuclide ventriculography.

A strong relationship between left ventricular ejection fraction and death after myocardial infarction has been demonstrated.[34, 84] A predischarge left ventricular ejection fraction of less than 0.40 was associated with an exponential increase in mortality rates. There was almost a 50 percent 1-year mortality rate in patients with a left ventricular ejection fraction of less than 0.20 (Fig. 32–3). The use of load-dependent measures of left ventricular function has limitations.[85] Alterations in the loading conditions of the heart can result in profound changes in the ejection fraction. This is the postulated mechanism for the wide variations in the left ventricular ejection fraction that have been observed in patients in the early convalescent phase of acute myocardial infarction.[86, 87] In these studies, despite sometimes marked variations in the left ventricular ejection, there were no associated changes in the clinical status or regional function and no correlation with any demographic variables measured.

The measurement of ventricular volumes, in particular, end-systolic volume, has been shown to provide additional important prognostic information.[88] Unfortunately, these applications have had only limited application for the study of patients after myocardial infarction using radionuclide ventriculography. Sanford and colleagues[89] found significantly increased end-systolic volumes in patients with Killip class III function who were studied within hours of admission. Corbett and associates[90] studied patients before discharge with the use of radionuclide ventriculography and the measurement of ventricular volumes. In these studies, patients with transmural infarcts generally had significantly larger end-systolic volumes than did patients with nontransmural infarcts, and patients with anterior transmural infarcts had the largest end-systolic volumes. Larger end-systolic volumes were noted among patients with poorer prognosis, especially among those who died or had persistent congestive heart failure or refractory angina.

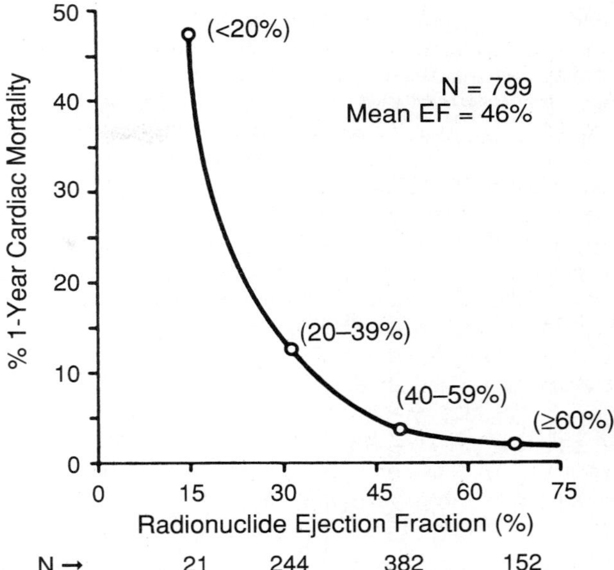

FIGURE 32–3 Prognostic importance of the predischarge left ventricular ejection fraction (EF) as measured with radionuclide ventriculography in patients with recent myocardial infarction. Note the exponential increase in mortality rate when the left ventricular EF falls to less than 0.40. (From Multicenter Postinfarction Research Group: Risk stratification and survival after myocardial infarction. N Engl J Med 309:331–336, 1983.)

Additional important information regarding the function of the left ventricle after acute myocardial infarction can be obtained by coupling radionuclide ventriculography with exercise. Corbett and associates[91] successfully used exercise radionuclide ventriculography for the risk stratification of patients at time of hospital discharge. Patients demonstrating depressed global left ventricular function at rest or an abnormal response to submaximal exercise (i.e., no change or decrease in ejection fraction, a rise in end-systolic volume, or a blunted response to systolic pressure/volume index) had a significantly higher evidence of future cardiac events, including death in the 6 to 24 months after hospital discharge (Fig. 32–4). Moderate or severely depressed ejection fraction (<0.35 to 0.40) either at rest or during submaximal exercise has been used to define populations of patients at an increased risk of subsequent death.[92–95]

An assessment of regional left ventricular function after myocardial infarction using radionuclide ventriculography also provides additional important prognostic information.[86, 96–98] Estimation of the left ventricular function without evaluation of regional function can be misleading. Several studies have analyzed serial changes in left ventricular function after acute myocardial infarction with the use of thrombolytic therapy. In these studies, changes in regional function often were not reflected by changes in the left ventricular ejection fraction. Studies with quantitative analysis of region wall motion during the acute phase of infarction before treatment and subsequently during the

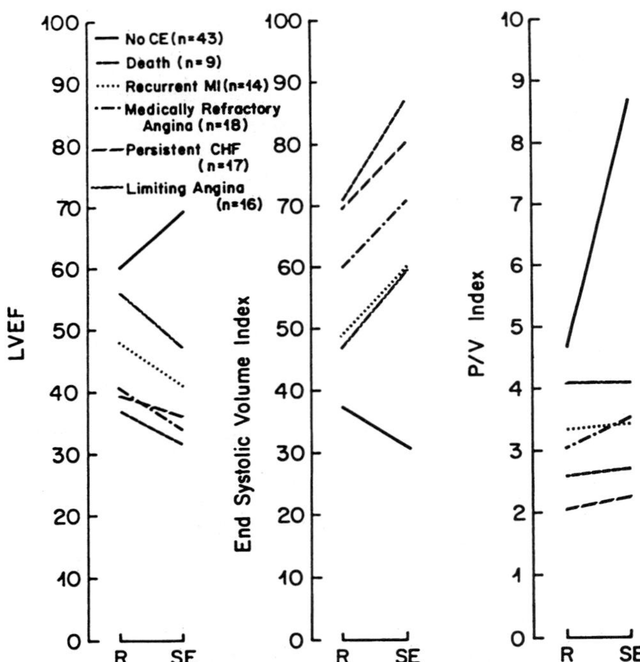

FIGURE 32–4 Prognostic importance of submaximal exercise radionuclide ventriculography in survivors of a recent myocardial infarction. Mean left ventricular ejection fraction (LVEF), end-systolic volume index, and systolic pressure/volume (P/V) index at rest (R) and at peak submaximal exercise (SE) according to specific cardiac events (CE) during follow-up. CHF, congestive heart failure; MI, myocardial infarction; n, number of patients. (From Corbett JR, Dehmer GJ, Lewis SE, et al: The prognostic value of submaximal exercise testing with radionuclide ventriculography before hospital discharge in patients with recent myocardial infarction. Circulation 64:535–544, 1981.)

convalescent phase have demonstrated a consistent evolutionary pattern that closely relates to the success of thrombolytic therapy.[99–101] Before treatment, the region supplied by the occluded vessel is severely reduced, whereas the noninvolved segments demonstrate compensatory hyperkinesis. After successful reperfusion, global ventricular function is generally preserved at follow-up. This is the net effect of improved function in the reperfused area and normalization of function in areas that were previously hyperkinetic[102] (Fig. 32–5). If reperfusion therapy is unsuccessful, there is little or no improvement in area subtended by the occluded vessel. As function returns to normal in the hypercontracting areas, there is a net deterioration in global function. Wackers and associates[86] demonstrated similar function patterns with the use of radionuclide ventriculography.

Alterations in left ventricular topography resulting from infarct expansion were originally described in a clinicopathologic study by Hutchins and Bulkley.[103] Meizlish and colleagues[104] used planar radionuclide ventriculography to detect areas of infarct expansion, "functional aneurysm" formation, in patients with a first anterior myocardial infarction. Despite no significant differences in the mean left ventricular ejection fraction or Killip classification in those with and without evidence of infarct expansion, there was a threefold excess in mortality rates in patients with functional aneurysm formation.

Assessment of Right Ventricular Function

The complex geometry of the right ventricle poses major problems for all imaging modalities. However, radionuclide techniques are less geometrically dependent than other conventional imaging techniques, such as contrast ventriculography or echocardiography, for the reasons discussed earlier. Three radionuclide techniques are used to assess right ventricular function.

The first-past technique, as described for the left ventricle, can be applied to the right ventricle.[105] This is probably the optimal technique for assessing right ventricular function but has the disadvantages discussed previously. The gated equilibrium technique can also be used, but overlap of the cardiac chambers is a significant limiting factor.[106–108] The right ventricular ejection fraction is calculated from the left anterior oblique projection because this affords best separation of the two ventricles; however, the right atrial and right ventricular overlap in this projection results in a systematic underestimation of the right ventricular ejection fraction. Despite this, there is a good correlation with other methods of assessing right ventricular function with the use of this technique.[109] A good compromise is the gated first-pass technique that involves the injection of a bolus of ^{99m}Tc pertechnetate; electrocardiographically gated scintigraphic data are acquired from the time the bolus is seen entering the superior vena cava until it leaves the main pulmonary artery.[110] This provides excellent spatial resolution of the right atrium and right ventricle with no background contamination from the lungs or left heart chambers. Radioisotopes of inert noble gases, ^{81}Kr and ^{133}Xe, have also been used to assess right ventricular function.[111–114] These radioisotopes are rapidly excreted during their first passage through the lungs, allowing repeated studies to be performed without significantly increasing the radiation burden to the patient or problems of increasing background activity.

Other Uses of Radionuclide Ventriculography

Valvular Heart Disease. Other than evaluation of ventricular function and estimation of the degree of valvular regurgitation, radionuclide ventriculography has a limited role to play in the patient with valvular heart disease. However, Bonow and associates[115] demonstrated that radionuclide ventriculography is useful in managing asymptomatic patients with aortic regurgitation. Asymptomatic patients with normal resting left ventricular systolic function have a benign prognosis with an annual mortality rate of less than 0.5 percent.[116, 117] Outcome after aortic valve replacement is dependent on the preoperative radionuclide left ventricular ejection fraction, the exercise tolerance of the patient, and the duration of left ventricular dysfunction.[118] Therefore, asymptomatic patients can be followed carefully with serial evaluation of left ventricular function and undergo valve replacement only after the onset of symptoms or a depressed left ventricular ejection fraction. The left ventricular ejection fraction response to exercise is nonspecific due to abnormal loading conditions on the left ventricle and is of limited value.[119]

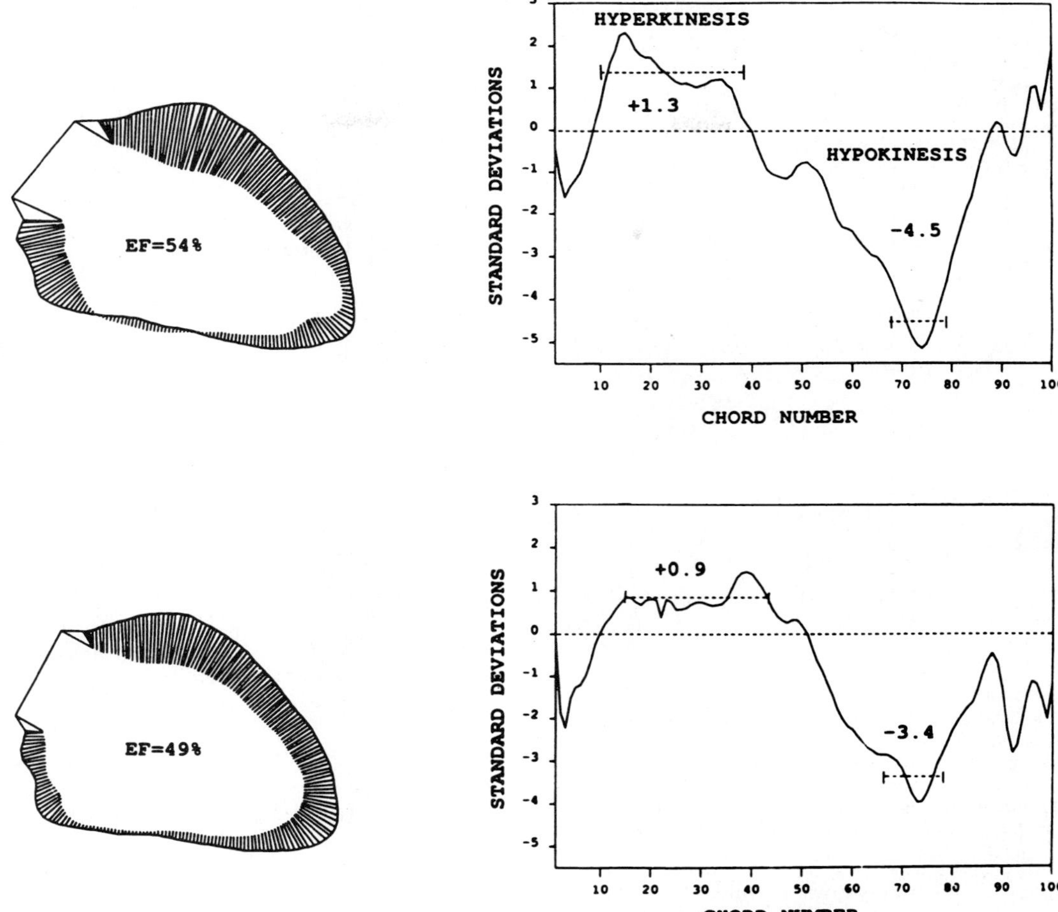

FIGURE 32–5 Assessment of regional ventricular function using the centerline method in a patient with acute myocardial infarction treated with thrombolytic therapy. Global left ventricular function improves due to the development of anterior hyperkinesis *(top)* despite a severe regional wall motion inferiorly in the region of the infarct. However, with time, there is a return to baseline level in the previously hyperkinetic region, leading to a slight reduction in the global ejection fraction despite functional recovery in the infarct region (see text for further details). (From Sheehan F: Cardiac angiography. *In* Marcus M, Schelbert HR, Skorton DJ, Wolf GL [eds]: Cardiac Imaging: A Companion to Braunwald's Heart Disease. pp. 109–148. Philadelphia: WB Saunders, 1991.)

Doxorubicin Toxicity. The chemotherapeutic agent doxorubicin is associated with the development of irreversible cardiotoxicity when given in doses of at least 450 mg/m^2. It is recommended that patients have a baseline measurement of their left ventricular ejection fraction before starting chemotherapy and again after receiving cumulative doses of 300 and 450 mg/m^2.[120] Exercise radionuclide ventriculography may improve the detection of patients at high risk of developing cardiotoxicity, but the specificity is so low that it is of doubtful clinical use.[121]

Positron Emission Tomography

Myocardial Perfusion Imaging

Clinical Application of Myocardial Perfusion Imaging With Positron Emission Tomography (PET)

Figure 32–6 shows the orientation of a three-dimensional topographic display of cardiac PET. These three-dimensional displays demonstrate more accurately spatial quantification and visualization of abnormalities compared with commonly used polar maps, which distort the spatial size and shape of perfusion defects.[122] Four views of the heart are shown in relation to the coronary arteries.

Plate 32–1 illustrates a clinical example of PET imaging using generator-produced ^{82}Rb.[123] The patient was a 53-year-old asymptomatic man with a normal ^{201}Tl and electrocardiography treadmill test 10 days and 1 year before the PET scan. Each panel of the topographic map views the left ventricle as if looking at the septum (top row, first panel), at the anterior wall (top row, second panel), at the left lateral wall (top row, third panel), or the inferior wall (top row, fourth panel). The dashed white line marks the upper limit of automated quantitative data because the membranous septum usually causes a normal defect at the atrioventricular ring. The black dashed lines delineate septal, anterior, lateral, and inferior quadrants, with the bottom dashed line delineating the apex. The rest study is shown in the top row (S1), and the dipyridamole study is shown in the bottom row (S2). Similar displays are shown for the

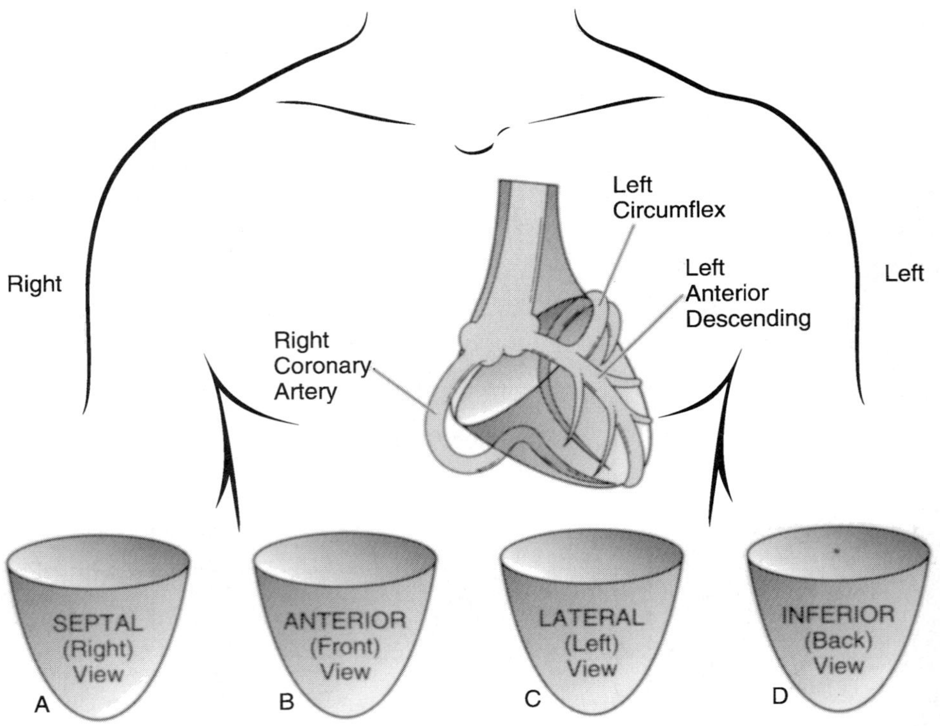

FIGURE 32–6 Orientation of three-dimensional topographic images viewed as if looking through the right ventricle at the septum or right side of the left ventricle **(A)**, at the anterior wall **(B)**, at the left lateral free wall **(C)**, and at the inferior wall **(D)**. The relation of coronary arterial distribution to these views is also illustrated.

absolute dipyridamole/rest ratio (ABS S2/S1, top row) and for the relative change dipyridamole/rest ratio (REL S2/S1, bottom row).

The rest image (top row) shows a mild small apical defect, suggesting a small, old, apical myocardial infarction despite the absence of symptoms, known coronary artery disease, or a clinical event. The dipyridamole image (bottom row) shows a large severe midproximal anterior and apical defect with definite but less severe defects of the proximal anterior septum and lateral wall. These results were interpreted as showing a very severe or occluded mid–left anterior descending coronary artery (LAD) stenosis, another more moderate LAD stenosis proximal to the first septal perforator, and a moderate stenosis of an artery to the lateral myocardial wall, probably a left circumflex stenosis. Left ventricular function was normal.

Accordingly, the patient was scheduled for simultaneous diagnostic catheterization and percutaneous transluminal coronary angioplasty (PTCA) of three stenoses with surgical backup at initial catheterization. Quantitative coronary arteriography confirmed significant stenoses of the proximal and mid-LAD and the mid-left circumflex artery. PTCA was carried out on these three lesions at the time of initial diagnostic catheterization due to severity of the disease involving a large extent of myocardium.

Plate 32–2 illustrates the dipyridamole PET images at baseline (top row) and after 15 months (bottom row) of vigorous cholesterol lowering and risk factor modification in a patient with coronary artery disease. At baseline, there is a severe inferior perfusion abnormality on the dipyridamole image. After the 15-month period of risk factor modification, coronary flow reserve in the inferior wall is markedly improved.

New Concepts in Myocardial Perfusion Imaging

For the comprehensive noninvasive diagnosis and management of coronary heart disease based on reversal treatment,[124, 125] the optimal diagnostic test must (1) be noninvasive other than an intravenous injection, (2) have high diagnostic accuracy that is definitive and comparable to or better than that of coronary arteriography to allow the decision regarding lifelong reversal treatment, (3) have proven accuracy in showing the progression or regression of coronary artery disease as well as or better than coronary arteriography, (4) have the capacity to quantify coronary artery function (specifically, resting and maximum coronary flow capacity) that may be impaired by diffuse disease before significant segmental stenoses, ischemia, symptoms, or contractile dysfunction develops, (5) be able to identify the effects of early atherosclerosis or abnormal endothelial function associated with diffuse atherosclerosis before coronary flow reserve is impaired, and (6) be able to quantify absolute myocardial perfusion and perfusion reserve (in ml/min/g) to identify balanced or diffuse three-vessel disease.

Noninvasive cardiac PET fulfills these criteria; it accurately detects localized and diffuse coronary artery disease and assesses its severity, thereby providing a reliable basis for lifelong reversal treatment.[124] PET identifies which coronary arteries are involved and the quantitative severity of disease and is accurate in both asymptomatic and symptomatic subjects. To follow changes in disease severity, either progression or regression, PET is as good or better than coronary arteriography.[124] Therefore, noninvasive diagnostic PET imaging has advanced to or beyond the accuracy and clinical utility of standard coronary arteriography for the principally noninvasive management of coronary artery disease.

Based on several new concepts in perfusion imaging that were developed in our laboratory, PET provides remarkable clinical insights into diffuse coronary artery disease, endothelial dysfunction, and stabilization-reversal treatment of coronary artery disease in individual patients.[124]

- The first of these new concepts in myocardial perfusion imaging is that diffuse coronary atherosclerosis causes a graded base-to-apex, longitudinal perfusion gradient along the long axis of the heart. Relative perfusion is best at the base of the heart, lower in midsections, and lowest at the apex in a continuous graded change, as illustrated by the schematic in Figure 32–7. This pattern of abnormal perfusion is distinctly different from the circumscribed, regional perfusion defects characterizing segmental coronary artery stenoses. Plate 32–3 is an example of a rest dipyridamole PET study in a patient with diffuse coronary atherosclerosis without hemodynamically significant segmental stenoses.
- The second new concept in perfusion imaging is that the endothelial dysfunction of the coronary microcirculation associated with coronary artery disease causes abnormal, inhomogeneous resting perfusion that improves after dipyridamole or adenosine stress.[124] Endothelium-derived nitric oxide maintains resting vasomotor tone and resting coronary blood flow. Smoking, hypercholesterolemia, hypertension, low high-density lipoprotein levels, and coronary atherosclerosis impair endothelial nitric oxide production, causing heterogeneous endothelial dysfunction, heterogeneous increased arteriolar vasoconstriction at resting conditions, and vasoconstrictive responses to stimuli normally causing vasodilation, such as acetylcholine and exercise. This heterogeneous endothelial dysfunction and resting vasomotor tone cause a "moth-eaten" appearance or, when severe, discrete, severe resting perfusion defects on PET images that improve, resulting in more homogeneous perfusion, after dipyridamole or adenosine stress, which are direct arteriolar vasodilators that are not dependent on endothelial nitric oxide (Plate 32–4). In addition, severe endothelial dysfunction may reduce coronary flow reserve, because the component of increased flow due to flow-sensitive, endothelium-mediated vasodilation is impaired.[124]

  After vigorous lipid treatment, endothelial healing begins within weeks to months, before anatomic regression occurs; resting PET perfusion abnormalities improve, reflecting improved endothelial function; stress perfusion defects diminish, reflecting anatomic regression of stenoses; symptoms diminish or disappear; and the risk of coronary events, death, or invasive procedures decreases markedly. Consequently, patients with endothelial dysfunction due to risk factors or due to early diffuse coronary atherosclerosis without significant circumscribed segmental perfusion defects or flow limiting stenoses should be vigorously treated because they are otherwise subject to plaque rupture and a high risk of coronary events.
- The final new concept is that PET perfusion imaging is as good or better than quantitative coronary arteriography for following progression or regression or coronary artery disease (Fig. 32–8).[124] Because coronary flow depends on arterial luminal radius raised to the fourth power, small changes in radii of severe stenoses or in diffuse disease that are difficult to measure with arteriography cause distinct changes on perfusion imaging. Perfusion also reflects the effects of multiple stenoses, diffuse narrowing, and endothelium-mediated vasomotor function of both epicardial arteries and the microcirculation. Consequently, PET perfusion imaging shows the cumulative anatomic and functional changes associated with progression or regression of the entire coronary vasculature more than the limited information obtained from the percent narrowing of one localized stenosis.

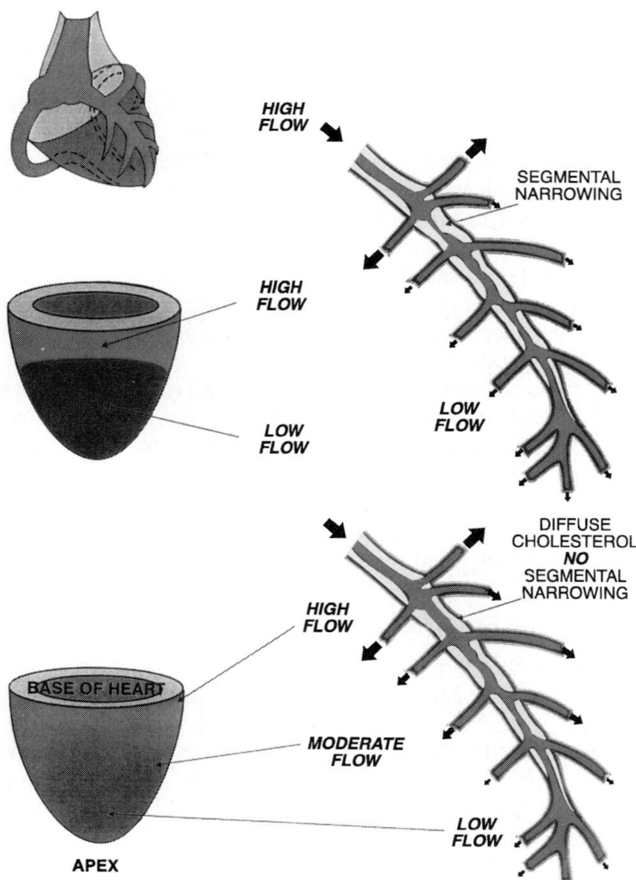

FIGURE 32–7 Schematic illustrates myocardial perfusion patterns with segmental and diffuse coronary artery disease.

Relationship of Positron Emission Tomography Perfusion Imaging to Plaque Rupture, Diffuse Coronary Atherosclerosis, Endothelial Dysfunction, and Prognosis

PET perfusion images must be interpreted in the context of recent extensive documentation of the role of endothelium and plaque rupture in the pathophysiology and treatment of coronary artery disease. *Diagnostic* interpretation of PET perfusion images must recognize and be influenced by the newer *therapeutic* options of treatment to stabilize or partially reverse coronary atherosclerosis based on intense risk factor management and cholesterol lowering.

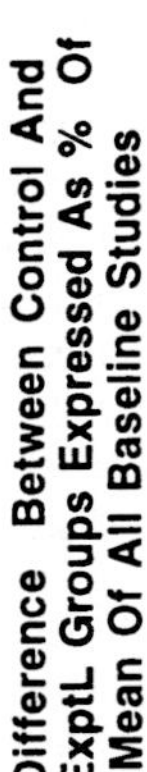

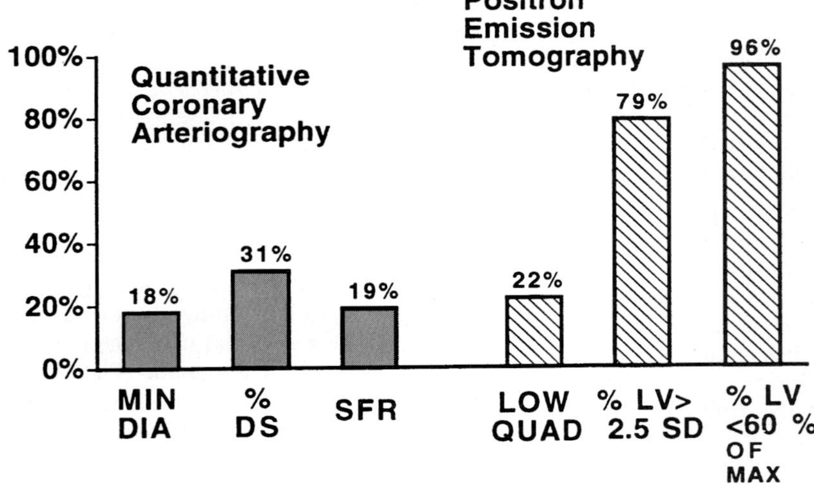

FIGURE 32–8 Myocardial perfusion by positron emission tomography after dipyridamole stress and quantitative coronary arteriography. (From Gould KL: Coronary Artery Stenosis and Reversing Heart Disease, 2nd ed. London: Arnold, 1998, distributed by Oxford University Press.)

Therefore, the guidelines for interpreting and applying PET perfusion imaging require a radical departure from traditional nuclear cardiology using standard SPECT imaging. These new guidelines for PET perfusion imaging are summarized[124]:

1. Owing to accurate attenuation correction, high resolution, and optimal counting statistics, PET perfusion imaging that is performed and viewed correctly is a definitive, stand-alone diagnostic procedure that does not require arteriographic confirmation.
2. The severity of perfusion abnormalities quantitatively reflects the severity of coronary artery disease and its changes with an accuracy at least equal to and usually better than that of arteriography, which fails to account for diffuse disease and the effects of multiple stenoses and is commonly misinterpreted in terms of severity of disease.
3. Severe perfusion abnormalities by PET do not in general require coronary arteriography and revascularization. They require reversal treatment as outlined elsewhere,[124, 125] with revascularization reserved for the minority who have progressive uncontrolled angina despite maximal reversal and antianginal treatment, including immediate vigorous cholesterol-lowering procedures, very low-fat food, and antianginal and antiplatelet drugs.[124, 125]
4. Mild perfusion abnormalities by PET indicate the substrate for plaque rupture and cardiovascular events that requires vigorous, lifelong reversal treatment.[124, 125] A mild perfusion defect by PET implies the same risk as a severe defect by virtue of identifying subjects with coronary artery disease who are subject to plaque rupture. Both mild and severe PET perfusion defects mandate equally vigorous cholesterol lowering and risk factor modification.
5. Coronary atherosclerosis is a diffuse disease with a graded range of severity of narrowing and a graded load of atherosclerosis in the arterial wall independent of luminal narrowing. PET perfusion imaging shows a corresponding range of abnormalities. Consequently, binary classification as normal or abnormal with an associated binary decision for or against coronary arteriography is not appropriate and poor medical practice in view of current knowledge about coronary plaque rupture, diffuse disease, endothelial function, prognosis, revascularization, and cholesterol lowering.
6. Changes in perfusion abnormalities by follow-up PET studies indicate progression or regression of coronary artery disease with an accuracy equal to or greater than that of arteriography due to perfusion reflecting diffuse changes throughout the length of the coronary arteries, perfusion depending on radius changes raised to the fourth power, and altered endothelium-mediated vasomotor function.
7. New approaches to interpreting PET perfusion images and measuring absolute perfusion (in ml/min/100 g) provide insights into diffuse coronary atherosclerosis, endothelial function, progression or regression, and collateral function for clinical management and reversal treatment that is definitive, not available by any other technology, and far beyond information from the standard arteriogram.[124]
8. Clinical reports of PET perfusion images must be written in a way that incorporates this new information while still recognizing the traditional viewpoints of most physicians (or patients) reading those PET reports, who may not be familiar with the implications of this integrated knowledge of coronary pathophysiology and its treatment.

Economics of Positron Emission Tomography

The total charge per PET study, which includes costs of setting up and operating PET centers with the ^{82}Rb generator for cardiac studies, is comparable to the total charges of standard SPECT with thallium or sestamibi. Moreover, the overall costs of cardiac care are reduced by PET due to fewer invasive procedures with comparable or lower adverse outcomes.[124]

Conclusions

Noninvasive management of coronary artery disease based on cardiac PET imaging and reversal treatment is a valid, safe, effective primary step or alternative to invasive procedures that requires patient and physician knowledge. Coronary artery disease should be treated immediately at the time of a firm diagnosis by simultaneous, vigorous risk factor management, low-fat food, and a statin class drug. For the control of high-density lipoproteins and triglycerides, other lipid active drugs should be added or substituted for statins if side effects prevent their use. Low-fat food and weight control through appropriate caloric-carbohydrate restriction are essential for reducing the highly atherogenic postprandial lipid surge that is not significantly reduced by statins. This vigorous reversal treatment, with aggressive antianginal and antiplatelet management as needed, should be used in *every* patient with diagnosed coronary artery disease before elective revascularization procedures are considered. In our experience, the majority of patients will pursue an effective reversal regimen when it is presented and managed appropriately with strong support by a knowledgeable participating physician providing sustained, intense guidance and pharmacologic control. PET can be used to follow progression or regression of disease. For the patients who do not respond to vigorous medical treatment and demonstrate progression of disease, coronary arteriography and revascularization procedures are then appropriate.

Assessment of Myocardial Viability

Flow Metabolism Patterns and Assessment of Cardiac Risk

Retrospective studies have demonstrated the value of flow metabolism patterns for predicting cardiac events. These studies include a total of 388 patients with average follow-up periods of 12 to 23 months.[126–129] Definitions of cardiac events vary among investigations and range from revascularization and unstable angina to hard events like nonfatal myocardial infarction or death. In one study, univariate analysis of various parameters in patients with relatively well preserved left ventricular performance identified the flow-metabolism mismatch as a predictor of future cardiac events.[126] Its predictive power exceeded that of ^{201}Tl stress redistribution scintigraphy. Other studies again confirm the value of the left ventricular ejection fraction as a predictor of cardiac death but again report a strong association between a flow-metabolism mismatch and future nonfatal myocardial infarction and unstable angina.[127] Finally, two additional investigations in patients with severely reduced left ventricular ejection fractions (<0.35) point to the flow metabolism pattern as a discriminator between high and low future cardiac morbidity.[127, 129] For instance, ischemic cardiomyopathy patients without mismatches revealed an about 82 percent survival rate over the 32-month observation period compared with only 50 percent in the presence of extensive flow-metabolism mismatches (Fig. 32–9). These observations are relevant for two reasons: they implicate the blood flow–glucose metabolism mismatch as a potentially unstable condition. The second one is the value of flow metabolism imaging in the clinical setting as a tool for assessing cardiac risk.

Impact of Flow Metabolism Imaging on Patient Management

Most useful has been the assessment of blood flow–metabolism patterns in patients with severely depressed left ventricular function or ischemic cardiomyopathy. In these patients, surgical revascularization is associated with a high perioperative risk, whereas before surgery, the outcome regarding congestive heart failure symptoms or long-term survival rates remains undetermined. It is in these patients when blood flow–metabolism imaging can significantly influence the risk-benefit ratio for surgical revascularization and, thus, aid in stratifying patients to the optimum treatment strategy (Fig. 32–10).

Perioperative Morbidity and Mortality Rates. A report in 76 patients with left ventricular ejection fractions of less than 0.35 suggests a direct impact of flow metabolism imaging on the perioperative mortality and morbidity rates.[130] Perioperative morbidity and mortality rates were compared between two patient groups. In one group, 34 of 41 patients had been selected for surgical revascularization based on flow-metabolism criteria, whereas the other group was selected by standard clinical and angiographic criteria. None of the flow-metabolism mismatch–based selected patients died within 30 days of surgery compared with four in-hospital deaths in the unselected patient group. Similarly, low cardiac output syndrome occurred in only 2.9 percent of patients selected for PET compared with 17.1 percent in unselected patients. A survey of the first postoperative year indicated similar findings. The 1-year mortality rate for PET-selected patients amounted to 2.9 percent but to 14.3 percent in the unselected group. Overall, two thirds of the selected compared with only one third of the unselected patients presented with an uncomplicated postoperative recovery. Although these observations await confirmation, they do imply a potentially important role of blood flow–metabolism imaging in ischemic cardiomyopathy patients for defining the risk-benefit ratio of surgical revascularization.

Revascularization and Clinical Symptoms. Several studies suggest an association between preoperatively demonstrated blood flow–metabolism patterns and postrevascularization changes in the congestive heart failure classification.[128, 129, 131] In one study, for example, 81 percent of patients with extensive blood flow–metabolism mismatches had improved from congestive heart failure class III or IV to class I or II compared with only 23 percent in patients with similar clinical characteristics and mismatches but treated only conservatively.[129] Other studies again reported an improved exercise performance in mismatched patients after revascularization.[132, 133] Another study explored a possible quantitative correlation between the extent of viable myocardium and the postsurgical improvement in physical activity.[131] This study queried patients with ischemic cardiomyopathy for the level of daily activity at the time of the initial blood flow–metabolism imaging study and 25 ± 14 months after surgery. Daily physical activities were converted into metabolic equivalents using a specific activity scale.[134] Of interest, the change in metabolic equivalents from before to after surgical revascularization correlated linearly with the extent of the blood flow mismatches expressed as a percentage of the entire left ventricular myocardium. Even in the absence of mismatches or the presence of only minor mismatches (<5 percent of the left ventricular myocardium), there was a statistically significant, although only very minor, improvement in physical activity, whereas in patients with large mismatches occupying at least 18 percent of the left ven-

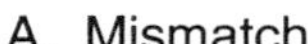

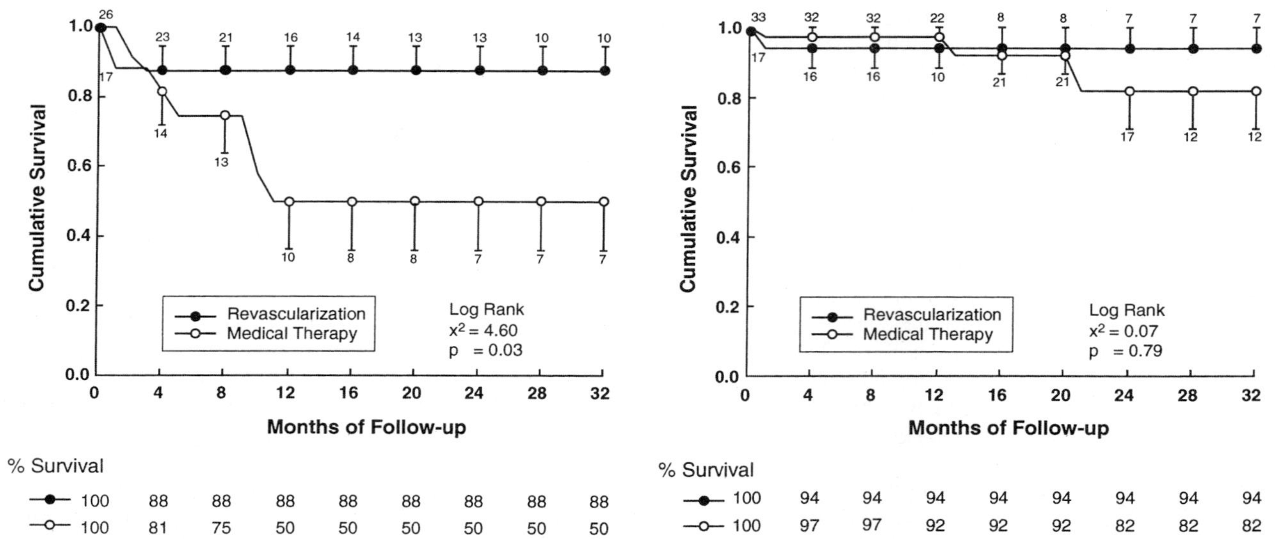

FIGURE 32–9 Survival of patients with severely reduced left ventricular ejection fraction according to the presence **(A)** or absence **(B)** of blood flow metabolism mismatches. The two patient groups are further divided into those undergoing conservative treatment *(open circles)* and those having undergone surgical revascularization *(filled circles).* Note the significant difference in survival rates of patients who have mismatches but were treated medically compared with those who received surgical revascularization. (**A** and **B,** From Di Carli M, Davidson M, Little R, et al: Value of metabolic imaging with positron emission tomography for evaluating prognosis in patients with coronary artery disease and left ventricular dysfunction. Am J Cardiol 73:527–533, 1994, copyright 1994, with permission from Excerpta Medica Inc.)

tricular myocardium, physical activity nearly doubled (Fig. 32–11). There were only moderate improvements in physical activity (by 6 percent on average) in patients with mismatches occupying 6 to 17 percent of the left ventricular myocardium. These observations suggest that the benefit of surgical revascularization on the patient's physical activity, and thus on the quality of life, might be predicted in more quantitative terms.

Survival After Surgical Revascularization. Early data from the Coronary Artery Surgery Study (CASS) reported a statistically significant increment in the 7-year survival rate after surgical revascularization compared with the survival rate in a comparable patient group treated only medically. Yet in the same study, there was no definitive difference in congestive heart failure between both groups. Another study again reports a modest postsurgical gain in left ventricular function in patients with severely impaired cardiac performance.[135] However, as reviewed in the previ-

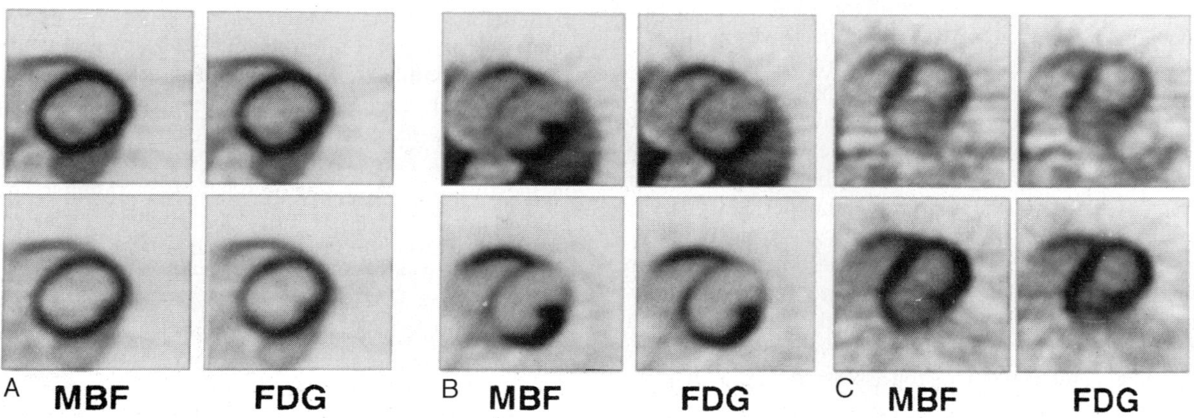

FIGURE 32–10 Blood flow (MBF) metabolism findings in patients with severely depressed left ventricular function. Short-axis cross-sectional images are shown. **A,** Note the homogeneous tracer distribution, consistent with idiopathic dilated cardiomyopathy (DCM). **B** and **C,** This is different from the findings in patients with ischemic heart disease, which demonstrate large, well-defined blood flow defects corresponding to the territory of the left anterior descending coronary artery. **B,** Associated with a concordant reduction in exogenous glucose utilization. **C,** Preserved or even enhanced glucose utilization. FDG, ^{18}F-deoxyglucose.

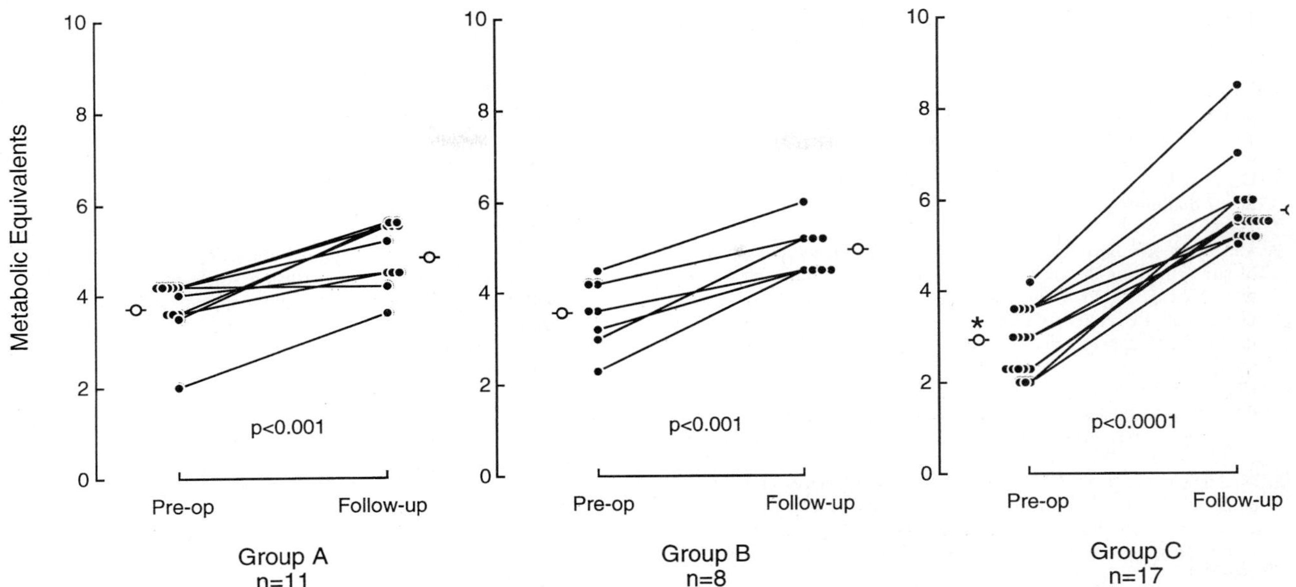

FIGURE 32–11 Amount of viable myocardium and postsurgical improvements in daily physical activities. The data were obtained from patients with left ventricular ejection fractions of less than 0.35. A small but statistically significant improvement occurred in patients with either no mismatch or only a small mismatch (less than 5 percent). Physical activity is expressed here in metabolic equivalents, or METS (see text). However, in patients with large blood flow metabolism mismatches, a marked improvement in physical activity was observed after revascularization. (From Di Carli M, Farbod A, Schelbert H, et al: Quantitative relation between myocardial viability and improvement in heart failure symptoms after revascularization in patients with ischemic cardiomyopathy. Circulation 92[12]:3436–3444, 1995.)

ous section, blood flow–metabolism imaging aided in predicting which patients would and which patients would not have an improvement in their left ventricular ejection fractions as well as congestive heart failure–related symptoms. Blood flow–metabolism imaging may prove equally useful in predicting the long-term survival rate.[129] Compared with medically treated patients with mismatches and an average 50 percent survival rate over 32 months after the PET study, patients with comparable hemodynamic impairments, heart failure symptoms, and mismatches who underwent revascularization demonstrated an 88 percent survival rate during the same time period (see Fig. 32–9). This then implies that the risk of cardiac complications and death associated with a blood flow–metabolism mismatch can be reduced by interventional revascularization.

Current and Future Developments

Much of the evidence presented in this discussion derives from observations made with pure PET. This is especially true for imaging of the myocardial glucose metabolism with ^{18}F-deoxyglucose (^{18}F-FDG), whereas some investigators evaluated regional myocardial blood flow with conventional single-photon–emitting tracers such as ^{201}Tl or ^{99m}Tc sestamibi.[136–138] This hybrid PET/SPECT approach begins to be replaced by a pure SPECT or SPECT-like approach. Comparison studies have demonstrated the feasibility of obtaining myocardial ^{18}F-FDG images with SPECT systems equipped with specifically designed high-energy photon collimators.[139–141] The image quality approached that available through dedicated PET imaging devices. Moreover, SPECT systems equipped with specifically designed high-energy photon collimators can be used for ^{18}F-FDG imaging as well as for depicting the relative distribution of myocardial blood flow using either ^{201}Tl or ^{99m}Tc sestamibi.[142] It appears that such approaches identify myocardial viability with an accuracy that approaches that available with PET. Furthermore, intrapatient comparisons between low dobutamine stress echocardiography and the SPECT-based flow metabolism imaging reported a somewhat superior predictive accuracy for SPECT-based flow metabolism imaging compared with low-dose dobutamine stress echocardiography. Other improvements in imaging instrumentation are in progress. One is the application of true positron emission coincidence detection systems to SPECT-like systems combined with correction of photon attenuation offering the potential for true quantitative imaging. These lower-cost imaging devices, together with the establishment of regional distribution centers for positron-emitting radiopharmaceutical agents in larger metropolitan areas, promise a more widespread availability of metabolic probes for the identification of myocardial viability and for risk assessment in patients with end-stage coronary artery disease.

REFERENCES

1. Hamilton GW: Myocardial imaging with thallium-201: controversy over its clinical usefulness in ischemic heart disease. J Nucl Med 20:1201–1205, 1979.
2. Hamilton GW, Trobaugh GB, Ritchie JL, et al: Myocardial imaging with 201-thallium: an analysis of clinical usefulness based on Bayes theorem. Semin Nucl Med 8:358–364, 1978.
3. Begg CB, Greenes RA: Assessment of diagnostic tests when disease verification is subject to selection bias. Biometrics 39:207–215, 1983.
4. Hlatky MA, Pryor DB, Harrell FE, et al: Factors affecting sensitivity and specificity of exercise electrocardiography: multivariate analysis. Am J Med 77:64–71, 1984.
5. Rozanski A, Diamond GA, Forrester JS, et al: Alternative referent standards for cardac normality: implications for diagnostic testing. Ann Intern Med 101:164–171, 1984.

6. Kotler TS, Diamond GA: Exercise thallium-201 scintigraphy in the diagnosis and prognosis of coronary artery disease. Ann Intern Med 113:684–702, 1990.
7. Tamaki N, Yonekura Y, Mukai T, et al: Stress thallium-201 transaxial emission computed tomography: quantitative versus qualitative analysis for evaluation of coronary artery disease. J Am Coll Cardiol 4:1213–1221, 1984.
8. Garcia EV, Van Train K, Maddahi J, et al: Quantification of rotational thallium-201 myocardial tomography. J Nucl Med 26:17–26, 1985.
9. Van Train KF, Berman DS, Garcia EV, et al: Quantitative analysis of stress thallium-201 myocardial scintigrams: a multicenter trial. J Nucl Med 27:17–25, 1986.
10. DePasquale EE, Nody AC, DePuey EG, et al: Quantitative rotational thallium-201 tomography for identifying and localizing coronary artery disease. Circulation 77:316–327, 1988.
11. Iskandrian AS, Heo J, Kong B, Lyons E: Effect of exercise level on the ability of thallium-201 tomographic imaging in detecting coronary artery disease: analysis of 461 patients. J Am Coll Cardiol 14:1477–1486, 1989.
12. Maddahi J, Van Train K, Prigent F, et al: Quantitative single photon emission computed thallium-201 tomography for detection and localization of coronary artery disease: optimization and prospective validation of a new technique. J Am Coll Cardiol 14:1689–1699, 1989.
12a. Mahmarian JJ, Pratt CM, Cocanougher MK, Verani MS: Altered myocardial perfusion in patients with angina pectoris or silent ischemia during exercise as assessed by quantitative thallium-201 single-photon emission computed tomography. Circulation 82:1305–1315, 1990.
13. Nguyen T, Heo J, Ogilby JD, Iskandrian AS: Single photon emission computed tomography with thallium-201 during adenosine-induced coronary hyperemia: correlation with coronary arteriography, exercise thallium imaging and two-dimensional echocardiography. J Am Coll Cardiol 16:1384–1386, 1990.
14. Nishimura S, Mahmanian JJ, Boyce TM, Verani MS: Quantitative thallium-201 single photon emission computed tomography during maximal pharmacologic coronary vasodilation with adenosine for assessing coronary artery disease. J Am Coll Cardiol 18:736–745, 1991.
15. Gupta NC, Esterbrooks DJ, Hilleman DE, Mohiuddin SM: Comparison of adenosine and exercise thallium-201 single-photon emission computed tomography (SPECT) myocardial perfusion imaging: the GE SPECT Multicenter Adenosine Study Group. J Am Coll Cardiol 19:248–257, 1992.
16. Quinones MA, Verani MS, Haichin RM, et al: Exercise echocardiography versus ^{201}T1 single-photon emission computed tomography in evaluation of coronary artery disease. Circulation 85:1025–1031, 1992.
17. Diamond GA, Forrester JS: Analysis of probability as an aid in the clinical diagnosis of coronary-artery disease. N Engl J Med 300:1350–1358, 1979.
18. Epstein SE, Quyyumi AA, Bonow RO: Sudden cardiac death without warning: possible mechanisms and implications for screening asymptomatic populations. N Engl J Med 320:320–323, 1989.
19. Brown KA: Prognostic value of thallium-201 myocardial perfusion imaging: a diagnostic tool comes of age. Circulation 83:364–381, 1991.
20. Brown KA, Boucher CA, Okada RD, et al: Prognostic value of exercise thallium-201 imaging in patients presenting for evaluation of chest pain. J Am Coll Cardiol 1:994–1001, 1983.
21. Landenheim ML, Pollack BH, Rozanski A, et al: Extent and severity of myocardial reperfusion as predictors of patients with suspected coronary artery disease. J Am Coll Cardiol 7:464–471, 1986.
22. Kaul S, Lilly DR, Gascho JA, et al: Prognostic utility of the exercise thallium-201 test in ambulatory patients with chest pain: comparison with cardiac catheterization. Circulation 77:745–758, 1988.
23. Kaul S, Finklestein DM, Homma S, et al: Superiority of quantitative exercise thallium-201 variables in determining long-term prognosis in ambulatory patients with chest pain: a comparison with cardiac catheterization. J Am Coll Cardiol 12:25–34, 1988.
24. Machecourt J, Longere P, Fagret D, et al: Prognostic value of thallium-201 single-photon emission computed tomographic myocardial perfusion imaging according to extent of myocardial defect: study in 1,926 patients with follow-up at 33 months. J Am Coll Cardiol 23:1096–1106, 1994.
25. Stratmann HG, Tamesis BR, Younis LT, et al: Prognostic value of dipyridamole technetium-99m sestamibi myocardial tomography in patients with stable chest pain who are unable to exercise. Am J Cardiol 73:647–652, 1994.
26. Stratmann HG, Younis LT, Wittry MD, et al: Exercise technetium-99m myocardial tomography for the risk stratification of men with medically treated unstable angina pectoris. Am J Cardiol 76:236–240, 1995.
27. Berman DS, Hachamovitch R, Kiat H, et al: Incremental value of prognostic testing in patients with known or suspected ischemic heart disease: a basis for optimal utilization of exercise technetium-99m sestamibi myocardial perfusion single-photon emission computed tomography [published erratum appears in J Am Coll Cardiol 1996 Mar 1;27(3):756]. J Am Coll Cardiol 26:639–647, 1995.
28. Berman DS, Hachamovitch R: Risk assessment in patients with stable coronary artery disease: incremental value of nuclear imaging. J Nucl Cardiol 3(6 pt 2):S41–S49, 1996.
29. Amanullah AM, Berman DS, Erel J, et al: Incremental prognostic value of adenosine myocardial perfusion single-photon emission computed tomography in women with suspected coronary artery disease. Am J Cardiol 82:725–730, 1998.
30. Hachamovitch R, Berman DS, Shaw LJ, et al: Incremental prognostic value of myocardial perfusion single photon emission computed tomography for the prediction of cardiac death: differential stratification for risk of cardiac death and myocardial infarction [published erratum appears in Circulation 1998 Jul 14;98(2):190]. Circulation 97:535–543, 1998.
31. Hachamovitch R, Berman DS, Kiat H, et al: Incremental prognostic value of adenosine stress myocardial perfusion single-photon emission computed tomography and impact on subsequent management in patients with or suspected of having myocardial ischemia. Am J Cardiol 80:426–433, 1997.
32. Brown KA: Prognostic value of thallium-201 myocardial perfusion imaging in patients with unstable angina who respond to medical treatment. J Am Coll Cardiol 17:1053–1057, 1991.
33. Marmur JD, Freeman MR, Langer A, Armstrong PW: Prognosis in medically stabilized unstable angina: early Holter ST-segment monitoring compared with predischarge thallium tomography. Ann Intern Med 114:336–337, 1991.
34. Greenberg H, McMaster P, Dwyer EM Jr: Left ventricular dysfunction after acute myocardial infarction: results of a multicenter study. J Am Coll Cardiol 4:867–874, 1984.
35. Bigger JT, Fleiss L, Miller JP, et al: The relationships among ventricular arrhythmias, left ventricular dysfunction, and mortality in the 2 years after myocardial infarction. Circulation 69:250–258, 1984.
36. Schuster EH, Bulkley BH: Early post-infarction angina: ischemia at a distance and ischemia in the infarct zone. N Engl J Med 305:1101–1105, 1981.
37. Theroux P, Waters DD, Halphen C, et al: Prognostic value of exercise testing soon after an uncomplicated myocardial infarction. N Engl J Med 301:341–345, 1979.
38. Cohn PF: The role of non-invasive testing after an uncomplicated myocardial infarction. N Engl J Med 309:90–93, 1983.
39. Gibson RS, Watson DD, Craddock GB, et al: Prediction of cardiac events after uncomplicated myocardial infarction: a prospective study comparing predischarge exercise thallium-201 scintigraphy and coronary angiography. Circulation 68:321–336, 1983.
40. Wilson WW, Gibson RS, Nygaard TW, et al: Acute myocardial infarction associated with single vessel disease: an analysis of clinical outcome and the prognostic importance of vessel patency and residual ischemic myocardium. J Am Coll Cardiol 11:223–234, 1988.
41. Hung J, Goris ML, Nash E, et al: Comparative value of maximal treadmill testing, exercise thallium myocardial perfusion scintigraphy and exercise radionuclide ventriculography for distinguishing high- and low-risk patients soon after acute myocardial infarction. Am J Cardiol 53:1221–1227, 1984.
42. Abraham RD, Freedman SB, Dunn RF, et al: Prediction of multivessel coronary artery disease and prognosis early after acute infarction by exercise electrocardiography and thallium-201 myocardial perfusion scanning. Am J Cardiol 58:423–427, 1986.
43. Leppo JA, O'Brien J, Rothendler JA, et al: Dipyridamole-thallium-201 scintigraphy in the prediction of future cardiac events after acute myocardial infarction. N Engl J Med 310:1014–1018, 1984.

44. Younis LT, Byers S, Shaw L, et al: Prognostic value of intravenous dipyridamole thallium scintigraphy after an acute ischemic event. Am J Cardiol 64:161–166, 1989.
45. Gimble LW, Hutter AM, Guiney TE, Boucher CA: Prognostic utility of predischarge dipyridamole-thallium imaging compared to predischarge submaximal exercise electrocardiography and maximal exercise thallium imaging after uncomplicated acute myocardial infarction. Am J Cardiol 64:1243–1248, 1989.
46. Brown KA, O'Meara J, Chambers CE, Plante DA: Ability of dipyridamole-thallium-201 imaging 1 to 4 days after acute myocardial infarction to predict in-hospital and late recurrent myocardial ischemic events. Am J Cardiol 65:160–167, 1990.
47. Tilkemeier PL, Guiney TE, LaRaia PJ, Boucher CA: Prognostic value of predischarge low-level exercise thallium testing after thrombolytic treatment of acute myocardial infarction. Am J Cardiol 66:1203–1207, 1990.
48. Sutton JM, Topol EJ: Significance of a negative exercise thallium test in the presence of a critical residual stenosis after thrombolysis for acute myocardial infarction. Circulation 83:1278–1286, 1991.
49. Miller TD, Gersh BJ, Christian TF, et al: Limited prognostic value of thallium-201 exercise treadmill testing early after myocardial infarction in patients treated with thrombolysis. Am Heart J 130:259–266, 1995.
50. Dakik HA, Mahmarian JJ, Kimball KT, et al: Prognostic value of exercise ^{201}Tl tomography in patients treated with thrombolytic therapy during acute myocardial infarction. Circulation 94:2735–2742, 1996.
51. Mahmarian JJ, Mahmarian AC, Marks GF, et al: Role of adenosine thallium-201 tomography for defining long-term risk in patients after acute myocardial infarction. J Am Coll Cardiol 25:1333–1340, 1995.
52. Tomatis NR, Frerens EE, Verbruyge GP: Evaluation of surgical risk in peripheral vascular disease by coronary arteriography: a series of 100 patients. Surgery 72:429–435, 1972.
53. Hertzer NR, Young JR, Kramer J, et al: Routine coronary arteriography prior to elective aortic reconstruction: results of selective myocardial revascularization in patients with peripheral vascular disease. Arch Surg 114:1336–1344, 1979.
54. Hertzer NR, Beven BG, Young JR, et al: Coronary artery disease in peripheral vascular patients: a classification of 1000 coronary angiograms and results of surgical management. Ann Surg 199:223–233, 1984.
55. Boucher CA, Brewster DC, Darling RC, et al: Determination of cardiac risk by dipyridamole-thallium imaging before peripheral vascular surgery. N Engl J Med 312:389–394, 1985.
56. Leppo J, Plaja J, Gionet M, et al: Noninvasive evaluation of cardaiac risk before elective vascular surgery. J Am Coll Cardiol 9:269–276, 1987.
57. Eagle KA, Singer DE, Brewster DC, et al: Dipyridamole-thallium scanning in patients undergoing vascular surgery: optimizing preoperative evaluation of cardiac risk. JAMA 257:2185–2189, 1987.
58. Eagle KA, Coley CM, Newell JB, et al: Combining clinical and thallium data optimizes preoperative assessment of cardiac risk before major vascular surgery. Ann Intern Med 110:895–866, 1989.
59. Mangano DT, London MJ, Tubua JF, et al: Dipyridamole thallium-201 scintigraphy as a preoperative screening tests. Circulation 84:493–502, 1991.
60. Baron JF, Mundler O, Bertrand M, et al: Dipyridamole-thallium scintigraphy and gated radionuclide angiography to assess cardiac risk before abdominal aortic surgery. N Engl J Med 330:663–669, 1994.
61. Eagle KA, Coley CM, Newell JB, et al: Combining clinical and thallium data optimizes preoperative assessment of cardiac risk before major vascular surgery. Ann Intern Med 110:895–866, 1989.
62. Brown KA, Rimmer J, Haisch C: Noninvasive cardiac risk stratification of diabetic and nondiabetic uremic renal allograft candidates using dipyridamole-thallium-201 imaging and radionuclide ventriculography. Am J Cardiol 64:1017–1021, 1989.
63. Camp AD, Garvin PJ, Hoff J, et al: Prognostic value of intravenous dipyridamole imaging in patients with diabetes mellitus considered for renal transplantation. Am J Cardiol 65:1495–1463, 1990.
64. Eagle KA, Brundage BH, Chaitman BR, et al: Guidelines for perioperative cardiovascular evaluation for noncardiac surgery: report of the American College of Cardiology/American Heart Association Task Force on Practice Guidelines. Committee on Perioperative Cardiovascular Evaluation for Noncardiac Surgery [see comments]. Circulation 93:1278–1317, 1996.
65. Stuckey TD, Burwell LR, Nygaard TW, et al: Quantitative exercise 201-Tl scintigraphy for predicting recurrence after percutaneous transluminal coronary angioplasty. Am J Cardiol 63:517–521, 1989.
66. Cloninger KG, DePuey EG, Garcia EV, et al: Incomplete redistribution in delayed thallium-201 single photon emission computed tomography (SPECT) images: an overestimation of myocardial scarring. J Am Coll Cardiol 12:955–963, 1988.
67. Breisblatt WM, Weiland FL, Spaccavento LF: Stress thallium-201 imaging after coronary angioplasty predicts restenosis and recurrent symptoms. J Am Coll Cardiol 12:1199–1204, 1988.
68. Jain A, Mahmarian JJ, Borges-Neto S, et al: Clinical significance of perfusion defects by thallium-201 single photon emission tomography following oral dipyridamole early after coronary angioplasty. J Am Coll Cardiol 11:970–976, 1988.
69. Ritchie JL, Harahara KA, Trobaugh GB, et al: Thallium-201 myocardial imaging before and after coronary revascularization: assessment of regional myocardial bloodflow and graft patency. Circulation 56:830–836, 1977.
70. Greenberg BH, Hart R, Botvinick EH, et al: Thallium-201 myocardial perfusion scintigraphy to evaluate patients after coronary bypass surgery. Am J Cardiol 42:167–176, 1978.
71. Kolibash AJ, Call TD, Bush CA, et al: Myocardial perfusion as an indicator of graft patency after coronary artery bypass surgery. Circulation 61:882–887, 1980.
72. Gibson RS, Watson DD, Taylor GJ, et al: Prospective assessment of regional myocardial perfusion before and after coronary revascularization surgery by quantitative thallium-201 scintigraphy. J Am Coll Cardiol 1:804–815, 1983.
73. Borer JS, Kent KM, Bacharach SL, et al: Sensitivity, specificity and predictive accuracy of radionuclide cineangiography during exercise in patients with coronary artery disease. Circulation 60:572–580, 1979.
74. Jones RH, McEwan P, Newman GE, et al: Accuracy of diagnosis of coronary artery disease by radionuclide measurement of left ventricular function during rest and exercise. Circulation 64:586–601, 1981.
75. Rozanski A, Diamond GA, Berman DS, et al: Declining specificity of exercise radionuclide ventriculography. N Engl J Med 309:518–522, 1983.
76. Harris PJ, Lee KL, Harrell FE, et al: Survival in medically tested coronary artery disease. Circulation 60:1259–1269, 1979.
77. Hammermeister KE, Rouen TA, Dodge HT: Variables predictive of survival in patients with coronary artery disease: selection by univariate and multivariate analysis from the clinical, electrocardiographic, exercise, arteriographic, and quantitative angiographic evaluations. Circulation 59:421–430, 1979.
78. Mock MB, Ringqvist I, Fisher LD, et al: Survival of medically treated patients in the Coronary Artery Surgery Study (CASS) registry. Circulation 66:562–568, 1982.
79. Jones RH, Floyd RD, Austin EH, et al: The role of radionuclide angiocardiography in the preoperative prediction of pain relief and prolonged survival following coronary artery bypass grafting. Ann Surg 197:743–753, 1983.
80. Bonow RO, Kent KM, Rosing DR, et al: Exercise-induced ischemia in mildly symptomatic patients with coronary artery disease and preserved left ventricular function: identification of subgroups at risk of death during medical therapy. N Engl J Med 311:1339–1345, 1984.
81. Miller TD, Taliercio CP, Zinsmeister AR, Gibbons RJ: Risk stratification of patients with single and double vessel disease and impaired left ventricular function during exercise radionuclide ventriculography. Am J Cardiol 65:1317–1321, 1990.
82. Rapaport E, Remedios P: The high risk patient after recovery from myocardial infarction: recognition and management. J Am Coll Cardiol 1:391–400, 1983.
83. Taylor GJ, Humphries JO, Mellits ED, et al: Predictors of clinical course, coronary anatomy and left ventricular function after recovery from acute myocardial infarction. Circulation 62:960–970, 1980.
84. Multicenter Postinfarction Research Group: Risk stratification and survival after myocardial infarction. N Engl J Med 309:331–336, 1983.
85. Sonnenblick EM, Strobeck JE: Derived indexes of ventricular and myocardial function. N Engl J Med 296:978–982, 1977.
86. Wackers FJ, Terrin ML, Kayden DS, et al: Quantitative radionuclide assessment of regional ventricular function after thrombolytic therapy for acute myocardial infarction: results of Phase I Thrombolysis

in Myocardial Infarction (TIMI) trial. J Am Coll Cardiol 13:998–1005, 1989.
87. Nemerovski M, Shah P, Pichler M, et al: Radionuclide assessment of sequential changes in left and right ventricular function following first acute myocardial infarction. Am Heart J 104:709–717, 1982.
88. White HD, Norris RM, Brown MA, et al: Left ventricular end-systolic volume as the major determinant of survival after recovery from myocardial infarction. Circulation 76:44–51, 1987.
89. Sanford CF, Corbett JR, Nicod P, et al: Value of radionuclide ventriculography in the immediate characterization of patients with acute myocardial infarction. Am J Cardiol 49:637–694, 1982.
90. Corbett JR, Nicod PH, Huxley RL, et al: Left ventricular functional alterations at rest and during submaximal exercise in patients with recent myocardial infarction. Am J Med 74:577–591, 1983.
91. Corbett JR, Dehmer GJ, Lewis SE, et al: The prognostic value of submaximal exercise testing with radionuclide ventriculography before hospital discharge in patients with recent myocardial infarction. Circulation 64:535–544, 1981.
92. Corbett JR, Nicod P, Lewis SE, et al: Prognostic value of submaximal exercise radionuclide ventriculography after myocardial infarction. Am J Cardiol 52:82A–91A, 1983.
93. Borer JS, Rosing DR, Miller RH, et al: Natural history of left ventricular function during the year after acute myocardial infarction: comparison with clinical, electrocardiographic and biochemical determinations. Am J Cardiol 46:1–12, 1980.
94. Dewhurst NG, Muir AL: Comparative prognostic value of radionuclide ventriculography at rest and during exercise in 100 patients after first myocardial infarction. Br Heart J 49:111–121, 1983.
95. Morris KG, Palmeri ST, Califf RM, et al: Value of radionuclide angiography for predicting specific cardiac events after acute myocardial infarction. Am J Cardiol 55:318–324, 1985.
96. Tamaki N, Yasuda T, Leinbach RC, et al: Spontaneous changes in regional wall motion abnormalities in acute myocardial infarction. Am J Cardiol 58:406–410, 1986.
97. Wynne J, Sayres M, Maddox DE, et al: Regional left ventricular ejection fraction: evaluation with quantitative radionuclide ventriculography. Am J Cardiol 45:220–209, 1980.
98. Buda AJ, Dubbin JD, Meindok H: Radionuclide assessment of regional left ventricular function in acute myocardial infarction. Am Heart J 111:36–41, 1986.
99. Sheehan FH, Mathey DG, Schofer J, et al: Effect of interventions in salvaging left ventricular function in acute myocardial infarction: a study of intracoronary streptokinase. Am J Cardiol 52:431–438, 1983.
100. Stack RS, Phillips HR, Grierson DS, et al: Functional improvement of jeopardized myocardium following intracoronary streptokinase infusion in acute myocardial infarction. J Clin Invest 72:84–95, 1983.
101. Serruys PW, Simoons ML, Suryapranata H, et al: Early preservation of global and regional ventricular left ventricular function after early thrombolysis in acute myocardial infarction. J Am Coll Cardiol 7:729–742, 1986.
102. Sheehan F: Cardiac angiography. *In* Marcus M, Schelbert HR, Skorton OJ, Wolf GL (eds): Cardiac Imaging—Principles and Practice. pp. 109–148. Philadelphia: WB Saunders, 1991.
103. Hutchins GM, Bulkley BH: Infarct expansion versus extension: two different complications of acute myocardial infarction. Am J Cardiol 41:1127–1132, 1978.
104. Meizlish JL, Berger HJ, Plankey M, et al: Functional aneurysm formation after acute anterior myocardial infarction. N Engl J Med 311:1001–1006, 1984.
105. Berger JH, Mathay RA, Pytlik LM, et al: First-pass radionuclide assessment of right and left ventricular performance in patients with cardiac and pulmonary disease. Semin Nucl Med 9:275–294, 1979.
106. Maddahi J, Berman DS, Masouka DT, et al: A new technique for assessing right ventricular ejection fraction using rapid multiple-gated equilibrium cardiac blood pool scintigraphy: description, validation and findings in chronic coronary artery disease. Circulation 60:581–589, 1979.
107. Rigo P, Murray M, Taylor D, et al: Right ventricular dysfunction in patients with acute inferior infarction. Circulation 32:268–274, 1975.
108. Slutsky R, Hooper W, Gerber K: Assessment of right ventricular function at rest and during exercise in patients with coronary heart disease: a new approach using equilibrium radionuclide ventriculography. Am J Cardiol 45:63–71, 1980.
109. Starling MR, Dell'Italia LJ, Chaudhuri TK, et al: First transit and equilibrium radionuclide angiocardiography in patients with inferior transmural myocardial infarction: criteria for diagnosis of associated hemodynamically significant right ventricular infarction. J Am Coll Cardiol 4:923–930, 1984.
110. Winzelberg CG, Boucher CA, Pohost GM, et al: Right ventricular function in aortic and mitral disease: relation of gated first-pass radionuclide angiography to clinical and hemodynamic findings. Chest 79:520–528, 1981.
111. Goldberg MJ, Mantel J, Freidin M, et al: Intravenous xenon-133 for determination of radionuclide first pass right ventricular ejection fraction. Am J Cardiol 47:626–630, 1981.
112. Martin W, Tweddel A, McGhie I, Hutton I: Gated xenon scans for right ventricular function. J Nucl Med 27:609–615, 1986.
113. McGhie I, Martin W, Tweddel A, Hutton I: Assessment of right ventricular function in acute inferior myocardial infarction using 133-xenon imaging. Int J Cardiol 22:195–202, 1989.
114. Ham HR, Piepz A, Vandevivere J, et al: The evaluation of right ventricular performance using krypton-81m. Clin Nucl Med 8:257–260, 1983.
115. Bonow RO: Radionuclide angiography in management of asymptomatic aortic regurgitation. Circulation 84(suppl I):I-296–I-302, 1991.
116. Bonow RO, Rosing DR, McIntosh CL, et al: The natural history of asymptomatic patients with aortic regurgitation and normal left ventricular function. Circulation 68:509–517, 1983.
117. Seimienczuk D, Greenberg B, Morris C, et al: Chronic aortic insufficiency: factors associated with progression to aortic valve replacement. Ann Intern Med 110:587–592, 1989.
118. Bonow RO, Dodd JT, Maron BJ, et al: Long-term serial changes in left ventricular function and reversal of ventricular dilatation after valve replacement for chronic aortic regurgitation. Circulation 78:1108–1120, 1988.
119. Kawanishi DT, McKay CR, Chandraratna AN, et al: Cardiovascular response to dynamic exercise in patients with chronic symptomatic mild-to-moderate and severe aortic regurgitation. Circulation 73:62–72, 1986.
120. Alexander J, Dainiak N, Berger HJ, et al: Serial assessment of doxorubicin cardiotoxicity in cancer patients with quantitative radionuclide angiocardiography. N Engl J Med 300:278–283, 1979.
121. McKillop JH, Bristow MR, Goris ML, et al: Sensitivity and specificity of radionuclide ejection fractions in doxorubicin cardiotoxicity. Am Heart J 106:1048–1056, 1983.
122. Hicks K, Ganti G, Mullani N, Gould KL: Automated quantitation of 3D cardiac PET for routine clinical use. J Nucl Med 30:1787–1797, 1989.
123. Gould KL: Coronary Artery Stenosis. New York: Elsevier Scientific, 1990.
124. Gould KL: Coronary Artery Stenosis and Reversing Heart Disease. 2nd Ed. London: Arnold, 1998, distributed by Oxford University Press.
125. Gould KL: Heal Your Heart: How to Prevent or Reverse Your Heart Disease. Rutgers University Press, 1998.
126. Tamaki N, Kawamoto M, Takahashi N, et al: Prognostic value of an increase in fluorine-18 deoxyglucose uptake in patients with myocardial infarction: comparison with stress thallium imaging. J Am Coll Cardiol 22:1621–1627, 1993.
127. Lee K, Marwick T, Cook S, et al: Prognosis of patients with left ventricular dysfunction, with and without viable myocardium after myocardial infarction. Circulation 90:2687–2694, 1994.
128. Eitzman D, Al-Aouar Z, Vom Dahl J, et al: Clinical outcome of patients with advanced coronary artery disease after viability studies with positron emission tomography. J Am Coll Cardiol 20:559–565, 1992.
129. Di Carli M, Davidson M, Little R, et al: Value of metabolic imaging with positron emission tomography for evaluating prognosis in patients with coronary artery disease and left ventricular dysfunction. Am J Cardiol 73:527–533, 1994.
130. Haas F, Haehnel C, Picker W, et al: Preoperative positron emission tomographic viability assessment and perioperative and postoperative risk in patients with advanced ischemic heart disease. J Am Coll Cardiol 30:1693–1700, 1997.
131. Di Carli M, Farbod A, Schelbert H, et al: Quantitative relation between myocardial viability and improvement in heart failure symptoms after revascularization in patients with ischemic cardiomyopathy. Circulation 92:3436–3444, 1995.

132. Carrel T, Jenni R, Haubold-Reuter S, et al: Improvement of severely reduced left ventricular function after surgical revascularization in patients with preoperative myocardial infarction. Eur J Cardiothorac Surg 6:479–484, 1992.
133. Marwick T, Nemec J, Lafont A, et al: Prediction by postexercise fluoro-18 deoxyglucose positron emission tomography of improvement in exercise capacity after revascularization. Am J Cardiol 69:854–859, 1992.
134. Goldman L, Hashimoto B, Cook E, Loscalzo A: Comparative reproducibility and validity of systems for assessing cardiovascular functional class: advantages of a new specific activity scale. Circulation 64:1227–1234, 1981.
135. Hausmann H, Ennker J, Topp H, et al: Coronary artery bypass grafting and heart transplantation in end-stage coronary artery disease: a comparison of hemodynamic improvement and ventricular function. J Card Surg 9:77–84, 1994.
136. Lucignani G, Paolini G, Landoni C, et al: Presurgical identification of hibernating myocardium by combined use of technetium-99m hexakis 2-methoxyisobutylisonitrile single photon emission tomography and fluorine-18 fluoro-2-deoxy-D-glucose positron emission tomography in patients with coronary artery disease. Eur J Nucl Med 19:874–881, 1992.
137. vom Dahl J, Altehoefer C, Sheehan F, et al: Recovery of regional left ventricular dysfunction after coronary revascularization: impact of myocardial viability assessed by nuclear imaging and vessel patency at follow-up angiography. J Am Coll Cardiol 28:948–958, 1996.
138. Schwarz E, Schaper J, vom Dahl J, et al: Myocyte degeneration and cell death in hibernating human myocardium. J Am Coll Cardiol 27:1577–1585, 1996.
139. Burt R, Perkins O, Oppenheim B, et al: Direct comparison of fluorine-18-FDG SPECT, fluorine-18-FDG SPECT, fluorine-18-FDG PET and rest thallium-201 SPECT for detection of myocardial viability. J Nucl Med 36:176–179, 1995.
140. Sandler M, Patton J: Fluorine 18-labeled fluorodeoxyglucose myocardial single-photon emission computed tomography: an alternative for determining myocardial viability. J Nucl Cardiol 3:342–349, 1996.
141. Bax J, Visser F, van Lingen A, et al: Feasibility of assessing regional myocardial uptake of ^{18}F-fluorodeoxyglucose using single photon emission computed tomography. Eur Heart J 14:1675–1682, 1993.
142. Bax J, Cornel J, Visser F, et al: Prediction of recovery of myocardial dysfunction after revascularization comparison of fluorine-18 fluorodeoxyglucose/thallium-201 SPECT, thallium-201 stress-reinjection SPECT and dobutamine echocardiography. J Am Coll Cardiol 28:558–564, 1996.

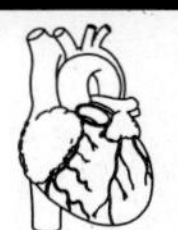

CHAPTER 33

NATURAL HISTORY

Chuichi Kawai and Yasuyuki Nakamura

CORONARY RISK FACTORS AND NATURAL HISTORY OF CORONARY ARTERY DISEASE
EFFECTS OF CORONARY ANATOMY AND LEFT VENTRICULAR FUNCTION ON NATURAL HISTORY
NATURAL HISTORY OF UNSTABLE ANGINA
NATURAL HISTORY OF VASOSPASTIC ANGINA
Long-Term Follow-Up Before the Introduction of Calcium Antagonists
Long-Term Follow-Up After the Introduction of Calcium Antagonists
TYPE AND LOCATION OF MYOCARDIAL INFARCTION AND THE NATURAL HISTORY
IMPACT OF THROMBOLYTIC THERAPY WITH OR WITHOUT ADJUNCT PHARMACOLOGIC AND MECHANICAL PROCEDURE AND PRIMARY MECHANICAL REPERFUSION APPROACH (INCLUDING ANGIOPLASTY AND STENTING) ON NATURAL HISTORY OF MYOCARDIAL INFARCTION
NONINVASIVE CARDIAC TESTS TO PREDICT PROGNOSIS
Rest Electrocardiography
Exercise Stress Electrocardiography
Holter Electrocardiography
Tests With Radionuclide Techniques

The major cause of death in industrialized countries is coronary artery disease (CAD). More than half of the deaths associated with acute myocardial infarction (MI) occur within 1 hour of the event, usually before the patient arrives at the hospital.[1] The cause of death is attributable to arrhythmias, most commonly, ventricular fibrillation. The majority of the studies on the natural history of CAD have been based on data obtained from patients who were able to reach medical facilities.

Data are no longer available on the true natural history of CAD because almost all patients with CAD receive some medical treatment. However, large-scale randomized clinical trials can provide comprehensive information on the relationships between baseline clinical characteristics and the outcome after coronary events because the number of control patients is often quite large. In addition, sophisticated statistical methods can help to identify independent factors that contribute to the natural history of CAD.

Initially, coronary artery bypass graft surgery (CABG) was believed to greatly alter the natural history of CAD. Its use improved survival rates and reduced the incidence of sudden death in certain high-risk subgroups of patients with symptomatic CAD.[2–5] However, in long-term follow-up studies of 5 and 10 years, it was demonstrated that CABG failed to reduce the overall incidence of MI. It did reduce the risk of death after MI, particularly during the first 30 days.[3, 6–8] Thrombolytic therapy may have a major influence on the early prognosis after acute MI. In this chapter, we present an overview of the factors that influence the natural history of CAD and discuss the impact of thrombolytic therapy and other revascularization procedures on the natural history of CAD, along with some of the noninvasive cardiac tests used to predict the prognosis.

CORONARY RISK FACTORS AND NATURAL HISTORY OF CORONARY ARTERY DISEASE

In general, *coronary risk factors* related to the incidence of CAD also contribute to the prognosis after a coronary event. In addition to these factors, clinical characteristics that are specific to the acute phase of CAD contribute to the natural history, as exemplified in a 9-year follow-up of the Perth Coronary Register, which was started in October 1979. Factors that affect the prognosis were assessed in 666 patients who survived for more than 28 days after acute MI of 1078 patients registered for the study. Only 0.3 percent were lost to follow-up.[9] The relationship between 54 variables and the survival rates of the patients was examined, and the following 9 variables were found by multivariate analysis to have important prognostic significance: history of MI, history of stroke, age, male gender, history of diabetes, history of hypertension, arrhythmias as a complication, systolic blood pressure of lower than 115 mm Hg, and heart rate of more than 104 beats/min at presentation. Smoking has been demonstrated to be one of the risk factors for CAD.[10] It was tested in this Perth Coronary Register study but was not found to be an important factor.

Another study showed similar findings. The post hoc study of Global Utilization of Streptokinase and Tissue Plasminogen Activator for Occluded Coronary Arteries (GUSTO-I) analyzed predictors of 30-day mortality after reperfusion for acute MI in 41,021 patients.[11] As shown in Figure 33–1, significant independent contributors to the 30-day outcome by a multivariate analysis were age, lower blood pressure at entry, worse Killip classification, higher heart rate at entry, anterior MI compared with inferior MI, previous MI, time to treatment, diabetes, previous CABG, history of hypertension, history of cerebrovascular disease, and choice of thrombolytic agents. In this study, smoking was associated with lower mortality rates. Other studies

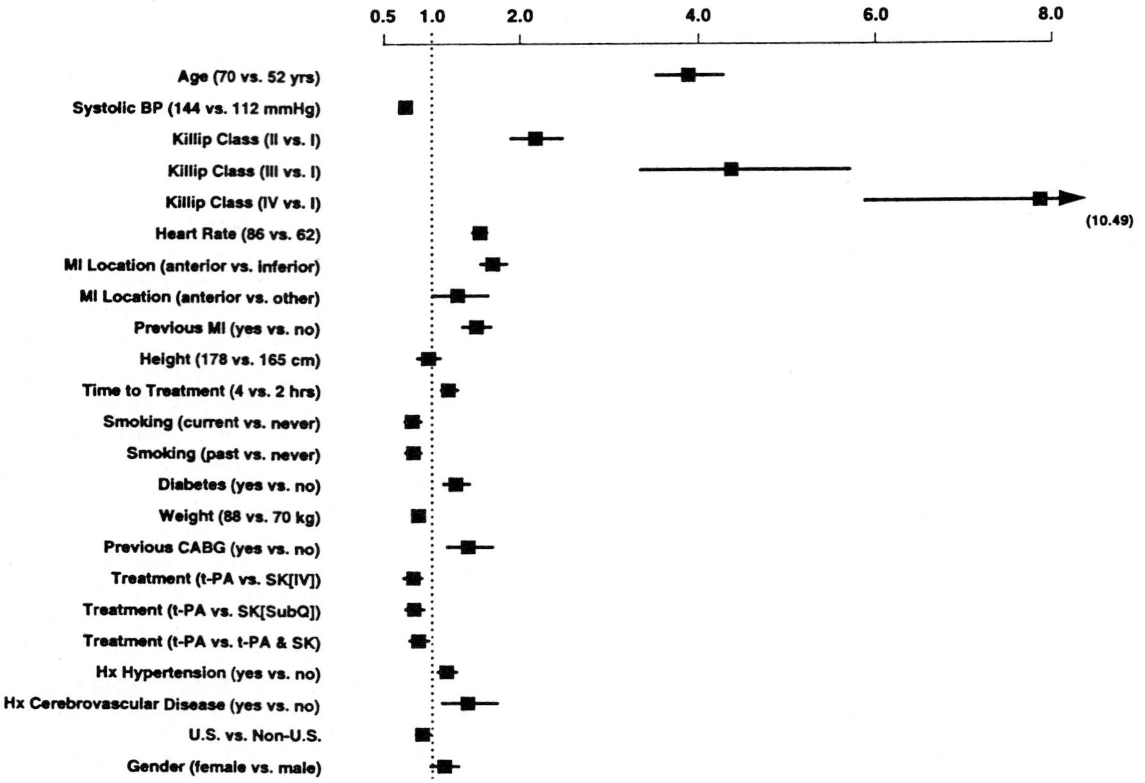

FIGURE 33–1 Relative risk (RR) and 95 percent confidence intervals for variables in the multivariate risk model. Each RR was calculated from a model containing all the factors listed on the left and is adjusted to account for the other variables in the model. BP, blood pressure; CABG, coronary artery bypass graft surgery; Hx, history; MI, myocardial infarction; SK, streptokinase; SubQ, subcutaneous; TPA (t-PA), accelerated tissue-type plasminogen activator. (From Lee KL, Woodlief LH, Topol EJ, et al: Predictors of 30 days mortality in the era of reperfusion for acute myocardial infarction: results from an international trial of 41,021 patients. Circulation 91:1659, 1995.)

have also reported lower mortality rates in patients with a history of smoking.[12, 13] Because abundant data have shown that cigarette smoking is one of the most potent risk factors for CAD, several important points should be taken into account before accepting these findings. As Ockene and Ockene[14] pointed out, a "smoker" in these studies is in fact not a smoker because almost no patients smoke in the hospital after an infarction and posthospitalization quit rates are high. In addition, the known propensity of smokers to die could have resulted in differences in preadmission mortality rates that might have removed a disproportionate number of sicker smokers from the study cohort. Therefore, patients should be strongly encouraged to quit smoking, and coronary events can be used as a window of opportunity.

Determinants of longer-term mortality rates were examined by Volpi and colleagues[15] with the Gruppo Italiano per lo Studio della Sopravvivenza nell'Infarto Miocardico 2 GISSI-2 database. Independent predictors of 6-month mortality rates among 10,219 hospital survivors by a Cox multivariate analysis were ineligibility for exercise test for cardiac or noncardiac reasons, early left ventricular (LV) failure, LV dysfunction in the recovery phase, age of more than 70 years, electrical instability, late LV failure, previous MI, and a history of hypertension. Predictors of long-term mortality rates after a first MI were studied by Kornowski and associates[16] with the Secondary Prevention Reinfarction Israeli Nifedipine Trial (SPRINT) database. A multivariate Cox analysis with a mean follow-up of 5.5 years among 3695 patients after their first MI revealed that age, previous stroke, congestive heart failure on admission, prior angina, and female gender were independent predictors of death from all causes.

Table 33–1 summarizes the results of these four studies. The Perth Coronary Register study and SPRINT were performed before the reperfusion era, whereas GUSTO-I and GISSI-2 were performed during the era of reperfusion. Several predictors are common to many studies, whereas predictors found in only one study may be either not examined or not available in other studies. Age was found to be a predictor of death in all four studies. Previous MI, history of cerebrovascular accident, and hypertension were predictors in three of the four studies. Previous MI was not analyzed in SPRINT because only first-MI patients were included in the analysis. Diabetes, lower blood pressure at entry, higher heart rate at entry, arrhythmia, and early LV failure were predictors of death in two of the four studies. In two studies, conflicting results were obtained regarding gender.

The importance of *gender* in the prognosis of acute MI has been a topic of considerable interest and controversy since before the era of reperfusion therapy.[17–19] Most studies have indicated that women have higher *unadjusted* rates of early and late death, as well as of cardiac events. The

TABLE 33-1 Predictors of Outcome After Myocardial Infarction

Perth Coronary Register	GUSTO-I	GISSI-2	SPRINT
Age	Age	Age	Age
Previous MI	Previous MI	Previous MI	
History of CVA	History of CVA		History of CVA
History of HTN	History of HTN	History of HTN	
Diabetes	Diabetes		
Lower BP at entry	Lower BP at entry		
Higher HR at entry	Higher HR at entry		
Arrhythmia		Electrical instability	
		Early LV failure	CHF on admission
Male			Female
	Worse Killip class		
	Previous CABG		
	Time to treatment		
	Thrombolytic agents		
	Anterior MI compared with inferior MI		
		Ineligibility for exercise test	
		Recovery phase LV dysfunction	
		Late LV failure	
			Prior angina

Abbreviations: BP, blood pressure; CABG, coronary artery bypass graft surgery; CHF, congestive heart failure; CVA, cerebrovascular accident; GISSI-2, Gruppo Italiano per lo Studio della Sopravvivenza Nell' Infarto Miocardico; GUSTO-I, Global Utilization of Streptokinase and Tissue Plasminogen Activator for Occluded Coronary Arteries; HR, heart rate; HTN, hypertension; LV, left ventricular; MI, myocardial infarction; SPRINT, Secondary Prevention Reinfarction Israeli Nifedipine Trial.

worse prognosis for women after acute MI did not change even after the introduction of reperfusion therapy. The apparently worse prognosis in women has been attributed to worse baseline characteristics such as older age and more frequent comorbidity, and the less frequent use of thrombolytic agents, percutaneous transluminal coronary angioplasty (PTCA), and CABG.[20–23] Studies have shown that women who have been treated with thrombolytic therapy for acute MI have the same mortality rates as men after correction for their worse baseline characteristics,[24–26] although one study showed that the incidence of hemorrhagic stroke was higher in women and another showed that the incidence of reinfarction was higher in women even after adjustment. Figure 33–2 shows the results of the Thrombolysis and Angioplasty in Myocardial Infarction (TAMI) trials, in which an apparent increase in the incidence of death and hemorrhagic stroke disappeared after adjustment for baseline characteristics.[25] However, in this study, the reinfarction rate in women was higher even after such adjustment.

Dyslipidemia, especially hypercholesterolemia, is clearly associated with an increased risk for CAD and affects the natural history of CAD. Pekkanen and associates[27] reported the importance of blood cholesterol level as one of the factors that affect the natural history of CAD. They studied 2541 white men, aged 40 to 69 years, for 10.1 years to determine the associations of total cholesterol, low-density lipoprotein (LDL), and high-density lipoprotein (HDL) cholesterol with death from CAD. Seventeen percent of the groups had cardiovascular disease, mostly CAD, at the initial examination. Multivariate analysis revealed that those with "high" blood cholesterol levels (>240 mg/dl) had a 3.45-fold higher risk of death from cardiovascular disease, including CAD, than did those with a "desirable" blood cholesterol level (<200 mg/dl). The corresponding risk ratios were 5.92 for LDL cholesterol levels above 160 mg/dl versus those below 130 mg/dl and 6.02 for HDL cholesterol levels below 35 mg/dl versus those above 45 mg/dl. All three lipid levels were also significant predictors of death from CAD (Fig. 33–3).

The beneficial effect of lowering cholesterol levels, particularly those of LDL cholesterol, with HMG-CoA reductase inhibitors on the secondary outcome of MI has been clearly demonstrated in large-scale clinical trials.[28, 29] It is unclear how low the LDL level should be kept to achieve a beneficial effect after MI. In a post hoc analysis of the

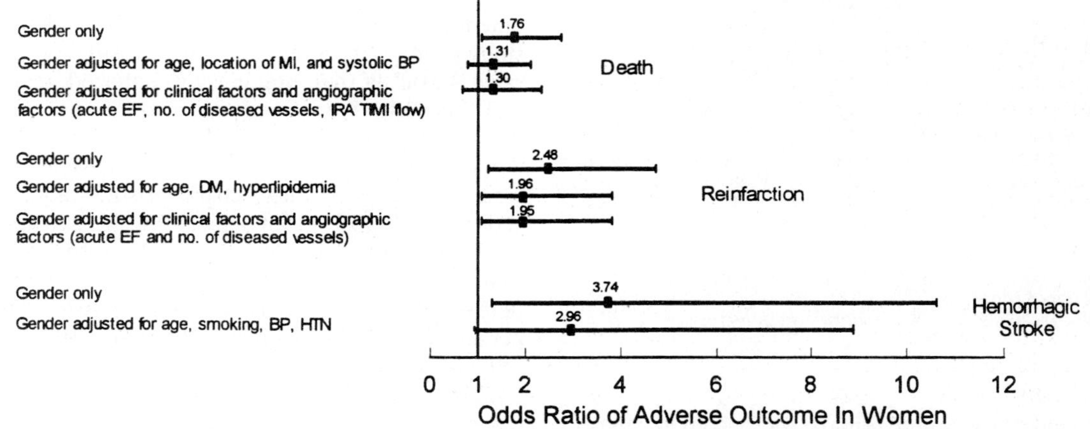

FIGURE 33–2 Multivariate model of the influence of female gender on mortality, reinfarction, and hemorrhagic stroke after acute myocardial infarction (MI), with adjustment for noninvasive clinical factors and angiographic variables. The relative risk of death or reinfarction in women compared with that in men is shown, along with 95 percent confidence intervals. BP, blood pressure; DM, diabetes mellitus; EF, ejection fraction; HTN, hypertension; IRA, infarct-related artery; TIMI, Thrombosis in Myocardial Infarction trial. (From Lincoff AM, Califf RM, Ellis SG, et al: Thrombolytic therapy for women with myocardial infarction: is there a gender gap? Reprinted with permission from the American College of Cardiology [Journal of the American College of Cardiology].)

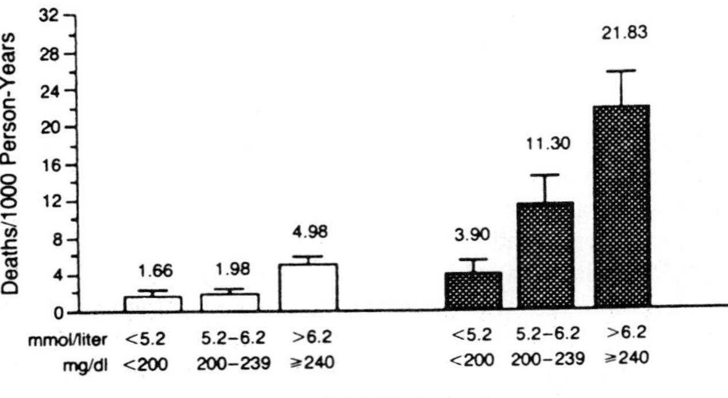

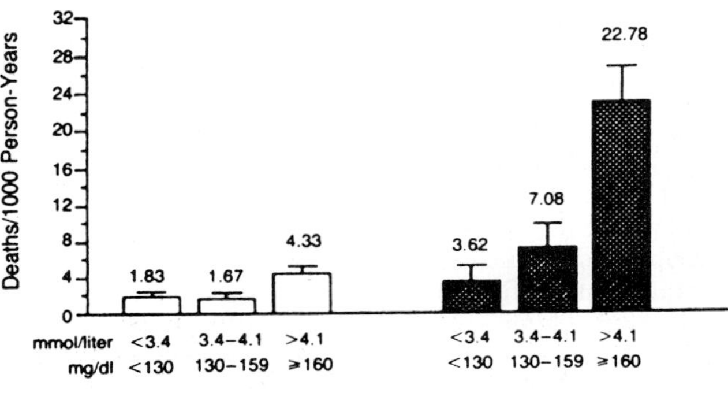

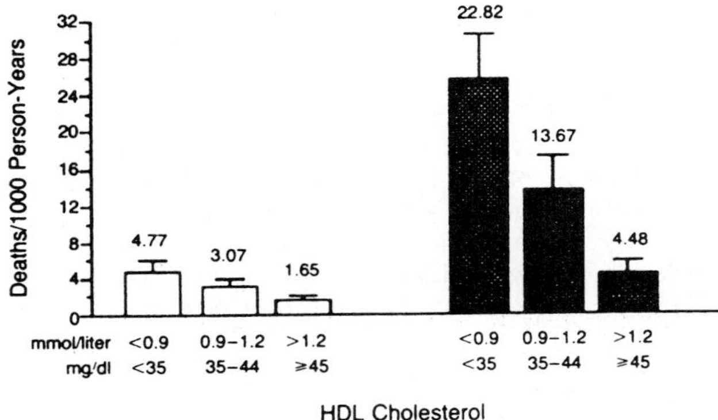

FIGURE 33–3 Age-adjusted rates of death from coronary heart disease per 1000 person-years of follow-up, according to lipid level, for men without evidence of cardiovascular disease at baseline. Men without cardiovascular disease at baseline are represented by *open bars,* and men with evidence of cardiovascular disease are represented by *shaded bars. T bars* indicate standard errors. HDL, high-density lipoprotein; LDL, low-density lipoprotein. (From Pekkanen J, Linn S, Heiss G, et al: Ten-year mortality from cardiovascular disease in relation to cholesterol level among men with and without pre-existing cardiovascular disease. Reprinted, by permission, from the New England Journal of Medicine, 322:1700, 1990. Copyright 1990, Massachusetts Medical Society. All rights reserved.)

Cholesterol and Recurrent Event (CARE) trial database, Sacks and colleagues[30] found that the LDL concentration achieved during treatment was associated with a reduction in coronary events to an LDL concentration of about 125 mg/dl. However, an LDL concentration below 125 mg/dl had little relationship to coronary events (Fig. 33–4).

The significance of *triglycerides* (TGs) as a risk factor for CAD has long been controversial. In general, TG levels predict CAD in univariate analyses, but this effect is often attenuated when other more powerful factors (e.g., HDL cholesterol, diabetes) are entered into the analysis.[31] However, several studies have revived interest in TGs (e.g., TG-rich lipoproteins have been discovered in atherosclerotic plaques,[32] and TGs or hydrolyzed TG-rich lipoproteins have been shown to predict the extent of CAD[33] and the progression of mild to moderate lesions[34]). The effect of TGs on the long-term outcome of CAD was evaluated in the Baltimore Coronary Observation Long Term Study (COLT), which is a retrospective cohort study in 350 patients with arteriographically documented CAD.[35] The subjects experienced 199 events (cardiac death, nonfatal MI, and revascularization) during the 18-year follow-up period. After adjustment for age, gender, and the use of beta-blockers, a Cox analysis revealed that diabetes mellitus (relative risk [RR], 2.1; 95 percent confidence interval [CI], 1.1 to 2.0), HDL cholesterol of less than 35 mg/dl (RR, 1.5; 95 percent CI, 1.1 to 2.0), and TGs of more than 100 mg/dl (RR, 1.5; 95 percent CI, 1.1 to 2.1) were the independent predictors of CAD events. TG levels that have previously been considered "normal" were predictive of new CAD events. The cutoff points for elevated TGs (>200 mg/dl) may have to be refined.

The significance of lipoprotein (a) (Lp [a]) as an independent risk factor for CAD has also been controversial,[36–39] and this controversy has been attributed to differences in study populations, the scarcity of prospective studies, and a lack of standardization for measurement methods and assays. Lp(a) has been shown to be a risk factor for the rapid angiographic coronary progression of CAD in small clinical studies.[40, 41] However, the effect of Lp(a) on the long-term outcome of CAD is not known.

Ethnic differences in the natural history of CAD have been noted since before the era of reperfusion therapy.[42, 43] The survival rate after MI has been reported to be particularly poor in black patients in the United States. A higher frequency of coronary risk factors and other comorbidities, prehospital delay, and the underuse of needed medical care have been suggested to contribute to this apparent poor outcome in black patients after MI.[44–46] The results of a study performed in the era of reperfusion therapy corroborated those of the previously published reports. Taylor and associates[47] analyzed the Thrombosis in Myocardial Infarction Phase II Trial (TIMI II) database, which included 2564 whites, 174 blacks, and 147 Hispanics. Differences were found in baseline characteristics among the three groups, including mean age (whites, 57.2 years; blacks, 54.8 years; Hispanics, 52.8 years, $P < .001$), female gender (whites, 17.6 percent; blacks, 28.7 percent; Hispanics, 14.3 percent; $P < .001$), current smoking status (whites, 11.9 percent; blacks, 22.4 percent; Hispanics, 19.7 percent; $P < .003$), history of hypertension (whites, 36.6 percent; blacks, 55.7 percent; Hispanics, 39.5 percent; $P < .001$), and diabetes mellitus (whites, 11.9 percent; blacks, 22.4 percent; Hispanics, 19.7 percent; $P < .001$). Mortality rates were similar in the white, black, and Hispanic patients during the first year after adjustment for baseline variables. Therefore, if the equal treatment is given and differences in baseline characteristics are taken into consideration, black

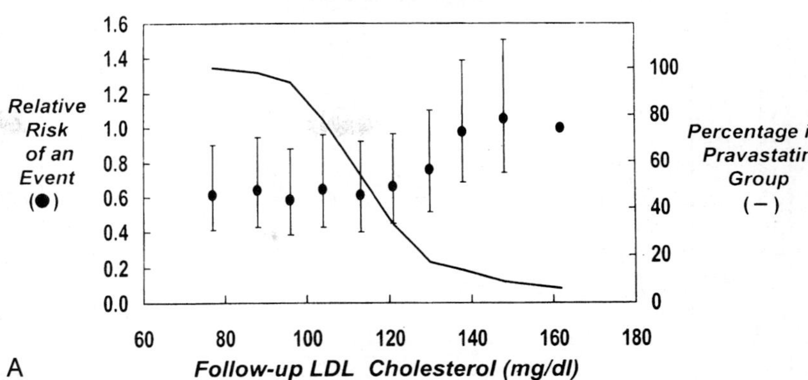

A

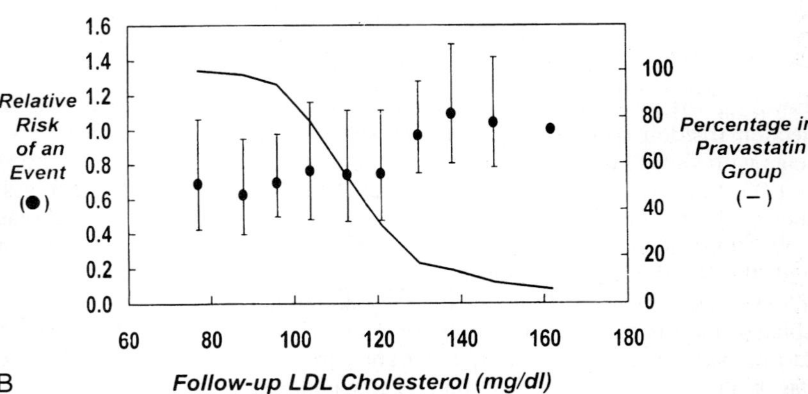

B

FIGURE 33–4 Low-density lipoprotein (LDL) cholesterol concentration during follow-up and coronary events. Placebo and pravastatin groups combined consisted of 4159 patients. **A,** Primary end point was coronary death or nonfatal myocardial infarction (n = 486 patients with end point, 55 in the 10th decile). **B,** Expanded end point consisted of coronary death or nonfatal myocardial infarction, bypass surgery, or angioplasty (n = 979 patients with end point, 111 in 10th decile). Relative risk was determined by a Cox proportional hazards analysis with time-dependent covariates. Data points show relative risks with 95 percent confidence intervals for coronary events for deciles of the follow-up for the LDL concentration. Percentages of patients in each decile of the LDL concentration who were in the pravastatin group are indicated by a *solid line,* corresponding to the right vertical axis. (**A** and **B,** From Sacks FM, Moye LA, Davis BR, et al: Relationship between plasma LDL concentrations during treatment with pravastatin and recurrent coronary events in the Cholesterol and Recurrent Events trial. Circulation 97:1446, 1998.)

patients can expect the same outcome as patients in the other ethnic groups after MI. However, patients in randomized clinical trials may not represent the current general situation, and the differences in unadjusted mortality rates among patients in different ethnic groups may actually be greater than those in these reports.

Recent interest in the association between *gene* polymorphism of several enzymes and the risk of CAD has resulted in several studies and reports. An earlier study of polymorphism of the angiotensin-converting enzyme gene by Cambien and colleagues[48] indicated that the *DD* genotype may be associated with an increased risk of MI. However, later studies could not confirm this finding.[49, 50] The relationship between polymorphism of the angiotensin-converting enzyme gene and the risk of and prognosis after MI was studied by Samani and associates.[51] They found that such polymorphism did not influence either the risk of or the short- to medium-term prognosis after MI. Other gene polymorphisms have been suggested to be associated with the risk of CAD; however, a consensus has not been achieved, and their effects on long-term outcome have not been studied.[50, 52, 53]

EFFECTS OF CORONARY ANATOMY AND LEFT VENTRICULAR FUNCTION ON NATURAL HISTORY

Except for lesions in the left main coronary artery, the extent of LV dysfunction is a more important prognostic predictor than the extent and severity of CAD. The 4-year survival rate for medically treated patients in the Coronary Artery Surgery Study (CASS) Registry was 97, 92, 84, and 68 percent in patients with zero-, one-, two-, and three-vessel disease, respectively[54] (Fig. 33–5). The presence of left main CAD decreased survival rates significantly, and the 4-year survival rate fell from 70 to 60 percent in patients with three-vessel disease when significant obstruction of the left main coronary artery was also present (Fig. 33–6). The survival rate of medically treated patients with CAD in Japan appears to be similar to that of the CASS data. Hiramori and Haze[55] reported that the 5-year survival rate of 1983 patients with angina was 97.7, 93, 88.6, and 84.6 percent in patients with zero-, one-, two-, and three-vessel or left main CAD, respectively (Fig. 33–7). As

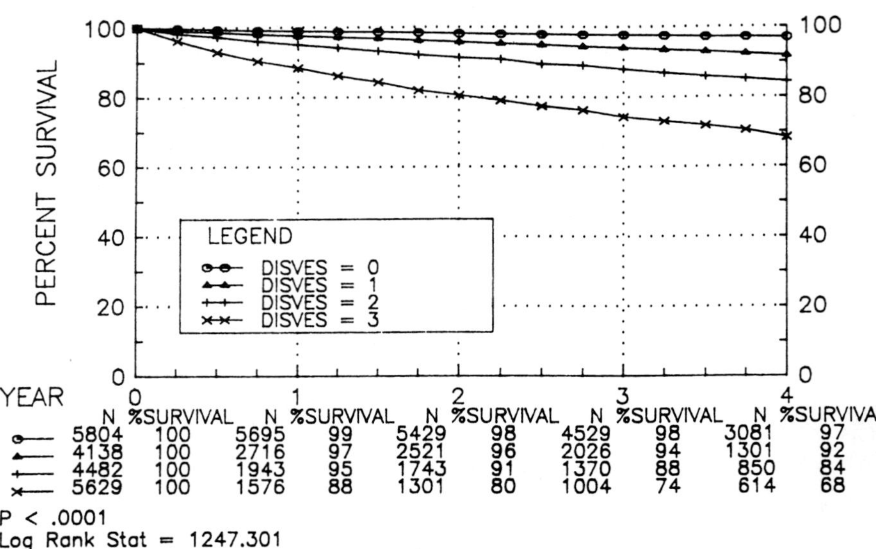

FIGURE 33–5 Cumulative 4-year survival rates for all of the medically treated Coronary Artery Surgery Study Registry patients. Four groups are shown on the basis of angiographic extent of coronary obstructive disease. DISVES, diseased vessels. (From Mock MB, Ringqvist I, Fisher LD, et al: Survival of medically treated patients in the Coronary Artery Surgery Study [CASS] Registry. Circulation 66:562, 1982.)

shown in Figure 33–8, taken from the CASS data, the ejection fraction is an important prognostic indicator. Patients with significant CAD and an ejection fraction of 0.50 to 1.00, 0.35 to 0.49, and 0 to 0.34 had 4-year survival rates of 92, 83, and 58 percent, respectively.

When the quantity of myocardium in jeopardy is considered, the location of the lesion becomes important. Califf and associates[56] analyzed the outcome in 688 patients with isolated stenosis of one major coronary artery. The survival rate of patients with disease of the right coronary artery was higher (96 percent) than that of patients with left anterior descending (LAD) or left circumflex coronary artery lesions, although the survival rates of all three anatomic subgroups were excellent (>90 percent at 5 years). The presence of a lesion proximal to the first septal perforator of the LAD was associated with a lower survival rate than the presence of a more distal lesion. Here, again, the LV ejection fraction was the baseline indicator most strongly associated with survival. In patients with one-vessel disease, the risk of a cardiac event was not related to the presence or absence of collateral channels.[57]

Natural History of Unstable Angina

The syndrome of unstable angina includes angina of new onset *(de novo angina),* angina occurring with increasing frequency *(crescendo angina),* anginal attacks occurring with progressively less effort *(changing pattern),* and an-

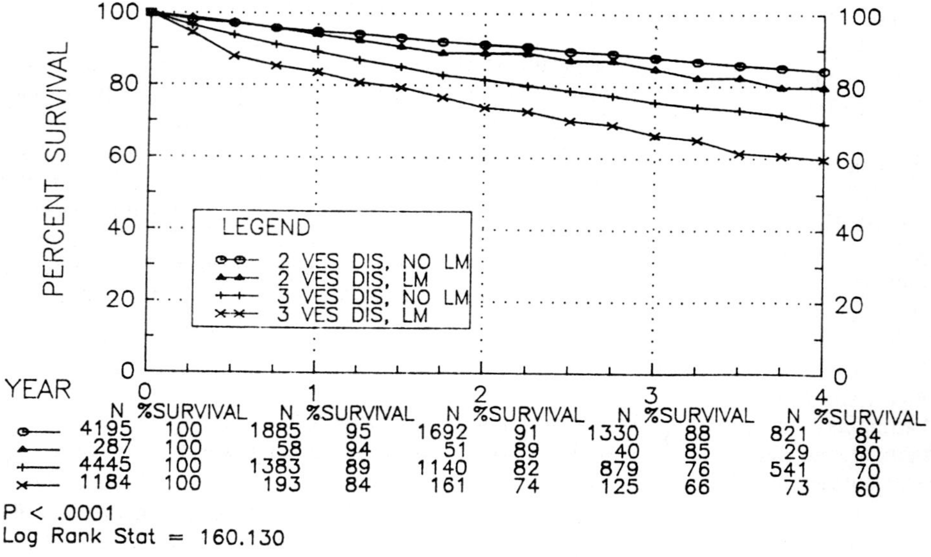

FIGURE 33–6 Cumulative 4-year survival rates of Coronary Artery Surgery Study Registry patients with two- and three-vessel disease (VES DIS) without left main coronary artery disease (LM) compared with the survival rates of patients with two- and three-vessel disease with left main coronary artery disease. (From Mock MB, Ringqvist I, Fisher LD, et al: Survival of medically treated patients in the Coronary Artery Surgery Study [CASS] Registry. Circulation 66:562, 1982.)

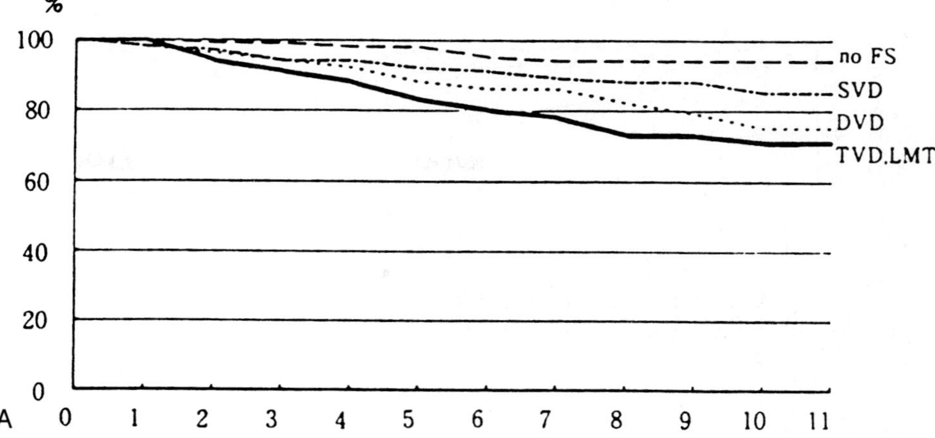

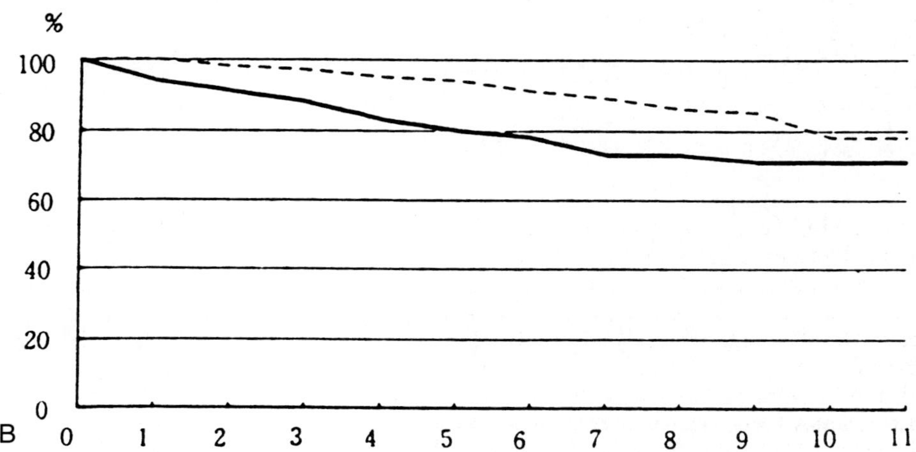

FIGURE 33–7 Cumulative survival curve after coronary angiography in patients with angina pectoris in Japan. **A,** Cumulative survival curve after coronary angiography in patients with angina pectoris. DVD, two-vessel coronary artery disease; LMT, left main coronary artery disease; no FS, no significant stenosis; SVD, one-vessel coronary artery disease; TVD, three-vessel coronary artery disease. **B,** Cumulative survival curves of patients with three-vessel coronary artery disease. Left main coronary artery disease treated medically *(solid line)* or surgically *(dashed line).* (From Hiramori K, Haze K: Pathophysiology, therapy and prognosis of angina pectoris. Jpn J Med 79:91, 1990.)

gina at rest. Patients with new-onset angina tended to have less severe CAD than those with chronic stable angina, but they were at an increased risk of a cardiac event (16 versus 7 percent at 1 year). There were no significant differences in survival rates between those with new-onset angina and those with chronic angina.[58] As a group, patients with unstable angina have an in-hospital mortality rate of about 1 percent and a 1-year mortality rate of 8 to 18 percent. Nonfatal MI occurs in 7 to 9 percent of patients in the hospital and in 14 to 22 percent by the end of 1 year.[58–60] The prognosis was worse in patients with unstable angina who did not respond to intensive medical treatment, in those with persistent ECG changes with symptoms, and in those with episodes of silent myocardial ischemia.[60, 61]

NATURAL HISTORY OF VASOSPASTIC ANGINA

This variant type of angina pectoris was first described by Prinzmetal and associates[62] and is characterized by recurrent attacks of chest pain at rest, often occurring at about the same time each day, associated with ST-segment elevation on electrocardiography (ECG). Its cause was initially considered to be a temporarily increased tonus of a large narrowed coronary artery,[62] but it is now known to be due to spasm of a major coronary artery,[63, 64] which can result in segmental vessel constriction.

Long-Term Follow-Up Before the Introduction of Calcium Antagonists

Before the era of calcium antagonists, Prinzmetal and associates[65] reported that at least 11 of 35 patients (30 percent) with the variant form of angina pectoris had MI. In a study of 59 patients with variant angina and without fixed coronary stenosis followed for an average of 5.9 years between 1962 and 1981, with calcium antagonist therapy used after 1976, MI occurred in 19 percent, but there were no cardiac deaths. Calcium antagonists controlled symptoms in 83 percent of patients unresponsive to nitrates.[66]

Long-Term Follow-Up After the Introduction of Calcium Antagonists

There are two studies[67, 68] of at least 200 patients with variant angina followed for 5 years or more: one from Canada and the other from Japan.

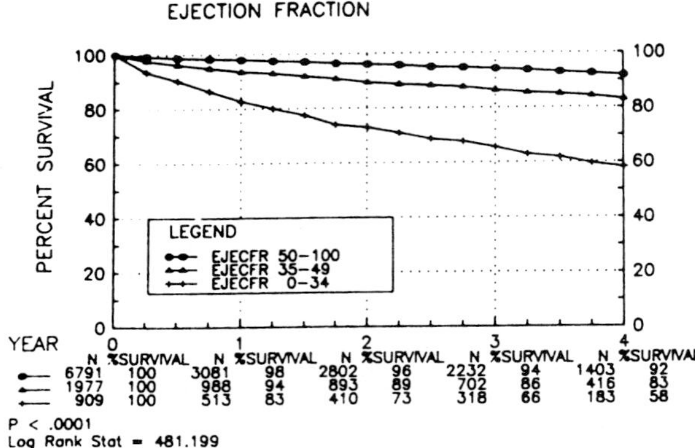

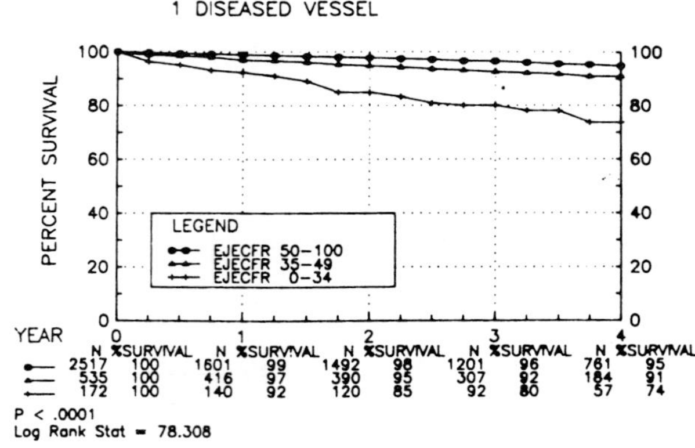

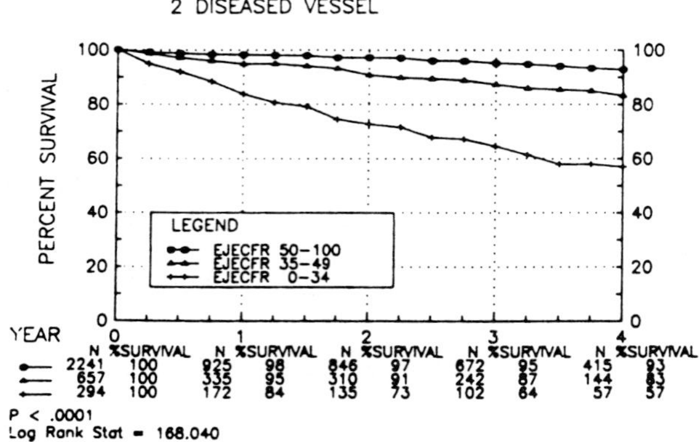

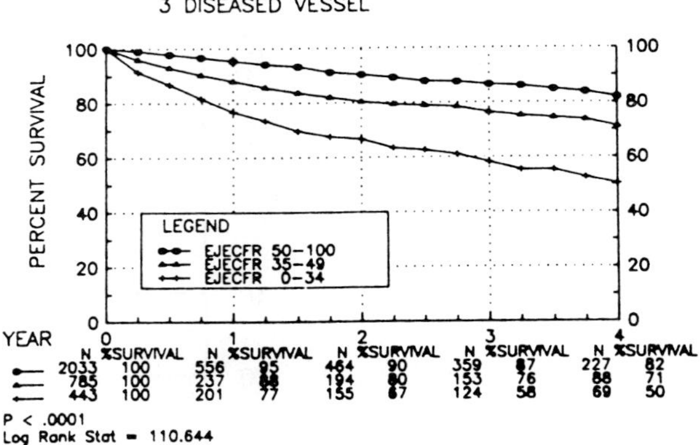

FIGURE 33–8 Four-year survival data for patients with at least one-vessel disease, less than 50 percent left main coronary artery obstruction, and a measured ejection fraction (EJECFR). (From Mock MB, Ringqvist I, Fisher LD, et al: Survival of medically treated patients in the Coronary Artery Surgery Study [CASS] Registry. Circulation 66:562, 1982.)

Survival Rate and Survival Rate Without Myocardial Infarction

The overall survival rate at 1, 3, and 5 years was 95, 92, and 89 percent, respectively, in Canada and 98, 97, and 97 percent, respectively, in Japan. The survival rate without MI at 1, 3, and 5 years was 83, 77, and 69 percent, respectively, in Canada and 86, 85, and 83 percent, respectively, in Japan (Fig. 33–9). In Canada, the 5-year survival rate was 94 percent or greater for patients with one-vessel disease and without significant stenosis but only 77 percent for those with multivessel disease.[67]

Cardiac death occurred in 30 patients (14 percent), and an additional 54 (25 percent) had a nonfatal MI in the Canadian study.[67] On the other hand, only 12 (5 percent) of 245 patients died from cardiovascular disease, and 32 patients (13 percent) developed nonfatal acute MI in the Japanese series.[68] Nine (30 percent) of 30 deaths in Canada and 5 (42 percent) of 12 deaths in Japan and 22 (41 percent) of 54 MIs in Canada and 15 (47 percent) of 32 MIs in Japan occurred during the first 3 months of follow-up.[67, 68] There is general agreement that regardless of ethnic differences, cardiac death and MI occur most often within 1 to 3 months[67–69] after the appearance of variant angina when vasospastic activity is high. Cardiac events, including cardiac deaths, appear to be less frequent among Japanese patients with variant angina treated with calcium antagonists.[68–70]

Factors Influencing the Prognosis

The extent and severity of CAD appear to be important prognostic determinants of survival and of survival without MI in patients with variant angina in studies of more than 100 patients.[71, 72] Although Yasue and colleagues[68] agreed that the extent and severity of CAD are significant independent predictors of survival without MI, in patients with variant angina, they demonstrated no significant association between the extent and severity of CAD and the overall survival rate. Six of 12 deaths occurred suddenly in patients who had no significant coronary stenosis.[68] Other authors,[70, 73] including those in the Japanese multicenter study, also found no association between sudden death and the extent and severity of CAD in patients with variant angina.

ST-segment elevation in both the anterior and inferior electrocardiographic leads during an attack was the most significant predictor of reduced survival by univariate analysis. Five of seven sudden deaths occurred in patients with multivessel coronary spasm.[68]

Because LV function correlated well with the severity and extent of CAD, this variable was a good predictor of survival without MI.[67, 68]

Treatment with calcium antagonists was a significant factor influencing survival without MI.[68, 70, 74] Calcium antagonists should not be discontinued, particularly in patients with multivessel coronary spasm and during the period of elevated disease activity.

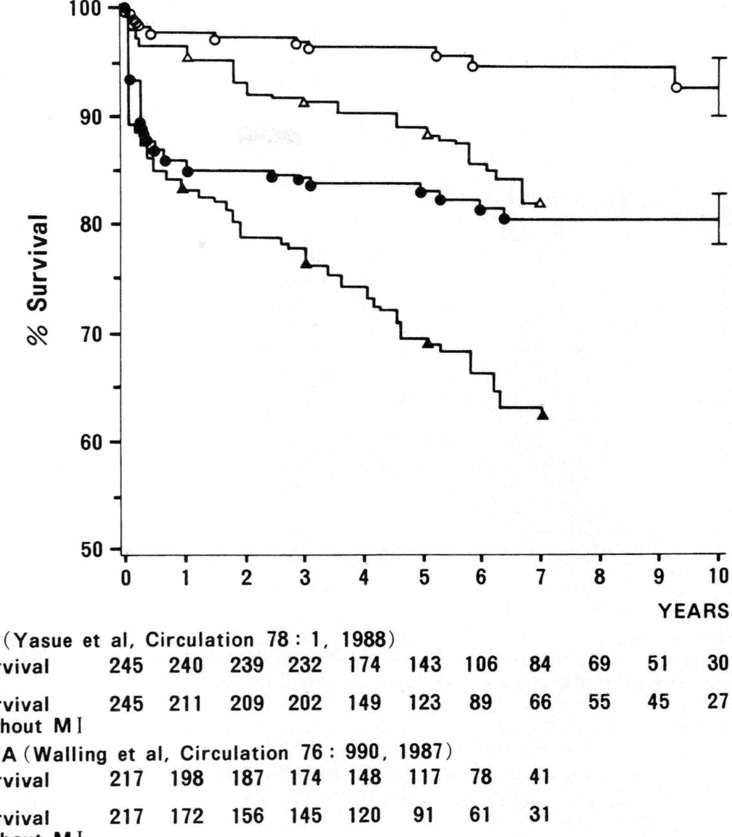

FIGURE 33–9 Comparison of survival and survival without myocardial infarction rates in patients with variant angina in Canada and Japan. Numbers at the bottom indicate numbers of patients at risk each year. *Vertical bars* indicate standard errors. MI, myocardial infarction. (Modified from Walling A, Waters DD, Miller DD, et al: Long-term prognosis of patients with variant angina. Circulation 76:990, 1987, and Yasue H, Takizawa A, Nagao M, et al: Long-term prognosis for patients with variant angina and influential factors. Circulation 78:1, 1988.)

Smoking and alcohol intake had adverse effects on survival rates in patients with variant angina. Sudden death has been reported to occur after the ingestion of large amounts of alcohol.

TYPE AND LOCATION OF MYOCARDIAL INFARCTION AND THE NATURAL HISTORY

Although earlier studies[75, 76] demonstrated that anterior MI carried a higher risk of death than inferior MI, one study[77] showed by both univariate and survival analyses the lack of a strong association between anterior MI and death. In that study, a low ejection fraction, ventricular ectopy of 10 or more depolarizations per hour, advanced New York Heart Association functional class before infarction, and rales heard in the upper two thirds of the lung fields while the patient was in the coronary care unit were the four risk factors independently predicting death (Fig. 33–10 and Table 33–2). These variables probably represent important functional information that is related to an unfavorable outcome in patients with anterior MI.

Although some studies have shown that the in-hospital mortality rate after acute non–Q wave infarction is higher than that after acute Q- wave MIs,[78] the majority of studies indicate that non–Q wave MI has a better prognosis in hospital but that this advantage is lost over time.[79, 80] It has been suggested that this is because patients with non–Q wave MIs have "incomplete infarctions" (i.e., they have more residual viable but unstable myocardium within the perfusion zone of the infarct-related vessel than do patients with acute Q-wave MIs). Therefore, it is not surprising that reinfarction, postinfarction angina, and the need for CABG appear to be higher in patients with non–Q wave MI.[80–86]

IMPACT OF THROMBOLYTIC THERAPY WITH OR WITHOUT ADJUNCT PHARMACOLOGIC AND MECHANICAL PROCEDURE AND PRIMARY MECHANICAL REPERFUSION APPROACH (INCLUDING ANGIOPLASTY AND STENTING) ON NATURAL HISTORY OF MYOCARDIAL INFARCTION

The most important factor in determining the clinical course after acute MI is undoubtedly the ultimate size of the infarct. It is therefore mandatory to maintain an optimal balance between myocardial oxygen supply and demand so as much of the jeopardized zone of the myocardium surrounding the necrotic zone of the infarct can be salvaged.

Thrombolytic therapy to recanalize occluded coronary arteries within the first several hours has been demonstrated

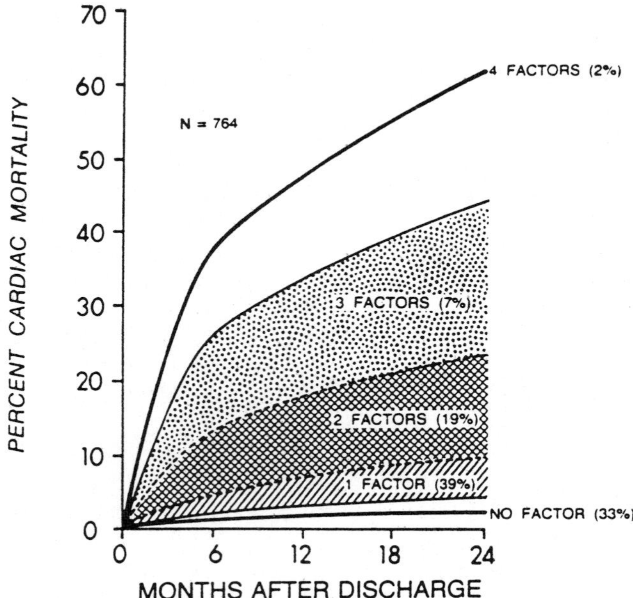

FIGURE 33–10 Mortality curves after discharge and zones of risk, according to number of risk factors. The risk factors were New York Heart Association functional classes II through IV before admission, pulmonary rales, occurrence of 10 or more ventricular ectopic depolarizations per hour, and a radionuclide ejection fraction of less than 0.40. The variation of risk within each zone reflects the spectrum of relative risk for individual factors (see Table 33–3) as well as the range of multiplicative risks for combinations of two and three factors. Numbers in parentheses denote the percentage of the population with the specified number of factors. (From the Multicenter Postinfarction Research Group: Risk stratification and survival after myocardial infarction. Reprinted, by permission, from the New England Journal of Medicine, 309:331, 1983. Copyright 1983 Massachusetts Medical Society. All rights reserved.)

to reduce infarct size, and thereby cardiac dysfunction and mortality rates. Although long-term follow-up has not yet been accomplished, it is evident that early reperfusion therapy has dramatically changed the natural course of acute MI.

The intravenous administration of thrombolytic agents such as streptokinase,[87, 88] recombinant tissue plasminogen activator (rt-PA),[89–95] anisolated plasminogen streptokinase complex,[96, 97] or recombinant prourokinase[98] within a few hours after the onset of chest pain has been proven to reduce short-term and in-hospital mortality rates. A few large scale trials have also demonstrated lower long-term mortality rates in patients followed for 1 year or longer.[88, 96, 99, 100]

Early coronary reocclusion after thrombolytic therapy, as well as reocclusion after PTCA, poses a serious problem in the management of acute MI. Because rethrombosis of the vessel tends to occur in those with severe residual coronary stenosis,[101] it is common practice in many institutions to carry out PTCA in those with suitable anatomy after thrombolytic therapy. However, the timing of rescue or prophylactic PTCA is still controversial because the risks of this therapeutic approach sometimes outweigh the benefits.

With 1636 patients randomly assigned to prophylactic PTCA if arteriography demonstrated suitable anatomy 18 to 48 hours after the administration of rt-PA, the TIMI-II study[102] concluded that the invasive prophylactic PTCA offered no advantages in the reduction in mortality or reinfarction rates, within the first 6 days and at 42 days, over a more conservative strategy in which PTCA was performed only in patients with spontaneous or exercise-induced ischemia. Immediate PTCA after thrombolytic therapy with rt-PA did not increase the ejection fraction more than PTCA performed 18 to 48 hours later, and it may even be harmful.[103] Similar results were obtained in several other large scale trials.[104–107] As a result, the general consensus up until the early 1990s seemed to support an approach that included the early intravenous administration of thrombolytic agents and deferred PTCA. However, because the importance of early[108, 109] and thorough[110] (TIMI grade 3) recanalization after the onset of acute MI has been advocated, the impact of a more aggressive approach,[111, 112] including the combination of thrombolytic therapy and immediate or rescue PTCA with or without stent deployment, on the natural history of patients with acute MI should be reappraised. The recent appearance of mutant t-PA,[113, 114] which can be administered via a single or double bolus intravenous injection, and improvements in interventional techniques and equipment have made a rapid and thorough recanalization after acute MI feasible.

Due to high recanalization rates (>90 percent), low in-hospital mortality rates (approximately 8 percent), and favorable 1-year survival rates (>90 percent), primary PTCA[115] has been advocated as the treatment of choice in patients with acute MI. Primary PTCA with or without stent deployment may also improve the natural history of MI. However, comparisons of primary PTCA and thrombolysis still provide controversial results in small numbers of patients[116–120] with relatively short-term effects. An ob-

TABLE 33–2 Contribution of the Preselected Risk Factors to the Final Survival Model

	Relative Risk*	χ Factor	*P* Value
Ejection fraction < 0.40	2.4 (1.5–3.7)	12.3	<.001
VED ≥ 10/h	1.6 (1.0–2.6)	3.8	<.05
Rales > bibasilar	3.3 (2.1–5.2)	20.5	<.001
NYHA class II–IV†	1.9 (1.2–3.0)	8.1	<.01
Time after hospitalization			
0–3 mo	4.0 (2.2–7.2)	33.5	<.001
3–6 mo	2.8 (1.6–5.1)		
6–12 mo	1.3 (0.8–2.4)		

Abbreviations: NYHA, New York Heart Association; VED, ventricular ectopic depolarization.

*Ratio of the risk of dying per unit of time (hazard rate) for patients with factor present to risk for patients with factor absent. For the time factors, the risk is relative to the probability of dying 12 to 36 mo after discharge. The relative risk ratios were derived from the survival analyses. Parentheses contain the 95 percent confidence intervals.

†NYHA functional classification 1 mo before entry. From The Multicenter Postinfarction Research Group: Risk stratification and survival after myocardial infarction. N Engl J Med 309:331, 1983. Copyright 1983 Massachusetts Medical Society. All rights reserved.

servational study[121] of more than 3000 patients in a community setting revealed that primary PTCA did not offer any benefit with regard to mortality rates or medical costs at the time of hospital discharge and after 3 years of follow-up. Moreover, in the same cohort of patients with acute MI, patients admitted to hospitals without on-site catheterization facilities who were managed with fewer procedures did not demonstrate any increase in long-term (3 years) mortality rates.[122] Therefore, the general consensus seems to be that the primary goal of treatment for patients with acute MI should be the rapid, complete, and sustained restoration of infarct-related coronary arterial flow and that the best therapy for an individual patient is that which can be applied most safely and expeditiously,[123, 124] regardless of whether it is thrombolytic treatment or primary PTCA with or without stent deployment.

The use of adjunct thrombolytic therapy for acute MI is also controversial. At 7 to 24 hours after the beginning of rt-PA infusion, 82 percent of the infarct-related arteries in 106 patients randomly assigned to immediate and then continuous intravenous heparin were patent compared with only 52 percent in the 99 patients assigned to immediate heparin therapy and then daily oral aspirin ($P < .0001$).[125] Subcutaneous calcium-heparin in patients treated with or without intravenous streptokinase reduced in-hospital mortality rates more than in the nonheparinized group (5.8 versus 9.9 percent; $P = .03$).[126] On the other hand, in 64 patients randomly assigned to receive t-PA (1.5 mg/kg/4 h) and a bolus of 10,000 units of heparin, the predischarge LV ejection fraction was not significantly greater than that in 70 patients receiving t-PA alone at the same dose. These authors concluded that early intravenous heparin does not facilitate the fibrinolytic effect of t-PA and that heparin therapy can be deferred for at least 60 to 90 minutes after t-PA has been initiated.[127] In another study,[128] after thrombolytic therapy with rt-PA and a bolus of 5000 units of heparin IV followed by 1000 U/h intravenous heparin IV for 24 hours, 202 patients were randomized to continue to receive intravenous heparin (99 patients) or to discontinue heparin therapy and begin oral aspirin and dipyridamole (300 mg/day of each; 103 patients). There were no differences between the two groups in patency rates of the infarct-related artery at 7 to 10 days or in LV ejection fraction at 1 month. It was concluded that heparin therapy can be discontinued 24 hours after rt-PA therapy and replaced with an oral antiplatelet medication. The GISSI[129] and ISIS-3[130] trials demonstrated a small but significant increased incidence of intracerebral hemorrhage and major noncerebral bleeding with the addition of heparin to the thrombolysis and aspirin regimen. Moreover, in a large cohort of older MI patients (6935 patients ≥ 65 years old) who did not undergo reperfusion therapy, the routine use of intravenous heparin was not associated with an improved 30-day mortality rate.[131]

A large-scale international trial[132] (41,021 patients with acute MI) documented a reduction in 30-day mortality rates with accelerated t-PA (*accelerated* refers to the administration of t-PA over a period of 90 minutes, with two thirds of the dose given in the first 30 minutes, rather than the conventional period of 3 hours) administered with aspirin and heparin IV by 14 percent compared with streptokinase, aspirin, and subcutaneous or intravenous heparin and by 10 percent compared with the combination of streptokinase, t-PA, aspirin, and intravenous heparin. The rate of hemorrhagic stroke was significantly increased with accelerated t-PA ($P = .03$) compared with that with streptokinase alone, but the incidence of the combined end point of death or disabling stroke was significantly lower in the accelerated t-PA group than in the streptokinase-only groups (6.9 versus 7.8 percent, $P = .006$). The 1-year mortality rate with accelerated t-PA (9.1 percent) was less than rates for streptokinase with subcutaneous heparin (10.1 percent, $P = .011$), streptokinase with heparin IV (10.1 percent, $P = .009$), and the combination of streptokinase and t-PA (9.9 percent, $P = .05$)[133] (Fig. 33–11).

The direct antithrombin agent hirudin, as adjunct therapy for thrombolysis in MI, provided a small advantage[134] or

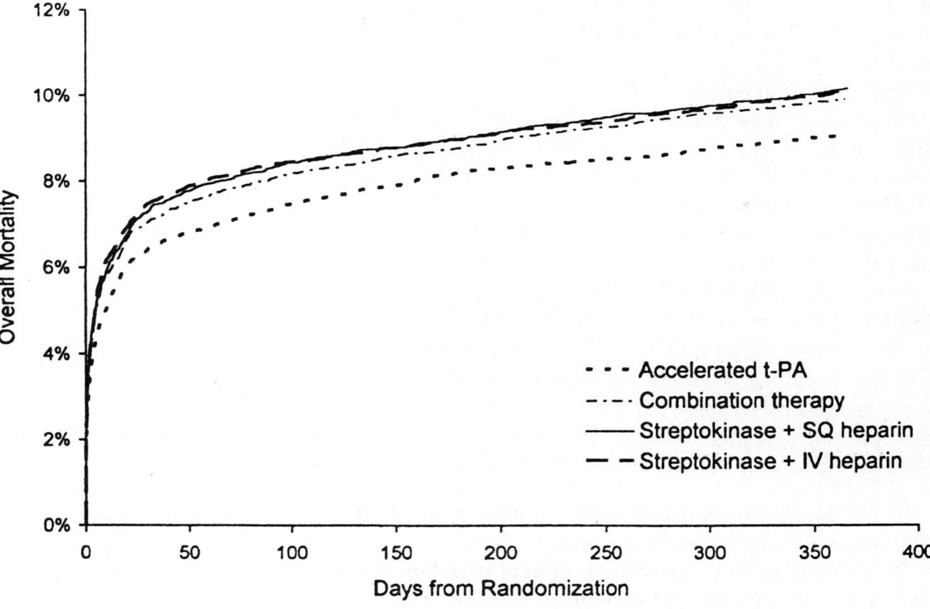

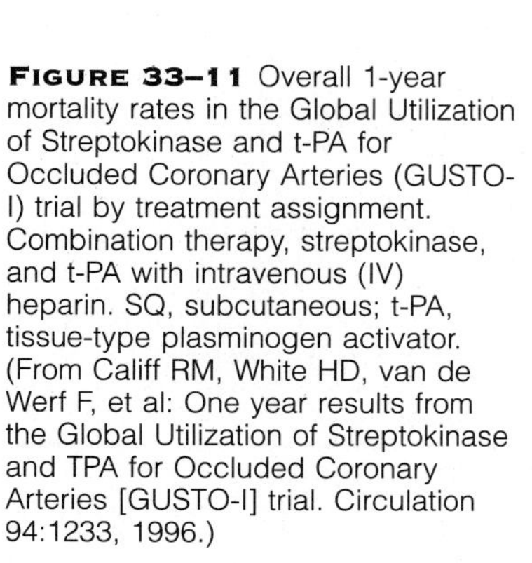
FIGURE 33–11 Overall 1-year mortality rates in the Global Utilization of Streptokinase and t-PA for Occluded Coronary Arteries (GUSTO-I) trial by treatment assignment. Combination therapy, streptokinase, and t-PA with intravenous (IV) heparin. SQ, subcutaneous; t-PA, tissue-type plasminogen activator. (From Califf RM, White HD, van de Werf F, et al: One year results from the Global Utilization of Streptokinase and TPA for Occluded Coronary Arteries [GUSTO-I] trial. Circulation 94:1233, 1996.)

had the same effect[135] compared with heparin for a primary end point of death or nonfatal MI at 30 days.

A low rate of recurrent ischemia along with low bleeding rates after treatment with a platelet glycoprotein (GP) IIb/IIIa receptor antagonist, m7E3 Fab (murine-derived monoclonal antibody 7E3 Fab), in patients receiving rt-PA[136] was confirmed in a relatively small and nonrandomized trial. In a recent study of a nonpeptide GP IIb/IIIa inhibitor, lamifiban reduced adverse ischemic events at 6 months compared with aspirin and heparin therapy in patients with unstable angina and non–Q wave infarction (PARAGON).[137] In addition, the optimal safe and effective dose of lamifiban for use in conjunction with thrombolysis was determined in 400 patients with acute MI (PARADIGM). Lamifiban has been demonstrated to reduce the incidence of death or nonfatal infarction at 1 month in 365 patients with unstable angina (8.1 percent of patients with placebo versus 2.5 percent of patients with two high doses of lamifiban, $P = .03$).[138]

In the Evaluation for the Prevention of Ischemic Complications (EPIC)[139] trial, c7E3, a monoclonal antibody Fab fragment to the platelet GP IIb/IIIa receptor, produced a 35 percent reduction ($P = .008$) in clinical events at 30 days among 2099 patients undergoing high-risk coronary angioplasty or directional atherectomy. This beneficial effect was maintained at 6 months of follow-up. However, this adjunct therapy carried a risk of bleeding complications. Subsequently, together with low-dose, weight-adjusted heparin, c7E3 markedly reduced the risk of acute ischemic complications at 30 days and throughout 6 months of follow-up in 2792 patients who underwent percutaneous coronary revascularization without increasing the risk of hemorrhage (Evaluation in PTCA to Improve Long-Term Outcome with Abciximab GP IIb/IIIa Blockade [EPILOG]).[140] In the initial 1050 patients with refractory unstable angina who were scheduled for PTCA, c7E3 also significantly reduced ($P < .0072$) the 30-day incidence of death, MI, or need for urgent intervention compared with the placebo control group (Chimeric 7E3 Antiplatelet Therapy in Unstable Angina Refractory to Standard Treatment [CAPTURE]).[141] Major bleeding rates were acceptably low (1.7 percent for placebo and 2.9 percent for 7E3 Fab; P = NS).

The loss of an early benefit in reducing ischemic complications after angioplasty with discontinuation of the 24- and 36-hour infusion of shorter-acting GP IIb/IIIa antagonists[142, 143] has necessitated prolonged GP IIb/IIIa inhibition, which could potentially be achieved by oral administration.[144] Large-scale trials are under way to assess the effectiveness of long-term oral GP IIb/IIIa antagonists on the natural history of MI as an adjunct therapy to thrombolysis, mechanical revascularization, or both.

The natural history of CAD has changed tremendously and will continue to change as new therapeutic approaches are introduced. Despite the promise of new thrombolytic therapies in MI, their ultimate effectiveness remains to be proved because of several unsolved problems:

1. Lack of long-term mortality rate studies for more than 5 years in major randomized trials
2. The potentially deleterious effects of reperfusion injury or lack of substantial benefit in patients presenting for treatment 6 to 24 hours after the onset of symptoms and in elderly patients who are usually not considered to be candidates for thrombolytic therapy
3. Lack of knowledge regarding the efficacy of primary, immediate, or rescue PTCA with or without stent deployment
4. Lack of knowledge about the best thrombolytic agent with or without adjunct therapies

The definitive answers to these questions must await the results of future studies.

NONINVASIVE CARDIAC TESTS TO PREDICT PROGNOSIS

Rest Electrocardiography

The prognosis of patients with high-degree atrioventricular block, intraventricular conduction disturbance, or both in the setting of acute MI is generally worse than that of patients without these complications—not only because patients with these complications frequently develop complete atrioventricular block and subsequent hemodynamic derangements secondary to marked bradycardia but also because the extent of MI tends to be larger when these complications are present.[145, 146] Hindman and associates[147] reported a greater risk of sudden death after discharge in patients with bundle branch block (BBB) than in those without BBB (Table 33–3). As seen in Table 33–3, when BBB was present, the risk of sudden death after discharge increased in patients with anterior or indeterminant MI, in patients without significant heart failure on admission, and in patients with a history of previous MI. The presence of BBB did not alter the prognosis in patients with inferior or

TABLE 33-3 Comparison of the Risk of Dying Suddenly After Discharge in Patients With Bundle Branch Block and in a Control Group of Patients Without Bundle Branch Block (No High-Degree Atrioventricular Block)

	Bundle Branch Block		No Bundle Branch Block		
Total Patients	***n* 248**	***SD (%)* 13**	***n* 708**	***SD (%)* 7**	***P* < .005**
Infarct location					
Anterior or indeterminant	190	15	394	8	<.001
Inferior or posterior	59	5	314	6	NS
P		<.05		NS	
Heart failure					
Killip class I or II	184	12	626	6	<.01
Killip class III or IV	65	17	82	14	NS
P		NS		<.01	
Previous myocardial infarction					
Yes	33	30	346	6	<.001
No	216	11	362	8	NS
P		<.001		NS	
Bundle branch block at discharge					
Yes	171	17	—	—	—
No	78	9	—	—	—
P		<.025			

Abbreviations: NS, not significant; SD, standard deviation.

From Hindman MC, Wagner GS, JaRo M, et al: The clinical significance of bundle branch block complicating acute myocardial infarction, 2: indications for temporary and permanent pacemaker insertion. Circulation 58:689, 1978.

posterior MI, in patients with overt heart failure, and in patients without a history of previous MI.

This trend has not changed after the introduction of reperfusion therapy. An analysis of 26,003 patients in the GUSTO-I trial in North America revealed that 420 patients (1.6 percent) had left (131 patients) or right (289 patients) BBB. These patients had higher 30-day mortality rates than matched control subjects (18 versus 11 percent, $P = .003$; RR, 1.8) and were more likely to experience cardiogenic shock (19 versus 11 percent, $P = .008$; RR, 1.78) or atrioventricular block or asystole (30 versus 19 percent, $P < .012$; RR, 1.57) and to require ventricular pacing (18 versus 11 percent, $P = .006$; RR, 1.74). BBB also carried an independent 53 percent higher risk for 30-day mortality.[148]

Exercise Stress Electrocardiography

The development of marked ST-segment depression in the early stage of exercise, poor exercise tolerance, a fall in blood pressure, and the development of severe angina indicate a poor prognosis.[149–151] The predischarge submaximal exercise test performed 7 to 10 days after acute MI is used to screen out high-risk patients who develop these abnormalities and exercise-induced arrhythmias.[152, 153] In such patients, a more intensive therapeutic strategy may be warranted.

Holter Electrocardiography

The severity of ventricular arrhythmias detected with Holter electrocardiographic monitoring, a measure of "irritability," has clear independent prognostic value.[77] In general, as the Lown grade increases, the risk of sudden death increases (Table 33–4).[154, 155] On the other hand, the prognostic value of the findings of electrical programmed[156–158] stimulation to test "vulnerability" has not been established.

Tests With Radionuclide Techniques

The importance of the LV ejection fraction in the prognosis of CAD was discussed earlier. In a number of studies that have demonstrated the value of radionuclide ventriculography, it has been used.[154, 159] Furthermore, radionuclide left ventriculography in conjunction with electrocardiographic monitoring during exercise may provide additional prognostic data. For example, in a study of 117 patients with mild symptoms and well preserved LV function, Bonow and colleagues[159] found that patients whose ejection fraction was unchanged or increased during exercise had a 4-year survival rate of 85 percent, whereas in those whose ejection fraction decreased during exercise, the survival rate was 65 percent. The electrocardiographic changes alone did not distinguish the high-risk population in this study.

Because of the high cost and lack of standardization of the technique, there have not been many studies to define the prognostic significance of the findings obtained from ^{201}Tl myocardial scintigraphy. Gibson and associates[160] reported that this technique was a better predictor than exercise ECG because it identified a group of high-risk patients and a group of very low-risk patients more clearly than did other tests (Fig. 33–12). However, soon after an acute MI, patients cannot undergo sufficient exercise stress, so the sensitivity of submaximal exercise ^{201}Tl imaging is less than ideal. Recently, dipyridamole ^{201}Tl imaging in the period 1 to 13 days after acute MI has been reported to be useful in assessing the prognosis.[161] Because the number of patients in this study was also very small, we must not draw conclusions about the prognostic value of this test until more definitive studies are performed.

A comprehensive study evaluated the clinical significance of silent and symptomatic myocardial ischemia detected by noninvasive testing in stable postcoronary patients.[162] In this study, noninvasive testing involved resting, ambulatory, and exercise ECG and stress ^{201}Tl scintigraphy in 936 patients (males, 76 percent; mean age, 58 years) who were clinically stable 1 to 6 months after hospitalization for acute MI or unstable angina. A Cox regression analysis was used to evaluate the association between the risk (hazard ratio) of first recurrent primary events (cardiac death, nonfatal infarction, or unstable angina) or restricted events (cardiac death or nonfatal infarction) and ischemic noninvasive test results. ST-segment depression on resting ECG was the only noninvasive test variable that was associated with a significantly increased risk ($P = .05$) for first recurrent primary events (hazard ratio; 95 percent confidence limits): rest ECG ST-segment depression (1.5; 1.00 and 2.25), ambulatory ECG ST-segment depression (0.86; 0.49 and 1.51), exercise ECG ST-segment depression (1.13; 0.82 and 1.56), and stress ^{201}Tl reversible defects (1.3; 0.96 and 1.74). The test results were similar for first recurrent restricted events and in patients with and without angina. The authors also evaluated ischemia detected by noninvasive testing with relevant components of the exercise tolerance test and of the stress ^{201}Tl study that reflect cardiac dysfunction. For the exercise test, there was a significant interaction ($P = .004$) between ST-segment depression and the duration of exercise for the primary end point; an increased risk was associated with exercise-induced ST-segment depression in patients with reduced exercise duration (hazard ratio, 3.4). There also was a significant interaction by ^{201}Tl scintigraphy ($P = .047$) between ischemia and lung uptake, with an increased risk

TABLE 33–4 Relation Between Lown Grade and Mortality in 400 Patients After Acute Myocardial Infarction

Lown Grade	Group Total	Deaths n	Deaths %
0	64	9	14
1	85	9	11
2	2	0	0
3	68	10	15
4A	44	9	20
4B	21	7	33
5	116	34	29
All	400	78	20

From Bigger JT, Weld FM: Analysis of prognostic significance of ventricular arrhythmias after myocardial infarction: shortcomings of Lown grading system. Br Heart J 45:717, 1981, with permission from the BMJ Publishing Group.

for primary end point events associated with a reversible defect only in patients with increased lung uptake (hazard ratio, 2.8) (Table 33–5). Because the number of patients in the high-risk subset identified by noninvasive testing was very small (23, or 2.5 percent study population by exercise ECG; and 20, or 2.2 percent of the study population by stress ^{201}Tl test), the authors concluded that the detection of silent or symptomatic myocardial ischemia by noninvasive testing in stable patients 1 to 6 months after an acute coronary event was not useful for identifying patients at increased risk for subsequent coronary events.

It has been shown that positron emission tomography can assess myocardial viability very accurately, so this technique may prove to be useful in predicting the prognosis and in selecting the best therapy for each patient.[163]

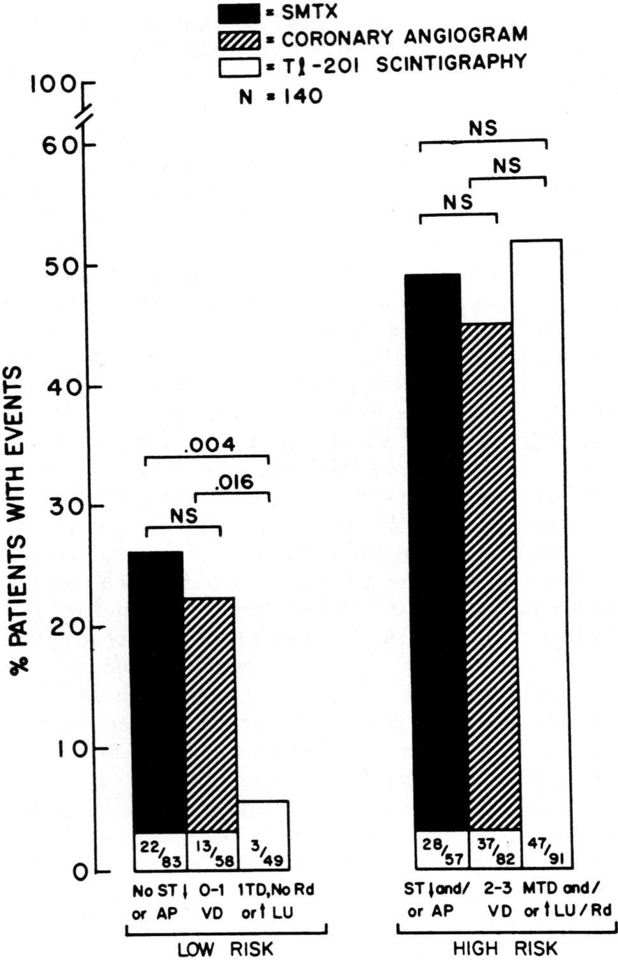

FIGURE 33–12 Proportion of patients with a subsequent cardiac event (cardiac death, recurrent infarction, class III or IV angina) related to the results of predischarge submaximal treadmill exercise testing (SMTX), coronary angiography, and ^{201}Tl scintigraphy after uncomplicated myocardial infarction. AP, angina pectoris; ↑LU, increased lung uptake of ^{201}Tl; MTD, thallium defects involving multiple vascular regions; Rd, redistribution; ST↓, ST-segment depression; 1TD, thallium defect in one vascular region; VD, vessel disease by angiography. (From Gibson RS, Watson DD, Craddock GB, et al: Prediction of cardiac events after uncomplicated myocardial infarction: a prospective study comparing predischarge exercise thallium-201 scintigraphy and coronary angiography. Circulation 68:321, 1983.)

TABLE 33–5 Interactions Between Relevant Components of the Exercise Tolerance Test and of Stress Thallium Scintigraphy for the Primary End Point

Exercise Tolerance Test	Hazard Ratio* Exercise Duration, min: <6	6–9	>9	Interaction P†
ST depression ≥0.1 mV (1.0 mm)				
Yes	3.4	1.9	1.1	< .01
No	0.8	0.9	1.0	
Stress Thallium Scintigraphy	**Lung Uptake: Increased**	**Not Increased**		
Reversible defect				
Yes	2.8	1.2		< .05
No	0.9	1.0		

*Ratio of the risk of primary end point events per unit of time among patients with the parameter of interest to that among patients with the reference parameter (unity value).

†Significance level for the lack of proportionally between the two rows of hazard ratios.

From Moss AJ, Goldstein RE, Hall WJ, et al: Detection and significance of myocardial ischemia in stable patients after recovery from an acute coronary event: Multicenter Myocardial Ischemia Research Group. JAMA 269:2379, 1993. Copyright 1993, American Medical Association.

REFERENCES

1. Kannel WB, Doyle JT, MacNamara PM, et al: Precursors of sudden coronary death: factors related to the incidence of sudden death. Circulation 51:606, 1975.
2. The Veterans Administration Coronary Artery Surgery Cooperative Study Group: Eleven-year survival in the veterans administration randomized trial of coronary bypass surgery for stable angina. N Engl J Med 311:1333, 1984.
3. Varnauskas E and the European Coronary Surgery Study Group: Survival, myocardial infarction, and employment status in a prospective randomized study of coronary bypass surgery. Circulation 72(suppl. V):V-90, 1985.
4. Passamani E, Davis KB, Gillespie MJ, Killip T, and the CASS Principal Investigators and Their Associates: A randomized trial of coronary artery bypass surgery: survival of patients with a low ejection fraction. N Engl J Med 312:1665, 1985.
5. Holmes DR Jr, Davis KB, Mock MB, et al: The effect of medical and surgical treatment on subsequent sudden cardiac death in patients with coronary artery disease: a report from the Coronary Artery Surgery Study. Circulation 73:1254, 1986.
6. Murphy ML, Meadows WR, Thomsen J, et al: The effect of coronary artery bypass surgery on the incidence of myocardial infarction and hospitalization. Prog Cardiovasc Dis 28:309, 1986.
7. CASS Principal Investigators and Their Associates: Myocardial infarction and mortality in the Coronary Artery Surgery Study (CASS) randomized trial. N Engl J Med 310:750, 1984.
8. Peduzzi P, Detre K, Murphy ML, et al: Ten-year incidence of myocardial infarction and prognosis after infarction: Department of Veterans Affairs Cooperative Study of Coronary Artery Bypass Surgery. Circulation 83:747, 1991.
9. Martin CA, Thompson PL, Armstrong BK, et al: Long-term prognosis after recovery from myocardial infarction: a nine year follow-up of the Perth Coronary Register. Circulation 68:961, 1983.
10. Vliestra RE, Frye RL, Kronmal RA, et al: Risk factors and angiographic coronary artery disease: a report from the Coronary Artery Surgery Study (CASS). Circulation 62:254, 1980.
11. Lee KL, Woodlief LH, Topol EJ, et al: Predictors of 30 days mortality in the era of reperfusion for acute myocardial infarction: results from an international trial of 41,021 patients. Circulation 91:1659, 1995.

12. Mueller HS, Cohen LS, Braunwald E, et al: Predictors of early morbidity and mortality after thrombolytic therapy of acute myocardial infarction: analyses of patient subgroups in the Thrombolysis in Myocardial Infarction (TIMI) Trial, Phase II. Circulation 85:1254, 1992.
13. Barbash GI, White HD, Modan M, et al: Significance of smoking in patients receiving thrombolytic therapy for acute myocardial infarction: experience gleaned from the International Tissue Plasminogen Activator/Streptokinase Mortality Trial. Circulation 87:535, 1993.
14. Ockene IS, Ockene JK. Smoking after acute myocardial infarction: a good thing? Circulation 87:297, 1993.
15. Volpi A, De Vita A, Franzosi MG, et al: Determinants of 6-month mortality in survivors of myocardial infarction after thrombolysis: results of the GISSI-2 data base. Circulation 88:416, 1993.
16. Kornowski R, Goldbourt U, Zion M, et al: Predictors and long-term prognostic significance of recurrent infarction in the year after a first myocardial infarction. Am J Cardiol 72:883, 1993.
17. Kannel WB, Sorlie P, McNamara PM: Prognosis after initial myocardial infarction: the Framingham Study. Am J Cardiol 44:53, 1979.
18. Greenland P, Reicher-Reiss H, Goldbourt U, et al: In hospital and 1-year mortality in 1524 women after myocardial infarction: comparison with 4315 men. Circulation 83:484, 1991.
19. Puletti M, Sunseri L, Curione M, et al: Acute myocardial infarction: sex-related difference in prognosis. Am Heart J 108:63, 1984.
20. Steingart RM, Packer M, Hamm P, et al: Sex difference in the management of coronary artery disease. N Engl J Med 325:226, 1991.
21. Maynard C, Althouse R, Cerqueira M, et al: Underutilization of thrombolytic therapy in eligible women with acute myocardial infarction. Am J Cardiol 68:529, 1991.
22. Krumholtz HM, Douglas PS, Lauer MS, et al: Selection of patients for coronary angiography and coronary revascularization early after myocardial infarction: is there evidence for gender bias? Ann Intern Med 115:173, 1991.
23. Ayanian JZ, Epstein AM: Difference in the use of procedures between women and men hospitalized for coronary heart disease. N Engl J Med 325:221, 1991.
24. White HD, Barbash GI, Modan M, et al: After correcting for worse baseline characteristics, women treated with thrombolytic therapy for acute myocardial infarction have the same mortality and morbidity as men except for a higher incidence of hemorrhagic stroke. Circulation 88(pt 1):2097, 1993.
25. Lincoff AM, Califf RM, Ellis SG, et al: Thrombolytic therapy for women with myocardial infarction: is there a gender gap? J Am Coll Cardiol 22:1780, 1993.
26. Becker RC, Terrin, M, Ross R, et al: Comparison of clinical outcomes for women and men after acute myocardial infarction. Ann Intern Med 120:638, 1994.
27. Pekkanen J, Linn S, Heiss G, et al: Ten-year mortality from cardiovascular disease in relation to cholesterol level among men with and without pre-existing cardiovascular disease. N Engl J Med 322:1700, 1990.
28. Scandinavian Simbastatin Survival Study Group: Randomized trial of cholesterol lowering in 4444 patients with coronary heart disease: the Scandinavian Simbastatin Survival Study (4S). Lancet 344:1383, 1994.
29. Sacks FM, Pfeffer MA, Moye LA, et al: The effect of pravastatin on coronary events after myocardial infarction in patients with average cholesterol levels. N Engl J Med 335:1001, 1996.
30. Sacks FM, Moye LA, Davis BR, et al: Relationship between plasma LDL concentrations during treatment with pravastatin and recurrent coronary events in the Cholesterol and Recurrent Events trial. Circulation 97:1446, 1998.
31. Hulley SB, Rosenman RH, Bawol RD, et al: Epidemiology as a guide to clinical decisions: the association between triglyceride and coronary heart disease. N Engl J Med 302:1383, 1980.
32. Rapp JH, Lespine A, Hamilton RL, et al: Triglyceride-rich lipoproteins isolated by selected affinity antiapolipoprotein B immunosorption from human atherosclerotic plaque. Arterioscler Thromb 14:1767, 1994.
33. Drexel H, Amann FW, Beran J, et al: Plasma triglycerides and three lipoprotein cholesterol fractions are independent predictors of the extent of coronary atherosclerosis. Circulation 90:2230, 1994.
34. Phillips NR, Waters D, Havel RJ: Plasma lipoproteins and progression of coronary artery disease evaluated by angiography and clinical events. Circulation 88:2762, 1993.
35. Miller M, Seidler A, Moalemi A, et al: Normal triglyceride levels and coronary artery disease events: the Baltimore Coronary Observation Long-Term Study. J Am Coll Cardiol 31:1252, 1998.
36. Rosengren A, Wilhelmsen L, Eriksson E, et al: Lipoprotein(a) and coronary heart disease: a prospective case-control study in a general population sample of middle-aged men. BMJ 301:1248, 1990.
37. Jauhiainen M, Koskinen P, Ehnholm C, et al: Lipoprotein(a) and coronary heart disease risk: a nested case-control study of the Helsinki Heart Study participants. Atherosclerosis 89:59, 1991.
38. Alfthan G, Pekkanen J, Jauhiainen M, et al: Relation of serum homocysteine and lipoprotein(a) concentrations to atherosclerotic disease in a prospective Finnish population-based study. Atherosclerosis 106:91, 1994.
39. Is lipoprotein(a) as independent risk factor for ischemic heart disease in men? The Quebec Cardiovascular Study. J Am Coll Cardiol 31:519, 1998.
40. Terres W, Tatsis E, Pfalzer B, et al: Rapid angiographic progression of coronary artery disease in patients with elevated lipoprotein(a). Circulation 91:948, 1995.
41. Tamura A, Watanabe T, Mikuriya Y, Nasu M: Serum lipoprotein(a) concentrations are related to coronary disease progression without new myocardial infarction. Br Heart J 74:365, 1995.
42. Gillum R, Liu KC: Coronary heart disease in black populations, I: mortality and morbidity. Am Heart J 104:839, 1982.
43. Tofler GH, Stone PH, Muller JE, et al: Effects of gender and race on prognosis after myocardial infarction: adverse prognosis for women, particularly black women. J Am Coll Cardiol 9:473, 1987.
44. Cooper RS, Simmons B, Castaner A, et al: Survival rates and prehospital delay during myocardial infarction among black persons. Am J Cardiol 57:208, 1986.
45. Wenneker MB, Epstein AM: Racial inequalities in the use of procedures for patients with ischemic heart disease. JAMA 261:253, 1989.
46. Blendon RJ, Aiken LH, Freeman HE, Corey CH: Access to medical care for black and white Americans: a matter of continuing concern. JAMA 261:278, 1989.
47. Taylor HA, Chaitman BR, Robers WJ, et al: Race and prognosis after myocardial infarction: results of the thrombolysis in Myocardial Infarction (TIMI) Phase II Trial. Circulation 88(pt 1):1484, 1993.
48. Cambien F, Poirier O, Lecerf L, et al: Deletion polymorphism in the gene for angiotensin-converting enzyme is a potent risk factor for myocardial infarction. Nature 359:641, 1992.
49. Lindpainter K, Pfeffer MA, Kreutz R, et al: A prospective evaluation of an angiotensin-converting-enzyme gene polymorphism and the risk of ischemic heart disease. N Engl J Med 332:706, 1995.
50. Katusya T, Koike G, Yee TW, et al: Association of angiotensinogen gene T235 variant with increased risk of coronary heart disease. Lancet 345:1600, 1995.
51. Samani NJ, O'Toole L, Martin D, et al: Insertion/deletion polymorphism in the angiotensin-converting enzyme gene and risk of and prognosis after myocardial infarction. J Am Coll Cardiol 28:338, 1996.
52. Kluijtman LA, van der Heuvel LP, Boers GH, et al: Molecular genetic analysis in mild hyperhomocysteinemia: a common mutation in the methylenetetrahydrofolate reductase gene is a genetic risk factor for cardiovascular disease. Am J Hum Genet 58:35, 1996.
53. Anderson JL, Gretchen JK, Thomas MJ, et al: A mutation in the methylenetetrahydrofolate reductase gene is not associated with increased risk for coronary artery disease of myocardial infarction. J Am Coll Cardiol 30:1206, 1997.
54. Mock MB, Ringqvist I, Fisher LD, et al: Survival of medically treated patients in the Coronary Artery Surgery Study (CASS) Registry. Circulation 66:562, 1982.
55. Hiramori K, Haze K: Pathophysiology, therapy and prognosis of angina pectoris. Jpn J Med 79:91, 1990.
56. Califf RM, Tomabechi Y, Lee KL, et al: Outcome in one-vessel coronary artery disease. Circulation 67:283, 1983.
57. Nestico PF, Hakki A, Meissner MD, et al: Effects of collateral vessels on prognosis in patients with one vessel coronary artery disease. J Am Coll Cardiol 6:1257, 1985.
58. Roberts KB, Califf RM, Harrell FE Jr, et al: The prognosis for patients with new-onset angina who have undergone cardiac catheterization. Circulation 68:970, 1983.

59. Gazes PC, Mobley EM Jr, Faris HM Jr, et al: Preinfarction (unstable) angina—a prospective study—ten year follow-up. Prognostic significance of electrocardiographic changes. Circulation 48:331, 1973.
60. Mulcahy R, Awadhi AHA, de Buitleor M, et al: Natural history and prognosis of unstable angina. Am Heart J 109:753, 1986.
61. Gottlieb SO, Weisfeldt ML, Ouyang P, et al: Silent ischemia as a marker for early unfavorable outcomes in patients with unstable angina. N Engl J Med 314:1214, 1986.
62. Prinzmetal M, Kennamer R, Merliss R, et al: Angina pectoris, I: a variant form of angina pectoris: preliminary report. Am J Med 27:375, 1959.
63. Oliva PB, Potts DE, Pluss RG: Coronary arterial spasm in Prinzmetal angina: documentation by coronary arteriography. N Engl J Med 288:745, 1973.
64. Yasue H, Touyama M, Kato H, et al: Prinzmetal's variant form of angina as a manifestation of alpha-adrenergic receptor mediated coronary artery spasm: documentation by coronary arteriography. Am Heart J 91:148, 1976.
65. Prinzmetal M, Ekmekci A, Kennamer R, et al: Variant form of angina pectoris: previously undelineated syndrome. JAMA 174:1794, 1960.
66. Bott-Silverman C, Heupler FA: Natural history of pure coronary artery spasm in patients treated medically. J Am Coll Cardiol 2:200, 1983.
67. Walling A, Waters DD, Miller DD, et al: Long-term prognosis of patients with variant angina. Circulation 76:990, 1987.
68. Yasue H, Takizawa A, Nagao M, et al: Long-term prognosis for patients with variant angina and influential factors. Circulation 78:1, 1988.
69. Waters DD, Szlachcic J, Miller D, Theroux P: Clinical characteristics of patients with variant angina complicated by myocardial infarction or death within 1 month. Am J Cardiol 49:658, 1982.
70. Nakamura M, Takeshita A, Nose Y: Clinical characteristics associated with myocardial infarction, arrhythmias, and sudden death in patients with vasospastic angina. Circulation 75:1110, 1987.
71. Waters DD, Miller DD, Szlachcic J, et al: Factors influencing the long-term prognosis of treated patients with variant angina. Circulation 68:258, 1983.
72. Severi S, Davies G, Maseri A, et al: Long-term prognosis of "variant" angina with medical treatment. Am J Cardiol 46:226, 1980.
73. Miller DD, Waters DD, Szlachcic J, Theroux P: Clinical characteristics associated with sudden death in patients with variant angina. Circulation 66:588, 1982.
74. Schroeder JS, Lamb IH, Bristow MR, et al: Prevention of cardiovascular events in variant angina by long-term diltiazem therapy. J Am Coll Cardiol 1:1507, 1983.
75. Luria MH, Knoke JD, Wachs JS, Luria MA: Survival after recovery from acute myocardial infarction: two and five year prognostic indices. Am J Med 67:7, 1979.
76. Davis HT, DeCamilla J, Bayer LW, Moss AJ: Survivorship patterns in the posthospital phase of myocardial infarction. Circulation 60:1252, 1979.
77. The Multicenter Postinfarction Research Group: Risk stratification and survival after myocardial infarction. N Engl J Med 309:331, 1983.
78. Edlavitch SA, Crow R, Burke GKL, Baxter J: Secular trends in Q wave and non-Q wave acute myocardial infarction: the Minnesota Heart Survey. Circulation 83:492, 1991.
79. Mahony C, Hindman MC, Aronin N, Wagner GS: Prognostic differences in subgroups of patients with electrographic evidence of subendocardial or transmural myocardial infarction: the favorable outlook for patients with an initially normal QRS complex. Am J Med 69:183, 1980.
80. Gibson RS, Beller GA, Gheorghiade M, et al: The prevalence and clinical significance of residual myocardial ischemia 2 weeks after uncomplicated non-Q wave infarction: a prospective natural history study. Circulation 73:1186, 1986.
81. Conolly DC, Elveback LR: Coronary heart disease in residents of Rochester, Minnesota, VI: hospital and posthospital course of patients with transmural and subendocradial myocardial infarction. Mayo Clin Proc 60:375, 1985.
82. Maisel AS, Ahnve S, Gilpin E, et al: Prognosis after extension of myocardial infarct: the role of Q wave or non-Q infarction. Circulation 71:211, 1985.
83. Cannom DS, Levy W, Cohen LS: The short- and long-term prognosis of patients with transmural and nontransmural myocardial infarction. Am J Med 61:452, 1976.
84. Hutter AM, DeSanctis RW, Flynn T, Yeatman LA: Nontransmural myocardial infarction: a comparison of hospital and late clinical course of patients with that of matched patients with transmural anterior and transmural inferior myocardial infarction. Am J Cardiol 48:595, 1981.
85. Marmor A, Sobel BE, Roberts R: Factors presaging early recurrent myocardial infarction ("extension"). Am J Cardiol 48:603, 1981.
86. Marmor A, Geltman EM, Schechtman K, et al: Recurrent myocardial infarction: clinical predictors and prognostic implications. Circulation 66:415, 1982.
87. The ISAM Study Group: A prospective trial of intravenous streptokinase in acute myocardial infarction (I.S.A.M): mortality, morbidity, and infarct size at 21 days. N Engl J Med 314:1465, 1986.
88. Kennedy JW, Martin GV, Davis KB, et al: The Western Washington Intravenous Streptokinase in Acute Myocardial Infarction randomized trial. Circulation 77:345, 1988.
89. The TIMI Study Group: The Thrombolysis in Myocardial Infarction (TIMI) trial: phase I findings. N Engl J Med 312:932, 1985.
90. Verstraete M, Bernard R, Bory M, et al: Randomized trial of intravenous recombinant tissue-type plasminogen activator versus intravenous streptokinase in acute myocardial infarction: report from the European Cooperative Study Group for Recombinant Tissue-type Plasminogen Activator. Lancet 1:842, 1985.
91. Van de Werf F, Arnold AER: Intravenous tissue plasminogen activator and size of infarct, left ventricular function, and survival in acute myocardial infarction. Br Med J 297:1374, 1988.
92. Wilcox RG, von der Lippe G, Olsson CG, et al: Trial of tissue plasminogen activator for mortality reduction in acute myocardial infarction: Anglo-Scandinavian Study of Early Thrombolysis (ASSET). Lancet 2:525, 1988.
93. Neuhaus KL, Tebbe U, Gottwik M, et al: Intravenous recombinant tissue plasminogen activator (rt-PA) and urokinase in acute myocardial infarction: results of the German Activator Urokinase Study (GAUS). J Am Coll Cardiol 12:581, 1988.
94. Armstrong PW, Baigrie RS, Daly PA, et al: Tissue plasminogen activator: Toronto (TPAT) placebo-controlled randomized trial in acute myocardial infarction. J Am Coll Cardiol 13:1469, 1989.
95. Magnani B for the PAIM Investigators: Plasminogen Activator Italian Multicenter Study (PAIMS): comparison of intravenous recombinant single-chain human tissue-type plasminogen activator (rt-PA) with intravenous streptokinase in acute myocardial infarction. J Am Coll Cardiol 13:19, 1989.
96. AMS Trial Study Group: Effect of intravenous APSAC on mortality after acute myocardial infarction: preliminary report of a placebo-controlled clinical trial. Lancet 1:545, 1988.
97. Anderson JL, Sorensen SG, Moreno FL, et al: Multicenter patency trial of intravenous anistreplase compared with streptokinase in acute myocardial infarction. Circulation 83:126, 1991.
98. PRIMI Trial Study Group: Randomised double-blind trial of recombinant pro-urokinase against streptokinase in acute myocardial infarction. Lancet 1:863, 1989.
99. Guppo Italiano per lo Studio della Streptochinasi nell'Infarto Miocardico (GISSI): Long-term effects of intravenous thrombolysis in acute myocardial infarction: final report of the GISSI study. Lancet 2:871, 1987.
100. ISIS-2 (Second International Study of Infarct Survival) Collaborative Group: Randomized trial of intravenous streptokinase, oral aspirin, both, or neither among 17,187 cases of suspected acute myocardial infarction: ISIS-2. J Am Coll Cardiol 12:3A, 1988.
101. Harrison DC, Ferguson DW, Collins SM, et al: Rethrombosis after reperfusion with streptokinase: importance of geometry of residual lesions. Circulation 69:991, 1984.
102. The TIMI Study Group: Comparison of invasive and conservative strategies after treatment with intravenous tissue plasminogen activator in acute myocardial infarction: results of the Thrombolysis in Myocardial Infarction (TIMI) Phase II Trial. N Engl J Med 320:618, 1989.
103. The TIMI Research Group: Immediate vs delayed catheterization and angioplasty following thrombolytic therapy for acute myocardial infarction: TIMI II A results. JAMA 260:2849, 1988.
104. Topol EJ, Califf RM, George BS, et al: A randomized trial of immediate versus delayed elective angioplasty after intravenous tissue plasminogen activator in acute myocardial infarction. N Engl J Med 317:581, 1987.

105. Guerci AD, Gerstenblith G, Brinker JA, et al: A randomized trial of intravenous tissue plasminogen activator for acute myocardial infarction with subsequent randomization to elective coronary angioplasty. N Engl J Med 317:1613, 1987.
106. Simoons ML, Arnold AER, Betriu A, et al: Thrombolysis with plasminogen activator in acute myocardial infarction: no additional benefit from immediate percutaneous coronary angioplasty. Lancet 1:197, 1988.
107. Arnold AER, Simoons ML, Van de Werf F, et al, the European Cooperative Study Group: Recombinant tissue-type plasminogen activator and immediate angioplasty in acute myocardial infarction: one-year follow-up. Circulation 86:111, 1992.
108. Boersma E, Maas AC, Deckers JW, Simoons ML: Early thrombolytic treatment in acute myocardial infarction: reappraisal of the golden hour. Lancet 348:771, 1996.
109. Newby LK, Rutsuch WR, Califf RM, et al: The GUSTO-I Investigators: Time from symptom onset to treatment and outcomes after thrombolytic therapy. J Am Coll Cardiol 27:1646, 1996.
110. Anderson JL, Karagounis LA, Becker LC, et al: TIMI perfusion grade 3 but not grade 2 results in improved outcome after thrombolysis for myocardial infarction: ventriculographic, enzymatic, and electrocardiographic evidence from the TEAM-3 study. Circulation 87:1829, 1993.
111. Califf RM, Topol EJ, Stack RS, et al: Evaluation of combination thrombolytic therapy and timing of cardiac catheterization in acute myocardial infarction: Results of Thrombolysis and Angioplasty in Myocardial Infarction-Phase 5 randomized trial. Circulation 83:1543, 1991.
112. Ellis SG, da Silva ER, Heyndrickx G, et al: The RESCUE investigators: Randomized comparison of rescue angioplasty with conservative management of patients with early failure of thrombolysis for acute anterior myocardial infarction. Circulation 90:2280, 1994.
113. Kawai C, Yui Y, Hosoda S, et al: E6010 study group: A prospective, randomized, double-blind multicenter trial of a single bolus injection of the novel modified t-PA E6010 in the treatment of acute myocardial infarction: comparison with native t-PA. J Am Coll Cardiol 29:1447, 1997.
114. Smalling RW, Bode C, Kalbfleisch J, et al: More rapid, complete, and stable coronary thrombolysis with bolus administration of reteplase compared with alteplase infusion in acute myocardial infarction. Circulation 91:2725, 1995.
115. O'Keefe JH, Bailey L, Rutherford BD, Hartzler GO: Primary angioplasty for acute myocardial infarction in 1,000 consecutive patients: results in an unselected population and high-risk groups. Am J Cardiol 72:107G, 1993.
116. Zijlstra F, Jan de Boer M, Hoorntje JC, et al: A comparison of immediate coronary angioplasty with intravenous streptokinase in acute myocardial infarction. N Engl J Med 328:680, 1993.
117. Gibbons RJ, Holmes DR, Reeder GS, et al: Randomized trial comparing immediate angioplasty to thrombolysis followed by conservative treatment for myocardial infarction. N Engl J Med 328:685, 1993.
118. Grines CL, Browne KF, Marco J, et al: A comparison of primary angioplasty with thrombolytic therapy for acute myocardial infarction. N Engl J Med 328:673, 1993.
119. Ribiero EE, Silva LA, Carneiro R, et al: Randomized trial of direct coronary angioplasty versus intravenous streptokinase in acute myocardial infarction. J Am Coll Cardiol 22:376, 1993.
120. Reeder GS, Bailey KR, Gersh BJ, et al: Cost comparison of immediate angioplasty versus thrombolysis followed by conservative therapy for acute myocardial infarction: a randomized prospective trial. Mayo Clin Proc 69:5, 1994.
121. Every NR, Parsons LS, Hlatky M, et al: A comparison of thrombolytic therapy with primary coronary angioplasty for acute myocardial infarction. N Engl J Med 335:1253, 1996.
122. Every NR, Parsons LS, Fihn SD, et al: Long-term outcome in acute myocardial infarction patients admitted to hospitals with and without on-site cardiac catheterization facilities. Circulation 96:1770, 1997.
123. Lange RA, Hillis LD: Immediate angioplasty for acute myocardial infarction. N Engl J Med 328:726, 1993.
124. Lange RA, Cigarroa JE, Hillis LD: Thrombolysis or primary PTCA for acute myocardial infarction. ACC Educational Highlights 12:1, 1997.
125. Hsia J, Hamilton WP, Kleiman N, et al: A comparison between heparin and low-dose aspirin as adjunctive therapy with tissue plasminogen activator for acute myocardial infarction. N Engl J Med 323:1433, 1990.
126. The SCATI (Studio Sulla Calciparina Nell'Angina E Nella Trombosi Ventricolare Nell'Infarto) Group: Randomised controlled trial of subcutaneous calcium-heparin in acute myocardial infarction. Lancet 2:182, 1989.
127. Topol EJ, George BS, Kereiakes DJ, et al: A randomized controlled trial of intravenous tissue plasminogen activator and early intravenous heparin in acute myocardial infarction. Circulation 79:281, 1989.
128. Thompson PL, Aylward PE, Federman J, et al: A randomized comparison of intravenous heparin with oral aspirin and dipyridamole 24 hours after recombinant tissue-type plasminogen activator for acute myocardial infarction. Circulation 83:1534, 1991.
129. Gruppo Italiano per lo Studio della Sopravvivenza nell'Infarto Miocardico: GISSI-2: a factorial randomised tiral of alteplase versus streptokinase and heparin versus no heparin among 12,490 patients with acute myocardial infarction. Lancet 336:65, 1990.
130. ISIS-3 Third International Study of Infarct Survival Collaborative Group. ISIS-3: a randomised comparison of streptokinase vs tissue plasminogen activator vs anistreplase and of aspirin plus heparin vs aspirin alone among 41,299 cases of suspected acute myocardial infarction. Lancet 339:753, 1992.
131. Krumholz HM, Hennen J, Ridker PM, et al: Use and effectiveness of intravenous heparin therapy for treatment of acute myocardial infarction in the elderly. J Am Coll Cardiol 31:973, 1998.
132. The GUSTO Investigators: An international randomized trial comparing four thrombolytic strategies for acute myocardial infarction. N Engl J Med 329:673, 1993.
133. Califf RM, White HD, van de Werf F, et al: One year results from the Global Utilization of Streptokinase and TPA for Occluded Coronary Arteries (GUSTO-I) trial. Circulation 94:1233, 1996.
134. The Global Use of Strategies to Open Occluded Coronary Arteries (GUSTO) IIb Investigators: A comparison of recombinant hirudin with heparin for the treatment of acute coronary syndromes. N Engl J Med 355:775, 1996.
135. Antman EM for the TIMI 9B Investigators: Hirudin in acute myocardial infarction: Thrombolysis and Thrombin Inhibition in Myocardial Infarction (TIMI) 9B trial. Circulation 94:911, 1996.
136. Kleiman N, Ohman M, Califf R, et al: Profound inhibition of platelet aggregation with monoclonal antibody 7E3 Fab after thrombolytic therapy: results of the Thrombolysis and Angioplasty in Myocardial Infarction (TAMI)-8 pilot study. J Am Coll Cardiol 22:381, 1993.
137. The PARAGON Investigators: International, ramdomized, controlled trial of lamifiban (a platelet glycoprotein IIb/IIIa inhibitor), heparin, or both in unstable angina. Circulation 97:2386, 1998.
138. Theroux P, Kouz S, Roy L, et al: Platelet membrane receptor glycoprotein IIb/IIIa antagonism in unstable angina: the Canadian Lamifiban study. Circulation 94:899, 1996.
139. Topol EJ, Califf RM, Weisman HF, et al: on behalf of the EPIC Investigators: Randomized trial of coronary intervention with antibody against platelet IIb/IIIa integrin for reduction of clinical restenosis: results at 6 months. Lancet 343:881, 1994.
140. The EPILOG Investigators: Platelet glycoprotein IIb/IIIa receptor blockade and low-dose heparin during percutaneous coronary revascularization. N Engl J Med 336:1689, 1997.
141. The CAPTURE Investigators: Randomized placebo-controlled trial of abciximab before and during coronary intervention in refractory unstable angina: the CAPTURE study. Lancet 349:1429, 1997.
142. The IMPACT-II Investigators: Randomized placebo-controlled trial of effect of eptifibatide on complications of percutaneous coronary intervention: IMPACT-II. Lancet 349:1422, 1997.
143. The RESTORE Investigators: The effects of platelet glycoprotein IIb/IIIa blockade with tirofiban on adverse cardiac events in patients with unstable angina or acute myocardial infarction undergoing coronary angioplasty. Circulation 96:1445, 1997.
144. Cannon CP, McCabe CH, Borzak S, et al: Randomized trial of an oral platelet glycoprotein IIb/IIIa antagonist, sibrafiban, in patients after an acute coronary syndrome: results of the TIMI 12 trial. Circulation 97:340, 1998.
145. Strasberg B, Pinchas A, Arditti A, et al: Left and right ventricular function in inferior acute myocardial infarction and significance of advanced atrioventricular block. Am J Cardiol 54:985, 1984.
146. Biddle TL, Ehrich DA, Yu PN, Hodges M: Relation of heart block and left ventricular dysfunction in acute myocardial infarction. Am J Cardiol 39:961, 1977.

147. Hindman MC, Wagner GS, JaRo M, et al: The clinical significance of bundle branch block complicating acute myocardial infarction, 2: indications for temporary and permanent pacemaker insertion. Circulation 58:689, 1978.
148. Sgarbossa EB, Pinski SL, Topol EJ, et al: Acute myocardial infarction and complete bundle branch block at hospital admission: clinical characteristics and outcome in the thrombolytic era. J Am Coll Cardiol 31:150, 1988.
149. Waters DD, Bosch X, Bouchard A, et al: Comparison of clinical variables and variables derived from a limited predischarge exercise test as predictors of early and late mortality after myocardial infarction. J Am Coll Cardiol 5:1, 1985.
150. Fioretti P, Brower RW, Simoons ML, et al: Prediction of mortality during the first year after acute myocardial infarction from clinical variables and stress test at hospital discharge. Am J Cardiol 55:1313, 1985.
151. Madsen EB, Gilpin E, Ahnve S, et al: Prediction of functional capacity and use of exercise testing for predicting risk after acute myocardial infarction. Am J Cardiol 56:839, 1985.
152. Krone RJ, Gillespie JA, Weld FM, et al: Low-level exercise testing after myocardial infarction: usefulness in enhancing clinical risk stratification. Circulation 71:80, 1985.
153. Starling MR, Crawford MH, Henry RL, et al: Prognostic value of electrocardiographic exercise testing and noninvasive assessment of left ventricular ejection fraction soon after acute myocardial infarction. Am J Cardiol 57:532, 1986.
154. Bigger JT, Weld FM: Analysis of prognostic significance of ventricular arrhythmias after myocardial infarction: shortcomings of Lown grading system. Br Heart J 45:717, 1981.
155. Ruberman W, Weinblatt E, Goldberg JD, et al: Ventricular premature complexes and sudden death after myocardial infarction. Circulation 64:297, 1981.
156. Dennis AR, Baaijens H, Cody DV, et al: Value of programmed stimulation and exercise testing in predicting one-year mortality after acute myocardial infarction. Am J Cardiol 56:1313, 1985.
157. Richards DA, Cody DV, Denniss AR, et al: Ventricular electrical instability: a predictor of death after myocardial infarction. Am J Cardiol 51:75, 1983.
158. Roy D, Marchand E, Theroux P, et al: Long-term reproducibility and significance of provokable ventricular arrhythmias after myocardial infarction. J Am Coll Cardiol 8:32, 1986.
159. Bonow RO, Kent KM, Rosing DR, et al: Exercise-induced ischemia in mildly symptomatic patients with coronary-artery disease and preserved left ventricular function: indication of subgroups at risk of death during medical therapy. N Engl J Med 311:1339, 1984.
160. Gibson RS, Watson DD, Craddock GB, et al: Prediction of cardiac events after uncomplicated myocardial infarction: a prospective study comparing predischarge exercise thallium-201 scintigraphy and coronary angiography. Circulation 68:321, 1983.
161. Okada RD, Glover DK, Leppo JA: Dipyridamole ^{201}T1 scintigraphy in the evaluation of prognosis after myocardial infarction. Circulation 84(suppl I):1-132, 1991.
162. Moss AJ, Goldstein RE, Hall WJ, et al: Detection and significance of myocardial ischemia in stable patients after recovery from an acute coronary event: Multicenter Myocardial Ischemia Research Group. JAMA 269:2379, 1993.
163. Shelbert HR: Positron emission tomography for the assessment of myocardial viability. Circulation 84(suppl I):1-122, 1991.

CHAPTER 34

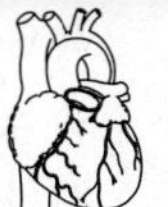

MEDICAL TREATMENT OF STABLE ANGINA

James T. Willerson

NITRATES
BETA-ADRENERGIC ANTAGONISTS
CALCIUM ANTAGONISTS
COMBINED THERAPY WITH A CALCIUM ANTAGONIST, NITRATES, AND A β-BLOCKER
PLATELET ANTAGONISTS
CLOPIDOGREL
REDUCING RISK FACTORS
AGGRESSIVE LIPID LOWERING COMPARED WITH ANGIOPLASTY IN STABLE CORONARY ARTERY DISEASE
ANGIOTENSIN-CONVERTING ENZYME INHIBITORS IN VASCULAR PROTECTION: HOPE TRIAL
Summary

Patients with stable angina usually have angina with effort, exercise, or emotion; after eating relatively large meals; or during other stressful circumstances that increase myocardial oxygen demand by increasing heart rate, contractile state, or ventricular wall tension. Cold exposure also causes angina as a result of increasing myocardial wall tension, as a consequence of increased blood pressure, and through coronary artery vasoconstriction.

Therapy is directed at reducing heart rate, blood pressure, and contractile responses to exercise and stress, so that myocardial oxygen demand for any given activity is reduced. Medication and interventions that increase coronary blood flow and oxygen delivery may also be useful. In individual patients, stable angina often develops in a predictable manner and at a level of activity or stress associated with a particular systolic blood pressure and heart rate. The heart rate–systolic blood pressure product provides an estimate of myocardial oxygen demand. Some patients have occasional episodes of angina at rest or with slight physical effort, possibly as a result of transient coronary artery vasoconstriction. In addition, the amount of effort required to cause angina may vary from time to time in individual patients. Some patients have angina as they begin exercise, which disappears as they exercise further ("walk-through angina"). Pharmacologic therapy used in the treatment of patients with stable angina is described later. However, the objectives of medical therapy are to reduce myocardial oxygen demand for any level of activity and to increase myocardial blood flow to vulnerable regions of the heart.

NITRATES

Stable angina can usually be relieved promptly and within 7 minutes by rest or nitroglycerin. The beneficial effects of nitroglycerin and other nitrates are the result of venodilatation of systemic veins and a decrease in venous return to the right heart, thereby reducing myocardial wall tension and oxygen demand, and a coronary vasodilator effect involving large and medium-sized coronary arteries, with a consequent increase in coronary blood flow to the subendocardial region where the imbalance between oxygen supply and demand exists (Fig. 34–1).[1–9] Nitrates increase oxygen delivery to the subendocardial region supplied by a severely narrowed coronary artery. Most other coronary vasodilators increase coronary blood flow and oxygen delivery to the epicardium or midmyocardium without directly changing oxygen availability within the subendocardial region itself. The coronary vasodilator effect of nitroglycerin is associated with an increase in endothelial guanylate cyclase activity and a consequent increase in cyclic guanosine monophosphate. The nitrates serve as a nitric oxide donor, increasing the availability of nitric oxide in the vasculature and contributing both to the vasodilator response and to reducing platelet aggregation and possibly inflammation, especially at sites of endothelial injury. The nitrate coronary vasodilator effect is *endothelium independent* (see Fig. 34–1).

The physiologic effects of nitrates to increase coronary blood flow and myocardial oxygen availability and decrease myocardial oxygen demand usually relieve angina promptly, that is, within 5 to 7 minutes. The commonly used and some recently developed nitrate preparations are listed in Table 34–1. Typically, relatively long-acting and orally administered nitrates, such as isosorbide dinitrate, are given at 6- to 8-hour intervals and isosorbide mononitrate once or twice during the day.[7–9] In high-risk patients, a nitroglycerin patch or paste is applied during the nighttime hours and removed the following morning after the patient arises. This approach provides the best opportunity presently available of using the "nitrate effect" to its maximal potential and avoiding the tolerance and loss of nitrate effect associated with continuous administration of the same preparation.[10, 11] It has been suggested that the antioxidant vitamins C and E may diminish tolerance to nitrates.

BETA-ADRENERGIC ANTAGONISTS

Beta-adrenergic antagonists attenuate heart rate, systolic blood pressure, and contractile responses at rest and during exercise (Tables 34–2 to 34–4). Reductions in heart rate–

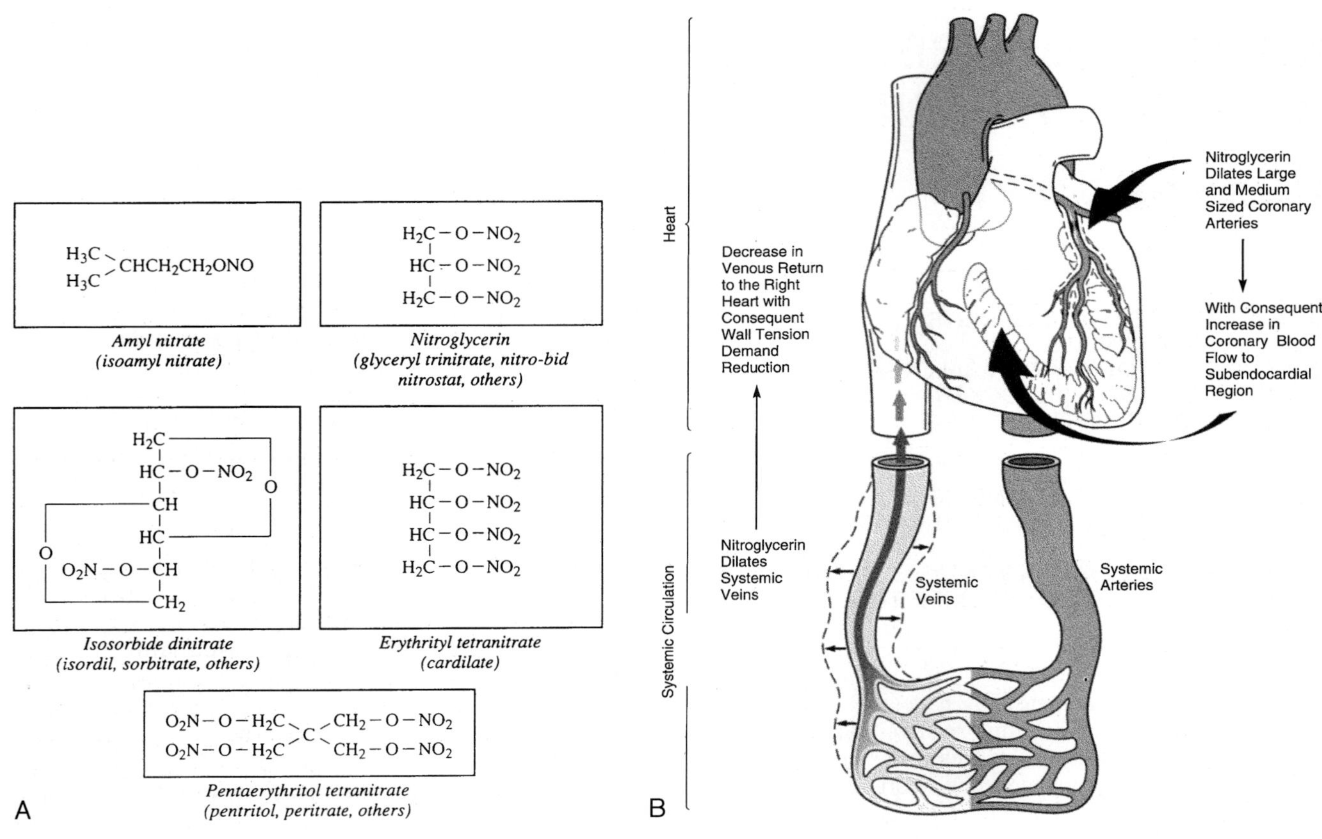

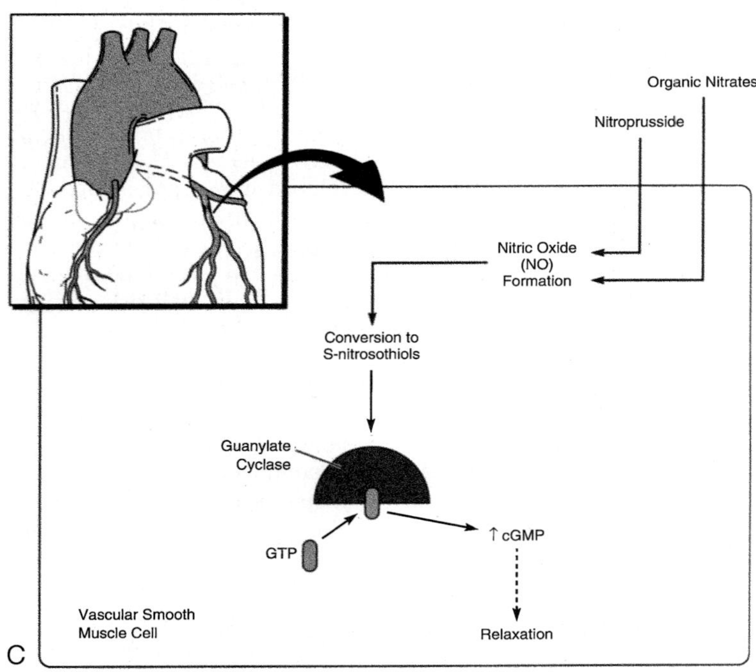

FIGURE 34–1 A, The chemical structures for selected nitrate preparations. **B,** Nitroglycerin's physiologic effects in the heart and in the peripheral venous system. Nitroglycerin dilates large and medium-sized coronary arteries and improves myocardial blood flow to the subendocardial region. In the systemic circulation, nitroglycerin is a venodilator; therefore, it decreases venous return to the right heart and diminishes preload and wall tension, thereby decreasing myocardial oxygen demand. **C,** The cellular biochemical effects of nitrates that correlate with their properties as coronary artery vasodilators. The nitrates increase guanylate cyclase activity, resulting in an increase in cyclic guanosine monophosphate (cGMP), which is associated with vasodilatation. It is believed that nitroglycerin exerts its endothelium-independent vasodilating effect through the activation of guanylate cyclase and the cellular increases in cGMP.

TABLE 34–1 **Nitrate Preparations Used in the Treatment of Angina Pectoris**

Preparation	Dosage	Duration of Effect	Frequency of Administration
Sublingual nitroglycerin	0.3–0.5 mg	15–30 min	For individual episodes
Sublingual or chewable isosorbide dinitrate	2.5–10 mg	30 min–1 h	May be used instead of nitroglycerin
Oral isosorbide dinitrate (Isordil)	5–30 mg	2 h	Every 2–3 h while patient is awake
Oral isosorbide mononitrate (Ismo)	10–20 mg	24 h	Daily
Oral isosorbide mononitrate (Imdur)	30–60 mg	24 h	Daily
Oral isosorbide dinitrate (Tembid), longer-acting preparation	40 mg	6–8 h	Every 6–8 h
Pentaerythritol tetranitrate (Peritrate)			
Oral	10–40 mg	3–4 h	Every 3–4 h
Sustained	80 mg	8–10 h	Every 8–10 h
Sustained-release oral nitroglycerin (Nitro-Bid)	2.5–6.5 mg	6 h	Every 6 h
Nitroglycerin ointment	Thin film on 1–2 inches over small area of anterior chest	4–6 h	Every 4–6 h
Nitroglycerin patches (sustained release)	0.1 mg/h, 0.2 mg/h, 0.4 mg/h	Approximately 12 h	Every 12–24 h
Nitroglycerin spray (Nitrolingual)	1 puff prn	Few minutes	Prn for chest pain

Modified from Willerson JT, Hillis LD, Buja LM (eds): Ischemic Heart Disease: Clinical and Pathophysiological Aspects. New York: Raven, 1982.

systolic blood pressure for any particular level of activity may reduce myocardial oxygen demand enough to allow a patient to engage in a particular activity without angina, whereas previously that was not possible. The beta-blockers most commonly used in the treatment of stable angina are listed in Table 34–5. β-Blockers are classified as β_1- or "nonspecific" β-blockers (Fig. 34–2; see also Table 34–5).[12–19] β_1-"Specific" blockers, such as metoprolol, alter heart rate and myocardial contractile responses but, at low doses, may interfere less with bronchial smooth muscle dilatation. At higher doses, the "selective" β-blockers have physiologic effects more like those of nonspecific β-blockers and may attenuate bronchial and smooth muscle dilatation and exacerbate bronchospasm. Nonspecific β-blockers, such as propranolol, reduce heart rate and myocardial contractile state and interfere with bronchial and vascular smooth muscle dilatation. Therefore, the β_1-specific blockers given in reduced dosage may have certain advantages in patients with chronic obstructive pulmonary diseases. They may also reduce insulin release less than nonspecific blockers and therefore may be of advantage in the treatment of selected patients with diabetes.

TABLE 34–2 **Side Effects of Beta-Adrenergic Antagonists**

- Easy fatigability
- Insomnia
- Dizziness or syncope
- Dyspnea with effort
- Sexual impotence
- Bronchospasm
- Bradycardia
- Heart block
- Hypotension
- More difficult to recognize hypoglycemia in the insulin-dependent diabetic

Modified from Willerson JT: Treatment of Heart Disease. New York: Gower Medical, 1993.

β-Blockers may cause bradycardia, bronchospasm, hypotension, atrioventricular (AV) block, and depression of myocardial contractility. They may also exacerbate coronary artery spasm and make it more frequent and severe. Therefore, they should not be used in patients with bradycardia, hypotension, AV block, or severe bronchopulmonary lung disease (especially in those with bronchospasm), or coronary artery spasm. They are used with great caution, and initially in very reduced doses, when they are used in patients with clinically important heart failure. They should also be used with caution in patients with important peripheral vascular disease and insulin-dependent diabetes mellitus, particularly when the blood glucose has been labile and difficult to control. Increasing in popularity are sustained-release β-blockers that can be administered once a day and have a sustained release into the systemic circulation, resulting in attenuation of β-adrenergic responses throughout the day (see Table 34–5). A β-blocker should be considered as therapy in the patient who experiences angina at a relatively low level of physical activity or stress. β-Blockers are often used in conjunction with nitrates to treat exercise- or stress-related angina.

Calcium Antagonists

Slow calcium channel antagonists alter slow calcium channel transport into the cell (Fig. 34–3 and Tables 34–6 to 34–8).[20–43] As a result, these agents cause vasodilatation of vascular smooth muscle and increase coronary blood flow.

TABLE 34–3 **Indications for Beta-Adrenergic Antagonists in Patients With Stable Angina**

- Prevent development of angina at relatively low heart rate–systolic blood pressure product
- Treat exercise-induced ventricular arrhythmias
- Treat systemic arterial hypertension

TABLE 34-4 Contraindications to the Administration of Beta-Adrenergic Antagonists

Severe congestive heart failure*	Severe peripheral vascular disease
Marked bradycardia (heart rate < 55 beats/min)	Insulin-dependent diabetes mellitus that is poorly controlled and labile
Advanced atrioventricular block (first-, second-, or third-degree)	Sexual impotence
Systemic arterial hypotension (systolic blood pressure < 90 mm Hg)	Bronchospasm
	Coronary artery spasm

*Selected patients with severe heart failure treated chronically with low and then very gradually increasing doses of beta-blockers are symptomatically improved during the course of weeks to months.

TABLE 34-5 Selected Beta-Adrenergic Antagonists

Name	Beta-Blockade Potency Ratio (Propranolol = 1.0)	Cardioselective	Usual Therapeutic Dose Range (mg/day)	Elimination Half-Life (h)	Route of Excretion
Propranolol (nonspecific)	1.0	0	80–480	3.5–6.0	Urine
Timolol	6.0	0	5–40	4–5	Urine
Oxprenolol	0.5–1.0	0	40–360	2	Urine
Sotalol	0.3	0	80–480	5–13	Urine
Metoprolol ($beta_1$)	1.0	+	Given IV at 5 mg in each of 3 doses at 2-min intervals, given orally at 100–800	3–4	Urine
Pindolol	6.0	0	2.5–30.0	3–4	Urine
Atenolol ($beta_1$)	1.0	+	100–400	6–9	Approximately 40% of unchanged drug in urine
Alprenolol	0.3	0	200–800	2–3	Urine
Acebutolol ($beta_1$)	0.3	+	400–800	8	Uncertain
Nadolol	0.5–1.0	0	40–80	20–24	Urine
Sotalol*	1	1	80–640	12	Urine
Esmolol† ($beta_1$)	0.025	+	Given IV at 25–300 mg/kg/min	12	Hydrolysis by plasma
Labetalol	0.3	Selective alpha- and nonselective beta-blockers	Given IV 0.25 mg/kg over 2 min and additional 40–80 mg at 1-h intervals, given orally 200–400	8–10	Urine and bile
Toprol		Selective long-acting metoprolol	50–100	24	

*Seen only at low dosage.
†Given intravenously for immediate control of supraventricular tachycardia or systemic arterial hypertension.
From Hillis LD, Firth BG, Willerson JT: Manual of Clinical Problems in Cardiology, 2nd ed. Boston: Little, Brown, 1984, with permission.

TABLE 34-6 Selected Prototype Slow Calcium Channel Blockers

	Dosage		Onset of Action		Therapeutic Plasma Concentration	Metabolism	Excretion
	Oral	*IV*	*Oral*	*IV*			
Diltiazem	30–90 μg	75–150 μg/kg (10–20 mg)	>30 min	>10 min	50–200 ng/ml	Deacetylation *N*-Demethylation *O*-Demethylation	60% fecal
Nifedipine (dihydropyridine calcium antagonist)	10–40 mg q 6–8 h	5–15 μg/kg	>20 min	>5 min (3 min SL)	25–100 ng/ml	Alpha-hydroxycarboxylic acid and alpha-lactone with no known activity	20–40% fecal 50–80% renal
Verapamil	80–120 mg q 6–12 h	150 μg/kg (10–20 mg)	>30 min	>5 min	<100 ng/ml	*N*-dealkylation *N*-demethylation Major hepatic first-pass effect	15% fecal 70% renal

Abbreviation: SL, sublingual.
Modified from Packer M, Frishman WH: Calcium Channel Antagonists in Cardiovascular Disease. East Norwalk, CT: Appleton-Century-Crofts, 1984.

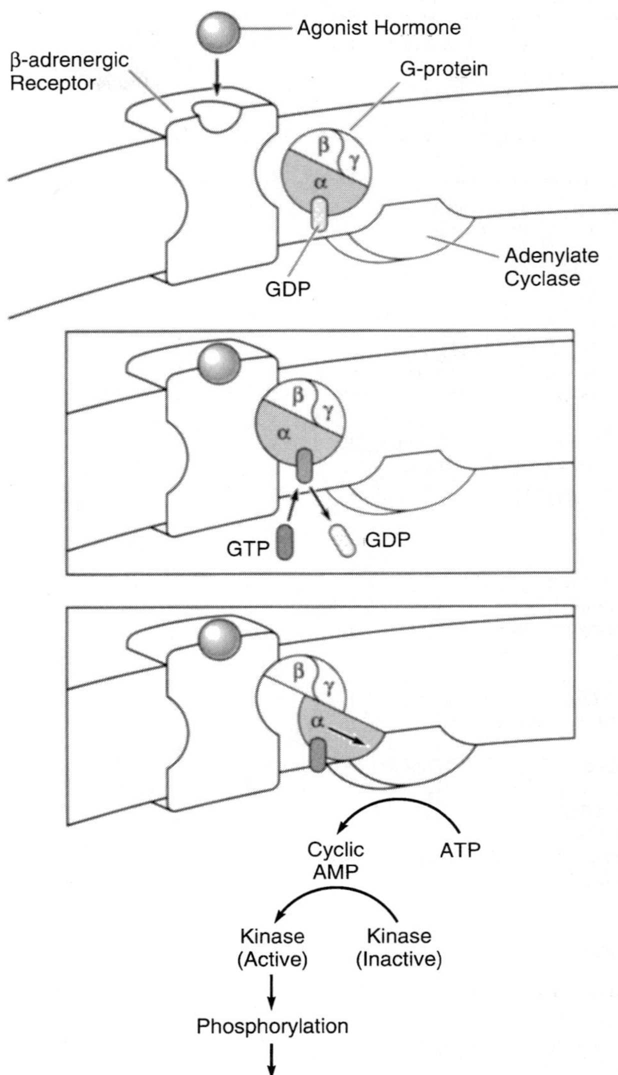

FIGURE 34–2 The cellular basis for the ability of beta-adrenergic antagonists to interfere with agonist stimulation of β-adrenergic receptors. Released from synaptic terminals, catecholamines enhance cardiac output and maintain arterial diffusion pressure. β-Adrenergic receptor binds the catecholamines. Catecholamines are released at the synapse, leading to enhanced heart rate and contractile force, through the following mechanisms: (1) sympathetic nerve terminals release norepinephrine, which binds to the β-adrenergic receptor, activating adenylate cyclase through the coupling effect of G proteins, (2) the increase in intracellular cyclic adenosine monophosphate (AMP) leads to activation of protein kinase A, and (3) protein kinase A phosphorylates a variety of proteins, which enhances their catalytic activity, promoting a calcium-dependent increase in cardiac contractility. ATP, adenosine triphosphate; GDP, guanosine diphosphate; GTP, guanosine triphosphate.

TABLE 34–7 Selected Newer Slow Channel Calcium Antagonists

Type	Dosage	Special Uses	Excretion
Nisoldipine (dihydropyridine)	10 mg PO q 12 h	Treat systemic arterial hypertension and angina	Renal
Felodipine (dihydropyridine)	5–10 mg PO q 24 h	Treat systemic arterial hypertension and angina	Renal
Nicardipine (dihydropyridine)	20–40 mg PO tid	Treat systemic arterial hypertension and angina	Renal
Nimodipine (dihydropyridine)	60 mg q 4 h PO for 21 days	Reduce cerebral vascular ischemia after subarachnoid hemorrhage	Renal
Isradipine (dihydropyridine)	2.5 mg PO bid increasing up to 20 mg PO qd	Hypertension	Renal
Amlodipine (dihydropyridine)	5–10 mg PO qd	Systemic arterial hypertension and angina	Bile and renal
Bepridil (Na^+ and Ca^{2+} channel blocker)	200 mg PO qd increasing to 400 mg PO qd	Angina	Renal and fecal

Modified from Packer M, Frishman WH: Calcium Channel Antagonists in Cardiovascular Disease. East Norwalk, CT: Appleton-Century-Crofts, 1984.

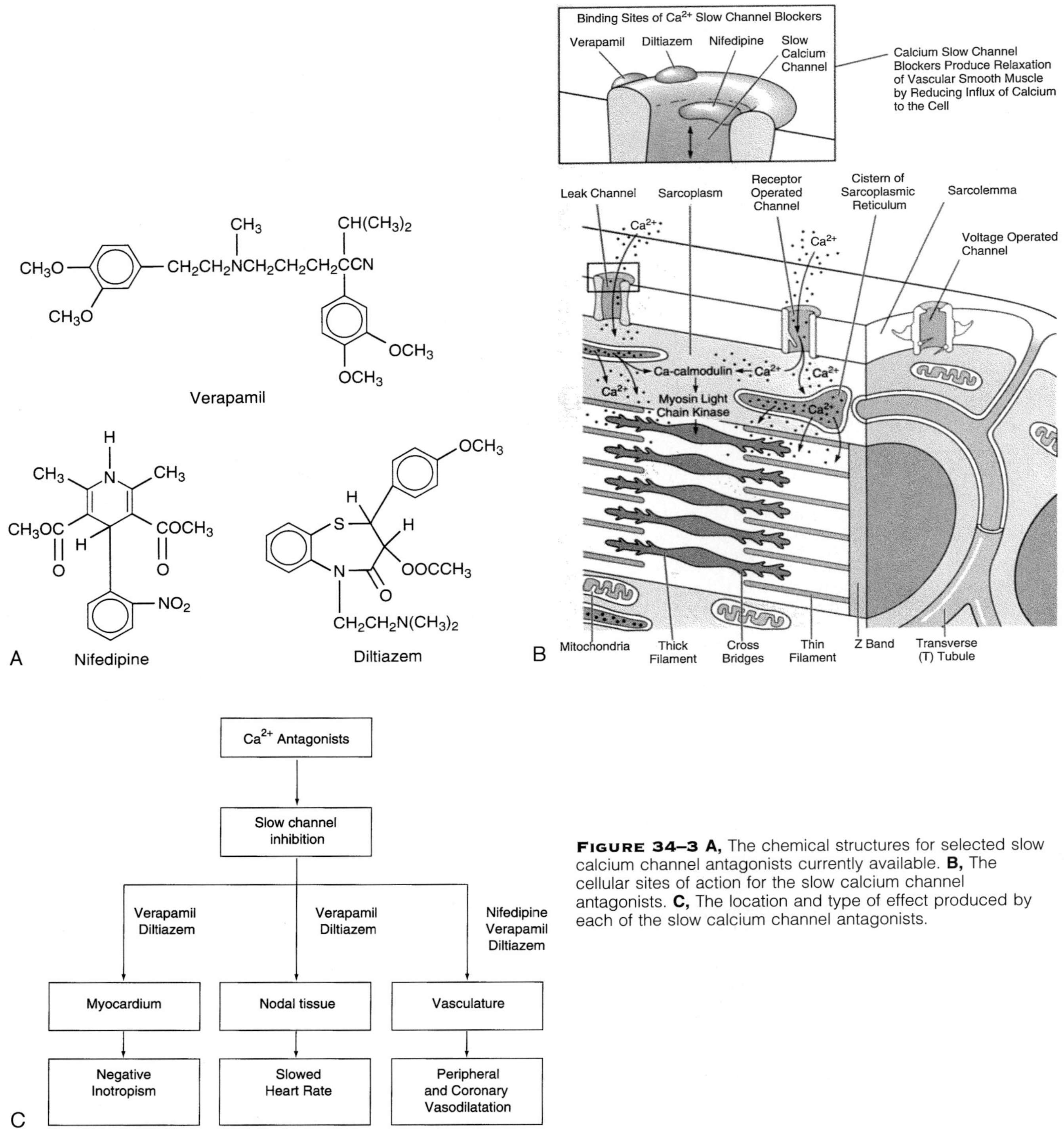

A

Verapamil

Nifedipine

Diltiazem

B

Binding Sites of Ca^{2+} Slow Channel Blockers

Verapamil Diltiazem Nifedipine Slow Calcium Channel

Calcium Slow Channel Blockers Produce Relaxation of Vascular Smooth Muscle by Reducing Influx of Calcium to the Cell

Leak Channel Sarcoplasm Receptor Operated Channel Cistern of Sarcoplasmic Reticulum Sarcolemma Voltage Operated Channel

Ca-calmodulin Myosin Light Chain Kinase

Mitochondria Thick Filament Cross Bridges Thin Filament Z Band Transverse (T) Tubule

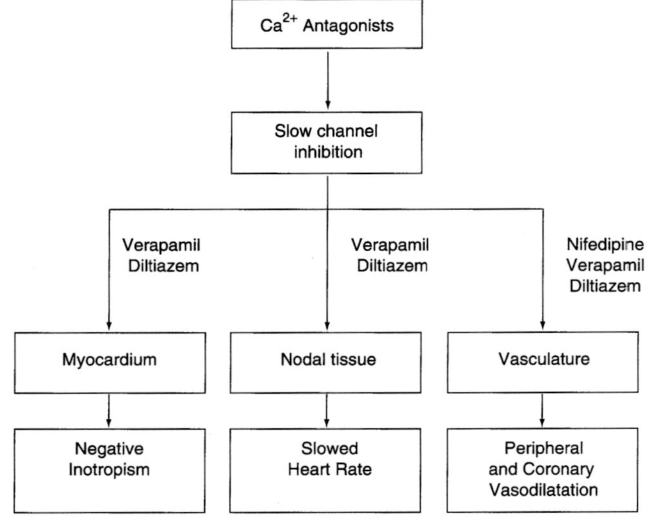

FIGURE 34–3 A, The chemical structures for selected slow calcium channel antagonists currently available. **B,** The cellular sites of action for the slow calcium channel antagonists. **C,** The location and type of effect produced by each of the slow calcium channel antagonists.

TABLE 34–8 Clinical Indications for Administration of Slow Calcium Channel Antagonists to Patients With Stable Angina

Treat the patient with chest pain at a relatively low level of exercise or stress. A calcium antagonist can be used alone or in combination with nitrates and/or a beta-blocker*
Treat the patient with systemic arterial hypertension
Treat the patient with atrial arrhythmias†
Treat the patient with exercise-induced ventricular tachycardia‡

*The safest combination of a calcium antagonist with a β-blocker is with a dihydropyridine calcium antagonist, such as nifedipine. Verapamil and a β-blocker given together may lead to bradycardia, hypotension, congestive heart failure, or atrioventricular block. Diltiazem and a β-blocker may lead to similar clinical problems. Therefore, verapamil and diltiazem should be used with great caution when combined with a β-blocker.

†Verapamil may convert paroxysmal supraventricular tachycardia to sinus rhythm when given intravenously, and verapamil or diltiazem may prevent its recurrence and/or control the ventricular rate in patients in whom the arrhythmia recurs. Verapamil and diltiazem help to control the ventricular rate in the patient with an atrial arrhythmia, such as atrial fibrillation or atrial flutter. Nifedipine has no protective effect against atrial arrhythmias.

‡The slow calcium channel antagonists often prevent exercise-induced ventricular tachycardia.

Two of the slow calcium channel antagonists, verapamil and diltiazem, slow the heart rate by decreasing sinus node impulse formation and AV conduction. Therefore, verapamil and diltiazem have some of the same hemodynamic effects as β-blockers in that they reduce myocardial oxygen demand at rest and during exercise by attenuating heart rate and contractile responses. However, they also increase coronary blood flow, primarily to epicardial regions supplied by severely narrowed coronary arteries.

Nifedipine, a dihydropyridine calcium antagonist, does not decrease impulse formation in the sinus node or delay AV conduction. Therefore, it does not decrease heart rate but may actually increase it. The dihydropyridine calcium antagonists are potent vasodilators, causing coronary artery vasodilatation. Nifedipine, as the prototype dihydropyridine calcium antagonist, dilates coronary arteries, increasing blood flow to the epicardial regions supplied by significantly narrowed coronary arteries. Nitrendipine has physiologic actions similar to those of nifedipine. Verapamil has a marked negative inotropic effect on the heart and should not be given to patients with clinically important congestive heart failure (CHF). Diltiazem has a lesser negative inotropic effect, but it should be given very carefully to patients with CHF. Great care should be used in combining diltiazem with another negative inotropic agent, such as a β-blocker, in the patient with clinically important CHF. Nifedipine may be given with relative safety to patients with important CHF. Its negative inotropic effect is masked by its ability to reduce systemic vascular resistance, which enables the heart to contract more effectively against a reduced afterload. As noted previously, β-blockers are used today in the treatment of selected patients with severe CHF, given in very small and slowly increasing doses.

Each of the slow calcium channel antagonists has important side effects (Table 34–9). With nifedipine administration, many patients describe a flushing sensation, dizziness, and palpitations, which are consequences of its systemic vasodilating effect. Peripheral edema occurs in patients who receive nifedipine (and other dihydropyridine calcium antagonists) and is probably the result of venodilatation. Constipation is the major side effect noted by patients taking verapamil, although symptoms related to CHF, bradycardia, or advanced AV block may also occur. The combination of verapamil with a β-blocker is particularly potent in reducing heart rate, systemic blood pressure, and contractile state. It should be used very carefully and not be given to patients with CHF, AV block, hypotension, or bradycardia. Diltiazem is usually the best tolerated of the slow calcium channel antagonists. When side effects occur, they are usually related to bradycardia or increasing CHF. A nondihydropyridine calcium antagonist can be used as an alternative to a β-blocker for treatment of the patient with stable angina. However, there has been considerable concern about potential adverse effects of the calcium antagonists in patients with coronary heart disease, especially in the patient with an acute coronary syndrome of unstable angina or myocardial infarction (MI) when relatively short-acting dihydropyridine calcium antagonists, such as nifedipine, are given in doses equaling or greater than 80 mg per day. There are data that suggest an increase in mortality and lack of clinical benefit when this agent is given in large doses to patients with acute coronary heart disease syndromes.[44]

COMBINED THERAPY WITH A CALCIUM ANTAGONIST, NITRATES, AND A β-BLOCKER

A calcium antagonist can be combined with nitrates and a β-blocker for treatment of the patient who experiences angina at low levels of effort. This combination of pharmacologic agents may be useful in enabling individual patients to be more active without having angina. Clinically, the safest combination of a β-blocker with a calcium antagonist is to use a dihydropyridine calcium antagonist, such as nifedipine. The next safest clinical combination is a β-blocker and diltiazem. One should initiate combined therapy with a β-blocker and diltiazem or verapamil using relatively small doses of the calcium antagonist and gradually increasing them as the patient demonstrates hemodynamic and clinical responses consistent with the safety of the combined regimen.

PLATELET ANTAGONISTS

When endothelial injury occurs, platelets aggregate after attaching to the subendothelial collagen and other matrix proteins exposed by the endothelial injury. Platelet aggrega-

TABLE 34–9 Side Effects of Slow Calcium Channel Antagonists

Verapamil or Diltiazem	*Nifedipine*
Marked bradycardia	Flushing sensation
Hypotension	Dizziness
Constipation	Hypotension
Congestive heart failure	Peripheral edema
Skin rash	Tachycardia
Heart block	Skin rash

tion may mechanically obstruct severely narrowed coronary arteries and is associated with the accumulation of mediators that promote further platelet aggregation and dynamic vasoconstriction, including thromboxane A_2, serotonin, thrombin, platelet-activating factor, adenosine diphosphate, oxygen-derived free radicals, tissue factor, and endothelin. In patients at increased risk for MI with known or suspected coronary artery disease, this risk may be reduced by the administration of aspirin.[45–48] Aspirin is an inhibitor of platelet and endothelial cyclooxygenase (COX 1 and COX 2) and thus reduces platelet thromboxane and endothelial cell prostacyclin formation (Fig. 34–4). Its effect on platelet cyclooxygenase is irreversible and persists for the lifetime of exposed platelets—approximately 11 days. With initial therapy, higher doses of aspirin are required to decrease endothelial cell cyclooxygenase activity; therefore, low-dose aspirin tends to reduce thromboxane more than prostacyclin concentration, but chronic administration of aspirin, even in a low dose, may reduce prostacyclin concentrations as well. Inhibiting release of thromboxane A_2 attenuates platelet aggregation in vivo. Aspirin's weaker effect to reduce COX 2 activity reduces inflammation, and at least some of its beneficial effects may be the result of its decreasing the vulnerability of unstable atherosclerotic plaques by its anti-inflammatory effects. The amount of aspirin required to protect patients is not well established. The Harvard Physicians' Study[45] suggested that 1 aspirin every other day reduced the risk for MI in male physicians believed to be at increased risk. However, a British study in which 1 aspirin per day was administered failed to show protection against the development of MI.[46]

Administration of aspirin to patients after MI reduces the risk of recurrent infarction and death, especially in patients with non–Q wave infarcts.[47] Although the optimal protective dose of aspirin in patients with coronary artery disease is not known, many physicians recommend administration of 1 (325 mg) aspirin every other day to 1 aspirin each day in individuals believed to be at risk for future coronary events. Ten large trials using platelet-inhibitor drugs in post-MI patients are available.[45–48] In eight of these trials, aspirin at a dose of 300 to 1500 mg daily was used alone or in combination with dipyridamole. Pooled analyses suggest significant reductions in mortality and reinfarction rates of 15 percent and 31 percent, respectively, in the aspirin-treatment groups.[46, 47] The chronic administration of aspirin, even at a low dose, may decrease vascular prostacyclin concentration. Theoretically, this may be disadvantageous over time, as prostacyclin is an endogenous endothelial vasodilator and an inhibitor of platelet aggregation. However, no adverse clinical consequence has been demonstrated.

The author recommends 1 aspirin every other day to 1 aspirin per day in patients believed to be at increased risk for future coronary events and in whom there is no contraindication (Table 34–10). Administration of aspirin with consequent cyclooxygenase inhibition and reduction

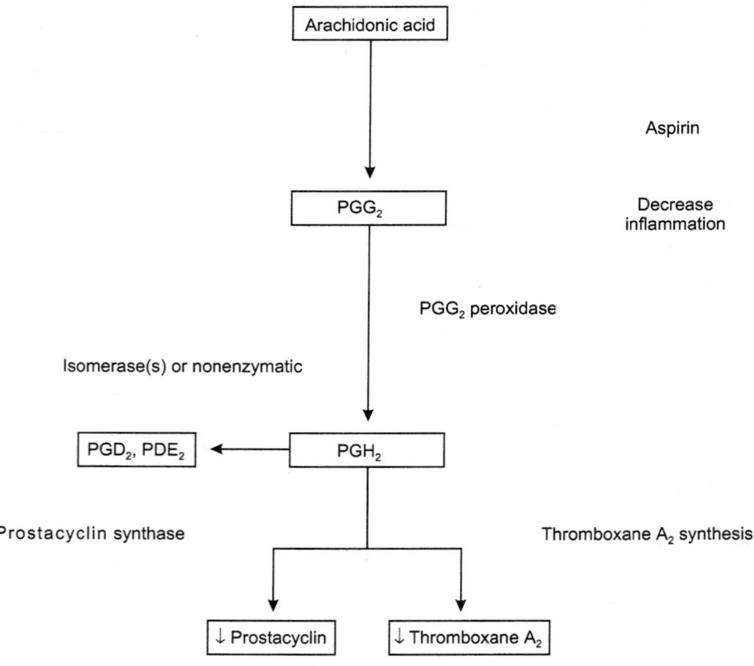

PGD_2 = The major prostaglandin produced by mast cells. Its effects include vasodilatation and contraction of nonvascular smooth muscle.
PGE_2 = An important prostaglandin having many effects. May cause smooth muscle to either contract or relax.
PGG_2 = A prostaglandin cyclic endoperoxide, an unstable intermediate.
PGH_2 = A prostaglandin cyclic endoperoxide formed from PGG_2. It is an unstable intermediate and can be converted to several important prostaglandins and thromboxanes.

FIGURE 34–4 The scheme for the synthesis of thromboxane A_2 (TXA_2) and prostacyclin (PGI_2) from arachidonic acid in platelets and endothelial cells. Aspirin's inhibitory effect is at the cyclooxygenase step, where it inhibits this enzyme and thereby diminishes the synthesis of both TXA_2 and prostacyclin. TXA_2 synthesis inhibitors interfere with the conversion of PGH_2 to TXA_2 through TXA_2 synthase. TXA_2 receptor antagonists simply antagonize the effects of TXA_2 on platelets and vascular tissue.

TABLE 34–10 Potential Side Effects of Aspirin

Gastritis
Stomach or gastrointestinal ulceration
Gastrointestinal bleeding
Easy bruising and bleeding with minor trauma
Asthma
Decline in renal function
Thrombocytopenia

in prostacyclin concentration may be associated with a reduction in renal blood flow and a rise in the serum blood urea nitrogen and creatinine. Nonsteroidal anti-inflammatory agents that are cyclooxygenase inhibitors may also cause a reduction of renal blood flow and a decline in renal function. Periodic measurements of blood urea nitrogen and creatinine concentrations are advised once aspirin therapy is begun. There is a risk for gastritis and gastrointestinal ulceration and bleeding when aspirin is administered. Some patients develop asthma. Therefore, patients should be selected and followed carefully with aspirin therapy.

CLOPIDOGREL

Clopidogrel, an analogue of ticoplidine, is an inhibitor of adenosine diphosphate activation of platelets by irreversibly and selectively blocking the binding of adenosine diphosphate to its receptor on the platelet surface. The protective effect of clopidogrel in patients at risk for vascular events was evaluated in a secondary prevention study comparing the effects of aspirin and clopidogrel in 19,185 patients with prior MI, ischemic stroke, or symptomatic peripheral arterial disease.[49] The Clopidogrel versus Aspirin in Patients at Risk for Ischaemic Events Trial (CAPRIE Trial) enrolled patients between 1992 and 1995 in 16 countries. At a mean follow-up of approximately 2 years, there was a 9 percent relative reduction in the composite of ischemic stroke, myocardial reinfarction, or vascular death with the use of clopidogrel. The annual occurrence of the primary endpoint was 5.8 percent in those treated with aspirin and 5.3 percent in those treated with clopidogrel (*P* = .04) (Fig. 34–5). Among the subgroup enrolled after MI, there was not a significant reduction in future vascular

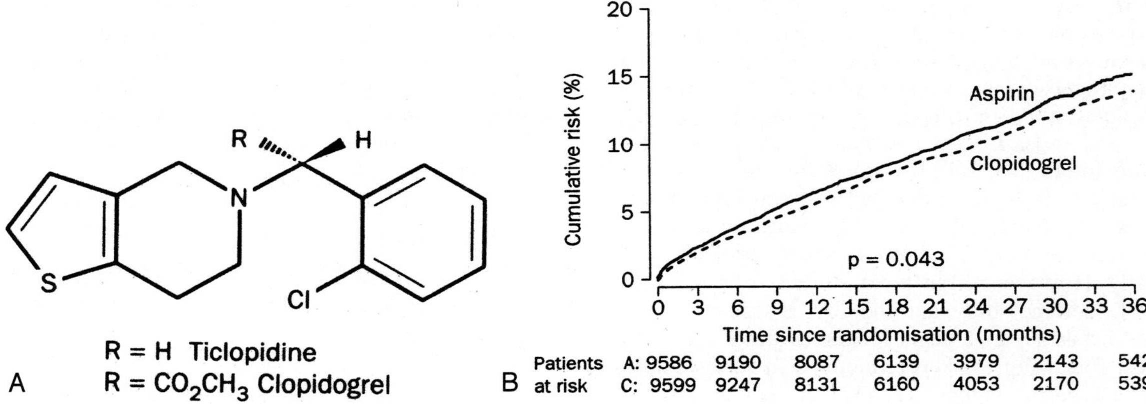

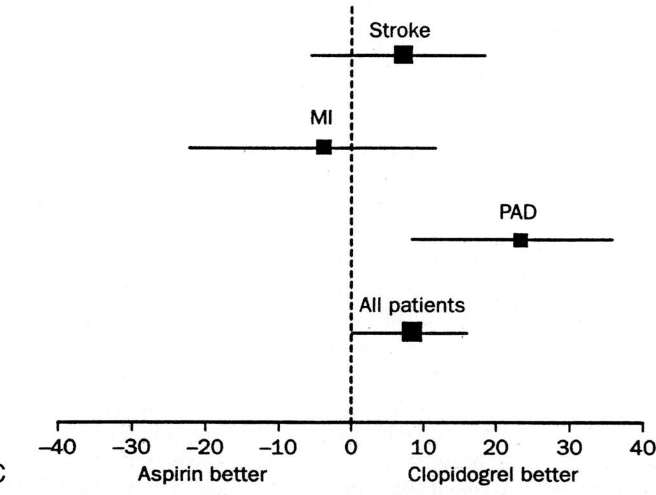

FIGURE 34–5 A, The chemical structure for ticlopidine and its analogue clopidogrel. **B,** The slight benefit of clopidogrel over aspirin in the Clopidogrel Versus Aspirin in Patients at Risk of Ischaemic Events (CAPRIE) trial in reducing future myocardial infarction, stroke, and vascular death. **C,** The influence of aspirin or clopidogrel in the CAPRIE trial by future event. PAD, peripheral artery disease. (**B** and **C,** From CAPRIE Steering Committee: A randomised, blinded, trial of clopidogrel versus aspirin in patients at risk of ischaemic events [CAPRIE]. Lancet 348[9038]:1329–1339, 1996, © by The Lancet Ltd. 1996.)

events in patients treated with clopidogrel. Many physician investigators, including the author, believe that a combination of aspirin and clopidogrel may be more protective than either intervention alone in preventing future acute coronary artery syndromes.

REDUCING RISK FACTORS

It is very important that patients with known or suspected coronary heart disease and stable angina do everything possible to reduce their risk of future coronary events. Specifically, cessation of smoking, rigorous control of serum cholesterol and low-density lipoprotein (LDL) and triglycerides, medical control of systemic arterial hypertension and hyperglycemia, regular exercise, and avoidance of ongoing stressful situations form the hallmark of preventive medical therapy in such individuals. The author believes that reduction in serum cholesterol and LDL to the lowest values possible provide the best protection. Three large multicenter clinical trials (the Scandinavian Simvastatin Survival Study [4S], the West of Scotland Study, and the Cholesterol and Recurrent Events [CARE] Trial) have demonstrated the value of 3-hydroxy-3-methylglutaryl coenzyme A–reductase inhibitors in lowering serum cholesterol and LDL values and reducing the risk of future coronary events in patients with coronary heart disease (Fig. 34–6).[50–52] Reductions in serum cholesterol to values below 200 mg/dl and in LDL values to below 125 mg/dl reduce the risk of future MI and the need for intervention or surgical therapy. In patients deemed to be at high risk for future coronary events, reducing LDL values to below 100 mg/dl may reduce the risk of future major vascular events substantially. However, these three studies—the 4S study, the West of Scotland study, and the CARE study—have all shown that it takes 1 to 2 years for the protective effect to be manifest following marked reductions in serum cholesterol and LDL serum values (see Fig. 34–6).

More recent studies have also shown that marked reduction of serum cholesterol and LDL values reduces the serum C-reactive protein concentration, itself a marker of risk for future coronary events in patients with coronary heart disease.[53] Thus, rigorous control of serum cholesterol and LDL concentrations by diet and medication may provide major protection against future coronary events. One would also like to raise serum high-density lipoprotein (HDL) values as much as possible, since very low HDL values are a risk factor for future coronary events. Very low HDL values, that is, less than 35 mg/dl, are found in patients with strong family histories of premature (earlier than 50 years of age) acute MI. Unfortunately, at the present time, it is difficult to raise serum HDL values. The most effective approaches have included regular exercise, weight loss, an occasional glass of red wine, and strict control of serum triglyceride and of total cholesterol and LDL concentrations; but all of these efforts together usually fail to substantially raise HDL values. There is an inverse relationship between serum triglyceride concentration and serum HDL values; thus, lowering serum triglycerides usually elevates serum HDL values modestly. Medications used to alter serum lipid values are reviewed elsewhere in this book (see Ch. 71, Atherosclerosis: Pathogenesis, Morphology, and Risk Factors, and Ch. 124, Cholesterol Disorders). We await the development of new medications and novel therapies that will substantially elevate serum HDL concentrations.

Figure 34–7 shows selected therapeutic options in the treatment of the patient with stable angina. It must be emphasized that when angina occurs at relatively low levels of effort or stress, or when it limits the lifestyle that a patient wishes to lead while he or she is receiving appropriate medical therapy, the patient should be referred for coronary arteriography and subsequently for coronary artery revascularization, either angioplasty, with or without stenting, atherectomy, or coronary artery bypass graft surgery, if the coronary anatomy is suitable. The same is true for the patient with objective evidence of myocardial ischemia, including classic ST-segment alteration (usually ST-segment depression but including ST-segment alteration), or reversible alterations in myocardial perfusion or function at low or moderate levels of stress (exercise or other form of stress myocardial scintigraphy or echocardiography) who is receiving appropriate medical therapy.[54–58] Patients with a significant (≥50 percent luminal diameter narrowing) left main coronary artery stenosis and those with significant three-vessel coronary artery disease (≥70 percent luminal diameter narrowing) and depressed left ventricular function should undergo life-prolonging coronary artery surgical bypass revascularization for the purpose of prolonging their survival, in conjunction with active reversal of all possible risk factors, as reviewed previously.[59–62]

AGGRESSIVE LIPID LOWERING COMPARED WITH ANGIOPLASTY IN STABLE CORONARY ARTERY DISEASE

Pitt and associates[63] studied 341 patients with stable coronary heart disease, relatively normal left ventricular function, asymptomatic or mild-to-moderate angina, and a serum level of LDL cholesterol of at least 115 mg/dl who were referred for percutaneous revascularization. These investigators randomly assigned the patients either to receive medical treatment with atorvastatin at 80 mg/day (164 patients) or to undergo the recommended percutaneous revascularization procedure (angioplasty) followed by the usual care, which could include lipid-lowering treatment (177 patients). The aggressive lipid-lowering treatment reduced mean serum LDL concentration to 77 mg/dl. Twenty-two (13 percent) of these patients had an ischemic event compared with 37 (21 percent) of the patients who had percutaneous transluminal coronary angioplasty (PTCA) during an 18-month follow-up. The PTCA-treated patients had a mean serum LDL concentration of 119 mg/dl. The incidence of ischemic events was 36 percent lower in the atorvastatin group ($P = .048$), and there was a significantly longer time to first ischemic event ($P = .03$). The reduction in events was fewer PTCAs, coronary artery bypass grafts, and hospitalizations for worsening angina. Thus, in low-risk patients, aggressive lipid-lowering therapy is at least as effective as PTCA and usual care in reducing future ischemic events.

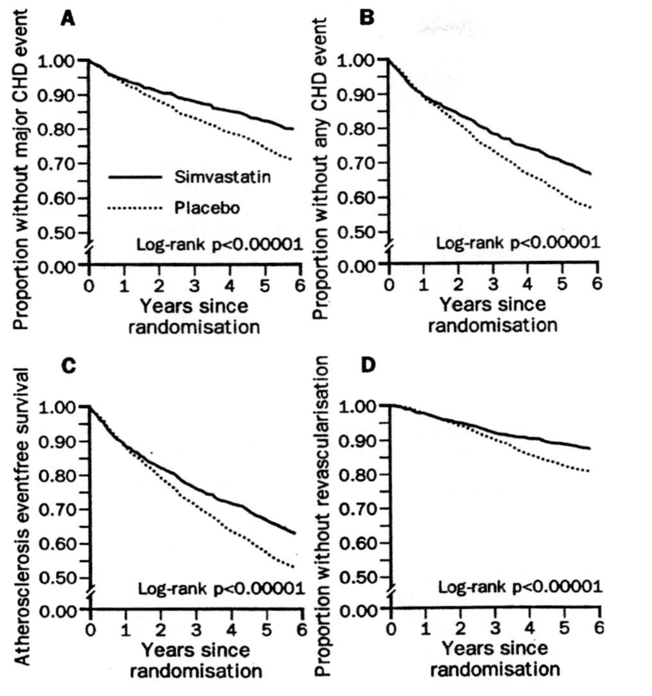

Kaplan-Meier curves for secondary and tertiary endpoints

A (A) major coronary events; (B) any coronary event; (C) survival free of any atherosclerotic event; (D) myocardial revascularisation procedures.

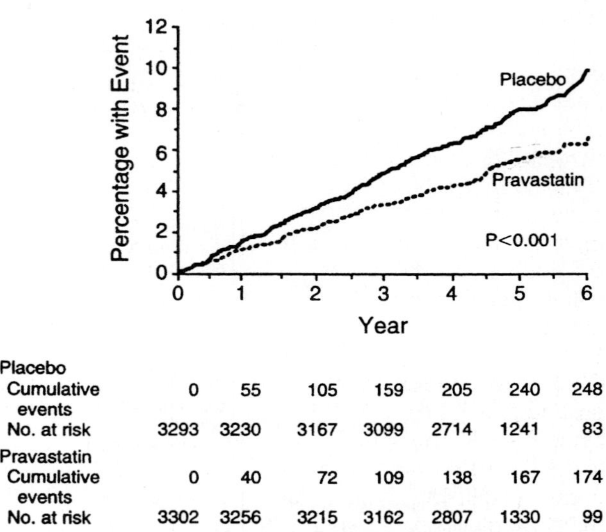

	0	1	2	3	4	5	6
Placebo							
Cumulative events	0	55	105	159	205	240	248
No. at risk	3293	3230	3167	3099	2714	1241	83
Pravastatin							
Cumulative events	0	40	72	109	138	167	174
No. at risk	3302	3256	3215	3162	2807	1330	99

B Kaplan–Meier Analysis of the Time to a Definite Nonfatal Myocardial Infarction or Death from Coronary Heart Disease, According to Treatment Group.

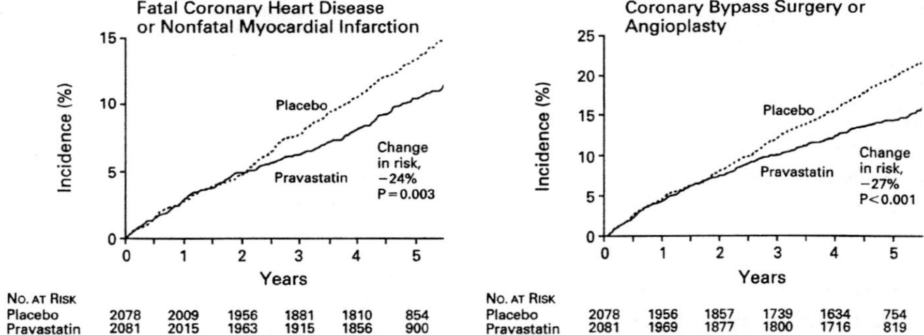

No. at Risk						
Placebo	2078	2009	1956	1881	1810	854
Pravastatin	2081	2015	1963	1915	1856	900

No. at Risk						
Placebo	2078	1956	1857	1739	1634	754
Pravastatin	2081	1969	1877	1800	1716	819

Kaplan–Meier Estimates of the Incidence of Coronary Events in the Pravastatin and Placebo Groups.

C The left-hand panel shows data for the primary end point — fatal coronary heart disease or nonfatal myocardial infarction. The right-hand panel shows data for coronary bypass surgery or angioplasty. Changes in risk are those attributable to pravastatin. P values and changes in risk are based on Cox proportional-hazards analysis.

FIGURE 34–6 **A,** The influence of simvastatin or placebo on future coronary events, survival, and need for revascularization procedure in the Scandinavian Simvastatin Survival Study (4S) trial. Note the beneficial effect of lipid lowering with simvastatin (Zocor) but also that between 1 and 2 years was required to begin to see the beneficial effect from lipid lowering on these variables. **B,** The beneficial effect of lipid lowering with the 3-hydroxy-3-methylglutaryl coenzyme A reductase inhibitor, pravastatin. Once again, 1 to 2 years of therapy was required to demonstrate the beneficial effect. **C,** The reduction in fatal coronary heart disease or nonfatal myocardial infarction *(left)* and need for coronary bypass surgery or angioplasty *(right)* with pravastatin or placebo in the Cholesterol and Related Events (CARE) trial. Note that the beneficial results from lipid-lowering therapy required nearly 2 years to be apparent. (**A,** From Scandinavian Simvastatin Survival Study Group: Randomised trial of cholesterol lowering in 4444 patients with coronary heart disease: the Scandinavian Simvastatin Survival Study [4S]. Lancet 344[8934]:1383–1389, 1994, © by The Lancet Ltd. 1994. **B,** From Shepherd J, Cobbe SM, Ford I, et al, for the West of Scotland Coronary Prevention Study Group: Prevention of coronary heart disease with pravastatin in men with hypercholesterolemia. N Engl J Med 333:1301–1307, 1995. Copyright © 1995 Massachusetts Medical Society. All rights reserved. **C,** From Sacks FM, Pfeffer MA, Moye LA, et al, for the Cholesterol and Recurrent Events Trial Investigators: The effect of pravastatin on coronary events after myocardial infarction in patients with average cholesterol levels. N Engl J Med 335:1001–1009, 1996. Copyright 1996 Massachusetts Medical Society. All rights reserved.)

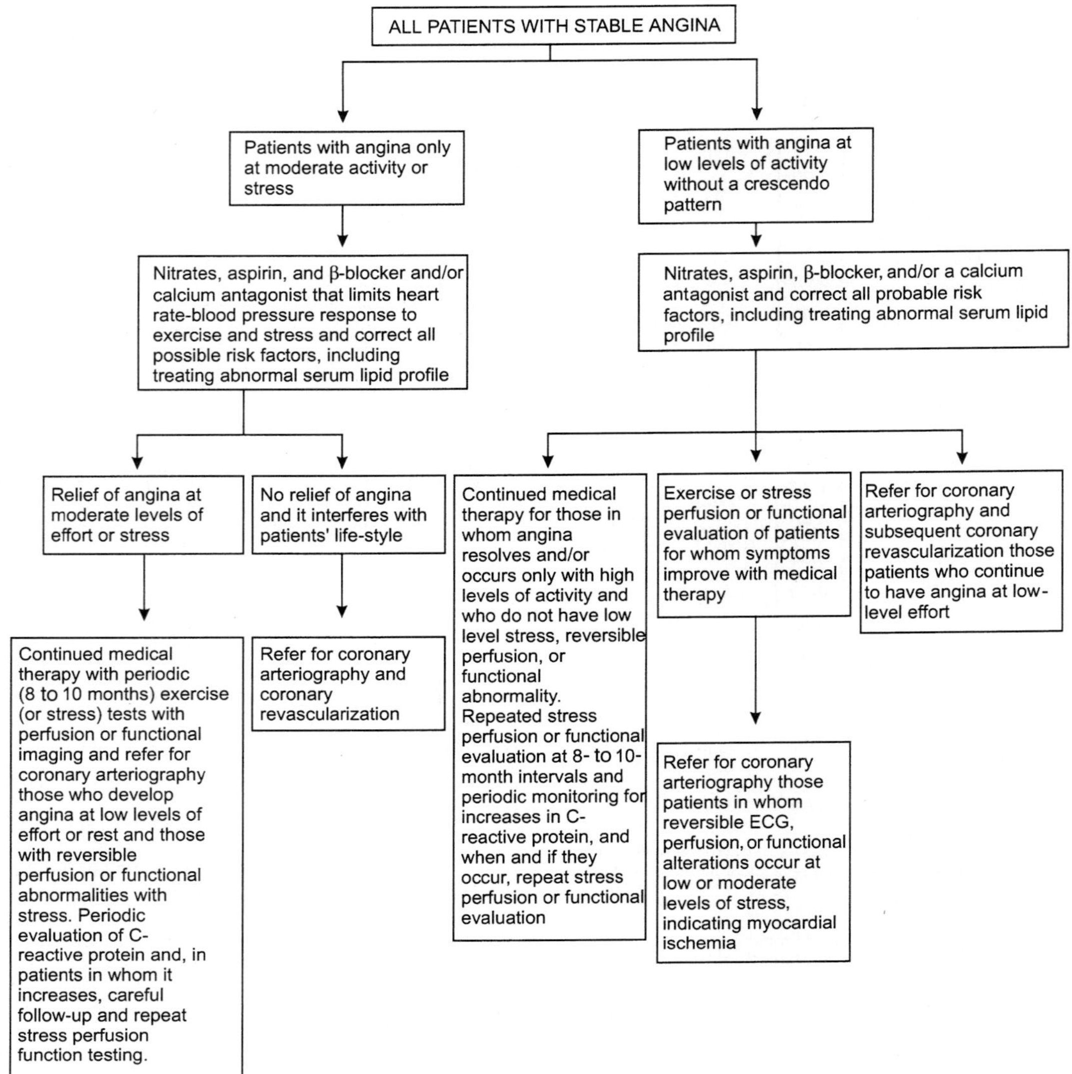

FIGURE 34–7 Author's schematic diagram of therapeutic options for the treatment of the patient with stable angina.

ANGIOTENSIN-CONVERTING ENZYME INHIBITORS IN VASCULAR PROTECTION: THE HEART OUTCOMES PREVENTION EVALUATION (HOPE) TRIAL

A large-scale multicenter (267 hospitals in 19 countries), randomized, placebo-controlled trial of angiotensin-converting enzyme (ACE) inhibitor therapy and vitamin E supplementation in patients at high risk for vascular events was performed.[64] Inclusion criteria included age greater than 55 years and evidence of vascular disease (coronary heart disease, stroke, or peripheral vascular disease) or diabetes and one other cardiovascular risk factor. Patients with heart failure, a low left ventricular ejection fraction, current ACE inhibitor or vitamin E therapy, or acute events within the previous 4 weeks were excluded. A total of 9541 qualifying patients were randomized in a 2 × 2 factorial design to ramipril (up to 10 mg/day) or placebo and vitamin E (400 IU/day) or placebo, and followed for 4 to 6 years. The primary endpoint of the study was the composite of cardiovascular death, MI, or stroke. Secondary endpoints included revascularization and the development of CHF, unstable angina, or complications of diabetes.

Vitamin E therapy was not associated with any significant clinical benefit. Composite primary outcome events occurred in 16 percent of the vitamin E group and 15 percent of the placebo group (P = NS). No specific clinical subgroups showed clinical benefit, and there were no benefits in any of the individual component endpoints or in any of the secondary outcome endpoints.

However, ramipril therapy was associated with a highly significant clinical benefit (Fig. 34–8). Composite primary outcome events occurred in 13.9 percent of the ramipril group and 17.5 percent of the placebo-treated group (risk ratio [RR] .78; P = .000002). There was also significant benefit in the individual endpoints of cardiovascular death (6.0 percent versus 8.0 percent; RR, .75; P = .002), MI

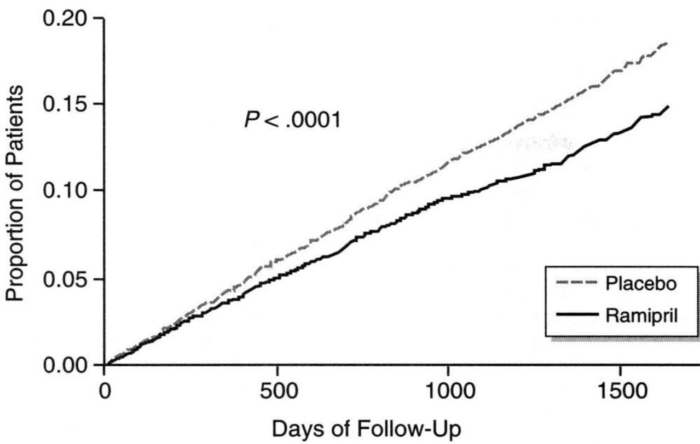

FIGURE 34–8 Kaplan-Meier estimates of the composite outcome of myocardial infarction, stroke, or death from cardiovascular causes in the ramipril group and the placebo group. The relative risk of the composite outcome in the ramipril group was 0.78 (95 percent confidence interval, 0.70 to 0.86). (From The Heart Outcomes Prevention Evaluation Study Investigators: Effects of an angiotensin converting enzyme inhibitor, ramipril, on death from cardiovascular causes, myocardial infarction, and stroke in high risk patients. N Engl J Med 342:145, 2000. Copyright © 2000 Massachusetts Medical Society. All rights reserved.)

(9.8 percent versus 12.0 percent; RR, .80; P = .0005), stroke (3.3 percent versus 4.8 percent; RR, .68; P = .0002), and total mortality (10.3 percent versus 12.2 percent; RR, .83, P = .035). There were no differences between groups in noncardiovascular death (4 percent versus 4 percent; P = NS). From the perspective of the secondary endpoints, there was no effect of ramipril therapy on the development of unstable angina, but there was a trend toward fewer heart failure hospitalizations and significantly fewer revascularizations (16.0 percent versus 18 percent; RR, .85; P = .0013).

There was also a striking benefit demonstrated in patients with documented normal left ventricular ejection fractions (n = 4676; mean ejection fraction 59 percent), with significant reductions in the primary outcome endpoint (13.6 percent versus 18.3 percent), cardiovascular death (5.0 percent versus 7.0 percent), MI (10.3 percent versus 13.5 percent), stroke (2.9 versus 4.2 percent), heart failure (8.3 percent versus 10.4 percent), and revascularization (19.8 percent versus 23.8 percent). In the overall population, the divergence of the primary endpoint was present in the first year, and the event curves continued to diverge through year 4. The clinical benefit was noted in virtually all of the major subgroups, including patients with or without cerebrovascular disease, diabetes, hypertension, coronary artery disease, peripheral vascular disease, men or women, and young or old.

Mechanistically, there was only a minor decrease in systolic (−2.17 mm Hg) and diastolic (−3.13 mm Hg) blood pressure, and the investigators speculated that although there was a strong relationship between clinical events and systolic blood pressure (but *not* diastolic blood pressure), the primary benefits of ramipril therapy were vascular rather than a blood pressure–lowering effect. In this population, the number of treated patients (4 years of therapy) needed to prevent 1 primary clinical event was 6; treating 1000 patients would prevent 170 adverse clinical events.

This study provides strong evidence that in patients at risk for vascular events, ACE inhibitor therapy with ramipril significantly reduces cardiovascular death, MI, stroke, heart failure, and revascularization, even in patients with documented normal left ventricular ejection fractions. Vitamin E therapy did not appear to be beneficial.

Earlier the TREND investigators showed that ACE inhibition with quinapril improved endothelial dysfunction in patients who were normotensive and who did not have severe hyperlipidemia or heart failure.[65] In this study, the authors postulated that the benefits of ACE inhibition are not likely due to attenuation of the controllable effects and superoxide generating effects of angiotensin II and to enhancement of endothelial cell release of nitric acid secondary to diminished breakdown of bradykinin.[65]

Summary

Thus, marked lowering of serum cholesterol and LDL values, the use of antithrombotic therapy with aspirin and/or clopidogrel, and the use of an ACE inhibitor appear to provide substantial clinical protection against future vascular events.

REFERENCES

1. Mason DT, Braunwald E: The effects of nitroglycerin and amyl nitrate on arteriolar and venous tone in the human forearm. Circulation 32:755, 1965.
2. Reichek N, Priest C, Zimrin D, et al: Antianginal effects of nitroglycerin patches. Am J Cardiol 54:1, 1984.
3. Parker JO, VanKoughnett KA, Fung HL: Transdermal isosorbide dinitrate in angina pectoris: effect of acute and sustained therapy. Am J Cardiol 54:8, 1984.
4. Glancy DL, Richter MA, Ellis EV, et al: Effect of swallowed isosorbide dinitrate on blood pressure, heart rate, and exercise capacity in patients with coronary artery disease. Am J Med 62:39, 1977.
5. Horowitz JD, Antman EM, Lorell BH, et al: Potentiation of the cardiovascular effects of nitroglycerin by *N*-acetylcysteine. Circulation 68:1247, 1983.
6. Murad F, Arnold WP, Mittal CK, Braughler JM: Properties and regulation of guanylate cyclase and some proposed functions of cyclic GMP. Cyclic Nucleotide Res 11:175, 1979.
7. Markis JE, Gorlin R, Mills RM, et al: Sustained effect of orally administered isosorbide dinitrate on exercise performance of patients with angina pectoris. Am J Cardiol 43:265, 1979.
8. Danahy DT, Aronow WS: Hemodynamics and antianginal effects of high dose oral isosorbide dinitrate after chronic use. Circulation 56:205, 1977.
9. Thadani U, Fung H-L, Darke AC, et al: Oral isosorbide dinitrate in angina pectoris: comparison of duration of action and dose-response relation during acute and sustained therapy. Am J Cardiol 49:411, 1982.
10. Needleman P, Johnson EM Jr: Mechanism of tolerance development to organic nitrates. J Pharmacol Exp Ther 184:709, 1973.
11. Abrams J: Nitrate tolerance and dependence. Am Heart J 99:113, 1980.
12. Frishman W: Clinical pharmacology of the new beta-adrenergic blocking drugs. IX. Nadolol: a new long-acting beta-adrenoceptor blocking drug. Am Heart J 99:124, 1980.
13. Moses JW, Borer JS: Beta-adrenergic antagonists in the treatment of patients with heart disease. Dis Mon 27:1, 1981.
14. Koch-Weser J: Metoprolol. N Engl J Med 301:698, 1979.
15. Koch-Weser J, Frishman WH: Beta-adrenoceptor antagonists: new drugs and new indications. N Engl J Med 305:500, 1981.

16. Opie LH: Drugs and the heart. I. Beta-blocking agents. Lancet 1:693, 1980.
17. Dreyfuss J, Brannick LJ, Vukovich RA, et al: Metabolic studies in patients with nadolol: oral and intravenous administration. J Clin Pharmacol 17:300, 1977.
18. Frishman W: Clinical pharmacology of the new beta-adrenergic blocking drugs. I. Pharmacodynamic and pharmacokinetic properties. Am Heart J 97:663, 1979.
19. Conolly ME, Kersting F, Dollery CT: The clinical pharmacology of beta-adrenoceptor-blocking drugs. Prog Cardiovasc Dis 19:203, 1976.
20. Forman R, Eng C, Kirk ES: Comparative effect of verapamil and nitroglycerin on collateral blood flow. Circulation 67:1200, 1983.
21. Muller JE, Gunther SJ: Nifedipine therapy for Prinzmetal's angina. Circulation 57:137, 1978.
22. Hugenholtz PG, Michels HR, Serruys PW, et al: Nifedipine in the treatment of unstable angina, coronary spasm and myocardial ischemia. Am J Cardiol 47:163, 1981.
23. Gunther S, Green L, Muller JE, et al: Prevention by nifedipine of abnormal coronary vasoconstriction in patients with coronary artery disease. Circulation 63:849, 1981.
24. Solberg LE, Nissen RG, Vlietstra RE, et al: Prinzmetal's variant angina—response to verapamil. Mayo Clin Proc 53:256, 1978.
25. Johnson SM, Mauritson DR, Willerson JT, Hillis LD: A controlled trial of verapamil for Prinzmetal's variant angina. N Engl J Med 304:862, 1981.
26. Freedman B, Dunn RF, Richmond DR, et al: Coronary artery spasm during exercise: treatment with verapamil. Circulation 64:68, 1981.
27. Hansen JF, Sando E: Treatment of Prinzmetal's angina due to coronary artery spasm using verapamil: a report of three cases. Eur J Cardiol 7:327, 1978.
28. Schroeder JS, Lamb IH, Ginsburg R, et al: Diltiazem for long-term therapy of coronary arterial spasm. Am J Cardiol 49:533, 1982.
29. Johnson SM, Mauritson DR, Willerson JT, et al: A comparison of verapamil and nifedipine in the treatment of variant angina pectoris. Am J Cardiol 47:1295, 1981.
30. Winniford MD, Johnson SM, Mauritson DR, et al: Verapamil therapy for Prinzmetal's variant angina: comparison with placebo and nifedipine. Am J Cardiol 50:913, 1982.
31. Hillis LD: The new coronary vasodilators: calcium blockers. J Cardiovasc Med 5:583, 1980.
32. Theroux P, Waters DD, Affaki GS, et al: Provocative testing with ergonovine to evaluate the efficacy of treatment with calcium antagonists in variant angina. Circulation 60:504, 1979.
33. Nagao T, Ikeo T, Sato M: Influence of calcium ions on responses to diltiazem in coronary arteries. Jpn J Pharmacol 27:330, 1977.
34. Weishaar R, Ashikawa K, Bing RJ: Effect of diltiazem, a calcium antagonist, on myocardial ischemia. Am J Cardiol 43:1137, 1979.
35. Previtali M, Salerno JA, Tavazzi L, et al: Treatment of angina at rest with nifedipine: a short-term controlled study. Am J Cardiol 45:825, 1980.
36. Heng MK, Singh BN, Roche AHG, et al: Effects of intravenous verapamil on cardiac arrhythmias and on the electrocardiogram. Am Heart J 90:487, 1975.
37. Schamroth L, Krinkler DM, Garreet C: Immediate effects of intravenous verapamil in cardiac arrhythmias. Cardiovasc Res 5:419, 1971.
38. Andreasen F, Boye E, Christoffersen E, et al: Assessment of verapamil in the treatment of angina pectoris. Eur J Cardiol 2:443, 1975.
39. Neumann M, Luisada AA: Double blind evaluation of orally administered iproveratril in patients with angina pectoris. Am J Med Sci 251:552, 1966.
40. Sandler G, Clayton GA, Thronicroft S: Clinical evaluation of verapamil in angina pectoris. BMJ 3:224, 1968.
41. Livesley B, Catley PF, Campbell RC, et al: Double-blind evaluation of verapamil, propranolol, and isosorbide dinitrate against a placebo in the treatment of angina pectoris. BMJ 1:375, 1973.
42. Balasubramian V, Khanna PK, Naryanan GR, et al: Verapamil in ischemic heart disease—quantitative assessment by serial multistage treadmill exercise. Postgrad Med J 52:143, 1976.
43. Johnson SM, Mauritson DR, Corbett JR, et al: Double-blind, randomized, placebo-controlled comparison of propranolol and verapamil in the treatment of patients with stable angina pectoris. Am J Med 71:443, 1981.
44. Furberg C, Psaty BM, Meyer JV: Nifedipine: dose-related increase in mortality in patients with coronary heart disease. Circulation 92:1326, 1995.
45. Steering Committee of the Physicians' Health Study Research Group: Final report on the aspirin component of the ongoing Physicians' Health Study. N Engl J Med 321:129, 1989.
46. Peto R, Gray R, Collins R, et al: Randomised trial of prophylactic daily aspirin in British male doctors. BMJ 296:13, 1988.
47. Secondary prevention of vascular disease by prolonged antiplatelet treatment: Antiplatelet trialists' collaboration. BMJ 296:320, 1988.
48. Klimt CR, Knatterud GL, Stamler J, Meier P: Persantine-aspirin reinfarction study. Part II. Secondary coronary prevention with Persantine and aspirin. J Am Coll Cardiol 7:251, 1986.
49. CAPRIE Study Organization: A randomised blinded trial of clopidogrel versus aspirin in patients at risk for ischaemic events (CAPRIE). Lancet 348:1329, 1996.
50. Scandinavian Simvastatin Survival Study Group: Randomised trial of cholesterol lowering in 4444 patients with coronary heart disease: the Scandinavian Simvastatin Survival Study (4S). Lancet 344:1383, 1994.
51. Shepard J, Cobb SM, Ford I, et al for the West of Scotland Coronary Prevention Study Group: Prevention of coronary heart disease with pravastatin in men with hypercholesterolemia. N Engl J Med 333:1301, 1995.
52. Sacks FM, Pfeffer MA, Moye LA, et al for the Cholesterol and Recurrent Events Trial Investigators: The effect of pravastatin on coronary events after myocardial infarction in patients with average cholesterol levels. N Engl J Med 335:1001, 1996.
53. Ridker PM, Rifai N, Pfeffer M, et al: Long term effects of pravastatin on plasma concentration of C-reactive protein. Circulation 100:230, 1999.
54. Borer J, Bacharach SL, Green MV, et al: Real time radionuclide cineangiography in the noninvasive evaluation of global and regional left ventricular function at rest and during exercise in patients with coronary artery disease. N Engl J Med 296:839, 1977.
55. Gibson RS, Watson DD, Craddock GB, et al: Prediction of cardiac events after uncomplicated myocardial infarction. Prospective study comparing predischarge exercise thallium-201 scintigraphy and coronary angiography. Circulation 68:321, 1983.
56. Ritchie JL, Trobaugh GB, Hamilton GW, et al: Myocardial imaging with thallium-201 at rest and during exercise: comparison with coronary arteriography and resting and stress electrocardiography. Circulation 56:66, 1977.
57. Corbett J, Dehmer GJ, Lewis SE, et al: The prognostic value of submaximal exercise testing with radionuclide ventriculography prior to hospital discharge in patients with recent myocardial infarction. Circulation 64:535, 1981.
58. Dehmer GJ, Lewis SE, Hillis LD, et al: Exercise induced alterations in left ventricular volumes in man: usefulness in predicting the relative extent of coronary artery disease. Circulation 63:1008, 1981.
59. Veterans Administration Coronary Artery Bypass Surgery Cooperative Study Group: Eleven-year survival in the Veterans Administration randomized trial of coronary bypass surgery for stable angina. N Engl J Med 311:1333, 1984.
60. Passamani E, Davis KB, Gillespie MJ, et al and the CASS Principal Investigators and Their Associates: A randomized trial of coronary artery bypass surgery. Survival of patients with a low ejection fraction. N Engl J Med 312:1665, 1985.
61. CASS Principal Investigators and Their Associates: Coronary Artery Surgery Study (CASS): a randomized trial of coronary artery bypass surgery: survival data. Circulation 68:939, 1983.
62. European Coronary Surgery Study Group: Coronary-artery bypass surgery in stable angina pectoris: survival at two years. Lancet 1:889, 1979.
63. Pitt B, Waters D, Brown WV, et al: Aggressive lipid-lowering therapy compared with angioplasty in stable coronary artery disease. N Engl J Med 341:70, 1999.
64. The Heart Outcomes Prevention Evaluation Study Investigators: Effects of an angiotensin-converting enzyme inhibitor, ramipril, on death from cardiovascular causes, myocardial infarction, and stroke in high-risk patients. N Engl J Med 342:145, 2000.
65. Mancini GBJ, Henry GC, Macaya C, et al: Angiotensin-converting enzyme inhibition with quinapril improves endothelial vasomotor dysfunction in patients with coronary artery disease: The TREND (Trial on Reversing Endothelial Dysfunction) study. Circulation 94:258, 1996.

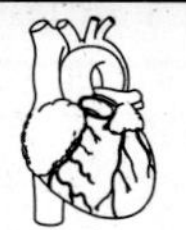

CHAPTER 35

MEDICAL TREATMENT OF UNSTABLE ANGINA AND NON–Q WAVE MYOCARDIAL INFARCTION

James T. Willerson

OVERVIEW
Specific Therapies
LOW-MOLECULAR-WEIGHT HEPARIN
Thrombosis in Myocardial Infarction II Study
ESSENCE Trial
Summary
PLATELET GLYCOPROTEIN IIb/IIIa ANTAGONISTS
CAPTURE Study
PURSUIT Trial
PRISM Study
PRISM-PLUS Study
Summary
Glycoprotein IIb/IIIa Receptor Antagonists Used With Interventional Therapies
GENERAL CONSIDERATIONS
CORONARY ARTERIAL SPASM (VARIANT ANGINA; PRINZMETAL'S ANGINA)
SUMMARY

OVERVIEW

The development of unstable angina with a crescendo or a rest anginal pattern, or both (Braunwald Classification IIIB and C, Table 35–1), should be considered a relative medical emergency and warrant hospitalization to rule out myocardial infarction (MI) and to initiate therapy that might prevent MI. Patients presenting with sustained and more severe chest pain, electrocardiographic changes of ST depression and T wave flattening or inversion, and elevated serum creatine kinase, the MB isoenzyme of creatine kinase, and troponin I concentrations have non–Q wave MI, and they are treated in the same ways as patients with unstable angina (Fig. 35–1). In the treatment regimen, one attempts to prevent persistent thrombus formation at the site of the unstable plaque and to relieve the associated vasoconstriction. Aspirin is begun immediately in patients without contraindication. Intravenous nitroglycerin is initiated beginning at doses of 1 to 2 μg/min with increases in dosage to one that reduces systolic blood pressure by at least 8 to 10 mm Hg while avoiding systemic arterial hypotension and/or that increases heart rate by 5 to 8 beats/min without increasing heart rate above 90 beats/min. Pain relief often occurs after complete bed rest and the institution of intravenous nitroglycerin and aspirin. Elevated blood pressure should be controlled with nitrates, calcium antagonists, and/or a beta blocker (see Tables 34–1, 34–2, and 34–6). Patients with rest angina should be given an antithrombin, such as heparin,[1] intravenously, typically beginning with a bolus dose of approximately 5000 units and followed by a sustained infusion of 900 to 1000 U/h. The partial thromboplastin time (PTT) (or activated coagulation time [ACT]) is followed at 8- to 12-hour intervals, and the heparin infusion rate is adjusted to maintain the PTT in the 60- to 80-second range or the ACT in the 250- to 350-second range. Alternatively, low-molecular-weight heparin might be given in appropriate dosage subcutaneously. Beta blockers should be added to this therapy in the patient without contraindications who has elevated blood pressure, increased heart rate due to pain or anxiety, or complex ventricular ectopy.

Specific Therapies

One to 4 aspirin per day reduces the risk of death and MI in the patient with unstable angina (Fig. 35–2).[1–3] Aspirin interferes with platelet aggregation and thromboxane A_2 synthesis and diminishes inflammation and platelet–white blood cell interaction. The combination of aspirin and heparin inhibits the effects of thromboxane A_2 and thrombin as potentiators of platelet aggregation leading to thrombosis and dynamic vasoconstriction. Their inhibition of thromboxane and thrombin improves regional myocardial blood flow and helps to prevent thrombosis. Heparin (and/or another thrombin antagonist) should be given to the patient with rest angina in whom there is no contraindication. Théroux and associates[1] have shown that the administration of heparin often relieves angina and reduces the risk for subsequent MI and death (see Fig. 35–2). In the Théroux and associates' study,[1] aspirin was also effective in the same patients in reducing fatal and nonfatal MI. Others have shown similar protective effects from aspirin therapy in these patients.[2–4] The combination of aspirin and heparin increased the risk of bleeding.[1] Abrupt withdrawal of heparin in the patient with unstable angina or MI may be associated with a heparin "rebound," with abrupt worsening of angina, the development of MI, or both.[5–7] When heparin and other thrombin inhibitors are discontinued in these patients, it should be done slowly over a period of several hours and with concomitant administration of aspirin or other antiplatelet therapy.

More specific thrombin inhibitors are being developed, and it is likely there will be a wider choice of thrombin antagonists in the future. Low-molecular-weight heparin or direct thrombin antagonists (hirudin, bivalirudin [Hirulog],

TABLE 35–1 Braunwald's Classification of Unstable Angina

Severity	Clinical Circumstances: A. Develops in Presence of Extracardiac Condition That Intensifies Myocardial Ischemia (Secondary UA)	B. Develops in Absence of Extracardiac Condition (Primary UA)	C. Develops Within 2 wk After AMI (Postinfarction UA)
I. New onset of severe angina or accelerated angina; no rest pain	IA	IB	IC
II. Angina at rest within past month but not within preceding 48 h (angina at rest, subacute)	IIA	IIB	IIC
III. Angina at rest within 48 h (angina at rest, acute)	IIIA	IIIB	IIIC

Abbreviations: AMI, acute myocardial infarction; UA, unstable angina.

Patients with UA may also be divided into three groups depending on whether UA occurs (1) in the absence of treatment for chronic stable angina, (2) during treatment for chronic stable angina, or (3) despite maximal anti-ischemic drug therapy. These three groups may be designated by subscripts 1, 2, or 3, respectively.

Patients with UA may be further divided into those with and without transient ST-T wave changes during pain.

From Braunwald E: Unstable angina: a classification. Circulation 80(2):410–414, 1989.

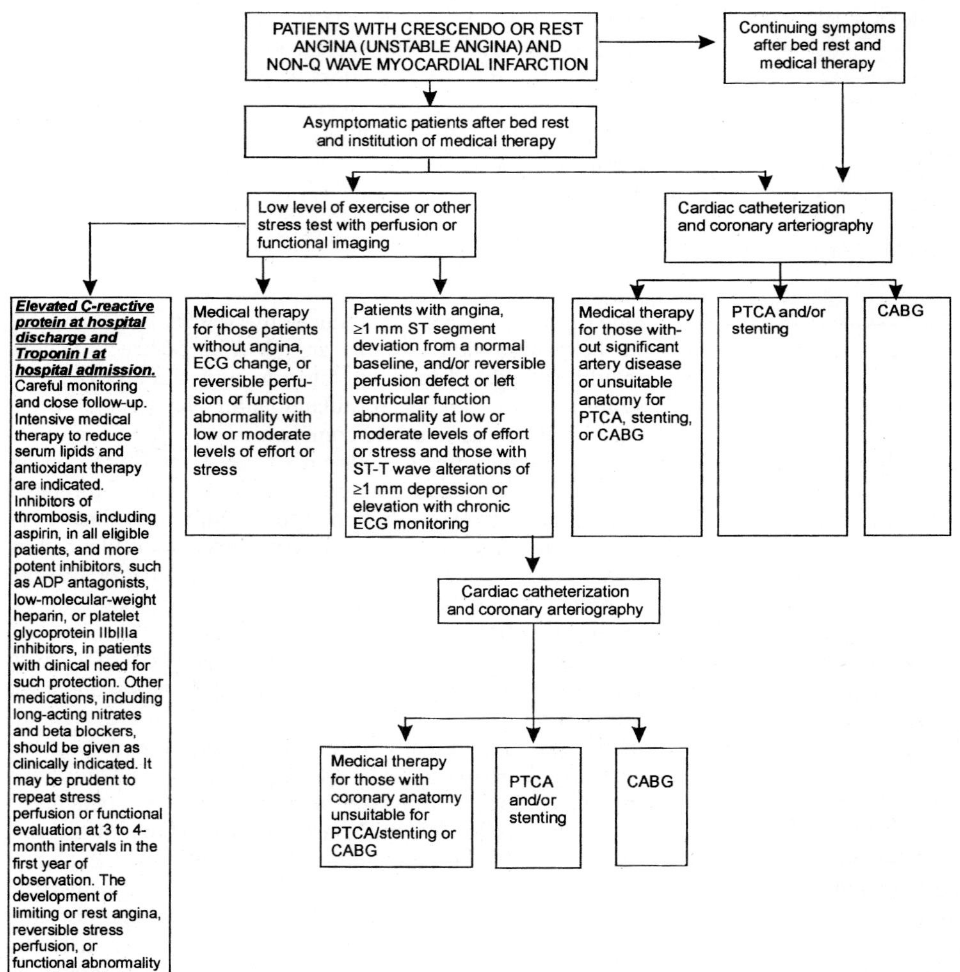

FIGURE 35–1 Schematic diagram demonstrates therapeutic alternatives for the treatment of patients with unstable angina pectoris and non–Q wave myocardial infarction. ADP, adenosine diphosphate; CABG, coronary artery bypass grafting; ECG, electrocardiogram; PTCA, percutaneous transluminal coronary angioplasty.

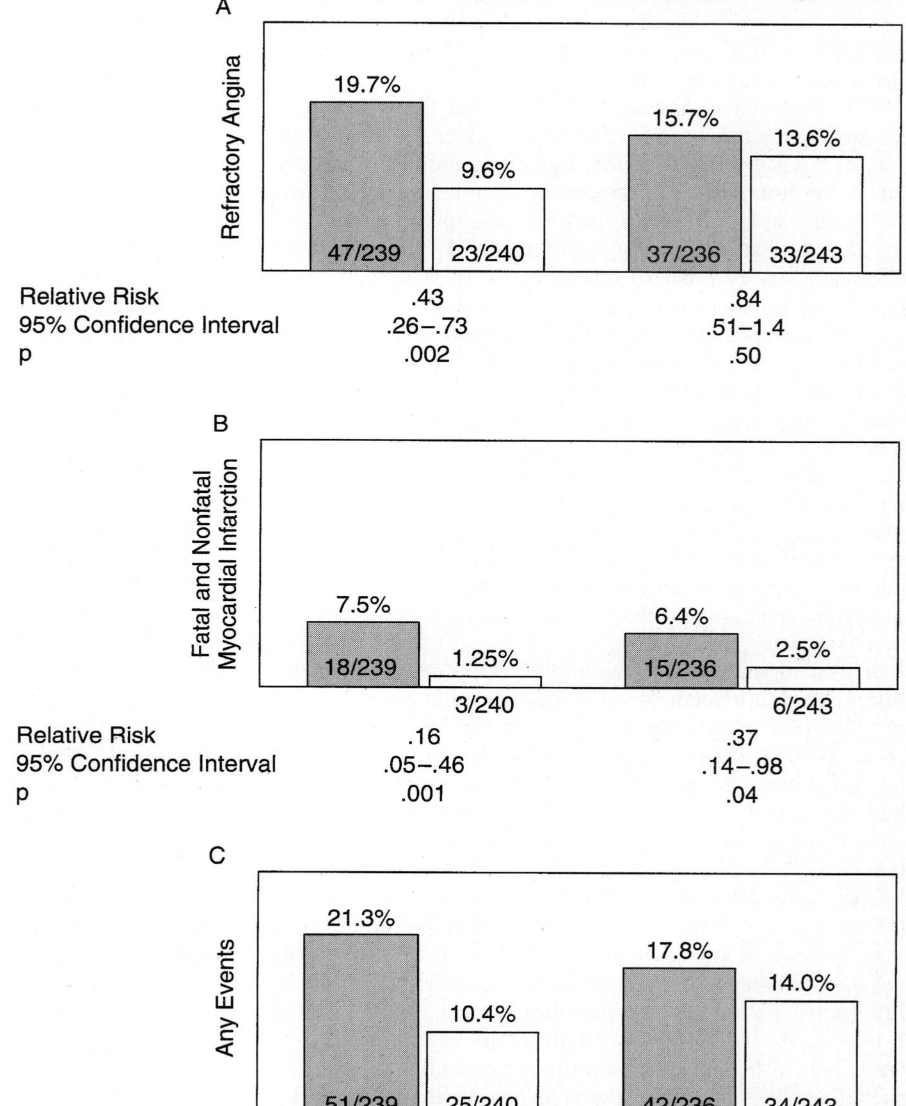

FIGURE 35–2 A–C, The influence of aspirin and heparin in the treatment of patients with unstable angina pectoris. **B,** Both aspirin and heparin reduce the risk for fatal and nonfatal myocardial infarction (MI). Heparin also reduces the frequency of important coronary events, including death, fatal and nonfatal MI, and continuing angina. The combination of heparin and aspirin was no more successful than heparin alone in this study. (**A–C,** Data from Théroux P, Ouimet H, McCann J, et al: Aspirin, heparin, or both to treat acute unstable angina. N Engl J Med 319:1105, 1988.)

and argatroban) should be useful alternatives to unfractionated heparin in the patient with unstable angina or non–Q wave MI. The direct thrombin antagonists will be useful to replace heparins in patients who develop thrombocytopenia and/or vascular thrombosis or bleeding as an allergic response to heparin administration—heparin-induced thrombocytopenia (HIT) and heparin-induced thrombosis syndromes (HITS) (see Ch. 108, Hematologic Disease and Heart Disease). The direct inhibitors of thrombin have more reliable and consistent effects on PTT than does heparin, allowing less frequent measurement of PTT or ACT. The use of low-molecular-weight inhibitors of heparin is discussed later in this chapter.

However, other mediators that promote thrombosis and are present at the site of a fissured or ulcerated plaque are not inhibited by this regimen, including adenosine diphosphate, serotonin, platelet activating factor, oxygen-derived free radicals, tissue factor, and endothelin (see Fig. 26–3 in Ch. 26, Pathophysiology and Clinical Recognition of Coronary Artery Disease Syndromes). If pain relief does not occur with bed rest and the use of these medications, the risk for subsequent MI, sudden death, and ventricular arrhythmias is increased. More comprehensive inhibitors of platelet aggregation than aspirin and heparin, inhibiting platelet aggregation in response to most or all of these mediators, can be useful in the treatment of these patients, including the addition of an adenosine diphosphate antagonist, such as ticlopidine or clopidogrel, or an inhibitor of platelet glycoprotein (GP) IIb/IIIa receptors, such as the monoclonal antibody, abciximab (ReoPro), the synthetic peptide, eptifibatide (Integrilin), or a low-molecular-weight inhibitor, such as tirofiban. These are discussed later in this chapter.

If rest angina persists, the addition of a calcium antagonist, such as diltiazem or verapamil, given in divided doses of 30 to 90 mg every 6 to 8 hours and 80 to 120 mg every 6 to 8 hours, respectively, and/or a β blocker is recommended. A platelet GP IIb/IIIa receptor antagonist may be added to this therapeutic regimen in the patient who continues to have rest angina despite this medical regimen, including those being referred for interventional therapy, percutaneous transluminal coronary angioplasty (PTCA), or stenting. One should consider the addition of intra-aortic balloon counterpulsation if rest angina persists despite the medical therapy outlined previously (Fig. 35–3). Intra-aortic balloon counterpulsation almost always relieves rest pain in the patient with unstable angina or non–Q wave MI. In patients with continuing rest angina requiring such intensive combined therapy, proceeding to coronary arteriography and PTCA, stenting, or coronary artery bypass graft surgery (CABG) is urgently needed.

Low-Molecular-Weight Heparin

As noted earlier, the disruption of an atherosclerotic plaque causes platelet activation, adhesion, and aggregation at the site of the injured plaque and activates the coagulation cascade through tissue factor release and the accumulation of multiple platelet and other cell-derived mediators of thrombosis. Tissue factor complexes with factor VIIa activating factor Xa, thereby catalyzing formation of thrombin (Fig. 35–4). Thrombin promotes further platelet aggregation, produces vasoconstriction at the site of vascular injury, and mediates the conversion of fibrinogen to fibrin. Since both platelet activation and thrombin generation are involved in the thrombotic process, there is obvious rationale for the use of inhibitors of both platelet aggregation and coagulation in the treatment of the patient with unstable angina or non–Q wave MI (and patients with acute Q wave MI). Low-molecular-weight heparin acts primarily through antithrombin III–mediated inhibition of factor Xa, but there is also some direct thrombin inhibition. As is true of conventional heparin, low-molecular-weight heparin promotes the release of tissue factor pathway inhibitor, which may contribute to its antithrombotic effects.[8–10]

Low-molecular-weight heparin is administered subcutaneously. It has a low degree of protein binding and a predictable anticoagulant response for a given dose without the need for laboratory monitoring.[8, 9] Therefore, one can provide a consistent anticoagulant and antithrombin effect by subcutaneous injections of fixed doses of low-molecular-weight heparin, generally on a two-times-per-day basis.[8–10]

The influence of low-molecular-weight heparin in patients with unstable angina pectoris or non–Q wave MI was evaluated in the Fragmin during Instability in Coronary Artery Disease (FRISC) Study.[8] In this double-blind trial, 1506 patients were randomly assigned to receive a low-molecular-weight heparin, subcutaneous dalteparin (Fragmin), 120 IU/kg body weight with a maximal dose of 10,000 IU given twice daily for 6 days, and then 7500 IU once daily for the next 35 to 45 days, or placebo. The primary endpoint was the rates of new MI and death during the first 6 days after beginning treatment. Secondary endpoints were rates of death and new MI after 40 days and 150 days, respectively; the frequency of revascularization procedures; the need for heparin infusion; and a composite endpoint.

Patients were recruited at 23 Swedish hospitals. Eligible patients were men older than 40 years and women more than 1 year after menopause admitted to the hospital with chest pain in the previous 72 hours. Eligibility for treatment required the patient to have newly developed or increased angina pectoris or angina at rest in the previous 2 months or persisting chest pain with the suspicion of MI and at least one of the following electrocardiographic criteria: transient or persistent ST-segment depression of 0.1 mV or more and T wave inversion of 0.1 mV or more in at least two adjacent leads without significant Q waves in these same leads. All patients without contraindications received aspirin, 75 mg daily after an initial dose of 300 mg, β blockers, and calcium antagonists and nitrates as needed. At the discretion of the attending physician, nitroglycerin was given intravenously.

The findings of the study are shown in Figure 35–5 and Table 35–2. Within the first 6 days, the rates of new MI and death were lower in the dalteparin group than in the placebo group (13 [1.8 percent] versus 36 [4.8 percent]; risk ratio, 0.37) (see Fig. 35–5). The frequency of the need for intravenous heparin and revascularization was also reduced by dalteparin treatment. The composite endpoint of death, MI, revascularization, and need for intravenous

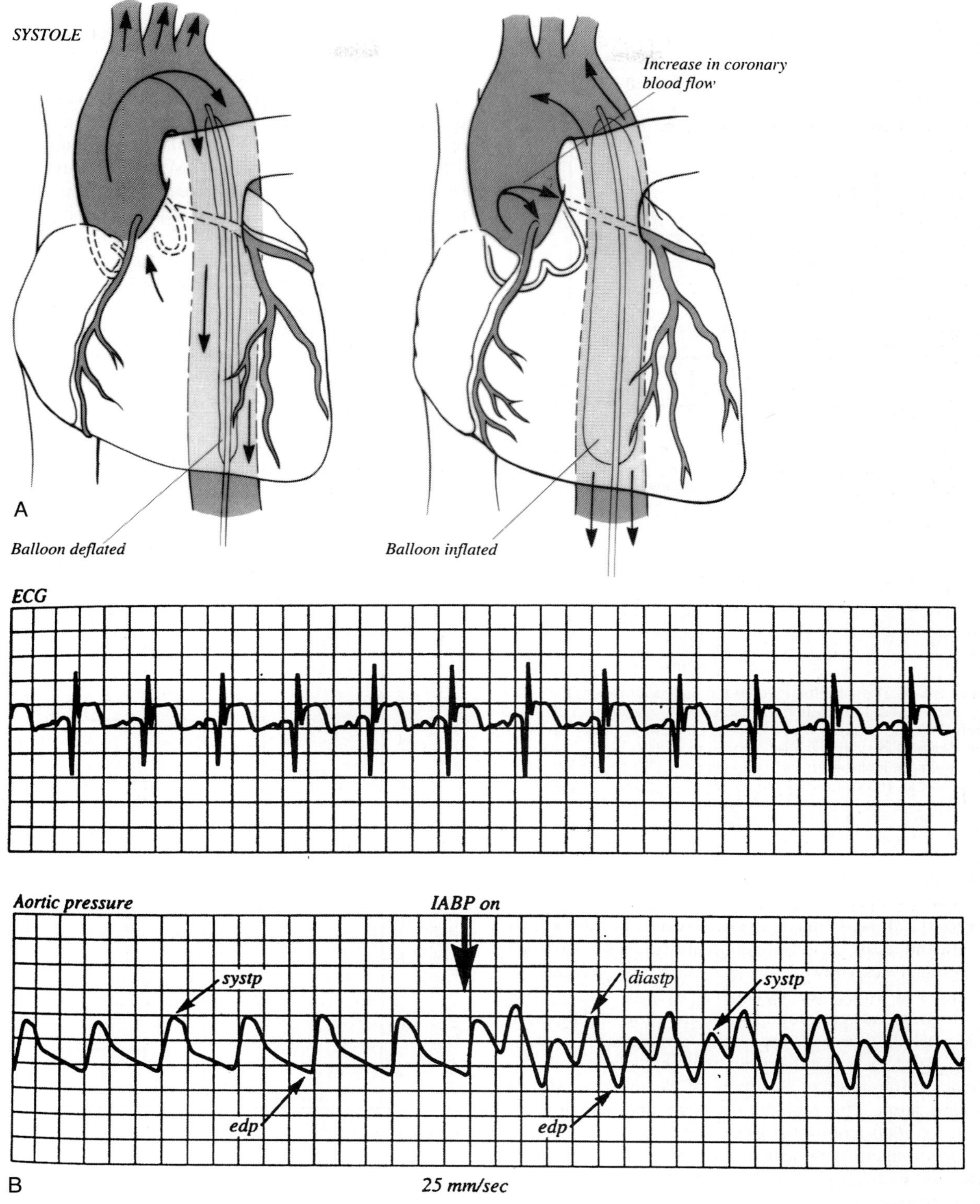

FIGURE 35–3 A, The position in which the intra-aortic balloon pump (IABP) is placed in the aorta. The balloon deflates during cardiac systole and inflates during cardiac diastole. The net results of this filling and collapsing action are to increase the diastolic blood pressure in the proximal aorta and consequently to increase coronary blood flow. The systolic collapse of the balloon reduces the work of the heart. **B,** The physiologic effects of the IABP. The increase in aortic diastolic blood pressure (diastp) associated with balloon inflation (IABP on) is shown. The electrocardiogram (ECG) is used to time cardiac systole and diastole. edp, end-diastolic pressure; systp, systolic blood pressure. (**A** and **B,** From Willerson JT: Treatment of Heart Disease. New York: Gower Medical, 1993.)

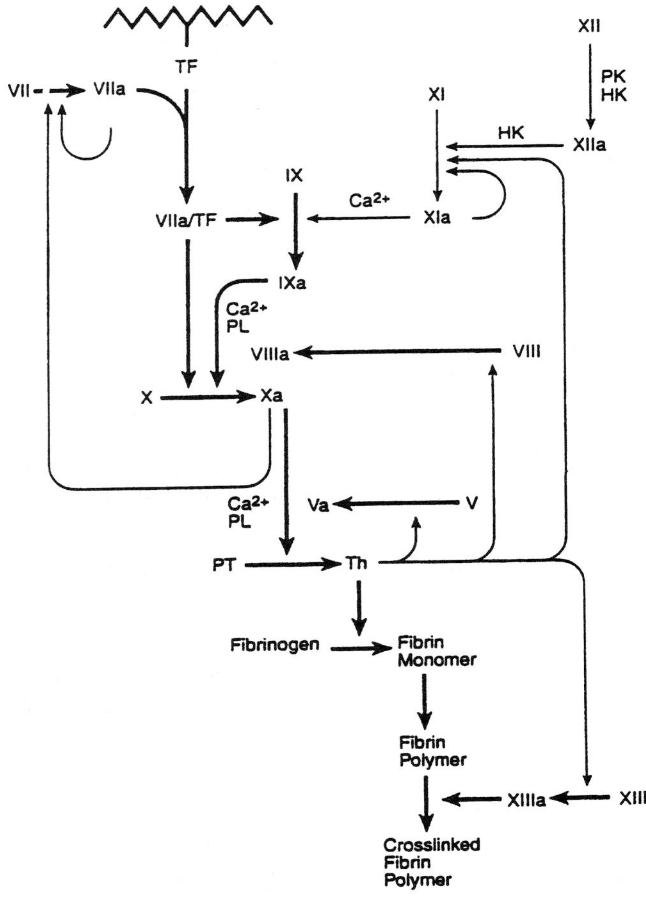

FIGURE 35–4 The scheme involved in tissue factor's (TF) participation in the coagulation cascade in the generation of thrombin (Th) and the role that thrombin plays in the development of fibrin crosslinking and platelet aggregation. HK, high-molecular-weight kininogen; PK, pre-kallikrein; PL, phospholipid; PT, prothrombin. (From Loscalzo J, Schafer AI [eds]: Thrombosis and Hemorrhage. p. 7. Oxford: Blackwell Scientific, 1994.)

heparin was also significantly reduced in favor of dalteparin (40 patients [4.5 percent] versus 78 patients [10.3 percent]; risk ratio, 0.52). At 40 days, the differences in rates of MI and death and in the composite endpoint persisted, although subgroup analyses showed that the effect was confined to nonsmokers at this time. Survival analysis showed a risk of reactivation and reinfarction when the dose of dalteparin was decreased; this was especially pronounced in nonsmokers. By 4 to 5 months after treatment, there were no significant differences in the rates of death, new MI, or revascularization. This regimen was safe, and patient compliance was good among the treated patients.

This study again demonstrates the benefits of thrombin inhibition in the treatment of patients with unstable angina pectoris and non–Q wave MI. However, a potential advantage of low-molecular-weight heparin therapy is the ability to continue it after hospital discharge with continued suppression of thrombin's effects. In this study, the effects of long-term treatment with low-molecular-weight heparin appeared to be primarily confined to the nonsmokers, which included 80 percent of the patient population. Efforts at reducing the dose of the low-molecular-weight inhibitor resulted in a risk of reinfarction that was most pronounced in nonsmokers.

The use of low-molecular-weight heparin is a potential alternative to unfractionated heparin in the patient with unstable angina and non–Q wave MI.[11, 12] There may be real advantages in continuing low-molecular-weight heparin after hospital discharge, particularly in patients who do not receive an interventional procedure, such as angioplasty or stenting, atherectomy, or surgical revascularization. There is an ongoing risk of MI or reinfarction in the subsequent 4 to 6 weeks in patients with unstable angina pectoris and non–Q wave infarction, probably related to the persistent presence of endothelial injury after plaque ulceration and fissuring and the time required for its repair. The author believes that as long as the endothelium remains anatomically disrupted, the patient has a continuing risk of unstable angina and MI and that these clinical entities represent aborted Q wave infarcts with transient rather than permanent thrombosis. Inhibition of thrombin during this period may be very useful; the FRISC Study suggests that this may be especially useful in nonsmokers.[8] One limitation, however, of the low-molecular-weight heparins is their relatively long duration of effect after their discontinuation (up to 24 hours) and the absence of an effective

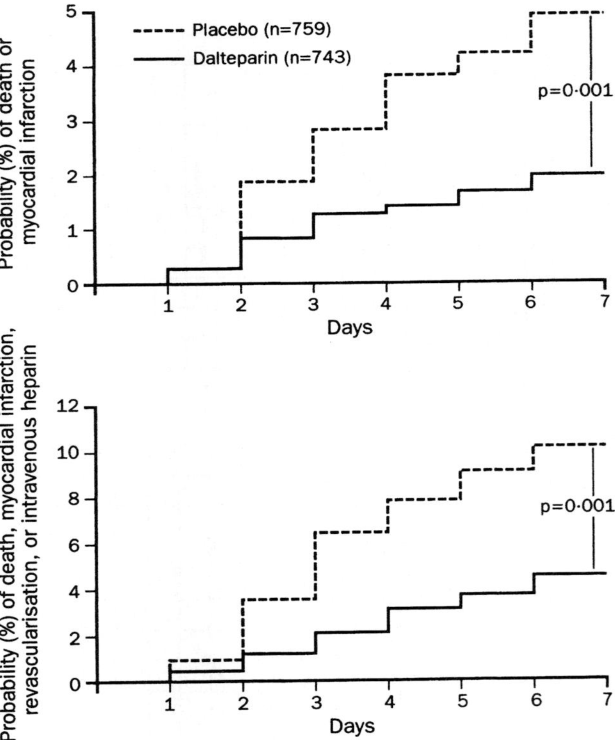

FIGURE 35–5 The protective effect of low-molecular-weight heparin in the form of dalteparin in the Fragmin during Instability in Coronary Artery Disease (FRISC) Study. The administration of dalteparin to patients with unstable angina and non–Q wave myocardial infarction reduced their risk of myocardial infarction **(top)** and of death, myocardial infarction, revascularization, or need for intravenous heparin **(bottom)**. See Table 35–2. (From Fragmin during Instability in Coronary Artery Disease [FRISC] Study: Low-molecular-weight heparin during instability in coronary artery disease. Lancet 347[9001]:561–568, © by The Lancet Ltd, 1996.)

TABLE 35–2 **Absolute Frequency of Primary and Separate Endpoints for Patients in the FRISC Study**

	Placebo (n = 749)	Dalteparin (n = 726)	Risk Ratio (95% CI)	*P*
Primary Endpoints				
Death or MI	116 (15.5%)	102 (14.0%)	0.90 (0.71–1.15)	0.41
Death, MI, or revascularization	326 (43.6%)	296 (40.6%)	0.92 (0.82–1.04)	0.18
Death, MI, revascularization, or intravenous heparin	337 (45.1%)	312 (42.7%)	0.94 (0.84–1.05)	0.28
Exclusion of Revascularization for Ischemia				
Death, MI, or revascularization because of angina	214 (28.7%)	175 (24.1%)	0.84 (0.70–0.99)	0.039
Death, MI, revascularization because of angina, or intravenous heparin	241 (32.3%)	204 (28.1%)	0.87 (0.74–1.01)	0.066
Separate Endpoints				
Death*	41 (5.5%)	39 (5.4%)	0.98 (0.64–1.50)	
MI*	98 (13.4%)	83 (11.7%)	0.86 (0.66–1.14)	0.30
Revascularization	254 (35.5%)	229 (32.9%)	0.92 (0.79–1.06)	0.23
Revascularization because of angina	131 (18.4%)	87 (12.5%)	0.68 (0.53–0.86)	0.002
Heparin infusion	121 (16.7%)	83 (11.9%)	0.71 (0.55–0.91)	0.008

Abbreviations: CI, confidence interval; MI, myocardial infarction.
*Separate statistical analyses of death and MI not planned in protocol.
From Fragmin during Instability in Coronary Artery Disease (FRISC) Study Group: Low-molecular-weight heparin during instability in coronary artery disease. Lancet 347(9001):561–568, © by The Lancet Ltd, 1996.

inhibitor of their effect. In patients with bleeding problems and those requiring emergent surgery, there are important limitations.

Thrombosis in Myocardial Infarction 11 Study

In the Thrombosis in Myocardial Infarction (TIMI) 11 Study, patients with unstable angina and non–Q wave MI were randomized to receive either (1) unfractionated heparin for approximately 3 days followed by placebo injections subcutaneously or (2) uninterrupted antithrombin therapy with enoxaparin during the acute phase (initial 30-mg intravenous bolus) followed by subcutaneous injections of 1.0 mg/kg every 12 hours and outpatient injections every 12 hours of 40 mg subcutaneously for patients less than 65 kg and 60 mg for those equal to or greater than 65 kg.[11] A total of 3910 patients were randomized in this study, and the primary endpoint was death, MI, or urgent revascularization. The primary endpoint occurred by 8 days in 14.5 percent of patients in the unfractionated heparin group and in 12.4 percent in the enoxaparin group (P = .048) and by 43 days in 19.7 percent of patients receiving unfractionated heparin and 17 percent of those receiving enoxaparin (P = .048) (Fig. 35–6). Throughout the initial hospitalization, there were no differences in the rate of major hemorrhage in the treatment groups. In the hospital, all patients received aspirin (100 to 325 mg daily). During the outpatient phase, major hemorrhage occurred in 1.5 percent of the group treated with placebo and 2.9 percent of the patients treated with enoxaparin (P = .02). From the TIMI 11 data, the authors concluded that enoxaparin is superior to unfractionated heparin for reducing a composite endpoint of death and serious cardiac ischemic events during the acute management of patients with unstable angina and non–Q wave MI without a significant increase in the rate of major hemorrhage. There was no further relative decrease in events with continuing treatment during the outpatient enoxaparin therapy, but there was an increase in the rate of major hemorrhage.

Efficacy and Safety of Subcutaneous Enoxaparin in Non–Q Wave Coronary Events Trial

The Efficacy and Safety of Subcutaneous Enoxaparin in Non–Q Wave Coronary Events (ESSENCE) Trial[12] randomly assigned 3171 patients with angina at rest or non–Q wave MI to receive either 1 mg/kg of low-molecular-weight heparin in the form of enoxaparin administered subcutaneously twice daily or continuous intravenous unfractionated heparin. Therapy was continued for a minimum of 48 hours to a maximum of 8 days. At 14 days, the risks of death, MI, and recurrent angina were significantly lower in the patients assigned to enoxaparin therapy (16.6 percent versus 19.8 percent, P = .019). At 30 days, the risk of this composite endpoint remained significantly lower in the enoxaparin group (19.8 percent versus 23 percent, P = .016). The need for revascularization procedures at 30 days was also significantly less frequent in patients assigned to enoxaparin (27 percent versus 32 percent, P = .001). The incidence of major bleeding complications at 30 days was 6.5 percent in the enoxaparin group and 7 percent in the unfractionated heparin group, but the incidence of bleeding overall was significantly higher in the enoxaparin group (18 percent versus 14 percent, P = .001), primarily because of ecchymoses at injection sites. The authors concluded from the data obtained in the ESSENCE Trial that antithrombotic therapy with enoxaparin plus aspirin was more effective than unfractionated heparin plus aspirin in reducing the incidence of ischemic events in patients with unstable angina or non–Q wave MI in the

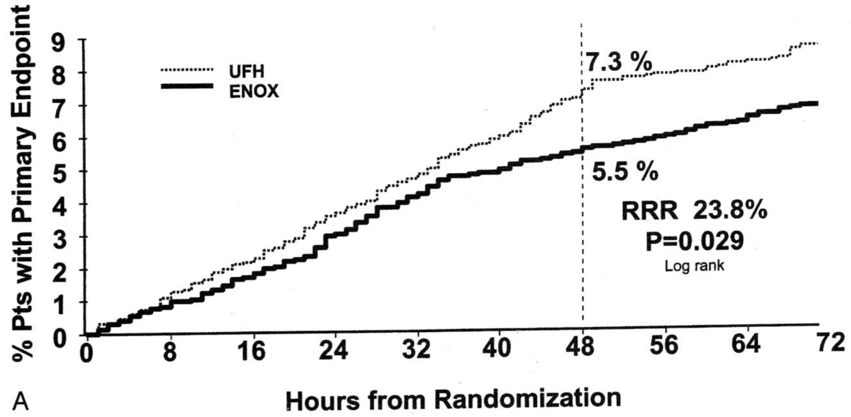

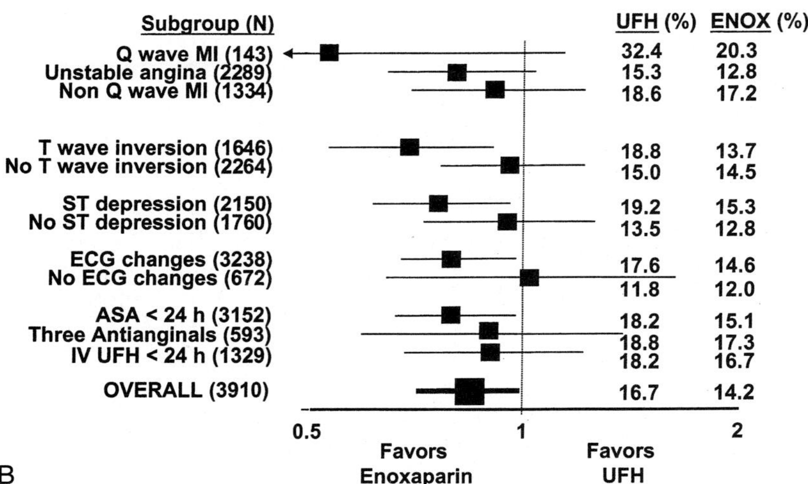

FIGURE 35–6 A, The reduction in primary endpoint (death, myocardial infarction, or urgent revascularization) in patients treated with low-molecular-weight heparin (Enoxaparin [ENOX]) in the Thrombolysis in Myocardial Infarction (TIMI) 11 study. RRR, relative risk reduction; UFH, unfractionated heparin. **B,** Subgroup analysis of patients in the TIMI 11 study shows that low-molecular-weight heparin reduces the primary endpoint better than unfractionated heparin in most patient subgroups with unstable angina and non–Q wave infarcts. ASA, acetylsalicylic acid; ECG, electrocardiogram; MI, myocardial infarction. (**A** and **B,** From Antman EM, McCabe CH, Gurfinkel EP, et al: Enoxaparin prevents death and cardiac ischemic events in unstable angina/non–Q wave myocardial infarction: results of the Thrombolysis in Myocardial Infarction [TIMI] 11B trial. Circulation 100:1597–1598, 1999.)

early phase of therapy. This benefit was achieved with an increase in minor but not major bleeding.

Summary

The FRISC, TIMI 11, and ESSENCE trials demonstrate the utility of low-molecular-weight heparin in the treatment of patients with unstable angina and non–Q wave MI. These trials suggest that low-molecular-weight heparin is clinically superior to unfractionated heparin in reducing the risk of MI and death and the need for revascularization in patients with unstable angina and non–Q wave MI. This benefit is achieved at some increase in risk of minor bleeding and, when continued in the outpatient phase, in minor-major bleeding. Thus, one should seriously consider the use of low-molecular-weight heparin in the treatment of these patients who are not allergic to heparin, most especially during the inpatient phase of therapy. In carefully selected patients, it may be protective to continue the subcutaneously administered low-molecular-weight heparin in the several weeks after hospital discharge, especially if the patient is deemed to be at increased risk after discharge. Bleeding with such therapy needs to be monitored so that it can be detected early and the low-molecular-weight heparin discontinued.

PLATELET GLYCOPROTEIN IIB/IIIA ANTAGONISTS

Figure 35–7 identifies the processes of platelet activation and aggregation and the inhibition of platelet aggregation by inhibitors of GP IIb/IIIa receptors. Platelet activation causes changes in the shape of platelets and conformational changes in the GP IIb/IIIa receptors, transforming the receptors from a ligand-unreceptive to a ligand-receptive state. Ligand-receptive GP IIb/IIIa receptors bind fibrinogen molecules, which form bridges between adjacent platelets and facilitate platelet aggregation. Inhibitors of GP IIb/IIIa receptors bind to the GP IIb/IIIa receptors blocking the binding of fibrinogen, thereby preventing platelet aggregation.

The GP IIb/IIIa receptor belongs to the integrin family of heterodimeric adhesion molecules formed by the noncovalent interaction of a series of alpha and beta subunits.[13] Integrins are found in almost all cell types and mediate a diversity of physiologic responses. Multiple integrins, including Ia/IIa, Ic, and IIa, are present on the surface of the platelet and play a role in platelet adhesion. The GP IIb/IIIa receptor is the most abundant on the platelet surface with approximately 50,000 copies per platelet.[14] The most important clinical interaction of the GP IIb/IIIa receptor is with fibrinogen, but this receptor has also been shown

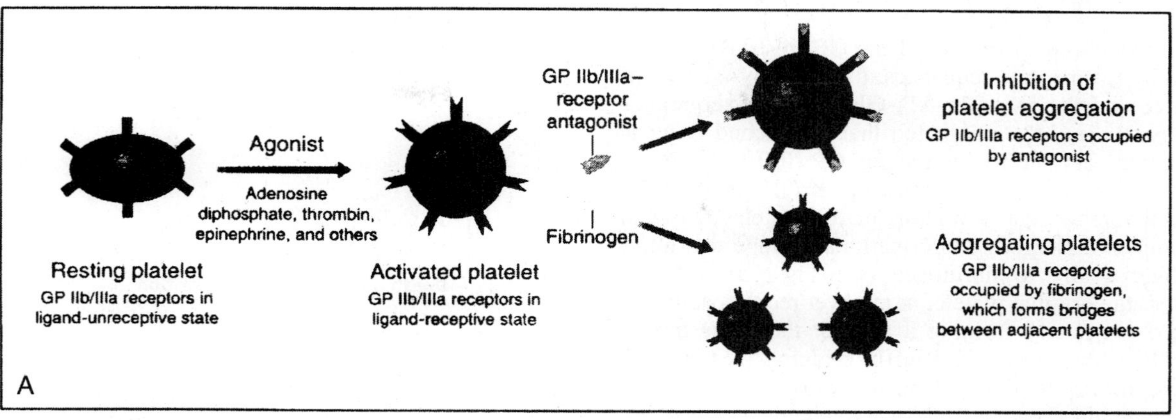

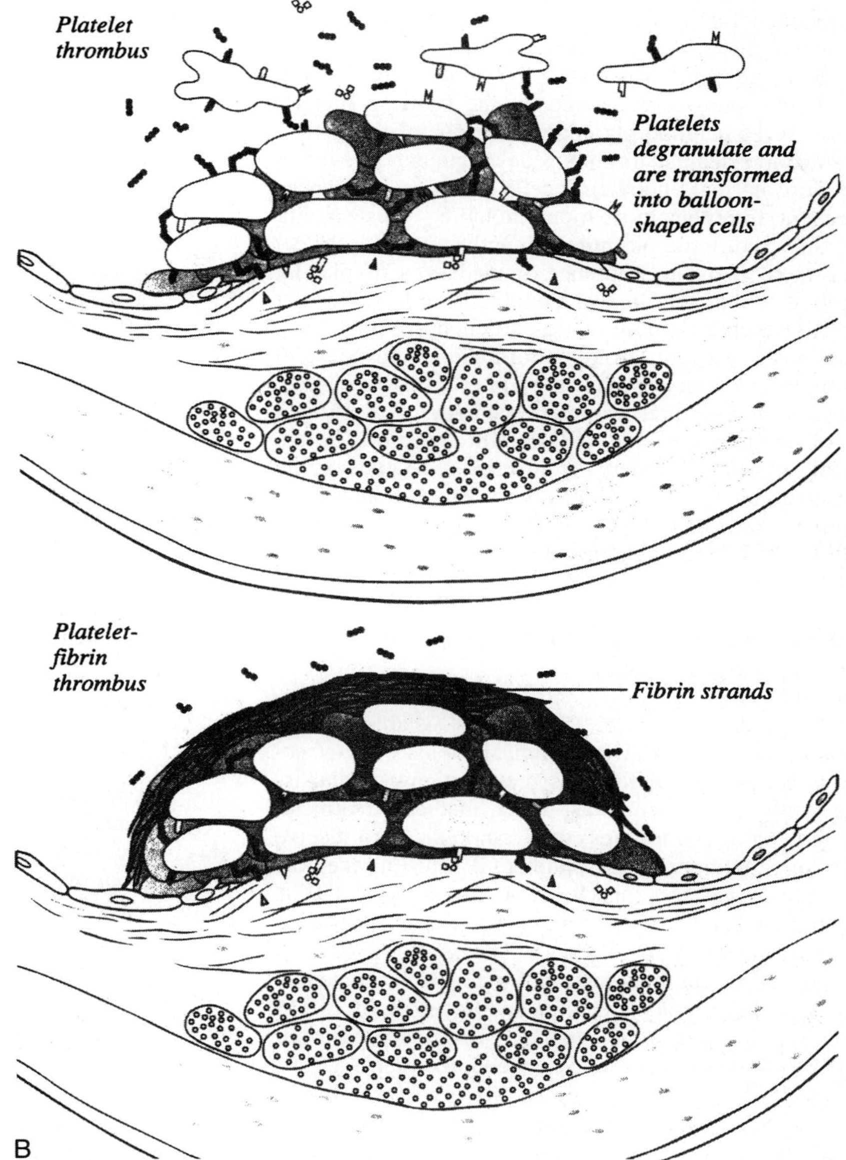

FIGURE 35–7 A, The activation of platelets, the expression of glycoprotein (GP) IIb/IIIa receptors in a ligand-receptive state, and the protective role played by GP IIb/IIIa receptor antagonists are demonstrated. Platelets aggregate by binding to one another through fibrinogen, which occupies the GP IIb/IIIa receptors, allowing platelets to aggregate in a fibrin mesh. **B,** Aggregating platelets develop thrombi at sites of endothelial injury. **Top,** As they aggregate, they degranulate and are transformed into balloon-shaped cells binding to one another through their GP IIb/IIIa–fibrinogen-binding sites. **Bottom,** A stable thrombus is formed. (**A,** From Lincoff AM, Topol EJ (eds): Platelet Glycoprotein IIb/IIIa Inhibitors in Cardiovascular Disease. p. 15. Totowa, NJ: Humana, 1999. **B,** From Willerson JT: Treatment of Heart Diseases. p. 1.43. New York: Gower Medical, 1992.)

to bind other adhesive proteins involved in aggregation, including fibronectin, vitronectin, and von Willebrand factor.[13]

The recognition specificity of the GP IIb/IIIa receptor is defined by two peptide sequences: the Arg-Gly-Asp (RGD) sequence and the Lys-Gln-Ala-Gly-Asp-Val sequence.[14] Previous studies have suggested that the second sequence is a predominant site for fibrinogen–GP IIb/IIIa binding.

Resting platelets do not express GP IIb/IIIa in a configuration suitable for ligand binding, but on platelet activation, this complex undergoes conformational change that allows it to bind avidly to fibrinogen (see Fig. 35–7).[15] Once activated, the original platelet monolayer recruits additional platelets, eventually forming a platelet thrombus through GP IIb/IIIa–fibrinogen–GP IIb/IIIa bridging (see Fig. 35–7). This process continues itself as new platelets enter the injured vascular bed, become activated by the mediators that are present locally, express GP IIb/IIIa receptors in the appropriate conformation, and become incorporated into the growing thrombus. An area of previously denuded endothelium resulting from fissuring or ulceration of an atherosclerotic plaque is covered by the growing platelet thrombus. If the neighboring endothelium is relatively normal, protection against thrombus development is exerted by the more normal endothelial cells secreting substances that prevent thrombus formation, including prostacyclin, nitric oxide, and tissue plasminogen activator.[16, 17]

Since there is a large number of mediators of platelet aggregation within the area of endothelial injury, platelet GP IIb/IIIa receptor inhibitors are particularly attractive as interventions to prevent thrombus formation in response to the multiple mediators because they interfere with platelet aggregation in the final common pathway. The clinical utility of inhibitors of the GP IIb/IIIa receptors in the treatment of acute coronary syndromes, unstable angina pectoris and non–Q wave MI, has been demonstrated. Representative examples of the protection afforded by inhibitors of GP IIb/IIIa receptors are reviewed subsequently.

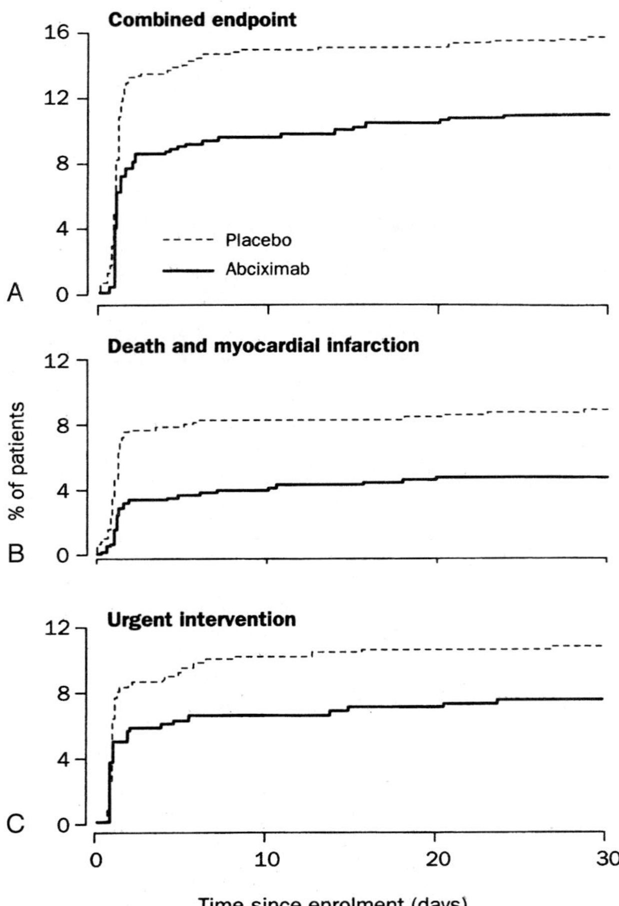

FIGURE 35–8 A–C, The protective effect of the monoclonal antibody directed against platelet GP IIb/IIIa receptors, abciximab, in reducing the composite endpoint **(A),** death and myocardial infarction **(B),** and the need for urgent intervention **(C)** in patients with unstable angina pectoris who were medically unstable. (**A–C,** From Marcel J, van den Brand BM, Simoons ML: The use of abciximab in therapy resistant unstable angina: clinical and angiographic results of the Capture Pilot and the Capture Study. *In* Lincoff AM, Topol EJ [eds]: Platelet Glycoprotein IIb/IIIa Inhibitors in Cardiovascular Disease. pp. 143–168. Totowa, NJ: Humana, 1999.)

c7E3 Fab Antiplatelet Therapy in Unstable Refractory Angina Study

In the c7E3 Fab Antiplatelet Therapy in Unstable Refractory Angina Study (CAPTURE) Study, patients with *refractory unstable angina* (defined as recurrent myocardial ischemia while the patient was under medical treatment, including heparin and nitrates) were randomized to receive a monoclonal antibody to the platelet GP IIb/IIIa receptors (abciximab) or placebo for 18 to 24 hours before PTCA and continuing for 1 hour afterward.[18, 19] The primary endpoint was the occurrence within 30 days after PTCA of death, MI, or urgent intervention for recurrent ischemia. By 30 days, the primary endpoint had occurred in 71 (11 percent) of 630 patients who received abciximab compared with 101 (16 percent) of 635 placebo recipients (P = .01) (Fig. 35–8). The frequency of MI was lower in the abciximab-treated patients than in the placebo-treated patients before PTCA (4 patients [0.6 percent] compared with 13 patients [2.1 percent], P = .029) and during PTCA (16 patients [2.6 percent] versus 34 patients [5.5 percent], P = .009). Major bleeding was infrequent, but it occurred more often with abciximab than with placebo (24 patients [3.8 percent] versus 12 patients [1.9 percent], P = .04). The protective effect of abciximab was not sustained after therapy, and at 6 months follow-up, death, MI, or repeat intervention had occurred in 193 patients in each group. Thus, this study demonstrates that in patients with refractory unstable angina, abciximab reduces the rate of thrombotic complications, especially MI before, during, and after PTCA, even in patients receiving nitrates and heparin. There was no evidence that this regimen influenced the rate of MI or the need for subsequent revascularization after the first few days following discontinuation of therapy.

Platelet Glycoprotein IIb/IIIa in Unstable Angina: Receptor Suppression in the Integrilin Therapy Trial

The Platelet Glycoprotein IIb/IIIa in Unstable Angina: Receptor Suppression Using Integrilin Therapy (PURSUIT)

Trial is the largest done to date involving a GP IIb/IIIa receptor antagonist in patients with unstable angina.[20] Between November 1995 and January 1997, 10,948 patients in 28 countries were randomized to one of two doses of eptifibatide (Integrilin) or placebo. All patients randomized to eptifibatide received a 180 μg/kg bolus and either a 1.3 μg/kg/min or a 2.0 μg/kg/min infusion for 72 hours. Eptifibatide is a synthetic peptide that competes for the GP IIb/IIIa receptor binding site. After 1487 patients received a moderate-dose infusion of 1.3 μg/kg/min of eptifibatide, this arm was discontinued because the higher-dose arm had a similarly acceptable safety profile. The primary endpoint of the trial was a composite all-cause mortality and nonfatal MI or reinfarction at 30 days after therapy. Secondary endpoints included death and MI or reinfarction at 30 days, the composite at 96 hours and 7 days, and safety and efficacy outcome in patients undergoing percutaneous coronary interventions. At the time of enrollment, 45 percent of the patients had a non–Q wave MI, and aspirin was administered to 93 percent and heparin to 90 percent of the patients in the study. Figure 35–9 shows the effect of eptifibatide on the cumulative incidence of death or nonfatal MI at 30 days. Eptifibatide reduced the composite endpoint from 15.7 to 14.2 percent, $P = .03$, a 10 percent relative reduction in death and nonfatal MI.

Platelet Receptor Inhibition in Ischemic Syndrome Management Study

In the Platelet Receptor Inhibition in Ischemic Syndrome Management (PRISM) Study, 3232 patients with unstable angina were randomized to received either intravenous tirofiban (a low-molecular-weight, nonpeptide, nonantibody inhibitor of the GP IIb/IIIa receptor) or heparin for 48 hours.[21] The primary endpoint was a composite of death, MI, or refractory ischemia. The incidence of the composite endpoint was 32 percent lower at 48 hours in patients who received tirofiban (3.8 percent versus 5.6 percent with heparin). Percutaneous revascularization was performed in 1.9 percent of the patients during the first 48 hours. At 30 days, the frequency of the composite endpoint with the addition of readmission for unstable angina was similar in the two groups (15.9 percent in the tirofiban group versus 17 percent in the heparin group). There was a trend toward a reduction in the rate of death or MI with tirofiban, 5.8 percent compared with 7 percent in the heparin group, but this did not reach statistical significance. Mortality was 2.3 percent in the tirofiban group compared with 3.6 percent in the heparin group ($P = .02$). Major bleeding occurred in 0.4 percent of the patients in both groups. Reversible thrombocytopenia occurred more frequently in tirofiban-treated patients than in heparin-treated patients (1.1 percent versus 0.4 percent, $P = .04$).

Platelet Receptor Inhibition in Ischemic Syndrome Management in Patients Limited by Unstable Signs and Symptoms (PRISM-PLUS) Study

In the Platelet Receptor Inhibition in Ischemic Syndrome Management in Patients Limited by Unstable Signs and Symptoms (PRISM-PLUS) Study, tirofiban was also given to patients with unstable angina and non–Q wave MI in 1915 patients randomly assigned in a double-blind manner to receive tirofiban, heparin, or tirofiban and heparin.[22] Patients received aspirin if its use was not contraindicated. The study drugs were infused for a mean of 71 ± 20 hours, during which time coronary angiography and angioplasty were performed after 48 hours when clinically indicated. The composite primary endpoint consisted of death, MI, and refractory ischemia within 7 days after randomization.

The study was stopped prematurely for the group receiving tirofiban alone because of an excess mortality at 7 days, 4.6 percent compared with 1.1 percent for the patients treated with heparin alone. The frequency of the composite primary endpoint at 7 days was lower among the patients who received tirofiban and heparin than among those who received heparin alone (12.9 percent versus 17.9 percent, risk ratio 0.68, $P = .004$) (Fig. 35–10). The composite endpoint for the tirofiban plus heparin group was also reduced compared with that in the heparin-only group at 30 days (18.5 percent versus 22 percent, $P = .03$) and at 6 months (27.7 percent versus 32 percent, $P = .02$). At 7 days, the frequency of death or MI was 4.9 percent in the tirofiban and heparin group as contrasted with 8 percent in the heparin-only group ($P = .006$). Comparable data at 30 days were 8.7 and 11.9 percent ($P = .03$), respectively, and at 6 months, 12 and 15 percent ($P = .06$). The protection from tirofiban and heparin was consistent in the various subgroups of patients, both in those treated medically and in those treated with PTCA. Major bleeding

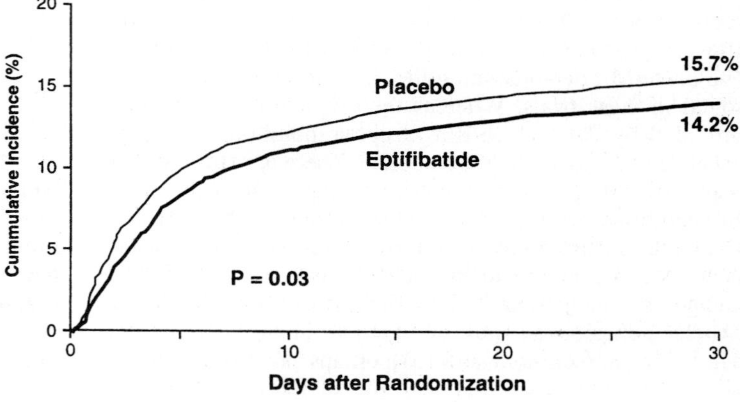

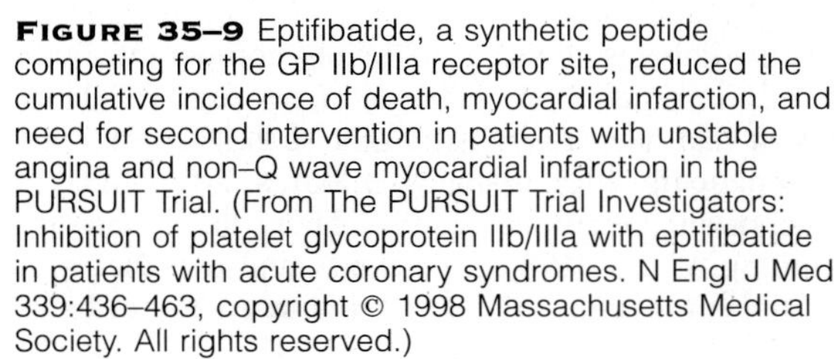
FIGURE 35–9 Eptifibatide, a synthetic peptide competing for the GP IIb/IIIa receptor site, reduced the cumulative incidence of death, myocardial infarction, and need for second intervention in patients with unstable angina and non–Q wave myocardial infarction in the PURSUIT Trial. (From The PURSUIT Trial Investigators: Inhibition of platelet glycoprotein IIb/IIIa with eptifibatide in patients with acute coronary syndromes. N Engl J Med 339:436–463, copyright © 1998 Massachusetts Medical Society. All rights reserved.)

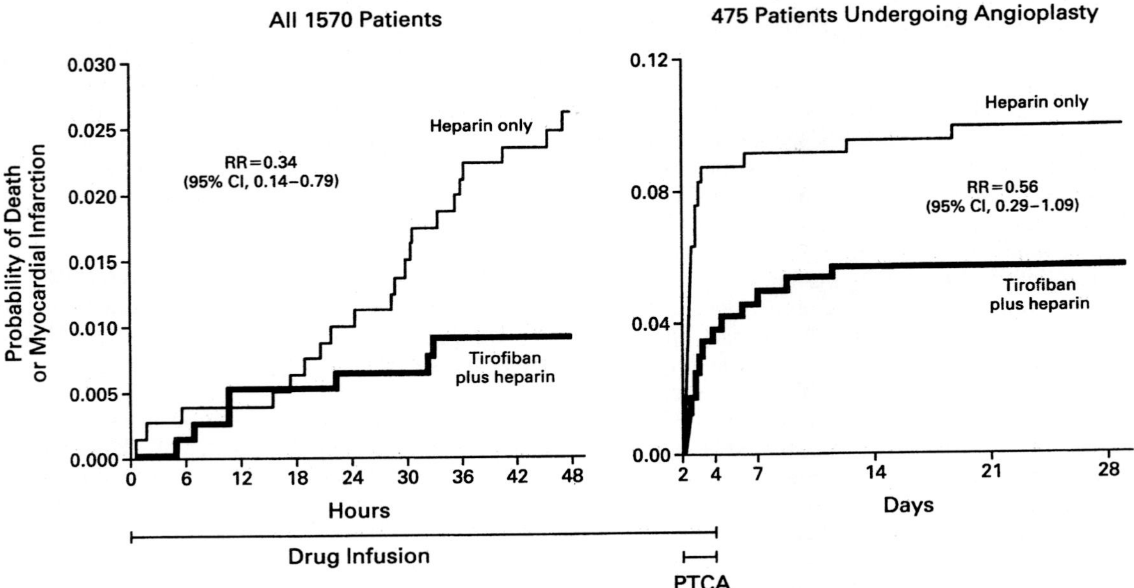

FIGURE 35–10 Left, The beneficial effect of a nonpeptide, nonantibody, small-molecular-weight inhibitor of GP IIb/IIIa receptors, tirofiban, and heparin compared with heparin alone in reducing the probability of death or myocardial infarction during the period of drug infusion. **Right,** The same protective effect of tirofiban and heparin is demonstrated in the patients admitted with unstable angina and non–Q wave infarction who subsequently had angioplasty. CI, confidence interval; PTCA, percutaneous transluminal coronary angioplasty; RR, risk ratio. (From Platelet Receptor Inhibition in Ischemic Syndrome Management in Patients Limited by Unstable Signs and Symptoms [PRISM-PLUS] Study Investigators: Inhibition of the platelet glycoprotein IIb/IIIa receptor with tirofiban in unstable angina and non–Q-wave myocardial infarction. N Engl J Med 338:1488, copyright © 1998 Massachusetts Medical Society. All rights reserved.)

occurred in 3 percent of the patients receiving heparin alone and 4 percent of the patients receiving combination therapy.

The conclusion of this study is that when administered with heparin and aspirin, the platelet GP IIb/IIIa receptor inhibitor, tirofiban, reduces the risk of death or MI in patients with unstable angina and non–Q wave MI.[22]

Summary

GP IIb/IIIa receptor antagonists, including the monoclonal antibody (abciximab), synthetic peptide (eptifibatide), and nonpeptide, low-molecular-weight inhibitor (tirofiban), when added to aspirin and heparin in patients with unstable angina pectoris and non–Q wave MI reduce the risks of MI, death, and need for interventional therapy during their administration and sometimes in the short time period thereafter (Fig. 35–11). Tables 35–3 and 35–4 provide a representative listing of clinical trials done with GP IIb/IIIa receptor antagonists in patients with unstable angina and acute MI, demonstrating the generally protective effect found in these trials. Whereas there is additive protection provided by the GP IIb/IIIa receptor inhibitors, it is also clear that protection is not complete. There are still patients that have MIs, recurrent unstable angina, and the need for additional intervention. Thus, antithrombotic therapy available still needs to be improved. Probable reasons for lack of more complete protection from the GP IIb/IIIa antagonists include that these agents do not inhibit (1) platelet adhesion at sites of vascular injury; (2) platelet activation or secretion; and (3) perhaps not the effects of thrombin bound to the thrombus or of tissue factor that is inaccessible within the thrombotic plaque.

Glycoprotein IIb/IIIa Receptor Antagonists Used With Interventional Therapies

Figure 35–11 and Table 35–5 demonstrate the effect of the GP IIb/IIIa inhibitors in patients requiring interventional procedures, including angioplasty and stents. These patients had strong medical reasons for interventional therapy, and many received interventional therapy after being hospitalized with unstable angina or non–Q wave MI. As the figure demonstrates, abciximab, eptifibatide, and low-molecular-weight inhibitors of GP IIb/IIIa receptors, as represented by tirofiban, exert beneficial effects and reduce composite endpoints of death, MI, or need for urgent revascularization at 30 days in these patients. Thus, the benefit of these interventions in patients treated medically for unstable angina and non–Q wave MI also occurs in patients who subsequently have angioplasty and stenting (see Fig. 35–11).

In the Evaluation of Platelet IIb/IIIa Inhibitor for Stenting (EPISTENT) Study, abciximab therapy reduced the risk of MI, death, and need for subsequent intervention in patients with diabetes mellitus to levels comparable with those found in nondiabetic patients (see Fig. 35–11).[23] Previously, it had been recognized that such interventional therapy in patients with diabetes mellitus often fails to provide important beneficial results. Thus, this is an important finding of the EPISTENT Study and one that may allow the diabetic patient to be treated with greater efficacy

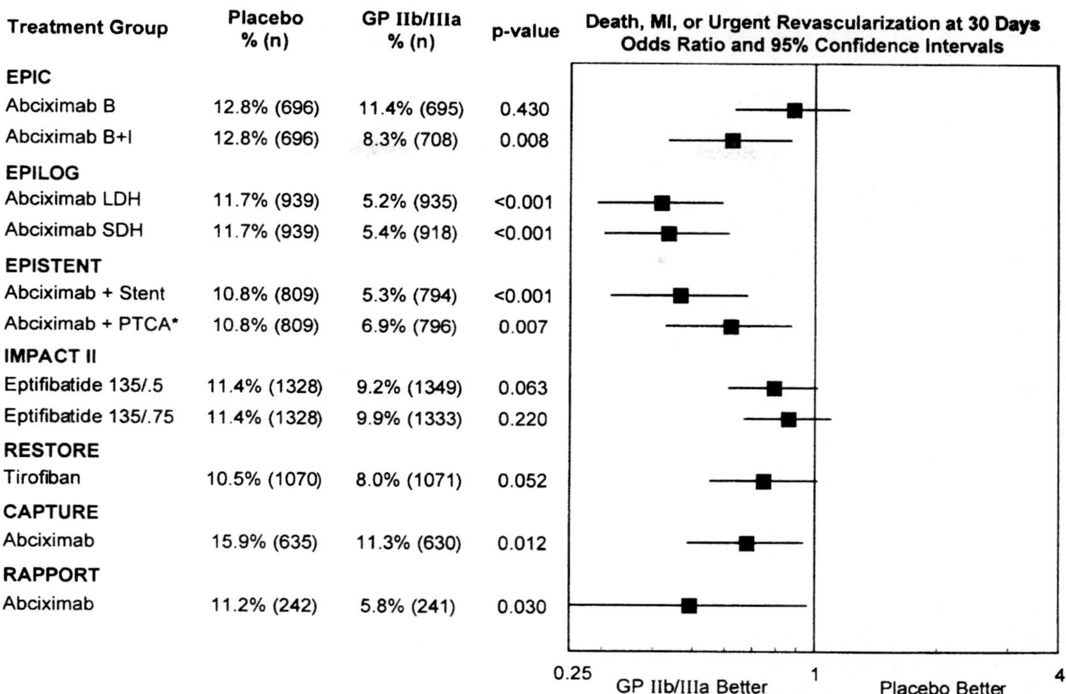

Treatment Group
Placebo % (n)
GP IIb/IIIa % (n)
p-value
Death, MI, or Urgent Revascularization at 30 Days
Odds Ratio and 95% Confidence Intervals
EPIC
Abciximab B 12.8% (696) 11.4% (695) 0.430
Abciximab B+I 12.8% (696) 8.3% (708) 0.008
EPILOG
Abciximab LDH 11.7% (939) 5.2% (935) <0.001
Abciximab SDH 11.7% (939) 5.4% (918) <0.001
EPISTENT
Abciximab + Stent 10.8% (809) 5.3% (794) <0.001
Abciximab + PTCA* 10.8% (809) 6.9% (796) 0.007
IMPACT II
Eptifibatide 135/.5 11.4% (1328) 9.2% (1349) 0.063
Eptifibatide 135/.75 11.4% (1328) 9.9% (1333) 0.220
RESTORE
Tirofiban 10.5% (1070) 8.0% (1071) 0.052
CAPTURE
Abciximab 15.9% (635) 11.3% (630) 0.012
RAPPORT
Abciximab 11.2% (242) 5.8% (241) 0.030
0.25
1
4
GP IIb/IIIa Better
Placebo Better

FIGURE 35–11 The results of randomized interventional trials in patients with unstable angina or non–Q wave myocardial infarction and other patients with limiting angina and complex coronary artery lesions who underwent an interventional procedure and were treated by GP IIb/IIIa antagonists. Composite endpoint data in each of these trials are shown. See Table 35–5. B, bolus; B+I, bolus and infusion; LDH, low dose heparin; SDH, standard dose heparin. (From Lincoff AM, Topol EJ [eds]: Overview of the glycoprotein IIb/IIIa inhibitor interventional trials. *In* Platelet Glycoprotein IIb/IIIa Inhibitors in Cardiovascular Disease. p. 179. Totowa, NJ: Humana, 1999.)

with angioplasty and stenting in the future. In addition, the Evaluation of PTCA to Improve Long-term Outcome by c7E3 GP IIb/IIIa Receptor Blockade (EPILOG) Study[24] demonstrated that the benefits of abciximab therapy in patients with coronary heart disease undergoing angioplasty extend to both low-risk and high-risk patients in a similar manner. The earlier Evaluation of IIb/IIIa Platelet Receptor Antagonist 7E3 in Preventing Ischemic Complications (EPIC) Study[25] had shown that abciximab therapy reduced the risk of subsequent MI, death, and need for a second intervention in high-risk patients undergoing PTCA. In the EPIC Study, high-risk patients were those with unstable angina, recent non–Q wave MI, and complicated coronary arterial lesions.[25]

TABLE 35-3 Study Design and Enrollment Details for the PARAGON, PRISM, PRISM-PLUS, and PURSUIT Trials in Which GP IIb/IIIa Antagonists Were Used to Treat Patients With Unstable Angina Pectoris and Non–Q Wave Myocardial Infarction

Characteristic	PARAGON	PRISM	PRISM-PLUS	PURSUIT
Enrollment dates	8/95–5/96	3/94–10/96	11/94–9/96	11/95–1/97
Age (y)	66	62	63	64
Female (%)	35	32	33	35
Diabetes (%)	18	21	23	22
Hypertension (%)	49	54	54	55
Hypercholesterolemia (%)	42	47	49	42
Current smoker (%)	23	26	NA	28
Prior MI (%)	35	47	43	32
Prior PTCA (%)	11	15	10	13
Prior CABG (%)	9	17	15	12
Presenting ECG				
ST depression (%)	52	32	58	50
ST elevation (%)	6	7	14	14
T wave inversion (%)	54	51	53	52
MI at enrollment (%)	36	25	45	45

Abbreviations: CABG, coronary artery bypass graft surgery; ECG, electrocardiogram; MI, myocardial infarction; PARAGON, Platelet IIb/IIIa Antagonism for the Reduction of Acute Coronary Syndrome Events in a Global Organization Network; PRISM, Platelet Receptor Inhibition in Ischemic Syndrome Management; PRISM-PLUS, Platelet Receptor Inhibition in Ischemic Syndrome Management in Patients Limited by Unstable Signs and Symptoms; PTCA, percutaneous transluminal coronary angioplasty; PURSUIT, Platelet Glycoprotein IIb/IIIa in Unstable Angina: Receptor Suppression Using Integrilin Therapy.

From Moliterno DJ, White H: Unstable angina: PARAGON, PURSUIT, PRISM, and PRISM-PLUS. *In* Lincoff AM, Topol EJ (eds): Platelet Glycoprotein IIb/IIIa Inhibitors in Cardiovascular Disease. p. 210. Totowa, NJ: Humana, 1999.

TABLE 35–4 **Clinical Outcomes of the PARAGON, PRISM, PRISM-PLUS, and PURSUIT Trials in Which GP IIb/IIIa Antagonists Were Used to Treat Patients With Unstable Angina Pectoris and Non–Q Wave Myocardial Infarction**

	PARAGON			PRISM		PRISM-PLUS			PURSUIT		
Characteristic	*Placebo*	*Lamifiban 1 μg/min ± Heparin*	*Lamifiban 5 μg/min ± Heparin*	*Heparin*	*Tirofiban 0.15 μg/kg-min*	*Heparin*	*Heparin + Tirofiban 0.10 μg/kg-min*	*Tirofiban 0.15 μg/kg-min*	*Placebo*	*Eptifibatide 1.3 μg/kg-min*	*Eptifibatide 20 μg/kg-min*
n	758	755	769	1616	1616	797	773	345	4739	1487	4722
30-Day outcome											
Death (%)	2.9	3.0	3.6	3.6	2.3	4.5	3.6	(6.1)	3.7	(3.4)	3.5
Nonfatal MI (%)	10.6	9.4	10.9	4.3	4.1	9.2	6.6	(9.0)	13.5	(12.0)	12.6
Death or MI (%)											
Overall	11.7	10.6	12.0	7.1	5.8	11.9	8.7	(13.6)	15.7	(13.4)	14.2
Relative reduction (%)		9	−6		18		27				10
PTCA patients				9.1	7.2	10.2	5.9		16.8		11.8
Non-PTCA patients				6.2	3.6	7.8	3.6		15.7		14.6
6-Month outcome											
Death (%)	6.6	5.2	6.8			7.0	6.9	(7.2)	6.2		6.4
Nonfatal MI (%)	14.3	10.8	12.9			10.5	8.3	(10.1)	15.7		14.7
Death or MI (%)	17.9	13.7	16.4			15.3	12.3	(15.9)	19.0		17.8
Relative reduction (%)		23	8				20				8
Major bleeding (%)*	3.0	3.0	6.0	0.4	0.4	0.8	1.4		1.3		3.0
Intracranial hemorrhage (%)	0	0	0.1	0.1	0.1	0	0		0.1		0.1
RBC transfusion (%)†	4.4	4.4	8.7	1.4	2.4	2.8	4.0		1.8		4.4
Thrombocytopenia (%)‡	1.1	1.5	1.3	0.1	0.4	0.3	0.5		0.4		0.6

Abbreviations: MI, myocardial infarction; PARAGON, Platelet IIb/IIIa Antagonism for the Reduction of Acute Coronary Syndrome Events in a Global Organization Network; PRISM, Platelet Receptor Inhibition in Ischemic Syndrome Management; PRISM-PLUS, Platelet Receptor Inhibition in Ischemic Syndrome Management in Patients Limited by Unstable Signs and Symptoms; PTCA, percutaneous transluminal coronary angioplasty; PURSUIT, Platelet Glycoprotein IIb/IIIa in Unstable Angina; Receptor Suppression Using Integrilin Therapy; RBC, red blood cell.

Numbers in parentheses are from discontinued treatment arms and are not contemporaneous; these are listed only for completeness, not direct comparisons.

*Major bleeding as defined by intracranial hemorrhage or decrease in hemoglobin ≥ 5 g/dl not associated with CABG.

†Transfusions reported are not associated with CABG, except for PARAGON.

‡Thrombocytopenia defined as platelet count ≤ 50,000 mm.

From Moliterno DJ, White H: Unstable angina: PARAGON, PURSUIT, PRISM, and PRISM-PLUS. *In* Lincoff AM, Topol EJ (eds): Platelet Glycoprotein IIb/IIIa Inhibitors in Cardiovascular Disease. p. 211. Totowa, NJ: Humana, 1999.

TABLE 35-5 Summary of Results of Randomized Interventional Trials in Patients With Unstable Angina/Non–Q Wave Myocardial Infarction and Other Patients With Limiting Angina and Complex Coronary Artery Lesions Who Underwent an Interventional Procedure and Were Treated by Glycoprotein IIb/IIIa Antagonists: 30-Day Efficacy Endpoint Figures

	Death (%)	MI (%)	Urgent PCI (%)	Urgent CABG (%)
EPIC Trial				
Placebo	1.7	8.6	4.5	3.6
Abciximab bolus	1.3	6.2	3.6	2.3
Abciximab bolus + infusion	1.7	5.2	0.8	2.4
EPILOG Trial				
Placebo	0.8	8.7	3.8	1.7
Abciximab + reduced heparin	0.3	3.7	1.2	0.4
Abciximab + standard heparin	0.4	3.8	1.5	0.9
EPISTENT Trial				
Placebo + stent	0.6	9.6	1.2	1.1
Abciximab + stent	0.3	4.5	0.6	
Abciximab + PTCA	0.8	5.3	1.3	0.6
IMPACT II Trial				
Placebo	1.1	8.1	2.8	2.8
Eptifibatide 135/0.5 dose	0.5	6.6	2.6	1.6
Eptifibatide 135/0.75 dose	0.8	6.9	2.9	2.0
RESTORE Trial*				
Placebo	0.7	5.7	4.0	1.4
Tirofiban	0.8	4.2	2.3	1.1
CAPTURE Trial				
Placebo	1.3	8.2	4.4	1.7
Abciximab	1.0	4.1	3.1	1.0
RAPPORT Trial†				
Placebo	2.1	4.1	5.4	1.2
Abciximab	2.5	3.3	1.7	0

Abbreviations: CABG, coronary artery bypass graft surgery; CAPTURE, c7E3 Fab Antiplatelet Therapy in Unstable Refractory Angina; EPIC, Evaluation of IIb/IIIa Platelet Receptor Antagonist 7E3 in Preventing Ischemic Complications; EPILOG, Evaluation of PTCA to Improve Long-term Outcome by c7E3 GP IIb/IIIa Receptor Blockade; EPISTENT, Evaluation of Platelet IIb/IIIa Inhibitor for Stenting; IMPACT, Integrilin (eptifibatide) to Minimize Platelet Aggregation and Coronary Thrombosis; MI, myocardial infarction; PCI, percutaneous coronary intervention; RAPPORT, ReoPro and Primary PTCA Organization and Randomized Trial; RESTORE, Randomized Efficacy Study of Tirofiban for Outcomes and REstenosis.

*RESTORE Trial endpoints listed here are for the published post hoc analysis including only *urgent* repeat revascularization for consistency with the other trials. The primary composite endpoint of RESTORE included *urgent or elective* repeat revascularization. RESTORE trial endpoints listed here differ from those of the other trials in that only patients in whom the lesion was successfully crossed with the guidewire were included in the efficacy analysis of RESTORE, providing a "treated patient" analysis rather than the "intenstion-to-treat" analysis utilized in the other studies.

†RAPPORT endpoints listed here are for the secondary composite of death, myocardial reinfarction, and urgent *target vessel* revascularization. This endpoint differs from those of the other trials in that it does not include urgent *nontarget vessel* revascularization procedures.

From Lincoff AM, Topol EJ: Overview of the glycoprotein IIb/IIIa inhibitor interventional trials. *In* Lincoff AM, Topol EJ (eds): Platelet Glycoprotein IIb/IIIa Inhibitors in Cardiovascular Disease. p. 181. Totowa, NJ: Humana, 1999.

In several of the previously mentioned interventional studies using abciximab, composite endpoints were favorable through 6 months and longer, even in the absence of continuing administration of the drug.

General Considerations

Coronary arteriography is often recommended for the patient with unstable angina and non–Q wave MI without other severe and life-threatening medical disease or very advanced age after the angina is controlled medically (see Fig. 35–1). Arteriography is absolutely indicated in patients with continuing rest angina in whom medical therapy does not prevent their pain (see Fig. 35–1). However, medical therapy initially, with subsequent referral for coronary arteriography and coronary revascularization of patients with continuing myocardial ischemia at low-level effort despite medical therapy, is a reasonable alternative (see Fig. 35–1). In the patient in whom rest angina recurs despite an appropriate medical regimen, coronary arteriography becomes mandatory. Ten to 15 percent of patients with unstable angina have significant left main coronary artery stenoses, including 50 percent or greater luminal diameter narrowing of the main left coronary artery.[26–30] Coronary artery bypass graft surgery (CABG) prolongs the lives of these patients.[29–32] Approximately 10 percent of patients with unstable angina have no angiographic evidence of significant coronary disease.[26–28] Therefore, in 25 percent of these patients, the angiographic findings help select an appropriate therapeutic approach. In the remaining patients, identifying the location and extent of coronary artery disease (CAD) is useful prognostically. In the patient with continuing angina at rest, the arteriographic findings allow the physician to consider PTCA and stenting or CABG (see Fig. 35–1).

In patients in whom angina is medically controlled and a conservative regimen is chosen, and in those in whom coronary angiographic findings do not suggest a need for immediate coronary artery revascularization, exercise (or some other form of stress) testing should be obtained (see Fig. 35–1). Submaximal exercise tests can usually be safely obtained several days after the relief of chest pain, followed several weeks later by maximal exercise tests. The addition of some form of nuclear, echocardiographic, or magnetic resonance perfusion or functional imaging cardiology testing with exercise or other stress improves its sensitivity and specificity for identification of patients with physiologically

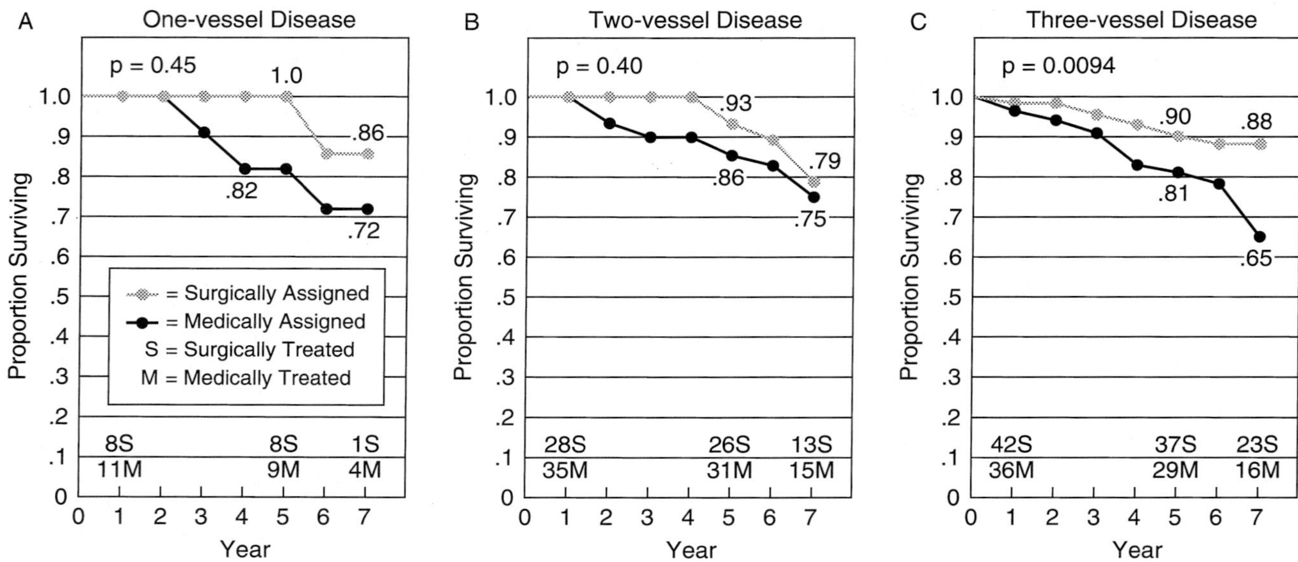

FIGURE 35–12 The influence of coronary artery bypass surgery compared with medical therapy in patients with significant one-vessel disease **(A),** two-vessel disease **(B),** and three-vessel disease **(C)**. As demonstrated, survival is better in patients with triple-vessel coronary disease who undergo coronary artery surgery **(C)**. (**A–C,** Data from Passamani E, Davis KB, Gillespie MJ, et al, and the CASS principal investigators and their associates: a randomized trial of coronary artery bypass surgery: survival of patients with a low ejection fraction. N Engl J Med 312:1665, 1985.)

important CAD.[33–37] Patients with continuing angina or objective evidence of myocardial ischemia at rest or at low levels of activity despite a good medical regimen, and those with significant left main and/or three-vessel coronary stenoses and depressed left ventricular function, should undergo coronary artery revascularization (Fig. 35–12).[29–32] Coronary artery revascularization relieves or markedly reduces the frequency of angina in the patient with continuing myocardial ischemia despite a good medical regimen, and CABG prolongs the lives of patients with significant left main and/or three-vessel coronary stenoses and depressed left ventricular function (see Fig. 35–12). In patients with unstable angina, CABG or PTCA and stenting usually relieves angina. CABG is also associated with a reduced risk for recurrent unstable angina compared with continuing medical therapy.[29–32] However, there is still no persuasive evidence that coronary artery revascularization reduces the risk for MI or prolongs the lives of patients with unstable angina who do not have significant left main coronary artery stenosis, three-vessel CAD, or severe two-vessel coronary artery disease, including 90 percent or greater proximal LAD stenosis above the first septal perforator artery, and reduced left ventricular function. A general scheme for the management of patients with unstable angina and non–Q wave MI is shown in Figure 35–1.

Coronary Arterial Spasm (Variant Angina; Prinzmetal's Angina)

The initial treatment of coronary artery spasm should utilize nitrates, a selected calcium antagonist, or both.[38–56] β-Blockers are avoided in patients with suspected or documented coronary artery spasm because they may cause more frequent and severe episodes of spasm. Patients with variant angina usually respond well to medical therapy with nitrates or one of the selected calcium antagonists (Fig. 35–13). Episodes of coronary artery spasm tend to be intermittent, occurring for a few days or weeks and then disappearing, sometimes to recur months or years later. In general, coronary artery revascularization and PTCA are not as useful in these patients as in those with other CAD syndromes. In patients with coronary artery spasm, PTCA itself may cause immediate and recurrent coronary artery spasm. The exceptions are patients with extensive coronary stenoses and superimposed coronary artery spasm in whom it may be necessary to treat both pathophysiologic mechanisms of CAD. Coronary artery revascularization may be necessary in the patient who has angina associated with low-level exercise or stress, an increased myocardial oxygen demand, and relative inability of the stenotic artery to deliver oxygen.[56] A calcium antagonist and/or nitrates are used to treat primary decreases in coronary blood flow caused by coronary artery spasm, even when they have been provoked by exercise or by cocaine.

Summary

In the management of patients with unstable angina and non–Q wave MI, several points are of critical importance. First, one should recognize that these two acute coronary syndromes are closely related one to the other and generally occur as a result of atherosclerotic plaque fissuring or ulceration allowing platelet aggregation, thrombosis, and dynamic vasoconstriction to occur at the site of the plaque injury. Unstable angina generally occurs when the periods of severe reduction in coronary blood flow persist for less than 20 minutes and non–Q wave MI occurs when the period of coronary occlusion lasts between 20 to 30 minutes and 1 to 2 hours. In both instances, the occlusive thrombus and dynamic vasoconstriction are transient and a

Q wave MI is prevented by the failure of the thrombus to remain permanently occlusive for longer periods of time. Patients with unstable angina and non–Q wave MI have a substantial risk of future coronary events within the subsequent 6 weeks as a result of persistent endothelial injury and recurrence of thrombosis and vasoconstriction. *The object of therapy in treating these syndromes acutely is to prevent the persistence of a thrombus with its associated vasoconstriction.* Thus, initial therapy depends on (1) the administration of nitrates, usually in the form of intravenous nitroglycerin; (2) antithrombotic therapies, most especially aspirin—an inhibitor of thromboxane A_2, of platelet–white blood cell complexes, and of inflammation; and (3) an inhibitor of thrombin, at present either unfractionated or low-molecular-weight heparin, but in the future possibly direct-acting antithrombins. In patients who continue to have rest angina or angina at mild-to-moderate effort, one may prescribe additional antithrombotic medication, including clopidogrel and/or platelet glycoprotein IIb/IIIa antagonists. Beta blockers should be added for patients with angina at limited effort, as well as those with elevated blood pressures or heart rates or considerable anxiety. They may also be useful in the treatment of complex ventricular ectopy.

In patients who still continue to have rest angina or angina at mild-to-moderate effort despite a good medical regimen, one recommends that the patient be taken to the cardiac catheterization laboratory for coronary arteriography to define the location and extent of the coronary disease and, ideally, the culprit lesion for some form of coronary artery revascularization, angioplasty, stenting, or both, or when the coronary stenoses are diffuse and severe, CABG. In patients who are to receive interventional therapies, such as angioplasty or stenting, the administration of a platelet glycoprotein IIb/IIIa receptor antagonist provides protection against the composite risks of MI, need for a second intervention, and death.

One of the major needs in contemporary cardiovascular medicine is to be able to identify those patients at risk for unstable angina/MI and their consequences generally and specifically in those patients who have had recent unstable angina or non–Q wave MI. Although it seems likely that one may need to evaluate coronary atherosclerotic plaques

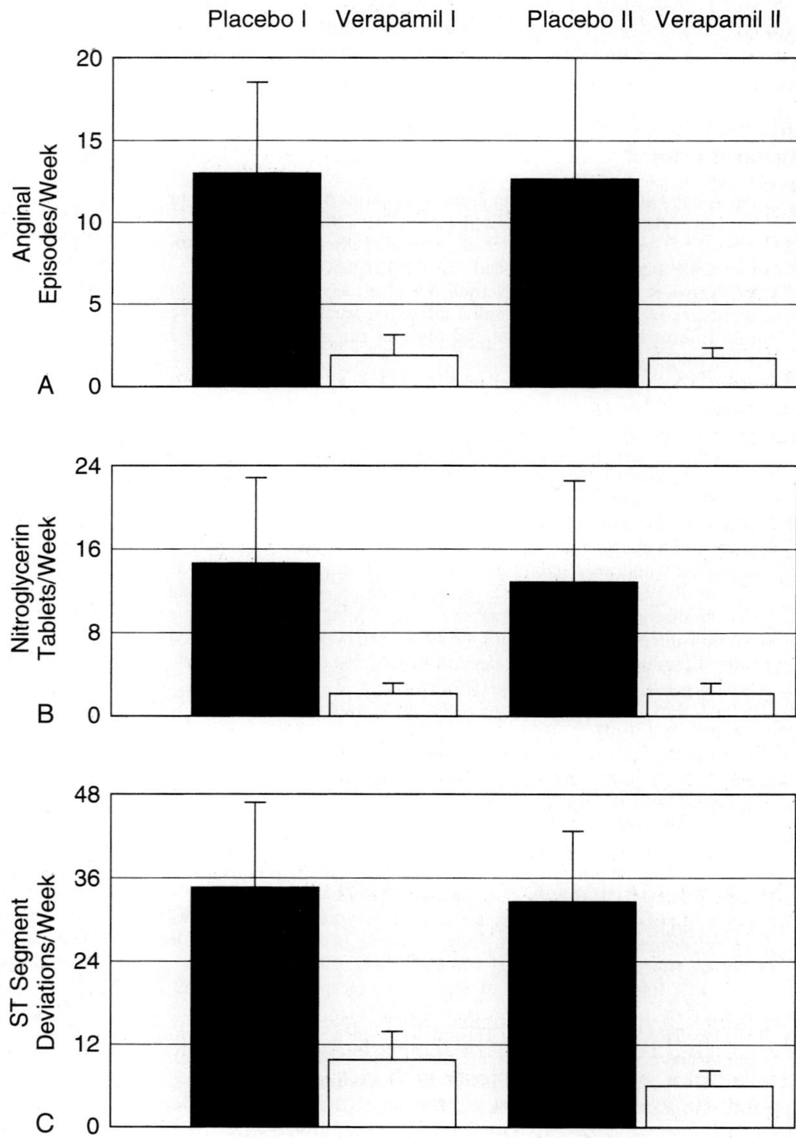

FIGURE 35–13 The beneficial effect of the slow channel calcium antagonist, verapamil, in patients with Prinzmetal's angina. In this study, verapamil reduced the number of anginal episodes per week **(A),** the number of nitroglycerin tablets consumed per week **(B),** and the electrocardiographic alterations detected by continuous 24-h Holter monitoring **(C)**. (**A–C,** From Johnson SM, Mauritson DR, Willerson JT, Hillis LD: A controlled trial of verapamil for Prinzmetal's variant angina. N Engl J Med 304:862, copyright © 1981 Massachusetts Medical Society. All rights reserved.)

directly for characteristics that identify their instability, at present one may use one of the following variables to identify patients at increased risk. Patients with increases in their troponin I or T with unstable angina/non–Q wave MI on admission are, in general, at increased risk for future unstable angina and MI. Similarly, patients with increases in their C-reactive protein on admission or at hospital discharge are also at increased risk for future unstable angina, MI, and their consequences. Patients with recurring ST-T wave changes consistent with recurrent myocardial ischemia are also at increased risk for future coronary events. Thus, one should have a low threshold for further evaluation of these patients, including possibly earlier coronary arteriography and some form of interventional therapy or CABG. One may also identify patients at increased risk by using low-level stress perfusion or functional evaluations within a few days after presentation of the patient with unstable angina or non–Q wave MI and at a time that the patient has become angina free. Reversible stress perfusion or function alterations in such patients identify those at increased risk for unstable angina/MI in the subsequent weeks to months and should lead to further evaluation of these patients with coronary arteriography and either intensified medical therapy or interventional therapy with coronary artery angioplasty/stenting or CABG when their coronary artery anatomy is suitable.

REFERENCES

1. Théroux P, Ouimet H, McCann J, et al: Aspirin, heparin, or both to treat acute unstable angina. N Engl J Med 319:1105, 1988.
2. Cairns JA, Gent M, Singer J, et al: Aspirin, sulfinpyrazone, or both in unstable angina. N Engl J Med 313:1369, 1985.
3. DeCaterina R, Giannessi D, Bernini W, et al: Low dose aspirin in patients recovering from myocardial infarction: evidence for selective inhibition of thromboxane-related platelet function. Eur Heart J 6:409, 1985.
4. Patrano C: Aspirin as an antiplatelet drug. N Engl J Med 330:1287, 1994.
5. Gold HK, Torres FW, Garabedian HD, et al: Evidence for a rebound coagulation phenomenon after cessation of a 4-hour infusion of a specific thrombin inhibitor in patients with unstable angina pectoris. J Am Coll Cardiol 21:1039, 1993.
6. Willerson JT, Casscells W: Thrombin inhibitors in the treatment of patients with unstable angina: rebound or continuation of angina after argatroban withdrawal [editorial]. J Am Coll Cardiol 21:1048, 1993.
7. Théroux P, Waters D, Lam J, et al: Reactivation of unstable angina after the discontinuation of heparin. N Engl J Med 327:141, 1992.
8. Fragmin during Instability in Coronary Artery Disease (FRISC) Study: Low-molecular-weight heparin during instability in coronary artery disease. Lancet 347:561, 1996.
9. Hirsh J, Levine MD: Low molecular weight heparin. J Am Soc Hematol 79:1, 1992.
10. Samama MM, Bara L, Garotziafas GT: Mechanisms for the antithrombotic activity in man of low molecular weight heparins (LMWHs). Hemostasis 24:105, 1994.
11. Antman EM, McCabe CH, Gurfinkel EP, et al: Enoxaparin prevents death and cardiac ischemic events in unstable angina/non–Q wave myocardial infarction: results of the Thrombolysis in Myocardial Infarction (TIMI) 11B trial. Circulation 100:1593, 1999.
12. Cohen M, Demers C, Gurfinkel EP, et al: A comparison of low-molecular-weight heparin with unfractionated heparin for unstable coronary artery disease. N Engl J Med 337:447, 1997.
13. Hynes RO: Integrins, a family of cell surface receptors. Cell 48:569, 1987.
14. Tolleson TR, Harrington RA: Thrombolysis in acute coronary syndromes and coronary interventions. *In* Lincoff AM, Topol EJ (eds): Platelet Glycoprotein IIb/IIIa Inhibitors in Cardiovascular Disease. pp. 3–20. Totowa, NJ: Humana, 1999.
15. Knoll MH, Harris TS, Moake JL, et al: VonWillebrand factor binding to platelet GpIB initiates signal for platelet activation. J Clin Invest 88:1568, 1991.
16. Shah PK: Pathophysiology of plaque rupture and the concept of plaque stabilization. Cardiol Clin 14:17, 1996.
17. Willerson JT, Golino P, Eidt J, et al: Specific platelet mediators and unstable coronary artery lesions: experimental evidence and potential clinical implications. Circulation 80:198, 1989.
18. Marcel J, van den Brand BM, Simoons ML: The use of abciximab in therapy resistant unstable angina. Clinical and angiographic results of the CAPTURE Pilot and the CAPTURE Study. *In* Lincoff AM, Topol EJ (eds): Platelet Glycoprotein IIb/IIIa Inhibitors in Cardiovascular Disease. pp. 143–168. Totowa, NJ: Humana, 1999.
19. The CAPTURE Investigators: Randomized placebo-controlled trial of abciximab before and during coronary intervention in refractory unstable angina: the CAPTURE study. Lancet 349:1429, 1997.
20. The PURSUIT Trial Investigators: Inhibition of platelet glycoprotein IIb/IIIa with eptifibatide in patients with acute coronary syndromes. N Engl J Med 339:436–463, 1998.
21. The Platelet Receptor Inhibition in Ischemic Syndrome Management (PRISM) Study Investigators: A comparison of aspirin plus tirofiban with aspirin plus heparin for unstable angina. N Engl J Med 338:1498, 1998.
22. Platelet Receptor Inhibition in Ischemic Syndrome Management in Patients Limited by Unstable Signs and Symptoms (PRISM-PLUS) Study Investigators: Inhibition of the platelet glycoprotein IIb/IIIa receptor with tirofiban in unstable angina and non–Q-wave myocardial infarction. N Engl J Med 338:1488, 1998.
23. The EPISTENT Investigators: Randomised placebo-controlled and balloon-angioplasty–controlled trial to assess safety of coronary stenting with use of platelet glycoprotein IIb/IIIa blockade. Lancet 352:87, 1998.
24. The EPILOG Investigators: Platelet glycoprotein IIb/IIIa blockade with abciximab with low-dose heparin during percutaneous coronary revascularization. N Engl J Med 336:1689, 1997.
25. EPIC Investigators: Use of a monoclonal antibody directed against the platelet glycoprotein IIb/IIIa receptor in high-risk coronary angioplasty. N Engl J Med 330:956, 1994.
26. Pugh B, Platt MR, Mills LJ, et al: Unstable angina pectoris: a randomized study of patients treated medically and surgically. Am J Cardiol 41:1291, 1978.
27. Luchi RJ, Scott SM, Deupree RH: Comparison of medical and surgical treatment for unstable angina pectoris. Results of a Veterans Administration Cooperative Study. N Engl J Med 316:977, 1987.
28. Conti CR, Hodges M, Hutter A, et al: Unstable angina—a national cooperative study comparing medical and surgical therapy. Cardiovasc Clin 8:167, 1977.
29. Veterans Administration Coronary Artery Bypass Surgery Cooperative Study Group: Eleven-year survival in the Veterans Administration randomized trial of coronary bypass surgery for stable angina. N Engl J Med 311:1333, 1984.
30. Passamani E, Davis KB, Gillespie MJ, et al and the CASS Principal Investigators and Their Associates: A randomized trial of coronary artery bypass surgery: survival of patients with a low ejection fraction. N Engl J Med 312:1665, 1985.
31. CASS Principal Investigators and Their Associates: Coronary Artery Surgery Study (CASS): a randomized trial of coronary artery bypass surgery: survival data. Circulation 68:939, 1983.
32. European Coronary Surgery Study Group: Coronary-artery bypass surgery in stable angina pectoris: survival at two years. Lancet 1:889, 1979.
33. Borer J, Bacharach SL, Green MV, et al: Real time radionuclide cineangiography in the noninvasive evaluation of global and regional left ventricular function at rest and during exercise in patients with coronary artery disease. N Engl J Med 296:839, 1977.
34. Gibson RS, Watson DD, Craddock GB, et al: Prediction of cardiac events after uncomplicated myocardial infarction. Prospective study comparing predischarge exercise thallium-201 scintigraphy and coronary angiography. Circulation 68:321, 1983.
35. Ritchie JL, Trobaugh GB, Hamilton GW, et al: Myocardial imaging with thallium-201 at rest and during exercise: comparison with coronary arteriography and resting and stress electrocardiography. Circulation 56:66, 1977.
36. Corbett J, Dehmer GJ, Lewis SE, et al: The prognostic value of submaximal exercise testing with radionuclide ventriculography prior

to hospital discharge in patients with recent myocardial infarction. Circulation 64:535, 1981.
37. Dehmer GJ, Lewis SE, Hillis LD, et al: Exercise induced alterations in left ventricular volumes in man: usefulness in predicting the relative extent of coronary artery disease. Circulation 63:1008, 1981.
38. Reichek N, Priest C, Zimrin D, et al: Antianginal effects of nitroglycerin patches. Am J Cardiol 54:1, 1984.
39. Parker JO, VanKoughnett KA, Fung HL: Transdermal isosorbide dinitrate in angina pectoris: effect of acute and sustained therapy. Am J Cardiol 54:8, 1984.
40. Glancy DL, Richter MA, Ellis EV, et al: Effect of swallowed isosorbide dinitrate on blood pressure, heart rate, and exercise capacity in patients with coronary artery disease. Am J Med 62:39, 1977.
41. Muller JE, Gunther SJ: Nifedipine therapy for Prinzmetal's angina. Circulation 57:137, 1978.
42. Hugenholtz PG, Michels HR, Serruys PW, et al: Nifedipine in the treatment of unstable angina, coronary spasm and myocardial ischemia. Am J Cardiol 47:163, 1981.
43. Gunther S, Green L, Muller JE, et al: Prevention by nifedipine of abnormal coronary vasoconstriction in patients with coronary artery disease. Circulation 63:849, 1981.
44. Solberg LE, Nissen RG, Vlietstra RE, et al: Prinzmetal's variant angina—response to verapamil. Mayo Clin Proc 53:256, 1978.
45. Johnson SM, Mauritson DR, Willerson JT, Hillis LD: A controlled trial of verapamil for Prinzmetal's variant angina. N Engl J Med 304:862, 1981.
46. Freedman B, Dunn RF, Richmond DR, et al: Coronary artery spasm during exercise: treatment with verapamil. Circulation 64:68, 1981.
47. Hansen JF, Sando E: Treatment of Prinzmetal's angina due to coronary artery spasm using verapamil: a report of three cases. Eur J Cardiol 7:327, 1978.
48. Schroeder JS, Lamb IH, Ginsburg R, et al: Diltiazem for long-term therapy of coronary arterial spasm. Am J Cardiol 49:533, 1982.
49. Johnson SM, Mauritson DR, Willerson JT, et al: A comparison of verapamil and nifedipine in the treatment of variant angina pectoris. Am J Cardiol 47:1295, 1981.
50. Winniford MD, Johnson SM, Mauritson DR, et al: Verapamil therapy for Prinzmetal's variant angina: comparison with placebo and nifedipine. Am J Cardiol 50:913, 1982.
51. Hillis LD: The new coronary vasodilators: calcium blockers. J Cardiovasc Med 5:583, 1980.
52. Théroux P, Waters DD, Affaki GS, et al: Provocative testing with ergonovine to evaluate the efficacy of treatment with calcium antagonists in variant angina. Circulation 60:504, 1979.
53. Nagao T, Ikeo T, Sato M: Influence of calcium ions on responses to diltiazem in coronary arteries. Jpn J Pharmacol 27:330, 1977.
54. Weishaar R, Ashikawa K, Bing RJ: Effect of diltiazem, a calcium antagonist, on myocardial ischemia. Am J Cardiol 43:1137, 1979.
55. Previtali M, Salerno JA, Tavazzi L, et al: Treatment of angina at rest with nifedipine: a short-term controlled study. Am J Cardiol 45:825, 1980.
56. DiPaolo C, Kerin NZ, Rubenfire M, Levin F: Surgical treatment of medically refractory variant angina pectoris: segmental coronary resection with aortocoronary bypass and plexectomy. Am J Cardiol 56:792, 1985.

CHAPTER 36

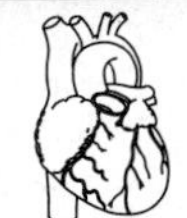

TREATMENT OF ACUTE Q WAVE MYOCARDIAL INFARCTION

Burton E. Sobel and James T. Willerson

THROMBOLYTIC THERAPY
Classification of Thrombolytic Agents
Development and Impact of Clot-Selective Agents
Differentiation Between First- and Second-Generation Agents With Respect to Clot Selectivity
First-Generation Agents
Second-Generation Agents
Principles Underlying Dose Regimens: Pharmacokinetics and Pharmacodynamics
Mechanisms Responsible for Effective Recanalization and Their Implications Regarding Dosing
Conjunctive Therapy
Administration of t-PA with Conjunctive and Adjunctive Agents
Studies with t-PA
Infarct Size and Left Ventricular Function
Survival and Its Dependence on Recanalization
Safety of Clot-Selective Agents
Anticipated Developments
Unresolved Issues
Comparison of Pharmacologic Coronary Thrombolysis With Primary Percutaneous Transluminal Coronary Angioplasty With or Without Stenting
Importance of Conjunctive Therapy
Pitfalls in the Interpretations of End Points
Ventricular Function
Survival
Results of Clinical Studies
Ventricular Function and the Extent of Infarction
Mortality
Safety
Recent Observations and Clinical Implications
LOOKING TO THE FUTURE: GP IIb/IIIa ANTAGONISTS/ THROMBOLYTIC THERAPY
Paradigm Trial
Assessment of Integrelin and Accelerated Tissue Plasminogen Activator: The IMPACT-AMI Study
TIMI 14 Trial
Treatment of the Survivor of Acute Myocardial Infarction

The patient with suspected or proven myocardial infarction (MI) should be admitted to a coronary care unit, where heart rate and rhythm can be monitored continuously. Unless there is an important contraindication, patients with ST segment elevation and Q wave infarcts evaluated within 6 hours of symptom onset should receive thrombolytic therapy as quickly as possible. Patients with continuing or recurrent chest pain believed to be part of continuing Q wave infarction and those with anterior Q wave MIs or inferior infarcts that also involve the true posterior, septal, lateral, or right ventricle should receive thrombolytic therapy, even 6 to 24 hours after MI.

Thrombolytic therapy should be given in association with a thrombin antagonist (i.e., intravenous heparin at present) and aspirin, one half (163 mg) to one aspirin (325 mg) given before or with the thrombolytic intervention. Aspirin therapy should be continued indefinitely. In the patient with an inferior infarct that also involves the right ventricle and/or the lateral or true posterior wall of the LV, the clinical prognosis is more similar to that of the patient with anterior MI. In patients without bradycardia, atrioventricular (AV) block, bronchospasm, or severe congestive heart failure (CHF), a beta-blocker can be given with the thrombolytic agent or a few days thereafter. When given initially with thrombolytic therapy, metoprolol reduces the frequency of new ischemic events in the first week after infarction, as shown in the Thrombolysis and Myocardial Infarction (TIMI-2B) trial.[1] In the TIMI-2B trial, a subset of patients with acute Q wave infarcts was treated with metoprolol, 5 mg IV at 2-minute intervals over 6 minutes for a total intravenous dose of 15 mg, followed by 50 mg orally every 12 hours in the first 24 hours and 100 mg orally every 12 hours thereafter. Doses were not given if systolic blood pressure fell below 100 mm Hg, heart rate decreased below 60 beats per minute, or CHF developed. Metoprolol given in this manner was associated with a reduction in the frequency of reinfarction and recurrent chest pain during the first 6 days of hospitalization.[1]

Beginning a specific or nonspecific β-blocker without beta-adrenergic agonist effect several days after infarction reduces the subsequent risk for MI and death in subsequent years.[2–4] In addition, the administration of an inhibitor of the renin-angiotensin system, usually an angiotension-converting enzyme (ACE) inhibitor or angiotensin receptor antagonist, reduces the remodeling of the infarct and the subsequent dilatation of the heart, especially with anterior and nonreperfused infarcts. Thus, we recommend the post-infarct administration of a β-blocker and/or an inhibitor of the renin-angiotensin system whenever possible and at doses of these agents that do not substantially reduce blood pressure or heart rate.

THROMBOLYTIC THERAPY

Classification of Thrombolytic Agents

Thrombolysis depends on conversion of plasminogen, a zymogen present in the circulation, to plasmin, a nonspecific proteolytic enzyme that degrades fibrin, among many other proteins. A useful distinction between available thrombolytic agents is based on their clot selectivity. The terms *clot selective, fibrin selective,* and *fibrin specific* are often used interchangeably. However, to be more specific, agents that are clot selective convert clot-associated plasminogen to clot-associated plasmin preferentially, that is, with higher affinity and at a greater rate compared with their action on free, circulating plasminogen. Fibrin selective means greater activity (activation of plasminogen) in the presence of fibrin than in the absence of fibrin and may reflect high affinity for, and/or higher binding affinity to, fibrin. Fibrin specific means that fibrin (or a biologically equivalent surface) is required for activation of plasminogen with or without binding.

First-generation fibrinolytic agents (streptokinase, urokinase, anistreplace [anisoylated plasminogen streptokinase activator complex, or APSAC]); reteplase, or rPA (a kringle 1 deletion mutant of tissue-type plasminogen activator [t-PA])[5–9]; and lanoteplase, or nPA,[10] a finger and epidermal growth factor domain deletion and point mutation mutant of t-PA, activate plasminogen comparably, whether it is free in the circulation or physically associated with fibrin. Second-generation agent plasminogen activators including t-PA, or alteplase (Activase); staphylokinase plasminogen activator recombinant[11–15]; duteplase, bat salivary gland t-PA (a kringle 2 deletion mutant)[16]; saruplase,[17, 18] single-chain urokinase (scu-PA), which is clot selective but converted to urokinase, which is not clot selective in vivo; and TNK–t-PA[19–22] activate plasminogen in the fibrin domain preferentially. In therapeutically effective doses after intravenous administration, all of these agents except scu-PA exhibit little or no activation of free plasminogen in the circulation. Investigational agents, designed for maximal fibrin and clot selectivity, include chimeras, such as t-PA/P-selectin and fibrin-targeted molecules.[23, 24]

Development and Impact of Clot-Selective Agents

Coronary thrombolysis is an established primary treatment for acute MI secondary to coronary thrombosis. Despite the discovery of the fibrinolytic system in 1903,[25] the extraction of an active fibrinolytic agent from streptococci (streptokinase [SIC]) in 1941,[26] and the identification of plasminogen in 1945,[27] coronary thrombolysis was not attempted until 1958.[28] Its entry into clinical practice was delayed for several decades, in part because of early controversy regarding the proximate cause of acute MI.

Several phenomena led to its acceptance including: (1) DeWoods'[29] pivotal angiographic study demonstrating the presence of intracoronary thrombi very early after the onset of infarction, resolving a long-standing controversy regarding its proximate cause; (2) maturation of coronary angiography permitting unequivocal demonstration of recanalization of occluded coronary arteries by thrombolytic agents[30]; and (3) development of clot-selective fibrinolytic agents, initially t-PA.[30–32] The only established mechanisms by which coronary thrombolysis confers benefit are prompt and durable recanalization of infarct-related arteries. Optimal benefit results when coronary thrombolysis restores patency promptly and persistently in patients[33–35] as well as in laboratory animals.[36, 37] Results in the landmark Gruppo Italiano per lo Studio della Streptochinasi nell'Infarto Miocardico (GISSI-1) trial demonstrated marked diminution of mortality in patients who were treated very early after the onset of infarction. Virtually no survival benefit accompanied treatment that was initiated more than 6 hours after the onset of symptoms. Results from the Myocardial Infarction Triage and Intervention (MITI) trial (1 percent mortality after very early treatment, compared with 10 percent mortality after later treatment) underscore the striking benefit of very prompt recanalization.[38]

Coronary thrombosis occurs most often on an active, lipid-laden atherosclerotic plaque replete with lipid (making up 40 percent or more of its volume) with a thin fibrous cap and substantial inflammation. The typical plaque is one prone to fissuring, intramural hemorrhage, and rupture, consequently predisposing to intraluminal thrombosis.[39] Such plaques may not give rise to high-grade obstruction until thrombotic occlusion occurs. Conversely, high-grade stenotic lesions are often characterized by fibrotic, relatively acellular plaques with a paucity of lipids and a thick fibrous cap. They are often associated with exercise-induced angina pectoris rather than with acute coronary syndromes precipitated by thrombotic occlusions, including unstable angina and acute MI.

Although acute coronary syndromes other than infarction, such as unstable angina[40] and angina at rest,[41–43] are associated with activation of the coagulation system and intermittent thrombosis,[44] fibrinolysis has not been particularly effective in these entities.[45] Its lack of efficacy in these disorders may be attributable in part to the extent and the severity of the underlying coronary artery disease (CAD)[46, 47] and the transient nature of the thrombosis.

Differentiation Between First- and Second-Generation Agents with Respect to Clot Selectivity

First-generation agents exhibit little or no clot selectivity. They activate plasminogen with equal alacrity, whether it is free in the circulation or associated with fibrin on the surface of and in the interstices of clots. Although the biochemical mechanisms of action differ among individual first-generation agents (SK, urokinase, APSAC, nPA, and retevase rPA being the most common), all first-generation agents share some common properties. In therapeutically effective doses given intravenously, they induce a systemic lytic state characterized by activation of circulating plasminogen to plasmin, depletion of circulating plasminogen, degradation of fibrinogen, generation of high concentrations of fibrinogen degradation products (FDPs),[48] degradation of procoagulant proteins, and consumption of alpha$_2$-antiplasmin.[32] The systemic lytic state is both a marker for an increased risk of bleeding and an indication that the induction of high concentrations of FDPs (moieties with anticoagulant properties) has occurred, thereby potentially diminishing the likelihood of early reocclusion after initially successful coronary thrombolysis in patients who are not optimally anticoagulated.

Second-generation or clot-selective fibrinolytic agents (t-PA, scu-PA, and TNK being the best known) activate clot- and fibrin-associated plasminogen preferentially to form plasmin, thereby targeting thrombi for lysis. They induce much less (as much as 1000-fold less) activation of plasminogen that is free in the circulation.[48] Therefore, at therapeutically effective doses, induction of a systemic lytic state is either absent or is more modest[49] than is the case with first-generation agents,[11–15, 19–22, 50] as reviewed by Fry and Sobel.[51] In view of the relative paucity of FDPs generated,[49] the particular need for concomitant anticoagulation when fibrin-selective agents are used is apparent.[52]

Although not often considered clinically, commercially available preparations of fibrinolytic agents have been compared biochemically. The ratio of active ingredient to total protein content differs markedly among them.[53] The plasminogen activator makes up 99.9 percent of total protein with clinically available t-PA, 55 percent with APSAC, 20 percent with urokinase, and 1 percent with SK. Some of the nonspecific effects that have been described after administration of SK and anistreplase, including hypotension, platelet aggregation,[54] and dissolution of collagen,[55] may be attributable in part to proteins in the preparation other than the plasminogen activator itself. Others reflect the nonspecificity of first-generation plasminogen activators, with generation of plasmin in the circulation and consequent activation of complement[56, 57] and of kinins, which can induce occasionally severe hypotension.[58]

The streptococci-derived plasminogen activator preparations, streptokinase and anistreplase, differ from other fibrinolytic agents in one important respect. Because the plasminogen activator is derived from extracts of streptococci with which many patients will have had clinical or subclinical encounters, interactions with preformed antibody are common. In approximately 15 percent of patients, interactions induce platelet aggregation, potentially impairing therapeutic efficacy.[54] Other immune-mediated phenomena, such as vasculitis (reported occasionally with APSAC)[59] and immediate hypersensitivity reactions with associated hypotension, can occur. Antigenicity is particularly important in patients who may require additional dosing within days to weeks after initial treatment. Under such circumstances, repeat dosing with SK or anistreplase may be ineffective because of an anamnestic immune response or may be dangerous. In addition, these agents are less able to lyse clots of moderate age (>4 to 6 hours) compared with clot-selective agents, particularly t-PA. As a result, it has been said that time is "running out" on their use.[60–62] Urokinase or t-PA is preferable for repeat dosing in a patient who has been treated with any fibrinolytic drug previously.[63]

Second-generation fibrinolytic agents were developed initially to facilitate clot lysis without concomitant induction of a systemic lytic state. Comparative studies with first- and second-generation agents soon demonstrated that transfusion requirements and the incidence of bleeding from vascular access and other sites were diminished with clot-selective agents.[64, 65] Nevertheless, all of the fibrinolytic agents in clinical use are safe when patient selection is appropriate and monitoring is judicious.

The 90-minute patency rate is greater with clot-selective compared with first-generation agents, as judged from direct comparisons in early small, random patient assignment trials (Table 36–1). A prospective recanalization trial in which occlusive thrombi were demonstrable in infarct-related arteries before treatment in every case and the efficacy of the thrombolytic agent in inducing recanalization could be documented definitively demonstrated the superiority of t-PA over streptokinase in heparinized patients.[66] More rapid and more frequent recanalization was found to occur with t-PA than with SK, regardless of the interval after the onset of treatment (up to a 6-hour maximum).[67] Similar results were obtained in a patency

TABLE 36–1 Angiographically Documented Patency in Infarct-Related Arteries 60 to 180 Minutes After the Start of Therapy in Patients With Acute Myocardial Infarction

Study	Dose	Mean Time to Treatment (h)	Reperfusion (n, %)	Angiographic End Point* (min)
Streptokinase				
Rogers et al	1 M, 45 min	6.8	7 of 16 (44)	75
Neuhaus et al	1.7 M	3.7	24 of 40 (60)	90
Schroder et al	0.5 M, 30 min	3.8	11 of 21 (52)	Up to 180
Alderman et al	0.725 M, 85 min	3.4	8 of 13 (62)	90
Spann et al	0.85–1.5 M	3.5	21 of 43 (49)	60
Hillis et al	1.5 M, 60 min	4.5	11 of 34 (32)	90
TIMI-I	1.5 M, 60 min	4.8	37 of 119 (31)	90
ECSG-I	1.5 M, 60 min	2.6	34 of 65 (55)	75 to 90
Total		4.1	153 of 351 (43)	
rt-PA				
Collen et al	TC, variable	4.7	25 of 33 (75)	90
Williams et al	TC, 50 mg/90 min	4.8	27 of 37 (68)	90
TIMI-I	TC, 50 mg/90 min	4.8	70 of 113 (62)	90
Gold et al	TC, 0.4–0.75 mg/kg, 60–120 min	3.0	24 of 29 (83)	60
TIMI-B	SC, 70 mg/90 min	4.6	59 of 83 (71)	90
TIMI-C	SC, 100 mg/90 min	4.6	42 of 62 (68)	90
ECSG-I	TC, 0.75 mg/kg, 90 min	3.0	43 of 64 (70)	75 to 90
Total		4.2	290 of 421 (69)	

Abbreviations: ECSG, European Cooperative Study Group; rt-PA, recombinant tissue-type plasminogen activator; M, mega (million) units; SC, single chain; TC, two chain; TIMI, Thrombolysis in Myocardial Infarction.

*Studies with angiography performed many hours or days after therapy have not been included in this analysis.

Adapted from Collen D: Coronary thrombolysis: streptokinase or recombinant tissue-type plasminogen activator? Ann Intern Med 112:529, 1990.

trial with angiography first performed 90 minutes after treatment.[68] One mechanism that may be responsible is the avoidance of plasminogen steal, discussed later.[69–71] The early benefit of t-PA on survival compared with SK has been sustained long term[72] and, in fact, amplified.[73] In a prodigious compilation of observational data from more than 354,000 patients in more than 1300 institutions, a remarkably low early mortality of 5.7 percent was evident in patients without age limitation and with bona fide infarction treated with t-PA, aspirin, and heparin in community hospitals.[74–76] Thus, despite cost differentials, with cost of clot-selective agents higher but well within the range assigned by health care economists to generally cost-effective modalities, the advantages of clot-selective agents have resulted in their becoming the agents of choice.[19, 77]

First-Generation Agents

SK is obtained as an extract of the fermentation of cultures of the hemolytic streptococcus. Urokinase, as its name implies, is obtained generally from extracts of urine. SK combines with plasminogen to form active complexes that circulate in the blood; undergo degradation of the SK and plasminogen portions, yielding complex mixtures with diverse proteolytic activity and diverse clearance; and activate plasminogen to form plasmin, the enzyme that attacks fibrin in clots. Plasmin is a nonspecific protease that acts also on fibrinogen to deplete it and to release fibrin split products, which have modest anticoagulant properties. The depletion of fibrinogen not only interferes with new clot formation but also lowers blood viscosity. By contrast, urokinase forms plasmin from plasminogen directly and stoichiometrically. Both agents and their congeners induce a systemic lytic state. Second-generation agents, which are fibrin selective, are less likely to impair hemostatic mechanisms. Early trials with them showed only modest reduction of the incidence of overall episodes of bleeding. In fact, t-PA appears to induce a small (0.1 percent) increase in the risk of cerebral hemorrhage compared with SK, with the risk related to advanced age and to sustained and uncontrolled hypertension.[78] The risk may reflect degradation of vascular wall elements by locally elaborated plasmin,[79, 80] particularly in a setting in which occult cerebral vasculopathy, such as hypertensive and beta-amyloid angiopathy, is present.[79]

Contrary to the conventional wisdom, proliferative retinopathy does not interdict the use of thrombolytic agents and confers little or no risk.[81] Menorrhagia is a risk in menstruating females but can be managed without requiring interdiction of thrombolytic agents.[82]

Many patients with acute MI have antistreptolysin antibodies as a result of previous infection with streptococci. It is therefore necessary to give a dose of SK large enough to neutralize levels of antibodies that exist in most patients.[83] The antigen-antibody reaction gives rise to "allergic" symptoms, such as rigors, backache, and, very rarely, anaphylactoid reactions. Hypotension is common. It appears to be attributable most often to activation of the vasodepressor kinin system.[34] When allergic rashes occur, hydrocortisone may be helpful.[34]

Unlike SK, urokinase is not allergenic. Although injection of SK elicits a further increase in antibody titers, and although the antibodies can neutralize fibrinolytic activity of SK, there does not appear to be a general relationship between the angiographic patency with SK or APSAC and the level of pretreatment antibody titer. Levels of antibody titer increase after administration of APSAC just as they do after administration of SK.[84] The increases persist for years.

SK is generally administered in a dose of 1.5 million U IV over 60 minutes with concomitant chewable aspirin (162 to 365 mg) and heparin. APSAC is given as 30 units IV over 5 minutes. Urokinase is given as 2 million units IV over 30 minutes.

The Efficacy of First-Generation Agents

Because most of the information available regarding efficacy pertains to SK, it is the focus of the following material. Because early meta-analysis[85] indicated a reduction in mortality, prospective trials were implemented. A 17-month trial performed in Italy in 1984 and 1985, the GISSI-1 Trial,[33] demonstrated the practicality and efficacy of intravenous (as opposed to previously used intracoronary) SK. A total of 11,806 patients (37 percent of those screened) were randomly assigned to SK (1.5 million U) or then conventional treatment without fibrinolytic drugs; 80 percent were given the drug within 6 hours after onset of chest pain. The risk of death in hospital (14 to 21 days) was reduced by 19 percent (from 13.0 to 10.7 percent; $P < .0002$) by SK. In a striking (but retrospective) analysis, risk reduction was 51 percent in the 1277 patients who had been randomly assigned within 1 hour of the onset of chest pain.

The ISIS-2 trial[34] was a placebo-controlled study that incorporated the use of aspirin (160 mg enteric coated, the first tablet chewed immediately, and then taken daily for 1 month) in a factorial design. Patients were randomly assigned to one of four groups; SK alone (1.5 million U IV over 1 hour); aspirin alone; both; or neither, with appropriate placebos.

Administration of aspirin daily for 1 month reduced 5-week mortality by approximately 20 percent. Effects of SK and aspirin were additive.[86] This may reflect potentiation of thrombolysis by aspirin secondary to attenuation of platelet-dependent thrombosis. Alternatively, the lack of inclusion of a qualifying electrocardiogram raises the possibility that the beneficial effects of aspirin were attributable to salutary effects in a subset of patients with unstable angina and that the apparently additive benefits of aspirin and SK were in part a reflection of the benefits of each agent in different subsets of patients, with fibrinolysis benefiting patients with bona fide infarction and aspirin benefiting those with unstable angina.

In ISIS-2, the incidence of major hemorrhage was not increased by concomitant aspirin. Minor bleeds were slightly more common with aspirin, but the overall stroke rate was reduced by about one half as a result of a diminution in the incidence of ischemic strokes. The beneficial effects of SK and of aspirin on survival were persistent throughout many years of follow up.

Results of both the GISSI and the ISIS-2 trials showed that treatment with SK was beneficial in older as well as younger patients. There was, however, a definite risk for adverse effects, especially cerebral hemorrhage. For most patients, the risk of death from acute MI was far from negligible. Results of the GISSI, ISIS-2, and Intravenous Streptokinase in Acute Myocardial Infarction (ISAM) trials showed that although the overall risk of stroke associated with treatment with a first-generation drug was not significantly increased, the incidence of intracranial bleeds (ICBs) was 1 to 2/1000 patients treated, and that of other major hemorrhage requiring transfusion was 3/1000 patients.[34] However, the risk of both was substantially less than the benefit conferred with respect to stroke-free survival.

Treatment with thrombolytic agents is associated with a risk of reinfarction because (1) underlying atherosclerotic coronary vascular disease is not obviated, (2) some patients who survive are at particularly high risk and would have succumbed without treatment with a thrombolytic drug, and (3) activation of platelets and of the coagulation system is induced as a result of endogenous factors (especially clot-associated factors) and exogenous factors (especially antiplatelet antibodies) with the use of SK and its congeners and plasminemia, particularly with first-generation compared with clot-selective agents. However, survivors of an index infarct can and should be managed aggressively to (1) ascertain risk of recurrence, (2) intervene with angioplasty and stenting as indicated, and (3) sustain an optimal medical regimen, including lipid lowering.

The Role of Anticoagulants

Most studies with streptokinase have been performed without protocol-mandated intravenous heparin given in dosages sufficient to induce systemic anticoagulation within the first 24 hours.[87] This approach may be ill advised. The efficacy of thrombolysis reflects a balance between clot lysis and interdiction of ongoing thrombosis that can both retard restoration of patency and predispose to early thrombotic reocclusion.[88–92]

The use of subcutaneous rather than protocol-mandated intravenous heparin in ISIS-2[89] and GISSI-2[93–95] was predicated on a concern regarding the need to minimize the incidence of cerebral hemorrhage and stroke and the recognition that SK, and, for that matter, all non–clot-selective plasminogen activators generate high concentrations of fibrinogen degradation products, themselves weak anticoagulants.[96] However, such reasoning is not well supported, as judged from data from numerous earlier studies.[97, 98]

There is no controversy regarding the fact that intravenous heparin is beneficial when no aspirin[99] or inadequate doses of aspirin[100] are used, as judged by assessment of coronary patency. When an adequate dose of aspirin is used, as in the European Cooperative Study Group trial,[101] the increase in patency (from 75 to 82 percent) appears to be more modest with non–clot-selective compared with clot-selective agents. As discussed later, use of heparin seems to be advisable even when aspirin is used with first-generation agents.

Second-Generation Agents

Results of Early Studies

Most studies with second-generation (fibrin- or clot-selective) agents have been performed with t-PA. However, principles delineated with this agent are applicable to other clot-selective agents, such as staphylokinase plasminogen activator recombinant[11–15] and TNK,[19–22] now being developed. After the initial purification of human t-PA in pharmacologic quantities, its potential advantages were demonstrated in studies of experimental animals with induced coronary thrombosis. Intravenously administered t-PA promptly induced lysis of the fibrin-rich thrombi without depleting fibrinogen from the circulation or inducing the systemic lytic state invariably encountered with therapeutically effective concentrations of first-generation agents.[102] Similar results were soon obtained with human t-PA produced by recombinant DNA technology.[103] In the first study of native t-PA in patients with thrombotic coronary occlusions, coronary thrombolysis was induced promptly without depletion of fibrinogen.[104] Soon thereafter, the efficacy of coronary thrombolysis with recombinant human t-PA was demonstrated in prospective, randomized, placebo-controlled cooperative trials.

These initial results suggested that clot-specific agents might be more effective than first-generation agents in promptly recanalizing infarct-related arteries. The Thrombolysis in Myocardial Infarction (TIMI)-I trial[105] was conducted by the National Heart, Lung, and Blood Institute to test this hypothesis directly. Its primary objective was delineation of the relative efficacy of t-PA compared with SK in promptly opening infarct-related arteries. Accordingly, all patients were evaluated angiographically before treatment to verify thrombotic coronary occlusion, randomly assigned subsequently in a double-blinded fashion to treatment with t-PA or SK, and studied angiographically 30 and 90 minutes after onset of treatment. A twofold greater incidence of angiographically documented recanalization in the first 90 minutes was seen with t-PA (62 percent), compared with SK (31 percent). Furthermore, effects of the agents on plasma fibrinogen were markedly different, with a much more striking depletion of fibrinogen seen with SK.

The primacy of prompt induction of coronary patency as the most powerful determinant of benefit of coronary thrombolysis is evident from seminal observations by Reimer and coworkers,[36] who studied morphologic changes in dog hearts subjected to ischemia for selected intervals before reperfusion. Others reached the same conclusions in tomographic studies of regional myocardial metabolism.[37] Large-scale multicenter clinical trials (GISSI-1[33], Second International Study of Infarct Survival [ISIS-2][34]) and studies of prehospital treatment (MITI trial[38, 106], European Myocardial Infarction Project [EMIP][107]) and registry data (Figure 36–1) demonstrate the same temporal dependence of benefit conferred on jeopardized myocardium include not only the rapidity, completeness, and persistence of recanalization of epicardial coronary arteries[108] but also the adequacy of tissue perfusion, dependent in part on avoidance of the "no reflow" phenomenon.[109–114]

Results of recanalization studies (with angiography both before and after treatment) and patency trials (with angiography only after treatment) are consistent in demonstrating the more rapid and more frequent induction of reperfusion with second- compared with first-generation drugs (Table 36–2). Therefore, as judged from results of 25 large clinical trials conducted between 1984 and 1988, intravenous ad-

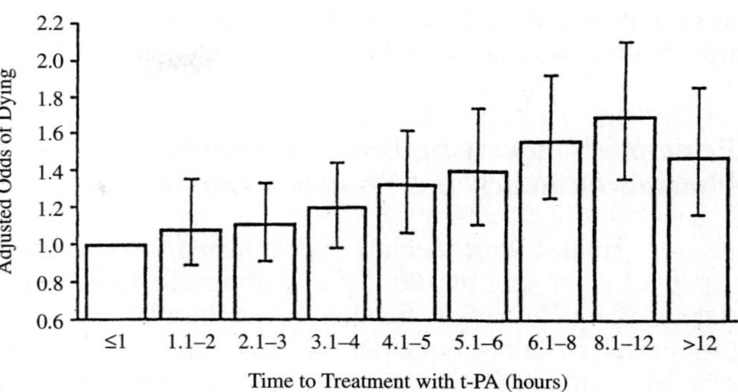

FIGURE 36–1 Multivariable adjusted odds of dying associated with time of administration of tissue-type plasminogen activator (t-PA) therapy and accompanying 95 percent confidence intervals: NRMI-2. (From Goldberg RJ, Mooradd M, Gurwitz JH, et al: Impact of time to treatment with tissue plasminogen activator on morbidity and mortality following acute myocardial infarction [The Second National Registry of Myocardial Infarction]. Am J Cardiol 82:259, 1998; copyright 1998, with permission from Excerpta Medica Inc.)

TABLE 36–2 Patency Shown by Coronary Angiography 60 to 180 Minutes After the Start of Therapy in Patients With Acute Myocardial Infarction

Study	Dose	Mean Time to Treatment (h)	Reperfusion (n, %)	Angiographic End Point* (min)
Streptokinase (SK)				
Taylor et al	0.85 M, 60 min	3.2	7 of 22 (77)	60
Schwarz et al	1.5 M, 90 min	2.5	25 of 55 (45)	90
Verstraete et al	1.5 M, 60 min	2.6	34 of 62 (55)	90
Cribier et al	1.5 M, 60 min	3.1	11 of 21 (52)	60
Brochier et al	1.5 M, 60 min	2.8	24 of 43 (56)	105
Monnier et al	1.5 M, 60 min	2.5	7 of 11 (64)	150
Chesebro et al	1.5 M, 60 min	4.7	61 of 146 (42)	90
Stack et al	1.5 M, 60 min	3.0	95 of 216 (44)	90
Lopez-Sendon et al	1.5 M, 60 min	2.9	14 of 24 (58)	90
Vogt et al			21 of 31 (72)	
PRIMI	1.5 M, 60 min	<4	124 of 194 (64)	90
Anderson	30 U APSAC, 2–4 min	3.4	59 of 115 (51)	90
	160,000 U SK, 60 min	3.4	67 of 111 (60)	60
Total		3.1	559 of 1051 (53)	
rt-PA				
Verstraete et al	TC, 0.75 mg/kg, 90 min	3.4	38 of 60 (61)	90
Verstraete et al	TC, 0.75 mg/kg, 90 min	3.0	43 of 61 (70)	90
Verstraete et al	TC, 40 mg/90 min	2.5	78 of 119 (66)	90
Topol et al	SC, 1.25 mg/kg, 3 h	4.0	27 of 38 (71)	90
Topol et al	SC, 150 mg, 6–8 h	3.9	288 of 386 (75)	90
Topol et al	SC, 150 mg, 6–8 h	3.8	60 of 89 (67)	90
		2.1	43 of 53 (81)	90
Topol et al	SC, 1.5 mg/kg, 3 h	2.8	104 of 131 (79)	90
Simoons et al	SC, 100 mg, 3 h	2.6	160 of 180 (89)	90
Johns et al	SC, 1 mg/kg, 90 min	<6	52 of 68 (76)	90
TIMI-IIA	SC, 100 mg, 90 min	2.8	47 of 62 (76)	120
	SC, 70 mg, 90 min	3.2	97 of 130 (75)	120
McNeill et al	TC, 100 mg, 90 min	2.3	14 of 17 (82)	90
Neuhaus et al	SC, 70 mg, 90 min	<6	43 of 62 (69)	
Neuhaus et al	SC, 100 mg, 90 min	2.8	30 of 35 (86)	90
TIMI-I	TC, 50 mg, 90 min	4.4	70 of 113 (62)	90
TIMI-II pilot	SC, 150 mg, 6 h	2.7	260 of 317 (82)	60
Johns Hopkins	TC, 80 to 100 mg, 3 h	3.2	48 of 72 (66)	120
Total		3.1	1502 of 1993 (75)	

Abbreviations: APSAC, anisoylated plasminogen streptokinase activator complex; M, mega units; PRIMI, Prourokinase in Myocardial Infarction; rt-PA, recombinant tissue-type plasminogen activator; SC, single chain; TC, two chain; TIMI, Thrombolysis in Myocardial Infarction.

*Studies with angiography done many hours or days after therapy have not been included in this analysis.

Modified from Collen, D: Coronary thrombolysis: streptokinase or recombinant tissue-type plasminogen activator? Ann Intern Med 112:529, 1990.

ministration of first-generation fibrinolytic drugs, even in large doses, induced early patency in only approximately 50 percent of patients compared with 75 percent or more in patients treated with second-generation agents, as judged from 90-minute patency delineated angiographically.[86]

Principles Underlying Dose Regimens: Pharmacokinetics and Pharmacodynamics

In early studies with recombinant human t-PA (produced as alteplase), a dose of 100 mg was administered over 3 to 6 hours, with a larger fraction given in the first hour. Computer-assisted simulations of the pharmacodynamics of t-PA, reflecting the complex kinetic interactions of changing concentrations of the large number of proteins involved in the fibrinolytic system, indicated that the duration of infusions, and hence the persistence of t-PA in the blood, would be a major determinant of clot selectivity and, presumably, of safety.[115]

The half-life of t-PA in the circulation is only a few minutes. Plasmin formed initially from activation of plasminogen in the blood (which occurs to some extent with the high pharmacologic concentrations of t-PA now used) is neutralized by circulating α_2-antiplasmin. However, if the duration of exposure of circulating plasminogen to pharmacologic concentrations of t-PA is prolonged, α_2-antiplasmin is consumed. Subsequently, the generation of additional plasmin elicits induction of a systemic lytic state. Accordingly, initially high concentrations of activator in blood with abbreviated infusions are desirable to optimize clot selectivity and safety. Conversely, the brevity of persistence in the circulation of intravenously administered t-PA is not associated with lack of persistence of fibrinolytic activity on already existing clots.[116] Nevertheless, continuing exposure to t-PA of a degrading clot is desirable, at least early in the evolution of thrombolysis, to ensure binding of t-PA to newly exposed lysine binding sites within the interstices of the fibrin mesh.[117] With the use of monoclonal antibodies to detect evolution of cross-linked products of fibrin degradation, we found that fibrinolysis proceeded for several hours after completion of intravenous infusions of t-PA, despite complete clearance of the administered t-PA from the circulation.[116] The persistence of lysis reflects the avid and prolonged juxtaposition of clot-bound t-PA to clot-bound plasminogen, with consequently persistent activation of clot-associated plasminogen yielding clot-associated plasmin-sustaining fibrinolysis.

Neuhaus and coworkers[118, 119] developed accelerated or front-loaded dose regimens that took advantage of these phenomena (an initial bolus of 15 mg followed by 50 mg in the next 30 minutes and 35 mg in the following hour) and elicited coronary patency in 91 percent of patients studied angiographically within 90 minutes of the onset of infusion, without inducing a systemic lytic state.[115] Modified front-loaded regimens being evaluated include bolus administration of 1 mg/kg (with patency rates as high as 82 percent)[120, 121] weight-adjusted modified Neuhaus regimens and repeated bolus administration of 50 mg 30 minutes apart. Extensive experience with the Neuhaus regimen justifies its use[122–124] as an alternative to earlier regimens. Although double-bolus regimens (50 mg at 30-minute intervals) appeared promising initially,[125] they have not been shown to be superior in a large, prospective, multicenter, randomized, patient assignment study.[126] Another novel regimen (20 mg bolus followed by 50 mg IV over 1 hour[127]) has elicited a very high incidence of TIMI 3 flow (280 percent), in an initial, dosage comparison study.

Mechanisms Responsible for Effective Recanalization and Their Implications Regarding Dosing

Results in early comparative studies between first- and second-generation fibrinolytic drugs indicated more rapid and more frequent induction of recanalization with clot-selective agents. Their superiority in this respect appears to depend, in part, on preservation of clot-associated plasminogen. We found that when clots are exposed to blood depleted of plasminogen, fibrin-associated plasminogen dissociates from the clots, thereby rendering them less susceptible to lyse despite exposure to a plasminogen activator.[69, 70] Plasminogen depletion from blood invariably occurs with first-generation agents. Its consequence, termed *plasminogen steal,* may account for the decreased efficacy of second- compared with first-generation fibrinolytic agents. The dependence of "lysability" of both venous and arterial thrombi on the plasminogen content in the clots has been confirmed by others,[71] as has the recruitment of plasminogen into clots from surrounding plasma (the obverse of plasminogen steal).[128] Furthermore, the preponderant mechanism responsible for dissolution of thrombi at pharmacologic concentrations of t-PA has been shown to be activation of plasminogen within the thrombus rather than of plasminogen in plasma.[129]

Compared with older clots, fresh clots lyse more rapidly with any given concentration of t-PA.[130] t-PA appears to retain activity against somewhat older clots in vivo, compared with SK, which becomes relatively ineffectual.[60–62] Factors involved in the increased susceptibility to lysis of fresh clots include the delayed incorporation of lysine-binding sites in relatively slowly formed fibrin cross-links compared with their consequently later diminished availability for binding of plasminogen. Clot retraction, potentiated by platelets, also contributes by diminishing access of fibrinolytic proteins to clot-bound plasminogen.[131] These considerations have practical implications. Optimal efficacy can be anticipated when coronary thrombolysis is initiated as early as possible after clot formation, not only because salvage of myocardium is dependent on the brevity of ischemia but also because the nascent clots are particularly susceptible to lysis. Front-loaded regimens of clot-selective agents provide a high concentration gradient for penetration of the plasminogen activator into thrombi. They are effective in part because the clot-associated activator continues to act long after clearance from the circulation is complete. Abbreviation of the total duration of infusion minimizes the induction of a lytic state, thereby presumably enhancing safety. Furthermore, initially higher concentrations of the plasminogen activator increase relative as well as absolute binding to fibrin. The preservation of plasminogen in the circulation that they afford may augment efficacy by diminishing the likelihood or the intensity of plasminogen steal.[117, 129]

Additional factors contributing to the superiority of clot-

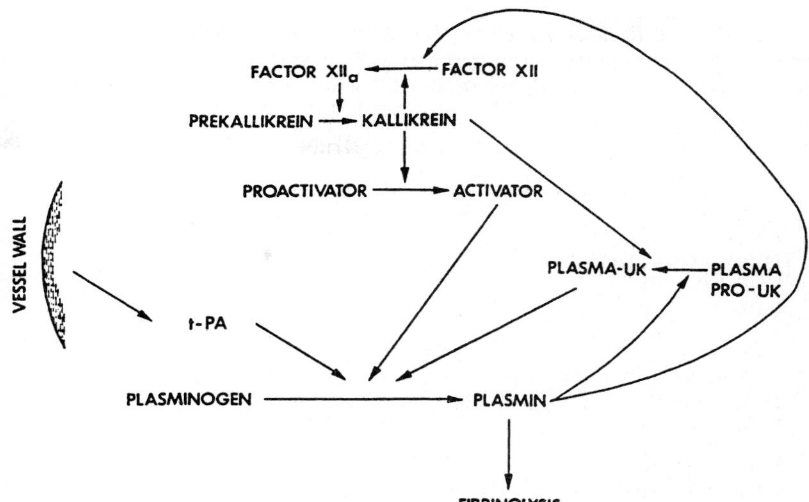

FIGURE 36–2 The plasminogen activating systems of blood and their interrelation. For details, see text. PRO-UK, prourokinase; t-PA, tissue-type plasminogen activator; UK, urokinase. (From Munkvad S, Jespersen J, Gram J, Kluft C: Long-lasting depression of the factor XII–dependent fibrinolytic system in patients with myocardial infarction undergoing thrombolytic therapy with recombinant tissue-type plasminogen activator: a randomized placebo-controlled study. J Am Coll Cardiol 17:957, 1991; with permission from The American College of Cardiology.)

selective compared with nonselective agents in inducing early patency appear to include their lack of a procoagulant effect and lack of degradation of clot-associated lysine binding sites on fibrin that facilitate targeting of plasminogen and endogenous as well as exogenous t-PA to the clot surface and its interstices. Thus, intravenous use of non–clot-selective agents results in plasminemia, which activates the coagulation system at multiple levels, including clearance of coagulation factors II, V, VII, and X to form IIa, Va, VIIa, and Xa.[132, 133] Particularly important is plasmin activation of factor XII to form XIIa, thereby initiating activation of the intrinsic limb of the coagulation cascade, normally quiescent in vivo yet activated ex vivo by contrast of blood with glass[133, 134] (Fig. 36–2). The result is not only a procoagulant effect, but also activation of the kallikrein and kinin systems. The capricious nature of plasmin's proteolytic effects gives rise to complement activation as well,[57, 135] potentially exacerbating myocardial injury.

Not only do first-generation drugs exert counterintuitive procoagulant effects despite lysing thrombi—effects that retard lysis and predispose to thrombotic reocclusion. They also inhibit (sic) fibrinolysis after its initial burst because of the elaboration of a protein called TAFI (thrombin-activated fibrinolytic inhibitor) and shown to be a plasmin activated procarboxypeptidase, resulting in carboxypeptidase N activity in blood.[136] The active carboxypeptidase cleaves lysine residues from fibrin and fibrin degradation products within and on clots, thereby paradoxically decreasing binding of plasminogen and endogenous and exogenous t-PA to fibrin and attenuating clot lysis.

In concert, plasminogen steal, procoagulant effects, and activation of procarboxypeptidase N appear to account for the slower rate and the lower incidence of induction of recanalization after administration of non–clot-selective compared with clot-selective fibrinolytic agents. In addition, in the case of SK and APSAC, platelet activation secondary to SK–anti-SK antibody interactions may potentiate thrombin generation markedly,[137–139] exacerbating procoagulation and further attenuating efficacy.

Conjunctive Therapy

Although desirable, initially rapid recanalization[32–35, 105] can be compromised by early thrombotic reocclusion,[112, 113] known to portend increased mortality. Ongoing thrombosis can limit the rapidity of recanalization as well.[31, 52, 91, 140, 141] Facilitation of optimal thrombolysis by attenuation of the adverse impact of occult, ongoing thrombosis is the objective of conjunctive therapy.[31, 52, 141, 142] In contrast to adjunctive therapy, which is designed to attenuate irreversible myocardial injury secondary to ischemia or reperfusion by diminishing myocardial oxygen requirements or inhibiting deleterious effects of noxious metabolites, among other mechanisms, conjunctive therapy is designed to accelerate recanalization, sustain recanalization, or both.

The importance of conjunctive therapy is supported by numerous observations. More than 90 percent of coronary thrombi occur on atherosclerotic plaques undergoing rupture.[143] Early reocclusion of an initially recanalized infarct-related artery is associated with substantial morbidity and mortality.[144] Fibrinolytic agents themselves activate the coagulation system by plasmin-mediated conversion of prothrombin to thrombin,[140] activation of factor X,[145] and consequent augmentation of thrombin activity.[146–149] Regardless of which of the plasminogen activators is used, generation of thrombin can limit efficacy.[150, 151] Thrombin generation persists despite inhibition of thrombin activity,[152, 153] giving rise to a rebound predisposition to thrombosis after cessation of anticoagulation,[153] or persistent thrombin activity despite the presence of antithrombin drugs in the circulation,[154, 155] both of which can exacerbate ischemia. Inhibition of their procoagulant effects, not only with heparin but also with direct-acting antithrombins and antiplatelet drugs, favors successful recanalization.[92, 147, 156, 157]

Results of clinical trials underscore the importance of attenuation of occult, concomitant thrombosis (Table 36–3). In studies of diverse fibrinolytic agents given to more than 40,000 patients, the use of intravenously administered heparin has been associated with substantial reduction of early mortality (Table 36–4). Reocclusion, attributable generally to thrombosis, is associated with as much as a 25 percent increase in mortality.[113] Fortunately, the incidence of reocclusion 24 hours or more after coronary thrombolysis can be diminished by the use of intravenous heparin (Table 36–5).

In addition to the generally used, readily titratable antithrombin agent with a rapid onset of action, heparin, other

TABLE 36–3 **Early Mortality in Trials With Thrombolytic Drugs Preceding GISSI-2 and the t-PA/SK International Trial**

	Placebo Group		First-Generation Drugs		Second-Generation Drugs	
Trial	***n***	***% mortality* (n)**	***n***	***% mortality* (n)**	***n***	***% mortality* (n)**
AIMS	502	12.2 (62)	502 (APSAC)	6.4 (32)		
GAUS			121 (UK)	4.1 (5)	124 (t-PA)	4.8 (6)
ISAM	463	7.1 (33)	477 (SK)	6.3 (30)		
PAIMS			85 (SK)	8.2 (7)	86 (t-PA)	4.7 (4)
PRIMI			203 (SK)	4.9 (10)	198 (scu-PA)	3.5 (7)
TIMI-I			147 (SK)	8.2 (12)	143 (t-PA)	4.9 (7)
TICO (Sydney/ Auckland)	71	5.6 (4)			74 (t-PA)	5.4 (4)
ECSG (1979)	106	30.6 (32)	125 (SK)	15.6 (20)		
ECSG-I (1985)			65 (SK)	4.6 (3)	64 (t-PA)	4.7 (3)
ECSG-II (1985)	65	6.2 (4)			64 (t-PA)	1.6 (1)
ECSG-III (1987)					123 (t-PA)	4.9 (6)
ECSG-IV (1988)					184 (t-PA)	3.0 (6)
					183 (t-PA + 2 h PTCA)	7.0 (13)
ECSG-V (1988)	366	5.7 (21)			355 (t-PA)	2.8 (18)
GISSI-1*	5852	13.0 (761)	5860 (SK)	10.7 (627)		
New Zealand I	93	12.9 (12)	79 (SK)	2.5 (2)		
New Zealand II			135 (SK)	7.4 (10)	135 (t-PA)	3.7 (5)
ISIS-2*†	8595	12.0 (1031)	8592 (SK)	9.2 (790)		
HART					106 (t-PA)	2.0 (2)
HART*					99 (t-PA)	3.0 (3)
SCATI			218 (SK + IV followed by SC heparin)	4.5 (10)		
			215 (SK w/o SC heparin)	8.8 (19)		
ASSET	2495	9.8 (245)			2516 (t-PA)	7.9 (181)
NHF Australia	71	2.8 (2)			73 (t-PA)	9.6 (7)
TIMI-II pilot					317 (t-PA)	4.4 (14)
TIMI-11a					195 (t-PA + 2 h PTCA)	5.2 (11)
					200 (t-PA + 24 h PTCA)	7.4 (15)
TIMI-IIb					3262 (t-PA)	4.9 (160)
Total	18,679	11.8 (2204)	16,824	9.4 (1577)	8501	5.6 (476)

Abbreviations: AIMS, APSAC (anisoylated plasminogen streptokinase activator complex) Intervention Mortality Study; ASSET, Anglo-Scandinavian Study of Early Thrombolysis; NHF, National Heart Foundation; ECSG, European Cooperative Study Group; GAUS, German Activator Urokinase Study; GISSI, Gruppo Italiano per lo Studio della Streptochinasi nell'Infarto Miocardio; HART, Heparin-Aspirin Reperfusion Trial; ISAM, Intravenous Streptokinase in Acute Myocardial Infarction; ISIS, Second International Study of Infarct Survival; PAIMS, Plasminogen Activator Italian Multicenter Study; PRIMI, Prourokinase in Myocardial Infarction Study; SCATI, Studio nella Calciparini nell'Angina nella Trombosi Ventriculaaire nell'Infarto; scu-PA, single chain urokinase plasminogen activator; SK, streptokinase; TICO, Thrombolysis in Acute Coronary Occlusion; t-PA, tissue-type plasminogen activator; UK, urokinase.

*Intravenous heparin was not included in the protocol.

†Intention to treat with intravenous heparin in a minority of treated patients.

From Tiefenbrunn AJ, Sobel BE: Thrombolysis and myocardial infarction. Fibrinolysis 5:1, 1991.

TABLE 36–4 **Coronary Patency in Patients Treated With t-PA (Alteplase) or scu-PA (Saruplase) With or Without Conjunctive Intravenous Heparin**

		Time of Angiography After Treatment (h)		Patency of the Infarct-Related Artery		
Study	**n**	***Mean***	***Range***	***With Heparin***	***Without Heparin***	**Drug**
HART	205	18	(7–24)	82% (−ASA)*	48% (+ASA)*	Alteplase
Bleich et al	83	57	(48–72)	71% (−ASA)*	44% (−ASA)*	Alteplase
ECSG-VI	609	81	(48–120)	84% (+ASA)*	75% (+ASA)*	Alteplase
Tebbe	118	8	(6–12)	81%	60%	Saruplase

Abbreviations: ASA, aspirin; ECSG, European Cooperative Study Group; HART, Heparin-Aspirin Reperfusion Trial.

*ASA refers to the use (+) or lack (−) of protocol-mandated aspirin.

From Sobel BE: Thrombolysis in the treatment of acute myocardial infarction. *In* Fuster V, Verstiaete M (eds): Thrombosis in Cardiovascular Diseases. p. 289. Philadelphia: WB Saunders, 1992.

TABLE 36–5 **Early Mortality (≤42 da) in Trials of Intravenous Thrombolytic Drugs Without Heparin**

Trial	Placebo Group		Treatment Group	
	n	*% Mortality* (n)	*n*	*% Mortality* (n)
GISSI-1				
Time to treatment				
≤12 h	5852	13.0 (761)	5860	10.7 (627)
≤1 h	642	15.4 (99)	635	8.2 (52)
≤3 h	3078	12.0 (369)	3016	9.2 (277)
3–6 h	1800	14.1 (254)	1849	11.7 (216)
6–9 h	659	14.1 (93)	693	12.6 (87)
GISSI-2/Intl t-PA/SK		N/A	10,364(t-PA)	8.9 (922)
			10,385 (SK)	8.5 (883)
ISIS-2	4300	13.2 (568)	1463(SK + ASA)	9.6 (140)
HART		N/A	99	3.0 (3)
SCATI		N/A	217	8.8 (19)
Total	16,331	13.1 (2,144)	34,581	9.3 (3226)

Abbreviations: ASA, aspirin; GISSI, Gruppo Italiano per lo Studio della Streptochinasi nell'Infarto Miocardico; HART, Heparin or Aspirin Reocclusion Trial; ISIS, International Study of Infarct Survival; SCATI, Studio sulla Calciparini nell'Angina nella Trombosi Ventriculare nell'Infarto; SK, streptokinase; t-PA, tissue-type plasminogen activator.

From Tiefenbrunn AJ, Sobel BE: Thrombolysis and myocardial infarction. Fibrinolysis 5:1, 1991.

conjunctive agents, including direct-acting antithrombins and antiplatelet agents, are being investigated vigorously.[88–90, 158–163] Low-molecular-weight heparin, which has superior bioavailability to that of unfractionated heparin,[89] is already commercially available worldwide. It appears to have several desirable properties (Fig. 36–3). Results in studies in experimental animals[164] and in patients[52, 148, 165–167] attest to the utility of heparin and diverse other agents (see Table 36–3). In general, the dosage of heparin is an intravenous bolus (5000 to 10,000 U) followed by a steady state infusion of 1000 to 1500 U/h.[48] The loading dose is required to saturate endothelial cell binding sites. Sustained infusion subsequently can maintain therapeutically effective concentrations of heparin in the circulation. Nevertheless, heparin is only moderately effective as a conjunctive agent because of incomplete saturation of endothelial cell binding sites with consequent subtherapeutic blood levels being attained, because of the relative inaccessibility of fibrin-bound thrombin to the heparin–antithrombin III complex and because of its failure to inhibit thrombin generated locally or released from clots undergoing lysis.[52] The duration of infusion of heparin required has been difficult to define. Results in studies of relatively small numbers of patients suggested that discontinuation after 24 hours is not necessarily deleterious. However, because of the slow resolution of thrombogenic vascular lesions underlying index infarctions, administration of intravenous heparin is generally continued for 48 to 72 hours or more.[168, 169]

As judged from results of diverse studies demonstrating enhanced patency with conjunctive heparin,[170] dosage should be sufficient to maintain the activated partial thromboplastin time at 1.5 to 2.0 times control values. Unfortunately, however, titration of dose based on this or analogous criteria (e.g., prolongation of the activated clotting time) may not obviate ongoing thrombosis evident with serial measurements of fibrinopeptide A.

Some investigators have championed the use of "conjunctive" agents, particularly megadoses of heparin (50,000 U [sic] as an IV bolus) as the sole treatment of thrombotic coronary occlusion,[171, 172] or of "low"-dose t-PA plus an antiplatelet agent.[92] Such an approach is predicated on the concept that endogenous fibrinolysis is sufficient to induce recanalization if coagulation is blocked completely. Although not established as a therapeutic alternative, the efficacy of megadose heparin underscores the essentiality of conjunctive treatment targeting coagulation and activated platelets,[173, 174] when fibrinolytic drugs are used. Alternative antithrombin agents are potentially attractive because, in contrast to heparin, they can inhibit thrombin associated with fibrin and fibrinogen degradation products independent of antithrombin III. Hirudin and its congeners, hirulog and hirugen[51, 175]; low-molecular-weight heparin[175]; argatroban; other serine protease inhibitors[175]; and antiplatelet agents[137, 138, 173, 176–178] are among them.

The potential value of antiplatelet agents is underscored by consideration of first principles, namely, the fact that activation of platelets augments thrombin generation by several orders of magnitude because of the pivotal role of the platelet surface in the assembly of the coagulation factor Xase and prothrombinase complexes.[137, 138] Concomitant use with plasminogen activators of antithrombin III to potentiate the action of heparin in subjects with antithrombin III deficiency, modulation of the protein C system,[175] and inhibition of generation of thrombin by inhibition of the extrinsic coagulation pathway with extrinsic pathway inhibitor[179] and of the common pathway with a factor Xa inhibitor, such as tick anticoagulation protein,[180] are being explored.

Inhibition of activation of platelets by thrombin generated by paradoxical activation of the coagulation system by plasmin[151–155, 181] increases as a result of the use of thrombolytic drugs.[181, 181a] It constitutes an important target for conjunctive therapy. Aspirin (60 to 300 mg daily) has proved to be helpful. However, platelets can be activated through diverse pathways, only some of which involve the cyclooxygenase inhibited by aspirin. Accordingly, effects of prostacyclin analogues,[182] thromboxane synthetase inhibitors and receptor antagonists,[183–186] inhibitors of platelet-activating factor,[187] inhibitors of the fibrinogen-binding adhesive platelet surface glycoprotein GP IIb/IIIa with

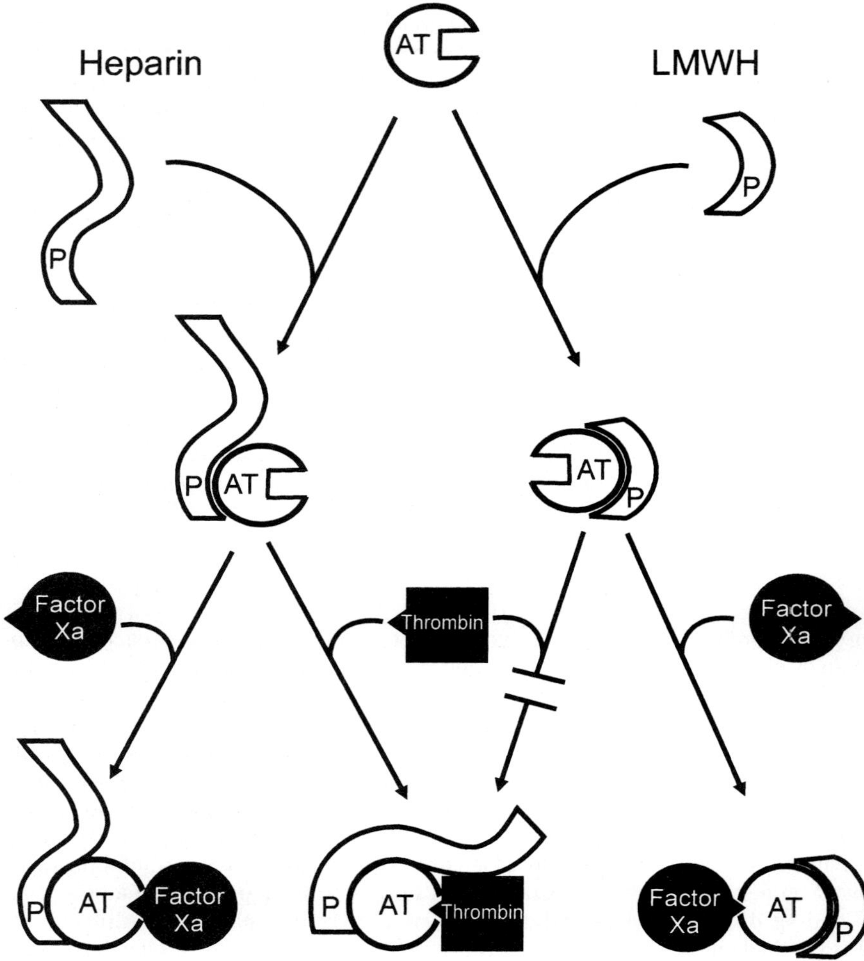

FIGURE 36–3 Mechanism of action of unfractionated heparin and low molecular weight heparin (LMWH). The interaction of unfractionated heparin and LMWH and antithrombin (AT) is mediated by their common pentasaccharide sequence (P). The heparin-antithrombin interaction produces conformational changes in antithrombin, accelerating its ability to inactivate thrombin and factor Xa. Because heparin catalysis of factor Xa inhibition by antithrombin does not require bridging between factor Xa and antithrombin, both unfractionated heparin and LMWH catalyse factor Xa inactivation by antithrombin. LMWH has less inhibitory activity against thrombin than against factor Xa, because only a small proportion of the LMWH chains are long enough to bridge antithrombin to thrombin. (From Bates SM, Weitz JI: The new heparins. Coron Artery Dis 9[2–3]:65–74, 1998.)

monoclonal antibodies, and small peptide mimics are being evaluated in strategies designed to optimize the benefit of thrombolysis by preventing early thrombotic reocclusion (Table 36–6). Such conjunctive measures may also be of benefit in diminishing the incidence of left ventricular (LV) thrombi.[187, 188]

Administration of t-PA with Conjunctive and Adjunctive Agents

Dose regimens for t-PA have varied from bolus intravenous injections of 1 mg/kg to infusions of 6-hour duration. Prolongation of persistence of t-PA in the circulation has been accomplished by concomitant administration of agents that interfere with mechanisms underlying its clearance in experimental animals[189] as well as by developing mutants with diminished clearance.[19–22, 50] The "front-loaded" regimens for t-PA have gained favor as a result of elucidation of principles underlying diverse dose regimens, use of conjunctive and adjunctive agents, and safety that have been reviewed extensively.[190] Front-loaded or "accelerated" regimens induce patency within 90 minutes in as many as 90 percent of patients. Risks of bleeding appear to be even less than those seen with conventional regimens. For example, the incidence of hemorrhagic stroke is approximately 0.4 to 0.7 percent, not markedly dissimilar from that in patients treated with anticoagulants alone. Most clinicians now use a 15 mg IV bolus of t-PA over 1 to 2 minutes, followed by 50 mg over the first 30 minutes and an additional 35 mg over the next 60 minutes. Thus, the total dose is 100 mg. Modifications have included weight-adjusted dosing with the initial bolus followed by 0.75 mg/kg over 30 minutes (not to exceed 50 mg) and 0.5 mg/kg over the next 60 minutes (not to exceed 35 mg).

In general, t-PA is given with intravenous heparin. Conventionally, a 5000-U intravenous bolus is administered (to saturate heparin-binding sites found ubiquitously on the surface of endothelial cells), followed by a steady state infusion of 1000 U/h. Variations include a higher bolus dose (10,000 U) and steady state infusions as high as 1500 U/h. Although some have titrated dosing in terms of activated partial thromboplastin time values, titration is not usually necessary. Heparin should be continued for 48 to 72 hours, even though results in formal studies have not conclusively demonstrated advantages beyond 24 hours, perhaps because of limited statistical power. Several alternative agents, including direct-acting antithrombins, have been studied as conjunctive agents. Unfortunately, when large trials have been initiated without detailed mechanistic information characterizing the nature and the extent of their interactions with lytic agents and elucidation of bleeding

TABLE 36-6 Adjunctive and Conjunctive Agents Under Investigation

Conjunctive Agents

Platelet Antagonists

- Thromboxane A_2 inhibitors
  - Cyclooxygenase inhibitor (aspirin)
  - Thromboxane A_2 receptor inhibitor
- Serotonin receptor inhibitor
- Eicosanoids (prostacyclin and prostaglandin E_1)
- Glycoprotein IIb/IIIa receptor blockers
  - Murine monoclonal antibody
  - Disintegrins
    - Synthetic arginine-glycine-aspartate peptides
    - Snake venom peptides
- Anti–von Willebrand factor, antiglycoprotein Ib–IX
- Ticlopidine and clopidogrel
- Eicosapentanoic acid
- Combined fibrinolytic drugs to augment fibrin degradation products

Thrombin Inhibitors

- Antithrombin III dependent (indirect)
  - Heparin
  - Heparin fragments
- Antithrombin III independent (direct)
  - Hirudin
  - Synthetic hirudin analogues (hirugen, hirulog, hirullin)
  - Arginine analogues (argatroban)
  - D-phenylalanyl-L-prolol-L-arginyl choloromethyl-ketone

Other Anticoagulants

- Activated protein C, thrombomodulin-like peptides, lipoprotein-associated coagulation factor
- Fibrinogen depletors (batroxibin, ancrod)
- Plasminogen activator inhibitor type 1 antagonists
- Factor Xa inhibitor (tick anticoagulant peptide)
- Factor XIII inhibitors

Adjunctive Agents

- β-Blockers
- Angiotensin-converting enzyme inhibitors
- Calcium channel blockers
- Oxygen free radical scavengers
  - Superoxide dismutase
  - Dimethylthiourea
  - Deferoxamine
  - Mercaptopropionyl
  - *N*-acetylcysteine

Neutrophil Inhibitors

- Adenosine
- Ibuprofen
- Perfluorochemicals
- Prostacyclin
- Leukocyte surface protein antibody

From Popma JJ, Topol EJ: Adjuncts to thrombolysis for myocardial reperfusion. Ann Intern Med 115:84, 1991.

risk, untoward complications, including ICBs, have been encountered.[158–163, 191] Nevertheless, direct-acting antithrombins and antiplatelet agents are likely to enhance results when dosages have been defined adequately.[88–90, 92, 156, 157, 191] Although such agents have been studied already in patients with acute MI or unstable angina and in those undergoing percutaneous coronary interventions, their use in combination with lytic drugs is just beginning to be explored thoroughly.

An additional conjunctive agent is aspirin. It is administered with an initial dose of 160 to 324 mg PO (chewable aspirin is preferred), followed by 81 to 324 mg PO daily.

As discussed later in the section on safety, use of conjunctive agents entails the risk of augmenting the incidence of bleeding, including that of intracranial hemorrhage.[191] Thus, mechanistic studies are required to rigorously define effects of combinations of agents that affect the fibrinolytic, coagulation, and platelet-dependent hemostatic systems in diverse fashions under diverse conditions.[191–193] Otherwise, untoward effects that may be avoidable with optimal dosing of all constituents of a regimen may be encountered.[158–163]

Clinicians should not neglect adjunctive measures designed to protect jeopardized, ischemic myocardium, including β-blockers (particularly in patients with demonstrable augmentation of sympathoadrenal tone manifested by an inappropriately high heart rate or frank tachycardia, diaphoresis, or transitory systolic hypertension). Atenolol (5 mg IV repeated once if well tolerated, followed by 50 mg PO daily) and metoprolol (5 mg IV repeated twice if well tolerated, followed by 50 mg PO twice daily) are used commonly. Vasodilators, such as nitroglycerin at an IV dose of 5 to 100 μg/min, titrated to lower systolic blood pressure modestly without inducing reflex tachycardia, are helpful. Thus, even though the use of nitroglycerin may modestly attenuate the intensity of thrombolysis, perhaps by increasing hepatic perfusion and clearance of the administered plasminogen activator,[194] the predominant effect appears to be favorable amelioration of myocardial ischemia during the evolution of thrombolysis. Support of the circulation with intra-aortic balloon counterpulsation or a left ventricular assist device is not contraindicated in patients who are being treated with thrombolytic agents and anticoagulants, even though some additional risk of bleeding may be encountered.

Studies with t-PA

Most clinical studies of fibrin-selective agents have been performed with t-PA. Because of the concrete nature of survival figures, mortality has been a primary end point. This has led to the use of the term *surrogate for mortality* for end points such as recanalization, early infarct-related artery patency, restoration of regional wall motion, reduction of infarct size, and other direct consequences of coronary thrombolysis that appear to underlie improved survival. In fact, such terminology is spurious. Mechanistically, the immediate objective of coronary thrombolysis is recanalization of thrombotically occluded coronary arteries. Beneficial effects on the heart and on the patient follow prompt and sustained recanalization.[195] Thus, results of mechanistic studies that delineate physiologic and biologic efficacy are particularly powerful in comparative assessments of diverse agents and approaches.

Care must be taken to avoid confusion between primary and secondary end points. For example, the paradoxical, inverse relationship between LV function and survival in groups of patients treated with thrombolytic agents compared with placebo has been explained by the observation that many treated patients who survived because they were given thrombolytic drugs are those with the most greatly impaired ventricular function. Accordingly, in group data, preservation of ventricular function has been related inversely to mortality, as shown by Van de Werf.[196] By the

TABLE 36–7 Ejection Fraction 3 Weeks After Myocardial Infarction

	n	Ejection Fraction SK or UK	t-PA
Studies Comparing Thrombolytic Agents			
White	270	58 ± 12	58 ± 12
PAIMS	171	53 ± 10	55 ± 11
GAUS	246	52 ± 14	53 ± 12
Thrombolysis With or Without Coronary Angioplasty		+PTCA	−PTCA
TAMI-1	386	53	56
ECSG	367	49	49
TIMI-IIa	389	50	49
TIMI-IIb	3262	50	50.4*
SWIFT	800	51.7 ± 15	50.7 ± 15
Adjunctive Agents		Treatment	Placebo
Captopril	38	52.4 ± 11.5	48.9 ± 13.8
Superoxide dismutase	120	52.4 ± 13.7	55.6 ± 12.6
Prostacyclin	50	48.0 ± 9.4	50.4 ± 9.8†
β-Blockers	1390	50.5	50
Nifedipine	149	54.0 ± 11	56.0 ± 15

Abbreviations: ECSG, European Cooperative Study Group; GAUS, German Activator Urokinase Study; PAIMS, Plasminogen Activator Italian Multicenter Study; PTCA (with) (without) percutaneous transluminal coronary artery angioplasty; SK, streptokinase; SWIFT, Should We Intervene Following Thrombolysis?; TAMI, Thrombolysis and Angioplasty in Myocardial Infarction; TIMI, Thrombolysis in Myocardial Infarction; t-PA, tissue-type plasminogen activator; UK, urokinase.

*By gated blood pool scintigraphy.

†Not randomized.

From Califf RM, Hamelson-Woodlief L, Topol EJ: Left ventricular ejection fraction may not be useful as an end point of thrombolytic therapy comparative trials. Circulation 82:1847, 1990. By permission of the American Heart Association, Inc.

same token, improved regional wall motion associated with prompt recanalization, as evident in sequential imaging procedures, is not usually accompanied by a comparable improvement in overall ejection fraction, in part because of the diminution of early compensatory hyperfunction in normally perfused zones. This contributes to the lack of observed differences in global ventricular function in treated compared with control groups, as pointed out by Califf and coworkers[196a] (Table 36–7). Interpretation of results of recanalization and patency studies is more straightforward.

In contrast to second-generation agents, with which recanalization occurs less frequently after intravenous administration than after intracoronary administration,[197] t-PA induces early recanalization with comparable frequency when given by either route.[198] Furthermore, as judged from results of the TIMI-1 (recanalization) and European Cooperative Study Group (patency) trials, t-PA induces recanalization within 90 minutes in 70 to 81 percent of patients, regardless of the interval between apparent onset of infarction and time to treatment (within the 6-hour window used) (Table 36–8). Results in patency trials (angiograms were obtained 60 to 190 minutes after initiation of treatment) are consistent with these observations (see Table 36–1). The incidence of prompt recanalization with scu-PA may be somewhat less than that with t-PA, perhaps because of its rapid conversion by plasmin in vivo to uPA and its consequent lack of clot selectivity.[17, 18, 199]

Infarct Size and Left Ventricular Function

A major impetus in the clinical development of coronary thrombolysis was the demonstrable reduction of infarct size by early reperfusion in experimental animals.[80, 108] In patients treated with t-PA, infarct size is reduced, as judged from serial changes in creatine kinase-MB.[200] Sequential assessments of regional wall motion by ventriculography, radioventriculography, and other modalities demonstrate improvement after administration of t-PA[35, 201–207] (reviewed by Fry and Sobel[51]). The benefit is greatest in patients who can be treated early and in whom recanalization is induced promptly. Beneficial effects persist and presage improved survival.[86, 208] In the absence of early treatment, differences between clot-selective and non–clot-selective drugs with respect to preservation of LV function may be obviated,[209] despite the superiority of clot-selective drugs, such as t-PA, compared with non–clot-selective agents, such as SK, in inducing patency earlier and more often.[57, 68]

Survival and Its Dependence on Recanalization

Early mortality in patients treated with second-generation fibrinolytic drugs is low (see Table 36–5). In comparison

TABLE 36–8 Relative Efficacy of rt-PA and Streptokinase for Coronary Thrombolysis in Patients With Acute Myocardial Infarction in Randomized Trials

Time From Onset of Symptoms to Therapy (h)	Study	rt-PA (n, %)	Streptokinase (n, %)	*P* Value
<3	ECSG	23 of 29 (79)	20 of 35 (57)	.06
	TIMI	11 of 13 (85)	11 of 21 (52)	.06
	Combined	34 of 42 (81)	31 of 56 (55)	<.01
3–6	ECSG	20 of 32 (62)	14 of 26 (54)	.51
	TIMI	89 of 130 (69)	50 of 125 (40)	<.001
	Combined	109 of 162 (67)	64 of 151 (42)	<.001
Overall	Combined	143 of 204 (70)	95 of 207 (46)	<.001

Abbreviations: ECSG, European Cooperative Study Group; rt-PA, recombinant tissue-type plasminogen activator; TIMI, Thrombolysis in Myocardial Infarction.

Data from Chesebro J, Knatterud G, Braunwald E: Thrombolytic therapy [letter]. N Engl J Med 319:1543, 1988.

From Collen, D: Coronary thrombolysis: streptokinase or recombinant tissue-type plasminogen activator? Ann Intern Med 112:529, 1990.

with an overall early mortality of 9.4 percent in studies completed in 1989 of first-generation drugs, mortality with second-generation drugs averaged 5.6 percent. The difference may be attributable not only to intrinsic differences in fibrinolytic agents but also to other determinants of early mortality, including the efficacy of prevention of reocclusion with conjunctive anticoagulants, differences in ages of patients studied in different trials, and differences in the time to treatment after the onset of the index infarcts. Nevertheless, before the publication of the ISIS-3 results, pooled data from several small randomized trials in which first- and second-generation drugs were administered had demonstrated a remarkably low early mortality with second-generation agents (Table 36–9), in keeping with their efficacy in inducing early recanalization. By contrast, the GISSI-2 and ISIS-3 studies failed to demonstrate differences in mortality between clot-selective and non–clot-selective agents.[116] Two factors may account for this: (1) lack of use of protocol-mandated intravenous heparin and (2) late time to treatment.[97, 98] The overall early mortality in both trials was high (e.g., 10.4 percent in ISIS-3), compatible with this interpretation.

Beneficial effects of thrombolytic agents usually have been sustained. In the landmark GISSI-1 study of SK compared with placebo, the reduction in mortality in patients treated early was sustained for years.[210] Sustained improvement of ventricular function has been demonstrated as well in studies performed by the Interuniversity Cardiology Institute of the Netherlands.[211] Long-term favorable effects on ventricular function[212] and electrophysiologic stability[213] have been demonstrated after administration of t-PA. Long-term benefits appear to depend on recanalization per se, as judged from the persistence of beneficial effects on LV function after coronary thrombolysis induced by SK given early after the onset of symptoms of acute infarction[214] and the high survival in high-risk subgroups (defined by age, magnitude of impairment of ventricular function, and extent of CAD) in patients treated successfully with t-PA followed by angioplasty or coronary artery bypass grafting when clinically indicated.[215] Comparisons

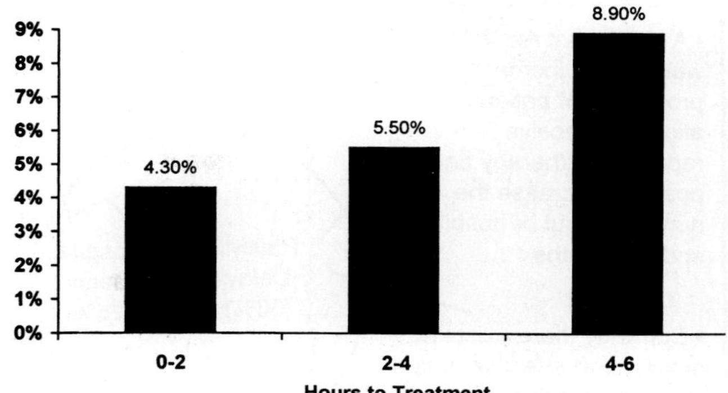

FIGURE 36–4 Mortality rate versus time to treatment in the GUSTO trial. Mortality increased 1%/h in the first 4 hours after symptom onset. (Data from the GUSTO Investigators and Weaver WD: Time to Thrombolytic Treatment: factors affecting delay and their influence on outcome. J Am Coll Cardiol 25 [suppl]:3S, 1995.)

of results among trials are fraught with difficulties, however, because of several confounding variables that can influence outcomes markedly. For example, differences in conjunctive regimens and time to treatment after onset of function, as well as regional differences in mortality,[216] can be confounders. Nevertheless, available information indicates that early and sustained recanalization and particularly avoidance of factors responsible for delay in implementing treatment, improve not only short-term but also long-term prognosis (Figs. 36–4 and 36–5).

TABLE 36–9 In-hospital Mortality in Randomized Studies With rt-PA Versus Streptokinase or Urokinase in Patients With Acute Myocardial Infarction*

Study	rt-PA	Nonfibrin-Specific Agent
ECSG-I	3/64	3/65 (SK)
TIMI-I	12/157	14/159 (SK)
White	5/135	10/135 (SK)
PAIMS	4/86	7/85 (SK)
TAMI-5	8/191	15/190 (UK)
GAUS	6/124	5/121 (UK)
TAPS	5/218	17/217 (APSAC)
Total	43/975 (4.4%)	71/972 (7.3%)

Abbreviations: ECSG, European Cooperative Study Group; GAUS, German Activator Urokinase Study; PAIMS, Plasminogen Activator Italian Multicenter Study; TAMI, Thrombolysis and Angioplasty in Myocardial Infarction; TAPS, rt-PA–APSAC Patency Study; TIMI, Thrombolysis in Myocardial Infarction.

*Heterogeneity index: χ^2 4.76; P = 0.57; odds ratio: 0.59 = 95% CI; 0.41–0.87). P value of the difference = 0.0067. For citations see Tiefenbrunn and Sobel.[86]

From Collen D, Linen HR: Basic and clinical aspects of fibrinolysis and thrombolysis. Blood 78:3114, 1991.

Safety of Clot-Selective Agents

The development of clot-selective drugs was stimulated by the expectation that avoidance of induction of a systemic lytic state would enhance patient safety. Early studies with t-PA demonstrated that the intravenous administration of the drug could elicit recanalization promptly, often without marked depletion of circulating fibrinogen or elevation of levels of circulating FDPs.[64, 217, 218] Bleeding was less common than that seen with first-generation drugs,[64] a phenomenon confirmed repeatedly in comparative trials.[93–95] Transfusion requirements have been generally lower as well.[65] One potentially hemorrhagic complication of treatment with any fibrinolytic agent that is catastrophic is cardiac rupture. However, as judged from the incidence of 58 cases of cardiac rupture among 1638 patients from four trials of thrombolytic drugs, early treatment (within 7 hours) actually reduces the incidence of rupture, presumably because early treatment salvages myocardium.[108] In contrast, late treatment (17 hours or more after onset of infarction) appears to increase the risk.[219]

With the use of all thrombolytic drugs, an early hazard phenomenon has been recognized, that is, a greater proportion of deaths occur early, in the first 24 hours, and especially in the first 6 hours,[220] compared with the corresponding fraction of deaths in patients with infarction who are not treated with lytic drugs. Contributing factors include possible reperfusion injury to myocardium with precipitation of congestive heart failure, lethal arrhythmias, cardiogenic shock, ventricular septal or free wall rupture, and

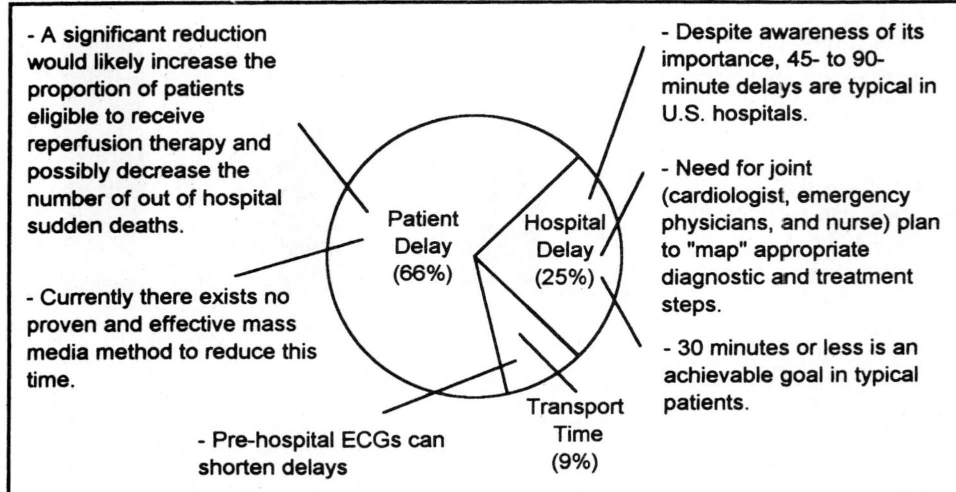
- A significant reduction would likely increase the proportion of patients eligible to receive reperfusion therapy and possibly decrease the number of out of hospital sudden deaths.
- Currently there exists no proven and effective mass media method to reduce this time.
Patient Delay (66%)
Hospital Delay (25%)
Transport Time (9%)
- Pre-hospital ECGs can shorten delays
- Despite awareness of its importance, 45- to 90-minute delays are typical in U.S. hospitals.
- Need for joint (cardiologist, emergency physicians, and nurse) plan to "map" appropriate diagnostic and treatment steps.
- 30 minutes or less is an achievable goal in typical patients.

FIGURE 36–5 Components of delay in management of patients with acute myocardial infarction. Two-thirds of delay is patient related, and 25% is hospital related. The times shown represent the experience in the Myocardial Infarction Triage and Intervention (MITI) acute myocardial infarction registry of 8000 patients in Seattle, Washington. ECGs, electrocardiograms. (From Weaver WD: Time to thrombolytic treatment: factors affecting delay and their influence on outcome. J Am Coll Cardiol 25 [suppl]:3S, 1995; with permission from The American College of Cardiology.)

increased incidence of ICBs.[221] Differences between clot-selective and non–clot-selective agents with respect to the risk of hemorrhagic complications are usually of only modest clinical importance. One exception is, of course, ICBs.

The overall incidence of cerebrovascular accidents (CVAs) (ischemia and hemorrhagic strokes) early after the onset of acute MI is approximately 1 percent, regardless of whether or not a fibrinolytic agent is used.[222] In patients treated with fibrinolytic drugs compared with those managed with anticoagulants alone, the fraction of CVAs attributable to hemorrhage as opposed to ischemia is somewhat higher, but little or no demonstrable increase in mortality can be ascribed to the shift. The incidence of ICBs is greater in elderly patients and in those with antecedent hypertension, but it is difficult to ascertain with certainty, even when surveillance with computed tomographic scanning plus autopsy is complete,[223] because of the similarity of hemorrhagic conversion of ischemic strokes to primary intracranial bleeding. As judged from results in the GISSI-2/International Study Group trial,[91] the incidence of intracranial bleeding is slightly greater when t-PA is used than when SK is used. Thus, the rate of intracranial bleeding was 0.4 percent in patients treated with t-PA, compared with 0.3 percent in those treated with SK. In the ISIS-3 trial,[93] the incidence of ICBs with t-PA was higher, 0.7 percent. However, the t-PA used in that trial was duteplase rather than the clinically used alteplase, and the duteplase was used in amounts (approximately 160 mg for an 80-kg patient) similar to amounts of t-PA shown previously by the TIMI investigators with alteplase (150 mg) to be associated with an increased risk of ICBs. Furthermore, the specific activity of duteplase and of alteplase (activity per milligram) is the same in kinetic, chromogenic substrate assays of fibrinolytic activity. Thus, it is not surprising that the incidence of intracranial bleeding with duteplase encountered in ISIS-3 exceeded that in the three largest trials with alteplase (GISSI-2/International Study Group trial,[94, 95] the TIMI-II trial[217]). In ISIS-3, the incidence of intracranial bleeding with APSAC was equivalent to that seen with t-PA.[93] Thus, it is difficult to implicate clot selectivity as a major determinant of risk of intracranial bleeding.

The adverse experience with duteplase in ISIS-3 differs not only from those in large trials with alteplase (GISSI-2, TIMI-II, and ASSET) but also from experience with alteplase in the treatment of more than 80,000 patients from more than 1300 institutions throughout the United States.[75] The incidence of total stroke in the t-PA–treated patients was approximately one third the incidence of total stroke encountered in the ISIS-3 trial with duteplase. The overall early mortality of t-PA–treated patients was 5.7 percent, approximately one half of that encountered in the ISIS-3 study.[224]

The risk for intracranial bleeding with any fibrinolytic agent is greater in patients of advanced age (especially older than 75 years) and in those with a history of CVA and hypertension,[225] as shown in Table 36–10. However, advanced age is associated with an increased risk of CVA in patients with MI who are not treated with lytic drugs as well. Because the risk of mortality is so much greater in the elderly, this segment of the population may experience the highest absolute benefit from coronary thrombolysis.[34, 93, 95, 226] Advanced age and protracted, severe hypertension and their sequelae constitute relative and absolute (previous

TABLE 36–10 TIMI-II: Determinants of Complications

Determinant	ICB Rate
BP_s > 180 mm Hg*	↑ 10-fold
BP_d > 120 mm Hg	↑ 10-fold
History of CVA (more than 6 mo earlier)*	↑ 7-fold
Age	
<50 yr	0.1%
60–75 yr	1.1%

Abbreviations: ASA, aspirin; BP, blood pressure; CVA, cerebrovascular accident; ICB, intracranial bleed; TIMI, Thrombolysis in Myocardial Infarction trial; t-PA tissue-type plasminogen activator.

*Before protocol change entailing decrease of dose of t-PA to 100 mg, initiation of ASA 24 h after thrombolysis, exclusion of any patient with any history of CVA or any BP reading ≥ 180 mm Hg systolic or 120 mm Hg diastolic.

From Gore JM, Sloan M, Price TR, et al: Intracerebral hemorrhage, cerebral infarction, and subdural hematoma after acute myocardial infarction and thrombolytic therapy in the Thrombolysis in Myocardial Infarction Study. Circulation 83:448, 1991. By permission of the American Heart Association, Inc.

CVA) contraindications. However, despite the higher absolute risks associated with the use of fibrinolytic agents in the elderly and the higher risk of mortality associated with infarction itself, the risk:benefit ratio (often estimated in terms of numbers of years of life saved per patient treated) is greatest in the elderly. Therefore, coronary thrombolysis should be employed in patients with ST elevation likely to portend Q wave infarction or new left bundle branch block[227] especially when the time to treatment is brief, the patient is physiologically intact, and the risks are well appreciated, despite advanced age of the patient.[228]

Another factor now known to be associated with an increased risk of intracranial bleeding in patients treated with lytic drugs is unusually lean body mass. Thus, for example, the risk of stroke in the LATE trial was 0.3 percent in patients 60 years or younger and body weight 60 kg or greater. By contrast, it was 3.4 percent in those older than 60 years of age with body weight less than 60 kg.[229] Accordingly, weight-adjusted dosage appears wise, especially for patients with exceptionally low body weight.

Anticipated Developments

In view of the high incidence of rapid recanalization of thrombotically occluded coronary arteries inducible with clot-selective agents and the remarkably low mortality (as low as 1 percent) in patients treated early after the onset of infarction (e.g., in the MITI trial[38]), it may be difficult to objectively demonstrate additional advantages of novel agents under development by judging from mortality alone. Therefore, despite the fact that approximately 200 molecular variants of t-PA have been synthesized and that genes for plasminogen activators from diverse species and organisms have been cloned, clinical validation of putative advantages of increased clot selectivity, altered half-life in the circulation, and decreased interactions with inhibitors may be difficult to acquire. Improved targeting of plasminogen activators to clots by conjugation to fibrin-specific antibody fragments,[230] construction of chimeras (e.g., scu-PA/t-PA[231]), or increasing the affinity of plasminogen activator to a platelet receptor (e.g., the GP IIb/IIIa surface glycoprotein[232]) is appealing, but the clinical advantages of these techniques have yet to be documented. Experience with alternative dose regimens[123, 233]; alternative routes of administration,[234] such as via the coronary sinus; and clot-selective plasminogen activators besides t-PA remains limited, albeit promising.[11, 16, 24, 50]

Both endogenous and pharmacologically induced fibrinolysis with t-PA can be attenuated by locally released naturally occurring inhibitors—particularly plasminogen activator inhibitor type-1. Because plasminogen activator inhibitor type-1 is elaborated in response to thrombin, platelet-associated growth factors,[235] and other products released from clots,[236–240] development of plasminogen activators rendered invisible to naturally occurring inhibitors and conjunctive interventions designed to inhibit the elaboration of inhibitors from endothelium, liver, and other tissues is promising.[65, 241–244]

Perhaps the most important improvements in treatment with fibrin-selective agents will entail the more effective use of conjunctive agents, including hirudin and other direct-acting antithrombins, titratable antiplatelet agents, and particularly anti–GP IIb/IIIa receptor agents and adenosine diphosphate receptor antagonists, including ticlopidine and clopidogrel, and inhibitors of procoagulant proteins. The introduction of such agents into clinical practice will require rigorous documentation of their safety at specific doses in combination with specific fibrinolytic agents.

One now discredited approach championed previously for maintaining patency of vessels initially recanalized with t-PA has involved combinations of first- and second-generation fibrinolytic agents[245–247]; this approach was predicated on the concept that the first-generation agent would elaborate high concentrations of FDPs, known to exert anticoagulant and antiplatelet effects. Unfortunately, the concomitant use of a first-generation fibrinolytic agent may induce plasminogen steal and hence limit the rapidity or the occurrence of early recanalization inducible with the fibrin-selective agent alone. In fact, results from the GUSTO trial[248] are consistent with the view that fibrin-selective agents are superior in terms of initiating early recanalization and conferring net clinical benefit compared with non-selective agents alone or in combination and that they are not associated with an increased incidence of early reocclusion in adequately anticoagulated patients.

In the late 1960s, early mortality associated with acute MI in hospitalized patients was approximately 30 percent. Treatment with t-PA in patients 75 years of age or less without contraindications to fibrinolytic drugs has been associated with early mortality as low as 5 percent.[32] Therefore, as was the case with the advent of coronary care units and immediate availability of defibrillation, which decreased hospital mortality by 50 percent, coronary thrombolysis with clot-selective drugs has contributed substantially to improved survival of hospitalized patients with acute MI.

Unresolved Issues

Prehospital Thrombolysis

Surprisingly, among all the constituents of delay time (the interval between onset of symptoms or signs of MI and initiation of treatment with fibrinolytic drugs), delays within the hospital rank highest.[249] Improvement has been made in recent years, but such delays remain unconscionable because they compromise the overall efficacy of strategies to induce recanalization at a time when myocardium can be salvaged and optimal benefit conferred.[250] An additional, and sometimes more important, delay is that occurring before hospitalization because of failure of recognition of the seriousness of symptoms by the patient or the patient's family, lack of rapid response of the medical surveillance system, or logistic considerations precluding prompt admission to emergency facilities. Such difficulties have led to consideration of the potential value of prehospital coronary thrombolysis.

Several trials, including the EMIP,[257] the MITI,[106] and the Grampian Region Early Anistreplase Trial (GREAT)[252] investigations, examined the potential value of prehospital coronary thrombolysis. Results from all three trials demonstrated the safety of the intervention. Unfortunately, however, the statistical power of each was insufficient to prove benefit. In the EMIP study, a 13 percent decrease in prehospital mortality was associated with the use of APSAC as opposed to placebo, with a reduction in cardiac mortality of 17 percent that was statistically significant. In the MITI study, the effect of treatment with t-PA within 1 hour after the onset of symptoms, regardless of whether the treatment was initiated inside or outside the hospital, was a reduction in mortality to less than 1 percent (as opposed to 10 percent) in patients treated 90 minutes or more after the onset of symptoms. In the GREAT study, early administration of APSAC by general practitioners in Scotland, compared with delay of administration until hospitalization of the patient, was associated with a 50 percent reduction in mortality that was statistically significant.

The results of these trials are consistent with a wealth of data from studies in experimental animals and mechanistic research in patients indicating that the single most powerful determinant of benefit after the onset of treatment with fibrinolytic drugs is the rapidity of initiation and persistence of recanalization.[250] Obviously, facilitation of processes within the hospital is important to reduce "door-to-needle" time as well.[249] The importance of hospitals' monitoring of their performance cannot be overemphasized.[249–254]

Comparison of Pharmacologic Coronary Thrombolysis with Primary Percutaneous Transluminal Coronary Angioplasty with or Without Stenting

Considerable controversy surrounds the questions that arise in comparisons between pharmacologic recanalization and primary angioplasty. Advantages of pharmacologic recanalization include the rapidity with which it can be initiated and its virtually universal applicability. Advantages of primary PTCA include induction of recanalization in a larger fraction of vessels, induction of patency of a greater extent (i.e., higher immediate incidence of TIMI 3 flow), and acquisition of definitive diagnostic information at the time of catheterization. The very understandable gratification experienced by the interventionalist who sees an occluded artery very rapidly become widely patent reinforces enthusiasm for primary angioplasty. Economic considerations, even if subconscious, sometimes play a role.

Regrettably, comparisons between these two modalities are much more difficult to interpret than seems likely at first blush. Based on a priori considerations, it seems irrational to seek to answer a question posed in the format of "which intervention is best?" Obviously, in patients with very-high-grade stenosis, luminal encroaching atherosclerotic plaques, and minimal clot burdens, angioplasty may be the preferred procedure. Conversely, in patients with minimal underlying vascular stenosis or plaque activity, as may be seen in women using oral contraceptive agents, for example, clot lysis would appear to be the preferred modality. Unfortunately, it is often not possible to determine, a priori, which type of lesion predominates in a given patient, although educated clinical guesses can often be helpful.

A second difficulty in developing meaningful comparisons is the presence of confounding variables. In patients who undergo angioplasty, an extensive network of support with highly skilled personnel, monitoring of pulmonary arterial wedge pressure, systemic arterial pressure, oximetry, and rhythm coupled with intra-aortic balloon counterpulsation or left ventricular assist devices are available and are generally implemented intensely. By contrast, patients undergoing coronary thrombolysis, even those in a coronary care unit, although closely monitored with respect to cardiac rhythm and vital signs, do not benefit from comparable minute-by-minute support, which can clearly modify prognosis (Fig. 36–6). Thus, one could argue that no valid comparison of primary angioplasty and pharmacologic thrombolysis has been made and, in fact, that one may never be made.

In view of the potential importance of confounding variables and the considerations mentioned earlier Lange and Hillis[255] approached the problem from a different perspective. They evaluated mortality in patients treated with primary angioplasty in centers with acknowledged expertise and compared it with mortality in patients treated primarily with pharmacologic agents in centers of comparable stature. Perhaps surprisingly, the mortality seen with the two approaches as initial approaches to treatment of acute coronary syndromes in large numbers of patients (well over 20,000) was indistinguishable. If any trend could be commented on, it was one favoring coronary thrombolysis.[255] Although prospective studies, such as the GUSTO IIb trial,[256] demonstrated an advantage in terms of early mortality associated with the use of PTCA, there was no difference in mortality 6 months after the index event in patients treated with t-PA as opposed to primary angioplasty.[256]

It is clear that the incidence of induction of widely patent infarct-related arteries is higher with primary PTCA than with pharmacologic thrombolysis,[257] and it appears that at least in some instances, the increased luminal cross-sectional area is associated with augmentation of myocardial perfusion, as assessed with the use of myocardial contrast echocardiography. However, the relative hypoperfusion seen distal to coronary arteries that exhibited TIMI 2 as opposed to TIMI 3 flow appears to be a result of microvascular injury manifested by edema, platelet plugging, and leukocyte adhesion and aggregation (the so-called no reflow phenomenon).[110, 111] Thus, the superior survival seen with TIMI 3 compared with TIMI 2 flow[73] may be misleading. In fact, the anticipated pretreatment mortality of patients who exhibit TIMI 2 flow after a coronary intervention may be much higher than that anticipated in patients

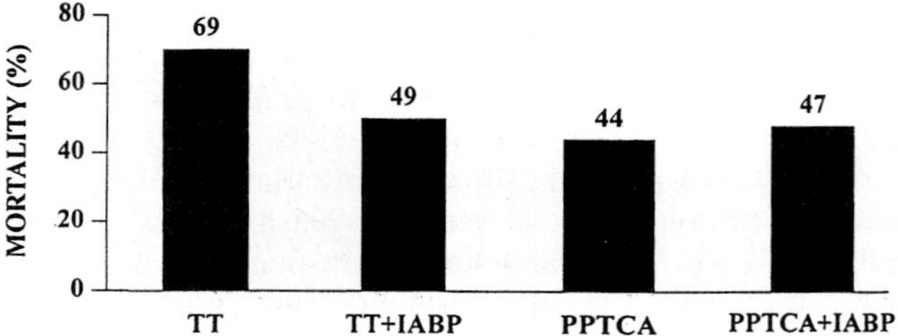

FIGURE 36–6 The use of intra-aortic balloon pump (IABP) in patients with acute myocardial infarction (AMI) complicated by cardiogenic shock is associated with a marked reduction in mortality when used in combination with thrombolytic therapy. However, the use of IABP is not associated with improved survival in patients undergoing PPTCA. (Adapted from Barron HV, Pirzada SR, Lomnitz DJ, et al: Use of intra-aortic balloon counterpulsation in patients with acute myocardial infarction complicated by cardiogenic shock. J Am Coll Cardiol 31 [suppl A]:1999, with permission from The American College of Cardiology.)

who exhibit TIMI 3 flow after treatment because of the nature of the underlying infarct, in turn responsible for the attenuation of flow and the appearance of the TIMI 2 flow after treatment. Accordingly, the argument that angioplasty is a preferred primary therapy because it results in greater dilatation of an infarct-related artery is not convincing.[111]

In one large subset of patients, namely those with insulin-resistance syndromes and particularly type 2 diabetes mellitus, who constitute as many as 50 percent of patients with acute MI under age 55 years, angioplasty has been shown to be accompanied by a remarkably high incidence of late mortality associated with restenosis after procedures performed electively in patients with an initial coronary event.[258] Thus, 5-year mortality after coronary surgery in such patients is almost 50 percent less than 5-year mortality after angioplasty,[259] and mortality with both interventions is twofold and fourfold greater than that seen in nondiabetic patients with comparable angiographically identified coronary artery disease. Thus, although it is well known that patients with type 2 diabetes experience higher mortality than that in nondiabetic subjects after infarction, including non–Q wave infarction[260] and that patients with type 2 diabetes are prone to a hypercoagulable state[261–263] as well as augmentation of thrombin generation associated with increased platelet aggregation,[264] coronary thrombolysis may well be the preferred treatment because of the very negative outcomes experienced after angioplasty with or without stenting[265] in diabetic patients.

In addition to the Lange and Hillis analysis mentioned earlier, the equivalent outcomes with respect to mortality after angioplasty and pharmacologic thrombolysis with t-PA has been recognized in observational studies involving large numbers of patients.[76, 266, 267] Prospective studies have shown similar results.[256, 268] One exception to the general equivalence appears to be in patients in shock. Results of several studies have suggested that primary angioplasty is more effective than thrombolysis in this cohort at very high risk.[76, 266, 269]

Until relatively recently, it was thought that angioplasty initiated after initial treatment with fibrinolytic drugs entailed high risk. In fact, its addition in an obligatory fashion did not increase survival beyond that obtained with pharmacologic thrombolysis but did increase the incidence of complications.[270] It has been demonstrated that rescue angioplasty after failed coronary thrombolysis can be performed safely,[271] with complication rates little different from those encountered with elective angioplasty. Mortality in patients undergoing angioplasty after failed coronary thrombolysis was more favorable than that in patients with failed coronary thrombolysis who did not undergo angioplasty but was less favorable than mortality in patients in whom pharmacologic thrombolysis was successful initially,[271] as shown by results in the GUSTO I angiographic trial, despite the lack of a similar conclusion in a meta-analysis.[272]

Taken together, these observations indicate that the decision to subject a patient to primary angioplasty or to pharmacologic thrombolysis should be based on (1) individual considerations, (2) availability of angiographic and interventional facilities sufficiently promptly so that the disparity between the time of implementation of pharmacologic thrombolysis and the time of implementation of angioplasty can be minimized, and (3) absence of specific characteristics of patients suggesting the utility of one intervention as opposed to the other (e.g., angioplasty for patients in shock and thrombolysis for patients with insulin resistance or type 2 diabetes).

The Plasminogen Activator Compatibility Trial (PACT) was undertaken to explore a novel and attractive hypothesis—namely, that sequential therapy with a relatively brief exposure to a clot-selective fibrinolytic drug followed by rescue angioplasty when indicated might be optimal.[273] The study was based on the concept that the higher patency rates achievable with angioplasty would be desirable, particularly in the context of selecting those patients who had failed thrombolysis. It was based also on the concept that implementing recanalization very early after the onset of symptoms with drugs would be desirable as well. The study design entailed initial treatment with a 50-mg dose of t-PA or placebo, aspirin, and heparin, followed by immediate transport of the patient to the catheterization laboratory. If the initial angiogram demonstrated TIMI 3 flow, no further therapy was implemented other than repeat administration of either t-PA or placebo. If the angiogram demonstrated a completely occluded vessel or TIMI 1 or 2 flow, angioplasty was performed immediately. End points included assessment of left ventricular function by ventriculography and ejection fraction 6 weeks after the index event as well as angiography 1 week after the index event.

In this remarkable study, results showed that when the initial angiogram was performed within 50 minutes of initial treatment, TIMI 3 flow was present in twice as many patients who had been treated with t-PA compared with placebo (33 percent compared with 15 percent) and that the combination of TIMI 2 and TIMI 3 flow was present in twice as many patients treated with t-PA also (66 percent and 34 percent). Induction of TIMI 3 flow by medication alone occurred in a median time of 51 minutes after the onset of chest pain, as demonstrated angiographically, in contrast to the 93-minute median when induction of TIMI 3 flow required implementation of angioplasty. The most striking observation was that the key determinant of functional benefit was the time to induction of TIMI 3 flow, regardless of how it was achieved. Thus, ejection fraction at 6 weeks was 62 percent in patients in whom TIMI 3 flow was present at the time of the initial angiogram and attributable to treatment with t-PA and was 58 percent when it was induced only after the initial angiography following t-PA. In patients in whom TIMI 3 flow could not be induced, 6-week ejection fraction was 55 percent. These characteristics of ventricular function were confirmed by regional wall motion, and results in each case differed from those in each other case significantly.

There was no greater incidence of complications in patients undergoing angioplasty who had been treated with t-PA compared than in those who had not. Angioplasty was successful 87 percent of the time in converting TIMI 2 to TIMI 3 flow.

In patients in whom TIMI 3 flow was achieved by angioplasty within 60 minutes from the onset of admission to the hospital, ventricular function was indistinguishable from that in patients in whom TIMI 3 flow had been induced by pharmacologic thrombolysis alone. There was no difference in the frequency of adverse events in any of the groups, and the overall mortality at 30 days was virtually identical, 3.3 percent and 3.6 percent in patients in whom TIMI 3 flow was induced by angioplasty and by pharmacologic thrombolysis alone, respectively.

Results of the PACT study indicate the importance of inducing recanalization promptly. They imply that additive advantages of each of the two modalities can be garnered when they are used in combination, and they suggest that a strategy of sequential intervention with pharmacologic agents followed by mechanical revascularization when indicated may indeed offer the most promise for a favorable outcome.

Non–Q Wave Myocardial Infarction

Conventional wisdom indicates that treatment of unstable angina or non–Q wave MI with fibrinolytic drugs is futile. This perspective is perhaps surprising in view of the clear involvement of the coagulation system and platelet activation in the pathogenesis of all acute coronary syndromes[274–276] and with impairment of fibrinolysis as a potential determinant[41] of such syndromes. The explanation for the lack of success may include the evanescent nature of thrombotic events in acute coronary syndromes other than Q wave infarction.[277] The issue cannot be considered to be closed, however, in view of results of some studies in which benefit appears to have been conferred to patients with unstable angina by treatment with fibrinolytic agents as well as anticoagulants[278] and on the basis of trends evident in prospective randomized patient assignment trials, including the GUSTO-1 study.[279] This is consistent with a more favorable outcome in patients with non–Q wave infarction with a patent compared with nonpatent infarct-related artery. The overriding principle may be that the presence of persistent, functionally significant ischemia is a necessary condition for justification of immediate revascularization, regardless of the nature of the coronary event.[276]

Costs of Agents and Mechanisms Responsible for Benefit

Controversy fueled by concerns focusing on high costs of second-generation agents and the lack of detection of thrombolytic drug-dependent differences in survival in the GISSI-2 and ISIS-3 trials has often been intense. In terms of mechanistic and clinical differences between agents, attention has focused on the proven pivotal role of rapidity, persistence, and completeness of opening of the infarct-related artery. In studies of experimental animals, myocardium becomes necrotic when perfusion is compromised for intervals as brief as 20 to 60 minutes. As a result, salvage of myocardium demonstrable by histologic analysis or positron emission tomography is directly dependent on the rapidity with which recanalization of occluded infarct-related arteries can be induced.[37] In human hearts, the impact of early recanalization as the major determinant of overall benefit conferred by coronary thrombolysis is well established. In the landmark GISSI-1 study, profound reduction of mortality was seen in patients treated with SK compared with placebo when treatment was initiated within 1 hour after the onset of symptoms. By contrast, survival was not improved in patients treated 6 hours or more after the onset of symptoms.[33] Similar results were obtained in the European Cooperative Study Group trials[68, 270] and in the ISIS-2 trials,[34] with the most striking reduction of mortality evident among patients who were treated early.

Beginning with observations obtained by the Western Washington study.[281] potential advantages of late recanalization have required consideration. Retrospective and subset analyses have indicated that patients who leave the hospital with an open infarct-related artery have a prognosis that is more favorable than that associated with discharge with an occluded artery. Electrophysiologic stability, facilitation of ventricular remodeling and healing, reduction of aneurysm formation, provision of a conduit for augmentation of collateral flow, and reduced LV wall stress have been postulated to be favorable consequences of late recanalization independent of salvage of myocardium per se.

Unfortunately, however, it is impossible to ascertain whether benefit does, in fact, occur under conditions in which only late recanalization is induced.[250] Clearly, some patients whose arteries are either spontaneously or pharmacologically recanalized relatively late after the onset of infarction will have had intermittent spontaneous recanalization earlier in its course. Therefore, the benefits associated with an infarct-related artery shown to be open when evaluated only late may be attributable to benefit in a subset of patients in whom occult, early intermittent, or sustained reperfusion had occurred (analogous to cyclic flow variations documented extensively in hearts of animals[280, 287]).

Regardless of whether or not late recanalization confers some benefit, the bulk of benefit conferred by coronary thrombolysis is attributable to early and sustained recanalization of infarct-related arteries. Perhaps no stronger evidence establishing its impact can be advanced than the results from the Myocardial Infarction Triage and Intervention (MITI) trial,[38] in which the mortality among patients treated within 60 minutes after seeking assistance was 1 percent (i.e., tenfold less than the 10 percent mortality in patients treated more than 60 minutes after an initial request for medical assistance).

Importance of Conjunctive Therapy

As noted in the discussion of fibrin-selective agents earlier in this chapter, several factors can compromise clinical benefit otherwise anticipated after initially successful coronary thrombolysis. None is more important than reocclusion. Induction of a procoagulant state secondary to plasminemia, a phenomenon encountered to some extent with conventional dosing of all clinically available fibrinolytic agents, including clot-selective agents, but more prominent with non–clot-selective drugs, can potentiate early reocclusion.[140, 146, 164] Furthermore, the persistence of an atherosclerotic plaque responsible for an initial coronary occlusive event constitutes a nidus for recurrent thrombosis and reocclusion. Accordingly, vigorous anticoagulation, implemented concomitantly with fibrinolysis, is necessary to sustain the benefits induced by early thrombolysis, regardless of which activator of the fibrinolytic system is used. Such measures, designed to potentiate or sustain clot lysis

TABLE 36-11 **Ninety-Minute Patency Rates of First- and Second-Generation Agents**

	Patency (%)	Hours to Treatment	n
First generation			
Duke	44	3.0	216
Anderson	51	3.4	115
Second generation			
TIMI-I	71	4.8	113
TAMI-1	75	2.9	386
TIMI-II pilot	82	2.7	317
Hopkins	66	3.2	72
TIMI-IIa	75	2.8	192

Abbreviations: TAMI, Thrombolysis and Angioplasty in Myocardial Infarction; TIMI, Thrombolysis in Myocardial Infarction.
Adapted from Tiefenbrunn AJ, Sobel BE: The impact of coronary thrombolysis on myocardial infarction. Fibrinolysis 3:1, 1989.

90 minutes after the onset of treatment with first-generation drugs administered intravenously are on the order of 50 percent. In contrast, they are about 75 to 80 percent with fibrin-selective agents. In relative terms, the difference is approximately 50 percent. Results in patency studies may be distorted by early reocclusion when vigorous anticoagulation with intravenous heparin is not implemented. In four angiographic studies with fibrin-selective agents that defined patency of the infarct-related artery at selected intervals relatively late after the onset of treatment, patency rates were significantly higher when intravenous heparin was used conjunctively. Because early (90-minute) patency rates are the same with or without intravenous heparin (79 percent in t-PA–treated patients with and without intravenous heparin in the Thrombolysis and Angioplasty in Myocardial Infarction [TAMI] study),[284] the later angiographic observations are best interpreted as demonstrating a high incidence of early reocclusion, when intravenous heparin is omitted, which can obscure interpretations of comparative studies of fibrinolytic agents. In the recombinant t-PA APSAC Patency Study (TAPS) that directly compared the two drugs, 90-minute patency in vigorously heparinized patients was greater with t-PA than with APSAC (84.4 percent compared with 70.3 percent). A correspondingly favorable early mortality difference of 2.4 percent compared with 8.1 percent was seen with t-PA compared with APSAC ($P < 0.01$).[287]

With first-generation agents, recanalization rates after intravenous administration are substantially lower than those seen after intracoronary administration.[51, 86] Therefore, results of recanalization trials with intravenous SK demonstrate that only approximately 50 percent of infarct-related arteries are recanalized,[288] compared with 75 percent with intracoronary administration of the drug.[289–295] In contrast, recanalization occurs with the same high frequency after intravenous as that achieved with intracoronary administration of fibrin-selective fibrinolytic agents.[86] Accordingly, early patency is evident considerably more often after intravenous administration of clot-selective agents than after nonselective agents.[198, 296–303]

Despite the generally similar rate of induction of recanalization seen with intracoronary administration of diverse fibrinolytic agents, the intrinsic capacity of clot-selective drugs to open thrombotically occluded arteries may exceed that of nonselective agents. In studies of experimental animals, 45-minute intracoronary infusions of t-PA and urokinase were compared at two doses of each agent. At the maximal dosages used, coronary thrombolysis was 43 percent greater with t-PA than with urokinase.[304] Similarly, in patients with thrombotic peripheral arterial disease, direct intra-arterial infusions of a fibrin-selective agent (t-PA) were more effective than infusions of SK in salvaging limbs (80 percent compared with 60 percent).[305]

The intrinsic advantages of clot-selective thrombolytic agents[57, 65, 86, 92, 104, 198, 199, 306–311] appear to depend on their specificity[312] and a consequent lack of depletion of the plasminogen associated with fibrin in clots necessary for clot dissolution.[69, 70] Effects of plasminemia seen particularly with first-generation agents on systems other than the coagulation and fibrinolytic systems include activation of complement[57] breakdown of collagen,[55] hypotension (secondary, in part, to activation of the kinin system),[56, 158] and activation of platelets by thrombin-dependent and thrombin-independent mechanisms.[140, 145–147, 181, 313–316]

Ventricular Function and the Extent of Infarction

The most compelling criteria indicative of favorable effects of coronary thrombolysis on ventricular function are changes in sequential measurements of regional wall motion in initially jeopardized ischemic myocardium in treated compared with control patients. In early studies with intracoronary SK, such measurements demonstrated benefit,[317, 318] particularly in patients treated early after the onset of infarction. Very early administration (within 1.5 hours of the onset of symptoms) of fibrinolytic agents given intravenously[319] was particularly effective. In the Intravenous Streptokinase in Acute Myocardial Infarction (ISAM)[320] study of intravenous SK, the improved global ventricular function seen in all treated patients compared with control patients was striking in those treated early (within 3 hours). Similar time-dependent benefit was evident in the New Zealand trial[321] and in the Western Washington study, particularly in patients with anterior infarction treated within 3 hours.[281]

Studies of sequential changes in ventricular performance have demonstrated benefit with fibrin-selective agents as well. Improvement was maximal when recanalization was maintained,[322] and particularly when treatment was initiated within the first few hours after the onset of symptoms.[35, 205, 323]

Results of the TIMI-I trial showed that improvement in ejection fraction depended not only on the time to treatment after the onset of symptoms but also on the rapidity of induction of recanalization after the onset of treatment.[206] Therefore, in patients in whom reperfusion was initiated within 90 minutes after the onset of treatment, regardless of which fibrinolytic agent was used, ejection fraction increased, particularly in patients with a robust collateral circulation supplying jeopardized myocardium.

In the Plasminogen Activator Italian Multicenter Study (PAIMS), which directly compared SK and t-PA in patients treated within 3 hours of the onset of symptoms,[207] global ventricular function improved more with t-PA. No drug-dependent differences were seen, however, in global ventricular function 3 weeks after infarction in the White-Norris study of t-PA and SK. However, short- and long-term survival rates favored t-PA (30-day mortality 3.7 percent versus 7.4 percent for t-PA versus SK; 9-month mortality 5.9 percent versus 8.9 percent, respectively).[321] In concert, available information indicates that administration of thrombolytic agents early in the course of MI improves regional wall motion and ventricular function, particularly in patients with anterior MI. Improvement appears to depend on the amount of jeopardized myocardium salvaged, which in turn is dependent on the rapidity of recanalization and its maintenance.[86, 205, 250, 323–325]

Improvement presages improved survival.[35, 206] In patients who can be treated very early after the onset of infarction, salvage of myocardium, preservation of regional ventricular function, and survival can be enhanced most markedly,[250] and drug-dependent differences in the rate of recanalization are likely to be particularly telling. Accordingly, the more rapid and more frequent early recanalization inducible with fibrin-selective as opposed to first-generation agents is likely to be particularly beneficial in patients who can be treated early after the onset of infarction.

Mortality

The dependence of improved survival on early induction of patency of infarct-related arteries is unequivocal.[33–35, 145, 326] Although exclusively late recanalization may be beneficial, as judged from meta-analyses,[326] the more modest reduction in mortality associated with late thrombolysis may reflect prevention of infarction in a subset of patients in whom bona fide infarction was not yet in progress or a subset in whom patency was induced or sustained in infarct-related arteries that had exhibited occult, intermittent, or sustained spontaneous recanalization.

The persistence of patency, potentiated by prompt, vigorous, and effective anticoagulation, previously generally requiring intravenous heparin, appears to be pivotal in reducing mortality (Table 36–12; see also Table 36–5).[327] An overall 69 percent increase in mortality (from 5.5 to 9.3 percent) is evident in pooled data comparisons of studies with and without conjunctive intravenous heparin (Table 36–13).

Analysis of all then available small, randomized, in-hospital studies of t-PA compared with non–fibrin-specific agents demonstrated a striking difference in mortality,[170] with a 66 percent greater mortality (7.3 percent compared with 4.4 percent) in patients treated with a first-generation compared with a fibrin-selective agent (Table 36–14). In studies in which intravenous heparin has been used with fibrin-selective agents,[169] their favorable effects are particularly evident. In the TAPS investigation,[93] the increased early patency after administration of t-PA with conjunctive heparin compared with anistreplase with heparin (84 percent versus 70 percent in 90 minutes) was associated with a highly favorable hospital mortality with the clot-selective agent (2.4 percent with front-loaded t-PA, as opposed to 8.1 percent with anistreplase; $P < .01$).

It had been anticipated by many that comparisons between first-generation and clot-selective agents in megatrials would yield analogous results. However, in the International t-PA/SK[95] and ISIS-3[93] studies, no thrombolytic drug-dependent differences in mortality were seen. Because of the large number of patients enrolled, such studies should be able to detect even small real differences. However, neither large sample sizes nor unambiguous end points such as mortality ensure valid conclusions if the efficacy

TABLE 36–12 **Early Mortality (≤42 da) in Trials of Intravenous Thrombolytic Drugs With Heparin**

Trial	Placebo Group		Treatment Group	
	n	*% Mortality* (n)	*n*	*% Mortality* (n)
ASSET	2495	9.8 (245)	2516	7.2 (181)
ECSG-I		N/A	64(t-PA)	4.7 (3)
			65(SK)	4.6 (3)
ECSG-II	65	6.2 (4)	64(t-PA)	1.6 (1)
ECSG-III			123(t-PA)	4.9 (6)
ECSG-IV		N/A	367	5.0 (18)
ECSG-V	366	5.7 (21)	355	2.8 (10)
HART			106	2.0 (2)
ISIS-2 ("intention to treat" with intravenous heparin)			1024(SK + ASA)	6.4 (66)
NHF Australia	71	2.8 (2)	73	9.6 (7)
New Zealand I	93	12.9 (12)	79	2.5 (2)
New Zealand II		N/A	135(t-PA)	3.7 (5)
			135(SK)	7.4 (10)
SCATI		N/A	218	4.5 (10)
TIMI-II pilot		N/A	317	4.4 (14)
TIMI-IIa			195(t-PA + 2 h PTCA)	5.2 (11)
			200(t-PA + 24 h PTCA)	7.4 (15)
TIMI-IIb		N/A	3262	4.9 (160)
Total	3,090	9.2 (284)	9298	5.5 (514)

Abbreviations: ASA, aspirin; ASSET, Anglo-Scandinavian Study of Early Thrombosis; ECSG, European Cooperative Study Group; HART, Heparin-Aspirin Reinfarction Trial; ISIS-2, Second International Study of Infarct Survival; NHF, National Heart Foundation; PTCA, percutaneous transluminal coronary angioplasty; SCATI, Studio Sulla Calciparini nell'Angina nella Trombosi Ventrialare nell'Infarto; SK, streptokinase; TIMI, Thrombolysis in Myocardial Infarction.

From Tiefenbrunn AJ, Sobel BE: Thrombolysis and myocardial infarction. Fibrinolysis 5:1, 1991.

TABLE 36–13 Pooled Data on Early Mortality (≤42 da) in Trials of Intravenous Thrombolytic Drugs With and Without Heparin

	Placebo Group		Treatment Group		Reduction in Mortality (Treatment Versus Placebo) (%)
	n	% *Mortality* (n)	*n*	% *Mortality* (n)	
With intravenous heparin	3090	9.2 (284)	9298	5.5 (514)	39
Without intravenous heparin	16,331	13.1 (2144)	34,581	9.3 (3226)	29

From Tiefenbrunn AJ, Sobel BE: Thrombolysis and myocardial infarction. Fibrinolysis 5:1, 1991.

of the agents tested is compromised by the trial design.[328] In both of these trials, overall mortality was high (8.7 percent in the International t-PA/SK and 10.5 percent in the ISIS-3 trial). Probable explanations are inclusion of many elderly patients, late onset of treatment, and omission of intravenous heparin.

Differences in age distribution of patients in the megatrials compared with those in earlier studies, such as TIMI-II,[270] do not appear to be responsible, as judged from the 37 percent lower mortality in patients 75 years or younger in TIMI-II compared with age-matched patients in ISIS-3 (4.9 percent versus 7.8 percent).[329] The severity of illness does not appear to be responsible either, because 95 percent of patients in the International Study group population[95] were Killip class 1 or 2. Delay in treatment onset may well have diminished the favorable impact of treatment with the drugs tested, in view of the median time to treatment in ISIS-2 of 4 hours. Very early treatment is most likely to lower mortality, as shown by the remarkably low mortality of 1 percent in patients treated within the first 90 minutes as opposed to 10 percent in those treated later in the MITI trial.[38]

A more compelling explanation that appears to account for both the high mortality and the lack of apparent thrombolytic drug-dependent differences in some megatrials is the omission of intravenous heparin. The heparin regimen used in ISIS-3 and GISSI-2 (12,500 U given subcutaneously every 12 hours)[93, 95] is known to generally fail to induce therapeutically effective blood levels for 24 hours or more.[330] To clarify the potential impact of omission of intravenous heparin, a meta-analysis was performed. Results in all studies with treatment arms comprising at least 150 patients with protocols including aspirin were considered. The analysis focused on patients less than 70 years of age who were treated within 6 hours of the onset of chest pain and who exhibited electrocardiographic ST segment elevation, because patients fulfilling these criteria are the ones most likely to benefit from coronary thrombolysis. In addition, masking of potential drug-dependent differences by lack of effect of treatment in patients without bona fide infarction and in those treated so late that substantial benefit could not be realistically anticipated was avoided. As can be seen in Table 36–15, intravenous heparin is associated with a 38 percent lower mortality in the treated patients younger than 70 years of age with ST elevation who are given t-PA within 6 hours of symptom onset ($P < .001$). A directionally similar trend is associated with intravenous heparin in patients treated with SK as well. In the absence of intravenous heparin, the mortality is identical, regardless of whether or not a fibrin-selective agent is used. In contrast, in patients given intravenous heparin, the mortality is 3.6 percent with t-PA and 5.2 percent with SK, a difference of 44 percent that is attributable to chance only six times out of a hundred. This analysis indicates that the mortality reduction that can be accomplished with clot-selective agents is compromised by a high incidence of early reocclusion when intravenous heparin or equivalent or superior anticoagulation is not used and that the compromise may obscure thrombolytic drug-dependent differences that would be apparent in well-anticoagulated patients.

The heparin regimens used in the International t-PA/SK and ISIS-3 studies do not induce therapeutic blood levels within the first 24 hours in most patients.[52, 170, 331, 332] Because first-generation thrombolytic agents elevate plasma concentrations of FDPs much more than clot-selective agents do, and because FDPs exert antithrombotic effects that may diminish the incidence of reocclusion,[108, 198] a high incidence of early reocclusion is particularly likely to compromise benefit in patients treated with clot-selective agents. Therefore, one interpretation of the lack of thrombolytic drug-dependent differences and the high mortality rates seen in the International t-PA/SK and ISIS-3 studies is that both reflect the deleterious impact of omission of protocol-mandated immediate administration of intrave-

TABLE 36–14 In-hospital Mortality in Randomized Assignment, Large-Scale Studies of rt-PA Versus Nonfibrin-Specific Thrombolytic Agents Combined With Immediate Intravenous Heparin for at Least 48 Hours in Patients With Acute Myocardial Infarction*

Study	rt-PA	Nonfibrin-Specific Agent
TIMI-I	12/157	14/159 (SK)
ECSG-I	3/64	3/65 (SK)
White et al	5/135	10/135 (SK)
PAIMS	4/86	7/85 (UK)
TAMI-5	8/191	5/190 UK)
GAUS	6/124	5/121 (UK)
TAPS	5/218	17/217 (ASPAC)
Total	43/975 (4.4%)	71/972 (all) (7.3%)

Abbreviations: APSAC, anisoylated plasminogen streptokinase activator complex; ECSG, European Cooperative Study Group; GAUS, German Activator Urokinase Study; PAIMS, Plasminogen Activator Italian Multicenter Study; rt-PA, recombinant tissue-type plasminogen activator; SK, streptokinase; TAMI, Thrombolysis and Angioplasty in Myocardial Infarction; TAPS, rt-PA–APSAC Patency Study; TIMI, Thrombolysis in Myocardial Infarction; UK, urokinase.

*Homogeneity index: $\chi^2 = 4.76$; $P = 0.57$; odds ratio: 0.59 (95% CI; 0.41–0.87), $P = 0.0067$.

From Sobel BE, Collen D: Questions unresolved by ISIS-3. Am J Cardiol 70:385, 1992; copyright 1992, reprinted with permission of Excerpta Medica Inc.

TABLE 36-15 Early Mortality in Aspirin-Treated Patients, <70 Yr of Age, Treated Within 6 h and Exhibiting ST-Segment Elevation*

	Intravenous Heparin			
	Yes	***No***	χ^2	***P* Value**
SK	ISAM: 37/730 (5.2%)	ISIS-2: 51/872 (5.8%)		
		ISG: 432/8005 (5.4%)		
		ISIS-3: 369/5855 (6.3%)		
	Total: 38/730 (5.2%)	Total: 852/14,732 (5.8%)	0.33	.57
rt-PA	ECSG-V: 10/355 (2.8%)	ISG: 469/7986 (5.8%)		
	TIMI-II: 55/1398 (3.9%)	ECSG-VI: 11/320 (3.4%)		
	ECSG-VI: 9/324 (2.8%)			
	Total: 74/2077 (3.6%)	Total: 479/8306 (5.8%)	15.6	<.001
χ^2	3.38	0.001		
P	0.06	0.98		

Abbreviations: ECSG, European Cooperative Study Group; ISAM, Intravenous Streptokinase in Acute Myocardial Infarction; ISG, International t-PA/SK Study Group; rt-PA, recombinant tissue-type plasminogen activator; SK, streptokinase; TIMI, Thrombolysis in Myocardial Infarction.

*χ^2 and *P* values on the right pertain to the effect of intravenous heparin with SK or rt-PA; χ^2 and *P* values on the bottom pertain to the effect of SK versus rt-PA with or without intravenous heparin.

From Sobel BE, Collen D: Questions unresolved by ISIS-3. Am J Cardiol 70:385, 1992; copyright 1992, reprinted with permission of Excerpta Medica Inc.

nous heparin. The results of those megatrials have confirmed the safety of fibrinolytic agents. However, they do not militate against the view that early recanalization, inducible more frequently with clot-selective agents, confers substantial clinical benefit.[328]

Safety

Clot-selective fibrinolytic agents were developed in part to decrease the risk of bleeding. Most bleeding with both types of fibrinolytic drugs occurs at vascular access sites.[108] Major bleeding requiring transfusion occurs less frequently with clot-selective than with first-generation agents (e.g., SK).[49, 68] In four trials that directly compared SK and t-PA,[66] the frequency of bleeding complications was similar in two[209, 333] and somewhat lower in the t-PA–treated patients in the other two.[68, 207] The incidence was lower with the clot-selective agent in the data pooled from all four trials.

Transfusion requirements were greater with SK compared with t-PA in the International t-PA/SK study but were modest with both agents. However, with the exception of intracranial hemorrhage, bleeding associated with all fibrinolytic drugs can be readily managed, and, accordingly, the practical implications of the more favorable experience with clot-selective agents are limited.

The absolute risk for bleeding is dependent on several factors, including the conjunctive regimens used for anticoagulation, the impact of antiplatelet drugs, the doses of fibrinolytic agents employed, the age of the patient, and the effects of thrombolytic agents not only on procoagulant proteins in blood but also on hemostatic plugs and vessel walls.

Unfortunately, no simple relationship exists between an easily measurable laboratory value and the risk of bleeding. Prolongation of the template bleeding time seems to correlate more closely with an increased risk of spontaneous bleeding than does any other conventionally measured variable.[334] Increased concentrations of FDPs in plasma have been associated with an increased risk of bleeding with both clot-selective[335] and non–clot-selective agents.[40]

The most serious bleeding complication associated with the use of fibrinolytic agents is intracranial bleeding. Even when thrombolytic agents are not used, patients with acute MI exhibit an incidence of CVAs approaching 1 percent.[222] The incidence is similar when fibrinolytic drugs are used. However, the fraction of episodes consisting of hemorrhage is somewhat higher. In the ASSET trial of t-PA, the incidence of stroke was 1.1 percent, virtually identical to the 1.0 percent incidence in placebo-treated controls.[336] In the more than 3000 patients first treated with conventional doses of t-PA in studies performed in the United States, the incidence was less than 0.5 percent.[86] Doses of t-PA of 150 mg combined with heparin were associated with a higher incidence of intracranial bleeding (1.6 percent,[337] compared with 0.36 percent in more than 3000 patients given 100 mg of t-PA, intravenous heparin, and aspirin in the TIMI-II trial[223]).

Elderly patients (>75 years), particularly those whose body weight is less than 60 kg,[229] are at an increased risk for intracranial hemorrhage associated with the use of both first-generation and clot-selective fibrinolytic drugs.[223, 338] Overall, the incidence of intracranial bleeding with 100 mg of t-PA and intravenous heparin was reported to be 0.5 percent in 6375 patients (3016 in the TIMI-II study and 3359 in eight other studies combined [including the European Cooperative Study Group-V, the Anglo-Scandinavian Study of Early Thrombolysis or ASSET, National Heart Foundation of Australia, Guerci, Raami, TAMI, the Thrombolysis in Acute Coronary Occlusion study or TICO, and TIMI-IIb trials]). With the exception of the ASSET trial, surveillance included either a computed tomographic scan or an autopsy in all instances. These figures are consistent with a low incidence of total stroke, hemorrhagic and ischemic, in registry data[74] and other large trials.[114]

The frequency of intracranial bleeding was virtually identical with t-PA and with SK in the International t-PA/SK GISSI-2 trial,[95] averaging 0.35 percent. A similar incidence was encountered in the SK-treated patients in

TABLE 36–16 **Frequency of Intracranial Hemorrhage in ISIS-3 and the International t-PA/SK Study, Two Megatrials Comparing Tissue-Type Plasminogen Activator and Streptokinase in Patients With Infarction**

Study	Intracranial Hemorrhage	Streptokinase	t-PA	*P* Value
International t-PA/SK Study n/n (%)	Definite hemorrhage	30/10,396 (0.3)*	44/10,372 (0.4)†	NS
ISIS-3, n/n (%)	Probable hemorrhage	39/12,848 (0.3)	94/12,841 (0.7)	<.001

Abbreviations: ISIS-3, Third International Study of Infarct Survival; NS, not significant; SK, streptokinase; t-PA, tissue-type plasminogen activator.
*No statistically significant difference compared with the streptokinase group in ISIS-3.
†n < .003 compared with the t-PA group in ISIS-3.
From Sobel BE, Collen D: Questions unresolved by ISIS-3. Am J Cardiol 70:385, 1992; copyright 1992, reprinted with permission of Excerpta Medica Inc.

ISIS-3 (Table 36–16). The incidence was greater in patients in ISIS-3 treated with duteplase, a different form of t-PA from that available clinically: 0.66 percent of patients were reported to have "probable" intracranial bleeding. As is evident from Table 36–16, the incidence with duteplase deviates from that seen with alteplase, the clinically available form of t-PA, and from that with SK.

Duteplase differs considerably from alteplase. The dose used in the ISIS-3 study was selected on the basis of assays of activity performed with a clot lysis assay and on the assumption that the amount given should correspond to that yielding comparable activity in the same assay of conventionally administered alteplase. For a typical 75-kg patient, this translated into a dose of 150 mg of duteplase. In view of the fact that the specific activities of duteplase and alteplase are the same in a kinetic chromogenic functional assay that reflects overall plasminogen activating activity in solutions in which fibrin stimulation is maximal (approximately 500,000 IU/mg), the 150-mg dose of duteplase used in ISIS-3 represents a substantially greater amount of kinetic assay unit activity and of mass than that employed with the standard dose of alteplase (100 mg).

A 150-mg dose of alteplase given in combination with intravenous heparin was found in the TIMI-2 trial to be associated with an incidence of intracranial bleeding of 1.6 percent,[339] which led the investigators to reduce the maximal dose to 100 mg and to the clinical abandonment of a dose of alteplase exceeding 100 mg. Therefore, the incidence of probable intracranial bleeding in ISIS-3 of 0.6 percent with 150 mg of dutaplase is not surprising, nor is it indicative of what can be anticipated with the conventional 100-mg dose of alteplase.[328]

The risk of bleeding is, of course, not completely avoidable with any fibrinolytic agent. By definition, clots that are serving a protective function are lysed along with those targeted for therapeutic intervention. Nevertheless, careful selection of patients and avoidance of administration of fibrinolytic agents to patients with contraindications can minimize risk (Table 36–17). Although a modest increase in the proportion of CVAs that are hemorrhagic can be anticipated in patients treated with thrombolytic agents, the overall beneficial impact of these drugs on survival far outweighs the negative impact of potential conversion of a small number of thromboembolic strokes to hemorrhagic strokes (Table 36–18).

In addition to differences related to the risk of bleeding, several differences distinguish clinically available clot-selective agents from non–clot-selective agents. From a biochemical point of view, commercially available fibrinolytic agents (e.g., alteplase [recombinant t-PA], streptokinase, urokinase, and anistreplase [APSAC]) differ markedly, as noted earlier, with respect to the fraction of active ingredient contained per total protein. For alteplase, the purity with respect to protein is 99.9 percent, in comparison with 1 percent for SK, 20 percent for urokinase, and 55 percent for anistreplase.[53]

The incidence of allergic reactions is virtually nil with t-PA (0.2 percent in the International t-PA/SK trial).[95] It is substantially higher with the SK preparations (SK and anistreplase [APSAC]), with urticaria, skin rash, eosinophilia, and fever occurring in 1.7 to 21 percent of patients. Vasculitis has been reported in 6 of 253 patients treated with APSAC,[59] and rare episodes of serum sickness and glomerulonephritis have been described after treatment with streptokinase.[340–344] Because of the possibility of severe allergic reactions, retreatment with any SK-based agent within 6 months to a year in patients given SK or APSAC is inadvisable. In contrast, retreatment with t-PA

TABLE 36–17 **Contraindications to Thrombolysis**

Absolute

- Active internal bleeding
- Aortic dissection
- Prolonged or traumatic cardiopulmonary resuscitation
- Recent head trauma or known intracranial neoplasm
- Diabetic hemorrhagic retinopathy or other hemorrhagic ophthalmic condition
- Pregnancy
- Previous allergic reaction to the thrombotic agent (streptokinase or anistreplase)
- Recorded blood pressure > 200/120 mm Hg
- History of cerebrovascular accident known to be hemorrhagic

Relative

- Recent trauma or surgery > 2 wk; trauma or surgery more recent than 2 wk, which could be a source of rebleeding, is an absolute contraindication
- History of chronic severe hypertension with or without drug therapy
- Active peptic ulcer
- History of cerebrovascular accident (many consider this to be an absolute contraindication)
- Known bleeding diathesis or current use of anticoagulants
- Significant liver dysfunction
- Prior exposure to streptokinase or anistreplase (this contraindication is particularly important in the initial 6- to 9-mo period after administration of either of these drugs and applies to reuse of any streptokinase-containing agent, but does not apply to repeat use of t-PA or urokinase regardless of the agent used initially)

From Sobel, BE: Thrombolysis in the treatment of acute myocardial infarction. *In* Fuster V, Verstraete M (eds): Thrombosis in Cardiovascular Diseases. p. 289. Philadelphia: WB Saunders, 1992.

TABLE 36–18 Incidence of Cerebrovascular Accidents in Patients Treated With Thrombolytic Agents or Managed With Anticoagulants Alone in Large Trials

Agents and Trials	Patients (n)	Events (n)	%
SK and APSAC (GISSI, PAIMS, ISIS-2)	14,954	126	0.84
SK and APSAC, placebo (GISSI, PAIMS, ISIS-2)	14,949	126	0.84
rt-PA (ASSET, ECSG [two trials], TIMI-II)	6500	50	0.76
rt-PA, placebo (ASSET, ECSG [two trials])	2861	27	0.94
TOTAL			
Active	21,454	176	0.82
Placebo	17,810	153	0.86

Abbreviations: APSAC, anisoylated plasminogen streptokinase activator complex; ASSET, Anglo-Scandinavian Study of Early Thrombolysis; ECSG, European Cooperative Study Group; GISSI, Gruppo Italiano per lo Studio della Streptochinasi nell'Infarto Miocardico; ISIS-2, Second International Study of Infarct Survival; PAIMS, Plasminogen Activator Italian Multicenter Study; rt-PA, recombinant tissue-type plasminogen activator; SK, streptokinase; TIMI-II, Thrombolysis in Myocardial Infarction Trial.

From Sobel, BE: Coronary thrombolysis and the new biology. J Am Coll Cardiol 14:850, 1989. Reprinted with permission from the American College of Cardiology.

is not contraindicated after any fibrinolytic agent and is often effective.[63]

Hypotension, sometimes associated with an allergic reaction but sometimes attributable to diminished viscosity of the blood, activation of the kinin system,[56] and other consequences of plasminemia, occurs in 2 to 22 percent of patients treated with APSAC or SK (package inserts for anistreplase and SK). It occurred in 10 percent of patients treated with streptokinase in ISIS-2.[34] Hypotension is less common and less severe in patients treated with t-PA,[93–94] and its incidence may not exceed that associated with the index infarction per se.

Recent Observations and Clinical Implications

Commercially available fibrinolytic agents differ markedly with respect to biochemical properties and purity, pharmacologic properties, and cost. Clot-selective agents induce recanalization of infarct-related arteries more frequently and more often than first-generation agents and are less prone to cause spontaneous bleeding. As noted earlier, drug-dependent differences in mortality have been evident as well in many prospective, randomized trials, in retrospective analyses of patients given the two types of fibrinolytic agents with intravenous heparin, and in a prospective, multicenter, large trial.[122, 131, 248, 345] Thus, reduction of mortality by fibrinolytic agents depends on the rapidity of induction of sustained patency early after onset of MI and the advantages of clot-selective compared with nonselective agents. Novel, highly clot-selective agents, such as TNK, perturb the coagulation system even less than t-PA does (Fig. 36–7) and have led to favorable clinical outcomes and a lower incidence of hemorrhage in some trials,[346] whereas less clot-selective drugs, such as nPA, have been associated with an increased incidence of intracranial hemorrhage.[347]

The primary end point in the pivotal, 40,000-patient GUSTO trial was "net clinical benefit," defined prospec-

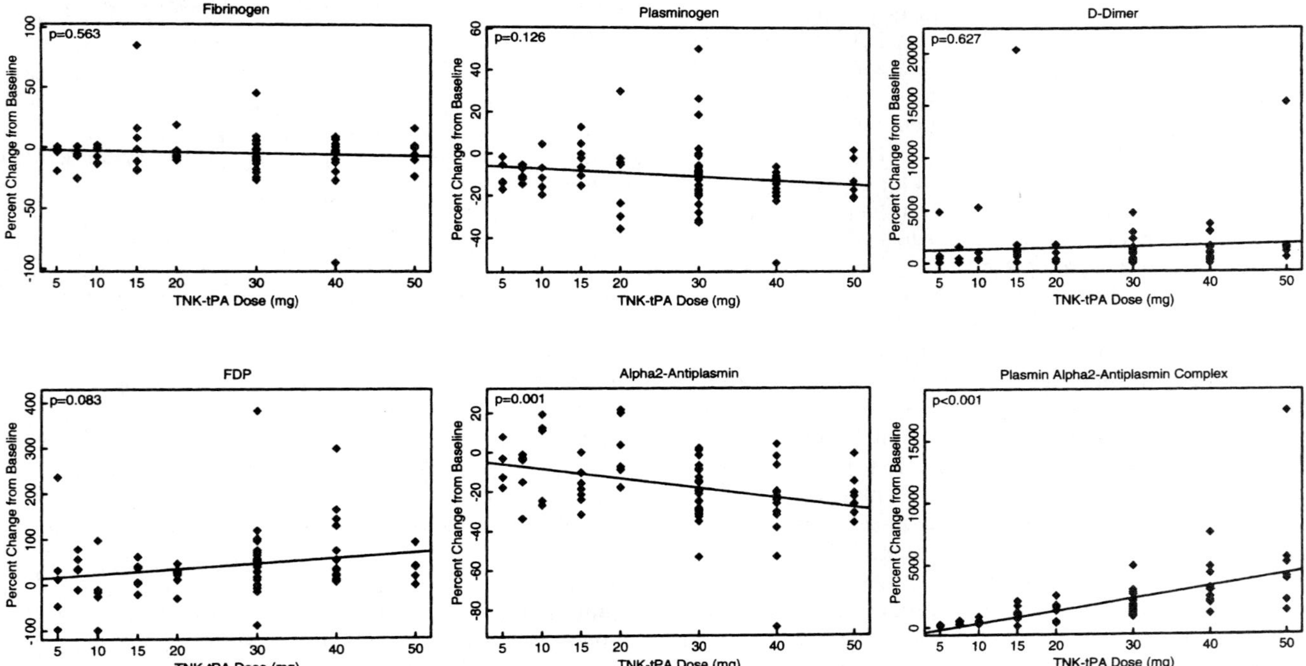

FIGURE 36–7 Effects of increasing doses of TNK-TPA on coagulation parameters. FDP, fibrin degradation products. (From Cannon CP, McCabe CH, Gibson CM, et al: TNK-tissue plasminogen activator in acute myocardial infarction. Results of the Thrombolysis in Myocardial Infarction [TIMI] 10A dose-ranging trial. Circulation 95[2]:351–356, 1997.)

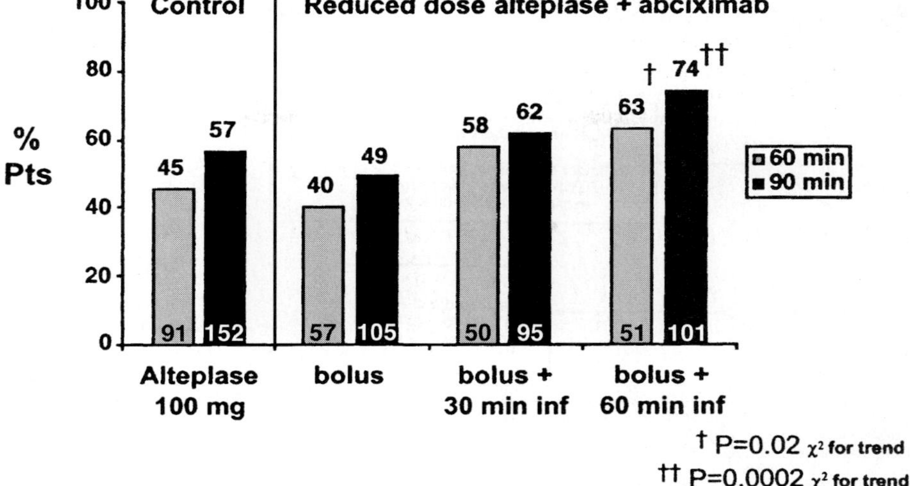

FIGURE 36–8 Impact of alteplase administration schedule on reperfusion of infarct-related artery. The percentage of patients (% Pts) achieving TIMI grade 3 flow at 60 minutes (*gray bars*) and 90 minutes (*black bars*) for different reperfusion regimens containing alteplase and abciximab tested during the dose finding phase is shown. Increasingly higher rates of TIMI 3 flow at both 60 and 90 minutes was seen with more prolonged duration of administration of alteplase. (From Antman EM, Giugliano RP, Gibson CM, et al: Abciximab facilitates the rate and extent of thrombolysis: results of the Thrombolysis in Myocardial Infarction [TIMI] 14 trial. The TIMI 14 Investigators. Circulation 99:2720, 1999. By permission of the American Heart Association, Inc.)

tively as survival and the absence of a disabling stroke. Overall mortality (at 24 hours and at 30 days) and net clinical benefit (at 30 days) with t-PA were significantly superior to those of IV or SC heparin and t-PA and SK. The relative 30-day mortality reduction by t-PA was 14 percent. The corresponding relative difference in net clinical benefit was 11.2 percent. The mortality reduction was the same as the relative risk reduction seen with CABG over a 10-year interval in the Coronary Artery Surgical Study (CASS) (14 percent relative risk reduction with surgery) that so profoundly changed medical practice more than a decade ago.

In the GUSTO angiographic substudy,[256] significant differences in early patency were seen with t-PA compared with SK (80.2 percent versus 58 percent), as were differences in preservation of ventricular function (with normal ventricular function evident in almost 50 percent more patients treated with t-PA than in those treated with SK). The incidence of reocclusion was not significantly different (range, 5 to 7 percent) with any of the four treatment regimens.

Reduction of mortality depended on the rapidity of onset of treatment and the nature of the plasminogen activator (clot selective or not). Thus, with t-PA, mortality in patients treated within the first 2 hours was 5.4 percent, compared with 6.6 percent in those treated 2 to 4 hours after the onset of symptoms and 9.4 percent in those treated 4 to 6 hours after symptom onset.

The advantages of fibrin selectivity were evident in the overall trial as well and were consistent across a wide range of patient demographic and clinical characteristics. In the trial as a whole, the excess incidence of disabling stroke attributable to t-PA compared with SK was 0.1 percent, an incidence more than offset by the more favorable mortality seen with t-PA compared with SK.

Conclusions from GUSTO are consistent with those of mechanistic trials and of laboratory studies of fibrinolytic agents. The results indicate that (1) mortality and net clinical benefit are significantly better with a clot-selective drug than with a non–clot-selective drug, (2) improved survival is dependent on the rapidity and the persistence of induction of patency in the infarct-related artery, (3) early patency is induced significantly more often by a clot-selective drug than with a non–clot-selective agent, and (4) optimal benefit results from the use of a fibrin-selective thrombolytic agent coupled with vigorous anticoagulation. Judicious combinations of reduced doses of a thrombolytic drug coupled with an antiplatelet agent may induce favorable outcomes and minimize bleeding[348] (Fig. 36–8). Accordingly, as judged from results of studies in laboratory animals, mechanistic clinical research, meta-analyses of rigorously controlled pilot studies of clot-selective compared with nonselective fibrinolytic agents, and large scale trials comparing both types of agents administered with vigorous, concomitant anticoagulation and antiplatelet drugs, clot-selective agents are more effective than nonselective agents in recanalizing infarct-related arteries promptly, reducing mortality, and conferring clinical benefit.

Taken together, the considerations presented support a management scheme for patients with suspected acute MI[349] (Fig. 36–9). Several specific considerations apply. First, the use of thrombolysis is well established for patients with Q wave infarction. Patients with ST depression rather than ST elevation (i.e., those with ischemia, subendocardial infarction in progress, or atypical Q wave infarction) are known to have a worse prognosis than that of patients with typical Q wave infarction preceded by ST segment elevation. Accordingly, benefits of thrombolysis in patients whose infarcts are manifest by ST depression have been difficult to demonstrate. Second, in patients with previous central nervous system insults, a bleeding diathesis or long-standing hypertension, or hypertension that has been inadequately controlled for a substantial inter-

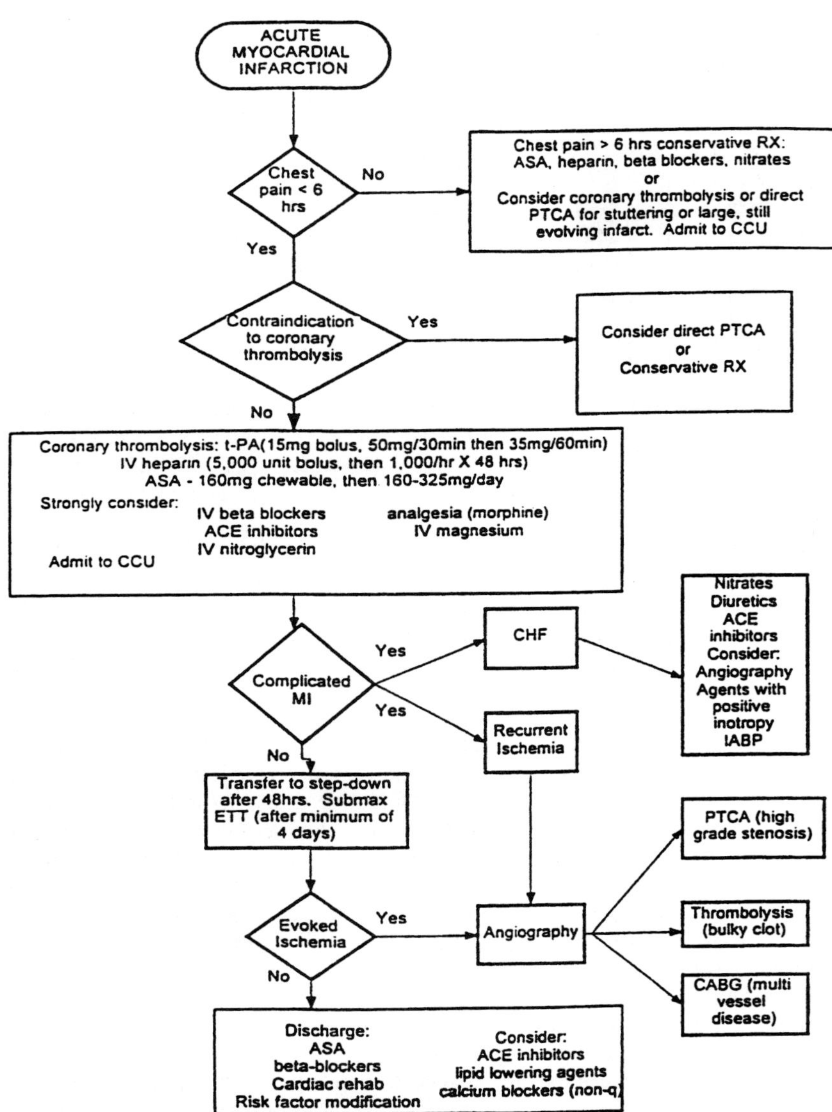

FIGURE 36–9 Flow diagram for the treatment of acute myocardial infarction. A management scheme pertinent to the optimal use of thrombolysis for patients presenting with suspected acute myocardial infarction. ACE, angiotensin-converting enzyme; ASA, acetylsalicylic acid; CABG, coronary artery bypass grafting; CCU, coronary care unit; CHF, congestive heart failure; ETT, exercise tolerance test; IABP, intra-aortic balloon pump; MI, myocardial infarction; PTCA, percutaneous transluminal coronary angioplasty; RX, therapy; Submax, submaximal; t-PA, tissue-type plasminogen activator. (From Battle RW, Sobel BE: Treatment of acute myocardial infarction. Contemp Treat Cardiovasc Dis 29:33, 1996.)

val before the index infarct, the risk of intracranial bleeding associated with the use of thrombolytic drugs is increased. Susceptibility of the cerebral vasculature to injury by proteolytic agents rather than lysis of a "protective" cerebral vascular clot appears to be responsible.[350, 351] Thus, when cerebral vasculopathy secondary to hypertension is demonstrably present or can be assumed to be present, thrombolysis is relatively or absolutely contraindicated (depending on the nature and the severity of the implicated risk factor), and angioplasty or other mechanical or surgical coronary interventions should supplant coronary thrombolysis. Hypertension per se in the absence of hypertensive vascular disease (i.e., an elevated blood pressure accompanying the index infarct but not associated with long-standing [>6 months], severe hypertension) is not a contraindication to coronary thrombolysis.

The flow diagram (see Fig. 36–9) indicates currently established medical regimens for induction of coronary thrombolysis. However, progress in the field is rapid. It appears highly likely that the use of low-molecular-weight heparin will supplant the use of unfractionated heparin as an anticoagulant. In addition, the use of antagonists to the GP IIb/IIIa platelet fibrinogen binding receptor, including intravenously administered agents, such as those used in association with angioplasty and orally administered drugs now becoming available, is likely to increase in combination with administration of thrombolytic drugs, in keeping with observations from the completed TIMI 14 trial.[348]

An important clinical issue is recognition of failed coronary thrombolysis. In a patient with ST elevation, chest pain at the time of onset of administration of a thrombolytic drug, as well as typical clinical sequelae of infarction in progress; rapid resolution of ST elevation, accelerated development of Q waves on the electrocardiogram; rapid resolution of pain; the appearance of so-called reperfusion arrhythmias, including idioventricular tachycardia; and improvement in hemodynamics all support the likelihood that reperfusion has been induced successfully. Changes in concentration in blood of biochemical markers consistent with this interpretation include rapid elevation of creatine kinase-MB or troponin T or I, consistent with accelerated washout of the biomarkers from ischemic myocardium undergoing reperfusion. Early peaking of biomarkers, such as creatine kinase-MB (within 8 to 10 hours as opposed to the more typical 12 to 16 hours), is typical of successful recanalization as well. In the absence of such electrocardiographic, clinical, hemodynamic, and biochemical phenomena, particularly when pain is persistent or recurrent and tachycardia, hypotension, pulmonary edema, or other manifestations of cardiac dysfunction persist, reperfusion is likely to have been unsuccessful. Prompt diagnostic evaluation in the cardiac catheterization laboratory is then indicated. If high-grade stenosis is identified, mechanical coronary intervention or surgery is obviously required. If a large clot burden is present, intracoronary administration of a fibrinolytic drug may be effective promptly, but if not, mechanical or surgical intervention should be implemented. No single algorithm can substitute for clinical judgment, particularly in a field in which the evolution of effective therapeutic approaches is so striking. The approach outlined in Figure 36–9 is designed to provide general guidelines that must be modified in keeping with individual circumstances and with progress in the development of even more clot-selective fibrinolytic agents and conjunctive antiplatelet and anticoagulant drugs.

Looking to the Future: Glycoprotein IIb/IIIa Antagonists/Thrombolytic Therapy

Paradigm Trial

This trial was designed to assess the safety, pharmacodynamics, and effects of reperfusion of the platelet GP IIb/IIIa receptor inhibitor lamifiban when given with thrombolysis to patients with ST segment elevation in acute MI.[352] Lamifiban is a selective, nonpeptide antagonist of the platelet GP IIb/IIIa receptor that provides dose-dependent inhibition of platelet aggregation in response to most or all known agonists. In this study, patients with ST segment elevation presenting within 12 hours of symptom onset who were treated with tissue plasminogen activator or streptokinase were enrolled in a three-part phase II dose exploration study. In part A, all patients received the GP IIb/IIIa receptor inhibitor lamifiban in an open-label, dose-escalation scheme. Parts B and C were a randomized, double-blind comparison of a bolus plus 24-hour infusion of lamifiban versus placebo with patients randomly assigned in a 2:1 ratio. The goal was to identify a dose of lamifiban that provided greater than 85 percent inhibition of adenosine diphosphate–induced platelet aggregation inhibition. A composite of angiographic, continuous electrocardiographic, and clinical markers of reperfusion was the primary efficacy end point, and bleeding was the primary safety end point. Platelet aggregation was inhibited by lamifiban in a dose-dependent manner, with the highest doses inducing 85 percent adenosine diphosphate–induced platelet aggregation inhibition. Lamifiban given with a thrombolytic agent induced more rapid reperfusion, as measured by all continuous electrocardiographic variables. More bleeding was associated with lamifiban with transfusions required in 16 percent of lamifiban-treated patients and in 10 percent of the placebo-treated patients. This preliminary study suggested that lamifiban given with thrombolytic therapy is associated with more rapid and complete reperfusion than placebo.

Assessment of Integrelin and Accelerated Tissue Plasminogen Activator: The IMPACT-AMI Study

One hundred thirty-two patients were randomly assigned in a 2:1 ratio to receive a bolus and continuous infusion of one of six integrelin doses or placebo.[353] All patients received accelerated alteplase, aspirin, and intravenous heparin infusion. Individuals 18 to 65 years of age were eligible if they were seen within 6 hours of acute MI onset with ST segment elevation. The primary end point was TIMI grade 3 flow at 90 minutes of angiography. Secondary end points were time to ST segment recovery and an in-hospital composite of death, reinfarction, stroke, revascularization procedures, new heart failure, and pulmonary edema and bleeding variables. The highest integrelin dose group had more complete reperfusion, with TIMI grade 3 flow of 66 percent versus 39 percent for placebo-treated patients ($P = .006$) and a shorter median time to ST segment recovery (65 minutes versus 116 minutes for placebo, $P = .05$). Bleeding was similar in the placebo and treated patients. The authors concluded that the incidence and the speed of reperfusion can be enhanced when a potent inhibitor of the platelet glycoprotein IIb/IIIa integrin receptor, such as integrelin, is combined with accelerated alteplase, aspirin, and intravenous heparin.

TIMI 14 Trial

The TIMI 14 trial tested the hypothesis that abciximab, a monoclonal antibody directed against the glycoprotein IIb/IIIa receptor, is a potent and safe addition to reduced-dose thrombolytic regimens in patients with acute ST segment elevation MI.[348] Eight hundred eighty-eight patients with ST segment elevation in MI presenting less than 12 hours from onset of symptoms were treated with aspirin and randomly assigned to either 100 mg of accelerated-dose alteplase or abciximab (bolus 0.25 mg/kg and 12-hour infusion of 0.125 μg/kg/min) alone or in combination with reduced doses of alteplase (20 to 65 mg) or streptokinase (500,000 U to 1.5 million U). Control patients received standard weight-adjusted heparin, whereas those with a treatment regimen, including abciximab, received low-dose heparin (60 U/kg bolus and infusion of 7 U/kg/h). TIMI 3 flow at 90 minutes for patients treated with accelerated alteplase alone was 57 percent, compared with 32 percent for abciximab alone TIMI 3 flow at 90 minutes was 34 to 46 percent for doses of SK between 500,000 U and 1.25 million U with abciximab. Higher rates of TIMI 3 flow both at 60 and 90 minutes were observed with increasing duration of the administration of alteplase progressing from a bolus alone to a bolus followed by either a 30- or a 60-minute infusion ($P < .02$) (see Fig. 36–8). The most promising regimen in this study was 50 mg of alteplase as a 15-mg bolus and infusion of 35 mg over 60 minutes, which produced a 76 percent rate of TIMI 3 flow at 90 minutes. It was tested subsequently in conjunction with either low-dose or very-low-dose heparin. TIMI 3 flow rates were significantly higher in the 50-mg alteplase plus abciximab group versus the alteplase-only group at both 60 minutes (72 percent versus 43 percent, $P = .0009$) and 90 minutes (77 percent versus 62 percent, $P = .02$). The rates of major hemorrhage were 6 percent in patients receiving alteplase alone, 3 percent with abciximab alone, 10 percent with SK plus abciximab, 7 percent with 50 mg of alteplase plus abciximab and low-dose heparin, and 1 percent with 50 mg of alteplase plus abciximab with very-low-dose heparin. The TIMI 14 study demonstrated that abciximab facilitates the rate and extent of thrombolysis, producing an early, marked increase in TIMI 3 flow when the drug is combined with half the usual dose of alteplase. This improvement in reperfusion with alteplase occurred without an increase in the risk of major bleeding. Substantial reductions in heparin dosing may reduce the risk of bleeding even further.

Treatment of the Survivor of Acute Myocardial Infarction

Because many of the complications of acute MI occur within the first 96 hours, the patient should remain in a coronary care unit for some part of this time period. Complete bed rest is recommended initially, followed by gradual mobilization of those who are clinically stable, so that patients are beginning to walk and sit in a chair within 2 to 3 days after the infarct. Emotional stimulation and strenuous physical effort should be avoided. Chest pain during the initial 24 hours is treated with opiates, usually intravenous morphine or meperidine. Thereafter, recurrent chest pain believed to represent angina is treated with nitrates, a calcium antagonist, aspirin, and/or β-blockers as is most appropriate for the individual patient. The patient with angina at rest or low-level effort despite nitrates, calcium antagonists, and/or β-blockers should be referred for coronary arteriography and subsequently coronary artery revascularization. Intravenous nitroglycerin can be used to relieve the chest pain and to stabilize the patient before angiography.[354–361]

During the initial hours after MI, oxygen is administered by mask or nasal cannula. Vital signs are checked frequently. Patients with new LV thrombi after MI are anticoagulated with intravenously administered heparin given as a 5000-U IV bolus, followed by 700 to 1400 U every hour to keep the prothrombin time in the 60- to 80-second range for 7 to 10 days. This regimen is followed by warfarin, usually administered as 2.5 to 10 mg every day to maintain the prothrombin time in the 18- to 20-second range and International Normalized Ratio (INR) in the 2- to 2.5-range for at least 6 months. Low-molecular-weight heparin may be given as an alternative to unfractionated heparin. Newly formed thrombi and those that appear to be freely mobile and/or to protrude into the LV cavity are those most likely to embolize. Thrombi present for several months usually become firmly adherent to the LV endocardium, and the risk of embolization becomes small. In patients with anterior Q wave infarcts, there is a 10 to 40 percent risk for the development of LV thrombi.[362–364]

β-Blockers

Several studies have shown that β-blockers without intrinsic sympathomimetic effect reduce the risk for future MI and death in patients with anterior Q wave infarcts and in patients with reversible LV failure, in those with moderate depression of LV ejection fraction, in older individuals, and in those with continuing myocardial ischemia at low levels of effort (Figs. 36–10 to 36–12).[365–371] Specifically, timolol, metoprolol, and propranolol reduce the risk for recurrent MI and death in patients after MI during follow-up periods of up to 6 years. β-Blockers with intrinsic sympathomimetic activity do not appear to reduce mortality and the risk for reinfarction. Prompt administration of a relatively selective β-blocker, metoprolol, reduces the incidence of recurrent myocardial ischemia and reinfarction during the first 6 days after Q wave infarction in patients who receive t-PA and heparin as a thrombolytic intervention.[371] β-Blockers should not be given to patients with

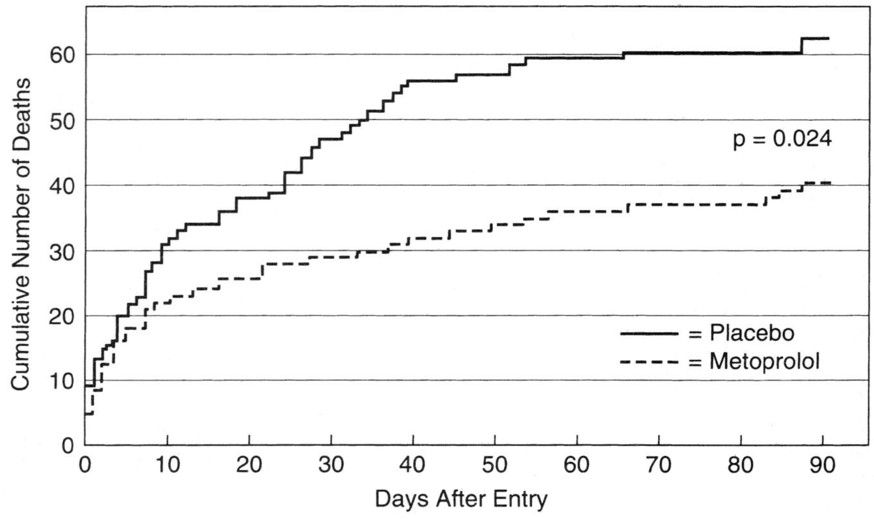

FIGURE 36–10 Influence of metoprolol administration on the cumulative number of deaths in patients after myocardial infarction. Metoprolol reduced mortality in patients after myocardial infarction. (From Hjalmarson A, Herlitz J, Malek I, et al: Effect on mortality of metoprolol in acute myocardial infarction. Lancet 2:823, 1981. © by the Lancet Ltd., 1981.)

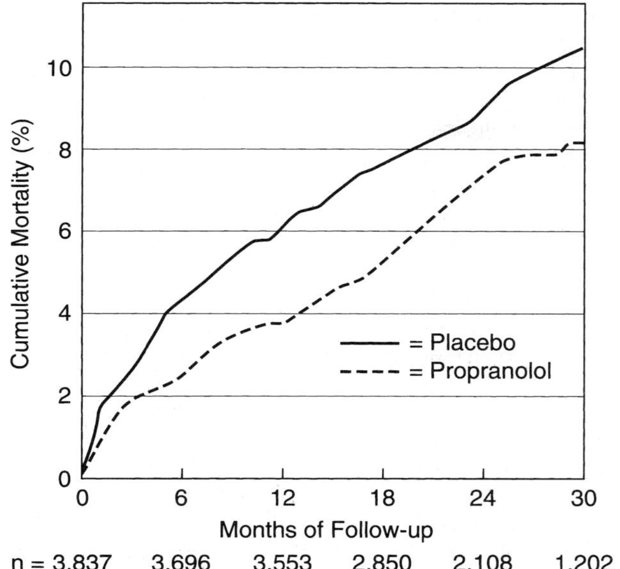

FIGURE 36–11 The influence of propranolol in reducing mortality in patients after myocardial infarction is shown in this figure. (From Beta-Blocker Heart Attack Study Group: The beta-blocker heart attack trial. JAMA 246:2073, 1981. Copyright 1981, American Medical Association.)

acute MI with marked bradycardia, AV block, clinically severe CHF, bronchospasm, and/or systemic arterial hypotension. They should also be used very carefully in the patient with insulin-dependent diabetes mellitus.

Schematic diagrams for therapeutic options in the management of patients after acute MI and their initial therapy are shown in Figure 36–13.

Treatment of Specific Complications of Myocardial Infarction

Cardiogenic shock is defined as systemic arterial hypotension caused by extensive infarction of the left or right ventricle with the amount of irreversible myocardial damage usually equal to or exceeding 40 percent of the muscle mass.[372] Prompt opening of the infarct-related artery should be attempted, preferably with PTCA, and if this is not feasible, with thrombolytic therapy. Immediate coronary artery bypass grafting is another alternative if one can perform it promptly. PTCA performed within 2 hours of symptom onset and resulting in opening the infarct-related artery may reverse cardiogenic shock.[373, 374] PTCA appears to be the most effective means to open the infarct-related artery in such patients, allowing approximately 50 percent to survive when they receive early reperfusion (i.e., within the first 2 hours of symptom onset).[373, 374] In patients in whom the infarct-related artery is not opened promptly, the risk for death is substantial. Patients in whom prompt opening of the infarct-related artery is not possible within the initial 2 hours can occasionally be saved by an aggressive regimen that includes inotropic agents, such as dobutamine, dopamine, or norepinephrine; diuresis; and mechanical circulatory assistance.[375–381] However, most patients die as the result of extensive heart muscle damage in the absence of an acute intervention that restores coronary blood flow. The further development of artificial heart devices that can be used indefinitely and/or the ability to utilize cardiac transplantation rapidly or after a period of cardiac assistance with an artificial heart device should result in enhanced survival of patients with extensive MI. Most patients with cardiogenic shock resulting from LV infarction either have anterior Q wave infarcts or have had several previous infarcts, making the location of the most recent infarct relatively less important.

Right Ventricular Infarcts

Cardiogenic shock occurs in some patients with extensive right ventricular (RV) infarction.[382–392] In almost every instance, these patients have inferior Q wave infarcts, elevated RV end-diastolic and right atrial pressures, low or normal mean pulmonary capillary wedge pressures, and

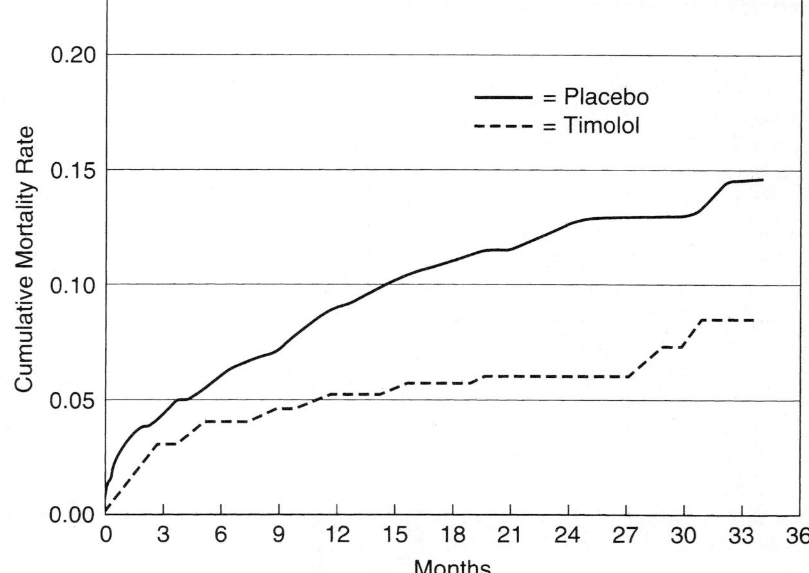

FIGURE 36–12 The influence of the nonspecific β-blocker, timolol, on cumulative mortality in patients after myocardial infarction. Administration of timolol significantly reduced mortality among the patients for more than 30 months after myocardial infarction. (From the Norwegian Multicenter Study Group: Timolol-induced reduction in mortality and reinfarction in patients surviving acute myocardial infarction. N Engl J Med 304:801, 1981. Copyright © 1981 Massachusetts Medical Society. All rights reserved.)

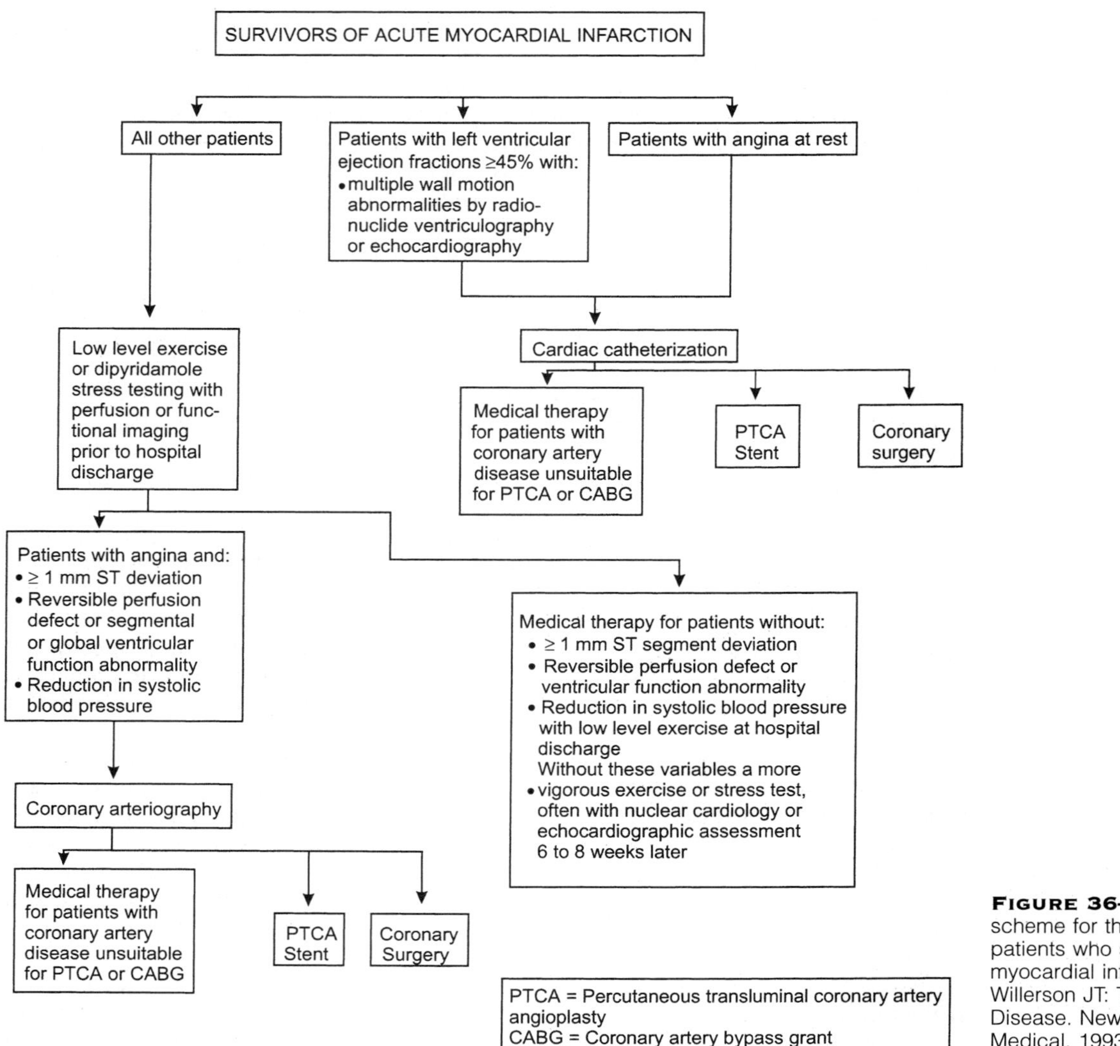

FIGURE 36–13 A suggested scheme for the management of patients who survive their myocardial infarcts. (From Willerson JT: Treatment of Heart Disease. New York: Gower Medical, 1993.)

preserved LV function. Clinically, these patients present with systemic arterial hypotension, tachycardia, elevated venous pressure, and clinical evidence of RV dysfunction, clear lungs, but relatively normal mean pulmonary capillary wedge pressures. They can usually be stabilized by promptly expanding their intravascular volume with saline and by raising their mean pulmonary capillary wedge pressures to values of 16 to 20 mm Hg, if necessary, to restore an adequate systemic arterial blood pressure. If hypotension is corrected rapidly, most of these patients survive. An alternative or additive therapy includes the administration of a thrombolytic agent or the use of PTCA to open the infarct-related artery promptly. RV infarction can be identified in patients with inferior Q wave infarcts by obtaining right precordial leads that show ST segment elevation in leads V_4R or V_4R to V_6R (Fig. 36–14).[390] RV infarction may be suggested also by two-dimensional echocardiography, radionuclide ventriculography, magnetic resonance imaging, or another imaging procedure that shows RV dysfunction in the patient with an inferior infarct.

Acute Ventricular Septal Defects

Acute ventricular septal defects (VSDs) usually occur in patients with Q wave infarcts, often anterior Q wave infarcts.[393–399] A new systolic murmur located at the lower left sternal border suggests the development of a VSD (or acute mitral insufficiency), which can occur within hours to 14 days after MI. If the VSD is large enough to allow a left-to-right shunt of 1.5 or greater, pressure and volume loads are placed on the heart, and ventricular failure often ensues. Acute VSDs are usually associated with a palpable systolic thrill and a holosystolic murmur located at the left sternal border. A flow-directed catheter demonstrates an oxygen step-up in the right heart, and with pulmonary-to-systemic flow ratios of approximately 2:1 or greater, there is a future risk for pulmonary hypertension. Defects of this size must be closed.[395–399] Subacute bacterial endocarditis is an additional risk in the patient with a VSD. With the development of a murmur consistent with possible VSD, a flow-directed catheter should be inserted so that one can identify an oxygen step-up in the right ventricle if it is present. A two-dimensional echocardiogram with Doppler can be used to identify the presence and the location of a VSD and to estimate the shunt size. These patients are given a diuretic and an unloading intervention, such as intravenous nitroprusside and/or an ACE inhibitor or angiotensin receptor blocker if their blood pressures allow. Initial doses of these agents depend on the systemic arterial blood pressure and the need to avoid hypotension and tachycardia, but they are typically 5 mg PO once a day, increasing to two to four times per day if necessary for enalapril, and 6.5 mg PO three times per day, increasing to 25 to 50 mg three times per day, if necessary, for captopril. There are several other ACE inhibitors that might be used as alternative therapies. However, with the earliest development of CHF (development of tachycardia, increase in respiratory rate, reduction in blood pressure, or development of radiographic evidence of CHF), the VSD should be promptly closed surgically today, but most likely by some type of clam-shell occluder in the future. With surgical closure of the VSD, coronary artery bypass grafting of the infarct-related artery and other importantly narrowed coronary arteries is usually accomplished at the same time. The operative risk for correcting a VSD immediately after MI is substantial, but failing to correct the defect and allowing CHF to progress often leads to death.

Acute Mitral Insufficiency

Acute mitral insufficiency may occur as a consequence of papillary muscle dysfunction or rupture.[400–407] With papillary muscle rupture, severe mitral insufficiency develops. Papillary muscle dysfunction usually leads to mild or moderate mitral insufficiency. In both circumstances, severe CHF may ensue. With mitral papillary muscle rupture, prompt surgical correction of the mitral insufficiency, either by primary repair or by replacement with a new valve, is mandatory if the patient is to survive. With papillary muscle rupture, there may be a soft apical systolic murmur or, on occasion, no audible murmur. Typically, there is a late-peaking systolic murmur at the cardiac apex in the patient with papillary muscle dysfunction. Third heart sounds are usually heard with moderate or severe mitral insufficiency, and the patient ordinarily has other evidence of CHF. Two-dimensional echocardiography with Doppler imaging enables detection and estimation of the severity of mitral insufficiency. A flow-directed catheter should permit demonstration of prominent V waves in the pulmonary capillary wedge tracing in the patient with acute mitral insufficiency. With papillary muscle dysfunction, medical therapy, including diuretics and/or systemic unloading interventions (e.g., intravenous nitroprusside), usually resolves the CHF.

Ventricular Aneurysms

A ventricular aneurysm is identified by the presence of systolic thinning of the infarcted segment during systole.[408–415] With large ventricular aneurysms, CHF may develop. Sustained ventricular tachycardia or embolic events from LV mural thrombi within the aneurysm are important potential complications.[416, 417] CHF is treated in a standard manner, including diuretics, digoxin, and unloading therapy with an ACE inhibitor, angiotensin receptor antagonist, or combined vasodilator and nitrates (e.g., hydralazine given as 25 to 50 mg PO every 6 to 8 hours and isosorbide dinitrate, 10 to 30 mg PO every 6 to 8 hours). Sustained ventricular tachycardia is treated by invasive electrophysiologic evaluation and an antiarrhythmic agent that is protective or by electrocardiographically guided surgical endocardial resection and coronary artery revascularization.[416, 417] Implantable automatic defibrillators are inserted in patients with recurrent ventricular tachycardia/ventricular fibrillation in whom no effective pharmacologic therapy has been identified and no completely successful surgical procedure can be employed. Systemic embolic events in patients with recently developed ventricular aneurysms are treated by heparin (usually for 10 to 14 days) and then with warfarin for at least 6 months. Six months or more after LV thrombi

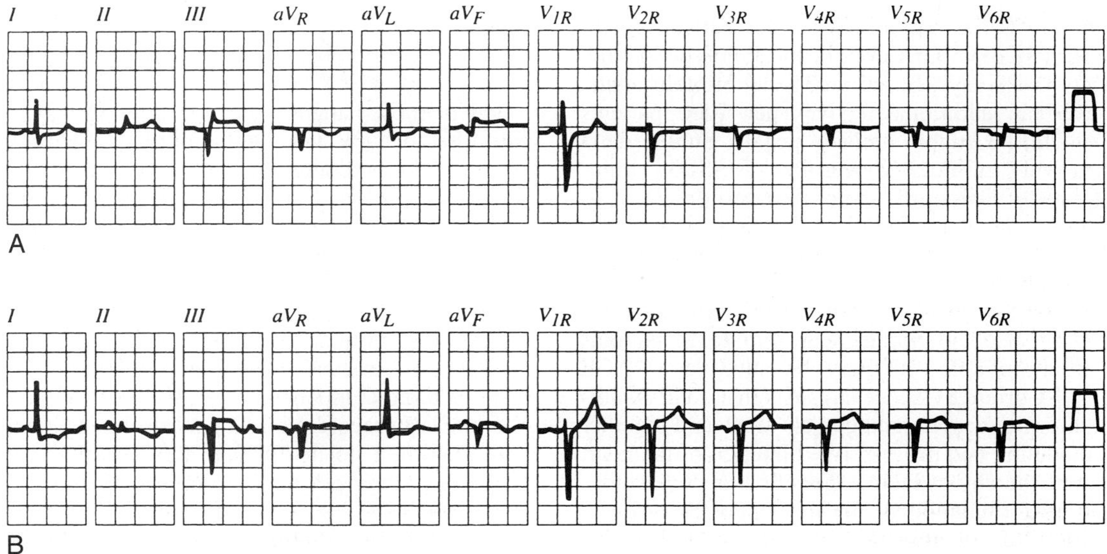

FIGURE 36–14 Electrocardiograms (ECGs) from two patients with inferior myocardial infarcts. **Top,** The right precordial leads (V_1R-V_6R) do not show important ST elevation. **Bottom,** ST-segment elevation is shown in the right precordial leads (V_3R-V_6R). The patient whose ECG is shown in the bottom panel had a right ventricular infarction, and the patient whose ECG is shown in the top panel did not.

form in ventricular aneurysms, they usually become firmly adherent to the LV endocardium, and the risk for systemic embolization is small. Anticoagulation therapy may no longer be necessary at that time.

Pseudoaneurysms

False ventricular aneurysms represent a partial rupture of the heart.[410–414, 418–420] The outer border of the aneurysm is the partial rupture and the pericardium. There is a serious risk for rupture of a false ventricular aneurysm, and it must be corrected surgically as soon as possible. A partial rupture of the heart is recognized by the identification of an enlarging pericardial effusion or pericardial tamponade in the patient after infarction. A two-dimensional echocardiogram with Doppler, a radionuclide ventriculogram, a magnetic resonance imaging study, or an LV angiogram often allows recognition of a false ventricular aneurysm, because these aneurysms typically communicate with the LV cavity through a narrow neck.[410, 411]

Angiotensin-Converting Enzyme Inhibitors to Treat Congestive Heart Failure and to Reduce Mortality

Studies have suggested that administration of an ACE inhibitor, such as captopril, in doses of 6.5 to 50 mg three times per day improves survival in patients after MI with LV dysfunction and LV failure and attenuates the development of progressive LV dilatation and CHF, especially in patients with anterior Q wave infarcts (SAVE Trial).[421] Other clinical trials, including the Consensus II and SOLVD trials, have demonstrated that enalapril in doses of 2.5 to 20 mg/day reduces the incidence of CHF in patients with recent infarction.[422, 423] The SOLVD trial demonstrated a reduction in mortality, incidence of reinfarction, and need for future hospitalizations for CHF in patients with reduced LV ejection fractions after MI (Fig. 36–15).[423] The Fourth International Study of Infarct Survival (ISIS-4) compared the effects of captopril with an oral controlled-release mononitrate, with intravenous magnesium, and with standard therapy in 58,000 patients who had had an MI.[424] Captopril was started within 1 hour of thrombolytic therapy and continued for 28 days. Based on 35-day mortality date, captopril saved an additional 5 lives per 1000 patients treated. The Third Gruppo Italiano per lo Studio della Sopravvienza Nell' Infarcto Miocardico (GISSI-3) evaluated the effects of lisinopril and/or nitrates on early (6 weeks) or late (6 months) mortality in patients with acute MI.[425] There was an 11 percent reduction in 6-week mortality after early therapy with lisinopril.[425]

Similar evidence is developing that angiotensin receptor antagonists may also ameliorate heart failure in patients with myocardial infarcts and may be additive to ACE inhibitors.[426, 427] Current evidence suggests that ACE inhibitors and angiotensin receptor antagonists alone and together attenuate remodeling and progressive dilatation of the heart after infarction, thereby reducing the subsequent development of CHF and dilatation of the heart and their consequences. There is also some evidence that the ACE inhibitors preserve vascular endothelial function. Thus, an appropriate ACE inhibitor and/or an angiotensin receptor antagonist should be given to patients without contraindication and beginning within hours or days after MI. Table 36–19 summarizes results of several ACE inhibitor trials in patients following myocardial infarction.

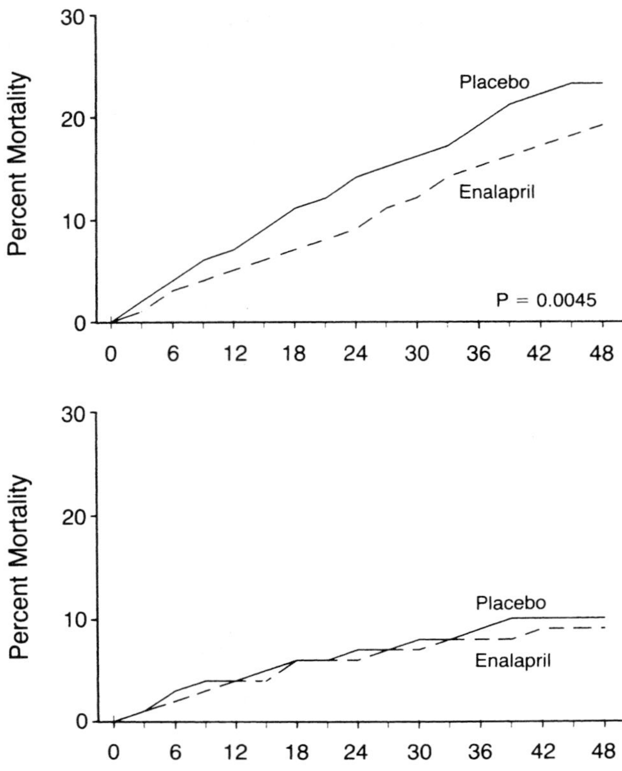

FIGURE 36–15 Mortality due to progressive heart failure **(A)** (P = .0045) and presumed to be due to an arrhythmia but not preceded by worsening congestive heart failure **(B)** (not significant) are shown. (Reprinted, by permission, from The SOLVD Investigators: N Engl J Med 327:685, 1992.)

Pericarditis

Acute pericarditis occurs commonly in patients with acute Q wave MIs.[428, 429] Histologic evidence of pericarditis is found in most patients who die after Q wave MI. Chest pain that occurs with pericarditis can be mistaken for angina and/or a continuing MI. However, if the patient is carefully questioned, it is common for the clinician to find that the quality of the pain has changed and that it now has a pleuritic quality (i.e., it is increased in severity or occurs primarily with respiration, turning, coughing, or sneezing). It is often made worse by assumption of the supine position and is partially relieved by sitting up. On occasion, a pericardial friction rub, which consists of a two- or three-component harsh leathery sound, is audible over the left precordium and persists during breath-holding. It is important not to mistake the pain of pericarditis for continuing angina after MI. In some patients, the chest pain associated with pericarditis responds well to moderate or large doses of aspirin (one to three buffered aspirin every 6 to 8 hours); however, the authors have found an even more beneficial response to small-to-moderate doses

TABLE 36–19 **Selected Studies of Therapy with Angiotensin-Converting Enzyme Inhibitors After Myocardial Infarction***

	Study (ref)	Patients Enrolled	Follow-Up	Event Rate (%) Drug	Event Rate (%) Placebo	Relative Risk of Death (CI, 95%)
Patients with Impaired LVEF	AIRE	2006	15 month	17.0	23.0	0.73 (0.69–0.89)
	SAVE	2231	42 month	20.4	24.6	0.81 (0.68–0.97)
	TRACE	1749	40 month	34.7	62.3	0.78 (0.70–0.86)
All Patients: No LVEF Screen	CONSENSUS II	6090	6 month	9.4	10.2	1.11 (0.93–1.29)
	ISIS-4	58,050	5 week	7.2	7.7	0.93 (0.87–0.99)
	GISSI-3	19,394	6 week	6.3	7.1	0.88 (0.79–0.99)

Abbreviations: ACE, angiotensin-converting enzyme; AIRE, Acute Infarction Ramipril Efficacy; CI, confidence interval; CONSENSUS, Cooperative New Scandinavian Enalapril Survival Study; EF, ejection fraction; GISSI, Gropo Italiano Per Lo Studio Della Streptochinasi Nell'Infarto Miocardico; ISIS, International Study of Infarct Survival; LVEF, left ventricular ejection fraction; MI, myocardial infarction; SAVE, Survival and Ventricular Enlargement; TRACE, Trandolapril Cardiac Evaluation.

*All trials except CONSENSUS II showed significant reductions in mortality in patients treated with ACE inhibitors. Patients with an impaired EF appeared to have a greater benefit.

of indomethacin (25 to 50 mg orally every 8 hours). In theory, indomethacin might cause problems when given to the patient with MI because its administration leads to coronary artery vasoconstriction, and, in animal models with infarction, it may interfere with infarct healing.[430] Nevertheless, it is usually very effective and has no obvious associated clinical problems when given to patients after acute infarction and in the weeks to months thereafter. Very rarely, steroid therapy is necessary to prevent disabling chest pain. However, it is desirable to avoid multidose and large-dose steroid therapy in patients soon after MI because this interferes with infarct healing, leads to a thinner scar, and is associated with increased risk for rupture of the heart.[431]

The patient with active pericarditis should not undergo anticoagulation unless there is a life-threatening condition that requires such therapy. There is a substantial risk for hemopericardium and pericardial tamponade in the patient who receives anticoagulant therapy during active pericarditis. The development of pericardial tamponade requires pericardiocentesis, and an indwelling pericardial catheter is often left in place for at least several days so that the chances for reaccumulation of a large pericardial effusion are lessened.

In some patients, pericarditis recurs after MI, requiring the use of long-term aspirin; nonsteroidal anti-inflammatory agents, such as indomethacin; or steroid therapy, or on occasion, when medical therapy does not provide pain relief, pericardial resection.

Infarct Extension

Infarct extension occurs generally when there is reinfarction after the acute event.[432, 433] Patients with systemic arterial hypertension, tachycardia, hypotension, and metabolic abnormalities, including hypoglycemia, are at risk for infarct extension (Table 36–20). In addition, patients who receive pharmacologic interventions that increase myocardial oxygen demand without increasing oxygen delivery are also at risk for infarct extension. Therefore, the use of powerful inotropic interventions that increase heart rate and/or contractile state substantially in the nonfailing heart

TABLE 36–20 **Univariate Analysis of Possible Risk Factors for Infarct Extension**

Risk Factor	Extension: Yes	Extension: No	P
Angina on the second hospital day	27/71 (38%)	177/777 (23%)	<.01
ST-segment depression on initial ECG	16/67 (24%)	97/755 (13%)	<.02
Previous myocardial infarction	24/71 (34%)	175/777 (23%)	<.04
Early peaking of MB creatine kinase (≤15 h)	25/70 (36%)	193/775 (25%)	<.05
History of diabetes mellitus	19/71 (27%)	138/770 (18%)	<.07
Obesity (body mass index > upper 25th percentile)	14/17 (20%)	197/773 (26%)	NS
Inferior ST-segment elevation or infarction on initial ECG	28/67 (42%)	388/755 (51%)	NS
Pretreatment left ventricular ejection fraction < 40%	28/62 (45%)	238/652 (37%)	NS
Angina > 3 wk before this episode	36/71 (51%)	344/777 (44%)	NS
Systolic pressure ≥ 150 mm Hg in first 48 h	51/71 (72%)	508/766 (66%)	NS
Anterior ST-segment elevation or infarction on initial ECG	27/67 (40%)	337/775 (45%)	NS
Diastolic pressure ≥ 90 mm Hg in first 48 h	59/70 (84%)	664/769 (86%)	NS
Heart rate > 100 in first 48 h	31/71 (44%)	325/769 (42%)	NS
Male sex	52/71 (73%)	564/777 (73%)	NS
Age (yr)	58.5 ± 1.1	56.7 ± 0.4	NS

Abbreviations: ECG, electrocardiogram; NS, not significant at .10 level.

From Muller JE, Rude RE, Braunwald E, et al: Myocardial infarct extension: incidence, outcome, and risk factors in MILIS study. Ann Intern Med 108:1, 1988.

should be avoided in attempts to preclude increasing myocardial oxygen demand above its availability, which may lead to consequent extension of the infarct. Reocclusion of the infarct-related artery after thrombolytic therapy may also cause infarct extension.

Infarct Expansion or "Remodeling"

Infarct expansion is caused by stress and strain relationships within the infarct area and very likely the release of certain proteases that cause the degradation of collagen and dilatation of the heart.[434–442] There is a topographic enlargement of the infarct area and an increase in LV diastolic and systolic dimensions after acute MI without any change in the extent of infarction. It is associated with progressive cardiac enlargement and deterioration of ventricular function, with increased morbidity and mortality.[434–447] Remodeling of the infarct is most likely to occur in patients with systemic arterial hypertension, in patients with anterior MIs, in patients with large infarcts, in patients with transmural extent of the infarct in those with an occluded infarct-related artery, and in older patients.[441–447] Ventricular remodeling is now recognized as one of the major dominant factors that determines long-term survival of patients who have had an MI. Clinical studies have suggested that an early assessment (day 31) of Doppler-derived mitral deceleration time provides a relatively simple and accurate means to predict late LV dilation after reperfused MI.[448] There appears to be a significant inverse relationship between deceleration time and changes in LV end-diastolic volume 6 months after MI.[448]

Pfeffer and colleagues[437] have shown that ACE inhibitors reduce infarct expansion and remodeling of the infarct. An open infarct-related artery also reduces the risk of infarct remodeling in subsequent months. Future studies are very likely to demonstrate that angiotensin receptor inhibitors exert the same beneficial effect. Control of systemic arterial hypertension is important in the patient with MI to reduce the risk for infarct expansion or extension and rupture of the heart. Rupture of the heart occurs most commonly in patients with their first infarcts, in elderly patients, and in patients who have systemic arterial hypertension during and after MI. Blood pressure control is also important in patients with recent MI to prevent the development of worsening CHF or new myocardial ischemia or infarction as a result of increased afterload, increasing LV wall tension, and myocardial oxygen demand. Agents chosen to treat systemic arterial hypertension during and after infarction should be those that do not importantly depress ventricular function or markedly increase heart rate. ACE inhibitors, selected calcium antagonists, and nitrates including intravenous nitroglycerin, nitroprusside, and β-blockers can be used in selected patients to control blood pressure and to prevent the complications mentioned earlier.

Heart Block

Heart block occurs as a consequence of acute or chronic CAD and with acute MI. Chapter 3, Chest Radiography, and Chapter 8, Pathophysiology, Clinical Recognition, and Treatment of Congenital Heart Disease, provide a detailed discussion of mechanisms, recognition, and treatment of heart block. First-degree heart block alone requires no therapy, although one should avoid medications that might further slow AV conduction. Second-degree heart block of the Mobitz I ("Wenckebach's") type occurs primarily in patients with acute inferior MIs (or recurrent inferior ischemia associated with a significant right or circumflex coronary artery stenosis). It also develops in patients who have degenerative conduction system disease, in those given excessive amounts of a cardiac glycoside, and in some highly trained athletes. It is usually an infrajunctional (AV nodal) form of heart block. Mobitz I heart block requires pacing only if the ventricular rate is slow enough to cause hemodynamic or electrical problems, including dizziness or syncope, progressive angina, or CHF, and/or if it predisposes to enhanced re-entry mechanisms and frequent or complex ventricular premature beats. Mobitz II heart block is an intraventricular block that is unstable and is usually associated with an acute anterior MI or degenerative conduction system disease. It is not caused by digitalis overdose. A temporary pacemaker should be inserted when this form of heart block develops, often followed later by a permanent pacemaker. Complete heart block may develop for many reasons, including acute MI, cardiac glycoside excess, and degenerative conduction system disease. When it complicates acute MI, a temporary pacemaker should be inserted, followed later by a permanent pacemaker if the heart block fails to resolve. In the patient with an acute inferior MI, complete heart block almost always resolves within 3 to 4 days, although sometimes up to 2 weeks. It rarely requires permanent pacing. With anterior infarcts, complete heart block often does not resolve, requiring permanent pacing.

Bundle Branch Block

The development of acute left bundle branch block with MI occurs in patients with large infarcts and infarcts often complicated by heart failure and/or shock. The risk for developing complete heart block is 20 to 40 percent, and prophylactic insertion of a temporary pacemaker is recommended. If AV block does not develop in the subsequent week, the pacemaker can be removed. In the patient who develops acute right bundle branch block, close monitoring should be provided, but the risk for developing complete heart block is only approximately 10 percent. The acute development of bilateral bundle branch block (left-axis deviation and right bundle branch block, right-axis deviation and right bundle branch block, first-degree AV block and left bundle branch block, or alternating left and right bundle branch block on the electrocardiogram) is associated with a large infarct. These infarcts are usually complicated by CHF, complete heart block, shock, and/or death. Complete heart block develops in approximately 40 to 60 percent of those patients not receiving thrombolytic therapy, and a temporary pacemaker should be inserted prophylactically. Early thrombolytic therapy or PTCA in these patients sometimes reverses the bilateral bundle branch block and reduces ultimate infarct size, thereby altering the otherwise expected adverse outcome. In patients who experience first-degree or greater AV block with bilateral bundle branch block, a permanent pacemaker should be inserted.

When left bundle, right bundle, or bilateral bundle branch block precedes an infarct, pacemaker insertion is not recommended prophylactically, unless other clinical indications suggest the need for this form of therapy.

Recurrent Myocardial Ischemia

Patients who have recurrent myocardial ischemia at rest or at low levels of activity after MI while receiving an appropriate medical regimen should be referred for coronary arteriography and PTCA or coronary artery revascularization if their coronary artery anatomy is suitable.[449–461] Submaximal exercise or stress perfusion or functional tests should be obtained 4 to 5 days after infarction to identify individuals with angina, ST segment deviation, reversible perfusion or functional responses, and/or life-threatening ventricular arrhythmias at low-level stress.[449–459, 461] Low-level exercise-induced arrhythmias are treated with appropriate antiarrhythmic agents, often β-blockers.

Patients with LV ejection fractions of 40 percent or less and more than 8 to 10 ventricular premature beats per hour, ventricular premature beat couplets, or runs of ventricular tachycardia have an increased risk for sudden death in the initial 6 months after myocardial infarction.[460] Reduction in systemic arterial blood pressure developing with low-level exercise in the patient after infarction and 3 mm or greater ST segment depression from a relatively normal electrocardiographic baseline suggest significant left main and/or important triple-vessel CAD.[451, 452, 459–461] Such patients should be evaluated by coronary arteriography. Patients with significant (≥50 percent luminal narrowing) left main coronary artery narrowing and in those with significant (≥70 percent or more luminal narrowing) three-vessel CAD, and those with severe proximal (≥90 percent narrowing) left anterior descending coronary artery and one other significant stenosis of an epicardial artery and LV dysfunction have their lives prolonged by coronary artery revascularization.

The addition of nuclear cardiology procedures, including perfusion scintigraphy with thallium 201 or technetium-labeled sestamibi, or other perfusion markers, or assessment of ventricular function by radionuclide ventriculography, MRI, or echocardiography with low-level exercise or other stress testing after infarction, allows identification of patients at risk for future important coronary events.[451, 458–460]

Additional Therapeutic Considerations

An open infarct-related artery is of benefit in reducing the risk of infarct remodeling and of sudden death in the subsequent months to year after MI. Thus, it may be in the patient's interest to consider opening the left anterior descending artery in the patient with a relatively recent Q wave MI, especially anterior Q wave MIs.[442, 444, 447, 461, 462]

In every patient, it is very important to correct all possible risk factors to reduce the risk of future coronary events. A reduction in total serum cholesterol and low-density lipoprotein levels, avoidance of cigarettes, control of hypertension, use of antioxidant vitamins and an inhibitor of platelet aggregation, control of weight, reduction in stress, and regular but careful exercise are critical issues in the physician's attempt to prevent recurrent MI. Cocaine use is a major hazard, and it must be prevented.[463] Cocaine promotes vasospasm and thrombosis, increases heart rate and systolic blood pressure, and may injure the vascular endothelium.[463] Thus, even a single exposure may cause the abrupt development of profound coronary artery vasoconstriction and/or thrombosis that leads to MI and/or sudden death.

The reader is referred to the websites of the American College of Cardiology (www.acc.org) and the American Heart Association (www.americanheart.org) for the ACC/AHA Guidelines for the Management of Patients with Acute Myocardial Infarction.

References

1. Roberts R, Rogers WJ, Mueller HS, et al, for the TIMI Investigators: Immediate versus deferred β-blockade following thrombolytic therapy in patients with acute myocardial infarction: results of the thrombolysis in myocardial infarction (TIMI) II-B Study. Circulation 83:422, 1991.
2. ISIS-I (First International Study of Infant Survival) Collaborative Group (1988): Mechanisms for the early mortality reduction produced by beta blockade started early in myocardial infarction. Lancet 1:921, 1988.
3. Ryden L, Ariniego R, Amman K, et al: A double blind trial of metoprolol in acute myocardial infarction: effects on ventricular tachyarrhythmias. N Engl J Med 308:614, 1983.
4. Rossi PRF, Yusuf S, Ramsdale D, et al: Reduction of ventricular arrhythmias by early intravenous atenolol in suspect acute myocardial infarction. BMJ 286:506, 1983.
5. Smalling RW, Bode C, Kalbfleisch J, et al: More rapid, complete, and stable coronary thrombolysis with bolus administration of reteplase compared with alteplase infusion in acute myocardial infarction. Circulation 91:2725, 1995.
6. Bode C, Smalling RW, Berg G, et al: Randomized comparison of coronary thrombolysis achieved with double-bolus reteplase (recombinant plasminogen activator) and front-loaded, accelerated alteplase (recombinant tissue plasminogen activator) in patients with acute myocardial infarction. Circulation 94:891, 1996.
7. Martin U, Sponer G, Strein K: Evaluation of thrombolytic and systemic effects of the novel recombinant plasminogen activator BM 06.022 compared with alteplase, anistreplase, streptokinase and urokinase in a canine model of coronary artery thrombosis. J Am Coll Cardiol 19:433, 1992.
8. International Joint Efficacy Comparison of Thrombolytics: Randomised, double-blind comparison of reteplase double-bolus administration with streptokinase in acute myocardial infarction (INJECT): trial to investigate equivalence. Lancet 346:329, 1995.
9. The Global Use of Strategies to Open Occluded Coronary Arteries (GUSTO III) Investigators: A comparison of reteplase with alteplase for acute myocardial infarction. N Engl J Med 337:1118, 1997.
10. InTIME Study Design. *In* Advances in Thrombolytic Therapy: Focus on Lanoteplase. p. 14. Slide Lecture Kit. Princeton, NJ: Bristol-Myers Squibb, 1998.
11. Lijnen HR, De Cock F, Matsuo O, Collen D: Comparative fibrinolytic and fibrinogenolytic properties of staphylokinase and streptokinase in plasma of different species in vitro. Fibrinolysis 6:33, 1992.
12. Collen D, Stockx L, Lacroix H, et al: Recombinant staphylokinase variants with altered immunoreactivity. IV: identification of variants with reduced antibody induction by intact potency. Circulation 95:463, 1997.
13. Collen D, De Cock F, Demarsin E, et al: Recombinant staphylokinase variants with altered immunoreactivity. III: species variability of antibody binding patterns. Circulation 95:455, 1997.
14. Vanderschueren S, Barrios L, Kerdsinchai P, et al: A randomized trial of recombinant staphylokinase versus alteplase for coronary artery patency in acute myocardial infarction. Circulation 92:2044, 1995.
15. Collen D, Lijnen HR, Vanderschueren S: Staphylokinase: fibrinolytic properties and current experience in patients with occlusive arterial thrombosis. Verh K Acad Geneeskd Blg 57:183, 1995.
16. Gulba DC, Bode C, Runge MS, Huber K: Thrombolytic agents: an overview. Ann Hematol 73(suppl I):S9, 1996.
17. Bar FW, Meyer J, Vermeer F, et al: Comparison of saruplase and

alteplase in acute myocardial infarction. Coron Artery Dis 79:727, 1997.

18. Teebe U, Michels R, Adgey J, et al: Randomized, double-blind study comparing saruplase with streptokinase therapy in acute myocardial infarction: the COMPASS equivalence trial. J Am Coll Cardiol 31:487, 1998.
19. Lee TH: A new, improved thrombolytic agent? J Watch Cardiol 3:33, 1997.
20. Keyt BA, Paoni NJ, Bennett WF: Site-directed mutagenesis of tissue-type plasminogen activator. *In* Cleland JL, Craik CS (eds): Protein Engineering: Principles and Practice. p. 435. Columbia, MO: Wiley-Liss, 1996.
21. Sasahara A, Loscalzo J: New therapeutic agents in thrombosis and thrombolysis. *In* McClusky ER, Keyt BA, Love TS (eds): TNK-tPA. New York: Marcel Dekker, 1996.
22. Cannon CP, McCabe CH, Gibson CM, et al: TNK-tissue plasminogen activator in acute myocardial infarction: results of the Thrombolysis in Myocardial Infarction (TIMI) 10A Dose-Ranging Trial. Circulation 95:351, 1997.
23. Fujise K, Revelle BM, Stacy L, et al: A tissue plasminogen activator/P-selectin fusion protein is an effective thrombolytic agent. Circulation 95:715, 1997.
24. Runge MS, Harker LA, Bode C, et al: Enhanced thrombolytic and antithrombotic potency of a fibrin-targeted plasminogen activator in baboons. Circulation 94:1412, 1996.
25. Delezonne C, Pozerski E: Action du sérum sanguin sur la gélatine en présence du chloroforme. C R Soc Biol (Paris) 55:327, 1903.
26. Milstone H: A factor in normal human blood which participates in streptococcal fibrinolysis. J Immunol 42:109, 1941.
27. Christensen LR: Streptococcal fibrinolysis: a proteolytic reaction due to a serum enzyme activated by streptococcal fibrinolysis. J Gen Physiol 28:363, 1945.
28. Sherry S, Fletcher AP, Alkjaersig N: Fibrinolysis and fibrinolytic activity in man. Physiol Rev 39:343, 1959.
29. DeWood MA, Spores J, Notske RN, et al: Prevalence of total coronary occlusion during the early hours of transmural myocardial infarction. N Engl J Med 303:897, 1980.
30. Tiefenbrunn AJ, Sobel BE: Factors contributing to the emergence of coronary thrombolysis. Cardiol Clin 5:49, 1987.
31. Rijken DL, Collen D: Purification and characterization of the plasminogen activator secreted by human melanoma cells in culture. J Biol Chem 256:7035, 1981.
32. Sobel BE: Thrombolysis in the treatment of acute myocardial infarction. *In* Fuster V, Verstraete M (eds): Thrombosis in Cardiovascular Diseases. p. 289. Philadelphia: WB Saunders, 1992.
33. Gruppo Italiano per lo Studio della Streptochinasi nell'Infarto Miocardico (GISSI): Effectiveness of intravenous thrombolytic treatment in acute myocardial infarction. Lancet 1:397, 1986.
34. ISIS-2 (Second International Study of Infarct Survival) Collaborative Group: Randomised trial of intravenous streptokinase, oral aspirin, both, or neither among 17,187 cases of suspected acute myocardial infarction: ISIS-2. Lancet 2:349, 1988.
35. van de Werf F, Arnold AER, for the European Cooperative Study Group for Recombinant Tissue-Type Plasminogen Activator: Effect of intravenous tissue plasminogen activator on infarct size, left ventricular function and survival in patients with acute myocardial infarction. BMJ 297:1374, 1988.
36. Reimer KA, Lowe JE, Tasmussen MM, Jennings RB: The wavefront phenomenon of ischemic cell death. I: myocardial infarct size vs duration of coronary occlusion in dogs. Circulation 56:786, 1977.
37. Bergmann SR, Lerch RA, Fox KAA, et al: Temporal dependence of beneficial effects of coronary thrombolysis characterized by positron tomography. Am J Med 73:573, 1982.
38. Weaver WD: Myocardial Infarction Triage and Intervention (MITI) trial of prehospital initiated thrombolysis: results. Presented at the American College of Cardiology National Meeting, Dallas, Texas, April 14, 1992.
39. Woolf N, Davies MJ: Interrelationships between atherosclerosis and thrombosis. *In* Fuster V, Verstraete M (eds): Thrombosis in Cardiovascular Diseases. p. 41. Philadelphia: WB Saunders, 1992.
40. Ogawa H, Yasue H, Oshima S, et al: Circadian variation of plasma fibrinopeptide A level in patients with variant angina. Circulation 80:1617, 1989.
41. Zalewski A, Shi Y, Nardone D, et al: Evidence for reduced fibrinolytic activity in unstable angina at rest. Circulation 83:1685, 1991.
42. Fitzgerald DJ: Platelet activation in the pathogenesis of unstable angina: importance in determining the response to plasminogen activators. Am J Cardiol 68:51B, 1991.
43. Chesebro JH, Zoldhelyi P, Fuster V: Pathogenesis of thrombosis in unstable angina. Am J Cardiol 68:2B, 1991.
44. Eisenberg PE, Sherman LA, Schechtman K, et al: Fibrinopeptide A: a marker of acute coronary thrombosis. Circulation 71:912, 1985.
45. DiSciascio G, Kohli RS, Goudreau E, et al: Intracoronary recombinant tissue-type plasminogen activator in unstable angina: a pilot angiographic study. Am Heart J 122:1, 1991.
46. Roberts WC: Qualitative and quantitative comparison of amounts of narrowing by atherosclerotic plaques in the major epicardial coronary arteries at necropsy in sudden coronary death, transmural acute myocardial infarction, transmural healed myocardial infarction and unstable angina pectoris. Am J Cardiol 64:324, 1989.
47. Roberts WC, Kragel AH, Gertz SD, et al: The heart in fatal unstable angina pectoris. Am J Cardiol 68:22B, 1991.
48. Collen D, Lijnen HR: The fibrinolytic system in man: an overview. *In* Collen D, Lijnen HR, Verstraete M (eds): Thrombolysis: Biological and Therapeutic Properties of New Thrombolytic Agents. p. 1. Edinburgh: Churchill Livingstone, 1985.
49. Collen D, Bounameaux H, De Cock F, et al: Analysis of coagulation and fibrinolysis during intravenous infusion of recombinant human tissue-type plasminogen activator in patients with acute myocardial infarction. Circulation 73:511, 1986.
50. Kawai C, Yui Y, Hosoda S, et al: A prospective, randomized, double-blind multicenter trial of a single bolus injection of the novel modified t-PA E6010 in the treatment of acute myocardial infarction: comparison with native t-PA. J Am Coll Cardiol 29:1447, 1997.
51. Fry ETA, Sobel BE: Coronary thrombolysis. Prog Cardiol 3/1:199, 1990.
52. Sobel BE, Hirsh J: Principles and practice of coronary thrombolysis and conjunctive treatment [editorial]. Am J Cardiol 68:382, 1991.
53. Werner RG, Bassarab S, Hoffman H, Schluter M: Quality aspects of fibrinolytic agents based on biochemical characterization. Arz Forsch 41:1196, 1991.
54. Vaughn DE, Vanhoutte E, Declerck PJ, Collen D: Streptokinase-induced platelet activation: prevalence and mechanisms. Circulation 84:84, 1991.
55. Peuhkurinen KJ, Risteli L, Melkko JT, et al: Thrombolytic therapy with streptokinase stimulates collagen breakdown. Circulation 83:1969, 1991.
56. Sundsmo JS, Fair DS: Relationships among the complement, kinin, coagulation, and fibrinolytic systems in the inflammatory reaction. Clin Physiol Biochem 1:225, 1983.
57. Munkvad S, Brandslund I, Gram J, Jespersen J: The complement system is activated by streptokinase, but not by recombinant tissue-type plasminogen activator (rt-PA) therapy in patients with myocardial infarction: a placebo-controlled study. Coron Artery Dis 2:889, 1991.
58. Goa KL, Henwood JM, Stolz JF, et al: Intravenous streptokinase: a reappraisal of its therapeutic use in acute myocardial infarction. Drugs 39:693, 1990.
59. Bucknall C, Darley C, Flax J, et al: Vasculitis complicating treatment with intravenous anisoylated plasminogen streptokinase activator complex in acute myocardial infarction. Br Heart J 59:9, 1988.
60. Sane DC, Little WC: Is time running out on streptokinase? J Am Coll Cardiol 31:780, 1998.
61. Taylor GL, Moses HW, Koester D, et al: A difference between front-loaded streptokinase and standard-dose recombinant tissue-type plasminogen activator in preserving left ventricular function after acute myocardial infarction (The Central Illinois Thrombolytic Therapy Study). Am J Cardiol 72:1010, 1993.
62. Steg PG, Laperche T, Golmard J-L, et al: Efficacy of streptokinase, but not tissue-type plasminogen activator, in achieving 90-minute patency after thrombolysis for acute myocardial infarction decreases with time to treatment. J Am Coll Cardiol 31:776, 1998.
63. Barbash GI, Hod H, Roth A, et al: Repeat infusion of recombinant tissue-type plasminogen activator in patients with acute myocardial infarction and early recurrent myocardial ischemia. J Am Coll Cardiol 16:779, 1990.
64. Sobel BE: Safety and efficacy of tissue-type plasminogen activator produced by recombinant DNA technology (rt-PA). J Am Coll Cardiol 10:40B, 1987.
65. Sobel BE: Coronary thrombolysis and the new biology. J Am Coll Cardiol 14:850, 1989.

66. Collen D: Coronary thrombolysis: streptokinase or recombinant tissue-type plasminogen activator? Ann Intern Med 112:529, 1990.
67. Chesebro JH, Knatterud G, Roberts R, et al: Thrombolysis in myocardial infarction (TIMI) trial, phase I: a comparison between intravenous tissue plasminogen activator and intravenous streptokinase. Circulation 76:142, 1987.
68. Verstraete M, Bernard R, Bory M, et al: Randomised trial of intravenous recombinant tissue-type plasminogen activator versus intravenous streptokinase in acute myocardial infarction. Lancet 1:842, 1985.
69. Sobel BE, Nachowiak DA, Fry ETA, et al: Paradoxical attenuation of fibrinolysis attributable to "plasminogen steal" and its implications for coronary thrombolysis. Coron Artery Dis 1:111, 1990.
70. Torr SR, Nachowiak DA, Fujii S, Sobel BE: "Plasminogen steal" and clot lysis. J Am Coll Cardiol 19:1085, 1992.
71. Potter van Loon BJ, Rijken DC, Brommer EJP, van der Maas APC: The amount of plasminogen, tissue-type plasminogen activator and plasminogen activator inhibitor type 1 in human thrombi and the relation to ex-vivo lysibility. Thromb Haemost 67:101, 1992.
72. Lamas GA, Flaker GC, Mitchell G, et al: Effect of infarct artery patency on prognosis after acute myocardial infarction. Circulation 92:1101, 1995.
73. Lenderink T, Simoons ML, Vans Es G-A, et al: Benefit of thrombolytic therapy is sustained throughout five years and is related to TIMI perfusion grade 3 but not grade 2 flow at discharge. Circulation 92:1110, 1995.
74. Barron HV, Bowlby LJ, Breen T, et al: Use of reperfusion therapy for acute myocardial infarction in the United States: data from the National Registry of Myocardial Infarction 2. Circulation 97:1150, 1998.
75. Rogers WJ, Tiefenbrunn AJ, French WJ, et al: National registry of myocardial infarction-phase I: 354,435 patients depicting evolving practice patterns in the United States. Eur Heart J 17 (suppl):25, 1996.
76. Tiefenbrunn AF, Chandra NC, French WJ, et al: Clinical experience with primary percutaneous transluminal coronary angioplasty compared with alteplase (recombinant tissue-type plasminogen activator) in patients with acute myocardial infarction. J Am Coll Cardiol 31:1240, 1998.
77. Roberts R: La différence: long-term benefit of one thrombolytic over another. Circulation 94:1203, 1996.
78. Selker HP, Beshansky JR, Schmid CH, et al: Presenting pulse pressure predicts thrombolytic therapy-related intracranial hemorrhage: Thrombolytic Predictive Instrument (TPI) project results. Circulation 90:1657, 1994.
79. Case Records of the Massachusetts General Hospital. N Engl J Med 335:192, 1996.
80. Shatos MA, Doherty JM, Penar PL, Sobel BE: Suppression of plasminogen activator inhibitor-1 release from human cerebral endothelium by plasminogen activators. Circulation 94:636, 1996.
81. Higgs ER, Parfitt VJ, Harney BA, Hartog M: Use of thrombolysis for acute myocardial infarction in the presence of diabetic retinopathy in the UK, and associated ocular haemorrhagic complications. Diabet Med 12:426, 1995.
82. Karnash SL, Granger CB, White HD, et al: Treating menstruating women with thrombolytic therapy: insights from the Global Utilization of Streptokinase and Tissue Plasminogen Activator for Occluded Coronary Arteries (GUSTO-I) trial. J Am Coll Cardiol 26:1651, 1995.
83. Verstraete M, Tygat G, Amera A, Vermylen J: Thrombolytic therapy with streptokinase using a standard dosage. Thromb Diath Haemorr 16 (suppl 21):494, 1966.
84. Fears R, Ferres H, Glasgow E, et al: Monitoring of streptokinase resistance titre in acute myocardial infarction patients up to 30 months after giving streptokinase or anistreplase and related studies to measure specific antistreptokinase IgG. Br Heart J 68:167, 1992.
85. Yusuf S, Collins R, Peto R, et al: Intravenous and intracoronary fibrinolytic therapy in acute myocardial infarction: overview of results on mortality, reinfarction and side effects from 33 randomized controlled trials. Eur Heart J 6:556, 1985.
86. Tiefenbrunn AJ, Sobel BE: The impact of coronary thrombolysis on myocardial infarction. Fibrinolysis 3:1, 1989.
87. Verstraete M, Arnold AER, Brower RW, et al: Acute coronary thrombolysis with recombinant tissue plasminogen activator: initial patency and influence of maintained infusion on reocclusion rate. Am J Cardiol 60:231, 1987.
88. Von Essen R, Zeymer U, Tebbe U, et al: HBW-23 (recombinant hirudin) for the acceleration of thrombolysis and prevention of coronary reocclusion in acute myocardial infarction: results of a dose-finding study (HIT-II) by the Arbeitsgemeinschaft Leitender Kardiologischer Krankenhausärzte. Coron Artery Dis 9:265, 1998.
89. Jun L, Arnout J, Vanhove P, et al: Comparison of a low-molecular-weight heparin (nadroparin calcium) and unfractionated heparin as adjunct to coronary thrombolysis with alteplase and aspirin in dogs. Coron Artery Dis 6:257, 1995.
90. Kleiman NS, Ohman EM, Califf RM, et al: Profound inhibition of platelet aggregation with monoclonal antibody 7E3 Fab after thrombolytic therapy: results of the Thrombolysis and Angioplasty in Myocardial Infarction (TAMI) 8 pilot study. J Am Coll Cardiol 22:381, 1993.
91. McKenzie CR, Abendschein DR, Eisenberg PR: Sustained inhibition of whole-blood clot procoagulant activity by inhibition of thrombus-associated factor Xa. Arterioscler Thromb Vasc Biol 16:1285, 1996.
92. Yasuda T, Gold HK, Leinbach RC, et al: Lysis of plasminogen activator-resistant platelet-rich coronary artery thrombus with combined bolus injection of recombinant tissue-type plasminogen activator and antiplatelet GPIIb/IIIa antibody. J Am Coll Cardiol 16:1728, 1990.
93. ISIS-3 (Third International Study of Infarct Survival Collaborative Group): A randomised comparison of streptokinase vs tissue plasminogen activator vs anistreplase and of aspirin plus heparin vs aspirin alone among 41,299 cases of suspected acute myocardial infarction. Lancet 339:753, 1992.
94. Gruppo Italiano Per Lo Studio Della Sopravvivenza Nell'infarcto Miocardico (GISSI-2): A factorial randomised trial of alteplase versus streptokinase and heparin versus no heparin among 12,490 patients with acute myocardial infarction. Lancet 336:65, 1990.
95. The International Study Group: In-hospital mortality and clinical course of 20,891 patients with suspected acute myocardial infarction randomized between alteplase and streptokinase with or without heparin. Lancet 336:71, 1990.
96. Sobel BE, Collen D: After ISIS-3. Lancet 339:1225, 1992.
97. Sobel BE, Collen D: Strokes, statistics, and sophistry in trials of thrombolysis for acute myocardial infarction. Am J Cardiol 71:424, 1993.
98. Sobel BE, Collen D: ISIS-3 and GISSI-2: critique of the meta-analysis. Am J Cardiol 71:1128, 1993.
99. Bleich SD, Nichols TC, Schumacher RR, et al: Effect of heparin on coronary arterial patency after thrombolysis with tissue plasminogen activator in acute myocardial infarction. Am J Cardiol 66:1412, 1990.
100. Hsia J, Hamilton WP, Kleiman N, et al: A comparison between heparin and low-dose aspirin as adjunctive therapy with tissue plasminogen activator for acute myocardial infarction. N Engl J Med 323:1433, 1990.
101. Bono DP, Simoons ML, Tijssen J, et al: Effect of early intravenous heparin on coronary patency, infarct size, and bleeding complications after alteplase thrombolysis: results of a randomised double blind European Cooperative Study Group trial. Br Heart J 67:122, 1992.
102. Bergmann SR, Fox KAA, Ter-Pogossian MM, et al: Clot-selective coronary thrombolysis with tissue-type plasminogen activator. Science 220:1181, 1983.
103. van de Werf F, Bergmann SR, Fox KAA, et al: Coronary thrombolysis with intravenously administered human tissue-type plasminogen activator produced by recombinant DNA technology. Circulation 69:605, 1984.
104. van de Werf F, Ludbrook PA, Bergmann SR, et al: Coronary thrombolysis with tissue-type plasminogen activator in patients with evolving myocardial infarction. N Engl J Med 310:609, 1984.
105. The TIMI Study Group: The Thrombolysis in Myocardial Infarction (TIMI) trial. N Engl J Med 312:932, 1985.
106. Weaver WD, Eisenberg MS, Martin JS, et al: Myocardial Infarction Triage and Intervention Project—Phase I: patient characteristics and feasibility of prehospital initiation of thrombolytic therapy. J Am Coll Cardiol 15:925, 1990.
107. Boissel J-P: European Myocardial Infarction Project (EMIP): Short-term mortality and nonfatal outcomes. Presented at the American College of Cardiology National Meeting, Dallas, TX, April 15, 1992.
108. Tiefenbrunn AJ, Sobel BE: Timing of coronary recanalization: paradigms, paradoxes, and pertinence. Circulation 85:2311, 1992.

109. White CW: Simplicity's virtue scorned: precision comes to TIMI flow grading and the results are . . . surprising. Circulation 93:853, 1996.
110. Iwakura K, Ito H, Takiuchi S, et al: Alternation in the coronary blood flow velocity pattern in patients with no reflow and reperfused acute myocardial infarction. Circulation 94:1269, 1996.
111. Sobel BE: Conundrums in coronary thrombolysis: the TIMI-II/TIMI-III flow dichotomy and the denominator problem. Coron Artery Dis 7:81, 1996.
112. Verheugt FWA, Meijer A, Lagrand WK, et al: Reocclusion: the flip side of coronary thrombolysis. J Am Coll Cardiol 27:766, 1996.
113. Brouwer MA, Bohncke JR, Veen G, et al: Adverse long-term effects of reocclusion after coronary thrombolysis. J Am Coll Cardiol 26:1440, 1995.
114. Maes A, Van de Werf F, Nuyts J, et al: Impaired myocardial tissue perfusion early after successful thrombolysis. Impact on myocardial flow, metabolism, and function at late follow-up. Circulation 92:2072, 1995.
115. Tiefenbrunn AJ, Graor RA, Robison AK, et al: Pharmacodynamics of tissue-type plasminogen activator (t-PA) characterized by computer-assisted simulation. Circulation 73:1291, 1986.
116. Eisenberg PR, Sherman LA, Tiefenbrunn AI, et al: Sustained fibrinolysis after administration of t-PA despite its short half life in the circulation. Thromb Haemost 57:35, 1987.
117. Sakharov DV, Rijken DC: Superficial accumulation of plasminogen during plasma clot lysis. Circulation 92:1883, 1995.
118. Neuhaus K-L, Feurer W, Jeep-Tebbe S, et al: Improved thrombolysis with a modified dose regimen of recombinant tissue-type plasminogen activator. J Am Coll Cardiol 14:1566, 1989.
119. Tanswell P, Tebbe U, Neuhaus K-L, et al: Pharmacokinetics and fibrin specificity of alteplase during accelerated infusions in acute myocardial infarction. J Am Coll Cardiol 19:1071, 1992.
120. Tebbe U, Tanswell P, Seifried E, et al: Single-bolus injection of recombinant tissue-type plasminogen activator in acute myocardial infarction. Am J Cardiol 64:448, 1989.
121. Tranchesi B, Verstraete M, Vanhove PH, et al: Intravenous bolus administration of recombinant tissue plasminogen activator to patients with acute myocardial infarction. Coron Artery Dis 1:83, 1990.
122. Wall TC, Califf RM, George BS, et al: Accelerated plasminogen activator dose regimens for coronary thrombolysis. J Am Coll Cardiol 19:482, 1992.
123. Vaughan DE, Braunwald E: Front-loaded accelerated infusions of tissue plasminogen activator: putting a better foot forward. J Am Coll Cardiol 19:1076, 1992.
124. Cannon CP, McCabe CH, Diver DJ, et al: Comparison of front-loaded recombinant tissue-type plasminogen activator, anistreplase and combination thrombolytic therapy for acute myocardial infarction: results of the Thrombolysis in Myocardial Infarction (TIMI) 4 Trial. J Am Coll Cardiol 24:1602, 1994.
125. Purvis JA, McNeill AJ, Siddiqui RA, et al: Efficacy of 100 mg of double-bolus alteplase in achieving complete perfusion in the treatment of acute myocardial infarction. J Am Coll Cardiol 23:6, 1994.
126. The Continuous Infusion versus Double-Bolus Administration of Alteplase (COBALT) Investigators: A comparison of continuous infusion of alteplase with double-bolus administration for acute myocardial infarction. N Engl J Med 337:1124, 1997.
127. Gulba DC, Tanswell P, Dechend R: Sixty-minute alteplase protocol: a new accelerated recombinant tissue-type plasminogen activator regimen for thrombolysis in acute myocardial infarction. J Am Coll Cardiol 30:1611, 1997.
128. Sabovic M, Lijnen HR, Keber D, Collen D: Effect of retraction on the lysis of human clots with fibrin-specific and nonfibrin-specific plasminogen activators. Thromb Haemost 62:1083, 1989.
129. Nishino N, Kakkar VV, Scully MF: Influence of intrinsic and extrinsic plasminogen upon the lysis of thrombi in vitro. Thromb Haemost 66:672, 1991.
130. Fox KAA, Robison AK, Knabb RM, et al: Prevention of coronary thrombosis with subthrombolytic doses of tissue-type plasminogen activator. Circulation 72:1346, 1985.
131. Kunitada S, FitzGerald GA, Fitzgerald DJ: Inhibition of clot lysis and decreased binding of tissue-type plasminogen activator as a consequence of clot retraction. Blood 79:1420, 1992.
132. Lee CD, Mann KG: Activation/inactivation of human factor V by plasmin. Blood 73:185, 1989.
133. Ewald GA, Eisenberg PR: Plasmin-mediated activation of contact system in response to pharmacological thrombolysis. Circulation 91:28, 1995.
134. Munkvad S, Jespersen J, Gram J, Kluft C: Long-lasting depression of the factor XII-dependent fibrinolytic system in patients with myocardial infarction undergoing thrombolytic therapy with recombinant tissue-type plasminogen activator: a randomized placebo-controlled study. J Am Coll Cardiol 17:957, 1991.
135. Schaiff WT, Eisenberg PR: Direct induction of complement activation by pharmacologic activation of plasminogen. Coron Artery Dis 8:9, 1997.
136. Loskutoff DJ: Carboxypeptidases: new regulators of plasminogen activation in vivo? J Clin Invest 96:2104, 1995.
137. Schneider DJ, Tracy PB, Sobel BE: Acute coronary syndromes. 1: the platelet's role. Hosp Pract 32:171, 1998.
138. Schneider DK, Tracy PB, Sobel BE: Acute coronary syndromes. 2: antiplatelet agents. Hosp Pract 33:107, 1998.
139. Vaughan DE, Kirshenbaum JM, Loscalzo J: Streptokinase-induced, antibody-mediated platelet aggregation: a potential cause of clot propagation in vivo. J Am Coll Cardiol 11:1343, 1988.
140. Eisenberg PR, Sobel BE, Jaffe AS: Activation of prothrombin accompanying thrombolysis with recombinant tissue-type plasminogen activator. J Am Coll Cardiol 19:1065, 1992.
141. Sobel BE: Coronary thrombolysis: editorial overview. Coron Artery Dis 1:3, 1990.
142. Garabedian HD, Gold HK: Coronary thrombolysis, conjunctive heparin, and the effect on systemic thrombin activity. Circulation 85:1205, 1992.
143. Qiao J-H, Fishbein MC: The severity of coronary atherosclerosis at sites of plaque rupture with occlusive thrombosis. J Am Coll Cardiol 17:1138, 1991.
144. Ohman EM, Califf RM, Topol EJ, et al: Consequences of reocclusion after successful reperfusion therapy in acute myocardial infarction. Circulation 82:781, 1990.
145. Eisenberg PR, Miletich JP, Sobel BE: Factors responsible for differential procoagulant effects of diverse plasminogen activators in plasma. Fibrinolysis 5:217, 1991.
146. Eisenberg PR, Miletich JE, Sobel BE, Jaffe AS: Differential effects of activation of prothrombin by streptokinase compared with urokinase and tissue-type plasminogen activator (t-PA). Thromb Res 50:707, 1988.
147. Eisenberg PR, Sherman L, Rich M, et al: Importance of continued activation of thrombin reflected by fibrinopeptide A to the efficacy of thrombolysis. J Am Coll Cardiol 7:1255, 1986.
148. Eisenberg PR, Sherman LA, Jaffe AS: Paradoxic elevation of fibrinopeptide A after streptokinase: evidence of continued thrombosis despite intense fibrinolysis. J Am Coll Cardiol 10:527, 1987.
149. Rapold HJ, deBono D, Arnold AER, et al: Plasma fibrinopeptide A levels in patients with acute myocardial infarction treated with alteplase: correlation with concomitant heparin, coronary artery patency, and recurrent ischemia. Circulation 85:928, 1992.
150. Gulba DC, Barthels M, Westhoff-Bleck M, et al: Increased thrombin levels during thrombolytic therapy in acute myocardial infarction. Circulation 83:937, 1991.
151. Merlini PA, Bauer KA, Oltrona L, et al: Thrombin generation and activity during thrombolysis and concomitant heparin therapy in patients with acute myocardial infarction. J Am Coll Cardiol 25:203, 1995.
152. Zoldhelyi P, Bichler J, Owen WG, et al: Persistent thrombin generation in humans during specific thrombin inhibition with hirudin. Circulation 90:2671, 1994.
153. Granger CB, Miller JM, Bovill EG, et al: Rebound increase in thrombin generation and activity after cessation of intravenous heparin in patients with acute coronary syndromes. Circulation 91:1929, 1995.
154. Galvani M, Abendschein DR, Ferrini D, et al: Failure of fixed dose intravenous heparin to suppress increases in thrombin activity after coronary thrombolysis with streptokinase. J Am Coll Cardiol 24:1445, 1994.
155. Oltrona L, Eisenberg PR, Lasala JM, et al: Association of heparin-resistant thrombin activity with acute ischemic complications of coronary interventions. Circulation 94:2064, 1996.
156. Theroux P, Perez-Villa F, Waters D, et al: Randomized double-blind comparison of two doses of hirulog with heparin as adjunctive therapy to streptokinase to promote early patency of the infarct-related artery in acute myocardial infarction. Circulation 91:2132, 1995.

157. White HD, Aylward PE, Frey MJ, et al: Randomized, double-blind comparison of hirulog versus heparin in patients receiving streptokinase and aspirin for acute myocardial infarction (HERO). Circulation 96:2155, 1997.
158. Neuhaus K-L, v Essen R, Tebbe U, et al: Safety observations from the pilot phase of the randomized r-hirudin for improvement of thrombolysis (HIT-III) study. Circulation 90:1638, 1994.
159. The Global Use of Strategies to Open Occluded Coronary Arteries (GUSTO) IIa Investigators: Randomized trial of intravenous heparin versus recombinant hirudin for acute coronary syndromes. Circulation 90:1631, 1994.
160. Cannon CP, Braunwald E: Hirudin: Initial results in acute myocardial infarction, unstable angina and angioplasty. J Am Coll Cardiol 25(suppl):30S, 1995.
161. Antman EM for the TIMI 9B Investigators: Hirudin in acute myocardial infarction: Thrombolysis and Thrombin Inhibition in Myocardial Infarction (TIMI) 9B trial. Circulation 94:911, 1996.
162. The Global Use of Strategies to Open Occluded Coronary Arteries (GUSTO) IIb Investigators: A comparison of recombinant hirudin with heparin for the treatment of acute coronary syndromes. N Engl J Med 335:775, 1996.
163. Antman EM for the TIMI 9A Investigators: Hirudin in acute myocardial infarction: safety report from the Thrombolysis and Thrombin Inhibition in Myocardial Infarction (TIMI) 9A trial. Circulation 90:1624, 1994.
164. Cannon CP, McCabe CH, Diver DJ, et al: Comparison of front-loaded recombinant tissue-type plasminogen activator, anistreplase and combination thrombolytic therapy for acute myocardial infarction: results of the Thrombolysis in Myocardial Infarction (TIMI) 4 Trial. J Am Coll Cardiol 24:1602, 1994.
165. Eisenberg PR: Mechanism of action of heparin and anticoagulation therapy: implications for the prevention of arterial thrombosis and the treatment of mural thrombosis. Coron Artery Dis 1:159, 1990.
166. Rapold HJ: Promotion of thrombin activity by simultaneous thrombolytic therapy without simultaneous anticoagulation. Lancet 1:481, 1990.
167. Scarfstein JS, Abendschein DR, Eisenberg PR, et al: Usefulness of fibrinogenolytic and procoagulant markers during thrombolytic therapy in predicting clinical outcomes in acute myocardial infarction. Am J Cardiol 78:503, 1996.
168. Thompson PL, Aylward PE, Federman J, et al: A randomized comparison of intravenous heparin with oral aspirin and dipyridamole 24 hours after recombinant tissue-type plasminogen activator for acute myocardial infarction. Circulation 83:1534, 1991.
169. Mahan EF, Chandler JW, Rogers WJ, et al: Heparin and infarct coronary artery patency after streptokinase in acute myocardial infarction. Am J Cardiol 65:967, 1990.
170. Hirsh J: Heparin. N Engl J Med 324:1565, 1991.
171. Verheugt FWA, Marsh RC, Veen G, et al: Megadose bolus heparin as reperfusion therapy for acute myocardial infarction: results of the HEAP pilot study. J Am Coll Cardiol (suppl A):11A, 1996.
172. Verheugt FWA, Liem A, Zijlstra F, et al: High dose bolus heparin as initial therapy before primary angioplasty for acute myocardial infarction: results of the Heparin in Early Patency (HEAP) pilot study. J Am Coll Cardiol 31:289, 1998.
173. Gurbel PA, Serebruany VL, Shustov AR, et al: Effects of reteplase and alteplase on platelet aggregation and major receptor expression during the first 24 hours of acute myocardial infarction treatment. J Am Coll Cardiol 31:1466, 1998.
174. Furman MI, Benoit SE, Barnard MR, et al: Increased platelet reactivity and circulating monocyte-platelet aggregates in patients with stable coronary artery disease. J Am Coll Cardiol 31:352, 1998.
175. Salzman EW: Low-molecular-weight heparin and other new antithrombotic drugs. N Engl J Med 326:1017, 1992.
176. Farrell TP, Hayes KB, Sobel BE, Schneider DJ: The lack of augmentation by aspirin of inhibition of platelet reactivity by ticlopidine. Am J Cardiol 83:770–774, 1999.
177. Holmes MB, Sobel BE, Howard DB, Schneider DJ: Differences between activation thresholds for platelet P-selectin and glycoprotein IIb-IIIa expression and their clinical implications. Thromb Res 95:75–82, 1999.
178. Cannon CP, McCabe CH, Borzak S, et al: Randomized trial of an oral platelet glycoprotein IIb/IIIa antagonist, sibrafiban, in patients after an acute coronary syndrome: results of the TIMI 12 trial. Circulation 97:340, 1998.
179. Haskel EJ, Torr SR, Day KC, et al: Prevention of arterial reocclusion after thrombolysis with recombinant lipoprotein-associated coagulation inhibitor. Circulation 84:821, 1991.
180. Vlasuk GP, Ramjit D, Fujita T, et al: Comparison of the in vivo anticoagulant properties of standard heparin and the highly selective factor Xa inhibitors antistasin and tick anticoagulant peptide (TAP) in a rabbit model of venous thrombosis. Thromb Haemost 65:257, 1991.
181. Watkins MW, Leutmer PA, Schneider DJ, et al: Determinants of rebound thrombin activity after cessation of heparin in patients undergoing coronary interventions. Cathet Cardiovasc Diagn 44:257, 1998.
181a. Torr SR, Eisenberg PR, Sobel BE: The dependence of activation of platelets by plasminogen activators on evolution of thrombin activity. Thromb Res 64:435, 1991.
182. Kerins DM, Roy L, Kunitada S, et al: Pharmacokinetics of tissue-type plasminogen activator during acute myocardial infarction in men: effect of a prostacyclin analogue. Circulation 85:526, 1992.
183. Ashton JH, Schmitz JM, Campbell WB, et al: Inhibition of cyclic flow variations in stenosed canine coronary arteries by thromboxane A2/prostaglandin H2 receptor antagonists. Circ Res 59:568, 1986.
184. Golino P, Yao SK, Rosolowsky M, et al: Simultaneous blockade of thromboxane A2 receptors and inhibition of thromboxane A2 synthase is more effective in enhancing thrombolysis and preventing reocclusion after tissue plasminogen activator than blockade of thromboxane A2 receptors alone [abstract]. Clin Res 37:518A, 1989.
185. Willerson JT, Golino P, Eidt J, et al: Specific platelet mediators and unstable coronary artery lesions: experimental evidence and potential clinical implications. Circulation 80:198, 1989.
186. Golino P, Ashton JH, Glas-Greenwalt P, et al: Mediation of reocclusion by thromboxane A2 and serotonin after thrombolysis with tissue-type plasminogen activator in a canine preparation of coronary thrombosis. Circulation 77:678, 1988.
187. Torr SR, Haskel EJ, VonVoightlander PF, et al: Inhibition of cyclic flow variations and reocclusion after thrombolysis in dogs by a novel antagonist of platelet-activating factor. J Am Coll Cardiol 18:1804, 1991.
188. Motro M, Barbash GI, Hod H, et al: Incidence of left ventricular thrombi formation after thrombolytic therapy with recombinant tissue plasminogen activator, heparin, and aspirin in patients with acute myocardial infarction. Am Heart J 122:23, 1991.
189. Noorman F, Rijken DC: Regulation of tissue-type plasminogen activator concentrations by clearance via the mannose receptor and other receptors. Fibrinolysis Proteolysis 11:183, 1997.
190. Sobel BE, Collen D (eds): Coronary Thrombolysis in Perspective: Principles Underlying Conjunctive and Adjunctive Therapy. New York: Marcel Dekker, 1993.
191. Sobel BE: Intracranial bleeding, fibrinolysis, and anticoagulation: causal connections and clinical implications. Circulation 90:2147, 1994.
192. Lefkowitz J, Horrigan MC: Direct thrombin inhibitors vs platelet GP IIB/IIIA antagonists: is the risk of intracerabral haemorrhage comparable? Presented at the 44th Annual Scientific Meeting of the Cardiac Society of Australia and New Zealand, Brisbane, Australia, August 1996.
193. Gold HK, Coller BS, Yasuda T, et al: Rapid and sustained coronary artery recanalization with combined bolus injection of recombinant tissue-type plasminogen activator and monoclonal antiplatelet GPIIb/IIIa antibody in a canine preparation. Circulation 77:670, 1988.
194. Nicolini FA, Ferrini D, Ottani F, et al: Concurrent nitroglycerin therapy impairs tissue-type plasminogen activator-induced thrombolysis in patients with acute myocardial infarction. Am J Cardiol 74:662, 1994.
195. Sobel BE, Furberg CD: Surrogates, semantics, and sensible public policy: special commentary. Circulation 95:1661, 1997.
196. van de Werf F: Discrepancies between the effects of coronary reperfusion on survival and left ventricular function. Lancet 1:1367, 1989.
196a. Califf RM, Hamelson-Woodlief L, Topol EJ: Left ventricular ejection fraction may not be useful as an end point of thrombolytic therapy comparative trials. Circulation 82:1847, 1990.
197. Rentrop KP: Thrombolytic therapy in patients with acute myocardial infarction. Circulation 71:627, 1985.
198. Collen D, Topol EJ, Tiefenbrunn AJ, et al: Coronary thrombolysis

with recombinant human tissue-type plasminogen activator: a prospective, randomized, placebo-controlled trial. Circulation 70:1012, 1984.
199. Loscalzo J, Wharton TP, Kirshenbaum JM, et al: Clot-selective coronary thrombolysis with pro-urokinase. Circulation 79:776, 1989.
200. Munkvad S, Gram J, Jespersen J, Grande P: Reduction of infarct size estimation enzymatically in patients with acute myocardial infarction after treatment with recombinant tissue-type plasminogen activator or after spontaneous coronary recanalisation: a randomised, placebo-controlled study. Fibrinolysis 4:95, 1990.
201. Wackers FJT, Terrin WL, Kayden DS, et al: Quantitative radionuclide assessment of regional ventricular function after thrombolytic therapy for acute myocardial infarction: results of phase I Thrombolysis in Myocardial Infarction (TIMI) trial. J Am Coll Cardiol 13:998, 1989.
202. Zaret BL, Wackers FJT, Terrin ML, et al: Assessment of global and regional left ventricular performance at rest and during exercise after thrombolytic therapy for acute myocardial infarction: results of the Thrombolysis in Myocardial Infarction (TIMI) II study. Am J Cardiol 69:1, 1992.
203. Feit F, Mueller HS, Braunwald E, et al: Thrombolysis in Myocardial Infarction (TIMI) phase II trial: outcome comparison of a "conservative strategy" in community versus tertiary hospitals. J Am Coll Cardiol 16:1529, 1990.
204. O'Rourke M, Baron D, Keogh A, et al: Limitation of myocardial infarction by early infusion of recombinant tissue-type plasminogen activator. Circulation 77:1311, 1988.
205. National Heart Foundation of Australia Coronary Thrombolysis Group: Coronary thrombolysis and myocardial salvage by tissue plasminogen activator given up to 4 hours after onset of myocardial infarction. Lancet 1:203, 1988.
206. Sheehan FH, Braunwald E, Canner P, et al: The effect of intravenous thrombolytic therapy on left ventricular function: a report on tissue-type plasminogen activator and streptokinase from the Thrombolysis in Myocardial Infarction (TIMI Phase I) trial. Circulation 75:817, 1987.
207. Magnani B for the PAIMS Investigators: Plasminogen Activator Italian Multicenter Study (PAIMS): comparison of intravenous recombinant single-chain human tissue-type plasminogen activator (rt-PA) with intravenous streptokinase in acute myocardial infarction. J Am Coll Cardiol 13:19, 1989.
208. Sheehan FH, Doerr R, Schmidt WG, et al: Early recovery of left ventricular function after thrombolytic therapy for acute myocardial infarction: an important determinant of survival. J Am Coll Cardiol 12:289, 1988.
209. White HD, Rivers JT, Maslowski AH, et al: Effects of intravenous streptokinase as compared with that of tissue plasminogen activator on left ventricular function after first myocardial infarction. N Engl J Med 320:817, 1989.
210. Gruppo Italiano Per Lo Studio Della Streptochinasi Nell'infarto Miocardico (GISSI): Long-term effects of intravenous thrombolysis in acute myocardial infarction: final report of the GISSI study. Lancet 2:871, 1987.
211. Simoons ML, Vos J, Tijssen JGP, et al: Long-term benefit of early thrombolytic therapy in patients with acute myocardial infarction: 5 year follow-up of a trial conducted by the Interuniversity Cardiology Institute of the Netherlands. J Am Coll Cardiol 14:1609, 1989.
212. Bonaduce D, Petretta M, Villari B, et al: Effects of late administration of tissue-type plasminogen activator on left ventricular remodeling and function after myocardial infarction. J Am Coll Cardiol 16:1561, 1990.
213. Gang ES, Lew AS, Hong M, et al: Decreased incidence of ventricular late potentials after successful thrombolytic therapy for acute myocardial infarction. N Engl J Med 321:712, 1989.
214. Voth E, Tebbe U, Schicha H, et al: Intravenous Streptokinase in Acute Myocardial Infarction (I.S.A.M.) trial: serial evaluation of left ventricular function up to 3 years after infarction estimated by radionuclide ventriculography. J Am Coll Cardiol 18:1610, 1991.
215. Califf RM, Topol EJ, George BS, et al: One-year outcome after therapy with tissue plasminogen activator: report from the Thrombolysis and Angioplasty in Myocardial Infarction trial. Am Heart J 119:777, 1990.
216. Barbash GI, Modan M, Goldbourt U, et al: comparative case fatality analysis of the International Tissue Plasminogen Activator/Streptokinase Mortality Trial: Variation by country beyond predictive profile. J Am Coll Cardiol 21:281, 1993.
217. Collen D, Bounameaux H, De Cock F, et al: Analysis of coagulation and fibrinolysis during intravenous infusion of recombinant human tissue-type plasminogen activator in patients with acute myocardial infarction. Circulation 73:511, 1986.
218. Rao AK, Pratt C, Berke A, et al: The Thrombolysis in Myocardial Infarction trial. Phase I: hemorrhagic manifestations, complications, and changes in plasma fibrinogen and fibrinolytic system. J Am Coll Cardiol 11:1, 1988.
219. Honan MB, Harrell FE, Reimer KA, et al: Cardiac rupture, mortality and the timing of thrombolytic therapy: a meta-analysis. J Am Coll Cardiol 16:359, 1990.
220. Mauri F, de Biase M, Franzosi MG, et al: In hospital causes of death in the patients admitted to the GISSI Study. Giorn Ital Cardiol 17:37, 1987.
221. Ohman EM, Topol EJ, Califf RM et al: An analysis of the cause of early mortality after administration of thrombolytic therapy. Coron Artery Dis 4:957, 1993.
222. Tiefenbrunn AJ, Ludbrook PA: Coronary thrombolysis: it's worth the risk. JAMA 261:2107, 1989.
223. Gore JM, Sloan M, Price TR, et al: Intracerebral hemorrhage, cerebral infarction, and subdural hematoma after acute myocardial infarction and thrombolytic therapy in the Thrombolysis in Myocardial Infarction Study. Circulation 83:448, 1991.
224. National Registry of Myocardial Infarction Data. Statistical Consultants, Lexington, KY, February, 1992.
225. Bovill EG, Terrin ML, Stump DC, et al: Hemorrhagic events during therapy with recombinant tissue-type plasminogen activator, heparin, and aspirin for acute myocardial infarction: results of the Thrombolysis in Myocardial Infarction (TIMI) Phase II Trial. Ann Intern Med 115:256, 1991.
226. Krumholz HM, Pasternak RC, Weinstein MC, et al: Cost effectiveness of thrombolytic therapy with streptokinase in elderly patients with suspected acute myocardial infarction. N Engl J Med 327:7, 1992.
227. White HD, Van de Werf FJJ: Thrombolysis for acute myocardial infarction. Circulation 97:1632, 1998.
228. Topol EJ, Califf RM: Thrombolytic therapy for elderly patients. N Engl J Med 327:45, 1992.
229. Aylward PG, Bett JHN for the LATE Steering Committee: The risk of stroke in patients with acute myocardial infarction admitted to LATE. Presented at the 42nd Annual Scientific Meeting of the Cardiac Society of Australia and New Zealand, Adelaide, Australia, August 1994.
230. Bode C, Runge MS, Schonermark S, et al: Conjugation to antifibrin Fab′ enhances fibrinolytic potency of single-chain urokinase plasminogen activator. Circulation 81:1974, 1990.
231. Nelles L, Lijnen HR, Van Nuffelen A, et al: Characterization of domain deletion and/or duplication mutants of a recombinant chimera of tissue-type plasminogen activator and urokinase-type plasminogen activator (rt-PA/u-PA). Thromb Haemost 64:53, 1990.
232. Bode C, Meinhardt G, Runge MS, et al: Platelet-targeted fibrinolysis enhances clot lysis and inhibits platelet aggregation. Circulation 84:805, 1991.
233. McKendall GR, Attubato MJ, Drew TM, et al: Safety and efficacy of a new regimen of intravenous recombinant tissue-type plasminogen activator potentially suitable for either prehospital or in-hospital administration. J Am Coll Cardiol 18:1774, 1991.
234. Miyazaki A, Tadokoro H, Drury K, et al: Retrograde coronary venous administration of recombinant tissue-type plasminogen activator: a unique and effective approach to coronary artery thrombolysis. J Am Coll Cardiol 18:613, 1991.
235. Hopkins WE, Fujii S, Sobel BE: Synergistic induction of plasminogen activator inhibitor type-1 in Hep G2 cells by thrombin and transforming growth factor-β. Blood 79:75, 1992.
236. Fujii S, Abendschein DR, Sobel BE: Augmentation of plasminogen activator inhibitor type 1 activity in plasma by thrombosis and by thrombolysis. J Am Coll Cardiol 18:1547, 1991.
237. Fujii S, Hopkins WE, Sobel BE: Mechanisms contributing to increased synthesis of plasminogen activator inhibitor type-1 in endothelial cells by constituents of platelets and their implications for thrombolysis. Circulation 83:645, 1991.
238. Hopkins WE, Westerhausen DR, Sobel BE, Billadello JJ: Transcriptional regulation of plasminogen activator inhibitor type-1 mRNA in Hep G2 cells by epidermal growth factor. Nucleic Acids Res 19:163, 1991.

239. Fujii S, Lucore CL, Hopkins WE, et al: Induction of synthesis of plasminogen activator inhibitor type-1 by tissue-type plasminogen activator in human hepatic and endothelial cells. Thromb Haemost 64:412, 1990.
240. Fujii S, Sobel BE: Induction of plasminogen activator inhibitor by products released from platelets. Circulation 82:1485, 1990.
241. Sane DC, Stump DC, Topol EJ, et al: Correlation between baseline plasminogen activator inhibitor levels and clinical outcome during therapy with tissue plasminogen activator for acute myocardial infarction. Thromb Haemost 65:275, 1991.
242. Fujii S, Lucore CL, Hopkins WE, et al: Potential attenuation of fibrinolysis by growth factors released from platelets and their pharmacologic implications. Am J Cardiol 63:1505, 1989.
243. Reilly CF, Mayer EJ, Sitko GR, et al: The effect of exogenous plasminogen activator inhibitor-1 in a canine model of occlusive thrombus formation. Fibrinolysis 5:99, 1991.
244. Prins MH, Hirsh J: A critical review of the relationship between impaired fibrinolysis and myocardial infarction. Am Heart J 122:545, 1991.
245. The Urokinase and Alteplase in Myocardial Infarction Collaborative Group: Combination of urokinase and alteplase in the treatment of myocardial infarction. Coron Artery Dis 2:225, 1991.
246. Califf RM, Topol EJ, Stack RS, et al: Evaluation of combination thrombolytic therapy and timing of cardiac catheterization in acute myocardial infarction: results of Thrombolysis and Angioplasty in Myocardial Infarction—Phase 5 Randomized Trial. Circulation 83:1543, 1991.
247. Grines CL, Nissen SE, Booth DC, et al: A prospective, randomized trial comparing combination half-dose tissue-type plasminogen activator and streptokinase with full-dose tissue-type plasminogen activator. Circulation 84:540, 1991.
248. The GUSTO Investigators: The global utilization of streptokinase and tissue plasminogen activator for occluded coronary arteries (GUSTO) trial. N Engl J Med 329:673–682, 1998.
249. Pell ACH, Miller HC, Robertson CE, Fox KAA: Effect of "fast track" admission for acute myocardial infarction on delay to thrombolysis. BMJ 304:83, 1992.
250. Tiefenbrunn AJ, Sobel BE: Timing of coronary recanalization: paradigms, paradoxes, and pertinence. Circulation 85:2311, 1992.
251. The European Myocardial Infarction Project (EMIP): Potential time saving with pre-hospital intervention in acute myocardial infarction: report of the European Myocardial Infarction Project (EMIP) Subcommittee. Eur Heart J 9:118, 1988.
252. GREAT Group: Feasibility, safety, and efficacy of domiciliary thrombolysis by general practitioners: Grampian Region Early Anistreplase Trial. BMJ 305:548, 1992.
253. Birkhead JS: Time delays in provision of thrombolytic treatment in six district hospitals. BMJ 305:445, 1992.
254. Hendra TJ, Marshall AJ: Increased prescription of thrombolytic treatment to elderly patients with suspected acute myocardial infarction associated with audit. BMJ 304:423, 1992.
255. Lange RA, Hillis LD: Use and overuse of angiography and revascularization for acute coronary syndromes. N Engl J Med 338:1838, 1998.
256. The Global Use of Strategies to Open Occluded Coronary Arteries in Acute Coronary Syndromes (GUSTO IIb) Angioplasty Substudy Investigators: A clinical trial comparing primary coronary angioplasty with tissue plasminogen activator for acute myocardial infarction. N Engl J Med 336:1621, 1997.
257. Agati L, Voci P, Hickle P, et al: Tissue-type plasminogen activator therapy versus primary coronary angioplasty: impact on myocardial tissue perfusion and regional function 1 month after uncomplicated myocardial infarction. J Am Coll Cardiol 31:228, 1998.
258. Weintraub WS, Stein B, Kosinski A, et al: Outcome of coronary bypass surgery versus coronary angioplasty in diabetic patients with multivessel coronary artery disease. J Am Coll Cardiol 31:10, 1998.
259. Faxon DP: Revascularization in diabetics: lessons from the BARI trial. Cardiol Rev 6:20, 1998.
260. Gowda MS, Vacek JL, Hallas D: One-year outcomes of diabetic versus nondiabetic patients with non-Q-wave acute myocardial infarction treated with percutaneous transluminal coronary angioplasty. Am J Cardiol 81:1067, 1998.
261. McGill JB, Schneider DJ, Arfken CL, et al: Factors responsible for impaired fibrinolysis in obese subjects and NIDDM patients. Diabetes 43:104, 1994.
262. Sobel BE, Woodcock-Mitchell J, Schneider DJ, et al: Increased plasminogen activator inhibitor type-1 in coronary artery atherectomy specimens from type 2 diabetic compared with nondiabetic patients: a potential factor predisposing to thrombosis and its persistence. Circulation 97:2213, 1998.
263. Schneider DJ, Sobel BE: Diabetes and thrombosis. *In* Johnstone MT (ed): Diabetes and Cardiovascular Disease. NJ: Totowa, Humana, 1999 (in press).
264. Aoki I, Shimoyama K, Aoki N, et al: Platelet-dependent thrombin generation in patients with diabetes mellitus: effects of glycemic control on coagulability in diabetes. J Am Coll Cardiol 27:560, 1996.
265. O'Neill WW: Multivessel balloon angioplasty should be abandoned in diabetic patients! J Am Coll Cardiol 31:20, 1998.
266. Eckman MH, Wong JB, Salem DN, Pauker SG: Direct angioplasty for acute myocardial infarction: a review of outcomes in clinical subsets. Ann Intern Med 117:667, 1992.
267. Rogers WJ, Dean LS, Moore PB, et al: Comparison of primary angioplasty versus thrombolytic therapy for acute myocardial infarction. Am J Cardiol 74:111, 1994.
268. Every NR, Parsons LS, Hlatky M, et al: A comparison of thrombolytic therapy with primary coronary angioplasty for acute myocardial infarction. N Engl J Med 335:1253, 1996.
269. Kovack PJ, Rasak MA, Bates ER, et al: Thrombolysis plus aortic counterpulsation: improved survival in patients who present to community hospitals with cardiogenic shock. J Am Coll Cardiol 29:1454, 1997.
270. The TIMI Study Group: Comparison of invasive and conservative strategies after treatment with intravenous tissue plasminogen activator in acute myocardial infarction. Results of the thrombolysis in myocardial infarction (TIMI) phase II trial. N Engl J Med 320:618, 1989.
271. Ross AM, Lundergan CF, Rohrbeck SC, et al: Rescue angioplasty after failed thrombolysis: technical and clinical outcomes in a large thrombolysis trial. J Am Coll Cardiol 31:1511, 1998.
272. Michels KB, Yusuf S: Does PTCA in acute myocardial infarction affect mortality and reinfarction rates? A quantitative overview (meta-analysis) of the randomized clinical trials. Circulation 91:476, 1995.
273. Ross A: Overview of PACT: results from the Plasminogen Activator-Angioplasty Compatibility Trial. Presented at the 47th Annual Scientific Session of the American College of Cardiology, Atlanta, GA, March 1998.
274. Wilensky RL, Bourdillon PDV, Vix VA, Zelleer JA: Intracoronary artery thrombus formation in unstable angina: a clinical, biochemical and angiographic correlation. J Am Coll Cardiol 21:692, 1993.
275. Theroux P, Fuster V: Acute coronary syndromes: unstable angina and non-Q-wave myocardial infarction. Circulation 97:1195, 1998.
276. Waters D: Acute coronary syndromes: is a unified management strategy emerging? J Am Coll Cardiol 31:103, 1998.
277. Chesebro JH, Fuster V: Thrombosis in unstable angina. N Engl J Med 327:192, 1992.
278. Romeo F, Rosano GMC, Martuschelli E, et al: Effectiveness of prolonged low dose recombinant tissue-type plasminogen activator for refractory unstable angina. J Am Coll Cardiol 25:1295, 1995.
279. Goodman SG, Langer A, Ross AM, et al: Non-Q-wave versus Q-wave myocardial infarction after thrombolytic therapy: angiographic and prognostic insights from the Global Utilization of Streptokinase and Tissue Plasminogen Activator for Occluded Coronary Arteries-I Angiographic Substudy. Circulation 97:444, 1998.
280. Collen D, Gold HK: Fibrin-specific thrombolytic agents and new approaches to coronary arterial thrombolysis. *In* Julian D, Kubler W, Norris RM, et al (eds): Thrombolysis in Cardiovascular Disease. p. 53. New York: Marcel Dekker, 1989.
281. Kennedy JW, Ritchie JL, Davis KB, Fritz JK: Western Washington randomized trial of intracoronary streptokinase in acute myocardial infarction. N Engl J Med 309:1477, 1983.
282. Folts J: An in vivo model of experimental arterial stenosis, intimal damage, and periodic thrombosis. Circulation 83 (suppl IV):IV-3, 1991.
283. Sobel BE, Hirsh J: Coronary Thrombolysis and Conjunctive Therapy: Principles and Practice. Hamilton, Ontario: Decker Periodicals, 1991.
284. Topol EJ, George BS, Kereiakes DJ, et al: A randomized controlled trial of intravenous tissue plasminogen activator and early intravenous heparin in acute myocardial infarction. Circulation 79:281, 1989.

285. Bleich SD, Nichols T, Schumacher R, et al: The role of heparin following coronary thrombolysis with tissue plasminogen activator (t-PA), abstracted. Circulation 80 (suppl II):II-113, 1989.
286. de Bono DP, Simoons ML, Tijssen I, et al: The effect of early intravenous heparin on coronary patency, infarct size and bleeding complications after alteplase thrombolysis: results of a randomised, double-blind European Cooperative Study Group trial. Br Heart J 67:122, 1992.
287. Neuhaus KL, von Essen R, Tebbe U, et al: Improved thrombolysis in acute myocardial infarction with front-loaded administration of alteplase: results of the rt-PA–APSAC Patency Study (TAPS). J Am Coll Cardiol 19:885, 1992.
288. Rentrop KP: Thrombolytic therapy in patients with acute myocardial infarction. Circulation 71:627, 1985.
289. Rentrop P, Balnke H, Karsch KR, et al: Selective intracoronary thrombolysis in acute myocardial infarction and unstable angina pectoris. Circulation 63:307, 1981.
290. Ganz W, Buchbinder N, Marcus H, et al: Intracoronary thrombolysis in evolving myocardial infarction. Am Heart J 101:4, 1981.
291. Mathey DG, Kuck K-H, Tilsner V, et al: Nonsurgical coronary artery recanalization in acute transmural myocardial infarction. Circulation 63:489, 1981.
292. Reduto LA, Smalling RW, Freund GC, Gould KL: Intracoronary infusion of streptokinase in patients with acute myocardial infarction: effects of reperfusion on left ventricular performance. Am J Cardiol 48:403, 1981.
293. Cowley MJ, Hastillo A, Vetrovic GWW, Hess ML: Effects of intracoronary streptokinase in acute myocardial infarction. Am Heart J 102:1149, 1981.
294. Schwarz F, Schuler G, Katus H, et al: Intracoronary thrombolysis in acute myocardial infarction: correlations among serum enzyme, scintigraphic and hemodynamic findings. Am J Cardiol 50:32, 1982.
295. Tennant SN, Dixon J, Venable TC, et al: Intracoronary thrombolysis in patients with acute myocardial infarction: comparison of the efficacy of urokinase with streptokinase. Circulation 69:756, 1984.
296. Mathey DG, Schofer J, Sheehan FH, et al: Intravenous urokinase in acute myocardial infarction. Am J Cardiol 55:878, 1985.
297. Timmis AD, Griffin B, Crick JCP, et al: An interim report of a double-blind placebo controlled recanalisation study of anisoylated plasminogen streptokinase activator complex in acute myocardial infarction. Drugs 33 (suppl 3):146, 1987.
298. Leizorovicz A, Durrieu G, Boissel JP: A randomised placebo-controlled pilot dose-response study with anisoylated plasminogen streptokinase activator complex in acute coronary occlusions. Drugs 33 (suppl 3):133, 1987.
299. Anderson JL, Rothbard RL, Hackworthy RA, et al: Multicenter reperfusion trial of intravenous anisoylated plasminogen streptokinase activator complex (APSAC) in acute myocardial infarction: controlled comparison with intracoronary streptokinase. J Am Coll Cardiol 11:1153, 1988.
300. Bonnier JJRM (Report of the Dutch Multicentre Invasive Reperfusion Study Group): Comparison of intravenous anisoylated plasminogen streptokinase activator complex with intracoronary streptokinase in acute myocardial infarction. Drugs 33(suppl 3):151, 1987.
301. Marder VJ, Rothbard RL, Fitzpatrick PG, et al: Dose-ranging studies of anisoylated plasminogen streptokinase activator complex: studies in healthy volunteers and in patients with acute myocardial infarction. Drugs 33 (suppl 3):124, 1987.
302. Passamani ER: Thrombolysis in myocardial infarction: the NHLBI experience. *In* Sobel BE, Collen D, Grossbard E (eds): Tissue Plasminogen Activator in Thrombolytic Therapy. p. 75. New York: Marcel Dekker, 1987.
303. Mueller HS, Rao AK, Forman SA: Thrombolysis in Myocardial Infarction (TIMI): Comparative studies of coronary reperfusion and systemic fibrinogenolysis with two forms of recombinant tissue-type plasminogen activator. J Am Coll Cardiol 10:479, 1987.
304. Gu S, Ducas J, Patton JN, et al: Coronary thrombolysis: comparative effects of intracoronary administration of recombinant tissue plasminogen activator and urokinase. Chest (in press).
305. Berridge DC, Gregson RHS, Hopkinson BR: Randomized trial of intra-arterial recombinant tissue plasminogen activator, intravenous recombinant tissue plasminogen activator and intra-arterial streptokinase in peripheral arterial thrombolysis. Br J Surg 78:988, 1991.
306. Belgian Saruplase Alteplase Trial Group: Effects of alteplase and saruplase on hemostatic variables: a single-blind, randomized trial in patients with acute myocardial infarction. Coron Artery Dis 2:349, 1991.
307. Abrams J: Nitrate tolerance and dependence. Am Heart J 99:113, 1980.
308. Sobel BE, Gross RW, Robison AK: Thrombolysis, clot selectivity, and kinetics. Circulation 70:160, 1984.
309. Sobel BE: Thrombolytic therapy with t-PA. *In* Kluft C (ed): Tissue-type Plasminogen Activator (t-PA): Physiological and Clinical Aspects. pp. 147–155. Boca Raton, FL: CRC Press, 1988.
310. Sobel BE, Collen D, Grossbard E (eds): Tissue Plasminogen Activator in Thrombolytic Therapy. New York: Marcel Dekker, 1987.
311. Tiefenbrunn AJ, Sobel BE: Pharmacodynamics of activation of plasminogen with t-PA. *In* Sobel BE, Collen D, Grossbard E (eds): Tissue Plasminogen Activator in Thrombolytic Therapy. p. 25. New York: Marcel Dekker, 1987.
312. Eisenberg PR, Sobel BE, Jaffe AS: Characterization in vivo of the fibrin specificity of activators of the fibrinolytic system. Circulation 78:592, 1988.
313. Haskel EH, Prager NA, Adams SP, et al: Relative efficacy of antithrombin compared with antiplatelet agents in accelerating coronary thrombolysis and preventing early reocclusion. Circulation 83:1048, 1991.
314. Torr SR, Winters KJ, Santoro SA, Sobel BE: The nature of interactions between tissue-type plasminogen activator and platelets. Thromb Res 59:279, 1990.
315. Fitzgerald DJ, Wright F, FitzGerald GA: Increased thromboxane biosynthesis during coronary thrombolysis. Evidence that platelet activation and thromboxane A2 modulate the response to tissue-type plasminogen activator in vivo. Circ Res 65:83, 1989.
316. Chesebro JH: Antithrombotic therapy in coronary artery disease: review in depth. Coron Artery Dis 2:147, 1990.
317. Anderson JL, Marshall HW, Bray BE, et al: A randomized trial of intracoronary streptokinase in the treatment of acute myocardial infarction. N Engl J Med 308:1312, 1983.
318. Van der Laarse A, Kerkhof PL, Vermeer F, et al: Relation between infarct size and left ventricular performance assessed in patients with first acute myocardial infarction randomized to intracoronary thrombolytic therapy or to conventional treatment. Am J Cardiol 61:1, 1988.
319. Koren G, Weiss AT, Hasin Y, et al: Prevention of myocardial damage in acute myocardial ischemia by early treatment with intravenous streptokinase. N Engl J Med 313:1384, 1985.
320. The ISAM Study Group: A prospective trial of Intravenous Streptokinase in Acute Myocardial infarction (ISAM): mortality, morbidity, and infarct size at 21 days. N Engl J Med 314:1465, 1986.
321. White HD, Norris RM, Brown MA, et al: Effect of intravenous streptokinase on left ventricular function and early survival after acute myocardial infarction. N Engl J Med 317:850, 1987.
322. Topol EJ, Weiss JL, Brinker JA, et al: Regional wall motion improvement after coronary thrombolysis with recombinant tissue plasminogen activator: importance of coronary angioplasty. J Am Coll Cardiol 6:426, 1985.
323. O'Rourke M, Baron D, Koegh A, et al: Limitation of myocardial infarction by early infusion of recombinant tissue-type plasminogen activator. Circulation 77:1311, 1988.
324. Cross DB, Ashton NG, Norris RM, et al: Comparison of the effects of streptokinase and tissue plasminogen activator on regional wall motion after first myocardial infarction: analysis by the centerline method with correction for area at risk. J Am Coll Cardiol 17:1039, 1991.
325. Guerci AD, Gerstenblith G, Brinker JA, et al: A randomized trial of intravenous tissue plasminogen activator for acute myocardial infarction with subsequent randomization to elective coronary angioplasty. N Engl J Med 317:1613, 1987.
326. Yusuf S, Collins R, Peto R et al: Intravenous and intracoronary fibrinolytic therapy in acute myocardial infarction: overview of results on mortality, reinfarction and side-effects from 33 randomised controlled trials. Eur Heart J 6:556, 1985.
327. Tiefenbrunn AJ, Sobel BE: Thrombolysis and myocardial infarction. Fibrinolysis 5:1, 1991.
328. Sobel BE, Collen D: Questions unresolved by ISIS-3. Am J Cardiol 70:385, 1992.
329. Rogers WJ: Update on recent clinical trials of thrombolytic therapy in myocardial infarction. J Invasive Cardiol 3 (suppl A):11A, 1991.
330. Turpie AGG, Robinson JH, Doule DJ, et al: Comparison of high-

dose with low-dose subcutaneous heparin to prevent left ventricular mural thrombus in patients with acute transmural anterior myocardial infarction. N Engl J Med 320:352, 1989.
331. Hull RD, Raskob GE, Hirsh J, et al: Continuous intravenous heparin compared with intermittent subcutaneous heparin in the initial treatment of proximal-vein thrombosis. N Engl J Med 315:1109, 1986.
332. Pini M, Pattachini C, Quintavalla R, et al: Subcutaneous vs intravenous heparin in the treatment of deep venous thrombosis: a randomized clinical trial. Thromb Haemost 64:222, 1990.
333. TIMI Study Group: The Thromobolysis In Myocardial Infarction (TIMI) trial. N Engl J Med 312:932, 1985.
334. Gimple LW, Gold HK, Leinbach RC, et al: Correlation between template bleeding times and spontaneous bleeding during treatment of acute myocardial infarction with recombinant tissue-type plasminogen activator. Circulation 80:581, 1989.
335. Arnold AER, Brower RW, Collen D, et al: Increased serum levels of fibrinogen degradation products due to treatment with recombinant tissue-type plasminogen activator for acute myocardial infarction are related to bleeding complications, but not to coronary patency. J Am Coll Cardiol 14:581, 1989.
336. Wilcox RG, von der Lippe G, Olsson CG, et al: Trial of tissue plasminogen activator for mortality reduction in acute myocardial infarction: Anglo-Scandinavian Study of Early Thrombolysis (ASSET). Lancet 2:525, 1988.
337. Braunwald E, Knatterud GL, Passamani E, et al: Update from the Thrombolysis in Myocardial Infarction Trial [letter]. J Am Coll Cardiol 10:970, 1987.
338. Lew AS, Hod H, Cercek B, et al: Mortality and morbidity rates of patients older and younger than 75 years with acute myocardial infarction treated with intravenous streptokinase. Am J Cardiol 59:1, 1987.
339. Braunwald E, Knatterud GL, Passamani E: Announcement of a protocol change in the Thrombolysis in Myocardial Infarction trial. J Am Coll Cardiol 9:467, 1997.
340. Alexopoulos D, Raine AEG, Cobbe SM: Serum sickness complicating intravenous streptokinase therapy in acute myocardial infarction. Eur Heart J 5:1010, 1984.
341. Totty WG, Romano T, Benian GM, et al: Serum sickness following streptokinase therapy. Am J Radiol 138:143, 1982.
342. Weatherbee C: Serum sickness following selective intracoronary streptokinase. Curr Ther Res 35:433, 1984.
343. Noel J, Rosenbaum LH, Gangadharan V, et al: Serum sickness-like illness and leukocytoclastic vasculitis following intracoronary arterial streptokinase. Am Heart J 113:395, 1987.
344. Murray N, Lyons J, Chappell M: Crescentic glomerulonephritis: a possible complication of streptokinase treatment for acute myocardial infarction. Br Heart J 56:483, 1986.
345. Ross AM, Coyne KS, Moreyra E, et al: Extended mortality benefit of early postinfarction reperfusion. Circulation 97:1549, 1998.
346. Fox NL, Cannon CP, Berioli S, et al: Rates of serious bleeding events requiring transfusion in AMI patients treated with TNK-tPA. J Am Coll Cardiol 33:353A, 1999.
347. Kostis JB, Lio W-C, Belerle FA, et al: Single bolus regimen of lanoteplase (nPA) in acute myocardial infarction: hemostatic evaluation vs TPA in the InTime Study. J Am Coll Cardiol 33:325A, 1999.
348. Antman EM, Giugliano RP, Gibson CM, et al: Abciximab facilitates the rate and extent of thrombolysis: results of Thrombolysis in Myocardial Infarction (TIMI) 14 trial. Circulation 99:2720, 1999.
349. Battle RW, Sobel BE: Treatment of acute myocardial infarction. Contemp Treat Cardiovasc Dis 1:33, 1996.
350. Shatos MA, Doherty JM, Penar PL, et al: Suppression of plasminogen activator inhibitor-1 release from human cerebral endothelium by plasminogen activators: a factor potentially predisposing to intracranial bleeding. Circulation 94:636, 1996.
351. Absher PM, Hendley E, Jaworski DM, et al: Impairment of the blood-brain barrier: a potential surrogate delineating determinants of cerebral bleeding caused by fibrinolytic drugs. Coron Artery Dis 10:413, 1999.
352. Moliterno DJ, Harrington RA, Newby K, et al: Pronounced reduction in long-term ischemic events with platelet IIbIIIa antagonism among diabetics with unstable angina: paragon 6 month results. Circulation 96:2646A, 1997.
353. Schulman SP, Goldschmidt-Clermont PJ, Topol EJ, et al: Effects of integrelin, a platelet lycoprotein llb/llla receptor antagonist in unstable angina: a randomized multicenter trial. Circulation 94:2083, 1996.
354. Gunnar RM, Lambrew CT, Abrams W, et al: Task Force IV: pharmacologic interventions. Am J Cardiol 50:393, 1982.
355. Bussmann WD, Passek D, Seidel W, Kaltenbach M: Reduction of CK and CK-MB indexes of infarct size by intravenous nitroglycerin. Circulation 63:615, 1981.
356. Jugdutt BI, Warnica JW: Intravenous nitroglycerin therapy to limit myocardial infarct size, expansion and complications: effect of timing, dosage and infarct location. Circulation 78:906, 1988.
357. Stockman MB, Verrier RL, Lown B: Effect of nitroglycerin on vulnerability to ventricular fibrillation during myocardial ischemia and reperfusion. Am J Cardiol 43:233, 1979.
358. Flaherty JT, Reid PR, Kelly DT, et al: Intravenous nitroglycerin in acute myocardial infarction. Circulation 51:132, 1975.
359. Borer JS, Redwood DR, Levit B, et al: Reduction in myocardial ischemia with nitroglycerin or nitroglycerin plus phenylephrine administered during acute myocardial infarction. N Engl J Med 293:1008, 1975.
360. Cottrell JE, Turndorf H: Intravenous nitroglycerin. Am Heart J 96:550, 1978.
361. Flaherty JT: Intravenous nitroglycerin. Johns Hopkins Med J 151:36, 1982.
362. Visser CA, Kan G, Lie KI, Durrer D: Incidence and one-year follow-up of left ventricular thrombus following acute myocardial infarction: an echocardiographic study. J Am Coll Cardiol 1:648, 1983.
363. Asinger RW, Mikell FE, Elspeyer J, Hodges M: Incidence of left ventricular thrombosis after acute transmural myocardial infarction: serial evaluation of two-dimensional echocardiography. N Engl J Med 305:297, 1981.
364. Meltzor RS, Visser CA, Fuster V: Intracardiac thrombi and systemic embolization. Ann Intern Med 104:689, 1986.
365. The Norwegian Multicenter Study Group: Timolol-induced reduction in mortality and reinfarction in patients surviving acute myocardial infarction. N Engl J Med 304:801, 1981.
366. Frishman WH, Furberg CD, Friedewald WT: Beta-adrenergic blockade for survivors of acute myocardial infarction. N Engl J Med 310:830, 1984.
367. Pederson TR for the Norwegian Multicenter Study Group: Six-year follow-up of the Norwegian multicenter study on timolol after acute myocardial infarction. N Engl J Med 313:1055, 1985.
368. Hjalmarson A, Herlitz J, Malek I, et al: Effect on mortality of metoprolol in acute myocardial infarction. Lancet 2:823, 1981.
369. Beta-Blocker Heart Attack Study Group: The beta-blocker heart attack trial. JAMA 246:2073, 1981.
370. Antman E, Dupont W, Bonalsky J, et al: Early treatment with intravenous metoprolol for suspected acute myocardial infarction. Int J Cardiol 23:185, 1989.
371. Roberts R, Rogers WJ, Mueller HS, et al: Immediate versus deferred beta-blockade following thrombolytic therapy in patients with acute myocardial infarction: results of the Thrombolysis in Myocardial Infarction (TIMI) II-B Study. Circulation 83:422, 1991.
372. Page DL, Caulfield JB, Kastor JA, et al: Myocardial changes associated with cardiogenic shock. N Engl J Med 285:133, 1971.
373. Lee L, Bates ER, Pitt B, et al: Percutaneous transluminal coronary angioplasty improves survival in acute myocardial infarction complicated by cardiogenic shock. Circulation 78:1345, 1988.
374. Willerson JT, Frazier OH: Reducing mortality in patients with extensive myocardial infarction [editorial]. N Engl J Med 325:1166, 1991.
375. McEnany MT, Kay HR, Buckley MJ, et al: Clinical experience with intraaortic balloon pump support in 723 patients. Circulation 58 (suppl 1):124, 1978.
376. Gold HK, Leinbach RC, Mundth ED, et al: Reversal of myocardial ischemia complicating acute infarction by intraaortic balloon pumping (IABP). Circ 45–46 (suppl II):22, 1972.
377. Willerson JT, Curry GC, Watson JT, et al: Intraaortic balloon counterpulsation in patients in cardiogenic shock, medically refractory left ventricular failure, and/or recurrent ventricular tachycardia. Am J Med 58:183, 1975.
378. Gutovitz AL, Sobel BE, Roberts R: Progressive nature of myocardial injury in selected patients with cardiogenic shock. Am J Cardiol 41:469, 1978.
379. Resnekov L: Cardiogenic shock. Chest 83:893, 1983.
380. Gunnar RM, Cruz A, Boswell J, et al: Myocardial infarction in shock: hemodynamic studies and results of therapy. Circulation 33:753, 1966.

381. Johnson SA, Scanlon PJ, Loeb HS, et al: Treatment of cardiogenic shock in myocardial infarction by intraaortic balloon counterpulsation and surgery. Am J Med 62:687, 1977.
382. Alonso DR, Scheidt S, Post M, Killip T: Pathophysiology of cardiogenic shock: quantification of myocardial necrosis, clinical, pathologic, and electrocardiographic correlation. Circulation 48:588, 1973.
383. Gewirtz H, Gold HK, Fallon JT, et al: Role of right ventricular infarction in cardiogenic shock associated with inferior myocardial infarction. Br Heart J 42Z:719, 1979.
384. Sharpe DN, Botvinick EH, Shames DM, et al: The noninvasive diagnosis of right ventricular infarction. Circulation 57:483, 1978.
385. Dell'Italia LD, Starling MR, Crawford MH, et al: Right ventricular infarction: identification by hemodynamic measurements before and after volume loading and correlation with noninvasive techniques. J Am Coll Cardiol 4:931, 1984.
386. Isner JM, Roberts WC: Right ventricular infarction complicating left ventricular infarction secondary to coronary heart disease: frequency, location, associated findings, and significance from analysis of 236 necropsy patients with acute or healed myocardial infarction. Am J Cardiol 42:885, 1978.
387. Cohn JN, Guiha NH, Broder MI, et al: Right ventricular infarction: clinical and hemodynamic features. Am J Cardiol 33:209, 1974.
388. Croft CH, Rude RE, Willerson JT: Right ventricular infarction: changing concepts. Prim Cardiol 9:21, 1983.
389. Coma-Canella L, Lopez-Sendon J, Gamallo C: Low output syndrome in right ventricular infarction. Am Heart J 98:613, 1979.
390. Croft CH, Nicod P, Corbett JR, et al: Detection of acute right ventricular infarction by right precordial electrocardiography. Am J Cardiol 50:421, 1982.
391. Lorell B, Leinbach RC, Pohost GM, et al: Right ventricular infarction: clinical diagnosis and differentiation from cardiac tamponade and pericardial constriction. Am J Cardiol 43:465, 1979.
392. Roberts N, Harrison DG, Reimer KA, et al: Right ventricular infarction with shock but without significant left ventricular infarction: a new clinical syndrome. Am Heart J 110:1047, 1985.
393. Radford MJ, Johnson RA, Daggett WM, et al: Ventricular septal rupture: a review of clinical and physiologic features and an analysis of survival. Circulation 64:454, 1981.
394. Matsui K, Kay JH, Mendez M, et al: Ventricular septal rupture secondary to myocardial infarction: clinical approach and surgical results. JAMA 245:1537, 1981.
395. Edwards BS, Edwards WD, Edwards JE: Ventricular septal rupture complicating acute myocardial infarction: identification of simple and complex types in 53 autopsied hearts. Am J Cardiol 54:1201, 1984.
396. Moore CA, Nygaard TW, Kaiser DL, et al: Post infarction ventricular septal rupture: the importance of location of infarction and right ventricular function in determining survival. Circulation 74:45, 1986.
397. Nishimura RA, Schaft HV, Gersh BJ, et al: Early repair of mechanical complications after acute myocardial infarction. JAMA 356:47, 1986.
398. Montoya A, McKeever L, Scanlon P, et al: Early repair of ventricular septal rupture after infarction. Am J Cardiol 45:345, 1980.
399. Vlodaver Z, Edwards JE: Rupture of ventricular septum or papillary muscle complicating myocardial infarction. Circulation 55:815, 1977.
400. Roberts WC, Cohen LD: Left ventricular papillary muscles: description of the normal and a survey of conditions causing them to be abnormal. Circulation 46:138, 1972.
401. Wei JY, Hutchins GM, Bulkley BH: Papillary muscle rupture in fatal acute myocardial infarction. Ann Intern Med 90:149, 1979.
402. Sanders CA, Armstrong PW, Willerson JT, Dinsmore RE: Etiology and differential diagnosis of acute mitral regurgitation. Prog Cardiovasc Dis 14:129, 1971.
403. Nichimura RA, Schaft HV, Shub C, et al: Papillary muscle rupture complicating acute myocardial infarction: analysis of 17 patients. Am J Cardiol 51:373, 1983.
404. Barbour DJ, Roberts WC: Rupture of a left ventricular papillary muscle during acute myocardial infarction: analysis of 22 necropsy patients. J Am Coll Cardiol 8:588, 1986.
405. Cheng TO: Some new observations on the syndrome of papillary muscle dysfunction. Am J Med 47:924, 1969.
406. Tepe NA, Edmunds LH: Operations for acute post infarction mitral insufficiency and cardiogenic shock. J Thorac Cardiovasc Surg 89:525, 1985.
407. Connolly MW, Gelbfish JS, Jacobowitz IJ, et al: Surgical results for mitral regurgitation from coronary artery disease. J Thorac Cardiovasc Surg 91:379, 1986.
408. Vlodaver Z, Coe JJ, Edwards JE: True and false aneurysms: propensity for the latter to rupture. Circulation 51:567, 1975.
409. Martin RH, Almond CH, Saab S, Watson LE: True and false aneurysms of the left ventricle following myocardial infarction. Am J Med 62:418, 1977.
410. Catherwood E, Mintz GS, Kotler MN, et al: Two-dimensional echocardiographic recognition of left ventricular pseudoaneurysm. Circulation 62:294, 1980.
411. Roelandt J, VandenBrand M, Vletter WB, et al: Echocardiographic diagnosis of pseudoaneurysm of the left ventricle. Circulation 52:466, 1975.
412. Gueron M, Wanderman KL, Hirsch M, Borman J: Pseudoaneurysm of the left ventricle after myocardial infarction: a curable form of myocardial rupture. J Thorac Cardiovasc Surg 69:736, 1975.
413. Roberts WC, Morrow AG: Pseudoaneurysm of the left ventricle: an unusual sequel of myocardial infarction and rupture of the heart. Am J Med 43:639, 1967.
414. Stratton JR, Resnick AD: Increased embolic risk in patients with left ventricular thrombi. Circulation 75:1004, 1987.
415. Weinrich DJ, Burke JF, Pauletto FJ: Left ventricular mural thrombi complicating acute myocardial infarction: long-term follow-up with serial echocardiography. Ann Intern Med 100:789, 1984.
416. Josephson ME, Harken AH, Horowitz LN: Endocardial excision: a new surgical technique for the treatment of recurrent ventricular tachycardia. Circulation 60:1430, 1979.
417. Miller JM, Marchlinski FE, Harken AH, et al: Subendocardial resection for sustained ventricular tachycardia in the early period after acute myocardial infarction. Am J Cardiol 55:980, 1985.
418. Van Tassel RA, Edwards JE: Rupture of the heart complicating myocardial infarction: analysis of 40 cases including nine examples of left ventricular false aneurysms. Chest 61:104, 1972.
419. Lewis AJ, Burchell HB, Titus JL: Clinical and pathologic features of post infarction cardiac rupture. Am J Cardiol 23:43, 1969.
420. Feneley MP, Chang VP, O'Rourke MF: Myocardial rupture after acute myocardial infarction: ten year review. Br Heart J 49:550, 1983.
421. Pfeffer MA, Braunwald E, Moye LA, et al: Effect of captopril on mortality and morbidity in patients with left ventricular dysfunction after myocardial infarction: results of the Survival and Ventricular Enlargement Trial. N Engl J Med 327:669, 1992.
422. Swedberg K, Held P, Kjekshus J, et al: on Behalf of the CONSENSUS II Study Group: Effects of the early administration of enalapril on mortality in patients with acute myocardial infarction: results of the Cooperative New Scandinavian Enalapril Survival Study II (Consensus II). N Engl J Med 327:678, 1992.
423. The SOLVD Investigators: Effect of enalapril on mortality and the development of heart failure in asymptomatic patients with reduced left ventricular ejection fractions. N Engl J Med 327:685, 1992.
424. ISIS-4 Collaborative Group: Fourth International Study of Infarct Survival: protocol for a large simple study of the effects of oral mononitrate, oral captopril, and of intravenous magnesium. Am J Cardiol 68:87D, 1991.
425. GISSI-3 Gruppo Italiano Per Lo Studio Della Supravvivenza Nell Infarcto Miocardico: Study protocol on the effects of lisinopril, of nitrates, and their association in patients with acute myocardial infarction. Am J Card 70:62C, 1992.
426. Lawrence B, Anand I, Cohen I, et al: Augmented short and long-term hemodynamic and hormonal effects of an angiotensin receptor blocker added to angiotensin converting enzyme inhibitor therapy in patients with heart failure. Circulation 99:2658, 1999.
427. Goodfield NER, Newby D, Ludham C, Flapan A: Effects of acute angiotensin II type I receptor antagonism and angiotensin converting enzyme inhibition on plasma fibrinolytic parameters in patients with heart failure. Circulation 99:2983, 1999.
428. Berman J, Haffajee CL, Alpert JS: Therapy of symptomatic pericarditis after myocardial infarction: retrospective and prospective studies of aspirin, indomethacin, prednisone, and spontaneous resolution. Am Heart J 101:750, 1981.
429. Fowler NO, Harbin AD III: Recurrent acute pericarditis: follow-up study of 31 patients. J Am Coll Cardiol 7:300, 1986.

430. Hannerman H, Kloner RA, Schoen FJ, et al: Indomethacin-induced scar thinning following experimental myocardial infarction. Circulation 67:1290, 1983.
431. Roberts R, deMello V, Sobel BE: Deleterious effects of methylprednisolone in patients with myocardial infarction. Circulation 53 (suppl I):204, 1976.
432. Muller JE, Rude RE, Braunwald E, et al: Myocardial infarct extension: incidence, outcome, and risk factors in the MILIS study. Ann Intern Med 108:1, 1988.
433. Marmor A, Sobel BE, Roberts R: Factors presaging early recurrent myocardial infarction ("extension"). Am J Cardiol 48:603, 1981.
434. Hammerman H, Schoen FJ, Braunwald E, et al: Drug-induced expansion of infarct: morphologic and functional correlations. Circulation 69:611, 1984.
435. Eaton LW, Weiss JL, Bulkley BH, et al: Regional cardiac dilatation after acute myocardial infarction: recognition by two-dimensional echocardiography. N Engl J Med 300:57, 1979.
436. McKay RG, Pfeffer MA, Pasternak RC, et al: Left ventricular remodeling after myocardial infarction: a corollary to infarct expansion. Circulation 74:693, 1986.
437. Pfeffer MA, Lamas GA, Vaughan DE, et al: Effect of captopril on progressive ventricular dilatation. N Engl J Med 319:80, 1988.
438. Hutchins GM, Bulkley BH: Infarct expansion versus extension: two different complications of acute myocardial infarction. Am J Cardiol 41:227, 1978.
439. Roan PG, Buja LM, Saffer S, et al: Effects of systemic hypertension on ischemic and non-ischemic regional left ventricular function in awake, unsedated dogs after experimental coronary occlusion. Circulation 65:115, 1982.
440. Hillis LD, Davis C, Brotherton S, et al: The effect of various degrees of systemic arterial hypertension on acute canine myocardial ischemia. Am J Physiol 9:H855, 1981.
441. Gaudron P, Eilles C, Kugler I, Ertl G: Progressive left ventricular dysfunction and remodeling after myocardial infarction: potential mechanisms and early predictors. Circulation 87:755, 1993.
442. Warren SE, Royal H, Markis JE, et al: Time course of left ventricular dilation after myocardial infarction: influence of infarct related artery and success of coronary thrombolysis. J Am Coll Cardiol 11:12, 1988.
443. Bolognese L, Cerisano G, Buonamici P, et al: Influence of infarct zone viability on left ventricular remodeling following acute myocardial infarction. Circulation 96:3353, 1997.
444. Jeremy RW, Hackworthy RA, Bautovich G, et al: Infarct artery perfusion and changes in left ventricular volume in the month after acute myocardial infarction. J Am Coll Cardiol 9:989, 1987.
445. Raya TE, Gay RG, Lancaster L, et al: Serial changes in left ventricular relaxation and chamber stiffness after large myocardial infarction in rats. Circulation 77:1424, 1988.
446. Pipilis A, Meyer TE, Ormerod D, et al: Early and late changes in left ventricular filling after acute myocardial infarction and the effect of infarct size. Am J Cardiol 70:1397, 1992.
447. Popovic Ad, Neskovic AN, Babic R, et al: Independent impact of thrombolytic therapy and vessel patency on left ventricular dilation after myocardial infarction: serial echocardiographic follow-up. Circulation 77:1424.
448. Cerisano G, Bolognese L, Carrabba N, et al: Doppler-derived mitral deceleration time: an early strong predictor of left ventricular remodeling after reperfused anterior acute myocardial infarction. Circulation 99:230, 1999.
449. DeBusk RF, Blomqvist CG, Kouchoukos NT, et al: Identification and treatment of low-risk patients after acute myocardial infarction and coronary artery bypass graft surgery. N Engl J Med 314:161, 1986.
450. Rapaport E, Remedios P: The high-risk patient after recovery from myocardial infarction: recognition and management. J Am Coll Cardiol 1:391, 1983.
451. Norris RM, Brandt PWT, Caughey DE, et al: A new coronary prognostic index. Lancet 1:274, 1969.
452. Tofler GH, Stone PH, Muller JE, et al: Effects of gender and race on prognosis after acute myocardial infarction: adverse prognosis for women, particularly black women. J Am Coll Cardiol 9:473, 1987.
453. Moss AJ, Bigger JT, Odoroff CL: Post infarction risk stratification. Prog Cardiovasc Dis 29:389, 1987.
454. Norris RM, Barnaby PF, Brandt PWT, et al: Prognosis after recovery from first acute myocardial infarction: determinants of reinfarction and sudden death. Am J Cardiol 53:408, 1984.
455. Smith J, Marcus FI, Serkoman R, with the Multicenter Postinfarction Research Group: Prognosis of patients with diabetes mellitus after acute myocardial infarction. Am J Cardiol 54:718, 1984.
456. Weiner DA, McCabe CH, Ryan TJ: Identification of patients with left main and three vessel coronary disease with clinical and exercise test variables. Am J Cardiol 46:21, 1980.
457. Hung J, Goris M, Nash E, et al: Comparative value of maximal treadmill testing, exercise thallium myocardial perfusion scintigraphy and exercise radionuclide ventriculography for distinguishing high- and low-risk patients soon after acute myocardial infarction. Am J Cardiol 53:1221, 1984.
458. Corbett JR, Nicod P, Lewis SE, et al: Prognostic value of submaximal exercise radionuclide ventriculography following acute transmural and nontransmural myocardial infarction. Am J Cardiol 52:82A, 1983.
459. Mukharji J, Rude RE, Poole WK, et al (Milis Study Group): Risk factors for sudden death after acute myocardial infarction: two-year follow-up. Am J Cardiol 54:31, 1984.
460. Dehmer GJ, Lewis SE, Hillis LD, et al: Exercise induced alterations in left ventricular volumes in man: usefulness in predicting the relative extent of coronary artery disease. Circulation 63:1008, 1981.
461. Banters C, Delomez M, VanBelle E, et al: Angiographically documented late reocclusion after successful coronary angioplasty in infarct-related lesion is a powerful predictor of long-term mortality. Circulation 99:2243, 1999.
462. Lamas GA, Flaker GC, Mitchell G, et al, for the Survival and Ventricular Enlargement Investigators: Effects of infarct artery patency on prognosis after acute myocardial infarction. Circulation 92:1101, 1995.
463. Mittleman M, Mintzer D, Maclure M, et al: Triggering of myocardial infarction by cocaine. Circulation 99:2737, 1999.
464. Popma JJ, Topol EJ: Adjuncts to thrombolysis for myocardial reperfusion. Ann Intern Med 115:84, 1991.
465. Collen D, Lijnen HR: Basic and clinical aspects of fibrinolysis and thrombolysis. Blood 78:3114, 1991.

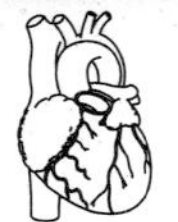

CHAPTER 37

PERCUTANEOUS CORONARY INTERVENTIONS FOR STABLE ANGINA PECTORIS

H. Vernon Anderson

MECHANISMS
Stents
Atherectomy
Combined Treatment
PATIENT SELECTION
Chronic Stable Angina
Long-Term Results
One-Vessel Disease
Multivessel Disease
RESTENOSIS
SUMMARY

The basic concept behind percutaneous coronary interventions arises from the knowledge that focal atherosclerotic narrowings in arteries limit the flow of blood through the vessel. This deprives the subtended organ (the heart) of adequate nutrient blood flow, especially under conditions of increased demand, such as strenuous physical activity, emotional distress, or other challenges. Enlargement of the arterial lumen at the stenotic site can restore blood flow to a more normal value. The idea of using a catheter to apply force from the inside of an artery to expand the narrowed region was developed and first reported by Dotter and Judkins.[1] In 1964, they described the use of rigid dilators to treat obstructions in peripheral arteries. Their method was effective, but numerous technical problems prevented its widespread clinical application. The sizes of dilators that could be introduced through an arterial puncture were limited, the relatively stiff dilators were difficult to maneuver through curved or twisted arterial segments, and unintentional vascular trauma was not infrequent.

In the early 1970s, Andreas Gruentzig experimented with the technique of Dotter and Judkins and made several important modifications. One of these was the development of a flexible, small-bore plastic catheter that had a nonelastic balloon at the distal end and contained an internal channel to inflate and deflate the balloon from the proximal end. This device could be introduced easily into a peripheral artery percutaneously and positioned at a stenotic site, and the balloon could be inflated for a few moments. The preformed, nonelastic balloon expanded to a known diameter and would remain at that diameter even as the pressure inside was increased. Sufficient force was developed to dilate the stenotic section of the vessel without overdistention of the adjacent normal vessel. In 1974, this new approach began to be applied quite successfully in peripheral arteries.[2] Further technical improvements then followed. Catheters and balloons were made much smaller. In 1977, the percutaneous transluminal dilatation technique was first applied to human coronary arteries, beginning the era of percutaneous transluminal coronary angioplasty (PTCA), and opening the way for a variety of subsequent techniques.[3, 4] As a group, these procedures are commonly called percutaneous transluminal coronary interventions (PTCIs); they encompass balloon dilatation angioplasty, rotational atherectomy, directional atherectomy, and the most important modification yet developed: stent deployment (Fig. 37–1). The application of these interventions for the treatment of stable angina pectoris is described here. Later chapters describe the use of PTCIs in the

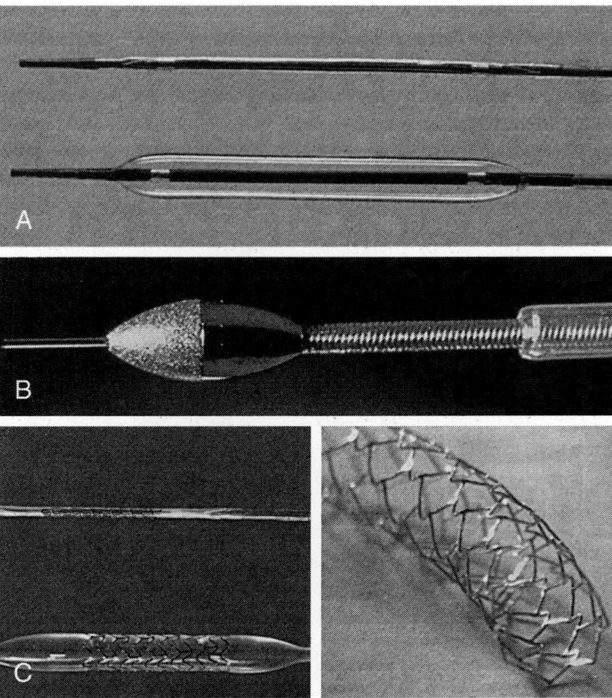

FIGURE 37–1 Devices for percutaneous transluminal coronary interventions. **A,** Coronary balloon. **B,** Rotational atherectomy burr (Rotablator). **C,** Coronary stent.

clinical settings of unstable angina pectoris and acute myocardial infarction.

Mechanisms

When it was originally developed—first in peripheral arteries and later extended to coronary arteries—balloon angioplasty was thought to produce enlargement of a vessel lumen mostly through the compression of atheromatous plaque by the distending force of the balloon (Fig. 37–2).[1,4] More extensive histologic research has revealed that the major mechanisms via which balloon dilatation achieves lumen enlargement are splitting or fracture of the atherosclerotic plaque, stretching of the media and adventitia of the arterial wall, and expansion of the overall diameter of the artery.[5,6] Balloon angioplasty, therefore, represents deliberate injury to the vessel wall. Most of the important complications that may occur with balloon angioplasty can be traced in large part to this injury. The technique of stent deployment (see later) was in fact originally developed to deal with two of the most common interrelated complications of balloon dilatation: extensive dissection with partially detached intimal flaps and the formation of occlusive thrombus. Interestingly, the early history of stenting was itself marked by problems of thrombosis, despite the use of complicated and intensive anticoagulation regimens. This stent-related thrombosis was subsequently found to be mostly due to inadequate stent expansion, with incomplete support of intimal dissection lines, as well as the presence of turbulent or static regions of blood flow between the outside edges of the stent and the intimal surface of the arterial wall. Once this problem was identified and resolved, and as the superior clinical outcomes of stents came to be appreciated, stenting became the preferred mode of interventional therapy.

Stents

In 1969, Charles Dotter developed a coil-spring endovascular prosthesis (stent) in an attempt to improve the long-term patency of atherosclerotic peripheral vessels treated with his method of dilatation.[7] Since the original description of Dotter's coil, there have been many variations on the original concept, including thermally shaped memory alloy coils, self-expanding steel spirals, balloon-expandable stainless steel mesh, balloon-expandable interdigitating coils, synthetic polymeric stents, and biodegradable stents.[8–13] These various devices differ greatly in their fundamental geometry (multiwire mesh or single wire), composition (metal or plastic), and mechanical behavior (active or passive expansion). Besides these fundamental differences, there are a variety of subtle differences that may also be important, such as filament thickness, alloy composition, electrostatic behavior, and coating.

Rationale for Stents

A stent helps optimize the dilatation process because it can "contain" the fractured irregular surface of the atherosclerotic plaque created by the disruptive action of the balloon.

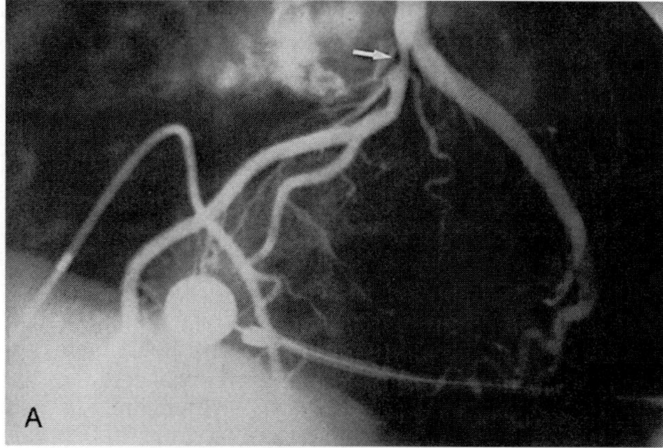

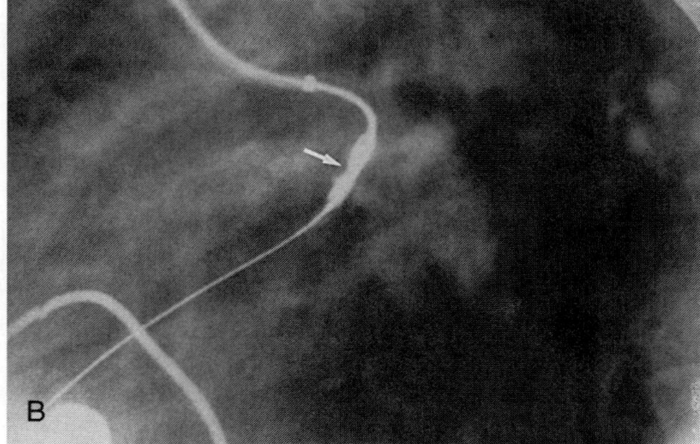

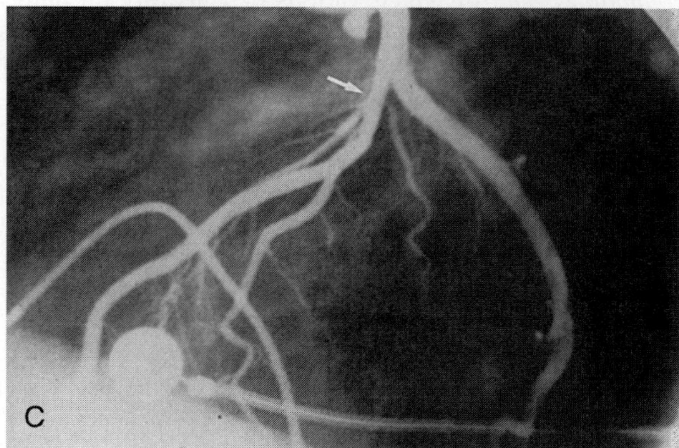

FIGURE 37–2 Selected frames from coronary arteriogram illustrate successful percutaneous transluminal coronary angioplasty in the left anterior oblique views. **A,** Stenosis (*arrow*) of the proximal left anterior descending coronary artery. **B,** During inflation of the angioplasty balloon. Note indentation of the balloon (*arrow*) by atherosclerotic plaque before full expansion. **C,** After balloon deflation and withdrawal. Luminal caliber (*arrow*) has been increased.

Two potential adverse effects of balloon dilatation—distal embolization of debris originating from the plaque and protruding obstructive flaps—are both checked by the stent acting as a scaffolding device. Elastic recoil of the artery, which is increasingly documented but probably still underestimated as a cause of abrupt closure and restenosis, is also prevented.[14] The stent has a smoothing effect, which reduces both the turbulent and laminar resistances to blood flow and so improves the immediate result. This might also be beneficial in preventing restenosis. Theoretical arguments have been proposed that assert how one particular stent design might be more effective than others in reducing recurrences. An attractive theoretical concept that favors the rigid stent is that limitation of vessel wall stress seems to be protective against atherogenesis. On the other hand, by stretching the vessel wall continuously (or at least over a long period), the self-expanding stent might have the countervailing effect of accelerating the neointimal proliferation of the restenosis process. Although there are experimental data from animal models to support both claims, there is little clinical evidence to support them, and they must be regarded as speculative. However, there is a wealth of data that indicate that stent implantation itself improves the immediate postdilatation result, producing a smooth, straight-bordered appearance of the treated arterial segment. This visual impression has been confirmed through quantitative analysis with both edge detection and videodensitometry techniques.[15]

Stents in Clinical Use

There are two different types of stent designs in clinical use. The first and less common stent type, and the first to be implanted in a human coronary artery, is a spring-like mesh design that is constrained to a small diameter around a delivery catheter and expands to a predetermined dimension when the constraint sheath is removed (*self-expanding stent*). The second and more common type is the *balloon-expandable stent*, of which various designs rely on deformation of the metal wire braids beyond their elastic limits to remain expanded. As mentioned, it is not clear whether there are important differences in these differing designs. The crucially important point about stents was the definitive reduction in adverse events that occurred when they were introduced into angioplasty practice. Before stents, the occurrence of abrupt closure of the treated artery was a feared and not infrequent complication. Table 37–1 lists the occurrences and outcomes of abrupt closure before and after the introduction of stents. In three large studies of the problem, involving more than 4300 procedures,[16–18] the incidence of abrupt closure was 6.4 percent. Only about one half (53 percent) of the closed arteries could be successfully reopened, and emergency coronary artery bypass graft surgery (CABG) was necessary in approximately one third (31 percent) of the patients. The in-hospital mortality rate was 4.6 percent. In several large studies of stenting as a treatment for abrupt closure (either actual or impending closure),[19–24] the success rate for reopening the arteries was 96 percent. Emergency CABG was necessary in only 3.1 percent of the patients, and the in-hospital mortality rate was reduced to 1.7 percent. In addition to these data, several large institutions reported their adverse event rates before and after the introduction of stents, without regard to abrupt closure (Table 37–2).[25–28] In more than 10,000 procedures performed at these institutions before the use of stents, the rate for emergency CABG was 3 percent, and the overall in-hospital mortality rate was 0.6 percent. Corresponding rates in more than 14,000 procedures performed after stent availability are 1.9 and 0.2 percent, respectively.

It then remained to be seen whether these dramatic improvements in short-term adverse event rates could be sustained over longer periods, and especially whether recurrence (*restenosis*) rates would be reduced. Although several nonrandomized reviews suggested that restenosis rates were lower with the use of stents than with the use of balloon angioplasty, doubt remained. There have been five randomized published studies that compare balloon angioplasty with stenting (Table 37–3).[29–35] Angiographic restenosis rates (in a comparison of only angiographic measures), as well as clinical event rates (for death, myocardial infarction, or repeat revascularization), have been found to be improved with the use of stents. Taken together, these data on acute complications and longer-term favorable outcomes have established stenting as the standard mode of therapy.

TABLE 37–1 Outcome of Abrupt Closure Before and After Stenting

	Patients		Outcome of Abrupt Closure (%)		
	PTCA	*With Abrupt Closure*	*Success*	*EmCABG*	*Death*
Before Stenting					
Sinclair et al[16]	1160	54 (4.7%)	57	33	1.9
Detre et al[17]	1801	122 (6.8%)	49	35	5.0
de Feyter et al[18]	1423	104 (7.3%)	54	30	6.0
Weighted average	4384	280 (6.4%)	53	31	4.6
After Stenting					
Roubin et al[19]	1338	115 (8.6%)	100	4.2	1.7
George et al[20]	NR	518	95	4.3	2.2
Schomig et al[21]	4959	339 (6.8%)	97	0	1.8
Eeckhout et al[22]	NR	101	100	0	0
Antoniucci et al[23]	697	120 (17%)	100	1	1
Dean et al[24]	4421	350 (7.9%)	92	6	1.7
Weighted average		1543	96	3.1	1.7

Abbreviations: EmCABG, emergency coronary artery bypass graft surgery; NR, not reported; PTCA, percutaneous transluminal coronary angioplasty.

TABLE 37–2 **Emergency Coronary Artery Bypass Graft Surgery and In-Hospital Mortality Rates Before and After the Introduction of Stenting**

Study	Before Stenting			After Stenting		
	PTCI	*EmCABG*	*Death*	*PTCI*	*EmCABG*	*Death*
Scott et al[25]	3448	64 (1.9%)	8 (0.2%)	3863	46 (1.2%)	4 (0.1%)
Lindsay et al[26]	3877	173 (4.5%)	NR	8484	207 (2.4%)	NR
Altmann et al[27]	1525	44 (2.9%)	16 (1.1%)	717	8 (1.1%)	5 (0.7%)
Stauffer et al[28]	1468	28 (1.9%)	13 (0.9%)	1615	13 (0.8%)	2 (0.1%)
Total procedures, weighted average	10,318	3%	0.6%	14,679	1.9%	0.2%

Abbreviations: EmCABG, emergency coronary artery bypass graft surgery; NR, not reported (not included in weighted averages); PTCI, percutaneous coronary artery intervention.

Atherectomy

Atherectomy refers to various methods that physically remove portions of obstructing lesions from the lumen of an artery. This tissue removal is also termed *ablative* or *debulking*. The initial impetus stemmed from the hope that by actually removing atheromatous material, rather than just compressing it and stretching the artery walls, both acute closure and restenosis might be curtailed. Several different types of atherectomy devices have been devised; two are in regular but infrequent clinical use.

Directional Coronary Atherectomy

The directional coronary atherectomy catheter consists of a flexible shaft with a 1-cm cutting chamber just behind a collecting chamber and a low-pressure balloon opposite the opening of the cutting chamber. The device is designed to be advanced into an atheromatous coronary lesion over a standard guide wire, followed by inflation of the balloon (which effectively presses the cutting window against the atheroma). Next, the rotary cutter is pulled back and then activated, spinning at approximately 1500 rpm. The rotating cutter is advanced across the cutting chamber window, shaving off atheroma and pushing the shaved material into the collecting chamber. The balloon is then deflated. The device is repositioned within the plaque, and the procedure is repeated, typically four to eight times. When it is finally withdrawn, all of the excised material comes out with the catheter because it is held within the front collecting chamber. Although the mechanism of action was initially thought to be solely atheroma extraction, it was subsequently found that the device also stretches the arterial wall while it excises plaque.[36–38] The angiographic improvement seen immediately after directional atherectomy is probably very much related to vessel and plaque stretching as well as to tissue extraction.

Directional Atherectomy Versus Balloon Angioplasty

Several studies have been conducted that compare directional atherectomy with balloon angioplasty. In general, the immediate- and long-term results of the two procedures are comparable, both in native coronary arteries and in saphenous vein bypass grafts (Table 37–4).[39–42] These findings are supported by analyses of combined data from two large registries of PTCIs, in which the results for balloon

TABLE 37–3 **Randomized Trials Comparing Balloon Angioplasty With Stenting**

Study	n	Procedure Success Rate (%)		Angiographic Restenosis Rate (%)		Clinical Events by 6 mo (%)		Clinical Events by 1 yr (%)	
		Balloon	*Stent*	*Balloon*	*Stent*	*Balloon*	*Stent*	*Balloon*	*Stent*
Stent Restenosis Study[29, 30]	407	90	96	42	32	16	15	26	21
BENESTENT[31, 32]	503	95	95	32	22	30	20	32	23
Versaci et al[33]	120	93	95	40	19	—	—	30	13
Rodriguez et al[34]†	66	100	100	73	21	75	21	—	—
Erbel et al[35]‡	354	93	99	32	18	28	16	—	—
Total procedures, weighted average	1450	93	96	37	23	30	19	31	23

*Lesions in proximal left anterior descending coronary artery only.
†Lesions with early recoil only.
‡Restenosis lesions only.
Abbreviations: BENESTENT, Belgium-Netherlands Stent Restenosis Study.

TABLE 37-4 **Randomized Trials of Directional Coronary Atherectomy Versus Balloon Angioplasty**

	Patients (n)		In-Hospital						6-mo TLR (%)	
			Angiographic Success (%)		*Death (%)*		*EmCABG (%)*			
Study	BAL	DCA	BAL	DCA	BAL	DCA	BAL	DCA	BAL	DCA
CAVEAT-I[39]	500	512	80	89	0.4	0	2	3	37	37
CCAT[40]	136	138	91	98	0	0	4.4	1.4	26	28
BOAT[41]*	492	497	97	99	0.4	0	2	1	20	17
CAVEAT-II[42]†	156	149	79	89	2	2	1	1	26	19

*TLR rates for BOAT are 1-yr rates.
†CAVEAT-II involved vein graft interventions only.
Abbreviations: BAL, balloon angioplasty; BOAT, Balloon vs. Optimal Atherectomy Trial; CAVEAT, Coronary Angioplasty Versus Excisional Atherectomy Trial; CCAT, Canadian Coronary Atherectomy Trial; DCA, directional coronary atherectomy; EmCABG, emergency coronary artery bypass graft surgery; TLR, target lesion revascularization.

angioplasty and directional atherectomy were almost identical.[43] Atherectomy results are improved if the cutting procedure itself is followed by balloon dilatation as an adjunctive maneuver at completion.[44] Directional atherectomy may be a useful procedure for eccentric lesions of a proximal large vessel or for some ostial or bifurcation lesions. Characteristics that are correlated with an adverse outcome include stenosis located on a bend (not dissimilar from coronary balloon angioplasty), vessels with significant tortuosity proximal to the attempted lesion, a relatively small vessel lumen diameter, and heavily calcified lesions. Directional atherectomy can also be performed before stent deployment.[45, 46] The same optimization that stenting provides to balloon angioplasty may be equally applicable to directional atherectomy.

High-Speed Rotational Atherectomy (Rotablator)

The Rotablator consists of a diamond-tipped, olive-shaped metal burr that traverses along a stainless steel monofilament guide wire (see Fig. 37–1). The burr is welded to a flexible drive shaft that is covered by a plastic sheath. Burr sizes range between 1 and 2.75 mm. The typical working speed of the burr is 150,000 to 180,000 rpm. The shaft is cooled and irrigated with pressurized saline. The Rotablator burr is advanced along the coronary guide wire, spinning at high speeds and differentially abrading the relatively hard atheroma while leaving the softer and more pliable normal vessel wall intact. One advantage of the Rotablator appears to be the ease with which it can reach the distal portions of diffusely diseased vessels. In addition, it can enlarge very hard calcified lesions, as well as some ostial lesions. As a sole treatment device, it has been found to be lacking. However, it was recognized early in clinical experience with the device that adjunctive balloon angioplasty after the use of the Rotablator was an acceptable and even favorable treatment strategy. In the original New Approaches to Coronary Intervention (NACI) Registry, Rotablator alone in 349 patients in whom it was attempted achieved a successful result 72 percent of the time. Success rates increased to 97 percent when adjunctive balloon angioplasty was performed.[47] Other studies have reported similar results, and Rotablator is almost always a "pretreatment" before balloon angioplasty or stenting, at least in larger vessels.[48–52]

Combined Treatment

As mentioned earlier, both types of atherectomy procedures are usually followed by adjunctive balloon angioplasty or stenting. The excellent results with this approach are increasingly recognized. Tables 37–5 and 37–6 illustrate the immediate- and long-term (9-month) clinical results of the combined approaches.[51, 52] The low rates of immediate adverse events, along with the lower recurrence rates, have made adjunctive treatment after atherectomy the favored strategy.

PATIENT SELECTION

Coronary interventions are performed in patients with the full spectrum of clinical syndromes, including chronic stable angina, unstable angina, and acute myocardial infarction. They are performed in native coronary arteries as well as in arterial or venous bypass grafts. The patients may have disease in one or multiple vessels, multiple stenoses within one vessel, or totally occluded arteries. Left ventricular function can be normal or compromised. Patients may or may not be candidates for CABG. In general, the main consideration is that the operator and the patient must be reasonably confident that the operator can successfully treat the culprit coronary lesion or lesions.

Chronic Stable Angina

One of the original specifications for coronary intervention was the presence of chronic stable angina pectoris of such severity that coronary bypass surgery was indicated. This generally meant grade III or IV angina according to the grading system of the Canadian Cardiovascular Society. In those early days, most patients would have had medical therapy instituted for their angina, with subsequent adjustments in doses, before undergoing diagnostic catheterization and the consideration of revascularization of any sort.

TABLE 37-5 **Procedural Success and In-Hospital Complication Rates for Combined Devices**

	Balloon Angioplasty	Ablative Device*	Balloon + Stent	Ablative Device* + Stent	*P*
n	1089	631	1029	364	—
Success (%)	89	95	98	96	<.001
Death (%)	0.9	0.8	0.4	1	.898
EmCABG (%)	2	1	0.5	0.6	.009

*Ablative device includes directional atherectomy, extractional atherectomy, rotational atherectomy, and laser angioplasty.
Abbreviation: EmCABG, emergency coronary artery bypass graft surgery.
From Lindsay J, Pinnow EE, Pichard AD: New devices enhance results of coronary angioplasty. Cathet Cardiovasc Diagn 43:1–6, 1998; copyright 1998. Reprinted by permission of Wiley-Liss, Inc., a subsidiary of John Wiley & Sons, Inc.

The advent of balloon angioplasty in 1977 began to change that approach. Patients who had experienced chronic stable angina for many years began to undergo catheterization and intervention without any precipitating change in symptoms or medication adjustments. In addition, even when they had relatively mild symptoms and stable patterns, patients with new-onset angina began to undergo catheterization and intervention much sooner. Excellent results were achieved with balloon coronary angioplasty in these settings.[53–55] Mortality rates were low, less than 0.05 percent overall, and the rates of myocardial infarction were approximately 2 to 4 percent. This was comparable to the results obtained with elective CABG undertaken at the time. The advent of stents in the early 1990s further improved the outcomes of PTCIs. As pointed out, although stents were originally developed and introduced into clinical practice to help combat the problem of abrupt closure, they rapidly came to be recognized as a superior procedure.

Long-Term Results

The primary goal of coronary interventions is to reduce or eliminate angina pectoris or other objective signs of myocardial ischemia. The secondary goal is to decrease the number of untoward cardiac events such as cardiac death or myocardial infarction that might otherwise occur during the years after significant coronary disease is first recognized and treated. Postponement or perhaps even elimination of the requirement for CABG is another secondary goal of PTCIs.

The clinical evidence that coronary interventions relieve chronic stable angina pectoris is so strong that only three relatively small randomized trials of traditional balloon angioplasty compared with medical therapy have been conducted.[56–58] Two of these trials were conducted in patients with one-vessel disease, whereas one trial involved patients with either one-vessel or some simple types of multivessel disease. Earlier work comparing CABG with medical therapy had already indicated that patients with multivessel coronary disease (especially three-vessel and left main disease) did not do as well with medical therapy as with surgical revascularization.[59–61] Therefore, it has not generally been thought appropriate to assign patients with severe multivessel disease to a medical therapy arm.

One-Vessel Disease

The first angioplasty-versus-medical therapy trial, the Department of Veterans Affairs Angioplasty Compared to Medicine (ACME) trial, randomly assigned 105 patients with one-vessel disease to receive balloon PTCA and 107 patients to receive medical therapy.[56] By 6 months later, more patients in the PTCA group were free of angina than were those in the medical therapy group (64 versus 46 percent, $P < .01$), and their duration of exercise on a treadmill was greater (increase of 2.1 versus 0.5 minute, $P < .0001$). The PTCA patients also had a greater improvement in physical and psychologic quality-of-life measures than did the medically treated patients.[62] At an extended follow-up 2 to 3 years later, the PTCA patients continued

TABLE 37-6 **Immediate and 9-Month Clinical Outcomes After Rotational Atherectomy, Stenting, or the Combination**

	Rotational Atherectomy	Stenting	Rotational Atherectomy + Stenting	*P*
n	147	103	56	—
Success (%)	99	98	98	—
Death (%)	0	1	1.8	—
EmCABG (%)	0.6	1	0	—
Events by 9 mo (%)				
Death	1	2	0	.44
MI	1	0	0	.58
TLR	28	21	15	.08

Abbreviations: EmCABG, emergency coronary artery bypass graft surgery; MI, myocardial infarction; TLR, target lesion revascularization.
From Hoffmann R, Mintz GS, Kent KM, et al: Comparative early and nine-month results of rotational atherectomy, stents, and the combination of both for calcified lesions in large coronary arteries. Am J Cardiol 81:552–557, 1998; with permission from Excerpta Medica, Inc.

to have a greater duration of exercise tolerance than the medically treated patients.[63] Interestingly, the use of revascularization procedures beyond the initial hospitalization during the 2- to 3-year follow-up was no different between the two groups.

The second trial, the Medicine, Angioplasty or Surgery Study (MASS), was conducted in Brazil.[57] In this trial, 214 patients with stable angina, normal left ventricular function, and a single stenosis of the proximal left anterior descending coronary artery were randomly assigned to medical therapy (n = 72), angioplasty (n = 72), or CABG (n = 70). End point events were death, myocardial infarction, or revascularization. At an average follow-up of 3.5 years, the probability of event-free survival was greatest in the surgical patients (97 percent) and lower but similar in both the angioplasty and medical therapy patients (76 and 83 percent, respectively). The two revascularization strategies were each superior to medical therapy for the suppression of angina at follow-up. Significantly more patients in the two revascularization groups had ischemia-free exercise tests than the medically treated patients.

The third trial, a pilot trial from the Department of Veterans Affairs, randomly assigned 328 male patients with stable angina and either one-vessel (n = 227) or two-vessel (n = 101) disease to PTCA or medical therapy.[58] In the one-vessel disease patients, PTCA was superior to medical therapy for suppression of angina, increase in exercise test duration, and improved quality of life scores at follow-up 6 months later. These relative benefits of PTCA over medical therapy were not as great in patients with two-vessel disease. The improvement in thallium perfusion imaging for ischemia was better for PTCA than for medical therapy only for one-vessel disease patients and was not improved or was worse in simple two-vessel disease patients.

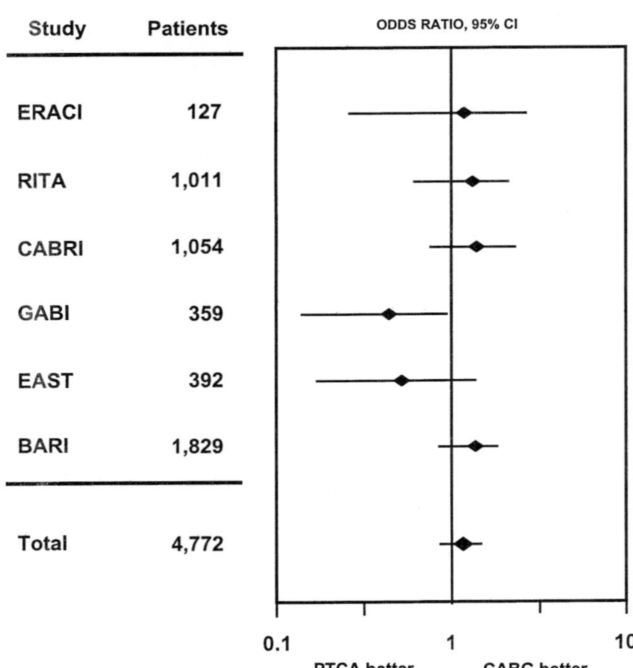

FIGURE 37–3 Overall combined risk for death and nonfatal myocardial infarction in six randomized trials comparing coronary angioplasty (PTCA) with coronary artery bypass graft surgery (CABG). See text for details. BARI, Bypass Angioplasty Revascularization Investigation trial; CABRI, Coronary Angioplasty versus Bypass Revascularization Investigation; EAST, Emory Angioplasty versus Surgery Trial; ERACI, Argentine Randomized Trial of Coronary Angioplasty versus Bypass Surgery in Multivessel Disease; GABI, German Angioplasty Bypass Surgery Investigation; RITA, Randomized Intervention Treatment of Angina.

Multivessel Disease

The aforementioned trials that compared CABG with medical therapy clearly established that revascularization was preferred when multivessel coronary disease was present. Revascularization with coronary angioplasty instead of CABG can in many cases be performed in multiple coronary arteries, raising the question of when each technique might be appropriately used. The multiple adjunctive techniques now available, and especially the improved safety profile obtained with stents, have highlighted this question even further.

There have been six moderately large trials comparing PTCA with CABG for patients with multivessel coronary disease (Table 37–7).[64–72] The overwhelming majority of patients assigned to angioplasty had traditional balloon PTCA only; adjunctive device use was extremely rare in these trials. The trials have differed somewhat in their patient enrollment specifications. All of them have included patients with multivessel coronary disease, yet the Randomized Intervention Treatment of Angina (RITA) trial also included some patients with one-vessel disease. Some of the trials have specified certain left ventricular functional requirements, but others have not. They also differ in the proportions of men and women enrolled, as well as in the proportions of patients with stable versus unstable coronary syndromes. By far the greatest difficulty with these trials is the small percentage of screened patients who were enrolled in them. Overall, only 5 percent of 91,730 patients who were evaluated were entered into the randomization arms. Patients were excluded on appropriate angiographic grounds, including left main disease, chronic total occlusions, and diffuse disease. In many cases, patients with infarctions (recent or even remote) or previous PTCA or CABG were excluded. This highly selective process limits the ability to extrapolate results from these trials to the broad general population of multivessel disease patients. Nevertheless, they are the only data available. The results, both individually and collectively (Fig. 37–3), indicate that there are no differences in death or myocardial infarction outcomes between angioplasty and CABG. It is important to note, however, that repeat revascularization was much more likely to be required during the first year after PTCA than in the first year after CABG (33.7 versus 3.3 percent).[73]

The Bypass Angioplasty Revascularization Investigation (BARI) trial was the only one that was sufficiently large to examine mortality differences in subgroups. Overall, at 5 years, cardiac mortality rates in patients randomized to PTCA were 8.0 compared with 4.9 percent in those randomized to CABG (Fig. 37–4).[71] This mortality rate difference was due entirely to the subgroup of patients with

TABLE 37-7 Randomized Trials of Coronary Angioplasty Versus Bypass Surgery

Study	Year Reported	Length of Follow-up (yr)	Patients Screened	Patients Enrolled	Enrollment (% of Screened)	Median Age (yr)	Men (% of Enrolled)	Diseased Vessels	LVEF (mean)
ERACI[64, 65]	1993	3	1409	127	9	58	85	≥2	0.61
RITA[66]	1993	2.5	27,975	1011	4	57	81	≥1	NR
CABRI[67]	1994	1	23,047	1054	5	61	78	≥2	0.63
GABI[68]	1994	1	8981	359	4	59	89	≥2	NR
EAST[69]	1994	3	5118	392	8	62	74	≥2	0.61
BARI[70–72]	1996	5	25,200	1829	7	62	73	≥2	0.57
Total		1–5	91,730	4772	5		80		

Abbreviations: BARI, Bypass Angioplasty Revascularization Investigation trial; CABRI, Coronary Angioplasty versus Bypass Revascularization Investigation; EAST, Emory Angioplasty versus Surgery Trial; ERACI, Argentine Randomized Trial of Coronary Angioplasty versus Bypass Surgery in Multivessel Disease; GABI, German Angioplasty Bypass Surgery Investigation; NR, not reported; RITA, Randomized Intervention Treatment of Angina.

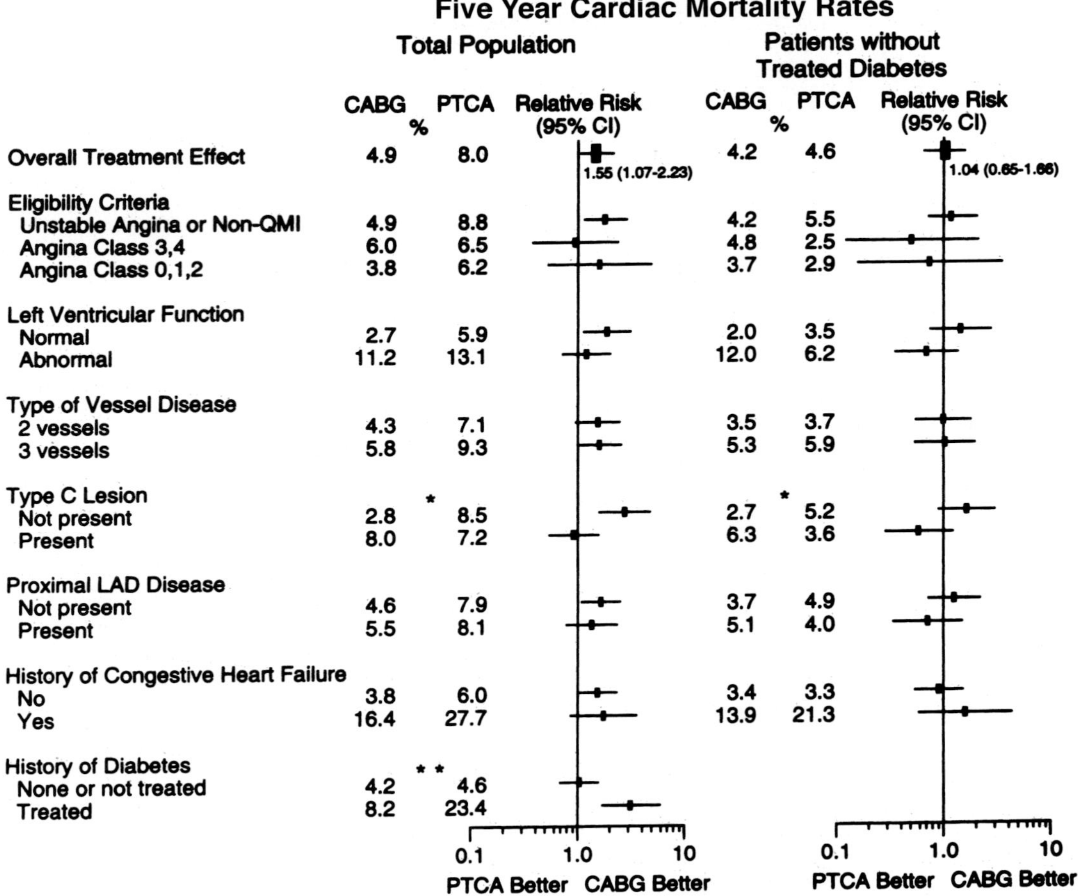

FIGURE 37–4 Five-year cardiac mortality rates in the Bypass Angioplasty Revascularization Investigation (BARI) trial. The relative risks with 95 percent confidence intervals (CI) are displayed for the overall effect and for subgroups of clinical interest. **Left,** Relative risks for the entire treated population. **Right,** Relative risks for the patients without diabetes mellitus. CABG, coronary artery bypass graft surgery; LAD, left anterior descending coronary artery; PTCA, percutaneous transluminal coronary angioplasty; QMI, Q wave myocardial infarction. (From Chaitman BR, Rosen AD, Williams DO, et al: Myocardial infarction and cardiac mortality in the Bypass Angioplasty Revascularization Investigation [BARI] randomized trial. Circulation 96:2162–2170, 1997.)

treated diabetes mellitus. In treated diabetics, those randomized to PTCA had a 5-year cardiac mortality rate of 23.4 percent compared with 8.2 percent in those randomized to CABG. In patients without treated diabetes, the 5-year cardiac mortality rates were similar and lower (4.6 versus 4.2 percent). These data have prompted a reevaluation of treatment strategies for diabetics with multivessel coronary artery disease.

TABLE 37–8 Repeat Angioplasty for First Restenosis

Study	Patients (n)	Procedural Success (%)	Additional Site Treated (%)	Complications (%) MI	EmCABG	Death	Angiographic Recurrent Restenosis (%)
Williams et al[74]	203	85	NR	1.5	2	0	34
Meier et al[75]	95	97	12	0	1	0	26
Rapold et al[76]	66	91	24	3	2	0	36
Schweiger et al[77]	51	100	10	NR	0	2	33
Quigley et al[78]	117	98	2	0	0	0.8	32
Glazier et al[79]	196	92	NR	NR	3	NR	26
Deligonul et al[80]	144	94	44	0	1	0	NR
Weintraub et al[81]	1051	96	17	0.8	2.5	0.1	51
Dimas et al[82]	465	97	23	0.9	1.5	0	NR
Total, weighted average	2388	95	19	0.8	2	0.1	38

Abbreviations: EmCABG, emergency coronary artery bypass graft surgery; MI, myocardial infarction; NR, not reported (not included in averages).

TABLE 37–9 **Long-Term Clinical Outcomes of Coronary Angioplasty**

Study	Patients (n)	Follow-up (yr)	Repeat PTCA (%)	CABG (%)	MI (%)	Death (%)
King and Schlumpf[86]	133	>10	23	23	NR	11
Ruygrok et al[87]	856	8–14	26	26	17	23
Hasdai et al[88]	611	10–16	38	33	15	23
Holmes et al[89]	1989	10	41	25	18	22
Total, weighted average	3589		36	27	17	22

Abbreviations: CABG, coronary artery bypass graft surgery; MI, myocardial infarction; NR, not reported; PTCA, percutaneous transluminal coronary angioplasty.

Restenosis

Coronary intervention as a long-term therapeutic treatment for atherosclerotic coronary disease remains limited by the problem of recurrence of the stenotic lesion (restenosis). This is counterbalanced by the fact that multiple repeat interventions, in general, can be performed relatively easily over a period of years, postponing CABG to a time later in life when graft longevity becomes a minor consideration. Restenosis appears to occur via a mechanism of hyperplastic intimal and medial response to the injury of dilatation. This process develops in the weeks after angioplasty and is generally completed within 4 to 6 months. If restenosis does occur, coronary intervention often can be repeated with excellent results (Table 37–8).[74–82] Procedural success rates are excellent. Interestingly, additional sites are often treated whenever patients undergo repeat angioplasty for restenosis. Complication rates are low, with emergency CABG needed in approximately 2 percent of patients, and an in-hospital mortality rate of only about 0.1 percent. In fact, the relative ease and lower risk with which repeat intervention can be done represent an argument in favor of its widespread application. Even so, restenosis rates after second or subsequent interventional procedures appear to be at least as high or higher than those for first-time angioplasty, averaging about 30 to 50 percent.[83–85]

The very long-term clinical outcomes after coronary angioplasty are beginning to be examined.[86–89] With follow-up extending beyond 10 years in more than 3500 patients, the results are quite favorable (Table 37–9). At least one repeat angioplasty was required in about one third of the patients (36 percent), about one fourth ultimately underwent CABG (27 percent), and an infarction had occurred in about one in six patients (17 percent). The crude mortality rate at 10 or more years was approximately 22 percent, unadjusted for age or comorbid conditions.

Summary

Coronary interventions are useful revascularization strategies in a variety of clinical situations but especially for chronic stable angina. In an integrated approach to coronary artery disease and its management, interventions are ideally suited to early disease detection. In the early stages of coronary disease, it is more likely to involve only single vessels and to have not yet produced infarction. Over the course of many years, several interventional procedures can be performed to treat the same or different coronary lesions. As the disease progresses to involve multiple sites in several vessels, additional procedures remain possible but become less attractive. CABG could be used at this stage for continued preservation of myocardial function. Should focal stenoses develop in bypass grafts, further interventional procedures may be required. Coupled with aggressive management of known risk factors, as well as an improved understanding of risk factor management in the future, revascularization with PTCIs will continue to play a major role in relieving symptoms and signs of myocardial ischemia and contribute greatly to the overall cardiovascular health of patients.

References

1. Dotter CT, Judkins MP: Transluminal treatment of atherosclerotic obstruction: description of a new technique and a preliminary report of its application. Circulation 30:654–658, 1964.
2. Gruentzig AR, Kumpe DA: Techniques of percutaneous transluminal angioplasty with the Gruentzig balloon catheter. AJR 132:547–552, 1979.
3. Gruentzig A: Transluminal dilatation of coronary artery stenosis. Lancet 1:263, 1978.
4. Gruentzig A, Senning A, Siegenthaler WE: Nonoperative dilatation of coronary artery stenosis: percutaneous transluminal coronary angioplasty. N Engl J Med 61:303–307, 1979.
5. Castaneda-Zuniga WR, Formarek A, Todavarthy M, Edwards JE: The mechanism of balloon angioplasty. Radiology 135:565–569, 1980.
6. Waller BF: Crackers, breakers, stretchers, drillers, scrapers, shavers, burners, welders and melters—the future treatment of atherosclerotic coronary artery disease? A clinical-morphological assessment. J Am Coll Cardiol 13:969–987, 1989.
7. Dotter CT: Transluminally placed coil-spring endarterial tube grafts: long-term patency in canine popliteal artery. Invest Radiol 4:329–332, 1969.
8. Cragg A, Lund G, Rysavy J, et al: Nonsurgical placement of arterial endoprostheses: a new technique using nitinol wire. Radiology 147:261–263, 1983.
9. Maass D, Zollikofer CL, Larglader F, Senning A: Radiological follow-up of transluminally inserted vascular endoprostheses: an experimental study using expanding spirals. Radiology 152:659–663, 1984.
10. Sigwart U, Puel J, Mirkovitch V, et al: Intravascular stents to prevent occlusion and restenosis after transluminal angioplasty. N Engl J Med 316:701–706, 1987.
11. Schatz RA, Palmaz JC, Tio FO, et al: Balloon-expandable intracoronary stents in the adult dog. Circulation 76:450–457, 1987.
12. Roubin GS, Robinson KA, King SB III, et al: Early and late results of intracoronary arterial stenting after coronary angiography in dogs. Circulation 76:891–897, 1987.
13. Slepina MJ, Schmidler A: Polymeric endoluminal paving/sealing: a bio-degradable alternative to intracoronary stenting. Circulation (suppl II):II-409, 1988.
14. Rensing BJ, Hermans WRM, Beatt KJ, et al: Quantitative angiographic assessment of elastic recoil after percutaneous transluminal coronary angioplasty. Am J Cardiol 66:1039–1044, 1990.
15. Strauss BH, Juilliere Y, Rensing BJ, et al: Edge detection versus

densitometry for assessing coronary stenting quantitatively. Am J Cardiol 67:484–490, 1991.

16. Sinclair IN, McCabe CH, Sipperly ME, Baim DS: Predictors, therapeutic options and long-term outcome of abrupt reclosure. Am J Cardiol 61:61G–66G, 1988.
17. Detre KM, Holmes DR, Holubkov R, et al: Incidence and consequences of periprocedural occlusion. Circulation 82:739–750, 1990.
18. de Feyter PJ, van den Brand M, Jaarman GJ, et al: Acute coronary artery occlusion during and after percutaneous transluminal coronary angioplasty. Circulation 83:927–936, 1991.
19. Roubin GS, Cannon AD, Agarwal SK, et al: Intracoronary stenting for acute and threatened closure complicating percutaneous transluminal coronary angioplasty. Circulation 85:916–927, 1992.
20. George BS, Voorhees WD, Roubin GS, et al: Multicenter investigation of coronary stenting to treat acute or threatened closure after percutaneous transluminal coronary angioplasty: clinical and angiographic outcomes. J Am Coll Cardiol 22:135–143, 1993.
21. Schomig A, Kastrati A, Mudra H, et al: Four-year experience with Palmaz-Schatz stenting in coronary angioplasty complicated by dissection with threatened or present vessel closure. Circulation 90:2716–2724, 1994.
22. Eeckhout E, Stauffer JC, Vogt P, et al: Unplanned use of intracoronary stents for the treatment of a suboptimal angiographic result after conventional balloon angioplasty. Am Heart J 130:1164–1167, 1995.
23. Antoniucci D, Valenti R, Santoro GM, et al: Bailout coronary stenting without anticoagulation or intravascular ultrasound guidance. Cathet Cardiovasc Diagn 41:14–19, 1997.
24. Dean LS, George CJ, Roubin GS, et al: Bailout and corrective use of Gianturco-Roubin flex stents after percutaneous transluminal coronary angioplasty. J Am Coll Cardiol 29:934–940, 1997.
25. Scott NA, Weintraub WS, Carlin SF, et al: Recent changes in the management and outcome of acute closure after percutaneous transluminal coronary angioplasty. Am J Cardiol 71:1159–1163, 1993.
26. Lindsay J, Hong MK, Pinnow EE, Pichard AD: Effects of endoluminal coronary stents on the frequency of coronary artery bypass grafting after unsuccessful percutaneous transluminal coronary revascularization. Am J Cardiol 77:647–649, 1996.
27. Altmann DB, Racz M, Battleman DS, et al: Reduction in angioplasty complications after the introduction of coronary stents. Am Heart J 132:503–507, 1996.
28. Stauffer JC, Eeckhout E, Vogt P, et al: Stand-by versus stent-by during percutaneous transluminal coronary angioplasty. Am Heart J 130:21–26, 1995.
29. Fischman DL, Leon MB, Baim DS, et al: A randomized comparison of coronary-stent placement and balloon angioplasty in the treatment of coronary artery disease. N Engl J Med 331:496–501, 1994.
30. George CJ, Baim DS, Brinker JA, et al: One-year follow-up of the Stent Restenosis (STRESS I) study. Am J Cardiol 81:860–865, 1998.
31. Serruys PW, de Jaegere P, Kiemeneij F, et al: A comparison of balloon-expandable-stent implantation with balloon angioplasty in patients with coronary artery disease. N Engl J Med 331:489–495, 1994.
32. Macaya C, Serruys PW, Ruygrok P, et al: Continued benefit of coronary stenting versus balloon angioplasty: one-year clinical follow-up of Benestent trial. J Am Coll Cardiol 27:255–261, 1996.
33. Versaci F, Gaspardone A, Tomai F, et al: A comparison of coronary-artery stenting with angioplasty for isolated stenosis of the proximal left anterior descending coronary artery. N Engl J Med 336:817–822, 1997.
34. Rodriguez AE, Santaera O, Larribau M, et al: Coronary stenting decreases restenosis in lesions with early loss in luminal diameter 24 hours after successful PTCA. Circulation 91:1397–1402, 1995.
35. Erbel R, Haude M, Hopp HW, et al: Coronary-artery stenting compared with balloon angioplasty for restenosis after initial balloon angioplasty. N Engl J Med 339:1672–1678, 1998.
36. Garratt KN, Edwards WD, Vlietstra RE, et al: Coronary morphology after percutaneous directional coronary atherectomy in humans: autopsy analysis of three patients. J Am Coll Cardiol 16:1432–1436, 1990.
37. Safian RD, Gelbfish JS, Erny RE, et al: Coronary atherectomy: clinical, angiographic, and histological findings and observations regarding potential mechanisms. Circulation 82:69–79, 1990.
38. Umans VA, Baptista J, di Mario C, et al: Angiographic, ultrasonic, and angioscopic assessment of the coronary artery wall and lumen area configuration after directional atherectomy: the mechanism revisited. Am Heart J 130:217–227, 1995.
39. Topol EJ, Leya F, Pinkerton CA, et al: A comparison of directional atherectomy with coronary angioplasty in patients with coronary artery disease. N Engl J Med 329:221–227, 1993.
40. Adelman AG, Cohen EA, Kimball BP, et al: A comparison of directional atherectomy with balloon angioplasty for lesions of the left anterior descending coronary artery. N Engl J Med 329:228–233, 1993.
41. Baim DS, Cutlip DE, Sharma SK, et al: Final results of the Balloon vs Optimal Atherectomy Trial (BOAT). Circulation 97:322–331, 1998.
42. Holmes DR, Topol EJ, Califf RM, et al: A multicenter, randomized trial of coronary angioplasty versus directional atherectomy for patients with saphenous vein bypass graft lesions. Circulation 91:1966–1974, 1995.
43. King SB, Yeh W, Holubkov R, et al: Balloon angioplasty versus new device intervention: clinical outcomes: a comparison of the NHLBI PTCA and NACI registries. J Am Coll Cardiol 31:558–566, 1998.
44. Simonton CA, Leon MB, Baim DS, et al: Optimal directional coronary atherectomy: final results of the Optimal Atherectomy Restenosis Study (OARS). Circulation 97:332–339, 1998.
45. Moussa I, Moses J, Di Mario C, et al: Stenting after Optimal Lesion Debulking (SOLD) registry: angiographic and clinical outcome. Circulation 98:1604–1609, 1998.
46. Bramucci E, Angoli L, Merlini PA, et al: Adjunctive stent implantation following directional coronary atherectomy in patients with coronary artery disease. J Am Coll Cardiol 32:1855–1860, 1998.
47. Baim DS, Kent KM, King SB, et al: Evaluating new devices: acute (in-hospital) results from the New Approaches to Coronary Intervention Registry. Circulation 89:471–481, 1994.
48. Ellis SG, Popma JJ, Buchbinder M, et al: Relation of clinical presentation, stenosis morphology, and operator technique to the procedural results of rotational atherectomy and rotational atherectomy-facilitated angioplasty. Circulation 89:882–892, 1994.
49. Safian RD, Freed M, Reddy V, et al: Do excimer laser angioplasty and rotational atherectomy facilitate balloon angioplasty? Implications for lesion-specific coronary intervention. J Am Coll Cardiol 27:552–559, 1996.
50. Reifart N, Vandormael M, Kracjar M, et al: Randomized comparison of angioplasty of complex coronary lesions at a single center: Excimer Laser, Rotational Atherectomy, and Balloon Angioplasty Comparison (ERBAC) study. Circulation 96:91–98, 1997.
51. Lindsay J, Pinnow EE, Pichard AD: New devices enhance results of coronary angioplasty. Cathet Cardiovasc Diagn 43:1–6, 1998.
52. Hoffmann R, Mintz GS, Kent KM, et al: Comparative early and nine-month results of rotational atherectomy, stents, and the combination of both for calcified lesions in large coronary arteries. Am J Cardiol 81:552–557, 1998.
53. Stammen F, Piessens J, Vrolix M, et al: Immediate and short-term results of a 1988–1989 coronary angioplasty registry. Am J Cardiol 67:253–258, 1991.
54. Tuzcu EM, Simpfendorfer C, Dorosti K, et al: Changing patterns in percutaneous transluminal coronary angioplasty. Am Heart J 117:1374–1377, 1989.
55. Kamp O, Beatt K, DeFeyter PJ, et al: Short-, medium-, and long-term follow-up after percutaneous transluminal coronary angioplasty for stable and unstable angina pectoris. Am Heart J 117:991–996, 1989.
56. Parisi AF, Folland ED, Hartigan P: A comparison of angioplasty with medical therapy in the treatment of single-vessel coronary artery disease. N Engl J Med 326:10–16, 1992.
57. Hueb WA, Belloti G, Almeida de Oliveira S, et al: The Medicine, Angioplasty or Surgery Study (MASS): a prospective, randomized trial of medical therapy, balloon angioplasty or bypass surgery for single proximal left anterior descending artery stenoses. J Am Coll Cardiol 26:1600–1605, 1995.
58. Folland ED, Hartigan PM, Parisi AF: Percutaneous transluminal coronary angioplasty versus medical therapy for stable angina pectoris. J Am Coll Cardiol 29:1505–1511, 1997.
59. Califf RM, Harrell FE, Lee KL, et al: The evolution of medical and surgical therapy for coronary artery disease: a 15-year perspective. JAMA 261:2077–2086, 1989.
60. Yusuf S, Zucker D, Peduzzi P, et al: Effect of coronary artery bypass graft surgery on survival: overview of 10-year results from randomised trials by the Coronary Artery Bypass Graft Surgery Trialists Collaboration. Lancet 344:563–570, 1994.
61. Mark DB, Nelson CL, Califf RM, et al: Continuing evolution of

therapy for coronary artery disease: initial results from the era of coronary angioplasty. Circulation 89:2015–2025, 1994.

62. Strauss WE, Fortin T, Hartigan P, et al: A comparison of quality of life scores in patients with angina pectoris after angioplasty compared with after medical therapy. Circulation 92:1710–1719, 1995.
63. Hartigan PM, Giacomini JC, Folland ED, Parisi AF: Two- to three-year follow-up of patients with single-vessel coronary artery disease randomized to PTCA or medical therapy (results of a VA cooperative study). Am J Cardiol 82:1445–1450, 1998.
64. Rodriguez A, Boullon F, Perez-Balino N, et al: Argentine randomized trial of percutaneous transluminal coronary angioplasty versus coronary artery bypass surgery in multivessel disease (ERACI): in-hospital results and 1-year follow-up. J Am Coll Cardiol 22:1060–1067, 1993.
65. Rodriguez A, Mele E, Peyregne E, et al: Three-year follow-up of the Argentine randomized trial of percutaneous transluminal coronary angioplasty versus coronary artery bypass surgery in multivessel disease (ERACI). J Am Coll Cardiol 27:1178–1184, 1996.
66. RITA trial participants: Coronary angioplasty versus coronary artery bypass surgery: the Randomized Intervention Treatment of Angina (RITA) trial. Lancet 341:573–580, 1993.
67. CABRI trial participants: First-year results of CABRI (Coronary Angioplasty versus Bypass Revascularisation Investigation). Lancet 346:1179–1184, 1995.
68. Hamm CW, Reimers J, Ischinger T, et al: A randomized study of coronary angioplasty compared with bypass surgery in patients with symptomatic multivessel coronary disease. N Engl J Med 331:1037–1043, 1994.
69. King SB, Lembo NJ, Weintraub WS, et al: A randomized trial comparing coronary angioplasty with coronary bypass surgery. N Engl J Med 331:1044–1050, 1994.
70. The Bypass Angioplasty Revascularization Investigation (BARI) Investigators: Comparison of coronary bypass surgery with angioplasty in patients with multivessel disease. N Engl J Med 335:217–225, 1996.
71. Chaitman BR, Rosen AD, Williams DO, et al: Myocardial infarction and cardiac mortality in the Bypass Angioplasty Revascularization Investigation (BARI) randomized trial. Circulation 96:2162–2170, 1997.
72. The Writing Group for the Bypass Angioplasty Revascularization Investigation (BARI) Investigators: Five-year clinical and functional outcome comparing bypass surgery and angioplasty in patients with multivessel coronary disease. JAMA 277:715–721, 1997.
73. Solomon AJ, Gersh BJ: Management of chronic stable angina: medical therapy, percutaneous transluminal coronary angioplasty, and coronary artery bypass graft surgery: lessons from the randomized trials. Ann Intern Med 128:216–223, 1998.
74. Williams DO, Gruentzig AR, Kent KM, et al: Efficacy of repeat percutaneous transluminal coronary angioplasty for coronary restenosis. Am J Cardiol 53:32C–35C, 1984.
75. Meier B, King SB, Gruentzig AR, et al: Repeat coronary angioplasty. J Am Coll Cardiol 463–466, 1984.
76. Rapold HJ, David PR, Guiteras Val P, et al: Restenosis and its determinants in first and repeat coronary angioplasty. Eur Heart J 8:575–586, 1987.
77. Schweiger MJ, Garb JL, Blank F, et al: Long-term follow-up and influence of symptom-free interval on restenosis after repeat percutaneous transluminal coronary angioplasty. Am J Cardiol 62:476–478, 1988.
78. Quigley PJ, Hlatky MA, Hinohara T, et al: Repeat percutaneous transluminal coronary angioplasty and predictors of recurrent restenosis. Am J Cardiol 63:409–413, 1989.
79. Glazier JJ, Varricchione TR, Ryan TJ, et al: Factors predicting recurrent restenosis after percutaneous transluminal coronary balloon angioplasty. Am J Cardiol 63:902–905, 1989.
80. Deligonul U, Vandormael M, Kern MJ, Galan K: Repeat coronary angioplasty for restenosis: results and predictors of follow-up clinical events. Am Heart J 117:997–1002, 1989.
81. Weintraub WS, Ghazzal ZMB, Douglas JS, et al: Initial management and long-term clinical outcome of restenosis after initially successful percutaneous transluminal coronary angioplasty. Am J Cardiol 70:47–55, 1992.
82. Dimas AP, Grigera F, Arora RR, et al: Repeat coronary angioplasty as treatment for restenosis. J Am Coll Cardiol 19:1310–1314, 1992.
83. Joly P, Bonan R, Palisaitis D, et al: Treatment of recurrent restenosis with repeat percutaneous transluminal coronary angioplasty. Am J Cardiol 61:906–908, 1988.
84. Teirstein PS, Hoover CA, Ligon RW, et al: Repeat coronary angioplasty: efficacy of a third angioplasty for a second restenosis. J Am Coll Cardiol 13:291–296, 1989.
85. Bauters C, McFadden EP, Lablanche JM, et al: Restenosis rate after multiple percutaneous transluminal coronary angioplasty procedures at the same site. Circulation 88:969–974, 1993.
86. King SB, Schlumpf M: Ten-year completed follow-up of percutaneous transluminal coronary angioplasty: the early Zurich experience. J Am Coll Cardiol 22:353–360, 1993.
87. Ruygrok PN, de Jaegere PPT, van Domburg RT, et al: Clinical outcome 10 years after attempted percutaneous transluminal coronary angioplasty in 856 patients. J Am Coll Cardiol 27:1669–1677, 1996.
88. Hasdai D, Bell MR, Grill DE, et al: Outcome 10 years after successful percutaneous transluminal coronary angioplasty. Am J Cardiol 1005–1011, 1997.
89. Holmes DR, Kip KE, Yeh W, et al: Long-term analysis of conventional coronary balloon angioplasty and an initial "stent-like" result. J Am Coll Cardiol 32:590–595, 1998.

CHAPTER 38

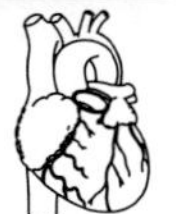

Percutaneous Coronary Intervention for Unstable Coronary Artery Disease

Pim J. de Feyter

PATHOPHYSIOLOGY OF THE UNSTABLE CORONARY PLAQUE
PROGNOSIS OF THE PATIENT WITH UNSTABLE ANGINA
RISK STRATIFICATION OF PERCUTANEOUS CORONARY INTERVENTION FOR UNSTABLE CORONARY ARTERY DISEASE
RATIONALE FOR PERCUTANEOUS CORONARY INTERVENTION
CORONARY BALLOON ANGIOPLASTY AND STENT IMPLANTATION
OTHER PERCUTANEOUS MODALITIES
ANTIPLATELET THERAPIES
CORONARY ANGIOPLASTY AND STENT IMPLANTATION FOR UNSTABLE ANGINA IN THE ELDERLY
TROPONIN T OR I TO GUIDE TREATMENT
INVASIVE TREATMENT STRATEGY VERSUS CONSERVATIVE STRATEGY
CONCLUSIONS
FUTURE

Unstable coronary artery disease (CAD), defined as unstable angina and non–Q wave myocardial infarction (MI), accounts for a large proportion of hospitalizations of patients suffering from CAD.[1] It is a serious, potentially dangerous condition that may herald acute myocardial (re)-infarction and subsequent cardiac death.

The common underlying pathophysiology of unstable CAD involves the rupture or erosion of a vulnerable coronary atherosclerotic plaque with subsequent mural or occlusive thrombus formation, severe enough to reduce antegrade coronary blood flow, thereby causing myocardial ischemia or necrosis.

Therapy for the various clinical manifestations of unstable CAD (new-onset angina, progressive angina at rest, post-MI angina, or non–Q wave MI) is similar, consisting of aspirin, intravenous heparin, and anti-ischemic medications.[2]

The majority of these patients will stabilize with this treatment and can be discharged with continued medical treatment. Prompt revascularization (percutaneous coronary intervention or coronary artery bypass graft surgery [CABG]) is deemed necessary in those patients who do not stabilize with medical treatment or who have signs of severe ischemic left ventricular dysfunction. Early revascularization is offered to patients with unstable angina at high risk of progression. Elective revascularization is recommended only for those patients with stress-induced ischemia. This chapter deals with the outcome of patients with unstable CAD who are referred for percutaneous coronary intervention. Currently, percutaneous coronary interventions are performed with the use of two major techniques: balloon angioplasty and intracoronary stent implantation.

Pathophysiology of the Unstable Coronary Plaque

The common factor precipitating an acute coronary ischemic event is coronary thrombosis (Fig. 38–1).[3–14] Coronary thrombosis occurs owing to (sudden) changes of the fibrous cap. The fibrous cap of an atherosclerotic plaque may undergo either erosion or plaque rupture. Erosion is more likely to occur in plaques that are rich in smooth muscle cells and proteoglycans and that do not contain a large lipid core.[12] Plaques prone to rupture have a large lipid core, often occupying more than 40 percent of the overall plaque volume.[10] The fibrous cap is thin and undermined by macrophages producing metalloproteinases that degrade collagen and have a low density of smooth muscle cells.[11] Erosion or rupture transforms the tissue factor–rich atheroma into a highly thrombogenic surface that leads to platelet adherence, activation and aggregation, and subsequent thrombosis.[15–19] In addition, erosion or rupture exposes subendothelial collagen, to which platelets adhere. Activated platelets externalize the glycoprotein IIb/IIIa receptor, which binds to adhesive macromolecules, such as fibrinogen and von Willebrand factor, and thus lead to platelet aggregation. The platelets are further activated owing to the high–shear rate forces induced by the coronary narrowing. At the site of the disrupted vessel wall, exposed tissue factor combines with factors VIIa and Xa to form the prothrombinase complex, which converts prothrombin to thrombin. Thrombin plays a crucial control role because it acts as a further stimulant for platelet activation and aggregation and converts fibrinogen into fibrin. An intracoronary thrombus develops with a component covering the plaque, the mural thrombus, predominantly consisting of platelets and a fibrin red cell–rich component building up in the coronary vessel, which may be subocclusive or totally occlusive.[8]

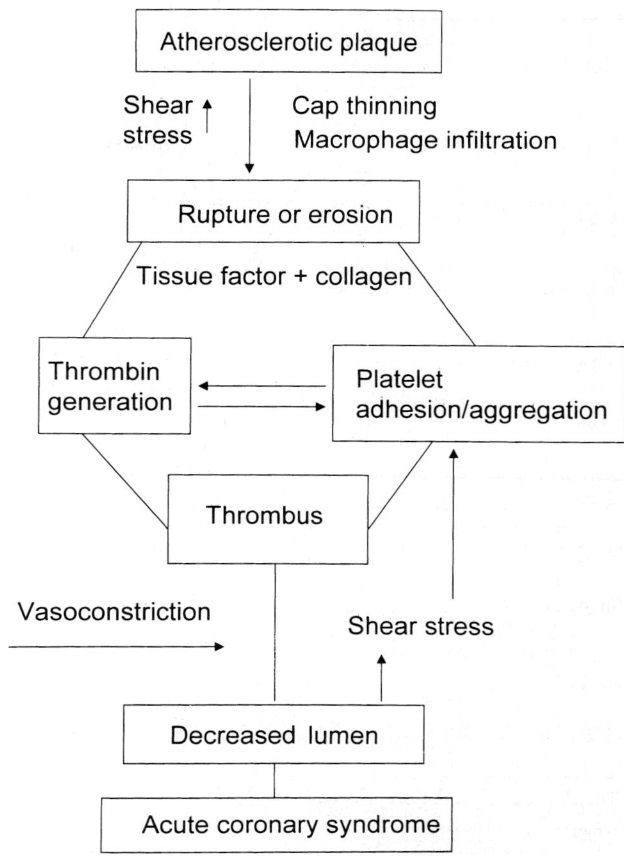

FIGURE 38–1 Physiopathologic mechanisms underlying acute coronary syndromes.

Autopsy studies have shown that the development of a major thrombus is more often associated with plaque rupture (60 percent of the cases) than with plaque erosion (30 percent of the cases).[8]

In addition to thrombosis, increased vasomotion plays an active role in the acute ischemic event.[20–22] Endothelial dysfunction at the lesion and production of vasoactive substances, such as thromboxane A_2, serotonin, endothelin, and thrombin, further contribute to threatening closure of the vessel. The intracoronary space-occupying thrombus formation and vasoconstriction cause a decrease of the lumen diameter, which, if critical, causes myocardial ischemia. Further luminal narrowing increases the shear stress, which stimulates platelet activation and aggregation, with von Willebrand factor relative to fibrinogen becoming more important at a high shear rate.

The resulting extent and duration of myocardial ischemia determine the subsequent clinical syndrome, which may range from no symptoms to stable angina, unstable angina, non–Q wave MI, Q wave MI, to sudden death.[23, 24]

During an unstable episode, there is often a marked progression of the angiographic severity of the "culprit" coronary lesion, often resulting in a critical lesion or even total occlusion.[25–28]

Prognosis of the Patient With Unstable Angina

Although many studies on the prognosis of unstable angina are available, it remains difficult to determine the precise prognosis of patients presenting with unstable angina.[29–56] This is due mainly to the wide heterogenicity of the patients studied and the differences of end points used in these studies. Many of these earlier studies are nowadays considered to be less representative owing to recent improvements in medical management, more aggressive use of coronary angiography, and subsequent use of revascularization (CABG or percutaneous transluminal coronary angioplasty [PTCA]). From recent large studies, prognostic information can be gleaned about patients presenting with unstable angina or non–Q wave MI, all of whom received standard treatment with combinations of aspirin and heparin and various anti-ischemic medications (Table 38–1). The overall mortality rates at 48 hours, 7 days, 30 days, and 6 months were, on average, 0.3 percent, 1.7 percent, 3.7 percent, and 6.4 percent, respectively.[57–64] The combined death and nonfatal MI rates are 2.4 percent (48 hours), 8.7 percent (7 days), 11.3 percent (30 days), and 16.3 percent (6 months).

However, these prognostic data are rather crude and represent the average prognosis of a heterogeneous group of patients with unstable CAD. It appears that the prognosis of unstable angina is mainly dependent on the clinical manifestation, the baseline electrocardiographic changes, the release of the cardiac-specific enzymes troponin T (TnT) and troponin I (TnI), and the intensity of medical treatment.

Braunwald[65] developed a classification in 1989 that has proved to be clinically useful and correlated with underlying coronary angiographic and histopathologic findings.[66, 67] The risk stratification is based on the severity of angina

TABLE 38–1 **Incidence of Death or Death/Myocardial Infarction in Unstable Angina or Non–Q Wave Myocardial Infarction (Acute Phase Treatment: Aspirin and Heparin)**

		48 Hours		7 Days		30 Days		6 Months	
Trial	**Patients (n)**	***Death (%)***	***Death/MI (%)***	***Death (%)***	***Death/MI (%)***	***Death (%)***	***Death/MI (%)***	***Death (%)***	***Death/MI (%)***
GUSTO-IIb[57]	4017		3.1			3.9	9.1		
FRISC[58]	757			1.1	4.8	3.0*	10.7	5.5†	15.5
FRIC[59]	731			0.4	3.6	2.0‡	4.7		
ESSENCE[60]	1564	0.4	1.3			3.6	7.8		
PRISM-PLUS[61]	797	0.3	2.6	1.9	8.3	4.5	11.9	7.0	15.3
PRISM[62]	1616	0.2	1.6	1.6	4.2	3.6	7.1		
PARAGON[63]	758					2.9	11.7	6.6	17.9
PURSUIT[64]	4739			2.0	11.6	3.7	15.7		
Total	14,979								
Weighted Average		0.3	2.4	1.7	8.7	3.7	11.3	6.4	16.3

Abbreviations: ESSENCE, Efficacy and Safety of Subcutaneous Enoxaparin in Non–Q-Wave Coronary Events Study Group; FRIC, Fragmin in Unstable Coronary Artery Disease Study; FRISC, Fragmin During Instability in Coronary Artery Disease; GUSTO-IIb, Global Use of Strategies to Open Occluded Arteries in Acute Coronary Syndromes; MI, myocardial infarction; PARAGON, Platelet IIb/IIIa Antagonism for the Reduction of Acute Coronary Syndrome Events in a Global Organization Network; PRISM, Platelet Receptor Inhibition in Ischemic Syndrome Management; PRISM-PLUS, Platelet Receptor Inhibition in Ischemic Syndrome Management in Patients Limited by Unstable Signs and Symptoms; PURSUIT, Platelet Glycoprotein IIb/IIIa in Unstable Angina: Receptor Suppression Using Integrilin Therapy.
*40 days.
†150 days.
‡Between 6 and 45 days.

and clinical circumstances in which unstable angina occurs (Table 38–2). Two prospective studies using this classification demonstrated that the risk of death and nonfatal MI at 3 months follow-up ranges from 5 percent in the lowest risk group to between 25 and 35 percent in the highest risk group.[68, 69]

Patients in Braunwald classes IB and IC are at low risk (<5 percent), those in Braunwald classes IIB and IIC are at intermediate risk (5 to 10 percent), and those in Braunwald classes IIIB and IIIC at highest risk (10 to 15 percent) of progression to nonfatal (re-)MI or death within the ensuing 6 months to 1 year.[31–56]

The Global Use of Strategies to Open Occluded Arteries in Acute Coronary Syndromes (GUSTO-IIb) trial demonstrated that in patients with unstable CAD and no ST-segment elevation, those patients with unstable angina fared better than those with non–Q wave MI. The 6-month and 1-year mortality rates of unstable angina versus non–Q wave MI patients were 5.0 percent and 7.0 percent versus 8.8 percent and 11 percent, respectively. The 6-month (re-)MI rates were 6.2 percent versus 9.8 percent.[70]

The baseline electrocardiogram is an important prognostic marker. In the GUSTO-IIb trial the 30-day incidence of death or (re-)MI was 5.5 percent in patients with T wave inversion, 9.4 percent in those with ST-segment elevation, 10.5 percent in those with ST-segment depression, and 12.4 percent in those with ST-segment depression and elevation.[71] In addition, mortality is influenced by the number of leads with ST changes and the extent of ST deflection (in millimeters).[43, 47, 48, 72]

The cardiac-specific proteins TnT and TnI are sensitive markers of myocardial cell injury and are highly predictive of adverse coronary events.[73–78] High levels of TnT or TnI release in patients with unstable CAD are associated with poor outcome (Table 38–3).

TABLE 38–2 **Braunwald Classification Adapted to the Practice of Percutaneous Coronary Intervention**

	Severity UA	B Primary UA	C Post-MI UA Within 2 wk After AMI
I	New onset of angina or accelerated angina; no rest pain	I B	I C
II	Angina at rest within past month but not within past 48 h	II B	II C
III	Angina at rest within 48 h	III B	III C

Abbreviations: AMI, acute myocardial infarction; MI, myocardial infarction; UA, unstable angina.

Risk Stratification of Percutaneous Coronary Intervention for Unstable Coronary Artery Disease

Patients with unstable angina and early post-MI unstable angina undergoing balloon angioplasty have a higher frequency of major procedural complications than do patients with stable angina (Fig. 38–2).[79–111] The difference in complication rate between unstable and stable angina patients became gradually less distinct owing to improvements in PTCA techniques, increased operator experience, availability of bail-out stenting, and use of potent antiplatelet therapy.[112]

In several large randomized studies, there was no remarkable difference in adverse outcome between patient groups considered at high or low risk of percutaneous coronary intervention (Table 38–4).[113–118] Of note is the fact

TABLE 38-3 **Baseline Troponin I or T as Prognostic Markers**

First Author	Disease	End-point	Follow-Up	Test Positivity	Troponin Marker +	Troponin Marker −
Lindahl[73]	UAP	Death/MI	5 mo	TnT > 0.06 μg/L	(51/399) 12.8%	(8/182) 4.4%
Antman[75]	UAP/non–Q wave MI	Death	42 d	TnI > 0.4 ng/ml	(21/573) 3.7%	(8/831) 1.0%
Hamm[76]	UAP/non–Q wave MI	Death/MI	30 d	TnI > 0.1 ng/ml	(32/171) 18.7%	(2/602) 0.4%
				TnT > 0.1 ng/ml	(27/123) 22%	(7/650) 1.1%
Holmvang[77]	UAP	Death/MI	30 d	TnT > 0.1 μg/L	(8/130) 6.2%	(6/209) 2.9%

Abbreviations: MI, myocardial infarction; Tn, troponin; UAP, unstable angina pectoris.

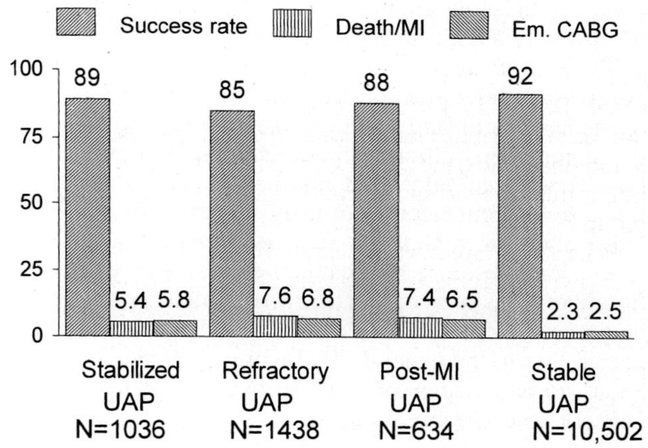

FIGURE 38–2 Success rate and in-hospital procedural major complication rate in patients with unstable (UAP) and stable angina pectoris. Em. CABG, emergent coronary artery bypass graft surgery; MI, myocardial infarction.

TABLE 38-4 **30-Day Outcome of Recent Randomized Trials (All Patients Treated With Aspirin and Heparin)**

Trial	Patient Category	Patients (n)	Death (%)	MI: *Q Wave (%)*	MI: *All (%)*	Urgent Revascularization (%)	Stent Use (%)
EPIC[113]	High risk	696	1.7	2.3	8.6	8.1	0.6
EPILOG[114]	Elective	939	0.8	0.8	8.7	5.2	13
IMPACT II[115]	UAP/elective	1328	1.1	1.6	8.1	5.6	1.4
RESTORE[116]	UAP	1070	0.7	NA	5.7	7.6	2.5
CAPTURE[117]	Refractory UAP	635	1.3	2.7	8.2	10.9	6.6
EPIC (substudy)[118]	UAP	156	3.3	4.6	9.2	5.9	NA

Abbreviations: CAPTURE, c7E3 Fab Antiplatelet Therapy in Unstable Refractory Angina; EPIC, Evaluation of IIb/IIIa Platelet Receptor Antagonist 7E3 in Preventing Ischemic Complications; EPILOG, Evaluation of PTCA to Improve Long-Term Outcome by c7E3 GP IIb/IIIa Receptor Blockade; IMPACT II, Integrilin (eptifibatide) to Minimize Platelet Aggregation and Coronary Thrombosis-II; NA, not available; RESTORE, Randomized Efficacy Study of Tirofiban for Outcomes and REstenosis; UAP, unstable angina pectoris.

that the majority of studies demonstrated a 30-day mortality rate between 1 and 2 percent and an MI rate between 6 and 9 percent. These adverse event rates are higher than usually reported and probably reflect the careful screening and high reliability of reporting of adverse events in randomized controlled trials.

However, the inclusion of highly heterogeneous population groups in these trials may have obscured the potential presence of a gradient of risk in patients undergoing percutaneous intervention for unstable angina. Indeed, in a few carefully conducted trials, it was shown that there are differences in risk profile among the various subgroups of patients presenting with unstable angina. In a subanalysis of the HELVETICA study, it was clear that the risk of major complication is lower for patients with unstable angina Braunwald class I, intermediate for Braunwald class II, and higher for Braunwald class III (Fig. 38–3).[119, 120] In the Hirulog angioplasty study, there was a slightly higher complication rate of death or MI in patients with postinfarction angina than in those with unstable angina.[121] This was further confirmed in a Thoraxcenter study, in which we demonstrated that the risk of major complication was lowest for coronary intervention for stable angina, intermediate for unstable angina Braunwald class II, and highest for unstable angina Braunwald class III (Fig. 38–4).[109]

The use of intracoronary stent implantation in combination with platelet glycoprotein (GP) IIb/IIIa receptor antagonists has significantly reduced the major complication rate of percutaneous coronary interventions. The procedure is now considered safer, and this has broadened the indications for percutaneous coronary intervention to include more high-risk pathology, such as complex, ulcerated lesions, long lesions, bifurcation lesions, calcified lesions, thrombotic lesions, or treatment of smaller vessel disease in patients with unstable CAD. It may therefore be expected that in the general "real world" practice of percutaneous coronary intervention, the overall complication rate will not considerably decrease.

Accordingly, we constructed a risk stratification classification based on the Braunwald classification for patients who are scheduled for coronary intervention for unstable CAD (Fig. 38–5). The risk of major complications—death, MI, urgent revascularization—was estimated between 2 and 5 percent for progressive angina (Braunwald class I), between 5 and 10 percent for angina at rest for more than 48 hours (Braunwald class II), and between 10 and 15 percent for angina at rest for less than 48 hours (Braunwald class III). Factors that additionally increase the risk in each category are the presence and extent of recent MI, presence of reversible electrocardiographic changes, the intensity of concomitant treatment, and the presence of high levels of TnT or TnI. Obviously, additional significant comorbidity increases the risk.

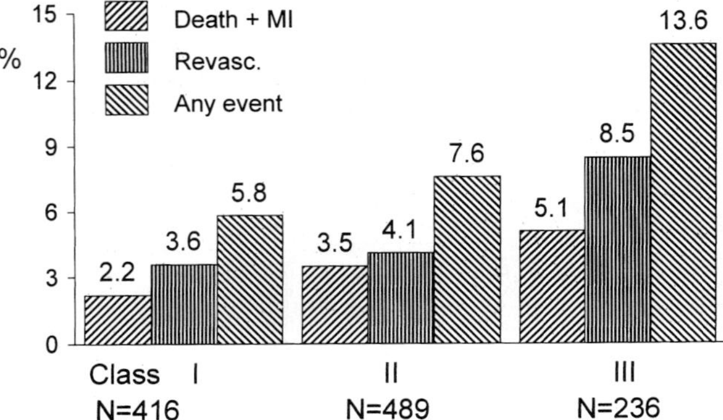

FIGURE 38–3 Major complication rate during percutaneous transluminal coronary angioplasty in patients with Braunwald unstable angina classes I, II, and III. MI, myocardial infarction; Revasc., urgent surgical revascularization. (Data from Serruys PW, Herrman JP, Simon R, et al: A comparison of hirudin with heparin in the prevention of restenosis after coronary angioplasty. Helvetica Investigators. N Engl J Med 333:757–763, 1995.)

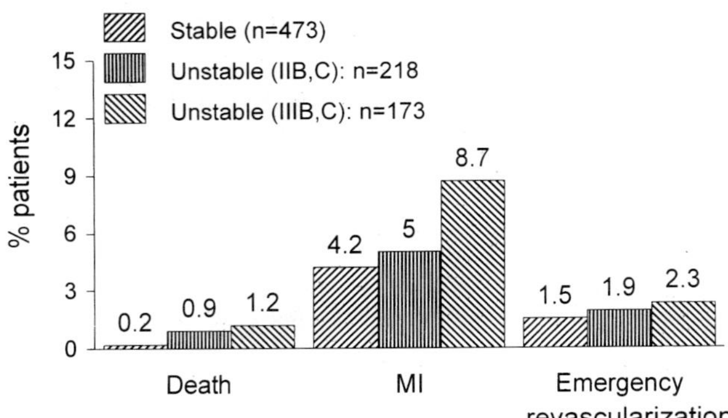

FIGURE 38–4 Major complication rate of consecutive series of patients with stable angina and unstable angina Braunwald classification IIb/IIc and IIIb/IIIc who underwent percutaneous transluminal coronary angioplasty at the Thoraxcenter in 1994. MI, myocardial infarction.

RATIONALE FOR PERCUTANEOUS CORONARY INTERVENTION

Plaque erosion preferentially occurs in coronary obstructive plaques, and plaque rupture preferentially occurs in nonobstructive or minimally obstructive plaques that, however, have a high propensity to progress rapidly to cause a severe coronary narrowing.[25–28]

Balloon angioplasty is an effective method to enlarge the lumen of a coronary narrowing by mechanical disruption of the media, increase of the vessel circumference, and dissolution of the (mural) intracoronary thrombus.[122–124] This restores normal blood flow and reduces the high shear rate–dependent platelet activation and aggregation. Additional balloon injury of "spontaneous" erosion or disruption of a coronary plaque may further intensify the ongoing thrombus formation and may lead to abrupt vessel closure and subsequent MI. Distal thrombotic embolization owing to balloon angioplasty may occur and cause myocardial necrosis. Intracoronary stent implantation does improve suboptimal angioplasty outcome and may prevent distal embolization of thrombotic material because intracoronary stent implantation scaffolds the disrupted plaque and friable thrombotic material. Thus, stenting creates an optimal coronary lumen and coronary flow hemodynamics that appear to effectively interrupt the thrombotic formation process and to form a platform from which healing and

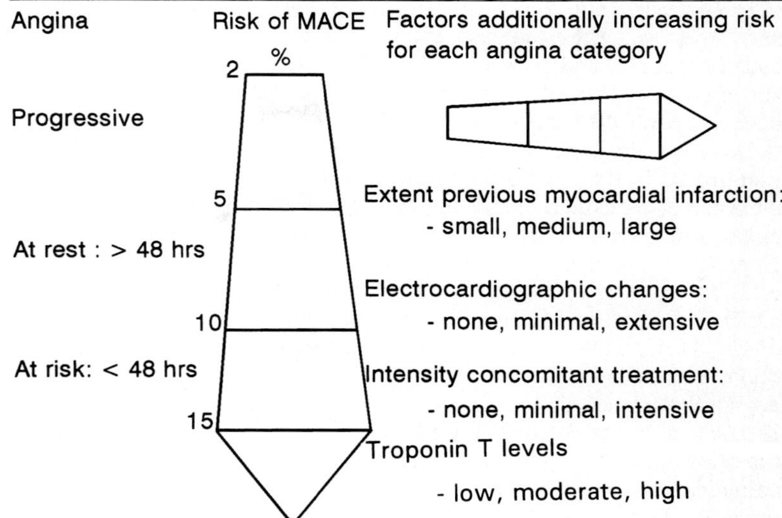

FIGURE 38–5 Stratification of risk of patients with unstable angina who undergo coronary angioplasty. MACE, major adverse coronary event.

stabilization occur. This is suggested by the finding that the elevated plasma levels of tissue-type plasminogen activator and von Willebrand factor, both associated with instability of the atheromatous plaque, decrease within 1 month after coronary intervention, probably reflecting plaque reendothelialization and stabilization.[125]

Coronary Balloon Angioplasty and Stent Implantation

Currently, percutaneous coronary intervention for patients with unstable CAD is performed using two major techniques: balloon angioplasty and stent implantation (Fig. 38–6).

Several nonrandomized observational studies have shown that balloon angioplasty and stent implantation are relatively safe procedures in patients with unstable CAD, even in patients who require multiple stent implantation (Table 38–5).[126–132] The occurrence of (sub)acute thrombotic stent occlusion has significantly decreased to less than 1 percent after treatment with aspirin and ticlopidine or clopidogrel.[133–135]

In the Evaluation of Platelet IIb/IIIa Inhibitor for Stenting (EPISTENT) trial, a subgroup analysis of patients with unstable angina for less than 48 hours, unstable angina for less than 7 days, and stable angina, stent implantation and adjunctive treatment with aspirin and heparin were associated with a 30-day composite end-point rate (death, MI, or need for urgent revascularization) of 14.8 percent, 11.1 percent, and 11.5 percent, respectively.[136]

In a subanalysis of the Benestent II trial, it was shown that stent implantation was significantly safer and more effective than balloon angioplasty in unstable angina patients (Table 38–6).[137]

The 6-month outcome in terms of cardiac death and nonfatal MI after coronary intervention for unstable angina is relatively good and does not appear to be much different from that in stable angina patients (Table 38–7). Several studies have indicated that the presence of "instability" at the time of a coronary intervention is a predictor of increased risk of clinical or angiographic restenosis.[138–147] It was hypothesized that a subsequent additional mechanical disruption of an initial precipitating plaque rupture would amplify the vascular injury response. Yet, the data concerning the restenosis rate in patients with balloon angioplasty for unstable angina compared with that for stable angina

TABLE 38–5 **Stent Implantation in Unstable Coronary Artery Disease**

Study	Patients (n)	Procedural Complications			
		Death (%)	*MI (%)*	*Abrupt Occlusion (%)*	*Emergency Surgery (%)*
Robinson[126]	83	0	2.7	3.6	7.2
TASTE-Registry[127]	461	2.6	4.3	—	1.9
Marzocchi[128]	132	0	4.5	6.8	4.5
Chauhan[129]	110	0	4.5	3.6	0.9
Alfonso[130]	86	6	6.0	1.0	0
Madan[131]	156	0.6	1.9	1.9	1.9
Kornowski[132]	334	1.0	0.6	0.6	3.0

Abbreviations: MI, myocardial infarction; TASTE, Ticlopidine Aspirin Stent Evaluation Study.

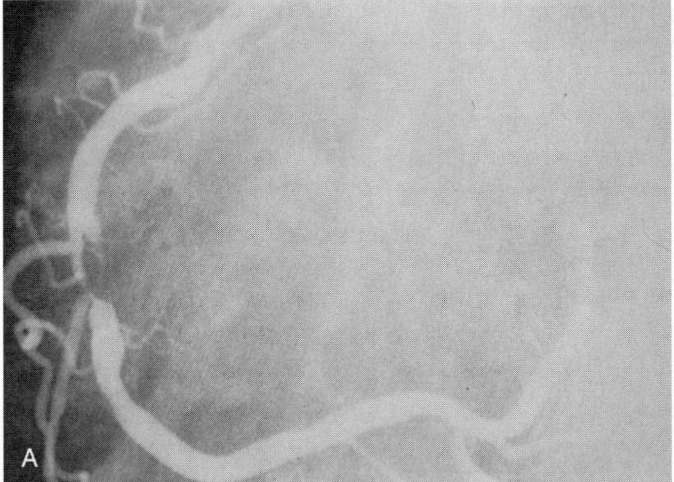

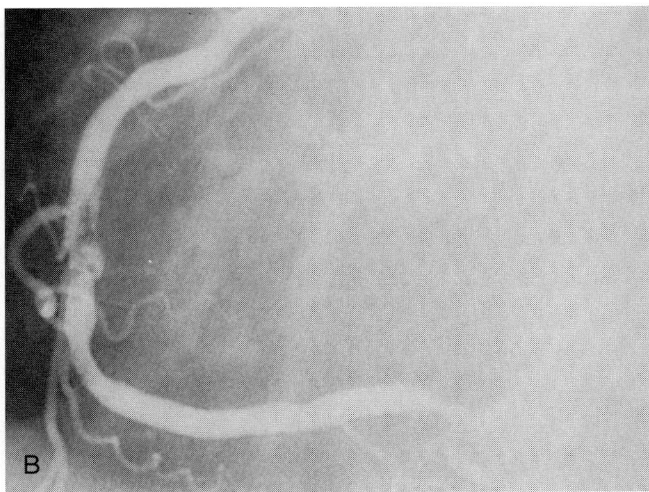

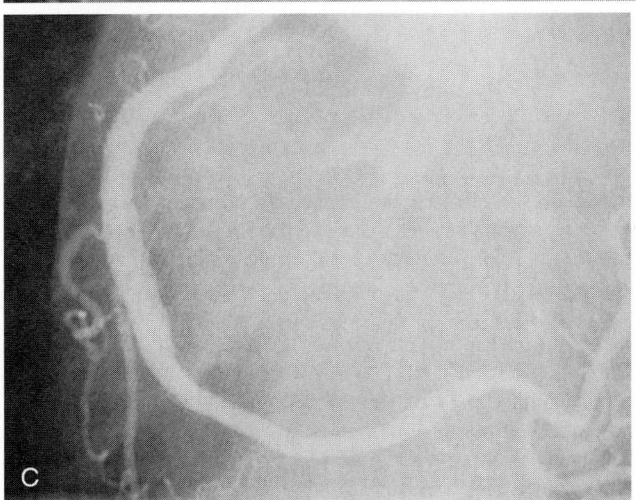

FIGURE 38–6 A, Coronary angiogram of the right coronary artery of a patient with unstable angina. A severe narrowing due to a complex thrombotic plaque is present in the midsegment. **B,** The angiographic result after balloon angioplasty is suboptimal owing to dissection and rupture of plaque caused by the barotrauma. **C,** Stent implantation results in a wide, regular, patent lumen.

are conflicting. In a quantitative angiographic study of 339 consecutive patients with angiographic follow-up of 85 percent, Luijten and colleagues[141] found that the restenosis rate was similar in 133 patients with unstable angina and 206 patients with stable angina. Rupprecht and coworkers[95] studied the restenosis rate in 379 patients with successful PTCA for stable angina and in 185 patients with successful PTCA for unstable angina. Control angiography was performed at a mean of 6 months in 73 percent of the lesions in the stable and 71 percent of the lesions in the unstable group. The restenosis rate was significantly higher—37 percent versus 24 percent ($P < .01$)—in patients with unstable angina compared with those with stable angina. Bauters and associates[145] demonstrated that the restenosis rate after repeat balloon angioplasty for a first restenosis was significantly higher in patients presenting with unstable angina than in those with stable angina (61 percent versus 43 percent, $P < .05$). Foley and colleagues[146] showed that restenosis, defined as recurrence of symptoms with more than 50 percent stenosis, occurred in 27 percent of unstable patients and 24 percent of stable patients.

TABLE 38–6 Stenting in Unstable Angina: Subanalysis Benestent II Trial

	Benestent II	
400 Days Follow-Up	***Balloon (79)***	***Stent (96)***
Composite end-point (death/MI/CABG/Re-PTCA)	21.5%	6.3%
Restenosis (>50%)	35%	18%

Abbreviations: CABG, coronary artery bypass graft surgery; MI, myocardial infarction; PTCA, percutaneous transluminal coronary angioplasty.

Stent implantation is expected to reduce the restenosis rate in patients with unstable CAD. In a matched control group of patients with balloon angioplasty who were compared with patients with stent implantation, the 6-month restenosis rate was 52 percent in the balloon group versus 27 percent in the stent group.[148] In another study, the target vessel revascularization was only 11 percent in 334 patients who underwent coronary stent implantation for early post-MI angina.[132] In a subanalysis of the Benestent II trial, it was demonstrated that the restenosis rate of patients with unstable angina undergoing stent implantation was significantly reduced compared with those undergoing balloon angioplasty (see Table 38–6).

Only few data are available about the long-term prognosis of percutaneous coronary intervention for unstable an-

TABLE 38–7 **Six-Month Outcome After Coronary Intervention in Stable and Unstable Angina**

Trial	Patient Category	Patients (n)	Death	MI	Repeat Revascularization
EPILOG[114]	Stable angina	939	1.7	9.9	18.1
EPIC[113]	Stable angina	408	—	—	21.3 (TVR)
	High risk (all)	696	3.4	10.5	22.3 (TVR)
EPIC (substudy)[118]	UAP	156	6.6	11.1	22.0 (TVR)
Hirulog Trial[121]	UAP/post MI-AP	1926	1.1	6.1	23.9
CAPTURE[117]	Refractory UAP	635	2.2	9.3	24.9
HELVETICA[119]	Unstable angina	1141	1.4	5.4	25.5

Abbreviations: AP, angina pectoris; CAPTURE, c7E3 Fab Antiplatelet Therapy in Unstable Refractory Angina; EPIC, Evaluation of IIb/IIIa Platelet Receptor Antagonist 7E3 in Preventing Ischemic Complications; EPILOG, Evaluation of PTCA to Improve Long-term Outcome by c7E3 GP IIb/IIIa Receptor Blockade; HELVETICA, Hirudin in a European Trial versus Heparin in the Prevention of Restenosis After PTCA; MI, myocardial infarction; TVR, target vessel revascularization; UAP, unstable angina pectoris.

gina. A study concerning the data from a single center revealed that the clinical outcome 10 years after percutaneous coronary intervention is good, and on an intention-to-treat analysis, there are only minimal differences in the clinical outcome of patients with stable and those with unstable angina (Fig. 38–7).[149]

Other Percutaneous Modalities

Directional coronary atherectomy in patients with unstable angina may remove the total "thrombogenic" plaque and may thus reduce the problem of abrupt thrombotic vessel occlusion.[150, 151] In a study performed in the Thoraxcenter,[152] we compared the success and complication rate of directional coronary atherectomy in 82 patients with stable and 68 patients with unstable angina. The overall success rate was 91 percent for stable and 88 percent for unstable angina. The in-hospital major complication rate was not significantly different, comparing the stable with the unstable group (9 percent versus 12 percent).

Abdelmeguid and coworkers[153] performed directional atherectomy in stable patients (group I = 77) and in 2 subgroups of patients with unstable angina: those with progressively worsening angina (group II = 110) and those with angina at rest or post-MI angina (group III = 100). These authors reported a higher major complication rate of 7.0 percent in group III versus 1.3 percent in group I and 0.9 percent in group II.

Transluminal extraction atherectomy as pretreatment for coronary intervention in acute ischemic syndromes may enhance the outcome. This was tested in a randomized multicenter trial comparing the use of transluminal extraction atherectomy versus balloon angioplasty in acute ischemic syndromes.[154] One hundred fifteen patients were assigned to transluminal extraction atherectomy and 135 patients to balloon angioplasty. There was no difference in death, emergent revascularization, or percentage of final diameter stenosis. The frequency of patients with an increase of creatine kinase (more than 3 times the upper limit of normal) was lower in transluminal extraction atherectomy (1.6 percent) than in PTCA (5.7 percent [P = .08]), suggesting that transluminal extraction atherectomy pretreatment enhances the safety of percutaneous intervention.

The role of atherectomy in unstable angina is not firmly established, but in certain thrombotic lesions, directional atherectomy may offer some advantage.

Antiplatelet Therapies

Platelets play a major role in the pathophysiology of unstable angina and non–Q wave MI, and there is accumulating

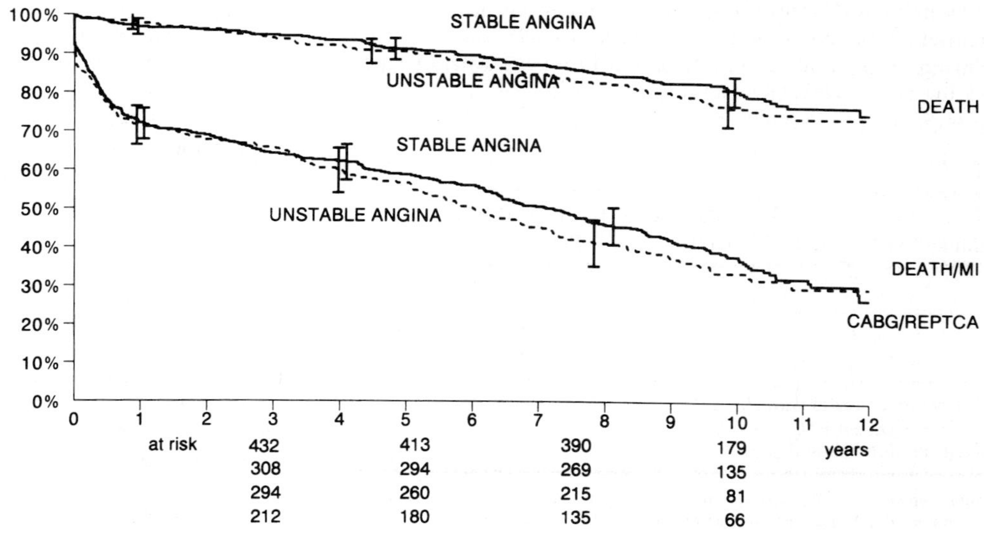

FIGURE 38–7 Long-term survival and event-free survival curves (Kaplan-Meier) of patients with stable and unstable angina who underwent coronary angioplasty. CABG, coronary artery bypass graft surgery; MI, myocardial infarction; REPTCA, repeat percutaneous transluminal coronary angioplasty. (Data from Ruygrok PN, de Jaegere PT, van Domburg RT, et al: Clinical outcome 10 years after attempted percutaneous transluminal coronary angioplasty in 856 patients. J Am Coll Cardiol 27:1669–1677, 1996.)

TABLE 38-8 **Efficacy of Antiplatelet Treatment After Stent Implantation**

First Author	End Point	Aspirin + Ticlopidine % (n)	Conventional A.C. % (n)	Aspirin Only % (n)
Schomig[133]	Death/MI Urgent revascularization	1.6 (257)	6.2* (260)	—
Bertrand[135]	Death/MI	5.7 (249)	8.3* (236)	—
Leon[134]	Death/MI Revascularization	0.5 (546)	2.7† (550)	3.6 (557)

Abbreviations: A.C., anticoagulation; MI, myocardial infarction.
*Heparin + aspirin + phenprocoumon.
†Aspirin + warfarin.

evidence that platelets also play a significant role in thrombotic major adverse events during percutaneous coronary intervention.

Aspirin in combination with heparin has always been considered as the key treatment to prevent acute thrombotic complications during percutaneous coronary intervention. Subacute thrombotic stent occlusion is effectively prevented by the combination of aspirin and ticlopidine (or clopidogrel) (Table 38–8).[133–135]

However, despite the use of aspirin, heparin, and ticlopidine, thrombotic complications continue to occur, and more potent platelet inhibitors, such as the platelet GP IIb/IIIa receptor antagonists, which block the final common pathway of platelet aggregation, may reduce this. Indeed, three major randomized trials—Evaluation of IIb/IIIa Platelet Receptor Antagonist 7E3 in Preventing Ischemic Complications (EPIC),[113] Evaluation of PTCA to Improve Long-term Outcome by c7E3 GP IIb/IIIa Receptor Blockade (EPILOG),[114] and c7E3 Fab Antiplatelet Therapy in Unstable Refractory Angina (CAPTURE)[117]—demonstrated convincingly that abciximab dramatically reduced the adverse major complications occurring during balloon angioplasty. This reduction in adverse procedural events was on the order of 30 to 50 percent, and this was achieved in patients at high risk or low risk of acute balloon angioplasty complications and in patients who underwent balloon angioplasty for stable or unstable angina.

A subanalysis of the EPIC trial examined the efficacy of abciximab in patients with unstable angina.[118] Here again, a significant decrease of major complications at 30 days in particular in the occurrence of Q wave MI was observed during treatment with abciximab (Table 38–9). A subanalysis of the EPILOG trial focused on the results in patients with unstable angina or recent MI undergoing balloon angioplasty.[114] Again, a dramatic decrease of major complications at 30 days was demonstrated (Table 38–10).

The CAPTURE trial investigated the efficacy of abciximab versus placebo in patients with unstable angina Braunwald class III.[117] Six hundred thirty-five patients were allocated to placebo and 630 patients to treatment with abciximab (ReoPro). A marked decrease in major ischemic complications at 30 days, especially in the development of MI during coronary intervention, was noted with the use of abciximab (Table 38–11). This beneficial effect, however, was much less striking at 6 months.

More modest reductions in the acute complication rates were observed in patients undergoing balloon angioplasty who were treated with eptifibatide (Integrilin [eptifibatide] to Minimize Platelet Aggregation and Coronary Thrombosis [IMPACT]-II trial)[115] or tirofiban (Randomized Efficacy Study of Tirofiban for Outcomes and REstenosis [RESTORE]).[116] The initial beneficial effects were virtually lost at 30 days. This may have been caused by the rather low dose of eptifibatide used in the IMPACT-II trial or possibly the short period of treatment (36 hours) in the RESTORE trial.

The Platelet Receptor Inhibition in Ischemic Syndrome Management in Patients Limited by Unstable Signs and Symptoms (PRISM-PLUS) trial demonstrated that patients who underwent angioplasty had fewer adverse events when treated with heparin and tirofiban (239 patients) compared with heparin alone (236 patients).[61] The death and MI rate at 30 days was 5.9 percent versus 10.2 percent (RR 0.56; CI 0.29 to 1.09). A similar trend was shown in the Platelet

TABLE 38-9 **Subanalysis EPIC: Unstable Angina at 30 Days End Point**

	Placebo (n = 156) %	Abciximab Bolus (n = 168) %	Abciximab Bolus + Infusion (n = 165) %	*P* Value
Death	3.2	0.6	1.2	.164
MI	9.0	4.2	1.8	.004
Q wave MI	4.5	0.6	0.0	.002
Non–Q wave MI	4.5	4.2	1.8	.197
Urgent PTCA or CABG	5.8	4.2	3.0	.223
Primary end point	12.8	7.8	4.8	.012

Abbreviations: CABG, coronary artery bypass graft surgery; EPIC, Evaluation of IIb/IIIa Platelet Receptor Antagonist 7E3 in Preventing Ischemic Complications; MI, myocardial infarction; PTCA, percutaneous transluminal coronary angioplasty.

TABLE 38–10 **EPILOG Trial: Subanalysis of Unstable Angina and Recent Myocardial Infarction**

	Placebo		ReoPro + Low-Dose Heparin		ReoPro + Standard-Dose Heparin	
30 Days End Point	*UAP (n = 474)*	*Recent MI (n = 189)*	*UAP (n = 434)*	*Recent MI (n = 200)*	*UAP (n = 420)*	*Recent MI (n = 190)*
Death/nonfatal MI or urgent revascularization (%)	12.2	11.1	4.8	7.5	5.0	4.2

Abbreviations: EPILOG, Evaluation of PTCA to Improve Long-term Outcome by c7E3 GP IIb/IIIa Receptor Blockade; GP, glycoprotein; MI, myocardial infarction; PTCA, percutaneous transluminal coronary angioplasty; UAP, unstable angina pectoris.

Receptor Inhibition in Ischemic Syndrome Management (PRISM) trial in which the heparin group patients (n = 352) and the tirofiban group patients (n = 348) underwent angioplasty.[62] The combined death and MI rate was 9.1 percent and 7.2 percent, respectively (not statistically significant).

In a subanalysis of prespecified groups of patients with unstable CAD enrolled in the Platelet Glycoprotein IIb/IIIa in Unstable Angina: Receptor Suppression Using Integrilin Therapy (PURSUIT) trial who underwent coronary angioplasty (50 percent of whom had stent implantation) within 72 hours after randomization, eptifibatide decreased the combined death and nonfatal MI rate, compared with placebo, from 16.7 percent to 11.6 percent, which is a relative reduction of 31 percent.[64]

Most importantly, both the CAPTURE trial and the PURSUIT trial demonstrated that there was already a significant decrease of adverse events in the period before scheduled coronary intervention in patients treated with GP IIb/IIIa antagonists compared with placebo; this beneficial effect was much greater during coronary intervention, but after the procedure, this effect was no longer apparent (Table 38–12). This suggests that patients at high risk, scheduled for percutaneous coronary intervention, should begin their treatment 12 to 24 hours before the procedure and continue during the procedure.

Inhibition of the platelet glycoprotein IIb/IIIA receptor with abciximab not only has been shown to be very effective in reducing balloon angioplasty–induced major complications but also appears highly effective in improving the outcome of coronary stenting. The EPISTENT trial[136] investigated the efficacy of abciximab as adjunctive treatment to heparin, aspirin, and ticlopidine. Three patient groups—stent plus placebo (I), stent plus abciximab (II), and balloon plus abciximab (III)—were compared. The primary end point was a combination of death, MI, and need for urgent revascularization in the first 30 days. The major adverse events were significantly reduced in all stented patients who received abciximab versus placebo (Table 38–13).[136] Furthermore, it was demonstrated that the primary event rate in the balloon plus abciximab group was lower than that in the stent plus placebo group (see Table 38–13). A subanalysis in a prespecified subgroup of patients with unstable angina for less than 48 hours or unstable angina for less than 7 days demonstrated a similar trend of the efficacy of abciximab to reduce the adverse events (see Table 38–13).[136] The EPISTENT trial also demonstrated a major protection in diabetic patients, with abciximab reducing their composite end point for PTCA and stent to one similar to the nondiabetic patients receiving the same procedure (Fig. 38–8).

Thus, it may be concluded that abciximab is highly recommended for patients with unstable angina undergoing balloon angioplasty or intracoronary stent implantation.

TABLE 38–11 **CAPTURE Trial: Unstable Angina (Braunwald Class III)**

	Placebo (%) (n = 635)	ReoPro (%) (n = 630)	*P* Value
30 Days End Point			
Death	1.3	1.0	>.1
Nonfatal MI	8.2	4.1	.002
Urgent intervention	10.9	7.8	.054
Any event	15.9	11.3	.012
6 Months End Point			
Death	2.2	2.8	N.S.
Nonfatal MI	9.3	6.6	N.S.
Revascularization	24.9	25.4	N.S.
Any event	30.8	31.0	N.S.

Abbreviations: CAPTURE, c7E3 Fab Antiplatelet Therapy in Unstable Refractory Angina; MI, myocardial infarction; N.S., not significant.

Coronary Angioplasty and Stent Implantation for Unstable Angina in the Elderly

In our industrialized world, the population continues to age. CAD affects 20 percent of elderly people and is the reason for approximately 25 percent of the morbidity and more than 50 percent of the mortality in this age group.[155] Therefore, the absolute number of elderly patients with CAD and, accordingly, the need for revascularization will continue to increase. Elderly people often have generalized atherosclerosis and are difficult to catheterize, thus presenting a particular challenge for coronary intervention. Over the years, a strategy has been developed in elderly patients who often have multivessel disease to dilate only the culprit lesion, a "minimal approach," rather than referring them to bypass surgery to undergo total revascularization, which is often associated with serious complications in the elderly.[156]

Studies have reported that coronary intervention in elderly patients is associated with an increased risk of major complications and a lower success rate, varying between

TABLE 38-12 **Efficacy of GPIIb/IIIa in Relation to Percutaneous Coronary Intervention**

	Before PTCA		During PTCA		After PTCA		
End Point: Death/MI	***Placebo (%)***	***GP IIb/IIIa (%)***	***Placebo (%)***	***GP IIb/IIIa (%)***	***Placebo (%)***	***GP IIb/IIIa (%)***	
CAPTURE[117]	2.1	0.6 (*P* = .03)	5.5	2.6 (*P* = .009)	0.9	1.0	(N.S.)
PURSUIT[64]	4.4	2.1 (*P* = .02)	7.1	3.1 (*P* = .001)	2.1	2.4	(N.S.)

Abbreviations: CAPTURE, c7E3 Fab Antiplatelet Therapy in Unstable Refractory Angina; GP, glycoprotein; MI, myocardial infarction; N.S., not significant; PTCA, percutaneous transluminal coronary angioplasty; PURSUIT, Platelet Glycoprotein IIb/IIIa in Unstable Angina: Receptor Suppression Using Integrilin Therapy.

TABLE 38-13 **EPISTENT Trial: 30-Day Primary Event Rate**

			Subgroups			
Treatment (n)	**All Patients**	***P* Value**	***UA < 48 h***	**P *Value***	***UA < 7 da***	**P *Value***
Stent + placebo (809)	10.8	—	14.8	—	11.1	—
Stent + abciximab (794)	5.3	<.001	4.5	.003	5.2	.036
Balloon + abciximab (796)	6.9	.007	7.3	.109	9.4	.69

Abbreviation: UA, unstable angina.

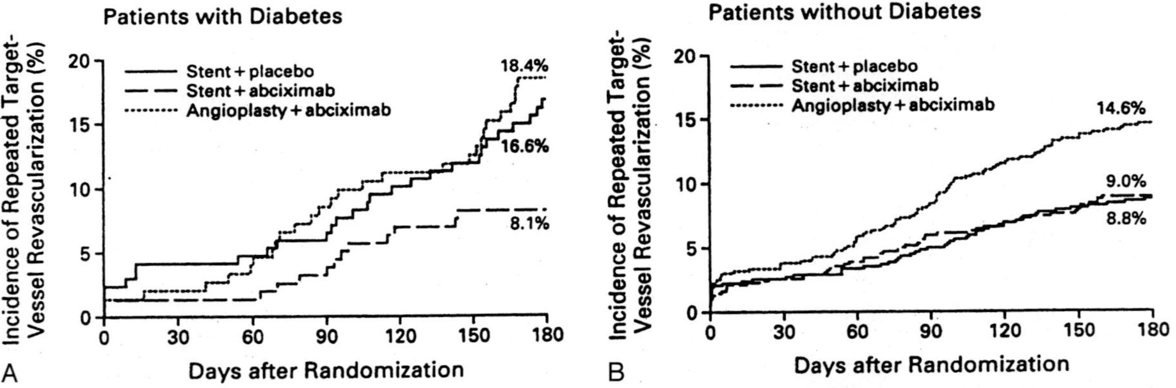

FIGURE 38–8 Kaplan-Meier estimates of the incidence of repeated target vessel revascularization within 6 months after randomization, according to treatment assignment, among patients with diabetes **(A)** and patients without diabetes **(B)**. **A,** Among patients with diabetes, *P* = .02 for the comparison between the stent-plus-abciximab group and the stent-plus-placebo group, *P* = .70 for the comparison between the angioplasty-plus-abciximab group and the stent-plus-placebo group, and *P* = .008 for the comparison between the stent-plus-abciximab group and the angioplasty-plus-abciximab group. **B,** Among patients without diabetes, *P* = .95 for the comparison between the stent-plus-abciximab group and the stent-plus-placebo group, *P* = .002 for the comparison between the angioplasty-plus-abciximab group and the stent-plus-placebo group, and *P* = .002 for the comparison between the stent-plus-abciximab group and the angioplasty-plus-abciximab group. (**A** and **B,** From The EPISTENT Investigators: Randomised placebo-controlled and balloon-angioplasty–controlled trial to assess safety of coronary stenting with use of platelet glycoprotein-IIb/IIIa blockade. Evaluation of Platelet IIb/IIIa Inhibitor for Stenting. Lancet 352:87–92, 1998. © The Lancet Ltd, 1998.)

TABLE 38–14 **PTCA for Unstable Angina in Elderly Patients**

First Author	Age (yr)	Patients (n)	Success (%)	Death (%)	Q Wave MI (%)	Em. CABG (%)
Simpfendorfer[157]	>70	212	93	0.9	0.9	2.8
Holt[158]	>70	54	80	0	4.0	6.0
Rizo-Patron[159]	>80	53	83	1.8	5.5	7.5
Reynen[160]	>70	102	84	4.0	5.0	n.a.
Eggeling[161]	>75	51	91	4	6	n.a.
Morrison[162]	>70	131	79	11*	n.a.	1.0
Thompson[163]	>65	768	93.5	1.4	2.2	1.4

Abbreviations: Em. CABG, emergency coronary artery bypass graft surgery; MI, myocardial infarction; n.a., not applicable; PTCA, percutaneous transluminal coronary angioplasty.
*Very high risk group; 62% of all patients were refused for surgery due to serious co-morbidity.

79 and 91 percent (Table 38–14).[157–163] In Morrison and associates' study,[162] the mortality was excessively high because these patients were a high cardiac risk group and had a high incidence of serious comorbidity.

Coronary stent implantation in elderly patients is also associated with a higher rate of procedure-related complications, including death, 2.2 percent; MI, 2.9 percent; and emergency CABG, 3.7 percent.[164]

Thus, despite the increased risk of major complications, percutaneous coronary intervention for elderly patients who present with unstable angina appears a reasonable therapeutic option for improvement of symptoms and, importantly, for improvement in quality of life.

Troponin T or I to Guide Treatment

It has been convincingly shown that the release of TnT or TnI is associated with a high likelihood of adverse events in patients with unstable CAD. Prestratification with measuring TnT or TnI release might open avenues to treat only high-risk patients, which may be more cost effective. The Fragmin during Instability in Coronary Artery Disease (FRISC) trial demonstrated that treatment with low-molecular-weight heparin of patients with a high TnT level reduced the incidence of death and MI to a figure comparable with that of patients with a low TnT level.[58] A subanalysis of the CAPTURE study evaluated the outcome of placebo-treated patients versus abciximab-treated patients who were classified according to TnT release into a low and high troponin T group (Fig. 38–9).[117] It appeared that the majority of adverse end points (death, MI) occurred in the high-risk group (TnT level > 0.1 ng/ml), and treatment with abciximab was associated with a striking decrease of adverse events compared with placebo. Indeed, in the low-risk group (TnT level ≤ 0.1 ng/ml), the frequency of adverse events was much less than in the high-risk group, and it was of note that the efficacy of abciximab to reduce adverse events was relatively smaller compared with its efficacy in the high-risk group.[165]

It may be concluded that the best cost-benefit ratio is obtained with treatment with abciximab in the high-risk group of patients with unstable angina who have a high level of TnT.

So far, it is still not defined what the optimal treatment strategy of unstable patients with high levels of TnT or TnI should be. Future studies may demonstrate that an early revascularization strategy in these patients may improve their poor outcome.

Invasive Treatment Strategy Versus Conservative Strategy

It was thought that an aggressive, invasive management strategy in patients with unstable angina or non–Q wave

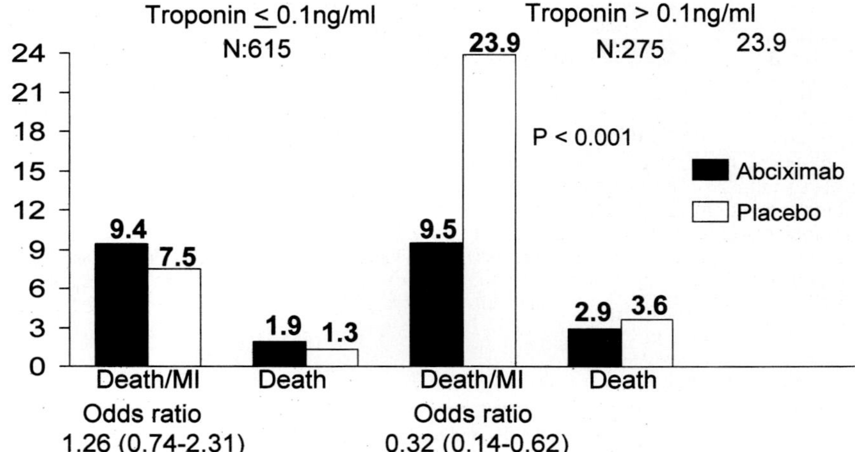

FIGURE 38–9 Relation of the occurrence of the combination of death and myocardial infarction (MI) at 6 months and release of troponin T in patients with refractory angina undergoing coronary angioplasty. A high-risk and a low-risk group can be identified.

TABLE 38-15 TIMI IIIB Trial: 6-Wk Outcome

Outcome	Early Invasive (%) (n = 740)	Early Conservative (%) (n = 733)
Coronary angiography	98	64
Revascularization	61	49
Death	2.4	2.5
Nonfatal MI	5.1	5.7
Positive 6-wk ETT	8.6	10.0
Total (primary end point)	16.2	18.1

Abbreviations: ETT, exercise stress test; MI, myocardial infarction; TIMI, Thrombolysis in Myocardial Infarction.

MI or after thrombolytic treatment for acute MI might be better than a conservative, ischemia-guided strategy. Three randomized trials have addressed this clinically important topic.

The Thrombolysis in Myocardial Infarction (TIMI) IIIB trial[166] was initiated to study the efficacy of an early invasive strategy versus a conservative strategy for the treatment of patients with suspected unstable angina or non–Q wave infarction. Early invasive strategy consisted of coronary angiography 18 to 48 hours after randomization followed by revascularization when indicated anatomically. In the early conservative strategy, patients underwent angiography followed by revascularization only if they had (1) recurrent ischemic pain with electrocardiographic changes, (2) more than 20 minutes of ischemic ST-segment deviation on 24-hour Holter electrocardiography in the hospital, (3) provokable ischemia (angina, ≥2-mm electrocardiographic deviation, or "high-risk" thallium) before completion of Bruce stage II or predischarge exercise stress test, or (4) post-discharge severe angina (angina at rest or Canadian class III or IV).

The main results of this important study are displayed in Table 38–15. There was no significant difference in the frequency of death or nonfatal MI and the frequency of a positive stress test at 6 weeks. However, the frequency of less serious events, such as the need for rehospitalization, residual angina, the need for multiple antianginal drugs, was lower in the early invasive strategy. The overall conclusion was that an early invasive strategy is suitable in patients if they have a high likelihood of failure of conservative strategy. These patients require access to a center with high-quality PTCA expertise. In all other clinical situations, early conservative strategy appears to be appropriate.

The Veterans Affairs Non–Q-Wave Infarction Strategies in Hospital (VANQWISH) trial was designed to answer the question whether an early invasive management strategy was equivalent to a conservative management strategy in survivors of a non–Q wave MI.[167] The combined primary end point was death from any cause or recurrent nonfatal MI during a minimum of 12 months of follow-up.

The invasive strategy consisted of early angiography in all patients and revascularization (CABG or PTCA) if deemed necessary. Conservative management consisted of medical therapy and noninvasive testing, with subsequent coronary angiography and revascularization in case of spontaneous or inducible ischemia within 72 hours or the onset of non–Q wave MI. A total of 920 patients were randomized. The patients were followed during an average period of 23 months. The outcome of the trial is tabulated in Table 38–16. Overall, the death and MI rate was higher (not statistically significant) in the invasive strategy group. At 1 year follow-up, this was significant, but the difference became smaller during longer follow-up. It may be concluded that in survivors of a non–Q wave MI, a conservative strategy, with invasive management guided by the occurrence of myocardial ischemia, is safe and effective.

The trials previously discussed can be criticized because the difference in actual revascularization rate in both the invasive arm and the conservative arm was so small that one may not expect to find a difference in outcome between the two strategies. Furthermore, the revascularization rate in the VANQWISH trial in the invasive strategy was only 44 percent, the operative mortality was high (11.9 percent), and the patients who were not revascularized had a very high adverse event rate, which might have been lower if they had received an appropriate revascularization procedure.

Of great interest is the very recently released FRISC-II (Fragmin and Fast Revascularization during Instability in Coronary Artery Disease) trial.[168] In the FRISC-II trial, high risk unstable patients were randomly allocated to an early invasive strategy or a conservative strategy. The patients were at high risk because they fulfilled these inclusion criteria: (1) randomized within 12 hours after chest

TABLE 38-16 VANQWISH Trial: Survivors of Non–Q Wave Myocardial Infarction

Outcome	Invasive Strategy (n = 462)	Conservative Strategy (n = 458)	*P* Value
Coronary angiography (%)	96	48	
Revascularization (%)	44	33	
CABG (NP)	95	87	
PTCA (NP)	98	55	
CABG + PTCA (NP)	11	10	
Primary end point	Death/MI (death)	Death/MI (death)	
In-hospital (NP)	36 (21)	15 (6)	0.004 (0.007)
1 mo (NP)	48 (23)	26 (9)	0.021 (0.021)
1 yr (NP)	111 (58)	85 (36)	0.05 (0.025)
Average 23 mo (12–44) (NP)	152 (80)	139 (59)	0.35

Abbreviations: CABG, coronary artery bypass surgery; MI, myocardial infarction; NP, number of patients; PTCA, percutaneous transluminal coronary angioplasty; VANQWISH, Veterans Affairs Non–Q Wave Infarction Strategies in Hospital.

TABLE 38–17 **FRISC-II Trial: Revascularization Strategies in High-Risk Unstable Angina Patients**

Outcome	Invasive Strategy (n = 1215) (%)	Conservative Strategy (n = 1229) (%)	*P* Value
Revascularization			
Within 10 da	71	9	
Within 6 mo	78	38	
Death/MI at 6 mo			
All patients	9.5	12	.04
Males	9.1	13.9	.002
Death at 6 mo			
All patients	1.9	3.0	.10
Males	1.5	3.2	.003
Females	2.9	2.6	.75

Abbreviations: FRISC, Fragmin during Instability in Coronary Artery Disease; MI, myocardial infarction.

pain, (2) ST-segment depression or T-wave changes, and (3) evidence of the release of the MB isoenzyme of creatine kinase or of TnT. Early revascularization (within 10 days) was achieved in 71 percent in the invasive strategy and 9 percent in the conservative strategy patients. The 6-month combined death and MI rate was statistically significant, less than 9.5 percent in the invasive arm compared with 12 percent in the noninvasive arm ($P < .04$) (Table 38–17). Noteworthy is the fact that this favorable effect was predominantly achieved in males only, and apparently no efficacy was noted in female patients. In the FRISC-II trial, if patients underwent revascularization, more patients were referred for coronary intervention than for CABG. The use of stents was 65 percent, a left internal mammary artery graft was used in 95 percent of the patients, and the overall procedural in-hospital mortality was 0.8 percent.

It may be concluded from the previously cited randomized trials that in high-risk unstable angina patients, an early invasive strategy, followed by immediate revascularization in the majority of patients, is recommended. A conservative strategy is recommended for those at medium risk or low risk according to which only those patients may undergo revascularization procedures who demonstrate evidence of stress-induced ischemia or (early) recurrence of ischemia.

CONCLUSIONS

Patients with unstable angina or non–Q wave MI should initially receive pharmacologic treatment aimed at stabilizing the plaque and at achieving prompt effective anti-ischemic response (Table 38–18).[1] The role of low-molecular-weight heparins and/or GP IIb/IIIa antagonists in stabilization of the plaque is emerging. Anti-ischemic medications should be individualized according to the response to medication. This initial approach is usually effective in the majority of patients. Prompt angiography and subsequent revascularization (percutaneous coronary intervention or CABG) is indicated in very high-risk patients in whom this initial medical approach fails and ischemic episodes continue or recur despite "full" medical treatment or who have signs of severe ischemic left ventricular dysfunction (Fig. 38–10).

Early coronary angiography and subsequent revascularization is indicated in high-risk patients who have a high likelihood of progression of disease (associated transient ST-T changes or high-release TnT).

Patients who initially stabilize (medium to low risk) should undergo stress testing, preferably before discharge.[169] Those with inducible ischemia should undergo coronary angiography with subsequent elective revascularization. Those without inducible ischemia require continued medical treatment including aspirin and cholesterol-lowering therapy.

The indications to proceed with either percutaneous coronary intervention or CABG are still controversial. In general, bypass surgery is indicated if there is (1) significant left main coronary artery disease or (2) significant three-vessel disease. An attempt should be made to maximally use arterial grafts. Percutaneous coronary intervention is indicated in patients with one- or two-vessel disease. Percutaneous intervention consists of balloon angioplasty and intracoronary stent implantation in case of threatening occlusion or suboptimal angioplasty result. In selected patients with multivessel disease, one might, to enhance safety, prefer to treat the ischemia-related vessel only, rather than to achieve complete revascularization by multiple interventions in one session. Patients who undergo percutaneous coronary intervention should receive antiplatelet treatment, including aspirin, ticlopidine, and GP IIb/IIIa receptor antagonists to reduce major complications.

Stent implantation has been shown to reduce the 6-month restenosis rate in patients with unstable CAD. All

TABLE 38–18 **Medical Treatment of Unstable Angina and Non–Q Wave Myocardial Infarction**

General management: bed rest (CCU) and sedation
Stabilization of plaque
- Aspirin and heparin (intravenous)
- LMWH or GP IIb/IIIa antagonists?

Anti-ischemic treatment with individual tailoring of agents
- β-Adrenergic blockade to achieve a resting pulse < 60 bpm
- Nitroglycerin and/or calcium antagonists to reduce preload and afterload (systolic aortic pressure < 110 mm Hg) and induce coronary vasodilatation

Elimination of precipitating factors (anemia, hypertension, tachycardia)

Abbreviations: CCU, coronary care unit; GP, glycoprotein; LMWH, low-molecular-weight heparin.

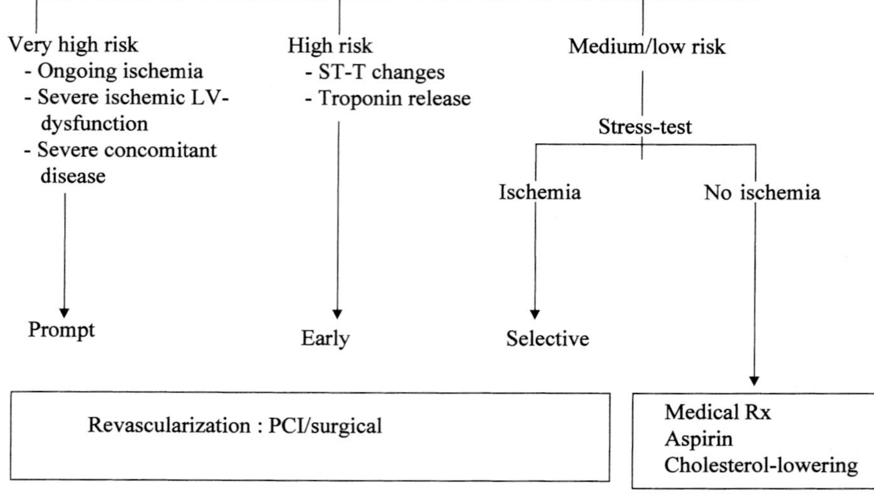

FIGURE 38–10 Management strategy of patients with unstable angina pectoris. LV, left ventricular; PCI, percutaneous coronary intervention; Rx, therapy.

patients who undergo percutaneous coronary intervention for unstable angina or non–Q wave MI should be offered cholesterol-modifying treatment and aspirin to prevent or reduce the occurrence of adverse long-term clinical events.

FUTURE

Further investigations are needed to help unravel the more precise causes of instability, to determine how to identify and stabilize an unstable plaque, and how to more effectively treat unstable patients so that their rather worse prognosis can be improved.

What will be the role of low-molecular-weight heparin in the setting of percutaneous intervention and unstable disease? Will it replace unfractionated heparin before and during the procedure? Should it be continued after the procedure, and for how long?

What will be the role of direct antithrombins or other antithrombotic approaches such as tissue factor antagonists? What will be the role of the von Willebrand factor in high–shear rate situations, and will blockade of the GP Ib or GP IIb/IIIa receptors decrease thrombotic procedural complications? Is an invasive aggressive strategy in patients with high TnT or TnI release more favorable than a conservative strategy?

REFERENCES

1. Braunwald E, Jones RH, Mark DB, et al: Diagnosing and managing unstable angina. Agency for Health Care Policy and Research. Circulation 90:613–622, 1994.
2. Oler A, Whooley MA, Oler J, Grady D: Adding heparin to aspirin reduces the incidence of myocardial infarction and death in patients with unstable angina. A meta-analysis. JAMA 276:811–815, 1996.
3. Sherman CT, Litvack F, Grundfest W, et al: Coronary angioscopy in patients with unstable angina pectoris. N Engl J Med 315:913–919, 1986.
4. DeWood MA, Spores J, Notske R, et al: Prevalence of total coronary occlusion during the early hours of transmural myocardial infarction. N Engl J Med 303:897–902, 1980.
5. Fuster V, Badimon L, Badimon JJ, Chesebro JH: The pathogenesis of coronary artery disease and the acute coronary syndromes (1). N Engl J Med 326:242–50, 1992.
6. Fuster V, Badimon L, Badimon JJ, Chesebro JH: The pathogenesis of coronary artery disease and the acute coronary syndromes (2). N Engl J Med 326:310–318, 1992.
7. Davies MJ, Thomas AC, Knapman PA, Hangartner JR: Intramyocardial platelet aggregation in patients with unstable angina suffering sudden ischemic cardiac death. Circulation 73:418–427, 1986.
8. Davies MJ: Stability and instability: two faces of coronary atherosclerosis. The Paul Dudley White Lecture 1995. Circulation 94:2013–2020, 1996.
9. van der Wal AC, Becker AE, van der Loos CM, Das PK: Site of intimal rupture or erosion of thrombosed coronary atherosclerotic plaques is characterized by an inflammatory process irrespective of the dominant plaque morphology. Circulation 89:36–44, 1994.
10. Mann JM, Davies MJ: Vulnerable plaque. Relation of characteristics to degree of stenosis in human coronary arteries. Circulation 94:928–931, 1996.
11. Libby P: Molecular bases of the acute coronary syndromes. Circulation 91:2844–2850, 1995.
12. Farb A, Burke AP, Tang AL, et al: Coronary plaque erosion without rupture into a lipid core. A frequent cause of coronary thrombosis in sudden coronary death. Circulation 93:1354–1363, 1996.
13. Falk E, Shah PK, Fuster V: Coronary plaque disruption. Circulation 92:657–671, 1995.
14. de Feyter PJ, Ozaki Y, Baptista J, et al: Ischemia-related lesion characteristics in patients with stable or unstable angina. A study with intracoronary angioscopy and ultrasound. Circulation 92:1408–1413, 1995.
15. Fernandez-Ortiz A, Badimon JJ, Falk E, et al: Characterization of the relative thrombogenicity of atherosclerotic plaque components: implications for consequences of plaque rupture. J Am Coll Cardiol 23:1562–1569, 1994.
16. Annex BH, Denning SM, Channon KM, et al: Differential expression of tissue factor protein in directional atherectomy specimens from patients with stable and unstable coronary syndromes. Circulation 91:619–622, 1995.
17. Marmur JD, Thiruvikraman SV, Fyfe BS, et al: Identification of active tissue factor in human coronary atheroma. Circulation 94:1226–1232, 1996.
18. Ardissino D, Merlini PA, Ariens R, et al: Tissue-factor antigen and activity in human coronary atherosclerotic plaques. Lancet 349:769–771, 1997.

19. Toschi V, Gallo R, Lettino M, et al: Tissue factor modulates the thrombogenicity of human atherosclerotic plaques. Circulation 95:594–599, 1997.
20. Maseri A, L'Abbate A, Baroldi G, et al: Coronary vasospasm as a possible cause of myocardial infarction. A conclusion derived from the study of "preinfarction" angina. N Engl J Med 299:1271–1277, 1978.
21. Ludmer PL, Selwyn AP, Shook TL, et al: Paradoxical vasoconstriction induced by acetylcholine in atherosclerotic coronary arteries. N Engl J Med 315:1046–1051, 1986.
22. Bogaty P, Hackett D, Davies G, Maseri A: Vasoreactivity of the culprit lesion in unstable angina. Circulation 90:5–11, 1994.
23. Ambrose JA: Plaque disruption and the acute coronary syndromes of unstable angina and myocardial infarction: if the substrate is similar, why is the clinical presentation different? J Am Coll Cardiol 19:1653–1658, 1992.
24. de Feyter PJ: Coronary angioplasty for unstable angina. Am Heart J 118:860–868, 1989.
25. Neill WA, Wharton TP Jr, Fluri-Lundeen J, Cohen IS: Acute coronary insufficiency–coronary occlusion after intermittent ischemic attacks. N Engl J Med 302:1157–1162, 1980.
26. Moise A, Theroux P, Taeymans Y, et al: Unstable angina and progression of coronary atherosclerosis. N Engl J Med 309:685–689, 1983.
27. Rafflenbeul W, Smith LR, Rogers WJ, et al: Quantitative coronary arteriography. Coronary anatomy of patients with unstable angina pectoris reexamined 1 year after optimal medical therapy. Am J Cardiol 43:699–707, 1979.
28. Kaski JC, Chester MR, Chen L, Katritsis D: Rapid angiographic progression of coronary artery disease in patients with angina pectoris. The role of complex stenosis morphology. Circulation 92:2058–2065, 1995.
29. Scanlon PJ: The intermediate coronary syndrome. Prog Cardiovasc Dis 23:351, 1982.
30. Plotnick GD: Approach to the management of unstable angina. Am Heart J 98:243–255, 1979.
31. Conti CR, Brawley RK, Griffith LS, et al: Unstable angina pectoris: morbidity and mortality in 57 consecutive patients evaluated angiographically. Am J Cardiol 32:745–750, 1973.
32. Betriu A, Heras M, Cohen M, Fuster V: Unstable angina: outcome according to clinical presentation. J Am Coll Cardiol 19:1659–1663, 1992.
33. Harris PJ, Harrell FE Jr, Lee KL, et al: Survival in medically treated coronary artery disease. Circulation 60:1259–1269, 1979.
34. Duncan B, Fulton M, Morrison SL, et al: Prognosis of new and worsening angina pectoris. BMJ 1:981–985, 1976.
35. Roberts KB, Califf RM, Harrell FE Jr, et al: The prognosis for patients with new-onset angina who have undergone cardiac catheterization. Circulation 68:970–978, 1983.
36. Heng MK, Norris RM, Singh BM, Partridge JB: Prognosis in unstable angina. Br Heart J 38:921–925, 1976.
37. Mulcahy R, Al Awadhi AH, de Buitleor M, et al: Natural history and prognosis of unstable angina. Am Heart J 109:753–758, 1985.
38. Krauss KR, Hutter AM Jr, DeSanctis RW: Acute coronary insufficiency. Course and follow-up. Arch Intern Med 129:808–813, 1972.
39. Severi S, Orsini E, Marraccini P, et al: The basal electrocardiogram and the exercise stress test in assessing prognosis in patients with unstable angina. Eur Heart J 9:441–446, 1988.
40. Gazes PC, Mobley EM Jr, Faris HM Jr, et al: Preinfarctional (unstable) angina—a prospective study—ten year follow-up. Prognostic significance of electrocardiographic changes. Circulation 48:331–337, 1973.
41. Bertolasi CA, Tronge JE, Riccitelli MA, et al: Natural history of unstable angina with medical or surgical therapy. Chest 70:596–605, 1976.
42. Olson HG, Lyons KP, Aronow WS, et al: The high-risk angina patient. Identification by clinical features, hospital course, electrocardiography and technetium-99m stannous pyrophosphate scintigraphy. Circulation 64:674–684, 1981.
43. Ouyang P, Brinker JA, Mellits ED, et al: Variables predictive of successful medical therapy in patients with unstable angina: selection by multivariate analysis from clinical, electrocardiographic, and angiographic evaluations. Circulation 70:367–376, 1984.
44. Cairns JA, Fantus IG, Klassen GA: Unstable angina pectoris. Am Heart J 92:373–386, 1976.
45. Mulcahy R, Conroy R, Katz R, Fitzpatrick M: Does intensive medical therapy influence the outcome in unstable angina? Clin Cardiol 13:687–689, 1990.
46. Wilcox I, Freedman SB, McCredie RJ, et al: Risk of adverse outcome in patients admitted to the coronary care unit with suspected unstable angina pectoris. Am J Cardiol 64:845–848, 1989.
47. Langer A, Freeman MR, Armstrong PW: ST segment shift in unstable angina: pathophysiology and association with coronary anatomy and hospital outcome. J Am Coll Cardiol 13:1495–1502, 1989.
48. Stenson RE, Flamm MD, Zaret BL, McGowan RL: Transient ST-segment elevation with postmyocardial infarction angina: prognostic significance. Am Heart J 89:449–454, 1975.
49. Fraker TD Jr, Wagner GS, Rosati RA: Extension of myocardial infarction: incidence and prognosis. Circulation 60:1126–1129, 1979.
50. Madigan NP, Rutherford BD, Frye RL: The clinical course, early prognosis and coronary anatomy of subendocardial infarction. Am J Med 60:634–641, 1976.
51. Marmor A, Sobel BE, Roberts R: Factors presaging early recurrent myocardial infarction ("extension"). Am J Cardiol 48:603–610, 1981.
52. Schuster EH, Bulkley BH: Early post-infarction angina. Ischemia at a distance and ischemia in the infarct zone. N Engl J Med 305:1101–1105, 1981.
53. Hutter AM Jr, DeSanctis RW, Flynn T, Yeatman LA: Nontransmural myocardial infarction: a comparison of hospital and late clinical course of patients with that of matched patients with transmural anterior and transmural inferior myocardial infarction. Am J Cardiol 48:595–602, 1981.
54. Fioretti P, Brower RW, Balakumaran K: Early post-infarction angina. Incidence and prognostic relevance. Eur Heart J 7(suppl C):73–77, 1986.
55. Gibson RS, Beller GA, Gheorghiade M, et al: The prevalence and clinical significance of residual myocardial ischemia 2 weeks after uncomplicated non–Q wave infarction: a prospective natural history study. Circulation 73:1186–1198, 1986.
56. Bosch X, Theroux P, Waters DD, et al: Early postinfarction ischemia: clinical, angiographic, and prognostic significance. Circulation 75:988–995, 1987.
57. A comparison of recombinant hirudin with heparin for the treatment of acute coronary syndromes. The Global Use of Strategies to Open Occluded Arteries (GUSTO) IIb Investigators. N Engl J Med 335:775–782, 1996.
58. Fragmin during Instability in Coronary Artery Disease (FRISC) Study Group: Low-molecular-weight heparin during instability in coronary artery disease. Lancet 347:561–568, 1996.
59. Klein W, Buchwald A, Hillis SE, et al: Comparison of low-molecular-weight heparin with unfractionated heparin acutely and with placebo for 6 weeks in the management of unstable coronary artery disease. Fragmin in Unstable Coronary Artery Disease (FRIC) Study. Circulation 96:61–68, 1997.
60. Cohen M, Demers C, Gurfinkel EP, et al: A comparison of low-molecular-weight heparin with unfractionated heparin for unstable coronary artery disease. Efficacy and Safety of Subcutaneous Enoxaparin in Non–Q-Wave Coronary Events (ESSENCE) Study Group. N Engl J Med 337:447–452, 1997.
61. Inhibition of the platelet glycoprotein IIb/IIIa Receptor with tirofiban in unstable angina and non-Q-wave myocardial infarction. Platelet Receptor Inhibition in Ischemic Syndrome Management in Patients Limited by Unstable Signs and Symptoms (PRISM-PLUS) Study Investigators. N Engl J Med 338:1488–1497, 1998.
62. A comparison of aspirin plus tirofiban with aspirin plus heparin for unstable angina. Platelet Receptor Inhibition in Ischemic Syndrome Management (PRISM) Study Investigators. N Engl J Med 338:1498–1505, 1998.
63. International, randomized, controlled trial of lamifiban (a platelet glycoprotein IIb/IIIa inhibitor), heparin, or both in unstable angina. The PARAGON Investigators. Platelet IIb/IIIa Antagonism for the Reduction of Acute coronary syndrome events in a Global Organization Network. Circulation 97:2386–2395, 1998.
64. Inhibition of platelet glycoprotein IIb/IIIa with eptifibatide in patients with acute coronary syndromes. The PURSUIT Trial Investigators. Platelet Glycoprotein IIb/IIIa in Unstable Angina: Receptor Suppression Using Integrilin Therapy. N Engl J Med 339:436–443, 1998.

65. Braunwald E: Unstable angina. A classification. Circulation 80:410–414, 1989.
66. Ahmed WH, Bittl JA, Braunwald E: Relation between clinical presentation and angiographic findings in unstable angina pectoris, and comparison with that in stable angina. Am J Cardiol 72:544–550, 1993.
67. Depre C, Wijns W, Robert AM, et al: Pathology of unstable plaque: correlation with the clinical severity of acute coronary syndromes. J Am Coll Cardiol 30:694–702, 1997.
68. van Miltenburg-van Zijl AJ, Simoons ML, Veerhoek RJ, Bossuyt PM: Incidence and follow-up of Braunwald subgroups in unstable angina pectoris. J Am Coll Cardiol 25:1286–1292, 1995.
69. Calvin JE, Klein LW, VandenBerg BJ, et al: Risk stratification in unstable angina. Prospective validation of the Braunwald classification. JAMA 273:136–141, 1995.
70. Armstrong PW, Fu Y, Chang WC, et al: Acute coronary syndromes in the GUSTO-IIb trial: prognostic insights and impact of recurrent ischemia. The GUSTO-IIb Investigators. Circulation 98:1860–1868, 1998.
71. Savonitto S, Ardissino D, Granger CB, et al: Prognostic value of the admission electrocardiogram in acute coronary syndromes [see comments]. JAMA 281:707–713, 1999.
72. Topol E: Patient stratification and its predictive value of cardiac events. Eur Heart J 19(suppl K):K5–K7, 1998.
73. Lindahl B, Venge P, Wallentin L: Relation between troponin T and the risk of subsequent cardiac events in unstable coronary artery disease. The FRISC Study Group. Circulation 93:1651–1657, 1996.
74. Ohman EM, Armstrong PW, Christenson RH, et al: Cardiac troponin T levels for risk stratification in acute myocardial ischemia. GUSTO-IIa Investigators. N Engl J Med 335:1333–1341, 1996.
75. Antman EM, Tanasijevic MJ, Thompson B, et al: Cardiac-specific troponin I levels to predict the risk of mortality in patients with acute coronary syndromes. N Engl J Med 335:1342–1349, 1996.
76. Hamm CW, Goldmann BU, Heeschen C, et al: Emergency room triage of patients with acute chest pain by means of rapid testing for cardiac troponin T or troponin I. N Engl J Med 337:1648–1653, 1997.
77. Holmvang L, Luscher MS, Clemmensen P, et al: Very early risk stratification using combined ECG and biochemical assessment in patients with unstable coronary artery disease (a thrombin inhibition in myocardial ischemia [TRIM] substudy). The TRIM Study Group. Circulation 98:2004–2009, 1998.
78. Newby LK, Christenson RH, Ohman EM, et al: Value of serial troponin T measures for early and late risk stratification in patients with acute coronary syndromes. The GUSTO-IIa Investigators. Circulation 98:1853–1859, 1998.
79. Gruntzig AR, Senning A, Siegenthaler WE: Nonoperative dilatation of coronary-artery stenosis: percutaneous transluminal coronary angioplasty. N Engl J Med 301:61–68, 1979.
80. Williams DO, Riley RS, Singh AK, et al: Evaluation of the role of coronary angioplasty in patients with unstable angina pectoris. Am Heart J 102:1–9, 1981.
81. Meyer J, Schmitz HJ, Kiesslich T, et al: Percutaneous transluminal coronary angioplasty in patients with stable and unstable angina pectoris: analysis of early and late results. Am Heart J 106:973–980, 1983.
82. Faxon DP, Detre KM, McCabe CH, et al: Role of percutaneous transluminal coronary angioplasty in the treatment of unstable angina. Report from the National Heart, Lung, and Blood Institute Percutaneous Transluminal Coronary Angioplasty and Coronary Artery Surgery Study Registries. Am J Cardiol 53:131C–135C, 1984.
83. de Feyter PJ, Serruys PW, van den Brand M, et al: Emergency coronary angioplasty in refractory unstable angina. N Engl J Med 313:342–346, 1985.
84. Quigley PJ, Erwin J, Maurer BJ, et al: Percutaneous transluminal coronary angioplasty in unstable angina: comparison with stable angina. Br Heart J 55:227–230, 1986.
85. de Feyter PJ, Serruys PW, Suryapranata H, et al: Coronary angioplasty early after diagnosis of unstable angina. Am Heart J 114:48–54, 1987.
86. Steffenino G, Meier B, Finci L, Rutishauser W: Follow up results of treatment of unstable angina by coronary angioplasty. Br Heart J 57:416–419, 1987.
87. Myler RK, Shaw RE, Stertzer SH, et al: Lesion morphology and coronary angioplasty: current experience and analysis. J Am Coll Cardiol 19:1641–1652, 1992.
88. Stammen F, De Scheerder I, Glazier JJ, et al: Immediate and follow-up results of the conservative coronary angioplasty strategy for unstable angina pectoris. Am J Cardiol 69:1533–1537, 1992.
89. Timmis AD, Griffin B, Crick JC, Sowton E: Early percutaneous transluminal coronary angioplasty in the management of unstable angina. Int J Cardiol 14:25–31, 1987.
90. de Feyter PJ, Suryapranata H, Serruys PW, et al: Coronary angioplasty for unstable angina: immediate and late results in 200 consecutive patients with identification of risk factors for unfavorable early and late outcome. J Am Coll Cardiol 12:324–333, 1988.
91. Thijs Plokker HW, Ernst SM, Bal ET, et al: Percutaneous transluminal coronary angioplasty in patients with unstable angina pectoris refractory to medical therapy: long-term clinical and angiographic results. Cathet Cardiovasc Diagn 14:15–18, 1988.
92. Sharma B, Wyeth RP, Kolath GS, et al: Percutaneous transluminal coronary angioplasty of one vessel for refractory unstable angina pectoris: efficacy in single and multivessel disease. Br Heart J 59:280–286, 1988.
93. Perry RA, Seth A, Hunt A, Shiu MF: Coronary angioplasty in unstable angina and stable angina: a comparison of success and complications. Br Heart J 60:367–372, 1988.
94. Morrison DA: Percutaneous transluminal coronary angioplasty for rest angina pectoris requiring intravenous nitroglycerin and intraaortic balloon counterpulsation. Am J Cardiol 66:168–171, 1990.
95. Rupprecht HJ, Brennecke R, Kottmeyer M, et al: Short- and long-term outcome after PTCA in patients with stable and unstable angina. Eur Heart J 11:964–973, 1990.
96. de Feyter PJ, Serruys PW, Soward A, et al: Coronary angioplasty for early postinfarction unstable angina. Circulation 74:1365–1370, 1986.
97. Holt GW, Gersh BJ, Holmes DR: The results of percutaneous transluminal coronary angioplasty (PTCA) in post infarction angina pectoris. J Am Coll Cardiol 7:62, 1986.
98. Gottlieb SO, Walford GD, Ouyang P, et al: Initial and late results of coronary angioplasty for early postinfarction unstable angina. Cathet Cardiovasc Diagn 13:93–99, 1987.
99. Safian RD, Snyder LD, Synder BA, et al: Usefulness of percutaneous transluminal coronary angioplasty for unstable angina pectoris after non–Q-wave acute myocardial infarction. Am J Cardiol 59:263–266, 1987.
100. Hopkins J, Savage M, Zalewski A, et al: Recurrent ischemia in the zone of prior myocardial infarction: results of coronary angioplasty of the infarct-related artery. Am Heart J 115:14–19, 1988.
101. Suryapranata H, Beatt K, de Feyter PJ, et al: Percutaneous transluminal coronary angioplasty for angina pectoris after a non–Q-wave acute myocardial infarction. Am J Cardiol 61:240–243, 1988.
102. Morrison DA: Coronary angioplasty for medically refractory unstable angina within 30 days of acute myocardial infarction. Am Heart J 120:256–261, 1990.
103. Comparison of invasive and conservative strategies after treatment with intravenous tissue plasminogen activator in acute myocardial infarction. Results of the Thrombolysis in Myocardial Infarction (TIMI) phase II trial. The TIMI Study Group. N Engl J Med 320:618–627, 1989.
104. Bredlau CE, Roubin GS, Leimgruber PP, et al: In-hospital morbidity and mortality in patients undergoing elective coronary angioplasty. Circulation 72:1044–1052, 1985.
105. Holmes DR Jr, Holubkov R, Vlietstra RE, et al: Comparison of complications during percutaneous transluminal coronary angioplasty from 1977 to 1981 and from 1985 to 1986: the National Heart, Lung, and Blood Institute Percutaneous Transluminal Coronary Angioplasty Registry. J Am Coll Cardiol 12:1149–1155, 1988.
106. Tuzcu EM, Simpfendorfer C, Badhwar K, et al: Determinants of primary success in elective percutaneous transluminal coronary angioplasty for significant narrowing of a single major coronary artery. Am J Cardiol 62:873–875, 1988.
107. de Feyter PJ, van den Brand M, Serruys PW: Increase of initial success and safety of single vessel PTCA in 1371 patients: a seven-years experience. J Interv Cardiol 1:1, 1988.
108. O'Keefe JH Jr, Reeder GS, Miller GA, et al: Safety and efficacy of percutaneous transluminal coronary angioplasty performed at time of diagnostic catheterization compared with that performed at other times. Am J Cardiol 63:27–29, 1989.
109. Ruygrok PN, de Jaegere PPT, Verploegh J: Immediate outcome following coronary angioplasty. Eur Heart J 16:124, 1995.

110. Bentivoglio LG, Detre K, Yeh W, et al: Outcome of percutaneous transluminal coronary angioplasty in subsets of unstable angina pectoris. A report of the 1985–1986 National Heart, Lung, and Blood Institute Percutaneous Transluminal Coronary Angioplasty Registry. J Am Coll Cardiol 24:1195–1206, 1994.
111. de Feyter PJ, Ruygrok PN: Coronary intervention: risk stratification and management of abrupt coronary occlusion. Eur Heart J 16:97, 1995.
112. Bittl JA: Advances in coronary angioplasty [published erratum appears in N Engl J Med 1997 Feb 27;336:670]. N Engl J Med 335:1290–1302, 1996.
113. Use of a monoclonal antibody directed against the platelet glycoprotein IIb/IIIa receptor in high-risk coronary angioplasty. The EPIC Investigation. N Engl J Med 330:956–961, 1994.
114. Platelet glycoprotein IIb/IIIa receptor blockade and low-dose heparin during percutaneous coronary revascularization. The EPILOG Investigators. N Engl J Med 336:1689–1696, 1997.
115. Randomised placebo-controlled trial of effect of eptifibatide on complications of percutaneous coronary intervention: IMPACT-II. Integrilin to Minimise Platelet Aggregation and Coronary Thrombosis-II. Lancet 349:1422–1428, 1997.
116. Effects of platelet glycoprotein IIb/IIIa blockade with tirofiban on adverse cardiac events in patients with unstable angina or acute myocardial infarction undergoing coronary angioplasty. The RESTORE Investigators. Randomized Efficacy Study of Tirofiban for Outcomes and REstenosis. Circulation 96:1445–1453, 1997.
117. Randomised placebo-controlled trial of abciximab before and during coronary intervention in refractory unstable angina: the CAPTURE Study. Lancet 349:1429–1435, 1997.
118. Lincoff AM, Califf RM, Anderson KM, et al: Evidence for prevention of death and myocardial infarction with platelet membrane glycoprotein IIb/IIIa receptor blockade by abciximab (c7E3 Fab) among patients with unstable angina undergoing percutaneous coronary revascularization. EPIC Investigators. Evaluation of 7E3 in Preventing Ischemic Complications. J Am Coll Cardiol 30:149–156, 1997.
119. Serruys PW, Herrman JP, Simon R, et al: A comparison of hirudin with heparin in the prevention of restenosis after coronary angioplasty. Helvetica Investigators. N Engl J Med 333:757–763, 1995.
120. Herrman JP, Simon R, Umans VA, et al: Evaluation of recombinant hirudin (CGP 39,393/TMREVASC) in the prevention of restenosis after percutaneous transluminal coronary angioplasty. Rationale and design of the HELVETICA trial, a multicentre randomized double blind heparin controlled study. Eur Heart J 16(suppl L):56–62, 1995.
121. Bittl JA, Strony J, Brinker JA, et al: Treatment with bivalirudin (Hirulog) as compared with heparin during coronary angioplasty for unstable or postinfarction angina. Hirulog Angioplasty Study Investigators. N Engl J Med 333:764–769, 1995.
122. Block PC, Myler RK, Stertzer S, Fallon JT: Morphology after transluminal angioplasty in human beings. N Engl J Med 305:382–385, 1981.
123. Waller BF: "Crackers, breakers, stretchers, drillers, scrapers, shavers, burners, welders and melters"—the future treatment of atherosclerotic coronary artery disease? A clinical-morphologic assessment. J Am Coll Cardiol 13:969–987, 1989.
124. Wilentz JR, Sanborn TA, Haudenschild CC, et al: Platelet accumulation in experimental angioplasty: time course and relation to vascular injury. Circulation 75:636–642, 1987.
125. Yazdani S, Simon AD, Kovar L, et al: Percutaneous interventions alter the hemostatic profile of patients with unstable versus stable angina. J Am Coll Cardiol 30:1284–1287, 1997.
126. Robinson NK, Thomas MR, Wainwright RJ: Is unstable angina a contra-indication to intracoronary stent insertion? J Invasive Cardiol 8:351, 1996.
127. Danchin N, Lablanche JM, Grollier G: Intracoronary stenting in patients with unstable angina. Results from the French TASTE Registry. Eur Heart J 18:389, 1997.
128. Marzocchi A, Piovaccari G, Marrozzini C, et al: Results of coronary stenting for unstable versus stable angina pectoris. Am J Cardiol 79:1314–1318, 1997.
129. Chauhan A, Vu E, Ricci DR, et al: Multiple coronary stenting in unstable angina: early and late clinical outcomes. Cathet Cardiovasc Diagn 43:11–16, 1998.
130. Alfonso F, Rodriguez P, Phillips P, et al: Clinical and angiographic implications of coronary stenting in thrombus-containing lesions. J Am Coll Cardiol 29:725–733, 1997.
131. Madan M, Marquis JF, de May MR, et al: Coronary stenting in unstable angina: early and late clinical outcomes. Can J Cardiol 14:1109–1114, 1998.
132. Kornowski R, Hong MK, Saucedo J, et al: Procedural results and long-term clinical outcomes following coronary stenting in perimyocardial infarction syndromes. Am J Cardiol 82:1163–1167, 1998.
133. Schomig A, Neumann FJ, Kastrati A, et al: A randomized comparison of antiplatelet and anticoagulant therapy after the placement of coronary-artery stents. N Engl J Med 334:1084–1089, 1996.
134. Leon MB, Baim DS, Popma JJ, et al: A clinical trial comparing three antithrombotic-drug regimens after coronary-artery stenting. Stent Anticoagulation Restenosis Study Investigators. N Engl J Med 339:1665–1671, 1998.
135. Bertrand ME, Legrand V, Boland J, et al: Randomized multicenter comparison of conventional anticoagulation versus antiplatelet therapy in unplanned and elective coronary stenting. The Full Anticoagulation Versus Aspirin and Ticlopidine (FANTASTIC) Study. Circulation 98:1597–1603, 1998.
136. The EPISTENT Investigators: Randomised placebo-controlled and balloon-angioplasty–controlled trial to assess safety of coronary stenting with use of platelet glycoprotein-IIb/IIIa blockade. Evaluation of Platelet IIb/IIIa Inhibitor for Stenting. Lancet 352:87–92, 1998.
137. Serruys PW, van Hout B, Bonnier H, et al: Randomised comparison of implantation of heparin-coated stents with balloon angioplasty in selected patients with coronary artery disease (Benestent II). Lancet 352:673–681, 1998.
138. Ellis SG, Roubin GS, King SB 3d, et al: Angiographic and clinical predictors of acute closure after native vessel coronary angioplasty. Circulation 77:372–379, 1988.
139. Detre KM, Holmes DR Jr, Holubkov R, et al: Incidence and consequences of periprocedural occlusion. The 1985–1986 National Heart, Lung, and Blood Institute Percutaneous Transluminal Coronary Angioplasty Registry. Circulation 82:739–750, 1990.
140. Tenaglia AN, Fortin DF, Califf RM, et al: Predicting the risk of abrupt vessel closure after angioplasty in an individual patient. J Am Coll Cardiol 24:1004–1011, 1994.
141. Luijten HE, Beatt KJ, de Feyter PJ, et al: Angioplasty for stable versus unstable angina pectoris: are unstable patients more likely to get restenosis? A quantitative angiographic study in 339 consecutive patients. Int J Card Imaging 3:87–97, 1988.
142. Hermans WR, Foley DP, Rensing BJ, et al: Usefulness of quantitative and qualitative angiographic lesion morphology, and clinical characteristics in predicting major adverse cardiac events during and after native coronary balloon angioplasty. CARPORT and MERCATOR Study Groups. Am J Cardiol 72:14–20, 1993.
143. Halon DA, Merdler A, Shefer A, et al: Identifying patients at high risk for restenosis after percutaneous transluminal coronary angioplasty for unstable angina pectoris. Am J Cardiol 64:289–293, 1989.
144. Bauters C, Khanoyan P, McFadden EP, et al: Restenosis after delayed coronary angioplasty of the culprit vessel in patients with a recent myocardial infarction treated by thrombolysis. Circulation 91:1410–1418, 1995.
145. Bauters C, Lablanche JM, McFadden EP, et al: Repeat percutaneous coronary angioplasty: clinical and angiographic follow-up in patients with stable or unstable angina pectoris. Eur Heart J 14:235–239, 1993.
146. Foley JB, Chisholm RJ, Common AA, et al: Aggressive clinical pattern of angina at restenosis following coronary angioplasty in unstable angina. Am Heart J 124:1174–1180, 1992.
147. Chen L, Leatham E, Chester M, et al: Aggressive pattern of angina after successful coronary angioplasty: the role of clinical and angiographic factors. Eur Heart J 16:1085–1091, 1995.
148. Bauters C, Lablanche JM, Van Belle E, et al: Effects of coronary stenting on restenosis and occlusion after angioplasty of the culprit vessel in patients with recent myocardial infarction. Circulation 96:2854–2858, 1997.
149. Ruygrok PN, de Jaegere PT, van Domburg RT, et al: Clinical outcome 10 years after attempted percutaneous transluminal coronary angioplasty in 856 patients. J Am Coll Cardiol 27:1669–1677, 1996.
150. Safian RD, Gelbfish JS, Erny RE, et al: Coronary atherectomy. Clinical, angiographic, and histological findings and observations regarding potential mechanisms. Circulation 82:69–79, 1990.

151. Hinohara T, Rowe MH, Robertson GC, et al: Effect of lesion characteristics on outcome of directional coronary atherectomy. J Am Coll Cardiol 17:1112–1120, 1991.
152. Umans VA, de Feyter PJ, Deckers JW, et al: Acute and long-term outcome of directional coronary atherectomy for stable and unstable angina. Am J Cardiol 74:641–646, 1994.
153. Abdelmeguid AE, Ellis SG, Sapp SK, et al: Directional coronary atherectomy in unstable angina. J Am Coll Cardiol 24:46–54, 1994.
154. Schreiber TL, Kaplan BM, Brown GC: Transluminal extraction atherectomy vs balloon angioplasty in acute ischemic syndromes (TOPIT). J Am Coll Cardiol 29:132A, 1997.
155. Gersh BJ, Kronmal RA, Frye RL, et al: Coronary arteriography and coronary artery bypass surgery: morbidity and mortality in patients ages 65 years or older. A report from the Coronary Artery Surgery Study. Circulation 67:483–491, 1983.
156. de Feyter PJ, Serruys PW, Arnold A, et al: Coronary angioplasty of the unstable angina related vessel in patients with multivessel disease. Eur Heart J 7:460–467, 1986.
157. Simpfendorfer C, Raymond R, Schraider J, et al: Early and long-term results of percutaneous transluminal coronary angioplasty in patients 70 years of age and older with angina pectoris. Am J Cardiol 62:959–961, 1988.
158. Holt GW, Sugrue DD, Bresnahan JF, et al: Results of percutaneous transluminal coronary angioplasty for unstable angina pectoris in patients 70 years of age and older. Am J Cardiol 61:994–997, 1988.
159. Rizo-Patron C, Hamad N, Paulus R, et al: Percutaneous transluminal coronary angioplasty in octogenarians with unstable coronary syndromes. Am J Cardiol 66:857–858, 1990.
160. Reynen K, Kunkel B, Bachmann K, et al: PTCA in elderly patients: acute results and long-term follow-up. Eur Heart J 14:1661–1668, 1993.
161. Eggeling T, Holz W, Osterhues HH, et al: Management of unstable angina in patients over 75 years old. Coron Artery Dis 6:891–896, 1995.
162. Morrison DA, Bies RD, Sacks J: Coronary angioplasty for elderly patients with "high risk" unstable angina: short-term outcomes and long-term survival. J Am Coll Cardiol 29:339–344, 1997.
163. Thompson RC, Holmes DR Jr, Grill DE, et al: Changing outcome of angioplasty in the elderly. J Am Coll Cardiol 27:8–14, 1996.
164. De Gregorio J, Kobayashi Y, Albiero R, et al: Coronary artery stenting in the elderly: short-term outcome and long-term angiographic and clinical follow-up. J Am Coll Cardiol 32:577–583, 1998.
165. Hamm CW, Heeschen C, Goldmann B, et al: Benefit of abciximab in patients with refractory unstable angina in relation to serum troponin T levels. c7E3 Fab Antiplatelet Therapy in Unstable Refractory Angina (CAPTURE) Study Investigators. N Engl J Med 340:1623–1629, 1999.
166. Effects of tissue plasminogen activator and a comparison of early invasive and conservative strategies in unstable angina and non–Q-wave myocardial infarction. Results of the TIMI IIIB Trial. Thrombolysis in Myocardial Ischemia. Circulation 89:1545–1556, 1994.
167. Boden WE, O'Rourke RA, Crawford MH, et al: Outcomes in patients with acute non–Q-wave myocardial infarction randomly assigned to an invasive as compared with a conservative management strategy. Veterans Affairs Non–Q-Wave Infarction Strategies in Hospital (VANQWISH) Trial Investigators. N Engl J Med 338:1785–1792, 1998.
168. FRISC-II Investigators: Invasive compared with non-invasive treatment in unstable coronary artery disease: FRISC-II prospective randomised multicentre study. Lancet 356:708–715, 1999.
169. Coplan NL, Wallach ID: The role of exercise testing for evaluating patients with unstable angina. Am Heart J 124:252–256, 1992.

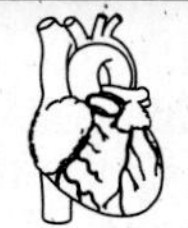

Percutaneous Coronary Intervention for Acute Myocardial Infarction

Richard W. Smalling and Ali Denktas

PATHOPHYSIOLOGY OF MYOCARDIAL INFARCTION AND SALVAGE
PLATEAU OF THROMBOLYTIC EFFICACY
PTCA VERSUS THROMBOLYSIS
STENTING VERSUS PTCA
ANTIPLATELET THERAPY PLUS STENTING
THROMBOLYSIS-FACILITATED PTCA FOR ACUTE MI
PREHOSPITAL THROMBOLYSIS
CARDIOGENIC SHOCK
SUMMARY

Pathophysiology of Myocardial Infarction and Salvage

Defining the optimal treatment for acute myocardial infarction (MI) has been aggressively pursued since the late 1970s in terms of interventional approaches. Falk and associates[1] nicely demonstrated that the pathophysiology of acute MI is associated with rupture of an atherosclerotic plaque with liberation of the lipid and collagen contents of the plaque into the lumen of the vessel. This intensely thrombogenic milieu subsequently leads to intense platelet activation followed by white and then red thrombus formation. This ruptured, or active, plaque remains thrombogenic even after successful thrombolysis for at least 1 month after the index event.[2] Performing interventions in vessels with ruptured plaques or persistent thrombus may be treacherous and is frequently associated with an increased incidence of late adverse events such as reclosure, reinfarction, and increased mortality.[3] These new mechanistic findings probably help explain the adverse effects seen in early trials of percutaneous transluminal coronary angioplasty (PTCA) after coronary thrombolysis.[4–6]

Early work by Reimer and Jennings[7] demonstrated that myocardial necrosis progresses from endocardium to epicardium after abrupt coronary occlusion, and this process occurs at a rapid pace such that most of the thickness of the myocardial wall in the risk or ischemic zone is irreversibly damaged within 3 hours after coronary occlusion. Conversely, if reperfusion can be achieved quickly, the zone of infarction is substantially minimized. The Myocardial Infarction Triage and Intervention Trial (MITI) investigators demonstrated that patients treated with intravenous thrombolysis within 70 minutes after onset of chest pain had a dramatic reduction in 30-day mortality compared with those who were treated somewhat later in their course (1.2 percent versus 8.5 percent)[8] (Fig. 39–1). There is some evidence in animal models that reperfusion relatively late in the course of ischemic injury can result in additional injury, secondary to white blood cell activation and free radical generation, as well as other mechanisms.[9] Various treatment cocktails have been shown to help minimize this additional damage in animals. However, to date, clinical trials with white blood cell antagonists and free radical scavengers have been disappointing.[10] Thus, the most important strategy for treating acute MI patients is early reperfusion followed by stabilization of the active plaque, in an attempt to achieve optimal myocardial salvage and prevent reinfarction and reocclusion.

Plateau of Thrombolytic Efficacy

The Global Utilization of Streptokinase and Tissue Plasminogen Activator for Occluded Coronary Arteries (GUSTO-I) angiographic investigators demonstrated a link

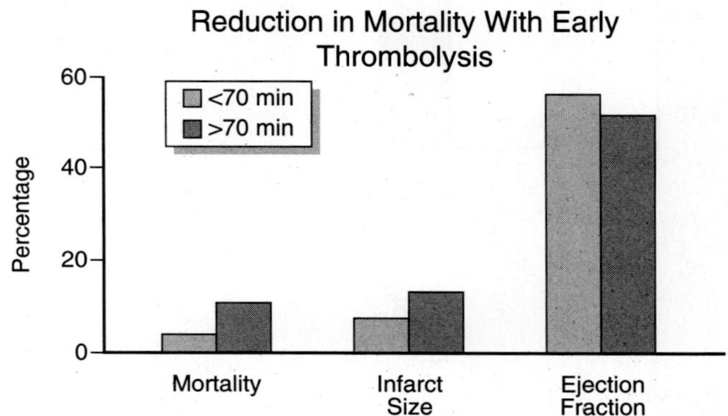

Figure 39–1 Reduction in mortality and infarct size and improvement in ejection fraction seen in patients receiving thrombolytics within 70 minutes after onset of chest pain. (Data from Weaver WD, Cerqueira M, Hallstrom AP, et al: Prehospital-initiated vs hospital-initiated thrombolytic therapy. The Myocardial Infarction Triage and Intervention Trial. JAMA 270:1211–1216, 1993.)

between restoration of normal infarct-related artery blood flow (so-called Thrombolysis in Myocardial Infarction Trial [TIMI] 3 flow) and improved survival after thrombolysis.[11] Intravenous tissue-type plasminogen activator (t-PA) achieved an incidence of TIMI 3 flow in 54 percent of patients at 90 minutes after onset of administration of the agent. In contrast, however, intravenous streptokinase achieved only a 32 percent incidence of TIMI 3 flow at 90 minutes (Fig. 39–2). This decrease in reperfusion efficacy was reflected by an increase in mortality and a decrease in left ventricular function. Many other investigators have demonstrated similar findings in this linkage between restoration of TIMI 3 flow and both left ventricular function and 30-day mortality. The low success in thrombolysis is disappointing and has led to the development of a number of other so-called designer thrombolytic agents.

Reteplase (r-PA) is a deletion mutant modification of the wild type t-PA molecule that was shown to achieve faster and more complete thrombolysis in a large number of patients when studied angiographically.[12, 13] This agent is given by two boluses of 10 MU, 30 minutes apart, and therefore is relatively simple to use. Despite the impressive angiographic results in the RAPID trials (Reteplase Angiographic Phase II International Dose-Finding Trial [RAPID-1] and Reteplase versus Alteplase Patency Investigation during Myocardial Infarction [RAPID-2]), the large megatrial Global Use of Strategies to Open Occluded Arteries (GUSTO-III) demonstrated identical outcomes in terms of mortality and stroke with t-PA and r-PA.[14] Subsequent angiographic analysis of the r-PA and t-PA patient subsets in GUSTO-III suggested that although r-PA was good at opening arteries quickly, if an emergency or rescue procedure intervention was not done relatively early in the patient's course, the infarct artery was perhaps at increased

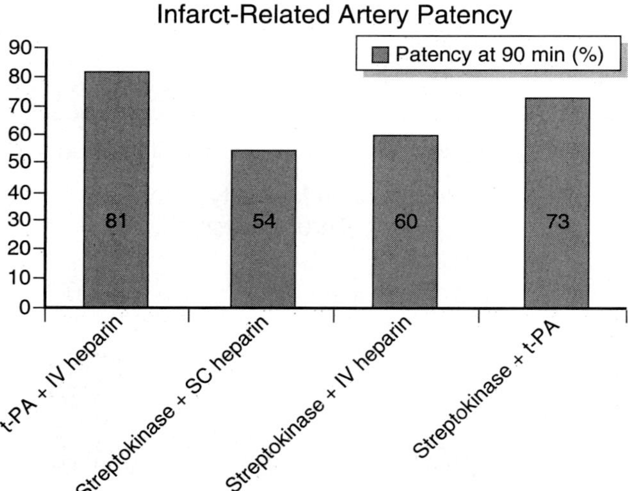

FIGURE 39–2 Infarct-related artery patency in the Global Utilization of Streptokinase and Tissue Plasminogen Activator for Occluded Arteries (GUSTO) I trial. The best patency rates were seen with tissue-type plasminogen activator (t-PA) and intravenous (IV) heparin. SC, subcutaneous. (Data from The GUSTO Angiographic Investigators: The effects of tissue plasminogen activator, streptokinase, or both on coronary-artery patency, ventricular function, and survival after acute myocardial infarction. N Engl J Med 329:1615–1622, 1993.)

risk for reclosure. At 24 hours, there was an equal incidence of TIMI 3 flow in both patient subgroups receiving r-PA and t-PA. Thus, it would appear that the newer designer drugs may be slightly more efficacious in opening arteries, but they may also be associated with a slightly increased risk of early reclosure that apparently negates their early advantage unless emergency angioplasty is performed or perhaps a concomitant glycoprotein IIb/IIIa receptor blocker is used.

Lanoteplase (n-PA) is a deletion and point mutation modification of wild-type t-PA that has a longer half-life and is able to be given in a single bolus. Angiographic analyses of patients treated with this agent compared with t-PA, were also favorable,[15] and a large mortality trial is under way. A new multiple point mutation modified t-PA (TNK-tPA) has also been evaluated. This agent also can be given as a single bolus but seems to be no faster than wild-type t-PA in achieving thrombolysis, and the percentage of patients with restoration of TIMI 3 flow is not different between wild-type t-PA and TNK-tPA.

Therefore, it appears that despite the best efforts of multiple investigators and pharmaceutical corporations, thrombolytics appear to have reached a plateau of efficacy. Although newer hybrid thrombolytics may be developed in the future, it is clear that, at the present time, a combined approach of thrombolysis, antiplatelet therapy, and coronary intervention will most likely be necessary.

PTCA Versus Thrombolysis

The complication of thrombolytic therapy for acute MI that causes the most concern is intracranial hemorrhage. Most physicians who favor PTCA over thrombolysis point out the very, very rare incidence of intracranial bleeding and stroke that is observed in patients treated with direct PTCA for acute MI. With current technologies in guide wires and PTCA balloons, the success in achieving infarct-related artery patency with direct angioplasty for acute MI is very high. Several randomized trials have compared direct angioplasty to thrombolysis, with varying results. The Primary Angioplasty in Myocardial Infarction (PAMI) investigators[16] and the group from Zwolle in the Netherlands have shown an apparent favorable outcome of PTCA for acute MI compared with intravenous thrombolysis[16–18] (Fig. 39–3). In a larger trial, the Global Use of Strategies to Open Occluded Arteries in Acute Coronary Syndromes (GUSTO-IIb) investigators found that there was not an apparent advantage of direct PTCA over thrombolysis, despite initial promising results. At 6 months, GUSTO-IIb subgroups with primary PTCA and thrombolysis had identical outcomes.[19] Some have suggested that once direct PTCA for acute MI is taken out of the larger, higher-volume, PTCA centers into community-oriented hospitals, the results are not as favorable. This concept seems to be mirrored by the outcome of a large registry of patients treated with thrombolysis or PTCA in the Seattle metropolitan area.[20] Weaver and colleagues have performed a meta-analysis of all the previously published trials, comparing thrombolysis with PTCA for acute MI. This analysis of the randomized trials suggests that there may be a slight advantage of PTCA over thrombolysis, but this is not a huge advantage.[21] As

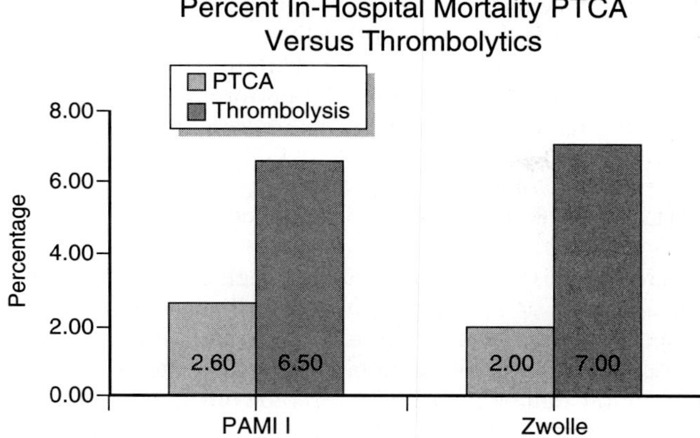

FIGURE 39–3 In-hospital mortality in post–percutaneous transluminal coronary angioplasty (PTCA) versus thrombolysis in acute myocardial infarction. PAMI, Primary Angioplasty in Myocardial Infarction. (Data from Grines CL, Browne KF, Marco J, et al: A comparison of immediate angioplasty with thrombolytic therapy for acute myocardial infarction. The Primary Angioplasty in Myocardial Infarction Study Group. N Engl J Med 328:673–679, 1993, and de Boer MJ, Hoorntje JC, Ottervanger JP, et al: Immediate coronary angioplasty versus intravenous streptokinase in acute myocardial infarction: left ventricular ejection fraction, hospital mortality and reinfarction. J Am Coll Cardiol 23:1004–1008, 1994.)

stated previously, one of the drawbacks behind direct PTCA of a thrombus-laden ruptured plaque is the relatively high incidence of early reclosure and late restenosis.[3] Therefore, other mechanical approaches may be advantageous.

Stenting Versus PTCA

Whereas there are a number of studies under way comparing direct PTCA for acute MI with coronary stenting for MI, the published results to date suggest a clear advantage of coronary stenting. Both Antoniucci and coworkers[22] and the Zwolle investigators[23] found an improved result when patients were treated with coronary stenting rather than PTCA for acute MI (Fig. 39–4). Mechanistically this makes sense, given the fact that coronary stents seem to remold and partially cover the ulcerated plaque and potentially provide a much larger lumen, which should in turn improve blood flow and further reduce the risk of rethrombosis. Obviously, patients treated with coronary stenting would also receive antiplatelet agents, and this may have been part of the reason the outcomes were better in stented patients than in those treated by PTCA alone.

Antiplatelet Therapy Plus Stenting

Recent advances in the understanding of blockade of the glycoprotein IIb/IIIa receptor of the platelet support the concept of a combined assault on the unstable plaque in order to optimize its passivation. Results from the Evaluation of IIb/IIIa Platelet Receptor Antagonist 7E3 in Preventing Ischemic Complications (EPIC) Trial suggested that abciximab (ReoPro) markedly reduced the adverse events associated with interventions in patients with complex coronary lesions. This effect was most marked in patients immediately after MI or with unstable angina, both patient groups that are most likely to have unstable plaques with lesion-associated thrombus.[3, 24] Subsequently, the Evaluation of Platelet IIb/IIIa Inhibitor for Stenting (EPISTENT) Trial confirmed that stenting with abciximab is safer and produces much better outcomes than PTCA alone or stenting alone.[25] Other shorter-acting IIb/IIIa receptor blockers have also demonstrated promising results; however, they have not been evaluated in the setting of acute intervention for MI or unstable angina. Given the prolonged affect of the abciximab, it is unclear how long the infusions of small molecule IIb/IIIa blockers will be needed or whether in fact, a relatively potent oral antiplatelet agent, such as clopidogrel, will be sufficient after initial intravenous therapy with a short-acting IIb/IIIa blocker. Oral IIb/IIIa blockers are also being evaluated, and this is an area that should be closely observed for further developments.

Thrombolysis-Facilitated PTCA for Acute MI

Despite the attractiveness of direct PTCA for acute MI, it is still hampered by the obligate need for mobilization of the catheterization laboratory personnel, as well as an operator skilled in acute coronary interventions. Ross and associates[26] proposed a different strategy that relies on a partial dose of thrombolytic on presentation to the emergency department, followed by rapid mobilization to the catheterization laboratory and emergency angiography with possible intervention as necessary to maintain the vessel with the maximal TIMI flow status. Preliminary results with this strategy have been very encouraging and suggest that a greater percentage of patients will have open arteries at the time of their acute coronary angioplasty, potentially improving the outcome and reducing the amount of infarcted myocardium in at least a substantial minority of

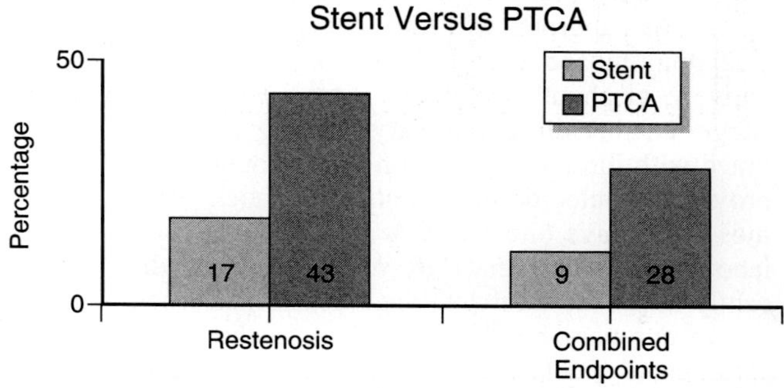

FIGURE 39–4 Improved outcome with stent use. PTCA, percutaneous transluminal coronary angioplasty. (Data from Antoniucci D, Santoro GM, Bolognese L, et al: A clinical trial comparing primary stenting of the infarct-related artery with optimal primary angioplasty for acute myocardial infarction: results from the Florence Randomized Elective Stenting in Acute Coronary Occlusions [FRESCO] trial. J Am Coll Cardiol 31:1234–1239, 1998.)

patients. This concept is being further enhanced by very early administration of a thrombolytic, plus a potent IIb/IIIa blocker, such as abciximab. In both the TIMI 14[27] and the Strategies for Patency Enhancement in the Emergency Department (SPEED) Trial,[28] initial results suggest that TIMI 3 flow rates approaching 80 percent at 60 minutes after initiation of therapy are achievable with this strategy. Emergency angiography might be safely delayed until the following morning if a patient is brought in in the middle of the night, given the relatively high probability that the patient would have an open vessel with the hybrid therapy. It is also possible that coronary interventions will not be necessary as often if patency can be restored and the IIb/IIIa blocker can successfully passivate the plaque over the course of several days. This is another area that will receive intense scrutiny in the coming years.

Prehospital Thrombolysis

A number of trials have suggested that prehospital thrombolysis can improve the number of patients treated within the so-called golden hour of MI (the initial hour) from approximately 20 percent to almost 70 percent. A multicenter trial performed by Weaver and colleagues[8] suggested that prehospital thrombolysis is clearly superior to routine thrombolysis in the emergency department in terms of reducing mortality. It is quite possible that combining prehospital administration of a potent antiplatelet agent with a partial dose of a thrombolytic agent will more promptly restore TIMI 3 flow in the infarct-related artery in the majority of patients. Those with persistent ST elevation or pain on arrival at the emergency department could then be sent directly to cardiac catheterization for angiography and possible rescue stenting. This strategy is an attractive one and should be relatively feasible in terms of implementation.

Cardiogenic Shock

Cardiogenic shock is becoming more rare in the thrombolytic era. Nonetheless, approximately 7 percent of patients with acute MI present with cardiogenic shock. The mortality in this subgroup with thrombolysis alone is uniformly disappointing and not different than patients treated conservatively, at about 80 percent. Antoniucci and associates[29] suggested that direct coronary stenting (presumably combined with intra-aortic balloon pump counterpulsation) improved the outcome in patients with shock compared with those who have direct PTCA alone. Studies in our animal laboratory suggest that left ventricular unloading significantly improves infarct salvage in animals when activated before coronary reperfusion. Thus, in those patients with cardiogenic shock, the intra-aortic balloon pump should be inserted before direct-infarct PTCA and stent to maximize the outcome. Ideally, the intra-aortic balloon pump should be maintained in position for at least 48 hours to unload the ventricle and give it a chance to recover after the acute intervention. It is quite possible that a combination of left ventricular unloading with the intra-aortic balloon pump, together with vigorous antiplatelet inhibition with a IIb/IIIa receptor blocker and coronary stent placement in the infarct-related artery, should produce an optimal result in patients with cardiogenic shock. This complex and aggressive approach, however, must be performed in institutions with full cardiovascular support and capability.[30]

Summary

The aggressive interventional approach for the treatment of acute MI is evolving. Key components, however, now appear to be very early thrombolysis with a partial reduced dose of thrombolytic combined with vigorous antiplatelet inhibition utilizing a IIb/IIIa receptor blocker. If pain and ST-segment elevation are not resolved promptly with this approach, then early angiography and coronary stenting of the infarct-related artery seem to produce the best results. In the presence of cardiogenic shock, left ventricular unloading before coronary stenting will produce the best results in terms of infarct salvage and improved survival. It is quite feasible, with the implementation of a prehospital treatment strategy—a combined approach of prehospital partial thrombolysis and vigorous antiplatelet therapy, followed by immediate coronary angiography and intervention—has the potential to reduce the mortality from acute MI to the 1 to 2 percent range from the current level of 6 to 8 percent. These types of therapy, however, require significant organization and most likely will necessitate designation of acute cardiovascular centers capable of administering such therapy, similar to Level I Trauma Centers, which are certified for taking care of the most critically injured patients.

References

1. Falk E: Plaque rupture with severe pre-existing stenosis precipitating coronary thrombosis. Characteristics of coronary atherosclerotic plaques underlying fatal occlusive thrombi. Br Heart J 50:127–134, 1983.
2. Van Belle E, Lablanche JM, Bauters C, et al: Coronary angioscopic findings in the infarct-related vessel within 1 month of acute myocardial infarction: natural history and the effect of thrombolysis. Circulation 97:26–33, 1998.
3. Feld S, Ganim M, Carell ES, et al: Comparison of angioscopy, intravascular ultrasound imaging and quantitative coronary angiography in predicting clinical outcome after coronary intervention in high risk patients. J Am Coll Cardiol 28:97–105, 1996.
4. The TIMI Study Group: Comparison of invasive and conservative strategies after treatment with intravenous tissue plasminogen activator in acute myocardial infarction. Results of the Thrombolysis in Myocardial Infarction (TIMI) phase II trial. N Engl J Med 320:618–627, 1989.
5. Topol EJ, Califf RM, George BS, et al: A randomized trial of immediate versus delayed elective angioplasty after intravenous tissue plasminogen activator in acute myocardial infarction. N Engl J Med 317:581–588, 1987.
6. Simoons ML, Arnold AE, Betriu A, et al: Thrombolysis with tissue plasminogen activator in acute myocardial infarction: no additional benefit from immediate percutaneous coronary angioplasty. Lancet 1:197–203, 1988.
7. Reimer KA, Jennings RB: The "wavefront phenomenon" of myocardial ischemic cell death. II. Transmural progression of necrosis within the framework of ischemic bed size (myocardium at risk) and collateral flow. Lab Invest 40:633–644, 1979.
8. Weaver WD, Cerqueira M, Hallstrom AP, et al: Prehospital-initiated vs hospital-initiated thrombolytic therapy. The Myocardial Infarction Triage and Intervention Trial. JAMA 270:1211–1216, 1993.
9. Stewart S: Current theories and therapies relating to acute myocardial

infarction and reperfusion injury. Intensive Crit Care Nurs 8:104–112, 1992.

10. Smalling RW: Clinical trials to limit reperfusion injury. Fibrinolysis Proteolysis 11:123–124, 1997.
11. The GUSTO Angiographic Investigators: The effects of tissue plasminogen activator, streptokinase, or both on coronary-artery patency, ventricular function, and survival after acute myocardial infarction. N Engl J Med 329:1615–1622, 1993.
12. Smalling RW, Bode C, Kalbfleisch J, et al: More rapid, complete, and stable coronary thrombolysis with bolus administration of reteplase compared with alteplase infusion in acute myocardial infarction. RAPID Investigators. Circulation 91:2725–2732, 1995.
13. Bode C, Smalling RW, Berg G, et al: Randomized comparison of coronary thrombolysis achieved with double-bolus reteplase (recombinant plasminogen activator) and front-loaded, accelerated alteplase (recombinant tissue plasminogen activator) in patients with acute myocardial infarction. The RAPID II Investigators. Circulation 94:891–898, 1996.
14. The Global Use of Strategies to Open Occluded Coronary Arteries (GUSTO III) Investigators: A comparison of reteplase with alteplase for acute myocardial infarction. N Engl J Med 337:1118–1123, 1997.
15. den Heijer P, Vermeer F, Ambrosioni E, et al: Evaluation of a weight-adjusted single-bolus plasminogen activator in patients with myocardial infarction: a double-blind, randomized angiographic trial of lanoteplase versus alteplase. Circulation 98:2117–2125, 1998.
16. Grines CL, Browne KF, Marco J, et al: A comparison of immediate angioplasty with thrombolytic therapy for acute myocardial infarction. The Primary Angioplasty in Myocardial Infarction Study Group. N Engl J Med 328:673–679, 1993.
17. Zijlstra F, de Boer MJ, Hoorntje JC, et al: A comparison of immediate coronary angioplasty with intravenous streptokinase in acute myocardial infarction. N Engl J Med 328:680–684, 1993.
18. de Boer MJ, Hoorntje JC, Ottervanger JP, et al: Immediate coronary angioplasty versus intravenous streptokinase in acute myocardial infarction: left ventricular ejection fraction, hospital mortality and reinfarction. J Am Coll Cardiol 23:1004–1008, 1994.
19. Armstrong PW, Fu Y, Chang WC, et al: Acute coronary syndromes in the GUSTO-IIb trial: prognostic insights and impact of recurrent ischemia. The GUSTO-IIb Investigators. Circulation 98:1860–1868, 1998.
20. Every NR, Parsons LS, Hlatky M, et al: A comparison of thrombolytic therapy with primary coronary angioplasty for acute myocardial infarction. Myocardial Infarction Triage and Intervention Investigators. N Engl J Med 335:1253–1260, 1996.
21. Weaver WD, Simes RJ, Betriu A, et al: Comparison of primary coronary angioplasty and intravenous thrombolytic therapy for acute myocardial infarction: a quantitative review. JAMA 278:2093–2098, 1997.
22. Antoniucci D, Santoro GM, Bolognese L, et al: A clinical trial comparing primary stenting of the infarct-related artery with optimal primary angioplasty for acute myocardial infarction: results from the Florence Randomized Elective Stenting in Acute Coronary Occlusions (FRESCO) trial. J Am Coll Cardiol 31:1234–1239, 1998.
23. Suryapranata H, van't Hof AW, Hoorntje JC, et al: Randomized comparison of coronary stenting with balloon angioplasty in selected patients with acute myocardial infarction. Circulation 97:2502–2505, 1998.
24. The EPIC Investigation: Use of a monoclonal antibody directed against the platelet glycoprotein IIb/IIIa receptor in high-risk coronary angioplasty. N Engl J Med 330:956–961, 1994.
25. The EPISTENT Investigators. Randomised placebo-controlled and balloon-angioplasty–controlled trial to assess safety of coronary stenting with use of platelet glycoprotein–IIb/IIIa blockade. Evaluation of Platelet IIb/IIIa Inhibitor for Stenting. Lancet 352:87–92, 1998.
26. Draus C, Ross A, Riba A: Is patient care facilitated or impeded by participation in an acute myocardial infarction research trial? J Am Coll Cardiol 33:346A, 1999.
27. Giugliano R, Antman E, McCabe C, et al: Abciximab + tPA improves coronary flow in a wide range of subgroups: results from TIMI 14. Circulation 98:I-560, 1998.
28. Ohman E, Lincoff A-M, Bode C, et al: Enhanced early reperfusion at 60 minutes with low-dose reteplase combined with full dose abciximab in acute myocardial infarction: preliminary results from the GUSTO-4 Pilot (SPEED) dose-ranging trial. Circulation 98:I-504, 1998.
29. Antoniucci D, Valenti R, Santoro GM, et al: Systematic direct angioplasty and stent-supported direct angioplasty therapy for cardiogenic shock complicating acute myocardial infarction: in-hospital and long-term survival. J Am Coll Cardiol 31:294–300, 1998.
30. Smalling RW, Sweeney M, Lachterman B, et al: Transvalvular left ventricular assistance in cardiogenic shock secondary to acute myocardial infarction. Evidence for recovery from near fatal myocardial stunning. J Am Coll Cardiol 23:637–644, 1994.

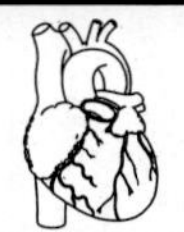

CHAPTER 40

RADIATION THERAPY

Paul S. Teirstein

RADIOTHERAPY IN ANIMAL MODELS OF RESTENOSIS
CLINICAL TRIALS
GAMMA VERSUS BETA RADIATION
Gamma Radiation
Beta Radiation
LONG-TERM CONSEQUENCES OF VASCULAR RADIOTHERAPY
VASCULAR RADIOTHERAPY DELIVERY SYSTEMS CURRENTLY UNDER DEVELOPMENT
Catheter-Based Line Sources
Radioactive-Filled Balloons
Beta-Emitting Radioactive Stents
ONGOING CLINICAL TRIALS
THE FUTURE

The need for repeat procedures owing to restenosis continues to be the Achilles heel of coronary angioplasty.[1] An enormous body of investigative work has been directed at potential restenosis therapies. Literally, scores of pharmaceutical agents have been tested in clinical trials.[2–4] Despite initial promising results in the animal laboratory, most clinical trials to date have been disappointing. Coronary stents are currently the only intervention proved to decrease restenosis. In the Stent Restenosis Study (STRESS) and the Benestent Trial, implantation of a single Palmaz-Schatz coronary stent was associated with a 30 percent reduction in restenosis rates.[5, 6]

Restenosis can be divided into two general concepts. The first, termed *recoil and remodeling,* refers to the mechanical collapse and constriction of the treated vessel. The second, termed *intimal hyperplasia,* refers to the proliferative response to injury and consists largely of smooth muscle cells and matrix formation.[7, 8] Coronary stents provide a luminal scaffolding that virtually eliminates classic recoil and remodeling, resulting in an approximately 30 percent reduction in angiographic and clinical restenosis.[5, 6] The impact of stents on restenosis, however, is purely mechanical.[7, 9] Stent implantation expands the vessel lumen farther than balloon angioplasty alone. This larger lumen creates more space for the still ubiquitous intimal proliferation. Stents do not diminish the cellular response to injury. In fact, the proliferative response, as measured by angiographic compromise in the luminal diameter (late loss) after the procedure, is actually increased by stents. Stents decrease restenosis by simply increasing the artery's capacity to tolerate intimal proliferation. Despite extensive clinical testing, to date no mechanical or pharmaceutical therapy has been shown to inhibit the proliferative component of restenosis.

Radiotherapy is one of the latest of a long line of potential antiproliferative agents to be enthusiastically tested as an adjunct to angioplasty. In over 100 years of clinical experience, radiotherapy has proved highly effective in inhibiting cellular proliferation, in both malignant and benign disease. Examples of benign hyperplastic entities effectively treated with radiotherapy include the exuberant fibroblastic activity of keloid scar formation, heterotopic ossification, desmoid/aggressive fibromatosis, Peyronie's disease, and pterygia.[10–14] In these benign proliferative disorders, doses of 700 to 1000 cGy in one treatment or fractionated treatments after the stimuli have proved effective in inhibiting fibroblastic activity without significantly interfering with the normal healing process.

RADIOTHERAPY IN ANIMAL MODELS OF RESTENOSIS

Wiedermann and coworkers[15, 16] and Waksman and associates[17–19] demonstrated significant reductions in intimal proliferation using radiotherapy in the swine model of restenosis. Wiedermann and coworkers[15, 16] used a swine balloon overstretch injury model of coronary injury to test iridium 192 (^{192}Ir, a gamma emitter), delivering 2000 cGy over a 30- to 45-minute dwell time. Morphometric analysis at 30 days demonstrated a maximal neointimal area of 0.84 ± 0.60 mm^2 in control animals compared with only 0.24 ± 0.13 mm^2 in treated animals (P = .001). At 6-month follow-up, these differences were 1.59 ± 0.78 mm^2 versus 0.46 ± 0.35 mm^2 ($P < .001$).[20]

Waksman and coworkers[17–19] used a similar model to deliver ^{192}Ir at three doses (3500, 7000, or 14,000 cGy). An additional group received 7000 cGy delayed 48 hours after balloon injury. Measurement of the proliferative response to injury was normalized by the ratio of intimal area to medial fracture length, in addition to quantitation of the maximal intimal thickness. At 14-day follow-up, all treated arteries demonstrated significantly decreased neointima formation compared with control arteries. In addition, as indicated in Figure 40–1, a dose-response effect was found. Interestingly, delaying the treatment by 48 hours appeared to augment the responses. Inhibition of proliferation continued to be observed at 6-month follow-up. These investigators found similar results when a beta source (strontium 90/yttrium 90[^{90}Sr/^{90}Y]) at 7000 to 56,000 cGy) was used in the same animal model.[21]

In another trial, Waksman and colleagues[22] provided insight into the target of vascular radiotherapy and its mechanism of action. Balloon injury was performed on

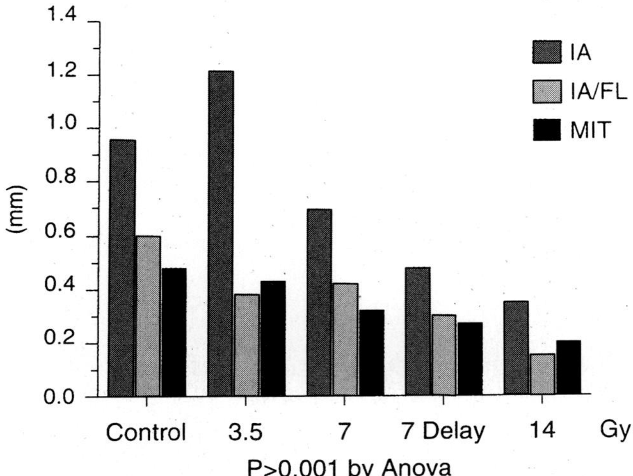

FIGURE 40–1 Effect of four doses of radiation (3.5 Gy, 7 Gy, 7 Gy delayed, and 14 Gy) on indices of neointima formation. IA, intimal area (mm²); IA/FL, intimal to fracture length ratio; MIT, maximal intimal thickness (mm). A significant inhibitory effect of radiation treatment on MIT, IA, and particularly IA/FL was observed. In addition, delay of radiation for 2 days after balloon injury suppressed neointima formation compared with the same dose at the time of injury.

swine coronary arteries, followed immediately by either $^{90}Sr/^{90}Y$ or ^{192}Ir sources designed to deliver 1400 or 2800 cGy at a depth of 2 mm from the source. Animals were sacrificed at 3, 7, or 14 days. Bromodeoxyuridine was administered 24 hours before euthanasia to label proliferating cells. On day 3, cellular proliferation was significantly reduced in both the adventitia and the media of treated vessels compared with those in controls. At 2 weeks after injury, there were fewer alpha-actin–positive myofibroblasts in the adventitia of treated compared with control animals, and morphometric analysis indicated that the vessel perimeter of treated vessels was significantly larger than that in controls. Apoptosis was estimated by terminal transferase deoxyuridine triphosphate (dUTP)–biotin nick-end labeling (TUNEL) at 3 and 7 days after injury. No differences in TUNEL-labeled cells were found between treated and control vessels. These studies suggest that intracoronary radiation primarily inhibits cellular proliferation in both the media and the adventitia and suggests a mechanism other than apoptosis. It also demonstrates a favorable effect on late remodeling, probably by preventing adventitial fibrosis at the injury site.

Numerous other investigators have demonstrated the efficacy of both gamma and beta radiation in various animal models of restenosis.[23–31] Others have successfully inhibited neointimal proliferation using beta-emitting radioactive stents.[32–38] Importantly, these animal models demonstrated efficacy without evidence of necrosis, significant fibrosis, or aneurysm formation.

CLINICAL TRIALS

Clinical trials of intravascular gamma radiation therapy to reduce restenosis are limited, but data are rapidly accumulating. In one very early study, Bottcher and coworkers[39, 40] used ^{192}Ir to treat 13 patients with angioplasty plus stent implantation for femoral artery restenosis. All 13 patients also received 12 Gy radiation immediately after the procedure. Clinical follow-up indicated no recurrent restenosis over 3 to 27 months. Steidl[41] also used ^{192}Ir to treat 24 patients after stent implantation for femoral artery stenosis. Percutaneous radiation therapy with 2.5 Gy per day for 5 days for a total of 12.5 Gy was administered to 11 of his 24 patients. Over a 7-month follow-up period, reocclusion occurred in 2 of 11 patients in the radiation group and 5 of 13 patients in the no-radiation group.

Condado and associates[42] treated 21 patients undergoing coronary angioplasty with ^{192}Ir. Although there was no control group, follow-up results were very encouraging, with a reported late loss index of 0.19 and a restenosis rate of 27.3 percent.

In the Scripps Coronary Radiation to Inhibit Proliferation Post-Stenting (SCRIPPS) trial, patients with previous restenosis and stent implantation were randomized to receive a 0.03-inch ribbon containing either ^{192}Ir sealed sources at its tip or placebo, inactive sources (Best Industries, Springfield, VA). ^{192}Ir dosimetry was calculated using intravascular ultrasound (IVUS) measurements. The radiation oncologist and physicist used information from the IVUS image to determine a dwell time that delivered 800 cGy to the internal elastic membrane farthest from the radiation source, provided that no more than 3000 cGy was delivered to the internal elastic membrane closest to the radiation source. All angiographic and IVUS measurements were performed at an independent core ultrasound laboratory by investigators blinded to procedural information and patient assignment.

Between 3/24/95 and 12/22/95, 55 patients were randomized; 26 were assigned to ^{192}Ir and 29 to placebo. Angiographic indices of restenosis at 6 months were markedly different in treated versus placebo patients (Fig. 40–2). Late luminal loss was significantly lower in the ^{192}Ir group (0.38 ± 1.06 mm versus 1.03 ± 0.97 mm, $P = .009$). Notably, the late lumen loss index (a sensitive measure of a therapy's ability to preserve the postprocedural luminal diameter) was significantly lower in the ^{192}Ir group (0.12 ± 0.63 versus 0.60 ± 0.43, $P = .002$). Using a dichotomous definition, angiographic restenosis ($\geq$50 percent diameter stenosis at follow-up) either within the stent or at the stent border (outside the stent but still covered by the study ribbon) was only 16.7 percent in the ^{192}Ir group compared with 53.6 percent for placebo patients ($P = .025$) (Fig. 40–3). Restenosis limited to the stented segment occurred in only 8.3 percent of the ^{192}Ir group compared with 35.7 percent of placebo patients ($P = .024$).

The angiographic results were supported by the independent IVUS analysis (Fig. 40–4). By IVUS analysis, there was no significant change in stent area or stent volume between the immediate postprocedure and the follow-up period. The decrease in mean lumen area at follow-up was smaller in the ^{192}Ir group (0.7 ± 1.0 mm^2 versus 2.2 ± 1.8 mm^2, $P = .003$), as was the increase in area of tissue growth within the stent struts (0.7 ± 0.9 mm^2 versus 2.2 ± 1.8 mm^2, $P = .003$). The decrease in lumen volume was also smaller in the ^{192}Ir group (16.4 ± 24.0 mm^3 versus 44.3 ± 34.6 mm^3, $P = .008$), as was the increase

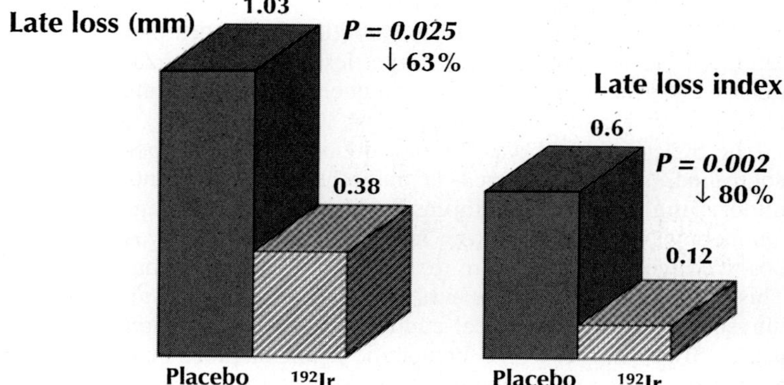

FIGURE 40–2 Comparison of late luminal loss and late loss index in placebo versus ^{192}Ir patients. Late loss was reduced by 63 percent, whereas the late loss index was reduced by 80 percent.

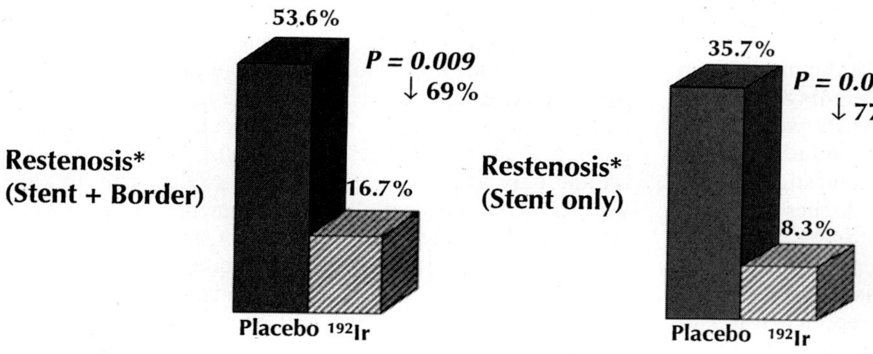

FIGURE 40–3 Comparison of a dichotomous definition of angiographic restenosis (≥50 percent diameter stenosis) between placebo and ^{192}Ir patients. Restenosis is reduced by 69 percent when both the stent and the stent border are included in the analysis. Restenosis is reduced by 77% when only the stented region is measured.

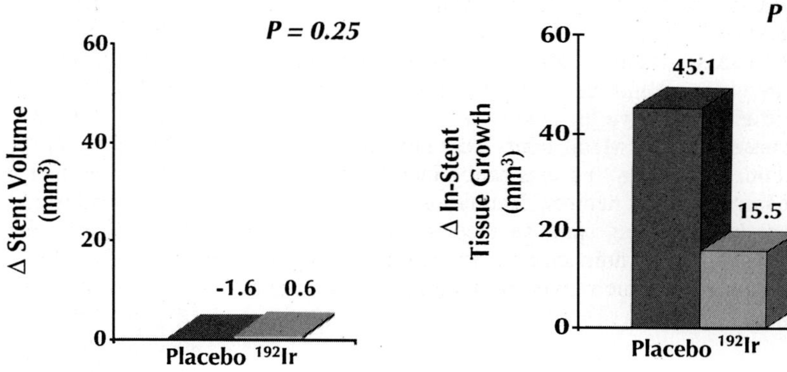

FIGURE 40–4 Intravascular ultrasound measurement of change in mean stent volume and in the volume of tissue growth over a 6-month period in placebo versus ^{192}Ir patients. The stent volume did not change in either placebo or treated patients. However, placebo patients demonstrated nearly three times the volume of tissue growth within stent struts at the follow-up examination.

in volume of tissue growth within stent struts (15.5 ± 22.7 mm^3 versus 45.1 ± 39.4 mm^3, P = .0091).

Clinical follow-up was obtained for all patients at the 2-year point. The difference in angiographic restenosis rates was supported by a reduction in target lesion revascularization in the ^{192}Ir group (11.5 percent versus 44.8 percent, P = .008). Composite clinical events (death, myocardial infarction, stent thrombosis, or target lesion revascularization) were also significantly less frequent in ^{192}Ir patients (15.4 percent versus 48.3 percent, P = .011).

The SCRIPPS Trial was the first double-blind, placebo-controlled, randomized trial of radiotherapy in patients undergoing coronary angioplasty. Although the patient numbers were small, a striking reduction in restenosis was observed when patients were treated with ^{192}Ir γ radiation. This reduction in restenosis was similar for angiographic, ultrasonographic, and clinical endpoints. Thus, γ radiation using ^{192}Ir is the very first therapeutic agent of more than 50 clinically tested to demonstrate an impact on neointima formation after angioplasty.[43]

β Emitters differ from the γ energy used in the trials previously discussed in that β energy is less penetrating and easily shielded, making these devices somewhat easier to handle in the catheterization laboratory environment. However, questions have been raised concerning the ability of a β emitter to provide therapeutic radiation doses to the required depth. The results to date are conflicting.[44] Verin and colleagues[45] treated 15 patients undergoing coronary angioplasty with ^{90}Y, a β emitter. The results were disappointing due to a loss index of 50 percent and a restenosis rate of 40 percent at 6 months. These investigators are currently pursuing subsequent trials using higher-dose prescriptions. King and coworkers[46] used ^{90}Sr/^{90}Y, also a β emitter, to treat 21 patients undergoing coronary angioplasty in the Beta Energy Restenosis Trial (BERT) I. Although there was no control group, the reported 6-month restenosis rate of 17 percent and loss index of 0.05 percent were very encouraging. In the expanded BERT II study,[47] 82 patients were treated with the same radiation delivery system. At 6-month follow-up, the restenosis rate was 17 percent and the late loss index was only 9 percent[47] (Novoste newswire, August 17, 1998). These favorable results have inspired an 1100-patient, multicenter, randomized trial (the Beta-Cath Trial) to definitively test this system's safety and efficacy.

Clearly, a dose-finding study with β radiotherapy is required, as well as continued studies using other emitters. One potentially effective β emitter is a radioactive, β-emitting coronary stent. Metal stents have been made radioactive by ion-implanting ^{31}P beneath the metal surface and then exposing them to neutron irradiation to convert ^{31}P into ^{32}P[48] or by activating stainless steel stents in a cyclotron.[34] The β-emitting radioactive stent is applied directly to the vessel wall, which may provide more favorable dosimetry.

Gamma Versus Beta Radiation

A fundamental component of any radiation delivery system is the radioisotope itself. Each isotope has important physical characteristics, such as energy and half-life. Perhaps the most important differentiating characteristics of a particular radiation source is its characterization as a γ or β energy source.[49] The differences between γ and β sources underlie one of the current "hot debates" in the vascular radiotherapy field.

Radiation probably inhibits the cellular proliferative response to injury after angioplasty by creating a double-stranded break in the cell's DNA, preventing cell division.[50] It is important to realize that our current understanding of the mechanism of action of the radiotherapy on the cell cycle is that once radiation energy is delivered to a dividing cell, its effects are independent of the source used. That is, cell division will be equally inhibited by γ and β energy. As long as the required energy is brought to the intended target, either γ or β radiation will probably be equally effective.

Gamma Radiation

γ Sources are photons and have several advantages when applied to vascular diseases. Early data from randomized trials indicate that γ sources will be effective, particularly for the treatment of in-stent restenosis. Data from the SCRIPPS Trial, a randomized, double-blind, placebo-controlled study, demonstrated a reduction in restenosis rates from 54 percent in the placebo group to 17 percent in patients treated with γ radiation (^{192}Ir).[51, 52] Currently, these are the only available controlled data. Of course, by 2000 we will have substantially more data and will be better able to evaluate the effectiveness of γ sources, particularly as they compare with β sources. γ Sources penetrate human tissues deeply. This makes γ energy ideal for treating large vessels, especially if a line source is used, and especially if this source is not centered. Finally, γ sources are not shielded by stents. This makes them ideal for the treatment of in-stent restenosis.

There are, however, numerous disadvantages to using γ sources. Photons are not blocked by the "usual" lead shields.[53] A heavy, 1-inch-thick lead shield is required. This is usually in the form of a very cumbersome lead device attached to rollers that allow it to be wheeled into the catheterization laboratory.[54] Owing to the presence of deeply penetrating ionizing radiation, when high-energy γ radiation is used in the catheterization laboratory, the procedure room must be cleared of all "nonessential" personnel. The patient is observed from the control room, which is protected by thick lead shielding. Also, the patient receives more radiation from a γ radiation procedure than from a β procedure. The radiation oncologist, who delivers the actual radiation sources, also receives additional radiation exposure. This problem of radiation exposure in the catheterization laboratory environment limits the maximal specific activity of the radiation sources. If the sources are of very high activity, the exposure to health care personnel in the control room will be unacceptably high. To circumvent this problem, lower specific activity sources must be used. This requires a longer dwell time (8 to 20 minutes) to achieve therapeutic doses than that required for most β sources (only 3 to 10 minutes).

Beta Radiation

β Sources are electrons that penetrate only several millimeters into the vessel wall.[55, 56] β Energy is easily shielded, even by thick plastics. The fact that exposure from β sources is limited allows the specific activity to be much higher than that of γ sources. This translates into very short dwell times, adding only 3 to 10 minutes to the angioplasty procedure. Radiation safety concerns surrounding the use of β sources are vastly reduced compared with those of γ radiation. Heath care personnel can ramain in the cardiac catheterization laboratory, and additional exposure to the patient and radiation oncologist is negligible.

The disadvantages of β energy for the treatment of vascular disease derive, for the most part, from our lack of data concerning its efficacy. Although results from the early BERT trials are encouraging,[46] at the present time, no results are available from randomized, controlled clinical trials. Such trials are currently in progress. Whereas the fact that β energy can be easily shielded and does not penetrate far is an advantage with respect to radiation safety, it is a potential disadvantage with respect to efficacy. β Energy delivered as a line source will probably not be able to treat large diameter vessels (>4 mm) or will probably require centering devices. Also, β energy has been shown to be partially shielded by metallic stents. Currently, it is not known whether this shielding effect will be clinically important, but it is possible that β radiation may not be an effective treatment for in-stent restenosis.

The debate concerning γ versus β energy will continue until adequate clinical data is available. Whereas β energy is clearly easier to work with in the clinical environment, γ radiation has now been routinely used in numerous catheterization laboratories for over 3 year without significant problems. Issues such as health care personnel exiting the catheterization room while the patient receives treatment have not been a practical problem. Patients have received excellent care, and if a nurse or physician is required to enter the catheterization laboratry urgently, the γ source can be withdrawn into a shielded container in under 20 seconds, allowing entry by all necessary personnel. Furthermore, the additional exposure to health care personnel by the use of γ radiation has been quite minimal. Cardiologists receive little or no additional exposure during γ radiation procedures because after delivering the afterloading catheter, they exit the room and receive no further radiation. Although the radiation oncologist receives extra radiation from γ radiotherapy, this exposure is minimal and relatively small compared with the exposure received by radiation oncologist during the other kinds of brachytherapy treatment routinely performed, such as the treatment of prostate, pelvic, and head and neck malignancies.

In the end, the debate between β and γ vascular radiotherapy will be won by the outcome of a relative efficacy analysis. β Energy is unquestionably easier to use. However, γ energy is not impractical, and if β sources prove to be ineffective, the medical community will embrace γ energy. Yet, if β energy is as effective or almost as effective, β radiation will prevail.

Long-Term Consequences of Vascular Radiotherapy

Although early safety and efficacy have been demonstrated in numerous animal studies and limited human trials, the long-term efficacy and, most importantly, safety of this technique have been questioned. The possibility of late untoward consequences such as aneurysm formation, perforation, or accelerated vascular disease is a significant concern.[18, 20] In addition, it is not known whether the beneficial effects of radiation therapy will be durable or whether radiation will only delay and not permanently reduce restenosis. With the exposure of increasing numbers of patients to intravascular radiation, it is essential to obtain long-term clinical follow-up.

At present, long-term follow-up of patients enrolled in clinical trials using vascular radiotherapy is very limited. Two-year angiographic follow-up after intracoronary γ radiation was reported by Condado and associates.[57] The restenosis rate was low at 28 percent, but this study lacked a control group for comparison. Several coronary aneurysms and one definite pseudoaneurysm were reported in the Condado and associates series, possibly because the vessels were potentially exposed to very high radiation doses (up to 9200 cGy) compared with the lower 800 to 5000 cGy used in most other series. In another report, long-term follow-up documented high patency rates after exposing femoropopliteal arteries undergoing angioplasty to intravascular γ radiation.[39–41]

Long-term adverse events after radiation therapy for nonvascular indications are well documented. Potential complications include accelerated vascular disease, coronary perforation (including pseudoaneurysm), and late malignancy. Accelerated vascular disease has been reported in patients irradiated for treatment of Hodgkin's disease followed beyond 9 years.[58] The morphology of radiation-induced coronary artery disease appears to involve smaller arteries (<0.5 mm) and is similar to that of spontaneous coronary artery disease.[59] Larger arteries (>0.5 mm) appear more resistant to radiation.[60–63] In intravascular brachytherapy, the volume of irradiation is small, with significant radial dose fall-off from the lumen to the adventitia. Additionally, only a single vessel is radiated over a limited longitudinal segment, with little exposure to the surrounding normal tissue. Therefore, the risk of radiation-induced fibrosis or atherosclerosis is believed to be much lower than that occurring with the treatment of Hodgkin's disease, in which a much larger volume of tissue is irradiated. High doses of radiation could also lead to arterial rupture.[64, 65] Perforation or pseudoaneurysm of coronary arteries would likely be detected in the first few months after treatment. In some studies, such as the SCRIPPS Trial, the careful avoidance of greater than 3000 cGy to any one part of the luminal surface, with much lower doses delivered to the adventitia layers, probably reduces the risk of vessel perforation.

Secondary malignancies after radiation range from leukemia to solid tumors. Hematologic malignancies are usually seen within the first 3 to 7 years in cancer patients who receive combination chemotherapy and are often immunocompromised.[66–69] Secondary solid tumors have a longer latent period of 7 to 10 years. These are occasionally soft tissue sarcomas but are more often epithelial tumors of irradiated organs. Again, it is emphasized that the volume of radiation in intravascular brachytherapy is extremely small, making secondary malignancy unlikely. The application of radiation therapy in modest doses in other benign proliferative disorders (i.e., heterotopic ossification and keloid scars) appears to be safe, with no apparent long-term complications.

Vascular Radiotherapy Delivery Systems Currently Under Development

Brachytherapy has been routinely used by radiation therapists for several decades. The concept of brachytherapy involves bringing the radioisotope in close proximity to the target, reducing the source to target distance (*brachy* from the Greek *brackus* meaning short). This minimizes undesired tissue exposure compared with treatment with external-beam radiation. A tremendous amount of creativity and innovation has been brought to bear on the development of intravascular radiation delivery systems. Whereas many traditional radiotherapy systems have been adapted for vascular use, a wide array of new concepts, specifically invented for coronary artery treatment, are currently under development. This new technology encompasses line sources, liquid sources, and gas and membrane sources, as well as stent-based delivery systems.

Catheter-Based Line Sources

Line sources are commonly employed to deliver radiation to a variety of benign and malignant disorders. These traditionally used devices can be easily adapted for the treatment of vascular disease. Radioactive sources such as ^{192}Ir, ^{32}P, ^{90}Sr, and ^{90}Sr/^{90}Y can be encapsulated and manufactured in 0.014- to 0.040-inch diameters that can easily pass through intracoronary catheters. Typically, after dilatation or stenting of the target lesion, a 3 to 5 French catheter containing a blind-end source delivery lumen is advanced over a guide wire and positioned across the target lesion. A wire (typically composed of nylon or nitinol) containing radioactive sources at its distal tip is then loaded into the source lumen of the catheter and advanced distally until the radioactive sources span the target lesion (Fig. 40–5). This process, called *afterloading,* can be accomplished either manually, by the radiation oncologist advancing the source wire by hand (Fig. 40–6),[51, 52] or automatically, by a motor-driven unit.[70–72] Remote automatic afterloaders can be programmed to advance and then withdraw the source wire at specific time intervals without the need for physician handling, thus reducing exposure to personnel (Fig. 40–7). One variation of the line source concept is a hydraulic delivery system (Novoste, Atlanta, GA), in which encapsulated sources are injected into a blind-end catheter by a syringe or automated pumping system[46] (Fig. 40–8).

Radiation delivery via a line source with a simple catheter can result in a source placed eccentrically within the vessel lumen. Assuming the target for radiotherapy is the adventitial border, a noncentered source will deliver a high radiation dose to the adventitia closest to the catheter and a low radiation dose to the adventitia farthest from the catheter. This dose heterogeneity (maximal/minimal dose) is almost 3:1 for most noncentered systems.[73] Alternatively, catheter centering systems, using either a segmented balloon (Fig. 40–9)[45] (Schneider, Minneapolis, MN) or a helical balloon (Fig. 40–10)[24, 28] that also allows perfusion while inflated (Guident, Santa Clara, CA), can reduce dose heterogeneity by maintaining the source in the center of the lumen. Although lumen centering does not center the source with respect to the adventitia, in noneccentric lesions lumen centering can lower dose heterogeneity from about a 3:1 to about a 2.5:1 ratio.[73]

Radioactive-Filled Balloons

One method of centering a radioactive source is to use a radioactive liquid to inflate a balloon catheter.[74, 75] Isotopes such as rhenium 188 and rhenium 189 provide a homogeneous dose distribution surrounding an inflated balloon.[53] The liquid-filled balloon provides excellent lumen centering of the device. Also, by bringing the radioisotope to the outer edge of the balloon, penetration of a β emitter deeper into the vessel wall may be achieved. Of course, a theoretical liability of a radioactive-filled balloon system is the very low but finite possibility of balloon or catheter leakage resulting in contamination of the catheterization laboratory or, worse, exposure to a patient's blood stream. A spill of ^{188}Re (half-life 20 hours) in the catheterization laboratory would require isolating the room for approximately 5 half-

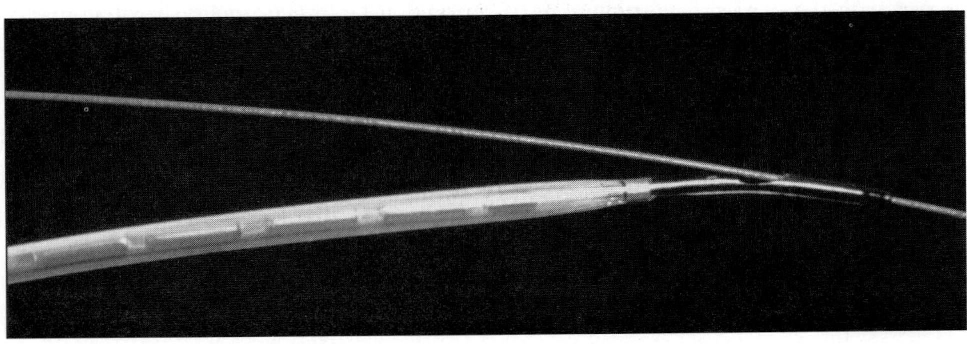

FIGURE 40–5 Hand-delivered distal monorail system. (Courtesy of Cordis, Miami, FL.)

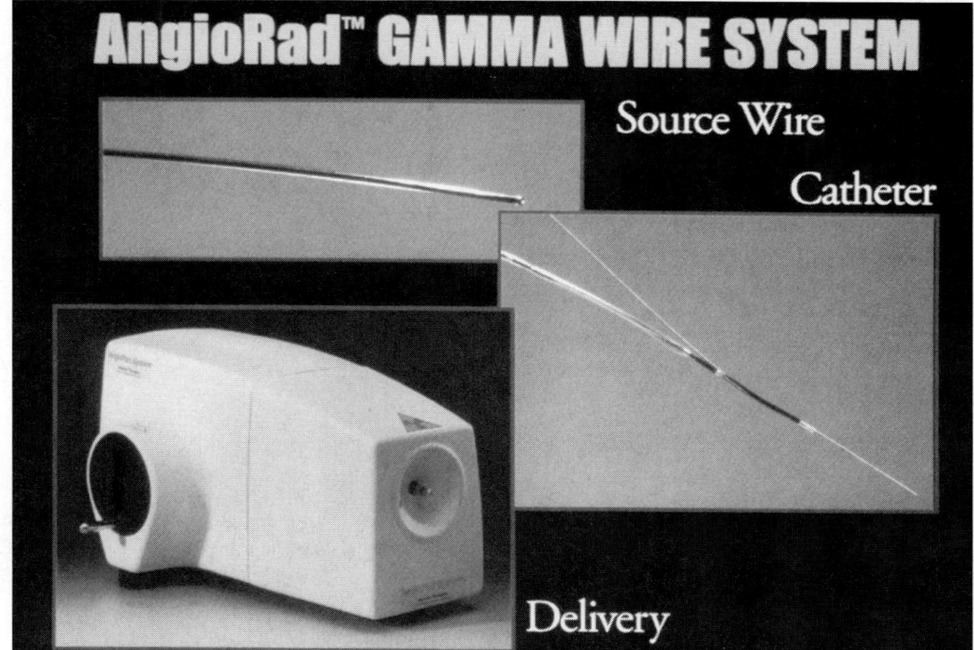

FIGURE 40–6 Manual, hand-crank, delivery device. The manual crank allows advancement and retraction of the source wire. This device is not available in the United States. (Courtesy of Vascular Therapies, Norwalk, CT. Currently being acquired by Interventional Therapies LLC.)

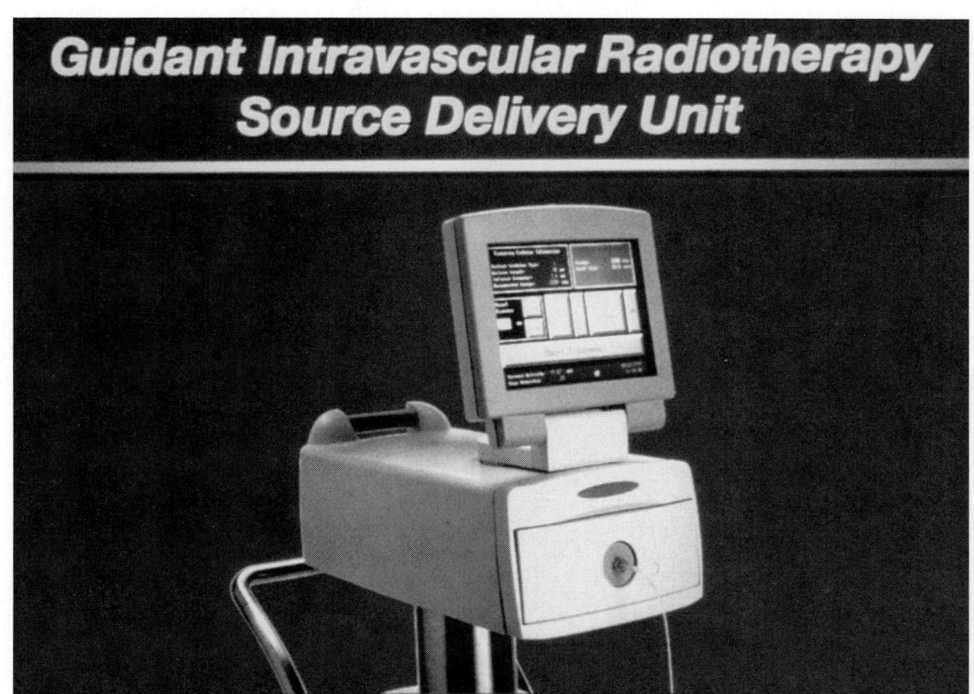

FIGURE 40–7 Remote afterloader is programmed to automatically deliver a radioactive line source for a specified dwell time. Limited by U.S. law to investigational use. (Courtesy of Guidant, Houston, TX.)

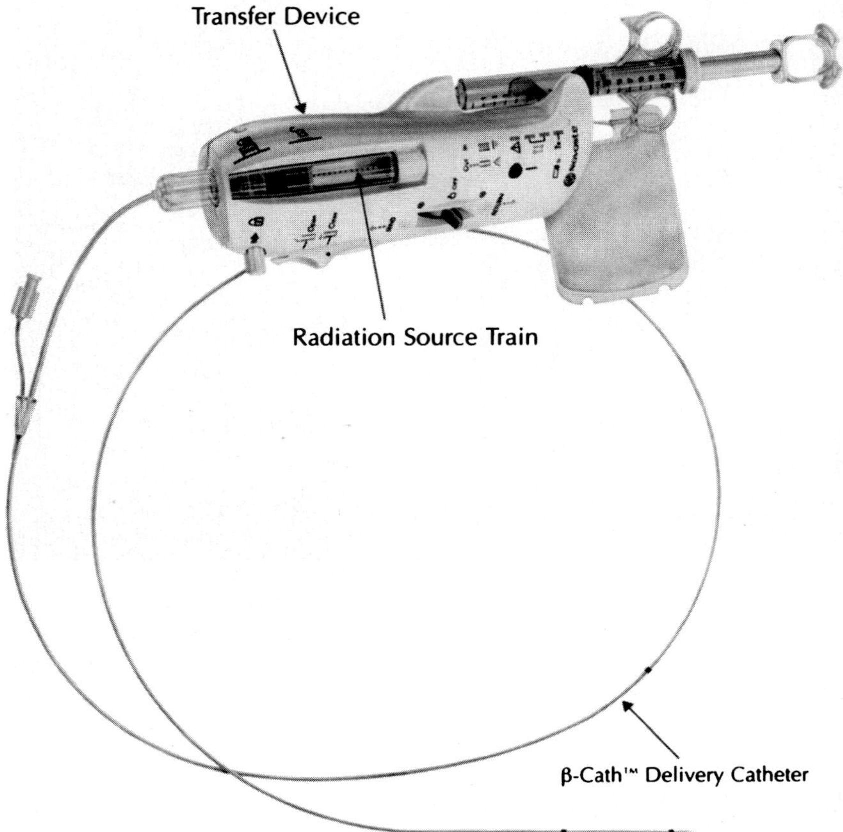

FIGURE 40–8 The Beta-Cath system delivers a "train" of cylindrical, sealed strontium 90 sources via a hydraulic delivery system. Not commercially available. (Courtesy of Novoste, Atlanta, GA.)

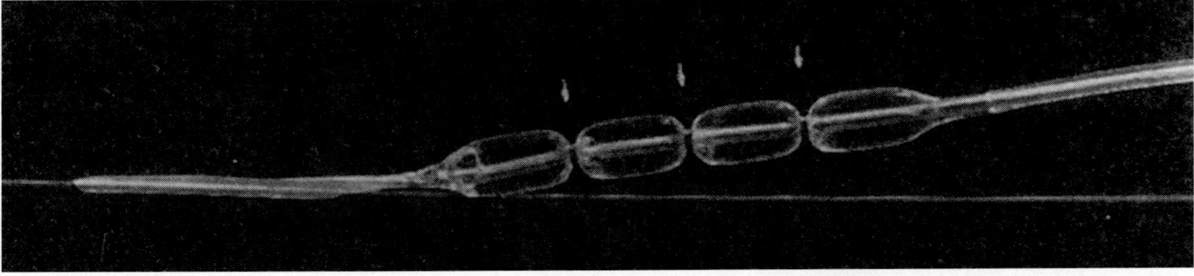

FIGURE 40–9 Segmented balloon centering catheter. Distal tip "monorail" design reduces profile. (Courtesy of Schneider, Minneapolis, MN.)

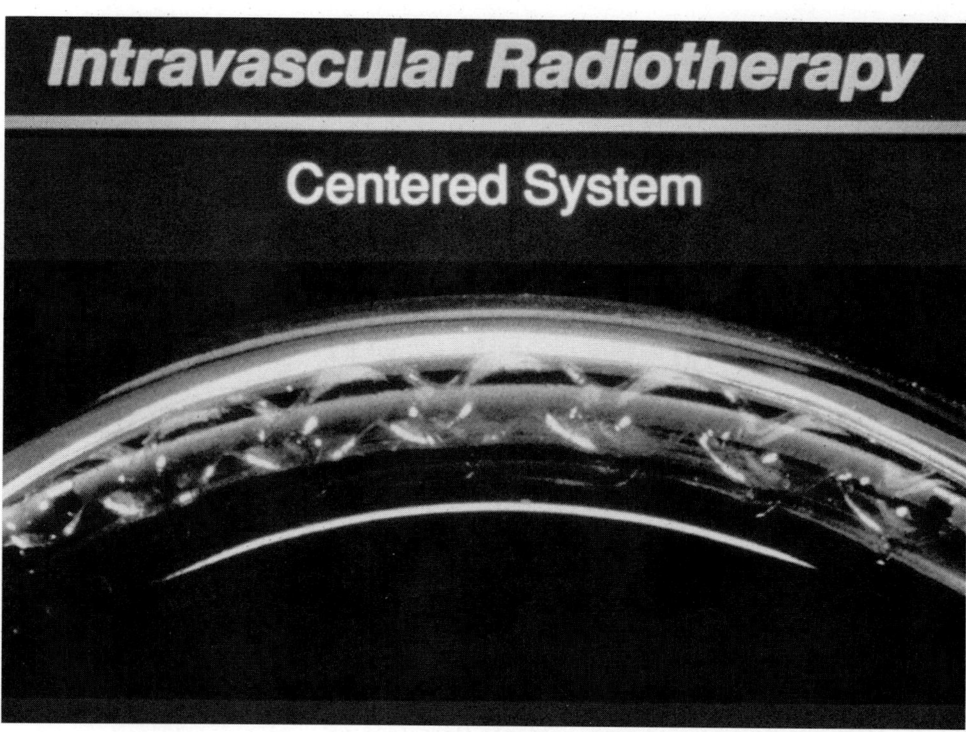

FIGURE 40–10 A spiral balloon catheter centering system. The source lumen is centered within the vessel lumen while the helical balloon allows perfusion. Limited by U.S. law to investigational use. (Courtesy of Guidant, Houston, TX.)

lives (i.e., about 3 days). Leakage of a radioactive liquid–filled balloon into a patient's blood stream can be managed by biochemically coupling the radioactive liquid to a substance that inhibits bone uptake and promotes renal excretion (i.e., mercaptoacetylglycylglyclglycine [MAG_3]. Although balloon breakage would still be undesirable, its consequences could be minimized with intravenous hydration, diuretics, and placement of an in-dwelling urethral catheter with a collection bag.

Another approach to a radioactive-filled balloon is to use a radioactive gas. Xenon 133, routinely used for ventilation scans, is a combination β and γ emitter.[76] Homogeneous dosimetry, similar to a liquid-filled balloon system, can be achieved with a gas-filled balloon system. Leakage of ^{133}Xe would likely be a less significant clinical and environmental problem because this radioactive gas would rapidly disperse into the atmosphere, resulting in very low local concentrations.

Beta-Emitting Radioactive Stents

Permanent implantation of a β-emitting radioactive stent has significant practical advantages over other radiation delivery systems. Currently, the majority of patients undergoing percutaneous coronary interventions receive coronary stents. Coupling the radiation delivery to the stent itself makes radiation delivery more efficient, obviating the need for a separate radiation delivery step. Several radioactive stent systems have been developed including ion implantation of ^{32}P[35, 77, 78] and activation of a stainless steel stent in a cyclotron, producing a spectrum of radioisotopes.[32–34, 37, 38, 79] Most clinical investigation has been undertaken with the ^{32}P β-emitting stent. Stents ion-implanted with ^{32}P containing a specific activity ranging from 0.5 to 20 μCi have a 14.3-day half-life, thereby effectively exposing the vessel to β radiation for about 45 days (approximately 3 half-lives). These stents are of extremely low activity and can be handled with the aid of a simple 1-cm-thick acrylic shield (Fig. 40–11). Establishing safe and effective dosimetry presents a technical challenge to radioactive stent design. As stent struts expand, they separate, increasing the intrastrut distance and creating gaps in dose delivery. These relative cold spots cannot be avoided. In contradistinction, when stent struts come together, the dose is amplified, creating a relative "hot" spot. Finding the appropriate dose requires establishing a therapeutic window broad enough to achieve effective inhibition of proliferation in the region where the stent struts are widely spread, without delivering a toxic dose in the region where stent struts come together.

ONGOING CLINICAL TRIALS

Numerous single and multicenter trials testing a variety of radiation delivery devices and isotopes for a wide spectrum of clinical indications are currently ongoing. The Beta-Cath (Novoste, Atlanta, GA) is testing a hydraulically delivered ^{90}Sr (β) line source in patients with de novo and restenotic lesions. The GAMMA-ONE and Washington Radiation for In-Stent Restenosis (WRIST) Trials (Cordis/Best, Miami, FL) are both testing a manually delivered ^{192}Ir (γ) line source in patients with in-stent restenosis. The Angiorad Radiation Technology for In-Stent restenosis Trial In native Coronaries (ARTISTIC) Trial (Vascular Therapies, Norwalk, CT) is testing a 0.014-inch ^{192}Ir (γ) line source manually delivered using a hand-crank system in patients with in-stent restenosis. The Angiorad Radiation for Restenosis (ARREST) Trial uses the same system for

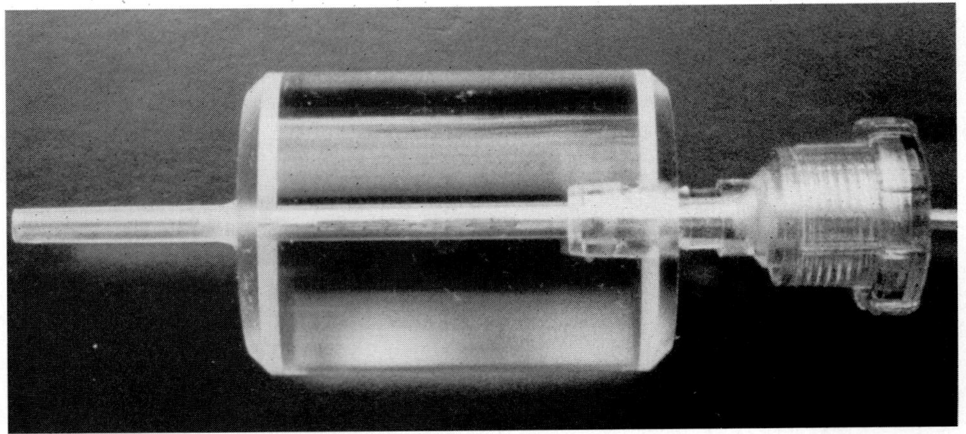

FIGURE 40–11 ^{32}P radioactive stent mounted on a stent delivery system and covered with a protective lucite shield to prevent radiation exposure to the operator. (Courtesy of Isostent, Belmont, CA.)

de novo native coronary stenoses. The Proliferation Reduction with Vascular Energy Trial (PREVENT) (Guidant/NeoCardiology, Houston, TX) is testing a ^{32}P (β) line source delivered via an automatic afterloader connected to a catheter incorporating a helical centering balloon in both de novo and restenotic native lesions. The INHIBIT Trial (Guidant/NeoCardiology, Houston, TX) uses the same system in patients with de novo native coronary stenoses. The RADIANT Trial (Vascular Therapies, Menlo Park, CA) is testing a ^{188}Re liquid-filled balloon (β) in native coronaries with in-stent restenosis.[74] The European Multicenter dose-finding study (Schneider, Europe AG) is testing a ^{90}Y β-emitting line source in a segmented centering balloon system. The Isostent for Restenosis Intervention Study Isostents (IRIS) feasibility trial (Isostent, San Carlos, CA) is testing escalating doses of a ^{32}P radioactive stent for patients with de novo native coronary stenoses.[80]

Most of these clinical studies benefit from a true double-blind randomized trial design. All include clinical as well as 6- to 9-month follow-up angiographic endpoints. When these trials reach completion (by 2000), data will be available for over 2000 randomized patients undergoing treatment with a variety of radiation delivery devices for a wide spectrum of clinical indications.

THE FUTURE

The work required to develop and refine clinically useful vascular radiotherapy systems is daunting. There are many unanswered questions. What will be the most practical catheter-based radiation system? Will β radiation penetrate deep enough into the diseased vessel wall to provide clinical efficacy? Will radioactive stents be effective or will they be limited by dose heterogeneity or other complications. If radiation is proved to have long-lasting efficacy, should it be used for all patients undergoing angioplasty or confined only to patients with restenosis or other subgroups? Will radiation therapy be so effective it replaces coronary stents or will it be used as an adjunct to a stenting strategy? These questions lay the foundation for the next decade of investigation.

ACKNOWLEDGMENT

The author is indebted to his colleagues in the Scripps Clinic Radiation Oncology Department, especially Vincent Massullo, M.D., Shirish Jani, M.D., and Prabhakar Tripuraneni, M.D., as well as to Krishnan Suthanthiran of Best Industries, Inc.

REFERENCES

1. Holmes DR Jr, Vliestra RE, Smith HC, et al: Restenosis after percutaneous transluminal coronary angioplasty (PTCA): a report from the PTCA Registry of the National Heart, Lung and Blood Institute. Am J Cardiol 53(suppl):77C–81C, 1984.
2. Popma JJ, Califf RM, Topol EJ: Clinical trials of restenosis after coronary angioplasty. Circulation 84:1426–1436, 1991.
3. Serruys PW, Klein W, Rutsch W, et al: PARK: the Post Angioplasty Restenosis Ketanserin Trial. J Am Coll Cardiol 21:322A, 1993.
4. Faxon D, Sprio T, Minor S, et al: Enoxaparin, a low molecular weight heparin, in the prevention of restenosis after angioplasty: results of a double-blind randomized trial. J Am Coll Cardiol 19:258A, 1992.
5. Serruys PW, de Jaegere P, Kiemeneij F, et al for the Benestent Study Group. A comparison of balloon-expandable stent implantation with balloon angioplasty in patients with coronary artery disease. N Engl J Med 331:489–495, 1994.
6. Fischman DL, Leon MB, Baim DS, et al for the Stent Restenosis Study Investigators: A randomized comparison of coronary stent placement and balloon angioplasty in the treatment of coronary artery disease. N Engl J Med 331:496–501, 1994.
7. Kuntz RE, Gibson CM, Nobuyoshi M, Baim DS: Generalized model of restenosis after conventional balloon angioplasty, stenting and directional atherectomy. J Am Coll Cardiol 21:15–25, 1993.
8. Mintz GS, Popma JJ, Pichard AD, et al: Arterial remodeling after coronary angioplasty. A serial intravascular ultrasound study. Circulation 94:35–43, 1996.
9. Kuntz RE, Safian RD, Levin MJ, et al: Novel approach to the analysis of restenosis after the use of three new coronary devices. J Am Coll Cardiol 19:1493–1499, 1992.
10. Reitamo JJ: The desmoid tumor IV. Choice of treatment results and complications. Arch Surg 118:1318–1322, 1983.
11. MacLennan I, Keys HM, Evarts CM, Rubin P: Usefulness of postoperative hip irradiation in the prevention of heterotopic bone formation in a high risk group of patients. Int J Radiat Oncol Biol Phys 10:49–53, 1984.
12. Enhamre A, Hammar H: Treatment of keloids with excision and postoperative x-ray irradiation. Dermatologica 167:90–93, 1983.
13. Alth G, Koren H, Gasser G, Edler R: On the therapy of indurated penis plastica by means of radium moulages. Strahlentherapie 161:30–34, 1985.
14. Bahrassa F, Datta R: Postoperative beta radiation treatment of pterygium. Int J Radiat Oncol Biol Phys 9:679–684, 1983.
15. Wiedermann JG, Marboe C, Amols H, et al: Intracoronary irradiation markedly reduces restenosis after balloon angioplasty in a porcine model. J Am Coll Cardiol 23:1491–1498, 1994.
16. Wiedermann J, Leavy J, Amols H: Intracoronary irradiation acutely impairs endothelial and smooth muscle function as assessed by intravascluar ultrasound [abstract]. Circulation 86(suppl 1):1–88, 1992.
17. Waksman R, Robinson K, Crocker I, et al: Intracoronary irradiation after angioplasty reduces restenosis in a swine model. J Am Coll Cardiol 23:3, 1998.

18. Waksman R, Robinson KA, Crocker IR, et al: Endovascular low-dose irradiation inhibits neointima formation after coronary artery balloon injury in swine. A possible role for radiation therapy in restenosis prevention. Circulation 91:1533–1539, 1995.
19. Waksman R, Robinson KA, Crocker IR, et al: Intracoronary radiation before stent implantation inhibits neointima formation in stented porcine coronary arteries. Circulation 92:1383–1386, 1995.
20. Wiedermann JG, Marboe C, Amols H, et al: Intracoronary irradiation markedly reduces neointimal proliferation after balloon angioplasty in swine: persistent benefit at 6-month follow-up. J Am Coll Cardiol 25:1451–1456, 1995.
21. Waksman R, Robinson KA, Crocker IR, et al: Intracoronary low-dose β-irradiation inhibits neointima formation after coronary artery balloon injury in the swine restenosis model. Cirulation 92:3025–3031, 1995.
22. Waksman R, Rodriguez JC, Robinson KA, et al: Effect of intravascular irradiation on cell proliferation, apoptosis, and vascular remodeling after balloon oversearch injury of porcine coronary arteries. Circulation 96:1944–1952, 1997.
23. Verin V, Popowski Y, Urban P, et al: Intra-arterial beta irradiation prevents neointimal hyperplasia in a hypercholesterolemic rabbit restenosis model. Circulation 92:2284–2290, 1995.
24. Mazur W, Ali MN, Dabaghi SF, et al: High-dose rate intracoronary radiation suppresses neointimal proliferation in the stented and ballooned model of porcine restenosis [abstract]. Circulation 90:1–652, 1994.
25. Mayberg MR, Lou Z, London S, et al: Radiation inhibition of intimal hyperplasia after arterial injury. Radiat Res 142:212–220, 1995.
26. Shimotakahara S, Mayberg MR: Gamma irradiation inhibits neointimal hyperplasia in rats after arterial injury. Stroke 25:424–428, 1994.
27. Abbas MA, Afshari NA, Standius ML, et al: External beam irradiation inhibits neointimal hyperplasia following balloon angioplasty. Int J Cardiol 44:191–202, 1994.
28. Mazur W, Ali MN, Khan MM, et al: High dose rate intracoronary radiation for inhibition of neointimal formation in the stented and balloon-injured porcine models of restenosis: angiographic morphometric and histopathologic analyses. Int J Radiat Oncol Biol Phys 36:777–778, 1996.
29. Wiedermann JG, Marboe C, Amols H, et al: Intracoronary irradiation fails to reduce neointimal proliferation after oversized stenting in a porcine model. Circulation 92:146, 1995.
30. Waksman R: Intracoronary radiation adjunct therapy to stenting. J Intervent Cardiol 10:2133–2136, 1977.
31. Waksman R, Robison K, Crocker I, et al: Intracoronary radiation decreases the second phase of intimal hyperplasia in a repeat balloon angioplasty swine model of restenosis. Int J Radiat Oncol Biol Phys 39:475–480, 1997.
32. Hehrlein C, Stintz M, Kinscherf R, et al: Pure β-particle emitting stents inhibit neointima formation in rabbits. Circulation 93:641–645, 1996.
33. Hehrlein C, Zimmermann J, Metz J, et al: Radioactive coronary stent implantation inhibits neointimal proliferation in nonatherosclerotic rabbits. Circulation 88:1–651, 1993.
34. Hehrlein C, Gollan C, Dönges K, et al: Low-dose radioactive endovascular stents prevent smooth muscle cell proliferation and neointimal hyperplasia in rabbits. Circulation 92:1570–1575, 1995.
35. Fischell TA, Kharma BK, Fischell DR, et al: Low-dose, β-particle emission from "stent" wire results in complete, localized inhibition of smooth muscle cell proliferation. Circulation 90:2956–2963, 1994.
36. Shefer A, Eigler NL, Whiting JS, Litvack FI: Suppression of intimal proliferation after balloon angioplasty with local beta irradiation in rabbits. [abstract]. J Am Coll Cordiol 21(suppl A):185A, 1993.
37. Hehrlein C, Donges K, Gollan C, et al: Low-dose radioactive Palmaz-Schatz stents prevent smooth muscle cell proliferation and neointimal hyperplasia in rabbits [abstract]. J Am Coll Cardiol 9A, 1995.
38. Hehrlein C, Kaiser S, Kollum N, et al: Effects of very low dose endovascular irradiation via an activated guide wire on neointima formation after stent implantation. Circulation 92:146, 1995.
39. Bottcher HD, Schopohl B, Liermann D, et al: Endovascular irradiation—a new method to avoid recurrent stenosis after stent implantation in peripheral arteries: technique and preliminary results. Int J Radiat Oncol Biol Phys 29:183–186, 1994.
40. Liermann DD, Boettcher HD, Kollatch J, et al: Prophylactic endovascular radiotherapy to prevent intimal hyperplasia after stent implantation in femoro-popliteal arteries. Cardiovasc Intervent Radiol 17:12–16, 1994.
41. Steidle B: Preventive percutaneous radiotherapy for avoiding hyperplasia of the intima following anigoplasty together with stent implantation [German]. Strahlenther Onkol 170:151–154, 1994.
42. Condado JA, Waksman R, Gurdiel O, et al: Long-term angiographic and clinical outcome after percutaneous transluminal coronary angioplasty and intracoronary radiation therapy in humans. Circulation 96:727–732, 1997.
43. Handley DA: Experimental therapeutics and clinical studies in (re)stenosis. Micron 26:51–68, 1995.
44. Teirstein P: β-radiation to reduce restenosis. Too little, too late. Circulation 95:1095–1097, 1997.
45. Verin V, Urban P, Popowski Y, et al: Feasibility of intracoronary β-irradiation to reduce restenosis after balloon angioplasty. A clinical pilot study. Circulation 95:1138–1144, 1997.
46. King SB III, Williams DO, Chougule P, et al: Endovascular β-radiation to reduce restenosis after coronary balloon angioplasty. Results of the Beta Energy Restenosis Trial (BERT). Circulation 97:2025–2030, 1998.
47. Novoste Newswire, August 17, 1998.
48. Laird JR, Carter AJ, Kufs WM, et al: Inhibition of neointimal proliferation with low-dose irradiation from a β-particle–emitting stent. Circulation 93:529–536, 1996.
49. Jani SK: Handbook of Dosimetry for Radiotherapy. p. 152. Boca Raton, FL: CRC, 1993.
50. Hall EJ: DNA strand breaks and chromosomal aberrations. *In* Hall EJ (ed): Radiobiology for the Radiologist. 4th ed. pp. 15–73. Philadelphia: JB Lippincott, 1994.
51. Teirstein PS, Massullo V, Jani S: Radiation therapy following coronary stenting—6-month follow-up of a randomized clinical trial. Circulation 94(suppl 1):1–210, 1996.
52. Massullo VM, Teirstein PS, Jani SK, et al: Endovascular brachytherapy to inhibit coronary artery restenosis: an introduction to the Scripps Coronary Radiation to Inhibit Proliferation Post Stenting Trial. Int J Radiat Oncol Biol Phys 36:973–975, 1996.
53. Amols HI, Reinstein LE, Weinberger J: Dosimetry of a radioactive coronary balloon dilatation catheter for treatment of neointimal hyperplasia. Med Phys 23:1783–1788, 1996.
54. Jani SK, Massullo VM, Teirstein PS, et al: Physics and safety aspects of a coronary irradiation pilot study to inhibit restenosis using manually loaded Ir-192 ribbons. Semin Intervent Cardiol 2:119–123, 1997.
55. Hall EJ: The physics and chemistry of radiation absorption. *In* Hall EJ (ed.): Radiobiology for the Radiologist. 4th ed. pp. 1–13. Philadelphia: JB lippincott, 1994.
56. Amols HI, Zaider M, Weinberger J, et al: Dosimeric considerations for catheter based beta and gamma emitters in the therapy of neointimal hyperplasia in human coronary arteries. Int J Radiat Oncol Biol Phys 36:913–921, 1996.
57. Condado JA, Saucedo JF, Caldera C, et al: Two year angiographic evaluation after intracoronary 192 iridium in humans [abstract]. Circulation 96(suppl):1–220, 1997.
58. Hancock SL, Tucker M, Hoppe RT: Factors affecting late mortality from heart disease after treatment of Hodgkin's disease. JAMA 270: 1949–1955, 1993.
59. Stewart JR, Fajardo LF, Gillette SM, Constine LS: Radiation injury to the heart. Int J Radiat Oncol Biol Phys 31:1205–1211, 1955.
60. Fajardo LP: Pathology of Radiation Injury. p. 192. New York: Masson, 1982.
61. Fajardo LF, Berthrong M: Vascular lesions following radiation. Pathol Annu 23:297–330, 1988.
62. Hopewell JW, Campling D, Calvo W, et al: Vascular irradiation damage: its cellular basis and likely consequences. Br J Cancer 53(suppl VII):181–191, 1986.
63. Reinhold HS, Fajardo LF, Hopewell JW: The vascular system. *In* Altman KJ (ed): Relative Radiosensitivity of Human Organ Systems. pp. 177–226, London: Academic, 1990.
64. Fajardo LF, Lee A: Rupture of major vessels after radiation. Cancer 36:904–913, 1975.
65. Fee WF Jr, Goffinet DR, Guthaner D, et al: Safety of ^{125}iodine and ^{192}iridium implants to the canine carotid artery: preliminary report. Laryngoscope 95:317–320, 1985.
66. Hancock SL, Hoppe RT: Long-term complications of treatment and causes of mortality after Hodgkin's disease. Semin Radiat Oncol 6:225–242, 1996.
67. Van Leeuwen FE, Klokman WJ, Stovall M, et al: Roles of radiotherapy and smoking in lung cancer following Hodgkin's disease. J Natl Cancer Inst 87:1530–1537, 1995.

68. Hancock SL, Tucker M, Hoppe RT: Breast cancer after treatment of Hodgkin's disease. J Natl Cancer Inst 85:25–31, 1993.
69. Birdwell SH, Hancock SL, Varghese A, et al: Gastrointestinal cancer after treatment of Hodgkin's disease. Int J Radiat Oncol Biol Phys 37:67–73, 1995.
70. Henschke UK, Hilaris BS, Mahan GD: Remote afterloadiong for intracavitary radiation therapy. Radiology 83:344–345, 1964.
71. Parikh S, Nori D: Endovascular brachytherapy: Current status and future trends. J Brachyther Int 13:167–177, 1997.
72. Jani SK, Massullo V, Teirstein P: The ^{192}Ir radioactive seed ribbon. *In* Waksman R, Serruys PW (eds): Handbook of Vascular Brachytherapy. pp. 27–32. London: Martin Dunitz, 1998.
73. Arbab-Zadeh A, Russo RJ, Bhargava V, et al: A comparison of centered vs noncentered source for intracoronary radiation therapy: observations from the SCRIPPS Trial [abstract]. Circulation 96:(suppl):1–219, 1997.
74. Mikkar R, Whiting J, Li A, et al: A β-emitting liquid isotope filled balloon markedly inhibits restenosis in stented porcine coronary arteries [abstract]. J Am Coll Cardiol 31(suppl):350A, 1998.
75. Giedd KN, Amols H, Marboe CC, et al: Effectiveness of a beta-emitting liquid-filled perfusion balloon to prevent restenosis [abstract]. Circulation 96(suppl):1–220, 1997.
76. Waksman R, Chan RC, Vodovotz Y, et al: Radioactive 133-Xenon gas-filled angioplasty balloon: a novel intracoronary radiation system to prevent restenosis [abstract]. J Am Coll Cardiol 31(suppl):356A, 1998.
77. Laird JR, Carter AJ, Kufs WM, et al: Inhibition of neointimal proliferation with a beta particle emitting stent [abstract]. J Am Coll Cardiol 287A:773, 1995.
78. Fischell TA, Abbas MA, Kallman RF: Low-dose irradiation inhibits clonal proliferation of smooth muscle cells: a new approach to restenosis [abstract]. Arterioscler. Thromb 11:1435a, 1991.
79. Hehrlein C, Zimmermann M, Metz J, et al: Radiactive stent implantation inhibits neointimal proliferation in non-atherosclerotic rabbits [abstract]. Circulation 88:1–65, 1993.
80. Moses JW, Ellis SG, Bailey SR, et al for the IRIS Investigators: Short-term (1 month) results of the dose response IRIS feasibility study of a beta-particle emitting radioisotope stent [abstract]. J Am Coll Cardiol 31(suppl):350A, 1998.

CHAPTER 41

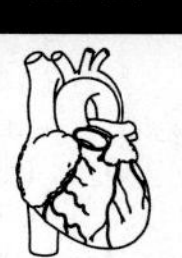

Surgical Treatment

Michael S. Sweeney, O. H. Frazier, and Denton A. Cooley

INDICATIONS
RISK FACTORS
MYOCARDIAL PRESERVATION
PREOPERATIVE EVALUATION
CONVENTIONAL SURGICAL TECHNIQUE
Right Coronary Artery
Left Anterior Descending Coronary Artery
SPECIAL CONSIDERATIONS
The Conduit
Sequential Grafts
Reoperation
WARM HEART SURGERY WITH A VENTRICULAR ASSIST DEVICE
MINIMALLY INVASIVE CORONARY ARTERY BYPASS GRAFT SURGERY
Technique
Advantages and Disadvantages
ENDARTERECTOMY
TRANSMYOCARDIAL LASER REVASCULARIZATION
SUMMARY

Coronary artery bypass graft surgery (CABG) remains a major invasive treatment for coronary artery occlusive disease, although percutaneous transluminal coronary angioplasty (PTCA) is also used to treat many patients who before the introduction of PTCA would have undergone a bypass procedure.

The first bypass procedure was performed by Sabiston in 1962. A bypass graft was made to the right coronary artery without the use of extracorporeal circulation. Unfortunately, the patient died of a cerebrovascular accident 3 days after the operation; a blood clot was found at the origin of the graft in the aorta. In 1965, Garrett and colleagues[1] performed the first successful CABG. While performing an endarterectomy, they encountered technical difficulties and were forced to bypass the left anterior descending coronary artery. Much of the pioneering work with CABG, however, was done by Favoloro and associates[2, 3] at the Cleveland Clinic in 1967 and by Johnson and associates[4] in Milwaukee in 1968. Hallman and colleagues[5] performed the first successful direct reconstruction of a congenital coronary artery anomaly with the use of a Dacron tube graft in 1963.

Since those early days, the operation has evolved significantly. This chapter describes our techniques for the performance of CABG.

Indications

The major indication for CABG remains the need for relief of myocardial ischemia and disabling angina pectoris, although CABG may also be performed as a concomitant procedure in patients with cardiac failure resulting from ventricular aneurysm, ventricular septal perforation, papillary muscle rupture, or valvular disease. In addition, CABG may be performed in a few patients with severe myocardial dysfunction who have sufficient areas of viable myocardium to support bypass grafts, in the hope of improving myocardial function.[6]

Risk Factors

Like other open heart surgery, CABG poses certain risks, some of which are related to the need for cardiopulmonary bypass (CPB).[7, 8] Potential CPB-related complications include neutrophil and complement activation, interstitial pulmonary edema, reduced oxygen delivery, impaired hemostasis, and cerebral microembolism. To avoid these problems, CABG may be performed without CPB in selected cases, as discussed in the next section.

Patient-related factors that increase the risk of CABG include calcification, small vessels, and diffuse coronary atherosclerosis. Diabetes mellitus, hypertension, collagen disease, long-term steroid use, advanced age, and female sex are additional risk factors, as is severe myocardial dysfunction. Arrhythmias related to ischemia or revascularization should be assessed before and during surgery and should be controlled with aggressive medical management. In these cases, temporary pacing or even an automatic internal defibrillator may be necessary.

Myocardial Preservation

Researchers are still trying to determine the best method of preserving the myocardium during CABG.[9, 10] The concept of delivering a protective energy substrate to the myocardium through the coronary sinus was suggested in the 1930s and 1940s by Beck and colleagues.[11] After the advent of CABG, laboratory investigations by Buckberg and others placed this concept on firm physiologic ground. Over the years, blood cardioplegia has proved to be superior to crystalloid cardioplegia.[12] Most surgeons still use the simple, potassium-enriched solutions developed during the 1970s.[13] They continue to debate the advantages of warm[14–16] versus cold,[15–19] continuous[15, 18] versus intermittent,[15, 16, 19] and antegrade[19, 20] versus retrograde[14, 20, 21] cardioplegia. As of 1995, approximately 60 percent of cardiac surgeons were using a combined antegrade/retrograde approach.[22] Although some studies[23, 24] have suggested that this approach provides the best myocardial protection, par-

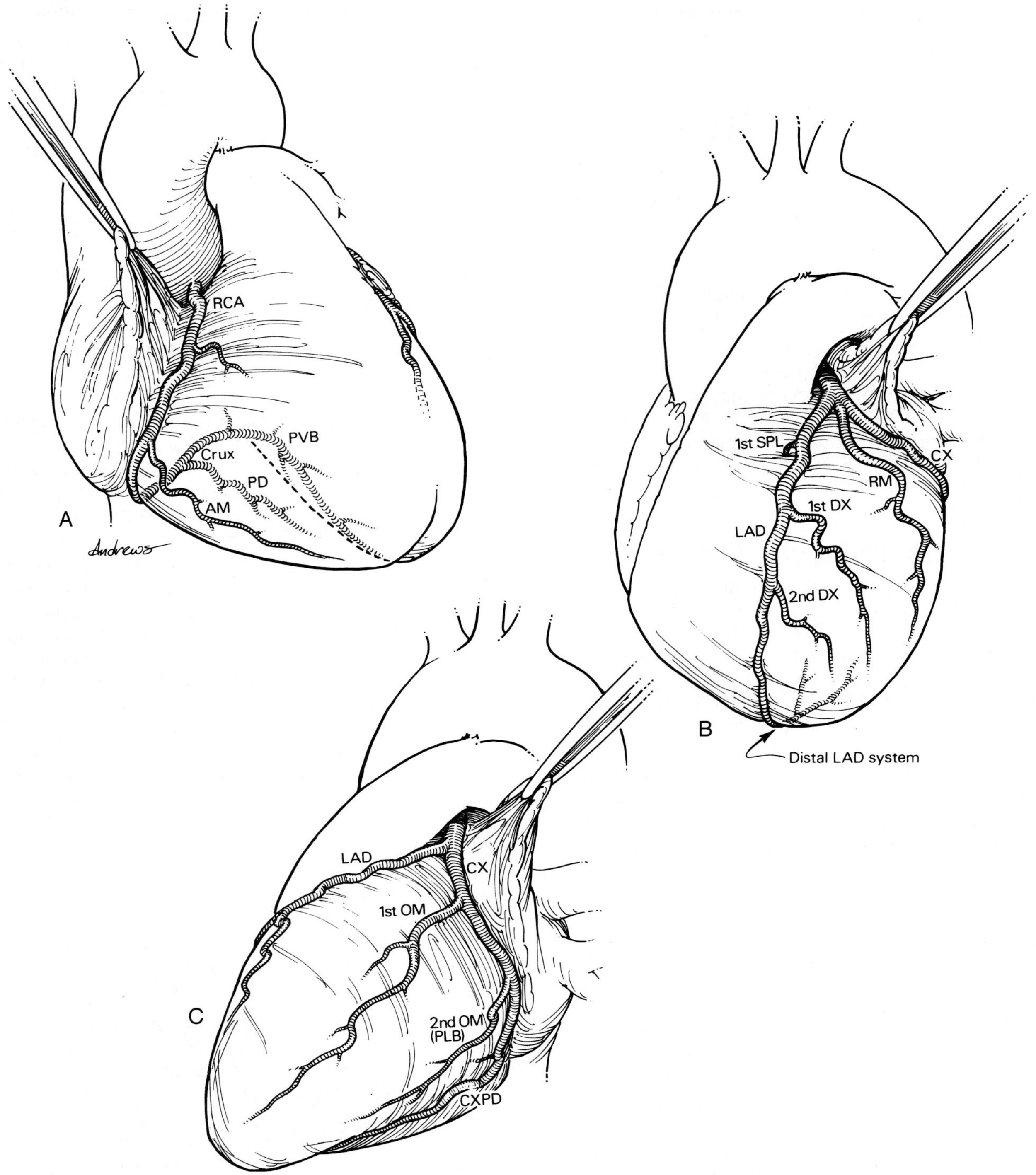

FIGURE 41–1 Surgical anatomy of the coronary system. **A,** The right coronary system has several branches that can be considered for bypass. In some instances, the acute marginal branch (AM) is bypassed, particularly if it has a large retrograde collateral blood supply to the left system. Most anastomoses are made at the area of the crux. The posterior ventricular branch (PVB), posterior descending branches (PD), or their distal branches may be grafted. The dotted line indicates the area of the interventricular septum as denoted by the right coronary vein. RCA, right coronary artery. **B,** In the left anterior descending coronary artery (LAD) system, the first septal perforator (1st SPL) is usually just opposite the first diagonal (1st DX) branch or is proximal to it. It descends posteriorly into the interventricular septum and may be an important artery. The 1st DX and second diagonal (2nd DX) branches arise from the LAD. The distal LAD usually supplies the apex of the left ventricle. The ramus medialis branch (RM) arises between the circumflex (CX) and the LAD and may be in the DX or obtuse marginal position. **C,** The circumflex (CX) coronary system shows the first branch as the first obtuse marginal (1st OM) and the second branch as the second obtuse marginal (2nd OM) or posterior lateral branch (PLB) of the CX system. The main CX trunk is in the atrioventricular groove in close association with the coronary sinus vein. (**A–C,** From Cooley DA: Revascularization of the ischemic myocardium. *In* Techniques in Cardiac Surgery. 2nd ed. pp. 221–258. Philadelphia: WB Saunders, 1984.)

ticularly in higher-risk patients, other studies have not shown that this technique necessarily confers any advantage.[25, 26] In general, the results of clinical studies that attempt to evaluate the relative merits of various cardioplegia delivery systems with regard to specific clinical outcomes should be interpreted with caution, and the choice of system should be tailored to the specific patient being treated.[27]

In 1992, we reported the concept of CABG without the induction of ischemic arrest.[28] Again, this is not a new concept, although it remains controversial. Warm heart surgery without ischemic arrest is especially useful in high-risk patients[16, 29, 30]; such patients include those who have very poor heart function or congestive heart failure and those who require urgent surgery after a serious heart attack or a failed balloon angioplasty procedure (see Warm Heart Surgery With a Ventricular Assist Device). This method is also used in patients with poor ventricular function who require long aortic cross-clamp times. The development of short-term beta blockers, which markedly slow the heart rate, has further improved the outcome in these patients.

Preoperative Evaluation

When CABG is indicated, the surgeon should review the preoperative coronary angiogram to determine which vessels to bypass and where to place the distal anastomoses (Fig. 41–1). The goal is to obtain the most complete revascularization possible. The three main coronary arterial systems (right, left anterior descending, and circumflex) should all be bypassed when 50 percent or more of the artery is occluded.[31–34] In general, vessels 1.5 mm or larger in diameter are suitable for bypass grafting if they are free of significant distal plaque. At times, diffuse disease of the vessel wall may be found in arteries 2.0 to 2.5 mm, or larger. In such cases, bypass to the large distal vessel should be performed despite the diffuse nature of the disease. In some patients, especially women, men of small stature, and those with diabetes, major coronary arteries of small size require revascularization, even though the operative risk is greater.

If necessary, carotid[35] or great vessel[36] occlusive disease may be treated at the same time as coronary artery disease with an acceptably low operative risk.

Patients with post-transplantation coronary artery disease represent a special group, in whom CABG should be used only for multivessel disease that involves patent distal vessels and preserved ventricular function.[37]

Conventional Surgical Technique

After systemic heparinization (approximately 3 mg/kg) is achieved, CPB is instituted by placing cannulae in the ascending aorta to return oxygenated blood from the extracorporeal circuit and in the right atrium to shunt venous blood into the extracorporeal circuit. Right atrial cannulation is accomplished through the insertion of a single, large cannula or, when concomitant intracardiac surgery is being considered, the insertion of two smaller cannulae that traverse the right atrium to lie directly in the superior and inferior venae cavae. When we use systemic cooling for myocardial protection, we usually cool to temperatures of 28° to 30°C; cooling to lower temperatures should be considered when a long pump run is anticipated.

When we plan to use coronary sinus perfusion, we place the pursestring suture before arrest of the heart. The os of the coronary sinus can be cannulated directly, or a closed loop can be created in the right atrium. With this method, solutions infused into the right atrium exit via the coronary sinus (Fig. 41–2).

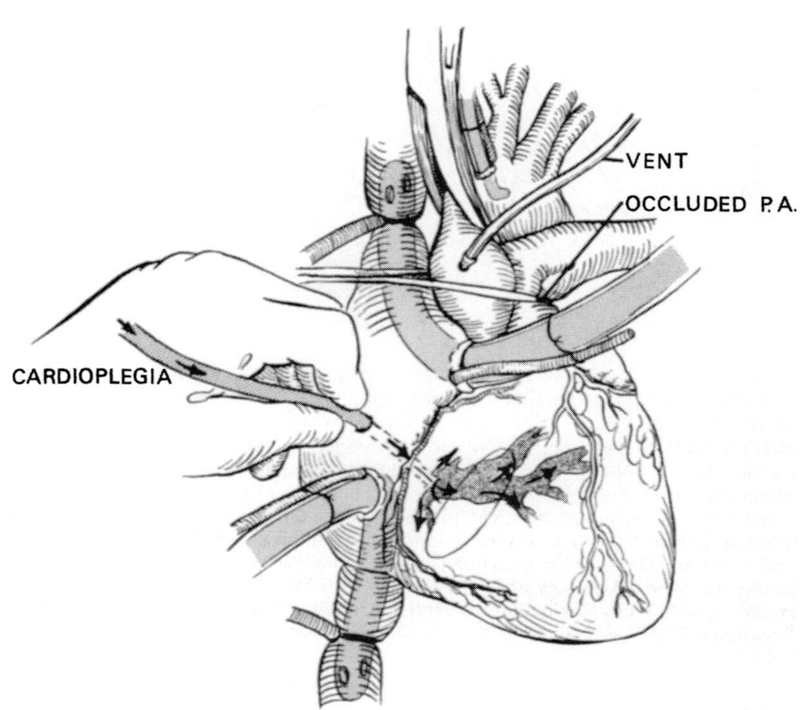

FIGURE 41–2 The coronary sinus is cannulated by making a small puncture in the right atrial free wall. When necessary, the atrium can be incised to place the cardioplegia line into the coronary sinus under direct vision. P.A., pulmonary artery. (From Frazier OH, Sweeney MS, Radovancevic B, Cooley DA: Surgical treatment of heart disease [coronary artery surgery]. *In* Willerson JT [ed]: Treatment of Heart Diseases. pp. 6.3–6.12. New York: Gower Medical Publishing, 1992.)

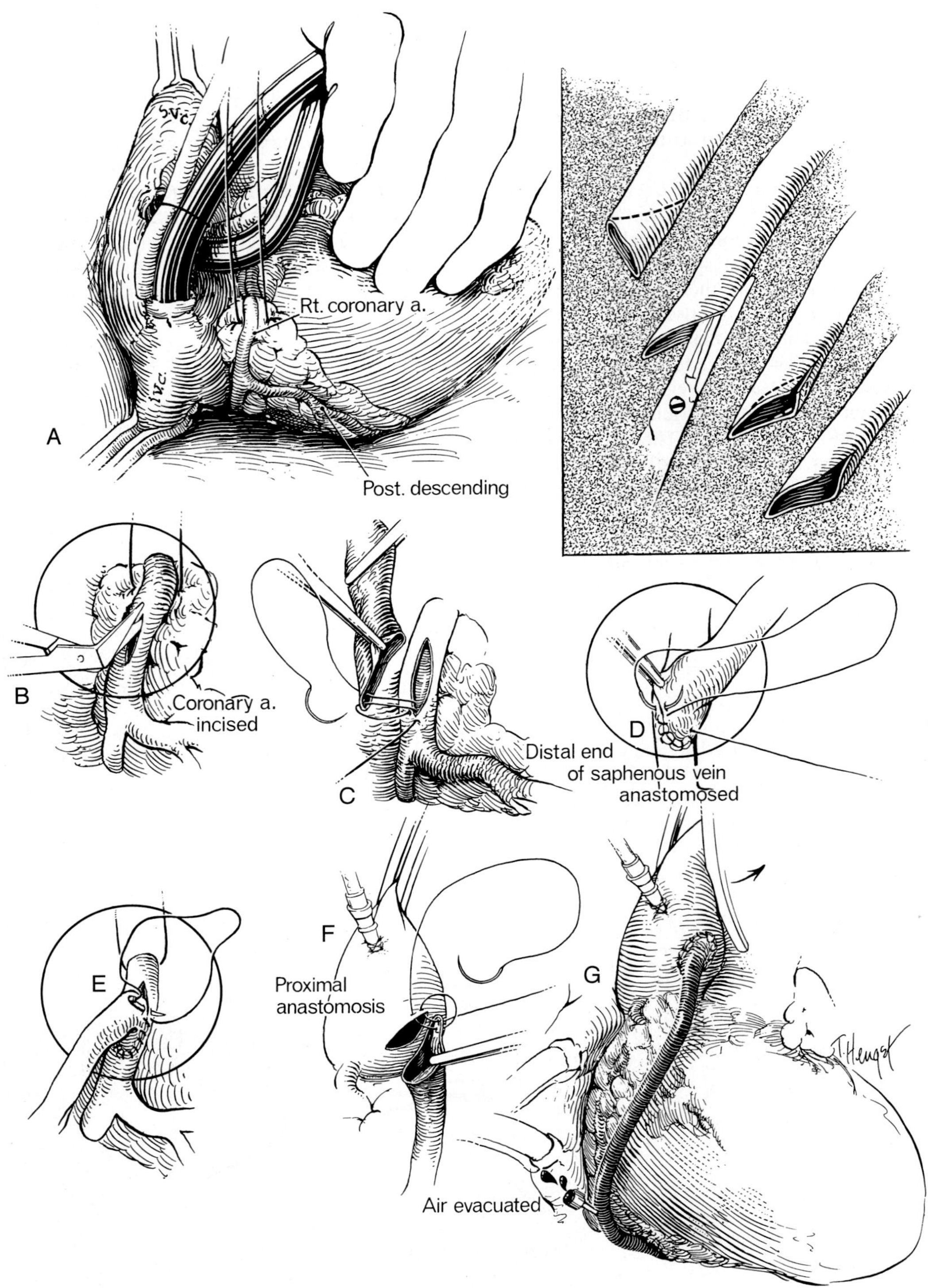

FIGURE 41–3 Saphenous vein graft to the right coronary artery. **A,** The right coronary artery is isolated by placing a traction suture in the myocardium beneath the right coronary artery. **Inset,** The vein is beveled, depending on the length of the anastomosis and the size of the vein. **B,** The coronary artery is incised, and the incision is extended with the use of Potts scissors. **C,** The right coronary anastomosis is begun at the distal portion of the artery and the toe of the vein graft. **D,** The anastomosis is sutured on the right side first, from the artery to the vein. **E,** The anastomosis is completed from the left side. The suture is usually tied at or to the right of the apex. **F,** The proximal anastomosis is completed with the aid of either complete or partial aortic occlusion. **G,** The clamp is removed, and air is evacuated from the vein graft. The vein graft may be clamped with a small bulldog clamp to avoid introducing more air into the coronary system. (**A–G,** From Cooley DA: Revascularization of the ischemic myocardium. *In* Techniques in Cardiac Surgery. 2nd ed. pp. 221–258. Philadelphia: WB Saunders, 1984.)

Before the heart is arrested, the surgeon should locate the coronary arteries to be bypassed. These arteries can be intramyocardial or obscured by epicardial fat or scarring. If the arteries are difficult to find, palpation of the anatomic area at the expected site of the distal anastomosis may help to locate the artery. The artery can be recognized by its whitish-yellow intima and thickened wall.

Right Coronary Artery

The right main coronary artery is often obscured by the atrioventricular groove on the right. Once the artery is located (Fig. 41–3A), we select a site for bypass grafting based on the size and quality of the artery. When the right coronary artery is dominant, we generally perform the bypass at the level of the crus or just above the crus at the level of the posterior descending and posterior ventricular branches. Branches of the coronary venous system may cross the right coronary artery at this level. If these branches are transected to expose the right coronary artery, they should be oversewn.

Occlusive disease often recurs at the level of the crus. When a large posterior descending branch arises from the right coronary artery, we usually place the anastomosis at this site. The posterior descending artery is usually smaller than the right main coronary artery and is free of disease. If all vessels are diseased, an endarterectomy may be indicated.

In general, the saphenous vein is used to bypass the right coronary artery. For the anastomosis, an incision is made in the middle of the artery with a small scalpel. The incision is extended with Potts scissors for 4 to 6 mm (see Fig. 41–3B). Care should be taken to avoid calcified areas of the artery. When possible, we gently dilate the artery (proximally and distally) with a small probe, which simplifies the anastomosis and makes it more accurate. A running 6-0 prolene suture is used (see Figs. 41–3C–E and 41–4). If no intimal calcification or atheroma is present, the arterial side of the anastomosis can be created from outside the vessel. However, when calcification or atheroma is present, the anastomosis should be created from inside the artery.

On completion of the anastomosis, the graft should be checked for bleeding, and any bleeding sites should be repaired. To determine the proper length of vein for a comfortable anastomosis with the ascending aorta, the vein is inflated under pressure (preferably with blood), and the length to the ascending aorta is measured. Obtaining an adequate length of vein is important because the saphenous vein tends to become fibrotic and to shorten with time.

The proximal anastomosis is completed with the aid of complete or partial aortic occlusion (see Figs. 41–3F, 41–5, and 41–6). After the clamp is removed, air is evacuated from the vein graft (see Fig. 41–3G).

Left Anterior Descending Coronary Artery

The left anterior descending coronary artery is usually found on the surface of the anterolateral aspect of the heart at the level of the septum. When this artery appears to have a straight rather than a tortuous course on the angiogram, an intramyocardial location should be suspected. If the artery is intramyocardial, its location can be assessed through visualization and palpation of the distal superficial branches before cardiac arrest. The vessel wall of an intramyocardial artery is typically thin and fragile. The surgeon can facilitate the anastomosis by using a fine needle and a 7-0 monofilament suture. The suture is passed through the

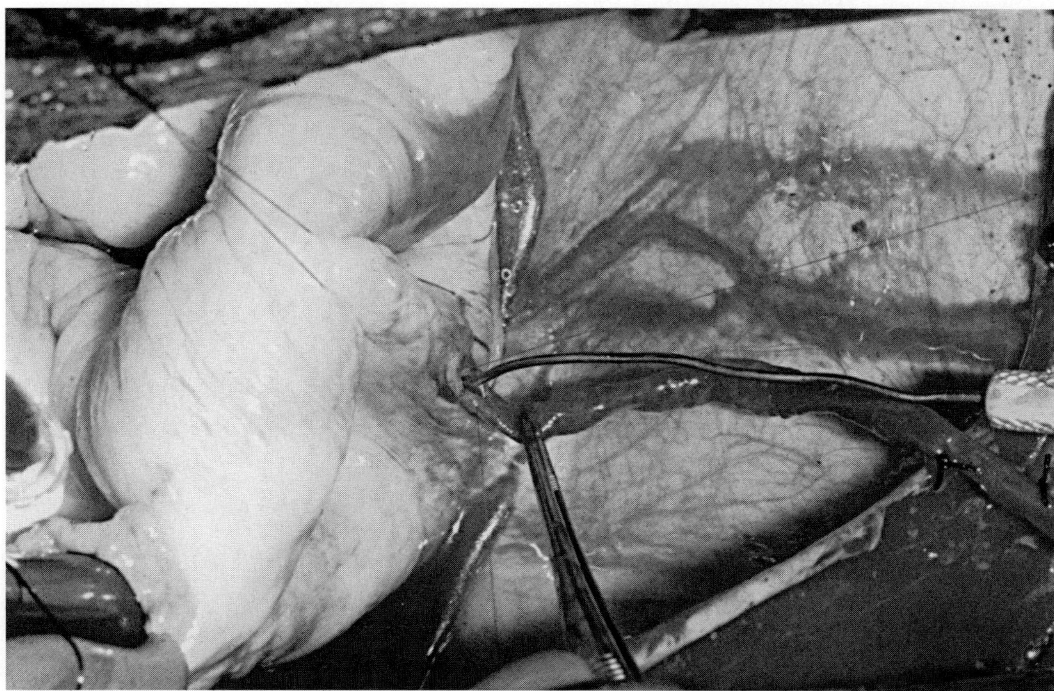

FIGURE 41–4 Coronary artery probe is being passed into the site of the distal right coronary anastomosis.

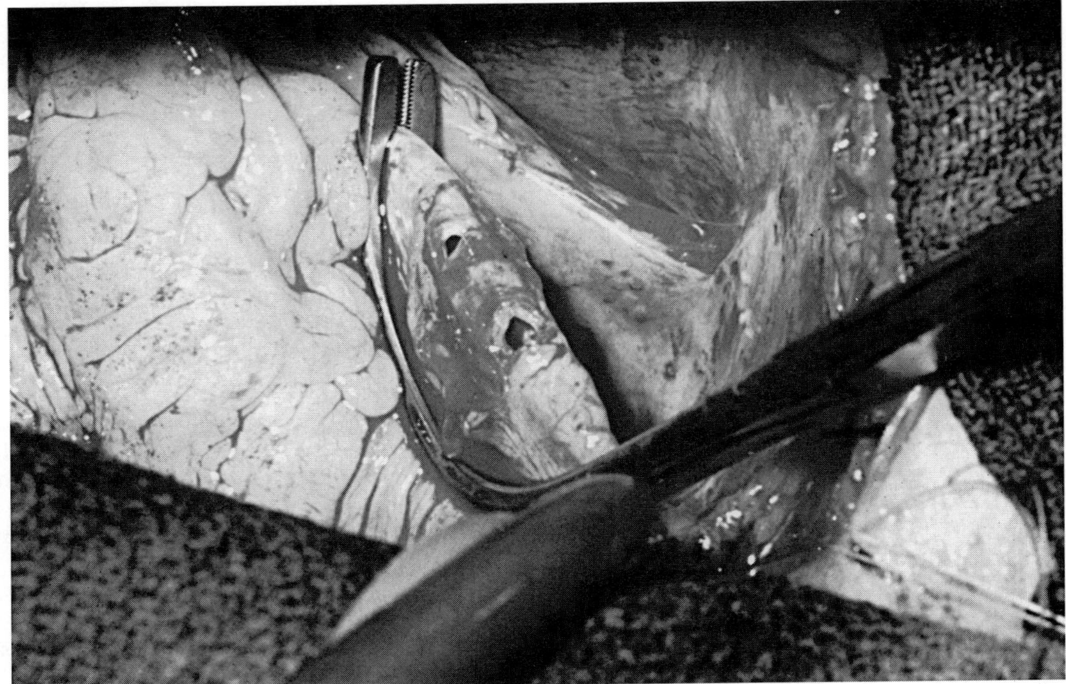

FIGURE 41–5 Incisions are made in the aorta for the proximal anastomoses.

fat and myocardium, as well as the arterial wall, to reinforce the suture line and to reduce the risk of bleeding or arterial laceration. The parallel vein, which is generally to the left of the left anterior descending coronary artery, can also serve as a guide to the location of that artery.

The usual site for bypass to the left anterior descending coronary artery is two thirds of the distance from the origin of that artery, just distal to the most significant obstruction. In this location, the artery can usually be seen as it emerges from the epicardial fat and tends to be sufficiently large for bypass.

To make the distal anastomosis, the left anterior descending coronary artery is incised in a manner similar to that described for the right coronary artery (Fig. 41–7A and B).

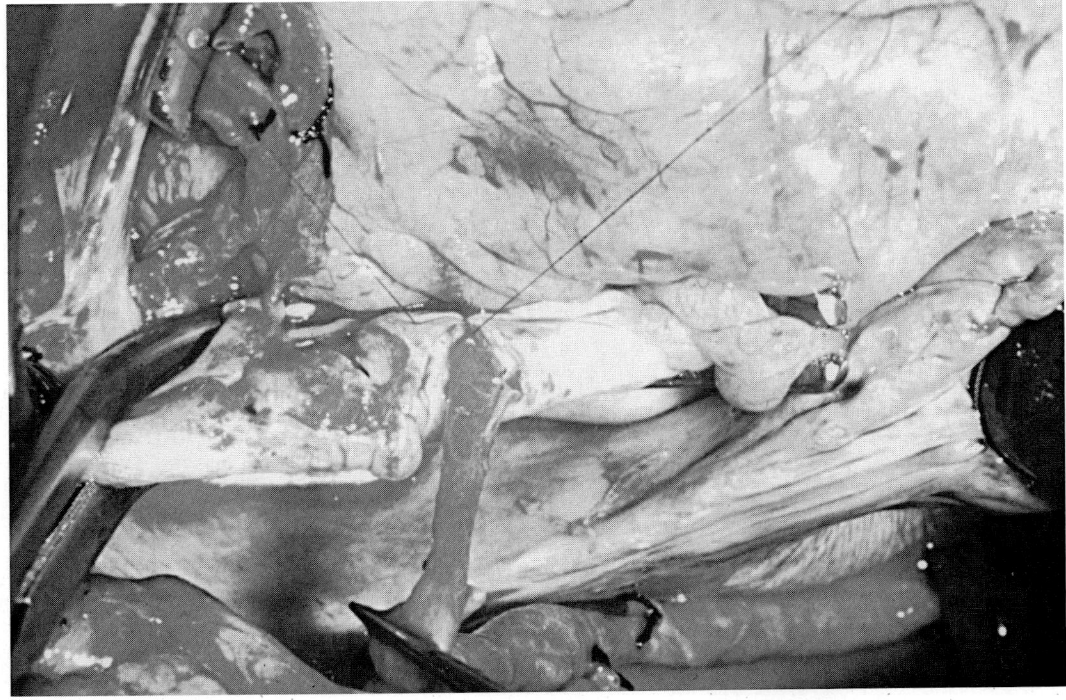

FIGURE 41–6 Proximal anastomosis of the right coronary artery bypass graft.

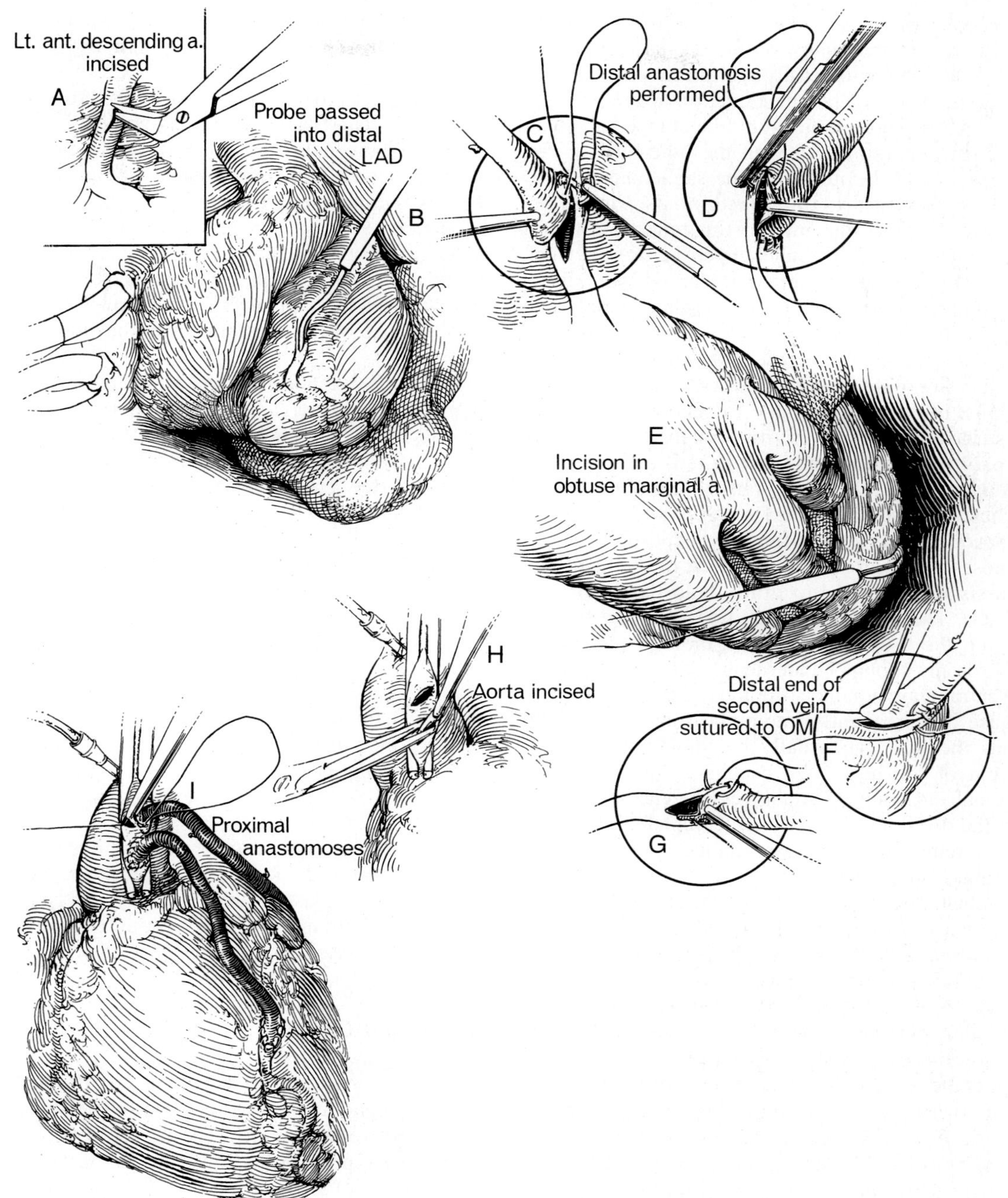

FIGURE 41–7 Saphenous vein graft to the left circumflex system. **A,** The left anterior descending coronary artery (LAD) is identified and incised. The incision is enlarged with Potts scissors. **B,** The probe is passed into the distal LAD to ensure patency. **C,** The distal anastomosis is created by attaching the heel of the graft to the proximal portion of the artery, from outside the artery to inside the vein. Left-side suturing is completed around the toe of the graft to approximately the midportion of the right side of the artery. **D,** The other end of the suture is then sutured from the heel of the graft, passing the vein to the artery. The graft is then tied in the midportion of the artery. **E,** To expose the obtuse marginal artery, the heart is retracted to the right by an assistant. The obtuse marginal branch is then incised. **F,** and **G,** Anastomosis of the obtuse marginal (OM) branch is begun at the proximal portion of the artery, placing the heel of the graft to the proximal portion of the artery. Suturing is accomplished on the left side of the graft, from outside the artery to inside the vein. The anastomosis is completed on the right side by suturing from outside the vein to inside the artery. The sutures are usually tied at or near the apex. **H,** The aorta is incised. **I,** The proximal anastomoses are completed. (**A–I,** From Cooley DA: Revascularization of the ischemic myocardium. *In* Techniques in Cardiac Surgery. 2nd ed. pp. 221–258. Philadelphia: WB Saunders, 1984.)

The anastomosis is begun at the heel of the incision and carried forward on the right side of the artery (see Fig. 41–7C and D). If the artery is large and free of intimal disease at the anastomotic site, the distal part of the anastomosis may be carried completely around to the left side of the artery. The lumen can be easily seen in this manner. If, however, there is a risk of plaque elevation at the level of the distal lumen, the suture line should be stopped short of the distal lumen and completed with the other end of the suture coming around the lumen. If the saphenous vein is used for the bypass graft, the anastomosis should be checked at this time. If the internal mammary artery is used for the bypass graft, it is unclamped before the final knot is tied. This places the artery under pressure from flowing blood and helps prevent pursestringing of the anastomosis when the knot is tied.

Bypass grafts can also be placed to the diagonal branch of the left anterior descending coronary artery, although the vessel must be sufficiently large to support the bypass graft and sufficiently important functionally to improve runoff. Bypass of the circumflex system is best accomplished through the placement of grafts to the obtuse marginal branches, because the circumflex artery, which lies in the atrioventricular groove, is difficult to expose. To make the anastomoses to the arteries on the back of the heart, an additional assistant is needed to firmly hold the heart (see Fig. 41–7E–G). The diagonal vessel, however, can be bypassed without the use of an assistant through the placement of laparotomy sponges underneath, and lateral to, the ventricle. The ramus medialis is the most difficult artery to locate because it is frequently intramyocardial. The origin of the ramus medialis can usually be found high on the obtuse margin of the heart. We usually bypass both the obtuse marginal and ramus medialis vessels with saphenous vein. When the distal anastomoses are completed, the arterial clamp is removed. The heart should spontaneously resume beating.

A partial occluding clamp is then placed on the aorta, and the proximal anastomoses are created (see Fig. 41–7H and I). If the aorta is thickened, an aortic punch (usually 5 mm) can be used to make the incision, thereby facilitating proximal flow. A punch should not be used, however, if the aorta is thin. We use a 5-0 Prolene suture for the proximal anastomoses. If the internal mammary artery is used to bypass the left anterior descending coronary artery, the saphenous vein bypasses on the left side of the heart are brought beneath the internal mammary artery. When the proximal anastomoses are completed, the proximal clamp is removed. If necessary, additional sutures are placed both proximally and distally before CPB is discontinued. When hemostasis is satisfactory, the patient is weaned from CPB.

SPECIAL CONSIDERATIONS

The Conduit

Various bypass conduits are available, and the best choice in any given case depends on numerous factors.[38–40] Autogenous saphenous vein is still the most plentifully available conduit for CABG. If the saphenous vein is damaged or has been removed, we use the lesser saphenous vein in the posterior calf or the cephalic or basilic veins from the arm. Care must be taken not to damage the bypass grafts during handling. Side branches should be ligated to prevent kinking and distortion, which would compromise flow through the lumen. We distend the grafts while we are ligating the side branches. Too vigorous distention, however, may cause intimal damage[41] and should be avoided.

We use the internal mammary artery to bypass the left anterior descending coronary artery (Figs. 41–8 and 41–9), because this vessel has been proven to be superior to the saphenous vein for long-term patency.[42, 43] When the left anterior descending coronary artery is small or calcified, patency of the graft can be enhanced by incision of the artery, placement of a vein patch over the incision, and performance of the anastomosis to the smooth edges of the vein patch.

Although we normally use only the left internal mammary artery (LIMA), the right internal mammary artery (RIMA) may be used as a graft through the transverse sinus to the obtuse marginal vessel or to the right coronary artery. A free graft, however, must be used to obtain adequate length to bypass the right coronary artery.

There are some instances in which the internal mammary artery is not the ideal conduit. Harvest of the mammary artery may decrease the blood supply to the sternum. Although there is no apparent increase in the rate of complications after the harvest of a single internal mammary artery, sternal infections and even dehiscence have been reported after bilateral harvest. Use of the radial artery from the nondominant wrist was reintroduced by Buxton and others[44–46]; the original results were poor because of graft failure attributed to vasospasm, but results have improved because of postoperative treatment with nitroglycerin and calcium channel blockers.

Other arteries can also be used as bypass grafts. Occasionally, we use the left gastroepiploic[47, 48] and the superior and inferior epigastric arteries as bypass conduits, mainly in patients without adequate venous conduits. In general, however, we use these arteries sparingly.

Sequential Grafts

Sequential anastomosis is performed for two reasons: to conserve conduits and to increase long-term graft patency through increased runoff. The presence of more than two distal anastomotic sites, however, decreases any advantage gained from runoff and may impair patency.

In the creation of sequential anastomoses to parallel obtuse marginal vessels, the most distal anastomosis should be performed first. The toe of the vein should be fitted to the heel of the artery, allowing for a gentle S curve. The side-to-side anastomosis can then be constructed to the more proximal vessel. For sequential anastomoses to the left anterior descending coronary and diagonal arteries, this sequencing is unnecessary (Fig. 41–10). In this case, the side-to-side anastomosis to the diagonal vessel should be made from the usual course of the left anterior descending vein.

Some surgeons advocate the creation of sequential anastomoses with mammary artery grafts. However, the impor-

Text continued on page 851

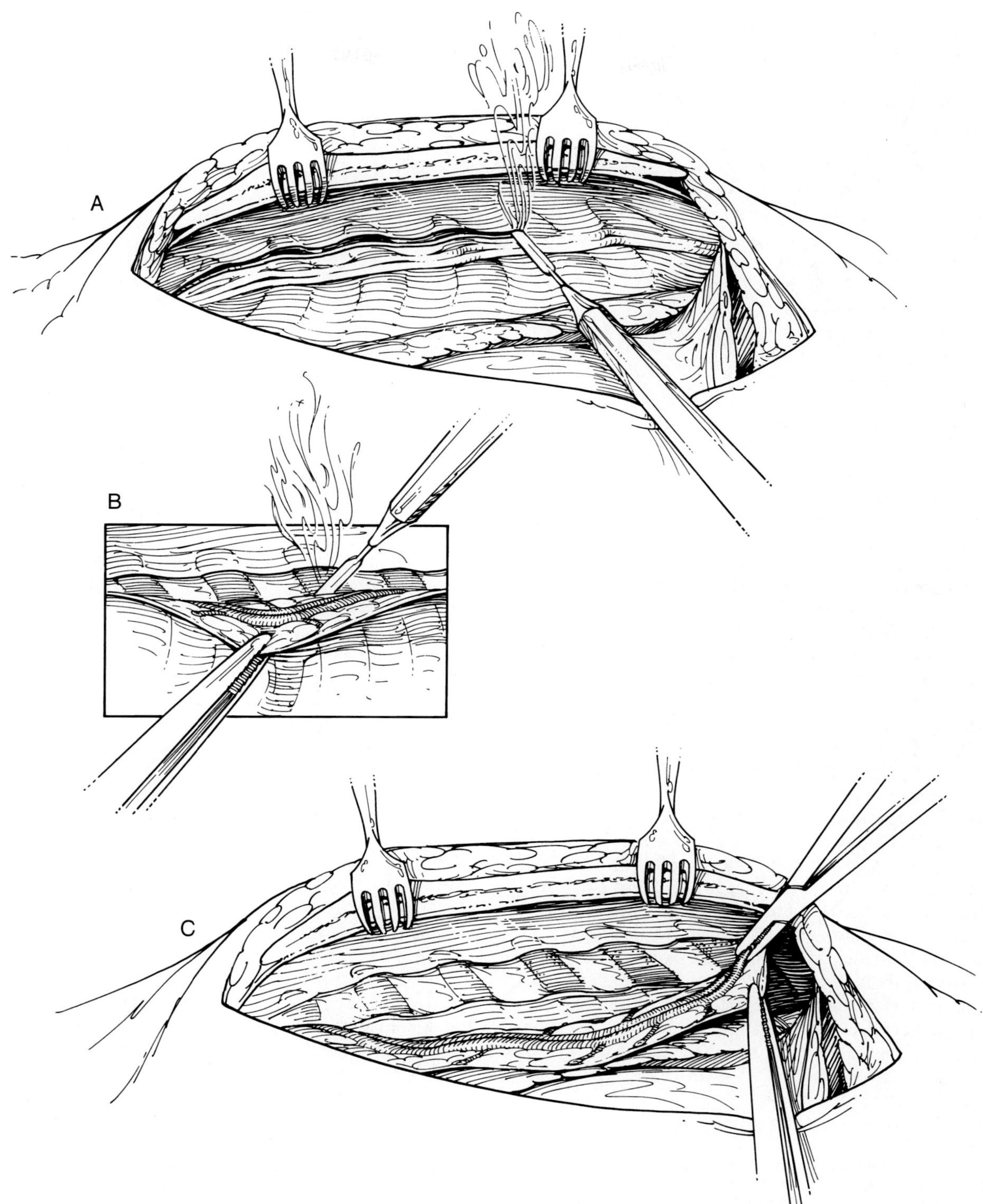

FIGURE 41–8 Technique for obtaining the internal mammary artery (IMA) for use as a bypass conduit. **A,** The IMA is mobilized from the chest wall with cautery. Parallel incisions are made on each side of the pedicle, which includes the vein, artery, lymphatics, fascia, and muscle. **B,** Only the tissue around the IMA should be handled with forceps. The distal intercostal arteries and branches are electrocoagulated. Metal clips or ligatures are placed on the proximal branches. **C,** The distal portion of the pedicle around the IMA has been removed, and a metal clip has been placed on the distal mammary artery. Metal clips are used to gain hemostasis of the pedicle without trauma to the artery.

Illustration continued on following page

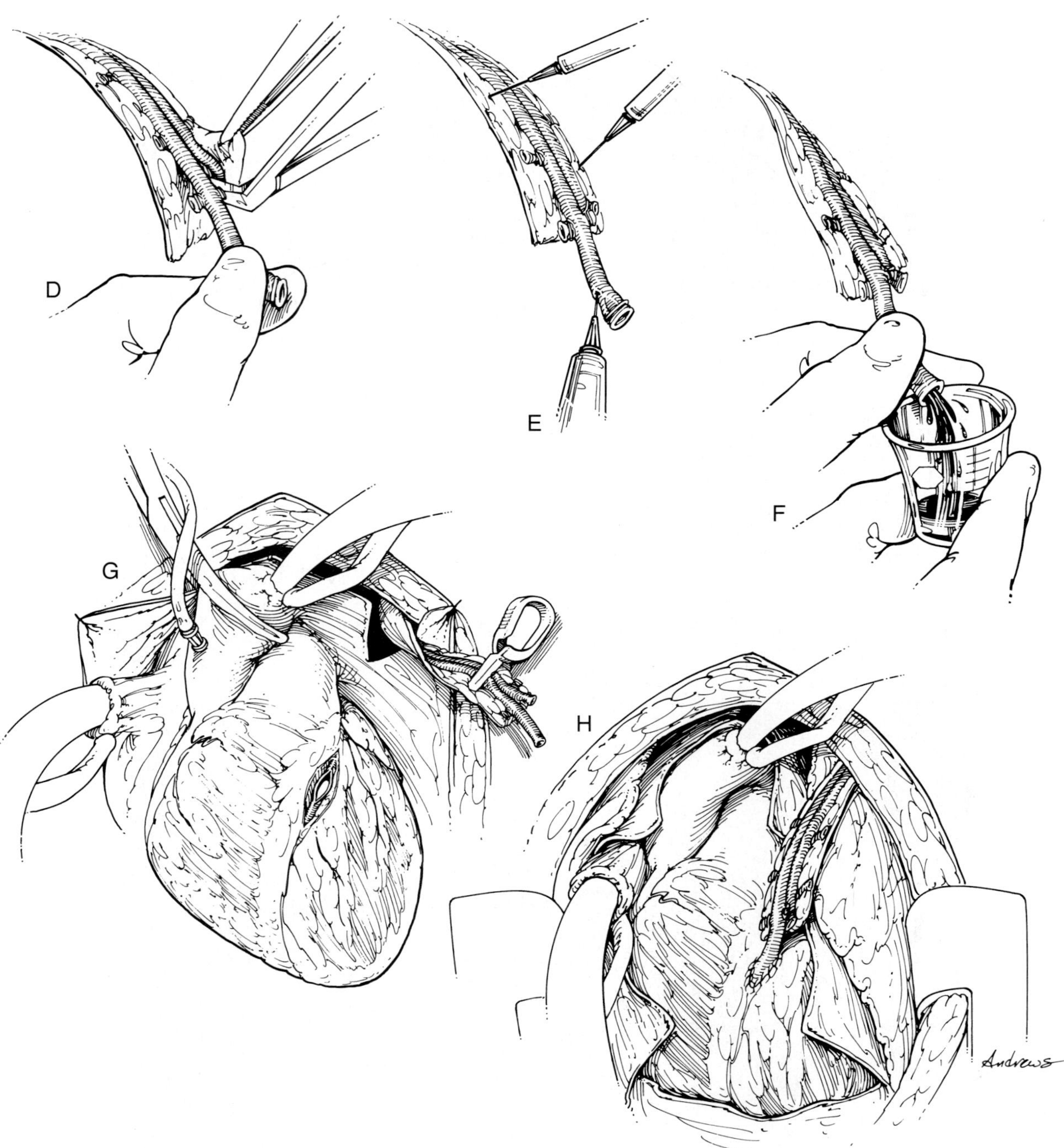

FIGURE 41–8 *Continued* **D,** The pedicle is cleaned of its distal portion, and the artery is exposed. **E,** A solution of papaverine (30 mg/100 ml) is injected into the mammary artery with a syringe. Papaverine solution is also applied to the pedicle. **F,** After the graft is dilated, flow is assessed. If flow is less than 60 to 100 ml/min, a more proximal portion with a higher flow rate should be obtained. **G,** The LAD is isolated, and the graft is aligned. **H,** The anastomosis is completed. Care must be taken to ensure proper alignment of the graft on the myocardium, especially with respect to the pericardium, the pleura, the lung, and the beating heart. (**A–H,** From Cooley DA: Revascularization of the ischemic myocardium. *In* Techniques in Cardiac Surgery. 2nd ed. pp. 221–258. Philadelphia: WB Saunders, 1984.)

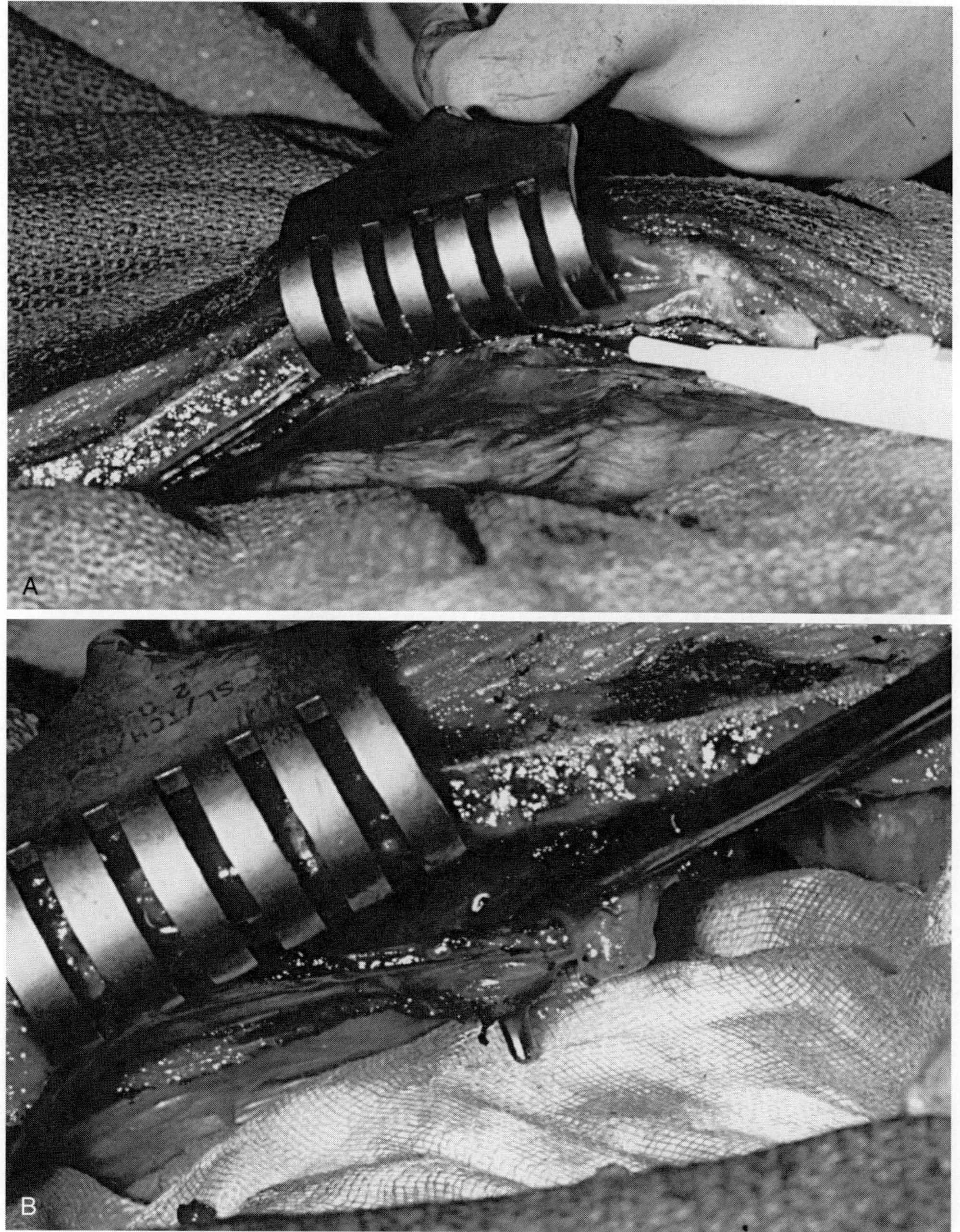

FIGURE 41–9 The IMA is used to bypass the LAD. **A** and **B,** Harvest.
Illustration continued on following page

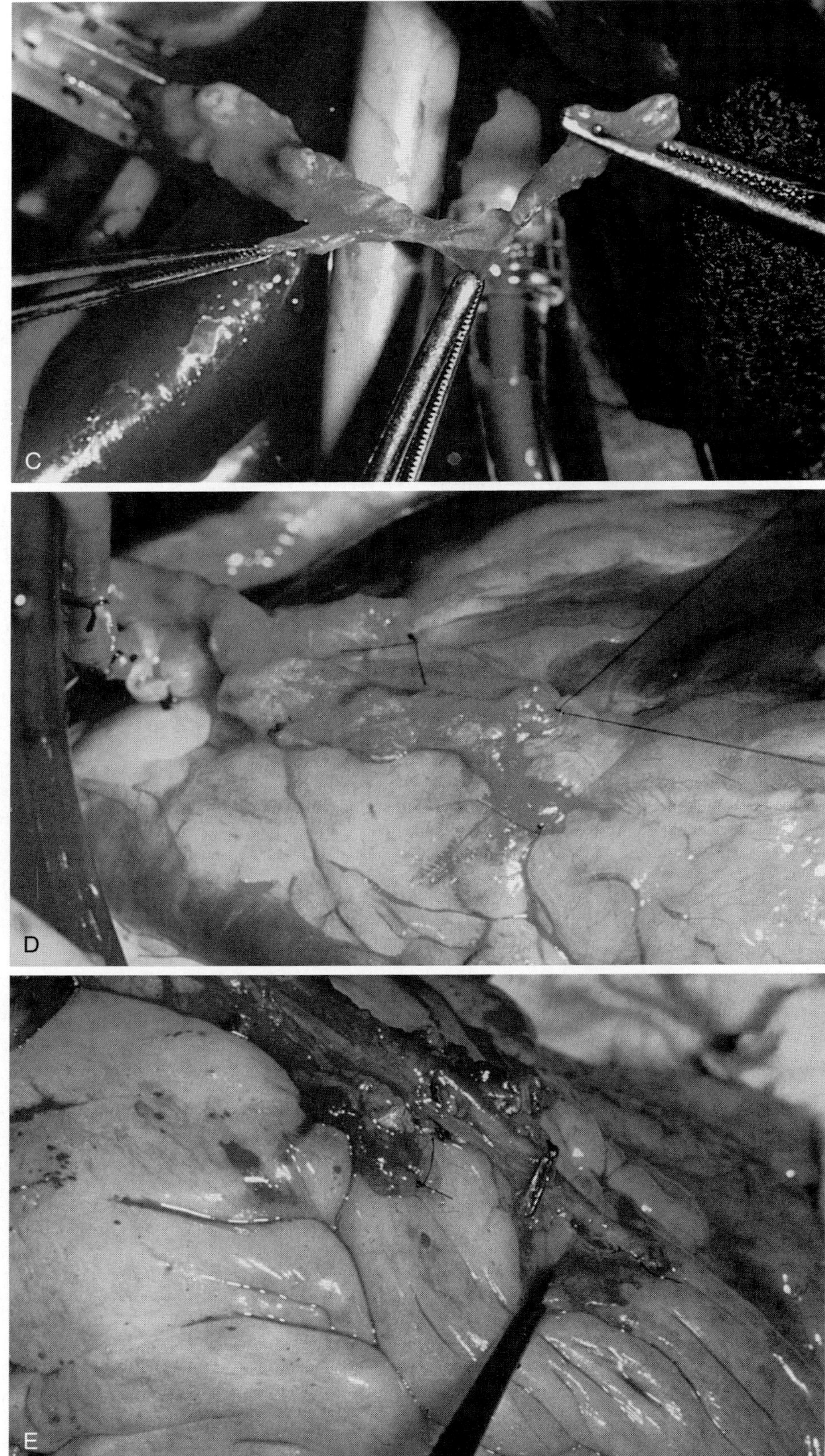

FIGURE 41–9 *Continued* **C,** Handling. **D,** Anastomosis. **E,** Completed anastomosis. (**A–E,** From Frazier OH, Sweeney MS, Radovancevic B, Cooley DA: Surgical treatment of heart disease [coronary artery surgery]. *In* Willerson JT [ed]: Treatment of Heart Diseases. pp. 6.3–6.12. New York: Gower Medical Publishing, 1992.)

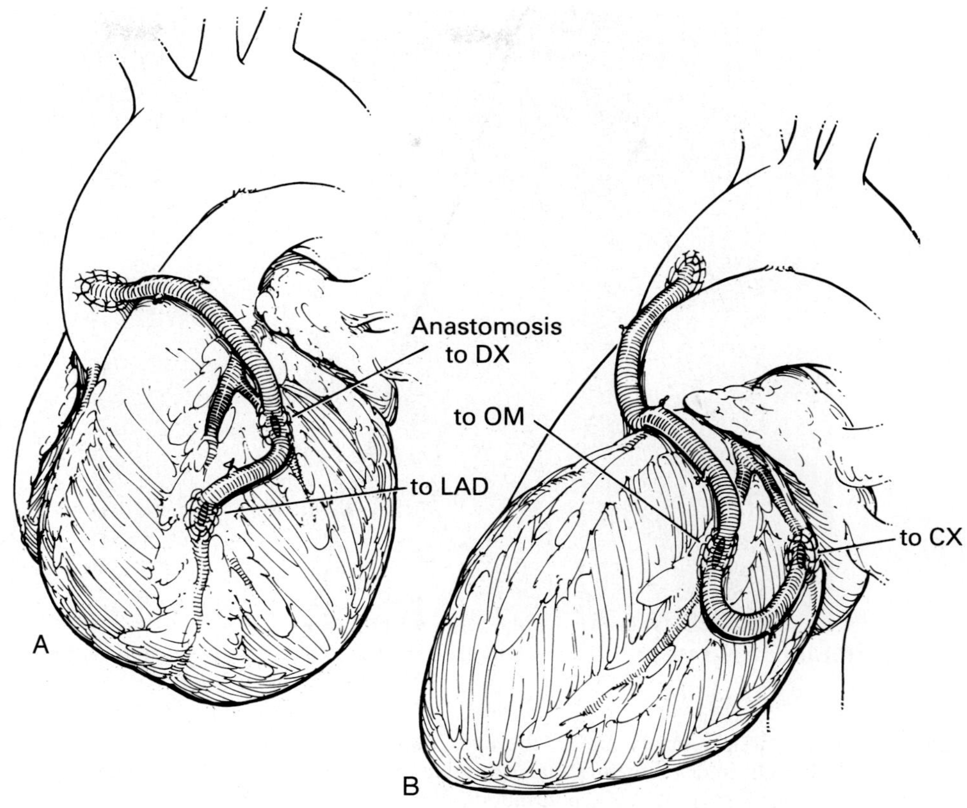

FIGURE 41–10 A, Antegrade, longitudinal sequential bypass graft to the left anterior descending coronary artery (LAD) and diagonal (DX) branches. Flow in the vein graft is directed toward the distal ends of the arteries. **B,** Retrograde, longitudinal sequential graft to the circumflex (CX) and obtuse marginal (OM) branches. The CX shows the vein directed in a retrograde fashion to allow for a gentle loop between the two anastomoses. Both incisions on the vein graft are fashioned longitudinally. This type of anastomosis avoids positioning of an S-shaped curve between both arteries, which would result if an antegrade-type anastomosis were done to the CX artery. (**A** and **B,** From Cooley DA: Revascularization of the ischemic myocardium. *In* Techniques in Cardiac Surgery. 2nd ed. pp. 221–258. Philadelphia: WB Saunders, 1984.)

tance of the left anterior descending anastomosis in this instance and the lower flow characteristics of the mammary artery seem to make sequencing of this important anastomosis a needless hazard. In the right coronary system, more than one bypass may be indicated. This goal is best achieved by creating a side-to-side anastomosis to the more proximal right main coronary artery.

Reoperation

A reoperation is obviously more difficult to perform technically than the initial bypass procedure. When the sternum is opened, care must be taken to avoid injuring the underlying right ventricle or the previous bypass grafts, especially internal mammary artery grafts, which may lie just beneath the sternum. We use a conventional sternal saw to open the sternum in patients undergoing reoperation, but we are careful to advance the instrument only 2 to 3 inches at a time, in a sawing-type motion, to avoid tearing the right ventricle. Once the sternum is opened, each side is carefully dissected from the underlying cardiac tissue. Usually, both pleural cavities must be opened.

After the underlying tissue has been freed from the sternum, a conventional sternal retractor is placed, and the heart is dissected free for cannulation. Once an adequate length of aorta and right atrium is exposed, cannulation is performed. Before the heart is arrested, however, all old patent saphenous vein grafts must be interrupted to prevent embolization of atheromatous plaque when cardioplegic solution is introduced through the ascending aorta. To keep patent vein grafts intact, high-dose potassium should be administered through a coronary sinus catheter. This technique arrests the heart without causing a coronary embolus.

The heart should be completely exposed before cardiac arrest occurs. In addition, before arrest of the heart, the surgeon should determine the approximate location of the bypass sites. This is not always easy, but the old, occluded vein grafts may help in location of the sites for the distal anastomoses.

Warm Heart Surgery With a Ventricular Assist Device

For emergency coronary bypass procedures and for high-risk patients, we developed a surgical technique of warm heart surgery that avoids myocardial ischemia.[28] The technique can be used with or without an oxygenator. Originally, we unloaded the left ventricular cavity with a Hemopump (Johnson & Johnson Interventional Systems, Warren, NJ). We then created anastomoses to the empty, but beating, left ventricular vessels while the patient's lungs served as an oxygenator. After our first four operations, the Hemopump became unavailable. The Biomedicus continuous-flow pump (Eden Prairie, MN) may be used for CABG, but it is fairly cumbersome. We have used the ABIOMED temporary left ventricular assist device (Danvers, MA) to unload the ventricle while performing CABG in high-risk patients. Researchers are developing newer pumps, expressly designed for CABG, that may be applicable in the future.

The aorta is cannulated in the usual manner, as is the right atrium. Additional cannulae are placed near the bifur-

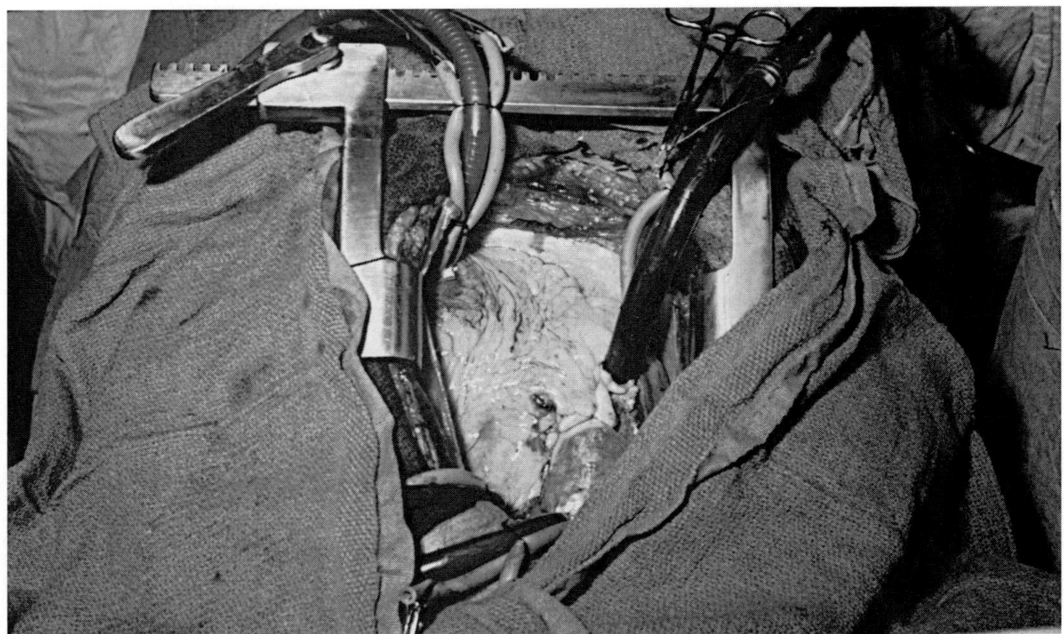

FIGURE 41–11 Completed setup for biventricular assistance during warm heart surgery without ischemic arrest.

cation of the pulmonary artery and at the apex of the left ventricle. Both right and left ventricular cannulae are then connected to separate Biomedicus continuous-flow pumps (Fig. 41–11). The Biomedicus pump is set at the maximum flow rate to bypass the ventricular cavities. Only minimal heparinization (1 to 1.5 mg/kg) is required because the patient's lungs are used as the oxygenator. Once the heart is satisfactorily decompressed, we administer a high dose of esmolol (a 10-mg/kg IV bolus, followed by a continuous infusion of 500 μg/kg/min) to further slow the heart rate. Esmolol, which clears rapidly, lowers vascular resistance and keeps the heart more flaccid. We also use an intraoperative autotransfusion device (Cell Saver; Cobe Laboratories, Inc., Lakewood, CA) to salvage blood during most operations.

At this point, CABG is performed in the usual manner. Once the proximal anastomoses are completed, flow through the Biomedicus pump is slowly decreased until decannulation can be achieved. If, however, native heart function is inadequate after the operation is completed, the left-sided cannulae can be left in place as a form of temporary ventricular assistance. In our experience, this step has rarely been required.

Minimally Invasive Coronary Artery Bypass Graft Surgery

Minimally invasive techniques have recently been introduced as a means of simplifying CABG and reducing morbidity rates. Minimally invasive coronary artery bypass graft surgery (MICABG) involves the use of a 7- to 10-cm skin incision (usually an anterior minithoracotomy) and may be performed on the beating heart, without the use of CPB.[49–51] In port-access procedures,[51–54] CPB may be used with the aid of multiple ports, peripheral cannulation, and video techniques, but the CPB time may be longer than that for conventional CABG. So far, MICABG has mainly been performed for bypass of the left anterior descending coronary or proximal right coronary artery. The circumflex and posterior descending coronary arteries, which lie on the far side of the heart, are difficult to access with current methods. As in conventional CABG, the internal mammary artery is the preferred bypass conduit.

We favor a ministernotomy technique,[55, 56] which is performed on the beating heart without CPB and is a safe, effective alternative to both conventional CABG and MICABG.

Technique

We perform a ministernotomy (division of only the lower part of the sternum, up to the manubrium) (Fig. 41–12A) or use a submammary approach (with or without division of costal cartilage). In a few patients, we extend the ministernotomy incision to one side, so as to form a T, by dividing the sternomanubrial junction to facilitate mobilization of the LIMA and RIMA, proximally. The heart rate is reduced to 40 to 60 beats/min with the intravenous administration of a beta blocker. Once the LIMA has been harvested (see Fig. 41–12B), the left anterior descending anastomosis is constructed with a single continuous 8-0 polypropylene suture (see Fig. 41–12C).

Our technique of bypassing the right coronary artery while off the pump, with the use of a reversed saphenous vein graft, has been described elsewhere.[57] Currently, a smaller incision is used for MICABG involving the RIMA or a reversed saphenous vein graft. In patients who have had previous CABG with bilateral internal mammary arteries, a reversed saphenous vein graft may be used to bypass

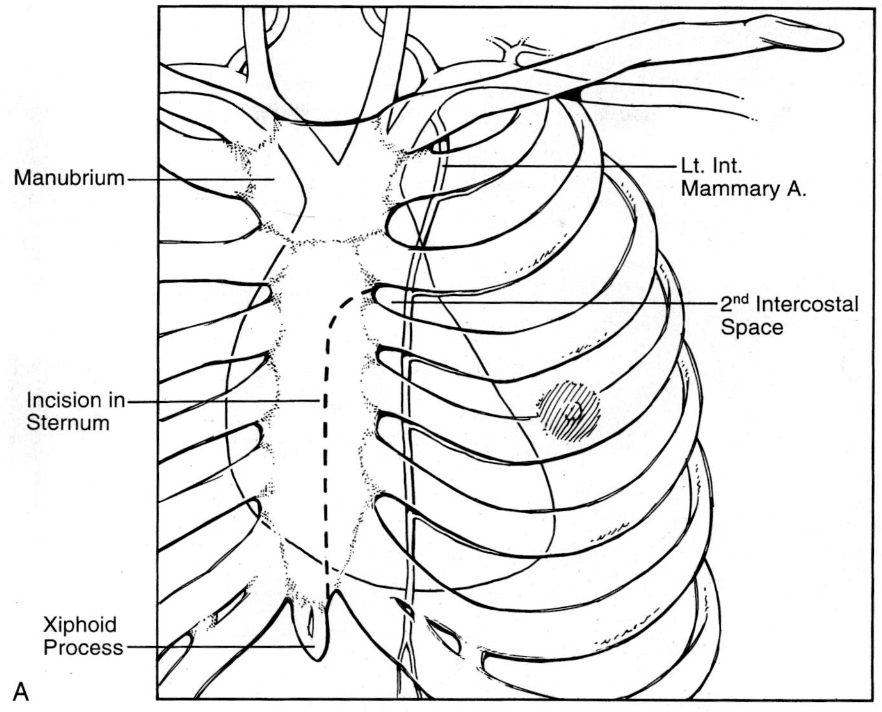

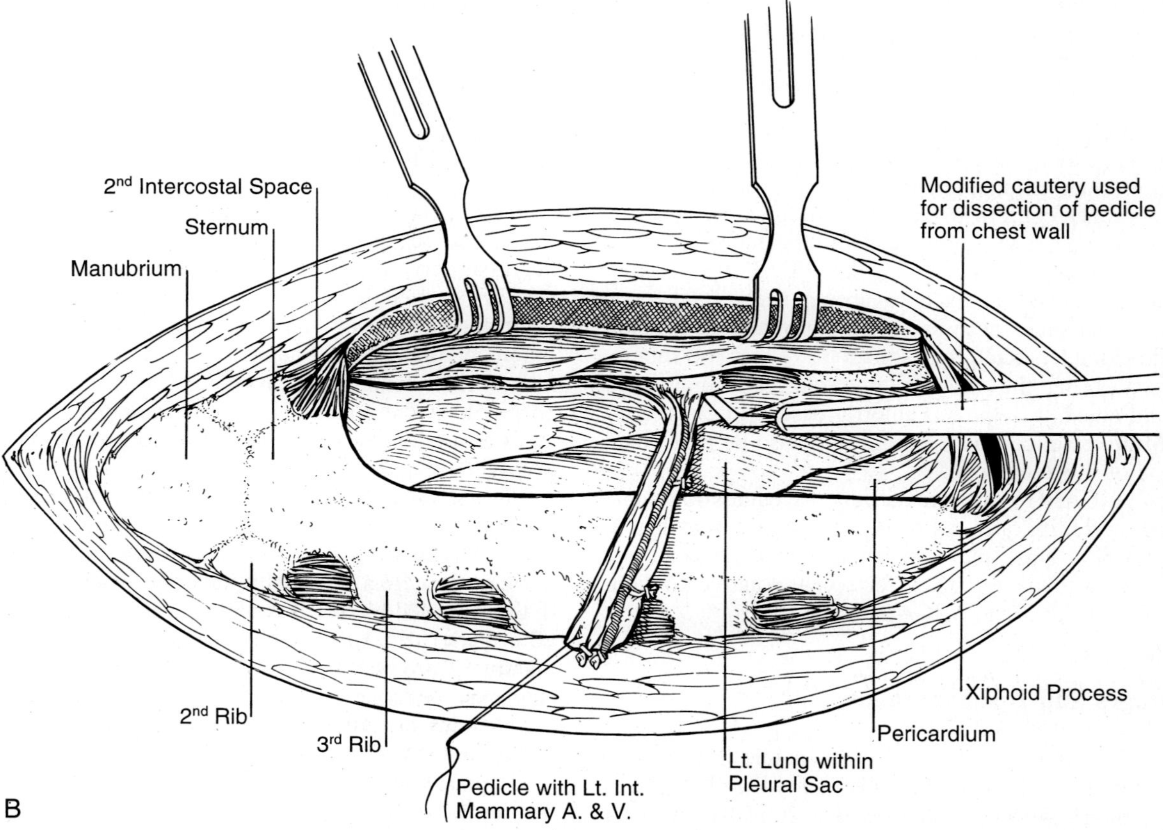

FIGURE 41–12 Coronary artery bypass of the LAD through a ministernotomy incision. **A,** The incision is extended to the second intercostal space. **B,** The IMA is mobilized with electrocautery.

Illustration continued on following page

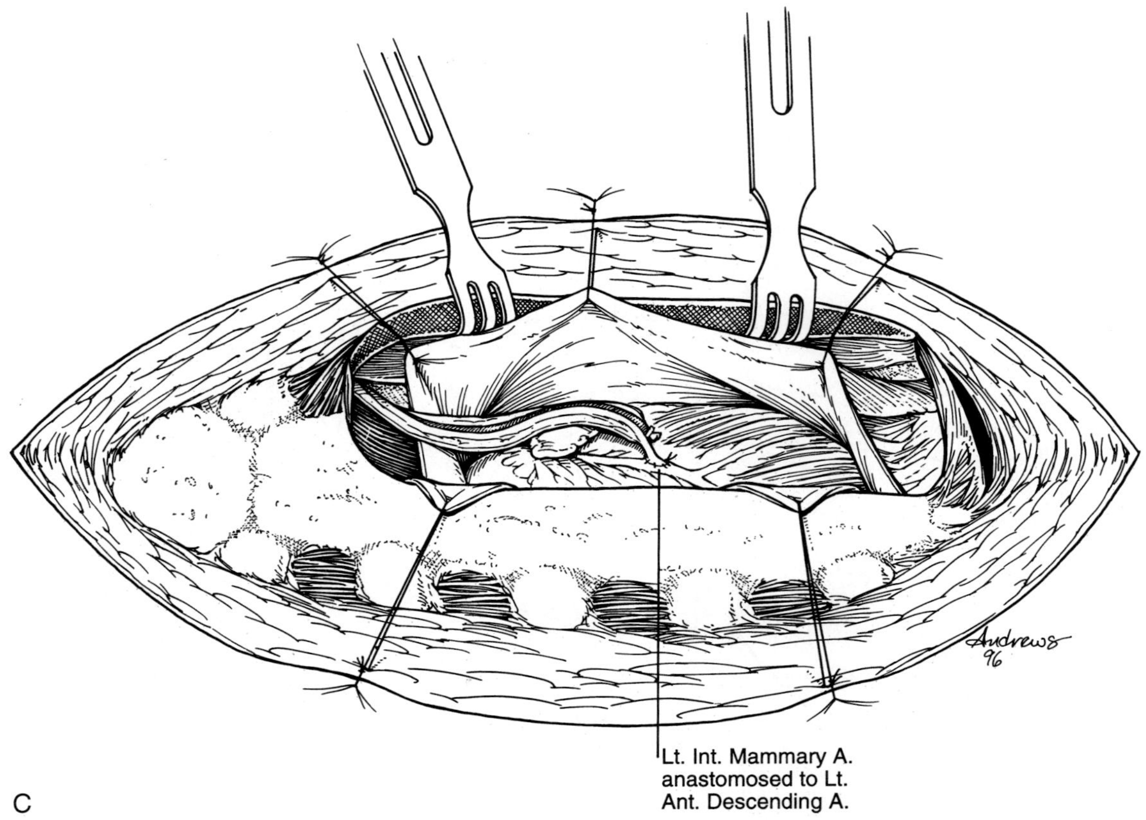

FIGURE 41–12 *Continued* **C,** The IMA is anastomosed to the LAD with a continuous 8-0 polypropylene suture.

the left anterior descending/right coronary artery from the left/right subclavian artery via an infraclavicular incision in addition to an inframammary incision during MICABG.

This approach confers an extra margin of safety because, if necessary, one may simply convert the incision into a conventional one and proceed with CPB. If the internal mammary artery is damaged or absent and a saphenous vein bypass becomes necessary, one can make an incision under the clavicle, attach the saphenous vein to the subclavian artery, bring the vein down through the intercostal space, and attach it to the left anterior descending coronary artery. Multivessel coronary bypass may also be performed by means of this technique.

Off-pump CABG via a ministernotomy entails low mortality and morbidity rates, a low need for blood transfusion, a short hospital stay, and a reasonable hospital cost. We have found it to be a safe, effective alternative to both conventional CABG and MICABG.

Advantages and Disadvantages

Because MICABG causes little hemodynamic disturbance, it can serve as an alternative means of myocardial protection for patients who have major risk factors and reduced ventricular function. In our experience, the myocardial protective effect of the beating heart in the absence of CPB has been reflected by the lack of intraoperative ventricular arrhythmias, reduced requirement for inotropic drugs, decreased incidence of postoperative arrhythmias, and early recovery.[55, 56] In our high-risk patients who have undergone MICABG, the operating time, blood loss, transfusion requirements, perioperative complications, ventilatory support, need for intensive care, and length of hospitalization have been acceptable. In patients who have had previous heart surgery, the epicardial adhesions seem to have a stabilizing effect locally, reducing the motion of the beating heart and facilitating anastomosis. Because cardiac cannulation and dissection of adhesions are unnecessary, manipulation of the heart can be avoided. These advantages markedly reduce the coagulopathy rate, amount of blood loss, and transfusion requirements in patients requiring reoperation.

Despite these advantages, the minimal access approach is applied to only 5 to 10 percent of patients undergoing CABG.[58] Creation of the anastomoses is technically more difficult through a minimally invasive incision, particularly if the diseased vessel is small, intramyocardial, diffusely atherosclerotic, or calcified. Dissection of the internal mammary artery may also be a challenge. Although this step may be done endoscopically, it involves the use of extra equipment that takes considerable time to manipulate. Other challenges may be posed by the presence of excessive epicardial fat. A survey of 162 cardiac surgeons[59] regarding the use of MICABG underscored concerns about the inferior quality of the anastomoses, unknown long-term outcome, and potentially high morbidity and mortality rates.

Some[60–63] advocate an integrated "hybrid" approach for selected patients with multivessel disease. In this two-stage

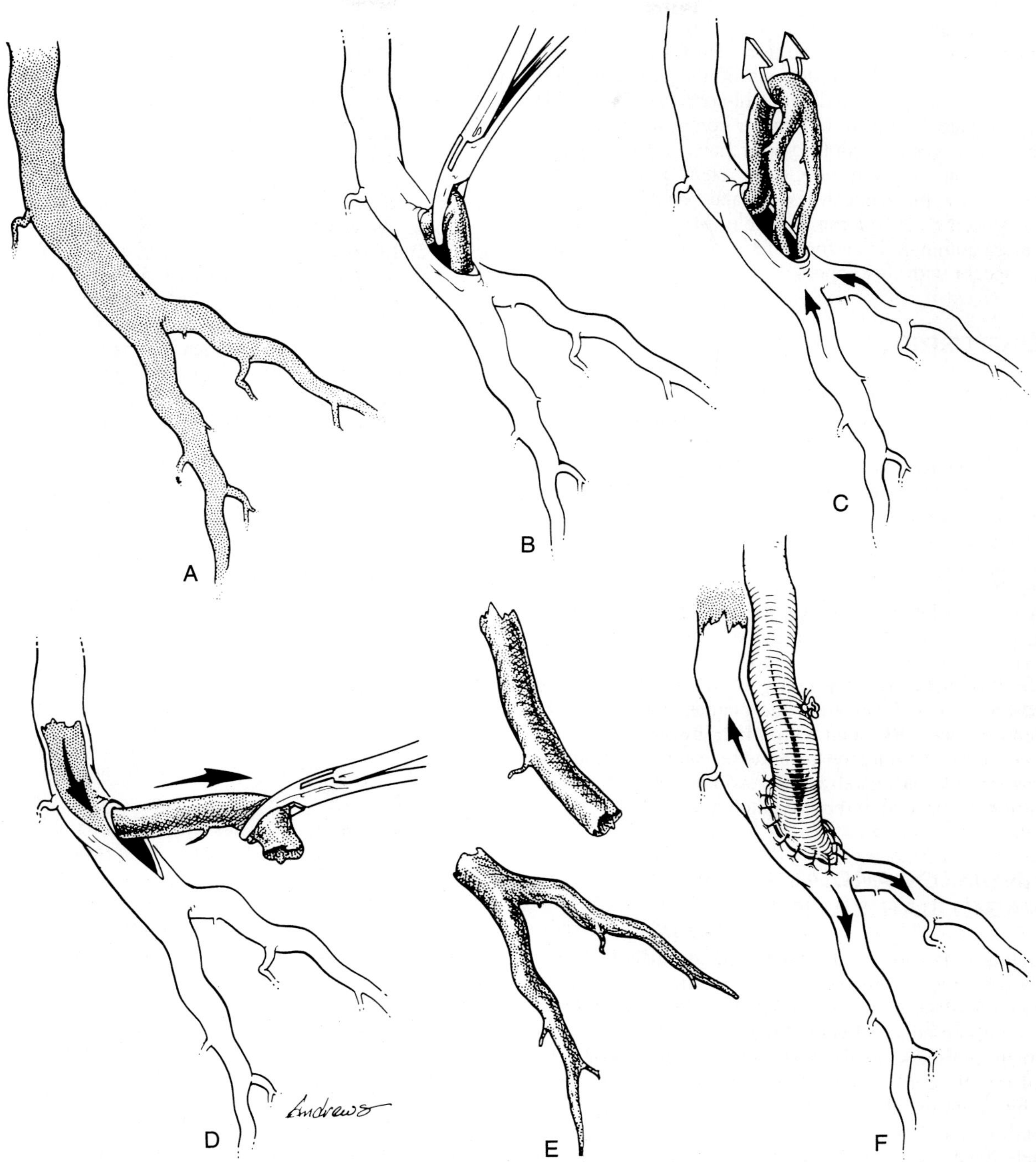

FIGURE 41–13 Technique for performing a right coronary endarterectomy. **A,** Occluded right coronary artery. **B,** Incision just above the crux. The core is brought out through the incision. Gentle traction is exerted on the distal portion while the artery is peeled back. **C** and **D,** The distal vessels should be cleared individually. The proximal portion is then removed by means of gentle traction until it breaks free from the proximal area. It is not important to obtain a clearly feathered proximal portion. **E,** A satisfactory specimen (i.e., the distal specimen and small branches have feathered ends). **F,** A vein graft is placed over the arteriotomy to ensure flow in both directions. (**A–F,** From Cooley DA: Revascularization of the ischemic myocardium. *In* Techniques in Cardiac Surgery. 2nd ed. pp. 221–258. Philadelphia: WB Saunders, 1984.)

approach, MICABG is used for left anterior descending/right coronary artery disease after PTCA/stenting of other coronary arteries has been performed. Both stages are completed during the same hospital admission.

We conclude that MICABG has a limited, but definite, role in the treatment of carefully selected patients. At our institution, it will continue to be indicated for patients with a calcific aorta or isolated stenosis of the left main, left anterior descending, or proximal right coronary artery. It is also appropriate for those with major comorbidities, a history of unsuccessful angioplasty, or recurrent coronary stenosis after one or more PTCA or stent procedures or CABG. As new mechanical devices and computer-assisted surgical systems[64, 65] become available, MICABG may become more common, even for patients with lesions that are hard to access with this approach.

Endarterectomy

Endarterectomy may be useful for improving the long-term patency of severely diseased and occluded coronary arteries, especially the left anterior descending coronary artery.[66–70] We have found endarterectomy to be most useful in two groups: patients with severely calcified vessels in which sutures cannot be satisfactorily placed and patients with such severe distal disease that an adequate lumen cannot be found. When performing an endarterectomy, the surgeon should make the incision as far proximal as possible. A proximal incision allows the endarterectomy to be performed with the least shearing effect on the smaller branches of the vessel (Fig. 41–13). Care must be taken not to pull on the plaque but rather to push the surrounding and attached tissue away from the plaque. An endarterectomy can also be performed with a long incision. The long incision allows the surgeon to remove plaque completely, both proximally and distally. After a long endarterectomy, however, the artery may require patching.

Transmyocardial Laser Revascularization

In patients with severe atherosclerotic occlusive disease that does not respond to conventional treatment, transmyocardial laser revascularization (TMLR) may be performed with or without concomitant CABG.[71–76] In TMLR, a laser instrument is used to drill a series of channels through the wall of the diseased left ventricle. This method appears to work by shunting blood from the left ventricle into the diseased myocardium. In extensive clinical trials, the laser channels have been strongly correlated with a subsequent long-term improvement in angina. However, because no causal relation has yet been established, the role and mechanism of TMLR are still debated.

The best candidates for TMLR are patients who have satisfactory systolic function, who lack severe arrhythmias, and whose predominant problem is angina unrelieved by conventional medical therapy. In most cases, TMLR has improved the patient's clinical status and exercise ability, but a corresponding improvement in overall cardiac function has been hard to document. Therefore, TMLR appears to increase the quality, rather than the length, of life. Although most experience has been gained with the carbon dioxide laser, clinical trials of TMLR with a holmium:yttrium aluminum garnet (Ho:YAG) laser are under way. Moreover, a catheter-based approach, with the Ho:YAG and xenon-chloride (excimer, Xe:CL) lasers, is also undergoing clinical evaluation.

Summary

In the final analysis, CABG remains an effective direct treatment for coronary artery occlusive disease. In 1996, about 598,000 bypass procedures were performed on 367,000 patients in the United States.[77] CABG has changed, however, as a result of the advent of balloon angioplasty; patients who now undergo CABG are older and sicker.[78] Nevertheless, the early mortality rate remains low, probably as a result of surgical experience and technical expertise. By means of the techniques described above, the mortality rates for CABG can be minimized, even in very-high-risk patients.

References

1. Garrett HE, Gartmill TB, Thiele JP, et al: Experimental evaluation of venous autografts as aorta to left ventricular myocardial shunts in revascularization of the heart: a preliminary report. Cardiovasc Res Center Bull 3:15, 1964.
2. Favaloro RG: Direct myocardial revascularization. Surg Clin North Am 51:1035, 1971.
3. Favaloro RG, Effler DB, Groves LK: Severe segmental obstruction of the left main coronary artery and its divisions: surgical treatment by the saphenous vein graft technic. J Thorac Cardiovasc Surg 60:469, 1970.
4. Johnson WD, Flemma RJ, Lepley D Jr, Ellison EH: Extended treatment of severe coronary artery disease: a total surgical approach. Ann Surg 170:460, 1969.
5. Hallman GL, Cooley DA, McNamara DG, et al: Single left coronary artery with fistula to right ventricle. Circulation 33:293, 1965.
6. Cooley DA, Frazier OH, Duncan JM, et al: Intracavitary repair of ventricular aneurysm and regional dyskinesia. Ann Surg 214:417, 1992.
7. Westaby S: Cardiopulmonary bypass for coronary artery surgery. *In* Buxton B, Frazier OH, Westaby S (eds): Ischemic Heart Disease: Surgical Management. pp. 103–112. London: Mosby, 1999.
8. Roach GW, Kanchuger M, Mangano CM, et al: Adverse cerebral outcomes after coronary bypass surgery. N Engl J Med 335:18, 1996.
9. Esmailian F, Athanasuleas CL, Buckberg GD: Myocardial preservation. *In* Buxton B, Frazier OH, Westaby S (eds): Ischemic Heart Disease: Surgical Management. pp. 113–119. London: Mosby, 1999.
10. Amrani M, Yacoub MH, Royston D: Myocardial protection for cardiac surgery: classical views and new trends. Int Anesthesiol Clin 37:39, 1999.
11. Beck CS, Stanton E, Batiuchok W, Leiter E: Revascularization of heart by graft of systemic artery into coronary sinus. JAMA 137:436, 1948.
12. Schlensak C, Doenst T, Beyersdorf F: Clinical experience with blood cardioplegia. Thorac Cardiovasc Surg 46(suppl 2):282, 1998.
13. Shiroishi MS: Myocardial protection: the rebirth of potassium-based cardioplegia. Tex Heart Inst J 26:71, 1999.
14. Kamlot A, Bellows SD, Simkhovich BZ, et al: Is warm retrograde blood cardioplegia better than cold for myocardial protection? Ann Thorac Surg 63:98, 1997.
15. Tofukuji M, Stamler A, Li J, et al: Comparative effects of continuous warm blood and intermittent cold blood cardioplegia on coronary reactivity. Ann Thorac Surg 64:1360, 1997.

16. Caputo M, Ascione R, Angelini GD, et al: The end of the cold era: from intermittent cold to intermittent warm blood cardioplegia. Eur J Cardiothorac Surg 14:467, 1998.
17. Jasinski M, Kadziola Z, Bachowski R, et al: Comparison of retrograde versus antegrade cold blood cardioplegia: randomized trial in elective coronary artery bypass patients. Eur J Cardiothorac Surg 12:620, 1997.
18. Louagie YA, Gonzalez E, Jamart J, et al: Assessment of continuous cold blood cardioplegia in coronary artery bypass grafting. Ann Thorac Surg 63:689, 1997.
19. Jacquet LM, Noirhomme PH, Van Dyck MJ, et al: Randomized trial of intermittent antegrade warm blood versus cold crystalloid cardioplegia. Ann Thorac Surg 67:471, 1999.
20. Casthely PA, Shah C, Mekhjian H, et al: Left ventricular diastolic function after coronary artery bypass grafting: a correlative study with three different myocardial protection techniques. J Thorac Cardiovasc Surg 114:254, 1997.
21. Arom KV, Emery RW, Petersen RJ, Bero JW: Evaluation of 7,000+ patients with two different routes of cardioplegia. Ann Thorac Surg 63:1619, 1997.
22. Aldea GS: Complementary use of antegrade and retrograde cardioplegia. Ann Thorac Surg 66:697, 1998.
23. Gates RN, Lee J, Laks H, et al: Evidence of improved microvascular perfusion when using antegrade and retrograde cardioplegia. Ann Thorac Surg 62:1388, 1996.
24. Tian G, Shen J, Sun J, et al: Does simultaneous antegrade/retrograde cardioplegia improve myocardial perfusion in the areas at risk? A magnetic resonance perfusion imaging study in isolated pig hearts. J Thorac Cardiovasc Surg 115:913, 1998.
25. Cernaianu AC, Flum DR, Maurer M, et al: Comparison of antegrade with antegrade/retrograde cold blood cardioplegia for myocardial revascularization. Tex Heart Inst J 23:9, 1996.
26. Honkonen EL, Kaukinen L, Pehkonen EJ, Kaukinen S: Combined antegrade-retrograde blood cardioplegia does not protect right ventricle better than either technique alone in patients with occluded right coronary artery. Scand Cardiovasc J 31:289, 1997.
27. Robinson LA, Schwartz GD, Goddard DB, et al: Myocardial protection for acquired heart disease surgery: results of a national survey. Ann Thorac Surg 59:361, 1995.
28. Sweeney MS, Frazier OH: Device-supported myocardial revascularization: safe help for sick hearts. Ann Thorac Surg 54:1065, 1992.
29. Lucchetti V, Caputo M, Suleiman MS, et al: Beating heart coronary revascularization without metabolic myocardial damage. Eur J Cardiothorac Surg 14:443, 1998.
30. Perrault LP, Menasche P, Peynet J, et al: On-pump, beating-heart coronary artery operations in high-risk patients: an acceptable trade-off? Ann Thorac Surg 64:1368, 1997.
31. Livesay JJ, Cooley DA: Which vessels should be grafted? *In* Wheatley D (ed): Surgery of Coronary Artery Disease. pp. 387–413. London: Chapman & Hall, 1986.
32. Jones EL, Craver JM, Guyton RA: Importance of complete revascularization in performance of the coronary bypass operation. Am J Cardiol 51:7, 1983.
33. Cooley DA: Revascularization of the ischemic myocardium. *In* Techniques of Cardiac Surgery. pp. 221–258. 2nd. ed. Philadelphia: WB Saunders, 1984.
34. Frazier OH, Sweeney MS, Radovancevic B, Cooley DA: Surgical treatment of heart disease (coronary artery surgery). *In* Willerson JT (ed): Treatment of Heart Diseases. pp. 6.3–6.12. New York: Gower Medical Publishing, 1992.
35. Takach TJ, Reul GJ Jr, Cooley DA, et al: Is an integrated approach warranted for concomitant carotid and coronary artery disease? Ann Thorac Surg 64:16, 1997.
36. Takach TJ, Reul GJ Jr, Cooley DA, et al: Concomitant occlusive disease of the coronary arteries and great vessels. Ann Thorac Surg 65:79, 1998.
37. Patel VS, Radovancevic B, Springer W, et al: Revascularization procedures in patients with transplant coronary artery disease. Eur J Cardiothorac Surg 11:895, 1997.
38. He GW: Arterial grafts for coronary artery bypass grafting: biological characteristics, functional classification, and clinical choice. Ann Thorac Surg 67:277, 1999.
39. Barner HB: Arterial grafting: techniques and conduits. Ann Thorac Surg 66(5 suppl):S2, 1998.
40. Reardon MJ, Conklin LD, Reardon PR, Baldwin JC: Coronary artery bypass conduits: review of current status. J Cardiovasc Surg (Torino) 38:201, 1997.
41. Ramos JR, Berger K, Mansfield PB, et al: Histological fate and endothelial changes of distended and nondistended vein grafts. Ann Surg 183:205, 1976.
42. Dougenis D, Brown AH: Long-term results of reoperations for recurrent angina with internal mammary artery versus saphenous vein grafts. Heart 80:9, 1998.
43. Lytle BW, Blackstone EH, Loop FD, et al: Two internal thoracic artery grafts are better than one. J Thorac Cardiovasc Surg 117:855, 1999.
44. Buxton B, Fuller J, Gaer J, et al: The radial artery as a bypass graft. Curr Opin Cardiol 11:591, 1996.
45. Buxton BF, Fuller JA, Tatoulis, J: Evolution of complete arterial grafting for coronary artery disease. Tex Heart Inst J 25:17, 1998.
46. Tatoulis J, Buxton BF, Fuller JA: Bilateral radial artery grafts in coronary reconstruction: technique and early results in 261 patients. Ann Thorac Surg 66:714, 1998.
47. Cooley DA: Coronary bypass grafting with bilateral internal thoracic arteries and the right gastroepiploic artery. Circulation 97:2384, 1998.
48. Bergsma TM, Grandjean JG, Voors AA, et al: Low recurrence of angina pectoris after coronary artery bypass graft surgery with bilateral internal thoracic and right gastroepiploic arteries. Circulation 97:2402, 1998.
49. Borst C, Santamore WP, Smedira NG, Bredee JJ: Minimally invasive coronary artery bypass grafting: on the beating heart and via limited access. Ann Thorac Surg 63(6 suppl):S1, 1997.
50. Mariani MA, Boonstra PW, Grandjean JG, et al: Minimally invasive coronary artery bypass grafting without cardiopulmonary bypass. Eur J Cardiothorac Surg 11:881, 1997.
51. Reichenspurner H, Boehm DH, Welz A, et al: Minimally invasive coronary artery bypass grafting: port-access approach versus off-pump techniques. Ann Thorac Surg 66:1036, 1998.
52. Galloway AC, Shemin RJ, Glower DD, et al: First report of the Port Access International Registry. Ann Thorac Surg 67:51, 1999.
53. Groh MA: Post-access coronary artery bypass grafting: technical strategies for multivessel complete revascularization. J Card Surg 13:297, 1998.
54. Reichenspurner H, Welz A, Gulielmos V, et al: Port-access cardiac surgery using endovascular cardiopulmonary bypass: theory, practice, and results. J Card Surg 13:275, 1998.
55. Talwalkar NG, Cooley DA, Ott DA, Livesay JJ: Limited-access coronary artery bypass grafting: the Texas Heart Institute experience. Tex Heart Inst J 25:175, 1998.
56. Talwalkar NG, Cooley DA: Minimally invasive coronary artery bypass grafting: a review. Cardiol Rev 6:345, 1998.
57. Favaloro RG: Current status of coronary artery bypass graft (CABG) surgery. Semin Thorac Cardiovasc Surg 6:67, 1994.
58. Cooley DA: Potential pitfalls of minimally invasive coronary artery bypass grafting. Cardiovasc Rev Rep (in press).
59. Shennib H, Mack MJ, Lee AGL: A survey on minimally invasive coronary artery bypass grafting. Ann Thorac Surg 64:110, 1997.
60. Angelini GD, Wilde P, Salerno TA, et al: Integrated anterior small thoracotomy and angioplasty for multivessel coronary artery revascularization. Lancet 347:757, 1996.
61. Calafiore AM, Angelini GD, Bergsland J, Salerno TA: Minimally invasive coronary artery bypass grafting. Ann Thorac Surg 62:1545, 1996.
62. Westaby S, Benetti F: Less invasive coronary surgery: consensus from the Oxford meeting. Ann Thorac Surg 62:924, 1996.
63. Subramanian VA: Less invasive arterial CABG on a beating heart. Ann Thorac Surg 63:S68, 1997.
64. Loulmet D, Carpentier A, d'Attellis N, et al: Endoscopic coronary artery bypass grafting with the aid of robotic assisted instruments. J Thorac Cardiovasc Surg 118:4, 1999.
65. Reichenspurner H, Damiano RJ, Mack M, et al: Use of the voice-controlled and computer-assisted surgical system Zeus for endoscopic coronary artery bypass grafting. J Thorac Cardiovasc Surg 118:11, 1999.
66. Asimakopoulos G, Taylor KM, Ratnatunga CP: Outcome of coronary endarterectomy: a case-control study. Ann Thorac Surg 67:989, 1999.
67. Plestis KA, Ke S, Jiang ZD, Howell JF: Combined carotid endarterectomy and coronary artery bypass: immediate and long-term results. Ann Vasc Surg 13:84, 1999.

68. Riggs PN, DeWeese JA: Carotid endarterectomy. Surg Clin North Am 78:881, 1998.
69. Dagenais F, Cartier R, Farinas JM, et al: Coronary endarterectomy revisited: mid-term angiographic results. Can J Cardiol 14:1121, 1998.
70. Mills NL: Coronary endarterectomy: surgical techniques for patients with extensive distal atherosclerotic coronary disease. Adv Card Surg 10:197, 1998.
71. Frazier OH, Kadipasaoglu KA, Cooley DA: Transmyocardial laser revascularization: does it have a role in the treatment of ischemic heart disease? Tex Heart Inst J 25:24, 1998.
72. Frazier OH, Kadipasaoglu KA: Transmyocardial laser revascularization as a new therapeutic option for refractory coronary artery occlusive disease. Eur Heart J 19:1420, 1998.
73. Frazier OH, Kadipasaoglu KA, Radovancevic B, et al: Transmyocardial laser revascularization in allograft coronary artery disease. Ann Thorac Surg 65:1138, 1998.
74. Schoebel FC, Frazier OH, Jesserun GA, et al: Refractory angina pectoris in end-stage coronary artery disease: evolving therapeutic concepts. Am Heart J 134:587, 1997.
75. Cooley DA, Frazier OH, Kadipasaoglu K, et al: Transmyocardial laser revascularization: clinical experience with 12-month follow-up. J Thorac Cardiovasc Surg 111:791, 1996.
76. Horvath KA, Cohn LH, Cooley DA, et al: Transmyocardial laser revascularization: results of a multicenter trial with transmyocardial laser revascularization used as sole therapy for end-stage coronary artery disease. J Thorac Cardiovasc Surg 113:645, 1997.
77. American Heart Association: 1999 Heart and Stroke Statistical Update. Retrieved July 1, 1999, from the World Wide Web: http://www.americanheart.org/statistics/09medicl.html.
78. Naunheim K, Fiore AC, Wadley JJ, et al: The changing profile of the patient undergoing coronary artery bypass surgery. J Am Coll Cardiol 11:494, 1988.

CHAPTER 42

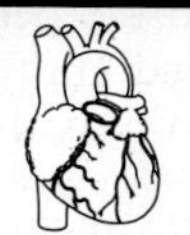

Coronary Artery Bypass Surgery and Percutaneous Coronary Intervention: Impact on Morbidity and Mortality in Patients With Coronary Artery Disease

James M. Wilson, James J. Ferguson, and Robert J. Hall

REVASCULARIZATION FOR CORONARY ARTERY DISEASE
History
Trials
Techniques
Summary of Surgical Bypass Trials
NONSURGICAL INTERVENTIONAL THERAPY FOR CORONARY ARTERY DISEASE
History
Trials Comparing PTCA to Medical Therapy
Trials Comparing PTCA to Coronary Bypass Surgery
The Impact of Diabetes Mellitus
The Natural History of a Balloon-Dilated Vessel
Stents
NONRANDOMIZED DATA
ACUTE CORONARY SYNDROMES
Surgery
Percutaneous Revascularization
TREATMENT OF SAPHENOUS VEIN GRAFT DISEASE
CONCLUSIONS

The goals of therapy for ischemic cardiovascular disease are to improve the physiologic consequences of myocardial ischemia (e.g., angina, heart failure) and to prevent the catastrophic events that may result from the evolution of coronary artery lesions (e.g., myocardial infarction or sudden death). Symptoms such as angina and heart failure and the chance of dying as a result of coronary atherosclerosis are clearly related to the amount of myocardium with nutrient blood flow that has been jeopardized by a coronary artery lesion and to the severity of limitation of the blood flow. Therefore, the ideal treatment for coronary atherosclerosis must prevent the progression of atherosclerotic lesions and must relieve coronary stenosis to restore normal myocardial perfusion.

For a large proportion of patients with symptomatic coronary artery disease, achieving the goals of therapy requires a strategy of medical therapy that affects the progression of atherosclerosis combined with mechanical therapy that treats existing, flow-limiting coronary lesions. Antianginal therapy reduces myocardial blood flow requirements, and medical therapy, such as administering aspirin and lowering cholesterol intake, reduces the risk of myocardial infarction; however, neither is able to normalize myocardial blood flow. Coronary bypass surgery and percutaneous angioplasty are safe, effective, and commonly used methods that improve myocardial perfusion and relieve the symptoms of myocardial ischemia. This chapter summarizes the development of these two procedures and their current place in the treatment of ischemic heart disease.

Revascularization for Coronary Artery Disease

History

The first suggestion that surgical therapy could be used to treat angina pectoris is attributed to François-Franck,[1, 2] a professor of physiology in Paris, who studied the effects on vascular structures of sympathetic nerve manipulations. In 1899, he suggested that interruption of the sympathetic fibers supplying the thorax would successfully eliminate angina. Indeed, sympathectomy, which interrupts sensory nerve fibers, was effective in relieving discomfort for many patients, and for a time the procedure enjoyed some measure of popularity, but symptom relief did not correlate with a beneficial impact on the course of disease.

From the end of the 18th century, coronary artery obstruction was recognized as the most probable source of angina pectoris.[2] Unfortunately, there appeared to be few options for therapy, save rest or perhaps sympathectomy, until Alexis Carrel[3] proposed the idea of vascular bypass. His pioneering work in developing methods of vascular anastomosis would set the stage for the eventual success of coronary bypass surgery. Claude Beck[4, 5] attempted a number of unsuccessful procedures to influence myocardial perfusion, including grafting a pedicle of pectoral muscle to the pericardium, obstructing coronary venous drainage, and grafting an artery from the aorta to the coronary sinus to provide retrograde blood flow.[4]

In 1945, Vineberg[6] proposed insertion of the internal mammary artery into ischemic myocardium, a procedure that would come to bear his name. He felt that the internal mammary artery, placed in this way, would create its own anastomoses with the rich network of small intramyocardial vessels.[6] His idea proved to have merit but was impractical for complete myocardial revascularization. It was soon abandoned in favor of coronary endarterectomy and later, aortocoronary bypass.

In 1958, Sones and associates[7, 8] performed the first selective coronary angiogram. This procedure vastly improved understanding of the natural history of coronary atherosclerosis and lit the way for successful revascularization of the heart. Prior to the development of selective coronary arteriography, the diagnosis of coronary atherosclerosis was made on clinical grounds, with objective confirmation being obtained through electrocardiography and exercise testing. Symptoms or signs prompting a diagnosis of coronary artery disease were associated with a survival expectation of about 10 years. There were few methods of improving prognosis estimation or of altering this natural history, and the obstacles to be overcome in improving myocardial perfusion in an individual patient were little more than guesswork.

Observational data derived from numerous patients undergoing coronary angiography revealed that a diagnosis of coronary artery disease made clinically is not invariably accompanied by severe coronary obstruction. Conversely, severe coronary obstruction may exist in the presence of deceivingly minor symptoms.[9, 10] Sones and coworkers[9, 10] showed that the most accurate diagnosis and estimate of prognosis could be obtained by performing selective coronary angiography. Using a rough estimate of disease severity (the number of major vessel regions with severe stenosis; Fig. 42–1) in combination with a similarly rough estimate of ventricular systolic function (normal, localized scar, or diffuse scar; Fig. 42–2), distinct populations with high, intermediate, or low risk of dying could be identified. The 5-year cardiac mortality rate ranged from 7 percent in patients with disease in only one vessel and normal ventricular function to 100 percent in those with left main coronary stenosis and severe contractile dysfunction[9, 10] (see Fig. 42–2). In addition to diagnostic and prognostic information, coronary angiography allowed detailed planning of surgical revascularization efforts.

Meanwhile, vascular surgeons who were frustrated by the limitations of coronary endarterectomy were returning to Carrel's idea of vascular bypass.[11] In 1962, David Sabiston[12] performed the first aorta-to–coronary artery bypass graft (CABG) surgery using a reversed segment of the greater saphenous vein. Although the patient died of a postoperative cerebrovascular accident, the bypass technique was considered successful. Two years later, the first

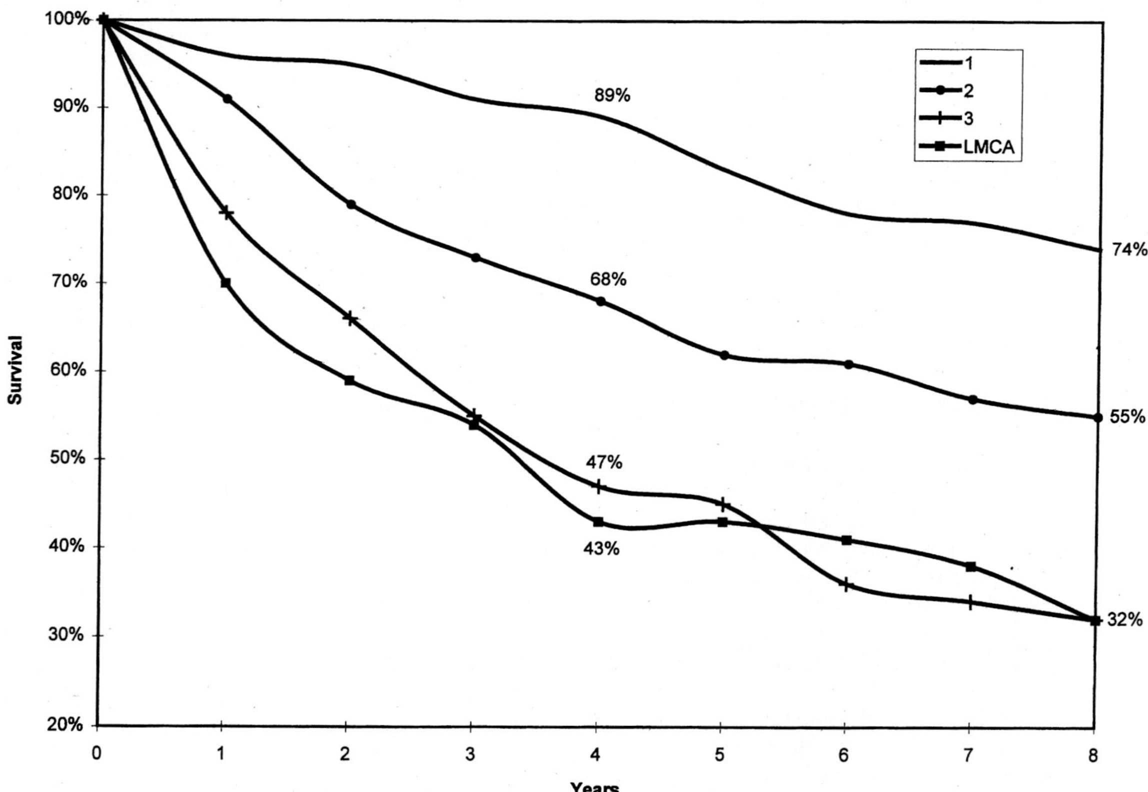

FIGURE 42–1 Survival according to number of major vessels diseased. In one of the first studies of its kind, Sones and coworkers described the natural history of coronary atherosclerosis. When patients were classified according to the number of major epicardial coronary arteries with severe stenosis, distinctly separate survival curves were seen; three-vessel and left main coronary artery (LMCA) stenosis displayed the worst prognosis. (From Bruschke AV, Proudfit WL, Sones FM Jr: Progress study of 590 consecutive nonsurgical cases of coronary disease followed 5–9 years. I. Arteriographic correlations. Circulation 47:1147–1153, 1973.)

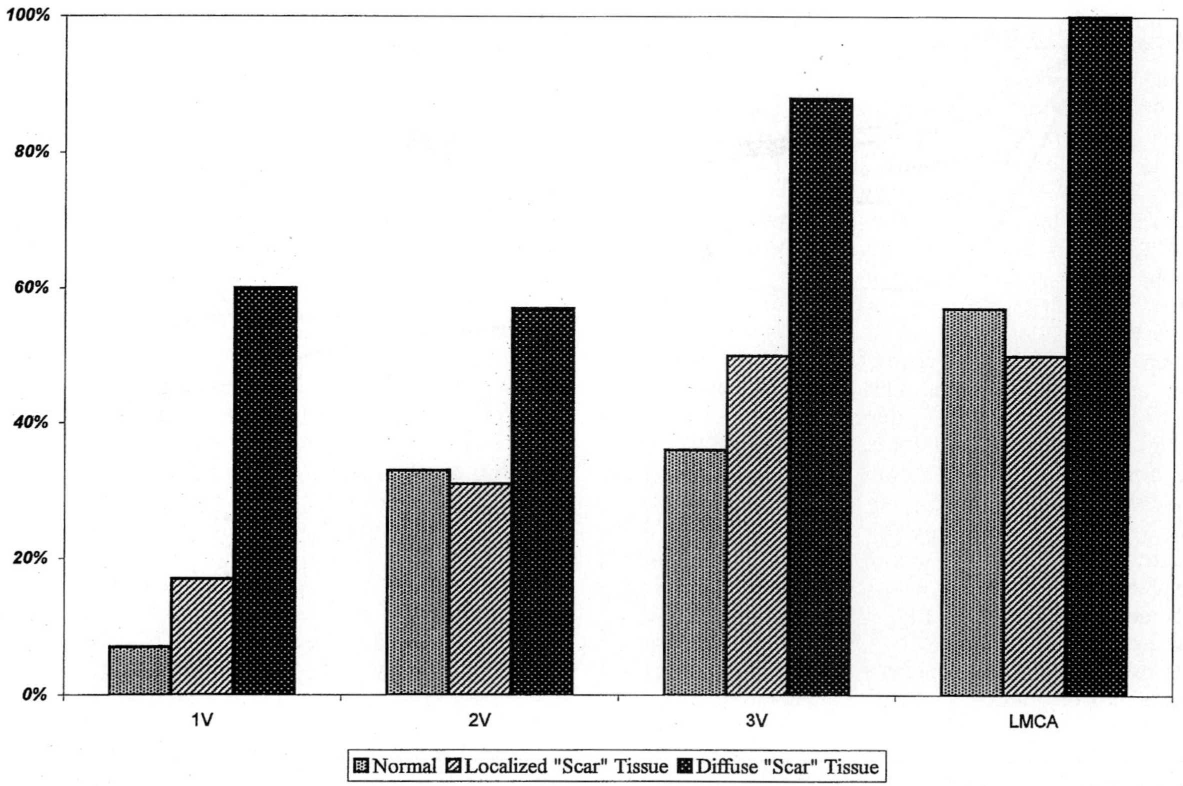

FIGURE 42–2 Survival according to number of major vessels diseased and left ventricular function. In addition to the number of major vessels with severe stenosis, the severity of left ventricular dysfunction proved to be a powerful predictor of 5-year survival in the population studied by Sones and coworkers. Left ventricular function remains one of the most useful measures for estimating prognosis in patients with ischemic heart disease. LMCA, left main coronary artery; V, vessel. (From Bruschke AV, Proudfit WL, Sones FM Jr: Progress study of 590 consecutive nonsurgical cases of coronary disease followed 5–9 years. II. Ventriculographic and other correlations. Circulation 47:1154–1163, 1973.)

completely successful aortocoronary saphenous vein graft procedure would go virtually unnoticed, performed as a result of a complicated endarterectomy.[13] Coronary bypass surgery using a reversed saphenous vein graft proved to be a practical revascularization procedure that could be performed with an acceptable risk. Its place in therapy quickly became a matter of discord among clinicians, many of whom were concerned about the procedural risk and troubled by the memory of sympathectomy and the ill-conceived internal mammary artery ligation procedure. Despite such arguments, supporters of the procedure such as René Favaloro and colleagues[14–16] perfected the use of reversed saphenous vein grafts for coronary revascularization and began treating multivessel disease.

Coronary bypass surgery was very effective in providing relief from angina pectoris. When observational studies similar to those reported by Sones and coworkers[9, 10] were repeated in the coronary bypass population, the first evidence of an impact on the natural history of coronary atherosclerosis was obtained (Fig. 42–3).[17–20] After coronary bypass surgery, the survival curves for each category of disease severity, which had been distinctly different, were almost superimposed on one another. Patients with coronary atherosclerosis of all grades of severity enjoyed a survival expectation somewhere between the previously reported values for unoperated patients with one- and two-vessel disease.

Many physicians questioned the accuracy of observational studies and called for randomized trials comparing surgical with medical therapy. Three large randomized trials were performed to assess the efficacy of surgical revascularization (Table 42–1). These landmark studies provided the first incontrovertible evidence that could guide decisions about revascularization. However, their data are frequently misinterpreted and misquoted. These trials compare two philosophies of therapy for coronary occlusive disease—referring patients for revascularization rather than medical management on recognition of disease and reserving revascularization for patients with unacceptable symptom control. The trials are not true comparisons between surgical therapy and medical therapy for coronary artery disease. In each study, patients assigned to the medical arm were allowed to undergo coronary bypass surgery if they or their physicians deemed it necessary. This is especially important when considering that at a time of apparent superiority of surgery over medicine for specific subgroups, between one third and slightly less than one half of the patients in the medical arm underwent coronary bypass surgery.

Trials

The Veterans Affairs Cooperative Study Trial

The Department of Veterans Affairs (VA) Cooperative Study of Coronary Artery Bypass Surgery was the first

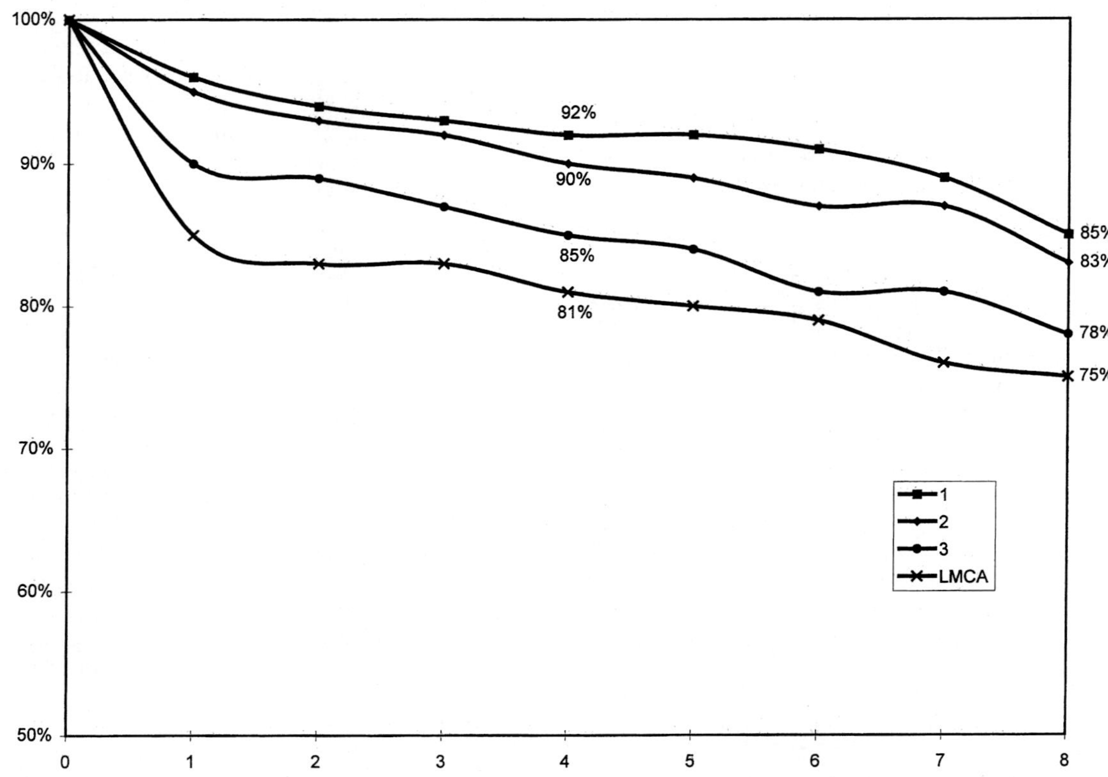

FIGURE 42–3 Survival according to number of major vessels diseased: the effect of surgical revascularization. One of several observational studies of the impact of surgical revascularization on patients with coronary disease, this study from Texas Heart Institute repeated the natural history study of Sones and coworkers in patients who had undergone bypass surgery. Survival over a period of 8 years is still stratified by disease severity, but survival in the most severely affected patients is markedly different from that reported by Sones and coworkers. This was among the first studies to establish a survival benefit of revascularization, and it suggested that angiographic risk stratification would be useful in identifying which patients would realize that benefit. LMCA, left main coronary artery. (Data from Hall RJ, Garcia E, Wukasch DC, et al: Long-term results of coronary artery bypass. Tex Heart Inst J 3:22–31, 1976.)

TABLE 42-1 The Three Major Surgery Trials

	VA						CASS		ECSS	
Number	686						780		768	
Date	72–74						74–79		73–76	
Angina										
Asymptomatic	0						26%		0	
Mild/moderate	42%						74%		57%	
Lesion requirement	≥50%						≥70%		≥50%	
Ejection fraction	>35%						>30%		>50%	
Operative mortality rate	5.8%						1.4%		3.3%	
	11 yr		**18 yr**		**22 yr**		**10 yr**		**12 yr**	
Survival M/S	M	S	M	S	M	S	M	S	M	S
All patients	58	58	33	30	25	20	79	82	67	71‡
2-Vessel disease	69	55	34	30	31†	24†	83	88	*	*NS
3-Vessel disease	50	56	32	25	—	—	75	76	68	78§
3-Vessel disease with low LVEF	39	51 ‡	21	24	11	12	57	75	—	—

Abbreviations: CASS, Coronary Artery Surgery Study[28]; ECSS, European Coronary Surgery Study[30]; LVEF, left ventricular ejection fraction; M, medical therapy; S, surgical therapy; VA, Veterans Affairs Cooperative Study of Surgery.[22, 23, 26]
*Number not reported, difference not statistically significant.
†Not high risk.
‡$P < .05$.
§$P = .01$.

large-scale randomized trial of CABG versus medical therapy. Between 1972 and 1974, 686 male patients with symptomatic coronary artery disease were enrolled in the study and randomized to either medical or surgical therapy (see Table 42–1). To qualify for the study, patients were required to have had stable angina for 6 months, including a 3-month trial of medical management, electrocardiographic evidence of a previous myocardial infarction or ischemic changes at rest or with exercise, and at least 50 percent diameter stenosis of at least one major coronary artery. Patients who were randomized to medical therapy were not prohibited from later bypass grafting if it was deemed necessary.[21] Follow-up after 22 years revealed that 66 percent of patients assigned to the medical therapy arm had undergone coronary bypass surgery.[22]

Almost 10 percent of patients randomized to initial surgical intervention suffered a perioperative myocardial infarction, and almost 6 percent died. However, surgery provided more complete relief of symptoms than did medical therapy, and by 2½ years, a survival benefit was apparent in patients with left main coronary artery stenosis.[23–25] Patients classified as being at high risk (stenosis of the three main vessel regions and an ejection fraction < 50 percent) had improved survival that was maximal at about 7 to 11 years as a result of early surgical bypass.[23, 26]

Extended follow-up revealed equalization of the two therapeutic philosophies.[22, 23] Actually, by 7 years, the benefit of surgery for symptom control began to diminish, becoming equal to medical therapy by 10 years.[24] The effect on survival followed suit: The two groups showed equal results at 18 years, and there was actually the suggestion of a harmful effect of early surgery at 22 years (Fig. 42–4).[22, 23] This was true even for the group of patients classified as high angiographic risk (survival 20 percent medical versus 15 percent surgical at 22 years). Freedom from myocardial infarction was marginally higher for the medically assigned group (51 percent surgical versus 59 percent medical) at 18 years and became significant at 22 years (41 percent surgical versus 57 percent medical).[22, 23] A strategy of early surgical referral was associated with a greater number of revascularization procedures without a survival benefit at 22 years (medical survival 25 percent versus surgical survival 20 percent, *P* = NS [not significant]). Patients with low angiographic risk randomized to early coronary bypass using only reversed saphenous vein grafts appeared to suffer an increased long-term mortality in comparison to their peers for whom surgical therapy was deferred.[22]

Angiographic follow-up studies demonstrated that atherosclerosis progressed much faster in the saphenous vein graft than in native coronary vessels.[23] At 1, 5, and 10 years, angiographic patency rates were 71 percent, 64 percent, and 50 percent, respectively. The observed decline in survival benefit with early surgery and increased late event rate mirrored saphenous vein graft behavior. Therefore, the VA trial, although beset by high operative mortality rates,

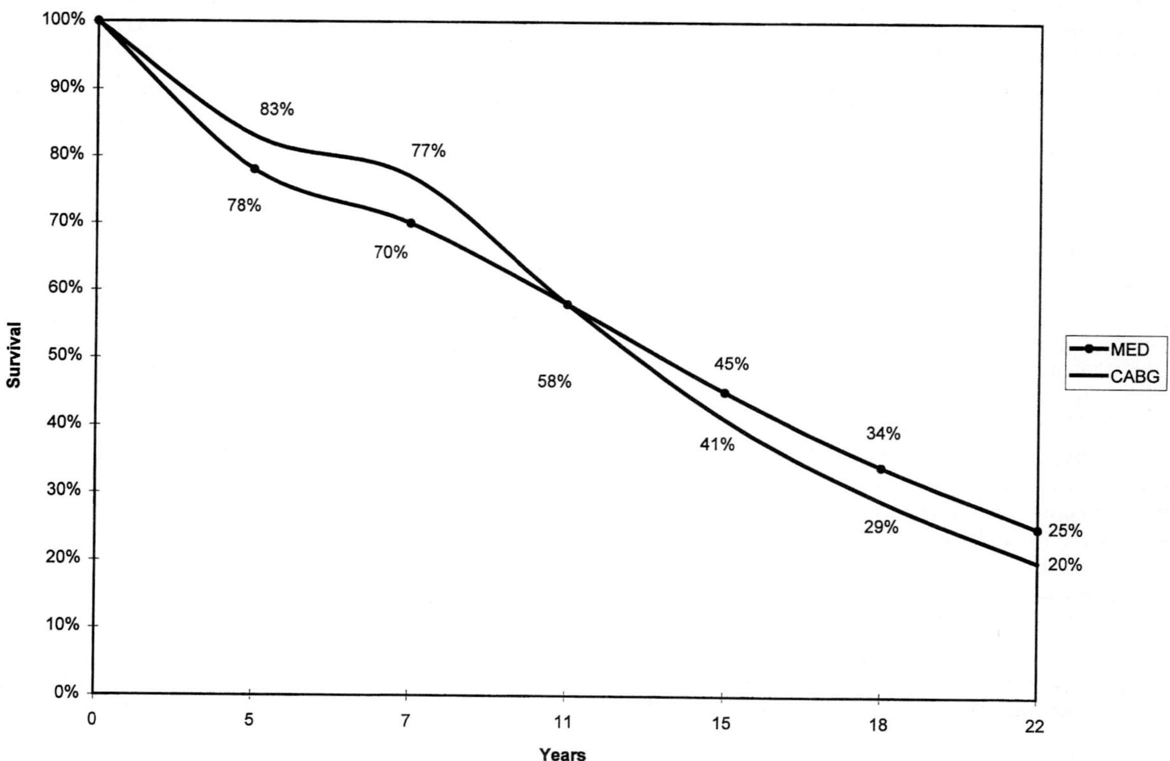

FIGURE 42–4 Veterans Affairs (VA) Cooperative Study trial: 22-year follow-up. The VA randomized trial established that surgical revascularization could improve the survival rate of patients with the most severe coronary disease. As the survival curves show, the temporary benefit of surgical revascularization gives way to an increased late hazard as saphenous vein graft atherosclerosis appears, resulting in myocardial infarction and the need for repeat revascularization procedures. CABG, coronary artery bypass graft; MED, medical therapy. (Reprinted from Am J Cardiol, Vol. 81, Peduzzi P, Kamina A, Detre K, Twenty-two-year follow-up in the VA Cooperative Study of Coronary Artery Bypass Surgery for Stable Angina, pp. 1393–1399, Copyright 1998, with permission from Excerpta Medica Inc.)

established that surgical revascularization in patients with clinically stable, symptomatic coronary artery disease temporarily improved the symptoms of coronary ischemia in most patients and survival of specific groups of patients (i.e., those with the most severe disease). Long-term follow-up data emphasize the merely palliative nature of revascularization procedures using the reversed saphenous vein graft because of its susceptibility to atherosclerosis and also the value of delaying surgical therapy when possible.

Coronary Artery Surgery Study

In 1974, the Coronary Artery Surgery Study (CASS) was initiated to compare the results of an initial strategy of surgical bypass combined with medical therapy versus medical therapy alone for the treatment of coronary artery disease accompanied by mild or no symptoms (see Table 42–1).[27, 28] The CASS consisted of two parts: a 15-center observational registry and an 11-center randomized trial. In order to be included in the study, patients had to have stenosis of more than 70 percent of the diameter of one or more coronary arteries. Exclusion criteria were Canadian Cardiovascular Society class 3 or 4 angina severity, prior coronary bypass surgery, age of more than 65 years, left main coronary artery stenosis of 70 percent or more, a left ventricular ejection fraction (LVEF) of less than 35 percent overt heart failure, and shock. The number of patients enrolled in the registry between July 1974 and May 1979 was 24,959; of those patients, 16,626 were considered to be candidates for participation in the randomized trial. After baseline coronary angiography, 2099 patients were offered the opportunity to participate; 780 agreed and were randomized to immediate surgery or to medical treatment.

Perioperative infarction occurred in 6.4 percent of the patients. Perioperative mortality was 1.4 percent. Analysis of 10 year follow-up data revealed that although surgery improved symptoms, there was no difference in cumulative survival (79 percent medical versus 82 percent surgical) or event-free survival (69 percent medical, 66 percent surgical).[28] Of the 390 patients randomized to the medical treatment strategy, 6 percent crossed over to surgery within 6 months; the percentage increased to 40 percent by 10 years (22 percent with single-vessel disease, 42 percent with double-vessel disease, and 53 percent with triple-vessel disease). Subgroup analysis uncovered significant benefits of a surgical strategy in specific patient populations, similar to the results of previously reported observational data (see Table 42–1). Patients with an LVEF of less than 50 percent benefited from early surgical referral, with a survival of 79 percent versus 61 percent among those who had had medical therapy. Patients with a combination of three-vessel disease and an LVEF of less than 50 percent saw the greatest benefit in terms of survival. Conversely, patients with an LVEF greater than 50 percent did better when surgery was reserved for the treatment of unacceptable symptoms (event-free survival was 75 percent with medical therapy versus 68 percent with surgery).

The CASS added to the findings of the VA cooperative trial by establishing that symptoms are an unreliable guide to disease severity and the need for revascularization. Severe disease marked by the presence of multivessel coronary stenosis and depressed left ventricular systolic function identified patients who benefited from revascularization regardless of their symptom control.[28]

The European Coronary Surgery Study

In the European Coronary Surgery Study (ECSS), 767 men under the age of 65 with mild or moderate angina and normal or minimally abnormal left ventricular function (Table 42–1) were randomized at 12 clinical centers to either medical or surgical treatment.[29, 30] To qualify for this study, patients had to have luminal diameter narrowing of 50 percent or more in at least two major coronary arteries and to have had symptoms for at least 3 months. The primary endpoints measured were symptoms, functional status, and survival.

Perioperative mortality was 3.2 percent. At 5 years there was a significantly higher survival rate in the surgical treatment group (92.4 percent versus 83.1 percent in the medical group).[29, 30] During the next 7 years of follow-up, mortality advanced somewhat more rapidly in the surgical group than in the medical group, although survival at 12 years favored the surgical group (70.6 percent versus 66.7 percent in the medical group). A total of 136 patients (36 percent) in the medical group had crossed over to surgery. There were 39 patients in the surgical group who required second operations, and 5 patients who required third operations.[30]

In addition to an overall beneficial effect of surgical bypass, the ECSS revealed the predictive power of physiologic testing (Fig. 42–5) and emphasized the importance of proximal stenosis of the left anterior descending coronary artery. In-depth analysis of the effect of coronary artery anatomy on survival revealed an insufficient power to detect a difference in survival in patients with left main coronary artery stenosis. A survival benefit was clear in patients with three vessel disease. When patients with and without proximal left anterior descending artery stenosis were compared, disease in this location seemed to have a detrimental effect on survival and to predict benefit from surgical revascularization. However, many of the patients with proximal left anterior descending artery stenosis had disease in all three major vessel regions. When multivariate analysis was performed, the impact of proximal left anterior descending artery stenosis still appeared to be important but did not reach statistical significance ($P = .07$).[30]

Meta-Analysis of Coronary Bypass Surgery Trials

The combined data of six major randomized studies that compared CABG and medical therapy in a total of 2499 patients have been studied.[31] Of those patients, 21 percent had an abnormal LVEF (less than 50 percent), 10 percent had single-vessel disease, 32 percent had two-vessel disease, 51 percent had three-vessel disease, and 7 percent had left main coronary artery disease. The internal mammary artery was used for only 10 percent of bypass grafts.

Early referral for surgical therapy provided a 33 percent reduction in 7-year mortality compared with medical therapy and provided a 70 percent reduction in mortality for

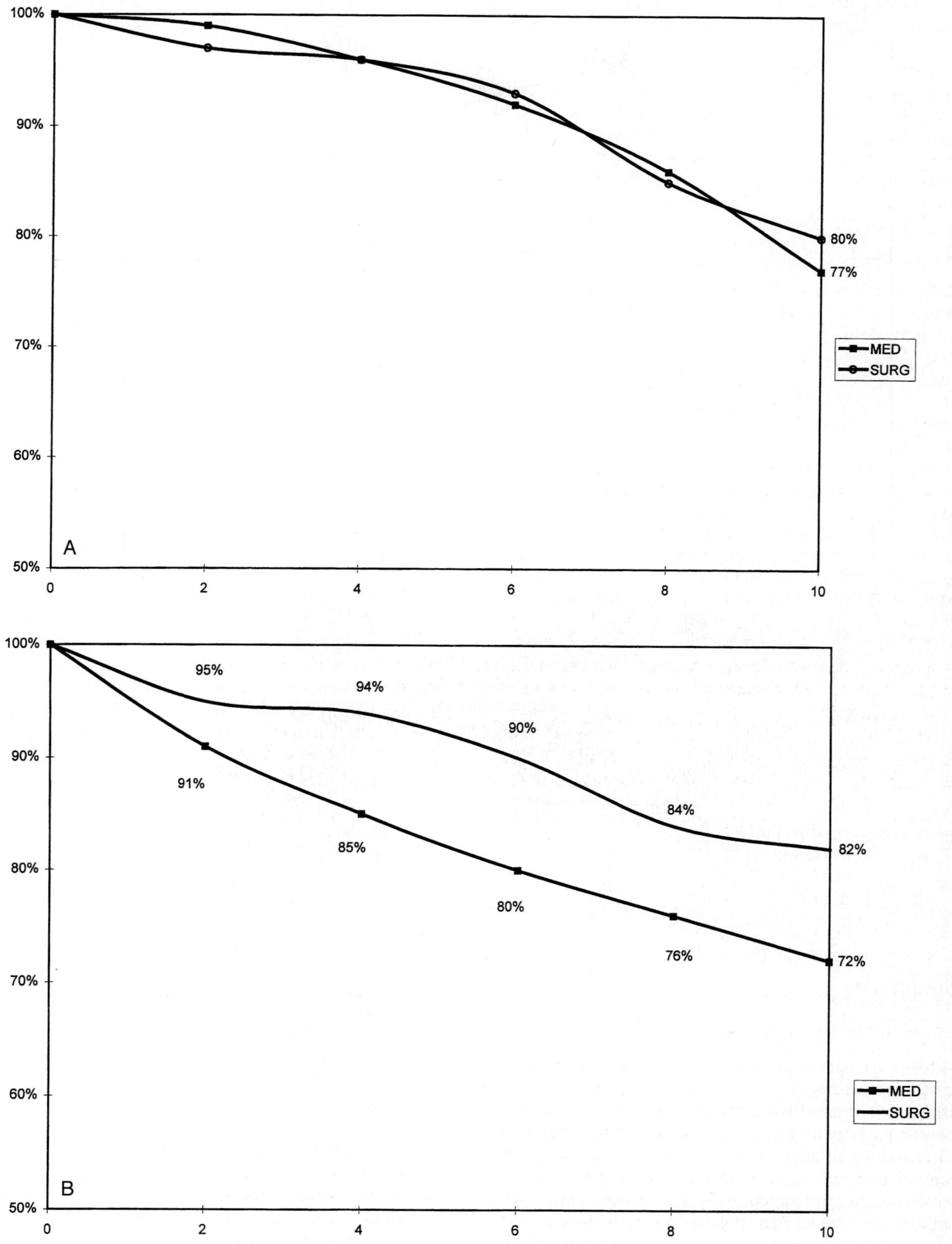

FIGURE 42–5 Physiologic testing and the effect of revascularization. In the European Cooperative Surgery Study, a survival benefit of coronary bypass surgery during a 10-year follow-up could be predicted by exercise test performance. **A,** A normal or slightly positive exercise test predicted no benefit. **B,** A positive exercise test predicted a survival benefit of early surgical referral.

Illustration continued on following page

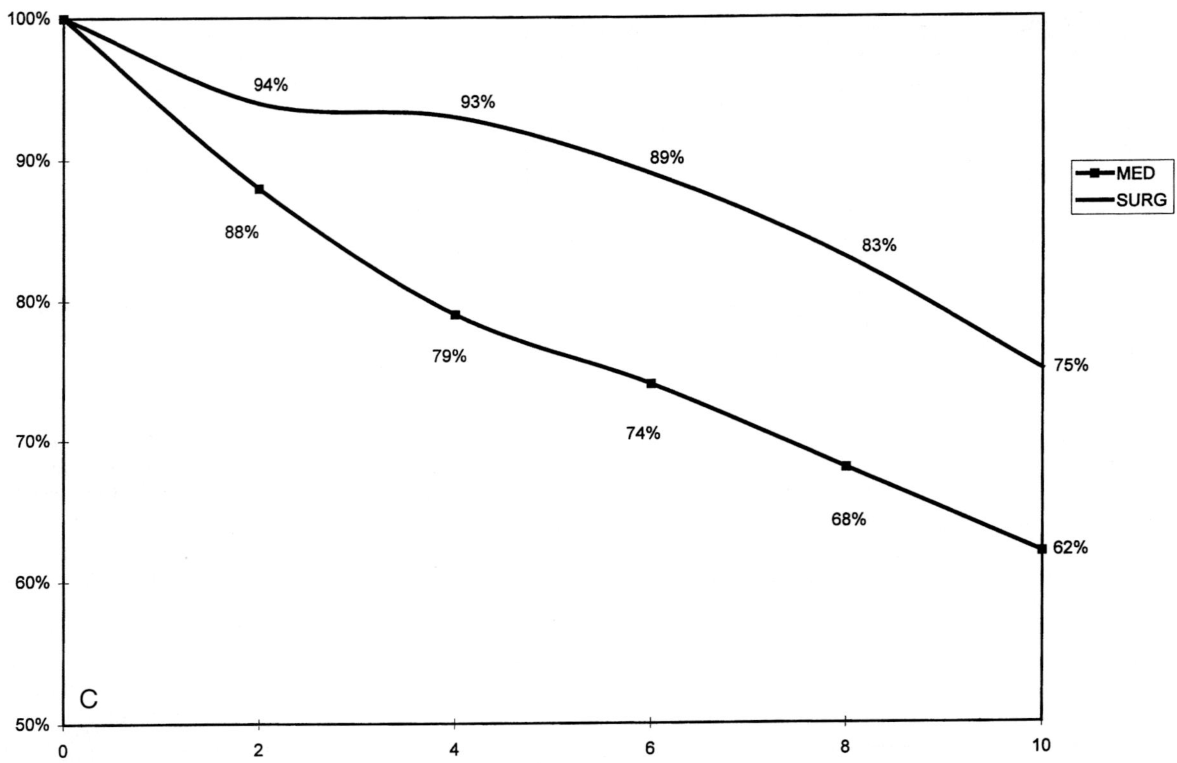

FIGURE 42–5 *Continued.* **C,** A strikingly positive test identified a very high risk population. A strikingly positive test was defined as the presence of two of three possible measures: a maximal heart rate ≤ 120 bpm, a maximal workload of ≤ 100 watt, and ST-segment depression ≥ 1.5 mm. bpm, beats per minute; MED, medical therapy; SURG, coronary bypass surgery. (**A–C,** From Varnauskas E: Twelve-year follow-up of survival in the European Coronary Surgery Study. N Engl J Med 319:332–337, 1988.)

patients with left main coronary artery stenosis. In three-vessel disease, there was a 45 percent reduction in mortality in the surgical group. In one-vessel and two-vessel disease groups, there were far fewer events, and the trend favoring surgery was much weaker, although certain high-risk subsets appeared to benefit. Patients with both low and normal LVEF appeared to benefit from surgery, with reductions in mortality of about 50 and 30 percent respectively. Physiologic testing predicted a survival benefit of early surgical referral. Symptom severity did not.

Techniques

The Saphenous Vein Graft

The life of a saphenous vein graft may be divided into three stages: a response to autotransplantation, fibrous transformation, and atherothrombotic evolution. The time course for each period is subject to individual variation. Careful handling of the saphenous vein graft during surgery is required to avoid injury and thrombosis that results in early closure after implantation.[32–35] Even when placed with meticulous care, the human saphenous vein is poorly suited to transmit blood under arterial pressure. The endothelium of the saphenous vein is quickly overwhelmed by arterial pressure and flow conditions. Platelets and fibrin begin to coat the vessel lumen, later to be replaced by smooth muscle cells that reinforce the vessel wall by producing ground substance and short elastic fibers. Chronic medial ischemia results in a loss of muscle cells and replacement by fibrous tissue. The evolution of fibrous medial replacement may alter the shape and flow characteristics of the graft through contraction, distortion, and increased rigidity. With time, the predominant appearance of the vessel wall is that of dense fibrous tissue. These early responses to saphenous vein autotransplantation combine to occlude 12 to 19 percent of vein graft bypasses within 1 year of surgery.[36, 37]

After fibrous transformation is complete, a period of relative histologic and clinical stability lasts for an average 5 to 6 years.[38, 39] Meanwhile, the proximal native vessel, which undergoes reduced flow requirements, suffers accelerated disease progression, often closing quietly and thus causing complete dependence on the bypass graft.[40] Following this "grace" period, aggressive atherosclerosis appears within the graft. Continued accumulation of intimal connective tissue, perhaps complicated by persistent endothelial dysfunction, provides a fertile ground for the development and progression of atherosclerosis. Maturation of this process eventually leads to thrombosis and produces acute or subacute graft closure.[32–34, 36, 39–54] At 5 years, the proportion of saphenous vein grafts that have closed has risen to 29 percent, reaching 51 percent at 12 years (Table 42–2).[36]

Declining patency of saphenous vein grafts is evident clinically in the return of symptoms in surgically bypassed patients after 5 years and in the increased morbidity that follows.[23, 36, 40–42, 44–48, 55, 56] The rate of clinical events such

TABLE 42–2 **The Occurrence of Saphenous Vein Graft Disease After Surgery**

	Early	1 yr	2.5 yr	5 yr	7.5 yr	10 yr	12.5 yr	≥15 yr
Number of grafts	4592	3706	469	1889	495	856	227	353
Occluded grafts	12%	19%	29%	25%	40%	40%	51%	50%
>50% DS	0%	2%	4%	16%	26%	26%	28%	28%
Mild	0%	3%	6%	20%	17%	20%	14%	12.5%
No stenosis	88%	76%	61%	39%	17%	14%	7%	9.5%

Abbreviations: DS, diameter stenosis; Y, year.

Adapted from Fitzgibbon GM, Kafka HP, Leach AJ, et al: Coronary bypass graft fate and patient outcome: angiographic follow-up of 5,065 grafts related to survival and reoperation in 1,388 patients during 25 years [see comments]. Reproduced with permission from the American Academy of Cardiology (J Am Coll Cardiol 28:616–626, 1996); and Fitzgibbon GM, Leach AJ, Kafka HP, Keon WJ: Coronary bypass graft fate: long-term angiographic study. Reproduced with permission from the American College of Cardiology (J Am Coll Cardiol 17:1075–1080, 1991).

as recurrent angina, repeat revascularization procedures, and mortality mirror the rate of graft occlusion. At 5 years after bypass, 2 percent of patients require a second procedure, and all-cause mortality is only 6 percent. By 12 years, one in five patients requires a second bypass surgery. In fact, less than one half of patients avoid myocardial infarction or a second surgery.[56]

Internal Mammary Artery

In 1967, Kolessov, a surgeon in the Soviet Union, dissected the internal mammary artery free of its normal anatomic course and attached the free end to the left anterior descending coronary artery.[57] His procedure was later simplified and popularized in the United States.[58, 59] In contrast to saphenous vein grafts, internal mammary conduits appear remarkably resistant to atherosclerosis and have 10-year patency rates of 80 to 95 percent (Fig. 42–6).[46, 58, 60–65] The internal mammary artery performs best when used to bypass the left anterior descending artery. Although it is used for a variety of bypasses, in other positions it may be no better than the saphenous vein.[66]

Low rates of disease progression and higher long-term patency translate into improved symptom control and survival.[63] Actuarial survival is improved with the use of internal mammary arteries versus saphenous veins in cases of disease in one, two, and three vessels [63, 67] (Fig. 42–7). The importance of stenosis of the left anterior descending coronary artery and the success of using the internal mammary artery to bypass it have led to the almost routine use of the internal mammary artery for bypass of the left anterior descending artery. Unfortunately, the time and technical constraints involved in emergency procedures do not always allow its use.

The use of bilateral internal mammary conduits has recently become popular in some centers and shows equally good patency rates.[66, 68–70] The accessibility of the internal mammary artery and the left anterior descending coronary artery has encouraged attempts at coronary bypass surgery that use smaller incisions, thus minimizing or avoiding median sternotomy. The immediate and long-term success of these limited-access procedures has not yet received intense scrutiny; therefore, the procedure cannot be considered the equivalent of the traditional operation.[71–75]

In addition to mammary vessels, the gastroepiploic and radial arteries may be used as bypass conduits. The exclusive use of arterial bypass conduits may improve the long-term success rate of coronary bypass surgery. Some questions remain about generalizability of the procedure, but it is a matter that deserves intense investigation.[68, 76, 77]

Summary of Surgical Bypass Trials

Patients with stable coronary disease, physiologic evidence confirming the significance of coronary lesions, or large

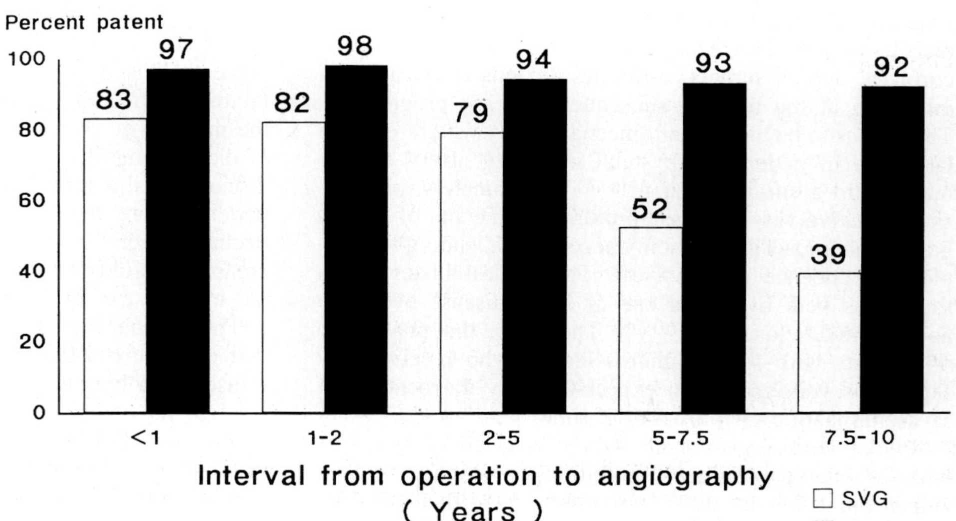

FIGURE 42–6 Internal mammary artery (IMA) and saphenous vein graft (SVG) patency. With time, the SVG will succumb to an accelerated form of atherosclerosis. The IMA is relatively resistant to this process. By 10 years, only 39 percent of vein grafts remain patent, compared with 92% of IMA grafts. (Adapted from Lytle BW, Loop FD, Cosgrove DM, et al: Long-term [5 to 12 years] serial studies of internal mammary artery and saphenous vein coronary bypass grafts. J Thorac Cardiovasc Surg 89:248–258, 1985.)

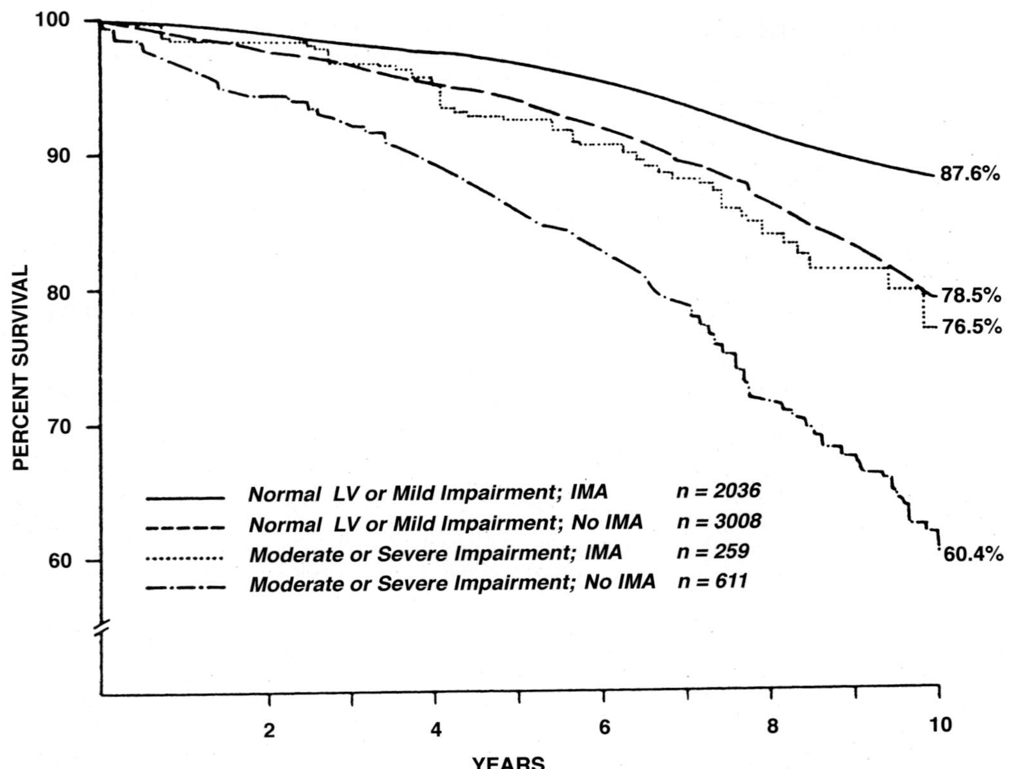

FIGURE 42–7 Internal mammary artery (IMA) and survival. The use of the IMA as a bypass conduit to the left anterior descending coronary artery provides a profound survival benefit. This benefit was apparent for patients with a left ventricular ejection fraction (LVEF) less than 50 percent ($P < .0001$) or more than 50% ($P = .0002$). In fact, patients with an LVEF below 50 percent who received an IMA bypass showed a survival rate comparable with that of patients with an LVEF above 50 percent who received only saphenous vein grafts. LV, left ventricle. (From Loop FD, Lytle BW, Cosgrove DM, et al: Influence of the internal-mammary-artery graft on 10-year survival and other cardiac events. N Engl J Med 314:1–6, 1986.)

territories of myocardium dependent upon severely diseased coronary arteries benefit from revascularization, regardless of symptom severity. Provision of alternative routes for perfusion of myocardium at risk diminishes the symptoms of myocardial ischemia, limits the extent of muscle injury at the time of infarction, and provides, albeit temporarily, a survival benefit for patients with the most severe disease.[23, 25, 27, 28, 30, 78, 79] Interestingly, coronary bypass surgery does not appear to reduce the risk of myocardial infarction. However, patients who have undergone coronary bypass surgery suffer less extensive myocardial infarction at the time of subsequent disease progression. This seems to be the primary mechanism by which revascularization in patients with stable coronary artery disease may afford a survival benefit.[78, 79] Unfortunately, progression of native vessel disease proximal to the site of bypass graft anastomosis is commonly accelerated, leading to complete dependence on the graft. The natural history of a saphenous vein bypass is one of rapid disease evolution and eventual closure.[41, 42, 79, 80] Therefore, the population of patients with severe atherosclerosis who receive only saphenous vein grafts can expect to enjoy the benefits of revascularization for only a brief time.

Randomized surgical trials were conducted in the 1970s when anesthetic techniques, monitoring, postoperative care, and medical therapy were less sophisticated than they are today. Improvements in surgical techniques and postoperative care have reduced the risk of perioperative myocardial infarction and death.[81] Even patients with the most severe ventricular dysfunction, who would not have been allowed entry into the randomized trials, have been shown to obtain benefit from surgical revascularization.[82, 83] Although the current population undergoing coronary bypass surgery is at higher risk than were the majority of patients entered in these trials, the expected operative mortality rate in patients undergoing a first coronary bypass surgery is about 1.5 percent. This is, of course, influenced by individual risk factors, such as the severity of left ventricular dysfunction, the number of vessels requiring bypass, age, the presence of diabetes mellitus, gender, coexistent peripheral vascular disease, renal insufficiency, and pulmonary disease. Among patients more than 70 years of age, who are normally excluded from randomized trials, the mortality rate increases twofold to threefold. Patients more than 80 years old have an expected mortality rate of 7 to 13 percent.[84–97]

The internal mammary artery has a history of durability that differs from that of the saphenous vein graft when it is used as a bypass conduit (see Fig. 42–6). It was rarely used in the major surgery trials. The use of the internal mammary artery and secondary prevention techniques has prolonged the life of bypass grafts and improved the long-term outcome of coronary bypass surgery.[36, 58, 60–62, 64, 65, 98–103]

Therefore, the magnitude of benefit reported in the randomized trials of coronary bypass surgery must be viewed today with these limitations in mind.

The number of patients who have improved survival expectation after coronary bypass surgery has almost certainly been increased by improved perioperative care and routine use of the internal mammary artery as a bypass conduit to the left anterior descending coronary artery. For example, the ECSS suggested that populations with proximal two-vessel coronary stenosis involving the left anterior descending coronary artery would benefit from coronary bypass surgery. Subsequent observational studies that included patients who received internal mammary bypass conduits lend credence to the nonsignificant trend reported in the ECSS.[104] In fact, populations with proximal single-vessel disease in a large left anterior descending coronary artery probably benefit from internal mammary–to–coronary artery bypass surgery as well.[104, 105]

In patients without proximal major-vessel stenosis and in those whose anatomy does not allow use of the internal mammary artery, early surgical referral carries a stiff penalty when native or saphenous vein graft disease later mandates additional revascularization efforts. Therefore, although surgery is clearly beneficial in patients with severe coronary obstruction, those with less severe disease and other alternatives for treatment should delay coronary bypass as long as possible.

Nonsurgical Interventional Therapy for Coronary Artery Disease

History

In 1929, Werner Forssman[106] inserted a catheter into his own basilic vein and advanced it into his right atrium. His stated intent was to develop "a safer approach for intracardiac drug injection."[106] Cardiac catheterization for diagnostic purposes was later truly developed by Cournand, Richards, Sones, Abrams, and Judkins.[7, 8, 107–110] The ability to obtain detailed information about coronary artery anatomy opened the door to bypass surgery and set the stage for percutaneous interventions.

In 1964, Dotter and Judkins[111] successfully dilated peripheral atherosclerotic lesions using progressively larger coaxial dilators. This technique, which they termed "transluminal angioplasty" was not widely accepted, in large part because of the formidable technical limitations and associated complications. However, European investigators continued to experiment with transluminal angioplasty, using the Dotter technique until 1974, when Andreas Gruentzig[112, 113] developed the double-lumen balloon catheter. These balloon catheters were used successfully in iliac, femoral, and popliteal arteries and, in 1976, were miniaturized for use in coronary arteries.[112, 114, 115] In 1977, Gruentzig[15] successfully performed the first percutaneous dilatation of a human coronary artery. The equipment used for percutaneous transluminal coronary angioplasty (PTCA) evolved rapidly as new technology was applied to the creation of guiding catheters, exchangeable over-the-wire catheters, new balloon materials, low-profile catheters, and autoperfusion systems. Techniques, such as directional atherectomy, rotational atherectomy, extraction atherectomy, and laser ablation, have been developed, each one finding a clinical niche.[116–131]

Balloon angioplasty reliably produces an increase in vessel lumen diameter. The chance of success depends greatly on the clinical situation and the lesion approached (Table 42–3).[132] In patients with stable angina, the mortality rate at 1 month after the procedure is only 1 percent.[133] Patients with limited disease and successful angioplasty enjoy a good prognosis, with the 5-year survival rate exceeding 95 percent.[133, 134] One third to slightly less than one half of successfully treated vessels renarrow by 6 months. However, only one fourth of patients report recurrent angina warranting investigation, and approximately 15% require coronary bypass surgery.[134]

In approximately 2 to 10 percent of angioplasty procedures, intimal dissection, thrombosis, and perhaps medial smooth muscle spasm combine to reocclude the treated vessel soon after balloon deflation.[134–136] This event, termed *abrupt closure,* may be successfully treated with repeat balloon inflation in about half of such cases.[136, 137] Intractable abrupt closure may be treated by stent placement or emergency coronary bypass surgery.[135–143] Even when percutaneous methods of managing abrupt closure are successful, patients are at increased risk of myocardial infarction.[143] It is the specter of abrupt closure and myocardial infarction or emergency bypass surgery and its attendant complications that has historically limited the application of balloon angioplasty.

Experience, improved balloon technology, stents, perfusion devices, and intraoperative cardiopulmonary bypass

TABLE 42-3 Classification of Coronary Artery Lesions According to the Relative Likelihood of Success With Routine Balloon Angioplasty

Type A Lesions (High Success, >85%; Low Risk)	
Discrete (<10 mm length)	Little or no calcification
Concentric	Less than totally occlusive
Readily accessible	Not ostial in location
Nonangulated segment, <45°	No major branch involvement
Smooth contour	Absence of thrombus
Type B Lesions (Moderate Success, 60–85%; Moderate Risk)	
Tubular (10–20 mm length)	Moderate to heavy calcification
Eccentric	Total occlusions < 3 mo old*
Moderate tortuosity of proximal segment	Ostial in location
Moderately angulated segment, >45° to <90°	Bifurcation lesions requiring double guide wires
Irregular contour	Some thrombus present
Type C Lesions (Low Success, <60%; High Risk)	
Diffuse (>2 cm length)	Total occlusion > 3 mo old
Excessive tortuosity of proximal segment	Inability to protect major side branches
Extremely angulated segments >90°	Degenerated vein grafts with friable lesions

*Although the risk of abrupt vessel closure is moderate, in certain instances the likelihood of a major complication may be low, as in dilatation of total occlusions < 3 mo old or when abundant collateral channels supply the distal vessel.

Reproduced with permission. From Guidelines for percutaneous transluminal coronary angioplasty. A report of the American College of Cardiology/American Heart Association Task Force on Assessment of Diagnostic and Therapeutic Cardiovascular Procedures (Subcommittee on Percutaneous Transluminal Coronary Angioplasty). J Am Coll Cardiol 12:529–545, 1988.

have expanded the population of patients who may be treated safely by percutaneous means. Reports include high-risk lesion morphology, multivessel disease with depressed LVEF, saphenous vein grafts, and in selected patients, left main coronary artery stenosis.[144–162] Multivessel angioplasty may be performed; there is a procedural mortality of 1 to 2 percent in patients with good left ventricular function. The 5-year survival rate in successfully treated patients is almost 90 percent.[163–176]

Randomized trials of early surgical revascularization are consistent in reporting that early surgical referral does not improve the survival rate of patients with one- or two-vessel disease and good ventricular function (but the high rate of eventual surgical bypass in the medically treated patients is to be noted). In these populations, the risk of adverse events associated with surgical bypass and the subsequent need for repeat procedures balances or may outweigh the benefit obtained from early referral for revascularization. Percutaneous procedures are associated with a lower risk of morbidity and are not associated with an increased risk should coronary bypass surgery or a repeat percutaneous procedure become necessary. Therefore, percutaneous coronary revascularization seems to be an ideal treatment for those patients with unacceptable symptoms in whom surgery will provide no clear survival benefit.

PTCA is effective for symptom relief. Available evidence from randomized trials does not suggest a survival benefit, but technological advances have continued to improve the safety and efficacy of percutaneous revascularization, calling into question the evidence of clinical trials. This is especially true for the coronary stent. The coronary stent represents a genuine advance over balloon angioplasty for routine percutaneous revascularization.[138, 141, 142, 144, 145, 152, 154, 177–191] The implantation of a permanent, expandable metal buttress limits arterial dissection and prevents prolapse of dissected tissue into the vessel lumen, allowing more aggressive vessel dilatation. Its availability has substantially improved the safety and long-term efficacy of percutaneous intervention.[178]

Trials Comparing PTCA to Medical Therapy

The Angioplasty Compared to Medicine Trial

The Angioplasty Compared to Medicine (ACME) trial evaluated the efficacy of PTCA compared with medicine in the treatment of symptomatic single-vessel coronary artery disease.[192] Entry criteria included a 70 to 90 percent narrowing of a single coronary artery and either stable angina, a strikingly positive exercise test (ST-segment depression of 3 mm or more or reversible thallium defect), or a history of myocardial infarction within 3 months of enrollment. Ultimately, 212 patients were randomized to either PTCA (n = 105) or medical therapy (n = 107). Follow-up continued through 6 months, when a scheduled exercise test was performed. The primary endpoints of the study were change in exercise tolerance from baseline, frequency of angina, and nitroglycerin usage.

Only 100 of the 105 patients randomized to PTCA actually underwent the procedure; the success rate was 80 percent. Of the patients undergoing PTCA, 4 experienced perioperative myocardial infarction. There were no deaths. At 6 months, 1 patient who had been randomized to medical therapy had died; 9 patients had suffered myocardial infarction (1 additional patient in the PTCA group, to total 5, and 3 in the medicine group); and 27 patients had undergone PTCA, 16 repeat procedures in the PTCA group and 11 first procedures in the medicine group. CABG was required more often in patients randomized to PTCA, with 7 operations performed (2 emergent), compared with none in the medical group. By 3 years of follow-up, 6.1 percent of patients randomized to medical therapy had died compared with 4.8 percent of patients undergoing PTCA (P = NS). The incidence of myocardial infarction and CABG was the same.[193]

PTCA was superior to medicine in relieving the symptoms of myocardial ischemia, with 64 percent of the PTCA patients free of angina at 6 months, compared with 46 percent of the medical patients. PTCA increased exercise duration by 1.6 minutes over medical therapy. Correlating with objective measures of ischemia, revascularized patients enjoyed a substantial improvement in their overall sense of well-being and quality of life.[194] The ACME investigators extended their observations in a small group of patients with two-vessel disease and found no significant difference in follow-up events and a trend toward better control of angina with revascularization.[195]

A second small study of single-vessel revascularization has been performed in patients who were asymptomatic or easily controlled with medication.[196] In that study, 88 patients with a mean single coronary artery stenosis of 86 percent were randomized to PTCA (n = 44) or were continued on medical therapy (n = 44). Patients with prior Q wave myocardial infarctions, treadmill tests positive at 50W, or diabetes mellitus were excluded. Patients were followed for 2 years, and no difference in survival rates were found.

These reports include small numbers of events and are inadequate to exclude a survival benefit for revascularization in patients with single-vessel coronary disease or to examine specific subgroups (such as proximal versus distal coronary stenosis). They establish that PTCA is an effective means of treating symptomatic ischemia and that a price must be paid in terms of procedural risk.

The Randomized Intervention Treatment of Angina (RITA-2) trial compared PTCA to medical therapy in 1018 patients with stable or unstable angina pectoris and no definite indication for coronary bypass surgery or urgent revascularization.[197] Medical therapy included a beta-blocker and a calcium channel blocker or a long-acting nitrate preparation. The use of lipid-lowering agents varied throughout the course of the study. At randomization, 20 percent of patients had functional class 3 or 4 angina, 40 percent had multivessel disease, and 45 percent had moderate to severe left ventricular wall motion abnormalities. At 2.7 years of follow-up, there was no difference in mortality among the groups. Myocardial infarction was recognized twice as frequently in the PTCA group, so that at completion of follow-up, the incidence of death or myocardial infarction was 6.3 percent in the PTCA group compared with 3.3 percent in medically treated patients (P = .02). In contrast, angina was better controlled in patients who underwent revascularization. In addition to improved control of angina, there was a trend toward a decreased frequency of congestive heart failure in patients treated with revascularization.

The Medicine, Angioplasty, or Surgery Study and the Asymptomatic Coronary Ischemia Pilot Study

Two other trials have compared any form of revascularization to medical therapy—the Medicine, Angioplasty, or Surgery Study (MASS) trial and the Asymptomatic Coronary Ischemia Pilot (ACIP) study.[198, 199] MASS compared strategies of medical therapy, angioplasty, or internal mammary bypass in patients with single-vessel coronary disease involving the proximal left anterior descending coronary artery. After 3.5 years of follow-up, 2.8 percent of patients treated medically suffered acute myocardial infarction and 9.7 percent required revascularization of some form. In the PTCA group, 2.8 percent experienced procedural complications requiring emergency coronary bypass surgery and 30 percent required an eventual second revascularization procedure. The group randomized to coronary bypass surgery had a 1.4 percent operative mortality. At follow-up, 98 percent of surgically treated patients, 82 percent of patients randomized to angioplasty, and only 32 percent of medically treated patients were free of angina. In summary, for patients with isolated stenosis of the proximal left anterior descending coronary artery, the strategies of medical therapy, angioplasty, or surgery may be equivalent in terms of mortality and the risk of myocardial infarction. However, revascularization is by far the most effective means of relieving angina, with coronary bypass outperforming balloon angioplasty.[1, 9, 8]

Although not specifically addressing the subgroup of patients with single-vessel coronary disease, the ACIP study was designed as a preliminary study to seek the most appropriate form of therapy for patients without definite indications for revascularization whose symptoms might be unreliable as a guide to ischemia severity. Patients with objective ischemia on physiologic study and at least one episode of asymptomatic ST-segment depression during 24-hour ambulatory electrocardiogram recording were randomized to medical therapy guided by symptoms, to medical therapy guided by objective ischemia, or to revascularization. The attending physician chose the mode of revascularization.[199] Of these patients, 16 percent had diabetes mellitus, 40 percent had a history of myocardial infarction, and 76 percent had multivessel disease. Of particular note is that 35 percent of patients had stenosis of the proximal left anterior descending coronary artery. In 192 patients randomized to revascularization, there were one myocardial infarction and two urgent coronary bypass procedures. All of these events occurred in patients undergoing PTCA. At 2 years, the mortality rate among patients receiving medical therapy guided by symptoms was 6.6 percent. Ischemia-guided medical therapy and revascularization resulted in a mortality rate of 4.4 percent and 1.1 percent, respectively.[200]

The differences in survival rates demonstrated in ACIP were a surprise. There are several possible explanations for this unexpected observation, but perhaps the most interesting arises from an analysis of diagnostic angiograms used to screen patients for ACIP. Patients who had silent ischemia that met the criteria for study entry were more likely to have proximal, discrete, complex coronary lesions.[201] The requirement for objective demonstration of silent ischemia may have unwittingly skewed the population to include patients at higher risk for cardiac events and death.

The observations arising from ACIP were foreshadowed by an in-depth angiographic analysis from CASS. Ringqvist and coworkers[202] reviewed angiographic anatomy and outcomes in 8773 patients included in the CASS registry. They found that in addition to the crude classification of number of vessels diseased and the severity of left ventricular dysfunction, the positions of lesions (i.e., proximal or nonproximal) were predictive of outcome (Fig. 42–8). For example, patients with moderate left ventricular dysfunction and proximal two-vessel disease demonstrated a survival rate that was virtually identical to that of patients with three-vessel disease and no proximal stenosis. The observed survival rate of patients with nonproximal single-vessel disease was virtually identical to that of patients with no disease.

The ACIP study population largely consisted of patients with multivessel coronary disease, many of whom appear to have had proximal stenoses that are associated with decreased survival expectancy. Regardless of how the population may have been skewed, ACIP provides the first evidence that revascularization (not just coronary bypass surgery) can improve the survival expectancy of patients with coronary artery disease who do not fit into the categories defined by the randomized surgical trials. The angiographic substudy adds to the findings of Ringqvist and coworkers and casts a shadow on simple classification by number of vessels diseased.[202]

Trials Comparing PTCA to Coronary Bypass Surgery

Many patients with symptomatic atherosclerosis have multivessel coronary disease and require revascularization for symptom control. The surgical trials defined select populations that enjoy survival advantage with surgical bypass. That survival advantage is temporary because of the inherent limitations of saphenous vein grafts. Meanwhile, percutaneous revascularization is successful in reducing angina and may have a lower risk of procedural morbidity and earlier return to normal activity. The profound psychological and physical effects of bypass surgery and the finite life span of a vein graft favor percutaneous interventions when feasible. However, patients with multivessel coronary disease in whom complete revascularization is not achieved may pay a price in terms of survival expectation. In addition, the frequent recurrence of lesions treated by PTCA and improved graft survival using the internal mammary artery and antiplatelet therapy suggest that surgical bypass may be more effective in the long run. Percutaneous and surgical revascularization methods have been compared in seven trials designed to identify the most effective and least costly treatment alternative (Table 42–4).[163, 165–169, 173, 175, 197, 203–205]

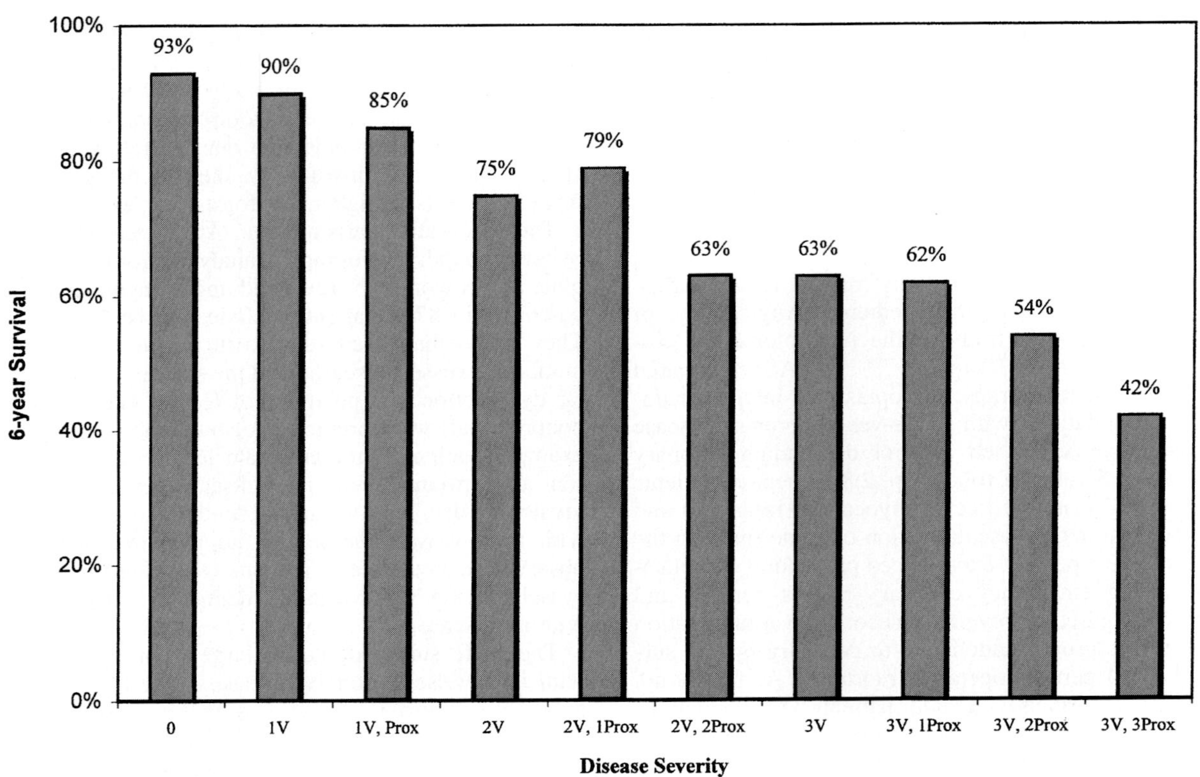

FIGURE 42–8 Anatomic description of disease severity. The anatomic description of the severity of coronary disease should express the quantity of myocardium that is or may become ischemic under hemodynamic stress. The first practical and successful scheme used the number of major vessel regions with critical stenosis and ventricular function. Including the position (proximal or nonproximal) of stenosis in the major vessel regions further refines the estimation of prognosis. Prox, proximal; V, vessel. (Data from Ringqvist I, Fisher LD, Mock M, et al: Prognostic value of angiographic indices of coronary artery disease from the Coronary Artery Surgery Study [CASS]. J Clin Invest 71:1854–1866, 1983.)

Emory Angioplasty Versus Surgery Trial

The Emory Angioplasty versus Surgery Trial (EAST) studied patients with multivessel coronary artery disease in need of revascularization therapy in whom angioplasty or surgery could be performed.[167] Among more than 5000 patients screened, only 842 were eligible for entry. Of those, 392 patients were randomized to bypass surgery or PTCA.

In 194 patients randomized to surgical treatment, 10 percent suffered perioperative myocardial infarction. The 30-day mortality rate was 1 percent. In the 198 patients randomized to PTCA, there was a similar 30-day mortality rate but a lower incidence (3.5 percent) of perioperative infarction. Follow-up through 3 years revealed no difference in mortality or myocardial infarction between the strategies. However, surgery was more effective in providing complete revascularization and freedom from a subsequent revascularization procedure (see Table 42–4). Both strategies performed well in improving quality of life, and the cost of medical care was no different.

The Randomized Intervention Treatment of Angina Trial

The Randomized Intervention Treatment of Angina (RITA) trial included 1011 patients with one or more coronary artery stenoses ranging from 70 percent to complete occlusion who were randomized to PTCA (n = 510) or CABG (n = 501) at 16 centers in the United Kingdom.[174, 203] At a median 6.5 years of follow-up, the mortality in the PTCA arm is 7.6 percent, which is not significantly different from the 9 percent mortality in the surgical arm (see Table 42–4). During the first 6 months of follow-up, 28 percent of PTCA patients required additional intervention (coronary bypass in 15 percent). Beyond year 3, the reintervention rate was 3 percent per year. Meanwhile, patients undergoing CABG had a reintervention rate of 2 percent per year. At 5 years, 47.7 percent of patients undergoing CABG were free of events and recurrent angina as opposed to 22.2 percent of patients undergoing initial PTCA. Although there were fewer physically active patients 1 month after CABG (38 percent) than after PTCA (52 percent), there was no difference at later time points. After 2 years, the cost of care for PTCA was 20 percent less than for CABG, but this difference virtually disappeared by 5 years.[174, 205]

German Angioplasty Bypass Investigation

The German Angioplasty Bypass Surgery Investigation (GABI) is a randomized, multicenter trial of PTCA versus CABG in eight clinical centers in Germany.[166] Eligibility criteria included an indication for revascularization of at least two major coronary vessels where either PTCA or CABG was considered technically feasible. The goal of

TABLE 42–4 Trials of Angioplasty Versus Surgery for Multivessel Disease

				Procedural			Follow-Up			
			n	*Death*	*Myocardial Infarction*	*Emergent Revascularization*	*Death*	*Myocardial Infarction*	*CABG*	*PTCA*
RITA	>50% stenosis of at least one coronary artery with an equal chance of successful revascularization; 2.5-year follow-up	PTCA	510	1.8	?	4.3%	3.1%	6.7%	1.9%	12%
		CABG	501	1.2%	?		3.6%	5.2%	0.8%	3.2%
GABI	≥70% stenosis of more than one coronary artery and severe angina; 1-year follow-up	PTCA	176	1.2%	2.4%	11.4%	0.6%	6%*	21%	23%
		CABG	161	2.5%	8.3%	1.9%	0.7%	13.5%*	1.0%	4.0%
ERACI	>70% stenosis of at least one coronary artery with revascularization judged necessary; 3-year follow-up	PTCA	63	1.5%	6.3%	1.5%	9.5%	7.8%	22.2%	14.5%
		CABG	64	4.6%	6.2%	1.5%	4.7%	7.8%	0%	4.9%
EAST	Two or more vessels with > 50% stenosis and an equal chance of successful revascularization; 3-year follow-up	PTCA	198	1%	3.0%	10%	7.1%	14.6%	22%	41%
		CABG	194	1%	10.3%	0%	6.2%	19.6%	1%	13%
CABRI	Two- or three-vessel disease with at least one vessel suitable for angioplasty; 1-year follow-up	PTCA	541	1.3%	NR	NR	3.9%	4.9%	15.7%	20.8%
		CABG	513	1.3%	NR	NR	2.7%	3.5%	0.8%	2.7%
BARI	≥50% stenosis of more than one coronary artery with angina or myocardial infarction; 5-year follow-up	PTCA	904	1.1%	2.1%	8.4%	13.7%	21.3%*	31%	34%
		CABG	892	1.3%	4.6%	0.1%	10.7%	19.6%*	1%	7%
Toulouse	≥70% stenosis of more than one coronary artery with +TMT or myocardial infarction; 5-year follow-up	PTCA	76	1.3%	3.9%	3.9%	13.2%	6%*	13.6%	15.2%
		CABG	76	1.3%	6.6%	1.3%	10.5%	1.5%*	0%	4.4%

Abbreviations: BARI, Bypass Angioplasty Revascularization Investigation; CABG, coronary artery bypass graft; CABRI, Coronary Angioplasty Bypass Revascularization Investigation; EAST, Emory Angioplasty versus Surgery Trial; ERACI, Argentine Randomized Trial of Percutaneous Transluminal Coronary Angioplasty versus Coronary Artery Bypass Surgery in Multivessel Disease; GABI, German Angioplasty Bypass Surgery Investigation; NR, not relevant; PTCA, percutaneous transluminal coronary angioplasty; RITA, Randomized Intervention Treatment of Angina; TMT, treadmill test; Toulouse, the Toulouse Trial.

*Death or Q wave myocardial infarction.

treatment was complete revascularization. The primary endpoint of the study was the presence of angina pectoris at 1 year. Internal mammary grafts were used in 35 percent of surgical cases. There was a 3 percent incidence of emergency CABG after PTCA (see Table 42–4). Bypass surgery was associated with an increased risk of myocardial infarction (8.1 versus 2.3 percent) and pneumonia (10.6 versus 1.1 percent); the difference in perioperative mortality (2.5 percent surgical versus 1.1 percent PTCA) did not reach statistical significance.

Reintervention prior to hospital discharge was required more often for patients treated with PTCA (11 versus 2 percent). In follow-up, this difference was magnified: 44 percent of the patients treated with initial PTCA required additional revascularization (one half undergoing surgical bypass) compared with 6 percent of the patients initially treated surgically. However, this did not have an impact on the number of patients returning to work, as both groups were equal in this regard.

A 6-month angiographic follow-up study found that 12 percent of saphenous vein grafts and 6.7 percent of internal mammary grafts were completely occluded. An additional 10 percent of saphenous vein grafts contained stenosis lesions larger than 50 percent in diameter. More than one third of native vessels receiving bypass grafts had progressed to complete occlusion.[37] These findings are comparable with those reported in older studies of bypass surgery.[36, 37, 42, 55]

Argentine Randomized Trial of PTCA Versus CABG in Multivessel Disease

The Argentine Randomized Trial of Percutaneous Transluminal Coronary Angioplasty versus Coronary Artery Bypass Graft in Multivessel Disease (ERACI) compared the costs and outcomes of early surgery with PTCA in 127 patients with multivessel disease and indications for revascularization therapy.[168, 169] Entry criteria included severely limiting stable angina despite maximal medical therapy, refractory rest angina, an extensive area of myocardium at risk as judged by exercise testing, and stenosis of 70 percent or more in more than one major coronary artery. The internal mammary artery was used for grafting in 76.5 percent of patients undergoing bypass surgery.[168]

There was no significant difference in the incidence of death, perioperative myocardial infarction, or requirement for emergency revascularization (CABG or PTCA). At 1 and 3 years of follow-up, overall survival and survival free of myocardial infarction were no different in the two groups. Surgical bypass was a more effective means of preventing angina, although the difference between the groups has narrowed with time (see Table 42–4). The total cost of care (including subsequent hospitalizations) for the PTCA group through 3 years was slightly over one half that for the surgery group ($474,000 versus $832,000, $P = .02$).[169]

Coronary Angioplasty Bypass Revascularization Investigation

The Coronary Angioplasty Bypass Revascularization Investigation (CABRI) is the European cooperative study of outcomes in patients with multivessel disease treated with bypass surgery or PTCA. Its design is similar to that of the other studies, although there was no effort to provide complete revascularization. Patients with multivessel disease and at least one lesion treatable with PTCA could be randomized. Results at 1-year follow-up are consistent with other reports, finding no difference in mortality or myocardial infarction but a more frequent need for additional revascularization procedures in patients treated with PTCA[173] (see Table 42–4). Cost of care was similar in both strategies.

Bypass Angioplasty Revascularization Investigation

The Bypass Angioplasty Revascularization Investigation (BARI) is a multicenter, prospective, randomized trial of PTCA and CABG in patients with multivessel coronary artery disease that was performed under the direction of the National Heart, Lung, and Blood Institute.[175, 204] Inclusion criteria were luminal narrowing of 50 percent or more in at least two coronary vessels that are equally suitable to revascularization by either procedure. The primary endpoint was mortality at 5 years (the time of maximal benefit from surgical revascularization and well past the period of lesion activity following PTCA).

In the BARI trial, 914 patients were randomized to coronary bypass surgery and 915 to PTCA. There was no difference in perioperative mortality. Q wave myocardial infarction was more than twice as frequent in patients undergoing surgery (4.6 versus 2.1 percent, $P < .01$). Almost 10 percent of patients randomized to PTCA required surgical bypass before hospital discharge. At a mean follow-up duration of 5.4 years, there was no difference in mortality or in the incidence of myocardial infarction. A repeat revascularization procedure was necessary more often in patients randomized to PTCA (see Table 42–4).

The Toulouse Trial

At a single center in Toulouse, France, 152 patients with multivessel coronary disease were randomized to surgical therapy (76 patients) or percutaneous therapy (76 patients).[163] The majority of patients had unstable symptoms: 30 percent of patients had three vessel disease, and 69 percent had disease involving the left anterior descending coronary artery; 97 percent of patients had normal ventricular function.

Procedural success rates were identical, but hospital stay was more than twice as long for patients undergoing bypass. At 5 years of follow-up, overall survival for the two groups was the same (CABG 89 percent, PTCA 87 percent), but survival free of recurrent angina, myocardial infarction, or repeat procedures was greater for CABG (82.9 percent) than for PTCA (68.4 percent).[163]

The Impact of Diabetes Mellitus

Diabetes mellitus is recognized as a risk factor for the development of atherosclerosis and for worse outcome when atherosclerosis is present. The presence of diabetes mellitus confers an increased risk of acute coronary events and increased mortality with their occurrence.[9, 206–209] Revascularization, whether percutaneous or surgical, is similarly affected.[171, 210–214] The mortality rate in diabetic patients undergoing coronary bypass surgery is greater than in the nondiabetic population (4.2 versus 1.8 percent). After successful revascularization, the 5-year survival rate, adjusted for various risk factors, is 75 percent, with 2.2 percent requiring reoperation.[214] Percutaneous treatment of multivessel disease in diabetics is associated with a similarly adjusted 5-year survival rate of 68 percent.[214] After coronary stent placement, the mortality observed at 30 days is nearly doubled (2.7 versus 1.4 percent) by the presence of diabetes mellitus.[211] In long-term follow-up after stent placement, the mortality rate, adjusted for risk factors, remains elevated (6.6 versus 4 percent). Stent restenosis occurs with a frequency of 37.5 percent, with 21.1 percent requiring repeat revascularization.[211]

An important subgroup analysis from BARI revealed that the survival rate of patients with treated diabetes mellitus who were randomized to PTCA was significantly worse than that of patients who underwent bypass surgery (65.5 versus 80 percent, $P = .003$).[210] In patients without diabetes mellitus, the follow-up mortality rate was identical. The CABRI trial and two nonrandomized studies support the findings of BARI, reporting an extremely high incidence of recurrent ischemic events or need for repeat procedures in diabetic patients treated with angioplasty.[215] However, EAST, whose patients underwent screening for recurrent ischemia, and RITA-1 did not find a difference in outcome between revascularization methods in their diabetic populations.

Diabetic patients tend to have more diffuse atherosclerosis and a greater prevalence of additional lesions in the treated vessel when compared to nondiabetics. Noncritical stenoses have prognostic significance as they reflect sites in the vessel that are severely diseased and harbor the potential for rapid evolution.[216] In a vessel with multiple noncritical lesions in addition to a severe stenosis, the ability of percutaneous therapy to provide reliable, complete revascularization may be impaired.[217] In fact, angiographic evidence of the extent of atherosclerosis may be more important than the diagnosis of diabetes mellitus in determining the long-term success of percutaneous revascularization. In an unpublished trial of angioplasty in diabetic patients, focal, discrete lesions amenable to complete revascularization predicted a comparable outcome with PTCA or surgery, regardless of the presence or absence of diabetes mellitus.[215] Therefore, the severity of disease and the lesion characteristics may be the true discriminating factors rather than the physiologic state of the diabetes mellitus.

The Natural History of a Balloon-Dilated Vessel

In the best of circumstances, percutaneous angioplasty results in near-total resolution of coronary artery stenosis; appearing to compress a malleable atheroma, angioplasty results in a vessel that has a smooth and regular angiographic appearance. In truth, the vessel's appearance at angiography may be quite deceptive.[218–227] Balloon angioplasty transmits increased intraluminal pressures circumferentially to the atherosclerotic vessel wall, which is noncompliant and often brittle. When exposed to mechanical stress, the intima fractures, allowing further balloon expansion and increases in luminal diameter.[218–226] The fracture of a lesion may extend through the intimal layer and allow the formation of dissection plane with an extension that is determined by the mechanical characteristics of the lesion. A dissection plane extending along the intima-media border may result in luminal displacement of the diseased intima and vessel occlusion. This is known as abrupt or acute closure. Although extensive dissection may produce luminal obstruction and abrupt closure, small or limited dissection is a requirement for successful balloon angioplasty.[172, 227] In addition to plaque fracture and dissection, the stretching of the plaque of a normal vessel wall and even some element of plaque compression may contribute to luminal enlargement after balloon angioplasty.[219, 220, 226]

On completion of the angioplasty procedure, the lesion, now devoid of endothelial protection and rich in thrombogenic material, attracts platelets and initiates the formation of a thrombus. Should the stimulus for clot formation overcome anticoagulation and antiplatelet agents that are routinely employed, a large platelet-fibrin clot may form, occluding the vessel. After a successful procedure (without extensive dissection or thrombus formation), platelet accumulation and thrombus formation is limited.

Platelet-rich mural thrombus is inevitable after manipulation of the coronary artery. It is believed to provide a stimulus and a framework for colonization by specialized vascular smooth muscle cells.[228–230] These cells synthesize connective tissue and reinforce the injured intima. The appearance of an abundance of vascular smooth muscle cells and newly formed connective tissue has been termed *intimal hyperplasia.* Eventually, the angioplasty site is recovered by endothelium and intimal hyperplasia gives way to collagen-rich connective tissue. Surrounding media and adventitia that have also been injured by the mechanical effects of angioplasty become fibrotic and may alter their conformation, or remodel, as the vessel heals.

Many times, after manipulation of the coronary arteries, intimal hyperplasia becomes bulky and extends well into the vessel lumen. The result is no different from the original obstructing atheroma.[228–230] Additionally, the media and adventitia may contract with healing and reduce the absolute cross-sectional area of the vessel. These two processes, intimal hyperplasia and vessel contracture, are the primary processes that produce restenosis after angioplasty.[231–233] Reoccurrence of stenosis that is 50 percent or more of the diameter of the vessel is present after 40 to 50 percent of PTCA procedures, almost always occurring within 6 months of the procedure.[132, 164, 212, 234–237] Patients with restenosis are at increased risk of myocardial infarction and are more likely to require coronary bypass surgery.[238] Restenosis almost certainly has an adverse effect on survival.[133]

Stents

Balloon angioplasty produces better results in certain types of atherosclerotic lesions than in others (see Table 42–3).[239] Attempts to extend percutaneous revascularization to high-risk lesions and to prevent abrupt closure and restenosis have resulted in the development of a variety of angioplasty devices, including atherectomy devices, laser ablation, and stents.[116–119, 121–127, 129, 131, 139–141, 147, 186, 188, 240, 241] Particular devices produce more favorable outcomes in specific situations or anatomies. However, only the coronary stent has been shown to improve the effectiveness of percutaneous angioplasty. Lesion characteristics retain their value for predicting an increased rate of restenosis, even with stents.[242]

The introduction of coronary stents has revolutionized percutaneous revascularization. The likelihood of untreatable abrupt closure and referral for emergency coronary bypass surgery has been reduced by almost 50 percent.[178] Meanwhile, in selected populations, angiographic evidence of restenosis and the need for repeat revascularization procedures is reduced.[144, 145, 154, 179, 181, 182, 185, 187, 189–191] Stents are more effective than routine balloon angioplasty for discrete, de novo coronary lesions, restenotic lesions, saphenous vein graft angioplasty, and chronic total occlusions and in the setting of acute myocardial infarction.[144, 145, 154, 177, 179, 182, 185, 187, 189–191, 243–245] There are several comparisons of the performance of routine stenting as opposed to balloon angioplasty. As in earlier trials of surgical bypass, the superiority of stent implantation in treating abrupt or threatened vessel closure was accepted and was allowed as a treatment option "if necessary" for the angioplasty group.

The Belgium Netherlands Stent Trial (Benestent) compared primary stent implantation to angioplasty in 520 patients with stable angina and new coronary lesions at 28 centers throughout Europe.[187] There was no significant difference in the incidence of death, Q wave myocardial infarction, or coronary bypass surgery. Defining restenosis as a greater than 50 percent luminal diameter narrowing at follow-up angiography, primary stenting was superior to angioplasty, showing a restenosis rate of 22 percent as compared with 32 percent, respectively. This was accompanied by a reduction in the need to repeat angioplasty procedures of almost 50 percent. This benefit was sustained out to 1 year.[182]

Stent Restenosis Study (STRESS) addressed the impact of stent implantation on angiographic evidence of restenosis in 410 patients with new coronary lesions in the United States and Canada.[154] Almost one half of the patients had an unstable coronary syndrome. There was no difference in the incidence of death or myocardial infarction or the need for coronary bypass surgery. Restenosis, using the same definition as the Benestent trial, was a bit higher for both groups, although better in the stented group (31.6 versus 42.1 percent, $P = .046$). Interestingly, the need for late, repeat target lesion revascularization did not reach statistical significance and was lower for both groups than that quoted in Benestent—10.2 percent for stenting versus 15.8 percent for angioplasty, $P = .06$.

Routine angioplasty has been compared with primary stent implantation in 120 patients with isolated stenosis of the proximal left anterior descending coronary artery.[191] The incidence of restenosis at follow-up angiography was reduced from 40 percent in the PTCA group to 19 percent in the stent group ($P = .02$). Similarly, the incidence of recurrent angina was reduced from 25 to 10 percent ($P = .05$).

At the time these trials were conducted, the implantation of coronary stents had not been completely refined. Using standard deployment methods and oral anticoagulation, thrombosis of the stent occurred in almost 3 percent of treated patients. Since then, the use of high balloon-inflation pressures to fully deploy the stent and the use of potent antiplatelet drugs have reduced this risk. Modern stent implantation with adjuvant, antiplatelet therapy is associated with a less than 1 percent risk of major adverse events at 1 month for most patients.[246–249] This fact, combined with a reduction in the need for repeat intervention, has resulted in an almost routine use of coronary stents for percutaneous revascularization at many centers in the United States.

The many successes of coronary stenting have led some to question the validity of published trials of percutaneous revascularization with respect to general practice. Trials comparing multivessel angioplasty using stents to coronary bypass surgery are under way.[250, 251] Preliminary results from the Argentine Randomized Study of Optimal Coronary Balloon Angioplasty and Stenting versus Coronary Bypass Surgery in Multivessel Disease (ERACI II) suggest that these concerns are well founded and that the use of coronary stents will alter the relationship between percutaneous and surgical therapy. In 440 patients randomized to percutaneous therapy or coronary bypass surgery, those undergoing angioplasty or stenting enjoyed a substantial reduction in in-hospital death and myocardial infarction (1.8 versus 11.6 percent, $P = .0002$). No patients required emergency coronary bypass surgery.[250] The ARTS (Arterial Revascularization Therapy Study) trial of multivessel stenting compared with coronary bypass surgery that enrolled 1200 patients reports an incidence of death, myocardial infarction, or stroke in 5 percent of stented patients and 6 percent of patients undergoing surgery.[251]

A note of caution is in order. A stent does not prevent accumulation of neointima after balloon dilatation.[239] The proliferative response of the body to the stent may, in fact, be enhanced. A consistent finding in all of the angiographic studies is that neointimal proliferation is greater in the stented population than in the angioplasty population but because the lumen size immediately after stenting is larger than after angioplasty alone, the final result is usually slightly larger.[154, 187, 239] The likelihood of restenosis within a stent has been shown to be proportional to the length of the lesion treated. In the Johnson & Johnson/Palmaz-Schatz coronary stent registry, the rate of restenosis after the placement of tandem stents is more than three times that of single stent placement for a de novo lesion.[240] When restenosis occurs within a stent it may be very difficult to treat. There are reports of successful treatment of in-stent restenosis with balloon, laser, rotational atherectomy, and local radiation.[128–130, 252–256] Local radiation therapy appears to be very promising but the best therapy and long-term outcome in these situations is unknown.[253, 255, 256]

Studies of coronary bypass surgery emphasize the importance of long-term follow-up data and the impact of treatment on subsequent treatment alternatives. Although long-term follow-up studies of coronary stent use extending through 6 years have been published, more experience is needed.[242, 257] The impact of stent implantation at various sites through many years and of total vessel reconstruction on later disease progression, percutaneous revascularization attempts, or the ability of the surgeon to construct a reliable anastomosis is unknown.

Nonrandomized Data

Many important questions that affect clinical reasoning are studied in a randomized, controlled format, which means that two similar and relatively homogeneous populations are given treatments that are identical or equivalent except for the treatment being studied. Coronary bypass surgery and the efforts undertaken to assess its utility set the standard of proof to which new devices and techniques are held. However, even these randomized trials are not without weakness. First and foremost, the population studied may influence the outcome. The selection process, requiring the consent of both the patient and the attending physician for study entry, inherently biases randomized trials. Patients enrolled have, therefore, been filtered by the patients' and the physicians' opinions regarding the most appropriate form of therapy. The EAST trial maintained a registry of screened patients who were not entered into the randomized trial because they or their physicians refused following the outcome of the treatment chosen by the attending physician. The survival rate of this cohort of patients was better than the rate of the patients entered into randomization. This suggests that patients' and physicians' judgments are important predictors of outcome.[258]

Perhaps the most important limitation in randomized trials is time. Individual studies follow a protocol for treatment that may become outdated as the trial progresses. Examples are clearly seen in trials of percutaneous angioplasty compared with surgical coronary bypass. After the design and implementation of these trials, the introduction of the coronary stent forever altered the performance of percutaneous revascularization. In addition, improvements in surgical technique, the use of the internal mammary artery conduit, the availability of angioplasty and stent implantation, and adjunctive medical care have certainly altered the balance of outcomes after early referral for revascularization and conservative care. However, no rigorously controlled randomized trial has addressed this question. Nonrandomized observational studies often have greater statistical power and are more current than their randomized counterparts and thus provide an easy, accessible source to use as a basis for evaluating clinical practice.

The Duke University database was used to examine the outcomes of 9263 patients whose treatment decisions in favor of medical therapy, percutaneous revascularization, or surgical coronary bypass were made according to individual clinical practice.[104] Patients were classified according to the anatomic severity of disease, and attempts were made to avoid bias by correcting for clinical features that might influence long-term survival. Revascularization therapy appeared to improve outcomes for all levels of coronary disease (Fig. 42–9). Percutaneous therapy (primarily PTCA) was most effective for patients with one-vessel disease, excluding subtotal occlusion of the proximal left anterior descending artery. Patients with two-vessel disease or subtotal occlusion of the left anterior descending artery were equally well treated by surgery or PTCA. Patients with three-vessel disease or two-vessel disease involving subtotal occlusion of the proximal left anterior descending artery fared better with surgical therapy.

Survival data for patients entered into the New York state CABG surgery and angioplasty registry were reviewed in an effort to uncover any differences in outcome between the two therapies.[105] Survival at 3 years was compared for 29,930 patients undergoing percutaneous angioplasty (about 12 percent received stents) and 29,646 patients undergoing coronary bypass surgery. Patients were classified according to anatomic subgroups (one-, two-, or three-vessel disease) and the position of stenosis in the left anterior descending coronary artery (proximal or nonproximal). The results suggest that PTCA is a superior treatment for patients with one-vessel disease, excluding disease of left anterior descending artery. Patients with nonproximal left anterior descending artery disease or two-vessel disease were equally well treated with angioplasty or surgery. Finally, patients with proximal left anterior descending artery disease or three-vessel coronary disease were better treated with coronary bypass surgery.

Acute Coronary Syndromes

Coronary artery atherosclerotic lesions have the potential to undergo rapid, thrombotic evolution, abruptly altering the dynamics of coronary blood flow.[49, 259–271] Complete vessel occlusion or severe narrowing may result in acute myocardial infarction and, in some instances, sudden death.[262–265, 272, 273] Restoration of flow results in the rapid resolution of symptoms and improved short- and long-term, complication-free survival.[274–287]

Realization of the importance of atheroma evolution and thrombus formation in unstable coronary syndromes has led to the use of aggressive antiplatelet and anticoagulation strategies and, in specific settings, the administration of thrombolytic agents.[282, 283, 287–302] All have been remarkably successful in treating unstable angina and myocardial infarction. Although heparin and aspirin are effective therapies for unstable angina pectoris, they do not dissolve a thrombus once it has formed. In some patients, they are unable to prevent the progression to myocardial infarction.[298] Thrombolytics are not uniformly effective; there is a significant risk of hemorrhage, they do not address the underlying coronary stenosis, and they have no proven value in patients without ST-segment elevation or new left bundle branch block.[282, 283, 293, 294, 299] Therefore, a prominent role remains for mechanical revascularization in the therapy of unstable coronary syndromes.[287]

Surgery

Surgical bypass reduces mortality and the extent of myocardial damage when it is employed in evolving (<6 hours) myocardial infarction.[274, 276] Indeed, this was once not an uncommon setting for emergency bypass surgery, the inciting event being failed PTCA. The surgical mortality rate increases, ranging from 2.9 to 38 percent in patients with cardiogenic shock requiring inotropes or an intra-aortic balloon pump.[276, 285] Furthermore, as with thrombosis, the

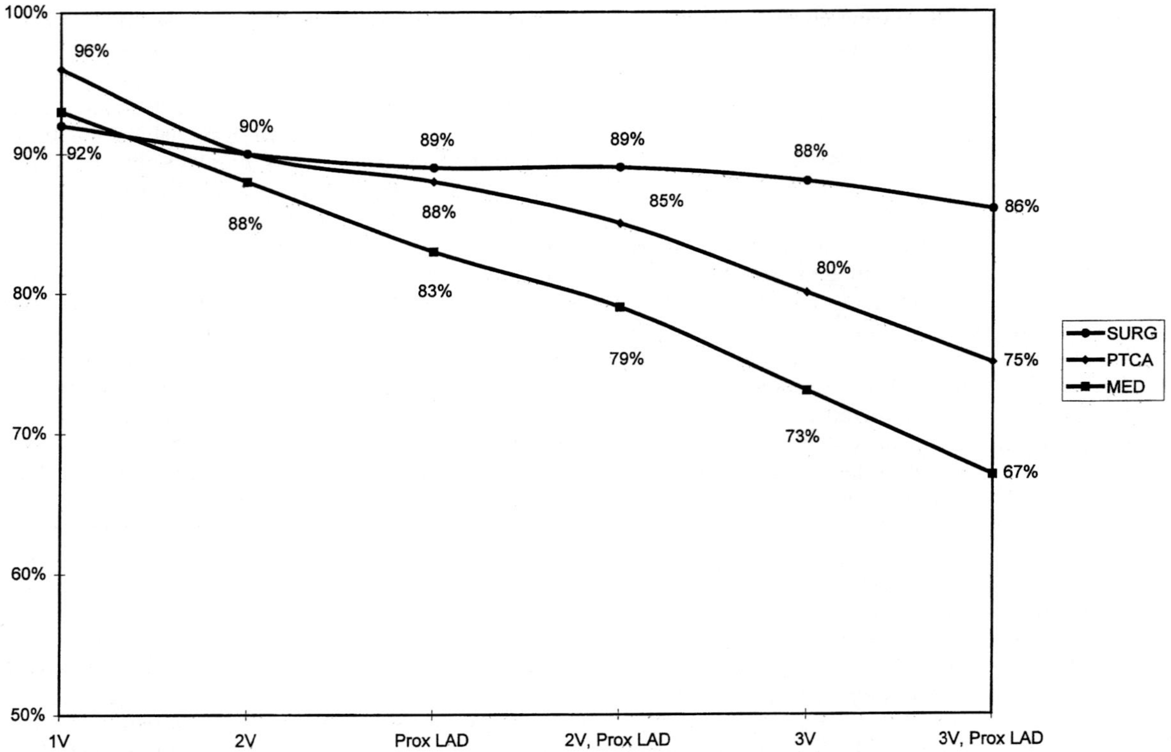

FIGURE 42–9 Survival benefit of any form of revascularization: nonrandomized data. A retrospective analysis of survival and treatment stratified by disease severity and highlighting the importance of stenosis in the proximal left anterior descending artery (LAD) suggests the survival benefit of any form of revascularization. Percutaneous revascularization appears to be most effective for patients with less severe disease. Survival benefits are most profound for patients with multivessel coronary stenosis involving the proximal LAD who undergo coronary bypass surgery. MED, medical therapy; Prox, proximal; PTCA, percutaneous transluminal coronary angioplasty; SURG, surgical therapy; V, vessel. (Data from Jones RH, Kesler K, Phillips HR, et al: Long-term survival benefits of coronary artery bypass grafting and percutaneous transluminal angioplasty in patients with coronary artery disease. J Thorac Cardiovasc Surg 111:1013–1125, 1996.)

benefit of surgery may be realized only if revascularization is achieved early.[274, 276] Emergency surgery may be performed with relative safety despite prior administration of thrombolytic agents.[286] There is, of course, an increased risk of hemorrhage and need for transfusion requirement. However, limited experience suggests that only 8 percent of patients so treated suffer sufficiently severe effects to warrant reexploration to search for the source of bleeding.[286]

When surgery is performed after the first 6 hours in the setting of acute myocardial infarction, the risk of death or complications is substantially increased[303] (Table 42–5). After 1 to 6 weeks, the risk of adverse events returns to normal. Therefore, in a patient who is stable after myocardial infarction but whose anatomy warrants referral for coronary bypass surgery, the procedure should be delayed for at least 1 week if possible.

Surgical bypass is effective in relieving symptoms of ischemia and improving the likelihood of survival of patients with refractory unstable angina pectoris.[285, 304–307] Operative mortality increases in the setting of unstable angina, left main, or three-vessel coronary artery disease.[285, 304, 305] Although the quoted perioperative mortality rate ranges from 1.7 to 5.7 percent, improvements in supportive care have produced a decline in the number of surgical deaths.[276, 285, 304, 305, 308] Similar to therapy for stable angina pectoris, surgical revascularization does not confer greater likelihood of survival on patients with one- and two-vessel coronary artery disease and normal LVEF.[285, 307] In the setting of impaired ventricular function, the benefits are profound (Fig. 42–10). Medically treated patients with an LVEF of less than 50 percent have a mortality rate of 17.6 percent at 3 years compared with 6.1 percent in patients who undergo bypass surgery.

TABLE 42–5 Coronary Artery Bypass Graft Surgery Mortality Rate in Patients With Acute Myocardial Infarction

Time From Infarction	Mortality (%)		
	Q Wave MI	*Non–Q Wave MI*	*Total Mortality*
<48 h	50.0	0	18.0
3–5 da	0	16.0	3.3
6–42 da	10.0	1.9	2.2

Reproduced with permission. Adapted from Eagle KA, Guyton RA, Davidoff R, et al: ACC/AHA Guidelines for Coronary Artery Bypass Graft Surgery: A Report of the American College of Cardiology/American Heart Association Task Force on Practice Guidelines (Committee to Revise the 1991 Guidelines for Coronary Artery Bypass Graft Surgery). J Am Coll Cardiol 34:1262–1347, 1999. © 1999 by the American College of Cardiology and the American Heart Association, Inc.

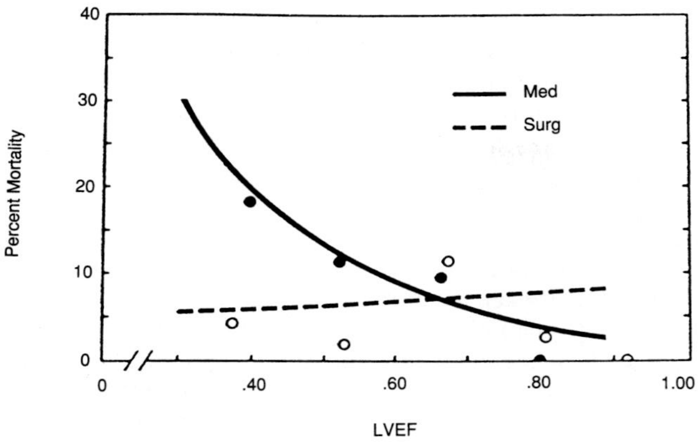

FIGURE 42–10 Surgical revascularization in unstable angina. Survival at 2 years after medical or surgical therapy for unstable angina pectoris reveals that mortality is increased with declining left ventricular function in the medical group (*solid line*). The relationship between mortality and left ventricular ejection fraction (LVEF) in the surgical group is almost horizontal (*dashed line*). This allows a significant survival benefit for surgical over medical therapy in patients with unstable angina and a depressed LVEF. Med, medical therapy; Surg, surgical therapy. (From Luchi RJ, Scott SM, Deupree RH: Comparison of medical and surgical treatment for unstable angina pectoris. Results of a Veterans Administration Cooperative Study. N Engl J Med 316:977–984, 1987.)

Percutaneous Revascularization

PTCA is a successful mode of therapy for acute coronary syndromes.[275, 277–279, 309–326] Successful PTCA within the first 6 hours of myocardial infarction is as effective as thrombolytic agents in limiting myocardial damage and improving in-hospital survival.[275, 277, 278, 309–311, 327] Beyond treating the intracoronary thrombus that is so often present, PTCA addresses the underlying coronary artery stenosis. The incidence of recurrent ischemia is reduced, and left ventricular function may be better preserved than when patients are treated with thrombolytic agents.[277, 278, 311] Furthermore, PTCA is not accompanied by a significant risk of intracranial hemorrhage.[278] Although direct angioplasty is successful in the vast majority of cases, failure may require emergency coronary bypass surgery and is accompanied by an increased risk of mortality.[328] This is, in part, a result of the diminished success rate of angioplasty in patients who are at high risk in any interventional procedure, such as those with multivessel coronary artery disease and those in cardiogenic shock. Patients undergoing urgent PTCA have a 20 to 40 percent risk of experiencing recurrent angina, restenosis, or the need for repeat revascularization.

Stents, which were initially avoided in arteries with a high probability of harboring thrombus, may actually be more effective than PTCA, especially when used in combination with a potent antiplatelet regimen.[177, 179, 243–245] The routine use of coronary stents in the setting of acute myocardial infarction is associated with a restenosis rate of 17 percent and a 6-month event-free survival rate of 83 to 95 percent.[179, 239, 243, 244]

In contrast to primary angioplasty for acute myocardial infarction, routine angioplasty following full-dose thrombolytic therapy is not uniformly beneficial. The incidence of complications and nonfatal myocardial infarction is increased in patients undergoing PTCA soon after thrombolytic therapy.[329–334] Following full-dose thrombolytic regimens, the injury produced by angioplasty may produce bleeding and intramural hematoma that may enlarge and obstruct flow.[221, 224, 335] Each approach to the treatment of myocardial infarction has specific strengths and weaknesses. Thrombolysis may be introduced rapidly upon confirming ongoing myocardial injury and may be made widely available. PTCA requires mobilization of a specially trained team and sophisticated equipment that may produce delays in effecting treatment. However, successful treatment of the culprit lesion reduces the incidence of late vessel closure and recurrent ischemic events. Preliminary data suggest that administration of low-dose tissue plasminogen activator (tPA) followed by angioplasty of significant residual lesions is a promising treatment.[336]

Balloon angioplasty is an effective form of therapy for patients with unstable angina.[315–324, 326, 336–341] Procedural success rates vary from 63 to 93 percent with an incidence of myocardial infarction of 7 to 8 percent and an in-hospital mortality rate of zero to .9 percent.[315–318, 324] Unstable angina is accompanied by an increased frequency of apparent thrombus that increases the risk of procedural complications and probably accounts for the higher incidence of myocardial infarction that accompanies PTCA in this setting.[266–271, 342–345] Adjunctive treatment with platelet glycoprotein IIb/IIIa antagonists substantially reduces the incidence of ischemic complications after PTCA or stent placement.[249, 302, 346–348] Long-term success rates are good. Restenosis rates may be similar to those of PTCA in stable angina, but reports differ on this point.[315, 320, 324, 349] When coronary stents are used, the restenosis rate is not substantially different in the setting of unstable angina.[183, 350] In fact, the routine use of stents with glycoprotein IIb/IIIa antagonists appears to provide the best short-term and long-term outcomes for patients undergoing percutaneous revascularization.[177, 351]

Treatment of Saphenous Vein Graft Disease

The development of atherosclerosis that produces luminal obstruction is almost certain in a saphenous vein bypass graft. With luminal obstruction, ischemic symptoms and the risk of infarction and death are present. Accelerated atherosclerosis in the native vessel proximal to the site of anastomosis commonly results in dependence upon the vein graft.[37, 41, 55] As a result, an increasing proportion of patients whose symptoms demand revascularization require treatment of saphenous vein graft atherosclerosis.[103]

Saphenous vein graft atherosclerosis differs from native vessel disease in that the recognition of significant stenosis is a reasonably good predictor of graft behavior. Unfortunately, the appropriate action in response to the recognition of advancing disease is unclear. An aged vein graft is diffusely diseased and fragile and is a perilous target for revascularization attempts.[352] Manipulation, whether surgical or percutaneous, is associated with a risk of cholesterol embolization and infarction that is not corrected by an open vessel. Repeat coronary bypass surgery is associated with a substantially greater risk of mortality or complica-

TABLE 42–6 Morbidity and Mortality With Primary Versus Reoperation

Mortality and Morbidity	Primary* (n = 16,996) (%)	Reoperation (n = 2509) (%)	*P* Value
Operative mortality	1.1	3.2	<.0001
Perioperative myocardial infarction	2.1	5.9	<.0001
Bleeding	4.8	6.2	<.0001
Respiratory insufficiency	2.0	3.9	<.0001
Neurologic deficit	1.6	1.8	NS
Wound complication	1.6	1.6	NS

Abbreviation: NS, not significant.
*First 1000 cases annually from 1971 to 1987.
From Loop FD, Lytle BW, Cosgrove DM, et al: Reoperation for coronary atherosclerosis: changing practice in 2509 patients. Ann Surg 212:378–386, 1990.

tion than is present in a primary procedure.[45, 103, 353–355] The risk of complications and adverse events with repeat surgical revascularization, although far better now than it was in the 1970s, remains higher than that of a first surgery (Table 42–6).[103, 353–357] Known risks for adverse outcomes are amplified at the time of a second surgery. A patient older than 70 years with severely depressed left ventricular function has a mortality risk approaching 20 percent.

Repeat coronary bypass, despite its increased operative risk, has a natural history almost identical to that of the primary procedure. After 5 years, 88 to 95 percent of patients are alive, 81 percent are free of myocardial infarction, and 55 percent are free of myocardial infarction, CABG, and PTCA. By 10 years, 51 percent remain alive, 69 percent of survivors are free of myocardial infarction, and 21 percent remain free of any event (Fig. 42–11).[45, 358] Patients with significant disease in the saphenous vein graft supplying the left anterior descending coronary artery appear to survive longer with surgical therapy, which leads some to recommend reoperation for these patients.[359]

PTCA has been used successfully to dilatate obstructing lesions in saphenous vein grafts and may provide a safer alternative to repeat surgery for some patients whose disease recurrence is symptomatic.[150, 151, 360–366] Time since surgery, location of the index lesion, and angiographic appearance provide useful indicators of the likelihood of initial success and subsequent restenosis with PTCA (Table 42–7).[150] Stent implantation is the preferred form of percutaneous revascularization in saphenous vein grafts; its use improves the short- and long-term success rates of the procedure.[145] Unfortunately, diseased grafts have a high probability of developing new lesions during follow-up, which reduces the long-term event-free survival rate (see Fig. 42–11). After stent implantation, the overall survival rate is 79 percent at 4 years, but the rate of survival free of myocardial infarction or a second revascularization procedure is only 29 percent.[152, 162, 180, 184, 272]

CONCLUSIONS

Appropriately applied revascularization therapy for coronary occlusive disease improves symptom control, quality of life, and likelihood of survival. During the thrombotic progression of atherosclerosis, timely revascularization may salvage myocardium and address an underlying obstructive coronary lesion. The beneficial effects on symptoms and survival are quickly realized. In patients with stable coronary artery disease, measurable myocardial salvage and improved survival rate must await subsequent disease progression. In the experience gained during the evolution and study of coronary bypass and angioplasty procedures, a central concept has surfaced: the risks of performing a revascularization procedure and its long-term effectiveness must be weighed against the estimated prognosis of coronary atherosclerosis using clinical, physiologic, and anatomic criteria. Innovation, technology, and new medical therapies are constantly improving the safety and reliability of revascularization methods and bettering the overall prognosis for patients with coronary atherosclerosis. This makes the task of providing strict guidelines for therapy difficult. Nevertheless, indications for performing revascularization (Table 42–8) and the most appropriate method to use (Table 42–9) are generally agreed upon.[367] The key principles used to make decisions are outlined in Table 42–10.

Patients with clear symptoms or physiologic evidence of occlusive coronary artery disease should be offered coronary angiography in order to assess the risk of and probable benefit from revascularization efforts. The extent of disease (preferably determined by using a scheme similar to that outlined by Ringqvist) and the lesions' characteristics guide the choice of therapy. Patients with left main coronary stenosis or multivessel stenosis (including the left anterior descending artery) caused by long lesions or accompanied by numerous noncritical stenoses are likely to see the best long-term outcome with surgical revascularization as opposed to percutaneous methods or medical therapy alone.

Percutaneous revascularization methods are effective but are less reliable than coronary bypass surgery. However, the comparatively lower perioperative complication rate, rapid recovery, and negligible impact on the risk of subse-

TABLE 42–7 Classification of Saphenous Vein Graft Lesions According to the Relative Likelihood of Success With Routine Balloon Angioplasty

Success Rate > 90%, Complication rate < 2%, Restenosis Rate 30%
Focal, short lesion
Graft < 4–6 years old
Single graft
Distal part sequential graft
Lesion at distal site
Success Rate > 90%, Complication Rate < 5%, Restenosis Rate 45–50%
Long lesion
Graft > 4–6 years old
Diffuse vein graft disease
Intragraft thrombus
Proximal part sequential graft
Lesion at proximal site
Lesion at body
Success Rate < 50%, Complication Rate > 10%, Restenosis Rate > 60%
Chronic totally occluded old vein grafts

From de Feyter PJ, van Suylen RJ, de Jaegere PP, et al: Balloon angioplasty for the treatment of lesions in saphenous vein bypass grafts. J Am Coll Cardiol 21:1539–1549, 1993.

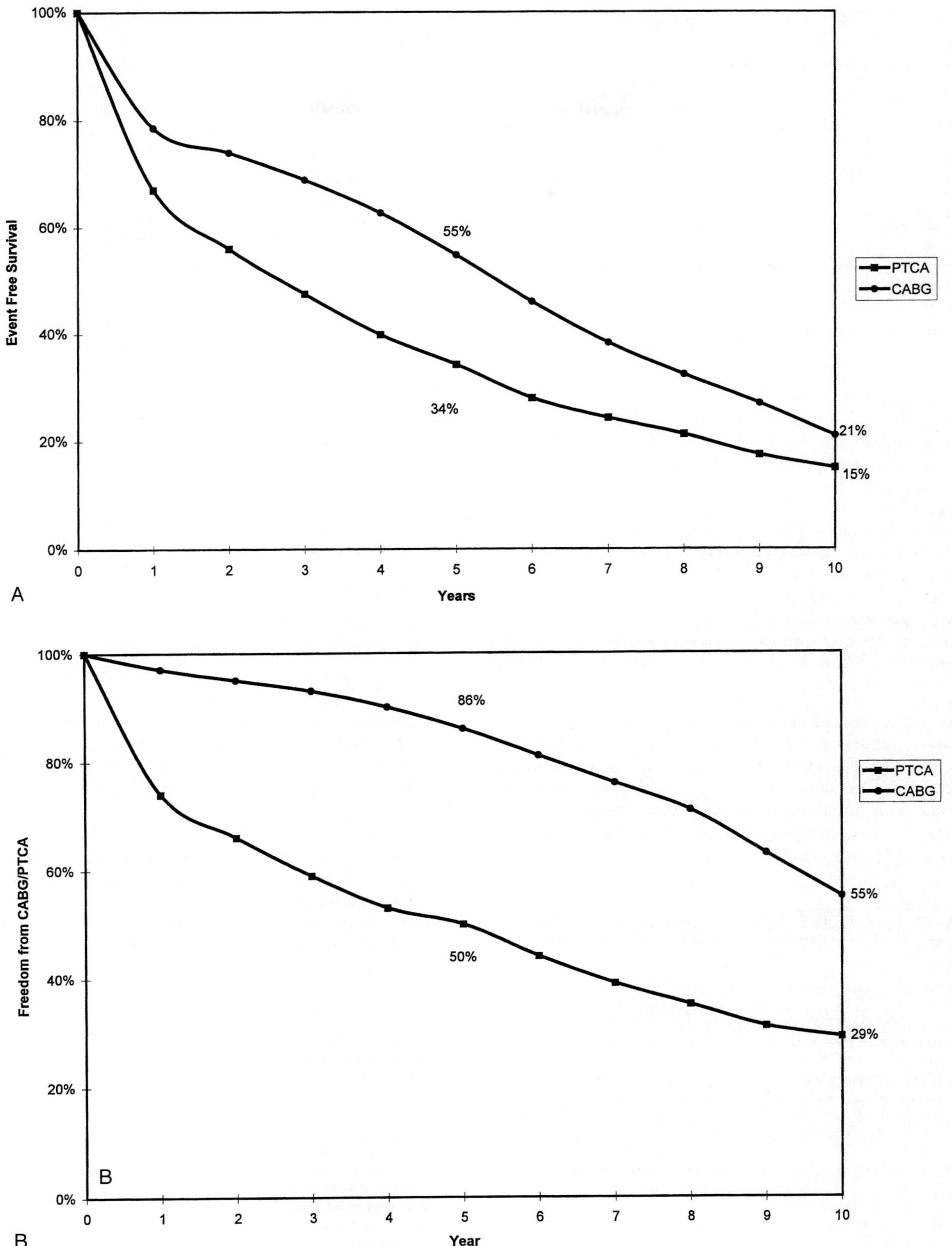

FIGURE 42–11 Revascularization for saphenous vein graft disease. A second coronary bypass surgery, despite its increased operative risk, has a natural history almost identical to that of the primary procedure. After 5 years, 88 to 95 percent of patients are alive, 81 percent are free of myocardial infarction, and 55 percent are free of myocardial infarction (MI), coronary artery bypass graft (CABG), and percutaneous transluminal coronary angioplasty (PTCA). **A,** By 10 years, 51 percent remain alive, 69 percent of survivors are free of MI, and 21 percent remain free of any event. **B,** When compared to repeat coronary bypass surgery, percutaneous revascularization is associated with an increased risk of requiring additional procedures.

Illustration continued on following page

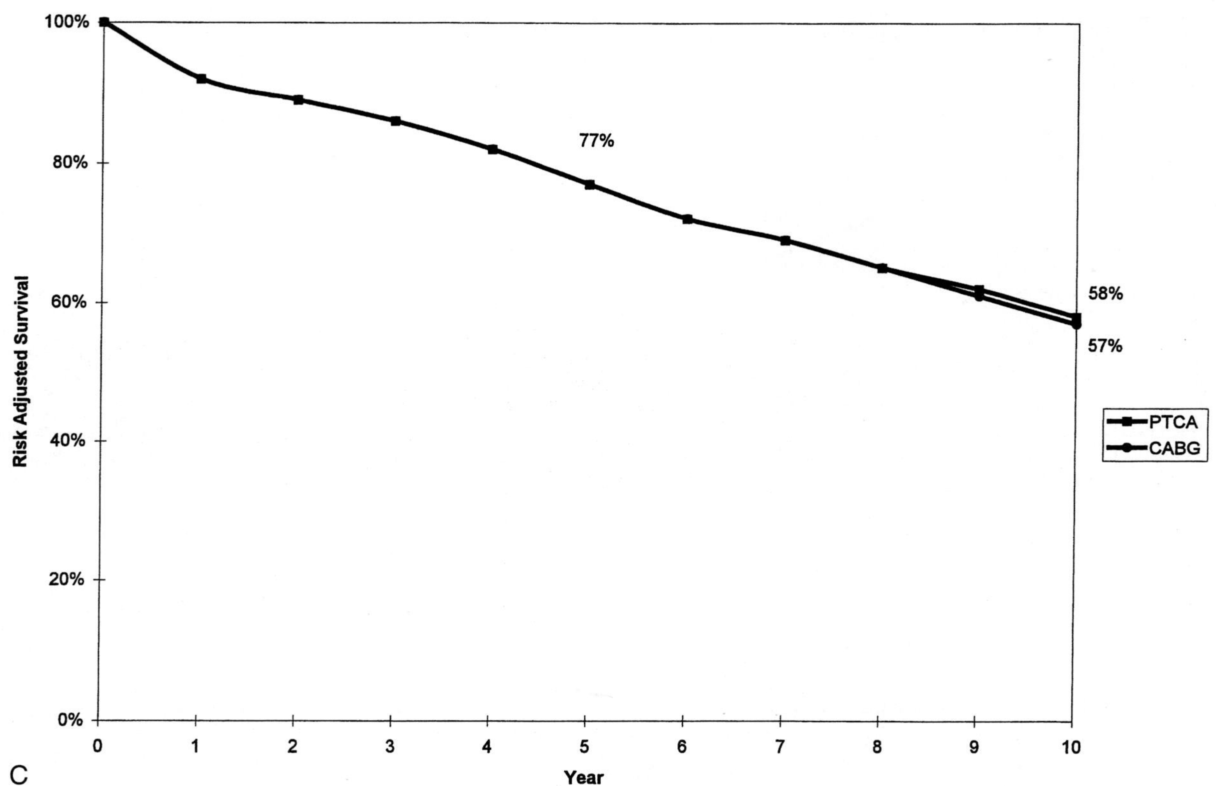

FIGURE 42–11 *Continued.* **C,** However, there was no measurable difference in survival. (**A–C,** From Weintraub WS, Jones EL, Morris DC, et al: Outcome of reoperative coronary bypass surgery versus coronary angioplasty after previous bypass surgery. Circulation 78:I158–I162, 1988.)

quent revascularization efforts make percutaneous methods the most attractive revascularization option for patients with less severe disease. Percutaneous revascularization is preferred for patients with single-vessel disease and for patients with multivessel disease and suitable coronary lesions or no opportunity to use the internal mammary artery as a bypass conduit.

TABLE 42–8 Indications for Revascularization

Definite

Left main coronary artery stenosis ≥ 50%
Coronary artery stenosis of three vessel regions with depressed left ventricular function (ejection fraction < 0.50), poor exercise tolerance or inducible ischemia with physiologic testing
Proximal significant stenosis of two coronary arteries (particularly the left anterior descending coronary artery) with depressed left ventricular function (ejection fraction < 0.50), poor exercise tolerance, or inducible ischemia with physiologic testing
Angina that impairs lifestyle or is unresponsive to medical therapy
Postinfarction angina
Unstable angina resistant to medical therapy

Possible

Acute myocardial infarction with a contraindication for thrombolytic therapy
Acute myocardial infarction with a failure of thrombolytic agents
Acute myocardial infarction with cardiogenic shock
Severely depressed left ventricular function with evidence of hibernating myocardium

Deferring revascularization is a reasonable and sometimes preferable treatment alternative for patients with limited disease, good functional status, and lesion characteristics that do not lend themselves to percutaneous methods. A good example of such a patient is one who is asymptomatic but comes to the attention of clinicians after a physiologic test is positive at high workload. An angiographic finding of complete single-vessel occlusion with excellent collateral-vessel blood supply and normal ventricular function should prompt appropriate medical therapy rather than revascularization attempts.

TABLE 42–9 Indications for Revascularization Where Surgery Is Preferred

Left main coronary artery stenosis
Three-vessel disease with depressed left ventricular ejection fraction
Intractable ischemia or evolving infarction complicating percutaneous transluminal coronary angioplasty (excluding patients with no-reflow phenomenon)
Acute myocardial infarction with cardiogenic shock in the setting of three-vessel disease or mechanical complication of myocardial infarction (ventricular septal defect, wall rupture, severe mitral regurgitation)
Angina impairing lifestyle and unresponsive to medical therapy with one or more coronary artery lesions that are not treatable using percutaneous techniques or that repeatedly recurs despite their use
Coronary stenosis accompanying a second cardiac lesion requiring cardiac surgery

TABLE 42-10 The Revascularization Decision

What proportion of viable myocardium is or may become ischemic under hemodynamic stress?
Is the magnitude of risk for injury to or dysfunction of the myocardial segment(s) high (e.g., a patient with unstable angina or non–Q wave myocardial infarction) or is dysfunction already present (i.e., stunning or hibernation)?
How does the risk of revascularization compare with the expected outcome of medical management?
What is the likelihood of long-term success of the revascularization procedure?
What comorbidities are present that may modify the rate or significance of disease progression, and how do they alter the risk of revascularization?
What are the patient's needs or wishes with respect to the risks and temporary disability accompanying surgery or the risk of requiring repeat revascularization with percutaneous procedures?

When surgical bypass is chosen, complete revascularization is the goal. Every coronary artery larger than 1.5 mm with a lesion causing 70 percent stenosis or more should receive a bypass. A caveat to this rule is that the estimation of coronary artery size may be difficult in the setting of complete vessel occlusion with poor collateral filling. Not infrequently, a vessel that is felt to be an inadequate target for bypass anastomosis is found to be a good target for bypass upon visual inspection at the time of surgery. Therefore, when percutaneous and surgical revascularization methods are being considered equally or when a patient has been referred for surgery, a completely occluded vessel that is poorly opacified by collateral filling should not be dismissed as a candidate for bypass anastomosis.

Patients with saphenous vein graft atherosclerosis are a unique, high-risk population. The presence of 50 percent stenosis or more in a saphenous vein graft indicates a significant risk of graft failure. Stent placement may be performed with a reasonable likelihood of success (noting a 10 to 20 percent risk of periprocedural myocardial infarction). Long-term freedom from recurrent events is unlikely because of the aggressive nature of saphenous vein graft disease. However, the mortality risk accompanying repeat bypass surgery is substantial. Therefore, a single diseased graft that supplies a small or moderately sized territory is best treated by percutaneous means if the graft is approachable. Patients with disease of multiple saphenous vein grafts must have low expectations of disease-free survival, even when stents are routinely used. When multiple grafts are diseased, especially if the graft responsible for the left anterior descending artery distribution is included, repeat coronary bypass surgery should be strongly considered. An exception may be made in a patient with a functioning internal mammary graft that may be injured during attempts at a second bypass procedure.

Revascularization procedures do not alter the natural history of atherosclerosis, only the likelihood of surviving as the disease progresses. Therefore, maintaining the benefit of revascularization requires that the disease process be arrested or substantially altered, a goal that has been realized only recently with the advent of potent lipid-lowering therapy. The limitations of revascularization as the sole treatment method for coronary occlusive disease are most evident in the long-term follow-up results of the VA Cooperative trial of surgical revascularization but exist no matter which revascularization method is chosen. This serves to emphasize the importance of applying appropriate medical therapy and advising on risk factor reduction before and after revascularization efforts are undertaken.

Acknowledgments

The authors acknowledge the invaluable assistance of Angie Esquivel and Linda Clifton in preparing this manuscript.

References

1. François-Franck C: Signification physiologique de la résection du sympathique dans le maladie de basedow, l'épilepsie, l'idiotie et le glaucome. Bull Acad Med Par 41:565, 1899.
2. Acierno LJ: A History of Cardiology. 1st ed. Pearl River, NY: Parthenon, 1994.
3. Carrel A: On the experimental surgery of the aorta and the heart. Ann Surg 52:83, 1910.
4. Beck CS: Principles underlying the operative approach to the treatment of myocardial ischemia. Ann Surg 118:788–806, 1943.
5. Beck CS, Leighninger DS: Operations for coronary artery lesions. Ann Surg 141:24–37, 1955.
6. Vineberg AM: Development of an anastamosis between coronary vessels and transplanted internal mammary artery. Can Med Assoc J 55:117–119, 1946.
7. Sones FMJ, Shirey EK, Proudfit WL, Wescott RN: Cine coronary arteriography. Circulation 20:773, 1959.
8. Sones FMJ, Shirey EK: Cine coronary arteriography. Mod Concepts Cardiovasc Dis 31:735, 1962.
9. Bruschke AV, Proudfit WL, Sones FM Jr: Progress study of 590 consecutive nonsurgical cases of coronary disease followed 5–9 years. II. Ventriculographic and other correlations. Circulation 47:1154–1163, 1973.
10. Bruschke AV, Proudfit WL, Sones FM Jr: Progress study of 590 consecutive nonsurgical cases of coronary disease followed 5–9 years. I. Arteriographic correlations. Circulation 47:1147–1153, 1973.
11. Favaloro RG: Critical analysis of coronary artery bypass graft surgery: a 30-year journey. J Am Coll Cardiol 31:1B–63B, 1998.
12. Sabiston DCJ: The coronary circulation. The William F. Reinhoff Lecture. John's Hopkins Med J 134:314, 1974.
13. Garrett HE, Dennis EW, DeBakey ME: Aortocoronary bypass with saphenous vein graft: seven-year follow-up. JAMA 223:792–794, 1973.
14. Favaloro RG, Effler DB, Groves LK, et al: Direct myocardial revascularization by saphenous vein graft: present operative technique and indications. Ann Thorac Surg 10:97–111, 1970.
15. Favaloro RG: Saphenous vein graft in the surgical treatment of coronary artery disease: operative technique. J Thorac Cardiovasc Surg 58:178–185, 1969.
16. Favaloro RG: Saphenous vein autograft replacement of severe segmental coronary artery occlusion: operative technique. Ann Thorac Surg 5:334–339, 1968.
17. Hall RJ, Garcia E, Wukasch DC, et al: Long-term results of coronary artery bypass. Texas Heart Inst 3:22–31, 1976.
18. Johnson WD, Flemma RJ, Lepley D Jr, Ellison EH: Extended treatment of severe coronary artery disease: a total surgical approach. Ann Surg 170:460–470, 1969.
19. Johnson WD, Flemma RJ, Lepley D Jr: Direct coronary surgery utilizing multiple-vein bypass grafts. Ann Thorac Surg 9:436–444, 1970.
20. Sheldon WC, Favaloro RG, Sones FM Jr, Effler DB: Reconstructive coronary artery surgery: venous autograft technique. JAMA 213:78–82, 1970.
21. Peduzzi P, Detre K, Gage A: Veterans Administration Cooperative Study of medical versus surgical treatment for stable angina: progress report: Section 2: design and baseline characteristics. Prog Cardiovasc Dis 28:219–228, 1985.
22. Peduzzi P, Kamina A, Detre K: Twenty-two-year follow-up in the

VA Cooperative Study of Coronary Artery Bypass Surgery for Stable Angina. Am J Cardiol 81:1393–1399, 1998.
23. The VA Coronary Artery Bypass Surgery Cooperative Study Group: Eighteen-year follow-up in the Veterans Affairs Cooperative Study of Coronary Artery Bypass Surgery for stable angina. Circulation 86:121–130, 1992.
24. Peduzzi P, Hultgren H, Thomsen J, Detre K: Ten-year effect of medical and surgical therapy on quality of life: Veterans Administration Cooperative Study of Coronary Artery Surgery. Am J Cardiol 59:1017–1023, 1987.
25. Takaro T, Hultgren HN, Lipton MJ, Detre KM: The VA cooperative randomized study of surgery for coronary arterial occlusive disease II. Subgroup with significant left main lesions. Circulation 54:III107–III117, 1976.
26. The Veterans Administration Coronary Artery Bypass Surgery Cooperative Study Group: Eleven-year survival in the Veterans Administration randomized trial of coronary bypass surgery for stable angina. N Engl J Med 311:1333–1339, 1984.
27. Rogers WJ, Coggin CJ, Gersh BJ, et al: Ten-year follow-up of quality of life in patients randomized to receive medical therapy or coronary artery bypass graft surgery. The Coronary Artery Surgery Study (CASS) [see comments]. Circulation 82:1647–1658, 1990.
28. Alderman EL, Bourassa MG, Cohen LS, et al: Ten-year follow-up of survival and myocardial infarction in the randomized Coronary Artery Surgery Study [comments]. Circulation 82:1629–1646, 1990.
29. European Coronary Surgery Study Group: Long-term results of prospective randomised study of coronary artery bypass surgery in stable angina pectoris. Lancet 2:1173–1180, 1982.
30. Varnauskas E: Twelve-year follow-up of survival in the randomized European Coronary Surgery Study. N Engl J Med 319:332–337, 1988.
31. Yusuf S, Zucker D, Peduzzi P, et al: Effect of coronary artery bypass graft surgery on survival: overview of 10-year results from randomised trials by the Coronary Artery Bypass Graft Surgery Trialists Collaboration. Lancet 1994;344:563–570.
32. Breyer RH, Spray TL, Kastl DG, Roberts WC: Histologic changes in saphenous vein aorta-coronary bypass grafts: the effect of the angle of the aortic anastomosis. J Thorac Cardiovasc Surg 72:916–924, 1976.
33. Kennedy JH, Wieting DW, Hwang NH, et al: Hydraulic and morphologic study of fibrous intimal hyperplasia in autogenous saphenous vein bypass grafts. J Thorac Cardiovasc Surg 67:805–813, 1974.
34. Storm FK, Gierson ED, Sparks FC, Barker WF: Autogenous vein bypass grafts: biological effects of mechanical dilatation and adventitial stripping in dogs. Surgery 77:261–267, 1975.
35. Grondin CM, Lepage G, Castonguay YR, et al: Aortocoronary bypass graft: initial blood flow through the graft and early postoperative patency. Circulation 44:815–819, 1971.
36. Fitzgibbon GM, Kafka HP, Leach AJ, et al: Coronary bypass graft fate and patient outcome: angiographic follow-up of 5,065 grafts related to survival and reoperation in 1,388 patients during 25 years. J Am Coll Cardiol 28:616–626, 1996.
37. Rupprecht HJ, Hamm C, Ischinger T, et al: Angiographic follow-up results of a randomized study on angioplasty versus bypass surgery (GABI trial). GABI Study Group. Eur Heart J 17:1192–1198, 1996.
38. Walts AE, Fishbein MC, Matloff JM: Thrombosed, ruptured atheromatous plaques in saphenous vein coronary artery bypass grafts: ten years' experience. Am Heart J 114:718–723, 1987.
39. Unni KK, Kottke BA, Titus JL, et al: Pathologic changes in aortocoronary saphenous vein grafts. Am J Cardiol 34:526–532, 1974.
40. Hamby RI, Aintablian A, Handler M, et al: Aortocoronary saphenous vein bypass grafts. Long-term patency, morphology and blood flow in patients with patent grafts early after surgery. Circulation 60:901–909, 1979.
41. Campeau L, Lesperance J, Hermann J, et al: Loss of the improvement of angina between 1 and 7 years after aortocoronary bypass surgery: correlations with changes in vein grafts and in coronary arteries. Circulation 60:1–5, 1979.
42. Campeau L, Enjalbert M, Lesperance J, et al: Atherosclerosis and late closure of aortocoronary saphenous vein grafts: sequential angiographic studies at 2 weeks, 1 year, 5 to 7 years, and 10 to 12 years after surgery. Circulation 68:II1–II7, 1983.
43. Bond MG, Hostetler JR, Karayannacos PE, et al: Intimal changes in arteriovenous bypass grafts. Effects of varying the angle of implantation at the proximal anastomosis and of producing stenosis in the distal runoff artery. J Thorac Cardiovasc Surg 71:907–916, 1976.
44. Grondin CM, Meere C, Castonguay Y, et al: Progressive and late obstruction of an aorto-coronary venous bypass graft. Circulation 43:698–702, 1971.
45. Loop FD, Cosgrove DM, Kramer JR, et al: Late clinical and arteriographic results in 500 coronary artery reoperations. J Thorac Cardiovasc Surg 81:675–685, 1981.
46. Lytle BW, Loop FD, Cosgrove DM, et al: Long-term (5 to 12 years) serial studies of internal mammary artery and saphenous vein coronary bypass grafts. J Thorac Cardiovasc Surg 89:248–258, 1985.
47. Fitzgibbon GM, Leach AJ, Kafka HP, Keon WJ: Coronary bypass graft fate: long-term angiographic study. J Am Coll Cardiol 17:1075–1080, 1991.
48. Frey RR, Bruschke AV, Vermeulen FE: Serial angiographic evaluation 1 year and 9 years after aorta-coronary bypass. A study of 55 patients chosen at random. J Thorac Cardiovasc Surg 87:167–174, 1984.
49. Bulkley BH, Hutchins GM: Accelerated "atherosclerosis": a morphologic study of 97 saphenous vein coronary artery bypass grafts. Circulation 55:163–169, 1977.
50. Brody WR, Angeli WW, Kosek JC: Histologic fate of the venous coronary artery bypass in dogs. Am J Pathol 66:111–130, 1972.
51. Jones M, Conkle DM, Ferrans VJ, et al: Lesions observed in arterial autogenous vein grafts. Light and electron microscopic evaluation. Circulation 48:III198–III221, 1973.
52. Kern WH, Dermer GB, Lindesmith GG: The intimal proliferation in aortic-coronary saphenous vein grafts. Light and electron microscopic studies. Am Heart J 84:771–777, 1972.
53. van der Wal AC, Becker AE, Elbers JR, Das PK. An immunocytochemical analysis of rapidly progressive atherosclerosis in human vein grafts. Eur J Cardiothorac Surg 6:469–473, 1992.
54. Vlodaver Z, Edwards JE. Pathologic changes in aortic-coronary arterial saphenous vein grafts. Circulation 44:719–728, 1971.
55. Spray TL, Roberts WC: Status of the grafts and the native coronary arteries proximal and distal to coronary anastomotic sites of aorto-coronary bypass grafts. Circulation 55:741–749, 1977.
56. Weintraub WS, Jones EL, Craver JM, Guyton RA: Frequency of repeat coronary bypass or coronary angioplasty after coronary artery bypass surgery using saphenous venous grafts. Am J Cardiol 73:103–112, 1994.
57. Kolessov VI: Mammary artery-coronary artery anastomosis as method of treatment for angina pectoris. J Thorac Cardiovasc Surg 54:535–544, 1967.
58. Loop FD, Lytle BW, Cosgrove DM, et al: Free (aorta-coronary) internal mammary artery graft. Late results. J Thorac Cardiovasc Surg 92:827–831, 1986.
59. Green GE, Stertzer SH, Gordon RB, Tice DA: Anastomosis of the internal mammary artery to the distal left anterior descending coronary artery. Circulation 41:II79–II85, 1970.
60. Singh RN, Sosa JA, Green GE: Long-term fate of the internal mammary artery and saphenous vein grafts. J Thorac Cardiovasc Surg 86:359–363, 1983.
61. Tector AJ, Schmahl TM, Janson B, et al: The internal mammary artery graft: its longevity after coronary bypass. JAMA 246:2181–2183, 1981.
62. Barner HB, Swartz MT, Mudd JG, Tyras DH: Late patency of the internal mammary artery as a coronary bypass conduit. Ann Thorac Surg 34:408–412, 1982.
63. Loop FD, Lytle BW, Cosgrove DM, et al: Influence of the internal-mammary-artery graft on 10-year survival and other cardiac events. N Engl J Med 314:1–6, 1986.
64. Grondin CM, Campeau L, Lesperance J, et al: Comparison of late changes in internal mammary artery and saphenous vein grafts in two consecutive series of patients 10 years after operation. Circulation 70:I208–I212, 1984.
65. Cameron AA, Green GE, Brogno DA, Thornton J: Internal thoracic artery grafts: 20-year clinical follow-up. J Am Coll Cardiol 25:188–192, 1995.
66. Huddleston CB, Stoney WS, Alford WC Jr, et al: Internal mammary artery grafts: technical factors influencing patency. Ann Thorac Surg 42:543–549, 1986.
67. Boylan MJ, Lytle BW, Loop FD, et al: Surgical treatment of isolated

left anterior descending coronary stenosis. Comparison of left internal mammary artery and venous autograft at 18 to 20 years of follow-up. J Thorac Cardiovasc Surg 107:657–662, 1994.
68. Bergsma TM, Grandjean JG, Voors AA, et al: Low recurrence of angina pectoris after coronary artery bypass graft surgery with bilateral internal thoracic and right gastroepiploic arteries [see comments]. Circulation 97:2402–2405, 1998.
69. Fiore AC, Naunheim KS, Dean P, et al: Results of internal thoracic artery grafting over 15 years: single versus double grafts. Ann Thorac Surg 49:202–209, 1990.
70. Galbut DL, Traad EA, Dorman MJ, et al: Twelve-year experience with bilateral internal mammary artery grafts. Ann Thorac Surg 40:264–270, 1985.
71. Diegeler A, Matin M, Falk V, et al: Coronary bypass grafting without cardiopulmonary bypass—technical considerations, clinical results, and follow-up. Thorac Cardiovasc Surg 47:14–18, 1999.
72. Holubkov R, Zenati M, Akin JJ, et al: MIDCAB characteristics and results: the Cardio Thoracic Systems (CTS) registry. Eur J Cardiothorac Surg 14 Suppl 1:S25–S30, 1998.
73. Izzat MB, Yim AP, El-Zufari MH: Minimally invasive left anterior descending coronary artery revascularization in high-risk patients with three-vessel disease. Ann Thorac Cardiovasc Surg 4:205–208, 1998.
74. Doty JR, Salazar JD, Fonger JD, et al: Reoperative MIDCAB grafting: 3-year clinical experience. Eur J Cardiothorac Surg 13:641–649, 1998.
75. Tatoulis J, Goldblatt JC, Skillington PD, Warren RJ: Minimally invasive coronary artery bypass surgery without cardiopulmonary bypass. Med J Aust 167:359–362, 1997.
76. Borger MA, Cohen G, Buth KJ, et al: Multiple arterial grafts: radial versus right internal thoracic arteries. Circulation 98:II7–II14, 1998.
77. Cooley DA: Coronary bypass grafting with bilateral internal thoracic arteries and the right gastroepiploic artery [editorial; comment]. Circulation 97:2384–2385, 1998.
78. Peduzzi P, Detre K, Murphy ML, et al: Ten-year incidence of myocardial infarction and prognosis after infarction. Department of Veterans Affairs Cooperative Study of Coronary Artery Bypass Surgery [see comments]. Circulation 83:747–755, 1991.
79. Crean PA, Waters DD, Bosch X, et al: Angiographic findings after myocardial infarction in patients with previous bypass surgery: explanations for smaller infarcts in this group compared with control patients. Circulation 71:693–698, 1985.
80. Bourassa MG, Campeau L, Lesperance J, Grondin CM: Changes in grafts and coronary arteries after saphenous vein aortocoronary bypass surgery: results at repeat angiography. Circulation 65:90–97, 1982.
81. Califf RM, Harrell FE Jr, Lee KL, et al: The evolution of medical and surgical therapy for coronary artery disease: a 15-year perspective [see comments]. JAMA 261:2077–2086, 1989.
82. Elefteriades JA, Morales DL, Gradel C, et al: Results of coronary artery bypass grafting by a single surgeon in patients with left ventricular ejection fractions or = 30%. Am J Cardiol 79:1573–1578, 1997.
83. Eltchaninoff H, Franco I, Whitlow PL: Late results of coronary angioplasty in patients with left ventricular ejection fractions or = 40%. Am J Cardiol 73:1047–1052, 1994.
84. Ivanov J, Weisel RD, David TE, Naylor CD: Fifteen-year trends in risk severity and operative mortality in elderly patients undergoing coronary artery bypass graft surgery. Circulation 97:673–680, 1998.
85. Gann D, Colin C, Hildner FJ, et al: Coronary artery bypass surgery in patients seventy years of age and older. J Thorac Cardiovasc Surg 73:237–241, 1977.
86. Knapp WS, Douglas JS Jr, Craver JM, et al: Efficacy of coronary artery bypass grafting in elderly patients with coronary artery disease. Am J Cardiol 47:923–930, 1981.
87. Gersh BJ, Kronmal RA, Frye RL, et al: Coronary arteriography and coronary artery bypass surgery: morbidity and mortality in patients ages 65 years or older. A report from the Coronary Artery Surgery Study. Circulation 67:483–491, 1983.
88. Hibler BA, Wright JO, Wright CB, et al: Coronary artery bypass surgery in the elderly. Arch Surg 118:402–404, 1983.
89. Hochberg MS, Levine FH, Daggett WM, et al: Isolated coronary artery bypass grafting in patients seventy years of age and older: early and late results. J Thorac Cardiovasc Surg 84:219–223, 1982.
90. Horneffer PJ, Gardner TJ, Manolio TA, et al: The effects of age on outcome after coronary bypass surgery. Circulation 76:V6–V12, 1987.
91. Horvath KA, DiSesa VJ, Peigh PS, et al: Favorable results of coronary artery bypass grafting in patients older than 75 years [comments]. J Thorac Cardiovasc Surg 99:92–96, 1990.
92. Freeman WK, Schaff HV, O'Brien PC, et al: Cardiac surgery in the octogenarian: perioperative outcome and clinical follow-up [see comments]. J Am Coll Cardiol 18:29–35, 1991.
93. Hannan EL, Burke J: Effect of age on mortality in coronary artery bypass surgery in New York, 1991–1992. Am Heart J 128:1184–1191, 1994.
94. Curtis JJ, Walls JT, Boley TM, et al: Coronary revascularization in the elderly: determinants of operative mortality. Ann Thorac Surg 58:1069–1072, 1994.
95. He GW, Ryan WH, Acuff TE, et al: Risk factors for operative mortality and sternal wound infection in bilateral internal mammary artery grafting. J Thorac Cardiovasc Surg 107:196–202, 1994.
96. Tsai TP, Nessim S, Kass RM, et al: Morbidity and mortality after coronary artery bypass in octogenarians. Ann Thorac Surg 51:983–986, 1991.
97. Ko W, Krieger KH, Lazenby WD, et al: Isolated coronary artery bypass grafting in one hundred consecutive octogenarian patients: a multivariate analysis. J Thorac Cardiovasc Surg 102:532–538, 1991.
98. The Post-Coronary Artery Bypass Graft Trial Investigators. The effect of aggressive lowering of low-density lipoprotein cholesterol levels and low-dose anticoagulation on obstructive changes in saphenous-vein coronary-artery bypass grafts. N Engl J Med 336:153–162, 1997.
99. Frick MH, Syvanne M, Nieminen MS, et al: Prevention of the angiographic progression of coronary and vein-graft atherosclerosis by gemfibrozil after coronary bypass surgery in men with low levels of HDL cholesterol. Lopid Coronary Angiography Trial (LOCAT) Study Group. Circulation 96:2137–2143, 1997.
100. Stein PD, Dalen JE, Goldman S, Theroux P: Antithrombotic therapy in patients with saphenous vein and internal mammary artery bypass grafts. Chest 114:658S–665S, 1998.
101. Cameron A, Davis KB, Green GE, et al: Clinical implications of internal mammary artery bypass grafts: the Coronary Artery Surgery Study experience. Circulation 77:815–819, 1988.
102. Buxton BF, Komeda M, Fuller JA, Gordon I: Bilateral internal thoracic artery grafting may improve outcome of coronary artery surgery. Risk-adjusted survival. Circulation 98:II1–II6, 1998.
103. Loop FD, Lytle BW, Cosgrove DM, et al: Reoperation for coronary atherosclerosis: changing practice in 2509 consecutive patients. Ann Surg 212:378–386, 1990.
104. Jones RH, Kesler K, Phillips HR, et al: Long-term survival benefits of coronary artery bypass grafting and percutaneous transluminal angioplasty in patients with coronary artery disease. J Thorac Cardiovasc Surg 111:1013–1125, 1996.
105. Hannan EL, Racz MJ, McCallister BD, et al: A comparison of three-year survival after coronary artery bypass graft surgery and percutaneous transluminal coronary angioplasty. J Am Coll Cardiol 33:63–72, 1999.
106. Forssman W: Die Sonderrung des rechten Hertzens. Klin Wochenschr 8:2085, 1929.
107. Cournand AF, Ranges HS: Catheterization of the right auricle in man. Proc Soc Exp Biol Med 45:462, 1941.
108. Richards DW: Cardiac output in the catheterization technique in various clinical conditions. Fed Proc 4:215, 1945.
109. Rickets JH, Abrams HL: Percutaneous selective coronary cine arteriography. JAMA 181:620, 1962.
110. Judkins MP: Selective coronary arteriography. I. A percutaneous transfemoral technic. Radiology 89:815–824, 1967.
111. Dotter CT, Judkins MP: Transluminal treatment of arteriosclerotic obstruction: description of a new technique and preliminary report of its application. Circulation 30:654, 1964.
112. Zeitler E, Schoop W, Zanhow W: The treatment of occlusive arterial disease by transluminal catheter angioplasty. Radiology 99:19–26, 1971.
113. Gruentzig AR: Die perkutane transluminale Rekanalisation chronischer arterieller Verschlusse (Dotter-Prinzip) mit einem doppellumigen Dilatations-Katheter. Fortschr Roentgenstr 124:80, 1976.
114. Gruentzig A: [Percutaneous dilatation of experimental coronary ar-

tery stenosis: description of a new catheter system]. Klin Wochenschr 54:543–545, 1976.
115. Gruentzig A: Transluminal dilatation of coronary-artery stenosis [letter]. Lancet 1:263, 1978.
116. Baim DS, Cutlip DE, Sharma SK, et al: Final results of the Balloon vs Optimal Atherectomy Trial (BOAT). Circulation 97:322–331, 1998.
117. Simonton CA, Leon MB, Baim DS, et al: "Optimal" directional coronary atherectomy: final results of the Optimal Atherectomy Restenosis Study (OARS). Circulation 97:332–339, 1998.
118. Topol EJ, Leya F, Pinkerton CA, et al: A comparison of directional atherectomy with coronary angioplasty in patients with coronary artery disease. The CAVEAT Study Group. N Engl J Med 329:221–227, 1993.
119. Adelman AG, Cohen EA, Kimball BP, et al: A comparison of directional atherectomy with balloon angioplasty for lesions of the left anterior descending coronary artery. N Engl J Med 329:228–233, 1993.
120. Fishman RF, Kuntz RE, Carrozza JP, et al: Long-term results of directional coronary atherectomy: predictors of restenosis. J Am Coll Cardiol 20:1101–1110, 1992.
121. Stertzer SH, Rosenblum J, Shaw RE, et al: Coronary rotational ablation: initial experience in 302 procedures. J Am Coll Cardiol 21:287–295, 1993.
122. Spears JR, Reyes VP, Wynne J, et al: Percutaneous coronary laser balloon angioplasty: initial results of a multicenter experience. J Am Coll Cardiol 16:293–303, 1990.
123. Sanborn TA, Faxon DP, Kellett MA, Ryan TJ: Percutaneous coronary laser thermal angioplasty. J Am Coll Cardiol 8:1437–1440, 1986.
124. Estella P, Ryan TJ Jr, Landzberg JS, Bittl JA: Excimer laser-assisted coronary angioplasty for lesions containing thrombus. J Am Coll Cardiol 21:1550–1556, 1993.
125. Popma JJ, Leon MB, Mintz GS, et al: Results of coronary angioplasty using the transluminal extraction catheter. Am J Cardiol 70:1526–1532, 1992.
126. Feld H, Schulhoff N, Lichstein E, et al: Coronary atherectomy versus angioplasty: the CAVA study. Am Heart J 126:31–38, 1993.
127. Litvack F, Grundfest W, Eigler N, et al: Percutaneous excimer laser coronary angioplasty [letter]. Lancet 2:102–103, 1989.
128. Topaz O, Vetrovec GW: The stenotic stent: mechanisms and revascularization options. Cathet Cardiovasc Diagn 37:293–299, 1996.
129. Stone GW: Rotational atherectomy for treatment of in-stent restenosis: role of intracoronary ultrasound guidance. Cathet Cardiovasc Diagn Suppl 3:73–77, 1996.
130. Sharma SK, Duvvuri S, Dangas G, et al: Rotational atherectomy for in-stent restenosis: acute and long-term results of the first 100 cases. J Am Coll Cardiol 32:1358–1365, 1998.
131. Gilmore PS, Bass TA, Conetta DA, et al: Single-site experience with high-speed coronary rotational atherectomy. Clin Cardiol 16:311–316, 1993.
132. Guidelines for percutaneous transluminal coronary angioplasty. A report of the American College of Cardiology/American Heart Association Task Force on Assessment of Diagnostic and Therapeutic Cardiovascular Procedures (Subcommittee on Percutaneous Transluminal Coronary Angioplasty). J Am Coll Cardiol 12:529–545, 1988.
133. Kadel C, Vallbracht C, Buss F, et al: Long-term follow-up after percutaneous transluminal coronary angioplasty in patients with single-vessel disease. Am Heart J 124:1159–1169, 1992.
134. Berger PB, Bell MR, Garratt KN, et al: Initial results and long-term outcome of coronary angioplasty in chronic mild angina pectoris. Am J Cardiol 71:1396–1401, 1993.
135. Detre KM, Holmes DR Jr, Holubkov R, et al: Incidence and consequences of periprocedural occlusion. The 1985–1986 National Heart, Lung, and Blood Institute Percutaneous Transluminal Coronary Angioplasty Registry. Circulation 82:739–750, 1990.
136. Sinclair IN, McCabe CH, Sipperly ME, Baim DS: Predictors, therapeutic options and long-term outcome of abrupt reclosure. Am J Cardiol 61:61G–66G, 1988.
137. Wilson JM, Silberman H, Ferguson JJ: Abrupt vascular closure. J Inv Cardiol 6:306–313, 1994.
138. Maiello L, Colombo A, Gianrossi R, et al: Coronary stenting for treatment of acute or threatened closure following dissection after coronary balloon angioplasty. Am Heart J 125:1570–1575, 1993.
139. Roubin GS, Cannon AD, Agrawal SK, et al: Intracoronary stenting for acute and threatened closure complicating percutaneous transluminal coronary angioplasty. Circulation 85:916–927, 1992.
140. Sutton JM, Ellis SG, Roubin GS, et al: Major clinical events after coronary stenting. The multicenter registry of acute and elective Gianturco-Roubin stent placement. The Gianturco-Roubin Intracoronary Stent Investigator Group. Circulation 89:1126–1137, 1994.
141. Herrmann HC, Buchbinder M, Clemen MW, et al: Emergent use of balloon-expandable coronary artery stenting for failed percutaneous transluminal coronary angioplasty. Circulation 86:812–819, 1992.
142. George BS, Voorhees WD, Roubin GS, et al: Multicenter investigation of coronary stenting to treat acute or threatened closure after percutaneous transluminal coronary angioplasty: clinical and angiographic outcomes. J Am Coll Cardiol 22:135–143, 1993.
143. Piana RN, Ahmed WH, Chaitman B, et al: Effect of transient abrupt vessel closure during otherwise successful angioplasty for unstable angina on clinical outcome at six months. Hirulog Angioplasty Study Investigators. J Am Coll Cardiol 33:73–78, 1999.
144. Savage MP, Fischman DL, Rake R, et al: Efficacy of coronary stenting versus balloon angioplasty in small coronary arteries. Stent Restenosis Study (STRESS) Investigators. J Am Coll Cardiol 31:307–311, 1998.
145. Savage MP, Douglas JS Jr, Fischman DL, et al: Stent placement compared with balloon angioplasty for obstructed coronary bypass grafts. Saphenous Vein De Novo Trial Investigators [see comments]. N Engl J Med 337:740–747, 1997.
146. Turi ZG, Campbell CA, Gottimukkala MV, Kloner RA: Preservation of distal coronary perfusion during prolonged balloon inflation with an autoperfusion angioplasty catheter. Circulation 75:1273–1280, 1987.
147. Turi ZG, Rezkalla S, Campbell CA, Kloner RA: Amelioration of ischemia during angioplasty of the left anterior descending coronary artery with an autoperfusion catheter. Am J Cardiol 62:513–517, 1988.
148. Vogel JH, Ruiz CE, Jahnke EJ, et al: Percutaneous (nonsurgical) supported angioplasty in unprotected left main disease and severe left ventricular dysfunction. Clin Cardiol 12:297–300, 1989.
149. Vogel RA, Shawl F, Tommaso C, et al: Initial report of the National Registry of Elective Cardiopulmonary Bypass Supported Coronary Angioplasty [see comments]. J Am Coll Cardiol 15:23–29, 1990.
150. de Feyter PJ, van Suylen RJ, de Jaegere PP, et al: Balloon angioplasty for the treatment of lesions in saphenous vein bypass grafts. J Am Coll Cardiol 21:1539–1549, 1993.
151. Dorros G, Johnson WD, Tector AJ, et al: Percutaneous transluminal coronary angioplasty in patients with prior coronary artery bypass grafting. J Thorac Cardiovasc Surg 87:17–26, 1984.
152. Eeckhout E, Goy JJ, Stauffer JC, et al: Endoluminal stenting of narrowed saphenous vein grafts: long-term clinical and angiographic follow-up [see comments]. Cathet Cardiovasc Diagn 32:139–146, 1994.
153. de Scheerder IK, Strauss BH, de Feyter PJ, et al: Stenting of venous bypass grafts: a new treatment modality for patients who are poor candidates for reintervention. Am Heart J 123:1046–1054, 1992.
154. Fischman DL, Leon MB, Baim DS, et al: A randomized comparison of coronary-stent placement and balloon angioplasty in the treatment of coronary artery disease. Stent Restenosis Study Investigators. N Engl J Med 331:496–501, 1994.
155. Erbel R, Clas W, Busch U, et al: New balloon catheter for prolonged percutaneous transluminal coronary angioplasty and bypass flow in occluded vessels. Cathet Cardiovasc Diagn 12:116–123, 1986.
156. Ellis SG, Tamai H, Nobuyoshi M, et al: Contemporary percutaneous treatment of unprotected left main coronary stenoses: initial results from a multicenter registry analysis 1994–1996. Circulation 96:3867–3872, 1997.
157. Lopez JJ, Ho KK, Stoler RC, et al: Percutaneous treatment of protected and unprotected left main coronary stenoses with new devices: immediate angiographic results and intermediate-term follow-up. J Am Coll Cardiol 29:345–352, 1997.
158. Nanto S, Nishida K, Hirayama A, et al: Supported angioplasty with synchronized retroperfusion in high-risk patients with left main trunk or near left main trunk obstruction. Am Heart J 125:301–309, 1993.
159. Park SJ, Park SW, Hong MK, et al: Stenting of unprotected left main coronary artery stenoses: immediate and late outcomes. J Am Coll Cardiol 31:37–42, 1998.

160. Tommaso CL, Vogel JH, Vogel RA: Coronary angioplasty in high-risk patients with left main coronary stenosis: results from the National Registry of Elective Supported Angioplasty. Cathet Cardiovasc Diagn 25:169–173, 1992.
161. Wong P, Wong CM, Ko P, Fong PC: Elective stenting of unprotected left main coronary disease. Cathet Cardiovasc Diagn 39:347–354, 1996.
162. Wong SC, Baim DS, Schatz RA, et al: Immediate results and late outcomes after stent implantation in saphenous vein graft lesions: the multicenter U.S. Palmaz-Schatz stent experience. The Palmaz-Schatz Stent Study Group. J Am Coll Cardiol 26:704–712, 1995.
163. Carrie D, Elbaz M, Puel J, et al: Five-year outcome after coronary angioplasty versus bypass surgery in multivessel coronary artery disease: results from the French Monocentric Study. Circulation 96:II1–II6, 1997.
164. Mabin TA, Holmes DR Jr, Smith HC, et al: Follow-up clinical results in patients undergoing percutaneous transluminal coronary angioplasty. Circulation 71:754–760, 1985.
165. Comparison of coronary bypass surgery with angioplasty in patients with multivessel disease. The Bypass Angioplasty Revascularization Investigation (BARI) Investigators. N Engl J Med 335:217–225, 1996.
166. Hamm CW, Reimers J, Ischinger T, et al: A randomized study of coronary angioplasty compared with bypass surgery in patients with symptomatic multivessel coronary disease. German Angioplasty Bypass Surgery Investigation (GABI). N Engl J Med 331:1037–1043, 1994.
167. King SB 3rd, Lembo NJ, Weintraub WS, et al: A randomized trial comparing coronary angioplasty with coronary bypass surgery. Emory Angioplasty versus Surgery Trial (EAST). N Engl J Med 331:1044–1050, 1994.
168. Rodriguez A, Boullon F, Perez-Balino N, et al: Argentine randomized trial of percutaneous transluminal coronary angioplasty versus coronary artery bypass surgery in multivessel disease (ERACI): in-hospital results and 1-year follow-up. ERACI Group. J Am Coll Cardiol 22:1060–1067, 1993.
169. Rodriguez A, Mele E, Peyregne E, et al: Three-year follow-up of the Argentine Randomized Trial of Percutaneous Transluminal Coronary Angioplasty Versus Coronary Artery Bypass Surgery in Multivessel Disease (ERACI). J Am Coll Cardiol 27:1178–1184, 1996.
170. O'Keefe JH Jr, Allan JJ, McCallister BD, et al: Angioplasty versus bypass surgery for multivessel coronary artery disease with left ventricular ejection fraction or = 40%. Am J Cardiol 71:897–901, 1993.
171. Vandormael M, Deligonul U, Taussig S, Kern MJ: Predictors of long-term cardiac survival in patients with multivessel coronary artery disease undergoing percutaneous transluminal coronary angioplasty. Am J Cardiol 67:1–6, 1991.
172. Cowley MJ, Vetrovec GW, Wolfgang TC: Efficacy of percutaneous transluminal coronary angioplasty: technique, patient selection, salutary results, limitations and complications. Am Heart J 101:272–280, 1981.
173. First-year results of CABRI (Coronary Angioplasty versus Bypass Revascularization Investigation). CABRI Trial Participants [see comments]. Lancet. 346:1179–1184, 1995.
174. Henderson RA, Pocock SJ, Sharp SJ, et al: Long-term results of RITA-1 trial: clinical and cost comparisons of coronary angioplasty and coronary-artery bypass grafting. Randomised Intervention Treatment of Angina [see comments]. Lancet 352:1419–1425, 1998.
175. Five-year clinical and functional outcome comparing bypass surgery and angioplasty in patients with multivessel coronary disease. A multicenter randomized trial. Writing Group for the Bypass Angioplasty Revascularization Investigation (BARI) Investigators [see comments]. JAMA 277:715–721, 1997.
176. Warner MF, DiSciascio G, Kohli RS, et al: Long-term efficacy of triple-vessel angioplasty in patients with severe three-vessel coronary artery disease. Am Heart J 124:1169–1174, 1992.
177. Randomised placebo-controlled and balloon-angioplasty-controlled trial to assess safety of coronary stenting with use of platelet glycoprotein IIb/IIIa blockade. The EPISTENT Investigators. Evaluation of Platelet IIb/IIIa Inhibitor for Stenting [comments]. Lancet 352:87–92,
178. Altmann DB, Racz M, Battleman DS, et al: Reduction in angioplasty complications after the introduction of coronary stents: results from a consecutive series of 2242 patients. Am Heart J 132:503–507, 1996.
179. Antoniucci D, Santoro GM, Bolognese L, et al: A clinical trial comparing primary stenting of the infarct-related artery with optimal primary angioplasty for acute myocardial infarction: results from the Florence Randomized Elective Stenting in Acute Coronary Occlusions (FRESCO) trial. J Am Coll Cardiol 31:1234–1239, 1998.
180. Brener SJ, Ellis SG, Apperson-Hansen C, et al: Comparison of stenting and balloon angioplasty for narrowings in aortocoronary saphenous vein conduits in place for more than five years. Am J Cardiol 79:13–18, 1997.
181. Cohen DJ, Krumholz HM, Sukin CA, et al: In-hospital and one-year economic outcomes after coronary stenting or balloon angioplasty. Results from a randomized clinical trial. Stent Restenosis Study Investigators. Circulation 92:2480–2487, 1995.
182. Macaya C, Serruys PW, Ruygrok P, et al: Continued benefit of coronary stenting versus balloon angioplasty: one-year clinical follow-up of Benestent trial. Benestent Study Group. J Am Coll Cardiol 27:255–261, 1996.
183. Malosky SA, Hirshfeld JW Jr, Herrmann HC: Comparison of results of intracoronary stenting in patients with unstable vs. stable angina. Cathet Cardiovasc Diagn 31:95–101, 1994.
184. Piana RN, Moscucci M, Cohen DJ, et al: Palmaz-Schatz stenting for treatment of focal vein graft stenosis: immediate results and long-term outcome. J Am Coll Cardiol 23:1296–1304, 1994.
185. Rubartelli P, Niccoli L, Verna E, et al: Stent implantation versus balloon angioplasty in chronic coronary occlusions: results from the GISSOC trial. Gruppo Italiano di Studio sullo Stent nelle Occlusioni Coronariche. J Am Coll Cardiol 32:90–96, 1998.
186. Schatz RA, Baim DS, Leon M, et al: Clinical experience with the Palmaz-Schatz coronary stent. Initial results of a multicenter study. Circulation 83:148–161, 1991.
187. Serruys PW, de Jaegere P, Kiemeneij F, et al: A comparison of balloon-expandable-stent implantation with balloon angioplasty in patients with coronary artery disease. Benestent Study Group. N Engl J Med 331:489–495, 1994.
188. Sigwart U, Puel J, Mirkovitch V, et al: Intravascular stents to prevent occlusion and restenosis after transluminal angioplasty. N Engl J Med 316:701–706, 1987.
189. Sirnes PA, Golf S, Myreng Y, et al: Stenting in Chronic Coronary Occlusion (SICCO): a randomized, controlled trial of adding stent implantation after successful angioplasty. J Am Coll Cardiol 28:1444–1451, 1996.
190. Sirnes PA, Golf S, Myreng Y, et al: Sustained benefit of stenting chronic coronary occlusion: long-term clinical follow-up of the Stenting in Chronic Coronary Occlusion (SICCO) study. J Am Coll Cardiol 32:305–310, 1998.
191. Versaci F, Gaspardone A, Tomai F, et al: A comparison of coronary-artery stenting with angioplasty for isolated stenosis of the proximal left anterior descending coronary artery [see comments]. N Engl J Med 336:817–822, 1997.
192. Parisi AF, Folland ED, Hartigan P: A comparison of angioplasty with medical therapy in the treatment of single-vessel coronary artery disease. Veterans Affairs ACME Investigators [see comments]. N Engl J Med 326:10–16, 1992.
193. Hartigan PM, Giacomini JC, Folland ED, Parisi AF: Two- to three-year follow-up of patients with single-vessel coronary artery disease randomized to PTCA or medical therapy (results of a VA cooperative study). Veterans Affairs Cooperative Studies Program ACME Investigators. Angioplasty Compared to Medicine. Am J Cardiol 82:1445–1450, 1998.
194. Strauss WE, Fortin T, Hartigan P, et al: A comparison of quality of life scores in patients with angina pectoris after angioplasty compared with after medical therapy. Outcomes of a randomized clinical trial. Veterans Affairs Study of Angioplasty Compared to Medical Therapy Investigators [see comments]. Circulation 92:1710–1719, 1995.
195. Folland ED, Hartigan PM, Parisi AF: Percutaneous transluminal coronary angioplasty versus medical therapy for stable angina pectoris: outcomes for patients with double-vessel versus single-vessel coronary artery disease in a Veterans Affairs Cooperative randomized trial. Veterans Affairs ACME Investigators [see comments]. J Am Coll Cardiol 29:1505–1511, 1997.

196. Sievers B, Hamm CW, Herzner A, Kuck KH: Medical therapy versus PTCA: a prospective randomized trial in patients with asymptomatic coronary single vessel disease. Circulation 88:297, 1993.
197. RITA-2 trial participants: Coronary angioplasty versus medical therapy for angina: the second Randomised Intervention Treatment of Angina (RITA-2) trial. Lancet 350:461–468, 1997.
198. Hueb WA, Bellotti G, de Oliveira SA, et al: The Medicine, Angioplasty or Surgery Study (MASS): a prospective, randomized trial of medical therapy, balloon angioplasty or bypass surgery for single proximal left anterior descending artery stenoses. J Am Coll Cardiol 26:1600–1605, 1995.
199. Pepine CJ, Geller NL, Knatterud GL, et al: The Asymptomatic Cardiac Ischemia Pilot (ACIP) study: design of a randomized clinical trial, baseline data and implications for a long-term outcome trial. J Am Coll Cardiol 24:1–10, 1994.
200. Davies RF, Goldberg AD, Forman S, et al: Asymptomatic Cardiac Ischemia Pilot (ACIP) study two-year follow-up: outcomes of patients randomized to initial strategies of medical therapy versus revascularization. Circulation 95:2037–2043, 1997.
201. Sharaf BL, Williams DO, Miele NJ, et al: A detailed angiographic analysis of patients with ambulatory electrocardiographic ischemia: results from the Asymptomatic Cardiac Ischemia Pilot (ACIP) study angiographic core laboratory. J Am Coll Cardiol 29:78–84, 1997.
202. Ringqvist I, Fisher LD, Mock M, et al: Prognostic value of angiographic indices of coronary artery disease from the Coronary Artery Surgery Study (CASS). J Clin Invest 71:1854–1866, 1983.
203. Coronary angioplasty versus coronary artery bypass surgery: the Randomized Intervention Treatment of Angina (RITA) trial. Lancet 341:573–580, 1993.
204. Comparison of coronary bypass surgery with angioplasty in patients with multivessel disease. The Bypass Angioplasty Revascularization Investigation (BARI) Investigators. N Engl J Med 335:217–225, 1996.
205. Sculpher MJ, Seed P, Henderson RA, et al: Health service costs of coronary angioplasty and coronary artery bypass surgery: the Randomised Intervention Treatment of Angina (RITA) trial [see comments]. Lancet 344:927–930, 1994.
206. Fava S, Azzopardi J, Agius-Muscat H: Outcome of unstable angina in patients with diabetes mellitus. Diabet Med 14:209–213, 1997.
207. Kornowski R, Goldbourt U, Zion M, et al: Predictors and long-term prognostic significance of recurrent infarction in the year after a first myocardial infarction. SPRINT Study Group. Am J Cardiol 72:883–888, 1993.
208. Mueller HS, Cohen LS, Braunwald E, et al: Predictors of early morbidity and mortality after thrombolytic therapy of acute myocardial infarction. Analyses of patient subgroups in the Thrombolysis in Myocardial Infarction (TIMI) trial, phase II. Circulation 85:1254–1264, 1992.
209. Zuanetti G, Latini R, Maggioni AP, et al: Influence of diabetes on mortality in acute myocardial infarction: data from the GISSI-2 study. J Am Coll Cardiol 22:1788–1794, 1993.
210. Influence of diabetes on 5-year mortality and morbidity in a randomized trial comparing CABG and PTCA in patients with multivessel disease: the Bypass Angioplasty Revascularization Investigation (BARI) [see comments]. Circulation 96:1761–1769, 1997.
211. Elezi S, Kastrati A, Pache J, et al: Diabetes mellitus and the clinical and angiographic outcome after coronary stent placement. J Am Coll Cardiol 32:1866–1873, 1998.
212. Myler RK, Shaw RE, Stertzer SH, et al: Recurrence after coronary angioplasty. Cathet Cardiovasc Diagn 13:77–86, 1987.
213. Stein B, Weintraub WS, Gebhart SP, et al: Influence of diabetes mellitus on early and late outcome after percutaneous transluminal coronary angioplasty. Circulation 91:979–989, 1995.
214. Weintraub WS, Stein B, Kosinski A, et al: Outcome of coronary bypass surgery versus coronary angioplasty in diabetic patients with multivessel coronary artery disease [see comments]. J Am Coll Cardiol 31:10–19, 1998.
215. Gum PA, O'Keefe JH Jr, Borkon AM, et al: Bypass surgery versus coronary angioplasty for revascularization of treated diabetic patients. Circulation 96:II7–II10, 1997.
216. Proudfit WL, Bruschke VG, Sones FM Jr: Clinical course of patients with normal or slightly or moderately abnormal coronary arteriograms: 10-year follow-up of 521 patients. Circulation 62:712–717, 1980.
217. Kuntz RE: Importance of considering atherosclerosis progression when choosing a coronary revascularization strategy: the diabetes–percutaneous transluminal coronary angioplasty dilemma. Circulation 99:847–851, 1999.
218. Naruko T, Ueda M, Becker AE, et al: Angiographic-pathologic correlations after elective percutaneous transluminal coronary angioplasty. Circulation 88:1558–1568, 1993.
219. Waller BF: Pathology of transluminal balloon angioplasty used in the treatment of coronary heart disease. Hum Pathol 18:476–484, 1987.
220. Waller BF: The eccentric coronary atherosclerotic plaque: morphologic observations and clinical relevance. Clin Cardiol 12:14–20, 1989.
221. Waller BF, Crowley MJ. Plaque hematoma and coronary dissection with percutaneous transluminal angioplasty (PTCA) of severely stenotic lesions: morphologic coronary observations in 5 men within 30 days of PTCA. Circulation 68:144, 1983.
222. Block PC, Myler RK, Stertzer S, Fallon JT: Morphology after transluminal angioplasty in human beings. N Engl J Med 305:382–385, 1981.
223. Baughman KL, Pasternak RC, Fallon JT, Block PC: Transluminal coronary angioplasty of postmortem human hearts. Am J Cardiol 48:1044–1047, 1981.
224. Colavita PG, Ideker RE, Reimer KA, et al: The spectrum of pathology associated with percutaneous transluminal coronary angioplasty during acute myocardial infarction. J Am Coll Cardiol 8:855–860, 1986.
225. Mizuno K, Kurita A, Imazeki N: Pathological findings after percutaneous transluminal coronary angioplasty. Br Heart J 52:588–590, 1984.
226. Block PC, Baughman KL, Pasternak RC, Fallon JT: Transluminal angioplasty: correlation of morphologic and angiographic findings in an experimental model. Circulation 61:778–785, 1980.
227. Castaneda-Zuniga WR, Formanek A, Tadavarthy M, et al: The mechanism of balloon angioplasty. Radiology 135:565–571, 1980.
228. Willerson JT, Yao SK, McNatt J, et al: Frequency and severity of cyclic flow alternations and platelet aggregation predict the severity of neointimal proliferation following experimental coronary stenosis and endothelial injury. Proc Natl Acad Sci U S A 88:10624–10628, 1991.
229. Forrester JS, Fishbein M, Helfant R, Fagin J: A paradigm for restenosis based on cell biology: clues for the development of new preventive therapies. J Am Coll Cardiol 17:758–769, 1991.
230. Liu MW, Roubin GS, King SB: Restenosis after coronary angioplasty. Potential biologic determinants and role of intimal hyperplasia. Circulation 79:1374–1387, 1989.
231. Schwartz RS, Holmes DR Jr, Topol EJ: The restenosis paradigm revisited: an alternative proposal for cellular mechanisms [editorial]. J Am Coll Cardiol 20:1284–1293, 1992.
232. Schwartz RS, Edwards DW, Huber KC et al: Coronary restenosis: prospects for solution and new perspectives from a porcine model. Mayo Clin Proc 68:54–62, 1993.
233. Austin GE, Ratliff NB, Hollman J, et al: Intimal proliferation of smooth muscle cells as an explanation for recurrent coronary artery stenosis after percutaneous transluminal coronary angioplasty. J Am Coll Cardiol 6:369–375, 1985.
234. Essed CE, Van den Brand M, Becker AE: Transluminal coronary angioplasty and early restenosis. Fibrocellular occlusion after wall laceration. Br Heart J 49:393–396, 1983.
235. Nobuyoshi M, Kimura T, Nosaka H, et al: Restenosis after successful percutaneous transluminal coronary angioplasty: serial angiographic follow-up of 229 patients. J Am Coll Cardiol 12:616–623, 1988.
236. Holmes DR Jr, Vlietstra RE, Smith HC, et al: Restenosis after percutaneous transluminal coronary angioplasty (PTCA): a report from the PTCA Registry of the National Heart, Lung, and Blood Institute. Am J Cardiol 53:77C–81C, 1984.
237. Serruys PW, Luijten HE, Beatt KJ, et al: Incidence of restenosis after successful coronary angioplasty: a time-related phenomenon. A quantitative angiographic study in 342 consecutive patients at 1, 2, 3, and 4 months. Circulation 77:361–371, 1988.
238. Weintraub WS, Ghazzal ZM, Douglas JS Jr, et al: Long-term clinical follow-up in patients with angiographic restudy after successful angioplasty. Circulation 87:831–840, 1993.
239. Bauters C, Hubert E, Prat A, et al: Predictors of restenosis after coronary stent implantation. J Am Coll Cardiol 31:1291–1298, 1998.

240. Ellis SG, Savage M, Fischman D, et al: Restenosis after placement of Palmaz-Schatz stents in native coronary arteries. Initial results of a multicenter experience. Circulation 86:1836–1844, 1992.
241. King SB 3rd, Yeh W, Holubkov R, et al: Balloon angioplasty versus new device intervention: clinical outcomes. A comparison of the NHLBI PTCA and NACI registries. J Am Coll Cardiol 31:558–566, 1998.
242. Laham RJ, Carrozza JP, Berger C, et al: Long-term (4- to 6-year) outcome of Palmaz-Schatz stenting: paucity of late clinical stent-related problems [see comments]. J Am Coll Cardiol 28:820–826, 1996.
243. Mahdi NA, Lopez J, Leon M, et al: Comparison of primary coronary stenting to primary balloon angioplasty with stent bailout for the treatment of patients with acute myocardial infarction. Am J Cardiol 1:957–963, 1998.
244. Rodriguez A, Bernardi V, Fernandez M, et al: In-hospital and late results of coronary stents versus conventional balloon angioplasty in acute myocardial infarction (GRAMI trial). Gianturco-Roubin in Acute Myocardial Infarction. Am J Cardiol 81:1286–1291, 1998.
245. Suryapranata H, van't Hof AW, Hoorntje JC, et al: Randomized comparison of coronary stenting with balloon angioplasty in selected patients with acute myocardial infarction [see comments]. Circulation 97:2502–2505, 1998.
246. Schuhlen H, Hadamitzky M, Walter H, et al: Major benefit from antiplatelet therapy for patients at high risk for adverse cardiac events after coronary Palmaz-Schatz stent placement: analysis of a prospective risk stratification protocol in the Intracoronary Stenting and Antithrombotic Regimen (ISAR) trial. Circulation 95:2015–2021, 1997.
247. Leon MB, Baim DS, Popma JJ, et al: A clinical trial comparing three antithrombotic-drug regimens after coronary-artery stenting. Stent Anticoagulation Restenosis Study Investigators [see comments]. N Engl J Med 339:1665–1671, 1998.
248. Schomig A, Neumann FJ, Kastrati A, et al: A randomized comparison of antiplatelet and anticoagulant therapy after the placement of coronary-artery stents [see comments]. N Engl J Med 334:1084–1089, 1996.
249. Use of a monoclonal antibody directed against the platelet glycoprotein IIb/IIIa receptor in high-risk coronary angioplasty. The EPIC Investigation [see comments]. N Engl J Med 330:956–961, 1994.
250. Rodriguez AE, Grinfeld L, Balino NP, et al: Argentine randomized study optimal coronary balloon angioplasty and stenting vs. coronary bypass surgery in multiple vessel disease (ERACI II): in hospital and 30-day results. J Am Coll Cardiol 33:33A, 1999.
251. Serruys P. ARTS. *In* Ferguson JJ (ed): 71st Scientific Sessions of the American Heart Association. pp. 2486–2491. Dallas: Circulation, 1999.
252. Baim DS, Levine MJ, Leon MB, et al: Management of restenosis within the Palmaz-Schatz coronary stent (the U.S. multicenter experience). The U.S. Palmaz-Schatz Stent Investigators. Am J Cardiol 71:364–366, 1993.
253. King SB 3rd: Radiation for restenosis: watchful waiting [editorial; comment]. Circulation 99:192–194, 1999.
254. Macander PJ, Roubin GS, Agrawal SK, et al: Balloon angioplasty for treatment of in-stent restenosis: feasibility, safety, and efficacy. Cathet Cardiovasc Diagn 32:125–131, 1994.
255. Meerkin D, Tardif JC, Crocker IR, et al: Effects of intracoronary beta-radiation therapy after coronary angioplasty: an intravascular ultrasound study. Circulation 99:1660–1665, 1999.
256. Teirstein PS, Massullo V, Jani S, et al: Two-year follow-up after catheter-based radiotherapy to inhibit coronary restenosis [see comments]. Circulation 99:243–247, 1999.
257. Kimura T, Yokoi H, Nakagawa Y, et al: Three-year follow-up after implantation of metallic coronary-artery stents [see comments]. N Engl J Med 334:561–566, 1996.
258. King SB 3rd, Barnhart HX, Kosinski AS, et al: Angioplasty or surgery for multivessel coronary artery disease: comparison of eligible registry and randomized patients in the EAST trial and influence of treatment selection on outcomes. Emory Angioplasty versus Surgery Trial Investigators. Am J Cardiol 79:1453–1459, 1997.
259. Fuster V, Badimon L, Badimon JJ, Chesebro JH: The pathogenesis of coronary artery disease and the acute coronary syndromes (1). N Engl J Med 326:242–250, 1992.
260. Fuster V, Badimon L, Badimon JJ, Chesebro JH: The pathogenesis of coronary artery disease and the acute coronary syndromes (2). N Engl J Med 326:310–318, 1992.
261. Ross R: The pathogenesis of atherosclerosis—an update. N Engl J Med 314:488–500, 1986.
262. Davies MJ, Thomas AC: Plaque fissuring—the cause of acute myocardial infarction, sudden ischaemic death, and crescendo angina. Br Heart J 53:363–373, 1985.
263. Davies MJ, Bland JM, Hangartner JR, et al: Factors influencing the presence or absence of acute coronary artery thrombi in sudden ischaemic death. Eur Heart J 10:203–208, 1989.
264. Falk E: Unstable angina with fatal outcome: dynamic coronary thrombosis leading to infarction and/or sudden death. Autopsy evidence of recurrent mural thrombosis with peripheral embolization culminating in total vascular occlusion. Circulation 71:699–708, 1985.
265. Willerson JT, Hillis LD, Winniford M, Buja LM: Speculation regarding mechanisms responsible for acute ischemic heart disease syndromes. J Am Coll Cardiol 8:245–250, 1986.
266. Holmes DR Jr, Hartzler GO, Smith HC, Fuster V: Coronary artery thrombosis in patients with unstable angina. Br Heart J 45:411–416, 1981.
267. Hombach V, Hoher M, Kochs M, et al: Pathophysiology of unstable angina pectoris—correlations with coronary angioscopic imaging. Eur Heart (suppl N):40–45, 1988.
268. Mizuno K, Satomura K, Miyamoto A, et al: Angioscopic evaluation of coronary-artery thrombi in acute coronary syndromes. N Engl J Med 326:287–291, 1992.
269. Vetrovec GW, Cowley MJ, Overton H, Richardson DW: Intracoronary thrombus in syndromes of unstable myocardial ischemia. Am Heart J 102:1202–1208, 1981.
270. Wilensky RL, Bourdillon PD, Vix VA, Zeller JA: Intracoronary artery thrombus formation in unstable angina: a clinical, biochemical and angiographic correlation. J Am Coll Cardiol 21:692–699, 1993.
271. Zack PM, Ischinger T, Aker UT, et al: The occurence of angiographically detected intracoronary thrombus in patients with unstable angina pectoris. Am Heart J 108:1408–1412, 1984.
272. Frimerman A, Rechavia E, Eigler N, et al: Long-term follow-up of a high-risk cohort after stent implantation in saphenous vein grafts. J Am Coll Cardiol 30:1277–1283, 1997.
273. Braunwald E: Unstable angina. A classification. Circulation 80:410–414, 1989.
274. Berg R Jr, Selinger SL, Leonard JJ, et al: Acute evolving myocardial infarction: a surgical emergency. J Thorac Cardiovasc Surg 88:902–906, 1984.
275. Lange RA, Hillis LD: Immediate angioplasty for acute myocardial infarction [editorial; comment]. N Engl J Med 328:726–728, 1993.
276. Phillips SJ, Zeff RH, Skinner JR, et al: Reperfusion protocol and results in 738 patients with evolving myocardial infarction. Ann Thorac Surg 41:119–125, 1986.
277. Zijlstra F, de Boer MJ, Hoorntje JC, et al: A comparison of immediate coronary angioplasty with intravenous streptokinase in acute myocardial infarction. N Engl J Med 328:680–684, 1993.
278. Grines CL, Browne KF, Marco J, et al: A comparison of immediate angioplasty with thrombolytic therapy for acute myocardial infarction. The Primary Angioplasty in Myocardial Infarction Study Group. N Engl J Med 328:673–679, 1993.
279. Gibbons RJ, Holmes DR, Reeder GS, et al: Immediate angioplasty compared with the administration of a thrombolytic agent followed by conservative treatment for myocardial infarction. The Mayo Coronary Care Unit and Catheterization Laboratory Groups [see comments]. N Engl J Med 328:685–691, 1993.
280. Simoons ML, Serruys PW, van den Brand M, et al: Early thrombolysis in acute myocardial infarction: limitation of infarct size and improved survival. J Am Coll Cardiol 7:717–728, 1986.
281. Schroder R, Neuhaus KL, Leizorovicz A, et al: A prospective placebo-controlled double-blind multicenter trial of intravenous streptokinase in acute myocardial infarction (ISAM): long-term mortality and morbidity. J Am Coll Cardiol 9:197–203, 1987.
282. Effectiveness of intravenous thrombolytic treatment in acute myocardial infarction. Gruppo Italiano per lo Studio della Streptochinasi nell'Infarto Miocardico (GISSI). Lancet 1:397–402, 1986.
283. Effect of intravenous APSAC on mortality after acute myocardial infarction: preliminary report of a placebo-controlled clinical trial. AIMS Trial Study Group. Lancet 1:545–549, 1988.

284. Randomised trial of intravenous streptokinase, oral aspirin, both, or neither among 17,187 cases of suspected acute myocardial infarction: ISIS-2. ISIS-2 (Second International Study of Infarct Survival) Collaborative Group. Lancet 2:349–360, 1988.
285. Luchi RJ, Scott SM, Deupree RH: Comparison of medical and surgical treatment for unstable angina pectoris. Results of a Veterans Administration Cooperative Study. N Engl J Med 316:977–984, 1987.
286. Kereiakes DJ, Topol EJ, George BS, et al: Emergency coronary artery bypass surgery preserves global and regional left ventricular function after intravenous tissue plasminogen activator therapy for acute myocardial infarction. J Am Coll Cardiol 11:899–907, 1988.
287. Ryan TJ, Anderson JL, Antman EM, et al: ACC/AHA guidelines for the management of patients with acute myocardial infarction. A report of the American College of Cardiology/American Heart Association Task Force on Practice Guidelines (Committee on Management of Acute Myocardial Infarction). J Am Coll Cardiol 28:1328–1428, 1996.
288. International, randomized, controlled trial of lamifiban (a platelet glycoprotein IIb/IIIa inhibitor), heparin, or both in unstable angina. The PARAGON Investigators. Platelet IIb/IIIa Antagonism for the Reduction of Acute coronary syndrome events in a Global Organization Network. Circulation 97:2386–2395, 1998.
289. Theroux P, Kouz S, Roy L, et al: Platelet membrane receptor glycoprotein IIb/IIIa antagonism in unstable angina. The Canadian Lamifiban Study [see comments]. Circulation 94:899–905, 1996.
290. Cannon CP, McCabe CH, Borzak S, et al: Randomized trial of an oral platelet glycoprotein IIb/IIIa antagonist, sibrafiban, in patients after an acute coronary syndrome: results of the TIMI 12 trial. Thrombolysis in Myocardial Infarction [see comments]. Circulation 97:340–349, 1998.
291. Randomized trial of intravenous heparin versus recombinant hirudin for acute coronary syndromes. The Global Use of Strategies to Open Occluded Coronary Arteries (GUSTO) IIa Investigators [see comments]. Circulation 90:1631–1637, 1994.
292. Gold HK, Johns JA, Leinbach RC, et al: A randomized, blinded, placebo-controlled trial of recombinant human tissue-type plasminogen activator in patients with unstable angina pectoris. Circulation 75:1192–1199, 1987.
293. Williams DO, Topol EJ, Califf RM, et al: Intravenous recombinant tissue-type plasminogen activator in patients with unstable angina pectoris. Results of a placebo-controlled, randomized trial. Circulation 82:376–383, 1990.
294. An international randomized trial comparing four thrombolytic strategies for acute myocardial infarction. The GUSTO investigators [see comments]. N Engl J Med 329:673–682, 1993.
295. Inhibition of platelet glycoprotein IIb/IIIa with eptifibatide in patients with acute coronary syndromes. The PURSUIT Trial Investigators. Platelet Glycoprotein IIb/IIIa in Unstable Angina: Receptor Suppression Using Integrilin Therapy. N Engl J Med 339:436–443, 1998.
296. A comparison of aspirin plus tirofiban with aspirin plus heparin for unstable angina. Platelet Receptor Inhibition in Ischemic Syndrome Management (PRISM) Study Investigators. N Engl J Med 338:1498–1505, 1998.
297. Inhibition of the platelet glycoprotein IIb/IIIa receptor with tirofiban in unstable angina and non-Q-wave myocardial infarction. Platelet Receptor Inhibition in Ischemic Syndrome Management in Patients Limited by Unstable Signs and Symptoms (PRISM-PLUS) Study Investigators. N Engl J Med 338:1488–1497, 1998.
298. Theroux P, Ouimet H, McCans J, et al: Aspirin, heparin, or both to treat acute unstable angina [see comments]. N Engl J Med 319:1105–1111, 1988.
299. de Zwaan C, Bar FW, Janssen JH, et al: Effects of thrombolytic therapy in unstable angina: clinical and angiographic results. J Am Coll Cardiol 12:301–309, 1988.
300. Nicklas JM, Topol EJ, Kander N, et al: Randomized, double-blind, placebo-controlled trial of tissue plasminogen activator in unstable angina. J Am Coll Cardiol 13:434–441, 1989.
301. Wilcox RG, von der Lippe G, Olsson CG, et al: Trial of tissue plasminogen activator for mortality reduction in acute myocardial infarction. Anglo-Scandinavian Study of Early Thrombolysis (ASSET). Lancet 2:525–530, 1988.
302. Randomised placebo-controlled trial of abciximab before and during coronary intervention in refractory unstable angina: the CAPTURE Study [see comments] [published erratum appears in Lancet 350:744, 1997]. Lancet 349:1429–1435, 1997.
303. Eagle KA, Guyton RA, Davidoff R, et al: ACC/AHA Guidelines for Coronary Artery Bypass Graft Surgery: A Report of the American College of Cardiology/American Heart Association Task Force on Practice Guidelines (Committee to Revise the 1991 Guidelines for Coronary Artery Bypass Graft Surgery). J Am Coll Cardiol 34:1262–1347, 1999.
304. McCormick JR, Schick EC Jr, McCabe CH, et al: Determinants of operative mortality and long-term survival in patients with unstable angina. The CASS experience. J Thorac Cardiovasc Surg 89:683–688, 1985.
305. Rahimtoola SH, Nunley D, Grunkemeier G, Ten-year survival after coronary bypass surgery for unstable angina. N Engl J Med 308:676–681, 1983.
306. Scott SM, Luchi RJ, Deupree RH: Veterans Administration Cooperative Study for treatment of patients with unstable angina. Results in patients with abnormal left ventricular function. Circulation 78:I113–I121, 1988.
307. Parisi AF, Khuri S, Deupree RH, et al: Medical compared with surgical management of unstable angina: 5-year mortality and morbidity in the Veterans Administration Study. Circulation 80:1176–1189, 1989.
308. Weintraub WS, Craver JM, Jones EL, et al: Improving cost and outcome of coronary surgery. Circulation 98:II23–II28, 1998.
309. Ribichini F, Steffenino G, Dellavalle A, et al: Comparison of thrombolytic therapy and primary coronary angioplasty with liberal stenting for inferior myocardial infarction with precordial ST-segment depression: immediate and long-term results of a randomized study. J Am Coll Cardiol 32:1687–1694, 1998.
310. Stone GW, Brodie BR, Griffin JJ, et al: Clinical and angiographic follow-up after primary stenting in acute myocardial infarction: the Primary Angioplasty in Myocardial Infarction (PAMI) stent pilot trial. Circulation 99:1548–1554, 1999.
311. The Global Use of Strategies to Open Occluded Coronary Arteries in Acute Coronary Syndromes (GUSTO IIb) Angioplasty Substudy Investigators: A clinical trial comparing primary coronary angioplasty with tissue plasminogen activator for acute myocardial infarction. N Engl J Med 336:1621–1628, 1997.
312. de Boer MJ, Hoorntje JC, Ottervanger JP, et al: Immediate coronary angioplasty versus intravenous streptokinase in acute myocardial infarction: left ventricular ejection fraction, hospital mortality and reinfarction. J Am Coll Cardiol 23:1004–1008, 1994.
313. Brodie BR, Grines CL, Ivanhoe R, et al: Six-month clinical and angiographic follow-up after direct angioplasty for acute myocardial infarction. Final results from the Primary Angioplasty Registry. Circulation 90:156–162, 1994.
314. Every NR, Parsons LS, Hlatky M, et al: A comparison of thrombolytic therapy with primary coronary angioplasty for acute myocardial infarction. Myocardial Infarction Triage and Intervention Investigators. N Engl J Med 335:1253–1260, 1996.
315. de Feyter PJ, Suryapranata H, Serruys PW, et al: Coronary angioplasty for unstable angina: immediate and late results in 200 consecutive patients with identification of risk factors for unfavorable early and late outcome. J Am Coll Cardiol 12:324–333, 1988.
316. de Feyter PJ, Serruys PW, van den Brand M, et al: Emergency coronary angioplasty in refractory unstable angina. N Engl J Med 313:342–346, 1985.
317. Meyer J, Schmitz H, Erbel R, et al: Treatment of unstable angina pectoris with percutaneous transluminal coronary angioplasty (PTCA). Cathet Cardiovasc Diagn 7:361–371, 1981.
318. Meyer J, Schmitz HJ, Kiesslich T, et al: Percutaneous transluminal coronary angioplasty in patients with stable and unstable angina pectoris: analysis of early and late results. Am Heart J 106:973–980, 1983.
319. Myler RK, Shaw RE, Stertzer SH, et al: Unstable angina and coronary angioplasty. Circulation 82:II88–II95, 1990.
320. Faxon DP, Detre KM, McCabe CH, et al: Role of percutaneous transluminal coronary angioplasty in the treatment of unstable angina. Report from the National Heart, Lung, and Blood Institute Percutaneous Transluminal Coronary Angioplasty and Coronary Artery Surgery Study Registries. Am J Cardiol 53:131C–135C, 1984.
321. Halon DA, Flugelman MY, Merdler A, et al: Long-term (10-year)

outcome in patients with unstable angina pectoris treated by coronary balloon angioplasty. J Am Coll Cardiol 32:1603–1609, 1998.
322. de Feyter PJ, Serruys PW, Arnold A, et al: Coronary angioplasty of the unstable angina related vessel in patients with multivessel disease. Eur Heart J 7:460–467, 1986.
323. de Feyter PJ, Serruys PW, Suryapranata H, et al: Coronary angioplasty early after diagnosis of unstable angina. Am Heart J 114:48–54, 1987.
324. Quigley PJ, Erwin J, Maurer BJ, et al: Percutaneous transluminal coronary angioplasty in unstable angina: comparison with stable angina. Br Heart J 55:227–230, 1986.
325. Tiefenbrunn AJ, Chandra NC, French WJ, et al: Clinical experience with primary percutaneous transluminal coronary angioplasty compared with alteplase (recombinant tissue-type plasminogen activator) in patients with acute myocardial infarction: a report from the Second National Registry of Myocardial Infarction (NRMI-2). J Am Coll Cardiol 31:1240–1245, 1998.
326. Invasive compared with noninvasive treatment in unstable coronary-artery disease: FRISC II prospective randomised multicentre study. FRagmin and Fast Revascularisation during InStability in Coronary artery disease Investigators [see comments]. Lancet 354:708–715, 1999.
327. Ribeiro EE, Silva LA, Carneiro R, et al: Randomized trial of direct coronary angioplasty versus intravenous streptokinase in acute myocardial infarction. J Am Coll Cardiol 22:376–380, 1993.
328. Bedotto JB, Kahn JK, Rutherford BD, et al: Failed direct coronary angioplasty for acute myocardial infarction: in-hospital outcome and predictors of death. J Am Coll Cardiol 22:690–694, 1993.
329. The TIMI Research Group immediate vs. delayed catheterization and angioplasty following thrombolytic therapy for acute myocardial infarction. TIMI II A results. JAMA 260:2849–2858, 1988.
330. SWIFT (Should We Intervene Following Thrombolysis?) Trial Study Group: SWIFT trial of delayed elective intervention v conservative treatment after thrombolysis with anistreplase in acute myocardial infarction. BMJ 302:555–560, 1991.
331. Ellis SG, Mooney MR, George BS, et al: Randomized trial of late elective angioplasty versus conservative management for patients with residual stenoses after thrombolytic treatment of myocardial infarction. Treatment of Post-Thrombolytic Stenoses (TOPS) Study Group. Circulation 86:1400–1406, 1992.
332. Simoons ML, Arnold AE, Betriu A, et al: Thrombolysis with tissue plasminogen activator in acute myocardial infarction: no additional benefit from immediate percutaneous coronary angioplasty. Lancet 1:197–203, 1988.
333. Topol EJ, Califf RM, George BS, et al: A randomized trial of immediate versus delayed elective angioplasty after intravenous tissue plasminogen activator in acute myocardial infarction. N Engl J Med 317:581–588, 1987.
334. Williams DO, Braunwald E, Knatterud G, et al: One-year results of the Thrombolysis in Myocardial Infarction investigation (TIMI) Phase II Trial [see comments]. Circulation 85:533–542, 1992.
335. Waller BF, Rothbaum DA, Pinkerton CA, et al: Status of the myocardium and infarct-related coronary artery in 19 necropsy patients with acute recanalization using pharmacologic (streptokinase, r-tissue plasminogen activator), mechanical (percutaneous transluminal coronary angioplasty) or combined types of reperfusion therapy. J Am Coll Cardiol 9:785–801, 1987.
336. Ferguson JJ: Meeting highlights: 42nd Annual Scientific Sessions, American College of Cardiology, March 14 to 18, 1993. Circulation 88:6–10, 1993.
337. Thijs Plokker HW, Ernst SM, Bal ET, et al: Percutaneous transluminal coronary angioplasty in patients with unstable angina pectoris refractory to medical therapy: long-term clinical and angiographic results. Cathet Cardiovasc Diagn 14:15–18, 1988.
338. Williams DO, Riley RS, Singh AK, et al: Evaluation of the role of coronary angioplasty in patients with unstable angina pectoris. Am Heart J 102:1–9, 1981.
339. Morrison DA, Sacks J, Grover F, Hammermeister KE: Effectiveness of percutaneous transluminal coronary angioplasty for patients with medically refractory test angina pectoris and high risk of adverse outcomes with coronary artery bypass grafting. Am J Cardiol 75:237–240, 1995.
340. Morrison DA, Bies RD, Sacks J: Coronary angioplasty for elderly patients with "high risk" unstable angina: short-term outcomes and long-term survival. J Am Coll Cardiol 29:339–344, 1997.
341. Williams DO, Braunwald E, Thompson B, et al: Results of percutaneous transluminal coronary angioplasty in unstable angina and non-Q-wave myocardial infarction. Observations from the TIMI IIIB Trial. Circulation 94:2749–2755, 1996.
342. Cools FJ, Vrints CJ, Snoeck JP: Angiographic coronary artery lesion morphology and pathogenetic mechanisms of myocardial ischemia in stable and unstable coronary artery disease syndromes. Acta Cardiol 47:13–30, 1992.
343. Bresnahan DR, Davis JL, Holmes DR Jr, Smith HC: Angiographic occurrence and clinical correlates of intraluminal coronary artery thrombus: role of unstable angina. J Am Coll Cardiol 6:285–289, 1985.
344. Capone G, Wolf NM, Meyer B, Meister SG: Frequency of intracoronary filling defects by angiography in angina pectoris at rest. Am J Cardiol 56:403–406, 1985.
345. Mabin TA, Holmes DR Jr, Smith HC, et al: Intracoronary thrombus: role in coronary occlusion complicating percutaneous transluminal coronary angioplasty. J Am Coll Cardiol 5:198–202, 1985.
346. Platelet glycoprotein IIb/IIIa receptor blockade and low-dose heparin during percutaneous coronary revascularization. The EPILOG Investigators. N Engl J Med 336:1689–1696, 1997.
347. Randomised placebo-controlled trial of effect of eptifibatide on complications of percutaneous coronary intervention: IMPACT-II. Integrilin to Minimise Platelet Aggregation and Coronary Thrombosis-II. Lancet 349:1422–1428, 1997.
348. Lincoff AM, Tcheng JE, Califf RM, et al: Sustained suppression of ischemic complications of coronary intervention by platelet GP IIb/IIIa blockade with abciximab: one-year outcome in the EPILOG trial. Circulation 99:1951–1958, 1999.
349. Bauters C, Lablanche JM, McFadden EP, et al: Repeat percutaneous coronary angioplasty; clinical and angiographic follow-up in patients with stable or unstable angina pectoris. Eur Heart J 14:235–239, 1993.
350. Marzocchi A, Piovaccari G, Marrozzini C, et al: Results of coronary stenting for unstable versus stable angina pectoris. Am J Cardiol 79:1314–1318, 1997.
351. Topol E, Lincoff AM: EPISTENT. *In* Ferguson JJ (ed): 71st Scientific Sessions of the American Heart Association. 99th ed. pp. 2486–2491. Dallas: Circulation, 1999.
352. Perrault L, Carrier M, Cartier R, et al: Morbidity and mortality of reoperation for coronary artery bypass grafting: significance of atheromatous vein grafts. Can J Cardiol 7:427–430, 1991.
353. Foster ED, Fisher LD, Kaiser GC, Myers WO: Comparison of operative mortality and morbidity for initial and repeat coronary artery bypass grafting: the Coronary Artery Surgery Study (CASS) registry experience. Ann Thorac Surg 38:563–570, 1984.
354. Kaul TK, Fields BL, Wyatt DA, et al: Reoperative coronary artery bypass surgery: early and late results and management in 1300 patients. J Cardiovasc Surg (Torino) 36:303–312, 1995.
355. Kron IL, Cope JT, Baker LD Jr, Spotnitz HM: The risks of reoperative coronary artery bypass in chronic ischemic cardiomyopathy: results of the CABG Patch Trial. Circulation 96:II21–II25, 1997.
356. Cameron A, Kemp HG Jr, Green GE: Reoperation for coronary artery disease: 10 years of clinical follow-up. Circulation 78:I158–I162, 1988.
357. Noppeney T, Eberlein U, Langhans L, von der Emde J: The influence of age and other risk factors on the results of coronary reoperation. Thorac Cardiovasc Surgeon 41:43–48, 1993.
358. Weintraub WS, Jones EL, Morris DC, et al: Outcome of reoperative coronary bypass surgery versus coronary angioplasty after previous bypass surgery. Circulation 95:868–877, 1997.
359. Lytle BW, Loop FD, Taylor PC, et al: The effect of coronary reoperation on the survival of patients with stenoses in saphenous vein bypass grafts to coronary arteries. J Thorac Cardiovasc Surg 105:605–614, 1993.
360. Block PC, Cowley MJ, Kaltenbach M, et al: Percutaneous angioplasty of stenoses of bypass grafts or of bypass graft anastomotic sites. Am J Cardiol 53:666–668, 1984.
361. Cooper I, Ineson N, Demirtas E, et al: Role of angioplasty in patients with previous coronary artery bypass surgery. Cathet Cardiovasc Diagn 16:81–86, 1989.
362. Douglas JS Jr, Gruentzig AR, King SB, et al: Percutaneous transluminal coronary angioplasty in patients with prior coronary bypass surgery. J Am Coll Cardiol 2:745–54, 1983.

363. Corbelli J, Franco I, Hollman J, et al: Percutaneous transluminal coronary angioplasty after previous coronary artery bypass surgery. Am J Cardiol 56:398–403, 1985.
364. El Gamal M, Bonnier H, Michels R, et al: Percutaneous transluminal angioplasty of stenosed aortocoronary bypass grafts. Br Heart J 52:617–620, 1984.
365. Ford WB, Wholey MH, Zikria EA, et al: Percutaneous transluminal angioplasty in the management of occlusive disease involving the coronary arteries and saphenous vein bypass grafts: preliminary results. J Thorac Cardiovasc Surg 79:1–11, 1980.
366. Dorros G, Lewin RF, Mathiak LM, et al: Percutaneous transluminal coronary angioplasty in patients with two or more previous coronary artery bypass grafting operations. Am J Cardiol 61:1243–1247, 1988.
367. Gibbons RJ, Chatterjee K, Daley J, et al: ACC/AHA/ACP-ASIM guidelines for the management of patients with chronic stable angina: a report of the American College of Cardiology/American Heart Association Task Force on Practice Guidelines (Committee on Management of Patients With Chronic Stable Angina). J Am Coll Cardiol 33:2092–2197, 1999.

CHAPTER 43

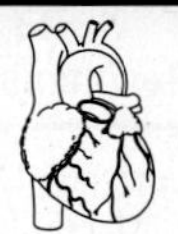

Cardiac Rehabilitation

Victor F. Froelicher

INFARCT SEVERITY
Risk Prediction
CARDIAC REHABILITATION
Early Ambulation
Animal Experiments
Bed Rest: Lack of Activity or Gravity
EARLY STUDIES OF PROGRESSIVE AMBULATION POST-MI
RANDOMIZED TRIALS OF EARLY AMBULATION
Exercise Testing Before Hospital Discharge
Exercise Prescription
Circuit Training
Intervention Studies
Meta-Analysis of the Cardiac Rehabilitation Studies
Complications During Exercise Training
Improved Exercise Capacity Owing to Cardiac Rehabilitation
Cardiac Changes Owing to Exercise Progress in Cardiac Patients
The Effect of Beta-Blockers on Exercise Training
Compliance
Patients With Left Ventricular Dysfunction
Patients With Right Ventricular Dysfunction
Elderly Patients
Exercise Programs for Patients After CABG
PERFEXT CABG Patients
Rehabilitation After PTCA
Return to Work
Risk Factor Modification
Predicting Outcome in Cardiac Rehabilitation Patients
Summary: Changes Owing to Economic Forces
FUTURE DIRECTIONS IN THE UNITED STATES
Reinventing Cardiac Rehabilitation: Implement Restructuring
Initiate Patient Contact Early
Reach a More Diverse Pool of Patients
Increase Physician Awareness
Include Underserved Populations
Expand Utilization
Highlight Potential Reduction in Mortality
Document Cost Efficacy
Implement Restructuring
Summary

Cardiac rehabilitation was conceived in the 1960s as a treatment for patients who had suffered a myocardial infarction (MI). Before the 1970s, the patient who suffered an MI was almost completely immobilized for 6 weeks or more and was even washed, shaved, and fed in order to keep the work of the heart to a minimum (Table 43–1). It was thought that this approach provided the heart with the opportunity to form a firm scar. Also, the patient was told not to expect to be able to return to a normal life. These were incorrect beliefs, particularly in the situation of an uncomplicated MI. Prolonged immobilization not only did not speed healing but also exposed the patient to the additional risks of venous thrombosis, pulmonary embolism, muscle atrophy, lung infections, and deconditioning. Equally serious was the psychological result of such an approach, often leading to psychological impairment.

Today, the physician's approach to the acute MI has completely changed.[1] A relatively brief period of time monitored by the high technology in the coronary care unit is followed by early mobilization, sitting at the bedside, graduated exercise, and in the uncomplicated patient, discharge from the hospital in less than a week. This policy has been shown by randomized trials to be safe from the point of view of cardiac complications. In-patient rehabilitation is brief, but educational videos and pamphlets can begin the patient's education. Iatrogenic deconditioning is not a problem because a walking program can begin very early. Psychological rehabilitation takes place in the doctor's office along with prescribing exercise and education. Certainly, all patients do not need all rehabilitative interventions, but exercise programs, educational sessions, group therapy, and psychological and vocational counseling are available in most communities for those who need them.

Hospital admission for an acute MI is a stressful experience with a powerful impact. But it must be remembered that hospital discharge, although less dramatic, can be equally stressful after the patient has been relying on the highly protective hospital support systems. Discharge into an uncertain future and to home and work, where one is considered damaged, can be as damaging to one's self-esteem as the acute event itself. The physician is faced with the difficult task not only of supervising the physical recovery of the patient but of maintaining morale, providing education, helping the family cope and provide support, and facilitating the return to a gratifying lifestyle. Cardiac rehabilitation can be considered the conservation of human life. Its goal is to restore the patient to optimal physiologic, psychological, and vocational status.

Cardiovascular diseases, largely atherosclerotic, are also the leading cause of activity limitation and disabled worker benefits in the United States and the fourth leading cause of days lost from work. In fact, coronary artery disease alone is responsible for almost one out of five disability allowances paid by the Social Security Administration. However, the total economic impact of the disability related to cardiovascular diseases results from the combination of

TABLE 43–1 A Review of Previous Textbook Recommendations for Bed Rest in Acute Myocardial Infarction

Lewis T: Diseases of the Heart. New York: Macmillan, 1937	8 wk bed rest
White PD: Heart Disease. 3rd ed. New York: Macmillan, 1945	4 wk bed rest
Wood P: Diseases of the Heart and Circulation. 2nd ed. London: Eyre & Spottiswoode, 1960	3–6 wk in bed
Friedberg CK: Diseases of the Heart. 3rd ed. Philadelphia: WB Saunders, 1966	2–3 wk minimum bed rest
Wood P: Diseases of the Heart and Circulation. 3rd ed. London: Eyre & Spottiswoode, 1968	2 wk in bed

Social Security benefits, welfare support, disability insurance income, unemployment compensation, loss of taxable revenue, and reduced worker productivity related to these diseases. Therefore, from a purely economic standpoint, it is essential that patients with coronary artery disease be rehabilitated as quickly and efficiently as possible to enable their return to renumerative employment. Just as important, however, is the psychosocial impact of heart disease, which cannot be measured in dollars lost. Clearly, therefore, improved quality of life, including lessened depression and an expedient return to pre-illness social roles in the family and community, should be another important goal in the effective rehabilitation of patients with heart disease.

With the addition of thrombolysis and acute catheter interventions to MI treatment, the disability incurred by a MI has been decreased. Today's standard practice is that 85 percent of MI patients undergo cardiac catheterization. Because of the functional benefits observed in cardiac rehabilitation, physicians have extended services to other groups of patients. These patients include those who have undergone interventions (percutaneous transluminal coronary angioplasty [PTCA] and coronary artery bypass graft surgery [CABG], pacemakers, transplantation, and valve surgery) as well as those limited by angina or congestive heart failure or whose heart disease is complicated by additional diseases such as diabetes and renal disease. But first, the pathophysiology of MI that relates to rehabilitation is reviewed.

INFARCT SEVERITY

MIs are divided basically into those that evolve Q waves and result in transmural myocardial cell death and those that do not evolve Q waves and result only in subendocardial cell death.[2] Subendocardial MI cannot be localized, whereas transmural MI can be roughly localized by the Q wave pattern. Attempts have been made to judge MI severity or size electrocardiographically by Q wave and R wave scores and even by utilizing body surface mapping, but these methods provide only rough estimates. In general, the greater the number of areas with Q waves and the greater the R wave loss, the larger the MI. Non–Q wave MIs are usually less associated with complications such as congestive heart failure or shock, but they can be complicated, particularly when a prior MI has taken place. The prognosis for patients is particularly good if they do not have prior MIs or a decreased ejection fraction. Because more myocardium has survived, patients with non–Q wave MIs are more likely to suffer ischemic events. Anterior Q wave MIs are usually larger than inferior infarcts and are more likely to be associated with congestive heart failure and cardiogenic shock. Anterior infarcts are more likely to cause aneurysms and a greater decrease in ejection fraction. Surprisingly, however, in follow-up they have a similar or not much poorer prognosis than Q wave inferior MIs.[3] Fifteen percent of patients with Q wave MI lose their Q waves over the following year but still have the same prognosis as those who do not lose their Q waves.

Risk Prediction

It is well known that morbidity and mortality in postinfarction patients who have complicated courses are much higher than in those with uncomplicated MIs. Diabetes doubles the mortality with any type of MI. The criteria for a complicated MI are listed in Table 43–2. The progressive ambulation program should be delayed until such individuals reach an uncomplicated status, and even then progressive ambulation should be slower.

There has been some controversy over the relative long-term risk of subendocardial versus transmural MI. Some of this difficulty has been due to whether or not prior MIs occurred, which raises the risk in both types. Estimation of the severity of a MI requires consideration of clinical findings and test results other than the electrocardiogram to judge a patient's risk and infarct size. Clinical findings, hemodynamic monitoring, the level of enzyme elevation, and the presence of congestive heart failure or shock, or both, should judge the severity of an infarction. The concept that a subendocardial infarction is "uncompleted" and poses an increased postdischarge risk has not been substantiated; however, they are more likely to be associated with postinfarction angina. The Mayo Clinic study[4] demonstrated that in the patient with a first MI, prognosis is much better in follow-up for a non–Q wave MI than for a Q wave MI. The recent Veterans Affairs Non–Q-Wave Infarction Strategies in Hospital (VANQWISH) trial demonstrated that acute intervention does not improve survival in all non–Q wave MI patients.[5]

Certain clinical features during a patient's immediate post-MI convalescence identify a higher risk for future

TABLE 43–2 The Presence of Any One or More of these Criteria Classifies a Myocardial Infarction as Complicated

- Prior myocardial infarction
- Continued cardiac ischemic (pain, late enzyme rise)
- Left ventricular failure (congestive heart failure, new murmurs, chest x-ray changes)
- Shock (blood pressure drop, pallor, oliguria)
- Important cardiac dysrhythmias (premature ventricular contractions greater than 6/min, atrial fibrillation)
- Conduction disturbances (bundle branch block, atrioventricular block, hemiblock)
- Severe pleurisy or pericarditis
- Complicating illnesses
- Marked enzyme rise without a noncardiac explanation
- Age greater than 75 yr
- Stroke or transient ischemic attacks

cardiac events or death, and mandate coronary angiography for consideration or coronary revascularization (PTCA or CABG). Ross and colleagues[6] developed a scheme for deciding which patients should undergo coronary angiography post-MI. If a patient manifests any spontaneous ischemia during hospitalization, he or she has an increased risk of 18 to 20 percent mortality in the first year post-MI and should be referred for diagnostic coronary angiography before discharge. If patients have had a previous MI and clinical or radiographic evidence of left ventricular failure, their projected mortality risk is 25 percent in the first year, and they should undergo coronary angiography as well. In those patients who are unable to exercise, a resting evaluation of ventricular function is recommended. Given that ventricular function is the most powerful predictor of prognosis in patients under the age of 70 years, patients with left ventricular ejection fractions between 20 and 40 percent would be classified as high risk (12 percent first-year mortality).[7]

It is estimated that for every 100 people who suffer an acute MI and survive their hospitalization, 10 will manifest spontaneous ischemia/angina, 20 will have evidence of diminished ventricular function, and an additional 10 patients will have probable ischemia on predischarge exercise testing and be identified at higher risk.[8] Klein and coworkers[9] studied 198 patients who survived an MI and underwent predischarge submaximal exercise testing and followed them for 2 years. They found that patients who had exercise-induced ST depression had a risk ratio for suffering reinfarction or death twice that of patients without ST depression. However, if the pretest electrocardiogram did not have diagnostic Q waves, the risk increased to 11 times for an abnormal ST-segment response. This suggests that the predischarge exercise test is an even more powerful predictor of risk in the patient who has suffered an acute non–Q wave MI. This is in agreement with Krone and associates,[10] who found that non–Q wave MI patients with exercise-induced ischemia (angina and/or ST depression) had a threefold higher incidence of cardiac events in the year after their infarction compared with those with a normal predischarge exercise test.

The invasive strategy of predischarge diagnostic coronary angiography to consider PTCA in patients with clinical evidence of reperfusion by thrombolytic therapy, but no evidence of spontaneous or residual ischemia, has been found to offer no benefit over a conservative strategy.[11–13] Despite these studies, nearly 85 percent of patients receive a heart catheterization at the time of their infarction. Benefits from thrombolysis appear to extend for 10 years.[14]

CARDIAC REHABILITATION

Early Ambulation

Before 1960, patients with acute MI were thought to require prolonged restriction of physical activity. The concern was that physical activity could lead to complications such as ventricular aneurysm formation, cardiac rupture, congestive heart failure, dysrhythmias, reinfarction, or sudden death.

Animal Experiments

Hammerman and colleagues[15] designed a study to evaluate the effect of early exercise on late scar formation in an MI animal model. After occlusion of the proximal left coronary artery, infarct extent was assessed 24 hours later by electrocardiographic criteria. They concluded that short-term swimming during the first week after an MI had effects on scar formation when assessed 2 weeks later. A similar study by Kloner and Kloner[16] with rats forced to swim 7 days post-MI reported the same results. However, the relevance to the clinical situation of rats forced to swim is uncertain. Hochman and Healy[17] performed similar experiments and found no signs in their rats of myocardial thinning or aneurysm formation.

Bed Rest: Lack of Activity or Gravity

There are definite hemodynamic alterations due to deconditioning, including a 20 to 25 percent decrease in maximal oxygen uptake. Other than decreased functional capacity, prolonged bed rest can result in orthostatic hypotension and venous thrombosis through a loss of blood volume, in which plasma loss exceeds red blood cell mass loss. Pulmonary function is decreased, and the patient can be in negative nitrogen and calcium balance.

At least four reasons support the concept that much of these alterations are due to loss of the upright exposure to gravity: (1) supine exercise does not prevent the deconditioning effects of being in bed; (2) there is both less and a slower decline in maximal oxygen consumption with chair rest than with bed rest; (3) there is a greater decrease in maximal oxygen uptake after a period of bed rest measured during upright exercise versus supine exercise; and (4) a lower body positive-pressure device decreases the deconditioning effect of bed rest.[18] Perhaps intermittent exposure to gravitational stress during the bed rest stage of hospital convalescence from surgery or MI may obviate much of the deterioration in cardiovascular performance that can follow these events.

Postdischarge activity recommendations have had little basis for their enforcement. Return to work, return to driving, and return to sex have been based on clinical judgments rather than physiologic assessments.[19] Because of this, physicians have left much of this up to their patients—allowing them to see how they respond symptom-wise—rather than the older, conservative approach, which can foster invalidism. These decisions should be made considering the consequence of the coronary event (ischemia or symptoms of congestive failure, dysrhythmias) and the nature of the activities (manual labor versus desk work, light driving versus congested freeway driving, sex with an established partner versus other relationships).

EARLY STUDIES OF PROGRESSIVE AMBULATION POST-MI

In 1961, Cain and coworkers[20] reported one of the first studies of the use of a progressive activity program for acute MI patients. They reported 335 patients with an uncomplicated MI who were at least 15 days' postinfarction. The electrocardiogram was monitored after the patient performed activities such as climbing stairs and walking up a grade. In 1964, Torkelson[21] reported results in 10 patients with an uncomplicated MI. On the sixth week of his in-hospital rehabilitation program, a low-level treadmill test was performed using 1.7 mph at a 10 percent grade. Sivarajan and associates[22] described 12 patients with an acute MI whose symptoms, signs, and hemodynamic and electrocardiographic responses during and after three activities were assessed. Activities included sitting upright, walking to the toilet, and walking on a treadmill done at 3, 6, and 10 days after infarction. These observational studies set the stage for the following randomized trials.

Randomized Trials of Early Ambulation

Hayes and colleagues[23] studied 189 patients with an uncomplicated MI selected at random for early or late mobilization and discharge from the hospital. Patients were admitted to the study after 48 hours in a coronary care unit if they were free of pain and showed no evidence of heart failure or significant dysrhythmias. One group of patients was mobilized immediately and discharged home after a total of 9 days in the hospital, and the second group was mobilized on the 9th day and discharged on the 16th day. At 6 weeks after admission, no significant differences were observed between the groups in terms of morbidity or mortality.

In a randomized study, Bloch and associates[24] studied the effects of early mobilization after uncomplicated MI. One hundred fifty-four patients under 70 years of age who were hospitalized for an acute MI and had no complications on day 1 or 2 were randomly assigned to two treatment groups. In the early mobilization group, patients were treated by a physical therapist with a progressive activity program that began on day 2 or 3 after infarction. In the control group, the patients underwent the traditional hospital regimen of strict bed rest for 3 or more weeks. The mean duration of hospitalization was 21 days for active patients and 33 days for the control group. There were no significant differences between the two groups, and on follow-up there was actually greater disability in the control than in the active group.

Sivarajan and coworkers[25] reported the effects of early supervised exercises in preventing deconditioning after an acute MI. Eighty-four patients were randomized to a control group, 174 to an exercise group. The exercise program began at an average of 4.5 days after admission. The mean discharge was 10 days after admission for both groups. There were no differences between the two groups in the clinical, hemodynamic, or electrocardiographic responses to a low-level treadmill test performed on the day before hospital discharge. Nor was there any significant difference between the two groups for the incidence of complications or death. These three randomized studies of patients with uncomplicated infarctions have demonstrated that the risks of early ambulation are minimal and that progressive mobilization during the early stages of an acute MI is recommended.

Exercise Testing Before Hospital Discharge

The low-level exercise test early after an acute MI (from 3 days to 3 weeks) has been shown to be safe. Today, it is a standard part of the treatment for MI patients in many hospitals. This test has many benefits, including clarification of the response to exercise and the work capacity, determination of an exercise prescription, and recognition of the need for medications or surgery. It appears to have a beneficial psychological impact on recovery and is an effective part of rehabilitation.

Exercise Prescription

Exercise training can be an important part of cardiac rehabilitation for returning a patient to a formerly active lifestyle, or as functional a lifestyle as possible, after an acute cardiac event. Cardiac rehabilitation is defined by the World Health Organization as "the sum of activities required to ensure them the best possible physical, mental, and social conditions so that they may, by their own efforts, resume as normal a place as possible in the life of the community . . . and that . . . rehabilitation cannot be regarded as an isolated form of therapy, but must be integrated into the whole treatment of which it constitutes only one facet."[26] The explicit details of exercise protocols/equipment, absolute and relative contraindications to exercise, warm-up and cool-down periods, guidelines for terminating exercise, are all outlined by the American College of Cardiology and the American Heart Association.[27]

In prescribing exercise, two basic physiologic principles should be considered. Myocardial oxygen consumption is the amount of oxygen required by the heart to maintain itself and do the work of pumping blood to the other organs. It cannot be measured directly without catheters but can be estimated by the product of systolic blood pressure and heart rate (double product). The higher the double product, the higher the myocardial oxygen consumption and vice versa. Patients usually have their angina at the same double product, unless affected by other facts such as catecholamine level, left ventricular end-diastolic volume, hemoglobin-oxygen dissociation as affected by acid-base balance, and coronary artery spasm.

The second consideration is ventilatory oxygen consumption (V_{O_2}), which is the amount of oxygen taken in from inspired air by the body to maintain itself and to do the work of muscular activity. Measuring V_{O_2} requires the collection of expired air, gas analyzers, and skilled technical help. However, it can be estimated from knowing the workload of various activities. Since the body's mechanical efficiency is relatively constant, estimates of the oxygen cost of various activities without using gas analysis can be applied between individuals. Many tables list the approximate oxygen cost of different activities. Since oxygen consumption is equal to arteriovenous oxygen difference ($V_{aO_2} - V_{vO_2}$) times cardiac output, and $V_{aO_2} - V_{vO_2}$ difference is roughly a constant at maximal exercise, maximal oxygen consumption can be an approximation of maximal cardiac output. However, patients with diseased hearts will often have a wider $Va_{O_2} - Vv_{O_2}$ difference, a lower cardiac output, and a lower V_{O_2} than normal subjects performing the same submaximal workload.

Another important physiologic concept of exercise is the type of work the body is performing. Dynamic work (bicycling, running, jogging) involves the movement of large muscle masses and requires a high blood flow and increased cardiac output. Since this movement is rhythmic, there is little resistance to flow, and in fact, there is a "milking" action that returns blood to the heart. The other type of muscular work is isometric work such as lifting a weight or squeezing a ball. Isometric activities involve a constant muscular contraction that limits blood flow. Instead of a cardiac response to increased cardiac output and blood flow, as during dynamic exercise, blood pressure must be increased to force blood into the active, contracting muscles. Pressure work demands much more oxygen by the heart than does flow work, and because coronary artery blood flow depends on cardiac output, the myocardial oxygen supply can become inadequate. Also, dynamic exercise is more easily controlled or graded so that myocardial oxygen consumption can be gradually increased, whereas isometric exercise can increase myocardial oxygen consumption needs very quickly. In addition, although isometric exercise is good for peripheral muscle tone and function, it does not result in the same beneficial cardiac and hemodynamic effects as dynamic exercise.

Circuit Training

Kelemen and colleagues[28] performed a prospective, randomized evaluation of the safety and efficacy of 10 weeks of circuit weight training in coronary disease patients, aged 35 to 70 years. Circuit weight training was safe and resulted in significant increases in aerobic endurance and musculoskeletal strength compared with traditional exercise used in cardiac rehabilitation programs. Sparling and coworkers[29] also demonstrated the safety and efficacy of circuit weight training in cardiac patients. In a 6-month study of 16 men, there was a 22 percent gain in strength without an increase in blood pressure. Weight training is now known to be safe for post-MI patients, an activity once thought to be dangerous.

Intervention Studies (Table 43–3)

Kallio and associates[30] were part of a World Health Organization coordinated project to assess the effects of a comprehensive rehabilitation and secondary prevention program on morbidity, mortality, return to work, and various clinical, medical, and psychosocial factors after an MI. The study included 375 consecutive patients under 65 years of age treated for acute MI from two urban areas in Finland between 1973 and 1975. On discharge, the patients were randomly allocated to an intervention or a control group, both of which were followed for 3 years. Patients in the control group were followed by their own doctors and were seen by the study team only once a year during the 3-year follow-up. The program for the intervention group was started 2 weeks after hospital discharge. An exercise prescription was determined from a bicycle test, and for most patients the program was supervised. After the 3-year follow-up, the cumulative coronary mortality was significantly smaller in the intervention group than in the controls (18.6 percent versus 29.4 percent). Of the intervention group and the controls, 18.1 percent and 11.2 percent, respectively, presented with nonfatal infarctions. Total mortality was 21.8 percent in the intervention group and 29.9 percent in the control group. Kentala[31] studied 298 consecutive males less than 65 years of age admitted to the University of Helsinki Hospital in 1969 with a diagnosis of acute MI. They were divided by the year of birth: Controls were from odd-numbered years (n = 146) and exercisers were from even-numbered years (n = 152). There was no difference in morbidity or mortality between the groups.

Palatsi's study[32] was a nonrandomized trial of 380 patients less than 65 years old recovering from MI. The first 100 patients were allocated to an exercise program and the second were the controls. Exercise training was begun 10 weeks after the MI and included breathing and relaxation exercises, calisthenics of all muscle groups, and walking that progressed to running in place. The author concluded that home training was not as effective as continual supervised programs, but still accelerated recovery of aerobic capacity. There was no group difference in symptoms, smoking habits, serum cholesterol, or return to work.

Wilhelmsen and colleagues'[33] study included patients born in 1913 or later and hospitalized for an MI between 1968 and 1970 in Goteborg, Sweden. Patients were randomized to a control (n = 157) or an exercise group (n = 158). The exercise group trained three times a week for 30 minutes a session. Calisthenics, cycling, and running were performed at 80 percent of the maximal age-predicted heart rate. After 1 year, the exercise group showed increased work capacity and lower blood pressure, but no difference in blood lipids. At 1 year, only 39 percent continued to come to the hospital to exercise, whereas 21 percent trained elsewhere. No significant differences were seen with respect to cause of death, type of death, or place of death.

The National Exercise and Heart Disease Project (NEHPD)[34] included 651 men post-MI enrolled in five centers in the United States. It was a randomized 3-year clinical trial of the effects of a prescribed supervised exercise program starting 2 to 36 months after MI (80 percent were more than 8 months postinfarction). In this study, 323 randomly selected patients performed exercise three times a week that was designed to increase their heart rate to 85 percent of the individual maximal heart rates achieved during treadmill testing, and 328 patients served as controls. The 3-year mortality rate was 7.3 percent (24 deaths) in the control group versus 4.6 percent (15 deaths) in the exercise group. Neither difference was statistically significant. The need for coronary artery surgery and hospitalization was equal in both groups. This study suggests a beneficial effect of cardiac rehabilitation, but insufficient participants owing to financial limitations and dropouts prevented a definitive conclusion.

The Ontario Study[35] included seven Canadian centers that collaborated in a randomized prospective trial. Seven

TABLE 43-3 Summary of the Major Randomized Trials of Cardiac Rehabilitation Assessing Cardiac Events, Mortality, or Both, in Patients With Coronary Disease

First Investigator	Population Randomized					Mean No. Months Entry After Myocardial Infarction	Mean Age (yr)	Follow-Up (yr)	Dropouts (%)		Return to Work (%)		Re–Myocardial Infarction		Mortality (%)					
															Sudden		*Cardiac*		*Total*	
	Total (n)	*Controls (n)*	*Exercised (n)*	*Exclusions (>yr)*	*Women (%)*				*Controls*	*Exercised*	*Controls*	*Exercised*	*Controls*	*Exercised*	Controls	Exercised	Controls	Exercised	Controls	Exercised
Kentala, 1972	158	81	77	>65	0	1.75	53	2			5	8	5	8			12	10	14	14
Wilhelmsen, 1975	315	157	158	>57	11	3	51	4		46			21	18			18	16	22	18
Palatsi, 1976	380	200	180	>65	19	2.5	52	2.5		35	33	36	15	12	3	6	14	10	14	10
Kallio, 1979	357	187	188	>65	19	3	55	3					11	18	14	6	29	19	30	22
Mayou, 1981	129	42	44	>60	0	1	51	1.5	25	25	30	57								
NEHDP, 1981	651	328	323		0	14	52	3	31	23			7	5			6	4	7	5
Carson, 1982	303	152	151	>70	0	1.5	52	2.1					7	8					14	8
Ontario, 1982	761	371	390	>54	0	6	48	3.3	45	46			10	9			4	4	7	10
Sivarajan, 1982	172	84	88	>70	20	0.13	56	0.50	13	15							2	4		
Bengtsson, 1983	171	90	81	>65	0	1.5	56	1			73	75	4	2					7	10
Carson, 1983	303	152	151	>70	0	1.5	51	3.5	6	17	81	81	7	7					14	8
Roman, 1983	193	100	93		10	2	55	9	4	4			23	17	7	4	17	10	24	14
Vermeulen, 1983	98	51	47	>55	0	1.75	49	5					18	9			10	4	10	4
Froelicher, 1984	146	74	76	>65	0	4	53	1	14	17			1	1					0	1
Hung, 1984	53	23	30	>70	0	0.75	55	0.5	7	9			7	9	0	0	3	0	3	0
Hedback, 1985	297	154	143	>65	15	1.5	57	1		45	59	66	16	5			8	8	8	9
Marra, 1985	167	83	84	>65		2		4.5					11	6			5	6	6	7
Hamalainen, 1989	375	187	188	>65	20	<1		10					19	26	23	13	47	35	52	44
DeBusk, 1994	585	292	293	>70	21	0.10	57	1	12	15			7	3			3	4	3	4

Abbreviation: NEHDP, National Exercise and Heart Disease Project.

hundred thirty-three post-MI males underwent random stratified allocation to either a high-intensity or a low-intensity exercise group. This continued for 8 weeks, after which they trained four times a week on their own. The low-intensity group trained once a week with relaxation exercises, volleyball, bowling, or swimming for 1 hour. They attempted to keep their heart rate at less than 50 percent of maximal oxygen uptake. Both groups were encouraged to stop smoking and control their weight. The authors found that the high-intensity exercise program had similar results to one designed to produce a minimal training effect and did not reduce the risk of reinfarction.

Bengtsson[36] reported on 171 MI patients under the age of 65 years who were randomized to a control and an exercise group. The rehabilitation program consisted of an outpatient examination supervised exercise (large muscle group interval training by use of bicycles, calisthenics, and jogging for 30 minutes, 2 days a week for 3 months at 90 percent of the maximal heart), and counseling. There were no reported differences between groups for age, gender, number of infarcts, highest enzyme, heart size, number of days in the hospital, number of admissions, angina, congestive heart failure, arrhythmia, or depression or hypochondriasis on the Minnesota Multiphasic Personality Inventory.

Carson and coworkers[37] performed their 3½-year study in a population of 1311 male MI patients. The exercise group trained in a gym two times a week for 12 weeks at 85 percent of the exercise-test–determined maximal heart rate or until symptoms of angina, shortness of breath, or a poor systolic blood pressure response developed. The authors concluded that the difference in fitness between the exercise and the control patients after completion of the study was highly significant. There was no significant decrease in mortality for the exercise group except for those with an inferior wall MI.

Vermeulen and associates[38] described a prospective randomized trial with a 5-year follow-up. Approximately 1 month after MI, patients underwent a symptom-limited exercise test. Their 6-week rehabilitation program was associated with a 50 percent decrease in progressive coronary artery disease when compared with the control group. Mortality and morbidity were 50 percent lower in the rehabilitation group.

Roman[39] reported on 139 patients, including 19 females who entered into their cardiac rehabilitation study. The exercisers trained 30 minutes, three times a week at 70 percent of maximal heart rate for an average of 42 months. At the 9-year follow-up, the mortality rate was 5.2 percent for the control group and 2.9 percent for the rehabilitation group. There was a significant decrease in angina in the exercise group.

Mayou[40] studied 129 men, 60 years of age or less, admitted with an MI. They were sequentially allocated to either normal treatment, exercise training, or counseling groups. The control group received standard inpatient care, advice booklets, and one to two visits as outpatients. The exercise group received the normal treatment plus eight sessions (twice a week) of circuit training in groups, written reminders, and reviews of their results. The advice group received normal treatment plus discussion groups, kept a daily activity diary, had couples therapy, and had three to four follow-up sessions. The three groups were comparable socially, medically, and psychologically. Evaluation was performed after 12 weeks using exercise testing and standard tests of psychological state and social adjustment. There were no differences among the groups in psychological outcome, physical activity, or satisfaction with leisure or work. At 18 months, the only significant findings were a better outcome in terms of overall satisfaction, hours of work, and frequency of sexual intercourse for the counseled group. There was no group difference in compliance with advice in smoking, diet, or exercise.

Hedback and colleagues' study in Sweden[41] was retrospective with a control group of 154 patients and an intervention group of 143 patients. Both groups were treated the same during their acute hospitalization. Training began 6 weeks after MI following a bicycle test. One year after the MI, there was no group difference in mortality, but the exercise group had a significantly lower rate of nonfatal reinfarction, fewer uncontrolled hypertensives, and fewer smokers. Goble and coworkers[42] found similar benefits from a low-level program compared with a high-level one.

Meta-Analysis of the Cardiac Rehabilitation Studies

Although not every single-center study has shown definitive differences between participants in exercise programs compared with controls in regard to physiologic or psychosocial variables, the overall benefits of cardiac rehabilitation are accepted. Because of the time and expense involved in conducting controlled studies with large numbers of patients, few such trials have been performed. We are left with numerous studies showing significant benefits in exercise capacity, and often psychosocial benefits, but usually only trends toward improved morbidity and mortality. Meta-analysis has gained popularity in recent years as a method of combining separate but similar studies, and this approach has yielded some very important information on the efficacy of cardiac rehabilitation. O'Connor and associates[43] performed a meta-analysis of 22 randomized trials of cardiac rehabilitation involving 4554 patients. They found a 20 percent reduction in risk for total mortality, a 22 percent reduction for cardiovascular mortality, and a 25 percent reduction in the risk for fatal reinfarction. Oldridge and colleagues[44] performed a similar meta-analysis with 10 randomized trials including 4347 patients and found a similar reduction for all-cause death and cardiovascular death in the patients undergoing cardiac rehabilitation.

Complications During Exercise Training

Haskell[45] surveyed 30 cardiac rehabilitation programs in North America using a questionnaire to assess major cardiovascular complications. This survey included approximately 14,000 patients for 1.6 million exercise-hours. Of 50 cardiopulmonary resuscitations (CPRs), 8 resulted in death, and of 7 MIs, 2 resulted in death. Exercise programs resulted in 4 other fatalities occurring after hospitalization. Thus, there was 1 nonfatal event per 35,000 patient-hours and 1 fatal event per 160,000 patient-hours. The complication rates were lower in electrocardiographically monitored programs. These programs reported a 4 percent annual mortality rate during exercise, which is a rate not different from that expected for such patients. Other programs have reported rates of CPRs ranging from 1 in 6000 to 1 in 25,000 person-hours of exercise. Such events are difficult to predict, can occur in patients with only single-vessel disease, and can occur at any time after being in a program.

A Seattle cardiac rehabilitation program (CAPRI, Cardiopulmonary Rehabilitation Institute)[46] reported the highest rate of 1 CPR in 6000 exercise hours. Of 15 patients requiring defibrillation, the CAPRI group successfully resuscitated all of them. Eleven had angiography, which showed single-vessel disease in 4 patients and multivessel disease in 7. Subsequently, the CAPRI record improved, and they have had experience with defibrillating 2 patients simultaneously; on another occasion, a physician monitoring an exercise class was defibrillated. Of 2464 patients observed during a 13-year period, 25 cardiac arrests occurred during 375,000 hours of supervised exercise, a rate of 1 arrest per 15,000 hours. The same incidence rate was reported in Toronto and in Atlanta, where 5 arrests occurred in 75,000 hours of exercise, and a similar rate of 1 arrest per 12,000 hours (total of 36,000 gymnasium-hours) was reported in Connecticut. In CAPRI, 12 of the 25 victims had been enrolled for 12 or more months. Fibrillation was recorded in 23 cases and ventricular tachycardia in 2. Prompt defibrillation was carried out and all patients survived. Each cardiac arrest was a "primary" arrhythmic event, and none was associated with acute MI. Eighteen of the 25 patients had ST-segment depression, and 5 had developed hypotension with prior exercise testing.

Van Camp and Peterson[47] obtained statistics from 167 randomly selected outpatient cardiac rehabilitation programs and found that the incidence rate for cardiac arrest was 8.9 per million patient-hours. Of these cardiac arrests, 86 percent were successfully resuscitated, giving an incidence rate for death of 1.3 per million patient-hours. This compares favorably with the estimated fatality rate for unselected joggers at 2.5 per million person-hours of jogging.[48] There also was no significant difference in cardiac event rate between rehabilitation programs with or without electrocardiographic monitoring.[49]

The incidence of exertion-related cardiac arrest in cardiac rehabilitation programs is small, and because of the availability of rapid defibrillation, death rarely occurs. Using an annual 10 percent incidence rate of sudden arrhythmic deaths during any activity (1 per 88,000 person-hours), the risk is one sixth that observed during participation in exercise programs. The majority of sudden deaths are temporally associated with routine activities of daily life and not with exercise. Exertion-related cardiac arrest is usually due to ventricular fibrillation or tachycardia, and exercise may increase its risk by 100 times.[50, 51]

Improved Exercise Capacity Owing to Cardiac Rehabilitation

In a comprehensive review, Greenland and Chu[52] analyzed eight controlled studies of supervised exercise programs and their effect on physical work capacity. In all the studies reviewed, exercise capacity improved after the intervention, whether the patients were in a control or an active intervention group. This suggests that either a patient's exercise capacity is artificially limited by the patient himself or herself or by the physicians providing care or there is a spontaneous improvement in exercise capacity as time passes from time of infarction. However, the exercise groups always had a greater exercise capacity than the control groups after the interventions—on the order of 20 to 25 percent better. Studies that failed to show any benefit may have been limited by exercise programs of inadequate duration, as it probably takes longer than 3 to 6 months for any improvement in cardiac adaptation, and also by compliance with the exercise prescription.

Cardiac Changes Owing to Exercise Progress in Cardiac Patients

When at the University of California, San Diego, I was funded by the National Institutes of Health to perform a study called PERFEXT (PERFusion, PERFormance, EXercise Trial).[53] The San Diego community was informed that we were recruiting male coronary heart disease patients between the ages of 35 and 65 years for a free exercise program. They were encouraged to accept randomization by being promised that if randomized to the control group, they could join the exercise classes after the 1-year study was completed. The patients were classified by the following criteria: (1) history of MI, (2) stable exertional angina pectoris, or (3) CABG. Disease stability was assured by careful history taking and by not allowing the patient to enter the study until at least 4 months after a cardiac event, a change in symptoms, or surgery. Of 146 patients randomized, 72 were in the training group and 74 in the control group. The patients randomized to the exercise intervention group began training in a continuous electrocardiographically monitored class. The initial training intensity was set at a minimal duration of 60 percent of the estimated maximal oxygen uptake from the initial treadmill test, and training intensity progressed in standard fashion throughout the year. Patients randomized to the control group were offered a low-intensity walking program. The distribution of patients is illustrated in Figure 43–1.

The decrease in their resting and submaximal heart rates, as well as the significant increase in the measured and estimated maximal oxygen uptake, evidenced a significant training effect in the intervention group. The control group showed a significant decrease in exercise capacity at least partially due to the lower maximal heart rate obtained at 1 year. The significant increase in estimated (18 percent) and measured (8.5 percent) $\dot{V}o_2max$ is similar to that in most studies.

Radionuclide ventriculography demonstrated a baseline increase in both end-systolic and end-diastolic volume in response to supine exercise. There were no significant differences at rest, during the three stages of exercise, or in the percent change from rest to exercise between the control and the trained group at 1 year in ejection fraction, end-diastolic volume, stroke volume, or cardiac output.

The PERFEXT exercise intervention group experienced a significant improvement in the exercise thallium images following the year, using the Atwood scoring system[54] as

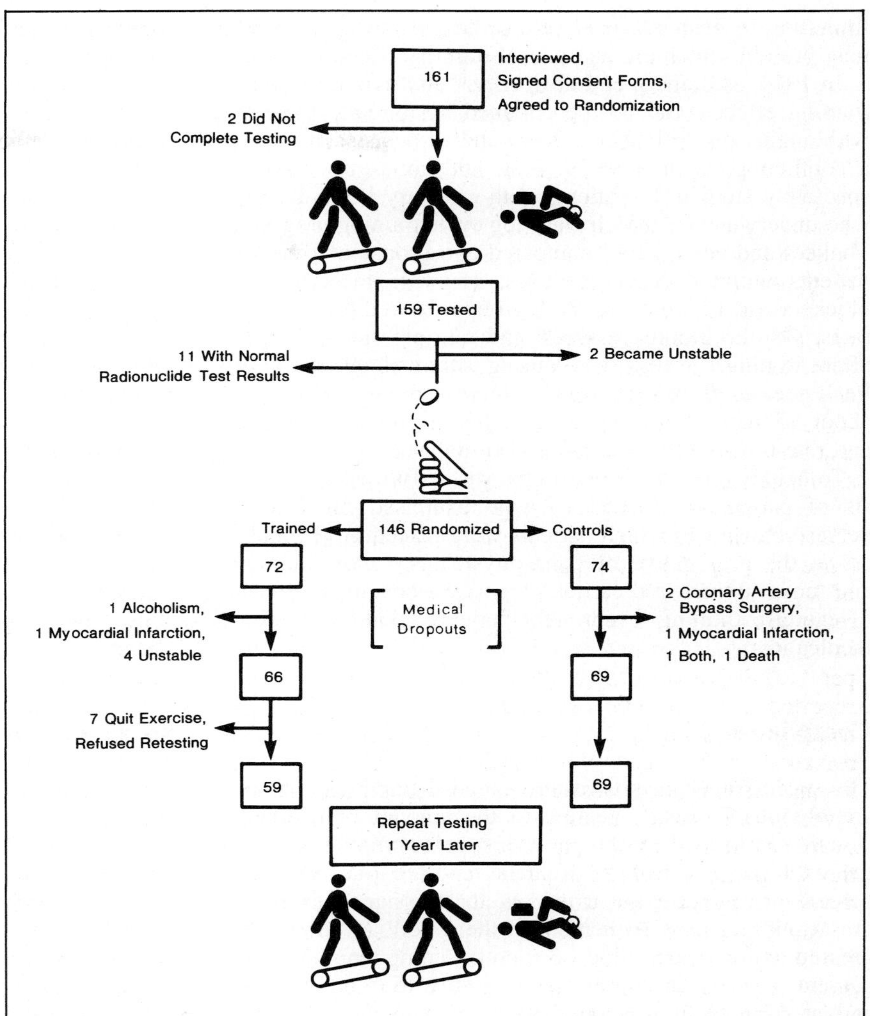

FIGURE 43–1 Patient distribution and flow in the PERFusion, PERFormance, EXercise Trial (PERFEXT). (From Froelicher V, Jensen D, Genter F, et al: A randomized trial of exercise training in patients with coronary heart disease. JAMA 252:1291–1297, 1984. Copyright 1984, American Medical Association.)

well as computer techniques.[55] However, comparing thallium scans side-by-side, which has been done effectively to evaluate surgical intervention, was not successful in the clinical assessment of changes in myocardial perfusion after an exercise program. Disappointingly, the ST-segment changes did not show an improvement nor did they agree with the thallium changes.[56]

One criticism might be that our patients did not exercise hard enough and that if they had, more definite improvements might have been possible. However, even if we chose those who trained the most intensely or had the highest exercise class attendance, we did not find greater changes. Surprisingly, there was a poor correlation between the intensity or attendance and the change in aerobic capacity or the radionuclide changes; in fact, there was a poor correlation between the change in aerobic capacity and the changes in the radionuclide tests. A paradox now exists regarding this. Although impressive cardiac changes have been reported in highly selected groups of cardiac patients with asymptomatic ST-segment depression exercised at very high levels,[57] the question remains whether the usual cardiac patient can be exercised safely at higher levels, and if so, whether more definite cardiac changes can be demonstrated.

The Effect of Beta-Blockers on Exercise Training

There is evidence that a functioning sympathetic nervous system may be necessary to achieve the beneficial hemodynamic alterations of training. In addition, the limitation in cardiac output due to beta-blockade may result in fatigue and reduce the intensity of training or compliance to exercise. Also, if ischemia (the major stimulus for collateral development), is lessened by β-blockade, this potential benefit of training could also be impeded. Beta-adrenergic blockade is widely used to treat patients with coronary heart disease, and aerobic exercise is now commonly prescribed as part of cardiac rehabilitation. However, one of the beneficial hemodynamic effects of both regular exercise and β-blockade is that heart rate at rest and submaximal workloads is decreased. If β-adrenergic stimulation is needed for the effects of exercise training to occur or if β-blockade lessens the ischemia necessary to promote collateralization, then β-blockade might be expected to interfere with the beneficial results of exercise. β-Blockade could also increase perceived exertion and fatigue, thus lessening the tolerance for higher exercise levels and adherence to an exercise program. Therefore, a pharmacologically imposed limitation in heart rate and cardiac output during exercise may prohibit obtaining an optimal training effect.

In 1974, Malmborg and coworkers[58] first reported that a training effect could not be obtained in coronary patients with angina on β-blockers. Obma and associates[59] reported a conflicting result in 1979. Pratt and colleagues[60] retrospectively studied 35 patients with coronary heart disease who underwent a 3-month walk-jog cycle training program. Vanhees and coworkers[61] compared two groups of post-MI patients without angina pectoris; 15 were receiving β-blockers and 15 were not. Both groups showed lower heart rates, systolic blood pressures, and rate pressure products after training, at rest, and during submaximal exercise. Peak measured oxygen uptake increased an average of about 35 percent in both groups, but maximal heart rate and rate-pressure product were also higher.

To help resolve these questions, we performed an analysis of patients in PERFEXT who exercised for 1 year versus controls, in which patients were placed on β-blockers at the prerogative of their physicians.[62] Our findings and those summarized earlier support the beneficial effects of exercise training in coronary patients taking β-blocker medication.

Compliance

The success and benefits of any exercise training program are obviously directly related to the amount of exercise actually performed by the patients—their compliance with the exercise prescription. Kentala reported that only 13 percent of his patients carried out their assigned exercise prescription at least 70 percent of the time.[31] As time progressed, compliance fell. At 3 months, compliance was 80 percent, 1 year later compliance was only 45 to 60 percent, and at 4 years, it was only 30 to 55 percent.[63] Several options are available to improve compliance behavior—reduce the waiting time; provide expert supervision; tailor the exercise prescription to avoid physical discomfort and/or frustration; use variable activities, including games; incorporate social events; recall absent patients; involve the patient's family or spouse in the program; and involve the patients in monitoring themselves and their progress.

Patients With Left Ventricular Dysfunction

Not long ago, patients with left ventricular dysfunction were thought to be poor candidates for exercise programs. This was out of concern for safety and the general thinking that they were unable to benefit from training. This has been dispelled, however, by a number of studies performed since the late 1980s. Squires and associates[64] studied 20 post-MI patients with left ventricular ejection fractions less than 25 percent in a supervised cardiac rehabilitation program. There was substantial improvement in exercise capacity in most patients, and a favorable trend was observed in performing desired activities and returning to work. Conn and colleagues[65] studied 10 patients with a history of prior MI and left ventricular ejection fractions of less than 27 percent. They found that with a cardiac rehabilitation program, the patients' exercise capacity increased from a mean of 7.0 metabolic equivalents of the task (METs) to 8.5 METs, and there was no exercise-related morbidity or mortality.

The controversy was reignited in 1988 when Judgutt and coworkers[66] reported 13 patients with anterior Q wave MIs using echocardiography before and after supervised low-level exercise training. They found that patients with evidence of greater left ventricular asynergy (akinesis or dyskinesis) had more detrimental ventricular shape distortion, with expansion and thinning of their left ventricle after exercise training. Several randomized trials have shown training not only improves exercise capacity but also reverses skeletal muscle metabolic derangement,[67] increases maximal cardiac output, and improves measures of quality of life in these patients.

Giannuzzi and associates[68] completed a multicenter controlled trial of exercise training in Italy. After 6 months, patients in both the trained and the control groups whose ejection fractions were 40 percent or lower demonstrated some degree of additional global and regional dilatation. Importantly, however, training had no effect on this response, and there was no effect in either group among patients with ejection fractions greater than 40 percent. More recently, these investigators[69] completed a larger randomized trial in patients with left ventricular dysfunction after an MI. After 6 months, patients in the control group demonstrated increases in both end-systolic and end-diastolic volumes and a worsening in both wall motion abnormalities and regional dilatation relative to patients in the exercise group. The latter study was the first to suggest that an exercise program may actually attenuate abnormal remodeling in patients with reduced ventricular function.

The data from Switzerland using magnetic resonance imaging confirm that exercise training in patients with reduced left ventricular function after an MI is effective in improving exercise capacity[70] and support the Agency for Health Care Policy and Research recommendations[71] that this modality is a useful adjunct to medical therapy in these patients. Training did not cause further myocardial damage (i.e., wall thinning, infarct expansion, changes in ejection fraction, or increases in ventricular volume), nor were there any long-term changes in these measures assessed using magnetic resonance imaging. The application of magnetic resonance imaging represents a significant advance in precision over previous studies.

Patients With Right Ventricular Dysfunction

Haines and colleagues[72] studied 61 patients after they had suffered an acute inferior or true posterior MI. Right ventricular dysfunction was determined to be none, moderate, or severe by blinded, subjective readings of gated-equilibrium blood pool images at rest. They found no significant differences in exercise tolerance as assessed by treadmill time or METs, at predischarge or 3 months post–discharge testing, between patients with and without right ventricular dysfunction. There also was no difference in exercise-induced ST-segment depression, chest pain, thallium 201 defects, medically refractory angina, reinfarction rate, or cardiac mortality. No attempt was made to standardize cardiac rehabilitation, other than usual care by the patient's own physicians. Crosby and coworkers[73] studied five patients who had suffered a hemodynamically significant right ventricular infarction and found an improvement in exercise capacity with cardiac rehabilitation similar to that of patients without right ventricular infarction.

Elderly Patients

Williams and associates[74] studied 361 patients grouped according to age, with 76 patients being 65 years of age or older, all of whom had acute MI or CABG, enrolled in a 12-week exercise program. They found that the improvement in physical capacity by the elderly group was the same as for the younger groups and that benefits from cardiac rehabilitation were unrelated to age. This is a very important result because, as was mentioned earlier, the majority of MIs occur in this age group.

Exercise Programs for Patients After CABG

Adams and colleagues[75] were the first to report a study of exercise training for CABG patients. They entered four male CABG patients into a training program with 45 sedentary normal males and 11 post-MI patients. After 3 months of walking and jogging at least 3 days a week, 40 minutes a day at a heart rate 75 to 85 percent of maximum, the bypass patients had exercise capacities equal to the trained post-infarction patients, and had shown an 11 percent increase in maximal oxygen uptake.

Oldridge and coworkers[76] conducted a study of the effects of an exercise program of 32 months' duration among post-CABG patients. Twenty-one patients with angina were given maximal treadmill tests 1 week before CABG and again 16 weeks after surgery. Six of these patients then entered a program of 45 to 60 minutes of exercise, three times a week, at heart rates 65 to 75 percent of their postoperative functional capacity. Treadmill tests were performed on the exercise subjects 32 months after training began, and 28 to 34 months after surgery in the control group. Maximal oxygen uptake increased by 28 percent in the exercisers, with only a 3 percent increase observed in the controls. The exercise group had also been tested after 4 months of exercise, and by that time 90 percent of the total improvement in functional capacity observed at the end of 32 months had already occurred.

Soloff[77] conducted a nonrandomized study of the effect of rehabilitation on mood and physical performance in 27 postbypass and 18 postinfarction patients. The postbypass patients significantly improved maximal oxygen uptake and maximal heart rate after an inpatient program of bedside exercise and early ambulation, followed by 6 weeks of monitored, three-times-weekly calisthenics and 20 minutes of bicycle ergometry.

In Ireland, Horgan and associates[78] exercised 51 patients three times a week, in a program that began 8 to 10 weeks after CABG. These patients exercised 16 minutes each session at 85 percent of their maximal heart rate. After 8 weeks of exercise, duration of exercise and maximal workload were increased.

Dornan and colleagues[79] reported 210 men who were referred consecutively to a rehabilitation program after CABG. The program involved submaximal exercise testing at 8 weeks with an intervening 12-week exercise program and a repeat exercise test. A retrospective analysis showed 50 percent of the patients to be on no medication throughout their rehabilitation, whereas the others were on medications likely to affect cardiac performance. Age and the extent of revascularization did not appear to influence exercise tolerance. After the 12-week exercise program, patients in both groups had improved significantly.

Fletcher and coworkers[80] retrospectively studied 22 patients who had undergone CABG. Group I (mean age 53 years) was currently enrolled in the rehabilitation program. The authors concluded that the CABG patients in their program had greater maximal oxygen uptake, smoked less, were less often rehospitalized, and were more often fully employed than those who dropped out.

A study by Nakai and associates[81] showed that physical exercise improved graft patency rate at 7 weeks post-CABG (98 percent patency in the exercise group versus 80 percent patency in the control group) documented by coronary angiography. Perk and colleagues[82] demonstrated less medication use and hospitalizations in CABG patients who participated in an exercise program.

PERFEXT CABG Patients

Analysis of the CABG patients in our randomized exercise trial included 53 CABG patients who were randomized, resulting in 28 in the exercise-intervention group and 25 in the control group.[83] The mean time from surgery to entry into the study was 2 years. Favorable training effects were observed, however, that were similar to the larger group, but no radionuclide changes were significant. The available studies demonstrate that exercise programs can improve the exercise capacity of patients who have undergone CABG.[84, 85]

Rehabilitation After PTCA

Fitzgerald and coworkers[86] showed that despite the minimal invasiveness of PTCA and the lack of any physical contraindications, some patients found it difficult to return to work because of low self-confidence, and only 81 percent of PTCA patients actually return to work.[87] It would therefore seem practical to offer cardiac rehabilitation to these patients so that they too can benefit from the improvement in exercise capacity.

Ben-Ari and coworkers[88] studied the effects of cardiac rehabilitation in patients post-PTCA and compared them with a group of matched patients who received usual-care post-PTCA without rehabilitation. They found a higher physical work capacity and ejection fraction in the rehabilitation group compared with controls, and a lower total cholesterol, lower low-density lipoprotein, and higher high-density lipoprotein as well. There was no difference in the rate of restenosis, however, at 5.5 months of follow-up. Further work by this group[89] documented a higher return to work after their program.

Return to Work

The presumed inability to resume gainful employment can contribute greatly to a patient's loss of self-esteem and perceived economic impotence. A concerted effort by the medical/rehabilitation team must be directed to allay these concerns.[90] A symptom-limited exercise test, if normal, can do much to encourage and reinstill confidence in the patient to resume job-related activities. On the other hand, an exercise test showing a lower exercise capacity can be used to guide a patient's level of activity at work.

Occupational evaluation and counseling was shown to be of benefit by Dennis and associates[91] who decreased the time interval between infarction and return to work by an average of 32 percent with counseling low-risk patients. Cost-benefit analysis of these same patients revealed that total medical costs per patient in the 6 months post-MI were lower by $502, and their occupational income in this same time period was $2,102 greater.[92] The facts that people are working longer into their later years and that 80 percent of patients under the age of 65 years eventually return to work after their MI underscore that the majority of post-MI patients can benefit from this type of counseling. A rehabilitation program has also been found to lower rehospitalization costs in 580 patients (58 percent post-CABG and 42 percent post MI) followed over 3 years.[93]

Risk Factor Modification

Given the recurrence rate of reinfarction and overall cardiovascular mortality in survivors of MI, theoretical benefits of risk factor modification, in this selected high-risk population, could be very significant.[94] As part of a World Health Organization study, Kallio and associates performed a multifactorial intervention combined with cardiac rehabilitation in post-MI patients beginning 2 weeks after their event.[26, 30] In the treated group, they found a decrease in blood pressure, lower body weight, and improved serum cholesterol and triglycerides; smoking decreased by 50 percent in both the treated and the control groups. The NEHDP[95] showed a reduction in low-density lipoprotein fractions. The analysis of 10-year mortality from cardiovascular disease in relation to cholesterol level by Pekkanen and colleagues[96] demonstrated the importance of serum cholesterol in men with preexisting cardiovascular disease. Hamalainen and coworkers[97] noted a reduction in sudden deaths by almost 50 percent in patients enrolled in an aggressive, multifactorial intervention program for 10 years post-MI. Their interventions included control of smoking, hypertension, and lipids and the use of antiarrhythmic agents in addition to β-blockers. The demonstration of regression and retarding progression of coronary artery disease,[98, 99] the demonstration of cardiac changes due to diet and exercise,[100, 101] and the development of the public health recommendations for physical activity rather than physical fitness all have an important impact on how health professionals counsel risk factor modification.[102] The multitude of studies demonstrating a 30 to 50 percent reduction in cardiac events in cardiac patients receiving a statin ensure their prominent role in rehabilitation.

Predicting Outcome in Cardiac Rehabilitation Patients

If a patient's likelihood of improving work capacity could be predicted on the basis of initial data, much time and money could be saved. Considering V_{O_2}max and other indicators of a training effect,[103] we asked the following questions: (1) Can clinical features before training predict whether or not beneficial changes occur with training? (2) Do initial treadmill and/or radionuclide measurements contribute information to improve this prediction? and (3) Does the intensity of training over the year predict beneficial changes? Our major finding was that a patient's success or failure in improving aerobic capacity after a 1-year aerobic exercise program was poorly predicted on the basis of initial clinical, treadmill, or radionuclide data. Correlation between initial parameters and outcome was poor. Training intensity had little to do with outcome. Those with ischemic markers (exercise test–induced angina, ST depression, or dropping ejection fraction) did not show a different degree of training effect than patients without ischemia; neither did those with markers of myocardial damage.

There was a trend for those who initially showed evidence of the poorest state of fitness (high resting or submaximal heart rate, low estimated maximal oxygen uptake) or high thallium ischemia scores to have the most improvement in the same respective parameter. However, initial measured maximal oxygen uptake, the best measure of aerobic capacity on entry, showed no relationship to any measure of training effect at the end of the year of training. Older patients showed only slightly less benefit than younger ones. Those with characteristics suggesting larger amounts of scar or ischemia did not have results significantly different from those with less. Multivariate analysis did not greatly improve the ability to predict outcome.

A detailed initial evaluation did not allow accurate prediction of who would train and who would not. Even those patients whose characteristics suggested they had the most ischemia or scar showed as much improvement from training as patients without such characteristics. Van Dixhoorn and associates[104] added psychosocial variables and were able to better predict "failure" to improve than success. Other investigators of this issue have observed mixed results.[105]

Summary: Changes Owing to Economic Forces

There are significant changes coming about in the United States regarding exercise testing and cardiac rehabilitation. The current wave of changes also includes care provider assessment by regulatory bodies and reimbursement for cognitive interactions, with a decrease in payment for procedures.[106, 107] Influential in this area is the Joint Commission on Accreditation of Health Care Organizations (JCAHO); hospital accreditation will depend on the assessment of physician diagnostic and treatment performance. The JCAHO plans a change of agenda from quality assurance (i.e., quality by inspection) to quality assessment.[108] Markers of performance must be utilized to evaluate quality of care and the implementation of guidelines. In an effort to shape these changes, medical associations (such as the American Heart Association, American College of Physicians, American College of Cardiology, AACVPR, and American College of Sports Medicine) are defining and refining guidelines for treatment and the use of technology and are becoming more involved in the accreditation of practitioners. Although not initially put into practice as hoped, they are now being used as a means of evaluating health organization and physician performance.[109, 110] They are even replacing "the standard of practice in the community" in legal matters.

The changes that are coming in regard to exercise testing and cardiac rehabilitation are the following:

1. Exercise testing will be performed more by family practitioners and internists than by cardiologists. In a American College of Physicians survey,[111] 50 percent of internists were performing exercise tests. The test will be used to decide which patients need to be referred to the cardiologist. It will serve as the "gatekeeper" to more expensive and invasive tests. A key need will be to educate these practitioners to do testing properly.
2. Cardiac rehabilitation is being accepted as standard practice in the United States. "In-hospital" programs must be implemented in order for hospitals to be accredited. Physical and occupational therapists are critical in this process. "Outpatient" programs are being greatly curtailed by declining reimbursement. No longer can they generate revenue by charging for electrocardiographic monitoring of patients who really do not need it. Guidelines have greatly limited the percentage of patients who are to receive the electrocardiographically monitored component. Each hospital has had its own outpatient program in order to compete with nearby hospitals, but eventually centralized programs responsible for a region will be the best approach. The practitioners are changing as well. It is much more practical and realistic to teach cardiology and exercise physiology to physical medicine rehabilitation physicians and to family practitioners than to expect cardiologists to perform cardiac rehabilitation. In addition, research has demonstrated that exercise programs can be safely carried out in selected low-risk patients in the home setting.[112] The Multi-Fit program tested in the health maintenance organization setting by DeBusk and colleagues[112] demonstrates that trained nurses can save health care costs by using computer algorithms and telephone surveillance methods.

Some of the problems of modern medicine can be explained by the imposition of technology between practitioners and patients. Cardiac rehabilitation can ensure that humanistic concerns reverse these problems. It may well be that the guise of our implementation of these goals is changing, and we should become part of the "outcome assessment" plan proposed by JCAHO. The three or four phases of cardiac rehabilitation were largely directed to the exercise goals at different time points of MI. With the in-hospital phase shortened to 3 to 5 days, phase 1 has all but disappeared and now applies only to patients with complications. Interventions including CABG and PTCA have also affected the early phases. Two factors are responsible for lessening the need for formal later phases: the public health emphasis on increasing levels of moderate physical activity rather than promoting fitness, and the fact that patients now experience less deconditioning with shorter hospital stays.

Future Directions in the United States

Cardiac rehabilitation professionals must continue to develop innovative means to deliver their services and to document what they are doing by using outcome assessment and cost control. They must gather evidence on consequences of care, not just at completion of formal treatment, but downstream and with assessment tools that are sensitive to lifestyle factors associated with disease risk and progression as well as quality of life. Their services must have a focus that is population based with a primary responsibility to manage capitated enrollees. Rather than respond to hospital directors, they must relate to executives responsible for managing primary care. Reengineering is critical. Cardiac rehabilitation professionals must start asking, "Do we really need this particular aspect of rehabilitation?," "Is there a better and cheaper way to deliver this service?," and "Which patients really need and benefit from a particular component?" No longer can each hospital or clinic have a program just to be competitive. One or two centers will be sufficient for each community. The following sections describe suggestions for the survival of cardiac rehabilitation.

Reinventing Cardiac Rehabilitation: Implement Restructuring

As our group[113] suggested, a new era requires a new model. The old model of a standard, fixed 36-session program in which every patient receives the same intervention, regardless of specific needs or characteristics, is outmoded and a disservice to patients. Part of the reason for adhering to the old model was failure to interact with third-party payers in the design of appropriate programs that met patient needs. The security of a "safe" and reliable means of obtaining reimbursement was the driving force behind this approach—and programs have been reluctant to make any change because of a fear that revenues would be lost. Some observations/suggestions follow and then recommendations of several models for consideration that are based on impressions of current trends and opportunities that exist today.

Initiate Patient Contact Early

Too many patients are leaving the inpatient setting without any contact with the cardiac rehabilitation specialists. Efforts must be intensified to ensure an early contact at the inpatient setting. The cardiac rehabilitation team must be integrated into the clinical pathway to work with these patients at this ideal time. Waiting until well after discharge has proved to be ineffective. The current trend is to reduce the length of both the hospital stay and the follow-up period as a method of cost saving. Thus, it becomes even more important that these patients be provided with an opportunity to interact with rehabilitation specialists who can assist them in their recovery. Practitioners must be more active in educating primary care physicians, managed care administrators, and consumers about the value of rehabilitation. Under a capitated system, they must be convinced that low-technology alternatives are in place to minimize costs. They also must be able to readily access services, so admissions occur at acceptable rates when appropriate cases arise. With cardiac rehabilitation care serving approximately 15 to 20 percent of eligible patients today, utilization is low.

Reach a More Diverse Pool of Patients

The treatment plan for patients with cardiovascular disease is really limited to a single diagnosis. It is unusual to find an older patient who is free of other diagnoses of chronic disease. It is likely that many patients with cardiac disease have one or more additional disease such as obesity, diabetes, chronic obstructive pulmonary disease, arthritis, or other complications that must be taken into account in the intervention plan. Yet few programs market their services to patients with these other diagnoses and thereby lose a key opportunity to serve the widest client base with a common set of interventional strategies applicable to the treatment of multiple disease. For instance, *weight control* is an important intervention in the treatment of those chronic diseases that are aggravated by obesity. *Dietary modification,* including a reduction of fat and cholesterol intake and an increase in complex carbohydrates in the form of whole grains, fresh fruits, and vegetables, is not only essential in clinical efforts to slow the progress of atherosclerotic lesions but also helps the diabetic, the arthritic, and the obese. The *benefits of exercise* to each of these chronic disease groups are well documented, as is the use of *relaxation* and cognitive strategies in *behavior change.* Cardiac rehabilitation needs to consider a new and broader identity and expand its scope of practice to include all chronic disease—especially as the aged segment of our patient population continues to grow, requiring the most costly services available in the health care system.

Increase Physician Awareness

There is a clear lack of awareness among those in the medical profession who are responsible for making decisions regarding the treatment options available to their patients in the community. It is a well-recognized fact that physicians infrequently counsel their patients regarding healthful behaviors, even though most would agree to the benefits. Whether it is a lack of awareness of the availability of these services or simply negligence, ignorance, or skepticism, the fact remains that few patients are being referred to rehabilitative programs. The critical step in any effort to change this pattern rests with the primary care physician, who now serves as a gatekeeper to these potential services. The primary care physicians must become an integral part of the treatment plan for their patients who are most likely to benefit from cardiac rehabilitation. They must become educated about the short- and long-term benefits; otherwise, without this collaborative treatment planning and consequent increase in clientele, it is unlikely that these programs can survive in the future. Since training in preventive strategies has never been an integral part of medical education, efforts must be made to convince current practitioners and medical students about the benefits to patients.

Include Underserved Populations

The misconception that cardiovascular disease predominantly afflicts men is a major deterrent to referrals of women to rehabilitative programs. Cardiovascular disease is still the major cause of death in women, and mortality rates are comparable between the genders. Other groups who are underserved owing to reasons of economics as well as misconception are the elderly, the poor/uneducated, and minorities. The population being served in most programs across the nation remains relatively young, white, professional, and male.

Expand Utilization

Less than 20 percent of all eligible cardiac patients are referred to cardiac rehabilitation programs; 100 percent of all eligible patients could benefit from some form of cardiac rehabilitation. One reason for this discrepancy may be a physician belief system that fails to incorporate secondary prevention (i.e., cardiac rehabilitation) into the patient's treatment plan. Physicians should become more familiar with alternatives to their current practice and utilize other health care professionals to efficiently and economically extend their capacity to treat their patients. Ideally, specialists who would determine their needs and individualize a program would see every patient at a rehabilitation center. All of the modalities of rehabilitation would be considered (home-based to monitored groups) without outside pressures to enter patients into expensive approaches. In addition, eligibility should be expanded to the elderly and patients with congestive heart failure and postsurgical intervention. In some circumstances, all the rehabilitation that is needed or available might be counseling by a primary care physician. Patients who are more successful in changing their lifestyle behaviors report that the physician's recommendation had a strong influence on their willingness to change. Physicians who are confident and have good counseling skills are more effective in changing the behavior of their patients. Physicians with good personal health habits and positive health beliefs are also more likely to have a positive influence on their patients' lifestyles. It has been suggested that the traditional physical examination in apparently healthy persons is a waste of physician and patient time—time that could better be spent on counseling regarding better lifestyle habits.

Highlight Potential Reduction in Mortality

Cardiac rehabilitation is successful, as demonstrated by two independent meta-analyses. These rigorous analyses collectively demonstrated a 25 percent reduction in cardiovascular mortality but no reduction in morbidity.[114, 115] Numerous studies have documented the benefits of lowering serum cholesterol using drugs. Angiographic studies have shown regression or stopping of progression, and a follow-up study found a 25 percent reduction in mortality and a 42 percent reduction in CABG. Since the recent studies of regression of coronary disease and decrease in events with cholesterol lowering using statins underscore the benefits of rehabilitation, the control of lipid abnormalities must be a key part of any rehabilitation program.

Document Cost Efficacy

Like all clinical interventions today, cardiac programs must demonstrate to hospital administrators that they are cost effective. Although such documentation is likely to exist for many if not most programs, few have made the effort to publish such data. There has been a proliferation of research methodologies in recent years that consider alternative ways of conducting economic evaluation of health care.[116] Although this has added some uncertainty of approach, standardization is coming and decision makers are beginning to consider these findings as they reformulate the scope of their health insurance coverage. Importantly, recent studies clearly demonstrate that cardiac rehabilitation is cost effective. Oldridge and coworkers[117] performed an economic evaluation of patients 1 year after randomization to either an 8-week rehabilitation intervention or usual care and revealed that cardiac rehabilitation is an efficient use of health care resources. Ades and associates[118] presented the results of a 3-year economic evaluation of patients undergoing 12 weeks of rehabilitation, which revealed that per-capita hospitalization charges for rehabilitation participants were $739 lower than for nonparticipants. Bondestam and colleagues[119] described the effects of early rehabilitation that relied totally on the primary health care system on consumption of medical care resources during the first year after acute MI in patients 65 years of age or older. Patients from one primary health care district were assigned to a rehabilitation program, and patients from a neighboring district constituted a control group. The rehabilitation measures were initiated very early after the infarction, with individual counseling in the home of the patient and later in the local health center, where 21 percent of the patients also joined a low-intensity exercise group. During the first 3 months, there was a significantly lower incidence of rehospitalization in the intervention group, expressed both in terms of percentage of patients and in days of rehospitalization. Visits to the emergency department without rehospitalization were also significantly lower in the intervention group. After 12 months, the differences still remained, with the exception of no intergroup difference in follow-up relative to days of rehospitalization. In the matched groups, the same result was seen. Whereas readmissions and emergency department visits were generally well justified in the intervention group, vague symptoms dominated among the controls. Levin and coworkers[120] presented the results of an economic evaluation of patients followed 5 years after rehabilitation intervention or usual care, which demonstrated that mean patient costs were $8,800 lower in the rehabilitation group.

Implement Restructuring

Cardiac rehabilitation needs to be restructured by adding newer cost-effective techniques to survive the current reformation of health care. Traditional rehabilitation will be best delivered at centers in the community rather than the current fragmented approach in which each hospital has a competitive program. Newer models involve the use of other medical and paramedical professionals, volunteers, and communication with patients via telephone, Internet, and the postal service. Four specific models with research documenting their efficacy are presented.

Center-Based Model

Physician referral could be improved as general practitioners become more responsible for triage and have the option of directing patients to a center with multidisciplinary specialists available. Health care managers must be convinced that cardiac rehabilitation is effective. The necessary components of this triaging approach include initial assessment by a team of specialists, risk stratification, exercise prescription (often just a walking program, with indirect supervision, when medically appropriate), dietary instruction, lipid abnormality classification and treatment, psychological and vocational counseling, education, and a discharge plan.

The center-based model is the classic model that was the prototype for the majority of the programs in recent history. Its major shortcoming is lack of adequate referral—physician referral could be improved if general practitioners became more responsible for triage and had the option of directing patients to a center with multidisciplinary specialists available. In addition, health care managers must be convinced that cardiac rehabilitation is as effective as yet less expensive than interventional cardiology.

Home-Based Model

This model has been in place since the late 1980s, and numerous studies in the literature have documented its effectiveness. This model has been validated at Stanford in a 1-year randomized clinical trial including 160 women and 197 men aged 50 to 65 years who were sedentary and free of cardiovascular disease.[121] It included physician referral, assessment, prescription, and multiple intervention. There was regular feedback and home visits to prevent relapses. The main outcomes measured were treadmill exercise performance, exercise participation rates, and cardiovascular disease risk factors. Compared with controls, subjects in all three exercise training conditions showed significant improvements in V_{O_2}max at both 6 and 12 months. Lower-intensity training achieved training changes comparable with those of higher-intensity training. Twelve-month exercise adherence rates were better for the two home-based exercise training conditions in comparison to the group-based exercise training condition. This community-based exercise training program improved fitness but not coronary heart disease risk factors among sedentary, healthy older adults. Home-based exercise was as effective as group exercise in producing these changes. Lower-intensity exercise training was as effective as higher-intensity exercise training in the home setting.

Volunteer Community Model

The volunteer community model is a unique approach that was developed by Lorig and colleagues[122] in patients with arthritis. These investigators trained nonmedical lay volunteers (who themselves had arthritis) to direct educational programs of self-management in the community to help patients with arthritis deal with their disease outside of a medical setting. Lorig and colleagues[122] have since expanded this model to include four chronic disorders (coronary heart disease, chronic obstructive pulmonary disease, stroke, and arthritis). After physician referral, there was assessment, prescription, and multiple intervention as in the center-based model, but utilizing an 8-week educational training program off-site. There was regular monitoring of behaviors as well as regular feedback and modification of intervention to prevent relapses. The program was 2 hours per week for 7 weeks and was taught by two lay leaders in small interactive groups. The processes taught included problem solving, cognitive symptom management, design of exercise programs, fatigue and sleep management, anger and depression management, appropriate use of medications, patient/physician communications, proper use of advanced directives, self-efficacy enhancement, skills mastery, modeling, and reinterpretation of symptoms. The patients developed self-confidence, understood symptom management, and learned how to solve problems.

Health Risk Appraisal Model

A randomized 12-month trial comparing claims data was performed in a large insured population.[123] After assessment with a health risk appraisal instrument accomplished via mail, feedback on risk factors and recommendations for change were provided again by mail using an educational packet of self-management materials. This study demonstrated a considerable cost trend reduction from a simple mail-based health promotion program. The insurance company was so pleased with the reduction in claims that the program has been continued.

Summary

Cardiac rehabilitation is going through the same type of dramatic metamorphosis as the entire health care system. However, its principles have become part of good medical practice. The emphasis on the health benefits of physical activity rather than physical fitness and the lessening of iatrogenic deconditioning have decreased the emphasis on exercise prescription and the phased approach.

References

1. Ryan TJ, Anderson JL, Antman EM, et al: ACC/AHA guidelines for the management of patients with acute myocardial infarction: executive summary. A report of the American College of Cardiology/American Heart Association Task Force on Practice Guidelines (Committee on Management of Acute Myocardial Infarction). Circulation 94:2341–2350, 1996.
2. Maisel AS, Ahnve S, Gilpin E, et al: Prognosis after extension of myocardial infarct: the role of Q wave or non–Q wave infarction. Circulation 71:211–217, 1985.
3. Maisel AS, Gilpin E, Hoit B, et al: Survival after hospital discharge in matched populations with inferior or anterior myocardial infarction. J Am Coll Cardiol 6:731–736, 1985.
4. Connolly DC, Elveback LR: Coronary heart disease in residents of Rochester, Minnesota. VI. Hospital and posthospital course of patients with transmural and subendocardial myocardial infarction. Mayo Clin Proc 60:375–381, 1985.
5. Boden WE, O'Rourke RA, Crawford MH, et al: Outcomes in patients with acute non–Q-wave myocardial infarction randomly assigned to an invasive as compared with a conservative management strategy. Veterans Affairs Non–Q-Wave Infarction Strategies in Hospital (VANQWISH) Trial Investigators. N Engl J Med 338:1785–1792, 1998.
6. Ross J, Gilpin EA, Madsen EB, et al: A decision scheme for coronary angiography after acute myocardial infarction. Circulation 79:292–303, 1989.
7. Ahnve S, Gilpin E, Ditrich H, et al: First myocardial infarction: age and ejection fraction identify a low-risk group. Am Heart J 116:925–932, 1988.
8. Guidelines for risk stratification after myocardial infarction. American College of Physicians. Ann Intern Med 126:556–560, 1997.
9. Klein J, Froelicher VF, Detrano R, et al: Does the rest electrocardiogram after myocardial infarction determine the predictive value of exercise-induced ST depression? A 2 year follow-up study in a Veteran population. J Am Coll Cardiol 14:305–311, 1989.
10. Krone RJ, Dwyer EM, Greenberg H, et al: Risk stratification in patients with first non–Q wave infarction: limited value of the early low level exercise test after uncomplicated infarct. The Multicenter Post-Infarction Research Group. J Am Coll Cardiol 14:31–37, 1989.
11. TIMI Study Group: Comparison of invasive and conservative strategies after treatment with intravenous tissue plasminogen activator in acute myocardial infarction. Results of the Thrombolysis in Myocardial Infarction (TIMI) Phase II Trial. N Engl J Med 320:618–627, 1989.
12. Simoons ML, Arnold AER, Betriu A, et al: Thrombolysis with tissue plasminogen activator in acute myocardial infarction: no additional benefit from immediate percutaneous coronary angioplasty. Lancet 1:197–203, 1988.
13. DeBono DP, for the SWIFT Investigators Group: Should we intervene following thrombolysis? The SWIFT study of intervention versus conservative management after anistreplase thrombolysis. Eur Heart J 10(suppl):253, 1989.
14. Franzosi MG, Santoro E, De Vita C, et al: Ten-year follow-up of the first megatrial testing thrombolytic therapy in patients with acute myocardial infarction: results of the Gruppo Italiano per lo Studio Della Sopravvivenza Nell'Infarto-1 study: Circulation 98:2659–2665, 1998.
15. Hammerman H, Schoen FJ, Kloner RA: Short-term exercise has a prolonged effect on scar formation after experimental acute myocardial infarction. J Am Coll Cardiol 2:979–982, 1983.
16. Kloner RA, Kloner JA: The effect of early exercise on myocardial infarct scar formation. Am Heart J 106:1009–1014, 1983.
17. Hochman JS, Healy B: Effect of exercise on acute myocardial infarction in rats. J Am Coll Cardiol 7:126–132, 1986.
18. Convertino VA: Effect of orthostatic stress on exercise performance after bed rest: relation to inhospital rehabilitation. J Card Rehabil 3:660–663, 1983.
19. DeBusk RF: Sexual activity triggering myocardial infarction. One less thing to worry about [editorial; comment]. JAMA 275:1447–1448, 1996.
20. Cain HD, Frasher WG, Stivelman R: Graded activity program for safe return to self-care after myocardial infarction. JAMA 177:111–120, 1961.

21. Torkelson LO: Rehabilitation of the patient with acute myocardial infarction. J Chron Dis 17:685–704, 1964.
22. Sivarajan ES, Snydsman A, Smith B, et al: Low-level treadmill testing of 41 patients with acute myocardial infarction prior to discharge from the hospital. Heart Lung 6:975–980, 1977.
23. Hayes MJ, Morris GK, Hampton JR: Comparison of mobilization after two and nine days in uncomplicated myocardial infarction. BMJ 3:10–13, 1974.
24. Bloch A, Maeder J, Haissly J, et al: Early mobilization after myocardial infarction. A controlled study. Am J Cardiol 34:152–157, 1974.
25. Sivarajan E, Bruce RA, Almes MJ, et al: In-hospital exercise after myocardial infarction does not improve treadmill performance. N Engl J Med 305:357–362, 1981.
26. World Health Organization (WHO), Report of Expert Committee: Rehabilitation of Patients With Cardiovascular Diseases. Technical Report No. 270. Geneva: WHO, 1964.
27. Fletcher GF, Balady G, Blair SN, et al: Statement on exercise: benefits and recommendations for physical activity programs for all Americans. A statement for health professionals by the Committee on Exercise and Cardiac Rehabilitation of the Council on Clinical Cardiology, American Heart Association, Dallas, TX 75231–4596, USA. Circulation 94:857–862, 1996.
28. Kelemen MH, Stewart KJ, Gillilan RE, et al: Circuit weight training in cardiac patients. J Am Coll Cardiol 7:38–42, 1986.
29. Sparling PB, Cantwell JD, Dolan CM, Niederman RK: Strength training in a cardiac rehabilitation program: a six-month follow-up. Arch Phys Med Rehabil 71:148, 1990.
30. Kallio V, Hamalainen H, Hakkila J, Luurila OJ: Reduction in sudden deaths by a multifactorial intervention programme after acute myocardial infarction. Lancet 2:1091–1094, 1979.
31. Kentala E: Physical fitness and feasibility of physical rehabilitation after myocardial infarction in men of working age. Ann Clin Res 4:1–25, 1972.
32. Palatsi I: Feasibility of physical training after myocardial infarction and its effect on return to work, morbidity, and mortality. Acta Med Scand Suppl 599:1–100, 1976.
33. Wilhelmsen L, Sanne H, Elmfeldt D, et al: A controlled trial of physical training after myocardial infarction. Prev Med 4:491–508, 1975.
34. Shaw LW: Effects of a prescribed supervised exercise program on mortality and cardiovascular mortality in patients after a myocardial infarction. Am J Cardiol 48:39–46, 1981.
35. Shepard RJ: Exercise regimens after myocardial infarction: rationale and results. Cardiovasc Clin 14:145–157, 1985.
36. Bengtsson K: Rehabilitation after myocardial infarction. Scand J Rehabil Med 15:1–9, 1983.
37. Carson P, Phillips R, Lloyd M, et al: Exercise after myocardial infarction: a controlled trial. J R Coll Physicians Lond 16:147–151, 1982.
38. Vermeulen A, Liew KI, Durrer D: Effects of cardiac rehabilitation after myocardial infarction: changes in coronary risk factors and long-term prognosis. Am Heart J 105:798–801, 1983.
39. Roman O: Do randomized trials support the use of cardiac rehabilitation? J Card Rehabil 5:93–96, 1985.
40. Mayou RA: A controlled trial of early rehabilitation after myocardial infarction. J Card Rehabil 3:397–402, 1983.
41. Hedback B, Perk J, Perski A: Effect of a post-myocardial infarction rehabilitation program on mortality, morbidity, and risk factors. J Cardiopulm Rehabil 5:576–583, 1985.
42. Goble AJ, Hare DL, Macdonald PS, et al: Effect of early programmes of high and low intensity exercise on physical performance after transmural acute myocardial infarction. Br Heart J 65:126–131, 1991.
43. O'Connor GT, Buring JE, Yusuf S, et al: An overview of randomized trials of rehabilitation with exercise after myocardial infarction. Circulation 80:234–244, 1989.
44. Oldridge NB, Guyatt GH, Fischer ME, Rimm AA: Cardiac rehabilitation after myocardial infarction. Combined experience of randomized clinical trials. JAMA 260:945–950, 1988.
45. Haskell WL: Cardiovascular complications during exercise training of cardiac patients. Circulation 57:920–924, 1978.
46. Hossack KF, Hartwig R: Cardiac arrest associated with supervised cardiac rehabilitation. J Card Rehabil 2:402–408, 1982.
47. Van Camp SP, Peterson RA: Cardiovascular complications of outpatient cardiac rehabilitation programs. JAMA 256:1160–1163, 1986.
48. Thompson PD, Funk EJ, Carleton RA, Sturner WQ: Incidence of death during jogging in Rhode Island from 1975 through 1980. JAMA 247:2535–2538, 1982.
49. Thompson PD: The benefits and risks of exercise training in patients with chronic coronary artery disease. JAMA 259:1537–1540, 1988.
50. Cobb LA, Weaver DW: Exercise: a risk for sudden death in patients with coronary heart disease. J Am Coll Cardiol 7:215, 1986.
51. Cantwell J: Exercise and the heart: current management of severe exercise-related cardiac events. Chest 93:1264–1269, 1988.
52. Greenland P, Chu JS: Efficacy of cardiac rehabilitation services. With emphasis on patients after myocardial infarction. Ann Intern Med 109:650–666, 1988.
53. Froelicher VF, Jensen D, Genter F, et al: A randomized trial of exercise training in patients with coronary heart disease. JAMA 252:1291–1297, 1984.
54. Atwood JE, Jensen D, Froelicher VF, et al: Agreement in human interpretation of analog thallium myocardial perfusion images. Circulation 64:601–609, 1981.
55. Sebrechts CP, Klein JL, Ahnve S, et al: Myocardial perfusion changes following 1 year of exercise training assessed by thallium-201 circumferential count profiles. Am Heart J 112:1217–1226, 1986.
56. Myers J, Ahnve S, Froelicher V, et al: A randomized trial of the effects of 1 year of exercise training on computer-measured ST segment displacement in patients with coronary artery disease. J Am Coll Cardiol 4:1094–1102, 1984.
57. Ehsani AA, Martin WH, Heath GW, Coyle EF: Cardiac effects of prolonged and intense exercise training in patients with coronary artery disease. Am J Cardiol 50:246–254, 1982.
58. Malmborg R, Isaccson S, Kallivroussis G: The effect of beta-blockade and/or physical training in patients with angina pectoris. Curr Ther Res 16:171, 1974.
59. Obma RT, Wilson PK, Goebel ME, Campbell DE: Effect of a conditioning program in patients taking propranolol for angina pectoris. Cardiology 64:365–371, 1979.
60. Pratt CM, Welton DE, Squired WG, et al: Demonstration of training effect during chronic beta-adrenergic blockade in patients with coronary artery disease. Circulation 64:1125–1129, 1981.
61. Vanhees L, Fagard R, Amery A: Influence of beta-adrenergic blockade on the hemodynamic effects of physical training in patients with ischemic heart disease. Am Heart J 108:270–275, 1984.
62. Froelicher VF, Sullivan M, Myers J, Jensen D: Can patients with coronary artery disease receiving beta blockers obtain a training effect? Am J Cardiol 55:155D–161D, 1985.
63. Rechnitzer PA, Cunningham DA, Andrew CM, et al: Relation of exercise to recurrence rate of myocardial infarction in men. Ontario Exercise-Heart Collaborative Study. Am J Cardiol 51:65–69, 1983.
64. Squires RW, Lavie CJ, Brandt TR, et al: Cardiac rehabilitation in patients with severe ischemic left ventricular dysfunction. Mayo Clin Proc 62:997–1002, 1987.
65. Conn EH, Williams RS, Wallace RG: Exercise responses before and after physical conditioning in patients with severely depressed left ventricular function. Am J Cardiol 49:296–300, 1982.
66. Judgutt BI, Michorowski BL, Kappagoda CT: Exercise training after anterior Q-wave myocardial infarction: importance of regional left ventricular function and topography. J Am Coll Cardiol 12:363–372, 1988.
67. Adampouls S, Coats AJS, Brunotte F, et al: Physical training improves skeletal muscle metabolism in patients with chronic heart failure. J Am Coll Cardiol 21:1101–1106, 1993.
68. Giannuzzi P, Tavazzi L, Temporelli PL, et al: Long-term physical training and left ventricular remodeling relative to infarct size. Circulation 92:S2041, 1995.
69. Giannuzzi P, Corra U, Gattone M, et al: Attenuation of unfavorable remodeling by exercise training in postinfarction patients with left ventricular dysfunction: results of the Exercise in Left Ventricular Dysfunction (ELVD) trial. Circulation 96:1790–1797, 1997.
70. Dubach P, Myers J, Dziekan G, et al: Effect of exercise training on myocardial remodeling in patients with reduced left ventricular function after myocardial infarction. Circulation 95:2060–2067, 1997.
71. Agency for Health Care Policy and Research Clinical Practice Guidelines: Cardiac rehabilitation. Washington, DC: U.S. Department of Health and Human Services, 1995.

72. Haines DE, Beller GA, Watson DD, et al: A prospective clinical, scintigraphic, angiographic, and functional evaluation of patients after inferior myocardial infarction with and without right ventricular dysfunction. J Am Coll Cardiol 6:995–1003, 1985.
73. Crosby L, Paternostro-Bayles M, Cottington E, Pifalo WB: Outpatient rehabilitation after right ventricular infarction. J Cardiopulmon Rehabil 7:286–291, 1989.
74. Williams MA, Maresh CM, Esterbrooks DJ, et al: Early exercise training in patients older than age 65 years compared with that in younger patients after acute myocardial infarction or coronary artery bypass grafting. Am J Cardiol 55:263–266, 1985.
75. Adams WC, McHenry MM, Bernauer EM: Long term physiologic adaptations to exercise with special reference to performance and cardiorespiratory function in health and disease. Am J Cardiol 33:765–775, 1974.
76. Oldridge NB, Nagle FJ, Balke B, et al: Aortocoronary bypass surgery: effects of surgery and 32 months of physical conditioning on treadmill performance. Arch Phys Med Rehabil 59:268–275, 1978.
77. Soloff PH: Medically and surgically treated coronary patients in cardiovascular rehabilitation: a comparative study. Int J Psychiatry Med 9:93–106, 1980.
78. Horgan JH, Teo KK, Murren KM, et al: The response to exercise training and vocational counselling in post-myocardial infarction and coronary artery bypass surgery patients. Ir Med J 74:463–469, 1980.
79. Dornan J, Rolko AF, Greenfield C: Factors affecting rehabilitation following aortocoronary bypass procedures. Can J Surg 25:677–680, 1982.
80. Fletcher BJ, Lloyd A, Fletcher GF: Outpatient rehabilitative training in patients with cardiovascular disease: emphasis on training method. Heart Lung 17:199–205, 1988.
81. Nakai Y, Kataoka Y, Bando M, et al: Effects of physical exercise training on cardiac function and graft patency after coronary artery bypass grafting. J Thorac Cardiovasc Surg 93:62–65, 1987.
82. Perk B, Hedback E, Engvall G: Effects of cardiac rehabilitation after CABS on readmissions, return to work, and physical fitness. Scand J Soc Med 18:45–53, 1990.
83. Froelicher VF, Jensen D, Sullivan M: A randomized trial of the effects of exercise training after coronary artery bypass surgery. Arch Intern Med 145:689–692, 1985.
84. Robinson G, Froelicher VF, Utley JR: Rehabilitation of the coronary artery bypass graft surgery patient. J Card Rehabil 4:74–86, 1984.
85. Foster C: Exercise training following cardiovascular surgery. Exerc Sport Sci Rev 14:303–323, 1986.
86. Fitzgerald ST, Becker DM, Celentano DP, et al: Return to work after percutaneous transluminal coronary angioplasty. Am J Cardiol 64:1108–1112, 1989.
87. Meier B, Gruentzig AR: Return to work after coronary artery bypass surgery in comparison to coronary angioplasty. *In* Walter PJ (ed): Return to Work After Coronary Bypass Surgery: Pychosocial and Economic Aspects. pp. 171–176. New York: Springer-Verlag, 1987.
88. Ben-Ari E, Rothbaum DA, Linnemeir TJ, et al: Benefits of a monitored rehabilitation program versus physician care after percutaneous transluminal coronary angioplasty: follow-up of risk factors and rate of restenosis. J Cardiopulm Rehabil 7:281–285, 1989.
89. Ben-Ari E, Rothbaum DA, Linnemeier TA, et al: Return to work after successful coronary angioplasty: comparison between a comprehensive rehabilitation program and patients receiving usual care. J Cardiopulm Rehabil 12:20–24, 1992.
90. Haskel WL: Restoration and maintenance of physical and psychosocial function in patients with ischemic heart disease. J Am Coll Cardiol 12:1090–1121, 1988.
91. Dennis C, Houston-Miller N, Schwartz RG, et al: Early return to work after uncomplicated myocardial infarction: results of a randomized trial. JAMA 260:214–220, 1988.
92. Picard MH, Dennis C, Schwartz RG, et al: Cost-benefit analysis of early return to work after uncomplicated acute myocardial infarction. Am J Cardiol 63:1308–1314, 1989.
93. Ades P, Huang D, Weaver SO: Cardiac rehabilitation participation predicts lower rehospitalization costs. Am Heart J 123:916–920, 1992.
94. Siegel D, Grady P, Browner WS, Hulley SB: Risk factor modification after myocardial infarction. Ann Intern Med 109:213–218, 1988.
95. LaRosa JC, Cleary P, Muesing RA, et al: Effect of long-term moderate physical exercise on plasma lipoproteins: the National Exercise and Heart Disease Project. Arch Intern Med 142:2269–2274, 1982.
96. Pekkanen J, Linn S, Heiss G, et al: Ten-year mortality from cardiovascular disease in relation to cholesterol level among men with and without preexisting cardiovascular disease. N Engl J Med 332:1700–1707, 1990.
97. Hamalainen H, Luurila OJ, Kallio V, et al: Long-term reduction in sudden deaths after a multifactorial intervention programme in patients with myocardial infarction: 10-year results of a controlled investigation. Eur Heart J 10:55–62, 1989.
98. Brown G, Albers JJ, Fisher LD, et al: Regression of coronary artery disease as a result of intensive lipid-lowering therapy in men with high levels of apolipoprotein B. N Engl J Med 323:1289–1298, 1990.
99. Schuler G, Hambrect R, Schlierf G, et al: Progression of coronary stenoses in patients on intensive physical exercise and low fat diet. Circulation 4:III-238, 1990.
100. Ornish D, Brown SE, Scherwitz LW, et al: Can lifestyle changes reverse coronary heart disease? Lancet 336:129–133, 1990.
101. Schuler G, Shlierf G, Wirth A, et al: Low-fat diet and regular, supervised physical exercise in patients with symptomatic coronary artery disease: reduction of stress-induced myocardial ischemia. Circulation 77:172, 1988.
102. McHenry PL, Ellestad MH, Fletcher GF, et al: A position statement for health professionals by the Committee on Exercise and Cardiac Rehabilitation of the Council on Clinical Cardiology, American Heart Association. Circulation 81:396–398, 1990.
103. Hammond KH, Kelly TL, Froelicher VF, Pewen W: Use of clinical data in predicting improvement in exercise capacity after cardiac rehabilitation. J Am Coll Cardiol 6:19–26, 1985.
104. Van Dixhoorn E, Duivenvoorden H, Pool G: Success and failure of exercise training after myocardial infarction: is the outcome predictable? J Am Coll Cardiol 15:974–980, 1990.
105. Myers J, Froelicher VF: Predicting outcome in cardiac rehabilitation. J Am Coll Cardiol 15:983–985, 1990.
106. Detsky AS, Naglie IG: A clinician's guide to cost-effectiveness analysis. Ann Intern Med 113:147–154, 1990.
107. Hadorn DC: The future of the American health care system. N Engl J Med 10:752, 1990.
108. JCAHO Report: Clinical outcomes: managing patients and the total cost of care. 1:1–8, 1990.
109. McGuire LB: A long run for a short jump: understanding clinical guidelines. Ann Intern Med 113:705–708, 1990 .
110. Audet AM, Greenfield S, Field M: Medical practice guidelines: current activities and future directions. Ann Intern Med 113:709–714, 1990.
111. Wigton RS, Nicolas JA, Blank LL: Procedural skills of the general internist: a survey of 2500 physicians. Ann Intern Med 111:1023–1034, 1990.
112. DeBusk FR, Haskell WL, Miller NH, et al: Medically directed at-home rehabilitation soon after clinically uncomplicated acute myocardial infarction: a new model for patient care. Am J Cardiol 55:251, 1985.
113. Froelicher VF, Herbert W, Myers J, Ribisl P: How cardiac rehabilitation is being influenced by changes in health-care delivery. J Cardiopulm Rehabil 16:151–159, 1996.
114. Oldridge NB, Guyatt GH, Fischer ME, Rimm AA: Cardiac rehabilitation after myocardial infarction: combined experience of randomized clinical trials. JAMA 260:945–950, 1988.
115. O'Conner GT, Buring JE, Yusaf S: Meta-analysis of the randomized trials for patients with heart disease. Circulation 80:234–244, 1989.
116. Drummond M, Brandt A, Luce B, Rovira J: Standardizing methodologies for economic evaluation in health care. Practice, problems, and potential. Int J Technol Assess Health Care 9:26–36, 1993.
117. Oldridge N, Furlong W, Feeny D, Guyatt GH: Economic evaluation of cardiac rehabilitation soon after acute myocardial infarction. Am J Cardiol 72:154–161, 1993.
118. Ades PA, Huang D, Weaver SO: Cardiac rehabilitation participation predicts lower rehospitalization costs. Am Heart J 123:916–921, 1992.
119. Bondestam E, Breikss A, Hartford M: Effects of early rehabilitation on consumption of medical care during the first year after acute myocardial infarction in patients 65 years of age or older. Am J Cardiol 75:767–771, 1995.

120. Levin LA, Perk J, Hedback B: Cardiac rehabilitation: a cost analysis. J Intern Med 230:427–434, 1991.
121. King AC, Haskell WL, Taylor CB, et al: Group versus home-based exercise training in healthy older men and women: a community-based clinical trial. JAMA 266:1535–1542, 1991.
122. Lorig K, Holman H, Sobel D, et al: Living a Healthy Life with Chronic Conditions: Self-Management of Heart Disease, Arthritis, Stroke, Diabetes, Asthma, Bronchitis, Emphysema. Palo Alto, CA: Bull Publishing, 1994.
123. Fries R, Long M, Forsythe D: Randomized controlled trial of cost reductions from a health education program. Am J Health Promotion 8:216, 1994.

SECTION V

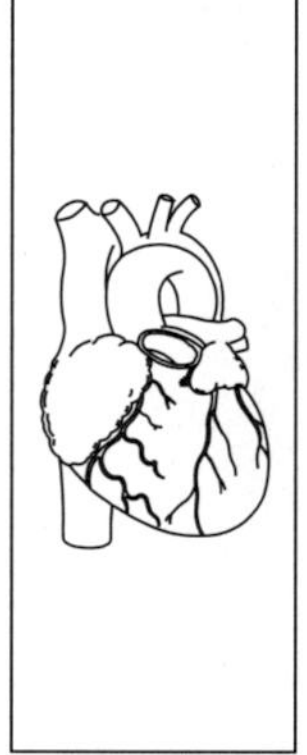

BASIC ASPECTS OF MYOCARDIAL FUNCTION, GROWTH, AND DEVELOPMENT

Cardiac Development: Toward a Molecular Basis for Congenital Heart Disease

Myocardial Metabolism

Cardiac Hypertrophy and Failure: Basic Aspects

Cardiac Hypertrophy: Physiologic and Clinical Considerations

Regulation of Cardiac Contraction and Relaxation

Clinical Abnormalities of Cardiac Relaxation

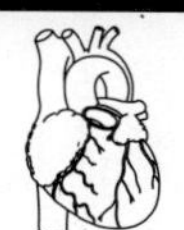

Cardiac Development: Toward a Molecular Basis for Congenital Heart Disease

Michael D. Schneider and Eric N. Olson

GENETIC APPROACHES TO CARDIOGENESIS
CARDIOGENIC TRANSCRIPTION FACTORS
Cardiac Morphogenesis
Myocyte Enhancer Factor-2
NK-2 Homeodomain Proteins
Iriquois-Related Homeobox Gene 4
GATA Factors
HAND Factors
Serum Response Factor
Transcriptional Enhancer Factor-1
T-Box 5
Evolutionary Conservation of the Cardiogenic Transcriptional Pathway
EXTRINSIC SIGNALS FOR EARLY HEART FORMATION
LEFT-RIGHT POSITION AND LOOPING MORPHOGENESIS
CARDIAC MYOCYTE PROLIFERATION
GENES IMPLICATED IN HUMAN CARDIAC MALFORMATIONS
Cardiofacial Syndromes
Hand-Heart Syndromes
Left-Right Axis Malformations
Atrial Septal Defects
IMPLICATIONS OF CARDIAC DEVELOPMENT FOR THE POSTNATAL HEART
Reactivation of Fetal Genes During Load-Induced Hypertrophy
Postmitotic Cardiac Phenotype
CONCLUSIONS AND PERSPECTIVES

Establishing precisely which molecules and pathways are essential for creation of the normal, mature, multichambered heart is, like the more general problem of how any adult organ arises from a lone initial cell, a topic of inherent fundamental interest. Moreover, congenital malformations of the heart are the most common cause of cardiac disease in children, with a frequency of 2 to 18 per 1000 live births (and perhaps a 10-fold greater prevalence in stillbirths).[1] Despite this, cardiac morphogenesis had until recently received scant attention from the molecular and cell biologists, despite compelling clinical needs to understand the mechanistic basis for congenital malformations of valves, septa, and cardiac muscle. Even in 1995, in the first edition of this textbook,[2] a genetic framework for cardiac development was only beginning to emerge. It would have been only a speculative possibility that human congenital heart defects might soon be reconciled with findings in model organisms—including flies, fish, and frogs, as well as genetically engineered mice.

In this chapter, we summarize the remarkably encouraging insights that have been gained in understanding the rules that govern heart formation, with an emphasis on several broad questions (Fig. 44–1). As totipotent daughter cells of the fertilized zygote proliferate, when (and how) does cell "fate" become restricted and a cardiac fate become acquired? As cardiac progenitor cells arise, and genes for cardiac-specific structural proteins are selectively induced, what is the role of cardiac-restricted transcription factors analogous to "determination" genes that trigger cell fate in skeletal muscle or other lineages? As committed cardiac myocytes migrate ventrally to create the linear heart tube, what controls the normal rightward direction of cardiac looping, the earliest anatomic sign of left-right asymmetry in the embryo? As later morphogenesis proceeds, what genes control the partitioning of the heart tube into a pulmonic and a systemic circulation and into discrete atrial and ventricular chambers? As heart cell number increases and the ventricle becomes trabeculated, what are the essential mitogens driving the proliferation of cardiac myocytes, and what developmental mechanisms later block the capacity for proliferative growth?

Throughout this discussion, findings and conclusions directly relevant to heart formation in humans are highlighted. A further discussion of genes implicated in human congenital heart disorders can be found in a complementary chapter by Dr. Dianna Milewicz, Chapter 118, Genetic Aspects of Congenital Heart Disease. For additional information, apart from specific cited references, the reader is directed to other overall reviews of cardiac development[3–5] and to a textbook devoted to this topic.[6] A glossary of terms is presented in Table 44–1.

Genetic Approaches to Cardiogenesis

Historically, one barrier to a mechanistic dissection of cardiac development has been that some simple organisms

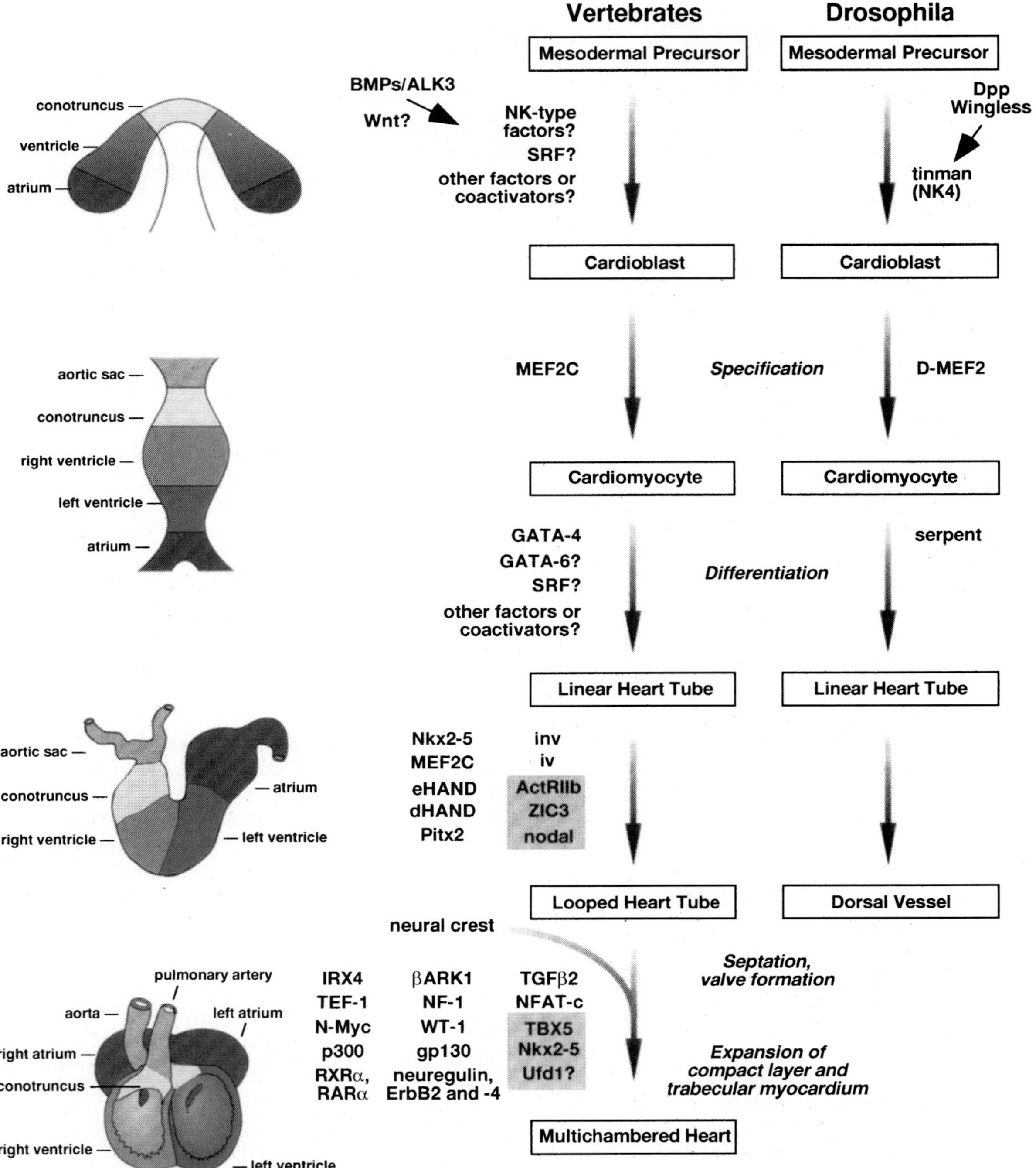

FIGURE 44–1 Schematic diagram of key stages and events in cardiac development. In response to inducing signals from adjacent endoderm, cardiogenic precursor cells in the cardiac crescent arise from anterior lateral mesoderm and migrate to the ventral midline of the embryo, forming the linear heart tube. In vertebrates, the heart tube undergoes rightward looping followed by septation and the development of atrioventricular valves, resulting in the mature, multichambered heart. Segments positioned along the anteroposterior axis of the heart tube give rise to the conotruncus (outflow tract), ventricles, atria, and inflow tract, respectively. In flies, the dorsal vessel, a rudimentary heart, parallels the early stages of heart formation in vertebrates. Several of the key molecules implicated at each step are shown; highlighted are single-gene defects that result in human congenital cardiac malformations.

TABLE 44-1 **Glossary**

Adaptor	Coactivator that can bind multiple transcription factors
Axonemal	Referring to the microtubules of cilia and flagellae
Basic-helix-loop-helix (bHLH)	Structure of the DNA-binding domain of MyoD-related transcription factors
Bigenic	Inheriting two different transgenes
Coactivators	Proteins that form complexes with the DNA-bound transcription factors and modulate their transcriptional activity
Dorsal vessel	Rudimentary, linear heart of the fly
Embryonic stem cells	Primitive, undifferentiated, totipotent cells
Enhancer	A DNA segment that controls the expression of the gene, often located far from the site where transcription begins; classically, functional even if inverted in orientation, and even if put adjacent to a heterologous promoter
Gain-of-function	Expressing more of a protein, or expressing it in an activated form
Gastrulation	Orchestrated cell movements in the early embryo, following subdivision of the zygote into blastomeres, giving rise to the three cell layers; ectoderm, mesoderm, and endoderm
Hemizygous	Having one copy of a given gene, not the usual two
Heterokaryon	Cell containing one or more exogenous nuclei
Homeodomain, homeobox	Shared region for DNA binding, common to the Hox superfamily of transcription factors, including Nkx2.5
Homologous recombination	Process of exchanging segments of DNA from one molecule to another, based on crossing over between shared regions, spontaneously or experimentally; used as the principal means to engineer gene deletions
Insertional mutagenesis	Creating mutations through random interpolation of foreign DNA (transgene, transposon, or retrovirus)
Juxtacrine	Secreted signals acting on adjacent cells
Lateral plate mesoderm	Source of cardiac progenitor cells in vertebrates
Loss of function	Expressing less or none of a protein, or expressing it in a less active form
MADS	Acronym for MCM1 (in yeast), *Agamous* and *Deficiens* (in flowering plants), and serum response factor; a family of transcription factors, also including MEF2
MyoD family	Four related transcription factors that control skeletal muscle formation in the embryo and later skeletal muscle gene expression; archetypes for the bHLH transcription factors, including eHAND and dHAND
OMIM (On-line Mendelian Inheritance in Man)	Internet database of human genes and genetic disorders (http://www.ncbi.nlm.nih.gov/Omim/)
Paracrine	Secreted signals acting over very short distances (unlike endocrine)
Promoter	A DNA segment that controls the expression of the gene, typically located close to the site where transcription begins
Retrovirus	Any RNA virus that creates a DNA copy, through reverse transcriptase, that gets inserted into chromosomal DNA of the infected cells
Ribozyme	An RNA that can catalyze the degradation of other RNAs
Syntenic	On the same chromosome, or the corresponding chromosome segment in another species
Totipotent	Capable of giving rise to all cell types found in the organism
Transcription factor	A protein that typically binds specific DNA sequences and activates or represses gene expression; may also refer to coactivators
Transgene	An exogenous gene introduced into the fertilized zygote (e.g., by microinjection or homologous recombination)
Transposon	Mobile DNA element that inserts randomly into chromosomal DNA, encoding an enzyme (transposase) that catalyzes the insertion

with especially tractable genetics, such as the nematode *Caenorhabditis elegans,* the first multicellular organism whose genome was completely sequenced,[7] lack structures equivalent in anatomy and function to the vertebrate heart. From this perspective, advances in the understanding of cardiac development have been spurred by the judicious use of a range of model organisms, whose strengths and limitations complement each other. Thus, progress has been marked in part by the recognition that at least the early steps of heart formation can be studied with the dorsal vessel in the fruit fly *Drosophila melanogaster,* despite the linear structure of this rudimentary organ.[8–10] This disadvantage is offset by the marked simplicity of the *Drosophila* genome (one *MEF2* gene versus four in mammals, an example discussed later)[9, 11] and by the technical feasibility of saturation mutagenesis.[12] In other words, rather than the pursuit of hypotheses based on a predefined specific candidate gene (encoding a known protein, expressed at the right time and place for a plausible role), *Drosophila* is amenable to a "genetically unbiased" approach. To implement such a strategy, all the genes of an organism are subjected to random mutagenesis, with the use of chemical mutagens like ethyl methanesulfonate, or insertional mutagenesis with exogenous DNA as transposons or retroviruses, and the resulting progeny are screened for relevant phenotypes. Through this genome-wide approach, which also has been applied to vertebrates in the case of zebrafish (*Danio rerio*), the obligatory functions of undiscovered genes can be disclosed.[12, 13] Like other organisms that develop external to the mother, such as birds or amphibians, zebrafish are more accessible than mice to physical manipulation of the embryo, such as for ablation studies of cell fate, for transplantation, or for microinjection of mRNA as one means of expressing an exogenous protein.

More than any other vertebrate, mice are amenable not only to the addition of a gene to the fertilized oocyte through microinjection of a transgene into the male pronucleus to increase the expression or activity of a protein but also to gene deletion, creating knockout mutations through the homologous recombination in embryonic stem cells. Thus, in mice, these genetic approaches to the dissection of cardiac and vascular development have enabled a systematic analysis of relevant candidate genes, testing Koch's postulates by creating gain- and loss-of-function mutations in putative regulators that are restricted or specific to these tissues. As a second, related source of information, many mutations that were engineered in ubiquitously expressed genes have unmasked the unexpectedly essential role of a protein in cardiac organogenesis. Third, genome-wide sequencing and the available markers of gene position are much more complete for the mouse than for any other vertebrate (apart from humans): this markedly expedites the pace to progress from identification of a random or spontaneous mutation to the actual cloning of the affected gene. In addition, methods for high-throughput mutagenesis exist that are applicable to mice, including gene trapping in embryonic stem cells[14] and targeted large-scale deletions in tandem with chemical mutagens.[15] However, genome-wide mutagenesis has not been coupled to a phenotypic screen for cardiovascular mutations in mice.

Cardiogenic Transcription Factors

Cardiac Morphogenesis

The heart is the first organ to form during vertebrate embryogenesis.[4, 13, 16] Heart formation begins at about embryonic day (E) 7.5 in the mouse, when cells within bilaterally symmetric regions of the anterior lateral plate mesoderm become committed to a cardiogenic fate in response to inductive signals from adjacent endoderm[17] (see Fig. 44–1). Cardiogenic precursor cells from this region, known as the cardiac crescent, converge along the ventral midline of the embryo to form the linear heart tube at about E8.0. Soon thereafter, the heart tube initiates rhythmic contractions and undergoes rightward looping, followed by chamber specification, septation, and valvulogenesis.

Although the embryologic events involved in heart formation have been carefully documented in a variety of organisms, little has been known of the transcriptional networks that control cardiac myogenesis or morphogenesis. However, several important cardiac transcription factors have been identified, and a few have been subjected to genetic analysis. Moreover, the realization that several key cardiac transcription factors are structurally and functionally conserved in vertebrates and invertebrates has made it possible to consider heart development in the context of an evolutionarily conserved transcriptional pathway and to gain insights into the complex events of cardiogenesis in vertebrates from studies of simpler, genetically more tractable organisms, such as *Drosophila*.[4, 18]

A common theme that has emerged is that cardiac gene expression is controlled through combinatorial mechanisms involving protein-protein interactions between cell type–restricted and widely expressed transcription factors. To date, no cardiac-specific transcription factors have been identified that are sufficient for the recruitment of heterologous cells to a cardiac "fate." This distinguishes cardiac from skeletal muscle development, in which members of the MyoD family of skeletal muscle-specific bHLH (basic helix-loop-helix) transcription factors can activate the complete program for skeletal muscle gene expression when expressed ectopically in nonmuscle cell types.[19] On the contrary, the results of *heterokaryon* experiments with cardiac and noncardiac cell types have suggested that the cardiac phenotype is actually recessive and can be extinguished by noncardiac factors.[20]

Most vertebrate transcription factors implicated in cardiac gene expression belong to *multigene* families in which closely related members are expressed in overlapping patterns in the developing heart. This has complicated genetic analyses of the functions of these factors in mice and zebrafish, the only two vertebrates in which experimental genetics can be practically pursued, because functional redundancy prevents the creation of complete loss-of-function phenotypes. Thus, most of our knowledge of the in vivo functions of cardiac transcription factors has come from studies in *Drosophila,* in which most cardiac transcription factors act singly. Later we describe the best characterized cardiac transcription factors, their biochemical functions, and their roles in a transcriptional hierarchy for cardiac myogenesis and morphogenesis. Based on the defects in cardiogenesis observed in *Drosophila* or mouse mutants lacking individual cardiac transcription factors, an outline of a transcriptional pathway for cardiac development can be envisioned (see Fig. 44–1).

Myocyte Enhancer Factor-2

The best understood cardiac transcription factor is myocyte enhancer factor-2 (MEF2), which belongs to the MADS (MCM1, *Agamous, Deficiens,* serum response factor [SRF]) box family of transcription factors. This family controls cell-specific transcription in organisms ranging from yeast and plants to humans.[11] There are four MEF2 genes in vertebrates, designated *MEF2A, MEF2B, MEF2C,* and *MEF2D* and a single *MEF2* gene in all invertebrates analyzed thus far. MEF2 proteins share homology in an amino-terminal MADS box, which mediates DNA binding and dimerization, and an adjacent MEF2-specific domain, which influences DNA binding affinity and cofactor interactions. MEF2 factors bind an A/T-rich DNA consensus sequence found in the control regions of the majority of cardiac, skeletal, and smooth muscle genes and activate transcription combinatorially with other factors.[21, 22]

During vertebrate embryogenesis, the four MEF2 genes are expressed in overlapping patterns in early developing muscle cell lineages before becoming more widely expressed after birth.[23–26] Within the developing heart, *MEF2B* and *MEF2C* are expressed in the cardiac crescent soon after specification of the cardiac lineage, and *MEF2A* and *MEF2D* are expressed about 1 day later as looping morphogenesis of the heart tube ensues.

Each of the four MEF2 genes has been inactivated in mice through homologous recombination, with only *MEF2C* showing an obvious function in the heart.[27] Mice lacking *MEF2C* die of apparent heart failure at about E9.5. Hearts from these mutants fail to form a right ventricular chamber and express only a subset of cardiac contractile protein genes, resulting in a sluggish and irregular heartbeat.[27] *MEF2C* mutants also exhibit severe vascular defects, characterized by failure of endothelial cells to organize into vessels and the absence of smooth muscle–specific gene expression.[28] *MEF2A* and *MEF2B* mutant mice are viable, whereas *MEF2D* mutants die before *gastrulation* (E. Olson, unpublished results). The creation of mice lacking different combinations of MEF2 genes, as was necessary to clarify the function of MyoD family members in skeletal muscle,[29, 30] will be of interest and is likely to reveal overlapping functions of the individual genes.

In *Drosophila,* there is only one MEF2 gene, referred to as *D-MEF2,* which encodes a protein closely related to its vertebrate counterparts.[31, 32] *D-MEF2* is expressed specifically in developing cardiac, skeletal, and visceral muscle cell lineages during embryogenesis; binds the same DNA sequence as the vertebrate MEF2 factors; and can activate transcription through the MEF2 site when expressed in mammalian cells, arguing for evolutionary conservation of function. Loss-of-function mutations of *D-MEF2* result in the complete absence of differentiated muscle cells in all three muscle lineages, but undifferentiated myoblasts are properly specified and positioned in mutant embryos.[9, 33, 34] These findings reveal a molecular commonality among different muscle cell types and demonstrate that MEF2 is a central component of the differentiation programs of all muscle cell types.

In the skeletal muscle lineage, MEF2 factors act combinatorially with members of the MyoD family of bHLH proteins to establish a combinatorial code that uniquely activates skeletal muscle–specific transcription.[22, 35, 36] By analogy, it is likely that a similar type of combinatorial mechanism provides the basis for cardiac and smooth muscle gene expression. Although no cardiac-specific partner for MEF2 has been identified thus far, this mechanism has been demonstrated to operate in cardiac muscle more generally, through pairwise interactions of other cardiogenic factors, as discussed later.

NK-2 Homeodomain Proteins

Several homeobox gene products belonging to the NK-2 subclass are expressed in the earliest cardiac cells in vertebrate and *Drosophila* embryos, with expression remaining largely, but not exclusively, restricted to the cardiac lineage throughout prenatal and postnatal development.[37] The prototype of these factors is tinman from *Drosophila,* which is essential for formation of the heartlike organ, the dorsal vessel, that lies along the dorsal midline of the organism and rhythmically pumps hemolymph throughout the open circulatory system of the embryo.[8, 38] At least five tinman-related genes, *Nkx2-3, Nkx2-5, Nkx2-6, Nkx2-7,* and *Nkx2-8,* have been identified in vertebrates, with each expressed predominantly in the developing heart, although expression is also seen in overlapping patterns in pharyngeal precursors and their derivatives, as well as in thyroid and stomach. The overlapping expression patterns of these genes have led to the concept of an Nkx code, in which cell fates are specified by unique combinations of these NK homeodomain proteins.[39]

Nkx2-5 is the only cardiac NK homeobox gene to be knocked out thus far in mice. In mice homozygous for an *Nkx2-5* null allele, cardiomyocytes differentiate and the linear heart tube forms normally, but looping morphogenesis is disrupted.[40] This relatively late function for *Nkx2-5* in cardiac morphogenesis contrasts with the early function of *tinman* in the specification of cardiac cell fate and suggests either that *Nkx2-5* and *tinman* are not functionally conserved or, more likely, that other cardiac-expressed NK homeobox genes substitute in the absence of *Nkx2-5.*

In an effort to determine whether Nkx2-5 has the ability to specify the cardiac lineage, cross-species transgenic rescue assays have been performed in which mouse Nkx2-5 was expressed in *Drosophila* embryos lacking tinman.[41, 42] These studies showed that Nkx2-5 cannot substitute for tinman, despite the fact that the two proteins bind the same DNA sequence. Thus, there must be at least two distinct steps in cardiogenic specification by these factors: they must recognize their downstream target genes in the cardiac pathway and then must activate transcription. The ability of tinman to activate cardiac transcription in the *Drosophila* embryo has been mapped to a unique 43–amino acid domain at the extreme amino terminus of tinman.[41] If this cardiac-inducing domain is tethered to Nkx2-5, it confers on Nkx2-5 the ability to induce the cardiac lineage in *Drosophila.* It is likely this domain mediates interaction with an essential cardiogenic cofactor.

Consistent with an early role for *Nkx2-5* in cardiomyocyte specification or differentiation, the forced expression of *Nkx2-5* in zebrafish or frog embryos expands the heart field and accelerates cardiac gene expression.[43–45] Conversely, if Nkx2-5 is fused to the *engrailed repressor domain,* it will block cardiogenesis in injected *Xenopus laevis* embryos,[46, 47] indicating that one or more Nkx family members are essential for this process.

In *Drosophila,* tinman has been shown to directly activate transcription of the *D-MEF2* gene by binding two sites in a cardiac-specific enhancer located several thousand nucleotides upstream of the gene.[48] Nkx2-5 has been shown to bind the same DNA consensus sequence in several cardiac structural genes, suggesting that these transcription factors activate multiple genes in the cardiac pathway.[49] As will be discussed, a wider range of targets for Nkx2-5 exists because this protein can be tethered to DNA at unrelated sites, as a "coactivator" physically associated with other DNA-bound factors.

Iriquois-Related Homeobox Gene 4

Iriquois-related homeobox gene 4 *(IRX4)* is a vertebrate homeobox gene, distinct from the NK-2 class, that is instead related to the *Iriquois* homeobox gene in *Drosophila.* Studies have demonstrated that *IRX4* is expressed in the ventricles but not in the atria or outflow tract of the developing chick heart.[50] Ventricle-specific expression was observed in the prospective ventricular region at the linear heart tube stage and was maintained throughout embryogenesis and in the adult heart. Misexpression of *IRX4* in the atria, through a retroviral expression system, was sufficient to activate ventricle-specific genes and repress atrial genes. Conversely, a dominant negative form of *IRX4* was able to inhibit ventricular gene expression and up-regulate atrial myosin heavy chain in the ventricle. These studies suggest that the atrial phenotype may be a default pathway for cardiac gene expression and that *IRX4* overrides this program by regulating ventricle-specific muscle structural genes.

GATA Factors

Six GATA transcription factors have been identified in vertebrates, each of which contains a highly conserved DNA binding domain consisting of two *zinc fingers* of the motif Cys-X_2-Cys-X_{17}-Cys-X_2-Cys.[51] Based on their expression patterns, the GATA proteins have been divided into two subfamilies. GATA-1, GATA-2, and GATA-3 are expressed in early hematopoietic progenitors, whereas GATA-4, GATA-5, and GATA-6 are expressed in mesodermal precursors that give rise to the heart, as well as in the endoderm of the gut epithelium.

Binding sites for GATA factors, (A/T)GATA(A/G), are essential for the expression of a number of cardiac structural genes, including alpha-myosin heavy chain, cardiac troponin-C (cTnC), atrial natriuretic factor (ANF), and brain natriuretic peptide (BNP).[52–54] Transcription of Nkx2-5 in the cardiac crescent and early heart tube has also been shown to be controlled by two GATA-dependent upstream enhancers, indicating that GATA factors play important roles throughout cardiac development.[55, 56] Further evidence for the involvement of GATA factors in cardiogenesis comes from studies in P19 embryonic carcinoma cells, which fail to differentiate into cardiomyocytes when transfected with an antisense GATA-4 expression vector.[57] The injection of GATA-4, GATA-5, or GATA-6 RNA into *Xenopus* embryos also induces premature activation of cardiac gene expression.[58] However, another study reported that overexpression of GATA-6 in *Xenopus* embryos caused a delay in cardiac differentiation, resulting in a substantially enlarged heart.[59] In this regard, GATA-4 has been shown to play an important role in cardiac hypertrophy and heart failure in the adult heart by interacting directly with the calcium-regulated transcription NFAT3 to establish a unique transcriptional code that reactivates fetal genes in the myocardium and evokes a hypertrophic response.[60] This pathway is discussed at greater length later, with others that may mediate the fetal gene program during cardiac hypertrophy.

Mice lacking GATA-4 die at about E8.5 of defects in ventral morphogenesis resulting in failure of the linear heart tube to form.[61, 62] Cardiomyocytes are correctly specified and can differentiate in GATA-4 mutant embryos, but they remain as parallel heart tubes on each side of the embryo and do not converge at the midline, a defect referred to as *cardia bifida*. GATA-6 mutant embryos die at gastrulation, presumably because of an essential role for GATA-6 in visceral endoderm.[63, 64]

GATA factors have a propensity to interact with other transcription factors, resulting in unique transcriptional complexes within cardiac cells. In addition to interaction with NFAT3,[60] GATA4 interacts with the cardiac homeodomain protein Nkx2-5 to activate the ANF and cardiac alpha-actin genes.[65–67] GATA factors also interact with the multitype zinc finger factor FOG-2, which can act as an activator or a repressor of cardiac genes, depending on cell background and the promoter.[68–70] This protein-protein interaction is likely to influence chamber-specific gene expression as well as cardiac growth in response to hypertrophic signaling.

HAND Factors

Skeletal muscle formation is dependent on the MyoD family of skeletal muscle-specific bHLH transcription factors, which act at multiple points in the skeletal muscle lineage to control myoblast determination and differentiation.[19] These myogenic regulators are not expressed in the heart; however, the bHLH proteins dHAND and eHAND are expressed during the early stages of cardiogenesis.[71–74] In the mouse, dHAND and eHAND are expressed in the cardiac crescent. dHAND is then expressed throughout the linear heart tube before becoming restricted to the right ventricular region. In contrast, eHAND expression becomes localized to two specific segments of the linear heart tube: the anterior-most segment, which gives rise to the conotruncus, and the more posterior region, which is fated to form the left ventricular region cardiogenesis.[71, 72, 75, 76] The HAND genes are the earliest known markers for the future right and left ventricular segments of the heart tube.

Mice heterozygous for either dHAND or eHAND null alleles are normal, whereas homozygous mutants for either gene die during embryogenesis and exhibit cardiac defects.[77–79] dHAND mutant mice die between E10.5 and E11.0 and display abnormalities in the mesodermal and neural crest–derived components of the heart.[77] The linear heart tube of the dHAND mutant undergoes incorrect looping, and the region of the heart tube that would normally give rise to the right ventricle does not develop. As a result, the heart is displaced to the left, and the ventricular region is reduced in size. These morphologic defects are localized to regions of the developing heart tube in which dHAND is normally expressed, and they demonstrate that dHAND is required for right ventricular development. eHAND continues to be expressed in the left region of the heart tube of dHAND mutant embryos, suggesting that left ventricular development is unperturbed by the absence of dHAND. How dHAND controls development of the future right ventricle is unclear, but possibly dHAND is required within the heart tube for expansion of the population of cardiogenic cells destined to form the right ventricular region or dHAND is required for specification of this population of cells.

In addition to their expression in the developing heart, dHAND and eHAND are expressed in cardiac neural crest cells. The aortic arch arteries, which are normally populated by neural crest cells, also fail to form in dHAND mutant embryos. dHAND is expressed in this neural crest cell population coincident with their aggregation at their destination within the branchial arches.[72, 80] This suggests that dHAND controls the differentiation or organization of neural crest cells into vessels, rather than their initial migration from the neural folds. Because the formations of the heart and outflow tract are interdependent and dHAND is expressed in both regions, it is difficult to distinguish which of the cardiovascular defects in dHAND mutant embryos are due to primary effects of dHAND in cardiomyocytes and neural crest cells and which defects might arise secondarily.

eHAND mutant mouse embryos also exhibit defects in cardiogenesis and die at about E9.0.[78, 79] However, these mutants also show abnormalities in extraembryonic membranes where eHAND is also expressed, which has made it difficult to specifically define the role of eHAND in cardiovascular development through conventional knockout approaches. Consistent with the notion that eHAND regulates left ventricular development, mice lacking the cardiac homeobox gene *Nkx2-5/Csx* do not express eHAND in the heart[75] and exhibit defects in looping morphogenesis.[40] Thus, eHAND may lie downstream from Nkx2-5 in a pathway for left ventricular development.

In contrast to their mutually exclusive expression patterns in the heart tube of the mouse, dHAND and eHAND are expressed homogeneously throughout the heart tube of the chick.[72] This may explain the finding that both genes must be inactivated by antisense oligonucleotides for cardiac defects in chick embryos to be observed.

The target genes for the HAND factors within the developing heart and neural crest are of particular interest. As discussed subsequently, one gene that is down-regulated in dHAND null embryos maps to the minimal deleted region for DiGeorge's syndrome (DGS) in humans and is a plausible candidate gene responsible for this disease, although this will require further confirmation.[81]

Serum Response Factor

The SRF is a MADS-box transcription factor that binds a consensus sequence referred to as a serum response element (SRE) or CArG box [CC(A/T)$_6$GG] in the regulatory regions of numerous cardiac structural genes. Although widely expressed in diverse cell types, SRF is highly enriched in developing cardiac, skeletal, and smooth muscle cell lineages during embryogenesis.[82, 83] SRF has been shown to be an important regulator of muscle gene expression based on mutations of SREs in muscle regulatory regions, which result in inactivation of the genes,[84, 85] as shown, likewise, for transcription of cardiac and skeletal α-actin in cardiac muscle cells.[86, 87] A dominant negative mutant of SRF has also been shown to block MyoD expression and skeletal muscle differentiation in vitro.[82, 88]

In addition to its essential role in the regulation of muscle gene expression, SRF confers serum inducibility to a variety of genes, at least in part by responding to mitogen-activated protein kinase signaling.[89, 90] How this transcription factor mediates both muscle-specific and serum-inducible transcription, which represent opposing gene regulatory programs, is an important unanswered question. The best explanation is that the pattern of SRF-dependent gene activation is dictated by interaction of SRF with other transcriptional cofactors. Indeed, studies have shown that SRF, like other MADS-box transcription factors, acts combinatorially with other factors, including Nkx2-5,[91] to activate cardiac transcription.

The single SRF gene in mice has been inactivated through homologous recombination, resulting in embryonic death at gastrulation, lacking a primitive streak or detectable mesoderm.[92] This early embryonic phenotype indicates that SRF plays a role in the formation of the germ layers and precludes an analysis of its role in the heart per se. Conditional gene ablation studies are required to address this issue.[93] There is a single SRF gene in *Drosophila* (DSRF). Homozygous mutants for this gene fail to develop a tracheal system, which mediates oxygen exchange and functions in a manner somewhat analogous to a respiratory system in vertebrates.[94] DSRF also is required for appropriate development of intervein tissue and to suppress ectopic vein formation in the *Drosophila* wing.[95] However, no defects in cardiac or skeletal muscle development have been noted in *Drosophila* mutants lacking SRF.

Transcriptional Enhancer Factor-1 Family

Members of the transcriptional enhancer factor-1 (TEF-1) family of transcription factors belong to a superfamily of transcriptional regulators that are implicated in muscle gene activation through a conserved sequence motif, referred to as an M-CAT site (CATTCCT), first identified in the promoter of the cTnT gene.[96] Subsequent studies revealed important roles for M-CAT sites in a wide range of cardiac and embryonic skeletal muscle genes.[87, 97, 98] Four members of the TEF-1 family have been identified in vertebrates, but there are likely to be more.[97, 99–101] NTEF-1 and RTEF-1 are highly enriched in skeletal muscle, DTEF-1 is most abundant in cardiac muscle, and ETEF-1 is confined largely to embryonic neural tissues. Alternative splicing of TEF-1 genes adds further complexity to the functions of this regulatory gene family. The TEF-1 isoforms differ in their transcriptional activity, which provides a mechanism for cell type specificity of gene activation.

TEF-1 proteins belong to the TEA class of transcription factors that includes yeast TEC-1, which regulates Ty1 enhancer activity; AbaA, which regulates sporulation-specific genes in *Aspergillus nidulans;* and *Drosophila* scalloped, which is required for neural differentiation. TEF-1 was cloned initially on the basis of its ability to bind the GTIIC and Sph motifs from the simian virus 40 (SV40) enhancer. The ability of TEF-1 proteins to activate widely expressed enhancers such as SV40, as well as muscle-specific enhancers, may be explained by the results of studies that have demonstrated that TEF-1 binding sites from muscle-specific genes differ from those of other TEF-1 target genes with respect to DNA flanking sequences that can dictate the activity of the M-CAT site.[102] This is most likely to occur through interactions with cell-specific TEF-1 cofactors.

The mouse NTEF-1 gene was inactivated serendipitously through a random retroviral gene trap insertion, resulting in embryonic death between E10.5 and E11.5, apparently due to cardiac abnormalities.[103] The heart tube forms normally in *NTEF-1* mutants, but there is poor trabeculation and reduced contractility, presumably because of a lack of expression of essential NTEF-1 target genes. Known NTEF-1 target genes, such as cTnT, cTnl, cTnC, and cardiac myosins, are expressed normally in NTEF-1 mutants, leaving the key NTEF-1 target genes unknown.

T-Box 5

The T-box transcription factor TBX5 is implicated in normal heart and limb development and is discussed later as a cause of Holt-Oram syndrome in humans.[104–106]

Evolutionary Conservation of the Cardiogenic Transcriptional Pathway

The phenotypes of mouse mutants defective in cardiogenic transcription factors have made it possible to begin to envision cardiogenesis within the framework of a multistep transcriptional pathway (see Fig. 44–1). Similarities in expression patterns and putative functions of many cardiogenic transcription factors also suggest that many of the early events in the pathway for cardiac development are evolutionarily ancient and conserved.

In *Drosophila,* tinman is at the top of hierarchy of cardiac transcription factors, being required for the expression of all cardiac genes and for specification of the cardiac lineage. In vertebrates, the five tinman-related NK-2 homeobox genes are expressed in early cardiogenic cells and are likely to play redundant roles in cardiac specification. Tinman directly activates transcription of *D-MEF2* in the dorsal vessel, and then *D-MEF2* is required to activate cardiac contractile genes. In vertebrate embryos, members of the MEF2 family are expressed concomitant with the cardiac NK-type homeobox genes, consistent with the notion that the regulatory relation between these two classes of cardiogenic genes has been conserved. It remains to be determined whether NK-type homeobox gene products directly activate the expression of MEF2 genes during vertebrate cardiogenesis, although this seems likely.

In vertebrates and fruit flies, differentiated cardiomyocytes become organized into a linear heart tube. This requires ventral folding of the vertebrate embryo, a process shown to be controlled by GATA-4. Dorsal-ventral polarity is reversed in fruit flies, such that dorsal folding brings together the parallel cardiogenic precursor cells along the dorsal midline; this process likewise is dependent on a GATA factor, serpent.[107] At this point, vertebrate cardiogenesis continues as the heart tube undergoes looping and chamber specification, whereas the fly heart does not develop beyond the linear heart tube stage. Intriguingly, it appears that some of the genes that have evolutionarily conserved roles in the early steps of cardiogenesis are reused at later stages in cardiogenesis in vertebrates. *Nkx2-5,* for example, would be expected to have a role in the specification of cardioblasts that is likely to be obscured due to functional redundancy with other members of this family, but it also has a role in cardiac looping, unique to vertebrates. Similarily, MEF2C is required for the activation of cardiac contractile protein genes in the mouse, which is similar to its function in differentiation of cardioblasts in *Drosophila.* However, MEF2C also has a role in cardiac looping and chamber maturation, which are unique to vertebrate cardiogenesis. Thus, although *Drosophila* has been and will continue to be a powerful system in which to uncover fundamental mechanisms of cardiogenesis without complications from genetic redundancy of multigene families, there are many aspects of cardiogenesis that can be understood only through the study of vertebrate model systems. Conversely, it will be interesting to determine whether cardiac transcription factors such as dHAND, eHAND, IRX4, and TBX5, which are required for these late steps in vertebrate cardiogenesis, have counterparts that participate in cardiogenesis in invertebrates.

EXTRINSIC SIGNALS FOR EARLY HEART FORMATION

Secreted factors as diffusible, paracrine signals provide one general mechanism for cell fate decisions, positional information, and other aspects of embryogenesis. Several distinct secreted factors are required for heart formation in *Drosophila.* The sustained expression of *tinman* in dorsal mesoderm requires the secretion of **decapentaplegic** (dpp) by dorsal ectoderm, a transforming growth factor-beta (TGFβ)–related protein in whose absence the maturation of dorsal mesoderm into cardiac and visceral mesoderm is arrested, resembling *tinman* mutants.[108] As a prerequisite for this action of dpp, the primitive mesodermal cells first must migrate dorsolaterally, a migration directed by *heartless,* a *Drosophila* fibroblast growth factor (FGF) receptor.[109] However, the later distinction between cardiac and visceral muscle requires additional signals. **Wingless** (wg), a secreted protein with diverse roles in embryonic patterning, including segmentation polarity, is necessary for this subsequent specialization to a cardiac fate but not for visceral mesoderm.[10] Heart development also requires two proteins that act downstream of wg in other cascades—*dishevelled,* a cytosolic adaptor protein, and *armadillo,* a beta-catenin homologue that functions as a transcriptional coactivator.[110] **Hedgehog** (hh), another segmentation-polarity protein secreted by the ectoderm in cell rows adjacent to those producing wg, likewise is essential for normal heart formation, although sporadic cells remain positive for cardiac markers.[110] Overexpression of wg can compensate for the absence of hh, but not vice versa.[110]

To what extent can these findings in *Drosophila* be extrapolated to the vertebrate heart? In part, this effort is confounded by the much greater genetic complexity of the homologous growth factor families, as discussed earlier for the heterogeneity and redundancy seen for transcription factors. In the mouse, there are at least 15 *Wnt* genes homologous to wg,[111] three varieties of hh (Sonic, Indian, and desert),[112] and 36 members of the TGF-β superfamily.

In avian explants derived from the heart-forming region, cardiac differentiation is mediated via a signal from anterior endoderm,[113] which can be reproduced by bone morphogenetic proteins (BMPs), although perhaps requiring FGFs in concert.[114, 115] In related experiments with target explants outside the normal heart-forming field, anterior endoderm can trigger ectopic cardiogenesis,[116] and BMPs suffice for ectopic induction of multiple cardiogenic transcription factors, including Nkx2-5, GATA-4, and MEF2C.[117, 118] Most importantly, perhaps, the inductive effect of anterior endoderm is prevented by noggin, an extracellular antagonist of BMPs, implicating endogenous BMPs as the normal signal provided by the endoderm.[9] The hypothesis that BMPs might be involved in the induction of the cardiac myocyte lineage also draws support from the spatial distribution of BMPs in the endoderm that lies adjacent to the cardiogenic region.[119] Thus, the *juxtacrine action* of BMPs as the inducer of Nkx-2.5 parallels the action of *dpp* as the inducer of tinman.[9]

In murine embryonic stem cells, cardiac differentiation, as measured by α-myosin heavy chain induction, has been triggered by activin A or BMP-4, with complex concentration-dependent effects on the nature of mesoderm that develops.[119] Similar results with activin A were seen in other systems, including *Xenopus* animal pole explants[120] and axolotl explants.[121] However, a functional role for activins in cardiac differentiation, like its role inferred for mesoderm formation more generally, is not supported by the genetic evidence available from mice lacking activin subunits, singly or in combination, or from mice lacking type II activin receptors.[122–125] (A possible role for the type IB activin receptor remains open because the conventional knockout is arrested at the egg cylinder stage, before gastrulation occurs[126]; a similar phenotype results in mice lacking Smad2, a transcription factor phosphorylated by and mediating the effect of type I receptors for activin and TGF-β.[127]

As for TGF-β, three isoforms exist in mammals. Each has been deleted singly, and it is still unknown whether combinatorial deletions of the isoforms would yield phenotypes that are more than merely additive. The absence of TGF-β1 can disrupt yolk sac vasculogenesis, with death in midgestation, but survivors develop normally, with inflammation in multiple organs after birth.[128, 129] Although the absence of TGF-β2 causes cardiac malformations such as tetralogy of Fallot (ventricular septal defects and defects of outflow tract septation),[130] cardiac myogenesis per se is not impaired, and the absence of TGF-β3 results in cleft palate.[131] A more compelling case can be made for the involvement of BMPs in early heart formation in mammals, given the absence of mesoderm, including cardiac mesoderm, in mice lacking the type I BMP receptor, ALK3[13]; the more variable failure of mesoderm formation in mice lacking BMP-4[14]; and the absence of the heart in some mice lacking BMP-2.[15]

LEFT-RIGHT POSITION AND LOOPING MORPHOGENESIS

The rightward looping of the linear heart tube is, as mentioned earlier, not only the earliest structural sign of a left-right body axis as the vertebrate embryo matures but also, arguably, the earliest step in heart formation that cannot be investigated through the surrogate of *Drosophila.* Defining a molecular basis for positional information in the embryo is one of the most fundamental and urgent questions posed in developmental biology. For the left-right axis, two sets of clues have proved to be especially helpful. First, detailed descriptive studies of the expression of some genes in the heart-forming regions and linear heart tube have made it clear that molecular asymmetries precede the earliest anatomic left-right differences. Second, in several cases, ectopic expression and blocking studies have provided evidence that the asymmetries in gene expression operate in a functional cascade for left-right determination.

The molecule discovered to be expressed preferentially with the left-right axis of the body was flectin, a 250-kDa component of extracellular matrix that was found in the left precardiac mesoderm of early chick embryos and continues to be expressed asymmetrically through the tubular heart stage.[132] In mice, flectin likewise is expressed asymmetrically in the tubular heart, with right-sided predominance in the outflow tract but left-sided predominance in the ventricular segment.[133] This identification of an asymmetrically distributed matrix molecule was consistent with earlier studies demonstrating that surgical and pharmacologic perturbations of extracellular matrix were sufficient to randomize left-right asymmetry in *Xenopus* embryos.[134, 135] In addition, this finding helped spur the search for specific matrix-associated proteins (notably, growth factors) that might confer the left-right axis.

Among TGF-β family members, several of which show asymmetric expression in the heart tube or progenitor regions, nodal is more conserved in its spatial pattern than others, predominating in left lateral plate mesoderm of *Xenopus,* chick, and mouse.[136–140] Exogenous expression of nodal homologues in the chick (cNR-1) and frog (Xnr-1) is sufficient to cause left-right anomalies [141, 142]; although four nodal-related genes are expressed during gastrulation in *Xenopus,* only *Xnr-1* is expressed later, preferentially, in left lateral plate mesoderm.[142] It has been postulated that dorsal midline structures, possibly the notochord, regulate the direction of cardiac looping by repressing the expression of *Xnr-1* in right lateral plate mesoderm.[143]

This consistency of expression across species is not true for activin. In birds, right-sided expression of activin induces right-sided expression of the activin type IIa receptor, which represses right-sided expression of Sonic hh; continued expression of Sonic hh on the left then causes asymmetric, left-sided expression of cNR-1.[136] Interestingly, despite the fact that no left-right difference in abundance has been shown for activin or its receptors in mice, deletion of the type IIB activin receptor results in cardiac laterality defects (predominantly right atrial isomerism), malposition of the great arteries, and atrial and ventricular septal defects.[125]

Novel TGF-β family members have been discovered, however, with left-sided expression in mice: *lefty-1* and *lefty-2.*[137, 139, 144, 145] A transcriptional basis for their asymmetric expression has been established—*lefty-2* via a left side–specific enhancer and *lefty-1* via bilateral enhancers and a right side–specific silencer.[146] In mice lacking *lefty-1,* other left-sided genes at first are expressed normally but then are expressed promiscuously, with a bilateral distribution, suggesting a diffusible signal that confers a left-sided identity to the right-sided regions.[145] Interestingly, the expression of all three murine genes—*nodal, lefty-1,* and *lefty-2*—and the transcriptional activity of both side-specific *lefty* control regions, in turn, are randomized or inverted in concordance with the anatomic phenotype in two murine mutations with altered situs.[137, 139, 144] In mice carrying the spontaneous mutation, *iv* (*situs inversus viscerum*), 30 percent of homozygotes have situs inversus (mirror-image reversal of all asymmetric organs), 30 percent have situs solitus (the normal left-right distribution), and 40 percent have situs ambiguus (partial asymmetry), resembling the distribution expected if the left-right position of the heart versus abdominal organs were determined solely by chance. The presumptive gene for *iv* has been identified as *left-right dynein,* an axonemal microtubule motor protein related to the principal cause of hereditary situs inversus in humans (see later).[147, 148] Insertional mutagenesis (disruption of a locus by interpolation of a transgene) resulted in the second mouse mutation, *inversion of embryonic turning* (*inv*), which is noteworthy for its nearly uniform reversal of left-right asymmetry in homozygotes.[149] Gene mapping, together with rescue experiments using yeast artificial chromosomes spanning portions of the disrupted region, led to the identification of inversin, a novel ankyrin-repeat protein, as the basis for this phenotype.[150, 151] Thus, each of three TGF-β family members lies downstream from two proteins whose ability to impart left-right asymmetry is not yet understood. A constitutively activating mutation of ALK5, the type I TGF-β receptor, blocks looping morphogenesis in mice, perhaps by overriding growth control or other functional asymmetries created by one or more of these related growth factors.[152] The endogenous receptors for *nodal, lefty-1,* and *lefty-2* remain to be identified, which has fed speculation that ActRIIb might function in that role.[125]

Perhaps the best lead for a signal that initiates the left-right axis, as opposed to downstream genes that implement the axis, comes from *Xenopus,* in which another TGF-β family protein, Vg1, can invert or randomize the left-right axis, respectively, when expressed in particular (right lateral versus right dorsomedial) cells of the vegetal pole in 16-cell embryos.[153] Exogenous activin had some of the same effects—heterotaxy but not inversion. A dominant-inhibitory activin receptor injected into the left side randomized organ position but is known to interfere not only with activin but also with Vg1 and BMPs. Blocking experiments with follistatin and noggin, extracellular antagonists for activin and BMPs, excluded both of these as the endogenous signal, thus implicating Vg1 itself. These results are striking not only for their severity (inversion, not randomization, after ectopic expression) but also for the unique ability of Vg1 to rescue the normal left-right axis in randomized embryos (right-sided conjoined twins).[153] As in other studies of Vg1 function, a chimeric BMP-Vg1 precursor was used. Possibly, the marked severity that was seen could also be due, in part, to greater plasticity at this 16-cell stage than in embryos of other species that are studied later in development.

What are the ultimate downstream effectors of these morphogenic cascades for left-right asymmetry? Because compound heterozygotes for nodal plus Smad2 have defects in left-right patterning (along with other anomalies), Smad2 may mediate nodal signal transduction for establishing the left-right axis and other developmental events.[127] Transcription factors that are asymmetrically expressed include transient left predominance of the hepatocyte nuclear factor/forkhead protein, HNF-3β,[136] and right predominance of cSnR, the chick snail-related zinc finger protein.[154] Only limited functional data are available for these, however. Antisense oligonucleotides to disrupt cSnR expression did randomize heart situs and the direction of embryonic turning.[154] Compound heterozygotes for *HNF-3*β and *nodal* have bilateral nodal transcription in lateral plate mesoderm, left-right anomalies, and a randomized direction of embryonic turning.[137]

More complete functional data are available for a third transcription factor, Pitx2. This bicoid-related homeodomain protein is expressed asymmetrically in frog, fish, chick, and mouse embryos, with a left-sided distribution in the heart tube, the later heart, and the developing gut.[155–159] Both *nodal* and *lefty* induce Pitx2 in chick left lateral plate mesoderm, but not vice versa, placing Pitx2 downstream of these[155]; unsurprisingly, taking this relation together with data discussed earlier, Pitx2 expression was randomized or inverted, respectively, by the mouse mutations *iv* and *inv.*[156, 157] Ectopic, right-sided expression of Pitx2, using a recombinant retrovirus, resulted in bilaterally symmetric hearts or an inverted direction of looping and body rotation.[155, 157] Pitx2 even inverted gut looping when introduced to the visceral progenitor region of chick right lateral plate mesoderm[155] or overexpressed in two-cell *Xenopus* embryos.[157] Although target genes for Pitx2 are not yet known, the randomization of situs in mice lacking HNF-4 was associated with a lack of left-right dynein, linking this defect to the known *iv* pathway.[160]

Cardiac Myocyte Proliferation

The proliferative cell cycle—progression from G1 to S phase for DNA synthesis and from G2 to M phase for mitosis—typically is driven by extracellular, secreted proteins (mitogenic growth factors), in whose absence cells are quiescent with respect to growth. Hence, to understand the expansion in cardiac cell number after the establishment of a cardiac fate, one paramount goal is to determine what peptide growth factors are essential mitogens for the developing heart. Although certain FGFs provoke cell cycle reentry in precardiac mesoderm[161] and even neonatal cardiac myocytes,[162, 163] an essential role in cardiac muscle is more difficult to show for this broad set of mitogens. First, at least 18 genes for FGFs are known, many of which are expressed in the heart.[164–167] Thus, knockout mutations for single FGFs can be unrevealing: for example, mice lacking FGF-2 have a normally formed heart and other organs but exhibit a functional defect in vascular tone.[168] Second, an essential role for FGFs in mesoderm induction or patterning results in very early death in the absence of the receptor FGFR1 during gastrulation.[169, 170] Thus, even though FGF receptors can be studied with lesser problems of redundancy than can FGFs themselves, premature death confounds the use of mouse genetics to discern a role for FGFs in the heart once it has formed. Here, the use of dominant-inhibitory, kinase-defective mutations of the FGF receptor has proved to be informative. A dominant-negative mutation that forms homodimers with each of the known FGFRs receptors was expressed in the embryonic chick ventricle with the use of a recombinant retrovirus and blocked clonal expansion of the infected myocytes, thus proving that endogenous FGF is necessary for the proliferation of embryonic ventricular myocytes.[171] Third, transplacental, maternal rescue can confound the "null" phenotype for secreted proteins, as seen with TGF-β 1.[172]

Despite these issues, success has been achieved, implicating a small number of peptide growth factors and receptors as essential for myocyte cell number in the mammalian heart, including the epidermal growth factor homologue neuregulin[173–175] and its receptors, Erb2 and Erb4.[176, 177] Ventricular trabeculation also was blocked in developing chick embryos, after retroviral delivery of a hammerhead ribozyme to block neuregulin expression.[178] Because neuregulin is expressed as multiple isoforms from a single gene, some of which are membrane anchored with a long cytoplasmic tail, domain-specific gene disruption was performed to test the possible role of this tail in bidirectional signaling (i.e., by Erb2 or Erb4 serving as ligand), a mechanism seen with other transmembrane growth factors.[175] Intriguingly, the loss of just the cytoplasmic tail was sufficient to cause ventricular hypoplasia but was ascribed to impaired proteolytic processing and release of the extracellular ligand domain, not the postulated bidirectional pathway.[175]

Loss of the receptor glycoprotein (gp) 130—the shared signaling partner for several heteroduplex receptors, including cardiotropin-1, interleukin-6 (IL-6), and leukemia inhibitory factor—likewise is sufficient for ventricular hypoplasia and death in mid to late gestation.[179] Given the role of this phenotype as a mediator common to multiple ligands, the question of which of the cytokines that signals through the protein is essential emerges. Neither IL-6 nor its specific receptor is expressed in embryonic myocardium. Thus, endogenous IL-6 is unlikely to be obligatory here, notwithstanding the dramatic increase in cardiac mass provoked by concomitant overexpression of both IL-6 and its receptor in bigenic mice.[180] A more plausible candidate, therefore, is cardiotrophin-1, a cytokine identified through an expression cloning strategy based on cardiac myocytes generated in vitro from pluripotent embryonic stem cells.[181, 182] Another property of cardiotrophin-1 is its ability to suppress cardiac myocyte apoptosis,[183] a useful reminder that hypoplasia need not signify a block to proliferation but can also arise from deficient recruitment and ingrowth or from excessive death.

Even cardiac growth was altered, together with other abnormalites, when the gene for gp130 was inactivated after birth with the use of a drug-inducible DNA recombinase, a strategy discussed in greater detail later. Although the deletion of gp130 was much less efficient in the heart (20 to 30 percent) than in liver or hematopoietic tissues, cell diameter was decreased in a subset of ventricular myocytes, with a corresponding reduction in ventricular wall thickness.[184] A related refinement of gene deletion was applied to the retinoid receptor RXR alpha, which likewise produces a thin-walled, hypoplastic ventricle.[185, 186] In this case, a cardiac-restricted deletion was created using the Cre recombinase to determine whether it was cardiac myocytes themselves or some alternative cell type that required this receptor for the ventricle to form normally.[187] Despite the 80 percent deletion of RXRα from ventricular myocytes, cardiac malformations did not occur, implicating this protein in another lineage altogether, with an indirect but obligatory function in ventricular myocyte development. Similarly, thin-walled myocardium has been reported in mice lacking beta-adrenergic receptor kinase-1,[188] the neurofibromatosis gene (*NF1*),[189, 190] Wilm's tumor protein (WT-1),[191] the proto-oncogene N-*Myc*,[192] the transcriptional adaptor p300,[193] or the transcription factor TEF-1,[103] as discussed earlier. TEF-1–deficient mice, arising from a random retroviral insertion, die between E11 and E12, with hypoplastic myocardium and defective trabeculation.[103] The deletion of N-*myc*, a member of the Myc proto-oncogene family, causes embryonic death around E11, with a hypoplastic ventricle, ventricular septal defects, and other abnormalities.[192] A compound heterozygote expressing N-*myc* at 15 percent of normal levels survives to E14, with a selective defect in the compact layer, corresponding to the region of myocardium in which N-*myc* is expressed.[192] A dilated, thin-walled heart with defective trabeculation also results from the lack of p300,[193] a transcriptional coactivator that is essential for MyoD function in skeletal muscle[194, 195] and is a target for dedifferentiation of cardiac myocytes by the adenoviral protein E1A.[196, 197] The expression of sarcomeric myosin heavy chains and alpha-actinin was severely impaired. Although the essential partners for p300 in cardiac muscle are unproved, p300 is known to serve as a coactivator in skeletal muscle for MEF2, as well as MyoD,[198] and defective MEF2 function was postulated to be the basis for this cardiac abnormality.[193]

Unlike the genes discussed previously, in the case of FKBP12, the outcome of gene targeting in mice resembles the human congenital malformation noncompaction of the left ventricle, which is characterized by a hypoplastic compact layer but markedly increased trabeculation.[199] This immunophilin-binding protein, a target for the immunosuppressants FK506 and rapamycin, regulates transcription via calcineurin and NFAT, as well as the cell cycle via mTOR. However, the endogenous proteins that are its presumptive natural ligands are not completely understood. Cellular proteins that bind FKBP12 include the cytoplasmic signaling domains of type 1 receptors for the TGF-β family,[200] the ryanodine receptor (sarcoplasmic reticulum calcium release channel),[201] inositol-1,4,5-triphosphate receptor,[201] and others. In agreement with mutational analysis showing that its interaction with FKBP12 was dispensable for TGF-β receptor function,[202] TGF-β signaling was not affected by the absence of FKBP12, whereas calcium release channel function was abnormal.[199, 203] Hence, the lack of *FKBP12* may disrupt normal cardiac growth by interfering with a calcium-dependent pathway.

GENES IMPLICATED IN HUMAN CARDIAC MALFORMATIONS

Cardiofacial Syndromes

Congenital heart defects, in particular those affecting the outflow tract and great vessels, can be associated with craniofacial abnormalities, presumably because of the shared role played by the neural crest in the formation of both regions. Although many inherited disorders arise from a single nucleotide change—alteration in a critical amino acid, causing premature termination of protein translation, or introduction of a frame-shift affecting all amino acids C-terminal to the mutation—microdeletions within chromosome 22 are seen in more than 80 percent of individuals with the cardiofacial defects known as DGS (Online Mendelian Inheritance in Man [OMIM] 188400), velocardiofacial syndrome (VCFS; OMIM 192430), and conotruncal anomaly face syndrome (CAFS; OMIM 217095). Thus, given the absence of approximately 2 million base pairs from this region, patients are expected to have only one functional copy of the gene or genes responsible for these defects (haploinsufficiency).

The minimal region of chromosome 22q11 that is most typically deleted, the DGS/VCFS critical region, has been subjected to systematic investigation in testing for mutations of candidate genes in humans and for consequences of the deletion of syntenic genes in mice, including the goosecoid-like homeobox gene, *Gsc1*.[204, 205] In principle, another way to create an animal model to pinpoint mechanisms for this disease is through large-scale chromosome engineering in mice via site-directed recombination,[206] with deletion of the critical region, which shows that this mimics the human phenotypes, and then more selective deletion of smaller portions of the region. A functional role for *HIRA,* a DGS candidate gene resembling certain histone-binding repressors of transcription in yeast, was suggested by studies using antisense oligonucleotides to reduce *HIRA* expression in chick neural crest explants, which were then returned to the embryo[207]: this increased the incidence of persistent truncus arteriosus, potentially implicating *HIRA* in DGS, yet at least one counter-example is known, with clinical features typical of the 2-megabase (Mb) deletion, no deletion of the *HIRA* gene, and normal expression of *HIRA* in the thymus.[81] Thus, no specific gene for cardiofacial syndromes has been borne out through these approaches.

An alternative strategy[81] relied on knowledge that dHAND, a bHLH protein discussed earlier, was essential for the normal development both of the right ventricle and of neural crest–derived structures (i.e., the branchial arches and aortic arch arteries). Suppressive subtraction hybridization in which wild-type and mutant mouse embryos were compared was used to directly clone genes whose expression was contingent on dHAND. One of these, *Ufd1,* maps to the DGS/VCFS critical region and is expressed in mice in the sites of dHAND expression, including branchial arches, craniofacial structures, aortic arches, conotruncus, and limb bud, composed of the tissues affected by deletion of the 2-Mb region. A de novo deletion of *Ufd1* was found in the patient cited, in whom no gross deletion was seen, supporting the provisional conclusion that hemizygosity for *Ufd1* might suffice to prevent normal cardiofacial development.[81] In yeast, *Ufd1* mediates the turnover of proteins flagged with ubiquitin, an amino-terminal degradation signal. Because ubiquitin-dependent protein degradation mediates cellular pathways, including those for apoptosis and proliferation, the causative role inferred for *Ufd1* is intriguing.

Hand-Heart Syndromes

The T-box transcription factor TBX5 has been identified as a gene responsible for Holt-Oram syndrome (HOS1, OMIM 142900), an autosomal dominant disorder of heart and limb development.[104–106] The characteristic cardiac findings are atrial or ventricular septal defects, with associated conduction abnormalities; the most typical skeletal involvement affects the left arm, with radial (thumb) defects. Once linkage studies and physical mapping defined an HOS locus in chromosome 12q2, exon trapping was used to unmask expressed sequences from this region, which contains no genes that were already known.[104, 105] The archetype for the T-box family of transcription factors is *Brachyury* (T), mutations of which cause a short tail phenotype if heterozygous and loss of the trunk and tail if homozygous[208–210]; Brachyury also is required for normal mesoderm formation in *Xenopus* and zebrafish.[211] At least 10 family members exist in mammals, including TBX5,[212] which, in humans, is highly expressed in the early embryonic myocardium.[105] The first identified mutations of TBX5 were premature stop codons and frame-shift mutations, predicted null alleles.[104, 105] Then, several point mutations of TBX5 were identified, which selectively impair heart or limb development in the affected families.[213] It is unknown whether these selective phenotypes are mediated by specificity of the mutations for DNA binding (preferentially affecting essential hand or heart genes), protein-protein associations (preferentially affecting essential hand or heart coactivators), or alternative properties of the respective mutant proteins.

Left-Right Axis Malformations

In humans, as in other vertebrates discussed earlier, deviations from the normal left-right anatomic pattern (situs solitus) can occur during embryogenesis. These deviations can include a complete mirror-image reversal of organ position and orientation (situs inversus, or situs inversus totalis), as well as partial inversions (situs ambiguus, partial situs inversus, or heterotaxy); situs inversus and situs ambiguus can coexist in the same family.[214] Often, these left-right abnormalities occur in syndromic association with other defects, of which the most common is Kartagener's syndrome (OMIM 244400), which involves situs inversus with immotile cilia syndrome due to abnormalities in the ciliary and flagellar protein dynein.

Only rarely has familial situs inversus been noted outside this context. Mutations in the zinc finger transcription factor ZIC3 have been reported to segregate with situs inversus in five families with X-linked visceral heterotaxy (HTX1, OMIM 306955) and in one sporadic case.[214, 215] *Zic* genes resemble the *Drosophila* segment polarity gene, *odd-paired (opa),* which is involved in signaling by *wg* and the TGF-β family member dpp. In *Xenopus, Zic3* is preferentially expressed in the prospective neural plate and then in dorsal regions of the forebrain and can redirect epidermal cells to a neural or neural crest cell fate.[216] In mice, all three *Zic* genes are predominantly expressed in dorsal neural tissue but also in paraxial mesenchyme and limb bud.[217] Hence, there are few clues suggesting a molecular mechanism for the action of ZIC3 in left-right positional information.

A third situs inversus gene for humans was found through a candidate gene approach, in which affected individuals were screened for mutations in the type IIB activin receptor, whose deletion causes abnormal left-right axis development in mice.[125, 218] Another plausible candidate gene, *nodal,* maps to the murine region syntenic with chromosome 10q21-q23, the site of a de novo chromosomal breakpoint in a patient with situs ambiguus and midline malformations; this deletion encompasses the human *NODAL* gene.[214] A missense mutation in the prodomain of *NODAL* has been reported in one patient with left-right axis malformations and the unaffected mother.[215]

Mutations of connexin43, a gap junction protein that mediates cell-cell communication and electrical connectivity, also have been implicated in human laterality defects[219]; however, two subsequent surveys with large numbers of affected individuals have not confirmed this association.[220, 221]

Atrial Septal Defects

The cardiac homeobox transcription factor NKX2-5 was shown to mutate in four families with autosomal dominant transmission of congenital heart disease (mainly, secundum atrial septal defects but also structural cardiac malformations and atrioventricular conduction delays). Linkage to chromosome 5q35 and the fact that NKX2-5 also mapped to this region suggested the intriguing hypothesis that this known regulator of cardiac organogenesis might also be responsible for congenital heart defects in humans. Direct sequencing of the gene in these four affected families revealed three different mutations in or immediately adjacent to the homeodomain, in residues that are essential not only for DNA binding but also for physical association with GATA-4[65, 66] and SRF.[222] Gln170ter and Thr178Met, affecting the homeodomain, would presumably impair DNA binding; Gln198ter, truncating the protein just C terminal to the homeodomain, removes the autoinhibitory region[49, 65] and was postulated to act as a potential aberrant activating mutation.[223] However, both truncations of NKX2-5 would delete a region C terminal to the homeodomain, which also mediates the binding of the protein to GATA-4. Interestingly, Gln198ter might therefore confer both a gain and a loss of function, acting differently at NKX2-5 versus GATA-4 sites.[49, 65] The net phenotype arising from any given mutation of NKX2-5 in vivo might plausibly reflect the aggregate impact on NKX2-5 binding to DNA, tethering by NKX2-5 of coactivators to its own binding site, and NKX2-5 recruitment to other DNA-bound factors.

That the cardiac phenotypes resulting from mutations of NKX2-5 in humans differ so extensively from the embryonic-lethal disruption of cardiac organogenesis seen in *Nkx2.5*-deficient mice, which are arrested during looping, poses an intriguing challenge. The lack of obvious cardiac abnormalities in mice hemizygous for *Nkx2.5* could be viewed as a second discrepancy, given the case for haploinsufficiency with two of the human mutations. Potential biologic explanations include differences between species not only in developmental mechanisms per se but also in the secondary or tertiary effects of altered cardiac gene transcription. Purely technical issues may also be germane. The initially reported "knockout" of *Nkx2.5* includes the deletion of an exon predicted to be essential[40] but might result in a residual protein with potential dominant negative effects, interfering, for example, with *Nkx2.6*[224, 225] or with unrelated cardiogenic proteins (e.g., by competing for essential coactivators). This possibility is strongly supported by the milder phenotype reported for a truly null allele that abolished the expression of *Nkx2.5*.[226]

Implications of Cardiac Development for the Post-Natal Heart

Reactivation of Fetal Genes During Load-Induced Hypertrophy

One setting in cardiology that has broadly benefited from the emerging information on transcriptional mechanisms in cardiac development has been the analysis of cardiac hypertrophy and the transition to heart failure, from the perspective of altered gene regulation. The "hypertrophic phenotype" can be construed as an ensemble of responses, including but not limited to the global increase in ventricular wall thickness and myocyte size. Superimposed on growth itself, and the corresponding generalized increase in RNA and protein content per se, characteristic changes in specific genes are seen, often designated with some oversimplification, as reactivation of a fetal gene program. Thus, the hallmark events for this phenomenon include reexpression of ANF and genes for fetal contractile proteins in the adult ventricle, such as skeletal α-actin, atrial myosin light chain-1, and β-myosin heavy chain, accompanied by down-regulation of several genes normally expressed at higher levels in the adult than the embryonic ventricle, such as α-myosin heavy chain and the sarcoplasmic reticulum calcium "pump," SERCA2a. Gene induction in cardiac hypertrophy also extends to multiple myocardial growth factors and cytokines, including TGF-β,[227] insulin-like growth factor-1,[228] angiotensinogen,[229] the precursor of angiotensin II, endothelin-1,[230] and cardiotropin-1,[231] which act directly on cardiac myocytes, evoking transcriptional responses similar to those induced by load itself.[162, 232–234]

Although one perspective on the hypertrophic phenotype has been to debate whether such changes are beneficial adaptations versus maladaptive responses that (at least ultimately) lead to impaired function, an alternative point of view has been to seek evidence for hierarchical mechanisms that might regulate this broad subset of cardiac genes in tandem. Although the actual mechanical sensor to detect and transduce an increase in wall stress remains a subject for speculation, much has been learned about the cytoplasmic cascades for signal transduction in hypertrophy,[235, 236] as well as how these proteins are coupled to transcription factors that mediate the fetal program. Proposed mechanisms include the up-regulation of transcription factors like Fos, Myc, and Jun, which are up-regulated with immediate-early kinetics within just a few minutes of subjecting cells to mitogenic stimulation, hypertrophic agonists, or passive mechanical stress.[237] At least in cell culture, exogenous Fos and Jun suffice for several hypertrophic responses, including the induction of skeletal α-actin,[238, 239] ANF,[240] and TGF-β.[241] Load-inducible transcription factors might activate responsive promoters by binding directly, by binding indirectly (as coactivators), or by inducing the responsible DNA-binding proteins. Cardiogenic transcription factors that are up-regulated in hypertrophy include Nkx2.5,[242] GATA-4,[53] and one or more MEF2 proteins.[243] In vivo promoter mapping through the injection of reporter genes into adult myocardium, has shown GATA-4 sites in β-myosin heavy chain and angiotensin type Ia receptor promoters to be essential for the induction of these genes via aortic banding.[244, 245]

Ultimately, a paradox results in trying to explain gene induction through up-regulation of a transcription factor. What up-regulates the regulator? If activation requires an even earlier gene, what induces the earliest inducer? A general biologic solution to this problem is the functional activation of preexisting transcription factors, present in the cell in latent form, sequestered by an inhibitor, tethered in the cytoplasm, or just transcriptionally inert. SRF is implicated in hypertrophic signaling in response to TGF-β,[87] $alpha_1$-adrenergic agonists,[246, 247] endothelin,[247] electrical stimulation,[240] and forced expression of Fos/Jun.[239,240] One mechanism coupling these signals to SRF appears to be p38-dependent phosphorylation of ATF6, a coactivator bound to the SRF transactivation domain[247] (D. Zhang and M. D. Schneider, unpublished observations). As a second transcription factor whose phosphorylation is generic to multiple forms of hypertrophy, STAT proteins are phosphorylated as a response to gp130-linked agonists,[248, 249] angiotensin,[250, 251] and mechanical load in vivo,[252] and the functional importance of this for hypertrophic signaling was shown using a nonphosphorylatable mutation of STAT3.[249]

Conversely, dephosphorylation is the trigger for function of other transcription factors. The calcium-dependent phosphatase calcineurin dephosphorylates the transcription factor NFAT (nuclear factor of activated T cells), resulting in its translocation to the nucleus.[60] NFAT interacts physically with GATA-4 and can function as a coactivator when bound to GATA-4 at promoters with GATA-4–binding sites. Constitutively activated forms of calcineurin and NFAT each provoke cardiac hypertrophy in transgenic mice.[60] Existing pharmacologic inhibitors of this pathway are effective in blocking several models of hypertrophy, although not all.[253–255] Features that make this calcium-dependent pathway especially attractive as a target for drug discovery include both the known elevation of intracellular calcium in cardiac myocytes as a response common to diverse hypertrophic signals and the multiple defects in calcium homeostasis seen in human failing myocytes.[256–258]

Postmitotic Cardiac Phenotype

After birth, both normal cardiac growth and growth in adaptation to an increased workload occur preponderantly via an increase in cell size (the very definition of hypertrophy), not an increase in cell number (hyperplasia). Although it is contended that the block to myocyte proliferation is not absolute,[259] much of the data provided to support such claims relate to DNA synthesis or nuclear division, and a survey of such studies concluded that myocyte proliferation per se, if it occurs at all, does so at a frequency too low to be consequential.[260] "Irreversible" cell cycle exit thus is one eventual feature of cardiac differentiation, although a mutually exclusive relation does not exist between proliferation and tissue-specific transcription at earlier stages, as it does in skeletal myocytes.[261, 262] What mechanisms impose this block, the "postmitotic" phenotype?

In general, cell cycle control is mediated via several interacting multigene families.[263, 264] These encode cyclins, proteins that are expressed and degraded cyclically throughout the cell cycle, cyclin-dependent protein kinases (Cdks), inhibitors of these kinases, and substrates for the kinases. The essential substrates for G1 Cdks (Cdk4/6) are growth-inhibitory, tumor suppressor proteins, for which the archetype is the retinoblastoma gene product Rb. Pocket proteins, in turn, bind the E2F family of transcription factors and prevent their ability to activate an array of E2F-dependent genes for DNA synthesis. Thus, Cdk inhibitors inhibit Cdks, which inhibit pocket proteins, which inhibit the E2F-dependent gene program.

Rb is more highly expressed in adult myocardium than in the embryo. A related protein, p107, is expressed reciprocally, and a second, p130, is expressed at both stages. Up-regulation of Rb also is seen during skeletal muscle differentiation,[265] and one proposed explanation for irreversible cell cycle exit in that form of striated muscle focused on the functional differences between Rb and p107.[266] Myocytes lacking Rb, but containing p107, remained able to reenter the cell cycle after a mitogenic challenge.[266] This model poses an apparent paradox because Rb function is wholly reversible by Cdk phosphorylation and therefore would seem unable, by itself, to establish an irreversible block to serum-induced cell cycling. However, one notes the marked developmental regulation of other cell cycle machinery in cardiac myocytes, including down-regulation of cyclins and Cdks,[267–269] concurrent with up-regulation of certain Cdk inhibitors, p21 and p27.[270–272] These inhibitors and a more distantly related protein, p57, act both upstream of Rb, on Cdk4/6, and downstream of Rb, on Cdk2. In contrast, a second family of Cdk inhibitors acts on Cdk4/6 preferentially, including p15 and p18, two that are expressed in myocardium.[273, 274] Thus, in the postmitotic heart, Rb might be shielded from rephosphorylation at the level of Cdk4/6. Even if this were not the case, the resulting disinhibition of E2F might be blocked at the level of Cdk2. In support of this latter model, hyperphosphorylation of Rb even in neonatal cardiac myocytes has been reported to occur without DNA synthesis, after α_1-adrenergic stimulation, angiotensin II, or mitogenic serum.[275, 276] Whether Rb phosphorylation likewise can occur in the adult heart is unknown.

Direct functional data for the importance of this cyclin-Cdk-pocket protein for cardiac growth arrest have come from the use of viral gene transfer, with E1A used to inactivate pocket proteins in cardiac myocytes or exogenous E2F-1 used to bypass them[196, 197, 277, 278]: this results in efficient G1 exit into S phase even in the adult myocardium[279] but does not suffice for progression beyond a checkpoint at the G2/M boundary. Additional inhibitory mechanisms are in place even at the G1/S checkpoint, because E1A mutations that are defective for pocket protein binding also drive DNA synthesis in ventricular muscle cells, via the transcription adaptor proteins p300 and CBP,[196, 278] as discussed earlier. That down-regulation of G1 cyclins contributes to the postmitotic state was shown by forced expression of cyclin D1 in the myocardium of transgenic mice, resulting in cardiac enlargement, multinucleation, and sustained DNA synthesis in ventricular myocytes[269]; this increase was large proportionally but small in absolute terms (0.05 percent).

Although knockout mutations have become a virtual "gold standard" for protein function in vivo, as highighted by many examples throughout this chapter, the conventional genomic knockout deletes a gene from all cells of the organism and thus may disclose only the earliest essential function of a protein: inherently, death at any early stage precludes the use of a knockout at any later stage. This limitation has prevented a direct test for the role of Rb in the postmitotic cardiac phenotype because Rb-deficient mice die in midgestation, with extraneous defects in neural differentiation and hematopoiesis.[280–282] For this reason, Rb is an especially attractive candidate for a "conditional" deletion.[93, 283, 284] To implement this approach, the target motif for a DNA recombinase (Cre or Flp) is placed as an innocuous tag within the introns flanking a critical gene segment through conventional homologous recombination with embryonic stem cells; this modified gene is expressed normally, and the resulting animal has no phenotype, in the absence of the recombinase. However, in progeny that coinherit a transgene for Cre or in organs receiving a virus for Cre, the tagged gene is deleted (i.e., exclusively in cells that express the recombinase). This approach can be used for temporal or cell-type control over recombination with the use of lineage-specific or drug-inducible promoters. A cardiac-restricted deletion of Rb has been implemented, resulting in cardiac enlargement and sustained DNA synthesis, similar to that resulting from forced expression of cyclin D1.[269, 285] Thus, both studies are equally consistent with the existence of inhibitors distal to Rb and with only an incomplete relief of pocket protein function.

Candidates for the former inhibitor include p21 and p27; candidates for the latter include both of these, plus p15 and p18. Although no developmental or anatomic differences occurred in p21-null mice,[286, 287] mice lacking p27 show increased body size, with proportional enlargement of the heart and other organs and a susceptibility to pituitary adenomas.[288–290] Thus, despite overlapping patterns of expression and in vitro functions, the net effect of these related Cdk inhibitors is discernibly different in vivo. A phenotype similar to the p27 knockout was seen in p18-deficient mice.[291] Like other settings discussed earlier in this chapter, the molecular basis for irreversible cell cycle exit—the last step in cardiac development—is a logical target for genetic dissection through combinatorial deletions of functionally redundant or functionally interrelated proteins.

Conclusions and Perspectives

The genetic dissection of cardiac organogenesis has yielded gratifying results. Although numerous questions remain to be answered, the use in particular of murine models, fish, and flies has dramatically accelerated the pace for novel insights and has disclosed an array of cardiogenic regulators whose precise targets, partners, and inducers have become key elements of the research agenda in this field. Our brief review, which focused on cardiac muscle, lacks the opportunity to discuss several complementary aspects of cardiovascular development, such as creation of the septa and cardiac valves[130, 292–296] and formation of the vasculature, including the coronary arteries.[297] Advances will be fueled by ongoing refinements in genetic technologies, including the more widespread use of conditional transgenes, conditional gene targeting, and viral gene transfer to create developmental phenotypes and of genome-wide expression profiling ("gene chip" studies) or other genetically unbiased methods to aid in decoding the phenotypes. The identification of single gene defects that cause human cardiac malformations—perhaps the least expected component of progress made since the previous edition of this text—has brought bench and bedside together more than even optimistic projections might have foretold.

References

1. Labarthe DA, Kosinetz C, Jones TM: Epidemiology. *In* Garson A Jr, Bricker JT, McNamara DG (eds): The Science and Practice of Pediatric Cardiology, Vol. 1 pp. 135–151. Philadelphia: Lea & Febiger, 1990.
2. Olson EN, Martin JF, Schneider MD: Cardiac growth and development. *In* Willerson JT, Cohn JN (eds): Cardiovascular Medicine. New York: Churchill Livingstone, 1995.
3. Lin Q, Srivastava D, Olson EN: A transcriptional pathway for cardiac development. Cold Spring Harb Symp Quant Biol 62:405–411, 1997.
4. Fishman MC, Olson EN: Parsing the heart: genetic modules for organ assembly. Cell 91:153–156, 1997.
5. Sucov HM: Molecular insights into cardiac development. Annu Rev Physiol 60:287–308, 1998.
6. Harvey RP, Rosenthal N (eds): Heart Development. San Diego: Academic Press, 1998.
7. The *C. elegans* Sequencing Consortium: Genome sequence of the nematode *C. elegans*: a platform for investigating biology. Science 282:2012–2018, 1998.
8. Bodmer R: The gene tinman is required for specification of the heart and visceral muscles in *Drosophila.* Development 118:719–729, 1993.
9. Lilly B, Zhao B, Ranganayakulu G, et al: Requirement of MADS domain transcription factor D-MEF2 for muscle formation in *Drosophila.* Science 267:688–693, 1995.
10. Wu XS, Golden K, Bodmer R: Heart development in *Drosophila* requires the segment polarity gene wingless. Dev Biol 169:619–628, 1995.
11. Black BL, Olson EN: Transcriptional control of muscle development by myocyte enhancer factor-2 (MEF2) proteins. Annu Rev Cell Dev Biol 14:167–196, 1998.
12. Nusslein-Volhard C: Of flies and fishes. Science 266:572–574, 1994.
13. Fishman MC, Chien KR: Fashioning the vertebrate heart: earliest embryonic decisions. Development 124:2099–2117, 1997.
14. Zambrowicz BP, et al: Disruption and sequence identification of 2,000 genes in mouse embryonic stem cells. Nature 392:608–611, 1998.
15. Justice MJ, Zheng B, Woychik RP, Bradley A: Using targeted large deletions and high-efficiency N-ethyl-N-nitrosourea mutagenesis for functional analyses of the mammalian genome. Methods 13:423–436, 1997.
16. Olson EN, Srivastava D: Molecular pathways controlling heart development. Science 272:671–676, 1996.
17. Nascone N, Mercola M: An inductive role for the endoderm in *Xenopus* cardiogenesis. Development 121:515–523, 1995.
18. Bodmer R, Venkatesh TV: Heart development in *Drosophila* and vertebrates: conservation of molecular mechanisms. Dev Genet 22:181–186, 1998.
19. Olson EN, Klein WH: bHLH factors in muscle development: deadlines and commitments, what to leave in and what to leave out. Genes Dev 8:1–8, 1994.
20. Evans SM, Tai LJ, Tan VP, et al: Heterokaryons of cardiac myocytes and fibroblasts reveal the lack of dominance of the cardiac muscle phenotype. Mol Cell Biol 14:4269–4279, 1994.

21. Gossett LA, Kelvin DJ, Sternberg EA, Olson EN: A new myocyte-specific enhancer-binding factor that recognizes a conserved element associated with multiple muscle-specific genes. Mol Cell Biol 9:5022–5033, 1989.
22. Molkentin JD, Olson EN: Combinatorial control of muscle development by basic helix-loop-helix and MADS-box transcription factors. Proc Natl Acad Sci U S A 93:9366–9373, 1996.
23. Edmondson DG, Lyons GE, Martin JF, Olson EN: Mef2 gene expression marks the cardiac and skeletal muscle lineages during mouse embryogenesis. Development 120:1251–1263, 1994.
24. Molkentin JD, Firulli AB, Black BL, et al: MEF2B is a potent transactivator expressed in early myogenic lineages. Mol Cell Biol 16:3814–3824, 1996.
25. Subramanian SV, Nadalginard B: Early expression of the different isoforms of the myocyte enhancer factor-2 (MEF2) protein in myogenic as well tps non-myogenic cell lineages during mouse embryogenesis. Mech Dev 57:103–112, 1996.
26. Ticho BS, Stainier DYR, Fishman MC, Breitbart RE: Three zebrafish MEF2 genes delineate somatic and cardiac muscle development in wild-type and mutant embryos. Mech Dev 59:205–218, 1996.
27. Lin Q, Schwarz J, Bucana C, Olson EN: Control of mouse cardiac morphogenesis and myogenesis by transcription factor MEF2C. Science 276:1404–1407, 1997.
28. Lin Q, Lu JR, Yanagisawa H, et al: Requirement of the MADS-box transcription factor MEF2C for vascular development. Development 125:4565–4574, 1998.
29. Rudnicki MA, Schnegelsberg PNJ, Stead RH, et al: MyoD or myf-5 is required for the formation of skeletal muscle. Cell 75:1351–1359, 1993.
30. Rawls A, Morris JH, Rudnicki M, et al: Myogenin's functions do not overlap with those of MyoD or Myf-5 during mouse embryogenesis. Dev Biol 172:37–50, 1995.
31. Lilly B, Galewsky S, Firulli AB, et al: D-MEF2: a MADS box transcription factor expressed in differentiating mesoderm and muscle cell lineages during *Drosophila* embryogenesis. Proc Natl Acad Sci U S A 91:5662–5666, 1994.
32. Nguyen HT, Bodmer R, Abmayr SM, et al: D-mef2: a *Drosophila* mesoderm-specific MADS box-containing gene with a biphasic expression profile during embryogenesis. Proc Natl Acad Sci U S A 91:7520–7524, 1994.
33. Ranganayakulu G, Zhao B, Dokidis A, et al: A series of mutations in the D-MEF2 transcription factor reveal multiple functions in larval and adult myogenesis in *Drosophila*. Dev Biol 171:169–181, 1995.
34. Bour BA, O'Brien MA, Lockwood WL, et al: *Drosophila* MEF2, a transcription factor that is essential for myogenesis. Genes Dev 9:730–741, 1995.
35. Molkentin JD, Black BL, Martin JF, Olson EN: Cooperative activation of muscle gene expression by MEF2 and myogenic bHLH proteins. Cell 83:1125–1136, 1995.
36. Kaushal S, Schneider JW, Nadalginard B, Mahdavi V: Activation of the myogenic lineage by MEF2A, a factor that induces and cooperates with MyoD. Science 266:1236–1240, 1994.
37. Harvey RP: NK-2 homeobox genes and heart development. Dev Biol 178:203–216 1996.
38. Azpiazu N, Frasch M: tinman and bagpipe: two homeo box genes that determine cell fates in the dorsal mesoderm of *Drosophila*. Genes Dev 7:1325–1340, 1993.
39. Reecy JM, Yamada M, Cummings K, et al: Chicken Nkx-2.8: a novel homeobox gene expressed in early heart progenitor cells and pharyngeal pouch-2 and -3 endoderm. Dev Biol 188:295–311, 1997.
40. Lyons I, Parsons LM, Hartley L, et al: Myogenic and morphogenetic defects in the heart tubes of murine embryos lacking the homeobox gene Nkx2-5. Genes Dev 9:1654–1666, 1995.
41. Ranganayakulu G, Elliott DA, Harvey RP, Olson EN: Divergent roles for NK-2 class homeobox genes in cardiogenesis in flies and mice. Development 125:3037–3048, 1998.
42. Park M, Lewis C, Turbay D, et al: Differential rescue of visceral and cardiac defects in *Drosophila* by vertebrate tinman-related genes. Proc Natl Acad Sci U S A 95:9366–9371, 1998.
43. Fu YC, Izumo S: Cardiac myogenesis: overexpression of XCsx2 or XMEF2A in whole *Xenopus* embryos induces the precocious expression of XMHC alpha gene. Roux Arch Dev Biol 205:198–202, 1995.
44. Chen JN, Fishman MC: Zebrafish tinman homolog demarcates the heart field and initiates myocardial differentiation. Development 122:3809–3816, 1996.
45. Cleaver OB, Patterson KD, Krieg PA: Overexpression of the tinman-related genes XNkx-2.5 and XNkx-2.3 in *Xenopus* embryos results in myocardial hyperplasia. Development 122:3549–3556, 1996.
46. Fu YC, Yan W, Mohun TJ, Evans SM: Vertebrate tinman homologues XNkx2-3 and XNkx2-5 are required for heart formation in a functionally redundant manner. Development 125:4439–4449, 1998.
47. Grow MW, Krieg PA: Tinman function is essential for vertebrate heart development: elimination of cardiac differentiation by dominant inhibitory mutants of the tinman-related genes, XNkx2-3 and XNkx2-5. Dev Biol 204:187–196, 1998.
48. Gajewski K, Kim Y, Lee YM, et al: D-mef2 is a target for tinman activation during *Drosophila* heart development. EMBO J 16:515–522, 1997.
49. Chen C-Y, Schwartz RJ: Identification of novel DNA binding targets and regulatory domains of a murine tinman homeodomain factor, nkx-2.5. J Biol Chem 270:15628–15633, 1995.
50. Bao ZZ, Bruneau BG, Seidman JG, et al: Regulation of chamber-specific gene expression in the developing heart by Irx4. Science 283:1161–1164, 1999.
51. Grepin C, Nemer G, Nemer M: Enhanced cardiogenesis in embryonic stem cells overexpressing the GATA-4 transcription factor. Development 124:2387–2395, 1997.
52. Ip HS, Wilson DB, Heikinheimo M, et al: The GATA-4 transcription factor transactivates the cardiac muscle-specific troponin C promoter-enhancer in nonmuscle cells. Mol Cell Biol 14:7517–7526, 1994.
53. Molkentin JD, Kalvakolanu DV, Markham BE: Transcription factor GATA-4 regulates cardiac muscle-specific expression of the alpha-myosin heavy-chain gene. Mol Cell Biol 14:4947–4957, 1994.
54. Thuerauf DJ, Hanford DS, Glembotski CC: Regulation of rat brain natriuretic peptide transcription. J Biol Chem 269:17772–17775, 1994.
55. Searcy RD, Vincent EB, Liberatore CM, Yutzey KE: A GATA-dependent Nkx-2.5 regulatory element activates early cardiac gene expression in transgenic mice. Development 125:4461–4470, 1998.
56. Lien CL, Wu C, Mercer B, et al: Control of early cardiac-specific transcription of Nkx2-5 by a GATA-dependent enhancer. Development 126:75–84, 1999.
57. Grepin C, Robitaille L, Antakly T, Nemer M: Inhibition of transcription factor GATA-4 expression blocks in vitro cardiac muscle differentiation. Mol Cell Biol 15:4095–4102, 1995.
58. Jiang YM, Evans T: The *Xenopus* GATA-4/5/6 genes are associated with cardiac specification and can regulate cardiac-specific transcription during embryogenesis. Dev Biol 174:258–270, 1996.
59. Gove C, Walmsley M, Nijjar S, et al: Over-expression of GATA-6 in *Xenopus* embryos blocks differentiation of heart precursors. EMBO J 16:1806–1807, 1997.
60. Molkentin JD, et al: A calcineurin-dependent transcriptional pathway for cardiac hypertrophy. Cell 93:215–228, 1998.
61. Kuo CT, Morrisey EE, Anandappa R, et al: GATA4 transcription factor is required for ventral morphogenesis and heart tube formation. Genes Dev 11:1048–1060, 1997.
62. Molkentin JD, Lin Q, Duncan SA, Olson EN: Requirement of the transcription factor GATA4 for heart tube formation and ventral morphogenesis. Genes Dev 11:1061–1072, 1997.
63. Morrisey EE, Tang ZH, Sigrist K, et al: GATA6 regulates HNF4 and is required for differentiation of visceral endoderm in the mouse embryo. Gene Dev 12:3579–3590, 1998.
64. Koutsourakis M, Langeveld A, Patient R, et al: The transcription factor GATA6 is essential for early extraembryonic development. Development 126:723–732, 1999.
65. Durocher D, Charron F, Warren R, et al: The cardiac transcription factors Nkx2-5 and GATA-4 are mutual cofactors. EMBO J 16:5687–5696, 1997.
66. Sepulveda JL, Belaguli N, Nigam V, et al: GATA-4 and Nkx-2.5 coactivate Nkx-2 DNA binding targets: role for regulating early cardiac gene expression. Mol Cell Biol 18:3405–3415, 1998.
67. Lee Y, Shioi T, Kasahara H, et al: The cardiac tissue-restricted homeobox protein Csx/Nkx2.5 physically associates with the zinc finger protein GATA4 and cooperatively activates atrial natriuretic factor gene expression. Mol Cell Biol 18:3120–3129, 1998.
68. Tevosian SG, Deconinck AE, Cantor AB, et al: FOG-2: a novel GATA-family cofactor related to multitype zinc-finger proteins

Friend of GATA-1 and U-shaped. Proc Natl Acad Sci U S A 96:950–955, 1999.
69. Svensson EC, Tufts RL, Polk CE, Leiden JM: Molecular cloning of FOG-2: a modulator of transcription factor GATA-4 in cardiomyocytes. Proc Natl Acad Sci U S A 96:956–961, 1999.
70. Lu J, McKinsey T, Xu H, et al: FOG-2: a cardiac- and brain-restricted cofactor for GATA transcription factors. Mol Cell Biol 19:4495–4502, 1999.
71. Cserjesi P, Brown D, Lyons GE, Olson EN: Expression of the novel basic helix-loop-helix gene eHAND in neural crest derivatives and extraembryonic membranes during mouse development. Dev Biol 170:664–678, 1995.
72. Srivastava D, Cserjesi P, Olson EN: A subclass of bHLH proteins required for cardiac morphogenesis. Science 270:1995–1999, 1995.
73. Hollenberg SM, Sternglanz R, Cheng PF, Weintraub H: Identification of a new family of tissue-specific basic helix-loop-helix proteins with a two-hybrid system. Mol Cell Biol 15:3813–3822, 1995.
74. Cross JC, Flannery ML, Blanar MA, et al: Hxt encodes a basic helix-loop-helix transcription factor that regulates trophoblast cell development. Development 121:2513–2523, 1995.
75. Biben C, Harvey RP: Homeodomain factor Nkx2-5 controls left/right asymmetric expression of bHLH gene eHand during murine heart development. Genes Dev 11:1357–1369, 1997.
76. Thomas T, Yamagishi H, Overbeek PA, et al: The bHLH factors, dHAND and eHAND, specify pulmonary and systemic cardiac ventricles independent of left-right sidedness. Dev Biol 196:228–236, 1998.
77. Srivastava D, Thomas T, Lin Q, et al: Regulation of cardiac mesodermal and neural crest development by the bHLH transcription factor, dHAND. Nat Genet 16:154–160, 1997.
78. Firulli AB, McFadden DG, Lin Q, et al: Heart and extra-embryonic mesodermal defects in mouse embryos lacking the bHLH transcription factor Hand1. Nat Genet 18:266–270, 1998.
79. Riley P, AnsonCartwright L, Cross JC: The Hand1 bHLH transcription factor is essential for placentation and cardiac morphogenesis. Nat Genet 18:271–275, 1998.
80. Thomas T, Kurihara H, Yamagishi H, et al: A signaling cascade involving endothelin-1, dHAND and msx1 regulates development of neural-crest-derived branchial arch mesenchyme. Development 125:3005–3014, 1998.
81. Yamagishi H, Garg V, Matsuoka R, et al: A molecular pathway revealing a genetic basis for human cardiac and craniofacial defects. Science 283:1158–1161, 1999.
82. Croissant JD, Kim JH, Eichele G, et al: Avian serum response factor expression restricted primarily to muscle cell lineages is required for alpha-actin gene transcription. Dev Biol 177:250–264, 1996.
83. Belaguli NS, Schildmeyer LA, Schwartz RJ: Organization and myogenic restricted expression of the murine serum response factor gene: a role for autoregulation. J Biol Chem 272:18222–18231, 1997.
84. Sartorelli V, Webster KA, Kedes L: Muscle-specific expression of the cardiac alpha-actin gene requires MyoD1, CArG-box binding factor, and Sp1. Genes Dev 4:1811–1822, 1990.
85. Lee TC, Chow KL, Fang P, Schwartz RJ: Activation of skeletal alpha-actin gene transcription: the cooperative formation of serum response factor-binding complexes over positive cis-acting promoter serum response elements displaces a negative-acting nuclear factor enriched in replicating myoblasts and nonmyogenic cells. Mol Cell Biol 11:5090–5100, 1991.
86. Sartorelli V, Hong NA, Bishopric NH, Kedes L: Myocardial activation of the human cardiac α-actin promoter by helix-loop-helix proteins. Proc Natl Acad Sci U S A 89:4047–4051, 1992.
87. MacLellan WR, Lee TC, Schwartz RJ, Schneider MD: Transforming growth factor-beta response elements of the skeletal alpha-actin gene: combinatorial action of serum response factor, YY1, and the SV40 enhancer-binding protein, TEF-1. J Biol Chem 269:16754–16760, 1994.
88. Gauthier-Rouviere C, Vandromme M, Tuil D, et al: Expression and activity of serum response factor is required for expression of the muscle-determining factor MyoD in both dividing and differentiating mouse C2C12 myoblasts. Mol Biol Cell 7:719–729, 1996.
89. Treisman R: Journey to the surface of the cell: fos regulation and the SRE. EMBO J 14:4905–4913, 1995.
90. Whitmarsh AJ, Yang SH, Su MSS, et al: Role of p38 and JNK mitogen-activated protein kinases in the activation of ternary complex factors. Mol Cell Biol 17:2360–2371, 1997.
91. Chen CY, Schwartz RJ: Association of murine tinman homologue, Nkx-2.5, with SRF activates the cardiac α-actin promoter [abstract]. Circulation 92(suppl I): I-369, 1995.
92. Arsenian S, Weinhold B, Oelgeschlager M, et al: Serum response factor is essential for mesoderm formation during mouse embryogenesis. EMBO J 17:6289–6299, 1998.
93. Agah R, Frenkel PA, French BA, et al: Gene recombination in postmitotic cells: targeted expression of Cre recombinase provokes cardiac-restricted, site-specific rearrangement in adult ventricular muscle in vivo. J Clin Invest 100:169–179, 1997.
94. Guillemin K, Groppe J, Ducker K, et al: The pruned gene encodes the *Drosophila* serum response factor and regulates cytoplasmic outgrowth during terminal branching of the tracheal system. Development 122:1353–1362, 1996.
95. Montagne J, Groppe J, Guillemin K, et al: The *Drosophila* serum response factor gene is required for the formation of intervein tissue of the wing and is allelic to blistered. Development 122:2589–2597, 1996.
96. Farrance IKG, Mar JH, Ordahl, CP: M-CAT binding factor is related to the SV40 enhancer binding factor, TEF-1. J Biol Chem 267:17234–17240, 1992.
97. Jacquemin P, Davidson I: The role of the TEF transcription factors in cardiogenesis and other developmental processes. Trends Cardiovasc Med 7:192–197, 1997.
98. Gupta MP, Amin CS, Gupta M, et al: Transcription enhancer factor 1 interacts with a basic helix-loop-helix zipper protein, max, for positive regulation of cardiac alpha-myosin heavy-chain gene expression. Mol Cell Biol 17:3924–3936, 1997.
99. Azakie A, Larkin SB, Farrance IK, et al: DTEF-1, a novel member of the transcription enhancer factor-1 (TEF-1) multigene family. J Biol Chem 271:8260–8265, 1996.
100. Jacquemin P, Hwang JJ, Martial JA, et al: A novel family of developmentally regulated mammalian transcription factors containing the TEA/ATTS DNA binding domain. J Biol Chem 271:21775–21785, 1996.
101. Stewart AF, Richard CW 3rd, Suzow J, et al: Cloning of human RTEF-1, a transcriptional enhancer factor-1-related gene preferentially expressed in skeletal muscle: evidence for an ancient multigene family. Genomics 37:68–76, 1996.
102. Larkin SB, Farrance IKG, Ordahl CP: Flanking sequences modulate the cell specificity of m-CAT elements. Mol Cell Biol 16:3742–3755, 1996.
103. Chen Z, Friedrich GA, Soriano P: Transcriptional enhancer factor 1 disruption by a retroviral gene trap leads to heart defects and embryonic lethality in mice. Genes Dev 8:2293–2301, 1994.
104. Basson CT, Bachinsky DR, Lin RC, et al: Mutations in human TBX5 cause limb and cardiac malformation in Holt-Oram syndrome. Nat Genet 15:30–35, 1997.
105. Li QY, NewburyEcob RA, Terrett JA, et al: Holt-Oram syndrome is caused by mutations in TBX5, a member of the Brachyury (T) gene family. Nat Genet 15:21–29, 1997.
106. On-line Mendelian Inheritance in Man. Baltimore: Johns Hopkins University.
107. Rehorn KP, Thelen H, Michelson AM, Reuter R: A molecular aspect of hematopoiesis and endoderm development common to vertebrates and *Drosophila*. Development 122:4023–4031, 1996.
108. Frasch M: Induction of visceral and cardiac mesoderm by ectodermal dpp in the early *Drosophila* embryo. Nature 374:464–467, 1995.
109. Gisselbrecht S, Skeath JB, Doe CQ, Michelson AM: Heartless encodes a fibroblast growth factor receptor (DFR1/DFGF-R2) involved in the directional migration of early mesodermal cells in the *Drosophila* embryo. Genes Dev 10:3003–3017, 1996.
110. Park MY, Wu XS, Golden K, et al: The wingless signaling pathway is directly involved in *Drosophila* heart development. Dev Biol 177:104–116, 1996.
111. Cadigan KM, Nusse R: Wnt signaling: a common theme in animal development. Genes Dev 11:3286–3305, 1997.
112. Hammerschmidt M, Brook A, McMahon AP: The world according to hedgehog. Trends Genet 13:14–21, 1997.
113. Sugi Y, Lough J: Anterior endoderm is a specific effector of terminal cardiac myocyte differentiation of cells from the embryonic heart forming region. Dev Dyn 200:155–162, 1994.
114. Lough J, Barron M, Brogley M, et al: Combined BMP-2 and FGF-4, but neither factor alone, induces cardiogenesis in non-precardiac embryonic mesoderm. Dev Biol 178:198–202, 1996.

115. Ladd AN, Yatskievych TA, Antin PB: Regulation of avian cardiac myogenesis by activin/TGF beta and bone morphogenetic proteins. Dev Biol 204:407–419, 1998.
116. Schultheiss TM, Xydas S, Lassar AB: Induction of avian cardiac myogenesis by anterior endoderm. Development 121:4203–4214, 1995.
117. Schultheiss TM, Burch JBE, Lassar AB: A role for bone morphogenetic proteins in the induction of cardiac myogenesis. Genes Dev 11:451–462, 1997.
118. Wang DZ, Reiter RS, Lin JL, et al: Requirement of a novel gene, Xin, in cardiac morphogenesis. Development 126:1281–1294, 1999.
119. Johansson BM, Wiles MV: Evidence for involvement of activin A and bone morphogenetic protein 4 in mammalian mesoderm and hematopoietic development. Mol Cell Biol 15:141–151, 1995.
120. Logan M, Mohun T: Induction of cardiac muscle differentiation in isolated animal pole explants of *Xenopus laevis* embryos. Development 118:865–875, 1993.
121. Mangiacapra FJ, Fransen ME, Lemanski LF: Activin A and transforming growth factor-beta stimulate heart formation in axolotls but do not rescue cardiac lethal mutants. Cell Tissue Res 282:227–236, 1995.
122. Vassalli A, Matzuk MM, Gardner HA, et al: Activin/inhibin beta B subunit gene disruption leads to defects in eyelid development and female reproduction. Genes Dev 8:414–427, 1994.
123. Matzuk MM, Kumar TR, Vassalli A, et al: Functional analysis of activins during mammalian development. Nature 374:354–356, 1995.
124. Matzuk MM, Kumar TR, Bradley A: Different phenotypes for mice deficient in either activins or activin receptor type II. Nature 374:356–360, 1995.
125. Oh SP, Li E: The signaling pathway mediated by the type IIB activin receptor controls axial patterning and lateral asymmetry in the mouse. Genes Dev 11:1812–1826, 1997.
126. Gu ZY, Nomura M, Simpson BB, et al: The type I activin receptor ActRIB is required for egg cylinder organization and gastrulation in the mouse. Genes Dev 12:844–857, 1998.
127. Nomura M, Li E: Smad2 role in mesoderm formation, left-right patterning and craniofacial development. Nature 393:786–790, 1998.
128. Dickson MC, Martin JS, Cousins FM, et al: Defective haematopoiesis and vasculogenesis in transforming growth factor-beta 1 knock out mice. Development 121:1845–1854, 1995.
129. Bonyadi M, Rusholme SAB, Cousins FM, et al: Mapping of a major genetic modifier of embryonic lethality in TGF beta 1 knockout mice. Nat Genet 15:207–211, 1997.
130. Sanford LP, Ormsby I, GittenbergerdeGroot AC, et al: TGF beta 2 knockout mice have multiple developmental defects that are non-overlapping with other TGF beta knockout phenotypes. Development 124:2659–2670, 1997.
131. Proetzel G, Pawlowski SA, Wiles MV, et al: Transforming growth factor-beta 3 is required for secondary palate fusion. Nat Genet 11:409–414, 1995.
132. Tsuda T, Philp N, Zile MH, Linask KK: Left-right asymmetric localization of flectin in the extracellular matrix during heart looping. Dev Biol 173:39–50, 1996.
133. Tsuda T, Majumder K, Linask KK: Differential expression of flectin in the extracellular matrix and left-right asymmetry in mouse embryonic heart during looping stages. Dev Genet 23:203–214, 1998.
134. Yost HJ: Inhibition of proteoglycan synthesis eliminates left-right asymmetry in *Xenopus laevis* cardiac looping. Development 110:865–874, 1990.
135. Yost HJ: Regulation of vertebrate left-right asymmetries by extracellular matrix. Nature 357:158–161, 1992.
136. Levin M, Johnson RL, Stern CD, et al: A molecular pathway determining left-right asymmetry in chick embryogenesis. Cell 82:803–814, 1995.
137. Collignon J, Varlet I, Robertson EJ: Relationship between asymmetric nodal expression and the direction of embryonic turning. Nature 381:155–158, 1996.
138. Hyatt BA, Lohr JL, Yost HJ: Initiation of vertebrate left-right axis formation by maternal Vg1. Nature 384:62–65, 1996.
139. Lowe LA, Supp DM, Sampath K, et al: Conserved left-right asymmetry of nodal expression and alterations in murine situs inversus. Nature 381:158–161, 1996.
140. Lustig KD, Kroll K, Sun E, et al: A *Xenopus* nodal-related gene that acts in synergy with noggin to induce complete secondary axis and notochord formation. Development 122:3275–3282, 1996.
141. Levin M, Pagan S, Roberts DJ, et al: Left/right patterning signals and the independent regulation of different aspects of situs in the chick embryo. Dev Biol 189:57–67, 1997.
142. Sampath K, Cheng AM, Frisch A, Wright CV: Functional differences among *Xenopus* nodal-related genes in left-right axis determination. Development 124:3293–3302, 1997.
143. Lohr JL, Danos MC, Yost HJ: Left-right asymmetry of a nodal-related gene is regulated by dorsoanterior midline structures during *Xenopus* development. Development 124:1465–1472, 1997.
144. Meno C, Saijoh Y, Fujii H, et al: Left-right asymmetric expression of the TGF beta-family member lefty in mouse embryos. Nature 381:151–155, 1996.
145. Meno C, Shimono A, Saijoh Y, et al: lefty-1 is required for left-right determination as a regulator of lefty-2 and nodal. Cell 94:287–297, 1998.
146. Saijoh Y, Adachi H, Mochida K, et al: Distinct transcriptional regulatory mechanisms underlie left-right asymmetric expression of lefty-1 and lefty-2. Genes Dev 13:259–269, 1999.
147. Brueckner M, D'Eustachio P, Horwich AL: Linkage mapping of a mouse gene, iv, that controls left-right asymmetry of the heart and viscera. Proc Natl Acad Sci U S A 86:5035–5038, 1989.
148. Supp DM, Witte DP, Potter SS, Brueckner M: Mutation of an axonemal dynein affects left-right asymmetry in *inversus viscerum* mice. Nature 389:963–966, 1997.
149. Yokoyama T, Copeland NG, Jenkins NA, et al: Reversal of left-right asymmetry: a situs inversus mutation. Science 260:679–682, 1993.
150. Mochizuki T, Saijoh Y, Tsuchiya K, et al: Cloning of inv, a gene that controls left/right asymmetry and kidney development. Nature 395:177–181, 1998.
151. Morgan D, Turnpenny L, Goodship J, et al: Inversin, a novel gene in the vertebrate left-right axis pathway, is partially deleted in the inv mouse. Nat Genet 20:149–156, 1998.
152. Charng MJ, Frenkel PA, Lin Q, et al: A constitutive mutation of ALK5 disrupts cardiac looping and morphogenesis in mice. Dev Biol 199:72–79, 1998.
153. Hyatt BA, Yost HJ: The left-right coordinator: the role of Vg1 in organizing left-right axis formation. Cell 93:37–46, 1998.
154. Isaac A, Sargent MG, Cooke J: Control of vertebrate left-right asymmetry by a snail-related zinc finger gene. Science 275:1301–1304, 1997.
155. Logan M, PaganWestphal SM, Smith DM, et al: The transcription factor Pitx2 mediates situs-specific morphogenesis in response to left-right asymmetric signals. Cell 94:307–317, 1998.
156. Piedra ME, Icardo JM, Albajar M, et al: Pitx2 participates in the late phase of the pathway controlling left-right asymmetry. Cell 94:319–324, 1998.
157. Ryan AK, Blumberg B, RodriguezEsteban C, et al: Pitx2 determines left-right asymmetry of internal organs in vertebrates. Nature 394:545–551, 1998.
158. Yoshioka H, Meno C, Koshiba K, et al: Pitx2, a bicoid-type homeobox gene, is involved in a lefty-signaling pathway in determination of left-right asymmetry. Cell 94:299–305, 1998.
159. Campione M, Steinbeisser H, Schweickert A, et al: The homeobox gene Pitx2: mediator of asymmetric left-right signaling in vertebrate heart and gut looping. Development 126:1225–1234, 1999.
160. Chen J, Knowles HJ, Hebert JL, Hackett BP: Mutation of the mouse hepatocyte nuclear factor/forkhead homologue 4 gene results in an absence of cilia and random left-right asymmetry. J Clin Invest 102:1077–1082, 1998.
161. Zhu XL, Sasse J, McAllister D, Lough J: Evidence that fibroblast growth factors 1 and 4 participate in regulation of cardiogenesis. Dev Dyn 207:429–438, 1996.
162. Parker TG, Packer SE, Schneider MD: Peptide growth factors can provoke "fetal" contractile protein gene expression in rat cardiac myocytes. J Clin Invest 85:507–514, 1990.
163. Pasumarthi KB, Kardami E, Cattini PA: High and low molecular weight fibroblast growth factor-2 increase proliferation of neonatal rat cardiac myocytes but have differential effects on binucleation and nuclear morphology: evidence for both paracrine and intracrine actions of fibroblast growth factor-2. Circ Res 78:126–136, 1996.
164. Weiner HL, Swain JL: Acidic fibroblast growth factor mRNA is expressed by cardiac myocytes in culture and the protein is localized to the extracellular matrix. Proc Natl Acad Sci U S A 86:2683–2687, 1989.
165. Hartung H, Feldman B, Lovec H, et al: Murine FGF-12 and FGF-

13: expression in embryonic nervous system, connective tissue and heart. Mech Dev 64:31–39, 1997.
166. Hu MCT, Qiu WR, Wang YP, et al: FGF-18, a novel member of the fibroblast growth factor family, stimulates hepatic and intestinal proliferation. Mol Cell Biol 18:6063–6074, 1998.
167. Kok LD, Tsui SK, Wayne M, et al: Cloning and characterization of a cDNA encoding a novel fibroblast growth factor preferentially expressed in human heart. Biochem Biophys Res Commun 255:717–721, 1999.
168. Zhou M, Sutliff RL, Paul RJ, et al: Fibroblast growth factor 2 control of vascular tone. Nat Med 4:201–207, 1998.
169. Deng C-X, Wynshaw-Boris A, Shen MM, et al: Murine FGFR-1 is required for early postimplantation growth and axial organization. Genes Dev 8:3045–3057, 1994.
170. Yamaguchi TP, Harpal K, Henkmeyer M, Rossant J: *fgfr*-1 is required for embryonic growth and mesodermal patterning during mouse gastrulation. Genes Dev 8:3032–3044, 1994.
171. Mima T, Ueno H, Fischman DA, et al: Fibroblast growth factor receptor is required for in vivo cardiac myocyte proliferation at early embryonic stages of heart development. Proc Natl Acad Sci U S A 92:467–471, 1995.
172. Letterio JJ, Geiser AG, Kulkarni AB, et al: Maternal rescue of transforming growth factor-beta 1 null mice. Science 264:1936–1938, 1994.
173. Meyer D, Birchmeier C: Multiple essential functions of neuregulin in development. Nature 378:386–390, 1995.
174. Kramer R, Bucay N, Kane DJ, et al: Neuregulins with an Ig-like domain are essential for mouse myocardial and neuronal development. Proc Natl Acad Sci U S A 93:4833–4838, 1996.
175. Liu X, Hwang H, Cao L, et al: Domain-specific gene disruption reveals critical regulation of neuregulin signaling by its cytoplasmic tail. Proc Natl Acad Sci U S A 95:13024–13029, 1998.
176. Lee KF, Simon H, Chen H, et al: Requirement for neuregulin receptor ErbB2 in neural and cardiac development. Nature 378:394–398, 1995.
177. Gassmann M, Casagranda F, Orioli D, et al: Aberrant neural and cardiac development in mice lacking the ErbB4 neuregulin receptor. Nature 378:390–394, 1995.
178. Zhao JJ, Lemke G: Selective disruption of neuregulin-1 function in vertebrate embryos using ribozyme-tRNA transgenes. Development 125:1899–1907, 1998.
179. Yoshida K, Taga T, Saito M, et al: Targeted disruption of gp130, a common signal transducer for the interleukin 6 family of cytokines, leads to myocardial and hematological disorders. Proc Natl Acad Sci U S A 93:407–411, 1996.
180. Hirota H, Yoshida K, Kishimoto T, Taga T: Continuous activation of gp130, a signal-transducing receptor component for interleukin 6-related cytokines, causes myocardial hypertrophy in mice. Proc Natl Acad Sci U S A 92:4862–4866, 1995.
181. Pennica D, King KL, Shaw KJ, et al: Expression cloning of cardiotrophin 1, a cytokine that induces cardiac myocyte hypertrophy. Proc Natl Acad Sci U S A 92:1142–1146, 1995.
182. Sheng ZL, Pennica D, Wood WI, Chien KR: Cardiotrophin-1 displays early expression in the murine heart tube and promotes cardiac myocyte survival. Development 122:419–428, 1996.
183. Sheng ZL, Knowlton K, Chen J, et al: Cardiotrophin 1 (CT-1) inhibition of cardiac myocyte apoptosis via a mitogen-activated protein kinase-dependent pathway: divergence from downstream CT-1 signals for myocardial cell hypertrophy. J Biol Chem 272:5783–5791, 1997.
184. Betz UAK, Bloch W, vandenBroek M, et al: Postnatally induced inactivation of gp130 in mice results in neurological, cardiac, hematopoietic, immunological, hepatic, and pulmonary defects. J Exp Med 188:1955–1965, 1998.
185. Sucov HM, Dyson E, Gumeringer CL, et al: RXR alpha mutant mice establish a genetic basis for vitamin A signaling in heart morphogenesis. Genes Dev 8:1007–1018, 1994.
186. Kastner P, Grondona JM, Mark M, et al: Genetic analysis of RXR alpha developmental function: convergence of RXR and RAR signaling pathways in heart and eye morphogenesis. Cell 78:987–1003, 1994.
187. Chen J, Kubalak SW, Chien KR: Ventricular muscle-restricted targeting of the RXR alpha gene reveals a non-cell-autonomous requirement in cardiac chamber morphogenesis. Development 125:1943–1949, 1998.
188. Jaber M, Koch WJ, Rockman H, et al: Essential role of beta-adrenergic receptor kinase 1 in cardiac development and function. Proc Natl Acad Sci U S A 93:12974–12979, 1996.
189. Jacks T, Shih TS, Schmitt EM, et al: Tumour predisposition in mice heterozygous for a targeted mutation in Nf1. Nat Genet 7:353–361, 1994.
190. Brannan CI, Perkins AS, Vogel KS, et al: Targeted disruption of the neurofibromatosis type-1 gene leads to developmental abnormalities in heart and various neural crest-derived tissues. Genes Dev 8:1019–1029, 1994.
191. Kreidberg JA, Sariola H, Loring JM, et al: WT-1 is required for early kidney development. Cell 74:679–691, 1993.
192. Moens CB, Stanton BR, Parada LF, Rossant J: Defects in heart and lung development in compound heterozygotes for two different targeted mutations at the N-myc locus. Development 119:485–499, 1993.
193. Yao TP, Oh SP, Fuchs M, et al: Gene dosage-dependent embryonic development and proliferation defects in mice lacking the transcriptional integrator p300. Cell 93:361–372, 1998.
194. Puri PL, Avantaggiati ML, Balsano C, et al: p300 is required for MyoD-dependent cell cycle arrest and muscle-specific gene transcription. EMBO J 16:369–383, 1997.
195. Puri PL, Sartorelli V, Yang XJ, et al: Differential roles of p300 and PCAF acetyltransferases in muscle differentiation. Mol Cell 1:35–45, 1997.
196. Kirshenbaum LA, Schneider MD: Adenovirus E1A represses cardiac gene transcription and reactivates DNA synthesis in ventricular myocytes, via alternative pocket protein- and p300-binding domains. J Biol Chem 270:7791–7794, 1995.
197. Bishopric NH, Zeng GQ, Sato B, Webster KA: Adenovirus E1A inhibits cardiac myocyte-specific gene expression through its amino terminus. J Biol Chem 272:20584–20594, 1997.
198. Sartorelli V, Huang J, Hamamori Y, Kedes L: Molecular mechanisms of myogenic coactivation by p300: direct interaction with the activation domain of MyoD and with the MADS box of MEF2C. Mol Cell Biol 17:1010–1026, 1997.
199. Shou WN, Aghdasi B, Armstrong DL, et al: Cardiac defects and altered ryanodine receptor function in mice lacking FKBP12. Nature 391:489–492, 1998.
200. Wang TW, Donahoe PK, Zervos AS: Specific interaction of type I receptors of the TGF-beta family with the immunophilin FKBP-12. Science 265:674–676, 1994.
201. Marks AR: Cellular functions of immunophilins. Physiol Rev 76:631–649, 1996.
202. Charng M-J, Kinnunen P, Hawker J, et al: FKBP-12 recognition is dispensable for signal generation by type I TGFβ receptors. J Biol Chem 271:22941–22944, 1996.
203. Bassing CH, Shou WN, Muir S, et al: FKBP12 is not required for the modulation of transforming growth factor beta receptor I signaling activity in embryonic fibroblasts and thymocytes. Cell Growth Differ 9:223–228, 1998.
204. Wakamiya M, Lindsay EA, Rivera-Perez JA, et al: Functional analysis of Gscl in the pathogenesis of the DiGeorge and velocardiofacial syndromes. Hum Mol Genet 7:1835–1840, 1998.
205. Saint-Jore B, Puech A, Heyer J, et al: Goosecoid-like (Gscl), a candidate gene for velocardiofacial syndrome, is not essential for normal mouse development. Hum Mol Genet 7:1841–1849, 1998.
206. Ramirez-Solis R, Liu P, Bradley A: Chromosome engineering in mice. Nature 378:720–724, 1995.
207. Farrell MJ, Stadt H, Wallis KT, et al: HIRA, a DiGeorge syndrome candidate gene, is required for cardiac outflow tract septation. Circ Res 84:127–135, 1999.
208. Kispert A, Koschorz B, Herrmann BG: The T protein encoded by brachyury is a tissue-specific transcription factor. EMBO J 14:4763–4772, 1995.
209. Smith J: Brachyury and the T-box genes. Curr Opin Genet Dev 7:474–480, 1997.
210. Papaioannou VE, Silver LM: The T-box gene family. Bioessays 20:9–19, 1998.
211. Conlon FL, Sedgwick SG, Weston KM, Smith JC: Inhibition of Xbra transcription activation causes defects in mesodermal patterning and reveals autoregulation of Xbra in dorsal mesoderm. Development 122:2427–2435, 1996.
212. Agulnik SI, Papaioannou VE, Silver LM: Cloning, mapping, and expression analysis of TBX15, a new member of the T-Box gene family. Genomics 51:68–75, 1998.

213. Basson CT, Huang TS, Lin RC, et al: Different TBX5 interactions in heart and limb defined by Holt-Oram syndrome mutations. Proc Natl Acad Sci U S A 96:2919–2924, 1999.
214. Casey B: Two rights make a wrong: human left-right malformations. Hum Mol Genet 7:1565–1571, 1998.
215. Gebbia M, Ferrero GB, Pilia G, et al: X-linked situs abnormalities result from mutations in ZIC3. Nat Genet 17:305–308, 1997.
216. Nakata K, Nagai T, Aruga J, Mikoshiba K: Xenopus Zic3, a primary regulator both in neural and neural crest development. Proc Natl Acad Sci U S A 94:11980–11985, 1997.
217. Nagai T, Aruga J, Takada S, et al: The expression of the mouse Zic1, Zic2, and Zic3 gene suggests an essential role for Zic genes in body pattern formation. Dev Biol 182:299–313, 1997.
218. Kosaki R, Gebbia M, Kosaki K, et al: Left-right axis malformations associated with mutations in ACVR2B, the gene for human activin receptor type IIB. Am J Med Genet 82:70–76, 1999.
219. Britz-Cunningham SH, Shah MM, Zuppan CW, Fletcher WH: Mutations of the Connexin 43 gap-junction gene in patients with heart malformations and defects of laterality. N Engl J Med 332:1323–1329, 1995.
220. Gebbia M, Towbin JA, Casey B: Failure to detect connexin43 mutations in 38 cases of sporadic and familial heterotaxy. Circulation 94:1909–1912, 1996.
221. Penman Splitt M, Tsai MY, Burn J, Goodship JA: Absence of mutations in the regulatory domain of the gap junction protein connexin 43 in patients with visceroatrial heterotaxy. Heart 77:369–370, 1997.
222. Chen CY, Schwartz RJ: Recruitment of the tinman homolog nkx-2.5 by serum response factor activates cardiac alpha-actin gene transcription. Mol Cell Biol 16:6372–6384, 1996.
223. Schott JJ, Benson DW, Basson CT, et al: Congenital heart disease caused by mutations in the transcription factor NKX2-5. Science 281:108–111, 1998.
224. Biben C, Hatzistavrou T, Harvey RP: Expression of NK-2 class homeobox gene Nkx2-6 in foregut endoderm and heart. Mech Dev 73:125–127, 1998.
225. Tanaka M, Kasahara H, Bartunkova S, et al: Vertebrate homologs of tinman and bagpipe: roles of the homeobox genes in cardiovascular development. Dev Genet 22:239–249, 1998.
226. Tanaka M, Chen Z, Bartunkova S, et al: The cardiac homeobox gene Csx/Nkx2.5 lies genetically upstream of multiple genes essential for heart development. Development 126:1269–1280, 1999.
227. Takahashi N, Calderone A, Izzo NJ, et al: Hypertrophic stimuli induce transforming growth factor-beta(1) expression in rat ventricular myocytes. J Clin Invest 94:1470–1476, 1994.
228. Donohue TJ, Dworkin LD, Ma JX, et al: Antihypertensive agents that limit ventricular hypertrophy inhibit cardiac expression of insulin-like growth factor-I. J Invest Med 45:584–591, 1997.
229. Baker KM, Chernin MI, Wixson SK, Aceto JF: Renin-angiotensin system involvement in pressure-overload cardiac hypertrophy in rats. Am J Physiol 259:H324–H332, 1990.
230. Yorikane R, Sakai S, Miyauchi T, et al: Increased production of endothelin-1 in the hypertrophied rat heart due to pressure overload. FEBS Lett 332:31–34, 1993.
231. Ishikawa M, Saito Y, Miyamoto Y, et al: cDNA cloning of rat cardiotrophin-1 (CT-1): augmented expression of CT-1 gene in ventricle of genetically hypertensive rats. Biochem Biophys Res Commun 219:377–381, 1996.
232. Parker TG, Chow K-L, Schwartz RJ, Schneider MD: Differential regulation of skeletal α-actin transcription in cardiac muscle by two fibroblast growth factors. Proc Natl Acad Sci U S A 87:7066–7070, 1990.
233. Shubeita HE, McDonough PM, Harris AN, et al: Endothelin induction of inositol phospholipid hydrolysis, sarcomere assembly, and cardiac gene expression in ventricular myocytes: a paracrine mechanism for myocardial cell hypertrophy. J Biol Chem 265:20555–20562, 1990.
234. Sadoshima J, Izumo S: Rapamycin selectively inhibits angiotensin II-induced increase in protein synthesis in cardiac myocytes in vitro: potential role of 70-kD S6 kinase in angiotensin II-induced cardiac hypertrophy. Circ Res 77:1040–1052, 1995.
235. Komuro I, Yazaki Y: Control of cardiac gene expression by mechanical stress. Annu Rev Physiol 55:55–75, 1993.
236. Sadoshima J, Izumo S: The cellular and molecular response of cardiac myocytes to mechanical stress. Annu Rev Physiol 59:551–571, 1997.
237. Parker TG, Schneider MD: Growth factors, proto-oncogenes, and plasticity of the cardiac phenotype. Annu Rev Physiol 53:179–200, 1991.
238. Bishopric NH, Jayasena V, Webster KA: Positive regulation of the skeletal alpha-actin gene by fos and jun in cardiac myocytes. J Biol Chem 267:25535–25540, 1992.
239. Paradis P, Maclellan WR, Belaguli NS, et al: Serum response factor mediates AP-1-dependent induction of the skeletal alpha-actin promoter in ventricular myocytes. J Biol Chem 271:10827–10833, 1996.
240. McDonough PM, Hanford DS, Sprenkle AB, et al: Collaborative roles for c-Jun N-terminal kinase, c-Jun, serum response factor, and Sp1 in calcium-regulated myocardial gene expression. J Biol Chem 272:24046–24053, 1997.
241. Kim SJ, Angel P, Lafyatis R, et al: Autoinduction of transforming growth factor beta 1 is mediated by the AP-1 complex. Mol Cell Biol 10:1492–1497, 1990.
242. Thompson JT, Rackley MS, O'Brien TX: Upregulation of the cardiac homeobox gene Nkx2-5 (CSX) in feline right ventricular pressure overload. Am J Physiol 43:H1569–H1573, 1998.
243. Molkentin JD, Markham BE: Myocyte-specific enhancer-binding factor (MEF-2) regulates alpha-cardiac myosin heavy chain gene expression in vitro and in vivo. J Biol Chem 268:19512–19520, 1993.
244. Hasegawa K, Lee SJ, Jobe SM, et al: cis-acting sequences that mediate induction of beta-myosin heavy chain gene expression during left ventricular hypertrophy due to aortic constriction. Circulation 96:3943–3953, 1997.
245. Herzig TC, Jobe SM, Aoki H, et al: Angiotensin II type(1a) receptor gene expression in the heart: AP-1 and GATA-4 participate in the response to pressure overload. Proc Natl Acad Sci U S A 94:7543–7548, 1997.
246. Karns LR, Kariya K, Simpson PC: M-CAT, CArG, and Sp1 elements are required for alpha(1)-adrenergic induction of the skeletal alpha-actin promoter during cardiac myocyte hypertrophy: transcriptional enhancer factor-1 and protein kinase C as conserved transducers of the fetal program in cardiac growth. J Biol Chem 270:410–417, 1995.
247. Thuerauf DJ, Arnold ND, Zechner D, et al: p38 mitogen-activated protein kinase mediates the transcriptional induction of the atrial natriuretic factor gene through a serum response element: a potential role for the transcription factor ATF6. J Biol Chem 273:20636–20643, 1998.
248. Kodama H, Fukuda K, Pan J, et al: Leukemia inhibitory factor, a potent cardiac hypertrophic cytokine, activates the JAK/STAT pathway in rat cardiomyocytes. Circ Res 81:656–663, 1997.
249. Kunisada K, Tone E, Fujio Y, et al: Activation of gp130 transduces hypertrophic signals via STAT3 in cardiac myocytes. Circulation 98:346–352, 1998.
250. Bhat GJ, Thekkumkara TJ, Thomas WG, et al: Angiotensin II stimulates sis-inducing factor-like DNA binding activity: evidence that the AT(1A) receptor activates transcription factor-Stat91 and/or a related protein. J Biol Chem 269:31443–31449, 1994.
251. Mascareno E, Dhar M, Siddiqui MA: Signal transduction and activator of transcription (STAT) protein-dependent activation of angiotensinogen promoter: a cellular signal for hypertrophy in cardiac muscle. Proc Natl Acad Sci U S A 95:5590–5594, 1998.
252. Pan J, Fukuda K, Kodama H, et al: Role of angiotensin II in activation of the JAK/STAT pathway induced by acute pressure overload in the rat heart. Circ Res 81:611–617, 1997.
253. Sussman MA, Lim HW, Gude N, et al: Prevention of cardiac hypertrophy in mice by calcineurin inhibition. Science 281:1690–1693, 1998.
254. Mende U, Kagen A, Cohen A, et al: Transient cardiac expression of constitutively active $G_{\alpha q}$ leads to hypertrophy and dilated cardiomyopathy by calcineurin-dependent and independent pathways. Proc Natl Acad Sci U S A 95:13893–13898, 1998.
255. Luo Z, Shyu KG, Gualberto A, Walsh K: Calcineurin inhibitors and cardiac hypertrophy. Nat Med 4:1092–1093, 1998.
256. Gwathmey JK, Copelas L, MacKinnon R, et al: Abnormal intracellular calcium handling in myocardium from patients with end-stage heart failure. Circ Res 61:70–76, 1987.
257. Beuckelmann DJ, Nabauer M, Erdmann E: Intracellular calcium handling in isolated ventricular myocytes from patients with terminal heart failure. Circulation 85:1046–1055, 1992.

258. Schroder F, Handrock R, Bueckelmann DJ, et al: Increased availability and open probability of single L-type calcium channels from failing compared with nonfailing human ventricle. Circulation 98:969–976, 1998.
259. Anversa P, Kajstura J: Ventricular myocytes are not terminally differentiated in the adult mammalian heart. Circ Res 83:1–14, 1998.
260. Soonpaa MH, Field LJ: Survey of studies examining mammalian cardiomyocyte DNA synthesis. Circ Res 83:15–26, 1998.
261. Olson EN: Interplay between proliferation and differentiation within the myogenic lineage. Dev Biol 154:261–272, 1992.
262. Lassar AB, Skapek SX, Novitch B: Regulatory mechanisms that coordinate skeletal muscle differentiation and cell cycle withdrawal. Curr Opin Cell Biol 6:788–794, 1994.
263. Stillman B: Cell cycle control of DNA replication. Science 274:1659–1664, 1996.
264. MacLellan WR, Schneider MD: The cardiac cell cycle. *In* Harvey R, Rosenthal N (eds): Cardiac Development. pp. 405–427. San Diego: Academic, 1998.
265. Gu W, Schneider JW, Condorelli G, et al: Interaction of myogenic factors and the retinoblastoma protein mediates muscle cell commitment and differentiation. Cell 72:309–324, 1993.
266. Schneider JW, Gu W, Zhu L, et al: Reversal of terminal differentiation mediated by p107 in Rb(−/−) muscle cells. Science 264:1467–1471, 1994.
267. Soonpaa MH, Kim KK, Pajak L, et al: Cardiomyocyte DNA synthesis and binucleation during murine development. Am J Physiol 271:H2183–H2189, 1996.
268. Kang MJ, Kim JS, Chae SW, et al: Cyclins and cyclin dependent kinases during cardiac development. Mol Cells 7:360–366, 1997.
269. Soonpaa MH, Koh GY, Pajak L, et al: Cyclin D1 overexpression promotes cardiomyocyte DNA synthesis and multinucleation in transgenic mice. J Clin Invest 99:2644–2654, 1997.
270. Brooks G, Poolman RA, McGill CJ, Li JM: Expression and activities of cyclins and cyclin dependent kinases in developing rat ventricular myocytes. J Mol Cell Cardiol 29:2261–2271, 1997.
271. Poolman RA, Brooks G: Expressions and activities of cell cycle regulatory molecules during the transition from myocyte hyperplasia to hypertrophy. J Mol Cell Cardiol 30:2121–2135, 1998.
272. Flink IL, Oana S, Maitra N, et al: Changes in E2F complexes containing retinoblastoma protein family members and increased cyclin-dependent kinase inhibitor activities during terminal differentiation of cardiomyocytes. J Mol Cell Cardiol 30:563–578, 1998.
273. Quelle DE, Ashmun RA, Hannon GJ, et al: Cloning and characterization of murine p16(INK4a) and p15(INK4b) genes. Oncogene 11:635–645, 1995.
274. Guan KL, Jenkins CW, Li Y, et al: Growth suppression by p18, a p16INK4/MTS1- and p14INK4B/MTS2-related CDK6 inhibitor, correlates with wild-type pRb function. Genes Dev 8:2939–2952, 1994.
275. Liu Q, Dawes NJ, Lu Y, et al: Alpha-adrenergic stimulation induces phosphorylation of retinoblastoma protein in neonatal rat ventricular myocytes. Biochem J 327:299–303, 1997.
276. Sadoshima J, Aoki H, Izumo S: Angiotensin II and serum differentially regulate expression of cyclins, activity of cyclin-dependent kinases, and phosphorylation of retinoblastoma gene product in neonatal cardiac myocytes. Circ Res 80:228–241, 1997.
277. Kirshenbaum LA, Abdellatif M, Chakraborty S, Schneider MD: Human E2F-1 reactivates cell cycle progression in ventricular myocytes and represses cardiac gene transcription. Dev Biol 179:402–411, 1996.
278. Liu Y, Kitsis RN: Induction of DNA synthesis and apoptosis in cardiac myocytes by E1A oncoprotein. J Cell Biol 133:325–334, 1996.
279. Agah R, Kirschenbaum LA, Truong LD, et al: Adenoviral delivery of E2F-1 directs cell cycle re-entry and p53-independent apoptosis in post-mitotic adult myocardium in vivo. J Clin Invest 100:2722–2728, 1997.
280. Clarke AR, Maandag ER, van Roon M, et al: Requirement for a functional Rb-1 gene in murine development. Nature 359:328–330, 1992.
281. Jacks T, Fazeli A, Schmitt EM, et al: Effects of an Rb mutation in the mouse. Nature 359:295–300, 1992.
282. Lee EYHP, Chang CY, Hu NP, et al: Mice deficient for Rb are nonviable and show defects in neurogenesis and haematopoiesis. Nature 359:288–294, 1992.
283. Rajewsky K, Gu H, Kuhn R, et al: Conditional gene targeting. J Clin Invest 98:600–603, 1996.
284. Rossant J, McMahon A: "Cre"-ating mouse mutants: a meeting review on conditional mouse genetics. Genes Dev 13:142–145, 1999.
285. MacLellan WR, Frenkel PA, Vooijs M, et al: Cardiac-restricted gene targeting of the retinoblastoma gene using the Cre/LoxP system. Circulation 98(suppl I):I-608, 1998.
286. Brugarolas J, Chandrasekaran C, Gordon JI, et al: Radiation-induced cell cycle arrest compromised by p21 deficiency. Nature 377:552–557, 1995.
287. Deng CX, Zhang PM, Harper JW, et al: Mice lacking p21(C/P1/WAF1) undergo normal development, but are defective in G1 checkpoint control. Cell 82:675–684, 1995.
288. Fero ML, Rivkin M, Tasch M, et al: A syndrome of multiorgan hyperplasia with features of gigantism, tumorigenesis, and female sterility in p27(Kip1)-deficient mice. Cell 85:733–744, 1996.
289. Kiyokawa H, Kineman RD, Manovatodorova KO, et al: Enhanced growth of mice lacking the cyclin-dependent kinase inhibitor function of p27(Kip1). Cell 85:721–732, 1996.
290. Nakayama K, Ishida N, Shirane M, et al: Mice lacking p27(Kip1) display increased body size, multiple organ hyperplasia, retinal dysplasia, and pituitary tumors. Cell 85:707–720, 1996.
291. Franklin DS, Godfrey VL, Lee HY, et al: CDK inhibitors p18(INK4c) and p27(Kip1) mediate two separate pathways to collaboratively suppress pituitary tumorigenesis. Gene Dev 12:2899–2911, 1998.
292. Potts JD, Dagle JM, Walder JA, et al: Epithelial-mesenchymal transformation of cardiac endothelial cells is inhibited by a modified antisense oligodesoxynucleotide to TGFβ3. Proc Natl Acad Sci U S A 88:1516–1520, 1991.
293. Brown CB, Boyer AS, Runyan RB, Barnett JV: Antibodies to the type II TGF beta receptor block cell activation and migration during atrioventricular cushion transformation in the heart. Dev Biol 174:248–257, 1996.
294. Ramsdell AF, Markwald RR: Induction of endocardial cushion tissue in the avian heart is regulated, in part, by TFG beta-3-mediated autocrine signaling. Dev Biol 188:64–74, 1997.
295. Nakajima Y, Yamagishi T, Nakamura H, et al: An autocrine function for transforming growth factor (TGF)-beta 3 in the transformation of atrioventricular canal endocardium into mesenchyme during chick heart development. Dev Biol 194:99–113, 1998.
296. de la Pompa JL, Timmerman LA, Takimoto H, et al: Role of the NF-ATc transcription factor in morphogenesis of cardiac valves and septum. Nature 392:182–186, 1998.
297. Cleaver O, Krieg PA: Molecular mechanisms of vascular development. *In* Harvey RP, Rosenthal N (eds): Heart Development. pp. 221–252. San Diego: Academic, 1998.

CHAPTER 45

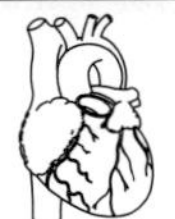

FUELS FOR THE HEART

Heinrich Taegtmeyer

BETWEEN GENOMICS AND ENERGETICS: FUEL METABOLISM IN PERSPECTIVE
HEART MUSCLE: CONSUMER AND PROVIDER OF ENERGY
ENERGY TRANSFER
METABOLIC PATHWAYS: THE HIGHWAYS OF ENERGY TRANSFER
"NUTRITION OF THE HEART"
SUBSTRATE COMPETITION
TRACING METABOLIC PATHWAYS
FUELS FOR THE HEART: METABOLISM OF THE MAJOR ENERGY-PROVIDING SUBSTRATES
Carbohydrates
Regulatory Sites of Glucose Metabolism
Fatty Acids
Ketone Bodies
Amino Acids
CONCLUSIONS
OUTLOOK

From the perspective of a practicing cardiologist, the advances of molecular biology have brought an important principle to light: Progress in the diagnosis and treatment of heart disease is directly related to the understanding of basic biologic concepts. What applies to the *chemistry* of gene regulation (the long-term regulation of cardiac function) also applies to the *chemistry* of fuel metabolism (the short-term regulation of cardiac function). Like any organ of the mammalian body, the heart consists of a complex system of interactive proteins, purine bases, energy-providing compounds, membranes, and signal molecules that are in a constant state of flux. In this dynamic system, the heart has retained its ability to adapt to a multitude of environmental changes, either by altering the synthesis of specific proteins[1–3] or by acutely changing flux through metabolic pathways to maintain its energy supply.[4] At a genomic level, we are now faced with the dilemma of a vast number of novel candidate genes and an inadequate understanding of underlying pathophysiologic events.[5] Fuel metabolism is perhaps the best example of a system in which a reductionist approach in vitro requires an understanding of the interaction of these gene products in the context of the whole organ. Unfortunately, there is only a small pool of scientists sufficiently trained to address these issues. Only the most severe environmental changes, such as those induced by an interruption of oxygen supply, create a clear-cut picture. They result in a collapse of energy production and, consequently, in a collapse of the circulation of blood.

BETWEEN GENOMICS AND ENERGETICS: FUEL METABOLISM IN PERSPECTIVE

Heart muscle derives its energy from the oxidative metabolism of fuels. The word metabolism was contrived by Theodore Schwann from the Greek word for change.[6] Not surprisingly, the central dogma of metabolism can also be traced to antiquity. In the 5th century BC, the historian Heraclitus already taught that all processes of life are in flux. In the 20th century, research on substrate metabolism has been the subject of intense research.[6] Progress in the understanding of metabolic regulation in heart muscle is closely linked to advances in biochemical and physiologic methods. Furthermore, research in cardiac metabolism has always been an integrative part of cardiac physiology. It is impossible to separate cardiac function from metabolism. As shown in the schematic in Figure 45–1, a decrease in the flux of metabolic energy results in a decrease in contractile function, and vice versa. It is not surprising that many of the advances in understanding of fuel metabolism in the heart have resulted from the introduction of new methods to assess metabolic activity in the intact, beating heart (such as nuclear magnetic resonance spectroscopy or magnetic resonance imaging [MRI]) or in the heart in vivo (such as positron emission tomography [PET]). A major feature of these new technologies is that they may permit a distinction

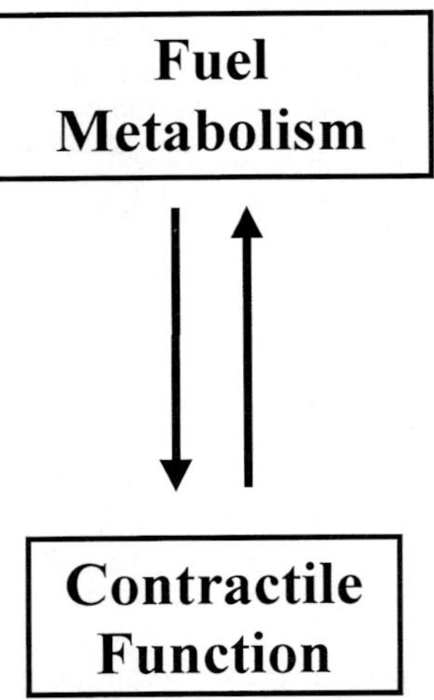

FIGURE 45–1 Fuels provide the energy for contraction of the heart. Fuel metabolism and contractile function are inseparably connected.

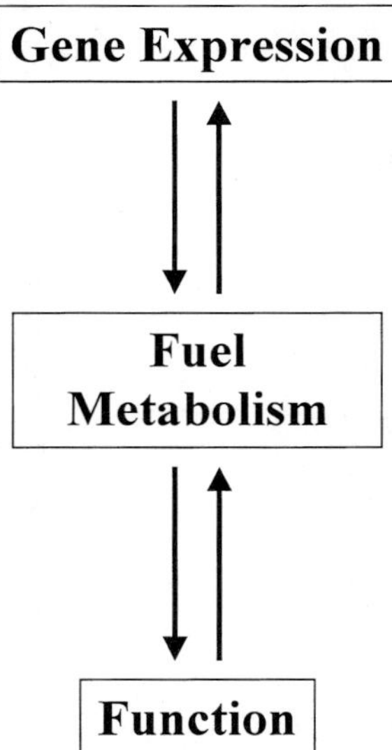

FIGURE 45–2 The enzymes of fuel metabolism are gene products. In this scheme, fuel metabolism is the link between gene expression and contractile function.

between heart muscle that is reversibly dysfunctional and heart muscle that is irreversibly damaged.

Research on biochemistry of the heart dates back to the end of the 19th century.[7] Many excellent and detailed papers on cardiac metabolism have appeared since the classical reviews by Evans[8] and Bing.[9] By measuring arteriovenous differences in the heart-lung preparation of the dog or in the human heart through cannulation of the coronary sinus, these two researchers have laid the foundation for our current understanding of myocardial substrate metabolism. The more recent reviews survey the knowledge gained through isolated heart preparations, isolated cell preparations, and isolated cell organelles.[10–15] Monographs on cardiac physiology and metabolism such as those of Opie,[16] of Langer,[17] and of Katz and colleagues,[18] as well as a collection of papers on myocardial energy metabolism from deJong,[19] serve as a repository of this knowledge. Since factual information can be gathered from these reviews, this chapter is limited to principles of cardiac metabolism as they may be relevant to the patient with heart disease. It is intended to provide a conceptual framework only. I shall place emphasis on the well-established concept that genes control enzymes[20] and on our more recent hypothesis[21] that metabolism links gene expression and function of the heart (Fig. 45–2). Important topics such as the metabolic responses to myocardial ischemia, signal transduction, membrane biochemistry, Ca^{2+} metabolism, myocardial protein turnover, and programmed cell death are discussed elsewhere in this book. We have recently reviewed metabolic aspects of programmed cell survival[22] and the concept of metabolic support for the reperfused heart that is gaining clinical acceptance.[23] However, what appeared at the time as a culmination of thought may be just a beginning. The present chapter must be read in this spirit.

HEART MUSCLE: CONSUMER AND PROVIDER OF ENERGY

The goal of cardiac metabolism is to maintain a dynamic state of equilibrium for efficient energy transfer in a highly specialized organ. Like the torch, familiar from the logo of the American Heart Association, heart muscle consumes energy locked in chemical bonds of fuels. In so doing, heart muscle converts chemical energy into physical energy. Unlike the torch, the physical energy of the heart consists of pump work (mechanical energy) that, in turn, distributes energy in the form of substrates and oxygen both to the heart itself and to the rest of the body. Thus, the heart has two important concepts, which must be considered. First, the heart is a "hot spot" of metabolic activity, continuously making and breaking adenosine triphosphate (ATP), the chemical energy available for conversion to mechanical energy at the contractile site (Fig. 45–3). The greater the work output, the higher the rate of ATP turnover, the higher the rate of oxygen consumption, and the higher the rate of substrate utilization. Second, when the heart's ability to convert chemical into mechanical energy is impaired for any reason,[24] the consequences lead to functional and metabolic abnormalities in the rest of the body, commonly referred to as *heart failure*. Although we distinguish between acute and chronic heart failure, both forms of heart failure are ultimately a systemic disease that begins and ends with the heart. Every organ in the human body is affected by an impairment of energy transfer in the heart. Understanding the regulation of energy transfer in the heart is the most important clue for understanding and treating heart failure.

Like other living organs, the human heart captures and uses energy in the form of ATP. The role of ATP as the main provider of chemical energy for the support of various cell functions was first postulated by Fritz Lipmann,[25] who drew attention to the biologic importance of the ATP–adenosine diphosphate (ADP) couple.[26] The rate of ATP turnover in the heart is far greater than in other organs of the body, and it is often underestimated. A simple calculation, based on measurements of myocardial oxygen consumption, indicates that during the course of a 24-hour period, the human heart produces (and uses) 5 kg of ATP (i.e., more than 10 times its own weight and 1000 times the amount of ATP stored in the heart). Another comparison comes to mind. Although the human heart makes up only 0.5 percent of total body weight, it claims 4 percent of total cardiac output and 10 percent of the body's oxygen

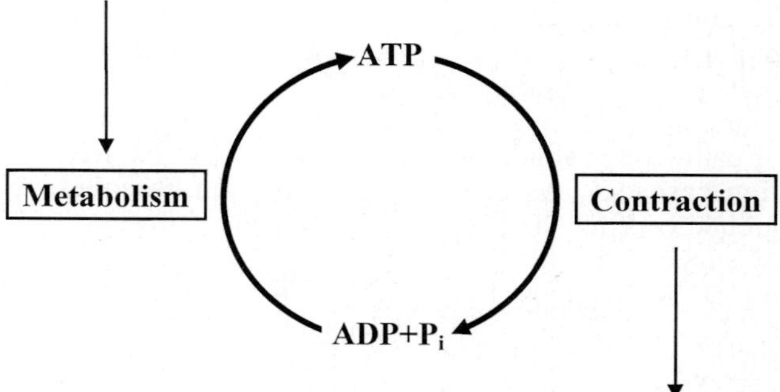

FIGURE 45–3 Adenosine triphosphate (ATP) cycle. Nature tends to conserve successful forms of energy production, including cycles such as the continuous cycle of ATP hydrolysis and resynthesis. In this way, the human heart produces (through oxidative phosphorylation) and uses many kilograms of ATP each day. ADP, adenosine diphosphate; P_i, inorganic phosphate. (Depre C, Taegtmeyer H: Metabolic aspects of programmed cell survival and cell death in the heart. Cardiovasc Res [in press].)

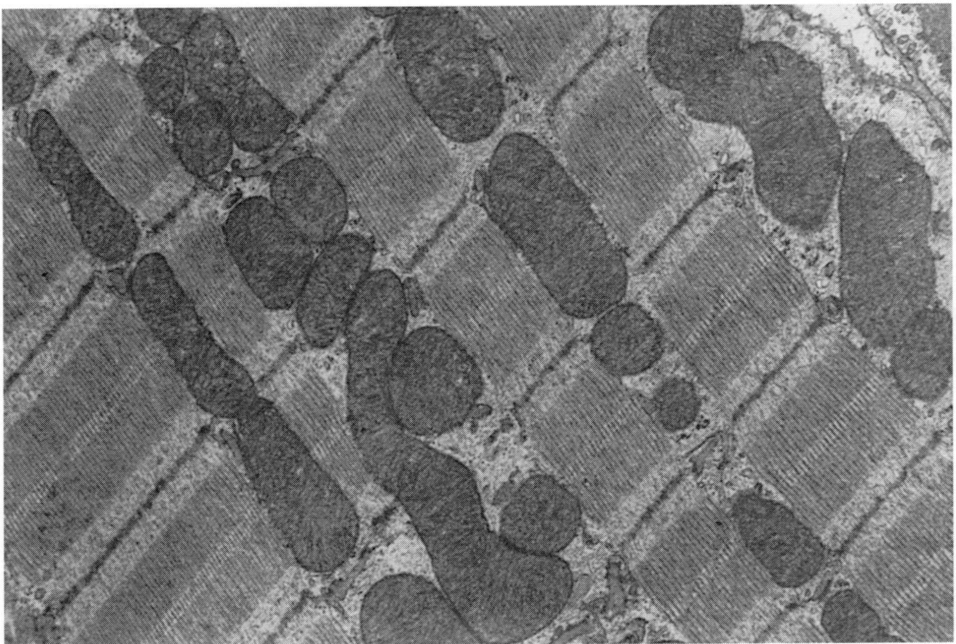

FIGURE 45–4 Ultrastructure of normal dog myocardium. The transmission electron micrograph shows, in addition to the regularly arranged contractile elements (sarcomeres), an abundance of mitochondria. Mitochondria are characterized by densely arranged cristae and constitute about 25 percent of the cell volume. A direct, positive correlation exists between the number of mitochondria, resting heart rate, and myocardial oxygen consumption. (×1800.) (Courtesy of Dr. W. Barry Van Winkle, Department of Pathology, University of Texas-Houston Medical School.)

consumption. Lastly, it is important to remember that it is the rate of energy turnover, and not the tissue content of ATP, that determines myocardial energy metabolism.[15, 27, 28] This statement holds true for an impaired creatine kinase system in failing hearts.[29]

The heart meets the bulk of its energy needs by oxidative phosphorylation of ADP. It is therefore not surprising that the capillary density in heart muscle is far greater than in other organs (2500 capillaries/mm^2 versus 400 capillaries/mm^2 in skeletal muscle)[30] and that heart muscle cells are filled with mitochondria, the cell organelles possessing the enzymes of oxidative metabolism (Fig. 45–4). A close correlation exists among mitochondrial volume fraction, heart rate, and total body oxygen consumption, with mitochondrial volume fractions ranging from 25 percent in humans to 38 percent in mice.[31] Not only are heart muscle mitochondria abundant, but they also contain a far greater number of cristae (the location of respiratory chain enzymes) than do mitochondria of other organs, such as liver, brain, or skeletal muscle.[32]

As stated earlier, energy metabolism of the heart cannot be considered separately from the transfer of energy in biologic systems. Defining the bewildering array of metabolic pathways in the cell (Fig. 45–5) is the result of many years of painstaking biochemical research. The unraveling of pathways is similar to the unraveling of signal transduction cascades. As in signal transduction cascades, the groundwork for the intertwined metabolic pathways is laid by enzyme-specific cardiac gene expression and by protein-protein interactions. Regulation of flux through the metabolic pathways is easy to understand with a basic knowledge of (1) energy transfer in biologic systems, (2) the nature of metabolic pathways, and (3) the purpose of enzyme-catalyzed reactions in heart muscle.

ENERGY TRANSFER

Energy transfer in biologic systems obeys the first and second laws of thermodynamics as defined by Helmholtz in 1845. The first law of thermodynamics states that within a closed system, energy can only be converted from one form into another. The second law of thermodynamics states that a process occurs spontaneously only if it is associated with an increase in randomness (or entropy) of the system.

Energy is captured from sunlight in the form of CH bonds in the process of photosynthesis, which also generates oxygen from water and carbon dioxide. The captured energy is, in turn, released through the reactions of intermediary metabolism that produce reducing equivalents (protons) to combine with molecular oxygen to form water (see later). Several important dehydrogenase reactions are linked to decarboxylation reactions (e.g., pyruvate dehydrogenase, isocitrate dehydrogenase, and 2-oxoglutarate dehydrogenase), resulting in the liberation of carbon dioxide. Carbon dioxide and water are, in turn, the substrates for photosynthesis. The description of this simple energy cycle emphasizes that heart muscle is an integral part of its biologic environment and that efficient energy transfer occurs through cyclic processes.

METABOLIC PATHWAYS: THE HIGHWAYS OF ENERGY TRANSFER

A characteristic property of all living cells, including heart muscle, is that complex chemical reactions can proceed rapidly at a relatively low temperature and at low substrate concentrations. The efficient transfer of energy occurs via enzyme-catalyzed pathways. At the center of these pathways are cycles. As is discussed, cycles have evolved as the most efficient form of energy transfer.[33] A *metabolic pathway* is defined as a series of enzyme-catalyzed reactions beginning with a flux-generating step (usually a reaction catalyzed by a nonequilibrium reaction or transport of

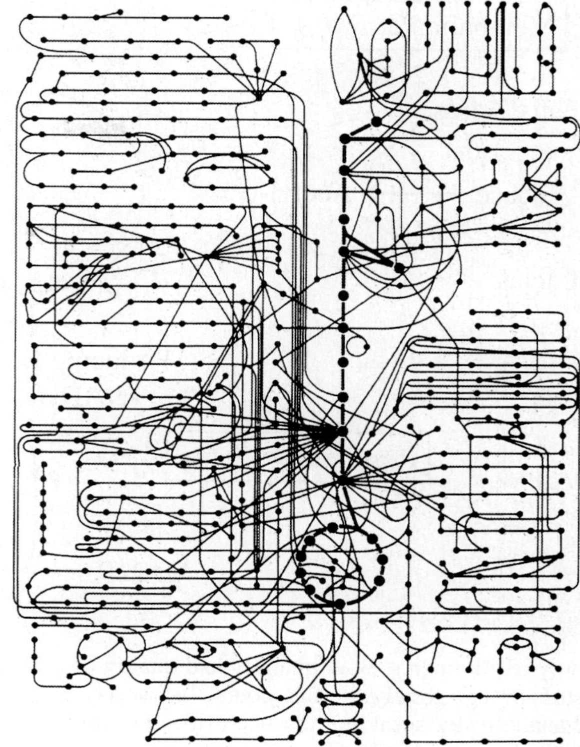

FIGURE 45–5 Representation of the maze of metabolic pathways. Each *dot* represents a metabolite and each *line* an enzyme. The glycolytic pathway, Krebs citric acid cycle, and respiratory chain are drawn in *heavy lines*. Like a chain reaction, the enzymes respond in concert to changes in the flux through a metabolic pathway. Although it has been the aim of biochemical research since the beginning of this century to define an unbroken sequence of reactions inside the cell, regulation of metabolic pathways is still not completely understood. (From Alberts B, Bray D, Lewis J, et al. Molecular Biology of the Cell. 3rd ed. p. 83. New York, Garland Publishing, 1994.)

the metabolite across a membrane) and ending with the removal of a product.[34, 35] Characteristic of most metabolic pathways is that once flux has been initiated, there is a rapid and concerted response of the entire pathway. In this system of flux, metabolite levels control enzyme activities and, in turn, enzyme activities control metabolite levels. It is important to distinguish between *control* and *regulation* of metabolism. *Metabolic control* is the power to change the state of metabolism in response to an external signal, whereas *metabolic regulation* is geared toward maintaining a constant internal state.[36] In such a system, large changes in the flux through metabolic pathways correspond to only very small changes in myocardial metabolite concentration.[37] Regulatory sites of metabolism, or *pacemaker enzymes,*[38] may become targets for the manipulation of metabolism with drugs.[21]

In the heart, the purpose of most enzyme-catalyzed reactions is catabolic: Substrates of high potential energy are broken down to products of lower potential energy. Synthetic or anabolic reactions, such as those serving protein, glycogen, or triglyceride synthesis, are quantitatively of lesser importance. In other words, heart muscle is endowed with an efficient system of energy transfer that liberates energy locked in chemical bonds by the generation of reducing equivalents and their reaction with molecular oxygen in the mitochondrial electron transport chain. *The main purpose of intermediary metabolism in normal heart muscle is therefore the production of reducing equivalents for ATP synthesis,*[39] in the course of which fuels are turned into carbon dioxide and water.

The breakdown of substrates can be divided into three stages (Fig. 45–6). The first stage consists of metabolic pathways that convert substrates to acetyl coenzyme A (acetyl-CoA); the second stage consists of the oxidation of acetyl-CoA in the Krebs cycle; and the third stage consists of the reaction of reducing equivalents with molecular oxygen in the respiratory chain, where electron transfer is coupled to rephosphorylation of ADP to ATP. As ATP production is tightly coupled to ATP utilization, so too is substrate oxidation coupled to cardiac work.[40–44] In the presence of adequate substrate supply, the maximal rate of substrate oxidation is determined by the capacity of the 2-oxoglutarate dehydrogenase reaction in the citric acid cycle and by the capacity of the respiratory chain.[45] The exact mechanism by which respiration is coupled to energy expenditure in vivo is, however, not known.[37, 39, 46] In contrast, the efficacy of oxidative phosphorylation for energy production is well established. For example, 1 mol of glucose, when oxidized, yields 36 mols of ATP, whereas the same amount of glucose yields only 2 mols of ATP when metabolized to lactate under anaerobic conditions.

"NUTRITION OF THE HEART"

Nutritional experiments (in the microorganism *Neurospora crassa*) are at the root of the fundamental discovery that genes provide the blueprints for enzymes.[20] Today, nutrition is often confused as a single issue. The recent interest in "heart-healthy" diets has focused almost exclusively on cholesterol because of its role in the development of coronary artery disease, even though there appears to be no direct correlation between dietary cholesterol and cholesterol levels in the blood.[47] Furthermore, the focus on cholesterol has shifted attention away from the fact that the heart requires large amounts of foodstuffs to meet its en-

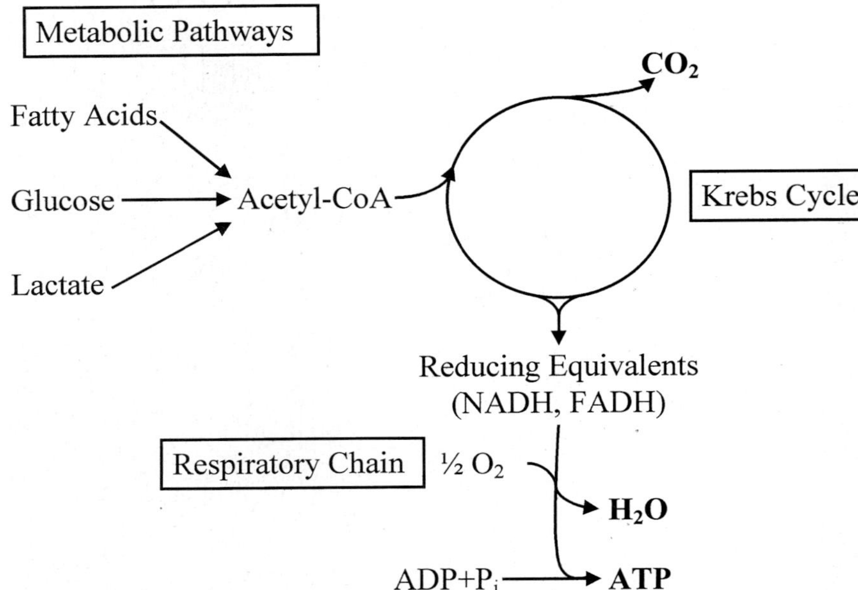

FIGURE 45–6 The three stages of fuel metabolism in the heart include metabolic pathways for the breakdown of fuels to acetyl-coenzyme A (CoA), the Krebs cycle for the generation of reducing equivalents, and the respiratory chain for the oxidation of reducing equivalents. Products (in **bold**) are adenosine triphosphate (ATP), CO_2, and H_2O. ADP, adenosine diphosphate; FADH, reduced flavin adenine dinucleotide; NADH, nicotinamide adenine dinucleotide, reduced form; P_i, inorganic phosphate.

ergy requirements. Both quantity and quality of these foodstuffs vary greatly in the course of a day (see later). Metabolically speaking, the heart does not differ from the body as a whole. The heart is an *omnivore* (i.e., an organ that has developed or retained its ability to oxidize a variety of different substrates).[48]

Myocardial cell function does not simply conform to the availability of substrate, but substrate utilization is regulated by the physiologic demands on the system. It is little appreciated that the heart stores endogenous substrates such as glycogen and triglycerides in response to changes in the dietary state[49, 50] and that the heart continuously synthesizes and degrades its own constituent proteins,[51] a process that requires energy[52] and is significantly slowed by myocardial ischemia.[53] The consequences of severe ischemia are the depletion of endogenous energy stores and the intracellular accumulation of toxic waste products.

SUBSTRATE COMPETITION

In the postprandial state and under resting conditions, long-chain fatty acids and glucose are the main fuels for respiration (Fig. 45–7). Fuel metabolism, oxidation, and utilization are finely regulated to match the energy requirements of the heart. Because of the omnivorous nature of the heart, glucose, lactate, fatty acids, ketone bodies, and under certain circumstances, amino acids compete with one another as fuels for respiration. The relative predominance of a fuel depends on the arterial substrate concentration, which can vary over a wide range, and on hormonal influences, workload, and oxygen supply. The utilization of specific substrates by the heart therefore varies with the physiologic state of its environment. When Bing[9] cannulated the coronary sinus and measured aorto–coronary sinus differences in substrate concentrations across the heart, he observed a proportional relationship between arterial substrate concentration and substrate uptake by the heart under steady state conditions, which changed with changes in the physiologic environment. Subsequent work by others[54] has established that the relative contribution of a substrate to the fuel for respiration depends on the physiologic state of the entire body, a parameter that can vary greatly, but that glucose uptake (16 to 31 percent) is relatively constant while the uptake of fatty acids plus ketone bodies and of lactate vary considerably (from 25 to 63 percent and from 5 to 61 percent, respectively). Although no systematic studies on the effects of competing substrates on the uptake of the clinically important glucose tracer analogue [^{18}F]-fluorodeoxyglucose (FDG) have been carried out as yet, the same general observation appears to be true for FDG.[55–58] Limitations to this approach are discussed in the following section (Tracing Metabolic Pathways).

Fatty acids are the preferred fuel for respiration in the fasted state,[59] but even when fatty acid or ketone body concentrations are high, a certain amount of glucose continues to be oxidized.[43, 60–62] Conversely, high lactate concentrations (as observed with strenuous exercise) can provide almost all[63] or at least the bulk of the fuel for respiration.[62] Even amino acids, when present in very high concentrations, can become a fuel for respiration in heart muscle.[9] A special characteristic of heart muscle is the preferential oxidation of glycogen in response to adrenergic stimulation.[60, 61] Glycogen is a source of energy, which is readily available from its stores inside the myocyte.

TRACING METABOLIC PATHWAYS

A detailed knowledge of the pathways of individual substrates for energy production is normally not required to diagnose or treat patients with heart disease. However, specific metabolic abnormalities must be considered when coronary arteries are not (or are no longer) obstructed and the heart fails to contract. This is the case, for example, in cardiomyopathies or in myocardium that is reperfused after

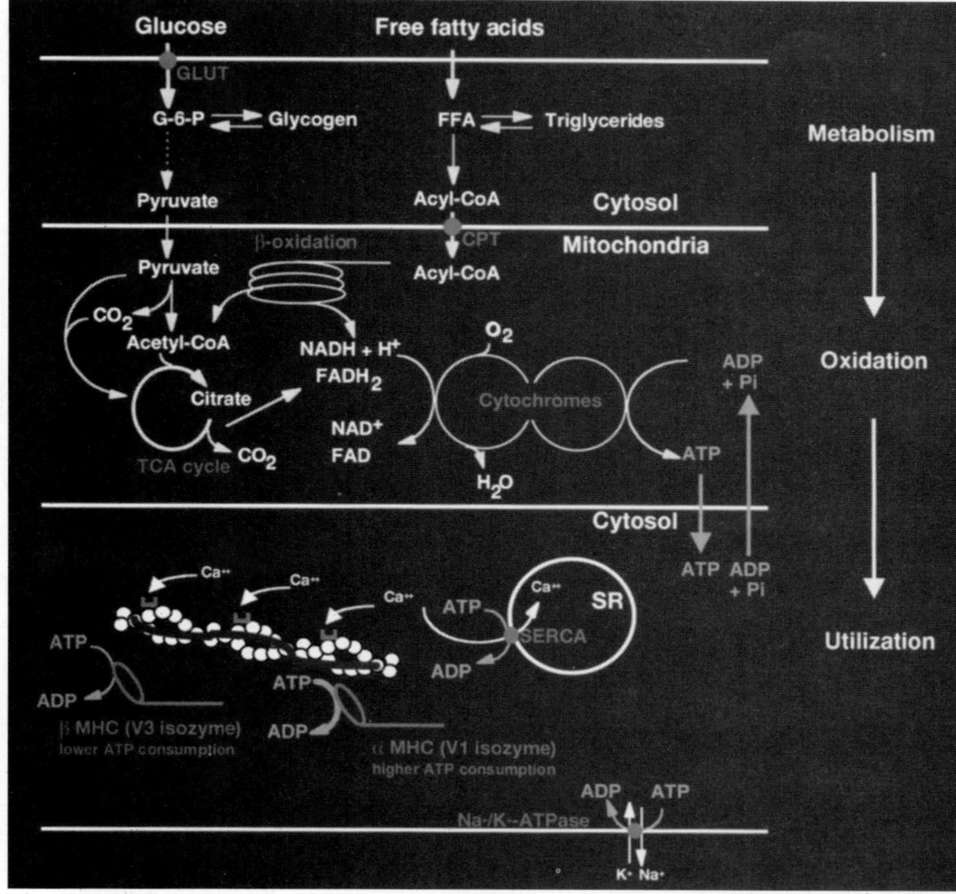

FIGURE 45–7 The main fuels for respiration in heart muscle uptake and oxidation of glucose and of long-chain fatty acids are tightly regulated to meet the energy needs for contraction of the heart. Acetyl-CoA, acetyl coenzyme A; Acyl-CoA, acyl coenzyme A; ADP, adenosine diphosphate; ATP, adenosine triphosphate; ATPase, adenosine triphosphatase; CPT, carnitine palmityl transferase; FAD, flavin adenine dinucleotide; $FADH_2$, flavin adenine dinucleotide, reduced form; FFA, free fatty acids; G-6-P, glucose 6-phosphate; GLUT, glucose transporter; MHC, major histocompatibility complex; NAD^+, nicotinamide adenine dinucleotide; NADH, nicotinamide adenine dinucleotide, reduced form; Pi, protease inhibitor; TCA, tricarboxylic acid; SERCA, sarcoendoplasmic reticulum ATPase; SR, sarcoplasmic reticulum.

complete coronary occlusion. Tracing of metabolic pathways can be accomplished qualitatively owing to the development of new, nondestructive imaging techniques such as nuclear magnetic resonance spectroscopy and PET, which permit the assessment of regional metabolic processes in the beating heart both in vitro and in vivo.[64–73]

Analysis of energy-rich phosphates in the beating heart by nuclear magnetic resonance spectroscopy of ^{31}P lends further support to the view that over a relatively wide range of work output, tissue content is not correlated with ATP turnover,[74] assessed by oxygen consumption or contractile performance of the heart. The recent adaptation of isotopomer analysis of ^{13}C natural abundance or ^{13}C-labeled compounds allows the analysis of flux through specific pathways, especially the Krebs citric acid cycle and glycogen turnover, to be studied quantitatively as serial spectra are obtained.[73, 75–78]

Tracing of metabolic pathways with short-lived positron-emitting tracers has been so successful in its clinical application because technology has been developed for the visual assessment of regional differences in metabolic activity of the heart and quantitative analysis of radioactivity in regions of interest.[72, 79] Two types of approaches can be distinguished and are depicted in Figure 45–8. The first approach is uptake and retention of a tracer analogue, such as FDG. The second approach is the uptake and clearance of tracers such as ^{11}C fatty acids, where the rapid phase of clearance from the tissue represents either beta-oxidation and oxidation in the Krebs citric acid cycle (in the case of long-chain fatty acids) or oxidation in the Krebs citric acid cycle alone (in the case of acetate). Uptake and retention of the tracer analogue FDG increase linearly with time (Fig. 45–9), whereas the clearance of a labeled fatty acid after an initial peak in tissue activity is biexponential.[80–82] Both types of approaches have been used clinically to

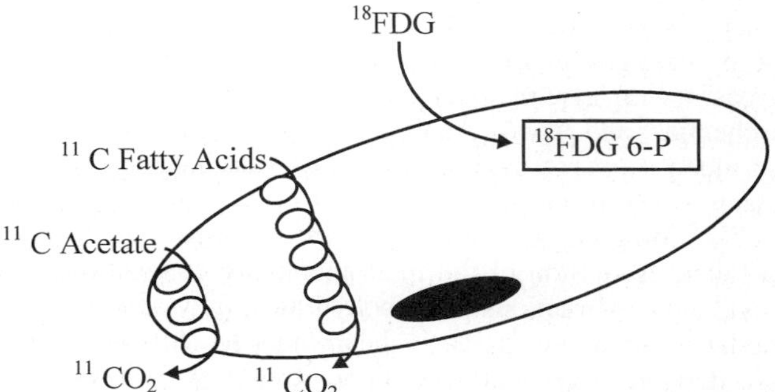

FIGURE 45–8 Schematic representation of representative positron emitting metabolic tracers (^{11}C) and tracer analogues (^{18}F). Tracers (fatty acids acetate) are taken up, metabolized, and cleared from the myocardium. Tracer analogues (e.g., fluorodeoxyglucose [FDG]) are taken up, metabolized, and retained by the myocardium. It is important to distinguish between uptake and clearance and uptake and retention because the time-activity curves differ substantially.

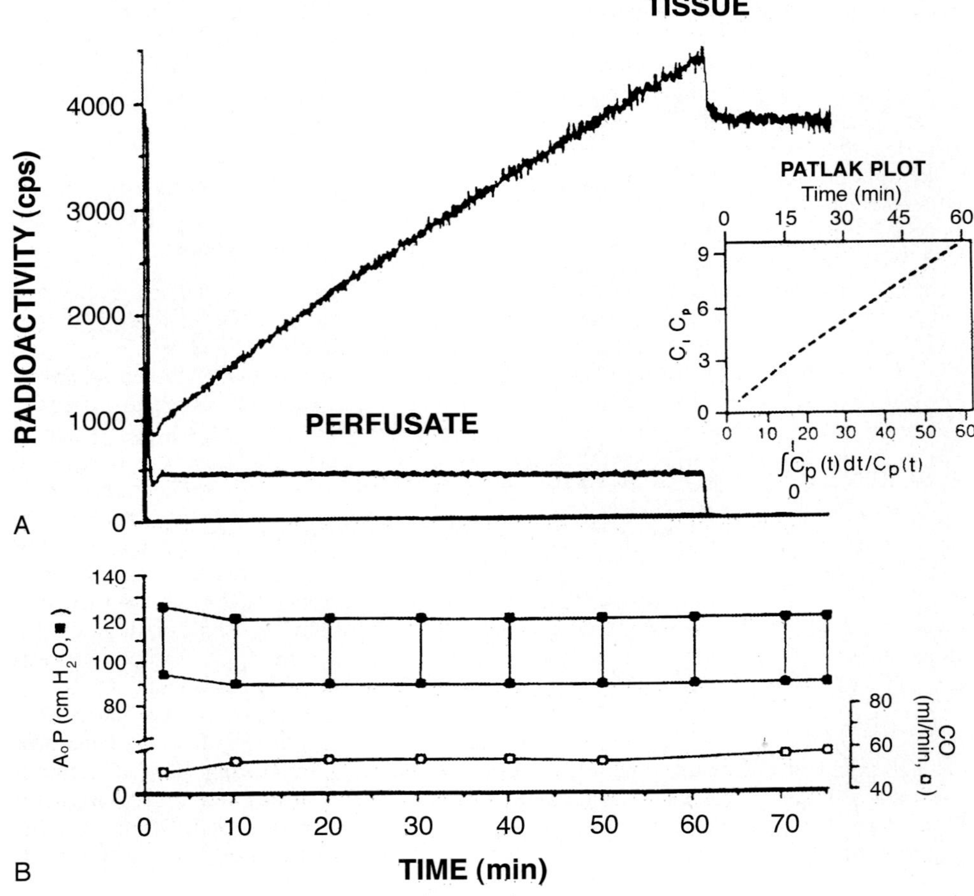

FIGURE 45–9 Fluorodeoxyglucose (FDG) accumulation by isolated working rat heart. Time-activity curves obtained for a heart perfused at a preload of 15 cm H_2O and an afterload of 100 cm H_2O with Krebs-Henseleit saline solution containing glucose (10 mM) plus 2-FDG (350 μCi/200 ml perfusate), recirculating for the first 60 min. **A,** *Top:* Myocardial retention of FDG. *Bottom:* 2-FDG activity in the perfusate curves is shown in the *inset.* **B,** Simultaneous recording of the physiologic performance of the heart (aortic pressure [AoP] and cardiac output [CO]). Note the stability of the preparation and the change of radioactive perfusate at 60 min to nonradioactive perfusate containing only glucose (10 mM). The tracer is retained by the tissue (see **A**). (**A** and **B,** From Nguyen VTB, Mossberg KA, Tewson TJ, et al: Temporal analysis of myocardial glucose metabolism by ^{18}F-2-deoxy-2-fluoro-D-glucose. Am J Physiol 259:H1022, 1990.)

assess substrate metabolism in normal and ischemic myocardium. Enhanced glucose uptake (assessed with FDG) or residual oxidative capacity (assessed by clearance of [^{11}C]-acetate) is used to identify reversible tissue injury in ischemic, reperfused, or "hibernating" myocardium.

However, a word of caution is in order. Quantitative assessment of myocardial glucose uptake by FDG depends on a correction factor, the lumped constant of Sokoloff.[83] The lumped constant is not a true constant, because the tracer/tracee ratio (uptake of FDG versus uptake of glucose) changes under non–steady state conditions. It decreases with insulin[84] and with reperfusion after low-flow ischemia[85] and would result in a spurious underestimation of glucose uptake unless a model of variable lumped constants is taken into account.[86]

The foregoing remarks highlight the need for a more detailed discussion of the main metabolic connections and regulatory interactions of carbohydrates, fatty acids, ketone bodies, and amino acids in heart muscle. All three fuels are derived either from the blood stream or from endogenous stores. Although the main fuels are fatty acids and carbohydrates, amino acid metabolism is included in the discussion because amino acids are not only building blocks of proteins but also active partners of intermediary metabolism. Amino acids play pivotal roles in the transfer of reducing equivalents from the cytosol to the mitochondria[87] and in the metabolic response to ischemia.[88, 89]

FUELS FOR THE HEART: METABOLISM OF THE MAJOR ENERGY-PROVIDING SUBSTRATES

Why does the heart use different fuels to make energy? The following analogy may be useful to explain this phenomenon. Metabolic pathways can be likened to a power grid, and the heart can be likened to a light bulb. Fuels are the various sources of energy (coal, water, natural gas, nuclear fission) that are all converted to electricity. A simple explanation for this redundancy is that different fuels are used whenever they are most readily available. All are converted to the same form of energy. In reality, the situation is more complex because the heart functions best when it oxidizes different substrates (sugars and fats) simultaneously, and we have even proposed a classification of carbohydrates as *essential* and of fatty acids as *nonessential* fuels for the heart.[12] The meaning of this classification will become apparent in the discussions later.

Carbohydrates

Carbohydrate fuels for the heart are glucose, lactate, and glycogen. Although long-chain fatty acids are normally the predominant fuel for energy production in the mammalian heart, glucose is the most reliable of all substrates.[90] Glucose is an anaplerotic substrate for the Krebs cycle,[43, 91] and glucose is essential for the initiation of fatty acid oxidation in heart.[92] Hypoglycemic newborns develop cardiomegaly and heart failure that are completely reversible with the administration of glucose.[93] Furthermore, isotope dilution studies[60, 94] have demonstrated that the normal human heart produces lactate at the same time it oxidizes lactate and that it takes up glucose to form glycogen when in the fasted, resting state.[91, 95] It appears that a large portion of exogenous glucose is shunted into glycogen rather than directly oxidized.[96, 97] Glucose and lactate extraction by the heart in vitro and in vivo increases with an increase in workload, even in the presence of competing substrates.[43, 98] This observation is of interest in view of the importance of pyruvate, which is the common metabolic product of glucose, glycogen, and lactate. As shown in Figure 45–10, pyruvate provides both acetyl-CoA (C_2 units) and oxaloacetate (C_4 units) for the Krebs citric acid cycle. Pyruvate becomes a critical intermediary when workload, and therefore turnover of the citric acid cycle, increases.

In keeping with the scheme presented earlier (see Fig. 45–6), there are three energy-yielding stages of glucose metabolism: the glycolytic pathway leading to pyruvate, oxaloacetate, and lactate; the Krebs cycle; and the respiratory chain. Each stage is regulated by its own set of controls, so that overall flux through the pathways (which may be assessed externally on a second-by-second timescale with the glucose tracer analogue FDG[44]) proceeds at a rate just sufficient to satisfy the heart's beat-to-beat needs for the final product, ATP. In other words, under physiologic conditions, the rate of ATP hydrolysis controls not only the rate of electron transfer along the respiratory chain but also the turnover rate of the Krebs cycle, the rate of pyruvate oxidation and carboxylation, and the rate of glucose utilization. Therefore, when ATP turnover is increased, the entire sequence of enzyme-catalyzed reactions and transport mechanisms moves into a higher gear.

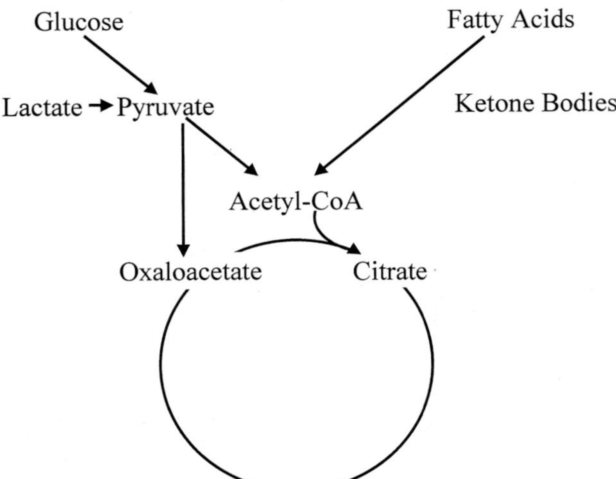

FIGURE 45–10 Differences in the metabolic fate of glucose and fatty acids as fuels for the heart. In contrast to fatty acids, glucose provides acetyl-coenzyme A (acetyl-CoA) plus oxaloacetate for the Krebs cycle. The formation of oxaloacetate replenishes citric acid cycle intermediates by a process termed *anaplerosis* (which means filling up of the cycle). Because of anaplerosis, the heart functions best when it oxidizes glucose or lactate together with fatty acids. High levels of acetyl-CoA stimulate the carboxylation of pyruvate to oxaloacetate.

Regulatory Sites of Glucose Metabolism

Glucose Transport and Phosphorylation

The first major regulatory site of the glycolytic pathway is glucose uptake, which is stereospecific and saturable and follows Mechaelis-Menten kinetics. Since the discovery of facilitated glucose transport across biologic membranes by Widdas and Wiedeman,[99] considerable effort has been invested in understanding the mechanism by which D-glucose crosses the plasma membrane. The transport of glucose into the cardiomyocyte occurs along a steep concentration gradient and is regulated by specific transporters.[100] The transporters display saturation kinetics and countertransport. The stereospecificity of the transporter for sugars of the carbon configuration is not matched by the same degree of selectivity, and various tracer analogues, including 2-deoxyglucose and FDG, are transported in the same way as glucose (Fig. 45–11; see also Figs. 45–7 and 45–8).

The transporters regulating glucose uptake belong to a family of glucose transporters (GLUT) that are conserved over a wide range of organisms, suggesting a common evolutionary origin.[101–104] The isoform that is predominantly expressed in adult cardiomyocytes is GLUT-4, the insulin-sensitive transporter also found in skeletal muscle and in adipose tissue.[101, 105] Heart muscle is an insulin-sensitive organ, and insulin has a multitude of hemodynamic effects.[106] Although insulin was discovered in the 1920s, we only recently began to understand the mechanisms by which insulin provides the uptake of glucose into the cells. Recruitment of GLUT-4 from a microsomal cytosolic pool to the sarcolemma by insulin (or ischemia or adrenergic stimulation)[107–110] increases the maximal velocity of glucose transport. Alpha-adrenergic stimulation uses the same signaling pathway as insulin to promote glucose uptake,[111] whereas the effects of ischemia, beta-receptor stimulation, and insulin on glucose uptake are additive.[112] In addition to GLUT-4, the cardiomyocyte expresses the GLUT-1 transporter isoform, which is presumably independent of insulin regulation and predominates in fetal myocardium.[102, 105] GLUT-1 is the first gene whose transcription is dually stimulated in response to hypoxia and inhibition of oxidative phosphorylation.[113] Both transporters have a K_m for glucose (i.e., the concentration at which the rate of glucose transport is half maximal) that is in the range of plasma glucose concentrations under fasting conditions.[114] The normal heart also expresses a low amount of GLUT-3, which has a K_m below the normal plasma glucose concentration.[115]

Cardiac work and substrate availability, as well as plasma glucose and insulin concentrations, act in concert as the most important factors determining glucose uptake.[116] Myocardial glucose uptake is also determined by the dietary state per se,[91, 117] by oxygen availability,[96, 118, 119] and by hormones, such as catecholamines, growth hormone, and cortisol, which, in addition to insulin and glucagon,

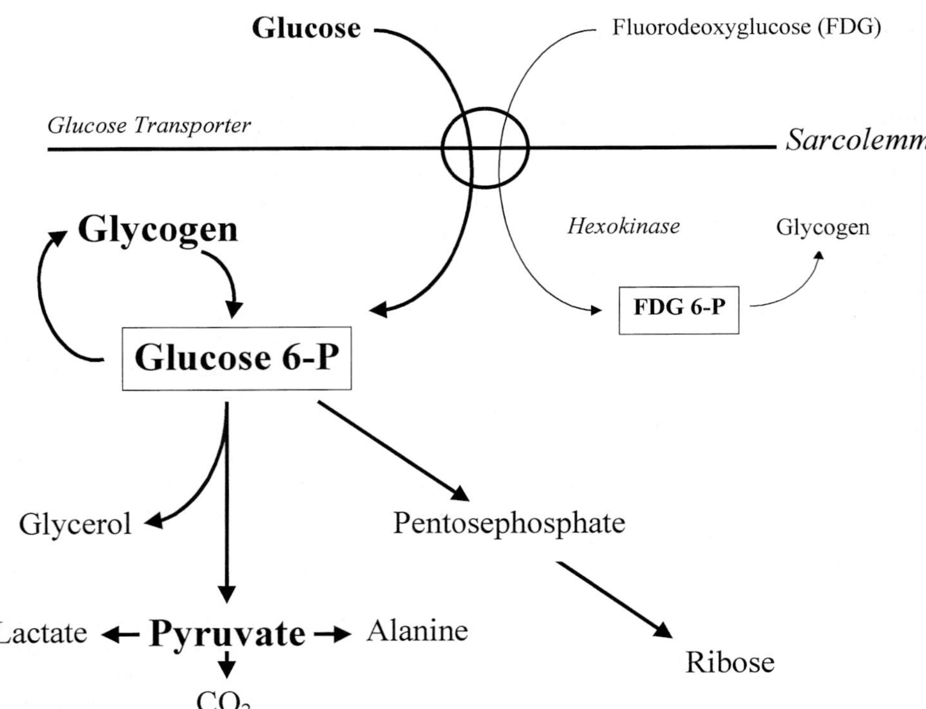

FIGURE 45–11 Initial steps in the glucose metabolic pathway. Glucose is immediately phosphorylated once it has entered the cell. Glucose 6-phosphate (6-P) is substrate for glycogen synthesis, the glycolytic pathway, and the pentose phosphate pathway. All major intermediates are given in **boldface**. Compared with the diverse metabolism of glucose, the metabolism of the glucose tracer analogue fluorodeoxyglucose (FDG) is simple and ends for the most part with FDG 6-P. A small amount of FDG finds its way into glycogen. Because there is no glucose 6-P in the heart, the accumulation of FDG under steady-state conditions is linear and in proportion to glucose uptake (see also Figs. 45–8 and 45–9).

may affect either K_m or V_{max} of glucose transport. Some of the intracellular signaling pathways are shared, and their regulation is currently under investigation.[112, 120, 121]

Phosphorylation of glucose by hexokinase becomes rate limiting for glycolysis at high rates of glucose transport. Rates of glucose phosphorylation measured in vitro are more than twice as high as the maximal measured rates of glucose utilization by the heart at a physiologic workload and with glucose as the only substrate.[122] Some evidence suggests that glucose, once inside the cell and phosphorylated, may preferentially enter the glycogen pool rather than the glycolytic pathway.[91, 97, 123] The intracellular glucose concentration of heart muscle rises during starvation, in diabetes, and with the concomitant oxidation of fatty acids, ketone bodies, or lactate, which indicates inhibition of the phosphorylation step. This is most likely to be due to accumulation of glucose-6-phosphate because of inhibition of the phosphofructokinase reaction.

Once glucose has been taken up by the heart muscle cell and phosphorylated, it is metabolized as glucose-6-phosphate, which is the substrate for several distinct enzyme systems (see Fig. 45–11). These systems include (1) degradation via the Embden-Meyerhof pathway (also termed the *glycolytic pathway* when it entails metabolism of glucose to lactate only), (2) conversion to glycogen via the glycogen synthase reaction, and (3) metabolism (oxidation) via the pentose-phosphate pathway, which yields ribose and the reduced form of nicotinamide adenine dinucleotide phosphate (NADPH). The latter pathway is of quantitatively lesser importance in heart muscle than are the former two. Of note is that most of these pathways are not available to the tracer analogue FDG 6-phosphate, which may, however, become a substrate for glycogen synthesis.[120] Hence, FDG traces glucose uptake and phosphorylation, but it lacks specificity with regard to the metabolic fate of glucose inside the cell.

Glycogen

The study of the pathways of glycogen synthesis and degradation in liver and muscle has contributed more to the understanding of enzyme regulation and the molecular basis of hormone action than any other known system of metabolic control.[124] It was in this system that the first example for the control of enzyme activity by an allosteric regulator (activation of phosphorylase by adenosine monophosphate [AMP]) was described,[125] enzyme regulation by covalent modification was discovered,[126] and the molecular basis of hormone action by signal transduction was elucidated through the discovery of cyclic adenosine monophosphate (cAMP).[127] Although glycogen is more abundant in cardiac than in skeletal muscle or in any other tissue except liver, the function of the large amount of glycogen in cardiac muscle (up to 2 percent of the cell volume) is not entirely clear.[32] The high concentration of glycogen in fetal cardiac muscle probably explains why the heart can maintain its contractile activity in the face of severe hypoxia[128] during birth. The high concentration of glycogen in the specialized conduction system of the heart was first described by Aschoff[129] at the beginning of the 20th century. The physiologic role of glycogen in the conduction system is not known, although it is tempting to speculate about its protective effect against ischemia. Collectively, there is good reason to assume that glycogen is more than an intracellular fuel store. Glycogen and glycogen phosphorylase are closely associated with the sarcoplasmic reticulum,[130] and in skeletal muscle a decreased glycogen content is closely associated with a reduction in force,

Ca^{2+} release from the sarcoplasmic reticulum, and contractile protein function.[131]

Glycogen synthesis and degradation occur in two separate pathways. The combined effects of protein phosphorylation and dephosphorylation on glycogen synthase and phosphorylase provide an interlocking system by which hormones (such as epinephrine) and mechanical activity (through Ca^{2+}) can control the net flux of glucose 1-P into and out of the intracellular glycogen stores.[77, 132] Epinephrine-induced cAMP formation promotes protein phosphorylation and simultaneously inhibits glycogen synthesis while stimulating glycogen breakdown, whereas stimulation of protein dephosphorylation shifts the balance toward glycogen synthesis. Although the interaction of the enzymes of glycogen breakdown and synthesis is more complex than this simple mechanism suggests,[133] the concept of a continuous turnover of the myocardial glycogen pool is relatively easy to grasp.

Excessive rates of glycogen breakdown during ischemia have been suggested to be deleterious for the recovery of contractile function because of the accumulation of lactate.[134] However, the heart subjected to low-flow ischemia continues to synthesize glycogen,[135, 136] and enhanced glycogen stores (and with them, high rates of glycogen breakdown) improve contractile function in the ischemic and reperfused myocardium,[137–141] in the exercised myocardium,[142] and in the ischemic heart.[143–145] The role of glycogen in the resistance to ischemia is seen most dramatically in amphibian myocardium, which is particularly rich in this compound.[146]

The importance of high preoperative levels of myocardial glycogen for myocardial preservation in patients undergoing cardiac surgery on cardiopulmonary bypass has been stressed.[147] Conversely, glycogen depletion before hypothermic ischemic arrest worsens contractile performance on reperfusion in isolated rabbit hearts.[148] Based on the collective experience of enhanced ischemia, tolerance in glycogen-rich hearts, and a decreased loss of proteins and cell constituents on reperfusion, it has been speculated that glycogen plays a physiologic role in addition to its role as fuel reserve. This physiologic role may rest in its function as an "anchoring molecule" for other macromolecular cell constituents, since the loss of marker proteins and adenine nucleotides from reperfused heart muscle is greatly diminished in glycogen-rich hearts compared with controls.[140]

Glycolysis

Lack of oxygen, clinically encountered in the context of ischemia, enhances flux through the glycolytic pathway that, in turn, augments substrate level phosphorylation of ADP and the formation of lactate as well as alanine.[88] Other stimulants of flux through the glycolytic pathway are increases in cardiac work, either acutely with exercise[98] or chronically with pressure overload,[149] and hypertrophy[150, 151] or sustained hypertension.[149]

Enhanced glycolytic flux was found to lessen ischemic tissue damage[144, 152] and indicates reversible ischemic injury.[153, 154] Although it is thought that the accumulation of glycolytic products may worsen the effects of ischemia[155, 156] and acute hyperglycemia may abolish ischemic preconditioning in vivo,[157] provision of glucose together with insulin and potassium improves contractile function in the acutely ischemic, reperfused myocardium.[112, 158, 159] The inotropic effect of insulin in the postischemic heart is additive to epinephrine and coupled to enhanced glucose uptake.[121] Glycolysis plays an essential role in the maintenance of intracellular calcium homeostasis during severe calcium overload.[160]

Glycolysis from extracellular glucose (and no other metabolic pathway) protects cardiac myocytes from hypoxic injury and subsequent apoptosis.[161] The first step committing glucose to the glycolytic pathway is 6-phospho-1-kinase (PFK-1), which catalyzes the phosphorylation of fructose 6-phosphate to fructose 1,6-bisphosphate. Because of the complex allosteric regulation of PFK, this is a rate-limiting step (pacemaker enzyme) for glycolysis.[162] ATP, citrate, and protons are negative allosteric effectors, whereas AMP and fructose 1,6-bisphosphate are positive effectors.[163–165] Fructose 2,6-bisphosphate is the main activator of PFK-1 in normoxic heart.

Further down in the glycolytic pathway, the oxidation of the triose-phosphate glyceraldehyde 3-phosphate to 1,3-diphosphoglycerate couples is the energy-conserving step in the glycolytic pathway that leads to the nonoxidative formation of ATP. The reaction is thought to be at near equilibrium. However, under conditions of high cardiac work[166] or ischemia,[167] when PFK becomes strongly activated, glycolysis is controlled at the triose-phosphate dehydrogenase step.

Pyruvate at the Crossroads: Oxidation, Carboxylation, Reduction, and Transamination

Just as the first committed intermediate of glycolytic pathway, glucose-6-phosphate, is at a branch point where several enzymes compete for it as substrate, so is the last committed intermediate, pyruvate (Fig. 45–12).

In heart muscle, pyruvate can be either reduced to lactate (which completes the glycolytic pathway), transaminated to alanine,[88] carboxylated to oxaloacetate or malate,[168, 169] or most importantly, oxidized to acetyl-CoA. Lactate and most of the alanine are formed in the cytosol by near-equilibrium reactions, and both metabolites may be washed out from the cell. In well-oxygenated, working heart muscle, however, the bulk of pyruvate enters the mitochondrion.

The inner mitochondrial membrane represents a barrier to the movement of charged molecules across it. Specific transport mechanisms are required to enable the transport of specific metabolites through the lipid bilayer, and since the early 1980s, an impressive number of carrier systems have been demonstrated for the transport of both anions and protons.[170] A specific carrier exists for transport of pyruvate into the mitochondrial matrix, as it has been most clearly demonstrated with the inhibitor 4-hydroxy-alpha-cyanocinnamate.[171]

Inside the mitochondrial matrix, pyruvate can be either decarboxylated to acetyl-CoA or carboxylated to oxaloacetate.[169, 172] The capture of metabolically produced carbon dioxide from the pyruvate dehydrogenase reaction to form oxaloacetate provides one example of the efficient use of one substrate supplying two precursors for citrate synthesis and efficient recycling of carbon dioxide.

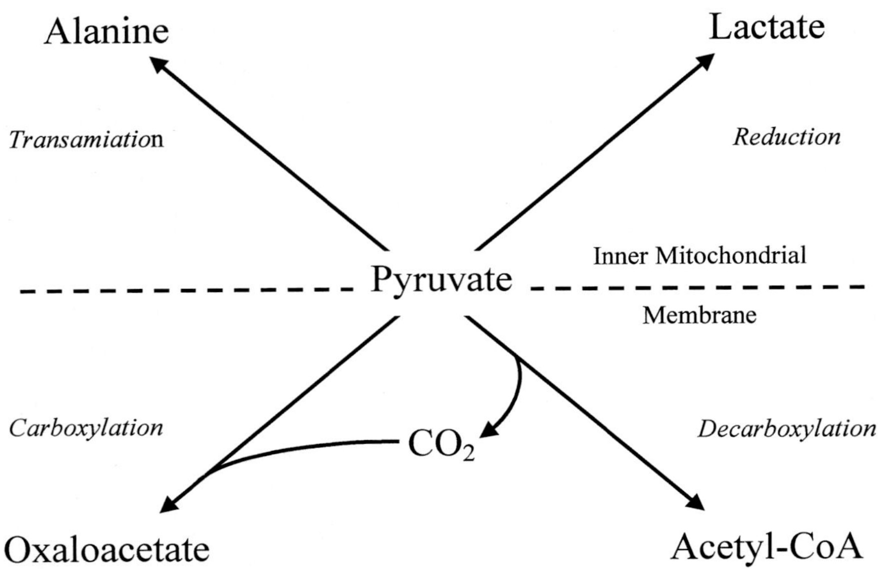

FIGURE 45–12 Pyruvate at crossroads. The central position of pyruvate in heart metabolism is often overlooked. Pyruvate can be decarboxylated, carboxylated, reduced, or transanimated. The physiologic environment controls the fate of pyruvate. Note the recycling of metabolic CO_2. Acetyl-coenzyme A, Acetyl-CoA.

Oxidative decarboxylation of pyruvate assumes a central position in the regulation of fuel supply to the heart. A system of intricate control mechanisms governs both activation and inactivation of the pyruvate dehydrogenase complex (PDC).[173] The conversion of pyruvate to acetyl-CoA requires the sequential action of three different enzymes: pyruvate dehydrogenase, dihydrolipoyl transacetylase, and dihydrolipoyl dehydrogenase. The reaction also requires five different coenzymes or prosthetic groups: thiamine pyrophosphate, lipoic acid, uncombined coenzyme A (CoA SH), FAD^+, and NAD^+. These enzymes and coenzymes are organized into a multienzyme cluster. The overall molecular weight of the PDC from heart tissue is about 8.5 million daltons (i.e., the size of a ribosome). The PDC complex is attached to the inner side of the inner mitochondrial membrane.

Much work has been done in the 1970s on the regulation of PDC by covalent modification through a phosphorylation and dephosphorylation cycle. Multisite phosphorylation of the pyruvate dehydrogenase component of the complex provides an indirect means by which the entire complex is regulated by the relative activities of the PDC kinase and phosphatase reactions. Like most mammalian tissues, heart muscle possesses both active (dephosphorylated) and inactive (phosphorylated) dehydrogenase. The total activity of both of these is approximately 30 U/g dry weight at 30°C,[174] of which normally about 20 percent is in the active form. The relative amount of active PDC increases with an increase in workload. Active PDC may decline to only 1 to 5 percent of total PDC during starvation or in alloxan diabetes[175] (i.e., when noncarbohydrate substrates become the main fuel for respiration). Both the protein kinase and the phosphoprotein phosphatase are probably active in vivo, and the relative proportion of active PDC must therefore be dependent on the relative activities of kinase and phosphatase as well as on the intramitochondrial concentration of the effectors of these enzymes.

Most of the known effectors of the phosphorylation-dephosphorylation cycle are also effectors of the kinase reaction. Of the metabolite pairs ATP-ADP, acetyl-CoA–Co ASH, NADH–NAD^+, and lactate-pyruvate, the first member either activates the kinase or serves as substrate, and the second member inhibits the enzyme. Ca^{2+} and Mg^{2+} both inhibit the kinase and activate the phosphatase reaction (i.e., lead to PDC activation). The effects of fatty acids or ketone body oxidation are likely to be mediated by the increase in acetyl-CoA[175] because the primary effect or the inhibition-inactivation of PDC by fatty acids or ketone bodies is the acetyl-CoA–CoA SH ratio.[175] Conversely, an increase in cardiac work may inhibit the PDC kinase owing to a decrease in NADH, acetyl-CoA, and ATP, leading to activation of PDC.[174]

Fatty Acids

Fatty acids, esterified as triglycerides, represent the body's main fuel reserve. Because oxidation of long-chain fatty acids releases more than six times as much energy as the oxidation of an equal mass of glucose, which is also readily converted into fatty acids (by the liver), fatty acids represent the predominant fuel for respiration in heart muscle. In spite of their preeminence as a source for energy, fatty acids are the only fuel capable of uncoupling oxidative phosphorylation.[176] This phenomenon lowers the efficiency of fatty acids as energy substrates. There is yet another unique feature of fatty acids. Fatty acids require oxygen for their catabolism, whereas glucose, glycogen, and certain amino acids can be catabolized in the absence of oxygen.

The predominant forms of fatty acids in the blood stream are the monounsaturated long-chain fatty acid oleate (C_{18}) and the saturated fatty acid palmitate (C_{16}). The pathway of long-chain fatty acid oxidation starts with the liberation of fatty acids from triglycerides in adipocytes and/or the albumin-bound transport of free fatty acids (FFAs) in the blood. It ends with the entry of acetyl-CoA into the citric acid cycle (Fig. 45–13). FFAs of any chain length cross the plasma membrane with the help of a carrier protein, fatty acid transport protein, that has been cloned and expressed in a variety of systems.[177] In the cytosol, long-chain fatty acids are bound by a fatty acid–binding protein[178, 179] and are activated on the outer mitochondrial membrane by esterification with CoA SH to form fatty acyl coenzyme A (acyl-CoA). Metabolism of long-chain fatty acids continues with fatty acyl transfer to carnitine, transport into the mitochondria in exchange for carnitine, reesterification with CoA SH, beta-oxidation, and finally, oxidation of acetyl-CoA (see Fig. 45–13). A variable amount of FFA taken up by heart muscle is esterified with glycerol in the cytosol to form triglycerides. Therefore, the fatty acyl-CoA formed on the outer mitochondrial membrane has two possible fates, either oxidation via the citric acid cycle in the mitochondria or conversion to triglycerides in the cytosol. Which pathway is taken depends on the rate of transfer of long-chain fatty acyl-CoA across the inner mitochondrial membrane and on the rate of esterification in the cytosol. Increased net triglyceride synthesis by the heart has been observed with starvation, diabetes, and ischemia. It is not known whether increased triglyceride levels are the result of increased rates of esterification or a decreased rate of lipolysis.

Carnitine Palmitoyl Transferase, Malonyl-CoA

Before the acyl group can be oxidized, it must be moved from the outer mitochondrial membrane into the mitochondrion. Transfer of long-chain fatty acyl-CoA into mitochondria requires a three-step membrane transport process, which is the rate-controlling step for long-chain fatty acid oxidation. The first step in this sequence is the transfer of the acyl group from CoA to carnitine, catalyzed by the enzyme carnitine palmitoyl transferase I (CPT I).

The CPT I system is inhibited by physiologic concentrations of malonyl-CoA, the product of acetyl-CoA carboxylation, and was first characterized in the liver, where malonyl-CoA serves as a signal regulating the relative rates of fatty acid oxidation, ketogenesis, and triglyceride synthesis.[180] Although the heart is not a lipogenic organ, it contains malonyl-CoA,[181] and the inhibition of cardiac CPT I by malonyl-CoA has been demonstrated.[182] A tissue-specific acetyl-CoA carboxylase has been identified for heart muscle.[183] Further studies are necessary to establish how malonyl-CoA synthesis is regulated in heart muscle and how the synthesis of malonyl-CoA might correlate with β-oxidation and Krebs citric acid cycle flux inside the

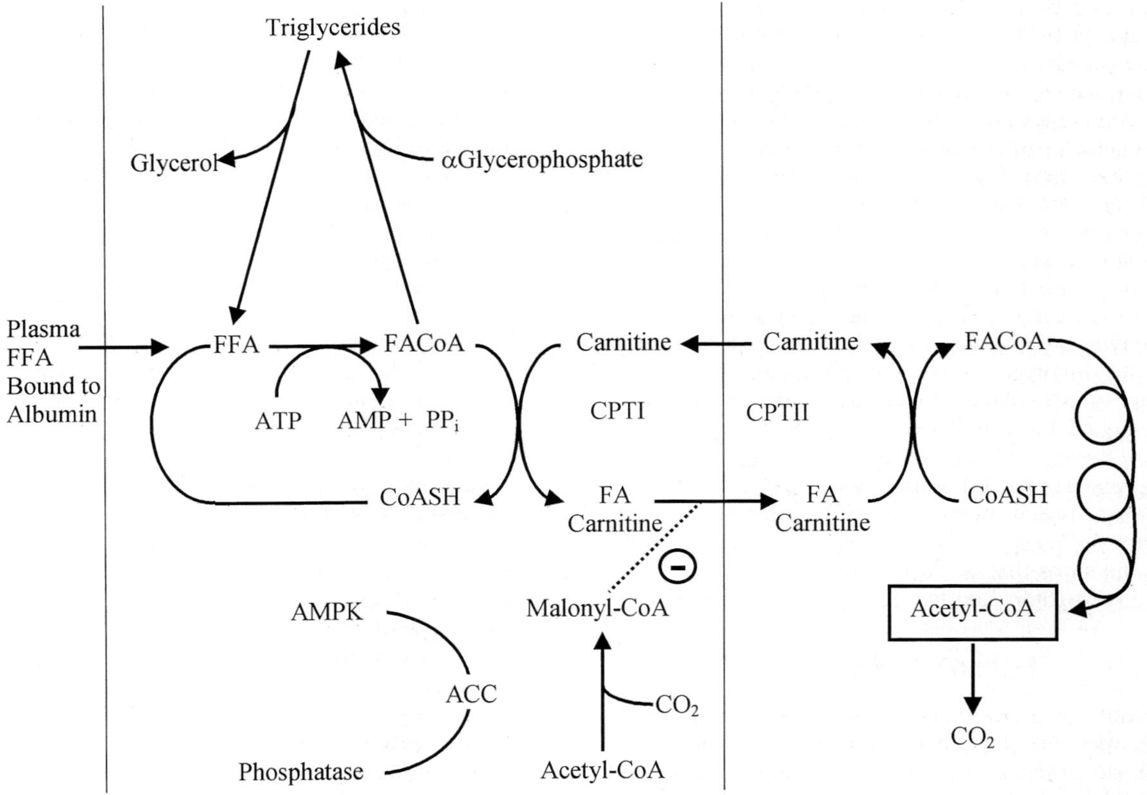

FIGURE 45–13 Simple scheme of long-chain fatty acid (FA) metabolism. FAs enter the myocyte through a fatty acid transporter protein (FATP), are bound to the heart-specific fatty acid binding protein (FABP) and activated to fatty acyl-coenzyme A (FACoA). FACoA is substrate for triglyceride synthesis and for carnitine palmitoyl-transferase I (CPTI), which regulates transport of FAs into mitochondria, where FAs undergo β-oxidation to acetyl-CoA and ultimately oxidation in the Krebs cycle. The rate of FA oxidation is controlled by CPTI and regulated by malonyl-CoA, which is an allosteric inhibitor of CPTI. Malonyl-CoA levels are, in turn, regulated by the rate of its synthesis by acetyl-CoA carboxylase (ACC) and degradation by malonyl-CoA decarboxylase. ACC is, in turn, regulated by a 5′ adenosine monophosphate–dependent kinase (AMPK) and by a phosphatase. AMPK has also been termed a *fuel gauge* of the myocyte because phosphorylation inactivates ACC, lowers malonyl-CoA, and increases rates of FA oxidation. AMPK is a target for drug development. In spite of the complexity of the scheme, note the cycling and recycling of metabolic intermediates. ATP, adenosine triphosphate; CoASH, xxx; CPTII, carnitine palmitoyl-transferase II; FFA, free fatty acids; PPi, inorganic pyrophosphate.

mitochondria. There is at least indirect evidence that malonyl-CoA plays an important role in substrate competition between fatty acids and glucose. It is noteworthy that in the isolated, perfused, working rat heart, glucose suppresses the oxidation of oleate.[43] The same suppression was not observed with octonoate, a short-chain fatty acid that does not require the CPT system for transport across the inner mitochondrial membrane.[184] It is also worth noting that ischemia reverses the inhibition of CPT I by malonyl-CoA, most probably through a modification in protein folding, thus making increased amounts of palmitoyl-carnitine for possible oxidation on reperfusion available.[185]

The carnitine-acyl unit traverses the inner mitochondrial membrane and is transferred to CoA SH inside the mitochondrial matrix by a second carnitine acyl-CoA transferase (CPT II) located at the inner surface of the inner mitochondrial membrane. Once inside the mitochondria, acyl-CoA is committed to oxidation by the system of beta-oxidation. The beta-oxidation pathway is controlled by fluctuations in the concentrations of substrates (acyl-CoA, NAD, and FAD)[186] or, expressed in more physiologic terms, by workload and oxygen supply of the heart. It is not yet clear how the rate of oxidation of FFA in the intact heart is related to citric acid cycle activity and the rate of oxidative phosphorylation. However, it is clear that fatty acid oxidation is arrested by ischemia and that the accumulation of long-chain acyl-CoA esters in ischemia inhibits the adenine nucleotide translocase in mitochondria.[187] This provides a possible explanation for contractile dysfunction.

The carnitine-acylcarnitine translocase system has been partially characterized in isolated heart mitochondria[188] and in the perfused heart itself.[189] An exchange reaction moves acyl-carnitine across the inner mitochondrial membrane in a stoichiometric exchange for carnitine. In the liver, and most probably also in heart muscle, CPT I is the regulatory site for fatty acid oxidation, with high concentrations of malonyl-CoA acting as an inhibitor of the enzyme during the carbohydrate-fed state. To explore the gene regulatory mechanisms involved in the metabolic control of long-chain fatty acid oxidation in the heart, the expression of muscle-type CPT-1 (mCPT-1) was recently characterized in primary cardiac myocytes after incubation with oleate, which regulates mCPT-1 expression via the peroxisome proliferator-activated receptor alpha.[190] Peroxisome proliferator-activated receptor-α is a nuclear receptor family with multiple functions that is currently attracting the attention of many investigators and the pharmaceutical industry.[191]

Defective Fatty Acid Metabolism

Inborn errors in myocardial fatty acid metabolism are increasingly recognized as important causes of cardiomyopathy and sudden death in children. Defects at nearly every step of the fatty acid oxidation pathway have been identified.[192] As reviewed by Kelly and Strauss,[192] the most common group of inherited defects involves the acyl-CoA dehydrogenase enzyme family, which catalyzes the initial reactions in mitochondrial β-oxidation of fatty acids.[194] In general, enzymatic defects involving long- and very-long-chain fatty acids (C_{14} or greater) or defects in cellular carnitine import of enzymes involved in the carnitine shuttle cause more severe clinical diseases, including cardiomyopathy, heart failure, and sudden death than with defects involving the metabolism of shorter-chain fatty acids.[195]

Clinical manifestations of inherited defects in fatty acid metabolism range from fasting hypoglycemia to frank cardiomyopathy or sudden death, most likely due to the accumulation of long-chain acyl-carnitines.[196, 197] A definitive diagnosis is not always easy because there is no correlation between in vitro enzyme assays in fibroblasts and clinical manifestations.[198] Although of rare incidence, systemic carnitine deficiency presents as familial endocardial fibroelastosis, which is associated with mitochondrial substrate deprivation and myocardial triglyceride accumulation.[199] As in experimental diphtheric cardiomyopathy,[200] the abnormality is reversible with the administration of L-carnitine, and it has therefore been recommended that plasma carnitine levels in all patients who present with familial cardiomyopathy be determined.[199] A chronic cardiomyopathy has been described in children who have a defect in carnitine uptake.[201]

Ketone Bodies

The ketone bodies, acetoacetate and beta-hydroxybutyrate, are produced by the liver when the supply of FFAs exceeds the liver's capacity for their complete oxidation in the citric acid cycle. They can be considered as "predigested fatty acids" with ready access to the enzymes of the citric acid cycle in the heart. As with carbohydrates and fatty acids, ketone bodies share in the supply of acetyl-CoA for energy production in heart muscle.[202] Compared with the complexity of glucose and long-chain fatty acid metabolism, the metabolism of ketone bodies requires only a few steps, none of which appears to be subject to any regulation.

Unique features of ketone body metabolism are the concentration-dependent linear uptake in vivo[203] and the activation of acetoacetate to acetoacetyl-CoA by succinyl-CoA, which itself is a citric acid cycle intermediate. The enzymes that degrade beta-hydroxybutyrate and acetoacetate to acetyl-CoA, beta-hydroxybutyrate dehydrogenase, 3-oxoacid-CoA transferase, and acetoacetyl-CoA thiolase are of comparatively high activity in heart muscle.[204] Ketone bodies, when present in relatively high concentrations, spare glucose utilization by the heart.[202] The ability of the heart to oxidize ketone bodies may constitute a buffer against qualitative changes in substrate supply when the relative proportions of oxidizable fuel are shifting as a result of changes in the dietary or hormonal state of the body. Even in physiologic situations, such as short-term starvation or exercise, ketone body concentrations in the plasma can rise by up to 50-fold.[13]

It is of interest that ketone bodies, when present as the only exogenous substrate for rat heart, do not sustain the full work output of the heart in vivo,[205] and their rate of oxidation in the citric acid cycle is insufficient to meet the energy needs of the heart in vitro.[43, 159, 170] This relative inhibition of the citric acid cycle occurs at the level of 2-oxoglutarate dehydrogenase and provides the first demonstration of a defect in metabolism that causes reversible contractile dysfunction of the heart.[43, 206] The inhibition is most probably related to sequestration of the enzyme's cofactor CoA SH, which is bound in the form of its thioester acetyl-CoA and as acetoacetyl-CoA, and is therefore not available for the reaction in the citric acid cycle.[91, 207] Whether or not this inhibition of the citric acid cycle is important in clinical situations, such as diabetic cardiomyopathy, is a matter of speculation.[208]

Observations in the isolated working rat heart perfused with ketone bodies have identified hitherto unknown mechanisms of the control of cardiac function by substrate metabolism. These include the reversible inhibition of contractile function by inhibited flux through the Krebs citric acid cycle, the operational control of substrate flux through citric acid cycle spans, and the importance of anaplerosis (i.e., the provision of oxaloacetate or other citric acid cycle intermediates in addition to acetyl-CoA for citrate synthesis for normal contractile function of the heart).[209] The importance of anaplerosis of the Krebs cycle in heart muscle is confirmed by improved cardiac function with propionyl-L-carnitine[210] and by stable isotope experiments using ^{13}C-nuclear magnetic resonance spectroscopy,[211] supporting the principle that the heart functions best when it oxidizes several substrates simultaneously.

Amino Acids

Not only are amino acids the "building blocks" of myocardial proteins, but, by their metabolism, they are also an integral part of myocardial energy metabolism. It cannot be emphasized strongly enough that each amino acid is different from the others with regard to control of its metabolism. Whereas many amino acids are either degraded or synthesized by heart muscle (e.g., glutamate, glutamine, aspartate, alanine, leucine), others are not metabolized at all (e.g., phenylalanine, tyrosine) and have therefore been used as tracers for myocardial protein synthesis and degradation.

In general, transamination is the first step of amino acid degradation in heart muscle. One of the functions of aminotransferases in heart muscle[212] is the provision of carbon skeletons for the citric acid cycle. The amino acids aspartate and glutamate also play an important role in the transfer of reducing equivalents across the mitochondrial membrane for oxidation of cytosolic NADH by the mitochondrial electron transport chain. Current evidence suggests that in heart muscle and liver, reducing equivalents are indirectly carried into the mitochondrial compartment by metabolic anions of the malate-aspartate cycle (see earlier). In the malate-aspartate cycle, cytosolic NADH, which cannot cross the inner mitochondrial membrane, is oxidized by the reduction of oxaloacetate to malate. Malate enters the mitochondrion and is oxidized to oxaloacetate, which is transaminated with glutamate to form 2-oxoglutarate and aspartate. The aspartate and 2-oxoglutarate leave the mitochondrion. Transamination of these metabolites regenerates oxaloacetate and glutamate in the cytosol, the net effect being a transfer of hydrogen ions across the mitochondrial membrane. A second postulated function for the malate-aspartate shuttle is the delivery of intermediates (malate) to the citric acid cycle, acting as a modulator of cycle activity.

Myocardial amino acid metabolism in vivo has been studied with both ^{14}N- and ^{11}C-labeled amino acids and PET.[213] Myocardial amino acid metabolism during hypoxia, ischemia, and reperfusion has been the subject of a number of studies in the intact and isolated heart muscle.[214–216] The amino acid alanine was found to be, like lactate, an end product of anaerobic glucose breakdown, arising through transamination of glutamate in the reaction:

$$\text{glutamate} + \text{pyruvate} \rightarrow \text{2-oxoglutarate} + \text{alanine}$$

This reaction is not the end of the pathway. Whereas alanine leaves the cell, 2-oxoglutarate is further metabolized and decarboxylated to succinate via substrate level phosphorylation in the citric acid cycle[89]:

$$\text{2-oxoglutarate} + NAD^+ + GDP + P_i \rightarrow \text{succinate} + CO_2 + NADH_2 + GTP$$

where NAD^+ is nicotinamide adenine dinucleotide, GDP is guanosine diphosphate, P_i is inorganic phosphate, and $NADH_2$ is reduced nicotinamide adenine dinucleotide. Since guanosine triphosphate (GTP) is readily transphosphorylated to ATP, this reaction is a source of anaerobic energy independent of lactate formation. Enhanced glutamate uptake in vivo has been shown by ^{13}N accumulation from labeled glutamate in ischemic heart muscle,[217] and glutamate enrichment has become a successful strategy to lessen the effects of ischemia with blood cardioplegia.[218] However, the neurotoxicity of glutamate precludes any systemic administration.

CONCLUSIONS

The heart is an omnivore that meets the bulk of its energy needs by oxidative phosphorylation of ADP. A bewildering array of enzyme-catalyzed reactions is responsible for the controlled transfer of energy from chemical bonds to mechanical work, which matches the energy requirements of the heart on a beat-to-beat basis. The groundwork for metabolic pathways is laid by enzyme-specific cardiac gene expression, and regulation of flux through the pathways is determined by a variety of environmental factors including workload, substrate supply, oxygen availability, and hormonal influences. Detailed biochemical analyses have identified a large number of factors that control regulatory enzymes in the different metabolic pathways, and the general principle of moiety-conserved cycles enhancing the efficiency of energy transfer has emerged.

Metabolism of energy-providing substrates by the heart therefore can no longer be regarded as a "black box." ATP turnover, not ATP content, determines the functional state of the heart. New methods for assessment of regional myocardial metabolism in vivo have effectively proved earlier concepts about the pathways of energy metabolism in the normal and ischemic heart. At the same time, studies performed in vitro have led to new concepts of metabolic control (such as mechanisms of substrate competition and the importance of myocardial glycogen metabolism) that will ultimately contribute to improved strategies for diagnosis and treatment of heart disease. Imaging of regional myocardial metabolism with positron-labeled tracers—now used with increasing frequency in the diagnosis of reversibly injured myocardium—and the treatment of certain forms of refractory heart failure by metabolic support with glucose, insulin, and potassium are two examples of how decades of painstaking basic research have resulted in potentially lifesaving new clinical strategies. In short: Understanding fuel metabolism of the heart provides essential clues to the understanding of ischemia and heart failure, the two most common manifestations of heart disease.

OUTLOOK

Improving energy transfer in the stressed heart through targeted metabolic interventions is an emerging goal of pharmacotherapy.[21] More importantly, there is reason to believe that the transcriptional regulation of "metabolic genes" is subject to modulation by metabolites per se, including oxygen, glucose, and fatty acids.[219] Metabolic regulation of cardiac gene expression and transcriptional modulators targeted at cardiac fuel metabolism[105, 220] usher in a new chapter in cardiac physiology.[221] Perhaps the most important challenge is to develop the right approaches to connect genes and cardiac function. Further study of the dynamics of cardiac fuel metabolism will be able to close this gap.

ACKNOWLEDGMENTS

I thank Rachel Ralston for help with preparation of the manuscript. Work from my laboratory was supported by NHLBI Grants RO1 HL61483 and 2 RO1 HL43133 and a grant from the American Heart Association National Center.

REFERENCES

1. Katz A: Molecular biology in cardiology, a paradigm shift. J Mol Cell Cardiol 20:355, 1988.
2. Roberts R: Molecular Basis of Cardiology. Oxford: Blackwell Scientific, 1993.
3. Chien KR (ed): Molecular Basis of Cardiovascular Disease. p. 637. Philadelphia: WB Saunders, 1999.
4. Goodwin GW, Taylor CS, Taegtmeyer H: Regulation of energy metabolism during acute increase in heart work. J Biol Chem 273:29530, 1998.
5. Pashmforoush M, Chien K: Tangled up in blue. Molecular cardiology in the post molecular era. Circulation 96:4126, 1997.
6. Holmes FL: Between Biology and Medicine: The Formation of Intermediary Metabolism. Berkeley: University of California at Berkeley, 1992.
7. Taegtmeyer H: One hundred years ago: Oscar Langendorff and the birth of cardiac metabolism. Can J Cardiol 11:1030, 1995.
8. Evans C: The metabolism of cardiac muscle. *In* Newton W (ed): Evans' Recent Advances in Physiology. 6th ed. p. 157. Philadelphia: Blakiston's, 1939.
9. Bing RJ: The metabolism of the heart. Harvey Lect 50:27, 1955.
10. Neely J, Morgan H: Relationship between carbohydrate and lipid metabolism and the energy balance of heart muscle. Annu Rev Physiol 36:413, 1974.
11. Randle P, Tubbs P: Carbohydrate and fatty acid metabolism. *In* Berne R, Sperelakis V, Geiger S (eds): Handbook of Physiology. The Cardiovascular System. p. 805. Bethesda, MD: American Physiological Society, 1979.
12. Taegtmeyer H: Energy metabolism of the heart: from basic concepts to clinical applications. Curr Probl Cardiol 19:57, 1994.
13. Taegtmeyer H: Six blind men explore an elephant: aspects of fuel metabolism and the control of tricarboxylic acid cycle activity in heart muscle. Basic Res Cardiol 79:322, 1984.
14. Taegtmeyer H: Carbohydrate interconversions and energy production. Circulation 72:1, 1985.
15. Balaban R, Kontor H, Katz L, et al: Relation between work and phosphate metabolite in the in vivo paced mammalian heart. Science 232:1121, 1986.
16. Opie L: Heart physiology from cell to circulation. 3rd ed. Philadelphia: Lippincott-Raven, 1998.
17. Langer G: The Myocardium. San Diego: Academic, 1997.
18. Katz EB, Stenbit AE, Hatton K, et al: Cardiac and adipose tissue abnormalities but no diabetes in mice deficient in GLUT4. Nature 377:151, 1995.
19. DeJong J: Myocardial Energy Metabolism. Dordrecht, The Netherlands: Martinus Nijhoff, 1988.
20. Beadle G, Tatum E: Genetic control of biochemical reactions in Neurospora. Proc Natl Acad Sci 27:499, 1941.
21. Taegtmeyer H, King L, Jones B: Energy substrate metabolism, myocardial ischemia, and targets for pharmacotherapy. Am J Cardiol 82:54K, 1998.
22. Depre C, Taegtmeyer H: Metabolic aspects of programmed cell survival and cell death in the heart. Cardiovasc Res (in press).
23. Taegtmeyer H, Goodwin GW, Doenst T, et al: Substrate metabolism as a determinant for postischemic functional recovery of the heart. Am J Cardiol 80:3A, 1997.
24. Katz A: Is the failing heart energy depleted? Cardiol Clin 16:633, 1998.
25. Lipmann F: Metabolic generation and utilization of phosphate bond energy. Adv Enzymol 1:99, 1941.
26. Soltoff S: ATP and the regulation of renal cell function. Annu Rev Physiol 48:9, 1986.
27. Taegtmeyer H, Roberts AFC, Rayne AEG: Energy metabolism in reperfused rat heart: return of function before normalization of ATP content. J Am Coll Cardiol 6:864, 1985.
28. Kupriyanov VV, Lakomkin VL, Kapelko VI, et al: Dissociation of adenosine triphosphate levels and contractile function in isovolumic hearts perfused with 2-deoxyglucose. J Mol Cell Cardiol 19:729, 1987.
29. Ingwall J: Is cardiac failure a consequence of decreased energy reserve? Circulation 87(suppl VII):VII-58, 1993.
30. Bassingthwaighte J, Ypintsoi T, Harvey R: Microvasculature of dog left ventricular myocardium. Microvasc Res 7:229, 1974.
31. Barth E, Stämmler G, Speiser B, et al: Ultrastructural quantitation of mitochondria and myofilaments in cardiac muscle from 10 different animal species including man. J Mol Cell Cardiol 24:669, 1992.
32. McNutt N, Fawcett D: Myocardial ultrastructure. *In* Lauger G, Brady A (eds): The Mammalian Myocardium. p. 1. New York: John Wiley & Sons, 1984.
33. Baldwin JE, Krebs HA: The evolution of metabolic cycles. Nature 291:381, 1981.
34. Newsholme E, Start C: Regulation in Metabolism. London: John Wiley & Sons, 1973.
35. Newsholme E, Leech A: Biochemistry for the Medical Sciences. Chichester, England: John Wiley & Sons, 1983.
36. Fell D: Understanding the Control of Metabolism. London: Portland, 1999.
37. Brown G: Control of respiration and ATP synthesis in mammalian mitochondria and cells. Biochem J 284:1, 1993.
38. Krebs H: Control of metabolic processes. Endeavour 16:125, 1957.
39. Hochachka P, Somero G: Strategies of Biochemical Adaptation. Philadelphia: WB Saunders, 1973.
40. Winterstein H: Ueber die Sauerstoffatmung des isolierten Säugetierherzens. Z Allg Physiol 4:333, 1904.
41. Evans CL: The effect of glucose on the gaseous metabolism of the isolated mammalian heart. J Physiol (Lond) 47:407, 1914.
42. Neely JR, Liebermeister H, Battersby EJ, et al: Effect of pressure development on oxygen consumption by isolated rat heart. Am J Physiol 212:804, 1967.
43. Taegtmeyer H, Hems R, Krebs HA: Utilization of energy providing substrates in the isolated working rat heart. Biochem J 186:701, 1980.
44. Nguyễn VTB, Mossberg KA, Tewson TJ, et al: Temporal analysis of myocardial glucose metabolism by ^{18}F-2-deoxy-2-fluoro-D-glucose. Am J Physiol 259:H1022, 1990.
45. Cooney G, Taegtmeyer H, Newsholme E: Tricarboxylic acid cycle flux and enzyme activities in the isolated working rat heart. Biochem J 200:701, 1981.
46. Balaban RS: Regulation of oxidative phosphorylation in the mammalian cell. Am J Physiol 258:C377, 1990.

47. Roseman R: Diet in haste: repent at leisure. Biochemist 14:6, 1992.
48. Jones B, Shan X, Park Y: Coordinated multisite regulation of cellular energy metabolism. Annu Rev Nutr 12:327, 1992.
49. Evans G: The glycogen content of the rat heart. J Physiol (Lond) 82:468, 1934.
50. Denton R, Randle P: Concentrations of glycerides and phospholipids in rat heart and gastrocnemius muscles. Biochem J 104:416, 1967.
51. Gevers W: Protein metabolism of the heart. J Mol Cell Cardiol 16:3, 1984.
52. Lesch M, Taegtmeyer H, Peterson M, et al: Studies on the mechanism of the inhibition of myocardial protein synthesis during oxygen deprivation. Am J Physiol 230:120, 1976.
53. Taegtmeyer H, Lesch M: Altered protein and amino acid metabolism in myocardial hypoxia and ischemia. Amsterdam: Elsevier/North Holland, 1980.
54. Keul J, Doll E, Steim H, et al: Über den Stoffwechsel des menschlichen Herzens I. Pflügers Arch Ges Physiol 282:1, 1965.
55. Merhige M, Ekas R, Mossberg K, et al: Catecholamine stimulation, substrate competition, and myocardial glucose uptake in conscious dogs assessed with positron emission tomography. Circ Res 61(suppl II):II-124, 1987.
56. Maki M, Luotolahti M, Nuutila P, et al: Glucose uptake in the chronically dysfunctional but viable myocardium. Circulation 93:1658, 1996.
57. Ng C, Soufer R, McNulty P: Effect of hyperinsulinemia on myocardial fluorine-18-FDG uptake. J Nucl Med 39:379, 1998.
58. Takala T, Nuutila P, Knuuti J, et al: Insulin action on heart and skeletal muscle glucose uptake in weight lifters and endurance athletes. Am J Physiol 276:E706, 1999.
59. Rothlin M, Bing R: Extraction and release of individual free fatty acids by the heart and fat deposits. J Clin Invest 40:1380, 1961.
60. Goodwin G, Taylor C, Taegtmeyer H: Regulation of energy metabolism of the heart during acute increase in heart work. J Biol Chem 273:29530, 1998.
61. Goodwin GW, Ahmad F, Doenst T, et al: Energy provision from glycogen, glucose and fatty acids upon adrenergic stimulation of isolated working rat heart. Am J Physiol 274:H1239, 1998.
62. Keul J, Doll E, Keppler D: Energy metabolism of human muscle. Basel: S Karger, 1972.
63. Drake AJ, Haines JR, Noble MM: Preferential uptake of lactate by the normal myocardium in dogs. Cardiovasc Res 14:65, 1980.
64. Gadian D, Hoult D, Radda G, et al: Phosphorous nuclear magnetic resonance studies in normoxic and ischemic cardiac tissue. Proc Natl Acad Sci U S A 73:291, 1976.
65. Weiss E, Hoffman E, Phelps M, et al: External detection and visualization of myocardial ischemia with ^{11}C substrates in vitro and in vivo. Circ Res 39:24, 1976.
66. Jacobus W, Taylor G, Hollis D, et al: Phosphorous nuclear magnetic resonance of perfused working rat hearts. Nature 265:756, 1977.
67. Ingwall J: Phosphorous nuclear magnetic resonance spectroscopy of cardiac and skeletal muscles. Am J Physiol 242:H729, 1982.
68. Bottomley P: Noninvasive study of high energy phosphate metabolism in human heart by depth-resolved ^{31}P NMR spectroscopy. Science 229:769, 1985.
69. Schelbert H: Assessment of myocardial metabolism by PET: a sophisticated dream or clinical reality? Eur J Nucl Med 12:570, 1986.
70. McMillin-Wood J: Biochemical approaches in metabolism: application to positron emission tomography. Circulation 72:IV-145, 1985.
71. Taegtmeyer H, Mossberg K, Nguyen V: Positron labelled tracers: A window for the assessment of energy metabolism in heart and skeletal muscle. Acta Radiol 376:40, 1991.
72. Schwaiger M, Hicks R: The clinical role of metabolic imaging of the heart by positron emission tomography. J Nucl Med 32:565, 1991.
73. Lewandowski ED: Nuclear magnetic resonance evaluation of metabolic and respiratory support of work load in intact rabbit hearts. Circ Res 70:576, 1992.
74. Russell R, Cline G, Guthrie P, et al: Regulation of exogenous and endogenous glucose metabolism by insulin and acetoacetate in isolated working rat heart: a three-tracer study of glycolysis, glycogen metabolism and glucose oxidation. J Clin Invest 100:2892, 1997.
75. Malloy C, Sherry A, Jeffrey F: Carbon flux through citric acid cycle pathways in perfused heart by ^{13}C NMR spectroscopy. FEBS Lett 212:58, 1987.
76. Weiss RG, Gloth ST, Kalil-Filho R, et al: Indexing tricarboxylic acid cycle flux in intact hearts by carbon-13 nuclear magnetic resonance. Circ Res 70:392, 1992.
77. Laughlin MR, Fleming Taylor J, Chesnik AS, et al: Regulation of glycogen metabolism in canine myocardium: effects of insulin and epinephrine in vivo. Am J Physiol 262:E875, 1992.
78. Malloy C, Jones J, Jeffrey F, et al: Contribution of various substrates to total citric acid cycle flux and anaplerosis as determined by ^{13}C isotopomer analysis and O_2 consumption in the heart. MAGMA 4:35, 1996.
79. Bergmann SR: Clinical applications of assessments of myocardial substrate utilization with positron emission tomography. Mol Cell Biochem 88:201, 1989.
80. Schelbert H, Henze E, Sochor H: Effects of substrate availability on myocardial ^{11}C palmitate kinetics by positron emission tomography in normal subjects and patients with ventricular dysfunction. Am Heart J 111:1055, 1986.
81. Brown M, Marshall D, Sobel B, et al: Delineation of myocardial oxygen utilization with carbon-11 labelled acetate. Circulation 76:687, 1987.
82. Buxton D, Schwaiger M, Nguyen N, et al: Radiolabelled acetate as a tracer of myocardial tricarboxylic acid cycle flux. Circ Res 63:628, 1988.
83. Sokoloff L, Reivich M, Kennedy C, et al: The [^{14}C] deoxyglucose method for the measurement of local cerebral glucose utilization: theory, procedure, and normal values in the conscious and anesthetized albino rat. J Neurochem 28:897, 1977.
84. Hariharan R, Bray MS, Ganim R, et al: Fundamental limitations of [^{18}F] 2-deoxy-2-fluoro-D-glucose for assessing myocardial glucose uptake. Circulation 91:2435, 1995.
85. Doenst T, Guthrie PH, Taegtmeyer H: Ischemic preconditioning in rat heart: no correlation between glycogen content and return of function. Mol Cell Biochem 180:153, 1998.
86. Botker H, Goodwin G, Holden J, et al: Myocardial glucose uptake measured with fluorodeoxyglucose: a proposed method to account for variable lumped constants. J Nucl Med 40:1186, 1999.
87. Safer B, Williamson J: Mitochondrial-cytosolic interactions in perfused rat heart: role of coupled transamination in repletion of citric acid cycle intermediates. J Biol Chem 248:2570, 1973.
88. Taegtmeyer H, Peterson MB, Ragavan VV, et al: De novo alanine synthesis in isolated oxygen-deprived rabbit myocardium. J Biol Chem 252:5010, 1977.
89. Taegtmeyer H: Metabolic responses to cardiac hypoxia: increased production of succinate by rabbit papillary muscles. Circ Res 43:808, 1978.
90. Depre C, Vanoverschelde J, Taegtmeyer H: Glucose for the heart. Circulation 99:578, 1999.
91. Russell RR, Taegtmeyer H: Coenzyme A sequestration in rat hearts oxidizing ketone bodies. J Clin Invest 89:968, 1992.
92. Tirosh R, Mishor T, Pinson A: Glucose is essential for the initiation of fatty acid oxidation in ATP-depleted cultured myocytes. Mol Cell Biochem 162:159, 1996.
93. Reid M, Reilly B, Murdock A, et al: Cardiomegaly in association with neonatal hypoglycaemia. Acta Paediatr Scand 60:295, 1971.
94. Gertz EW, Wisneski JA, Neese RA, et al: Myocardial lactate metabolism: evidence of lactate release during net chemical extraction in man. Circulation 63:1273, 1981.
95. Goodwin G, Ahmad F, Taegtmeyer H: Preferential oxidation of glycogen in isolated working rat heart. J Clin Invest 97:1409, 1996.
96. Wisneski JA, Gertz EW, Neese RA, et al: Metabolic fate of extracted glucose in normal human myocardium. J Clin Invest 76:1819, 1985.
97. Wisneski J, Stanley W, Neese R, et al: Effects of acute hyperglycemia on myocardial glycolytic activity in humans. J Clin Invest 85:1648, 1990.
98. Gertz EW, Wisneski JA, Stanley WC, et al: Myocardial substrate utilization during exercise in humans. J Clin Invest 82:2017, 1988.
99. Widdas W, Wiedeman M: Facilitated transfer of hexoses across the human erythrocyte membrane architecture. Handbook of Physiology, Section 2: The Cardiovascular System. Vol. IV: Microcirculation, part 1. 125, 1954
100. Gould G: Facilitative glucose transporters. Landes Comp., Georgetown, TX: Chapman & Hall, 1997.
101. Pessin JE, Bell GI: Mammalian facilitative glucose transporter family: structure and molecular regulation. Annu Rev Physiol 54:911, 1992.

102. Gould GW, Holman GD: The glucose transporter family: structure, function and tissue-specific expression. Biochem J 295:329, 1993.
103. Mueckler M: Facilitative glucose transporters. Eur J Biochem 219:713, 1994.
104. Shepherd P, Kahn B: Glucose transporters and insulin action: implications for insulin resistance and diabetes mellitus. N Engl J Med 341:248, 1999.
105. Depre C, Shipley G, Chen W, et al: Unloaded heart in vivo replicates fetal gene expression of cardiac hypertrophy. Nature Med 4:1269, 1998.
106. Baron AD: Hemodynamic actions of insulin. Am J Physiol 267:E187, 1994.
107. Cushman S, Wardzala L: Potential mechanism of insulin action on glucose transport in the isolated rat adipose cell. J Biol Chem 255:4755, 1980.
108. Wheeler TJ: Translocation of glucose transporters in response to anoxia in heart. J Biol Chem 263:19447, 1988.
109. Sun D, Nguyen N, Delgrado TR, et al: Ischemia induces translocation of the insulin-responsive glucose transporter GLUT 4 to the plasma membrane of cardiac myocytes. Circulation 89:793, 1994.
110. Russell R, Yin R, Caplan M, et al: Ischemia on myocardial GLUT1 and GLUT4 translocation in vivo. Circulation 98:2180, 1998.
111. Doenst T, Taegtmeyer H: α-Adrenergic stimulation mediates glucose uptake through phosphatidylinositol 3-kinase in rat heart. Circ Res 84:467, 1999.
112. Doenst T, Taegtmeyer H: Ischemia-stimulated glucose uptake does not require catecholamines in rat heart. J Mol Cell Cardiol 31:435, 1999.
113. Behrooz A, Ismail-Beigi F: Stimulation of glucose transport by hypoxia: signals and mechanisms. News Physiol Sci 14:105, 1999.
114. Nishimura H, Pallardo FV, Seidner GA, et al: Kinetics of GLUT1 and GLUT4 glucose transporters expressed in *Xenopus* oocytes. J Biol Chem 268:8514, 1993.
115. Shephard P, Gould G, Colville C, et al: Distribution of GLUT3 glucose transporter in human tissues. Biochem Biophys Res Comm 188:149, 1992.
116. Barrett E, Schwartz R, Francis C, et al: Regulation by insulin of myocardial glucose and fatty acid metabolism in the conscious dog. J Clin Invest 74:1073, 1984.
117. Russell RR, Nguyễn VTB, Mrus JM, et al: Fasting and lactate unmask insulin responsiveness in the isolated working rat heart. Am J Physiol 263:E556, 1992.
118. Morgan HE, Henderson MJ, Regen DM, et al: Regulation of glucose uptake in muscle. I. The effects of insulin and anoxia on glucose transport and phosphorylation in the isolated perfused heart of normal rats. J Biol Chem 236:253, 1961.
119. Schwaiger M, Neese R, Araujo L, et al: Sustained nonoxidative glucose utilization and depletion of glycogen in reperfused canine myocardium. J Am Coll Cardiol 13:745, 1989.
120. Doenst T, Taegtmeyer H: Profound underestimation of glucose uptake by [18F]2-deoxy-2-fluoroglucose in reperfused rat heart muscle. Circulation 97:2454, 1998.
121. Doenst T, Richwine R, Bray M, et al: Insulin improves functional and metabolic recovery of reperfused working rat heart. Ann Thorac Surg 67:1682, 1999.
122. Newsholme E, Crabtree B: Theoretical principles in the approaches to the control of metabolic pathways and their application to glycolysis in muscle. J Mol Cell Cardiol 11:839, 1979.
123. Camici P, Ferrannini E, Opie L: Myocardial metabolism in ischemic heart disease: basic principles and application to imaging by positron emission tomography. Progr Cardiovasc Dis 32:217, 1989.
124. Cohen P: Control of Enzyme Activity. London: Chapman & Hall, 1976.
125. Cori G, Colowick S, Cori C: The action of nucleotides on the disruptive phosphorylation of glycogen. J Biol Chem 123:381, 1938.
126. Krebs E, Fischer E: The phosphorylase b to a converting enzyme of rabbit skeletal muscle. Biochim Biophys Acta 20:150, 1956.
127. Robison G, Butcher R, Sutherland E: Cyclic AMP. London: Academic, 1971.
128. Johnson M, Everott B (eds): Essential Reproduction. 3rd ed. p. 275. Oxford: Blackwell Scientific, 1988.
129. Aschoff L: Ueber den glykogengehalt des reizleitungssystems des sangetierherzens. Verh Dtsch Pathol Ges 12:150, 1908.
130. Entman ML, Kanike K, Goldstein MA, et al: Association of glycogenolysis with cardiac sarcoplasmic reticulum. J Biol Chem 251:3140, 1976.
131. Chin E, Allen D: Effects of reduced muscle glycogen concentration on force, Ca^{2+} release and contractile protein function in intact mouse skeletal muscle. J Physiol (Lond) 498:17, 1997.
132. Laughlin M, Petit W, Dizon J, et al: NMR measurements of in vivo myocardial glycogen metabolism. J Biol Chem 263:2285, 1988.
133. Cohen P: The hormonal control of glycogen metabolism in mammalian muscle by multisite phosphorylation. Biochem Soc Trans 7:459, 1979.
134. Tillisch J, Brunker R, Marshall R: Reversibility of cardiac wall-motion abnormalities predicted by positron emission tomography. N Engl J Med 314:884, 1986.
135. Bolukoglu H, Goodwin GW, Guthrie PH, et al: Metabolic fate of glucose in reversible low-flow ischemia of the isolated working rat heart. Am J Physiol 270:H817, 1996.
136. Chen TM, Goodwin GW, Guthrie PH, et al: Effects of insulin on glucose uptake by rat hearts during and after coronary flow reduction. Am J Physiol 273:H2170, 1997.
137. Scheuer J, Stezoski SW: Protective role of increased myocardial glycogen stores in cardiac anoxia in the rat. Circ Res 27:835, 1970.
138. Hearse DJ, Chain EB: The role of glucose in the survival and "recovery" of the anoxic isolated perfused rat heart. Biochem J 128:1125, 1972.
139. McElroy DD, Walker WE, Taegtmeyer H: Glycogen loading improves left ventricular function of the rabbit heart after hypothermic ischemic arrest. J Appl Cardiol 4:455, 1989.
140. Schneider CA, Nguyễn VTB, Taegtmeyer H: Feeding and fasting determine postischemic glucose utilization in isolated working rat hearts. Am J Physiol 260:H542, 1991.
141. Schneider CA, Taegtmeyer H: Fasting in vivo delays myocardial cell damage after brief periods of ischemia in the isolated working rat heart. Circ Res 68:1045, 1991.
142. Conlee R, Tipton C: Cardiac glycogen depletion after exercise: influence of synthase and glucose 6-P. J Appl Physiol 42:240, 1977.
143. Opie L: The glucose hypothesis: relation to acute myocardial ischemia. J Mol Cell Cardiol 1:107, 1970.
144. Apstein CS, Gravino FN, Haudenschild CC: Determinants of a protective effect of glucose and insulin on the ischemic myocardium. Effects on contractile function, diastolic compliance, metabolism, and ultrastructure during ischemia and reperfusion. Circ Res 52:515, 1983.
145. Doenst T, Guthrie P, Chemnitius J-M, et al: Fasting, lactate, and insulin improve ischemia tolerance: a comparison with ischemic preconditioning. Am J Physiol 270:H1607, 1996.
146. Wasser J, Meinertz E, Chang S, et al: Metabolic and cardiodynamic responses of isolated turtle hearts to ischemia and reperfusion. Am J Physiol 262:H437, 1992.
147. Lolley DM, Ray JF, Myers WO, et al: Importance of preoperative myocardial glycogen levels in human cardiac preservation. Cardiovasc Surg 78:678, 1979.
148. Lagerstrom CF, Walker WE, Taegtmeyer H: Failure of glycogen depletion to improve left ventricular function of the rabbit heart after hypothermic ischemic arrest. Circ Res 63:81, 1988.
149. Taegtmeyer H, Overturf ML: Effects of moderate hypertension on cardiac function and metabolism in the rabbit. Hypertension 11:416, 1988.
150. Bishop S, Altschuld R: Increased glycolytic metabolism in cardiac hypertrophy and congestive heart failure. Am J Physiol 218:153, 1970.
151. Allard MF, Emanuel PG, Russell JA, et al: Preischemic glycogen reduction or glycolytic inhibition improves postischemic recovery of hypertrophied rat heart. Am J Physiol 267:H66, 1994.
152. Eberli FR, Weinberg EO, Grice WN, et al: Protective effect of increased glycolytic substrate against systolic and diastolic dysfunction and increased coronary resistance from prolonged global underperfusion and reperfusion in isolated rabbit hearts perfused with erythrocyte suspensions. Circ Res 68:466, 1991.
153. Marshall RC, Tillisch JH, Phelps ME, et al: Identification and differentiation of resting myocardial ischemia and infarction in man with positron computer tomography, ^{18}F-labeled fluorodeoxyglucose and ^{13}N ammonia. Circulation 67:766, 1983.

154. Tillisch J, Brunken R, Marshall R, et al: Prediction of reversibility of cardiac wall motion abnormalities predicted by positron tomography, ^{18}fluoro-deoxyglucose, and $^{13}NH_3$. N Engl J Med 314:884–888, 1986.
155. Neely JR, Grotyohann LW: Role of glycolytic products in damage to myocardium: dissociation of adenosine triphosphate levels and recovery of function of reperfused canine myocardium. Circ Res 55:816, 1984.
156. Kersten J, Schmeling T, Orth K, et al: Acute hyperglycemia abolishes ischemic preconditioning in vivo. Am J Physiol 275:H721, 1998.
157. Gradinak S, Coleman GM, Taegtmeyer H, et al: Improved cardiac function with glucose-insulin-potassium after coronary bypass surgery. Ann Thorac Surg 48:484, 1989.
158. Taegtmeyer H: The use of hypertonic glucose, insulin, and potassium (GIK) in myocardial preservation. J Appl Cardiol 6:255, 1991.
159. Aasum E, Lathrop D, Henden T, et al: The role of glycolysis in myocardial calcium control. J Mol Cell Cardiol 30:1703, 1998.
160. Malhotra R, Brosius F: Glucose uptake and glycolysis reduce hypoxia-induced apoptosis in cultured neonatal rat cardiac myocytes. J Biol Chem 274:12567, 1999.
161. Uyeda K: Phosphofructokinase. Adv Enzymol 48:193, 1979.
162. Passonneau JV, Lowry OH: Phosphofructokinase and the Pasteur effect. Biochem Biophys Res Comm 7:10, 1962.
163. Hue L, Rider MH: Role of fructose 2,6-bisphosphate in the control of glycolysis in mammalian tissues. Biochem J 245:313, 1987.
164. Depre C, Rider MH, Veitch K, et al: Role of fructose 2,6-bisphosphate in the control of heart glycolysis. J Biol Chem 268:13274, 1993.
165. Kobayashi K, Neely J: Control of maximum rates of glycolysis in rat cardiac muscle. Circ Res 44:166, 1979.
166. Rovetto M, Lamberton W, Neely J: Mechanisms of glycolytic inhibition in ischemic rat heart. Circ Res 37:742, 1975.
167. Nuutila P, Koivisto VA, Knuuti J, et al: Glucose-free fatty acid cycle operates in human heart and skeletal muscle in vivo. J Clin Invest 89:1767, 1992.
168. Peuhkurinen KJ, Hassinen IE: Pyruvate carboxylation as an anaplerotic mechanism in the isolated perfused rat heart. Biochem J 202:67, 1982.
169. Russell RR, Taegtmeyer H: Pyruvate carboxylation prevents the decline in contractile function of rat hearts oxidizing acetoacetate. Am J Physiol 261:H1756, 1991.
170. LaNoue K, Schoolwerth A: Metabolite transport in mitochondria. Annu Rev Biochem 48:871, 1979.
171. Denton R, Halestrap A: Regulations of pyruvate metabolism in mammalian tissues. Essays Biochem 15:37, 1979.
172. Randle P, Sugden P, Kerbey A, et al: Regulation of pyruvate oxidation and the conservation of glucose. Biochem Soc Symp 43:47, 1978.
173. Randle P: Regulation of glycolysis and pyruvate oxidation in cardiac muscle. Circ Res 38:I8, 1976.
174. Kerbey AL, Randle PJ, Cooper RH, et al: Regulation of pyruvate dehydrogenase in rat heart. Biochem J 154:327, 1976.
175. Olson M, Dennis S, DeBuysere M, et al: The regulation of pyruvate dehydrogenase in the isolated perfused rat heart. J Biol Chem 253:7369, 1978.
176. Borst P, Loos J, Christ E, et al: Uncoupling activity of long-chain fatty acids. Biochem Biophys Acta 62:509, 1962.
177. Schaffer JE, Lodish HF: Expression cloning and characterization of a novel adipocyte long chain fatty acid transport protein. 79:427, 1994.
178. van der Vusse G, Groot M: Interrelationship between lactate and cardiac fatty acid metabolism. Mol Cell Biochem 116:11, 1992.
179. Bass N: The cellular fatty acid binding proteins. Int Rev Cytol 111:143, 1988.
180. McGarry J, Mannaerts G, Foster D: A possible role for malonyl-CoA in the regulation of hepatic fatty acid oxidation and ketogenesis. J Clin Invest 60:265, 1977.
181. McGarry J, Mills S, Long C, et al: Observations on the affinity for carnitine and malonyl-CoA sensitivity of carnitine palmitoyl transferase I in animal and human tissues. Demonstration of the presence of malonyl-CoA in non-hepatic tissues of the rat. Biochem J 214:21, 1983.
182. Paulson D, Ward K, Shug A: Malonyl-CoA inhibition of carnitine palmitoyl transferase. FEBS Lett 176:381, 1984.
183. Bianchi A, Evans J, Iverson A, et al: Identification of an isozymic form of acetyl-CoA carboxylase. J Biol Chem 265:1502, 1990.
184. Forsey R, Reid K, Brosnan J: Competition between fatty acids and carbohydrate or ketone bodies as metabolic fuels for the isolated perfused heart. Can J Physiol Pharmacol 65:401, 1987.
185. Pauly D, Kirk K, McMillin J: Carnitine palmitoyl transferase in cardiac ischemia. A potential site for altered fatty acid metabolism. Circ Res 68:1085, 1991.
186. Bremer J, Wojtzak A: Factors controlling the role of fatty acid beta oxidation in rat liver mitochondria. Biochem Biophys Acta 280:515, 1972.
187. Shrago E, Shug AL, Sul H, et al: Control of energy production in myocardial ischemia. Circ Res 38:75, 1976.
188. Saggerson D, Ghadiminejad J, Awan M: Regulation of mitochondrial carnitine palmitoyl transferases from liver and extrahepatic tissues. Adv Enzyme Regul 32:285, 1992.
189. Oram J, Bennetch S, Neely J: Regulation of fatty acid utilization in isolated perfused rat hearts. J Biol Chem 248:5299, 1973.
190. Brandt J, Djouadi F, Kelly D: Fatty acids activate transcription of the muscle carnitine palmitoyltransferase I gene in cardiac myocytes via the peroxisome proliferator-activated receptor alpha. J Biol Chem 273:23786, 1998.
191. Vamecq J, Latruffe N: Medical significance of peroxisome proliferator-activated receptors. Lancet 354:141, 1999.
192. Coates P, Stanley C: Inherited disorders of mitochondrial fatty acid oxidation. Prog Liver Dis 10:123, 1992.
193. Kelly D, Strauss A: Inherited cardiomyopathies. N Engl J Med 330:913, 1994.
194. Hale D, Stanley C, Coates P: The long-chain acyl-CoA dehydrogenase deficiency. Prog Clin Biol Res 321:303, 1990.
195. Hale D, Bennet M: Fatty acid oxidation disorders: a new class of metabolic diseases. J Pediatr 121:1, 1992.
196. Naylor I, Mosovich L, Guthrie R, et al: Intermittent non-ketotic dicarboxylic aciduria in two siblings with hypoglycemia: an apparent defect in β-oxidation of fatty acids. J Inherit Metab Dis 3:19, 1980.
197. Schwenk W, Hale D, Haymond M: Decreased fasting free fatty acids with L-carnitine in children with carnitine deficiency. Pediatr Res 23:491, 1988.
198. Amendt B, Moon A, Teel L, et al: Long-chain acyl-coenzyme A dehydrogenase deficiency: biochemical studies in fibroblasts from three patients. Pediatr Res 23:603, 1988.
199. Tripp M, Katcher M, Peters H, et al: Systemic carnitine deficiency presenting as familial endomyocardial fibroelastosis. N Engl J Med 303:385, 1981.
200. Challoner D, Pols H: Fatty acid concentration and carnitine levels in diphtheric guinea pig myocardium. J Clin Invest 51:2071, 1972.
201. Stanley C, DeLeeuw S, Coats P, et al: Chronic cardiomyopathy and weakness or acute coma in children with a defect in carnitine uptake. Ann Neurol 30:709, 1991.
202. Williamson J, Krebs H: Acetoacetate as fuel of respiration in the perfused rat heart. Biochem J 80:540, 1961.
203. Rudolph W, Haas D, Richter J, et al: Uber die Bedeutung von Acetoacetat und β-Hydroxybutyrat im Stoffwechel der menschlichen Herzens. Klin Wochenscher 43:445, 1965.
204. Williamson D, Bates M, Page M, et al: Activities of enzymes involved in acetoacetate utilization in adult mammalian tissue. Biochem J 121:41, 1971.
205. Zimmermann A, Meijler F, Hülsmann W: The inhibitory effect of acetoacetate on myocardial contraction. Lancet 2:757, 1962.
206. Taegtmeyer H, Russell R: Control of cardiac function by substrate flux through Krebs cycle spans: a new concept for the relationship between metabolism and contraction. J Mol Cell Cardiol 23:S25, 1991.
207. Russell RR III, Taegtmeyer H: Coenzyme A sequestration in rat hearts oxidating ketone bodies. J Clin Invest 89:968, 1992.
208. Taegtmeyer H, Passmore JM: Defective energy metabolism of the heart in diabetes. Lancet 1:139, 1985.
209. Russell RR III, Taegtmeyer H: Pyruvate carboxylation prevents the decline in contractile function of rat hearts oxidating acetoacetate. Am J Physiol 261:H1756, 1991.
210. Russell RR, Mommessin JI, Taegtmeyer H: Propionyl-L-carnitine–mediated improvement in contractile function of rat hearts oxidizing acetoacetate. Am J Physiol 268:H441, 1995.
211. Cohen D, Bergman R: Improved estimation of anaplerosis in heart using ^{13}C NMR. Am J Physiol 273:E1228, 1997.

212. Krebs HA: Some aspects of the regulation of fuel supply in omnivorous animals. Adv Enzyme Regul 10:397, 1972.
213. Henze E, Schelbert H, Barrio J, et al: Evaluation of myocardial metabolism with ^{13}N and ^{11}C labelled amino acids and positron computed tomography. J Nucl Med 23:671, 1982.
214. Taegtmeyer H, Ferguson A, Lesch M: Protein degradation and amino acid metabolism in autolyzing rabbit myocardium. Exp Mol Pathol 26:52, 1977.
215. Mudge G, Mills R, Taegtmeyer H, et al: Alterations of myocardial amino acid metabolism in chronic ischemic heart disease. J Clin Invest 58:1185, 1976.
216. Bittl J, Shine K: Protection of ischemic rabbit myocardium by glutamic acid. Am J Physiol 245:H406, 1983.
217. Knapp W, Helus F, Ostertag H, et al: Uptake and turnover of L-[^{13}N] glutamate in the normal human heart and patients with coronary artery disease. Eur J Nucl Med 7:211, 1982.
218. Robertson J, Vinten-Johansen J, Buckberg G, et al: Safety of prolonged aortic clamping with blood cardioplegia: glutamate enrichment in normal hearts. J Thorac Cardiovasc Surg 88:402, 1984.
219. Van Bilsen M, Van Der Vusse G, Reneman R: Transcriptional regulation of metabolic processes: implications for cardiac metabolism. Pflugers Arch Eur J Physiol 437:2, 1998.
220. Zarain-Herzberg A, Rupp H: Transcriptional modulators targeted at fuel metabolism of hypertrophied heart. Am J Cardiol 83:31H, 1999.
221. Taegtmeyer H, Dietze GE: A symposium: from increased energy metabolism to cardiac hypertrophy and failure: mediators and molecular mechanisms. Am J Cardiol 83:1H, 1999.

CHAPTER 46

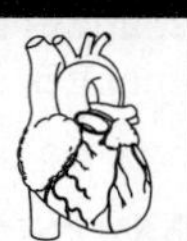

Cardiac Hypertrophy and Failure: Basic Aspects

Bernard Swynghedauw and Edouard Coraboeuf†

MYOCARDIAL ADAPTATION TO MECHANICAL OVERLOAD
Biologic Process of Adaptation
Energy Metabolism
GROWTH SIGNALS AND INITIATION OF THE HYPERTROPHIC PROCESS
Sensors
Transduction Systems
DNA Targets
Transgenic Technology
Transient Changes in Gene Expression
Permanent Changes in Gene Expression
CELLULAR CHANGES
Cell Division
Cell Death
BIOLOGIC DETERMINANTS OF SYSTOLIC DYSFUNCTION
Energy Metabolism
Contractile Apparatus
Membrane Proteins
Excitation-Contraction Coupling
Ca^{2+} Transient
Cytoskeleton
BIOLOGIC DETERMINANTS OF DIASTOLIC DYSFUNCTION
Intrinsic Myocardial Stiffness and Fibrosis
Active Relaxation
Atrial Contraction
ENDOCRINE FUNCTION OF THE HEART
Atrial Natriuretic Peptides
Renin-Angiotensin, Renin-Angiotensin System, and Aldosterone System
Other Vasoactive Compounds
ELECTROPHYSIOLOGIC ASPECTS
Basis of Cardiac Cellular Electrical Activity
Resting and Action Potentials in Cardiac Hypertrophy
Outward Currents
Inward Currents
Electrophysiologic Consequences of Cardiac Dilatation
Changes in Genetic Expression
Arrhythmias
BIOLOGIC MARKERS FOR CARDIAC FAILURE
SUMMARY

The physiologic alterations in cardiac mechanics that occur during chronic mechanical overload are the direct consequences of structural modifications. The hypertrophic process obviously results from an activation of the overall genetic expression. It was discovered in 1979, in our laboratory,[1] that the expression of isogenes coding for isomyosins was shifted during mechanical overload and therefore that the myocardium was also qualitatively modified. Subsequently, qualitative changes in the genetic expression of the cardiocyte have been documented at other levels, including the membrane proteins.[2]

The study of molecular and cell biology has not transformed the landscape of cardiac insufficiency but rather has allowed researchers to realize that hypertrophy is initially beneficial; that it is the physiologic adaptation of the heart to a disease, and not a disease by itself; and that failure indicates the limits and imperfections of the adaptational process.[3] Another idea emerging is that most of the targets for drugs could in fact be modified through the process of biologic adaptation, both in the heart and on vessels. For example, the shift in the phenotypic expression of the Na^+,K^+-ATPase,[4] which has been observed in experimental cardiac overload, explains, at least in part, the abnormal sensitivity of the isolated hypertrophied heart to ouabain.[5] Another good example is the enhanced angiotensin II receptor density during senescence (a good model of cardiac overload), which may allow these patients to be sensitive to converting enzyme inhibition with an extremely low plasma level of angiotensin II.[6]

This chapter concentrates on cardiac remodeling due to mechanical overload. Advances concerning cardiomyopathies and in particular the cardiomyopathies of genetic origin have been excluded. Also discussed are developments in molecular biology, energetics, and electrophysiology.

Remodeling qualifies changes that result in the rearrangement of normally existing structures[7] and was initially restricted to the remodeling that occurs after myocardial infarction. The meaning of the word has been extended and is used to qualify a variety of conditions, including pure mechanical overload, as well as hypertensive, valvular cardiopathy and familial hypertrophic and dilated cardiomyopathy. During cardiac remodeling, the permanent changes in molecular structure and their physiologic consequences are a complex issue and includes not only the general process of adaptation and its deleterious consequences that mainly occurs at the myocyte level but also fibrosis and the various forms of cell death that are multifactorial, the trophic effects of various hormones and peptides (the neuroendocrine factors), and specific structural

†In memoriam.

changes linked to etiology (ischemia, for example, induces changes in genetic expression[8]).

MYOCARDIAL ADAPTATION TO MECHANICAL OVERLOAD

Biologic Process of Adaptation

Biologic adaptation is a very general process by which a cell or an organ adapts to a change in the environment. There are several types of biologic adaptation: some do not involve the genome itself. During evolution, mutations and polymorphism (i.e., changes in the gene structure) may facilitate adaptation to new environmental requirements. Cardiac hypertrophy due to mechanical overload is a consequence of a change in the expression of the cardiac genome and is characterized by changes in genetic expression (i.e., modifications in several mRNAs and in their corresponding proteins). Advances in genome-based technology allows the study of the overall expression of mRNAs in a given tissue,[9] and showed that in processes such as mechanical overload, there are modifications at nearly every level of the cell structure.

To satisfy the new environmental requirements, the genome uses any new genetic programs available. The biologic adaptation of the heart results in modifications in gene expression and in the corresponding physiologic functions. Nevertheless, because the process is randomly governed, the changes observed at the mRNA level are not always translated in terms of protein or physiologic function. The inventory of the various changes in genetic expression that have been published strongly support the idea that the new genetic program is the fetal one (Table 46–1), probably simply because this program is the only one available in the heart.[10–33] In skeletal muscle, which possesses both an embryonic and a fetal program, hypertrophy is associated with the reexpression of the two programs. Adaptation necessarily means an improved thermodynamic status as a consequence of both quantitative and qualitative modifications.[34, 35] Hypertrophy is beneficial because it multiplies the number of contractile units and normalizes the wall stress. The slowing of V_{max}, the maximum shortening velocity of an unloaded muscle, is the most important qualitative change because it allows the cardiac fiber to produce more tension at a lesser cost. It is associated with or caused by the increased duration of both the action potential and calcium transient, which in turn are consequences of membrane protein modifications. The process is randomly governed, and the beneficial effects are inevitably associated with deleterious modifications: the slowing of V_{max} is also obviously detrimental at the organ level because it will finally be one of the determinants of the diminution of cardiac output; the prolongation of both the action potential and the Ca^{2+} transient is arrhythmogenic (the first favors afterpotentials and the second creates automaticity[36]).

As far as the adaptational process is concerned, cardiac failure indicates the limits of the genetic program of adaptation. From an experimental point of view, the failing heart is a poor model for basic studies, and the various neuroendocrine changes that occur when the pump starts to be depressed have secondary trophic effects on the genetic expression, which renders interpretation of the results extremely tenuous. The experimental approach indeed is only advantageous when it separates the various parameters at the origin of a disease, not when it results in a mixture of the factors.

TABLE 46–1 Changes in Myocardial Genetic Expression in Cardiac Hypertrophy: The Fetal Program

Hypertrophy (cardiocytes, fibroblasts, and extracellular matrix) is due to an overall increase in protein synthesis.* Fibrosis, which is an increased collagen concentration, does not participate in the adaptational process, whereas an increased collagen mass does.
Isogene shifts (from an adult to a fetal isoform)
- Sarcomeric protein
  - Myosin heavy chain (from α to β)[1, 14, 15, 16]†‡
  - Embryonic myosin light chains expressed in ventricles[17, 18]
  - Troponin T (to TnT 2; controversial)[19]
- Membrane proteins
  - Na^+,K^+-ATPase (from α2 to α3)[4, 5, 20]†‡
  - IVS3A calcium channel isoform[21]
- Energy metabolism
  - Mitochondria are more numerous and smaller[11]
  - Switch from fatty acid oxidation to glycolysis[22]
  - Lactate dehydrogenase (from H to M?)[23]
  - Creatine kinase (from M to B)[24]‡

Noninductions (genes are not activated)§
- Ca^{2+}-ATPase of sarcoplasmic reticulum[25]
- Ryanodine receptors[26]
- β_1-Adrenergic receptors[12, 27, 28]‡
- Muscarinic receptors[9, 12, 28]‡
- Kv 4.2 (early transient K^+ current, I_{to})[29, 30]
- Myoglobin[31]

Specific inductions
- Atrial natriuretic factors[32]

*The cellular density of a number of proteins, including the Ca^{2+} channels,[10] mitochondrial proteins,[11] and $G_{\alpha s}$,[12] is unchanged, which means that the synthesis of these specific proteins is activated in parallel.
†Tissue specific.
‡Species specific.
§Because the heart is bigger, the corresponding mRNAs and proteins become diluted. Their concentration diminishes in proportion to hypertrophy.

Energy Metabolism

The fundamental basis of adaptation is an improvement in the thermodynamic status of the heart at the cellular level. Although the beneficial effect of the process of hypertrophy is well documented in the papillary muscle,[34] it is not clear whether such an improved economy also exists in the whole organ, mainly because there are no techniques that allow such a determination to be made in situ. When a muscle is suddenly mechanically overloaded, it is not necessary to develop a complex mechanical approach to understand why this muscle, induced to lift an afterload greater than that to which it is accustomed, instantaneously contracts at a speed slower than normal.[34, 35] The immediate consequence is a fall in the economy of the system, with the muscle using more adenosine triphosphate (ATP) (or oxygen) per gram of developed tension than normal. This can be expressed through an analogy with mechanics. An automobile has an optimal speed, a speed for which the economy (the number of liters of gasoline burned per kilometer) is optimal. On either side of this optimum, the yield drops.

Changes in the biologic structure of the myocardium will allow the heart to continue to contract slowly but with a normalized economy (Table 46–2) through the use of another shortening velocity-afterload relation. In other words, if we want to continue to drive our automobile economically with an increased load, we have to change its motor; the only difference between mechanics and biology is that in the latter, the process is gradual. The final result at the cellular level is an improved economy (i.e., an improvement in the ratio of the mechanical performance of the muscle normalized for the energy flux). Efficiency, which is work normalized for the energy flux, is also improved, but this notion is more useful at the level of the working organ than at the level of the cell.[34]

In isometric conditions (see Table 46–2), there are two variables that allow one to quantify economy: the force-time integral and heat production.[34]

1. The activated muscle develops a certain amount of force per unit of time. The resulting force-time integral of an entire papillary muscle represents the sum of the force-time integrals developed by each of the muscular units (i.e., by each of the cross-bridges).
2. The heat produced by the muscle is the inevitable loss of the energy flux that occurs during any energy transduction, including mechanical transduction and various metabolic interventions, according to Carnot's principles. The heat produced during mechanical activity is proportional to work.

The myocardium uses energy for several purposes:

- Basic processes responsible for the simple survival of the tissue, which include ionic homeostasis and protein synthesis; the corresponding heat is called *resting heat.*
- Contraction, including ATP hydrolysis for cross-bridge cycling and excitation–contraction coupling; the corresponding heats are called *tension-dependent* and *tension-independent heat,* respectively. Total activity-related heat is the sum of *tension-dependent and tension-independent heat.*
- Mitochondrial resynthesis of the high-energy phosphate stores, which is responsible for the *recovery heat.*

The development of low-capacity thermopile permitted Alpert and associates[34] to analyze in detail cardiac heat production on a beat-to-beat basis. It also made it possible to partition the different heats according to their origin. The resting heat is measured at a steady state. Through incubation of the muscle in a 2,3-butanedione monoxime mannitol solution, which arrests the heart and maintains normal Ca^{2+} movements, the heat produced by tension development and that produced by the activity of the membrane pumps that maintain calcium homeostasis in the cell can be partitioned. The recovery heat is calculated through extrapolation from the curve obtained after the contractile cycle.

These variables have been measured in cardiac hypertrophy (see Table 46–2). The hypertrophied heart produces more tension (the tension-time integral is increased) at a slower velocity (indirectly appreciated by measuring dP/dt, which is not strictly speaking a velocity—a length unit per time). The total activity-related heat is reduced, but the reduction is mainly a consequence of a diminution of both tension-dependent and -independent heat. The recovery heat is likely to be normal, as is the corresponding oxidation/phosphorylation process in mitochondria (see later). As a consequence, both the overall economy and the contractile economy of the hypertrophied cardiac fiber are not only normalized but also strongly improved. An important finding is that the Ca^{2+} cycled per beat is also diminished from 50 to 20 nmol/g. This indirect measurement, together with the fact that both tension-dependent and -independent heat were improved, suggests that the biologic determinants of the adaptational process are located at the level of both the contractile apparatus and that of the various components of the membrane that play a role in calcium movements. Both systems function more economically in cardiac hypertrophy and in end-stage cardiac failure in humans.[34, 35]

TABLE 46–2 Energy Transduction in the Papillary Muscle in Compensated Cardiac Hypertrophy

	Hypertrophy (% of controls)
Cardiac hypertrophy	+45**
Force-time integral*	+17**
dP/dt_{max}†	−48**
Resting heat‡	+1
Total activity-related heat§	−41**
Force-dependent heat	−54**
Force-independent heat	−60**
Ca^{2+} cycled per beat‖	−59**
Overall economy¶	+99**
Contractile economy	+156**

*Under isometric conditions, expressed in $mN/s/mm^2$.
†Same results with V_{max} or time to peak tension.
‡Heat production is expressed in mJ/g and is measured with a thermopile. Resting heat is produced by an arrested heart.
§The total activity-related heat is composed of initial heat and recovery heat. Initial heat can be partitioned into force-dependent and -independent heats by incubation of muscle in 2,3-butanedione monoxime-mannitol solution, which eliminates force development without interfering with the various mechanisms used by the cell for Ca^{2+} cycling.
‖Calculated from the measurement of the force-independent heat and with the following assumptions: there is a coupling ratio of 2 Ca^{2+}/mol creatine phosphate hydrolyzed, the enthalpy of creatine phosphate hydrolysis is 35 kJ/m, and 13 percent of the heat is used for Na^+ removal.
¶Economy of isometric force development is the ratio of the force-time integral normalized for the total activity-related heat (overall economy) or the force-dependent heat (contractile economy).
**$P < .01$ as compared with control values.
From Alpert NR, Mulieri LA, Hasenfuss G: Myocardial chemo-receptor energy transduction. *In* Fozzard HA, Haber E, Jennings RB (eds): The Heart and Cardiovascular System. p. 111. New York: Raven, 1991.

Growth Signals and Initiation of the Hypertrophic Process

Cardiac remodeling can be triggered by different factors, including active tension, stretch, vasoactive peptides, and hormones, and requires a cascade of events that includes sensors that receive the information, transduction systems, DNA targets, transient changes in the expression of genes encoding different growth signals, and permanent modifications of the gene expression, which represent the final phenoconversion. Due to the explosive development of the field of molecular biology, this topic is becoming very popular, and the scheme is still extremely complicated.

Sensors

Several sensors that can activate protein synthesis have been identified, including neurotransmitters and hormonal and mechanical signals. It is well established that the local or circulating concentrations of several hormones or peptides (including catecholamines, endothelin, and angiotensin II) are increased as a consequence of the hemodynamic conditions that may play an additional role in promoting hypertrophy.

It is also clear from various experimental data that stretching or pressure overload can stimulate gene expression in the absence of any hormonal stimuli. The idea that mechanics may directly influence gene expression has been rather unorthodox for a long time but is now well documented not only in smooth and striated muscles but also in other tissues, such as fibroblasts, neurons (mechanical stretching of an axon to 100 μm/h or of a fibroblast has atrophic effect), bacteria, and plants (for a review, see Erdös and colleagues[37]). In isolated cardiac cells, protein synthesis is activated to a greater extent when the cells are adhesive and thus under tension; in adhering skeletal myocytes, the mechanical stretching of the support on which the cells are attached further activates amino acid incorporation.[38] Passive stretch of the heart both activates protein synthesis and modulates myocardial genetic expression in isolated adult and neonatal cardiocytes, in papillary muscle, and on isolated coronary perfused heart (in the latter, stretch is obtained through the Gregg effect—sarcomere stretching due to excessive coronary distention).[39]

The endothelium plays a particular role in this process. The endothelium is located at the interface between blood flow and the vascular or cardiac wall and functions as a mechanical sensor that is permanently exposed to pressure and stretch forces, as well as to high fluid shear stress.[40] Nevertheless, the endothelium is not unique in responding to mechanical forces; nearly every cell accommodates such a trigger.

Mechanosensing is still a controversial issue:

1. Pressure stretch can activate ion channels.[41] Such channels are likely to play a role in the genesis of arrhythmias during acute cardiac distension.
2. Shear stretch on endothelial cells activates the formation of endothelin-1, basic fibroblast growth factor, and nitric oxide and then modifies nuclear transcription.
3. Evidence suggests that through integrins and focal adhesion kinases, the cytoskeleton may act as a sensor.[42]
4. Another possibility would involve the mechanically induced production of a variety of hormones, including the myocardial or vascular renin-angiotensin system, endothelin, and several cytokines through autocrine or paracrine mechanisms.[43]

Transduction Systems

Several different transduction systems are likely to be involved after cardiac remodeling. The pioneer work of Yazaki and associates (Komuro and coworkers[43] and Hefti and colleagues[44]) has demonstrated that stretching of attached embryonic cardiac cells in culture simultaneously stimulates the c-*fos* gene expression and increases the production of several phosphatidylinositol cycle intermediates. Several cross-links are well characterized between these pathways, and the scheme is becoming an incredibly complicated puzzle.

The mitogen-activated protein kinase (MAPK) pathway is the best-documented pathway that can mediate both the stretch-induced hypertrophy and the trophic effects of angiotensin II.

- Transfection experiments have demonstrated that protein kinase C (PKC) is involved in the strech-induced expression of several oncogenes through a consensus DNA sequence located upstream from the oncogene and called serum-responsive element. PKC isoforms might be the second messenger in the signaling pathway between the mechanical stimulus and angiotensin II, and the nuclear response.
- PKC is a kinase, which in turn phosphorylates a low-molecular-weight guanosine triphosphate (GTP)-binding protein, p21 Ras, and then a cascade of phosphorylations of another group of kinases, including *Raf-1* (which is an oncogene), MAPK kinase kinase, MAPK kinase, and MAPK.
- The last component of this cascade translocates into the nucleus, where it activates transcription through *Jun*, *Elk-1*, and other oncogenes (for a review, see Hefti and colleagues).[44]

The receptors of most growth factors are transmembrane tyrosine kinases. When activated by the ligand, the receptors specifically autophosphorylate and bind several signaling proteins, including phosphatidylinositol 3-kinase, which activates mitogenesis; phospholipase Cγ, which activates phosphatidylinositol hydrolysis (and consequently increases the intracellular Ca^{2+} concentration); and GTP-bound Ras. Ras plays a central role and transmits the signal through several pathways, including the MAPK pathway, the mitogen-activated extracellular signal-regulated kinase (MEK) pathway, and several others.[44] Transfection experiments have demonstrated that several DNA sequences of the c-*fos* promoter are necessary for this induction; however, it is very unlikely that this transduction system is unique, and there are experiments favoring the role of cAMP or of intracellular Na^+ or Ca^{2+} transients. For example, in the papillary muscle of the ferret, load activates, in parallel, protein synthesis and $^{24}Na^+$ uptake. In addition, protein synthesis was both activated by Na^+ flux enhancers and attenuated by Na^+ flux inhibitors.[41]

DNA Targets

The target has to be one or several sequences of the genome, located upstream of the genes in the region of the promoter or enhancer. It is possible to transform an undifferentiated cell, such as a fibroblast, in a skeletal myoblast by introducing a single factor, MyoD. Such a factor is a nuclear protein (a transcription factor) that binds specific consensus DNA sequences and acts on the transcriptional process to coordinate the expression of several genes to make an entirely new differentiated cell (a similar process occurs during morphogenesis).

MyoD is absent from the heart, and in contrast to skeletal muscle, the genetic program regulating cardiac development is complex, combinatorial, and multifactorial. There are, for the moment, three transcription factors that have been identified in the heart: CATF, which binds the specific DNA consensus sequence CARE and transactivates atrial natriuretic factor (ANF) gene expression; MEF2, which belongs to the MADS motif family and regulates the expression of the gene encoding a specific cardiac myosin light chain; and the GATA motif, which is present on a variety of zinc finger transcription factors and is present on both the promoter of the beta-myosin heavy chain and that of angiotensin receptor subtype 1A. Mutagenesis experiments were made after aortic banding in rats and demonstrated that GATA4 mediates the hypertrophic responsiveness. For the moment, GATA4 is the only transcription factor that directly regulates cardiac hypertrophy. Other potential candidates include a DNA binding dimerization motif termed *helix-loop-helix*, which is found in MyoD1, myogenin, E12, and E47; the leucine zipper that binds DNA to several proto-oncogenes; the helix-turn-helix motif, which is found in SOX, and an activator protein termed AP-2 (for a review, see Grépin and associates[45]).

Transgenic Technology

Transgenic technology allows the generation of new strains of mice with either several types of cardiac hypertrophy or failure or specific cardiac dysfunction (for a review, see Swynghedauw[46]). Several models of cardiac hypertrophy without failure have been developed using genes encoding various transcriptional factors or cytokines, including c-*myc* (a 20-fold increase produces hypertrophy in 46 percent), v-*fps* (the overexpression of v-*fps* provokes cardiac fibrosis), *p-21 ras* (cardiac hypertrophy is then accompanied by diastolic dysfunction), and interleukin (IL)-6 plus IL-6 receptor. In contrast, ectopic expression of skeletal myogenic regulators or viral constructs have pronounced deleterious effects. The targeted expression of *bmyf5* or *MyoD* in the mouse heart activates the expression of several skeletal muscle–specific proteins in the myocardium and results in either pronounced cardiac necrosis and fibrosis with severe failure or embryonic lethality due to severe cardiac abnormalities. Models that associate both cardiac and skeletal myopathy, and as such resemble muscular dystrophies in humans, were achieved in mice by targeting the simian virus tsA58 to the heart and skeletal muscle. Other transgenic models of cardiac failure have been obtained with the use of other viral constructs, such as an early gene of polyomavirus (large T-antigen) or the Epstein-Barr virus nuclear antigen–leader protein. Finally, the targeted overexpression or disruption of genes known to play a critical role during the cardiac cycle results in specific modifications of various cardiac functions, such as relaxation, contraction, heart rate variability, sensitivity to isoproterenol, or tolerance to ischemia.

Transient Changes in Gene Expression

The expression of some genes is only transient. Most of the genes that belong to this category code for growth signals.

- A single stretch of an isolated cardiocyte is able to induce the expression of several proto-oncogenes. The same result is obtained in vivo a few minutes or hours after aortic banding or in an isolated heart under increased aortic pressure.[47] At least two groups of oncogenes are expressed: c-*myc*, which is a nuclear oncogene that has a role during mitosis and may be a candidate for activation of the mitotic division of the nonmuscular cardiac cells, and c-*fos*/c-*jun*, which codes for a rather complex group of oncoproteins and acts in synergy to induce gene expression in a rather nonspecific way.
- Another group consists of the heat-shock proteins (HSP), or stress proteins, which are expressed in the rat heart in vivo a few days after aortic stenosis or incompetence. They probably play a role in preservation of the mRNAs.[48]
- Polypeptide growth factors are present in the myocardium and have a role during development.[49] Transforming growth factor-β (TGFβ) is up-regulated more than sixfold after myocardial infarction in the rat. Data concerning the effects of aortic stenosis on polypeptide growth factor expression remain scarce. An interesting hypothesis is that the increased expression of growth factors relates to cardiac hypertrophy, which compensates for a decrease in mass, as occurs in myocardial infarction; this is the opposite of cardiac hypertrophy, which occurs as a reaction to stretch.
- A transient remodeling of the microtubular network occurs during the first days after aortic stenosis and can play the role of a guide in the shift in myosin isogene expression.[42] It is accompanied by the transient coexpression of the mRNA coding for the skeletal isoform of alpha-actin.[50]
- As explained, there are arguments favoring a superimposed post-transcriptional regulation. Such mechanisms may involve the expression of genes coding for translational factors, such as elongation factors. This avenue has not yet been really explored, and the only relevant suggestion is the finding of an early increase of ribosomal protein synthesis after mechanical overloading.[51]

Permanent Changes in Gene Expression

The main characteristics of the permanent modification of genetic expression are as follows (see Table 46–1):

- From a quantitative point of view, there is an overall increase in the cardiac expression of most of the genes that finally lead to hypertrophy. The concentration of the corresponding mRNAs and proteins remains unchanged, but the amount per ventricle is increased. Contractile proteins, including total myosin,[52] Ca^{2+} channels, and mitochondrial proteins, belong to this group.
- There is an enlarging group of membrane proteins whose density diminishes in cardiac hypertrophy. The concentrations of the protein and corresponding mRNA drop in parallel to the extent of hypertrophy. Ca^{2+}-ATPase of

the sarcoplasmic reticulum (SR) and the beta$_1$-adrenergic receptor belongs to this group of proteins,[12, 25, 27, 28] which suggests that the gene is not activated and that the corresponding products are diluted in the hypertrophied tissue.

- The concentration of other proteins can be in excess relative to the tissue mass. Such an excessive accumulation can correspond to the activation via the mechanics of certain genes such as the atrial natriuretic factor in the ventricle.[32]
- Qualitative changes in the gene expression mainly involve a shift in the expression of several isogenes toward another genetic program. This occurs not only in the sarcomere of the rat ventricle, where it was initially discovered,[1] but also in the external membrane and in other species, including human.[14] It is reversible.[14]
- Fibrosis (the increased concentration in extracellular matrix components, including collagen and fibronectin) is multifactorial and is not induced by the mechanical stress but rather by senescence, ischemia, inflammatory diseases, hormones, or vasoactive peptides. Depending on the cause, collagen synthesis can be transcriptionally or translationally regulated.[53] (Fibrosis is discussed later.)

CELLULAR CHANGES

Cell Division

The heart is normally composed of 50 percent myocytes and 50 percent of nonmuscular cells, including fibroblasts and endothelial cells. Nevertheless, the size of these two groups of cells is very different; the myocytes are indeed much bigger and represent more than 80 percent of the total cellular volume. Normal cardiocytes can be multinucleated in certain species, as in the pig, or have a polyploid nucleus, as in humans. In rats, these cells are either mononucleated or binucleated.[54] During cardiac hypertrophy in adults, the myocytes become bigger but usually do not divide. By contrast, it has been firmly established that the nonmuscular cells hypertrophy and multiply through mitotic division. Prelabeling shows an increased incorporation of DNA precursors in nonmuscular cells and no incorporation in cardiocytes during cardiac hypertrophy in rats.[55] Consequently, during cardiac hypertrophy, the total number of contractile cells is unchanged.

The nuclei are modified. In most species, there is an increased number of nucleoli, mainly at the beginning of overload. In certain species, as in humans, the degree of polyploidy is enhanced, and 32n and 64n nuclei are frequently observed in very enlarged hearts.[56] During childhood or in young animals, the myocytes are still able to divide, and mitoses are frequently seen in these cells.[57] In addition, there is evidence based on quantitative morphometry that, at least in human hearts (but it is nearly impossible to experimentally obtain very bulky hearts[58]), severe degrees of cardiac hypertrophy are accompanied by cardiocyte proliferation.[59] There also are convincing data showing mitotic images in atrial and ventricular cardiocytes during cardiac failure in humans and in the region adjacent to the necrotic area in both human hearts and experimental models of myocardial infarction.[60, 61] With a morphometric approach, the mitotic index for cardiocyte nuclei was rather high in the end-stage failing hearts compared with fetal hearts and was increased in the surviving tissue bordering the acute infarction. However, mitotic images observed during cardiac failure may not necessarily be indicative of cell division but could be a prerequisite for polyploidy, multinucleation, DNA repair, and even DNA fragmentation and cell death.[60] Cardiac hypertrophy is essentially caused by myocyte hypertrophy and hyperplasia of the nonmuscle cells; nevertheless, adult cardiocytes may not all be terminally differentiated cells, and mitotic divisions of the myocytes may constitute a growth reserve for severely damaged myocardium.

Cell Death

Cell death is a prominent feature in cardiac failure, especially in humans, because of the loss of contractile material. It is also responsible for compensatory hypertrophy of myocardial cells and reparative fibrosis.[62, 63] The main mechanisms of cell death are necrosis and apoptosis, but there are strong indications that other, unknown mechanisms also exist. As opposed to apoptotic cells, necrotic cells lose their membrane structures and become permeable to high molecular components such as radioactive monoclonal antibodies raised against myosin. Uninjured cells remain unlabeled. Apoptotic cells have a normal membrane structure. Apoptosis is an active process sensitive to mRNA or protein synthesis inhibitors that qualifies a genetically programmed cell death due to the activation of an endogenous endonuclease through a complex cascade of events. The resulting DNA fragmentation produces a characteristic "ladder" pattern when size-fractionated via electrophoresis. DNA fragmentation can also be identified with the terminal deoxynucleotidyl transferase biotin-dUTP nick end labeling technique. Apoptosis is associated with the expression of a number of antiapoptotic or proapoptotic regulatory genes commonly used as markers of apoptosis, such as *Bcl2*, a proto-oncogene, and *Fas*. In contrast to necrosis, apoptosis requires de novo gene expression. This topic is becoming very popular in cardiology, and there is evidence that the apoptotic process is activated in the myocardium during development[64] and ischemia,[65] after overstretch,[66] and in the failing heart.[67, 68] Apoptosis in the normal senescent heart is still a controversial issue.

In vitro studies with cultured neonatal cardiocytes exposed to hypoxia clearly demonstrate a mixed phenotype that associates necrotic and apoptotic cells. Apoptotic cells are observed during the anoxic period but are more abundant once normal oxygen and glucose conditions (which is equivalent to reperfusion) are restored.[65] In vivo experimental and clinical investigations have confirmed these findings, strongly suggesting that apoptosis could be, in association with necrosis, an important consequence of acute myocardial infarction.[69] Studies of myocardial samples from patients who died of acute myocardial infarction showed typical apoptotic myocytes, mainly in the border zone of the infarcted myocardium, and confirmed the predominance of apoptotic compared with necrotic cells.[70]

The involvement of apoptosis after thoracic aortic banding in rats was first demonstrated by Teiger and coworkers.[71] Cardiac hypertrophy without failure is accompanied by a wave of apoptosis that peaks by the seventh day, suggesting that apoptosis may participate in the initiation of the hypertrophic process. Apoptosis, as a consequence of stretch,[66] may result from hemodynamic overload. Recent experimental and clinical reports have shown an increased number of apoptotic cardiocytes in the failing heart, including dilated cardiomyopathy and myocardial infarction in humans and aged SHRs.[67, 68]

Biologic Determinants of Systolic Dysfunction

The shortening velocity of the hypertrophied fiber can be modified very early if the appropriate technique is used. Obviously, the reasons for discrepancies among clinical investigations and experimental findings reside in the fact that under clinical conditions, in the human heart, it is difficult to distinguish between pump and muscle, and thus from a clinical point of view, it is virtually impossible to estimate V_{max}. In both rat and guinea pig, banding of the abdominal aorta results in a 30 to 50 percent left ventricular hypertrophy and a decrease in papillary muscle V_{max}, which is the main determinant of the adaptational process. In addition, in the rat, both time to peak force and time to peak shortening are prolonged, allowing more force to be developed. By contrast, in the guinea pig, both variables are diminished; changes in systolic function are therefore in part species specific.[72]

Whether systolic failure is caused by a defect in energy production or a deficit in energy utilization is a continuing debate.[73, 74] There are two extreme conditions: (1) acute failure due to anoxia, which is obviously caused by a deficit in the production of energy, and (2) failure occurring a few weeks after a massive myocardial infarction, which is obviously caused by a deficit in energy utilization due to the loss in contractile material. Nevertheless, these are rather rare situations that are unrelated to cardiac remodeling as it usually occurs in clinical practice. The real concern is whether during the compensatory stage, modifications in the cellular apparatus that are responsible for energy production (mitochondria or anaerobic energy pathways) could account for further impairment in myocardial function or, conversely, whether failure could be more easily explained by a deficit in energy utilization at the level of the contractile machinery.

Energy Metabolism

Myoglobin transports oxygen from erythrocytes to mitochondria and is the first partner involved in energy metabolism in striated muscles. The myoglobin content in myocardium is well documented in cardiac failure[75] and affects the energy flux in the myocardium.

In every model of compensated cardiac hypertrophy, mitochondria adapt to the new situation by increasing their number and decreasing their size. Such fragmentation has a beneficial effect by enlarging the surface area for oxygen exchange. The mitochondrial mass increases via activation of mitochondrial DNA replication.[76, 77] Mitochondrial oxygen function and coupling,[74] as well as heat recovery (see earlier) and myocardial oxygen uptake,[34] are normal. Studies by Ingwall and colleagues[78] showed no significant differences in either the content or the turnover rates of the phosphoryl group.

The normal myocardium is mainly aerobic, and the main source of energy is the catabolism of fatty acids. The chronically overloaded heart becomes progressively more anaerobic with a shift of the overall metabolism to glycolysis. There is a shift in the lactate dehydrogenase isoenzymes toward the skeletal muscle type (M subunits), at least in humans.[79] Several detailed studies on cardiac metabolism in compensated cardiac hypertrophy demonstrated increased glucose utilization and pronounced enhancement in the activity of several enzymes that control glycolysis, together with diminished activity of enzymes responsible for ketone body metabolism.[80, 81] A gene-regulatory mechanism involved in the reexpression of the gene encoding medium-chain acyl-CoA dehydrogenase has been identified. This mechanism is controlled via members of the Sp and (COUP-TF)/erbA–related protein families of transcription factors.[82]

In congestive cardiac failure, early studies suggested that energy depletion was a consequence, and not the cause, of systolic dysfunction.[83] Later investigations have contradicted these findings. The mitochondrial function is clearly altered during end-stage heart failure, and oxidation of fatty acids is depressed.[84, 85] The failing heart is "energy starved,"[86] and its capacity to synthesize ATP and phosphocreatine via the creatine kinase system is impaired.[78, 87] An isoenzymic shift resulting in an increased amount of the B subunit is also observed. The ratio of myocardial creatine phosphate to ATP can be more directly assessed in situ on beating hearts with the use of nuclear magnetic resonance spectroscopy. This ratio is reduced in the noninfarcted area after myocardial infarction. In addition, calculations have shown that phosphoryl transfer via creatine kinase does not limit contractile performances during baseline conditions, but performances will be impaired during acute stress.[88, 89]

It is evident that there is an energy deficit in the failing heart. Nevertheless, it is for the moment impossible to conclude whether such a deficit originates early during the development of the adaptational process and is caused by the mechanical stress or is only created or aggravated by other external factors such as ischemia or the neurohormonal response during cardiac failure.

Contractile Apparatus

Figure 46–1 summarizes the general scheme of muscular contraction. One of the most important points is the dual role of ATP. ATP is not only the source of energy but also the initial (and main) determinant of relaxation.[90] When contraction stops, the recovery process reestablishes ATP stores and allows this compound to dissociate actin from myosin and then to relax the muscle. The ATPase activity of myosin proceeds in two steps with different time constants, a fast and a slow component, that correlate to each other.[91] The fast reaction is physiologic and lasts for the duration of the mechanical event (<1 second); ATP hydrolysis and the energy transduction occur at this moment. Therefore, a low myosin ATPase activity will slow the

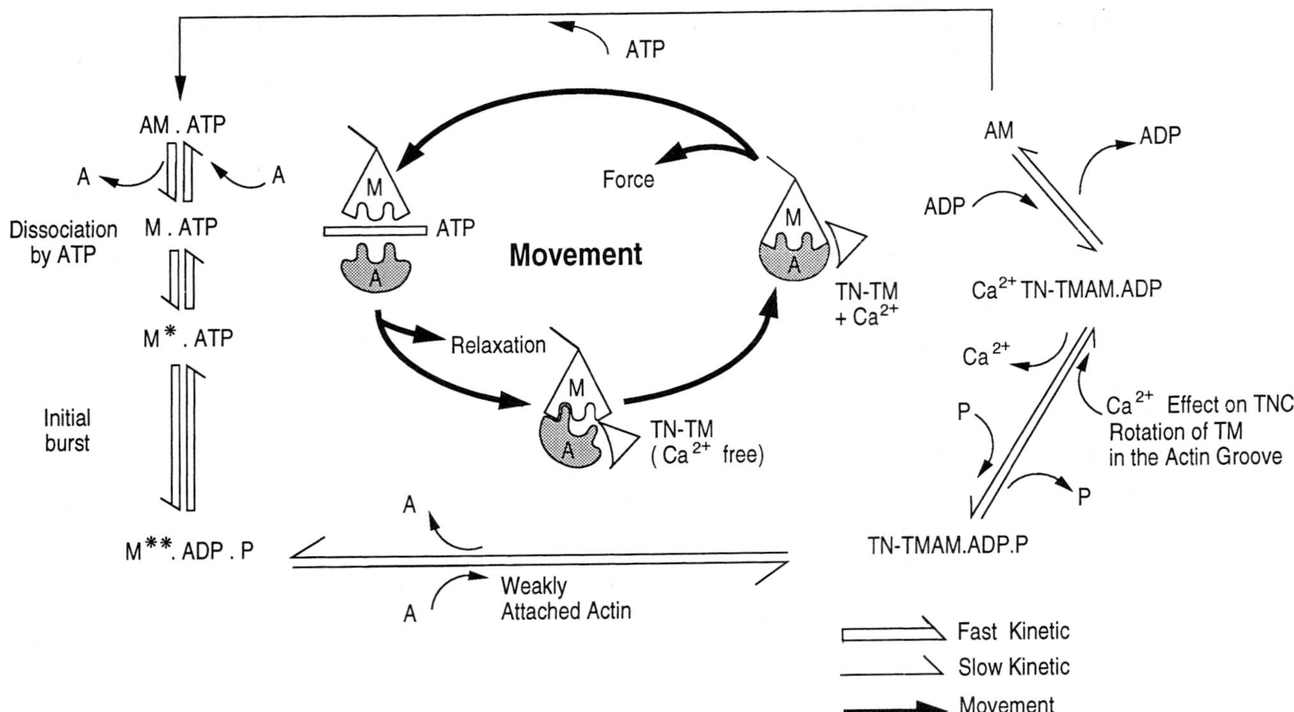

FIGURE 46–1 Steps of contraction in a striated muscle. **Middle,** the different steps of the movement are indicated. In the periphery, the enzymatic reaction by which adenosine triphosphate (ATP) is hydrolyzed by myosin (M) is described. First, a high concentration of ATP inhibits (or weakens) the M-actin (A) binding and relaxes the muscle. ATP binds M, whose conformation changes. Second, ATP is then very rapidly hydrolyzed (burst), which allows M to weakly bind A. Third, troponin complex (TN) is bound to A and can now regulate contraction. When the intracellular Ca^{2+} transient increases, Ca^{2+} reaches TN and then reinforces the A-M relationships and creates movement. At the same time, the ATP hydrolysis is completed, and the hydrolytic products are released. ADP, adenosine diphosphate; AM, actomyosin; M.ATP or M.ADP.P, ATP or ADP and P remain bound to the protein; P, inorganic phosphorus; TM, tropomyosin; *asterisks,* conformational changes in the myosin structure as shown by spin-labeling. TN-TMAM is also called natural actomyosin because actomyosin is naturally associated with TN and TM. TNC is one of the three components of the troponin complex—the one that specifically binds calcium.

movement. When ATP has been hydrolyzed, actin can bind myosin, albeit weakly, and by this means, the troponin-tropomyosin complex can influence the system. When calcium reaches the sarcomere, it binds troponin and then both reinforces the actin-myosin relation and accelerates the rotation of the system (the cross-bridge cycling). Consequently, a slower intracellular Ca^{2+} movement will also slow the contraction cycle.

A decrease in V_{max} may result either from a modification in the contractile protein apparatus that is the final target for Ca^{2+} or from a slowing of the intracellular Ca^{2+} transient as a consequence of a change in membrane protein composition. In several animal species (rat, mouse, rabbit), both are determinant. In such species, V_{max} remains depressed when the cardiac fibers are skinned (i.e., when all the membrane structures that are responsible for the intracellular Ca^{2+} transient have been removed).[92] In addition, an improvement in heat production has been observed in mechanically active muscle and when mechanical activity has been arrested (with the use of 2,3-butane-dione monoxime mannitol) while the intracellular Ca^{2+} movements are maintained (see Table 46–2).

In these models, there is a shift in the expression (in terms of proteins) of the two isogenes coding for the cardiac myosin heavy chains: from the alpha chain, which is the main component of the V_1 type, the fast isomyosin, to the β chain, which is the main component of the V_3 type, the slow isomyosin that has a slow ATPase. The shift explains why myosin ATPase is depressed in the rat ventricle 6 weeks after aortic banding and correlates with V_{max}, as it does in phylogeny of skeletal muscles.[14] Nevertheless, even in rats, it accounts for only half of the process of adaptation.[1, 34] The isomyosin shift has also been observed in all mammalian atria, including human atria[94] (Table 46–3; see also Table 46–1).

In the human ventricle, several early reports with histochemical techniques demonstrated a few cardiocytes that were immunostained with an anti–α myosin antibody; these myocytes were not found in the failing heart,[97] and it is commonly admitted that such changes have no physiologic significance. Nevertheless, the question is not fully resolved despite its importance. The correlation between cross-linked actomyosin ATPase and V_{max} is indeed more valid on a semilogarithmic than on a linear scale, showing that in a slow muscle (e.g., the normal human ventricle compared with the rat or the failing human heart compared with controls), a smaller change in myosin ATPase and in isomyosin profile is necessary to induce a significant modification of V_{max}.[98] Recently, a group of investigators demonstrated a considerable amount (≈30 percent) of α-myosin heavy chain mRNA in a large group of patients with nonfailing hearts or that exhibited donor heart dys-

TABLE 46–3 Sarcomeric Changes in Overloaded Human Ventricle: the Contractile Proteins in Human Hypertrophied or Failing Heart

Modifications	Meaning
Decline in crude myofibrillar ATPase	Repeatedly reported and still unexplained[14, 19, 34, 95]
Unchanged myosin ATPase and reconstituted actomyosin super-ATPase	Changes in Ca^{2+} transient and membrane proteins are unique determinants of the depressed contractility[98]
Disappearance of 2 to 8% of the α-myosin heavy chains (the fast myosin isoform)[97, 99]	May have an effect because the myosin ATPase/V_{max} relation is not linear[98]
No changes in isomyosin subtypes β1, β2, or β3	Other changes in isomyosin are unlikely[96, 97]
Higher α-myosin heavy chain mRNA in control than in failing heart	May explain the decreased V_{max}, if translated into proteins[15, 16]
Reexpression of a fetal/atrial myosin light chain	Change is limited, and its meaning unknown in term of physiologic function[17, 100]
Degree of phosphorylation of the myosin light chain[101]	Unexplored in humans
A shift in TnT isoforms to TnT 2	Could explain the diminution in myofibrillar ATPase[19]; controversial
Sensitivity to calcium of skinned fibers is unchanged	At least in the ventricle[93]

From Swynghedauw B: Development and functional adaptation of contractile proteins in cardiac and skeletal muscles. Physiol Rev 66:710, 1986.

function.[15] In cardiac failure, α-myosin heavy chain mRNA was down-regulated and β-myosin heavy chain mRNA was up-regulated, suggesting that an alteration in myosin, if translated, may be a major determinant of systolic dysfunction.[15, 16] For the moment, the question is still controversial because such findings have not been confirmed in terms of proteins (see Table 46–3).

Membrane Proteins

Changes in the Na^+,K^+-ATPase (the Na^+ pump), the key enzyme that is responsible for the Na^+/K^+ homeostasis and that specifically binds glycosides, are complex and species specific. This enzyme is a tetramer, and the main subunit, alpha, is polymorphic. In the normal rat heart, α1 and α2 are predominant, whereas with cardiac overload, α2 is replaced by a fetal isoform, α3 (see Table 46–1).[4] This shift may account for several modifications of the kinetic properties of the enzyme and pharmacologic characteristics of the heart with regard to glycoside, such as a shift from the isoform with low affinity for ouabain to a form with high affinity.[20, 102, 103] The situation is clearly species specific and is different in humans. In the failing human heart, the activity of the Na^+,K^+-ATPase is reduced and becomes less sensitive to Na^+.[104] Molecular biologic studies on the α subunit of the enzyme, made in a limited number of cases, showed a shift from the α1 to the α3 isoform. Because the human heart possesses an α1 subunit with low affinity for Na^+, one can conclude that in humans, as in rats, the final result is a diminution of the affinity of Na^+ for the enzyme and a slight accumulation of Na^+ below the membrane surface.

In the heart, Na^+,K^+-ATPase and Na^+/Ca^{2+} exchange are functionally coupled; they are both modified by the hypertrophic process, which probably means that the system in charge of extruding calcium out of the cell is altered. The activity of the Na^+/Ca^{2+} exchanger has been a controversial issue. Pioneer studies in rats with isolated membrane vesicles concluded that the activity of the exchanger was depressed in cardiac hypertrophy.[105, 106] Such results have been contradicted; it has been generally accepted that the molecular density of the Na^+/Ca^{2+} exchanger is increased in this condition.[107] Nevertheless, from a functional point of view, the situation is different. The Na^+/Ca^{2+} exchanger is an electrogenic transporter that generates a current, and the corresponding potential, $E_{Na\text{-}Ca}$, becomes increasingly positive as intracellular Ca^{2+} concentration $[Ca^{2+}]_i$ increases, and the exchanger generates an inward depolarizing current during almost the entire duration of the action potential (see Electrophysiologic Aspects). It is thought that the activity of the exchanger is both lengthened and attenuated by the slightest increase in intracellular Na^+, and it is likely that the changes in the protein density are more a consequence of the modification of the current than a cause.

At the level of the SR, it has been well established that the activity of Ca^{2+}-ATPase is depressed because the density of the molecule is diminished (as for the β-adrenergic receptor). As a consequence, the capacity of SR to pump and release calcium is hampered. Because SR Ca^{2+}-ATPase activity is almost absent in fetal rat hearts and increases substantially at the end of the fetal life,[25] it is generally accepted that the diminished concentration observed during cardiac overload participates in the reexpression of the fetal program (see Table 46–1). The reduction in the concentration of the enzyme is progressive and is linked to the progression of cardiac hypertrophy, which in turn is correlated with the appearance of symptoms of congestive cardiac failure, at least in the experimental models, which by definition are untreated animals. A reduced level of ATPase has therefore been proposed as a marker of cardiac failure.[108] The ryanodine channels are Ca^{2+} channels responsible for the Ca^{2+}-induced Ca^{2+} release phenomenon. In compensatory hypertrophy, their density also diminishes in parallel with that of Ca^{2+}-ATPase.[26] In end-stage failure in humans, several groups of researchers found a decreased mRNA content and an unchanged protein level with a twofold increase in the number of high-affinity sites,[109, 110] suggesting that during cardiac failure, additional regulatory factors affect the ryanodine-binding properties.

In the compensatory phase of cardiac hypertrophy the β_1-adrenergic and M2 muscarinic receptors are down-regulated, which means that even their density per unit of cell surface drops. In fact, the genes are not activated; consequently, the corresponding mRNAs and proteins are diluted in the hypertrophied heart[12, 27, 28] (see Table 46–1). During cardiac failure, a true homologous "down-regulation" occurs when the plasma catecholamine concentration increases and is superimposed on the precedent heterologous regulation.[15, 111] There is evidence that the process is species specific. A prominent feature in cardiac failure in humans is the existence of a 75 percent increase in $G_{\alpha i\text{-}2}$, and it is generally accepted that there is a transcriptional cross-regulation of G protein pathways due to the increased plasma catecholamines.[112]

Cardiac reactive hypertrophy occurring after a myocardial infarction is associated with an almost twofold increase in angiotensin II receptor (ATR) subtype 1a and 2 densities.[113] Results concerning other models of compensated hypertrophy are more controversial. A pronounced loss of ATR1, but not ATR2, occurs in end-stage cardiac failure in humans.[114] The drop in ATR1 density correlates with a decrease in β_1-adrenergic density, suggesting that the two phenomena may be related to the increased plasma levels of the corresponding agonists.[115]

Excitation-Contraction Coupling

The Ca^{2+}-induced Ca^{2+} release through the ryanodine receptors is facilitated by the close proximity of the sarcolemmal Ca^{2+} channels and ryanodine receptors in the dyads and can be directly observed in the confocal microscope as Ca^{2+} sparks. A direct estimation of the coupling consists of evaluation of the ability of the transmembrane inward Ca^{2+} current to provoke Ca^{2+} release over a fixed time period through measurement of the number of Ca^{2+} sparks and integration of I_{CaL} during a voltage-clamp pulse.[116] Isolated cardiocytes from a hypertensive strain of rats with compensated cardiac hypertrophy had weak contraction, reduced Ca^{2+} transient, and normal inward Ca^{2+} current that was associated with a markedly reduced ability to evoke Ca^{2+} sparks. The proposed explanation for such an uncoupling was based on ultrastructural data suggesting that the distance between the Ca^{2+} channels and SR structures was increased. Similar observations have been made in a model of cardiac failure.

Nevertheless, such an uncoupling is most probably species and model specific. It has been excluded, for example, in guinea pigs; in this model, the systolic dysfunction results in impaired myocyte contraction that is closely linked to the depressed $[Ca^{2+}]_i$ movements.[117] Other mechanisms could include modifications of proteins such as annexins, which are known to modify the ryanodine receptor properties.

Calcium Transient

The intracellular Ca^{2+} transient follows the electrical activity and precedes the mechanical movement. Figure 46–2 summarizes the main determinants of the $[Ca^{2+}]_i$ transient. Obviously, a slowing of this transient can cause a slowing of the shortening velocity of a given muscle, whereas a diminution of the peak of $[Ca^{2+}]_i$ may result in a lower maximum active tension. Calcium movements are modified in cardiac hypertrophy and failure. Whether such a slowing in calcium movement is a primary event or results from changes in the electrical activity is not known.

1. During compensatory hypertrophy, $[Ca^{2+}]_i$ is normal during diastole (by definition, the diastolic compliance of the ventricle is unchanged); nevertheless, the transient is prolonged to allow the heart to contract more slowly and to maintain its normal economy, as previously explained. Nevertheless, the cell is likely to be unable to control any abnormal influx of calcium that occurs under extreme conditions. For example, during ischemia or after strong inotropic interventions, stress, or maximum exercising, $[Ca^{2+}]_i$ accumulates, causes an increased diastolic stiffness and arrhythmias, and hampers systolic ejection.[118] The lengthening of the transient is explained by the slowing in activity of the SR (at the levels of both calcium uptake and release). In addition, at the external membrane level, the calcium influx increases in proportion with the degree of cardiac hypertrophy,[119] whereas the prolongation of the Ca^{2+} transient lengthens $I_{Na\text{-}Ca}$ (which aggravates prolongation of the duration of the action potential).
2. During cardiac insufficiency, various factors with a different trophic activity, including ischemia, aging, catecholamines, angiotensin II, and endothelin, strongly modifies the hypertrophic phenotype, and these modifications may have different consequences. The peak of the Ca^{2+} transient is now generally decreased, and the density of the Ca^{2+} channels is generally depressed, which worsens calcium homeostasis.[7] At the level of the SR, Ca^{2+}-ATPase is increasingly depressed, and unexplained modifications occur in the ryanodine receptor.

Cytoskeleton

A transient increase in the microtubular network of cardiocytes was observed 2 to 4 days after aortic stenosis in our laboratory in 1984.[120] It was suggested that the microtubules may play the role of a guideline in the phenotypic modifications affecting these cells.

Permanent changes in the microtubules were reported by the group of G. Cooper.[121] Both the microtubular network and tubulin concentration were enhanced in overloaded cat ventricles at 2 weeks to 6 months after pulmonary artery stenosis in association with the contractile deficit. Colchicine exposure depolymerizes the microtubular network and, in parallel, normalizes the contractile dysfunction. In addition, direct measurement of the extramyofibrillar cell stiffness and viscosity with the use of magnetic twisting cytometry showed that the increased amount and polymerization of tubulin have major consequences on myocyte function. It then was proposed that the microtubule network imposes a resistive intracellular load on sarcomere shortening and, when in excess, impedes sarcomere motion.[121]

Other cytoskeletal proteins could also play a role in the maintenance of cardiocyte stiffness. Titin, desmin, and vinculi protein expression are enhanced both in experimental decompensated cardiac hypertrophy in the guinea pig and in the failing human heart and may participate in the impairment of contractility.[122] Changes in cytoskeleton components have been observed only with the use of immunolabeling, and it currently is impossible to determine whether the cytoskeleton components became apparent because of the high degree of cellular disorganization or whether they represent a compensatory mechanism, thereby maintaining the cell shape.

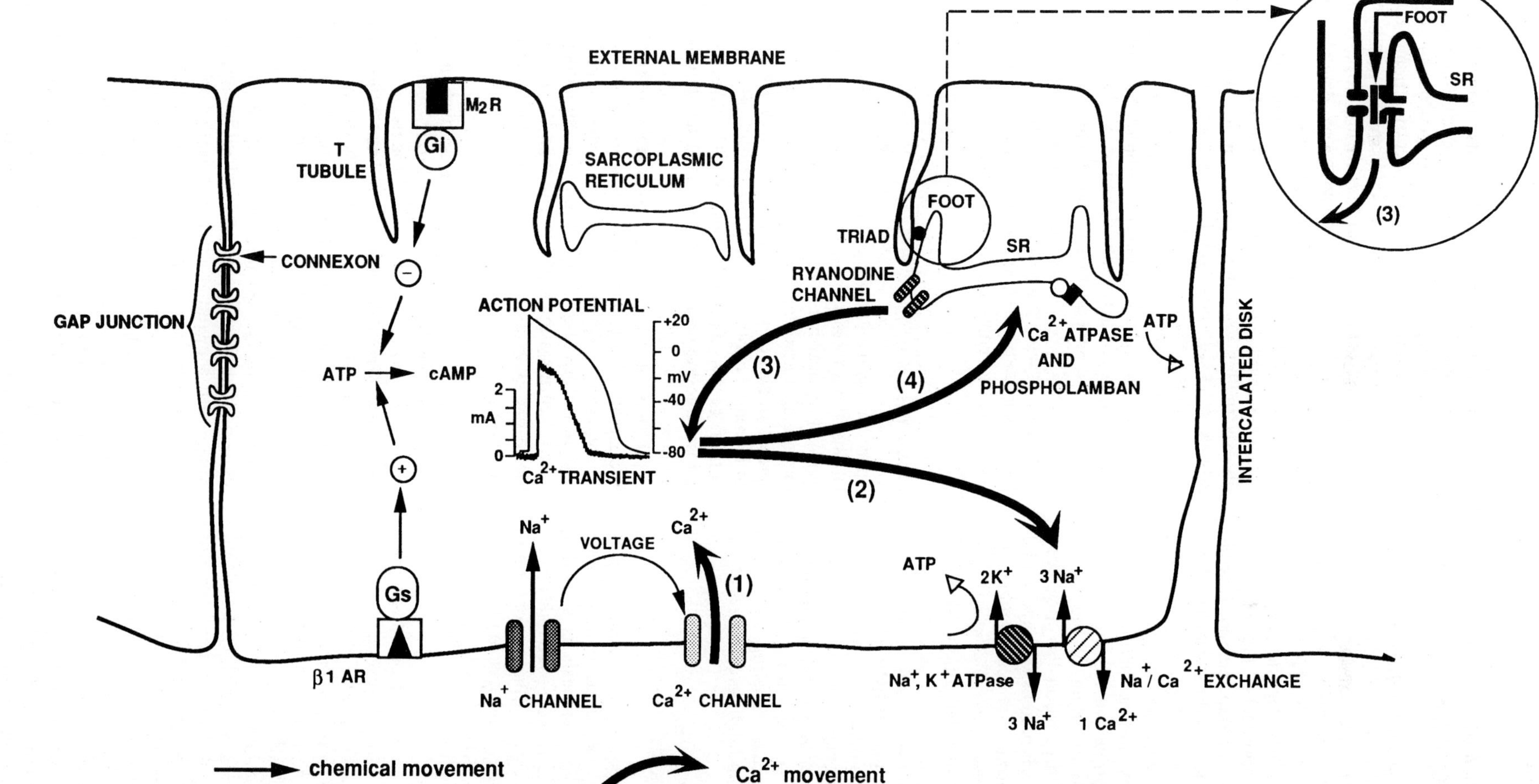

FIGURE 46–2 Membrane proteins and Ca^{2+} movements in a normal cardiac myocyte. The scheme is applicable to most mammalian ventricles, including humans, rat, and rabbit. Nevertheless, in the rat, the internal Ca^{2+} movements going from and to the sarcoplasmic reticulum (SR) are more important than those in other species. The intracellular Ca^{2+} transient (**middle**) follows the action potential and precedes the mechanical movement; it constitutes the main element of the excitation-contraction coupling. **Right,** The system in charge of permanently regulating the contraction-relaxation cycle (i.e., the intracellular Ca^{2+} movements). (1) Slow inward calcium current. The corresponding Ca^{2+} channel is inhibited by Ca^{2+} blockers and is voltage dependent. Its opening is triggered by the voltage change that follows the opening of the Na^+ channel. (2) The release of Ca^{2+} out of the cell occurs through the Na^+/Ca^{2+} exchanger, which is electrogenic and is functionally coupled to an enzyme, Na^+, K^+-ATPase (adenosine triphosphatase). (3) The SR is an internal store of Ca^{2+} that is able to concentrate Ca^{2+} against the normal gradient through the Ca^{2+}-ATPase of SR. (4) The release of Ca^{2+} through the ryanodine channels out of the SR is an autocatalytic process that is triggered by intracellular Ca^{2+}. **Left,** The systems that must inform the cell regarding outside events. The beta$_1$-adrenergic receptor (β1AR) and muscarinic receptor (M_2R) transduce the β_1-agonist signal into chemical information that controls the production of cyclic adenosine monophosphate, which may in turn, through phosphorylation, control the opening of the Ca^{2+} channels, the activity of Ca^{2+}-ATPase of SR (through phospholamban), and the affinity of troponin for calcium. At the level of the sinus node, the two receptors regulate heart rate. The cross-talk between two adjacent cells is secured by channels called *connexons,* which are made of connexins. ATP, adenosine triphosphate; Gi and Gs, inhibitory and stimulatory G proteins (made up of three different and polymorphic subunits). The Ca^{2+} transient is measured with the use of specific fluorescent markers. The results are expressed in milliamperes. FOOT is a protein located within the triad.

Biologic Determinants of Diastolic Dysfunction

Intrinsic Myocardial Stiffness and Fibrosis

Left ventricular chamber stiffness increases during the development of pressure overload hypertrophy; this is due to both increased wall thickness and fibrosis, which enhances the intrinsic myocardial stiffness (the tensile strength of collagen is 50 to 100 MPa and approaches that of steel), as assessed with the diastolic stress-strain relation. In general, a good correlation has been reported between myocardial stiffness and the myocardial content in collagen. From a purely clinical point of view, it is possible to separate patients with cardiac hypertrophy due to valvular disease into two groups: those with a normal muscle stiffness and those with a significant shift to the right of the elastic stiffness-stress curve.[123] Such a distinction has also been made in experimental models. Hypertensive myocardial hypertrophy in the nonhuman primate is accompanied by remodeling of the collagen network, a rapid increase in total collagen concentration, and a small augmentation of isocollagen III.

Collagen is the main component of the extracellular matrix (ECM) and constitutes a fibrillar network that embeds myofibers, maintains the alignment of myocytes and vessels, and prevents myocyte slippage during contraction. During systole, it acts as a force transducer that facilitates relengthening. ECM not only is an inert material but also plays an active role in transmembrane signaling, as a mediator of growth factor, and in modulating cell phenotype during development.

Origin of Myocardial Fibrosis

There are converging reports suggesting that collagen mass (not collagen concentration) increases in parallel with cardiac hypertrophy and that collagen synthesis is activated very early during the process of mechanical overload.[53, 124, 125] However, fibrosis that is an increased collagen concentration occurs as an additional process and has multiple origins. Fibrosis is multifactorial; it is not directly induced by stretch or mechanical overload and does not participate in the adaptational process.

The wound-healing response of the myocardium after myocardial infarction involves both the scar and reactive fibrosis in the noninfarcted area. The initial modifications of the ECM are increased collagen degradation and disorganization of the normal collagen network in the ischemic area, which provides a cellular basis for infarct expansion and myocyte slippage. Significant amounts of new collagen fibers appear in the infarcted area a few days later, and definitively constituted scar appears as a three-layered structure.[126] Significant amounts of fibrosis are observed after a left ventricular infarction, both in the right ventricle and in the noninfarcted area of the left ventricle and parallels compensatory myocyte hypertrophy.[127]

Catecholamines and several vasoactive peptides, including angiotensin II and endothelin, are fibrogenic. Nevertheless, fibrosis due to these compounds is much more complicated than previously expected because angiotensin II, for example, is a potent vasoconstrictor, has a direct trophic effect on the myocytes, activates collagen synthesis, and possesses a proliferative effect on the fibroblasts.[128] Aldosterone infusion induces both perivascular and interstitial necrosis and fibrosis in the two ventricles and atria and around the large vessels.[128–132] Clinical investigations have demonstrated systemic organ fibrosis in autopsy-confirmed adrenal adenoma. Long-term androgen treatment is also associated with fibrous tissue deposits.

Myocardial fibrosis is a consistent finding in healthy senescent hearts in both rats and humans.[133, 134] Cardiac fibrosis in this condition is at least in part a reparative process related to myocyte death, predominates in the subendocardium, and is associated with a decreased collagenase activity.[129] Nevertheless, the regulation of myocardial concentration during aging is a complex phenomenon.

Fibrosis is not inevitably linked to mechanical overload, and there are several experimental and clinical models of mechanically overloaded hearts with unchanged myocardial stiffness and collagen content, including volume overload.[13] There also are models of pressure overload hypertrophy without ventricular fibrosis, such as infrarenal aortic banding.[128]

Other Components of Fibrosis

There has been autoradiographic detection of large accumulations of angiotensin-converting enzyme at sites of various types of myocardial fibrosis.[125] ATR1 and bradykinin receptors are also associated with myocardial fibrosis after myocardial infarction. Data from our laboratory demonstrated an increased expression of ATRs, with a differential regulation of the two main subtypes—ATR1 and ATR2—in both aldosterone-induced cardiac fibrosis and fibrotic senescent rat heart.

Fibronectin accumulation precedes collagen accumulation during fibrillogenesis (for a review, see Farhadian and colleagues[135]). The FN-IIIA+ fibronectin isoform is the unique isoform expressed in most of the models of hypertensive cardiopathy. Laminin and type IV collagen contribute to the ECM assembly during healing after myocardial infarction.

Active Relaxation

Active relaxation is impaired during cardiac hypertrophy in parallel with the changes in contraction velocity, with important species differences.

This certainly is one of the first applicable results of the study of molecular biology in cardiology—to provide a rational basis to impaired relaxation in hypertrophy by showing that chronic cardiac overload is consistently associated with a quantitative change in the SR Ca^{2+}-ATPase that impairs Ca^{2+} reuptake by SR. Its role during relaxation varies among animal species or among tissues. In skeletal muscle, in which contraction is triggered only by the Ca^{2+} release from SR, Ca^{2+}-ATPase plays a major role. In frog ventricle, contraction depends only on the inward Ca^{2+} current through plasma membrane, and this enzyme is absent. In most species, including humans, the ventricular tissues are in an intermediary situation. In the hypertrophied heart, the reduction in functionally active Ca^{2+}-

ATPase molecules[25] (see Table 46–1) should be compensated at the external membrane level. Nevertheless, the entire adaptational process is still not understood because, for example, in a model of compensated hypertrophy, the senescent rat heart, the relaxation velocity correlates better with the isomyosin change than with the content in Ca^{2+}-ATPase of SR[134] (Table 46–4).

Atrial Contraction

Atrial contraction is another active participant in the ventricular filling, and it is well known that in hypertensive cardiopathy increased atrial contraction is a compensatory mechanism that maintains a normal ventricular filling.[123] Contraction of normal atria is more rapid than that of ventricles, and accordingly, the atrial isomyosin composition is almost 100% V_1, the fast isoform of myosin, compared with the ventricles, which in mammalians are mostly V_3, the slow isoform. It has been shown by researchers at several different laboratories, including ours[94] (see Table 46–3) that in atria, chronic cardiac overloading results in a shift from V_1 to V_3. This shift correlates with the size of the atria as quantified with echocardiography,[94] which can reasonably be considered as an adaptational process that allows the atria to tolerate the new working conditions in terms of thermodynamic requirements.

Endocrine Function of The Heart

The heart is an endocrine tissue that is able to produce atrial natriuretic peptides (ANPs), angiotensin II, aldosterone, and catecholamine. There is evidence that the first two are activated during mechanical overloading and that cardiac catecholamine stores are depleted.

Atrial Natriuretic Peptides

ANF, which was discovered by the group of P. Y. Hatt in 1976,[136] is normally expressed only in atria. ANF, and other ANPs (especially the brain isoform) is expressed in overloaded ventricles and secreted into the plasma in various experimental models of cardiac overload and in humans[32]; it is considered to be the best biologic marker of ventricular overload. ANF interacts with particulate guanylate cyclase in target cells to produce cGMP, and an increased urinary cGMP level is an easily measurable marker of the severity of the cardiac overload.[137]

TABLE 46–4 **Main Models of Experimental Cardiac Hypertrophy and Failure (Small Laboratory Animals)**

Model, Animal Species	Advantages	Disadvantages
Rat	Cheap, widely used, easy blood pressure measurement	Ca^{2+} metabolism different from that of humans
Abdominal aortic stenosis	Analogous to a Goldblatt (⇑ angiotensin II), widely used	Poorly reproducible
Thoracic aortic stenosis in young	Very enlarged heart, acutely overloaded, failure after 3 to 4 mo	Young animals (mitosis)
Aortic insufficiency	No fibrosis, no thoracotomy, no hormonal changes	Volume overload plus pressure component
Aortocaval fistula	Pure volume overload	Requires 3 to 4 mo
Myocardial infarction (chronic)	Diastolic dysfunction, cardiac failure, widely used in pharmacology	High mortality rates
Goldblatt hypertension	Fibrosis, hormonal changes	Requires training
DOCA-salt hypertension	Very easy to create	Very artificial model (⇓ renin-angiotensin)
Chronic infusions with angiotensin II or aldosterone	Monofactorial, atraumatic	Expensive, restricted use
Aortic stenosis and insufficiency	Good model of cardiac failure	High mortality rates
SHRs	Easy to obtain	Hypertension is associated with cardiomyopathy
Aged SHRs	Good model of cardiac failure, well documented	Expensive, fibrosis
Senescent Wistar rat	Easy to obtain, permanent arrhythmias	Expensive, fibrosis
Guinea Pig	Same electrophysiologic characteristics as in human heart	Fragile animal, high mortality rates
Aortic stenosis	Frequent subacute failure	Pronounced cellular damages
DOCA-salt hypertension	Same as in rat	Not widely used
Mice	Can become transgenic	Small size
Thoracic aortic stenosis		Difficult
Transgenic Models (mice)	Permanent strains, some are commercially available	Far from the clinical situation
Endogenous growth promotors	Cardiac hypertrophy, no failure	Not well documented
Ectopic growth promotors (skeletal or viral)	Cardiac failure	May be lethal
Overexpression of α_{1B}-adrenergic receptor	Cardiac hypertrophy + ⇑ atrial natriuretic factor	Not well documented
Rabbit	Size, allows easy hemodynamic blood sampling	Needs space
Abdominal aortic stenosis	Easy	Poorly reproducible
Thoracic aortic stenosis	Very reproducible	Serious thoracic damages
Aortic insufficiency	Enormous hearts after 12 mo	

Abbreviation: DOCA = deoxycorticosterone acetate–salt; SHRs, spontaneously hypertensive rats.

Renin-Angiotensin, Renin-Angiotensin System, and Aldosterone System

In cardiac failure, activation of the circulating renin-angiotensin system (RAS) and aldosterone production are major factors that adapt the peripheral circulation to the hemodynamic conditions. Tissue RAS and aldosterone production have been demonstrated in both normal vessels and myocardium, and normal isolated hearts produce angiotensinogen, angiotensin II, aldosterone, and corticosterone.[138, 139] In humans, but not in rats, the myocardial production of angiotensin II uses two different pathways: angiotensin-converting enzyme and a chymase.

Both the myocardial RAS and aldosterone production are activated by mechanical stretch.[43, 44] The direct assessment of angiotensin II levels in myocardial interstitial fluid showed levels more than 100-fold higher than plasma levels, suggesting that angiotensin II production in the heart may play an important local role.[140]

Aldosterone is mainly secreted by the adrenal cortex, but there is evidence that aldosterone can also be synthesized and regulated in the myocardium[139] through the RAS pathway.

Other Vasoactive Compounds

Catecholamines

Myocardial endothelin-1 and preproendothelin-1 mRNA are significantly increased in several experimental models of cardiac overload. In humans, the elevation of plasma endothelin-1 became significant in patients with moderate cardiac insufficiency.[141]

Basal circulating nitric oxide (NO) levels nearly double in idiopathic dilated cardiomyopathy. Inducible NO synthase (an isoform of NO synthase) mRNA and protein are not present in the normal human heart, but they are coexpressed with ANF in the myocardium of patients with cardiac failure, which raises the possibility that autocrine and paracrine actions of inducible NO synthase may be of physiopathologic importance.[142]

It is well known that plasma catecholamines increase in proportion to the severity of cardiac failure. Such an augmentation is associated with a depletion of norepinephrine stores, as initially shown by Chidsey and coworkers[143]; such a depletion is under local rather than systemic control and is accompanied by an increased cardiac interstitial level of norepinephrine.[144]

Cytokines

An increasing body of evidence supports the existence of paracrine and autocrine growth pathways in the myocardium; however, it is impossible to decide whether such an activation has a functional significance. The first suggestion of an autocrine myocardial growth factor system was made by Corda and colleagues,[145] who demonstrated in the pericardial fluid (which is an ultrafiltrate of the plasma) collected from patients undergoing cardiac surgery high concentrations of fibroblast growth factor-2 in proportion to the ventricular mass, suggesting a myocardial autocrine production of growth factor at the origin of hypertrophy.

Overexpression of tumor necrosis factor-alpha (TNF-α) a proinflammatory cytokine, in the heart as demonstrated with the use of transgenic technology, leads to cardiomegaly, suggesting that such a cytokine actively participates in end-terminal myocardial deterioration. TNF-α is present in the heart, and its level increases in cardiac failure. The plasma level of both TNF-α and IL-6 is enhanced in advanced congestive failure regardless of whether the patients are cachectic.[146]

ELECTROPHYSIOLOGIC ASPECTS

Basis of Cardiac Cellular Electrical Activity

In the heart, mechanical activity is triggered and controlled by a long-lasting phase of regenerative and propagated systolic depolarization, the action potential, starting from the diastolic resting potential. When a cell is at rest, the inside of the membrane is negative (−80 mV) compared with the outside. During the action potential, the inside of the membrane becomes transiently positive (+20 to +30 mV).

Resting Potential

The resting potential, E_R (E indicates the potential; E_m, membrane potential; E_R, value of E_m at rest), results from a dominant background membrane conductance for K^+, gK (a conductance, g, is the electrical result of an ionic permeability). If the resting membrane is impermeable, or almost impermeable, to any ion other than K^+, the resting potential equals, or nearly equals, the equilibrium potential for K^+, E_K (E_K = −90 mV). Usually, the resting potential is less negative than E_K. This is the result of the existence of a non-negligible background conductance for ions other than K^+, such as Na^+ or, to a lesser extent, Ca^{2+}. In cardiac cells, E_R is generally less negative than E_K by only a few millivolts at a normal extracellular K^+ concentration because the background gNa is small compared with the background gK. Electrogenic membrane systems are not passive conductances and can also generate transmembrane currents. For example, the Na^+ pump (Na^+,K^+-ATPase), which generates an outward repolarizing current, can participate in the buildup of the resting potential.

Under normal conditions, the diastolic or background gK of cardiac cells is mainly due to a conductance gK1 that is very large at potentials close to or more negative than E_K but that decreases considerably at potentials less negative than E_K. This large decrease in gK1 occurring when the cell is depolarized (during the action potential) is termed *abnormal*, or *inward*, *rectification* of gK1. Other sources of background current exist in cardiac cells (e.g., K^+ current resulting from muscarinic receptor activation, K^+ current normally inhibited by internal ATP, cAMP-activated chloride current, and so on).

Action Potential

The action potential is triggered by a diastolic phase of slow depolarization (the pacemaker potential) that is sufficiently large to be, in its final phase, a biologic stimulus

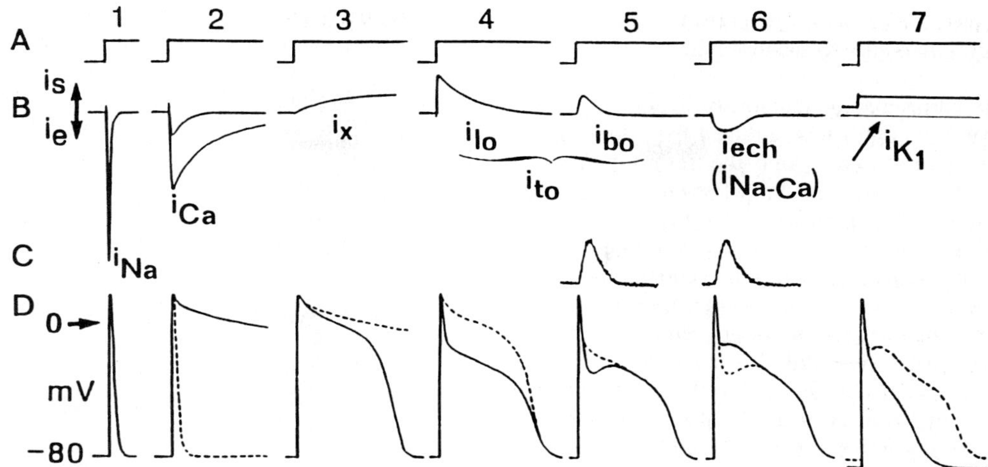

FIGURE 46–3 Sequential participation (from 1 to 7) of different transmembrane currents to the cardiac action potential development. **A,** Potential steps triggering currents during voltage-clamp experiments. **B,** Triggered currents. **C,** Calcium transients. **D,** Action potentials recorded in non–voltage-clamped cells and generated by the currents shown in **B.** If a membrane has only Na^+ channels, giving rise to i_{Na}, it generates a spike as in 1. If Ca^{2+} currents, i_{CaT} and i_{CaL}, are added, a long-lasting plateau develops (2). A delayed K^+ current, i_x, shortens the plateau (3). Additional transient outward currents, i_{lo} and i_{bo} i_{to}, induce a depressed (4) and a notched (5) plateau. In the presence of Na^+/Ca^{2+} exchange current, i_{ech} ($i_{Na\text{-}Ca}$), the plateau amplitude is enhanced (6). An increase in background current, i_{k1} (or an increase in either muscarinic K^+ current or K_{ATP} current), hyperpolarizes the cell and shortens the plateau (7).

(spontaneous activity) or by the action potential upstroke of neighboring cells with a similar but much faster stimulating role (propagated activity).

Action potentials from different parts of the heart differ in shape, amplitude, and duration. They also differ among species. They are generally composed of a fast upstroke followed by a long-lasting plateau. The *upstroke*, or rapid phase of depolarization, is highest and fastest in Purkinje fibers. In contrast, in most animal species, the plateau is higher in the ventricle (in the rat, however, the ventricular action potential often has a sigmoidal decay with a fast initial peak, an early brief plateau phase, and a late plateau phase of low amplitude). In humans, as in most other mammals, cardiac action potential differs in shape and duration among tissues.[147–150] In some animal species, the epicardial action potential differs from the endocardial action potential.[151]

In the most simple case, the cardiac action potential results from the opening of two membrane ionic conductances: a fast and brief conductance for Na^+, gNa, and a smaller and more prolonged conductance for Ca^{2+}, gCa. Action potential ends with the opening of a delayed conductance for K^+, gK or gx. In contrast to background conductances, these three conductances are not open at rest. They are activated by the depolarization process: gNa is activated by the stimulus-induced depolarization, whereas gCa is usually activated by the gNa-induced depolarization. When Na^+ and Ca^{2+} enter the cell through gNa and gCa, they bring positive charges on the internal face of the membrane, which becomes depolarized. In contrast, when K^+ leaves the cell through gx, it brings positive charges on the external face of the membrane, which becomes repolarized. In many types of cardiac cells, several conductances other than gNa, gCa, and gx and electrogenic systems, such as the Na^+/Ca^{2+} exchanger, participate in the modulation of the action potential (Fig. 46–3). Background ion conductances (generally activated by ligand-operated receptors) and electrogenic systems known to control the diastolic potential can also strongly modify the duration of the action potential because they deliver current during the entire cardiac cycle, (i.e., also during the action potential).

All of the these mechanisms do not necessarily coexist in a given type of cardiac tissue or in the same tissue among different species. For example, action potentials with a somewhat rectangular plateau (as in the frog or guinea pig ventricle) do not possess sizeable transient outward K^+ currents. In contrast, the existence of a sigmoidal or notched plateau (as in rat ventricle or in Purkinje fibers from different species) is a clue suggesting the presence of such K^+ currents. The rat ventricle also has an important $I_{Na\text{-}Ca}$, which is responsible for the lower component of the plateau (Fig. 46–4), whereas this current prolongs the plateau in the guinea pig ventricle.

Resting and Action Potentials in Cardiac Hypertrophy

The lengthening of the action potential duration has been consistently reported in various experimental models of

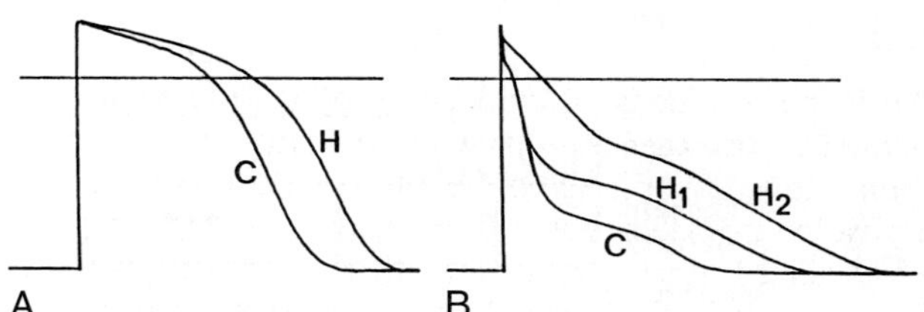

FIGURE 46–4 Schematic of hypertrophy-induced action potential lengthening in two characteristic types of ventricular tissue. **A,** Rounded plateau (cat or guinea pig ventricles). **B,** Sigmoidal plateau (rat heart). C, Control; H, H_1, and H_2, hypertrophied; H_1, lengthening is limited to the slower component of the plateau; H_2, global plateau lengthening.

cardiac hypertrophy, such as right hypertrophy and failure after chronic pulmonary artery banding in cats[152, 154] and left ventricular hypertrophy in various models of arterial hypertension, including the spontaneously hypertensive rat strain[153] and renal[155, 156] or DOCA-induced hypertension[157]; during thyroxine intoxication[156]; and the cardiomyopathic Syrian hamster with focal lesions and compensatory hypertrophy.[158] Such lengthening is proportional to the degree of hypertrophy and persists in isolated hypertrophied myocytes, as shown in guinea pig ventricular cells[159] (see Fig. 50–34). In rats, after myocardial infarction, treatment with angiotensin-converting enzyme inhibitors reduces in parallel both cardiac hypertrophy and the lengthening of the action potential.[160] Because the T wave of the electrocardiogram results from differences in action potential duration among parts of the heart (endocardium and epicardium, base and apex), the hypertrophy-induced action potential lengthening is likely to be the main cause of the T wave inversion often observed in the hypertrophied human heart.

In 1981, Aronson[161] observed that in rats with renal hypertension and cardiac hypertrophy (+33%), the action potential prolongation was not uniform. In epicardial fibers, it developed mainly in the latter half of repolarization, whereas the entire course of repolarization was prolonged in endocardial and papillary muscle fibers. Thollon and colleagues[162] showed that in severe hypertrophy, the action potential lengthening was much less marked in the epicardial fibers of rats subjected to volume overload (where it was also restricted to the later half of repolarization) than in the endocardium of rats with pressure overload (where the entire action potential was lengthened), although the heart weight–to–body weight ratio was larger in the former than in the latter. These observations indicate that when hypertrophy is associated with cardiac dilatation, the lengthening of the action potential does not occur during the initial part of the repolarization phase.

Outward Currents

In most mammals, including rats, hamsters, ferrets, dogs, rabbits, and even humans, the transient outward current, I_{t0}, is the main determinant of the repolarization process, and its specific inhibition by 4-aminopyridine results in a lengthening of the action potential duration (Fig. 46–5). The possibility that this current may be reduced in hypertrophied myocytes and then cause lengthening of the action potential was first suggested by the observation of apparent increases in Ca^{2+} current density that no longer appeared after cell dialysis with cesium, a well known inhibitor of K^+ currents.[163] Direct measurements of the transient outward current showed an almost 40 percent decrease compared with normal in myocytes from acromegalic rats.[164] A decrease in I_{t0} density was also observed in several other models of cardiac hypertrophy, including abdominal aortic stenosis and high altitude in rats,[165] right ventricular hypertrophy in ferret,[166] myocardial infarction in dogs,[167] and hypertension due to perinephritis in rabbit.[168] I_{t0} is reduced in the failing heart in humans, and this reduction is associated with a diminution of I_{K1}.[169, 170]

The participation of outward currents to hypertrophy-induced alterations of the action potential depend on the species studied. The normal ventricle of guinea pig does not possess any I_{t0} current, and in this species, the lengthening of the action potential is due to changes in the inactivation curve of I_{CaL} that result in a prolongation of the corresponding current and a pronounced augmentation (+100%) of $I_{Na\text{-}Ca}$.[171] In the cat, the action potential lengthening might result mainly from the slowing of delayed K^+ current activation.

The delayed K^+ current is reduced in amplitude in hypertrophied feline cardiocytes, and its activation is slowed.[172, 173] Although Kleiman and Houser[173] found that these effects were statistically significant only at a positive

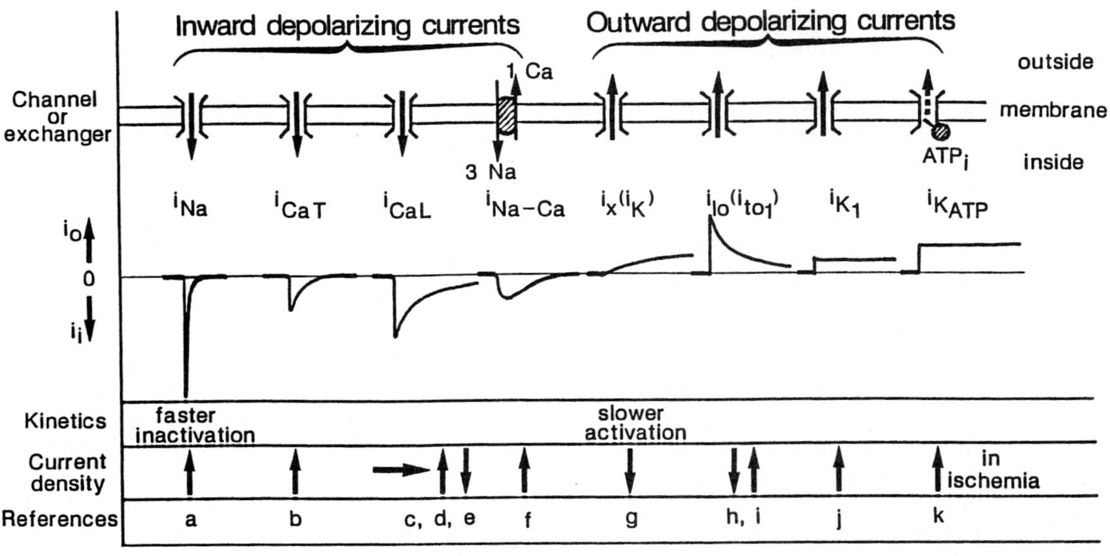

FIGURE 46–5 Effects of hypertrophy on different transmembrane current kinetics and densities. i_o, outward current; i_i, inward current. *Upward, horizontal,* and *downward arrows* indicate increased, unchanged, and decreased current densities, respectively. K_{ATP} channels are closed by internal adenosine triphosphate (ATP_i) and therefore opened during ischemia or hypoxia when ATP_i concentration decreases.

potential of +40 mV, they may contribute to the prolonged action potential duration of hypertrophied myocardium.

Several authors have previously found a larger background inward rectifier K^+ current (I_{K1}) in the hypertrophied feline myocytes.[172, 173] Such an increase in I_{K1} density should result in a shortening, rather than a lengthening, of action potential duration. It is therefore necessary that a decrease in other outward repolarizing currents, an increase in inward depolarizing currents, or both occur to reverse the shortening effect of the increase in I_{K1}. In contrast, in rabbits, cardiac hypertrophy is accompanied by a reduction of I_{K1} that can then participate in lengthening of the action potential.[168]

Background repolarizing currents can participate in both the building up of the resting potential and the repolarization of the action potential under either normal or abnormal conditions. Information is still largely lacking about the role of most of these currents in hypertrophied tissues; however, the ATP-sensitive K^+ channels are altered in hypertrophied feline myocytes and their sensitivity to ATP is reduced, with the half-maximal inhibition of channel activity induced by 250 μM intracellular ATP in hypertrophied versus 75 μM in normal myocytes.[174] Thus, for a given reduction in cellular ATP, the repolarizing activity of these K^+ channels is larger in hypertrophied than in normal cells, which can explain why action potentials are longer than in control under normal conditions but become as short as in control after 30-minute hypoxia in glucose-free medium.[175] Although ATP-sensitive K^+ channels are altered in hypertrophy, the effects of sulfonylurea derivatives, known as selective blockers of these channels, were the same in hypertrophied and normal cells.[176]

Inward Currents

Any increase in long-lasting inward current may result a priori in lengthening of the action potential (see Fig. 46–5). Among the possible candidates, a maintained component of the tetrodotoxin-sensitive Na^+ current has been excluded because after action of the toxin, the action potential of hypertrophied rats remains prolonged.[156] In addition, in cells from hypertrophied right ventricles of cats, the time constant for the slow inactivation of the Na^+ current is unchanged or slightly decreased at membrane potentials positive to −10 mV (i.e., the current inactivation was faster than in normal cells) despite an increase in peak Na^+ current density.

A more plausible candidate is the slow inward Ca^{2+} current, I_{CaL}, because this current triggers contractility. However, the total number of dihydropyridine-binding sites per heart is increased in both rat and guinea pig 5 days after aortic stenosis and remains elevated in chronically hypertrophied hearts. The ratio of the total number of dihydropyridine-binding sites per gram of tissue remains constant, suggesting that the density of Ca^{2+} channels per cell is normal.[10, 177] Such an observation was fully confirmed in three different reports in which direct measurements of the L-type Ca^{2+} current density was performed under conditions that excluded any participation of outward currents. In right ventricular hypertrophy in cats 10 weeks after pulmonary artery constriction and in rats 4 to 5 weeks after aortic stenosis, no significant changes in current density were observed.[173] A similar result was reported in rats with growth hormone–secreting tumors, inducing a marked prolongation of the ventricular action potential duration.[178]

Different results were reported in other models. In the Goldblatt renovascular hypertensive rat (8 to 12 weeks after the animals developed hypertension), the peak density of calcium current, measured after suppression of K^+ currents, was increased by more than 200 percent.[179] In contrast, in right hypertrophy in the ferret, a significant decrease (by −50 percent) in L-type Ca^{2+} current density was unmasked after the suppression of Na^+ and K^+ currents.[180] These results suggest that the hypertrophy-induced Ca^{2+} channel synthesis that appears to be most often adequately adapted to the increased area of cardiac cell membrane can, in some models and under the influence of presently unknown factors, escape the mechanisms involved in its control,[7] as discussed earlier.

No relevant information is available concerning a possible role of the fast T-type Ca^{2+} current in ventricular action potential lengthening. The fact that atrial myocytes from rats with growth hormone–secreting tumors showed a threefold increase in I_{CaT} density[178] is of little significance because this current is too short compared with most ventricular action potential durations (it inactivates almost completely in 40 milliseconds).[181] Nevertheless, it is possible that the ventricular expression of various genes coding for ion channels specific for the sinus node favor abnormal automaticity in cardiac hypertrophy, as suggested by Cerbai and associates.[182]

Among the other inward currents, the best candidate as a source of hypertrophy-induced action potential lengthening is the current generated by the Na^+/Ca^{2+} exchanger. This exchanger has an enhanced activity (at least in its "reverse" mode) in the hypertrophied ferret heart.[183] Although $I_{Na\text{-}Ca}$ can indeed reverse (and then it becomes an outward current) when the membrane is depolarized beyond its reversal potential, $E_{Na\text{-}Ca}$, such an event rarely occurs during the action potential plateau. It is generally assumed that $E_{Na\text{-}Ca} = 3\ E_{Na} - 2\ E_{Ca}$. As a result, $E_{Na\text{-}Ca}$ (whose value during diastole is −40 mV) becomes increasingly positive as the $[Ca^{2+}]_i$ rises, so during the systolic Ca^{2+} transient, $E_{Na\text{-}Ca}$ reaches values (+40 to +80 mV) much more positive than that of the action potential plateau.[184] For this reason, the exchanger can generate an inward depolarizing current during almost the entire length of the cardiac action potential, and any conditions leading to a prolongation of the intracellular Ca^{2+} transient will also prolong the inward current generated by the exchanger and therefore induce a lengthening of the plateau. Such a prolongation of the Ca^{2+} transient has been observed in the ferret heart with pressure overload hypertrophy,[102] in cells from cardiomyopathic Syrian hamster heart, and in the intact perfused hypertrophied ferret heart,[185] confirming that in these species, the rate of calcium sequestration by the SR is decreased in hypertrophy. In contrast, no lengthening—only a depression of the Ca^{2+} transient—was observed in ventricular cells from the hypertrophied guinea pig,[117] a species in which the participation of $I_{Na\text{-}Ca}$ to the genesis of the plateau is not absent.[186]

The fact that $I_{Na\text{-}Ca}$ is, at least in some species, in part responsible for the hypertrophy-induced lengthening of the action potential was suggested by experiments demonstrating that this lengthening disappears when the depolarizing influence of the Na^+/Ca^{2+} exchanger is depressed or suppressed. This has indeed been observed in rats when the external Ca^{2+} concentration is increased, which makes E_{Na-Ca} more negative,[161] and after caffeine-induced suppression of the calcium transient.[187] More direct results were obtained in cardiomyopathic Syrian hamster cardiac cells.[96] In these cells, the prolonged Ca^{2+} transient was associated with the development of a long-lasting slow inward current that disappeared after either suppression of external Na^+ or depletion of intracellular Ca^{2+} stores, indicating that it was generated by the Na^+/Ca^{2+} exchanger. However, when the Na^+/Ca^{2+} exchange current, I_{Na-Ca}, was triggered by a sudden caffeine-induced release of Ca^{2+} from the SR, the I_{Na-Ca} amplitude was similar in both normal and cardiomyopathic myocytes. Therefore, the enhancement of I_{Na-Ca} in cardiomyopathic myocytes is not caused by overexpression of the Na^+/Ca^{2+} exchanger but rather results from altered calcium sequestration.[188]

The prolongation of the Ca^{2+} transient does not necessarily result from lengthening of the Ca^{2+} release from the SR. It might also result from the entry into the cell of external calcium through gCa. Normally, the increase in systolic calcium due to gCa constitutes a fast but small component of the Ca^{2+} transient.[189] The situation is different in the human hypertrophied ventricle. In samples of transplanted cardiomyopathic hearts, the relatively brief peak ($\approx$150 milliseconds) of Ca^{2+} transient labeled L1, similar to that recorded in control organ donors, was followed by a huge plateau-like long-lasting component ($\approx$800 milliseconds) of intracellular Ca^{2+} increase labeled L2.[190] Such a delayed L2 component of Ca^{2+} transient did not occur in control samples unless the extracellular Ca^{2+} concentration was raised to 16 mM, whereas in the hypertrophied sample, it was already very large at an external Ca^{2+} concentration of 2 mM. Similar L1 and L2 components occurred at a normal Ca^{2+} concentration in samples obtained from patients with dilated cardiomyopathy; nevertheless, the L2 component is smaller than that in the hypertrophied cardiomyopathy. Interestingly, 1 to 3 $\times$ 10^{-6} M ryanodine, which prevents the systolic release of Ca^{2+} from the SR, also suppressed L1. The known calcium current blocker, verapamil, at 10^{-6} M, suppressed the L2 component. Therefore, the abnormal L2 component is likely to result from entry of Ca^{2+} into the cell through gCa. Under normal conditions, these ions would be rapidly extruded from the cell, whereas in cardiomyopathic human tissues, such an extrusion appears to have dramatically slowed down.[99]

These results show that the hypertrophy-induced alterations of the Ca^{2+} transient may differ among species or models and that the resulting participation of the Na^+/Ca^{2+} exchange current in action potential alterations can be quite important.

Electrophysiologic Consequences of Cardiac Dilatation

Action potential lengthening is not the only electrophysiologic change associated with the development of experimental hypertrophy. Three days after partial pulmonary artery occlusion in the cat, a surprisingly marked decrease in the action potential plateau amplitude was detected in the five cell layers below the endocardial surface, so that at that time, myocardial action potentials resembled those of conducting fibers.[191, 192] Such a plateau depression remains for 7 to 10 days before recovery to a normal shape. The mechanisms remains unclear.

However, during the first days after coarctation of aorta in the rat, marked ventricular dilatation occurs before the compensatory hypertrophy stage. In dilated human atria, the action potential plateau is markedly reduced as a result of a severe depression in Ca^{2+} current density,[193] suggesting that the decrease in plateau amplitude described in the hypertrophied right ventricle of the cat[191] is also due, at least in part, to a dilatation-induced decrease in Ca^{2+} current. If this is true, a similar decrease in Ca^{2+} current might also occur as a result of dilatation when compensated hypertrophy leads to failure, and a decrease in plateau amplitude due to Ca^{2+} current depression might be superimposed on the hypertrophy-induced plateau lengthening previously described.

Changes in Genetic Expression

Advances in the genetics of the long QT syndrome have clearly demonstrated several mutations at the origin of the electrocardiographic phenotype in genes encoding ion channels. Simultaneously, it was shown that the above-described acquired modifications of the ion currents do in fact reflect changes in genetic expression, which are likely to participate in the adaptational process. K^+ channel genes (called Kv 1.3, 4.1, and so on; 17 different Kv genes have been identified so far in the ferret heart) constitute a highly polymorphic family, and such a polymorphism is still aggravated by the fact that the K^+ channels are themselves made with several different subunits; therefore, it is not surprising that changes in genetic expression at this level play an important role in the process of adaptation.

I_{t0} is mainly encoded by Kv 4.3 in humans and dog and by Kv 4.3 and 4.2 in rat. It was shown by Gidh-Jain and associates[30] that the electrophysiologic modifications of I_{t0} were indeed accompanied in parallel with changes in the genetic expression of the corresponding K^+ channels at the level of both the protein and the mRNA. The expressions of Kv 1.5, Kv 2.1, and Kv 4.2 are decreased by 25, 55, and 52 percent, respectively, suggesting that the diminution of I_{t0} and the corresponding lengthening of both action potential and that of the QT interval are in fact transcriptionally (or at the least pretranslationally) regulated. Such a reduction is likely to participate in the reexpression of the fetal program because, at least in the human atria, I_{t0} is developmentally regulated and its density is twice that found in the atria of young subjects (see Table 46–1).

Such conclusions were reinforced by experiments with gene transfer technology.[7] In the canine tachycardia-induced model of cardiac failure, isolated cardiocytes have prolonged action potentials, which are due to a reduction in I_{t0}. Failing cardiocytes were infected with a genetic construct made with a prototype of the voltage-dependent class of K^+ channels with the genetic construct. Two days after infection, the action potentials were dramatically shortened in a dose-dependent manner, and the contraction velocity returned to control values, suggesting that the electrophysiologic modifications were in fact a primary event.

Arrhythmias

The hypertrophied heart is arrhythmogenic regardless of whether hypertrophy is associated with coronary insufficiency. Failure, of course, aggravates the incidence of arrhythmias, but arrhythmias are also a major concern in compensated cardiac hypertrophy.[36, 194] Several attempts have been made to predict severe arrhythmias through the use of various indices, including heart rate, heart rate variability, and QT interval.

The biologic substrate for arrhythmogenicity is a complex issue.[36, 194] Fibrosis and changes in the membrane protein composition are both essential during the compensated phase, but additional factors such as plasma catecholamines and ventricular dilatation are involved in the failing phase.

Three basic mechanisms can generate arrhythmias: reentry, triggered activity, and abnormal automaticity. Attempts to separate fibrosis from the other biologic determinants of arrhythmias were made by Chevalier and colleagues.[195] The degree of cardiac hypertrophy and the percentage of ventricular fibrosis are linked to each other; nevertheless, correspondence analysis shows that fibrosis and cardiac hypertrophy are independent arrhythmogenic factors.

1. Reentry is directly linked to fibrosis and to the changes in connexon isoforms. *Connexons* are components of the gap junctions that establish cell-to-cell electrical coupling. There is evidence for a rearrangement of connexon distribution in cardiac hypertrophy with a shift from connexon 43 to connexon 40. Because connexon 40 has a greater unitary conductance than connexon 43, the shift may favor arrhythmogenicity.[196] Fibrosis creates the alternative pathway and conduction block and slows the conduction.
2. Triggered ventricular arrhythmias after myocardial infarction are likely to be generated and maintained by fibrosis, and the amount of fibrosis correlates with abnormal propagation. During senescence and in patients with hypertrophic or dilated cardiomyopathy, an alternative explanation, called the *zig-zag mechanism*, has been proposed.[197, 198]
3. Two different biologic substrates may explain the increased automaticity of hypertrophied hearts.
   - A diminished capacity to restore a low resting Ca^{2+} level during diastole due to alterations in calcium handling by the SR leads to an increased cytosolic Ca^{2+} level, which in turn generates oscillating electrical currents sufficiently strong to cause recurrent action potentials.[199] Aronson[155, 161] showed that the hypertrophied rat heart has a greater propensity to develop both delayed and early afterdepolarizations. Such a scheme requires substrates, such as therapy with digitalis or adrenergic agonists, hypokalemia, stress, ischemia, and anoxia. Besides arrhythmias, there is another good example of such fragility: the anoxia-induced increase in diastolic stiffness is exaggerated in experimental models of cardiac hypertrophy.[118]
   - The other mechanism involves the expression of ion channels that normally initiate the pacemaker activity in the sinus node,[182] as previously explained.

It is worth noting that the induction of arrhythmias does not require that a large proportion of cardiac cells undergo abnormal activation; rather, a small number of calcium-overloaded or otherwise altered myocytes is sufficient to act as an ectopic focus. For example, a zone of developing necrosis can temporarily trigger depolarization-induced activity, whereas ischemic areas can be the source of reentry and fibrillation due to marked shortening of the action potential. It has been shown that ischemia induces a more dramatic shortening of the action potential and a greater susceptibility to ventricular fibrillation in the hypertrophied rat heart than in the normal heart.[175]

Contraction-excitation feedback is defined as the changes in the mechanical state that precede or alter the transmembrane potential and that occur during cardiac failure.[200] It consists of the direct effects of stretch on action potential duration, increased dispersion of ventricular repolarization, and electrical instability, all of which are linked to the state of decompensation.[201]

Finally, cardiac decompensation is also associated with modifications of the autonomic nervous system that favor arrhythmias. Heart rate variability, one of the best noninvasive indicators of autonomic nervous system activity, is both reduced and less chaotic and reflects neural damage due to the enhanced plasma catecholamine level and the previously described down-regulation of the adrenergic receptors.

Biologic Markers for Cardiac Failure

The definition of cardiac failure is fully clinical, and the search for a biologic marker of cardiac failure may be considered nonsensical. Nevertheless, this search has been so frequently proposed that we cannot avoid or ignore it. From a basic point of view, cardiac failure may indicate the thermodynamic limits of the adaptational process. Nevertheless, myocardial fibrosis, regardless of the cause, can play a crucial role, even if the adaptational process does not reach its limits. Finally, failure can be caused by the loss of contractile material due to cell death. These three parameters are usually associated, although to varying degrees.

There are no biologic markers for cardiac failure because the hemodynamic consequences of the myocardial primary deficit can be entirely masked by the peripheral compensation. In addition, failure depends on the entire activity of the cells and cannot be ascribed as the result of a single abnormality caused by a unique molecule. There are only a few experimental models that allow study of the transition process; these include aging SHRs,[202] Dahl salt-sensitive rats fed with high-salt diet, stenosis of the descending aorta in guinea pigs, myocardial infarction in young rats,[203] two-step mechanical overloading models in rat or rabbit (aortic stenosis plus aortic incompetence[1]), and tachycardia-induced cardiac failure in dogs[204] (see Table 46–4).

The only markers of failure are probes specific for the ECM components, including fibronectin and collagen isoforms, suggesting that failure occurs through this pathway when fibrosis reaches a certain level.[202] Another biologic marker of the transient that has been proposed is the disappearance of the sensitivity to beta agonists.[111] The markers can differ from one model to another; in guinea pig, for example, Ca^{2+} ATPase of SR remains unchanged in compensated hypertrophy and is modified only in cardiac failure.[108]

SUMMARY

Hypertrophy is initially the physiologic adaptation of the heart to a disease and not a disease by itself. Failure indicates the limits and imperfections of the adaptational process. At a molecular and cellular level, hypertrophy due to mechanical overload (including compensatory hypertrophy after myocardial infarction) is a consequence of a change in the expression of the cardiac genome and requires a cascade of events, including a sensor that receives information from the outside, a transduction system, a DNA target, transient changes in the expression of genes coding for growth signals, and permanent modifications in gene expression, which represent the final phenoconversion.

The basis for adaptation is an improvement in the thermodynamic status of the heart; the hypertrophied papillary muscle contracts more slowly and produces less heat per gram of tension than normal muscle. Such an improvement results from species- and tissue-specific quantitative and qualitative modifications in genetic expression and is associated with a shift in the energy metabolism to a more anaerobic pathway.

Depending on the animal species, the modifications of systolic ejection are determined either by isomyosin shift or by modifications of membrane proteins, including a shift to the fetal isoform of the Na^+ pump and K^+ channel responsible for I_{to} and diminished density of Ca^{2+}-ATPase of SR and several receptors. In addition, systolic dysfunction is aggravated by cell death caused by necrosis or apoptosis. The major determinant of diastolic dysfunction is ventricular fibrosis, which has a multifactorial origin and a complex regulation. In addition, abnormal active relaxation depends on the same factors as systolic dysfunction, and the enhanced atrial filling is associated with an atrial isomyosin shift that maintains the atrial economy in a normal range.

From an electrophysiologic point of view, the main effect of hypertrophy on the action potential in different animal species is a marked increase in amplitude and duration of the plateau. The mechanisms involved are species specific. In most species, including humans, decreased transient outward K^+ current, I_{to}, due to diminished expression of the corresponding genes is likely to be the main determinant of the prolonged action potential. Nevertheless, in other animal species, such as guinea pig, which normally expresses such a current, other ionic currents are involved. Concerning the inward depolarizing currents, the Ca^{2+} current density is generally considered as being maintained at a normal value, whereas the current generated by the Na^+/Ca^{2+} exchanger is likely to be augmented, at least in its duration, as a result of the prolonged intracellular systolic Ca^{2+} transient. The high incidence of arrhythmias in both compensated and decompensated cardiac hypertrophy has multiple origins, including fibrosis, which causes both reentry and triggered arrhythmias, and change in calcium metabolism, which is the main determinant for increased automaticity.

REFERENCES

1. Lompré AM, Schwartz K, Albis A, et al: Myosin isozymes redistribution in chronic heart overloading. Nature 282:105, 1979.
2. Swynghedauw B: Cardiac Hypertrophy and Failure. Paris: INSERM–J Libbey, 1990.
3. Lecarpentier Y, Bugaisky LB, Chemal D, et al: Coordinated changes in contractility, energetics and isomyosins after aortic stenosis. Am J Physiol 252:H275, 1987.
4. Charlemagne D, Maixent JM, Preteseille M, Lelièvre L: Ouabain-binding sites and (Na^+, K^+)-ATPase activity in rat cardiac hypertrophy: expression of the neonatal form. J Biol Chem 261:185, 1986.
5. Chevalier B, Berrebi-Bertrand I, Leliévre LG, et al: Diminished toxicity of ouabain in hypertrophied rat heart. Pflügers Arch 414:311, 1989.
6. Heymes C, Silvestre JS, Llorens-Cortes C, et al: Cardiac senescence is associated with enhanced expression of angiotensin II receptor subtypes. Endocrinology 139:2579, 1998.
7. Swynghedauw B: Molecular mechanisms of myocardial remodelling. Physiol Rev 79:215, 1999.
8. Assayag P, Charlemagne D, Marty I, et al: Effects of sustained low-flow ischemia on myocardial function and calcium-regulating proteins in adult and senescent hearts. Cardiovasc Res 38:169, 1998.
9. Hwang DM, Dempsey AA, Wang RX, et al: A genome-based resource for molecular cardiovascular medicine: toward a compendium of cardiovascular genes. Circulation 96:4146, 1997.
10. Mayoux E, Callens F, Swynghedauw B, Charlemagne D: Adaptational process of the cardiac Ca^{2+} channels to pressure overload: biochemical and physiological properties of the dihydropyridine receptors in normal and hypertrophied rat hearts. J Cardiovasc Pharmacol 12:390, 1988.
11. Rajamanickam C, Merten S, Kwiatkowska-Patzer B, et al: Changes in mitochondrial DNA in cardiac hypertrophy in the rat. Circ Res 45:505, 1979.
12. Moalic JM, Bourgeois F, Mansier P, et al: β1-Adrenergic receptor and $G_{\alpha s}$ in the rat heart as a function of mechanical overload and thyroxine intoxication. Cardiovasc Res 27:231, 1993.
13. Apstein CS, Lecarpentier Y, Mercadier JJ, et al: Changes in LV papillary muscle performance and myosin composition with aortic insufficiency in rats. Am J Physiol 253:H1005, 1987.
14. Swynghedauw B: Developmental and functional adaptation of contractile proteins in cardiac and skeletal muscles. Physiol Rev 66:710, 1986.
15. Lowes BD, Minobe W, Abraham WT, et al: Changes in gene expression in the intact human heart: downregulation of alpha-myosin heavy chain in hypertrophied, failing ventricular myocardium. J Clin Invest 100:2315, 1997.
16. Nakao K, Minobe W, Roden R, et al: Myosin heavy chain gene expression in human heart failure. J Clin Invest 100:2362, 1997.
17. Hirzel H, Tuchsmid C, Sneider J, et al: Relationship between myosin isoenzyme composition, hemodynamics and myocardial structure in various forms of human cardiac hypertrophy. Circ Res 57:729–740, 1985.
18. Cummins P: Transitions in human atrial and ventricular myosin light-chain isoenzymes in response to cardiac-pressure-overload-induced hypertrophy. Biochem J 205:195, 1982.
19. Anderson PAW, Malouf NN, Oakeley AF, et al: Troponin T isoform

expression in humans: a comparison among normal and failing adult heart; fetal heart and fetal skeletal muscle. Circ Res 69:1226, 1991.

20. Lelièvre L, Maixent JM, Lorente P, et al: Prolonged responsiveness to ouabaïn in hypertrophied rat heart: physiological and biological evidence. Am J Physiol 250:H923, 1986.
21. Gidh-Jain M, Huang B, Jain P, et al: Reemergence of the foetal pattern of L-type calcium channel gene expression in noninfarcted myocardium during left ventricular remodeling. Biochem Biophys Res Commun 216:892, 1995.
22. Taegtmeyer H, Overturf ML: Effects of moderate hypertension on cardiac function and metabolism in the rabbit. Hypertension 11:416, 1988.
23. Revis NW, Thomson RY, Cameron AJV: Lactate dehydrogenase isoenzymes in the human hypertrophic heart. Cardiovasc Res 11:172, 1977.
24. Younes A, Schneider JM, Bercovici J, Swynghedauw B: Creatine kinase isoenzymes redistribution in chronically overloaded myocardium. Cardiovasc Res 19:15, 1985.
25. Bastie de la D, Levitsky D, Rappaport L, et al: Function of the sarcoplasmic reticulum and expression of its CA^{2+}ATPase gene in pressure overload-induced cardiac hypertrophy in the rat. Circ Res 66:554, 1990.
26. Naudin V, Oliviero P, Rannou F, et al: Ryanodine receptors in pressure-overload induced cardiac hypertrophy in the rat. FEBS Lett 285:135, 1991.
27. Chevalier B, Mansier P, Callens-El Amrani F, Swynghedauw B: The beta adrenergic system is modified in compensatory pressure cardiac overload in rats: physiological and biochemical evidence. J Cardiovasc Pharmacol 13:412, 1989.
28. Brodde OE: β1- And β2-adrenoceptors in the human heart: properties, function, and alterations in chronic heart failure. Pharmacol Rev 43:204, 1991.
29. Benitah JP, Gomez AM, Bailly P, et al: Heterogenicity of the early outward current in ventricular cells isolated from normal and hypertrophied rat ventricles. J Physiol (Lond) 469:11, 1993.
30. Gidh-Jain M, Huang B, Jain P, El-Sherif N: Differential expression of voltage-gated K^+ channel genes in left ventricular remodeled myocardium after experimental myocardial infarction. Circ Res 79:669, 1996.
31. O'Brien PJ, Gwathmey JK: Myocardial Ca^{2+}- and ATP-cycling imbalances in end-stage dilated and ischemic cardiomyopathies. Cardiovasc Res 30:394, 1995.
32. Mercadier JJ, Samuel JL, Michel JB, et al: Atrial natriuretic factor gene expression in rat ventricle during experimental hypertension. Am J Physiol 257:H979, 1989.
33. Sonnenblick EH: Force velocity relations in mammalian heart muscle. Am J Physiol 205:931, 1962.
34. Alpert NR, Mulieri LA, Hasenfuss G: Myocardial chemo-mechanical energy transduction. *In* Fozzard HA, Haber E, Jennings RB (eds): The Heart and Cardiovascular System. p. 111. New York: Raven, 1991.
35. Hasenfuss G, Holubarsch, C, Just H, Alpert NR (eds): Cellular and Molecular Alterations in the Failing Human Heart. Darmstadt: Steinkopff, 1992.
36. Assayag P, Carré F, Chevalier B, et al: Compensated cardiac hypertrophy: the new myocardial phenotype in relation with arrhythmogenicity: part 1: fibrosis. Cardiovasc Res 34:439, 1997.
37. Erdös T, Butler-Browne GS, Rappaport L: Mechanogenetic regulation of transcription. Biochimie (Paris) 73:1219, 1991.
38. Vandenburgh H, Kaufman S: In vitro model for stretch-induced hypertrophy of skeletal muscle. Science 203:265, 1979.
39. Delcayre C, Klug D, Thiem NV, et al: Aortic perfusion pressure as early determinant of β-isomyosin expression in perfused hearts. Am J Physiol 263:H1537, 1992.
40. Davies PF, Tripathi SC: Mechanical stress mechanisms and the cell: an endothelial paradigm. Circ Res 72:239, 1993.
41. Kent RL, Hoober JK, Cooper G IV: Load responsiveness of protein synthesis in adult mammalian myocardium: role of cardiac deformation linked to sodium influx. Circ Res 64:74, 1989.
42. Rappaport L, Samuel JL: Microtubules in cardiac myocytes. Int Rev Cytol 113:101, 1988.
43. Komuro I, Katoh Y, Kaida T, et al: Mechanical loading stimulates cell hypertrophy and specific gene expression in cultured rat cardiac myocytes. J Biol Chem 266:1265, 1991.
44. Hefti MA, Harder BA, Eppenberger HM, et al: Signaling pathways in cardiac myocyte hypertrophy. J Mol Cell Cardiol 299:2873, 1997.
45. Grépin C, Durocher D, Nemer M: Le coeur: un programme unique de transcription et de différenciation musculaire. Médecine/Sciences (Paris) 11:395, 1995.
46. Swynghedauw B: Transgenic models of myocardial dysfunction. Heart Failure Rev 1:277, 1997.
47. Bauters C, Moalic JM, Bercovici J, et al: Coronary flow as a determinant of *c-myc* and *c-fos* proto-oncogene expression in an isolated adult rat heart. J Mol Cell Cardiol 20:97, 1988.
48. Delcayre C, Samuel JL, Marotte F, et al: Synthesis of stress protein in rat cardiac myocytes 2–4 days after imposition of hemodynamic overload. J Clin Invest 82:460, 1988.
49. Schneider MD, Parker TG: Cardiac growth factors. MDS/Prog Growth Factor Res 1, 1991.
50. Schwartz K, Bastie de la D, Bouveret P, et al: α-Skeletal muscle actin mRNAs accumulate in hypertrophied adult rat hearts. Circ Res 59:551, 1986.
51. Ray A, Aumont MC, Aussedat J, et al: Protein and 28S ribosomal RNA fractional turnover rates in the rat heart after abdominal aortic stenosis. Cardiovasc Res 21:587, 1987.
52. Morkin E, Kimata S, Skillman JJ: Myosin synthesis and degradation during development of cardiac hypertrophy in the rabbit. Circ Res 30:690, 1972.
53. Weber KT, Brilla CG: Pathological hypertrophy and cardiac interstitium: fibrosis and renin-angiotensin system. Circulation 83:1849, 1991.
54. Hatt PY, Rakusan K, Gastineau P, Laplace M: Morphometry and ultrastructure of heart hypertrophy induced by chronic volume overload (aorto-caval fistula in the rat). J Mol Cell Cardiol 11:989, 1979.
55. Nair KG, Cutilletta F, Zak R, et al: Biochemical correlates of cardiac hypertrophy, I: experimental model, changes in heart weight, RNA content and nuclear RNA polymerase activity. Circ Res 23:451, 1968.
56. Linzbach AJ: Heart failure from the point of view of quantitative anatomy. Am J Cardiol 5:370, 1960.
57. Grimm AF, Kubota R, Whitehorn WV: Properties of the myocardium in cardiomegaly. Circ Res 12:118, 1963.
58. Hatt PY: Experimental models. *In* Swynghedauw B (ed): Cardiac Hypertrophy and Failure. p. 9. Paris: INSERM–J Libbey, 1990.
59. Astorri E, Bolognesi R, Colla B, et al: Left ventricular hypertrophy: a cytometric study on 42 human hearts. J Mol Cell Cardiol 9:763, 1977.
60. Quaini F, Cigola E, Lagrasta C, et al: End-stage cardiac failure in humans is coupled with the induction of proliferating cell nuclear antigen and nuclear mitotic division in ventricular myocytes. Circ Res 75:1050, 1994.
61. Rumyantsev PP: DNA synthesis and nuclear division in embryonal and postnatal histogenesis of myocardium (autoradiographic study). Fed Proc 24:899, 1965.
62. Pagani ED, Alonsi AA, Grant AM, et al: Changes in myofibrillar content and Mg-ATPase activity in ventricular tissues from patients with heart failure caused by coronary artery disease, cardiomyopathy or mitral valve insufficiency. Circ Res 63:380, 1988.
63. Schäper J, Meiser E, Stämmler G: Ultrastructure morphometric analysis of myocardium from dogs, rats, hamsters, mice and human hearts. Circ Res 56:377, 1985.
64. James TN: Normal and abnormal consequences of apoptosis in the human heart: from postnatal morphogenesis to paroxysmal arrhythmias. Circulation 90:556, 1994.
65. Umansky SR, Cueno GM, Khutzian SS, et al: Post-ischemic apoptotic death of rat neonatal myocytes. Cell Growth Differ 2:235, 1995.
66. Cheng W, Li B, Kajstura J, et al: Stretch-induced programmed myocyte cell death. J Clin Invest 96:2247, 1995.
67. Narula J, Haider N, Virmani R, et al: Apoptosis in end-stage heart failure. N Engl J Med 335:1182, 1996.
68. Li Z, Bing OHL, Long X, et al: Increased cardiomyocyte apoptosis during the transition from hypertrophy to heart failure in the spontaneously hypertensive rat. Am J Physiol 272:H2313, 1997.
69. Kajstura J, Cheng W, Reiss K, et al: Apoptotic and necrotic myocyte cell deaths are independent contributing variables of infarct size in rats. Lab Invest 74:86, 1996.
70. Saraste A, Pulkki K, Kallajoki M, et al: Apoptosis in human acute myocardial infarction. Circulation 95:320, 1997.
71. Teiger E, Dam T-V, Richard L, et al: Apoptosis in pressure-overload-induced heart hypertrophy in the rat. J Clin Invest 97:2891, 1996.
72. Lecarpentier Y, Waldenström A, Clergue M, et al: Major alterations

in relaxation during cardiac hypertrophy induced by aortic stenosis in guinea pig. Circ Res 61:107, 1987.

73. Meerson FZ: The myocardium in hyperfunction, hypertrophy, and heart failure. Circ Res 25(suppl II):1, 1969.
74. Swynghedauw B, Delcayre C: Biology of cardiac overload. Pathobiol Ann 12:137, 1982.
75. O'Brien PJ, O'Grady M, McCutcheon LJ, et al: Myocardial myoglobin deficiency in various models of congestive heart failure. J Mol Cell Cardiol 24:721, 1992.
76. Hatt PY, Berjal G, Moravec J, Swynghedauw B: Heart failure: an electron microscopic study of the left ventricular papillary muscle in aortic insufficiency in the rabbit. J Mol Cell Cardiol 1:235, 1970.
77. Rajamanickam C, Merten S, Kwiatkowska-Patzer B, et al: Changes in mitochondrial DNA in cardiac hypertrophy in the rat. Circ Res 45:505, 1979.
78. Ingwall JS, Kramer MF, Fifer M, et al: The creatine kinase system in normal and diseased human myocardium. N Engl J Med 313:1050, 1985.
79. Revis NW, Cameron ASV: The relationship between fibrosis and lactate dehydrogenase isozymes in experimental hypertrophic heart of rabbits. Cardiovasc Res 12:348, 1978.
80. Kagaya Y, Kanno Y, Takeyama D, et al: Effects of long-term pressure overload on regional myocardial glucose and free fatty acid uptake in rats: a quantitative autoradiographic study. Circulation 81:1353, 1990.
81. Taegtmeyer H, Overturf ML: Effects of moderate hypertension on cardiac function and metabolism in the rabbit. Hypertension 11:416, 1988.
82. Sack MN, Disch DL, Rockman HA, Kelly DP: A role for Sp and nuclear receptor transcription factors in a cardiac hypertrophy growth program. Proc Natl Acad Sci U S A 94:6438, 1997.
83. Pool PE, Chandler BM, Sonnenblick EH, Braunwald E: Integrity of energy stores in cat papillary muscle. Circ Res 22:213, 1968.
84. Peters TJ, Wells G, Oakley CM, et al: Enzymic analysis of endomyocardial biopsy specimens from patients with cardiomyopathies. Br Heart J 39:1333, 1977.
85. Wittels B, Spann JF Jr: Defective lipid metabolism in the failing heart. J Clin Invest 47:1781, 1968.
86. Katz AM: Cardiomyopathy of overload: a major determinant of prognosis in congestive heart failure. N Engl J Med 322:100, 1990.
87. Nascimben L, Ingwall JS, Pauletto P, et al: Creatine kinase system in failing and nonfailing human myocardium. Circulation 94:1894, 1996.
88. McDonald KM, Yoshiyama M, Francis GS, et al: Myocardial bioenergetic abnormalities in a canine model of left ventricular dysfunction. J Am Coll Cardiol 23:786, 1994.
89. Neubauer S, Horn M, Naumann A, et al: Impairment of energy metabolism in intact residual myocardium of rat hearts with chronic myocardial infarction. J Clin Invest 95:1092–1100, 1995.
90. Swynghedauw B, Cheav SL, Callens-ElAmrani F: The biological basis of the diastolic dysfunction of the hypertensive heart: a review. Eur Heart J 13(suppl D):2, 1992.
91. Thiem NV, Lacombe G, Swynghedauw B: Early phosphate burst of heart myosin: phylogenic variations. Eur J Biochem 91:243, 1978.
92. Clapier-Ventura R, Mekhfi H, Oliviero P, Swynghedauw B: Pressure overload changes cardiac skinned fiber mechanics in rats, not in guinea pigs. Am J Physiol 254:H517, 1988.
93. Swynghedauw B, Schwartz K, Lecarpentier Y, et al: Species-specificity of the isomyosin shift in cardiac overload. J Appl Cardiol 3:133, 1988.
94. Mercadier JJ, de la Bastie D, Ménasché P, et al: Alpha-myosin heavy chain isoform and atrial size in patients with various types of mitral valve dysfunction: a quantitative study. J Am Coll Cardiol 9:1024, 1987.
95. Leclercq JF, Swynghedauw B: Myofibrillar ATPase, DNA and hydroxyproline content of human hypertrophied heart. Eur J Clin Invest 6:27, 1976.
96. Mercadier JJ, Bouveret P, Gorza L, et al: Myosin isoenzymes in normal and hypertrophied human ventricular myocardium. Circ Res 53:52, 1983.
97. Bouvagnet P, Léger JOC, Dechesne CA, et al: Local changes in myosin types in diseased human atrial myocardium: a quantitative immunofluorescence study. Circulation 72:272, 1985.
98. Lauer B, Nguyen VT, Swynghedauw B: The ATPase activity of the cross-linked complex between cardiac myosin subfragment1 and actin in several models of chronic overloading: a new approach to the biochemistry of contractility. Circ Res 64:1106, 1989.
99. Tsuchimochi A, Sugi M, Kuro-o M, et al: Isozymic changes in myosin of human atrial myocardium induced by overload. J Clin Invest 74:662, 1984.
100. Cummins P: Transitions in human atrial and ventricular myosin light-chain isoenzymes in response to cardiac pressure-overload-induced hypertrophy. Biochem J 205:195, 1982.
101. Winegrad S, Weisberg A: Isozyme specific modification of myosin ATPase by cAMP in rat heart. Circ Res 60:384, 1987.
102. Gwathmey JK, Morgan JP: Altered calcium handling in experimental pressure-overload hypertrophy in the ferret. Circ Res 57:836, 1985.
103. Charlemagne D, Orlowski J, Oliviero P, et al: Alteration of (Na^+, K^+)-ATPase subunit mRNA and protein levels in hypertrophied heart. J Biol Chem 269:1541, 1994.
104. Shamraj OI, Grupp IL, Grupp G, et al: Characterization of Na/K-ATPase, its isoforms, and the inotropic response to ouabain in isolated failing human hearts. Cardiovasc Res 27:2229, 1993.
105. Hanf R, Durubaix I, Leliévre L: Rat cardiac hypertrophy: altered sodium-calcium exchange activity in sarcolemmal vesicles. FEBS Lett 236:145, 1988.
106. Heyliger CE, Prakash AR, McNeill JH: Alterations in membrane Na^+-Ca^{2+} exchange in the aging myocardium. Age 11:1, 1988.
107. Studer R, Reinecke H, Bilger J, et al: Gene expression of the cardiac Na^+/Ca^{2+} exchanger in end-stage human heart failure. Circ Res 75:443, 1994.
108. Kiss E, Ball NA, Kranias EG, Walsh RA: Differential changes in cardiac phospholamban and sarcoplasmic reticular Ca^{2+}-ATPase protein levels. Circ Res 77:759, 1995.
109. D'Agnolo, MD, Luciani, GB, Mazzucco A, et al: Contractile properties and Ca^{2+} release activity of the sarcoplasmic reticulum in dilated cardiomyopathy. Circ Res 85:518, 1992.
110. Sainte-Beuve C, Allen PD, Dambrin G, et al: Cardiac calcium release channel (ryanodine receptor) in control and cardiomyopathic human hearts: mRNA and protein contents are differentially regulated. J Mol Cell Cardiol 29:1237, 1997.
111. Bristow MR, Ginsburg R, Minobe W, et al: Decreased catecholamine sensitivity and beta-adrenergic receptor density in failing human heart. N Engl J Med 307:205, 1982.
112. Eschenhagen T, Mende U, Nose M, et al: Increased messenger RNA level of the inhibitory G protein alpha–subunit $G_{i\alpha-2}$ in human end-stage heart failure. Circ Res 70:688, 1992.
113. Nio Y, Matsubara H, Murasawa S, et al: Regulation of gene transcription of angiotensin II receptors subtypes in myocardial infarction. J Clin Invest 95:46, 1995.
114. Regitz-Zagrosek V, Friedel N, Heymann A, et al: Regulation, chamber localization, and subtype distribution of angiotensin II receptors in human hearts. Circulation 91:1461, 1995.
115. Asano K, Dutcher DL, Port D, et al: Selective downregulation of the angiotensin II AT1-receptor subtype in failing human ventricular myocardium. Circulation 95:113, 1997.
116. Gomez AM, Valvidia HH, Cheng H, et al: Defective excitation-contraction coupling in experimental cardiac hypertrophy and heart failure. Science 276:800, 1997.
117. Siri FM, Krueger J, Nordin C, et al: Depressed intracellular calcium transients and contraction in myocytes from hypertrophied and failing guinea pig hearts. Am J Physiol 261:H514, 1991.
118. Callens-El Amrani F, Snoeckx L, Swynghedauw B: Anoxia-induced changes in ventricular diastolic compliance in two models of hypertension in rats. J Hypertens 10:229, 1992.
119. Scamps F, Mayoux E, Charlemagne D, Vassort G: Calcium current in single cells isolated from normal and hypertrophied rat heart. Circ Res 67:199, 1990
120. Samuel JL, Bertier B, Bugaisky L, et al: Different distributions of microtubules, desmin filaments and isomyosins during the onset of cardiac hypertrophy in the rat. Eur J Cell Biol 34:300, 1984.
121. Tsutsui H, Ishihara K, Cooper G IV: Cytoskeletal role in the contractile dysfunction of hypertrophied myocardium. Science 260:682, 1993.
122. Schaper J, Froede TA, Hein S, et al: Impairment of the myocardial ultrastructure and changes of the cytoskeleton in dilated cardiomyopathy. Circulation 83:504, 1991.
123. Gaasch WH, Apstein CS, Levine HJ: Diastolic properties of the left ventricle. *In* Levine HJ, Gaasch WH (eds): The Ventricle: Basic and Clinical Aspect. p. 143. Boston: Martinus Nijhoff, 1985.

124. Schaper J, Speiser B: The extracellular matrix in the failing human heart. *In* Hasenfuss G, Holubarsch C, Just H, Alpert NR (eds): Cellular and Molecular Alterations in the Failing Human Heart. p. 303. Darmstadt: Steinkopff, 1992.
125. Weber KT (ed): Wound Healing in Cardiovascular Disease. Armonk, NY: Futura, 1995.
126. Vivaldi MT, Eyre DR, Kloner RA, Schoen SJ: Effects of methylprednisolone on collagen biosynthesis in healing acute myocardial infarction. Am J Cardiol 60:424, 1987.
127. Cleutjens JPM, Kandala JC, Guntaka RV, Weber KT: Regulation of collagen degradation in the rat myocardium after infarction. J Mol Cell Cardiol 27:1281, 1995.
128. Brilla CG, Pick R, Tan LB, et al: Remodeling of the rat right and left ventricles in experimental hypertension. Circ Res 67:1355, 1990.
129. Robert R, Besse S, Sabri A, et al: Differential regulation of matrix metalloproteinases associated with aging and hypertension in the rat heart. Lab Invest 76:729, 1997.
130. Robert V, Silvestre JS, Charlemagne D, et al: Biological determinants of aldosterone-induced cardiac fibrosis in rat. Hypertension 26:971, 1995.
131. Sun Y, Weber KT: Angiotensin II receptor binding following myocardial infarction in the rat. Cardiovasc Res 28:1623, 1994.
132. Young M, Fullerton M, Dilley R, Funder J: Mineralocorticoids, hypertension and cardiac fibrosis. J Clin Invest 93:2578, 1994.
133. Anversa P, Palackal T, Sonnenblick EH, et al: Myocyte cell loss and myocyte cellular hyperplasia in the hypertrophied aging rat heart. Circ Res 67:871, 1990.
134. Besse S, Assayag P, Delcayre C, et al: Normal and hypertrophied senescent rat heart: mechanical and molecular characteristics. Am J Physiol 265:H183, 1993.
135. Farhadian F, Contard F, Sabr A, et al: Fibronectin and basement membrane in cardiovascular organogenesis and disease pathogenesis. Cardiovasc Res 32:433, 1996.
136. Marie JP, Guillemot H, Hatt PY: Le degré de granulation des cardiocytes auriculaires: étude planimétrique au cours des différents apports d'eau et de sodium chez le rat. Pathol Biol (Paris) 24:549, 1976.
137. Michel JB, Mercadier JJ, Galen FX, et al: Urinary cyclic guanosine monophosphate as an indicator of experimental congestive heart failure in rats. Cardiovasc Res 24:946, 1990.
138. Lindpainter K, Jin M, Niedermaier N: Cardiac angiotensinogen and its local activation in the isolated perfused beating heart. Circ Res 67:564, 1990.
139. Silvestre JS, Robert V, Heymes C, et al: Myocardial production of aldosterone and corticosterone in the rat: physiological regulation. J Biol Chem 273:4883, 1998.
140. Dell'italia LJ, Meng QC, Balcells E, et al: Compartmentalization of angiotensin II generation in the dog heart: evidence for independent mechanisms in intravascular and interstitial spaces. J Clin Invest 100:253, 1997.
141. Wei CM, Lerman A, Rodeheffer RJ, et al: Endothelin in human congestive heart failure. Circulation 89:1580, 1994.
142. Haywood GA, Tsao PS, Von Der Leyen HE, et al: Expression of inducible nitric oxide synthase in human heart failure. Circulation 93:1087, 1996.
143. Chidsey CA, Sonnenblick EH, Morrow AG, Braunwald E: Norepinephrine stores and contractility force of papillary muscle from the failing heart. Circulation 33:43, 1966.
144. Bristow MR, Minobe W, Rasmussen R, et al: β-Adrenergic neuroeffector abnormalities in the failing human heart are produced by local rather than systemic mechanisms. J Clin Invest 89:803, 1992.
145. Corda S, Mebazaa A, Gandolfini MP, et al: Trophic effect of human pericardial fluid on adult myocytes: differential role of fibroblast growth factor-2 and factors related to ventricular hypertrophy. Circ Res 181:679, 1997.
146. Anker SD, Chua TP, Ponikowski P, et al: Hormonal changes and catabolic/anabolic imbalance in chronic heart failure and their importance for cardiac cachexia. Circulation 96:526, 1997.
147. Trautwein W, Kassebaum DG, Nelson RM, Hecht HH: Electrophysiological study of human heart muscle. Circ Res 10:306, 1962.
148. Dangman KH, Danielo DP, Hordoff AJ, et al: Electrophysiologic characteristics of human ventricular and Purkinje fibers. Circ Res 65:362, 1982.
149. Christé G: Effects of low $[K]_o$ on the electrical activity of human cardiac ventricular and Purkinje cells. Cardiovasc Res 17:243, 1983.
150. Escande D, Loisance D, Planche C, Coraboeuf E: Age-related changes of action potential plateau shape in isolated human atrial fibers. Am J Physiol 249:H843, 1985.
151. Antzelevitch C, Sicouri S, Litovsky SH, et al: Heterogeneity within the ventricular wall. Circ Res 69:1427, 1991.
152. Gelband H, Bassett AL: Depressed transmembrane potentials during experimentally induced ventricular failure in cats. Circ Res 32:625, 1973.
153. Hayashi H, Shibata S: Electrical properties of cardiac cell membrane of spontaneously hypertensive rat. Eur J Pharmacol 27:355, 1974.
154. Tritthart H, Luedcke H, Bayer R, et al: Right ventricular hypertrophy in the cat: an electrophysiological and anatomical study. J Mol Cell Cardiol 7:163, 1975.
155. Aronson RS: Characteristics of action potentials of hypertrophied myocardium from rats with renal hypertension. Circ Res 47:443, 1980.
156. Gülch RW, Baumann R, Jacob R: Analysis of myocardial action potential in left ventricular hypertrophy of the Goldblatt rats. Basic Res Cardiol 74:69, 1979.
157. Coulombe A, Momtaz A, Richer P, et al: Reduction of calcium-independent transient outward potassium current density in DOCA-salt hypertrophied rat ventricle myocytes. Pflügers Arch 427:47, 1994.
158. Rossner KL, Sachs HG: Electrophysiological study of Syrian hamster hereditary cardiomyopathy. Cardiovasc Res 12:436, 1978.
159. Nordin C, Siri F, Aronson RS: Electrophysiologic characteristics of single myocytes isolated from hypertrophied guinea-pig hearts. J Mol Cell Cardiol 21:729, 1989.
160. Thollon C, Kreher P, Charlon V, Rossi A: Hypertrophy induced alteration of action potential and effects of the inhibition of angiotensin converting enzyme by perindopril in infarcted rat hearts. Cardiovasc Res 23:224, 1989.
161. Aronson RS: Afterpotentials and triggered activity in hypertrophied myocardium from rats with renal hypertension. Circ Res 48:720, 1981.
162. Thollon C, Aussedat J, Verdetti J, Kreher P: Absence chez le coeur de rat hypertrophié par fistule aorto-cave de certaines altérations métaboliques et éléctrophysiologiques observées dans le cas d'autres modèles d'hypertrophie. C R Acad Sci (Paris) 300 (série III):607, 1985.
163. Kleiman RB, Houser SR: Calcium currents in normal and hypertrophied isolated feline ventricular myocytes. Am J Physiol 255:H1424, 1988.
164. Xu X, Best PM: Decreased transient outward K^+ current in ventricular myocytes from acromegalic rats. Am J Physiol 260:H935, 1991.
165. Chouabe C, Espinosa L, Megas P, et al: Reduction of I_{CaL} and I_{t01} density in hypertrophied right ventricular cells by simulated high altitude in adult rats. J Mol Cell Cardiol 29:193, 1997.
166. Potreau D, Gomez JP, Fares N: Depressed transient outward current in single hypertrophied cardiomyocytes isolated from the right ventricle of ferret heart. Cardiovasc Res 30:440, 1995.
167. Lue WM, Boyden PA: Abnormal electrical properties of myocytes from chronically infarcted canine heart. Circulation 85:1175, 1992.
168. McIntosh MA, Cobbe SM, Kane KA, Rankin AC: Action potential prolongation and potassium currents in left-ventricular myocytes isolated from hypertrophied rabbit hearts. J Mol Cell Cardiol 30:43, 1998.
169. Beuckelmann DJ, Näbauer M, Erdmann E: Intracellular calcium handling in isolated ventricular myocytes from patients with terminal heart failure. Circulation 85:1046, 1992.
170. Beuckelmann DJ, Näbauer M, Erdmann E: Alterations of K^+ currents in isolated human ventricular myocytes from patients with terminal heart failure. Circ Res 73:379, 1993.
171. Ryder KO, Bryant SM, Hart G: Membrane current changes in left ventricular myocytes isolated from guinea pigs after abdominal aortic coarctation. Cardiovasc Res 27:1278, 1993.
172. Ten Eick R, Gelband H, Kahn J, Bassett A: Changes in outward transmembrane currents of papillary muscle of cats with right ventricular hypertrophy [abstract]. Circulation 55/56(suppl III):III-47, 1977.
173. Kleiman RB, Houser SR: Outward currents in normal and hypertrophied feline ventricular myocytes. Am J Physiol 256:H1450, 1989.
174. Cameron JS, Kimura S, Jackson-Burns DA, et al: ATP-sensitive K^+ channels are altered in hypertrophied ventricular myocytes. Am J Physiol 255:H1254, 1988.

175. Kohya T, Kimura S, Myerburg RJ, Bassett AL: Susceptibility of hypertrophied rat hearts to ventricular fibrillation during acute ischemia. J Mol Cell Cardiol 20:159, 1988.
176. Ciampollino F, Tung DE, Cameron JS: Effects of diazoxide and glyburide on ATP-sensitive K^+ channels from hypertrophied ventricular myocytes. J Pharmacol Exp Ther 260:254, 1992.
177. Primot I, Mayoux E, Olivero P, Charlemagne D: Effect of pressure overload on cardiac Ca^{2+} antagonist binding sites of guinea pig: comparison with the adaptational response of the hypertrophied rat heart. Cardiovasc Res 25:875, 1991.
178. Xu X, Best PM: Increase in T-type calcium current in atrial myocytes from adult rats with growth hormone-secreting tumors. Proc Natl Acad Sci U S A 87:4655, 1990.
179. Keung EC: Calcium current is increased in isolated adult myocytes from hypertrophied rat myocardium. Circ Res 64:753, 1989.
180. Bouron A, Potreau A, Raymond G: The L type calcium current in single hypertrophied cardiomyocytes isolated from right ventricle of ferret heart. Cardiovasc Res 26:662, 1992.
181. Richard S, Tiaho F, Charnet P, et al: Two pathways for Ca^{2+} channel gating differentially modulated by physiological stimuli. Am J Physiol 258:H1872, 1990.
182. Cerbai E, Barbieri M, Mugelli A: Characterization of the hyperpolarisation-activated current I_f in ventricular myocytes isolated from hypertensive rats. J Physiol (Lond) 481:585, 1994.
183. Baudet S, Noireaud J, Leoty C: Intracellular Na activity measurements in the control and hypertrophied heart of the ferret: an ion-sensitive micro-electrode study. Pflügers Arch 418:313, 1991.
184. Noble D: Sodium-calcium exchange and its role in generating electric current. *In* Nathan RD (ed): Cardiac Muscle: The Regulation of Excitation and Contraction. p. 171. Orlando, FL: Academic, 1986.
185. Bentivegna LA, Ablin LAW, Kihara Y, Morgan JP: Altered calcium handling in left ventricular pressure-overload hypertrophy as detected with aequorin in the isolated, perfused ferret heart. Circ Res 69:1538, 1991.
186. Mitchell MR, Powell T, Terrar DA, Twist VW: The effects of ryanodine, EGTA and low-sodium on action potentials in rat and guinea-pig ventricular myocytes: evidence for two inward currents during the plateau. Br J Pharmacol 81:543, 1984.
187. Thollon C, Kreher P: Altered electrical response to caffeine exposure in hypertrophied rat myocardium. Can J Physiol Pharmacol 67:1471, 1989.
188. Hatem SN, Sham JKS, Morad M: Enhanced Na^+-Ca^{2+} exchange activity in cardiomyopathic Syrian hamster heart. Circ Res 74:253, 1994.
189. Callewaert G, Lipp L, Pott L, Carmeliet E: High-resolution measurement and calibration of Ca^{2+} transients using indo-1 in guinea-pig atrial myocytes under voltage clamp. Cell Calcium 12:269, 1991.
190. Gwathmey JK, Copelas L, MacKinnon R, et al: Abnormal intracellular calcium handling in myocardium from patients with end-stage heart failure. Circ Res 61:70, 1987.
191. Bassett AL, Gelband H: Chronic partial occlusion of the pulmonary artery in cats. Circ Res 32:15, 1973.
192. Cameron JS, Gaide MS, Epstein K, et al: Regional distribution of action potential abnormalities induced by subacute right ventricular pressure overload. J Mol Cell Cardiol 16:321, 1984.
193. Le Grand B, Hatem S, Deroubaix E, et al: Depressed transient outward and calcium currents in dilated human atria. Cardiovasc Res 28:548, 1994.
194. Swynghedauw B, Chevalier B, Charlemagne D, et al: Cardiac hypertrophy: arrhythmogenicity and the new myocardial phenotype: part 2: the cellular adaptational process. Cardiovasc Res 35:6, 1997.
195. Chevalier B, Heudes D, Heymes C, et al: Trandolapril decreases prevalence of ventricular ectopic activity in middle-aged SHR. Circulation 92:1947, 1995.
196. Peters NS, Green CR, Poole-Wilson PA, Severs NJ: Reduced content of connexin43 gap junctions in ventricular myocardium from hypertrophied and ischemic human hearts. Circulation 88:864, 1993.
197. Anderson KP, Walker R, Urie P, et al: Myocardial electrical propagation in patients with idiopathic dilated cardiomyopathy. J Clin Invest 92:122, 1993.
198. Spach MS, Dolber PC: Relating extracellular potentials and their derivatives to anisotropic propagation at a microscopic level in human cardic muscle: evidence for electrical uncoupling of side-to-side fiber connections with increasing age. Circ Res 58:356, 1986.
199. Fabiato A, Fabiato F: Contractions induced by a calcium-triggered release of calcium from the sarcoplasmic reticulum of single skinned cardiac cells. J Physiol (Lond) 249:469, 1975.
200. Lab MJ: Contraction-excitation feed-back in myocardium: physiological basis and clinical relevance. Circ Res 50:757, 1982.
201. Qin D, Zhang ZH, Caref EB, et al: Cellular and ionic basis of arrhythmias in postinfarction remodeled ventricular myocardium. Circ Res 79:461, 1996.
202. Bolyut MO, O'Neill L, Meredith AL, et al: Alterations in cardiac gene expression during the transition from stable hypertrophy to heart failure: marked upregulation of genes encoding extracellular matrix components. Circ Res 75:23, 1994.
203. Pfeffer MA, Braunwald E: Ventricular remodeling after myocardial infarction. Circulation 81:1161, 1990.
204. Zellner JL, Spinale FG, Eble DK, et al: Alterations in myocyte shape and basement membrane attachment with tachycardia-induced heart failure. Circ Res 69:590, 1991.

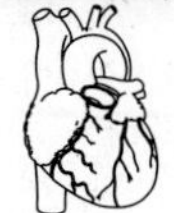

CARDIAC HYPERTROPHY: PHYSIOLOGIC AND CLINICAL CONSIDERATIONS

Sheldon E. Litwin, Andrew Thorburn, and William H. Barry

PATHOPHYSIOLOGY
Definition and Types of Hypertrophy
Signal Transduction Processes Involved in the Initiation of Cardiac Hypertrophy
Myocyte Functional Alterations Occurring as a Result of Hypertrophy
CLINICAL AND LABORATORY FINDINGS IN HYPERTROPHY
NATURAL HISTORY OF HYPERTROPHY
TREATMENT OF LEFT VENTRICULAR HYPERTROPHY
CONCLUSIONS

PATHOPHYSIOLOGY

Definition and Types of Hypertrophy

Hypertrophy is broadly defined as an increase in the bulk of part or all of an organ or a structure. Often, this definition is restricted to denote greater bulk through an increase in size, but not in number, of the individual tissue elements. In the case of the heart, hypertrophy is commonly defined as an increase in the total mass of one or more chambers. Because heart size varies widely depending on age, gender, and body size, chamber weight is often normalized for these variables. Gender- and age-specific ranges of normal cardiac chamber weights and dimensions have been previously established.[1] Although there is no general agreement on the best way to normalize left ventricular (LV) mass (e.g., total body weight, lean body weight, body surface area, height, and so on), the use of height or lean body mass may be superior because these references do not obscure the effects of obesity.[1]

Although there is some controversy on the subject,[2] it is widely believed that cardiac myocytes become terminally differentiated within days to weeks after birth. Cardiac enlargement occurs in large part through the process of myocyte hypertrophy rather than hyperplasia. The cardiac myocyte has a remarkable ability to hypertrophy during normal maturation. For example, heart weight increases from approximately 40 mg at birth to approximately 1600 mg in the adult rat. Although heart weight may double in the first week of life due purely to cellular hyperplasia, myocyte volume increases by approximately 30- to 35-fold thereafter.[3] Even after reaching normal adult size, myocytes retain a varying ability to further hypertrophy. Some data suggest that the hypertrophic reserve of cardiac myocytes declines with advancing age.[4] Interestingly, despite huge differences in body mass, the size of normal cardiac myocytes is quite similar across a large number of animal species, from mouse to humans.[5]

Once the adult body size has been reached, changes in cardiac mass usually occur in response to alterations in loading conditions. Cardiac hypertrophy has been described as a "compensatory" process that allows the heart to adapt to changing demands.[6] This view is strongly supported by experiments performed in the 1960s in which rabbits were subjected to constriction of the ascending aorta—an experimental technique that increased LV afterload.[7, 8] Increased protein synthesis could be demonstrated in the heart within hours after aortic banding. Over a period of days to weeks, animals with aortic constriction developed increased LV mass and showed no evidence of hemodynamic compromise. However, when aortic banding was followed by a protein-free diet or treatment with actinomycin D (an inhibitor of RNA synthesis), protein synthesis in the heart was blocked and a high percentage of animals developed signs of cardiac failure. These early experiments demonstrated the fundamental importance of cardiac hypertrophy as a means to handle increased load. Moreover, they underscore the notion that hypertrophy per se is an adaptation, not necessarily a disease. From a clinical perspective, hypertrophy of the left ventricle has received more attention than hypertrophy of the other chambers. Enlargement or hypertrophy of all of the cardiac chambers probably occurs with equal frequency; however, hypertrophy of the left ventricle has been studied much more intensively—perhaps because the complex geometry of the atria and right ventricle makes it quite difficult to model their structures. The main focus of this chapter is on left ventricular hypertrophy (LVH).

LVH has been classified according to the alterations in chamber geometry. The simplest schemes divide hypertrophy into concentric and eccentric categories. *Concentric* hypertrophy is considered to be present when there is a predominant increase in LV wall thickness with lesser changes in LV cavity size. Hypertrophy is considered *eccentric* when LV cavity volume increases to a greater extent than wall thickness. Several variations on this theme have been proposed. For example, Ganau and colleagues[9] described three different patterns of LV geometry in patients with hypertension based on the relative changes in

TABLE 47–1 Patterns of Left Ventricular Geometry in Patients With Arterial Hypertension

Chamber Geometry	Left Ventricular Mass	Relative Wall Thickness	With Pattern (%)
Normal	↔	↔	52
Concentric remodeling	↔	↑	13
Eccentric hypertrophy	↑	↔ or ↓	27
Concentric hypertrophy	↑	↑	8

Key: ↔, Normal or unchanged; ↑, increased; ↓, decreased; pattern, percent of hypertensive population showing each pattern of chamber geometry.

Adapted from Ganau A, Devereux RB, Roman MJ, et al: Patterns of left ventricular hypertrophy and geometric remodeling in essential hypertension. Adapted with permission from the American College of Cardiology (J Am Coll Cardiol, 1992, Vol. 19, pp. 1550–1558).

LV wall thickness and cavity size (Table 47–1). Pattern 1, referred to as *concentric remodeling,* is characterized by an increase in relative wall thickness (wall thickness/cavity dimension) but a normal LV mass. This pattern was seen in 13 percent of the patients of Ganau and colleagues.[9] Twenty-seven percent of their patients had increased LV mass with normal relative wall thickness (pattern 2: *eccentric hypertrophy*). Only 8 percent of their cohort had the "typical" pattern of *concentric hypertrophy* with increases in both LV mass and relative wall thickness (pattern 3). Interestingly, 52 percent of their patients had normal LV mass and chamber geometry. Other data support the notion that up to 50 percent of patients with increased afterload (i.e., aortic stenosis) do not meet conventional criteria for LVH.[10] The reasons for the lack of chamber hypertrophy in some patients with sustained pressure overload are unclear; additional discussion of this issue is provided later in this chapter.

The geometric pattern of LVH varies depending on the different hypertrophic stimuli. For example, long-term physical training is often associated with an increase in LV mass in which a normal relationship between wall thickness and cavity volume is maintained.[11] The increase in LV mass in the athlete's heart has been referred to as *physiological hypertrophy* because both systolic and diastolic functions are normal and the long-term prognosis appears to be excellent.[12] Concentric hypertrophy is typically due to chronic pressure overload from arterial hypertension or valvular aortic stenosis. Some forms of inherited hypertrophic cardiomyopathy also may fit this morphologic pattern. In concentric hypertrophy, wall stress is normal or low,[13] and contractile function of the ventricle is usually normal or increased. Individuals with concentric hypertrophy are often asymptomatic for extended periods of time. Eccentric hypertrophy involves an increase in cavity size, often with normal or minimally increased wall thickness. Eccentric hypertrophy is seen in pure volume overload (i.e., mitral or aortic regurgitation), after myocardial infarction, or in primary dilated cardiomyopathy. In this form of LVH, wall stress is typically increased (especially diastolic wall stress), and systolic function is variably depressed. In dilated cardiomyopathy or after transmural myocardial infarction, there is LV dilatation, but initially there may be little change in total LV mass because wall thickness may actually decrease. This architectural change has therefore been referred to as LV *remodeling* rather than LVH.[14] Increased LV internal dimensions or volumes in patients with pathological LV remodeling are a strong predictor of subsequent death.[15, 16] Combinations of the various patterns of chamber hypertrophy often occur because patients have coexisting disease processes (e.g., arterial hypertension and mitral regurgitation).

Patterns of hypertrophy at the cellular level generally parallel those seen in the intact organ. For example, myocytes from concentrically hypertrophied hearts usually show predominant increases in cell width, with small changes in cell length.[17] In contrast, eccentric hypertrophy is usually due to increases in myocyte length with lesser increases in cell width (Fig. 47–1).[18] The fact that resting sarcomere length is generally unchanged in either form of hypertrophy suggests that the increased cell size results from parallel or series addition of sarcomeres.[19] In addition to myocyte hypertrophy, side-to-side slippage of adjacent myocytes due to disruption of the collagen network may also contribute to the dilated chamber, particularly when myocardial infarction is the cause of eccentric hypertrophy.[20] Importantly, it is possible to have a dissociation between myocyte sizes and chamber mass. For example, after transmural myocardial infarction, significant portions of the LV wall are replaced by scar tissue that is much thinner than normal myocardium. Thus, even though surviving myocytes become hypertrophied, total LV mass may remain within the normal range.[18] Myocytes from infarcted hearts typically show significant increases in length with small or no changes in cell width.[18, 21] The fact that wall stress is often increased in the dilated, postinfarction heart has been taken as evidence of "inadequate hypertrophy."[18]

Control

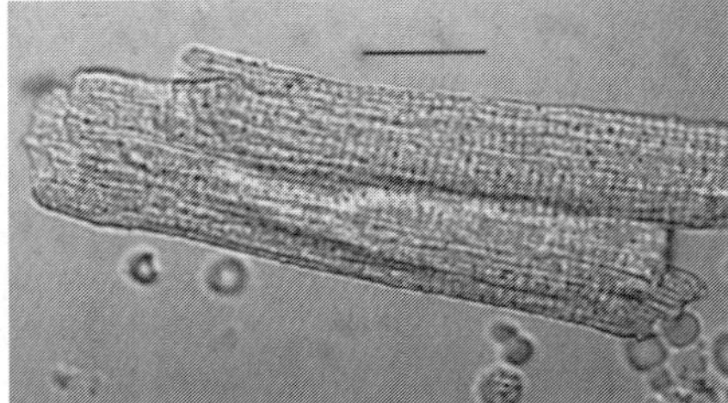

Myocardial Infarction

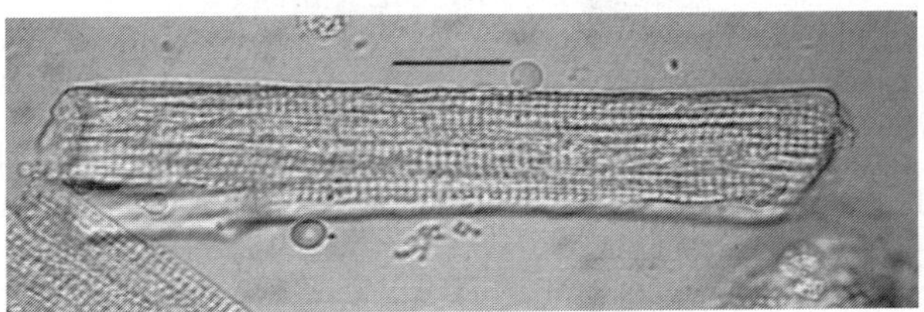

FIGURE 47–1 Examples of single left ventricular myocytes from a control rabbit **(top)** and a rabbit with postinfarction left ventricular remodeling/dilatation **(bottom)**. As in this example, myocytes from infarcted hearts typically show a pattern of eccentric hypertrophy at the cellular level with a predominant increase in cell length. Bar, 20 μm. (From Litwin SE, Bridge JHB: Enhanced Na^+-Ca^{2+} exchange in the infarcted heart: implications for excitation-contraction coupling. Circ Res 81[6]:1083–1093, 1997.)

At an ultrastructural level, hypertrophied myocytes show varying changes compared with normal myocytes.[3] In compensated hypertrophy, myocyte ultrastructure is usually normal except that the volume percent of mitochondria may be increased.[3] In decompensated hypertrophy and failure, mitochondria are smaller and the volume percent is diminished.[3] The volume percent of myofibrils has also been reported to decrease in decompensated hypertrophy and failure.[3, 22] In this condition, electron microscopy reveals enlarged areas of cytoplasm within myocytes that are devoid of contractile proteins or organelles. Decreased protein synthesis or increased degradation in the overloaded heart is responsible for the loss of contractile proteins.

LVH often involves alterations in the cardiac interstitium, as well as increases in myocyte size. The most commonly observed change is an increase in the amount of connective tissue between myocytes.[23] Although increased interstitial collagen may contribute significantly to the overall increase in LV mass, this is not usually the main component of cardiac hypertrophy. However, in patients with infiltrative disorders such as cardiac amyloidosis, deposition of amyloid protein in the interstitial space may produce dramatic increases in LV wall thickness (Fig. 47–2).

Signal Transduction Processes Involved in the Initiation of Cardiac Hypertrophy

There is tremendous interest in the signal transduction processes that mediate the development of myocyte and myocardial hypertrophy. There are several important questions under investigation. (1) What are the extracellular factors or stimuli that regulate cell growth? (2) What are the involved intracellular signaling pathways? (3) How do genetic mutations cause hypertrophy? Despite extensive work and much progress in each of these areas, complete answers have remained elusive. For this discussion, we approach each of these questions individually.

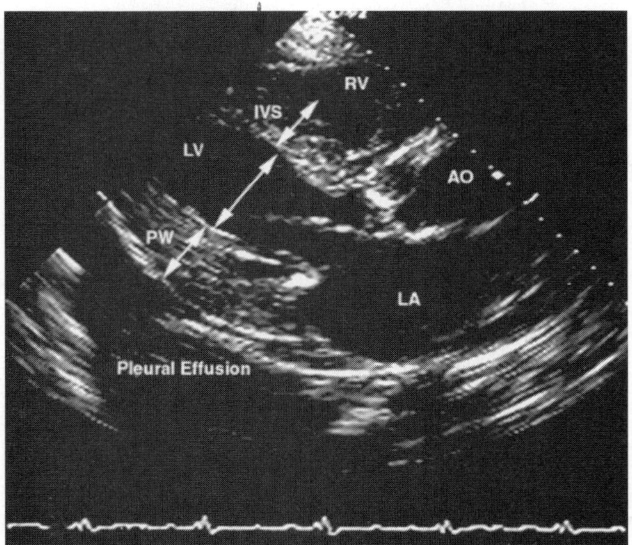

FIGURE 47–2 Example of a two-dimensional echocardiographic image from a patient with cardiac amyloidosis. This parasternal long-axis view shows typical concentric hypertrophy (IVS thickness, 22 mm; PW thickness, 26 mm). A pleural effusion also is present. AO, aortic root; IVS, interventricular septum; LA, left atrium; LV, left ventricular cavity; PW, posterior wall; RV, right ventricle.

What Are the Extracellular Factors or Stimuli That Regulate Cell Growth?

There are two main schools of thought on this topic. One group holds that cellular loading conditions (e.g., wall stress) are the major factors that regulate cell growth. The second group proposes a biochemical basis (e.g., neurohormones or growth factors) for the regulation of cell growth. In intact animals or patients, it is difficult or impossible to distinguish between these possibilities. However, in vitro experimentation allows the different possible components to be dissected. Available evidence suggests that both hypotheses are at least partially correct. For example, cultured cardiac myocytes exhibit striking hypertrophy and phenotypic alterations when exposed to the alpha-adrenergic agonist phenylephrine or angiotensin II.[24, 25] These findings support the biochemical point of view. However, other data show that simply stretching cardiac myocytes in culture can also induce cellular hypertrophy—evidence in favor of the "load" theory.[26] It has been hypothesized that a membrane ion channel is the most likely candidate for the "mechanosensor" underlying stretch-induced hypertrophy.[27] Finally, there is evidence that both load and humoral factors may interact to produce hypertrophy. Elegant work by Izumo and colleagues[28] suggests that increased load may mediate cellular hypertrophy by activating local production of angiotensin II.

At least part of the difficulty in reconciling the findings of different studies is due to the fact that myocytes seem to have multiple redundant pathways for the regulation of cell growth. As mentioned earlier, there is compelling evidence that angiotensin II is a key factor in the development of myocyte hypertrophy, at least in cultured myocytes.[25] The in vitro observations seem to be corroborated by clinical data showing that angiotensin-converting enzyme (ACE) inhibitors are highly effective in causing the regression of LVH in a variety of clinical situations.[29] However, data show that the development of hypertrophy in response to pressure overload is unabated in transgenic mice lacking the angiotensin II type 1 (AT_1) receptor.[30] Moreover, stretch-induced hypertrophy can occur in cultured myocytes from mice lacking AT_1 receptors.[31] Thus, AT_1 receptor stimulation is sufficient but not necessary for the cardiac growth response.

Intracellular Signaling Pathways Mediating the Hypertrophic Response

Studies have revealed a great deal about the biochemical signaling mechanisms that can lead to hypertrophic growth of cardiac muscle cells (Fig. 47–3). Much of this work has involved the use of model systems in which neonatal myocytes from rats were studied in tissue culture. However, in some cases, studies were extended into whole animals as a result of the use of transgenic mice.

Many hypertrophic stimuli work through cell surface

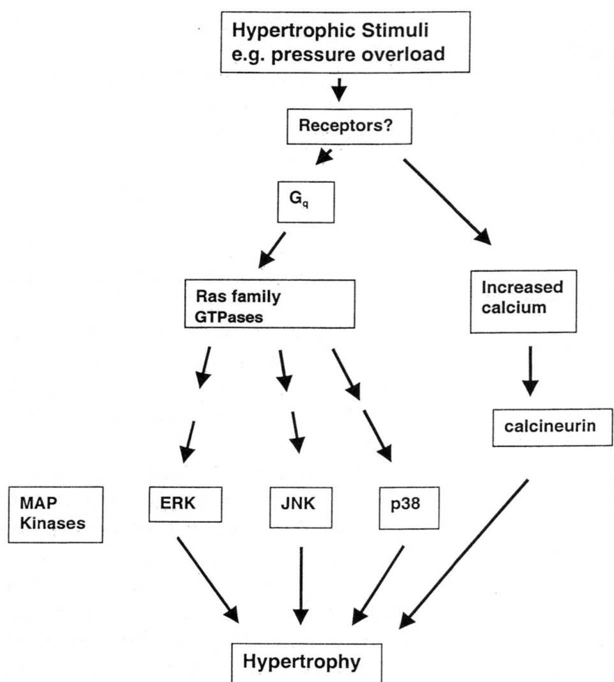

FIGURE 47–3 Simplified schematic of signal transduction pathways that influence cardiac hypertrophy. The interactions between these pathways and the mechanisms through which they each contribute to the various phenotypic changes that are associated with cardiac hypertrophy remain to be completely clarified. The various enzymes that are involved in these pathways represent targets for small molecule inhibitors that might allow therapeutic manipulation of the hypertrophic response.

receptors that are coupled to heterotrimeric G proteins, especially G_q. Inhibition of G_q-dependent signaling can prevent hypertrophy as a result of pressure overload in a mouse model.[32] Conversely, active G_q can induce hypertrophy in mice.[33, 34] In the in vitro models, a large number of studies have addressed G_q-dependent signaling pathways after the treatment of cells with adrenergic agonists or peptides such as angiotensin II or endothelin. G_q-coupled receptors activate numerous signaling pathways, including those leading to activation of protein kinase C and, particularly in heart muscle cells, the small GTPase Ras, which is a key regulator of hypertrophic responses in vitro[35–37] and in vivo.[38]

Active Ras and similar small GTPases, such as Rac and Rho,[39] can stimulate many downstream pathways, the best characterized of which is that leading to activation of mitogen-activated protein kinases (MAPKs). Mammalian cells contain at least three MAPK pathways that lead to activation of ERK, JNK, and p38 family MAPKs. All three of these MAPK families consist of several members (there are at least 10 JNKs, for example), and they appear to have both specific and common roles. During the past 5 years, a significant body of work has accumulated regarding the roles of MAPKs in cardiac muscle cells. Many, perhaps all, of the stimuli that lead to cardiac hypertrophy activate one or more of the MAPK cascades; however, there is considerable confusion as to their roles in hypertrophy. Some studies suggest that activation of the ERK pathway is necessary and sufficient to induce atrial natriuretic factor gene expression and hypertrophic morphology.[40, 41] This view has been challenged in other studies.[42–44] Similar confusion exists regarding the JNK pathway because some investigators have shown that JNK induces hypertrophy,[44, 45] whereas other investigators have found that this enzyme actually inhibited some hypertrophic responses.[46] Other data suggest that a third mammalian MAPK pathway, which leads to p38 activation, is sufficient to induce myocyte hypertrophy,[47–50] but there is some confusion here, too, because it seems that different isoforms of p38 may have different effects, such as induction of myocyte apoptosis.[49, 51] Taken together, the studies that have been performed to date indicate that the various MAPK pathways play a role in hypertrophy, but it is still difficult to define exactly the role of each molecule for any given stimulus. It is important to be able to define these roles because the various components of these signaling pathways are the subject of intense research efforts in the pharmaceutical industry to develop specific inhibitors that may prove to be useful drugs.

We are just beginning to understand the relationship between these signaling pathways and other biochemical signaling pathways that play a role in the hypertrophic response. For example, another important pathway may involve an increase in intracellular Ca^{2+} concentration ($[Ca^{2+}]_i$) and, thus, increased calcineurin activity (see Fig. 47–3). Calcineurin is a Ca^{2+}-dependent protein phosphatase that has been best characterized as a regulator of lymphocyte activation. This protein and its downstream target NFAT-3 are also sufficient to induce cardiac hypertrophy,[52] and the inhibition of calcineurin activity may prevent pressure overload-induced hypertrophy in some[53] but not all[54] models. It seems likely that we will soon be able to clarify the relationships between these and other signaling pathways that mediate hypertrophic responses. Such knowledge will provide important opportunities to design rational therapeutic approaches to limit hypertrophic responses in vivo.

Genetic Causes of Hypertrophy

A number of different genetic mutations have been identified in patients with hypertrophic cardiomyopathy. All of the mutations have been localized to contractile proteins, with a large number occurring in the gene for the myosin heavy chain. It is unclear exactly how these mutations produce the characteristic cardiac phenotype. It has been proposed that impaired force development at the sarcomeric level may be one stimulus leading to cardiac hypertrophy.[55, 56] The demonstration that transgenic animals with genetic alterations in various contractile[56] and cytoskeletal proteins[57] develop cardiac hypertrophy, heart failure, or both provides additional evidence that abnormal sarcomeric function may play a primary role in the initiation of the hypertrophy. Decreased force development induced by these abnormalities may lead to impaired ejection of blood during systole, with increased diastolic stretch and, hence, induction of further hypertrophy by the mechanisms described earlier.

Myocyte Functional Alterations Occurring as a Result of Hypertrophy

It has long been recognized that in patients with chronic pressure or volume overload of the heart, a syndrome of progressive ventricular dysfunction can develop.[58] Hypertrophy initially normalizes wall stress,[13] but eventually ventricular dilation occurs, resulting in a secondary increase in wall stress due to ventricular remodeling and associated increase in the radius of curvature of the ventricle. This increase in wall stress is proposed to cause further deterioration of ventricular function through a progressive sequence (Fig. 47–4). This sequence of events may also account for the progressive nature of the ventricular enlargement and remodeling that can occur after the loss of a significant component of functioning myocardium or a reduction in the number of myocytes as caused, for example, by myocardial infarction or myocarditis. The negative influence of depressed ventricular function and cardiac dilation on prognosis in patients with valvular disease, cardiomyopathy, and ischemic heart disease may be due in part to this process.

The potential causes of ventricular chamber dysfunction in patients with advanced hypertrophy include altered energetics, myocyte "drop out" caused by necrosis and/or apoptosis, alterations in the ventricular connective tissue matrix, and hypertrophy-induced changes in expression of myocyte genes and resulting alterations in myocyte protein constituents that lead to a decrease in myocyte function.[58, 59] Work from many laboratories has shown that hypertrophy in animals is associated with switch to a fetal pattern of gene expression,[60] including changes in actin and myosin isoforms, an increase in atrial natriuretic factor levels, a decrease in sarcoplasmic reticulum (SR) Ca^{2+}-ATPase, and an increase in Na^+/Ca^{2+} exchanger expression. The latter two effects might be expected to alter Ca^{2+} homeostasis in the myocyte.[61] Studies have shown that hypertrophy and failure in humans can be associated with similar changes in myocyte expression of genes or protein levels for the sarcoplasmic reticulum Ca^{2+}-ATPase,[62, 63] the Na^+/Ca^{2+} exchanger,[64] and contractile protein components of the myofilaments.[65]

A decrease in SR Ca^{2+}-ATPase activity could lead to decreased SR Ca^{2+} content and impaired Ca^{2+} increase from the SR during excitation-contraction coupling, causing a reduction in the Ca^{2+} transient.[66] Increased expression of the Na^+/Ca^{2+} exchanger could lead to enhanced Ca^{2+} extrusion from the cell[61] and thus also reduce the Ca^{2+} transient. However, enhanced Na^+/Ca^{2+} exchanger activity can also result in enhanced Ca^{2+} influx[67] and thus may help to maintain SR Ca^{2+} loading in hypertrophy.[21, 68] Studies in mice in which SR Ca^{2+} release and the Ca^{2+} transient are reduced by overexpression of the SR Ca^{2+} binding protein calsequestrin[69, 70] or by the administration of ryanodine, which partially blocks the SR Ca^{2+} release channel,[71] have indicated that a reduction in SR Ca^{2+} release, and thus in the Ca^{2+} transient, may be sufficient to induce hypertrophy. An alteration in the Ca^{2+} transient induced by hypertrophy may cause more hypertrophy and contribute to the progressive dysfunction (see Fig. 47–4).

Hypertrophy or sarcolemmal stress-induced decreases in the L-type Ca^{2+} current[72] and alterations in the cellular microdomains involved in coupling of the Ca^{2+} current to release of Ca^{2+} from the SR[73] may account for the frequently reported increase in the time to peak of the $[Ca^{2+}]_i$ transient noted in hypertrophied myocardium[74, 75] and contribute to a decrease in the $[Ca^{2+}]_i$ transient. There also are electrophysiologic changes associated with myocyte hypertrophy; the most prominent is an increase in the duration of the action potential that seems to be at least in part attributable to a decrease in the transient outward potassium current, I_{to}. Other K^+ currents may be altered as well.[76] This electrophysiologic change probably accounts, at least in part, for the increase in duration of the contraction and the $[Ca^{2+}]_i$ transient noted consistently in hypertrophy.[74, 75]

It is important to note that the changes in function in hypertrophied or overloaded myocytes may be reversible. Dipla and coworkers[77] have shown that myocytes isolated from hearts with end-stage dilated failure caused by both ischemic and idiopathic dilated cardiomyopathy, in which a LV assist device was used for an extended period of time to unload the ventricle, had significantly improved contraction, relaxation, and catecholamine responsiveness relative to hypertrophied myocytes isolated from the hearts of patients who did not undergo a period of ventricular unloading before heart transplantation. Preliminary data suggest that this improvement in function reflects changes in calcium homeostasis. This observation provides evidence that it is possible for load reduction through medical or surgical interventions (e.g., antihypertensive medication, valve replacement [see later]) in patients with ventricular dysfunction associated with hypertrophy to cause sufficient improvement in myocyte function to allow re-establishment of cardiac compensation and thus avoid or retard the progressive deterioration that complicates the management of heart failure.

Progression of Hypertrophy to Failure

↑ Load

↓

Hypertrophy

↓

Impaired Myocyte Function

↓

Ventricular Dilation

↓

↑ Load

FIGURE 47–4 Outline of the possible sequence of events leading to progressive ventricular dysfunction in hypertrophy (see text).

CLINICAL AND LABORATORY FINDINGS IN HYPERTROPHY

There are no historical features that are sensitive or specific for this condition. The majority of patients with physiologic or concentric LVH are asymptomatic. Although resting LV function is usually normal, exertional dyspnea may occur in patients with LVH as a result of impaired diastolic filling due to increased wall thickness and reduced chamber compliance. Patients with eccentric hypertrophy are more likely to have symptoms suggesting increased LV filling pressures, such as dyspnea on exertion or paroxysmal nocturnal dyspnea; however, these symptoms are associated with a wide variety of other conditions (i.e., pulmonary disease). Patients with LVH may also experience angina pectoris even in the absence of significant epicardial coronary artery obstruction. In this setting, angina is believed to result from subendocardial hypoperfusion. Decreased myocardial perfusion in the setting of LVH may reflect increased LV wall stress or decreased capillary density.[78] Because LV hypertrophy may increase the risk of arrhythmias, associated symptoms such as palpitations, lightheadedness, or syncope could be manifestations of LVH.[79] Again, these symptoms are nonspecific.

On physical examination, findings depend in large part on the type of hypertrophy that is present and the degree of hemodynamic compensation. The cardiac examination may be entirely normal in patients with physiologic hypertrophy. Patients with concentric LVH may have a laterally displaced or unusually forceful and sustained point of maximal impulse. A fourth heart sound is commonly present in such patients. In patients with eccentric hypertrophy, enlargement and lateral or downward displacement of a sustained PMI are likely to be present, as may signs of LV failure. There also may be evidence of right heart failure if LVH or LV dysfunction is severe or of significant duration. Indirect signs of LVH might include paradoxical splitting of the second heart sound due to the development of left bundle-branch block.

The standard chest radiograph is of only modest use in the diagnosis of LVH. The limitations of conventional radiography arise because only the epicardial contours of the heart are seen, so this technique is of little use in concentric LVH. Eccentric hypertrophy is likely to be present if the radiograph shows clear evidence of LV chamber enlargement (i.e., increased cardiothoracic ratio or abnormal contour of the LV free wall). However, considerable LV chamber enlargement may exist with a normal cardiac silhouette.

One of the most common methods for diagnosing LVH is the surface electrocardiogram. A number of different electrocardiographic criteria for LVH have been proposed.[80] These criteria usually center around the finding of increased QRS voltage in the precordial and, less often, the limb leads. Other criteria include the presence of p wave abnormalities suggesting left atrial enlargement, QRS widening, and characteristic ST-T abnormalities referred to as a "strain" pattern. Unfortunately, the electrocardiographic diagnosis of LVH has poor sensitivity and specificity,[81] and the use of electrocardiography for diagnosing LVH has dwindled in the echocardiography era.

Transthoracic echocardiography probably is the most reliable tool for diagnosing and quantifying LVH that is readily accessible to most physicians. Echocardiography is safe, noninvasive, fairly accurate, and reasonably reproducible. Measurements of LV wall thickness and cavity size are usually made from M-mode tracings (Fig. 47–5). Although M-mode measurements have good temporal resolution and reproducibility, it is sometimes difficult to clearly determine which lines represent endocardial and epicardial surfaces. Moreover, if the alignment of the M-mode beam is not perpendicular to the long axis of the heart, wall thickness will be overestimated. Another problem with the calculation of LV mass from M-mode measurements is that it requires assumptions about the geometry of the ventricle. In most commercially available software, the ventricle is modeled as a sphere or a prolate ellipsoid. These assumptions are not valid in the setting of asymmetric alterations in wall thickness or cavity radius (i.e., with segmental infarctions). LV mass can also be calculated from measurements performed on still-frame, two-dimensional images. Fewer assumptions about LV geometry are required for these calculations because measurements can be made in more than one plane and the long-axis dimension of the

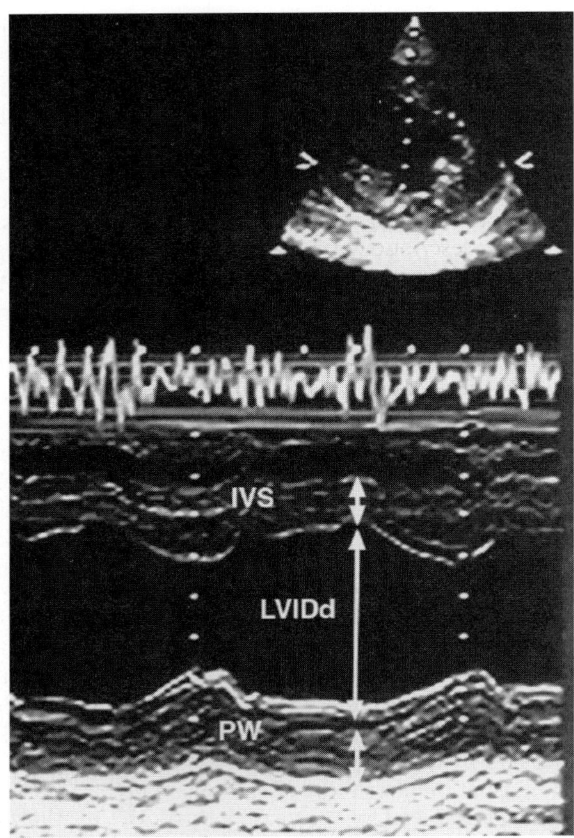

FIGURE 47–5 Example of an M-mode image obtained from the mid–left ventricular (LV) short-axis view. LV mass can be calculated from this routine clinical data with the use of a simple geometric cube formula (assumes spherical LV geometry). Previous work has shown that LV mass is more reliably calculated with an empirically derived correction to the cube formula:

$$\text{LV mass (g)} = 1.04\,([\text{LVIDd} + \text{PWT} + \text{IVST}]^3) - \text{LVIDd}^3) \times 0.8 + 0.6$$

where IVST is interventricular septal thickness (end-diastolic); LVIDd is left ventricular internal diastolic dimension; PWT is posterior wall thickness (end-diastolic); 1.04 is the specific gravity of muscle; and 0.8 is the correction factor. (From Devereux RB, Reichek N: Echocardiographic determination of left ventricular mass in man: anatomic validation of the method. Circulation 55[4]:613–618, 1977.)

heart can be directly measured. These approaches have been validated against actual LV mass measured at necropsy; the correlations are generally good.[82] Although the calculation of LV mass may be reliable in the hands of experienced and careful echocardiographers, because of the additional time required to make the measurements, quantification of LV mass often is not included as part of a routine echocardiographic examination. Rather, semiquantitative descriptions of the extent of LVH (i.e., mild, moderate, or severe) are often based strictly on the M-mode measurements of LV wall thickness. This approach is somewhat useful in the setting of concentric hypertrophy but is largely meaningless in the other patterns of hypertrophy. Some physicians have advocated the routine use of echocardiography in patients with hypertension to estimate LV mass. This approach has not been prospectively evaluated, and we believe it is unlikely to prove cost effective.

Newer imaging techniques such as ultrafast cine computed tomography and magnetic resonance imaging are very promising methods for the measurement of LV mass.[12] The identification of endocardial and epicardial borders is very reliable, and the axial resolution is quite good. Minimal or no geometric assumptions are required. Unfortunately, the cost of these tests are too high to make them applicable to large populations, so ultrafast computed tomography and magnetic resonance imaging are used predominantly as research tools in the evaluation of LVH.

Natural History of Hypertrophy

There are strong data showing that an increase in LV mass is associated with increased mortality rates.[79] LV chamber dilatation (but not necessarily an increase in LV mass) is also clearly associated with increased mortality rates in patients with prior myocardial infarction.[15] Available evidence suggests that increased LV mass in any geometric pattern is associated with increased mortality rates.[83] There are only limited data available regarding the prognostic implications of the different patterns of LVH. M-mode echocardiograms on patients in the Framingham Heart Study database suggest that a concentric pattern of LVH is associated with a worse prognosis than is concentric remodeling or eccentric LVH.[83] However, when corrected for the severity of LVH, the geometric pattern was no longer significant. Furthermore, this study included only persons who were free of cardiovascular disease at the time of enrollment. The results of another study also suggested that concentric LVH carries a high adverse risk.[84] At variance with the literature on this topic are the clinical observations that patients with compensated LVH often remain asymptomatic for many years, whereas patients with dilated hearts tend to be more symptomatic. Therefore, it seems possible that the prognosis for patients with established eccentric hypertrophy might be worse than that for patients with concentric hypertrophy.

As mentioned previously, hypertrophy is a compensatory response that allows the heart to adapt to increased workload. In many cases, however, the adaptation is incomplete, and after variable periods, heart failure develops. Determination of the nature of the transition from compensated hypertrophy to heart failure has been one of the "holy grails" of cardiovascular research. The onset of heart failure almost certainly is related to the abruptness and severity of the abnormal load imposed on the heart. However, a variety of other factors are probably important as well. One possibility is that the extent of hypertrophy is inadequate to normalize wall stress in some individuals or under some conditions.[22] Experimental evidence supports the notions that certain individuals have a greater ability to develop hypertrophy than others and that a greater degree of hypertrophy confers protective effects during cardiac overload.[85, 86] The basis of the differences in hypertrophic reserve among different patients is not known, but there may be a genetic component.[87] Interestingly, pharmacologic stimulation of myocardial hypertrophy beyond that which would normally occur also seems to be beneficial in the infarcted heart.[88, 89] Another potential cause of the transition from a compensated to a decompensated state is a decrease in myocyte contractile function due to hypertrophy-associated changes in excitation-contraction coupling and Ca^{2+} homeostasis as described earlier. A progressive loss of myocytes due to apoptosis[90, 91] may also be involved. These hypotheses may provide potential targets for new therapeutic interventions in patients with LVH.

Treatment of Left Ventricular Hypertrophy

Because LVH is a marker of increased mortality rates, it seems intuitive that regression of LVH would have beneficial effects; there is accumulating evidence that this is the case.[92, 93] However, there are no data from large-scale studies showing the prognostic implications of the regression of LVH. Such studies are planned and will be extremely important for understanding the pathophysiology of ventricular hypertrophy.

There are substantial data from experimental models of pressure-overload hypertrophy on the effects of different pharmacologic interventions. In most cases, lowered blood pressure produces regression of LVH. This holds true for treatment with multiple classes of drugs, including beta-adrenergic receptor–blocking agents, calcium channel blockers, ACE inhibitors, angiotensin II receptor blockers, α-adrenergic receptor antagonists, centrally acting agents, and diuretics.[94] Interestingly, the ability to control abnormal elevations of blood pressure does not always correlate with the ability of a given agent to reduce LV mass. The prototypical example of this dissociation is the direct vasodilator minoxidil. Although minoxidil has potent antihypertensive effects, LV mass may actually increase during long-term treatment.[95] This paradoxical effect most likely results from the strong reflex sympathetic activation that occurs with minoxidil and other direct vasodilators. Conversely, some treatments have been reported to produce regression of LVH when given in doses so low that they do not produce an antihypertensive effect. The best examples of this phenomenon involve the ACE inhibitors[96]; regression of LVH has been attributed to inhibition of local renin-angiotensin systems within the heart.

Mechanical relief of LV overload has also been shown to induce regression of LVH. The largest amount of data relates to the replacement of stenotic aortic valves.[97] Serial observations in patients with aortic valve replacement have produced important insights into the time course of the regression process. The regression of myocyte hypertrophy after aortic valve replacement occurs over months to years, but resolution of interstitial fibrosis may lag significantly behind. The replacement or repair of regurgitant mitral valves also may lead to decreases in LV mass. The use of implanted LV assist devices in patients with end-stage heart failure has been shown to reduce myocyte hypertrophy.[98]

As discussed previously, there may be cases in which it is desirable to enhance, rather than to regress, hypertrophy. This may be particularly true in conditions characterized by LV dilatation with little increase in wall thickness (e.g., postinfarction remodeling or dilated cardiomyopathy). Experimentally, inhibitors of long-chain fatty acid oxidation, thyroid hormone, and growth hormone have all been shown to be capable of enhancing hypertrophy in these settings.[88, 89, 99] Moreover, augmentation of the hypertrophic process has been associated with a reduction in pathologic remodeling and an improvement in hemodynamics. Clinical trials testing the concept of therapeutic hypertrophy are under way.

CONCLUSIONS

LVH is a complicated and dynamic response of the myocardium that serves primarily as a mechanism for adaptation to long-term changes in cardiac demand. The primary means of increasing LV mass is by increasing the size of individual myocytes. Different geometric patterns of hypertrophy develop, depending on the inciting stimulus. The different patterns of hypertrophy may have different functional and prognostic consequences. Hypertrophy is usually reversible on removal of the initiating signal. A great deal of progress has been made, but much remains to be discovered regarding the cellular and molecular signaling mechanisms responsible for myocyte hypertrophy and how they may be manipulated to improve cardiac function and prognosis in various disease states.

REFERENCES

1. Lauer MS, Larson MG, Levy D: Gender-specific reference M-mode values in adults: population-derived values with consideration of the impact of height. J Am Coll Cardiol 26:1039–1046, 1995.
2. Anversa P, Kajstura J: Ventricular myocytes are not terminally differentiated in the adult mammalian heart. Circ Res 83:1–14, 1998.
3. Bishop S: Ultrastructure of the myocardium in physiologic and pathologic hypertrophy in experimental animals. *In* Alpert NR (ed): Myocardial Hypertrophy and Failure. pp. 127–147. New York: Raven Press, 1983.
4. Isoyama S, Wei JY, Izumo S, et al: Effect of age on the development of cardiac hypertrophy produced by aortic constriction in the rat. Circ Res 61:337–345, 1987.
5. Su Z, Bridge JHB, Philipson KD, et al: Quantitation of Na/Ca exchanger function in single ventricular myocytes. J Mol Cell Cardiol 31:1125–1135, 1999.
6. Meerson FZ: Compensatory hyperfunction of the heart and cardiac insufficiency. Circ Res 10:250–258, 1962.
7. Meerson FZ, Kalebina NS, Malov GA, et al: Effect of actinomycin D on the development of the compensatory hyperfunction of the myocardium, kidney and liver. Acta Biol Acad Sci Hung 15:375–382, 1965.
8. Zuhlke V, Du Mesnil de Rochemont, Gubjarnason S, Bing RJ: Inhibition of protein synthesis in cardiac hypertrophy and its relation to myocardial failure. Circ Res 18:558–572, 1966.
9. Ganau A, Devereux RB, Roman MJ, et al: Patterns of left ventricular hypertrophy and geometric remodeling in essential hypertension. J Am Coll Cardiol 19:1550–1558, 1992.
10. Douglas PS, Otto CM, Mickel MC, et al: Gender differences in left ventricle geometry and function in patients undergoing balloon dilatation of the aortic valve for isolated aortic stenosis: NHLBI Balloon Valvuloplasty Registry. Br Heart J 73:548–554, 1995.
11. Douglas PS, O'Toole ML, Katz SE, et al: Left ventricular hypertrophy in athletes. Am J Cardiol 80:1384–1388, 1997.
12. Pluim BM, Lamb HJ, Kayser HW, et al: Functional and metabolic evaluation of the athlete's heart by magnetic resonance imaging and dobutamine stress magnetic resonance spectroscopy. Circulation 97:666–672, 1998.
13. Grossman W, Jones D, McLaurin LP: Wall stress and patterns of hypertrophy in the human left ventricle. J Clin Invest 56:56–64, 1975.
14. McKay RG, Pfeffer MA, Pasternak RC, et al: Left ventricular remodeling after myocardial infarction: a corollary to infarct expansion. Circulation 74:693–702, 1986.
15. White HD, Norris RM, Brown MA, et al: Left ventricular end-systolic volume as the major determinant of survival after recovery from myocardial infarction. Circulation 76:44–51, 1987.
16. St. John Sutton M, Pfeffer MA, Plappert T, et al: Quantitative two-dimensional echocardiographic measurements are major predictors of adverse cardiovascular events after acute myocardial infarction: the protective effects of captopril. Circulation 89:68–75, 1994.
17. Smith SH, Bishop SP: Regional myocyte size in compensated right ventricular hypertrophy in the ferret. J Mol Cell Cardiol 17:1005–1011, 1985.
18. Olivetti G, Capasso JM, Meggs LG, et al: Cellular basis of chronic ventricular remodeling after myocardial infarction in rats. Circ Res 68:856–869, 1991.
19. Julian FJ, Morgan DL, Moss RL, et al: Myocyte growth without physiological impairment in gradually induced rat cardiac hypertrophy. Circ Res 49:1300–1310, 1981.
20. Olivetti G, Capasso J, Sonnenblick EH, et al: Side-to-side slippage of myocytes participates in ventricular wall remodeling acutely after myocardial infarction in rats. Circ Res 67:23–34, 1990.
21. Litwin SE, Bridge JHB: Enhanced Na^+-Ca^{2+} exchange in the infarcted heart: implications for excitation-contraction coupling. Circ Res 81:1083–1093, 1997.
22. Urabe Y, Mann DL, Kent RL, et al: Cellular and ventricular contractile dysfunction in experimental canine mitral regurgitation. Circ Res 70:131–147, 1992.
23. Weber KT, Anversa P, Armstrong PW, et al: Remodeling and reparation of the cardiovascular system. J Am Coll Cardiol 20:3–16, 1992.
24. Simpson P: Stimulation of hypertrophy of cultured neonatal rat heart cells through an $alpha_1$-adrenergic receptor and induction of beating and through an $alpha_1$- and $beta_1$-adrenergic receptor interaction: evidence of independent regulation of growth and beating. Circ Res 56:884–894, 1985.
25. Sadoshima J, Izumo S: Molecular characterization of angiotensin II-induced hypertrophy of cardiac myocytes and hyperplasia of cardiac fibroblasts: critical role of the AT1 receptor. Circ Res 73:413–423, 1993.
26. Mann DL, Kent RL, Cooper G: Load regulation of the properties of adult feline cardiocytes: growth induction by cellular deformation. Circ Res 64:1079–1090, 1989.
27. Kent RL, Hoober JK, Cooper G: Load responsiveness of protein synthesis in adult mammalian myocardium: role of cardiac deformation linked to sodium influx. Circ Res 64:74–85, 1989.
28. Sadoshima J, Xu Y, Slayter HS, et al: Autocrine release of angiotensin II mediates stretch-induced hypertrophy of cardiac myocytes in vitro. Cell 75:977–984, 1993.
29. Schlaich MP, Schmieder RE: Left ventricular hypertrophy and its regression: pathophysiology and therapeutic approach: focus on treatment by antihypertensive agents. Am J Hypertens 11:1394–1404, 1998.
30. Hamawaki M, Coffman TM, Lashus A, et al: Pressure-overload hypertrophy is unabated in mice devoid of AT1A receptors. Am J Physiol 274:H868–H873, 1998.
31. Kudoh S, Komuro I, Hiroi Y, et al: Mechanical stretch induces hypertrophic responses in cardiac myocytes of angiotensin II type 1a receptor knockout mice. J Biol Chem 273:24037–24043, 1998.

32. Akhter SA, Luttrell LM, Rockman HA, et al: Targeting the receptor-G_q interface to inhibit in vivo pressure overload myocardial hypertrophy. Science 280:574–577, 1998.
33. Adams JW, Sakata Y, Davis MG, et al: Enhanced Gq signaling: a common pathway mediates cardiac hypertrophy and apoptotic heart failure. Proc Natl Acad Sci U S A 95:10140–10145, 1998.
34. Mende U, Kagen A, Cohen A, et al: Transient cardiac expression of constitutively active Gq leads to hypertrophy and dilated cardiomyopathy by calcineurin-dependent and independent pathways. Proc Natl Acad Sci U S A 95:13893–13898, 1998.
35. Hines WA, Thorburn A: Ras and rho are required for Gq-induced hypertrophic gene expression in neonatal rat cardiac myocytes. J Mol Cell Cardiol 30:485–494, 1998.
36. Sadoshima J, Izumo S: The heterotrimeric G_q protein-coupled angiotensin II receptor activates $p21^{ras}$ via the tyrosine kinase-Shc-Grb2-Sos pathway in cardiac myocytes. EMBO J 15:775–787, 1996.
37. Thorburn A, Thorburn J, Chen S-Y, et al: HRas dependent pathways can activate morphological and genetic markers of cardiac cell hypertrophy. J Biol Chem 268:2244–2249, 1993.
38. Hunter JJ, Tanaka N, Rockman HA, et al: Ventricular expression of a MLC-2v-ras fusion gene induces cardiac hypertrophy and selective diastolic dysfunction in transgenic mice. J Biol Chem 270:23173–23178, 1995.
39. Aikawa R, Komuro I, Yamazaki T, et al: Rho family small G proteins play critical roles in mechanical stress-induced hypertrophic responses in cardiac myocytes. Circ Res 84:458–466, 1999.
40. Gillespie-Brown J, Fuller SJ, Bogoyevitch MA, et al: The mitogen-activated protein kinase kinase MEK1 stimulates a pattern of gene expression typical of the hypertrophic phenotype in rat ventricular cardiomyocytes. J Biol Chem 270:28092–28096, 1995.
41. Glennon PE, Kaddoura S, Sale EM, et al: Depletion of mitogen-activated protein kinase using an antisense oligodeoxynucleotide approach downregulates the phenylephrine-induced hypertrophic response in cardiac myocytes. Circ Res 78:954–961, 1996.
42. Post GR, Goldstein D, Thuerauf DJ, et al: Dissociation of p44 and p42 mitogen-activated protein kinase activation from receptor-induced hypertrophy in neonatal rat ventricular myocytes. J Biol Chem 271:8452–8457, 1996.
43. Thorburn J, Carlson M, Mansour SJ, et al: Inhibition of a signaling pathway in cardiac muscle cells by active mitogen-activated protein kinase kinase. Mol Biol Cell 6:1479–1490, 1995.
44. Thorburn J, Xu A, Thorburn A: MAP kinase- and Rho-dependent signals interact to regulate gene expression but not actin morphology in cardiac muscle cells. EMBO J 16:1888–1900, 1997.
45. Wang Y, Su B, Sah VP, et al: Cardiac hypertrophy induced by mitogen-activated protein kinase kinase 7, a specific activator for c-Jun NH2-terminal kinase in ventricular muscle cells. J Biol Chem 273:5423–5426, 1998.
46. Nemoto S, Sheng Z, Lin A: Opposing effects of Jun kinase and p38 mitogen-activated protein kinases on cardiomyocyte hypertrophy. Mol Cell Biol 18:3518–3526, 1998.
47. Clerk A, Michael A, Sugden PH: Stimulation of the p38 mitogen-activated protein kinase pathway in neonatal rat ventricular myocytes by the G protein-coupled receptor agonists, endothelin-1 and phenylephrine: a role in cardiac myocyte hypertrophy? J Cell Biol 142:523–535, 1998.
48. Hines WA, Thorburn J, Thorburn A: A low-affinity serum response element allows other transcription factors to activate inducible gene expression in cardiac myocytes. Mol Cell Biol 19:1841–1852, 1999.
49. Wang Y, Huang S, Sah VP, et al: Cardiac muscle cell hypertrophy and apoptosis induced by distinct members of the p38 mitogen-activated protein kinase family. J Biol Chem 273:2161–2168, 1998.
50. Zechner D, Thuerauf DJ, Hanford DS, et al: A role for the p38 mitogen-activated protein kinase pathway in myocardial cell growth, sarcomeric organization and cardiac-specific gene expression. J Cell Biol 139:115–127, 1997.
51. Mackay K, Mochly-Rosen D: An inhibitor of p38 mitogen-activated protein kinase protects neonatal cardiac myocytes from ischemia. J Biol Chem 274:6272–6279, 1999.
52. Molkentin JD, Lu J-R, Antos CL, et al: A calcineurin-dependent transcription pathway for cardiac hypertrophy. Cell 93:215–228, 1998.
53. Sussman MA, Lim HW, Gude N, et al: Prevention of cardiac hypertrophy in mice by calcineurin inhibition. Science 281:1690–1693, 1998.
54. Ding B, Price RL, Borg TK, et al: Pressure overload induces severe hypertrophy in mice treated with cyclosporine, an inhibitor of calcineurin. Circ Res 84:729–734, 1999.
55. Bonne G, Carrier L, Richard P, et al: Familial hypertrophic cardiomyopathy: from mutations to functional defects. Circ Res 83:580–593, 1998.
56. Blanchard E, Seidman C, Seidman JG, et al: Altered crossbridge kinetics in the $MHC^{403/+}$ mouse model of familial hypertrophic cardiomyopathy. Circ Res 84:475–483, 1999.
57. Arber S, Hunter JJ, Ross J, et al: MLP-deficient mice exhibit a disruption of cardiac cytoarchitectural organization, dilated cardiomyopathy and heart failure. Cell 88:393–403, 1997.
58. Katz AM: Cardiomyopathy of overload: a major determinant of prognosis in congestive heart failure. N Engl J Med 322:100–110, 1990.
59. Barry WH: Load-dependent myocyte dysfunction. Circulation 97:2297–2298, 1998.
60. Chien KR, Grace AA, Hunter JJ: Molecular basis of cardiac hypertrophy and heart failure. *In* Chien KR (ed): Molecular Basis of Heart Disease. pp. 211–250. Philadelphia: WB Saunders, 1998.
61. Barry WH, Bridge JHB: Intracellular calcium homeostasis in cardiac myocytes. Circulation 87:1806–1815, 1993.
62. Arai M, Alpert NR, MacLennan DH, et al: Alterations in sarcoplasmic reticulum gene expression in human heart failure: a possible mechanism for alterations in systolic and diastolic properties of the failing myocardium. Circ Res 72:463–469, 1993.
63. Hasenfuss G, Reinecke H, Studer R, et al: Relation between myocardial function and expression of sarcoplasmic reticulum Ca^{2+}-ATPase in failing and nonfailing human myocardium. Circ Res 75:434–442, 1994.
64. Studer R, Reinecke H, Bilger J, et al: Gene expression of the cardiac Na^{+}-Ca^{2+} exchange in end-stage human heart failure. Circ Res 75:443–453, 1994.
65. Lowes BD, Minobe W, Abraham WT, et al: Changes in gene expression in the intact human heart: downregulation of α-myosin heavy chain in hypertrophied, failing ventricular myocardium. J Clin Invest 100:2315–2324, 1997.
66. Linder M, Erdmann E, Beuckelmann DJ: Calcium content of the sarcoplasmic reticulum in isolated ventricular myocytes from patients with terminal heart failure. J Mol Cell Cardiol 30:743–749, 1998.
67. Yao A, Nonaka A, Su Z, et al: The effects of overexpression of the Na/Ca exchanger on $[Ca^{2+}]_i$ transients in murine ventricular myocytes. Circ Res 82:657–665, 1998.
68. Dipla K, Mattiello JA, Margulies KB, et al: The sarcoplasmic reticulum and the Na^{+}/Ca^{2+} exchanger both contribute to the Ca^{2+} transient of failing human ventricular myocytes. Circ Res 84:435–444, 1999.
69. Jones LR, Suzuki YJ, Wang W, et al: Regulation of Ca^{2+} signaling in transgenic mouse cardiac myocytes overexpressing calsequestrin. J Clin Invest 101:1385–1393, 1998.
70. Sato Y, Ferguson DG, Sako D, et al: Cardiac-specific overexpression of mouse cardiac calsequestrin is associated with depressed cardiovascular function and hypertrophy in transgenic mice. J Biol Chem 273:28470–28477, 1998.
71. Meyer M, Trost SU, Bluhm WF, et al: Impaired sarcoplasmic reticulum function causes heart failure and cardiac hypertrophy in mice. Circulation 98(suppl I):I-490, 1998.
72. Nuss HB, Houser SR: Voltage dependence of contraction and calcium current in severely hypertrophied feline ventricular myocytes. J Mol Cell Cardiol 23:717–726, 1991.
73. Gomez AM, Valdivia H, Cheng H, et al: Defective excitation-contraction coupling in experimental cardiac hypertrophy and heart failure. Science 276:800–806, 1997.
74. Marban E: Calcium and heart failure. Cardiovasc Res 37:277–278, 1998.
75. Houser SR, Lakatta EG: Function of the cardiac myocyte in the conundrum of end-stage, dilated human heart failure. Circulation 99:600–604, 1999.
76. Wickenden AD, Kaprielian R, Kassiri Z, et al: The role of action potential prolongation and altered intracellular calcium handling in the pathogenesis of heart failure. Cardiovasc Res 37:312–323, 1998.
77. Dipla K, Mattiello JA, Jeevanandam V, et al: Myocyte recovery after mechanical circulatory support in humans with end-stage heart failure. Circulation 97:2316–2322, 1998.
78. Julius BK, Spillman M, Vassalli G, et al: Angina pectoris in patients with aortic stenosis and normal coronary arteries. Circulation 95:892–898, 1997.

79. Haider AW, Larson MG, Benjamin EJ, et al: Increased left ventricular mass and hypertrophy are associated with increased risk for sudden death. J Am Coll Cardiol 32:1454–1459, 1998.
80. Chou TC: Left ventricular hypertrophy. *In* Electrocardiography in Clinical Practice. pp. 37–52. 3rd ed. Philadelphia: WB Saunders, 1991.
81. Surawicz B: Stretching the limits of the electrocardiogram's diagnostic utility. J Am Coll Cardiol 32:483–485, 1998.
82. Devereux RB, Reichek N: Echocardiographic determination of left ventricular mass in man: anatomic validation of the method. Circulation 55:613–618, 1977.
83. Krumholz HM, Larson M, Levy D: Prognosis of left ventricular geometric patterns in the Framingham Heart Study. J Am Coll Cardiol 25:879–884, 1995.
84. Ghali JK, Liao Y, Cooper RS: Influence of left ventricular geometric patterns on prognosis in patients with or without coronary artery disease. J Am Coll Cardiol 31:1635–1640, 1998.
85. Ginzton LE, Conant R, Rodrigues DM, et al: Functional significance of hypertrophy of the noninfarcted myocardium after myocardial infarction. Circulation 80:816–822, 1989.
86. Koide M, Nagatsu M, Zile MR, et al: Premorbid determinants of left ventricular dysfunction in a novel model of gradually induced pressure overload in the adult canine. Circulation 95:1601–1610, 1997.
87. Post WS, Larson MG, Myers RH, et al: Heritability of left ventricular mass: the Framingham Heart Study. Hypertension 30:1025–1028, 1997.
88. Litwin S, Raya TE, Anderson PG, et al: Induction of myocardial hypertrophy after coronary ligation in rats decreases ventricular dilatation and improves systolic function. Circulation 84:1819–1827, 1991.
89. Cittadini A, Grossman JD, Napoli R, et al: Growth hormone attenuates early left ventricular remodeling and improves cardiac function in rats with large myocardial infarction. J Am Coll Cardiol 29:1109–1116, 1997.
90. Adams JW, Sakata Y, Davis MG, et al: Enhanced Gq signaling: a common pathway mediates cardiac hypertrophy and apoptotic heart failure. Proc Natl Acad Sci U S A 95:10140–10145, 1998.
91. Hirota H, Chen J, Betz UAK, et al: Loss of a gp 130 cardiac muscle cell survival pathway is a critical event in the onset of heart failure during biomechanical stress. Cell 97:189–198, 1999.
92. Rials SJ, Wu Y, Xu X, et al: Regression of left ventricular hypertrophy with captopril restores normal ventricular action potential duration, dispersion of refractoriness, and vulnerability to inducible ventricular fibrillation. Circulation 96:1330–1336, 1997.
93. Verdecchia P, Schillaci G, Borgioni C, et al: Prognostic significance of serial changes in left ventricular mass in essential hypertension. Circulation 97:48–54, 1998.
94. Schmieder RE, Martus P, Klingbeil A: Reversal of left ventricular hypertrophy in essential hypertension: a meta-analysis of randomized double-blind studies. JAMA 275:1507–1513, 1996.
95. Moravec CS, Ruhe T, Cifani JR, et al: Structural and functional consequences of minoxidil-induced cardiac hypertrophy. J Pharmacol Exp Ther 269:290–296, 1994.
96. Baker KM, Chernin MI, Wixson SK, et al: Renin-angiotensin system involvement in pressure-overload cardiac hypertrophy in rats. Am J Physiol 259:H324–H332, 1990.
97. Krayenbuehl HP, Hess OM, Monrad ES, et al: Left ventricular myocardial structure in aortic valve disease before, intermediate, and late after aortic valve replacement. Circulation 79:744–755, 1989.
98. Zafeiridis A, Jeevanandam V, Houser SR, et al: Regression of cellular hypertrophy after left ventricular assist device support. Circulation 98:656–662, 1998.
99. Gay R, Gustafson TA, Goldman S, et al: Effects of L-thyroxine in rats with chronic heart failure after myocardial infarction. Am J Physiol 253:H341–H346, 1987.

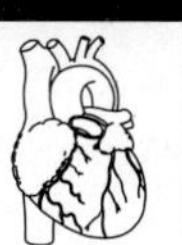

CHAPTER 48

Regulation of Cardiac Contraction and Relaxation

Arnold M. Katz

THE CONTRACTILE PROTEINS
Myosin
Actin
Tropomyosin
The Troponin Complex
CHEMISTRY OF THE INTERACTIONS AMONG ACTIN, MYOSIN, AND ADENOSINE TRIPHOSPHATE
Response of the Contractile Proteins to Calcium Ions
EXCITATION-CONTRACTION COUPLING
The Plasma Membrane
The Dyad
The Sarcoplasmic Reticulum
OVERVIEW OF THE CALCIUM FLUXES DURING EXCITATION-CONTRACTION COUPLING AND RELAXATION
THE ENERGY-STARVED HEART
Inadequate Substrate Levels
Allosteric Effects
Reduced Free Energy of Adenosine Triphosphate Hydrolysis

The pumping of the heart results from interactions between the contractile proteins in its muscular walls. These interactions transform chemical energy derived from the high-energy phosphate bonds of adenosine triphosphate (ATP) into the mechanical work that moves blood under pressure from the great veins into the pulmonary artery and from the pulmonary veins into the aorta. The interactions between the contractile proteins are, in turn, controlled by calcium, which serves as the final mediator of a complex signaling process called excitation-contraction coupling. This chapter provides a review of the properties of the contractile proteins of the heart and their control by calcium, with an emphasis on certain features of these basic aspects of myocardial function that shed light on the pathophysiology of human disease.

The Contractile Proteins

Myocardial contraction and its control can be understood in terms of the interactions among seven proteins (Table 48–1) that are found in the thick and thin filaments of the sarcomere, the fundamental unit of striated muscle, which is made up of the A-band and adjacent two half I-bands (Fig. 48–1). The thick filaments are localized in the A-band, and the thin filaments project from the Z-bands on either side of the sarcomere. When assembled in vitro, these seven proteins exhibit properties that reflect the three salient features of cardiac contraction: they hydrolyze ATP and thus are able to liberate chemical energy; when they hydrolyze ATP, they undergo physicochemical changes that are manifestations of tension development and shortening in living muscle; and their interactions are controlled by Ca^{2+} in a manner that reflects the processes of excitation-contraction coupling.

Myosin

Myosin, the major protein of the thick filament of muscle, is a large molecule containing a filamentous "tail" that is woven into the rigid backbone of the thick filament and a globular "head" that projects as the crossbridge that interacts with actin to effect muscle contraction (Fig. 48–2). In resting muscle, the crossbridges are almost perpendicular to the long axis of the thick filament, whereas in active muscle, their tips shift toward the center of the sarcomere. This conformational change, which uses energy derived from ATP hydrolysis, "rows" the thin filaments toward the center of the sarcomere, causing the sarcomere to shorten and, if the muscle is loaded, to develop tension.

Purified myosin has two important biologic properties: the ability to hydrolyze ATP so as to release its chemical energy and the ability to interact with actin in a manner that generates tension and shortening. Each myosin molecule

TABLE 48–1 **Contractile Proteins of the Heart**

Protein	Location	Salient Properties
Myosin	Thick filament	Hydrolyzes ATP, interacts with actin
Actin	Thin filament	Activates myosin ATPase, interacts with myosin
Tropomyosin	Thin filament	Modulates actin-myosin interaction
Troponin C	Thin filament	Binds calcium
Troponin I	Thin filament	Inhibits actin-myosin interactions
Troponin T	Thin filament	Binds troponin complex to tropomyosin

Abbreviations: ATP, adenosine triphosphate; ATPase, adenosine triphosphatase.
Modified from Katz AM: Physiology of the Heart. 2nd ed. New York: Raven, 1992.

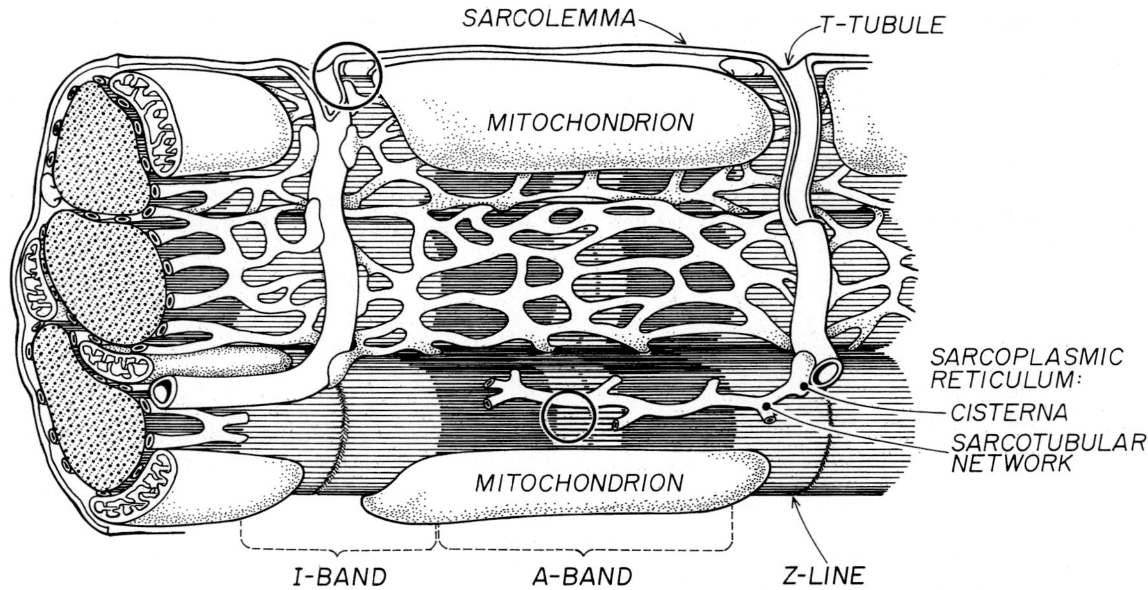

FIGURE 48–1 Ultrastructure of the working myocardial cell. Contractile proteins are arranged in a regular array of thick and thin filaments (seen in cross section at the left). The A-band represents the region of the sarcomere occupied by the thick filaments into which thin filaments extend from either side. The I-band is the region of the sarcomere occupied by only thin filaments; these extend toward the center of the sarcomere from the Z-lines, which bisect each I-band. The sarcoplasmic reticulum, a membrane network that surrounds the contractile proteins, consists of the sarcotubular network at the center of the sarcomere and the cisternae, which abut on the T-tubules and the sarcolemma. The transverse tubule system (T-tubule) is lined by a membrane that extends from the sarcolemma and carries the extracellular space into the myocardial cell. Mitochondria are shown in the central sarcomere and in cross section (left). (From Katz AM: Congestive heart failure: role of altered myocardial cellular control. N Engl J Med 293:1184, 1975. Copyright © 1975 Massachusetts Medical Society. All rights reserved.)

contains two heavy chains that extend through both head and tail and four light chains that are associated with the head of the molecule (see Fig. 48–2). The heavy chains are the major determinants of myosin ATPase activity in vitro and of shortening velocity in the living muscle. Both the myosin heavy chains and light chains are members of multigene families whose isoforms are found in different muscles and in the same muscle at different stages of development. Isoform shifts involving the myosin heavy chains occur in the chronically overloaded heart, where they participate in both the adaptive and the maladaptive response to chronic overloading. Myosin heavy chain isoforms can also change with endocrine abnormalities, notably thyroid disorders, and with aging.

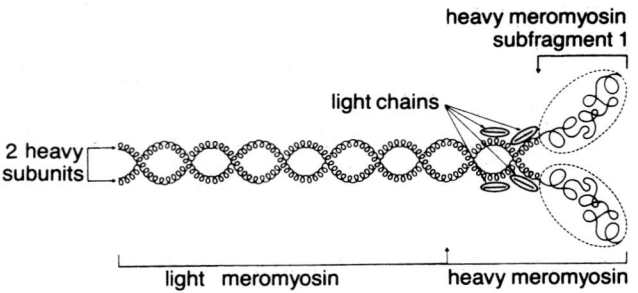

FIGURE 48–2 Myosin is an elongated molecule consisting of two heavy subunits and four light subunits. The "tail" of the molecule (left) is a coiled coil (two α-helical chains wound around each other) that extends into the paired globular "head" of the molecule (right). The latter projects from the thick filament as the crossbridges that interact with actin in the thin filament. The meromyosins are enzymatic products released through the digestion of this molecule. (From Katz AM: Physiology of the Heart. 2nd ed. New York: Raven, 1992.)

Rodent atria and ventricles contain high and low ATPase heavy chain isoforms. The high ATPase myosin heavy chain allows the myocardium to shorten rapidly, whereas the low ATPase myosin is associated with a lower contractility but greater efficiency when shortening against a heavy load. The high ATPase heavy chains are called alpha, or V_1, heavy chains, and the lower-ATPase, slower ventricular myosin heavy chains are called beta, or V_3. Small amounts of hybrid myosins, containing one alpha and one beta heavy chain (V_2) are also found. The human ventricle contains mainly the slow myosin heavy chain, but both fast and slow isoforms are found in human atria.

Each myosin molecule also contains two pairs of light chains. These are related to the calcium-binding proteins described later, although in most cases, these light chains have lost the amino acid sequence responsible for high-affinity calcium binding. In smooth muscle, myosin light chains participate in calcium signaling by serving as substrate for calcium-calmodulin–activated protein kinases that activate smooth muscle contraction. Some cardiac myosin light chains can also be phosphorylated by calcium-calmodulin–activated protein kinases, but the functional role of these phosphorylations remains unclear. There is some evidence that myosin light chain phosphorylation amplifies force development during systole.

Actin

Actin, which is much smaller than myosin, is a globular protein that makes up the backbone of the thin filaments of the sarcomere. Like myosin, actin is present as several isoforms. Human hearts contain mainly α-cardiac actin, along with a smaller amount of α-skeletal actin. The basic structure of the thin filament is a double-stranded macromolecular helix made up of two strands of actin monomers (Fig. 48–3). Actomyosins made from highly purified actin and myosin are able to liberate chemical energy from ATP and undergo physicochemical changes that provide in vitro models of the cardiac contractile process.

Tropomyosin

Tropomyosin is an elongated molecule that is found along with actin in the thin filament, where one tropomyosin molecule lies in each of the two longitudinal grooves between the two strands of actin. The tropomyosin molecule, which is made up of two α-helical peptide chains linked by a single disulfide bridge, can be a homodimer or heterodimer containing either or both of two isoforms: α and β. The major function of tropomyosin is to regulate the interactions between actin and myosin.

The Troponin Complex

The troponin complex is made up of three discrete proteins. One component, *troponin I*, in concert with tropomyosin, regulates the interactions between actin and myosin. *Troponin T* serves primarily to bind the troponin complex to tropomyosin, and *troponin C* contains the calcium-binding sites that, when occupied by this activator cation, activate cardiac contraction. Several isoforms exist for each of the troponin components.

Each troponin C molecule contains four similar amino acid sequences that are members of the extended family of calcium-binding proteins that includes calmodulin and the myosin light chains. In mammalian cardiac troponin C, only one of these four amino acid sequences binds calcium reversibly; this sequence represents the physiologic calcium receptor that activates the cardiac contractile proteins. Troponin I, in combination with tropomyosin, inhibits actin-myosin interactions. As is true for the other contractile proteins, there are many troponin I isoforms. Cardiac muscle troponin I contains a serine residue that, when phosphorylated by a cyclic AMP (cAMP)-dependent protein kinase, reduces the calcium affinity of troponin C. The resulting desensitization of the response of the myocardium to calcium favors relaxation in the heart under the influence of β-adrenergic agonists.

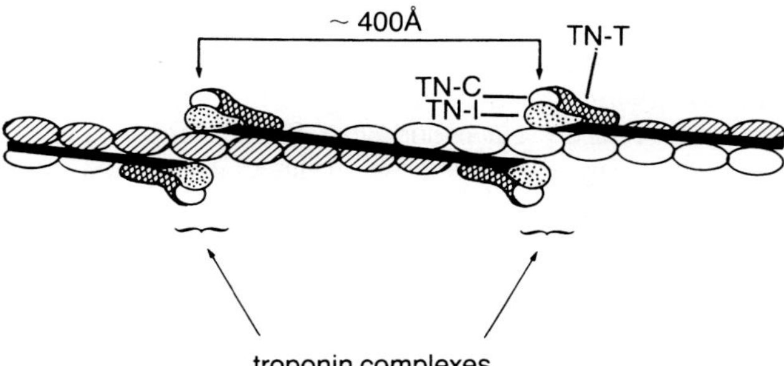

FIGURE 48–3 Schematic of the proteins of the thin filament shows troponin complexes (TN-T, TN-C, TN-I) distributed along with actin and tropomyosin at 400-Å intervals. (From Katz AM: Physiology of the Heart. 2nd ed. New York: Raven, 1992.)

Troponin T, which binds the troponin complex to tropomyosin, exists as more than 30 isoforms that can be produced through alternate gene splicing. Although troponin T itself does not bind calcium, isoform switches involving this protein appear to modify the calcium sensitivity of tension development. One such change may play a role in the desensitization of the contractile proteins in the chronically overloaded heart.

Chemistry of the Interactions Among Actin, Myosin, and Adenosine Triphosphate

Actomyosins reconstituted from highly purified actin and myosin can utilize high-energy phosphate bond energy, derived from ATP hydrolysis, to generate physicochemical changes analogous to those that lead to tension development and shortening in the intact muscle. However, ATP is not simply an energy donor, because ATP has a second effect on the interactions between the contractile proteins that reflects a very different role of this nucleotide. Even at very low concentrations, ATP saturates the substrate sites that provide the energy-consuming reactions that allow the heart to contract. At high concentrations, ATP also exerts regulatory (*allosteric*) effects that dissociate actin and myosin and thus inhibit ATPase activity. The normally high ATP concentrations in the living heart more than suffice to saturate the hydrolytic sites on myosin that provide energy for the actin-myosin interactions involved in contraction. However, the relaxing effect of ATP is more vulnerable than the substrate effect to attenuation in the energy-starved heart. The loss of the allosteric relaxing effect of high ATP concentrations probably contributes to impaired relaxation in the ischemic and chronically failing heart.

Physiologic control of the interactions between actin and myosin, of course, is brought about by variations in the calcium concentration around the myofibrils. At low cytosolic calcium concentrations, where troponin C is not bound to calcium, actin-myosin interactions are inhibited and the muscle is in the resting state. Calcium delivery to the cytosol and its subsequent binding to troponin C therefore represent key steps in the activation of cardiac systole.

Response of the Contractile Proteins to Calcium Ions

The ability of calcium binding to troponin C to initiate myocardial contraction occurs when calcium reverses an inhibitory effect of tropomyosin and the troponin complex. This activation of the contractile proteins of the heart by calcium involves a series of cooperative interactions among calcium, troponin C, troponin I, troponin T, and tropomyosin that modify the ability of actin in the thin filament to interact with the myosin crossbridges in the thick filament. In resting muscle, where calcium is not available to bind

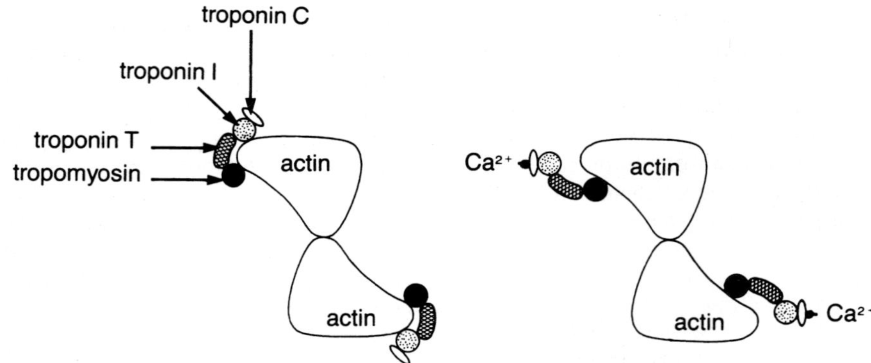

FIGURE 48–4 Cross section of a thin filament in the resting (diastole) **(left)** and active (systole) **(right)** states. At rest, the troponin complex holds the tropomyosin molecules toward the periphery of the groove between adjacent actin strands in a manner that prevents actin from interacting with the myosin crossbridges. In active muscle, calcium binding to troponin C weakens the bond linking troponin I to actin, causing a structural rearrangement of the regulatory proteins that shifts the tropomyosin deeper into the groove between the strands of actin. This rearrangement exposes active sites on actin for interaction with the myosin crossbridges. (From Katz AM: Physiology of the Heart. 2nd ed. New York: Raven, 1992.)

to troponin C, the tropomyosin filaments lie toward the outside of the grooves between the two chains of actin, where they block the development of actin-myosin interactions (Fig. 48–4). Binding of calcium to troponin C weakens the bond connecting troponin I to actin, causing a rearrangement of the proteins of the thin filament, which shifts the tropomyosin molecules toward the center of the groove between the two strands of actin. By moving tropomyosin away from its blocking position, these rearrangements enable the myosin crossbridges to interact with the active sites on actin, thereby initiating systole. The heart returns to its relaxed state when calcium removal from troponin C returns tropomyosin to its inhibitory position in the thin filament.

EXCITATION-CONTRACTION COUPLING

As noted, the heart uses calcium as the final signal in excitation-contraction coupling, the process by which depolarization of the cell surface membrane initiates the interactions between the contractile proteins that lead to tension development and shortening in the walls of the heart. Excitation-contraction coupling encompasses a complex sequence of steps that begins when an action potential depolarizes the plasma membrane and ends when the binding of calcium to troponin C causes the rearrangements in the proteins of the thin filament described earlier. Key structures involved in excitation-contraction coupling and relaxation are depicted in Figure 48–5A, and their functions are listed in Table 48–2.

The key to understanding the important energetics of excitation-contraction coupling is the fact that the level of ionized calcium in the extracellular fluid and within the sarcoplasmic reticulum (SR), the sources of this activator, is about 1 mM, whereas the calcium concentration needed to saturate troponin is about 100-fold less (<10 μM). Both are much higher than cytosolic calcium concentration in the resting heart, which is approximately 0.2 μM. This means that activation of contraction is due to passive calcium fluxes, in which this activator moves downhill to reach its binding sites on troponin C. Relaxation, on the other hand, requires that energy be expended to move calcium uphill, out of the cytosol.

Excitation-contraction coupling and relaxation are effected by interlocked systems of calcium channels and

TABLE 48–2 Structures That Participate in Cardiac Excitation-Contraction Coupling and Relaxation

Structure	Excitation-Contraction Coupling	Relaxation
Plasma Membrane		
Sarcolemma		
Na channel	Depolarization Open plasma membrane Ca channels	
Ca channel	Action potential plateau Open intracellular Ca-release channels	
Ca pump		Ca removal
Na/Ca exchanger	Ca entry in systole	Ca removal in diastole
Na pump		Establish Na gradient
Transverse Tubule		
Na channel	Propagate action potential into cell	
Ca channel	Open intracellular Ca-release channels	
Sarcoplasmic Reticulum		
Subsarcolemmal Cisternae		
Ca-release channel	Ca release for binding to troponin C	
Calsequestrin	Ca storage	
Sarcotubular Network		
Ca pump		Ca removal
Myofilaments		
Actin and myosin	Contraction	
Troponin C	Ca receptor	
Tropomyosin, troponins I and T	Allosteric regulation	

Modified from Katz AM: Physiology of the Heart. 2nd ed. New York: Raven, 1992.

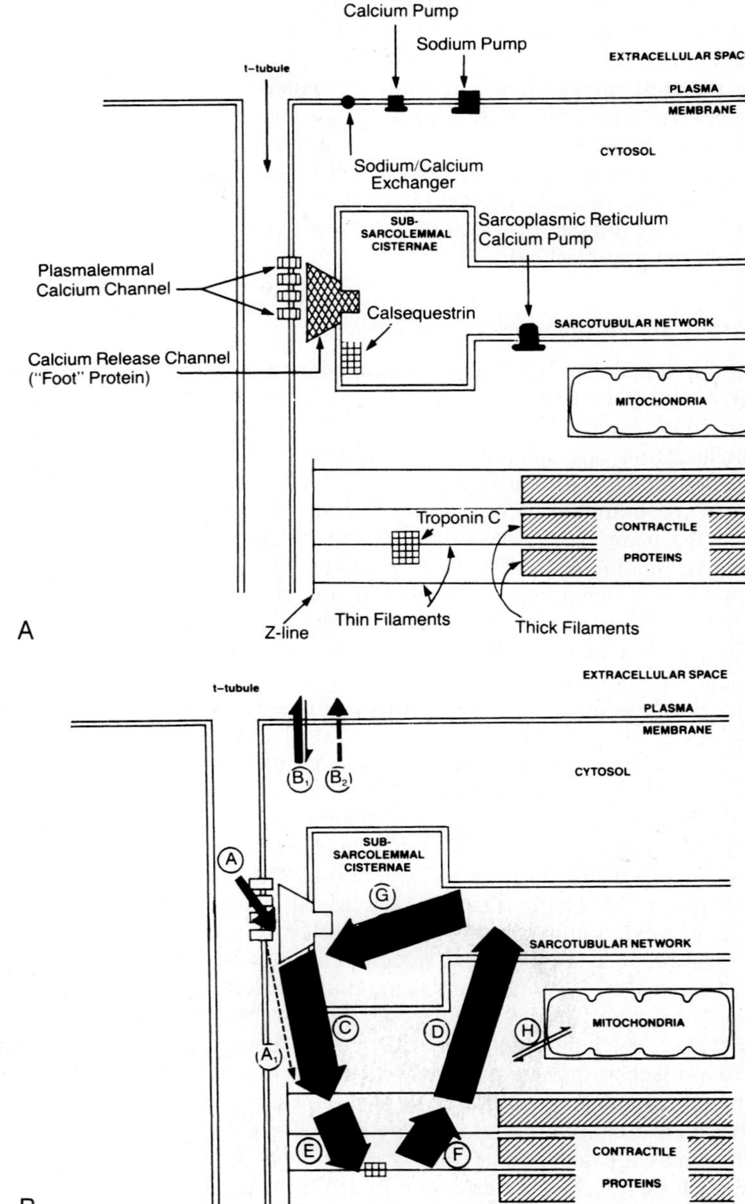

FIGURE 48–5 Schematic shows key structures **(A)** and major calcium fluxes **(B)** involved in cardiac excitation-contraction coupling. The thickness of the *arrows* indicates the magnitude of the calcium fluxes, and their directions represent the "energetics" of the calcium fluxes. *Downward arrows* represent passive calcium fluxes, and *upward arrows* represent energy-dependent calcium transport. Calcium enters the cell from the extracellular fluid via plasma membrane calcium channels (A); although most of this calcium triggers calcium release from the sarcoplasmic reticulum, a small portion directly activates the contractile proteins (A_1). Calcium transport back into the extracellular fluid involves two plasma membrane systems: sodium-calcium exchange (B_1) and the plasma membrane calcium pump (B_2). The sarcoplasmic reticulum membrane regulates two calcium fluxes: calcium release from the subsarcolemmal cisternae (C) and active calcium uptake by the calcium pump of the sarcotubular network (D). Calcium diffuses within the sarcoplasmic reticulum in a third calcium flux (G), returning to the subsarcolemmal cisternae, where it is stored in complex with calsequestrin and other calcium-binding proteins. Binding (E) and dissociation (F) of calcium with the high-affinity calcium-binding sites of troponin C define its affinity for calcium: the ratio of E to F. Movements of calcium into and out of mitochondria (H) buffer the cytosolic Ca^{2+} concentration. (**A** and **B**, From Katz AM: Physiology of the Heart. 2nd ed. New York: Raven, 1992.)

calcium pumps (see Fig. 48–5B). Control of these membrane systems enables the heart to adjust its mechanical behavior to a variety of physiologic, pharmacologic, and pathophysiologic stimuli that fine tune the systems that participate in the delivery and subsequent removal of activator calcium.

The Plasma Membrane

The plasma membrane of the heart, which separates the cytosol from the extracellular fluid, consists of the sarcolemma, unspecialized regions of the membrane that separate the cell interior from the extracellular space, and at least two specialized membranes. The first of the latter is the intercalated disc, which provides mechanical linkages between adjacent cells and contains nonselective nexus (gap junction) channels through which electrical current and small molecules flow from one cell to another. The second specialized regions of this membrane line the transverse tubular system (t-tubules), which are extensions of the sarcolemma that penetrate into the myocardial cell (see Fig. 48–1). As the lumen of the t-tubules opens to the extracellular space, the composition of the fluid within these tubules is similar to that of the extracellular fluid. The t-tubules transmit the action potential into the cell interior, thereby facilitating uniform activation of the muscle cell. Composite structures, called *dyads*, are formed between the membranes of the SR and those of either the sarcolemma or the t-system (see later).

The plasma membrane plays a complex role in excitation-contraction coupling, participating in both electrical activation (depolarization) and release of activator calcium into the cytosol. The electrical signal that initiates the contractile process begins when an action potential depolarizes the plasma membrane surrounding the myocardial cell. In the working cells of the atria and ventricles, action potentials begin with a depolarizing sodium current that initiates a second inward current carried by calcium ions. The latter, as discussed later, provides a key signal that triggers the release of calcium into the cytosol of the activated myocardial cell.

Plasma Membrane Calcium Channels

The calcium channels in the plasma membrane of the heart serve a number of functions. The first is to carry positive charge into the cell, which, as pointed out, contributes to depolarization and maintains the plateau of the cardiac action potential. This calcium entry, which also plays a key role in the initiation of cardiac contraction, is accelerated when the heart is activated through sympathetic stimulation. The binding of β-adrenergic agonists to their receptors in the plasma membrane of the heart increases the opening of these calcium channels via two mechanisms: a direct action of the receptor-agonist complex that is mediated by plasma membrane G proteins and phosphorylation of the channels by cAMP-dependent protein kinase (protein kinase A).

Calcium entry through the plasma membrane calcium channels in the adult mammalian heart provides only a small amount of activator calcium for binding to troponin C. This is due in part to the fact that much of this calcium is taken up and stored by the SR, where it contributes to the internal store of calcium that can be released in subsequent contractions. A more important role of calcium entry through the plasma membrane calcium channels is to trigger the release of a much larger amount of calcium from the internal stores in the SR (see later).

Because calcium enters the cell during each cardiac systole, mechanisms are required to remove this activator from the cell during diastole. As calcium enters the cell down both a concentration and an electrical gradient, calcium removal is an uphill process that involves the expenditure of energy. This process is effected by two different mechanisms. The first is an ATP-dependent calcium pump that uses the energy derived from ATP hydrolysis for the chemiosmotic work involved in the active transport of calcium. The second is a sodium-calcium exchanger that uses the energy of the sodium gradient across the plasma membrane to transport calcium out of the cell.

Plasma Membrane Calcium Pump

The plasma membrane calcium pump has many similarities to the calcium pump of the SR described below; however, these two related membrane calcium pumps are regulated differently. The plasma membrane calcium pump is stimulated by direct binding of the calcium-calmodulin complex, whereas the most important mechanism that activates the calcium pump of the SR is a phosphorylation reaction catalyzed by a cAMP-dependent protein kinase. Stimulation of calcium efflux when the calcium-calmodulin complex binds to the plasma membrane calcium pump allows elevated intracellular calcium concentration to increase the removal of this activator, thereby providing a negative feedback that avoids calcium overload by allowing excessive calcium entry to stimulate calcium efflux.

Sodium-Calcium Exchanger

Most of the calcium that enters the cardiac cell during each action potential is removed by an ion exchanger in the plasma membrane, which can carry either sodium or calcium in both directions across the plasma membrane. The relative amounts of these two ions that are carried in either direction are determined by their relative concentrations on the two sides of the membrane. This occurs because sodium and calcium compete for the transport site on this exchanger.

The major driving force for calcium efflux via sodium-calcium exchange is provided by the passive flux of sodium down a gradient across the plasma membrane that is established by the Na^+, K^+-ATPase (see later). Thus, the ultimate energy source for the uphill calcium transport out of the cell via the sodium-calcium exchanger is the ATP hydrolyzed by the sodium pump to establish the sodium gradient across the plasma membrane.

The sodium-calcium exchanger is electrogenic because it transports three sodium ions in one direction across the membrane in exchange for a single calcium ion that moves in the opposite direction. This exchange of three monovalent sodium ions for one divalent calcium ion generates a net movement of charge across the plasma membrane. The relationship between the current generated by this exchange and the directions of the ion fluxes is complex; unlike calcium flux through a calcium channel, where calcium and positive charge move in the same direction, the sodium-calcium exchanger moves charge in a direction opposite that of the calcium flux. This is because charge movement follows the flux of sodium rather than that of calcium, when three monovalent sodium ions are exchanged for one divalent calcium ion.

Because sodium-calcium exchange is associated with a charge movement, not only does the exchanger influence membrane potential but also membrane potential influences the ion exchange. In the resting cell, the negative intracellular potential tends to "pull" the net charge carried by the three sodium ions into the cell, which means that the exchanger favors calcium efflux during diastole. The reversal of membrane potential during the plateau of the action potential, when the inside of the cell becomes positively charged, has the opposite effect and so favors calcium influx. This electrogenic ion exchange also influences membrane potential, but the currents generated by sodium-calcium exchange are small and probably contribute less than a few millivolts to membrane potential.

The positive inotropic effects of agents that inhibit sodium efflux or increase sodium entry into myocardial cells are due to a gain in intracellular calcium brought about by the sodium-calcium exchanger. The cardiac glycosides, for example, exert their inotropic effects via direct inhibition of the Na^+, K^+-ATPase that inhibits sodium efflux. The resulting gain in cytosolic sodium provides more of this ion to compete for efflux via the intracellular cation binding site on the sodium-calcium exchanger. The result is reduced calcium efflux via the exchanger, leading to a net gain in intracellular calcium, which increases myocardial contractility.

Sodium Pump

The plasma membrane Na^+, K^+-ATPase, or sodium pump, uses energy derived from ATP hydrolysis to generate a sodium gradient across the plasma membrane. This gradient represents a store of potential energy that provides the driving force for the sodium currents that depolarize the working cells of the atria and ventricles and the rapidly conducting cells of the His-Purkinje system. As noted earlier, this gradient also energizes calcium efflux via the sodium-calcium exchanger.

The sodium pump exchanges the small amount of sodium that enters the cell during each action potential for the small amount of potassium lost from the cytosol during repolarization. Thus, the electrochemical work of this pump is minimized as the sodium pump moves positively charged ions in opposite directions across the membrane. However, the amounts of sodium and potassium moved in opposite directions during each turnover of the pump are not the same; instead, three sodium ions are transported out of the cell in exchange for only two potassium ions. This means that like the sodium-calcium exchanger, the sodium pump is electrogenic, generating a small, outward (repolarizing) current, which is normally less than 10 mV.

Sodium-Hydrogen Exchange

The plasma membrane of the heart also contains a sodium-hydrogen exchanger that, like the sodium-calcium exchanger, uses the energy of the sodium gradient to pump protons out of the cell. The sodium-hydrogen exchanger participates in the regulation of both intracellular sodium concentration and intracellular pH. In conditions such as ischemia, in which accelerated glycolysis and ATP hydrolysis cause a fall in intracellular pH, the sodium-hydrogen exchanger helps to rid the cell of excess hydrogen ions.

The Dyad

The plasma membrane of the heart forms composite structures with the internal membranes of the SR that play a key role in excitation-contraction coupling. This structure, the *dyad*, is composed of two membranes (Fig. 48–6), each of which contains one of two proteins that control the release of the activator calcium that initiates systole. The first protein is the plasma membrane calcium channel discussed earlier. This protein is often referred to as the *dihydropyridine receptor* because it binds tightly to calcium channel–blocking drugs. The second is the calcium-release channel of the SR, which is also referred to as the *foot protein*, or *ryanodine receptor*. The latter contains the channel through which calcium enters the cytosol from stores within the SR.

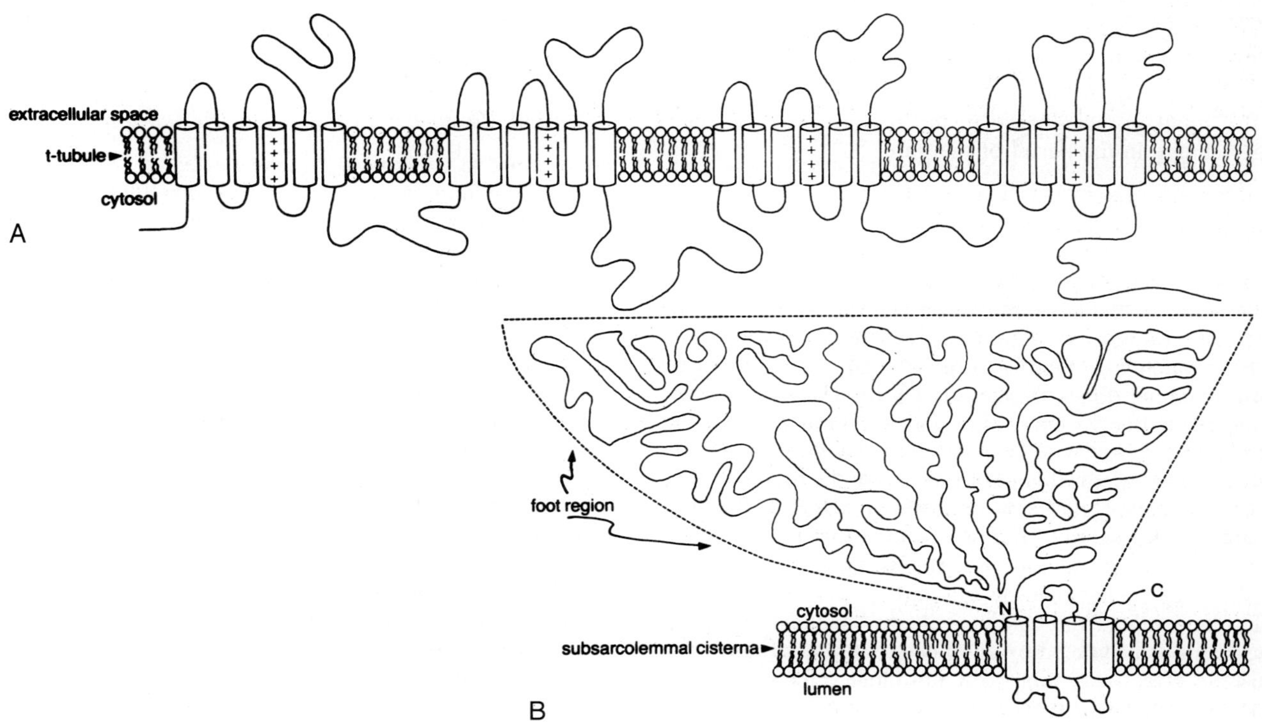

FIGURE 48–6 Structure of the dyad. The membrane of the t-tubule is above and that of the subsarcolemmal cisternae is below. One subunit of the dihydropyridine receptor (calcium channel) is shown in the t-tubule membrane **(A)**, and one ryanodine receptor (calcium release channel subunit) is shown in the membrane of the subsarcolemmal cisterna **(B)**. Both of these proteins are made up of four subunits. In the case of the dihydropyridine receptor, each subunit contains six membrane-spanning domains; one of these membrane-spanning domains is rich in positively charged amino acids and is believed to be the voltage sensor that opens that channel when the t-tubule is depolarized. The ryanodine receptor is also made up of four subunits, each of which contains four membrane-spanning domains and a large cytoplasmic peptide chain that is seen in the electron microscope as the foot protein. (**A** and **B,** From Katz AM: Physiology of the Heart. 2nd ed. New York: Raven, 1992.)

The Sarcoplasmic Reticulum

The SR is an intracellular membrane system whose major function is to regulate cytosolic calcium concentration by taking up, storing, and releasing calcium. Because the amount of calcium released for binding to the cardiac contractile proteins is central to the control of myocardial contractility, regulation of calcium release from the SR is a major determinant of the mechanical performance of the heart.

The SR of the heart can be divided into two regions (see Fig. 48–5). The subsarcolemmal cisternae are dilated extensions of the SR that contain the channels through which calcium flows to initiate systole; the channel proteins, as noted above, are visible in the electron microscope as the foot proteins of the dyad. The subsarcolemmal cisternae also store this activator, mostly bound to a protein called calsequestrin (see later). The more extensive sarcotubular network surrounds the contractile proteins in the center of the sarcomere; this region of the SR contains a densely packed array of the calcium pump ATPase proteins that actively transport calcium out of the cytosol so as to relax the heart.

It is generally agreed that calcium release from the cardiac SR is initiated by the small amount of calcium that enters the cell during the plateau of the action potential through calcium channels in the plasma membrane (dihydropyridine receptors). This calcium then triggers the opening of the calcium-release channels (ryanodine receptors) in the subsarcolemmal cisternae, which release a much larger amount of calcium from stores within the SR. This process, called calcium-triggered calcium release, resembles the firing of an old flintlock musket, where explosion of the small primer charge in the pan sets off the much larger charge in the barrel of the gun.

Calcium-Release Channels

As noted earlier, the morphologically described foot protein is known to be the calcium-release channel of the SR. This membrane protein is a tetrameric structure, of which each subunit contains a huge cytosolic domain and four membrane-spanning domains (see Fig. 48–6). The four subunits of the ryanodine receptor surround a central channel that appears to connect with radial channels within each of the four projections of this molecule into the cytosol (Fig. 48–7). A second class of intracellular calcium channels, which are structurally similar to those that participate in calcium-triggered calcium release, is opened by inositol trisphosphate rather than by calcium.

The opening of the calcium-release channels of the SR by calcium is promoted by an allosteric effect of ATP. This allosteric effect is similar to many other effects of a high ATP concentration that stimulate ion pumps and favor the opening of ion channels. The opening of cardiac calcium-release channels is inhibited by the calcium-calmodulin complex; this response, by further inhibiting calcium release from the SR, helps the heart to avoid an excessive increase in cytosolic calcium. A similar safety mechanism was described earlier, in which the calcium-calmodulin complex was seen to stimulate the ATP-dependent calcium pump of the plasma membrane, thereby promoting calcium removal from the cytosol of the calcium-overloaded heart.

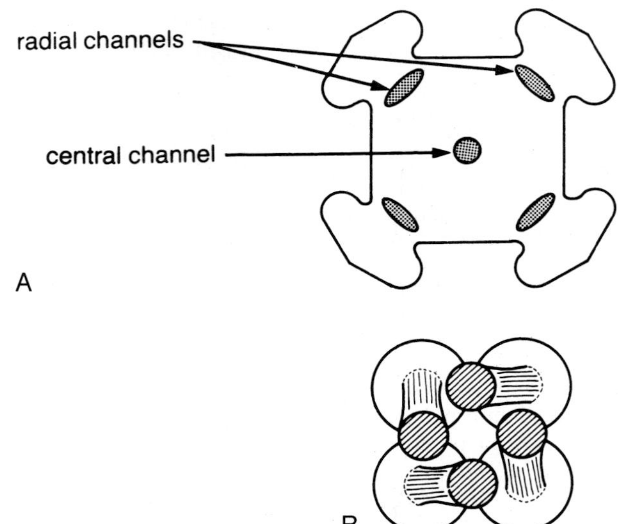

FIGURE 48–7 Schematic of the calcium-release channel of the sarcoplasmic reticulum. **A,** Image based on negative staining data shows a central channel surrounded by four radial channels. **B,** From within the lumen of the subsarcolemmal cisternae, the foot protein can be viewed as a structure made up of four subunits that resemble mushrooms. The putative central channel is surrounded by the four "stems," which correspond to the membrane-spanning helices, whereas the four radial channels are represented by the "caps." (**A** and **B,** From Katz AM: Physiology of the Heart. 2nd ed. New York: Raven, 1992.)

Calcium Pump of Sarcoplasmic Reticulum

In contrast to excitation, which is effected by the passive flux of calcium into the cytosol, relaxation requires the active transport of this cation into the SR. This uphill process is effected by an ATP-dependent calcium pump (Fig. 48–8), which, like the plasma membrane calcium pump described earlier, uses energy liberated through hydrolysis of the high-energy phosphate bonds of ATP to pump calcium against its concentration gradient from the cytosol into the sarcoplasmic reticulum.

The calcium pump of the SR (Fig. 48–9), like that of the plasma membrane described earlier, couples hydrolysis of the terminal phosphate of ATP to active ion transport. The SR calcium pump, which is a slightly smaller molecule than that of the plasma membrane, can be encoded by at least three genes, which, through alternate splicing, generate at least five isoforms of this ion pump.

Although the downhill flux of calcium through the calcium-release channels (ryanodine receptors) appears to occur through preformed channels (see Fig. 48–7), calcium transport via the calcium pump requires that this cation bind with high affinity to charged amino acids in the membrane-spanning helices of the pump protein. Conformational changes in this calcium-binding domain then raise the activity of the bound cation, much like a system of locks raises a ship in a canal. The absence of a preformed channel in the SR calcium pump is consistent with the much slower rate of calcium transport by the ion pump

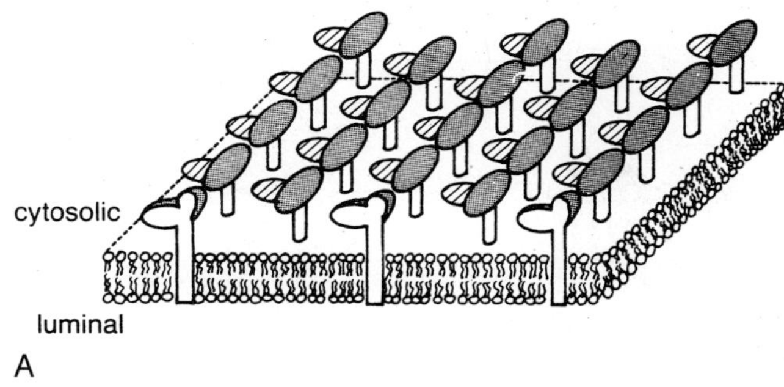

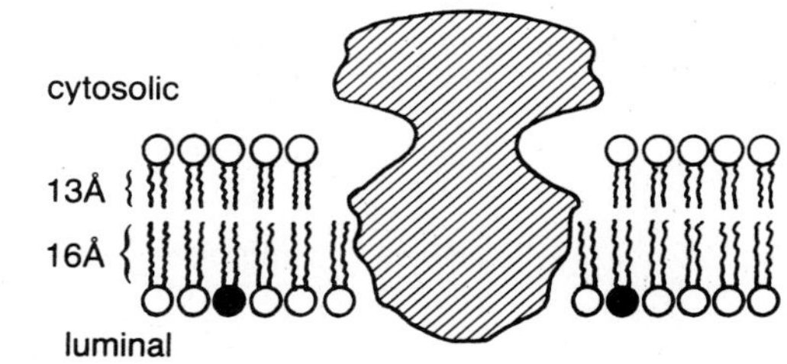

FIGURE 48–8 Structure of the sarcoplasmic reticulum membrane. **A,** Three-dimensional depiction of the sarcoplasmic reticulum. The cytosolic surface of the membrane is above the membrane, and the lumen into which calcium is pumped is below. The calcium pump ATPase molecules are packed in the bilayer, probably as dimers, in which a large portion of the mass projects from the cytosolic surface of the membrane. **B,** Cross section through the bilayer shows the cylindrically averaged mass of a single calcium pump ATPase unit; again, the cytosolic surface of the membrane is at the top. The average length of the fatty acyl chains is slightly longer in the cytosolic leaflet of the bilayer than in the luminal leaflet, and there are more phospholipid molecules in the latter (depicted as phospholipid with black head groups). (**A** and **B,** From Katz AM: Physiology of the Heart. 2nd ed. New York: Raven, 1992.)

than that of the passive calcium flux through the channel (see below).

The most important regulator of calcium transport by the SR is calcium itself; when this ion occupies the high-affinity calcium-binding site of the pump, it increases the rate of calcium transport. Therefore, even a slight increase in cytosolic calcium concentration directly accelerates calcium transport from the cytosol into the SR. A rise in cytosolic calcium also has an indirect effect to stimulate this calcium pump by activating a calcium-calmodulin–dependent protein kinase (see later).

As in the case of actomyosin, ATP has a dual effect on the calcium pump of the SR. Low concentrations of this nucleotide provide the energy required for active calcium transport, whereas the turnover of the fully energized calcium pump is also stimulated by an allosteric effect of high concentrations of ATP. These dual effects reflect the presence of two types of ATP-binding sites in these membranes: a high-affinity catalytic site that is half-saturated at micromolar ATP concentrations and a low-affinity regulatory site that is half-saturated at ATP concentrations of about 100 μM. Attenuation of the regulatory effects of ATP may play a role in the slowing of relaxation in the energy-starved heart.

The response of the heart to the sympathetic nervous system, which is mediated by cAMP, includes stimulation of calcium transport by the SR. The phosphodiesterase inhibitors, which inhibit cAMP breakdown, also increase calcium uptake into the SR. Increased cytosolic levels of cAMP stimulate the SR by activating a cAMP-dependent protein kinase that phosphorylates phospholamban, a small protein that in its dephosphorylated state inhibits this calcium pump (Fig. 48–10). Reversal of this inhibition when phospholamban is phosphorylated by either protein kinase A or the calcium-calmodulin–activated protein kinase described earlier increases both the calcium sensitivity and the calcium turnover of the pump. The inhibition reappears when phospholamban is dephosphorylated by a phosphoprotein phosphatase. These reactions enable sympathetic stimulation to promote relaxation by accelerating calcium transport into the SR. Phosphorylation of phospholamban also increases myocardial contractility by favoring retention of activator calcium in intracellular stores at the expense of calcium efflux via the plasma membrane calcium pump and sodium-calcium exchange.

The physiologic importance of the ability of cAMP-dependent protein kinase to stimulate calcium transport into the cardiac SR is related to the powerful effect of sympathetic stimulation in increasing myocardial contractility, which is mediated by increased calcium entry through the plasma membrane calcium channels (dihydropyridine receptors). At the same time, sympathetic stimulation markedly increases heart rate and therefore shortens diastole. Together, these responses require that a greater amount of calcium be pumped back into the SR in a shorter time period to allow the ventricle to fill. This is accomplished

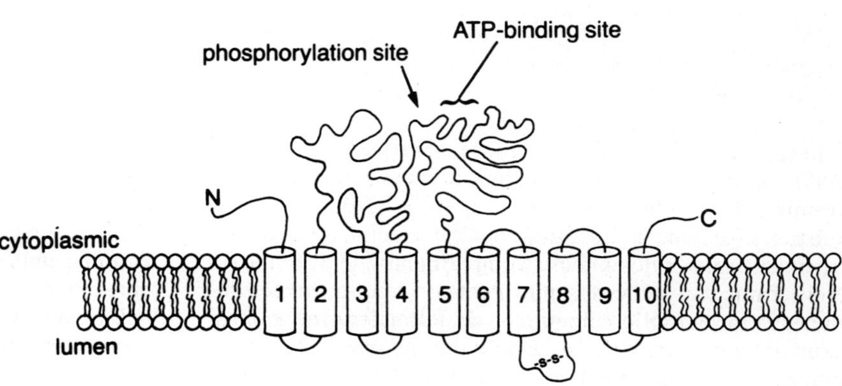

FIGURE 48–9 Depiction of the sarcoplasmic reticulum calcium pump ATPase, which contains 10 membrane-spanning helices (M1 through M10) and two large cytoplasmic loops. The latter forms the large projections of the protein shown in Figure 48–7.The sites for ATP binding and phosphorylation are in the large cytoplasmic loop between M4 and M5, whereas calcium binds to polar amino acids in the membrane-spanning helices, which participates in the actual transfer of calcium across the membrane bilayer. (From Katz AM: Physiology of the Heart. 2nd ed. New York: Raven, 1992.)

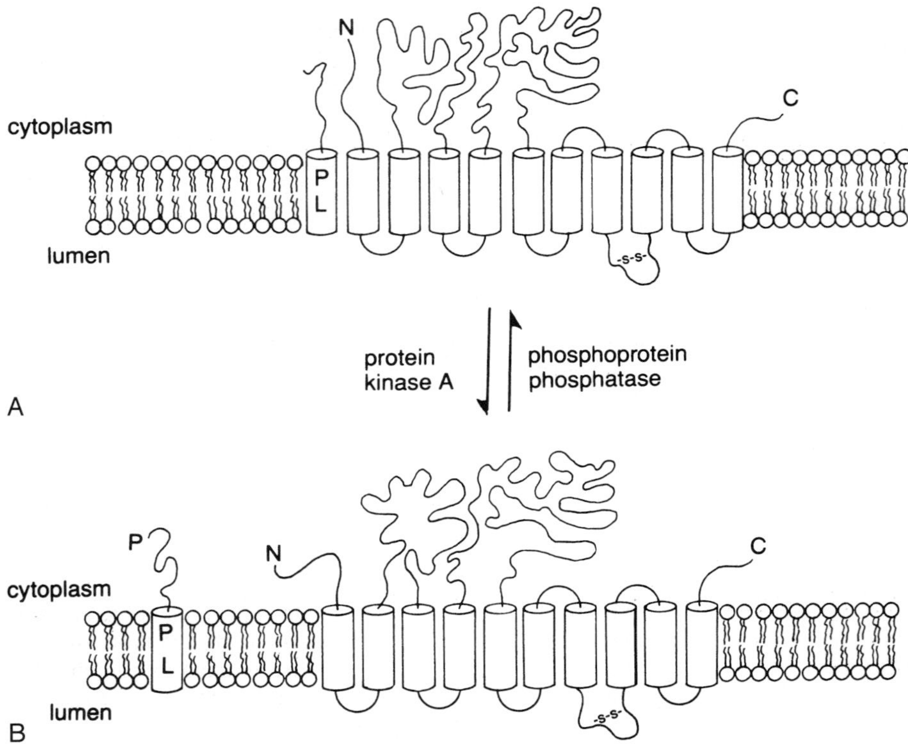

FIGURE 48–10 Schematic of the effects of phospholamban on the calcium pump of the cardiac sarcoplasmic reticulum. **A,** Phospholamban in the dephosphorylated form interacts with the calcium pump to decrease the calcium sensitivity of calcium transport and slow its turnover. **B,** These inhibitory effects are abolished when phospholamban is phosphorylated, which functionally dissociates this regulatory protein from the calcium pump. (**A** and **B,** From Katz AM: Physiology of the Heart. 2nd ed. New York: Raven, 1992.)

through two phosphorylation reactions: phospholamban phosphorylation, which increases both the rate and the calcium sensitivity of calcium transport into the cardiac SR, and troponin I phosphorylation, which decreases the calcium sensitivity of the heart's contractile proteins.

Calcium Retention Within the Sarcoplasmic Reticulum

Although much of the calcium taken up by the SR is stored as the free cation, some of the retained calcium is associated with calcium-binding proteins within this internal membrane system. Most important of the latter is calsequestrin, which traps calcium within the subsarcolemmal cisternae; this maintains a calcium store that can be readily released through the calcium-release channels that are also located in this region of the SR.

Overview of the Calcium Fluxes During Excitation-Contraction Coupling and Relaxation

This chapter has described excitation-contraction coupling and relaxation in terms of calcium movements among five compartments within the heart: extracellular space, SR, cytosol, troponin, and mitochondria (see Fig. 48–5). The calcium fluxes among these compartments, which initiate and terminate systole and play a major role in the regulation of myocardial contractility and filling, can be viewed as two distinct circulations of calcium: an external circulation across the plasma membrane and an internal circulation within the cell. As shown by the thicknesses of the arrows in Figure 48–5B, the amount of calcium that circulates within the cell during each cardiac cycle is much greater than that entering and leaving the cell.

The external circulation of calcium across the plasma membrane is described (see Fig. 48–5B) by the three arrows (A, B, and C). Calcium entry through the plasma membrane calcium channels (dihydropyridine receptors) (A) initiates calcium-triggered calcium release from the SR and makes a small contribution to calcium delivery to the contractile proteins (A_1). Although calcium can enter the cytosol via sodium-calcium exchange (B_1), this countertransport, like the plasma membrane calcium pump (B_2), serves mainly to transport calcium out of the cytosol. The internal circulation of calcium is described (see Fig. 48–5B) by the five arrows C, D, E, F, and G. Arrows C and D represent calcium fluxes across the SR membrane; arrow G describes the return of calcium from within the sarcotubular network to the subsarcolemmal cisternae. Arrows E and F describe the binding and dissociation of calcium from troponin C. The buffering role of the mitochondria is shown by the double arrow H.

A rough depiction of the energetics of the calcium fluxes involved in excitation-contraction is also provided in Fig. 48–5B. The downward arrows A and C represent the rapid passive calcium fluxes that are energized by diffusion, whereas rapid calcium binding to the contractile proteins (E) occurs when the cation becomes associated with high-affinity calcium-binding sites on troponin C. The corresponding uphill calcium fluxes, shown by arrows D and F, represent the much slower dissociation of calcium from troponin C and calcium uptake into the SR. Calcium return from the sarcotubular network to the subsarcolemmal cisternae occurs via diffusion; as the calcium concentration gradient within this membrane structure is small, arrow G is nearly horizontal. The two components of arrow H are also drawn nearly horizontal because the calcium concentration within the mitochondria, which plays little or no role in calcium fluxes in the normal heart, is normally low.

THE ENERGY-STARVED HEART

The consequences of cardiac energy depletion are of considerable importance in cardiology. In ischemic heart disease, oxidative energy production ceases within 1 minute after total coronary occlusion, and there is solid evidence that the failing heart is in an energy-starved state. The immediate consequences of impaired ATP production include slowed and incomplete relaxation, depressed contractility, and arrhythmias. Potential causes of these functional abnormalities include inadequate levels of ATP to provide the substrate for energy-consuming reactions, allosteric effects caused by a fall in ATP concentration, and reduced free energy of ATP hydrolysis (Table 48–3).

TABLE 48–3 **Possible Mechanisms by Which Energy Starvation Modifies Cardiac Function**

Lack of substrate ATP for energy-consuming reactions
Attenuation of allosteric effects of ATP
Reduced free energy of ATP hydrolysis

Abbreviation: ATP, adenosine triphosphate.

Inadequate Substrate Levels

Reduced ATP concentration could impair delivery of the high-energy phosphate needed to energize the many energy-consuming reactions involved in contraction, relaxation, and excitation-contraction coupling. However, normal ATP levels are very high, exceeding the ATP concentrations needed to saturate most substrate-binding sites by several orders of magnitude. Although it is not possible to determine precisely the ATP concentration (mol/L cytosol) in the normal heart, measurements of ATP content (mol/g tissue weight) are consistent with an "average" ATP concentration between 5 and 10 mM. Because the substrate-binding sites of most ATP-hydrolyzing systems are saturated at ATP concentrations below 1 μM, it is unlikely that this mechanism plays an important role in most clinical states of energy starvation, except in the dying heart.

Allosteric Effects

High ATP concentrations exert allosteric effects that accelerate ion pumps, ion exchangers, passive ion fluxes through membrane channels, and the interactions between the thick and thin filaments. These regulatory effects, which do not require hydrolysis of this nucleotide, therefore resemble those of a "lubricant." Allosteric effects of ATP accelerate the passive (downhill) calcium fluxes through calcium channels in the sarcolemma and sarcoplasmic reticulum, and so are inotropic. More important are the lusitropic effects, which stimulate active (uphill) transport of calcium out of the cytosol by calcium pump ATPases in the SR and plasma membrane and by the sodium-calcium exchanger. Perhaps the most important allosteric effect of ATP facilitates dissociation of actin and myosin during diastole, so attenuation of this "plasticizing effect" can allow even a modest decrease in ATP concentration to increase diastolic stiffness in an energy-starved heart. The Na^+, K^+-ATPase (sodium pump), which exchanges intracellular sodium for extracellular potassium, is also stimulated by an allosteric effect of ATP, so energy starvation causes plasma membrane depolarization by reducing intracellular potassium. This effect is arrhythmogenic because the lowered resting potential slows impulse conduction and so favors re-entry.

Reduced Free Energy of Adenosine Triphosphate Hydrolysis

Probably the most important consequences of energy starvation are caused by slowed rephosphorylation of ADP and accumulation of inorganic phosphate (P_i), both of which reduce the free energy made available through hydrolysis of the terminal (high-energy) phosphate bond of ATP. This free energy is proportional to the phosphorylation potential, which is defined as the ratio ATP/(ADP $\times$ P_i).

ADP levels in the normal heart are much lower than those of ATP, so even a relatively minor decrease in ATP content in an energy-starved heart causes a much greater rise in ADP levels. The resulting decrease in the ATP/ADP ratio reduces the free energy available for energy-consuming reactions, which can seriously impair the ability of ATP to power key cellular function. Because there is very little reserve in the phosphorylation potential of the heart, even a 15 to 25% reduction in this ratio can inhibit ATP-dependent reactions. The SR calcium pump is especially sensitive to reduced free energy release from ATP, which may explain why relaxation is more sensitive to energy starvation than is contraction.

REFERENCES

1. Katz AM: Congestive heart failure: role of altered myocardial cellular control. N Engl J Med 293:1187, 1975.
2. Katz AM: Physiology of the Heart. 2nd ed. New York: Raven, 1992.
3. Fozzard H, Haber E, Katz A, et al (eds): The Heart and Circulation. 2nd ed. New York: Raven Press, 1991.

SUGGESTED READINGS

OVERVIEW AND HEART FAILURE

Katz AM: Heart failure. Pathophysiology, molecular biology, clinical management. Philadelphia: Lippincott Williams & Wilkins, 2000.
Opie LH: The Heart. Physiology, from Cell to Circulation. Philadelphia: Lippincott-Raven, 1998.

THE CONTRACTILE PROTEINS

Huxley AF: Crossbridge tilting confirmed. Nature 375:631, 1995.
Schwartz K, de la Bastie K, Mercadier J-J, et al (ed): The biochemistry and molecular biology of the sarcomere. *In* Swynghedauw B (ed):

Cardiac Hypertrophy and Failure. pp. 105–135. London: John Libby, 1990.

Swynghedauw B: Developmental and functional adaptation of contractile proteins in cardiac and skeletal muscles. Physiol Rev 66:710, 1986.

Zot AS, Potter JD: Structural aspects of troponin-tropomyosin regulation of skeletal muscle contraction. Annu Rev Biophys Biophys Chem 16:535, 1987.

Excitation-Contraction Coupling

Bers DM: Excitation-Contraction Coupling and Cardiac Contractile Force. Dordrecht: Kluwer, 1991.

Blaustein MP, Lederer WJ: Sodium/calcium exchange: its physiological implications. Physiol Rev 79:763–854, 1999.

Carafoli E: Calcium pump of the plasma membrane. Physiol Rev 71:129, 1991.

Clapham DE: Calcium signaling. Cell 80:259, 1995.

Johnson RG Jr, Kranias EG: Cardiac sarcoplasmic reticulum function and regulation of contraction. Introduction. Ann N Y Acad Sci 853:xi–xvi, 1998.

Karmayzn M, Gan XT, Humphreys RA, et al: The myocardial Na^+/H^+ exchange. Structure, regulation, and its role in disease. Circ Res 85:777–786, 1999.

Katz AM: Calcium channel diversity in the cardiovascular system. J Am Coll Cardiol 28:522, 1996.

Langer GA (ed): The Myocardium. San Diego: Academic, 1997.

Sachs G (ed): Symposium on ion motive ATPases. Acta Physiol Scand 163(suppl 643), 1998.

The Energy-Starved Heart

Kammermeier H, Schmidt P, Jüngling E: Free energy change of ATP-hydrolysis: a causal factor of early hypoxic failure of the myocardium? J Mol Cell Cardiol 14:267, 1982.

Katz AM: Is the failing heart energy-depleted? Med Clin North Am 16:633, 1998.

Jacobus WE: Respiratory control and the integration of heart high-energy metabolism by mitochondrial creatine kinase. Annu Rev Physiol 47:707, 1985.

Tian R, Ingwall JS: Energetic basis for reduced contractile reserve in isolated rat hearts. Am J Physiol 270(Heart Circ Physiol 39):H1207, 1996.

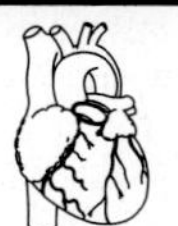

CHAPTER 49

Clinical Abnormalities of Cardiac Relaxation

Beverly H. Lorell

ANALYSIS OF CLINICAL DIASTOLIC DYSFUNCTION
LEFT VENTRICULAR RELAXATION
INTERACTION OF RELAXATION AND LOAD
INTERACTION OF RELAXATION AND EARLY DIASTOLIC FILLING
EXTRINSIC FACTORS THAT MODIFY DIASTOLIC FUNCTION
THE AGING HEART
THE ISCHEMIC HEART
THE HYPERTROPHIED HEART
DILATED CARDIOMYOPATHY
SUMMARY

Abnormalities of left ventricular (LV) relaxation are a major cause of the syndrome of congestive heart failure (CHF). The syndrome of CHF related to the elevation of left heart filling pressures can occur during predominant LV systolic dysfunction when the ventricle is presented with an excessive load during systolic ejection or when myocardial contractility is depressed due to myocardial cell loss or injury. CHF can also be due to predominant diastolic dysfunction when the left ventricle cannot fill with blood and maintain a normal low level of pressure during diastolic filling. When the resistance to LV filling is modest, the only hemodynamic manifestation may be the elevation of LV and pulmonary capillary pressures at rest or during stress. In this circumstance, the extent of diastolic filling and left ventricular fiber stretch (preload) is likely to be normal, such that stroke volume and cardiac output are preserved. However, because systolic and diastolic functions are closely coupled via the Frank-Starling relationship, severe impairment of LV relaxation and filling may affect the capability to adequately eject blood in systole. Thus, severe resistance of diastolic filling of the ventricle may directly lead to an incomplete extent of diastolic filling and the depression of stroke volume and cardiac output.

The recognition of predominant diastolic dysfunction is important because it is the predominant pathogenic mechanism in as many as 40 percent of patients with the clinical syndrome of CHF.[1, 2] Furthermore, the recognition of diastolic heart failure is critical for therapy because therapy that is directed toward the stimulation of ventricular ejection may be unhelpful or actually worsen pulmonary congestion. This chapter discusses the mechanisms that cause diastolic dysfunction, with an emphasis on the common conditions of aging, ischemia, and hypertrophy.

Analysis of Clinical Diastolic Dysfunction

In this discussion, we use a broad definition of diastole as the period of each cardiac cycle between aortic valve closure and mitral valve closure. Diastole can be divided into the periods of isovolumic relaxation between aortic valve closure and mitral valve opening, rapid early diastolic filling, diastasis (plateau phase of diastolic filling), and atrial contraction. Although isovolumic relaxation, early diastolic filling, and atrial transport are usually impaired in primary diastolic failure, these abnormalities are not the direct cause of pulmonary venous congestion, which occurs in response to the elevation of LV diastolic pressure and the secondary elevation of left atrial (LA) and pulmonary venous pressures. For this reason, it is helpful for the clinician to identify the hemodynamic cause of heart failure by examining the relationship between LV pressure and volume throughout the cardiac cycle.

In the normal left ventricle, the pressure at end systole just before mitral valve opening is usually 10 mm Hg or less in association with an end-systolic volume of about 12 to 18 ml/m^2. Immediately after mitral valve opening, the left atrium rapidly empties and the left ventricle rapidly fills, followed by a phase of much slower filling (diastasis) and the final contribution to ventricular filling by atrial contraction. At end diastole when the mitral valve closes, the LV diastolic pressure is 12 mm Hg or less in association with an end-diastolic volume of about 55 to 87 ml/m^2. The LV pressure-volume relationship is illustrated in Figure 49–1. Predominant diastolic failure can be recognized by an upward shift of the LV diastolic pressure-volume relationship in the presence of normal LV end-systolic (early diastolic) and end-diastolic volumes (see Fig. 49–1, *right*). In contrast, predominant systolic failure is characterized by the presence of an increase in LV end-systolic volume and a reduction in the extent of systolic emptying (stroke volume) (see Fig. 49–1, *left*). In this instance, LV end-diastolic pressure is elevated because LV end-diastolic volume is increased, and the diastolic portion of the pressure-volume curve has simply shifted upward and to the right. In this illustrative example, the level of the elevated LV end-diastolic pressure is comparable in the patient with systolic failure and the patient with diastolic failure. There have been many attempts to use mathematical models to quantify the curvilinear diastolic pressure-volume relationship,[3–5] including the calculation of LV chamber stiffness by defining

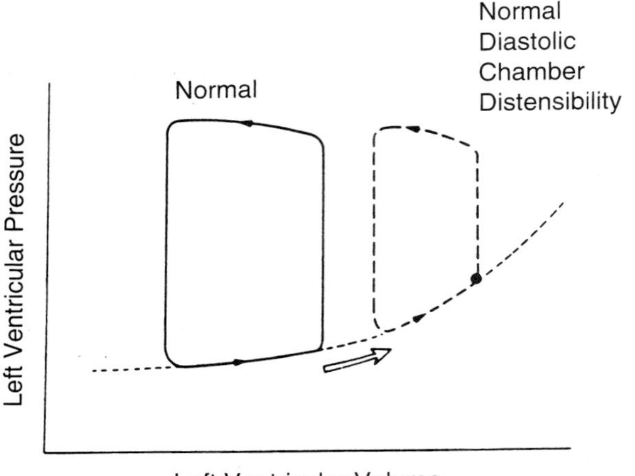

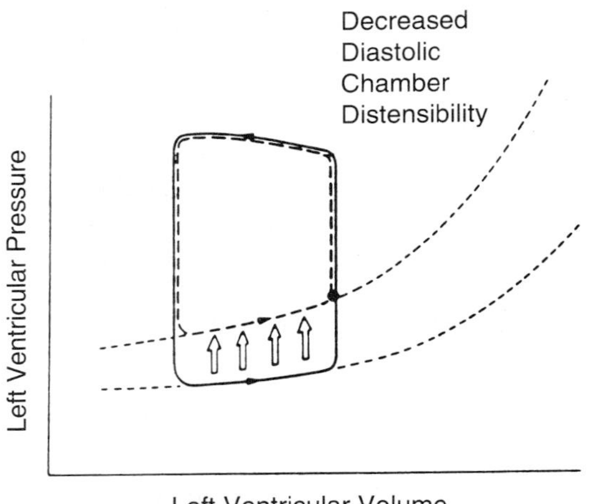

FIGURE 49–1 Left, Schematized left ventricular (LV) pressure-volume relation from a patient with primary systolic failure. A normal LV pressure-volume loop *(solid loop)* is shown on the left portion of the curve, whereas the transition to systolic failure *(dashed loop)* is shown on the right portion of the curve. Systolic dysfunction is manifest as an increase in LV end-systolic volume and as a reduction in the extent of ejection (stroke volume). Left ventricular end-diastolic pressure (LVEDP) is increased because LV volume is increased. The diastolic portion of the pressure-volume loop has simply shifted upward and to the right along the same diastolic pressure-volume relation *(arrow)*. No change in the distensibility of the left ventricle has occurred. **Right,** LV pressure-volume relation from a patient with primary diastolic failure *(dashed loop)*. The LVEDP is the same as that in the patient with primary systolic failure, as denoted by the *black circle* on the pressure-volume loops. Here, this is related to an upward shift of the LV diastolic pressure-volume relation *(arrows)*. This indicates a decrease in LV diastolic chamber distensibility such that a higher diastolic pressure is required to achieve the same diastolic volume. In this patient, no change in end-diastolic volume or systolic shortening has occurred. (Adapted from Lorell BH: Left ventricular diastolic pressure-volume relations: understanding and managing congestive heart failure. Heart Failure 4:206, 1988.)

the slope of a tangent of the diastolic pressure-volume relation (dP/dV). Because the diastolic pressure-volume relationship is highly curvilinear, the slope of this tangent varies throughout diastolic filling, and comparisons in the same patient or between patients must be made at a common ventricular volume and in the same portion of the filling curve. In the controlled experimental setting in normal animals, the diastolic pressure-volume curve can be tightly fitted to modified exponential models. However, in intact animals and in humans with diseased hearts, the actual diastolic pressure-volume points often deviate from an exponential fit. The term *myocardial stiffness* is used as an estimate of the resistance of the myofibrils themselves, rather than of the chamber, to passive stretch. The estimation of myocardial stiffness requires simultaneous measurements of LV pressure and wall thickness and the choice of a model of LV geometry to calculate the ventricular stress-strain relationship and its slope. Because of the complexity involved in the derivation of these indices, the need has arisen to describe the LV diastolic pressure-volume relationship in a way that is clinically understandable and useful in patient management. This has led to the use of the term *diastolic chamber distensibility* to describe the actual behavior of the diastolic pressure-volume relation in patients. Thus, a decrease in LV chamber distensibility describes an upward shift in the diastolic pressure-volume relationship and carries the meaning that LV diastolic pressure must be abnormally elevated to promote a normal diastolic volume. The concept of LV diastolic chamber distensibility includes the notion that almost-parallel upward shifts of the LV diastolic pressure-volume relationship can occur without major changes in slope. As is discussed later, such dynamic shifts in the diastolic pressure-volume relationship are characteristic of patients who experience severe and transient ischemia.

In clinical research studies performed in the cardiac catheterization laboratory, the LV diastolic pressure-volume relationship can be assessed by making simultaneous measurements of LV pressure with a high-fidelity micromanometer catheter and of LV volume with cine angiography at a fast frame rate with synchronized time markers. In the clinical research setting, synchronized measurements of high-fidelity LV pressure and LV volume estimated with echocardiography or radionuclide ventriculography at a fast acquisition speed can also be used. In clinical practice in the coronary care unit or catheterization suite, this precise technique is impractical. In everyday clinical practice, the LV diastolic pressure-volume relationship can be estimated by relating measurements of LV end-systolic (early diastolic) and end-diastolic volumes obtained with conventional echocardiography to measurements of LV end-systolic and end-diastolic pressures. (The phasic pulmonary capillary wedge pressure is a poor "surrogate" for LV diastolic pressure because of problems of pressure damping and poor frequency response that are characteristic of these catheters.) The measurements of LV pressure and volume must be made almost simultaneously. If severe mitral regurgitation is absent, the finding of clear-cut elevation of LV end-systolic (i.e., early diastolic) and end-diastolic pressures in the presence of normal end-systolic and end-diastolic volumes suggests that LV diastolic dysfunction is present.

LEFT VENTRICULAR RELAXATION

Patients do not complain of "abnormal cardiac relaxation," and clinicians cannot directly measure myofibrillar relaxation. As described later, there is indirect evidence that slowed rate and extent of myocardial relaxation are key factors that contribute to the elevation of LV diastolic pressure in common clinical disorders, such as ischemia and hypertrophy. In intact hearts, the time course of the fall of isovolumic LV pressure is assumed to reflect in part the process of myocardial relaxation (i.e., the dissociation of force-bearing myofibrillar crossbridges after systolic contraction to a basal level of crossbridge cycling and "tone"). In hemodynamic research studies, simultaneous measurements of high-fidelity LV pressure versus time are obtained at 2- to 5-millisecond intervals during the interval between aortic valve closure and mitral valve opening. These points are then fitted to an exponential function with a nonzero asymptote to derive the time constant, tau, of left ventricular relaxation.[6, 7] In the normal heart, there is an excellent fit of exponential models to actual data points of LV pressure decay, and the time course of LV pressure decay is nearly complete by mitral valve opening. In contrast, this approach has limitations in patients with diseased hearts because the time course of pressure decay often grossly deviates from an exponential fit and because the active process of LV relaxation may be very prolonged and may extend well beyond mitral valve opening. Even in the normal heart, an LV isovolumic pressure fall after certain interventions, such as extrasystoles, is not exponential.[7] Therefore, these factors limit efforts to obtain a simple single index of "LV relaxation" in patients. Nevertheless, abnormalities of the time course and extent of LV isovolumic pressure decay do provide some clues that the underlying process of myocardial relaxation is disturbed.

Isolated cardiac muscle experiments demonstrate that the process of myocardial relaxation is energy dependent and is modified by both cytosolic Ca^{2+} uptake and the magnitude and timing of load imposed on the muscle.[8] To achieve rapid and complete filling of the ventricle, systolic force development must be very rapidly inactivated after each contraction. The normal myocardium does not relax to a completely flaccid state but instead relaxes to a basal state of diastolic crossbridge cycling characterized by a basal level of heat production and energy use. Current models indicate that the control of excitation-contraction-relaxation coupling depends on the adenosine triphosphate (ATP)–dependent regulation of free cytosolic Ca^{2+}. After sarcolemmal depolarization, Ca^{2+} entry via the voltage-dependent slow channels triggers Ca^{2+} release from the intracellular storage site of the sarcoplasmic reticulum (SR), whose Ca^{2+} concentration is in the range of 100 to 700 μmol/L.[9, 10] Therefore, the movements of Ca^{2+} into the myocyte and from Ca^{2+} release channels in the SR into the cytosol are energy-favorable "downhill" fluxes, which result in an increase in cytosolic Ca^{2+} from basal diastolic concentration in the range of 0.1 to 0.2 μmol/L to systolic concentration in the range of 0.6 to 1.0 μmol/L. In late diastole, strong crossbridge formation between actin and myosin is blocked by the position of the regulatory protein tropomyosin on actin thin filaments. The increase in intracellular Ca^{2+} favors the binding of Ca^{2+} to the regulatory subunit troponin C (cTnC), which triggers a conformational change in the inhibitory regulatory protein cTnI that weakens its interaction with actin and tropomyosin. As this interaction is weakened, tropomyosin moves on the thin filament, causing a transition from weak to strong crossbridge attachment and cycling between adjacent actin sites and myosin heads of the thick filament.[11, 12] The crossbridge attachment between actin and myosin is cooperative, such that the initiation of attachment favors further crossbridge attachment, which is enhanced at high muscle loads and modified by regulatory proteins, including tropomyosin.

The termination of systolic force development and ongoing crossbridge cycling requires the rapid reduction of cytosolic Ca^{2+} to basal levels, which must occur via the ATP-dependent transport of Ca^{2} "uphill" against gradients between the cytosol and the SR and between the cytosol and the outside of the myocyte. The initial rapid fall of cytosolic Ca^{2+} is accomplished by the high-affinity and high-capacity system of the ATP-dependent SR pumps (SERCA-2). The process of restoring diastolic Ca^{2+} homeostasis is fragile because the passive process of Ca^{2+} entry down the Ca^{2+} concentration gradient is about 100,000 times more rapid than Ca^{2+} reuptake. Furthermore, optimum kinetics of SR Ca^{2+} uptake depend on the maintenance of a high level of ATP-dependent energy charge (free energy).[9, 13] Therefore, slight falls in energy charge slow Ca^{2+} removal, whereas when energy charge falls to critically low levels, SR Ca^{2+} transport becomes profoundly depressed and a conformational change occurs in the contractile proteins that promotes a latch state of ongoing crossbridge attachment. The function of the SR and the rate of both contraction and relaxation are also modified by the abundance and magnitude of phosphorylation of the SR regulatory protein phospholamban.[14] Developmentally, the duration of contraction is shorter and relaxation is faster in normal adult cardiac ventricular muscle than in neonatal muscle, and this appears to be directly related to enhanced SR Ca^{2+} uptake secondary to both increased expression of SR Ca^{2+}-ATPase pumps and phosphorylation state of phospholamban.[15]

There is a secondary slower phase of myocardial relaxation associated with the extrusion of the trigger Ca^{2+} that entered the cell during depolarization that depends on the low-affinity, high-capacity sarcolemmal Na^{+}-Ca^{2+} exchanger.[16] The directionality and magnitude of Ca^{2+} transport by the Na^{+}-Ca^{2+} exchanger are modified by the ATP-dependent regulation of the sarcolemmal Na^{+} gradient by the Na^{+}-K^{+} pump, membrane potential, and pH.[17] The contribution of the Na^{+}-Ca^{2+} exchanger to Ca^{2+} extrusion has been substantiated by recent experiments in transgenic animals,[18] and removal of Ca^{2+} by this exchanger relative to SR reuptake is more important in humans than in small mammals with very rapid resting heart rates, such as the rat.[19] The calmodulin-dependent Ca^{2+}-ATPase pump does not appear to contribute significantly to Ca^{2+} extrusion in normal adult cardiac myocytes.[20] Distinct from this sarcolemmal extrusion of Ca^{2+}, an additional mechanism that regulates diastolic properties has been identified. The diastolic stiffness of both muscle preparations and sarcomeres increases during diastole when intracellular Ca^{2+} is declining to very low levels and appears to involve an association between titin and the actin thin filament.[21]

Myocardial relaxation is also profoundly modified by changes in the Ca^{2+} sensitivity of the myofibers, such that a decrease in Ca^{2+} sensitivity usually promotes more rapid crossbridge detachment during diastole and enhances relaxation. Changes in regulatory proteins of the contractile apparatus modify the kinetics of both contraction and relaxation, but it is not yet known which regulatory proteins are dominant in either the normal or diseased heart. For example, the expression of excess skeletal relative to cardiac tropomyosin isoforms slows rates of both contraction and relaxation.[22] In addition, the increased expression of beta-myosin heavy chain isoform relative to alpha-myosin heavy chain isoform slows the rate of relaxation as well as the rate of force development.[23, 24] Myofibrillar Ca^{2+} sensitivity is decreased by mild intracellular acidification and the elevation of inorganic phosphate. Conversely, intracellular alkalosis, α-adrenergic stimulation, and increases in sarcomere length (fiber stretch) increase myofibrillar Ca^{2+} sensitivity and tend to slow relaxation. Studies show that myocardial relaxation is slowed by an increase in adenosine diphosphate (ADP) concentration, independent of ATP content, possibly by slowing of the rate of crossbridge detachment.[25]

Multiple pharmacologic interventions relevant to normal cardiac function as well as the therapy of patients with heart failure can modify this complex process of relaxation. For example, β-adrenergic stimulation increases cyclic adenosine monophosphate (cAMP), which decreases myofibrillar Ca^{2+} sensitivity and promotes phosphorylation of phospholamban, which stimulates SR Ca^{2+} reuptake. These lusitropic effects are offset by β-adrenergic stimulation of slow channel Ca^{2+} entry and tachycardia. In normal hearts, the net effect is an increase in both systolic force development, shortening of the duration of contraction, and the acceleration of relaxation. In the normal adult human heart, these effects of β-adrenergic stimulation contribute to the integrated exercise response, which is characterized by an increase in ejection fraction as well as an increase in relaxation rate, early diastolic filling, and the total amount of diastolic filling despite a shorter duration of diastole. Nitroglycerin, nitroprusside, and other nitric oxide donors have very different effects on contraction and relaxation and tend to promote a shorter duration of contraction and earlier onset of relaxation. These effects are observed in experimental muscle preparations[26] and have been clearly demonstrated in humans.[27] These actions appear to be related in part to the intracellular cyclic guanosine monophosphate signaling pathway and a secondary reduction in myofilament Ca^{2+} sensitivity caused by mild intracellular acidification.[28]

Interaction of Relaxation and Load

Myocardial relaxation is also modified by the magnitude and timing of a load imposed on cardiac muscle during the cycle of crossbridge cycling and detachment. Much of the insight into the effects of load is derived from the work of cardiac muscle physiologists, with more recent attempts to unravel the effects of load in the intact animal and human heart.[8, 29–31] In isolated cardiac muscles, the consequences of imposing a load differ when the load is imposed early during systolic contraction versus late in systole or during the transition from contraction to relaxation. In general, the imposition of an increased load early in systole delays the onset and prolongs the time course of relaxation. During the transition from contraction to relaxation in late systole, the imposition of an increased load tends to cause premature force decay, albeit at a slower rate. In contrast, the imposition of a load late in relaxation tends to accelerate relaxation, whereas the abrupt reduction of load late in relaxation tends to slow it. What are the effects of alterations of load in the intact heart in animal studies that may be relevant to patients? In general, moderate alterations in preload in the intact heart tend to have little effect on either the onset or the rate of relaxation. In contrast, augmentation of afterload by administration of arterial vasoconstrictors tends to delay the onset and prolong the time course of relaxation.[29–31]

Alterations in the time course of relaxation can modify both the diastolic pressure-volume relationship and the dynamics of early diastolic filling after mitral valve opening. After mitral valve opening, the rate of muscle lengthening depends on the rate and completeness of myofilament relaxation (residual crossbridge cycling) and on the load imposed by the increase in ventricular wall stress as a consequence of both ventricular filling and diastolic blood flow into the intramyocardial coronary vascular bed. In the normal heart, the increase in ventricular wall stress during early diastolic filling tends to accelerate crossbridge detachment during the final phase of active relaxation. Thus, an increase in the early diastolic filling load tends to accelerate relaxation, which can occur in the clinical situation of mitral regurgitation. Conversely, if the time course of relaxation itself is modestly prolonged, the early portion of the diastolic pressure-volume relationship is shifted up, with minimal effect on late diastole. If the extent of relaxation is incomplete, the early and late portions of the diastolic pressure-volume relationship would be expected to shift upward. As discussed later, this mechanism is believed to contribute to the striking upward shifts of the diastolic pressure-volume relationship that occur in patients who develop angina.

Interaction of Relaxation and Early Diastolic Filling

Because of conceptual and practical limitations in the assessment of LV relaxation in everyday practice in patients, it is common to study diastolic function by using noninvasive techniques to assess the dynamics of LV filling and infer underlying changes in isovolumic relaxation and the stiffness of the myocardium. In classic studies, Bonow and colleagues[32] and other investigators[33] developed the use of radionuclide angiography to obtain a time-activity curve of labeled red blood cells to describe several variables of diastolic filling, including

- The early diastolic peak filling rate
- The filling fraction during the early filling phase and atrial contraction
- The time interval from end systole to the time of peak early diastolic filling

In office practice and clinical investigation, Doppler echocardiographic techniques are more commonly used to assess *transmitral valve flow velocity curves,* which reflect left atrial emptying and diastolic filling, including (1) the phase of maximal acceleration of mitral inflow coinciding with the time of peak early diastolic filling (E-point), (2) the deceleration of initial mitral inflow, (3) the reacceleration of mitral flow during atrial contraction in end diastole

(A-point), and (4) the ratio of initial and late diastolic transmitral flow velocities (E/A ratio).[5, 34–37]

The major factors that modify early diastolic filling are now well understood. In the normal heart, LV pressure decay continues after mitral valve opening such that LV pressure reaches its lowest point just after the mitral valve opens and ventricular filling begins. This final fall of LV pressure to its lowest level in the cardiac cycle is due both to active myocardial relaxation and to cardiac restoring force, which is sometimes labeled as "diastolic suction."[38, 39] In the normal heart, vigorous systolic contraction of the heart to a volume below its equilibrium volume creates a measurable restoring force (diastolic suction) that contributes to the continued fall of LV pressure after mitral valve opening, promotes a downward shift of the early diastolic pressure-volume relationship, and accelerates early diastolic filling.[39] This critical period during which LV pressure is still rapidly falling during ventricular filling immediately after mitral valve opening has been labeled as the "relaxation filling period." The rate of initial LA emptying (measured by the transmitral flow velocity in early diastole) and early diastolic ventricular filling is directly determined by the pressure gradient across the mitral valve during this relaxation filling period in early diastole. This transmitral pressure gradient is determined by the LA pressure in early diastole and by the rate and magnitude of the rapid fall of LV pressure to its nadir in early diastole after mitral valve opening.

What are the effects of hemodynamic perturbations on early diastolic filling? In the normal heart, tachycardia has the complex effect of accelerating myocardial relaxation simultaneous with a decrease in LA pressure and shortening of the duration of the relaxation filling period. An abrupt increase in preload has minimal effect on relaxation rate but causes an increase in LA pressure, with the net effect of increasing early diastolic filling rate. In contrast, an abrupt increase in left ventricular and arterial pressure (afterload) tends to slow relaxation, lengthen the relaxation filling period, and increase left atrial pressure, such that there is minimal net change in the transmitral gradient and diastolic filling rate. The pattern of diastolic filling also modifies the diastolic filling curve due to viscoelastic forces. When ventricular filling occurs predominantly in early diastole, the decay of initial viscous forces promotes a lower diastolic pressure in mid and late diastole.[40]

In patients with diseased hearts, a depressed LV relaxation rate, which would itself cause slowed mitral valve flow and diastolic filling in early diastole, may be offset by the elevation of LA pressure, causing a "normal" or even accelerated rate of early ventricular filling. For these reasons, noninvasive filling indices suggestive of "diastolic failure" in individual patients must be interpreted cautiously with consideration of heart rate, an estimate of LA pressure and the transmitral pressure gradient in early diastole, and corroborative evidence of underlying heart disease. In a recent comprehensive review, Little and Downes[5] emphasized that three patterns of LV filling assessed with Doppler flow velocity curves generally indicate progressively worse diastolic dysfunction:

1. Reduced early diastolic filling with a compensatory increase in LA filling (decreased E/A ratio), suggesting slowed relaxation
2. "Pseudonormalization," with most filling in early diastole but a very rapid deceleration of early mitral flow
3. A "restrictive" pattern with nearly all filling occurring in very early diastole in association with a very short deceleration time

This pattern is often accompanied by the auscultatory finding of an S3 gallop and increased and prolonged left atrial regurgitant flow into the pulmonary veins. These patterns of mitral flow velocity and pulmonary flow velocity are illustrated in Figure 49–2. The duration of early filling deceleration is mainly determined by the stiffness (distensibility) of the left ventricle. Although these patterns can change in individual patients in response to changes in volume overload, a restrictive filling pattern with a short deceleration time predicts a poor prognosis.[35, 36] In healthy middle-aged adults, Doppler filling indices change during and immediately after exercise and must not be misinterpreted as diastolic dysfunction. For example, in normal healthy 50-year-old men and women, there is a decrease in the E/A ratio without a change in deceleration time that persists for 15 minutes after exercise in women and up to 1 hour in men.[41] In healthy subjects, Doppler filling indices after exercise are closely and independently related to filling indices at rest and heart rate. There is intense interest in the development of novel noninvasive techniques to assess ventricular wall dynamics, including M-mode color and tissue Doppler imaging[36, 42] and cine magnetic resonance imaging,[43] which may provide more complete information about regional and global diastolic function in both healthy adults and patients.

Normative data for the assessment of diastolic function in children, adolescents, and young adults are available and should be considered in the interpretation of Doppler flow velocity curves in young patients.[44, 45] Diastolic function also changes in normal human pregnancy, a natural state of volume overload; reference values are available.[46] In association with increases in heart rate, stroke volume, the reduction of systemic vascular resistance, and the increase in LV mass, women in their first trimester have an increase in early diastolic mitral flow velocity and shorter deceleration time, whereas during the second and third trimesters, the contribution of atrial contraction to ventricular filling progressively increases in association with an increase in pulmonary vein reverse flow velocity. These changes in diastolic filling indices rapidly reverse in the postpartum period, whereas LV mass regresses over several months.

Extrinsic Factors That Modify Diastolic Function

Factors extrinsic to the relaxation process of myofiber crossbridge detachment can also modify the diastolic pressure-volume relationship and the level of LV diastolic pressure in patients. Pericardial constraint is an important factor that modifies diastolic function via *ventricular interaction*, the process in which changes in ventricular contraction and volume modify function of the other ventricle.[47] The normal pericardium limits cardiac filling and distention of the heart and modifies the LV diastolic pressure-volume relation. This role of the pericardium is easily appreciated in

	E/A	E Decel Time	PVa>A Duration	PV S/D	PVa Velocity	IVRT
A. Normal—Young	>1	150–240 ms	No	S≈D	<25 cm/s	70–100 ms
—Old	<1.5		No	S>D	<25 cm/s	
B. Impaired or Delayed Relaxation	<1	>250 ms	Yes or No	S>>D	>25 cm/s	>100 ms
C. Pseudonormal: Abnormal Relaxation and Increased LA Pressure	1–1.5	150–240 ms	Yes	S<D	>25 cm/s	65–100 ms
D. Restrictive Filling Pattern: Stiff LV and Increased LA Pressure	>1.5	<150 ms	Yes	S<<D	>25 cm/s	<70 ms

A. B. C. D.

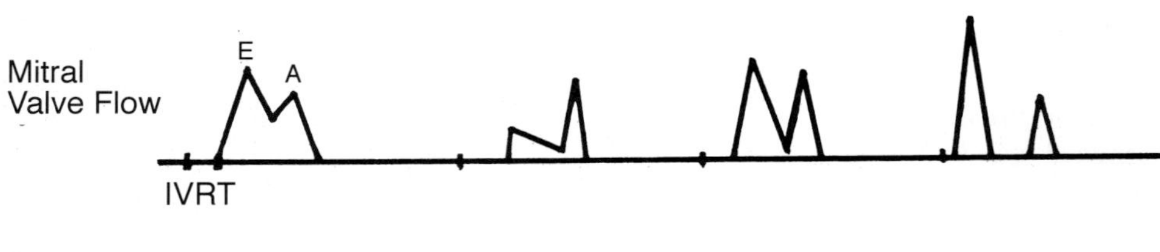

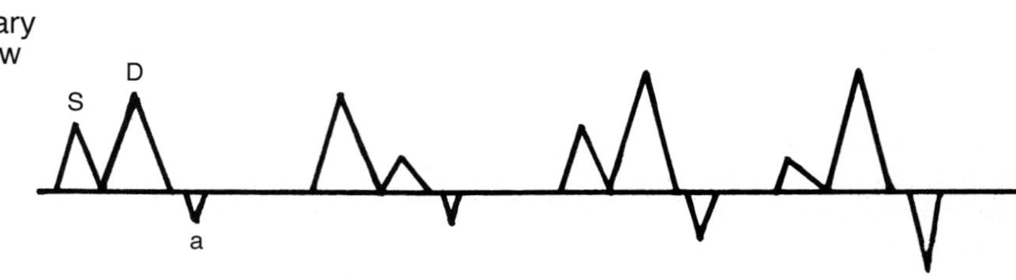

FIGURE 49–2 Echocardiographic Doppler assessment of left ventricular diastolic function. **Top,** Quantitative values of parameters used to assess diastolic function for each of the four types of filling patterns. In practice, not all variables may be measured, and there is often an overlap between categories. **Bottom,** Schematic flow velocity recordings corresponding to each of the four filling patterns. Mitral and pulmonary venous flows are temporarily aligned. A, late diastolic flow; D, diastolic component of pulmonary venous flow; E, early diastolic flow; E Decel, E deceleration; IVRT, isovolumic relaxation time; PVa, pulmonary venous a wave; and S, systolic component of pulmonary venous flow. (Courtesy of Pamela S. Douglas, M.D.)

constrictive pericarditis, in which an abnormally stiff and thick pericardium causes the elevation and equilibration of diastolic pressures in the right and left ventricles. In the presence of a normal pericardium, acute changes in total intrapericardial volume cause an upward shift of the diastolic pressure-volume relationship. This effect of pericardial constraint on ventricular interaction is particularly important when the right ventricle is distended with elevated RV diastolic pressure. In the presence of an intact pericardium, ventricular interaction is minimal when RV diastolic pressure is between 0 and 5 mm Hg; however, when RV diastolic pressure increases from 10 to 15 mm Hg, ventricular coupling is present and changes in RV diastolic pressure increase LV diastolic pressure and constrain its filling.[48] This effect is less but still present if RV diastolic pressure is elevated when the pericardium is opened due to septum-mediated interaction. Pericardial constraint and ventricular interaction account in large part for the ability of vasodilator drugs to reduce intracardiac filling pressures in patients with heart failure. Classic hemodynamic studies demonstrated that nitroprusside and nitroglycerin, which cause systemic venodilatation, promote a downward shift in the diastolic pressure-volume relationship by reducing RV distention and pericardial constraint pressure, and this effect is minimal when the pericardium is absent.[49, 50] Pericardial constraint associated with RV distention appears to mediate the striking upward shifts in RV and LV filling pressures during acute RV infarction[51] and during the development of acute mitral regurgitation.[52] In patients with advanced heart failure, diastolic ventricular interaction is important and often unrecognized. In these patients, Atherton and colleagues[53] showed that abrupt reductions in RV volume and diastolic pressure cause acute increases in LV diastolic filling and volume; in some patients, this abrupt increase in LV filling is sufficient to stimulate baroreceptor activity and promote systemic vasodilation.

Changes in the geometry and structural composition of the ventricular wall also change diastolic function.[54, 55] Both the quantity and characteristics of collagen deposition modify the development of diastolic heart failure.[55–57] Correlative studies of hemodynamic data and histologic analyses of myocardial biopsy samples in patients suggest that the extent of myocardial fibrosis correlates closely with indices of myocardial stiffness once the relative amount of fibrous tissue exceeds about 20 percent.[57] Other rare conditions that produce interstitial infiltrates and displace normal myocytes also give rise to elevation of diastolic pressure and severe impairment of ventricular filling, including cardiac amyloidosis, hemosiderosis, glycogen storage diseases, and Fabry's disease. Dynamic physiologic changes in the geometry and matrix structure of the ventricular wall also influence diastolic function. *Coronary turgor*, the degree of engorgement and pressurization of the coronary vasculature, influences the distensibility of the left ventricle. During diastole, the engorgement of the coronary vascular bed accounts for about 10 to 25 percent of the thickness of the LV wall, and experimental animals studies have shown that increments in coronary flow and pressure cause an upward shift in the diastolic pressure-volume relationship.[58] It is not known whether coronary turgor plays an important role in the regional or global diastolic behavior of the left ventricle in patients. There is good evidence that myocardial edema, which can occur during conditions such as hypoproteinemia, promotes diastolic dysfunction evident as slowing of LV isovolumic relaxation and the elevation of the diastolic pressure-volume relationship.[59]

Effects of Aging on Diastolic Function

The effect of aging on diastolic function in otherwise healthy adults is controversial, and a consideration of aging is critically important in the clinical assessment of diastolic dysfunction as a potential cause of the symptoms of dyspnea and exercise intolerance in the individual elderly patient. Studies of human atrial (not ventricular) trabeculae obtained from patients of 45 to 75 years old who are undergoing bypass surgery suggest that the ratio of SERCA-2 to phospholamban is decreased in senescent muscle.[60] In functional studies of these muscles, there was no age-related difference in basal measurements of force development and relaxation, whereas these indices were more abnormal during the stress of ischemia and reperfusion in senescent compared with young muscles.[60] These observations might lead to the speculation that aging in normal adults is associated with pathologic changes in gene expression that beget impaired myocardial relaxation. However, recent invasive hemodynamic measurements in normal subjects from 20 to 77 years old suggest that in the absence of coronary disease, systemic hypertension, or hypertrophy, LV isovolumic relaxation remains unchanged, at least until the eighth decade.[61] In contrast, LV filling rates decline with aging both at rest and during exercise in healthy conditioned adults from 20 to 90 years old, and filling rates are predictive of submaximal and maximal oxygen consumption during exercise.[62] Doppler mitral flow velocity studies also demonstrate that age and heart rate are independently associated with parameters of LV diastolic filling in healthy nonathletic adults, and there is a weaker but persistent association of age and diastolic function in patients with heart failure.[63]

Characterization of diastolic function in the elderly is confounded by the high prevalence of both hypertension and hypertrophy in otherwise healthy and asymptomatic aging adults. Diastolic function was analyzed with Doppler echocardiography in 2239 men and 2962 women in the multicenter Cardiovascular Health Study of community-dwelling elderly people.[64] Early diastolic peak filling velocity decreased and late diastolic (atrial) peak filling velocity increased with age by multivariate analysis, distinct from the separate variables of gender, heart rate, and blood pressure. Early and late filling velocities both increased with elevation of systolic blood pressure and decreased with increases in diastolic blood pressure. The subset of patients with hypertension had the lowest early-to-late diastolic peak velocity ratio, suggestive of an abnormal relaxation pattern, whereas the patient subset with heart failure had the highest ratio, suggestive of a "restrictive" filling pattern indicative of high LA pressure and a high left atrium–to–left ventricle early diastolic pressure gradient. In ambulatory hypertensive patients between 50 to 80 years old, Zabalgoitia and associates[65] reported that the predominant mitral flow pattern in older hypertensive people is the "impaired relaxation" pattern (reduced E/A peak flow velocity ratio and prominent A wave), which increases in prevalence with age, occurring in 89 percent of men and 91 percent of asymptomatic hypertensive patients older than 65 years. In this setting, systolic function indices tend to be preserved. In contrast, the frequency of a "restrictive" pattern of diastolic filling is extremely low (<1 percent) in ambulatory asymptomatic hypertensive older patients. In ambulatory older hypertensive patients without heart failure symptoms, hypertrophy is present in about 65 percent, but the prevalence of normal, impaired relaxation, and restrictive filling patterns does not differ in the presence or absence of LV hypertrophy (20, 79.5, and 0.5 percent versus 24, 75.5, and 0.5 percent).[66]

Thus, in *individual* elderly patients, a Doppler filling pattern of "impaired relaxation" may not distinguish pathologic changes of diastolic function due to pressure overload from the process of aging itself. These human studies also clearly show that diastolic filling indices cannot be used in isolation as the basis of a diagnosis of "diastolic heart failure" in the individual patient with the symptom of dyspnea or exercise intolerance. In healthy older adults as well as young people, LV diastolic function can be modified by exercise training. Spina and colleagues[67] found that men older than 65 years who underwent several months of aerobic exercise training showed a striking increase in exercise capacity related to an increase in systolic contractile function indices as well as enhanced early diastolic filling normalized for heart rate; importantly, these benefits were abolished with acute β-adrenergic blockade, which suggests an underlying mechanism of enhanced responsiveness to catecholamines.[67] These data support the speculation that the reduction in early diastolic filling velocity and increased dependence on atrial transport that occur in otherwise healthy aging adults may be predominantly related to complex changes in β-adrenergic signaling that accompany senescence.[68]

Effects of Ischemia on Diastolic Function

The process of myocardial relaxation is energy dependent; therefore, myocardial ischemia can impair the rate and extent of relaxation and can cause both the slowing of early diastolic filling and an upward shift in the diastolic pressure-volume relationship. In patients with coronary artery disease, the development of transient ischemia can cause abrupt and reversible increases in LV diastolic and pulmonary venous pressures via this mechanism. There are major differences in the effects of global no-flow ischemia (*supply ischemia*) versus severe low-flow ischemia associated with continued cardiac work (*demand ischemia*). In isolated beating hearts, studies performed a decade ago with intracellular Ca^{2+} probes and nuclear magnetic resonance (NMR) spectroscopy support the hypothesis that ischemia is associated with a prompt increase in cytosolic diastolic Ca^{2+} levels.[69–71] However, paradoxically, despite the increase in cytosolic Ca^{2+}, the imposition of abrupt global no-flow ischemia is associated with the cessation of contractile function within a few minutes and with an immediate *fall* in LV diastolic pressure and a downward shift of the diastolic pressure-volume relationship.[72] In hearts with global low-flow ischemia, resting diastolic pressure does not increase until after a delay of about 10 to 15 minutes. In this setting, it appears that initial effects of an increase in intracellular Ca^{2+} on diastolic pressure are offset by the loss of coronary turgor as well as the accumulation of intracellular protons and inorganic phosphate, which reduce myofiber Ca^{2+} sensitivity. The delayed and gradual increase in resting diastolic tone appears to be related to an increase in myofilament Ca^{2+} sensitivity as ATP levels fall and ADP levels rise, whereas prolonged ischemia results in the development of rigor and a "latch" state caused by the fall of ATP to critically low levels. In contrast, acute and reversible *demand ischemia* causes increases in diastolic pressure and slowing of relaxation, which can be demonstrated in both experimental animal models and patients who experience angina during transient ischemia in response to the stress of exercise or tachycardia in the presence of a preserved but reduced level of coronary flow. In isolated beating hearts exposed to global low-flow ischemia, systolic contractile function immediately decreases to a lower but preserved level of function, whereas diastolic pressure shows a delayed but gradual rise that is in part reversible.[73, 74] Notably, the imposition of tachycardia during global low-flow ischemia causes an immediate and reversible upward shift of diastolic pressure relative to volume.[74] During demand ischemia, the precarious state of diastolic Ca^{2+} homeostasis is likely to be exacerbated by tachycardia which promotes Ca^{2+} entry both via the slow channel and via Na^+-Ca^{2+} exchange. In support of this notion, inhibition of the Na^+-K^+ pump with ouabain strikingly worsens the upward shift of the diastolic pressure-volume relationship during global low-flow ischemia, whereas equi-inotropic levels of isoproterenol do not have this effect.[75] Drugs such as lidocaine, which affect Na^+-Ca^{2+} exchange, also dramatically aggravate diastolic dysfunction and aggravate the upward shift of the diastolic pressure-volume relation during demand ischemia.[76] The ATP produced by anaerobic glycolysis in the cytosol contributes to the preservation of diastolic function during low-flow ischemia, and the stimulation of glycolytic ATP production appears to protect against the ischemic depression of myocardial relaxation.[77, 78]

The effects of transient ischemia on diastolic function in humans have been elucidated in classic studies of patients with coronary artery disease undergoing cardiac catheterization in whom angina pectoris was induced by exercise or pacing tachycardia.[79–82] Such studies have demonstrated that demand ischemia results in an abrupt and reversible increase in LV diastolic pressure that is related to the prolongation of isovolumic LV relaxation (time constant τ) and an upward shift of the diastolic pressure-volume relation. As shown in Figure 49–3, which illustrates changes in the diastolic pressure-volume relation during pacing tachycardia and during transient coronary occlusion with an angioplasty balloon, these ischemic changes in diastolic function can occur in the presence of variable degrees of depression of LV systolic function, and global LV ejection fraction may be preserved. The magnitude of the acute depression of diastolic function, as well as the degree of depression of ejection fraction, is related to the extent of the ischemic territory and the duration of ischemia. The importance of heterogeneity of the diastolic function of ischemic and nonischemic regions has been shown in several clinical studies. Sasayama and coworkers[81] have elegantly shown that pacing-induced angina in patients causes an upward shift of the pressure-segment length relations of ischemic regions, whereas the overall increase in LV diastolic chamber pressure causes the nonischemic regions to "slide upward and to the right" on a higher portion of their baseline pressure-segment length relations. Pouleur and associates[82] showed that demand ischemia profoundly depresses diastolic relaxation in ischemic regions compared with nonischemic segments in patients with demand ischemia, and Bonow[83] identified the importance of diastolic heterogeneity with the use of radionuclide ventriculography techniques.

The comparative effects of regional pacing-induced ischemia and balloon coronary occlusion on LV diastolic function have also been studied.[84–86] In patients with one-vessel left anterior descending coronary artery disease, the upward shift in the global LV diastolic pressure-volume relation is more pronounced in response to pacing-induced ischemia than in response to transient balloon occlusion of the left coronary artery (see Fig. 49–3).[84] Furthermore, global LV ejection fraction is usually well preserved during pacing-induced angina but decreases substantially during transient balloon occlusion. Regionally, pacing-induced demand ischemia causes a marked upward shift of the pressure-segment length relationship that correlates with the presence of persistent systolic shortening, whereas balloon occlusion tends to cause a rightward shift of the pressure-segment length relationship (indicative of passive diastolic distention) associated with profound depression of systolic segmental shortening or frank systolic bulging. Comparative studies of changes in cardiac metabolism during pacing-induced ischemia and balloon occlusion show that washout of protons is maintained during pacing-induced ischemia, whereas regional accumulation of protons and myocardial acidosis occurs during balloon occlusion.[85] This transient tissue acidosis reduces myofilament Ca^{2+} sensitivity, which contributes to the large depression of systolic function and attenuates the rise in LV diastolic pressure that occurs during transient balloon occlusion in comparison with demand ischemia. The comparative effects of transient regional demand ischemia versus coronary occlusion on Doppler filling indices have not been as well studied. Solomon and associates[87] examined transmitral flow velocity patterns during regional ischemia caused by transient coronary occlusion and showed that regional is-

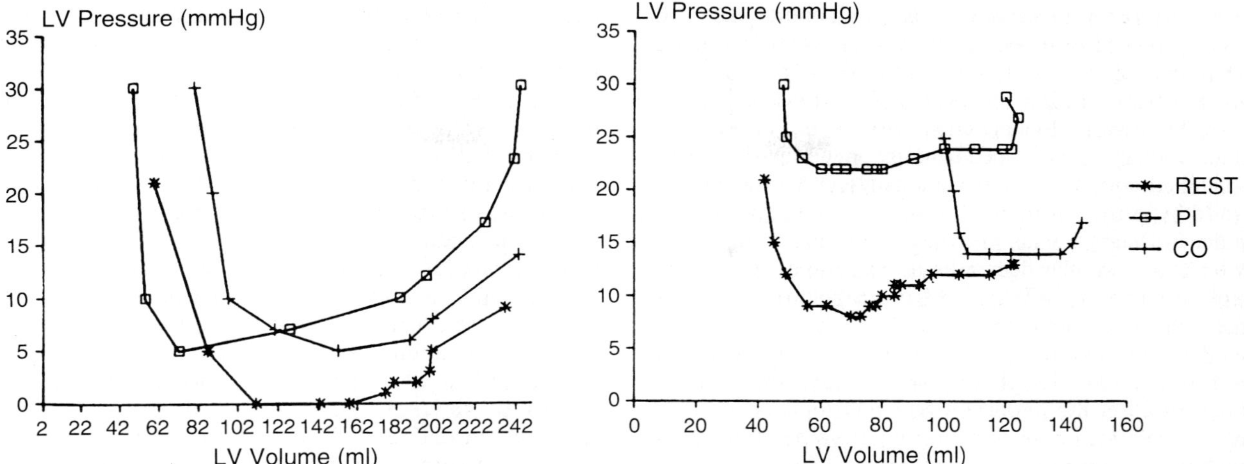

FIGURE 49–3 Diastolic left ventricular (LV) pressure-volume relations at rest, during pacing-induced ischemia (PI), and at the end of angioplasty balloon coronary occlusion (CO) in two different patients with left anterior coronary artery disease, representing the extremes of responses to coronary occlusion. **Left,** In this patient, systolic shortening was preserved at the end of coronary occlusion. Both pacing-induced ischemia and coronary occlusion caused the diastolic LV pressure-volume relation to shift upward. **Right,** In this patient, the ejection fraction was greatly reduced at the end of transient coronary occlusion compared with the rest baseline. Note that the diastolic LV pressure-volume relation during pacing-induced ischemia was shifted upward; in contrast, the relation at the end of coronary occlusion was shifted to the right and superimposable on the terminal portion of diastolic LV pressure-volume relation at rest. (Adapted from Bronzwaer JGF, de Bruyne B, Ascoop CAPL, Paulus WJ: Comparative effects of pacing-induced and balloon coronary occlusion ischemia on left ventricular diastolic function in man. Circulation 84:211, 1991.)

chemia modified two determinants of early diastolic filling: relaxation, which slowed, and LV chamber stiffness, which increased. These changes were associated with a depression of early transmitral flow that was shorter in duration and a minimal change in late diastolic flow; notably, increases in heart rate tended to accelerate relaxation and to mask these effects on early diastolic filling.

In acute myocardial infarction, extensive study of patients during cardiac catheterization has shown that the elevation of LV diastolic pressure (or its surrogate, pulmonary capillary wedge pressure) is common and expected. In this setting, mechanisms of the elevation of diastolic pressure are multiple and include ischemic depression of relaxation, an upward shift of the diastolic pressure-volume relationship, acute volume overload, and ischemic papillary muscle dysfunction causing acute mitral regurgitation. Acute coronary reperfusion by angioplasty is well recognized to be associated with delayed recovery of systolic function of viable myocardium, but it is less well understood if "diastolic stunning" occurs or if its mechanism or time course is similar to systolic myocardial stunning. Importantly, Doppler indices of diastolic function early after reperfused myocardial infarction appear to predict adverse LV remodeling. Cerisano and colleagues[88] studied such patients at 3 days and then 6 months after reperfused anterior infarction and showed through multiple regression analysis that a "restrictive filling pattern" and an abnormally short mitral deceleration time are highly predictive of late remodeling with LV volume expansion.

In summary, transient demand ischemia in the presence of restricted but preserved coronary flow is a major cause of severe and reversible depression of relaxation and the elevation of diastolic pressure. During exercise testing, the development of transient diastolic dysfunction during demand ischemia is supported by the development of transient rales, the appearance of a "restrictive pattern" of diastolic flow velocity signals detected by Doppler, or the transient appearance of thallium in the lungs during the immediate postexercise scan. The role of ischemia and occult coronary artery disease should always be rigorously evaluated in patients who present with "unexplained" episodes of congestive heart failure despite the presence of normal heart size and LV ejection fraction on baseline noninvasive imaging studies.

DIASTOLIC FUNCTION AND THE HYPERTROPHIED HEART

LV hypertrophy is characterized by the elevation of LV diastolic pressure in the presence of normal or small ventricular chamber size and well-preserved systolic contractile function. In response to chronic pressure overload due to hypertension or aortic stenosis, the LV remodels in the geometric pattern of *concentric hypertrophy,* in which there is an increase in wall thickness relative to cavity size associated with multiple changes in LV gene expression that recapitulate an immature fetal pattern. Taken together, these complex and coordinated changes in gene expression initially preserve normal systolic wall stress via geometric remodeling and preserve the magnitude of systolic shortening (ejection fraction) and force development, albeit at a slower rate, at a favorable myothermal economy.[89]

The pattern of hypertrophic remodeling appears to be influenced by the stimulus for hypertrophy as well as gender. Diastolic function has been well studied in young adult athletes. Moderate hypertrophy, characterized by an increase in LV diastolic chamber dimension with an increase in wall thickness that results in a normal or increased mass-to-volume ratio, is common in athletes and is likely to be an adaptation to an intermittent high output state.[90] In athletes with mild-to-moderate hypertrophy, there usually is no evidence of altered systolic contractile properties or Doppler diastolic filling indices.[90] A functional and metabolic evaluation of athlete cyclists with the use of magnetic resonance imaging and spectroscopy in comparison with age-matched normal subjects demonstrated that the athletes had mild hypertrophy but no differences in ejection fraction or indices of early versus late diastolic filling, and the two groups showed similar decreases in the ratio of myocardial phosphocreatine to ATP (reflecting myocardial energy charge) during dobutamine stress.[91]

Gender also modifies the evolution of pressure-overload hypertrophy. In hypertrophy due to hypertension or valvular heart disease, the evolution of hypertrophy appears to differ in older men and women. Older women with pressure-overload hypertrophy tend to have smaller LV systolic dimensions, thicker LV walls (more concentric remodeling), higher endocardial and midwall fractional shortening, and lower end-systolic wall stress compared with men, whereas both men and women tend to have a filling pattern of "impaired relaxation."[65] In hypertensive patients, LV mass and Doppler peak mitral inflow velocity are highly predictive of exercise capacity (peak oxygen consumption and workload) in men but not in women, suggesting gender-based differences in the contribution of diastolic filling to exercise capacity.[92] In an experimental model of aortic stenosis, Douglas and associates[93] demonstrated gender differences in the response to pressure overload and both systolic and diastolic functions.[93] Despite similar extent of hypertrophy, male, but not female, animals showed an early transition to failure characterized by LV dilatation and loss of concentric remodeling, elevated systolic wall stress, and more severe change in the deceleration of rapid diastolic filling. Recent studies in this model suggest that these gender-related functional differences are associated with the better preservation of a normal adult pattern of LV gene expression in females.[94]

Although multiple changes in gene expression occur in pressure overload, the most extensively studied molecular switches that are postulated to modify contractile function are the down-regulation of SERCA-2, which modifies the capacity for SR Ca^{2+} uptake, and the increased expression of β-myosin heavy chain isoenzyme relative to α-myosin heavy chain isoenzyme, which results in a slower myosin ATPase rate. These changes in gene expression have been observed in multiple animal models of pressure overload,[95–98] whereas the expression of these genes in human pressure-overload hypertrophy in the *absence* of heart failure has not been as well studied. In pressure-overload hypertrophy, the reduction in SERCA-2 pumps may favor prolonged availability of Ca^{2+} to activate the crossbridge cycling in systole and thus facilitate systolic force generation against an increased load. In diastole, the reduction in SERCA-2 expression and protein levels has been postulated to invariably lead to severe prolongation of relaxation and elevation of diastolic Ca^{2+} levels in hypertrophied muscle.[99] Studies in rat models of pressure-overload hypertrophy demonstrate that the down-regulation of SERCA-2 often does not occur in early adaptive hypertrophy, but it is a marker of later progression to early failure.[98, 100] In addition, studies of rat models of pressure-overload hypertrophy demonstrate that changes in diastolic relaxation in vivo and in isolated myocytes can be dissociated from levels of SERCA-2 message and protein.[100, 101] McCall and colleagues[101] studied Ca^{2+} fluxes in hypertrophied adult myocytes from aortic-banded rats with down-regulation of SERCA-2; despite a reduction in myocyte shortening amplitude, the SR Ca^{2+} content and rate of Ca^{2+} decline in diastole due to SR uptake were similar in hypertrophied and normal cells. However, the "gain" of fractional SR Ca^{2+} release due to the trigger Ca^{2+} that enters during depolarization was reduced. These results suggest that factors other than SERCA-2 down-regulation may contribute to subtle alterations in myocardial contraction and relaxation observed in compensated hypertrophy before the onset of heart failure.[100]

The upregulation of β-myosin heavy chain isoform is observed in both early and late hypertrophy and may contribute more than previously recognized to slowed relaxation in both compensated and decompensated hypertrophy. The kinetics of relaxation and the rate of crossbridge detachment are much slower in myocardium expressing predominantly β-myosin heavy chain in comparison with α-myosin heavy chain.[23, 24] Cardiac hypertrophy is also associated with complex changes in gene expression that modify energy reserve, including a depressed capacity of the creatine kinase system, a "stress" pathway that serves to rapidly regenerate ATP during rapid ATP turnover and to "buffer" and maintain ADP at low levels critical for normal crossbridge dissociation.[13, 102, 103] Tian and associates[103] showed a close association between intracellular ADP concentration and impaired relaxation in hypertrophied hearts and suggested that decreased energy reserve via the creatine kinase reaction may contribute to abnormal diastolic function in hypertrophied hearts. In support of a role of altered myocardial energetics in diastolic dysfunction in hypertrophy, NMR spectroscopy studies in patients with hypertensive hypertrophy and normal systolic function in comparison with normal subjects demonstrated that human LV hypertrophy is associated with depressed myocardial phosphocreatine/ATP ratios both at rest and during stress, and these energetic abnormalities are associated with abnormal early deceleration.[104]

Other mechanisms contribute to slowed relaxation and abnormal diastolic chamber distensibility in hypertrophied hearts, including altered passive distensibility properties of the thick chamber wall and changes in the type and amount of collagen deposition.[56, 57, 105] Increases in myocardial stiffness in hypertrophied hearts appear to be related to enhanced collagen cross-linking in addition to changes in total collagen or the proportion of type I to type II collagen.[105] Serial studies in patients with aortic stenosis before and after valve replacement have greatly enhanced our understanding of the relative contributions of myocyte hypertrophy and collagen deposition to diastolic dysfunction in patients with pressure-overload hypertrophy.[106] Early after load reduction by aortic valve replacement (22 months), LV mass decreased by about 35 percent, and LV relaxation, which was prolonged before surgery, improved. However, diastolic myocardial stiffness increased secondary to an increase in the proportion of collagen in the myocardium. Late after load reduction (~80 months), both diastolic stiffness and relaxation were normalized due to regression in both myocardial hypertrophy and fibrosis. These extraordinary data clearly show that normalization of diastolic function occurs after the relief of pressure overload and that it depends on both the regression of hypertrophy and the slower regression of fibrosis. In rare patients with acromegaly, cardiac hypertrophy develops in association with growth hormone and insulin growth factor I hypersecretion. Even in the absence of hypertension or depression of ejection fraction, acromegaly in young adults is associated with increased LV mass, prolonged isovolumic relaxation time, and reduced early diastolic mitral flow velocity in comparison with age-matched control subjects.[107, 108] These findings argue for a direct relationship between growth hormone and insulin growth factor I and cardiac hypertrophy with associated diastolic dysfunction independent of hypertension.

Abnormalities of slowed LV isovolumic relaxation, slowed early diastolic ventricular filling, and the elevation of LV diastolic pressure relative to a normal LV diastolic volume are common in patients with hypertrophic cardiomyopathy[109] and most patients with adaptive pressure-overload hypertrophy due to aortic stenosis or systemic hypertension.[92, 106, 110–114] In these patients, the impairment of diastolic function does not depend on the presence of coexisting depression of ejection fraction and occurs in both adults and children compared with age-matched control subjects.[115, 116] More subtle abnormalities of systolic function, including depressed LV midwall shortening, may be present in patients with hypertrophy and normal ejection fraction, and depressed LV midwall shortening is predictive of LV diastolic abnormalities of early diastolic filling.[117] There is a high prevalence of concentric hypertrophy in patients with isolated systolic hypertension,[118] and early diastolic filling abnormalities, including a Doppler filling pattern of "impaired relaxation," are present in more than 80 percent of older hypertensive patients.[65, 66] Diastolic dysfunction with a preserved LV ejection fraction is the underlying cause of episodic congestive heart failure in elderly patients with hypertension-induced chronic hypertrophy, an entity often called *hypertensive hypertrophic cardiomyopathy.*[119] In patients with slowed relaxation and reduced early diastolic filling, the ability of the ventricle to fill rapidly in diastole is impaired, which results in an increased dependence on the contribution of atrial contraction to filling of the stiff left ventricle. For this reason, the conversion from normal sinus rhythm to atrial fibrillation is commonly associated with clinical deterioration. In patients with cardiac hypertrophy and new-onset atrial fibrillation, efforts should be made to restore and maintain normal sinus rhythm.

The interrelationship between the adequacy of the rate and the extent of diastolic filling on systolic pump function is particularly important during exercise-induced tachycardia, when the time available for diastolic filling is abbreviated. The hypertrophied left ventricle also appears to be extremely susceptible to development of diastolic dysfunction during ischemic stress. Patients with advanced hypertrophy due to hypertension, aortic stenosis, or hypertrophic cardiomyopathy frequently develop exercise-induced angina with pulmonary congestion. Patients with chronic hypertrophy are vulnerable to development of ischemia from both coexisting coronary artery disease and impaired coronary vascular reserve.[120] Hemodynamic studies performed in animals and in isolated beating hearts with experimental pressure-overload hypertrophy show that the hypertrophied heart develops severe slowing of relaxation and elevation of LV diastolic pressure more rapidly in response to brief hypoxia or ischemia.[73, 121, 122] Invasive hemodynamic studies have shown that patients with hypertrophy who develop angina during pacing tachycardia develop severe diastolic dysfunction with a striking increase in LV diastolic pressure, which is related to the slowing of LV relaxation and an upward shift in the diastolic pressure-volume relation.[114, 123]

Impaired Diastolic Function in Dilated Cardiomyopathy

The hallmarks of dilated ischemic and nonischemic cardiomyopathies are the presence of increased LV end-systolic and end-diastolic volumes in association with depressed LV ejection fraction. In some patients with dilated cardiomyopathy, the presence of an increased LV end-diastolic pressure is simply related to the presence of volume overload and to an upward and rightward shift of the diastolic pressure-volume curve. In many patients, isovolumic relaxation is depressed and LV chamber distensibility is decreased, suggesting an alteration in diastolic properties of the ventricle as well.[124–126] The mechanisms of diastolic dysfunction in patients with dilated cardiomyopathy are incompletely understood. Multiple factors extrinsic to the myocyte may contribute, including RV distention and increased pericardial constraint and intermittent subendocardial ischemia due to abnormal coronary vascular reserve. Absolute levels of collagen and collagen volume fraction vary in dilated cardiomyopathy, but changes in myocardial stiffness also correlate with changes in collagen structure and the nonuniformity of collagen deposition, as well as the amount of collagen.[127] At the level of the myocyte, the issue is complex; end-stage dilated cardiomyopathy is characterized by a heterogeneous population of normal and "failing" myocytes, as well as by cell loss from necrosis and apoptosis, with a resultant increased load on residual myocytes and secondary hypertrophy.

The factors that contribute to impaired relaxation at the cellular level are likely to be similar to many of the abnormalities described in myocardial hypertrophy, including abnormalities in the regulation of cytosolic Ca^{2+} related to altered expression of SERCA-2 and the Na^{+}-Ca^{2+} exchanger; changes in myofibrillar crossbridge formation and detachment due to altered β-myosin ATPase activity, troponin I phosphorylation, or changes in TnT isoform expression; and impaired cyclic AMP signaling due to the downregulation of β-adrenergic receptors and changes in their regulation.[128, 129] In end-stage human heart failure due to dilated cardiomyopathy, there is intense interest in the role of SERCA-2 and other Ca^{2+} regulatory pumps in the genesis of both systolic and diastolic dysfunction. Most, but not all, investigators have found a reduction in message and protein levels of SERCA-2 in cardiac tissue from patients with end-stage heart failure undergoing cardiac transplantation.[130–133] In end-stage dilated cardiomyopathy in humans[133] and in dogs with pacing-induced cardiomyopathy,[134, 135] decreased levels of SERCA-2 may be partially compensated by increased expression of the Na^+-Ca^{2+} exchanger.

In muscle strips obtained from human failing myocardium paced at a rate of 60 times per minute, about 50 percent of the Ca^{2+} required for force development is derived from the SR and about 50 percent is derived from sarcolemmal influx, which is extruded in diastole via the Na^+-Ca^{2+} exchanger.[136] This contrasts with small rodents, such as the rat, in which the Na^+-Ca^{2+} exchanger normally accounts for less than 10 percent of Ca^{2+} movement during a twitch. In failing human myocardium, this dependence on sarcolemmal Ca^{2+} influx and efflux increases at higher frequency rates, implying that the failing human heart is exquisitely sensitive to the contribution of the Na^+-Ca^{2+} exchanger at rest and during exercise to sustain normal diastolic Ca^{2+} efflux and relaxation.[136] Hasenfuss and associates[137] examined diastolic properties in cardiac muscle strips from failing human hearts and found that frequency-dependent increases in diastolic force and depression of the rate of force decline were most pronounced in hearts with decreased protein levels of SERCA-2 and unchanged levels of the Na^+-Ca^{2+} exchanger, whereas hearts with increased expression of the Na^+-Ca^{2+} exchanger and normal levels of SERCA-2 had nearly normal diastolic function. Experiments in transgenic mice demonstrate that SERCA-2 overexpression is associated with an acceleration in the rate of contraction and relaxation[138]; however, it remains to be shown whether overexpression of SERCA-2 is sufficient to rescue severe diastolic dysfunction in experimental heart failure in the presence of other abnormalities of gene expression that accompany cardiac failure.

Regardless of the underlying cellular mechanisms, both human dilated cardiomyopathy and cardiomyopathy due to severe mitral regurgitation and pacing-induced experimental cardiomyopathy are frequently associated with slowed relaxation and a "restrictive" pattern of left ventricular filling with a decrease in early diastolic filling and a short deceleration time.[5, 139] Studies in dogs with pacing-induced cardiomyopathy indicate that the restrictive filling pattern may result in part from the dilated ventricle being forced to operate on the "steep" portion of the diastolic pressure-volume relation to maintain stroke volume, whereas the impairment in systolic contractility results in the inability to contract to an end-systolic volume smaller than equilibrium volume so that the failing heart cannot use elastic recoil (restoring forces) to enhance early diastolic filling.[140] In addition, tethering of the mitral valve with restricted mitral leaflet opening may also contribute to impaired early diastolic filling in patients with dilated ventricles.[141] The presence of impaired diastolic filling in patients with dilated cardiomyopathy is highly predictive of the magnitude of impairment of exercise capacity measured as peak oxygen consumption ($\dot{V}O_2$), whereas indices of systolic function, including ejection fraction, are not.[142] In patients with dilated cardiomyopathy, the presence of a "restrictive" pattern of dilated filling is also predictive of diastolic ventricular interaction such that reduction in RV filling and volume results in enhanced LV diastolic filling.[143] Thus, the identification of this severe pattern of impaired diastolic filling may identify patients who are likely to benefit from additional diuretic or vasodilator therapy. Interestingly, the elevation of plasma levels of brain natriuretic peptide, which is upregulated and secreted by the left ventricle in heart failure, appears to be highly predictive of the elevation in LV diastolic pressure independent of changes in other plasma neurohormones.[144] If this is substantiated, the measurement of brain natriuretic peptide may have a role as an adjunct to noninvasive Doppler studies to estimate LV diastolic pressure and follow its evolution in response to individual therapies.

Treatment of Heart Failure Due to Diastolic Dysfunction

There are no national consensus guidelines for the treatment of diastolic heart failure, and diastolic dysfunction is not yet recognized as an indication for U.S. Food and Drug Administration drug approval. Nevertheless, several guiding principles based on the biology of diastolic function apply to all causes of diastolic heart failure. In all patients, management should include the identification and prevention of myocardial ischemia due to known or occult coronary artery disease. Therapies aimed at blunting exercise-induced tachycardia and prolonging the duration of diastole for diastolic emptying and ventricular filling are usually beneficial in patients with poor exercise tolerance. For this reason, the use of β-adrenergic blockers and Ca^{2+} channel blockers may be beneficial. In patients with hypertrophic cardiomyopathy with or without outflow obstruction, verapamil and other Ca^{2+} channel blockers are sometimes effective in improving diastolic filling and palliating dyspnea.[109, 145] However, despite an early enthusiasm for the theoretic rationale of use of Ca^{2+} channel blockers to relieve "Ca^{2+}" overload, there still is no evidence to support this pharmacologic mechanism in patients with diastolic failure of any cause.[146] The judicious use of diuretics and vasodilators has a role in severe heart failure due to diastolic failure of all causes; because of the steep rise of the LV diastolic pressure-volume relationship, very small reductions in volume may result in large reductions in elevated LV diastolic pressure with little or no adverse effect on preload and stroke volume. Digoxin, which increases contractility via the augmentation of cytosolic Ca^{2+}, has no demonstrated role in diastolic failure due to acute ischemia or hypertrophy distinct from its use to control ventricular rate in atrial fibrillation. In patients with dilated nonischemic and ischemic cardiomyopathy, digoxin has been shown to modestly improve exercise tolerance, and consensus guidelines advise its use in these patients. In a trial of long-term use of digoxin in comparison with placebo, cardiomyopathy patients treated with digoxin showed a slight prolongation of relaxation time and a marked decrease in the rate and extent of early diastolic filling.[147] However, this apparent change in diastolic function did not interfere with a net favorable effect on outcome including survival.

In patients with hypertrophy and diastolic failure, the serial clinical investigations in patients with aortic valvular disease and valve replacement demonstrate that *the most effective short- and long-term therapy for improving diastolic function is the rigorous reduction in systolic pressure overload that results in early and long-term regression of both hypertrophy and collagen deposition.*[106] The failure to consistently observe these dramatic results in many hypertension trials is likely to be related to incomplete normalization of systolic blood pressure rather than to fundamental differences in the biology of hypertrophy. There is a strong theoretic rationale for the use of angiotensin-converting enzyme (ACE) inhibitors, and potentially angiotensin AT_1 receptor blockers, in the treatment of diastolic heart failure associated with hypertrophy. The expression of LV tissue ACE is upregulated in experimental hypertrophy[148] with an increased cardiac activation of angiotensin I to angiotensin II, and this pathologic change in cardiac gene expression has been demonstrated in humans with heart failure and hypertrophy.[149] The increase in ACE activity and local production of angiotensin II causes acute deterioration of diastolic function in experimental hypertrophy,[148] although the mechanism is still uncertain and not directly related to acute changes in diastolic Ca^{2+}.[150]

Friedrich and colleagues[151] demonstrated that intracardiac ACE inhibition via intracoronary infusion in patients with hypertrophy due to aortic stenosis acutely improves relaxation rate, myocardial stiffness, and ventricular filling properties. In subsequent studies, acute improvement in LV relaxation and diastolic distensibility in response to ACE inhibitors and AT_1 receptor blockers has been observed in dogs with hypertensive hypertrophy.[152, 153] In patients with hypertrophic obstructive cardiomyopathy, intracardiac ACE inhibition via intracoronary administration also decreases LV diastolic pressure, accelerates LV isovolumic relaxation, and reduces LV outflow gradient (possibly via enhanced LV diastolic filling).[154] In contrast, in these hypertrophic cardiomyopathy patients, systemic ACE inhibition that is sufficient to cause a large reduction in aortic pressure aggravates these hemodynamic abnormalities.[154] Taken together, these studies strongly suggest that cardiac ACE inhibition acutely improves diastolic dysfunction in hypertrophied hearts. The mechanism is uncertain and may be related in part to the pharmacologic action of ACE inhibition to amplify bradykinin–nitric oxide signaling. As discussed earlier in this chapter, nitric oxide donors acutely abbreviate systolic contraction and promote earlier diastolic relaxation. In patients with severe pressure-overload hypertrophy, intracoronary nitric oxide donors (nitroglycerin and nitroprusside) caused a marked fall in elevated LV diastolic pressure and decrease in chamber stiffness in the absence of change in heart rate or ejection fraction.[155] There is the potential to chronically augment nitric oxide production with L-arginine supplements, but this pharmacologic strategy has not yet been tested in humans with diastolic failure.

In patients with dilated cardiomyopathy, ACE inhibitors are the cornerstone of national consensus guidelines for the treatment of heart failure based on randomized clinical trials that have demonstrated benefits in survival rates and reduction in hospitalization time, as well as modification of LV remodeling.[156, 157] In the dog model of pacing-induced cardiomyopathy, subpressor doses of angiotensin II have little effect in control animals but greatly increase myocardial stiffness and LV diastolic pressure in cardiomyopathic hearts in association with activation of metalloproteinases and myocardial fibrosis.[158] Spinale and associates[159] demonstrated that angiotensin II receptor blockers failed to modify fractional shortening or diastolic dimension in this model, whereas treatment with an ACE inhibitor or the combined use of angiotensin II receptor blocker and ACE inhibitor increased fractional shortening and reduced LV diastolic dimension in association with the reduction in other plasma hormones, including endothelin.[159] Taken together, these data provide further rationale for ACE inhibition in patients with diastolic dysfunction and cardiomyopathy and suggest that the effects of ACE inhibition on remodeling and diastolic dysfunction are likely to be related to mechanisms in addition to changes in angiotensin II production. Clinical trials are under way for the treatment of heart failure due to dilated ischemic and nonischemic cardiomyopathies that will provide insight into the effects of aldosterone inhibitors, neutral endopeptidase inhibitors, endothelin receptor blockers, and β-adrenergic blockers on diastolic and systolic function and survival.

SUMMARY

In patients with the syndrome of heart failure, it is important to identify whether the cause is primary diastolic failure, which can be identified with an upward shift in the LV diastolic pressure-volume relationship. The diagnosis is supported by Doppler flow velocity studies that show a "restrictive" filling pattern and increased pulmonary vein flow during atrial contraction, whereas an "impaired relaxation" pattern can occur during aging in otherwise healthy adults. Multiple mechanisms may promote diastolic dysfunction including disturbances of cytosolic Ca^{2+} regulation, changes in myosin ATPase, and alterations in the geometry and structural composition of the ventricle. Diastolic dysfunction is a cause of heart failure in patients with the common conditions of transient ischemia in coronary artery disease as well as hypertrophic heart disease due to pressure overload. Once the underlying mechanisms and cause are identified, treatment can be aimed at the improvement of diastolic function rather than the stimulation of cardiac contractility. In patients with cardiac hypertrophy or dilated cardiomyopathy, the definitive therapy may depend on the promotion of the regression of cardiac remodeling and on new insights from molecular biology regarding the subcellular control of contraction-relaxation.

REFERENCES

1. Dougherty AH, Naccarelli GV, Gray E, et al: Congestive heart failure with normal systolic function. Am J Cardiol 54:778, 1984.
2. Soufer R, Wohlgelernter D, Vita NA, et al: Intact systolic left ventricular function in clinical congestive heart failure. Am J Cardiol 55:1032, 1985.
3. Gilbert JC, Glantz SA: Determinants of left ventricular filling and of the diastolic pressure-volume relation. Circ Res 64:827. 1989.
4. Mirsky I: Assessment of diastolic function: suggested methods and future considerations. Circulation 69:836, 1984.
5. Little WC, Downes TR: Clinical evaluation of left ventricular diastolic performance. Prog Cardiovasc Dis 32:273, 1990.
6. Craig WE, Murgo JP, Pasipoularides A: Evaluation of time course of left ventricular isovolumic relaxation in humans. *In* Grossman W, Lorell BH (eds): Diastolic Relaxation of the Heart. p. 11. Boston: Martinus-Nijhoff, 1987.
7. Courtois M, Barzilai B, Hall AF, et al: Postextrasystolic left ventricular isovolumic pressure decay is not monoexponential. Cardiovasc Res 35:206, 1997.

8. Brutsaert DL, Sys SV: Relaxation and diastole of the heart. Physiol Rev 69:1228, 1989.
9. Shannon TR, Bers DM: Assessment of intra-SR free [Ca] and buffering in rat heart. Biophys J 73:1524, 1997.
10. Bassani RA, Bers DM: Rate of diastolic Ca release from the sarcoplasmic reticulum of intact rabbit and rat ventricular myocytes. Biophys J 68:2015, 1995.
11. Solaro JR, Rarick HM: Troponin and tropomyosin: proteins that switch on and tune in the activity of cardiac myofilaments [review]. Circ Res 83:471, 1998.
12. Moss RL: Plasticity in the dynamics of myocardial contraction: calcium, crossbridge kinetics, or molecular cooperation. Circ Res 84:862, 1999.
13. Ingwall JS: Is cardiac failure a consequence of decreased energy reserve? Circulation 87(suppl II):VII-58, 1993.
14. Lorenz JN, Kranias EG: Regulatory effects of phospholamban on cardiac function in intact mice. Am J Physiol 273:H2826, 1997.
15. Gombosova I, Boknik P, Kirchhefer U, et al: Postnatal changes in contractile time parameters, calcium regulatory proteins, and phosphatases. Am J Physiol 274:H2123, 1998.
16. Yao A, Matsui H, Spitzer KW, et al: Sarcoplasmic reticulum and Na/Ca exchanger function during early and late relaxation in ventricular myocytes. Am J Physiol 273:H2765, 1997.
17. Bridge JHB, Smolley JR, Spitzer KW: The relationship between charge movements associated with I_{ca} and $I_{\text{NaûCa}}$ in cardiac myocytes. Science 248:376, 1990.
18. Yao A, Su Z, Nonaka A, et al: Effects of overexpression of the Na-Ca exchanger on $[Ca^{2+}]_i$ transients in murine ventricular myocytes. Circ Res 82:657, 1998.
19. Bassani JW, Bassani RA, Bers DM: Relaxation in rabbit and rat cardiac cells: species-dependent differences in cellular mechanisms. J Physiol (Lond) 476:279, 1994.
20. Hammes A, Oberdorf-Maass S, Rother T, et al: Overexpression of the sarcolemmal calcium pump in the myocardium of transgenic rats. Circ Res 83:877, 1998.
21. Stuyvers BD, Miura M, Jin JP, et al: Ca(2+) dependence of diastolic properties of cardiac sarcomeres: involvement of titin. Prog Biophys Mol Biol 69:425, 1998.
22. Wolska BM, Keller RS, Evans CC, et al: Correlation between myofilament response to Ca^{2+} and altered dynamics of contraction and relaxation in transgenic cardiac cells that express β-tropomyosin. Circ Res 84:745, 1999.
23. Fitzsimons DP, Patel JR, Moss RL: Role of myosin heavy chain composition in kinetics of force development and relaxation in rat myocardium. J Physiol (Lond) 513:171, 1998.
24. Schiaffino S, Reggiani C: Molecular diversity of myofibrillar proteins: gene regulation and functional significance. Physiol Rev 76:371, 1996.
25. Tian R, Christe ME, Spindler M, et al: Role of Mg ADP in the development of diastolic dysfunction in the intact beating rat heart. J Clin Invest 99:745, 1997.
26. Smith JA, Shah AM, Lewis MJ: Factors released from endocardium of the ferret and pig modulate myocardial contraction. J Physiol (Lond) 439:1, 1991.
27. Paulus WJ, Vantrimpont P, Shah AM: Acute effects of nitric oxide on left ventricular relaxation and diastolic distensibility in humans. Circulation 89:2070. 1994.
28. Ito N, Bartunek J, Spitzer KW, et al: Effects of the nitric oxide donor nitroprusside on intracellular pH and contraction in hypertrophied myocytes. Circulation 95:2303, 1997.
29. Zile MR, Gaasch WH: Mechanical loads and the isovolumic and filling indices of left ventricular relaxation. Prog Cardiovasc Dis 32;333, 1990.
30. Cheng C-P, Freeman GL, Santamore WP, et al: Effect of loading conditions, contractile state, and heart rate on early left ventricular filling in conscious dogs. Circ Res 66:814, 1990.
31. Paulus WJ, Heyndrickx GR, Buyl P, et al: Wide-range load shift of combined aortic valvuloplasty-arterial vasodilation slows isovolumic relaxation of the hypertrophied left ventricle. Circulation 81:886, 1990.
32. Bonow RO, Bacharach SL, Green MV, et al: Impaired left ventricular diastolic filling in patients with coronary artery disease: assessment with radionuclide angiography. Circulation 64:315, 1981.
33. Magorien DJ, Shaffer P, Bush C, et al: Hemodynamic correlation for timing intervals, ejection rate and filling rate derived from the radionuclide angiographic volume curve. Am J Cardiol 53:567, 1984.
34. Appleton CP, Hatle LK, Popp RL: Relation of transmitral flow velocity patterns to left ventricular diastolic function: new insights from a combined hemodynamic and Doppler echocardiographic study. J Am Coll Cardiol 12:42, 1988.
35. Little WC, Warner JG Jr, Rankin KM, et al: Evaluation of left ventricular diastolic function from the pattern of left ventricular filling. Clin Cardiol 21:5, 1998.
36. Vitarelli A, Gheorghiade M: Diastolic heart failure: standard Doppler approach and beyond. Am J Cardiol 81:115G, 1998.
37. Nishimura RA, Tajik AJ: Evaluation of diastolic filling of left ventricle in health and disease: Doppler echocardiography is the clinician's Rosetta Stone. J Am Coll Cardiol 30:8, 1997.
38. Brecher GA: Experimental evidence of ventricular diastolic suction. Circ Res 4:513, 1956.
39. Bell SP, Fabian J, LeWinter MM: Effects of dobutamine on left ventricular restoring forces. Am J Physiol 275:H190, 1998.
40. Fraites TJ Jr, Saeki A, Kass DA: Effect of altering filling pattern on diastolic pressure-volume curve. Circulation 96:4408, 1997.
41. Kangro T, Henriksen E, Jonason T, et al: Doppler indexes of left ventricular filling after exercise in 50 year-old healthy persons. Am J Cardiol 79:1507, 1997.
42. Garcia MJ, Thomas JD, Klein AL: New Doppler echocardiographic applications for the study of diastolic function. J Am Coll Cardiol 32:865, 1998.
43. Kudelka AM, Turner DA, Liebson PR, et al: Comparison of cine magnetic resonance imaging and Doppler echocardiography for evaluation of left ventricular diastolic function. Am J Cardiol 80:384, 1997.
44. Schmitz L, Koch H, Bein G, et al: Left ventricular diastolic function in infants, children, and adolescents: reference values and analysis of morphologic and physiologic determinants of echocardiographic Doppler flow signals during growth and maturation. J Am Coll Cardiol 32:1441, 1998.
45. O'Leary PW, Durongpisitkul K, Cordes TM, et al: Diastolic ventricular function in children: a Doppler echocardiographic study establishing normal values and predictors of increased ventricular end-diastolic pressure. Mayo Clin Proc 73:616, 1998.
46. Mesa A, Jessurun C, Hernandez A, et al: Left ventricular diastolic function in normal human pregnancy. Circulation 99:522, 1999.
47. Santamore WP, Dell'Italia LJ: Ventricular interdependence: significant left ventricular contributions to right ventricular systolic function. Prog Cardiovasc Dis 40:289, 1998.
48. Baker AE, Dani R, Smith ER, et al: Quantitative assessment of independent contributions of pericardium and septum to direct ventricular interaction. Am J Physiol 275:H476, 1998.
49. Smiseth OA, Manyari DE, Lima JA, et al: Modulation of vascular capacitance by angiotensin and nitroprusside: a mechanism of changes in pericardial pressure. Circulation 76:875, 1987.
50. Wong CY, Spotnitz HM: Effects of nitroprusside on end-diastolic pressure-diameter relations of the human left ventricle after pericardiotomy. J Thorac Cardiovasc Surg 82:350, 1981.
51. Lorell B, Leinbach RC, Pohost GM, et al: Right ventricular infarction. Am J Cardiol 43:465, 1979.
52. Bartle SH, Hermann HJ: Acute mitral regurgitation in man. Hemodynamic evidence and observations indicating an early role for the pericardium. Circulation 36:839, 1967.
53. Atherton JJ, Thomson HL, Moore TD, et al: Diastolic ventricular interaction: a possible mechanism for abnormal vascular responses during volume unloading in heart failure. Circulation 96:4273, 1997.
54. Grossman W, McLaurin LP, Moos SP, et al: Wall thickness and diastolic properties of the left ventricle. Circulation 49:129, 1974.
55. Thiedemann KU, Holubarsch CH, Medugorac I, et al: Connective tissue content and myocardial stiffness in pressure overload hypertrophy: a combined study of morphologic, morphometric, biochemical and mechanical parameters. Basic Res Cardiol 78:140, 1983.
56. Weber KT: Cardiac interstitium in health and disease: the fibrillar collagen network. J Am Coll Cardiol 13:1627, 1989.
57. Villari B, Campbell SE, Hess OM, et al: Influence of collagen network on left ventricular systolic and diastolic function in aortic valve disease. J Am Coll Cardiol 22:1477, 1993.
58. Vogel WM, Apstein CS, Briggs LL, et al: Acute alterations in left ventricular diastolic chamber stiffness: role of the "erectile" effect of coronary arterial pressure and flow in normal and damaged hearts. Circ Res 51:465, 1982.

59. Miyamoto M, McClure DE, Schertel ER, et al: Effects of hypoproteinemia-induced myocardial edema on left ventricular function. Am J Physiol 274:H937, 1998.
60. Cain BS, Meldrum DR, Joo KS, et al: Human SERCA2a levels correlate inversely with age in senescent human myocardium. J Am Coll Cardiol 32:458, 1998.
61. Yamakado T, Takagi E, Okubo S, et al: Effects of aging on left ventricular isovolumic pressure decay. Circulation 95:917, 1997.
62. Schulman SP, Lakatta EG, Fleg JL, et al: Age-related decline in left ventricular filling at rest and exercise. Am J Physiol 263:H1937, 1992.
63. Yu CM, Sanderson JE: Right and left diastolic function in patients with and without heart failure: effect of age, sex, heart rate, and respiration on Doppler-derived measurements. Am Heart J134:426. 1997.
64. Gardin JM, Arnold AM, Bild DE, et al: Left ventricular diastolic filling in the elderly: the cardiovascular health study. Am J Cardiol 82:345, 1998.
65. Zabalgoitia M, Rahman SN, Haley WE, et al: Comparison in systemic hypertension of left ventricular mass and geometry with systolic and diastolic function in patients $<$ 65 to $>$ or $=$ 65 years of age. Am J Cardiol 82:604, 1998.
66. Zabalgoitia M, Ur Rahman SN, Haley WE, et al: Role of left ventricular hypertrophy in diastolic dysfunction in aged hypertensive patients. J Hypertens 15:1175, 1997.
67. Spina RJ, Turner MJ, Ehsani AA: Beta-adrenergic-mediated improvement in left ventricular function by exercise training in older men. Am J Physiol 274:H397, 1998.
68. Xiao RP, Tomhave ED, Wang DJ, et al: Age-associated reductions in cardiac beta 1- and beta 2-adrenergic responses without changes in inhibitory G proteins or receptor kinases. J Clin Invest 101:1273, 1998.
69. Lee H-C, Mohabir R, Smith N, et al: Effect of ischemia on calcium-dependent fluorescence transients in rabbit hearts containing indo 1: correlation with monophasic action potentials and contraction. Circulation 78:1047, 1988.
70. Kihara Y, Grossman W, Morgan JP: Direct measurement of changes in Ca^{2+} during hypoxia, ischemia, and reperfusion of the intact mammalian heart. Circ Res 65:1029, 1989.
71. Steenbergen C, Murphy E, Levy L, et al: Elevation in cytosolic free calcium concentration early in myocardial ischemia in perfused rat heart. Circ Res 60:700, 1987.
72. Wexler LF, Weinberg EO, Ingwall JS, et al: Acute alterations in diastolic left ventricular chamber distensibility: mechanistic differences between hypoxemia and ischemia in isolated perfused rabbit and rat hearts. Circ Res 59:515, 1986.
73. Eberli FR, Apstein CS, Ngoy S, Lorell BH: Exacerbation of left ventricular ischemic diastolic dysfunction by pressure overload hypertrophy: modification by specific inhibition of cardiac angiotensin converting enzyme. Circ Res 70:931, 1992.
74. Isoyama S, Apstein CS, Wexler LF, et al: Acute decrease in left ventricular diastolic chamber distensibility during simulated angina in isolated hearts. Circ Res 61:925, 1987.
75. Lorell BH, Isoyama S, Grice WN, et al: Effects of ouabain and isoproterenol on left ventricular diastolic function during low-flow ischemia in isolated, blood-perfused rabbit hearts. Circ Res 63:457, 1988.
76. Tayama M, Solomon SB, Glantz SA: Effect of lidocaine on left ventricular pressure-volume curves during demand ischemia in pigs. Am J Physiol 274:H21, 1998.
77. Owen P, Dennis S, Opie LH: Glucose flux regulates rate of ischemic contracture in globally underperfused rat hearts. Circ Res 66:406, 1990.
78. Eberli FR, Weinberg EO, Grice WN, et al: Protective effect of increased glycolytic substrate against systolic and diastolic dysfunction and reperfusion in isolated rabbit heart perfused with erythrocyte suspensions. Circ Res 68:466, 1991.
79. Mann T, Brodie BR, Grossman W, et al: Effect of angina on the left ventricular diastolic pressure-volume relationship. Circulation 55:761, 1977.
80. Carroll JD, Hess OM, Hirzel HO, et al: Exercise-induced ischemia: the influence of altered relaxation on early diastolic pressures. Circulation 67:521, 1983.
81. Sasayama S, Nonogi H, Miyazaki S, et al: Changes in diastolic properties of the regional myocardium during pacing-induced ischemia in human subjects. J Am Coll Cardiol 5:599, 1985.
82. Pouleur H, Rousseau MF, Van Eyll C, et al: Assessment of regional left ventricular relaxation in patients with coronary disease: importance of geometric factors and change in wall thickness. Circulation 69:696, 1984.
83. Bonow RO: Regional left ventricular non-uniformity. Effects of left ventricular diastolic function in ischemic heart disease, hypertrophic cardiomyopathy, and the normal heart. Circulation 81(suppl III):III-54, 1990.
84. Bronzwaer JGF, de Bruyne B, Ascoop CAPL, Paulus WJ: Comparative effects of pacing-induced and balloon coronary occlusion ischemia on left ventricular diastolic function in man. Circulation 84:211, 1991.
85. deBruyne B, Bronzwaer JG, Hendrickx GR, et al: Comparative effects of ischemia and hypoxemia on left ventricular systolic and diastolic function in humans. Circulation 88:461, 1993.
86. Wijns W, Serruys PW, Slager CJ: Effect of coronary occlusion during percutaneous transluminal angioplasty in humans on left ventricular chamber stiffness and regional diastolic pressure-radius relations. J Am Coll Cardiol 7:455, 1986.
87. Solomon SB, Barbier P, Glantz SA: Changes in porcine transmitral flow pattern and its diastolic determinants during partial coronary occlusion. J Am Coll Cardiol 33:854, 1999.
88. Cerisano G, Bolognese L, Carrabba N, et al: Doppler-derived mitral deceleration time: an early strong predictor of left ventricular remodeling after reperfused anterior acute myocardial infarction. Circulation 99:230, 1999.
89. Morgan HE, Baker KM: Cardiac hypertrophy: mechanical, neural, and endocrine dependence. Circulation 83:13, 1991.
90. Colan SD: Mechanics of left ventricular systolic and diastolic function in physiologic hypertrophy of the athlete's heart. Cardiol Clin 15:355, 1997.
91. Zwinderman AH, van der Laarse A, Vliegen HW, et al: Functional and metabolic evaluation of the athlete's heart by magnetic resonance imaging and dobutamine stress magnetic resonance spectroscopy. Circulation 97:666, 1998.
92. Gharavi AG, Diamond JA, Goldman AY, et al: Resting diastolic function and left ventricular mass are related to exercise capacity in hypertensive men but not in women. Am J Hypertens 11:1252, 1998.
93. Douglas PS, Katz SE, Weinberg EO, et al: Hypertrophic remodeling: gender differences in the early response to left ventricular pressure overload. J Am Coll Cardiol 32:1118, 1998.
94. Weinberg EO, Thienelt CD, Katz SE, et al: Gender differences in molecular remodeling in pressure overload hypertrophy. J Am Coll Cardiol 34:264, 1999.
95. De la Bastie D, Levitsky DD, Rappaport L, et al: Function of the sarcoplasmic reticulum and expression of its Ca^{2+}ATPase gene in pressure overload induced cardiac hypertrophy in the rat. Circ Res 66:554, 1990.
96. Lompre A-M, Schwartz K, d'Albis A, et al: Myosin isoenzyme redistribution in chronic heart overload. Nature 282:105, 1979.
97. Nagai R, Zarain-Herzberg A, Brandl CJ, et al: Regulation of myocardial Ca ATPase and phospholamban mRNA expression in response to pressure overload and thyroid hormone. Proc Natl Acad Sci U S A 86:2966, 1989.
98. Feldman AM, Weinberg EO, Ray PE, Lorell BH: Selective changes in cardiac gene expression during compensated hypertrophy and the transition to cardiac decompensation in rats with chronic aortic banding. Circ Res 73:184, 1993.
99. Gwathmey JK, Morgan JP: Altered calcium handling in experimental pressure-overload hypertrophy in the ferret. Circ Res 57:836, 1985.
100. Qi M, Shannon TR, Euler DE, et al: Downregulation of sarcoplasmic reticulum Ca^{2+}-ATPase during progression of left ventricular hypertrophy. Am J Physiol 272:H2416, 1997.
101. McCall E, Ginsburg KS, Bassani RA, et al: Ca flux, contractility, and excitation-contraction coupling in hypertrophy rat ventricular myocytes. Am J Physiol 274:H1348, 1998.
102. Smith SH, Kramer MF, Reis I, et al: Regional changes in creatine kinase and myocyte size in hypertensive and nonhypertensive cardiac hypertrophy. Circ Res 67:1334, 1990.
103. Tian R, Nascimben L, Ingwall JS, et al: Failure to maintain a low ADP concentration impairs diastolic function in hypertrophied rat hearts. Circulation 96:1313, 1997.
104. Lamb HJ, Beyerbacht HP, van der Laarse A, et al: Diastolic dysfunction in hypertensive heart disease is associated with altered myocardial metabolism. Circulation 99:2261, 1999.

105. Norton GR, Tsotetsi J, Trifunovic B, et al: Myocardial stiffness is attributed to alterations in cross-linked collagen rather than total collagen or phenotypes in spontaneously hypertensive rats. Circulation 96:1991, 1997.
106. Villari B, Vassalli G, Monrad ES, et al: Normalization of diastolic dysfunction in aortic stenosis late after valve replacement. Circulation 91:2352, 1995.
107. Minniti G, Jaffrain-Rea ML, Moroni CM, et al: Echocardiographic evidence for a direct effect of GH/IGF-I hypersecretion on cardiac mass and function in young acromegalics. Clin Endocrinol 49:101, 1998.
108. Lopez-Velasco R, Escobar-Morreale HF, Vega B, et al: Cardiac involvement in acromegaly: specific myocardiopathy or consequence of systemic hypertension? J Clin Endocrinol Metab 82:1047, 1997.
109. Bonow RO, Rosing DR, Bacharach SL, et al: Effects of verapamil on left ventricular systolic function and diastolic filling in patients with hypertrophic cardiomyopathy. Circulation 64:787, 1981.
110. Paulus WJ, Sys SU, Nellens P, et al: Postextrasystolic potentiation worsens fast filling of the hypertrophied left ventricle in aortic stenosis and hypertrophic cardiomyopathy. Circulation 78:928, 1988.
111. Peterson KL, Tsugi J, Johnson A, et al: Diastolic left ventricular pressure-volume and stress-strain relations in patients with valvular aortic stenosis and left ventricular hypertrophy. Circulation 58:77, 1978.
112. Eichhorn P, Grimm J, Koch R, et al: Left ventricular relaxation in patients with left ventricular hypertrophy secondary to aortic valve disease. Circulation 65:1395, 1982.
113. Diver DJ, Royal HD, Aroesty JM, et al: Diastolic function in patients with aortic stenosis: influence of left ventricular load reduction. J Am Coll Cardiol 12:642, 1988.
114. Fifer MA, Bourdillon PD, Lorell BH: Altered left ventricular diastolic properties during pacing-induced angina in patients with aortic stenosis. Circulation 74:675, 1986.
115. Fifer M, Borow K, Colan S, Lorell BH: Early diastolic left ventricular function in children and adults with aortic stenosis. J Am Coll Cardiol 5:1147, 1985.
116. Banerjee A, Mendelsohn AM, Knilans TK, et al: Effect of myocardial hypertrophy on systolic and diastolic function in children: insights from the force-frequency and relaxation-frequency relationships. J Am Coll Cardiol 32:1088, 1998.
117. Schussheim AE, Diamond JA, Jhang JS, et al: Midwall fractional shortening is an independent predictor of left ventricular diastolic dysfunction in asymptomatic patients with systemic hypertension. Am J Cardiol 82:1056, 1998.
118. Heesen WF, Beltman FW, May JF, et al: High prevalence of concentric remodeling in elderly individuals with isolated systolic hypertension from a population survey. Hypertension 29:539, 1997.
119. Topol EJ, Trail TA, Fortuin NJ: Hypertensive hypertrophic cardiomyopathy of the elderly. N Engl J Med 312:277, 1985.
120. Julius BK, Spillman M, Vassalli G, et al: Angina pectoris in patients with aortic stenosis and normal coronary arteries: mechanisms and pathophysiologic concepts. Circulation 95:892, 1997.
121. Wexler LF, Lorell BH, Momomura S, et al: Enhanced sensitivity to hypoxia-induced diastolic dysfunction in pressure-overload left ventricular hypertrophy in rats: role of high-energy phosphate depletion. Circ Res 62:766, 1988.
122. Gaasch WH, Zile MR, Hoshino PK, et al: Tolerance of the hypertrophic heart to ischemia: studies in compensated and failing dog hearts with pressure overload hypertrophy. Circulation 81:1644, 1990.
123. Udelson JE, Cannon RO III, Bacharach SL, et al: Beta-adrenergic stimulation with isoproterenol enhances left ventricular diastolic performance in hypertrophic cardiomyopathy despite potentiation of myocardial ischemia: comparison to rapid atrial pacing. Circulation 79:371, 1989.
124. Grossman W, McLaurin LP, Rolett EL: Alterations in left ventricular relaxation and diastolic compliance in congestive cardiomyopathy. Cardiovasc Res 13:514, 1979.
125. Fifer MA, Colucci WS, Lorell BH, et al: Inotropic, vascular, and endocrine effects of nifedipine in heart failure: comparison with nitroprusside. J Am Coll Cardiol 5:731, 1985.
126. Carroll JD, Lang RM, Neumann AL, et al: The differential effects of positive inotropic and vasodilator therapy on diastolic properties in patients with congestive cardiomyopathy. Circulation 74:815, 1986.
127. Neumann T, Vollmer A, Schaffner T, et al: Diastolic dysfunction and collagen structure in canine pacing-induced heart failure. J Mol Cell Cardiol 31:179, 1999.
128. Mittman C, Eschenhagen T, Scholz H: Cellular and molecular aspects of contractile dysfunction in heart failure. Cardiovasc Res 39:267, 1998.
129. Bristow MR, Hershberger RE, Port JD, et al: Beta-adrenergic pathways in non-failing and failing human myocardium. Circulation 82(suppl I):I-12, 1990.
130. Feldman AM, Ray PE, Silan CM, et al: Selective gene expression in failing human heart: quantification of steady-state levels of messenger RNA in endomyocardial biopsies using the polymerase chain reaction. Circulation 83:1866, 1991.
131. Beuckelman DJ, Nabauer M, Erdmann E: Intracellular calcium handling in isolated ventricular myocardium. Circulation 85:1046, 1992.
132. Schmidt U, Hajjar RJ, Helm PA, et al: Contribution of abnormal sarcoplasmic reticulum ATPase activity to systolic and diastolic dysfunction in human heart failure. J Mol Cell Cardiol 30:1929, 1998.
133. Hasenfuss G: Alterations of calcium regulatory proteins in heart failure. Cardiovasc Res 37:279, 1998.
134. Gupta RC, Shimoyama H, Tanimura M, et al: SR Ca^{2+}-ATPase activity and expression in ventricular myocardium of dogs with heart failure. Am J Physiol 273:H12, 1997.
135. O'Rourke B, Kass DA, Tomaselli GF, et al: Mechanism of altered excitation-contraction coupling in canine tachycardia-induced heart failure, I. Circ Res 84:562, 1999.
136. Schotthauer K, Schottmann J, Bers DM, et al: Frequency-dependent changes in the contribution of SR Ca^{2+} to Ca^{2+} transients in failing human myocardium assessed with ryanodine. J Mol Cell Cardiol 30:1285, 1998.
137. Hasenfuss G, Schillinger W, Lehnart SE, et al: Relationship between Na^{+}-Ca^{2+} exchanger protein levels and diastolic function of failing human myocardium. Circulation 99:641, 1999.
138. He H, Giordano FJ, Hilal-Dandan R, et al: Overexpression of the rat sarcoplasmic reticulum Ca^{2+} ATPase gene in the heart of transgenic mice accelerates calcium transients and cardiac relaxation. J Clin Invest 100:380, 1997.
139. Sadaniantz A, Miller G, Hadi BJ, et al: Effects of left ventricular systolic function of left ventricular diastolic filling patterns in severe mitral regurgitation. Am J Cardiol 79:1488, 1998.
140. Solomon SB, Nikolic SD, Glantz SA, et al: Left ventricular diastolic function of remodeled myocardium in dogs with pacing-induced heart failure. Am J Physiol 274:H945, 1998.
141. Otsuji Y, Gilon D, Jiang L, et al: Restricted diastolic opening of the mitral leaflets in patients with left ventricular dysfunction: evidence for increased valve tethering. J Am Coll Cardiol 32:398, 1998.
142. Lapu-Bula R, Robert A, de Kick M, et al: Relation of exercise capacity to left ventricular systolic function and diastolic filling in idiopathic or ischemic dilated cardiomyopathy. Am J Cardiol 83:728, 1999.
143. Atherton JJ, Moore TD, Thomson HL, et al: Restrictive left ventricular filling patterns are predictive of diastolic ventricular interaction in chronic heart failure. J Am Coll Cardiol 31:413, 1998.
144. Maeda K, Tsutamoto T, Wada A, et al: Plasma brain natriuretic peptide as a biochemical marker of high left ventricular end-diastolic pressure in patients with symptomatic left ventricular dysfunction. Am Heart J 135:825, 1998.
145. Bonow RO, Vitale DF, Maron BJ, et al: Regional left ventricular asynchrony and impaired global left ventricular filling in hypertrophic cardiomyopathy: effect of verapamil. J Am Coll Cardiol 9:1108, 1987.
146. Mahon N, McKenna WJ: Calcium channel blockers in cardiac failure. Prog Cardiovasc Dis 41:191, 1998.
147. Hassapoyannes CA, Bergh ME, Movahed MR, et al: Diastolic effects of chronic digitalization in systolic heart failure. Am Heart J 136:688, 1998.
148. Schunkert H, Dzau VJ, Tang SS, et al: Increased rat cardiac angiotensin-converting enzyme activity and mRNA levels in pressure overload left ventricular hypertrophy: effects on coronary resistance, contractility and relaxation. J Clin Invest 86:1913, 1990.
149. Struder R, Reinecke H, Muller B, et al: Increased angiotensin-I converting enzyme gene expression in the failing human heart: quantification by competitive RNA polymerase chain reaction. J Clin Invest 94:301, 1994.
150. Ito N, Kagaya Y, Weinberg EO, et al: Endothelin and angiotensin II

stimulation of Na^+-H^+ exchange is impaired in cardiac hypertrophy. J Clin Invest 99:125, 1997.

151. Friedrich SP, Lorell BH, Rousseau MF, et al: Intracardiac angiotensin-converting enzyme inhibition improves diastolic function in patients with left ventricular hypertrophy due to aortic stenosis. Circulation 90:2761, 1994.
152. Hayashida W, Donckier J, Van Mechelen H, et al: Load-insensitive diastolic relaxation in hypertrophied left ventricles. Am J Physiol 274:H609, 1998.
153. Hayashida W, Donckier J, Van Mechelen H, et al: Diastolic properties in canine hypertensive left ventricular hypertrophy: effects of angiotensin converting enzyme inhibition and angiotensin II type-1 receptor blockade. Cardiovasc Res 33:54, 1997.
154. Kyriakidis M, Triposkiadis F, Dernellis J, et al: Effects of cardiac versus circulatory angiotensin-converting enzyme inhibition on left ventricular diastolic function and coronary blood flow in hypertrophic obstructive cardiomyopathy. Circulation 97:1342, 1998.
155. Matter CM, Mandinov L, Kaufman PA, et al: Effect of NO donors on LV diastolic function in patients with severe pressure-overload hypertrophy. Circulation 99:2396, 1999.
156. The SOLVD Investigators: Effect on enalapril on survival in patients with reduced left ventricular ejection fractions and congestive heart failure. N Engl J Med 325:293, 1991.
157. Pfeffer MA, Braunwald E, Moye LA, et al, on behalf of the SAVE Investigators: effect of captopril on mortality and morbidity in patients with left ventricular dysfunction after myocardial infarction. N Engl J Med 327:669, 1992.
158. Sensaki H, Gluzband YA, Pak PH, et al: Synergistic exacerbation of diastolic stiffness from short-term tachycardia-induced cardiodepression and angiotensin II. Circ Res 82:503, 1998.
159. Spinale FG, de Gasparo M, Whitebread S, et al: Modulation of the renin-angiotensin pathway through enzyme inhibition and specific receptor blockade in pacing-induced heart failure, I: effects of left ventricular performance and neurohormonal systems. Circulation 96:2385, 1887.

SECTION VI

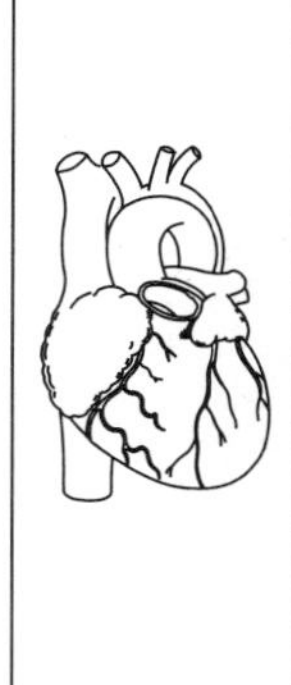

MYOCARDIAL DISEASE

Anatomic Abnormalities

Dilated Cardiomyopathy

Hypertrophic Cardiomyopathy

Restrictive Cardiomyopathy

Other Cardiomyopathies

Myocarditis

Cardiac Catheterization

Echocardiography

Radionuclide Techniques in Cardiomyopathies and Myocarditis

Pathophysiology and Clinical Recognition of Heart Failure

The Management of Heart Failure

Heart Transplantation: Indications, Outcome, and Long-Term Complications

Heart Transplantation: Pathogenesis, Immunosuppression, and Diagnosis and Treatment of Rejection

Surgical Treatment of Advanced Heart Failure

CHAPTER 50

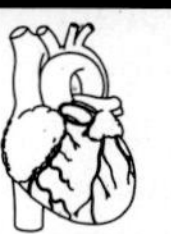

Anatomic Abnormalities

Hugh A. McAllister, Jr., L. Maximilian Buja, and Victor J. Ferrans

ANATOMIC ABNORMALITIES
DILATED CARDIOMYOPATHY
HYPERTROPHIC CARDIOMYOPATHY
RESTRICTIVE CARDIOMYOPATHY
OTHER CARDIOMYOPATHIES
MYOCARDITIS
CARDIAC CATHETERIZATION
ECHOCARDIOGRAPHY
RADIONUCLIDE TECHNIQUES IN CARDIOMYOPATHIES AND MYOCARDITIS
PATHOPHYSIOLOGY AND CLINICAL RECOGNITION OF HEART FAILURE
MANAGEMENT OF HEART FAILURE
HEART TRANSPLANTATION: INDICATIONS, OUTCOME, AND LONG-TERM COMPLICATIONS
HEART TRANSPLANTATION: PATHOGENESIS, IMMUNOSUPPRESSION, AND DIAGNOSIS AND TREATMENT OF REJECTION
SURGICAL TREATMENT OF ADVANCED HEART FAILURE
MYOCARDIAL BIOPSIES
CARDIAC HYPERTROPHY AND FIBROSIS
HYPERTROPHIC CARDIOMYOPATHY
DILATED CARDIOMYOPATHY
RESTRICTIVE CARDIOMYOPATHY
MYOCARDITIS
RHEUMATIC MYOCARDITIS AND ASCHOFF NODULES
CARDIAC TRANSPLANTATION–MONITORING REJECTION
METABOLIC AND STORAGE DISEASES
MURAL ENDOCARDIUM
MYOCARDIAL ISCHEMIA
CARDIAC ANEURYSMS
Pseudoaneurysm of the Heart
Annular Subvalvular Left Ventricular Aneurysms

Myocardial Biopsies

Procedures used to obtain myocardial tissue include operative resection (infundibular tissue in patients with muscular obstruction to right ventricular outflow, ventricular septal muscle in patients with hypertrophic obstructive cardiomyopathy, left atrial appendage in patients with mitral valvular disease); operative biopsies; and removal with the use of various types of bioptome catheters, which can be used to obtain samples of ventricular endocardium and subjacent myocardium. In the right ventricle, catheter biopsy samples are usually taken from the septal wall; in the left ventricle, they are taken from the free wall. Multiple samples can be obtained, each measuring about $3 \times 2 \times 2$ mm. Because of the risk of perforation of a thin chamber wall, catheter biopsy samples are not usually taken from the atrial walls or the free wall of the right ventricle. Transmural samples of ventricular wall also have been obtained (percutaneously or at open thoracotomy) with the use of biopsy needles.

Regardless of the method used to obtain tissue, myocardial biopsy samples show artifacts related to the unopposed contraction that the free edges of the tissue undergo as a response to cutting. These artifacts are manifested as hypercontraction bands and are most pronounced in a peripheral zone that extends for 100 to 200 pm into the depth of the tissue. They constitute a significant drawback to the use of needles for biopsies, particularly needles with small internal diameters. Operative biopsy samples also may show artifacts (especially in mitochondria) related to elective cardiac arrest and cardiopulmonary bypass.

Endomyocardial biopsy specimens are to be evaluated systematically to include the following:

1. Endocardium (thickness, cell type and number, stroma, contiguity, and thrombus)
2. Cardiac myocytes (size, arrangement, degeneration, storage deposits, sarcoplasmic membrane changes, nuclear changes, organisms such as *Toxoplasma* or trypanosomes, or cytomegalovirus inclusions)
3. Myocardial interstitium (cell type and number, stromal composition, storage deposits such as amyloid, organisms such as fungi)
4. Blood vessels (endothelium, basement membrane, wall thickness and composition, thrombus or embolic materials, and organisms such as rickettsiae)

Myocardial biopsy specimens must be properly oriented to include endocardium in the plane of sectioning. For electron microscopic processing, this should be done before tissues are darkened by postfixation with osmium tetroxide.

Light microscopic stains that are routinely used to study formalin-fixed myocardial biopsies are hematoxylin and eosin and Masson's trichrome. Movat's pentachrome method, periodic acid–Schiff reaction, Congo red, Prussian blue reaction for iron, and stains for organisms are used as needed. For immunohistochemical or biochemical studies, unfixed tissue must be frozen rapidly and kept under the appropriate storage conditions. A variety of antibodies can be used for the identification of subtypes of lymphocytes in frozen sections (and, in some instances, in paraffin sections) of myocardium. In addition, a large number of monoclonal and polyclonal antibodies can be used for immunohistochemical studies to evaluate the degree of immunoreactivity of many normal and abnormal myocardial components. These techniques can be applied to myocardial biopsy specimens, as indicated by clinical or pathologic features, for either diagnostic or research purposes. Tissue should not be rinsed with saline before fixation because this results in severe artifacts. If electron microscopic study is to be performed, the tissue can be fixed either with 2.5 or 3% glutaraldehyde or with a mixture of 1% glutaraldehyde and 4% formaldehyde in 0.1 M phosphate buffer, pH 7.4 (McDowell's fixative). Fixation with this solution allows satisfactory preparations to be made for both light and electron microscopic study. Staining en bloc with uranyl acetate is not necessary for ultrastructural study and may interfere with the staining of glycogen particles.

Cardiac Hypertrophy and Fibrosis

Hypertrophy is evaluated with the use of light microscopy on the basis of the transverse diameters of the muscle cells (normally < 15 mm) and nuclear morphology. If necessary, additional evaluation is made with electron microscopy, which is useful in the determination of the presence and severity of degenerative changes that occur in the late stages of hypertrophy.[1] Structural alterations resulting from hypertrophy alone are increased size of the nuclei, Golgi complexes, and T-tubules; increased degrees of convolution of intercalated discs; increased numbers of ribosomes; focal accumulations of Z-band material; variability in mitochondrial size; and large accumulations of glycogen granules and mitochondria in perinuclear areas.

Degenerative changes in hypertrophied myocardium may involve almost every type of subcellular organelle and can occur in hypertrophy of any cause. The enlarged, dilated atria of patients with mitral valvular disease and atrial fibrillation show the most severe cellular degeneration. Perhaps the most important degenerative change is myofibrillar lysis, which results in loss of myofibrils and usually involves the thick (myosin) filaments more than the thin (actin) filaments. Thus, in the muscle cells, myofibrillar lysis often leaves numerous actin filaments that are no longer associated with myosin filaments. Z-bands are much wider than normal and actually may become confluent. Some of these Z-bands have a highly organized substructure similar to that seen in skeletal and cardiac muscle in nemaline myopathy. In cells undergoing myofibrillar loss, the sarcoplasmic reticulum (SR) can undergo proliferation and formation of various types of aggregates of SR tubules and cisterns. Other changes indicative of degeneration of cardiac muscle cells include intranuclear tubules, intramitochondrial and intranuclear deposits of glycogen (these also can occur in nondegenerated cells), accumulation of tangled masses of intermediate or cytoskeletal (100 Å in diameter) cytoplasmic filaments, dilatation and disorganization of T-tubules, formation of electron-dense concentric lamellae (myelin figures), dissociation of intercellular junctions and development of unusual (intracytoplasmic) junctions formed by two parts of the plasma membrane of the same cell (rather than by the plasma membranes of two different cells), thickening of the basal laminae of the muscle cells[1] and formation of spherical microparticles derived from the plasma membrane, particularly in junctional areas. These spherical microparticles should not be confused with viral particles.

Two types of *myocardial fibrosis* are recognizable. The first, *interstitial fibrosis*, is often associated with myocardial hypertrophy and is characterized by bands of fibrous connective tissue that encircle the cardiac muscle cells and separate them from adjacent cells. The second, *replacement fibrosis*, is associated with the healing of muscle cell necrosis and is characterized by patches of fibrous connective tissue in which cardiac muscle cells are either very scarce or absent. Ultrastructurally, both types consist of collagen fibrils, spicules, and stellate granules of proteoglycan material, small elastic fibers, and connective tissue microfibrils. The relative amounts of these components are variable.

Hypertrophic Cardiomyopathy

The term *hypertrophic cardiomyopathy* designates a group of cardiac disorders that are characterized by generalized, concentric cardiac hypertrophy (Fig. 50–1), which may be associated with asymmetric hypertrophy of the ventricular septum and with obstruction of left ventricular outflow.[2, 3] Studies have demonstrated that the majority of cases of these disorders involve mutations in the structure of various contractile proteins of the heart.[4, 5] However, the relationship among the biochemical, anatomic, and functional abnormalities in these disorders remains unclear. Several forms of hypertrophic cardiomyopathy are recognized anatomically according to whether obstruction of left ventricular outflow and asymmetric hypertrophy of the ventricular septum are present.[3] In most of the patients, the asymmetric thickening is maximal in the middle third of the ventricular septum. In a minority of patients, the mass of asymetrically

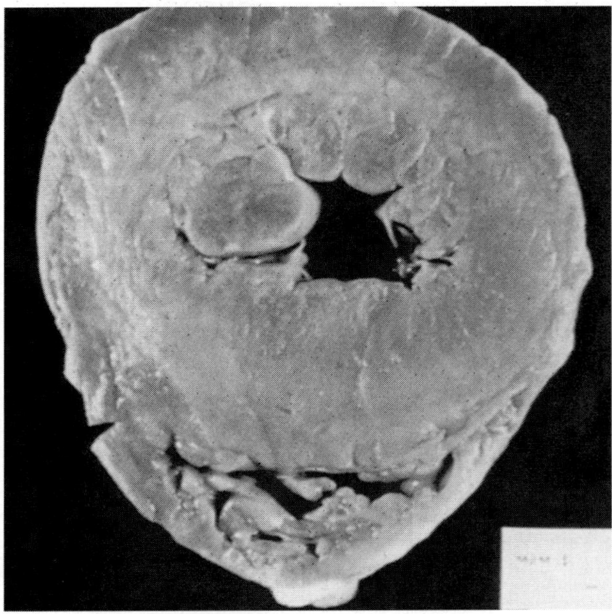

FIGURE 50–1 Concentric hypertrophy, left ventricle. Note the massive, concentric, symmetric hypertrophy of the left ventricle, including the ventricular septum and papillary muscles.

hypertrophied ventricular septal tissue is localized to the apical region of the left ventricle (apical hypertrophic cardiomyopathy). In a few patients, the obstruction is localized to the middle portion of the ventricular cavity (midventricular type of hypertrophic obstructive cardiomyopathy) and may be due to massive enlargement, with or without anomalous insertion, of the left ventricular papillary muscles. In many patients with the usual form of obstructive hypertrophic cardiomyopathy, the mitral valve, particularly the ventricular surface of the anterior leaflet, is thickened by fibrous and elastic tissue.[2, 3] A plaque of similar fibroelastotic thickening is present on the endocardium of the septal wall of the left ventricular outflow tract (Fig. 50–2). This plaque, which is thought to result from contact between the septal surface and the anterior mitral leaflet (as a consequence of systolic anterior motion of this leaflet), is removed during left ventricular myotomy-myectomy. Concentric cardiac hypertrophy, without asymmetric thickening of the ventricular septum, has been reported in patients with family members who had hypertrophic obstructive cardiomyopathy.[3] This concentric hypertrophy has been thought to represent another variant of hypertrophic cardiomyopathy.

The ventricular muscle in hypertrophic cardiomyopathy shows severe hypertrophy and foci of disarray, in which cells are arranged in whorls instead of in parallel and the myofibrils are oriented in different directions (Fig. 50–3). This disarray tends to be most prevalent in the ventricular septum and in the anterior and posterior free walls of the left ventricle. Quantitative studies have shown that in most patients, this disarray involves more than 5 percent of the total area of the ventricular septum and the left ventricular free walls.[6] Disarray is most pronounced in the central third of the septum, an area in which samples cannot be taken for endomyocardial biopsy. Myocardial fiber disarray is very frequently observed in myocardial biopsy samples from patients with hypertrophic cardiomyopathy; however, it is not specific for this disorder in a qualitative sense because it occurs focally, with involvement of less than 5 percent of the myocytes, in patients with various other disorders.[6] The diagnosis of hypertrophic cardiomyopathy should be neither made nor ruled out based only on the findings in the small areas of tissue included in myocardial biopsy samples.

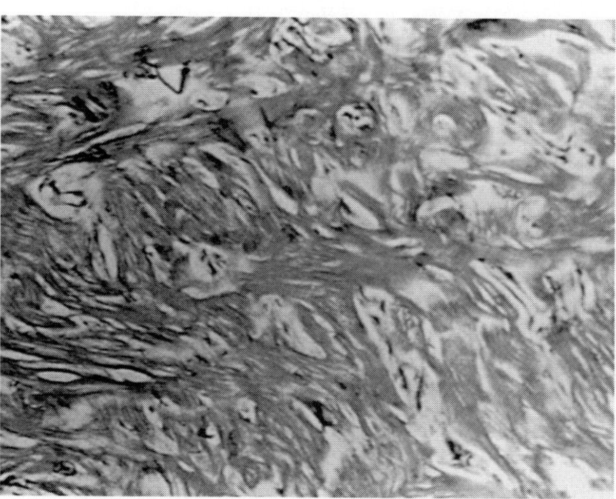

FIGURE 50–3 Asymmetric septal hypertrophy. Cardiac muscle shows marked hypertrophy with foci of disarray in which cells are arranged in whorls instead of in parallel and their myofibrils are oriented in various directions. This disarray is present in the ventricular septum and in the anterior and posterior free walls of the left ventricle (H&E, ×120).

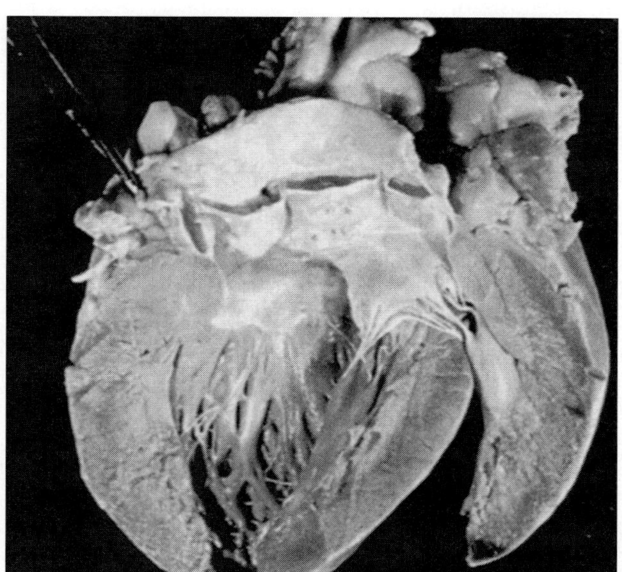

FIGURE 50–2 Asymmetric septal hypertrophy (idiopathic hypertrophic subaortic stenosis). Note the asymmetric hypertrophy of the upper and middle thirds of the ventricular septum (left). There is focal endocardial fibrosis (contact patch) involving the ventricular septum immediately below the aortic valve.

The small intramyocardial arterioles in many patients with hypertrophic cardiomyopathy, especially patients in the older age groups, may show severe degrees of thickening and narrowing by fibromuscular initimal proliferation and medial fibrosis.[3] In myocardial biopsy samples, such changes may be difficult to distinguish from those caused by artifactual contraction of the tissue at the time when the specimen is obtained.

DILATED CARDIOMYOPATHY

The term *dilated cardiomyopathy* designates a heterogeneous group of syndromes that are characterized anatomically by marked cardiac dilatation, mild or no thickening of the ventricular walls, mural thrombosis, atrioventricular valvular regurgitation due to displacement of the papillary muscles toward the apex, and varying degrees of fibrosis and myocardial cellular degeneration (Figs. 50–4 and 50–5). Foci of myocytolysis also may be present. The nonspecific nature of the histologic and ultrastructural changes precludes making the diagnosis of dilated cardiomyopathy on the basis of biopsy findings alone.[1] The histologic, immunohistochemical, and ultrastructural findings in dilated cardiomyopathy may be of clinical predictive value. Much attention is being given at the present time to the possibility that, in many cases, dilated cardiomyopathy develops as a consequence of myocarditis in which most of the initial inflammatory reaction has subsided, leaving myocyte damage and interstitial fibrosis. Dilated cardiomyopathy of unknown cause, with or without lymphocytic infiltrates, has been reported in some patients with acquired immune deficiency syndrome.

Peripartal cardiomyopathy and *alcoholic cardiomyopathy* are two syndromes of dilated cardiomyopathy that do not have specific microscopic features,[2, 7] although they are clinically distinct. Alcoholic cardiomyopathy may be complicated by thiamine deficiency (this can be determined only with biochemical studies). A significant number of patients with peripartal cardiomyopathy actually have lymphocytic myocarditis; therefore, endomyocardial biopsy is necessary to establish the proper diagnosis. *Anthracycline cardiomyopathy* is induced by the administration of daunorubicin or doxorubicin, two antibiotics used in cancer therapy. It is characterized microscopically by myofibrillar loss and by striking dilatation of the SR, which imparts a characteristic vacuolated appearance to the affected myocytes (Fig. 50–6).[8] The severity of these changes can be assessed in a semiquantitative manner in myocardial biopsies.[9, 10] This assessment is of value in deciding whether to continue the administration of these agents to patients suspected of developing anthracycline-induced cardiomyopathy.

Infantile cardiomyopathy with histiocytoid change is another type of cardiomyopathy with distinctive morphologic features,[11] which consist of yellow nodules composed of large, round, or elongated cardiac muscle cells that have lost practically all their contractile elements; are filled with mitochondria, lipid droplets, and glycogen; and show varying degrees of dissociation of their intercellular junctions. Thus far, these features have been reported only in small children presenting with the sudden onset of recurrent ventricular tachyarrhythmias, which have been fatal in many cases. The cause of this disorder remains unknown.

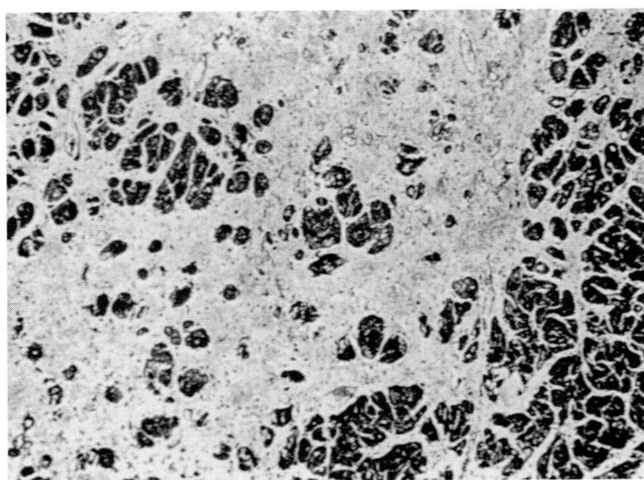

FIGURE 50–5 Dilated (congestive) cardiomyopathy. There is extensive myocardial cellular degeneration with replacement fibrosis (myocytes are dark; fibrosis is light). The remaining myocytes reflect compensatory hypertrophy with diffuse interstitial fibrosis (H&E, ×200).

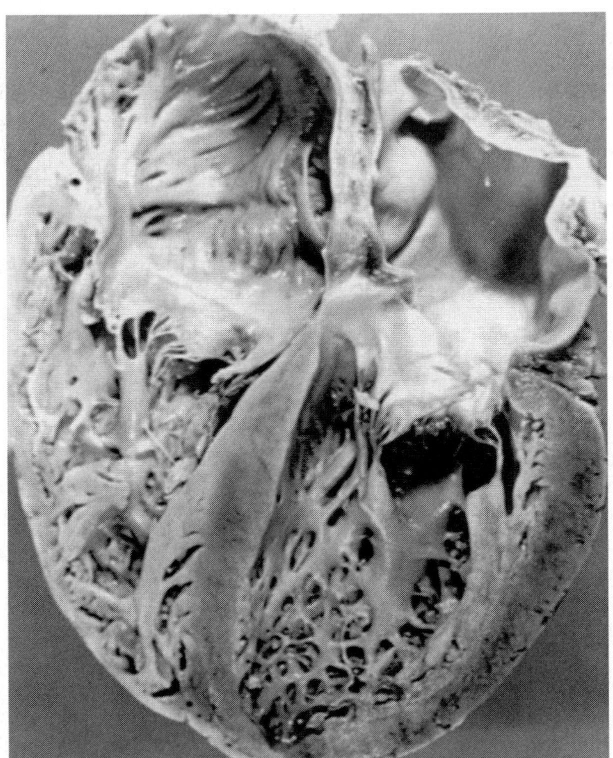

FIGURE 50–4 Dilated (congestive) cardiomyopathy. Note the marked dilatation of all cardiac chambers. The papillary muscles are thinned and displaced toward the apex, resulting in atrioventricular valvular regurgitation.

RESTRICTIVE CARDIOMYOPATHY

The diagnosis of restrictive cardiomyopathy is based primarily on the clinical and hemodynamic findings. The disorder can be caused by a variety of pathologic conditions, including the amyloidoses, hemochromatosis, chloroquine toxicity, and incompletely characterized diseases associated with abnormalities of desmin.[12] However, many patients with restrictive cardiomyopathy show only nonspecific changes of interstitial fibrosis on myocardial biopsy.[13] Myocardial biopsy samples from patients with restrictive cardiomyopathies associated with deposits of desmin have shown that this polypeptide forms large masses of granulofilamentous electron-dense material rather than the normal 10-nm filaments that normally interconnect adjacent

TABLE 50-1 Causes of Lymphocytic Myocarditis

Infection (viral, fungal, protozoal, rickettsial, bacterial, chlamydial, mycoplasmal)
Infectious mononucleosis
Aberrant immune response (postviral, Kawasaki disease, polymyositis, systemic lupus erythematosus, mixed connective tissue disease, other collagen-vascular diseases)
Drug reaction (hypersensitivity, drug-induced lupus, other)
Sarcoidosis (and other causes of granulomatous myocarditis)
Cardiac allograft rejection
Idiopathic process

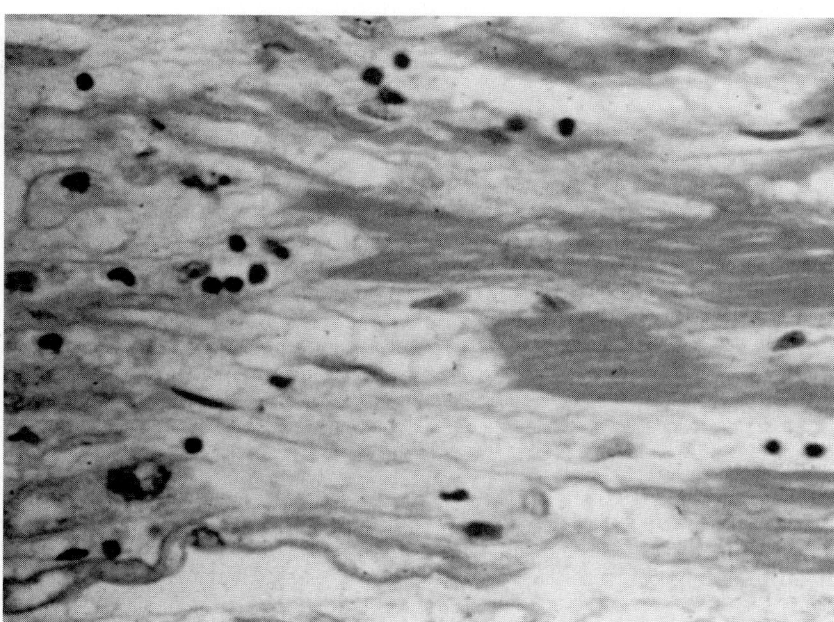

FIGURE 50–6 Toxic cardiomyopathy. Myocytolysis characterized by myofibrillar loss and by striking dilatation of the sarcoplasmic reticulum, which imparts a characteristic vacuolated appearance to the affected cells. An associated inflammatory cell response is minimal.

Z-bands.[12] Thus, staining for desmin should be performed in myocardial biopsy samples from patients with restrictive cardiomyopathy, particularly when this disorder is associated with skeletal myopathy.

MYOCARDITIS

Inflammatory cell infiltrates and myocyte damage or degeneration serve as the basis for the diagnosis of myocarditis,[14] which can be acute (infiltrates composed of polymorphonuclear leukocytes, lymphocytes, or both) or chronic (also including plasma cells, macrophages, and usually some degree of fibrosis). The timing of the endomyocardial biopsy with respect to the onset of the myocarditis is crucial to diagnosis and, perhaps, to therapeutic outcome. The interstitial cell population changes with time, as demonstrated in studies of animal models of viral myocarditis. In patients with progressive disease, decreasing numbers of lymphocytes and increasing numbers of fibroblasts have been observed with electron microscopy in serial endomyocardial biopsy samples.[14] Myocarditis can be caused by a wide variety of disorders, which usually present in predictable morphologic patterns, including inflammatory cell infiltrates characterized predominantly by granulomas, eosinophils, neutrophils, or lymphocytes. The morphologic types of myocarditis and their causes are summarized in Tables 50–1 through 50–4.

The most common type of myocarditis recognized by endomyocardial biopsy is lymphocytic myocarditis, which is presumed in most cases to be postviral and to be mediated by an aberrant immune response (Fig. 50–7). However, the histologic criteria for the diagnosis of lymphocytic myocarditis are controversial, largely because numerous types of mononuclear cells (which are connective tissue cells) in the myocardial interstitium resemble lymphocytes on conventional light microscopy (Table 50–5).

The identification of lymphocytes alone is not sufficient to establish the diagnosis of myocarditis. The presence of lymphocytes close to the sarcolemmal membranes of degenerating cardiac myocytes is helpful to establish the diagnosis of lymphocytic myocarditis.[14] Lymphocytes may be found in the myocardium of apparently normal individuals[15] and may be present in patients with such conditions as drug-associated myocardial damage (drug hypersensitivity or toxicity),[16] at the periphery of other types of lesions such as a granulomas,[17–19] or in ischemic lesions in the process of healing. Some disorders (e.g., lymphomas, leukemia, and so on) are associated with increased numbers

TABLE 50–2 Causes of Granulomatous Myocarditis

- Collagen-vascular disease (rheumatic fever, rheumatoid arthritis, ankylosing spondylitis, Wegener's granulomatosis)
- Metabolic disorder (Farber's disease, gout, oxalosis, granulomatous disease of childhood)
- Proliferative disorders of the mononuclear-phagocyte system (juvenile xanthogranuloma, Chester-Erdheim disease, malignant histiocytosis)
- Infection (bacterial, mycobacterial, fungal, parasitic, rickettsial, Whipple's disease)
- Sarcoidosis
- Hypersensitivity
- Foreign body granulomas
- Idiopathic

TABLE 50–3 Causes of Eosinophilic Myocarditis

- Drug hypersensitivity
- Disseminated eosinophilic collagen-vascular disease (Loeffler's syndrome)
- Parasitic infestation
- Wegener's granulomatosis
- Cardiac allograft rejection
- Idiopathic process

TABLE 50–4 Causes of Neutrophilic Myocarditis

Infarction
Infection
Direct (bacterial)
Indirect (toxic, as in diphtheria, or septic)
Leukoclastic vasculitis (collagen-vascular disease)

TABLE 50–5 Types of Mononuclear Cells in the Myocardial Interstitium

Lymphocytes	Perithelial cells
Plasma cells	Cardiac histiocytes
Mast cells	Macrophages
Schwann cells	Fibroblasts
Smooth muscle cells	Undifferentiated mesenchymal cells
Endothelial cells	

of lymphocytes in the heart without evidence of myocyte damage. Large numbers of myocardial lymphocytes may be present in these disorders, but this usually indicates a noninflammatory or neoplastic condition.

In such cases, an intensive search with the use of cultures, serologic studies, and appropriate tissue stains must be made for specific etiologic agents such as viruses, rickettsiae, bacteria, fungi, and parasites. Viruses are considered the most frequent cause of myocarditis but seldom are specifically identified. The value of viral cultures of myocardial biopsy specimens has not yet been established.

Rheumatic Myocarditis and Aschoff Nodules

Aschoff nodules, located in the endocardium or in perivascular areas, provide the basis for the diagnosis of the rheumatic process. They undergo a gradual evolution, during only part of which they show specific diagnostic features (Aschoff cells and fibrinoid necrosis) (see Fig. 17–4). Aschoff cells are large, mononucleated or multinucleated cells that contain serrated chromatin bars located in the central third of the nucleus, possess amphophilic cytoplasm, and have indistinct cytoplasmic borders. These cells differ from Anitschkow cells, which also have nuclear chromatin bars but are small and elongated, have a scanty cytoplasm lacking basophilia, and constitute a totally nonspecific finding.[1] A nonspecific lymphocytic myocarditis is frequently found in patients with rheumatic fever. In the absence of Aschoff nodules in a biopsy specimen, this rheumatic myocarditis cannot be accurately distinguished from that due to other causes.

Myocardial inflammatory reactions also occur in collagen-vascular diseases and in sarcoidosis. Lesions in collagen-vascular diseases include the following:

1. Nonspecific myocarditis, which occurs in dermatomyositis (with lymphocytic infiltrates) (Fig. 50–8) and systemic lupus erythematosus (often in association with fibrinoid necrosis, vasculitis, and pericardial and endocardial lesions)
2. Fibrosis, which occurs in scleroderma without being associated with a significant inflammatory reaction (Plate 50–1)
3. Rheumatoid nodules and less distinctive granulomatous lesions, which are found in rheumatoid arthritis (Plate 50–2)
4. Myocardial necrosis associated with vascular lesions, which occur in periarteritis nodosa, Wegener's granulomatosis (Plate 50–3), and thrombotic thrombocytopenic purpura[20]

The lesions in myocardial sarcoidosis consist of noncaseating granulomas with epithelioid cells and multinu-

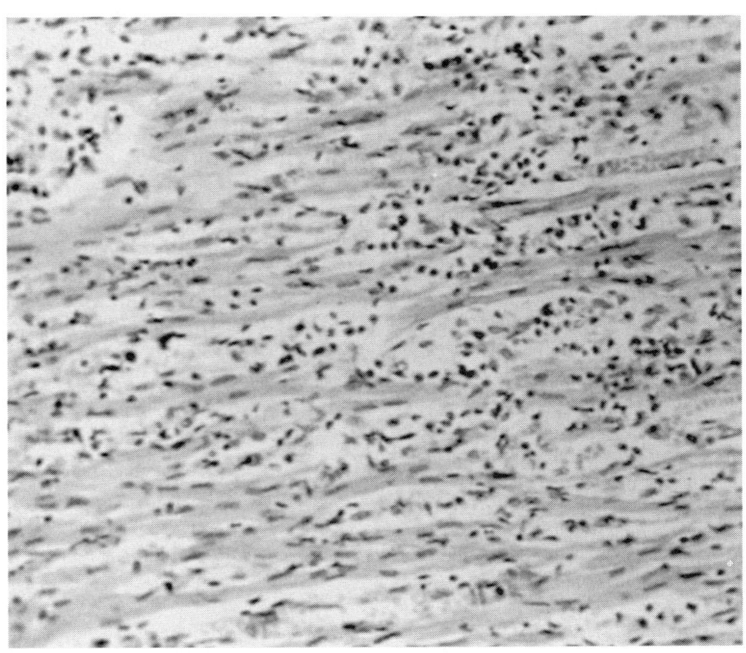

Figure 50–7 Lymphocytic myocarditis. Numerous lymphocytes are present close to the sarcolemmal membranes of degenerating cardiac myocytes (H&E, ×175).

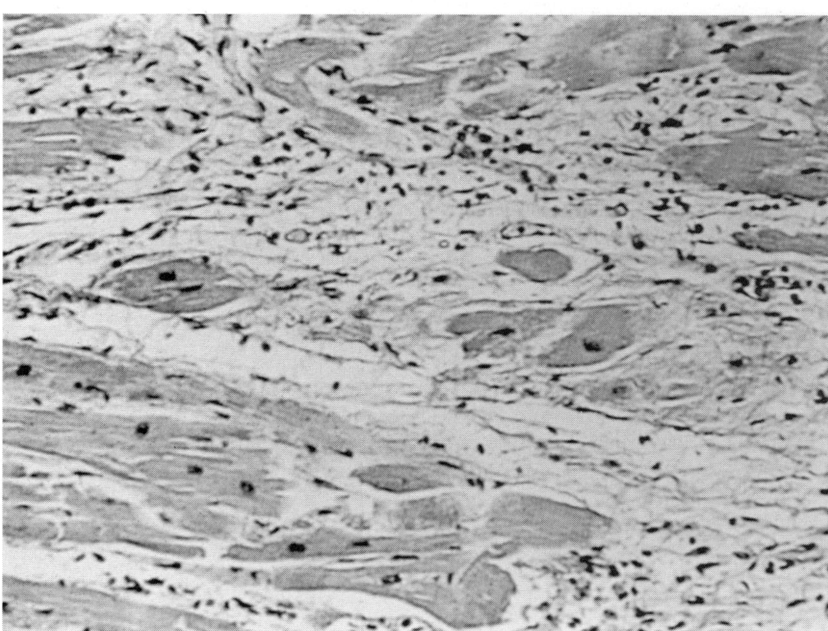

FIGURE 50–8 Polymyositis. This section of heart is from a patient with lymphocytic myocarditis with focal myocyte loss and replacement fibrosis. This evolution of lymphocytic myocarditis into dilated cardiomyopathy is referred to as *chronic myocarditis* (H&E, ×250).

cleated giant cells (Plates 50–4 and 50–5). Such lesions must be distinguished from other types of myocardial granulomatous processes and from giant cell myocarditis (Fig. 50–9 and Table 50–2).[14]

CARDIAC TRANSPLANTATION–MONITORING REJECTION

Percutaneous transvenous endomyocardial biopsy remains the most reliable means of detecting acute cardiac rejection and has contributed greatly to the increased survival rates of patients undergoing cardiac transplantations. Several systems have been used to grade the degree of cardiac allograft rejection.[21, 22] The Stanford system describes rejection as mild, moderate, or severe. At the Texas Heart Institute, cardiac allograft rejection is evaluated on a numerical scale ranging from 0 to 10 (Table 50–6). This scale was developed to provide numerical objectivity to the degree of cardiac allograft rejection and to enhance communication among the pathologist, surgeon, and cardiologist.[22] The prime determinant of higher grades of allograft rejection is the extent of cardiac myocyte degeneration (Figs. 50–10 and 50–11). By plotting the numerical value and the date of the patient's previous endomyocardial biopsies on the 0 to 10 scale, one can accurately determine

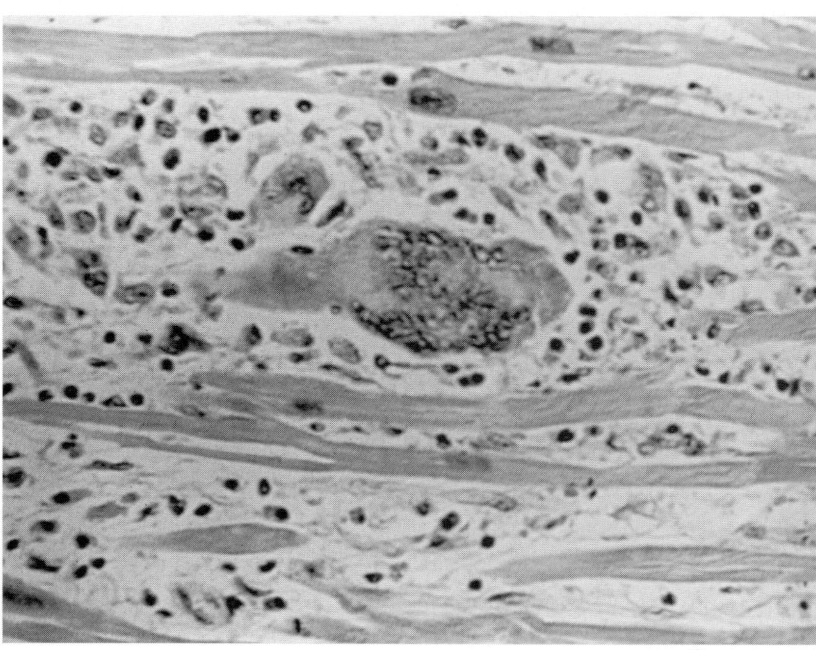

FIGURE 50–9 Lymphocytic myocarditis, myogenic giant cell. In rare patients with myocarditis, there is an abortive attempt by cardiac myocytes to regenerate, resulting in multiple nuclei accumulating in swollen portions of the myocytes. This condition should not be confused with cardiac sarcoid or other forms of granulomatous myocarditis (H&E, ×400).

TABLE 50–6 Texas Heart Institute Evaluation of Cardiac Allograft Rejection by Endomyocardial Biopsy

0	No evidence of rejection
1–2	Perivascular aggregates of mononuclear cells
3	Perivascular aggregates of mononuclear cells with extension into the interstitium
4–8	Interstitial mononuclear cells with cardiac myocyte degeneration of increasing severity
9–10	Extensive cardiac myocyte degeneration, interstitial mononuclear cells, and polymorphonuclear leukocytes

the degree of cardiac allograft rejection, the direction of change, and the speed of change. These parameters are important in determination of the patient's immunosuppressive regimen and the cardiac allograft biopsy interval.[22] Because of the differences between quantitative[23] and qualitative[24] systems, the International Society for Heart Transplantation convened an international meeting of pathologists from large, established transplantation centers to establish a universal grading system for biopsy interpretation.[25] The purpose of the consensus was not necessarily to change the grading systems in individual centers but rather to identify a system to which most other systems might be extrapolated for use in publications and multicenter drug trials. A comparison of the Texas Heart Institute, Stanford, and International Society for Heart Transplantation grading systems of cardiac allograft rejection is illustrated in Figure 50–12.

It also is important to consider the *differential diagnosis* of acute rejection in the interpretation of endomyocardial biopsy samples from these patients. During the first 2 weeks after transplantation, *ischemic injury* secondary to reperfusion is commonly encountered and is characterized by focal myocytolysis, with an infiltrate of macrophages and neutrophils rather than the predominantly lymphocytic infiltrate of acute rejection. Repeat biopsy samples frequently demonstrate the phenomena of healing at a previous biopsy site, including separation and disorganization of the myocytes by fibrin, granulation tissue, and, eventually, fibrosis. *Infection* (myocarditis) may also be seen in these immunocompromised patients and usually will produce a mixed inflammatory infiltrate rather than a purely mononuclear one; the organisms responsible (cytomegalovirus, *Toxoplasma*, various fungi) may or may not be identified in the biopsy specimen (Plate 50–6). Eosinophils may be a marker of infection but also are seen after treatment with cyclosporin in the absence of infection. *Resolving rejection* after the treatment of an acute rejection episode is characterized by resorption of necrotic myocytes and their replacement by hemosiderin-laden macrophages and fibroblasts. *Chronic rejection* is rarely encountered in endomyocardial biopsy material and is essentially a vascular phenomenon, with intimal proliferation and adventitial inflammatory infiltration in small and large coronary arteries.

METABOLIC AND STORAGE DISEASES

The diagnosis of glycogen storage disease should be based not only on the morphologic demonstration of increased amounts of glycogen but also on biochemical analysis of the glycogen structure and on identification of the enzymatic defect (in leukocytes, liver biopsy, or tissue culture of skin fibroblasts). Myocardial involvement is most severe in the infantile form (Pompe's disease) of type II glycogenosis but also occurs in types III and IV. In type II, the glycogen is morphologically and biochemically normal. In heart muscle, it is stored both within lysosomes and in the main cytoplasmic compartment. These deposits are associated with massive cardiomegaly and with a typical

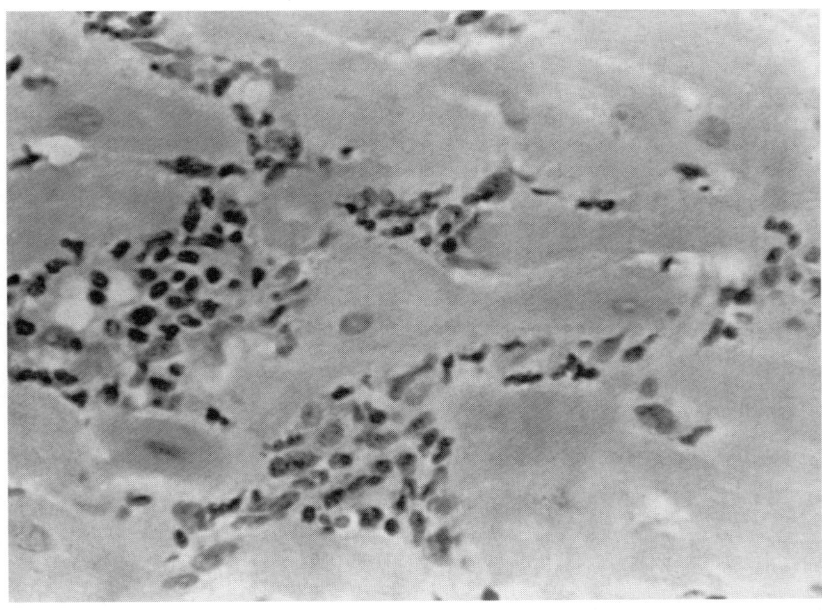

FIGURE 50–10 Cardiac allograft rejection, Texas Heart Institute (THI) grade 4. There is only occasional cardiac myocyte degeneration with associated lymphocytes in the sections available for examination. The pattern of lymphocytes close to the sarcolemmal membranes of degenerating cardiac myocytes appears to be identical to that of lymphocytic myocarditis (H&E, ×200).

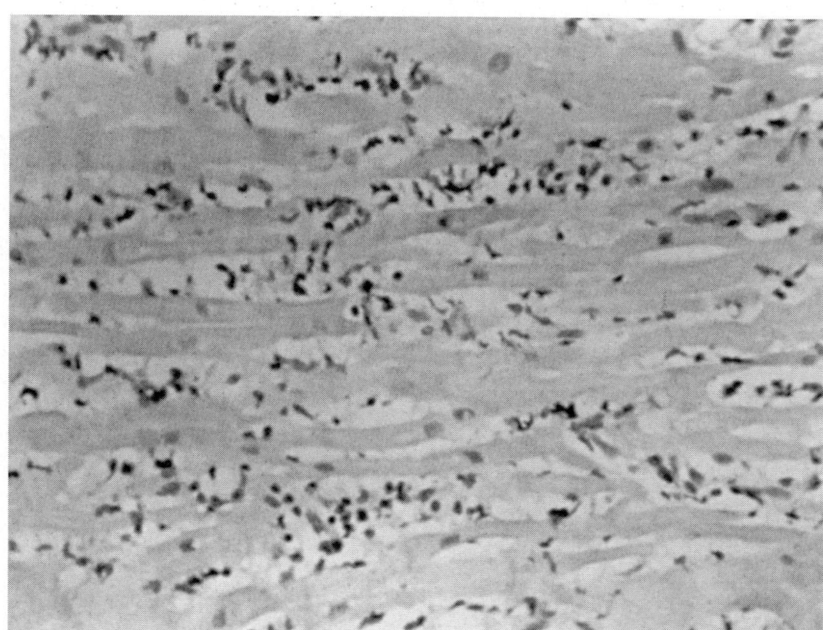

FIGURE 50–11 Cardiac allograft rejection, THI grade 8. There is extensive cardiac myocyte degeneration intimately associated with lymphocytes. Scattered eosinophils may also be present (H&E, ×200).

lacework appearance of the muscle cells (Fig. 50–13). In type III, the glycogen is morphologically normal but biochemically abnormal, and it is free in the cytoplasm. In type IV, the glycogen is both biochemically and morphologically abnormal; it is basophilic, free in the cytoplasm, and very slowly degraded by amylase, and it forms fibrils that measure about 40 to 50 Å in diameter that are ultrastructurally similar to those that occur in cardiac muscle cells in *basophilic degeneration* (a frequent, nonspecific incidental finding in the hearts of elderly individuals) and in the Lafora type of myoclonic epilepsy.[1, 26] Patients with phosphofructokinase deficiency, glycogen storage disease, and cardiac involvement have been reported.[27, 28] Two patients with glycogen storage disease limited to the heart and associated with deficient activity of cardiac phosphorylase kinase have been described.[29, 30] Two necessary notes of caution are that myocardial biopsy specimens often contain strikingly prominent pools of glycogen in perinuclear regions of the muscle cells (especially compared with necropsy specimens) and that glutaraldehyde fixation produces a marked artifactual increase in the intensity of the periodic acid–Schiff reaction.

Cardiovascular lesions in the *mucopolysaccharidoses* consist of deposits of acid mucopolysaccharides and often also of glycolipids (which have not been fully characterized) in pleomorphic (usually vacuolated) inclusions in cardiac muscle cells and in connective tissue and smooth muscle cells in endocardium, valves, and vessels. The large, extramural coronary arteries may display severe intimal thickening. Distinction between the cardiovascular morphologic findings in the various types of mucopolysaccharidoses and mucolipidoses is extremely difficult, and these findings should be closely correlated with extracardiac anatomic, clinical, and biochemical observations. The lesions in these disorders also must be distinguished[21] from those in GM$_1$ gangliosidosis, Sandhoff's disease (a type of G~ gangliosidosis), and Farber's disease (lipogranulomatosis).

Other disorders associated with lipid storage phenomena within cardiac muscle cells or cardiac connective tissue cells include *Fabry's disease*, in which the deposits contain glycolipids that show strong birefringence (Plate 50–7), are soluble in lipid solvents, and form parallel or concentric electron-dense lamellae with a regular periodicity (these

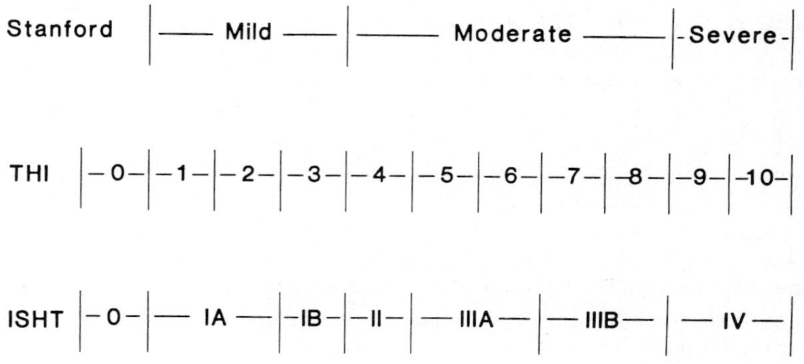

Stanford | — Mild — | — Moderate — | - Severe - |

THI | - 0 - | - 1 - | - 2 - | - 3 - | - 4 - | - 5 - | - 6 - | - 7 - | - 8 - | - 9 - | - 10 - |

ISHT | - 0 - | — IA — | - IB - | - II - | — IIIA — | — IIIB — | — IV — |

FIGURE 50–12 Comparison of Stanford, THI, and International Society for Heart Transplantation (ISHT) grading of cardiac allograft rejection.

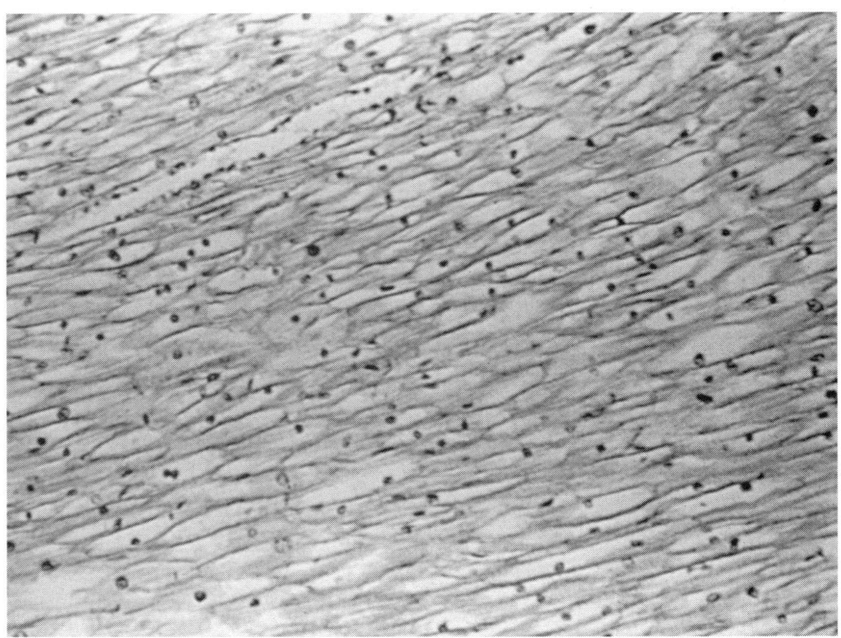

FIGURE 50–13 Pompe's disease. Note the extensive vacuolated appearance of the cardiac myocytes with nuclei that appear normal. The clear areas contain deposits of glycogen both within lysosomes and in the main cytoplasmic compartment, resulting in massive cardiomegaly and a typical lacework appearance of the muscle cells (H&E, ×150).

deposits also involve coronary endothelium and smooth muscle); *type I and type III hyperlipoproteinemia*, in which foam cells (containing neutral lipids) can form yellow patches in endocardium; homozygous *type II hyperlipoproteinemia*, in which cholesterol-rich foam cells can infiltrate the endocardium and coronary arteries; and *Gaucher's disease* and *Niemann-Pick disease*, in which foam cells (containing glucocerebroside and sphingomyelin, respectively) occasionally infiltrate the myocardial interstitium.[26] Lipid deposits containing cholesterol and triglycerides have been found not only in myocardium but also in valvular fibroblasts, in patients with Tangier's disease.[31] The lamellar deposits in the cytoplasm of cardiac myocytes in Fabry's disease and other metabolic disorders must be distinguished from those that occur in *chloroquine toxicity*. In the latter disorder, such deposits are associated with curvilinear bodies.[32, 33] *Triglyceride deposits* within cardiac muscle cells are found in numerous disorders, including carnitine deficiency, hypoxia and ischemia, alcoholic cardiomyopathy, Reye's syndrome, thyrotoxicosis, diabetes mellitus, prolonged hypotension, and conditions related to the toxicity of drugs and chemical agents.[26]

Other disease entities that must be considered in the differential diagnosis of myocardial storage disorders are hemochromatosis, hemosiderosis, oxalosis, and amyloidosis.[26, 34, 35] In *hemochromatosis and hemosiderosis*, the deposits show positive histochemical reactions for iron (Plate 50–8). In the various syndromes of primary and secondary oxalosis, the oxalate crystals can be identified in myocardium by polarization microscopy of routine paraffin sections and by specific histochemical staining (Plate 50–9). The green birefringence of Congo red–stained amyloid deposits and the identification of amyloid fibrils by electron microscopy establish the diagnosis of cardiac involvement in *amyloidosis* (Plate 50–10). Immunohistochemical staining with specific antibodies is useful to distinguish the different types of proteins involved in the formation of amyloid deposits.[36] Myocardium, endocardium, valves, and vessels (mainly intramural coronary arteries and arterioles) are involved to some extent in the majority of the syndromes of amyloidosis. Amyloid fibrils in myocardium must be distinguished from connective tissue microfibrils, which are larger in diameter (120 to 150 Å) than amyloid fibrils (100 Å), have a beaded appearance, and can be very numerous in fibrotic hearts. Amorphous deposits of electron-dense material have been found ultrastructurally in endocardium, myocardium, and blood in light chain disease associated with restrictive cardiomyopathy. Such deposits do not show the staining reactions typical of amyloid and can be recognized only by ultrastructural study or by immunohistochemical demonstration of the presence of immunoglobulin light chains.[37]

The cardiomyopathy in the *Duchenne type of progressive muscular dystrophy* is characterized by myocardial fibrosis that is preferentially distributed in subepicardial areas. Negative immunohistochemical staining for dystrophy is typically found in skeletal and cardiac muscle of patients with the disorder. Furthermore, such staining is patchy and discontinous in patients with the Becker type of muscular dystrophy.[38] Cardiac involvement without distinctive anatomic changes occurs in numerous other genetic neuromuscular disorders.[26]

Myocardial fiber atrophy, interstitial edema, and, rarely, inflammatory cell infiltrates have been described in obese patients who have severe, often fatal ventricular arrhythmias while ingesting a modified *liquid protein diet* as part of a weight-reduction program.[26]

Cardiac morphologic lesions reported in *endocrine disorders*[39] include myocardial hypertrophy and fibrosis in acromegaly, basophilic degeneration of the muscle cells in myxedema, focal myocarditis and myocytolysis in pheochromocytoma, observed vessel fiber calcification in hypercalcemia, focal vacuolization and hyalinization of the muscle cells in Cushing's syndrome (and also in hypokalemia of other causes), and hypertrophy in hyperthyroidism. Dilated cardiomyopathy has been reported in association with diabetes mellitus, but morphologic findings have been variable and nonspecific.[39] The basement membranes of myocardial capillaries have been reported to be thicker in diabetic and myxedematous patients than in control patients.[40]

Mural Endocardium

Mural endocardium in biopsy or surgical material should be evaluated with respect to (1) overall thickness, (2) layered arrangement, (3) type and number of cells present, (4) presence of overlying thrombus, and (5) relative amounts of extracellular components of connective tissue (i.e., collagen, elastic fibers, and proteoglycans). The pathologic reactions of mural endocardium to injury generally lead to endocardial thickening, of which several types are recognized on the basis of the predominant changes in the cellular and extracellular components of the endocardium.[1] Regional differences in normal endocardial thickness and layered structure must be taken into account: endocardium is much thicker and contains a much better developed layer of smooth muscle cells in the left atrium than elsewhere.

In *congenital endocardial fibroelastosis*, the thickness of ventricular and atrial endocardium is markedly increased, and the elastic fibers are very numerous and larger than normal. It should be noted that congenital endocardial fibroelastosis can be associated with carnitine deficiency.[41] Acquired endocardial fibroelastosis can be diffuse (a nonspecific finding in many conditions associated with ventricular dilatation) or focal (friction lesions, contact lesions, jet lesions); in these lesions, the elastic fibers are small, and the relative amounts of elastic fibers and collagen are variable.[1] The mural and valvular endocardial lesions in endomyocardial fibrosis and carcinoid heart diseases are described in the section on valves. Selective calcification of elastic fibers, which often assume a characteristic curled appearance, occurs in the mural endocardium and systemic vessels of patients with pseudoxanthoma elasticum.[26] Small, flat plaques containing amyloid deposits have been described in the mural endocardium in amyloidosis. Fibrous rings present in the left ventricular outflow tract of patients with fixed outlet subaortic stenosis have the usual layered structure of endocardium.[42] Pacing catheters inserted into the right ventricle become attached to mural endocardium by a small thrombus, which also forms a thin layer over the catheter surface. Organization of this thrombus leads to the formation of a tightly adherent white fibrous sheath composed of collagen, microfibrils, fibrin, and connective tissue cells.[1]

Myocardial Ischemia

Anatomic changes involving the myocardium in ischemic heart disease are

1. Cardiac muscle cell damage, necrosis, and associated inflammatory reaction
2. Myocardial fibrosis
3. Complications such as perforation of the ventricular septum or a ventricular free wall, various forms of papillary muscle dysfunction (which show variable degrees of necrosis, fibrosis, atrophy, and calcification), ventricular aneurysms, and embolic phenomena related to mural thrombi

Necrosis occurs in two main forms: (1) coagulation necrosis, which is basically limited to central regions of infarcts and is characterized by a relaxed appearance of the sarcomeres and by intramitochondrial flocculent deposits, and (2) necrosis with contraction bands, which is found in peripheral regions of infarcts and is characterized by deeply eosinophilic hypercontraction bands, intramitochondrial calcific deposits, and progression to myocytolysis.[43] Necrosis with contraction bands is thought to result from reperfusion of the ischemic area surrounding the central zone of coagulation necrosis. This type of necrosis is also observed in patients dying soon after cardiac operations (circumferential hemorrhagic necrosis), and it is characteristically severe in the stone heart syndrome. However, it is a nonspecific lesion, which can also be seen in other conditions, including prolonged hypotension, toxicity of endogenous or exogenous catecholamines, accidental and iatrogenic electrical injury, and myocarditis.

Apoptosis (programmed cell death) has been recently found to occur in cardiac myocytes, in addition to the two forms of myocardial necrosis (coagulation necrosis and necrosis with contraction bands) just described. It is characterized by nuclear and cytoplasmic condensation (rather than swelling), fragmentation of the chromatin and cleavage of the DNA into nucleosomes, and formation of apoptotic bodies derived from cellular breakdown. Apoptosis is associated with reperfusion injury of ischemic myocardium but also has been reported in myocardial immune rejection, dilated cardiomyopathy, arrhythmogenic right ventricular dysplasia, and viral myocarditis. Microscopically, apoptosis can be suggested by the finding of dark, condensed, hyperchromatic nuclei and cytoplasm. It can be identified by specific staining methods.[44] The implications of the finding of apoptosis in myocardium remain to be fully assessed.

The association of contraction band necrosis with coagulation necrosis in a myocardial biopsy specimen should suggest the possibility of acute myocardial infarction, particularly when lymphocytes are not a significant feature of the inflammatory infiltrate. Fibrosis associated with the healing of myocardial infarcts may lead to formation of ventricular aneurysms. Ventricular aneurysms and resected left ventricular papillary muscle (from patients undergoing mitral valve replacement for papillary muscle dysfunction) are the most common surgical pathology specimens related to ischemic heart disease.

Cardiac Aneurysms

The term *cardiac aneurysm* designates a spectrum of gross and microscopic changes associated with aneurysmal bulging of a segment of the ventricular wall. These changes consist of overall thinning of the ventricular wall, endocardial thickening by fibrous and elastic tissue, a decrease in the amount of cardiac muscle, and a corresponding increase in the amount of fibrous connective tissue in the wall (Fig. 50–14). In their most severe form, these changes lead to

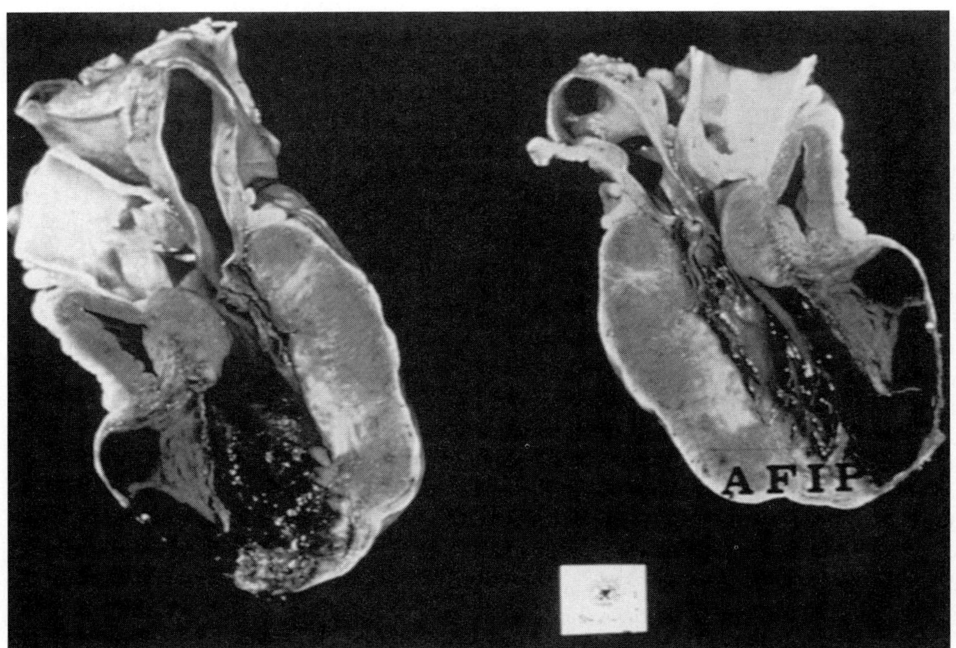

FIGURE 50–14 Cardiac aneurysm secondary to myocardial infarction. The aneurysmal sac is large and thin walled, contains minimal cardiac muscle, is partially filled with thrombus, and communicates via a large orifice with the main portion of the left ventricular cavity.

the formation of large aneurysmal sacs, which are thin walled, contain very little cardiac muscle in their walls, may be partially filled by laminated thrombi, and communicate via a large orifice with the main portion of the left ventricular cavity. Calcific deposits may be present in the aneurysmal wall. In less severe forms, the affected areas of the wall show lesser degrees of thinning, fibrosis, and endocardial thickening and contain more numerous cardiac muscle cells. The latter often show degenerative changes. The transition between fibrous aneurysmal wall and uninvolved myocardial wall may be gradual, and the borders of the ventricular aneurysm may be poorly demarcated.

The most common cause of true cardiac aneurysms is infarction of the anterior wall of the left ventricle. Apical aneurysms, however, are characteristically found in Chagas' disease.[45] They are formed by progressively severe thinning of the ventricular wall so that the aneurysmal wall contains practically only endocardium and visceral pericardium; such aneurysms also occur in idiopathic dilated cardiomyopathy[46] and, rarely, in hypertrophic cardiomyopathy.[47]

Pseudoaneurysm of the Heart

A pseudoaneurysm results when the myocardial wall ruptures, but the rupture is contained by adherent thrombus or by pericardial adhesions. The diagnosis is based on the following findings: (1) the orifice by which the pseudoaneurysm communicates with the cardiac chamber is small compared with the pseudoaneurysmal cavity, and (2) myocardial fibers are not present in the wall, which is a fibrous sac derived from parietal pericardium, organizing thrombus, or both. The latter distinction is best made through an examination of the borders of the resected specimen. The most common causes of cardiac pseudoaneurysm are (1) transmural myocardial infarction with cardiac rupture, (2) cardiac operations in which incisions are made in the left ventricular wall (or even in the ventricular septum, as in the myotomy-myectomy procedure for hypertrophic obstructive cardiomyopathy), and (3) various forms of trauma. Pseudoaneurysms are much more likely to rupture than are true cardiac aneurysms.

Annular Subvalvular Left Ventricular Aneurysms

Annular subvalvular aneurysms arise from the left ventricular cavity in the area of junction between the fibrous rings of the heart (most commonly the mitral and less frequently the aortic) and the left ventricular myocardium. These aneurysms are outpockets that extend through the tissue just below the ring toward the ventricular septum, the left atrium, or the epicardium.[48] They may contain laminated thrombus. They have a small circular opening with a rim fibrous tissue, and their walls usually are formed by collagenous tissue and may be partially calcified. They are not related to ischemic heart disease, and their cause is unknown.[48]

REFERENCES

1. Ferrans VJ, Butany JW: Ultrastructural pathology of the heart. *In* Trump BF, Jones RT (eds): Diagnostic Electron Microscopy. Vol 4. p. 319. New York: Churchill Livingstone, 1983.
2. Ferrans VJ, Rodriguez ER: The pathology of the cardiomyopathies. *In* Giles TD, Sander GE (eds): Cardiomyopathy. p. 15. Littleton, MA: PSG, 1988.
3. Maron BJ, Spirito P: Implications of left ventricular remodeling in hypertrophic cardiomyopathy. Am J Cardiol 81:1339–1344, 1998.
4. Schwartz K, Carrier L, Guicheney P, Komajda M: Molecular basis of familial cardiomyopathies. Circulation 91:532–540, 1995.
5. Charron P, Dubourg O, Desnos M, et al: Clinical features and prognostic implications of familial hypertrophic cardiomyopathy related

to the cardiac myosin-binding protein C gene. Circulation 97:230–236, 1998.

6. Maron BJ, Roberts WC: Quantitative analysis of cardiac muscle cell disorganization in the ventricular septum of patients with hypertrophic cardiomyopathy. Circulation 59:689, 1979.
7. Ferrans VJ, Buja LIM, Roberts WC: Cardiac morphologic changes produced by ethanol. *In* Rothschild MA, Oratz M, Schreiber S (eds): Alcohol and Abnormal Protein Biosynthesis. p. 139. New York: Pergamon, 1974.
8. Ferrans VJ: Overview of cardiac pathology in relation to anthracycline cardiotoxicity. Cancer Treat Rev 62:955, 1978.
9. Legha SS, Benjamin RS, Mackey B, et al: Reduction of doxorubicin cardiotoxicity by prolonged continuous intravenous infusion. Ann Intern Med 96:133, 1982.
10. Billingham ME, Mason JW, Brostow MR, Daniels JR: Anthracycline cardiomyopathy monitored by morphologic changes. Cancer Treat Rev 62:865, 1978.
11. Ferrans VJ, McAllister HA Jr, Haese WH: Infantile cardiomyopathy with histiocytoid change in cardiac muscle cells: report of six patients. Circulation 53:708, 1976.
12. Arbustini E, Morbini P, Grasso M, et al: Restrictive cardiomyopathy, atrioventricular block and mild to subclinical myopathy in patients with desmin-immunoreactive material deposits. J Am Coll Cardiol 31:645–653, 1998.
13. Arbustini E, Buonanno C, Trevi G, et al: Cardiac ultrastructure in primary restrictive cardiomyopathy. Chest 84:236–238, 1983.
14. McAllister HA Jr: Myocarditis: some current perspectives and future directions. Tex Heart Inst J 14:331, 1987.
15. Billingham M: The diagnostic criteria of myocarditis by endomyocardial biopsy. Heart Vessels 1 (suppl):133, 1985.
16. McAllister HA Jr, Hall RJ: Iatrogenic heart disease. *In* Cheng TO (ed): The International Textbook of Cardiology. p. 871. New York: Pergamon, 1986.
17. McAllister HA Jr, Ferrans VJ: Granulomas of the heart and major blood vessels. *In* Ioachim HL (ed): Differential Diagnosis of Granulomas. p. 75. New York: Raven, 1982.
18. McAllister HA Jr, Ferrans VJ: Eosinophilic and granulomatous inflammation of the heart. *In* Kapoor AS (ed): Cancer and the Heart: A Textbook of Cardiac Oncology. p. 246. New York: Springer-Verlag, 1986.
19. Edwards WD, Holmes DR Jr, Reeder GS: Diagnosis of active lymphocytic myocarditis by endomyocardial biopsy: quantitative criteria for light microscopy. Mayo Clin Proc 57:419, 1982.
20. McAllister HA Jr: Collagen diseases and the cardiovascular system. *In* Silver MD (ed): Cardiovascular Pathology. p. 1151. New York: Churchill Livingstone, 1991.
21. Billingham ME: Diagnosis of cardiac rejection by endomyocardial biopsy. Heart Transplant 1:25, 1982.
22. McAllister HA Jr, Schnee JM, Radovancevic B, Frazier OH: A system for grading cardiac allograft rejection. Tex Heart Inst J 13:1, 1986.
23. McAllister HA Jr: Histologic grading of cardiac allograft rejection: a quantitative approach. J Heart Transplant 9:277, 1990.
24. Billingham ME: Dilemma of variety of histopathologic grading systems for acute cardiac allograft rejection by endomyocardial biopsy. J Heart Transplant 9:272, 1990.
25. Billingham ME, Cary NRB, Hammand ME, et al: A working formulation for the standardization of nomenclature in the diagnosis of heart and lung rejection: Heart Rejection Study Group. J Heart Transplant 9:587, 1990.
26. Ferrans VJ: Metabolic and familial diseases. *In* Silver MD (ed): Cardiovascular Pathology. p. 1073. New York: Churchill Livingstone, 1991.
27. Hays AP, Hallett M, Delfs J, et al: Muscle phosphofructokinase deficiency: abnormal polysaccharide in a case of late-onset myopathy. Neurology 31:1077, 1981.
28. Amit R, Bashan N, Abarbanel JM, et al: Fatal familial infantile glycogen storage disease: multisystem phosphofructokinase deficiency. Muscle Nerve 15:455–458, 1992.
29. Elleder M, Shin YS, Zuntova A, et al: Fatal infantile hypertrophic cardiomyopathy secondary to deficiency of heart specific phosphorylase β kinase. 423:303–307, 1993.
30. Eishi Y, Takemura T, Sone R, et al: Glycogen storage disease confined to the heart with deficient activity of cardiac phosphorylase kinase: a new type of glycogen storage disease. Hum Pathol 16:193, 1985.
31. Mautner SL, Sanchez JA, Rader DJ, et al: The heart in Tangier disease. J Clin Pathol 98:191–198, 1992.
32. McAllister HA Jr, Ferrans VJ, Hall RJ, et al: Chloroquine-induced cardiomyopathy. Arch Pathol Lab Med 111:953, 1987.
33. Ratliff NB, Estes ML, Myles JL, et al: The diagnosis of chloroquine cardiomyopathy by endomyocardial biopsy. N Engl J Med 316:191, 1987.
34. Buja LM, Roberts WC: Iron in the heart: etiology and clinical significance. Am J Med 51:209, 1971.
35. Buja LM, Khoi NB, Roberts WC: Clinically significant cardiac amyloidosis. Am J Cardiol 26:394, 1970.
36. Arbustini E, Merlini G, Gavazzi A, et al: Cardiac immunocyte-derived (AL) amyloidosis: an endomyocardial biopsy study in 11 patients. Am Heart J 130:528–536, 1995.
37. McAllister HA Jr, Bossart M, Ferrans VJ, et al: Restrictive cardiomyopathy with kappa light chain deposits in myocardium as a complication of multiple myeloma: histochemical and electron microscopic observations. Arch Pathol Lab Med 112:1151, 1988.
38. Anan R, Higuchi I, Ichinari K, et al: Myocardial patchy staining of dystrophin in Becker's muscular dystrophy associated with cardiomyopathy. Am Heart J 123:1088–1089, 1992.
39. McAllister HA Jr: Pathology of the heart in endocrine disorders. *In* Silver MD (ed): Cardiovascular Pathology. p. 1181. New York: Churchill Livingstone, 1991.
40. Silver MD, Huckell VF, Lorber M: Basement membranes of small cardiac vessels in patients with diabetes and myxedema: preliminary observations. Pathology 7:213, 1977.
41. Bennett MJ, Hale DE, Pollitt RJ, et al: Endocardial fibroelastosis and primary carnitine deficiency due to a defect in the plasma membrane carnitine transporter [clinical conference]. Clin Cardiol 19:243–246, 1996.
42. Ferrans VJ, Muna WFT, Jones M, et al: Ultrastructure of the fibrous ring in patients with discrete subaortic stenosis. Lab Invest 39:30, 1978.
43. Jennings RB, Ganote CE: Ultrastructural changes in myocardium during acute ischemia. Circ Res 35 (suppl 3):156, 1974.
44. Anversa P, Leri A, Beltrami CA, et al: Myocyte death and growth in the failing heart. Lab Invest 78:767, 1998.
45. Santos-Buch CA: American trypanosomiasis: Chagas' disease. Int Rev Exp Pathol 19:63, 1979.
46. Alday LE, Moreyra E, Quiroga C, et al: Cardiomyopathy complicated by left ventricular aneurysms in children. Br Heart J 38:162, 1976.
47. Macma G, Singh A, Drew TM, et al: Asymmetric myocardial hypertrophy, left ventricular aneurysm, mural thrombus, and sudden death. Am Heart J 111:175, 1986.
48. Barbaresi F, Longhini C, Brunazzi C, et al: Idiopathic apical left ventricular aneurysm in hypertrophic cardiomyopathy: report of 3 cases, and review of the literature. Jpn Heart J 26:481, 1985.

CHAPTER 51

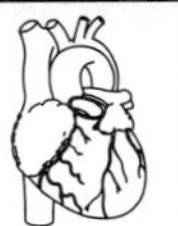

DILATED CARDIOMYOPATHY

Biykem Bozkurt and Douglas L. Mann

DEFINITION
EPIDEMIOLOGY
NATURAL HISTORY
Ischemic Cardiomyopathy Versus DCM
PATHOPHYSIOLOGY
ANATOMIC ABNORMALITIES
MYOCARDIAL DISEASES PRESENTING AS DCM
Idiopathic DCM
Familial Cardiomyopathy
Alcoholic or Toxic Cardiomyopathy
Inflammation-Induced Cardiomyopathy
Acquired Cardiomyopathy
Physical Agents
Autoimmune Mechanisms
CLINICAL RECOGNITION
Diagnostic Evaluation
TREATMENT STRATEGIES
Immunosuppression and Immunomodulation
Growth Hormone

DEFINITION

The term *dilated cardiomyopathy* (DCM) refers to a spectrum of heterogeneous myocardial disorders (Table 51–1) that are characterized by left ventricular (LV) dilatation or biventricular dilatation and depressed myocardial contractility.[1, 2] The DCMs constitute the largest group of myopathic disorders that are responsible for systolic heart failure. Indeed, more than 75 specific diseases can produce clinical manifestations that present with a DCM phenotype. Thus, DCM can be envisioned as the final common pathway for a myriad of cardiac disorders that either damage the heart muscle or, alternatively, disrupt the ability of the myocardium to generate force.

EPIDEMIOLOGY

The reported incidence of DCM varies annually from about 5 to 8 cases per 100,000 population. The true incidence may be underestimated owing to underreporting or underdetection of asymptomatic cases of DCM, which may occur in as many as 50 to 60 percent of patients. The age-adjusted prevalence of DCM in the United States averages 36 cases per 100,000 population and DCM accounts for 10,000 deaths annually.[3–5]

Compared with whites, African Americans have almost a threefold increase in risk for developing DCM. This increased risk is not explained by differences in hypertension, cigarette smoking, alcohol use, or socioeconomic factors. Moreover, African Americans have approximately a 1.5- to 2.0-fold higher risk of dying from DCM when compared with age-matched whites with DCM. Although the reasons for these differences are not known, there are several potential explanations including differences in the number of risk factors for development of heart failure, in the rate of progression of heart failure, the etiology of heart failure, responses to medical treatment, or access to medical care.

In general, heart failure is more common in men than in women. However, the overall effect of female gender on the prognosis of heart failure is not clear at this time, in large measure because many of the early clinical trials in heart failure have been composed predominantly of male subjects. For example, the treatment arm of the Studies on Left Ventricular Dysfunction (SOLVD), in which only 15 percent of the patients were women, reported no difference in gender-related survival in either the placebo or the enalapril group.[6] However, the SOLVD registry, which included approximately 20 percent female patients, suggested that women had a significantly higher annual risk of heart failure–related mortality and higher rates of hospitalization than did age-matched male subjects.[7] In the Italian Multicenter Cardiomyopathy Registry, women with idiopathic DCM tended to present with more advanced heart failure. However, the overall survival for woman was not statistically worse than for men, although there was a trend toward worse survival.[8] Thus, further studies are necessary to define the role of gender on the prognosis of heart failure.

Advancing age is a risk factor for mortality in heart failure. As reported in the SOLVD registry, the risk of death at 1 year for a person over the age of 64 years with heart failure was 1.5 times greater than for subjects who were less than 64 years of age.[7] Advancing age has been reported as an independent risk factor for mortality in DCM in several studies.[9, 10] Indeed, Sugrue and associates[11] reported that the relative risk of dying from heart failure increases by 0.51 with every 10 years of increase in age.

NATURAL HISTORY

The natural history of DCM is not well established for two reasons: (1) as noted at the outset, DCM represents a heterogeneous spectrum of myocardial disorders that may each progress at different rates, and (2) the onset of the disease may be insidious, particularly in the case of familial or idiopathic DCMs. Indeed, approximately 4 to 13 percent

TABLE 51–1 Etiologies of Dilated Cardiomyopathy

Idiopathic	
Idiopathic dilated cardiomyopathy	Idiopathic arrythmogenic right ventricular dysplasia
Familial (Hereditary)	
Duchenne's muscular dystrophy	Kearns-Sayre syndrome
Fascioscapulohumeral muscular dystrophy	Nemaline cardiomyopathy
Myotonic dystrophy	Multicore cardiomyopathy
Friedreich's ataxia	Erb's limb-girdle dystrophy
Alcoholic/Toxic	
Ethanol	Carbon monoxide
Cocaine	Lead
Adriamycin	Lithium
Catecholamine excess	Cyclophosphamide
Phenothiazines, antidepressants	Methysergide
Cobalt	
Inflammatory: Infectious	
Viral (coxsackievirus, cytomegalovirus, human immunodeficiency virus)	Spirochete
	Parasitic (toxoplasmosis, trichinosis, Chagas' disease)
Inflammatory: Noninfectious Etiology	
Collagen vascular disease: (scleroderma, lupus erythematosus, dermatomyositis)	Kawasaki's disease
	Hypersensitivity myocarditis
Miscellaneous Acquired Cardiomyopathy	
Postpartum cardiomyopathy	Obesity
Metabolic/Nutritional	
Thiamine	Hypervitaminosis D
Kwashiorkor	Selenium deficiency
Pellagra	Carnitine deficiency
Scurvy	
Endocrine	
Acromegaly	Cushing's disease
Thyrotoxicosis	Pheochromocytoma
Myxedema	Diabetes mellitus
Uremia	
Electrolyte Imbalance	
Hypophosphatemia	Hypocalcemia
Physiologic Agents	
Tachycardia	Hypothermia
Heat stroke	Radiation
Autoimmune Disorders	

of the patients with DCM will present with asymptomatic LV dysfunction and LV dilatation. For these patients, the overall prognosis is unclear. However, once DCM patients become symptomatic, the available evidence suggests that the prognosis is relatively poor, with a 25 percent mortality at 1 year and a 50 percent mortality at 5 years (Fig. 51–1).[12] The cause of death appears to be primarily pump failure in approximately 70 percent of patients with DCM, and sudden cardiac death accounts for approximately 30 percent of all deaths in patients with DCM.[13–15] However, it should be recognized that many of the natural history studies of DCM were performed before angiotensin-converting enzyme (ACE) inhibitors and beta blockers were routinely used. More recent studies suggest that the prognosis for patients with DCM and mild LV dilatation may be more favorable, perhaps reflecting earlier diagnosis and better

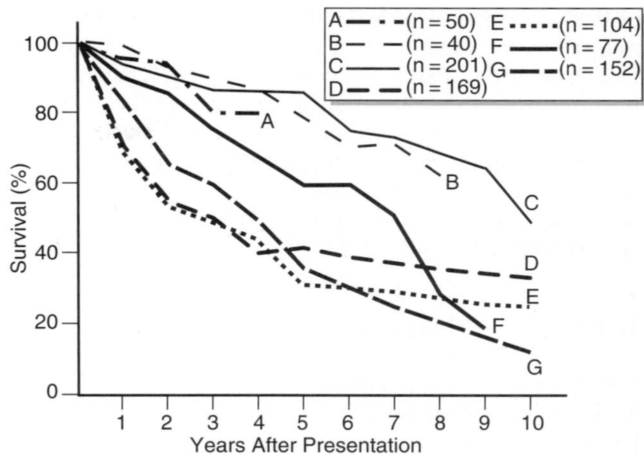

FIGURE 51–1 Survival of patients with idiopathic dilated cardiomyopathy in seven published series (A to G). n, number of patients enrolled. To identify each specific series, please refer to the article by Dec and Fuster.[12] (From Dec GW, Fuster V: Idiopathic dilated cardiomyopathy. N Engl J Med 331:1564–1575, 1994. Copyright © 1994 Massachusetts Medical Society. All rights reserved.)

treatment.[11] Furthermore, approximately 25 percent of DCM patients with the recent onset of symptoms of heart failure will improve spontaneously, including those who have been referred for cardiac transplantation.[16, 17] This statement notwithstanding, patients with symptoms lasting more than 3 months who present with severe clinical decompensation generally have less chance of recovery.[17]

As shown in Table 51–2, a number of other parameters predict a poor prognosis in patients with DCM, including left and right ventricular enlargement,[10, 18–20] persistent third heart sound (S_3) gallop, right-sided heart failure, pulmonary hypertension, electrocardiographic findings of first- or second-degree atrioventricular (AV) block or left bundle branch block, recurrent ventricular tachycardia,[21] myocytolysis on endomyocardial biopsy,[22, 23] elevated levels of neurohormones (norepinephrine, plasma renin activity, atrial natriuretic peptide, and endothelin-1), elevated levels of cytokines (tumor necrosis factor-alpha and interleukin-

TABLE 51–2 Factors Predicting a Poor Prognosis in Patients With Dilated Cardiomyopathy

Left ventricular enlargement[10, 18, 19]
Right ventricular enlargement[20]
Persistent S_3 gallop
Right-sided heart failure
Pulmonary hypertension
ECG findings: first- or second-degree atrioventricular block or LBBB
Recurrent ventricular tachycardia[21]
Myocytolysis on endomyocardial biopsy[22, 23]
Elevated levels of neurohormones (NE, PRA, ANF, and ET-1)
Elevated levels of cytokines (TNF-α and IL-6)[24, 25]
Peak oxygen consumption < 10–12 ml/kg/min[26–28]
Serum sodium < 137 mmol/L[29]
Advanced age (>64 yr)[7]

Abbreviations: ANF, atrial natriuretic factor; ECG, electrocardiographic; ET-1, endothelin-1; IL-6, interleukin-6; LBBB, left bundle branch block; NE, norepinephrine; PRA, plasma renin activity; S_3, third heart sound; TNF-α, tumor necrosis factor-α.

6),[24, 25] peak oxygen consumption less than 10 to 12 ml/kg/min,[26–28] serum sodium less than 137 mmol/L,[29] and age greater than 64 years.[7] Concomitant renal or hepatic dysfunction is likely to have an impact on prognosis that is not easily elucidated, insofar as these may limit the use of optimal diuretics or ACE inhibitors. Finally, it should be emphasized that comorbid conditions, such as diabetes and hypertension, increase the risk of developing heart failure approximately fivefold.

Ischemic Cardiomyopathy Versus DCM

The differential treatment benefit seen in DCM patients compared with patients with ischemic cardiomyopathy that has been observed in several randomized clinical trials suggests that patients with DCM have a better prognosis than patients with ischemic cardiomyopathy.[30, 31] However, although existing clinical studies suggest that patients with idiopathic DCM have a lower total mortality, the risk of sudden cardiac death appears to be relatively higher in patients with DCM in some studies.

PATHOPHYSIOLOGY

Figure 51–2 provides a general conceptual framework for discussing the development and progression of DCM. As shown, DCM may be viewed as a progressive disorder that is initiated after an "index event" either damages the heart muscle, with a resultant loss of functioning cardiac myocytes, or alternatively, disrupts the ability of the myocardium to generate force, thereby preventing the heart from contracting normally. This index event may have an abrupt onset, as in the case of acute exposure to toxins; or it may have a gradual or insidious onset, as in the case hemodynamic pressure or volume overloading; or it may be hereditary, as in the case of many of the familial cardiomyopathies. Regardless of the nature of the inciting event, the feature that is common to each of these index events is that they all, in some manner, produce a decline in pumping capacity of the heart. In most instances, patients will remain asymptomatic or minimally symptomatic after the initial decline in pumping capacity of the heart, or they will develop symptoms only after the dysfunction has been present for some time.

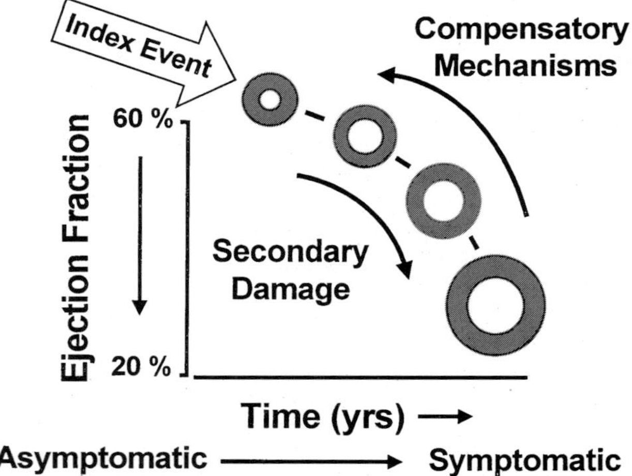

FIGURE 51–2 Pathogenesis of heart failure. Heart failure begins after an "index event" produces an initial decline in the pumping capacity of the heart. After this initial decline in the pumping capacity of the heart, a variety of compensatory mechanisms are activated, including the adrenergic nervous system, the renin angiotensin system, and the cytokine system. In the short term, these systems are able to restore cardiovascular function to a normal homeostatic range, with the result that the patient remains asymptomatic. However, with time, the sustained activation of these systems can lead to secondary end-organ damage within the ventricle, with worsening left ventricular remodeling and subsequent cardiac decompensation. Because of resultant worsening left ventricular remodeling and cardiac decompensation, patients undergo the transition from asymptomatic to symptomatic heart failure.

Although the precise reasons why patients with LV dysfunction remain asymptomatic is not certain, one potential explanation is that a number of compensatory mechanisms become activated in the setting of cardiac injury or depressed cardiac output that appear to be able to sustain and modulate LV function for a period of days to months to years. The portfolio of compensatory mechanisms that have been described include early activation of the sympathetic nervous system and salt- and water-retaining systems in order to preserve cardiac output,[32, 33] as well as activation of a family of vasodilatory molecules, including prostaglandins (PGE_2 and PGI_2)[34, 35] cytokines,[36, 37] and nitric oxide.[34, 35] However, it bears emphasis that our understanding of the family of molecules that may be involved in this process is far from complete. Moreover, we have very little information with respect to how genetic background, gender, age, or environment affects these compensatory mechanisms.

As shown in Figure 51–2, the compensatory mechanisms that are activated after the initial decline in the pumping capacity of the heart are able to modulate LV function within a physiologic or homeostatic range, such that the functional capacity of the patient is preserved or is depressed only minimally. Thus, patients may remain asymptomatic or minimally symptomatic for a period of years. However, at some point, patients will become overtly symptomatic, with a resultant striking increase in morbidity and mortality. Why this transition to symptomatic heart failure occurs, exactly how this transition occurs, and whether it occurs in all patients with LV dysfunction remain unknown. What is known, however, is that the transition to symptomatic heart failure is accompanied by further activation of neurohormonal and cytokine systems, as well as further LV remodeling.

ANATOMIC ABNORMALITIES

Patients with DCM generally present with dilatation of all four chambers of the heart (Fig. 51–3). Despite the fact that there is thinning of the LV wall in patients with DCM, there is massive hypertrophy at the level of the intact heart, as well as at the level of the cardiac myocyte, which has a characteristic elongated appearance that is observed in myocytes obtained from hearts subjected to chronic volume overload (Fig. 51–4). The coronary arteries are usually normal in DCM, although it should be emphasized that the

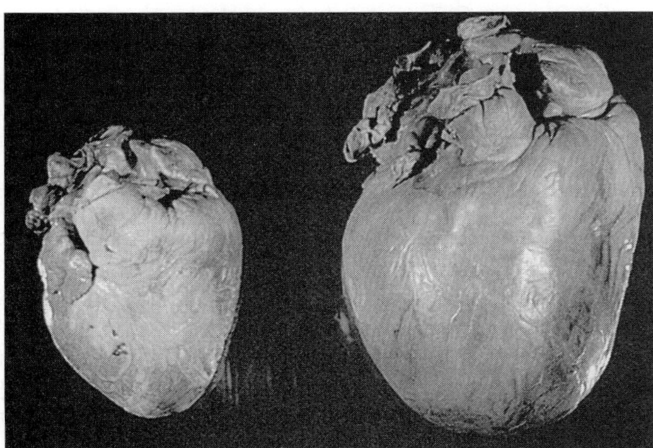

FIGURE 51–3 Pathology of a normal heart (*left*) and a dilated cardiomyopathic ventricle (*right*). The dilated cardiomyopathic ventricle is characterized by enlargement of all four cardiac chambers and a more spherical shape than the normal ventricle. (From Schumacher B, Luderitz B: Rate issues in atrial fibrillation: consequences of tachycardia and therapy for rate control. Am J Cardiol 82:29N–36N, 1998; reproduced with permission from Excerpta Medica Inc.)

end-stage "ischemic cardiomyopathies" may also present with a dilated phenotype. The cardiac valves are anatomically normal; however, there is usually tricuspid and mitral annular dilatation owing to cavity enlargement, distortion of subvalvular apparatus, and stretching of the papillary muscles giving rise to valvular regurgitation. Intracavitary thrombi are common usually in the ventricular apex.

The changes previously discussed that occur within the dilated left ventricle have been referred to collectively as *left ventricular remodeling*.[38, 39] Whereas the complex changes that occur in the heart during LV remodeling have been traditionally described in strict anatomic terms, as

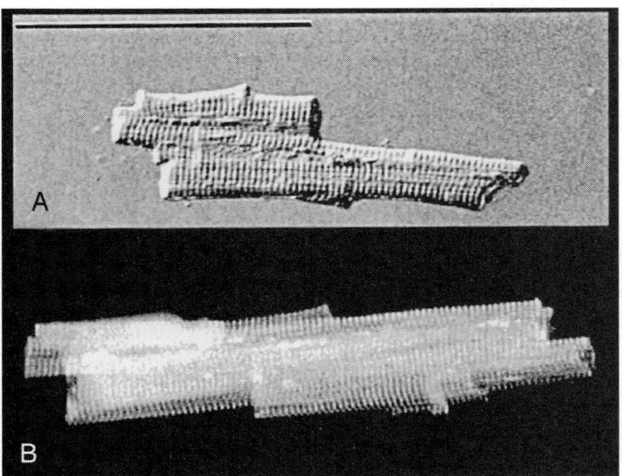

FIGURE 51–4 Cardiac myocyte structure in normal myocardium **(A)** and in dilated cardiomyopathy **(B)**. Cardiac myocytes isolated from the myocardium from patients with dilated cardiomyopathy are elongated as the result of the sarcomeres being formed in series. (**A** and **B,** From Fazio S, Sabatini D, Capaldo B, et al: A preliminary study of growth hormone in the treatment of dilated cardiomyopathy. N Engl J Med 334:809–814, 1996. Copyright 1996, Massachusetts Medical Society. All rights reserved.)

TABLE 51–3 Overview of Left Ventricular Remodeling

Alterations in Myocyte Biology
Excitation-contraction coupling
Myosin heavy chain (fetal) gene expression
ß-Adrenergic desensitization
Hypertrophy with loss of myofilaments
Cytoskeletal proteins
Myocardial Changes
Myocyte loss
Necrosis
Apoptosis
Alterations in extracellular matrix
Matrix degradation
Replacement fibrosis
Alterations in Left Ventricular Chamber Geometry
Increased wall stress
Mitral valve incompetence
Wall thinning with afterload mismatch

shown in Table 51–3, it is now recognized that the process of LV remodeling also has an important impact on the biology of the cardiac myocyte, on changes in the volume of myocyte and nonmyocyte components of the myocardium, and on the geometry and architecture of the LV chamber. Although each of these various components of the remodeling process may contribute importantly to the overall development and progression of heart failure, it is extremely unlikely that any single aspect of the remodeling process itself will satisfactorily explain the progressive cardiac decompensation that occurs as heart failure advances. The changes that occur at the level of the cardiac myocyte include changes in excitation-contraction coupling,[40] decreased alpha-myosin heavy chain gene expression with a concomitant increase in beta-myosin heavy chain expression,[41] progressive loss of myofilaments in cardiac myocytes,[42] alterations in cytoskeletal proteins,[42] as well as desensitization of beta-adrenergic signaling.[43] The changes that occur at the level of myocardial tissue include myocyte loss secondary to necrosis and apoptosis,[44–48] as well as alterations in the extracellular matrix such as matrix degradation and replacement fibrosis.[49–51] Lastly, the changes that occur at the level of the intact left ventricle include increased sphericity, LV dilatation, and LV wall thinning. It should be emphasized that the changes in the remodeled ventricle create a number of de novo mechanical burdens for the ventricle, including increased end-diastolic wall stress (secondary to increased LV volume) and increased hemodynamic overloading (secondary to functional mitral regurgitation). Taken together, the mechanical burdens that are engendered by LV remodeling might be expected to lead to worsening heart failure. Indeed, natural history studies have shown repeatedly that increases in LV volume and mass have been closely linked to future deterioration in LV performance and a less favorable clinical course.[39, 52, 53]

Myocardial Diseases Presenting as DCM

As shown in Figure 51–5, the most common causes of DCM are idiopathic, familial, alcoholic or toxic, viral, and

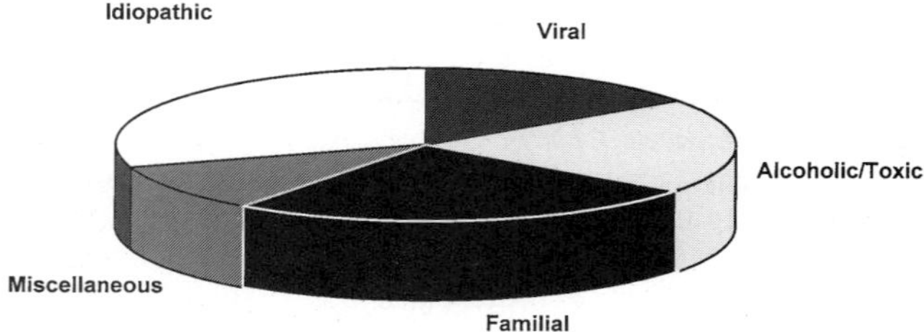

FIGURE 51–5 Etiologies of dilated cardiomyopathy. As shown, the most frequent causes of dilated cardiomyopathy, in descending order of frequency, are idiopathic, familial, alcoholic/toxic, viral, and miscellaneous others (inflammatory noninfectious, acquired, metabolic, and nutritional).

miscellaneous other causes (inflammatory noninfectious, acquired, metabolic, and nutritional). However, it should be recognized that the exact prevalence of the various forms of DCM will vary based on the demographics of the patient population. In this section, we review the etiologies that lead to the development of DCM.

Idiopathic DCM

Although the term *idiopathic dilated cardiomyopathy* has become synonymous with that of DCM in some heart failure parlance, the term *idiopathic* was originally intended to characterize the subset of DCM patients in whom no known etiology for ventricular dilatation and depressed myocardial contractility was apparent. However, with increasing sophistication in diagnostic testing, clinicians have become aware that many cases of so-called idiopathic DCM may occur as the result of inherited or spontaneous mutations of genes that regulate cardiac structure or function, such as the genes for cytoskeletal proteins. Thus, it is likely that many cases of so-called idiopathic DCM will prove to have a genetic basis. Furthermore, it is very likely that many cases of idiopathic DCM may occur in patients with undiagnosed hypertension, undiagnosed viral illness, or undiagnosed toxin exposure. Nonetheless, in the context of the present chapter, we use the terminology of *idiopathic dilated cardiomyopathy* to refer to those patients with DCM whose etiology remains unknown. As shown in Figure 51–5, idiopathic DCM represents the largest subset of patients with DCM; however, as alluded to immediately previously, it is likely that the proportion of patients with idiopathic DCM will diminish with increased sophistication in diagnostic testing.

Familial Cardiomyopathy

There is growing evidence that many cases of previously diagnosed "idiopathic" DCMs have a genetic basis. Indeed, although the familial occurrence of idiopathic DCM was first recognized by Battersby and Glenner in 1961,[53] it has not been until recently that investigators have been able to delineate the molecular basis for genetic cardiomyopathies. It is estimated that at least 20 to 30 percent of DCM cases are familial.[54] The pattern of inheritance of genetic cardiomyopathies is largely autosomal dominant; however, X-linked and autosomal recessive modes of inheritance have also been described.

Table 51–4 presents an overview of the known familial DCMs. It should be recognized that there will undoubtedly be other genes that will be linked to the development of cardiomyopathy as well. As discussed later, many of the genetic defects that have been identified in familial cardiomyopathy are related to defects in cytoskeletal proteins, including dystrophin and actin,[55–58] suggesting that defects in proteins that enable the myocardium to contract or

TABLE 51–4 Genetic Basis for Familial Cardiomyopathy

Author	Chromosomal Location	Gene Abnormality	Disease
Autosomal Dominant			
Kass et al[59]	1p1-1q1	Unknown	FDCM
Krajinovic et al[172]	9q13-q22	Unknown	FDCM
Durand et al[55]	1q32	Unknown	FDCM
Olson et al[58]	3p22-p25	Cardiac actin	FDCM
Bowles et al[173]	10q21-q23	Unknown	FDCM
Rampazzo et al[174]	1q42-q43	Actinin	ARVD
Rampazzo et al[174]	14q23-q24	Actinin	ARVD
X-Linked			
Towbin et al[57]	Xp21	Dystrophin	XLCM
Muntoni et al[175]	Xp21	Dystrophin	XLCM
Bolhuis et al[176]	Xq28	G4.5 gene	Barth's syndrome
D'Adamo et al[64]	Xq28	G4.5 gene	X-linked EFib
D'Adamo et al[64]	Xq28	G4.5 gene	Severe XLCM
Zeviani et al[178]	Mitochondrial	mtDNA gene	XLCM
Suomalainen et al[177]			
Hoffman et al[179]	Xp21	Dystrophin	Duchenne's MD
Gold et al[63]	Xp21	Dystrophin	Becker's MD
Autosomal Recessive			
Goldblatt et al[180]	Unknown	Unknown	FDCM
Michaud et al[181]	Unknown	Unknown	Alström's syndrome

Abbreviations: ARVD, arrhythmogenic right ventricular dysplasia; EFib, endocardial fibrosis; FDCM, familial dilated cardiomyopathy; MD, muscular dystrophy; XLCM, X-linked cardiomyopathy.

generate force will lead to the development of a DCM phenotype.

Autosomal Dominant Cardiomyopathy

The precise molecular causes of the majority of DCMs that have an autosomal dominant mode of inheritance are not known. However, as shown in Table 51–4, a number of laboratories have identified the chromosomes that harbor the mutations that are thought to be linked to the observed DCM phenotypes. For example, linkage analysis has mapped a family with DCM and conduction system disturbances to chromosome 1 (1p1-1q1).[59] However, the precise genes that are responsible for this disorder are not known at present. More recently, two unrelated families with DCM have been identified in which there is a missense mutation of the cardiac actin gene.[58] Both mutations affected conserved domains of the actin molecule that are responsible for attaching actin to the Z bands and the intercalated discs. Individuals in both families had a variable age (1 to 41 years) at the time of diagnosis.[58] Heart biopsy samples from these patients revealed histologic features characteristic of DCM.

X-Linked Familial Cardiomyopathy

Some families with DCM show convincing evidence of an X-linked cardiomyopathy. An X-linked mode of inheritance of DCM is suggested by the early onset in males, late onset in females, and lack of male-to-male transmission. The late onset of the disease in females, in contrast to the early onset in hemizygous males, is compatible with heterozygosity for the mutant allele. Since many cases of genetically lethal X-linked syndromes appear to be sporadic, for every case of "idiopathic" DCM in which X-linked inheritance can be confirmed from family information, it is possible that the development of the cardiomyopathy may be related to a new mutation.[60]

Duchenne's and Becker's Dystrophies

Duchenne's and Becker's dystrophies are X-linked disorders that represent a group of progressive skeletal muscle disorders that present primarily as a skeletal muscle myopathy with pseudohypertrophy of the affected limb muscles. Classic *Duchenne's muscular dystrophy* is transmitted from the mother to half of her sons as a manifest disease and to half of her daughters as a carrier state. The incidence of Duchenne's muscular dystrophy is 1 in 3500 males, making Duchenne's muscular dystrophy the most common X-linked disease in humans. The prevalence of the disease reflects the relatively high sporadic mutation rate and is thought to account for approximately one third of the new cases of the disease. Duchenne's muscular dystrophy is caused by abnormalities of a gene located at the Xp21 locus of the short arm of the X chromosome. The Duchenne muscular dystrophy gene has been cloned and identified as a cytoskeletal gene termed *dystrophin.* Dystrophin is a high-molecular-weight (156-kD) glycoprotein that links the cytoskeleton of the myocyte to the extracellular matrix and may thus stabilize the membrane. Overt clinical manifestations of Duchenne's muscular dystrophy begin in the second year of life. Creatine kinase elevations from skeletal muscle leak are present at birth and precede the onset of the clinical disease. The disease typically presents in children as walking difficulty and a clumsy, waddling gait. Cardiac involvement is a frequent occurrence in Duchenne's muscular dystrophy (>80 percent), although actual heart failure represents a terminal event in only a minority ($\approx$10 percent) of affected boys.[61] Female carriers of Duchenne's muscular dystrophy may have cardiac symptoms as well,[62] and DCM may be the presenting manifestation in affected carrier females.

Becker's muscular dystrophy is considered to be a milder allelic variant of Duchenne's muscular dystrophy; however, the clinical phenotype, including the cardiac involvement, is considered to be much more variable. In general, Becker's muscular dystrophy is later in onset and slower in progression than is Duchenne's dystrophy. The severity of cardiomyopathy is generally not related to age, and cardiomyopathy may be the presenting symptom of Becker's muscular dystrophy in rare instances.[63] Patients who reach adulthood will generally present with a DCM and may die as a result of complications arising from the cardiomyopathy.

Barth's Syndrome

Barth's syndrome is an X-linked disorder characterized clinically by the associated features of cardiac and skeletal myopathy, short stature, and neutropenia. The clinical manifestations of the disease are, in general, quite variable, but cardiac failure as a consequence of cardiac dilatation and hypertrophy is a constant finding and the most common cause of death in the first months of life. As shown in Table 51–4, the phenotype has been linked to markers at Xq28. X-linked cardiomyopathies with clinical manifestations similar to those of Barth's syndrome have been reported, and it has been proposed that they may be allelic. Molecular genetic studies have linked together what were formerly considered three different conditions and have shown that abnormalities of the G4.5 gene are responsible for Barth's syndrome, X-linked endocardial fibroelastosis, and severe X-linked cardiomyopathy. Very severe cardiac phenotypes may be associated with null mutations in the gene, whereas mutations in alternative portions or missense mutations may give rise to a phenotype that is less severe.[64]

Autosomal Recessive Cardiomyopathy

Although the number of DCMs that have been linked to an autosomal recessive mode of inheritance are relatively few, as shown in Table 51–4 at least two DCM phenotypes appear to have this mode of inheritance.

Alcoholic or Toxic Cardiomyopathy

Alcoholic Cardiomyopathy

Chronic alcoholism is one of the most important causes of DCM worldwide.[65] It is estimated that two thirds of the adult population use alcohol to some extent, and more than 10 percent are heavy users.[66] A large proportion of chronic alcoholics demonstrate impairment of cardiac function. The clinical diagnosis of alcoholic cardiomyopathy can be made when biventricular dysfunction and dilatation are persistently observed in a heavy drinker in the absence of other known causes for myocardial disease.[67] Thus, the diagnosis of alcoholic cardiomyopathy remains a diagnosis of exclusion. In some series, as many as 21 percent of subjects with excessive alcohol intake were reported to have clinical evidence of heart failure.[68] Alcoholic cardiomyopathy most commonly occurs in men 30 to 55 years of age who have been heavy consumers of alcohol for more than 10 years.[69] Even before the clinically overt heart failure, LV contractile dysfunction can be demonstrated in alcoholics. Although chronic alcoholic liver disease and heart failure are not usually observed clinically in the same patient, cirrhotic patients may present with asymptomatic LV dysfunction, in which case atrial fibrillation is usually the initial presenting manifestation of cardiac dysfunction.[70]

The risk of developing alcoholic cardiomyopathy is related to both the mean daily alcohol intake and the duration of drinking. Most patients in whom alcoholic cardiomyopathy develops have been drinking over 80 g/da for more than 5 years. However, it bears emphasis that there is significant individual susceptibility to the toxic effects of alcohol. For example, it is not known whether the persistent DCM that develops in only 1 to 2 percent of chronic drinkers occurs because of genetic predisposition or the presence of synergistic cardiovascular risk factors.

Studies in experimental animals have demonstrated that both acute and chronic ethanol administration impairs cardiac contractility. Alcohol results in acute as well as chronic depression of myocardial contractility even when ingested by normal individuals in quantities consumed during social drinking.[71] Compensatory mechanisms, such as vasodilatation or sympathetic stimulation, may mask the direct acute myocardial depressant effects of alcohol.[72] Despite the known deleterious effects of alcohol, it has been difficult to produce heart failure in animal models in which ethanol has been administered. Thus, the direct causal relationship between alcohol consumption and the development of cardiomyopathy has not been rigorously demonstrated in experimental models, despite the long-recognized clinical relationship between alcohol consumption and the development of DCM.

The potential mechanisms that have been invoked to explain the depressed myocardial function include the direct toxic effects of alcohol on striated muscle, because most alcoholics have manifestations of skeletal myopathy and cardiomyopathy.[73, 74] Alcohol and its metabolite acetaldehyde can also cause alterations in cellular calcium, magnesium, or phosphate homeostasis. The toxic effects of acetaldehyde or the formation of fatty acid ethyl esters may also impair mitochondrial oxidative phosphorylation. In acute ethanol toxicity, free radical damage or ischemia may occur, possibly due to increased xanthine oxidase activity or β-adrenergic stimulation, respectively.[75] In addition, ethanol and its metabolites interfere with numerous membrane and cellular functions such as transport and binding of calcium, mitochondrial respiration, lipid metabolism, myocardial protein synthesis, signal transduction, and excitation-contraction coupling.[66, 73, 76] Thus, the cardiomyopathy that develops after chronic alcohol consumption may be multifactorial in origin. Both autopsy and endomyocardial biopsy specimens from alcoholic cardiomyopathy patients reveal marked mitochondrial swelling, with fragmentation of cristae, swelling of endoplasmic reticulum, cytoskeletal disorganization, and destruction of myofibrils.[75] Several studies suggest that heavy drinking alters both lymphocyte and granulocyte production and function, raising the possibility that myocardial damage secondary to prolonged alcohol consumption might initiate autoreactive mechanisms comparable with those observed in viral or idiopathic myocarditis. In addition, nutritional deficiencies, commonly thiamine deficiency, may play an additive role to the direct myocardial damage of ethanol.[72]

The management of patients with alcohol cardiomyopathy begins with total abstinence from alcohol, in addition to the conventional management of heart failure, as described later. Numerous reports detail the reversibility of depressed LV dysfunction after the cessation of drinking.[77, 78] Even if the depressed LV function does not normalize completely, the symptoms and signs of congestive heart failure improve after abstinence.[78] However, the overall prognosis remains poor, with a mortality of 40 to 50 percent within 3 to 6 years, if the patient continues to drink despite being symptomatic with heart failure.[70]

Cocaine Cardiomyopathy

A detailed description of the toxic effects of cocaine on the myocardium are described in Chapter 105, Substance Abuse and the Heart, of this text. It bears emphasis that long-term cocaine use may eventuate in a DCM in previously healthy individuals. In 84 asymptomatic cocaine abusers studied at least 2 weeks after abstinence from the drug, Bertolet and colleagues[79] found that 7 percent had LV dysfunction. These patients were young and did not have evidence of myocardial infarction or coronary arterial disease.[79] Chakko and coworkers noted depressed LV function (left ventricular ejection fraction [LVEF] < 45 percent) in 4 percent of asymptomatic cocaine abusers hospitalized for rehabilitation.[80] As discussed in Chapter 105, Substance Abuse and the Heart, of this text, cocaine may produce LV dysfunction through direct toxic effects on the myocardium, by provoking coronary arterial spasm (and hence myocardial ischemia), and by causing increased release of catecholamines, which may be directly toxic to cardiac myocytes.[81] Myocarditis with inflammatory lymphocyte and eosinophils has also been reported in 20 percent of patients dying of natural or homicidal causes in whom cocaine was detected, raising the possibility of hypersensitivity myocarditis owing to cocaine or associated contaminants.[82] Alternatively, the myocarditis may occur directly in response to the necrosis that is caused by cocaine.

Other than abstinence, very little is known about the treatment of cocaine-induced cardiac dysfunction. Indeed, there are case reports of reversibility of cardiac function after cessation of drug use.[83] Given that some of the toxicity of cocaine is caused by catecholamine excess or myocardial ischemia, the use of β-adrenergic blocking agents may prove to be beneficial, both in terms of preventing further disease progression and for treating the ventricular arrhythmias that are prone to develop in this setting.

Anthracycline

Anthracyclines, such as doxorubicin (Adriamycin) and daunorubicin, produce cardiac toxicity possibly by increasing oxygen free radical generation, platelet-activating factor, prostaglandins, histamine, calcium, and ^{13}C hydroxy metabolites, or by interfering with the sarcolemmal sodium-potassium pump and mitochondrial electron transport chain.[84] Acute anthracycline toxicity generally has a fulminant course and may be fatal in some cases. The prognosis of mild to moderate heart failure with anthracycline-induced cardiomyopathy relates to the time course of treatment and preexisting additional risk factors for myocardial injury, such as radiation, coexisting coronary artery disease, and preexisting cardiac dysfunction. In general, patients with anthracylcine-induced cardiomyopathy generally have a worse survival than that seen with idiopathic DCM. Among children treated with anthracyclines, females are more sensitive to cardiotoxic effects of this agent than are males, although the reason is unknown.[85]

The most powerful predictor of anthracycline toxicity is the total cumulative dose administered. Clinically apparent cardiotoxicity is rare (>3 percent) below cumulative doses of 400 mg/m^2; however, toxicity becomes increasing more frequent with higher doses. Nonetheless, subclinical cardiac toxicity can be demonstrated at lower doses. For example, Bristow and associates[86] demonstrated evidence of myocyte damage on endomyocardial biopsy in 93 percent of the patients who received greater than 272 mg/m^2 and in 3 percent of the patients who received as little as 45 mg/m^2.

The current guidelines for administration and monitoring of patients receiving doxorubicin is as follows: doxorubicin should *not* be administered to patients with a baseline LVEF of 30 percent or less. If the baseline LVEF is between 30 and 50 percent, LV function should be assessed before each subsequent dose, and doxorubicin therapy should be discontinued if LVEF declines by 10 percent or more or to a value less than 30 percent. If, on the other hand, the patient has a baseline LVEF of 50 percent or greater, an assessment of LVEF should be repeated after the patient has received a total dose of 300 to 350 mg/m^2, and then again after each subsequent dose of doxorubicin. Therapy should be discontinued if LVEF declines by 10 percent or more or to a value less than 50 percent. The use of continuous infusion of doxorubicin, rather than bolus dosing, or the coadministration of antioxidants or free radical scavengers may reduce cardiotoxicity is some patients.[87] In addition to the guidelines for administration of doxorubicin outlined previously, patients who develop heart failure should be managed with conventional heart failure management (see later), which may lead to symptomatic improvement in 65 to 87 percent of patients.[88] Indeed, complete reversal of LV dysfunction has been reported in anecdotal cases.[89]

Other Myocardial Toxins

In addition to the classic toxins described previously, as shown in Table 51–1, a number of other toxic agents may lead to LV dysfunction and heart failure, including cobalt and catecholamines.

Inflammation-Induced Cardiomyopathy

Since the mid-1980s, increasing evidence suggests that inflammation or inflammatory processes may contribute to the overall pathogenesis of DCM. Moreover, there is increasing evidence that biologic properties of inflammatory mediators, such as proinflammatory cytokines, are also sufficient to produce a DCM phenotype.[90, 91] As discussed later, both infectious and noninfectious inflammatory processes may lead to the development of DCM. Although a great many infectious and noninfectious processes may affect the myocardium and may transiently lead to systolic dysfunction and congestive symptoms, the great majority of these infectious and noninfectious processes do not lead to the development of DCM. Therefore, in the section that follows, we focus primarily on those disease states that are considered to lead to DCM.

Infectious Causes

VIRAL CARDIOMYOPATHY

The subject of viral myocarditis is covered in detail in Chapter 55, Myocarditis. As shown in Table 51–5, the list of the viruses known to involve the myocardium is extensive. However, of the viral infections that affect the heart, the Coxsackie group of enteroviruses is associated with the highest incidence of cardiac involvement. The overall prevalence of myocarditis in patients with suspected viral illness ranges from 2.3 to 5 percent.[92] However, the true incidence of viral myocarditis is difficult to determine because of the limited methods for identification of viral infection of the heart.

The mechanisms by which the viruses produce myocardial damage are not at all clear. Potential mechanisms include direct cytopathogenetic effects of the invading virus, or viral persistence; spasm of the coronary microvasculature; and immunologic mechanisms involving macrophages, natural killer cells, T lymphocytes, autoantibodies directed against myosin, and cytokines such as interleukin-1-beta and tumor necrosis factor-α.[93] Each of these mecha-

TABLE 51–5 Viral Causes of Dilated Cardiomyopathy

Coxsackievirus types A and B
Poliomyelitis virus
Influenza virus types A and B
Human immunodeficiency virus
Adenovirus
Enteric cytopathogenic human orphan (ECHO) virus
Cytomegalovirus
Epstein-Barr virus
Rubeola virus
Mumps virus
Respiratory syncytial virus
Varicella-zoster virus
Rabies virus
Hepatitis virus
Yellow fever virus
Smallpox virus
Lymphocytic choriomeningitis virus
Epidemic hemorrhagic fever virus
Dengue virus

nisms may act singly or in combination to produce direct toxic effects on the myocardium.[94] Although activation of the immune system is initially beneficial because it limits the spread of infection, the immune response may act as a double-edged sword, insofar as excessive immune responses can lead to disease progression independent of the initial viral infection.

Both clinical and experimental data suggest that viral myocarditis is biphasic. The initial phase is infective with myocytolysis, lymphocytic infiltration, and a humoral immune response. The second phase is associated with a persistent antigen-antibody reaction between the virus and the myocardium. Myocarditis may be *acute* with lymphocytic infiltration and myocytolysis; *persistent active,* with continuing changes including inflammatory infiltrates, myocyte necrosis, and interstitial fibrosis; *healing,* with persistent inflammatory cell infiltrates but no myocyte necrosis; and *healed,* with the absence of necrosis and of inflammatory cell infiltrates but with interstitial fibrosis. This state is indistinguishable from DCM. The benefit from any therapeutic intervention is unlikely to occur when myocarditis is healed. Lymphocytic inflammatory cell infiltration alone is not sufficient indication for such therapy because such infiltration may be found in DCM and also in toxic myocarditis resulting from drug use.[95]

The presentation of viral myocarditis is quite variable, ranging from a clinically unapparent or relatively benign illness to acute progressive heart failure and death. The long-term follow-up studies of patients with suspected viral myocarditis reveal progression to DCM in a significant number of cases. The overall prognosis for patients with viral myocarditis is relatively benign, with the majority (50 to 60 percent) recovering spontaneously.[96] However, if there is persistent LV dysfunction, the overall prognosis is somewhat worse. Although the results of the Myocarditis Treatment Trial[97] suggest that there was a 5 to 10 percent increase in ejection fraction (over 28 weeks) in patients recovering from lymphocytic viral myocarditis, the overall mortality for the patients in this trial was still 20 percent at 1 year and 56 percent at 4.3 years. In contrast to patients with lymphocytic viral myocarditis, the results of a recent multicenter database study suggest that the natural history of giant cell myocarditis has a distinctly worse prognosis. In this retrospective database analysis of 66 patients with giant cell myocarditis, the rate of death or cardiac transplantation was approximately 90 percent, with a median survival of 5.5 months from the onset of symptoms.[98]

The clinical diagnosis of viral myocarditis should be suspected in a patient who presents with signs and symptoms referable to DCM with no apparent cause and whose clinical history suggests an antecedent viral illness within the preceding weeks to months before the onset of heart failure symptoms. The diagnosis of viral myocarditis is supported by the presence of myocarditis or viral genomic DNA on endomyocardial biopsy or by the identification of virus in stool, throat washings, blood, or pericardial fluid. A fourfold increase in virus neutralizing antibody, complement fixation, or hemagglutination inhibition titers is also supportive, although these tests are not routinely performed in most clinical settings. Although examination of the endomyocardial biopsy specimen is helpful for confirming the clinical diagnosis of myocarditis, the sampling error and differences in histologic interpretation decrease the overall specificity and sensitivity. In addition, the current "gold standard" for diagnosing myocarditis, the Dallas criteria (Table 51–6), may be too specific and therefore lack inherent sensitivity.[99] That is, the Dallas criteria require that both myocyte necrosis and degeneration are associated with an inflammatory infiltrate that is adjacent to the area of myocyte injury. To overcome this inherent limitation, the presence or absence of viral genomic DNA in myocardial samples is currently undergoing evaluation as a more sensitive means for diagnosing viral myocarditis. Indeed, enteroviral RNA has been detected in the myocardium of patients at all stages of the disease process, including acute myocarditis and chronic DCM. Persistence of viral RNA, particularly of enteroviral RNA, has been implicated in progression to DCM. Koide and colleagues[100] detected enteroviral RNA sequences in human endomyocardial biopsy samples in 32 percent of patients with clinical DCM and in 33 percent of patients with clinical myocarditis, using polymerase chain reaction (PCR) technology. In their study, patients who had histologic findings of myocarditis and clinical features resembling DCM had a high incidence ($\approx$85 percent) of enteroviral RNA sequences detected by PCR. Importantly, approximately 25 percent of patients with DCM who had no histologic findings of active myocarditis also had enteroviral RNA sequences detected by PCR. However, there is significant variability in frequency of detection of enteroviral RNA in endomyocardial tissue samples, with values ranging from 0 to 42 percent.[101] Thus, the validation of PCR technology as a reliable means for diagnosing viral myocarditis requires further refinement and study.

At the time of this writing, the therapy for viral myocarditis is primarily supportive. Although most of the agents

TABLE 51–6 Dallas Criteria for Diagnosing Myocarditis*

First Biopsy

Myocarditis with/without fibrosis
Borderline myocarditis
No myocarditis

Subsequent Biopsies

Ongoing (persistent) myocarditis with or without fibrosis
Resolving (healing) myocarditis with or without fibrosis
Resolved (healed) myocarditis with or without fibrosis

Inflammatory Infiltrate Classified as

Lymphocytic (mild, moderate, severe, focal, confluent)
Eosinophilic
Neutrophilic
Giant cell
Granulomatous
Mixed

*According to the Dallas criteria,[99] the diagnosis of *myocarditis* can be made only if myocyte necrosis, degeneration, or both, are associated with an inflammatory infiltrate adjacent to the degenerating or necrotic myocytes. *Borderline myocarditis* implies that the inflammatory infiltrate is too sparse and the damage to myocytes is not demonstrable. In borderline cases, additional levels of tissue or additional biopsies are recommended to further clarify the diagnosis. According to the Dallas criteria, the diagnosis of ongoing or persistent myocarditis can be made if myocarditis is associated with persistent myocyte damage and necrosis. The Dallas criteria further characterizes the inflammatory infiltrate based on the cell type and quantifies the infiltrate as mild, moderate, or severe and its distribution as focal, confluent, or diffuse.

that are traditionally used to treat patients with DCM are quite effective in treating the symptoms referable to viral-induced DCM, the use of digitalis has been proscribed during the acute phase of the illness because of the concern over aggravating potentially lethal ventricular arrhythmias. Whereas numerous anecdotal and small case series suggested that patients with viral myocarditis might benefit from early steroid or immunosuppressive therapy, the results of the Myocarditis Treatment Trial suggested that treating patients with the histopathologic diagnosis of myocarditis and a LVEF below 45 percent with a 24-week regimen of immunosuppressive therapy for 28 weeks (prednisone plus cyclosporine or prednisone plus azathioprine) did not result in an improvement in ejection fraction when compared with conventional therapy alone.[97] However, the major limitation of this study was the unexpectedly low rate of positive biopsies (less than 10 percent) and the extension of enrollment to 2 years after the initial clinical presentation. Accordingly, it is possible that in a substantial number of patients the disease had already progressed from the phase of acute myocarditis to the phase of DCM and that any form of therapy may not have been effective in this setting.[97] Nonetheless, on the basis of this study, routine immunosuppressive therapy is no longer recommended for myocarditis patients with a stable clinical course. However, many clinicians still recommend aggressive immunosuppressive therapy for patients with fulminant myocarditis or a deteriorating clinical course. The results of a multicenter database study of patients with giant cell myocarditis showed that the 22 patients with giant cell myocarditis who were treated with corticosteroids and cyclosporine, azathioprine, or both therapies survived for an average of 12.3 months, compared with an average of 3.0 months for the 30 patients who received no immunosuppressive therapy.[98] Of the 34 patients who underwent heart transplantation in this study, 9 (26 percent) had a giant cell infiltrate in the transplanted heart and 1 patient died of recurrent giant cell myocarditis. Thus, in addition to immunosuppressive therapy, the results of this study suggest that cardiac transplantation may be performed in patients with fulminant myocarditis.

ACQUIRED IMMUNODEFICIENCY SYNDROME

The subject of AIDS myocarditis is covered in Chapter 55, Myocarditis. Several investigators have reported that there is an association between AIDS and DCM. In a long-term echocardiographic follow-up by Barbaro and coworkers,[102] 8 percent of initially asymptomatic human immunodeficiency virus (HIV)–positive patients were diagnosed with DCM during the 60-month follow-up. All patients with DCM were in New York Heart Association functional class III (84 percent) or IV (16 percent). The mean annual incidence rate was 15.9 cases per 1000 patients. The extent of immunodeficiency of the patients, as assessed by the CD4 count, influenced the incidence of DCM. Specifically, there was a higher incidence among patients with a CD4 count of less than 400 cells/mm^3.

Although some authors have described an association between the use of antiretroviral therapy with zidovudine and the development of cardiomyopathy,[103, 104] the extent of immunodeficiency probably has a major role in the development of cardiomyopathy. In fact, among the patients who received zidovudine, the incidence of cardiomyopathy was greater in those with a CD4 count less than 300 cells/mm^3. Similarly, the difference observed in the incidence of DCM among the risk groups was influenced more by the extent of immunodeficiency than by the type of antiretroviral treatment.[102]

Current hypotheses concerning the pathogenesis of cardiomyopathy associated with infection with HIV include infection of myocardial cells with HIV1 or coinfection with other cardiotropic viruses, postviral cardiac autoimmunity, autonomic dysfunction, and cardiotoxicity from illicit drugs and pharmacologic agents (such as nucleoside analogues and pentamidine). The role of myocarditis in the development of DCM in HIV has not been fully characterized.[105] Lymphocytic myocarditis can be found at autopsy in 46 to 52 percent of patients with AIDS, as reported in a review of the literature.[106] Autopsy series of persons dying from AIDS-related illnesses demonstrate histologic evidence of myocarditis in approximately 50 percent of the patients. Symptomatic heart failure is seen in approximately half of these patients with myocardial involvement. Treatment with zidovudine appears to have little influence on the development or course of cardiac function; however, only a very small fraction of AIDS patients die from heart failure.

The increasing occurrence of HIV-associated cardiomyopathy detected by autopsy studies and by echocardiographic findings strongly suggests that a careful cardiovascular evaluation should be performed to detect early involvement of the heart in HIV-positive patients. Whether early treatment with ACE inhibitors or β-blockers will prevent or retard disease progression in these patients is unknown at this time. The treatment of patients with symptomatic HIV cardiomyopathy is the same as the conventional treatment for patients with DCM.

CHAGAS' DISEASE

Although Chagas' disease is a relatively uncommon cause of DCM in North America, Chagas' disease remains a leading cause of death in many areas of Central and South America. Indeed, 50,000 people die of Chagas' disease each year.[107] *Trypanosoma cruzi,* the causative organism for Chagas' disease, is found only in the Western Hemisphere, where it primarily infects wild and domestic mammals and insects. Humans become involved when infected vectors infest the simple houses that are common in Latin America. It is estimated that 16 to 18 million people have chronic *T. cruzi* infection.

The three different clinical and pathophysiologic phases of disease are the acute, indeterminate, and chronic phases. Sudden cardiac death can occur during each phase; however, DCM is a late manifestation of the disease and is generally seen during the chronic phase. Acute Chagas' disease is usually a mild illness with a case fatality rate less than 5 percent. The systemic spread of the parasites from the site of entry and their initial multiplication may be accompanied by fever, malaise, and edema of the face and lower extremities, as well as generalized lymphadenopathy and hepatosplenomegaly. Muscles, including the heart, are often heavily parasitized, and severe myocarditis develops in a small proportion of patients. The acute illness resolves spontaneously over a period of 4 to 6 weeks in most patients, who then enter the indeterminate phase of *T. cruzi* infection. In this phase, there are no symptoms, but there are lifelong, low-grade parasitemias in association with antibodies to many *T. cruzi* antigens. Many people in this phase have subtle signs of cardiac or gastrointestinal involvement long before the disease becomes symptomatic. Most infected people remain in the indeterminate phase for life. However, this carrier state can be a major cause of transfusion-associated transmission of the parasite.[108] Symptomatic chronic Chagas' disease develops in an estimated 10 to 30 percent of infected persons, years or even decades after the *T. cruzi* infection is acquired. The heart is most commonly affected, and the pathologic changes may include biventricular enlargement, thinning of ventricular walls, apical aneurysms, and mural thrombi. Widespread lymphocytic infiltration is often seen in stained specimens of cardiac tissue, as well as diffuse interstitial fibrosis and atrophy of myocardial cells. The conduction system is often affected, typically resulting in right bundle branch block, left anterior fascicular block, or complete AV block. The symptoms reflect the dysrhythmias, cardiomyopathy, and thromboembolism that develop over time. Death usually results from rhythm disturbances (≈40 percent of the patients) or progressive heart failure (≈60 percent of the patients). The overall prognosis for patients with Chagas' cardiomyopathy and heart failure is poor, with 50 percent dying within 47 months. The presence of complete heart block, atrial fibrillation, left bundle branch block, and complex ventricular ectopy augur a poor prognosis.

The pharmacologic treatment for *T. cruzi* infection remains unsatisfactory. Extensive clinical experience has been accumulated with two drugs, benznidazole and nifurtimox. Both shorten the acute phase of *T. cruzi* infection and decrease mortality, but they achieve parasitologic cures in only about 50 percent of treated patients. Moreover, these drugs cause substantial toxicity. There is no evidence that drug treatment of persons with chronic *T. cruzi* infection alters the natural course of the disease, and a sizable proportion of such patients remain positive for parasites indefinitely.[109]

Noninfectious Causes

HYPERSENSITIVITY MYOCARDITIS

Hypersensitivity to a variety of agents may result in allergic reactions that involve the myocardium, characterized by peripheral eosinophilia, and a perivascular infiltration of the myocardium by eosinophils, lymphocytes, and histiocytes. These infiltrates may occasionally be associated with necrosis. A variety of drugs—most commonly the sulfonamides, penicillins, methyldopa, and other agents such as amphotericin B, streptomycin, phenytoin, isoniazid, tetanus toxoid, hydrochlorothiazide, and chlorthalidone—have been reported to cause allergic hypersensitivity myocarditis. Most patients are not clinically ill but may die suddenly, presumably secondary to an arrhythmia. Hypersensitivity myocarditis is only rarely recognized clinically, but it may be sufficient to produce global or regional myocardial dysfunction detected by noninvasive methods. This entity is often first diagnosed on postmortem examination and, occasionally, on endomyocardial biopsy.

SYSTEMIC LUPUS ERYTHEMATOSUS

Although a number of cardiac abnormalities have been reported in patients with systemic lupus erythematosus, the development of DCM is not a prominent manifestation of this disease process. Global LV dysfunction has been reported in 5 percent of patients with systemic lupus erythematosus, whereas segmental LV wall motion abnormalities were observed in 4 percent of patients and right ventricular enlargement in 4 percent. In general, the abnormalities in cardiac function usually correlate with disease activity.

SCLERODERMA

The development of DCM is rare in patients with scleroderma. An echocardiographic study showed that although there was no difference in LV dimensions or fractional shortening in patients with scleroderma, there was indication of systolic impairment by systolic time intervals with an increased pre-ejection period:LV ejection time ratio and also an increased isovolumic contraction time:LV ejection time ratio in the majority of patients.[110] A distinctive focal myocardial lesion ranging from contraction band necrosis to replacement fibrosis without morphologic abnormalities of the coronary arteries is noted in approximately half of the patients with scleroderma. This is postulated to be due to intermittent vascular spasm with intramyocardial Raynaud's phenomenon.[111] Thus, progressive systemic sclerosis can lead to conduction abnormalities, arrhythmias, heart failure, angina pectoris with normal coronary arteries, myocardial fibrosis, pericarditis, and sudden death. Cardiac involvement in systemic sclerosis portends an ominous prognosis and is probably most directly related to the extent of myocardial fibrosis.

RHEUMATOID ARTHRITIS

Cardiac involvement in rheumatoid arthritis generally results from the development of myocarditis or pericarditis. However, the development of DCM is rare in these patients. In a retrospective study of 172 patients with juvenile rheumatoid arthritis, symptomatic cardiac involvement—including pericarditis, perimyocarditis, and myocarditis—occurred in 7.6 percent of patients. Both myocarditis and pericarditis are regarded as poor prognostic factors in rheumatoid arthritis.[112] Myocardial involvement in rheumatoid arthritis is thought to result from disturbances in the microcirculation secondary to microvasculitis and occurs in the absence of any clinical symptoms of electrocardiographic changes.

KAWASAKI'S DISEASE

Kawasaki's disease is an acute febrile illness associated with mucosal inflammation, skin rash, and cervical lymphadenopathy. This disease is recognized most often in children less than 4 years of age. Kawasaki's disease represents an acute vasculitic syndrome of unknown etiology that primarily affects small and medium-sized arteries, including coronary arteries. Coronary arterial aneurysms are seen in 25 to 55 percent of the acute Kawasaki cases. Of these, 4.7 percent progress to premature atherosclerotic ischemic heart disease. Myocardial infarction is noted in approximately 2 percent of patients, and cardiovascular death is reported in 0.8 percent. Although the development of DCM is not typical for Kawasaki's disease, repetitive infarctions secondary to coronary artery aneurysms may lead to a DCM phenotype.

Acquired Cardiomyopathy

Peripartum Cardiomyopathy

Peripartum cardiomyopathy is a disease of unknown cause in which severe LV dysfunction occurs during the last trimester of pregnancy or the early puerperium. It is reported to occur in 1 in 1300 to 4000 live births. In the past, the diagnosis of this entity was made on clinical grounds. However, modern two-dimensional echocardiographic techniques have allowed more accurate diagnoses by excluding cases of diseases that mimic the clinical symptoms and signs of heart failure. Risk factors for peripartum cardiomyopathy include advanced maternal age, multiparity, African descent, twinning, and long-term tocolysis. Anticoagulation is strongly recommended, especially if LV dysfunction is persistent. Although the etiology of peripartum cardiomyopathy remains unknown, most theories have focused on the hemodynamic[113] and immunologic stresses of pregnancy.[114] An immune pathogenesis is supported by the frequent finding of lymphocytic myocarditis on myocardial biopsy,[115, 116] and the fact that multiparity or previous exposure to fetal antigens is a significant risk factor.[117]

The prognosis of peripartum cardiomyopathy is related to the recovery of LV function. In contrast to the persistent LV dysfunction observed in patients with idiopathic DCM, significant improvement in myocardial function is observed in 30 to 50 percent of patients in the first 6 months after presentation.[117] However, for those patients who do not recover to normal or near-normal LV function, the prognosis is similar to that for other forms of DCM.[118] Cardiomegaly that persists for more than 4 months after diagnosis indicates a poor prognosis, with a 50 percent mortality reported at 6 years. If a woman already carries the diagnosis of peripartum cardiomyopathy, caution is advised in recommending subsequent pregnancy, especially if the LV dysfunction is persistent. Heart failure recurs during subsequent pregnancies in more than 50 percent of the patients.[114]

Obesity

Heart failure in the markedly obese usually develops over a long period of time and can be directly related to the duration of obesity. Initially, the dyspnea and edema in these patients are simply related to alterations in LV compliance with resultant elevated filling pressures. However, with chronicity, these patients will develop a DCM phenotype with further worsening of the patient's volume overload status. Although the precise reasons for obesity-related heart failure are not known, it is thought that the chronic increase in cardiac work and chronic increase in systemic blood pressure ultimately lead to myocardial failure. In addition, there is an increased prevalence of hypertension and coronary artery disease in obese patients, which may also contribute to the development of DCM in these patients. Although there are anecdotal reports regarding symptomatic improvement after weight reduction in obesity-induced heart failure, large scale clinical trials have not yet been performed.

Physical Agents

Tachycardia-Induced DCM

The concept that incessant or chronic tachycardia can lead to reversible LV dysfunction is supported by both animal models of chronic pacing and human studies documenting improvement in ventricular function with tachycardia rate or rhythm control. Sustained rapid pacing in experimental animal models can produce severe biventricular systolic dysfunction.[119–121] In humans, descriptions of reversal of cardiomyopathy with rate or rhythm control of incessant or chronic tachycardias have been reported with atrial tachycardias, accessory pathway reciprocating tachycardias, AV node re-entry, and atrial fibrillation with rapid ventricular responses.[122] Control of the rapid ventricular responses in atrial fibrillation has been shown to improve ventricular function following conversion to sinus rhythm, pharmacologic ventricular rate control and AV junction ablation, and permanent ventricular pacing.[123, 124] The investigation of potential tachycardia-induced cardiomyopathy in patients with heart failure requires further prospective confirmation in larger numbers of patients, with study of mechanisms, patient groups affected, and optimal therapies. Tachycardia-induced cardiomyopathy may be a more common mechanism of LV dysfunction than is recognized, and aggressive treatment of the arrhythmia should be considered.

Autoimmune Mechanisms

At the time of this writing, it is not clear whether abnormalities in cellular and humoral immune-mediated mechanisms are the cause or the consequence of DCM. Circulating autoantibodies to a variety of cardiac antigens including those to β-adrenergic receptors, mitochondrial antigens, adenosine diphosphate, adenosine triphosphate carrier proteins, and cardiac myosin heavy chain have been identified.[125–127] In this regard, it is interesting to note that immunization with certain cardiac (but not skeletal) muscle antigens such as α-myosin heavy chain can result in the development of a dilated cardiac phenotype in certain susceptible strains of mice. Moreover, a recent meta-analysis has shown that there is increased expression of the antigens of genes located at the major histocompatibility complex (MHC) on chromosome 6, which is the locus that is responsible for regulating immune responses. This study showed that human leukocyte antigen (HLA) class II antigens such as DR4 or DQw4 were present in 63 percent of the patients with cardiomyopathy compared with 26 percent in the control subjects.[128] Features that support an autoimmune etiology in patients who present with myocarditis and DCM include familial aggregation, a weak association with HLA-DR4 haplotype, abnormal expression of HLA class II antigens in cardiac tissue, and detection of organ-specific and disease-specific cardiac autoantibodies by immunofluorescence and immunoabsorption techniques.

CLINICAL RECOGNITION

The most common initial presenting manifestations of DCM are related to the presence of left heart failure and include progressive exertional dyspnea, fatigue, weakness, diminished exercise capacity, orthopnea, paroxysmal nocturnal dyspnea, and nocturnal cough. With the development of right heart failure, abdominal distension, right upper quadrant pain, early satiety, postprandial fullness, and nausea appear. Some cases will eventually develop cardiac cachexia and wasting from advanced heart failure. Systemic embolization and pulmonary emboli can be seen in 1 to 4 percent of cases and are more commonly seen with cardiomegaly. Palpitations can occur with atrial fibrillation and ventricular arrhythmias. Ventricular arrhythmias are common toward advanced stages of cardiomyopathy; however, syncope and sudden cardiac death are rare initial presentations.

Diagnostic Evaluation

Physical Examination

Patients with DCM may present with a resting or inappropriate tachycardia. The pulse may also reflect irregularities suggesting atrial fibrillation or premature beats with ventricular ectopy. In severe LV failure, pulsus alternans may be present and may even progress to low-volume, thready pulse in advanced heart failure. In the advanced stages of heart failure, the systolic blood pressure is usually normal or low and pulse pressure is narrow, suggesting a diminished stroke volume. In the setting of congestion or volume overload, tachypnea with exertion or at rest may be observed. The patient may be orthopneic to the point where he or she cannot remain in the recumbent position for more than a few seconds.

GENERAL APPEARANCE

The patient's appearance will vary depending on how far the disease process has advanced. Patients with advanced heart failure will appear chronically ill, weak, edematous, and sometimes cachectic. They may demonstrate anxious or depressed affect. The skin may reveal cold and clammy extremities, especially in cases of advanced heart failure with low output failure.

PHYSICAL EXAMINATION

Jugular venous distention may be present and should be sought in all patients presenting with shortness of breath or fatigue. The presence of prominent V waves in the neck veins suggests tricuspid regurgitation. Hepatojugular reflux is usually present in the setting of right ventricular volume overload. The precordium may be completely normal in the early phases of DCM. However, in the advanced stages of heart failure, both LV and right ventricular heaves may be palpated. The apical impulse is displaced laterally and downward, reflecting LV enlargement. Although the LV impulse may be prominent early on, it gradually becomes less prominent and less sustained as the disease progresses. The first heart sound (S_1) may be variable in intensity depending on the tachycardia or presence of a bundle branch block. The second heart sound (S_2) is usually physiologically split but may be paradoxically split in the presence of a left bundle branch block. The pulmonary component of the second heart sound (P_2) is accentuated in the setting of pulmonary hypertension that frequently accompanies advanced heart failure. A presystolic gallop (S_4) can be auscultated in early phases, usually preceding overt congestive heart failure, suggesting elevated LV end-diastolic filling pressures. S_3 is usually present and is best heard with the patient in the left lateral decubitus position. S_3 is usually of LV origin but can occasionally be detected over the right ventricle as well. S_3 and S_4 may overlap to produce a so-called summation gallop or gallop rhythm when the heart rate exceeds 100 to 110 beats/min. Low-grade systolic murmurs are common and are usually the result of tricuspid or mitral regurgitation. Pulmonary alveolar edema is usually detectable as fine crepitant rales. However, interstitial pulmonary edema may be clinically silent, but it may be sufficient to cause the patient to feel dyspneic. If pleural effusions are present, breath sounds may be absent or diminished and may be accompanied by dullness to percussion over the lung fields. Wheezing resulting from bronchospasm may be found as a consequence of bronchial hyperresponsiveness. In advanced stages of DCM, the liver may be enlarged, tender to palpation, and even pulsatile. With sufficient volume overload and right ventricular failure, it is not uncommon to detect ascites. In the final stages of DCM, a low output state may lead to mesenteric ischemia with diffuse or localized abdominal tenderness or tympanic distention from the resulting ileus. The extremities are remarkable for the presence of pitting peripheral edema in the setting of volume overload and may be dusky and cool to the touch in the setting of low output failure. Chronic venous stasis can lead to atrophic changes and discoloration of the skin.

Laboratory Testing

INITIAL LABORATORY TESTS

Initial screening laboratory studies for DCM patients should include a routine assessment of serum electrolytes, liver function tests, white blood cell count, and hemoglobin and hematocrit. Beyond these routine tests, the positive predictive value or utility of additional laboratory studies remains low unless supported by specific elements of the history and physical examination. One possible exception to this statement is the use of natriuretic peptides, such as N-terminal atrial natriuretic peptide and brain natriuretic peptide, as biochemical markers for identifying patients with asymptomatic LV systolic dysfunction.[129–131] Some studies have shown that elevated levels of these markers have a sensitivity of approximately 80 to 90 percent and a specificity of approximately 70 to 90 percent for detecting patients with ejection fractions less than 30 percent.[131] Although N-terminal atrial natriuretic peptide and brain natriuretic peptide levels may not be useful in assessing patients with known DCM, these markers may be useful in screening asymptomatic members of families with hereditary cardiomyopathies.

CHEST RADIOGRAPHY

In the early phases of DCM, cardiac enlargement may be minimal and may not be detected by chest radiography. However, in general, the chest radiograph usually reveals LV enlargement or generalized cardiomegaly that involves all four cardiac chambers. Depending on the patient's volume status, there may or may not be findings of pulmonary congestion. Cephalization of blood flow and pulmonary vascular redistribution are early signs of volume overload, followed by the development of interstitial edema with appearance of Kerley B lines and fluid in the interlobar fissures, followed by frank alveolar edema in advanced volume overload. Pleural effusions may be present, and the azygos vein and superior vena cava may be dilated, especially with right ventricular failure.

ELECTROCARDIOGRAPHY

If the patient with DCM presents with signs or symptoms referable to heart failure, the electrocardiogram usually reveals sinus tachycardia. However, sinus bradycardia may also be present in many patients with end-stage DCM. The electrocardiographic morphology is seldom normal and often shows nonspecific repolarization or ST segment abnormalities. Conduction abnormalities—especially left bundle branch block, left anterior hemiblock, and nonspecific intraventricular conduction delays, occasionally first-degree AV block—are common in patients with long-standing symptoms, and they may be markers of increasing interstitial fibrosis or myocyte hypertrophy. Right bundle branch block is rare.[132] Left atrial or biatrial enlargement may be present. Pathologic anterior, anterolateral, or diffuse Q waves mimicking myocardial infarction or poor R wave progression may be seen with viral myocarditis or when there is extensive LV fibrosis even without a discrete myocardial scar.[132] A variety of atrial and ventricular tachyarrhythmias and AV conduction disturbances may also be seen. Atrial fibrillation develops in approximately 20 percent of the patients. Premature ventricular contractions are not an uncommon finding on routine electrocardiograms in patients with DCM.

AMBULATORY ELECTROCARDIOGRAPHIC (HOLTER) MONITORING

There is an inverse relationship between the severity of ventricular arrhythmia and the LVEF.[133, 134] Thus, it is perhaps not surprising that the majority of DCM patients will have premature ventricular contractions when monitored over a 24-hour period. Moreover, approximately half of the patients with DCM will have nonsustained ventricular tachycardia on routine ambulatory 24-hour Holter monitoring. However, the predictive value of ambulatory Holter monitoring as a routine screening tool in asymptomatic patients for identification of risk for sudden cardiac death has not been validated. There are conflicting data from studies involving small groups of patients regarding the role of routine ambulatory electrocardiographic monitoring as a significant independent risk factor for sudden cardiac death.[135–137] Thus, at the present time, routine screening with Holter monitoring in asymptomatic heart failure patients is not recommended as a reliable means to predict those patients who will develop sudden cardiac death.

SIGNAL-AVERAGED ELECTROCARDIOGRAPHY

In patients with syncope or coronary artery disease, the presence of late potentials on a signal-averaged electrocardiogram (SAECG) identifies those patients at high risk for developing ventricular tachycardia and sudden death. Although late potentials are less frequent in patients with DCM, the current evidence suggests that an abnormal SAECG predicts ventricular arrhythmias and sudden cardiac death in patients with DCM as well (Fig. 51–6). However, not all studies have found that an abnormal SAECG predicts ventricular tachycardia or sudden cardiac death. Indeed, the sensitivity of the SAECG varies between 22 and 100 percent and the specificity ranges from 45 to 96 percent in various studies.[137–141] Thus, although the SAECG may be useful for predicting future events in some patients with DCM, the inherent problems with the sensitivity, specificity, and predictive value suggest that the SAECG may not be a reliable tool for screening asymptomatic patients who are at high risk for sudden cardiac death.

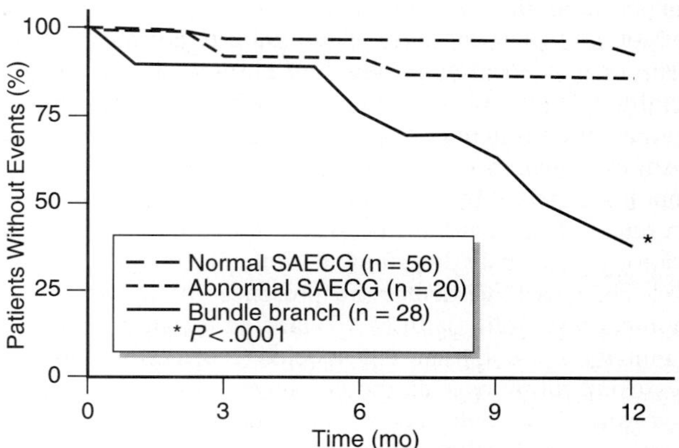

FIGURE 51–6 Role of signal-averaged electrocardiograms (SAECGs) in predicting future events in patients with dilated cardiomyopathy. Patients with positive SAECGs suffered significantly more events than patients with a normal electrocardiogram or with bundle branch block. (From Ikegawa T, Chino M, Hasegawa H, et al: Prognostic significance of 24-hour ambulatory electrocardiographic monitoring in patients with dilative cardiomyopathy: a prospective study. Clin Cardiol 10:78–82, 1987.)

TWO-DIMENSIONAL AND DOPPLER ECHOCARDIOGRAPHY

Two-dimensional and Doppler echocardiography are extremely useful techniques for assessing LV function, LV dimensions, and valvular structures in DCM patients. Generally, patients will have global LV dilatation, LV wall thinning, global hypokinesis, and an LVEF less than 35 to 40 percent. Segmental wall motion abnormalities may be seen with altered regional wall stress due to elevated filling pressures and depressed contractility or with acute myocarditis due to segmental myocardial injury. Interestingly, the presence of segmental wall motion abnormalities suggests a more favorable outcome than if global hypokinesis is present.[142] LV apical thrombi can be identified in as many as 40 percent of the patients with DCM.[143] A small pericardial effusion can sometimes be demonstrated, especially if an infectious or noninfectious inflammatory etiology is responsible for producing the DCM.

Doppler echocardiography usually reveals mild degrees of mitral and tricuspid regurgitation and sometimes trace pulmonary insufficiency. The mechanisms of mitral and tricuspid regurgitation have been attributed to ventricular enlargement, annular dilatation, lengthening of chordae tendineae, abnormalities in contractility of the papillary muscles, and displacement of the coaptation point of the mitral leaflets. The Doppler mitral inflow patterns can also provide useful information on elevated LV filling pressures, which are suggested by the appearance of high E/A ratio ("pseudonormalization") and short isovolumic relaxation time and deceleration time.[144, 145] The elevated early filling wave results from an elevated left atrial pressure, whereas the rapid deceleration time reflects a further decrease in LV compliance. These Doppler findings have been associated with a poor prognosis in DCM.

RADIONUCLIDE TECHNIQUES

Multigated radionuclide angiocardiography is a useful test for the initial assessment of LVEF in patients with DCM. Both the right ventricular ejection fraction and the LVEF can be quantified reliably with this technique. Moreover, the interobserver and inter-test variability appear to be less than with echocardiography.[147] Thallium 201 myocardial scintigraphy is not a reliable technique for differentiating patients with ischemic heart disease from those with DCM, insofar as patients with DCM may have both reversible and fixed perfusion abnormalities that are related to the presence of myocardial fibrosis.[148] In addition to the methodology previously described, radionuclide techniques have also been used to detect the presence of myocardial inflammation. Both gallium 67–labeled (a marker for inflammation) and indium 111–labeled (a marker for myocyte necrosis) antimyosin antibodies have been used to detect myocarditis in small uncontrolled studies.[149, 150] These techniques are supportive of the diagnosis of myocarditis when clinically suspected but do not have the specificity nor the sensitivity to be used reliably as screening tools for patients with myocarditis.[150]

CARDIAC CATHETERIZATION

Coronary arteriography is primarily used as a basis for planning further treatment options in patients who have ischemic heart disease. In the majority of patients with DCM, the coronary arteries are normal with no atherosclerotic lesions. However, a small portion may have evidence of mild, nonobstructive, isolated atherosclerotic lesions that may not be sufficient to explain the extent of cardiomyopathy. Therefore, in these cases, other etiologies for the cardiomyopathy should be sought. The ventriculogram generally reveals a dilated ventricle with depressed contractility. The LV end-diastolic pressures are usually elevated. Right heart catheterization is a useful means for adjusting medical therapy in patients with advanced symptoms,[151] especially when they are considered for vasodilator or inotropic or mechanical support, or for assessing the suitability of certain patients for cardiac transplantation.

ENDOMYOCARDIAL BIOPSY

The routine use of right ventricular endomyocardial biopsy as a diagnostic tool for evaluating patients with newly diagnosed DCM has fallen out of favor in many laboratories because of the apparent lack of benefit of immunosuppressive therapy in patients with myocarditis.[96] Moreover, as alluded to previously, the current criteria for diagnosing myocarditis by myocardial biopsy may be overly specific and lack sensitivity (see Table 51–6). Indeed, the reported incidence of biopsy-verified myocarditis ranges from 1 to 70 percent, with an average detection rate of 10 percent. The countervailing argument that has been raised in support of the use of endomyocardial biopsy in DCM is that this technique may yield a new diagnosis (i.e., different from idiopathic DCM) in up to 20 percent of patients and may provide a potentially new or beneficial form of therapy in 5 percent.[151, 152] Thus, myocardial biopsy should be considered in patients with suspected treatable systemic or infiltrative myocardial diseases, such as sarcoidosis, hypereosinophilic syndrome, hypersensitivity myocarditis, amyloidosis, hemachromatosis, doxorubicin-induced cardiomyopathy, or fulminant myocarditis. Moreover, as noted previously, in certain types of fulminant myocarditis, especially giant cell myocarditis, there is the suggestion that aggressive immunosuppression may attenuate disease progression.[98] Therefore, endomyocardial biopsies may be extremely useful in diagnosing patients who present with a fulminant course or who progressively decompensate despite optimal medical therapy.

In experienced laboratories, the risk of perforation of the heart from the biopsy is approximately 1 in 200 (0.5 percent) and the risk of death from the procedure is 3 in 10,000 (0.03 percent).[122] Therefore, in electing to perform a myocardial biopsy, the clinician must weigh the potential benefits of rendering a new diagnosis for which a specific form of therapy exists against the risks associated with performing myocardial biopsy in her or his institution.[152]

TREATMENT STRATEGIES

The first priority in implementing treatment strategies for patients with DCM is to determine whether the condition has an etiology for which there is a specific form of treatment. Table 51–7 lists a number of "etiology-specific" strategies designed to treat the underlying disease process

TABLE 51-7 **Primary Treatment Approaches to Dilated Cardiomyopathies**

Etiology	Primary Treatment
Alcoholic	Abstinence
Cocaine	Abstinence, ? β-blockers
Anthracycline	Cessation of anthracycline therapy
Systemic lupus erythematosus	Steroids, cytotoxic agents
Viral myocarditis	Prednisone and immunosuppressant therapy for fulminant course
Chagas' disease	Benznidazole, Nifurtimox
Scleroderma	Steroids, calcium channel blockers for Raynaud's syndrome
Kawasaki's disease	IV immunoglobulin
Thiamine, selenium, or carnitine deficiency	Replacement
Hyperthyroidism/hypothyroidism	Achieve euthyroid state
AIDS	Increase CD4 count
Uremia	Dialysis
Pheochromocytoma	Removal of tumor
Tachycardia induced	Atrioventricular nodal ablation, β-blockers

Abbreviation: AIDS, acquired immunodeficiency disease.

responsible for causing the DCM. The second priority in implementing treatment strategies for DCM is to initiate supportive "heart failure" therapy, the goals of which should be to (1) improve the quality of life, (2) avoid the need for future hospitalizations, (3) prolong life, and (4) prevent heart failure progression. Given that the general management for heart failure patients is discussed in detail in Chapter 60, in the section that follows we discuss only those strategies that appear (at the time of this writing) to be unique to the treatment of heart failure for patients with DCM.

Although existing studies suggest that both patients with ischemic cardiomyopathy and those with DCM benefit from the use of ACE inhibitors and β-blockers,[153–161] the results of the large multicenter randomized Digitalis Investigation Group (DIG) Trial suggest that DCM patients had a more favorable response to digitalis than patients with ischemic heart disease did. That is, patients with DCM were noted to have a 33 percent risk reduction in the combined endpoint of death and hospitalization attributable to worsening heart failure compared with a 21 percent risk reduction in patients with ischemic cardiomyopathy.[162] Although there is good clinical evidence that the use of first-generation calcium antagonists (diltiazem, verapamil, and nifedipine) in heart failure is potentially harmful in all patients with heart failure,[163] studies with the second-generation calcium channel blockers, such as amlodipine and felodipine, suggest that these agents are safe.[30, 164] Moreover, there is suggestive evidence that the use of amlodipine might confer a survival benefit for patients with DCM.[30] Another area in which there may be important differences in the treatment response between ischemic cardiomyopathy and DCM is the treatment of ventricular arrhythmias. For example, in the Survival Trial of Antiarrhythmic Therapy in Congestive Heart Failure with Amiodarone (CHF-STAT),[165] only patients with nonischemic DCM had significant reduction in the combined endpoint of cardiac death and hospitalization. However, this difference between ischemic cardiomyopathy and DCM was not observed in the randomized trial of low-dose amiodarone in severe congestive heart failure by Grupo de Estudio de la Sobrevida en la Insuficiencia Cardiaca en Argentina (GESICA),[166] in which patients with dilated nonischemic cardiomyopathy and ischemic cardiomyopathy patients both had reductions in total mortality, sudden death, and death due to progressive heart failure.[166]

Immunosuppression and Immunomodulation

Although an autoimmune pathogenesis has been postulated for DCM, immunosuppressive therapy has not been shown to be effective in clinical trials. The failure of the Myocarditis Treatment Trial to show a significant benefit for immunosuppressive therapy has been alluded to previously.[97] However, numerous anecdotal small case series suggest that patients with acute fulminant viral myocarditis may benefit from early steroid or immunosuppressive therapy.[98] Therefore, conventional medical therapy should be used to alleviate symptoms in patients with myocarditis of uncertain duration, whereas immunosuppressive agents should be reserved for myocarditis patients with progressive deterioration or a fulminant presentation. Immune modulatory therapy with immunoglobulin is effective for Kawasaki's disease in children, and it has been demonstrated to improve ventricular function in children with new-onset DCM.[167] There has been a report on the effectiveness of intravenous immunoglobulin therapy in the treatment of myocarditis and acute cardiomyopathy.[168]

Growth Hormone

There has been growing enthusiasm for the use of growth hormone in patients with DCM, based on the rationale that there may be inadequate compensatory cardiac hypertrophy in this disorder. Fazio and associates,[169] treated seven DCM patients with recombinant human growth hormone over 3 months. Growth hormone therapy was reported to increase myocardial mass and reduce the size of the LV chamber, resulting in improvement in hemodynamics, myocardial energy metabolism, and the clinical status of the patients.[169] More recently, a double-blind, randomized, placebo-controlled trial of recombinant human growth hormone in 50 patients treated for a minimum of 12 weeks was shown to increase LV mass but had no significant effect on LV systolic wall stress, mean blood pressure, systemic vascular resistance, New York Heart Association functional class, LVEF, or distance walked on a 6-minute walk test.[170] Whether longer-term treatment with recombinant growth hormone would have resulted in an improved clinical outcome in the patients with DCM is unknown.[171–181]

References

1. WHO/ISFC: Report of the WHO/ISFC Task Force on the Definition of Cardiomyopathies. Br Heart J 44:672–673, 1980.
2. Richardson P, McKenna W, Bristow M, et al: Report of the 1995 World Health Organization/International Society and Federation of Cardiology Task Force on the Definition and Classification of Cardiomyopathies. Circulation 93:841–842, 1996.
3. Gillum RF: Idiopathic cardiomyopathy in the United States, 1970–1982. Am Heart J 111:752–755, 1986.
4. Codd MB, Sugrue DD, Gersh BJ, Melton LJ III: Epidemiology of idiopathic dilated and hypertrophic cardiomyopathy. A population-based study in Olmsted County, Minnesota, 1975–1984. Circulation 80:564–572, 1989.
5. Manolio TA, Baughman KL, Rodeheffer R, et al: Prevalence and etiology of idiopathic dilated cardiomyopathy. Am J Cardiol 69:1458–1466, 1992.
6. SOLVD Investigators: Effect of enalapril on survival in patients with reduced left ventricular ejection fractions and congestive heart failure. N Engl J Med 325:293, 1991.
7. Bourassa MG, Gurne O, Bangdiwala SI, et al: Natural history and patterns of current practice in heart failure. The Studies of Left Ventricular Dysfunction (SOLVD) investigators. J Am Coll Cardiol 22:14A–19A, 1993.
8. DeMaria R, Gavazzi A, Recalcati F, et al: Comparison of clinical findings in idiopathic dilated cardiomyopathy in women versus men. Am J Cardiol 72:580, 1993.
9. Dec GW, Fuster V: Medical progress: idiopathic dilated cardiomyopathy. N Engl J Med 331:1564, 1994.
10. Fuster V, Gersch BJ, Giuliani ER, et al: The natural history of idiopathic dilated cardiomyopathy. Am J Cardiol 47:525–531, 1993.
11. Sugrue DD, Rodeheffer RJ, Codd MB, et al: The clinical course of idiopathic dilated cardiomyopathy: a population based study. Ann Intern Med 117:117–123, 1992.
12. Dec GW, Fuster V: Idiopathic dilated cardiomyopathy. N Engl J Med 331:1564–1575, 1994.
13. Middlekauff HR, Stevenson WG, Stevenson LW, Saxon LA: Syncope in advanced heart failure: high risk of sudden death regardless of origin of syncope. J Am Coll Cardiol 21:110–116, 1993.
14. Neri R, Mestroni L, Salvi A, Camerini F: Arrhythmias in dilated cardiomyopathy. Postgrad Med J 62:593–597, 1986.
15. Romeo F, Pelliccia F, Cianfrocca C, et al: Predictors of sudden death in idiopathic dilated cardiomyopathy. Am J Cardiol 63:138–140, 1989.
16. Stevenson LW, Perloff JK: The dilated cardiomyopathies: clinical aspects. Cardiol Clin 6:187–218, 1988.
17. Steimle AE, Stevenson LW, Fonarow GC, et al: Prediction of improvement in recent onset cardiomyopathy after referral for heart transplantation. J Am Coll Cardiol 23:553–559, 1994.
18. Ikram H, Williamson HG, Won M, et al: The course of idiopathic dilated cardiomyopathy in New Zealand. Br Heart J 57:521–527, 1987.
19. Romeo F, Pelliccia F, Cianfrocca C, et al: Determinants of end stage idiopathic dilated cardiomyopathy: a multivariate analysis of 104 patients. Clin Cardiol 12:387–392, 1989.
20. Lewis JF, Webber JD, Sutton LL, et al: Discordance in degree of left ventricular dilation in patients with dilated cardiomyopathy: recognition and clinical implications. J Am Coll Cardiol 21:649–654, 1993.
21. Unverferth DV, Magorien RD, Moeschberger ML, et al: Factors influencing the one-year mortality of dilated cardiomyopathy. Am J Cardiol 54:147–152, 1984.
22. Figulla HR, Rahlf G, Nieger M, et al: Spontaneous hemodynamic improvement or stabilization and associated biopsy findings in patients with congestive cardiomyopathy. Circulation 71:1095–1104, 1985.
23. Hammond EH, Menlove RL, Anderson JL: Predictive value of immunofluorescence and electron microscopic evaluation of endomyocardial biopsies in the diagnosis and prognosis of myocarditis and idiopathic dilated cardiomyopathy. Am Heart J 114:1055–1065, 1987.
24. Seta Y, Shan K, Bozkurt B, et al: Basic mechanisms in heart failure: the cytokine hypothesis. J Card Fail 2:243–249, 1996.
25. Tsutamoto T, Hisanaga T, Wada A, et al: Interleukin-6 spillover in the peripheral circulation increases with the severity of heart failure, and the high plasma level of interleukin-6 is an important prognostic predictor in patients with congestive heart failure. J Am Coll Cardiol 31:391–398, 1998.
26. Likoff MJ, Chandler SL, Kay HR: Clinical determinants of mortality in chronic congestive heart failure secondary to idiopathic dilated or ischemic cardiomyopathy. Am J Cardiol 59:634–638, 1987.
27. Cohn JN, Johnson G, Shabetai R, et al: Ejection fraction, peak exercise oxygen consumption, cardiothoracic ratio, ventricular arrhythmias, and plasma norepinephrine as determinants of prognosis in heart failure. Circulation 87:V15–V16, 1993.
28. Mancini DM, Eisen H, Kussmaul W, et al: Value of peak exercise oxygen consumption for optimal timing of cardiac transplantation in ambulatory patients with heart failure. Circulation 83:778–786, 1991.
29. Lee WH, Packer M: Prognostic importance of serum sodium concentration and its modification by converting-enzyme inhibition in patients with severe chronic heart failure. Circulation 73:257–267, 1986.
30. Packer M, O'Connor CM, Ghali JK, et al: Effect of amlodipine on morbidity and mortality in severe chronic heart failure. N Engl J Med 335:1107–1114, 1996.
31. CIBIS Investigators and Committee: A randomized trial of β-blockade in heart failure: the Cardiac Insufficiency Bisoprolol Study (CIBIS). Circulation 90:1765–1773, 1994.
32. Eisenhofer G, Friberg P, Rundqvist B, et al: Cardiac sympathetic nerve function in congestive heart failure. Circulation 93:1667–1676, 1996.
33. Hasking GJ, Esler MD, Jennings GL, et al: Norepinephrine spillover to plasma in patients with congestive heart failure: evidence of increased overall and cardiorenal sympathetic nervous activity. Circulation 73:615–621, 1986.
34. Dzau VJ, Packer M, Lilly LS, et al: Prostaglandins in severe congestive heart failure: relation to activation of the renin-angiotensin system and hyponatremia. N Engl J Med 310:347–352, 1984.
35. Dzau VJ, Colucci WS, Hollenberg NK, Williams GH: Relation of the renin-angiotensin-aldosterone system to clinical state in congestive heart failure. Circulation 63:645–651, 1981.
36. Torre-Amione G, Kapadia S, Lee J, et al: Tumor necrosis factor-α and tumor necrosis factor receptors in the failing human heart. Circulation 93:704–711, 1996.
37. Torre-Amione G, Kapadia S, Benedict C, et al: Proinflammatory cytokine levels in patients with depressed left ventricular ejection fraction: a report from the Studies of Left Ventricular Dysfunction (SOLVD). J Am Coll Cardiol 27:1201–1206, 1996.
38. Linzbach AJ: Heart failure from the point of view of quantitative anatomy. Am J Cardiol 69:370–382, 1960.
39. Cohn JN: Structural basis for heart failure: ventricular remodeling and its pharmacological inhibition. Circulation 91:2504–2507, 1995.
40. Beuckelmann DJ, Nabauer M, Erdmann E: Intracellular calcium handling in isolated ventricular myocytes from patients with terminal heart failure. Circulation 85:1046–1055, 1992.
41. Lowes BD, Minobe W, Abraham WT, et al: Changes in gene expression in the intact human heart. Downregulation of α-myosin heavy chain in hypertrophied, failing ventricular myocardium. J Clin Invest 100:2315–2324, 1997.
42. Schaper J, Froede R, Hein S, et al: Impairment of the myocardial ultrastructure and changes of the cytoskeleton in dilated cardiomyopathy. Circulation 83:504–514, 1991.
43. Leskinen M: Left ventricular responses to experimental aortic coarctation in growing puppies. Acta Physiol Scand 141:391–398, 1991.
44. Julian FJ, Moss RL: Effects of calcium and ionic strength on shortening velocity and tension development in frog skinned muscle fibres. J Physiol 311:179–199, 1981.
45. Josue O: Hypertrophie cardioque causée par l'adrenaline et la toxine typhique. C R Soc Biol (Paris) 63:285–290, 1907.
46. Bristow MR, Ginsburg R: $Beta_2$ receptors on myocardial cells in human ventricular myocardium. Am J Cardiol 57:3F–6F, 1986.
47. Narula J, Haider N, Virmani R, et al: Apoptosis in myocytes in end-stage heart failure. N Engl J Med 335:1182–1189, 1996.
48. Olivetti G, Abbi R, Quaini F, et al: Apoptosis in the failing human heart. N Engl J Med 336:1131–1141, 1997.
49. Thomas CV, Coker ML, Zellner JL, et al: Increased matrix metalloproteinase activity and selective upregulation in LV myocardium from patients with end-stage heart failure. Circulation 97:1708–1715, 1998.

50. Tyagi SC, Kumar S, Voelker DJ, et al: Differential gene expression of extracellular matrix components in dilated cardiomyopathy. J Cell Biochem 63:185–198, 1996.
51. Tyagi SC, Campbell SE, Reddy HK, et al: Matrix metalloproteinase activity expression in infarcted, noninfarcted and dilated cardiomyopathic human hearts. Mol Cell Biochem 155:13–21, 1996.
52. Douglas PS, Morrow R, Ioli A, Reicheck N: Left ventricular shape, afterload, and survival in idiopathic dilated cardiomyopathy. J Am Coll Cardiol 13:311–315, 1989.
53. Vasan RS, Larson MG, Benjamin EJ, et al: Left ventricular dilation and the risk of congestive heart failure in people without myocardial infarction. N Engl J Med 336:1350–1355, 1997.
54. Michels VV, Moll PP, Miller FA, et al: The frequency of familial dilated cardiomyopathy in a series of patients with idiopathic dilated cardiomyopathy. N Engl J Med 326:77–82, 1992.
55. Durand JB, Bachinski LL, Bieling LC, et al: Localization of a gene responsible for familial dilated cardiomyopathy to chromosome 1q32. Circulation 92:3387–3389, 1995.
56. Ortiz-Lopez R, Li H, Su J, et al: Evidence for a dystrophin missense mutation as a cause of X-linked dilated cardiomyopathy. Circulation 95:2434–2440, 1997.
57. Towbin JA, Hejtmancik JF, Brink P, et al: X-linked dilated cardiomyopathy—molecular genetic evidence of linkage to the Duchenne muscular dystrophy (dystrophin) gene at the Xp21 locus. Circulation 87:1854–1865, 1993.
58. Olson TM, Michels VV, Thibodeau SN, et al: Actin mutations in dilated cardiomyopathy, a heritable form of heart failure. Science 280:750–752, 1998.
59. Kass S, MacRae C, Graber HL, et al: A gene defect that causes conduction system disease and dilated cardiomyopathy maps to chromosome 1p1-1q1. Nat Genet 7:546–551, 1994.
60. Berko BA, Swift M: X-linked dilated cardiomyopathy. N Engl J Med 316:1186–1191, 1987.
61. Hunsaker RH, Fulkerson PK, Barry FJ, et al: Cardiac function in Duchenne's muscular dystrophy. Results of 10-year follow-up study and noninvasive tests. Am J Med 73:235–238, 1982.
62. Anonymous: [abstract]. MMWR 47:633–637, 1998.
63. Gold R, Kress W, Meurers B, et al: Becker muscular dystrophy: detection of unusual disease courses by combined approach to dystrophin analysis. Muscle Nerve15:214–218, 1992.
64. D'Adamo P, Fassone L, Gedeon A, et al: The X-linked gene G4.5 is responsible for different infantile dilated cardiomyopathies. Am J Hum Genet 61:862–867, 1997.
65. Walsh TK, Vacek JL: Ethanol and heart disease. An underestimated contributing factor. Postgrad Med 79:60–63, 1986.
66. Preedy VR, Atkinson LM, Richardson PJ, Peters TJ: Mechanisms of ethanol-induced cardiac damage. Br Heart J 69:197–200, 1993.
67. Wilke A, Kaiser A, Ferency I, Maisch B: Alcohol and myocarditis. Herz 21:248–257, 1996.
68. Schenk KA, Cohen J: The heart in chronic alcoholism. Clinical and pathological findings. Pathol Microbiol 35:96–104, 1970.
69. Cerqueira MD, Harp GD, Ritchie JL, et al: Rarity of preclinical alcoholic cardiomyopathy in chronic alcoholics less than 40 years of age. Am J Cardiol 67:183–187, 1991.
70. Regan TJ: Alcohol and the cardiovascular system. JAMA 264:377–381, 1990.
71. Lang RM, Borrow KM, Neumann A, Feldman T: Adverse cardiac effects of acute alcohol ingestion in young adults. Ann Intern Med 102:742–747, 1985.
72. McCall D: Alcohol and the cardiovascular system. Curr Probl Cardiol 12:1–414, 1987.
73. Diamond I: Alcoholic myopathy and cardiomyopathy. N Engl J Med 320:458–460, 1989.
74. Fernandez-Sola J, Estruch R, Grau JM, et al: The relation of alcoholic myopathy to cardiomyopathy. Ann Intern Med 120:529–536, 1994.
75. Patel VB, Why HJ, Richardson PJ, Preedy VR: The effects of alcohol on the heart. Adverse Drug React Toxicol Rev 16:15–43, 1997.
76. Guarnieri T, Lakatta EG: Mechanism of myocardial contractile depression by clinical concentrations of ethanol: a study in ferret papillary muscles. J Clin Invest 85:1462–1467, 1990.
77. Pavan D, Nicolosi GL, Lestuzzi C, et al: Normalization of variables of left ventricular function in patients with alcoholic cardiomyopathy after cessation of excessive alcohol intake: an echocardiographic study. Eur Heart J 85:535–540, 1987.
78. Nethala V, Brown EJ Jr, Timson CR, Patcha R: Reversal of alcoholic cardiomyopathy in a patient with severe coronary artery disease. Chest 104:626, 1993.
79. Bertolet BD, Freund G, Martin CA, et al: Unrecognized left ventricular dysfunction in an apparently healthy cocaine abuse population. Clin Cardiol 13:323–328, 1990.
80. Chakko S, Fernandez A, Mellman TA, et al: Cardiac manifestations of cocaine abuse: a cross-sectional study of asymptomatic men with a history of long-term abuse of "crack" cocaine. J Am Coll Cardiol 20:1168–1174, 1992.
81. Mann DL, Kent RL, Parsons B, Cooper G IV: Adrenergic effects on the biology of the adult mammalian cardiocyte. Circulation 85:790–804, 1992.
82. Virmani R, Robinowitz M, Smialek JE, Smyth DF: Cardiovascular effects of cocaine: an autopsy study of 40 patients. Am Heart J 115:1068–1076, 1988.
83. Henzlova MJ, Smith SH, Prchal VM, Helmcke FR: Apparent reversibility of cocaine-induced congestive cardiomyopathy. Am Heart J 122:577–579, 1991.
84. Olson RD, Mushlin PS: Doxorubicin cardiotoxicity: analysis of prevailing hypotheses. FASEB J 4:3076–3086, 1990.
85. Lipshultz SE, Lipsitz SR, Mone SM, et al: Female sex and drug dose as risk factors for late cardiotoxic effects of doxorubicin therapy for childhood cancer. N Engl J Med 332:1738–1743, 1995.
86. Bristow MR, Mason JW, Billingham ME, Daniels JR: Doxorubicin cardiomyopathy: evaluation by phonocardiography, endomyocardial biopsy, and cardiac catheterization. Ann Intern Med 88:168–175, 1978.
87. Doroshow JH: Doxorubicin-induced cardiac toxicity. N Engl J Med 324:843–845, 1991.
88. Moreb JS, Oblon DJ: Outcome of clinical congestive heart failure induced by anthracycline chemotherapy. Cancer 70:2637–2641, 1992.
89. Saini J, Rich MW, Lyss AP: Reversibility of severe left ventricular dysfunction due to doxorubicin cardiotoxicity. Report of three cases. Ann Intern Med 106:814–816, 1987.
90. Bozkurt B, Kribbs S, Clubb FJ Jr, et al: Pathophysiologically relevant concentrations of tumor necrosis factor-alpha promote progressive left ventricular dysfunction and remodeling in rats. Circulation 97:1382–1391, 1998.
91. Kubota T, McTiernan CF, Frye CS, et al: Dilated cardiomyopathy in transgenic mice with cardiac specific overexpression of tumor necrosis factor-alpha. Circ Res 81:627–635, 1997.
92. Kishimoto C, Kurnick JT, Fallon JT, et al: Characteristics of lymphocytes cultured from murine viral myocarditis specimens. J Am Coll Cardiol 14:799–802, 1989.
93. Martino TA, Liu P, Sole MJ: Viral infection and the pathogenesis of dilated cardiomyopathy. Circ Res 74:182–188, 1994.
94. Woodruff JF: Viral myocarditis. Am J Pathol 101:427–479, 1980.
95. Richardson PJ: Clinical aspects of myocarditis. Heart Vessels Suppl 1:97–100, 1985.
96. Quigley PJ, Richardson PJ, Meany BT: Long term follow up of acute myocarditis. Correlation of ventricular function and outcome. Eur Heart J 8(suppl):39–42, 1987.
97. Mason JW, O'Connel JB, Herskowitz A, et al: A clinical trial of immunosuppressive therapy for myocarditis. N Engl J Med 333:269–275, 1995.
98. Cooper LT Jr, Berry GJ, Shabetai R: Idiopathic giant-cell myocarditis—natural history and treatment. N Engl J Med 336:1860–1866, 1997.
99. Aretz HT: Myocarditis: the Dallas criteria. Hum Pathol 18:619–624, 1994.
100. Koide H, Kitaura Y, Deguchi H, et al: Genomic detection of enteroviruses in the myocardium—studies on animal hearts and coxsackievirus B3 myocarditis and endomyocardial biopsies from patients with myocarditis and dilated cardiomyopathy. Jpn Circ J 56:1081–1093, 1992.
101. Giacca M, Severini GM, Mestroni L, et al: Low frequency of detection by nested polymerase chain reaction of enterovirus ribonucleic acid in endomyocardial tissue of patients with idiopathic dilated cardiomyopathy. J Am Coll Cardiol 24:1033–1040, 1994.
102. Barbaro G, Di Lorenzo G, Grisorio B, Barbarini G: Incidence of dilated cardiomyopathy and detection of HIV in myocardial cells of HIV-positive patients. Gruppo Italiano per lo Studio Cardiologico dei Pazienti Affetti da AIDS. N Engl J Med 339:1093–1099, 1998.

103. Herskowitz A, Willoughby SB, Baughman KL, et al: Cardiomyopathy associated with antiretroviral therapy in patients with HIV infection: a report of six cases. Ann Intern Med 116:311–313, 1992.
104. Domanski MJ, Sloas MM, Follmann DA, et al: Effect of zidovudine and didanosine treatment on heart function in children infected with human immunodeficiency virus. J Pediatr 127:137–146, 1995.
105. Herskowitz A, Wu T-C, Willoughby SB, et al: Myocarditis and cardiotropic viral infection associated with severe left ventricular dysfunction in late-stage infection with human immunodeficiency virus. J Am Coll Cardiol 24:1025–1032, 1994.
106. Kaul S, Fishbein MC, Siegel RJ: Cardiac manifestations of acquired immune deficiency syndrome: a 1991 update. Am Heart J 122:535–544, 1991.
107. Control of Chagas disease: report of a WHO expert committee [abstract]. World Health Organ Tech Rep Ser 811:1–95, 1991.
108. Kirchhoff LV: Current concepts: American trypanosomiasis (Chagas' disease)—a tropical disease now in the United States. N Engl J Med 329:639–644, 1993.
109. Marr JJ, Docampo R: Chemotherapy for Chagas' disease: a perspective on current therapy and considerations for future research. Rev Infect Dis 8:884–903, 1986.
110. Kazzam E, Caidahl K, Hallgren R, et al: Non-invasive assessment of systolic left ventricular function in systemic sclerosis. Eur Heart J 12:151–156, 1991.
111. Bulkley BH, Ridolfi RL, Salyer WR, Hutchins GM: Myocardial lesions of progressive systemic sclerosis. A cause of cardiac dysfunction. Circulation 53:483–490, 1976.
112. Goldenberg J, Ferraz MB, Pessoa AP, et al: Symptomatic cardiac involvement in juvenile rheumatoid arthritis. Int J Cardiol 34:57–62, 1992.
113. Marin-Neto JA, Maciel BC, Urbanetz LL, et al: High output failure in patients with peripartum cardiomyopathy: a comparative study with dilated cardiomyopathy. Am Heart J 121:134–140, 1991.
114. Lampert MB, Lang RM: Peripartum cardiomyopathy. Am Heart J 130:860–870, 1995.
115. Melvin KR, Richardson PJ, Olsen EG, et al: Peripartum cardiomyopathy due to myocarditis. N Engl J Med 307:731–734, 1982.
116. Midei MG, DeMent SH, Feldman AM, et al: Peripartum myocarditis and cardiomyopathy. Circulation 81:922–928, 1990.
117. Demakis JG, Rahimtoola SH, Sutton GC, et al: Natural course of peripartum cardiomyopathy. Circulation 44:1053–1061, 1971.
118. O'Connell JB, Costanzo-Nordin MR, Subramanian R, et al: Peripartum cardiomyopathy: clinical, hemodynamic, histologic and prognostic characteristics. J Am Coll Cardiol 8:52–56, 1986.
119. Spinale FG, Tomita M, Zellner JL, et al: Collagen remodeling and changes in LV function during development and recovery from supraventricular tachycardia. Am J Physiol 261:H308–H318, 1991.
120. Spinale FG, Zellner JL, Tomita M, et al: Relationship between ventricular and myocyte remodeling with the development and regression of supraventricular tachycardia-induced cardiomyopathy. Circ Res 69:1058–1067, 1991.
121. Mukherjee R, Crawford FA, Hewett KW, Spinale FG: Cell and sarcomere contractile performance from the same cardiocyte using video microscopy. J Appl Physiol 74:2023–2033, 1993.
122. Shinbane JS, Wood MA, Jensen DN, et al: Tachycardia-induced cardiomyopathy: a review of animal models and clinical studies. J Am Coll Cardiol 29:709–715, 1997.
123. Schumacher B, Luderitz B: Rate issues in atrial fibrillation: consequences of tachycardia and therapy for rate control. Am J Cardiol 82:29N–36N, 1998.
124. Luchsinger JA, Steinberg JS: Resolution of cardiomyopathy after ablation of atrial flutter. J Am Coll Cardiol 32:205–210, 1998.
125. Limas CJ, Goldenberg IF, Limas C: Autoantibodies against β-adrenoceptors in human idiopathic dilated cardiomyopathy. Circ Res 64:97–103, 1989.
126. Ansari AA, Wang YC, Danner DJ, et al: Abnormal expression of histocompatibility and mitochondrial antigens by cardiac tissue from patients with myocarditis and dilated cardiomyopathy. Am J Pathol 139:337–354, 1991.
127. Caforio AL, Grazzini M, Mann JM, et al: Identification of alpha- and beta-cardiac myosin heavy chain isoforms as major autoantigens in dilated cardiomyopathy. Circulation 85:1734–1742, 1992.
128. Carlquist JF, Menlove RL, Murray MB, et al: HLA class II (DR and DQ) antigen associations in idiopathic dilated cardiomyopathy. Circulation 83:515–522, 1991.
129. Cowie MR, Struthers AD, Wood DA, et al: Value of natriuretic peptides in assessment of patients with possible new heart failure in primary care. Lancet 350:1349–1353, 1997.
130. McDonagh TA, Robb SD, Murdoch DR, et al: Biochemical detection of left-ventricular systolic dysfunction [see comments]. Lancet 351:9–13, 1998.
131. Davis M, Espiner E, Richards G, et al: Plasma brain natriuretic peptide in assessment of acute dyspnoea [see comments]. Lancet 343:440–444, 1994.
132. Wilensky RL, Yudelman P, Cohen AI, et al: Serial electrocardiographic changes in idiopathic dilated cardiomyopathy confirmed at necropsy. Am J Cardiol 62:276–283, 1988.
133. Meinertz T, Hofmann T, Kasper W, et al: Significance of ventricular arrhythmias in idiopathic dilated cardiomyopathy. Am J Cardiol 53:902–907, 1984.
134. Mestroni L, Miani D, Neri R, et al: Ambulatory ECG in cardiomyopathies. G Ital Cardiol 17:1139–1144, 1987.
135. Kron J, Hart M, Schual-Berke S, et al: Idiopathic dilated cardiomyopathy. Role of programmed electrical stimulation and Holter monitoring in predicting those at risk of sudden death. Chest 93:85–90, 1988.
136. Olshausen KV, Stienen U, Schwarz F, et al: Long-term prognostic significance of ventricular arrhythmias in idiopathic dilated cardiomyopathy. Am J Cardiol 61:146–151, 1988.
137. Ikegawa T, Chino M, Hasegawa H, et al: Prognostic significance of 24-hour ambulatory electrocardiographic monitoring in patients with dilative cardiomyopathy: a prospective study. Clin Cardiol 10:78–82, 1987.
138. Mancini DM, Wong KL, Simson MB: Prognostic value of an abnormal signal-averaged electrocardiogram in patients with nonischemic congestive cardiomyopathy [see comments]. Circulation 87:1083–1092, 1993.
139. Keeling PJ, Kulakowski P, Yi G, et al: Usefulness of signal-averaged electrocardiogram in idiopathic dilated cardiomyopathy for identifying patients with ventricular arrhythmias. Am J Cardiol 72:78–84, 1993.
140. Middlekauff HR, Stevenson WG, Woo MA, et al: Comparison of frequency of late potentials in idiopathic dilated cardiomyopathy and ischemic cardiomyopathy with advanced congestive heart failure and their usefulness in predicting sudden death. Am J Cardiol 66:1113–1117, 1990.
141. Meinertz T, Treese N, Kasper W, et al: Determinants of prognosis in idiopathic dilated cardiomyopathy as determined by programmed electrical stimulation. Am J Cardiol 56:337–341, 1985.
142. Wallis DE, O'Connell JB, Henkin RE, et al: Segmental wall motion abnormalities in dilated cardiomyopathy. J Am Coll Cardiol 13:311–315, 1989.
143. Takamoto T, Kim D, Urie PM, et al: Comparative recognition of left ventricular thrombi by echocardiography and cineangiography. Br Heart J 53:36–42, 1985.
144. Kono T, Sabbah HN, Rosman H, et al: Left atrial contribution to ventricular filling during the course of evolving heart failure. Circulation 86:1317–1322, 1992.
145. Nagueh SF, Kopelen HA, Zoghbi WA: Feasibility and accuracy of Doppler echocardiographic estimation of pulmonary artery occlusive pressure in the intensive care unit. Am J Cardiol 75:1256–1262, 1995.
146. Poisner AM: Regulation of utero-placental prorenin. Adv Exp Med Biol 377:411–426, 1995.
147. Pohost GM, Fallon JT, Strauss HW: The role of radionuclide techniques in patients with myocardial disease. Cardiovasc Clin 10:149–163, 1979.
148. Glamann DB, Lange RA, Corbett JR, Hillis LD: Utility of various radionuclide techniques for distinguishing ischemic from nonischemic dilated cardiomyopathy. Arch Intern Med 152:769–772, 1992.
149. O'Connell JB, Henkin RE, Robinson JA, et al: Gallium-67 imaging in patients with dilated cardiomyopathy and biopsy-proven myocarditis. Circulation 70:58–62, 1984.
150. Dec GW, Palacios I, Yasuda T, et al: Antimyosin antibody cardiac imaging: its role in the diagnosis of myocarditis. J Am Coll Cardiol 16:97–104, 1990.
151. Stevenson LW: Heart transplant centers: no longer the end of the road for heart failure. J Am Coll Cardiol 27:1198–1200, 1996.
152. Mason JW: Clinical merit of endomyocardial biopsy. Circulation 79:971–979, 1989.

153. Nagi KS, Joshi R, Thakur RK: Cardiac manifestations of Lyme disease: a review. Can J Cardiol 12:503–506, 1996.
154. Young JB, Leon CA, Weilbacher DA: Endomyocardial biopsy in critically ill patients: the procedure and diagnostic and prognostic potential. *In* Majid P, Kirby RR, Taylor RW (eds): Problems in Critical Care: Advances in Interventional Cardiology. pp. 433–443. Philadelphia: JB Lippincott, 1988.
155. Massie BM: 15 years of heart-failure trials: what have we learned? Lancet 352(suppl 1):29–33, 1998.
156. Bristow MR, Gilbert EM, Abraham WT, et al: Carvedilol produces dose-related improvements in left ventricular function and survival in subjects with chronic heart failure. Circulation 94:2807–2816, 1996.
157. Packer M, Colucci WS, Sackner-Bernstein JD, et al: Double-blind, placebo-controlled study of the effects of carvedilol in patients with moderate to severe heart failure. Circulation 94:2793–2799, 1996.
158. The SOLVD Investigators: Effect of enalapril on mortality and the development of heart failure in asymptomatic patients with reduced left ventricular ejection fraction. N Engl J Med 327:685–691, 1992.
159. The SOLVD Investigators: Effect of enalapril on survival in patients with reduced left ventricular ejection fractions and congestive heart failure. N Engl J Med 325:293–302, 1991.
160. Cohn JN, Johnson G, Ziesche S, et al: A comparison of enalapril with hydralazine-isosorbide dinitrate in the treatment of chronic congestive heart failure. N Engl J Med 325:303–310, 1991.
161. Cohn JN, Archibald DG, Ziesche S, et al: Effect of vasodilating therapy on mortality in chronic congestive heart failure: results of a Veterans Administration Cooperative Study. N Engl J Med 314:1547–1552, 1986.
162. Digitalis Investigation Group: The effect of digoxin on mortality and morbidity in patients with heart failure. N Engl J Med 336:525–533, 1997.
163. Packer M, Kessler PD, Lee WH: Calcium-channel blockade in the management of severe chronic congestive failure: a bridge too far. Circulation 75(suppl V):V-56–V-64, 1987.
164. Cohn JN, Ziesche S, Smith R, et al: Effect of the calcium antagonist felodipine as supplementary vasodilator therapy in patients with chronic heart failure treated with enalapril V-HeFT III. Circulation 96:856–863, 1997.
165. Singh S, Fletcher RD, Fisher SG, et al: Amiodarone in patients with congestive heart failure and asymptomatic ventricular arrhythmia. N Engl J Med 333:77–82, 1995.
166. Doval HC, Nul DR, Grancelli HO, et al: Randomised trial of low-dose amiodarone in severe congestive heart failure. Lancet 344:493–498, 1994.
167. Drucker NA, Colan SD, Lewis AB, et al: Gamma-globulin treatment of acute myocarditis in the pediatric population. Circulation 89:252–257, 1994.
168. McNamara DM, Rosenblum WD, Janosko KM, et al: Intravenous immune globulin in the therapy of myocarditis and acute cardiomyopathy. Circulation 95:2476–2478, 1997.
169. Fazio S, Sabatini D, Capaldo B, et al: A preliminary study of growth hormone in the treatment of dilated cardiomyopathy. N Engl J Med 334:809–814, 1996.
170. Pinamonti B, Zecchin M, di Lenarda A, et al: Persistence of restrictive left ventricular filling pattern in dilated cardiomyopathy: an ominous prognostic sign. J Am Coll Cardiol 29:604–612, 1997.
171. Gerdes AM, Kellerman SE, Moore JA, et al: Structural remodeling of cardiac myocytes in patients with ischemic cardiomyopathy. Circulation 86:426–430, 1992.
172. Krajinovic M, Pinamonti B, Sinagra G, et al: Linkage of familial dilated cardiomyopathy to chromosome 9. Heart muscle disease study group. Am J Hum Genet 57:846–852, 1995.
173. Bowles KR, Gajarski R, Porter P, et al: Gene mapping of familial autosomal dominant dilated cardiomyopathy to chromosome 10q21-23. J Clin Invest 98:1355–1360, 1996.
174. Rampazzo A, Nava A, Erne P, et al: A new locus for arrhythmogenic right ventricular cardiomyopathy (ARVD2) maps to chromosome 1q42-q43. Hum Mol Genet 4:2151–2154, 1995.
175. Muntoni F, Cau M, Ganau A, et al: Brief report: deletion of the dystrophin muscle-promoter region associated with X-linked dilated cardiomyopathy. N Engl J Med 329:921–925, 1993.
176. Bolhuis PA, Hensels GW, Hulsebos TJ, et al: Mapping of the locus for X-linked cardioskeletal myopathy with neutropenia and abnormal mitochondria (Barth syndrome) to Xq28. Am J Hum Genet 48:481–485, 1991.
177. Suomalainen A, Paetau A, Leinonen H, et al: Inherited idiopathic dilated cardiomyopathy with multiple deletions of mitochondrial DNA. Lancet 340:1319–1320, 1992.
178. Zeviani M, Gellera C, Antozzi C, et al: Maternally inherited myopathy and cardiomyopathy: association with mutation in mitochondrial DNA tRNA(Leu)(UUR). Lancet 338:143–147, 1991.
179. Hoffman EP, Brown RH Jr, Kunkel LM: Dystrophin: the protein product of the Duchenne muscular dystrophy locus. Cell 51:919–928, 1987.
180. Goldblatt J, Melmed J, Rose AG: Autosomal recessive inheritance of idiopathic dilated cardiomyopathy in a Madeira Portuguese kindred. Clin Genet 31:249–254, 1987.
181. Michaud JL, Heon E, Guilbert F, et al: Natural history of Alström syndrome in early childhood: onset with dilated cardiomyopathy. J Pediatr 128:225–229, 1996.

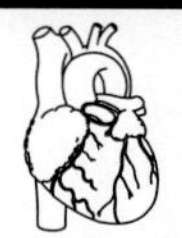

CHAPTER 52

HYPERTROPHIC CARDIOMYOPATHY

Diane Fatkin, J. G. Seidman, and Christine E. Seidman

PATHOGENESIS
Genetic Linkage Analyses
HCM Disease Genes
In Vitro Studies of Sarcomere Structure and Function
Mouse Models of HCM
Sarcomere Dysfunction Causes Cardiac Remodeling
Dominant Negative Versus Haploinsufficiency
LV Pathophysiology in HCM
CLINICAL EVALUATION
Clinical History
Physical Examination
Electrocardiography
Chest X-Ray
Echocardiography
Electrophysiologic Studies
Other Investigations
Genetic Studies
NATURAL HISTORY
TREATMENT
Genotype-Positive, Phenotype-Negative Individuals
Asymptomatic and Mildly Symptomatic Individuals
Heart Failure in Obstructive and Nonobstructive HCM
Prevention of Sudden Death

Hypertrophic cardiomyopathy (HCM) is a primary disorder of the myocardium characterized by ventricular hypertrophy in the absence of identifiable precipitating factors such as hypertension and aortic stenosis. Myocardial hypertrophy may affect either ventricle but usually involves the left. The hallmark diagnostic feature of HCM is asymmetric hypertrophy of the interventricular septum (Plate 52–1). However, two-dimensional echocardiographic studies have demonstrated that the distribution and severity of left ventricular (LV) hypertrophy may vary widely.[1–3] Ventricular septal hypertrophy may be associated with systolic anterior motion (SAM) of the mitral valve and subaortic obstruction of the left ventricular outflow tract (LVOT). Histologic examination of ventricular myocardium typically shows myocyte hypertrophy, myocyte and myofibrillar disarray, and interstitial fibrosis (Plate 52–2).

The clinical manifestations of HCM range from minor symptoms such as palpitations and dizziness to syncope and sudden death. HCM is particularly important as a cause of sudden death in young adults.[4] The differential diagnosis of myocardial hypertrophy in young adults may be difficult, particularly in those engaged in competitive athletic activities. The occurrence of sudden death in a number of elite athletes with HCM has focused considerable medical and media attention on this disease. Although initially considered to be a relatively uncommon disorder, some observations have estimated the prevalence of HCM in the general population to be 1 in 500.[5]

Since the first description of HCM in 1869,[6] numerous clinical and hemodynamic studies have been performed in attempts to elucidate its pathophysiology. The various names ascribed over this time reflect the traditional emphasis on the anatomic and hemodynamic features of the interventricular septum and LVOT: hypertrophic obstructive cardiomyopathy, asymmetric septal hypertrophy, and idiopathic hypertrophic subaortic stenosis. Since the late 1980s, the results of molecular genetic studies have revealed fundamental insights that challenge previous concepts of the pathogenesis of HCM. The discovery that HCM is caused by mutations in genes that encode sarcomere proteins has provided an important new framework for understanding the diverse pathologic and clinical manifestations of HCM and a basis for new strategies for diagnosis, prognostic stratification and therapy. HCM is one of the first examples of an inherited heart disease caused by a single gene defect and thus serves as a paradigm for the study of cardiovascular genetic disorders. Current concepts of the pathogenesis, clinical evaluation, natural history, and treatment of HCM are reviewed in this chapter.

PATHOGENESIS

Genetic Linkage Analyses

HCM is a familial disorder that is inherited as an autosomal dominant trait. Hence, the chance that a child of an affected parent will develop HCM is 50 percent, and males and females are equally likely to be affected (Fig. 52–1). Sporadic cases of HCM may occur,[7,8] arising presumably from de novo gene mutations. Individuals with sporadic disease also have a 50 percent likelihood of transmitting HCM to each of their offspring. To date, nine distinct chromosomal regions or loci have been identified to contain HCM gene mutations,[9–16] thereby defining HCM as a genetically heterogeneous disorder (Table 52–1).

HCM Disease Genes

The disease genes have been found in eight of the nine mapped HCM loci.[14–20] All of these genes have been shown

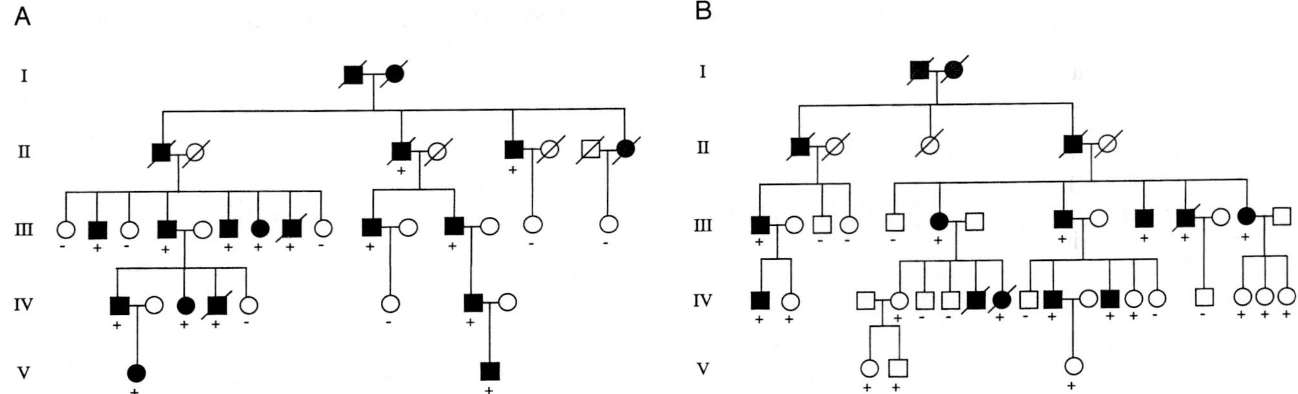

FIGURE 52–1 Pedigrees in two families with hypertrophic cardiomyopathy (HCM) caused by mutations in the beta myosin heavy chain (β-MHC) gene **(A)** and cardiac myosin binding protein C gene **(B)**. Generation numbers are indicated in *roman numerals. Squares* denote male family members, and *circles* denote females. Affected individuals are indicated by *black symbols,* unaffected individuals by *white symbols,* and individuals for whom the affected status is unknown are indicated by *gray symbols. Diagonal slashes* denote deceased family members. Individuals who have the disease (affected) haplotype in genetic linkage analyses are shown by *plus signs,* whereas those without the disease haplotype are shown by *minus signs.* In families with β-MHC gene mutations, the disease penetrance is high; that is, the majority of genotype-positive individuals are also phenotype-positive. In families with cardiac myosin binding protein C gene mutations, symptoms and signs of HCM may not appear until late adulthood. Consequently, some individuals in younger generations may be genotype-positive but phenotype-negative.

to encode sarcomere proteins (Plate 52–3; see also Table 52–1). The first HCM disease gene described was the beta myosin heavy chain (MHC) gene that mapped to chromosome 14q11.[17] Mutations in families with HCM have been found subsequently in two additional genes that encode thick filament proteins: essential myosin light chain (MLC) (chromosome 3p21) and regulatory MLC (chromosome 12q23). Mutations have also been found in four genes that encode thin filament proteins—cardiac troponin T (chromosome 1q32), cardiac troponin I (chromosome 19q13), alpha tropomyosin (chromosome 15q22), and cardiac actin (chromosome 15q14)—and in one gene that encodes a myosin binding protein: cardiac myosin binding protein C (chromosome 11p11). The disease gene at one locus (chromosome 7q3) has not as yet been identified.[13] Families that map to this locus have an unusual phenotype that includes both HCM and pre-excitation (Wolff-Parkinson-White) syndrome.

β-*Myosin Heavy Chain Gene*

Cardiac myosin is a hexamer composed of two MHCs, two essential light chains, and two regulatory light chains. MHCs contain a globular head connected through a neck region to a rodlike tail. The myosin heads contain binding sites for actin and adenosine triphosphate (ATP) and constitute the motor domain of the myosin molecule.[21, 22] In the myosin rod, the two MHCs are intertwined to form an alpha helical-coiled coil structure with repeats of 7 and 28 residues.

Cardiac MHC has two isoforms, β and α, that differ in expression pattern and adenosine triphosphatase (ATPase) activity. β-MHC, although expressed in fetal heart, becomes the major isoform in the adult human ventricle. β-MHC is expressed, to a lesser extent, in the adult human atrium and in slow skeletal muscle, such as the soleus.[23] The α-MHC isoform is expressed in the adult human atrium, but in rodents, it is the predominant MHC isoform

TABLE 52–1 Hypertrophic Cardiomyopathy Disease Genes

Chromosome Locus	Gene	Protein	Prevalence (%)	Mutation Type*
14q12	*MYH7*	β-MHC	>30	Missense (deletions, termination)
11p11.2	*MYBPC3*	Cardiac MyBP-C	>15	Truncation, missense (insertions, deletions, splicing variants)
1q32	*TNNT2*	Cardiac troponin T	15	Missense (deletion, splicing variants)
19q13.4	*TNNI3*	Cardiac troponin I	<10	Missense (deletion)
15q22.1	*TPM1*	α-Tropomyosin	<3	Missense
12q23-q24.3	*MYL2*	Regulatory MLC	<3	Missense
3p21.2-p21.3	*MYL3*	Essential MLC	<1	Missense
15q14	*ACTC*	Cardiac actin	<1	Missense
7q3	?	?	?	?

Abbreviations: MHC, myosin heavy chain; MLC, myosin light chain; MyBP-C, myosin-binding protein C.
*Less frequent mutation types are shown in parentheses.

in adult hearts. The genes encoding β-MHC (MYH7) and α-MHC (MYH6) are located in tandem 4-kb apart. MYH7 consists of approximately 23 kb of genomic DNA and has 41 exons, 38 of which encode a protein of 1935 amino acids.[24, 25]

Mutations in MYH7 have been estimated to account for 30 percent of cases of HCM.[26] Over 50 mutations in MYH7 have been reported.[27, 28] The majority are missense mutations that result in single nucleotide substitutions. "Hot spots" for MYH7 missense mutations have been found at codons 403,[17, 29] 719,[30, 31] and 741.[32, 33] Three deletions and one termination codon in MYH7 have also been found in families with HCM.[34–36]

Cardiac Myosin Binding Protein C Gene

Cardiac myosin binding protein C is one of three myosin binding protein C isoforms and is expressed solely in cardiac tissue.[23] The cardiac myosin binding protein C gene (MYBPC3) consists of 24 kb of genomic DNA and has 37 exons that encode a protein of 1274 amino acids.[37, 38] Mutations in MYBPC3 account for approximately 15 percent of cases of HCM.[38] Twenty-seven mutations have been reported, including missense mutations, insertions, deletions, and splice mutations. At least 17 of these mutations cause truncation of the encoded protein with loss of the myosin and titin binding domains.[15, 19, 20, 37–41]

Cardiac Troponin T Gene

Troponin T is one of three subunits of the troponin complex that also includes troponin C and troponin I. The cardiac troponin T isoform is expressed in fetal and adult heart and developing skeletal muscle.[23] The cardiac troponin T gene (TNNT2) consists of 17 kb of genomic DNA and has 17 exons.[42] Multiple different protein isoforms arise owing to alternate splicing of exons or acceptor sites. Mutations in TNNT2 have been estimated to account for approximately 15 percent of cases of HCM.[26] Eleven TNNT2 missense mutations, 1 splice donor site mutation, and a single codon deletion have been reported.[18, 26, 42–44]

Cardiac Troponin I Gene

Cardiac troponin I is expressed only in cardiac tissue.[23] The cardiac troponin I gene (TNNI3) consists of 6.2 kb of genomic DNA and has 8 exons that encode a protein of 210 amino acids.[45] Six mutations in TNNI3 have been reported[15]; five of these mutations were missense mutations, the remaining mutation was a single codon deletion that did not change the reading frame. Three of the missense mutations were associated with a typical HCM phenotype, and two mutations resulted in an unusual form of HCM characterized by hypertrophy of the LV apex.

α Tropomyosin Gene

Tropomyosin proteins form α helical-coiled coil dimers and lie in a head-to-tail arrangement in the major groove of actin filaments, spanning 7 actin monomers. α Tropomyosin is expressed in ventricular myocardium and in fast skeletal muscle.[23] The α tropomyosin gene (TPM1) consists of 15 exons; 5 exons are present in all transcripts, and 10 exons are alternatively spliced in a tissue-specific manner.[46] Ten TPM1 exons are expressed in cardiac tissue. The encoded protein consists of 284 amino acids and has two troponin T binding domains. Mutations in TPM1 have been estimated to account for less than 3 percent of cases of HCM[26]; four missense mutations in TPM1 have been reported in exons encoding troponin T binding domains.[18, 47, 48]

Myosin Regulatory Light Chain Gene

Two regulatory (or phosphorylatable) MLC isoforms have been recognized in cardiac muscle. The ventricular isoform, myosin light chain-2 slow (MLC-2s) is also expressed in slow skeletal muscle; the other isoform (MLC-2a) is expressed in atrial myocardium.[23] The MLC-2s gene (MYL2) consists of seven exons that encode a protein of 166 amino acids.[28] Five mutations in MYL2 have been reported.[14, 49] Two mutations (Ala13Thr, Glu22Lys) were associated with the same unusual form of HCM (midcavity obstruction) observed in individuals with MYL3 mutations.

Myosin Essential Light Chain Gene

The MLCs are arranged in tandem in the neck of the myosin molecule. Both essential and regulatory MLCs belong to a superfamily of calcium binding proteins that includes troponin C and calmodulin. This protein family is characterized by the presence of helix-loop-helix calcium binding sites (EF hands).[23] Two of the five essential (or alkali) light chain isoforms are expressed in cardiac muscle. The myosin light chain-1 slow/ventricular isoform (MLC-1 s/v) is expressed in ventricular myocardium and slow skeletal muscle fibers.[23] The MLC-1 s/v gene (MYL3) consists of seven exons, six of which encode a protein of 195 amino acids.[50]

Mutations in MYL3 are an uncommon cause of HCM. In a cohort of 383 unrelated HCM families, Poetter and colleagues[14] found one MYL3 missense mutation (Met149-Val) in a single family. Six of 13 affected family members had a distinct pattern of LV hypertrophy with midchamber thickening. Screening of an additional 16 unrelated individuals with this same phenotype revealed a second MYL3 missense mutation (Arg154His) in a young male with massive midventricular obstruction.

Cardiac Actin Gene

Four of the 20 actin genes present in the human genome are muscle isoforms that are expressed in cardiac, skeletal, and smooth muscles.[23] The cardiac actin and skeletal actin isoforms are coexpressed in both cardiac and skeletal muscle. The human cardiac actin gene (ACTC) has six exons that encode a protein of 375 amino acids.[51] Cardiac actin has two important functional domains: the amino terminal end of the actin filament forms crossbridges with myosin; the other end of the actin filament has binding domains for actinin, a protein in Z bands, and dystrophin, a protein that links myofibrils to the extracellular matrix.

One missense mutation (Ala295Ser) in cardiac actin has recently been identified in a family with HCM.[16] This mutation is located at the surface of the actin filament in proximity to a putative myosin binding site. Interestingly, mutations in ACTC have also been reported to cause dilated cardiomyopathy in two small, unrelated families.[52] Both of these mutations were missense mutations, located in the immobilized end of actin that attaches to the Z bands and intercalated discs. These observations demonstrate that mutations in separate functional domains of the same gene may cause different clinical phenotypes. Mutations in the cardiac actin gene that impair force generation cause HCM, whereas those that impair force transmission to adjacent sarcomeres and the extracellular matrix cause dilated cardiomyopathy.

In Vitro Studies of Sarcomere Structure and Function

In order to determine the consequences of HCM gene mutations, an understanding of normal sarcomere structure and function is first required. The sarcomere is the fundamental structural and functional unit of cardiac muscle that consists of an interdigitating system of thick and thin filaments. A widely accepted theory to explain the mechanism of muscle contraction is the crossbridge hypothesis. In this model, force generation results from the cyclical attachment and detachment of crossbridges between actin and myosin filaments. ATP binds to the myosin head during the crossbridge attachment phase. Hydrolysis of ATP then provides energy for the detachment and subsequent reattachment of the crossbridge that causes a steplike displacement of the actin filament relative to the myosin filament.[21] The troponin-tropomyosin complex constitutes the calcium-sensitive switch that regulates this process. Troponin I is an inhibitory component of the troponin-tropomyosin complex that binds actin and inhibits actomyosin ATPase activity in the absence of calcium. Calcium binding to troponin C causes the troponin-tropomyosin complex to release the myosin binding domain of actin, permitting the interaction of actin and myosin heads.[53] The MLCs are thought to be required to maintain optimal speed and efficiency of crossbridge cycling.[54–56] Myosin binding protein C is located in the A bands of the sarcomere where it is arrayed in a series of seven to nine transverse stripes spaced at 43-nm intervals. Myosin binding protein C has binding sites for myosin and titin and is thought to contribute to the organization and assembly of thick filaments.[57–60] Myosin binding protein C may also exert a modulatory effect on muscle contraction. Phosphorylation of myosin binding protein C influences crossbridge function by regulating the position of the myosin head relative to the thin filament.[61–63]

A major advance in understanding the mechanisms whereby HCM mutations perturb sarcomere function has been the recognition of the importance of the location of mutant residues on individual sarcomere protein molecules (Plate 52–4). β-MHC mutations have been studied in the greatest detail. Rayment and coworkers[64] mapped 29 missense β-MHC mutations on the three-dimensional structure of chicken skeletal myosin S1, which is highly similar to human myosin. Twenty-four of these mutations were found to be clustered at four important structural domains in the myosin head, specifically, at (1) the actin binding interface, (2) the nucleotide binding site, (3) adjacent to the region connecting two reactive cysteine residues, and (4) near the interface of the heavy chain and the essential light chain. The 5 remaining mutations were located in the myosin rod. Since primarily the myosin head determines force generation, it was proposed that rod mutations might reduce transmission of force to the thick filament array by alterations in thick filament assembly or stability.

A variety of in vitro studies have confirmed the predicted deleterious functional effects of β-MHC gene mutations on crossbridge kinetics and force generation. A widely used method of assessment of the rate of crossbridge cycling is the in vitro motility assay that measures the velocity of translocation of single actin filaments by single myosin filaments bound to a nitrocellulose-coated surface. Reduced actin sliding velocities have been demonstrated for nine β-MHC gene mutations.[65–67] In the study by Cuda and associates,[67] the greatest extent of inhibition of actin translocation was observed with the Arg403Gln and Tyr167Cys β-MHC gene mutations. These two mutations both occur in highly conserved residues that are located at the actin-myosin interface and in the nucleotide binding pocket, respectively. The least inhibition was observed with Gly256Glu and Thr124Ile β-MHC gene mutations. These mutations are located at the top of the nucleotide binding pocket and are thought to contribute to the structure of the pocket itself rather than to participate directly in ATP binding. Lankford and colleagues[68] performed mechanical studies on single-skinned soleus muscle fibers obtained from HCM patients with three different β-MHC gene mutations. Muscle fibers with Gly741Arg and Arg403Gln β-MHC gene mutations showed reductions in isometric force generation. In addition, the Arg403Gln fibers showed a decrease in the force:stiffness ratio, indicative of reduced force generation by individual crossbridges. Fibers with the Gly256Glu β-MHC gene mutation had mechanical properties that were indistinguishable from normal.

Two studies have demonstrated reduced sarcomere function with cardiac troponin T mutations. In one study, the introduction of a truncated cardiac troponin T into quail myotubes resulted in a reduction of the calcium-activated force of contraction.[69] In another study, mutant (Arg92Gln) human cardiac TnT expressed in adult feline cardiac myocytes demonstrated decreased fractional shortening and peak velocity of shortening when compared with control myocytes.[70]

Although the majority of HCM mutations studied using in vitro motility assays have demonstrated reduced contractile function, two mutations have been shown to increase the rate of actin translocation; Met179Val in the myosin essential light chain and Arg719Gln in β-MHC.[14] The latter mutation lies in a short α helix of the β-MHC that forms an interface with the essential light chain. One possible interpretation of these findings is that both increased and reduced actin translocation may cause similar detrimental effects on sarcomere function.

The reported effects of HCM mutant proteins on sarcomere structure have differed according to the various model systems used. In one study, the introduction of human β-MHC with the Arg403Gln mutation into adult feline cardiac myocytes caused disruption of sarcomere assembly.[71]

However, other authors[72] found sarcomere assembly was unchanged when this same mutation was introduced into neonatal rat cardiac myocytes. Regional sarcomere disruption was found in 14 to 21 percent of quail myotubes transfected with mutant (truncated) human cardiac troponin T,[69] but normal sarcomeres were observed with expression of mutant (Arg92Gln) human cardiac troponin T in adult feline cardiac myocytes.[70]

Mouse Models of HCM

The creation of genetically engineered mouse models has enabled the effects of the various HCM gene mutations on sarcomere structure and function to be examined in vivo. In the first mouse model of HCM, an Arg403Gln point mutation was introduced into the mouse α-MHC gene using homologous recombination.[73] Heterozygous mice (those bearing one normal and one mutant allele) exhibited LV diastolic dysfunction by 5 weeks of age, before any detectable histologic abnormalities. Myocyte hypertrophy and disarray, similar to that observed in human HCM, developed by 15 weeks of age. In isolated, isovolumic heart preparations from heterozygous Arg403Gln α-MHC (α-$MHC^{403/+}$) mutant mice, Spindler and coworkers[74] also found impaired diastolic function during inotropic stimulation and a depressed energetic state. Two studies performed with LV papillary muscle strips from α-$MHC^{403/+}$ mouse hearts have shown depression of crossbridge kinetics[75] and a reduction in developed force at high stimulation rates.[76] Interestingly, homozygous Arg403Gln α-MHC mutant mice demonstrate dilated cardiomyopathy at birth and die within the first 8 days of life.[77]

Two mouse models with cardiac troponin T mutations have been developed. Adult mice expressing an Arg92Gln cardiac troponin T transgene exhibited normal systolic LV function, diastolic dysfunction, and histologic evidence of myocyte disarray.[78] Mice expressing a truncated cardiac troponin T transgene were found to have mild systolic dysfunction, markedly abnormal diastolic function and myocellular disarray.[79] LV hypertrophy was not observed in either of these models. The mouse hearts expressing the truncated cardiac troponin T transgene were actually smaller than wild-type hearts and demonstrated a reduction in the number and size of myocytes.

Recently, two mouse models with cardiac myosin binding protein C mutations have been reported. One of these models was generated by expression of an Arg92Gln cardiac myosin binding C transgene that encoded a truncated protein lacking the myosin and titin binding domains.[80] The mutant protein was stable but did not incorporate efficiently into sarcomeres, resulting in a striking pattern of sarcomere disorganization. Functional studies of the transgenic muscle fibers demonstrated a leftward shift in the pCa^{2+}-force curve and reduced power output. In a second model, a truncated protein was created by insertion of a 2-kb fragment into exon 30 of the cardiac myosin binding protein C gene.[81] Heterozygous mice developed progressive LV hypertrophy with age (unpublished data). Homozygous mice with a truncated cardiac myosin binding protein C gene exhibited dilated cardiomyopathy from birth with subsequent development of progressive LV hypertrophy, myofibrillar disarray, and fibrosis. On electron microscopy, sarcomere assembly appeared normal with the exception of absence of the M bands. In vivo hemodynamic studies in the homozygous mice demonstrated significant impairment of both systolic and diastolic LV function.

Sarcomere Dysfunction Causes Cardiac Remodeling

Collectively, current data demonstrate that aberrant crossbridge kinetics and reduced force generation are the principal consequences of HCM gene mutations. The presence of dilated cardiomyopathy in homozygous α-$MHC^{403/403}$ mice and homozygous cardiac myosin binding protein C mutant mice[77, 81] suggests there may be a gene-dosage effect for the deleterious effects of mutant peptide on sarcomere function. Experimental evidence of sarcomere dysfunction provides a basis for the current concept that LV hypertrophy in HCM is a "compensatory" rather than a primary phenomenon. The pathways linking sarcomere dysfunction and the development of myocardial hypertrophy are likely to be complex and remain to be elucidated in detail. Although myocardial hypertrophy may be considered a "final common pathway" in response to sarcomere dysfunction associated with various gene mutations, there is considerable diversity in the extent of hypertrophy observed in murine models and in humans with different mutations or within families with the same mutation. These observations highlight the modifying role of other genes and environmental factors in the hypertrophic response. The angiotensin-converting enzyme gene deletion/insertion polymorphism is one such potential genetic modifier.[82]

Dominant Negative Versus Haploinsufficiency

One important question in understanding the pathogenesis of HCM is determination of the mechanism by which a defect in a single gene allele produces a dominant phenotype. Since the majority of HCM mutations are missense mutations, the mechanism by which these cause disease has been assumed to be through dominant negative actions. In this model, the mutant protein is incorporated into the sarcomere but prevents appropriate assembly or function of myofibrils by acting as a "poison polypeptide." An alternative hypothesis is that these mutations function as null alleles ("haploinsufficiency"), which results in an imbalance of stoichiometry of sarcomere proteins. The haploinsufficiency model has been proposed as a potential mechanism to explain HCM caused by gene mutations that encode truncated proteins, such as cardiac troponin T and cardiac myosin binding protein C.

A growing body of evidence has emerged in support of the dominant negative mode of action. Mutations in β-MHC are analogous to missense mutations in the unc54 MHC gene of *C. elegans*. In the nematode, mutant MHC are stable and are incorporated into myofibrils but disrupt normal sarcomere assembly.[83] In vitro motility assays performed with a mixture of wild-type and mutant (Arg403Gln) β-MHC demonstrate reductions in wild-type

MHC function with a disproportionate slowing of actin translocation as the proportion of mutant myosin is increased.[65] Finally, in several mouse models, relatively low levels of transgene expression (<10 percent) have been sufficient to elicit histologic and functional changes similar to those observed in HCM.[78, 79, 84]

LV Pathophysiology in HCM

Systolic Function

LV systolic function in HCM is usually normal or hyperdynamic. Reduced systolic function and wall thinning may occur in patients with long-standing chronic disease ("burnt out" HCM) owing to replacement of myocytes by myocardial fibrosis. HCM may be classified as *obstructive* or *nonobstructive* depending on the presence or absence of a systolic pressure gradient across the LVOT. Obstructive HCM occurs in less than 25 percent of cases. The subaortic gradient results from a mechanical impediment to LV outflow produced by the combination of (1) asymmetric hypertrophy of the proximal interventricular septum and (2) SAM of the mitral valve with subsequent mitral leaflet–septal contact. The mechanism of SAM has been controversial,[2] but it has been postulated that the anterior mitral valve leaflet is drawn upward toward the septum by a Venturi effect produced by high-velocity blood flow through the narrowed outflow tract.[85, 86] Subaortic obstruction to LV blood outflow gives rise to the "spike-and-dome" pattern on arterial pulse tracings. This waveform is characterized by a brisk upstroke due to rapid early ejection of blood from the left ventricle, a decline in pressure with the onset of obstruction to outflow, then a secondary pressure rise with late systolic ejection of the residual LV blood volume. Angulation and SAM of the anterior mitral valve leaflet also cause the mitral leaflets to coapt in the body of the leaflets rather than at the leaflet tips. A funnel-shaped opening created by the distal portions of both leaflets results in a posterior-directed jet of mitral regurgitation during midsystole and late systole.[87] The severity of mitral regurgitation has been shown to correlate with the length over which the mitral leaflets coapt, the relative mismatch of anterior to posterior leaflet length, and decreasing posterior leaflet mobility.[88]

The subaortic gradient in HCM has been described as "dynamic" because the magnitude of the pressure gradient can be varied by provocative maneuvers. The outflow tract obstruction is increased by maneuvers that reduce LV preload or afterload or that increase myocardial contractility (such as standing from a sitting or squatting position, Valsalva maneuver, exercise, or pharmacologic interventions such as administration of nitroglycerin or amyl nitrate). Conversely, the outflow tract obstruction is reduced by maneuvers that increase LV preload or afterload or that reduce myocardial contractility (such as squatting, passive leg elevation, handgrip, administration of phenylephrine or beta-blocking drugs).[86] In asymptomatic individuals, provocative maneuvers may be used to unmask latent obstruction.

Although obstructive HCM is caused by proximal ventricular septal hypertrophy in the majority of cases, a minority of individuals may exhibit midventricular obstruction owing to midventricular hypertrophy at the level of the papillary muscles. LV preload, afterload, and contractility influence the severity of midventricular obstruction. Other features of subaortic obstruction such as the spike-and-dome arterial pulse waveforms and mitral regurgitation are not observed with midventricular obstruction, however.[86]

Diastolic Function

Impaired diastolic relaxation is a characteristic feature of human HCM that has been reproduced in mouse models.[73–75, 78, 79, 81] The diastolic dysfunction has been attributed to a combination of prolonged LV relaxation and increased LV chamber stiffness. Studies in mouse models of HCM have provided insights into both of these processes. First, the detection of diastolic dysfunction prior to overt evidence of histologic change in mutant mice suggests that this physiologic abnormality is a primary consequence of sarcomere gene mutations. Slowed crossbridge cycling rates in mutant sarcomeres may directly lead to prolonged activation of the thin filament and reduced diastolic relaxation.[74] Increased or prolonged calcium availability to the myofibril may also prolong diastolic relaxation. Both increased intracellular calcium concentrations and increased sensitivity to calcium levels have been found in vitro muscle preparations from affected individuals with HCM and α-MHC$^{403/+}$ mice.[74–76, 89] The mechanism of altered calcium homeostasis in mutant sarcomeres is not yet known. LV relaxation is influenced also by load-dependent factors that may be abnormal in HCM, including end-systolic LV pressure and volume, wall stress, coronary artery blood flow-and regional asynchrony of LV wall motion.[85]

The secondary development of structural changes, such as hypertrophy and fibrosis, causes LV chamber remodeling and increased chamber stiffness that further exacerbate diastolic filling. Georgakopoulos and associates[90] performed sequential in vivo hemodynamic studies in α-MHC$^{403/+}$ mice and found delayed pressure development in mice aged 6 weeks; by 20 weeks, reductions of cardiac output and increased end-systolic chamber stiffness were also present, coincident with the development of LV hypertrophy and fibrosis (Fig. 52–2). Blanchard and colleagues[75] also demonstrated increased diastolic stiffness in resting LV papillary muscle strips from α-MHC$^{403/+}$ mice. Intracellular calcium overload and myocardial ischemia are two factors that may contribute to myocyte dysfunction and, ultimately, to myocyte death. Myocyte loss and replacement fibrosis have been observed to a greater extent in homozygous (α-MHC$^{403/403}$) than in heterozygous α-MHC$^{403/+}$ mutant mice, suggesting that there may be a threshold level for cell viability with increases in the proportion of mutant protein.[77]

Elevated LV end-diastolic pressures due to diastolic dysfunction, increased end-systolic pressure with LV outflow obstruction, and mitral regurgitation may contribute to elevation of left atrial pressure, left atrial enlargement, and a subsequent increased risk for the development of atrial fibrillation. The onset of atrial fibrillation may precipitate severe hemodynamic compromise in individuals with LV diastolic dysfunction, since LV filling is reliant to a greater extent on left atrial contraction. Atrial fibrillation is also

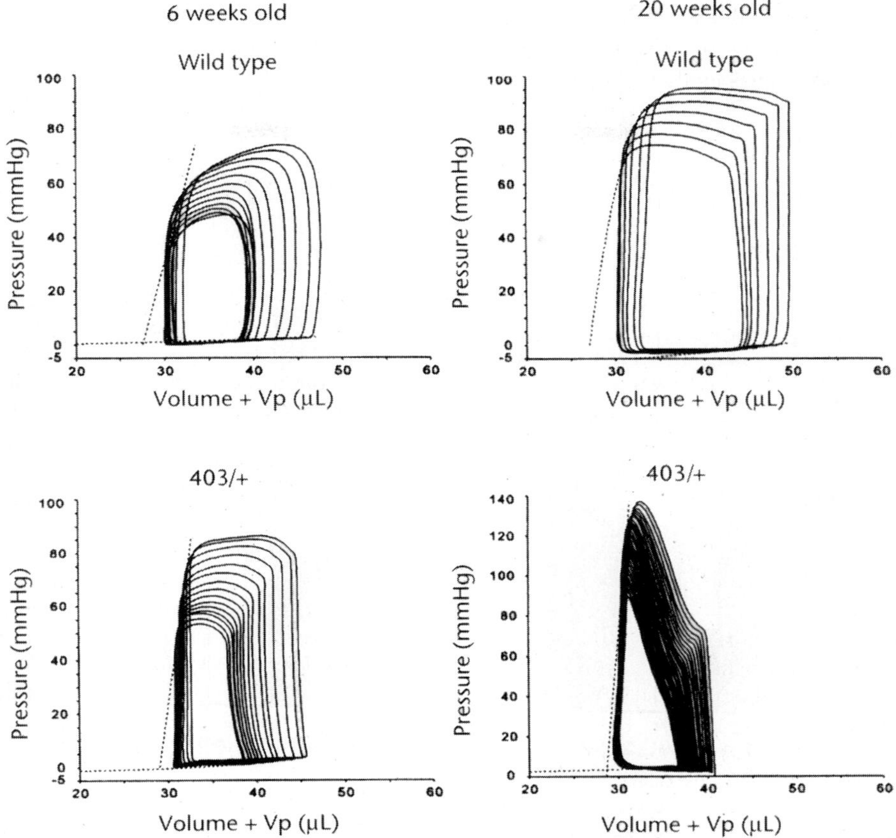

FIGURE 52–2 In vivo left ventricular pressure-volume relations measured during transient reduction of cardiac preload in wild-type and alpha myosin heavy chain (α-MHC)$^{403/+}$ mutant mice. At 6 weeks (left), data for wild-type and α-MHC$^{403/+}$ mice were similar. At 20 weeks (right), α-MHC$^{403/+}$ mice showed a change in loop shape with systolic pressure elevation during ejection and a substantial increase in the end-systolic elastance (*dashed vertical line*), consistent with an increase in systolic stiffness. (From Georgakopoulos D, Christe ME, Giewat M, et al: The pathogenesis of familial hypertrophic cardiomyopathy: early and evolving effects from an α cardiac myosin heavy chain missense mutation. Nat Med 5:327, 1999.)

associated with an increased risk of thromboembolic events.

Myocardial Ischemia

Myocardial ischemia may occur in both obstructive and nonobstructive HCM. Several mechanisms for myocardial ischemia in HCM have been proposed, including (1) increased myocardial oxygen demand due to increased LV mass and wall stress and (2) reduced myocardial oxygen supply due to decreased coronary perfusion pressure secondary to LV outflow obstruction, elevated diastolic filling pressures, systolic compression of large intramural coronary arteries, myocardial bridging, reduced capillary density and abnormally narrowed small intramural coronary arteries.[85, 86] Symptoms of myocardial ischemia in HCM are precipitated frequently by exertion, which causes further imbalance of the myocardial oxygen demand and supply ratio.

CLINICAL EVALUATION

Clinical History

Genotype-positive individuals with HCM may be asymptomatic or may experience symptoms ranging from mild dizziness and palpitations to sudden death. The most common presenting features are exertional dyspnea, angina pectoris, fatigue, and presyncope or syncope. Since a variety of pathophysiologic mechanisms contribute to symptoms in HCM, including LV subaortic outflow obstruction, LV diastolic dysfunction, and myocardial ischemia (see the previous section), the severity of symptoms generally does not correlate well with single factors such as the extent of LV hypertrophy or the magnitude of the LVOT pressure gradient.[85, 86] In individuals with LV diastolic dysfunction, symptoms and signs of congestive cardiac failure—such as paroxysmal nocturnal dyspnea, orthopnea, and peripheral edema—may be precipitated by atrial tachyarrhythmias. Syncope and sudden death may result from ventricular arrhythmias.

The age of onset of symptoms differs between HCM disease genes. For example, individuals with β-MHC gene mutations generally present in the first two decades of life. In contrast, individuals with cardiac myosin binding protein C gene mutations may be asymptomatic until the fifth or sixth decades of life (Fig. 52–3).[38, 91] A detailed family history is an essential component of the clinical history in HCM. Identification of young affected family members is particularly important in families that have mutations with a malignant course characterized by a high incidence of

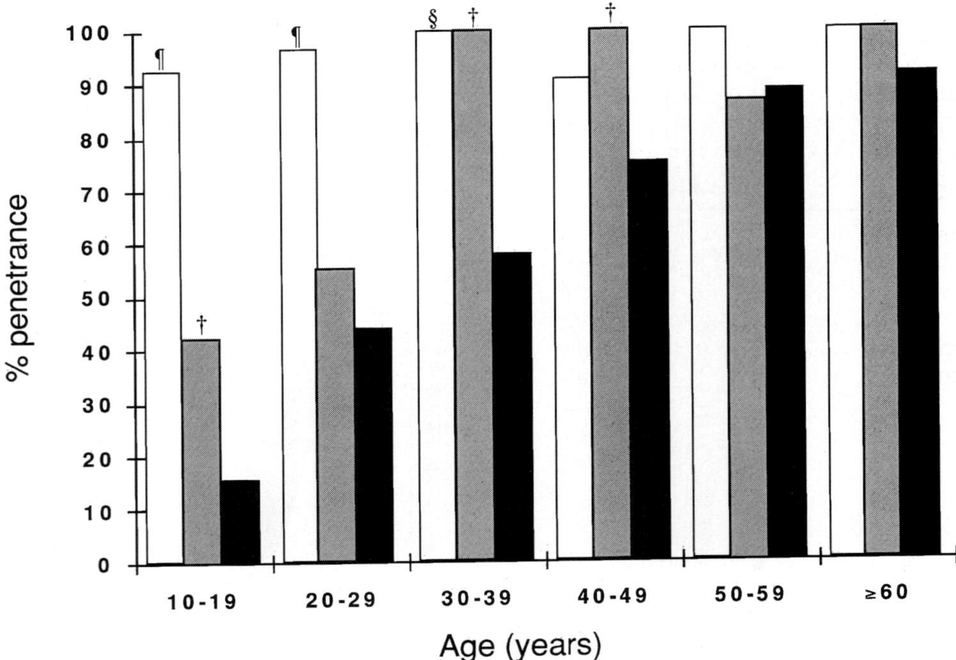

FIGURE 52–3 Age-related penetrance of HCM caused by mutations in the genes for β-MHC, cardiac troponin T, and cardiac myosin binding protein C. *Solid bars* denote the percentage of phenotype-positive individuals within the total population of genotype-positive individuals. In HCM caused by β-MHC and cardiac troponin T gene mutations, the onset of left ventricular hypertrophy is observed in early adulthood. In contrast, in HCM caused by cardiac myosin binding protein C gene mutations, the onset of left ventricular hypertrophy may be delayed until late adulthood. Significant differences in the penetrance of HCM caused by β-MHC, cardiac troponin T, and cardiac myosin binding C gene mutations are indicated as follows: *daggers,* $P < .05$; *section marks,* $P < .005$; *paragraph symbols,* $P < .001$. (From Niimura H, Bachinski LL, Sangwatanaroj S, et al: Mutations in the gene for cardiac myosin-binding protein C and late-onset familial hypertrophic cardiomyopathy. N Engl J Med 338:1248, 1998. Copyright 1998 Massachusetts Medical Society. All rights reserved.)

sudden death. In elderly individuals, although a positive family history for HCM may not be obtained, this diagnosis should be considered, particularly if the symptoms and signs cannot be accounted for by the presence of other pathologic processes, such as coronary artery disease or hypertension. It should be noted also that in the elderly, HCM may coexist with other pathologies. The absence of a positive family history in an individual with symptoms and signs of HCM suggests the possibility of a sporadic gene mutation.

Physical Examination

Physical findings may be unremarkable in the absence of LVOT obstruction. On examination of the precordium, the LV apex may be forceful and is variably displaced. A double, or triple, apical impulse may be present with the addition of a palpable left-sided fourth heart sound and/or forceful late systolic LV contraction. With extensive LV hypertrophy, the jugular venous pulse may have a prominent A wave due to reduced right ventricular compliance, and a bouncing carotid pulse may be present, analogous to the spike-and-dome pattern on arterial pressure tracings.

On auscultation, the first heart sound is generally normal. The second heart sound may have a narrow split or reversed splitting if LV contraction is prolonged by severe LV outflow obstruction. A loud fourth heart sound is often present and is due to augmented LV filling during left atrial systole when LV diastolic relaxation is prolonged. A systolic crescendo-decrescendo ejection murmur caused by turbulent blood flow through the LVOT may be audible between the left sternal border and the apex. This murmur can be distinguished from valvular aortic stenosis by its response to provocative maneuvers that increase or reduce the extent of LV outflow obstruction (see the previous section). In addition to the systolic ejection murmur, a pansystolic, blowing murmur due to mitral regurgitation may also be audible at the apex, with radiation to the axilla.

Electrocardiography

Electrocardiographic abnormalities are present in the majority of individuals with HCM and may occur in the absence of echocardiographic evidence of LV hypertrophy.[92] An example of an abnormal electrocardiogram found in a young genotype-positive, phenotype-negative individual is shown in Figure 52–4. Voltage criteria for the presence of LV hypertrophy have been defined according to the height of the QRS complexes, particularly in the precordial leads.[93] ST segment and T wave changes are observed commonly. Giant negative T waves in leads V_4 to V_6 are characteristically found with the apical pattern of LV hypertrophy observed predominantly in Japanese patients with HCM.[94, 95] A pseudoinfarction pattern with prominent Q waves may be present in the inferior (II, III, aVF) and precordial (V_2 to V_6) leads.[96, 97] The etiology of these Q waves is uncertain because a close correspondence with ventricular septal hypertrophy has not been observed. Abnormal P wave morphology may be present if the left atrium is dilated. Atrial tachyarrhythmias (atrial fibrillation, atrial flutter), accessory atrioventricular pathways (including Wolff-Parkinson-White syndrome), and ventricular arrhythmias may also be found.

Chest X-Ray

The chest X-ray in HCM may be normal or may demonstrate an abnormal cardiac silhouette owing to LV or left atrial enlargement. Infrequently, anterior ventricular septal hypertrophy may cause a bulge along the left heart border. Redistribution of pulmonary vascular markings and enlargement of the right ventricle and right atrium may be observed with secondary pulmonary hypertension or right ventricular hypertrophy.

Echocardiography

Transthoracic echocardiography is the primary diagnostic modality for evaluation of individuals with suspected HCM. Two-dimensional echocardiographic imaging provides assessment of LV and right ventricular hypertrophy, ventricular and atrial chamber size, and systolic contractile function. The presence of a LVOT gradient and LV diastolic dysfunction can be identified by color-flow Doppler studies. Both two-dimensional echocardiographic imaging and color-flow Doppler are used to examine valvular morphology and function. Although HCM is primarily a myocardial disorder, structural abnormalities of the mitral valve and subvalvular apparatus be present, including increased leaflet area, elongation and prolapse of leaflets, and anomalous papillary muscle insertion directly into the anterior leaflet.[98, 99] Mitral regurgitation is a relatively frequent finding that results primarily from abnormal coaptation of the mitral valve leaflets.[87, 88] Transesophageal echocardiography is indicated for (1) more precise delineation of mitral valve morphology and function, (2) exclusion of left atrial thrombus and spontaneous echo contrast in patients with atrial fibrillation and/or recent thromboembolic events, (3) intraoperative monitoring during surgical myectomy-myotomy, and (4) technically inadequate transthoracic echocardiographic images. Stress echocardiography may be useful to investigate individuals with symptoms suggestive of myocardial ischemia (Fig. 52–5).[100]

Asymmetric septal hypertrophy has been considered the sine qua non of HCM, with a septal:posterior wall ratio of 1.3:1 or greater regarded as diagnostic.[101] Transthoracic echocardiographic studies performed in large populations

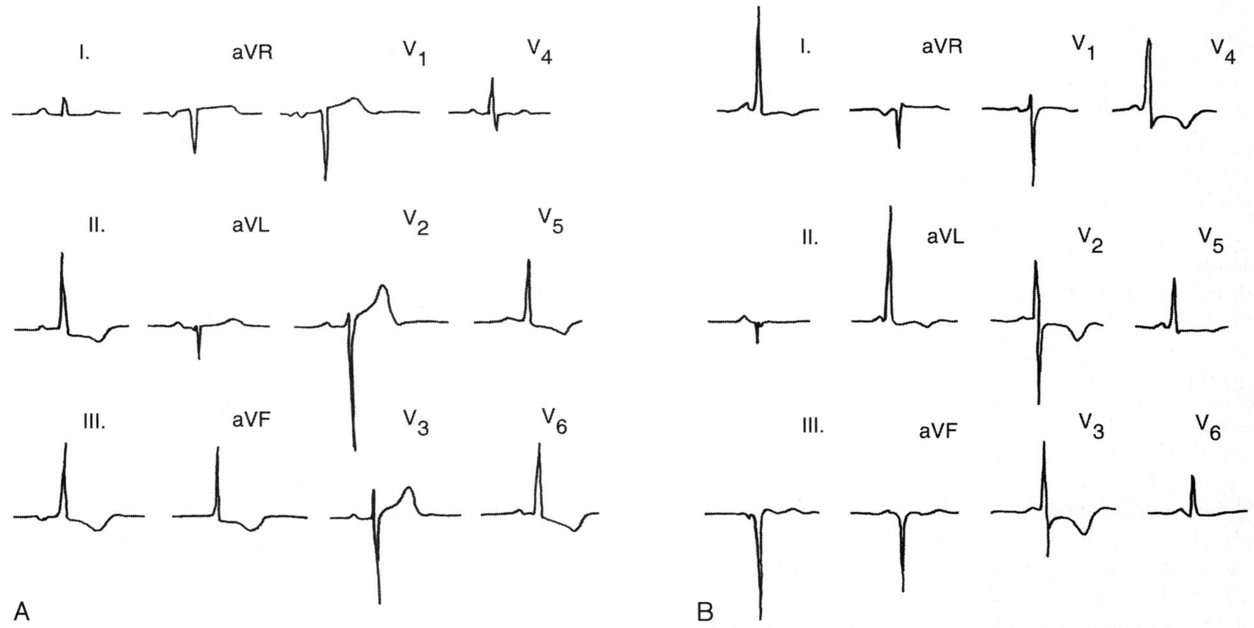

FIGURE 52–4 Twelve-lead electrocardiographic tracings from two individuals with HCM who were genotype-positive, phenotype-negative **(A)** and genotype-positive, phenotype-positive **(B)**. **A,** The electrocardiogram (ECG) was recorded from a 17-year-old male who was asymptomatic but had a positive family history of HCM. His echocardiogram was normal. This ECG shows inferolateral T wave inversion and voltage criteria for left ventricular hypertrophy. **B,** The ECG was recorded from a 32-year-old woman with symptoms and signs of HCM, including echocardiographic evidence of left ventricular hypertrophy. This ECG shows anterior and inferior Q waves, anterolateral T wave inversion, and voltage criteria for left ventricular hypertrophy.

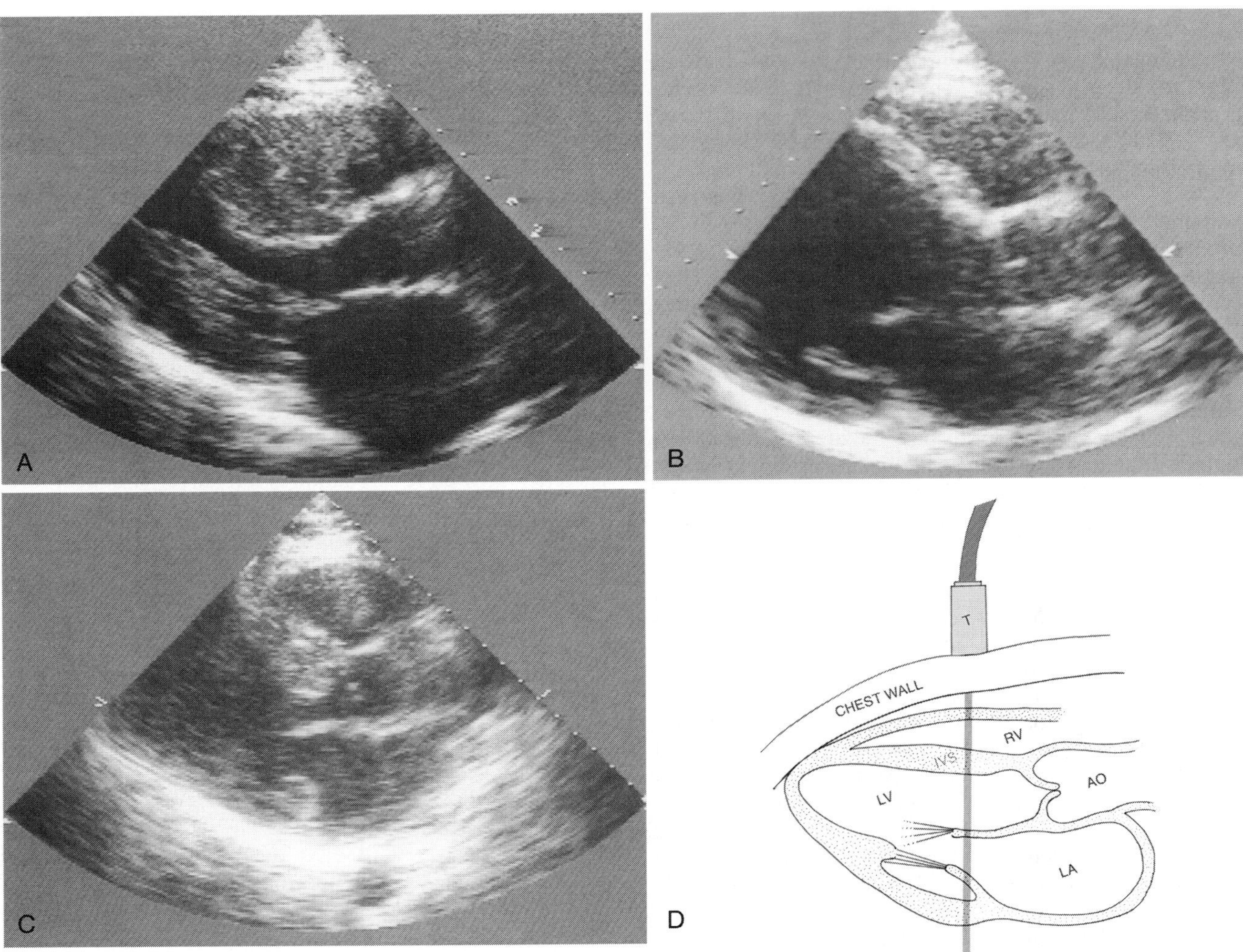

FIGURE 52–5 Two-dimensional echocardiographic images in the parasternal long-axis view from three individuals with HCM. **A,** A 20-year-old woman presented to the emergency room after a syncopal episode. A positive family history of HCM was elicited. On auscultation of the precordium, a systolic ejection murmur was audible. Echocardiography showed asymmetric hypertrophy of the interventricular septum, systolic anterior motion of the mitral valve, and left atrial dilatation. **B,** An asymptomatic 35-year-old man was evaluated after the sudden death of his sister. Postmortem examination of the deceased sister's heart had revealed histologic evidence of HCM. Echocardiography showed left ventricular dilatation and reduced fractional shortening, consistent with dilated cardiomyopathy. **C,** A 30-year-old man presented with presyncope after repeated episodes of standing from a squatting position. Echocardiography showed marked hypertrophy of the proximal interventricular septum, with systolic anterior motion of the mitral valve and left ventricular outflow tract obstruction (gradient, 90 mm Hg). Highly echogenic foci present in the septal myocardium caused a "groundglass" appearance. An echogenic plaque at the site of anterior mitral valve leaflet–septal contact was also noted. **D,** Schematic of the cardiac chambers visualized by two-dimensional echocardiography in the parasternal long-axis view. AO, aorta; IVS, interventricular septum; LA, left atrium; LV, left ventricle; RV, right ventricle.

with HCM have demonstrated, however, that although LV hypertrophy in the vast majority of cases is asymmetric, a variety of patterns of LV hypertrophy, ranging from extensive and diffuse to mild and segmental, can be found.[1, 2, 102–105] Such data indicate not only that traditional diagnostic criteria lack sensitivity and specificity but also that no single morphologic pattern can be considered pathognomonic for diagnosis of this disease.

Genotype-phenotype analyses have demonstrated that genetic heterogeneity contributes to phenotypic heterogeneity in HCM. For example, LV hypertrophy in β-MHC gene mutations may be moderate or severe, whereas LV hypertrophy in cardiac troponin T gene mutations is generally only mild.[26, 43, 91, 104] Cardiac troponin I and MLC gene mutations cause unusual forms of LV hypertrophy localized to the LV apex or midventricular cavity, respectively.[14, 15] Clinical evaluation of large families highlights the variable expressivity of HCM. Young genotype-positive individuals may have only mild thickening of LV wall segments, whereas older members of the same family may exhibit severe LV hypertrophy. In young individuals, the diagnosis of cardiac hypertrophy may be made more reliably by comparison of LV wall thickness measurements with unaffected siblings rather than with conventional HCM wall thickness criteria. Age-related penetrance also varies with different HCM disease genes. For example, individuals with β-MHC gene mutations are likely to develop LV hypertrophy within the first or second decades of life. In contrast, individuals with cardiac myosin binding protein C gene mutations may have normal echocardiograms until the fifth or sixth decades of life (see Fig. 52–3).[38, 91] In any HCM pedigree, a small number of nonpenetrant genotype-positive individuals may be found who do not exhibit LV hypertrophy at any age. In individuals with a family history but unknown genotype, a positive echocardiogram can confirm HCM, but a negative echocardiogram does not necessarily exclude this diagnosis. Genotype-phenotype correlations in large numbers of affected individuals are required to accurately define patterns of LV hypertrophy across the spectrum of HCM gene mutations. Genetic heterogeneity is unlikely to account fully for phenotypic heterogeneity in HCM. The role of additional genetic factors and environmental factors such as blood pressure, exercise, diet, and body mass need to be considered when assessing LV hypertrophy in individuals with HCM.

Electrophysiologic Studies

Individuals with HCM who experience syncopal episodes should be evaluated noninvasively with Holter monitoring to identify sustained or potentially lethal ventricular arrhythmias.[106–109] Whereas other techniques may be appropriate for investigation of syncope, including signal-averaged electrocardiography,[110–113] heart rate variability determination,[114, 115] and assessment of blood pressure response to exercise, the use of provocative studies such as tilt-table testing has great potential for precipitating hemodynamic compromise in patients with HCM. Histopathologic changes in HCM may cause variation in conduction properties with dispersion of conduction velocity throughout the myocardium. Assessment of QT dispersion may be a useful component in risk assessment for ventricular arrhythmias.[116] Invasive electrophysiologic studies have been used to identify spontaneous and provocable arrhythmias in patients at high risk of sudden death, including those with a strong family history or syncope or survivors of sudden death. The predictive value of inducible ventricular arrhythmias in HCM has, however, been found to be low.[109, 117–120]

Other Investigations

Radionuclide scanning with tomographic imaging (single-photon emission computed tomography) or magnetic resonance imaging are useful techniques to delineate the location and extent of LV hypertrophy if the technical quality of transthoracic echocardiographic images is inadequate.[121–124] Stress thallium studies may be useful to identify reversible defects caused by myocardial ischemia.[125–127] Myocardial blood flow and metabolism may also be assessed using positron emission tomography.[128–132] Gated radionuclide ventriculography is an alternative to echocardiography for assessing LV size and contractile function.[133] Cardiac catheterization and angiography are generally reserved for assessment of myocardial ischemia and for evaluation before surgical procedures such as myectomy and cardiac transplantation.

Genetic Studies

Genotype-phenotype correlations in large populations will provide important data for diagnostic and prognostic evaluation in HCM. Genotyping may be particularly useful in cases in which the clinical diagnosis is ambiguous, such as in individuals with borderline LV hypertrophy, including trained athletes, or in individuals with hypertension and suspected HCM.[134] Currently, DNA testing is limited predominantly to families with known mutations. Identification of mutations by conventional linkage analysis techniques in families in which the HCM disease gene is unknown is time-consuming, expensive, and available in few centers. The future development of automated screening methods such as DNA chips containing a comprehensive range of mutations in all the HCM disease genes will greatly facilitate the application of genetic information to clinical medicine.

The availability of genetic testing creates a number of psychosocial, ethical, and medicolegal issues. Although a genotype-positive diagnosis may stimulate beneficial lifestyle changes and therapeutic interventions, it may also create patient anxiety about having a genetic disorder and may potentially lead to discrimination by employers and insurance companies. Identification of genotype-positive, phenotype-negative individuals creates particular difficulties because the clinical significance of this diagnosis is uncertain. Many of these questions will be resolved over time as genetically oriented research studies provide a better understanding of the clinical implications of genetic diagnoses. From a community perspective, this genetic data will need to be viewed in the context of an appropriate ethical and legal framework.

NATURAL HISTORY

The natural history of HCM is variable; whereas some individuals remain asymptomatic throughout life, others have progression of symptoms with or without development of heart failure. A significant number of individuals die suddenly, often without premonitory symptoms. Estimated mortality rates in HCM differ according to the population studied. In hospital-based referral centers in which a large proportion of cases have moderate or severe symptoms, annual mortality rates of 3 to 6 percent have been found.[135–144] In contrast, studies performed in community clinics have emphasized the relatively mild symptoms and good survival in unselected populations with annual mortality rates of 1 percent or less.[145–149]

Longitudinal echocardiographic studies have demonstrated that LV remodeling may occur during the course of this disease. Progressive increases in LV wall thickness are observed predominantly in adolescents and young adults with HCM. In later adult life, LV wall thickness generally remains stable or decreases.[150–154] It is notable that the majority of studies that have examined the natural history of LV hypertrophy in HCM have been performed in patients whose genotype is unknown. We have observed progression of LV hypertrophy in selected subgroups of genotyped individuals over the age of 40 years, such as those with myosin binding protein C mutations[38] or the

Arg663His β-MHC mutation (Fig. 52–6).[155] LV wall thinning in individuals with long-standing disease may result from myocyte loss and fibrosis. Approximately 10 to 20 percent of individuals with HCM may ultimately develop symptoms and signs of dilated cardiomyopathy.[153, 156] Disease progression in HCM may also include the onset of atrial fibrillation. The prevalence of atrial fibrillation in affected individuals has been estimated to be 10 to 16 percent.[105, 157] Some HCM gene mutations or morphologic variants appear to have an increased propensity for atrial fibrillation. For example, we observed a high incidence of atrial fibrillation (47 percent) and proximal septal hypertrophy in a family with the Arg663His β-MHC mutation (see Fig. 52–6).[155]

Sudden death is the most devastating complication of HCM and may occur in young asymptomatic individuals or in those with chronic heart failure. Ventricular tachyarrhythmias are the cause of sudden death in the majority of cases. A complex interaction of electrical and hemodynamic factors may trigger ventricular tachyarrhythmias in HCM, including re-entrant depolarization pathways around foci of myofibrillar disarray and fibrosis, supraventricular tachyarrhythmias, LVOT obstruction, LV diastolic dysfunction, myocardial ischemia, and systemic arterial hypotension.[85, 158, 159] Bradyarrhythmias related to sinus node and atrioventricular node conduction abnormalities may cause sudden death in some individuals.[160–162] Given the complexity of mechanisms that may precipitate ventricular arrhythmias, it is not surprising that few clinical parameters have been found to reliably predict individuals at increased risk for sudden death. Most investigators agree that "high-risk" patients include survivors of a cardiac arrest with documented ventricular fibrillation and young patients (<30 years) with a strong family history of sudden death.[26, 85, 86, 141, 163–167]

For the large proportion of individuals who do not fall into the high-risk category, consideration of the risk associated with other clinical parameters is relevant. In various study populations, however, conflicting results have been found for the positive predictive value of factors such as young age at diagnosis, history of syncope, severity of symptoms, LVOT gradient, LV wall thickness, left atrial size, and atrial fibrillation.[86, 141, 146, 147, 149] Although these clinical variables may not identify individuals at increased risk for sudden death, their high negative predictive value does enable identification of individuals at low risk for sudden death. Adult individuals with HCM can be categorized as "low risk" if they are asymptomatic or have mild symptoms and also have none of the following: a family history of premature death due to HCM, nonsustained ventricular tachycardia on ambulatory monitoring, a marked LVOT gradient, substantial LV hypertrophy (>20 mm), marked left atrial dilatation, and an abnormal blood pressure response during exercise.[159]

Genotype determination may be the single most important component of risk stratification in HCM. It is likely that the majority of individuals considered at high risk due to a strong family history of sudden death also have a high-risk HCM gene mutation. It has been demonstrated that prognosis varies considerably between different HCM gene mutations. For example, some β-MHC mutations, such as Arg403Gln and Arg453Cys, are associated with a reduced life expectancy and high incidence of sudden death, whereas other β-MHC mutations, such as Val606-Met, have a relatively benign course.[164] Reduced survival has been shown with cardiac troponin T mutations and some α-tropomyosin mutations (Ala63Val, Lys70Thr).[26, 43, 44, 48] Survival was reduced in one family with the Asp175Asn α-tropomyosin mutation[48] but was normal in three other families with the same mutation,[168] suggesting that genetic susceptibility may be modified by other genetic or environmental factors.

The location of a HCM gene mutation in the sarcomere has been proposed as an important determinant of the degree of sarcomere dysfunction and the severity of clinical outcome. HCM mutations that alter amino acid charge have been associated with poor outcomes.[164] However, whereas mutations that do not alter amino acid charge usually have a benign clinical course, some mutations that do alter amino acid charge also have a good prognosis.[27] Electrophysiologic studies in mouse models may provide important clues into mechanisms and differential propensity for sudden death between HCM gene mutations.

TREATMENT

The overall strategy for treatment of individuals with HCM is shown in Figure 52–7. In general, the approach to treatment varies according to the classification of an individual patient into one of four categories: (1) genotype-positive, phenotype-negative, (2) asymptomatic and mildly

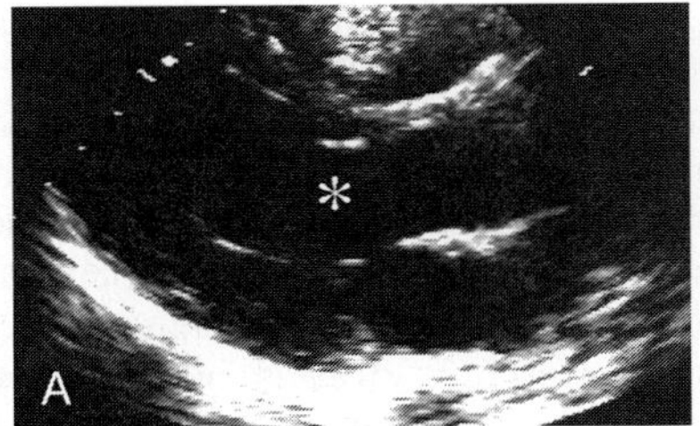

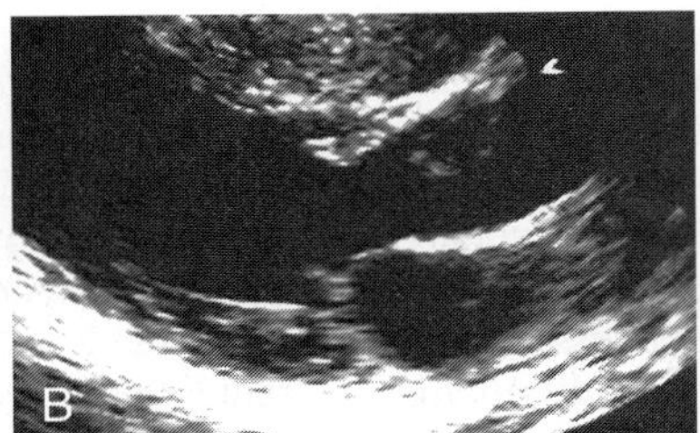

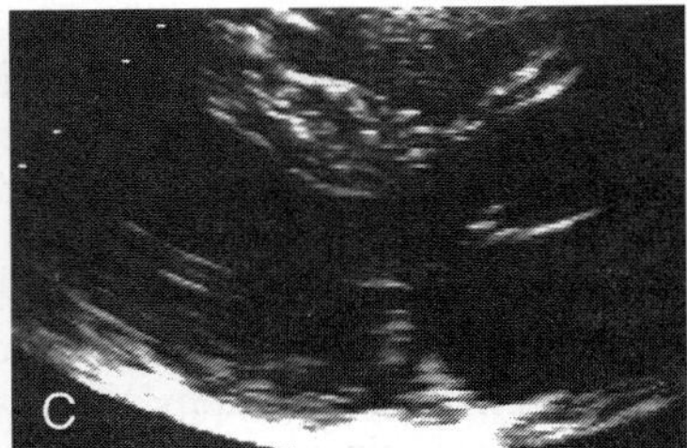

FIGURE 52–6 Two-dimensional echocardiographic images in the parasternal long-axis view demonstrate progressive left ventricular morphologic changes caused by the β-MHC Arg663His missense mutation. **A,** Mild proximal septal thickening (maximal wall thickness < 1.3 cm). *Asterisk* indicates focal proximal septal hypertrophy. **B,** Focal proximal septal hypertrophy. **C,** Predominant proximal septal hypertrophy with additional midseptal hypertrophy. (**A–C,** Reprinted from Am J Cardiol, Vol. 83, Gruver EJ, Fatkin D, Dodds GA, et al, Familial hypertrophic cardiomyopathy and atrial fibrillation caused by Arg663His β-cardiac myosin heavy chain mutation, pp. 13H–18H, Copyright 1999, with permission from Excerpta Medica Inc.)

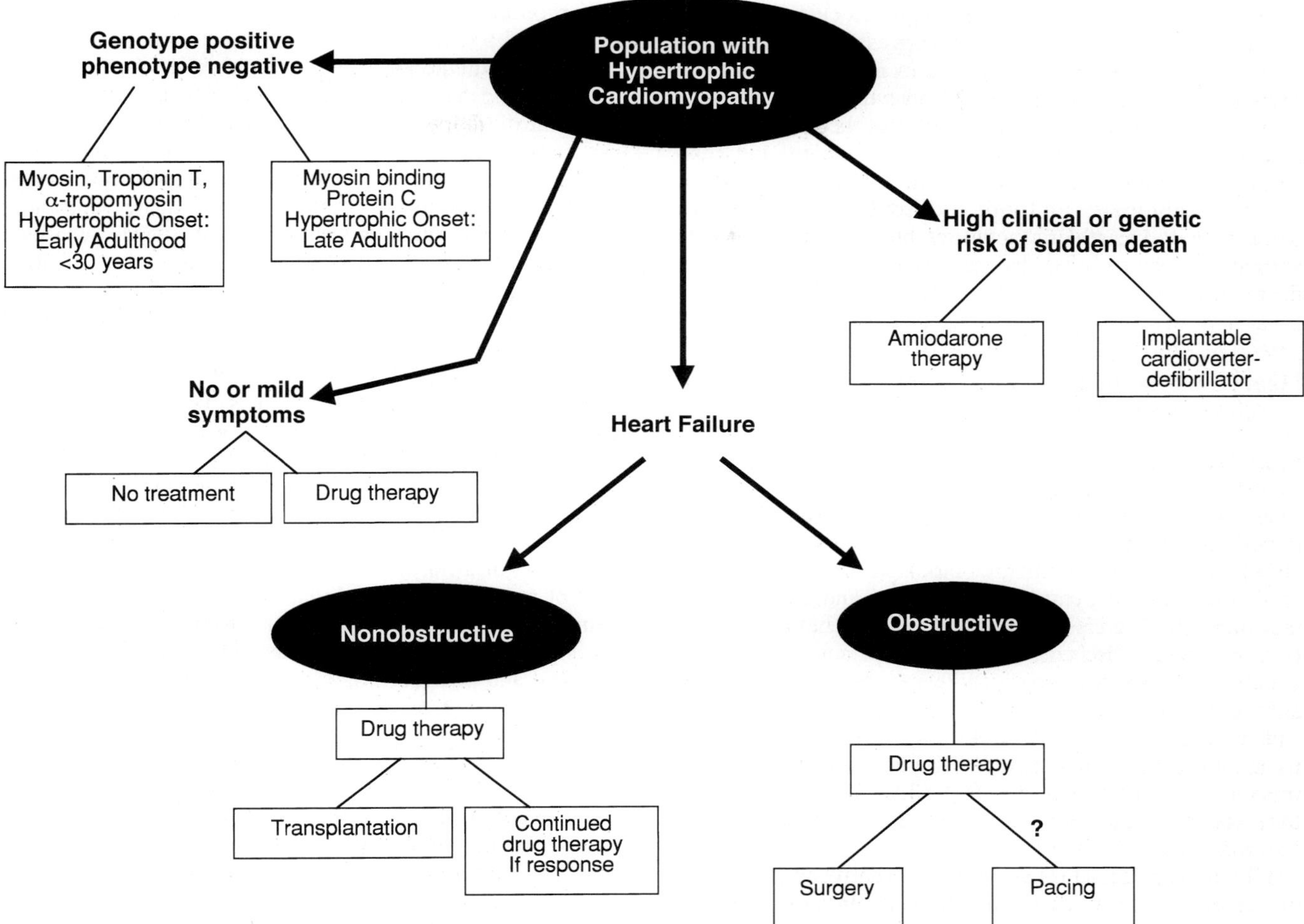

FIGURE 52–7 Schematic of the four principal clinical presentations of HCM with corresponding treatment strategies. (Modified from Spirito P, Seidman CE, McKenna WJ, et al: The management of hypertrophic cardiomyopathy. N Engl J Med 336:775, 1997. Copyright 1997 Massachusetts Medical Society. All rights reserved.)

symptomatic, (3) obstructive or nonobstructive HCM with heart failure, and (4) high clinical or genetic risk for sudden death.

Genotype-Positive, Phenotype-Negative Individuals

Genetic testing has led to the identification of a subgroup of individuals who are genotype-positive for HCM gene mutations but who have no clinical evidence of disease (phenotype-negative). Most of these individuals ultimately develop symptoms and signs of HCM. Young genotype-positive members of families in which a β-MHC mutation has been found should undergo longitudinal follow-up with serial echocardiograms throughout adolescence and early adult life. Genotype-positive members of families with known cardiac myosin binding protein C mutations should have serial echocardiograms throughout life. At present, there are no data to suggest that pharmacologic treatment of genotype-positive, phenotype-negative individuals will delay or prevent the onset of LV hypertrophy or complications such as sudden death. However, periodic assessment of clinically silent arrhythmias appears warranted in individuals with mutations associated with a high incidence of sudden death. The clinical implications of genetic abnormalities in the small percentage of individuals who remain nonpenetrant are not known.

Asymptomatic and Mildly Symptomatic Individuals

Genetic testing has also led to the identification of a large number of genotype-positive, phenotype-positive individuals who are asymptomatic. Further, community-based studies have shown that a significant proportion of individuals with HCM have only mild symptoms.[145–149] These observations suggest that asymptomatic and mildly symptomatic individuals account for the majority of the total HCM population.[159] Pharmacologic therapy is indicated for relief of mild symptoms but is generally not required in asymptomatic individuals. One possible exception is the young asymptomatic patient with massive LV hypertrophy or significant LVOT gradient, in whom the onset of symptoms would appear inevitable.[159] There is no evidence that prophylactic treatment with β-adrenergic blocking drugs or calcium antagonists will prevent progression of disease or improve prognosis in asymptomatic or mildly symptomatic individuals.[159] It should be noted, however, that prospective trials of prophylactic therapy have not been performed, largely because of the small study populations and relatively infrequent clinical endpoints. Asymptomatic or mildly symptomatic individuals should be discouraged from competitive athletic activities but may participate in recreational sports provided that risk factors for sudden death are absent (see the previous section).[169]

Heart Failure in Obstructive and Nonobstructive HCM

Drug Therapy

Pharmacologic therapy is indicated for relief of symptoms in patients with heart failure in both obstructive and nonobstructive HCM. β-Adrenergic blocking drugs are useful predominantly for symptoms of angina and dyspnea and may improve exercise performance. The beneficial effects of β-adrenergic blockers are mediated principally by their negative chronotropic effect, with reduced heart rates resulting in prolongation of the LV diastolic filling time.[170–172] The negative inotropic effect of these drugs also contributes to a reduction of myocardial oxygen demand and may prevent increases in severity of the LVOT gradient, which may occur during exercise when sympathetic tone is increased.[171–173]

Calcium antagonist drugs are an alternative to β-adrenergic blocking drugs for treatment of symptoms in HCM. Patients who do not respond to β-adrenergic blockers may experience symptomatic improvement with calcium antagonists. There is no evidence that the combined use of these two drug classes has synergistic effects. Verapamil has been the most widely used of the calcium antagonist drugs. Verapamil improves symptoms by increasing LV relaxation and diastolic filling.[174–180] The vasodilatory effects of verapamil improve myocardial blood flow but may also potentially exacerbate LVOT gradients in patients with obstructive HCM and precipitate hypotension and pulmonary edema in patients with elevated pulmonary pressures. The negative inotropic effects of verapamil may decrease LVOT gradients but may also contribute to the development of heart failure. Other adverse effects of verapamil include suppression of sinus node automaticity and inhibition of atrioventricular conduction. Nifedipine causes less depression of atrioventricular conduction but has a more potent vasodilatory action and may be particularly harmful in patients with obstructive HCM.[181] Diltiazem has been used less frequently in HCM but may improve LV diastolic function.[182, 183]

Disopyramide is a class IA antiarrhythmic drug that blocks the fast sodium channel and prolongs action potential duration. Disopyramide may improve symptoms in obstructive HCM by exerting a negative inotropic effect.[184] Disadvantages of disopyramide include anticholinergic side effects and prolongation of the QT interval, which increases the propensity for ventricular arrhythmias such as torsades de pointes. A reduction of hemodynamic benefits with prolonged use of disopyramide has also been observed.[86]

Patients with nonobstructive HCM who develop heart failure should be treated with standard therapeutic agents, including diuretics, angiotensin-converting enzyme inhibitors, and digitalis. These drugs should be administered with caution in patients with severe LV diastolic dysfunction who require high filling pressures for adequate ventricular filling and in patients with obstructive HCM. Although obstructive HCM has been regarded as a contraindication for these drugs, some data suggest that diuretics may reduce symptoms of pulmonary congestion when combined with β-adrenergic blockers or calcium antagonists.[185] A subset of patients with long-standing HCM and dilated cardiomyopathy who have severe heart failure that is inadequately controlled by medical therapy may ultimately become candidates for cardiac transplantation.

Atrial Fibrillation

Prevention of atrial fibrillation is an ideal goal in management of patients with HCM that may be difficult to achieve owing to the persistence of risk factors for arrhythmia development, particularly increased left atrial size. Both electrical and pharmacologic cardioversion may be used to restore sinus rhythm in patients with paroxysmal episodes of atrial fibrillation, but the risk of recurrence is high. Amiodarone is currently considered to be the most effective antiarrhythmic agent for prevention of recurrence in paroxysmal atrial fibrillation.[107, 186–189] Because of the serious side effects of amiodarone, however, alternative drugs such as sotalol are often used in younger patients. Both β-adrenergic blockers and verapamil may be used for rate control in patients with chronic atrial fibrillation.[85, 86, 186] In patients with rapid atrial fibrillation that is refractory to pharmacologic treatment, ablation of the atrioventricular node and insertion of a permanent pacemaker may be required. Aspirin therapy should be considered for all HCM patients with echocardiographic evidence of left atrial enlargement; for those with paroxysmal and chronic atrial fibrillation, anticoagulation is recommended to reduce the risk of thromboembolism.

Surgical Procedures

Surgical procedures may be required in patients who have high LVOT gradients (>50 mm Hg) and severe symptoms that are inadequately controlled by medical therapy.[85, 86] The most commonly performed procedure is the myotomy-myectomy, in which a wedge of muscle is removed from the hypertrophied basal septum.[190–199] Mitral valve replacement with a low-profile prosthesis has been used as an adjunct or alternative to myotomy-myectomy.[193, 200, 201] Other mitral valve procedures that have been combined with myotomy-myectomy include mitral valvuloplasty or plication of the anterior mitral valve leaflet.[202–204] Coronary artery bypass graft surgery is also performed in some cases. Intraoperative transesophageal echocardiography during myotomy-myectomy may be particularly helpful in planning the extent of resection, assessing the immediate result, and detecting complications.[87] In experienced surgical centers, the operative mortality of myotomy-myectomy is less than 2 percent.[86, 192, 194, 196, 198, 199] Operative mortality may be greater in elderly patients and in those in whom combined procedures are performed.[199, 205] Myotomy-myectomy improves symptoms in obstructive HCM by reducing or abolishing SAM of the mitral valve and the LVOT gradient, with consequent reductions in mitral regurgitation and LV pressures and increases in LV filling and myocardial perfusion.[86, 125, 206–209] Symptomatic improvement persists for 5 or more years after surgery in approximately 70 percent of patients.[191–199] The effects of myotomy-myectomy on long-term survival are unknown.

Nonsurgical Techniques for Reduction of LVOT Gradients

Insertion of a dual-chamber pacemaker has been used as an alternative to myotomy-myectomy in patients with severe symptoms due to LVOT obstruction. The benefits of pacing have been attributed to pre-excitation of the right ventricle, which causes paradoxical motion of the interventricular septum and reduction of the LVOT gradient. Initial observations in nonrandomized, unblinded studies reported that dual-chamber pacing caused substantial reductions in both the LV outflow gradient and symptoms.[210, 211] Subsequent more stringent evaluation has found the effects of pacing to be less favorable. In one randomized, double-blind, crossover study, the average decrease in gradient was small (25 percent) and variable. Subjective improvement in symptoms and objective measurements of exercise capacity after 2 to 3 months were reported with and without pacing.[212] Other studies have suggested that reductions in LVOT gradients produced by dual-chamber pacing may have adverse effects on LV filling and cardiac output.[213, 214] Currently, the indications for dual-chamber pacing are unclear. There are no data to suggest that pacing either alters the course of the disease or reduces the risk of sudden death.

Another method to reduce LVOT gradients in HCM is the use of alcohol injection into the first major septal coronary artery.[215] This procedure reduces septal thickness by induction of a limited myocardial infarction. Further studies are required to fully evaluate this technique.

Prevention of Sudden Death

Patients with high clinical or genetic risk for sudden death due to ventricular arrhythmias may be treated with amiodarone (100 to 300 mg/da) or an implantable cardioverter-defibrillator.[216–223] Two large clinical trials, Antiarrhythmics Versus Implantable Defibrillators (AVID)[224] and Multicenter Automatic Defibrillator Implantation Trial (MADIT),[225] have shown survival advantages with the use of implantable cardioverter-defibrillators compared with antiarrhythmic drug therapy in selected populations of patients at high risk of life-threatening ventricular arrhythmias. Neither of these studies specifically examined individuals with HCM. Patients enrolled in the AVID study were survivors of episodes of ventricular fibrillation or ventricular tachycardia associated with hemodynamic compromise. Those enrolled in MADIT had episodes of nonsustained ventricular tachycardia, low ejection fractions, and inducible, nonsuppressible ventricular arrhythmias during electrophysiologic testing. While clinical trials examining the efficacy of implantable cardioverter-defibrillators for primary and secondary prevention of sudden death in various other patient subgroups are currently ongoing, studies do not specifically address the use of these devices in HCM. Empirical use of antiarrhythmic drugs or implantable cardioverter-defibrillators in HCM must therefore reflect careful risk stratification based on an individual's symptoms, family history, and genotype. Anticipated event rates, availability, and cost will certainly influence these decisions. Although a small number of individuals who do not fall into the high-risk category may experience sudden death, it is difficult to identify these individuals on the basis of clinical parameters. Further, since the majority of individuals with HCM do not die suddenly, and given the side effects and expense of current therapies, prophylactic treatment to prevent sudden death in all genotype-positive individuals is not indicated.

References

1. Maron BJ, Gottdiener JS, Epstein SE: Patterns and significance of distribution of left ventricular hypertrophy in hypertrophic cardiomyopathy: a wide angle, two dimensional echocardiographic study of 125 patients. Am J Cardiol 48:418, 1981.
2. Shapiro LM, McKenna WJ: Distribution of left ventricular hypertrophy in hypertrophic cardiomyopathy: a two-dimensional echocardiographic study. J Am Coll Cardiol 2:437, 1983.
3. McKenna WJ, Kleinebenne A, Nihoyannopoulos P, et al: Echocardiographic measurement of right ventricular wall thickness in hypertrophic cardiomyopathy: relation to clinical and prognostic features. J Am Coll Cardiol 11:351, 1988.
4. Maron BJ, Epstein SE, Roberts WC: Causes of sudden death in young athletes. J Am Coll Cardiol 7:204, 1986.
5. Maron BJ, Gardin JM, Flack JM, et al: Prevalence of hypertrophic cardiomyopathy in a general population of young adults: echocardiographic analysis of 4111 subjects in the CARDIA study: Coronary Artery Risk Development in (Young) Adults. Circulation 92:785, 1995.
6. Hallopeau M: Retrecissement ventriculo-aortique. Gazette Med Paris 24:683, 1869.
7. Watkins H, Thierfelder L, Hwang D-S, et al: Sporadic hypertrophic cardiomyopathy due to de novo myosin mutations. J Clin Invest 90:1666, 1992.
8. Greve G, Bachinski L, Friedman DL, et al: Isolation of a de novo mutant myocardial βMHC protein in a pedigree with hypertrophic cardiomyopathy. Hum Mol Genet 3:2073, 1994.
9. Jarcho JA, McKenna W, Pare JAP, et al: Mapping a gene for familial hypertrophic cardiomyopathy to chromosome 14q1. N Engl J Med 321:1372, 1989.
10. Watkins H, MacRae C, Thierfelder L, et al: A disease locus for familial hypertrophic cardiomyopathy maps to chromosome 1q3. Nat Genet 3:333, 1993.
11. Thierfelder L, MacRae C, Watkins H, et al: A familial hypertrophic cardiomyopathy locus maps to chromosome 15q2. Proc Natl Acad Sci U S A 90:6270, 1993.
12. Carrier L, Hengstenberg C, Beckmann JS, et al: Mapping of a novel gene for familial hypertrophic cardiomyopathy to chromosome 11. Nat Genet 4:311, 1993.
13. MacRae CA, Ghaisas N, Kass S, et al: Familial hypertrophic cardiomyopathy with Wolff-Parkinson-White syndrome maps to a locus on chromosome 7q3. J Clin Invest 96:1216, 1995.
14. Poetter K, Jiang H, Hassanzadeh S, et al: Mutations in either the essential or regulatory light chains of myosin are associated with a rare myopathy in human heart and skeletal muscle. Nat Genet 13:63, 1996.
15. Kimura A, Harada H, Park JE, et al: Mutations in the cardiac troponin I gene associated with hypertrophic cardiomyopathy. Nat Genet 16:379, 1997.
16. Mogensen J, Klausen IC, Pedersen AK, et al: α-Cardiac actin is a

novel disease gene in familial hypertrophic cardiomyopathy. J Clin Invest 103:R39, 1999.

17. Geisterfer-Lowrance AAT, Kass S, Tanigawa G, et al: A molecular basis for familial hypertrophic cardiomyopathy: a β cardiac myosin heavy chain gene missense mutation. Cell 62:999, 1990.
18. Thierfelder L, Watkins H, MacRae C, et al: α-Tropomyosin and cardiac troponin T mutations cause familial hypertrophic cardiomyopathy: a disease of the sarcomere. Cell 77:701, 1994.
19. Watkins H, Conner D, Thierfelder L, et al: Mutations in the cardiac myosin binding protein-C gene on chromosome 11 cause familial hypertrophic cardiomyopathy. Nat Genet 11:434, 1995.
20. Bonne G, Carrier L, Bercovici J, et al: Cardiac myosin binding protein-C gene splice acceptor site mutation is associated with familial hypertrophic cardiomyopathy. Nat Genet 11:438, 1995.
21. Rayment I, Holden HM, Whittaker M, et al: Structure of the actin-myosin complex and its implications for muscle contraction. Science 261:58, 1993.
22. Sata M, Stafford WF, Mabuchi K, et al: The motor domain and the regulatory domain of myosin solely dictate enzymatic activity and phosphorylation-dependent regulation, respectively. Proc Natl Acad Sci U S A 94:91, 1997.
23. Schiaffino S, Reggiani C: Molecular diversity of myofibrillar proteins: gene regulation and functional significance. Physiol Rev 76:371, 1996.
24. Jaenicke T, Diederich KW, Haas W, et al: The complete sequence of the human β-myosin heavy chain gene and a comparative analysis of its product. Genomics 8:194, 1990.
25. Liew CC, Sole MJ, Yamauchi-Takihara K, et al: Complete sequence and organization of the human cardiac β-myosin heavy chain gene. Nucleic Acids Res 18:3647, 1990.
26. Watkins H, McKenna WJ, Thierfelder L, et al: Mutations in the genes for cardiac troponin T and α-tropomyosin in hypertrophic cardiomyopathy. N Engl J Med 332:1058, 1995.
27. Vikstrom KL, Leinwand LA: Contractile protein mutations and heart disease. Curr Opin Cell Biol 8:97, 1996.
28. Bonne G, Carrier L, Richard P, et al: Familial hypertrophic cardiomyopathy. From mutations to functional deficits. Circ Res 83:580, 1998.
29. Dausse E, Komajda M, Dubourg O, et al: Familial hypertrophic cardiomyopathy: microsatellite haplotyping and identification of a hot-spot for mutations in the β-myosin heavy chain gene. J Clin Invest 92:2807, 1993.
30. Anan R, Greve G, Thierfelder L, et al: Prognostic implications of novel β-myosin heavy chain gene mutations that cause familial hypertrophic cardiomyopathy. J Clin Invest 93:280, 1994.
31. Consevage M, Salada GC, Baylen BG, et al: A new missense mutation, Arg719Gln, in the β-cardiac heavy chain myosin gene of patients with familial hypertrophic cardiomyopathy. Hum Mol Genet 3:1025, 1994.
32. Fananapazir L, Dalakas MC, Cyran F, et al: Missense mutations in the β myosin heavy chain gene cause central core disease in hypertrophic cardiomyopathy. Proc Natl Acad Sci U S A 90:3993, 1993.
33. Arai S, Matsuoka R, Hirayama K, et al: Missense mutation of the β-cardiac myosin heavy chain gene in hypertrophic cardiomyopathy. Am J Med Genet 58:267, 1995.
34. Nakajima-Taniguchi C, Matsui H, Eguchi N, et al: A novel deletion mutation in the β-myosin heavy chain gene found in Japanese patients with hypertrophic cardiomyopathy. J Mol Cell Cardiol 27:2607, 1995.
35. Marian AJ, Yu QT, Mares A, et al: Detection of a new mutation in the β-myosin heavy chain gene in an individual with hypertrophic cardiomyopathy. J Clin Invest 90:2156, 1992.
36. Nishi H, Kimura A, Harada H, et al: A myosin missense mutation, not a null allele, causes familial hypertrophic cardiomyopathy. Circulation 91:2911, 1995.
37. Carrier L, Bonne G, Bahrend E, et al: Organization and sequence of human cardiac myosin binding protein C gene (MYBPC3) and identification of mutations predicted to produce truncated proteins in familial hypertrophic cardiomyopathy. Circ Res 80:427, 1997.
38. Niimura H, Bachinski LL, Sangwatanaroj S, et al: Mutations in the gene for cardiac myosin-binding protein C and late-onset familial hypertrophic cardiomyopathy. N Engl J Med 338:1248, 1998.
39. Rottbauer W, Gautel M, Zehelein J, et al: Novel splice donor site mutation in the cardiac myosin binding protein C gene in familial hypertrophic cardiomyopathy: characterization of cardiac transcript and protein. J Clin Invest 100:475, 1997.
40. Yu B, French JA, Carrier L, et al: Molecular pathology of familial hypertrophic cardiomyopathy caused by mutations in the myosin binding protein C gene. J Med Genet 35:205, 1998.
41. Moolman-Smook JC, Mayosi B, Brink P, et al: Identification of a new missense mutation in MyBP-C associated with hypertrophic cardiomyopathy. J Med Genet 35:253, 1998.
42. Forissier JF, Carrier L, Farza H, et al: Codon 102 of the cardiac troponin T gene is a putative hot spot for mutations in familial hypertrophic cardiomyopathy. Circulation 94:3069, 1996.
43. Moolman JC, Corfield VA, Posen B, et al: Sudden death due to troponin T mutations. J Am Coll Cardiol 29:549, 1997.
44. Nakajima-Taniguchi C, Matsui H, Fujio Y, et al: Novel missense mutation in cardiac troponin T gene found in Japanese patient with hypertrophic cardiomyopathy. J Mol Cell Cardiol 29:839, 1997.
45. Bhavsar PK, Brand NJ, Yacoub MH, et al: Isolation and characterization of the human cardiac troponin I gene (TNNI3). Genomics 35:11, 1996.
46. Lees-Miller JP, Helfman DM: The molecular basis for tropomyosin isoform diversity. Bioessays 13:429, 1991.
47. Nakajima-Taniguchi C, Matsui H, Nagata S, et al: Novel missense mutation in α-tropomyosin gene found in Japanese patients with hypertrophic cardiomyopathy. J Mol Cell Cardiol 27:2053, 1995.
48. Yamauchi-Takihara K, Nakajima-Taniguchi C, Matsui H, et al: Clinical implications of hypertrophic cardiomyopathy associated with mutations in the α-tropomyosin gene. Heart 76:63, 1996.
49. Flavigny J, Richard P, Isnard R, et al: Identification of two novel mutations in the ventricular regulatory myosin light chain gene (MYL2) associated with familial and classical forms of hypertrophic cardiomyopathy. J Mol Med 76:208, 1998.
50. Fodor WL, Darras B, Seharaseyon J, et al: Human ventricular/slow twitch myosin alkali light chain gene: characterization, sequence, and chromosomal location. J Biol Chem 264:2143, 1989.
51. Hamada H, Petrino MG, Kakunaga T: Molecular structure and evolutionary origin of human cardiac muscle actin gene. Proc Natl Acad Sci U S A 79:5901, 1982.
52. Olson TM, Michels VV, Thibodeau SN, et al: Actin mutations in dilated cardiomyopathy, a heritable form of heart failure. Science 280:750, 1998.
53. Zot AS, Potter JD: Structural aspects of troponin-tropomyosin regulation of skeletal muscle contraction. Annu Rev Biophys Biophys Chem 16:535, 1987.
54. Lowey S, Waller GS, Trybus KM: Skeletal muscle myosin light chains are essential for physiological speeds of shortening. Nature 365:454, 1993.
55. Trybus KM: Role of myosin light chains. J Muscle Res Cell Motil 15:587, 1994.
56. Sweeney HL, Bowman BF, Stull JT: Myosin light chain phosphorylation in vertebrate striated muscle: regulation and function. Am J Physiol 264:C1085, 1993.
57. Obinata T, Reinach FC, Bader DM, et al: Immunochemical analysis of C-protein isoform transitions during the development of chicken skeletal muscle. Dev Biol 101:116, 1984.
58. Schultheiss T, Lin Z, Lu MH, et al: Differential distribution of subsets of myofibrillar proteins in cardiac nonstriated and striated myofibrils. J Cell Biol 110:1159, 1990.
59. Seiler SH, Fischman DA, Leinwand LA: Modulation of myosin filament organization by C-protein family members. Mol Biol Cell 7:113, 1996.
60. Freiburg A, Gautel M: A molecular map of the interactions between titin and myosin-binding protein C. Implications for sarcomeric assembly in familial hypertrophic cardiomyopathy. Eur J Biochem 235:317, 1996.
61. Gautel M, Zuffardi O, Freiburg A, et al: Phosphorylation switches specific for the cardiac isoform of myosin binding protein C: a modulator of cardiac contraction? EMBO J 14:1952, 1995.
62. Weisberg A, Winegrad S: Alteration of myosin cross bridges by phosphorylation of myosin binding protein C in cardiac muscle. Proc Natl Acad Sci U S A 93:8999, 1996.
63. Weisberg A, Winegrad S: Relations between crossbridge structure and actomyosin ATPase activity in rat heart. Circ Res 83:60, 1998.
64. Rayment I, Holden HM, Sellarse JR, et al: Structural interpretation of the mutations in the β-cardiac myosin that have been implicated in familial hypertrophic cardiomyopathy. Proc Natl Acad Sci U S A 92:3864, 1995.
65. Sweeney HL, Straceski AJ, Leinwand LA, et al: Heterologous ex-

pression of a cardiomyopathic myosin that is defective in its actin interaction. J Biol Chem 269:1603, 1994.
66. Sata M, Ikebe M: Functional analysis of the mutations in the human cardiac β-myosin that are responsible for familial hypertrophic cardiomyopathy. J Clin Invest 98:2866, 1996.
67. Cuda G, Fananapazir L, Epstein ND, et al: The in vitro motility activity of β-cardiac myosin depends on the nature of the β-myosin heavy chain gene mutation in hypertrophic cardiomyopathy. J Muscle Res Cell Motil 18:275, 1997.
68. Lankford EB, Epstein ND, Fananapazir L, et al: Abnormal contractile properties of muscle fibers expressing β-myosin heavy chain gene mutations in patients with hypertrophic cardiomyopathy. J Clin Invest 95:1409, 1995.
69. Watkins H, Seidman CE, Seidman JG, et al: Expression and functional assessment of a truncated cardiac troponin T that causes hypertrophic cardiomyopathy. J Clin Invest 98:2456, 1996.
70. Marian AJ, Zhao G, Seta Y, et al: Expression of a mutant (Arg92Gln) human cardiac troponin T, known to cause hypertrophic cardiomyopathy, impairs adult cardiac myocyte contractility. Circ Res 81:76, 1997.
71. Marian AJ, Yu Q-T, Mann DL, et al: Expression of a mutation causing hypertrophic cardiomyopathy disrupts sarcomere assembly in adult feline cardiac myocytes. Circ Res 77:98, 1995.
72. Becker KD, Gottshall KR, Hickey R, et al: Point mutations in human β cardiac myosin heavy chain have differential effects on sarcomeric structure and assembly: an ATP binding site change disrupts both thick and thin filaments, whereas hypertrophic cardiomyopathy mutations display normal assembly. J Cell Biol 137:131, 1997.
73. Geisterfer-Lowrance AAT, Christe M, Connor DA, et al: A mouse model of familial hypertrophic cardiomyopathy. Science 272:731, 1996.
74. Spindler M, Saupe KW, Christe ME, et al: Diastolic dysfunction and altered energetics in the $\alpha MHC^{403/+}$ mouse model of familial hypertrophic cardiomyopathy. J Clin Invest 101:1775, 1998.
75. Blanchard E, Seidman CE, Seidman JG, et al: Altered crossbridge kinetics in the α $MHC^{403/+}$ mouse model of familial hypertrophic cardiomyopathy. Circ Res 84:475, 1999.
76. Gao WD, Perez NG, Seidman CE, et al: Altered cardiac excitation-contraction coupling in mutant mice with familial hypertrophic cardiomyopathy. J Clin Invest 103:661, 1999.
77. Fatkin D, Christe ME, Aristizabal O, et al: Neonatal cardiomyopathy in mice homozygous for the Arg403Gln mutation in the α cardiac myosin heavy chain gene. J Clin Invest 103:147, 1999.
78. Oberst L, Zhao G, Park JT, et al: Dominant-negative effect of a mutant cardiac troponin T on cardiac structure and function in transgenic mice. J Clin Invest 102:1498, 1998.
79. Tardiff JC, Factor SM, Tompkins BD, et al: A truncated cardiac troponin T molecule in transgenic mice suggests multiple cellular mechanisms for familial hypertrophic cardiomyopathy. J Clin Invest 101:2800, 1998.
80. Yang Q, Sanbe A, Osinka H, et al: A mouse model of myosin binding protein C human familial hypertrophic cardiomyopathy. J Clin Invest 102:1292, 1998.
81. McConnell BK, Jones K, Fatkin D, et al: Mice with a mutant myosin binding protein C gene provide a model for familial hypertrophic cardiomyopathy. Circulation 98(suppl I):I-625, 1998.
82. Tesson F, Dufour C, Moolman JC, et al: The influence of the angiotensin I converting enzyme genotype in familial hypertrophic cardiomyopathy varies with the disease gene mutation. J Mol Cell Cardiol 29:831, 1997.
83. Bejsovec A, Anderson P: Functions of the myosin ATP and actin binding sites are required for *C. elegans* thick filament assembly. Cell 60:133, 1990.
84. Vikstrom KL, Factor SM, Leinwand LA: Mice expressing mutant myosin heavy chains are a model for familial hypertrophic cardiomyopathy. Mol Med 2:556, 1996.
85. Maron BJ, Bonow RO, Cannon RO, et al: Hypertrophic cardiomyopathy. Interrelations of clinical manifestations, pathophysiology and therapy. N Engl J Med 316:780, 844, 1987.
86. Wigle ED, Rakowski H, Kimball BP, et al: Hypertrophic cardiomyopathy. Clinical spectrum and treatment. Circulation 92:1680, 1995.
87. Grigg LE, Wigle ED, Williams WG, et al: Transesophageal Doppler echocardiography in obstructive hypertrophic cardiomyopathy: clarification of pathophysiology and importance in intraoperative decision making. J Am Coll Cardiol 20:42, 1992.
88. Schwammenthal E, Nakatani S, He S, et al: Mechanism of mitral regurgitation in hypertrophic cardiomyopathy. Mismatch of posterior to anterior leaflet length and mobility. Circulation 98:856, 1998.
89. Gwathmey JK, Warren SE, Briggs GM, et al: Diastolic dysfunction in hypertrophic cardiomyopathy. Effect on active force generation during systole. J Clin Invest 87:1023, 1991.
90. Georgakopoulos D, Christe ME, Giewat M, et al: The pathogenesis of familial hypertrophic cardiomyopathy: early and evolving effects from an α cardiac myosin heavy chain missense mutation. Nat Med 5:327, 1999.
91. Charron P, Dubourg O, Desnos M, et al: Clinical features and prognostic implications of familial hypertrophic cardiomyopathy related to the cardiac myosin-binding protein C gene. Circulation 97:2230, 1998.
92. McKenna WJ, Stewart JT, Nihoyannopoulos P, et al: Hypertrophic cardiomyopathy without hypertrophy: two families with myocardial disarray in the absence of increased myocardial mass. Br Heart J 63:287, 1990.
93. Schamroth L: Ventricular hypertrophy. *In* An Introduction to Electrocardiography. 5th ed. p. 68. Oxford, Blackwell Scientific, 1976.
94. Sakamoto T, Tei C, Murayama M, et al: Giant negative T-wave inversion as a manifestation of asymmetric apical hypertrophy (AAH) of the left ventricle: echocardiographic and ultrasono-cardiotomographic study. Jpn Heart J 17:611, 1976.
95. Yamaguchi H, Ishimura T, Nishiyama S, et al: Hypertrophic nonobstructive cardiomyopathy with giant negative T-waves (apical hypertrophy): ventriculographic and echocardiographic features in 30 patients. Am J Cardiol 44:401, 1979.
96. Lemery R, Kleinebenne A, Nihoyannopoulos P, et al: Q waves in hypertrophic cardiomyopathy in relation to the distribution and severity of right and left ventricular hypertrophy. J Am Coll Cardiol 16:368, 1990.
97. Maron BJ: Q waves in hypertrophic cardiomyopathy: a reassessment. J Am Coll Cardiol 16:375, 1990.
98. Petrone RK, Klues HG, Panza JA, et al: Significance of the occurrence of mitral valve prolapse in patients with hypertrophic cardiomyopathy. J Am Coll Cardiol 20:55, 1992.
99. Klues HG, Maron BJ, Dollar AL, et al: Diversity of structural mitral valve alterations in hypertrophic cardiomyopathy. Circulation 85:1651, 1992.
100. Lazzeroni E, Picano E, Dodi C, et al: Dipyridamole echocardiography for diagnosis of coexistent coronary artery disease in hypertrophic cardiomyopathy. Am J Cardiol 75:810, 1995.
101. Epstein SE, Henry WL, Clark CE, et al: Asymmetric septal hypertrophy. Ann Intern Med 81:650, 1974.
102. Maron BJ, Wolfson JK, Ciro E, et al: Relation of electrocardiographic abnormalities and patterns of left ventricular hypertrophy identified by 2-dimensional echocardiography in patients with hypertrophic cardiomyopathy. Am J Cardiol 51:189, 1983.
103. Lever HM, Karam RF, Currie PJ, et al: Hypertrophic cardiomyopathy in the elderly: distinctions from the young based on cardiac shape. Circulation 79:580, 1989.
104. Solomon SD, Wolff S, Watkins H, et al: Left ventricular hypertrophy and morphology in familial hypertrophic cardiomyopathy associated with mutations of the beta-myosin heavy chain gene. J Am Coll Cardiol 22:498, 1993.
105. Klues HG, Schiffers A, Maron BJ: Phenotypic spectrum and patterns of left ventricular hypertrophy in hypertrophic cardiomyopathy: morphologic observations and significance as assessed by two-dimensional echocardiography in 600 patients. J Am Coll Cardiol 26:1699, 1995.
106. Lazzeroni E, Domenicucci S, Finardi A, et al: Severity of arrhythmias and extent of hypertrophy in hypertrophic cardiomyopathy. Am Heart J 118:734, 1989.
107. McKenna WJ, England D, Doi YL, et al: Arrhythmia in hypertrophic cardiomyopathy, I: influence on prognosis. Br Heart J 46:168, 1981.
108. Maron BJ, Savage DD, Wolfson JK, et al: Prognostic significance of 24 hour ambulatory electrocardiographic monitoring in patients with hypertrophic cardiomyopathy: a prospective study. Am J Cardiol 48:252, 1981.
109. Fananapazir L, Chang AC, Epstein SE, et al: Prognostic determinants in hypertrophic cardiomyopathy: prospective evaluation of a therapeutic strategy based on clinical, Holter, hemodynamic, and electrophysiological findings. Circulation 86:730, 1992.
110. Kulakowski P, Counihan PJ, Camm AJ, et al: The value of time and

frequency domain, and spectral temporal mapping analysis of the signal-averaged electrocardiogram in identification of patients with hypertrophic cardiomyopathy at increased risk of sudden death. Eur Heart J 14:941, 1993.

111. Gavaghan TP, Keely RP, Kuchar DL, et al: The prevalence of arrhythmias in hypertrophic cardiomyopathy: role of ambulatory monitoring and signal-averaged electrocardiography. Aust N Z J Med 16:666, 1986.
112. Fauchier JP, Cosnay P, Moquet B, et al: Late ventricular potentials and spontaneous and induced ventricular arrhythmias in dilated or hypertrophic cardiomyopathies: a prospective study about 83 patients. Pacing Clin Electrophysiol 11:1974, 1988.
113. Cripps TR, Counihan PJ, Frenneaux MP, et al: Signal-averaged electrocardiography in hypertrophic cardiomyopathy. J Am Coll Cardiol 15: 956, 1990
114. Ajiki K, Murakawa Y, Yanagisawa-Miwa A, et al: Autonomic nervous system activity in idiopathic dilated cardiomyopathy and in hypertrophic cardiomyopathy. Am J Cardiol 71:1316, 1993.
115. Counihan PJ, Fei L, Bashir Y, et al: Assessment of heart rate variability in hypertrophic cardiomyopathy. Association with clinical and prognostic features. Circulation 88:1682, 1993.
116. Posma JL, van der Wall EE, Blanksma PK, et al: New diagnostic options in hypertrophic cardiomyopathy. Am Heart J 132:1031, 1996.
117. Geibel A, Brugada P, Zehender M, et al: Value of programmed electrical stimulation using a standardized ventricular stimulation protocol in hypertrophic cardiomyopathy. Am J Cardiol 60:738, 1987.
118. Kuck K-H, Kunze KP, Schluter M, et al: Programmed electrical stimulation in hypertrophic cardiomyopathy: results in patients with and without cardiac arrest or syncope. Eur Heart J 9:177, 1988.
119. Wellens HJ, Brugada P, Stevenson WG: Programmed electrical stimulation of the heart in patients with life-threatening arrhythmias: what is the significance of induced arrhythmias and what is the correct stimulation protocol? Circulation 72:1, 1985.
120. Maron BJ, Cecchi F, McKenna WJ: Risk factors and stratification for sudden death in patients with hypertrophic cardiomyopathy. Br Heart J 72:S13, 1994.
121. Higgins CB, Byrd BF, Stark D, et al: Magnetic resonance imaging in hypertrophic cardiomyopathy. Am J Cardiol 55:1121, 1985.
122. Suzuki J, Watanabe F, Takenaka K, et al: New subtype of apical hypertrophic cardiomyopathy identified with nuclear magnetic resonance imaging as an underlying cause of markedly inverted T-waves. J Am Coll Cardiol 22:1175, 1993.
123. Webb JG, Sasson Z, Rakowski H, et al: Apical hypertrophic cardiomyopathy: clinical follow-up and diagnostic correlates. J Am Coll Cardiol 15:83, 1990.
124. Gaudio C, Pellicia F, Tanzilli G, et al: Magnetic resonance imaging for assessment of apical hypertrophy in hypertrophic cardiomyopathy. Clin Cardiol 15:164, 1992.
125. Cannon RO, Dilsizian V, O'Gara PT, et al: Impact of operative relief of outflow obstruction on thallium perfusion abnormalities in hypertrophic cardiomyopathy. Circulation 85:1039, 1992.
126. Takata J, Counihan PJ, Gane JN, et al: Regional thallium-201 washout and myocardial hypertrophy in hypertrophic cardiomyopathy and its relation to exertional chest pain. Am J Cardiol 72:211, 1993.
127. Dilsizian V, Bonow RO, Epstein SE, et al: Myocardial ischemia detected by thallium scintigraphy is frequently related to cardiac arrest and syncope in young patients with hypertrophic cardiomyopathy. J Am Coll Cardiol 22:796, 1993.
128. Niemeyer MG, Kuijper AFM, Gerhards LJ, et al: Nitrogen 13 ammonia perfusion imaging: relation to metabolic imaging. Am Heart J 125:848, 1993.
129. Camici PG: State of the art in cardiac positron emission tomography. *In* Van der Wall EE, Blanksma PK, Niemyer MG, Paans AMJ (eds): Cardiac Positron Emission Tomography: Viability, Perfusion, Receptors and Cardiomyopathy. pp. 1–14. Dordrecht, The Netherlands: Kluwer Academic, 1995.
130. Camici P, Chiriatti G, Lorenzoni R, et al: Coronary vasodilatation is impaired in both hypertrophied and nonhypertrophied myocardium of patients with hypertrophic cardiomyopathy: a study with nitrogen-13 ammonia and positron emission tomography. J Am Coll Cardiol 17:879, 1991.
131. Gistri R, Cecchi F, Choudhury L, et al: Effect of verapamil on absolute myocardial blood flow in hypertrophic cardiomyopathy. Am J Cardiol 74:363, 1994.
132. Nienaber CA, Gambhir SS, Vaghaiwalla Mody F, et al: Regional myocardial blood flow and glucose utilization in symptomatic patients with hypertrophic cardiomyopathy. Circulation 87:1580, 1993.
133. Chikamori T, Dickie S, Poloniecki JD, et al: Prognostic significance of radionuclide-assessed diastolic function in hypertrophic cardiomyopathy. Am J Cardiol 65:478, 1990.
134. Maron BJ, Moller JH, Seidman CE, et al: Impact of laboratory molecular diagnosis on contemporary diagnostic criteria for genetically transmitted cardiovascular diseases: hypertrophic cardiomyopathy, long-QT syndrome, and Marfan syndrome. Circulation 98:1460, 1998.
135. Frank S, Braunwald E: Idiopathic hypertrophic subaortic stenosis: clinical analysis of 126 patients with emphasis on the natural history. Circulation 37:759, 1968.
136. Shah PM, Adelman AG, Wigle ED, et al: The natural (and unnatural) history of hypertrophic obstructive cardiomyopathy. Circ Res 35(suppl 2):179, 1974.
137. Swan DA, Bell B, Oakley C, et al: Analysis of symptomatic course and prognosis and treatment of hypertrophic obstructive cardiomyopathy. Br Heart J 33:671, 1971.
138. Adelman AG, Wigle ED, Ranganathan N, et al: The clinical course in muscular subaortic stenosis: a retrospective and prospective study of 60 hemodynamically proved cases. Ann Intern Med 77:515, 1972.
139. Hardarson T, de la Calzada CS, Curiel R, et al: Prognosis and mortality of hypertrophic obstructive cardiomyopathy. Lancet 2:1462, 1973.
140. McKenna WJ, Deanfield JE: Hypertrophic cardiomyopathy: an important cause of sudden death. Arch Dis Child 59:971, 1984.
141. McKenna W, Deanfield J, Faruqui A, et al: Prognosis of hypertrophic cardiomyopathy: role of age and clinical, electrocardiographic and hemodynamic features. Am J Cardiol 47:532, 1981.
142. Fiddler GI, Tajik AJ, Weidman WH, et al: Idiopathic hypertrophic subaortic stenosis in the young. Am J Cardiol 42:793, 1978.
143. Maron BJ, Henry WL, Clark CE, et al: Asymmetric septal hypertrophy in childhood. Circulation 53:9, 1976.
144. Maron BJ, Cecchi F, McKenna WJ: Risk factors and stratification for sudden cardiac death in patients with hypertrophic cardiomyopathy. Br Heart J 72(suppl):S13, 1994.
145. Spirito P, Chiarella F, Carratino L, et al: Clinical course and prognosis of hypertrophic cardiomyopathy in an outpatient population. N Engl J Med 320:749, 1989.
146. Kofflard MJ, Waldstein DJ, Vos J, et al: Prognosis in hypertrophic cardiomyopathy observed in a large clinic. Am J Cardiol 72:939, 1993.
147. Cannan CR, Reeder GS, Bailey KR, et al: Natural history of hypertrophic cardiomyopathy. A population-based study, 1976 through 1990. Circulation 92:2488, 1995.
148. Cecchi F, Olivotto I, Montereggi A, et al: Hypertrophic cardiomyopathy in Tuscany: clinical course and outcome in an unselected regional population. J Am Coll Cardiol 26:1529, 1995.
149. Maron BJ, Casey SA, Poliac LC, et al: Clinical course of hypertrophic cardiomyopathy in a regional United States cohort. JAMA 281:650, 1999.
150. Maron BJ, Spirito P, Wesley Y, et al: Development and progression of left ventricular hypertrophy in children with hypertrophic cardiomyopathy. N Engl J Med 315:610, 1986.
151. Spirito P, Maron BJ: Absence of progression of left ventricular hypertrophy in adult patients with hypertrophic cardiomyopathy. J Am Coll Cardiol 9:1013, 1987.
152. Spirito P, Maron BJ: Relation between extent of left ventricular hypertrophy and age in hypertrophic cardiomyopathy. J Am Coll Cardiol 13:820, 1989.
153. Spirito P, Bellone P: Natural history of hypertrophic cardiomyopathy. Br Heart J 72(suppl):S10, 1994.
154. Semsarian C, French J, Trent RJ, et al: The natural history of left ventricular wall thickening in hypertrophic cardiomyopathy. Aust N Z J Med 27:51, 1997.
155. Gruver EJ, Fatkin D, Dodds GA, et al: Familial hypertrophic cardiomyopathy and atrial fibrillation caused by Arg663His β-cardiac myosin heavy chain mutation. Am J Cardiol 83:13H–18H, 1999.
156. Hina K, Kusachi S, Iwasaki K, et al: Progression of left ventricular enlargement in patients with hypertrophic cardiomyopathy: incidence and prognostic value. Clin Cardiol 16:403, 1993.
157. Cecchi F, Montereggi A, Olivotto I, et al: Risk for atrial fibrillation in patients with hypertrophic cardiomyopathy assessed by signal averaged P wave duration. Heart 78:44, 1997.

158. McKenna WJ, Camm AJ: Sudden death in hypertrophic cardiomyopathy. Assessment of patients at high risk. Circulation 80:1489, 1989.
159. Spirito P, Seidman CE, McKenna WJ, et al: The management of hypertrophic cardiomyopathy. N Engl J Med 336:775, 1997.
160. Joseph S, Balcon R, McDonald L: Syncope in hypertrophic obstructive cardiomyopathy due to asystole. Br Heart J 34:974, 1972.
161. Chmielewzki CA, Riley RS, Mahendran A, et al: Complete heart block as a cause of syncope in asymmetric septal hypertrophy. Am Heart J 93:91, 1977.
162. Gilligan DM, Nihoyannopoulos P, Chan WL, et al: Investigation of a hemodynamic basis for syncope in hypertrophic cardiomyopathy: use of a head-up tilt test. Circulation 85:2140, 1992.
163. Louie EK, Edwards LC III: Hypertrophic cardiomyopathy. Prog Cardiovasc Dis 36:275, 1994.
164. Watkins H, Rosenzweig A, Hwang D-S, et al: Characteristics and prognostic implications of myosin missense mutations in familial hypertrophic cardiomyopathy. N Engl J Med 326:1108, 1992.
165. DeRose JJ Jr, Banas JS Jr, Winters SL: Current perspectives on sudden cardiac death in hypertrophic cardiomyopathy. Prog Cardiovasc Dis 36:475, 1994.
166. Maron BJ, Lipson LC, Roberts WC, et al: "Malignant" hypertrophic cardiomyopathy: identification of a subgroup of families with unusually frequent premature death. Am J Cardiol 41:1133, 1978.
167. Vassalli G, Seiler C, Hess OM: Risk stratification in hypertrophic cardiomyopathy. Curr Opin Cardiol 9:330, 1994.
168. Coviello DA, Maron BJ, Spirito P, et al: Clinical features of hypertrophic cardiomyopathy caused by mutation of a "hot spot" in the alpha-tropomyosin gene. J Am Coll Cardiol 29:635, 1997.
169. Maron BJ, Isner JM, McKenna WJ: Recommendations for determining eligibility for competition in athletes with cardiovascular abnormalities: Task Force 3: hypertrophic cardiomyopathy, myocarditis and other myo-pericardial diseases and mitral valve prolapse. J Am Coll Cardiol 24:880, 1994.
170. Thompson DS, Naqvi N, Juul SM, et al: Effects of propranolol on myocardial oxygen consumption, substrate extraction, and haemodynamics in hypertrophic obstructive cardiomyopathy. Br Heart J 44:488, 1980.
171. Harrison DC, Braunwald E, Glick G, et al: Effects of beta adrenergic blockade on the circulation, with particular reference to observations in patients with hypertrophic subaortic stenosis. Circulation 29:84, 1964.
172. Cohen LS, Braunwald E: Amelioration of angina pectoris in idiopathic hypertrophic subaortic stenosis with beta-adrenergic blockade. Circulation 35:847, 1967.
173. Flamm MD, Harrison DC, Hancock EW: Muscular subaortic stenosis: prevention of outflow obstruction with propranolol. Circulation 38:846, 1968.
174. Rosing DR, Kent KM, Maron BJ, et al: Verapamil therapy: a new approach to the pharmacologic treatment of hypertrophic cardiomyopathy. II. Effects on exercise capacity and symptomatic status. Circulation 60:1208, 1979.
175. Hanrath P, Mathey DG, Kremer P, et al: Effect of verapamil on left ventricular isovolumic relaxation time and regional left ventricular filling in hypertrophic cardiomyopathy. Am J Cardiol 45:1258, 1980.
176. Bonow RO, Rosing DR, Bacharach SL, et al: Effects of verapamil on left ventricular systolic function and diastolic filling in patients with hypertrophic cardiomyopathy. Circulation 64:787, 1981.
177. ten Cate FJ, Serruys PW, Mey S, et al: Effects of short-term administration of verapamil on left ventricular relaxation and filling dynamics measured by a combined hemodynamic-ultrasonic technique in patients with hypertrophic cardiomyopathy. Circulation 68:1274, 1983.
178. Bonow RO, Dilsizian V, Rosing DR, et al: Verapamil-induced improvement in left ventricular diastolic filling and increased exercise tolerance in patients with hypertrophic cardiomyopathy: short- and long-term effects. Circulation 72:853, 1985.
179. Hess OM, Murakami T, Krayenbuehl HP: Does verapamil improve left ventricular relaxation in patients with myocardial hypertrophy? Circulation 74:530, 1986.
180. Udelson JE, Bonow RO, O'Gara PT, et al: Verapamil prevents silent myocardial perfusion abnormalities during exercise in asymptomatic patients with hypertrophic cardiomyopathy. Circulation 79:1052, 1989.
181. Lorell BH, Paulus WJ, Grossman W, et al: Modification of abnormal left ventricular diastolic properties by nifedipine in patients with hypertrophic cardiomyopathy. Circulation 65:499, 1982.
182. Iwase M, Sotobata I, Takagi S, et al: Effects of diltiazem on left ventricular diastolic behavior in patients with hypertrophic cardiomyopathy: evaluation with exercise pulsed Doppler echocardiography. J Am Coll Cardiol 9:1099, 1987.
183. Betocchi S, Piscione F, Losi MA, et al: Effects of diltiazem on left ventricular systolic and diastolic function in hypertrophic cardiomyopathy. Am J Cardiol 78:451, 1996.
184. Pollick C: Muscular subaortic stenosis: hemodynamic and clinical improvement after disopyramide. N Engl J Med 307:997, 1982.
185. Gilligan DM, Chan WL, Stewart R, et al: Cardiac responses assessed by echocardiography to changes in preload in hypertrophic cardiomyopathy. Am J Cardiol 73:312, 1994.
186. Robinson K, Frenneaux MP, Stockins B, et al: Atrial fibrillation in hypertrophic cardiomyopathy: a longitudinal study. J Am Coll Cardiol 15:1279, 1990.
187. McKenna WJ, Harris L, Rowland E, et al: Amiodarone for long-term management of patients with hypertrophic cardiomyopathy. Am J Cardiol 54:802, 1984.
188. Gosselink AT, Crijns HJ, Van Gelder IC, et al: Low-dose amiodarone for maintenance of sinus rhythm after cardioversion of atrial fibrillation or flutter. JAMA 267:3289, 1992.
189. Prystowsky EN, Benson DW Jr, Fuster V, et al: Management of patients with atrial fibrillation: a statement for healthcare professionals from the Subcommittee on Electrocardiography and Electrophysiology, American Heart Association. Circulation 93:1262, 1996.
190. Morrow AG, Reitz BA, Epstein SE, et al: Operative treatment in hypertrophic subaortic stenosis: techniques, and the results of pre- and post-operative assessments in 83 patients. Circulation 52:88, 1975.
191. Maron BJ, Merrill WH, Freier PA, et al: Long-term clinical course and symptomatic status of patients after operation for hypertrophic subaortic stenosis. Circulation 57:1205, 1978.
192. Williams WG, Wigle ED, Rakowski H, et al: Results of surgery for hypertrophic obstructive cardiomyopathy. Circulation 76(suppl V):V-104, 1987.
193. McIntosh CL, Maron BJ: Current operative treatment of obstructive hypertrophic cardiomyopathy. Circulation 78:487, 1988.
194. Cohn LH, Trehan H, Collins JJ Jr: Long-term follow-up of patients undergoing myotomy/myectomy for obstructive hypertrophic cardiomyopathy. Am J Cardiol 70:657, 1992.
195. Schulte HD, Bircks WH, Loesse B, et al: Prognosis of patients with hypertrophic obstructive cardiomyopathy after transaortic myectomy: late results up to twenty-five years. J Thorac Cardiovasc Surg 106:709, 1993.
196. ten Berg JM, Suttorp MJ, Knaepen PJ, et al: Hypertrophic obstructive cardiomyopathy: initial results and long-term follow-up after Morrow septal myectomy. Circulation 90:1781, 1994.
197. Heric B, Lytle BW, Miller DP, et al: Surgical management of hypertrophic obstructive cardiomyopathy: early and late results. J Thorac Cardiovasc Surg 110:195, 1994.
198. Robbins RC, Stinson EB: Long-term results of left ventricular myotomy and myectomy for obstructive hypertrophic cardiomyopathy. J Thorac Cardiovasc Surg 111:586, 1996.
199. McCully RB, Nishimura RA, Tajik AJ, et al: Extent of clinical improvement after surgical treatment of hypertrophic obstructive cardiomyopathy. Circulation 94:467, 1996.
200. Cooley DA, Leachman RD, Hallman GL, et al: Idiopathic hypertrophic subaortic stenosis: surgical treatment including mitral valve replacement. Arch Surg 103:606, 1971.
201. McIntosh CL, Greenberg GJ, Maron BJ, et al: Clinical and hemodynamic results after mitral valve replacement in patients with obstructive hypertrophic cardiomyopathy. Ann Thorac Surg 47:236, 1989.
202. McIntosh CL, Maron BJ, Cannon RO III, et al: Initial results of combined anterior mitral leaflet plication and ventricular septal myotomy-myectomy for relief of left ventricular outflow tract obstruction in patients with hypertrophic cardiomyopathy. Circulation 86(suppl II):II-60, 1992.
203. Schoendube FA, Klues HG, Reith S, et al: Long-term clinical and echocardiographic follow-up after surgical correction of hypertrophic obstructive cardiomyopathy with extended myectomy and reconstruction of the subvalvular mitral apparatus. Circulation 92(suppl II):II-122, 1995.
204. Kofflard MJ, van Herwerden LA, Waldstein DJ, et al: Initial results

of combined anterior mitral leaflet extension and myectomy in patients with obstructive hypertrophic cardiomyopathy. J Am Coll Cardiol 28:197, 1996.
205. Cooper MM, McIntosh CL, Tucker E, et al: Operation for hypertrophic subaortic stenosis in the aged. Ann Thorac Surg 44:370, 1987.
206. Shah PM, Gramiak R, Adelman AG, et al: Echocardiographic assessment of the effects of surgery and propranolol on the dynamics of outflow obstruction on hypertrophic subaortic stenosis. Circulation 45:516, 1972.
207. Schapira JN, Stemple DR, Martin RP, et al: Single and two-dimensional echocardiographic visualization of the effects of septal myectomy in idiopathic hypertrophic subaortic stenosis. Circulation 58:850, 1978.
208. Spirito P, Maron BJ, Rosing DR: Morphologic determinants of hemodynamic state after ventricular septal myotomy-myectomy in patients with obstructive hypertrophic cardiomyopathy: M-mode and two-dimensional echocardiographic assessment. Circulation 70:984, 1984.
209. Cannon RO III, McIntosh CL, Schenke WH, et al: Effect of surgical reduction of left ventricular outflow obstruction on hemodynamics, coronary flow and myocardial metabolism in hypertrophic cardiomyopathy. Circulation 79:766, 1989.
210. Jeanrenaud X, Goy JJ, Kappenberger L: Effects of dual-chamber pacing in hypertrophic obstructive cardiomyopathy. Lancet 339:1318, 1992.
211. Fananapazir L, Epstein ND, Curiel RV, et al: Long-term results of dual-chamber (DDD) pacing in obstructive hypertrophic cardiomyopathy: evidence for progressive symptomatic and hemodynamic improvement and reduction of left ventricular hypertrophy. Circulation 90:2731, 1994.
212. Nishimura RA, Trusty JM, Hayes DL, et al: Dual-chamber pacing for hypertrophic obstructive cardiomyopathy: a randomized, double-blind, crossover study. J Am Coll Cardiol 29:435, 1997.
213. Nishimura RA, Hayes DL, Ilstrup DM, et al: Effects of dual-chamber pacing on systolic and diastolic function in patients with hypertrophic cardiomyopathy: acute Doppler echocardiographic and catheterization hemodynamic study. J Am Coll Cardiol 27:421, 1996.
214. Betocchi S, Losi MA, Piscione F, et al: Effects of dual-chamber pacing in hypertrophic cardiomyopathy on left ventricular outflow tract obstruction and on diastolic function. Am J Cardiol 77:498, 1996.
215. Sigwart U: Non-surgical myocardial reduction for hypertrophic obstructive cardiomyopathy. Lancet 346:211, 1995.
216. Mirowski M, Reid PR, Mower MM, et al: Termination of malignant ventricular arrhythmias with an implanted automatic defibrillator in human beings. N Engl J Med 303:322, 1980.
217. Powell AC, Fuchs P, Finkelstein DM, et al: Influence of implantable cardioverter-defibrillators on the long-term prognosis of survivors of out-of-hospital cardiac arrest. Circulation 88:1083, 1993.
218. Nunain SO, Roelke M, Trouton T, et al: Limitations and late complications of third-generation automatic cardioverter-defibrillators. Circulation 91:2204, 1995.
219. Zipes DP: Are implantable cardioverter-defibrillators better than conventional antiarrhythmic drugs for survivors of cardiac arrest? Circulation 91:2115, 1995.
220. Ceremuzynski L, Kleczar E, Krzeminska-Pakula M, et al: Effect of amiodarone on mortality after myocardial infarction: a double-blind, placebo-controlled, pilot study. J Am Coll Cardiol 20:1056, 1992.
221. The CASCADE Investigators: Randomized antiarrhythmic drug therapy in survivors of cardiac arrest (the CASCADE Study). Am J Cardiol 72:280, 1993.
222. The Cardiac Arrhythmia Suppression Trial (CAST) Investigators: Effect of encainide and flecainide on mortality in a randomized trial of arrhythmia suppression after myocardial infarction. N Engl J Med 321:406, 1989.
223. McKenna WJ, Oakley CM, Krikler DM, et al: Improved survival with amiodarone in patients with hypertrophic cardiomyopathy and ventricular tachycardia. Br Heart J 53:412, 1985.
224. The Antiarrhythmics versus Implantable Defibrillators (AVID) Investigators: A comparison of antiarrhythmic-drug therapy with implantable defibrillators in patients resuscitated from near-fatal ventricular arrhythmias. N Engl J Med 337:1576, 1997.
225. Moss AJ, Hall WJ, Cannom DS, et al: Improved survival with an implanted defibrillator in patients with coronary disease at high risk for ventricular arrhythmia. N Engl J Med 335:1933, 1996.

CHAPTER 53

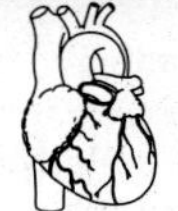

Restrictive Cardiomyopathy

James T. Willerson and John F. Goodwin

PATHOPHYSIOLOGY
THE EOSINOPHIL IN HEART DISEASE
CLINICAL RECOGNITION
History and Physical Examination
Laboratory Examination
TREATMENT
AMYLOID HEART DISEASE
Pathophysiology
Clinical Recognition
Physical Examination
Differential Diagnosis
Treatment
HEMOCHROMATOSIS
Pathophysiology
Clinical Recognition
Treatment
RADIATION-INDUCED HEART DISEASE
Pathophysiology
Clinical Recognition
Differential Diagnosis
Treatment

Restrictive cardiomyopathy (RCM) is the term used to describe the third and least common member of the cardiomyopathies that are defined as *heart muscle diseases of unknown cause* (see Chs. 51, Dilated Cardiomyopathy, and 52, Hypertrophic Cardiomyopathy).

RCM is defined as "organic interference with filling of the ventricles as the result of endocardial or myocardial disease or a combination of both with rapid early but slow late ventricular filling."[1–23] RCM is a component of the syndrome known as *diastolic heart disease*, which includes hypertrophy, amyloidosis, hemochromatosis, and constrictive pericarditis. Diastolic heart disease is defined as "heart disease initially and predominantly involving diastolic rather than systolic function." It does not refer to the most common causes of diastolic impairment (e.g., preceding impairment of systolic function due to conditions such as systemic hypertension, coronary artery, and valvular heart disease).[21]

Pathophysiology

The most common cause of RCM is endomyocardial fibrosis (EMF), now known as *eosinophilic endomyocardial disease*. Other causes include cryptogenic EMF without eosinophilia, hemochromatosis, amyloid heart disease, and radiation-induced heart muscle disease.

Constrictive pericarditis represents diastolic heart disease in its purest form. The impairment of ventricular filling is the result of the tight compression of the ventricles by the restricting pericardium, with the myocardium remaining normal in all except severe and prolonged cases. The tight pericardium permits rapid early filling without restriction, but as the ventricles expand against the rigid pericardium, mid and late filling is suddenly slowed and then halted. Systolic function remains normal until the late stages. In other restrictive diseases, thickening and rigidity of the endocardium and myocardium have much the same pathophysiologic effect whether the resistance to inflow and stiffening of the myocardium is due to infiltration with amyloid tissue or another substance or to fibrosis.[22, 23] It is characteristic of hypertrophic cardiomyopathy (HCM) that the massive hypertrophy, together with the fibrosis and myofibrillar disarray, produces similar functional defects. There are, of course, many differences between HCM and EMF, but increased myocardial stiffness associated with disturbed relaxation and prolongation of ventricular filling is common to both (see later).

There are important differences between constrictive pericarditis and RCM, which are dependent on the differing effects of generalized constriction in constrictive pericarditis and regional areas of endomyocardial disease that affect one or both ventricles in a patchy manner in RCM. These differences are discussed later.

The Eosinophil in Heart Disease

The disorder involving EMF described by Loeffler as *endocarditis parietalis fibroplastica* is associated with hypereosinophilia and occurs in temperate climates. A similar condition, *tropical endomyocardial fibrosis*, occurs in hot, humid climates but without an obvious association with hypereosinophilia. At the present, tropical EMF and Loeffler's eosinophilic endomyocardial disease are considered to represent the same process.[24] The Churg-Strauss syndrome also combines hypereosinophilia with heart disease, but instead of EMF there is a dilated form of heart muscle disease, frequently with pericardial effusion and often with bronchial asthma. The eosinophilia-myalgia syndrome associated with the ingestion of L-tryptophan tablets produces lesions in the coronary arteries and conduction system.[25]

The pathologic findings in EMF and Loeffler's disease are essentially identical, although there are physical differences due to geography, climate, culture, associated illnesses, and genetic influences.[26, 27] *Hypereosinophilic syn-*

TABLE 53–1 Stages of Eosinophilic Endomyocardial Disease

Pathologic Stage	Clinical Stage
Acute inflammatory	Recurrent fever Paroxysmal atrial fibrillation Episodic heart failure (embolism rare)
Organizing fibrotic (pericardial effusion mainly in tropical EMF)	Heart failure Tricuspid and mitral regurgitation Embolism
↓ ↑	
Thrombotic	Heart failure Embolism Tricuspid and mitral regurgitation

Abbreviation: EMF, endomyocardial fibrosis.

drome[28] is a term used to describe multiple organ involvement in association with hypereosinophilia and with cardiac involvement in 95 percent of cases. Hypereosinophilic disease may present with cardiac features that may be later associated with involvement of other systems; it may present with extracardiac features and then involve the heart; or it may involve the heart only.[29, 30]

Available evidence strongly suggests that hypereosinophilic endomyocardial disease is caused by the abnormal behavior of eosinophils.[26, 31, 32] Qualitatively abnormal eosinophils actively damage the endocardium and myocardium. Counts of such cells are usually around 1.510/mm^3,[1] and they show degranulation and vacuolation. They exude a cationic protein, which is thrombogenic and damages the endocardium. An increase in Fc receptors causes more effective binding to Ig- and C3B-coated particles to produce a cytotoxic response. In addition to damaging the endocardium, the abnormal eosinophils infiltrate the myocardium and may degranulate, causing myocardial lesions.[31] Eosinophil granular protein can be detected in acute thrombotic and necrotic myocardial lesions in acute necrotizing eosinophilic myocarditis.

There are three principal stages in eosinophilic endomyocardial disease. The first is an acute inflammatory action in the endomyocardium, with intense infiltration by eosinophils. The second is one of organization with endocardial and myocardial fibrosis and endarteritis obliterans of myocardial arterioles; eosinophils progressively disappear from the lesions. The third stage is one of thrombosis. The three stages are not always clear cut, and they may overlap (Table 53–1 and Figs. 53–1 to 53–3).

The cause of the abnormality in the eosinophil is not known. A viral infection might be responsible, but there is no direct evidence for this, and no virus has been isolated. There seems to be little doubt that the cationic protein is responsible for the inflammatory reaction in the endomyocardium, so the heart disease may, in a sense, be regarded as the result of a hematologic disorder. Because the eosinophilic disorder is cryptogenic, it is logical to consider EMF as a cardiomyopathy, although when other organs are involved, as in the hypereosinophilic syndrome, it could be regarded as a form of specific heart muscle disease.[21]

The abnormal eosinophils are not usually associated with bone marrow precursors that would suggest a leukemic process; however, eosinophilic leukemia can produce deposits in the heart, although it does not usually cause endomyocardial disease. EMF in Africa and in other tropical areas has not been found to be associated with hypereosinophilia, probably for two reasons. First, increased eosinophil counts are common in patients in Africa due to helminthic infestation independent of EMF. Second, the eosinophils have not usually been examined for degranulation or vacuolation.

The distribution of eosinophilic endomyocardial disease is characteristic, essentially involving the inflow tracts of the ventricles. Either or both ventricles can be involved, with the endocardial fibrosis gradually obliterating the cavity from the apex and leaving only a small area of outflow tract beneath the pulmonary valve (see Figs. 53–2 and 53–3). There usually is a plaque of fibrous tissue on the left atrial (LA) endocardium; otherwise, the atria are not

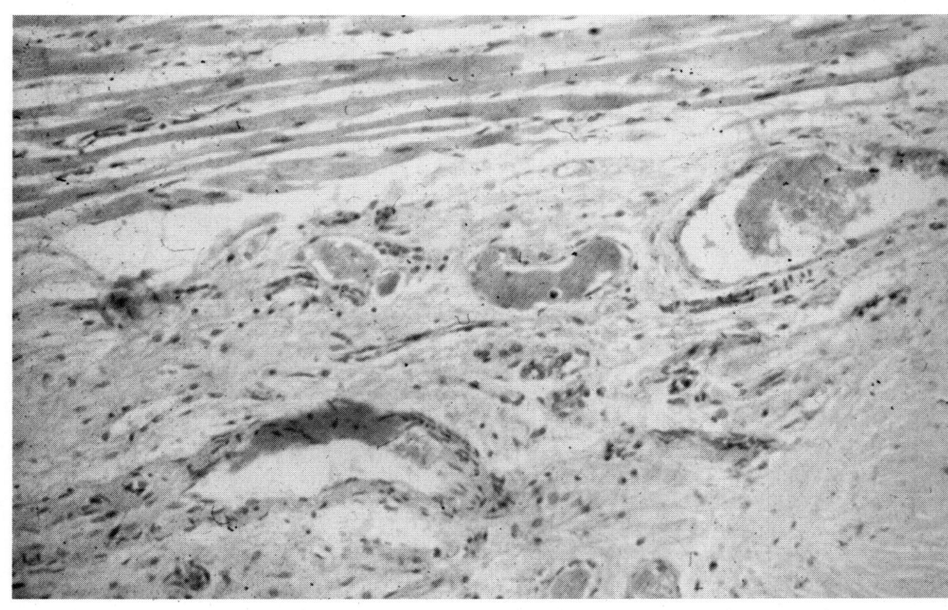

FIGURE 53–1 Photomicrograph of ventricular myocardium in stage 2 endomyocardial fibrosis shows extensive fibrosis but no eosinophilic infiltration. (Courtesy of E. Olsen, M.D.)

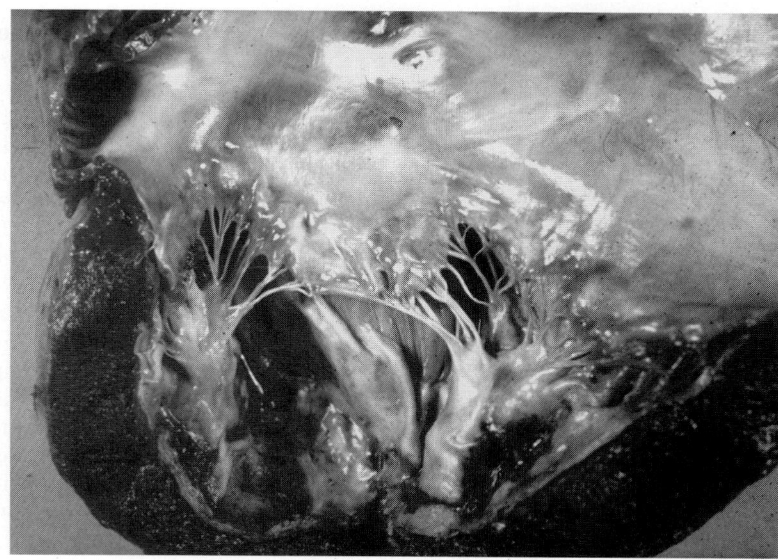

FIGURE 53–2 Heart with left ventricular endomyocardial fibrosis. There is extensive fibrosis involving the endocardium and the anterior, but not the posterior, mitral valve apparatus. Widespread antemortem thrombus overlies the endocardial fibrosis. (Courtesy of E. Olsen, M.D.)

involved directly but become enlarged as a result of the ventricular disease and of atrioventricular (AV) valvular regurgitation.

In the tropics, EMF can account for 10 percent of pediatric patients with cardiologic disease.[33] A study[34, 35] compared the incidence of EMF in the tropics with EMF in temperate climates and found that patients in the United Kingdom tended to be older, were mainly males, and often had a systemic illness.[28, 29] Tropical patients tended to be younger, had an equal male/female ratio, and often came from poor, undernourished families with heavy parasitic infestation, especially with filariasis. Abnormal eosinophil morphology has not thus far been seen. In the tropics, the involvement of both ventricles occurs in only 51 percent of patients, whereas biventricular disease is more common in temperate climates. However, endomyocardial biopsy abnormalities are identical, although half of the patients in the United Kingdom present in the acute early necrotic (stage 1) phase, whereas most patients in the tropics present in the late fibrotic state.

Clinical Recognition

History and Physical Examination

The inflammatory first stage of the illness is marked by episodes of palpitation and dyspnea due to atrial fibrilla-

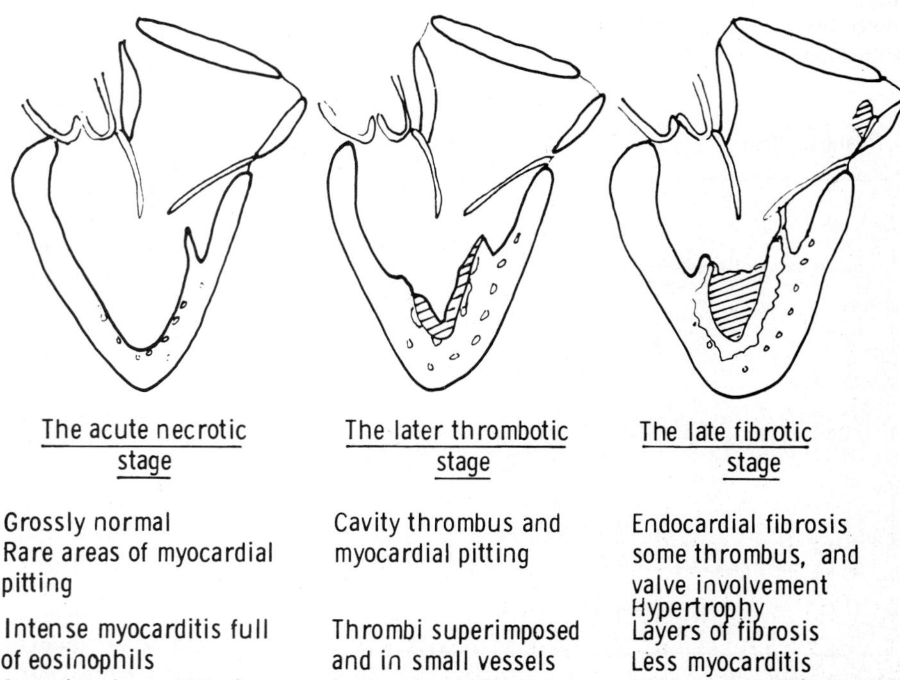

FIGURE 53–3 Diagrams of cardiac lesion in eosinophilic endomyocardial disease. (Courtesy of Professor I. Brockington, J. Davies, M.D., and E. Olsen, M.D.)

tion, periods of fever, progressive lassitude, and general malaise. The fibrotic second stage is notable for symptoms of heart failure and of AV valvular regurgitation, with progressive fatigue, increasing dyspnea, and swelling of the ankles and abdomen (see Table 53–1). When left-sided disease is dominant, dyspnea, which may be paroxysmal, is notable, whereas with right-sided involvement, the emphasis is on fatigue, swelling of the ankles and abdomen, and tightness of the throat due to the high jugular venous pressure. Despite reduced effort tolerance because of the low cardiac output, patients may remain reasonably ambulant until the very late stages. At any stage, however, embolism to the lungs may occur, producing hemoptysis.

The physical signs depend on the site and extent of the disease. In right-sided disease, there is peripheral edema, hepatomegaly, and ascites. The jugular venous pressure is raised, often to the angle of the jaw up to 20 cm above the sternal angle. Tricuspid regurgitation is common, especially when there is atrial fibrillation, producing a dominant systolic (S) wave in the jugular venous pulse with a normal *y* descent. The external jugular vein may exhibit palpable systolic pulsation. The very high venous pressure may produce a "moon face" and even proptosis. In early cases, the jugular venous pulse shows the characteristic dip-and-plateau configuration, with prominent A and V waves and *x* and *y* descents typical of RCM. The jugular venous pressure may rise on inspiration, giving a positive Kussmaul sign. The arterial pulse is small in volume and thready because when the right ventricle is extensively obliterated, the entire cardiac output depends on right atrial function. Arterial paradox may be present. When there is a large pericardial effusion, the cardiac impulse is quiet and cardiac pulsation is obscured, but otherwise the very large right atrium may produce pulsation to the right of the sternum. The heart sounds are faint, and gallop rhythm is common (Fig. 53–4). A systolic murmur that increases on inspiration may be heard in the tricuspid area as a result of tricuspid regurgitation. The abdomen is distended with ascites, and the liver is enlarged and pulsating. In addition,

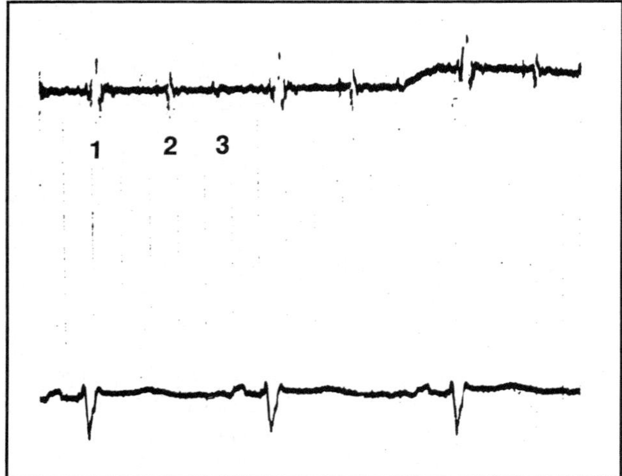

FIGURE 53–4 Phonocardiogram shows third heart sound (3) in eosinophilic endomyocardial disease.

there often is generalized muscular wasting due to tissue hypoxia resulting from the low cardiac output.

In left-sided disease, the emphasis is often but not always on mitral regurgitation. The arterial pulse is small in volume and poorly sustained. The cardiac impulse is left ventricular (LV) and may be displaced outside the midclavicular line. The jugular venous pressure may be unremarkable or show a dominant a wave (if there is sinus rhythm) due to pulmonary hypertension. Auscultation also may be unremarkable, apart from a third heart sound and (in sinus rhythm) a fourth sound. Tachycardia is common, and summation gallop of third and fourth heart sounds is usual. When mitral regurgitation is present, there is a holosystolic murmur at the cardiac apex, conducted usually to the axilla. The murmur tends to diminish in intensity toward the end of systole as the anterior chordae of the mitral valve that are relatively free of disease (see Fig. 53–2) render the valve competent. Pulmonary valve closure is accentuated when there is pulmonary hypertension due to the high LA pressure. Eventually, signs of right heart failure develop. Systemic embolism may occur at any time and is encouraged by the presence of paroxysmal or established atrial fibrillation.

In both right- and left-sided types, systemic blood pressure and pulse tend to be low, and tachycardia is invariable in well-advanced cases because an increase in heart rate is the only way the patient can maintain cardiac output.

Laboratory Examination

A moderate degree of anemia is common, but the striking feature in eosinophilic endomyocardial disease is the elevated eosinophil count. This alone, however, does not cause EMF, as demonstrated in the case of a patient with progressive renal failure and hypertensive heart failure with uremic pericarditis and with 84 percent eosinophils of a total white blood count of 38,000 but without any evidence of endomyocardial disease.[36] Therefore, although the total eosinophil count is raised for one reason or another, it appears that the eosinophil must first become activated to discharge the granules and cationic protein to cause the endomyocardial damage.[36] If more than 20 percent of eosinophils contain vacuoles and more than 15 percent are degranulated, endomyocardial damage is almost invariably confirmed by biopsy.[31] Therefore, EMF depends on the number of degranulated eosinophils rather than on the total count.

There are no specific biochemical blood changes. Liver function tests can be abnormal as the result of heart failure, with very high jugular venous pressure. Hypokalemia may result from the use of diuretics.

Radiology

In right-sided EMF, prominence of the right atrium is the main feature. When there is a pericardial effusion, the cardiac silhouette may be enormous, with marked enlargement to the right of the sternum. The lung fields tend to be clear unless pulmonary embolism has reduced the vascular markings or produced pulmonary infarction. The pulmonary arteries are not usually prominent. In left-sided disease, the

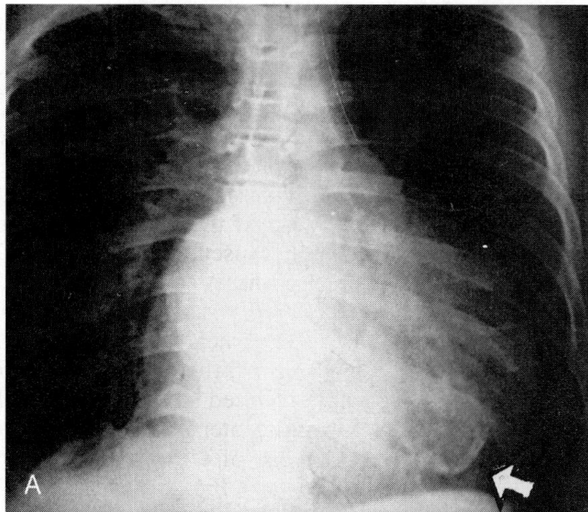

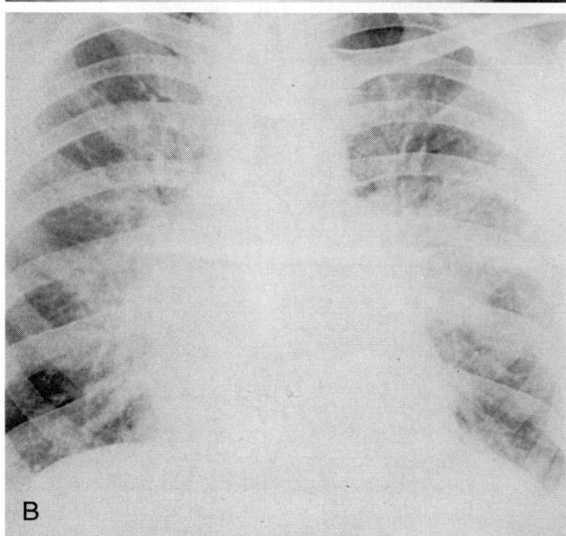

FIGURE 53–5 **A,** Six-foot posteroanterior chest radiograph in endomyocardial fibrosis shows linear calcification (*arrow*) in the region of the left ventricle. **B,** Acute massive pulmonary edema in left ventricular endomyocardial fibrosis.

left ventricle is enlarged, especially when there is mitral regurgitation, as is the left atrium. There is often a linear strip of calcification along the left border of the heart, which is characteristic of calcification in endocardial thrombus (Fig. 53–5A). The lung fields may show evidence of raised LA pressure, with reduction in caliber of lower lobe vessels and interstitial costophrenic lines. In advanced cases, there may be frank pulmonary edema (see Fig. 53–5B).

Electrocardiography

The electrocardiogram is not specific. In right-sided disease, right-axis deviation can be expected and right atrial enlargement is shown by augmented, pointed right atrial P waves. There may be first-degree AV block or right bundle-branch block.

Low-voltage QRS complexes and flat T waves are seen when there is a significant pericardial effusion. In left-sided disease, increased QRS voltage and T-wave inversion signal LV hypertrophy, and bifid P waves indicate LA enlargement. Ventricular arrhythmias tend to occur in the later stages and may be related more to heart failure than the fibrotic process.

Echocardiography

In the inflammatory first stage, the M-mode echocardiogram may show only increased ventricular dimensions and reduced contractility. On two-dimensional echocardiography, thrombus may be seen at the apex of either ventricle, especially in the apical four-chamber view (Fig. 53–6).

In the fibrotic second stage, two-dimensional studies show only slightly dilated ventricles with dilated atria, and patches of fibrosis on the ventricular endocardium, apical and inflow tracts, or AV valves. Isolated valvular lesions limited to the inflow valve and not involving the intervening myocardium may be seen.[37]

Apical ventricular contraction is usually preserved even in the presence of thrombus. Bright, sparkling echoes are often seen from the endocardial surfaces and myocardium but are not diagnostic, being representative only of high reflective echoes due to fibrosis (see Fig. 53–6).

Transesophageal echocardiography provides a useful posterior window on the left atrium and is helpful in demonstrating mitral and tricuspid regurgitation. Assessment of the extent and severity of the disease is facilitated by the use of color-coded and amplitude-processed echo imaging.

Doppler studies in diastolic heart disease do not necessarily reveal any specific features of eosinophilic endomyocardial disease except the characteristic patchy endocardial fibrosis and the apical ventricular obliteration. The restrictive process leads to impairment of ventricular compliance, with a large increment of early diastolic filling pressure for a small increase in volume as ventricular filling is halted in the first half of diastole. Pulsed Doppler records at the tip of the mitral or tricuspid valves show normal or increased peak E wave velocity and shortened deceleration time of the early filling E wave (Fig. 53–7).

Rapid filling is shortened and LV isovolumetric relaxation time is diminished.[37] These Doppler findings are not

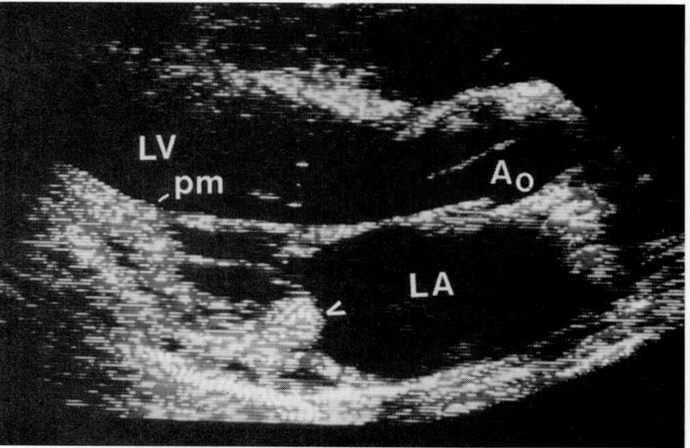

FIGURE 53–6 Color-coded two-dimensional echocardiogram in eosinophilic endomyocardial disease shows bright echoes (see text). *Arrowhead* indicates probable thrombus. A_o, aorta; LA, left atrium; LV, left ventricle; pm, papillary muscle. (Courtesy of Derek Gibson, M.D.)

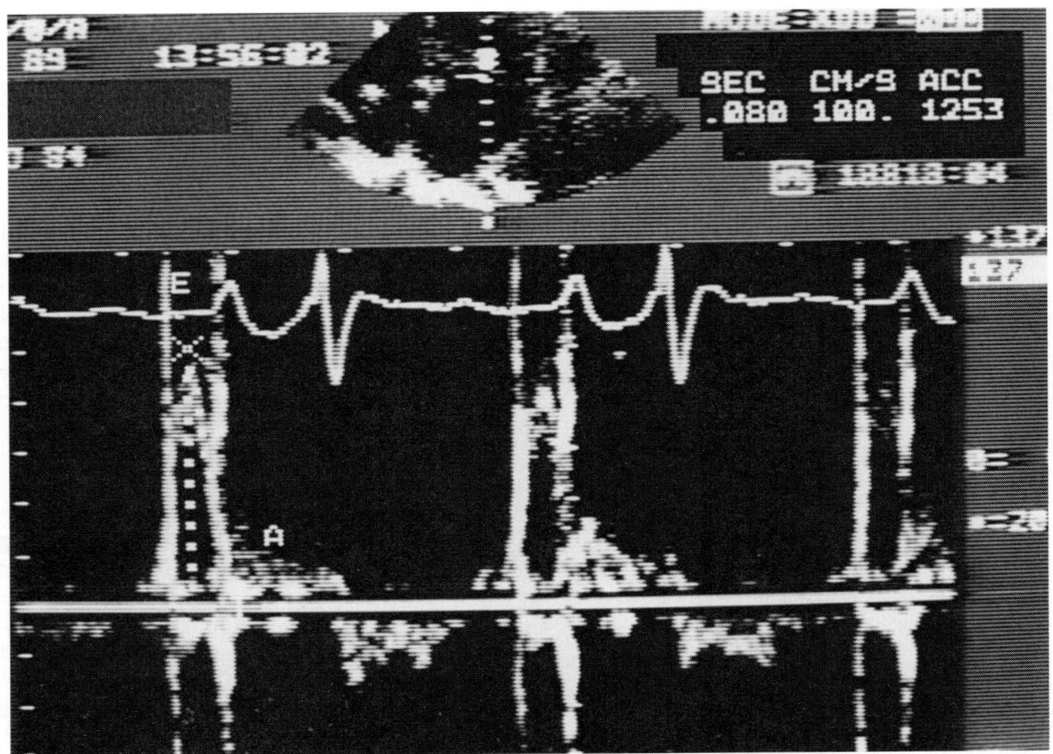

FIGURE 53–7 Pulsed Doppler record of mitral valve inflow velocity shows a restrictive pattern in endomyocardial fibrosis. High-peak early E inflow velocity (100 mm/s), short deceleration time (80 mm/s), and small peak atrial (A) inflow velocity (25 mm/s) are shown. E/A ratio is increased to 4. (From Acquatella H: Doppler-echocardiographic investigations in restrictive cardiomyopathy. *In* Goodwin JF, Olsen EGJ [eds]: Cardiomyopathies: Realisations and Expectations. Berlin: Springer-Verlag, 1992.)

specific to EMF or RCM. They are similar in other forms of diastolic heart disease and also in other forms of LV disease characterized by increased stiffness, including HCM and coronary artery disease.[36] Occasionally, advanced cases of dilated cardiomyopathy with marked myocardial fibrosis and endocardial thickening resulting from prolonged heart failure may show similar but less severe findings.

The most useful application of echocardiography in the diagnosis and assessment of eosinophilic endomyocardial disease is the two-dimensional technique demonstrating endocardial patches of thickening and obliteration of the apical ventricular cavities, supported by Doppler evidence of AV valve regurgitation. These techniques are also valuable in differentiation of EMF from other forms of RCM.

Cardiac Catheterization and Angiocardiography

In all types of RCM, the characteristic rapid early ventricular filling and slow or absent late ventricular filling produce a significant hemodynamic pattern and ventricular and atrial pressure curves. The rapid inflow produces an early low ventricular diastolic pressure, with a dip followed by rapid leveling off to a high end-diastolic level. The LV systolic pressure is often low due to the ventricular damage and heart failure. Right ventricular systolic pressure tends to be elevated because of LV disease. Because the disease is patchy and may involve left and right ventricles to different degrees, the early diastolic pressures in both ventricles differ (Fig. 53–8), in contrast to constrictive pericarditis in which, because the constrictive effect is generalized and equally affects both ventricles, the early and late diastolic pressures are identical (see Fig. 53–8).

Atrial pressure pulses best noted in the jugular venous pressure waveform show dominant A and V waves, with rapid *x* and *y* descents. The *x* descent represents the rapid inflow. The V wave summit marks the end of ventricular systole and is prominent because of the elevated ventricular filling pressure.

Angiocardiography

In EMF, angiocardiography demonstrates restriction of filling of the ventricles and the enlargement of the atria. Late in the right-sided form, the right atrium is enormous and the right ventricle is reduced to a small sinus beneath the pulmonary valve (Fig. 53–9A). If a pericardial effusion is present, a clear gap will be seen between the contrast medium outlining the outer border of the right atrium and the pericardium. In left-sided EMF, the apex of the left ventricle is seen to be blunted by a fibrothrombus (see Fig. 53–9B). The appearances have been likened to a boxing glove. There may be mitral regurgitation into the enlarged left atrium. The calcification of the LV thrombus noted on a plain radiograph may be visible (see Fig. 53–5A).

Angiocardiography is less valuable than echocardiography in the diagnosis and assessment of RCM. Echocardiography provides more detail, is noninvasive, is free of risk, and can be used repeatedly to judge progression.

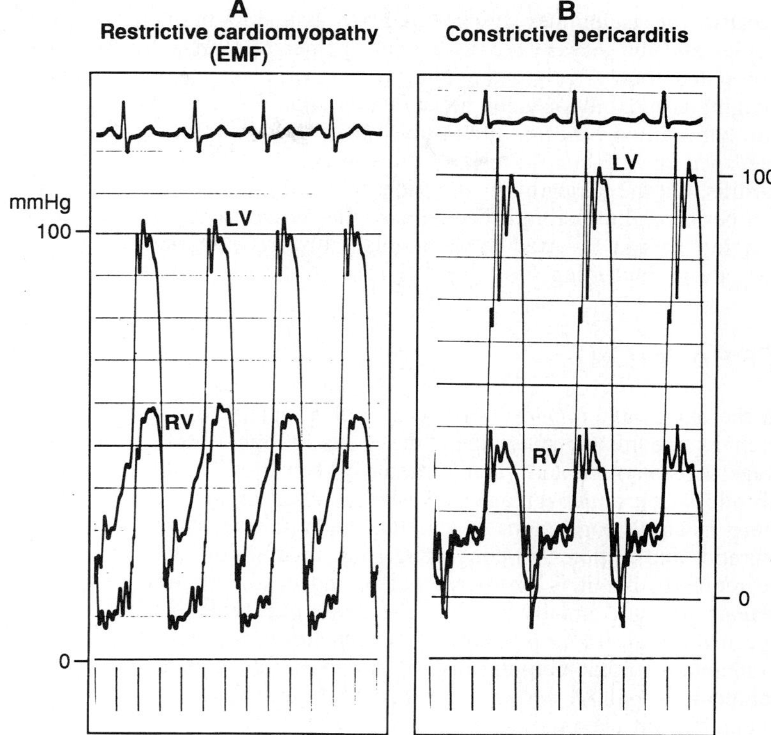

FIGURE 53–8 Ventricular pressure pulses in restrictive cardiomyopathy (endomyocardial fibrosis [EMF]) **(A)** and constrictive pericarditis **(B)**. The left ventricular (LV) systolic pressure is low. In endomyocardial fibrosis, the early and end-diastolic pressures are raised in both ventricles, and the right ventricular (RV) systolic pressure is 48/50 mm Hg. In constrictive pericarditis, the diastolic pressures are identical in both ventricles, the early diastolic pressure falls below zero, the end-diastolic pressure is normal, and the RV systolic pressure is not elevated.

Endomyocardial Biopsy

Endomyocardial biopsy is useful in the detection of the typical eosinophil infiltration in the inflammatory stage and the myocardial fibrosis in the later stage, although if eosinophils are absent the biopsy may not provide an exact diagnosis of the cause of the fibrosis, and the demonstration of characteristically abnormal eosinophils in the blood therefore may be of considerable importance. Biopsy carries a risk of embolism due to dislodgment of recent thrombus from the ventricle and therefore should be undertaken only with strong indications. Usually, a diagnosis of eosinophilic endomyocardial disease can be made by the combination of the clinical features suggestive of RCM with the demonstration of degranulating eosinophils in the peripheral blood and the characteristic echocardiographic features supported by hemodynamic studies. Clinically, the possibility of RCM should be considered in any patient with a high jugular venous pressure and a third heart sound but little or no cardiomegaly.

Ambulatory Electrocardiography

Ambulatory electrocardiographic monitoring can be useful in revealing arrhythmias, especially paroxysmal atrial fibrillation, ventricular tachycardia, and ectopic beats, and also in the detection of conduction defects. Therefore, the results are helpful in guiding antiarrhythmic therapy or in justifying the need for a pacemaker.

Radionuclide Studies

Radionuclide studies do not have an important place in the diagnosis of RCM, and few data are available on EMF

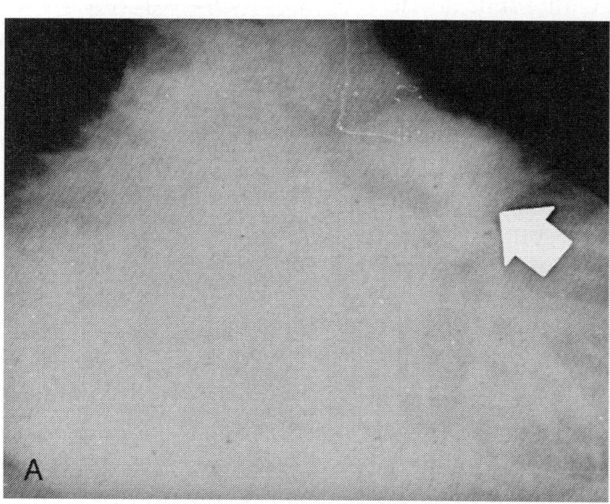

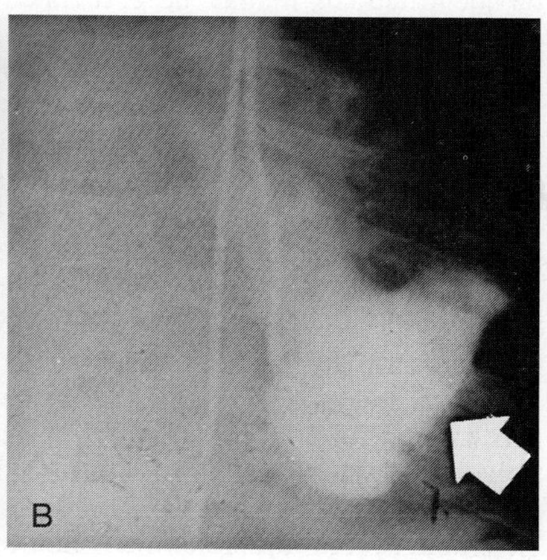

FIGURE 53–9 A, Anteroposterior angiogram in right-sided tropical endomyocardial fibrosis. The right atrium is greatly enlarged, and the right ventricular volume is reduced to a small "sinus" beneath the pulmonary valve (*arrow*). **B,** Anteroposterior left ventricular angiogram in left-sided tropical zone endomyocardial fibrosis. The left ventricular apex has been blunted by thrombus obliterating the apical cavity (*arrow*). (**A** and **B,** Courtesy of Professor I. Brockington.)

because the techniques are not usually available in the tropics and the disease is very rare in temperate climates. Computed tomography scanning and magnetic resonance imaging are mainly of value in providing a definite distinction between constrictive pericarditis and RCM. The thickened pericardium can be clearly seen in constrictive pericarditis, but the pericardium is normal in RCM unless there is a pericardial effusion, in which case magnetic resonance imaging should be used to distinguish this from fibrous pericardial thickening.

TREATMENT

In the acute inflammatory stage, anti-inflammatory agents such as prednisone may delay the onset of the fibrotic stage; hydroxyurea and vincristine have been tried. In the fibrotic stage, anticoagulants are needed, as is digitalis if there is atrial fibrillation. In the late heart failure stage, diuretics and angiotensin-converting enzyme inhibitors will be required, but it is important not to reduce the central venous pressure greatly or slow the heart rate too much because a high-filling pressure and tachycardia are needed to maintain cardiac output. Surgical methods include endocardectomy and AV valve repair and replacement. Transplantation has been used.

AMYLOID HEART DISEASE

Amyloid heart disease is a form of RCM and is classified as a diastolic heart disease, but it has important differences from other forms of RCM and therefore deserves a separate heading. In addition, it occupies a position in the classification of heart muscle disease between the cardiomyopathies and specific heart muscle disease, as defined in the section on dilated cardiomyopathy. When amyloid disease is confined to the heart, it is included in the restrictive group of cardiomyopathies, but when it is more widespread and involves organs other than the heart, it deserves to be classified as specific heart muscle disease.

Amyloidosis is a disorder of protein metabolism in which the abnormal fibrillar amyloid protein is laid down intercellularly. Some amyloid AL fibrils are derived from monoclonal macroglobulin light chains. Amyloid disease may be primary (cryptogenic), in which the cause cannot be identified, or it may be associated with multiple myeloma and B-lymphocyte lymphoma. It also occurs in a familial form, including Mediterranean fever, in which the major protein component of amyloid is not macroglobulin. "Reactive" amyloidosis is a complication of long-standing wasting illness (e.g., malignancy, chronic infection, tuberculosis, rheumatoid arthritis). Senile amyloidosis is found accidentally at autopsy in elderly subjects, some of whom have had heart failure that may have been caused or exacerbated by the amyloid process (Tables 53–2 and 53–3).

In primary amyloidosis, the process may be confined to the heart or may also involve mucous membranes, connective tissue, tendon sheaths, the tongue, and peripheral nerves. The amyloid deposits may be massive, leading to organ dysfunction and failure, including postural hypotension and severe and relentless cardiac, renal, or hepatic failure. The tongue may be so large as to prevent the patient from being able to speak normally or swallow easily. Small capillaries may also be infiltrated, leading to the classic "scratch petechiae" or purpura induced by gentle stroking of the eyelids, cheeks, or anterior chest. In macroglobulinemia, non-Hodgkin's lymphoma, and myeloma, amyloid may involve the heart, bone marrow, kidney, and peripheral nerves or skeletal muscles. Often, these amyloid deposits are scattered and small in amount. In the familial type, amyloid involves the nervous system and kidneys. In the senile type, only the heart is attacked, and the protein involved is different from that in macroglobulinemia.[38]

TABLE 53–2 Types of Amyloid Disease

Primary cryptogenic amyloid	Heart Mucous membranes Tendon sheaths Tongue, connective tissue Nerves, Kidney, Spleen, Liver } rarely
Non-Hodgkin's lymphoma	Heart Bone marrow Kidneys, skeletal muscles Nerves
Multiple myeloma	Heart Bone marrow Kidneys, skeletal muscles Nerves
Medullary thyroid carcinoma	Thyroid
Familial Mediterranean fever	Heart Kidneys Nerves
Reactive secondary to chronic disease	Liver Spleen Kidneys
Senile	Heart

Pathophysiology

Amyloid AL fibrils are deposited in and around the walls of capillaries, arterioles, and venules. The characteristic

TABLE 53–3 Classification of Amyloidosis

- Primary amyloidosis (AL type) with no evidence of preexisting or coexisting disease
- Amyloidosis associated with multiple myeloma (also AL type)
- Reactive amyloidosis associated with chronic infectious diseases such as osteomyelitis, tuberculosis, ulcerative colitis, or other chronic inflammatory disease (AA type)
- Herediofamilial amyloidosis, neuropathic (AF transthyretin or prealbumin type), and the amyloidosis associated with familial Mediterranean fever (AA type)
- Local amyloidosis with focal, tumor-like deposits that occur in isolated organs without evidence of systemic involvement
- Amyloidosis associated with aging, especially in the heart and the brain
- Amyloidosis associated with long-term hemodialysis
- Amyloidosis of endocrine tissues (e.g., precalcitonin in medullary carcinoma of the thyroid gland)

Abbreviations: AL, Amyloid-light chain type; AA, protein A; AF, amyloid fibril.

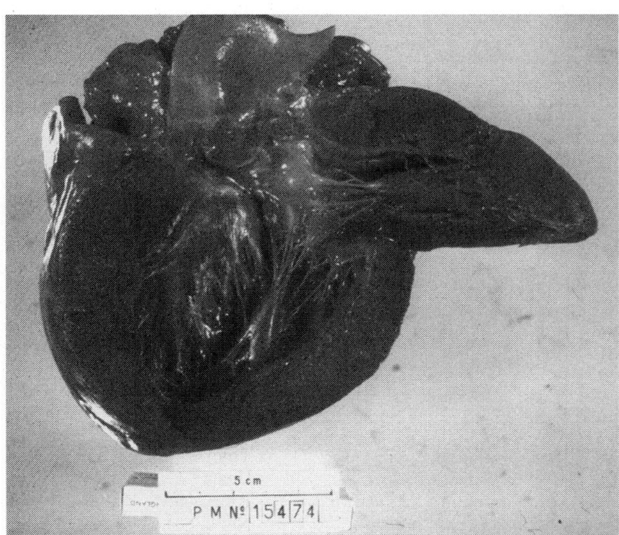

FIGURE 53–10 The heart in amyloid disease. There is ventricular hypertrophy but no obvious dilatation.

iodine reaction may be negative, but amyloid stains apple green with Congo red under polarized light and gives a metachromatic reaction to methyl violet. Staining techniques and light microscopy may occasionally be negative in tissue from endomyocardial biopsy samples, but the use of electron microscopy will show the characteristic irregularly arranged deposition of protein.

The gross pathology of the heart shows thickened, firm, rubbery ventricular muscle (Fig. 53–10), with atrial enlargement and sometimes thrombi in the appendages. The ventricular septum can be disproportionately hypertrophied and the papillary muscles exaggerated, resembling HCM. Amyloid deposits are found between the myocardial fibers and papillary muscles, as well as in surrounding blood vessels, which may be compressed. Endocardial and atrial involvement can occur. The valves may be thickened, and focal pericardial deposits of amyloid tissue can also be found. Amyloid deposits are not infrequently detected in the conducting tissue. The pathologic processes account for the common triad of angina, heart failure, and arrhythmia.

When present, the stiff, poorly compliant ventricular muscle and the endocardial involvement account for the restrictive features of the disease. These are discussed later.

Clinical Recognition

Amyloid heart disease is more common in men than women and is rare before the age of 30 years.[38] Symptoms include cardiac pain, dyspnea, and swelling of the legs and abdomen due to heart failure, with palpitations or syncope due to tachyarrhythmias or bradyarrhythmias. Heart failure is often due to impairment of both systolic and diastolic function, although it may also be caused by selective systolic or diastolic dysfunction.[39] Orthostatic hypotension is common as a result of autonomic, adrenal, or cardiac infiltration.

Physical Examination

On examination, the patient usually looks ill and tired and may have lost weight. A trace of icterus may be present. When heart failure is severe, the jugular venous pressure is increased, showing the characteristic tall A and V waves and sharp *x* and *y* descents unless there is tricuspid regurgitation or atrial fibrillation. The heart may not appear to be obviously enlarged. There often is a systolic murmur caused by tricuspid or mitral regurgitation. An LV third sound is usually absent[38, 40] because of a lack of sufficiently rapid LV filling, but a right ventricular third sound may be heard that increases in intensity with inspiration. Ascites, hepatomegaly, and edema of the legs are common.

Extracardiac involvement includes lymph gland enlargement, mononeuritis, and gastrointestinal symptoms. Occasionally, the patient presents with a rash due to infiltration of the skin. Periorbital hematomas are well recognized although rare. In the primary form of amyloidosis, the tongue is thickened and rubbery, and the mucous membranes may be erythematous and thickened, especially the conjunctiva (Fig. 53–11). Carpal tunnel syndrome may occur due to involvement of the palmar fascia.

Chest Radiography

There usually is little or no cardiac enlargement, but changes of pulmonary venous congestion due to the high filling pressure in the left ventricle are marked. Pericardial effusion may increase apparent cardiomegaly.

Electrocardiography

There usually is a generalized low-voltage electrocardiogram resembling pericardial effusion due to the myocardial disease (Fig. 53–12). Sinus rhythm is usual, although atrial fibrillation may occur. There often are ectopic beats. Fascicular blocks are not uncommon. Various degrees of heart block may occur. T-wave inversion is frequent, and large Q waves may be seen (Fig. 53–13).

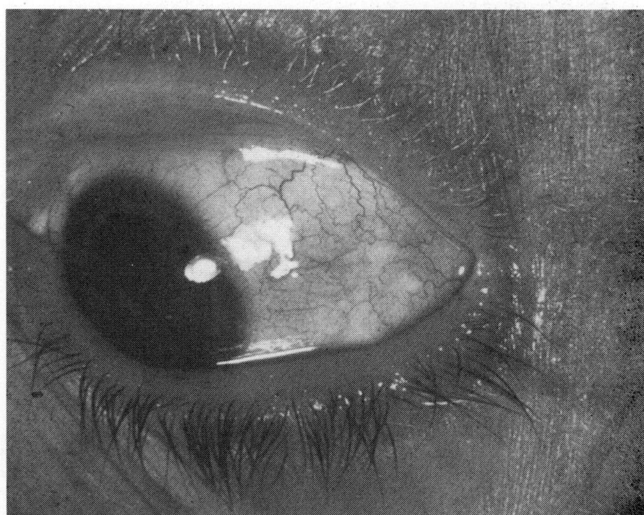

FIGURE 53–11 Erythematous and thickened palpebral conjunctiva in primary amyloid disease.

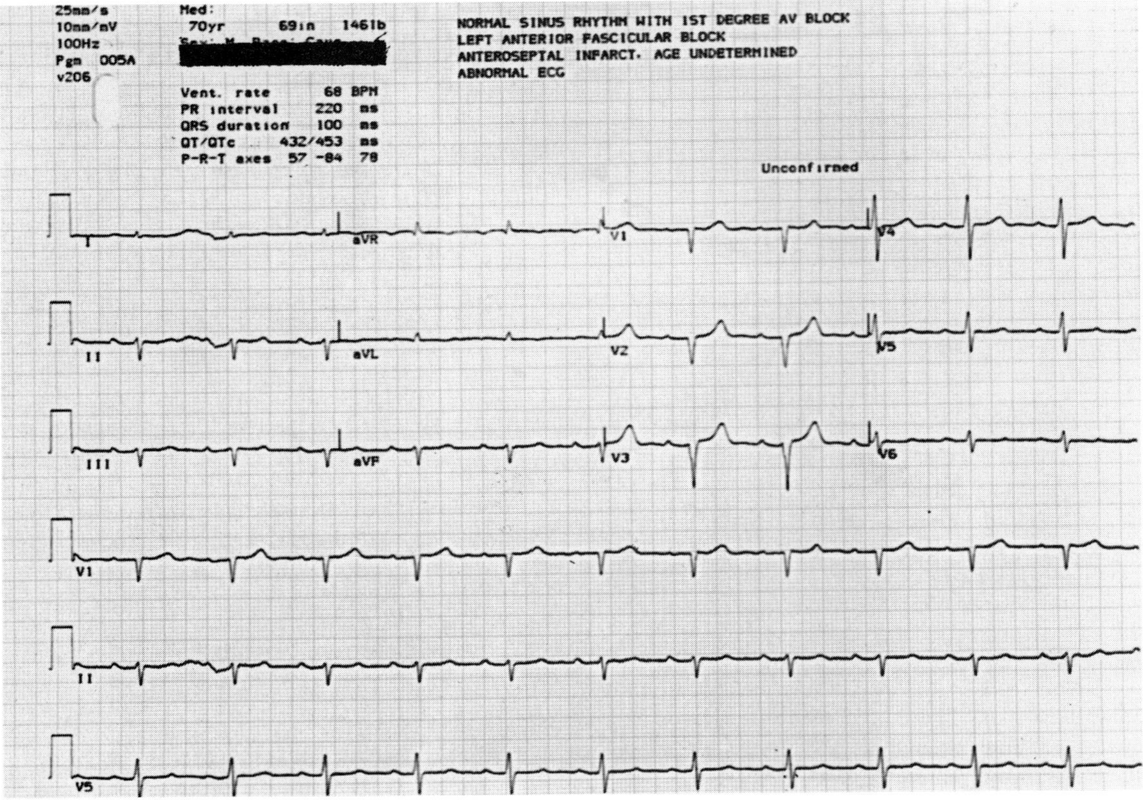

FIGURE 53–12 On electrocardiography, there often is low voltage due to myocardial disease, resembling pericardial effusion. Note the Q waves. (See the text for details.)

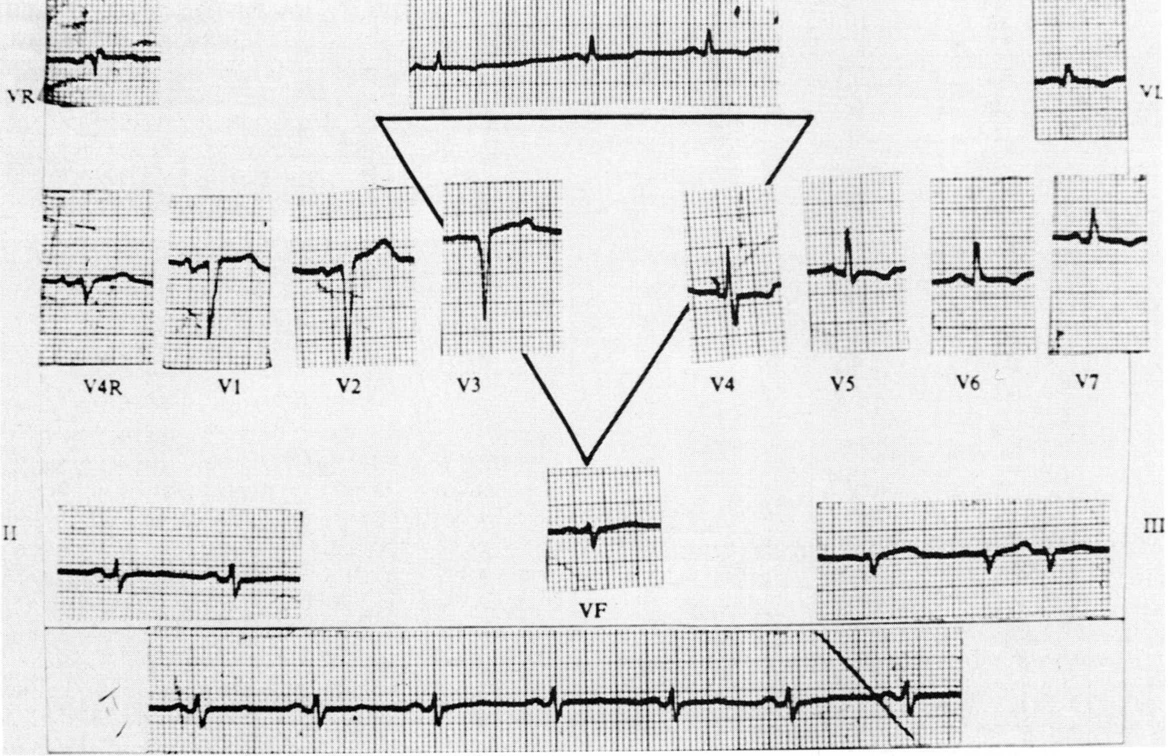

FIGURE 53–13 Twelve-lead electrocardiogram in cardiac amyloidosis shows precordial Q waves mimicking anterior myocardial infarction.

Echocardiography

M-mode studies reveal reduced size of the left ventricle, increased right ventricular wall thickness, and hypertrophy of the ventricular septum and LV posterior wall. An important sign is thickening of the atrial septum.

Bright, sparkling echoes in the ventricular muscle merely reflect increased echo density and are not specific for amyloid disease. The mitral valve may be thickened.[41] In advanced disease, Doppler studies show a shortened deceleration time, normal ventricular isovolumic relaxation time, and a normal or increased peak E velocity, producing an increase in the E/A ratio.[37]

Angiocardiography and Cardiac Catheterization

Ventriculography does not usually show dramatic abnormalities, but the end-diastolic volume is reduced and the internal aspect of the ventricles appears "shaggy." Mitral regurgitation may be seen. The major coronary arteries are normal.

The hemodynamics reflect the restrictive phenomena caused by the splinting effect of the amyloid infiltration on the heart muscle. Stroke and minute volume are reduced. The diastolic pressures in both ventricles are substantially increased but more so in the left than in the right ventricle. The characteristic dip-and-plateau pattern is modified; there is a slow rise from early diastolic pressure to end-diastolic pressure because filling is slow throughout diastole, and the normal early rapid filling phase seen in constrictive pericarditis and EMF is not present.[41] Pressure-volume curves show higher pressures at lower LV volumes than normal (i.e., a reduced compliance) (Fig. 53–14).

Biopsy Studies

Biopsy studies of rectal and gingival tissues may reveal amyloid deposits when the disease is generalized, but cardiac biopsy is necessary to prove cardiac involvement unless a combination of clinical, hemodynamic, and echocardiographic data is sufficient for secure diagnosis. The presence of amyloid in other tissues does not guarantee its presence in the heart. Even though there is no specific treatment for amyloid disease, a tissue diagnosis is important to rule out conditions that are treatable (see later). Electron microscopic examination is helpful in the detection of amyloid deposits with certainty.

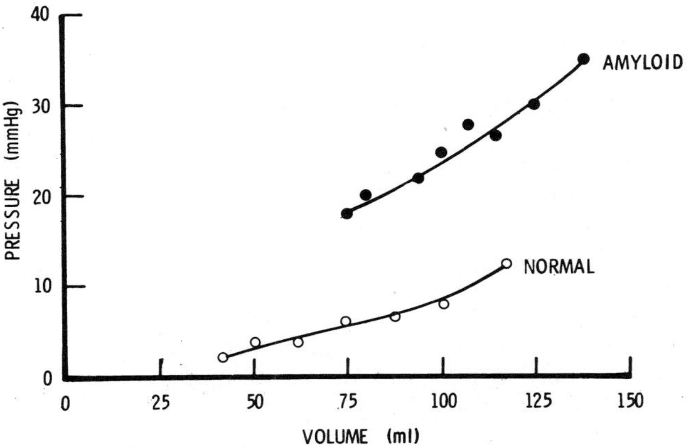

FIGURE 53–14 Pressure-volume curves in the left ventricle in diastole in a patient with amyloid disease and in a control subject with chest pain but normal coronary arteries. There is much greater pressure for an equivalent volume in the patient with amyloid disease than in the normal subject, reflecting the increased stiffness in the left ventricle in the former. (From Chew C, Ziady GM, Rafael MJ, et al: The functional defect in amyloid heart disease. Am J Cardiol 36:438, 1975.)

Rapid-Speed Computed Tomography and Magnetic Resonance Imaging

Computed tomography scans suggest amyloid when diffuse ventricular thickening is associated with radiographic myocardial density lower than that when myocardial hypertrophy exists alone.[42] The main value of computed tomography is to distinguish RCM and amyloidosis with normal pericardial structure from constrictive pericarditis. Magnetic resonance imaging provides more detail of myocardial and pericardial structure than computed tomography, but experience is limited.

Radionuclide Studies

Scintigraphy with ^{99m}Tc pyrophosphate or with an antibody directed against cardiac myosin shows extensive uptake in the myocardium in severe cases, but false-negative results can occur.[43, 44]

Differential Diagnosis

The principal disorders that deserve consideration are HCM, EMF, constrictive pericarditis, and coronary artery disease. When heart failure exists, both HCM and amyloid disease may closely resemble each other, although in the absence of heart failure there is usually no difficulty in distinguishing the two. With failure in HCM and amyloid heart disease, there is a high jugular venous pressure with LV enlargement. Systolic murmurs of AV valvular regurgitation are common, but an LV third sound is usually absent in the restrictive form of amyloid heart disease. The characteristic late onset of the systolic murmur and the jerky quality of the arterial pulse in HCM may be lost in heart failure, and if atrial fibrillation is present, there will be no fourth heart sound.

Echocardiographic results in amyloid heart disease may closely resemble those in HCM, showing an immobile hypertrophied ventricular septum and asymmetric septal hypertrophy.[45] Bright, sparkling echoes may be seen in both HCM and amyloid disease. Definite differentiation in life may be impossible without an endomyocardial biopsy. The finding of periorbital hematomas or evidence of amyloid elsewhere in the body may clarify the situation. HCM and amyloid disease may coexist, but this combination is very unusual.

Clinical differentiation of amyloidosis of the heart from EMF rests mainly on the absence of the LV third sound in amyloid disease and the characteristic echocardiographic and angiographic features of EMF aided by electron microscopic endomyocardial biopsy findings. In constrictive pericarditis, the absence of evidence of systolic myocardial disorder and of significant LV hypertrophy are important differential points.

A history of angina and the presence of Q waves (pseudoinfarct pattern) on the electrocardiogram occur in some patients with amyloid heart disease.

Amyloidosis of the heart can be suspected on the basis of significantly elevated jugular venous pressure, with the characteristic M-shaped pattern suggesting a degree of myocardial stiffness in excess of that found in coronary artery disease. Absolute confirmation often depends on myocardial biopsy.

Cardiac amyloidosis in familial Mediterranean fever should not cause difficulty because of the association of episodes of abdominal pain, fever, pleurisy, and arthritis occurring in Levantine people on a genetic basis. This form of amyloid deposition is the only one susceptible to medical therapy; the administration of colchicine appears to delay the progression of amyloid deposition.

The most important factor in the diagnosis of amyloid heart disease is to keep the possibility in mind, particularly when the combination of a high jugular venous pressure with a restrictive pattern and unimpressive cardiomegaly is seen. Observation of this combination should result in an initial provisional diagnosis of "diastolic heart disease," and steps should then be taken to narrow the field to the appropriate condition.

Treatment

Apart from the amyloidosis associated with familial Mediterranean fever, there is no effective drug therapy. Amyloidosis associated with chronic inflammatory conditions might be stabilized with effective therapy and cure for the chronic inflammatory condition. In patients with primary amyloidosis and extensive cardiac involvement, heart failure is usually progressive, with death occurring within 14 months. Transient improvement in symptoms may be associated with the addition of a diuretic and salt restriction and, in some patients, the judicious use of cardiac glycosides. Cardiac glycosides should be used with caution in amyloidosis because some patients seem to be extremely sensitive to their effects. Furthermore, when the problem is primarily diastolic dysfunction, it is difficult to imagine that cardiac glycosides would be particularly useful. In addition, some clinicians believe the patient with cardiac amyloidosis to be extremely sensitive to cardiac glycosides.

Chemotherapy and Stem Cell Replacement in the Treatment of Amyloidosis

Comenzo and colleagues[46] have evaluated the potential efficacy of dose-intensive melphalan with blood stem cell support in the treatment of AL amyloidosis. Their radionale for using such therapy is that autologous stem cell transplantation is effective therapy for multiple myeloma. They treated patients with adequate cardiac, pulmonary, and renal function with stem cells mobilized with granulocyte colony–stimulating factor. In this study, blood stem cells were mobilized with granulocyte colony–stimulating factor, collected and evaluated as described previously.[47] Dose-intensive melphalan was administered intravenously over 2 days and at 4 and 3 days before the infusion of stem cells. Stem cells were infused 72 hours later. Patients received antibody prophylaxis with an oral quinolone and acyclovir beginning on day 3 after stem cell infusion. Hematopoietic activity was determined by daily blood counts and defined as days from stem cell infusion to recovery of neutrophils. Overall recovery and survival by category or organ involvement is shown in Figure 53–15. The patients were treated with dose-intensive intravenous melphalan (200 mg/m^2). These authors enrolled 25 patients (median age 48 years, range 29–60 years), all of whom had biopsy-proven amyloidosis with clonal plasma cell disorders. Twenty-two patients (88 percent) were Southwest Oncology Group performance status 1 or 2 within a year of diagnosis and 16 (64 percent) had received no prior therapy. Amyloid-related organ involvement included cardiac (n = 8), renal (n = 7), hepatic (n = 6), neuropathic (n = 3), and lymphatic (n = 1). Fifteen patients had one or two organ systems involved, and 10 had three or more organ systems with amyloid deposition and dysfunction. With a median follow-up of 24 months and a range of 12 to 38 months, 17 of 25 patients (68 percent) were alive, and the median survival had not yet been reached. Thirteen of 21 patients (62 percent) evaluated 3 months post-transplant had complete response of their clonal plasma cell disorders. Two thirds of the surviving patients had experienced improvement in amyloid-related organ involvement in all systems, and 4 of 17 had stable disease. The improvement in the median performance status of the 17 survivors at follow-up was statistically significant versus baseline. Among these patients, the negative prognostic factors for overall survival included amyloid involvement of more than two major organ systems and predominantly cardiac involvement. Three patients had relapses of the clonal plasma cell disorders at 12 and 24 months. These findings suggest that dose-intensive therapy should be considered as a treatment for patients with light chain amyloidosis who meet functional criteria for autologous transplantation of their stem cells.

HEMOCHROMATOSIS

Pathophysiology

Hemochromatosis is associated with excessive deposition of iron in the heart and other organs, including the liver, pancreas, and skin. It occurs as either a familial or an idiopathic disorder. However, it is also found in association with defects in hemoglobin synthesis, with chronic liver disease, and with excessive oral or parenteral intake of iron over many years. The severity of myocardial dysfunction varies widely in patients with hemochromatosis, but it is associated with diastolic dysfunction and RCM, although some patients also have evidence of important systolic dysfunction.

Myocardial iron deposits are found within the sarcoplasmic reticulum and are primarily located in the subepicardial region. They are also present in the subendocardial region and are least common in the midmyocardium. The iron deposition is usually more prominent in ventricular than atrial myocardium, and it may involve the cardiac conduc-

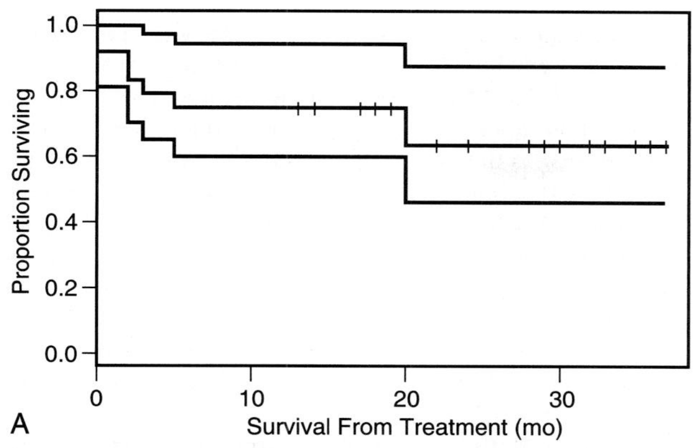

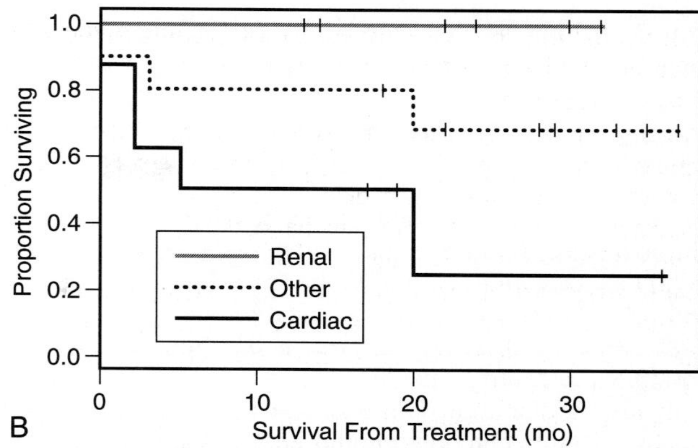

FIGURE 53–15 Overall survival and survival by category or organ involvement. With median follow-up of 24 months (12 to 38), 17 of 25 patients (68 percent) survived, and the median survival has not yet been reached as depicted in **(A),** a Kaplan-Meier plot showing the 95 percent confidence interval (proportional survival 0.65, 95 percent CI 0.48 to 0.88). **B,** Survival by predominant organ involvement. Total and mean times of follow-up for the three cohorts are 149 and 21.3 months (renal, n = 7), 225 and 22.5 months (other, n = 10), and 101 and 12.6 months (cardiac, n = 8). Patients without predominant cardiac involvement had better overall survival than cardiac patients (one-tailed Fisher's exact test, $P < .05$). (**A** and **B,** From Comenzo RL, Vosburgh E, Falk RH, et al: Dose-intensive melphalan with blood stem-cell support for the treatment of AL [amyloid light-chain] amyloidosis: survival and responses in 25 patients. Blood 91:3662–3670, 1998. Copyright 1998 American Society of Hematology.)

tion system. Patients with cardiac deposition of excessive iron usually have heart failure. Patients who receive more than 100 blood transfusions without associated iron loss with bleeding are at risk for the development of cardiac hemochromatosis.

Clinical Recognition

Some patients demonstrate the classic clinical signs of "bronze diabetes," including a grayish discoloration of the skin, the development of carbohydrate intolerance, the development of liver disease with prominent liver function abnormalities progressing to cirrhosis, and heart failure. However, in individual patients, one or more of the organ dysfunctions may be more prominent, and in some patients, only heart failure is evident initially. One makes a diagnosis of hemochromatosis by finding elevated plasma iron levels in the range of 180 to 300 mg/dl and markedly elevated values for saturation of transferrin (the iron-binding protein) to 80 to 100 percent (normal, 22 to 46 percent). Urine iron concentrations are often elevated and in the range of 9 to 23 mg/24-h samples, with the normal values being 2 mg or less. Liver iron concentrations are also increased into the range of 600 to 1800 g/100 mg dry weight, with normal values being 30 to 140 g/100 mg dry weight.

Hemochromatosis is a disease of men and of postmenopausal women because the woman who is menstruating has an obligate source of iron loss. However, women who have ceased menstruation or who have never menstruated are also at risk for the disease.

The diagnosis is usually made through a biopsy of the skin, liver, or heart, and the demonstration of excessive iron content is made through direct measurement and the use of the Prussian blue stain, which demonstrates the massive iron overload.

Radiography

As is true of other forms of restrictive heart muscle disease, hemochromatosis should be suspected when there is clinical evidence of heart failure with a small or normal-sized heart in a man or in a woman who is not menstruating and who may also have carbohydrate intolerance, liver function abnormalities, or a change in skin color.

Electrocardiography

Low voltage on the electrocardiogram is found in patients with restrictive cardiac muscle diseases based on infiltrative cardiomyopathies, including hemochromatosis. Low voltage is defined as less than 5 mm of voltage in the frontal QRS leads (i.e., leads I–aVF). There are many other causes of low voltage on the electrocardiogram, including obesity, emphysema, hypothyroidism, extensive coronary artery disease, and pericardial or pleural effusions, but RCM should always be considered.

Echocardiography

As is true for other RCMs, one expects to find evidence of diastolic dysfunction as reflected in delayed LV filling and diastolic relaxation of the left or right ventricle, or both. The ventricles may be hypertrophied, and regional areas of hypokinesis may be found in the patient with prominent systolic dysfunction.

Angiocardiography

Typically, one may find elevated LV and LA filling pressures in association with small or normal end-diastolic volumes. In the patient with systolic dysfunction as well, the ejection fraction will be reduced, segmental or global hypokinesis will be found, and the end-systolic volume may be elevated.

Endomyocardial Biopsy

The findings from the endomyocardial biopsy should be diagnostic and should demonstrate evidence of excessive iron deposition in the heart both through direct measurement and with Prussian blue staining.

Computed Tomography Scanning and Magnetic Resonance Imaging

Experience with these techniques in patients with hemochromatosis is limited to date. However, one would expect to find abnormalities similar to those found in other patients with RCMs. If tissue characterization becomes possible with either of these techniques in the future, it may be possible to identify specific abnormalities in the patient with myocardial iron overload that allow it to be distinguished. Both techniques should help in the differentiation of constrictive pericarditis from restrictive myocardial disease by demonstrating the absence of a thickened pericardium.

Radionuclide Studies

These are not of specific use in patients with cardiac hemochromatosis.

Treatment

When detected reasonably early, the myocardial physiologic abnormalities and some of the liver function abnormalities can be reversed with repeated phlebotomy, beginning on a once-weekly basis and progressing to once monthly after a period of several weeks to months. Clinical evidence of heart failure and severe abnormalities of liver function may disappear with the use of this therapy. The value of iron chelators, such as desferrioxamine, has also been suggested, and they represent the only alternative for the severely anemic patient who may have hemochromatosis or hemosiderosis on the basis of a very large number of blood transfusions as a therapy for chronic anemia. This compound has a high affinity for iron, it is administered parenterally, and most of the chelated iron is excreted in the urine within 4 hours of the injection. The addition of oral ascorbic acid increases iron excretion in association with the administration of an iron chelator. However, the administration of ascorbic acid not only makes more cellular iron available for chelation but also liberates free intracellular iron, which may cause the generation of free oxygen radicals and lead to myocardial damage. Therefore, one has to worry about induction of myocardial injury by the simultaneous administration of an iron chelator and ascorbic acid. Perhaps, this can be avoided by the administration of ascorbate after the patient has been started on chelation therapy. The patient with myocardial hemochromatosis may develop heart failure, conduction disturbances, and life-threatening or fatal arrhythmias.

Radiation-Induced Heart Disease

Pathophysiology

Ionizing radiation as administered during radiotherapy may lead to myocardial fibrosis and restrictive myocardial disease. It may also cause pericardial injury with pericardial effusion, tamponade, or constriction. The coronary arteries and myocardial valves may also be injured by excessive radiation, leading to coronary artery fibrosis and valvular abnormalities. Patients receiving radiotherapy to the mediastinum as part of the treatment for lung cancer, lymphoma, or other mediastinal neoplasm are at particular risk, especially when more than 1800 rads is delivered in the region of the heart.

Radiation damage may also occur in small microvessels, which leads to capillary rupture and microthrombi. This may cause myocardial ischemia and lead to additional myocardial fibrosis.

Myocardial, coronary artery, and valvular heart damage occur less commonly after radiation than damage to the pericardium. With radiation therapy, some patients complain of symptoms of acute pericarditis. Transient and asymptomatic depression of LV function may be found early after radiation therapy. The development of myocardial fibrosis, injury to coronary arteries or heart valves, and the development of constrictive pericarditis may become clinically apparent months or years after the initial exposure.

Clinical Recognition

One should be aware of the risks of pericardial, myocardial, coronary artery, and valvular heart damage in patients who receive radiotherapy or other forms of ionizing radiation in the heart region in the amounts mentioned. Every effort should be made to protect the heart when radiotherapy is used to treat a mediastinal neoplasm. Clinical recognition follows the understanding of the pathophysiology of the injury produced, and the acute or more chronic development of heart enlargement, pericardial effusion, evidence of restrictive myocardial or pericardial disease, angina, or new heart murmurs provides evidence for an injurious effect of irradiation.

Imaging Studies

These studies are useful in patients with radiation-induced myocardial injury by demonstrating the presence of diastolic dysfunction associated with myocardial fibrosis, valvular regurgitation or obstruction, a pericardial effusion, or constrictive pericarditis.

Endomyocardial Biopsy

In the months to years after the administration of ionizing radiation, a demonstration of myocardial fibrosis for patients receiving mediastinal radiation in the range of 1800 to 2000 rads or more could provide evidence of a radiation-induced myocardial abnormality.

Differential Diagnosis

For the restrictive myocardial diseases, it is the other RCMs, including amyloidosis, hemochromatosis, endomyocardial fibroelastosis, and the heart failure associated with each of these abnormalities, that must be considered.

Treatment

The best treatment is to do everything possible to prevent radiation-induced injury to the heart by limiting the amount of radiation the heart receives.

References

1. Shabetai R: Pathophysiology and differential diagnosis of restrictive cardiomyopathy. Cardiovasc Clin 19:123, 1988.
2. Child JS, Perloff JK: The restrictive cardiomyopathies. Cardiol Clin 6:289, 1988.
3. Schoenfeld MH, Supple EW, Dec DW, et al: Restrictive cardiomyopathy versus constrictive pericarditis: role of endomyocardial biopsy in avoiding unnecessary thoracotomy. Circulation 75:1012, 1987.
4. Gertz MA, Kyle RA: Primary systemic amyloidosis—a diagnostic primer. Mayo Clin Proc 64:1505, 1989.
5. Olson LJ, Gertz MA, Edwards WD, et al: Senile cardiac amyloidosis with myocardial dysfunction: diagnosis by endomyocardial biopsy and immunohistochemistry. N Engl J Med 317:738, 1987.
6. Plehn JF, Friedman BJ: Diastolic dysfunction in amyloid heart disease: restrictive cardiomyopathy or not? J Am Coll Cardiol 13:54, 1989.
7. Falk RH, Plehn JF, Deering T, et al: Sensitivity and specificity of the echocardiographic features of cardiac amyloidosis. Am J Cardiol 59:418, 1987.
8. Cueto-Garcia L, Reeder GS, Kyle RH, et al: Echocardiographic findings in systemic amyloidosis: spectrum of cardiac involvement and relation to survival. J Am Coll Cardiol 6:737, 1985.
9. Klein AL, Hatle LK, Burstow DJ, et al: Doppler characterization of left ventricular diastolic function in cardiac amyloidosis. J Am Coll Cardiol 13:1017, 1989.
10. Hongo M, Hirayama J, Fujii T, et al: Early identification of amyloid heart disease by technetium-99m-pyrophosphate scintigraphy: a study of familial amyloid polyneuropathy. Am Heart J 113:654, 1987.
11. Arnold M, McGuire L, Lee JC: Loeffler's fibroplastic endocarditis. Pathology 20:79, 1988.
12. Tai PC, Ackerman SJ, Spry CJ, et al: Deposits of eosinophil granule proteins in cardiac tissues of patients with eosinophilic endomyocardial disease. Lancet 21:643, 1987.
13. Lengyel M, Arvay A, Palik I: Massive endocardial calcification associated with endomyocardial fibrosis. Am J Cardiol 56:815, 1985.
14. Gupta PN, Valiathan MS, Balakrishnan KG, et al: Clinical course of endomyocardial fibrosis. Br Heart J 62:450, 1989.
15. Olsen EGJ, Spry CJF: Relation between eosinophilia and endomyocardial disease. Prog Cardiovasc Dis 27:241, 1985.
16. Dabestani A, Child JS, Henze E, et al: Primary hemochromatosis: anatomic and physiologic characteristics of the cardiac ventricles and their response to phlebotomy. Am J Cardiol 54:153, 1984.
17. Powell LW, Isselbacher KJ: Hemochromatosis. *In* Wilson JD (ed): Harrison's Principles of Internal Medicine. p. 1825. New York: McGraw-Hill, 1990.
18. Olson LJ, Edwards WD, McCall JT, et al: Cardiac iron deposition in idiopathic hemochromatosis: histologic and analytic assessment of 14 hearts from autopsy. J Am Coll Cardiol 10:1239, 1987.
19. Rahko PS, Salerni R, Uretsky BF: Successful reversal by chelation therapy of congestive cardiomyopathy due to iron overload. J Am Coll Cardiol 8:436, 1986.
20. Goodwin JF: Cardiomyopathies and specific heart muscle disease: definition, terminology and classification. *In* Goodwin JF (ed): Heart Muscle Disease. pp. 1–5. Lancaster, England: MTP, 1985.
21. Restrictive cardiomyopathy. *In* Goodwin JF, Olsen EGJ (eds): Cardiomyopathies: Realisations and Expectations. Berlin: Springer-Verlag, 1992.
22. Wilmshurst PT, Katritsis D: Restrictive cardiomyopathy [editorial]. Br Heart J 63:323, 1990.
23. Katritsis D, Wilmshurst PT, Wendon JA, et al: Primary restrictive cardiomyopathy: clinical and pathological characteristics. J Am Coll Cardiol 18:1230, 1991.
24. Report of WHO Expert Committee: Cardiomyopathies. Technical Report Series No. 697. Geneva: WHO, 1984.
25. James TN, Kamb ML, Sandberg GA, et al: Postmortem studies of the heart in three fatal cases of the eosinophilia-myalgia syndrome. Ann Intern Med 115:102, 1991.
26. Olsen EGJ, Spry CJF: The pathogenesis of Loeffler's endomyocardial disease and its relationship to endomyocardial fibrosis. *In* Yu PN, Goodwin JF (eds): Progress in Cardiology. Vol. 8. pp. 281–303. Philadelphia: Lea & Febiger, 1979.
27. Report of the WHO/ISFC Task Force on the Definition and Classification of Cardiomyopathies. Br Heart J 44:672, 1980.
28. Chusid MJ, Dale DC, West BC, et al: The hypereosinophilic syndrome: analysis of 14 cases with review of the literature. Medicine (Baltimore) 54:1, 1975.
29. Spry CJF, Davies J, Tai PC, et al: Clinical features of 15 patients with the hypereosinophilic syndrome. Q J Med 52:1, 1983.
30. Davies J, Spry CJF, Sapsford R, et al: Cardiovascular features of 11 patients with eosinophilic endomyocardial disease. Q J Med 52:23, 1983.
31. Olsen EGJ: Morphological overview and pathogenetic mechanisms in endomyocardial fibrosis associated with eosinophilia. *In* Olsen EGJ, Sekiguchi M (eds): Cardiomyopathy Update 3. Restrictive Cardiomyopathy and Arrhythmias. pp. 1–7. Tokyo: University of Tokyo Press, 1990.
32. Tai P-C, Spry CJF: Eosinophil effector mechanism: studies in the ways in which eosinophils induce endomyocardial fibrosis. *In* Olsen EGJ, Sekiguchi M (eds): Cardiomyopathy Update 3. Restrictive Cardiomyopathy and Arrhythmias. pp. 99–107. Tokyo: University of Tokyo Press, 1990.
33. Nair DV: Endomyocardial fibrosis in Kerala state. Indian Heart J Teaching Series 6:249, 1980.
34. Vijayarghavan G, Davies J, Sadanandan S, et al: Echocardiographic features of tropical endomyocardial disease in South India. Br Heart J 50:450, 1983.
35. Davies J: Restrictive cardiomyopathy. *In* Goodwin JF (eds): Heart Muscle Disease. pp. 87–94. Lancaster, England: MTP, 1985.
36. Andy JJ: The relationship of microfilaria and other helminthic worms to tropical endomyocardial fibrosis (EMF): a review. *In* Olsen EGJ, Sekiguchi M (eds): Cardiomyopathy Update. No. 3. Restrictive Cardiomyopathy. Tokyo: University of Tokyo Press, 1990.
37. Acquatella H: Doppler-echocardiographic investigations in restrictive cardiomyopathy. *In* Goodwin JF, Olsen EGJ (eds): Cardiomyopathies: Realisations and Expectations. Berlin: Springer-Verlag, 1992.
38. Oakley CM: Amyloid heart disease. *In* Symons C, Evans T, Mitchell AG (eds): Specific Heart Muscle Disease. pp. 13–23. Bristol, England: PSG Wright, 1983.
39. Roberts WC, Waller BF: Cardiac amyloidosis causing cardiac dysfunction: analysis of 54 autopsy patients. Am J Cardiol 52:137, 1983.
40. Chew C, Ziady GM, Rafael MJ, et al: The functional defect in amyloid heart disease. Am J Cardiol 36:438, 1975.
41. Oakley CM: Amyloid heart disease. *In* Goodwin JF (ed): Heart Muscle Disease. pp. 141–153. Lancaster, England: MTP, 1985.
42. Sekiya T, Foster CJ, Isherwood I, et al: Computerized tomographic appearances of cardiac amyloidosis. Br Heart J 51:519, 1984.
43. Wynne J, Braunwald E: The cardiomyopathies and myocarditides. *In* Braunwald E (ed): Heart Disease. pp. 1431–1434. Philadelphia: WB Saunders, 1988.
44. Falk RH, Lee VW, Rubinow A, et al: Sensitivity of technetium 99m pyrophosphate scintigraphy in diagnosis of cardiac amyloidosis. Am J Cardiol 51:826, 1983.
45. Griffiths BE, Hughes P, Dowdle R, et al: Cardiac amyloidosis with asymmetrical septal hypertrophy and deterioration after nifedipine. Thorax 37:177, 1982.
46. Comenzo RL, Vosburgh E, Falk RH, et al: Dose-intensive melphalan with blood stem-cell support for the treatment of AL (amyloid light-chain) amyloidosis: survival and responses in 25 patients. Blood 91:3662–3670, 1998.
47. Comenzo RL, Vosburgh E, Weintraub LR, et al: Collection of mobilized blood progenitor cells of hematopoietic rescue by large-volume leukapheresis. Transfusion 35:493, 1995.

CHAPTER 54

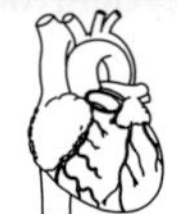

OTHER CARDIOMYOPATHIES

James T. Willerson

WHIPPLE'S DISEASE
FABRY'S DISEASE
GAUCHER'S DISEASE
METABOLIC ABNORMALITIES AND MYOCARDIAL DISEASE
Thiamine Deficiency
Carnitine Deficiency
Selenium/Taurine Deficiency
Starvation
Electrolyte Abnormalities
ALLERGIC AND HYPERSENSITIVITY MYOCARDIAL INJURY
Wasp Stings and Spider Bites
Snake Bites
Drugs
Giant Cell Myocarditis
OTHER CAUSES OF HEART MUSCLE INJURY
Carcinoid Heart Disease
Hyperthermia
Hypothermia

WHIPPLE'S DISEASE

Whipple's disease, intestinal lipodystrophy, is sometimes associated with an infiltrative myocarditis, with periodic acid–Schiff–positive macrophages in the myocardium, pericardium, and heart valves.[1–4] Some patients with this abnormality develop vasculitis and myocarditis. Valvular involvement may be of sufficient severity to cause aortic and mitral valve lesions, including aortic regurgitation and mitral stenosis. Overt clinical evidence of pericarditis and of congestive heart failure (CHF) develops in some patients. Electron microscopy has demonstrated the same rod-shaped structures in the myocardium as are found in the small intestine. Antibiotic treatment with parenteral penicillin and streptomycin followed by 1 year of trimethoprim/sulfamethoxazole or oral trimethoprim/sulfamethoxazole alone for 1 year appears to be effective in treating disease in some individuals, but relapses are frequent.

FABRY'S DISEASE

Fabry's disease is an X-linked disorder of glycosphingolipid metabolism resulting from a deficiency in the enzyme ceramide trihexosidase.[5–9] With this enzyme deficiency, there is an intracellular accumulation of a neutral glycolipid, with prominent involvement of the skin and kidneys as well as the myocardium. There may be widespread involvement of the myocardium, conducting tissues, valves, and vascular endothelium, especially the mitral valve. Involvement of small vessels may result in their occlusion. Accumulation of the glycolipid in the lysosomes of cardiac tissues is associated with CHF. Symptomatic cardiovascular involvement occurs in most affected males, whereas female carriers are usually asymptomatic or only minimally symptomatic. Patients with this disease have increased left ventricular (LV) wall thickness as a result of the glycolipid deposition, which may simulate hypertrophic cardiomyopathy. Some of these patients have mitral valve prolapse. Differentiation from other restrictive or hypertrophic processes can be accomplished by endomyocardial biopsy. A low alpha-galactosidase activity in leukocytes enables the correct diagnosis to be made biochemically. Recent studies suggest that magnetic resonance imaging may also provide a means to differentiate Fabry's disease from other restrictive cardiomyopathies.

GAUCHER'S DISEASE

Gaucher's disease is an inherited disorder of glycoceramide metabolism caused by a deficiency of the enzyme beta-glucosidase, resulting in the accumulation of cerebrosides in the myocardium, liver, spleen, bone marrow, lymph nodes, and brain. Interstitial infiltration of the left ventricle by cells laden with cerebroside develops, causing reduced LV compliance and cardiac output. LV dysfunction and hemorrhage, and pericardial effusion occurring in association with increases in LV wall mass and calcification of the left heart valves, have been described. This disease, usually diagnosed in childhood, may lead to early death.[10–12]

METABOLIC ABNORMALITIES AND MYOCARDIAL DISEASE

Thiamine Deficiency

Thiamine deficiency persisting for at least 3 months leads to a disorder known as *beri-beri heart disease*.[13–17] This abnormality is most common in the Far East, but it can be found anywhere in the world where individuals drink heavily and eat poorly, as well as in areas where the general diet consists predominantly of polished rice, which is deficient in thiamine. The presence of thiamine in the flour used to make white bread has diminished the incidence of this disease in the United States and Western Europe, except in alcoholics and those who consume unusual diets especially high in carbohydrates. In individuals who consume high-carbohydrate diets, including those who drink large quantities of beer and eat foods with a high carbohydrate content, there is an increased demand for thiamine and they may become thiamine deficient (Table 54–1).

Beri-beri occurs in "wet" and "dry" forms. In the Far East, patients often present with edema, fatigue, high-output heart failure associated with reductions in systemic resistance, and increased venous return to the heart. Treatment with thiamine reduces cardiac output, heart rate, and stroke volume and increases peripheral vascular resistance.

Dry beri-beri is found more commonly in patients in Western countries who also have a high-output state, appear malnourished, and may have peripheral neuropathy with sensory and motor defects, paresthesias, painful glossitis, anemia of iron or folate deficiency, and hyperkeratinized skin lesions.

Beri-beri heart disease is initially characterized by a high-output state with bounding peripheral pulses, increased cardiac output and stroke volume, biventricular failure, sinus tachycardia, and edema in its wet form. In the late stages of heart failure, the high-output state may convert to a low-output state with peripheral vasoconstriction. Third heart sounds and apical holosystolic murmurs of mitral insufficiency and tricuspid insufficiency are often found.

Electrocardiographic alterations consist of sinus tachycardia, low voltage of the QRS complex, prolongation of the QT interval, and inversion of T waves. Imaging procedures demonstrate generalized cardiomegaly, pulmonary vascular congestion, and pleural effusions. In the early stages of beri-beri heart disease, one expects increased cardiac output and cardiac index and LV ejection fraction, but in the later stages, especially in alcoholics, severely reduced ejection fraction may be found by the various imaging modalities used to make these measurements.

The diagnosis of thiamine deficiency can be made by demonstrating increased serum pyruvate and lactate levels in association with a reduced red blood cell transketolase level. Thiamine concentrations are low in biologic fluids. Postmortem examination in patients who succumb demonstrates dilatation of the heart, with edema and otherwise nonspecific changes.

CHF in individuals with beri-beri may develop abruptly, with patients dying in the first few days. A particular type of beri-beri in the Far East and Africa, known as *Shoshin beri-beri,* is usually a fulminating and rapidly progressive form of the disease, with profound hypotension, tachycardia, and lactic acidosis leading to death.

The therapy of beri-beri heart disease depends on the early administration of thiamine and, in the alcoholic, absolute abstinence from alcohol. Diets high in carbohydrates and low in thiamine should be corrected. Patients with beri-beri heart disease usually fail to respond well to diuretics and digitalis alone, but they improve once thiamine administration has begun, usually as 100 mg IV acutely, followed by 25 mg/da orally for at least 1 to 2 weeks.

TABLE 54-1 Metabolic/Nutritional Causes of Cardiomyopathy

Thiamine deficiency	Selenium deficiency
Pellagra	Starvation
Scurvy	Obesity
Carnitine deficiency	

Carnitine Deficiency

Carnitine is an essential cofactor for the oxidation of fatty acids. Deficiencies of carnitine result in a dilated cardiomyopathy or, sometimes, hypertrophic cardiomyopathy in children. Therefore, determination of serum carnitine levels is important in children with unexplained heart failure and cardiomyopathy. Carnitine supplementation may lead to symptomatic and functional improvement in children for whom this is the etiology of heart failure.[18, 19]

Selenium/Taurine Deficiency

Dietary deficiency of selenium or possibly taurine may result in a dilated cardiomyopathy.[20–22] It is usually found in rural areas in China. It affects primarily children and young women, and selenium deficiency can be prevented by the prophylactic administration of sodium selenite tablets. Relative selenium deficiency has also been described in populations subjected to prolonged parenteral hyperalimentation.[21, 22]

Starvation

Extreme malnutrition has been associated with development of a dilated cardiomyopathy and chronic CHF.[18–21] Severe malnutrition has been called *kwashiorkor* and is caused primarily by protein calorie deficiency. *Marasmus* is another malnutrition state that may occur in infants weaned early and in those individuals who follow fad diets deficient in calories, proteins, and other essential nutrients. Cardiac output and systemic blood pressure are usually low in these individuals, and there may be marked and generalized edema. Atrophy of the heart and reductions in ventricular function have been found. The severe electrolyte abnormalities associated with these malnutrition states may alter the PR-QRS-QT segments of the electrocardiogram in various ways, depending on the dominant electrolyte abnormality. The electrolyte abnormalities and malnutrition may be associated with atrial and ventricular arrhythmias, heart block, and sudden death. Plasma albumin and amino acid levels are generally low, as are serum concentrations of sodium, magnesium, phosphorus, and glucose. Hypocalcemia, hypomagnesemia, and hypokalemia increase the QT interval on the electrocardiogram and may contribute to reduced cardiac function and the risk of arrhythmias. CHF may occur, and it may develop in the early refeeding phases.

Electrolyte Abnormalities

Hypocalcemia

Profound reductions in myocardial calcium concentration depress myocardial contractility, prolong the QT interval, and may lead to heart block or ventricular arrhythmias, including ventricular arrhythmias of the torsades de pointes type. These patients may have depressed contractile responses to catecholamines and to cardiac glycosides. Chronic CHF may occur, resolving only when serum calcium is restored to normal.

Profound hypocalcemia may develop under conditions of malabsorption, in association with hypoparathyroidism, with rapid transfusion of citrated blood, and with severe chronic renal failure.

Hypomagnesemia

In patients with hypomagnesemia, focal myocardial necrosis may occur, especially in those who are also toxic from digitalis administration. Supraventricular and ventricular arrhythmias often develop, including serious ventricular arrhythmias. These patients also have prolonged QT intervals on their electrocardiograms. Repletion of magnesium usually corrects these arrhythmias.

Hypophosphatemia

Reversible LV dysfunction is found in some patients with severe hypophosphatemia. Correction of the serum phosphate level usually restores normal LV function.

Allergic and Hypersensitivity Myocardial Injury

Insect bites and stings may cause hypotension, anaphylaxis, and occasionally, signs and symptoms that suggest acute myocardial infarction.[23–29] Scorpion venom is neurotoxic, and a sting usually elicits neurotoxicity, but fatal cardiac injury has been described, especially in children. The hearts of such individuals may demonstrate interstitial edema, mononuclear cell infiltrate, and necrosis of heart muscle fibers, particularly in the subendocardial regions. Some individuals abruptly develop hypotension and pulmonary edema, whereas others experience serious cardiac arrhythmias. Protection against these problems and their treatment includes the use of specific antivenins. When arrhythmias, tachycardia, diaphoresis, and increases in blood pressure develop, the use of adrenergic blocking agents may be useful.

Wasp Stings and Spider Bites

Wasp stings and spider bites may cause hypotension and anaphylaxis. Some patients develop chest pain and clinical findings suggestive of myocardial infarction.

Snake Bites

The venom of most snakes is primarily neurotoxic and injurious to vessels. However, transient electrocardiographic abnormalities have been noted after some snake bites, and death from profound hypotension and vascular thrombosis, including coronary artery thrombosis or vasospasm, has been described.

Drugs

Many drugs may elicit hypersensitivity responses, including hypersensitivity myocarditis in susceptible individuals. Included are antibiotics, diuretics, anticonvulsants, antituberculous drugs, antineoplastic agents, and vaccines.[30–37]

Among the antibiotics for which hypersensitivity myocarditis has been described, penicillin, tetracycline, sulfonamides, chloramphenicol, streptomycin, the sulfonamides, and amphotericin B deserve mention. Allergic reactions occur in susceptible patients with all of these agents and myocardial involvement may develop, including hypersensitivity vasculitis, interstitial infiltrates in the myocardium composed of eosinophils and mononuclear cells, granulomas, heart block, arrhythmias, myocardial necrosis, and circulatory collapse. Occasionally, a patient develops severe chest pain that proves to be due to either myocardial infarction or pericarditis as a consequence of the hypersensitivity reaction. Diuretics that have been associated with the development of hypersensitivity myocarditis include acetazolamide, hydrochlorothiazide, and spironolactone.

Anticonvulsants associated with hypersensitivity myocarditis include phenytoin, carbamazepine, and phenindione. The development of CHF has been reported after the use of anticonvulsants, especially phenindione, with a clinical picture similar to that of dilated cardiomyopathy.

Antituberculous drugs that have been associated with the development of a hypersensitivity myocarditis include isoniazid and aminosalicylic acid. Some patients treated with these agents have developed inflammatory myocarditis, arrhythmias, hypotension, and CHF.

Chemotherapeutic Agents

The antineoplastic agents associated with development of myocardial injury include cyclophosphamide, 5-fluorouracil, daunorubicin, and doxorubicin (Adriamycin). High doses of cyclophosphamide have been associated with hemorrhagic myocarditis. The myocardial damage is sometimes caused by injury to the endothelium with the development of thrombosis. This is a serious abnormality and is associated with death in approximately one fourth of the patients. Decreases in systolic function and reductions in QRS voltage usually occur with this abnormality. 5-Fluorouracil administration has been associated with the development of an inflammatory infiltrate in the subendocardium, edema, and arrhythmias. Doxorubicin causes a dose-related injury to the heart that leads to a dilated cardiomyopathy. Doses of 450 mg/m^2 or larger of doxorubicin often lead to a decline in LV ejection fraction, an increase in LV end-systolic and end-diastolic volumes, and the development of severe CHF. Clinically manifest CHF has been observed from 0 to 231 days after the last dose of doxorubicin, with a mean duration of 33 days. The prognosis with the development of CHF is poor. The lowest risk of CHF occurs in patients on a weekly schedule of drug administration. The risk of developing CHF is increased in older individuals and in patients who have previously received mediastinal radiotherapy or additional cyclophosphamide therapy. One should monitor LV ejection fraction before and during doxorubicin therapy and discontinue the medication when the LV ejection fraction declines to values of 45 to 50 percent. If that is done, the LV ejection fraction often improves, allowing one to very carefully give additional doses of doxorubicin, if necessary.

Certain antihypertensive agents have also been associated with development of a hypersensitivity myocarditis, including methyldopa. Patients who develop hypersensitivity myocarditis usually have an inflammatory infiltrate consisting of eosinophils and mononuclear cells, a vasculitis, and focal myocardial necrosis. Arrhythmias and heart block may also develop, and sudden death has been described.

Giant Cell Myocarditis

Giant cell myocarditis is characterized by multinucleated giant cells in the myocardium. Its etiology is not yet elucidated, but it is likely to be of hypersensitivity or autoimmune origin.[33–35] Multinucleated giant cells are found in the myocardium, especially at the margins of myocardial necrosis, coexisting with an inflammatory infiltrate composed of eosinophils and histiocytes. The clinical course is often rapid and fatal, and it leads to the development of cardiomegaly and fulminant heart failure. Young and middle-aged adults are affected most commonly. Fever is usually prominent, and arrhythmias, heart block, and bundle branch blocks also occur. Giant cell myocarditis has been associated with other systemic diseases, including systemic lupus erythematosus, thyrotoxicosis, and thymomas, but it also occurs in individuals with no other underlying disease.

Therapeutic efforts have been disappointing to date. Corticosteroids and immunosuppressive agents have been used but have not been uniformly successful.

Other Causes of Heart Muscle Injury

Carcinoid Heart Disease

Pathophysiology

Carcinoid tumors are found most commonly in the appendix, but some originate in the ileum, stomach, duodenum, or bronchus.[38, 39] Carcinoid tumors of the ileum are those most likely to metastasize, with involvement of the liver and regional lymph nodes. Carcinoid tumors that invade the liver are usually the ones that may also result in carcinoid heart disease. Release of large quantities of serotonin, bradykinin, and possibly other substances usually inactivated by the liver or lungs may lead to cardiac injury. The carcinoid syndrome is characterized by wheezing, spontaneous flushing, diarrhea, and endocardial plaques that are fibrotic in nature and involve the tricuspid and pulmonary valves. Clinically severe right ventricular involvement, including tricuspid regurgitation and sometimes stenosis and pulmonic valvular stenosis and/or insufficiency, may occur, leading to CHF.[40–43] Rarely, left-sided valvular heart disease develops, although one expects inactivation of the humoral substances released by this tumor in the lungs.

Clinical Recognition

Typical spells of intermittent flushing with bronchoconstriction and tachycardia associated with diarrhea suggest the presence of carcinoid tumors. The murmurs of tricuspid insufficiency or stenosis and/or pulmonic stenosis and/or insufficiency suggest cardiac involvement by the carcinoid tumor. When these valvular lesions are significant, the right ventricle and right atrium may enlarge, and important right ventricular failure may develop. The electrocardiogram may demonstrate evidence of right atrial and right ventricular enlargement, along with evidence of intraventricular conduction defects. Echocardiography may demonstrate tricuspid or pulmonic valve dysfunction.

Treatment

Patients with important CHF are treated with diuretics and digitalis. Surgical replacement of the tricuspid or pulmonic valve or valvuloplasty may be beneficial in some patients. Flushing, wheezing, and diarrhea can be treated with antiserotonin agents, including receptor antagonists, or with alpha-adrenergic blockers.

Hyperthermia

Hyperthermia or "heat stroke" results from exposure to relatively high temperatures, such as may be associated with profound exercise under hot, humid conditions without adequate rehydration and rest.[44–48] This condition is a serious concern for young athletes, especially football players, exercising for long periods of time in heat and high humidity. The hyperthermic patient reacts as though there has been damage to a thermoregulatory center and exhibits other manifestations of central nervous system injury, including coma and seizures. Cardiovascular abnormalities, especially pulmonary edema, hypotension, dilatation of the right side of the heart, and right ventricular dysfunction are found in some of these patients. Subendocardial hemorrhages are present at autopsy. Sinus tachycardia is usually present, and conduction abnormalities, including prolongation of the QT interval, may be found. Evidence of rhabdomyolysis and myocardial injury, reflected by increases in the associated enzymes and substances released from injured heart and skeletal muscle cells, are often found. The best therapy for hyperthermia is its prevention by avoidance of excessively prolonged periods of exercise under hot, humid conditions without adequate rehydration.

Hypothermia

Profound hypothermia causes a slowing of all cardiac pacemakers and the development of a sinus bradycardia, ectopic nodal and ventricular arrhythmias, advanced heart block, and ultimately, asystole or ventricular fibrillation.[49–53] Profoundly low ambient temperatures for prolonged periods

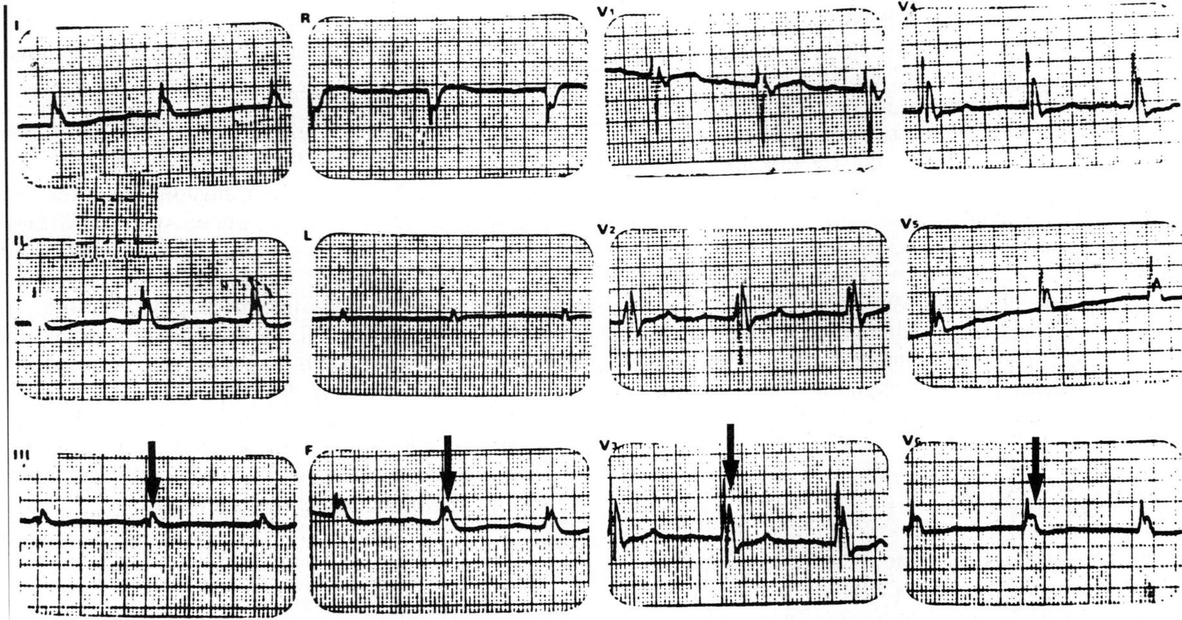

FIGURE 54–1 The positive deflection immediately following the R wave associated with severe hypothermia and known as an *Osborne wave* is marked by *arrows*. (From Solomon A, Barish RA, Browne B, Tso E: The electrocardiographic features of hypothermia. J Emerg Med 7:169, 1989.)

of time may also lead to myocardial damage, with subendocardial hemorrhage and microinfarcts associated with circulatory collapse, hemoconcentration, and reduced myocardial blood flow. In the patient with profound hypothermia, a characteristic deflection of the terminal portion of the QRS pattern, known as an *Osborne wave,* may be found (Fig. 54–1).

REFERENCES

1. Feldman M: Whipple's disease. Am J Med Sci 291:56, 1986.
2. Sossai P, DeBoni M, Cielo R: The heart and Whipple's disease [letter]. Int J Cardiol 23:275, 1989.
3. Southern JF, Moscicki RA, Magro C, et al: Lymphedema, lymphocytic myocarditis, and sarcoid-like granulomatosis. Manifestations of Whipple's disease. JAMA 261:1467, 1989.
4. Keinath RD, Merrell DE, Vlietstra R, Dobbins WO III: Antibiotic treatment and relapse in Whipple's disease. Long-term follow-up of 88 patients. Gastroenterology 88:1867, 1985.
5. Sakurabab H, Yanagawa Y, Igarashi T, et al: Cardiovascular manifestations in Fabry's disease. Clin Genet 29:276, 1986.
6. Tanaka H, Adachi K, Yamashita Y, et al: Four cases of Fabry's disease mimicking hypertrophic cardiomyopathy. J Cardiol 18:705, 1988.
7. Kramer W, Thormann J, Mueller K, Frenzel H: Progressive cardiac involvement by Fabry's disease despite successful renal allotransplantation. Int J Cardiol 7:72, 1985.
8. Goldman ME, Cantor R, Schwartz MF, et al: Echocardiographic abnormalities and disease severity in Fabry's disease. J Am Coll Cardiol 7:1157, 1986.
9. Matsui S, Murakami E, Takekoshi N, et al: Myocardial tissue characterization by magnetic resonance imaging in Fabry's disease. Am Heart J 117:472, 1989.
10. Laks Y, Passwell J: The varied clinical and laboratory manifestations of type II Gaucher's disease. Acta Paediatr Scand 76:378, 1987.
11. Wilson ER, Barton NW, Barranger JH: Vascular involvement in type 3 neuromyopathic Gaucher's disease. Arch Pathol Lab Med 109:82, 1985.
12. Platzker Y, Pisman EZ, Pines A, Kellermann J: Unusual echocardiographic pattern in Gaucher's disease. Cardiology 72:144, 1985.
13. Burwell CS, Dexter L: Beriberi heart disease. Trans Assoc Am Physicians 60:59, 1947.
14. Carson P: Alcoholic cardiac beriberi. BMJ 284:1817, 1982.
15. Akbarian M, Yankopoulos NA, Abelmann WH: Hemodynamic studies in beriberi heart disease. Am J Med 41:197, 1966.
16. Akram H, Maslowski AH, Smith BL, Nichols MG: The haemodynamic, histopathological and hormonal features of alcoholic beriberi. Q J Med 50:359, 1981.
17. Akbarian M, Dreyfus PM: Blood trans-ketolase activity in beriberi heart disease. JAMA 203:23, 1968.
18. Ino T, Sherwood WG, Benson LN, et al: Cardiac manifestations in disorders of fat and carnitine metabolism in infancy. J Am Coll Cardiol 11:1301, 1988.
19. Bautista J, Rafel E, Martinez A, et al: Familial hypertrophic cardiomyopathy and muscle carnitine deficiency. Muscle Nerve 13;192, 1990.
20. Tenaglia A, Cody R: Evidence for a taurine-deficiency cardiomyopathy. Am J Cardiol 62:136, 1988.
21. Reeves WC, Marcuard SP, Willis SE, Movahed A: Reversible cardiomyopathy due to selenium deficiency. J Parenter Enter Nutr 13:663, 1989.
22. Yang G, Ge K, Chen J, Chen X: Selenium-related endemic disease and the daily selenium requirement of humans. World Rev Nutr Diet 55:98, 1988.
23. Kounis NG, Zavras GM, Soufras, GD, Kitrou MP: Hypersensitivity myocarditis. Ann Allergy 62:71, 1989.
24. Amitai Y, Mines Y, Aker M, Goitein K: Scorpion sting in children. A review of 51 cases. Clin Pediatr 24:136, 1985.
25. Jones E, Joy M: Acute myocardial infarction after a wasp sting. Br Heart J 59:506, 1988.
26. Santhanakrishnan BR, Gajalakshmi BS: Pathogenesis of cardiovascular complications in children following scorpion envenoming. Ann Trop Paediatr 6:117, 1986.
27. Tibballs J, Sutherland S, Kerr S: Studies on Australian snake venoms. Part 1: the haemodynamic effects of brown snake (*Pseudonaja*) species in the dog. Anaesth Intensive Care 17:466, 1989.
28. Brand A, Keren A, Kerem E, et al: Myocardial damage after a scorpion sting: long-term echocardiographic follow-up. Pediatr Cardiol 9:59, 1988.
29. Lee SY, Lee CY, Chen YM, Kochva E: Coronary vasospasm as the primary cause of death due to the venom of the burrowing asp, *Atractaspis engaddensis*. Toxicon 24:285, 1986.
30. Taliercio CP, Olney BA, Lie JT: Myocarditis related to drug hypersensitivity. Mayo Clin Proc 60:463, 1985.

31. Martin M, Diaz-Rubio E, Furio V, et al: Lethal cardiac toxicity after cisplatin and 5-fluorouracil chemotherapy. Report of a case with necropsy study. Am J Clin Oncol 12:229, 1989.
32. Kantrowitz NE, Bristow MR: Cardiotoxicity of antitumor agents. Prog Cardiovasc Dis 27:195, 1984.
33. Wilson MS, Barth RF, Baker PB, et al: Giant cell myocarditis. Am J Med 79:647, 1985.
34. McFalls EO, Hosenpud JD, McAnulty JH, et al: Granulomatous myocarditis. Diagnosis by endomyocardial biopsy and response to corticosteroids in two patients. Chest 89:509, 1986.
35. Davidoff R, Palacios I, Southern J, et al: Giant cell versus lymphocytic myocarditis: a comparison of their clinical features and long-term outcomes. Circulation 83:953, 1991.
36. Nariman S: Adverse reactions to drugs used in the treatment of tuberculosis. Adv Drug React Acute Poison Rev 7:207, 1988.
37. Rabson AB, Schoen FJ, Warhol MJ, et al: Giant cell myocarditis after mitral valve replacement: case report and studies of the nature of giant cells. Hum Pathol 15:585, 1984.
38. Ross EM, Roberts WC: The carcinoid syndrome: comparison of 21 necropsy subjects with carcinoid heart disease to 15 necropsy subjects without carcinoid heart disease. Am J Med 79:339, 1985.
39. Lundin L, Funa K, Hansson HE, et al: Histochemical and immunohistochemical morphology of carcinoid heart disease. Pathol Res Pract 187:73, 1991.
40. Tornebrandt K, Eskilsson J, Nobin H: Heart involvement in metastatic carcinoid disease. Clin Cardiol 9:13, 1986.
41. Lundin L, Norheim I, Landelius J, et al: Carcinoid heart disease: relationship of circulating vasoactive substances to ultrasound-detectable cardiac abnormalities. Circulation 77:264, 1988.
42. Lundin L, Landelius J, Andren B, Oberg K: Transesophageal echocardiography improves the value of cardiac ultrasound in patients with carcinoid heart disease. Br Heart J 64:190, 1990.
43. Lundin L, Hansson HE, Landelius J, Oberg K: Surgical treatment of carcinoid heart disease. J Thorac Cardiovasc Surg 100:552, 1990.
44. Zahger D, Moses A, Weiss AT: Evidence of prolonged myocardial dysfunction in heat stroke. Chest 95:1089, 1989.
45. Gronert GA: Malignant hyperthermia. Anesthesiology 53:395, 1980.
46. Penn AS: Myoglobin and myoglobinuria. Handb Clin Neurol 41:259, 1979.
47. Frank JR, Harcti Y, Butler IJ, et al: Central core disease and malignant hyperthermia syndrome. Ann Neurol 7:11, 1980.
48. Willner JH, Wood DS, Cerri L, Britt B: Increased myophosphorylase a in malignant hyperthermia. N Engl J Med 303:138, 1980.
49. Solomon A, Barish RA, Browne B, Tso E: The electrocardiographic features of hypothermia. J Emerg Med 7:169, 1989.
50. Marius P: Laboratory comparison of techniques rewarming hypothermia casualties. Aviat Space Environ Med 49:652, 1978.
51. Soung LS, Swank L, Ing TS, et al: Treatment of accidental hypothermia with peritoneal dialysis. J Can Med Assoc 117:1415, 1990.
52. Morrison JB, Conn ML, Hayward JS: Thermal increment provided by inhalation rewarming from hypothermia. J Appl Physiol Respirat Environ Exercise Physiol 46:1061, 1979.
53. Jessen K, Hagelsten JO: Peritoneal dialysis in the treatment of profound accidental hypothermia. Aviat Space Environ Med 49:426, 1978.

CHAPTER 55

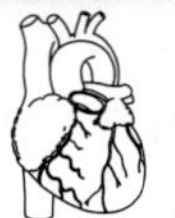

MYOCARDITIS

Sanjeev Trehan, Dale G. Renlund, and Jay W. Mason

ETIOLOGY AND EPIDEMIOLOGY
Bacterial Myocarditis
Other Causative Infectious Agents
Other Noninfectious Causes
PATHOPHYSIOLOGY OF VIRAL MYOCARDITIS
Animal Models
Role of Cellular Immunity
Role of Humoral Immunity
Role of Cytokines
Significance of Animal Models
CLINICAL FEATURES AND APPROACH TO DIAGNOSIS
Clinical Presentation
Physical Examination
Laboratory Findings
Electrocardiography, Echocardiography, and Cardiac Scintigraphy
Endomyocardial Biopsy and Cardiac Catheterization
Natural History of Myocarditis
TREATMENT
General Supportive Measures
Conventional Therapy
Immunosuppressive Therapy
Cardiac Transplantation
OTHER VARIANTS OF INFECTIOUS MYOCARDITIS
Human Immunodeficiency Virus and Myocarditis
Nonviral Infectious Myocarditis
NONINFECTIOUS MYOCARDITIS
Giant Cell Myocarditis
Eosinophilic Myocarditis
Cardiac Sarcoidosis
Peripartum Myocarditis/Cardiomyopathy

Although myocarditis was recognized over two centuries ago, accurate diagnosis and treatment are still elusive. As expressed by Senac in 1772: "The inflammation of the heart is difficult to diagnose and when we have diagnosed it, can we then treat it better?"[1] After Sobernheim in 1837[2] defined myocarditis as any inflammation or degeneration of the heart, the term *myocarditis* was used for nonvalvular myocardial diseases, including ischemic and hypertensive cardiomyopathies. Nearly a century later, White[3] suggested that the term *myocarditis* be restricted to "true inflammation of the myocardium." The last half century has seen the development of endomyocardial biopsy techniques and histologic criteria to diagnose myocarditis, and as our knowledge of the immunopathologic mechanisms evolves, it is hoped that therapeutic strategies may also develop.

The World Health Organization/International Society and Federation of Cardiology Task Force on Cardiomyopathies[4] classified cardiomyopathies whenever possible by etiologic/pathogenetic factors. This classification recognizes chronic viral, postinfectious autoimmune, and primary autoimmune forms of dilated cardiomyopathy (DCM). Although the classification states that "myocarditis is diagnosed by established histological, immunological and immunohistochemical criteria," only the Dallas criteria[5] provide consensus-derived guidance. Whereas the Dallas criteria require "an inflammatory infiltrate of the myocardium with necrosis and/or degeneration of adjacent myocytes not typical of ischemic damage associated with coronary artery disease" for diagnosis, additional immunologic and immunohistochemical criteria can be used productively. Myocarditis, irrespective of the etiopathologic factors, remains an inflammatory cardiomyopathy associated with cardiac dysfunction.

ETIOLOGY AND EPIDEMIOLOGY

A wide variety of infectious and noninfectious causes are associated with myocarditis (Tables 55–1 to 55–3). Several epidemiologic observations linking these agents with myocarditis have now been corroborated by application of serologic, polymerase chain reaction, or in situ hybridization methods. The incidence of infectious myocarditis in the general population is largely undetermined. In a prospective study[6] over several years, in a predefined subpopulation, an incidence of 0.02 percent was found. These cases were confirmed by myocardial enzyme leak and characteristic electrocardiographic (ECG) changes.[6] ECG

TABLE 55–1 **Common Etiologies of Myocarditis**

Infections	*Hypersensitivity Reactions to Drugs*
Adenovirus	Hydrochlorothiazide
Coxsackievirus	Methyldopa
Cytomegalovirus	Penicillins
Epstein-Barr virus	Sulfadiazine
Human immunodeficiency virus type 1	Sulfamethoxazole
Borrelia (Lyme disease)	*Systemic Diseases*
Toxoplasmosis	Crohn's disease
Drugs	Kawasaki's disease
Amphetamines	Sarcoidosis
Anthracyclines (especially doxorubicin [Adriamycin])	Systemic lupus erythematosus
Catecholamines	Ulcerative colitis
Cocaine	Cardiac rejection
Cyclophosphamide	Giant cell myocarditis
Interleukin-2	Peripartum myocarditis

TABLE 55-2 Uncommon Infectious Etiologies of Myocarditis

Viral

- Arbovirus (dengue fever, yellow fever)
- Arenavirus (Lassa fever)
- Coronavirus
- Echovirus
- Encephalomyocarditis virus
- Hepatitis B
- Herpesvirus
- Influenzavirus
- Junin virus
- Mumps virus
- Polio virus
- Rabies virus
- Respiratory syncytial virus
- Rubella virus
- Rubeola virus
- Vaccinia virus
- Varicella-zoster virus
- Variola virus

Bacterial

- *Brucella*
- *Campylobacter jejuni*
- *Chlamydia psittaci*
- *Chlamydia trachomatis*
- *Clostridia*
- *Corynebacterium diphtheriae*
- *Francisella tularensis*
- *Gonococcus*
- *Haemophilus*
- *Legionella*
- *Listeria*
- *Meningococcus*
- *Mycobacteria (tuberculosis, avium-intercellulare, leprae)*
- *Mycoplasma*
- *Pneumococcus*
- *Salmonella*
- *Staphylococcus*
- *Streptococcus*
- *Tropheryma whippelii* (Whipple's disease)

Fungal

- *Actinomyces*
- *Aspergillus*
- *Blastomyces*
- *Candida*
- *Coccidioides*
- *Cryptococcus*
- *Fusarium oxysporum*
- *Histoplasma*
- *Mucor*
- *Nocardia*
- *Sporothrix*

Rickettsial

- *Coxiella burnetti* (Q fever)
- *Rickettsia typhi* (typhus)
- *Rickettsia rickettsii* (Rocky Mountain spotted fever)
- *Rickettsia tsutsugamushi* (scrub typhus)

Spirochetal

- *Leptospira*
- *Treponema pallidum* (syphilis)

Helminthic

- *Cysticercus*
- *Echinococcus*
- *Schistosoma*
- *Toxocara* (visceral larva migrans)
- *Trichinella*

Protozoal

- *Entamoeba*
- *Leishmania*

abnormalities suggesting asymptomatic myocardial involvement, in the absence of enzyme release, have been noted in 1.2 percent of military transcripts during the course of other acute infectious diseases.[7] During an epidemic of influenza A, the incidence rose to 7.7 percent.[8] In a prospective trial of 2310 consecutive patients admitted to a large infectious disease hospital in Sweden, 8 percent showed ECG abnormalities suggestive of myocarditis.[9] The exact incidence of myocarditis is difficult to estimate, but approximately 5 percent of a virus-infected population may experience symptoms suggestive of cardiac involvement. The incidence of myocarditis associated with nonviral infections is even more difficult to estimate. Although the list of possible etiologic agents is large, the enteroviruses, specifically coxsackievirus B, are the most commonly identified etiologic agents of inflammatory cardiomyopathy; among healthy active adults, at least 50 percent have detectable serum antibodies indicating prior infection with coxsackievirus B.[10, 11] The World Health Organization has surveyed viral infections related to cardiovascular disease globally. In a 10-year period from 1975 to 1985, coxsackievirus B had the highest incidence of cardiovascular disease (34.6 cases per 1000 population), followed by influenza B (17.4 cases), influenza A (11.7 cases), coxsackievirus A (9.1 cases), and cytomegalovirus (CMV) (8.0 cases).[12]

The predominance of enteroviruses among myocarditis-associated agents has been substantiated by several laboratory and clinical studies.[13–15] Using serologic methods, Vikerfors and associates[13] reported that nearly 50 percent of consecutively studied myocarditis patients had enterovirus immunoglobulin (Ig) M. Frisk and coworkers[14] found a similar incidence of coxsackievirus B IgM antibodies by reverse radio immunoassay. Other agents such as adenoviruses, Epstein-Barr virus, *Mycoplasma,* and *Chlamydia* have also been associated with myocarditis. Martin and colleagues[15] demonstrated specific viral genome sequences in endomyocardial biopsies in 26 of 38 patients (68 percent) with acute myocarditis: adenovirus in 15 patients, enterovirus in 8, herpes simplex in 2, and CMV in 1 patient. The control group did not demonstrate any viral genome sequences. Others have refuted these findings and questioned the diagnostic value of enteroviral serologic and molecular genetic assays. Whereas there is a high incidence

TABLE 55-3 Uncommon Noninfectious Causes of Myocarditis

Drugs

Toxic Myocarditis

- Amphetamines
- Arsenic
- Chloroquine
- Emetine
- 5-Fluorouracil
- Interferon-alpha
- Lithium
- Paracetamol
- Thyroid hormone

Hypersensitivity Myocarditis

- Acetazolamide
- Allopurinol
- Amphotericin B
- Carbamazepine
- Cephalothin
- Chlorthalidone
- Colchicine
- Diclofenac
- Diphenhydramine
- Furosemide
- Indomethacin
- Isoniazid
- Lidocaine
- Methysergide
- Oxyphenbutazone
- Para-aminosalicyclic acid
- Phenindione
- Phenylbutazone
- Phenytoin
- Procainamide
- Pyribenzamine
- Ranitidine
- Reserpine
- Spironolactone
- Streptomycin
- Tetracycline
- Trimethoprim

Toxins

- Arsenic
- Carbon monoxide
- Copper
- Iron
- Lead
- Mercury
- Phosphorus
- Scorpion stings
- Snake venom
- Spider bites
- Wasp stings

Systemic Diseases

- Arteritis (giant cell, Takayasu's)
- Beta-thalassemia major
- Churg-Strauss vasculitis
- Cryoglobulinemia
- Dermatomyositis
- Diabetes mellitus
- Hashimoto's thyroiditis
- Mixed connective tissue disease
- Myasthenia gravis
- Periarteritis nodosa
- Pernicious anemia
- Pheochromocytoma
- Polymyositis
- Rheumatoid arthritis
- Scleroderma
- Sjögren's syndrome
- Thymoma
- Wegener's granulomatosis

Other

- Eosinophilic myocarditis
- Genetic
- Granulomatous myocarditis
- Head trauma
- Hypothermia
- Hyperpyrexia
- Ionizing radiation
- Mononuclear myocarditis

of IgM antibodies against enteroviruses in patients with myocarditis and DCM, the enteroviral genomic sequences are seldom isolated (6 to 15 percent) from myocardial tissue.[16, 17]

CMV is a recognized cause of acute infectious myocarditis, although it is rare in healthy individuals.[18, 19] Maisch and associates[19a] demonstrated, using in situ hybridization techniques, CMV-specific nucleotide sequences in 15 percent of patients with acute myopericarditis. Certainly in transplant recipients, CMV infection is fairly common and has been reported to affect the transplanted heart.[20, 21] Hepatitis C virus infection is frequently noted in patients with DCM,[22] and hepatitis C virus RNA has also been recovered from lymphocytes infiltrating the myocardium in chronic active myocarditis.[23]

Bacterial Myocarditis

Myocarditis is a well-recognized complication of *Corynebacterium diphtheriae* infection, although this is now rare in the Western world.[24] Myocardial dysfunction is also seen in association with *Salmonella* septicemia, although it is rarely clinically severe.[25, 26] Myocardial dysfunction is mostly related to the toxemia of the severe infection, which is also noted with meningococcal and nonrheumatic streptococcal infections.

Perhaps the best-recognized bacterial agent thought to be responsible for myocarditis is the beta-hemolytic streptococcus that produces rheumatic fever. Fortunately, rheumatic fever is seen in the Western world with only a low frequency of sporadic cases in regional clusters. The incidence in the United States is less than 2 per 100,000, but in the developing world, rheumatic heart disease continues to be the leading cause of cardiac hospitalization in the 5- to 25-year-old age group.[27] Although the inflammatory component of rheumatic carditis is largely restricted to the valves, it has been believed to cause myocardial dysfunction.

Myocarditis is a well-documented complication with *Borrelia burgdorferi* infection (Lyme disease) and is reported in up to 8 percent of cases. Cardiac involvement is often characterized by the development of atrioventricular (AV) block and rarely progresses to left ventricular dysfunction and cardiomegaly.[28] *Mycoplasma pneumoniae* infection has also been associated with myocarditis. Lewes and coworkers[29] demonstrated asymptomatic myocardial involvement as documented by ECG changes in a third of the cases with acute *Mycoplasma* infection. Six percent of military conscripts with clinical myocarditis were found to have active *M. pneumoniae* infection.[30] *Chlamydia* infections have also been associated with myocarditis, especially among small children, often having fatal outcomes.[31] *C. pneumoniae* infection has also been noted in a few cases of mild myocarditis[32] and has been found with respiratory infection associated with myocarditis, resulting in sudden death in a young athlete.[33] *Chlamydia psittaci* infection may be associated with myocarditis in 5 to 15 percent of those affected, usually with minimal clinical signs or symptoms.[31] Pericarditis is more frequent and likely to cause cardiac morbidity with ornithosis.[34]

Other Causative Infectious Agents

Rickettsial infections, like Rocky Mountain spotted fever and scrub typhus, are frequently accompanied by myocardial involvement, although vasculitis is more prominent with these infections.[35] Q fever may also be associated with myocarditis.[36] *Trypanosoma cruzi* (Chagas' disease) is a well-recognized cause of myocarditis in cardiomyopathy in South America.[37] *Toxoplasma gondii* poses a significant problem among cardiac transplant recipients because a large number of the recipients lack antibodies against this agent, which may cause myocarditis.[38] Toxoplasmosis also poses a major threat to patients with AIDS, and myocarditis has frequently been seen in human immunodeficiency virus (HIV)–infected populations with or without concomitant *Toxoplasma* infection.[39, 40] In two autopsy studies of AIDS patients, myocarditis was found in almost half of the cases; in another study, 54 percent of 102 prospectively studied patients with AIDS had echocardiographic evidence of myocardial dysfunction.[41, 42] Myocarditis may also occur in patients with AIDS with T-cell restitution after antiviral therapy.[43]

Myocarditis can also be seen with parasitic infections such as *Trichinella spiralis,* which has an affinity for striated muscle, including the heart.[44]

Other Noninfectious Causes

Noninfectious causes of myocarditis include drug-induced hypersensitivity,[45–54] direct toxicity of specific pharmaceutical agents,[55–58] and systemic collagen vascular disorders.[59–66] Eosinophilic myocarditis[67–70] and giant cell myocarditis (GCM)[71–75] are distinct forms of inflammatory myocarditis of uncertain etiology.

Microorganisms are rarely isolated or demonstrated in heart muscle; hence, identification of a specific infectious etiologic agent depends on recognition of its systemic manifestations. Once specific noninfectious and nonviral infectious agents are excluded, myocarditis is often assumed to be of viral etiology. Although definitive serologic evidence of viral infection can be obtained in many patients, it is absent in the majority of patients with presumed myocarditis. A significant number of cases of myocarditis are due to autoimmune phenomena either induced by a viral infection or resulting from systemic autoimmune disease. Since there is ambiguity in establishment of a definitive etiologic diagnosis, the terms *viral myocarditis, idiopathic myocarditis, lymphocytic myocarditis, autoimmune myocarditis,* and *interstitial myocarditis* are frequently used interchangeably.

Pathophysiology of Viral Myocarditis

Animal Models

The most widely accepted models for the study of human myocarditis are those of enteroviral myocarditis induced by coxsackievirus B3 (CVB3) and the encephalomyocarditis virus. Induction of chronic murine myocarditis by CVB3 requires the virus to have a cardiovirulence capacity and murine strains of certain genetic background.[76, 77] Infection of syngeneic weanling mice with CVB3 results in brief cardiac infection lasting about a week, beyond which the virus cannot be cultured. However, viral RNA persists for several months after the initial infection.[78, 79] Several mechanisms have been hypothesized to explain the initiation of chronic inflammatory response in myocytes by the viral infection.

1. Dysregulatory processes that stimulate inflammation and result in myocyte destruction may be provoked by persistent infection of the cell by the replicating virus or even remnant virions.[80]
2. The virus-induced myocyte injury releases or exposes hitherto hidden or cryptic antigens to immune cells, leading to autoimmune effector molecule synthesis and maintained inflammatory response.[81, 82]
3. The CVB3 virion or other viral proteins share epitopes with internal or plasma membrane proteins of normal cells (molecular mimicry) and stimulate immune responses that participate in autoimmune reactions.[83]

These three mechanisms are not mutually restrictive and all may be simultaneously operative. The CVB3 and CVB4 share epitopes with human cardiac myocyte sarcolemmal proteins,[84, 85] human and mouse cardiac myosins,[86, 87] streptococcal M protein,[86] adenine nucleotide translocator protein,[88] and other proteins on normal mouse myocytes and fibroblasts.[89] A large number of target epitopes have been proposed, including the beta-adrenergic receptor,[90] laminin,[91] branched chain ketoacid dehydrogenase,[92] and heat shock protein 60.[93] Although antibodies to these antigens are frequently identified in association with myocarditis, the clinical significance and causal relationship are yet unresolved. It is quite possible that this antibody response may be just an epiphenomenon existing adjunctively to the cardinal pathologic processes.

Cytotoxic lymphocytes (CTLs) from mice with CVB3-induced myocarditis have been demonstrated to possess the ability to recognize and kill in vitro neonatal myocytes, fibroblasts, and endothelial cells infected with the same strain of the virus,[94] suggesting that the recognition of a novel tissue antigen is induced by the infection. There is also evidence for cross-reactive concurrent recognition of unrelated cardiac epitopes because CTLs also lyse uninfected myocytes in vitro.[95] The production of perforin, a pore-forming protein, has been proposed as one of the mechanisms for cytolysis induced by the lymphocytes. Perforins, when inserted into myocyte membrane, induce a lethal augmentation in cell permeability that results in cellular edema and death.[96] Perforin-independent mechanisms have also been proposed including a Fas (CD95/Apo1)–based inositol 1,4,5 triphosphate–mediated cytolysis that can be demonstrated in perforin-deficient gene-knockout mice.[97] Coxsackievirus-infected mice also develop additional immune sensitization to cardiac heavy chain myosin, possibly owing to the release of the sequestered myosin antigens from the virus-damaged cells. Immunization of mice with the heavy chain myosin and an adjuvant produces a histomorphologically similar picture to the CVB3-induced myocarditis. Experimental autoimmune myocarditis can also be produced by adoptive transfer of splenocytes after myocardial infarction in syngeneic rats. The sensitized lymphocytes when transferred to normal rats cause cardiac-specific cellular infiltration with accompanying myocyte necrosis.[98] The genetic susceptibility, kinetics, and cellular composition of the infiltrates in these models are similar and suggest the role of endogenous antigens as an epitope for the inflammatory response.[99]

Role of Cellular Immunity

The pathways and cellular participants in the immunopathogenesis of experimental viral myocarditis are well recognized and illustrated in Figure 55–1. The replicating

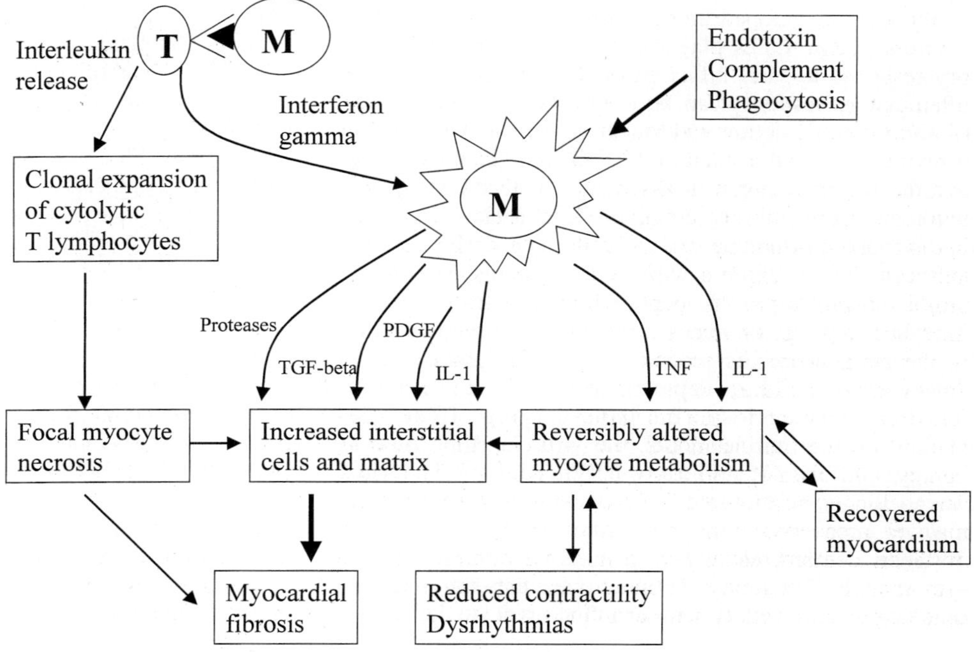

FIGURE 55–1 Cellular pathways mediating reversible and irreversible immune injury to the heart. T, T lymphocyte; M, macrophages; TGF-beta, transforming growth factor-beta; PDGF, platelet-derived growth factor; IL-1, interleukin-1; TNF, tumor necrosis factor. (From Lange LG, Schreiner GF: Immune mechanisms of cardiac disease. N Engl J Med 330:1129–1135, 1994. Copyright © 1994 Massachusetts Medical Society. All rights reserved.)

viral particles can be readily identified in cardiac myocytes within a few hours of inoculation of CVB3 into mice.[100, 101] The viral particles reach a numerical peak in 3 to 4 days, and usually at 7 to 10 days they are no longer detectable.[102] The inflammatory infiltrate is detectable by day 5 and reaches a plateau by days 7 to 10. The early inflammatory infiltrate consists of lymphocytes, macrophages, neutrophils, natural killer cells, and the associated cytokines and humoral effectors.[103–106] The natural killer cells are the first to appear and are detected in the activated state in 3 to 4 days. These cells are capable of lysing virus-infected cells in vitro.[106] The T lymphocytes and macrophages follow the natural killer cells in the temporal sequence and become the predominant cells infiltrating the myocardium in 7 to 10 days. Although CVB3 replicates readily in myocytes in vitro, the cells are resistant to lysis in comparison with other cultured cell lines. Direct myocytolysis appears to play a minimal role in cell lines derived from normal mice.[107, 108]

The immunodeficient severe combined immunodeficiency (SCID) mouse model has provided valuable insight into the early immune activity in response to the viral infection. The SCID mice lack mature T- and B-lymphocyte function and develop extensive myocardial necrosis with pleomorphic infiltrates, rapid viral proliferation, and profound virus-associated myocytolysis when inoculated with CVB3.[109] The macrophage and natural killer cell activity is unaffected in the SCID mouse model and may participate in the myocytolytic activity, although direct viral myocytolysis predominates. Pharmacologically immunosuppressed mice demonstrate similar characteristics, with higher viral loads, delayed clearance, and extensive myocyte necrosis, although direct viral myocytolysis is not frequent in immunocompetent mice.[94, 102, 110–112] Even noncardiovirulent strains may have sufficient time to replicate and transform into quasicardiovirulent species in the absence of a functional antiviral immune response, which can then result in fatal myocarditis.[113] This may also explain the clinical observation that many severe and fatal cases of myocarditis develop in young children with immature and incompletely developed immune systems.[114]

Virus-specific CTLs play a major role in the inflammatory response to viral infection of the myocyte.[102, 112] The inflammatory response can be diminished significantly by T-lymphocyte depletion with either antithymocyte globulin or thymectomy and irradiation.[101, 115] The CTLs must recognize the foreign antigen in association with the syngeneic major histocompatibility complex (MHC) class I antigen that is found on immune-derived cells. The CVB3-infected cells can readily express MHC class I antigens.[116] MHC class I molecules provide peptide-binding sites that evoke effector responses on recognition of the foreign peptide by the antigen-specific receptors of the T lymphocyte.[117] However, T-lymphocyte depletion and specific immunosuppression using cyclosporine have varying effects, depending on the murine model, the virus, and the time of therapy, and are not uniformly beneficial.[118–120] The virus can no longer be cultured from cells after 7 to 10 days; however, areas of inflammatory infiltrate and myocyte necrosis do demonstrate persistence of viral RNA and the virus-specific CTLs may continue to see these as immunologic targets and, hence, perpetuate the myocyte damage.[121]

The infected myocyte can still remain a target for the CTLs, even if the viral antigens are cleared, owing to expression of "neoantigens" either induced by the virus or unsequestered due to the injury.[122, 123] Even nonviral antigens on infected myocytes can react with CTLs, such as those induced by actinomycin D,[123] and new glycoproteins have been identified on the surface of CVB3-infected cells that can be recognized by CTLs from other syngeneic-infected mice.[124] Recent observations suggest that costimulatory molecules B7-1, B7-2, and CD-40 may be expressed on myocytes in patients with myocarditis and may make the myocytes into antigen-presenting cells for CTLs and natural killer cells, thereby playing an important role in the direct myocardial damage by these lytic cells.[125]

Role of Humoral Immunity

Another mechanism for ongoing myocyte damage is the antibody-mediated autoimmune response. Since the majority of the proteins identified as cardiac autoantigens are intracellular, it is unclear how these antibodies could harm normal intact myocytes. There are several proposed mechanisms: one suggests that after the antibody response is initiated, the circulating antibodies to intracellular antigens cross-react with the native membrane cardiac tissue proteins. Thus, after a small number of myocytes are damaged by the viral infection and release intracellular antigens, the resulting antibody response may affect normal myocytes, leading to global myocardial dysfunction. This hypothesis is supported by the demonstration of a number of cross-reacting antibodies.[84–93] Also, the antibodies against the intracellular mitochondrial adenine nucleotide transferase protein cross-react with the myocyte sarcolemmal calcium ion channel protein, and binding of these channels can physiologically alter the metabolism and contractile function of the myocyte.[126]

Another theory holds that CTLs and antibodies target uninfected myocytes by recognition of self-antigens that were previously sequestered from immune surveillance. The processing and presentation of the self-immunogenic peptides complexed with the MHC is a prerequisite for this hypothesis. Normal human cardiac myocytes do not express detectable levels of MHC class II antigens, and their constitutive expression of MHC class I molecules remains controversial.[127] A significant increase in the expression of MHC class I and class II antigens by the myocytes has been demonstrated in association with myocardial inflammation, such as that seen with viral myocarditis or transplant rejection.[128–130] The increased MHC expression has also been demonstrated in endomyocardial biopsy specimens from patients with idiopathic DCM and myocarditis,[131–133] and there may be a genetic predisposition to immune regulatory dysfunction.[134] There is also evidence for aberrant expression of intracellular antigens, such as adenine nucleotide translocator (ANT) and branched-chain alpha-keto acid dehydrogenase (BCKD), on the surface of the myocytes.[133]

The formation of anti-idiotypic antibodies is an additional mechanism of immune regulation in which an antibody is formed to the idiotypic determinants (antigen recognition site) of the primary antibody. The anti-idiotypic antibody may cross-react with unoccupied viral receptor sites on uninfected myocytes. This phenomenon has been reported with the reovirus, polyomavirus, and coxsackievirus B models of myocarditis.[135–137] The passive transfer of anti-idiotypic B cells from a CVB3 myocarditic mouse to a syngeneic mouse can cause nonviral myocarditis.[138]

Role of Cytokines

The presence of a complex, cytokine-rich microenvironment is suggested by the heterogeneous inflammatory cell populations in the hearts of infected mice. The cytokines perform myriad immunomodulatory functions, including regulation of antibody production, preservation of self-tolerance,[139, 140] conscription of ancillary cells in the inflammatory milieu,[141, 142] and maintenance of clonal expansion of CTLs.[143, 144] Certain cytokines regulate the collagenogenic and collagenolytic activity of fibroblasts.[145] Although mounting evidence supports the negative inotropic effects and/or the blunting of catecholamine response in myocytes exposed to various cytokines, there is no direct evidence to suggest that the cytokines are directly responsible for myocytolysis.[146] In an in vitro model, Barry[146] demonstrated that high concentrations of interleukin (IL)-1, tumor necrosis factor-alpha (TNF-α), interferon-gamma (INF-γ), and IL-4 have no effect on myocyte survival over 24 hours, whereas the CTLs from a mixed lymphocyte reaction cause virtually 100 percent killing.

Gulick and colleagues[147] demonstrated that cultured neonatal myocytes, when exposed to macrophage-derived IL-1 and TNF-α, have reduced levels of cyclic adenosine monophosphate and have a reduced inotropic response to catecholamines. The mechanism for decreased responsiveness to catecholamines is believed to be modulated by increases in nitric oxide production mediated by increased inducible nitric oxide synthase (iNOS) activity, and the blunting of the catecholamine response can be inhibited by the L-arginine analogue N^G-monomethyl-L-arginine (L-NMMA).[148] The decreased contractile response of cardiac myocytes to β-adrenergic agonists following induction of iNOS also requires the presence of insulin and the coinduction of enzymes responsible for the production of tetrahydrobiopterin, a cofactor for nitric oxide synthase.[149] The role of iNOS remains controversial because increased expression of iNOS mRNA and that of other proinflammatory cytokines is evident and is associated with contractile dysfunction.[150] There is evidence to support that iNOS induction is crucial for the host response to CVB3 infection and iNOS-deficient mice have significantly increased viral loads with extensive myocardial damage.[151]

Other investigators have suggested that inflammatory cytokines may have direct negative inotropic effects, independent of the responsiveness to the β-adrenergic agonists. High doses of IL-2 during chemotherapy have been reported to result in depression of myocardial function.[152] Exposure of cardiac myocytes to endotoxin results in increased nitric oxide production and direct depression of contractility owing to increased levels of cyclic guanosine monophosphate.[153] Further, TNF-α may induce direct negative inotropic effects by decreasing the Ca^{2+} transient, with no change in the L-type Ca^{2+} current and independent of nitric oxide synthesis.[154] Although the extent to which cytokines cause direct negative inotropic effects or attenuation of endogenous β-adrenergic agonist activity remains unclear, they do produce myocyte dysfunction and cardiac decompensation. Transgenic mice with overexpression of TNF-α develop biventricular dilatation and cardiac failure, resulting in premature death. Pathologic specimens from these mice reveal globular dilated hearts and transmural myocarditis with myocyte apoptosis.[155]

Increased levels of intracellular adhesion molecule (ICAM-1), IL-1-alpha, IL-1-beta, TNF-α, and macrophage-stimulating factor have been demonstrated in patients with myocarditis and idiopathic DCM.[156, 157] Furthermore, the susceptibility of mice in the CVB3 myocarditis model can be increased by pretreatment with these cytokines.[158] Transforming growth factor-beta is identifiable by immunohistochemistry in the prenecrotic regions of infiltrates in the murine myocardium and decreases when the macrophages and fibroblasts migrate to the necrotic foci. These growth factors may be responsible for recruitment of the immunologic effectors and may directly affect cardiac function.[159] An intriguing feature of cytokine activity remains their role in the secondary development of myocyte hypertrophy and interstitial fibrosis, characteristic of dilated cardiomyopathy.[160] Among animals with different forms of viral myocarditis associated with similar intensity of initial myocyte necrosis, only those animals with persistent inflammation develop interstitial fibrosis, reflected by fibroblast proliferation and an increase in the extracellular matrix. Myocardial fibrosis correlates well with the presence of T lymphocytes and macrophages, which in their activated state release fibrogenic cytokines such as fibroblast growth factor and transforming growth factor-β.[161]

Significance of Animal Models

The lymphocytic myocarditis models in animals have conclusively demonstrated the association of viral infection and myocarditis, but the strength of this association in humans remains nebulous. The myocardial damage in murine models of viral myocarditis occurs in two distinct phases: an early phase of direct viral cytotoxicity in which virus-specific T-lymphocyte– and antibody-mediated cytotoxicity predominate; and a late or chronic phase in which the persistent viral genome, reactive CTLs, autoantibodies, cytokines, and microvascular damage mediate myocyte damage and dysfunction. The hypothetical mechanisms of virus-induced autoimmune heart disease are presented in Figure 55–2.

The recognition that immune responses to specific viruses are consequential in the development of myocyte injury has led to exhaustive research to exploit the possibility of designing immunomodulatory and antiviral therapies. The pretreatment of mice with inactivated virus vaccine prevents the manifestations of encephalomyocarditis virus myocarditis.[162] The administration of antiviral therapies reduces the viral load and attenuates the histologic findings of myocarditis.[163, 164] The antiviral response can be augmented by INF-α or the exogenous administration of IL-6.[165, 166] Recombinant murine INF-γ has also been demonstrated to improve the prognosis of acute murine

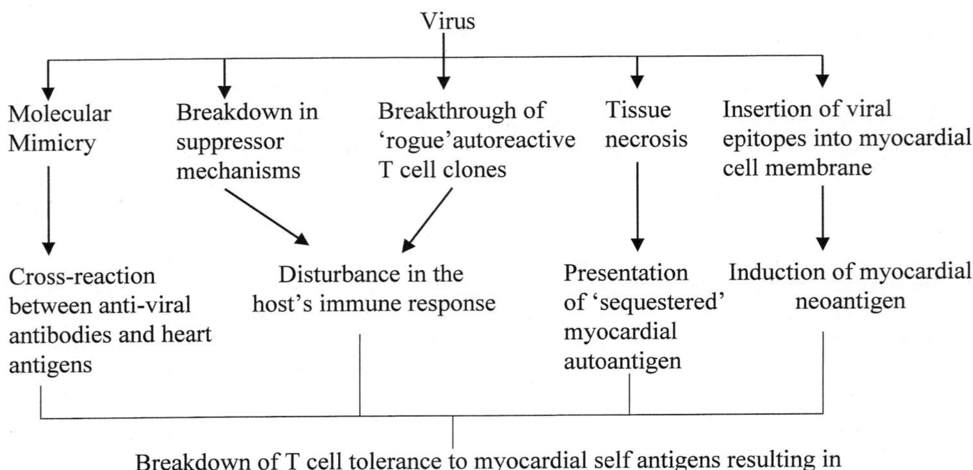

FIGURE 55–2 Hypothetical mechanisms of virus-induced or precipitated autoimmune heart disease. (From Caforio ALP: Postviral autoimmune heart disease—fact or fiction? Eur Heart J 18:1051–1055, 1997.)

myocarditis caused by ECM virus by suppressing virus replication.[167]

The murine model has also been the subject of intensive study with clinically applied immunosuppressants, such as corticosteroids,[168] nonsteroidal anti-inflammatory agents,[169, 170] and cyclophosphamide,[171] all of which have demonstrated deleterious effects when given in the acute viremic phase. Cyclosporine, when administered in the early viremic phase, worsens myocardial injury but, in the late immune phase, has a beneficial effect.[172–174] Similar results have been reported with tacrolimus,[175] and survival improves significantly when immunosuppressants such as cyclosporine, azathioprine, and 15-deoxyspergualin are used in adjunct to immunomodulators, such as INF-α.[176] Antibodies to TNF-α have been demonstrated to improve survival and reduce myocardial injury.[177] Cytokine inhibitors have had promising results in animal models, but human clinical trials have been inconsistent. Vesnarinone, a phosphodiesterase III inhibitor, has demonstrated beneficial hemodynamic effects and inhibits the production of TNF-α and favorably modulates induction of iNOS.[178] Amlodipine has also been shown to increase survival of mice with viral myocarditis by inhibiting expression of iNOS and production of nitric oxide in vivo and in vitro.[179]

CLINICAL FEATURES AND APPROACH TO DIAGNOSIS

Clinical Presentation

The diversity of immunopathogenetic mechanisms and variability in the severity of observed disease in the murine model are only a preview to the potpourri of clinical manifestations of myocarditis in humans. The presentation of unexplained progressive cardiac dysfunction or ventricular arrhythmias should lead to the suspicion of myocarditis, especially when routine cardiac diagnostic studies do not reveal an etiology. The history of an antecedent viral infection or prodrome is often sought but seldom reported and rarely confirmed by convalescent serologies. The presence of mild MB isoenzyme of creatine kinase (CK-MB) or troponin elevation, leukocytosis, or ECG changes may further underscore the possibility of myocarditis.

The majority of patients with myocarditis likely remain asymptomatic and never seek medical attention. The high frequency of exposure to cardiotropic viruses and the observation of a fairly high incidence of ECG abnormalities in apparently healthy individuals support this speculation.[9] The incidence of myocarditis in an autopsy series following traumatic deaths in previously healthy individuals has been reported at 2.2 percent.[180] Others have reported incidences ranging from 0.11 percent to as high as 5 percent in unselected autopsy series.[181, 182] These studies may suggest that at any given time, a significant percentage of the asymptomatic general population has myocarditis.

The most common presentation of myocarditis is an acute febrile syndrome associated with pericardial and systemic complaints. Cardiotropic viruses may cause pericardial inflammation, and patients often present with a syndrome of myopericarditis. Chest pain is the most common symptom and is secondary to pericarditis or myocardial injury.[183] A rather dramatic presentation of myocarditis is one indistinguishable from an acute myocardial infarction, complete with chest pain, ECG features suggesting acute ischemic injury, enzymatic evidence of myocardial damage, and echocardiographic or ventriculographic regional wall motion abnormalities but, on endomyocardial biopsy, myocarditis is confirmed.[184–186] Most patients presenting with this acute syndrome will have complete recovery, although there are isolated instances where progressive myocyte loss and cardiac failure or sudden arrhythmic death is reported.[187] The segmental wall motion abnormalities result from virus-mediated injury, although local coronary arteritis and vasospasm have been suggested as possible culprits.[188, 189]

Symptoms of right and left ventricular failure and even cardiogenic shock are frequently found in patients with biopsy-proven myocarditis, since it is these symptoms that lead to medical attention. However, the true incidence of heart failure in patients with myocarditis is probably much lower. In patients presenting with recent-onset heart failure and biopsy-proven myocarditis, 50 to 60 percent have had an antecedent flulike illness.[187]

Neonatal myocarditis is often a fulminant syndrome consisting of fever, tachycardia, tachypnea, cyanosis, and rapid progression to circulatory collapse.[190] Mortality rates are the highest in this subpopulation, approaching as high as 50 percent. Children are known to present with syncope due to heart block.[191] Other atrial arrhythmias described with myocarditis include sinoatrial block, atrial standstill, AV block, intra-atrial conduction abnormalities, atrial tachycardia, flutter, and fibrillation.[192–197] Histologic evidence of possible myocarditis has been described in up to two thirds of patients with lone atrial fibrillation.[198] Complete heart block has also been described in certain viral infections, such as Epstein-Barr virus or mumps, and also with rickettsiae.[199–201]

Ventricular arrhythmias are frequently encountered with myocarditis, ranging from innocuous premature ventricular contractions to malignant and incessant ventricular tachycardia.[202–204] Myocarditis has been incriminated as a cause of ventricular repolarization abnormalities in athletes with or without arrhythmias.[204, 205] Ventricular arrhythmias may also be precursors to sudden cardiac death in young athletes with occult myocarditis.[206] In autopsy series, myocarditis accounts for 17 to 25 percent of sudden deaths in young, healthy people.[207, 208] In a population-based retrospective study from Turin, Italy, an incidence of only 0.53 percent was reported among 17,162 autopsies performed over three decades,[209] but the application of standardized systematic histologic examination tends to give a higher incidence, in the range of 5 percent, among autopsies performed at a general hospital.[210] Wesslen and associates[211] reported signs of active, healing, or healed myocarditis in 12 of 16 cases of sudden death in young Swedes. Among high-performance athletes, sudden death due to undiagnosed myocarditis often stirs media attention.[212] Myocarditis is also not uncommonly noted in sudden infant death syndrome.[213]

Myocarditis may also manifest as myocardial thickening and fibrosis presenting as diastolic dysfunction or restrictive cardiomyopathy and asymmetric septal thickening resembling hypertrophic cardiomyopathy.[214–216] Lieberman and coworkers[217] proposed a clinicopathologic description of myocarditis based on the initial manifestations, endomyocardial biopsy, and recovery (fulminant, acute, chronic active, or chronic persistent myocarditis).

Physical Examination

The physical findings in acute myocarditis are dependent on the extent of myocardial or pericardial involvement, inciting agent (cardiotropic virus), and other factors. Fever occurs occasionally, and in the Myocarditis Treatment Trial (MTT),[218] it was noted in 18 percent of patients with myocarditis. Sinus tachycardia may frequently accompany the febrile state but is often out of proportion to the fever and is more likely adrenergically mediated owing to the hemodynamic alterations of the failing heart. Significant ventricular dysfunction may also be associated with hypotension, gallops, murmurs of regurgitation, rales, jugular venous distention, hepatomegaly, ascites, pleural effusions, and peripheral edema. Pericardial involvement may result in a friction rub. The physical findings are not specific for myocarditis.

Laboratory Findings

Patients with myocarditis will frequently have serologic evidence of an inflammatory state with elevation of nonspecific markers of inflammation, such as erythrocyte sedimentation rate, C-reactive protein, and leukocyte counts. A fourfold increase in virus-specific IgG titers in the convalescent period is considered reliable evidence of recent infection and is found in 20 percent of patients with myocarditis.[219, 220] In the MTT, more than half of the patients with biopsy-proven myocarditis had an elevated sedimentation rate.[218] Other markers noted to be elevated in myocarditis include TNF-α, ICAM-1, vascular cell adhesion molecule-1, interleukins, and soluble Fas.[156, 157, 221, 222] Unfortunately, these markers are not specific for myocarditis.

Myocarditis, although associated with myocyte damage and necrosis, results in CK-MB elevation in only 12 percent of patients with biopsy-proven myocarditis.[223] More recently, Lauer and colleagues[224] reported on CK-MB elevation in only one of five patients with histologic evidence of myocarditis, but cardiac troponin T (cTnT), which is extremely specific for myocardial damage, was elevated in all five. Additionally, cTnT was elevated in 28 patients, of whom 26 had immunohistologic evidence of myocarditis. Thus, cTnT elevation appears to be highly predictive for myocarditis.[224] In an analysis of stored sera on 88 patients from the MTT,[218] cardiac troponin I (cTnI) was elevated in 34 percent of patients (18 of 53) with myocarditis, compared with 11 percent (4 of 35) without myocarditis. In contrast, CK-MB values were elevated in only 5.7 percent patients (3 of 53) with myocarditis. Further, the cTnI elevations correlated with less than 1 month's duration of heart failure symptoms.[225]

Electrocardiography, Echocardiography, and Cardiac Scintigraphy

Historically, acute myocarditis was diagnosed with the constellation of clinical symptoms, physical signs, and ECG abnormalities. Although no particular feature on the electrocardiogram is pathognomonic of acute myocarditis, sinus tachycardia, repolarization abnormalities, conduction abnormalities, and arrhythmias are common findings. In a series of 45 patients with biopsy-proven myocarditis, Morgera and associates[226] noted an abnormal QRS duration in 45 percent; abnormal Q waves in 18 percent; left bundle branch block (LBBB) and right bundle branch block (RBBB) patterns in 18 percent and 13 percent, respectively; ST elevation in 16 percent; T wave inversions in 16 percent; and advanced AV block in 16 percent. In patients presenting earlier in the course of the disease, with symptoms of less than 1 month's duration, 31 percent had advanced AV block and 47 percent had ST elevation with T-wave inversions. The latter finding has been noted to portend a poorer prognosis. Other predictors of poor outcome include LBBB, RBBB, and other conduction abnormalities, which seem to suggest active, severe, and extensive myocarditis.[227] Patients may present with sustained ventricular tachycardia, and continuous ECG monitoring of patients with myocarditis often reveals complex ventricular ectopy and nonsustained ventricular tachycardia.[202, 228]

Echocardiography is useful in assessing the extent of left ventricular systolic dysfunction, which may range from mild segmental hypokinesis to severe global hypokinesis or akinesis associated with severe congestive heart failure (CHF).[229] Patients presenting with chest pain or arrhythmias without CHF often have normal echocardiograms. The ventricular dimensions may remain normal or may be only mildly enlarged. There may be an increase in left ventricular sphericity and right ventricular elongation and an increase in wall thickness and left ventricular mass with the interstitial edema and compensatory hypertrophy.[230, 231] Restrictive filling patterns in the left ventricle identifying diastolic dysfunction have been reported consistently in biopsy-proven myocarditis.[231] Mural thrombi in diffusely hypokinetic ventricles have been reported frequently.[232] Hyperrefractile myocardium and other qualitative and quantitative analyses of myocardial texture have been described to assess the degree of active myocardial inflammation.[233] Pericardial effusions are reported in 10 percent of patients with myocarditis, but hemodynamic compromise with cardiac tamponade is infrequent.[233]

Cardiac scintigraphy has been proposed as a convenient, noninvasive test with high sensitivity to diagnose active myocarditis. Gallium 67 imaging, which identifies areas of increased inflammation, has been studied in clinical settings and noted to have sensitivity and specificity of 83 and 86 percent respectively, with a negative predictive value of 98 percent for the diagnosis of myocarditis.[234] Indium 111 antimyosin monoclonal antibodies have been extensively studied to identify areas of myocyte damage in acute myocarditis.[235, 236] This technique has extremely high sensitivity and often detects myocarditis that, on endomyocardial biopsy, is not seen by routine histologic assessment but is detected by immunohistochemistry.[237] Dec and coworkers[238] studied 74 patients with DCM with radiolabeled antimyosin antibody and endomyocardial biopsy. Thirty-nine patients had abnormal antimyosin scans, but only 11 of 39 had evidence for myocarditis (predictive value of 33 percent). However, functional improvement was more likely in antimyosin scan–positive patients irrespective of the biopsy. The left ventricular ejection fraction (LVEF) improved significantly in both concordant-positive (scan and biopsy both positive) and discordant-positive (scan positive, biopsy negative) patients, but it did not markedly improve in the negative scan–negative biopsy subset. The investigators proposed that discordant-positive scans represented patients with myocarditis in whom there may have been a sampling error on biopsy, hence missing the diagnosis.[238]

Contrast media–enhanced magnetic resonance imaging in patients with myocarditis has also been demonstrated to be an excellent tool in visualizing the location, activity, and extent of inflammation. Early in myocarditis (day 2), the enhancement on magnetic resonance imaging signals is accentuated and focal, whereas later (day 84), this seems to be attenuated and more diffuse.[239] Myocardial phosphorus 31–magnetic resonance spectroscopy has been utilized in assessing abnormalities in cardiac high-energy phosphate metabolism in patients with DCM and allograft rejection, but its role in the diagnosis of active myocarditis remains to be elucidated.[240, 241]

Endomyocardial Biopsy and Cardiac Catheterization

The antemortem diagnosis of myocarditis was made feasible by the development of endomyocardial biopsy technique. Myocardial samples could be obtained via a transvascular approach with minimal discomfort to the patient and a low complication rate. Whereas other approaches for acquiring myocardial tissue included percutaneous biopsy and mediastinotomy,[242, 243] these were fraught with complications, precluding their acceptance into clinical practice. The safe and successful transvascular endomyocardial biopsy first described by Sakakibara and Konno[244] was readily accepted for surveillance of cardiac allograft rejection in transplant recipients. The use of endomyocardial biopsy for the diagnosis and management of myocarditis was first reported in 1980.[245] Subsequently, many reports[246–274] documented myocarditis in patients presenting with unexplained heart failure or ventricular arrhythmias (Table 55–4). However, there was considerable incongruity in the diagnostic criteria used in these largely anecdotal reports. The Dallas criteria were developed in preparation for a large, randomized, multicenter clinical trial of immunosuppressive therapy in myocarditis.[218] These criteria define *active* myocarditis as "an inflammatory infiltrate of the myocardium with necrosis and/or degeneration of adjacent myocytes not typical of ischemic damage associated with

TABLE 55-4 Myocarditis by Biopsy

Investigators	Year	Biopsies (n)	Myocarditis (n [%])
In Unexplained Heart Failure			
Mason et al[245]	1980	400	7 (2)
Baandrup and Olsen[246]	1981	201	8 (4)
Fenoglio et al[247]	1983	135	34 (25)
Rose et al[248]	1984	76	0 (0)
Daly et al[249]	1984	69	12 (17)
Parillo et al[250]	1984	74	19 (26)
Regitz et al[251]	1985	150	41 (27)
Cassling et al[252]	1985	80	6 (7)
Salvi et al[253]	1985	74	13 (18)
Dec et al[254]	1985	27	18 (67)
Mortensen et al[255]	1985	65	12 (18)
Hammond et al[256]	1987	79	14 (18)
Meany et al[257]	1987	123	40 (32)
Chow et al[258]	1988	90	4 (4)
Maisch et al[259]	1988	123	10 (8)
Hobbs et al[260]	1989	148	31 (21)
Popma et al[261]	1989	61	8 (13)
Vasiljevic et al[262]	1990	85	10 (12)
Lieberman et al[263]	1991	348	60 (17)
Herskowitz et al[264]	1993	534	38 (26)
Kuhl et al[265]	1996	170	9 (5)
Arbustini et al[266]	1997	601	26 (4.3)
In Unexplained Ventricular Arrhythmias			
Strain et al[267]	1983	18	3 (17)
Sugrue et al[268]	1984	12	1 (8)
Take et al[269]	1985	241	21 (9)
Hosenpud et al[270]	1986	12	4 (33)
Yoshizato et al[271]	1990	8	2 (25)
Sekiguchi et al[272]	1992	43	9 (21)
Wiles et al[273]	1992	33	3 (9)
Thongtang et al[274]	1993	53	18 (36)

coronary artery disease." Furthermore, other causes of inflammation (e.g., connective tissue disorders, infection, drugs) should be excluded.[5, 275] The Dallas criteria also defined *borderline* myocarditis as an inflammatory infiltrate that is sparse and lacks myocyte injury, and often (67 percent) on repeat biopsy, borderline myocarditis will histologically progress to active myocarditis.[276]

A possible limitation of endomyocardial biopsy is sampling error. The inflammation in myocarditis may be patchy or focal, unlike allograft rejection, which is a relatively diffuse process. Although obtaining four samples from the right ventricular septum provides a high sensitivity for detection of allograft rejection in transplant recipients,[277] this may not hold true for myocarditis. In an autopsy study of the right ventricular biopsy technique (10 samples taken from the apical septum), only 6 of 11 patients dying of myocarditis were correctly identified. Left ventricular biopsy missed the diagnosis in 8 of 11.[278] In another study using the standard four to six samples, the sensitivity of right ventricular endomyocardial biopsy was reported at 50 percent.[279] Dec and colleagues[276] reported that employing repeat left and right ventricular biopsies in patients with suspected myocarditis with an initial negative biopsy increases the yield by 15 percent. Because an ideal study to evaluate sampling error has not been done, the true yield is unknown, but clearly, a negative biopsy does not exclude active myocarditis. In the MTT, only 10 percent of patients screened had histologic evidence of myocarditis. The European Study of Epidemiology and Treatment of Cardiac Inflammatory Disease (ESETCID)[280] demonstrated a 20 percent incidence of biopsy-proven myocarditis by expanding the Dallas criteria with the use of newer techniques of polymerase chain reaction and in situ hybridization.

Coronary arteriography is usually normal, although in animal models, coronary vasculitis has been reported. The one major exception is Kawasaki's disease, in which coronary artery aneurysms are frequently seen in association with myocarditis.[281] Ventriculograms may demonstrate global or regional ventricular dysfunction, associated valvular regurgitation, and mural thrombi.[282] Localized ventricular aneurysms with normal global systolic function have also been reported.[283]

The hemodynamic profiles of patients with acute myocarditis are representative of the extent of myocardial and pericardial involvement. In patients with significant ventricular dysfunction, elevated filling pressures with depressed cardiac output and stroke work indices are seen. A restrictive hemodynamic profile can be seen and must be differentiated from that seen with postviral constrictive pericarditis.

Natural History of Myocarditis

The true natural history of myocarditis is largely unknown because the great majority of cases are perhaps subclinical and resolve without any significant residual cardiac dysfunction. Clinically apparent myocardial dysfunction as seen with acute coxsackievirus B infections also resolves without any adverse sequelae in most cases. It has been estimated that only 12 percent of patients with clinically suspected acute myocarditis will proceed to develop DCM,[284] but the true incidence is unknown. The murine myocarditis models frequently develop a pathologic process indistinguishable from that of the human form of idiopathic DCM.

The direct link among viral infection, myocarditis, and DCM has not been conclusively proven. The definitive proof would be the isolation of infectious virus from the heart tissue as per Koch's postulates, but this has been achieved in only a few cases of acute fulminant myocarditis in neonates or infants.[285, 286] The indirect evidence of viral etiology of DCM relies on (1) the experimental animal models of virus-induced cardiomyopathy progressing to DCM, (2) apparent progression of myocarditis in some patients to DCM, and (3) increased enteroviral antibody titers in patients with DCM. The major limitations are that the relevance of disease in mice to humans is suspect, most cases of DCM are not preceded by documented myocarditis, and interpretation of epidemiologic serologic data is fraught with uncertainty. Whereas coxsackievirus B IgM antibodies are detected with greater frequency in patients with DCM than in normal controls, the frequency is similar to matched community controls and household contacts.[287] Enteroviral genomic sequences are detected in the myocardium of 8 to 70 percent of patients with active myocarditis and in 0 to 45 percent of patients with DCM, but in data derived from most published studies, the average detection frequencies are 25 percent for active myocarditis, 15 percent for DCM, and not significantly different from 15 percent among healthy controls.[288] In a meta-analysis of the association of enteroviruses with human heart disease, Baboonian and Treasure concluded that although the causative role of enteroviruses in acute myocarditis, particularly in children, was supported by an overall odds ratio of 4.4 (confidence interval [CI] 2.4 to 8.2), the association of DCM was only suggested by an overall odds ratio of 3.8 (CI 2.1 to 4.6).[289]

Although the link between myocarditis and DCM is unclear, certain prognostic factors are identifiable. The presence of an abnormal QRS complex on electrocardiography correlates with more severe left ventricular damage and is an independent predictor of survival. Left atrial enlargement, atrial fibrillation, and LBBB are also associated with increased mortality.[226] Higher baseline LVEF is positively associated with survival, whereas intensity of conventional therapy at baseline is negatively associated with survival.[218] The presence of right ventricular dysfunction, as evidenced by abnormal right ventricular systolic shortening on echocardiography, was shown to be the most important predictor of death or need for cardiac transplantation in a group of 23 patients with biopsy-proven myocarditis who were followed long term.[290] In addition, a net increase in LVEF (between initial and final ejection fraction) was associated with improved survival, whereas baseline ejection fraction was not predictive of outcome. The presence and degree of left ventricular regional wall motion abnormalities did not affect the clinical course.[290]

Light microscopic findings on biopsy have not been found to predict outcome in myocarditis. However, higher baseline serum antibodies to cardiac IgG by indirect immunofluorescence was associated with a better LVEF and a smaller left ventricular end-diastolic dimension.[218]

TREATMENT

General Supportive Measures

General supportive measures for patients with myocarditis include a low-sodium diet, discontinuation of ethanol, and fluid restriction, especially in the presence of heart failure. Patients with myopericarditis may need analgesics for pain control. Recommendations for the limitation of physical activity are based on the murine model of CVB3 myocarditis, in which forced exercise during the acute phase of illness was associated with higher titers of infectious virus, increased inflammatory and necrotic lesions, and mortality.[285, 291, 292] Ibuprofen, indomethacin, and salicylates administered to mice after inoculation with CVB3 also resulted in increased viral titers, increased histologic severity of myocarditis, and increased mortality.[293] This led to the suggestion that even nonsteroidal anti-inflammatory drugs should be avoided in patients with active acute myocarditis. The American College of Cardiology Task Force on myopericardial diseases recommends a convalescent period of approximately 6 months after onset of clinical manifestations before a return to competitive sports.[294]

Conventional Therapy

The management of patients with presumed or confirmed myocarditis is primarily directed toward treatment of CHF, arrhythmias, and symptoms from pericardial disease. Diuretics, vasodilators, and digoxin should be administered to patients with mild-to-moderate systolic dysfunction. Inotropic therapy and mechanical support with intra-aortic balloon pump or ventricular-assist devices may be required for patients in refractory cardiogenic shock. Cardiac transplantation is reserved for those patients who do not improve despite the measures described previously.

Although there are multiple studies on the use of angiotensin-converting enzyme inhibitors (ACEIs) in heart failure,[295] the utility of ACEIs in myocarditis has been studied only in the murine model. Early treatment with captopril in a CVB3 myocarditis model resulted in less inflammatory infiltrate, myocardial necrosis, and calcification. Heart weight, heart/body weight ratio, and liver congestion diminished. Even with delayed therapy, a reduction in left ventricular mass and liver congestion was evident.[296] ACEIs exert a potent vasodilator response, improve pump function, prevent ventricular remodeling, and may have antiarrhythmic properties. Hence, all patients with systolic dysfunction, including those with myocarditis, should be placed on maximally tolerated doses of ACEIs.

The use of beta-blockers in patients with mild-to-moderate heart failure due to DCM has been reported to be beneficial,[297] but once again, no trials in humans with myocarditis have been performed. Metoprolol-treated mice in an acute CVB3 murine myocarditis model have increased viral replication, myocyte necrosis, and 30-day mortality rates.[298] Carteolol, a nonselective β-blocker, has been studied in a chronic myocarditis model and found to have beneficial effects with improved histologic scores, reduced heart weight and volume, and liver congestion.[299] It appears that in the acute setting, β-blockers should be avoided, and in the chronic heart failure stage, the nonselective β-blockers may be beneficial.

Antiarrhythmic therapy may be needed for control of ventricular and supraventricular dysrhythmias. Although the data from clinical trials of antiarrhythmic therapy in heart failure have not shown a primary mortality benefit, patients with active myocarditis were excluded in these trials. Since immunosuppression is probably not helpful in myocarditis[218] and no other specific therapy is available, one might consider treating the arrhythmias in the usual fashion, but there appears to be a rationale for making the diagnosis of myocarditis in patients who do not have profound ventricular dysfunction along with their arrhythmia. First, the majority of patients with myocarditis will have spontaneous resolution. Second, current antiarrhythmic therapy of ventricular tachyarrhythmias is exacting, involving electrophysiologic studies and use of potentially toxic drugs and/or implantable defibrillators. The benefit of making the diagnosis of myocarditis is that the patient may require only short-term protection while the underlying process resolves, which can be provided by using amiodarone, a very effective pharmacologic agent for control of refractory ventricular arrhythmia, for a period of 3 months. If myocarditis resolves, antiarrhythmic therapy can be withdrawn. Patients whose arrhythmias fail to improve despite histologic resolution of myocarditis may be candidates for aggressive electrophysiologic approaches and implantable defibrillators.[300] Temporary and permanent pacemakers may be required in patients presenting with conduction system abnormalities.

Immunosuppressive Therapy

Clinical trials of immunosuppressive therapy were first reported in children with clinical evidence of myocarditis, prior to the introduction of endomyocardial biopsy. In two series, in a total of eight children presenting with acute onset of severe CHF, rapid improvement and survival were noted with adrenocorticotropic hormone or hydrocortisone treatment.[301, 302] Mason and associates[245] reported 10 patients with biopsy-proven myocarditis, half of whom improved with azathioprine and prednisone. Gagliardi and coworkers[303] followed 20 children with biopsy-proven myocarditis who were treated with cyclosporine and prednisone. At 1 year, 10 of 20 patients still had histologic evidence of myocarditis. No patient died or required transplantation. However, there was no control group. The data supporting an immunologic basis of myocarditis resulted in multiple treatment trials using immunosuppressants (Table 55–5). The average proportion of patients showing improvement with a variety of immunosuppressants was 54 percent.[304] A large number of the trials predated the development of the Dallas criteria; thus, the histologic definition of myocarditis was not uniform. Immunosuppressive regimens were arbitrary, and the lack of control groups made interpretation of these trials arduous. It was unclear whether immunosuppression was beneficial in those patients with myocarditis, as they can improve spontaneously. Further, the infectious complications of immunosuppression were frequently seen and occasionally reported.[245, 305]

The conflicting results from these nonrandomized obser-

TABLE 55-5 **Selected Nonrandomized Trials of Immunosuppressive Treatment in Myocarditis**

Investigators	Year	Patient Treated (n)	Treatment	Improved (n [%])
Mason et al[245]	1980	8	P + (A, P)	4 (50)
Fenoglio et al[247]	1983	18	P, (A, P)	7 (39)
Daly et al[249]	1984	1	P	0
Dec et al[254]	1985	9	A + P	4 (44)
Mortensen et al[255]	1985	12	A + P, CyA	8 (67)
Hobbs et al[259]	1989	34	A + P, P, CyA	25 (74)

**Abbreviations:* A, azathioprine; P, prednisone; CyA, cyclosporine.

vations led to the MTT.[218] In a multicenter, prospective, randomized design, the MTT enrolled patients with heart failure of recent onset (<2 years), left ventricular dysfunction (LVEF < 45 percent), and biopsy-proven myocarditis (per the Dallas criteria). The study screened 2333 patients; 214 (10 percent) had endomyocardial biopsy evidence of myocarditis, and 111 patients had a qualifying LVEF of less than 45 percent and agreed to enrollment. Patients were randomized to three treatment arms: prednisone and cyclosporine, prednisone and azathioprine, and no immunosuppressant treatment. All patients received conventional therapy for heart failure. The prednisone and azathioprine group was subsequently eliminated owing to low patient recruitment in the trial. Patients were treated for 24 weeks, and the primary endpoint was comparison of the mean increase in LVEF at 28 weeks. Secondary analysis of other markers of left ventricular function, survival, and several immune parameters was performed.

At both 28 and 52 weeks, no difference in LVEF was observed in immunosuppressive-treated patients compared with untreated patients (Fig. 55–3). At 1 and 5 years, there was no difference in survival or need for cardiac transplantation between groups (Fig. 55–4). On multivariate analysis, better baseline LVEF, less intensive conventional therapy, and shorter illness duration were independent predictors of improvement in LVEF during follow-up. Analysis of immunologic variables (cardiac IgG, circulating IgG, natural killer and macrophage activity, helper T-cell level) suggested an association between better outcome and a more robust immune response. A higher level of cardiac IgG was associated with a higher LVEF and a smaller left ventricular size. The mortality rate for the entire trial was 20 percent at 1 year and 56 percent at 4.3 years. The results of the MTT were important for diagnostic management because the authors recommended that in patients with unexplained CHF, the performance of endomyocardial biopsy for the sole purpose of instituting immunosuppressive therapy was not warranted.

Nonetheless, certain subgroups may benefit from immunosuppressant therapy, including those with GCM, hypersensitivity myocarditis, or cardiac sarcoidosis. Using a multicenter database, Cooper and colleagues[306] reviewed 63 patients with GCM. The rate of death or cardiac transplantation was 89 percent. Median survival was 5.5 months from symptom onset to death or transplantation. The median survival in patients treated with corticosteroids was 3.8 months versus 3.0 months in untreated patients. However, patients treated with corticosteroids and azathioprine had an average survival of 11.5 months. Cyclosporine in combination with corticosteroids, corticosteroids and azathioprine, and corticosteroids, azathioprine, and Orthoclone survived an average of 12.6 months. The uncontrolled nature of this report decreases the reliability of its conclusions.

Patients with myocarditis associated with a known im-

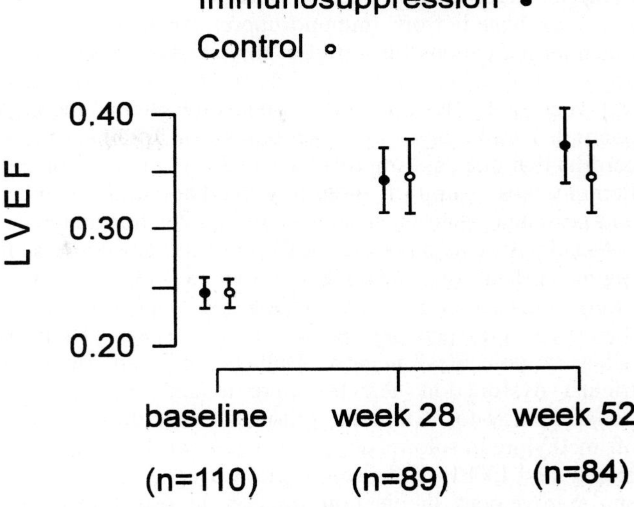

FIGURE 55–3 Changes in left ventricular ejection fraction (LVEF) in the Myocarditis Treatment Trial. (Adapted from Mason JW, O'Connell JB, Herskowitz A, et al: A clinical trial of immunosuppressive therapy for myocarditis. N Engl J Med 333:269–275, 1995.)

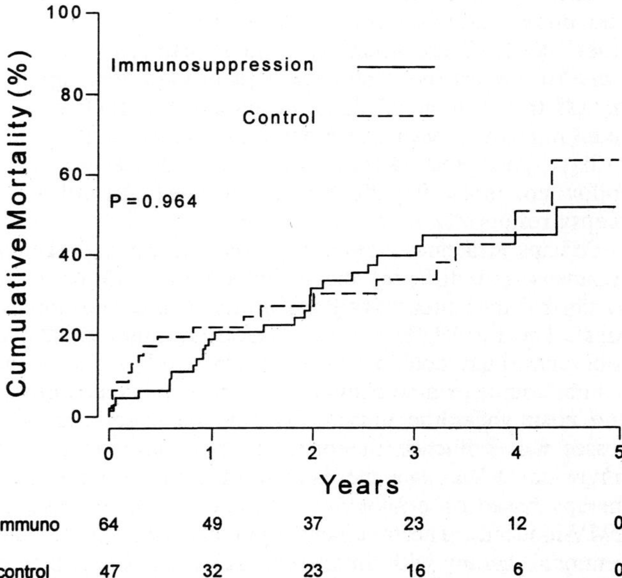

FIGURE 55–4 Cumulative mortality in the Myocarditis Treatment Trial. (Adapted from Mason JW, O'Connell JB, Herskowitz A, et al: A clinical trial of immunosuppressive therapy for myocarditis. N Engl J Med 333:269–275, 1995.)

mune-mediated disease, such as systemic lupus erythematosus, may benefit from immunosuppressive therapy. Other potential indications for a trial of immunosuppressant therapy include failure of myocarditis to resolve, progressive left ventricular dysfunction despite conventional therapy, continued active myocarditis on biopsy, or fulminant myocarditis that does not improve within 24 to 72 hours of full hemodynamic support, including mechanical assistance, and persistent ventricular tachycardia and/or fibrillation.

Smaller studies have used differing immunosuppressant regimens. Kühl and Schultheiss[307] treated 31 patients with biopsies classified as immunohistologically positive (more then two cells per high-power field and expression of adhesion molecules), negative Dallas criteria, and left ventricular dysfunction. Patients were treated with conventional therapy for 3 months, followed by gradual tapering of methylprednisolone doses over 24 weeks (following biopsy and LVEF response). Therapy was associated with an improvement in ejection fraction in 64 percent and improved New York Heart Association functional class in 77 percent. Four patients (12 percent) had no change in ejection fraction despite improvement in inflammatory infiltrates. However, study conclusions are limited by the absence of a control group.

Drucker and coworkers[308] retrospectively reviewed 46 children with congestive cardiomyopathy and Dallas criteria of borderline or definite myocarditis. Twenty-one patients were treated with intravenous IgG (2 g/kg over 24 hours) and were compared to 25 historical controls. Overall survival was not improved, although there was a trend toward improvement in 1-year survival rates in the treated group. In the intravenous IgG group, the left ventricular function was improved and persisted after adjustment for age, biopsy status, and use of ACEIs and inotropes.

In a comparative study of INF-α, thymomodulin, and conventional therapy in patients with biopsy-proven myocarditis or idiopathic DCM, an improvement in the active treatment groups was reported for ejection fraction (at rest and during exercise), maximal exercise time, functional class, and ECG abnormalities.[309] In 10 patients with CHF, New York Heart Association class III or IV, with symptoms of less than 6 months' duration, intravenous IgG resulted in an improvement in LVEF and a functional improvement to New York Heart Association class I or II at 1 year of follow-up, in all 9 patients who survived, regardless of biopsy results.[310]

Perhaps strategies with alternative immunosuppressive regimens and different diagnostic criteria will be more successful in demonstrating the utility of immunosuppressants. The ESETCID[280] is a prospective multicenter, placebo-controlled, double-blind study intended to address the natural course of myocarditis, myopericarditis, pericarditis, and postmyocarditic muscle disease; the underlying processes that influence the progression to chronic disease states or DCM; and the benefit of immunosuppressant therapy based on etiology (autoimmune-, enterovirus-, or CMV-induced). The treatment regimens will include conventional therapy with diuretics, ACEIs, digoxin, and antiarrhythmics or defibrillators, specific therapy for CMV and enteroviral myocarditis, and prednisolone and azathioprine for myocarditis without detectable virus. The duration of blinded therapy is 6 months, with follow-up for 24 months.

Cardiac Transplantation

In a small series (n = 12) composed predominantly of female patients (75 percent), the outcome of patients with active lymphocytic myocarditis confirmed by histologic examination of the explanted heart was significantly worse than in controls undergoing transplantation for other diagnoses.[311] This concern has not been validated in the analysis of outcome of 14,055 cardiac transplant recipients in the registry of the International Society for Heart and Lung Transplantation. One-year actuarial survival in all groups transplanted (idiopathic DCM, myocarditis, peripartum cardiomyopathy, versus other diagnoses) was 80 percent.[312] Nonetheless, myocarditis may recur in the transplanted heart.[313]

Other Variants of Infectious Myocarditis

Human Immunodeficiency Virus and Myocarditis

The advances in treatment strategies for HIV-infected patients have successfully resulted in prolonged survival times, and noninfectious complications of AIDS, such as dementia and heart disease, have become increasingly prevalent. Early in the history of the AIDS epidemic, reports emerged of a rapidly fatal DCM affecting HIV-infected patients.[314, 315] Since the early reports, several clinical and echocardiographic series[316–321] have suggested that a subgroup of HIV-infected patients are predisposed to development of progressive heart disease. In a prospective echocardiographic survey of 296 HIV-infected adults over a period of 4 years, 44 patients were found to have significant cardiac dysfunction. DCM occurred in 13 of 44 and was strongly associated with a CD4 count of less than 100/mm^3 and poorer survival.[321] It has been estimated by some authors that clinically significant cardiac disease occurs in 6 to 7 percent of HIV-seropositive individuals.[322]

An interesting hypothesis to explain the high frequency of dilated heart muscle disease is the presence of myocarditis in HIV-infected patients with left ventricular dysfunction. Reilly and colleagues[323] reported in an autopsy series of 58 consecutive AIDS patients a significantly higher incidence of myocarditis in those with clinically apparent cardiac disease or DCM. There have been other reports of higher prevalence of myocarditis in endomyocardial biopsy series of HIV-seropositive patients compared with those without risk factors for HIV who were biopsied for suspected myocarditis.[324]

HIV-related myocarditis has unique and atypical immunopathogenic features. It is characterized by increased CD8 T lymphocytes and sole induction of MHC class I, perhaps as a part of the systemic depletion of CD4 T cells. The myocarditis may not be readily apparent on histology owing to the accompanying lymphopenia, and special immunohistology and histochemistry techniques may need to be employed.[325] Although in situ hybridization techniques have demonstrated HIV-1 transcripts in cardiac myocytes, interstitial dendritic cells, and endothelial cells, the pathologic significance of this finding is still unclear because patients with evident transcripts may or may not have clinical disease. Also, it is not evident that myocyte injury is a result of direct cytotoxicity of the virus, transcripts, cytokines, or other cardiotropic viruses.[326] A large number of HIV-seropositive patients with left ventricular dysfunction also manifest evidence of nonpermissive or latent infection of myocytes with CMV immediate-early (CMV IE-2) genes. Although evidence for classic intranuclear inclusions of active lytic CMV infection is rarely found, there is increasing speculation that the latent viral infection may be responsible for enhanced MHC expression and provide stimulus for ongoing immune injury, as seen with most models of myocarditis.[327]

A role for direct cytokine-mediated cardiac injury has also been proposed in HIV-infected populations with myocardial dysfunction. TNF-α and IL-6, known to be elevated in HIV infection, directly inhibit cardiac contractility in vitro,[328] and the former has been implicated in causing myocardial dysfunction. Increased catecholamines may be responsible for microvascular spasm and chronic ischemic dysfunction.

The clinical management of patients with HIV-related myocarditis and cardiomyopathy is targeted toward improving congestive symptoms, afterload reduction, and digitalis for improved neurohormonal axis. A specific role for antiviral therapies is controversial, since medications like zidovudine and INF-α are themselves recognized as cardiotoxins. Zidovudine has been known to result in premature termination of myocyte mitochondrial DNA chain replication.[329]

Nonviral Infectious Myocarditis

Bacterial Myocarditis

Bacterial infection of the myocardium occurs frequently in association with infective endocarditis, usually in the form of myocardial abscesses adjacent to the valve ring (see Ch. 3, Chest Radiography). Myocardial involvement has also been reported in association with a wide range of bacterial pathogens in the absence of endocarditis.[330–337] With most of these agents, myocardial involvement is uncommon and occurs principally in the setting of overwhelming systemic infection.

STREPTOCOCCUS

Cardiac involvement after streptococcal infection is usually manifested as acute rheumatic fever, which develops 2 to 3 weeks after onset of pharyngitis and has a distinctive histologic appearance (see Ch. 3, Chest Radiography). Streptococcal pharyngitis may also be associated with a nonrheumatic form of myocarditis that occurs concurrently with the febrile illness.[338–341] The most common clinical manifestations are chest pain and marked ST-segment and T-wave abnormalities on the electrocardiogram, which correlate with segmental wall motion abnormalities observed with echocardiography.[338] Cardiomegaly and CHF are uncommon. Histologic examination reveals lymphocytic infiltrates and myocyte necrosis in the absence of Aschoff bodies, similar to the findings in viral or idiopathic myocarditis.[341] Bacteria are not present in the myocardium, and it is hypothesized that inflammation is caused by streptococcal exotoxins in a manner similar to that in diphtheritic myocarditis.

DIPHTHERIA

Although vaccination has virtually eliminated diphtheria in most Western nations, it remains an important public health problem in many underdeveloped countries.[342] Infection with *C. diphtheriae* is usually confined to the respiratory mucosa. Systemic manifestations are due to secretion of a potent exotoxin. ECG abnormalities suggesting myocardial involvement are present in a high proportion of patients,[343] but clinical evidence of cardiac dysfunction occurs in only 10 to 25 percent of cases. Nevertheless, cardiac involvement is the most common cause of death in fatal infections.[344] Disturbances of AV conduction, including bundle branch blocks and complete AV block, are observed frequently in affected patients and are associated with a mortality rate of 60 to 90 percent. Patients may also present with progressive cardiac dilatation and CHF. Histologic study reveals diffuse mononuclear cell infiltrates associated with myocyte necrosis.[345] Corticosteroid therapy does not appear to be effective in the prevention or treatment of diphtheritic myocarditis, although only one prospective trial has been performed.[346] One report suggested that administration of carnitine may decrease the incidence and severity of cardiac involvement.[347]

Spirochetal Myocardial Disease

LYME DISEASE

Lyme disease is caused by the spirochetal organism *B. burgdorferi*, which is transmitted to humans by certain species of deer ticks in endemic areas of North America, Europe, and Asia. The acute phase of the illness is characterized by fever, myalgia, lymphadenopathy, and a characteristic rash known as *erythema chronicum migrans*.[348] The organism persists in many tissues, and chronic manifestations include arthritis and a variety of neurologic syndromes. Manifestations of cardiac involvement develop in 4 to 10 percent of patients at an average of 4.8 weeks (range 4 days to 7 months) after the acute illness.[349–351] Disturbances of AV conduction are the most common manifestations, occurring in 87 percent of cases, with complete or high-grade block in more than 50 percent. AV block is usually supra-Hisian, with a narrow complex escape rhythm.[352] Temporary transvenous pacing is required frequently, but AV block almost always resolves within 7 to 10 days. Endomyocardial biopsy may reveal lymphocytic infiltrates with associated myocyte necrosis,[352] and spirochetes may be identified in biopsy specimens. Lyme carditis occasionally develops in patients without a preceding rash or other symptoms of acute Lyme disease.[353]

Therapy with a brief course of corticosteroids and either intravenous penicillin or oral tetracycline is recommended for patients with Lyme carditis.[349, 351] Antibiotic therapy has proved effective in the prevention and treatment of chronic arthritic and neurologic syndromes, but its use in cardiac disease has not been tested prospectively. Evidence of diffuse myocardial involvement is common, including evolving ST-segment and T-wave abnormalities on the electrocardiogram, reversible abnormalities of left ventricular wall motion,[349] and diffuse myocardial uptake on gallium scan.[352] One fatal case of pancarditis has been reported, but frank heart failure is uncommon.

A high incidence of positive serologies for *B. burgdorferi* was reported in European patients with chronic DCM, and in two patients, the organism was cultured from myocardial biopsies.[354, 355] It has been suggested that unrecognized Lyme carditis may be responsible for a small but significant proportion of cases of idiopathic DCM.

LEPTOSPIROSIS AND RELAPSING FEVER

Evidence of severe myocarditis is present at autopsy in a high proportion of fatal cases of leptospirosis and relapsing fever.[356–358] Nonspecific ECG abnormalities are common in these diseases, but clinical evidence of left ventricular dysfunction is rare.

Fungal Myocarditis

Although previously uncommon, the incidence of fungal infections of the heart has increased markedly since the early 1970s. This increased incidence is due to several factors, including the increasing use of antibiotics, immunosuppressive agents for transplantation, and chemotherapy, as well as increasing application of cardiac surgery and increasing prevalence of intravenous drug abuse.[359]

CANDIDA INFECTION

The most common fungal organisms causing cardiac infection are *Candida* species. *Candida* endocarditis occurs most frequently after thoracic surgery and in intravenous drug abusers. Immunocompromised patients, on the other hand, are more likely to develop *Candida* myocarditis without involvement of the valves or endocardium, usually in the setting of disseminated systemic infection.[360–362] Autopsy studies reveal extensive myocardial involvement in 10 to 63 percent of patients who die of systemic candidiasis.

Histologically, *Candida* myocarditis is characterized by focal abscesses (usually microscopic, although gross nodules may be present) interspersed with areas of normal myocardium. Clinical manifestations typically include nonspecific ECG abnormalities, disturbances of AV conduction, including complete heart block, and tachyarrhythmias.[360] Cardiomegaly and CHF are rare. Myocardial involvement is usually not recognized antemortem.

ASPERGILLUS INFECTION

Myocardial involvement is present in 22 percent of patients with disseminated aspergillosis,[363] and myocardial invasion is almost always present in patients with *Aspergillus* endocarditis. As in other tissues, histology is characterized by microscopic and macroscopic abscess formation.[363, 364] Extensive vascular invasion by fungal hyphae results in thrombosis and coagulation necrosis. Although *Aspergillus* endocarditis has been treated successfully, myocarditis is uniformly fatal.

ACTINOMYCES INFECTION

Cardiac involvement in actinomycosis occurs in only 2 percent of cases and usually develops by direct extension from a contiguous focus of pulmonary or mediastinal infection.[365–367] Hematogenous seeding of the myocardium occurs occasionally. Myocardial involvement is characterized by necrotizing abscess formation with masses of mycelial bodies and characteristic sulfur granules. In many cases, cardiac symptoms are absent, but patients may present with chest pain characteristic of pericarditis,[366] pericardial tamponade,[367] or CHF.[365]

OTHER MYCOSES

Myocardial involvement has rarely been reported in immunocompromised patients with disseminated coccidioidomycosis and cryptococcosis.[368–371] Cardiac involvement is usually not clinically apparent antemortem, although death due to progressive CHF has been reported.[371] Cardiac involvement with blastomycosis and histoplasmosis is extremely uncommon and usually results from direct extension from a contiguous intrathoracic focus.

Rickettsial Myocarditis

Rocky Mountain spotted fever caused by infection with *Rickettsia rickettsii* is characterized by a diffuse vasculitis, and in fatal cases, death is usually due to vascular collapse. Vasculitis of the coronary vessels may also be present, and lymphocytic infiltrates with myocyte necrosis are present in approximately 50 percent of fatal cases.[372, 373] Although cardiac dilatation and cardiogenic pulmonary edema occur infrequently,[374] echocardiography demonstrates systolic left ventricular dysfunction in the majority of patients.[375, 376] Clinical evidence of myocarditis has been reported in association with scrub typhus due to *R. tsutsugamushi*, whereas Q fever (*Coxiella burnetii*) usually causes endocarditis in its chronic form.

Protozoal Myocarditis

AMERICAN TRYPANOSOMIASIS (CHAGAS' DISEASE)

It is estimated that 10 to 18 million people in South and Central America are infected with *T. cruzi*, and Chagas' cardiomyopathy resulting from this infection is the most common cause of CHF and cardiac death in these endemic areas.[377, 378] The parasite is transferred to humans by triatomine insects known as *reduviid bugs*. The clinical course of infection is characterized by an acute phase, an indeterminate or latent phase of variable duration, and a chronic phase.[378, 379]

After inoculation, parasites are disseminated throughout the body, with the highest concentrations appearing in striated and cardiac muscle and autonomic ganglia. A lesion may appear at the point of entry, and an acute illness develops characterized by fever, myalgia, edema of the face and lower extremities, hepatomegaly, and generalized lymphadenopathy. Because of the nonspecific nature of the symptoms, the acute phase of the disease is usually unrecognized.

Rarely, acute inflammatory myocarditis develops during the acute phase, with ECG abnormalities, cardiomegaly, and CHF. Histologic examination in these cases demonstrates inflammatory infiltrates adjacent to myocytes containing large numbers of intracellular parasites. These findings suggest that cardiac manifestations during the acute phase of the illness may be due to direct lysis of myocytes by parasites.[380, 381]

The acute illness resolves over a period of weeks to months, and patients enter the indeterminate phase. These patients are asymptomatic, with low-level parasitemia, and antibodies to *T. cruzi* are present. Although the electrocardiogram is normal, echocardiography and left ventricular cine angiography demonstrate focal wall motion abnormalities in a high proportion of cases, most commonly involving the left ventricular apex and posterior wall. Endomyocardial biopsy is frequently normal but may reveal hypertrophy, fibrosis, and inflammatory infiltrates in up to 37 percent of patients without clinical manifestations.[382, 383]

Manifestations of chronic Chagas' disease develop in 30 to 70 percent of infected patients after a highly variable period, which may be as long as 50 years.[377, 381] Involvement of autonomic ganglia may cause megacolon or megaesophagus, but the heart is the organ most commonly affected. Histology is characterized by focal areas of inflammation or fibrosis interspersed with areas of normal myocardium. Endomyocardial biopsy reveals myocarditis in approximately 60 percent of patients.[384, 385] This process frequently involves the specialized conducting tissue, and therefore disturbances of AV conduction, especially RBBB with or without associated left anterior fascicular block, are present in up to 60 percent of patients. Complete heart block may require permanent transvenous pacing. Ventricular arrhythmias are also frequent, and the initial manifestation of the disease may be sudden death due to ventricular tachyarrhythmia or complete heart block. Decreased ventricular function is present in almost all patients with chronic Chagas' disease, and in its most advanced form, Chagas' disease presents as a congestive cardiomyopathy with four-chamber dilatation. A characteristic apical aneurysm is usually present.[386–388] Left ventricular thrombus is frequently observed, and systemic embolization is common.[389, 390] This advanced form of the disease is usually fatal within a few years.

Diagnosis of chronic Chagas' cardiomyopathy is dependent on detection of circulating antibodies to *T. cruzi* by one of several serologic methods. Parasites are usually not detected in the myocardium, but low-level parasitemia can be demonstrated by hemoculture or xenodiagnosis, using uninfected reduviid bugs allowed to ingest the patient's blood.[378]

The pathogenic mechanisms leading to myocardial injury, in some patients many years after the initial infection, are poorly understood. The presence of inflammatory infiltrates in the absence of detectable parasites suggests the possibility of autoimmune injury, as postulated for viral and idiopathic myocarditis. Support for this hypothesis includes the demonstration of antibodies to *T. cruzi* as well as anti-idiotypic antibodies that cross-react with myocyte antigens.[391, 392] Histologic studies demonstrate loss of autonomic ganglia, and physiologic studies are suggestive of marked autonomic dysfunction.[393–395]

Withdrawal of parasympathetic tone may lead to excess sympathetic stimulation, which can cause cardiomyopathy. Histologic studies also demonstrate abnormalities of the microvascular bed,[379, 396] and in vitro experiments demonstrate altered endothelial cell function and increased platelet–endothelial cell adhesion.[379, 397] All three reports suggest that progressive focal myocardial disease is the result of ischemia due to obstruction of the microvascular bed.

Treatment of chronic Chagas' cardiomyopathy is supportive, with the use of standard therapy for CHF. Dynamic cardiomyoplasty has resulted in symptomatic improvement in some patients. The role for left ventricular reduction or the commonly known Batista procedure is controversial.[398] Antiarrhythmic therapy may be indicated for sustained ventricular tachyarrhythmias, and a permanent pacemaker should be implanted in patients with high-degree AV block.

Two antiparasitic drugs are available for the treatment of American trypanosomiasis. Both nifurtimox and benznidazole decrease the level and duration of parasitemia and decrease mortality in patients with acute Chagas' disease.[378] Low-level parasitemia persists in most treated patients, however, and it is unclear whether therapy in the acute phase decreases the incidence of subsequent progression to chronic Chagas' disease. Whereas earlier studies with these drugs have not been shown to decrease progression from latent phase to chronic disease or to decrease symptoms or improve cardiac function in patients with chronic disease,[378, 399] the recent studies with itraconazole and allopurinol have shown partial success with parasitologic cure and normalization of ECG changes in nearly half the patients.[400] In a randomized, placebo-controlled trial of benznidazole, there was successful negative seroconversion of 55 percent of patients with early chronic disease as manifested by seropositivity for *T. cruzi*–specific antibodies after treatment for 60 days.[401] Immunosuppressive therapy in patients with malignancies or after organ transplantation has been associated with reactivation causing acute Chagas' disease.[402, 403] Reactivation of Chagas' disease in this setting has usually responded promptly to therapy.[404–406]

AFRICAN TRYPANOSOMIASIS

African trypanosomiasis is caused by *Trypanosoma gambiense* or *T. rhodanese* and characteristically presents with progressive somnolence owing to central nervous system involvement. Autopsy studies demonstrate a pancarditis involving the mural and valvular endocardium as well as the myocardium in up to 50 percent of fatal cases.[407–410] The conduction system and autonomic ganglia may also be involved. Nonspecific abnormalities are often present on the electrocardiogram, but other clinical manifestations of the frequent cardiac involvement are apparently uncommon.

TOXOPLASMOSIS

Patients with acute infection by *T. gondii* are usually asymptomatic, but they may have a transient syndrome of fever and lymphadenopathy. The infection usually persists in a latent phase, with cysts deposited predominantly in the brain and myocardium. Immunosuppression after chemotherapy, in transplant recipients, and in patients with AIDS may be associated with disseminated infection characterized by severe encephalitis and myocarditis.[411–414] Myocarditis after transplantation occurs frequently in seronegative recipients of hearts from seropositive donors.[412–414] Endomyocardial biopsy demonstrates intracellular *Toxoplasma* pseudocysts and a mixed interstitial infiltrate, frequently including eosinophils. *Toxoplasma* myocarditis can be successfully treated with pyrimethamine and sulfadiazine.

Metazoal Myocardial Infection

Cardiac involvement in metazoal infections is uncommon. Up to 2 percent of patients with echinococcosis have cardiac cysts.[415–417] These patients may present with pericardial or atypical chest pain, CHF owing to inflow or outflow obstruction, ventricular arrhythmias, or pulmonary hypertension owing to diffuse pulmonary embolization of scolices. The diagnosis is usually documented by two-dimensional echocardiography, and surgical excision is indicated, when possible, even in asymptomatic patients.

Trichinosis, caused by the parasite *T. spiralis,* is usually a benign syndrome characterized by fever, myositis, and eosinophilia. Mild, asymptomatic myocardial involvement is probably common, as suggested by frequent ECG abnormalities and pericardial effusion noted by echocardiography.[418] Rarely, a severe myocarditis develops, which is the apparent cause of death in most fatal cases.[419–421] Eosinophils are prominent in the interstitial infiltrate. *T. spiralis* does not become encysted in the heart, and larvae are seldom identified in the myocardium. Myocardial injury is thought to be immune mediated, and therapy with corticosteroids is generally recommended, although prospective trials have not been performed owing to the infrequent occurrence of this syndrome.

KAWASAKI'S DISEASE

The mucocutaneous lymph node syndrome or Kawasaki's disease occurs predominantly in children under the age of 10 years and is most prevalent in Japan.[422, 423] It has been recognized worldwide, and in the United States and the developed world it has replaced rheumatic fever as the most common cause of acquired heart disease in children. It is widely believed to have an infectious etiology, but no agent has yet been identified. Its diagnosis is based on recognition of clinical features of the illness, which include remittent high-spiking fever with distinctive conjunctival injection, anterior uveitis, strawberry tongue with erythema, dryness, fissuring and peeling of the lips and mouth, erythematous truncal rash, redness of palms and soles with periungual desquamation, and cervical lymphadenopathy.[424] The principal cardiovascular manifestation of the disease is a multisystem arteritis with frequent involvement of the coronary arteries.[425] Coronary arteritis leads to aneurysm formation and thrombosis. The most common cause of death is myocardial infarction due to aneurysm rupture or coronary occlusion. Myocardium obtained by endomyocardial biopsy or at autopsy reveals histologic evidence of myocarditis in a high proportion of patients.[425–429] Segmental wall motion abnormalities and nonspecific ECG changes are frequently present in the absence of coronary aneurysms.[430, 431] These findings have been attributed to myocarditis, but they might also reflect ischemia due to small vessel arteritis. CHF in the absence of infarction is uncommon. Intravenous gamma-globulin and high-dose aspirin are effective in the prevention of coronary aneurysms and thrombosis,[432] but their effect on myocarditis is not known.

NONINFECTIOUS MYOCARDITIS

Giant Cell Myocarditis

GCM is a rare but frequently fatal disorder. It is defined histologically by extensive but patchy myocyte necrosis with areas of intense multicellular inflammatory infiltration that includes histiocytes, lymphocytes, and the characteristic multinucleated giant cells (Fig. 55–5).[433–436] There has been a great deal of controversy as to whether GCM and cardiac sarcoidosis are distinct pathologic entities because multinucleated giant cells in GCM seldom organize to form granulomas.[437, 438] Litovsky and associates[438] showed that GCM is characterized by myocytic destruction mediated by cytotoxic T cells, macrophagic giant cells, and eosinophils. In contrast, cardiac sarcoid is an interstitial granulomatous disease without myocytic necrosis.[439]

Although the etiology of GCM is unknown, it has been associated with a medley of autoimmune disorders and perhaps is immunologically mediated. Thymomas, systemic lupus, rheumatoid arthritis, Wegener's granulomatosis, ulcerative colitis, chronic hepatitis, myasthenia gravis, myositis, pernicious anemia, Takayasu's arteritis, and lymphomas have been associated with GCM.[440–448] The clinical presentation of GCM may mimic lymphocytic myocarditis, although arrhythmias and heart failure are usually more severe and rapidly progressive.[449, 450] Frequently, patients with GCM will present with conduction system abnormalities, ventricular tachycardia, or even sudden cardiac death.[440, 451–453] GCM has also been reported to present as asymmetric septal hypertrophy.[453]

The natural history of GCM is obscure owing to its rare occurrence, but the isolated reports in literature suggest that it carries a poor prognosis. Davidoff and coworkers[454] reported that 70 percent of patients with GCM required cardiac transplantation or died during a 4-year follow-up period compared with the 29 percent of patients with lymphocytic myocarditis. Cooper and colleagues[455] more recently reported on 63 patients with GCM collected in a worldwide registry. The registry patients had an 89 percent rate of death or need for transplantation, which was significantly worse than that for the 111 patients with lymphocytic myocarditis seen in the MTT. The median survival with GCM was 5.5 months. The patients treated with immunosuppressive regimens including cyclosporine, azathioprine, and prednisone had an average cardiac survival of 12.3 months compared with 3.0 months for the untreated patients. The rate of recurrent GCM in the transplanted patients was 26 percent (9 of 36).

The role of immunosuppressive therapy for GCM is unknown, but at least anecdotal and registry reports suggest

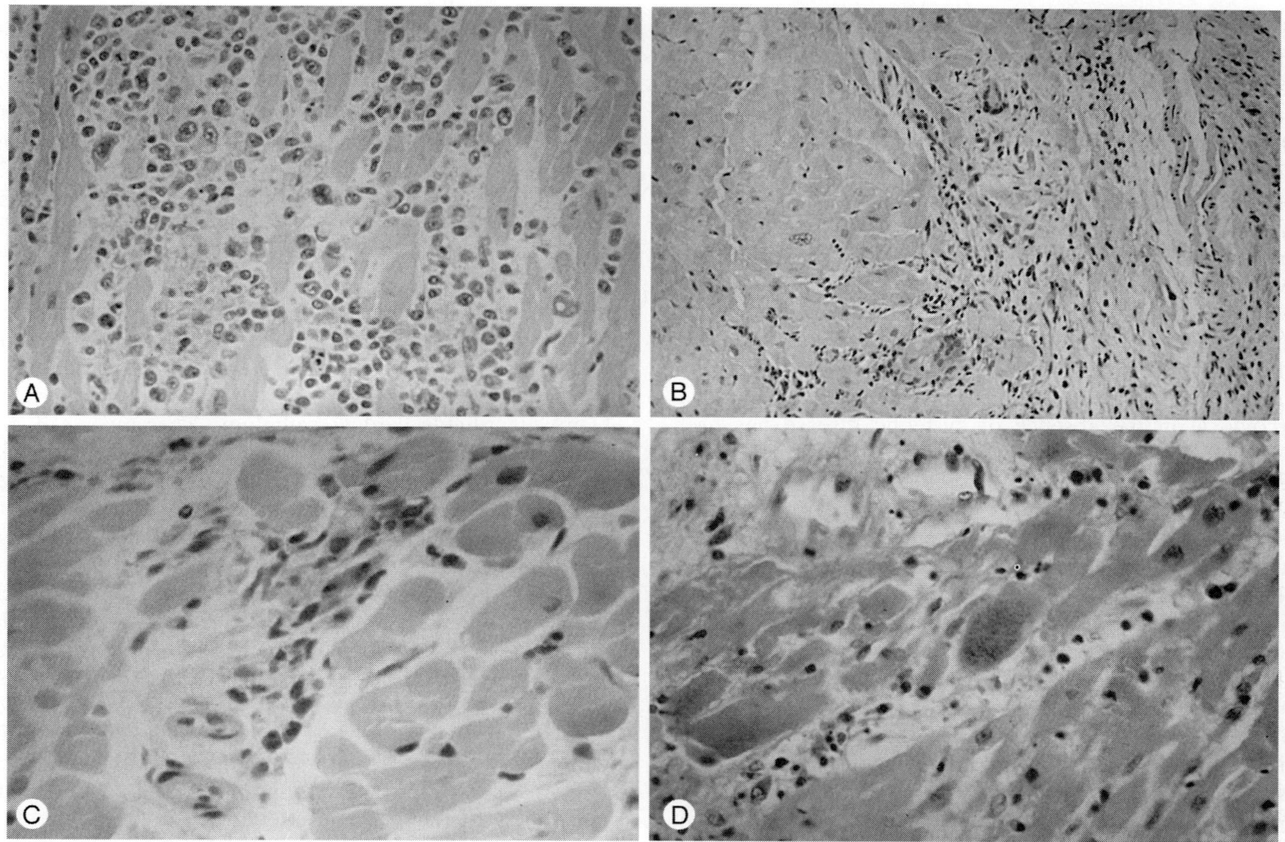

FIGURE 5–5 **A,** Lymphocytic myocarditis. **B,** Giant cell myocarditis. **C,** Eosinophilic myocarditis. **D,** *Toxoplasma* myocarditis. H&E. (**A–D,** Courtesy of Elizabeth H. Hammond, M.D., and Robert F. Yowell, M.D., Department of Pathology, Latter Day Saints, Hospital and the Utah Cardiac Transplant Program, Salt Lake City, Utah.)

possible benefit of cyclosporine and prednisone with or without azathioprine. Cardiac transplantation remains the last therapeutic resort for these patients, although there is risk of recurrent disease,[455–457] which seems to be associated with abatement of immunosuppressive therapy after transplantation[458] and may represent atypical rejection in the allograft.[459] It usually resolves with intensification of the immunosuppressive regimen.

Eosinophilic Myocarditis

The association of eosinophils with cardiac disease was first described by Loffler,[460] who reported "endocarditis parietalis fibroplastica" in association with eosinophilia. The endocardial disease with eosinophilia is well recognized and extensively reviewed elsewhere.[461, 462] Myocardial involvement is rare and frequently fatal; hence, diagnosis is often made postmortem. Endomyocardial biopsy is essential to the antemortem diagnosis of eosinophilic myocarditis.[463] It is believed that myocarditis may represent a more fulminant and necrotic form of the endocardial disease.[464]

Eosinophils have the ability to secrete highly toxic cationic proteins into areas of inflammation and to produce harmful oxygen radicals and potent lipid mediators, leading to myocyte necrosis as seen in proximity of degranulating eosinophils.[465, 466] Animal experiments have confirmed that exposure of myocytes to eosinophil granule proteins is lethal, and there is a reduction in ventricular function in hypereosinophilic states in intact hearts.[467] Eosinophilic myocardial infiltrates have been reported in association with profound eosinophilia caused by an allergic diathesis, parasitic infection, drug hypersensitivity, vasculitis, or Churg-Strauss syndrome,[468–470] but eosinophilic myocarditis can occur in the absence of profound eosinophilia.[471] Further, eosinophilic myocarditis may present as acute myocardial infarction, sudden death, cardiogenic shock, or nonspecific chest pain and dyspnea.

The natural history of eosinophilic myocarditis is usually swift and ominous with rapid evolution to refractory heart failure or intractable arrhythmias, leading to death. Early biopsy-aided histologic confirmation is fundamental to antemortem diagnosis. Clinical improvement may occur with corticosteroid therapy.[471]

Cardiac Sarcoidosis

Sarcoidosis is a multiorgan, noncaseating granulomatous disorder of unknown etiology. Histologically, it may involve the lung, lymph nodes, skin, liver, spleen, parotid glands, and heart.[472] Right heart failure owing to pulmonary manifestations of pulmonary hypertension and pulmonary fibrosis is the predominant cardiac finding.[473] Asymptomatic cardiac involvement is common, with a quarter of the patients having sarcoid granulomas in the heart at autopsy.[474] Characteristically, the noncaseating granulomas infiltrate the ventricular walls and become fibrotic. They may involve the conduction system, although there is no definite predilection for specialized tissues. There may be transmural involvement with fibrous replacement of portions of the myocardium and aneurysm formation.[475] The fibrous transition of granulomas may result in early diastolic dysfunction, but as the disease progresses and with extensive involvement, systolic impairment occurs. Whereas cardiac involvement in sarcoidosis commonly occurs as part of the systemic affliction, isolated cardiac sarcoidosis in the absence of systemic disease has been described.[476]

The clinical presentation of cardiac sarcoidosis is variable and may depend on the amount of myocardium replaced with granulomas and the amount and location of scar tissue. Rhythm abnormalities and conduction disorders predominate,[477] although asymptomatic patients with mildly restrictive filling patterns may elude medical attention. Patients with CHF may show clinical features of restrictive cardiomyopathy or DCM.[478] Papillary dysfunction with mitral regurgitation and pericardial involvement with effusive-constrictive disease have also been described.[477] Radionuclide myocardial imaging with thallium 201 and gallium 67 is helpful in identifying patients with myocardial involvement.[479] Magnetic resonance imaging has also been proposed as a diagnostic modality.[480, 481] Histologic diagnosis with endomyocardial biopsy is corroborative, but a negative biopsy does not rule out the possibility, owing to sampling error.

The finding of pulmonary involvement with bilateral hilar adenopathy and evidence of myocardial disease may suggest cardiac sarcoidosis in a young person. Corticosteroids are indicated when myocardial involvement, conduction abnormalities, and ventricular arrhythmias are present.[482] Patients with scintigraphic uptake of gallium 67 may be more responsive to corticosteroid therapy.[483] Permanent pacemakers may be needed to treat the conduction abnormalities. Implantable defibrillators may be utilized in the prevention of sudden death.[484] Heart failure is treated in the conventional manner, whereas heart transplantation is reserved for intractable heart failure.[485] Heart-lung transplants are performed infrequently for patients with pulmonary involvement, but there is a significant risk of recurrent disease.[485]

Peripartum Myocarditis/Cardiomyopathy

Virchow and Porak first reported the association of pregnancy with DCM in 1870 in an autopsy series.[486] Peripartum myocarditis/cardiomyopathy occurs in 1 of every 3000 to 15,000 pregnancies. The incidence is higher in Africa, and it increases with older age, multiparity, multiple gestations, and prior history of peripartum myocarditis/cardiomyopathy. Peripartum cardiomyopathy is currently believed to be a myocarditis of unknown etiology, perhaps an infectious, autoimmune, or idiopathic process. The viral myocarditis hypothesis stems from the observations that pregnant mice are more susceptible to cardiotropic viruses, with increased viral replication,[487] and with the increased hemodynamic burden of pregnancy, the myocardial lesions worsen.[488] Recently, it has been postulated that after delivery, the rapid degeneration of the uterus results in fragmentation of tropocollagen by enzymatic degradation. This releases actin, myosin, and their metabolites, and antibodies are formed that then cross-react with the myocardium.[486] An association between tocolytic therapy and cardiomyopathy has also been reported.[489]

The diagnosis of peripartum myocarditis/cardiomyopathy must be made within 1 month before delivery of the fetus or 5 months hence. The presentation is usually of decompensated ventricular systolic failure in the absence of any identifiable cardiac pathology. Therapy is tailored to the decompensated state with diuretics, digoxin, and vasodilators (ACEIs are contraindicated in pregnancy). Inotropic therapy may be needed for supporting those in cardiogenic shock, along with use of mechanical circulatory-assist devices. Although there are anecdotal reports of benefit of immunosuppressive therapy,[490] the routine use of these agents cannot be recommended; in fact, the only indication would be biopsy-proven fulminant myocarditis. Cardiac transplantation is an alternative therapeutic option and may be offered to those with intractable heart failure, but it is preferred that transplantation be delayed. The early outcome after transplantation in these patients is often unfavorable, with increased allograft rejection, and the natural history of peripartum myocarditis/cardiomyopathy suggests that more than half of the patients have spontaneous resolution.[491] There are perhaps two different subgroups. One presents with a rapidly progressive, fulminant course with often near-complete resolution of myocardial dysfunction within days and excellent long-term prognosis.[490] The other group has late, insidious onset and presents with progressively worsening heart failure with poor prognosis. It is often difficult to differentiate this from the common variety of DCM.

References

1. Senac JB: Traité de la structure du Couer, de Son Action et de Ses Maladies. 1772.
2. Sobernheim JF: Praktisch Diagnostik der Inneren Kronkheiten mit Vorzuegli der Ruecksicht und pathologische Anatomie. Berlin: Hirschwald, 1837.
3. White PD: Heart Disease. New York: Macmillan, 1931.
4. Richardson P, McKenna WJ, Bristow M, et al: Report of the 1995 World Health Organization/International Society and Federation of Cardiology Task Force on the Definition and Classification of Cardiomyopathies. Circulation 93:841–842, 1996.
5. Aretz HT, Billingham ME, Edwards WD, et al: Myocarditis: histopathologic definition and classification. Am J Cardiovasc Pathol 1:3–14, 1987.
6. Karjalainen J, Heikkila J, Nieminen M, et al: Etiology of mild acute infectious myocarditis. Relation to clinical features. Acta Med Scand 213:65–73, 1983.
7. Sahi T, Karjalainen J, Viitasalo MT, et al: Myocarditis in connection with viral infections in Finnish conscripts. Ann Med Milit Finn 57:198–203, 1982.
8. Karjalainen J, Nieminen M, Heikkila J: Influenza AI myocarditis in conscripts. Acta Med Scand 207:27–30, 1980.
9. Bengtsson E: Electrocardiographic studies in patients with abnormalities in serial examinations with standard leads during acute infectious diseases. 1. Occurrence of abnormalities in STT complex of chest leads in resting electrocardiograms suggestive of localized myocardial lesions. Acta Med Scand 159:395, 1957.

10. Walterson AP: Virological investigations in congestive cardiomyopathy. Postgrad Med 54:505–507, 1978.
11. Kitaura Y: Virological study of idiopathic cardiomyopathy. Jpn Circ J 45:279–294, 1981.
12. Grist NR, Reid D: Epidemiology of viral infections of the heart. *In* Banatvala JE (ed): Viral Infections of the Heart. pp. 23–31. London: Hodder & Stoughton, 1993.
13. Vikerfors T, Stjerna A, Olcen P, et al: Acute myocarditis. Serologic diagnosis, clinical findings and follow-up. Acta Med Scand 223:45–52, 1988.
14. Frisk G, Torfason EG, Diderholm H: Reverse radioimmune assays of IgM and IgG antibodies to Coxsackie B viruses in patients with acute pericarditis. J Med Virol 14:191–200, 1984.
15. Martin AB, Webber S, Fricker FJ, et al: Acute myocarditis. Rapid diagnosis by PCR in children. Circulation 19:330–339, 1994.
16. Muir P, Nicholson F, Illavia SJ, et al: Serological and molecular evidence of enterovirus infection in patients with end-stage dilated cardiomyopathy. Heart 76:243–249, 1996.
17. Tracy S, Chapman NM, McManus BM, et al: A molecular and serological evaluation of enteroviral involvement in human myocarditis. J Mol Cell Cardiol 22:403–414, 1990.
18. Wilson RSE, Morris TH, Russell RJ: Cytomegalovirus myocarditis. Br Heart J 34:865–868, 1972.
19. Wink K, Schmitz H: Cytomegalovirus myocarditis. Am Heart J 100:667–672, 1980.
19a. Maisch B, Schonian U, Crombach M, et al: Cytomegalovirus associated inflammatory heart muscle disease. Scand J Infect Dis 88(suppl):135–148, 1993.
20. Wreghitt T, Cary N: Virus infections in heart transplant recipients and evidence for involvement of the heart. *In* Banatvala JE (ed): Viral Infections of the Heart. pp. 240–250. London: Hodder & Stoughton, 1993.
21. Partanen J, Nieminen MS, Jrogerus L, et al: Cytomegalovirus myocarditis in transplanted heart verified by endomyocardial biopsy. Clin Cardiol 14:846–849, 1991.
22. Matsumori A, Matoba Y, Sasayama S: Dilated cardiomyopathy associated with hepatitis C virus infection. Circulation 92:2519–2525, 1995.
23. Okabe M, Fukuda K, Arakawa K, et al: Chronic variant of myocarditis associated with hepatitis C virus infection. Circulation 96:22–24, 1997.
24. Havaldar PV: Diphtheria in the 80s: experience in a South Indian district hospital. J Indian Med Assoc 19:155–156, 1992.
25. Burt CR, Proudfoot JC, Roberts M, et al: Fatal myocarditis secondary to *Salmonella* septicemia in a young adult. J Emerg Med 8:295–297, 1990.
26. Baysal K, Sancak R, Ozturk F, et al: Cardiac involvement due to *Salmonella typhi* infections in children. Ann Trop Paediatr 18:23–25, 1998.
27. Ledford DK: Immunologic aspects of vasculitis and cardiovascular disease. JAMA 278:1962–1971, 1997.
28. McCallister HF, Klementowica PT, Andrew C, et al: Lyme carditis: an important cause of reversible heart block. Ann Intern Med 110:339–345, 1989.
29. Lewes D, Rainford DJ, Lane WF: Symptomless myocarditis and myalgia in viral and *Mycoplasma pneumoniae* infections. Br Heart J 36:924–932, 1974.
30. Karjalainen J: A loud third heart sound and asymptomatic myocarditis during *Mycoplasma pneumoniae* infection. Eur Heart J 11:960–963, 1990.
31. Odeh M, Oliven A: Chlamydial infections of the heart. Eur J Microbiol Infect Dis 11:885–893, 1992.
32. Fryden A, Kihlstrom E, Maller R, et al: A clinical and epidemiological study of "ornithosis" caused by *Chlamydia psittaci* and *Chlamydia pneumoniae* (strain TWAR). Scand J Infect Dis 21:681–691, 1989.
33. Wesslen L, Pahlson C, Friman G, et al: Myocarditis caused by *Chlamydia pneumoniae* (TWAR) and sudden unexpected death in a Swedish elect orienteer. Lancet 340:427–428, 1992.
34. Page SR, Stewart JT, Bernstein JJ: A progressive pericardial effusion caused by psittacosis. Br Heart J 60:87, 1988.
35. Marin-Garcia J, Mirvis DM: Myocardial disease in Rocky Mountain spotted fever: clinical, functional, and pathologic findings. Pediatr Cardiol 5:149–154, 1984.
36. Schmeer N, Krauss H, Werth D, et al: Serodiagnosis of Q-fever by enzyme-linked immunosorbent assay (ELISA). Zentralbl Bakteriol Mikrobiol Hyg 267:57, 1987.
37. Parada H, Carrasco HA, Anez N, et al: Cardiac involvement is a constant finding in acute Chagas' disease: a clinical, parasitological and histopathological study. Int J Cardiol 60:49–54, 1997.
38. Speirs GE, Hakim M, Calne RY, et al: Relative risk of donor transmitted *Toxoplasma gondii* infection in heart, liver and kidney transplant patients. Clin Transplant 2:257–60, 1988.
39. Albrecht H, Stellbrink HJ, Fenske S, et al: Successful treatment of *Toxoplasma gondii* myocarditis in an AIDS patient. Eur J Microbiol Infect Dis 13:500–504, 1994.
40. Hofman P, Drici MD, Gibelin P, et al: Prevalence of *Toxoplasma* myocarditis in patients with acquired immunodeficiency syndrome. Br Heart J 70:376–381, 1993.
41. Anderson DW, Virmani R, Reilly JM, et al: Prevalent myocarditis at necropsy in acquired immune deficiency syndrome. J Am Coll Cardiol 11:792–799, 1988.
42. Corallo S, Mutimelli MR, Moroni M, et al: Echocardiography detects myocardial damage in AIDS: prospective study in 102 patients. Eur Heart J 9:887–892, 1988.
43. Herskowitz A, Willoughby SB, Baughman KL, et al: Cardiomyopathy associated with anti-retroviral therapy in patients with HIV infection: a report of six cases. Ann Intern Med 116:311–313, 1992.
44. Compton SJ, Celum CL, Lee C, et al: Trichinosis with ventilatory failure and persistent myocarditis. Clin Infect Dis 16:500–504, 1993.
45. French AJ, Weller CV: Interstitial myocarditis following the clinical and experimental use of sulfonamide drugs. Am J Pathol 18:109, 1942.
46. Judge KW, Ward NE: Fatal azide-induced cardiomyopathy presenting as acute myocardial infarction. Am J Cardiol 64:830, 1989.
47. Gravanis MB, Hertzler GL, Franch RH, et al: Hypersensitivity myocarditis in heart transplant candidates. J Heart Lung Transplant 10:688, 1991.
48. Getz MA, Subramanian R, Logemann T, Ballantyne F: Acute necrotizing eosinophilic myocarditis as a manifestation of severe hypersensitivity myocarditis. Antemortem diagnosis and successful treatment. Ann Intern Med 115:201, 1991.
49. Kounis NG, Zavras GM, Soufras GD, Kitrou MP: Hypersensitivity myocarditis. Ann Allergy 62:71, 1989.
50. Burke AP, Saenger J, Mullick F, et al: Hypersensitivity myocarditis. Arch Pathol Lab Med 115:764, 1991.
51. Garty BZ, Offer I, Livni E, Danon YL: Erythema multiforme and hypersensitivity myocarditis caused by ampicillin. Ann Pharmacother 28:730, 1994.
52. Taliercio CP, Olney BA, Lie JT: Myocarditis related to drug hypersensitivity. Mayo Clin Proc 60:463, 1985.
53. Samlowski WE, Ward JH, Craven CM, Freedman RA: Severe myocarditis following high dose interleukin-2 therapy. Am J Med 88:438, 1990.
54. Nariman S: Adverse reactions to drugs used in the treatment of tuberculosis. Adverse Drug React Toxicol Rev 7:207, 1988.
55. Fagan E, Forbes A, Williams R: Toxic myocarditis in paracetamol poisoning. BMJ 296:63, 1988.
56. Misset B, Escudier B, Leclercq B, et al: Acute myocardiotoxicity during 5-fluorouracil therapy. Intensive Care Med 16:210, 1990.
57. Martin M, Diaz-Rubio E, Furio V, et al: Lethal cardiac toxicity after cisplatin and 5-fluorouracil chemotherapy. Report of a case with necropsy study. Am J Clin Oncol 12:229, 1989.
58. Rowinsky EK, Eisenhauer EA, Chaudhry V, et al: Clinical toxicities encountered with paclitaxel (Taxol). Semin Oncol 20:1, 1993.
59. Mandell BF: Cardiovascular involvement in systemic lupus erythematosus. Semin Arthritis Rheum 17:126–141, 1987.
60. Doherty NE, Siegel RJ: Cardiovascular manifestations of systemic lupus erythematosus. Am Heart J 110:1257–1265, 1985.
61. Bacon PA, Gibson DG: Cardiac involvement in rheumatoid arthritis. An echocardiographic study. Ann Rheum Dis 33:20–24, 1974.
62. Botstein GR, LeRoy EC: Primary heart disease in systemic sclerosis (scleroderma): advances in clinical and pathologic features, pathogenesis, and new therapeutic approaches. Am Heart J 102:913–919, 1981.
63. Dalakas MC: Polymyositis, dermatomyositis, and inclusion-body myositis. N Engl J Med 325:1487–1498, 1991.
64. Oka M, Raasakka T: Cardiac involvement in polymyositis. Scand J Rheum 7:203–208, 1978.
65. Graham DC, Smythe HA: The carditis and aortitis of ankylosing spondylitis. Bull Rheum Dis 9:171–175, 1958.

66. Bergfeldt L: HLA B27 associated cardiac disease. Ann Intern Med 127:621–629, 1997.
67. Fauci AS, Harley JG, Roberts WC, et al: The idiopathic hypereosinophilic syndrome: clinical, pathophysiologic and therapeutic considerations. Ann Intern Med 97:78, 1982.
68. Parrillo JE, Borer JS, Henry WL, et al: The cardiovascular manifestations of hypereosinophilic syndrome: prospective study of 26 patients, with review of literature. Am J Med 67:572, 1979.
69. Parrillo JE: Heart disease and the eosinophil. N Engl J Med 323:1560–1561, 1990.
70. Brockington IF, Olsen EGJ: Loffler's endocarditis and Davies' endomyocardial fibrosis. Am Heart J 85:308, 1973.
71. Dilling NV: Giant cell myocarditis. J Pathol Bacteriol 71:295, 1956.
72. Fukahara T, Morino M, Sakoda S, et al: Myocarditis with multinucleated giant cells detected in biopsy specimens. Clin Cardiol 11:341, 1988.
73. Wilson MS, Barth RF, Baker PB, et al: Giant cell myocarditis. Am J Med 79:647, 1985.
74. Mason JW: Distinct forms of myocarditis. Circulation 83:1110, 1990.
75. McFalls EO, Hosenpud JD, McAnulty JH, et al: Granulomatous myocarditis: diagnosis by endomyocardial biopsy and response to corticosteroids in two patients. Chest 89:509, 1986.
76. Gauntt C, Higdon A, Bowers D, et al: What lessons can be learned from the animal model studies in viral heart diseases? Scand J Infect Dis 88(suppl):49–65, 1993.
77. Herskowitz A, Wolfgram LJ, Rose NR, Beisel KW: Coxsackievirus B3 murine myocarditis: a pathologic spectrum of myocarditis in genetically defined inbred strains. J Am Coll Cardiol 9:1311–1319, 1987.
78. Kyu B-S, Matsumori A, Sato Y, et al: Cardiac persistence of cardioviral RNA detected by polymerase chain reaction in a murine model of dilated cardiomyopathy. Circulation 86:522–530, 1992.
79. Wee L, Liu P, Penn L, et al: Persistence of viral genome into late stages of murine myocarditis detected by polymerase chain reaction. Circulation 86:1605–1614, 1992.
80. Kandolf R, Ameis D, Kirschner P, et al: In situ detection of enteroviral genomes in myocardial cells by nucleic acid hybridization: an approach to the diagnosis of viral heart disease. Proc Natl Acad Sci U S A 84:6272–6276, 1987.
81. Wolfgram LJ, Rose NR: Coxsackie virus infection as a trigger of cardiac autoimmunity. Immunol Res 8:61–80, 1989.
82. Neumann DA, Rose NR, Ansari AA, et al: Induction of multiple heart autoantibodies in mice with coxsackievirus B3 and cardiac myosin induced autoimmune myocarditis. J Immunol 152:343–350, 1994.
83. Oldstone MBA: Molecular mimicry and autoimmune disease. Cell 50:819, 1987.
84. Beisel KW, Srinivasappa J, Prabhakar BS: Identification of a putative shared epitope between coxsackievirus B4 and alpha cardiac myosin heavy chain. Clin Exp Immunol 86:49–55, 1991.
85. Maisch B, Bauer E, Cirst M, et al: Cytolytic crossreactive antibodies directed against cardiac membranes and viral proteins in coxsackievirus B3 and B4 myocarditis. Characterization and pathogenetic relevance. Circulation 87(suppl IV):IV-49–IV-65, 1993.
86. Cunningham MW, Antone SM, Gulizia JM, et al: Cytotoxic and viral neutralizing antibodies crossreact with streptococcal M protein, enteroviruses and human cardiac myosin. Proc Natl Acad Sci U S A 89:1320–1324, 1992.
87. Gauntt CJ, Higdon AL, Arizpe HM, et al: Epitopes shared between coxsackievirus B3 (CVB3) and normal heart tissue contribute to CVB3-induced murine myocarditis. Clin Immunol Immunopathol 68:129–134, 1993.
88. Schwimmbeck PL, Schwimmbeck NK, Schultheiss HP, et al: Mapping of antigenic determinants of adenine nucleotide translocator and coxsackie B3 virus with synthetic peptides: use for the diagnosis of viral heart disease. Clin Immunol Immunopathol 68:135–140, 1993.
89. Weller AH, Simpson K, Herzum M, et al: Coxsackie B3 induced myocarditis: virus receptor antibodies modulate myocarditis. J Immunol 143:1843–1850, 1989.
90. Limas CJ, Goldenberg IF, Limas C: Autoantibodies against beta-adrenoreceptors in human dilated cardiomyopathy. Circ Res 64:97–103, 1989.
91. Wolff PG, Kuhl U, Schultheiss HP: Laminin distribution and autoantibodies to laminin in dilated cardiomyopathy and myocarditis. Am Heart J 117:1303–1309, 1989.
92. Ansari AA, Herskowitz A, Danner DJ: Identification of mitochondrial proteins that serve as targets for autoimmunity [abstract]. Circulation 78(suppl):457, 1988.
93. Latif N, Baker CS, Dunn MJ, et al: Frequency and specificity of antiheart antibodies in patients with dilated cardiomyopathy detected using SDS-PAGE and Western blotting. J Am Coll Cardiol 22:1378–1384, 1993.
94. Huber SA, Job LP, Woodruff JF: Lysis of infected myofibers by coxsackievirus B3 immune T lymphocytes. Am J Pathol 98:681–694, 1980.
95. Huber SA, Lodge PA: Coxsackievirus B3 in Balb/c mice: evidence for autoimmunity to myocyte antigens. Am J Pathol 116:21–29, 1984.
96. Seko Y, Shinkai Y, Kawasaki A, et al: Expression of perforins in infiltrating cells in murine hearts with acute myocarditis caused by coxsackievirus B3. Circulation 84:788–795, 1991.
97. Felzen B, Shilkrut M, Less H, et al: Fas (CD95/Apo1)–mediated damage to ventricular myocytes induced by cytotoxic T lymphocytes from perforin deficient mice: a major role for inositol 1,4,5-triphosphate. Circ Res 82:438–450, 1998.
98. Maisel A, Cesario D, Baird S, et al: Experimental autoimmune myocarditis produced by adoptive transfer of splenocytes after myocardial infarction. Circ Res 82:458–463, 1998.
99. Neu N, Rose NR, Biesel KW, et al: Cardiac-myosin induces myocarditis in genetically predisposed mice. J Immunol 139:3630–3636, 1987.
100. Adesanya CO, Goldberg AH, Phear WPC, et al: Heart muscle performance after experimental viral myocarditis. J Clin Invest 57:569–575, 1976.
101. Woodruff JF, Woodruff JJ: Involvement of T lymphocytes in the pathogenesis of Coxsackie virus B3 heart disease. J Immunol 113:1726–1734, 1974.
102. Woodruff JF, Kilbourne ED: The influence of quantitated post-weaning undernutrition on coxsackievirus B3 infection of adult mice. I. Viral persistence and increased severity of lesions. J Infect Dis 121:137–163, 1970.
103. Godeny EK, Gauntt CJ: Interferon and natural killer cell activity in coxsackievirus B3 induced murine myocarditis. Eur Heart J 8(suppl J):433–435, 1987.
104. Godeny EK, Gauntt CJ: In situ immune autoradiographic identification of cells in heart tissues of mice with coxsackievirus B3–induced myocarditis. Am J Pathol 129:267–276, 1987.
105. Entman ML, Youker K, Shoji T, et al: Neutrophil induced oxidative injury of cardiac myocytes. J Clin Invest 90:1335–1345, 1992.
106. Godeny EK, Gauntt CJ: Murine natural killer cells limit coxsackievirus B3 replication. J Immunol 139:913–918, 1987.
107. Huber SA: Viral and immune mechanisms in cardiac disease. *In* Spry CJF (ed): Immunology and Molecular Biology of Cardiovascular Disease. pp. 143–159. Boston: MTP, 1987.
108. Landau BJ: Replication of coxsackievirus B3 in primary mouse cell cultures of cardiac origin. Abstracts of the Annual Meeting of the American Society of Microbiology, 1978. p. 233. Washington, DC: American Society of Microbiology, 1978.
109. Chow LH, Beisel KW, McManus BM: Enteroviral infection of mice with severe combined immunodeficiency: evidence for direct viral pathogenesis of myocardial injury. Lab Invest 66:24–31, 1992.
110. Rager-Zisman B, Allison AC: Effects of immunosuppression on Coxsackie B3 virus in mice and passive protection by circulating antibody. J Gen Virol 19:339–351, 1973.
111. Kilbourne ED, Wilson CB, Perrier D: The induction of gross myocardial lesions by Coxsackie (pleurodynia) virus and cortisone. J Clin Invest 35:362–370, 1956.
112. Wong CY, Woodruff JJ, Woodruff JF: Generation of cytotoxic T lymphocytes during coxsackievirus B3 infection. II. Characterization of effector cells and demonstration of cytotoxicity against viral infected myofibers. J Immunol 118:1165–1169, 1977.
113. Hufnagel G, Chapman N, Tracy S: A noncardiovirulent strain of coxsackievirus B3 causes myocarditis in mice with severe combined immunodeficiency syndrome. Eur Heart J 16(suppl O):18–19, 1995.
114. Modlin J: Coxsackieviruses, echoviruses, and newer enteroviruses. *In* Mandell G, Douglas R, Bennett J (eds): Principles and Practice of Infectious Diseases. New York: Churchill Livingstone, 1990.
115. Lodge PA, Herzum M, Olszewski J, et al: Coxsackievirus B3 myo-

carditis: acute and chronic forms of the disease caused by different immunopathogenic mechanisms. Am J Pathol 128:455–463, 1987.

116. Seko Y, Tsuchimochi H, Nakamura T, et al: Expression of major histocompatibility complex class I antigen in murine ventricular myocytes infected with coxsackievirus B3. Circ Res 67:360–367, 1990.
117. Germain RN: MHC dependent antigen processing and peptide presentation: providing ligands for T lymphocyte activation. Cell 76:287–289, 1994.
118. Monrad ES, Matsumori A, Murphy JC, et al: Cyclosporine therapy in experimental murine myocarditis with encephalomyocarditis virus. Circulation 73:1058–1064, 1986.
119. O'Connell JB, Reap EA, Robinson JA: The effects of cyclosporine on acute murine Coxsackie B3 myocarditis. Circulation 73:353–359, 1986.
120. Estrin M, Smith C, Huber S: Coxsackievirus B3 myocarditis. T-cell autoimmunity to heart antigens is resistant to cyclosporin-A treatment. Am J Pathol 125:244–251, 1986.
121. Klingel K, Hohenadl C, Canu A, et al: Ongoing enterovirus induced myocarditis is associated with persistent heart muscle infection: quantitative analysis of virus replication, tissue damage, and inflammation. Proc Natl Acad Sci U S A 89:314–318, 1992.
122. Wilson FM, Miranda QR, Chason JL, et al: Residual pathologic changes following murine Coxsackie A and B myocarditis. Am J Pathol 55:253–265, 1969.
123. Huber SA, Heintz N, Tracy R: Coxsackievirus B3 induced myocarditis: virus and actinomycin D treatment of myocytes induces novel antigens recognized by cytolytic T lymphocytes. J Immunol 141:3214–3219, 1988.
124. Lutton CW, Gauntt CJ: Coxsackievirus B3 infection alters the plasma membrane of neonatal skin fibroblasts. J Virol 60:294–296, 1986.
125. Kawai S, Azuma M, Yagita H, et al: Expression of co-stimulatory molecules B7-1, B7-2, and CD40 in the heart of patients with acute myocarditis and dilated cardiomyopathy. Circulation 97:637–639, 1998.
126. Morad M, Davies NW, Ulrich G, et al: Antibodies against ADP-ATP carrier enhance Ca^{2+} current in isolated cardiac myocytes. Am J Physiol 255:H960–H964, 1988.
127. Rose ML, Coles MI, Griffin RJ, et al: Expression of class I and class II major histocompatibility antigens in normal and transplanted human heart. Transplantation 41:776–780, 1986.
128. Herskowitz A, Ansari AA, Neumann DA, et al: Induction of major histocompatibility complex (MHC) antigens within the myocardium of patients with active myocarditis: a nonhistologic marker of myocarditis. J Am Coll Cardiol 15:624–632, 1990.
129. Ahmed-Ansari A, Tadros TS, Knopf WD, et al: Major histocompatibility complex class I and class II expression by myocytes in cardiac biopsies posttransplantation. Transplantation 45:972–978, 1988.
130. Hammond EH, Menlove RL, Yowell RL, et al: Vascular HLA-DR expression correlates with pathologic changes suggestive of ischemia in idiopathic dilated cardiomyopathy. Clin Immunol Immunopathol 68:197–203, 1993.
131. Hammond EH, Menlove RL, Anderson JL: Predictive value of immunofluorescence and electron microscopic evaluation of endomyocardial biopsies in the diagnosis and prognosis of myocarditis and idiopathic dilated cardiomyopathy. Am Heart J 114:1055–1065, 1987.
132. Wang YC, Herskowitz A, Gu LB, et al: Influence of cytokines and immunosuppressive drugs on major histocompatibility complex class I/II expression by human cardiac myocytes in vitro. Hum Immunol 31:1–11, 1991.
133. Ansari AA, Wang YC, Danner DJ, et al: Abnormal expression of histocompatibility and mitochondrial antigens by cardiac tissue from patients with myocarditis and dilated cardiomyopathy. Am J Pathol 139:337–354, 1991.
134. Carlquist JF, Menlove RL, Murray MB, et al: HLA class II (DR and DQ) antigen associations in idiopathic dilated cardiomyopathy. Circulation 83:515–522, 1991.
135. Marriott SJ, Roeder DJ, Consigli RA: Anti-idiotypic antibodies to a polyomavirus monoclonal antibody recognize cell surface components of mouse kidney cells and prevent polyomavirus infection. J Virol 61:2747–2753, 1987.
136. Erlanger BF, Cleveland WL, Wasserman NH, et al: Auto-anti-idiotype: a basis for autoimmunity and a strategy for anti-receptor antibodies. Immunol Rev 94:23–37, 1986.
137. Weremeichik H, Moraska A, Herzum M, et al: Naturally occurring anti-idiotypic antibodies: mechanisms of autoimmunity and immunoregulation? Eur Heart J 12(suppl D):154–157, 1991.
138. Paque RE, Miller R: Anti-idiotype pulsed B cells in the induction and expression of autoimmune myocarditis. Clin Immunol Immunopathol 68:111–117, 1993.
139. Neumann, Lane JR, Allen GS, et al: Viral myocarditis leading to cardiomyopathy: do cytokines contribute to pathogenesis? Clin Immunol Immunopathol 68:181–190, 1993.
140. Kroemer G, Martinez AC: Cytokines and auto-immune disease. Clin Immunol Immunopathol 61:275–295, 1991.
141. Entman ML, Youker K, Shappel SB, et al: Neutrophil adherence to isolated adult canine myocytes. J Clin Invest 85:1497–1506, 1990.
142. Baggiolini M, Walz A, Kunkel SL: Neutrophil activating peptide-1/interleukin 8, a novel cytokine that activates neutrophils. J Clin Invest 84:1045–1049, 1989.
143. Smith KA: Interleukin-2: inception, impact and implication. Science 240:1169–1176, 1988.
144. Arai K, Lee F, Miyajima A, et al: Cytokines: coordinators of immune and inflammatory responses. Annu Rev Biochem 59:783–836, 1990.
145. Postlewaite AE, Kang AH: Induction of fibroblast proliferation by human mononuclear leukocyte derived protein. Arthritis Rheum 26:22–27, 1983.
146. Barry WH: Mechanisms of immune-mediated myocyte injury. Circulation 89:2421–2432, 1994.
147. Gulick T, Pieper ST, Murphy MA, et al: Interleukin 1 and tumor necrosis factor inhibit cardiac myocyte beta adrenergic responsiveness. Proc Natl Acad Sci U S A 86:6753–6757, 1989.
148. Balligand JL, Ungureanu D, Kelly RA, et al: Abnormal contractile function due to induction of nitric oxide synthesis in rat cardiac myocytes follows exposure to activated macrophage-conditioned medium. J Clin Invest 91:2314–2319, 1993.
149. Smith TW, Balligand JL, Kaye DM, et al: The role of NO pathway in the control of cardiac function. J Cardiac Fail 2:S141–S148, 1996.
150. Freeman GL, Colston JT, Zabalgoitia M, et al: Contractile depression and expression of proinflammatory cytokines and iNOS in viral myocarditis. Am J Physiol 274:H249–H258, 1998.
151. Zaragoza C, Ocampo C, Saura M, et al: The role of inducible nitric oxide synthase in the host response to coxsackievirus myocarditis. Proc Natl Acad Sci U S A 95:2469–2474, 1998.
152. Beck AC, Ward JH, Hammond EH, et al: Cardiomyopathy associated with high-dose interleukin-2 therapy. West J Med 155:293–296, 1991.
153. Brady AJ, Poole-Wilson PA, Harding SE, et al: Nitric oxide production within cardiac myocytes reduces their contractility in endotoxemia. Am J Physiol 263:H1963–H1966, 1992.
154. Yokoyama T, Vaca L, Rossen RD, et al: Cellular basis for the negative inotropic effects of tumor necrosis factor-alpha in the adult mammalian heart. J Clin Invest 92:2303–2312, 1993.
155. Bryant D, Becker L, Richardson J, et al: Cardiac failure in transgenic mice with myocardial expression of tumor necrosis factor-alpha. Circulation 97:1375–1381, 1998.
156. Toyozaki T, Saito T, Takano H, et al: Increased serum levels of circulating intercellular adhesion molecule-1 in patients with myocarditis. Cardiology 87:189–193, 1996.
157. Matsumori A, Yamada T, Suzuki H, et al: Increased circulating cytokines in patients with myocarditis and cardiomyopathy. Br Heart J 72:561–566, 1994.
158. Huber SA, Polgar J, Schultheiss P, Schwimmbeck P: Augmentation of pathogenesis of coxsackievirus B3 infections in mice by exogenous administration of interleukin-1 and interleukin-2. J Virol 68:195–206, 1994.
159. Ishido S, Sakaue M, Asaka K, Maeda S: Detection of transforming growth factor-β1 in Coxsackie B3 virus-induced murine myocarditis. Acta Histochem Cytochem 28:137–142, 1995.
160. Herskowitz A, Neumann DA, Ansari AA: Concepts of autoimmunity applied to idiopathic dilated cardiomyopathy. J Am Coll Cardiol 22:1385–1388, 1993.
161. Leslie KO, Schwarz J, Simpson K, et al: Progressive interstitial collagen deposition in coxsackievirus B3 myocarditis. Am J Pathol 136:683–693, 1990.
162. Matsumori A, Crumpacker CS, Abelmann WH: Prevention of encephalomyocarditis virus myocarditis in mice by inactivated virus vaccine. *In* Sekiguchi M, Olsen EGJ, Goodwin JF (eds): Myocarditis and Related Disorders. pp. 228–229. Tokyo: Springer-Verlag, 1995.

163. Matsumori A, Wang H, Abelmann WH, Crumpacker CS: Treatment of viral myocarditis with ribavirin in an animal preparation. Circulation 71:834–839, 1985.
164. Kishimoto C, Crumpacker CS, Abelmann WH: Ribavirin treatment of murine coxsackievirus B3 myocarditis with analyses of lymphocyte subsets. J Am Coll Cardiol 12:1334–1341, 1988.
165. Matsumori A, Crumpacker CS, Abelmann WH: Prevention of viral myocarditis with recombinant human leukocyte interferon alpha A/D in a murine model. J Am Coll Cardiol 9:1320–1325, 1987.
166. Kanda T, McManus JEW, Nagai R, et al: Modification of viral myocarditis in mice by interleukin-6. Circ Res 78:848–856, 1996.
167. Yamamoto N, Shibamori M, Ogura M, et al: Effects of intranasal administration of recombinant murine interferon-gamma on murine acute myocarditis caused by encephalomyocarditis virus. Circulation 97:1017–1023, 1998.
168. Tomioka N, Kishimoto C, Matsumori A, Kawai C: Effects of prednisolone on acute viral myocarditis in mice. J Am Coll Cardiol 7:868–872, 1986.
169. Costanzo-Nordin MR, Reap EA, O'Connell JB, et al: A nonsteroid antiinflammatory drug exacerbates Coxsackie B3 murine myocarditis. J Am Coll Cardiol 6:1078–1082, 1985.
170. Rezkalla S, Khatib G, Khatib R: Coxsackievirus B3 murine myocarditis: deleterious effects of nonsteroidal anti-inflammatory agents. J Lab Clin Med 107:393–395, 1986.
171. Kishimoto C, Thorp KA, Abelmann WH: Immunosuppression with high doses of cyclophosphamide reduces the severity of myocarditis but increases the mortality in murine coxsackievirus B3 myocarditis. Circulation 82:982–989, 1990.
172. O'Connell JB, Reap EA, Robinson JA: The effects of cyclosporine on acute murine Coxsackie B3 myocarditis. Circulation 73:353–359, 1986.
173. Monrad ES, Matsumori A, Murphy JC, et al: Therapy with cyclosporine in experimental murine myocarditis with encephalomyocarditis virus. Circulation 73:1058–1064, 1986.
174. Rezkalla S, Kloner RA, Khatib G, Khatib R: Effect of delayed cyclosporine therapy on left ventricular mass and myonecrosis during acute coxsackievirus murine myocarditis. Am Heart J 120:1377–1380, 1990.
175. McManus BM, Caruso HR, Stratta RJ, Wilson JE: Impact of FK 506 on myocarditis in the enteroviral murine model. Transplant Proc 23:3365–3367, 1991.
176. Kanda T, Nagaoka H, Kaneko K, et al: Synergistic effects of tacrolimus and human interferon-α A/D in murine viral myocarditis. J Pharmacol Exp Ther 274:487–493, 1995.
177. Yamada T, Matsumori A, Sasayama S: Therapeutic effect of anti-tumor necrosis factor-α antibody on the murine model of viral myocarditis induced by encephalomyocarditis virus. Circulation 89:846–851, 1994.
178. Matsui S, Matsumori A, Matoba Y, et al: Treatment of virus-induced myocardial injury with a novel immunomodulating agent, vesnarinone. J Clin Invest 94:1212–1217, 1994.
179. Matsumori A: The use of cytokine inhibitors. A new therapeutic insight into heart failure. Int J Cardiol 62(suppl 1):S3–S12, 1997.
180. Stevens PJ, Ground KE: Occurrence and significance of myocarditis in trauma. Aerosp Med 41:776–780, 1970.
181. Gore I, Saphir O: Myocarditis. A classification of 1402 cases. Am Heart J 34:827, 1947.
182. Okada R, Wakafuji S: Myocarditis in autopsy. *In* Sekiguchi M, Olsen EGJ, Goodwin JF (eds): Myocarditis and Related Disorders. pp. 23–29. Berlin: Springer-Verlag, 1985.
183. Gardiner AJS: Four faces of acute myopericarditis. Br Heart J 35:433, 1973.
184. Dec GW, Waldman H, Southern J, et al: Viral myocarditis mimicking acute myocardial infarction. J Am Coll Cardiol 20:85–89, 1992.
185. Costanzo-Nordin MR, O'Connell JB, Subramanian R: Myocarditis confirmed by biopsy presenting as acute myocardial infarction. Br Heart J 53:25–29, 1985.
186. Saffitz JE, Schwartz DJ, Southworth W, et al: Coxsackie viral myocarditis causing transmural right and left ventricular infarction without coronary narrowing. Am J Cardiol 52:644–647, 1983.
187. Herskowitz A, Campbell S, Deckers J, et al: Demographic features and prevalence of idiopathic myocarditis in patients undergoing endomyocardial biopsy. Am J Cardiol 71:982–986, 1993.
188. Burch GE, Shewey LL: Viral coronary arteritis and myocardial infarction. Am Heart J 92:11–14, 1976.
189. Ferguson DW, Farwell AP, Bradley WA, Rollings RC: Coronary artery vasospasm complicating acute myocarditis: a rare association. West J Med 148:664–669, 1988.
190. Friedman RA, Duff DF: Myocarditis. *In* Feig RD, Cherry JD (eds): Textbook of Pediatric Infectious Diseases. pp. 393–413. Philadelphia: WB Saunders, 1987.
191. Onoughi Z, Haba S, Kiyosawa N, et al: Stokes-Adams attacks due to acute nonspecific myocarditis in childhood. Jpn Heart J 21:307–315, 1980.
192. Frustaci A, Cameli S, Zeppilli P: Biopsy evidence of atrial myocarditis in an athlete developing transient sinoatrial disease. Chest 108:1460–1462, 1995.
193. Talwar KK, Radhakrishnan S, Chopra P: Myocarditis manifesting as persistent atrial standstill. Int J Cardiol 20:283–286, 1988.
194. Straumanis JP, Wiles HB, Case CL: Resolution of atrial standstill in a child with myocarditis. Pacing Clin Electrophysiol 16:2196–2201, 1993.
195. Nakazato Y, Nakata Y, Hisaoka T, et al: Clinical and electrophysiological characteristics of atrial standstill. Pacing Clin Electrophysiol 18:1244–1254, 1995.
196. Liao PK, Seward JB, Hagler DJ, et al: Acute myocarditis associated with transient marked myocardial thickening and complete atrioventricular block. Clin Cardiol 7:356–362, 1984.
197. Shah SS, Hellenbrand WE, Gallagher PG: Atrial flutter complicating neonatal Coxsackie B2 myocarditis. Pediatr Cardiol 19:185–186, 1998.
198. Frustaci A, Chimenti C, Bellocci F, et al: Histological substrate of atrial biopsies in patients with lone atrial fibrillation. Circulation 96:1180–1184, 1997.
199. Reitman MJ, Zirin HJ, DeAngelis CJ: Complete heart block in Epstein-Barr myocarditis. Pediatrics 62:847–849, 1978.
200. Arita M, Ueno Y, Masuyama Y: Complete heart block in mumps myocarditis. Br Heart J 46:342–344, 1981.
201. Salvi A, Grazia ED, Silvestri F, Camerini F: Acute rickettsial myocarditis and advanced atrioventricular block: diagnosis and treatment aided by endomyocardial biopsy. Int J Cardiol 7:405–409, 1985.
202. Karjalainen J, Viitasalo M, Kala R, Heikkila J: 24-hour electrocardiographic recordings in mild acute infectious myocarditis. Ann Clin Res 16:34–39, 1984.
203. Tai Y-T, Law C-P, Fong P-C, et al: Incessant automatic ventricular tachycardia complicating acute Coxsackie B myocarditis. Cardiology 30:339–344, 1992.
204. Zeppilli P, Santini C, Cameli S, et al: Brief report: healed myocarditis as a cause of ventricular repolarization abnormalities in athlete's heart. Int J Sports Med 18:213–216, 1997.
205. Zeppilli P, Santini C, Palmieri V, et al: Role of myocarditis in athletes with minor arrhythmias and/or echocardiographic abnormalities. Chest 106:373–380, 1994.
206. Maron BJ, Shirani J, Poliac LC, et al: Sudden death in young competitive athletes. Clinical, demographic, and pathological profiles. JAMA 276:199–204, 1996.
207. Phillips M, Robinowitz M, Higgins JR, et al: Sudden cardiac death in Air Force recruits: a 20-year review. JAMA 256:2696–2699, 1986.
208. Gravanis MB, Sternby NH: Incidence of myocarditis: a 10-year autopsy study from Malmo, Sweden. Arch Pathol Lab Med 115:390–392, 1991.
209. Passarino G, Burlo P, Ciccone G, et al: Prevalence of myocarditis at autopsy in Turin, Italy. Arch Pathol Lab Med 121:619–622, 1997.
210. Burlo P, Comino A, Di Gioia V, et al: [Adult myocarditis in a general hospital: observations on 605 autopsies]. Pathologica 87:646–649, 1995.
211. Wesslen L, Pahlson C, Lindquist O, et al: An increase in sudden unexpected cardiac deaths among young Swedish orienteers during 1979–1992. Eur Heart J 17:902–910, 1996.
212. Maron BJ: Sudden death in young athletes. Lessons from the Hank Gathers affair. N Engl J Med 329:55–57, 1993.
213. Shatz A, Hiss J, Arensburg B: Myocarditis misdiagnosed as sudden infant death syndrome (SIDS). Med Sci Law 37:16–18, 1997.
214. Arvan S, Manalo E: Sudden increase in left ventricular mass secondary to acute myocarditis. Am Heart J 116:200–202, 1988.
215. James KB, Lee K, Thomas JD, et al: Left ventricular diastolic dysfunction in lymphocytic myocarditis as assessed by Doppler echocardiography. Am J Cardiol 73:282–285, 1994.
216. Kondo M, Takahashi M, Shimono Y, et al: Reversible asymmetric

septal hypertrophy in acute myocarditis: serial findings of two-dimensional echocardiogram and thallium-201 scintigram. Jpn Circ J 49:589–593, 1985.
217. Lieberman EB, Herskowitz A, Rose NR, Baughman KL: A clinicopathologic description of myocarditis. Clin Immunol Immunopathol 68:191–196, 1993.
218. Mason JW, O'Connell JB, Herskowitz A, et al: A clinical trial of immunosuppressive therapy for myocarditis. N Engl J Med 333:269–275, 1995.
219. Grist NR, Bell EJ: A six year study of Coxsackie B virus infections in heart disease. J Hyg [Lond] 73:165–172, 1974.
220. Smith WG: Coxsackie B myopericarditis in adults. Am Heart J 80:34–46, 1970.
221. Wojnicz R, Kozielska K, Szczurek J, et al: HLA, ICAM-1 and VCAM-1 molecules in the endomyocardial biopsy specimens—patients with clinically suspected myocarditis [abstract]. Eur Heart J 18(suppl):594, 1997.
222. Toyozaki T, Hiroe M, Saito T, et al: Levels of soluble Fas in patients with myocarditis, heart failure of unknown origin, and in healthy volunteers. Am J Cardiol 81:798–800, 1998.
223. Myocarditis Treatment Trial (MTT) Investigators: Incidence and clinical characteristics of myocarditis [abstract]. Circulation 84(suppl II):II-2, 1991.
224. Lauer B, Niederau C, Kuhl U, et al: Cardiac troponin T in patients with clinically suspected myocarditis. J Am Coll Cardiol 30:1354–1359, 1997.
225. Smith SC, Ladenson JH, Mason JW, et al: Elevations of cardiac troponin I associated with myocarditis. Experimental and clinical correlates. Circulation 95:163–168, 1997.
226. Morgera T, DiLenarda A, Dreas L, et al: Electrocardiography of myocarditis revisited: clinical and prognostic significance of electrocardiographic changes. Am Heart J 124:455–467, 1992.
227. Take M, Sekiguchi M, Hiroe M, et al: Long-term follow-up of electrocardiographic findings in patients with acute myocarditis proven by endomyocardial biopsy. Jpn Circ J 46:1227–1234, 1982.
228. Vignola PA, Aounuma K, Swaye PS, et al: Lymphocytic myocarditis presenting as unexplained ventricular arrhythmias: diagnosis with endomyocardial biopsy and response to immunosuppression. J Am Coll Cardiol 4:812, 1984.
229. Nieminen MS, Heikkla J, Karjalainen J: Echocardiography in acute infectious myocarditis: relation to clinical and echocardiographic findings. Am J Cardiol 53:1331–1337, 1984.
230. Mendes LA, Picard MH, Dec GW, et al: Discordance of right and left ventricular remodeling in active myocarditis. J Am Coll Cardiol 23:365A, 1994.
231. James KB, Lee K, Thomas JD, et al: Left ventricular diastolic dysfunction in lymphocytic myocarditis as assessed by Doppler echocardiography. Am J Cardiol 73:282–285, 1994.
232. Kojima J, Miyazaki S, Fujiwara H, et al: Recurrent left ventricular mural thrombi in a patient with acute myocarditis. Heart Vessels 4:120–122, 1988.
233. Pinamonti B, Alberti E, Cigalotto A, et al: Echocardiographic findings in myocarditis. Am J Cardiol 62:285–291, 1988.
234. O'Connell JB, Henkin RE, Robinson JA, et al: Gallium-67 imaging in patients with dilated cardiomyopathy and biopsy proven myocarditis. Circulation 70:58–62, 1984.
235. Yasuda T, Palacios IF, Dec GW, et al: Indium-111 monoclonal antimyosin antibody imaging in the diagnosis of acute myocarditis. Circulation 76:306–311, 1987.
236. Khaw BA, Narula J: Non-invasive detection of myocyte necrosis in myocarditis and dilated cardiomyopathy with radiolabelled antimyosin. Eur Heart J 16(suppl O):119–123, 1995.
237. Lauer B, Kuhl U, Souvatzoglu M, et al: Correlation of antimyosin-scintigraphy with histological and immunohistological findings in the endomyocardial biopsy in patients with clinically suspected myocarditis [abstract]. J Am Coll Cardiol 31(suppl A)110A, 1998.
238. Dec GW, Palacios I, Yasuda T, et al: Antimyosin antibody cardiac imaging: its role in the diagnosis of myocarditis. J Am Coll Cardiol 13:97–104, 1989.
239. Friedrich MG, Strohm O, Schulz-Menger J, et al: Contrast media–enhanced magnetic resonance imaging visualizes myocardial changes in the course of viral myocarditis. Circulation 97:1802–1809, 1998.
240. Neubauer S, Horn M, Pabst T, et al: Contributions of ^{31}P-magnetic resonance spectroscopy to the understanding of dilated heart muscle disease. Eur Heart J 16(suppl O):115–118, 1995.
241. Van Dobbenburgh JO, de Jonge N, Klopping C, et al: Altered myocardial energy metabolism in heart transplant patients: consequences of rejection or post-ischemic phenomena. *In* Proceedings of the 12th Annual Meeting of the Society of Magnetic Resonance in Medicine, August 14–20, 1993. p. 1093. New York: SMRM, 1993.
242. Shirey EK, Hawk WA, Mukerji D, et al: Percutaneous myocardial biopsy of the left ventricle. Experience in 198 patients. Circulation 46:112–122, 1972.
243. Sutton GC, Driscoll JF, Gunnar RM, et al: Exploratory mediastinotomy in primary myocardial disease. Prog Cardiovasc Dis 7:83–97, 1964.
244. Sakakibara S, Konno S: Endomyocardial biopsy. Jpn Heart J 3:537–543, 1962.
245. Mason JW, Billingham ME, Ricci DR: Treatment of acute inflammatory myocarditis assisted by endomyocardial biopsy. Am J Cardiol 45:1037–1044, 1980.
246. Baandrup U, Olsen EGJ: Critical analysis of endomyocardial biopsies from patients suspected of having cardiomyopathy. I: morphological and morphometric aspects. Br Heart J 45:475–486, 1981.
247. Fenoglio JJ, Ursell PC, Kellogg CF, et al: Diagnosis and classification of myocarditis by endomyocardial biopsy. N Engl J Med 308:12–18, 1983.
248. Rose AG, Fraser RC, Beck W: Absence of evidence of myocarditis in endomyocardial biopsy specimens from patients with dilated (congestive) cardiomyopathy. S Afr Med J 66:871–874, 1984.
249. Daly K, Richardson PJ, Olsen EGJ, et al: Acute myocarditis. Role of histological and virological examination in the diagnosis and assessment of immunosuppressive treatment. Br Heart J 51:30–35, 1984.
250. Parrillo JE, Aretz HT, Palacios I, et al: The results of transvenous endomyocardial biopsy can frequently be used to diagnose myocardial diseases in patients with idiopathic heart failure. Circulation 69:93–101, 1984.
251. Regitz V, Olsen EGJ, Rudolph W: Histologisch nachweisbare Myokarditis bei Patienten mit eingeschrankter linksventrikularer Funktion. Herz 10:27–35, 1985.
252. Cassling RS, Linder J, Sears TD, et al: Quantitative evaluation of inflammation in biopsy specimens from idiopathically failing or irritable hearts: experience in 80 pediatric and adult patients. Am Heart J 110:713–720, 1985.
253. Salvi A, Silvestri F, Gori D, et al: Endomyocardial biopsy: initial experience in 156 patients. G Ital Cardiol 15:251–259, 1985.
254. Dec GW, Palacios IF, Fallon JT, et al: Active myocarditis in the spectrum of acute dilated cardiomyopathies. Clinical features, histologic correlates, and clinical outcomes. N Engl J Med 312:885–890, 1985.
255. Mortensen SA, Baandrup U, Buck J, et al: Immunosuppressive therapy of biopsy proven myocarditis: experiences with corticosteroids and cyclosporin. Int J Immunotherapy 1:35–45, 1985.
256. Hammond EH, Menlove RL, Anderson JL: Predictive value of immunofluorescence and electron microscopic evaluation of endomyocardial biopsies in the diagnosis and prognosis of myocarditis and idiopathic dilated cardiomyopathy. Am Heart J 114:1055–1065, 1987.
257. Meany BT, Quigley PJ, Olsen EGJ, et al: Recent experience of endomyocardial biopsy in the diagnosis of myocarditis. Eur Heart J 8:17–18, 1987.
258. Chow LC, Dittrich HC, Shabetai R: Endomyocardial biopsy in patients with unexplained congestive heart failure. Ann Intern Med 109:535–539, 1988.
259. Maisch B, Bauer E, Hufnagel G, et al: The use of endomyocardial biopsy in heart failure. Eur Heart J 9:59–71, 1988.
260. Hobbs RE, Pelegrin D, Ratliff NB, et al: Lymphocytic myocarditis and dilated cardiomyopathy: Treatment with immunosuppressive agents. Cleve Clin J Med 56:628–635, 1989.
261. Popma JJ, Cigarroa RG, Buja LM, Hillis LD: Diagnostic and prognostic utility of right-sided catheterization and endomyocardial biopsy in idiopathic dilated cardiomyopathy. Am J Cardiol 63:955–958, 1989.
262. Vasiljevic JD, Kanjuh V, Seferovic P, et al: The incidence of myocarditis in endomyocardial biopsy samples from patients with congestive heart failure. Am Heart J 120:1370–1377, 1990.
263. Lieberman EB, Hutchins GM, Herskowitz A, et al: Clinicopathologic description of myocarditis. J Am Coll Cardiol 18:1617–1626, 1991.

264. Herskowitz A, Campbell S, Deckers J, et al: Demographic features and prevalence of idiopathic myocarditis in patients undergoing endomyocardial biopsy. Am J Cardiol 71:982–986, 1993.
265. Kuhl U, Noutsias M, Seeberg B, Schultheiss H-P: Immunohistological evidence for a chronic intramyocardial inflammatory process in dilated cardiomyopathy. Heart 75:295–300, 1996.
266. Arbustini E, Gavazzi A, Dal Bello B, et al: Ten-year experience with endomyocardial biopsy in myocarditis presenting with congestive heart failure: frequency, pathologic characteristics, treatment and follow-up. G Ital Cardiol 27:209–223, 1997.
267. Strain JE, Grose RM, Factor SM, et al: Results of endomyocardial biopsy in patients with spontaneous ventricular tachycardia but without apparent structural heart disease. Circulation 68:1171–1181, 1983.
268. Sugrue DD, Holmes DR Jr, Gersh BJ, et al: Cardiac histologic findings in patients with life-threatening ventricular arrhythmias of unknown origin. J Am Coll Cardiol 4:952–957, 1984.
269. Take M, Sekiguchi M, Hiroe M, et al: A clinicopathologic study on a cause of idiopathic cardiomyopathy and arrhythmia and conduction disturbance employing endomyocardial biopsy. Heart Vessels Suppl 1:159–164, 1985.
270. Hosenpud JD, McAnulty JH, Niles NR: Unexpected myocardial disease in patients with life threatening arrhythmias. Br Heart J 56:55–61, 1986.
271. Yoshizato T, Edwards WD, Alboliras ET, et al: Safety and utility of endomyocardial biopsy in infants, children and adolescents: a review of 66 procedures in 53 patients. J Am Coll Cardiol15:436–442, 1990.
272. Sekiguchi M, Nishizawa M, Nunoda S, et al: Endomyocardial biopsy approach in cases with ventricular arrhythmias. Postgrad Med J 68(suppl 1):S40–S43, 1992.
273. Wiles HB, Gillette PC, Harley RA, et al: Cardiomyopathy and myocarditis in children with ventricular ectopic rhythm. J Am Coll Cardiol 20:359–362, 1992.
274. Thongtang V, Chiathiraphan S, Ratanarapee S, et al: Prevalence of myocarditis in idiopathic dysrhythmias: role of endomyocardial biopsy and efficacy of steroid therapy. J Med Assoc Thai 76:368–373, 1993.
275. Aretz HT, Billingham ME, Edwards WD, et al: The utility of the Dallas Criteria for the histopathological diagnosis of myocarditis in endomyocardial biopsy specimens [abstract]. Circulation 88(suppl I):I-552, 1993.
276. Dec GW, Fallon JT, Southern JF, Palacios I: "Borderline" myocarditis: an indication for repeat endomyocardial biopsy. J Am Coll Cardiol 15:283–289, 1990.
277. Billingham ME: Endomyocardial biopsy detection of acute rejection in cardiac allograft recipients. Heart Vessels Suppl 1:86–90, 1985.
278. Hauck AJ, Kearney DL, Edwards WD: Evaluation of postmortem endomyocardial biopsy specimens from 38 patients with lymphocytic myocarditis: implications for role of sampling error. Mayo Clin Proc 64:1235–1245, 1989.
279. Chow LH, Radio SJ, Sears TE, et al: Insensitivity of right ventricular endomyocardial biopsy in the diagnosis of myocarditis. J Am Coll Cardiol 14:915–920, 1989.
280. Hufnagel G, Maisch B: The European Study of Epidemiology and Treatment of Cardiac Inflammatory Disease (ESETCID)—first epidemiological results [abstract]. Eur Heart J 18(suppl):594, 1997.
281. Kato H, Ichinose E, Kawasaki T: Myocardial infarction in Kawasaki disease: clinical analysis in 195 cases. J Pediatr 108:923–927, 1986.
282. Hasumi M, Sekiguchi M, Morimoto S, et al: Ventriculographic findings in the convalescent stage in eleven cases with acute myocarditis. Jpn Circ J 47:1310–1316, 1983.
283. Frustaci A, Maseri A: Localized left ventricular aneurysms with normal global function caused by myocarditis. Am J Cardiol 70:1221–1224, 1992.
284. O'Connell JB, Mason JW: Diagnosing and treating active myocarditis. West J Med 150:431–435, 1989.
285. Woodruff JF: Viral myocarditis. A review. Am J Pathol 101:425–484, 1980.
286. Martin AB, Webber S, Fricker J, et al: Acute myocarditis. Rapid diagnosis by PCR in children. Circulation 90:330–339, 1994.
287. Keeling PJ, Lukaszyk A, Poloniecki J, et al: A prospective case control study of antibodies to Coxsackie B virus in idiopathic dilated cardiomyopathy. J Am Coll Cardiol 23:593–8, 1994.
288. Martino TA, Liu P, Sole MJ: Enterovirus myocarditis and dilated cardiomyopathy: a review of clinical and experimental studies. *In* Rotbart HA (ed): Human Enterovirus Infections. pp. 291–350. Washington, DC: American Society of Microbiology, 1995.
289. Baboonian C, Treasure T: Meta-analysis of the association of enteroviruses with human heart disease. Heart 78:539–543, 1997.
290. Mendes LA, Dec GW, Picard MH, et al: Right ventricular dysfunction: an independent predictor of adverse outcome in patients with myocarditis. Am Heart J 128:301–307, 1994.
291. Ilbäck N-G, Fohlman J, Friman G: Exercise in coxsackie B3 myocarditis: effects on heart lymphocyte subpopulations and the inflammatory reaction. Am Heart J 117:1298–1302, 1989.
292. Reyes MP, Lerner AM: Coxsackievirus myocarditis—with special reference to acute and chronic effects. Prog Cardiovasc Dis 27:373, 1985.
293. Costanzo-Nordin MR, Reap EA, O'Connell JB, et al: A non-steroidal anti-inflammatory drug exacerbates coxsackievirus B3 murine myocarditis. J Am Coll Cardiol 6:1078, 1985.
294. Maron BJ, Isner JM, McKenna WJ: Task Force 3: hypertrophic cardiomyopathy, myocarditis and other myopericardial diseases and mitral valve prolapse. J Am Coll Cardiol 24:845–899, 1994.
295. Cohn JN: ACE inhibitors in non-ischemic heart failure: results from the MEGA trials. Eur Heart J 16(suppl O):133–6, 1995.
296. Rezkalla S, Kloner RA, Khatib G, Khatib R: Beneficial effects of captopril in acute coxsackievirus B3 murine myocarditis. Circulation 81:1039–1046, 1990.
297. Waagstein F: Adrenergic beta-blocking agents in congestive heart failure due to idiopathic dilated cardiomyopathy. Eur Heart J 16(suppl O):128–132, 1995.
298. Rezkalla S, Kloner RA, Khatib G, et al: Effect of metoprolol in coxsackie virus B3 murine myocarditis. J Am Coll Cardiol 12:412–414, 1988.
299. Tominaga M, Matsumori A, Okada I, et al: β-Blocker treatment of dilated cardiomyopathy. Beneficial effect of carteolol in mice. Circulation 83:2021–2028, 1991.
300. Mason JW: Arrhythmias associated with myocarditis. Cardiac Electrophysiol Rev 1/2:268–269, 1997.
301. Garrison RF, Swisher RC: Myocarditis of unknown etiology (Fiedler's) treated with ACTH. J Pediatr 42:591, 1953.
302. Aingler LE: Acute aseptic myocarditis: corticosteroid therapy. J Pediatr 64:716, 1964.
303. Gagliardi MG, Bevilacqua M, Squitieri C, et al: Dilated cardiomyopathy caused by acute myocarditis in pediatric patients: evolution of myocardial damage in a group of potential heart transplant candidates. J Heart Lung Transplant 12:S224–S229, 1993.
304. O'Connell JB, Mason JW: Immunosuppressive therapy in experimental and clinical myocarditis. Pathol Immunopathol Res 7:292, 1988.
305. Hosenpud JD, McAnulty JH, Niles NR: Lack of objective improvement in ventricular systolic function in patients with myocarditis treated with azathioprine and prednisone. J Am Coll Cardiol 6:797, 1985.
306. Cooper LT, Berry GJ, Shabetai R: Idiopathic giant-cell myocarditis—natural history and treatment. Multicenter Giant Cell Myocarditis Study Group Investigators. N Engl J Med 336:1860–1866, 1997.
307. Kühl U, Schultheiss H-P: Treatment of chronic myocarditis with corticosteroids. Eur Heart J 16:168–172, 1995.
308. Drucker NA, Colan SD, Lewis AB, et al: Gamma-globulin treatment of acute myocarditis in the pediatric population. Circulation 89:252–257, 1994.
309. Miric M, Vasiljevic J, Bojic M, et al. Long-term follow-up of patients with dilated heart muscle disease treated with human leucocytic interferon alpha or thymic hormones: initial results. Heart 75:596–601, 1996.
310. McNamara DM, Rosenblum WD, Janosko KM, et al: Intravenous immune globulin in the therapy of myocarditis and acute cardiomyopathy. Circulation 95:2476–2478, 1997.
311. O'Connell JB, Dec GW, Goldenberg IF, et al: Results of heart transplantation for active lymphocytic myocarditis. J Heart Lung Transplant 9:351–356, 1990.
312. O'Connell JB, Breen TJ, Hosenpud JD: Heart transplantation in dilated heart muscle disease and myocarditis. Eur Heart J 16(suppl O):137–139, 1995.
313. Grant SC: Recurrent giant cell myocarditis after transplantation. J Heart Lung Transplant 12:155–156, 1993.
314. Autran BR, Gorin I, Lerbowitch M: AIDS in a Haitian woman with

cardiac Kaposi's sarcoma and Whipple's disease. Lancet 1:767–768, 1983.
315. Himelman RB, Chung WS, Chernoff DN, et al: Cardiac manifestations of human immunodeficiency virus infection: a two dimensional echocardiographic study. J Am Coll Cardiol 13:1030–1036, 1989.
316. Monseuz JJ, Kinney EL, Vittecoq D, et al: Comparison among acquired immuno-deficiency syndrome patients with and without clinical evidence of cardiac disease. Am J Cardiol 62:1311–1313, 1988.
317. Levy WS, Simon GL, Rios JC, et al: Prevalence of cardiac abnormalities in human immunodeficiency virus infection. Am J Cardiol 63:86–89, 1989.
318. Hsia J, Adams S, Mohanty N, et al: Human immunodeficiency virus related heart disease during 560 patient-years of follow-up [abstract]. Circulation 86(suppl 1):I-795, 1992.
319. Herskowitz A, Vlahov D, Willoughby SB, et al: Prevalence and incidence of left ventricular dysfunction in patients with human immuno-deficiency virus infection. Am J Cardiol 71:955–958, 1993.
320. Herskowitz A, Willoughby SB, Baughman KL, et al: Cardiomyopathy associated with anti-retroviral therapy in patients with human immuno-deficiency virus infection: a report of six cases. Ann Intern Med 116:311–313, 1992.
321. Currie PF, Jacob AJ, Foreman AR, et al: Heart muscle disease related to HIV infection: prognostic implications. BMJ 309:1605–1607, 1994.
322. Anderson DW, Virmani R. Emerging patterns of heart disease in human immunodeficiency virus infection. Hum Pathol 21:253–259, 1990.
323. Reilly JM, Cunnion RE, Anderson DW, et al: Frequency of myocarditis, left ventricular dysfunction and ventricular tachycardia in the acquired immuno-deficiency syndrome. Am J Cardiol 62:789–793, 1988.
324. Herskowitz A, Willoughby SB, Vlahov D, et al: Dilated heart muscle disease associated with HIV infection. Eur Heart J 16(suppl O):50–55, 1995.
325. Beschorner WE, Baughman KL, Turnicky RP, et al: HIV-associated myocarditis: pathology and immunopathology. Am J Pathol 137:1365–1371, 1990.
326. Herskowitz A, Willoughby SB, Wu TC, et al: Immunopathogenesis of HIV-1 associated cardiomyopathy. Clin Immunol Immunopathol 68:234–241, 1993.
327. Wu TC, Pizzorno MC, Hayward GS, et al: In situ detection of human cytomegalovirus immediate-early gene transcripts within cardiac myocytes of patients with HIV-associated cardiomyopathy. AIDS 6:777–785, 1992.
328. Finkel MS, Oddis CV, Jacob TD, et al: Negative inotropic effects of cytokines on the heart mediated by nitric oxide. Science 257:387–390, 1992.
329. Benbrik E, Chariot P, Bonavaud S, et al: Cellular and mitochondrial toxicity of zidovudine (AZT), didanosine (ddI) and zalcitabine (ddC) on cultured human muscle cells. J Neurol Sci 149:19–25, 1997.
330. Shalit M, Braverman AJ, Eliakim M: Congestive heart failure in the course of typhoid fever. J Infect 4:81, 1982.
331. Brasier AR, Macklis JD, Vaughan D, et al: Myopericarditis as an initial presentation of meningococcemia. Am J Med 82:64, 1987.
332. Gross D, Willens H, Zeldis SM: Myocarditis in legionnaires' disease. Chest 79:232, 1981.
333. McCue MJ, Moore EE: Myocarditis with microabscess formation caused by *Listeria monocytogenes* associated with myocardial infarction. Hum Pathol 10:469, 1979.
334. Chen SC, Tsai CC, Nouri S: Carditis associated with *Mycoplasma pneumoniae* infection. Am J Dis Child 140:471, 1986.
335. Le-Van-Diem AK: Typhoid fever with myocarditis. Am J Trop Med Hyg 23:218, 1974.
336. Lewes D, Rainford DJ, Lane WF: Symptomless myocarditis and myalgia in viral and *Mycoplasma pneumoniae* infection. Br Heart J 36:924, 1974.
337. Ringel RE, Brenner JI, Rennels MB, et al: Serologic evidence for *Chlamydia trachomatis* myocarditis. Pediatrics 70:54, 1982.
338. Karjalainen J: Streptococcal tonsillitis and acute nonrheumatic myopericarditis. Chest 95:359, 1989.
339. Caraco J, Arnon R, Raz I: Atrioventricular block complicating acute streptococcal tonsillitis. Br Heart J 59:389, 1988.
340. Putterman C, Caraco Y, Shalit M: Acute nonrheumatic perimyocarditis complicating streptococcal tonsillitis. Cardiology 78:156, 1991.
341. Gore I, Saphir O: Myocarditis associated with acute nasopharyngitis and acute tonsillitis. Am Heart J 34:831, 1947.
342. MacGregor RR: *Corynebacterium diphtheriae*. *In* Mandell GL, Douglas RG, Bennett JE (eds): Principles and Practice of Infectious Diseases. pp. 1574–1581. New York: Churchill Livingstone, 1990.
343. Boyer NH, Weinstein L: Diphtheritic myocarditis. N Engl J Med 239:913, 1948.
344. Morgan BC: Cardiac complications of diphtheria. Pediatrics 32:549, 1963.
345. Burch GE, Sun S-C, Sohal R, et al: Diphtheritic myocarditis: a histochemical and electron microscopic study. Am J Cardiol 21:261, 1968.
346. Thisyakorn U, Wongvanich J, Kumpeng V: Failure of corticosteroid therapy to prevent diphtheritic myocarditis or neuritis. Pediatr Infect Dis 3:126, 1984.
347. Ramos ACMF, Elias PRP, Barrucand L, Da Silva JAF: The protective effect of carnitine in human diphtheric myocarditis. Pediatr Res 18:815, 1984.
348. Duray PH: Clinical pathologic correlations of Lyme disease. Rev Infect Dis 11(suppl 6):S1487, 1989.
349. Steere AC, Batsford WP, Weingerg M, et al: Lyme carditis: abnormalities of Lyme disease. Ann Intern Med 93:8, 1980.
350. McCalister HF, Klementowicz PT, Andrews C, et al: Lyme carditis: an important cause of reversible heart block. Ann Intern Med 110:339, 1989.
351. Olson LJ, Okafor EC, Clements IP: Cardiac involvement in Lyme disease: manifestations and management. Mayo Clin Proc 61:745, 1986.
352. Reznick JW, Braunstein DB, Walsh RL, et al: Lyme carditis. Am J Med 81:923, 1985.
353. Kimball SA, Janson PA, LaRaia PJ: Complete heart block as the sole presentation of Lyme disease. Arch Intern Med 149:1897, 1989.
354. Stanek G, Klein J, Bittner R, Glogar D: Isolation of *Borrelia burgdorferi* from the myocardium of a patient with longstanding cardiomyopathy. N Engl J Med 322:249, 1990.
355. Klein J, Stanek G, Bittner R, et al: Lyme borreliosis as a cause of myocarditis and heart muscle disease. Eur Heart J 12(suppl D):73, 1991.
356. Farrar WE: *Leptospira* species (leptospirosis). *In* Mandell GL, Douglas RG, Bennett JE (eds): Principles and Practice of Infectious Diseases. pp. 1813–1816. New York: Churchill Livingstone, 1990.
357. Arean VM: The pathologic anatomy and pathogenesis of fatal human leptospirosis (Weil's disease). Am J Pathol 40:393, 1962.
358. Southern PM Jr, Sanford JP: Relapsing fever: a clinical and microbiological review. Medicine 48:129, 1969.
359. Atkinson JB, Connor DH, Robinowitz M, et al: Cardiac fungal infections: review of autopsy findings in 60 patients. Hum Pathol 15:935, 1984.
360. Franklin WG, Simon AB, Sodeman TM: *Candida* myocarditis without valvulitis. Am J Cardiol 38:924, 1976.
361. Ihde DC, Roberts WC, Marr KC, et al: Cardiac candidiasis in cancer patients. Cancer 41:2364, 1978.
362. Parker JC: The potentially lethal problem of cardiac candidiases: Am J Clin Pathol 73:356, 1980.
363. Schwartz DA: *Aspergillus* pancarditis following bone marrow transplantation for chronic myelogenous leukemia. Chest 95:1338, 1989.
364. Williams A: *Aspergillus* myocarditis. Am J Clin Pathol 61:247, 1974.
365. Dutton WP, Inclan AP: Cardiac actinomycosis. Chest 54:463, 1968.
366. Cole FH, Larrett CL: Primary actinomycosis of the pericardium. South Med J 75:1028, 1982.
367. Slutzker AD, Claypool WD: Pericardial actinomycosis with cardiac tamponade from a contiguous thoracic lesion. Thorax 44:442, 1989.
368. Vartivarian SE, Coudron PE, Markowitz SM: Disseminated coccidioidomycosis. Am J Med 83:949, 1987.
369. Lafont A, Wolff M, Marche C, et al: Overwhelming myocarditis due to *Cryptococcus neoformans* in an AIDS patient. Lancet 2:1145, 1987.
370. Lewis W, Lipsick J, Cammarosano C: Cryptococcal myocarditis in acquired immune deficiency syndrome. Am J Cardiol 55:1240, 1985.
371. Hagar JM, Rahimtoola SH: Chagas' heart disease in the United States. N Engl J Med 325:763, 1991.
372. Bradford W, Hackel DB: Myocardial involvement in Rocky Mountain spotted fever. Arch Pathol Lab Med 102:357, 1978.
373. Marin-Garcia J, Gooch WM, Coury DL: Cardiac manifestations of Rocky Mountain spotted fever. Pediatrics 67:358, 1981.

374. Lankford HV, Glauser FL: Cardiopulmonary dynamics in a severe case of Rocky Mountain spotted fever. Arch Intern Med 140:1357, 1980.
375. Marin-Garcia J, Barrett FF: Myocardial function in Rocky Mountain spotted fever. Am J Cardiol 51:341, 1983.
376. Feltes TF, Wilcox WD, Feldman WE, et al: M-mode echocardiographic abnormalities in Rocky Mountain spotted fever. South Med J 77:1130, 1984.
377. Dias JCP: The indeterminate form of human chronic Chagas' disease: a clinical epidemiological review. Rev Soc Bras Med Trop 22:147, 1988.
378. Kirchhoff LV: Trypanosoma species (American trypanosomiasis, Chagas' disease): biology of trypanosomes. *In* Mandell GL, Douglas RG, Bennett JE (eds): Principles and Practice of Infectious Diseases. pp. 2077–2084. New York: Churchill Livingstone, 1990.
379. Morris SA, Tanowitz HB, Wittner M, et al: Pathophysiological insights into the cardiomyopathy of Chagas' disease. Circulation 82:1900, 1990.
380. Molina HA, Kierszenbaum F: Eosinophil activation in acute and chronic chagasic myocardial lesions and deposition of toxic eosinophil granule proteins on heart myofibers. J Parasitol 75:129, 1989.
381. Palacios-Pru E, Carrasco H, Scorza C, Espinoza R: Ultrastructural characteristics of different stages of human chagasic myocarditis. Am J Trop Med Hyg 1:29, 1989.
382. Barretto ACP, Mady C, Arteaga-Fernandez E, et al: Right ventricular endomyocardial biopsy in chronic Chagas' disease. Am Heart J 111:307, 1986.
383. Guerra HAC, Palacios-Pru E, de Scorza CD, et al: Clinical, histochemical, and ultrastructural correlation in septal endomyocardial biopsies from chronic chagasic patients: detection of early myocardial damage. Am Heart J 113:716, 1987.
384. Pimenta J, Miranda M, Pereira CB: Electrophysiologic findings in long-term asymptomatic chagasic individuals. Am Heart J 106:374, 1983.
385. Maguire JH, Hoff R, Sherloci I, et al: Cardiac morbidity and mortality due to Chagas' disease: prospective electrocardiographic study of a Brazilian community. Circulation 75:1140, 1987.
386. Acquatella H, Schiller NB, Puigbo JJ, et al: M-mode and two-dimensional echocardiography in chronic Chagas' heart disease: a clinical and pathologic study. Circulation 62:787, 1980.
387. Combellas I, Puigbo JJ, Acquatella H, et al: Echocardiographic features of impaired left ventricular diastolic function in Chagas' heart disease. Br Heart J 53:298, 1985.
388. Carrasco HA, Barboza JS, Inglessis G, et al: Left ventricular cineangiography in Chagas' disease: detection of early myocardial damage. Am Heart J 104:595, 1982.
389. Bestetti RB, Oliveira JSM: A hitherto neglected cause of myocardial infarction associated with normal coronary arteries: chronic Chagas' heart disease [letter]. Am J Cardiol 63:766, 1988.
390. De Morais CF, Higuchi ML, Lage S: Chagas' heart disease and myocardial infarct. Incidence and report of four necropsy cases. Ann Trop Med Parasitol 83:207, 1989.
391. Sadigursky M, von Kreuter BF, Ling P-Y, Santos-Buch CA: Association of elevated anti-sarcolemma, anti-idiotype antibody levels with the clinical and pathologic expression of chronic Chagas myocarditis. Circulation 80:1269, 1989.
392. Mesri EA, Levitus G, Hontebeyrie-Joskowicz M, et al: Major *Trypanosoma cruzi* antigenic determinant in Chagas' heart disease shares homology with the systemic lupus erythematosus ribosomal P protein epitope. J Clin Microbiol 28:1219, 1990.
393. Oliveira JSM, dos Santos M, Muccillo G, Ferreira AL: Increased capacity of the coronary arteries in chronic Chagas' heart disease: further support for the neurogenic pathogenesis concept. Am Heart J 109:304, 1985.
394. Gallo L, Filho JM, Maciel BC, et al: Functional evaluation of sympathetic and parasympathetic system in Chagas' disease using dynamic exercise. Cardiovasc Res 21:922, 1987.
395. Iosa C, DeQuattro V, Lee DD-P, et al: Plasma norepinephrine in Chagas' cardioneuromyopathy: a marker of progressive dysautonomia. Am Heart J 117:882, 1989.
396. Rossi MA: Microvascular changes as a cause of chronic cardiomyopathy in Chagas' disease. Am Heart J 120:233, 1990.
397. Tanowitz HB, Burns ER, Sinha AK, et al: Enhanced platelet adherence and aggregation in Chagas' disease: a potential pathogenic mechanism for cardiomyopathy. Am J Trop Med Hyg 43:274, 1990.
398. Marr JJ, Docampo R: Chemotherapy for Chagas' disease: a perspective of current therapy and considerations for future research. Rev Infect Dis 8:884, 1986.
399. Brener Z: Present status of chemotherapy and chemoprophylaxis of human trypanosomiasis in the Western hemisphere. Pharmacol Ther 7:71, 1979.
400. Apt W, Aguilera X, Arribada A, et al: Treatment of chronic Chagas' disease with itraconazole and allopurinol. Am J Trop Med Hyg 59:133–138, 1998.
401. de Andrade AL, Zicker F, de Oliveira RM, et al: Randomised trial of efficacy of benznidazole in treatment of early *Trypanosoma cruzi* infection. Lancet 348:1407–1413, 1996.
402. Kohl S, Pickering LK, Frankel LS, Yaeger RG: Reactivation of Chagas' disease during therapy of acute lymphocytic leukemia. Cancer 50:827, 1982.
403. Lopez-Blanco OA, Cavalli NH, Jasovich A, et al: Kidney transplantation and Chagas' disease. Transplantation 36:211, 1983.
404. Aulet F, Riarte A, Pattin M, et al: Chagas disease and kidney transplantation. Transplant Proc 23:2653, 1991.
405. Lopez Blanco OA, Muller LA, Cavalli NH, et al: Chronic intracellular protozoan infections and kidney transplantation. Transplantation 52:377, 1991.
406. Stolf NAG, Higushi L, Bocchi E, et al: Heart transplantation in patients with Chagas' disease cardiomyopathy. J Heart Transplant 6:307, 1987.
407. Poltera AA, Cox JN, Owor R: Pancarditis affecting the conducting system and all valves in human African trypanosomiasis. Br Heart J 38:827, 1976.
408. Bertrand E, Baudin L, Vacher P, et al: Heart involvement in 100 cases of African trypanosomiasis caused by *T. gambiense*. WHO/FAO Publication-Tryp/Inf 24:2, 1967.
409. Kirchoff LV: Agents of African trypanosomiasis (sleeping sickness). *In* Mandell GL, Douglas RG, Bennett JE (eds): Principles and Practice of Infectious Diseases. pp. 2085–2089. New York: Churchill Livingstone, 1990.
410. Adair OV, Randive N, Krasnow N: Isolated *Toxoplasma* myocarditis in acquired immune deficiency syndrome. Am Heart J 118:856, 1989.
411. Jehn U, Fink M, Gundlach P et al: Lethal cardiac and cerebral toxoplasmosis in a patient with acute myeloid leukemia after successful allogeneic bone marrow transplantation. Transplantation 4:430–433, 1984.
412. Luft BJ, Billingham M, Remington JS: Endomyocardial biopsy in the diagnosis of toxoplasmic myocarditis. Transplant Proc 18:1871, 1986.
413. Luft BJ, Naot Y, Araujo FG, et al: Primary and reactivated *Toxoplasma* infection in patients with cardiac transplants. Ann Intern Med 99:27, 1983.
414. Hakim M, Esmore D, Wallwork J, et al: Toxoplasmosis in cardiac transplantation. BMJ 292:1108, 1986.
415. Perez-Gomez F, Duran H, Tamames S, et al: Cardiac echinococcosis: clinical picture and complications. Br Heart J 35:1326, 1973.
416. Oliver JM, Sotillo JF, Domingues FJ, Lopez de Sa E: Two-dimensional echocardiographic features of echinococcosis of the heart and great blood vessels: clinical and surgical implications. Circulation 78:327, 1988.
417. Russo G, Tamburino C, Cuscuna S, et al: Cardiac hydatid cyst with clinical features resembling subaortic stenosis. Am Heart J 117:1385, 1989.
418. Bessoudo R, Marrie TJ, Smith WR: Cardiac involvement in trichinosis. Chest 79:698, 1981.
419. Gray DF, Morse BS, Phillips WF: Trichinosis with neurologic and cardiac involvement. Ann Intern Med 57:230, 1962.
420. Ursell PC, Habib A, Babchick O, et al: Myocarditis caused by *Trichinella spiralis*. Arch Pathol Lab Med 108:4, 1984.
421. Kaimal KP, Beyt BE Jr: Cardiac dysfunction in trichinosis. N Engl J Med 307:374, 1982.
422. Melish ME, Hicks RV: Kawasaki syndrome: clinical features. Pathophysiology, etiology and therapy. J Rheumatol 17(suppl 24):2, 1990.
423. Gersony WM: Diagnosis and management of Kawasaki disease. JAMA 265:2699, 1991.
424. Rowley AH, Shulman ST: Kawasaki syndrome. Clin Microbiol Rev 11:405–414, 1998.
425. Rose V: Kawasaki syndrome—cardiovascular manifestations. J Rheumatol 17(suppl 24):11, 1990.

426. Takahashi M: Myocarditis in Kawasaki syndrome: a minor villain? Circulation 79:1398, 1989.
427. Yutani C, Go S, Kamiya T, et al: Cardiac biopsy of Kawasaki disease. Arch Pathol Lab Med 105:470, 1981.
428. Fujiwara H, Hamashima Y: Pathology of the heart in Kawasaki disease. Pediatrics 61:100, 1978.
429. Fujiwara H, Kawai C, Hamashima Y: Clinicopathologic study of the conduction systems in 10 patients with Kawasaki's disease (mucocutaneous lymph node syndrome). Am Heart J 96:744, 1978.
430. Matsuura H, Ishikita T, Yamamoto S, et al: Gallium-67 myocardial imaging for the detection of myocarditis in the acute phase of Kawasaki disease (mucocutaneous lymph node syndrome): the usefulness of single photon emission computed tomography. Br Heart J 58:385, 1987.
431. Ino T, Akimoto K, Nishimoto K, et al: Myocarditis in Kawasaki disease. Am Heart J 117:1400, 1989.
432. Furusho K, Nakano H, Shinomiya K, et al: High-dose intravenous gammaglobulin for Kawasaki disease. Lancet 2:1055, 1984.
433. Theaker JM, Gatter KC, Heryet A, et al: Giant cell myocarditis: evidence for the macrophage origin of the giant cells. J Clin Pathol 38:160–164, 1985.
434. Fukuhara T, Morino M, Sakoda S, et al: Myocarditis with multinucleated giant cells detected in biopsy specimens. Clin Cardiol 11:341–344, 1988.
435. Humbert P, Faivre R, Fellman D, et al: Giant cell myocarditis: an autoimmune disease? Am Heart J 115:485–487, 1988.
436. Roberts WC, McAllister HA Jr, Ferrans VJ: Sarcoidosis of the heart. A clinicopathologic study of 35 necropsy patients (group I) and review of 78 previously described necropsy patients (group II). Am J Med 63:86–108, 1977.
437. Johansen A: Isolated myocarditis versus myocardial sarcoidosis. Acta Pathol Microbiol Scand 67:15–26, 1966.
438. Litovsky SH, Burke AP, Virmani R: Giant cell myocarditis: an entity distinct from sarcoidosis characterized by multiphasic myocyte destruction by cytotoxic T cells and histiocytic giant cells. Mod Pathol 9:1126–1134, 1996.
439. de Jongste MJ, Oosterhuis HJ, Lie KI: Intractable ventricular tachycardia in a patient with giant cell myocarditis, thymoma and myasthenia gravis. Int J Cardiol 13:374–378, 1986.
440. Kilgallen CM, Jackson E, Bankoff M, et al: A case of giant cell myocarditis and malignant thymoma: a postmortem diagnosis by needle biopsy. Clin Cardiol 21:48–51, 1998.
441. Leib ML, Odel JG, Cooney MJ: Orbital polymyositis and giant cell myocarditis. Ophthalmology 101:950–954, 1994.
442. Stevens AW, Grossman ME, Barr ML, et al: Orbital myositis, vitiligo, and giant cell myocarditis. J Am Acad Dermatol 35:310–312, 1996.
443. Weidhase A, Grone HJ, Unterberg C, et al: Severe granulomatous giant cell myocarditis in Wegener's granulomatosis. Klin Wochenschr 68:880–885, 1990.
444. McKeon J, Haagsma B, Bett JH, et al: Fatal giant cell myocarditis after colectomy for ulcerative colitis. Am Heart J 111:1208–1209, 1986.
445. Ariza A, Lopez MD, Mate JL, et al: Giant cell myocarditis: monocytic immunophenotype of giant cells in a case associated with ulcerative colitis. Hum Pathol 26:121–123, 1995.
446. Kloin JE: Pernicious anemia and giant cell myocarditis. New association. Am J Med 78:355–360, 1985.
447. Hales SA, Theaker JM, Gatter KC: Giant cell myocarditis associated with lymphoma: an immunocytochemical study. J Clin Pathol 40:1310–1313, 1987.
448. Singham KT, Azizah NW, Goh TH: Complete atrioventricular block due to giant cell myocarditis. Postgrad Med J 56:194–196, 1980.
449. Desjardins V, Pelletier G, Leung TK, et al: Successful treatment of severe heart failure caused by idiopathic giant cell myocarditis. Can J Cardiol 8:788–792, 1992.
450. Nieminen MS, Salminen US, Taskinen E, et al: Treatment of serious heart failure by transplantation in giant cell myocarditis diagnosed by endomyocardial biopsy. J Heart Lung Transplant 13:543–545, 1994.
451. Lindvall K, Edhag O, Erhardt LR, et al: Complete heart block due to granulomatous giant cell myocarditis: report of 3 cases. Eur J Cardiol 8:349–358, 1978.
452. Piette M, Timperman J: Sudden death in idiopathic giant cell myocarditis. Med Sci Law 30:280–284, 1990.
453. Hori T, Fujiwara H, Tanaka M, et al: Idiopathic giant cell myocarditis accompanied by asymmetric septal hypertrophy. Jpn Circ J 51:153–156, 1987.
454. Davidoff R, Palacios I, Southern J, et al: Giant cell versus lymphocytic myocarditis. A comparison of their clinical features and long-term outcomes. Circulation 83:953–961, 1991.
455. Cooper LT Jr, Berry GJ, Shabetai R: Idiopathic giant-cell myocarditis—natural history and treatment. Multicenter Giant Cell Myocarditis Study Group Investigators. N Engl J Med 336:1860–1866, 1997.
456. Grant SC: Giant cell myocarditis in a transplanted heart. Eur Heart J 14:1437, 1993.
457. Kong G, Madden B, Spyrou N, et al: Response of recurrent giant cell myocarditis in a transplanted heart to intensive immunosuppression. Eur Heart J 12:554–557, 1991.
458. Gries W, Farkas D, Winters GL, et al: Giant cell myocarditis: first report of disease recurrence in the transplanted heart. J Heart Lung Transplant 11:370–374, 1992.
459. Wolfsohn AL, Davies RA, Smith CO, et al: Giant cell myocarditis-like appearance after transplantation: an atypical manifestation of rejection? J Heart Lung Transplant 13:731–733, 1994.
460. Loffler W: Endocarditis parietalis fibroplastica mit Bluteosinophilie, ein eigenartiges Krankheitsbild. Schweiz Med Wochenschr 66:817–820, 1936.
461. Spry CJ, Take M, Tai PC: Eosinophilic disorders affecting the myocardium and endocardium: a review. Heart Vessels Suppl 1:240–242, 1985.
462. Oakley CM, Olsen EGJ: Eosinophilia and heart disease [editorial]. Br Heart J 39:233–237, 1977.
463. Herzog CA, Snover DC, Staley NA: Acute necrotising eosinophilic myocarditis. Br Heart J 52:343–348, 1984.
464. Olsen EG, Spry CJ: Relation between eosinophilia and endomyocardial disease. Prog Cardiovasc Dis 27:241–254, 1985.
465. Spry CJ: The pathogenesis of endomyocardial fibrosis: the role of the eosinophil. Springer Semin Immunopathol 11:417–477, 1989.
466. Nakayama Y, Kohriyama T, Yamamoto S, et al: Electron-microscopic and immunohistochemical studies on endomyocardial biopsies from a patient with eosinophilic endomyocardial disease. Heart Vessels Suppl 1:250–255, 1985.
467. Tai PC, Hayes DJ, Clark JB, et al: Toxic effects of human eosinophil products on isolated rat heart cells in vitro. Biochem J 204:75–80, 1982.
468. Terasaki F, Hayashi T, Hirota Y, et al: Evolution to dilated cardiomyopathy from acute eosinophilic pancarditis in Churg-Strauss syndrome. Heart Vessels 12:43–48, 1997.
469. Getz MA, Subramanian R, Logemann T, et al: Acute necrotizing eosinophilic myocarditis as a manifestation of severe hypersensitivity myocarditis. Antemortem diagnosis and successful treatment. Ann Intern Med 115:201–202, 1991.
470. Schuchter LM, Hendricks CB, Holland KH, et al: Eosinophilic myocarditis associated with high-dose interleukin-2 therapy. Am J Med 88:439–440, 1990.
471. Galiuto L, Enriquez-Sarano M, Reeder GS, et al: Eosinophilic myocarditis manifesting as myocardial infarction: early diagnosis and successful treatment. Mayo Clin Proc 72:603–610, 1997.
472. Newman LS, Rose CS, Maier LA: Sarcoidosis. N Engl J Med 336:1224–1234, 1997.
473. Rizzato G, Pezzano A, Sala G, et al: Right heart impairment in sarcoidosis: hemodynamic and echocardiographic study. Eur J Respir Dis 64:121–128, 1983.
474. Silverman KJ, Hutchins GM, Bulkley BH: Cardiac sarcoid: a clinicopathologic study of 84 unselected patients with systemic sarcoidosis. Circulation 58:1204–1211, 1978.
475. Jain A, Starek PJ, Delany DL: Ventricular tachycardia and ventricular aneurysm due to unrecognized sarcoidosis. Clin Cardiol 13:738–740, 1990.
476. Bohle W, Schaefer HE: Predominant myocardial sarcoidosis. Pathol Res Pract 190:212–217, 1994.
477. Yazaki Y, Isobe M, Hiramitsu S, et al: Comparison of clinical features and prognosis of cardiac sarcoidosis and idiopathic dilated cardiomyopathy. Am J Cardiol 82:537–540, 1998.
478. Sharma OP, Maheshwari A, Thaker K: Myocardial sarcoidosis. Chest 103:253–258, 1993.
479. Hirose Y, Ishida Y, Hayashida K, et al: Myocardial involvement in patients with sarcoidosis. An analysis of 75 patients. Clin Nucl Med 19:522–526, 1994.

480. Chandra M, Silverman ME, Oshinski J, et al: Diagnosis of cardiac sarcoidosis aided by MRI. Chest 110:562–565, 1996.
481. Eliasch H, Juhlin-Dannfelt A, Sjogren I, et al: Magnetic resonance imaging as an aid to the diagnosis and treatment evaluation of suspected myocardial sarcoidosis in a fighter pilot. Aviat Space Environ Med 66:1010–1013, 1995.
482. Shammas RL, Movahed A: Sarcoidosis of the heart. Clin Cardiol 16:462–472, 1993.
483. Okayama K, Kurata C, Tawarahara K, et al: Diagnostic and prognostic value of myocardial scintigraphy with thallium-201 and gallium-67 in cardiac sarcoidosis. Chest 107:330–334, 1995.
484. Bajaj AK, Kopelman HA, Echt DS: Cardiac sarcoidosis with sudden death: treatment with the automatic implantable cardioverter defibrillator. Am Heart J 116:557–560, 1988.
485. Padilla ML, Schilero GJ, Teirstein AS: Sarcoidosis and transplantation. Sarcoidosis Vasc Diffuse Lung Dis 14:16–22, 1997.
486. Brown CS, Bertolet BD: Peripartum cardiomyopathy: a comprehensive review. Am J Obstet Gynecol 178:409–414, 1998.
487. Farber PA, Glasgow LA: Factors modulating host resistance to virus infection, II: enhanced susceptibility of mice to encephalomyocarditis virus infection during pregnancy. Am J Pathol 53:463–478, 1968.
488. Takatsu T, Kitamura Y, Morita H, et al: Viral myocarditis and cardiomyopathy. *In* Sekigushi M, Olsen EGJ (eds): Cardiomyopathy. pp. 34–35. Tokyo: University of Tokyo Press, 1978.
489. Lampert MB, Hibbard J, Weinest L, et al: Peripartum heart failure associated with prolonged tocolytic therapy. Am J Obstet Gynecol 168:493–495, 1993.
490. Midei MG, DeMent SH, Feldman AM, et al: Peripartum myocarditis and cardiomyopathy. Circulation 81:922–928, 1990.
491. O'Connell JB, Costanzo-Nordin MR, Subramanian R, et al: Peripartum cardiomyopathy: clinical, hemodynamic, histologic and prognostic characteristics. J Am Coll Cardiol 8:52–56, 1986.

C H A P T E R **56**

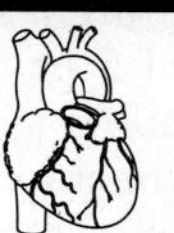

Cardiac Catheterization

James J. Ferguson

GENERAL HEMODYNAMIC ASSESSMENT
DILATED CARDIOMYOPATHY
RESTRICTIVE CARDIOMYOPATHY
HYPERTROPHIC CARDIOMYOPATHY
ENDOMYOCARDIAL BIOPSY

Cardiomyopathies are a group of diseases of unknown etiology that are characterized primarily by involvement of heart muscle in the disease process.[1–3] There are three general categories of cardiomyopathies (Table 56–1): *dilated cardiomyopathies* (otherwise known as congestive cardiomyopathies); *restrictive* or *infiltrative cardiomyopathies* (with scarring and fibrosis of the ventricle and diastolic dysfunction); and *obstructive*, or *hypertrophic, cardiomyopathies*, (HCMs), characterized by left ventricular (LV) hypertrophy with normal or supernormal systolic function and usually abnormal diastolic function.[1–3] There may be areas of overlap among these three general categories, such as patients with extreme hypertrophy who manifest restrictive diastolic abnormalities.

Hypertensive heart disease, valvular heart disease, congenital heart disease, pericardial disease, and ischemic heart disease are not usually included among the cardiomyopathies. The term *ischemic cardiomyopathy* has been applied to the LV chamber dilatation and heart failure resulting from multiple myocardial infarctions with associated diffuse fibrosis and LV dysfunction.[4] However, ischemic cardiomyopathy is not usually included among the cardiomyopathies.

It is also possible to classify the cardiomyopathies on the basis of etiology. *Primary cardiomyopathies* have an underlying pathologic process involving the heart muscle that does not involve other organs or the cause of which is unknown. *Secondary cardiomyopathies* involve a known systemic disease or disease process, one manifestation of which is cardiac involvement (such as amyloidosis and hemochromatosis).[3]

This section describes the hemodynamics and cardiac catheterization laboratory findings in the cardiomyopathies. The hemodynamic pictures of dilated, restrictive, and obstructive cardiomyopathies are discussed, as well as the role of endomyocardial biopsy.

General Hemodynamic Assessment

In general, the complete hemodynamic assessment of a patient with cardiomyopathy should include right and left heart catheterization, with measurements of cardiac output, intracardiac pressures, and pulmonary and systemic vascular resistances. When the left ventricle and right ventricle are entered with catheters for pressure measurement, care should be taken not to provoke ventricular arrhythmias, which may be very poorly tolerated in patients with compromised LV function. The pressure measurement system should be designed to provide the highest possible frequency response and optimal damping. The highest natural frequency for a pressure measurement system is obtained by using a stiff, short, wide-bore catheter directly connected to a pressure transducer without stopcocks or tubing; rigorous attention must be paid to avoid air bubbles in the measurement system.[5]

Superior vena cava (SVC), inferior vena cava (IVC), right atrial, right ventricular (RV), and pulmonary arterial oxygen saturations should be measured to detect right-to-left shunting. A saturation step-up of 7 percent or greater between SVC/IVC and the right atrium should be considered abnormal and indicates the presence of a significant left-to-right shunt at the atrial level. A saturation step-up of 5 percent or greater between the right atrium and the right ventricle indicates the presence of a significant left-

TABLE **56–1** **Usual Features Characterizing Dilated, Restrictive, and Hypertrophic Cardiomyopathy**

	Dilated Cardiomyopathy	Restrictive Cardiomyopathy	Hypertrophic Cardiomyopathy
Chamber size	↑↑	Normal	↓ normal, or ↑
Systolic function	Impaired	Normal or ↓	Hyperdynamic
Diastolic function	Elevated filling pressures Passive congestion	Impaired (throughout diastole, L → R may be brought out by exercise)	Impaired (may be similar to restrictive if hypertrophy severe)
Wall thickness	↓	Increased	Increased (may be very increased), sometimes with further asymmetric septal thickening

to-right shunt at the ventricular level. A saturation step-up of 5 percent or greater between the right ventricle and the pulmonary artery indicates the presence of a left-to-right shunt at the level of the great vessels.[6] Coronary angiography, biplanar left ventriculography, and endomyocardial biopsy (discussed later) are also considered as part of the usual evaluation of patients with cardiomyopathy, although the need for contrast studies should be individually tailored to the patient's medical status and the diagnosis being considered. In some situations (such as restrictive cardiomyopathy), hemodynamic monitoring during supine bicycle exercise may be a valuable part of the diagnostic evaluation in order to elicit otherwise inapparent hemodynamic abnormalities.

Dilated Cardiomyopathy

Dilated cardiomyopathy, otherwise known as congestive cardiomyopathy, is characterized by cardiac enlargement and LV systolic dysfunction, usually resulting in congestive heart failure. Although the underlying cause is often not identifiable, this syndrome probably represents the end-stage of a variety of causes for myocardial damage, some of which may be reversible and some of which are not reversible.

Underlying inciting factors for dilated cardiomyopathy include metabolic causes (e.g., uremia, hypophosphatemia, hypocalcemia), toxic causes (e.g., alcohol, cobalt), and infectious causes (e.g., myocarditis). The course of dilated cardiomyopathy is usually progressively downhill (unless a reversible cause can be identified), and 75 percent of patients will be dead within 5 years of the onset of symptoms.[7]

The hemodynamic findings in dilated cardiomyopathy are fairly nonspecific. Cardiac catheterization usually demonstrates elevated left-sided filling pressures, including elevations in the LV end-diastolic left atrial and pulmonary capillary wedge pressures[8] (Fig. 56–1). Moderate pulmonary hypertension is often present. As the disease progresses and the degree of congestive heart failure worsens, right-sided hemodynamic abnormalities may also develop, including elevations in the RV end-diastolic, right atrial, and central venous pressures.

Left ventriculography shows a dilated, diffusely hypokinetic left ventricle. Although focal wall-motion abnormalities (mimicking coronary artery disease) can be found,[8, 9] the usual picture is one of global LV systolic dysfunction, with reduction of the ejection fraction and increases in the absolute LV end-diastolic and end-systolic volumes. Mitral regurgitation may be present on the basis of LV dilatation and chamber distortion; LV thrombi may also be present. Again, as the disease progresses to include right-sided involvement, there will be RV dilatation and perhaps associated tricuspid regurgitation.

Coronary arteriography is an important part of the diagnostic evaluation to exclude ischemic causes, particularly if focal wall-motion abnormalities are present. Coronary angiography is usually normal in patients with dilated cardiomyopathy,[8] although coronary artery vasodilator reserve may be impaired[10] and the potential exists for coronary emboli arising from an LV thrombus.

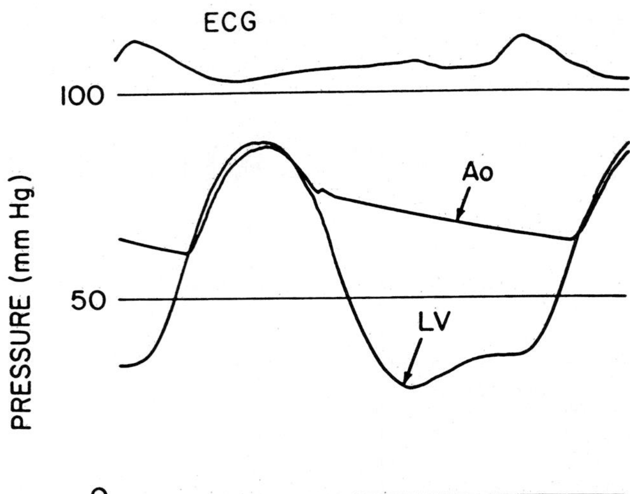

Figure 56–1 Simultaneous left ventricular (LV) and aortic (Ao) pressures in a 68-year-old patient with dilated cardiomyopathy. Note the deviation of LV diastolic pressure and the slow systolic rise and fall of LV pressure, giving it a triangular configuration. ECG, electrocardiogram. (From Grossman W: Profiles in dilated and hypertrophic cardiomyopathies. *In* Grossman W [ed]: Cardiac Catheterization and Angiography. 4th ed. pp. 618–632. Philadelphia: Lea & Febiger, 1991.)

Restrictive Cardiomyopathy

The characteristic abnormality in restrictive cardiomyopathy is diastolic dysfunction resulting in impaired ventricular filling.[11, 12] In contrast to the dilated cardiomyopathies with abnormal systolic function, systolic function in restrictive cardiomyopathy is usually normal or near normal. There are a number of specific pathologic causes for restrictive cardiomyopathy (Table 56–2), and the abnormal diastolic dysfunction is usually the result of infiltration, fibrosis, or hypertrophy. However, the exact etiology of the underlying pathologic process frequently remains unknown.[13] The many potential primary causes of restrictive cardiomyopathy include amyloidosis, hemochromatosis, endomyocardial fibrosis, glycogen storage diseases, sarcoid (and other collagen vascular diseases), fibroelastosis, and pseudoxanthoma elasticum.[13, 14]

The hemodynamic features of restrictive cardiomyopathy can be very similar to those of constrictive pericarditis, and close attention should be paid in the cardiac catheterization laboratory to obtaining accurate hemodynamic tracings. Outside of the catheterization laboratory, other tests, including rapid-speed computed tomographic scanning, and particularly magnetic resonance imaging, may be useful in distinguishing between restrictive cardiomyopathy and con-

TABLE 56–2 Usual Primary Causes of Restrictive Cardiomyopathy

Amyloid	Glycogen storage disease
Hemochromatosis	Mucopolysaccharidoses
Endomyocardial fibroelastosis	

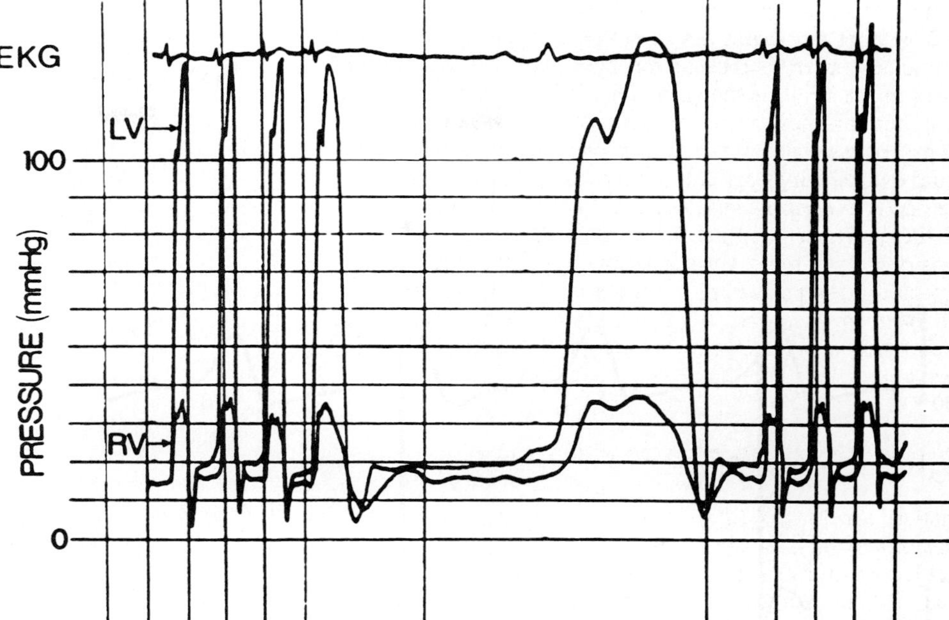

FIGURE 56–2 Simultaneously right ventricular (RV) and left ventricular (LV) pressure tracings in a 43-year-old patient with restrictive cardiomyopathy. Note prominent dip and plateau of both pressure recordings. There is more of a divergence of diastolic pressures in late diastole with the LV pressure significantly higher than the RV pressure. EKG, electrocardiogram. (From Benotti JR, Grossman W, Cohn PF: The clinical profile of restrictive cardiomyopathy. Circulation 61(5):1206–1210, 1980.)

strictive pericarditis[15, 16] by demonstrating the presence or absence of increased pericardial thickness. In the catheterization laboratory, both syndromes manifest as a diastolic filling abnormality.[13] The diastolic abnormality in constrictive pericarditis involves left and right ventricles equally and begins in early to mid-diastole, with normal or supranormal early filling, whereas in restrictive cardiomyopathy, the diastolic abnormality persists throughout diastole and the left ventricle may be more involved than the right ventricle (Fig. 56–2). Both syndromes are characterized by a rapid early decline in ventricular pressure at the onset of diastole, with a subsequent rapid plateau, the so-called square root sign (Fig. 56–3), although some high-fidelity LV diastolic pressure recordings do not show a clear-cut early diastolic dip (Fig. 56–4).[17] On atrial and central (or pulmonary) venous tracings, rapid early diastolic filling of the ventricles will be expressed as a prominent *y* descent (see Fig. 56–3). Both syndromes are also usually associated with elevations in pulmonary and systemic venous pressures. One major clinical feature distinguishing the two is that in restrictive cardiomyopathy with infiltrative involvement of both ventricles (left more than right because of its greater mass), there is usually a divergence between LV and RV pressures, with left exceeding right by at least 5 mm Hg, especially with exercise (see Fig. 56–2). In contrast, in constrictive pericarditis, the RV and LV diastolic pressures are usually within 5 mm Hg of each other, and often there is a relative equalization of pressures such that the mean right atrial, RV end-diastolic, pulmonary artery diastolic, and mean pulmonary wedge pressures are almost identical.

Other hemodynamic features can help to distinguish restrictive cardiomyopathy from constrictive pericarditis.[18] Pulmonary artery systolic pressure can often be greater than 45 mm Hg in restrictive cardiomyopathy but less than 45 mm Hg in constrictive pericarditis. Finally, the height of the RV diastolic plateau is often less than one third of the RV peak systolic pressure in restrictive cardiomyopathy, whereas in constrictive pericarditis, it is usually greater than one third of the RV peak systolic pressure (Table 56–3).

HYPERTROPHIC CARDIOMYOPATHY

The characteristic feature of HCM is myocardial hypertrophy in a nondilated ventricle, which often involves the interventricular septum.[19, 20] A subaortic pressure gradient has been noted in a subset of these patients, giving rise to the terms *idiopathic hypertrophic subaortic stenosis, muscular subaortic stenosis*, and hypertrophic obstructive cardiomyopathy.[21] Although some patients may exhibit a distinct gradient (Fig. 56–5), many patients show no evidence of LV outflow obstruction at rest. There is a strong genetic linkage of this disorder, with approximately 25

TABLE 56–3 Usual Hemodynamic Features of Restrictive Cardiomyopathy and Constrictive Pericarditis

	Restrictive Cardiomyopathy	Constrictive Pericarditis
Diastolic filling	Dip and plateau	Dip and plateau
Venous	Prominent *y* descent	Prominent *y* descent
Diastolic pressures	LV exceeds RV by at least 5 mm Hg	LV within 5 mm Hg of RV
PA systolic pressure	>45 mm Hg	<45 mm Hg
RV pressure	Plateau < ⅓ of RV systolic pressure	Plateau > ⅓ of RV systolic pressure

Abbreviations: LV, left ventricle; PA, pulmonary artery; RV, right ventricle.

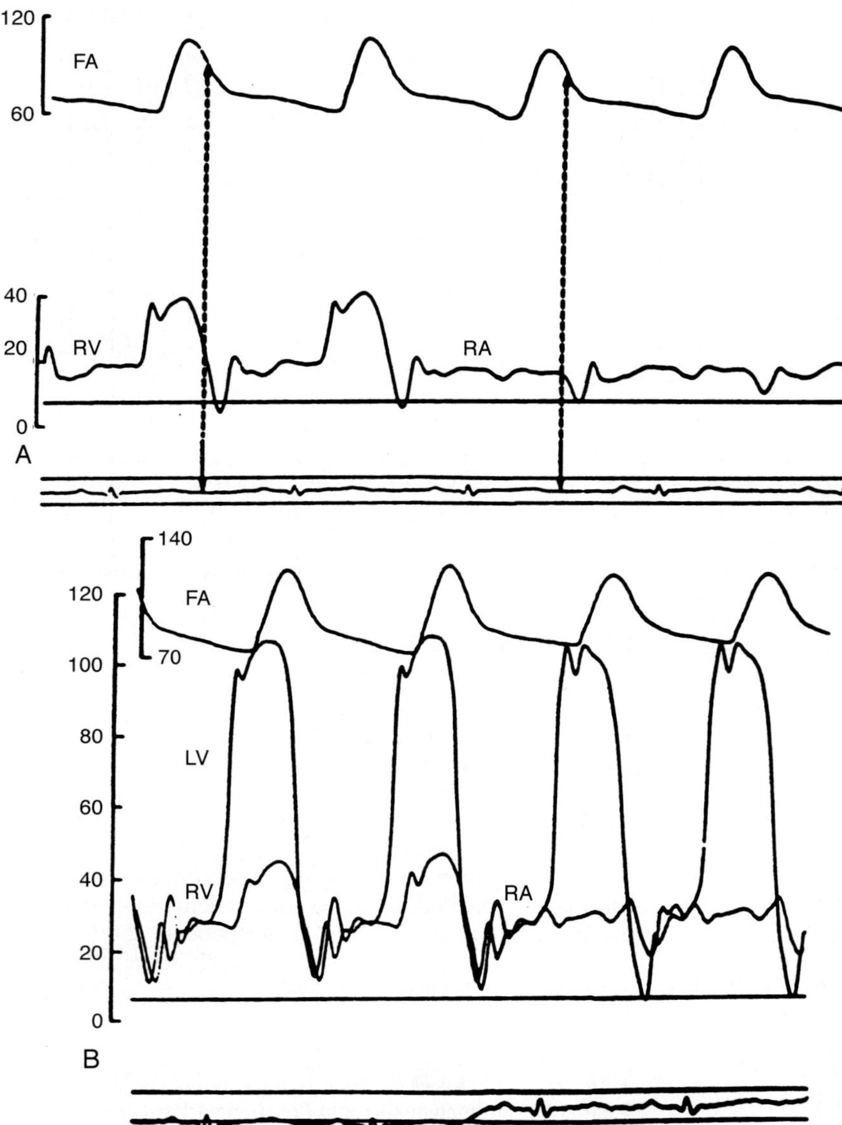

FIGURE 56–3 Prominent *y* descent on a right atrial pressure tracing in a patient with restrictive cardiomyopathy. **A,** Simultaneous pressures in the femoral artery (FA) and right ventricle (RV) pulled back to the right atrium (RA) show rapid *y* descent. **B,** Superimposed left ventricular (LV) pressure demonstrates a square root configuration. (**A** and **B,** From Olney BA: Restrictive myocardial disease. *In* Giuliani ER, Fuster V, Gersh BJ, et al [eds]: Cardiology: Fundamentals and Practice. pp. 1775–1791. St. Louis: Mosby–Year Book, 1991.)

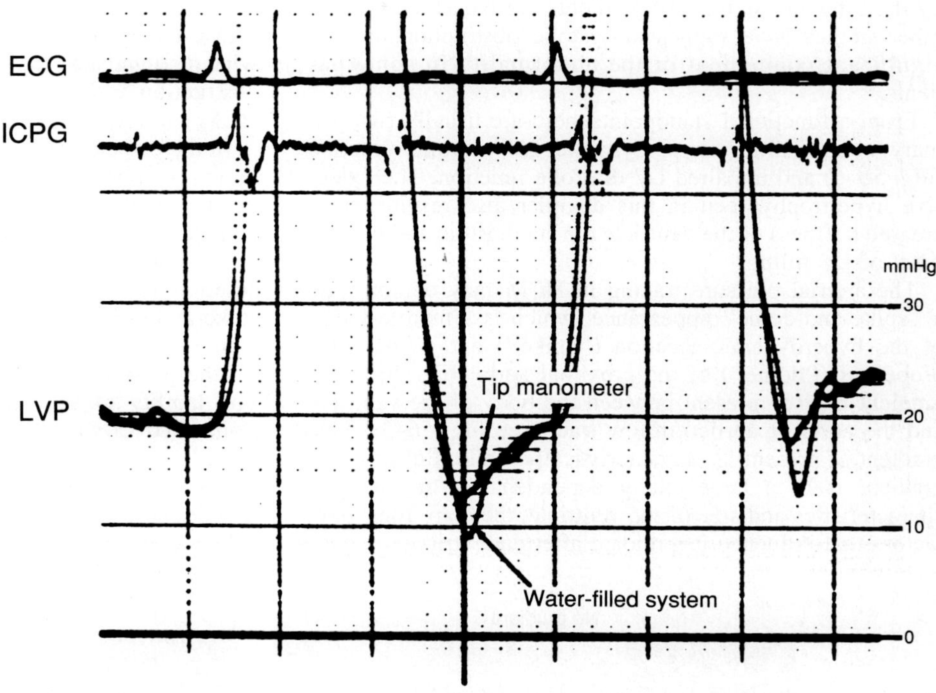

FIGURE 56–4 Simultaneous left ventricular pressure (LVP) recordings with a fluid-filled catheter and a catheter tip manometer in a patient with restrictive cardiomyopathy. Although there appears to be an early diastolic dip and diastolic plateau with the fluid-filled catheter, the micromanometer recordings do not confirm the presence of an early diastolic dip. ECG, electrocardiogram; ICPG, intracardiac phonocardiogram. (From Hirota Y, Kohriyama T, Hayashi T, et al: Idiopathic restrictive cardiomyopathy: differences of left ventricular relaxation and diastolic wave forms from constrictive pericarditis. Am J Cardiol 52:421, 1983.)

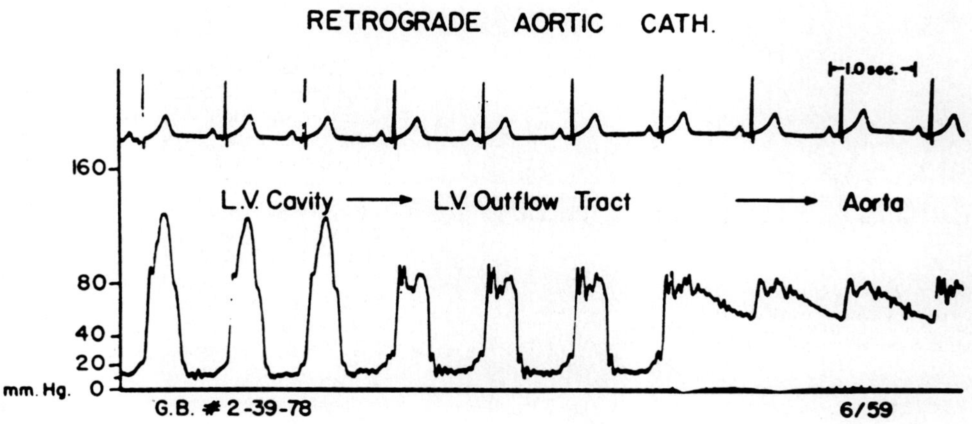

FIGURE 56–5 Continuous pressure recording during pullback of a fluid-filled catheter from the left ventricle to the aorta in a patient with hypertrophic cardiomyopathy. There is a gradient within the body of the left ventricle. The aortic pressure recordings also show a spike-and-dome appearance. LV, left ventricular. (From Braunwald E, Lambrew CT, Rockoff SD, et al: Idiopathic hypertrophic subaortic stenosis. Circulation 29/30 [suppl IV]: 1, 1964.)

percent of the first-degree relatives of patients with HCM exhibiting some evidence of the disease.[22] It is inherited as an autosomal dominant trait with incomplete penetrance, and the gene responsible has been shown to be present on chromosome 14.[23, 24]

The issue of "obstruction" continues to engender significant controversy; there are experimental data indicating that most of the ventricular ejection has already taken place by the time any significant gradients are measured,[25–29] but other studies have suggested systolic obstruction to be a significant component of the abnormality in some patients.[30–34]

From a functional standpoint, there are usually two primary abnormalities: hyperdynamic LV systolic function (Fig. 56–6) and impaired LV diastolic function. The extensive hypertrophy seen in this disorder also results in increased stiffness of the ventricle during diastole and impairment of LV filling.

The arterial pressure tracing in HCM may demonstrate a "spike-and-dome" appearance, which is a manifestation of the hyperdynamic ejection ("spike") and Windkessel properties ("dome") of the proximal aorta (Fig. 56–7). A gradient may be present between the body of the ventricle and the aorta or aortic outflow tract (see Fig. 56–5). This gradient, if present, is characteristically labile. Because this gradient is to a large extent dependent on the ejection characteristics and size of the ventricle, there are four main factors that influence it: preload, afterload, atrioventricular synchrony, and contractility.[20, 35] Provocations that decrease preload (Valsalva maneuver), decrease afterload (nitroglycerin), and increase contractility (isoproterenol), or any positive inotropic intervention (including cardiac glycosides) all increase the gradient, although most provocative maneuvers can have mixed effects on preload, afterload, and contractility. Similarly, maneuvers that increase preload (Mueller maneuver), increase afterload (handgrip or squatting down), and decrease contractility (beta-blockade) decrease the gradient. The lability of the gradient is usually what distinguishes HCM from other fixed forms of outflow obstruction, although some patients with otherwise classic HCM can have a fixed gradient.

In the catheterization laboratory, postextrasystolic potentiation is one of the best techniques for provoking an otherwise inapparent gradient. The postextrasystolic augmentation of contractility far outweighs the increase in preload, and a gradient (and murmur) may be recorded. In addition to provocation of a gradient, the characteristic spike-and-dome arterial pressure waveform becomes more manifest, and there is no change in (or even a narrowing of) the pulse pressure (Brockenbrough sign) (Fig. 56–8).[36] The lability of the gradient is what distinguishes HCM from fixed valvular aortic stenosis, as well as the fact that in valvular aortic stenosis, the postextrasystolic arterial pressure contour will be unchanged, and the pulse pressure will be increased.

In measuring LV pressure, care must be taken to avoid

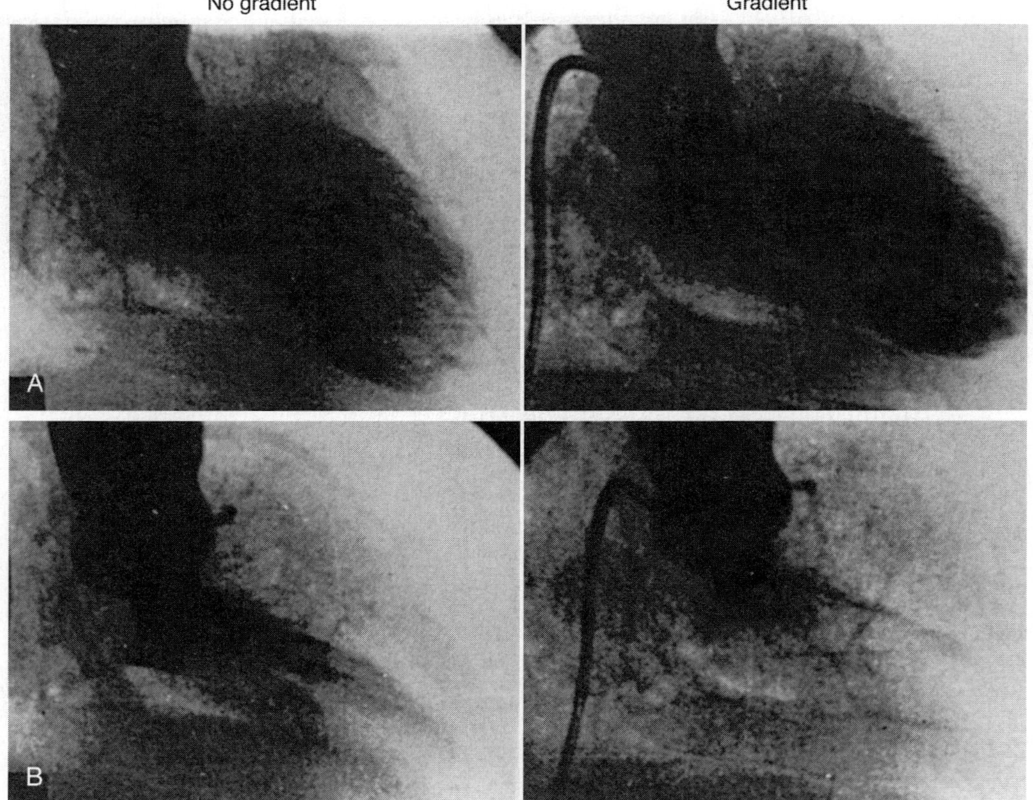

FIGURE 56–6 Right anterior oblique contrast ventriculograms in a patient with hypertrophic cardiomyopathy. End-diastolic **(A)** and end-systolic **(B)** frames with no gradient *(left)* and after induction of an 87 mm Hg gradient with nitroprusside *(right).* In both studies, there is obliteration of the left ventricular cavity, more so after nitroprusside administration. (**A** and **B,** From Siegel RJ, Criley JM: Comparison of ventricular emptying with and without a pressure gradient in patients with hypertrophic cardiomyopathy. Br Heart J 53:283, 1985.)

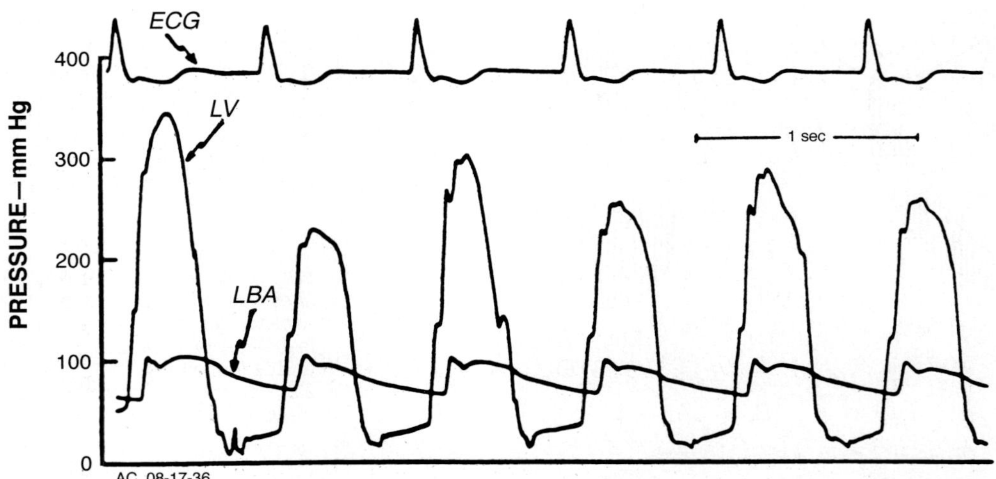

FIGURE 56–7 Simultaneous left ventricle (LV) and left brachial artery (LBA) pressure tracings in a patient with hypertrophic cardiomyopathy after a premature ventricular contraction (not shown). Note the prominent spike-and-dome appearance on the LBA pressure recording. ECG, electrocardiogram. (From Glancy DL, Shephard RL, Beiser GD, Epstein SE: The dynamic nature of left ventricular outflow obstructions in idiopathic hypertrophic subaortic stenosis. Ann Intern Med 75:589, 1971.)

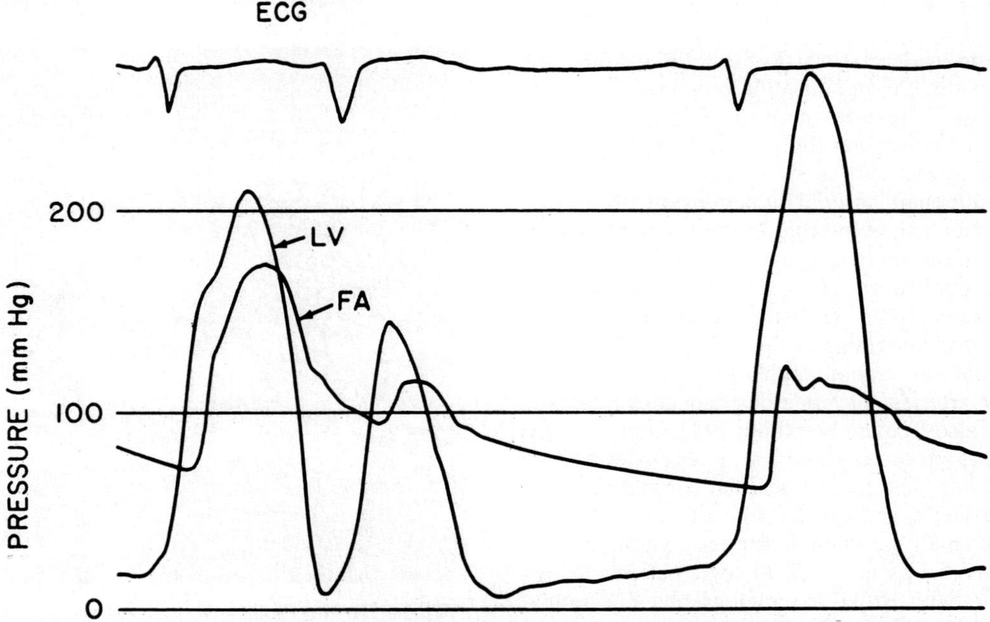

FIGURE 56–8 Simultaneous left ventricle (LV) and femoral artery (FA) pressure tracings in a patient with hypertrophic cardiomyopathy. Note that after the extrasystolic beat, there is an increase in the gradient, a more prominent spike-and-dome configuration to the peripheral pulse contour, and narrowing of the pulse pressure. ECG, electrocardiogram. (From Grossman W: Profiles in dilated and hypertrophic cardiomyopathies. *In* Grossman W [ed]: Cardiac Catheterization and Angiography. 4th ed. pp. 618–632. Philadelphia: Lea & Febiger, 1991.)

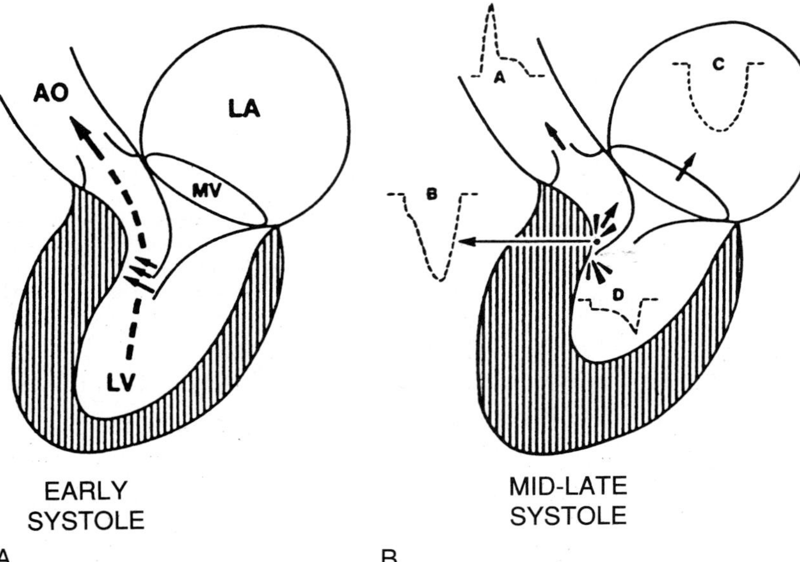

FIGURE 56–9 Schematic representation of the dynamics of mitral leaflet systolic anterior motion, outflow obstruction, and mitral regurgitation in hypertrophic cardiomyopathy. **A,** Outflow tract is narrowed owing to septal hypertrophy, and ejection velocity is increased. The resulting Venturi forces draw the anterior and posterior mitral leaflet toward the septum, ultimately resulting in anterior leaflet septal contact. AO, aorta; LA, left atrium; LV, left ventricle; MV, mitral valve. **B,** Septal contact results in outflow obstruction and mitral regurgitation. The *dashed lines* illustrate Doppler velocity recordings at the ascending aorta (A), at the level of mitral leaflet–septal contact (B), in the left atrium (C), and at the left ventricular apex (D). (From Wigle ED: Hypertrophic cardiomyopathy: a 1987 viewpoint. Circulation 75[2]:311–322, 1987.)

catheter entrapment (particularly with end-hole catheters), which may produce an artifactual gradient. Left ventriculography usually demonstrates a small LV cavity with vigorous contraction that may obliterate the LV cavity, and hypertrophied walls with prominent papillary muscles. However, the left ventricle may be very large in some patients. The mitral valve often moves anteriorly during systole (systolic anterior motion pattern), impinging on the LV outflow tract, with associated mitral regurgitation (Fig. 56–9), also generating a characteristic echocardiographic pattern (Fig. 56–10).

There is often evidence of LV diastolic dysfunction, with elevation of the LV end-diastolic pressure or even an abnormal LV diastolic pressure contour. With impaired LV filling, there are resulting elevations in LA and pulmonary capillary wedge pressures. Approximately 25 percent of patients have pulmonary arterial hypertension. Moreover, dynamic obstruction can be present in the RV outflow tract as well and has been reported in as many as 15 percent of patients with LV outflow gradients.[20, 37] Visualization of the interventricular septum can be facilitated by simultaneous right and left ventriculograms obtained in a left anterior oblique projection with cranial angulation.

The coronary arteries may demonstrate atherosclerotic obstructions but also frequently exhibit "blanching" of the septal vessels and intramyocardial left anterior descending artery during systole. The large epicardial coronary arteries in patients with HCM are usually free of atherosclerotic obstruction, but small intramural arteries exhibit intimal thickening and medial hypertrophy in some patients.[38] Furthermore, patients with HCM and angiographically normal epicardial coronary arteries still exhibit regional myocardial thallium 201 defects and metabolic evidence of myocardial ischemia during rapid atrial pacing.[39]

ENDOMYOCARDIAL BIOPSY

Nonsurgical biopsies of the heart were initially obtained in the early 1960s using percutaneous needle techniques similar to those utilized for liver or kidney biopsy.[40, 41] These procedures had an approximately 10 percent incidence of major complications. In 1962, Sakakibara and Konno[42] developed a flexible transvenous endomyocardial biopsy

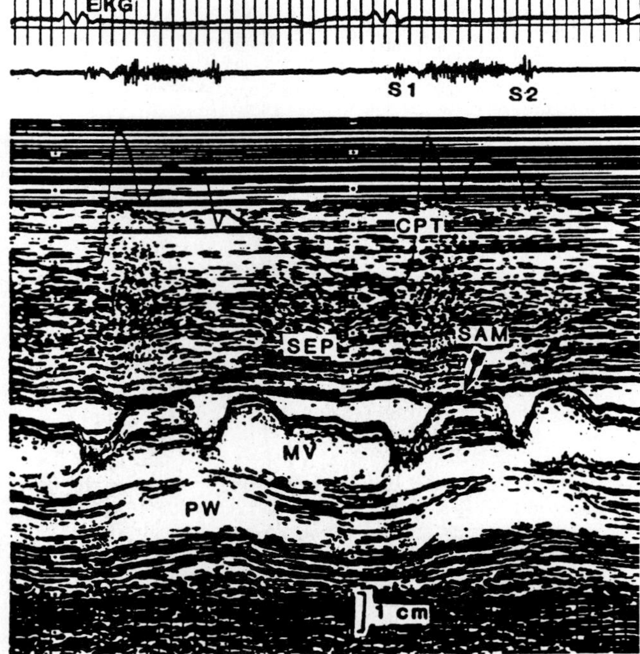

FIGURE 56–10 Simultaneous carotid pulse tracing (CPT), phonocardiogram, and M-mode echocardiographic recording at the level of the mitral valve (MV) in a patient with hypertrophic cardiomyopathy. The septum (SEP) is disproportionately thickened, there is systolic anterior motion (SAM) of the mitral valve, there is systolic retraction on the CPT, and a systolic murmur is noted. EKG, electrocardiogram; PW, posterior wall; S_1, S_2, first and second heart sounds. (From Come PC: Echocardiographic evaluation of the cardiomyopathies and specific heart muscle diseases. *In* Diagnostic Cardiology: Noninvasive Imaging Techniques. p. 375. Philadelphia: JB Lippincott, 1985.)

device that allowed much safer access to myocardial tissue. Since that time, there have been considerable technical improvements in the devices and technique, to the point where transvenous endomyocardial biopsy is a standard procedure that can be performed as part of the diagnostic evaluation in most catheterization laboratories.[43]

Biopsy specimens can be obtained from both the right and the left ventricle. Multiple biopsy specimens should be obtained because of the nonhomogeneous nature of some disease processes. The routine use of endomyocardial biopsy in patients with cardiomyopathies remains controversial, but it can clearly be of benefit in identifying specific causes of cardiac pathology.[43, 44] As a general rule, endomyocardial biopsy is most helpful (1) in myocarditis, (2) in diagnosis of cardiac involvement in systemic disease processes, such as amyloidosis, hemochromatosis, and sarcoid, (3) in distinguishing restrictive cardiomyopathy from constrictive pericarditis, (4) in postcardiac transplant evaluation for identification of rejection, (5) in cardiac tumors, and (6) in identification of cardiotoxic effects of agents such as Adriamycin. Therefore, the use of endomyocardial biopsy can help to facilitate the diagnosis of underlying causes for cardiomyopathy, particularly myocarditis and infiltrative disorders.

REFERENCES

1. Brigden W: Uncommon myocardial diseases: the non-coronary cardiomyopathies. Lancet 2:1179, 1957.
2. Report of the WHO/ISFC Task Force on the Definition and Classification of Cardiomyopathies. Br Heart J 44:672, 1980.
3. Abelmann WH: Classification and natural history of primary myocardial disease. Prog Cardiovasc Dis 27:73, 1984.
4. Pantely GA, Gristow JD: Ischemic cardiomyopathy. Prog Cardiovasc Dis 27:95, 1984.
5. Grossman W: Pressure measurement. *In* Grossman W (ed): Cardiac Catheterization and Angiography. 4th ed. pp. 123–142. Philadelphia: Lea & Febiger, 1991.
6. Antman EM, Marsh JD, Green LH, Grossman W: Blood oxygen measurements in the assessment of intracardiac left to right shunts: a critical appraisal of methodology. Am J Cardiol 46:265, 1980.
7. Fuster V, Gersh BJ, Giuliani ER, et al: The natural history of idiopathic dilated cardiomyopathy. Am J Cardiol 47:525, 1981.
8. Johnson RA, Palacios I: Dilated cardiomyopathies of the adult. Parts I & II. N Engl J Med 307:1051, 1119, 1982.
9. Wallis DE, O'Connell JB, Henkin RE, et al: Segmental wall motion abnormalities in dilated cardiomyopathy: a common finding and good prognostic sign. J Am Coll Cardiol 4:674, 1984.
10. Opherk D, Schwarz F, Mall G, et al: Coronary dilatory capacity in idiopathic dilated cardiomyopathy: analysis of 16 patients. Am J Cardiol 51:1657, 1983.
11. Hosenpud JD, Niles NR: Clinical, hemodynamic and endomyocardial biopsy findings in idiopathic restrictive cardiomyopathy. West J Med 144:303, 1986.
12. Benotti JR, Grossman W, Cohn PF: The clinical profile of restrictive cardiomyopathy. Circulation 61:1206, 1980.
13. Siegel RJ, Shah PK, Fishbein MC: Idiopathic restrictive cardiomyopathy. Circulation 70:165, 1984.
14. Benotti JR, Grossman W: Restrictive cardiomyopathy. Annu Rev Med 35:113, 1984.
15. Soulen RD, Stark DD, Higgins CB, et al: Magnetic resonance imaging of constrictive pericardial disease. Am J Cardiol 55:480, 1985.
16. Sutton FJ, Whitley NO, Applefeld MM, et al: The role of echocardiography and computed tomography in evaluation of constrictive pericarditis. Am Heart J 109:350, 1985.
17. Hirota Y, Kohriyama T, Hayashi T, et al: Idiopathic restrictive cardiomyopathy: differences of left ventricular relaxation and diastolic wave forms from constrictive pericarditis. Am J Cardiol 52:421, 1983.
18. Lorell BH, Grossman W: Profiles in constrictive pericarditis, restrictive cardiomyopathy, and cardiac tamponade. *In* Grossman W (ed): Cardiac Catheterization and Angiography. 4th ed. pp. 633–653. Philadelphia: Lea & Febiger, 1991.
19. Goodwin JF: The frontiers of cardiomyopathy. Br Heart J 48:1, 1982.
20. Braunwald E, Lambrew CT, Rockoff SD, et al: Idiopathic hypertrophic subaortic stenosis. Circulation 29/30(suppl IV):1, 1964.
21. Maron BJ, Epstein SE: Hypertrophic cardiomyopathy: a discussion of nomenclature. Am J Cardiol 43:1242, 1979.
22. Maron BJ, Nichols PF III, Pickle LW, et al: Patterns of inheritance in hypertrophic cardiomyopathy: assessment by M-mode and two-dimensional echocardiography. Am J Cardiol 53:1087, 1984.
23. Jarcho JA, McKenna W, Pare JA, et al: Mapping a gene for familial hypertrophic cardiomyopathy to chromosome 14q1. N Engl J Med 321:1372, 1989.
24. Hejtmancik JF, Brink PA, Towbin J, et al: Localization of gene for familial hypertrophic cardiomyopathy to chromosome 14q1 in a diverse US population. Circulation 83:1592, 1991.
25. Murgo JP, Alter BR, Dorethy JF, et al: Dynamics of left ventricular ejection in obstructive and nonobstructive hypertrophic cardiomyopathy. J Clin Invest 66:1369, 1980.
26. Murgo JP: Does outflow obstruction exist in hypertrophic cardiomyopathy? N Engl J Med 307:1008, 1982.
27. Criley JM, Siegel RJ: Has "obstruction" hindered our understanding of hypertrophic cardiomyopathy? Circulation 72:1148, 1985.
28. Criley JM, Lewis KB, White RI, Ross RS: Pressure gradients without obstruction: a new concept of "hypertrophic subaortic stenosis." Circulation 22:881, 1965.
29. White RI, Criley JM, Lewis KB, Ross RS: Experimental production of intracavity pressure differences: possible significance in the interpretation of human hemodynamic studies. Am J Cardiol 19:806, 1967.
30. Levine RA, Weyman AE: Dynamic subaortic obstruction in hypertrophic cardiomyopathy: criteria and controversy. J Am Coll Cardiol 6:16, 1985.
31. Maron BJ, Gottdiener JS, Arco J, et al: Dynamic subaortic obstruction in hypertrophic cardiomyopathy: analysis by pulsed Doppler echocardiography. J Am Coll Cardiol 6:1, 1985.
32. Wigle ED, Auger P, Marquis Y: Muscular subaortic stenosis. The direct relation between the intraventricular pressure difference and the left ventricular ejection time. Circulation 36:36, 1967.
33. Sasson Z, Henderson M, Wilansky S, et al: Causal relation between the pressure gradient and left ventricular ejection time in hypertrophic cardiomyopathy. J Am Coll Cardiol 13:1275, 1989.
34. Bonow RO: Left ventricular ejection dynamics and outflow obstruction in hypertrophic cardiomyopathy. J Am Coll Cardiol 13:1280, 1989.
35. Glancy DL, Shephard RL, Beiser GD, Epstein SE: The dynamic nature of left ventricular outflow obstructions in idiopathic hypertrophic subaortic stenosis. Ann Intern Med 75:589, 1971.
36. Brockenbrough EC, Braunwald E, Morrow AG: A hemodynamic technique for the detection of hypertrophic subaortic stenosis. Circulation 23:189, 1961.
37. Frank S, Braunwald E: Idiopathic hypertrophic subaortic stenosis. Clinical analysis of 126 patients with emphasis on the natural history. Circulation 37:759, 1968.
38. Maron BJ, Wolfson JK, Epstein SE, Roberts WC: Intramural ("small vessel") coronary artery disease in hypertrophic cardiomyopathy. J Am Coll Cardiol 8:545, 1986.
39. Cannon RO III, Dilsizian V, O'Gara PT, et al: Myocardial metabolic, hemodynamic, and electrocardiographic significance of reversible thallium-201 abnormalities in hypertrophic cardiomyopathy. Circulation 83:1660, 1991.
40. Shugoll GI: Percutaneous myocardial and pericardial biopsy with Menghini needle. Am Heart J 85:35, 1973.
41. Shirey EK, Hawk WA, Mukerji D, Effler DB: Percutaneous myocardial biopsy of the left ventricle: experience in 198 patients. Circulation 46:112, 1972.
42. Sakakibara S, Konno S: Endomyocardial biopsy. Jpn Heart J 3:537, 1962.
43. Fowles RE, Mason JW: Endomyocardial biopsy. Ann Intern Med 97:885, 1982.
44. Mason JW: Endomyocardial biopsy: the balance of success and failure. Circulation 71:185, 1985.

45. Grossman W: Profiles in dilated and hypertrophic cardiomyopathies. *In* Grossman W (ed): Cardiac Catheterization and Angiography. 4th ed. pp. 618–632. Philadelphia: Lea & Febiger, 1991.
46. Olney BA: Restrictive myocardial disease. *In* Giuliani ER, Fuster V, Gersh BJ, et al (eds). Cardiology. Fundamentals and Practice. pp. 1775–1791. St. Louis: Mosby–Year Book, 1991.
47. Siegel RJ, Criley JM: Comparison of ventricular emptying with and without a pressure gradient in patients with hypertrophic cardiomyopathy. Br Heart J 53:283, 1985.
48. Wigle ED: Hypertrophic cardiomyopathy: a 1987 viewpoint. Circulation 75:311, 1987.
49. Come PC: Echocardiographic evaluation of the cardiomyopathies and specific heart muscle diseases. *In* Diagnostic Cardiology: Noninvasive Imaging Techniques. p. 375. Philadelphia: JB Lippincott, 1985.

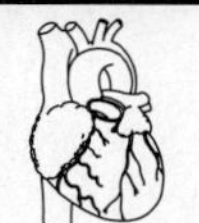

CHAPTER 57

ECHOCARDIOGRAPHY

Francis T. Thandroyen and Eddy Barasch

HYPERTROPHIC CARDIOMYOPATHY
Hypertrophy
Systolic Anterior Motion of the Mitral Valve
Doppler Analysis of LVOT Gradient
Mitral Regurgitation
LV Size and Function
DILATED CARDIOMYOPATHY
Ventricular Dilatation and Impaired Function
Differential Diagnosis
Mitral and Tricuspid Regurgitation
Thrombus
RESTRICTIVE CARDIOMYOPATHY
Amyloidosis
Hemochromatosis
Sarcoidosis

HYPERTROPHIC CARDIOMYOPATHY

Hypertrophy

The characteristic feature of hypertrophic cardiomyopathy is asymmetric left ventricular (LV) hypertrophy.[1] The typical site of hypertrophy is the interventricular septum, the septal thickness being disproportionately increased to that of the posterior wall thickness. Asymmetric septal hypertrophy (Fig. 57–1) is defined echocardiographically by a septal wall thickness of at least 15 mm and a ratio of septal thickness/posterior wall thickness of 1.31 or greater. Hypertrophy of the interventricular septum may be localized to the proximal segment, the midsegment, or the distal segment.[1] Although the specificity of asymmetric septal hypertrophy for hypertrophic cardiomyopathy is approximately 90 percent, other conditions in which asymmetric septal hypertrophy may occur include (1) hypertension or aortic stenosis, (2) pulmonary hypertension, (3) infiltrative diseases such as amyloid, and (4) tumor invasion by lymphoma. Two-dimensional echocardiography may identify sites of hypertrophy other than the interventricular septum (e.g., hypertrophy localized to either the free wall, the midportion, or the apex of the left ventricle).[2] Rarely, hypertrophic cardiomyopathy may be associated with concentric LV hypertrophy or hypertrophy localized to the right ventricle. Hypertrophic cardiomyopathy commonly manifests with asymmetric LV hypertrophy and LV diastolic dysfunction; left ventricular outflow tract (LVOT) or intraventricular obstruction is not present. Less commonly, hypertrophic cardiomyopathy manifests with asymmetric LV hypertrophy, LVOT or intraventricular obstruction, and LV diastolic dysfunction.

Systolic Anterior Motion of the Mitral Valve

M-mode and two-dimensional echocardiography characterize the presence or absence of systolic anterior motion (SAM) of the mitral valve. SAM may involve the anterior leaflet, posterior leaflet, both leaflets, or the chordae.[3] Two-dimensional (Fig. 57–2) and M-mode (Fig. 57–3) echocardiography best illustrate the anterior motion of the mitral valve toward the interventricular septum during systole. SAM of the mitral valve results in narrowing of the LVOT, thereby causing dynamic obstruction and the generation of a late systolic pressure gradient.[4] A temporal relationship has been shown between the onset of apposition of the anterior mitral leaflet with the septum and the onset of a systolic gradient in the LVOT. Patients without SAM of the mitral valve usually have no LVOT gradient, whereas patients with severe SAM (Fig. 57–4) of the mitral valve usually have a resting gradient.

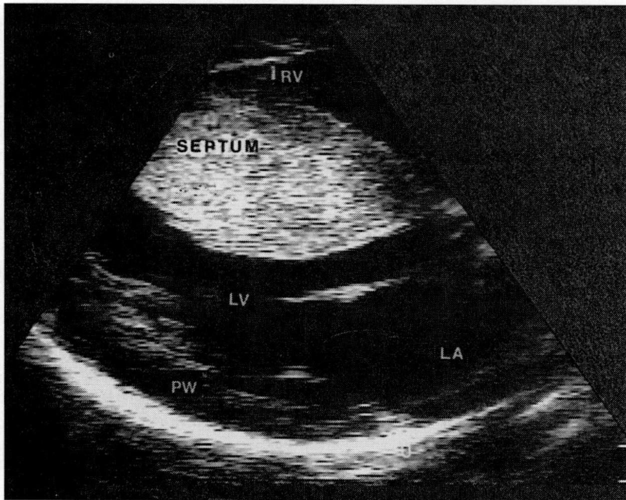

FIGURE 57–1 Parasternal long-axis view of a two-dimensional echocardiogram of a patient with hypertrophic cardiomyopathy illustrates the markedly thickened interventricular septum. In contrast, the thickness of the posterior wall of the left ventricle (LV) is normal. The disproportionate increase of the septal to posterior wall thickness is termed *asymmetric septal hypertrophy.* The left ventricular cavity size is normal. LA, left atrium; PW, posterior wall of LV; RV, right ventricle.

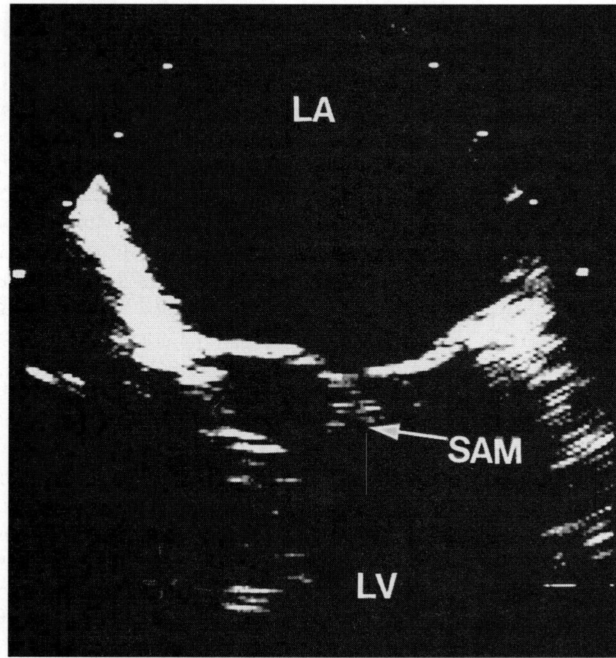

FIGURE 57–2 Transesophageal two-dimensional echocardiogram of a patient with hypertrophic cardiomyopathy. The anterior leaflet of the mitral valve is displaced toward the interventricular septum (SAM), resulting in narrowing of the left ventricular outflow tract. LA, left atrium; LV, left ventricle; SAM, systolic anterior motion of the mitral valve.

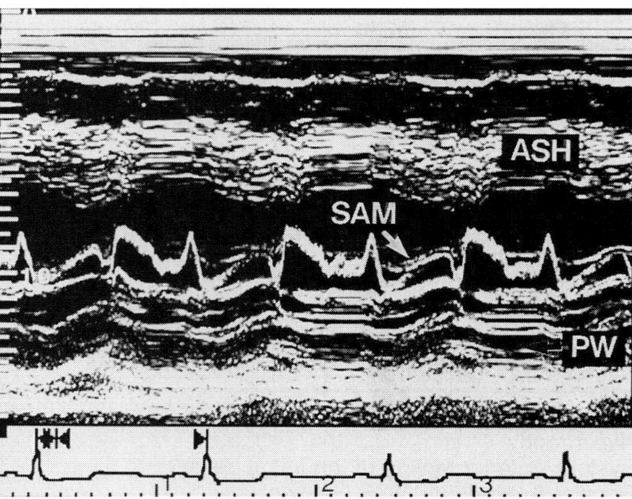

FIGURE 57–3 M-mode recording of a patient with hypertrophic cardiomyopathy demonstrates asymmetric septal hypertrophy (ASH). During systole, there is systolic anterior movement of the mitral leaflet (SAM) toward the interventricular septum. In this figure, there is no apposition of the anterior mitral leaflet with the interventricular septum. PW, posterior wall of the left ventricle.

Doppler Analysis of LVOT Gradient

Pulsed-wave Doppler and high-pulse repetition frequency analysis from the apex of the left ventricle to the LVOT delineate the site of dynamic obstruction and provide an accurate estimation of the magnitude of the LVOT gradient.[5] As the site of the obstruction is approached, there is acceleration of blood flow, as well as aliasing of blood flow; the highest flow velocity is recorded at the site of obstruction. The characteristic Doppler spectral profile of LVOT obstruction is increased peak flow velocity with late systolic peaking (Fig. 57–5). The latter profile has been characterized as a saber pattern. Factors that either decrease the volume of the left ventricle (amyl nitrite) or increase the contractility (isoproterenol or a postextrasystolic beat) increase the magnitude of the gradient, whereas factors that increase the volume of the left ventricle (beta-receptor antagonists) or decrease the contractility decrease the mag-

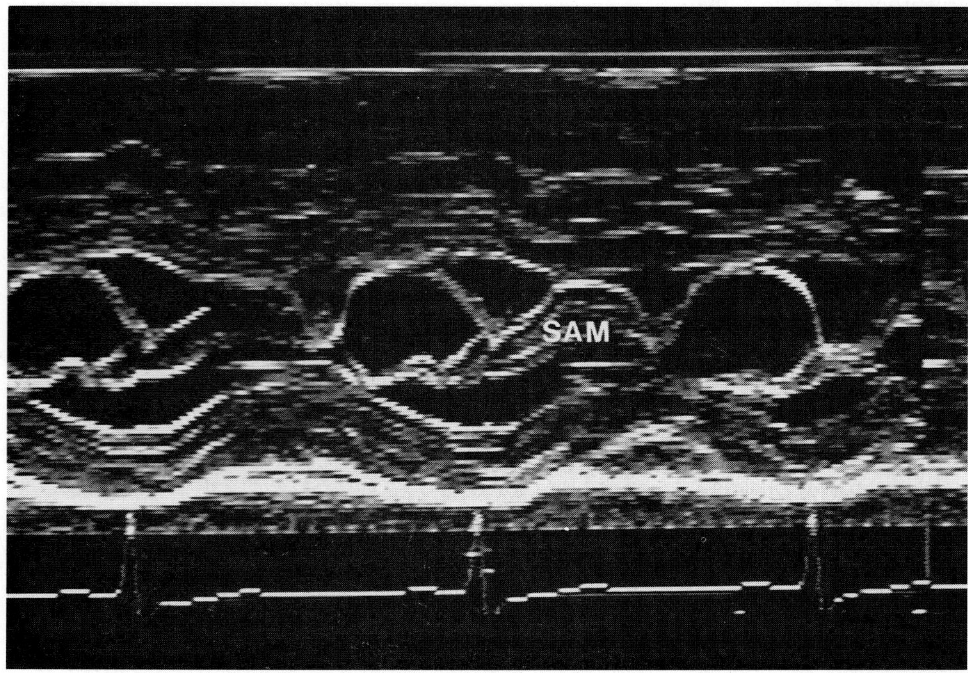

FIGURE 57–4 M-mode recording demonstrates systolic anterior movement of the mitral leaflets (SAM) with prolonged apposition of the mitral valve with the interventricular septum through systole. These cases usually have a resting systolic gradient.

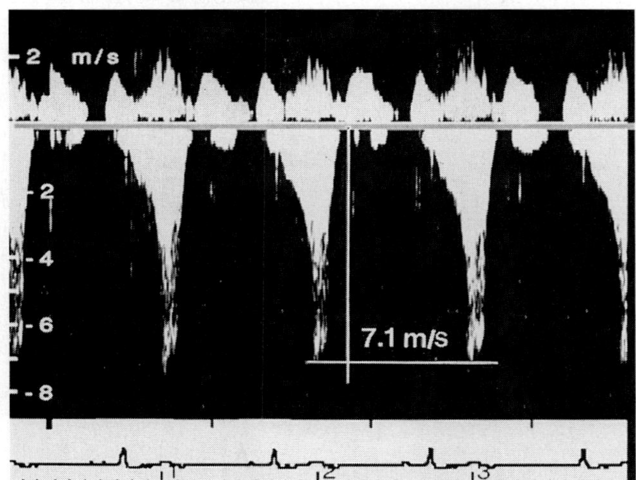

FIGURE 57–5 Continuous-wave Doppler in the left ventricular outflow tract (LVOT) of a patient with hypertrophic cardiomyopathy demonstrates a marked increase in the peak flow velocity (7.1 m/s) with late systolic peaking.

nitude of the gradient. The duration of the SAM septal contact (see Fig. 57–4) has been correlated with the extent of the LVOT gradient. SAM septal contact has also been correlated with deceleration of flow in the aorta and the development of premature closure of the aortic valve in midsystole. The premature closure may involve one or two leaflets. Color-flow Doppler may also delineate the site of LVOT obstruction by illustrating a mosaic of color in the LVOT (Plates 57–1 and 57–2) during systole, indicative of turbulent flow below the level of the aortic valve.[6]

Recent evidence shows significant daily variability in the LVOT gradient. In view of this, accurate measurement of the gradient can be obtained only by repeated measurements on different days.[7]

Mitral Regurgitation

Dynamic obstruction of the LVOT is usually accompanied by a posteriorly directed jet of mitral regurgitation (see Plate 57–2). Mitral regurgitation is considered to result from the abnormal position of the mitral valve in the LVOT. A recent report[8] explains the interindividual differences in the severity of mitral regurgitation for comparable degrees of SAM. Limitation of motion of posterior mitral leaflet and decreased length over which the leaflets coapt directly correlate with the severity of regurgitation.[8] Imaging from the apical views may illustrate overlap of two high-velocity jets on the Doppler spectral display (Fig. 57–6). Distinguishing between the two high-velocity jets of LVOT obstruction and mitral regurgitation is important to avoid incorrect interpretation. The spectral Doppler trace of LVOT obstruction is characterized by late systolic peaking; in contrast, the Doppler velocity trace of mitral regurgitation is characterized by early systolic peaking, with attainment of the peak velocity usually within the first third of systole. In addition, the mitral regurgitation jet can be identified by its onset in the isovolumic contraction period and ending after aortic valve closure.

LV Size and Function

The LV cavity size is either small or normal, and systolic function is usually normal. When hypercontractile systolic function with cavitary obliteration occurs, the intraventricular Doppler flow pattern during systole may reveal increased peak flow velocity with late systolic peaking, a pattern similar to that of LVOT obstruction. A peculiar Doppler spectral profile of diastolic blood flow from apex

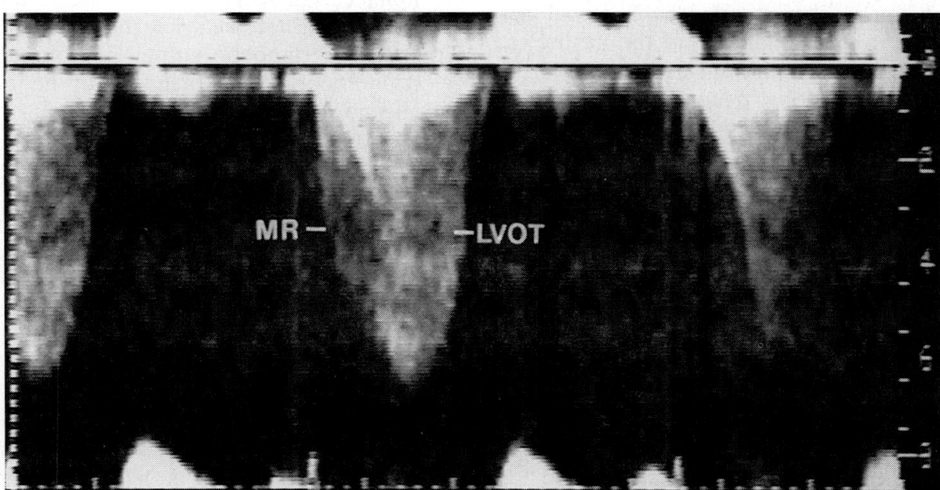

FIGURE 57–6 Imaging from the apical views may illustrate overlap of the spectral display of two high-velocity jets (middle of three traces). Distinguishing between the two high-velocity jets is of importance to obviate incorrect interpretation of the spectral trace of mitral regurgitation (MR) as the trace of left ventricular outflow tract (LVOT) obstruction. The spectral Doppler trace of LVOT obstruction is characterized by late systolic peaking (seen alone in the third trace). In contrast, the Doppler flow velocity trace of MR is characterized by early systolic peaking, with attainment of the peak velocity usually within the first third of systole.

to base of the left ventricle can be seen in patients in whom the apex undergoes cavity obliteration during systole. LV diastolic dysfunction is associated with hypertrophic cardiomyopathy.[9] Pulsed-wave analysis of the mitral inflow velocity, pulmonic veins, transmitral color M-mode, and Doppler tissue imaging of the mitral annulus or myocardial walls have been utilized to analyze diastolic function.[10] In general, at the early stages of the disease, an impaired relaxation pattern of LV filling is observed, whereas at more advanced stages, a pseudonormalized and, finally, a restrictive pattern can occur. In a study evaluating the validity of deceleration time (DT) of the transmitral E wave to predict mean left atrial pressure (LAP), no significant correlation was found between mean LAP and DT in a group of 55 patients with hypertrophic cardiomyopathy compared with a group of patients with dilated cardiomyopathy.[11] Doppler echocardiography has an important role in the selection of patients who might benefit from surgical or nonsurgical septal reduction. For those patients for whom septal myotomy/myectomy is envisioned, preoperative variables of asymmetric hypertrophy, severe SAM, and prolonged isovolumic relaxation time can identify patients who are most likely to benefit from this procedure.[12] Anomalous papillary muscle insertion into the anterior mitral leaflet has been recently described as a cause for muscular midcavitary obstruction requiring another surgical technique for relief of LVOT obstruction than the classic ventricular septal myotomy/myectomy.[13] Myocardial contrast echocardiography has been shown to be very valuable to identify the target vessel in addition to probatory balloon occlusion in patients undergoing percutaneous transluminal septal ablation.[14, 15]

DILATED CARDIOMYOPATHY

Ventricular Dilatation and Impaired Function

Dilated cardiomyopathy is characterized by a global decrease in systolic function and dilatation of the ventricles. The characteristic echocardiographic manifestations of dilated cardiomyopathy are a global decrease in ventricular contraction, dilatation of the left ventricle, and dilatation of the right ventricle (Figs. 57–7 and 57–8).[16, 17] Left atrial and right atrial dilatation may occur owing to ventricular dysfunction and/or valvular regurgitation, producing four-chamber dilatation (see Fig. 57–7). The LV wall thickness is usually normal but may be decreased from muscle loss and replacement by fibrosis or increased from hypertrophy. In contrast, total LV mass is usually increased.

M-mode echocardiography delineates an increase in the E point septal distance (see Fig. 57–8) (indicative of an increase in the residual volume) and also reveals increases in the LV end-diastolic and end-systolic dimensions indicative of elevated end-diastolic and end-systolic volumes, respectively.[16, 17] The measured indices of systolic function from M-mode echocardiograms, such as percentage fractional shortening of the left ventricle and calculated ejection fraction, are reduced. Such parameters of ventricular function can be estimated, as dilated cardiomyopathy is usually associated with a symmetric global decrease in the ventricular function. Real-time two-dimensional echocardiography shows symmetric global impairment in systolic function. Reduction in the rate of rise of LV pressure development (LV dP/dt) can be estimated from continuous-wave Doppler analysis of the mitral regurgitant jet. With severe impairment in LV function, M-mode echocardiography may show decreased excursion of the mitral and aortic leaflets secondary to a reduced cardiac output.

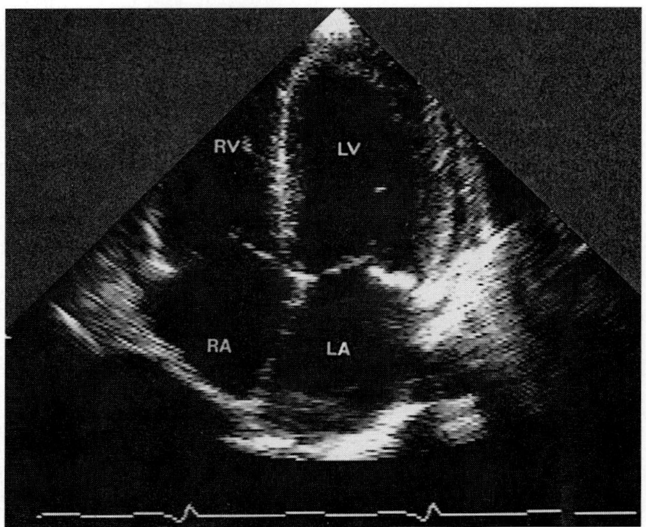

FIGURE 57–7 Two-dimensional echocardiogram of a patient with a dilated cardiomyopathy. The apical four-chamber view reveals dilatation of both the left and the right ventricles as well as dilatation of both the left and the right atria. LA, left atrium; LV, left ventricle; RA, right atrium; RV, right ventricle.

Pulsed-wave Doppler analysis may reveal a restrictive mitral inflow velocity profile[18] in which the characteristic findings are a tall E wave with a short DT (indicative of rapid ventricular filling and rapid equilibration of LV and left atrial pressures) and a small A wave. The latter mitral flow profile is representative of marked impairment in LV compliance. In a number of studies, the diastolic filling pattern of the left ventricle has been shown to have an important prognostic value. Combining left ventricular ejection fraction (LVEF) and DT of the transmitral E wave, Rihal and colleagues[19] found that an LVEF less than 25 percent and DT less than 130 ms yielded a 2-year survival of 35 percent in contrast to those patients with LVEF less than 25 percent and DT greater than 130 ms who had a 2-year survival of 72 percent, and those with LVEF greater than 25 percent who had a 2-year survival of 95 percent regardless of DT. Another group of investigators, analyzing by Doppler echocardiography 100 patients with congestive heart failure with LVEF less than 40 percent, found that those patients with a transmitral E wave DT of 140 ms and $E/A \geq 2$ or $E/A = 1$ to 2 had a mortality at 1 and 2 years of 19 percent and 51 percent, respectively, in contrast to the nonrestrictive group DT greater than 140 ms and $E/A \leq 1$ or $E/A = 1$ to 2 who had a mortality of 5 percent at both follow-up periods.[20]

Differential Diagnosis

The previously mentioned echocardiographic features are suggestive but not diagnostic of dilated cardiomyopathy

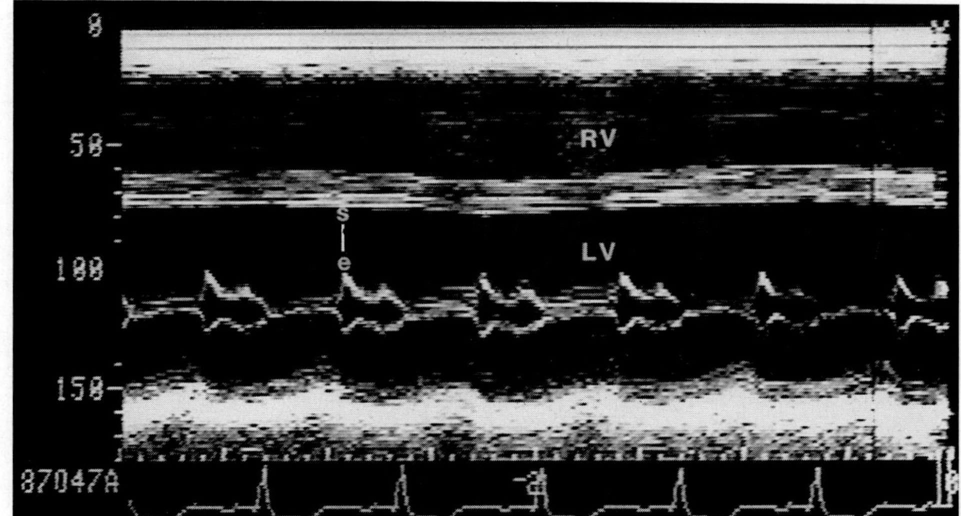

FIGURE 57–8 M-mode echocardiogram of a patient with a dilated cardiomyopathy. The left ventricle (LV) is dilated with an increase in the E point septal distance, the interventricular septum is akinetic, and the posterior wall is hypokinetic. The right ventricle (RV) is dilated.

and do not allow for differentiation as to the etiology of the underlying heart disease. For example, in some patients with ischemic heart disease, the extensive loss of muscle from multiple myocardial infarcts may result in marked ventricular dilatation and global impairment of systolic function, echocardiographic features of a dilated cardiomyopathy. In addition, in patients with long-standing severe mitral regurgitation, ventricular dilatation and severe global impairment in ventricular function may occur, thereby simulating the echocardiographic features of dilated cardiomyopathy. Finally, in cases of cardiomyopathy secondary to alcohol or myocarditis, or in cardiomyopathies complicated by coronary emboli, regional wall motion abnormalities may occur and simulate echocardiographic features of ischemic heart disease.

Mitral and Tricuspid Regurgitation

Color-flow Doppler echocardiography provides semiquantitative analysis of mitral regurgitation. Such mitral regurgitation may occur as a result of mitral annular dilatation, changes in the LV geometry, which becomes more globular, or papillary muscle dysfunction. Apparently, there is a decrease in both midsystolic regurgitant flow rate and mitral orifice area, which are strongly correlated with the dynamic changes in the transmitral pressure, which ultimately is responsible for the valve closure.[21] The development of mitral regurgitation may augment previously depressed wall motion, especially the septum. Color-flow Doppler echocardiography also provides semiquantitative analysis of tricuspid regurgitation, and spectral Doppler analysis defines the peak flow velocity of the tricuspid regurgitant jet. Using the modified Bernoulli equation, right ventricular (RV) systolic pressure can be accurately estimated from the peak flow velocity of the tricuspid regurgitant jet.

Thrombus

Two-dimensional echocardiography may demonstrate decreased blood flow within the ventricular cavity as spontaneous echo contrast. In addition, two-dimensional analysis may illustrate thrombus in the left ventricle or, less commonly, in the right ventricle. It has been shown on transesophageal echocardiography that in patients in sinus rhythm, a marked elevation in the LAP can reduce the left atrial appendage peak emptying wave velocities, which may explain a higher incidence of thrombus formation in the left atrial appendage compared with subjects with normal or only mildly elevated LAPs.[22]

RESTRICTIVE CARDIOMYOPATHY

The characteristic features of restrictive cardiomyopathy are abnormal compliance of the ventricles with restriction to ventricular filling and elevated ventricular filling pressures. LV systolic function is normal or decreased, and diastolic dysfunction is usually present. The echocardiography usually shows biatrial dilatation in the presence of thickened wall ventricles and dilated systemic and pulmonic veins. Although the LV systolic function is in general preserved, the transmitral Doppler, pulmonic vein flow, and isovolumic relaxation time show the restrictive pattern in general in the late stages of the disease. Doppler tissue imaging of the mitral annulus has been shown to be able to differentiate between restrictive and constrictive physiology, an early diastolic peak velocity of 8 cm/s can differentiate between restriction and constriction (<8 cm/s and >8 cm/s, respectively).[23]

Amyloidosis

Amyloid heart disease is the most frequent type of infiltrative or restrictive cardiomyopathy. The amyloid protein is deposited between myofibrils, within papillary muscles, or in the conduction system, valvular structures, or atrial septum.

The characteristic two-dimensional and M-mode findings[24] are of a normal-sized LV or RV cavity with increased

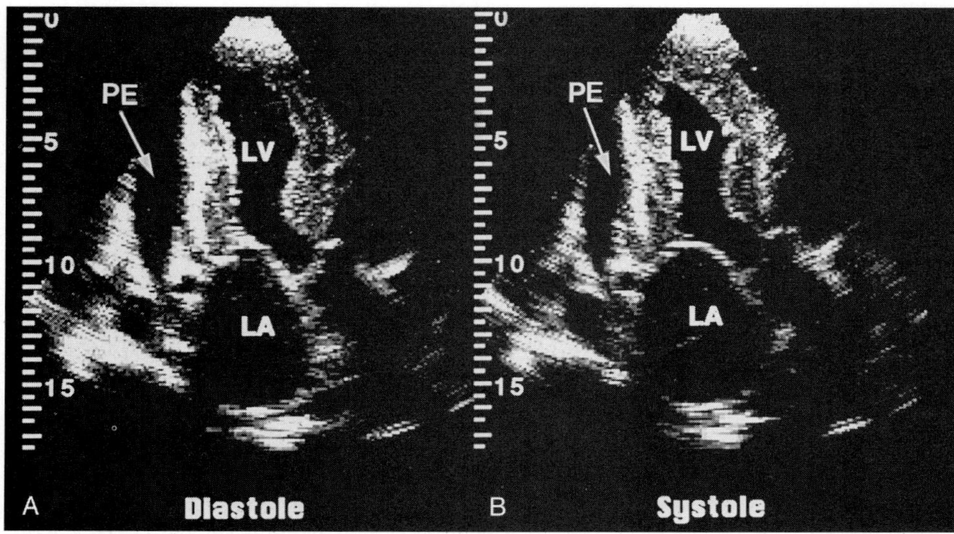

FIGURE 57–9 Two-dimensional echocardiogram of a patient with amyloidosis. **A,** Diastole. **B,** Systole. The apical three-chamber view reveals a small-sized left ventricular cavity with marked increase in the thickness of the walls of the left ventricle (LV). There is dilatation of the left atrium (LA) and a moderate pericardial effusion (PE).

wall thickness that may involve the left ventricle (Fig. 57–9) and right ventricle (Fig. 57–10). Increased wall thickness may precede clinical manifestations of cardiac disease, and progressive increase of wall thickness has been associated with a worse prognosis. A speckled or granular appearance to the myocardium may be visualized on two-dimensional echocardiographic images; however, this appearance is not specific for amyloid. Left atrial (see Fig. 57–9) or biatrial dilatation (see Fig. 57–10) is common and usually results from abnormal diastolic compliance of the ventricles, with its attendant restriction to ventricular filling. Amyloid infiltration produces thickening of valvular structures. The mitral and tricuspid valves are the most commonly involved and may manifest as mild mitral or tricuspid regurgitation (Plate 57–3). Atrioventricular regurgitation may contribute to atrial dilatation. LV systolic function is either normal or mildly reduced (Fig. 57–11). Progressive reduction in systolic function has been associated with an adverse prognosis. Small or moderate pericardial effusions (see Fig. 57–11 and Plates 57–1 and 57–2) are detected in up to 30 percent of patients. Hypertrophy of the interatrial septum may occur from infiltration by amyloid; the differential diagnosis is of lipomatous infiltration. The duration of pulmonary venous atrial reversal was found to be longer than that of mitral A wave in patients with amyloidosis, signifying the presence of LV end-diastolic pressure greater than 15 mm Hg in this group of patients when compared with normal subjects.[25] In patients with primary cardiac amyloidosis, the RV dilatation (LV/RV area ratio ≤ 2) brings a poor prognosis, with a median survival of 4 months.[26] Increased wall thickness on echocardiography in association with low voltage on the electro-

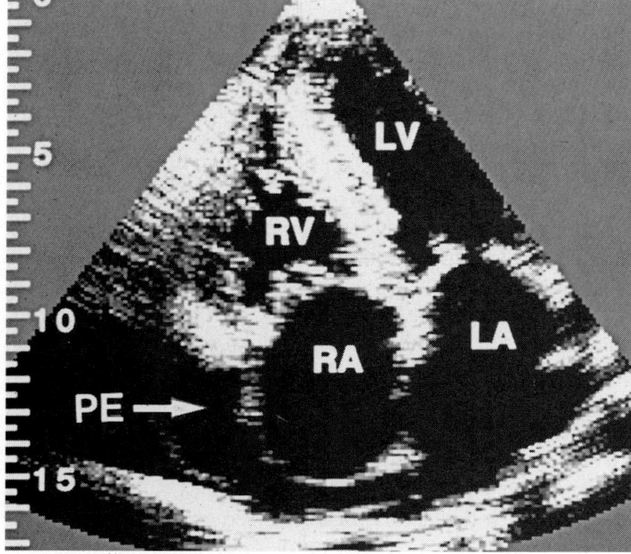

FIGURE 57–10 Two-dimensional echocardiogram of a patient with amyloidosis diastole. The apical four-chamber view reveals a small right ventricular cavity with marked increase in the thickness of the walls of the right ventricle (RV). There is biatrial dilatation and a moderate-sized pericardial effusion (PE) anterior to the right atrium (RA). LA, left atrium; LV, left ventricle.

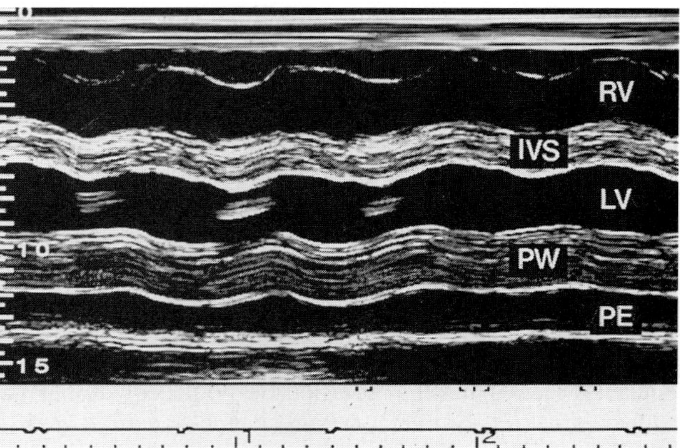

FIGURE 57–11 M-mode echocardiogram of a patient with amyloidosis. The characteristic features are a small left ventricular cavity with marked increase in the thickness of the interventricular septum (IVS) and the posterior wall (PW). There is not a marked difference in the internal dimensions of the ventricular cavity during systole and diastole indicative of impaired ventricular function. There is a moderate pericardial effusion (PE). LV, left ventricle; RV, right ventricle.

cardiogram is strongly suggestive of amyloid, but the definitive diagnosis of amyloid is ultimately dependent on tissue biopsy.

Hemochromatosis

The characteristic echocardiographic features of primary and secondary hemochromatosis include dilatation of the ventricular chambers in association with biatrial dilatation. LV systolic function exhibits mild to severe impairment because of deposition of iron within the ventricular myocytes and myocyte injury. Secondary hemochromatosis has been associated with increased wall thickness.

Sarcoidosis

Sarcoid granulomas occur within the myocardium, especially in the interventricular septum. M-mode and two-dimensional echocardiography show regional wall motion abnormalities, especially involving the interventricular septum. LV cavity size is dilated, with impairment in systolic function; diastolic dysfunction may occur. Two-dimensional echocardiography may reveal segmental wall thinning. Rarely, an apical aneurysm of the left ventricle may be detected.

References

1. Henry WL, Clark CE, Epstein SE: Asymmetric septal hypertrophy: the unifying link in the IHSS disease spectrum: observation regarding its pathogenesis, pathophysiology and course. Circulation 47:827, 1973.
2. Maron BJ, Gottdiener JS, Epstein SE: Patterns and significance of distribution of left ventricular hypertrophy in hypertrophic cardiomyopathy: a wide angle, two-dimensional echocardiographic study of 125 patients. Am J Cardiol 48:418, 1981.
3. Ballester M, Rickards A, Rees S, et al: Systolic anterior motion of the mitral valve in hypertrophic cardiomyopathy. A cross sectional echocardiographic study. Eur Heart J 4:846, 1983.
4. Polick C, Morgan CD, Gilbert BW, et al: Muscular subaortic stenosis: the temporal relationship between systolic anterior motion of the anterior mitral leaflet and the pressure gradient. Circulation 66:1087, 1982.
5. Maron BJ, Gottdiener JS, Arce J, et al: Dynamic subaortic obstruction in hypertrophic cardiomyopathy: analysis by pulsed Doppler echocardiography. J Am Coll Cardiol 6:1, 1985.
6. Hoit BD, Penonen E, Dalton N, et al: Doppler color flow mapping studies of jet formation and spatial orientation in obstructive hypertrophic cardiomyopathy. Am Heart J 117:1119, 1989.
7. Kizilbash AM, Heinle SK, Grayburn PA: Spontaneous variability of left ventricular pressure gradient in hypertrophic obstructive cardiomyopathy. Circulation 97:461, 1998.
8. Schwammenthal E, Nakatani S, He S, et al: Mechanism of mitral regurgitation in hypertrophic cardiomyopathy: mismatch of posterior to anterior septal leaflet length and mobility. Circulation 98:856, 1998.
9. Spirito P, Maron BJ: Relation between extent of left ventricular hypertrophy and diastolic filling abnormalities in hypertrophic cardiomyopathy. J Am Coll Cardiol 15:811, 1990.
10. Severino S, Caso P, Galderisi M, et al: Use of pulsed Doppler tissue imaging to assess regional left ventricular diastolic dysfunction in hypertrophic cardiomyopathy. Am J Cardiol 82:1394, 1998.
11. Nishimura RA, Appleton CP, Redfield MM, et al: Noninvasive Doppler echocardiographic evaluation of left ventricular filling pressures in patients with cardiomyopathies: a simultaneous Doppler echocardiographic and cardiac catheterization study. J Am Coll Cardiol 28:1226, 1996.
12. McCully RB, Nishimura RA, Bailey KR, et al: Hypertrophic obstructive cardiomyopathy: preoperative echocardiographic predictors of outcome after septal myectomy. J Am Coll Cardiol 27:1491, 1996.
13. Baron BJ, Nishimura RA, Danielson GK: Pitfalls in clinical recognition and a novel operative approach for hypertrophic cardiomyopathy with severe outflow obstruction due to anomalous papillary muscle. Circulation 98:2505, 1998.
14. Nagueh SF, Lakkis NM, He ZX, et al: Role of myocardial contrast echocardiography during nonsurgical septal reduction therapy for hypertrophic obstructive cardiomyopathy. J Am Coll Cardiol 32:225, 1998.
15. Faber L, Seggewiss H, Gleichmann U: Percutaneous transluminal septal myocardial ablation in hypertrophic obstructive cardiomyopathy: results with respect to intraprocedural myocardial contrast echocardiography. Circulation 98:2451, 1998.
16. Johnson RA, Palacios I: Dilated cardiomyopathies of the adult. N Engl J Med 307:1051, 1982.
17. Shah PM: Echocardiography in congested or dilated cardiomyopathy. J Am Soc Echocardiogr 1:20, 1988.
18. Appleton CP, Hatle LV, Popp RL: Demonstration of restrictive ventricular physiology by Doppler echocardiography. J Am Coll Cardiol 11:757, 1988.
19. Rihal CS, Nishimura RA, Hatle LK, et al: Systolic and diastolic dysfunction in patients with clinical diagnosis of dilated cardiomyopathy. Relation to symptoms and prognosis. Circulation 90:2772, 1994.
20. Xie GY, Berk MR, Smith MD, et al: Prognostic value of Doppler transmitral flow patterns in patients with congestive heart failure. J Am Coll Cardiol 24:132, 1994.
21. Hung J, Otsuji Y, Handschumacher MD, et al: Mechanism of dynamic regurgitant orifice area variation in functional mitral regurgitation: physiologic insights from the proximal flow convergence technique. J Am Coll Cardiol 33:538, 1999.
22. Tabata T, Oki T, Fukuda N, et al: Influence of left atrial pressure on left atrial appendage flow velocity patterns in patients in sinus rhythm. J Am Soc Echocardiogr 9:857, 1996.
23. Garcia MJ, Rodriguez L, Ares MA, et al: Differentiation of constrictive pericarditis from restrictive cardiomyopathy: assessment of left ventricular diastolic velocities in the longitudinal axis by Doppler tissue imaging. J Am Coll Cardiol 27:108, 1996.
24. Picano E, Pinamonti B, Ferdeghini EM, et al: Two dimensional echocardiography in myocardial amyloidosis. Echocardiography 8:253, 1991.
25. Abdalla I, Murray RD, Lee JC, et al: Duration of pulmonary venous atrial reversal flow velocity and mitral inflow a wave: new measure of severity of cardiac amyloidosis. J Am Soc Echocardiogr 11:1125, 1998.
26. Patel AR, Dubrey SW, Mendes LA, et al: Right ventricular dilatation in primary amyloidosis: an independent predictor of survival. Am J Cardiol 80:486, 1997.

CHAPTER 58

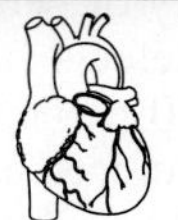

Radionuclide Techniques in Cardiomyopathies and Myocarditis

A. Iain McGhie

DILATED CARDIOMYOPATHY
HYPERTROPHIC CARDIOMYOPATHY
RESTRICTIVE CARDIOMYOPATHY
MYOCARDITIS
CARDIAC ALLOGRAFT REJECTION

Dilated Cardiomyopathy

Radionuclide ventriculography is widely used in the evaluation of patients with dilated cardiomyopathy for calculation of indices of left ventricular function (e.g., ejection fraction and end-systolic and end-diastolic volumes). Typically, there is dilatation of all four cardiac chambers with diffuse, nonsegmental regional dysfunction. However, regional wall motion abnormalities are not infrequent in the absence of atherosclerotic coronary artery disease and are associated with less global ventricular dysfunction and more benign prognoses.[1]

Determination of the functional status of the right ventricle can provide additional important information in patients with cardiac failure. The predictive value of left ventricular function in terms of prognosis and functional status is low in patients with dilated cardiomyopathy.[2] However, the presence of coexistent right ventricular dysfunction in patients with congestive heart failure related to dilated cardiomyopathy or coronary artery disease is associated with a poor prognosis.[3,4] Despite lack of correlation between the extent of left ventricular dysfunction and exercise capacity, right ventricular dysfunction is associated with reduced exercise tolerance in patients with congestive heart failure.[5,6] Normal right ventricular function in patients with heart failure makes it more likely that the etiology results from underlying coronary artery disease.[7] In a study of 90 patients with cardiac failure, patients with primary cardiomyopathy had significantly lower right ventricular ejection fractions (29 ± 12 percent) than those with underlying coronary artery disease (38 ± 16 percent) despite similar left ventricular ejection fractions, 22 ± 6 percent and 21 ± 6 percent, respectively.[7] However, the predictive value of the right ventricular ejection fraction and the presence or absence of regional wall motion abnormalities in determining the etiology of cardiac failure in any individual patient is limited because of the overlap between the two groups of patients.[8]

Dipyridamole ^{201}Tl imaging has been used to differentiate patients with a primary cardiomyopathy from those with coronary artery disease.[9] Patients with primary dilated cardiomyopathy had more homogeneous myocardial perfusion and smaller perfusion abnormalities (25 ± 11 percent versus 6 ± 6 percent of the left ventricle, $P < .001$) than patients with underlying coronary artery disease. In this study, quantitative ^{201}Tl imaging correctly predicted the etiology of left dysfunction in 20 of 22 (91 percent) patients. Schelbert and colleagues[10] reported similar findings using positron emission tomography. Using ^{13}N-ammonia and ^{18}F-fluorodeoxyglucose, they also reported more homogeneous distribution of these radiopharmaceuticals in patients with primary cardiomyopathy. The diagnostic accuracy of visual image analysis for distinguishing between the two groups was 85 percent. However, when quantitative image analysis was used, positron emission tomography had a sensitivity and specificity of 100 percent and 80 percent, respectively.

Hypertrophic Cardiomyopathy

The radionuclide ventriculogram of a patient with hypertrophic cardiomyopathy characteristically reveals an extremely vigorously contracting left ventricle with a "supernormal" ejection fraction with a very small end-systolic volume. In addition, myocardial hypertrophy is often evident from the prominent myocardial silhouette surrounding the cardiac blood pool. Furthermore, radionuclide ventriculography provides a noninvasive means to determine diastolic ventricular function. Abnormal diastolic function in these patients is common, resulting primarily from underlying myocardial hypertrophy, cellular disarray, and fibrosis. Diastolic dysfunction is a key factor in the pathophysiology of hypertrophic cardiomyopathy and an important determinant of exercise tolerance and prognosis.[11–13] The beneficial effects of pharmacologic interventions on diastolic function in these patients have been demonstrated using radionuclide ventriculography.[14]

^{201}Tl perfusion defects are common in patients with hypertrophic cardiomyopathy. In a study of 72 patients using exercise-redistribution ^{201}Tl imaging, regional perfusion defects were identified in 57 percent of patients.[15] The majority of patients (82 percent) with fixed or partially reversible defects had left ventricular ejection fractions of less than 50 percent. In contrast, patients with completely reversible defects had left ventricular ejection fractions greater than 50 percent. In a significant number of reversible perfusion defects (41 percent), the myocardium was moderate-to-markedly increased in thickness. The authors hypothesized that reversible perfusion defects reflected ischemia in areas of hypertrophied myocardium. In a subsequent study, they tested this hypothesis by studying 50 patients with hypertrophic cardiomyopathy using exercise-redistribution ^{201}Tl imaging and measurement of myocardial lactate metabolism and hemodynamics during atrial pacing.[16] Thirty-seven (73 percent) patients had reversible perfusion defects, of which 27 of 37 (73 percent) had metabolic evidence of ischemia during pacing, compared with 4 of 13 (31 percent) patients with normal ^{201}Tl imaging. Cavity dilatation during ^{201}Tl imaging was seen in 11 patients, which was associated with significantly higher postpacing left ventricular end-diastolic pressures. In contrast, ST-segment changes with exercise and systolic compression of coronary arteries on angiography were found to be unreliable indicators of inducible myocardial ischemia.

Restrictive Cardiomyopathy

Differentiation between restrictive cardiomyopathy and constrictive pericarditis often poses a diagnostic problem. Aroney and associates[17] reported on the utility of radionuclide ventriculography to differentiate between these entities using diastolic parameters of left ventricular function. They studied 12 patients with hemodynamic features of constriction (Table 58–1). Five patients had restrictive cardiomyopathy, 5 had pericardial constriction, and 2 had combined pericardial constriction and restrictive cardiomyopathy. The authors were able to differentiate between patients with pericardial constriction, with restrictive cardiomyopathy, and with combined pathologic states using the time-to–peak filling rate, the peak filling rate normalized to stroke volume, and the atrial contribution to left ventricular filling.

Time to peak filling rate in patients with pericardial constriction was shorter (110 ± 4 ms) compared with those with restrictive cardiomyopathy (195 ± 45 ms) or in normal subjects (173 ± 32 ms) (Fig. 58–1). The peak filling rate normalized to stroke volume was significantly greater in patients with pericardial constriction (5.09 ± 0.97) than in restrictive cardiomyopathy or normal subjects, 3.52 ± 0.43 ml/ms and 3.98 ± 0.70 ml/ms, respectively. Atrial contribution to left ventricular filling was higher in those with restrictive cardiomyopathy (45 ± 17 percent) than in those with pericardial constriction or in normal subjects, 21 ± 6 percent and 24 ± 9 percent, respectively. Others have also demonstrated the utility of radionuclide ventriculography in differentiating between these conditions.[18]

TABLE 58–1 Hemodynamic Features Suggestive of Constrictive Physiology

Equalization of RV and LV diastolic pressures < 5 mm Hg
Mean atrial or ventricular diastolic pressure ≥ 10 mm Hg
"Dip-and-plateau" pattern of ventricular pressure curve
Prominent Y descent in RA pressure
RVEDP > ⅓ RVSP
LVEF > 40 percent

Abbreviations: LV, left ventricular; LVEF, left ventricular ejection fraction; RA, right atrial; RV, right ventricular; RVEDP, right ventricular end-diastolic pressure; RVSP, right ventricular systolic pressure.

Adapted from Aroney CN, Ruddy TD, Dighero H, et al: Differentiation of restrictive cardiomyopathy from pericardial constriction: assessment of diastolic function by radionuclide angiography. Adapted with permission from the American College of Cardiology (J Am Coll Cardiol, 1989, Vol. 13, pp. 1007–1014).

Myocarditis

Differentiation of myocarditis from primary cardiomyopathy can be a clinical dilemma in a patient presenting de novo with cardiac failure. At present, the "gold standard" for diagnosis of myocarditis is histologic evidence of myocardial inflammation and myocyte injury in myocardial tissue obtained by right ventricular biopsy. In contrast, primary cardiomyopathy is characterized by myofibrillar degeneration and fibrosis with little or no inflammatory changes. However, right ventricular endomyocardial biopsy has significant limitations.[19] These include sampling error resulting from the focal or multifocal nature of the disease process and differences in the criteria for the interpretation of histologic findings. This has led to the development of imaging techniques to diagnose this condition noninvasively.

Radiolabeled antimyosin imaging has been used to detect the myocardial necrosis associated with myocarditis.[20–22] In one study[20] of 28 patients evaluated within 1 year of presentation with dilated cardiomyopathy, there was concordance in 20 of 28 patients between findings from antimyosin imaging and those from right ventricular endomyocardial biopsy (9 patients with positive and 11 with negative findings). A spontaneous increase in the left ventricular ejection fraction was observed in 4 of 8 patients with positive antimyosin findings but negative endomyocardial biopsies. It was postulated that improvement in ventricular function in this latter group of patients was consistent with healing of focal areas of myocarditis that went undetected by endomyocardial biopsy. In a larger study,[21] by the same group of investigators, the technique was evaluated in patients with suspected myocarditis (n = 82), including patients with dilated cardiomyopathy (92 percent), chest pain syndromes (6 percent) and life-threatening arrhythmias (2 percent). Fifteen of 18 patients with myocarditis on right ventricular endomyocardial biopsy had abnormal antimyosin scans. Thirty patients with no evidence of myocarditis on biopsy had an abnormal scan. Using the findings from right ventricular endomyocardial biopsy as the gold standard, a normal scan had a predictive value of 92 percent, and an abnormal scan had a predictive value of 33 percent. Another group used ^{67}Ga imaging both for diagnosis of myocarditis and for predicting response to immunosuppressive therapy.[23, 24] They reported a sensitivity of 36 percent and a specificity of 98 percent for this technique. This method differs from antimyosin imaging in

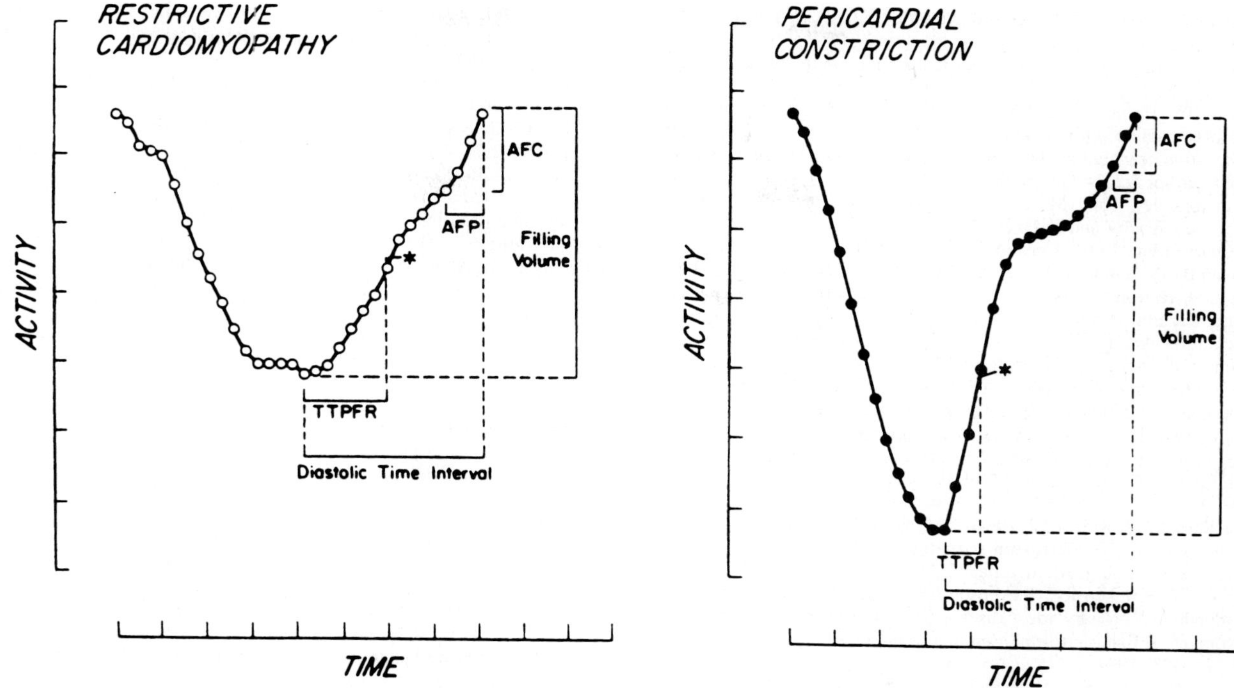

FIGURE 58–1 Time-activity curves from a patient with restrictive cardiomyopathy **(A)** and a patient with pericardial constriction **(B)**. *Asterisk* shows peak filling rate. AFC, atrial filling contribution; AFP, atrial filling period; TFPFR, time to peak filling rate. (**A** and **B**, Adapted from Aroney CN, Ruddy TD, Dighero H, et al: Differentiation of restrictive cardiomyopathy from pericardial constriction: assessment of diastolic function by radionuclide angiography. Adapted with permission from the American College of Cardiology [J Am Coll Cardiol, 1989, Vol. 13, pp. 1007–1014].)

that it identifies areas of inflammation rather than necrosis. To date, there have been no studies investigating the clinical utility of using both of these complementary techniques in the diagnosis of myocarditis.

Cardiac Allograft Rejection

Survival after cardiac transplantation has consistently improved since the late 1980s, with current 1-year and 5-year survival rates of 80 to 90 percent and 60 to 70 percent, respectively.[25] This has led to an increasing use of cardiac transplantation in the management of patients with end-stage cardiac disease. Two of the most important clinical problems in the post-transplant period are detection and management of rejection. At present, detection and quantification of cardiac allograft rejection require serial endomyocardial biopsies to obtain tissue for histologic analysis.[26, 27]

Use of indices of systolic function are known to be of no value in identification of allograft rejection.[28, 29] Others have used indices of diastolic function in an attempt to detect rejection with either radionuclide ventriculography or echocardiography and Doppler techniques.[29–31] These studies reported variable results, possibly related to the multifactorial etiology of diastolic dysfunction after transplantation.[32–34]

More encouraging preliminary results have been reported with nuclear imaging techniques using radiolabeled monoclonal antibodies to detect abnormal antigens in rejecting cardiac allografts. Several studies have shown that moderate-to-severe rejection after cardiac allograft transplantation can be detected using radiolabeled monoclonal antibody to myosin both in experimental models[35–38] and also in patients.[39, 40] These studies have shown a reasonably good correlation between scintigraphic findings using ^{111}In-labeled antimyosin antibody and the histologic extent of myocyte necrosis after transplantation. In patients with cardiac allografts, radiolabeled antimyosin antibody uptake is reported to have a reasonable sensitivity (range 80 to 95 percent); however, the specificity (range 33 to 80 percent) for the detection of allograft rejection was very variable.[41]

The immunoglobulin superfamily of adhesion receptors, including the major histocompatibility complex molecules and the intercellular adhesion molecule-1, are expressed in rejecting myocardium and may have an important role in the pathophysiology of allograft rejection.[42–45] Preliminary studies using animal models of cardiac transplantation have shown that it is feasible to detect cardiac rejection using radiolabeled monoclonal antibodies to major histocompatibility complex class II antigens and intercellular adhesion molecule-1.[46–48] These imaging techniques may prove to be more specific. In addition, they may be more sensitive, as expression of these surface molecules occurs before the irreversible process of myocyte necrosis does.

References

1. Wallis DE, O'Connell JB, Henkin RE, et al: Segmental wall motion abnormalities in dilated cardiomyopathy: a common finding and good prognostic sign. J Am Coll Cardiol 4:674–679, 1984.

2. Natural history of dilated cardiomyopathy [editorial]. Lancet 1:248–249, 1986.
3. Oakley C: Importance of right ventricular function in congestive heart failure. Am J Cardiol 32:14A–19A, 1988.
4. Polak JF, Holman BL, Wynne J, Colucci WS: Right ventricular ejection fraction: an indicator of increased mortality in patients with congestive heart failure associated with coronary artery disease. J Am Coll Cardiol 2:217–224, 1983.
5. Franciosa JA, Park M, Levine TB: Lack of correlation between exercise capacity and indexes of resting left ventricular performance in heart failure. Am J Cardiol 47:33–39, 1981.
6. Baker BJ, Wilen MM, Boyd CM, et al: Relation of right ventricular ejection fraction to exercise capacity in chronic left ventricular failure. Am J Cardiol 54:596–599, 1984.
7. Iskandrian AS, Helfeld H, Lemlek J, et al: Differentiation between primary dilated cardiomyopathy and ischemia cardiomyopathy based on right ventricular function. Am Heart J 123:768–773, 1992.
8. Greenberg JM, Murphy JH, Okada RD, et al: Value and limitations of radionuclide angiography in determining the cause of reduced left ventricular ejection fraction: comparison of idiopathic dilated cardiomyopathy and coronary artery disease. Am J Cardiol 55:541–544, 1985.
9. Eichhorn EJ, Kosinski EJ, Lewis SM, et al: Usefulness of dipyridamole-thallium-201 perfusion scanning for distinguishing ischemic from nonischemic cardiomyopathy. Am J Cardiol 62:945–951, 1988.
10. Mody FV, Brunken RC, Stevenson LW, et al: Differentiating cardiomyopathy of coronary artery disease from nonischemic dilated cardiomyopathy utilizing positron emission tomography. J Am Coll Cardiol 17:373–383, 1991.
11. Bonow RO, Dilsizian V, Rosing DR, et al: Verapamil-induced improvement in left ventricular filling and increased exercise tolerance in patients with hypertrophic cardiomyopathy: short- and long-term effects. Circulation 72:853–864, 1985.
12. Newman H, Sugrue D, Oakley CM, et al: Relation of left ventricular function and prognosis in hypertrophic cardiomyopathy: an angiographic study. J Am Coll Cardiol 5:1064–1074, 1985.
13. Chikamori T, Dickie S, Poloniecki JD, et al: Prognostic significance of radionuclide-assessed diastolic function in hypertrophic cardiomyopathy. Am J Cardiol 65:478–482, 1990.
14. Hanrath P, Schluter M, Sonntag F, et al: Influence of verapamil therapy on left ventricular performance at rest and during exercise in hypertrophic cardiomyopathy. Am J Cardiol 52:544–548, 1983.
15. O'Gara PT, Bonow RO, Maron BJ, et al: Myocardial perfusion abnormalities in patients with hypertrophic cardiomyopathy: assessment with thallium-201 emission computed tomography. Circulation 76:1214–1223, 1987.
16. Cannon RO, Dilsizian V, O'Gara PT, et al: Myocardial metabolic, hemodynamic, and electrocardiographic significance of reversible thallium-201 abnormalities in hypertrophic cardiomyopathy. Circulation 83:1660–1667, 1991.
17. Aroney CN, Ruddy TD, Dighero H, et al: Differentiation of restrictive cardiomyopathy from pericardial constriction: assessment of diastolic function by radionuclide angiography. J Am Coll Cardiol 13:1007–1014, 1989.
18. Greson MC, Colthar MS, Fowler NO: Differentiation of constrictive pericarditis and restrictive cardiomyopathy by radionuclide ventriculography. Am Heart J 118:114–120, 1989.
19. Billingham M: Acute myocarditis: a diagnostic dilemma. Br Heart J 58:6–8, 1987.
20. Yasuda T, Palacios IF, Dec GW, et al: Indium-111 monoclonal antimyosin antibody imaging in diagnosis of acute myocarditis. Circulation 76:306–311, 1987.
21. Dec GW, Palacios I, Yasuda T, et al: Antimyosin antibody cardiac imaging: its role in the diagnosis of myocarditis. J Am Coll Cardiol 16:97–104, 1990.
22. Narula J, Khaw BA, Dec GW, et al: Brief report: recognition of acute myocarditis masquerading as acute myocardial infarction. N Engl J Med 328:100–104, 1993.
23. O'Connell JB, Henjin RE, Robinson JA, et al: Gallium-67 imaging in patients with dilated cardiomyopathy and biopsy-proven myocarditis. Circulation 70:58–62, 1984.
24. O'Connell JB, Robinson JA, Henkin RE, Gunnar RM: Immunosuppressive therapy in patients with congestive cardiomyopathy and uptake of gallium-67. Circulation 64:780–786, 1981.
25. Kriett JM, Kaye MP: The registry of the International Society for Heart and Lung Transplantation: eighth official report—1991. J Heart Lung Transplant 10:491–498, 1991.
26. Caves PK, Schulz WP, Dong E, et al: New instrument for transvenous cardiac biopsy. Am J Cardiol 33:264–267, 1974.
27. Rose AG. Endocardial biopsy diagnosis for cardiac rejection. Heart Failure 2:64–72, 1986.
28. Stinson EB, Techklenberg PL, Hollingsworth JF, et al: Changes in left ventricular mechanical and hemodynamic function during acute rejection of orthopically transplanted hearts in dogs. J Thorac Cardiovasc Surg 68:783–791, 1974.
29. Paulsen W, Magid N, Sagar K, et al: Left ventricular function of heart allografts during acute rejection: an echocardiographic assessment. J Heart Transplant 4:525–529, 1985.
30. Tatum JL, Thompson JA, Prasad U, et al: Radionuclide detection of abnormal ventricular filling patterns in rejecting human allografts. Clin Nucl Med 14:175–178, 1989.
31. Haverich A, Kemnitz J, Fieguth HG, et al: Non-invasive parameters for detection of allograft rejection. Clin Transplant 1:151–158, 1987.
32. Valantine HA, Appleton CP, Hatle LK, et al: A hemodynamic and Doppler echocardiographic study of ventricular function in long-term cardiac allograft recipients: etiology and prognosis of restrictive-constrictive physiology. Circulation 79:66–75, 1989.
33. Young JB, Leon CA, Short ID, et al: Evolution of hemodynamics after orthotopic heart and heart-lung transplantation. J Heart Transplant 6:34–43, 1987.
34. Hosenpud JD, Pantely GA, Morton MJ, et al: Relation between recipient:donor body size match and hemodynamics three months after heart transplantation. J Heart Transplant 8:241–243, 1989.
35. Hall TS, Baumgarter WA, Borkon AM, et al: Diagnosis of acute cardiac rejection with antimyosin monoclonal antibody, phosphorous nuclear magnetic resonance imaging, two-dimensional echocardiography, and endocardial biopsy. J Heart Transplant 5:419–424, 1986.
36. Addonizio LJ, Michler RE, Marboe C, et al: Imaging of cardiac allograft rejection in dogs using indium-111 monoclonal antimyosin Fab. J Am Coll Cardiol 9:555–564, 1987.
37. Isobe M, Haber E, Khaw BA: Early detection of rejection and assessment of cyclosporine therapy in ^{111}In antimyosin imaging in mouse heart allografts. Circulation 84:1246–1255, 1991.
38. Takeda K, Ueda K, Scheffel U, et al: Indium-111 myosin-specific antibodies and technetium-99m pyrophosphate in the detection of acute cardiac rejection of transplanted hearts: studies in a heterotopic heart model. Eur J Nucl Med 18:461–466, 1991.
39. Frist W. Yasuda T, Segall G, et al: Noninvasive detection of human cardiac transplant rejection with indium-111 antimyosin (Fab) imaging. Circulation 76:81–85, 1987.
40. Ballester M, Obrador D, Carrio I, et al: Early postoperative reduction of monoclonal antimyosin antibody uptake is associated with absent rejection-related complications after heart transplantation. Circulation 85:61–68, 1992.
41. Hosenpud JD: Noninvasive diagnosis of cardiac allograft rejection. Circulation 85:368–371, 1992.
42. Rose ML, Coles MI, Griffin RJ, et al: Expression of class I and class II major histocompatibility antigens in normal and transplanted human heart. Transplantation 41:776–782, 1986.
43. Carlquist JF, Hammond ME, Yowell RL, et al: Correlation between class II antigen (DR) expression and interleukin-2–induced lymphocyte proliferation during the acute cardiac allograft rejection. Transplantation 50:582–588, 1990.
44. Steinhoff G, Behrend M, Haverich A: Signs of endothelial inflammation in human heart allografts. Eur Heart J 12(suppl D):141–143, 1991.
45. Rose M, Page C, Hengstenberg C, Yacoub M: Immunocytochemical markers of activation in cardiac transplant rejection. Eur Heart J 12(suppl D):147–150, 1991.
46. Mitsuaki I, Narula J, Southern JF, et al: Imaging the rejecting heart: in vivo detection of major histocompatibility complex class II antigen induction. Circulation 85:738–746, 1992.
47. Ohtani H, Southern JF, Strauss HW, Isobe M: Imaging of ICAM-1 induction in rejecting heart: a new scintigraphic approach to detect early allograft rejection [abstract]. Circulation 86:I–37, 1992.
48. McGhie AI, Radovancevic B, Capek P, et al: MHC class II antigen expression in rejecting cardiac allografts: detection using in vivo imaging with radiolabeled monoclonal antibody. Circulation 96:1605–1611, 1997.

CHAPTER 59

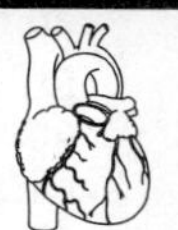

PATHOPHYSIOLOGY AND CLINICAL RECOGNITION OF HEART FAILURE

Jay N. Cohn

PATHOPHYSIOLOGY
Definitions
ETIOLOGY
Myocardial or Ventricular Dysfunction
Ischemic Heart Disease
Cardiomyopathy
Abnormal Myocardial Load
Pressure Overload
Volume Overload
Restrictive Disease
Electrical Abnormalities
PATHOPHYSIOLOGY
Left Ventricular Dysfunction
Systolic Dysfunction
Diastolic Dysfunction
Ventricular Remodeling
Infarct Expansion
Myocyte Lengthening
Myocyte Thickening
Fiber Slippage
Neurohormonal Activation
Sympathetic Nervous System
Renin-Angiotensin-Aldosterone System
Vasopressin System
Endothelium
Cytokines
Natriuretic Peptides
CLINICAL RECOGNITION OF HEART FAILURE
History
Physical Examination
Laboratory Tests
ASSESSMENT OF SEVERITY
PROGNOSIS
Ejection Fraction
Exercise Capacity
Cardiac Enlargement and the Right Ventricle
Ventricular Arrhythmias
Plasma Hormone Levels
CLINICAL COURSE OF HEART FAILURE

PATHOPHYSIOLOGY

Heart failure is a syndrome characterized by exertional fatigue, exertional dyspnea, or both related to cardiac usually left ventricular (LV) dysfunction.[1] It is commonly accompanied by circulatory congestion manifested by edema in the lungs or extremities and by ventricular arrhythmias (Fig. 59–1). Heart failure may be precipitated by acute events that disturb the structure or function of the ventricular chambers or by chronic cardiac disease that eventuates in the clinical syndrome. The distinction between cardiac and noncardiac causes of the symptomatology depends on the clinical demonstration of altered cardiac structure or impaired cardiac function. This may be accomplished at the bedside, in the cardiac catheterization laboratory, or by the use of a variety of imaging techniques.

Heart failure is a syndrome of growing prevalence. There are at least three reasons for this growing prevalence:

1. *Aging of the population.* The incidence of heart failure rises dramatically with age, affecting more than 10 percent of the population over 70 years of age. The mechanism of this age-dependent increase in the incidence of heart failure is probably multifactorial, but it may be related to aging of the myocardium associated in particular with abnormalities of ventricular relaxation, aging of the vasculature that places

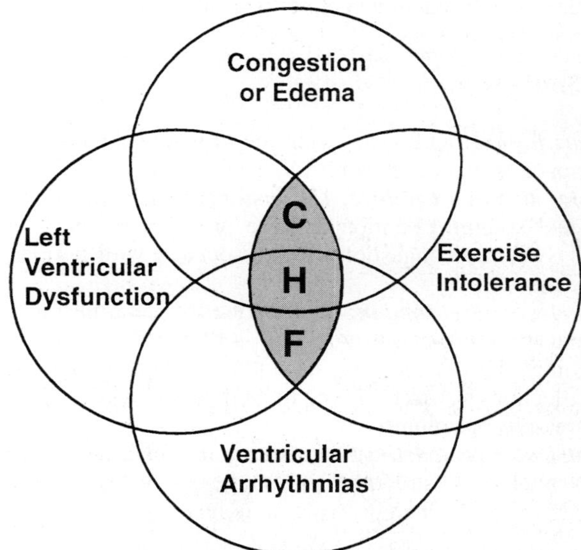

FIGURE 59–1 Clinical heart failure (CHF) represents the coexistence of left ventricular dysfunction and exercise intolerance. It frequently is accompanied by congestion or edema, and the majority of patients exhibit ventricular arrhythmias.

an impedance load on the left ventricle, and increased prevalence of myocardial ischemia due to coronary artery disease. Furthermore, subtle degrees of myocardial disease may exist for many years and eventually produce symptoms in the elderly.

2. *Increased survival from acute myocardial infarction* (MI). The case fatality rate of acute MI has dropped remarkably in the past 20 years because of the more effective management of acute myocardial ischemia with aggressive medical and interventional techniques. Survival of patients who have sustained an MI provides a reservoir of individuals with ventricular dysfunction who may eventually progress to the stage of overt heart failure.
3. *Improved management of heart failure.* Recognition and effective treatment of patients with early manifestations of heart failure may improve their survival and thus contribute to the increased prevalence of the disease over time. This prolongation of life leads to a further reservoir of patients who consume health care dollars and increase the overall cost of medical care.

The precision with which the diagnosis of heart failure is made often is inadequate. Fatigue and dyspnea may be attributed to aging and deconditioning; thus, an early diagnosis may not be made, and appropriate therapy may be delayed. On the other hand, other clinical conditions may mimic the symptoms of heart failure even if cardiac function is normal. For example, fluid overload,[2] severe anemia,[3] and mitral stenosis[4] may produce dyspnea and fatigue with normal ventricular function. To maintain mechanistic uniformity to the terms *heart failure* or *cardiac failure,* those conditions not associated with impairment of systolic or diastolic ventricular pump function should not be identified as heart failure. In addition, a distinction must be made between asymptomatic abnormalities of cardiac function and the diagnosis of the clinical syndrome of heart failure, which requires symptoms of dyspnea or fatigue.

Definitions

Heart failure: a clinical syndrome in which exercise intolerance is associated with LV dysfunction

Congestive heart failure: LV dysfunction accompanied by renal sodium retention and the presence of pulmonary or systemic congestion often associated with peripheral edema

Ventricular dysfunction: an abnormality of cardiac performance such that LV emptying is impaired, LV chamber compliance is reduced, or both; it is manifested by a reduction in stroke volume or an increase in end-diastolic pressure or volume

Ventricular remodeling: a condition in which the ventricle is altered in structure and shape so that its mass is increased, its chamber volume is increased, or both

ETIOLOGY

Heart failure may be a consequence of all forms of cardiac disease. In the strictest sense, the diagnosis should be restricted to individuals who have developed cardiac dysfunction as a consequence of myocardial disease. In most instances, the mechanism of the global cardiac dysfunction resulting in this syndrome is not well understood. In sustained hypertension, hypertrophy supports LV dysfunction against a high impedance for many months or years until chamber dilatation and reduced wall motion or chamber stiffness with impaired filling herald the onset of symptomatic heart failure.[5, 6] In valvular heart disease in which a pressure or volume overload burdens the left ventricle, systolic ventricular function may remain normal for years until the process of dilatation and reduced wall motion develops.[7] In the setting of acute MI, a regional wall motion abnormality may not adversely affect global LV systolic function until months or years later, when ventricular chamber dilatation and reduced wall motion begin to develop.[8] Acute inflammatory processes involving the myocardium or toxic insults to the myocardium also may develop subtly and result in symptoms only after chamber dilatation supervenes. Furthermore, the structural changes in the myocardium characteristic of heart failure may develop many months or years before symptoms of the syndrome become apparent.[9] Therefore, the full-blown syndrome of heart failure appears to require not only the structural changes of the left ventricle but also the interaction of systemic neuroendocrine and vasomotor changes that contribute to symptomatology.[10]

The ventricular pump dysfunction that causes heart failure usually has its origin in the left ventricle. Pure right ventricular (RV) failure may develop acutely in response to diseases such as RV infarction[11] and may occur chronically in response to pulmonary vascular obstructive processes.[12] However, even in these instances of right-sided cardiac involvement, abnormalities of LV function may contribute to the clinical symptomatology. RV dysfunction in the absence of disease involving the pulmonary vasculature or the free wall or septum of the left ventricle are often so well tolerated that symptoms of heart failure do not develop.[13] Nevertheless, RV dysfunction developing as a consequence of disturbed function of the left ventricle appears to be an important contributor to the symptoms of heart failure.[14] Whether such a structural remodeling of the right ventricle is a consequence of increased RV workload or other factors activated in the heart failure process remains unknown.

The cardiac dysfunction that initiates the syndrome of heart failure can be divided into conditions that directly affect myocardial or ventricular function and those that place an abnormal load on the myocardium, resulting in impairment of cardiac function (Table 59–1).

Myocardial or Ventricular Dysfunction

Primary dysfunction of the heart may result from a variety of conditions, including myocyte loss, impaired myocyte function, interstitial or pericardial structural alterations that affect ventricular function, and electrical dyssynergy that impairs pump function. Coronary artery disease (CAD) is the most common cause of myocardial dysfunction in Western society, but primary myocardial processes, including cardiomyopathies, are prevalent in some areas of the

TABLE 59–1 Causes of Heart Failure

Primary myocardial or ventricular dysfunction
- Ischemic heart disease
  - Acute myocardial infarction
  - Myocardial "stunning"
  - Myocardial "hibernation"
  - Ventricular remodeling after myocardial infarction
- Cardiomyopathy
  - Idiopathic
  - Genetic
  - Infectious/inflammatory
  - Metabolic
  - Toxic
  - Infiltrative
  - Aging

Increased ventricular load
- Pressure load
  - Hypertension
  - Aortic stenosis
  - Hypertrophic subaortic
- Volume load
  - Mitral regurgitation
  - Aortic regurgitation
  - Arteriovenous fistula

Restrictive diseases
- Pericardium
  - Constrictive pericarditis
  - Pericardial effusion
- Myocardium
  - Decreased myocardial distensibility
  - Restrictive myocardial disease
  - Endocardial fibroelastosis

Electrical abnormalities
- Tachycardias
- Ventricular dyssynergy

world and constitute a growing cause of heart failure in most countries.

Ischemic Heart Disease

CAD can produce a number of ventricular functional abnormalities that can precipitate heart failure. The most subtle is ischemia in the absence of infarction and sometimes in the absence of symptoms of inadequate coronary perfusion.[15] The most dramatic is the pump dysfunction that complicates an acute MI.[16]

Myocardial ischemia causes both diastolic and systolic ventricular dysfunction.[17–19] Transient loss of nutritional support for myocardial relaxation and contraction can result in rather prolonged functional impairment without loss of cellular integrity. The functional abnormality of this reversible *stunning* may be mistaken for an MI.[15, 20] Similarly, a chronic modest inadequacy of regional coronary perfusion may result in a reversible down-regulation of myocardial function classified as *hibernation*.[21, 22] After a localized MI, changes in both the flow-deprived and remote areas of the ventricle may contribute to pump dysfunction. Akinesis or dyskinesis in the infarcted zone may reduce stroke output, particularly if the infarct zone becomes aneurysmal or if the residual myocardium cannot functionally compensate for the disturbed regional function.[23] The uninvolved myocardium may undergo structural changes that eventuate in remodeling and global ventricular dysfunction[24] (see later).

Cardiomyopathy

A wide variety of known and unknown agents may directly attack the myocardium and induce myocyte loss or impairment of myocardial contractile function. Diabetes,[25, 26] excess alcohol intake,[27, 28] and viral diseases[29] are the most prevalent acquired causes of cardiomyopathy. Genetic forms of cardiomyopathy may be more common than was previously suspected.[30, 31] Most of these primary myocardial processes involve diffuse or focal myocyte loss, replacement fibrosis, hypertrophy of remaining myocytes, and dilatation of the ventricular chamber. Aging also appears to be associated with myocyte loss[32] that might contribute to the high incidence of heart failure in the elderly.

Abnormal Myocardial Load

Hypertension and valvular heart disease are the most common causes of a chronic increase in cardiac load that can result in heart failure or contribute to the syndrome when primary myocardial disease coexists.

Pressure Overload

A sustained increase in systolic blood pressure results in an increased systolic wall stress during LV ejection.[33] Essential hypertension, isolated systolic hypertension, and aortic stenosis are common causes of this phenomenon. The ventricular response to this pressure overload is concentric hypertrophy, which should normalize wall stress by laying down new sarcomeres in parallel within the myocardial fibers.[34]

Volume Overload

Mitral valvular regurgitation, aortic insufficiency, arteriovenous fistulae, and other high-output circulatory states place a volume load on the ventricle that results in chamber remodeling and dilatation. The dilatation represents at least in part the lengthening of myocytes by the laying down of new sarcomeres in series within the myocardial fiber.[35]

Restrictive Disease

Infiltrative processes in the myocardium or pericardium may reduce the distensibility of these structures and therefore impair the ability of the ventricle to fill. This process usually affects both ventricles and results in an increased cardiac filling pressure (right atrium and left atrium) and symptoms of congestion.[36] A precise diagnosis of the mechanism of this restricted filling is essential because the therapeutic approaches to these diverse processes may vary widely. Exclusion of pericardial tamponade that can be drained is critical. Constrictive pericarditis may be surgically corrected. Infiltrative processes may have very unique therapeutic approaches.

Electrical Abnormalities

LV emptying is dependent on a well orchestrated process of excitation-contraction coupling. Heterogeneity of the contraction process in the left ventricle may result from dyssynchronous electrical depolarization or delayed contraction. When the left ventricle is dilated, especially when there are areas of scar or inflammation, the electrical depolarization may become circuitous and some areas of the ventricle may contract out of sequence with other areas.[37] The result of this dyssynchrony may be a reduced stroke volume and impaired diastolic relaxation and filling. The role of electrical abnormalities in the development or progression of heart failure can be documented only if interventions to correct this problem prove effective. Studies are currently being carried out with various multisite pacing procedures in an attempt to improve the synchrony of LV contraction.[38, 39]

PATHOPHYSIOLOGY

Left Ventricular Dysfunction

LV pump dysfunction can be predominantly systolic or predominantly diastolic. Abnormal function of the left ventricle as a precipitating cause of symptoms of heart failure implies that the left ventricle is unable adequately to augment stroke volume in response to the increased cardiac output demand of exercise or is able to augment stroke volume only in the face of an inappropriately large increase in end-diastolic pressure or volume that precipitates a rise in pulmonary capillary wedge pressure (Fig. 59–2). In most patients with heart failure, some degree of systolic dysfunction coexists with some degree of diastolic dysfunction. Although these two pathophysiologic entities are

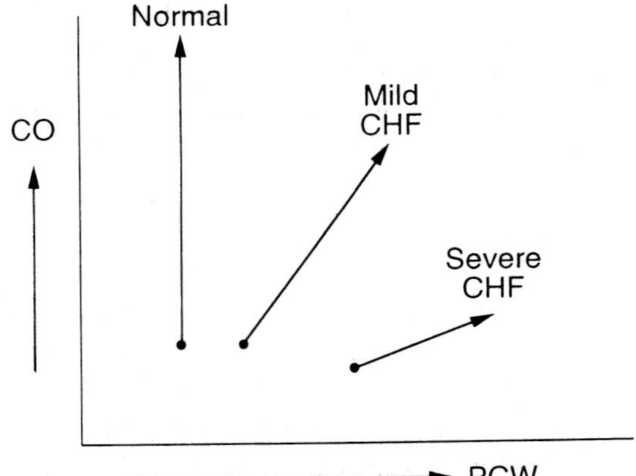

FIGURE 59–2 The hemodynamic hallmark of the syndrome is an abnormal response to exercise in which peak cardiac output is reduced and pulmonary capillary wedge pressure (PCW) (left ventricular filling pressure) rises inappropriately. CHF, congestive heart failure; CO, cardiac output.

TABLE 59–2 Mechanisms of Reduced Left Ventricular Systolic Contraction

Myocardial factors
Myocyte loss
Myocardial scar
Myocardial ischemia*
Myocardial "stunning," "hibernation"*
Myocardial inflammation*
Decreased cytosol calcium concentration*
Decreased excitation-contraction coupling*
Decreased contractility/beta-receptor responsiveness*
Left ventricular structural dilatation
Peripheral factors
Increased arterial vascular resistance*
Decreased arterial vascular compliance*
Increased total arterial impedance*

*Potentially reversible.

therefore not independent, they are considered separately in the next section.

Systolic Dysfunction

Ventricular systolic function is the result of shortening of sarcomeres, which are the contractile elements within myocardial cells or myocytes that make up myocardial fibers. The velocity and extent of sarcomere shortening are dependent on loading conditions before and during shortening[40] and on cytosol calcium concentration that couples excitation to contraction.[41] Reduced systolic shortening of cardiac muscle may therefore result from a global or regional reduction of contractility or a high impedance to LV ejection (Table 59–2).

Modest lengthening of sarcomeres (preload) will augment ventricular end-diastolic volume and increase contractile force (Frank-Starling mechanism).[42] Such an augmentation of preload can provide short-term compensation for reductions in contractility or increases in impedance that might otherwise reduce sarcomere shortening.[43] Longer-term compensation usually involves myocardial hypertrophy, which results from the laying down of new sarcomeres that increase the width (concentric) or the length (eccentric) of myocytes.[35]

Another factor contributing to reduced sarcomere shortening is the process of structural remodeling of the myocardium (see later). If myocytes lengthen or fibers slip against neighboring fibers, the resultant larger chamber volume will require less sarcomere shortening to generate an adequate stroke volume. Therefore, in some circumstances a reduction in sarcomere shortening can be viewed as a compensatory response to a dilated chamber rather than necessarily as the primary deficit in the process. In addition, however, this lesser sarcomere shortening results in a greater end-systolic volume and a larger chamber radius of curvature, resulting in a higher sustained ventricular wall stress. The metabolic, functional, and protein synthetic effects of this increased wall stress may exert profound effects on the myocardium.

Under any of these circumstances of reduced fiber shortening, the LV ejection fraction (EF) (i.e., the fraction of end-diastolic volume ejected during systole) will be reduced and the end-systolic volume will be increased. Some of the causes of diminished systolic contraction are reversible, and some appear to be largely irreversible. Management of the systolic dysfunction therefore includes efforts to treat the reversible causes in hopes that systolic function will improve and to deal pharmacologically with the irreversible causes by administering agents that can favorably affect LV systolic function either acutely or chronically. Because muscle contraction is an energy-consuming process, it must be recognized that interventions that increase myocardial oxygen consumption may aggravate systolic dysfunction if the energy supply to the myocardium is limited.

Diastolic Dysfunction

The ability of the left ventricle to relax during diastole to allow rapid filling from the atrium is also an energy-dependent process.[44] Cytosolic calcium uptake into sarcoplasmic reticulum is a critical factor in the rate of muscle relaxation, and this process may be influenced by primary myocardial diseases.[45] Chamber relaxation also is related to the myocardial mass, collagen content, and extrinsic forces, such as the pericardium, that may impede filling.[46, 47] The process of myocardial and ventricular relaxation is therefore under the influence of a variety of pathophysiologic processes that can induce diastolic dysfunction. Furthermore, the measurement of diastolic dysfunction is considerably more complex than that of systolic dysfunction and cannot easily be assessed in clinical practice.[48, 49] Therefore, for practical purposes, the demonstration of an elevation in LV end-diastolic pressure (LVEDP) or left atrial pressure, particularly when the ventricle is not grossly dilated, can be accepted as evidence of a role for diastolic dysfunction in the heart failure syndrome.[50–52] Therapy to alter diastolic performance of the ventricle also is not satisfactory. When ischemia plays a role, coronary reperfusion or a reduction in myocardial oxygen consumption may be an effective form of therapy.[18, 53, 54] When extrinsic mechanical factors, such as constrictive pericarditis or pericardial effusion, produce a structural impingement on ventricular filling, surgical management may be required.[55] Efforts to relieve diastolic dysfunction by pharmacologic interventions that affect structure or function of the myocardium have not been uniformly successful.

Ventricular Remodeling

A key factor in the syndrome of heart failure is a process of ventricular remodeling that appears to accompany most cardiac diseases. This process is characterized by a progressive change in shape of the left ventricle and a progressive increase of ventricular volume, associated with a progressive increase of LV muscle mass. The remodeling process may be the primary mechanism for a reduction in LV wall motion that accompanies a reduced LVEF. Thus, the systolic dysfunction described above may often result not from a primary deficit of contraction but rather an enlargement of the chamber as a result of remodeling.

The remodeling process involves both the myocyte and interstitial elements of the myocardium. An increase in myocyte volume and an increase in myocyte length accompany most processes of ventricular dilation.[56] Concentric hypertrophy is associated with an increase in myocyte width rather than length. In heart failure, cellular hypertrophy often is characterized by an increase in both myocyte length and width. Interstitial changes usually are manifested by an increase in collagen content.[57] This alteration in collagen may contribute to impaired systolic contraction but most often is associated with reduced ventricular compliance and impaired ventricular filling.

The process of remodeling may also be accompanied by myocyte loss or apoptosis.[58] The magnitude and mechanism of apoptosis in heart failure and cardiac remodeling are controversial. Considerable molecular research in this area is under way in multiple laboratories around the world.

Infarct Expansion

Necrosis of myocytes and dissolution of the collagen support network in an area of MI lead to a bulging out of this nonfunctional segment and a change in the geometry and volume of the left ventricle.[59–61] This process appears to be initiated early after an acute MI and probably is complete within days to weeks.

Myocyte Lengthening

The process of protein synthesis in the myocardium leads to laying down of new sarcomeres that enlarge the myocyte. When this hypertrophy process occurs in series in an individual myocardial fiber, the fiber lengthens and allows an enlargement of the ventricular chamber volume.[35] This eccentric hypertrophy is characteristic of volume overload states and may also occur over time when myocardial wall stress is increased.

Myocyte Thickening

When new sarcomeres are laid down in parallel, the myocardial fiber and the ventricular wall are thickened.[62] This concentric hypertrophy is a characteristic response to pressure overload and may initially result in a thick-walled chamber with impaired diastolic relaxation.

Fiber Slippage

Another mechanism purported to account for chamber enlargement is the slippage of myocytes[35] or sarcomeres within the myocyte[63] so that the total length of the myocardium is increased and the chamber is enlarged. The nature of this process is not well understood but may relate, at least in part, to the loss of the constraining collagen network that tends to hold myocytes together.[64]

Chamber dilatation has a potential physiologic advantage in the setting of a reduced myocardial contractility because it allows the left ventricle to eject an adequate stroke

TABLE 59–3 Consequences of Left Ventricular Remodeling

Increased systolic wall tension/stress
Increased myocardial oxygen consumption
Reduced myocyte shortening
Increased diastolic wall tension/stress
Reduced subendocardial perfusion
Dyssynchronous depolarization/contraction
Mitral regurgitation
Ventricular arrhythmias
Ventricular fibrillation

volume with considerably less muscle shortening. A disadvantage of this process, however, is that the wall stress (i.e., the pressure multiplied by the radius of curvature as defined by the Laplace relation) is increased. Because wall stress is a critical determinant of myocardial oxygen consumption,[65] this process of remodeling may place the ventricle at a metabolic disadvantage that can result in further ischemic dysfunction. A number of other physiologic consequences of ventricular chamber enlargement are listed (Table 59–3).

Neurohormonal Activation

Increased sympathetic nervous system (SNS) activity and activation of a wide variety of circulating and tissue hormonal systems are characteristic of the heart failure syndrome. The mechanism by which these neural and endocrine systems are activated in heart failure remains incompletely understood. Carotid and aortic baroreceptors are stimulated by stretch that inhibits central sympathetic discharge. Reduced stretch resulting from a decrease in arterial pressure, pulse pressure, or stroke volume could contribute to sympathetic activation.[66] Skeletal muscle afferent receptors stimulated by ischemia[67] or stretch[68] increase sympathetic outflow and may be activated in heart failure. In addition, structural and functional abnormalities in the responsiveness of afferent receptors have been identified in experimental and clinical heart failure.[69–73] These abnormalities could contribute to activation of the SNS or to failure to inhibit the system in response to compensatory physiologic adjustments such as volume expansion.

Regardless of the stimulatory mechanism, these systems may contribute importantly to structural and functional alterations in the myocardium and peripheral vasculature. Among these effects are redistribution of regional blood flow, changes in tone and structure of the vasculature that increase impedance to LV ejection, reduction in myocardial contractility, myocardial growth and chamber remodeling, loss of myocytes, increase in collagen deposition, and metabolic abnormalities in the myocardium. Most of the activated neurohormonal systems produce vasoconstriction and cardiovascular tissue growth. Vascular growth and remodeling reduce the compliance or distensibility of the arterial vasculature[74] and increase the impedance load on the left ventricle.[75] This impedance load consists of two components: (1) reduced capacitance of the conduit arteries that reduces their storage capacity during systole and (2) increased reflectance that results in rapid return to the left ventricle in late systole of reflected waves generated in the periphery. Both of these effects increase the afterload on the left ventricle and decrease fiber shortening of a dysfunctional left ventricle (Fig. 59–3).[76–79]

Cardiovascular tissue growth also involves the myocyte and interstitium of the myocardium. LV hypertrophy and remodeling may result from the hemodynamic load placed on the left ventricle by the increased impedance and by the direct effect of neurohormonal stimulation on myocardial growth.

Sympathetic Nervous System

Activation of the SNS occurs early and consistently in the heart failure syndrome.[80–82] Plasma norepinephrine (PNE) is elevated even in patients who are asymptomatic with dilated, remodeled ventricles.[83] Sympathetic nerve traffic is increased,[82] thus confirming that the elevated PNE is not due primarily to reduced clearance but rather to enhanced spillover of norepinephrine from the synaptic cleft into which it is secreted by nerve terminals.[84] One factor that may contribute to SNS activation is the failure of the normal suppression of sympathetic activity associated with baroreceptor stimulation.[69–71] Because the level of PNE is predictive of mortality rates, it is reasonable to assume that the degree of SNS activation serves as a marker for the severity of the syndrome.[85]

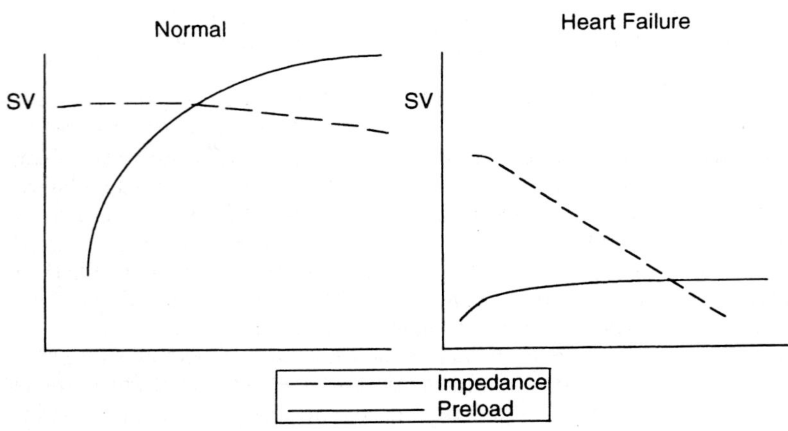

FIGURE 59–3 Left, The normal heart exhibits a rising stroke volume as ventricular filling is augmented and only a modest fall in stroke volume (SV) as impedance to ejection is increased. **Right,** The failing heart exhibits little response to augmented filling and a marked reduction in stroke volume as impedance is increased.

percent of rejections are asymptomatic. The possible signs and symptoms of rejection are subtle and nonspecific and include malaise, fatigue, low-grade fevers, arrhythmias, unexplained tachycardia, chest pain, pericardial rubs, and manifestations of congestive heart failure. Rejection with hemodynamic compromise occurs in about 5 to 8 percent of recipients, especially those who are diabetic, black, or female.[122] The prognosis is much poorer, with only 60 percent surviving 3 months after rejection.

Diagnosis by Endomyocardial Biopsy

The "gold standard" for the diagnosis of acute cellular rejection is histologic assessment of right ventricular endomyocardial biopsies. Endomyocardial tissue from the right ventricular septum is obtained using a transvenous bioptome. This is placed through an internal jugular sheath and the bioptome is directed with fluoroscopic or echocardiographic guidance[123] to the septum. Because the rejection process can be patchy, four to six specimens are obtained at each collection to improve sensitivity and specificity. The procedure is well tolerated with limited morbidity and very rare mortality rates.[124, 125] Complications include injury at the vascular access site, arrhythmias, vasovagal episodes, bundle-branch block, and pneumothorax. Tricuspid regurgitation may result from inadvertent damage to the chordae tendineae of the tricuspid valve during biopsy.[126]

Rejection does not progress in a uniform stepwise manner, and waiting until there are signs of graft dysfunction is very hazardous, as it may be very hard to reverse. Recent data have shown that the mortality rate associated with an episode of acute rejection accompanied by hemodynamic compromise may be as high as 40 percent.[122] This has led to the standard of performing protocol biopsies at predetermined intervals in heart transplant recipients to detect rejection before it causes graft dysfunction. Most patients undergo an average of 10 to 12 biopsies in the first year after transplantation for surveillance purposes. Endomyocardial biopsies are performed weekly for the first month, then biweekly for 1 month, then monthly for approximately 3 months, and then every 2 to 3 months. After approximately 24 months, endomyocardial biopsies are performed when rejection is suspected and once per year, typically at the annual visit. In most patients, the frequency of rejection decreases over time, and the value of surveillance biopsies diminishes.[127] Unfortunately, over time, the yield of acceptable specimens can decrease because recurrent sampling leads to scarring of the septum.

Treatment of Acute Rejection

There are many options for the treatment of acute rejection. Treatment is tailored for each individual based on the ISHLT score, time since transplant, previous rejection history, clinical presentation (graft dysfunction), and type and severity of coexisting morbidities such as diabetes, osteoporosis, or active infection. The majority of rejection episodes occur within the first 3 months, and this portends a worse long-term prognosis.[128] Hence, treatment regimens are slightly more aggressive for early compared with later episodes.[129]

Most agree that treatment is not required for ISHLT grades 0, 1A, and 1B, in which inflammation, if present, typically resolves spontaneously. However, there is substantial debate and deviation among institutions on an approach to focal moderate rejection (ISHLT score 2 and even ISHLT score 3A). In one study involving 161 transplant patients, approximately 20 percent of those with ISHLT grade 2 biopsies progressed to ISHLT grade 3 or 4.[130] These authors concluded that more judicious monitoring and early intervention might reduce the incidence of high-grade rejection. On the other hand, there are several reports of spontaneous clearing of infiltrates in endomyocardial biopsies with ISHLT grades 1 through 3A without bolus immunosuppressive therapy.[131–133] In a series of 208 heart transplants, 85 percent of cases of ISHLT grade 2 resolved, with only 15 percent progressing to a higher grade. There was no difference in survival between those that progressed and those that did not. These investigators concluded that intensive treatment of focal moderate rejection is not warranted. The recent rapamycin trial of treatment of rejection in patients for longer than 6 months after transplantation included a placebo arm and showed that nearly 50 percent of grade 2 and 40 percent of 3A rejections cleared without therapy.[134] The benign course for the patients with rejection episodes scored 2 and 3A raises further questions about treatment based on the degree of mononuclear infiltration.

There is more consensus regarding the treatment of moderate and severe rejections (ISHLT grades 3 and 4). In the first 3 months after transplantation, ISHLT grade 3 episodes are typically treated with pulse steroids. For clinical instability with signs of heart failure, arrhythmias, or evidence of elevated filling pressures on right heart catheterization, then intravenous methylprednisolone (0.5 to 1.0 g/day for 3 to 5 days) is used and immunosuppression is optimized at higher levels. For ISHLT grade 3B with clinical instability or ISHLT grade 4, antibody strategies targeting the T cell such as ATG (horse antithymocyte globulin) or OKT-3 (murine anti-CD3) are added. Repeat biopsy is performed approximately every 7 days until there are two acceptable (grade $\leq$ 1B) biopsies. Recurrent and resistant rejection with persistent clinical instability or endomyocardial histology without evidence of resolution is often treated with ATG or OKT-3.[135] Cyclosporine drug levels are optimized, and often the third agent in the triple drug program is replaced with one of the newer immunosuppressive agents (FK-506, mofetil, or rapamycin).[136, 137]

Antibody-Mediated Forms of Rejection

The overwhelming majority (>90 percent) of biopsies read as rejection represent pure cellular rejection. Antibody-mediated forms of rejection are considered when there are significant immunoglobulin, fibrinogen, or complement deposits observed in the graft vasculature. This form of rejection is also referred to as humoral or acute vascular rejection.[120, 138–141] These patients present with acute graft dysfunction associated with extensive endothelial injury but without substantial parenchymal leukocyte infiltration.[142] Based on these clinical features, it is widely believed that this form of rejection is mediated by a humoral immune response that dominates over the cellular immune response.

However, occasionally, patients have evidence of both cellular and antibody-mediated rejection.

Pathogenesis of Antibody-Mediated Rejection

Humoral or antibody-mediated rejection usually occurs in the first month after transplantation in recipients for whom there was positive donor cross-match, elevated PRA levels, or human antimouse antibodies after OKT-3 treatment.[143] One additional source of sensitization is blood transfusion, and any patient who receives a transfusion before transplantation should have a PRA screen measured within 3 weeks of transfusion to detect new antibody formation. Humoral rejection may also be common in multiparous women whose sensitization was at the time of parturition. The antibody titer in these women may be falsely negative at the time of listing by routine PRA testing, due to the remoteness of the sensitization. However, memory cells remain viable and will produce a brisk anamnestic antibody response if the same antigens are present on the allograft.

Diagnosis of Antibody-Mediated Rejection

The diagnosis of antibody-mediated rejection is made on the finding of lymphocytic arteritis on routine histologic examination of the vascular endothelium of heart biopsy and positive immunofluorescent staining for immunoglobulin and complement in the absence of significant cellular infiltrates (ISHLT scores of < 1).

Prognosis of Antibody-Mediated Rejection

In general, antibody-mediated forms of rejection are associated with a poorer prognosis both early and late after heart transplantation.[119, 122] Early morbidity and mortality rates associated with acute graft dysfunction are related to protracted hypotension. There have been some reports that antibody-mediated or acute vascular rejection is more likely to be associated with myocyte necrosis than cellular rejection,[144] which may explain the ventricular dysfunction. However, there also is an increased risk of accelerated development of cardiac vasculopathy in patients with evidence of antibody-mediated forms of rejection.[141, 120]

Treatment

High-dose corticosteroids, ATG, and OKT-3 and even short courses of cyclophosphamide and plasmapheresis have been used as treatment with varying success.[119]

Chronic Rejection With Graft Vasculopathy

After the first year of heart transplantation, pathology studies have shown that graft vascular disease, myocardial hypertrophy, and fibrosis develop.[145] The term *chronic rejection* is used to describe gradual deterioration in solid organ allografts (particularly kidney) manifest with parenchymal fibrosis and vascular obliteration from a concentric fibrosis. *Chronic rejection after heart transplantation* is an ill-defined term that has fallen out of favor. The dominant problem is obliteration of the coronary arteries. There is increasing information on the potentially important role of antigen-independent mechanisms (see Ch. 61, Heart Transplantation: Indications, Outcomes, and Long-Term Complications). An accelerated neointimal expansion develops in a longitudinal fashion in a spectrum of coronary vessels in the transplanted heart. The expanded neointima is composed of infiltrating mononuclear cells, smooth muscle cells, increases and alterations in extracellular matrix, and increased quantity of lipids.[146] This occlusive disease is the leading cause of late cardiac graft failure.[97] Of the many terms applied to describe this occlusive process, *cardiac allograft vasculopathy* is used in this textbook. A detailed review of the features, diagnosis, and treatment of graft vascular disease is given in Chapter 61, Heart Transplantation: Indications, Outcomes, and Long-Term Complications.

Noninvasive Testing for Heart Rejection

Since the first heart transplant, efforts have been ongoing to identify alternative noninvasive measures, indicators, or surrogate markers of various forms of rejection. Although highly sensitive, endomyocardial biopsies are invasive, sampling is restricted to the septum, and the inflammation and injury that serve as a measure of rejection are not specific. Noninvasive testing often does not identify cardiac rejection. First, the heart transplant is denervated and, hence, recipients have few cardiac symptoms. Second, focal abnormalities are easiest to identify with most of the noninvasive modalities, but early forms of rejection tend to be diffuse and patchy. Cardiac imaging, cardiac electrophysiology, cytoimmunologic monitoring, and serologic assays are actively being evaluated as surrogate measures of rejection. Echocardiographic studies have included measures of wall thickening, mass, and dimension; of left ventricular filling by pulsed Doppler; and of peak relaxation and systolic velocities by Doppler tissue imaging.[147, 148] Most of these small studies did not correlate with rejection or correlated only with high-grade rejection that was clinically evident. Hence, improved sensitivity for earlier diagnosis has yet to be demonstrated.

Electrocardiographic studies have examined the usefulness of the corrected QT interval, signal-averaged electrocardiograms, and even paced epimyocardial electrograms, with some usefulness shown in very small studies.[149–154] Among the nuclear medicine studies that have been evaluated, imaging with the use of antimyosin antibody did identify rejection-associated injury to the myocardium but lacked sensitivity.[155] However, studies in which annexin V was used as a marker of rejection-associated apoptosis identified rejection at earlier time points in transplant models.[156]

The identification of serologic markers continues to be a priority because of the ease in obtaining blood. A multitude of factors have been evaluated, including cytokines, activation products, MHC antigens, and myocardial proteins (e.g., troponin T).[110, 157–160] The disadvantage is that factors produced at high local levels within the graft are diluted in the systemic circulation and differences fall below the sensitivity required to clearly identify a rejection episode.

One way to obviate this is to measure levels from coronary sinus blood,[161] but this involves an invasive procedure.

Immunologic Testing

Pretransplantation Immunologic Evaluation

Before solid allograft transplantation, potential recipients undergo immunologic testing that includes blood group antigen typing (ABO), RH status, PRA screening, and HLA typing. The major purpose of testing in heart transplantation is to identify incompatible matches likely to lead to hyperacute or humoral rejection. However, as more rapid and sensitive assay techniques are developed, a future goal might be to identify the most compatible donor/recipient matches.

Heart transplantation is performed between ABO-compatible, if not ABO-identical, donors and recipients. First, blood group antigens (ABO) may produce clinically significant histoincompatibility. Major ABO and even Lewis incompatibility between donors and recipients produces higher rates of rejection. Second, donor (as opposed to recipient) lymphocytes may produce antibodies against recipient blood group antigens (ABO, Rh, and Lew). The presence of an antibody response leads to reactions against the donor as well as to transfused blood products.

Serum PRA is a screening test to determine whether the recipient has preformed cytotoxic antidonor antibodies. Microlymphocytotoxicity assays are completed with the use of recipient sera. A panel of lymphocytes representing a range of high-frequency HLA types is incubated with recipient sera. The addition of complement results in lysis of donor lymphocytes bound with antibodies in the recipient sera. Percent PRA denotes the percentage of panel of lymphocyte HLA subtypes in which lysis occurred. Higher percent PRA values indicate the presence of an increased number of anti-HLA antibodies and a high chance of a positive cross-match. The identification of an acceptable donor is even harder in this situation, and the use of plasmapheresis or immunosuppression before transplantation would be considered to reduce the PRA.[162] There is very high structural homology between epitopes on HLA antigens, which may lead to cross-reactivity of a single antibody. PRA of more than 10 percent is associated with an adverse outcome in heart transplantation.[163–166] Only IgG isotype, not IgM, antibodies are considered clinically relevant.

Cross-matching is performed between specific potential donors and recipients to identify the presence of antidonor antibodies. Recipient serum is incubated with donor target cells (mononuclear cells), complement is added, and cell lysis is assessed. Variations on the cross-match test include the use of flow cytometry without complement, performance of T- and B-cell cross-matches, and measurement for the presence of IgM autoantibodies. Transplantation is not performed in recipients with positive donor cross-matches because of the high risk of hyperacute rejection. Flow cytometry has been used in heart transplantation and is associated with improved sensitivity.[167]

In heart transplantation, HLA typing is not typically completed prospectively because of time constraints. For heart and lung transplantation, ischemic times of longer than 4 hours are associated with intramyocardial injury and poorer outcomes. In kidney transplantation, in which timing permits an analysis of HLA phenotype between donors and recipients, the number of matched HLA loci correlates with improved graft survival. A similar trend with improved survival with mismatches of two or less has been reported after heart transplantation, but the data are limited because the majority of grafts have at least four mismatches.[168–171]

After heart transplantation, a number of immunologic parameters can be followed to predict rejection. Peripheral blood lymphocyte subsets, soluble MHC I and II,[172] cytokines[173] and their receptors (IL-2 receptor, IL-6, IL-8),[106–108, 174] and donor-specific antibodies[175, 176] have all been linked in small-scale studies to increases in high grades of rejection. Active research continues on these and other potential surrogate markers of rejection in an effort to identify methods that detect rejection at earlier time points.

CONCLUSION

The type and severity of rejection are determined by the duration, intensity, and characteristics of alloimmune responses that arise between the transplanted heart and the recipient. Future treatments for rejection will evolve as the immunopathogenesis of the various types and stages of rejection is elucidated. First, diagnostic screening that identifies rejection in earlier phases based on specific molecular pathways is on the horizon. Second, therapies will be developed that target precise molecular pathways overcoming some of the nonspecific effects of general immunosuppression. Third, therapy will be tailored based on an individual recipient's immune phenotype. In characterizing the cytokine phenotype of heart transplant recipient, it has been demonstrated that those with high TNF-α and low IL-10 production are at a higher risk of rejection.[173, 177] These studies have been carried one step further with the demonstration that phenotype can be completed at the genetic level.[178] Further study of the elaborate cytokine and growth factor expression patterns may allow stratification of patient risk and target therapy to attenuate the response in a more directed manner.

The control of rejection involves therapeutic strategies that induce a state of general immunosuppression. One future goal would be to develop donor antigen-specific immunosuppressive strategies. The avoidance of general immunosuppression could eliminate many forms of drug toxicity and reduce infection and malignancy. However, the ultimate goal would be to attain a state of "tolerance" in which graft function is maintained without the need to administer immunosuppression therapy.[178] This concept of graft acceptance has been inspired by reports of stable graft function in patients in whom immunosuppression had been erroneously curtailed or discontinued. Along these lines, many researchers are evaluating methods to modify the recipient's immune system through the use of hematopoietic transplantation.[179, 180] Studies in animal models have shown that by inducing a state of chimerism with hematopoietic stem cell transfusion, graft survival is prolonged without immunosuppression. It is unclear whether this level of tolerance considered acceptable in the animal models will be sufficient in the clinical arena. A second area of promise is to modify donor antigenicity. Of the many efforts in this arena, advances have been made in the application of gene therapy to heart transplantation.[181, 182] In many ways, the transplanted heart is an ideal mode for the use of gene therapy. First, time from harvest until implantation can be used as dwell time for the targeted genes. By infusing at the time of harvest, the entire donor vasculature may be exposed to gene transduction. The problem of inflammation associated with gene therapy might be obviated by the immunosuppression used to allow engraftment of the heart, and the transient nature of expression after gene therapy may be acceptable for the induction of tolerance. Heart transplantation continues to be a dynamic and evolving field, providing those with end-stage heart failure a second chance at life. Its therapeutic potential will expand as the forces that produce rejection are unraveled and selective therapies are developed to ameliorate the destructive alloimmune responses.

References

1. Abbas AK, Lichtman AH, Pober JS: General properties of immune responses. *In* Cellular and Molecular Immunolology. 3rd ed. Philadelphia: WB Saunders, 1997.
2. VanBuskirk AM, Pidwell DJ, Adams PW, Orosz CG: Transplantation immunology: primer on allergic and immunologic diseases. JAMA 278:1993–1999, 1997.
3. Jewell DA, Wilson IA: Structure and function of MHC class I and class II. *In* Hames BD, Glover DM (eds): Molecular Immunology. Oxford: IRL, 1996.
4. Gorer P, Lyman S, Snell GD: Studies on the genetic and antigenic basis of tumor transplantation: linkage between histocompatibility gene and "fused" in mice. Proc R Soc B135:499, 1948.
5. Graff RJ, Silvers WK, Billingham RE, Hildemann WH: The cumulative effect of histocompatibility antigens. Transplantation 4:605, 1966.
6. Warrens AN, Lombardi G, Lechler RI: Presentation and recognition of major and minor histocompatibility antigens. Transplant Immunol 2:103, 1994.
7. Sayegh MH, Carpenter CB: Role of indirect allorecognition in allograft rejection. Int Rev Immunol 13:221, 1996.
8. Halloran PF: Rethinking immunosuppression in terms of the redundant and nonredundant steps in the immune response. Transplant Proc 28:11–18, 1996.
9. Bluestone JA: Costimulation and its role in organ transplantation. Clin Transplant 10:104–109, 1996.
10. Sayegh MH, Turka LA: The role of T-cell costimulatory activation pathways in transplant rejection. N Engl J Med 338:1813–1821, 1998.
11. Wells AD, Turka LA: Individual T-cells hold unexpected clues to the nature of anergy and memory. Immunol Res 17:261–268, 1998.
12. Waterhouse P, Penninger JM, Timms E: Lymphoproliferative disorders with early lethality in mice deficient in CLTA-4 [see comments]. Science 270:985, 1995.
13. Healy JI, Goodnow CC: Positive versus negative signaling by lymphocyte antigen receptors. Annu Rev Immunol 16:645, 1998.
14. Mosmann TR, Sad S: The expanding universe of T-cell subsets: Th1, Th2, and more [see comments]. Immunol Today 17:138, 1996.
15. Abbas AK, Murphy KM, Sher A: Functional diversity of helper T lymphocytes. Nature 383:787, 1996.
16. Halloran PF, Batiuk TD, Goes NB, Campbell P: Strategies to improve the immunologic management of organ transplants. Clin Transplant 9:227–236, 1995.
17. Kahan BD: The three fates of immunosuppression in the next millennium: selectivity, synergy, and specificity [editorial]. Transplant Int 96:527–534, 1996.
18. Eisen HJ: Targeting the alloimmune response for prevention of chronic graft loss: efficacy of new immunosuppressive drugs. Transplant Proc 29:29S–31S, 1997.
19. Halloran PF: Immunosuppressive agents in clinical trials in transplantation. Am J Med Sci 313:283–288, 1997.
20. Cardenas ME, Zhu D, Heitman J: Molecular mechanisms of immunosuppression by cyclosporine, FK506, and rapamycin. Curr Opin Nephrol Hypertens 4:472–477, 1995.
21. Morris RE: Mechanisms of action of new immunosuppressive drugs. Ther Drug Monit 17:564–569, 1995.
22. Halloran PF: The effect of immunosuppressive drugs on T cell signalling pathways: non-redundant steps in the T cell response. Kidney Blood Press Res 19:174–176, 1996.
23. Borel JF, Baumann G, Chapman I, et al: In vivo pharmacological effects of cyclosporin and some analogues. Adv Pharmacol 35:115–246, 1996.
24. Stepkowski SM, Tian L, Wang ME, et al: Sirolimus in transplantation. Arch Immunol Ther Exp 45:383–390, 1997.
25. Spencer CM, Goa KL, Gillis JC: Tacrolimus: an update of its pharmacology and clinical efficacy in the management of organ transplantation. Drugs 54:925–975, 1997.
26. Salomon DR: Rationale and mechanisms of immunosuppression. Kidney Int Suppl 58:S48–S50, 1997.
27. Kahan BD, Chang JY, Sehgal SN: Preclinical evaluation of a new potent immunosuppressive agent, rapamycin. Transplantation 52:185–191, 1991.
28. Morris RE: Rapamycins: antifungal, antitumor, antiproliferative, and immunosuppressive macrolides. Transplant Rev 6:39–87, 1992.
29. Marx SO, Jayaraman TG, Loewe O, Marks AR: Rapamycin-FkBp inhibits cell cycle regulators of proliferation in vascular smooth muscle cells. Circ Res 76:412–417, 1995.
30. Gregory CR, Huie P, Billingham ME, Morris RE: Rapamycin inhibits arterial intimal thickening caused by both alloimmune and mechanical injury: its effect on cellular, growth factor, and cytokine responses in injured vessels. Transplantation 55:1409–1418, 1993.
31. Morris RE, Hoyt EG, Murphy MP, et al: Mycophenolic acid morpholinoethylester (RS-61443) is a new immunosuppressant that prevents and halts heart allograft rejection by selective inhibition of T- and B-cell purine synthesis. Transplant Proc 22:1659–1662, 1990.
32. Morris RE: Mechanisms of new immunosuppressive drugs. Kidney Int 53:526–538, 1996.
33. Taylor DO, Bristow MR, O'Connell JB: A prospective, randomized comparison of cyclophosphamide and azathioprine for early rejection prophylaxis after cardiac transplantation. Transplantation 58:645, 1994.
34. Wagoner LE, Olsen S, Bristow M, et al: Cyclophosphamide as an alternative to azathioprine in cardiac transplant recipients with suspected azathioprine-induced hepatotoxicity. Transplantation 56:1415–1418, 1993.
35. Costanzo MR, Koch DM, Fisher SG, et al: Effects of methotrexate on acute rejection and cardiac allograft vasculopathy in heart transplant recipients. J Heart Lung Transplant 16:169, 1997.
36. Sanchez ER: Hsp56: a novel heat shock protein associated with untransformed steroid receptor complexes. J Biol Chem 265:22067–22070, 1990.
37. Miyata Y, Yahara I: Cytoplasmic 8 S glucocorticoid receptor binds to actin filaments through the 90-kDa heat shock protein moiety. J Biol Chem 266:8779–8783, 1991.
38. Vacca A, Felli MP, Farina AR: Glucocorticoid receptor-mediated suppression of the interleukin 2 gene expression through impairment of the cooperativity between nuclear factor of activated T cells and AP-1 enhancer elements. J Exp Med 175:637–646, 1992.
39. Lee JI, Burchkart GJ: Nuclear factor kappa B: important transcription factor and therapeutic target. J Clin Pharmacol 38:981–993, 1998.
40. Ettenger RB, Yadin O: The potential role of therapeutic antibodies in the regulation of rejection. Transplant Proc 27(suppl 1):13–17, 1995.
41. Chatenoud L: Biological immunosuppressants: the way to clinical transplantation tolerance. Transplant Proc 29:51–55, 1997.
42. Strom TB, Steele AW, Nicols J: Genetically engineered proteins for immunoregulation. Transplant Proc 27(suppl 1):18–20, 1995.
43. Helderman JH: Review and previous of anti-T-cell antibodies. Transplant Proc 27(suppl 1):8, 1995.
44. Norman DJ. Mechanisms of action and overview of OKT3. Ther Drug Monit 17:615–620, 1995.
45. Bonnefoy-Berard N, Revillard JP: Mechanisms of immunosuppres-

sion induced by antithymocyte globulins and OKT3. J Heart Lung Transplant 15:435–442, 1996.
46. Masroor S, Schroeder TJ, Michler RE, et al: Monoclonal antibodies in organ transplantation: an overview. Transplant Immunol 2:176–189, 1994.
47. Copeland JG, Icenogle TB, Williams RJ, et al: Rabbit antithymocyte globulin: a 10-year experience in cardiac transplantation. J Thorac Cardiovasc Surg 99:852–860, 1990.
48. Taylor DO, Kfoury AG, Pisani B, et al: Antilymphocyte-antibody prophylaxis: review of the adult experience in heart transplantation. Transplant Proc 29:13S–15S, 1997.
49. Terhorst C: Structure and function of the T-cell receptor/T3 complex. Transplant Proc 18:931–936, 1986.
50. Bristow M, Gilbert EM, Renlund D, et al: Use of OKT3 monoclonal antibody in heart transplantation: review of the initial experience. J Heart Lung Transplant 7:1–11, 1988.
51. Norman DJ: The clinical role of OKT3. Immunol Allergy Clin North Am 9:97–105, 1989.
52. Jaffers GJ, Colvin RB, Cosimi AB, et al: The human immune response to murine OKT3 monoclonal antibody. Transplant Proc 15:646–648, 1983.
53. Chatenoud L, Legendre C, Ferran C, et al: Corticosteroid inhibition of the OKT3-induced cytokine-related syndrome—dosage and kinetics prerequisites. Transplantation 51:334–338, 1991.
54. First R, Schroeder TJ, Hariharan S, et al: The effect of indomethacin on the febrile response following OKT3 therapy. Transplantation 53:91–94, 1992.
55. Pascual M, Rubin RH, Cosimi AB: Minimizing the toxicity of antilymphocyte antibody therapy. Transplant Proc 28:2113–2114, 1996.
56. Shaw LM, Kaplan B, Kaufman D: Toxic effects of immunosuppressive drugs: mechanisms and strategies for controlling them. Clin Chem 42:1316–1321, 1996.
57. Hammond E, Wittwer CT, Greenwood J, et al: Relationship of OKT3 sensitization and vascular rejection in cardiac transplant patients receiving OKT3 rejection prophylaxis. Transplantation 50:776–782, 1990.
58. Soulillou JP: Relevant targets for therapy with monoclonal antibodies in allograft transplantation. Kidney Int 46:540–553, 1994.
59. Cosimi AB: Current and future application of monoclonal antibodies in clinical immunosuppressive protocols. Clin Transplant 9:219–226, 1995.
60. Halloran PF, Prommool S: Humanized monoclonals and other biological initiatives. Clin Biochem 31:353–357, 1998.
61. Costanzo MR: New monoclonal antibodies. Curr Opin Cardiol 11:204–207, 1996.
62. Turka LA: What's new in transplant immunology: problems and prospects. Ann Intern Med 128:946–948, 1998.
63. Waldmann TA, O'Shea J: The use of antibodies against the IL-2 receptor in transplantation. Curr Opin Immunol 10:507–512, 1998.
64. Alegre ML, Lenschow DJ, Bluestone JA: Immunomodulation of transplant rejection using monoclonal antibodies and soluble receptors. Dig Dis Sci 40:58–64, 1995.
65. Vincenti F, Kirkman R, Light S, et al: Interleukin-2 receptor blockade with daclizumab to prevent acute rejection in renal transplantation. N Engl J Med 338:161–165, 1998.
66. Cardi G, Ciardelli TL, Ernstoff MS: Therapeutic applications of cytokines for immunostimulation and immunosuppression: an update. Prog Drug Res 47:211–250, 1996.
67. Orosz C, Huang EH, Bergese SD: Prevention of acute murine cardiac allograft rejection: anti-CD4 or anti-vascular cell adhesion molecular one monoclonal antibodies block acute rejection but permit persistent graft-reactive alloimmunity and chronic tissue remodelling. J Heart Lung Transplant 16:889–904, 1999.
68. Schaub M, Stadlbauer TH, Chandraker A, et al: Comparative strategies to induce long-term graft acceptance in fully allogeneic renal versus cardiac allograft models by CD28-B7 T cell costimulatory blockade: role of thymus and spleen. J Am Soc Nephrol 9:891–898, 1998.
69. Zheng XG, Turka LA: Blocking T-cell costimulation to prevent transplant rejection. Transplant Proc 30:2146–2149, 1998.
70. Pearson TC, Alexander DZ, Hendrix R: CTLA4-lg plus bond marrow induces long-term allograft survival and donor specific unresponsiveness in the murine model: evidence for hematopoietic chimerism. Transplantation 61:991, 1996.
71. Russell ME, Hancock WW, Akalin E: Chronic cardiac rejection in the LEW to F34 rat model: blockade of CD28-B7 costimulation by CTLA41g modulates T cell and macrophage activation and attenuates arteriosclerosis. J Clin Invest 97:833, 1996.
72. Guinan EC, Boussiotis VA, Neuberg D, et al: Transplantation of anergic histoincompatible bone marrow allografts. N Engl J Med 340:1704–1714, 1999.
73. Costanzo-Nordin MR, Hubbell EA, O'Sullivan EJ, et al: Successful treatment of heart transplant rejection with photopheresis. Transplantation 53:S808–S815, 1992.
74. DeNofrio D, Rosengard B, Reynolds C, et al: Rescue photochemotherapy for the treatment of acute cardiac rejection in the absence of cyclosporine maintenance therapy. J Heart Lung Transplant 17:1036–1037, 1998.
75. Wieland M, Thiede VL, Strauss RG: Treatment of severe cardiac allograft rejection with extracorporeal photochemotherapy. J Clin Apheresis 9:S171–S175, 1994.
76. Meiser BM, Kur F, Reichenspurner H: Reduction of the incidence of rejection by adjunct immunosuppression with photochemotherapy after heart transplantation. Transplantation 57:S563–S568, 1994.
77. Dall'Amico R, McLaughlin SN, Murphy MP: Benefits of photopheresis in the treatment of heart transplant patients with multiple/refractory rejection. Transplant Proc 29:S609–S611, 1997.
78. Barr ML: Photopheresis in transplantation: future research and directions. Transplant Proc 30:2248–2250, 1998.
79. Ratkovec RM, Hammond EH, O'Connell JB: Outcome of cardiac transplant recipients with a positive donor-specific crossmatch—preliminary results with plasmapheresis. Transplantation 54:651, 1992.
80. Trachiotis GD, Johnston TS, Vega JD: Single-field total lymphoid irradiation in the treatment of refractory rejection after heart transplantation. J Heart Lung Transplant 17:1045, 1998.
81. Kaufman CL, Colson YL, Wren SM, et al: Phenotypic characterization of a novel bone-marrow derived cell that facilitates engraftment of allogeneic bone marrow stem cells. Blood 84:2436, 1994.
82. Zouboulis CC, Schmuth M, Doepfmer S, et al: Extracorporeal photopheresis of cutaneous T-cell lymphoma is associated with reduction of peripheral $CD4^+$ T lymphocytes. Dermatology 196:305–308, 1998.
83. Barr ML, Meiser BM, Eisen HJ, et al: Photopheresis for the prevention of rejection in cardiac transplantation. N Engl J Med 339:1744–1751, 1998.
84. Wieland M, Theide VL, Strauss RG: Treatment of severe cardiac allograft rejection with extracorporeal photochemotherapy. J Clin Apheresis 9:171, 1994.
85. Valantine HA: Individualizing immunosuppression for heart transplantation: strategies for the next decade. Transplant Proc 29:5S–8S, 1997.
86. Kobashigawa JA: Advances in immunosuppression for heart transplantation. Adv Card Surg 10:155–174, 1999.
87. Meiser BM, Reichart B: New trends in clinical immunosuppression. Transplant Proc 26:3181–3183, 1994.
88. Miller LW: Optimal use of cyclosporine in cardiac transplantation. Transplant Proc 26:2700–2703, 1994.
89. Kahan BD: Cyclosporine. N Engl J Med 321:1725–1738, 1989.
90. Lake KD, Canafax DM: Important interactions of drugs with immunosuppressive agents used in transplant recipients. J Antimicrob Chemother 36(suppl B):11–22, 1995.
91. Mignat C: Clinically significant drug interactions with new immunosuppressive agents. Drug Safety 16:267–278, 1997.
92. Philip AT, Gerson B: Toxicology and adverse effects of drugs used for immunosuppression in organ transplantation. Clin Lab Med 18:755–765, 1998.
93. Miller LW: Cyclosporine-associated neurotoxicity. The need for a better guide for immunosuppressive therapy [editorial; comment]. Circulation 94:1209, 1996.
94. Winkler M, Christians U: A risk-benefit assessment of tacrolimus in transplantation. Drug Safety 12:348–357, 1995.
95. Taylor DO, Barr ML, Radovancevic B: A randomized, multicenter comparison of tacrolimus and cyclosporine immunosuppressive regimens in cardiac transplantation: decreased hyperlipidemia and hypertension with tacrolimus. J Heart Lung Transplant 18:336, 1999.
96. Kobashigawa J, Miller L, Renlund D: A randomized active-controlled trial of mycophenolate mofetil in heart transplant recipients. Transplantation 66:507, 1998.

97. Hosenpud JD, Bennett LE, Keck BM, et al: The Registry of the International Society for Heart and Lung Transplantation: fifteenth Official Report—1998. J Heart Lung Transplant 17:656–668, 1998.
98. Sharples LD, Caine N, Mullins P: Risk factor analysis for the major hazards following heart transplantation—rejection, infection, and coronary occlusive disease. Transplantation 52:244, 1991.
99. Kubo SH, Naftel DC, Mills RM Jr, et al: Risk factors for late recurrent rejection after heart transplantation: a multiinstitutional, multivariable analysis. J Heart Lung Transplant 14:409–418, 1995.
100. Billingham ME, Cary NR, Hammond ME: A working formulation for the standardization of nomenclature in the diagnosis of heart and lung rejection: Heart Rejection Study Group. J Heart Lung Transplant 9:587, 1990.
101. Winters GL, Marboe CC, Billingham ME: The International Society for Heart and Lung Transplantation grading system for heart transplant biopsy specimens: clarification and commentary. J Heart Lung Transplant 17:754, 1998.
102. Durham JR, Nakhleh RE, Levine A, Levine TB: Persistence of interstitial inflammation after episodes of cardiac rejection associated with systemic infection. J Heart Lung Transplant 14:774, 1995.
103. Fyfe B, Loh E, Winters GL, et al: Heart transplantation-associated perioperative ischemic myocardial injury: morphological features and clinical significance. Circulation 93:1133, 1996.
104. Briscoe DM, Yeung AC, Schoen FJ: Predictive value of inducible endothelial cell adhesion molecule expression for acute rejection of human cardiac allograft. Transplantation 60:204, 1995.
105. Torry RJ, Labarrere CA, Torry DS, et al: Vascular endothelial growth factor expression in transplanted human hearts. Transplantation 60:1451, 1995.
106. George JF, Kirklin JK, Naftel DC, et al: Serial measurements of interleukin-6, interleukin-8, tumor necrosis factor-α, and soluble vascular cell adhesion molecule-1 in the peripheral blood plasma of human cardiac allograft recipients. J Heart Lung Transplant 16:1046–1053, 1997.
107. Roodman ST, Miller LW, Tsai CC: Role of interleukin 2 receptors in immunologic monitoring following cardiac transplantation. Transplantation 45:1050–1056, 1988.
108. Young JB, Windsor NT, Kleiman NS, Lawrence EC: Relationship of soluble interleukin-2 receptor levels to allograft arteriopathy after heart transplantation. J Heart Lung Transplant 11:S79–S82, 1992.
109. Grant SC, Guy SP, Lamb WR, et al: Expression of cytokine messenger RNA after heart transplantation: relationship with rejection and serum cytokines. Transplantation 62:910, 1996.
110. Azzawi M, Grant SD, Hasleton PS: TNF alpha mRNA and protein in cardiac transplant biopsies: comparison with serum TNF alpha levels. Cardiovasc Res 32:551, 1996.
111. Utans U, Quist WC, McManus BM: Allograft inflammatory factor-1: a cytokine-responsive macrophage molecular expressed in transplanted human hearts. Transplantation 61:1387, 1996.
112. Strehlau J, Pavlakis M, Lipman M, et al: Quantitative detection of immune activation transcripts as a diagnostic tool in kidney transplantation. Proc Natl Acad Sci U S A 94:695–700, 1997.
113. Labarrere CA, Pitts D, Halbrook H, Faulk WP: Tissue plasminogen activator, plasminogen activator inhibitor-1, and fibrin as indexes of clinical course in cardiac allograft recipients: an immunocytochemical study. Circulation 89:1599, 1994.
114. Reul RM, Fang JC, Denton MD: CD40 and CD40 ligand (CD154) are coexpressed on microvessels in vivo in human cardiac allograft rejection. Transplantation 64:1765, 1997.
115. Azzawi M, Hasleton PS, Geraghty PJ: RANTES chemokine expression is related to acute cardiac cellular rejection and infiltration by CD45RO T-lymphocytes and macrophages. J Heart Lung Transplant 17:881, 1998.
116. Cerilli J, Brasile L, Galouzis T, et al: Vascular endothelial cell antigen system. Transplantation 39:286–289, 1985.
117. Trento A, Hardesty RL, Griffith BP, Bahnson HT: Role of the antibody to vascular endothelial cells in hyperacute rejection in patients undergoing cardiac transplantation. J Thorac Cardiovasc Surg 95:37–41, 1988.
118. Cerilli J, Brasile L, Karmody A: Role of the vascular endothelial cell antigen system in the etiology of atherosclerosis. Ann Surg 202:329–334, 1985.
119. Olsen SL, Wagoner LE, Hammond EH: Vascular rejection in heart transplantation: clinical correlation, treatment options, and future considerations. J Heart Lung Transplant 12:S135, 1993.
120. Grauhan O, Baeyer H, Volk H, et al: Treatment of humoral rejection after heart transplantation. J Heart Lung Transplant 17:S1184–S1194, 1998.
121. Kubo SH, Naftel DC, Mills RM: Risk factors for late recurrent rejection after heart transplantation: a multiinstitutional, multivariable analysis. J Heart Lung Transplant 14:409, 1995.
122. Mills RM, Naftel DC, Kirklin JK, Bourge RC: Heart transplant rejection with hemodynamic compromise: a multiinstitutional study of the role of endomyocardial cellular infiltrate. J Heart Lung Transplant 16:813–821, 1997.
123. Miller LW, Labovitz AJ, McBride LA, et al: Echocardiography-guided endomyocardial biopsy: a five year experience. Circulation 78(suppl III):III-99–III-102, 1988.
124. Anastassiou-Nana MI, O'Connell JB, Nanas JN, et al: Relative efficiency and risk of endomyocardial biopsy: comparisons in heart transplant and nontransplant patients. Cathet Cardiovasc Diagn 18:7, 1989.
125. Baraldi-Junkins C, Levin HR, Kasper EK, et al: Complications of endomyocardial biopsy in heart transplant patients [see comments]. J Heart Lung Transplant 12:63, 1993.
126. Hausen B, Albes JM, Rohde R, et al: Tricuspid valve regurgitation attributable to endomyocardial biopsies and rejection in heart transplantation. Ann Thorac Surg 59:1134, 1995.
127. Heimansohn DA, Robison RJ, Paris JM, et al: Routine surveillance endomyocardial biopsy: late rejection after heart transplantation [see comments]. Ann Thorac Surg 64:1231, 1997.
128. Kobashigawa JA, Miller LW, Yeung AC, Wiederman J: Does acute rejection correlate with the development of transplant coronary artery disease? A multicenter study using intravascular ultrasound. J Heart Lung Transplant 14:S221–S226, 1995.
129. Kobashigawa JA: Treatment of nonhemodynamic compromising rejection: conventional approaches vs individualization/new immunosuppressive drugs. Transplant Proc 29:37S–39S, 1997.
130. Brunner-La Rocca H, Sutsch G, Schneider J, et al: Natural course of moderate cardiac allograft rejection (International Society for Heart Transplantation grade 2) early and late after transplantation. Circulation 94:1334, 1996.
131. Yeoh T-K, Frist WH, Eastburn TE, Atkinson J: Clinical significance of mild rejection of the cardiac allograft. Circulation 86(suppl II):267–271, 1992.
132. Fishbein MC, Bell G, Lones MA, et al: Grade 2 cellular heart rejection: does it exist? J Heart Lung Transplant 13:1051–1057, 1994.
133. Lloveras J-J, Escourrou G, Delisle MB, et al: Evolution of untreated mild rejection in heart transplant recipients. J Heart Lung Transplant 11:751–756, 1992.
134. Valantine HA, Brozena SC, Hobbs R, et al: A randomized double blind, placebo-controlled dose-response study to assess the safety and efficacy of oral sirolimus (rapamycin) in the treatment of acute grade 2 or grade 3A cardiac allograft rejection. Circulation (in press).
135. Cantarovich M, Latter DA, Leortscher R: Treatment of steroid-resistant and recurrent acute cardiac transplant rejection with a short course of antibody therapy. Clin Transplant 11:316, 1997.
136. Mentzer RM, Jahania MS, Lasley RD: Tacrolimus as a rescue immunosuppressant after heart and lung transplantation: the U.S. Multicenter FK506 Study Group. Transplantation 65:109, 1998.
137. Kirklin JK, Bourge RC, McGiffin DC: Recurrent or persistent cardiac allograft rejection: therapeutic options and recommendations. Transplant Proc 29:40S–44S, 1997.
138. Miller LW, Wesp A, Jennison SH: Vascular rejection in heart transplant recipients. J Heart Lung Transplant 12:S147, 1993.
139. Yowell RL, Hammond EH, Bristow MR, et al: Acute vascular rejection involving the major coronary arteries of a cardiac allograft. J Heart Transplant 7:191, 1988.
140. Hammond EH, Yowell RL, Nunoda S: Vascular (humoral) rejection in heart transplantation: pathologic observations and clinical implications. J Heart Transplant 8:430, 1989.
141. Ma H, Hammond EH, Taylor DO: The repetitive histologic pattern of vascular cardiac allograft rejection: increased incidence associated with longer exposure to prophylactic murine monoclonal anti-CD3 antibody (OKT3). Transplantation 62:205, 1996.
142. Normann SJ, Salomon DR, Leelachaikul P: Acute vascular rejection of the coronary arteries in human heart transplantation: pathology and correlations with immunosuppression and cytomegalovirus infection. J Heart Lung Transplant 10:674, 1991.

143. Cherry R, Nielsen H, Reed E, et al: Vascular (humoral) rejection in human cardiac allograft biopsies: relation to circulating anti-HLA antibodies. J Heart Lung Transplant 11:24, 1992.
144. Hook S, Caple JF, McMahon JT, et al: Comparison of myocardial cell injury in acute cellular rejection versus acute vascular rejection in cyclosporine-treated heart transplants. J Heart Lung Transplant 14:351, 1995.
145. Pucci AM, Forbes RD, Billingham ME: Pathologic features in long-term cardiac allografts. J Heart Lung Transplant 9:339, 1990.
146. McDonald PC, Kenyon JA, McManus BM: The role of lipids in transplant vascular disease. Lab Invest 78:1187, 1998.
147. Lieback E, Meyer R, Nawrocki M, et al: Noninvasive diagnosis of cardiac rejection through echocardiographic tissue characterization. Ann Thorac Surg 57:1164, 1994.
148. Puleo JA, Aranda JM, Weston MW: Noninvasive detection of allograft rejection in heart transplant recipients by use of Doppler tissue imaging. J Heart Lung Transplant 17:176, 1998.
149. Warnecke H, Muller J, Cohnert T: Clinical heart transplantation without routine endomyocardial biopsy. J Heart Lung Transplant 11:1093, 1992.
150. Graceffo MA, O'Rourke RA: Cardiac transplant rejection is associated with a decrease in the high-frequency components of the highest-resolution, signal-averaged electrocardiogram. Am Heart J 132:820, 1996.
151. Richartz BM, Radovancevic B, Bologna MT, Frazier OH: Usefulness of the QTc interval in predicting acute allograft rejection. Thorac Cardiovasc Surg 46:217, 1998.
152. Bourge R, Eisen H, Hershberger R: Noninvasive rejection monitoring of cardiac transplants using high resolution intramyocardial electrograms: initial US multicenter experience. Pacing Clin Electrophysiol 21:2338, 1998.
153. Grasser B, Iberer F, Schreier G: Intramyocardial electrogram variability in the monitoring of graft rejection after heart transplantation. Pacing Clin Electrophysiol 21:2345, 1998.
154. Volgman AS, Winkel EM, Pinski SL, et al: Characteristics of the signal-averaged P wave in orthotopic heart transplant recipients. Pacing Clin Electrophysiol 21:2327, 1998.
155. Frist W, Yasuda T, Segall G: Noninvasive detection of human cardiac transplant rejection with indium-111 antimyosin (Fab) imaging. Circulation 76(suppl V):V-81, 1987.
156. Blankenberg FG, Katsikis PD, Tait JF: In vivo detection and imaging of phosphatidylserine expression during programmed cell death. Proc Natl Acad Sci U S A 95:6349, 1998.
157. DeVito-Haynes LD, Jankowska-Gan E, Heisey D: Donor-derived human leukocyte antigen class I proteins in the serum of heart transplant recipients. J Heart Lung Transplant 15:1012, 1996.
158. Grant SC, Lamb WR, Brooks NH, et al: Serum cytokines in human heart transplant recipients: is there a relationship to rejection? Transplantation 62:480, 1996.
159. Dengler TJ, Zimmerman R, Braun K: Elevated serum concentrations of cardiac troponin T in acute allograft rejection after human heart transplantation. J Am Coll Cardiol 32:405, 1998.
160. Laguens RP, Vigliano CA, Argel MI: Anti-skeletal muscle glycolipid antibodies in human heart transplantation as predictors of acute rejection: comparison with other risk factors. Transplantation 65:1345, 1998.
161. Fyfe A, Daly P, Galligan L, et al: Coronary sinus sampling of cytokines after heart transplantation: evidence for macrophage activation and interleukin-4 production within the graft [see comments]. J Am Coll Cardiol 21:171, 1993.
162. De Marco T, Damon L, Colombe B, et al: Successful immunomodulation with intravenous gamma globulin and cyclophosphamide in an alloimmunized heart transplant recipient. J Heart Lung Transplant 16:360–365, 1997.
163. Herzberg G, Rossi A, Courtney M, Gelb B: The effects of HLA mismatching and immunosuppressive therapy on early rejection outcome in pediatric heart transplant recipients. J Heart Lung Transplant 17:S1195–S1200, 1998.
164. Fenoglio J, Ho E, Reed E, et al: Anti-HLA antibodies and heart allograft survival. Transplant Proc 21:807–809, 1998.
165. Lavee J, Kormos RL, Duquesnoy RJ, et al: Influence of panel-reactive antibody and lymphocytoxic crossmatch on survival after heart transplantation. J Heart Lung Transplant 10:921–930, 1991.
166. Crisp SJ, Dunn MJ, Rose ML, et al: Antiendothelial antibodies after heart transplantation: the accelerating factor in transplant-associated coronary artery disease? J Heart Lung Transplant 13:81–92, 1994.
167. Kerman RH, Susskind B, Kerman D, et al: Comparison of PRA-STAT, sHLA-EIA, and anti-human globulin-panel reactive antibody to identify alloreactivity in pretransplantation sera of heart transplant recipients: correlation to rejection and posttransplantation coronary artery disease. J Heart Lung Transplant 17:S789–S794, 1998.
168. Smith JD, Rose ML, Pomerance A, et al: Reduction of cellular rejection and increase in longer-term survival after heart transplantation after HLA-DR matching [see comments]. Lancet 345:1318, 1995.
169. Taylor CJ, Smith SI, Sharples LD: Human leukocyte antigen compatibility in heart transplantation: evidence for a differential role of HLA matching on short- and medium-term patient survival. Transplantation 63:1346, 1997.
170. Costanzo MR: Role of histoincompatibility in cardiac allograft vasculopathy. J Heart Lung Transplant 14:S180–S184, 1995.
171. Opelz G, Wujciak T: Influence of HLA compatibility on graft survival after heart transplantation. N Engl J Med 330:816–819, 1994.
172. Sell KW, Tadros T, Wang YC: Studies of major histocompatibility complex class I/II expression on sequential human heart biopsy specimens after transplantation. J Heart Transplant 7:407, 1988.
173. Baan CC, Weimer W: Intragraft cytokine gene expression: implications for clinical transplantation. Transplant Int 11:169–180, 1998.
174. Kimball PM, Radovancevic B, Isom T, et al: The paradox of cytokine monitoring-predictor of immunologic activity as well as immunologic silence following cardiac transplantation. Transplantation 61:909, 1996.
175. Christiaans MH, Overhof-de Roos R, Nieman R, et al: Donor-specific antibodies after transplantation by flow cytometry: relative change in fluorescence ratio most sensitive risk factor for graft survival. Transplantation 65:427, 1998.
176. Itescu S, Tung TC, Burke EM, et al: Preformed IgG antibodies against major histocompatibility complex class II antigens are major risk factors for high-grade cellular rejection in recipients of heart transplantation. Circulation 98:786–793, 1998.
177. Turner D, Grant SC, Yonan N: Cytokine gene polymorphism and heart transplant rejection. Transplantation 64:776, 1997.
178. Starzl TE, Zinkernagel RM: Antigen localization and migration in immunity and tolerance. N Engl J Med 339:1905, 1998.
179. Pham SM, Kennan RJ, Rao AS: Perioperative donor bone marrow infusion augments chimerism in heart and lung transplant recipients. Ann Thorac Surg 60:1015, 1995.
180. Gandy KL, Weissman IL: Tolerance of allogeneic heart grafts in mice simultaneously reconstitute with purified allogeneic hematopoietic stem cells. Transplantation 65:295, 1998.
181. Hullett DA: Gene therapy in transplantation. J Heart Lung Transplant 15:857–962, 1996.
182. Khachigian LM, Lindner V, Williams AJ, Collins T: Egr-1-incuded endothelial gene expression: a common theme in vascular injury. Science 271:1427–1431, 1996.

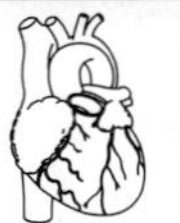

CHAPTER 63

SURGICAL TREATMENT OF ADVANCED HEART FAILURE

O. H. Frazier, Michael P. Macris, Denton A. Cooley, and Michael S. Sweeney

HEART TRANSPLANTATION
Preoperative Considerations
Surgical Techniques
Early Postoperative Management
Clinical Results
MECHANICAL CIRCULATORY SUPPORT
The HeartMate Left Ventricular Assist Device
CONTINUING RESEARCH
Total Artificial Hearts
Investigative Surgical Techniques
CONCLUSION

Because of improved medical therapy, a growing number of patients are surviving hypertension, acute myocardial infarction, and other previously fatal cardiovascular conditions. However, many of these patients later succumb to heart failure, which is assuming epidemic proportions in the United States. Until recently, heart transplantation was considered the only definitive treatment for advanced heart failure. However, advances in mechanical circulatory support are now expanding the options for treating this critical condition.

Since the late 1960s, surgeons at the Texas Heart Institute have gained extensive clinical experience in both heart transplantation and mechanical circulatory support. We describe this experience, as well as our techniques for heart transplantation and for implantation of the HeartMate left ventricular assist device (LVAD) (Thermo Cardiosystems Inc., Woburn, MA), a pump designed for long-term circulatory support. New, alternative options for treating end-stage heart disease are also discussed.

HEART TRANSPLANTATION

Shortly after Barnard[1] performed the first successful clinical heart transplant in 1967, a number of medical centers throughout the world established heart transplant programs.[2, 3] At that time, however, the promise of transplantation for treating end-stage heart disease was not fulfilled. Because little was known about transplant immunology and immunosuppression, most transplant recipients died of allograft rejection or opportunistic infection soon after surgery. Therefore, in the early 1970s, only a few centers, including Stanford, continued to perform heart transplants.

The 1980s saw a renewed interest in heart transplantation because of the advent of cyclosporine. This potent immunosuppressant made it possible to combat rejection while minimizing the risk of infection.[4] Since then, techniques for detecting[5] and grading[6–8] the extent of rejection have been refined, and immunosuppressive protocols have been improved.[9–16] Cyclosporine has become available in a microemulsion formula (Neoral) that improves drug absorption and has more predictable pharmacokinetics.[14] Moreover, a newer immunosuppressant, tacrolimus (formerly FK 506), is being used as a substitute for cyclosporine in selected patients.[11, 13, 15] As we enter the 21st century, cardiac transplantation remains the best hope for many patients with end-stage heart failure.[17–20]

Preoperative Considerations

Recipient and Donor Selection

Most patients referred for heart transplantation have an ischemic or idiopathic cardiomyopathy. Other indications include refractory valvular disease, congenital heart disease, primary myocardial diseases (e.g., sarcoidosis, amyloidosis), infection (e.g., Chagas' disease), or drug-induced myocardial disease. In general, patients on the transplant waiting list are in New York Heart Association (NYHA) functional class IV and have a life expectancy of less than 1 year. Class III patients at risk for sudden death related to malignant arrhythmias can also be placed on the waiting list.

Additional selection criteria for transplant recipients vary from center to center. Over the years, the original criteria have been broadened, so that an increasing number of patients are deemed appropriate candidates. For example, two previously excluded categories, patients aged 60 years or older[21, 22] and those with diabetes mellitus,[23, 24] now have outcomes that compare favorably with those of routine transplant patients. However, patients with terminal illnesses besides advanced heart disease are still ineligible for a transplant.

Donors are matched with recipients based on ABO blood-type compatibility and, when necessary, other histocompatibility markers.[25] The criteria for donor selection have been expanded to include suitable donors 60 years of age or older.[26] In some urgent circumstances, donors receiving high doses of inotropic agents, or donors who were potentially infected have been accepted,[27, 28] usually without adverse effects.

Immunosuppression

At our institution, the immunosuppressive regimen is based on triple-drug therapy, consisting of cyclosporine, azathioprine, and steroids. After transplantation, we taper steroid dosages to avoid side effects.[29] The monoclonal antibody OKT3 is used to induce immunosuppression in patients with renal dysfunction or to treat acute allograft rejection episodes.[30]

Surgical Techniques

Through the years, the basic techniques for heart transplantation have remained the same.[31–33] In the majority of cases, orthotopic transplantation (Fig. 63–1) is performed, but in selected patients, heterotopic transplantation (Fig. 63–2) may be necessary.[34, 35] High pulmonary vascular resistance in the recipient or other conditions that might compromise donor heart function (e.g., a size mismatch in which the donor's weight is 30 percent less than the recipient's) may warrant heterotopic transplantation. The native heart can then assist the donor heart during the initial period after transplantation.

Orthotopic Technique

DONOR

In the case of multiorgan donation, the heart procurement team works along with kidney, liver, and lung procurement teams. After a median sternotomy and pericardial incision have been performed, the superior and inferior venae cavae are dissected up to the pericardial reflections, and 2-0 silk sutures are placed around the superior vena cava. At this point, the procurement team carefully evaluates the myocardial function and inspects the heart for abnormalities. Then the other teams dissect the remaining organs to be donated. After heparinization (3 mg/kg) has been achieved, the superior vena cava is ligated, and the inferior vena cava is transected. Next, the aorta is crossclamped, and cardioplegic solution (4°C) is infused to induce cardiac arrest. During the operation, the myocardium is protected by means of topical cooling with 4°C saline solution.

The right superior pulmonary vein or the left atrial appendage is incised to decompress the heart. Then the heart is removed, beginning with transection of the intrapericardial pulmonary veins, followed by transection of the left and right pulmonary arteries (just distal to the bifurcation) and the aortic root (at the level of the innominate artery). The pulmonary arteries and aortic root must be long enough to be anastomosed to the recipient's vessels.

The heart is placed in a basin with ice-cold saline solution and prepared for transplantation. The left pulmonary veins are connected to create a common left atrial opening (see Fig. 63–1B and C), and the pulmonary artery is incised at the bifurcation. The lateral aspect of the right atrium is then incised from the opening of the inferior vena cava to the right atrial appendage. Care is taken to avoid injuring the sinoatrial node and atrioventricular conduction pathways. Finally, the heart is placed in double plastic bags containing ice-cold saline solution and then in an ice chest for transport to the recipient.

RECIPIENT

After a median sternotomy and a pericardial incision have been performed, heparin (3 mg/kg) is administered intravenously. Cardiopulmonary bypass cannulas are placed in the ascending aorta at the base of the innominate artery and in the venae cavae via the right atrium. The caval cannulas should be close to the atriocaval junction but posterior enough to allow for the right atrial anastomosis. Cardiopulmonary bypass is instituted, and the operation is performed with the aid of systemic hypothermia (28° to 30°C). Tourniquets around the venae cavae are tightened, and the aorta is crossclamped.

The native heart is excised at the midlevel of the atria, just distal to the aortic and pulmonary valves (see Fig. 63–1A), and the donor heart is brought to the operative field (see Fig. 63–1B). The donor and recipient left atria are anastomosed with a continuous 3-0 monofilament polypropylene suture, beginning at the left lateral margin of the free wall and continuing toward the septum. The right atria are anastomosed in the same manner, beginning at the septum and continuing toward the free wall. While systemic warming is begun, the pulmonary artery and the ascending aorta are anastomosed end-to-end with 3-0 polypropylene sutures. The heart is then aspirated, and blood flow is restored by removing the aortic crossclamp and releasing the caval tourniquets.

If the donor heart fails to resume normal sinus rhythm, electrical cardioversion should be performed. If the heart rate is slow, isoproterenol should be infused; if necessary, a temporary pacing wire should be placed on the right ventricle (100 beats/min). If pulmonary vascular resistance is high, the isoproterenol infusion is continued. The patient is gradually weaned from cardiopulmonary bypass, and the cardiopulmonary bypass cannulas are removed. Protamine sulfate is administered to reverse the effects of heparin, and the operation is completed in the usual manner.

Heterotopic Technique

DONOR

The main difference in removing the donor heart for heterotopic transplantation is that the superior vena cava is ligated at the level of the innominate vein, allowing a larger opening to be created for the right atrial anastomosis (see Fig. 63–2A). To prepare the donor heart for heterotopic transplantation, the inferior vena cava and the right pulmonary veins are closed with double-layer 5-0 polypropylene sutures. The bridge of tissue between the left pulmonary veins is incised to form a common opening into the left atrium. At the time of transplantation, an incision is made in the posterior right atrium and extended to the superior vena cava.

RECIPIENT

After a median sternotomy has been performed, the pericardium is opened to the left of midline, and the incision is extended toward the right phrenic nerve. A rectangular flap is formed to allow the right lung to be isolated. Heparin is given, and the aorta is cannulated proximal to the origin of the innominate artery. The superior vena cava is cannulated

Text continued on page 1230

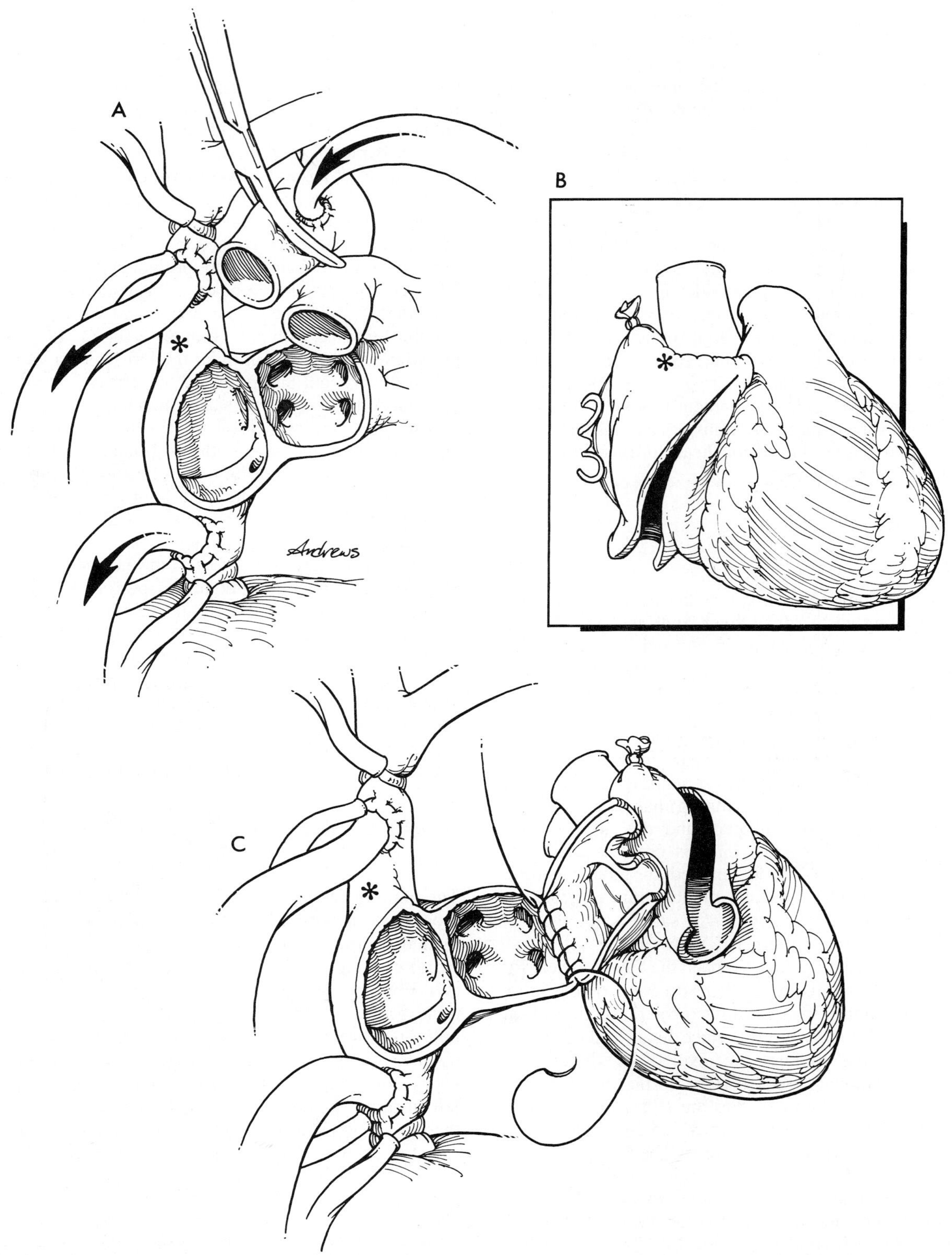

FIGURE 63–1 Technique for orthotopic heart transplantation. **A,** Excision of the native heart. **B,** Preparation of the donor heart. **C,** Left atrial anastomosis, beginning at the free wall.

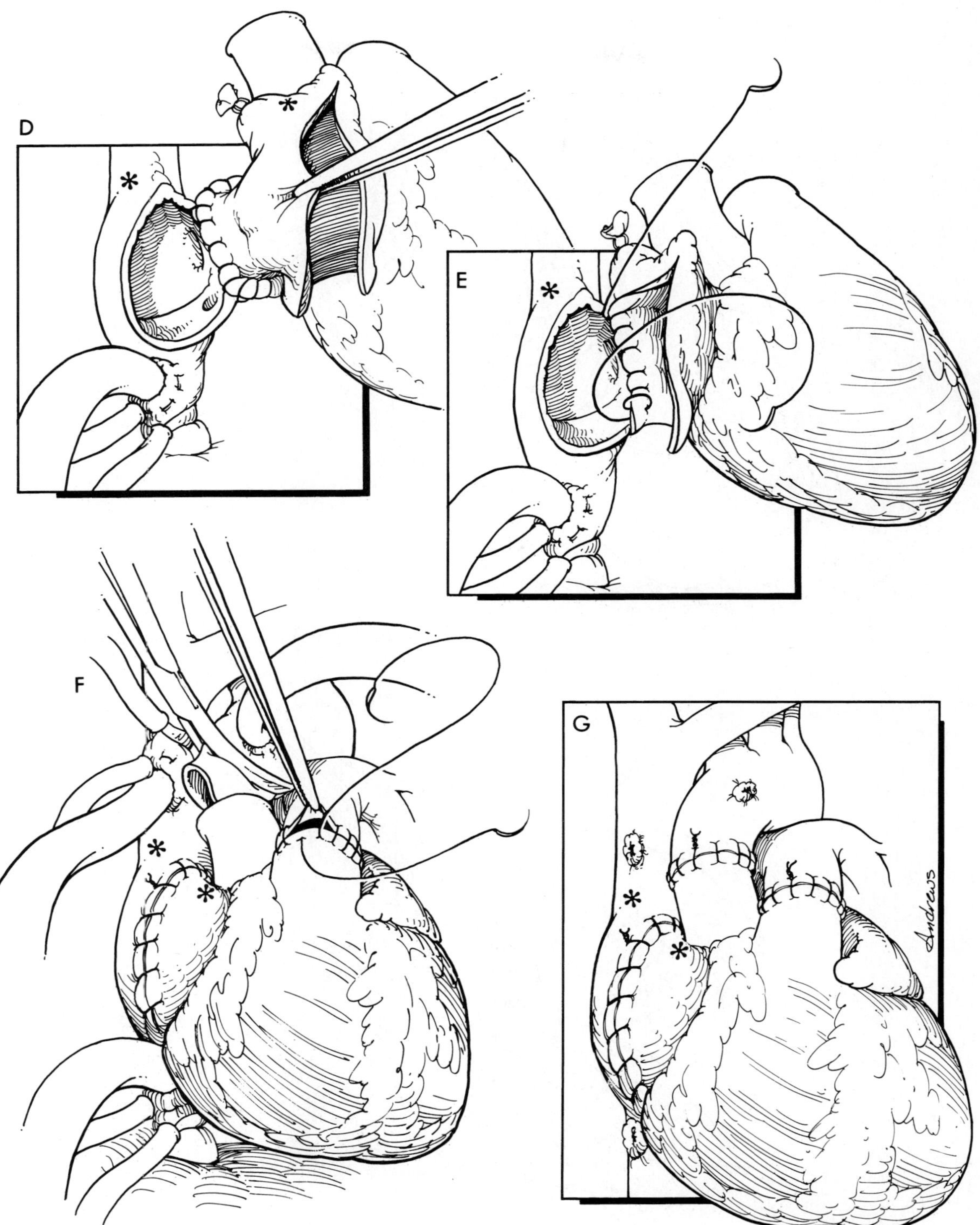

FIGURE 63–1 *Continued.* **D,** Completed left atrial anastomosis. **E,** Right atrial anastomosis, beginning at the interatrial septum. **F,** Pulmonary artery and aortic anastomoses. **G,** Completed transplant. The *asterisk* represents the sinoatrial node. (**A–G,** From Cooley DA: Cardiac and cardiopulmonary transplantation and the mechanical heart. *In* Cooley DA [ed]: Techniques in Cardiac Surgery. 2nd ed. pp. 369–385. Philadelphia: WB Saunders, 1984.)

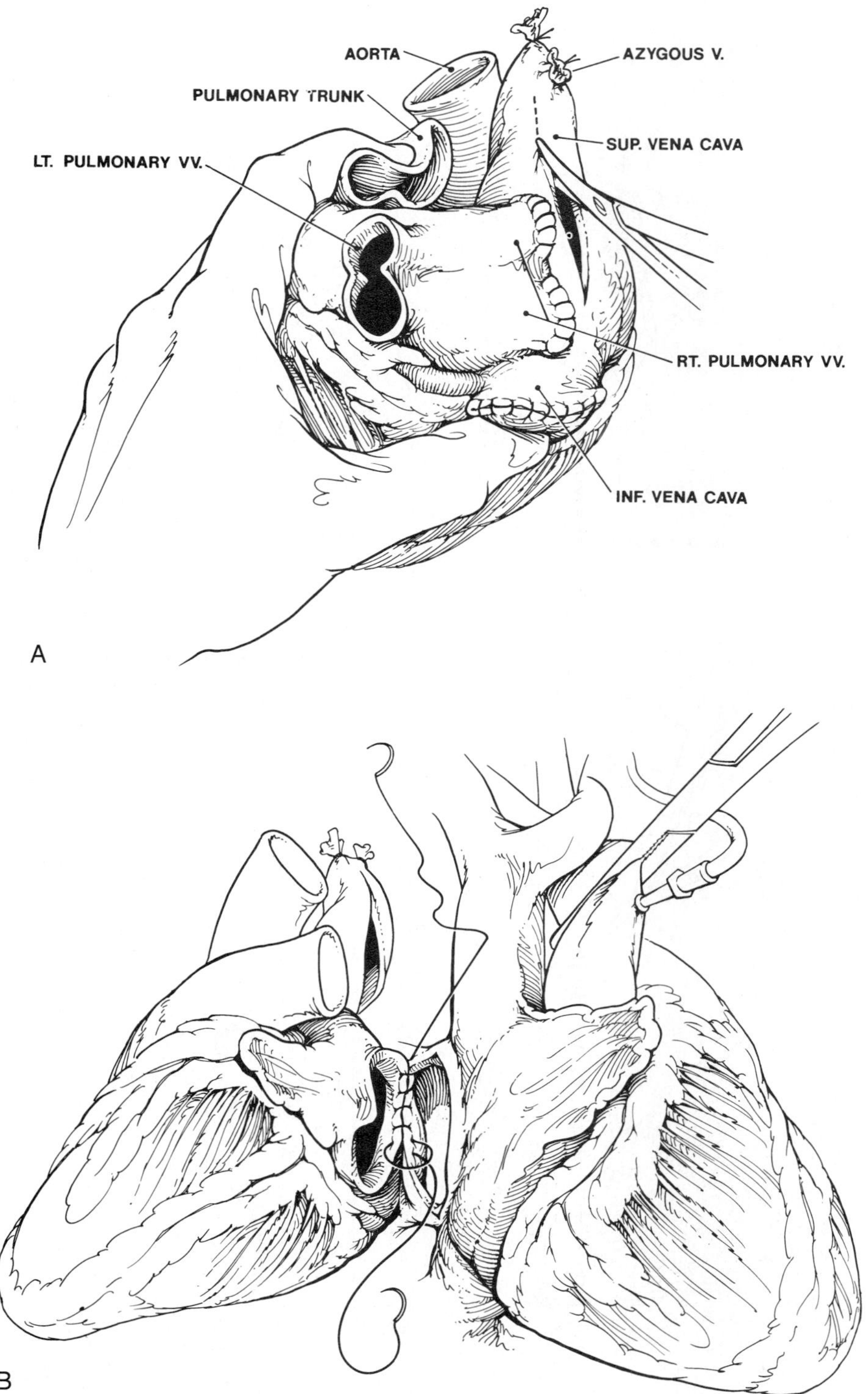

FIGURE 63–2 Technique for heterotopic heart transplantation. **A,** Preparation of the donor heart. **B,** Left atrial anastomosis.

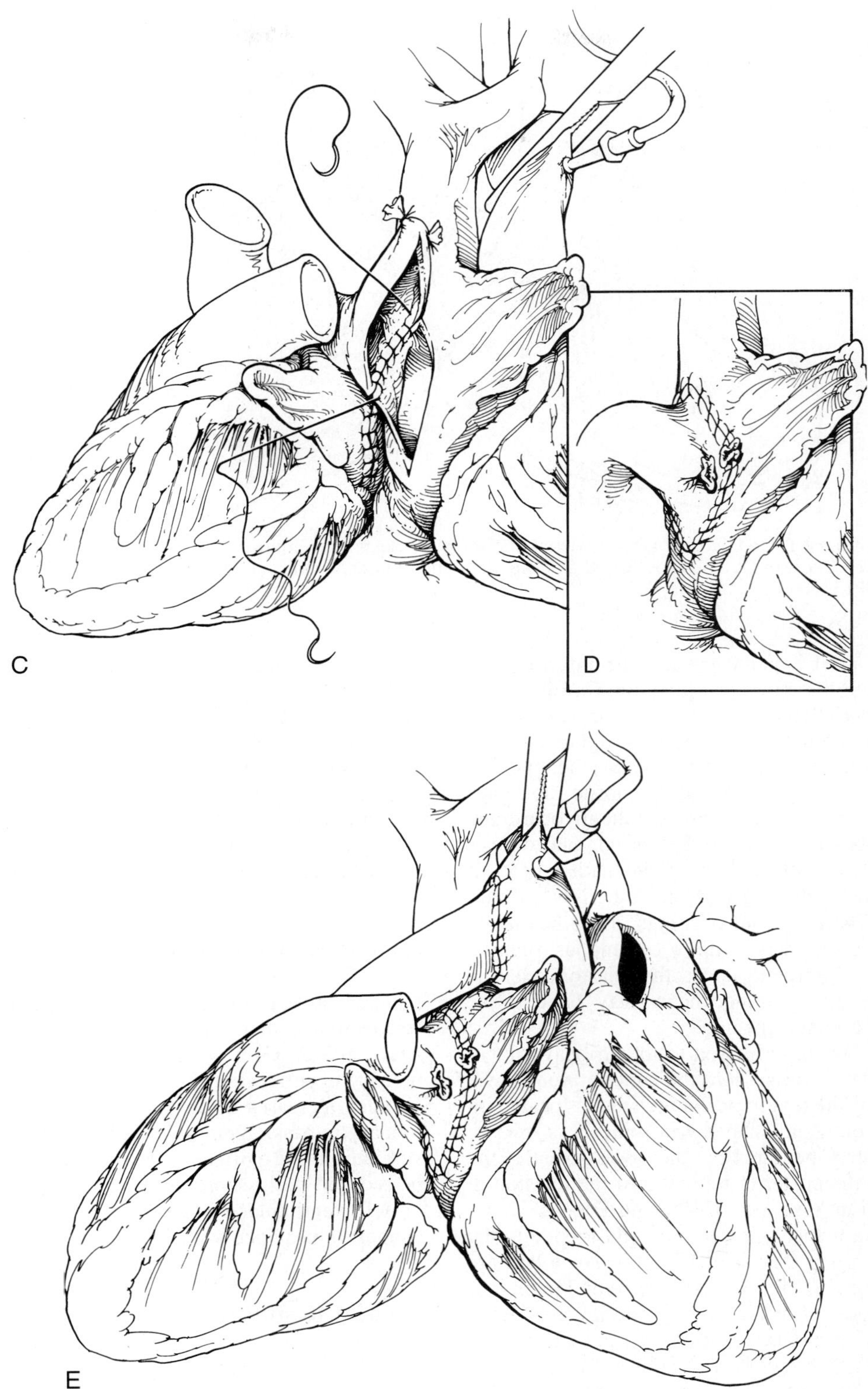

FIGURE 63–2 *Continued.* **C,** Right atrial anastomosis. **D,** Completed right atrial anastomosis. **E,** Aortic anastomosis.
Illustration continued on following page

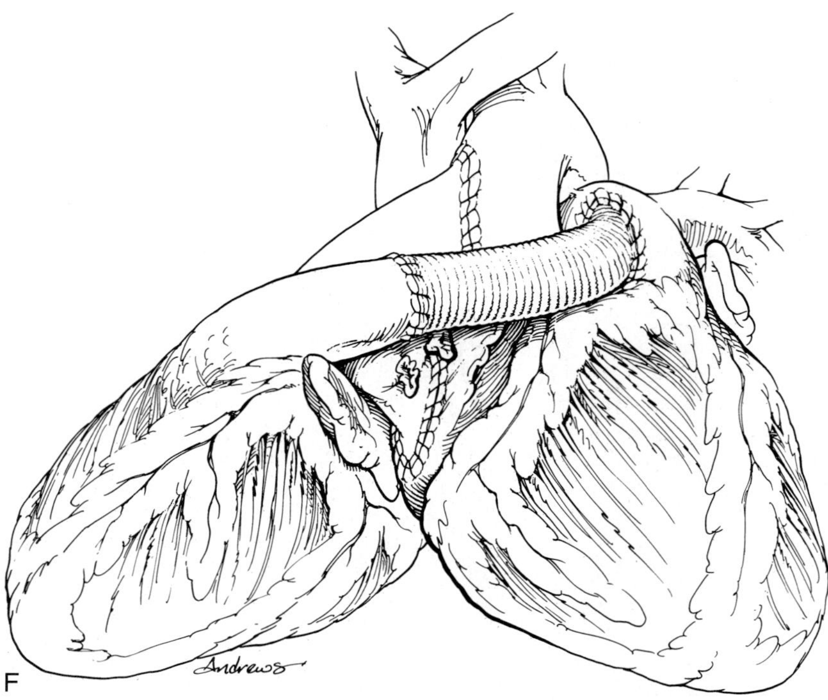

FIGURE 63–2 *Continued.* **F,** Dacron graft sewn to donor and recipient pulmonary arteries to complete the heterotopic heart transplant. (**A–F,** From Frazier OH, Okereke OUJ, Cooley DA, et al: Heterotopic heart transplantation in three patients at the Texas Heart Institute. Tex Heart Inst J 18:221, 1985.)

through the right atrial appendage, and the inferior vena cava is cannulated at the atriocaval junction. Cardiopulmonary bypass is started, the ascending aorta is crossclamped, and tourniquets around the venae cavae are tightened. Systemic hypothermia is induced, and the heart is stopped by infusing cardioplegic solution through the aortic root. During the operation, topical cooling protects the myocardium.

The transplant begins with the left atrial anastomosis (see Fig. 63–2B). The left atrium of the native heart is incised between the right superior and the right inferior pulmonary veins. The left atrial openings of the hearts are joined, beginning posteriorly, with a continuous running suture. To prevent a gradient across the anastomosis, the left atrial incision in the donor heart may have to be extended to create a wider opening.

The native right atrium is incised to the atriocaval junction. The incision is continued into the superior vena cava, so that two thirds of the length of the incision is located on the cava. A large diamond-shaped anastomosis is created between the right atria, beginning at the lowest point of the donor incision and the posterior midpoint of the incision in the native right atrium (see Fig. 63–2C and D).

The donor's aorta is then anastomosed end-to-side to the native ascending aorta (see Fig. 63–2E). An adequate length of donor aorta is necessary to prevent kinking of the atrial anastomoses. The pulmonary arteries are joined with a preclotted 22-mm Dacron graft. The graft is anastomosed end-to-side to the recipient pulmonary artery trunk, then end-to-end to the donor's pulmonary artery (see Fig. 63–2F).

Air is removed from both hearts, and blood flow is restored. The function of both hearts must be checked before cardiopulmonary bypass is stopped. Finally, temporary pacing wires are placed on both hearts to establish a satisfactory rhythm and to monitor electrocardiographic activity. Using a dual-chamber pacemaker with adjustable atrioventricular delay, one can easily institute counterpulsation to treat hemodynamic instability and minimize inotropic drug use immediately after heterotopic heart transplantation. Moreover, long-term linked pacing may lead to improvements in native heart function and, thus, offer better backup support in case of allograft dysfunction.[36]

Early Postoperative Management

Patients are carefully monitored for hyperacute allograft rejection or other complications that could cause donor heart failure. Right ventricular failure can result from pulmonary hypertension. Therefore, if pulmonary vascular resistance increases at the time of weaning from cardiopulmonary bypass, aggressive measures are taken to increase ventilation and correct acidosis. Pulmonary pressure may be reduced with isoproterenol or prostaglandin E_1. If right or left ventricular failure occurs, mechanical circulatory support is provided with an appropriate assist device.[37–39]

Clinical Results

Most heart transplant recipients enjoy a good quality of life,[40] and most of them (particularly the older ones) have a reasonable life expectancy. In following up 43,936 adult heart transplant recipients from 1967 through 1999, the Registry of the International Society for Heart and Lung Transplantation[41] reported overall actuarial survival rates of

79.4 percent at 1 year, 65.2 percent at 5 years, and 45.8 percent at 10 years. Early mortality (within 30 days of transplantation) ranges from 9 to 10 percent.

To further improve long-term survival, transplant researchers have begun to focus on analyzing and preventing allograft coronary atherosclerosis.[42–44] This disease, which is one of the primary causes of death after transplantation, seems to be associated with allograft rejection. Furthermore, since the number of donor hearts has remained fairly constant (2340 in 1998[45]), researchers are seeking ways to increase the donor pool and optimize the use of available hearts.[46, 47] Nonetheless, donor scarcity will continue to limit the number of patients who can undergo heart transplantation. Moreover, a large number of patients with end-stage heart disease do not meet the transplant selection criteria. Advances in long-term mechanical circulatory support are offering hope for solving these dilemmas.

Mechanical Circulatory Support

The history of mechanical circulatory support has paralleled, and often overlapped, that of heart transplantation. Experience with the total artificial heart (TAH) has stimulated the evolution of ventricular assist devices and vice versa.

In 1969, Cooley and colleagues[48] performed the first clinical implant of a TAH (Fig. 63–3). The pump served as a bridge to transplantation in a 47-year-old man who could not be weaned from cardiopulmonary bypass. After 64 hours, the patient underwent a successful heart transplant but died of *Pseudomonas* pneumonia and overwhelming sepsis 32 hours later. In retrospect, compared with later TAH recipients, this patient appears to have had the best surgical outcome. He was extubated shortly after surgery and had minimal bleeding. Immune suppression with the panimmunosuppressant azathioprine (Imuran) was begun at the time of TAH implantation; by the time of the transplant, the patient's leukocyte count had decreased to 2000/μL.

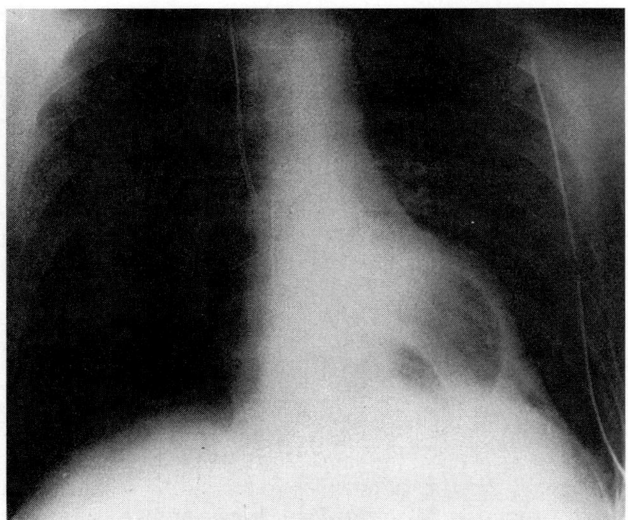

FIGURE 63–3 Roentgenogram obtained after the first clinical implantation of a total artificial heart in 1969 by Cooley.

Twelve years would pass before another TAH was implanted, again by Cooley and coworkers.[49] In this case, the TAH was used as a bridge to transplantation in a 36-year-old man who had had severe cardiac dysfunction after undergoing double-valve replacement. The patient was supported by the TAH for approximately 30 hours and then underwent transplantation. He survived for another 7½ days before succumbing to overwhelming sepsis.

The third Texas Heart Institute patient to receive a TAH as a bridge to transplantation was a 41-year-old man,[50] who was supported by a Jarvik-7 TAH for 31 days. Despite infectious complications that arose soon after the transplant, the patient recovered, was discharged from the hospital, and lived for 2 years.

In 1982, DeVries[51] performed the first of five permanent Jarvik-7 TAH implantations. Although the TAH was able to provide total circulatory support for prolonged periods, the patients had to remain hospitalized, tethered to control consoles. In addition, device-related complications, particularly infections and strokes, supervened. Only 2 of the 5 patients to receive permanent TAHs lived for more than 1 year.[52] In 1988, the smaller Jarvik 7-70 TAH model was introduced, and 75 implantations were performed that year.[33] By 1991, a total of 230 TAHs had been implanted in 226 patients, including the 5 patients who received the device on a permanent basis. Today, the successor of the Jarvik-7 TAH, now known as the *CardioWest pump* (CardioWest Technology, Tucson, AR), is being used as a bridge to transplantation.

In the 1970s, problems related to TAH development and cardiac transplantation stimulated interest in long-term left ventricular assistance. Several research centers began to work on pumps for treating patients with advanced heart disease characterized primarily by left ventricular failure. This effort was stimulated by the work of DeBakey and associates,[53] who first used the LVAD as a bridge to recovery in 1963. By 1978, Texas Heart Institute investigators[54] were conducting clinical tests of an abdominally implanted pneumatic LVAD in patients with cardiogenic shock. One patient, a 21-year-old man with "stone heart" syndrome, was supported for 5 days before transplantation, proving that the LVAD could maintain circulation in the absence of left and right ventricular function.[55] In the 1980s, with the emergence of cardiac replacement as the standard of treatment for end-stage heart failure, LVADs became widely used as bridges to transplantation. Increasing clinical experience led to the introduction of improved devices, including the fully implantable HeartMate LVAD, which has been the focus of long-term testing at our institution.

The HeartMate Left Ventricular Assist Device

Designed for long-term or permanent left ventricular support, the HeartMate is available in a pneumatically and an electrically powered version, each of which has an identical pump.[56, 57] Clinical trials in bridge-to-transplant patients were initiated for the pneumatic model in 1986 and for the electric model in 1991. On the basis of these trials, the

U.S. Food and Drug Administration later approved both models for commercial use.

The intra-abdominally implanted HeartMate pumps blood from the left ventricle into the ascending aorta. The titanium pump, which measures 11.2 × 4.0 cm, is divided by a flexible diaphragm into a blood chamber and a pumping chamber. It has a maximal stroke volume of 83 mL and can provide flows of up to 11.6 L/min. For pneumatic support, the pump is controlled with an external portable console; for electric support, transcutaneous electric leads are attached to rechargeable batteries, which are worn in a shoulder holster. With the electric HeartMate, patients who achieve NYHA class I status are able to await cardiac transplantation at home, even returning to full-time employment in some cases. One patient lived comfortably for more than 500 days with this device.[58, 59]

Unique to the HeartMate are its specially textured surfaces within the blood chamber. As blood flows through the chamber, elements from the blood adhere to the surfaces, so that, within a few days of pump implantation, a smooth biologic coagulum begins to form.[60, 61] As a result, strokes—which have hindered long-term support with other devices—have been minimized. Moreover, patients can be maintained on antiplatelet therapy, consisting of dipyridamole (75 mg tid) and aspirin (80 mg/day), without the need for other anticoagulants.

Although infection can be a problem with any type of LVAD, this complication does not preclude survival to transplantation or reduce the survival rate after transplantation.[62, 63]

Indications

The indication for HeartMate implantation is a rapid deterioration in hemodynamic status despite maximal pharmacologic support, intra-aortic balloon support, or both. Specific selection criteria include a pulmonary capillary wedge pressure of 20 mm Hg or greater, a cardiac index of 2 L/min/m^2 or less, and a systolic blood pressure of 80 mm Hg or less.

Conditions that preclude HeartMate treatment include severe pulmonary hypertension, irreversible renal dysfunction, hepatic dysfunction, or a small body surface area (<1.5 m^2).

Surgical Techniques

IMPLANT OPERATION

The pump is implanted through a median sternotomy incision that extends to the umbilicus (Fig. 63–4A).[64] After heparin (3 mg/kg) has been administered, cardiopulmonary bypass is instituted. We have found that using a BioMedicus pump (Medtronic-BioMedicus, Inc., Eden Prairie, MN) and a cell saver helps prevent damage to platelets and clotting factors. The right atrium and ascending aorta are cannulated for cardiopulmonary bypass. Alternatively, the femoral artery can be cannulated to provide arterial return, which then frees the ascending aorta for anastomosis of the outflow graft. Administering low-dose prostaglandin E_1 before the start of cardiopulmonary bypass helps prevent increased pulmonary vascular resistance and resultant right ventricular failure. The introduction of nitric oxide has helped to reduce pulmonary vascular resistance without causing the systemic effects produced by prostaglandins.

After cardiopulmonary bypass has been instituted, the ascending aorta is crossclamped, and cold cardioplegic solution is rapidly infused. Systemic hypothermia is maintained at 28°C, and cold saline solution is applied topically to protect the heart during the operation.

The pump is positioned intraperitoneally or extraperitoneally in the left upper quadrant of the abdomen (see Fig. 63–4C). The pump inflow and outflow conduits are attached to the device with rotatable joints so that the conduits can be adjusted to fit the patient. Each conduit contains a 25-mm porcine valve to produce unidirectional flow.

The left ventricular apex is cored with a special circular knife (see Fig. 63–4B). A Teflon-covered, reinforced Silastic sewing ring is then sutured to the opening with interrupted, pledgeted sutures (see Fig. 63–4D and E). Next, the inflow and outflow conduits are connected to the blood pump (see Fig. 63–4F and G). The inlet conduit is tunneled through an incision in the diaphragm, is aligned with the mitral valve, and is then secured to the sewing ring. The outflow conduit, a polyester graft, is anastomosed end-to-side to the ascending aorta with a running 4-0 polypropylene suture. To ensure proper seating of the device, the outflow graft must be trimmed to an appropriate length. The percutaneous driveline is exteriorized and the device is positioned before the graft is cut. The driveline is tunneled subcutaneously from the left lower quadrant to the right upper quadrant exit site. The long tunnel may help to prevent serious driveline infections. The graft is cut so that it lies over the diaphragm, just to the right of the median sternotomy. Proper placement of the graft helps prevent complications during the resternotomy for transplantation.

If the pump is placed intraperitoneally, the omentum is wrapped around the pump and the intraperitoneal portion of the driveline to prevent bowel adhesion, and the pump is secured to the abdominal wall (see Fig. 63–4H and I).

Before LVAD pumping is initiated, the patient is placed in the Trendelenburg position. The outflow graft is crossclamped near the anastomosis, and air is slowly vented from the system with a 19-gauge needle placed in the outflow graft. Pump flow is started and gradually increased, while cardiopulmonary bypass flow is gradually decreased. Transesophageal echocardiography helps confirm proper placement of the inflow graft.

The unloading action of the LVAD introduces a new physiologic state in which the left atrial pressure decreases to below normal while the right atrial pressure remains high. In patients with a previously asymptomatic patent foramen ovale, LVAD pumping may cause the foramen to become symptomatic and produce significant shunting. Such an opening, which is best detected with transesophageal echocardiography, must be closed before the patient leaves the operating room.

At the end of the operation, the effect of heparin is reversed, thoracic drainage tubes are placed, and the sternotomy and laparotomy incisions are closed.

EXPLANT OPERATION

At transplantation, cardiopulmonary bypass is instituted; cannulation may be done via the femoral artery to allow

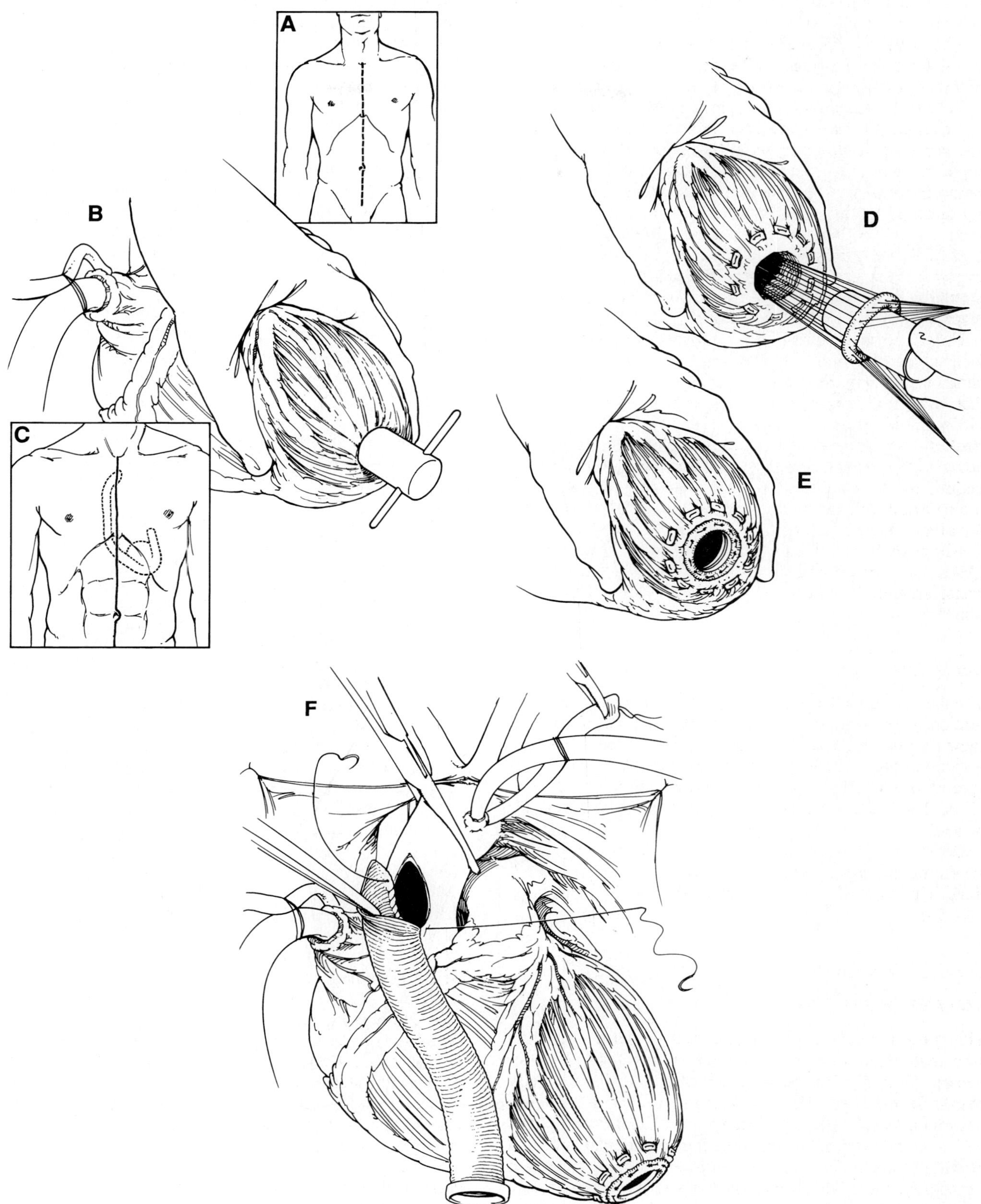

FIGURE 63–4 Implantation of the HeartMate left ventricular assist device. **A,** Extended median sternotomy incision. **B,** Coring of the left ventricular apex. **C,** Anatomic placement of the pump. **D,** Sewing ring sutured to apical opening with interrupted pledgeted sutures. **E,** Sewing ring in place. **F,** Polyester outflow graft anastomosed to ascending aorta.

Illustration continued on following page

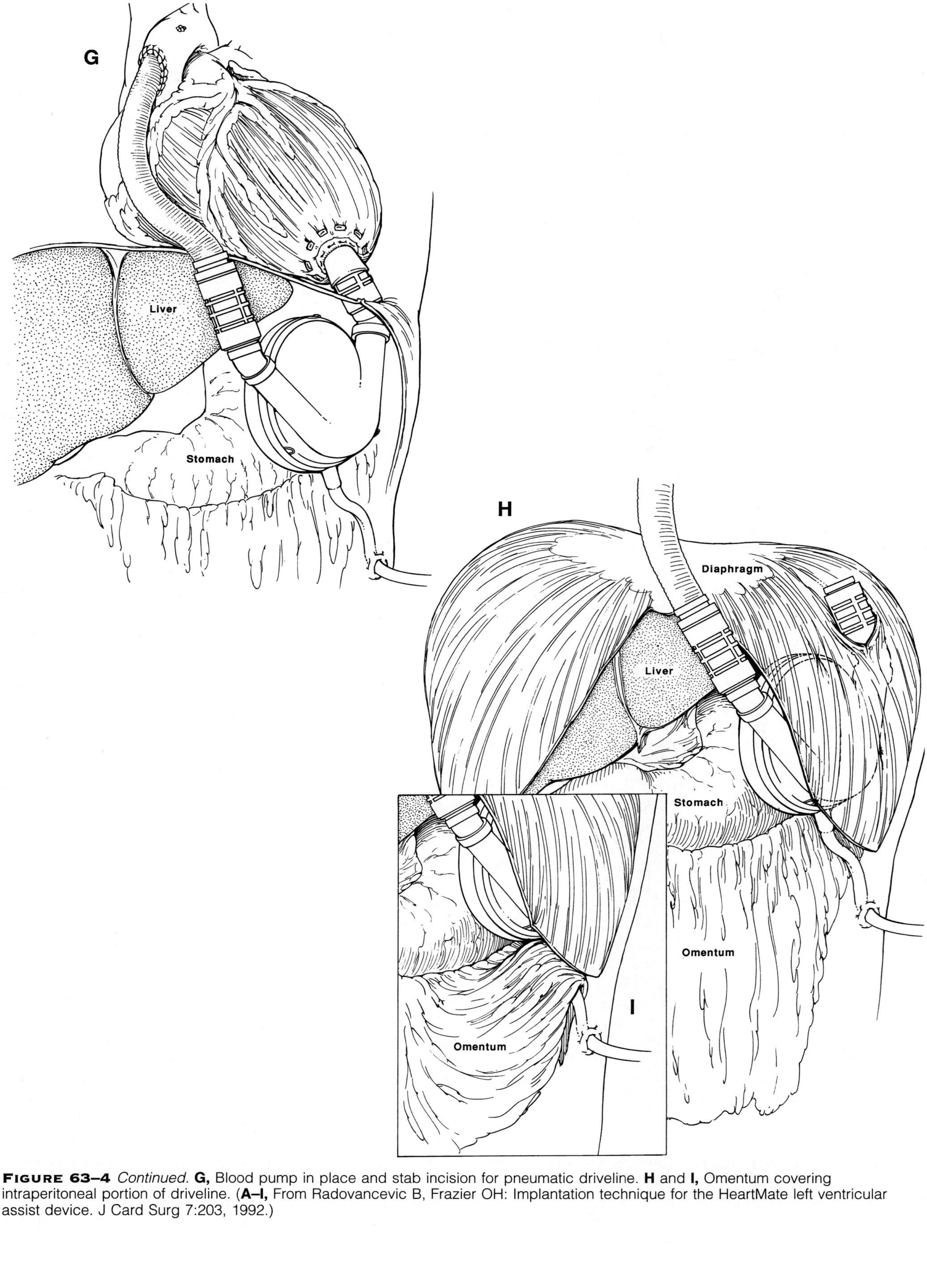

G

Liver

Stomach

H

Diaphragm

Liver

Stomach

Omentum

I

Omentum

FIGURE 63–4 *Continued.* **G,** Blood pump in place and stab incision for pneumatic driveline. **H** and **I,** Omentum covering intraperitoneal portion of driveline. (**A–I,** From Radovancevic B, Frazier OH: Implantation technique for the HeartMate left ventricular assist device. J Card Surg 7:203, 1992.)

more room for the aortic anastomosis. The native heart is excised in routine fashion, and the outflow graft is completely removed to prevent infection. If a heterotopic procedure is planned, the left ventricular apex is oversewn with a Dacron patch and pledgeted sutures. After the pump has been removed, the transplant is performed routinely.

Clinical Results

As of July 1998, the HeartMate had been implanted in 1387 bridge-to-transplant patients at 122 hospitals around the world.[56] The pneumatic model was implanted in 971 cases (70 percent), and the electric model in 416 cases (30 percent). Many of the patients required prolonged support (>30 days). Both HeartMate models substantially improved the clinical status of these patients.[65, 66] In most instances, those in NYHA class IV returned to class I within 3 to 4 weeks after LVAD implantation. In a nonrandomized multicenter trial involving 75 pneumatic HeartMate recipients and 33 non-LVAD patients,[65] the HeartMate reduced the pretransplant mortality by 55 percent; 1 year after transplantation, the survival rate was 90 percent versus 67 percent for the HeartMate and control groups, respectively. This is the only study that used a concomitant control group, consisting of patients who met the criteria for LVAD implantation but for whom the device was not available. In the control group, survival was achieved only by means of cardiac transplantation; the average waiting time for a donor heart was 12 days.

As the universal waiting period for donor hearts has increased, circulatory assistance has become necessary for longer periods. In many cases, long-term LVAD support has resulted in the recovery of native heart function.[67–70] Such recovery was originally observed in the first recipient of a long-term, untethered LVAD, who was supported by the device for 505 days.[58, 59] Cardiac recovery was suggested by anatomic, physiologic, and histologic improvements that were evident on device removal at transplantation.[71] Other investigators later documented improved function at the cellular and subcellular levels, as characterized by normalization of the deranged calcium transport characteristic of advanced heart failure,[72] improvement in tumor necrosis factor levels (G. Torre-Amione, M.D., personal communication), and improved glucose transport and energy utilization (H. Taegtmeyer, M.D., personal communication). In addition, left ventricular unloading improves (1) the heart failure–related changes in gene expression that involve an increase in ventricular expression of atrial natriuretic factor and a decrease in sarcoplasmic reticulum Ca^{2+} adenosine triphosphatase[73] and (2) beta-adrenergic density and the contractility of cardiac muscle in response to isoproterenol stimulation.[74]

Because experience in the bridge-to-transplant population has been so successful, the HeartMate is now being tested in patients with end-stage heart failure who are not candidates for transplantation. A National Heart, Lung, and Blood Institute–sponsored trial, known as *REMATCH* (Randomized Evaluation of Mechanical Assistance and Treatment of Congestive Heart Failure), is seeking to determine whether combined LVAD and medical treatment is superior to optimal medical treatment alone.[75, 76] So far, the results of the combined regimen have been encouraging.

CONTINUING RESEARCH

Unfortunately, a safe, reliable TAH has not yet become available. Having learned from past clinical experience, investigators are trying to develop more compact, biocompatible TAHs for treating patients ineligible for transplantation or LVAD support.

Total Artificial Hearts

At present, only two centers in the United States—the Texas Heart Institute, working with the ABIOMED heart (ABIOMED, Danvers, MA), and the Hershey Medical Center in Pennsylvania, working with the Sarns/3M heart (Sarns/3M, Ann Arbor, MI)—are receiving federal funding for research on TAHs. The new devices differ from previous models in a number of ways, the most important being an emphasis on electric or electrohydraulic power sources. Ultimately, these power sources will allow total implantation of the device and its driveline, so that patients are no longer tethered to a drive console. Freedom from an external power source not only will improve the patients' quality of life but also will reduce the long-term threat of infection. These developments may allow investigators to achieve the original goal of this research—the use of TAHs for long-term therapy.

A mechanical assist device for smaller patients is urgently needed, as the current devices are hindered by limitations in blood flow rate, anatomic size, and space for device implantation. Therefore, new pumps, intended for permanent support, are being developed with these patients in mind. Our institution is collaborating with Jarvik Heart, Inc. (New York, NY) in conducting preclinical studies of the Jarvik-2000, an implantable, intraventricular axial-flow pump that can provide blood flows of up to 10 L/min.[77, 78] Because of this device's small dimensions (2.5 × 10 cm), it is suitable for both large and small adults and for pediatric patients. In addition, ABIOMED is performing preclinical studies of a small pneumatic TAH designed to generate flows of 1.5 to 3.5 L/min in pediatric patients.

Investigative Surgical Techniques

Cardiomyoplasty

Another option being investigated for the treatment of end-stage heart failure is dynamic cardiomyoplasty, in which the transposed latissimus dorsi muscle is wrapped around the heart and then electrically stimulated to augment systolic function.[79] Techniques for cardiomyoplasty and biomechanical cardiac assistance are based on the concept of muscle plasticity, in which prolonged electrical pacing of skeletal muscle gradually alters the fundamental structure of the muscle and strengthens it against fatigue.[80] Dynamic cardiomyoplasty is mainly used for treating ischemic and dilated cardiomyopathies involving isolated left ventricular failure. The operative procedure is demanding and time-consuming, lasting for 7 to 8 hours. Because muscle conditioning takes up to 3 months postoperatively, cardiac improvement does not occur immediately. To prevent possibly fatal dysrhythmias, patients must take antidysrhythmic agents; in some cases, an implantable cardioverter defibrillator is needed. Moreover, the underlying cardiovascular problem remains uncorrected.

As of early 1999, dynamic cardiomyoplasty had been performed in about 600 patients worldwide, using a variety of wrapping techniques.[81, 82] Although many of these patients had subsequent improvements in functional status and quality of life, these improvements were not always confirmable by objective measurements.[82] Therefore, the clinical application of cardiomyoplasty remains limited, and randomized trials designed to determine the proper role of this therapy are needed. Such trials would help clarify the value of biomechanical assistance and the ability of the skeletal muscle to perform adequately on a long-term basis.

Partial Left Ventriculectomy

In heart failure patients, the compensatory mechanism of ventricular dilatation causes increased ventricular wall stress, leading to a vicious circle of myocardial cell death and fibrosis. Once most of the myocardial cells have been replaced by fibrotic tissue, the chances for recovery are minimal, no matter what form of treatment is instituted. However, if ventricular dilatation can be reversed in time, further myocardial cell death may be prevented, and hypertrophied cells may resume their normal function.

Partial left ventriculectomy, as introduced by Batista and coauthors in Brazil,[83] is an alternative therapy being used to treat end-stage heart disease in selected cases. This procedure is also known as *left ventricular reduction surgery.* It involves resecting a segment of the enlarged myocardium to restore normal size and function, thereby reducing the afterload and improving ventricular ejection. The mitral valve is also repaired or replaced, and coronary artery bypass may be performed if necessary.

The indications for this procedure are still being studied. Partial left ventriculectomy may be performed as an alternative to a bridge-to-transplant operation. It may be valuable in poorly developed countries, where other methods may be unavailable. Moreover, partial left ventriculectomy may be applied early, before irreversible cellular changes have occurred. In the United States, the results have been uneven: postoperatively, some patients have had worsening heart failure, whereas others have had a stable improvement in cardiac function.[84, 85] Eventually, it may be possible to predict which patients will be most likely to benefit from this procedure. Meanwhile, partial left ventriculectomy remains controversial, although several pilot studies are being continued in the United States, Europe, and Japan.

CONCLUSION

As we enter the 21st century, heart failure can be expected to take a growing toll, especially as the average age of the population continues to increase. Although advanced heart failure entails a poor prognosis, treatment options have expanded with the advent of cardiac transplantation, mechanical circulatory support systems, and other innovative surgical procedures. Eventually, the underlying conditions responsible for heart failure may become amenable to medical therapy. Meanwhile, although current treatments are limited, an increasing range of surgical strategies are being assessed for application to larger numbers of heart failure patients.

REFERENCES

1. Barnard CN: A human cardiac transplantation: an interim report of a successful operation performed at Groote Schuur Hospital, Capetown. S Afr Med J 41:1271, 1967.
2. Cooley DA, Hallman GL, Bloodwell RD, et al: Human heart transplantation: experience with twelve cases. Am J Cardiol 22:804, 1968.
3. Shumway NE, Stinson EB, Dong E: Cardiac homotransplantation in man. Transplant Proc 1:739, 1969.
4. Kahan BD: Cyclosporin A: a new advance in transplantation. Tex Heart Inst J 9:253, 1982.
5. Lowry RW, Young JB: Noninvasive techniques for detection of heart allograft rejection. *In* Frazier OH, Macris MP, Radovancevic B (eds): Support and Replacement of the Failing Heart. pp. 213–231. Philadelphia: Lippincott-Raven, 1996.
6. McAllister HA, Schnee MJ, Radovancevic B, et al: System for grading cardiac allograft rejection. Tex Heart Inst J 13:1,1986.
7. Billingham ME, Cary NRB, Hammond NE, et al: A working formulation for the standardization of nomenclature in the diagnosis of heart and lung rejection: Heart Rejection Study Group. J Heart Transplant 9:587, 1990.
8. McAllister HA Jr: Endomyocardial biopsy, conditions leading to heart transplantation, and the evaluation of cardiac allograft rejection: morphologic considerations. *In* Frazier OH, Macris MP, Radovancevic B (eds): Support and Replacement of the Failing Heart. pp. 121–145. Philadelphia: Lippincott-Raven, 1996.
9. Kahan BD, Van Buren CT: The new immunosuppressants. *In* Frazier OH, Macris MP, Radovancevic B (eds): Support and Replacement of the Failing Heart. pp. 309–326. Philadelphia: Lippincott-Raven, 1996.
10. Kobashigawa JA: Advances in immunosuppression for heart transplantation. Adv Card Surg 10:155, 1998.
11. Kobashigawa JA: Controversies in heart and lung transplantation immunosuppression: tacrolimus versus cyclosporine. Transplant Proc 30:1095, 1998.
12. Doty JR, Walinsky PL, Salazar JD, et al: Conservative management of late rejection after heart transplantation: a 10-year analysis. Ann Surg 228:395, 1998.
13. Reichart B, Meiser B, Vigano M, et al: European Multicenter Tacrolimus (FK506) Heart Pilot Study: one-year results—European Tacrolimus Multicenter Heart Study Group. J Heart Lung Transplant 17:775, 1998.
14. White M, Pelletier BG, Tan A, et al: Pharmacokinetic, hemodynamic, and metabolic effects of cyclosporine Sandimmune versus the microemulsion Neoral in heart transplant recipients. J Heart Lung Transplant 16:787, 1997.
15. Gerber DA, Bonham CA, Thomson AW: Immunosuppressive agents: recent developments in molecular action and clinical application. Transplant Proc 30:1573, 1998.
16. Land W: Future challenges in immunosuppression. Transplant Proc 30:1580, 1998.
17. Young JB: Cardiac transplantation: three decades of experience define our challenge. Transplant Proc 30:1885, 1998.
18. Bernabeu M: Meeting the challenges of transplantation in the 21st century. Transplant Proc 30:1619, 1998.
19. Hunt SA: Current status of cardiac transplantation. JAMA 19:1692, 1998.
20. Radovancevic B, Frazier OH: Heart transplantation: approaching a new century. Tex Heart Inst J 26:60, 1999.
21. Frazier OH, Macris MP, Duncan JM, et al: Cardiac transplantation in patients over 60 years of age. Ann Thorac Surg 45:129, 1988.
22. Bull DA, Karwande SV, Hawkins JA: Long-term results of cardiac transplantation in patients older than sixty years. UTAH Cardiac Transplant Program. J Thorac Cardiovasc Surg 111:423, 1996.
23. Munoz E, Lonquist JL, Radovancevic B, et al: Long-term results in diabetic patients undergoing heart transplantation. J Heart Lung Transplant 11:943, 1992.

24. Aleksic I, Czer LS, Freimark D, et al: Heart transplantation in patients with diabetic end-organ damage before transplantation. Thorac Cardiovasc Surg 44:282, 1996.
25. Macris MP: Donor selection and management. *In* Frazier OH, Macris MP, Radovancevic B (eds): Support and Replacement of the Failing Heart. pp. 87–98. Philadelphia: Lippincott-Raven, 1996.
26. Tenderich G, Koerner MM, Stuttgen, et al: Extended donor criteria: hemodynamic follow-up of heart transplant recipients receiving a cardiac allograft from donors > or = 60 years of age. Transplantation 66:1109, 1998.
27. Lammermeier DE, Sweeney MS, Haupt HE, et al: Use of potentially infected donor hearts for cardiac transplantation. Ann Thorac Surg 50:222, 1990.
28. Alexander JW, Zola JC: Expanding the donor pool: use of marginal donors for solid organ transplantation. Clin Transplant 10:1, 1996.
29. Lonquist JL, Radovancevic B, Vega JD, et al: Re-evaluation of steroid tapering after steroid pulse therapy for heart rejection. J Heart Lung Transplant 11:913, 1992.
30. Macris MP, Frazier OH, Lammermeier D, et al: Clinical experience with muromonab-CD3 monoclonal antibody (OKT3) in heart transplantation. J Heart Transplant 8:281, 1989.
31. Cass MH, Brock R: Heart excision and replacement. Guys Hosp Rep 108:285, 1959.
32. Cooley DA: Cardiac and cardiopulmonary transplantation and the mechanical heart. *In* Cooley DA (ed): Techniques in Cardiac Surgery. 2nd ed. pp. 369–385. Philadelphia: WB Saunders, 1984.
33. Macris MP, Frazier OH: Techniques of heart transplantation. *In* Frazier OH, Macris MP, Radovancevic B (eds): Support and Replacement of the Failing Heart. pp. 169–196. Philadelphia: Lippincott-Raven, 1996.
34. Frazier OH, Okereke OUJ, Cooley DA, et al: Heterotopic heart transplantation in three patients at the Texas Heart Institute. Tex Heart Inst J 18:221, 1985.
35. Nakatani T, Frazier OH, Lammermeier DE, et al: Heterotopic heart transplantation: a reliable option for a select group of high-risk patients. J Heart Transplant 8:40, 1989.
36. Beyer E, Vatcharasiritham C, Sweeney M, et al: Linked pacing after heterotopic heart transplantation with concurrent left ventricular reduction of the native heart. Tex Heart Inst J 25:299, 1998.
37. Radovancevic B, Nakatani T, Frazier OH, et al: Mechanical circulatory support for perioperative donor heart failure. ASAIO Trans 35:539, 1989.
38. Nakatani T, Radovancevic B, Frazier OH: Right heart assist for acute right ventricular failure after orthotopic heart transplantation. Trans Am Soc Artif Intern Organs 33:695, 1987.
39. Tenderich G, Koerner MM, Stuttgen B, et al: Mechanical circulatory support after orthotopic heart transplantation. Int J Artif Organs 21:414, 1998.
40. Grady KL, Jalowiec A, White-Williams C: Improvement in quality of life in patients with heart failure who undergo transplantation. J Heart Lung Transplant 15:749, 1996.
41. International Society for Heart and Lung Transplantation: Fifteenth Annual Data Report. Survival statistics: adult heart survival. Retrieved July 8, 1999, from the World Wide Web: http://www.ishlt.org/ishlt_99/surv_1.html#overall.
42. Hayry P: Chronic allograft vasculopathy: new strategies for drug development. Transplant Proc 30:3989, 1998.
43. Isobe M, Suzuki J: New approaches to the management of acute and chronic cardiac allograft rejection. Jpn Circ J 62:315, 1998.
44. Orbaek Andersen H: Heart allograft vascular disease: an obliterative vascular disease in transplanted hearts. Atherosclerosis 142:243, 1999.
45. United Network for Organ Sharing: UNOS critical data: number of transplants performed in 1997. Retrieved July 8, 1999, from the World Wide Web: http://www. unos. org./Newsroom/critdata_main.htm.
46. Young JB, Naftel DC, Bourge RC, et al: Matching the heart donor and heart transplant recipient. Clues for successful expansion of the donor pool: a multivariable, multiinstitutional report. The Cardiac Transplant Research Database Group. J Heart Lung Transplant 13:353, 1994.
47. Briganti EM, Bergin PJ, Rosenfeldt FL, et al: Successful long-term outcome with prolonged ischemic time cardiac allografts. J Heart Lung Transplant 14:840, 1995.
48. Cooley DA, Liotta D, Hallman GL, et al: Orthotopic cardiac prosthesis for two-staged cardiac replacement. Am J Cardiol 24:723, 1969.
49. Cooley DA, Akutsu T, Norman JC, et al: Total artificial heart in two-staged cardiac transplantation. Cardiovasc Dis Bull Tex Heart Inst 8:305, 1981.
50. Frazier OH, Cooley DA: Use of cardiac assist devices as bridges to cardiac transplantation: review of current status and report of the Texas Heart Institute's experience. *In* Unger F (ed): Assisted Circulation 3. pp. 247–259. Berlin: Springer-Verlag, 1989.
51. DeVries WC: The permanent artificial heart: four case reports. JAMA 259:849, 1988.
52. Johnson KE, Liska MB, Joyce LD, Emery RW: Use of total artificial hearts: summary of world experience, 1969–1991. ASAIO J 38:M486, 1992.
53. Hall CW, Liotta D, Henly WS, et al: Development of artificial intrathoracic circulatory pumps. Am J Surg 108:685, 1964.
54. Norman JC, Duncan JM, Frazier OH, et al: Intracorporeal (abdominal) left ventricular assist devices or partial artificial hearts: a five-year clinical experience. Arch Surg 116:1441, 1981.
55. Norman JC, Cooley DA, Kahan BD, et al: Total support of the circulation of a patient with postcardiotomy stone-heart syndrome by a partial artificial heart (ALVAD) for 5 days followed by heart and kidney transplantation. Lancet 1:1125, 1978.
56. Frazier OH, Myers TJ, Radovancevic B: The HeartMate left ventricular assist system. Overview and 12-year experience. Tex Heart Inst J 25:265, 1998.
57. McCarthy PM, Smedira NO, Vargo RL, et al: One hundred patients with the HeartMate left ventricular assist device: evolving concepts and technology. J Thorac Cardiovasc Surg 115:904, 1998.
58. Myers TJ, Dasse KA, Macris MP, et al: Use of a left ventricular assist device in an outpatient setting. ASAIO J 40:M471, 1994.
59. Myers TJ, Catanese KA, Vargo RL, et al: Extended cardiac support with a portable left ventricular assist system in the home. ASAIO J 42:M576, 1996.
60. Menconi MJ, Pockwinse S, Owen TA, et al: Properties of blood-contacting surfaces of clinically implanted cardiac assist devices: gene expression, matrix composition, and ultrastructural characterization of cellular linings. J Cell Biochem 57:557, 1995.
61. Slater JP, Rose EA, Levin HR, et al: Low thromboembolic risk without anticoagulation using advanced-design left ventricular assist devices. Ann Thorac Surg 62:1321, 1996.
62. Springer WE, Wasler A, Radovancevic B, et al: Retrospective analysis of infection in patients undergoing support with left ventricular assist systems. ASAIO J 42:M763, 1996.
63. Myers TJ, McGee MG, Zeluff B, et al: Frequency and significance of infections in patients receiving prolonged LVAD support. ASAIO Trans 37:M425, 1991.
64. Radovancevic B, Frazier OH: Implantation technique for the HeartMate left ventricular assist device. J Card Surg 7:203, 1992.
65. Frazier OH, Rose EA, McCarthy P, et al: Improved mortality and rehabilitation of transplant candidates treated with a long-term implantable left ventricular assist system. Ann Surg 222:327, 1995.
66. DeRose JJ Jr, Umana JP, Argenziano M, et al: Implantable left ventricular assist devices provide an excellent outpatient bridge to transplantation and recovery. J Am Coll Cardiol 30:1773, 1997.
67. Rose EA, Frazier OH: Resurrection after mechanical circulatory support. Circulation 96:393, 1997.
68. Frazier OH, Benedict CR, Radovancevic B, et al: Improved left ventricular function after chronic left ventricular unloading. Ann Thorac Surg 62:675, 1996.
69. Nishimura M, Radovancevic B, Odegaard P, et al: Exercise capacity recovers slowly but fully in patients with a left ventricular assist device. ASAIO J 42:M568, 1996.
70. Westaby S, Jin XY, Katsumata T, et al: Mechanical support in dilated cardiomyopathy: signs of early left ventricular recovery. Ann Thorac Surg 64:1303, 1997.
71. Scheinin SA, Capek P, Radovancevic B, et al: The effect of prolonged left ventricular support on myocardial histopathology in patients with end-stage cardiomyopathy. ASAIO J 38:M271, 1992.
72. Bick RJ, Poindexter BJ, Buja LM, et al: Improved sarcoplasmic reticulum function after mechanical left ventricular unloading. Cardiovasc Pathobiol 2:159, 1998.
73. Dilulio NA, DiPaola NR, Smedira NG, et al: Reversal of the heart failure phenotype by mechanical unloading [abstract]. J Heart Lung Transplant 18:89, 1999.
74. Ogletree-Hughes ML, Barrett-Stull L, Smedira NG, et al: Mechanical unloading restores beta-adrenergic responsiveness in the failing human heart. J Heart Lung Transplant 18:63, 1999.

75. Skolnick AA: Using ventricular assist devices as long-term therapy for heart failure. JAMA 279:1509, 1998.
76. Westaby S, Coats AJ: Mechanical bridge to myocardial recovery. Eur Heart J 19:541, 1998.
77. Westaby S, Katsumata T, Houel R, et al: Jarvik 2000 Heart: potential for bridge to myocyte recovery. Circulation 98:1568, 1998.
78. Westaby S: The need for artificial hearts. Heart 76:200, 1996.
79. Frazier OH: Surgical therapy for severe heart failure. Curr Prob Cardiol 23:721, 1998.
80. Magovern GJ: Introduction to the history and development of skeletal muscle plasticity and its clinical application to cardiomyoplasty and skeletal muscle ventricle. Semin Thorac Cardiovasc Surg 3:95, 1991.
81. Lehmann A, Faust K, Boldt J, et al: Dynamic cardiomyoplasty in patients with end-stage heart failure: anesthetic considerations. Br J Anaesth 82:140, 1999.
82. Delahaye F, Jegaden O: Cardiomyoplasty in severe heart failure: where do we stand? Eur Heart J 19:202, 1998.
83. Batista RJV, Santos JLV, Takeshita N, et al: Partial left ventriculectomy to improve left ventricular function in end-stage heart disease. J Card Surg 11:96, 1996.
84. Gorcsan J III, Feldman AM, Kormos RL, et al: Heterogeneous immediate effects of partial left ventriculectomy on cardiac performance. Circulation 97:839, 1998.
85. Konertz W, Khoynezhad A, Sidiropoulos A, et al: Early and intermediate results of left ventricular reduction surgery. Eur J Cardiothorac Surg 15(suppl 1):S26, 1999.

CHAPTER 64

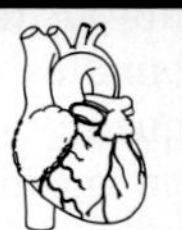

Anatomic Abnormalities

Hugh A. McAllister, Jr., L. Maximilian Buja, and Victor J. Ferrans

PERICARDIAL FLUID
PERICARDITIS
PERICARDIAL CYSTS
PERICARDIAL TUMORS
MESOTHELIAL HYPERPLASIA

The important diagnostic features of specimens from biopsy procedures or operative resections of the pericardium are (1) the overall thickness of the pericardium, (2) the presence and type of cellular infiltrates (acute or chronic inflammatory cells, granulomas, or neoplastic cells), (3) morphology of the mesothelial lining cells, (4) infective agents (including appropriate culture and staining procedures), and (5) extracellular deposits (calcium, fibrin, thrombus, or amyloid), either on the surface or within the tissue itself.

Pericardial Fluid

To correctly interpret the morphologic findings, one must know the cytologic, microbiologic, and chemical characteristics of the pericardial fluid that is removed when the tissue sample is obtained. Serous fluid can be found in patients with congestive heart failure, hypoalbuminemia, or irradiation-induced injury. Bloody fluid (hematocrit > 10 percent) can be due to cardiac surgery, penetrating or nonpenetrating injury (including the complications of cardiac catheterization), coagulopathies, overdoses of anticoagulants, complications of chemotherapy (cyclophosphamide), acute myocardial infarction, rupture of the heart or a major vessel, neoplasms, tuberculosis, or chronic renal disease (uremic pericarditis). Fluid that contains lymph or chyle can result from pericardial neoplasms or obstruction (due to neoplasm, iatrogenic injury, or other causes) of the thoracic duct, pulmonary hilum, or superior vena cava. Pericardial, pleural, and peritoneal chylous effusions also have been reported in patients with pulmonary lymphangiomyomatosis.[1] Some cases of idiopathic or primary chylopericardium have also been reported.[2] Cholesterol-rich fluid ("gold paint") is the hallmark of cholesterol pericarditis, which has been reported in patients with myxedema, rheumatoid arthritis, tuberculosis, and other conditions.[3] Purulent pericardial fluid can be caused by bacterial, fungal, or parasitic infections of the pericardium.

Pericarditis

Pericarditis can be infectious or noninfectious. The most common causes of *bacterial pericarditis* are infection with staphylococci, streptococci, pneumococci, or *Pseudomonas* species Nontuberculous infective pericarditis most often occurs as a complication of cardiothoracic surgery, disseminated infections in patients receiving immunosuppressive or antineoplastic therapy, rupture of the esophagus (as a consequence of a neoplasm) into the pericardial cavity, or infective endocarditis (associated with a septic coronary embolus or the rupture of a ring abscess or a myocardial abscess).

Tuberculous pericarditis continues to be clinically important. Four stages of this disorder have been described:

1. A fibrinous stage, which is associated with a granulomatous reaction (caseating granulomas)
2. A stage of effusion (which can be serous, serosanguineous, or bloody)
3. A stage of pericardial thickening by fibrous tissue and granulomas
4. A stage of cardiac constriction, in which the pericardial space is obliterated by fibrous adhesions

In the fourth stage, the granulomas may disappear completely and be replaced by fibrous tissue, with or without accompanying calcium deposits.[3]

A number of *parasites* have been reported to invade the pericardial cavity.[4] The most commonly encountered is *Entamoeba histolytica.* Among *fungi, Coccidioides, Actinomyces, Histoplasma,*[7] and *Candida*[8, 9] are known causes of pericarditis.

Pericarditis, usually serofibrinous but occasionally bloody, also occurs in association with *viral diseases,* including infectious mononucleosis, mumps, measles, smallpox, and influenza. Coxsackieviruses are considered the most common cause of viral pericarditis and probably account for the majority of the cases of idiopathic pericarditis.

Pericardial involvement, ranging from fibrinous exudation (Plates 64–1 and 64–2) to large, bloody effusions, occurs in collagen vascular diseases,[10] including acute rheumatic fever, rheumatoid arthritis, scleroderma, and systemic lupus erythematosus, as well as in chronic renal disease (uremic pericarditis).[11, 12] Bloody effusions also have been reported in patients with Gaucher's disease.

Fibrous thickening of the pericardium can occur with or without focal or diffuse adhesions (obliterative pericarditis) forming between the visceral and parietal pericardium (Plate 64–3). Morphologic examination reveals that the fibrous thickening results from the presence of large, coarse bundles of collagen, which often are hyalinized. Very frequently, however, the cause of the scarring is not evident on morphologic examination. Amyloid deposits can be a cause of constrictive or restrictive pericardial and myocardial disease and should be specifically sought in biopsy specimens from patients with these clinical syndromes. Chronic fibrous pericarditis also can result from the healing of hemopericardium in the presence of serosal injury, irradiation, chronic renal disease, rheumatoid arthritis, systemic lupus erythematosus, scleroderma, or infectious agents, particularly tuberculosis. In nearly all these processes, the fibrous thickening can be associated with calcium deposits (fibrocalcific pericarditis).

Pericardial thickening also can be associated with granulomatous inflammation (granulomatous pericarditis) (Plate 64–4).[4] The granulomas may be caused by infective agents (*Mycobacterium tuberculosis,* fungi, or parasites), cholesterol, talc or starch (particularly in patients undergoing thoracic surgical procedures), rheumatoid arthritis (in which they bear a resemblance to rheumatoid nodules), and sarcoidosis (Figs. 64–1 and 64–2).[13] Examination of tissue sections by polarized light microscopy can be helpful in the identification of deposits of cholesterol, talc, and starch. Healed granulomas also can undergo considerable degrees of calcification.

Obliterative and fibrocalcific pericarditis may be associated with the clinical syndromes of subacute pericarditis and chronic constrictive pericarditis. The latter condition is more often idiopathic than tuberculous in origin.

Pericardial Cysts

Although most pericardial cysts are attached to the parietal pericardium along the border of the right side of the heart, usually at the right costophrenic angle, approximately 25 percent are present along the border of the left side of the heart. Eight percent project into the posterior or anterior superior mediastinum.[14, 15] The cysts range in diameter from 1 to 15 cm or larger. They commonly appear multilocular

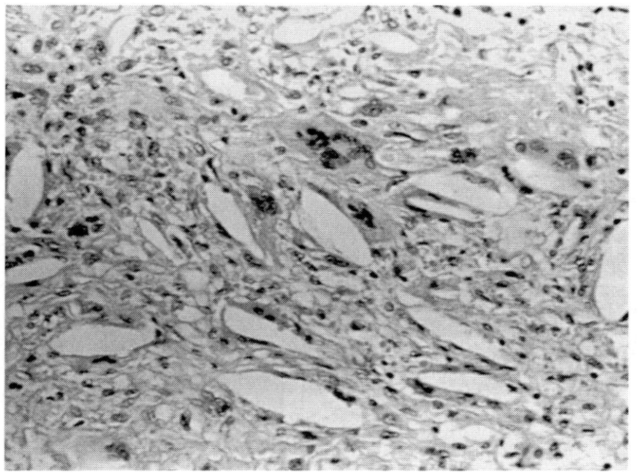

Figure 64–1 Cholesterol pericarditis. Note the "cholesterol clefts," many of which have contiguous foreign body–type giant cells. (H&E, ×250.)

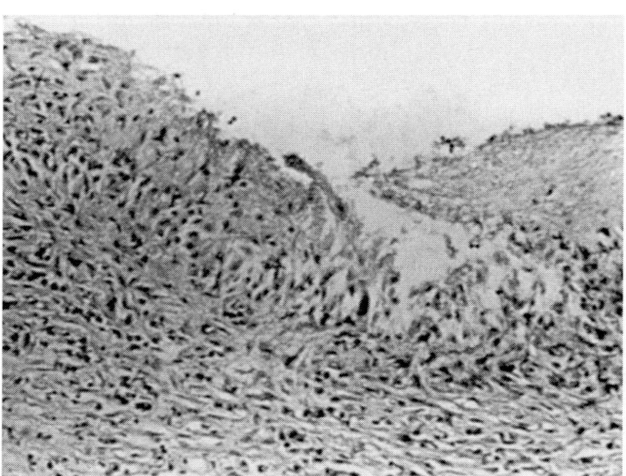

Figure 64–2 Rheumatoid pericarditis. Although any portion of the heart may be involved in patients with rheumatoid arthritis, the pericardium is the most common. Note that the fibrous thickening of the pericardium contains a microscopic lesion with palisading histiocytes and central necrobiosis suggestive of a rheumatoid granuloma. (H&E, ×250.)

externally; however, although the cyst lining is occasionally trabeculated, most cysts are unilocular. They contain clear yellow fluid and occasionally communicate with the pericardial sac. The wall of the cyst is composed mainly of collagen with scattered elastic fibers and is lined by mesothelial cells. Although these mesothelial cells usually form a single layer, foci or hyperplastic mesothelial cells are occasionally encountered. Rarely, foci of calcification and accumulations of lymphocytes and plasma cells are present.

The pericardial cyst and the pericardial diverticulum are microscopically similar, and both probably originate as persistent, blind-ending parietal pericardial recesses.

Pericardial cysts may be detected in patients from childhood to old age, although the majority are discovered during the third or fourth decade of life. Some tumors of the pericardium, such as lipoma, hemangioma, or lymphangioma, may simulate the clinical and radiologic picture of pericardial cysts.[14, 15] Ultrasonic diagnosis and computed tomography may be helpful in the differentiation of pericardial cysts from solid tumors of the pericardium.

Pericardial Tumors

The pericardium is involved much more frequently with metastatic neoplasms than with primary neoplasms, and carcinomatous invasion is more common than sarcomatous invasion. The most common primary malignant tumor of the pericardium is mesothelioma. The majority of pericardial mesotheliomas diffusely cover the parietal and visceral pericardium, encasing the heart. Solitary or localized pericardial mesotheliomas are distinctly rare. Histologically, localized mesotheliomas are identical to diffuse mesotheliomas and may be of the epithelioid or fibrous type.[14, 16]

Microscopically, mesotheliomas are characterized by cellular regularity and histologic variability. They consist of either tubules or solid cords of malignant cells (in a tubular or tubulopapillary pattern) or of spindle-shaped cells with a connective tissue stroma (fibrous pattern). Frequently, both patterns are present in the same tumor. In either histologic pattern, the cells usually are strikingly regular in appearance, and the nuclei most frequently are large, rounded, and vesicular, with prominent nucleoli. Cellular pleomorphism and anaplasia are unusual, and atypical mitoses are rare, although multinucleated cells and occasional mitoses may be seen. Fibrous or mixed fibrous and epithelioid mesotheliomas predominate in the pericardium, as in the pleura.

Mesotheliomas, whether nodular or sheetlike, only superficially invade contiguous structures, including the heart. This is an important differential diagnostic point, in that other primary cardiac sarcomas, most notably angiosarcomas, can diffusely involve the pericardium but almost invariably have a significant intramyocardial or intracavitary component.[14, 16]

Pericardial mesotheliomas frequently spread to the adjacent pleura and mediastinum and may involve the mediastinal lymph nodes. Occasionally, pericardial mesotheliomas spread through the diaphragm and involve the peritoneum. Distant metastases are extremely unusual.[14]

Mesothelial Hyperplasia

Mesothelial hyperplasia may be focal or diffuse and is found most frequently in patients with underlying heart disease (i.e., chronic pericarditis or rheumatic heart disease). The mesothelial cells may form tumor-like masses within the pericardial space. More frequently, mesothelial hyperplasia is diffuse along the parietal or visceral pericardium. Reactive mesothelial cells are multilayered, and nests of mesothelial cells often lie within the pericardial stroma. Again, the cells are remarkably uniform in appearance, with minimal pleomorphism. Mitoses may be seen.[14] Differential special staining of mesothelial cells and carcinoma cells, together with the clinical history, should distinguish mesothelial hyperplasia from metastatic carcinoma involving the pericardium.

Mesothelial hyperplasia may be a complication of treatment with radiotherapy for patients with carcinoma, or it may develop secondary to the pericarditis that sometimes follows the spread of carcinoma to the pericardium. Thus, because of the known coexistence of the two conditions, the diagnosis of metastatic carcinoma involving the pericardium is not excluded by the finding of mesothelial hyperplasia alone.[14]

References

1. Taylor JR, Ruy J, Colby TV, et al: Lymphangioleiomyomatosis: clinical course in 32 patients. N Engl J Med 323:1254–1260, 1990.
2. Ferrans VJ, Roberts WC: Pathology of pericardial effusion. *In* Reddy PS, Leon DF, Shaver JA (eds): Pericardial Disease. p. 77. New York: Raven, 1982.
3. Roberts WC, Ferrans VJ: A survey of the causes and consequences of pericardial heart disease. *In* Reddy PS, Leon DF, Shaver JA (eds): Pericardial Diseases. p. 49. New York: Raven, 1982.
4. McAllister HA Jr, Ferrans VJ: Granulomas of the heart and major blood vessels. *In* Ioachim HL (ed): Pathology of Granulomas. p. 75. New York: Raven, 1982.
5. Reingold JM: Myocardial lesions in disseminated coccidiomycosis. Am J Clin Pathol 20:1044, 1950.
6. Kasper JA, Pinner M: Actinomycosis of heart: report of case with actinomycotic emboli. Arch Pathol 10:687, 1930.
7. Crawford SE, Crook WF, Harrison WW, Somervill B: Histoplasmosis as a cause of acute myocarditis and pericarditis. Pediatrics 28:92, 1961.
8. McAllister HA Jr, Mullick FG: The cardiovascular system. *In* Riddell R (ed): Pathology of Drug Induced and Toxic Diseases. p. 201. New York: Churchill Livingstone, 1982.
9. Parker JC Jr: The potentially lethal problem of cardiac candidosis. Am J Clin Pathol 73:356, 1980.
10. McAllister HA Jr: Collagen diseases and the cardiovascular system. *In* Silver MD (ed): Cardiovascular Pathology. p. 1151. New York: Churchill Livingstone, 1991.
11. Buja LM, Friedman CA, Roberts WC: Hemorrhagic pericarditis in uremia. Arch Pathol 90:325, 1970.
12. McAllister HA Jr: Pathology of the cardiovascular system in chronic renal failure. *In* Laventhol DT, Pennock RL, Likoff W, et al (eds): Management of Cardiovascular Disease in Renal Failure. p. 1. Philadelphia: FA Davis, 1981.
13. Roberts WC, McAllister HA Jr, Ferrans VJ: Sarcoidosis of the heart: a clinicopathologic study of 35 necropsy patients (group I) and review of 78 previously described necropsy patients (group II). Am J Med 63:86, 1977.
14. McAllister HA Jr, Fenogho JJ Jr: Tumors of the Cardiovascular System: Atlas of Tumor Pathology, Second Series, Fascicle 15. Washington, DC: Armed Forces Institute of Pathology, 1974.
15. Feigin DS, Fenogho JJ, McAllister HA Jr, Madewell JE: Pericardial cysts: a radiologic-pathologic correlation and review. Radiology 125:15, 1977.
16. McAllister HA Jr: Tumors of the heart and blood vessels. *In* Silver MD (ed): Cardiovascular Pathology. p. 1297. New York: Churchill Livingstone, 1991.

CHAPTER **65**

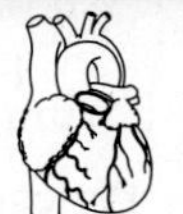

ETIOLOGY, PATHOPHYSIOLOGY, CLINICAL RECOGNITION, AND TREATMENT

Ralph Shabetai

GENERAL CONSIDERATIONS
ETIOLOGY
Idiopathic Pericardial Disease
Viral Infections
Bacterial Infections
Other Infections
Degenerative Disease
Trauma
Radiation
Neoplasia
Metabolic Disorders
Collagen Vascular and Immune Disorders
Myocardial Infarction
Drug-Induced Pericardial Disease
Chylopericardium
PATHOPHYSIOLOGY, CLINICAL RECOGNITION, AND TREATMENT
Pericardial Effusion
Chronic Effusive Pericarditis
Cardiac Tamponade
Constrictive Pericarditis
Acute Pericarditis
Recurrent Pericarditis

GENERAL CONSIDERATIONS

Pericardial heart disease is much less common than hypertensive heart disease or than heart disease originating from primary disorders of the coronary arteries, the myocardium, or the cardiac valves. On the other hand, the pericardium can become involved in a far greater number of systemic diseases than affect the myocardium; furthermore, diseases that may affect both myocardium and pericardium almost always affect the latter more often than the former. In many disorders, such as AIDS and myocardial infarction, pericardial involvement is often occult and therefore not detected unless specifically sought—usually through the use of echocardiography. In other instances, because the pericardium may be the source of pain resembling myocardial ischemia or of dyspnea and edema resembling heart failure, it may come to dominate the clinical picture of a widespread systemic disorder. It is a small wonder, then, that the diagnosis of pericardial disease is often missed, and when it is diagnosed, it is only after other, incorrect diagnoses have been made. Examples include the incorrect diagnosis of hepatic cirrhosis when the correct diagnosis is constrictive pericarditis, heart failure when the correct diagnosis is constrictive pericarditis, cardiomegaly when the correct diagnosis is pericardial effusion, and pulmonary embolism or acute myocardial infarction when the correct diagnosis is acute pericarditis. Confusion between restrictive cardiomyopathy and constrictive pericarditis occurs in many patients who have either of these two disorders.

When a patient with constrictive pericarditis is treated for nonexistent cirrhosis, restrictive cardiomyopathy, tricuspid valve disease, or heart failure, the opportunity to relieve symptoms and prevent complications and death is delayed or lost forever. Cardiac tamponade, as a complication of cardiac surgery,[1] is an important cause of postoperative death because it is not recognized or is thought of too late. All too often, the case of a patient in whom the possibility of cardiac tamponade is not thought of until late in the course of cardiopulmonary resuscitation or in whom cardiac tamponade is not discovered until postmortem examination ends up in a court of law. The thread that connects these seemingly disparate medical misadventures is that pericardial heart disease, being so much less common than other forms of heart disease, is often not considered until late in the patient's course or is omitted altogether from the differential diagnosis. The key to successful recognition and management, therefore, lies in a high index of suspicion; when cardiovascular and hemodynamic abnormalities, particularly edema, dyspnea, chest pain, and cardiomegaly, are not readily explained, the possibility of pericarditis or cardiac tamponade must be included in the differential diagnosis. This consideration usually means that appropriate tests should be performed to establish or exclude the diagnosis of pericardial disease. This consideration may sound trite, but if all of the physicians who treat patients recognized and adhered to the need for a high index of suspicion of pericardial disease, much of the remainder of this chapter would be redundant. Thus far, we have not advanced to the point at which Sir William Osler's[2] statements no longer apply:

> Even with copious effusions, the onset and course may be so insidious that no suspicion of the true nature of the disease is aroused.
>
> Probably no serious disease is so frequently overlooked by the practitioner. Postmortem experience

shows how often pericarditis is not recognized, or goes on to resolution and adhesion without attracting notice.

Pericardial heart disease and pericardial disease present a number of highly distinctive clinical syndromes. What is meant by the term *pericardial heart disease* is an abnormality of the heart and circulation secondary to an abnormality of the pericardium, whereas *pericardial disease* is disease limited to the pericardium that does not exert any cardiovascular manifestations. The major entities include pericardial effusion, cardiac tamponade, constrictive pericarditis, and acute fibrinous pericarditis including recurrent pericarditis. These clinical entities do not bear a strong relationship to cause because many forms of pericarditis and pericardiopathy may be associated with effusion, and effusion of any cause may progress to cardiac tamponade. Furthermore, although progression to constrictive pericarditis is uncommon in some causes of pericardial disorder, examples of constrictive pericarditis have been reported after pericardial disease of almost every known cause.

ETIOLOGY

Because of the large number of systemic disorders that may involve the pericardium, it should not come as a surprise that the list of possible causes is quite formidable. The clinician can best deal with this problem through two approaches:

1. Separate the common from the unusual and rare causes of pericardial disease.
2. Use the time-honored classification of disease into the categories of congenital, inflammatory, degenerative, neoplastic, traumatic, collagen vascular, allergic, metabolic, and drug induced.

Some causes are more commonly associated with particular clinical syndromes of acute pericarditis, or pericardial effusion, or constrictive pericarditis; however, there is considerable overlap. It is preferable to deal with the general topic of cause before a discussion of specific syndromes is undertaken. Causes commonly associated with particular syndromes of pericardial disease and pericardial heart disease are considered in subsequent chapter sections.

Idiopathic Pericardial Disease

Despite complete clinical and laboratory investigation, many cases of pericardial disease remain idiopathic. It is generally believed that a significant number of cases of idiopathic acute pericarditis are secondary to an undetected viral infection. The same consideration applies to a lesser percentage of cases with large pericardial effusion. In the instance of constrictive pericarditis, in which many cases unfortunately must still be considered idiopathic, a number are probably related to unrecognized prior tuberculosis or other infection or to remote trauma. The syndrome of effusive-constrictive pericarditis is often associated with tuberculous pericarditis. This syndrome may also occur in neoplastic pericardial disease after mediastinal radiation and in idiopathic and viral pericarditis.

Viral Infections

Infections constitute an important cause of pericarditis. Viral infection, for the most part, causes an illness indistinguishable from acute idiopathic pericarditis. The major offenders include coxsackievirus A, coxsackievirus B, and echovirus; less common offenders are adenovirus, mumps virus, infectious mononucleosis, hepatitis B, and varicella. Influenza A is an important pathogen in the acute pericarditis of infants and children. Lymphogranuloma venereum and *Mycoplasma pneumoniae* have been reported as causes of acute pericarditis.

Of particular importance in the present era is pericarditis associated with AIDS.[3] These pericarditides are usually caused by commensal infection with such organisms as avian tubercle bacillus and *Mycobacterium tuberculosis*, but hybridization studies have proved that the AIDS virus itself can infect the pericardium.

Bacterial Infections

Bacterial infections are an important cause of purulent pericarditis.[4] As with so many other bacterial infections, the clinical spectrum has changed as a consequence of the widespread use of potent antibiotics and, to a lesser extent, of immunosuppressive agents. Thus, *Pneumococcus* and *Streptococcus*, which in the past were frequent causes of acute pericarditis, often with a fatal resolution, are less common, having been replaced to some extent by such organisms as coagulase-positive staphylococci.[5] Pneumococcal pericarditis secondary to empyema, which continues to have a high mortality rate, remains an important cause of purulent pericarditis and is due, at least in part, to late recognition. Other bacterial infections include meningococci, *Haemophilus influenzae*, and *Legionella pneumophila*. Pericarditis can occur in the course of psittacosis. Even salmonella infection can involve the pericardium. Tuberculosis, which was in the past a most important and quite frequent cause of pericarditis, remains important but occurs much less frequently in developed countries; however, with the incidence of tuberculosis on the rise and the greater prevalence of drug-resistant infection,[6] this fortunate circumstance may not endure.

Other Infections

Pericarditis may occur as a result of fungal infection—notably, histoplasmosis, blastomycosis, coccidioidomycosis, and *Candida albicans*. Aspergillosis and rickettsial pericarditis have been well described. The pericardium may be infected in toxoplasmosis, amebiasis, *Mycoplasma*, *Nocardia*, actinomycosis, echinococcosis, and Lyme disease.[7]

Degenerative Disease

An example of a degenerative disease of the pericardium is amyloidosis.

Trauma

A very important cause of pericardial disease is trauma; examples include blunt[8] and sharp chest trauma, as well as a number of iatrogenic causes, including surgical pericardiotomy,[9] transseptal cardiac catheterization, intramyocardial contrast injection, perforation from a pacing[10] or central[11, 12] venous catheter, implantation of epicardial and defibrillating devices, and electric cardioversion.[13]

Radiation

An important example of the cause of noninfectious acute and chronic inflammation is radiation.[14, 15]

Neoplasia

The pericardium is frequently involved in neoplastic disease.[16–19] Primary tumors are uncommon, but the most common primary tumor is mesothelioma. Less common are teratoma, fibroma, lipoma, angioma, and leiomyofibroma. Metastatic neoplasm involving the pericardium is an important and quite frequent problem encountered in the practice of internal medicine. The major primary sources are carcinoma of the lung and carcinoma of the breast; also of extreme importance are lymphoma and leukemia.

Metabolic Disorders

Of the metabolic causes of pericardial disease, pericarditis associated with chronic renal disease[20, 21] is the most common. Usually, this refers to pericarditis associated with chronic dialysis, but a few cases associated with severe uremia are still encountered. Effusive pericarditis in patients with myxedema is a less frequent metabolic example of pericarditis.

Collagen Vascular and Immune Disorders

The autoimmune disorders quite frequently involve the pericardium.[22, 23] Acute pericarditis is a feature of acute rheumatic carditis. Pericarditis with or without effusion, and sometimes progressing to constrictive pericarditis, may be found in lupus erythematosus, rheumatoid arthritis, scleroderma, mixed connective tissue disease, Wegener's granulomatosis, polyarteritis nodosa, dermatomyositis, and vasculitis.

Myocardial Infarction

Pericarditis, with or without effusion,[24, 25] may occur in the course of acute myocardial infarction[26] in the form of either acute contiguous pericarditis or delayed pericardial effusion (i.e., Dressler's syndrome), which is, along with the postpericardiotomy syndrome and traumatic pericardial disease, an example of the postpericardial injury syndrome.[27, 28]

Drug-Induced Pericardial Disease

Anticoagulant drugs may cause or facilitate the appearance of pericarditis, usually hemorrhagic. Other drug-induced pericarditides can occur with the use of such agents as procainamide, hydralazine, methysergide, isoniazid, doxorubicin, and diphenylhydantoin.

Chylopericardium

Chylopericardium may be idiopathic[29] but more commonly is traumatic or arises as a complication of thoracic surgery[30] in which the thoracic duct or one of its tributaries is injured. Chylopericardium may complicate cardiac transplantation.[31] Chylopericardium should not be confused with *cholesterol pericarditis*, a complication of chronic pericarditis with or without effusion in which cholesterol crystals are deposited in the pericardial tissue and fluid. In this condition, the fluid is not milky but has an exceedingly high cholesterol content.

Pathophysiology, Clinical Recognition, and Treatment

Pericardial Effusion

Pericardial effusion may be small or large, hemodynamically benign or life threatening, and transudative, exudative, sanguinous, or chylous. Pericardial effusion may develop from what in the classic literature, written before the era of echocardiography, was described as dry or fibrinous pericarditis. The clinician's approach to pericardial effusion should be a logical progression from recognition of its presence to determination of the cause and its hemodynamic significance to appropriate treatment.

Recognition of Pericardial Effusion

Pericardial effusion must first be suspected, after which its presence or absence must be definitely established. Pericardial effusion is suspected when a patient has one of the diseases that may be associated with pericardial involvement or when a finding, such as the appearance of a pericardial friction rub or unexpected radiographic cardiomegaly, alerts the physician to the possibility of a pericardial effusion. In some instances, the patient is known or found to have a disease that can affect the pericardium, and a search for pericardial involvement is instituted. In other cases, the patient is found to have evidence of pericarditis, and the attending systemic disease is discovered during the course of a search for the cause of pericarditis. Usually, once pericardial effusion is suspected, its presence is definitively documented through echocardiography, which unquestionably is the most common as well as the most reliable means of establishing the presence of a pericardial effusion (Fig. 65–1).

Physical Examination

Older textbooks have emphasized physical findings, such as the ability to percuss cardiac dullness beyond the cardiac

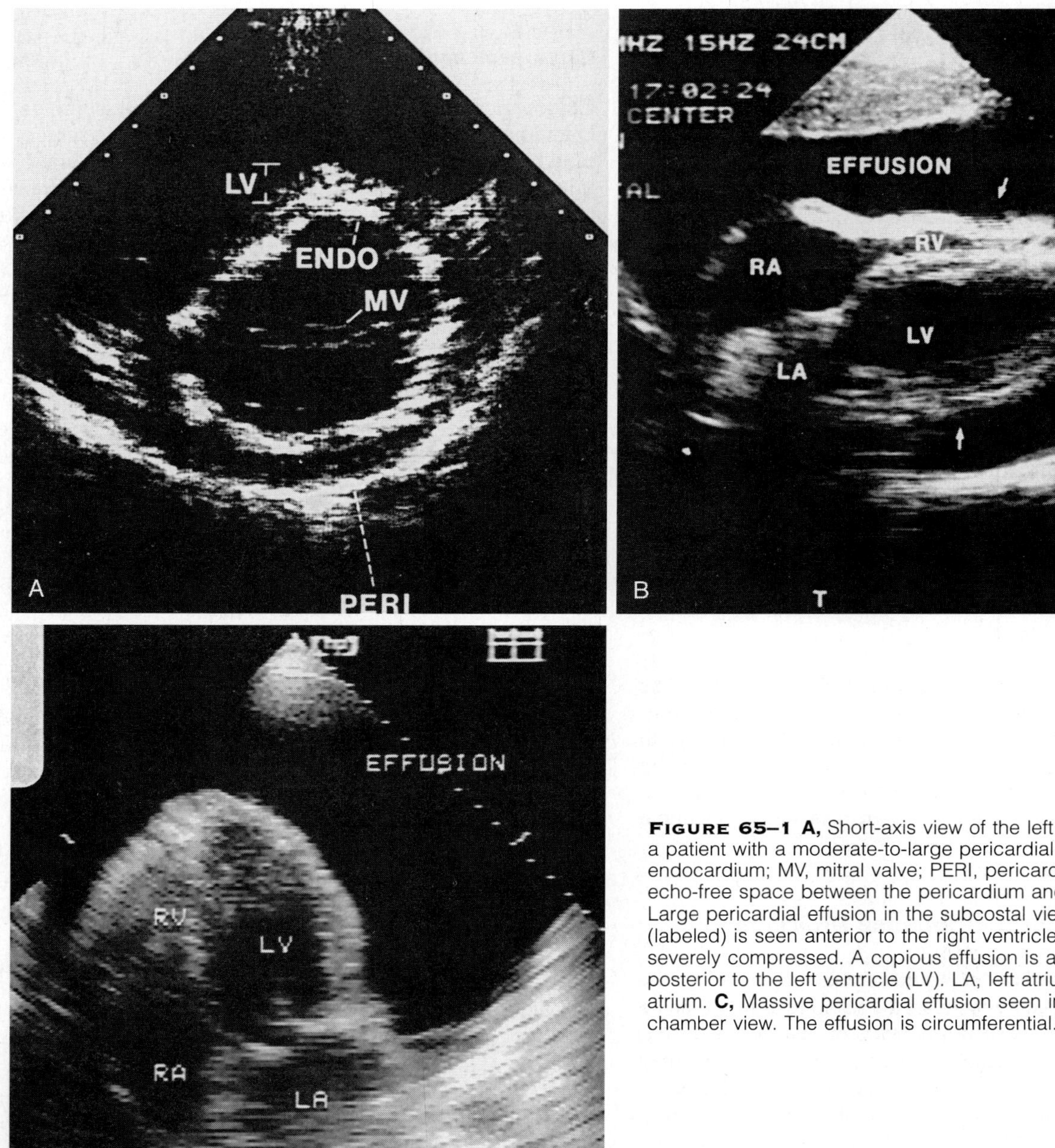

FIGURE 65–1 **A,** Short-axis view of the left ventricle (LV) in a patient with a moderate-to-large pericardial effusion. ENDO, endocardium; MV, mitral valve; PERI, pericardium. Note the echo-free space between the pericardium and the heart. **B,** Large pericardial effusion in the subcostal view. The effusion (labeled) is seen anterior to the right ventricle (RV), which is severely compressed. A copious effusion is also visible posterior to the left ventricle (LV). LA, left atrium; RA, right atrium. **C,** Massive pericardial effusion seen in the four-chamber view. The effusion is circumferential.

apex and a dullness in Ewing triangle, but these signs are so unreliable and so seldom sought that they are virtually worthless.

Laboratory Examination

CHEST RADIOGRAPHY

The unexpected development of cardiomegaly on the chest radiogram of a patient in whom prior chest radiograms showed a normal-sized heart can be strong evidence of the probability of a pericardial effusion, especially if the heart is somewhat flask shaped and if the lung fields are clearer than would have been anticipated with cardiomegaly due to heart failure. In this connection, however, it should be mentioned that severe heart failure complicated by tricuspid regurgitation may show massive cardiomegaly with clear lung fields. The explanation for this phenomenon is that blood that would have congested the lungs regurgitates into the systemic circulation. Massive cardiomegaly may occur in large volume-overload situations of the heart, such as severe aortic regurgitation or mitral regurgitation. When these abnormal loading conditions of the heart are present without heart failure, the heart appears large on the chest radiogram but the lungs remain clear, or relatively so.

In a minority of cases, the lucency created by subepicardial fat separates the cardiac from the pericardial density, thereby betraying the true nature of apparent cardiomegaly.

SCINTIGRAPHY

When the heart is imaged, for instance, for a radionuclide ventriculogram, the scintigram shows a clear zone of pericardial effusion, separating the radioactivity in the heart from that in the liver.

Any of these circumstances, together with any reasonable suspicion that a pericardial effusion may be present, particularly if it is thought that the effusion may be of clinical importance, should lead to echocardiography, which will reveal the presence or absence of pericardial effusion with a sensitivity and specificity rarely achieved with any test used in clinical practice.

ECHOCARDIOGRAPHY

Echocardiography is, without doubt, the best tool for establishing the presence of pericardial effusion. Not only can the presence or absence of pericardial effusion be established with remarkable certainty,[32] but in addition, one can make a reliable estimate as to whether the effusion is trivial, small, medium, large, or massive. More precise quantification is, for clinical purposes, not possible, nor is it needed. Beyond providing a good estimate of the size of a pericardial effusion, the study can identify whether it is likely that cardiac tamponade is present and, if so, whether it is mild, moderate, or severe. Evidence strongly supporting cardiac tamponade includes an inspiratory increase in the right ventricular area with a parallel decrease in the left ventricular area and compression of the right atrial border such that its normal convexity is reversed and the chamber appears to have a concave outer wall. Collapse of the right ventricle in early diastole is another indication that cardiac tamponade may be present. Furthermore, the longer into diastole that this collapse can be seen, the more severe the tamponade is likely to be. A number of lesser signs of cardiac tamponade can be identified echocardiographically, but these are discussed in the section on cardiac tamponade. Most pericardial effusions surround the heart, but echocardiography may show that the pericardial effusion is localized. Localized pericardial effusion is particularly common after cardiac surgery. When pericardial effusion begins to organize with the deposition of fibrin, this change is often recognizable by the appearance of opacities within the pericardial fluid image.[33] Smaller pericardial effusions may not be visible behind the left atrium; the large effusions are seen here well, as they are around the remainder of the heart.

Pericardial effusion is imaged as an echo lucent region surrounding the heart and separating the echo dense epicardium from the echo dense mediastinal structures. Experienced echocardiographers do not encounter difficulties in the differential diagnosis of pericardial effusion from pleural effusion, excessive epicardial fat, a giant left atrium, cysts, tumors, and diaphragmatic hernia. Pleural effusion lies posterior to the descending aorta, whereas in patients with combined pleural and pericardial effusion, echo-free spaces are seen both behind the back of the left ventricle and descending aorta and behind the ascending aorta. Care must be taken to distinguish between pericardial fluid behind the left atrium and a left pleural effusion. Almost all of these potential difficulties were significant when echocardiography was limited to the M-mode technique but have largely been resolved by two-dimensional echocardiography. With a particularly large pericardial effusion, the heart demonstrates a rocking or pendular motion within the motionless pericardial space.[34] This finding appears to be more common with malignant pericardial effusion and has also been associated with cardiac tamponade. On the electrocardiogram, this pendular motion may be reflected as electric alternans.

Doppler interrogation often shows increased respiratory variation in the velocity of inflow through the mitral and tricuspid valves and the velocity of ejection through the aortic and pulmonary valves. With the advent of cardiac tamponade, this finding becomes even more marked.

The extent of the echocardiographic or echocardiographic Doppler examination should be tailored to the clinical need. In some patients, a brief examination to document whether pericardial effusion is present and in roughly what amount may be all that is required, whereas in others, as for example when the diagnosis of cardiac tamponade is suspected, a comprehensive echocardiographic Doppler examination should be performed and should include imaging of the inferior vena cava and hepatic veins that are distended and, when the venous pressure is greatly elevated, fail to show the decrease in dimension during inspiration or with a sniff.

Extremely useful information may accrue when radiographic cardiomegaly is further investigated through echocardiography. In the case of an uncomplicated pericardial effusion, the examination will document the presence and extent of pericardial effusion and will quickly identify whether all cardiac chambers are of a normal size and exhibit normal systolic and diastolic function. When pericardial effusion occurs in the presence of dilated heart failure, the contribution of each can be assessed by judging the size of the pericardial effusion and the extent of hypokinesis and the dimensions of the cardiac chambers. The examination, in such cases, would not be expected to show significant regional wall motion abnormalities or evidence of valvular heart disease. In the case of cardiac tamponade with severe compression of the heart, left ventricular wall thickness may appear to be abnormally increased, but in reality, the apparent increase is merely a reflection of the reduction in cardiac volume.

Echocardiography may demonstrate clinically unsuspected pericardial effusion. Serial echocardiography in pregnant women has shown that a benign pericardial effusion is not uncommon in normal pregnancy.[35] Likewise, serial echocardiography after acute myocardial infarction will reveal pericardial effusion in a number of patients without pericardial friction rub or other evidence of pericarditis. In patients with AIDS,[36] pericardial effusion can be found even in patients with no cardiovascular complaints, or as a further complication in those who develop dilated heart failure. At autopsy, congestive heart failure is considered the leading cause of pericardial effusion, but clinically, this finding is distinctly uncommon. Innumerable patients have been entered into heart failure studies in which serial echocardiography is used, yet pericardial effusions are rarely encountered.

PERICARDIOSCOPY

Pericardioscopy allows the operator to view the epicardium and to select the loci for biopsy.[37] Both rigid instruments and fiberoptic instruments have been used—the former in the operating room.

Etiology

All of the causes of pericarditis may cause pericardial effusion. In the practice of internal medicine, the more common causes are bronchogenic carcinoma, mammary carcinoma, lymphoma, idiopathic pericarditis, dialysis-related pericarditis, and collagen vascular disease. In the setting of the emergency department, common causes include sharp trauma, as occurs with bullets and sharp instruments, and blunt trauma,[38] as is often inflicted by the steering wheel in a motor vehicle accident. Rupture of an aortic aneurysm or a dissecting hematoma of the aorta into the pericardial space is often first encountered in the emergency department. Rupture of the myocardial infarction is more likely to be encountered in the coronary care unit because this event usually occurs around the third day after acute infarction. Strictly speaking, these massive hemorrhages into the pericardium are not effusions, but they have the same pathophysiology and are potent causes of cardiac tamponade. In surgical practice, cardiac tamponade is an ever present danger after cardiac surgery. This complication, which is reviewed in detail,[39] usually occurs when the patient is still in the surgical intensive care unit or even in the recovery room, but can be delayed and may not develop until after the patient has been sent to a regular surgical ward or even discharged home.[40] A high index of suspicion that cardiac tamponade may be present is mandatory in any postoperative cardiac patient with unexplained dyspnea, cardiomegaly, increased jugular venous pressure, or other evidence of hemodynamic compromise.

When the common causes of pericardial effusion have been ruled out, a detailed history and extensive physical examination, with the latter often repeated as the patient is observed for days or weeks, should be carried out to identify one of the systemic disorders that can be associated with pericardial disease. In practically all patients, tests should include routine blood chemistry, erythrocyte sedimentation rate or C-reactive protein, viral titers, and a tuberculin skin test. A screen of the plasma proteins, including rheumatoid factor and antinuclear antibodies, is performed in many patients, particularly those with arthralgia or other evidence suggesting collagen vascular disease or vasculitis. Suggestive abnormality of the blood count should be followed up for the possibility of leukemia or lymphoma. In older patients, neoplasm, especially of the breast or lung, must be carefully considered, and it must be recalled that many other neoplasms can metastasize to the mediastinum, including the pericardium. Pericardial effusion is common in severe myxedema but is much less common in mild hypothyroidism, as commonly diagnosed.[41] No simple rule of thumb regarding the extent of investigation for neoplasm can be provided here; that would depend on the individual clinical circumstances. Although at first the task of making a correct etiologic diagnosis appears daunting, in many instances it is straightforward. For example, a previously healthy young person with a short history of malaise followed by chest pain and the discovery of a pericardial effusion probably has idiopathic or viral pericarditis. An elderly patient with an abnormal opacity in the lung field probably has malignant pericardial effusion, secondary to carcinoma of the lung. A young adult with splenomegaly, fever, and enlarged lymph nodes, especially mediastinal nodes, is liable to have pericardial effusion from lymphoma. Dermatologic, muscular, and articular abnormalities may quickly lead to the diagnosis of rheumatoid or lupus pericardial disease.

EXAMINATION OF PERICARDIAL FLUID AND TISSUE

When exhaustive and appropriate laboratory evaluations have failed to disclose the cause of pericardial effusion, the question often arises of whether a diagnostic pericardial tap or pericardial biopsy should then be undertaken. It should be remembered that the so-called diagnostic pericardial tap or pericardiocentesis has a remarkably low diagnostic yield, whereas the so-called therapeutic tap, which is usually performed for the relief of cardiac tamponade or because the clinician strongly suspects the presence of pus in the pericardium, has a high diagnostic yield.[42] In the former category, malignant cells often lead to the diagnosis of neoplastic pericardial effusion, and in the latter category, the suspected pus is often found. Thus, in the absence of a therapeutic need to drain the pericardium and when the clinician does not suspect pus in the pericardium, pericardiocentesis or surgical pericardial drainage should be delayed[43] or not performed. It is usually futile to seek the cause of a pericardial effusion in a patient with normal venous pressure and no symptoms or signs of infection.

However, some recommend that a pericardial effusion that persists unchanged or increases after 3 weeks merits a diagnostic tap, and if this tap does not prove to be of diagnostic value, pericardial biopsy is suggested. The decision of whether to perform these low-yield and slightly hazardous procedures rests to some extent on whether the circumstances permit close long-term follow-up. If the patient can be observed at appropriate intervals with careful determination of the jugular venous pressure, chest radiograph, and echocardiogram and with renewed efforts to uncover an underlying disorder, invasive procedures can be delayed or avoided altogether.

Chronic Effusive Pericarditis

Periodically, patients present with a moderate or large pericardial effusion, normal jugular venous and systemic arterial blood pressures, and the absence of pulsus paradoxus or echocardiographic signs of cardiac tamponade. Such patients are often asymptomatic or may have symptoms related to some other disorder. When an extensive investigation fails to uncover the cause of pericardial effusion and effusion persists in varying amounts for months or years, the patient may be considered to have chronic effusive pericarditis.[44] Many recommend that pericardiectomy be performed,[45] which certainly abolishes the chronic pericardial effusion, but whether the patient is rewarded with the relief of previously unnoticed symptoms or with increased exercise tolerance is a moot point. On the other hand, even after several years, an etiologic diagnosis, such as tuberculosis, may be established in a small proportion of such patients. In my practice, when these patients are entirely asymptomatic and can demonstrate good exercise tolerance, I do not recommend pericardiectomy provided good and regular follow-up can be ensured. If they cannot, pericardiectomy, which is a safe operation under these circumstances, should be recommended.

Purulent pericarditis and cardiac tamponade are considered in more detail later.

Cardiac Tamponade

Cardiac tamponade is best defined as the compression of the heart by pericardial fluid under increased pressure. As such, until the end-stage, it is a disorder of impaired venous return and impedance to diastolic filling of the ventricles. Clinically, this definition translates into central venous, atrial, and ventricular diastolic pressures governed not by their normal determinants but rather by the intrapericardial pressure. When intrapericardial pressure is measured in a patient after pericardiocentesis or in an animal in which the physiologic pericardial effusion has not been aspirated, the pressure is a few millimeters of mercury less than the venous and atrial pressures, being slightly subatmospheric. When effusion or blood (or air) accumulates in sufficient quantity and at sufficient speed in the pericardial space, intrapericardial pressure rises, soon equaling the right atrial and central systemic venous pressures. At this stage, cardiac tamponade can be considered to have begun, but there may well be no symptoms or abnormal physical findings. In such a situation, the right atrial and intrapericardial pressures may have equilibrated at 4 or 5 mm Hg. If further fluid accumulation occurs, intrapericardial pressure rises further,[46] with the degree of increase being highly dependent on the rate of further effusion or bleeding. At this point, right atrial and pericardial pressures may have risen to approximately 8 to 10 mm Hg. The patient may continue to be asymptomatic and the blood pressure and pulse remain normal, but abnormal elevation of the jugular venous pressure is apparent on the bedside examination. By this time, cardiomegaly is usually apparent on the chest radiogram unless the fluid collection was hyperacute.

When the intrapericardial pressure rises to exceed the preexisting left atrial and pulmonary wedge pressures, pericardial and right and left atrial pressures become equal to each other and to diastolic pressures in the ventricles and the pulmonary artery. Moderately severe classic cardiac tamponade is present, with the pressures equilibrated at approximately 10 mm Hg. Before the full spectrum of cardiac tamponade had been appreciated by clinicians, the diagnosis of cardiac tamponade was seldom, if ever, made before this stage had appeared.

In severe tamponade, the intrapericardial pressure rises to or exceeds approximately 15 mm Hg with a corresponding increase in the venous pressures on both sides of the circulation. In this situation, pulsus paradoxus is likely to appear, and there may be a significant, but not profound, drop in systemic arterial pressure. Dyspnea and fatigue may appear, indicating some decrease in cardiac output. For the most severe cardiac tamponade, pericardial and intracardiac pressures may increase to 20 mm Hg or even higher. When this degree of tamponade has developed, severe decompensation occurs with a profound drop in arterial pressure and a major decrease in cardiac output with dyspnea, chest discomfort, and decreased renal function.

Physical Examination

The key physical finding is the jugular venous pressure. When this pressure remains normal and there is no reason, such as major hemorrhage, for profound hypovolemia, cardiac tamponade is either absent or of such a mild degree that no treatment for the condition per se is warranted. With more severe cardiac tamponade, bedside examination shows an increase in the jugular venous pressure. At the stage of moderate cardiac tamponade, the venous pressure may approximate 10 to 12 mm Hg and falls slightly in the normal manner during inspiration.

A skilled observer can also detect an abnormality of the waveform of the jugular venous pulsations. In normal subjects, venous pressure falls during the period of early rapid filling of the ventricle. This nadir in the jugular pulse is referred to as the *y* descent. At the time of its inscription, the tricuspid valve is open, so right atrial and ventricular diastolic pressures are equal. In early diastole, the ventricle is dilating rapidly with a resulting dip in pressure during the early rapid filling period. The tricuspid valve being open, this dip is accurately reflected in the jugular venous pressure as the *y* descent. In cardiac tamponade, the *y* descent is attenuated in mild cases and absent in moderate or severe cases (Fig. 65–2). The absence of the *y* descent

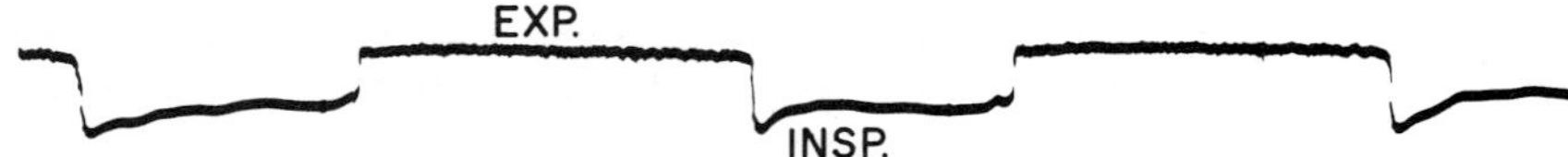

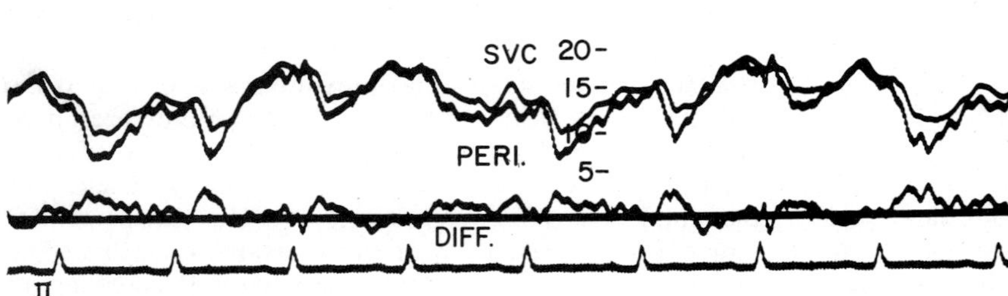

FIGURE 65–2 Pericardial (PERI.) and superior vena caval (SVC) pressures recorded by means of a differential transducer during catheterization and pericardiocentesis in a patient with severe cardiac tamponade. The two pressures are virtually identical, and both are severely elevated. Pressure falls during inspiration (INSP.). EXP., expiration. The waveform shows a dominant *x* but no *y* descent. The phase of respiration is indicated by a thermistor tracing at the top of the figure. The difference between the pressures (DIFF.) is shown fluctuating around the zero baseline.

could be interpreted as an abnormality of ventricular relaxation but more likely is related to the dynamics of pericardial volume. Consider that the pericardium is distended by an abnormal collection of fluid under increased pressure. Within that pericardial space lies the heart, the size of which is at its maximum in diastole but decreases during ventricular ejection, which is more rapid than cardiac filling. Thus, during ventricular ejection, intrapericardial pressure is slightly reduced; this is when venous return takes place. Venous return to the heart therefore occurs during the period of ventricular ejection with no further contribution during ventricular diastole. This monophasic pattern of venous return is reflected in the jugular venous pulse by a single nadir, the *x* descent, instead of the normal two nadirs, the *x* and *y* descents. In normal physiology, systemic venous return is bimodal, with one component occurring during ventricular systole, which creates a brief suction effect on the venous reservoir, pulling blood toward the heart, and a second component occurring in early diastole as soon as the tricuspid valve opens (Fig. 65–3).

In mild cases, systemic arterial pressure, the peripheral pulses, and the heart rate remain normal. Once pericardial and right and left atrial pressures are elevated and equalized, the phenomenon of pulsus paradoxus usually appears. Pulsus paradoxus can be defined as an abnormally large decrease in systemic arterial pressure during inspiration. In normal physiology, systemic blood pressure declines slightly, but this decline, although easily measured via a catheter in a systemic artery, is too small to be perceptible to clinical examination, especially during normal breathing. Arbitrarily, the maximum fall in arterial pressure with inspiration has been set at 10 mm Hg, although it is frequently considerably less than that. Pulsus paradoxus can be appreciated, on clinical examination, as a decreased force of the pulse synchronous with inspiration. In the most severe cases, the pulse disappears altogether during inspiration, hence the term *pulsus paradoxus* is used, with the paradox being a regular heartbeat but an apparently irregular peripheral pulse. In the most severe cases, when hypotension has developed, pulsus paradoxus may be hard to detect in the radial pulse but often is still apparent in the carotid and femoral pulses.

Pulsus paradoxus can be semiquantified through sphygmomanometry. It is observed that the first blood pressure sound can be heard when the patient is breathing out, only to disappear when the patient breathes in. As the cuff is

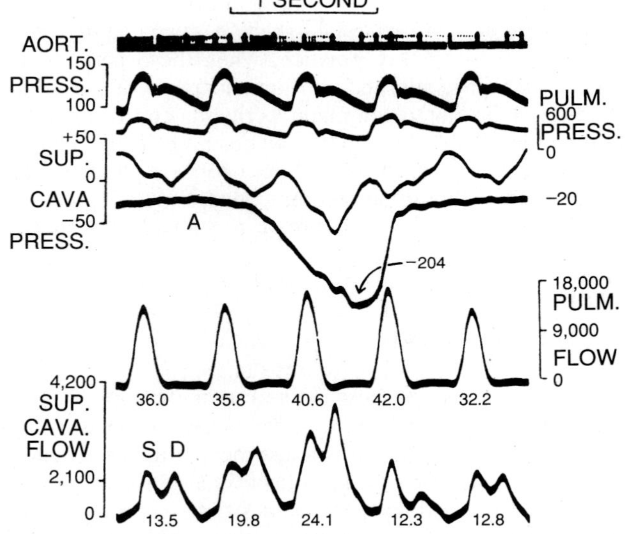

FIGURE 65–3 Effects of inspiration on the hemodynamics of an instrumented dog with closed chest spontaneous breathing. Tracings from top down: aortic pressure (AORT. PRESS.; mm Hg); pressures in the pulmonary artery (PULM. PRESS.), superior vena cava (SUP. CAVA PRESS.), and pleural cavity (A) (cm H_2O); and flow in the pulmonary artery (PULM. FLOW) and superior vena cava (SUP. CAVA FLOW; ml/stroke). With inspiration, pressures fall in the aorta, pulmonary artery, and superior vena cava, but venous return increases. Note that the increased stroke flow in the superior vena cava precedes that in the pulmonary artery by one beat. Right heart volume therefore increases during inspiration. Venous return increases during inspiration despite an increase in pulmonary vascular resistance. (From Brecher GA, Hubay CA: Pulmonary blood flow and venous return during spontaneous respiration. Circ Res 3:210–214, 1955.)

slowly deflated and the phase of respiration is monitored by eye or with a hand on the chest, there comes a point when the first blood pressure sound is audible throughout the respiratory cycle. The difference in systolic blood pressure between the level at which the first blood pressure sound can be heard only during expiration to the pressure at which it can be heard all the time provides a clinical estimate of the degree of pulsus paradoxus.

Laboratory Examination

ECHOCARDIOGRAPHY

Cardiac tamponade is a clinical syndrome that can be recognized and classified as to severity at the bedside. However, the echocardiographic features of cardiac tamponade are highly characteristic and therefore also are of great help in establishing the diagnosis and assessing its severity. In some cases, the diagnosis is first established on clinical grounds, but in others, it is first suspected after echocardiography. Despite the frequency with which the relative merits of the echocardiographic versus the clinical criteria are debated, arguing whether cardiac tamponade should be a clinical or an echocardiographic diagnosis is a futile exercise because the two modalities complement each other. In complex cases, such as those with additional atrial septal defect, aortic regurgitation, heart failure, shock, or pulmonary hypertension, tamponade may be difficult to diagnose with confidence at the bedside. On the other hand, the echocardiographic signs of cardiac tamponade may be absent in specific cases, particularly when complicated by another cardiac condition. Furthermore, signs normally diagnostic of cardiac tamponade may be found in the echocardiogram of patients with pericardial effusion but no tamponade. Thus, the diagnosis may be made on clinical or echocardiographic grounds. Ideally, echocardiographic and clinical information is synthesized.

A number of echocardiographic abnormalities have been described as evidence of cardiac tamponade.[47] Of these, the three most important are right atrial compression,[48, 49] right ventricular diastolic collapse,[50] and increased respiratory variation in atrioventricular inflow velocity and in blood velocity through the semilunar valves.[51, 52] Other abnormalities, which were described earlier, are less pathognomonic. Whenever cardiac tamponade is a reasonable diagnostic possibility, the obvious datum that must be acquired is whether the patient has a pericardial effusion. Again, it is emphasized that suspicion of the possibility of cardiac tamponade almost invariably demands that an echocardiogram be obtained. If pericardial effusion is absent, the diagnosis of tamponade cannot be entertained.

When the presence of pericardial effusion is confirmed with the echocardiogram, its amount is usually at least moderate and often large when tamponade exists. The effusion is recognized as a motionless echo-free space surrounding the heart and can be detected on both M-mode and two-dimensional echocardiograms. The two-dimensional echocardiogram provides a more reliable estimate of the distribution of the effusion.

Under normal physiologic conditions, pericardial pressure is slightly subatmospheric, whereas right atrial pressure is a few millimeters of mercury above atmospheric, providing a significantly positive transmural atrial pressure. The free wall of the normally distended right atrium is seen in the four-chamber view and the subcostal view as a convex structure. With cardiac tamponade, this normal positive transmural pressure is abolished, becoming zero or even slightly negative so that the right atrial free wall becomes concave.[53] This finding has been termed *right atrial compression* and, in the presence of pericardial effusion, is a reliable sign of cardiac tamponade. However, when there is pulmonary hypertension, heart failure, or tricuspid valve disease, right atrial pressure may be substantially higher than pericardial pressure even when cardiac tamponade exists. Naturally, under those circumstances, right atrial compression is absent and the right atrium maintains its normal convexity.

In early diastole, right ventricular diastolic pressure is at its lowest point. In cardiac tamponade, therefore, right ventricular diastolic pressure falls below intrapericardial pressure during early diastole. This occurrence of transient negative right ventricular transmural diastolic pressure causes the cavity of the right ventricle to collapse during early diastole.[54] With the most severe grades of cardiac tamponade, heart rate is rapid and the reversed transmural right ventricular diastolic pressure persists longer into diastole. Therefore, the more severe the cardiac tamponade, the longer into diastole does the diastolic collapse of the right ventricle persist.

The ability to assess right ventricular collapse requires skill and experience in echocardiography. When using real-time images, it is essential to use a stop-frame technique to ensure the collapse indeed occurs during diastole. M-mode images are easier to interpret for this particular finding because from appropriate scans, diminishing right ventricular dimension is easily seen to occur when the mitral valve is open, when the aortic valve is closed, or after the T wave of the electrocardiogram (Fig. 65–4).

Right ventricular diastolic collapse has been observed in some patients without cardiac tamponade. Likewise, right ventricular diastolic collapse fails to appear when there is right ventricular failure or hypertrophy of any cause. Collapse of the right ventricular outflow tract during early diastole can be recognized by M-mode echocardiography and was indeed first described before the advent of the two-dimensional technique. Atrial compression usually occurs earlier than right ventricular diastolic collapse in the course of cardiac tamponade.[53] Right ventricular diastolic collapse occurs earlier when blood volume is decreased[55] and is associated with a significant decline in cardiac output, although it precedes marked hypotension and pulsus paradoxus.[56] Much less commonly, left atrial compression and even left ventricular diastolic collapse may be seen.[57, 58]

Perhaps the next most important echocardiographic sign of cardiac tamponade is a highly exaggerated respiratory variation in the relative size of the two ventricles.[59] In normal subjects, inspiration augments systemic venous return, thereby dilating the right atrium and right ventricle. In the absence of cardiac tamponade, increased right ventricular volume involves all of the walls of the chamber and is not limited to the interventricular septum. In the presence of cardiac tamponade, however, the free walls of the right ventricle are constrained by the pericardial effusion. Cardiac tamponade does not prevent the augmentation

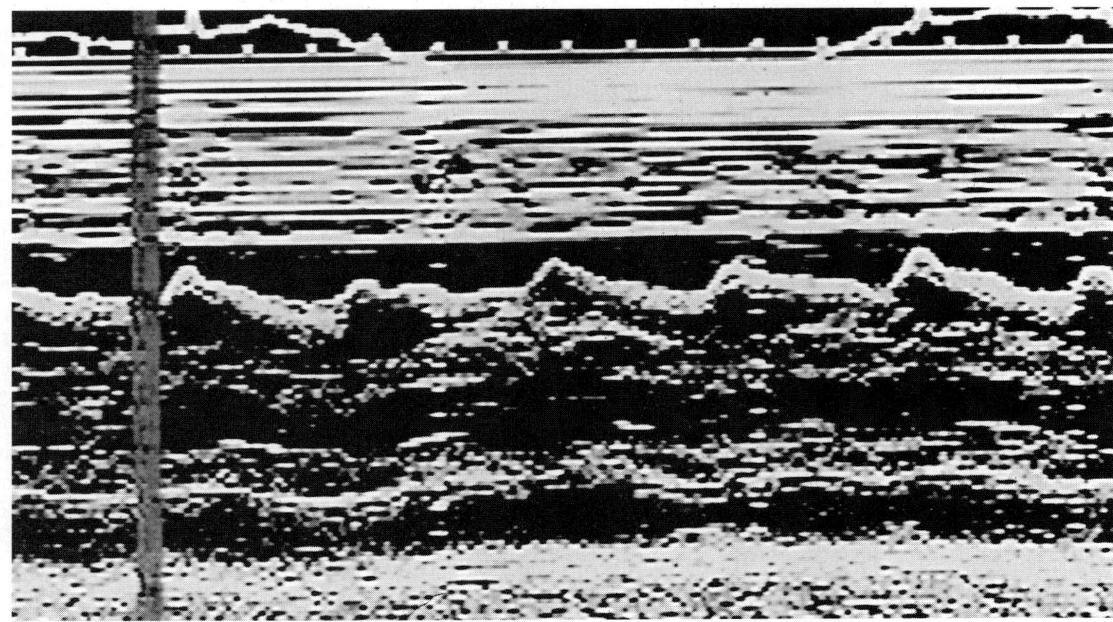

FIGURE 65–4 M-mode echocardiogram from a patient with cardiac tamponade. A large pericardial effusion is present anteriorly and posteriorly. The right ventricular free wall (topmost moving image) moves toward the interventricular septum during diastole, indicating right ventricular diastolic collapse.

of systemic venous return during inspiration,[60] but now the increase in right ventricular volume is accommodated primarily or entirely by the interventricular septum, which is bowed toward the left ventricle, with the result that the dimension of the right ventricle increases while that of the left ventricle decreases. A small amount of this respiratory variation in the relative dimensions of two ventricles is seen in normal subjects, but the phenomenon is diagnostically valuable because it is greatly exaggerated in cardiac tamponade.

In normal subjects during quiet respiration, tricuspid peak inflow velocity increases by approximately 15 percent and mitral peak inflow velocity decreases by a maximum of 10 percent. With cardiac tamponade, however, the degree of respiratory variation is greatly exaggerated and becomes obvious on the Doppler tracings of ventricular inflow velocities.[51] Inspiration is characterized by a dramatic increase in tricuspid blood flow velocity and decrease in mitral blood flow velocity of 25 to 30 percent. These exaggerated respiratory variations of blood flow velocity appear early, certainly before the advent of pulsus paradoxus. They can be detected even in what is usually considered to be a hemodynamically insignificant pericardial effusion, the so-called lax pericardial effusion.[61, 62]

Cardiac tamponade diminishes the volume of the ventricles, which therefore appear to have thicker walls. Not surprisingly, diminution in ventricular volume creates the substrate for prolapse of the mitral valve. This pseudoprolapse is one of the minor echocardiographic signs of cardiac tamponade. Inspiration normally reduces the caliber of the inferior vena cava; this finding is attenuated by cardiac tamponade.[63]

In some patients with tamponade and a very large, usually malignant pericardial effusion, the whole heart appears to swing dramatically in the large echo-free space. The rate of the swinging motion is often exactly half the heart rate. The occurrence of this phenomenon has been explained on hemodynamic grounds, but the event has also been modeled using nonlinear dynamics. Although this phenomenon is most easily observed on two-dimensional echocardiogram, the changing position of the heart is also readily apparent on the M-mode echocardiogram. The large shift in the mechanical position of the heart influences its electric axis, accounting for the frequent association of electric alternans with abnormal pendular motion of the heart in cardiac tamponade.

ECHOCARDIOGRAPHIC CLINICAL BALANCE

A confident diagnosis of cardiac tamponade in need of relief through the removal of fluid can be made when the presence of a pericardial effusion is documented echocardiographically; the clinical examination demonstrates a raised jugular pressure with the x descent dominant, pulsus paradoxus, dyspnea, and a degree of hypotension, and right heart compression is seen echocardiographically. But what if the echocardiographic signs are prominent but the patient is not in distress and has normal venous and arterial pressures? Alternatively, what if the patient has all or most of the classic features of cardiac tamponade but no right heart compression?

Successful management is based on understanding that cardiac compression can sometimes occur when tamponade is relatively mild and possibly can be managed conservatively. Second, false-positive compression can occur from, for example, a massive pleural effusion. Third, severe cardiac tamponade can exist in the absence of echocardiographic right heart compression or pulsus paradoxus, especially but not exclusively when there is preexisting heart disease and after cardiac surgery. Pericardiocentesis or open drainage should almost never be performed on a patient who is not in cardiorespiratory distress and lacks the clinical findings of cardiac tamponade, simply because an echocardiographic report, especially one issued by a physician who has not examined the patient, states that the study shows cardiac tamponade.

For years, the question of whether cardiac tamponade is a clinical or an echocardiographic diagnosis was debated, but the debate was foolish. The diagnosis and assessment of severity are based on both sets of criteria. When one set is lacking, a good clinician can usually determine why and thus can decide whether evacuation of the fluid is indicated. When the effusion is large, central venous pressure is high, and pulsus paradoxus is pronounced, removal of the fluid is almost always necessary, even when the echocardiogram does not show chamber compression. This is only one of the many examples of the folly of affixing labels such as "ruled in" or "ruled out" and basing treatment on that label instead of on an integrated evaluation of all available clinical and laboratory information.

ELECTROCARDIOGRAM

In the majority of cases, the electrocardiogram is not particularly useful. Sometimes the electrocardiogram remains normal, and often, when abnormalities are present, they are not specific; sinus tachycardia, low voltage, or ST-segment and T-wave changes may not be detected. Rarely, the tracing may demonstrate the characteristic abnormalities of acute pericarditis with widespread elevation of the ST segment and sometimes depression of the PR segment. As discussed earlier, very large pericardial effusion may be associated with electric alternans. Alternans of the P, QRS, and T is virtually pathognomonic of a large pericardial effusion.[64] However, this form of alternans, although highly specific, is not at all sensitive.[65]

CHEST RADIOGRAM

Some degree of enlargement of the cardiopericardial silhouette is to be expected in cardiac tamponade. Acute effusion or hemorrhage induces severe cardiac tamponade after a relatively small accumulation. In such cases, cardiac enlargement is modest. Cardiac tamponade, secondary to many disorders such as neoplasm and viral or tuberculous pericarditis, in which fluid accumulation is slower, allowing the pericardium time to stretch, is associated with the considerably larger cardiopericardial silhouette. Because the left and right sides of the heart are equally constrained, pulmonary congestion is less pronounced in association with apparent cardiomegaly from cardiac tamponade than it is in most cases with cardiomegaly as a manifestation of heart failure.

CARDIAC CATHETERIZATION

In the vast majority of cases, the diagnosis of cardiac tamponade can be established without resorting to cardiac catheterization. However, except in extraordinary emergencies, monitoring of at least the right atrial and systemic arterial pressures should be part of pericardiocentesis. In some cases, the procedure is limited to right heart catheterization performed in an intensive care unit or a comparable environment or in the operating room. In others, a more formal cardiac catheterization is performed in the cardiac catheterization laboratory.

Simple Right Heart Catheterization. When a diagnosis of cardiac tamponade is made or strongly suspected and drainage of the fluid is considered necessary, a minimum of three pressures should be recorded: right atrial, systemic arterial, and intrapericardial. The measurement of cardiac output is desirable but less important in most of the cases.

Commonly, a Swan-Ganz catheter is used. Because equalization of filling pressure on the two sides of the heart is so crucial to the hemodynamic diagnosis of cardiac tamponade, one should not rely on sequential pressure measurements recorded as the catheter is pulled back from the pulmonary wedge position to the right atrium. Rather, advantage should be taken of the two lumina of the catheter to simultaneously record right atrial and pulmonary wedge pressures. If the right atrial and pulmonary wedge pressures are separated by more than 5 mm Hg, provided the transducers have been properly leveled to the same height, the diagnosis of uncomplicated cardiac tamponade comes into serious question. In cardiac tamponade, the right atrial pressure is elevated, with the magnitude of the elevation depending on the severity of cardiac tamponade. Close inspection of the tracing reveals that the pressure drops slightly during inspiration. The tracing also should confirm the clinical observation that the *y* descent is attenuated in mild cases and absent in moderate or severe cases. There is a single descent: the *x* wave. The pulmonary wedge pressure may vary more with respiration than does the right atrial pressure; therefore, equilibration between the two pressures may not be exact throughout the respiratory cycle.

In mild cardiac tamponade, the cardiac output is normal but falls progressively with increasing severity of cardiac tamponade. Likewise, there may be little discernible abnormality in the tracing of systemic arterial pressure, but with increasing severity of cardiac tamponade, the pressure begins to fall and pulsus paradoxus begins to make its appearance. When pulsus paradoxus is evaluated from a direct tracing of arterial pressure, it is observed that inspiration is accompanied not only by a decline in peak systolic pressure but also by a decline in pulse pressure. The latter reflects diminished stroke volume during inspiration.

In the most severe cases, central venous pressure is elevated to the range of 20 mm Hg or higher. Severe respiratory distress, as may occur with the most severe grades of cardiac tamponade, superimposes large swings of pulmonary wedge pressure during the cardiac cycle. This grossly exaggerated respiratory variation of pressure reflects large changes in intrathoracic pressure in patients with respiratory distress.

Blood gas analysis shows a progressive drop in mixed venous oxygen saturation from its normal value of around 75 percent to values in extreme cases that may be as low as the teens. More commonly, mixed venous oxygen saturation around 50 to 60 percent is observed.

In many cases, pericardiocentesis is performed in the cardiac catheterization laboratory; less often, it is performed in the operating room. Increasingly, however, the procedure is carried out in an intensive care unit with echocardiographic rather than fluoroscopic monitoring.[66] It is highly desirable to have available a multichannel pressure recording system so that at least two, and preferably three, pressures can be simultaneously monitored and recorded. The transducer used to measure intrapericardial pressure must be at the same hydrostatic level as the transducer measuring right atrial pressure. In cardiac tamponade, intrapericardial pressure is, by definition, elevated and equal to the right atrial pressure. In more severe cases, intrapericardial, right atrial, and pulmonary wedge pressures are all more or less equal (to within 3 or 4 mm Hg).

Formal Cardiac Catheterization. The cardiac catheterization laboratory is the ideal place in which to record hemodynamics in patients who have, or are suspected of having, cardiac tamponade, but are likely to have coexistent heart disease, especially when coronary arteriography is also required. The advantages of this location include the ability to carry out cardiac fluoroscopy and to determine the correct location of an intrapericardial catheter through visualization of its position within the cardiac silhouette and observation of the fate of a small volume of contrast agent injected into the catheter. When the catheter is intrapericardial, the contrast does not circulate but instead pools in the most dependent portion of the pericardial cavity. If a cardiac chamber has been inadvertently catheterized, the contrast will be seen to disappear as a puff into the pulmonary circulation. Correct positioning of the needle or catheter in the pericardium can alternatively be verified through the injection of agitated saline and the observation that the bubble contrast is confined to the pericardium.

When the patient undergoes fluoroscopy, the lack of normal convexity of the right atrial border is easily observed in the anterior posterior projection and better so in a shallow right anterior oblique projection. If a Cournand, a National Institutes of Health, or a multipurpose catheter is advanced into the right atrium and its tip is made to engage the endocardium, the catheter tip will be seen to be separated from the edge of the cardiac silhouette by the width of the pericardial effusion.

The cardiac catheterization laboratory has further advantages. The pressure recording equipment is usually more sophisticated, allowing for the simultaneous recording of several pressures and electrograms at varying chart speeds. In this setting, one expects right atrial and intrapericardial pressures to be just about identical throughout the respiratory cycle. These two pressures should be recorded simultaneously with the pulmonary wedge pressure; right atrial and pulmonary wedge pressures should not differ by more than 2 or 3 mm Hg from intrapericardial pressure. Once the baseline pressures have been recorded, the measurements can be repeated while aliquots of pericardial fluid are removed, minimally at the beginning and end of the procedure. In uncomplicated cardiac tamponade, all pressures return to normal, and pericardial pressure is below right atrial and pulmonary wedge pressures throughout the cardiac and respiratory cycles.

Echocardiographic rather than fluoroscopic monitoring has much to commend it, even when pericardiocentesis is performed in the cardiac catheterization laboratory.

HEMODYNAMIC ASSESSMENT OF RESULTS

The pericardial volume relation is J shaped[67] and thus extremely steep at greatly elevated intrapericardial pressure. Thus, after the removal of the first 100 ml of pericardial fluid, one can anticipate a dramatic fall in right atrial and pulmonary wedge pressures, a substantial increase in systemic arterial pressure, a diminution in the severity of pulsus paradoxus, and sometimes a decrease in heart rate. The withdrawal of intrapericardial fluid progressively lessens the severity of cardiac tamponade; therefore, pericardial pressure progressively declines. The drop in right atrial and pulmonary wedge pressure is identical to that in pericardial pressure, with the result that all three pressures remain in equilibration.[68]

After pericardial pressure has been reduced to a level lower than the preexisting pulmonary wedge pressure (e.g., 10 mm Hg), further pericardiocentesis has no additional effect on pulmonary wedge pressure, but right atrial and pericardial pressures remain identical until the normal right atrial pressure is reached, at which point pericardial pressure declines below right atrial pressure. The former becomes subatmospheric, and the latter levels off around 5 mm Hg.[68]

The sequence of hemodynamic events described in the preceding paragraphs applies to uncomplicated cardiac tamponade in a patient without preexisting heart disease or constrictive pericarditis. When there is preexisting increase in left ventricular end-diastolic and pulmonary wedge pressures, these pressures may be higher than intrapericardial and right atrial pressures measured before the removal of a significant quantity of pericardial fluid. Pericardiocentesis would normalize pericardial and right atrial pressures, but pulmonary wedge pressure would remain elevated. In patients with right heart failure, pericardiocentesis may normalize the pericardial pressure, but right atrial pressure would remain elevated. Likewise, if there is effusive-constrictive pericarditis, a condition characterized by pericardial fluid under pressure combined with cardiac constriction by the visceral layer of the pericardium, right atrial and pulmonary wedge pressures would both remain elevated and equal each other, even after pericardial pressure had been restored to normal.[69] If a patient has severe tricuspid regurgitation, large systolic waves may be present in the right atrial pressure but not in the pericardial pressure. Thus, after pericardiocentesis, if right atrial pressure remains abnormal, the clinician should consider effusive-constrictive pericarditis, right heart failure, and tricuspid valve disease. If the patient has effusive-constrictive pericarditis, the characteristic hemodynamic findings (vide infra) are unmasked by pericardiocentesis. Tricuspid regurgitation can be documented by performing a right ventriculogram or by Doppler echocardiography. Tricuspid stenosis can be documented with careful simultaneous pressure recordings of the right atrial and right ventricular pressures or by Doppler. The right atrial tracing will show a dominant A wave, and there will be a diastolic pressure gradient across the tricuspid valve that increases with inspiration. If there is right heart failure, impaired function of the right ventricle can be demonstrated by the right ventriculogram or by Doppler echocardiography. The ability to carry out these additional investigations as the need becomes apparent is another major advantage of performing pericardiocentesis in a cardiac catheterization laboratory and not in a coronary care unit. The advantages of having echo-Doppler capabilities in the cardiac catheterization laboratory should be apparent.

PATHOPHYSIOLOGIC EXPLANATION OF HEMODYNAMICS

It was mentioned earlier that in cardiac tamponade, the *y* descent of right atrial pressure is absent because venous return to the heart is limited to the period of ventricular ejection when intracardiac volume is minimal. In normal physiology, the *y* descent marking early rapid ventricular filling occurs during the period of active ventricular relaxation. When there is cardiac tamponade, the period of early rapid filling is abolished, and therefore an early diastolic dip of ventricular pressure does not occur and the *y* descent of atrial pressure is correspondingly absent.[70] The dip-and-plateau phenomenon of ventricular pressure thus is a feature of constrictive pericarditis but does not occur in cardiac tamponade. In cardiac tamponade, there is slow filling of the ventricle throughout diastole such that the diastolic pressure is elevated throughout diastole and increases steadily from early to end diastole. In the majority of cases of cardiac tamponade, in the absence of preexisting heart disease, ventricular function is normal or supranormal.[71] Increased ejection fraction and heart rate partially compensate for reduced end-diastolic ventricular volume. In most cases, angiocardiography is not required but should be carried out when there is suspicion of coexisting cardiomyopathy or heart failure. When these conditions are absent, and opaque contrast medium is injected at the junction of the superior vena cava and right atrium, the motionless fluid density of the pericardial effusion is in stark contrast to the hyperdynamic action of the cardiac ventricles. If left ventriculography is performed, the chamber volume is found to be normal or reduced depending on the severity of tamponade, the ejection fraction above normal, and segmental wall motion relatively normal, although a small degree of regional abnormality may be present. When left ventricular ejection fraction is depressed, the most common explanation is preexisting myocardial disease, but this finding may also occur at the very end-stages of cardiac tamponade when cardiac compression is so severe that it impedes the coronary circulation. This latter finding is uncommon outside the experimental laboratory.

In previous years, it was customary to inject air, or preferably carbon dioxide, into the evacuated pericardial sac to delineate the thickness of the parietal pericardium (Fig. 65–5). With the advent of satisfactory techniques for imaging the heart and pericardium, particularly computed tomography and magnetic resonance imaging, this practice has greatly declined. In some laboratories, the diagnostic evaluation of pericardial effusion and cardiac tamponade includes pericardioscopy.[72] The technique permits visualization of the epicardium, fibrin deposits, and areas suitable for biopsy.

Treatment

Because cardiac tamponade should be viewed as a spectrum ranging from a pericardial pressure elevated a few millimeters of mercury above normal to extreme cases with pericardial pressure in the range of 25 to 30 mm Hg, it follows that treatment is not the same for all cases. In general, although the treatment of cardiac tamponade is to evacuate pericardial fluid with the object of lowering pericardial and thus intracardiac atrial and ventricular diastolic pressures toward normal, there are variations. For instance, a patient brought to the emergency department in extremis after a motor vehicle accident, in whom the physician has reason to suspect cardiac tamponade, may have to

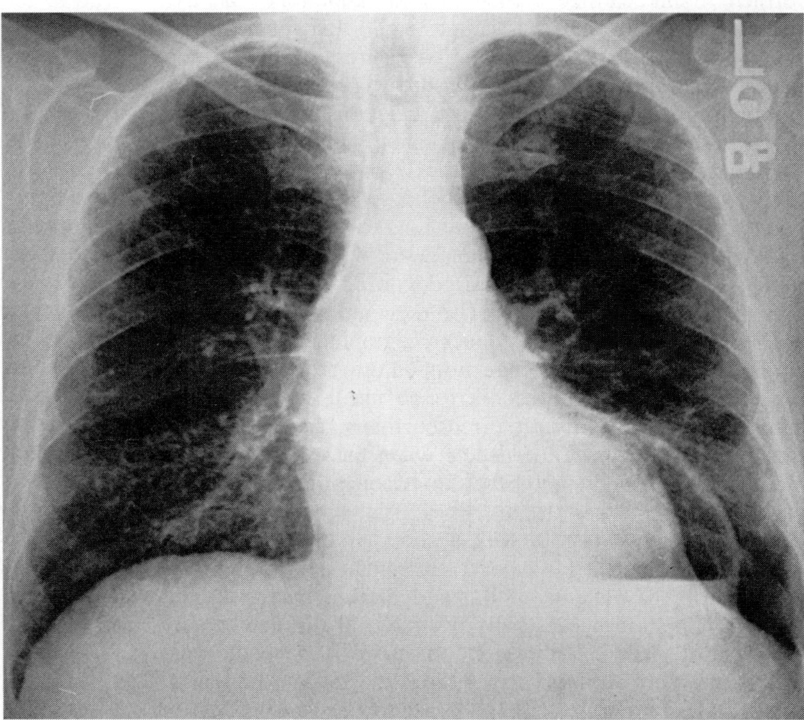

FIGURE 65–5 Chest radiograph immediately after aspiration of a large pericardial effusion, followed by the instillation of carbon dioxide. The pericardium is well imaged. This technique is less often used since the introduction of noninvasive imaging.

have a needle placed into the pericardial sac with minimal prior investigation. In the most extreme cases, there may not be time even to obtain an echocardiogram, a prerequisite in all other cases. At the other end of the spectrum, a patient without clinical evidence of cardiovascular compromise, except a modest increase in jugular venous pressure to the range of 5 to 7 mm Hg, may not require evacuation of pericardial fluid, especially if the likely cause is idiopathic or viral pericarditis, which would be expected to respond to anti-inflammatory treatment. Such patients, however, should be observed in the hospital in case the hemodynamic situation deteriorates, indicating the need for removal of the pericardial fluid.

Between the extremes mentioned previously lie the majority of patients who have moderate or severe but not end-stage or decompensated cardiac tamponade. These patients require elective, planned removal of pericardial fluid via pericardiocentesis or surgical pericardiotomy or, less commonly, via balloon pericardiostomy. Which of the techniques should be selected is largely a matter of local preference, the facilities available, and the training, interests, and expertise of the medical and surgical staff. Pericardiocentesis has the advantages of being less expensive and less invasive and allows the optimal measurement of hemodynamic parameters. Surgical pericardiostomy has the advantages of being performed under direct vision and facilitating the procurement of adequate pericardial biopsy material. It has been suggested that a better diagnostic yield is attained when surgical pericardiectomy is supplemented with intraoperative pericardioscopy.[73] Balloon techniques are in the development stage but appear to be promising, especially for malignant pericardial effusion.[74, 75]

PERICARDIOCENTESIS

For reasons described here, pericardiocentesis is best performed in the cardiac catheterization laboratory. Ideally, before pericardiocentesis is begun, right heart catheterization, including the simultaneous measurement of pulmonary wedge and right atrial pressures, is carried out, and right atrial pressure is monitored throughout the procedure. A reliable arterial pressure cannula should be placed before commencing pericardiocentesis. Before the decision to carry out pericardiocentesis, an echocardiogram will have been performed, but it is advantageous to have an echocardiograph available in the laboratory to make a final determination of the distribution of pericardial fluid when the patient is in the laboratory.[76] The procedure can be safely and effectively monitored echocardiographically. Often, it is desirable to have the thorax propped upward, particularly if the subxiphoid approach is to be used. Although the subxiphoid approach is preferred by many, the final selection of where to place the needle when the effusion is not large can be based on where the echocardiogram shows effusion to be closest to the skin. The procedure is best performed with a needle with a short bevel; long, large-bore needles with a long bevel are dangerous because in the majority of patients, if the pericardium has not been reached and fluid successfully aspirated at the depth of a few centimeters from the skin, the tip of the needle has missed the pericardium or punctured the myocardium. As soon as it is apparent that the pericardial space has been entered, pericardial pressure along with pulmonary wedge and right atrial pressures should be measured before the removal of a substantial volume of pericardial fluid. If the fluid is deeply sanguinous, pressure should immediately be measured to ensure the needle does not lie within the cavity of the right ventricle. If a venous type of pressure is recorded, it may still be necessary to distinguish between right atrial and pericardial location because the two pressures will be identical. The hematocrit of blood in the right atrium and fluid from the pericardium can be compared quickly, but the quickest and easiest way to distinguish between these two sites is to inject contrast through the needle, provided the fluid or blood can be aspirated freely throughout the cardiac and respiratory cycles.

Constrictive Pericarditis

Constrictive pericarditis is another of the major pericardial causes of compressive disease of the heart. It therefore shares some important characteristics with cardiac tamponade, but nevertheless important clinical and pathophysiologic differences clearly distinguish between the two conditions. Constrictive pericarditis can be subacute or chronic but seldom acute.

Pathophysiology

Constrictive pericarditis is a condition in which the pericardium, responding to prior insult, becomes scarred and loses all, or virtually all, of its normal compliance. Venous return to the heart and diastolic filling of the ventricles are therefore impeded. In the most severe cases, not only is diastolic expansion of cardiac volume severely limited but also the heart is compressed so the end-diastolic volume of the ventricles is appreciably decreased, thereby limiting stroke volume despite a normal or increased ventricular ejection fraction. Impeded venous return and ventricular volume lead to abnormally increased ventricular diastolic pressures on both sides of the heart, and thereby to increased pulmonary venous and systemic venous pressures with resulting congestion of the lungs and systemic tissues. In the majority of cases, systemic congestion is more profound and more apparent on clinical examination than is pulmonary congestion. The combination of increased ventricular and venous pressures on both sides of the heart, together with low stroke volume and tachycardia, simulates the clinical picture of congestive heart failure. However, because ventricular systolic function is normal[77] and ventricular diastolic dysfunction is due to decreased pericardial, not myocardial, stiffness, it is misleading to consider constrictive pericarditis as a form of congestive heart failure. Congestive heart failure results from overload of the heart, whereas in constrictive pericarditis, the heart is underloaded and only the circulation is overloaded.[56] Therefore, although the use of diuretics is appropriate treatment for both conditions, preload and afterload reduction and drugs with positive inotropic action have little, if any, place in the treatment of constrictive pericarditis.

CHARACTERISTICS COMMON TO CONSTRICTIVE PERICARDITIS AND CARDIAC TAMPONADE

Under both conditions, systolic function of the left ventricle is preserved and may be supranormal. In the vast majority of cases of both constrictive pericarditis and cardiac tamponade, the abnormal external constraint around the heart is global, so all chambers are equally affected. In both disorders, therefore, one anticipates elevation and equalization of the left and right ventricular diastolic pressures with each other and with the pressures in the two atria. Under both conditions, equilibration occurs between pulmonary wedge and right atrial pressures in at least one portion of the respiratory cycle, and pulmonary arterial diastolic pressure is close to or equal to biventricular diastolic pressure. Elevated jugular pressure is a feature of both disorders, and in both, pulmonary hypertension is commensurate with the elevated left ventricular diastolic pressure and thus seldom exceeds 35 to 45 mm Hg. Both constrictive pericarditis and cardiac tamponade can be localized, creating atypical syndromes. Atypical syndromes of cardiac tamponade were discussed earlier, and atypical syndromes of constrictive pericarditis are discussed later.

Greatly enhanced ventricular interaction is a critical component of the pathophysiology of cardiac tamponade and constrictive pericarditis. Ventricular interaction is the influence that changes in the pressure and volume of one ventricle exert on the opposite ventricle. Here, we are concerned with diastolic interaction. In the absence of the pericardium, ventricular interaction is present but weak. It is somewhat strengthened by a normal pericardium and greatly so by increased external constraint such as tamponade or constriction. When one side of the heart enlarges, the other must shrink. This interaction underlies the mechanism of pulsus paradoxus and the echo-Doppler and hemodynamic signs of tamponade and constriction.

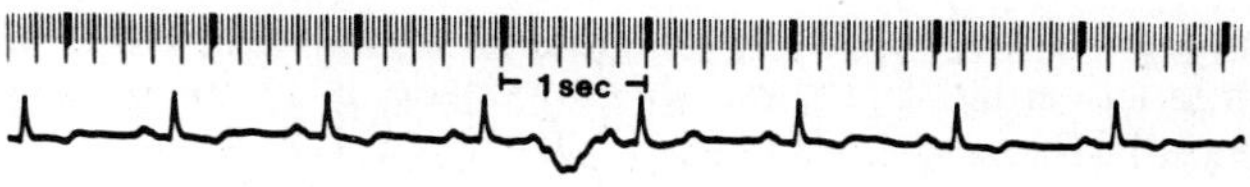

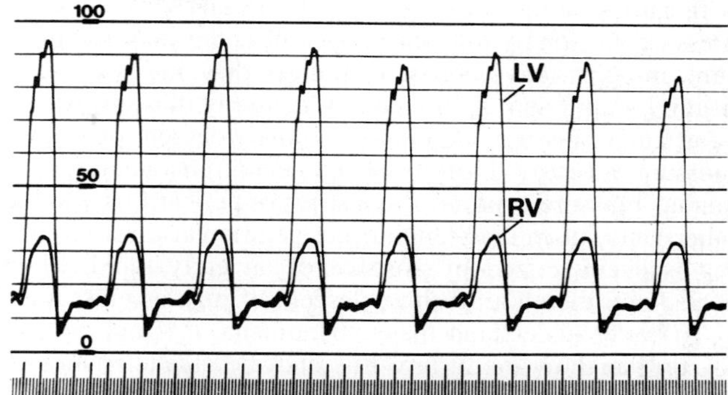

FIGURE 65–6 Pressures recorded simultaneously from right (RV) and left (LV) ventricles in a patient with constrictive pericarditis. Note the dip-and-plateau configuration of the diastolic pressures, which are elevated to 15 mm Hg and are equilibrated. Respiratory variation in left and right ventricular peak systolic pressures is neither in-phase nor exactly 180 degrees out-of-phase.

PATHOPHYSIOLOGIC CHARACTERISTICS THAT DISTINGUISH CONSTRICTIVE PERICARDITIS FROM CARDIAC TAMPONADE

The most important feature that distinguishes the pathophysiology of constrictive pericarditis from that of cardiac tamponade relates to the pattern of ventricular filling. In constrictive pericarditis, the velocity of early rapid filling is considerably faster than normal, but once early rapid filling has been completed, the ventricles attain their largest possible volume, having engaged the pericardium, and therefore cannot increase in volume after the end of the early rapid filling period. The most likely explanation for this phenomenon is the combination of impeded venous return with a small rapidly recoiling ventricle.[78] This pattern of ventricular filling confined to early diastole is reflected in the configuration of ventricular pressure in the two ventricles. The early rapid phase of filling is represented by a sharp dip in early diastolic pressure. The period of diastasis that constitutes the remainder of diastole is represented by a plateau of pressure. In the normal ventricle, ventricular diastolic pressure increases gradually from early to end diastole. In constrictive pericarditis, ventricular diastolic pressure is constant from the end of early rapid filling until end diastole (Fig. 65–6). This phenomenon is referred to in the literature as the dip-and-plateau phenomenon,[79] or the square-root sign.

The pattern of ventricular filling in constrictive pericarditis is in marked contrast with that occurring in cardiac tamponade. The absence of an early diastolic rapid filling phase characterizes the pattern of ventricular filling in cardiac tamponade; therefore, the dip-and-plateau phenomenon does not occur in this condition. Ventricular pressure is elevated throughout diastole and rises steeply from early to late diastole in a smooth, progressive fashion (Fig. 65–7). In constrictive pericarditis, the limitation of ventricular filling after the end of the early rapid filling period is absolute, whereas in cardiac tamponade, the ventricle can

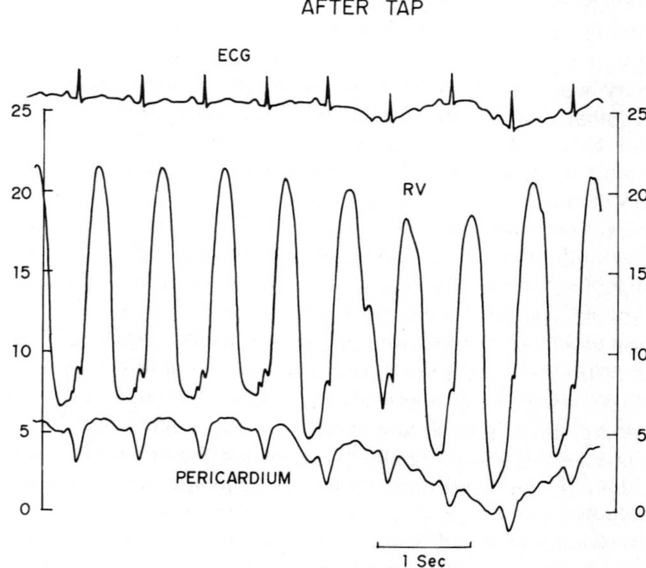

FIGURE 65–7 Simultaneous recording of right ventricular (RV) and pericardial pressures immediately after pericardiocentesis. Note that ventricular diastolic pressure exceeds pericardial pressure throughout the respiratory and cardiac cycles. Also, there is a fall in pericardial pressure coincident with ventricular ejection. ECG, electrocardiogram.

enlarge throughout diastole but at the expense of increasing intrapericardial pressure, so tamponade is at its peak at end diastole.

The patterns of atrial filling and pressure also differ in important ways when constrictive pericarditis is compared with cardiac tamponade.[70] During ventricular diastole, atrial pressure is strongly influenced by ventricular diastolic pressure. In constrictive pericarditis, early diastolic ventricular filling is rapid and is reflected by the early diastolic dip of ventricular pressure. Consequently, the *y* descent of venous pressure, an early diastolic phenomenon, characterizes the venous pressure contour of constrictive pericarditis. On the other hand, in cardiac tamponade, ventricular diastolic filling is characterized by absence of an early rapid filling period and therefore of the *y* descent of jugular pressure.

To better understand these phenomena, it is appropriate to consider how the atrium fills and the characteristics of its pressure contour when the heart and pericardium are normal. The act of ventricular ejection causes the mitral and tricuspid atrioventricular rings to descend at the time when their respective valves are closed. This piston effect aspirates blood from the venous reservoirs to the atria. In addition, cardiac volume is minimal during ventricular ejection, and therefore pericardial pressure is lowered as can be readily recognized from a pressure tracing from the pericardial cavity that shows a distinct drop during ventricular systole (see Fig. 65–7). The two events—descent of the atrioventricular rings and lowered intrapericardial pressure—accelerate venous return. Superior vena caval and pulmonary venous flow therefore increase during ventricular systole. Tracings of blood flow velocity through these veins show a clear peak, whereas simultaneous pressure tracings show a sharp nadir, both of which are manifestations of the suction-piston effect of ventricular ejection on venous return. In constrictive pericarditis, this systolic component of venous return is maintained, and therefore the right atrial, systemic venous, and pulmonary venous pressure tracings maintain a normal *x* descent, as well as the deep, sharp *y* descent that is characteristic of constrictive pericarditis. In a sense, then, the venous pressure waveform of constrictive pericarditis is an exaggeration of the normal, whereas that of cardiac tamponade is a distinctly abnormal waveform, because the *y* descent is missing.

It was stressed in the discussion of cardiac tamponade that although difficult to see clinically because of the high venous pressure, the normal inspiratory decline in systemic venous and right atrial pressures is maintained and is easily documented on intravascular and intracardiac tracings.[60] In constrictive pericarditis, however, this inspiratory decrease in systemic venous pressure is greatly attenuated or absent (Fig. 65–8). When right atrial pressure tracings are carefully scrutinized, it is apparent that the whole curve varies little, if at all, during respiration, although the *y* descent becomes sharper and deeper. Thus, respiratory variation of systemic venous pressure in constrictive pericarditis is limited to the *y* descent, which corresponds to the exaggerated early rapid filling phase of ventricular filling. The older literature stressed a paradoxical increase in systemic venous pressure and jugular venous pressure, as observed at the bedside, as an important feature that assists in the diagnosis of constrictive pericarditis. First described by

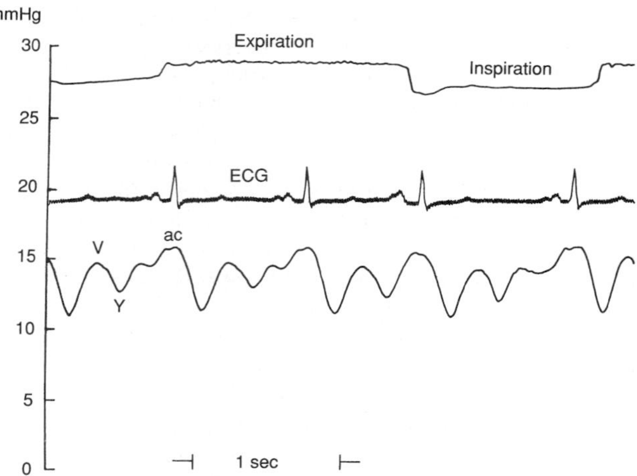

FIGURE 65–8 Right atrial pressure tracing recorded from a patient with moderate-to-severe constrictive pericarditis. Both the *x* and the *y* descents are prominent. In this case, the *x* descent is more prominent than the *y* descent. Respiratory variation is absent. ECG, electrocardiogram.

Kussmaul,[80] this sign still bears his name. However, the Kussmaul sign is very rarely overt in constrictive pericarditis when the patient is breathing normally or as near normally as the pericardial heart disease permits. When the patient is asked to take slow, very deep breaths during which intra-abdominal and inferior vena caval pressures increase, the true Kussmaul sign can sometimes be elicited, but it is not diagnostic of constrictive pericarditis[81] because the behavior of the systemic venous pressure tracing is similar, if not identical, in constrictive pericarditis, restrictive cardiomyopathy or, indeed, right heart failure of any cause, or tricuspid regurgitation.

A discussion of differences in systemic venous pressure between the two compressive diseases of the heart under consideration leads to another fundamental difference between these two conditions—pericardial pressure. In cardiac tamponade, pericardial pressure is elevated. It can be measured, and its pressure waveform can be accurately depicted. From measurements of intrapericardial pressure in cardiac tamponade, several fundamentally important observations have been made. The first is that during inspiration, intrapericardial pressure decreases slightly (e.g., in a severe case, from 20 to 17 mm Hg during quiet breathing). Second, in addition to intrapericardial pressure variations coupled to the respiratory cycle, variations coupled to the cardiac cycle are easily documented, the most notable of which is a sharp but small drop in intrapericardial pressure coincident with ventricular ejection. Last, transmural pericardial pressure (i.e., pericardial minus intrathoracic pressure) increases slightly during cardiac tamponade, from which one may conclude that the drop in intrathoracic pressure during inspiration is transmitted to the pericardial space, but its effect on pericardial pressure is slightly attenuated by the increase it creates in right heart volume. These respiratory and cardiac cycle–related variations in intrapericardial pressure have important effects on hemodynamics, many of which have been emphasized in preceding sections of this chapter.

The situation in constrictive pericarditis is altogether

different. Instead of a fluid-filled space in which hydrostatic pressures can be measured, the pericardial space is obliterated and there is no place in which to measure either fluid or contact pressure; therefore, the decline in intrathoracic pressure accompanying inspiration is not transmitted across the rigid, noncompliant pericardial scar into the intrapericardial portion of the venae cavae or the right atrium. In this situation, any increase in venous return that can occur with inspiration must be accommodated in the right atrium and right ventricle by bulging of the intra-atrial and interventricular septa from the right-sided to the left-sided chamber, because any expansion of the free walls of these chambers is prevented by the pericardial scar. This situation differs fundamentally from that pertaining in cardiac tamponade, in which increased venous return is accommodated partly by bowing of the septum but also by distention of the free wall. Proof of the latter is the increase in transmural pericardial pressure associated with inspiration in cardiac tamponade. In normal physiology, intrapericardial and intrapleural pressures change equally during inspiration, and therefore no change in transmural pressure of the pericardium is registered.

A number of clinical observations fit the pathophysiology described. Postextrasystolic beats fail to show an increased end-diastolic pressure.[82] The large A wave of right atrial pressure may exceed pulmonary arterial diastolic pressure, causing the pulmonary valve to open prematurely in presystole.[83] An effect that would not be predicted is that in the last trimester of pregnancy, cardiac output increases when the patient is turned into the left lateral decubitus position.[84] The proposed mechanism is a fall in arteriolar vascular resistance because under this condition, cardiac output is not influenced by increases in central venous pressure. Right atrial pressure is characteristically greatly elevated in severe cases, but atrial distention is characteristically limited compared with heart failure. The stimulus to atrial natriuretic peptide secretion is therefore lacking, which contributes to severe salt and water retention.[85]

The pathophysiology of constrictive pericarditis and cardiac tamponade has been emphasized and treated at some length because it is so important in understanding the clinical and hemodynamic features of these conditions and of restrictive cardiomyopathy. Furthermore, a clear understanding of what is known and what is not known about the pathophysiology of these three conditions serves as a guide to the many publications claiming to have established a single foolproof test to distinguish between restrictive cardiomyopathy and constrictive pericarditis.

Etiology

It is probably wise to assume that any cause of pericarditis, with the probable exception of rheumatic heart disease, may eventually result in constrictive pericarditis, but the more common causes should always be considered first.[86] These more common causes include *neoplastic pericardial disease*, usually secondary to carcinoma of the breast or lung, and *postradiation pericardiopathy*, which must always be considered in patients who have received extensive radiation for such conditions as lymphoma or malignant disease with metastatic thoracic involvement. *Trauma* is a significant etiologic factor that requires that any patient with constrictive pericarditis be questioned carefully about prior thoracic trauma, which, in many of the cases, occurred some years earlier. It is regrettable that *infections* may still be the cause of constrictive pericarditis, although in many instances, this undesirable sequel to purulent pericarditis can be avoided through prompt and adequate medical or surgical treatment. *Tuberculosis*[87, 88] can still cause constrictive pericarditis; although tuberculous pericarditis is relatively uncommon in the United States and western Europe, it is still rampant in many parts of the world, where it remains an important cause of effusive-constrictive pericarditis that results in chronic constrictive pericarditis if not adequately managed. *H. influenzae* can cause constrictive pericarditis, especially in children, and is often subacute. *Collagen vascular diseases* often involve the pericardium and may eventually develop into constrictive pericarditis.[89] Rheumatoid arthritis is the most common offender among this group; again, this is a form of constrictive pericarditis that may be subacute rather than chronic.[90] Rarely, constrictive pericarditis is *drug induced*, with the most notorious example perhaps being that of methysergide.[91] Constrictive pericarditis may be *iatrogenic*; the most common of this form of pericarditis occurs after intracardiac surgery.[92] Fortunately, this complication of intracardiac surgery is far less common than one might have anticipated, considering the trauma to which the pericardium is exposed. It is thought to occur after 0.1 to 0.3 percent of cardiac operations. Nevertheless, despite its low prevalence, constrictive pericarditis must be included in the differential diagnosis of any patient who, after cardiac surgery, demonstrates signs suggestive of right heart failure. When there is no apparent cause for right heart failure, such as left heart failure, whether systolic or diastolic, malfunction of a prosthesis, or severe ischemia, postoperative constrictive pericarditis must be considered. Evaluation may require imaging of the pericardium, as well as hemodynamic studies, which should demonstrate the findings discussed in preceding paragraphs. In some of these cases, it may be difficult to distinguish between postoperative pericarditis and the postoperative development of restrictive cardiomyopathy. Therefore, when such patients are investigated, endomyocardial biopsy should be considered at the time of hemodynamic study. Cases have been reported after the placement of patch electrodes for implantable defibrillators[93] and after asbestos exposure.[94]

History

The history of any condition known to be associated with pericarditis, particularly those mentioned in the preceding paragraph, is of great importance in establishing the diagnosis. The symptoms are similar to those of right heart failure, notably edema, increased abdominal girth, increased weight, breathlessness, and fatigue. Right-sided congestion usually predominates over left. When the condition is chronic, these symptoms are progressive. Unfortunately, by the time many of the patients consult a physician, these complaints are long-standing and far advanced.

Clinical Examination

The findings on clinical examination clearly depend on the severity and chronicity of constrictive pericarditis. The most important physical finding, the critical nature of which cannot be overemphasized, is the abnormal jugular venous pressure. In severe cases, the jugular venous pressure is often elevated to as much as 20 cm H_2O. To appreciate elevated jugular venous pressure of this severity, the patient must be examined sitting upright or standing up, as the characteristic jugular venous pulsations are damped when the patient is examined in a semirecumbent posture. Frequently, the external jugular vein is distended and prominent, but it is still desirable to evaluate the jugular venous pulse whenever possible. As described earlier, the dominant abnormality is the rapid deep *y* descent of the jugular venous pulse. The correct timing of this event is determined by palpating the contralateral carotid artery, enabling the clinician to be satisfied that the inward movement of the jugular pulse, being out of phase with the carotid pulse, is in fact a *y* descent. In less extreme cases, the jugular venous pressure may best be determined with the patient's thorax elevated to 30, 45, or 70 degrees from the horizontal, depending on the severity of increase in central venous pressure. The examiner should constantly change the posture of the patient's thorax to determine the optimal angle at which to assess the central venous pressure from the jugular pulse. Many clinicians try to elicit the Kussmaul sign when examining the venous pressure in constrictive pericarditis, but this procedure is of little diagnostic value. Atrial fibrillation is an almost invariable sequel in chronic cases. In mild, moderate, and early cases, sinus rhythm is the rule.

In the more severe and chronic cases, edema is impressive and may extend to the thighs; in males, it may involve the scrotum, which may become huge. In addition, in far advanced cases, ascites, often tense, can be diagnosed at the bedside through the usual maneuvers. In the most severe cases, dullness and decreased volume of breath sounds may indicate pleural effusion, which is common in long-standing constrictive pericarditis. Its origin is hemodynamic, and it does not imply, in most cases, associated pleural disease. In milder cases, signs of ascites and pleural effusion are usually absent, and edema may be less impressive and, in the mildest cases, even absent. In these mild cases, the jugular venous pressure is usually only about 7 or 8 cm H_2O, although the characteristic *y* descent is readily elicited.

One might anticipate that constrictive pericarditis may render the cardiac impulse impalpable; however, although this is sometimes the case, often it is not. Likewise, the heart sounds are not necessarily diminished in amplitude. In some case, there is retraction of the chest wall such that an inward motion accompanies the apex beat. In other cases, palpation of the heart does not reveal abnormal findings.

Examination of the abdomen is particularly important in constrictive pericarditis, because not only must the possibility of ascites be assessed but also the liver must be carefully examined. In severe cases, it is enlarged and usually pulsates (Fig. 65–9). The pulsation is caused by the high pressure and dominant *y* descent occurring in the hepatic veins, just as they do in the jugular veins.

There is no murmur characteristic of constrictive pericarditis, but the condition does not prevent auscultation of preexisting murmurs, such as that of aortic stenosis or sclerosis or that of mitral or tricuspid regurgitation. Characteristically, there is a loud third heart sound occurring approximately 100 ms after the second heart sound *(pericardial knock)*, and thus at a time comparable to that of the third heart sound of heart failure, and the opening snap of mitral stenosis.

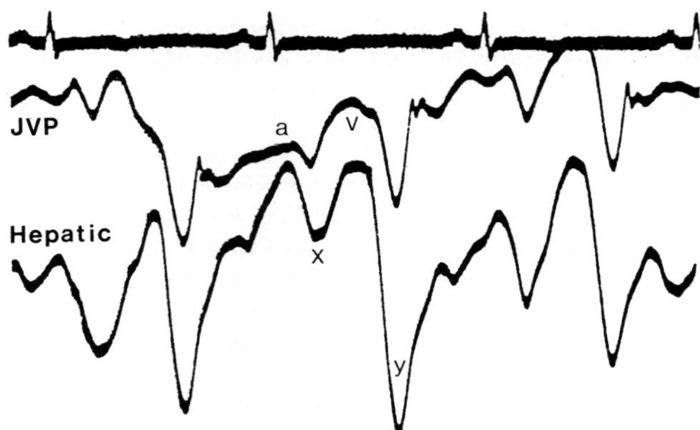

FIGURE 65–9 Noninvasive recordings of jugular venous (JVP) and hepatic pulsations in a patient with severe constrictive pericarditis. **Top,** Electrocardiogram. Displacement transducers were placed over the jugular and hepatic pulsations. Note the close correspondence in waveform. (From Manga P, Vythilingom S, Mitha A: Pulsatile hepatomegaly in constrictive pericarditis. Br Heart J 52:465, 1984.)

Laboratory Findings

In severe cases, routine clinical laboratory investigation discloses considerable metabolic derangement. The plasma concentration of sodium, chloride, and potassium may be decreased, especially in patients receiving large doses of diuretic. The blood urea nitrogen and serum creatinine concentrations are elevated, and creatinine clearance is markedly diminished. Liver function tests are abnormal, showing increased levels of bilirubin and enzymes, secondary to hepatic congestion. Hepatic congestion is also largely responsible for decreased levels of serum albumin, although in severe cases, protein-losing enteropathy may contribute to this phenomenon.[95] Additional laboratory abnormalities may be those associated with the underlying cause of constrictive pericarditis, such as collagen vascular disease or infection.

ELECTROCARDIOGRAM

The electrocardiogram characteristically shows no abnormality of ventricular depolarization, but nonspecific ST-segment and T-wave changes are common.[96] Rarely, depolarization changes, such as bundle branch block, may occur and have been attributed to involvement of the epicardial coronary arteries in the scar process.[97] Atrial fibrillation is common in long-standing cases. Other arrhythmias are uncommon. P mitrale is common in patients in whom sinus rhythm is preserved.

CHEST RADIOGRAM

One might anticipate that the heart would appear small on the chest radiogram. Although this is often true, it is by no means a universal finding. In some cases, cardiac enlargement preexisted from valvular or other disease of the heart. Sometimes, heart size is difficult to evaluate because of pleural effusion and a high diaphragm. In some cases, especially the more chronic and those due to tuberculosis, calcification of the pericardium is easily seen (Fig. 65–10). Its presence is best evaluated in a lateral or oblique projection. Calcification is also easily recognized on the chest computed tomogram (Fig. 65–11). Small areas of calcification may be seen in the pericardium of patients who have no evidence of pericarditis, constrictive or otherwise. The appearance of calcification in constrictive pericarditis is that of a complete or nearly complete ring (see Fig. 65–10). Calcification of the pericardium can be appreciated at cardiac fluoroscopy. Severe pulmonary hypertension does not develop, and impairment of the right ventricle is the same as that of the left. These features may explain why pulmonary venous congestion is less apparent in constrictive pericarditis than in patients with heart failure who have the same or similar elevation of pulmonary venous pressure.

ECHOCARDIOGRAPHY

Although the echocardiogram is the best laboratory test for pericardial effusion, it has not proved to be particularly helpful in providing a diagnostic image of the pericardium in constrictive pericarditis.[98] In very severe cases, the increased thickness and calcification of the pericardium are reasonably apparent on the M-mode and two-dimensional echocardiogram,[99] but in many proven cases of constrictive pericarditis, these findings are doubtful or absent. Careful inspection of diastole may show that ventricular volume increases rapidly in early diastole but remains static during the remainder of diastole. This finding is somewhat subjective and, in any case, does not differentiate between restrictive cardiomyopathy and constrictive pericarditis. Abnormal notching of the interventricular septum[100] related to atrial systole[98] has been described, but the finding, although fairly specific, is highly insensitive. By and large, echocardiography is disappointing as a tool with which to evaluate the anatomy and pathology of the pericardium in constrictive pericarditis. However, Doppler echocardiography is a most important tool in the evaluation of this condition, as is discussed under the context of the differential diagnosis of constrictive pericarditis and restrictive cardiomyopathy.

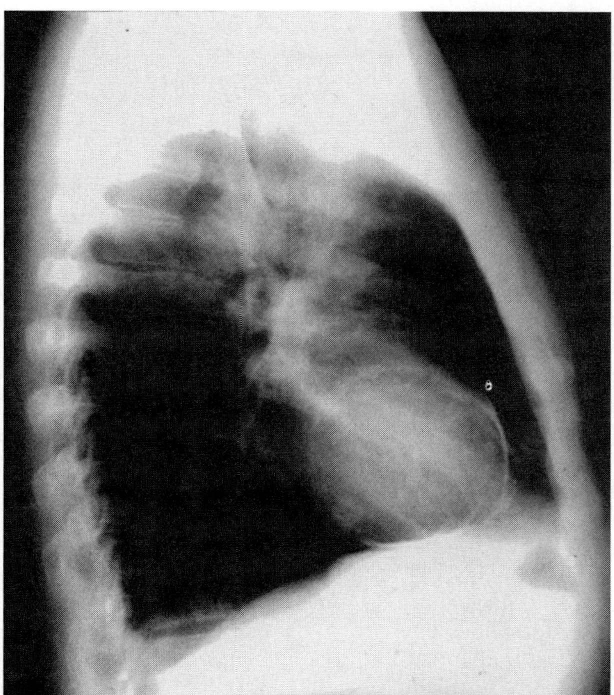

FIGURE 65–10 Lateral chest radiogram of a patient with chronic calcific pericarditis. The ring of calcium is clearly seen.

OTHER IMAGING MODALITIES

The pericardium is imaged well with computed tomography.[101, 102] In normal subjects, it either is invisible or appears as a thin line not exceeding 2 mm in thickness. In many cases of constrictive pericarditis, the pericardial thickness is greatly increased, sometimes to as much as 1 cm or more (see Fig. 65–11). Calcification can be identified when present. Unfortunately, in some cases, the scarred visceral pericardium forms a very tight skin around the heart but is not particularly increased in thickness. Thus, although the detection of increased pericardial thickness is of great value in the diagnosis and in the differential diagnosis from restrictive cardiomyopathy, false-negative results do occur.

Magnetic resonance imaging is another technique that provides highly satisfactory images of an abnormally thickened pericardium (Fig. 65–12).[103] Some consider magnetic resonance imaging superior to computed tomography as a tool to image the pericardium. Either one of these techniques is indicated in any case in which the diagnosis of constrictive pericarditis is reasonable.

CARDIAC CATHETERIZATION

In many cases, the diagnosis of constrictive pericarditis can be reached on the basis of clinical and noninvasive laboratory studies. Two major indications for cardiac catheterizations are doubt as to whether the patient has constrictive pericarditis or restrictive cardiomyopathy and evaluation for pericardiectomy. In the former case, endomyocardial biopsy performed during cardiac catheterization may be of critical value in the differential diagnosis,[104] and in the latter, assessment of the coronary arteries is important. The findings have been described in detail under the discussion of pathophysiology. The right atrial pressure shows absence of significant respiratory variation and prominence of the x and y descents, and the ventricular pressures are characterized by the early diastolic dip followed by the mid and late diastolic plateau (Fig. 65–13). Equilibration of pressures in diastole on the left and right sides of the heart is characteristic. The coronary arteries may show lack of the normal accordion effect[105] and an abnormal profile of blood flow.[106] Furthermore, the vessels do not appear to lie on the surface of the cardiopericardial silhouette in any fluoroscopic projection. When studying patients for signs of constrictive pericarditis, extra attention should be given to obtaining tracings as nearly critically damped as possible. Otherwise, damping artifact may be difficult to distinguish from the true dip and plateau. Extra care should also be directed to ensuring that the transducers

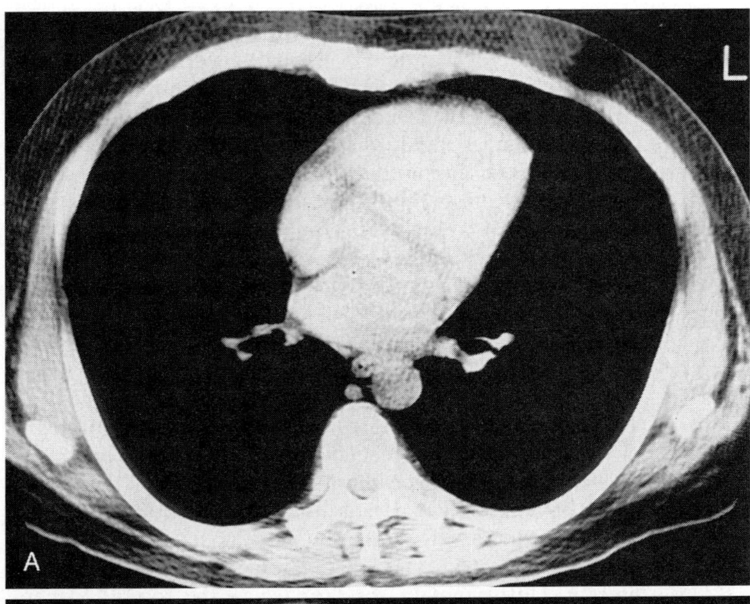

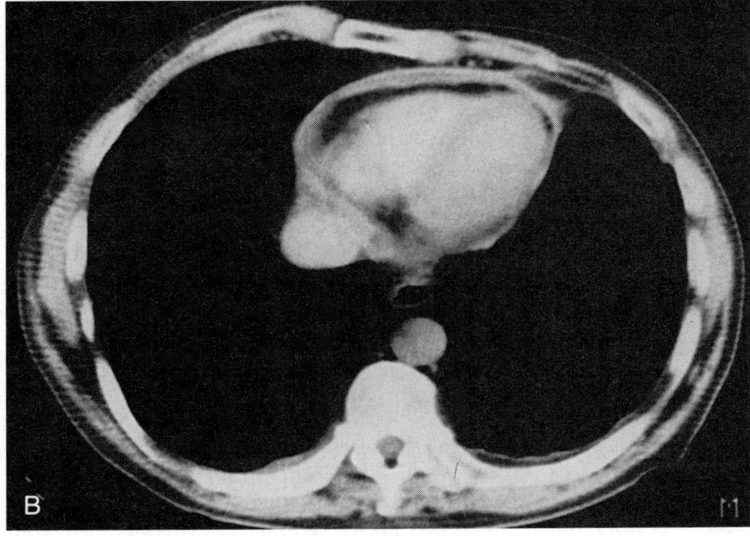

FIGURE 65–11 **A,** Computed tomogram from a patient without pericardial disease. **B,** Computed tomogram of a patient with calcified constrictive pericarditis. The calcification is clearly seen with use of this technique.

are leveled at the same height and that the pressure recordings are truly equisensitive. If the patient is thought to have constrictive pericarditis and the diastolic pressure of one ventricle during diastasis significantly exceeds that of the other, the attachments of the left and right ventricular catheters to transducers should be reversed. This technique will rapidly distinguish a true intraventricular diastolic pressure difference from a recording artifact.

It is important to recall that pulmonary wedge pressure varies normally, often in an exaggerated way during the respiratory cycle, whereas right atrial pressure varies little, if at all, with respiration. Therefore, the much-sought-after equilibration between pulmonary wedge and right atrial pressures may not be present throughout the respiratory cycle but is instead confined to inspiration (see Fig. 65–13).

It has been pointed out earlier that tight ventricular interaction and insulation of the cardiac chambers from variation of intrathoracic pressure during the respiratory cycle are two key mechanisms underlying the pathophysiology of constrictive pericarditis.[107] These mechanisms explain why respiratory variation of peak systolic pressures in the two ventricles is out of phase in constrictive pericarditis (with maximal left ventricular pressure occurring when right ventricular pressure is minimal) and why with inspiration pulmonary venous pressure declines but left ventricular diastolic pressure remains constant. The consequence of a smaller pulmonary venous–to–left ventricular diastolic pressure gradient is an inspiratory decline in left ventricular filling and a smaller ventricle. The right ventricle therefore fills more, and its systolic pressure increases. Another consequence is that any tricuspid regurgitation that may be present increases in magnitude and velocity in the first beat after the onset of inspiration.[108] In restrictive cardiomyopathy, ventricular interaction is not increased above normal, and the left ventricle is not insulated from respiratory fluctuations of thoracic pressure. The diastolic pressure gradient from the pulmonary vein to the left ventricle does not decline significantly during inspiration, the left and right ventricular peak systolic pressures are in phase, right ventricular systolic pressure declines during

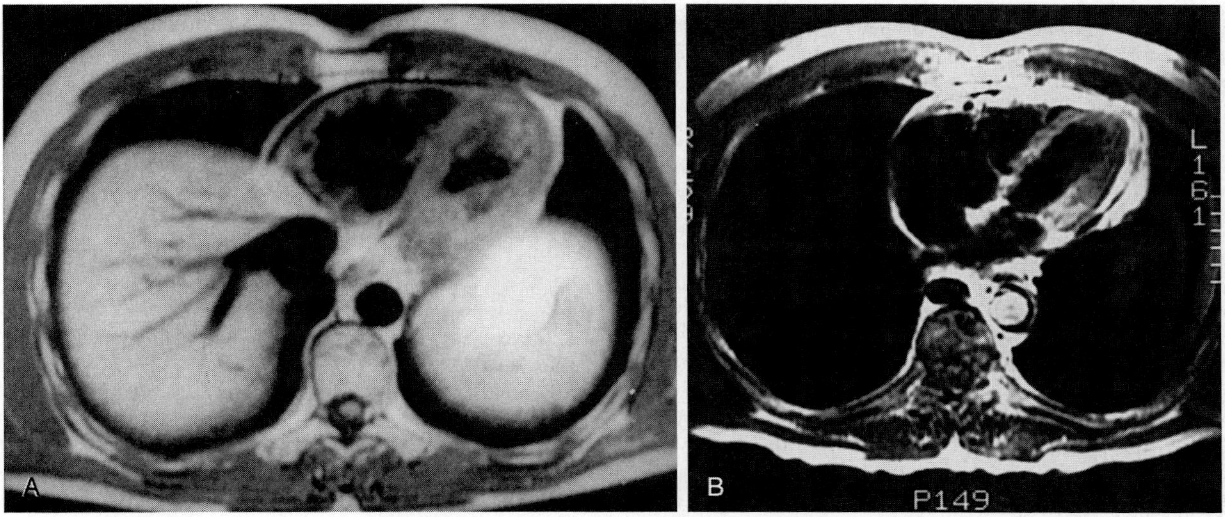

FIGURE 65–12 A, Magnetic resonance image of a patient without pericardial disease. The pericardium is visualized at the top of the image as a thin, dark, curved line. **B,** Magnetic resonance image from a patient with constrictive pericarditis secondary to tuberculosis. The dark area (top right) is a grossly thickened and calcified pericardium. The low-intensity line around the thick-walled left ventricle is pericardium with epicardial and pericardial fat.

inspiration, and tricuspid regurgitation does not increase in velocity and magnitude in the first beat after inspiration.

If ventriculography is performed, some degree of mitral and tricuspid regurgitation may be observed. Filling confined to early diastole can be suspected from the gross appearance of the ventriculogram but is best documented by a digital frame-by-frame analysis of ventricular volume throughout diastole. Endomyocardial biopsy is particularly safe when the patient has constrictive pericarditis because it is virtually impossible to create intrapericardial bleeding.

Diagnosis

As is true for pericardial disease in general, the key to successful diagnosis is a high index of suspicion. The possibility of constrictive pericarditis should be considered in any patient with fluid retention and a high jugular venous pressure when these findings are not readily explained. When evaluating patients with fluid retention, the determination of the jugular or central venous pressure is of paramount importance. If the patient has ascites and edema but a normal jugular venous pressure, it is at once clear that the cause is neither cardiac nor pericardial. Attention must then be directed away from the cardiovascular system to diseases of the liver, kidneys, and lymphatic systems. When the jugular venous pressure is indeed high, the distinction is between cardiac disease and pericardial disease. Pericardial disease becomes a serious consideration when no etiologic factor suggesting heart disease is present, whereas possible causes of pericardial disease are present or occurred in the prior history. Significant cardiac murmurs, calcification of cardiac valves, abnormal depolarization patterns of electrocardiogram, and evidence of ventricular systolic dysfunction are absent. Here, the echocardiogram plays an important role. Although it was mentioned earlier that this tool is disappointing as a means to image the pericardium itself, it is important in distinguishing between heart disease and constrictive pericarditis. In the former, ventricular systolic function may be documented as severely depressed, and major abnormalities of valvular structure and function can readily be documented. Tricuspid valve disease must also be ruled out before arriving at a diagnosis of constrictive pericarditis. Tricuspid regurgitation can be the cause of massive fluid retention,

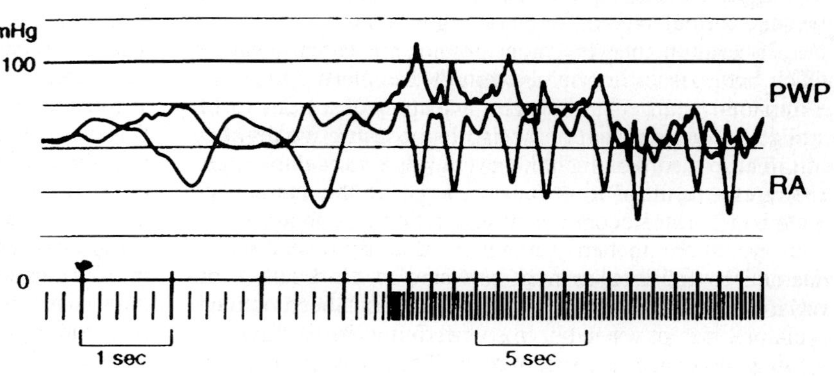

FIGURE 65–13 Simultaneously recorded pulmonary wedge (PWP) and right atrial (RA) pressures in a patient with surgically proven constrictive pericarditis. Note that respiratory variation of RA pressure is small, whereas that of the PWP is more marked. Hence, the pressures are closer to each other during inspiration. Both pressures are substantially elevated.

greatly elevated jugular venous pressure, a jugular venous waveform characterized by the absence of respiratory variation and a sharp *y* descent, and by an enlarged pulsating liver.

In clinical practice, confusion of constrictive pericarditis with cirrhosis of the liver is a considerably more common problem than confusion with heart disease. Common to both constrictive pericarditis and heart failure is massive edema and ascites, sometimes with a pleural effusion, and an enlarged pulsating liver with abnormal liver function tests. Not surprisingly, a significant number of such patients are referred to a gastroenterology department for further evaluation. That evaluation is often extensive and includes abdominal scanning, evaluation of portal hypertension, and sometimes liver biopsy. The lesson is that had the venous pressure been evaluated by the referring physician, the patient would have been sent not to a gastroenterologist but rather to a cardiologist, and had the gastroenterologist recognized the high jugular venous pressure, that physician would have quickly referred the patient to a cardiologist. When a patient is first seen with anasarca, the most important step is to evaluate the central venous pressure. In the vast majority of cases, this can be done during simple bedside examination. In the few cases in which it cannot, a catheter can be placed into the superior vena cava or right atrium to establish the pressure. This procedure is simple and of low cost, and its results are rewarding.

Differentiation From Restrictive Cardiomyopathy

One of the more difficult problems faced by the clinician evaluating a patient with clinical features consistent with constrictive pericarditis is to exclude the alternative possibility of restrictive cardiomyopathy.[109, 110] In some cases, this distinction is straightforward and easily made; in a minority, it is difficult to make the distinction without extensive laboratory investigation; and finally, there are some patients in whom the distinction can by made only during surgery. It should also be recalled that some patients have a combination of myocardial disease and constrictive pericarditis. In these cases, the clinician's function is to assess the relative contributions of myocardial and pericardial pathology, because some patients may benefit from pericardiectomy despite some degree of myocardial involvement. Radiation injury is an important cause of combined cardiomyopathy and constrictive pericarditis. Patients who have constrictive pericarditis as a complication of prior cardiac surgery may also have sustained intraoperative myocardial injury. Neoplasm more commonly affects the pericardium than the myocardium, but cases occur in which both tissues are involved in the neoplastic process.

Impaired ventricular filling is a feature of a number of cardiac conditions that do not simulate constrictive pericarditis. These disorders include severe left ventricular hypertrophy as a result of hypertension, hypertrophic cardiomyopathy, or aortic stenosis. Ventricular filling is abnormal in other conditions that may impair ventricular relaxation or diastolic compliance, as may be found in heart failure of many causes. Restrictive cardiomyopathy has been defined in many different ways, but in connection with the differential diagnosis from constrictive pericarditis, a specific and clinically useful definition is needed. Thus, restrictive cardiomyopathy can be defined as an idiopathic cardiomyopathy or systemic myocardial disorder in which the clinical picture strongly simulates constrictive pericarditis. Significant ventricular hypertrophy or dilatation and systolic dysfunction are absent or mild. The clinical approach to the differential diagnosis of restrictive cardiomyopathy, so defined, and constrictive pericarditis is outlined in the next paragraphs.

HISTORY

The history may be of great value. Prior acute pericarditis, tuberculosis, rheumatoid arthritis, radiation therapy, malignancy, trauma, or other disease that frequently involves the pericardium strongly favors constrictive pericarditis. A history of a disease such as amyloidosis, of hemochromatosis, or of cardiac transplantation[111] that may involve the myocardium would point strongly to restrictive cardiomyopathy, although it is important to bear in mind that restrictive cardiomyopathy may be idiopathic. Restrictive cardiomyopathy may occur after orthotopic cardiac transplantation, in which it may be a transient phenomenon in the early weeks after the procedure but uncommonly may persist indefinitely.

PHYSICAL EXAMINATION

The foregoing definition of restrictive cardiomyopathy requires that the physical findings closely simulate those of constrictive pericarditis. It stands to reason, therefore, that clinical examination is not helpful in the differential diagnosis. Both conditions are characterized by an elevated jugular venous pressure, with the venous pulse displaying a prominent *y* descent. Edema, hepatomegaly, and other manifestations of systemic congestion are present in both disorders. It is not possible to distinguish reliably between a pericardial knock and a third heart sound that may be present in restrictive cardiomyopathy. In both conditions, if the cardiac impulse is palpable, evidence for cardiac enlargement may be lacking, but as mentioned earlier, the heart size is not necessarily normal in constrictive pericarditis and in restrictive cardiomyopathy massive atrial enlargement may cause radiologic, if not clinical, cardiomegaly. Prominent systolic murmurs are unusual in either condition, and diastolic murmurs should not occur at all unless caused by an unrelated valvular lesion.

ELECTROCARDIOGRAM

The electrocardiogram of constrictive pericarditis has been described in an earlier paragraph. It shows nonspecific ST-segment and T-wave changes. In more advanced cases, the P wave is wide in lead II and biphasic in lead V_1 and thus indistinguishable from the P mitrale of mitral stenosis. In the later stages, atrial fibrillation supervenes. As may be anticipated, depolarization changes are present in restrictive cardiomyopathy in addition to the repolarization changes that characterize constrictive pericarditis. The most common is left bundle branch block, although in some cases, right bundle branch block or a nonspecific interventricular conduction defect is found. Other cases may show left ventricular hypertrophy with attendant repolarization abnormalities. Delayed atrial ventricular conduction may also be present. In addition to atrial fibrillation, other arrhythmias are common; they include ventricular extrasystoles from numerous sites, ventricular tachycardia, and an assortment of atrial tachycardias. In some cases, sinus rhythm or sinus tachycardia is dominant. Abnormal Q waves simulating myocardial infarction are found in the minority of cases despite a normal coronary arteriogram. In a minority of cases of constrictive pericarditis, conduction and depolarization changes similar to those of myocardial disease may be encountered.[97] Abnormalities of depolarization or conduction very strongly favor myocardial over pericardial disease, but abnormalities confined to repolarization are equally likely in myocardial or pericardial disease and therefore are entirely unhelpful in their differential diagnosis.

CHEST RADIOGRAM

The only chest radiographic finding likely to be helpful in the differential diagnosis is calcification of the pericardium as may occur in the most chronic cases. However, in many cases of severe constrictive pericarditis, calcification is absent. Minor degrees of calcification can be detected in the pericardium by fluoroscopy or with greater sensitivity by computed tomography. However, these minor degrees of calcification are for the most part unrelated to constrictive pericarditis. Significant calcification of the pericardium is absent in restrictive cardiomyopathy. Thus, the finding of a dense ring of calcium on the chest radiogram virtually ensures the diagnosis of constrictive pericarditis, but its absence is equally compatible with constrictive pericarditis or restrictive cardiomyopathy.

IMAGING MODALITIES

A thick pericardium demonstrated by an imaging technique can be interpreted as strong supportive evidence for constrictive pericarditis compared with restrictive cardiomyopathy. The thickness of the pericardium can be measured by transesophageal echocardiography, which in addition may show increased echogenicity. Unfortunately, the transthoracic echocardiogram is not a sensitive tool with which to detect increased thickness of the pericardium. The normal sliding of the heart on the pericardium best seen in the subcostal views is absent in constrictive pericarditis. Transesophageal echocardiography provides accurate measurements of pericardial thickness.[66] More reliable than transthoracic echocardiography are computed tomography and magnetic resonance imaging. In some cases of constrictive pericarditis, particularly those primarily involving the visceral pericardium, the appearance of the pericardium may be normal. Nevertheless, imaging of the pericardium remains a useful tool because false-negative results are uncommon.[109]

DOPPLER ECHOCARDIOGRAPHY

Doppler echocardiography is a noninvasive reliable method to help distinguish constrictive pericarditis from restrictive cardiomyopathy.[112] The underlying pathophysiologic mechanisms are that constrictive pericarditis increases coupling between the two ventricles[113] and that the myocardium comprising the ventricular septum is abnormal in cardiomyopathy but uninvolved by constrictive pericarditis. Thus, it is posited that respiratory variations in ventricular filling and emptying velocities are much greater in patients with constrictive pericarditis than in those with restrictive cardiomyopathy.[51] Common to both conditions is abnormally fast early rapid diastolic filling of the left and right ventricles. This factor, together with early equilibration of atrial and ventricular pressures, shortens the deceleration time of the early rapid filling wave from its normal lower limit of 150 ms. In restrictive cardiomyopathy, but not in constrictive pericarditis, inspiration further abbreviates the shortened deceleration time of early rapid ventricular filling.

In normal subjects breathing quietly, the peak rate of early rapid left ventricular filling may decline by up to 10 percent during inspiration, and the velocity of early rapid filling of the right ventricle may increase by up to about 15 percent during inspiration.[114] This relatively small reciprocal variation with respiration in early rapid filling of the two ventricles appears rather inconspicuous on Doppler interrogation. A number of investigators have found that in patients with constrictive pericarditis, these reciprocal variations in the rates of left and right ventricular filling related to the respiratory cycle are greatly exaggerated.[51, 112] When constrictive pericarditis is strongly suspected but exaggerated respiratory variation in transmitral and transtricuspid blood flow velocities is not detected, the patient can be reexamined in the head-up tilt position to bring out this Doppler sign. Ejection through the semilunar valves shows similar reciprocal variation. However, many investigators have found that pulsus paradoxus is unusual in constrictive pericarditis.[115] In restrictive cardiomyopathy, respiratory variation in the rate of ventricular filling during early diastole is not increased above normal.

Pulmonary venous and superior vena caval pressures in normal subjects show predominance of the x over the y descent and, accordingly, systolic inflow velocity that exceeds diastolic. Respiratory variation in diastolic pulmonary venous return is small. In both constrictive pericarditis and restrictive cardiomyopathy, diastolic inflow velocity may exceed systolic and may show increased respiratory variation. Retrograde flow during atrial systole may be found in restrictive cardiomyopathy but does not occur to any significant extent in normal subjects and is reported to be less common in patients with constrictive pericarditis. Satisfactory evaluation of pulmonary venous blood flow velocity may require the use of transesophageal echocardiography. In both constrictive pericarditis and restrictive cardiomyopathy, the velocity profile of systemic venous return resembles that of pulmonary venous return.

Acute Pericarditis

Acute pericarditis may take many forms, such as acute cardiac tamponade or subacute constrictive pericarditis. The term, however, is commonly reserved for what has been called *acute fibrinous*, or *dry, pericarditis*, a syndrome consisting of chest pain, pericardial friction rub, and diffuse electrocardiographic ST-segment elevation.

Etiology

Acute pericarditis is often idiopathic or secondary to viral infection. Many of the idiopathic cases may in reality be secondary to viral infection, but this cause can only be presumed unless acute and chronic viral titers establish that there has been recent infection with a virus, especially one that tends to infect the heart and pericardium. Any of the causes of pericarditis listed earlier in the chapter may be responsible for the acute syndrome. More common causes include myocardial infarction, leukemia, and neoplasm; somewhat less frequent are rheumatic carditis, collagen vascular disease, uremia, and drug-induced illness.

Pathology

The pathology is that of acute inflammation. The pericardium is slightly thickened owing to edema. *Acute fibrinous pericarditis* owes its name to the widespread shaggy coat of fibrin noted at autopsy or surgical exploration. This feature is particularly noticeable in patients with hemodialysis-related acute pericarditis, which also tends to have a hemorrhagic appearance.

Symptoms

In the case of viral pericarditis, the specific findings of pericarditis are often preceded by a nonspecific influenza-like prodromal syndrome. The most common major presenting complaint is chest pain that frequently has features resembling both myocardial ischemic pain and pleuritic pain. It is commonly retrosternal and somewhat crushing in nature but is often aggravated by inspiration and coughing and may be relieved by sitting up. It tends not to radiate in a manner characteristic of myocardial ischemic pain, but its crushing nature can lead to an initial misdiagnosis of acute myocardial infarction. A characteristic site of radiation is the trapezius ridge, especially the left. The chest pain is sometimes accompanied by dysphagia. As in pleurisy, respiration may be shallow and rapid, causing the patient to complain of dyspnea. Additionally, symptoms of viremia and toxemia may be present, as may symptoms of the underlying cause.

Clinical Examination

Clinical examination frequently shows a patient with fever in varying degrees of acute distress, such as tachycardia, sweating, and flushing. The pathognomonic physical finding is the pericardial friction rub. This abnormal auscultatory feature commonly is best heard along the mid to lower left sternal edge, between the sternal edge and apex, or at the apex itself. However, it may be widespread and audible over the entire precordium. It has a superficial scratching character and seems to the examiner to originate closer to the patient's skin than do heart sounds and murmurs. It is usually fairly fine and high pitched, but in some cases, especially those associated with uremia, it may be lower pitched and more coarse and may even be palpable. The friction rub may vary in distribution and intensity from time to time. In acute pericarditis after myocardial infarction, the rub is often inconstant and is not detected unless the patient is carefully auscultated on frequent occasions. The intensity and character of the pericardial friction rub are apt to change with patient posture and in many cases become louder during inspiration. When the murmur is heard only during inspiration, it is frequently referred to as a *pleuropericardial rub*. The rub is usually heard better with the diaphragm chest piece of the stethoscope. Firm pressure with the diaphragm over the chest facilitates recognition of the pericardial friction rub. The friction may obscure cardiac murmurs that may be present. This problem can be particularly difficult in children with acute rheumatic pancarditis and in pregnant women with acute viral pericarditis.

The classic pericardial friction rub has three components: atrial systolic, ventricular systolic, and diastolic.[116] Sometimes only the systolic and diastolic components are present, in which case the clinician must be careful to differentiate it from a to-and-fro murmur, such as that of aortic regurgitation. Less commonly, the pericardial friction rub is confined to systole and then must be differentiated from various causes of systolic murmurs. Mediastinal air may simulate the pericardial friction rub; in addition, in some thin patients with a hyperactive precordium, an artifactual sound caused by the skin rubbing on the chest piece of the stethoscope may be confused with a pericardial friction rub. A pericardial friction rub is almost routinely audible for the first several days after cardiac surgery. It is important to reemphasize that the presence of a large pericardial effusion does not prevent the development of a pericardial friction rub, a common observation that suggests that the mechanism of production of pericardial friction rubs is more complex than the rubbing of the epicardium against the parietal pericardium.

ELECTROCARDIOGRAM

Electrocardiogram of acute pericarditis is characterized by diffuse elevation of the ST segment.[117] Myocardial ischemia, unlike acute pericarditis, is not likely to cause elevation of the ST segment in leads I, II, III, and aVF. The ST segment in acute pericarditis is usually depressed; however, it is elevated in leads aVR and V_1. In contrast to the pattern of evolving myocardial infarction, the T wave remains upright at the time that the ST segment is elevated. Depression of the PR segment is a specific but nonsensitive sign of acute pericarditis (Fig. 65–14). If one has the opportunity to observe the patient over several days, one may observe that as the ST segment moves toward the baseline, the electrocardiogram may become normal before showing the findings of more chronic pericarditis (i.e., an isoelectric ST segment with T-wave inversion).[96]

CLINICAL LABORATORY FINDINGS

There usually is elevation of the erythrocyte sedimentation rate and leukocytosis, as expected in an acute viral infection. If acute pericarditis is a manifestation of a systemic disease, such as uremia, rheumatoid arthritis, or myocardial infarction, the laboratory data will help in determination of the underlying cause of pericarditis. Mild elevation of the creatine kinase–MB and troponins I and T may be present when there is no other evidence of myocarditis. However,

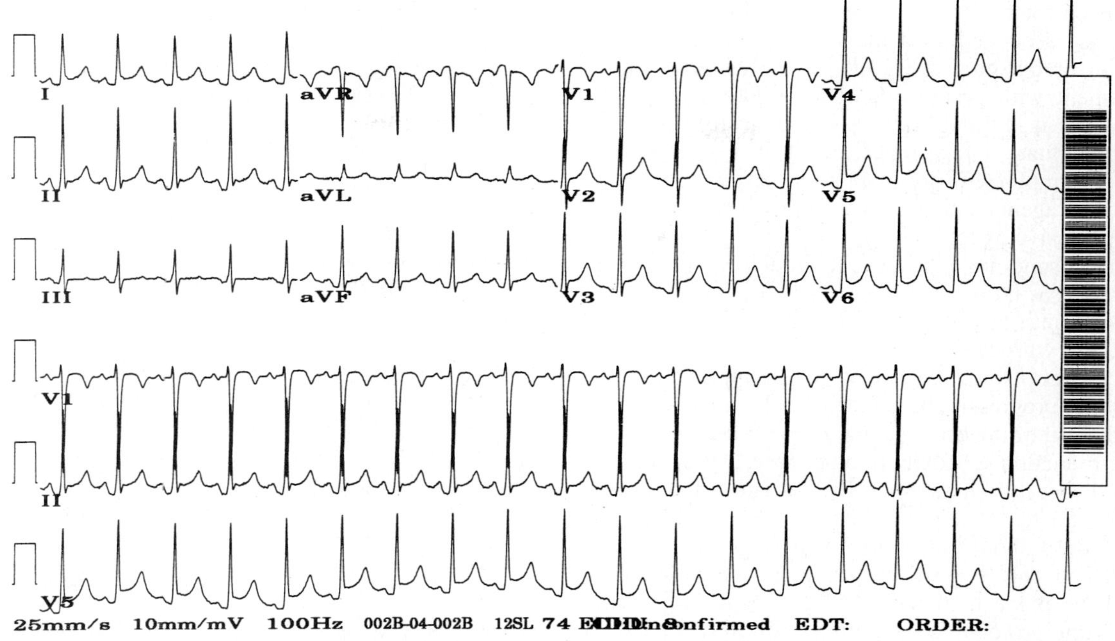

FIGURE 65–14 Electrocardiogram from a patient with acute viral or idiopathic pericarditis. Note ST-segment elevation in leads I, aVF, aVL, and V_4 through V_6 and PR-segment depression in leads I and II and in leads V_3 through V_6. The ST segment is depressed in lead aVR.

some cases of acute pericarditis are indeed a manifestation of acute myopericarditis.

ECHOCARDIOGRAM

Echocardiography is quite often carried out to confirm the clinical diagnosis of acute pericarditis or to establish it in more doubtful cases, such as those in whom a pericardial friction rub has never been heard or in whom the electrocardiogram is atypical. In some of these cases, the study will show a small, clinically unsuspected pericardial effusion. This finding is a useful confirmation of pericarditis in patients in whom a clinical diagnosis has not been established before echocardiography was performed. Patients with a small pericardial effusion are still considered to have "dry" pericarditis. Unless the effusion is growing large or causing cardiac tamponade, it should be managed in the same way as in patients without a pericardial effusion. The absence of pericardial effusion by no means excludes the diagnosis of pericarditis, which may indeed be dry. In uncomplicated cases, the echocardiogram confirms the absence of myocardial or valvular disease and demonstrates normal size and function of the cardiac chambers.

CHEST RADIOGRAM

Radiographically, the chest usually appears normal, but in some cases an associated parenchymal opacity or pleural effusion may be detected.

Clinical Course

The majority of patients have a benign course. The initial treatment consists of an anti-inflammatory agent. Aspirin may be used for this purpose, but more commonly, a nonsteroidal anti-inflammatory agent such as indomethacin is prescribed. With this treatment, most patients are free from pain and fever within 24 to 48 hours. Treatment is usually continued for 1 or 2 weeks. In a few patients, this treatment is unsuccessful. Colchicine (1 to 2 mg/day) may then be effective with or without continuation of the other anti-inflammatory agent, the dose of which can be escalated if necessary. Only when these therapies fail should prednisone be used.

Some patients with acute pericarditis will progress to acute cardiac tamponade, and some will present initially with this syndrome. Rarely, acute pericarditis may lead to constrictive pericarditis.

Recurrent Pericarditis

The most important complication of acute pericarditis is recurrent or relapsing pericarditis. This syndrome may follow an episode of idiopathic or viral pericarditis. It may also follow Dressler's syndrome: pericarditis after trauma and postpericardiotomy syndrome. The latter is a form of pericarditis seen after the pericardium has been opened for cardiac surgery; it takes the form of acute pericarditis with or without effusion.

Relapsing pericarditis is uncommon but is an extremely troublesome and difficult syndrome to manage.[118] Recurrences may occur for a few weeks or months, but in many cases for years, sometimes many years. The principles of treatment are similar to those for an initial episode of acute pericarditis but unfortunately the condition may be more resistant to nonsteroidal anti-inflammatory agents. Again, colchicine has been proposed as a means to prevent or lessen the need for prednisone treatment.[119] Because of the complications associated with the frequent administration of high-dose prednisone, every effort should be made to avoid treatment with prednisone. This is particularly important because it is thought that withdrawal from prednisone can precipitate a recurrence. Nevertheless, there are patients who simply will not respond to any combination of nonsteroidal agents, and recourse to prednisone or other immunosuppressive agents must be had.[120]

When prednisone must be used, it should be initiated in high dose, such as 60 or 75 mg/day. This high dose should be maintained until all symptoms and signs of pericarditis, including the erythrocyte sedimentation rate, have returned to normal. After 1 or 2 weeks of total suppression, the dose should be progressively reduced. In the most successful cases, the use of the drug can be discontinued at the end of the dose-reduction schedule. In other cases, symptoms or signs may reoccur, such as when the patient has achieved a drop from 60 to 10 mg/day. In such cases, the lowest suppressing dose should be reinstituted (e.g., 15 mg/day) and maintained for 3 or 4 weeks, after which another attempt can be made to reduce the dose or to stop treatment. The same protocol is continued until all evidence of pericarditis disappears. After an interval of weeks, months, or, occasionally, years, the syndrome may recur, in which case treatment must begin all over again. Patients who do require prednisone must be watched carefully for osteoporosis or other evidence of major prednisone toxicity. When these symptoms occur or when it is clear that prednisone is not having the desired effect, consideration should be given to pericardiectomy. Unfortunately, although this operation sometimes cures the patient, relapses may still occur; in many such cases, recurrences are fewer and milder, and the syndrome probably burns out faster than it would have without the operation.

References

1. Russo AM, O'Connor WH, Waxman HL: Atypical presentations and echocardiographic findings in patients with cardiac tamponade occurring early and late after cardiac surgery. Chest 104:71–78, 1993.
2. Osler W: The Principles and Practice of Medicine. New York: Appleton, 1892.
3. Heidenreich PA, Eisenberg MJ, Kee LL, et al: Pericardial effusion in AIDS: incidence and survival. Circulation 92:3229, 1995.
4. Brook I, Frazier EH: Microbiology of acute purulent pericarditis: a 12-year experience in a military hospital. Arch Intern Med 156:1857, 1996.
5. Demey HE, Eycken M, Vandermast M, et al: Purulent pericarditis due to methicillin-resistant *Staphylococcus aureus*. Acta Cardiol 46:485, 1991.
6. Iseman MD, Cohn DL, Sbarbaro JA: Directly observed treatment of tuberculosis. N Engl J Med 328:576, 1993.
7. Horowitz HW, Belkin RN: Acute myopericarditis resulting from Lyme disease. Am Heart J 130:176, 1995.
8. Fulda G, Brathwaite CEM, Rodriguez A, et al: Blunt traumatic rupture of the heart and pericardium: a ten-year experience (1979–1989). J Trauma 31:167, 1991.
9. Cohen MV, Greenberg MA: Constrictive pericarditis: early and late complication of cardiac surgery. Am J Cardiol 43:657, 1979.
10. Schwartz DJ, Thanavaro S, Kleiger RE, et al: Epicardial pacemaker complicated by cardiac tamponade and constrictive pericarditis. Chest 76:226, 1979.
11. Jiha JG, Weinberg GL, Laurito CE: Intraoperative cardiac tamponade after central venous cannulation. Anesth Analg 82:664, 1996.
12. Lubliner J, Ghosh PK, Vidne BA: Cardiac tamponade and central venous catheter. Int Surg 70:79, 1985.
13. Jessurun GAJ, Crijns HJGM, van Wijngaarden J: An unusual case of cardiac tamponade following electrical cardioversion. Int J Cardiol 53:317, 1996.
14. Veinot JP, Edwards WD: Pathology of radiation-induced heart disease: a surgical and autopsy study of 27 cases. Hum Pathol 27:766, 1996.
15. Benoff LJ, Schweitzer P: Radiation therapy-induced cardiac injury. Am Heart J 129:1193, 1995.
16. Wilkes JD, Fidias P, Valckus L, et al: Malignancy-related pericardial effusion. 127 cases from the Roswell Park Cancer Institute. Cancer 76:1377, 1995.
17. Stewart JR, Fajardo LP, Gillette SM, et al: Radiation injury to the heart. Int J Radiat Oncol Biol Phys 31:1205, 1995.
18. Lashevsky I, Yosef RB, Rinkevich D, et al: Intrapericardial minocycline sclerosis for malignant pericardial effusion. Chest 109:1452, 1996.
19. Liu G, Crump M, Goss PE, et al: Prospective comparison of the sclerosing agents doxycycline and bleomycin for the primary management of malignant pericardial effusion and cardiac tamponade. J Clin Oncol 14:3141, 1996.
20. Kumar S, Lesch M: Pericarditis in renal disease. Prog Cardiovasc Dis 22:357, 1980.
21. Rutsky EA, Rostand SG: Treatment of uremic pericarditis and pericardial effusion. Am J Kidney Dis 10:2, 1987.
22. Kahl LE: The spectrum of pericardial tamponade in systemic lupus erythematosus: report of ten patients. Arthritis Rheum 35:1343, 1992.
23. Panchal P, Adams E, Hsieh A: Calcific constrictive pericarditis: a rare complication of CREST syndrome. Arthritis Rheum 39:347, 1996.
24. Galve E, Garcia-Del-Castillo H, Evangelista A, et al: Pericardial effusion in the course of myocardial infarction: incidence, natural history, and clinical relevance. Circulation 73:294, 1986.
25. Pierard LA, Albert A, Henrard L, et al: Incidence and significance of pericardial effusion in acute myocardial infarction as determined by two-dimensional echocardiography. J Am Coll Cardiol 8:517, 1986.
26. Marsa R, Mehta S, Willis N, et al: Constrictive pericarditis after myocardial revascularization: report of three cases. Am J Cardiol 44:177, 1979.
27. Bartels C, Honig R, Burger G, et al: The significance of anticardiolipin antibodies and anti-heart muscle antibodies for the diagnosis of postpericardiotomy syndrome. Eur Heart J 5:494, 1994.
28. Prabhu AS, Ross RD, Heinert MR, et al: Decreased incidence of postoperative pericardial effusions after cardiac surgery for congenital heart disease. Am J Cardiol 77:774, 1996.
29. Mewis C, Kühlkamp V, Sokiranski R, et al: Primary chylopericardium due to partial aplasia of the thoracic duct. Eur Heart J 18:880, 1997.
30. Tchervenkov CI, Dobell ARC: Chylopericardium following cardiac surgery. Can J Surg 28:542, 1985.
31. Mailander L, Van Meter C, Ventura H, et al: Chylopericardium after orthotopic heart transplantation. J Heart Lung Transplant 11:587, 1992.
32. Engel PJ: Echocardiographic findings in pericardial disease. *In* Fowler NO (ed): The Pericardium in Health and Disease. p. 99. New York: Futura, 1985.
33. Sinha PR, Singh BP, Jaipuria N, et al: Intrapericardial echogenic images and development of constrictive pericarditis in patients with pericardial effusion. Am Heart J 132:1268, 1996.
34. Rigney DR, Goldberger AL: Nonlinear mechanics of the heart's swinging during pericardial effusion. Am J Physiol 257:H1292, 1989.
35. Haiat R, Halpern L: Pericardial effusion in later pregnancy: a new entity. Cardiovasc Intervent Radiol 7:267, 1984.
36. Turco M, Seneff M, McGrath BJ, et al: Cardiac tamponade in the acquired immunodeficiency syndrome. Am Heart J 120:1467, 1990.
37. Maisch B, Drude L: Pericardioscopy—a new diagnostic tool in inflammatory diseases of the pericardium. Eur Heart J 12(suppl D):2, 1991.
38. Parmley LF, Manion WC, Mattingly TW: Non-penetrating traumatic injury of the heart. Circulation 18:371, 1958.
39. D'Cruz IA, Overton DH, Ganesh MP: Pericardial complications of cardiac surgery: emphasis on the diagnostic role of echocardiography. J Card Surg 7:257, 1992.

40. Nottestad SY, Mascette AM: Loculated pericardial effusion and cardiac tamponade late after cardiac surgery. Chest 101:852, 1992.
41. Kabadi UM, Kumar SP: Pericardial effusion in primary hypothyroidism. Am Heart J 120:1393, 1990.
42. Permanyer-Miralda G, Sagrista-Sauleda J, Soler-Soler J: Primary acute pericardial disease: a prospective series of 231 consecutive patients. Am J Cardiol 56:623, 1985.
43. Merce J, Sagrista-Sauleda J, Permanyer-Miralda G, et al: Should pericardial drainage be performed routinely in patients who have a large pericardial effusion without tamponade? Am J Med 105:106, 1998.
44. Colombo A, Olson HG, Egan J, et al: Etiology and prognostic implications of a large pericardial effusion in men. Clin Cardiol 11:389, 1988.
45. Olsen PS, Sorensen C, Andersen HO: Surgical treatment of large pericardial effusions: etiology and long-term survival. Eur J Cardiothorac Surg 5:430, 1991.
46. Reddy PS, Curtiss EI, Uretsky BF: Spectrum of hemodynamic changes in cardiac tamponade. Am J Cardiol 66:1487, 1990.
47. D'Cruz IA, Cohen HC, Ravindra P, et al: Diagnosis of cardiac tamponade by echocardiography: changes in mitral valve motion and ventricular dimensions, with special reference to paradoxical pulse. Circulation 52:460, 1975.
48. Kronzon I, Cohen ML, Winer HE: Diastolic atrial compression: a sensitive echocardiographic sign of cardiac tamponade. J Am Coll Cardiol 2:770, 1983.
49. Gillam LD, Guyer DE, Gibson TC, et al: Hydrodynamic compression of the right atrium: a new echocardiographic sign of cardiac tamponade. Circulation 68:294, 1983.
50. Schiller NB, Botvinick EH: Right ventricular compression as a sign of cardiac tamponade: an analysis of echocardiographic ventricular dimensions and their clinical implications. Circulation 56:774, 1977.
51. Appleton CP, Hatle LK, Popp RL: Cardiac tamponade and pericardial effusion: respiratory variation in transvalvular flow velocities studied by Doppler echocardiography. J Am Coll Cardiol 11:1020, 1988.
52. Fowler NO: The significance of echocardiographic-Doppler studies in cardiac tamponade. J Am Coll Cardiol 11:1031, 1988.
53. Singh S, Wann LS, Schuchard GH, et al: Right ventricular and right atrial collapse in patients with cardiac tamponade—a combined echocardiographic and hemodynamic study. Circulation 70:966, 1984.
54. Leimgruber PP, Klopfenstein HS, Wann LS, et al: The hemodynamic derangement associated with right ventricular diastolic collapse in cardiac tamponade: an experimental echocardiographic study. Circulation 68:612, 1983.
55. Klopfenstein HS, Cogswell TL, Bernath GA, et al: Alterations in intravascular volume affect the relation between right ventricular diastolic collapse and the hemodynamic severity of cardiac tamponade. J Am Coll Cardiol 6:1057, 1985.
56. Klopfenstein HS, Schuchard GH, Wann LS, et al: The relative merits of pulsus paradoxus and right ventricular diastolic collapse in the early detection of cardiac tamponade: an experimental echocardiographic study. Circulation 71:829, 1985.
57. Fusman B, Schwinger ME, Charney R, et al: Isolated collapse of left-sided heart chambers in cardiac tamponade: demonstration by two-dimensional echocardiography. Am Heart J 121:613, 1991.
58. D'Cruz IA, Kensey K, Campbell C, et al: Two-dimensional echocardiography in cardiac tamponade occurring after cardiac surgery. J Am Coll Cardiol 5:1250, 1985.
59. Settle HP, Adolph RJ, Fowler NO, et al: Echocardiographic study of cardiac tamponade. Circulation 56:951, 1977.
60. Shabetai R, Fowler NO, Fenton JC, et al: Pulsus paradoxus. J Clin Invest 44:1882, 1965.
61. Wayne VS, Bishop RL, Spodick DH: Dynamic effects of pericardial effusion without tamponade: respiratory responses in the absence of pulsus paradoxus. Br Heart J 51:202, 1984.
62. Firestein G, Hensley C, Varghese PJ: Left ventricular function in presence of small pericardial effusion: echocardiographic study. Br Heart J 43:382, 1980.
63. Himelman RB, Kircher B, Rockey DC, et al: Inferior vena cava plethora with blunted respiratory response: a sensitive echocardiographic sign of cardiac tamponade. J Am Coll Cardiol 12:1470, 1988.
64. Littmann D, Spodick DH: Total electrical alternation in pericardial disease. Circulation 17:912, 1958.
65. Spodick DH: Electric alternation of the heart: its relation to the kinetics and physiology of the heart during cardiac tamponade. Am J Cardiol 10:155, 1962.
66. Sohn DW, Shin GJ, Oh JK, et al: Role of transesophageal echocardiography in hemodynamically unstable patients. Mayo Clin Proc 70:925, 1995.
67. Holt JP, Rhode EA, Kines H: Pericardial and ventricular pressure. Circ Res 8:1171, 1960.
68. Reddy PS, Curtiss EI, O'Toole JD, et al: Cardiac tamponade: hemodynamic observations in man. Circulation 58:265, 1978.
69. Hancock EW: Subacute effusive-constrictive pericarditis. Circulation 43:183, 1971.
70. Shabetai R, Fowler NO, Guntheroth WG: The hemodynamics of cardiac tamponade and constrictive pericarditis. Am J Cardiol 26:480, 1970.
71. Gaasch WH, Peterson KL, Shabetai R: Left ventricular function in chronic constrictive pericarditis. Am J Cardiol 34:107, 1974.
72. Millaire A, Wurtz A, de Groote P, et al: Malignant pericardial effusions: usefulness of pericardioscopy. Am Heart J 124:1030, 1992.
73. Nugue O, Millaire A, Porte H, et al: Pericardioscopy in the etiologic diagnosis of pericardial effusion in 141 consecutive patients. Circulation 94:1635, 1996.
74. Bertrand O, Legrand V, Kulbertus H: Percutaneous balloon pericardiotomy: a case report and analysis of mechanism of action. Cathet Cardiovasc Diag 38:180, 1996.
75. Devlin GP, Smyth D, Charleson HA, et al: Balloon pericardiostomy: a new therapeutic option for malignant pericardial effusion. Aust N Z J Med 26:556, 1996.
76. Clarke DP, Cosgrove DO: Real-time ultrasound scanning in the planning and guidance of pericardiocentesis. Clin Radiol 38:119, 1987.
77. Lewis BS, Gotsman MS: Left ventricular function in systole and diastole in constrictive pericarditis. Am Heart J 86:23, 1973.
78. Brecher GA: Venous Return. New York: Grune & Stratton, 1956.
79. Hansen AT, Eskildsen P, Gotzsche H: Pressure curves from the right auricle and the right ventricle in chronic constrictive pericarditis. Circulation 3:881, 1951.
80. Kussmaul A: Ueber schwielige Mediastino-Pericarditis und den paradoxen Puls. Berl Klin Wochenschr 10:461, 1878.
81. Meyer TE, Sareli P, Marcus RH, et al: Mechanism underlying Kussmaul's sign in chronic constrictive pericarditis. Am J Cardiol 64:1069, 1989.
82. Kaul U, Gupta CD, Anand IS, et al: Characteristic postextrasystolic ventricular pressure response in constrictive pericarditis. Am Heart J 102:461, 1981.
83. Tanaka C, Nishimoto M, Takeuchi K, et al: Presystolic pulmonary valve opening in constrictive pericarditis. Jpn Heart J 20:419, 1979.
84. Blake S, Bonar F, McCarthy C, et al: The effect of posture on cardiac output in late pregnancy complicated by pericardial constriction. Am J Obstet Gynecol 146:865, 1983.
85. Anand IS, Ferrari R, Kalra GS, et al: Pathogenesis of edema in constrictive pericarditis. Circulation 83:1880, 1991.
86. Fowler NO: Constrictive pericarditis: its history and current status. Clin Cardiol 18:341, 1995.
87. Cegielski JP, Lwakatare J, Dukes CS, et al: Tuberculous pericarditis in Tanzanian patients with and without HIV infection. Tuber Lung Dis 75:429, 1994.
88. Seino Y, Ikeda U, Kawaguchi K, et al: Tuberculous pericarditis presumably diagnosed by polymerase chain reaction analysis. Am Heart J 126:249, 1993.
89. Kahl LE: The spectrum of pericardial tamponade in systemic lupus erythematosus: report of ten patients. Arthritis Rheum 35:1343, 1992.
90. Thould AK: Constrictive pericarditis in rheumatoid arthritis. Ann Rheum Dis 45:89, 1986.
91. Harbin AD, Gerson MC, O'Connell JB: Simulation of acute myopericarditis by constrictive pericardial disease with endomyocardial fibrosis due to methysergide therapy. J Am Coll Cardiol 4:196, 1984.
92. Ribeiro P, Sapsford R, Evans T, et al: Constrictive pericarditis as a complication of coronary artery bypass surgery. Br Heart J 51:205, 1984.
93. Almassi GH, Chapman PD, Troup PJ, et al: Constrictive pericarditis associated with patch electrodes of the automatic implantable cardioverter-defibrillator. Chest 92:369, 1987.

94. Fischbein L, Namade M, Sachs RN, et al: Chronic constrictive pericarditis associated with asbestosis. Chest 94:646, 1988.
95. Kumpe DA, Jaffe RB, Waldmann TA, et al: Constrictive pericarditis and protein-losing enteropathy: an imitator of intestinal lymphangiectasia. AJR 124:365, 1975.
96. Surawicz B, Lasseter KC: Electrocardiogram in pericarditis. Am J Cardiol 26:471, 1970.
97. Levine HD: Myocardial fibrosis in constrictive pericarditis: electrocardiographic and pathologic observations. Circulation 48:1268, 1973.
98. Tei C, Child JS, Tanaka H, et al: Atrial systolic notch on the interventricular septal echogram: an echocardiographic sign of constrictive pericarditis. J Am Coll Cardiol 1:907, 1983.
99. Candell-Riera J, Garcia-Del-Castillo H, Permanyer-Miralda G, et al: Echocardiographic features of the interventricular septum in chronic constrictive pericarditis. Circulation 57:1154, 1978.
100. Gibson TC, Grossman W, McLaurin LP, et al: An echocardiographic study of the interventricular septum in constrictive pericarditis. Br Heart J 38:738, 1976.
101. Isner JM, Carter BL, Bankoff MS, et al: Differentiation of constrictive pericarditis from restrictive cardiomyopathy by computed tomographic imaging. Am Heart J 105:1019, 1983.
102. Silverman PM, Harell GS, Korobkin M: Computed tomography of the abnormal pericardium. AJR 140:1125, 1983.
103. White CS: MR evaluation of the pericardium. Topics Magn Reson Imaging 7:258, 1995.
104. Schoenfeld MH, Supple EW, Dec GW Jr, et al: Restrictive cardiomyopathy versus constrictive pericarditis: role of endomyocardial biopsy in avoiding unnecessary thoracotomy. Circulation 75:1017, 1987.
105. Soto B, Shin MS, Arciniegas J, et al: The septal arteries in the differential diagnosis of constrictive pericarditis. Am Heart J 108:332, 1984.
106. Akasaka T, Yoshida K, Yamamuro A, et al: Phasic coronary flow characteristics in patients with constrictive pericarditis: comparison with restrictive cardiomyopathy. Circulation 96:1874, 1997.
107. Hurrell DG, Nishimura RA, Higano ST, et al: Value of dynamic respiratory changes in left and right ventricular pressures for the diagnosis of constrictive pericarditis. Circulation 93:2007, 1996.
108. Klodas E, Nishimura RA, Appleton CP, et al: Doppler evaluation of patients with constrictive pericarditis: use of tricuspid regurgitation velocity curves to determine enhanced ventricular interaction. J Am Coll Cardiol 28:652, 1996.
109. Vaitkus PT, Kussmaul WG: Constrictive pericarditis versus restrictive cardiomyopathy: a reappraisal and update of diagnostic criteria. Am Heart J 122:1431, 1991.
110. Kushwaha SS, Fallon JT, Fuster V: Restrictive cardiomyopathy. N Engl Med J 336:267, 1997.
111. Hinkamp TJ, Sullivan HJ, Montoya A, et al: Chronic cardiac rejection masking as constrictive pericarditis. Ann Thorac Surg 57:1579, 1994.
112. Hatle LK, Appleton CP, Popp RL: Differentiation of constrictive pericarditis and restrictive cardiomyopathy by Doppler echocardiography. Circulation 79:357, 1989.
113. Santamore WP, Bartlett R, Van Buren SJ, et al: Ventricular coupling in constrictive pericarditis. Circulation 74:597, 1986.
114. Brecher GA, Hubay CA: Pulmonary blood flow and venous return during spontaneous respiration. Circ Res 3:210, 1955.
115. Shabetai R, Fowler NO, Guntheroth WG: The hemodynamics of cardiac tamponade and constrictive pericarditis. Am J Cardiol 26:480, 1970.
116. Spodick DH: Acoustic phenomena in pericardial disease. Am Heart J 81:114, 1971.
117. Spodick DH: Diagnostic electrocardiographic sequences in acute pericarditis: significance of PR segment and PR vector changes. Circulation 48:575, 1973.
118. Fowler NO, Harbin AD III: Recurrent acute pericarditis: follow-up study of 31 patients. J Am Coll Cardiol 7:300, 1986.
119. Adler Y, Finkelstein Y, Guindo J, et al: Colchicine Treatment for recurrent pericarditis: a decade of experience. Circulation 97:2183, 1998.
120. Marcolongo R, Russo R, Laveder F, et al: Immunosuppressive therapy prevents recurrent pericarditis. J Am Coll Cardiol 26:1276, 1995.

SECTION VIII

VASCULAR MEDICINE

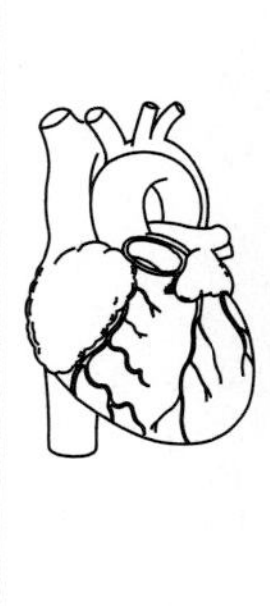

Molecular and Cellular Physiology of Differentiated Vascular Smooth Muscle

Circulatory Regulation: Basic Considerations

Circulatory Regulation: The Role of Vascular Remodeling

Vascular Endothelial Cell Function and Thrombosis

Atherosclerosis: Pathologic Anatomy

Atherosclerosis: Pathogenesis, Morphology, and Risk Factors

Diseases of the Aorta

Peripheral Vascular Diseases

Gene Therapy

Interventional Procedures for Vascular Disease

B-Mode Ultrasound: A Noninvasive Method for Assessing Atherosclerosis

Intravascular Ultrasound

Intravascular Ultrasound: Clinical Applications

Arterial Compliance

Hypertension

Shock

Autonomic Dysfunction and Hypotension

C H A P T E R **66**

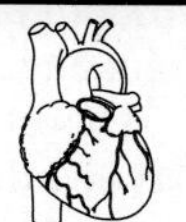

Molecular and Cellular Physiology of Differentiated Vascular Smooth Muscle

Jürgen R. Sindermann, Leonard P. Adam, and Keith L. March

SUBCELLULAR STRUCTURE OF VASCULAR MYOCYTES
THE BIOCHEMICAL MECHANISM OF CONTRACTION
Contractile Proteins
Regulation of Crossbridge Cycling by Light Chain Phosphorylation
The Latch State
Other Regulatory Proteins
EXCITATION-CONTRACTION COUPLING
Electrochemical Gradient and Muscle Activation
Mechanisms That Regulate Cytoplasmic Ca^{2+} Levels
Signal Transduction
CONCLUSION

Our understanding of the basic functions of blood vessels has evolved and matured since the early studies of Harvey.[1] In addition to serving as simple conduits, blood vessels are multicellular organs that contract, regenerate, and secrete vasoactive substances. Moreover, at the level of the capillaries, blood vessels specialize in the vital exchange of oxygen, nutrients, and fluids.

Blood vessels are composed of three major layers: adventitia, media, and intima (Fig. 66–1). The endothelium lines the intraluminal surface, which contributes to hemostatic, barrier, and vasoreactive properties of the blood vessel. The three principal layers vary considerably in extent within the vascular tree. For example, muscular arteries are composed of at least 50 percent media, whereas veins may have only one or two layers of smooth muscle cells. Capillaries have no adventitia or media, although smooth muscle–like cells (pericytes) are sparsely distributed along the extraluminal surface.

The layers of the blood vessel have specialized functions. For example, the media, which is composed of smooth muscle cells enmeshed in collagen and elastin fibrils, generates active tension in response to neural, hormonal, or pharmacologic stimulation. Based on the behavior of isolated preparations, smooth muscle can be divided into tonic muscle, as is found in large arteries, and into phasic muscle, which is found in some veins and in most nonvascular smooth muscle.[2] The adventitia consists of collagen, elastin, and other extracellular matrix proteins interspersed with fibroblasts. Separating the adventitia and media is a layer of interconnected elastin fibrils—the external elastic lamina. Much of the compliance of the blood vessel is determined by the composition and thickness of the adventitia. For example, aortic muscle, which is relatively inelastic, has a thick adventitia. Similarly, the pulmonary arteries have a thick adventitia, although the proportion of elastin versus collagen fibrils is greater and these arteries are considerably more compliant than the aorta. Finally, the intima is generally quite small and is bordered by the internal elastic lamina on the medial side and the endothelium on the luminal side. In disease states or in response to injury, the intima may fill with proliferating

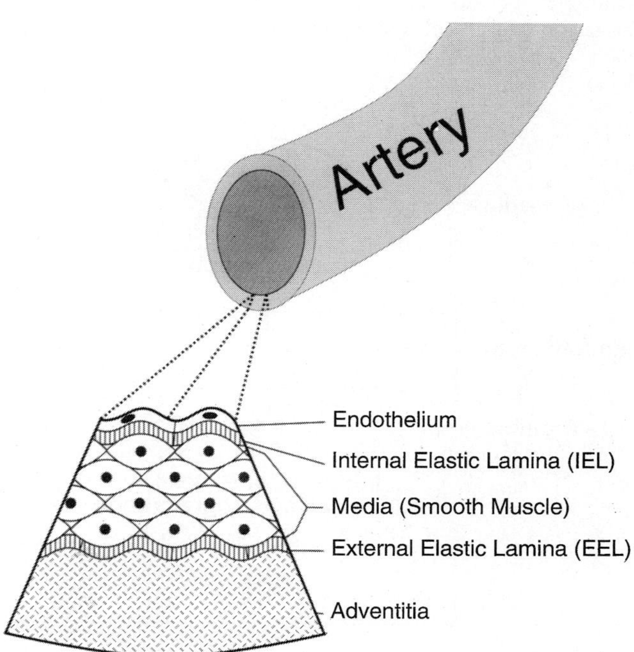

FIGURE 66–1 Major layers of the arterial wall. The intima is composed of the endothelial cell layer lining the internal aspect of the artery, the internal elastic lamina, and a basement membrane secreted by the endothelium. In disease processes such as atherosclerosis, the intima may become quite large owing to the proliferation of smooth muscle cells and deposition of extracellular matrix material.

smooth muscle cells and monocytes, giving rise to a greatly thickened neointima.

The endothelium is discussed separately in Chapter 50, Myocardial Metabolism. Nevertheless, it is an integral part of the structure and function of the blood vessel, serving as a barrier, as a hemostatic and anticoagulant surface, and as a secretory organ for modulation of vascular contractility. As a barrier, the endothelium can modulate transmural flux of fluid and proteins, and this capacity can be dynamically regulated. In addition, the membranes of endothelial cells elaborate anticoagulants, cellular adhesion molecules, and various autocoids that permit complex interactions with blood clotting factors and platelets and leukocytes. Finally, the endothelium releases powerful vasodilators (e.g., prostacyclin and nitric oxide) and vasoconstrictors (e.g., endothelin) in response to hemodynamic, hormonal, or pharmacologic stimulation (Fig. 66–2).

SUBCELLULAR STRUCTURE OF VASCULAR MYOCYTES

Vascular myocytes are elongated and spindle shaped. Within muscle, these cells form interdigitating layers and are enveloped in a weave of connective tissue. Myocytes form junctions with one another (i.e., tight junctions and desmosomes) and possess pathways of low electrical resistance, especially near the ends (i.e., gap junctions). Thus, vascular muscle is a functional syncytium. The gap junctions or connexons are composed of specialized proteins that form intercellular pores that allow the passage of ions and small molecules up to molecular weight 1000. Moreover, because ions can move from cell to cell, depolarization of one cell can spread to another.[3]

One of the most notable features of vascular smooth muscle, compared with cardiac and skeletal muscles, is the general absence of an obviously well organized subcellular structure. However, several structures common to all muscles are present (Fig. 66–3). First, there are filaments that tend to run parallel to the long axis of the myocyte. Thin filaments are composed of actin and several associated proteins, and thick filaments consist of myosin. Interspersed throughout the cytoplasm are many intermediate filaments composed of the proteins desmin or vimentin, or both. Second, surrounding each thick filament are six thin filaments. The spaces between the thick filaments contain many more thin filaments than striated muscle; thus, the ratio of thin to thick filaments is 16 to 20:1. In striated muscle, this ratio is just 6:1. Studies on protein content also confirm that vascular muscle contains a higher mass ratio of actin to myosin and, generally, less myosin per cell.[3]

Thin filaments insert into two structures. At the cellular membrane, these filaments enter membrane plaques, which tend to be concentrated near the ends of cells. In the cytoplasm, thin filaments attach to the dense bodies. The latter structures are analogous to the Z-lines of striated muscle and contain many of the same proteins such as alpha-actin. It has been suggested that intermediate filaments also course through the dense bodies and may therefore serve as a subcellular scaffold for the contractile elements.[3]

The nucleus of the myocyte is centrally located; sparsely scattered throughout the cytoplasm are other familiar organelles, such as mitochondria and lysosomes. A sarcoplasmic reticulum (SR) lies near the inner surface of the sarcolemma. Invaginations of the sarcolemma, caveolae, may make contact with the underlying sarcoplasmic reticulum.

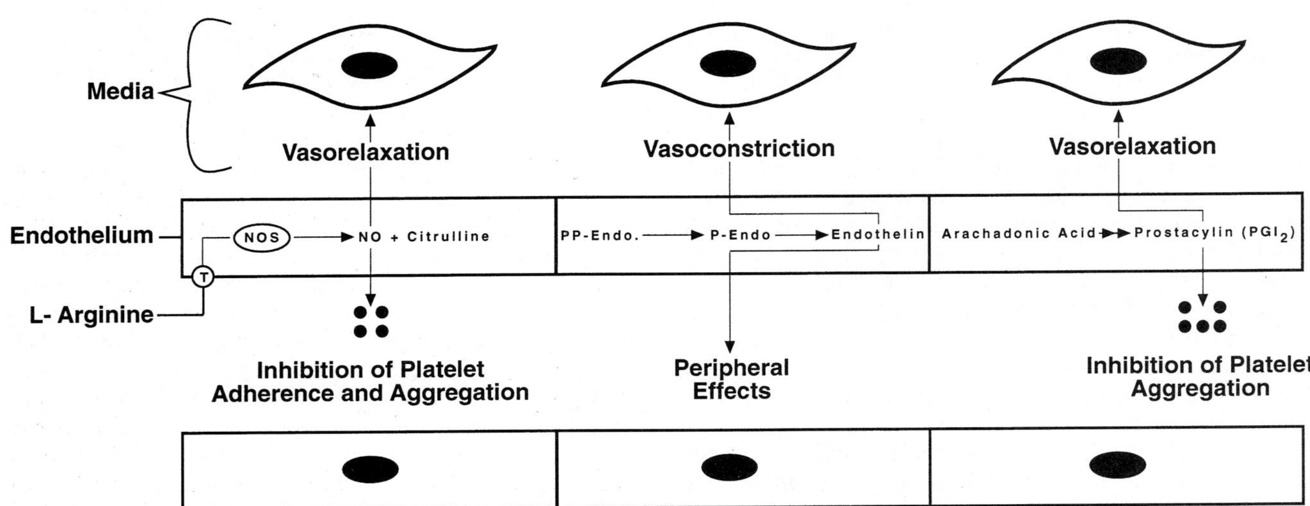

FIGURE 66–2 Vasoactive substances released by the endothelium. A major vasodilator elaborated by endothelium is nitric oxide (NO) or endothelium-derived relaxing factor. Arginine is the precursor for NO. Although cells can synthesize arginine, another important source is the arginine circulating in the blood, which can be taken into endothelial cells through specific transport molecules (T). Nitric oxide synthase (NOS) converts arginine to NO plus citrulline. In addition to vasorelaxation, NO inhibits platelet adherence and aggregation. Endothelin is a peptide vasoconstrictor. It is processed from a much larger precursor, preproendothelin (PP-Endo), to a smaller form, proendothelin (P-Endo), and finally to the fully active, 21-amino-acid hormone endothelin. Endothelin contracts blood vessels both locally and at distinct sites. Prostacyclin is another potent vasorelaxant molecule that is produced from arachidonic acid and is an inhibitor of platelet aggregation.

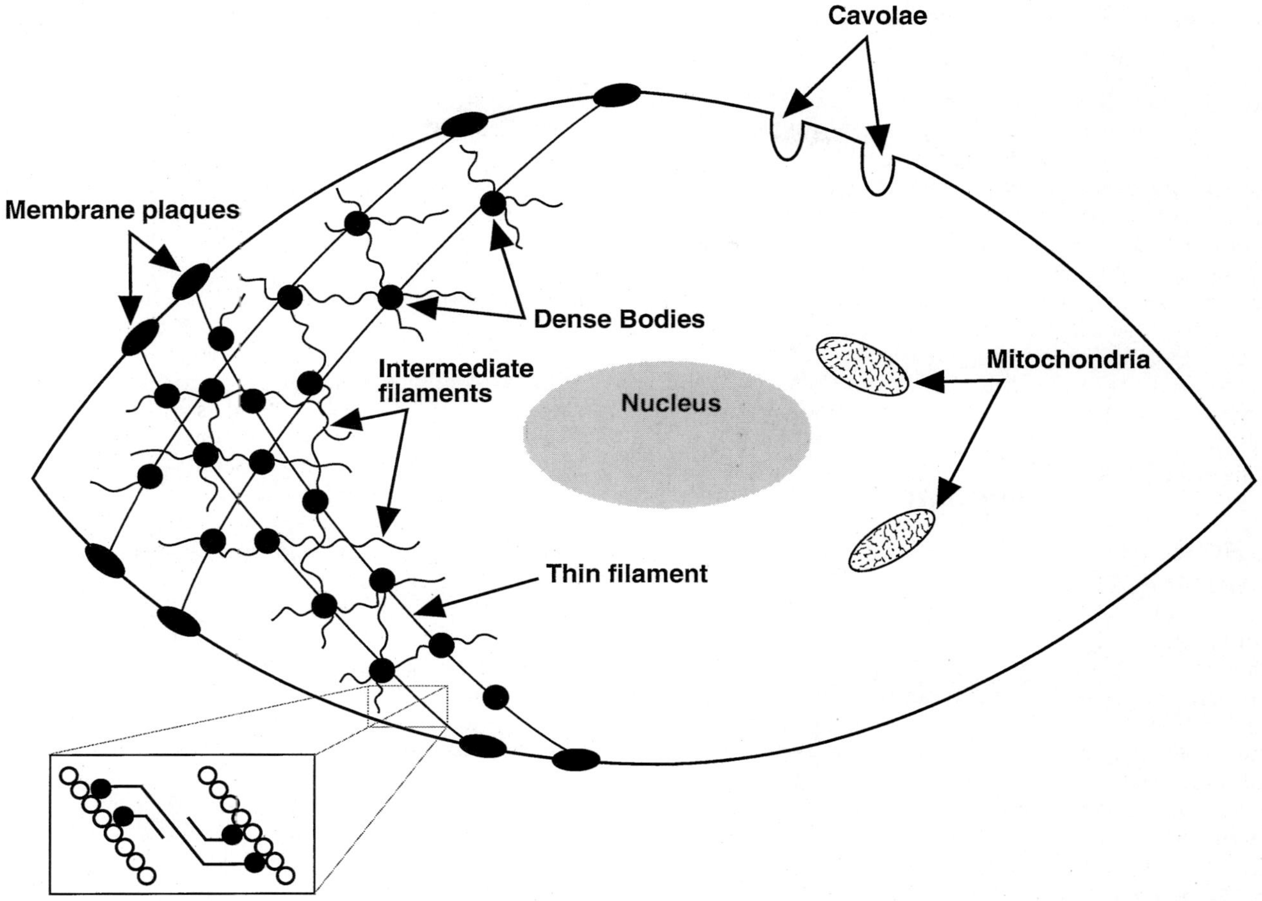

FIGURE 66–3 Filament systems and other structures in vascular myocytes. Thin filaments are composed of actin, tropomyosin, and certain proteins such as caldesmon and calponin. As shown in the magnification, myosin (thick) filaments are associated with the thin filaments. Thin filaments are connected by dense bodies that are similar in composition to the Z lines of striated muscle. In addition, the attachment sites for thin filaments on the outer membrane (sarcolemma) are membrane plaques. These are similar to dense bodies but contain other proteins such as vinculin. Another filament network is composed of intermediate filaments. These filaments course through dense bodies and may determine the spatial array. Intermediate filaments are composed of vimentin, desmin, or both. The nuclei of smooth muscle cells are centrally located. Caveolae are invaginations of the sarcolemma that may play an important rôle in excitation-contraction coupling.

These structures are most likely involved in excitation-contraction coupling and may be analogous to the T tubules of striated muscle sarcolemma.

THE BIOCHEMICAL MECHANISM OF CONTRACTION

Contractile Proteins

The contractile proteins are packed into thick and thin filaments (Fig. 66–4). Thin filaments are composed of actin, tropomyosin, and specific thin filament–binding proteins. Actin is a globular protein of molecular weight 40,000 that polymerizes to form long helical chains or cables. Vascular muscle contains a unique α isoform of actin that differs from the α-actins of striated muscle largely owing to a few amino acid substitutions at the amino terminus of the molecule. Tropomyosin, an elongated molecule of molecular weight 36,000, forms dimers that lie in the grooves of the helical actin cables. One tropomyosin dimer spans seven actin monomers. Several additional proteins are bound to thin filaments, including myosin light chain kinase, caldesmon, and calponin.[3, 4]

Thick filaments are composed of myosin. Myosin molecules are actually hexamers that consist of two heavy chains and two sets each of two dissimilar light chain subunits. In the contractile phenotype of vascular muscle, the expression of a single myosin heavy chain gene predominates, although four variants, resulting from alternative RNA splicing, are present. The significance of these variants to overall contractile function is unknown. One of the sets of light chains, the 20,000-Da or regulatory light chains, plays a central role in the dynamic regulation of the crossbridge cycle, the basic mechanism of muscle contraction. The other set of light chains, known as the essential or 17,000-Da light chains, lies in proximity to the adenosine triphosphate (ATP)-binding sites on the myosin heads (i.e., crossbridges) and may be one important determinant of the maximal rate at which crossbridges can cycle.

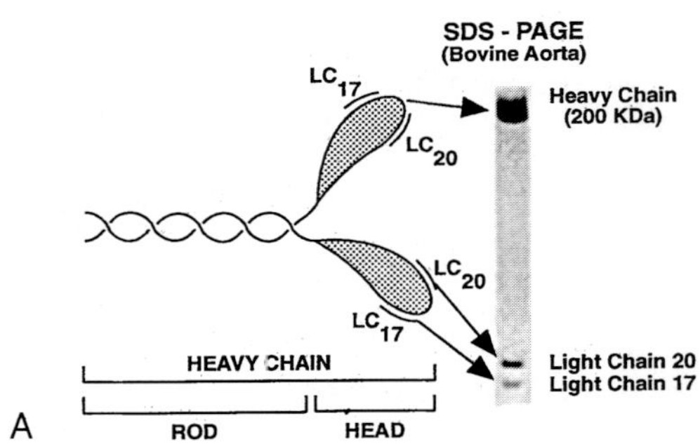

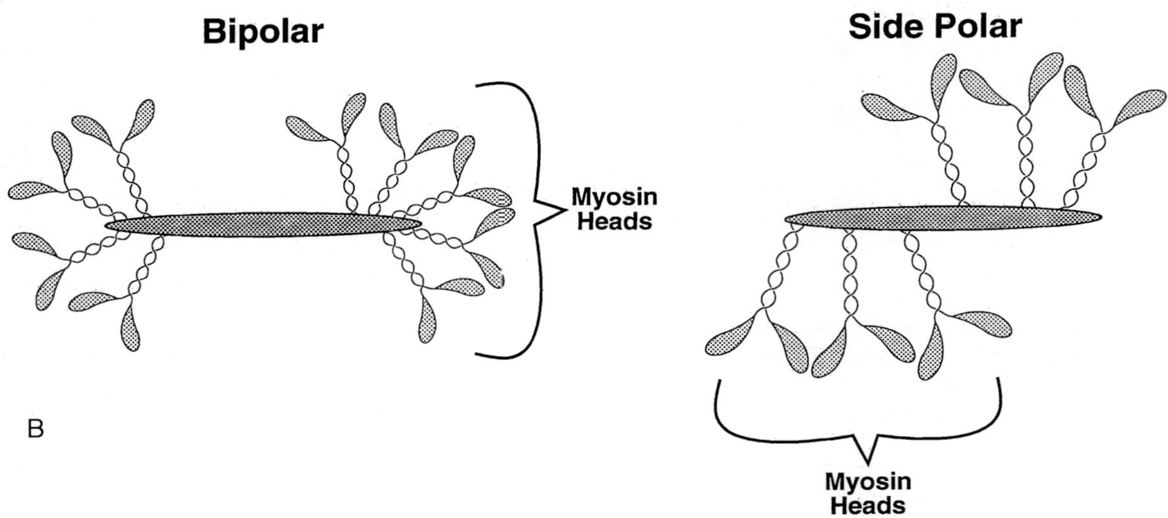

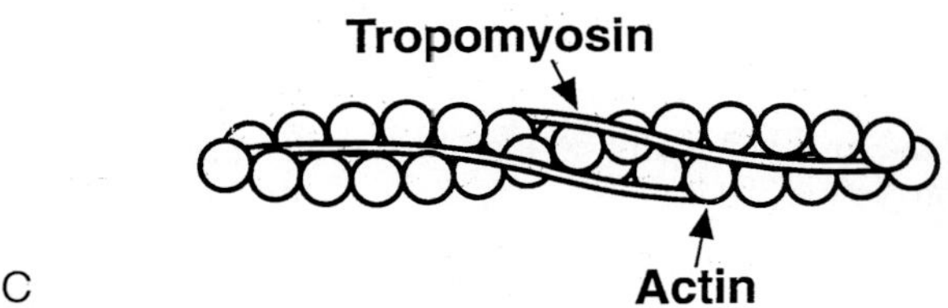

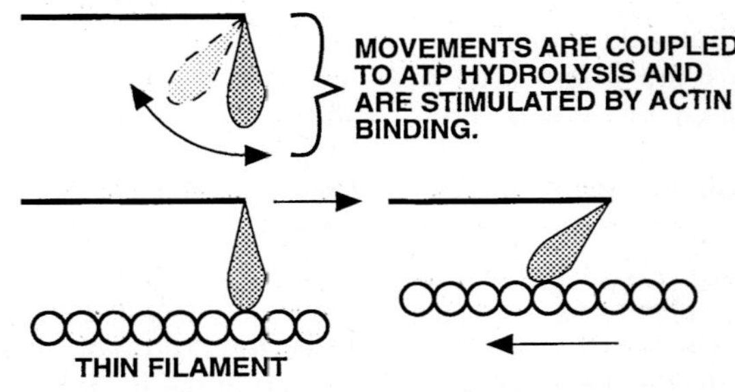

FIGURE 66–4 *See legend on opposite page*

Two isoforms of these light chains have been identified that arise from the same gene but differ slightly as a result of alternative RNA splicing.

Regulation of Crossbridge Cycling by Light Chain Phosphorylation

The regulatory light chains of vascular smooth muscle myosin undergo phosphorylation in response to an increase in intracellular Ca^{2+} (for a review, see Somlyo and Somlyo[5]). The specific mechanism involves the binding of Ca^{2+} to the protein calmodulin and the subsequent binding of the Ca^{2+}-calmodulin complex to the enzyme myosin light chain kinase (Fig. 66–5). The binding of Ca^{2+}-calmodulin to myosin light chain kinase activates the kinase, which in turn phosphorylates the regulatory light chains of myosin. Specifically, phosphate is transferred from ATP to Ser-19 of the light chains. When the regulatory light chains are phosphorylated, myosin molecules can undergo repeated cycles of binding and release from actin. This cyclical binding is accompanied by energy-dependent movements of the myosin heads. The heads of myosin are capable of angular motion, so the hydrolysis of ATP is coupled to displacements of the heads. It is the displacement of myosin heads that are attached to actin that generates tension or produces shortening of the muscle.

As long as the regulatory light chains remain phosphorylated, the crossbridges continue to cycle. However, vascular muscle also contains a phosphoprotein phosphatase that can remove phosphate from the regulatory light chains, thereby restoring crossbridges to the resting or relaxed state. Studies have shown that myosin phosphatase is a heterotrimeric protein consisting of a catalytic subunit and two regulatory subunits, one of which targets the phosphatase to myosin. Myosin phosphatase is subject to regulation via the low-molecular-weight guanosine triphosphate (GTP)-binding protein rhoA. rhoA is activated by the binding of GTP and in turn activates a 160,000-Da kinase called rho-kinase. rho-kinase phosphorylates and thereby inactivates myosin phosphatase. When myosin phosphatase is inactive, it no longer can remove phosphate from the regulatory subunits of myosin, thus promoting crossbridge cycling and contraction. Conversely, the inhibition of rho-kinase by the low-molecular-weight compound Y-27632 results in enhanced myosin phosphatase activity and subsequent relaxation of the muscle.[6] When the muscle is stimulated by neurohumoral agonists, Ca^{2+} is mobilized to turn on the activity of myosin light chain kinase, and the rhoA pathway is activated to inhibit myosin phosphatase. Independent regulation of myosin light chain kinase and myosin phosphatase by different contractile agonists could provide a mechanism for modulation of the Ca^{2+} sensitivity of vascular muscle tone.[7]

The Latch State

Many types of smooth muscle, including vascular smooth muscle, possess a unique mechanism for maintaining tone. After a brief period of accelerated crossbridge cycling, when a maximum level of tone has been achieved, the crossbridges begin to cycle very slowly but support full levels of tension. Because tension depends directly on the total numbers of attached (high-affinity) crossbridges, this change in cycling kinetics requires parallel reductions in the rates of both crossbridge formation and detachment. During this period, intracellular levels of Ca^{2+} fall to near basal levels, and ATP utilization drops in parallel with the decrease in crossbridge cycling. Clearly, this is a highly efficient mechanism for maintaining tension because tension is maintained with minimal ATP utilization. Skeletal and cardiac muscles have no analogous mechanism for conserving energy and must depend on ATP-consuming crossbridge cycling to maintain contractile force. As originally described, this unique state of the crossbridge in smooth muscle was referred to as the *latch state,* because the phenomenon behaved as if the myosin heads had become stuck or latched to actin filaments. However, the latch state model is still a matter of discussion. It has been suggested that the latch state contributes to force production via dephosphorylation of attached and phosphorylated crossbridges while in the high-affinity state. Although the specific molecular mechanisms remain unknown, it seems clear that crossbridges attach and detach at much slower rates in the latch state. Moreover, the latch state is dynamic, meaning that it can be turned on and off. Finally, the existence of the latch state provides a mechanism in vascular muscle for maintaining tone at low levels of energy expenditure. This mechanism is especially well suited to the function of the vasculature, which must maintain some level of tone throughout the entire life span of the organism.[4]

Other Regulatory Proteins

Although the classic mechanism of regulatory light chain phosphorylation-dephosphorylation is the paradigm for understanding how vascular muscle undergoes phasic contraction and relaxation, it is likely that most vascular tone in humans is maintained via gradations of the latch mechanism. Thus, a key biochemical mechanism remains incompletely understood. Two other proteins present in abundance and associated with thin filaments have been isolated

FIGURE 66–4 The contractile proteins. **A,** The myosin molecule is a hexamer composed of two heavy chains (molecular weight, 200,000) and two sets each of two different light chains (molecular weights, 20,000 and 17,000). SDS-PAGE, sodium dodecyl sulfate–polyacrylamide gel electrophoresis. **B,** Myosin molecules are assembled into thick filaments; these may be either bipolar or side polar. The heads of myosin molecules extend from the thick filaments to form crossbridges. **C,** Thin filaments are composed of actin, tropomyosin, and an array of other proteins. Actin forms a helical structure, and tropomyosin molecules lie in the grooves of the helix. **D,** Myosin is a chemomechanical protein. On association with actin, it converts chemical energy (e.g., adenosine triphosphate [ATP]) into movements of the heads or crossbridges. Through the exertion of force on thin filaments, tension or movement is produced.

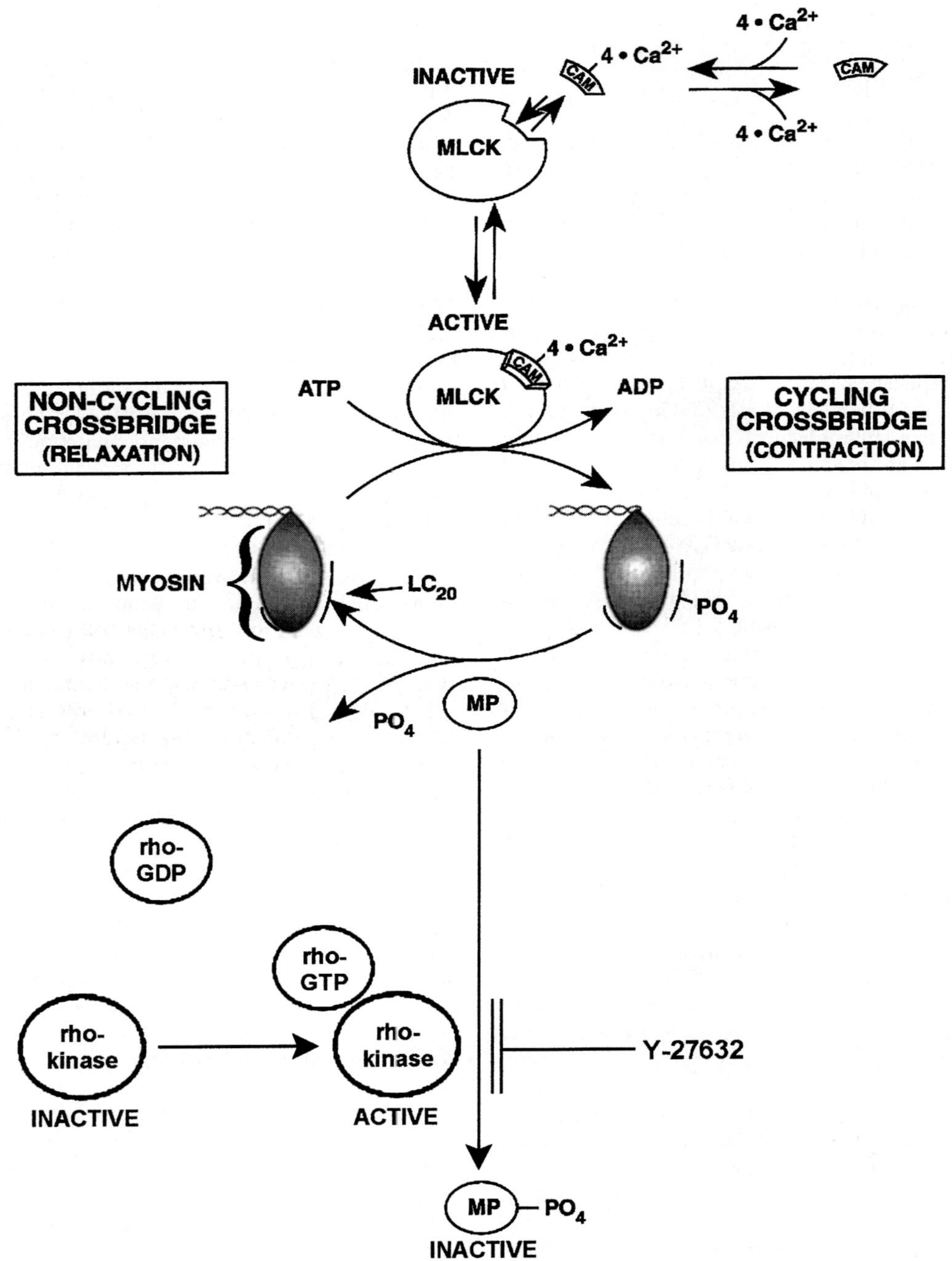

FIGURE 66–5 The switch that turns on vascular contraction. The enzyme myosin light chain kinase (MLCK) catalyzes the transfer of phosphate from adenosine triphosphate (ATP) to the 20,000-Da light chain subunits of myosin (LC_{20}). This reaction or phosphorylation of LC_{20} induces the cyclic binding of myosin heads to actin (i.e., crossbridge cycling). MLCK is activated on binding of calmodulin that is saturated with Ca^{2+}. Calmodulin has four Ca^{2+}-binding sites. MLCK can be inactivated by the removal of Ca^{2+}-calmodulin. The cessation of crossbridge cycling occurs when phosphate is removed from LC_{20} by another enzyme, myosin phosphatase (MP). MP is also regulated by phosphorylation. When MP is phosphorylated by active rho-kinase, MP is inactivated. Rho-kinase is activated by the low-molecular-weight G protein rhoA when rhoA is complexed with guanosine triphosphate (GTP). Rho-kinase is inactivated by the specific kinase inhibitor Y-27632. ADP, adenosine diphosphate; GDP, guanosine diphosphate.

from smooth muscle: caldesmon and calponin. Two isoforms of caldesmon exist that result from the alternative splicing of a single gene. One isoform has a molecular weight of 93,000 and is exclusively expressed in smooth muscle of the contractile phenotype. The other isoform, with molecular weight 60,000, lacks a central helical portion of the molecule and is expressed more broadly. The high-molecular-weight isoform of caldesmon is present in varying amounts in different smooth muscles. In fact, the content seems to parallel the amount of myosin such that the ratio of caldesmon to myosin is approximately 1:1. Caldesmon has two sticky ends; the amino terminus binds to actin and tropomyosin. It may act, therefore, as a cross-linking protein in muscle. In addition, caldesmon is phosphorylated in response to stimulation by several contractile agonists and reversibly binds Ca^{2+}-calmodulin. On the basis of these observations, caldesmon is thought to play a role in contractile regulation, but the nature of this participation has not been elucidated.[3]

Calponin is a 34,000-Da actin-binding protein that is abundant in vascular muscle. Calponin inhibits actomyosin activity, and this inhibition is reversed by binding of Ca^{2+}-calmodulin in vitro. It seems possible that calponin is analogous to the troponin components of striated muscle, but its function in vascular muscle physiology is unclear.

EXCITATION-CONTRACTION COUPLING

Electrochemical Gradient and Muscle Activation

Vascular cells possess unique electrophysiologic properties compared with cardiac and skeletal myocytes. For example, the resting membrane potential (E_M) of vascular myocytes is approximately −40 to −50 mV, which is more positive than that of striated muscles. In the latter, the E_M is quite close to the equilibrium potential for K^+ (E_K). This departure of E_M from E_K is due to a lower permeability of vascular membranes to K^+ as well as to contributions of the equilibrium potentials for Na^+ and Cl^-. In addition, smooth muscle membranes do not contain tetrodotoxin-sensitive, fast Na^+ channels. Although depolarization in response to neurohumoral stimulation does occur, the inward current is carried by Ca^{2+} that enters largely through voltage-gated or L-type Ca^{2+} channels and, also to a lesser extent, through T-type Ca^{2+} channels. Finally, Ca^{2+} can be released from intracellular stores via mechanisms that do not necessitate membrane depolarization, although contractile mechanisms are nevertheless activated (Fig. 66–6).

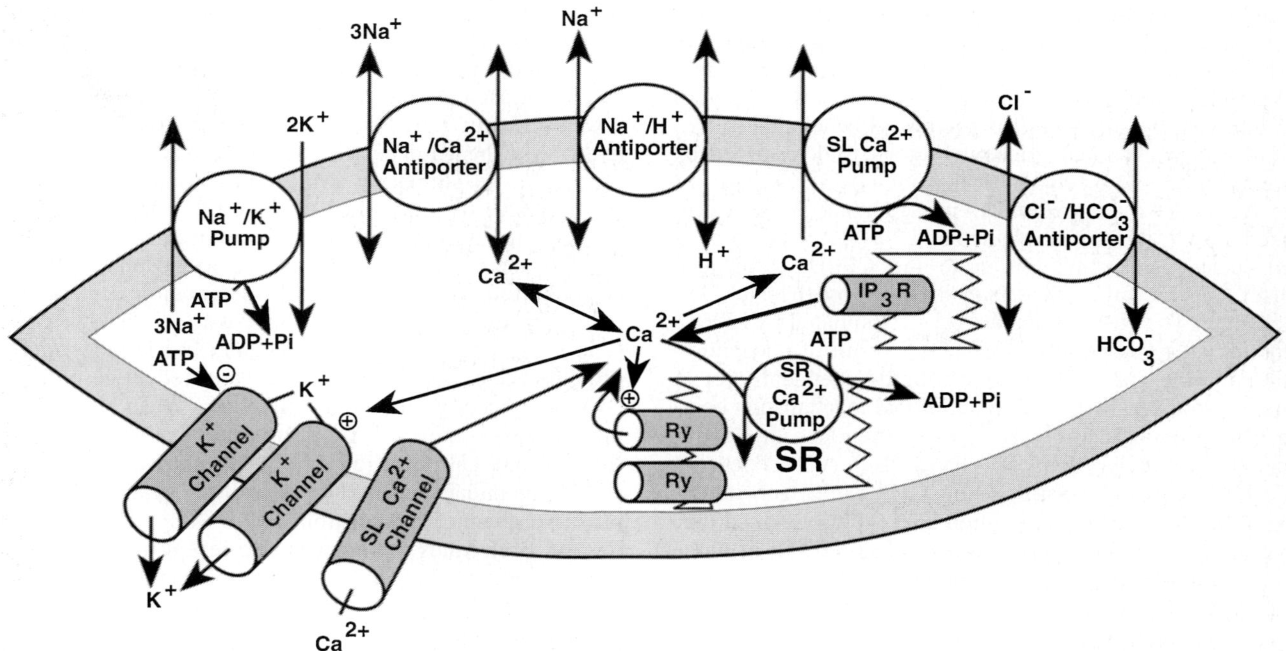

FIGURE 66–6 Ion channels, antiporters, and pumps. The electrochemical gradient in vascular cells is maintained through active and passive processes. The Na^+/K^+ pump extrudes Na^+ and imports K^+ in an energy-requiring process (i.e., adenosine triphosphate [ATP] is hydrolyzed). Cytoplasmic Ca^{2+} levels are maintained in the resting state at less than 10^{-6} M by a sarcolemmal Ca^{2+} pump (SL Ca^{2+} pump) that extrudes Ca^{2+} and by a sarcoplasmic reticulum Ca^{2+} pump (SR Ca^{2+} pump) that imports Ca^{2+} into an intracellular membrane system, the SR. Both Ca^{2+} pumps require energy for activity (e.g., ATP). Antiporters, also called *exchangers,* move ions across the sarcolemma in either direction but do not require energy. Nevertheless, the binding of ions to these structures can be dynamically regulated via second messengers or protein phosphorylation. In addition to a contribution to the electrochemical gradient of ions, intracellular pH regulation is an especially important function of the Na^+/H^+ and Cl^-/HCO^-_3 antiporters. Vascular smooth muscle cells lack Na^+ channels but possess an array of K^+ channels. Two important K^+ channels are shown. One is activated by Ca^{2+} (+), and the other is inhibited by ATP (−). There are several different types of Ca^{2+} channels. One sarcolemmal Ca^{2+} channel (SL Ca^{2+} channel) allows influx of Ca^{2+} at membrane potentials of −40 to −45 mV but is inhibited at more negative values. In addition to exhibition of this voltage dependence, these L-type Ca^{2+} channels are the targets of several kinds of Ca^{2+}-blocking drugs (e.g., dihydropyridines). Two kinds of internal Ca^{2+} channels have been identified in vascular muscle: the SR Ca^{2+} release channels or ryanodine receptors (Ry), and the 1,4,5-inositol triphosphate receptor (IP_3R). Both release stored Ca^{2+} into the cytoplasm. Ca^{2+} stimulates the release of Ca^{2+} from Ry, whereas IP_3 stimulates Ca^{2+} release from IP_3R. ADP, adenose diphosphate.

This latter phenomenon has been called *pharmacomechanical coupling* and is linked to the receptor-mediated enzymatic hydrolysis of membrane phosphoinositides.[7] Common neurohumoral transmitters for vascular muscle include norepinephrine released locally from sympathetic nerve endings, angiotensin II, and endothelin. Although action potentials per se are not generated in tonic vascular smooth muscle, the stimulation of α-adrenergic receptors by norepinephrine does increase the frequency and open time of voltage-gated, L-type Ca^{2+} channels. Ca^{2+} entering via this mechanism may act directly on the myofilaments, and it most likely stimulates the release of Ca^{2+} from sarcoplasmic reticulum.

Repolarization (i.e., restoration of E_M) or membrane hyperpolarization is determined by changes in K^+ permeability. Several different types of K^+ channels have been described in vascular smooth muscle cells, including Ca^{2+}-activated, delayed rectifier, and ATP-sensitive K^+ channels. An increase in the negativity of E_M effectively inhibits the effects of agonists that are dependent on membrane depolarization for their action (e.g., neurohumoral agonists), because the movement of Ca^{2+} through voltage-dependent Ca^{2+} channels is diminished. Ca^{2+}-activated K^+ channels can be inhibited by certain agents such as charybdotoxin and tetraethylammonium ions. ATP-sensitive K^+ channels are activated by several pharmacologic agents, including pinacidil, nicorandil, minoxidil, and diazoxide. Predictably, all of the latter are vasodilators, because an increase in K^+ conductance diminishes L-type Ca^{2-} channel activity. On the other hand, ATP-sensitive K^+ channels are inhibited by sulfonylureas such as glibenclamide.[8]

The electrochemical gradient of ions is determined by several additional mechanisms that include various pumps and exchangers. For example, intracellular Cl^- is maintained via Cl^--HCO^-_3 exchange and $Na^+/K^+/Cl^-$ cotransport mechanisms. In addition to the Cl^-/HCO^-_3 transporter, intracellular $[H^+]$ is controlled by the Na^+-H^+ exchanger. The Na^+-H^+ exchanger is stimulated by several contractile agonists and mitogens as a result of phosphorylation by the Ca^{2+}- and phospholipid-dependent protein kinase, protein kinase C. Two additional mechanisms operate to adjust intracellular Na^+ concentrations: an electrogenic (i.e., activity that can change E_M) ATP-dependent Na^+-K^+ pump and a passive Na^+-Ca^{2+} exchanger. Inhibition of the Na^+-K^+ pump by high concentrations of cardiac glycosides can induce vasoconstriction as a result of a rise in intracellular Na^+, the subsequent increase in Na^+-Ca^+ exchange, and an increase in intracellular $[Ca^{2+}]$.[3]

Mechanisms That Regulate Cytoplasmic Ca^{2+} Levels

Several different mechanisms modulate levels of intracellular Ca^{2+} in vascular myocytes (see Fig. 66–6). Both L- and T-type Ca^{2+} channels permit transsarcolemmal Ca^{2+} influx. The former are particularly important sites of drug action: L-type Ca^{2+} channel blockers (i.e., dihydropyridines, verapamil, diltiazem) inhibit contraction by preventing Ca^{2+} entry. Passive exchange mechanisms can also increase intracellular Ca^{2+}. For example, a rise in intracellular H^+ can lead to an increase in Na^+ via Na^+-H^+ exchange. The intracellular Na^+ can then be extruded by the Na^+-Ca^{2+} exchanger with a net increase in cytoplasmic Ca^{2+}. The diuretic amiloride inhibits the Na^+-H^+ exchanger at low concentrations and the Na^+-Ca^{2+} exchanger at high concentrations.[3]

At least two mechanisms exist for the release of Ca^{2+} from internal stores. First, vascular muscle contains an SR with ryanodine-sensitive Ca^{2+}-release channels. In striated muscles, a rise in cytoplasmic Ca^{2+} stimulates the release of Ca^{2+} from SR via these Ca^{2+}-release channels. Such a mechanism probably also exists in vascular muscle. This is referred to as the Ca^{2+}-induced Ca^{2+}-release, a mechanism that is pH sensitive in that increased pH increases the sensitivity of the channel to Ca^{2+}, similar to the mechanisms found for skeletal and cardiac muscle. Studies on guinea pig urinary bladder smooth muscle cells have shown that this mechanism accounts for 70 percent of the total depolarization-induced increase of intracellular Ca^{2+}.[9] The SR contains a Ca^{2+} pump that actively imports Ca^{2+} into the SR lumen as well as Ca^{2+}-binding proteins (e.g., calsequestrin) that serve as an intraluminal Ca^{2+}-buffering system. The affinity of the Ca^{2+} pump for Ca^{2+} is regulated by the SR membrane protein phospholamban. Phosphorylation of phospholamban by cyclic AMP (cAMP)- or cyclic GMP (cGMP)-dependent protein kinases stimulates the Ca^{2+} pump and facilitates relaxation by reducing cytoplasmic Ca^{2+}.[3, 4] Smooth muscle contains an SR Ca^{2+} pump (Ca^{2+}, Mg^{2+}-ATPase), SERCA2b, that differs structurally and functionally from that expressed in skeletal and cardiac muscle (SERCA2a). Although SERCA2b has a lower turnover rate for Ca^{2+} transport and for the ATP hydrolysis, the pH dependence of SERCA2b and SERCA2a appears to be similar in that acidic conditions would directly reduce the pump rate of the Ca^{2+}, Mg^{2+}-ATPase.[2]

A second mechanism that mediates internal Ca^{2+} release involves the messenger inositol-1,4,5-triphosphate (IP_3). IP_3 is generated from L-α-phosphatidylinositol diphosphate (PIP_2) by the action of phospholipase C.[10] Phospholipase C is subject to regulation by guanine nucleotide–binding proteins (G proteins), which are activated in response to hormone receptor stimulation. IP_3 binds to an IP_3 receptor that is also a kind of Ca^{2+} channel that releases Ca^{2+} from an internal pool (Fig. 66–7). IP_3-gated channels have similar secondary and tertiary structures as the ryanodine-sensitive channels responsible for the Ca^{2+}-induced Ca^{2+} release. Both kinds of channels also reveal functional similarities because they have a similar dependence on Ca^{2+} and are sensitive to adenine nucleotides.[2] Pharmacomechanical coupling, which is contraction in the absence of a change in membrane potential, may occur via IP_3-mediated Ca^{2+}-release.[7, 10]

Finally, Ca^{2+} can be actively extruded from the cell via a sarcolemmal Ca^{2+} pump. In addition to requiring ATP for activity, this pump is subject to regulation by cAMP. Beta-adrenergic agents may produce a portion of their relaxing effects on vascular muscle by stimulating the active extrusion of Ca^{2+} from the cell.[4]

Signal Transduction

An understanding of the multiplicity and regulation of signaling mechanisms in vascular smooth muscle is still

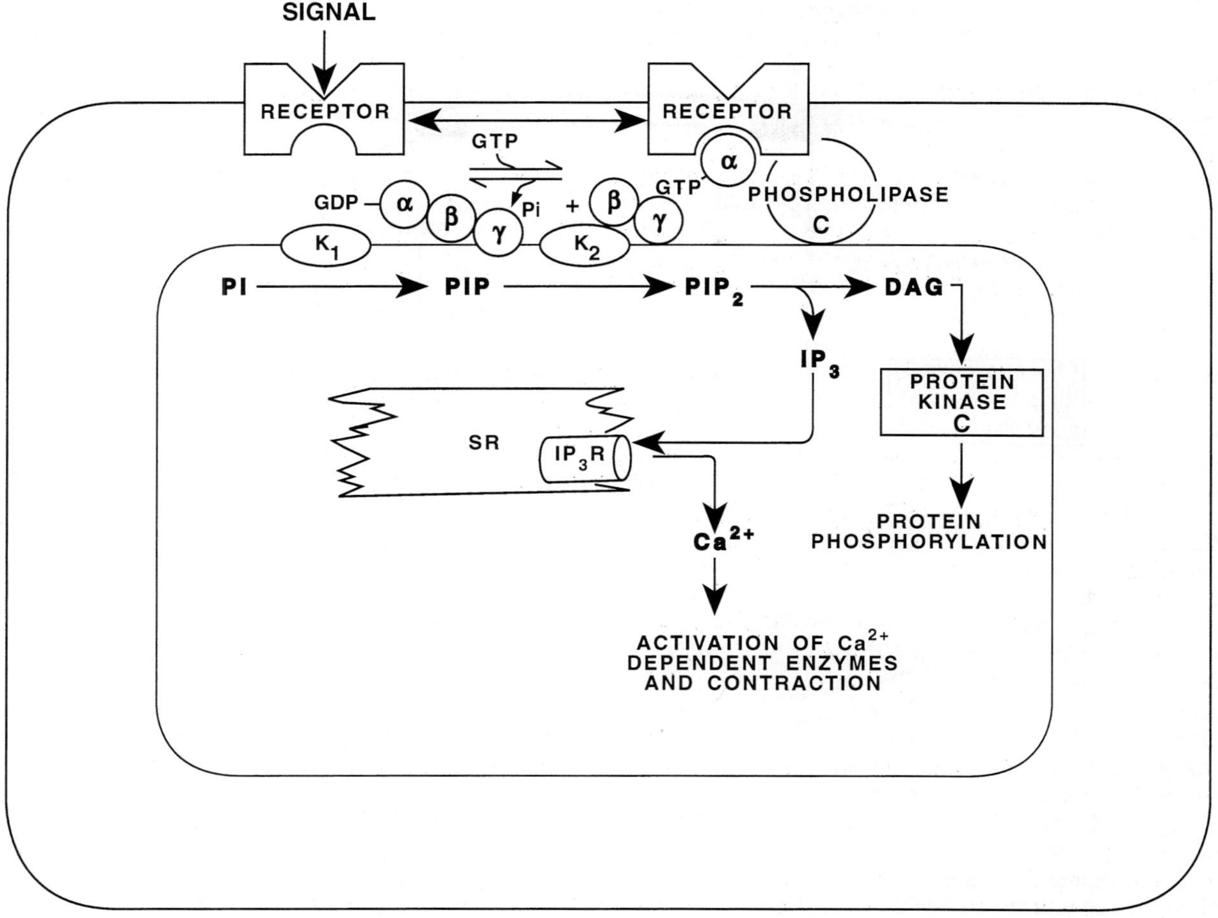

FIGURE 66–7 The phosphoinositide pathway and G proteins. Many receptors are activated by a process that involves binding of a hormone to a receptor and subsequent binding of the α-subunit of the G proteins. This process also requires binding of guanosine triphosphate (GTP) to the α subunit of the G protein complex and dissolution of the α-subunit from the βγ complex. The G protein/receptor complex can activate many processes or enzymes. One important cascade in vascular muscle is the phosphoinositide pathway. G protein/receptor complexes activate the enzyme phospholipase C, which catalyzes the conversion of L-α-phosphatidylinositol diphosphate (PIP_2) to diacylglycerol (DAG) and 1,4,5-inositol triphosphate (IP_3). IP_3 binds to an intracellular receptor (IP_3R) located in some regions of the sarcoplasmic reticulum (SR). The IP_3R is a Ca^{2+} channel, and its stimulation causes the release of Ca^{2+} into the cytoplasm and the subsequent activation of many Ca^{2+}-dependent processes. PI, phosphatidylinositol.

evolving. Nevertheless, it is clear that the process of signal transduction begins with the binding of a ligand (e.g., hormone, drug, extracellular matrix protein) to a membrane receptor on the exterior of the cell. These receptor proteins span the cellular membrane and are coupled to effectors that transduce agonist binding into a specific biochemical message (Fig. 66–8). There are at least two major effector systems in vascular muscle that couple to membrane receptor binding: G proteins and intrinsic receptor kinases. Two major classes of G proteins have been identified: heterotrimeric G proteins and low-molecular-weight G proteins that resemble the proto-oncogene *ras* (i.e., *ras*-like proteins). Heterotrimeric G proteins consist of α, β, and γ subunits. Multiple forms of each exist, but the greatest polymorphism resides in the α-subunit as a result of several unique genes that encode this protein.[10] The binding of a hormone to a receptor results in the following sequence of events: (1) association of the receptor with the G protein, (2) activation of the α-subunit by binding the GTP, (3) dissociation of the α-subunit from the βγ-subunit complex, (4) activation of the effector system by binding of the α-subunit, (5) hydrolysis of GTP and inactivation of the α-subunit, and (6) reversal of the sequence of molecular events (see Fig. 66–7). Although this has been the dogma for activation of intracellular events via heterotrimeric G proteins, a growing body of evidence exists to show that the βγ dimer may also directly act on effector proteins.

The low-molecular-weight G proteins are similar in structure to the isolated α-subunits of the heterotrimeric G proteins. Several different types have been identified in vascular muscle, although the prototype of this family is the proto-oncogene product *ras*.[12] The *ras* family of proteins is also activated by GTP binding and deactivated by hydrolysis of GTP to GDP. The rate of GTP hydrolysis can be stimulated by GAP proteins (i.e., GTPase-activating proteins). Such stimulation abbreviates the action of the *ras*-like proteins. In addition, another regulatory protein stimulates the release of GDP (guanine nucleotide–releasing protein), allowing for the subsequent binding of GTP and an enhancement of activity. *Ras* and its family of

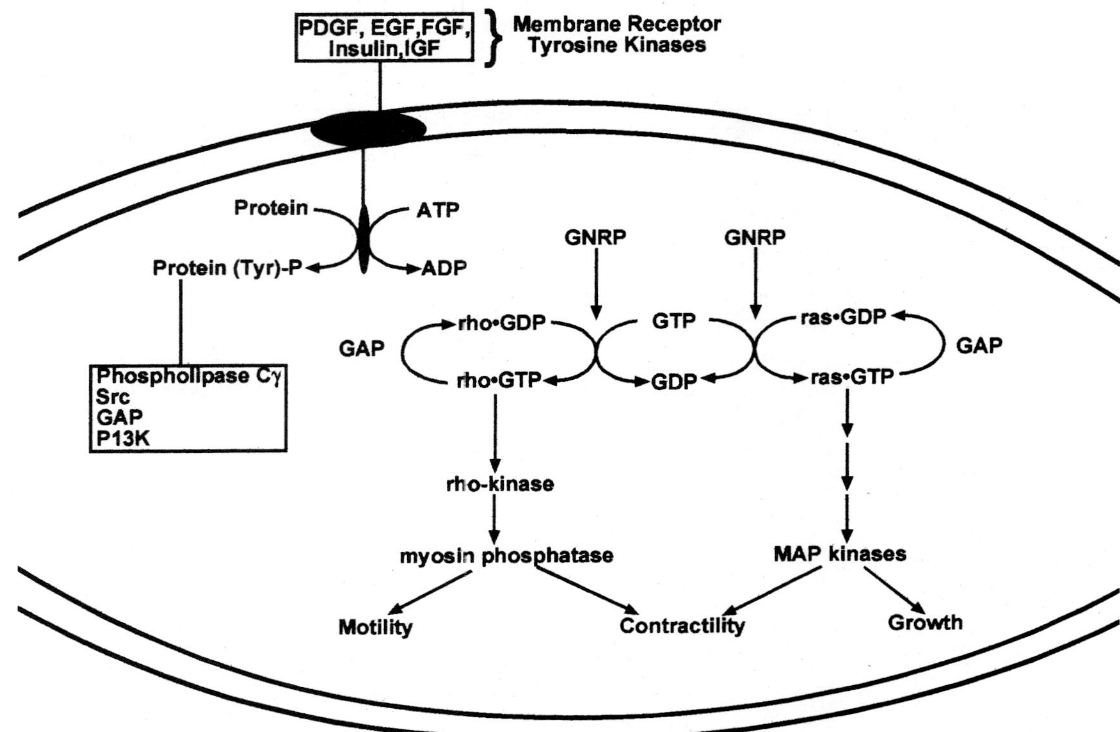

FIGURE 66–8 Membrane receptor tyrosine kinases and the small (*ras*-like) guanosine triphosphate (GTP)-binding proteins. Several different kinds of peptide hormones or growth factors possess tyrosine kinase activity in the cytoplasmic domain of the receptor protein. The tyrosine kinase domain is activated on binding to the receptor, and phosphate is transferred from adenosine triphosphate (ATP) to a tyrosine residue on a specific substrate protein. For example, phospholipase Cγ, the tyrosine kinase *src,* the GTPase-activating protein (GAP), and phosphatidylinositol-3 kinase (PI_3K) are all phosphorylated on tyrosine residues by the platelet-derived growth factor (PDGF) receptor. Other hormone or growth factor receptors (i.e., epidermal growth factor [EGF], fibroblast growth factor [FGF], insulin-like growth factor [IGF], and insulin) have a separate and unique array of substrates. The small GTP-binding proteins identified in smooth muscle are similar to the proto-oncogene *ras* and include *ras* and *rhoA.* These proteins resemble the α subunit of heterotrimeric G proteins. The active forms of *ras* or *rho* bind GTP and in this state can activate a number of processes or enzyme cascades, including the activation of mitogen-activating protein (MAP) kinase (for *ras*) and myosin phosphatase (for *rho*). Both *ras* and *rho* are inactivated by hydrolysis of GTP (i.e., to form *ras*-GDP or *rho*-GDP). This reaction is stimulated by a G protein–specific GTPase-activating protein (GAP). Certain GAP proteins may be inactivated through tyrosine phosphorylation by the PDGF receptor. Both *ras* and *rho* are activated by the exchange of guanosine diphosphate (GDP) for GTP, which is stimulated by the guanine nucleotide–releasing protein (GNRP). The activation of myosin phosphatase or MAP kinases may alter several functional properties of smooth muscle, including motility, growth, and contractility. ADP, adenosine diphosphate.

proteins are involved in several cellular functions, including intracellular trafficking of transport vesicles and activation of selected protein kinase cascades.[12]

Finally, the receptor tyrosine kinases are protein kinases that reside in the cytoplasmic domains of several peptide hormone and growth factor receptors (see Fig. 66–8). These are named tyrosine kinases because they transfer phosphate from ATP to tyrosine residues on target proteins in response to receptor stimulation.[13] Tyrosine phosphorylation serves as a switch to turn on the activity of several important enzymes, including phospholipase C, phosphatidylinositol-3-phosphate kinase, and the *ras*-type G proteins. There is growing evidence that tyrosine phosphorylation is a mechanism for coupling receptor activation of vascular smooth muscle cells to increases in intracellular Ca^{2+} and contraction.[14]

Beyond the effector systems are the second messengers or tertiary targets. These include three basic systems that are activated by the G proteins or via tyrosine phosphorylation: the synthesis and hydrolysis of membrane phosphoinositides, the nucleotide cyclases, and specific protein kinases and phosphatases. L-α-Phosphatidylinositol is a major constituent of cellular membranes. Sequential phosphorylation of L-α-phosphatidylinositol yields PIP_2. Hydrolysis of PIP_2 by phospholipase C generates IP_3 and diacylglycerol (see Fig. 66–7). The former stimulates Ca^{2+} release from an internal pool, whereas the latter, in concert with Ca^{2+}, activates the enzyme protein kinase C. Protein kinase C can phosphorylate and thereby modulate the activity of several key enzyme cascades.[3] For example, phosphorylation of the Na^+-H^+ exchanger enhances H^+ extrusion, resulting in intracellular alkalization. In addition, phosphorylation of L-type Ca^{2+} channels alters the opening probability and mean open time of the individual channel molecules. Finally, protein kinase C is involved in adrenergic receptor down-regulation, modulation of the activity of heterotrimeric G proteins and the *ras* family of proteins, and modulation of the activity of ion channels and exchangers.

The nucleotide cyclases convert either ATP to cAMP (adenylyl cyclase) or GTP to cGMP (guanylyl cyclase). Adenylyl cyclase is coupled to beta$_2$-adrenergic receptors via G proteins.[15] The cAMP generated activates a cAMP-dependent protein kinase. The latter phosphorylates several proteins, such as phospholamban of the SR, as well as the Ca^{2+} pump of the sarcolemma. The net effect is to reduce intracellular Ca^{2+} concentrations and promote relaxation. Guanylyl cyclase can be activated by nitric oxide that is either produced by the endothelium or administered in the form of a nitric oxide donor such as nitroglycerin, sodium nitroprusside, or diazoxide.[16] In addition, a sarcolemma-bound form of guanylyl cyclase is a receptor for atrial natriuretic peptide. cGMP, which is generated from GTP by guanylyl cyclase, activates a specific cGMP-dependent protein kinase. The activation of cGMP-dependent protein kinase results in a reduced level of intracellular Ca^{2+}, thus accounting for the potent vascular relaxant effects of exogenously administered nitric oxide donors.

As mentioned previously, vascular smooth muscle contains a rhoA-regulated rho-kinase that phosphorylates and inactivates myosin phosphatase. Alterations in rhoA activity, by virtue of the subsequent alteration of myosin phosphatase activity, result in either a change in contractility in smooth muscle cells of the contractile phenotype or a change in motility of cultured smooth muscle cells. In addition, other protein kinases activated in vascular myocytes in response to several agonists include the mitogen-activated protein (MAP) kinases.[17] MAP kinases can phosphorylate caldesmon or myosin light chain kinase, thereby altering contractility; however, they also phosphorylate various nuclear proteins involved in cell growth and proliferation. Membrane receptor tyrosine kinases provide a separate limb in the activation of MAP kinases, although it appears that receptor tyrosine kinases produce their effects by activating *ras* or other low-molecular-weight G proteins. Importantly, both growth factors (e.g., platelet-derived growth factor) and contractile agonists can initiate the cascades that ultimately lead to MAP kinase activation and myosin phosphatase inhibition. Therefore, regulation of growth, motility, and contractility in a smooth muscle cell is ultimately controlled by a number of neurohumoral and protein/peptide factors acting in concert on different membrane receptors of the same cell.[17, 18]

CONCLUSION

Research in the 1980s and 1990s has elucidated many of the key molecular mechanisms that underlie vascular smooth muscle contraction. This information has provided a clearer picture of the mechanisms underlying drug action and raises many intriguing possibilities for future strategies aimed at the modulation of vascular tone. In addition, the setting is obviously ripe for exploration of the molecular pathophysiology of hypertension, vasospastic disorders, and atherosclerosis at the level of the endothelium and vascular myocyte. With the new tools provided by molecular biology, the solid foundation in basic mechanisms already established, and the continuing need to provide specific therapies for the most prevalent diseases of the industrialized world, the current multidisciplinary focus on blood vessel function is likely to yield new strategies for treating the patient with blood vessel disease.

REFERENCES

1. Hathaway DR, March KL: Molecular cardiology: new avenues for the diagnosis and treatment of cardiovascular disease. J Am Coll Cardiol 13:265, 1989.
2. Smith GL, Austin C, Crichton C, Wray S: A review of the actions and control of intracellular pH in vascular smooth muscle. Cardiovasc Res 38:316, 1998.
3. Somlyo AP, Somlyo AV: Smooth muscle structure and function. *In* Fozzard HA, et al (eds): The Heart and Cardiovascular System. pp. 1295–1324. New York: Raven, 1992.
4. Hathaway DR, March KL, Lash JA, et al: Vascular smooth muscle: a review of the molecular basis of contractility. Circulation 83:382, 1991.
5. Somlyo AP, Somlyo AV: Signal transduction and regulation in smooth muscle. Nature 372:231, 1994.
6. Uehata M, Ishizaki T, Satoh H, et al: Calcium sensitization of smooth muscle mediated by a Rho-associated protein kinase in hypertension. Nature 389:990, 1997.
7. Somlyo AP, Somlyo AV: From pharmacomechanical coupling to G-proteins and myosin phosphatase. Acta Physiol Scand 164:437, 1998.
8. Knot HJ, Brayden JE, Nelson MT: Calcium channels and potassium channels. pp. 203–219. *In* Barany M (ed): Biochemistry of Smooth Muscle Contraction. San Diego: Academic, 1996.
9. Ganitkevich VY, Isenberg G: Contribution of Ca^{2+}-induced Ca^{2+}-release to the $[Ca^{2+}]_i$ transients in myocytes from guinea pig urinary bladder. J Physiol 458:119, 1992.
10. Berridge MJ: Inositol triphosphate and calcium signaling. Nature 361:315, 1993.
11. Simon SI, Strathmann MP, Gautam N: Diversity of G-proteins in signal transduction. Science 252:802, 1991.
12. Satoh T, Nakafuku M, Kuziro Y: Function of ras as a molecular switch in signal transduction. J Biol Chem 267:24149, 1992.
13. Yarden Y, Ullrich A: Growth factor receptor tyrosine kinases. Annu Rev Biochem 57:443, 1987.
14. Di Salvo J, Nelson SR, Kaplan N: Protein tyrosine phosphorylation in smooth muscle: a potential coupling mechanism between receptor activation and intracellular calcium. Proc Soc Exp Biol Med 214:285, 1997.
15. Gilman AG, Tang WJ: Adenylyl cyclases. Cell 70:869, 1992.
16. Lincoln TM, Cornwell TL, Komalavilas P, et al: *In* Barany M (ed): Biochemistry of Smooth Muscle Contraction. pp. 257–268. San Diego: Academic, 1996.
17. Adam LP: Mitogen-activated protein kinase. *In* Barany M (ed): Biochemistry of Smooth Muscle Contraction. pp. 167–177. San Diego: Academic, 1996.
18. Pelech SL, Sanghera JS: MAP kinases: charting the regulatory pathways. Science 257:1355, 1992.

C H A P T E R **67**

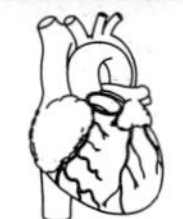

Circulatory Regulation: Basic Considerations

John T. Shepherd, Thomas F. Lüscher, and Giuseppe Mancia

NORMAL CIRCULATORY REGULATION
Local Factors
Autonomic Nerves, Neurotransmitters, and Vascular Receptors
Cardiovascular Reflexes
Interactions Between Neurotransmitters and Endothelial Cells
Hormones
Aging
Orthostatic Stress
Mental Stress
Muscular Exercise
CIRCULATORY DYSFUNCTION
Vasovagal Syncope
Smoking
Obesity
Diabetes
Hypertension
Heart Failure
Hypercholesterolemia
Atherosclerosis
Gene Transfer

The cardiovascular system is regulated to ensure there is appropriate perfusion of the tissues and organs of the body to fulfill their metabolic requirements and to maintain proper thermoregulation. This demands complex interactions of local, humoral, and nervous factors to adjust the performance of the heart and blood vessels to meet the changing stresses of daily life. In diseases of the cardiovascular system, these regulatory mechanisms are disturbed with resultant abnormalities in circulatory control.

Normal Circulatory Regulation

Local Factors

The endothelium forms vascular relaxing and contracting factors that act locally to alter the tone of the underlying smooth muscle. The major relaxing factor is nitric oxide (NO); others are prostaglandin I_2 (also termed prostacyclin), endothelium-derived hyperpolarizing factor,[1] and C-type natriuretic peptide (CNP). The major contracting factor is endothelin (ET)-1; others are angiotensin II (Ang II) and vasoconstrictor metabolites of arachidonic acid. These locally formed substances also modulate the response of the underlying vascular smooth muscle to hormones, neurotransmitters, and platelet products (Fig. 67–1).

Endothelium-Derived Relaxing Factors

In the endothelial cells, the constitutive enzyme nitric oxide synthase (eNOS) converts L-arginine to L-citrulline with a release of NO. A cofactor, tetrahydrobiopterin, is required for activation of nitric oxide synthase (NOS).[2] NO activates soluble guanylate cyclase in the underlying smooth muscle, and the resultant increase in cyclic guanosine monophosphate causes its relaxation. The NO is inactivated within a few seconds by superoxide anions.

NO not only is a potent vasodilator but also inhibits platelet aggregation and leukocyte adhesion to endothelial cells and suppresses the proliferation and migration of vascular smooth muscle cells. The expression of eNOS is regulated by the action of shear stress on the endothelial cells and by cyclic circumferential stretch of the blood vessels.[3] Unidirectional shear stress increases eNOS mRNA expression via a transcriptional mechanism, whereas oscillatory shear stress and cyclic stretch do this through post-transcriptional regulatory events.[4] The earliest mechanochemical signal transduction is activation of specific G proteins in the endothelium within 1 second of flow-induced signaling.[5]

The biologic effects of NO are determined by the amount released and its inactivation by superoxide anions (O_2^-). The endothelial cells are a source of superoxide, and NOS can produce superoxide.[6] Tetrahydrobiopterin determines the balance of O_2^- and NO production from eNOS after prolonged stretch of human aortic endothelial cells.[7]

NOS also may catalyze formation of hydrogen peroxide (H_2O_2). This is favored by low endogenous concentrations of L-arginine, tetrahydrobiopterin, or both. Although H_2O_2 is a potent vasodilator, prolonged increased concentrations of H_2O_2 may be harmful to endothelial and smooth muscle cells, leading to a shift in the balance between the production of protective NO and deleterious O_2^-.[8, 9] In addition, O_2^- from the adventitia of the blood vessel can inactivate NO.[10]

Oxygen-derived free radicals have been implicated in the pathogenesis of atherosclerosis and restenosis. Hypercholesterolemia, diabetes, and ischemia followed by reperfusion are also associated with increased vascular O_2^- production. Native low-density lipoprotein and Ang II have been reported to stimulate O_2^- production from endothelial

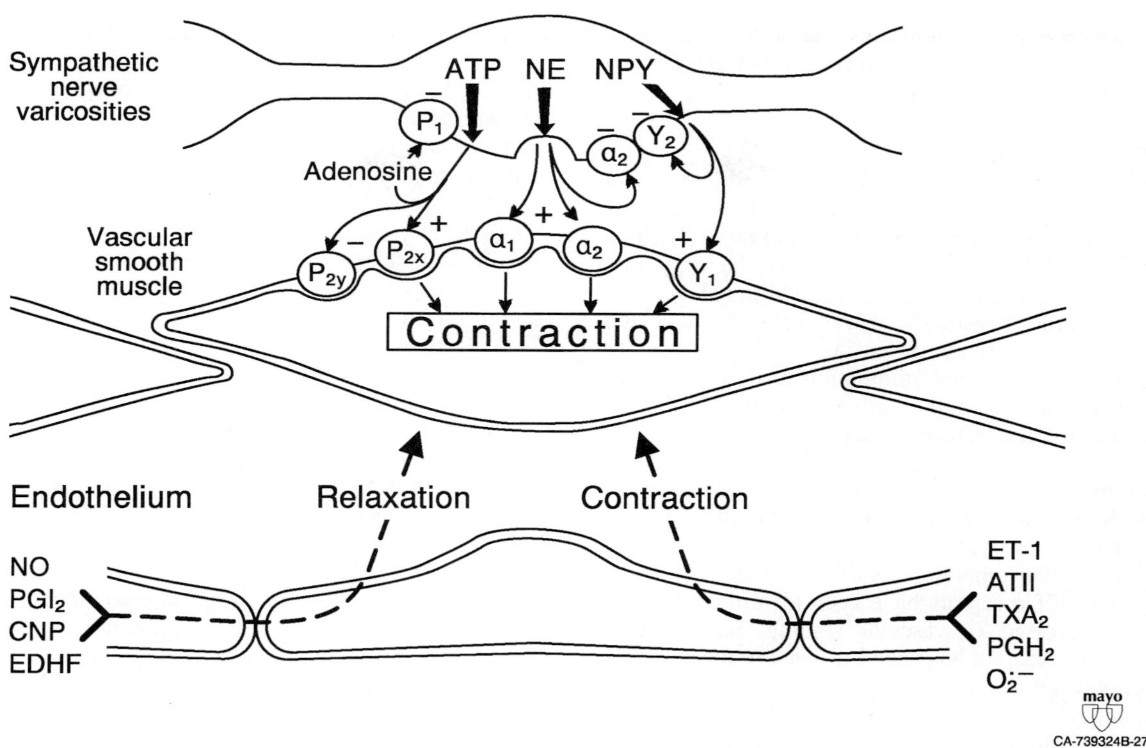

FIGURE 67–1 Control of systemic resistance blood vessels by neurotransmitters and endothelium-derived vasoactive factors. The neurotransmitters released from the sympathetic nerves—norepinephrine (NE), adenosine triphosphate (ATP), and neuropeptide Y (NPY)—cause contraction of the arterial resistance vessels by NE-activating alpha$_1$- and alpha$_2$-adrenoceptors, ATP-activating P_{2x} receptors, and NPY-activating Y_1 receptors. Some of the ATP may activate a vasodilator P_{2y} receptor, but the vasoconstriction predominates. Some of the NE can activate an α_2-adrenoceptor (α_2) on the endothelial cells. The resultant release of NO can attenuate the vasoconstriction. In contrast, in the coronary arteries, the simultaneous activation of beta-adrenergic and P_{2y} receptors results in their dilatation. NPY also enhances the activity of NE and ATP on their receptors. The α_2, Y_2, and P_1 receptors also are present on the sympathetic nerve varicosities. If these are activated by NE and NPY and, in the case of P_1, by the metabolism of ATP to adenosine in the synaptic cleft, there is decreased output from the nerves of NE and ATP. The release of NO from nitroxidergic nerves will cause vasorelaxation. The normal resting endothelial cells continuously release NO to relax the underlying smooth muscle. The other endothelium-derived relaxation factors are prostacyclin (PGI_2), C-type natriuretic peptide (CNP), and endothelium-derived hyperpolarizing factor (EDHF). The endothelial cells also have the potential to release vasoconstrictor substances: endothelin-1 (ET), angiotensin II (ATII), thromboxane A_2 (TXA_2), and oxygen-derived free radicals ($O_2^{\cdot-}$). PGH_2, cyclic endoperoxides.

and vascular smooth muscle cells. Moreover, the proliferative response of smooth muscle cells to platelet-derived growth factor is mediated by H_2O_2. Pulsatile stretch applied to human coronary artery smooth muscle cells causes their proliferation, which is associated with increased oxidative stress. This increase promotes DNA synthesis in these muscles.[11]

NO forms complexes with various biomolecular carriers such as nitrosothiol (RS-NO) that retain biologic activity. Studies on the forearm resistance vessels of normal humans indicate that RS-NO contributes to vascular smooth muscle relaxation.[12] Basal and flow-induced release of NO from vascular endothelium can be mediated via local cholinergic mechanisms. The flow may cause acetylcholine release from certain endothelial cells, which stimulates NO release from these cells or from neighboring endothelial cells.[13]

There are numerous receptors in the endothelial cells that, if activated, cause a release of NO. Some of the norepinephrine released when the sympathetic nerves are activated stimulates alpha$_2$-adrenoceptors on the endothelial cells. The resultant release of NO attenuates the vasoconstriction.[14] Other agonists include bradykinin, histamine, and substances released from platelets (adenosine triphosphate, 5-hydroxytryptamine [serotonin], and thromboxane A_2).

NO, but not prostacyclin, is essential for flow-mediated dilatation of large human arteries.[15]

There are two other important roles for NO: first, to maintain a balance in the kidney between oxygen consumption and sodium reabsorption.[16] Second, NO released from the vascular endothelium has an important role in the regulation of tissue mitochondrial respiration in skeletal muscle[17] and in the regulation of cardiac contractile function.[18]

Another important finding is that in healthy conscious adults, the pulmonary vascular resistance is maintained in part through the continuous local production of NO.[19]

Pulsatile stretch in coronary arteries also can release endothelium-derived hyperpolarizing factor.[20] CNP is produced in endothelial cells and has been proposed to mediate vascular relaxation by causing endothelium-dependent hyperpolarization. To study this in porcine coronary arteries, the endothelium-dependent relaxations and hyperpolarization of CNP and bradykinin were compared. In contrast to bradykinin, CNP induced endothelium-independent and weaker relaxation and hyperpolarization of coronary artery vascular smooth muscle, suggesting that it is an unlikely mediator of endothelium-dependent hyperpolarization of porcine coronary arteries.[21]

Endothelium-Derived Contracting Factors

ET-1, which is produced by endothelial cells of blood vessels, is a potent vasoconstrictor peptide. It is a member of a family of 21-amino-acid peptides consisting of three isoforms: ET-1, ET-2, and ET-3. ET-1 is the only one produced by endothelial cells. It has additional actions, including interactions with the sympathetic nervous and renin-angiotensin systems, potentiation of responses to other constrictor agents, and stimulation of mitogenesis of vascular smooth muscle cells and cardiomyocytes. It also appears to have major effects on cardiac, renal, and cerebral functions.[22]

The mechanism of ET-mediated vasoconstriction involves binding to specific receptors on vascular smooth muscle and direct activation of voltage-operated calcium channels in vascular smooth muscle membrane. Two distinct cDNAs of ET receptors have been identified; the ET_A receptor is expressed in vascular smooth muscle cells, whereas the ET_B receptor has been localized to the endothelial and smooth muscle cells. The ET_B receptor may have a dual vasoconstrictive and vasodilatory effect.[23]

An $ET_{A/B}$ receptor antagonist decreases peripheral vascular resistance and, to a lesser extent, arterial blood pressure. It increases circulating ET concentrations and blocks forearm vasoconstriction to exogenous ET-1. These results suggest that the endogenous generation of ET-1 plays an important physiologic role in the maintenance of peripheral vascular tone and blood pressure in humans.[24]

Selective ET_A receptor antagonism causes vasodilatation of human forearm resistance vessels in vivo due mostly to increased NO generation. ET_B receptor antagonism causes local vasoconstriction, indicating that these receptors in blood vessels respond to ET-1 predominantly by causing vasodilatation.[25]

Acute elevations in plasma ET-1 concentrations in the coronary artery within a pathophysiologic range do not impair blood flow to normal or collateral vessel–dependent myocardium. This is because increased prostacyclin production in response counteracts the vasoconstrictor properties of ET-1.[26]

There are complex interactions between endothelium-derived substances, including ET-1 and NO. ET-1 induces the formation of NO, which is believed to mediate its vasodepressor action. Furthermore, endothelium-derived NO inhibits the synthesis and may also counteract the vasoconstrictor and vasopressor actions of ET-1. In addition, both NO and ET-1 have been implicated in the regulation of blood and plasma volume and albumin extravasation in various vascular beds.[27]

Other endothelium-derived contracting factors that are less important than ET-1 are Ang II, thromboxane A_2, prostaglandin H_2, and oxygen-derived free radicals (see Fig. 67–1).[28]

Autonomic Nerves, Neurotransmitters, and Vascular Receptors

In 1946, Von Euler demonstrated that norepinephrine was released on activation of the sympathetic nerves. Adenosine triphosphate and neuropeptide Y are cotransmitters in these nerves. In the smooth muscle of the systemic vessels, norepinephrine excites α_1- and α_2-adrenoceptors, adenosine triphosphate P_{2x} purinoceptors, and neuropeptide Y_1 receptors to cause vasoconstriction (see Fig. 67–1).[29] In contrast, in the coronary arteries, the simultaneous activation of beta-adrenoceptors and P_{2y} receptors results in their dilation. Neuropeptide Y also enhances the activity of norepinephrine and adenosine triphosphate on their receptors.[30] α_2-Adrenoceptors and neuropeptide Y_2 receptors also are present on the sympathetic nerve varicosities (see Fig. 67–1). If these are activated, there is a decrease in the output of norepinephrine and adenosine triphosphate.

Interactions of the sympathetic and parasympathetic nerves at the heart have traditionally been defined in terms of their classic neurotransmitters: norepinephrine and acetylcholine. It is known that neuropeptides, which are released from the sympathetic nerves during their activation, have powerful and long-lasting inhibitory actions on vagal transmission in the heart.[31] Long-term sympathectomy causes a decrease in eNOS, 5-hydroxytryptamine, and substance P and an increase in ET-1 immunoreactivity in the thoracic aortic endothelium of the rat.[32]

In addition, nerves that function by releasing NO have been discovered (*nitroxidergic,* or *nitrergic,* nerves) and, in the vessels from different species so far examined, are distributed to the cerebral, femoral, mesenteric, penile, renal, and retinal arteries.[33, 34]

A local sympathetic venoarteriolar axon reflex has been identified that contributes to the maintenance of arterial blood pressure in humans on assumption of the upright position.[35]

Cardiovascular Reflexes

Changes in sympathetic outflow are governed by arterial baroreceptors and chemoreceptors, cardiopulmonary mechanoreceptors, and receptors in skeletal muscles that are activated by muscular contraction. Changes in sympathetic outflow also can occur due to primary changes in the activity of particular centers in the brain. To meet the various stresses to which the body is subjected, the sympathetic outflow occurs in a differentiated pattern. Thus, in response to reflex or central stimuli, the efferent sympathetic activity varies among the different organs and tissues and, in the same organ or tissue, can vary between resistance and capacitance vessels. In some instances, sympathetic activity may increase in some organs and decrease in others. For example, in essential hypertension, obesity, and congestive heart failure (CHF), sympathetic nerve activity is increased to muscle, but not to skin, vessels.[36]

Arterial blood pressure and heart rate change not only in relation to behavioral and environmental factors but also as a result of regular fluctuations unrelated to external stimuli. Blood pressure variability includes rhythmic and nonrhythmic fluctuations.[37] Physical training improves the baroreceptor control of the systemic circulation via the sympathetic nervous system, and this effect may be different from the concomitant effect of training on arterial or baroreceptor control of cardiac sympathetic activity.[38]

In addition to the importance of local factors at the site of the mechanoreceptors in the carotid sinus and aortic arch in regulation of the autonomic outflow to the heart and circulation, studies in conscious rabbits have shown that NO in the brain stem plays an important role in the rapid central adaptation of baroreflex control of sympathetic nerve activity.[39] Also, an elevated level of Ang II is critical for the inhibitory effect of NO on the sympathetic outflow.[40]

Mechanoreceptors in the heart and lungs are important in the reflex control of the circulation. In humans, this reflex influence includes vascular resistance, plasma renin activity, and plasma vasopressin levels, indicating a role for these receptors in both blood volume and blood pressure control (Fig. 67–2).[41]

Nitroxidergic (Nitrergic) Nerves

Nitroxidergic nerves have a constitutive neuronal isoform of NOS and cause vasodilatation through the release of NO. Because NO is a labile free radical, unlike other transmitters, it is not stored in synaptic vesicles and is not released by exocytosis but instead diffuses from the nerve terminals into adjacent cells.[33, 34, 42]

Interactions Between Neurotransmitters and Endothelial Cells

Are the actions on the vascular system of the neurotransmitters and the endothelium-derived vasoactive substances the sum of their separate effects, or are they modified by interactions between them? This depends on the ability of any neurotransmitter to diffuse through the vascular wall and to affect the specific endothelial receptor.[43] In the coronary arteries, acetylcholine released from the vagal nerves causes their dilatation through the activation of a muscarinic receptor on the endothelial cells, leading to a release of NO.[44]

In other studies to examine whether autonomic influences modulate vascular NO-mediated vasodilatation or even directly contribute to production of NO via nitroxidergic fibers, it was found that tonic NO-dependent vasodilatation can normally be maintained in the unanesthetized,

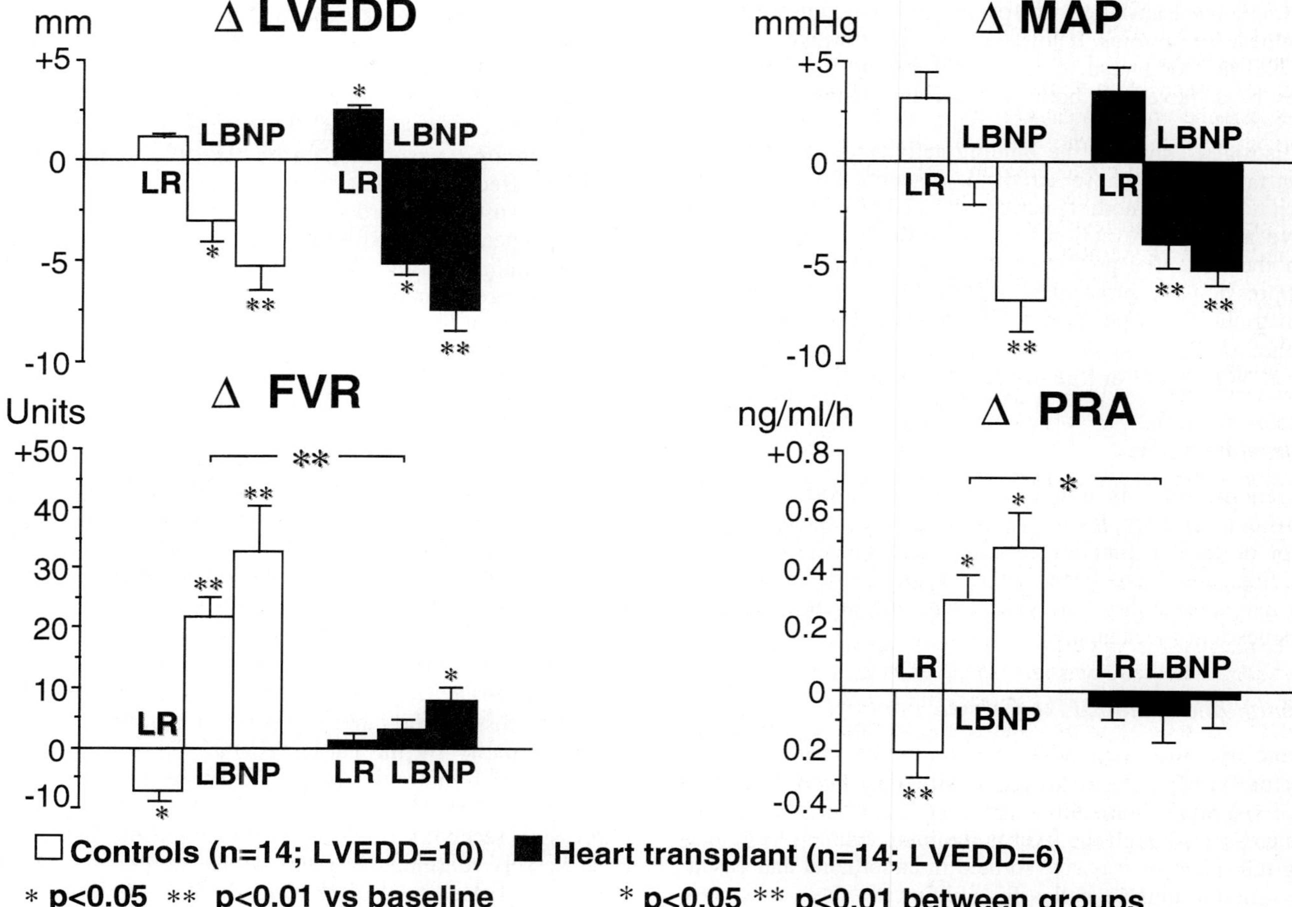

FIGURE 67–2 Changes in left ventricular end-diastolic diameter (Δ LVEDD, echocardiography), mean arterial pressure (Δ MAP), forearm vascular resistance (Δ FVR), and plasma renin activity (Δ PRA) induced by cardiopulmonary receptor stimulation (leg raising [LR]) and deactivation (lower body negative pressure [LBNP]) in control subjects *(open columns)* and in heart transplant recipients *(solid columns)*. (Modified from Giannattasio C, Del Bo A, Cattaneo BM, et al: Reflex vasopressin and renin modulation by cardiac receptors in humans. Hypertension 21:461–469, 1993.)

unrestrained rat regardless of autonomic or humoral adrenergic influences.[45]

Hormones

Angiotensin II

The vasoconstrictor peptide Ang II plays an important role in the control of systemic blood pressure. In addition to its direct action on the blood vessels, it facilitates the sympathetic influences on the cardiovascular system.

It seems that Ang II can stimulate the synthesis of eNOS and hence enhance the production of NO. It is suggested that in the kidney, this protects the preglomerular vessels from the constrictor effect of Ang II.[46] In patients with coronary artery disease, angiotensin-converting enzyme (ACE) inhibition attenuates sympathetic coronary vasoconstriction.[47]

Estrogen

Both endothelial and vascular smooth muscle cells possess estrogen receptors. Estrogen regulates the transcription of numerous genes, and its cellular actions are mediated through the translation of specific mRNA transcripts and synthesis of proteins. It stimulates the constitutive synthesis of NO in blood vessels, heart, and skeletal muscles. This may be achieved via both genomic and nongenomic pathways.[48, 49]

Estrogen enhances the binding activity of the transcription factor Sp1, whose activity is essential for eNOS transcription. Even modest increases in eNOS expression may have a protective action against cardiovascular disease.[50] Another potential protective mechanism of estrogen is the suppression of a prostaglandin H synthase–dependent vasoconstriction.[51] In perimenopausal women, estrogen supplementation reduced arterial blood pressure and enhanced basal NO release in forearm resistance arteries.[52]

Adrenomedullin

Adrenomedullin is a newly identified vasorelaxing and natriuretic peptide. It may function as an endogenous regulator of cardiac function, because adrenomedullin and its binding sites have been found in the heart. It enhances cardiac contractility via cyclic adenosine monophosphate–independent mechanisms.[53]

Insulin and Insulin-Like Growth Factor-I

There are three peptide hormones in the insulin growth factor family—insulin and insulin-like growth factors (IGFs)-I and -II. Insulin is produced and secreted by the pancreas. Although the liver is the main source of circulating IGF-I levels, it is also formed in endothelial and vascular smooth muscle cells. In addition to their metabolic and growth-promoting actions, these peptides have both vasoconstrictor and vasodilator actions on the vascular system.[54, 55]

Some studies suggest that endothelium-derived NO mediates the vasodilator actions of insulin and IGF-I,[56] but others have disagreed. We must recognize, however, the heterogeneity of endothelium-mediated responses in different arteries and veins, even within the same species. In isolated porcine coronary arteries, both insulin and IGF-I caused non–endothelium-dependent coronary relaxation, probably through a mechanism involving the activation of potassium channels.[57]

Aging

Primary aging produces a number of changes in the cardiovascular system in humans.[58] Findings provide support for the concept that cardiopulmonary and integrative baroreflex control of sympathetic nerve activity during acute hypovolemia is enhanced rather than depressed in healthy older humans. This may help minimize the functional impact of a marked age-related reduction in peripheral vasoconstrictor responsiveness to sympathetic neural stimulation and contribute to the effective regulation of arterial blood pressure in older adults during orthostatic challenge.[59] Aging in humans, however, is associated with an impairment of arterial blood pressure homeostasis. This is reflected by an increased pressure lability and a greater decrease in pressure during orthostatic stress compared with younger subjects. This impairment is explained in part by a decreased buffering role of the arterial baroreflex.[37] Cigarette smoking, on the other hand, increases sympathetic outflow.[60] In contrast, sodium restriction in the diet may impair the arterial baroreflex, and thus oppose, through sympathetically mediated vasoconstriction, the blood pressure–lowering effect of the diet.[61]

Several vascular disorders, including a diminished endothelium-dependent vasodilatation, have been demonstrated in aging humans.[62] In aging rats, eNOS activity and NO production are reduced, which could explain the observations in humans.[63, 64]

Orthostatic Stress

Gravitational stresses, which are common daily events for humans, result in a diminution in central blood volume due to the displacement of blood to the lower parts of the body. Complex adjustments in the cardiovascular system are required to offset the decrease in cardiac filling pressure. Such changes are necessary to sustain arterial blood pressure at an appropriate level so there is adequate perfusion of vital organs, especially the brain. These adjustments must compensate for both the initial and sustained orthostatic stresses. The rapid short-term adaptations are mediated primarily by the cardiovascular reflexes, with humoral agents reinforcing these reflexes during severe and prolonged orthostatic stress.

Pressure receptors (mechanoreceptors) in the heart and great vessels continuously relay information on the blood pressure in these areas to the cardiovascular centers in the brain stem. A decrease in pressure excites the centers with a resultant increase in sympathetic and decrease in vagal outflow and vice versa. An increase in the sympathetic outflow to the heart and blood vessels and decrease in cardiac vagal activity cause an increase in heart rate and cardiac output and constriction of resistance vessels in skeletal muscle, kidney, and splanchnic bed and of the venous capacitance vessels in the splanchnic bed. The latter contributes importantly to maintenance of the cardiac filling pressures and, hence, the stroke volume. The great sensitivity and rapidity of the reflex responses of the splanchnic capacitance vessels to very low frequency of sympathetic discharge indicate their importance in regulation of the stroke volume. An important adjunct to the central activation of the vasomotor outflow is the local sympathetic venoarteriolar axon reflex. In addition, if the orthostatic stress is accompanied by contraction of the postural muscles, the decrease in vagal and increase in sympathetic outflow can be augmented and sustained by two mechanisms. One is a "central command" related to the motor signals from higher brain centers that stimulates the brain stem cardiovascular centers, and the other is a feedback reflex from the contracting muscles due to activation of their mechanoreceptors and metaboreceptors. The three principal humoral factors involved in the maintenance of cardiovascular homeostasis during prolonged orthostatic stress are the renin-angiotensin-aldosterone system, vasopressin, and atrial natriuretic factor.[65]

Mental Stress

Mental stress in humans results in arterial hypertension and tachycardia. In the offspring of hypertensive parents, sympathetic activation during mental stress is increased compared with the offspring of normotensive parents.[66] Mental stress also causes a neurogenically mediated vasodilatation in the skeletal muscles. The dilation is absent after surgical sympathectomy and is blunted after intra-arterial infusions of atropine. It has been shown that NO plays a key role in the autonomic control of the circulation during stress, with most of the NO release being due to autonomic nerve cholinergic stimulation of the vascular endothelium in the muscles.[67]

Muscular Exercise

Muscular exercise constitutes the major recurrent normal stress on the cardiovascular system, and numerous books have been written on the complexity of events that involve the regulation and integration of multiple systems, such as dilatation of the resistance vessels in the active muscles to provide the additional blood to meet their increased metabolic demand. The mechanisms are still undetermined after investigations that started in the 19th century. The muscle vasodilatation is accompanied by the appropriate increase in cardiac output. As exercise increases in severity, it is necessary to decrease the blood flow to other vascular beds to permit the arterial blood pressure to increase. This is accomplished via the input to the central nervous system from the arterial and cardiopulmonary mechanoreceptors and via ergoreceptors and chemoreceptors in the active muscles. In addition, a so-called central command modulates the autonomic outflow. The venous return, and hence the stroke volume, is sustained by the skeletal muscle pump and the reflex constriction of the splanchnic capacitance vessels. When static versus rhythmic exercise is performed, the so-called blood pressure–raising reflex is evoked from the active muscles.[68]

Although NO from the vascular endothelium may have a modest role in exercise hyperemia, in humans its presence is not essential for a nearly normal vasodilatation in skeletal muscles.[69] In the heart of the dog, it is estimated that NO is able to produce about one fourth of the coronary vasodilatation that occurred in response to exercise when all vasodilator systems were intact.[70] However, although NO production by the coronary circulation is increased with exercise, it does not affect levels of coronary blood flow because it shifts the relationship between cardiac work and myocardial oxygen consumption, suggesting that endogenous NO modulates myocardial metabolism.[71]

Chronic exercise in dogs increases eNOS gene expression, presumably by increasing endothelial shear stress, and this may contribute to the benefit of sustained exercise on the cardiovascular system.[72]

Circulatory Dysfunction

Vasovagal Syncope

During vasovagal syncope, profound bradycardia and hypotension occur. Atropine administration can prevent the bradycardia but not the hypotension, suggesting that marked peripheral vasodilation is a major cause of the fall in arterial pressure. This concept has been confirmed, because vasovagal syncope can be seen in patients who have undergone heart transplantation and in patients subjected to cardiac pacing. In both cases, there is no bradycardia but there is hypotension during the syncopal attacks. The major site of the vasodilation is in skeletal muscle, and muscle sympathetic nerve activity is suppressed just before and during vasovagal attacks, indicating that sympathetic withdrawal contributes to the dilation. However, the skeletal muscle vasodilation seen during syncope is greater than that caused by sympathetic withdrawal alone, and it is absent in limbs that have undergone surgical sympathectomy or local anesthetic nerve block. These observations suggest a role for neurally mediated "active" vasodilation during syncope. The afferent neural pathways that evoke the profound vasodilation during vasovagal attacks remain the subject of debate. The neural pathways responsible for the active component of the dilation are also unknown. Recent evidence has demonstrated that cholinergic, β-adrenergic, and nitroxidergic (NO) vasodilator mechanisms are not essential for the dilation.[73]

Patients with orthostatic vasovagal reactions have impaired vagal baroreflex responses to arterial pressure changes below resting levels but normal initial responses to upright tilt. Subtle vasovagal physiology begins before overt presyncope. The final trigger of human orthostatic vasovagal reactions appears to be the abrupt disappearance of muscle sympathetic nerve activity.[74]

In patients with sympathetic denervation due to primary autonomic failure, increased blood flow (due to excessive vasodilatation, lack of sympathetic restraint, or both) in leg muscle during and after exercise in combination with impaired splanchnic vasoconstriction in the early stages of exercise may have contributed to exercise-induced hypotension.[75]

Smoking

Baroreflex sensitivity is impaired in habitual smokers, which may contribute to the smoking-related increase in arterial blood pressure and heart rate and the decrease in heart rate variability during smoking.[76]

Long-term cigarette smoking is associated with impaired endothelium-dependent coronary vasodilation regardless of the presence or absence of coronary atherosclerotic lesions[77]; this is due to a deficiency in NO bioactivity.[73] The antioxidant vitamin C, as well as a potent reducing agent, tetrahydrobiopterin, improves endothelium-dependent responses in chronic smokers.[79] This observation supports the concept that endothelial dysfunction in chronic smokers is at least in part mediated by enhanced formation of oxygen-derived free radicals.[80] Coronary endothelial dysfunction also may occur in passive as well as in active smokers.[81]

Obesity

Human obesity is characterized by marked changes in the hemodynamic and metabolic states. In normotensive obese subjects, the postganglionic sympathetic nerve firing rate to the leg muscles was twice that seen in lean control subjects. This sympathetic activation occurs in the absence of arterial blood pressure regulation. The mechanism is unknown, but it may be one of the factors facilitating, in the long term, the development of hypertension, which is much more frequent in overweight than nonobese people.[82] However, later studies have found that obesity alone, in the absence of obstructive sleep apnea, is not accompanied by increased sympathetic activity to muscle blood vessels.[83]

In obese normotensive subjects, a reduction in body weight induced by a hypocaloric diet with normal sodium content exerts a marked reduction in sympathetic activity due to central sympathoinhibition (Fig. 67–3). This can be the consequence of an increased insulin sensitivity but also a restoration of the baroreflex control of the cardiovascular system with weight loss. This has clinical implications because the removal of the sympathetic activation through the loss of body weight may eliminate a factor that is involved in the high prevalence of hypertension, CHF, ischemic heart disease, and sudden death typical of obese persons. The suppression of sympathetic activity associated with the correction of an overweight condition may not have an entirely favorable significance because in obese subjects, a sympathetic activation may favor energy consumption and thus oppose further body weight increase; its suppression by body weight loss thus predisposes to a weight regain.[84]

Diabetes

There appears to be diminished basal NO production in diabetes. Decreases in endothelium-dependent relaxation are common in both conduit and resistant arteries of chemically induced experimental diabetic animals. In humans, endothelial dysfunction was first reported in penile corpora cavernosa of patients with insulin-dependent and non–insulin-dependent diabetes mellitus, but it is not yet known whether the response of the vascular smooth muscle to NO is compromised.[85] The time of onset of these changes due to diabetes is not yet established. There may be enhanced endothelial function early in the disease that changes later to dysfunction. In addition, diabetes is associated with an enhanced production of endothelium-derived contracting factors derived from the cyclooxygenase pathway.[86]

Changes in prostaglandin synthesis may alter NO production or reactivity to NO, but this may not be obligatory for the impaired endothelial function in diabetes. Arginine, via an unknown mechanism, appears to provide protection from alterations in vascular function caused by elevated glucose concentration.[87]

In isolated blood vessels, exposure to elevated glucose causes endothelial dysfunction. Concerning the mechanism, a prolonged exposure of human aortic endothelial cells to high glucose levels increases eNOS gene expression, protein expression, and NO release. However, the up-regulation of eNOS and NO release is associated with a marked increase in O_2^- production. The resulting imbalance between NO and O_2^- may explain the impaired endothelial function in diabetic vascular disease.[88]

Vitamin C selectively restores the impaired endothelium-dependent vasodilation in the forearm resistance vessels of patients with insulin-dependent diabetes mellitus. These findings indicate that NO degradation by oxygen-derived free radicals contributes to abnormal vascular reactivity in humans with this disease.[89]

Hypertension

The baroreceptor modulation of heart rate is impaired in patients with either essential or secondary hypertension, but there is controversy as to whether there are changes in the modulation of vasomotor tone due to the impairment of sympathetic control of systemic vascular resistance. In moderate and more severe essential hypertensive subjects, the stimulation and deactivation of baroreceptors by alteration of arterial blood pressure through vasoactive drug infusions caused much less reflex bradycardia and tachycardia, respectively, than in age-matched normotensive subjects. However, the concomitant reflex inhibition and excitation of muscle sympathetic nerve traffic were superimposable in the normotensive and hypertensive groups. Thus, in essential hypertension, the well-known impairment of the baroreflex ability to modulate the sinus node is not accompanied by any similar impairment of the baroreflex sympathetic modulation, which is of fundamental importance for the main baroreflex function (i.e., homeostatic blood pressure control).[90]

Concerning the role of NO, in studies with spontaneously hypertensive rats, it appears that the L-arginine–NO pathway in the rostral ventrolateral medulla is impaired, and this may contribute to the increase in arterial pressure.[91]

Concerning the arterial vessels, studies in the human forearm circulation have shown that the release of NO is

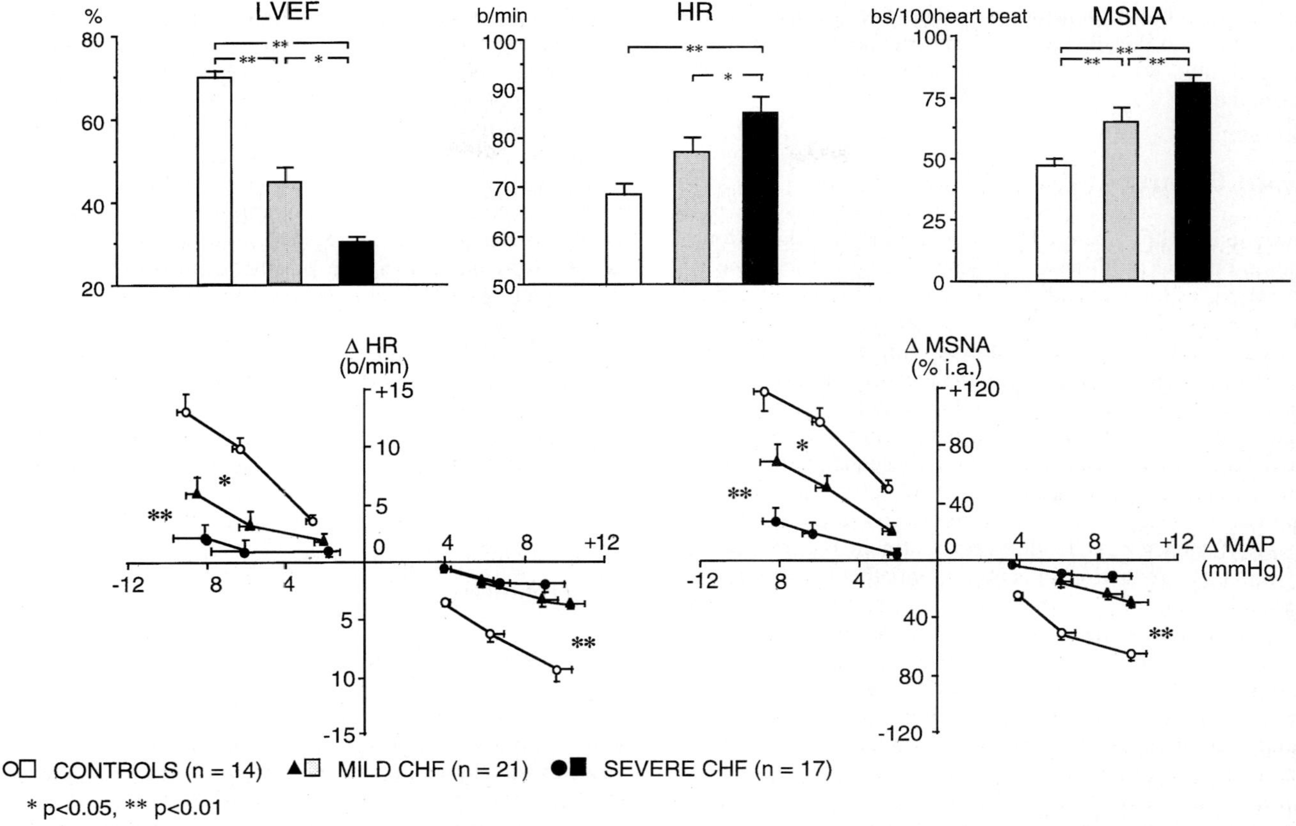

FIGURE 67–3 Left ventricular ejection fraction (LVEF), heart rate (HR), muscle sympathetic nerve activity (MSNA), and baroreflex HR and MSNA modulation in control subjects *(open columns)*, subjects with mild congestive heart failure (CHF) *(shaded columns)*, and subjects with severe CHF *(solid columns)*. (Modified from Grassi G, Seravalle G, Cattaneo BM, et al: Sympathetic activation and loss of reflex sympathetic control in mild congestive heart failure. Circulation 92[11]:3206–3211, 1995.)

reduced in patients with uncomplicated essential hypertension.[92] In prehypertensive rats, dysfunctional constitutive nitric oxide synthase (cNOS) may be a source of O_2 and contribute to the development of hypertension.[93] This also may explain why eNOS expression and function are increased rather than decreased despite normal endothelial function in spontaneously hypertensive rats.[94]

As mentioned previously, a cofactor, tetrahydrobiopterin, is required for activation of NOS and the release of NO. Tetrahydrobiopterin is also a potent reducing agent, and it is possible that prolonged oxidative stress may change the redox environment in endothelium and vascular smooth muscle cells, leading to a depletion of reduced tetrahydrobiopterin. As a consequence, there may be an impairment of NOS and hence of NO production.[95] Endothelial relaxations also are reduced because of endothelium-dependent production of vasoconstrictor prostanoids. Antihypertensive therapy improves endothelium-dependent hyperpolarization in spontaneously hypertensive rats.[96] In Sprague-Dawley rats, Ang II–mediated hypertension is associated with an enhanced production of ET-1 in vivo.[97] ET-1 partially mediates Ang II–induced vascular changes in vivo. Studies with Wistar-Kyoto rats suggest that angiotensin type 1 (AT_1) receptor antagonists, but not calcium antagonists, modulate tissue ET-1.[98] In the rat, chronic ET_A receptor blockade partially prevents Ang II–induced hypertension and the alterations in the endothelial function.[99]

In asymptomatic elderly hypertensive patients with the *ACE DD* genotype, it is speculated that the *ACE D* allele is a risk factor for the development of hypertension associated with endothelial cell damage.[100]

Concerning the role of genetic versus environmental factors in essential hypertension, it has been shown that handgrip exercise resulted in a sustained ET-1 release into the blood stream during recovery in the normotensive young male offspring of hypertensive parents compared with the offspring of normotensive parents.[101]

The endothelial dysfunction observed in hypertensive blood vessels is likely to be a consequence rather than a cause of the disease process.[102]

In epidemiologic and clinical studies, essential hypertension has been correlated with insulin resistance and hyperinsulinemia in humans. However, the results of studies in obese hypertensive patients argue against the hypothesis of a causal pressor effect of insulin as the "missing link" between insulin resistance and essential hypertension.[103] In rats, AT_1 receptors have a determinant role in the pathogenesis of insulin-induced hypertension.[104]

It appears that endogenous dopamine and renal D_{1A} receptors have an important role in the regulation of sodium and body volume homeostasis. There is evidence that a defective renal dopaminergic receptor signaling system contributes to the development and maintenance of hypertension, but the nature of the defect in this system is unsolved.[105]

Heart Failure

In patients with severe CHF, the baroreceptor regulation of the autonomic outflow to the heart and systemic vessels is impaired; as a consequence, the sympathetic nerve activity is increased. Studies have shown that compared with age-matched control subjects, patients with mild symptoms of CHF and only a limited impairment of cardiac function have increased sympathetic nerve activity. This indicates that in this disease, there is an early impairment of reflex sympathetic restraint, possibly as a consequence of a reduction in arterial compliance, with a resultant decreased responsiveness of the baroreceptors to pressure stimuli (Fig. 67–4).[106] Chronic ACE inhibitor treatment is accompanied by a marked reduction in central sympathetic outflow. This reduction may depend on a persistent restoration of baroreflex restraint on the sympathetic neural drive.[107]

In the peripheral resistance arteries in patients with CHF, endothelial dysfunction has been documented. There is an impaired flow-dependent, endothelium-mediated dilation of conduit arteries, and the formation and basal release of NO are decreased in the coronary circulation in the absence of coronary artery disease.[108] Physical training restores endothelium-mediated flow-dependent dilatation in these patients, possibly via enhanced endothelial release of NO.[109] Vitamin C improves endothelium-mediated dilation of conduit arteries as a result of increased availability of NO.[110]

ET may participate in the adaptations to acute reductions in perfusion pressure in CHF. The kidney, lung, heart, and peripheral vasculature are sites of ET mRNA expression that may contribute to its elevation. The mechanisms contributing to its increase in CHF probably include increased atrial and venous pressures and reduced perfusion pressure and shear stress. The vasoconstrictor action of ET may be beneficial early in CHF, augmenting cardiac preload via venoconstriction and increasing systemic vascular resistance to maintain adequate perfusion pressure despite the counteraction of NO and atrial natriuretic factor. However, as the heart failure continues, the increasing action of ET contributes to the deterioration of cardiac function.[111]

Concerning the role of ET receptors in CHF, ET_A receptors exert a pathophysiologic vasoconstrictive effect, whereas ET_B receptors generally have a vasodilative action. Hence, for the treatment of CHF, it seems that a selective ET_A receptor antagonist may offer therapeutic benefits.[112]

Hypercholesterolemia

The induction of hypercholesterolemia in animals with high-fat or high-cholesterol diets impairs endothelium-dependent relaxations. This impairment is also seen in genetically hyperlipidemic rabbits and in humans with atherosclerosis, hypercholesterolemia, or both.[113] In the pig, experimental hypercholesterolemia is characterized by enhanced coronary vasoconstriction and attenuated NO activity. This is associated with a decrease in eNOS immunoreactivity without a change in ET receptor density or binding affinity.[114]

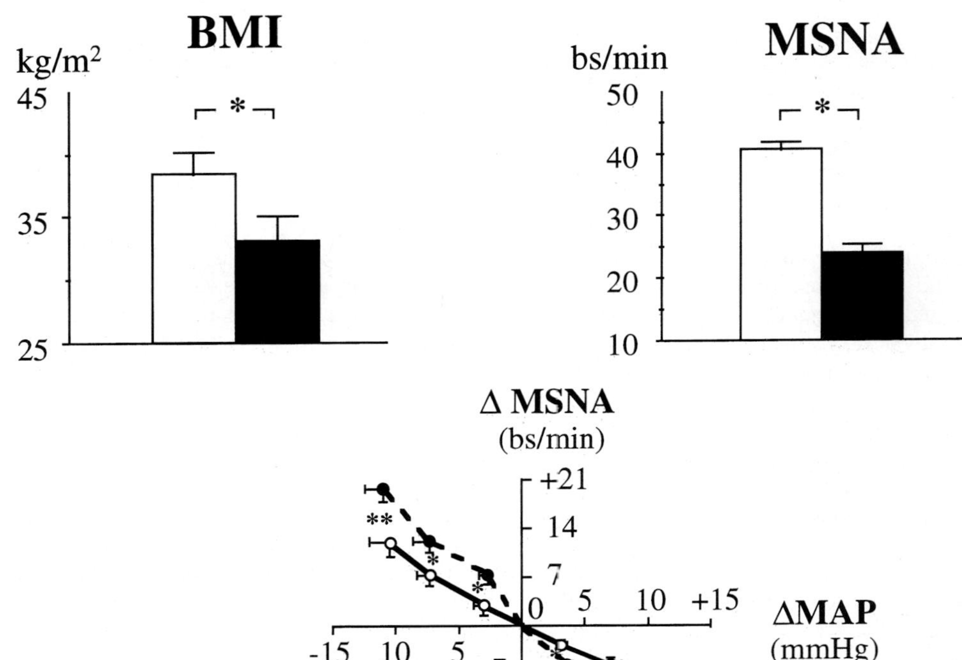

FIGURE 67–4 Effects of a 16-week low-calorie diet on body mass index (BMI) and muscle sympathetic nerve activity (MSNA) in 10 obese subjects. MAP, mean arterial blood pressure. (Modified from Grassi G, Seravalle G, Colombo M, et al: Body weight reduction, sympathetic nerve traffic, and arterial baroreflex in obese normotensive humans. Circulation 97[20]:2037–2042, 1998.)

Atherosclerosis

Oxidized low-density lipoproteins (LDLs) at high plasma concentrations are a major risk factor for the development of atherosclerosis. They may contribute to this via various mechanisms, including being a chemoattractant for monocytes, enhancing lipid accumulation by monocytes, impairing metabolic activity of vascular cells, and altering endothelial function. Concerning the latter, in addition to causing vasodilatation, NO inhibits platelet adherence and aggregation, vascular smooth muscle proliferation, and endothelial cell–leukocyte interactions. Thus, a reduction in NO synthesis in endothelial cells or in its release may be involved in the development of atherosclerosis. It seems that an oxidized form of LDL specifically impairs endothelium-dependent vasodilatation by reducing NO synthesis through enhanced production of superoxide anion and a consequent reduction in the cellular level of L-arginine.[115] This may explain why eNOS expression, as well as NO production, is reduced in atherosclerotic human arteries.[116]

Gene Transfer

Gene therapy involves the transfer of a functional gene into host cells to correct the malfunction of a specific gene or to alleviate the symptoms of a disease. Vascular gene transfer refers to the introduction of genes into relevant cells of the blood vessel wall. For gene transfer to the cardiovascular system, adenoviral vectors are the most efficient means of transfer.

Enzyme Nitric Oxide Synthase Gene Transfer

eNOS genes have been expressed in dog basilar arteries, mediated by a replication-incompetent adenovirus. The expression of recombinant eNOS in endothelial cells may prove useful in the site-specific therapy of vascular diseases characterized by endothelial dysfunction, such as atherosclerosis and hypertension. In addition, adventitial fibroblasts differentiate into myofibroblasts and migrate into the intima. Because recombinant eNOS can be targeted to these fibroblasts, this might inhibit cellular proliferation.[117]

In pigs, percutaneous adenovirus-mediated NOS gene transfer after angioplasty in coronary arteries restored NO production.[118] In canine basilar arteries affected by subarachnoid hemorrhage, after successful eNOS gene transfer to the spastic vessel, the impaired NO-mediated relaxation was partially restored through the local (adventitial) production of NO.[119] In humans, internal mammary artery bypass grafts have a higher patency than saphenous vein grafts. Intimal proliferation in the latter is due to smooth muscle proliferation and migration. In isolated smooth muscle cells from these vessels, platelet-derived growth factor increased mitogen-activated protein kinase only in the vein muscle and down-regulated cell cycle inhibitor in the vein muscle. These findings may contribute to the longer patency of arterial versus venous grafts.[120] The question may be asked as to whether eNOS gene transfer in the latter would improve their patency. To add to the complexity, functional thrombin receptors are present on the endothelium and smooth muscle cells of human coronary bypass vessels, both internal mammary artery and saphenous vein. These receptors on the endothelium mediate relaxation in the artery but not in the vein. In addition, thrombin causes greater contraction and proliferation in the smooth muscle cells of the saphenous vein.[121]

A deletion polymorphism in the *ACE* gene is associated with a high serum level of ACE, with the resultant risk of myocardial infarction. Ang II receptors include at least two different subtypes: AT_1 and AT_2. In Sprague-Dawley rats, antisense oligodeoxynucleotides directed at AT_1 receptor mRNA prevented an increase in plasma Ang II immediately after ischemia-reperfusion.[122]

REFERENCES

1. Cohen RA, Vanhoutte PM: Endothelium-dependent hyperpolarization: beyond nitric oxide and cyclic GMP. Circulation 92:3334–3349, 1995.
2. Cosentino F, Katusic Z: Tetrahydrobiopterin and dysfunction of endothelial nitric oxide synthase in coronary arteries. Circulation 91:139–144, 1995.
3. Davies PF: Flow-mediated endothelial mechanotransduction. Physiol Rev 75:519–560, 1995.
4. Ziegler T, Silacci P, Harrison VJ, et al: Nitric oxide synthase expression in endothelial cells exposed to mechanical forces. Hypertension 32:351–355, 1998.
5. Gudi SRP, Clark CB, Frangos JA: Fluid flow rapidly activates G proteins in human endothelial cells. Circ Res 79:834–839, 1996.
6. Pou S, Pou WS, Bread DS, et al: Generation of superoxide by purified brain nitric oxide synthase. J Biol Chem 267:24173–24176, 1992.
7. Hishikawa K, Lüscher T: Pulsatile stretch stimulates superoxide production in human aortic endothelial cells. Circulation 96:3610–3616, 1997.
8. Katusic ZS, Cosentino F: Nitric oxide synthase: from molecular biology to cerebrovascular physiology. News Physiol Sci 9:64–67, 1994.
9. Cosentino F, Lüscher T: Tetrahydrobiopterin and endothelial function. Eur Heart J 19(suppl G):G3–G8, 1998.
10. Wang HD, Pagano PJ, Du Y, et al: Superoxide anion from the adventitia of the rat thoracic aorta inactivates nitric oxide. Circ Res 82:810–818, 1998.
11. Hishikawa K, Oemar BS, Yang Z, et al: Pulsatile stretch stimulates superoxide production and activates nuclear factor-κB in human coronary smooth muscle. Circ Res 81:797–803, 1997.
12. Creager MA, Roddy M-A, Boles K, et al: *N*-Acetylcysteine does not influence the activity of endothelium-derived relaxing factor in vivo. Hypertension 29:668–672, 1997.
13. Martin CM, Beltran-Del-Rio A, Albrecht A, et al: Local cholinergic mechanisms mediate nitric oxide-dependent flow-induced vasorelaxation in vitro. Am J Physiol 270:H442–H446, 1996.
14. Miller VM, Vanhoutte PM: Endothelial α_2-adrenoceptors in canine pulmonary and systemic blood vessels. Eur J Pharmacol 118:123–129, 1985.
15. Joannides R, Haefeli WE, Linder L, et al: Nitric oxide is responsible for flow-dependent dilatation of human peripheral conduit arteries in vivo. Circulation 91:1314–1319, 1995.
16. Laycock SK, Vogel T, Forfia PR, et al: Role of nitric oxide in the control of renal oxygen consumption and the regulation of chemical work in the kidney. Circ Res 82:1263–1271, 1998.
17. Shen W, Hintze TH, Wolin MS: Nitric oxide: an important signaling mechanism between vascular endothelium and parenchymal cells in the regulation of oxygen consumption. Circulation 92:3505–3512, 1995.
18. Kelly RA, Balligand J-L, Smith TW: Nitric oxide and cardiac function. Circ Res 79:363–380, 1996.
19. Cooper CJ, Landzberg MJ, Anderson TJ, et al: Role of nitric oxide in the local regulation of pulmonary vascular resistance in humans. Circulation 93:266–271, 1996.
20. Popp R, Fleming I, Busse R: Pulsatile stretch in coronary arteries elicits release of endothelium-derived hyperpolarizing factor: a modulator of arterial compliance. Circ Res 82:696–703, 1998.

21. Barton M, Bény J-L, d'Uscio LV, et al: Endothelium-independent relaxation and hyperpolarization to C-type natriuretic peptide in porcine coronary arteries. J Cardiovasc Pharmacol 31:377–383, 1998.
22. Parris RJ, Webb DJ: The endothelin system in cardiovascular physiology and pathophysiology. Vasc Med 2:31–43, 1997.
23. Cannan CR, Burnett JC Jr, Brandt RR, et al: Endothelin at pathophysiological concentrations mediates coronary vasoconstriction via the endothelin-A receptor. Circulation 92:3312–3317, 1995.
24. Haynes WG, Ferro CJ, O'Kane KPJ, et al: Systemic endothelin receptor blockade decreases peripheral vascular resistance and blood pressure in humans. Circulation 93:1860–1870, 1996.
25. Verhaar MC, Strachan FE, Newby DE, et al: Endothelin-A receptor antagonist-mediated vasodilatation is attenuated by inhibition of nitric oxide synthesis and by endothelin-B receptor blockade. Circulation 97:752–756, 1998.
26. Traverse JH, Judd D, Bache RJ: Dose-dependent effect of endothelin-1 on blood flow to normal and collateral-dependent myocardium. Circulation 93:558–566, 1996.
27. Filep JG: Endogenous endothelin modulates blood pressure, plasma volume, and albumin escape after systemic nitric oxide blockade. Hypertension 30:22–28, 1997.
28. Katusic ZS, Shepherd JT: Endothelium-derived vasoactive factors, II: endothelium-dependent contraction. Hypertension 18(suppl III):III-86–III-92, 1991.
29. Burnstock G, Ralevic V: Cotransmission. *In* Garland CJ, Angus J (eds): The Pharmacology of Smooth Muscle. Oxford: Oxford University Press, 1996.
30. Westfall TC, Yang CL, Curfam-Falvey M: Neuropeptide-Y-ATP interactions at the vascular sympathetic neuroeffector junction. J Cardiovasc Pharmacol 26:682–687, 1995.
31. Potter EK, Ulman LG: Neuropeptides in sympathetic nerves affect vagal regulation of the heart. News Physiol Sci 9:174, 1994.
32. Aliev G, Ralevic V, Burnstock G: Depression of endothelial nitric oxide synthase but increased expression of endothelin-1 immunoreactivity in rat thoracic aortic endothelium associated with long-term, but not short-term, sympathectomy. Circ Res 79:317–323, 1996.
33. Okamura T, Yoshida K, Toda N: Nitroxidergic innervation in dog and monkey renal arteries. Hypertension 25:1090–1095, 1995.
34. Toda N, Okamura T: Nitroxidergic nerve: regulation of vascular tone and blood flow in the brain. J Hypertens 14:423–434, 1996.
35. Henriksen O: Circulatory studies: local sympathetic veno-arteriolar axon "reflex" in the sympathoadrenal system. *In* Christensen NJ, Henriksen O, Lassen NA (eds): The Sympathoadrenal System, Physiology and Pathophysiology. pp. 67–80. Copenhagen: Munksgaard, 1986.
36. Grassi G, Seravalle G, Colombo M, et al: Body weight reduction, sympathetic nerve traffic, and arterial baroreflex in obese normotensive humans. Circulation 97:2037–2042, 1998.
37. Parati G, Saul JS, Di Rienzo M, et al: Spectral analysis of blood pressure and heart rate variability in evaluating cardiovascular regulation: a critical appraisal. Hypertension 25:1276–1286, 1995.
38. Grassi G, Seravalle G, Calhoun DA, et al: Physical training and baroreceptor control of sympathetic nerve activity in humans. Hypertension 23:294–301, 1994.
39. Hironaga K, Hirooka Y, Matsuo I, et al: Role of endogenous nitric oxide in the brain stem on the rapid adaptation of baroreflex. Hypertension 31:27–31, 1998.
40. Liu J-L, Murakami H, Zucker IH: Angiotensin II–nitric oxide interaction on sympathetic outflow in conscious rabbits. Circ Res 82:496–502, 1998.
41. Giannattasio C, Del Bo A, Cattaneo BM, et al: Reflex vasopressin and renin modulation by cardiac receptors in humans. Hypertension 21:461–469, 1993.
42. Rand MJ, Lie CG: Nitric oxide as a neurotransmitter in peripheral nerves: nature of transmitter and mechanism of transmission. Annu Rev Physiol 57:659–682, 1995.
43. Shepherd JT: Perivascular nerves and endothelial cells: normal actions and interactions and changes in hypertension. High Blood Press 5:124–138, 1996.
44. Feigl EO: Neural control of coronary blood flow. J Vasc Res 35:85–92, 1998.
45. Radelli A, Mircoli L, Perlini S, et al: Lack of autonomic contributions to tonic nitric oxide-mediated vasodilatation in unanesthetized free-moving rats. J Hypertens 16:55–61, 1998.
46. Hennington BS, Zhang H, Miller MT, et al: Angiotensin II stimulates synthesis of endothelial nitric oxide synthase. Hypertension 31:283–288, 1998.
47. Perondi R, Saino A, Tio RA, et al: ACE inhibition attenuates sympathetic coronary vasoconstriction in patients with coronary artery disease. Circulation 85:2004–2013, 1992.
48. Weiner CP, Lizasoain I, Bayliss SA, et al: Induction of calcium-dependent nitric oxide synthases by sex hormones. Proc Natl Acad Sci U S A 91:5212–5216, 1994.
49. White CR, Darley-Usmar V, Oparil S: No role for NO in estrogen-mediated vasoprotection? Circulation 96:2769–2771, 1997.
50. Kleinert H, Wallerath T, Euchenhofer C, et al: Estrogens increase transcription of the human endothelial NO synthase gene: analysis of the transcription factors involved. Hypertension 31:582–588, 1998.
51. Davidge ST, Zhang Y: Estrogen replacement suppresses a prostaglandin H synthase-dependent vasoconstrictor in rat mesenteric arteries. Circ Res 83:388–395, 1998.
52. Sudhir K, Jennings GL, Funder JW, et al: Estrogen enhances basal nitric oxide release in the forearm vasculature in perimenopausal women. Hypertension 28:330–334, 1996.
53. Szokodi I, Kinnunen P, Tavi P, et al: Evidence for cAMP-independent mechanisms mediating the effects of adrenomedullin, a new inotropic peptide. Circulation 97:1062–1070, 1998.
54. Creager MA, Liang CS, Coffman JD, et al: Beta adrenergic-mediated vasodilator response to insulin in the human forearm. J Pharmacol Exp Ther 235:709–714, 1985.
55. Wu H, Jeng YY, Yue C, et al: Endothelial-dependent vascular effects of insulin and insulin-like growth factor-1 in the perfused rat mesenteric artery and aortic ring. Diabetes 43:1027–1032, 1994.
56. Scherrer U, Randin D, Vollenweider P, et al: Nitric oxide release accounts for insulin's vascular effects in humans. J Clin Invest 94:2511–2515, 1994.
57. Hasdai D, Rizza RA, Holmes DR Jr: Insulin and insulin-like growth factor-I cause coronary vasorelaxation in vitro. Hypertension 32:228–234, 1998.
58. Folkow B, Svanborg A: Physiology of cardiovascular aging. Physiol Rev 73:725–764, 1993.
59. Davy KP, Seals DR, Tanaka H: Augmented cardiopulmonary and integrative sympathetic baroreflexes but attenuated peripheral vasoconstriction with age. Hypertension 32:298–304, 1998.
60. Narkiewicz K, van de Borne PJH, Hausberg M, et al: Cigarette smoking increases sympathetic outflow in humans. Circulation 98:528–534, 1998.
61. Grassi G, Cattaneo BM, Seravalle G, et al: Baroreflex impairment by low sodium diet in mild or moderate essential hypertension. Hypertension 29:802–807, 1997.
62. Gerhard M, Roddy M, Creager SJ, et al: Aging progressively impairs endothelium-dependent vasodilatation in forearm resistance vessels of humans. Hypertension 27:849–853, 1996.
63. Tschudi MR, Barton M, Bersinger NA, et al: Effect of age on kinetics of nitric oxide release in rat aorta and pulmonary artery. J Clin Invest 98:899–905, 1996.
64. Cernadas MR, Sánchez de Miguel L, García-Durán M, et al: Expression of constitutive and inducible nitric oxide synthases in the vascular wall of young and aging rats. Circ Res 83:279–286, 1998.
65. Wieling W, Shepherd JT: Initial and delayed circulatory responses to orthostatic stress in normal humans and in subjects with orthostatic intolerance. Int Angiol II:69–82, 1992.
66. Noll G, Wenzel RR, Schneider M, et al: Increased activation of sympathetic nervous system and endothelin by mental stress in normotensive offspring of hypertensive parents. Circulation 93:866–869, 1996.
67. Dietz NM, Rivera JM, Eggener SE, et al: Nitric oxide contributes to the rise in forearm blood flow during mental stress in humans. J Physiol 480:2, 1994.
68. Mitchell JH, Shepherd JT: Control of the circulation during exercise. *In* Hill P (ed): Exercise—The Physiological Challenge. Ch. 5. Auckland, New Zealand: Conference Publishing, 1993.
69. Dyke CK, Proctor DN, Dietz NM, et al: Role of nitric oxide in exercise hyperaemia during prolonged rhythmic handgripping in humans. J Physiol (Lond) 488:259–265, 1995.
70. Ishibashi Y, Duncker DJ, Zhang J, et al: ATP-sensitive K^+ channels, adenosine, and nitric oxide-mediated mechanisms account for coronary vasodilation during exercise. Circ Res 82:346–359, 1998.
71. Bernstein RD, Ochoa FY, Xu X, et al: Function and production of

nitric oxide in the coronary circulation of the conscious dog during exercise. Circ Res 79:840–848, 1996.

72. Sessa WC, Pritchard K, Seyedi N, et al: Chronic exercise in dogs increases coronary vascular nitric oxide production and endothelial cell nitric oxide synthase gene expression. Circ Res 74:349–353, 1994.
73. Dietz NM, Joyner MJ, Shepherd JT: Vasovagal syncope and skeletal muscle vasodilatation: the continuing conundrum. Pacing Clin Electrophysiol 20:775–780, 1997.
74. Morillo CA, Eckberg DL, Ellenbogen KA, et al: Vagal and sympathetic mechanisms in patients with orthostatic vasovagal syncope. Circulation 96:2509–2513, 1997.
75. Puvi-Rajasingham S, Smith GDP, Akinola A, et al: Abnormal regional blood flow responses during and after exercise in human sympathetic denervation. J Physiol 505:841–849, 1997.
76. Mancia G, Groppelli A, Di Rienzo M, et al: Smoking impairs baroreflex sensitivity in humans. Am J Physiol 42:H1555–H1560, 1997.
77. Zeiher AM, Schächinger V, Minners J: Long-term cigarette smoking impairs endothelium-dependent coronary arterial vasodilator function. Circulation 92:1094–1100, 1995.
78. Kugiyama K, Yasue H, Ohgushi M, et al: Deficiency in nitric oxide bioactivity in epicardial coronary arteries of cigarette smokers. J Am Coll Cardiol 28:1161–1167, 1996.
79. Higman DJ, Strachan AMJ, Buttery L, et al: Smoking impairs the activity of endothelial nitric oxide synthase in saphenous vein. Arterioscler Thromb Vasc Biol 16:546–552, 1996.
80. Heitzer T, Just H, Münzel T: Antioxidant vitamin C improves endothelial dysfunction in chronic smokers. Circulation 94:6–9, 1996.
81. Sumida H, Watanabe H, Kugiyama K: Does passive smoking impair endothelium-dependent coronary artery dilation in women? J Am Coll Cardiol 31:811–815, 1998.
82. Grassi G, Seravalle G, Cattaneo BM, et al: Sympathetic activation in obese normotensive subjects. Hypertension 25:560–563, 1995.
83. Narkiewicz K, van de Borne PJH, Cooley RL, et al: Sympathetic activity in obese subjects with and without obstructive sleep apnea. Circulation 98:772–776, 1998.
84. Grassi G, Colombo M, Seravalle G, et al: Dissociation between muscle and skin sympathetic nerve activity in essential hypertension, obesity, and congestive heart failure. Hypertension 31:64–67, 1998.
85. De Tejada IS, Goldstein I, Azadzol K, et al: Impaired neurogenic and endothelium-mediated relaxation of penile smooth muscle from diabetic men with impotence. N Engl J Med 320:1025–1030, 1989.
86. Tesfamariam B, Jakubowski JA, Cohen RA. Contraction of diabetic rabbit aorta due to endothelium-derived PGH/TXA. Am J Physiol 257:1327–1333, 1989.
87. Pieper G: Review of alterations in endothelial nitric oxide production in diabetes: protective role of arginine on endothelial dysfunction. Hypertension 31:1047–1060, 1998.
88. Cosentino F, Hishikawa K, Katusic ZS, et al: High glucose increases nitric oxide synthase expression and superoxide anion generation in human aortic endothelial cells. Circulation 96:25–28, 1997.
89. Timimi FK, Ting HH, Haley EA, et al: Vitamin C improves endothelium-dependent vasodilation in patients with insulin-dependent diabetes mellitus. J Am Coll Cardiol 31:552–571, 1998.
90. Grassi G, Cattaneo BM, Seravalle G, et al: Baroreflex control of sympathetic nerve activity in essential and secondary hypertension. Hypertension 31:68–72, 1998.
91. Kagiyama S, Tsuchihashi T, Abe I, et al: Enhanced depressor response to nitric oxide in the rostral ventrolateral medulla of spontaneously hypertensive rats. Hypertension 31:1030–1034, 1998.
92. Linder L, Kiowski W, Bühler FR, et al: Indirect evidence for release of endothelium-derived relaxing factor in human forearm circulation in vivo: blunted response in essential hypertension. Circulation 81:1762–1767, 1990.
93. Cosentino F, Patton S, d'Uscio LV, et al: Tetrahydrobiopterin alters superoxide and nitric oxide release in prehypertensive rats. J Clin Invest 101:1530–1537, 1998.
94. Nava E, Farré AL, Moreno C, et al: Alterations to the nitric oxide pathway in the spontaneously hypertensive rat. J Hypertens 16:609–615, 1998.
95. Kinoshita H, Tsutsui M, Milstien S, et al: Tetrahydrobiopterin, nitric oxide and regulation of cerebral arterial tone. Prog Neurobiol 52:295–302, 1997.
96. Onaka U, Fujii K, Abe I, et al: Antihypertensive treatment improves endothelium-dependent hyperpolarization in the mesenteric artery of spontaneously hypertensive rats. Circulation 98:175–182, 1998.
97. Rajagopalan S, Laursen JB, Borthayre A, et al: Role for endothelin-1 in angiotensin II–mediated hypertension. Hypertension 30:29–34, 1997.
98. d'Uscio LV, Shaw S, Barton M, et al: Losartan but not verapamil inhibits angiotensin II–induced tissue endothelin-1 increase: role of blood pressure and endothelial function. Hypertension 31:1305–1310, 1998.
99. d'Uscio LV, Moreau P, Shaw S, et al: Effects of chronic ET_A-receptor blockade in angiotensin II–induced hypertension. Hypertension 29:435–441, 1997.
100. Kario K, Matsuo T, Kobayashi H, et al: Endothelial cell damage and angiotensin-converting enzyme insertion/deletion in elderly hypertensive patients. J Am Coll Cardiol 32:444–450, 1998.
101. Mangieri E, Tanzilli G, Barilla F, et al: Handgrip increases endothelin-1 secretion in normotensive young male offspring of hypertensive parents. J Am Coll Cardiol 31:1362–1366, 1998.
102. Vanhoutte PM: Endothelial dysfunction in hypertension. J Hypertens 14(suppl 5):84, 1996.
103. Heise T, Magnusson K, Heinemann L, et al: Insulin resistance and the effect of insulin on blood pressure in essential hypertension. Hypertension 32:243–248, 1998.
104. Fang T-C, Huang W-C: Angiotensin receptor blockade blunts hyperinsulinemia-induced hypertension in rats. Hypertension 32:235–242, 1998.
105. Hussain T, Lokhandwala MF: Renal dopamine receptor function in hypertension. Hypertension 32:187–197, 1998.
106. Grassi G, Seravalle G, Cattaneo BM, et al: Sympathetic activation and loss of reflex sympathetic control in mild congestive heart failure. Circulation 92:3206–3211, 1995.
107. Grassi G, Cattaneo BM, Seravalle G, et al: Effects of chronic ACE inhibition on sympathetic nerve traffic and baroreflex control of circulation in heart failure. Circulation 96:1173–1179, 1997.
108. Hayoz D, Drexler H, Münzel T, et al: Flow-mediated arteriolar dilation is abnormal in congestive heart failure. Circulation 87(suppl VII):VII-92–VII-96, 1993.
109. Hornig B, Maier V, Drexler H: Physical training improves endothelial function in patients with chronic heart failure. Circulation 93:210–214, 1996.
110. Hornig B, Arakawa N, Kohler C, et al: Vitamin C improves endothelial function of conduit arteries in patients with chronic heart failure. Circulation 97:363–368, 1998.
111. Clavell A, Stingo A, Margulies K, et al: Physiological significance of endothelin: its role in congestive heart failure. Circulation 87(suppl V):V-45–V-50, 1993.
112. Wada A, Tsutamoto T, Fukai D, et al: Comparison of the effects of selective endothelin ET_A and ET_B receptor antagonists in congestive heart failure. J Am Coll Cardiol 30:1385–1392, 1997.
113. Vanhoutte PM, Perrault LP, Vilaine JP: Endothelial dysfunction and vascular disease. *In* Rubanyi GM, Dzau VJ (eds): The Endothelium in Clinical Practice. Ch. 9. p. 265. New York: Marcel Dekker, 1997.
114. Verghese M, Cannan CR, Miller VM, et al: Enhanced endothelin-mediated coronary vasoconstriction and attenuated basal nitric oxide activity in experimental hypercholesterolemia. Circulation 96:1930–1936, 1997.
115. Hein TW, Kuo L: LDLs impair vasomotor function of the coronary microcirculation: role of superoxide anions. Circ Res 83:404–414, 1998.
116. Oemar BS, Tschudi MR, Godoy N, et al: Reduced endothelial nitric oxide synthase expression and production in human atherosclerosis. Circulation 997:2494–2498, 1998.
117. Chen AFY, O'Brien T, Katusic ZS: Transfer and expression of recombinant nitric oxide synthase genes in the cardiovascular system. Trends Pharmacol Sci 19:276, 1998.
118. Varenne O, Pislaru S, Gillijns H, et al: Local adenovirus-mediated transfer of human endothelial nitric oxide synthase reduces luminal narrowing after coronary angioplasty in pigs. Circulation 98:919–926, 1998.
119. Onoue H, Tsutsui M, Smith L, et al: Expression and function of recombinant endothelial nitric oxide synthase gene in canine basilar artery after experimental subarachnoid hemorrhage. Stroke 29:1959–1966, 1998.

120. Yang Z, Oemar BS, Carrel T, et al: Different proliferative properties of smooth muscle cells of human arterial and venous bypass-vessels: role of PDGF receptors, mitogen-activated protein kinase, and cyclin-dependent kinase inhibitors. Circulation 97:181–187, 1998.
121. Yang Z, Ruschitzka F, Rabelink TJ, et al: Different effects of thrombin receptor activation on endothelium and smooth muscle cells of human coronary bypass vessels: implications for venous bypass graft failure. Circulation 95:1870–1876, 1997.
122. Yang BC, Phillips MI, Zhang YC, et al: Critical role of AT_1 receptor expression after ischemia/reperfusion in isolated rat hearts: beneficial effect of antisense oligodeoxynucleotides directed at AT_1 receptor mRNA. Circ Res 83:552–559, 1998.

CHAPTER 68

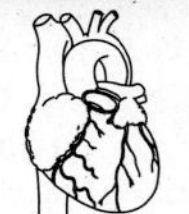

Circulatory Regulation: The Role of Vascular Remodeling

Victor J. Dzau and Christian M. Matter

THE BIOLOGIC PROCESS OF BLOOD VESSEL REMODELING
Vascular Growth Promoters
Vascular Growth Inhibitors
Modulators of Vascular Cell Apoptosis
Vasoactive Substances With Growth Regulatory Properties
PHYSIOLOGIC VASCULAR REMODELING
Acute Response to Flow: Vasodilatation
Chronic Response to Flow: Vascular Remodeling
DISORDERS OF VASCULAR STRUCTURE (PATHOLOGIC VASCULAR REMODELING)
Hypertension
Atherosclerosis
Restenosis
SUMMARY

Traditional understanding of circulatory regulation emphasizes the control of vascular tone and cardiac contractility. As described in Chapter 48, Regulation of Cardiac Contraction and Relaxation, cardiac contractility is determined by intrinsic properties of the myocardium, loading conditions of the ventricle, and neurohormonal factors. Similarly, vascular tone is regulated by myogenic and viscoelastic properties of the blood vessel, neurohormonal systems, and endogenous vasoactive substances released by the vasculature. This subject is reviewed in detail later in this chapter.

An emerging concept in circulatory regulation is the contribution of cardiovascular structural changes. The long-term adaptive changes of the circulation to chronic burdens of pressure or volume overload, altered shear stress, turbulent flow, hormonal activation, and so forth involve cardiac and vascular remodeling that consequently maintain systemic or local homeostasis (Fig. 68–1). However, these structural changes may become maladaptive, thereby contributing to the pathogenesis of cardiovascular complications, such as cardiac hypertrophy/dilatation, cardiac failure, hypertensive vascular hypertrophy, atherosclerosis, and restenosis. The pathophysiology of cardiac remodeling is discussed in detail elsewhere in this book (Ch. 46, Cardiac Hypertrophy and Failure: Basic Aspects). This section of the chapter deals primarily with the role of vascular structural changes in circulatory regulation and cardiovascular disorders.

The blood vessel is a biologically active organ capable of sensing changes in its environment, of synthesizing a myriad of biologically active mediators, and of modifying its own contractility and structure.[1] All cellular components of the vessel wall participate in the functional and structural changes. The endothelium plays a particularly prominent role. It is capable of producing potent vasorelaxing factors, such as nitric oxide (NO), prostacyclin, and hyperpolarizing factor, as well as powerful vasoconstrictive factors, such as endothelin and angiotensin II (AII). At basal conditions, these opposing forces achieve a state of equilibrium, and normal vascular tone is maintained. Alterations in hemodynamic conditions of humoral factors may result in an imbalance of these modulating forces, thereby favoring vasoconstriction or vasodilatation.

As discussed, it is now clear that the changes in vascular resistance to hemodynamic/humoral stimuli are relatively short-term adaptations. However, the long-term adaptive responses to sustained alterations in physiologic or pathophysiologic conditions are mediated primarily by changes in vascular structure. This is accomplished by an active remodeling of the blood vessel that involves cell growth or apoptosis, extracellular matrix expansion or contraction, and activation or inhibition of specific proteolytic enzymes or glycosidases.[2–4] Vascular remodeling is usually an adaptive process that occurs in response to long-term changes in hemodynamic conditions, but it may subsequently contribute to the pathophysiology of vascular diseases and circulatory disorders.

The Biologic Process of Blood Vessel Remodeling

The spectrum of structural alterations of the blood vessel is illustrated in Figure 68–2.[2] In response to increased arterial pressure, the vessel structure is altered such that the wall-to-lumen ratio is increased by either an increase in muscle mass (see Fig. 68–2, vessel a) or rearrangements of cellular and non–cellular elements (see Fig. 68–2, vessel b). These changes contribute to a modest increase in basal peripheral resistance but markedly amplify the contractile response to vasoconstrictive agents in hypertension.[5–7] Another form of vascular remodeling involves changes primarily in lumen dimensions (see Fig. 68–2, vessels c and d). In this example, an active restructuring of the cellular

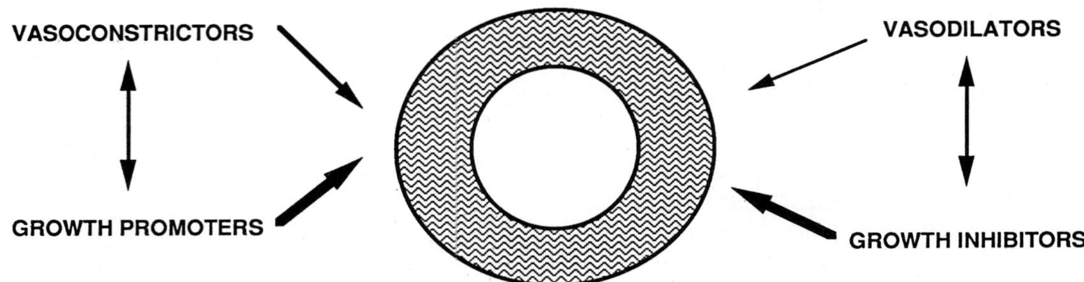

FIGURE 68–1 Modulation of vascular function by opposing forces. The short-term control of vascular tone is regulated by the balance between vasoconstrictive and vasodilatory substances. The long-term regulation of vasculature structure is controlled by endogenous growth-promoting versus growth-inhibiting agents. Note that vasoactive substances possess growth regulatory properties and vice versa. (Adapted from Dzau VJ: Role of endothelium-derived vasoactive substances in the regulation of vascular tone via structural remodeling of blood vessels. *In* Ryan US, Rubanyi GM [eds]: Endothelial Regulation of Vascular Tone. pp. 331–339. New York: Marcel Dekker, 1992. Courtesy of Marcel Dekker Inc.)

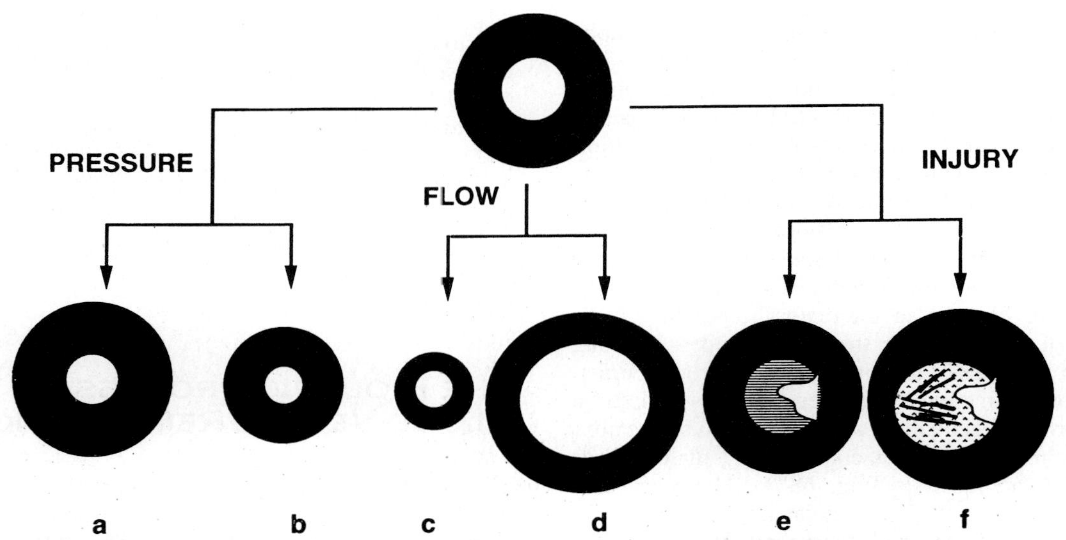

FIGURE 68–2 Different types of vascular remodeling **a,** Vascular hypertrophy in hypertensive vascular disease with thickened medial layer and reduction in lumen diameter. **b,** Reduction in lumen diameter in hypertensive vascular disease without medial hypertrophy. **c,** Decreased vessel dimension in response to a chronic decrease in flow. **d,** Increased vessel dimensions in response to a chronic increase in flow. **e,** Myointimal hyperplasia (migration and proliferation of vascular smooth muscle). **f,** Atherosclerosis in response to vascular injury in conduit vessels. (Adapted from Gibbons GH, Dzau VJ: The emerging concept of vascular remodeling. N Engl J Med 330:1431–1438, 1994.)

and noncellular components of the vessel wall results in changes in lumen dimensions with relatively small changes in medial thickness. Clinical examples of this form of remodeling include the vascular dilatation associated with a sustained rate of high blood flow (see Fig. 68–2, vessel d) (e.g., artenovenous fistula). Conversely, a reduction in the vessel mass and caliber results from a chronic reduction in blood flow (see Fig. 68–2, vessel c). Indeed, rarefaction of the microcirculation (capillary loss) resulting from apoptosis is another form of vascular remodeling that is observed with hypertension and may promote increased vascular resistance and tissue ischemia.[8] The architecture of the vessel wall is also markedly altered in response to vascular injury (see Fig. 68–2, vessels e and f). The neointima forms as part of a reparative response to injury that involves thrombosis, vascular cell migration and proliferation, matrix modification, and inflammatory cell adhesion and infiltration.

The biologic process of vascular remodeling may be divided into the following components: (1) *sensor*—the detection of signals emanating from changes in hemodynamic conditions and humoral factors; (2) *transducer*—the relay of signals within the cell and adjacent cells; (3) *mediator*—the synthesis and release or activation of substances that influence cell growth and death, cell migration, or composition of the extracellular matrix; and (4) *response*—the resultant structural changes in the vessel wall involving cellular and/or noncellular components.

The endothelium participates in the process of vascular remodeling as the sensor and the transducer of the changes in the circulation. In addition, it is capable of producing biologic mediators of vascular remodeling. Endothelial cells (ECs) can participate directly in vascular remodeling by the release or activation of substances that can influence growth, death, and migration of cellular elements and/or can modulate the status of the extracellular matrix. These components of the vessel wall interact closely, and their relation ultimately determines the geometry of the blood vessel. The endothelium-derived growth factors that regulate cellular growth are listed in Table 68–1. These factors can be divided into growth promoters and growth inhibitors, proapoptic and antiapoptic agents, and vasoactive substances with growth-regulatory properties. This classification is not rigid, because it has been shown that a single factor may manifest multiple properties, depending on experimental conditions. For example, it has been shown that peptide growth factors, such as platelet-derived growth factor (PDGF) and epidermal growth factor, possess vasoconstrictive properties. Conversely, vasoactive substances can regulate vascular smooth muscle cell (VSMC) growth. A growth promoter may also act paradoxically as a growth inhibitor under appropriate conditions. Indeed, transforming growth factor beta-1 (TGF-β1) and AII both have been shown to exert bifunctional effects on cell growth.[9–11] Furthermore, these vasoactive mediators may exert proapoptotic action on one type of vascular cell but have an antiapoptotic effect on another cell type. For example, NO induces VSMC apoptosis[12] but protects ECs from apoptosis in response to serum withdrawal.[13]

TABLE 68–1 Vessel Wall–Derived Growth Factors

Growth-Promoting Substances
Platelet-derived growth factors AA, AB, BB
Acidic and basic fibroblast growth factors
Insulin-like growth factor-1
Vascular endothelium-derived growth factor
Interleukin-1
Angiotensin II*
Endothelin
Growth-Inhibitory Substances
Prostacyclin
Nitric oxide
Heparin sulfate
TGF-β1*
Vasoactive Substances With Growth-Regulatory Properties
Angiotensin II*
Endothelin
Bradykinin
Nitric oxide
Prostacyclin
Type C natriuretic peptide
Vascular Substances With Proapoptotic Properties
Nitric oxide (VSMC)†
Angiotensin II (EC)†
TGF-β1 (EC)†
Vascular Substances With Antiapoptotic Properties
Nitric oxide (EC)†
Angiotensin II (VSMC)†
TGF-β1 (VSMC)†
Insulin-like growth factor-1
Vascular endothelium-derived growth factor

Abbreviations: EC, endothelial cell; TGF-β1, transforming growth factor beta-1; VSMC, vascular smooth muscle cell.
*Bifunctional growth response.
†Cell-specific effect; parentheses denote target cell.

Vascular Growth Promoters

The vessel wall produces several growth-promoting factors, such as PDGF, basic fibroblast growth factor (bFGF), insulin-like growth factor-1 (IGF-1) and interleukin 1 (IL-1).[14–16]

Both the A and the B chains of PDGF are synthesized by the endothelium, VSMCs, and macrophages. All three dimeric isoforms of PDGF (AA, AB, BB) may be produced and secreted in the vessel wall. This may be significant because there are two PDGF receptors, alpha (α) and beta (β), that have different binding affinities for each isoform.[17] Production of either the AB or the BB isoform promotes VSMC migration and proliferation and may play a role in some forms of vascular remodeling. Both PDGF A- and B-chain messenger RNA levels are increased in microvascular endothelium in response to phorbol esters, thrombin, and TGF-β1. This response appears primarily to be due to an effect on the transcription rate. Tumor necrosis factor, IL-1, and endotoxin (possibly mediated by IL-1) also promote the secretion of PDGF by EC.[18]

The cytokine IL-1 is expressed by endothelium and may play a role in vascular remodeling associated with inflammation. Endothelial IL-1 expression is increased by proinflammatory substances, such as endotoxin and tumor necrosis factor. The administration of IL-1 to cultured VSMCs induces proliferation only during prostaglandin synthesis blockade.[19] The IL-1 proliferative response appears to be mediated by the induction of autocrine production of PDGF AA.[20] Studies of cultured ECs suggest that IL-1 inhibits EC proliferation and angiogenesis. Interestingly, increased autocrine expression of IL-1 is associated with EC senescence. This decrease in proliferative capacity can be reversed by antisense oligonucleotides directed against IL-1 production.[21] Although IL-1 lacks a signal peptide, these studies suggest that in addition to paracrine effects on VSMC growth, the autocrine expression of IL-1 may modulate EC growth and differentiation.

The growth factor IGF-1 participates in the regulation of EC and VSMC growth. Several reports suggest that it plays an autocrine growth-promoting role in microvascular ECs.[22, 23] In VSMCs, IGF-1 acts as a growth progression factor for quiescent cells rendered "competent" to proceed through the cell cycle toward DNA synthesis by growth factors such as PDGF and bFGF.[24] In the absence of other growth factors, IGF-1 promotes VSMC hypertrophy and matrix production.[25] The growth effects of IGF-1 also are modulated by IGF binding proteins that may either inhibit or potentiate its activity, depending on experimental conditions.[26]

Basic FGF is a potent autocrine growth factor for ECs and is a potent VSMC mitogen.[27, 28] In vitro studies with neutralizing antibodies suggest that bFGF plays a critical role in EC proliferation, cell migration, cell invasion, matrix alterations, and angiogenesis.[16, 28] bFGF lacks a classic signal peptide and is primarily cell associated but can be recovered from the extracellular matrix.[16] The peptide contains a nuclear localization sequence that, when deleted by site-directed mutagenesis, abolishes its mitogenic properties. Indeed, labeling studies of the peptide have documented rapid nuclear localization. These findings suggest that bFGF may behave as an intracrine growth factor. In addition to these intracellular actions, bFGF is bound to heparin sulfate within the matrix. The matrix acts as a reservoir that binds bFGF released during cell wounding/lysis and may release it in response to proteases, such as heparinitase, released by platelets and leukocytes.[16] Although regulation of its function is still poorly defined, bFGF has profound effects on vascular structure. VEGF is an endothelial-specific growth factor that has no effect on VSMC, fibroblasts, or other vascular cells. VEGF has been shown to induce EC proliferation, stimulate cell migration,[29, 30] and inhibit apoptosis.[31, 32] In vivo, VEGF plays a central role in vasculogenesis and angiogenesis in response to tissue hypoxia.[33] Because of the latter effect, VEGF is gaining increasing attention as a therapeutic tool to induce postnatal angiogenesis in ischemic conditions.[34]

Vascular Growth Inhibitors

Campbell and Campbell[35] and Castellot and colleagues[36] have observed that confluent ECs secrete growth-inhibitory substances that appear to promote the expression of certain characteristics exhibited by the most quiescent, differentiated-appearing VSMC phenotype. Other studies suggest that heparin sulfate produced by ECs inhibits VSMC growth and migration.[37, 38] Studies demonstrate that the endothelium VSMC and macrophage also produce TGF-β1.[39–41] This multifunctional growth factor promotes angiogenesis and inhibits EC proliferation and migration.[40, 42, 43] TGF-β1 has a bifunctional effect on VSMC growth in that it either inhibits mitogen-induced proliferation or stimulates VSMC proliferation that is mediated by the autocrine production of PDGF AA.[14, 15, 44] Based on the available data, we would speculate that TGF-β1 and heparin participate in vascular remodeling. Factors such as TGF-β1 may be particularly important in structural changes in which the vessel lumen size decreases or blood vessels undergo rarefaction or regression, that is, settings in which cell loss and matrix production are important. As is discussed later, several endothelium-derived vasodilator substances, such as prostacyclin and NO, appear to possess growth-inhibitory properties. These substances are released in response to hemodynamic stimuli and play a role in the long-term modulation of vascular structure.

Modulators of Vascular Cell Apoptosis

The knowledge about regulators and signaling mechanisms of apoptosis is expanding rapidly. Indeed, an increasing number of vascular substances have been identified that exert bifunctional effects on cell fate by modulating cell growth as well as cell death. Furthermore, it is noteworthy that the effect on apoptosis depends highly on the target cell type and its environment.

For example, NO has been shown to have antiproliferative effects in VSMCs[45] and to induce apoptosis in the same cell type.[12] Opposite findings have been reported in ECs. Administration of "physiologic" levels of an NO donor diminishes apoptosis in human ECs.[46] This effect has been reproduced by exposing the cells to shear stress.[13] In addition, shear stress–induced endothelial nitric oxide synthase activation in ECs has been found to involve Akt-dependent phosphorylation.[47, 48] The relevance of NO-mediated apoptosis in the context of vascular remodeling remains to be defined.

AII has also been demonstrated to exhibit bifunctional effects on the fate of vascular cells. This peptide has been shown to promote apoptosis in ECs.[49] Its effect on VSMCs depends on activation of its specific receptor. Binding to angiotensin type I receptor mediates antiapoptotic effects in VSMCs,[12] whereas activation of its type 2 receptor confers proapoptotic properties.[50, 51] Currently, there is only indirect evidence supporting the antiapoptotic action mediated by the angiotensin type 1 receptor on VSMC fate in vivo. A decrease in vascular hypertrophy has been observed in response to normalization of blood pressure in previously hypertensive rats.[52] This regression of hypertensive remodeling was associated with an increase in medial VSMC apoptosis.

TGF-β1 has also been shown to play a dual role in the context of vascular cell apoptosis. Although it has been shown to promote EC apoptosis, it exerts antiapoptotic effects on VSMCs.[53]

Finally, IGF-1 has been shown to diminish VSMC apoptosis involving an Akt-dependent pathway.[54] The same survival pathway has been implied for VEGF-induced antiapoptotic effects in ECs.[32]

Vasoactive Substances With Growth Regulatory Properties

As noted earlier, classic mitogens, such as PDGF and epidermal growth factors, have vasomotor effects, whereas vasoactive substances, such as AII and serotonin, can be mitogenic.[55, 56] These data suggest that vasoactive agents and growth factors share overlapping signal transduction pathways. In confluent quiescent VSMCs in culture, AII induces cellular hypertrophy.[57] We have shown that the hypertrophic response is associated with increased messenger RNA (mRNA) levels of proto-oncogene c-*fos*, c-*jun*, and c-*myc* and the autocrine growth factors PDGF A chain, bFGF, and TGF-β1.[58] These autocrine growth factors may mediate angiotensin-induced hypertrophy. We have demonstrated further that AII-induced PDGF and bFGF production is responsible in large part for the VSMC proliferative growth response.[58]

On the other hand, AII-induced TGF-β1 production is responsible for modulating the mitogenic effect of PDGF and bFGF because blockade of the TGF-β1 effect by specific antibodies or antisense oligonucleotide resulted in AII-induced DNA synthesis and cell proliferation.[58, 59] Thus, angiotensin is a bifunctional growth factor able to activate proliferative (PDGF, bFGF) and antiproliferative (TGF-β1) cellular mechanisms simultaneously. The latter is dependent on the activation of a protein kinase C–dependent pathway. In addition to its direct effects on VSMCs, AII also can interact with other growth factors in the vessel wall. Angiotensin may potentiate serum-, bFGF-, and PDGF-induced DNA synthesis.[9, 60] These findings suggest that angiotensin may modulate the proliferative response to autocrine/paracrine growth factors. Moreover, alterations in VSMC phenotype may modulate the AII-induced growth response by altering the susceptibility to proliferative versus antiproliferative factors.

Similar to the response to AII, we and others have shown that endothelin also can induce an increased expression of c-*myc* in association with VSMC proliferation.[61] Growth-promoting effects on VSMCs also have been described for many other vasoconstrictors, for example, norepinephrine, thromboxane, leukotrienes, vasopressin, substance K, and serotonin.[56, 62–65] The sympathetic nervous system appears to exert a trophic effect on the vasculature to promote growth and remodeling.[65, 66] Removal of this neural input attenuates the structural responses of the vasculature. The growth effects of catecholamines may be mediated by the autocrine production of PDGF AA.[67] These growth effects of vasoactive substances also are associated with effects on VSMC migration. AII, serotonin, and norepinephrine have been shown to enhance cell migration as well as stimulate growth.[68, 69] In contrast, endogenous vasodilators that activate adenylate cyclase, such as prostacyclin, prostaglandin E_2, and adenosine, or vasodilators that activate guanylate cyclase, such as NO and atrial natriuretic peptide, inhibit VSMC growth.[45, 70–72] The effects of vasodilators on VSMC migration are not well defined.

The effect of vasoactive substances on EC growth is not as well characterized. It has been reported that catecholamines, histamine, and adenosine enhance serum-stimulated cell proliferation.[73–75] The growth stimulation of adenosine appears to be potentiated in the setting of hypoxia.[75] Conversely, activation of guanylate cyclase inhibits the proliferation of conduit vessel endothelium, and protein kinase C activation inhibits microvascular endothelial proliferation.[76, 77] The effects on endothelial growth usually are associated with other functional changes, such as alterations in cell movement. It has been reported that AII, serotonin, norepinephrine, and histamine inhibit EC migration in vitro.[68, 69]

These data suggest that circulating or locally produced vasoactive substances may influence VSMC and EC growth and migration and thereby modulate vascular structure. Given that ECs generate prostacyclin, nitrovasodilators, angiotensin, and endothelin locally, these substances may modulate each other's effect on vascular tone, cell growth, and migration. These vasoactive agents appear to interact with endogenously produced growth factors in the regulation of vascular cell growth (see Fig. 68–1). Thus, it is important to recognize that circulatory regulation is achieved in the short term by controlling vascular tone and in the long term by influencing vascular structure through remodeling.

Physiologic Vascular Remodeling

Some studies suggest that exercise may alter vascular structure and/or reactivity. Studies using various animal models from rats to monkeys have demonstrated enlargement in the diameter of coronary arteries of animals performing vigorous endurance-type exercise. Epicardial coronary arteries are enlarged in physically active rats compared with sedentary litter mates.[78–81] Short-term exercise training of dogs produces a significant increase in the diameter of their epicardial coronary arteries,[82] and 42 months of endurance training of monkeys results in increased cardiac mass and larger coronary artery size compared with sedentary controls.[81]

Men who reportedly have physically active occupations[83, 84] have larger than expected coronary arteries. Frequently cited is the case report based on the autopsy of the marathon runner Clarence De Mar, in which his epicardial vessels were found to be "two or three times the normal size."[85] Mann and colleagues[86] found that vigorously active Masai tribesmen dying of noncardiovascular causes and with no clinical evidence of coronary disease had as much coronary atherosclerosis at autopsy as American men but had patent arterial lumens because of the large size of their epicardial vessels. Rose and associates[83] at autopsy studied the hearts of a group of men and women with and without infarction and found an association between increasing physical activity of occupation and increasing coronary artery diameter. Schuler and coworkers[87] used quantitative angiography to find that an exercise program reduced the progression of coronary artery disease.

Coronary artery diameter has been shown to increase in proportion to increases in cardiac mass. O'Keefe and colleagues[88] reported a positive correlation between left ventricular mass and coronary artery cross-sectional area in 40 patients with valvular heart disease or normal valvular and ventricular function. Similar results have been reported by other investigators from angiographic[89] and autopsy[90] observations. However, the exercise-induced increase in vessel diameter is out of proportion to the hypertrophy of the end-organ supplied by the vessel. The results of several cross-sectional[91, 92] and exercise-training[93, 94] studies have demonstrated that in trained men and women, there is significantly greater hyperemic blood flow in the calf and forearm, even after correction for differences in muscle mass. These results are consistent with a greater capacity for dilatation in the vasculature of trained skeletal muscle unrelated to muscle hypertrophy. The results appear to be due to adaptation of the vascular structure, possibly an increase in the caliber and/or the number of resistance arterioles. The beneficial effects of exercise training are likely mediated by biologic effects, including changes in lipoprotein, glucose, and insulin levels; reduced neurohormonal activation and myocardial oxygen demands; and increased efficacy of substrate utilization. We propose that one of the major mechanisms by which exercise training reduces the manifestations of coronary artery disease is via flow-induced changes in vascular structure and reactivity.

Clinical observations suggest that changes in coronary blood flow result in changes in vascular structure. Coronary blood flow is dramatically increased in patients with coronary arteriovenous fistulas, and this abnormality is associated with marked enlargement and tortuosity of the vessel segment involved in the fistula.[95] Although the phenomenon of coronary vascular remodeling is most striking in the unusual clinical condition of arteriovenous fistula, less dramatic manifestations of this process are widespread. In their studies of human coronary arteries at autopsy, Glagov and associates[96] found that many atherosclerotic vessels with significant atheroma had maintained a normal lumen diameter via enlargement of the vessel wall. They proposed that as the lumen is narrowed by increasing atheroma, the resulting increase in shear stress may also affect vascular reactivity. Miller and colleagues[97] increased femoral arterial flow long term in dogs by means of a surgically induced arteriovenous fistula. After 6 weeks, the femoral arteries were harvested for studies of vascular reactivity. Endothelial responsiveness was augmented in the vessel exposed to increased flow. Conversely, a chronic decrease in flow that results from a low cardiac output in heart failure models is associated with a decrease in endothelium-dependent relaxation.[98, 99] These studies suggest that chronic changes in blood flow may alter vascular reactivity. To summarize, clinical and experimental observations suggest that the vessel wall is capable of responding to increase in shear stress via changes in vascular structure and/or reactivity. Research in studying the mechanism by which the vessel wall senses and responds to increased flow has focused on the role of the endothelium.

Acute Response to Flow: Vasodilatation

As blood flow increases, the conduit vessel dilates. This flow-induced vasodilatation is mediated by the endothelium, and in conduit vessels (including the coronary artery), it is largely due to the release of endothelium-derived vasodilators such as NO.[100–103] In the microvasculature, prostanoids play a greater role[104]; in the cerebral circulation, neither NO nor prostanoids are involved.[105] An endothelium-dependent hyperpolarizing factor may also contribute.[106] The mechanism by which the endothelium transduces the stimulus of flow remains undetermined. However, Olesen and colleagues[107] found that flow activates an endothelial potassium channel. Subsequently, we found that the release of NO by flow requires an endothelial channel of the K_{ca2+} type.[108] We propose that the endothelial potassium channel is required to transduce the flow stimulus, whereas NO is the major effector of the vasodilatation. As discussed earlier, NO, known to be derived from the metabolism of L-arginine,[109–111] is a potent vasodilator and also inhibits vascular smooth muscle cell growth. Because of its effect on cell growth, it may be involved in vascular remodeling.

Chronic Response to Flow: Vascular Remodeling

Just as flow-mediated vasodilatation is dependent on the endothelium, so is flow-induced vascular remodeling. Langille and O'Donnell[112] have shown that a chronic decrease in flow through the rabbit carotid artery induces a decrease in vessel caliber. This chronic effect appears to be due to a *structural* rather than a functional modification of the arterial wall. Furthermore, this shrinkage remodeling has been shown to depend on the integrity of the endothelial layer because the change in vessel architecture can be abolished by removal of the endothelium.[112] The endothelial mechanism mediating these structural effects remains undefined. We hypothesize that the endothelium induces changes in vessel structure by producing mediators that regulate cell growth, extracellular matrix production, and proteolysis. Although many mediators may be involved in vascular remodeling, experimental evidence from our laboratory and others has established that flow stimulates the release of NO, PDGF, and TGF-β1.

The importance of NO in flow-induced shrinkage remodeling has been further documented by a study using endothelial nitric oxide synthase (eNOS) knockout mice.[113] A reduction in blood flow induced an increase in wall thickness in eNOS knockout mice compared to the wild-type strain, suggesting eNOS as an important regulator of flow-induced shrinkage remodeling. However, the molecular pathways involved in this response remain to be defined.

The obligatory role of endothelial NO in flow-induced enlargement remodeling in response to a chronic increase in flow has been documented in a rabbit arteriovenous fistula model by Tronc and colleagues.[114] The adaptive enlargement remodeling was abolished after administration of the nitric oxide synthase inhibitor *NG*-nitro-L-arginine methylester. Similar effects have been reported in a rat model of combined unilateral external and internal carotid ligation.[115] These investigators have shown a flow-induced adaptive remodeling in the contralateral artery with increased flow.

Disorders of Vascular Structure (Pathologic Vascular Remodeling)

One of the outcomes of an imbalance of the production and/or the action of endogenous growth promoters and inhibitors is abnormal vascular structure. Disorders that involve altered vascular structure include hypertensive vascular hypertrophy, atherosclerosis, and restenosis. Although the pathophysiologic processes of these disorders are complex and involve the participation of multiple cell types, biologically active molecules, extracellular matrix modulation, and so forth, a consistent feature of all these processes is abnormal smooth muscle growth.

Hypertension

The hemodynamic alterations in hypertension initiate adaptive changes in the conduit and resistance vessels that are characterized by medial smooth muscle hypertrophy or hyperplasia, increased extracellular matrix, reduced compliance, and increased resistance.[46] This adaptive remodeling response normalizes the wall stress and confers an increase in basal vascular reactivity, may contribute to the amplification of vasoconstriction and the perpetuation of hypertension, and may promote the development of vascular complications, such as atherosclerosis. Research has focused on these vessel wall changes and the cellular and molecular mechanisms of vascular hypertrophy in hypertension.[116, 117] A series of interesting experiments on this subject using several models of hypertension have been performed. Hypertension induced by the administration of deoxycorticosterone acetate and a high-salt diet (deoxycorticosterone acetate [DOCA]-salt) results in a fourfold increase in the steady-state levels of TGF-β1 gene expressions in the aorta.[118] Changes in the gene expression of growth factor receptors such as the PDGF receptor[119] have also been recognized to play an important role in this context. These investigators have demonstrated that PDGF-β receptor mRNA levels are increased severalfold in the aortas of DOCA-salt–treated rats, spontaneously hypertensive rats, and aging animals.

In addition to alterations in cell growth, vascular remodeling in hypertension involves changes in the extracellular matrix. The onset of hypertension induced by either DOCA-salt or AII infusion resulted in a severalfold increase in fibronectin mRNA levels that reverted to basal levels after correction of hypertension.[120] Pulse-chase experiments and Western blot analysis also demonstrated increased secretion of fibronectin into the extracellular matrix of hypertensive vessels. Based on the finding that fibronectin influences VSMC growth in vitro,[120] these observations suggest that the modification of matrix composition associated with the hypertensive state may influence the vascular cell growth response to increases in blood pressure.

It is well established that hypertension enhances the development of atherosclerosis in humans. In the presence of hypercholesterolemia, the vascular complications of hypertension are markedly potentiated. Animal models of concomitant hypertension and hypercholesterolemia may be particularly useful for the studies of the pathophysiologic mechanisms of accelerated vascular disease. Indeed, the production of renovascular hypertension in hyperlipidemic animal models results in an increase in atherosclerotic lesions that are directly attributable to elevations in blood pressure.[121] Thus, changes in the extracellular matrix, autocrine/paracrine growth factor expression, and growth factor receptor expression that accompany the vascular response to hypertension may also influence the response to other forms of vascular injury, such as hyperlipidemia. These findings provide an understanding of the potential molecular mechanisms that are responsible for the long-standing clinical observations that the interaction of risk factors promotes the development of vascular disease.

Atherosclerosis

In atherosclerosis, endothelial dysfunction has been demonstrated as impaired endothelium-dependent relaxation and paradoxical vasoconstriction in response to acetylcholine and increased blood flow (both are stimuli of NO release).[122, 123] These abnormalities have been reported in human and animal coronary arteries, peripheral vasculature, and the aorta. The endothelium of atherosclerotic arteries also exhibits enhanced expression of adhesion molecules, cytokines, and growth factors.[124] In fact, impaired endothelium-dependent relaxation has been observed in human forearm vasculature, epicardial coronary artery, coronary microvasculature of subjects with hypercholesterolemia, or hypertension without obvious atherosclerosis.[125–128] Thus, it is hypothesized that an early initiating event of atherogenesis is endothelial "injury"[129] by hypercholesterolemia and other risk factors.

The evolution of atherosclerotic vascular disease involves the infiltration of leukocytes into the vessel wall, alterations in lipid metabolism, and cell migration through the extracellular matrix.[129] The early development of this disease (as induced by hypercholesterolemia) is associated with the expression of specific molecules on ECs that promotes monocyte migration and adhesion. Exposure of cultured ECs to minimally modified low-density lipid (LDL) cholesterol induces the EC expression of monocyte chemotactic protein.[130] Furthermore, immunohistochemical studies documented the presence of a monocyte adhesive protein related to vascular cell adhesion molecule-1 on ECs overlying foamy macrophages in hypercholesterolemic rabbits and in the LDL receptor–deficient Watanabe rabbit during the development of foam lesions. These results suggest that this adhesion molecule may be an EC mediator and/or marker for early atherogenesis and may be potentially involved in the development of the initial fatty streak lesion.[131]

Clinical studies have clearly established the link between elevated LDL cholesterol levels and the development of atherosclerotic lesions.[132] Once inflammatory cells have invaded the vessel wall, their function is modulated by the local milieu created by abnormalities in lipid metabolism. The monocyte that invades the vascular wall may be transformed into a foamy macrophage within a fatty streak lesion. This transformation can occur as the macrophage takes up modified (acetylated or oxidized) LDL. Oxidatively modified LDL may be generated by ECs, smooth muscle cells, or macrophages. The oxidative modification process may involve the release of superoxide anions from the cells or by the transfer of oxidized cell lipids to LDL. The oxidation of LDL may be linked to the activity of the lipoxygenase pathway. In situ hybridization studies show that 15-lipoxygenase mRNA and protein are present at high levels in macrophage-rich lesions of the Watanabe rabbit.[133] The activated macrophages synthesize and release cytokines and growth factors. These macrophage-derived substances, especially IL-Iβ, subsequently stimulate medial and intimal VSMCs. Activated VSMCs express autocrine growth factor (e.g., PDGF-A) and undergo cellular proliferation and migration into the intima, eventually resulting in the development of intimal hyperplasia, an important component of atherosclerosis.

Restenosis

In response to injury induced by interventional procedures such as balloon angioplasty, a reparative process is activated that may lead to restenosis. This process involves cellular and noncellular events that may be divided into three phases (Table 68–2), according to the sequence of events compiled from studies of several animal models and analysis of human histologic, angiographic, and intravascular ultrasound data. Thus, the duration of these phases is arbitrary because there is substantial overlap among the events and potentially significant variability among patients.

Phase I: Acute Injury and Release of Mediators

Balloon angioplasty causes local vascular injury, including endothelial denudation, rupture of the internal elastic lamina, lysis of some medial VSMCs, and fracture of the atherosclerotic plaque. With further stretching, medial dissection may result in subsequent dilatation of the outer media and adventitia. Initiated by this mechanical injury, phase I is characterized by interaction of platelets and thrombin with the vessel wall (phase IA) and release of numerous biologically active mediators (phase IB). These events occur over minutes to hours after injury.

PHASE IA: ACTIVATION OF PLATELETS AND THROMBIN

Exposure of the subintimal layers and collagen to bloodborne elements leads to activation of the homeostatic system with extensive platelet deposition and fibrin formation.[134] Platelet aggregation is mediated by release of adenosine diphosphate, serotonin, thromboxane A^2, fibrinogen, fibronectin, and von Willebrand factor. Platelets make contact with subendothelial layers and other platelets by glycoprotein Ib and IIb/IIIa receptors. Interestingly, the thickness of the deposited platelet layer and the predisposition to thrombus formation are proportional to the amount of subendothelial injury. With severe injury, thrombus formation ultimately may contribute to an organized fibrocellular plug. These initial events begin within minutes after injury, peak 4 to 12 hours later, and are sustained for at least 24 to 48 hours. Thrombin generation (through the intrinsic and extrinsic pathways) can promote platelet aggregation and fibrin production. Thrombin generation by apoptotic VSMCs has also been described.[135] This may be important in light of reports describing significant VSMC apoptosis immediately after balloon injury.[136, 137] Thrombin has been shown to stimulate growth factor release, VSMC proliferation, and alterations in extracellular matrix composition.[138, 139] Fibrin is also chemotactic for VSMCs in vitro. Therefore, the activation of thrombin and the coagulation cascade are likely to contribute to the development of neointimal hyperplasia.

PHASE IB: RELEASE OF GROWTH FACTORS AND CYTOKINES

A number of vasoconstrictors (e.g., thromboxane and serotonin) and mitogens are released by activated platelets, the most important of which are PDGF, epidermal growth factor, and TGF-β1.[140] As a chemotactic and mitogenic agent, PDGF is a potent stimulus to VSMC migration and proliferation. A polyclonal antibody to PDGF has been shown to attenuate neointima formation in rats. Mechanical injury itself may lead to VSMC proliferation by resulting in denudation of the endothelium and release of growth factors from ECs and VSMCs. Fibroblast growth factor appears to be one such mitogen for ECs and VSMCs.[141, 142] Destruction of the intact endothelium by angioplasty also halts production of growth inhibitors (e.g., NO and prostacyclin). Reduction in the levels of these important inhibitors of VSMC growth and migration contributes to the initial process of neointima formation.

Phase II: Smooth Muscle Replication and Inflammation

The intermediate phase is characterized by initial activation and replication of medial VSMCs followed by migration

TABLE 68–2 Phases Leading to Restenosis

Phase	Events	Duration
I. Acute injury and release of mediators	Endothelial denudation; interaction of platelets and thrombin with the vessel wall; release of growth factors and cytokines	Minutes to hours
II. Smooth muscle replication and inflammation	A. Activation and replication of medial VSMCs; migration of medial VSMCs to intima	Days to weeks
	B. Replication of intimal VSMCs	Days to months
	C. Leukocyte infiltration and replication	Days to months
III. Vascular remodeling	Modulation of extracellular matrix and shrinkage remodeling	Weeks to months

Abbreviation: VSMCs, vascular smooth muscle cells.

of VSMCs from the media to the subintima (phase IIA) over days to weeks. This is followed by VSMC replication initiating the development of neointimal hyperplasia (phase IIB) over days to months. Concomitant to these processes is the infiltration of leukocytes brought into the area by cytokines and chemotactic agents as well as adhesion molecules and the proliferation of these inflammatory cells (phase IIC).

PHASE IIA: MEDIAL SMOOTH MUSCLE CELL REPLICATION AND MIGRATION

Stimulated by PDGF (released from platelets, macrophages, injured ECs, and VSMCs), thrombin, fibroblast growth factor (from injured ECs and VSMCs), and other factors, approximately 30 percent of medial VSMCs become activated within the first few days after balloon angioplasty.[143] These cells increase DNA synthesis, express the "synthetic" phenotype, and begin to replicate.[144, 145] With extensive injury, up to 30 percent of the medial VSMCs may migrate to the subintimal space[146] and subsequently replicate, usually beginning in the first few days after angioplasty.[147] Although PDGF appears to be a principal growth factor stimulating cells to migrate, fibroblast growth factor, AII, and changes in the extracellular matrix (with expression of proteolytic enzymes) may also participate.

PHASE IIB: REPLICATION OF INTIMAL VSMC

This phase is characterized by "autoreplication" of VSMCs now present in the intima. In humans, intimal hyperplasia can be detected by the second to third week and appears to plateau by the third to fourth month after coronary angioplasty.[145, 147] During this proliferative phase, intimal VSMCs, fibroblasts, and macrophages express autocrine and paracrine growth factors, including PDGF, fibroblast growth factor, IGF-1, TGF-β, and AII. These local factors play an important role in stimulating VSMC proliferation.

Phase III: Vascular Remodeling

An active process of extracellular matrix modulation occurs in restenosis. There is evidence for both matrix deposition and degradation. Fibroblast and inflammatory cells contribute to these processes. As the intimal VSMCs lose their capacity to replicate, they also produce large amounts of extracellular matrix proteoglycan. Experimental and clinical studies, especially those using intravascular ultrasound, have suggested that a reduction in vessel caliber resulting from vascular remodeling may play an important role in the ultimate narrowing of the restenotic segment.[148] Although metalloproteinase inhibitors have been shown to affect the early response after rat balloon injury by influencing smooth muscle cell migration, they have not been shown to affect restenosis.[149]

With the increased use of stents after angioplasty, the lesion of restenosis has become primarily neointimal hyperplasia mediated by phase I to II because vascular remodeling is counteracted by the scaffolding of the stent.[150, 151] Neointima formation in this context is the sum of the proliferative stimuli resulting from initial balloon injury and foreign body reaction to the stent.[152]

SUMMARY

An important aspect of circulatory regulation is cardiovascular structural adaptation mediated by the process of cardiac and vascular remodeling. Remodeling occurs as a physiologic process in response to chronic alterations in hemodynamic or humoral conditions. Thus, in response to sustained increases in blood flow associated with exercise or arteriovenous fistula, the blood vessel can structurally enlarge in caliber. In hypertension, the chronic increase in blood pressure can elicit cardiac and/or vascular hypertrophy. Although the structural changes are usually adaptive responses, cardiac and vascular remodeling may contribute to the pathophysiology of cardiovascular disorders, such as cardiac failure, atherosclerosis, and restenosis. Future progress in the research of structural remodeling of the vasculature and the heart will provide a better understanding of the process of circulatory regulation and the pathobiology of cardiovascular diseases.

REFERENCES

1. Dzau VJ, Gibbons GH, Cooke JP, Omoigui N: Vascular biology and medicine in the 1990s: scope, concepts, potentials, and perspectives. Circulation 87:705–719, 1993.
2. Gibbons GH, Dzau VJ: The emerging concept of vascular remodeling. N Engl J Med 330:1431–1438, 1994.
3. Dzau VJ, Gibbons GH: Endothelium and growth factors in vascular remodeling of hypertension. Hypertension 18:III115–III121, 1991.
4. Dzau VJ, Gibbons GH: The role of the endothelium in vascular remodeling. *In* Rubanyi GM (ed): Cardiovascular Significance of Endothelium-Derived Vasoactive Factors. pp. 281–291. New York: Futura, 1991.
5. Mulvany MJ: The fourth Sir George Pickering memorial lecture: the structure of the resistance vasculature in essential hypertension. J Hypertens 5:129–136, 1987.
6. Owens GK: Control of hypertrophic versus hyperplastic growth of vascular smooth muscle cells. Am J Physiol 257:H1755–H1765, 1989.
7. Baumbach GL, Heistad DD: Remodeling of cerebral arterioles in chronic hypertension. Hypertension 13:968–972, 1989.
8. Greene AS, Tonellato PJ, Zhang Z, et al: Effect of microvascular rarefaction on tissue oxygen delivery in hypertension. Am J Physiol 262:H1486–H1493, 1992.
9. Battegay EJ, Raines EW, Seifert RA, et al: TGF-beta induces bimodal proliferation of connective tissue cells via complex control of an autocrine PDGF loop. Cell 63:515–524, 1990.
10. Owens GK, Geisterfer AA, Yang YW, Komoriya A: Transforming growth factor-beta-induced growth inhibition and cellular hypertrophy in cultured vascular smooth muscle cells. J Cell Biol 107:771–780, 1988.
11. Gibbons GH, Pratt RE, Dzau VJ: Angiotensin II is a bifunctional vascular smooth muscle cell growth factor [abstract]. Hypertension 14:358, 1989.
12. Pollman MJ, Yamada T, Horiuchi M, Gibbons GH: Vasoactive substances regulate vascular smooth muscle cell apoptosis: countervailing influences of nitric oxide and angiotensin II. Circ Res 79:748–756, 1996.
13. Dimmeler S, Haendeler J, Nehls M, Zeiher AM: Suppression of apoptosis by nitric oxide via inhibition of interleukin-1beta–converting enzyme (ICE)–like and cysteine protease protein (CPP)-32-like proteases. J Exp Med 185:601–607, 1997.
14. Starksen NF, Harsh GR4th, Gibbs VC, Williams LT: Regulated expression of the platelet-derived growth factor A chain gene in microvascular endothelial cells. J Biol Chem 262:14381–14384, 1987.

15. Hansson HA, Jennische E, Skottner A: Regenerating endothelial cells express insulin-like growth factor-I immunoreactivity after arterial injury. Cell Tissue Res 250:499–505, 1987.
16. Saksela O, Rifkin DB: Release of basic fibroblast growth factor-heparan sulfate complexes from endothelial cells by plasminogen activator-mediated proteolytic activity. J Cell Biol 110:767–775, 1990.
17. Hart CE, Forstrom JW, Kelly JD, et al: Two classes of PDGF receptor recognize different isoforms of PDGF. Science 240:1529–1531, 1988.
18. Hajjar KA, Hajjar DP, Silverstein RL, Nachman RL: Tumor necrosis factor-mediated release of platelet-derived growth factor from cultured endothelial cells. J Exp Med 166:235–245, 1987.
19. Libby P, Warner SJ, Friedman GB: Interleukin 1: a mitogen for human vascular smooth muscle cells that induces the release of growth-inhibitory prostanoids. J Clin Invest 81:487–498, 1988.
20. Raines EW, Dower SK, Ross R: Interleukin-1 mitogenic activity for fibroblasts and smooth muscle cells is due to PDGF-AA. Science 243:393–396, 1989.
21. Maier JA, Voulalas P, Roeder D, Maciag T: Extension of the life-span of human endothelial cells by an interleukin-1 alpha antisense oligomer. Science 249:1570–1574, 1990.
22. Bar RS, Boes M, Booth BA, et al: The effects of platelet-derived growth factor in cultured microvessel endothelial cells. Endocrinology 124:1841–1848, 1989.
23. King GL, Goodman AD, Buzney S, et al: Receptors and growth-promoting effects of insulin and insulinlike growth factors on cells from bovine retinal capillaries and aorta. J Clin Invest 75:1028–1036, 1985.
24. Clemmons DR: Interaction of circulating cell-derived and plasma growth factors in stimulating cultured smooth muscle cell replication. J Cell Physiol 121:425–430, 1984.
25. Badesch DB, Lee PD, Parks WC, Stenmark KR: Insulin-like growth factor I stimulates elastin synthesis by bovine pulmonary arterial smooth muscle cells. Biochem Biophys Res Commun 160:382–387, 1989.
26. Clemmons DR, Gardner LI: A factor contained in plasma is required for IGF binding protein-1 to potentiate the effect of IGF-I on smooth muscle cell DNA synthesis. J Cell Physiol 145:129–135, 1990.
27. Burgess WH, Maciag T: The heparin-binding (fibroblast) growth factor family of proteins. Annu Rev Biochem 58:575–606, 1989.
28. Mignatti P, Tsuboi R, Robbins E, Rifkin DB: In vitro angiogenesis on the human amniotic membrane: requirement for basic fibroblast growth factor-induced proteinases. J Cell Biol 108:671–682, 1989.
29. Leung DW, Cachianes G, Kuang WJ, et al: Vascular endothelial growth factor is a secreted angiogenic mitogen. Science 246:1306–1309, 1989.
30. Keck PJ, Hauser SD, Krivi G, et al: Vascular permeability factor, an endothelial cell mitogen related to PDGF. Science 246:1309–1312, 1989.
31. Spyridopoulos I, Brogi E, Kearney M, et al: Vascular endothelial growth factor inhibits endothelial cell apoptosis induced by tumor necrosis factor-alpha: balance between growth and death signals. J Mol Cell Cardiol 29:1321–1330, 1997.
32. Gerber HP, McMurtrey A, Kowalski J, et al: Vascular endothelial growth factor regulates endothelial cell survival through the phosphatidylinositol 3′-kinase/Akt signal transduction pathway: requirement for Flk-1/KDR activation. J Biol Chem 273:30336–30343, 1998.
33. Shweiki D, Itin A, Soffer D, Keshet E: Vascular endothelial growth factor induced by hypoxia may mediate hypoxia-initiated angiogenesis. Nature 359:843–845, 1992.
34. Isner JM, Pieczek A, Schainfeld R, et al: Clinical evidence of angiogenesis after arterial gene transfer of phVEGF165 in patient with ischaemic limb. Lancet 348:370–374, 1996.
35. Campbell JH, Campbell GR: Endothelial cell influences on vascular smooth muscle phenotype. Annu Rev Physiol 48:295–306, 1986.
36. Castellot JJ Jr, Favreau LV, Karnovsky MJ, Rosenberg RD: Inhibition of vascular smooth muscle cell growth by endothelial cell–derived heparin: possible role of a platelet endoglycosidase. J Biol Chem 257:11256–11260, 1982.
37. Majack RA, Clowes AW: Inhibition of vascular smooth muscle cell migration by heparin-like glycosaminoglycans. J Cell Physiol 118:253–256, 1984.
38. Imamura T, Engleka K, Zhan X, et al: Recovery of mitogenic activity of a growth factor mutant with a nuclear translocation sequence. Science 249:1567–1570, 1990.
39. Antonelli-Orlidge A, Saunders KB, Smith SR, D'Amore PA: An activated form of transforming growth factor beta is produced by cocultures of endothelial cells and pericytes. Proc Natl Acad Sci U S A 86:4544–4548, 1989.
40. Sato Y, Rifkin DB: Inhibition of endothelial cell movement by pericytes and smooth muscle cells: activation of a latent transforming growth factor-beta 1–like molecule by plasmin during co-culture. J Cell Biol 109:309–315, 1989.
41. Sato Y, Tsuboi R, Lyons R, et al: Characterization of the activation of latent TGF-beta by co-cultures of endothelial cells and pericytes or smooth muscle cells: a self-regulating system. J Cell Biol 111:757–763, 1990.
42. Heimark RL, Twardzik DR, Schwartz SM: Inhibition of endothelial regeneration by type-beta transforming growth factor from platelets. Science 233:1078–1080, 1986.
43. Yang EY, Moses HL: Transforming growth factor beta 1-induced changes in cell migration, proliferation, and angiogenesis in the chicken chorioallantoic membrane. J Cell Biol 111:731–741, 1990.
44. Assoian RK, Sporn MB: Type beta transforming growth factor in human platelets: release during platelet degranulation and action on vascular smooth muscle cells. J Cell Biol 102:1217–1223, 1986.
45. Garg UC, Hassid A: Nitric oxide-generating vasodilators and 8-bromo-cyclic guanosine monophosphate inhibit mitogenesis and proliferation of cultured rat vascular smooth muscle cells. J Clin Invest 83:1774–1777, 1989.
46. Haendeler J, Dimmeler S, Nehls M, Zeiher AM: Nitric oxide inhibits TNF-α–induced apoptosis of human endothelial cells: role of interleukin-1 β converting enzyme like proteases. Circulation 94:I–155, 1996.
47. Dimmeler S, Fleming I, Fisslthaler B, et al: Activation of nitric oxide synthase in endothelial cells by Akt-dependent phosphorylation. Nature 399:601–605, 1999.
48. Fulton D, Gratton JP, McCabe TJ, et al: Regulation of endothelium-derived nitric oxide production by the protein kinase Akt. Nature 399:597–601, 1999.
49. Dimmeler S, Rippmann V, Weiland U, et al: Angiotensin II induces apoptosis of human endothelial cells: protective effect of nitric oxide. Circ Res 81:970–976, 1997.
50. Yamada T, Horiuchi M, Dzau VJ: Angiotensin II type 2 receptor mediates programmed cell death. Proc Natl Acad Sci U S A 93:156–160, 1996.
51. Horiuchi M, Hayashida W, Akishita M, et al: Stimulation of different subtypes of angiotensin II receptors, AT1 and AT2 receptors, regulates STAT activation by negative crosstalk. Circ Res 84:876–882, 1999.
52. deBlois D, Tea BS, Than VD, et al: Smooth muscle apoptosis during vascular regression in spontaneously hypertensive rats. Hypertension 29:340–349, 1997.
53. Pollman MJ, Naumovski L, Gibbons GH: Vascular cell apoptosis: cell type–specific modulation by transforming growth factor-beta1 in endothelial cells versus smooth muscle cells. Circulation 99:2019–2026, 1999.
54. Bai H, Pollman MJ, Inishi Y, Gibbons GH: Regulation of vascular smooth muscle cell apoptosis: modulation of bad by a phosphatidylinositol 3-kinase-dependent pathway. Circ Res 85:229–237, 1999.
55. Campbell-Boswell M, Robertson AL Jr: Effects of angiotensin II and vasopressin on human smooth muscle cells in vitro. Exp Mol Pathol 35:265–276, 1981.
56. Nemecek GM, Coughlin SR, Handley DA, Moskowitz MA: Stimulation of aortic smooth muscle cell mitogenesis by serotonin. Proc Natl Acad Sci U S A 83:674–678, 1986.
57. Naftilan AJ, Pratt RE, Dzau VJ: Induction of platelet-derived growth factor A-chain and c-*myc* gene expressions by angiotensin II in cultured rat vascular smooth muscle cells. J Clin Invest 83:1419–424, 1989.
58. Itoh H, Mukoyama M, Pratt RE, et al: Multiple autocrine growth factors modulate vascular smooth muscle cell growth response to angiotensin II. J Clin Invest 91:2268–2274, 1993.
59. Gibbons GH, Pratt RE, Dzau VJ: Vascular smooth muscle cell hypertrophy vs. hyperplasia: autocrine transforming growth factor-beta 1 expression determines growth response to angiotensin II. J Clin Invest 90:456–461, 1992.
60. Bobik A, Grinpukel S, Little PJ, et al: Angiotensin II and noradrena-

line increase PDGF-BB receptors and potentiate PDGF-BB stimulated DNA synthesis in vascular smooth muscle. Biochem Biophys Res Commun 166:580–588, 1990.

61. Dubin D, Pratt RE, Cooke JP, Dzau VJ: Endothelin, a potent vasoconstrictor, is a vascular smooth muscle mitogen. J Vasc Med Biol 1:150, 1989.
62. Ishimitsu T, Uehara Y, Ishii M, et al: Thromboxane and vascular smooth muscle cell growth in genetically hypertensive rats. Hypertension 12:46–51, 1988.
63. Palmberg L, Claesson HE, Thyberg J: Leukotrienes stimulate initiation of DNA synthesis in cultured arterial smooth muscle cells. J Cell Sci 88:151–159, 1987.
64. Nilsson J, von Euler AM, Dalsgaard CJ: Stimulation of connective tissue cell growth by substance P and substance K. Nature 315:61–63, 1985.
65. Nakaki T, Nakayama M, Yamamoto S, Kato R: Alpha 1-adrenergic stimulation and beta 2-adrenergic inhibition of DNA synthesis in vascular smooth muscle cells. Mol Pharmacol 37:30–36, 1990.
66. Bevan RD: Trophic effects of peripheral adrenergic nerves on vascular structure. Hypertension 6:III19–III26, 1984.
67. Majesky MW, Daemen MJ, Schwartz SM: Alpha 1-adrenergic stimulation of platelet-derived growth factor A-chain gene expression in rat aorta. J Biol Chem 265:1082–1088, 1990.
68. Bell L, Madri JA: Effect of platelet factors on migration of cultured bovine aortic endothelial and smooth muscle cells. Circ Res 65:1057–1065, 1989.
69. Bell L, Madri JA: Influence of the angiotensin system on endothelial and smooth muscle cell migration. Am J Pathol 137:7–12, 1990.
70. Jonzon B, Nilsson J, Fredholm BB: Adenosine receptor-mediated changes in cyclic AMP production and DNA synthesis in cultured arterial smooth muscle cells. J Cell Physiol 124:451–456, 1985.
71. Nilsson J, Olsson AG: Prostaglandin E1 inhibits DNA synthesis in arterial smooth muscle cells stimulated with platelet-derived growth factor. Atherosclerosis 53:77–82, 1984.
72. Kariya K, Kawahara Y, Araki S, et al: Antiproliferative action of cyclic GMP-elevating vasodilators in cultured rabbit aortic smooth muscle cells. Atherosclerosis 80:143–147, 1989.
73. Sherline P, Mascardo R: Catecholamines are mitogenic in 3T3 and bovine aortic endothelial cells. J Clin Invest 74:483–487, 1984.
74. Marks RM, Roche WR, Czerniecki M, et al: Mast cell granules cause proliferation of human microvascular endothelial cells. Lab Invest 55:289–294, 1986.
75. Meininger CJ, Schelling ME, Granger HJ: Adenosine and hypoxia stimulate proliferation and migration of endothelial cells. Am J Physiol 255:H554–H562, 1988.
76. Leitman DC, Fiscus RR, Murad F: Forskolin, phosphodiesterase inhibitors, and cyclic AMP analogs inhibit proliferation of cultured bovine aortic endothelial cells. J Cell Physiol 127:237–243, 1986.
77. Doctrow SR, Folkman J: Protein kinase C activators suppress stimulation of capillary endothelial cell growth by angiogenic endothelial mitogens. J Cell Biol 104:679–687, 1987.
78. Tepperman J, Perlman D: Effect of exercise and anemia on coronary arteries of small animals as revealed by the corrosion-cast technique. Circ Res 9:576–584, 1961.
79. Leon AS, Bloor CM: Effects of exercise and its cessation on the heart and its blood supply. J Appl Physiol 24:485–490, 1968.
80. Bloor CM, Leon AS: Interaction of age and exercise on the heart and its blood supply. Lab Invest 22:160–165, 1970.
81. Kramsch DM, Aspen AJ, Abramowitz BM, et al: Reduction of coronary atherosclerosis by moderate conditioning exercise in monkeys on an atherogenic diet. N Engl J Med 305:1483–1489, 1981.
82. Wyatt HL, Mitchell J: Influences of physical conditioning and deconditioning on coronary vasculature of dogs. J Appl Physiol 45:619–625, 1978.
83. Rose G, Prineas RJ, Mitchell JR: Myocardial infarction and the intrinsic calibre of coronary arteries. Br Heart J 29:548–552, 1967.
84. Norris JN, Crawford MD: Coronary heart disease and physical activity of work: evidence of a national necropsy survey. Br Med J 5111:1485–1496, 1958.
85. Currens JH, White PD: Half century of running: clinical, physiologic and autopsy findings in the case of Clarence DeMar ("Mr. Marathon"). N Engl J Med 265:988–993, 1961.
86. Mann GV, Spoerry A, Gray M, Jarashow D: Atherosclerosis in the Masai. Am J Epidemiol 95:26–37, 1972.
87. Schuler G, Hambrecht R, Schlierf G, et al: Regular physical exercise and low-fat diet: effects on progression of coronary artery disease. Circulation 86:1–11, 1992.
88. O'Keefe JH Jr, Owen RM, Bove AA: Influence of left ventricular mass on coronary artery cross-sectional area. Am J Cardiol 59:1395–1397, 1987.
89. Koiwa Y, Bahn RC, Ritman EL: Regional myocardial volume perfused by the coronary artery branch: estimation in vivo. Circulation 74:157–163, 1986.
90. Roberts CS, Roberts WC: Cross-sectional area of the proximal portions of the three major epicardial coronary arteries in 98 necropsy patients with different coronary events: relationship to heart weight, age and sex. Circulation 62:953–959, 1980.
91. Snell PG, Martin WH, Buckey JC, Blomqvist CG: Maximal vascular leg conductance in trained and untrained men. J Appl Physiol 62:606–610, 1987.
92. Martin WH 3rd, Montgomery J, Snell PG, et al: Cardiovascular adaptations to intense swim training in sedentary middle-aged men and women. Circulation, 75:323–330, 1987.
93. Sinoway LI, Shenberger J, Wilson J, McLaughlin D, Musch T, Zelis R: A 30-day forearm work protocol increases maximal forearm blood flow. J Appl Physiol 62:1063–1067, 1987.
94. Martin WH3rd, Kohrt WM, Malley MT, et al: Exercise training enhances leg vasodilatory capacity of 65-yr-old men and women. J Appl Physiol 69:1804–1809, 1990.
95. Gasul BM, Arcilla RA, Fell EH, et al: Congenital coronary arteriovenous fistula: clinical, phonocardiographic, angiocardiographic and hemodynamic studies in five patients. Pediatrics 25:531–560, 1960.
96. Glagov S, Weisenberg E, Zarins CK, et al: Compensatory enlargement of human atherosclerotic coronary arteries. N Engl J Med 316:1371–1375, 1987.
97. Miller VM, Aarhus LL, Vanhoutte PM: Modulation of endothelium-dependent responses by chronic alterations of blood flow. Am J Physiol 251:H520–H527, 1986.
98. Kaiser L, Spickard RC, Olivier NB: Heart failure depresses endothelium-dependent responses in canine femoral artery. Am J Physiol 256:H962–H967, 1989.
99. Treasure CB, Vita JA, Cox DA, et al: Endothelium-dependent dilation of the coronary microvasculature is impaired in dilated cardiomyopathy. Circulation 81:772–779, 1990.
100. Pohl U, Holtz J, Busse R, Bassenge E: Crucial role of endothelium in the vasodilator response to increased flow in vivo. Hypertension 8:37–44, 1986.
101. Rubanyi GM, Romero JC, Vanhoutte PM: Flow-induced release of endothelium-derived relaxing factor. Am J Physiol 250:H1145–H1149, 1986.
102. Young MA, Vatner SF: Blood flow- and endothelium-mediated vasomotion of iliac arteries in conscious dogs. Circ Res 61:II88–II893, 1987.
103. Cooke JP, Stamler J, Andon N, et al: Flow stimulates endothelial cells to release a nitrovasodilator that is potentiated by reduced thiol. Am J Physiol 259:H804–H812, 1990.
104. Koller A, Kaley G: Prostaglandins mediate arteriolar dilation to increased blood flow velocity in skeletal muscle microcirculation. Circ Res 67:529–534, 1990.
105. Faraci FM, Heistad DD: Regulation of cerebral blood vessels by humoral and endothelium-dependent mechanisms: update on humoral regulation of vascular tone. Hypertension 17:917–922, 1991.
106. Feletou M, Vanhoutte PM: Endothelium-dependent hyperpolarization of canine coronary smooth muscle. Br J Pharmacol 93:515–524, 1988.
107. Olesen SP, Clapham DE, Davies PF: Haemodynamic shear stress activates a K^+ current in vascular endothelial cells. Nature 331:168–170, 1988.
108. Cooke JP, Rossitch E Jr, Andon NA, et al: Flow activates an endothelial potassium channel to release an endogenous nitrovasodilator. J Clin Invest 88:1663–1671, 1991.
109. Ignarro LJ, Byrns RE, Buga GM, Wood KS: Endothelium-derived relaxing factor from pulmonary artery and vein possesses pharmacologic and chemical properties identical to those of nitric oxide radical. Circ Res 61:866–879, 1987.
110. Palmer RM, Ferrige AG, Moncada S: Nitric oxide release accounts for the biological activity of endothelium-derived relaxing factor. Nature 327:524–526, 1987.
111. Palmer RM, Ashton DS, Moncada S: Vascular endothelial cells synthesize nitric oxide from L-arginine. Nature 333:664–666, 1988.

112. Langille BL, O'Donnell F: Reductions in arterial diameter produced by chronic decreases in blood flow are endothelium-dependent. Science 231:405–407, 1986.
113. Rudic RD, Shesely EG, Maeda N, et al: Direct evidence for the importance of endothelium-derived nitric oxide in vascular remodeling. J Clin Invest 101:731–736, 1998.
114. Tronc F, Wassef M, Esposito B, et al: Role of NO in flow-induced remodeling of the rabbit common carotid artery. Arterioscler Thromb Vasc Biol 16:1256–1262, 1996.
115. Miyashiro JK, Poppa V, Berk BC: Flow-induced vascular remodeling in the rat carotid artery diminishes with age. Circ Res 81:311–319, 1997.
116. Dzau VJ, Gibbons GH: Endothelium and growth factors in vascular remodeling of hypertension. Hypertension 18(5 suppl):III115–III121, 1991.
117. Krieger JE, Dzau VJ: Molecular biology of hypertension. Hypertension 18(3 suppl):I3–I17, 1991.
118. Sarzani R, Brecher P, Chobanian AV: Growth factor expression in aorta of normotensive and hypertensive rats. J Clin Invest 83:1404–1408, 1989.
119. Sarzani R, Claffey KP, Chobanian AV, Brecher P: Hypertension induces tissue-specific gene suppression of a fatty acid binding protein in rat aorta. Proc Natl Acad Sci U S A 85:7777–7781, 1988.
120. Takasaki I, Chobanian AV, Brecher P: Biosynthesis of fibronectin by rabbit aorta. J Biol Chem 266:17686–17694, 1991.
121. Hollander W, Madoff I, Paddock J, Kirkpatrick B: Aggravation of atherosclerosis by hypertension in a subhuman primate model with coarctation of the aorta. Circ Res 38:63–72, 1976.
122. Ludmer PL, Selwyn AP, Shook TL, et al: Paradoxical vasoconstriction induced by acetylcholine in atherosclerotic coronary arteries. N Engl J Med 315:1046–1051, 1986.
123. Ganz P, Vekshtein VI, Yeung AC: Impaired endothelial vasodilator function in human coronary arteries. *In* Rubanyi GM (ed): Cardiovascular Significance of Endothelium-Derived Vasoactive Factors. pp. 115–123. New York: Futura, 1991.
124. Ross R: Atherosclerosis: an inflammatory disease. N Engl J Med 340:115–126, 1999.
125. Creager MA, Cooke JP, Mendelsohn ME, et al: Impaired vasodilation of forearm resistance vessels in hypercholesterolemic humans. J Clin Invest 86:228–234, 1990.
126. Pieper GM, Gross GJ: Endothelial dysfunction in diabetes. *In* Rubanyi GM (ed): Cardiovascular Significane of Endothelium-Derived Vasoactive Factors. pp. 223–249. New York: Futura, 1991.
127. Drexler H, Zeiher AM: Endothelial function in human coronary arteries in vivo: focus on hypercholesterolemia. Hypertension 18:II90–II99, 1991.
128. Luscher TF, Vanhoutte PM, Boulanger C, et al: Endothelial dysfunction in hypertension. *In* Rubanyi GM (ed): Cardiovascular Significance of Endothelium-Derived Vasoactive Factors. pp. 199–221. New York: Futura, 1991.
129. Ross R: The pathogenesis of atherosclerosis: a perspective for the 1990s. Nature 362:801–809, 1993.
130. Berliner JA, Territo MC, Sevanian A, et al: Minimally modified low density lipoprotein stimulates monocyte endothelial interactions. J Clin Invest 85:1260–1266, 1990.
131. Cybulsky MI, Gimbrone MA Jr: Endothelial expression of a mononuclear leukocyte adhesion molecule during atherogenesis. Science 251:788–791, 1991.
132. Steinberg D: Low density lipoprotein oxidation and its pathobiological significance. J Biol Chem 272:20963–20966, 1997.
133. Yla-Herttuala S, Rosenfeld ME, Parthasarathy S, et al: Colocalization of 15-lipoxygenase mRNA and protein with epitopes of oxidized low density lipoprotein in macrophage-rich areas of atherosclerotic lesions. Proc Natl Acad Sci U S A 87:6959–6963, 1990.
134. Steele PM, Chesebro JH, Stanson AW, et al: Balloon angioplasty: natural history of the pathophysiological response to injury in a pig model. Circ Res 57:105–112, 1985.
135. Flynn PD, Byrne CD, Baglin TP, et al: Thrombin generation by apoptotic vascular smooth muscle cells. Blood 89:4378–4384, 1997.
136. Perlman H, Maillard L, Krasinski K, Walsh K: Evidence for the rapid onset of apoptosis in medial smooth muscle cells after balloon injury. Circulation 95:981–987, 1997.
137. Pollman MJ, Hall JL, Gibbons GH: Determinants of vascular smooth muscle cell apoptosis after balloon angioplasty injury: influence of redox state and cell phenotype. Circ Res 84:113–121, 1999.
138. Okazaki H, Majesky MW, Harker LA, Schwartz SM: Regulation of platelet-derived growth factor ligand and receptor gene expression by alpha-thrombin in vascular smooth muscle cells. Circ Res 71:1285–1293, 1992.
139. Graham DJ, Alexander JJ: The effects of thrombin on bovine aortic endothelial and smooth muscle cells. J Vasc Surg 11:307–312; discussion 312–313, 1990.
140. Ross R: Platelet-derived growth factor. Lancet 1:1179–1182, 1989.
141. Lindner V, Majack RA, Reidy MA: Basic fibroblast growth factor stimulates endothelial regrowth and proliferation in denuded arteries. J Clin Invest 85:2004–2008, 1990.
142. Lindner V, Reidy MA: Proliferation of smooth muscle cells after vascular injury is inhibited by an antibody against basic fibroblast growth factor. Proc Natl Acad Sci U S A 88:3739–3743, 1991.
143. Clowes AW, Schwartz SM: Significance of quiescent smooth muscle migration in the injured rat carotid artery. Circ Res 56:139–145, 1985.
144. Campbell GR, Campbell JH: Smooth muscle phenotypic changes in arterial wall homeostasis: implications for the pathogenesis of atherosclerosis. Exp Mol Pathol 42:139–162, 1985.
145. Schwartz SM: Smooth muscle migration in atherosclerosis and restenosis. J Clin Invest 100:S87–S89, 1997.
146. Ip JH, Fuster V, Israel D, et al: The role of platelets, thrombin and hyperplasia in restenosis after coronary angioplasty. J Am Coll Cardiol 17:77B–88B, 1991.
147. Gravanis MB, Roubin GS: Histopathologic phenomena at the site of percutaneous transluminal coronary angioplasty: the problem of restenosis. Hum Pathol 20:477–485, 1989.
148. Post MJ, Borst C, Kuntz RE: The relative importance of arterial remodeling compared with intimal hyperplasia in lumen renarrowing after balloon angioplasty: a study in the normal rabbit and the hypercholesterolemic Yucatan micropig. Circulation 89:2816–2821, 1994.
149. Prescott MF, Sawyer WK, Von Linden-Reed J, et al: Effect of matrix metalloproteinase inhibition on progression of atherosclerosis and aneurysm in LDL receptor-deficient mice overexpressing MMP-3, MMP-12, and MMP-13 and on restenosis in rats after balloon injury. Ann N Y Acad Sci 878:179–190, 1999.
150. Mintz GS, Popma JJ, Hong MK, et al: Intravascular ultrasound to discern device-specific effects and mechanisms of restenosis. Am J Cardiol 78:18–22, 1996.
151. Post MJ, de Smet BJ, van der Helm Y, et al: Arterial remodeling after balloon angioplasty or stenting in an atherosclerotic experimental model. Circulation 96:996–1003, 1997.
152. Rogers C, Tseng DY, Squire JC, Edelman ER: Balloon-artery interactions during stent placement: a finite element analysis approach to pressure, compliance, and stent design as contributors to vascular injury. Circ Res 84:378–383, 1999.

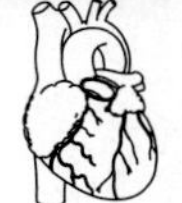

Vascular Endothelial Cell Function and Thrombosis

H. Roger Lijnen, Jef Arnout, and Désiré Collen

FIBRINOLYTIC SYSTEM
Protein Structure of Plasminogen Activators and Plasminogen Activator Inhibitors
Regulation of Plasminogen Activator Production
Regulation of Plasminogen Activator Inhibitor Production
Assembly of Fibrinolytic Components at the (Endothelial) Cell Surface
Pathophysiologic Aspects
COAGULATION SYSTEM
Structure of the Main Procoagulant and Anticoagulant Proteins
Procoagulant Mechanisms
Anticoagulant Mechanisms

Integrity of the vascular wall is necessary for normal functioning blood vessels and to maintain a nonthrombotic state. When the continuity of the vascular endothelium is disrupted, platelets and fibrin seal off the defect, and the fibrinolytic system subsequently dissolves the blood clot. The endothelial cells, which form a monolayer that lines the inner surface of blood vessels, synthesize and release activators as well as inhibitors of platelet aggregation, blood coagulation, and fibrinolysis and thus play an active role in the regulation of these systems by providing both procoagulant and anticoagulant substances.

Fibrinolytic System

The fibrinolytic system in mammalian blood plays an important role in the dissolution of blood clots and in the maintenance of a patent vascular system. The fibrinolytic system (Fig. 69–1) consists of an inactive proenzyme, plasminogen, that can be converted to the active enzyme, plasmin, that degrades fibrin into soluble fibrin degradation products. Two immunologically distinct physiologic plasminogen activators have been identified in blood: tissue-type plasminogen activator (t-PA) and urokinase-type plasminogen activator (u-PA). Inhibition of the fibrinolytic system may occur either at the level of the plasminogen activators, by specific plasminogen activator inhibitors (PAI-1 and PAI-2), or at the level of plasmin, mainly by alpha$_2$-antiplasmin. t-PA–mediated plasminogen activation is primarily involved in the dissolution of fibrin in the circulation.[1] u-PA binds to a specific cellular receptor (u-PAR), resulting in enhanced activation of cell-bound plasminogen. The main role of u-PA appears to be in the induction of pericellular proteolysis during events such as tissue remodeling and repair, macrophage function, and tumor invasion.[2]

Regulation and control of the fibrinolytic system are mediated by specific molecular interactions between its main components and by the controlled synthesis and release of plasminogen activators and plasminogen activator inhibitors, primarily from endothelial cells. Furthermore, the endothelial cell surface may serve as a focal point for the assembly of components of the fibrinolytic system, resulting in local stimulation of fibrinolytic activity.

The physiologic importance of the fibrinolytic system is demonstrated by the association between abnormal fibrinolysis and a tendency toward bleeding or thrombosis.[3–6]

Protein Structure of Plasminogen Activators and Plasminogen Activator Inhibitors

t-PA is a 70-kD serine proteinase, originally isolated as a single polypeptide chain of 527 amino acids.[7] It was subsequently shown that native t-PA contains an NH$_2$-terminal extension of three amino acids (Gly-Ala-Arg-). t-PA is converted by plasmin to a two-chain form by hydrolysis of the Arg^{275}-Ile^{276} peptide bond. The NH$_2$-terminal region is composed of several domains with homologies to other proteins: a finger domain composed of residues 4 to 50, a growth factor domain composed of residues 50 to 87, and two kringles composed of residues 87 to 176 and 176 to 262. The region constituted by residues 276 to 527 represents the serine proteinase part with the catalytic site, composed of His^{322}, Asp^{371}, and Ser^{478}. The t-PA molecule is composed of three potential *N*-glycosylation sites, at Asn^{117}, Asn^{184}, and Asn^{448}. t-PA preparations usually contain a mixture of variant I (with the three sites glycosylated) and variant II (lacking carbohydrate at Asn^{184}).[7] These distinct domains in t-PA are involved in several functions of the enzyme, including its binding to fibrin, fibrin-specific plasminogen activation, rapid clearance in vivo, and binding to endothelial cell receptors (for references, see Lijnen and Collen[8]).

u-PA is secreted as a single-chain 54-kD glycoprotein (scu-PA) containing 411 amino acids.[9] On proteolytic cleavage of the Lys^{158}-Ile^{159} peptide bond, the molecule is converted to a two-chain derivative (tcu-PA). The catalytic triad is located in the COOH-terminal polypeptide chain and is composed of Asp^{255}, His^{204}, and Ser^{356}. The NH$_2$-

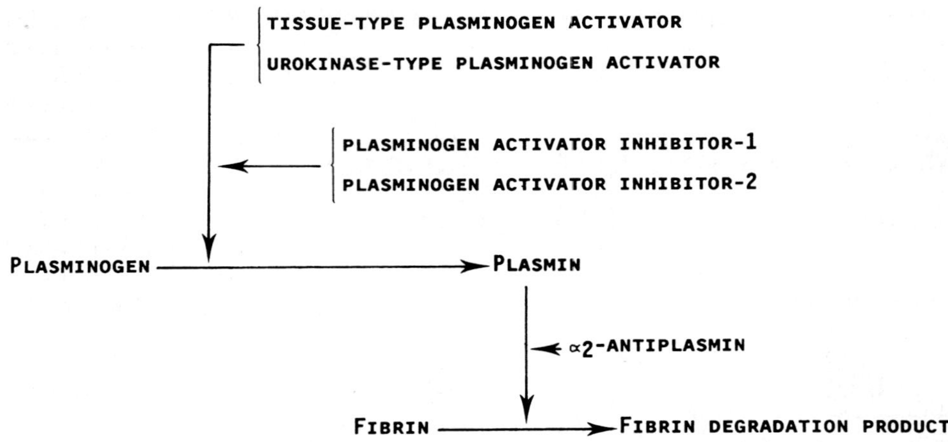

FIGURE 69–1 Schematic representation of the fibrinolytic system. The proenzyme plasminogen is activated to the active enzyme plasmin by tissue-type or urokinase-type plasminogen activator. Plasmin degrades fibrin into soluble fibrin degradation products. Inhibition of the fibrinolytic system may occur at the level of the plasminogen activators, by plasminogen activator inhibitors, or at the level of plasmin, mainly by alpha$_2$-antiplasmin.

terminal chain contains an epidermal growth factor domain (residues 5 to 49) and one kringle domain. A low-molecular-weight tcu-PA (33 kD) can be generated with plasmin through hydrolysis of the Lys^{135}-Lys^{136} peptide bond in tcu-PA.

PAI-1 is a 52-kD single-chain glycoprotein consisting of 379 amino acids; it is a serpin with reactive site peptide bond Arg^{346}-Met^{347}.[10] It inhibits both t-PA and tcu-PA very rapidly through the formation of a 1:1 stoichiometric complex. PAI-1 is stabilized by binding to S protein or vitronectin.[11]

PAI-2 exists in two different forms with comparable kinetic properties: a 47-kD intracellular nonglycosylated form with pI 5.0 and a 60-kD secreted glycosylated form with pI 4.4.[12] PAI-2 is a serpin[13] that contains 393 amino acids with reactive site Arg^{358}-Thr^{359}. The precise (patho)-physiologic role of PAI-2 remains to be determined.

Regulation of Plasminogen Activator Production

Vascular endothelial cells synthesize and secrete t-PA into the circulating blood,[14] yielding a concentration of about 5 ng/ml, of which a significant part is complexed to PAI-1. Although the synthesis of t-PA occurs mainly in endothelial cells, immunocytochemical staining of tissues indicates that many cells of different origin (e.g., fibroblasts, epithelial cells, pneumocytes) produce u-PA.[15] The u-PA concentration in human plasma is about 10 to 20 ng/ml.

The stimulation of vascular endothelium by venous occlusion, infusion of desmopressin acetate and epinephrine, or physical exercise results in a rapid release (within minutes) of t-PA.[16] This response is too rapid to represent increased synthesis and may reflect release from cellular storage pools, although such a storage pool has not been conclusively identified. The L-arginine/nitric oxide pathway may contribute to the acute release of t-PA in vivo in humans, as suggested by the finding that the administration of a nitric oxide synthase inhibitor results in impaired release of t-PA from the forearm.[17]

A variety of agents have been shown to increase the synthesis of t-PA by cultured endothelial cells, including thrombin,[18, 19] histamine,[19] dexamethasone,[20] butyrate,[21] phorbol-12-myristate-13-acetate (PMA),[22] basic fibroblast growth factor,[23] activated protein C,[24] butanol and alcohol derivatives,[25] and retinoids.[26, 27] Agents such as thrombin that stimulate the release of t-PA from endothelial cells also stimulate the secretion of PAI-1.[18, 19] Dexamethasone increases t-PA antigen levels in hepatoma cells moderately but increases PAI-1 antigen levels to a greater extent, resulting in inhibition of t-PA activity.[28] Only histamine, butyrate, or a combination of cyclic adenosine monophosphate with protein kinase C agonists exclusively stimulates t-PA synthesis without affecting PAI-1 synthesis.

The mechanisms involved in the stimulatory effect of these various agents on t-PA synthesis appear to be different and are gradually being elucidated. Vitamin A, retinoic acid, and some of its analogues induce t-PA–related antigen secretion by human umbilical vein endothelial cells in vitro[26] but also in the plasma and specific tissues of vitamin A–deficient rats,[26] suggesting that circulating retinoic acid may regulate t-PA expression in the vessel wall. The receptors for these agents are members of the nuclear receptor superfamily, a class of transcription factors that specifically bind to *cis*-elements in the gene regulatory region. Recently, a functional retinoic acid–response element, which consists of a direct repeat of the GGTCA motif spaced by five nucleotides (DR5), has been localized 7.3 kb upstream for the transcription start site of the human *t-PA* gene. This element mediates the direct regulation by retinoic acid in human fibrosarcoma, endothelial, and neuroblastoma cells.[29] This t-PA/DR5-retinoic acid–response element is part of a multihormone responsive enhancer covering an upstream fragment that contains a complex glucocorticoid responsive unit composed of four binding sites for the receptor.[30] The induction of t-PA by retinoic acid in human umbilical vein endothelial cells involves a two-step mechanism, requiring induction of retinoic acid receptor beta$_2$ via retinoic acid receptor alpha$_1$, followed by induction of t-PA synthesis via retinoic acid receptor β_2.[31]

Vasoactive substances, such as histamine and thrombin, bind to specific receptors and activate phospholipase C, which acts on phosphatidylinositol biphosphate to produce diacylglycerol. Diacylglycerol activates membrane-bound protein kinase C, which plays an important role in the regulation of t-PA synthesis. This is suggested by the findings that direct activation of protein kinase C by phorbol esters induces t-PA synthesis, whereas suppression of protein kinase C impairs the increase in t-PA synthesis by histamine and by PMA.[32] The increase of t-PA induced by histamine, thrombin, and PMA in endothelial cells is paralleled by increased levels of mRNA, as a result of enhanced transcription of the *t-PA* gene.[33] Very little is known, however, about the regulation of human *t-PA* gene transcription. Two *cis*-elements (a cyclic adenosine monophosphate response element in the proximal promoter and an activator protein-2–binding site in exon 1) have been identified that are involved in basal expression and induction of human *t-PA* gene transcription by cyclic adenosine monophosphate and phorbol esters.[34] In vivo footprinting analysis revealed that specificity protein-1 binds the t-PA promoter at two proximal sites, of which one overlaps with the activator protein-2 site in exon 1.[35]

Overexpression of t-PA in endothelial cells in vitro using a retroviral expression vector has been achieved without altering the morphology, attachment, proliferation, migration, or invasion. Potentially, such *t-PA*–transduced cells could increase local fibrinolysis and may be useful for in vivo therapeutic interventions.[36] Interestingly, plasmin inhibits the biosynthesis of t-PA antigen by human umbilical vein endothelial cells in a dose-dependent manner, possibly through the signal transduction pathway involving one or more protein kinases.[37]

Regulation of Plasminogen Activator Inhibitor Production

PAI-1 mRNA has been demonstrated in a large variety of tissues, suggesting that common cells in these tissues, such as endothelial or smooth muscle cells, are the site of production. PAI-1 is, however, also synthesized by hepatocytes, fibroblasts, certain tumor cells, and adipocytes.[38–40] PAI-1 is found in plasma, platelets, placenta, and in the extracellular matrix. In blood, platelets constitute the main PAI-1 reservoir (essentially in an inactive form), whereas the plasma concentration is about 10 ng/ml. Plasma PAI-1 most likely originates from synthesis by and release from vascular endothelial cells.[41] For unknown reasons, PAI-1 exhibits a circadian variation; its plasma concentration is highest in the morning and lowest in the late afternoon and evening, whereas t-PA exhibits an opposite diurnal variation.

The synthesis and secretion of PAI-1 can be modulated by various agonists, such as hormones, growth factors, endotoxin, cytokines, and phorbol esters.[42] Although post-transcriptional regulation of *PAI-1* mRNA levels has been suggested,[43–45] most studies on the regulation of PAI-1 expression demonstrated an effect at the transcriptional level.[46–49] Alterations in mRNA stability may also contribute to increased PAI-1 levels in some cells.[38] In endothelial cells, *PAI-1* gene expression is stimulated by lipopolysaccharide,[44, 50–53] interleukin-1,[52–54] tumor necrosis factor-α (TNF-α),[44, 55, 56] transforming growth factor-β (TGF-β),[57] basic fibroblast growth factor,[57] phorbol esters,[49, 58, 59] thrombin,[18, 19, 60] very low density lipoprotein,[61, 62] lipoprotein(a),[63] insulin[48] or proinsulin,[64] glucose,[65] unsaturated fatty acids,[66] recombinant human erythropoietin,[67] and angiotensin II.[68, 69] Angiotensin II–induced PAI-1 expression in cultured endothelial cells is mediated via angiotensin receptors.[68, 70] Captopril, an inhibitor of the angiotensin-converting enzyme, reduces PAI-1 expression in the vessel wall in vivo by blocking the receptor pathways.[71] Forskolin,[58, 72] endothelial cell growth factor supplement combined with heparin,[73] gemfibrozil (a lipid-lowering drug),[74] and herpes simplex virus infection[75] have been reported to down-regulate PAI-1 expression in endothelial cells.

Adipocytes are important contributors to the elevated PAI-1 levels observed in the plasma under obese conditions.[39, 40, 76–78] Moreover, TGF-β administered in vivo increases PAI-1 activity in mouse plasma and *PAI-1* mRNA expression in adipose tissue.[39, 79]

The local production of PAI-1 by smooth muscle cells can modulate the local PA activity and affect smooth muscle cell migration.[80] Thrombin,[81] plasminogen,[82] angiotensin II,[68, 83] platelet-derived growth factor, and TGF-β[84, 85] increase PAI-1 expression in cultured smooth muscle cells.

In endothelial cells juxtaposed to thrombi, in smooth muscle cells adjacent to the neointima, and in macrophages, PAI-1 mRNA is increased and PAI-1 protein is detectable. This augmented arterial wall expression of PAI-1 induced by thrombosis may shift the local balance between fibrinolysis and thrombosis toward the latter.[86]

Despite the numerous reports describing the regulation of PAI-1 at the level of antigen secretion and mRNA synthesis, little is known about the regulation of *PAI-1* gene transcription. Several *cis*-responsive elements in the *PAI-1* promoter have been described. The 5′-flanking region of the human *PAI-1* gene contains a major TGF-β responsive element and a minor element upstream from the cap site, both of which are active in HepG2 cells.[87] Two transcription factors, a CCAAT-binding transcription factor/nuclear factor 1 and an ubiquitous factor of the β-helix-loop-helix family, have been shown to bind specifically to sequences in the major TGF-β responsive element and to be important for the TGF-β response.[88]

There are four putative activation protein-1–like binding sites that closely resemble the consensus PMA-responsive element, TGAg/cTCA, in the 5′-flanking region of the human *PAI-1* gene: two proximal sites and two distal sites.[89–91] Two proximal sites are required for PMA response,[91] whereas the two distal sites are involved in the induction of PAI-1 by TGF-β.[87] Binding of the c-jun homodimer to a PMA-responsive element is important in the basal activity and PMA induction of the *PAI-1* promoter in HeLa cells,[90] HepG2 cells,[92] and some human breast carcinoma cells.[91] p53, a tumor suppressor, transactivates the human *PAI-1* gene promoter through binding to a region that is highly similar to the p53 consensus binding sequence, whereas p53 represses transcription from the enhancer and promoter of the human *u-PA* and *t-PA* genes through a non–DNA-binding mechanism.[93]

PAI-2 has been identified in human placenta and in pregnancy plasma; it is also secreted by leukocytes and by fibrosarcoma cells. Secretion of PAI-2 is regulated by endotoxin and by phorbol esters, which stimulate the gene transcription of PAI-2 (for references, see Belin,[94] Schleef and Loskutoff,[95] and Kruithof[96]).

Assembly of Fibrinolytic Components at the (Endothelial) Cell Surface

Analogies have been recognized between the role of fibrin and that of cell surfaces in plasminogen activation.[97] Many cell types bind plasminogen activators and plasminogen, resulting in enhanced plasminogen activation[98–101] and protection of bound plasmin from inhibition by α_2-antiplasmin.[102, 103]

Binding of plasminogen to cultured human umbilical vein endothelial cells was reported with a dissociation constant (K_D) of 310 nM and approximately 10^6 binding sites per cell.[99] Other studies report that most cells bind plasminogen via its lysine binding sites with a high capacity ($>10^7$ sites per cell) but a relatively low affinity ($K_D \sim$ 1 μM). Gangliosides,[104] as well as a class of membrane proteins with COOH-terminal lysine residues such as α-enolase,[105] play an important role in the binding of plasminogen to cells. The catalytic efficiency of t-PA for activation of cell-bound plasminogen is about 10-fold higher than that in solution, possibly as a result of conversion of the plasminogen conformation to the more readily activatable "Lys-plasminogen" structure.[106] Alternatively, it was shown that vascular cells have the capacity to regulate pericellular fibrinolysis by modulating the expression of plasminogen receptors; enhanced receptor occupancy results in enhanced plasminogen activation by t-PA.[107]

Binding of t-PA to human umbilical vein endothelial cells is specific, saturable, and reversible.[98, 108] A high-affinity binding site with a low number of sites and a lower-affinity binding site with a high number of sites have been identified. With ligand blot techniques, a 40-kD membrane protein was identified (annexin II) that may represent a functional t-PA receptor.[109] Cell surface–bound t-PA retains its enzymatic activity and is protected from inhibition by PAI-1. Assembly of plasminogen and plasminogen activators at the endothelial cell surface thus provides a focal point for plasmin generation and may play an important role in maintaining blood fluidity and nonthrombogenicity (Fig. 69–2).

Lipoprotein(a) competes with plasminogen for binding

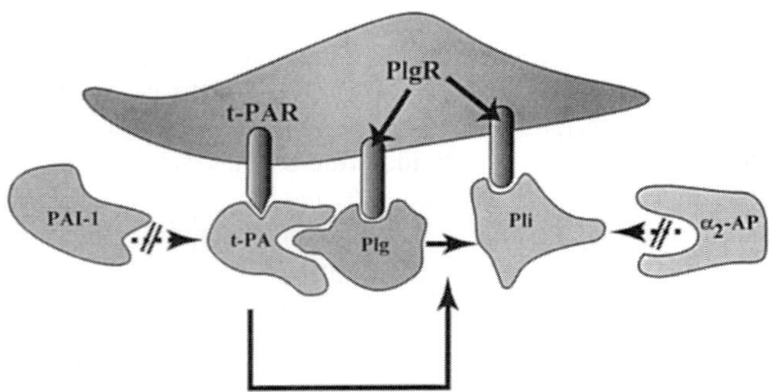

FIGURE 69–2 Schematic representation of the molecular interactions that regulate tissue-type plasminogen activator (t-PA)–mediated plasminogen activation at the cell surface. t-PA bound to its cellular receptor or receptors (t-PAR) is protected from inhibition by plasminogen activator inhibitor-1 (PAI-1) and efficiently converts plasminogen (Plg) bound to its cellular receptor or receptors (PlgR) to plasmin (Pli), which is protected from inhibition by alpha$_2$-antiplasmin (α_2-AP).

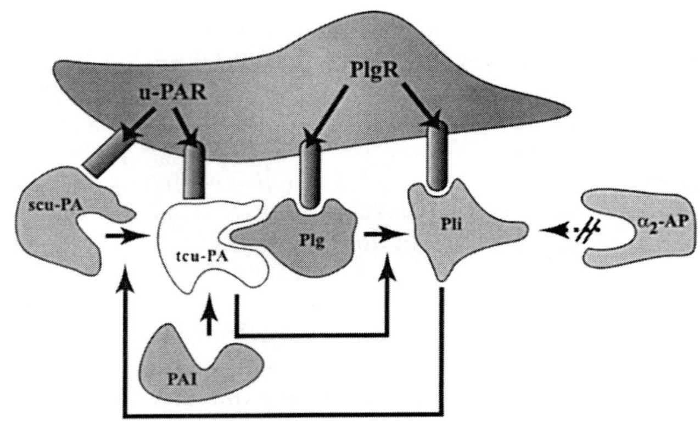

FIGURE 69–3 Schematic representation of the molecular interactions that regulate urokinase-type plasminogen activator (u-PA)–mediated plasminogen activation at the cell surface. Two-chain u-PA (tcu-PA) bound to its cellular receptor (u-PAR) activates plasminogen (Plg), bound to its receptor or receptors (PlgR), to plasmin (Pli), which is protected from inhibition by alpha$_2$-antiplasmin (α_2-AP). Plasmin converts u-PAR–bound single-chain u-PA (scu-PA) to tcu-PA, resulting in enhanced plasminogen activation. The u-PAR–bound tcu-PA, but not scu-PA, is inhibited by plasminogen activator inhibitors-1 and -2 (PAI).

to endothelial cells, resulting in down-regulated activation of cell surface–bound plasminogen by t-PA. Thus, lipoprotein(a) may play a role in the regulation of fibrinolysis at the endothelial cell surface.[110]

Cellular receptors may not only be important for the localization of proteolytic activity at the cell surface but also play a role in the rapid clearance of t-PA from the circulation. Circulating t-PA (half-life of 5 to 6 minutes in humans) may interact with several receptor systems in the liver. Liver endothelial cells have a receptor that recognizes the high mannose-type carbohydrate antenna on kringle 1 of t-PA. Liver parenchymal cells contain a calcium-dependent receptor that interacts with the finger or growth factor domains of t-PA.[111] They also contain a high-affinity receptor for the uptake and degradation of t-PA/PAI-1 complexes that binds free t-PA, albeit with lower affinity; this receptor, termed low-density lipoprotein receptor–related protein, is identical to the α_2-macroglobulin receptor.[112]

The binding of u-PA to its specific receptor (u-PAR) at the cell surface plays a role in regulating its activity under physiologic conditions. u-PAR is a heterogeneously glycosylated protein of 50 to 60 kD, synthesized as a 313-amino-acid polypeptide, anchored to the plasma membrane by a glycosyl phosphatidylinositol moiety that is attached at amino acid 282, 283, or 284. The u-PAR molecule is composed of three distantly related structural domains, of which the NH_2-terminal domain binds u-PA (for references, see Lijnen and associates[113]); it binds all forms of u-PA containing an intact growth factor domain. Binding of u-PA to u-PAR results in a strongly enhanced plasmin generation due to effects on both the activation of plasminogen[114] and the feedback activation of scu-PA to tcu-PA by generated plasmin.[115] Both of these effects are also critically dependent on the cellular binding of plasminogen. Cell-associated plasmin is protected from rapid inhibition by α_2-antiplasmin, which further favors the activation of receptor-bound scu-PA. This system can, however, be efficiently inhibited by both PAI-1 and PAI-2 (Fig. 69–3).[116] The observation that direct anchorage of u-PA to the cell surface (using a glycosyl phosphatidylinositol–anchored u-PA mutant) leads to a potentiation of plasmin generation equivalent to that observed in the presence of u-PAR suggests that u-PAR mainly functions to localize u-PA at the cell surface.[117] Furthermore, a u-PAR–independent function of u-PA has been demonstrated in fibrin clearance and in arterial neointima formation in mice.[118, 119]

Pathophysiologic Aspects

Impairment of fibrinolysis may be associated with thrombosis. It may be due to a defective synthesis or release of t-PA from the vessel wall, to a deficiency or functional defect in the plasminogen molecule, or to increased levels of inhibitors of t-PA or of plasmin. Defective release of t-PA from the vessel wall during venous occlusion or a decreased t-PA content in walls of superficial veins was found in about 70 percent of patients with idiopathic recurrent venous thrombosis.[120] In addition, resistance to activated protein C, caused by Arg^{506} to Gln mutation in factor V, is a strong risk factor for venous thrombosis and may explain a significant portion of previously unexplained cases of thrombophilia.[121]

Defective fibrinolysis in patients with venous thrombosis may be due to a low concentration of t-PA or to an increased level of PAI-1. In 35 percent of patients with spontaneous or recurrent deep vein thrombosis, a poor fibrinolytic response to venous occlusion was observed, which was due to deficient t-PA release in 25 percent and to increased PAI-1 levels in 75 percent of these cases.[122]

In six studies with healthy subjects as controls, an impaired fibrinolytic capacity after venous occlusion was observed in patients with thrombotic episodes,[123] whereas in the Physician's Health Study,[124] PAI-1 levels in patients who developed venous thrombosis during a 5-year follow-up were not different from those of control subjects. The association between enhanced PAI-1 levels and symptomatic venous thrombosis thus apparently requires further study.

In patients with acute myocardial infarction or unstable angina, high plasma PAI-1 levels were found to be predictive for recurrent (within 3 years) myocardial infarction in some studies[125, 126] but not in others.[127, 128] In the prospective European Concerted Action on Thrombosis (ECAT) study, 10 fibrinolytic variables were measured in 3043 patients with angina pectoris recruited from 18 European centers.[129, 130] A first analysis after adjustment for other nonfibrinolytic coronary risk factors (body mass index, triglyceride levels, diabetes, systolic blood pressure) revealed that an increased risk of coronary events within 2 years was associated with higher baseline concentrations of t-PA antigen but not of PAI-1 activity and antigen levels. However, after separate adjustment for clusters of markers of insulin resistance, inflammation, or endothelial cell damage, it appeared that factors involved in the insulin resistance syndrome strongly affected PAI-1 and, to a lesser extent, t-PA antigen; the latter was primarily influenced by inflammation and endothelial cell damage.[131] Thus, t-PA antigen levels may constitute a biologic marker of coronary heart disease, influenced by a variety of pathophysiologic pathways, including inflammation. In contrast, PAI levels that determine fibrinolytic activity and are mainly dependent on the metabolic status emerge as a risk factor predictive for the future development of atherothrombosis.

Evidence has been provided for a regulation of PAI-1 synthesis at the transcriptional level. Genetic variation at a polymorphic locus of the *PAI-1* gene is associated with differences in plasma PAI-1 levels,[132] and a single guanosine insertion/deletion (4G/5G) polymorphism in the PAI-1 promoter region has been suggested to play an important role in the regulation of the expression of the *PAI-1* gene.[133] A *4G* allele of this polymorphism was claimed to be a risk factor for myocardial infarction,[134] although this was not confirmed in the Etude Cas-Temoins de l'Infarctus du Myocarde (ECTIM) study.[135] Thus, the homozygous form of the *4G* allele is associated with increased PAI-1 antigen levels, but the relation with thrombotic disease remains to be established.

Coagulation System

Blood coagulation has classically been divided into an extrinsic and an intrinsic pathway.[136] This model, although valuable for laboratory diagnosis of coagulation abnormalities, has been revised.[137] The main basis for this revision was the discovery of tissue factor pathway inhibitor (TFPI)[138, 139] and the finding that factor XI can be activated by thrombin.[140, 141] In the current model (Fig. 69–4), the extrinsic tenase reaction initiates coagulation. Once critical amounts of factor Xa, which are required for the initiation of thrombin generation, are formed, the extrinsic tenase reaction is efficiently turned off by TFPI and further formation of thrombin is maintained via positive feedback mechanisms involving thrombin-induced activation of factors V, VIII, and XI. Excess thrombin is efficiently inhibited by its physiologic inhibitor antithrombin and down-regulates its own generation via stimulation of the protein C pathway. Endothelium plays a crucial role in the regulation of both procoagulant and anticoagulant mechanisms.

Structure of the Main Procoagulant and Anticoagulant Proteins

Procoagulant and anticoagulant proteins are composed of multiple domains, which have a high degree of structural and functional homology (Table 69–1) (for references, see Colman and colleagues[142] and Bloom and associates[143]).

Signal Peptide

Both procoagulant and anticoagulant proteins in plasma are initially synthesized with a signal peptide. This short, usually very hydrophobic peptide, which is required for translocation of the growing polypeptide chain into the endoplasmic reticulum, is cleaved off before secretion.

Propeptide/Carboxyglutamic Acid–Rich Domain

All vitamin K–dependent proteins; prothrombin; factors VII, IX, and X; and proteins C and S contain a gamma-

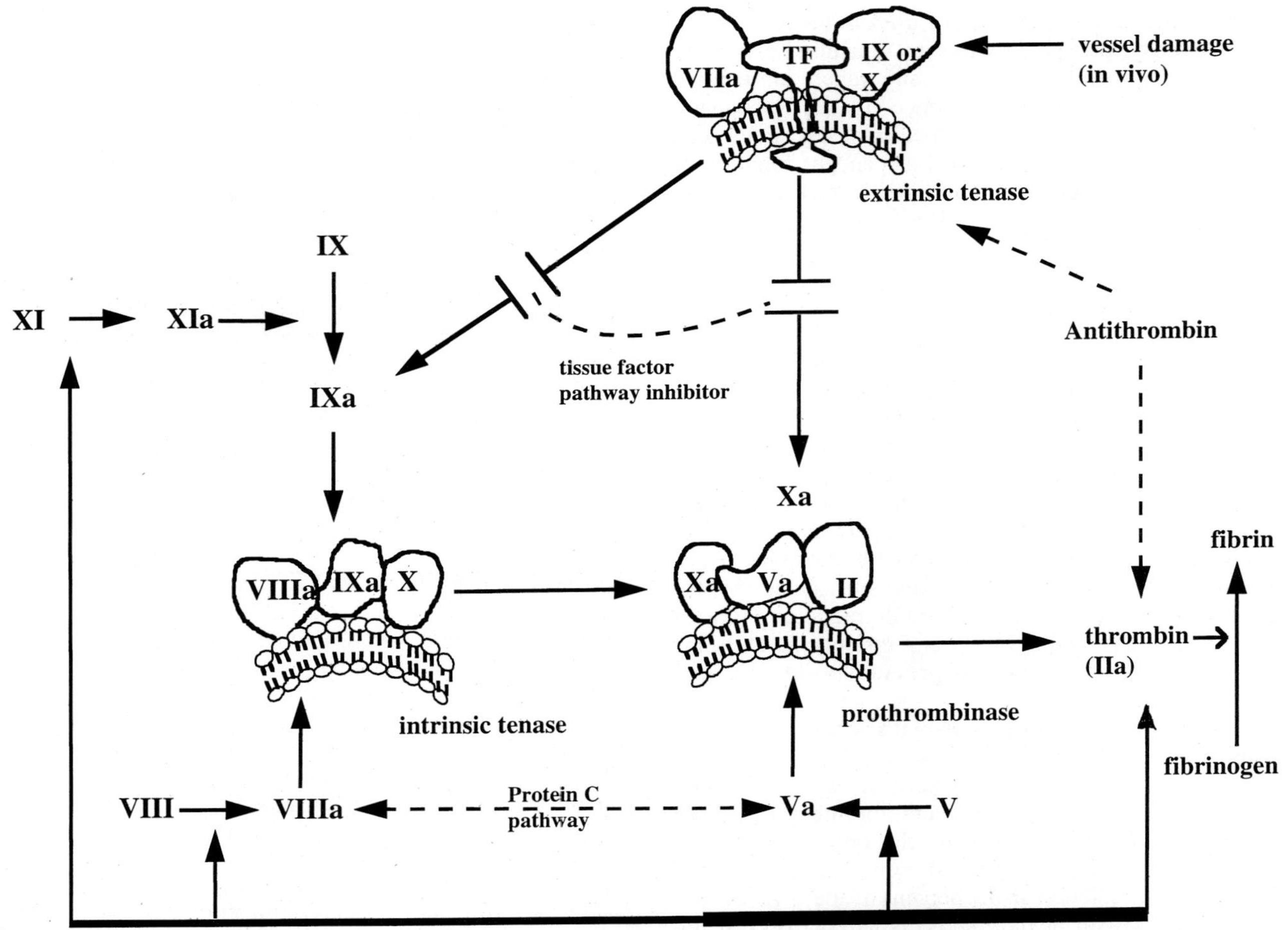

FIGURE 69–4 Simplified scheme of procoagulant and anticoagulant pathways of coagulation. On vascular injury, blood coagulation is initiated by the extrinsic tenase reaction. Once critical amounts of factor Xa, as required for the initiation of coagulation, are generated, the extrinsic tenase reaction is efficiently turned off by the tissue factor (TF) pathway inhibitor and probably by antithrombin; further formation of thrombin is maintained via positive feedback mechanisms involving thrombin-induced activation of factors V, VIII, and XI. Thrombin is efficiently inhibited by its physiologic inhibitor antithrombin and down-regulates its own generation via stimulation of the protein C pathway.

carboxylation recognition site located on the propeptide domain between the signal peptide and the γ-carboxyglutamic acid–rich domain (Gla domain). This site directs γ-carboxylation of the γ-carboxyglutamic acid residues located in the adjacent approximately 40-residue-long Gla domain. After carboxylation of the Gla domain, which is crucial for the Ca^{2+}-mediated binding of vitamin K–dependent proteins to negatively charged membranes, the propeptide is cleaved off.

Epidermal Growth Factor Domain

Several procoagulant and anticoagulant proteins contain two or more epidermal growth factor (EGF)-like domains. These domains consist of about 43 to 50 amino acid residues, and their structure is determined by three characteristic disulfide bonds. The function of EGF-like domains in many coagulation proteins, although not fully understood, appears to be in the formation of protein complexes. The EGF-like domains in factor VII are important for the binding to tissue factor. The second EGF-like domain of factor IX contains a binding site for activated factor VIII. The second EGF-like domain of protein C is involved in the binding of protein S. The binding sites on thrombomodulin for protein C and thrombin are located on the fourth and fifth EGF-like domains, respectively.

Kringle Domain

Kringle domains consist of about 100 amino acids, and their structure is determined by three disulfide bonds. These domains are involved in interaction with other proteins. Only two procoagulant proteins, prothrombin and factor XII, contain kringle domains. The second kringle of prothrombin probably contains the main binding site for activated factor V.

Catalytic Domain

The catalytic domain of all procoagulant enzymes contains an active site and an internal core that is similar to that of trypsin. Conversion of an inactive proenzyme to an active enzyme depends on limited proteolysis and for some proteins on cleavage of so-called activation peptides. The

TABLE 69-1 **Overview of the Main Procoagulant and Anticoagulant Proteins With Some of Their Properties**

	Function or Main Substrate of the Active Form	Molecular Weight (kD)	Chain Composition	Plasma Concentration (μg/ml)	$t_{1/2}$ (hr)	Domain				
						Gla	*EGF*	*Kringle*	*Catalytic*	*Other*
Zymogen										
Prothrombin	Fibrinogen, factor XIII	72	sc, 581 AA	100	72	10 AA	None	2	Ser proteinase	
Factor VII	Factor X, factor IX	50	sc, 406 AA	0.5	5	10 AA	2	None	Ser proteinase	
Factor X	Prothrombin	59	tc, 254 AA, 139 AA	8	32	11 AA	2	None	Ser proteinase	
Factor IX	Factor X	56	sc, 415 AA	5	24	12 AA	2	None	Ser proteinase	
Factor XI	Factor IX	160	tc, 607 AA each	5	72	None	None	None	Ser proteinase	
Factor XII	Factor XI	80	sc, 596 AA	30	60	None	2	1	Ser proteinase	
Protein C	Factor Va, factor VIIIa	62	tc, 262 AA, 155 AA	3–5	7	9 AA	2	None	Ser proteinase	
Cofactor										
Tissue factor	Extrinsic tenase cofactor	45	sc, 263 AA	Cell bound		None	None	None		Two barrel-like structures, transmembrane module, cytoplasmic tail
Factor V	Prothrombinase cofactor	330	sc, 2196 AA	7–10	12	None	None	None		A1, A2, B, A3, C1, C2
Factor VIII	Intrinsic tenase cofactor	280	tc, 1313 AA, 684 AA	0.2	12	None	None	None		A1, A2, B, A3, C1, C2
Protein S	Cofactor for activated protein C	75	sc, 635 AA	20	42	11 AA	4	None		Sex hormone–binding globulin-like module
Thrombomodulin	Cofactor for protein C activation	60	sc, 557 AA	Cell bound		None	6	None		Lectin-like module, hydrophobic region, transmembrane module, cytoplasmic tail
Inhibitor										
Antithrombin	Inhibitor of thrombin and factor Xa	58	sc, 432 AA	125	48	None	None	None		
Tissue factor pathway inhibitor	Inhibitor of extrinsic tenase and factor Xa	42	sc, 276 AA	0.1						Kunitz domains 1, 2, and 3

Abbreviations: AA, amino acids; sc, single chain; tc, two chain.

active site of all clotting (serine) proteinases contains a serine, an aspartic acid, and a histidine residue.

Pseudosubstrates

The natural inhibitors of coagulation, antithrombin and TFPI, are pseudosubstrates with high affinity for their specific target enzymes. Antithrombin is a single-chain globular molecule that depends on heparin to obtain its optimal inhibitory conformation required for docking and locking the catalytic center of its target enzymes thrombin and factor Xa. It forms 1:1 stoichiometric complexes that are rapidly cleared from the circulation. TFPI is a single-chain molecule characterized by the presence of three Kunitz domains. These domains contain about 58 residues, and their structure is determined by three characteristic disulfide bonds. They act as pseudosubstrates for their target serine proteinases. The first Kunitz domain of TFPI inhibits the factor VIIa/tissue factor complex, whereas the second Kunitz domain inhibits factor Xa; the function of the third Kunitz domain is unknown.

Procoagulant Mechanisms

Tissue factor is the vascular trigger required to initiate coagulation.[144] In healthy blood vessels, tissue factor is mainly located in the extracellular matrix beneath and between endothelial cells and therefore appears to form a protective lining around blood vessels capable of activating blood coagulation after vascular injury.[145] Endothelial cells themselves have little or no tissue factor activity,[146] but the level can be strongly induced by endotoxin, thrombin, fibrin, and several cytokines, as well as by shear and hypoxia.[144, 147–149] Both monocytes and natural killer cells have also been found to up-regulate tissue factor expression in endothelial cells.[150] Tissue factor is highly concentrated in the areas surrounding the cholesterol clefts of diseased coronary vessels and initiates thrombus formation after plaque rupture.[147]

Tissue factor binds to factor VIIa and accelerates the activation of factor IX and factor X by factor VIIa.[144] At high tissue factor concentrations, factor X is mainly activated by the factor VIIa/tissue factor complex, whereas at low tissue factor concentrations, factor IXa/factor VIIIa–dependent activation of factor X becomes more pronounced.[151, 152] Studies show that factor Xa generation via the intrinsic tenase reaction occurs after that of the extrinsic tenase reaction, as it requires thrombin-dependent activation of factor VIII.[153] Association of tissue factor with phospholipids is required to exhibit significant procoagulant activity.[147] Relipidation experiments with recombinant tissue factor have shown that both phosphatidyl choline and phosphatidyl ethanolamine support the procoagulant properties of tissue factor, whereas phosphatidyl serine is inactive. The physiologic importance of tissue factor has been confirmed by the finding that disruption of the *tissue factor* gene in mice is associated with impaired vascular development and lethal embryonic bleeding.[154, 155]

Activated endothelial cells not only express tissue factor but also promote coagulation by releasing and binding certain clotting factors and by providing a catalytic surface for the prothrombinase and intrinsic tenase reactions. Endothelial cells synthesize and bind factor V, and its expression on the endothelial cell surface is enhanced by mechanical injury.[156] Endothelial cells also contain factor VIII[157]; although its cellular localization is not clearly identified, it is conceivable that factor VIII is stored in the Weibel-Palade bodies associated with von Willebrand factor, because both are concomitantly released on infusion of desmopressin acetate. Thrombin-activated endothelial cells release von Willebrand factor that plays a role in platelet adhesion, whereas the concomitant release of factor VIII may cause an increased concentration at the site of thrombus formation.

Factor Xa bound to its recently described high-affinity receptor appears to be involved in the prothrombinase reaction.[158] Factor IXa interacts with a binding protein of 140 kD on endothelial cells, through γ-carboxyglutamic acid and through its epidermal growth factor domain.[159] Binding and activity of factor IXa are enhanced by factors VIII, X, and V, and cell-bound factor IXa is severalfold more active than that in solution. Three different receptors have been identified that may be involved in activation of endothelial cells by thrombin.[160, 161] Thrombin receptors are high-affinity G protein–coupled proteins called protease-activated receptors, which are activated when the new extracellular NH_2-terminal, formed after thrombin cleavage, binds to sites in the second extracellular loop. Thrombin activation triggers both procoagulant and anticoagulant pathways. Thrombin-induced procoagulant pathways include tissue factor expression, release of PAI-1 and von Willebrand factor, and expression of procoagulant phospholipid surfaces.

Thrombin activation also causes the expression of negatively charged phospholipids on the cell surface and the shedding of procoagulant phospholipid vesicles, providing a catalytic surface for coagulation reactions. Activated endothelial cell membranes appear to be a better surface for the intrinsic tenase reaction than phospholipid vesicles in solution,[162] whereas prothrombinase activity is not associated with the cell surface but rather with the procoagulant phospholipid surface shed in the fluid phase.[163]

Anticoagulant Mechanisms

The formation of thrombin and the deposition of fibrin on the surface of quiescent endothelial cells are impaired by several inhibitory pathways.

The extrinsic tenase activity is inhibited by the Kunitz-type inhibitor TFPI[138, 139, 164] and by the serine protease inhibitor antithrombin.[144, 165] Both inhibitors neutralize factor VIIa only when it is bound to tissue factor. The mature full-length TFPI is a 43-kD protein with an acidic NH_2-terminal region followed by three tandem Kunitz-type proteinase inhibitory domains and a basic COOH-terminal region. TFPI inhibits the extrinsic tenase reaction via a two-step mechanism. In the first step, factor Xa is inhibited by binding to an arginine residue in the reactive center of the second Kunitz domain. In the second step, the TFPI/factor Xa complex forms a quaternary complex with factor VIIa/tissue factor, in which factor VIIa binds to a lysine residue in the reactive center of the first Kunitz domain.

TFPI is predominantly located in the endothelial cell extracellular matrix, where it is bound to heparan sulfate or to other glycosaminoglycans. The plasma concentration of TFPI (2 nM) is increased severalfold after the intravenous injection of heparin. Plasma TFPI has a lower molecular weight (34 to 41 kD) than its endothelium-bound form and appears to be truncated at the COOH-terminal end. It circulates bound to lipoproteins and has substantially lower factor Xa inhibitory activity than the full-length form. The physiologic importance of TFPI has been extensively studied in animal models. The infusion of high concentrations of TFPI prevents thrombosis and intravascular coagulation after tissue factor or endotoxin infusion in rabbits.[164] The neutralization of TFPI by polyclonal antibodies promotes tissue factor–induced intravascular coagulation.[144, 164] Targeted *TFPI* gene disruption has been shown to cause intrauterine lethality in mice owing to yolk sac hemorrhages or fatal bleeding, compatible with a consumptive coagulopathy.[166]

Antithrombin, in the presence of heparin, rapidly inhibits the extrinsic tenase reaction.[164, 165, 167] In solution, this inhibitory pathway is probably equivalent to the TFPI-dependent inhibition of factor VIIa/tissue factor, whereas on cell surfaces, TFPI-dependent inhibition is much faster.[164, 165]

Antithrombin is the major thrombin-inactivating protein.[168] This serine proteinase inhibitor also inactivates factors Xa, IXa, and XIa and kallikrein. Antithrombin displays its full inhibitory activity only in the presence of heparin or other sulfated glycosaminoglycans that are synthesized and expressed by endothelial cells. Some cell surface heparan sulfate proteoglycans may be involved in thrombin-antithrombin interactions.[169] Heparan sulfate proteoglycans are also a major constituent of the extracellular matrix, which explains why the thrombogenicity of balloon-injured vessels can be abolished by treatment with antithrombin, whereas heparin is ineffective.[170]

Another endothelial cell–dependent anticoagulant pathway involves the integral membrane glycoprotein thrombomodulin.[171] Its physiologic importance is well established and supported by gene disruption studies.[172] Thrombomodulin consists of a lectin-like NH_2-terminal domain, followed by six EGF-like domains, a serine/threonine-rich domain, a transmembrane domain, and a short cytoplasmic tail. The fifth and sixth EGF-like domains are essential for thrombin binding, whereas the calcium-dependent binding of protein C requires the linker region between the third and fourth EGF-like domains. Thrombomodulin has both direct and indirect anticoagulant properties. The direct anticoagulant function of thrombomodulin involves binding, neutralization, and degradation of thrombin.[171] Thrombomodulin accounts for about half of the thrombin-binding sites on endothelial cells. Agents such as endotoxin, interleukin-1, and TNF, which stimulate tissue factor activity, down-regulate thrombomodulin activity by suppressing its transcription. Thrombomodulin-bound thrombin cannot cleave fibrinogen; cannot activate factor V, factor XIII, or platelets; and is rapidly endocytosed and degraded.[171, 173] The indirect anticoagulant function of thrombomodulin involves the generation of activated protein C.[174] The zymogen protein C, a vitamin K–dependent protein, is activated by thrombin, and this activation is accelerated up to 20,000-fold by thrombomodulin. Activated protein C has anticoagulant properties by inhibiting factors Va and VIIIa. This reaction is moderately catalyzed at the endothelial cell surface by protein S, another vitamin K–dependent cofactor protein that is synthesized and expressed by endothelial cells in the liver.[175] Protein S binds to the endothelial cell membrane and to protein C, forming a cell surface–bound complex. Owing to the exposure of negatively charged phospholipids, activated platelets may provide the appropriate surface for the inactivation of factors Va and VIIIa. However, activated protein C is also active on endothelial cells, probably involving the described endothelial cell protein C receptor.[176] Protein S not only functions as a cofactor in the protein C pathway but also directly inhibits the prothrombinase and tenase reactions on phospholipid vesicles, platelets, and human endothelial cells or matrices.[177–180]

Other potential anticoagulant proteins include annexin V, protease nexin (PN)-1, and PN-2, whose roles as endothelial anticoagulants are, however, not firmly established. Annexins are a family of nonglycosylated proteins that bind calcium and phospholipids. Annexin V is localized in the endothelium of venous and arterial blood vessels[181]; it preferentially binds to phosphatidyl serine, thereby preventing the assembly of activated coagulation factors on phospholipid surfaces. Anticoagulant properties of annexin V have been reported on phospholipid vesicles, platelets, and endothelial cells. PN-1 is a serpin that inhibits thrombin, plasmin, urokinase, activated protein C, kallikrein, factor Xa, and trypsin.[182] PN-1 is localized on the surface of vascular endothelial cells, fibroblasts, and platelets. PN-1 bound to cell surfaces or endothelial cell matrix retains its inhibitory properties for thrombin but not for urokinase or plasmin. Inhibition of thrombin and factor Xa by PN-1 is accelerated by heparin, whereas that of plasmin is not. PN-2 is the secreted form of the transmembrane amyloid β-protein precursor. It is abundantly present in the α-granules of platelets but also in monocytes and endothelial cells.[183] PN-2 is a much more potent inhibitor of factors IXa and XIa than of thrombin and may be involved in the regulation of the intrinsic tenase reaction on endothelium.[184]

References

1. Collen D, Lijnen HR: Basic and clinical aspects of fibrinolysis and thrombolysis. Blood 78:3114, 1991.
2. Blasi F: Urokinase and urokinase receptor: a paracrine/autocrine system regulating cell migration and invasiveness. Bioessays 15:105, 1993.
3. Lijnen HR, Collen D: Congenital and acquired deficiencies of components of the fibrinolytic system and their relation to bleeding or thrombosis. Fibrinolysis 3:67, 1989.
4. Wiman B, Hamsten A: The fibrinolytic enzyme system and its role in the etiology of thromboembolic disease. Semin Thromb Hemost 16:207, 1990.
5. Declerck PJ, Juhan-Vague I, Felez J, Wiman B: Pathophysiology of fibrinolysis. J Int Med 236:425, 1994.
6. Lijnen HR, Collen D: Impaired fibrinolysis and the risk for coronary heart disease. Circulation 94:2052, 1996.
7. Pennica D, Holmes WE, Kohr WJ, et al: Cloning and expression of human tissue-type plasminogen activator cDNA in *E. coli.* Nature 301:214, 1983.
8. Lijnen HR, Collen D: Strategies for the improvement of thrombolytic agents. Thromb Haemost 66:88, 1991.
9. Holmes WE, Pennica D, Blaber M, et al: Cloning and expression

of the gene for pro-urokinase in *Escherichia coli*. Biotechnology 3:923, 1985.
10. Pannekoek H, Veerman H, Lambers H, et al: Endothelial plasminogen activator inhibitor (PAI): a new member of the serpin gene family. EMBO J 5:2539, 1986.
11. Declerck PJ, De Mol M, Alessi MC, et al: Purification and characterization of a plasminogen activator inhibitor-1-binding protein from human plasma: identification as a multimeric form of S protein (vitronectin). J Biol Chem 263:15454, 1988.
12. Genton C, Kruithof EKO, Schleuning WD: Phorbol ester induces the biosynthesis of glycosylated and nonglycosylated plasminogen activator inhibitor 2 in high excess over urokinase-type plasminogen activator in human U-937 lymphoma cells. J Cell Biol 104:705, 1987.
13. Ye RD, Wun TC, Sadler JE: cDNA cloning and expression in *Escherichia coli* of a plasminogen activator inhibitor from human placenta. J Biol Chem 262: 3718, 1987.
14. Van Hinsbergh VWM, Kooistra T, Emeis JJ, Koolwijk P: Regulation of plasminogen activator production by endothelial cells: role in fibrinolysis and local proteolysis. Int J Rad Biol 60:261, 1991.
15. Larsson LI, Skriver L, Nielsen LS, et al: Distribution of urokinase-type plasminogen activator immunoreactivity in the mouse. J Cell Biol 98:894, 1984.
16. Smith D, Gilbert M, Owen WG: Tissue plasminogen activator release in vivo in response to vasoactive agents. Blood 66:835, 1985.
17. Newby DE, Wright RA, Dawson P, et al: The L-arginine/nitric oxide pathway contributes to the acute release of tissue plasminogen activator in vivo in man. Cardiovasc Res 38:485, 1998.
18. Gelehrter TD, Sznycer-Laszuk R: Thrombin induction of plasminogen activator-inhibitor in cultured human endothelial cells. J Clin Invest 77:165, 1986.
19. Hanss M, Collen D: Secretion of tissue-type plasminogen activator and plasminogen activator inhibitor by cultured human endothelial cells: modulation by thrombin, endotoxin and histamine. J Lab Clin Med 109:97, 1987.
20. Medcalf RL, Van den Berg E, Schleuning WD: Glucocorticoid-modulated gene expression of tissue- and urinary-type plasminogen activator and plasminogen activator inhibitor 1 and 2. J Cell Biol 106:971, 1988.
21. Kooistra T, Van den Berg J, Töns A, et al: Butyrate stimulates tissue-type plasminogen activator synthesis in cultured human endothelial cells. Biochem J 247:605, 1987.
22. Moscatelli D: Urokinase-type and tissue-type plasminogen activators have different distributions in cultured bovine capillary endothelial cells. J Cell Biochem 30:19, 1986.
23. Montesano R, Vassalli JD, Baird A, et al: Basic fibroblast growth factor induces angiogenesis in vitro. Proc Natl Acad Sci U S A 83:7297, 1986.
24. Sakata Y, Curriden S, Lawrence D, et al: Activated protein C stimulates the fibrinolytic activity of cultured endothelial cells and decreases antiactivator activity. Proc Natl Acad Sci U S A 82:1121, 1985.
25. Laug WE: Ethyl alcohol enhances plasminogen activator secretion by endothelial cells. JAMA 250:772, 1983.
26. Kooistra T, Opdenberg JP, Toet K, et al: Stimulation of tissue-type plasminogen activator synthesis by retinoids in cultured human endothelial cells and rat tissues in vivo. Thromb Haemost 65:565, 1991.
27. Thompson EA, Nelles L, Collen D: Effect of retinoic acid on the synthesis of tissue-type plasminogen activator and plasminogen activator inhibitor-1 in human endothelial cells. Eur J Biochem 201:627, 1991.
28. Gelehrter TD, Sznycer-Laszuk R, Zeheb R, et al: Dexamethasone inhibition of tissue-type plasminogen activator (t-PA) activity: paradoxical induction of both t-PA antigen and plasminogen activator inhibitor. Mol Endocrinol 1:97, 1987.
29. Bulens F, Ibanez-Tallon I, Van Acker P, et al: Retinoic acid induction of human tissue-type plasminogen activator (t-PA) gene expression via a direct repeat element (DR5) located at −7 kilobases. J Biol Chem 270:7167, 1995.
30. Bulens F, Merchiers P, Ibanes-Tallon I, et al: Identification of a multihormone responsive enhancer far upstream from the human tissue-type plasminogen activator gene. J Biol Chem 272:663, 1997.
31. Lansink M, Kooistra T: Stimulation of tissue-type plasminogen activator expression by retinoic acid in human endothelial cells requires retinoic acid receptor β_2 induction. Blood 88:531, 1996.
32. Levin EG, Santell L: Stimulation and desensitization of tissue plasminogen activator release from human endothelial cells. J Biol Chem 263:9360, 1988.
33. Levin EG, Marotti KR, Santell L: Protein kinase C and the stimulation of tissue plasminogen activator release from human endothelial cells: dependence on the elevation of messenger RNA. J Biol Chem 264:16030, 1989.
34. Medcalf RL, Ruegg M, Schleuning WD: A DNA motif related to the cAMP-responsive element and an exon-located activator protein-2 binding site in the human tissue-type plasminogen activator gene promoter cooperate in basal expression and convey activation by phorbol ester and cAMP. J Biol Chem 265:14618, 1990.
35. Arts J, Herr I, Lansink M, et al: Cell-type specific DNA-protein interactions at the tissue-type plasminogen activator promoter in human endothelial and HeLa cells in vivo and in vitro. Nucleic Acids Res 25:311, 1997.
36. Jaklitsch MT, Biro S, Casscells W, Dichek DA: Transduced endothelial cells expressing high levels of tissue plasminogen activator have an unaltered phenotype in vitro. J Cell Physiol 154:207, 1993.
37. Shi GY, Hau JS, Wang SJ, et al: Plasmin and the regulation of tissue-type plasminogen activator biosynthesis in human endothelial cells. J Biol Chem 267:19363, 1992.
38. Loskutoff DJ: Regulation of PAI-1 gene expression. Fibrinolysis 5:197, 1991.
39. Samad F, Yamamoto K, Loskutoff D: Distribution and regulation of plasminogen activator inhibitor-1 in murine adipose tissue in vivo: induction by tumor necrosis factor alpha and lipopolysaccharide. J Clin Invest 97:37, 1996.
40. Lundgren C, Brown S, Nordt T, et al: Elaboration of type-1 plasminogen activator inhibitor from adipocytes: a potential pathogenic link between obesity and cardiovascular disease. Circulation 93:106, 1996.
41. van Meijer M, Pannekoek H: Structure of plasminogen activator inhibitor 1 (PAI-1) and its function in fibrinolysis: an update. Fibrinolysis 9:263, 1995.
42. Krishnamurti C, Alving BM: Plasminogen activator inhibitor type 1: biochemistry and evidence for modulation of fibrinolysis in vivo. Semin Thromb Hemost 18:67, 1992.
43. Ginsburg D, Zeheb R, Yang AY, et al: cDNA cloning of human plasminogen activator-inhibitor from endothelial cells. J Clin Invest 78:1673, 1986.
44. van den Berg EA, Sprengers ED, Jaye M, et al: Regulation of plasminogen activator inhibitor-1 mRNA in human endothelial cells. Thromb Haemost 60:63, 1988.
45. Konkle BA, Kollros PR, Kelly MD: Heparin-binding growth factor-1 modulation of plasminogen activator inhibitor-1 expression. J Biol Chem 265:21867, 1990.
46. Medcalf RL, Kruithof EK, Schleuning WD: Plasminogen activator inhibitor 1 and 2 are tumor necrosis factor/cachectin-responsive genes. J Exp Med 168:751, 1988.
47. Keski-Oja J, Raghow R, Sawdey M, et al: Regulation of mRNAs for type-1 plasminogen activator inhibitor, fibronectin, and type 1 procollagen by transforming growth factor-β. J Biol Chem 263:3111, 1988.
48. Kooistra T, Bosma PJ, Töns HAM, et al: Plasminogen activator inhibitor 1: biosynthesis and mRNA level are increased by insulin in cultured human hepatocytes. Thromb Haemost 62:723, 1989.
49. Bosma PJ, Kooistra T: Different induction of two plasminogen activator inhibitor 1 mRNA species by phorbol ester in human hepatoma cells. J Biol Chem 266:17845, 1991.
50. Colucci M, Paramo JA, Collen D: Generation in plasma of a fast-acting inhibitor of plasminogen activator in response to endotoxin stimulation. J Clin Invest 75:818, 1985.
51. Crutchley DJ, Conanan LB: Endotoxin induction of an inhibitor of plasminogen activator in bovine pulmonary artery endothelial cells. J Biol Chem 261:154, 1986.
52. Medina R, Socher SH, Han JH, Friedman PA: Interleukin-1, endotoxin or tumor necrosis factor/cachectin enhance the level of plasminogen activator inhibitor messenger RNA in bovine aortic endothelial cells. Thromb Res 54:41, 1989.
53. Emeis JJ, Kooistra T: Interleukin 1 and lipopolysaccharide induce an inhibitor of tissue-type plasminogen activator in vivo and in cultured endothelial cells. J Exp Med 163:1260, 1986.
54. Bevilacqua MP, Schleef RR, Gimbrone MA Jr, Loskutoff DJ: Regulation of the fibrinolytic system of cultured human vascular endothelium by interleukin 1. J Clin Invest 78:587, 1986.

55. van Hinsbergh VW, Kooistra T, van den Berg EA, et al: Tumor necrosis factor increases the production of plasminogen activator inhibitor in human endothelial cells in vitro and in rats in vivo. Blood 72:1467, 1988.
56. Schleef RR, Bevilacqua MP, Sawdey M, et al: Cytokine activation of vascular endothelium: effects on tissue-type plasminogen activator and type 1 plasminogen activator inhibitor. J Biol Chem 263:5797, 1988.
57. Saksela O, Moscatelli D, Rifkin DB: The opposing effects of basic fibroblast growth factor and transforming growth factor beta on the regulation of plasminogen activator activity in capillary endothelial cells. J Cell Biol 105:957, 1987.
58. Santell L, Levin EC: Cyclic AMP potentiates phorbol ester stimulation of tissue plasminogen activator release and inhibits secretion of plasminogen activator inhibitor-1 from human endothelial cells. J Biol Chem 263:16802, 1988.
59. Scarpati EM, Sadler JE: Regulation of endothelial cell coagulant properties: modulation of tissue factor, plasminogen activator inhibitors, and thrombomodulin by phorbol 12-myristate 13-acetate and tumor necrosis factor. J Biol Chem 264:20705, 1989.
60. Dichek D, Quertermous T: Thrombin regulation of mRNA levels of tissue plasminogen activator and plasminogen activator inhibitor-1 in cultured human umbilical vein endothelial cells. Blood 74:222, 1989.
61. Stiko-Rahm A, Wiman B, Hamsten A, Nilsson J: Secretion of plasminogen activator inhibitor-1 from cultured human umbilical vein endothelial cells is induced by very low density lipoprotein. Arteriosclerosis 10:1067, 1990.
62. Tremoli E, Camera M, Maderna P, et al: Increased synthesis of plasminogen activator inhibitor-1 by cultured human endothelial cells exposed to native and modified LDLs: an LDL receptor-independent phenomenon. Arterioscler Thromb 13:338, 1993.
63. Etingin OR, Hajjar DP, Hajjar KA, et al: Lipoprotein (a) regulates plasminogen activator inhibitor-1 expression in endothelial cells: a potential mechanism in thrombogenesis. J Biol Chem 266:2459, 1991.
64. Schneider DJ, Nordt TK, Sobel BE: Stimulation by proinsulin of expression of plasminogen activator inhibitor type-1 in endothelial cells. Diabetes 41:890, 1992.
65. Nordt TK, Klassen KJ, Schneider DJ, Sobel BE: Augmentation of synthesis of plasminogen activator inhibitor type-1 in arterial endothelial cells by glucose and its implications for local fibrinolysis. Arterioscler Thromb 13:1822, 1993.
66. Kariko K, Rosenbaum H, Kuo A, et al: Stimulatory effect of unsaturated fatty acids on the level of plasminogen activator inhibitor-1 mRNA in cultured human endothelial cells. FEBS Lett 361:118, 1995.
67. Nagai T, Akizawa T, Kohjiro S, et al: rHuEPO enhances the production of plasminogen activator inhibitor-1 in cultured endothelial cells. Kidney Int 50:102, 1996.
68. Feener EP, Northrup JM, Aiello LP, King GL: Angiotensin II induces plasminogen activator inhibitor-1 and -2 expression in vascular endothelial and smooth muscle cells. J Clin Invest 95:1353, 1995.
69. Vaughan DE, Lazos SA, Tong K: Angiotensin II regulates the expression of plasminogen activator inhibitor-1 in cultured endothelial cells: a potential link between the renin-angiotensin system and thrombosis. J Clin Invest 95:995, 1995.
70. Kerins DM, Hao Q, Vaughan DE: Angiotensin induction of PAI-1 expression in endothelial cells is mediated by the hexapeptide angiotensin IV. J Clin Invest 96:2515, 1995.
71. Hamdan AD, Quist WC, Gagne JB, Feener EP: Angiotensin-converting enzyme inhibition suppresses plasminogen activator inhibitor-1 expression in the neointima of balloon-injured rat aorta. Circulation 93:1073, 1996.
72. Georg B, Riccio A, Andreasen P: Forskolin down-regulates type-1 plasminogen activator inhibitor and tissue-type plasminogen activator and their mRNAs in human fibrosarcoma cells. Mol Cell Endocrinol 72:103, 1990.
73. Konkle BA, Ginsburg D: The addition of endothelial cell growth factor and heparin to human umbilical vein endothelial cell cultures decreases plasminogen activator inhibitor-1 expression. J Clin Invest 82:579, 1988.
74. Fujii S, Sawa H, Sobel BE: Inhibition of endothelial cell expression of plasminogen activator inhibitor type-1 by gemfibrozil. Thromb Haemost 70:642, 1993.
75. Bok RA, Jacob HS, Balla J, et al: Herpes simplex virus decreases endothelial cell plasminogen activator inhibitor. Thromb Haemost 69:253, 1993.
76. Alessi MC, Peiretti F, Morange P, et al: Production of plasminogen activator inhibitor 1 by human adipose tissue: possible link between visceral fat accumulation and vascular disease. Diabetes 46:860, 1997.
77. Shimomura I, Funahashi T, Takahashi M, et al: Enhanced expression of PAI-1 in visceral fat: possible contributor to vascular disease in obesity. Nat Med 2:800, 1996.
78. Juhan-Vague I, Alessi MC, Declerck PJ: Pathophysiology of fibrinolysis. Baillieres Clin Haematol 8:329, 1995.
79. Samad F, Yamamoto K, Pandey M, Loskutoff DJ: Elevated expression of transforming growth factor-beta in adipose tissue from obese mice. Mol Med 3:37, 1997.
80. van Leeuwen RTJ: Extracellular proteolysis and the migrating vascular smooth muscle cell. Fibrinolysis 10:263, 1995.
81. Wojta J, Gallicchio M, Zoellner H, et al: Thrombin stimulates expression of tissue-type plasminogen activator and plasminogen activator inhibitor type 1 in cultured human vascular smooth muscle cells. Thromb Haemost 70:469, 1993.
82. Lee E, Vaughan DE, Parikh SH, et al: Regulation of matrix metalloproteinases and plasminogen activator inhibitor-1 synthesis by plasminogen in cultured human vascular smooth muscle cells. Circ Res 78:44, 1996.
83. van Leeuwen RT, Kol A, Andreotti F, et al: Angiotensin II increases plasminogen activator inhibitor type 1 and tissue-type plasminogen activator messenger RNA in cultured rat aortic smooth muscle cells. Circulation 90:362, 1994.
84. Reilly CF, McFall RC: Platelet-derived growth factor and transforming growth factor-beta regulate plasminogen activator inhibitor-1 synthesis in vascular smooth muscle cells. J Biol Chem 266:9419, 1991.
85. Reilly CF, Broski JE: Differential effects of PDGF and PDGF-BB on vascular smooth muscle cells. Biochem Biophys Res Commun 160:1047, 1989.
86. Sawa H, Fujii S, Sobel BE: Augmented arterial wall expression of type-1 plasminogen activator inhibitor induced by thrombosis. Arterioscler Thromb 12:1507, 1992.
87. Westerhausen DR, Hopkins WE, Billadello JJ: Multiple transforming growth factor-beta-inducible elements regulate expression of the plasminogen activator inhibitor type-1 gene in HepG2 cells. J Biol Chem 266:1092, 1991.
88. Riccio A, Pedone P, Lund L, et al: Transforming growth factor beta-1 responsive element: closely associated binding sites for USF and CCAAT-binding transcription factor-nuclear factor I in the type 1 plasminogen activator inhibitor gene. Mol Cell Biol 12:1846, 1992.
89. Bosma PJ, van den Berg EA, Kooistra T, et al: Human plasminogen activator inhibitor-1 gene: promoter and structural gene nucleotide sequences. J Biol Chem 263:9129, 1988.
90. Descheemaeker KA, Wijns S, Nelles L, et al: Interaction of AP-1-like, AP-2-like and Sp1-like proteins with two distinct sites in the upstream regulatory region of the plasminogen activator inhibitor-1 gene mediates the phorbol 12-myristate 13-acetate response. J Biol Chem 267:15086, 1992.
91. Knudsen H, Olesen T, Riccio A, et al: A common response element mediates differential effects of phorbol esters and forskolin on type-1 plasminogen activator inhibitor gene expression in human breast carcinoma cells. Eur J Biochem 220:63, 1994.
92. Arts J, Grimbergen J, Bosma PJ, et al: Role of c-Jun and proximal phorbol 12-myristate-13-acetate-(PMA)-responsive elements in the regulation of basal and PMA-stimulated plasminogen-activator inhibitor-1 gene expression in HepG2. Eur J Biochem 241:393, 1996.
93. Kunz C, Pebler S, Otte J, von-der-Ahe D: Differential regulation of plasminogen activator and inhibitor gene transcription by the tumor suppressor p53. Nucleic Acids Res 23:3710, 1995.
94. Belin D: Biology and facultative secretion of plasminogen activator inhibitor-2. Thromb Haemost 70:144, 1993.
95. Schleef RR, Loskutoff DJ: Fibrinolytic system of vascular endothelial cells: role of plasminogen activator inhibitors. Haemostasis 18:328, 1988.
96. Kruithof EKO: Plasminogen activator inhibitors: a review. Enzyme 40:113, 1988.
97. Plow EF, Felez J, Miles LA: Cellular regulation of fibrinolysis. Thromb Haemost 66:32, 1991.

98. Hajjar KA, Hamel NM, Harpel PC, Nachman RL: Binding of tissue plasminogen activator to cultured human endothelial cells. J Clin Invest 80:1712–1719, 1987.
99. Hajjar KA, Harpel PC, Jaffe EA, Nachman RL: Binding of plasminogen to cultured human endothelial cells. J Biol Chem 261:11656, 1986.
100. Miles LA, Plow EF: Binding and activation of plasminogen on the platelet surface. J Biol Chem 260:4303, 1985.
101. Stephens RW, Pöllänen J, Tapiovaara H, et al: Activation of pro-urokinase and plasminogen on human sarcoma cells: a proteolytic system with surface-bound reactants. J Cell Biol 108:1987, 1989.
102. Miles LA, Plow EF: Plasminogen receptors: ubiquitous sites for cellular regulation of fibrinolysis. Fibrinolysis 2:61, 1988.
103. Plow EF, Freaney DE, Plescia J, Miles LA: The plasminogen system and cell surfaces: evidence for plasminogen and urokinase receptors on the same cell type. J Cell Biol 103:2411, 1986.
104. Miles LA, Dahlberg CM, Levin EG, Plow EF: Gangliosides interact directly with plasminogen and urokinase and may mediate binding of these fibrinolytic components to cells. Biochemistry 28:9337, 1989.
105. Miles LA, Dahlberg CM, Plescia J, et al: Role of cell-surface lysines in plasminogen binding to cells: identification of alpha-enolase as a candidate plasminogen receptor. Biochemistry 30:1682, 1991.
106. Hajjar KA, Nachman RL: Endothelial cell-mediated conversion of Glu-plasminogen to Lys-plasminogen: further evidence for assembly of the fibrinolytic system on the endothelial cell surface. J Clin Invest 82:1769, 1988.
107. Félez J, Miles LA, Fàbregas P, et al: Characterization of cellular binding sites and interactive regions within reactants required for enhancement of plasminogen activation by t-PA on the surface of leukocytic cells. Thromb Haemost 76:577, 1996.
108. Barnathan ES, Kuo A, Van der Keyl H, et al: Tissue-type plasminogen activator binding to human endothelial cells: evidence for two distinct binding sites. J Biol Chem 263:7792, 1988.
109. Hajjar KA, Jacovina AT, Chacko J: An endothelial cell receptor for plasminogen/tissue plasminogen activator, I: identity with annexin II. J Biol Chem 269:21191, 1994.
110. Nachman RL, Hajjar KA: Endothelial cell fibrinolytic assembly. Ann N Y Acad Sci 614:240, 1991.
111. Otter M, Zocková P, Kuiper J, et al: Isolation and characterization of the mannose receptor from human liver potentially involved in the plasma clearance of tissue-type plasminogen activator. Hepatology 16:54, 1992.
112. Strickland DK, Kounnas MZ, Williams SE, et al: LDL receptor-related protein (LRP): a multiligand receptor. Fibrinolysis 8(suppl 1):204, 1994.
113. Lijnen HR, Bachmann F, Collen D, et al: Mechanisms of plasminogen activation. J Int Med 236:415, 1994.
114. Ellis V, Behrendt N, Danø K: Plasminogen activation by receptor-bound urokinase: a kinetic study with both cell-associated and isolated receptor. J Biol Chem 266:12752, 1991.
115. Ellis V, Scully MF, Kakkar VV: Plasminogen activation initiated by single-chain urokinase-type plasminogen activator: potentiation by U937 monocytes. J Biol Chem 264:2185, 1989.
116. Ellis V, Wun TC, Behrendt N, et al: Inhibition of receptor-bound urokinase by plasminogen-activator inhibitors. J Biol Chem 265: 9904, 1990.
117. Lee SW, Ellis V, Dichek DA: Characterization of plasminogen activation by glycosylphosphatidylinositol-anchored urokinase. J Biol Chem 269:2411, 1994.
118. Carmeliet P, Collen D: Gene manipulation and transfer of the plasminogen and coagulation system in mice. Semin Thromb Hemost 22:525, 1996.
119. Bugge TH, Flick MJ, Danton MJS, et al: Urokinase-type plasminogen activator is effective in fibrin clearance in the absence of its receptor or tissue-type plasminogen activator. Proc Natl Acad Sci U S A 93:5899, 1996.
120. Nilsson IM, Ljungner H, Tengborn L: Two different mechanisms in patients with venous thrombosis and defective fibrinolysis: low concentration of plasminogen activator or increased concentration of plasminogen activator inhibitor. BMJ 290:1453, 1985.
121. Dahlbäck B: New molecular insights into the genetics of thrombophilia: resistance to activated protein C caused by Arg^{506} to Gln mutation in factor V as a pathogenic risk factor for venous thrombosis. Thromb Haemost 74:139, 1995.
122. Juhan-Vague I, Valadier J, Alessi MC, et al: Deficient t-PA release and elevated PA inhibitor levels in patients with spontaneous or recurrent deep venous thrombosis. Thromb Haemost 57:67, 1987.
123. Prins MH, Hirsh J: A critical review of the evidence supporting a relationship between impaired fibrinolytic activity and venous thromboembolism. Arch Intern Med 151:1721, 1991.
124. Ridker PM, Vaughan DE, Stampfer MJ, et al: Baseline fibrinolytic state and the risk of future venous thrombosis: a prospective study of endogenous tissue-type plasminogen activator and plasminogen activator inhibitor. Circulation 85:1822, 1992.
125. Hamsten A, De Faire U, Walldius G, et al: Plasminogen activator inhibitor in plasma: risk factor for recurrent myocardial infarction. Lancet 2:3, 1987.
126. Gram J, Jespersen J: A selective depression of tissue plasminogen activator (t-PA) activity in euglobulins characterises a risk group among survivors of acute myocardial infarction. Thromb Haemost 57:137, 1987.
127. Cimmiello C: Tissue type plasminogen activator and risk of myocardial infarction. Lancet 342:48, 1993.
128. Jansson JH, Nilsson TK, Johnson O: Von Willebrand factor in plasma: a novel risk factor for recurrent myocardial infarction and death. BMJ 66:351, 1991.
129. Van de Loo JCW, Haverkate F, Thompson SG: Hemostatic factors and the risk of myocardial infarction. N Engl J Med 332:389, 1995.
130. Thompson SG, Kienast J, Pyke SDM, et al: Hemostatic factors and the risk of myocardial infarction or sudden death in patients with angina pectoris. N Engl J Med 332:635, 1995.
131. Juhan-Vague I, Pyke SDM, Alessi M-C, et al: Fibrinolytic factors and the risk of myocardial infarction or sudden death in patients with angina pectoris. Circulation 94:2057, 1996.
132. Dawson S, Hamsten A, Wiman B, et al: Genetic variation at the plasminogen activator inhibitor-1 locus is associated with altered levels of plasma plasminogen activator inhibitor-1 activity. Arterioscl Thromb 11:183, 1991.
133. Dawson SJ, Wiman B, Hamsten A, et al: The two allele sequences of a common polymorphism in the promoter of the plasminogen activator inhibitor-1 (PAI-1) gene respond differently to interleukin-1 in HepG2 cells. J Biol Chem 268:10739, 1993.
134. Eriksson P, Kallin B, van't Hooft FM, et al: Allele-specific increase in basal transcription of the plasminogen-activator inhibitor 1 gene is associated with myocardial infarction. Proc Natl Acad Sci U S A 92:1851, 1995.
135. Ye S, Green FR, Scarabin PY, et al: The 4G/5G genetic polymorphism in the promoter of the plasminogen activator inhibitor-1 (PAI-1) gene is associated with differences in plasma PAI-1 activity but not with risk of myocardial infarction in the ECTIM study. Thromb Haemost 74:837, 1995.
136. MacFarlane RG: An enzyme cascade in the blood clotting mechanism, and its function as a biochemical amplifier. Nature 202:498, 1964.
137. Broze GJ Jr: Tissue factor pathway inhibitor and the revised theory of coagulation. Annu Rev Med 46:103, 1995.
138. Rapaport SI: Inhibition of factor VIIa/tissue factor-induced blood coagulation with particular emphasis upon a factor Xa-dependent inhibitory mechanism. Blood 73:359, 1989.
139. Broze GJ Jr, Girard TJ, Novotny WF: Regulation of coagulation by a multivalent Kunitz-type inhibitor. Biochemistry 29:7539, 1990.
140. Naito K, Fujikawa K: Activation of human blood coagulation factor XI independent of factor XII: factor XI is activated by thrombin and factor XIa in the presence of negatively charged surfaces. J Biol Chem 266:7353, 1991.
141. Gailani D, Broze GJ: Factor XI activation in a revised model of blood coagulation. Science 253:909, 1991.
142. Colman RW, Hirsh J, Marder VJ, Salzman E (eds): Hemostasis and Thrombosis: Basic Principles and Clinical Practice. 3rd ed. Philadelphia: JB Lippincott, 1994.
143. Bloom AL, Forbes CD, Thomas DP, Tuddenham EGD (eds): Haemostasis and Thrombosis. 3rd ed. Edinburgh: Churchill Livingstone, 1994.
144. Rapaport SI, Rao VM: The tissue factor pathway: how it has become a "prima ballerina." Thromb Haemost 74:7, 1995.
145. Ryan J, Brett J, Tijburg P, et al: Tumor necrosis factor-induced endothelial tissue factor is associated with subendothelial matrix vesicles but is not expressed on the apical surface. Blood 80:966, 1992.

146. Drake TA, Morrisey JH, Edgington TS: Selective cellular expression of tissue factor in human tissues: implications for disorders of hemostasis and thrombosis. Am J Pathol 134:1087, 1989.
147. Nemerson Y: Tissue factor: then and now. Thromb Haemost 74:180, 1995.
148. Contrino J, Goralnick S, Qi J, et al: Fibrin induction of tissue factor expression in human vascular endothelial cells. Circulation 96:605, 1997.
149. Lin MC, Almus-Jacobs F, Chen HH, et al: Shear stress induction of the tissue factor gene. J Clin Invest 99:737, 1997.
150. Napoleone E, Di Santo A, Lorenzet R: Monocytes upregulate endothelial cell expression of tissue factor: a role for cell-cell contact and cross-talk. Blood 89:541, 1997.
151. Osterud B, Rapaport SI: Activation of factor IX by the reaction product of tissue factor and factor VII: additional pathway of human blood coagulation. Proc Natl Acad Sci U S A 74:5260, 1977.
152. Marlar RA, Kleiss AJ, Griffin JH: An alternative pathway of human blood coagulation. Blood 60:1353, 1982.
153. Butenas S, van't Veer C, Mann KG: Evaluation of the initiation phase of blood coagulation using ultrasensitive assays for serine proteases. J Biol Chem 272:21527, 1997.
154. Carmeliet P, Mackman N, Moons L, et al: Role of tissue factor in embryonic blood vessel development. Nature 383:73, 1996.
155. Bugge TH, Xiao Q, Kormbrinck KW, et al: Fatal embryonic bleeding events in mice lacking tissue factor, the cell-associated initiation of blood coagulation. Proc Natl Acad Sci U S A 93:6258, 1996.
156. Annamalia AE, Stewart GJ, Hansel B, et al: Expression of factor V on human umbilical vein endothelial cells is modulated by cell injury. Arteriosclerosis 6:196, 1986.
157. Kadhom N, Wolfrom C, Gautier M, et al: Factor VIII procoagulant antigen in human tissues. Thromb Haemost 59:289, 1988.
158. Bono F, Herault JP, Avril C, et al: Human umbilical vein endothelial cells express high affinity receptors for factor Xa. J Cell Physiol 172:36, 1997.
159. Ryan J, Wolitzky B, Heimer E, et al: Structural determinants of the factor IX molecule mediating interaction with the endothelial cell binding site are distinct from those involved in phospholipid binding. J Biol Chem 264:20283, 1989.
160. Brass LF, Molino M: Protease-activated G protein-coupled receptors on human platelets and endothelial cells. Thromb Haemost 78:234, 1997.
161. Ishihara H, Connoly AJ, Zeng D, et al: Protease-activated receptor 3 is a second thrombin receptor in humans. Nature 386:502, 1997.
162. Brinkman HJ, Koster P, Mertens K, van Mourik JA: Dissimilar interaction of factor VIII with endothelial cells and lipid vesicles during factor X activation. Biochem J 323:735, 1997.
163. Shoen P, Reutelingsperger C, Lindhout T: Activation of prothrombin in the presence of human umbilical-vein endothelial cells. Biochem J 281:661, 1992.
164. Broze GJ Jr: Tissue factor pathway inhibitor. Thromb Haemost 74:90-93, 1995.
165. van't Veer C, Mann KG: Regulation of tissue factor initiated thrombin generation by the stoichiometric inhibitors tissue factor pathway inhibitor, antithrombin-III, and heparin cofactor II. J Biol Chem 272:4367, 1997.
166. Huang ZF, Higuchi D, Lasky N, Broze GJ Jr: Tissue factor pathway inhibitor gene disruption produces intrauterine lethality in mice. Blood 90:944, 1997.
167. Lawson JH, Butenas S, Ribarik N, Mann KG: Complex-dependent inhibition of factor VIIa by antithrombin III and heparin. J Biol Chem 268:767, 1993.
168. Beresford CH, Owen MC: Antithrombin III. Int J Biochem 22:121, 1990.
169. Mertens G, Cassiman JJ, van den Berghe H, et al: Cell surface heparin sulfate proteoglycans from human vascular endothelial cells: core protein characterization and antithrombin III binding properties. J Biol Chem 267:20435, 1992.
170. Frebelius S, Hedin U, Swedenborg J: Thrombogenicity of the injured vessel wall: role of antithrombin and heparin. Thromb Haemost 71:147, 1994.
171. Esmon CT: Thrombomodulin as a model of molecular mechanisms that modulate protease specificity and function at the vessel surface. FASEB J 9:946, 1995.
172. Rosenberg RD: Thrombomodulin gene disruption and mutation in mice. Thromb Haemost 78:705, 1997.
173. Esmon CT: Molecular events that control the protein C anticoagulant pathway. Thromb Haemost 70:29, 1993.
174. Esmon CT: The roles of protein C and thrombomodulin in the regulation of blood coagulation. J Biol Chem 264:4743, 1989.
175. Dahlback B: Protein S and C4b-binding protein: components involved in the regulation of the protein C anticoagulant system. Thromb Haemost 66:49, 1991.
176. Fukudome K, Esmon CT: Identification, cloning and regulation of a novel endothelial cell protein C/activated protein C receptor. J Biol Chem 269:26486, 1994.
177. Heeb MJ, Mesters RM, Tans G, et al: Binding of protein S to factor Va associated with inhibition of prothrombinase that is independent of activated protein C. J Biol Chem 268:2872, 1993.
178. Heeb MJ, Rosing J, Bakker HM, et al: Protein S binds to and inhibits factor Xa. Proc Natl Acad Sci U S A 91:2728, 1994.
179. Koppelman SJ, Hackeng TM, Sixma JJ, Bouma BN: Inhibition of the intrinsic factor X activating complex by protein S: evidence for a specific binding of protein S to factor VIII. Blood 86:1062, 1995.
180. van Wijnen M, Stam JG, van't Veer C, et al: The interaction of protein S with the phospholipid surface is essential for the activated protein C-independent activity of protein S. Thromb Haemost 76:397, 1996.
181. van Heerde WL, de Groot PG, Reutelingsperger CPM: The complexity of the phospholipid binding protein annexin V. Thromb Haemost 73:172, 1995.
182. Bombeli T, Mueller M, Haeberli A: Anticoagulant properties of the vascular endothelium. Thromb Haemost 77: 408, 1997.
183. van Nostrand WE, Schmaier AH, Wagner SL: Potential role of protease nexin-2/amyloid beta-protein precursor as a cerebral anticoagulant. Ann N Y Acad Sci 674:243, 1992.
184. Schmaier AH, Dahl LD, Hasan AA, et al: Protease nexin-2/amyloid beta-protein precursor: a tight binding inhibitor of coagulation factor IXa. J Clin Invest 92:2540, 1993.

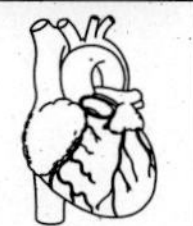

CHAPTER 70

ATHEROSCLEROSIS: PATHOLOGIC ANATOMY

L. Maximilian Buja

GENERAL ASPECTS OF VASCULAR DISEASE
PATHOLOGIC ANATOMY OF VASCULAR LESIONS
EARLY EVENTS IN ATHEROSCLEROSIS
LEUKOCYTE-ENDOTHELIAL INTERACTIONS
PLAQUE GROWTH

GENERAL ASPECTS OF VASCULAR DISEASE

Vascular diseases develop as responses of vessels to injury.[1–8] *Arteriosclerosis* is a generic term for processes that cause hardening and thickening of the arteries. The term encompasses several conditions, including arteriolosclerosis, Mönckeberg's medial calcific sclerosis, and atherosclerosis. *Arteriolosclerosis* is a term for thickening and narrowing of the small arteries and arterioles, which develops in hypertension, diabetes mellitus, and amyloidosis. *Mönckeberg's medial calcific sclerosis* is an age-related change characterized by fibrosis and calcification of certain medium-sized to small muscular arteries, including the femoral, tibial, radial, and ulnar arteries and arteries of the male and female genital tracts. *Atherosclerosis,* which is the most important form of arteriosclerosis, is a disease of the elastic arteries, including the aorta and iliac arteries, and of large and medium-sized muscular arteries, including the coronary, carotid, intracerebral, and femoropopliteal arteries. The term *atherosclerosis* emphasizes the nature of the intimal lesions, which are composed of mixtures of fibrous tissue and fatty material and are known as *plaque.*[9–13]

Atherosclerosis and its complications constitute the leading cause of disability and death in the United States and other developed countries,[14–16] and the incidence of atherosclerotic diseases is on the increase in developing countries.[17] Atherosclerosis is a dynamic process with potential for regression as well as progression. However, the clinical manifestations of atherosclerosis result from progressive growth of plaques and secondary changes in the plaques. These changes *(complications)* can lead to luminal stenosis, thrombosis, embolization, aneurysm formation, and vessel rupture. The resultant clinical manifestations include ischemic heart disease, stroke, and peripheral vascular disease. Because net progression of the disease tends to occur over time, age is a significant risk factor for the clinical expression of disease. The progression of atherosclerosis also is influenced by well defined genetic defects, such as familial hypercholesterolemia, as well as by more heterogeneous genetic factors, which contribute to a positive family history of disease.[18] In addition, a large body of epidemiologic work has confirmed the existence of four major risk factors: hypertension, hyperlipidemia, cigarette smoking, and diabetes mellitus.[14–18] These factors, which are treatable, clearly modulate the progression of disease, even though not all of the mechanisms involved have been clearly defined.[1–8] Epidemiologic and basic studies have focused attention on a number of "nontraditional" risk factors, including altered coagulation factors,[19, 20] increased blood level of homocysteine,[21–23] and exposure to infectious organisms, particularly herpesviruses and *Chlamydia.*[24–29] These studies indicate that the progression of atherosclerosis also can be influenced by a broad array of metabolic, immunologic, and inflammatory factors.

PATHOLOGIC ANATOMY OF VASCULAR LESIONS

Arteries consist of an adventitia of connective tissue, a muscularis containing smooth muscle cells, and an intima. In newborns, the intima is exceedingly thin and consists of endothelium overlying the internal elastic lamella with only rare intervening connective tissue elements. Diffuse intimal thickening occurs over time due to the accumulation of smooth muscle cells and connective tissue matrix. Early vascular lesions consist of focal alterations superimposed on the diffusely thickened intima.[9–13]

Gray gelatinous lesions are focal areas of excess fluid accumulation in the intima.[9, 10] *Fatty streaks* are zones of lipid accumulation that produce minimal additional thickening of the intima.[9–13] The lipid usually has a predominantly intracellular localization but may be partially or exclusively extracellular. The lipid-containing foam cells are macrophages derived from blood monocytes and smooth muscle cells derived from the vessel wall. The intracellular lipid consists of cholesterol esters, and the extracellular lipid is composed of free cholesterol, phospholipid, and intact lipoprotein. Both the intracellular and extracellular lipids are derived primarily from low-density lipoprotein (LDL) from the blood.[1–6] Microthrombi, composed of platelets and fibrin, constitute another type of lesion that may be observed in the early stages of disease.[9–13] In addition, fibrinogen, fibrin, and fibrin products can be identified as components of lesions.[30]

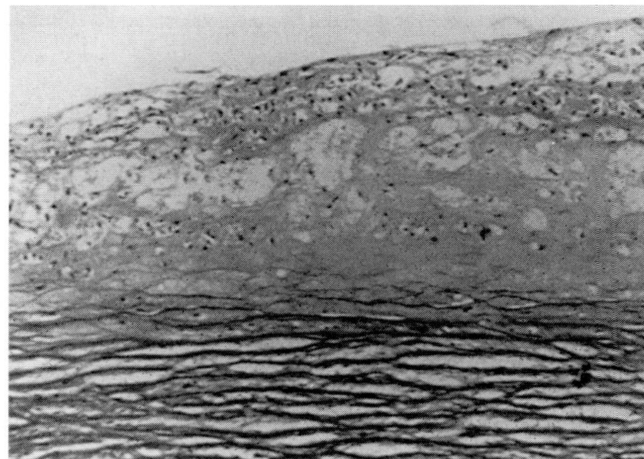

FIGURE 70–1 Atherosclerotic plaque from the aorta of a 4-year-old boy with homozygous familial hypercholesterolemia is composed of fibrous tissue, lipid-laden foam cells, and extracellular lipid deposits. The latter appear as clear spaces owing to lipid extraction during preparation of the paraffin sections. Patients with familial hypercholesterolemia are prone to accelerated atherosclerosis but develop typical atherosclerotic plaques that are similar to those in patients without the genetic disorder (H & E stain, ×37). (From Willerson JT, Hillis LD, Buja LM: Pathogenesis and pathology of ischemic heart disease. *In* Ischemic Heart Disease: Clinical and Pathophysiological Aspects. pp. 7–83. New York: Raven, 1982.)

The lesions of established atherosclerosis are atherosclerotic plaques.[9–13] These are raised intimal lesions composed of variable combinations of lipid, cells, and connective tissue matrix (Figs. 70–1 to 70–4). The variable compositions of the lesions are reflected by the different designations for various subtypes, including fibrofatty plaques, fibrous plaques, and atheromatous plaques. Typical lesions have a fibrous capsule and a central core of lipid-rich material. The fibrous capsule is completely or partially lined by endothelium and is composed of smooth muscle

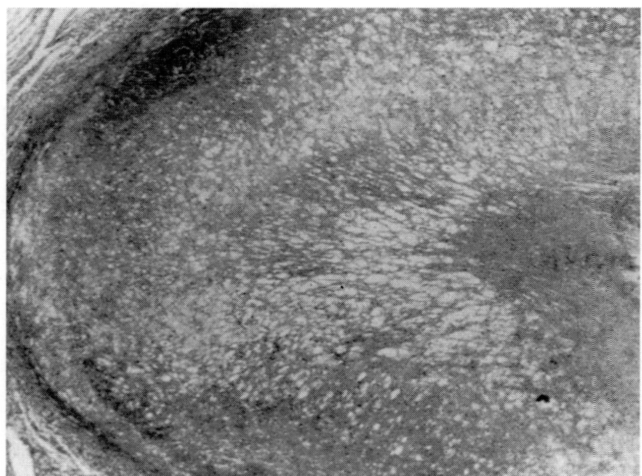

FIGURE 70–2 Atherosclerotic plaque produces severe stenosis of the lumen of coronary artery from a 4-year-old child with homozygous familial hypercholesterolemia. This lesion contains abundant foam cells and lipid deposits (H & E stain, ×92). (From Willerson JT, Hillis LD, Buja LM: Pathogenesis and pathology of ischemic heart disease. *In* Ischemic Heart Disease: Clinical and Pathophysiological Aspects. pp. 7–83. New York: Raven, 1982.)

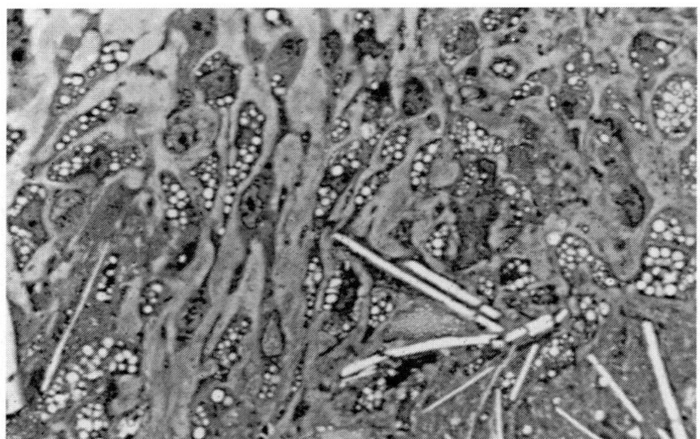

FIGURE 70–3 Aortic plaque from a 9-year-old child with homozygous familial hypercholesterolemia. Foam cells in the plaque contain lipid droplets rich in cholesteryl ester. Crystals of free cholesterol are present in the center of the plaque (epoxy section stained with toluidine blue, ×500). (From Buja LM, Kovanen PT, Bilheimer DW: Cellular pathology of homozygous familial hypercholesterolemia. Am J Pathol 97:327–357, 1979.)

cells, collagen fibers, glycosaminoglycans, and few elastic fibers. Peripheral and deep portions of the lesions are composed of similar tissue. Lipid-laden foam cells of macrophage and smooth muscle origin also are present in the connective tissue matrix, especially adjacent to the central core. The lesions also contain lymphocytes, predominantly of the T-cell type. The central core contains necrotic debris, is rich in extracellular lipid, and often is vascularized by an ingrowth of vessels from the vasa vasorum. Atherosclerotic plaques are associated with medial degeneration and weakening, as well as adventitial fibrosis with lymphocytic infiltrates. Thus, established atherosclerosis involves all three layers of the vessel wall. The inflammatory component of the lesions is of biologic and potential clinical significance.[31]

The relationship of the early lesions to the plaques of established atherosclerosis is a complex phenomenon.[1–13] The early vascular lesions do not produce significant focal thickening, lack necrosis, and are reversible. In contrast, plaques produce focal intimal thickening, usually have necrotic cores, and are less easily reversible. A plausible hypothesis is that some fatty streaks progress to intermediate fibrofatty lesions and then into atherosclerotic plaques. There is a general similarity in the distribution of preatherosclerotic lesions and initial stages of atherosclerosis. The lesions tend to form around branch points and in other areas of nonlaminar blood flow. This emphasizes the influence of hemodynamic factors in pathogenesis. Early atherosclerotic lesions tend to form in areas of low shear stress adjacent to zones of high shear. It is thought that activation of blood cells may occur in zones of high shear and turbulent flow and that the activated cells are primed to interact with endothelium in areas of reduced blood movement in zones of low shear and flow.[32, 33]

EARLY EVENTS IN ATHEROSCLEROSIS

Atherogenesis involves complex interactions between the vessel wall and soluble and formed elements of the blood

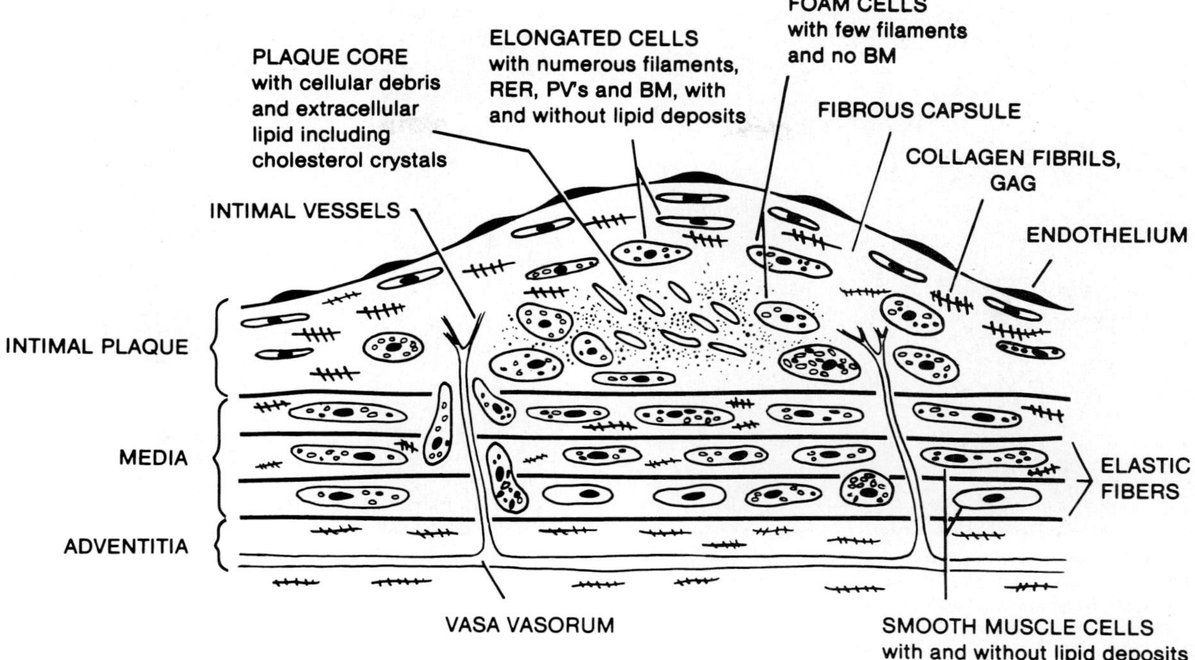

FIGURE 70–4 Diagram of an atherosclerotic plaque. The plaque is lined with endothelial cells and is composed of a fibrous capsule and a core containing necrotic tissue and extracellular lipid. The plaque is vascularized by vessels derived from the vasa vasorum. Lipid deposits are present in elongated cells, which are typical of altered smooth muscle cells. These cells have numerous filaments, rough-surface endoplasmic reticulum (RER), pinocytotic vessels (PVs), and a basement membrane (BM). Lipid deposits are also present in ovoid foam cells, which have few filaments and no basement membrane, consistent with macrophage origin. Medial smooth muscle cells also may contain lipid deposits. Extracellular components of the plaque include numerous collagen fibrils and deposits of glycosaminoglycans (GAG) and some elastic fibers. (From Buja LM, Kovanen PT, Bilheimer DW: Cellular pathology of homozygous familial hypercholesterolemia. Am J Pathol 97:327–357, 1979.)

(Figs. 70–5 to 70–9).[1–8] Important factors in the initiation and growth of plaques are (1) endothelial injury or dysfunction, (2) monocyte/macrophage accumulation, (3) influx of T-lymphocytes, (4) platelet aggregation and attachment, (5) smooth muscle proliferation, (6) influx of plasma LDL, (7) oxidation and/or other local modification of LDL, (8) progressive lipid accumulation in foam cells from uptake of modified LDL and secondary extracellular lipid deposition, and (9) hemodynamic influences related to blood pressure and pattern of blood flow.

The response to injury hypothesis, as synthesized by Ross,[3, 4] represents a contemporary integration of the insudation theory of Virchow and the encrustation theory of Rokitansky. This hypothesis emphasizes a primary role for endothelial injury. An alternate theory, proposed by Benditt, has emphasized a primary role for monoclonal smooth muscle proliferation induced by mutagenic events.[34, 35] The evidence supports an important role for smooth muscle proliferation but not necessarily on a monoclonal basis.[36–38] Previous concepts of early atherogenesis, which were based

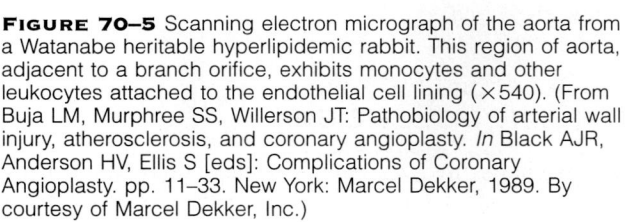

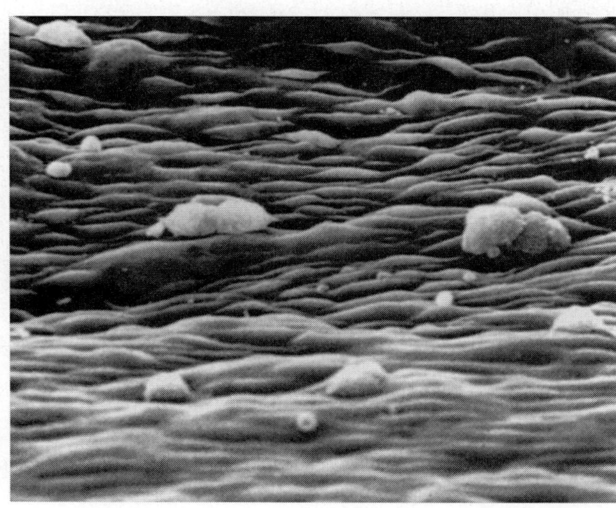

FIGURE 70–5 Scanning electron micrograph of the aorta from a Watanabe heritable hyperlipidemic rabbit. This region of aorta, adjacent to a branch orifice, exhibits monocytes and other leukocytes attached to the endothelial cell lining (×540). (From Buja LM, Murphree SS, Willerson JT: Pathobiology of arterial wall injury, atherosclerosis, and coronary angioplasty. *In* Black AJR, Anderson HV, Ellis S [eds]: Complications of Coronary Angioplasty. pp. 11–33. New York: Marcel Dekker, 1989. By courtesy of Marcel Dekker, Inc.)

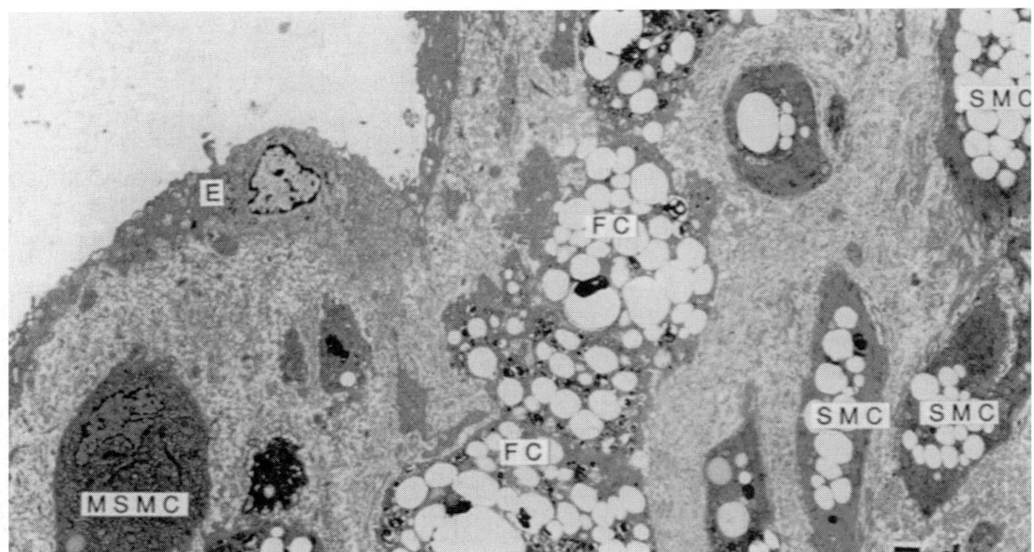

FIGURE 70–6 Electron micrograph of an advanced intimal lesion from a 6-month-old Watanabe heritable hyperlipidemic rabbit. The lesion is lined with endothelium (E). The lesion contains typical smooth muscle cells (SMC) with lipid deposits, foam cells (FC), and a modified smooth muscle cell (MSMC). Bar, 1μm. (From Buja LM, Kita T, Goldstein JL, et al: Cellular pathology of progressive atherosclerosis in the WHHL rabbit, an animal model of familial hypercholesterolemia. Arteriosclerosis 3:87, 1983.)

on models of traumatic endothelial denudation, have been supplanted by concepts derived from models that involve more subtle forms of endothelial injury. Early endothelial injury is generally characterized by modulation of endothelial cell function without loss of cells. Chronic repetitive endothelial injury is important in lesion progression. Injurious factors can include hypertension[39]; high circulating levels of LDL, lipoprotein(a), and other atherogenic lipids,[1–6, 18, 40–46] components of cigarette smoke,[1–6] high levels of homocysteine,[21–23] immunologic mechanisms,[47–50] and inflammatory injury induced by herpesviruses and *Chlamydia.*[24–29] Considerable information has come from studies of hypercholesterolemic animals, including cholesterol-fed animals and the Watanabe heritable hyperlipidemia rabbit, an animal model of human familial hypercholesterolemia[1, 11–13] (see Figs. 70–5 to 70–8).

Vascular integrity is critically dependent on endothelial function, which is complex and multifactorial. The endothelium is a major source of humoral mediators,[3–8] including antithrombotic as well as prothrombotic factors[19, 20]; cytokines, growth factors, and vasodilatory factors, including prostacyclin and endothelium-derived relaxing factor (EDRF) (i.e., nitric oxide [NO]); and vasoconstrictors, including endothelin[51–54] (Tables 70–1 to 70–3). The regulation of these mediators of opposing functions is related to the constitutive state of the endothelium versus an activated

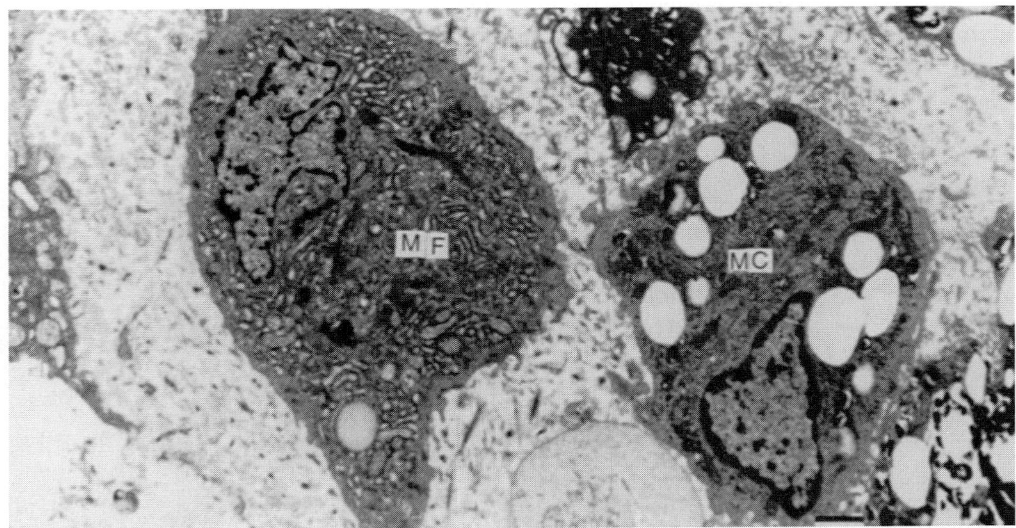

FIGURE 70–7 Modified smooth muscle cell (MF) and macrophage (MC) form aortic lesion of a Watanabe heritable hyperlipidemic rabbit. Both cells exhibit early lipid accumulation.

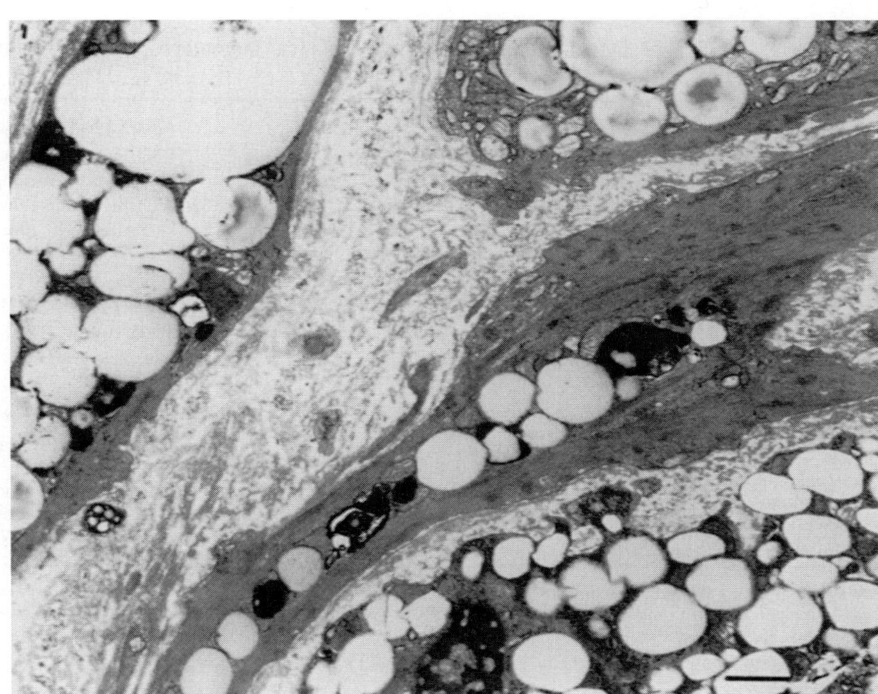

FIGURE 70–8 Smooth muscle cells containing lipid droplets from aortic lesion of a Watanabe heritable hyperlipidemic rabbit. Bar, 1 μm.

state that can be induced by various mediators (Table 70–4). In general, normal endothelium tends to be in a mode favoring vasodilation, antithrombosis, and fibrinolysis.[5, 19, 20] Conversely, in diseased arteries, endothelial injury can focally shift the balance toward vasoconstriction and thrombosis. In such arteries, the thrombotic process is initiated by platelet aggregation with secondary activation of the coagulation cascade. Complex interactions among the endothelium, platelets, and coagulation factors then follow. For example, activation of thrombin receptors can stimulate further platelet aggregation.

Mechanisms of gene activation involved in endothelial function are under active investigation.[55–57] Activation of the transcription factor nuclear factor-kappa B is a key

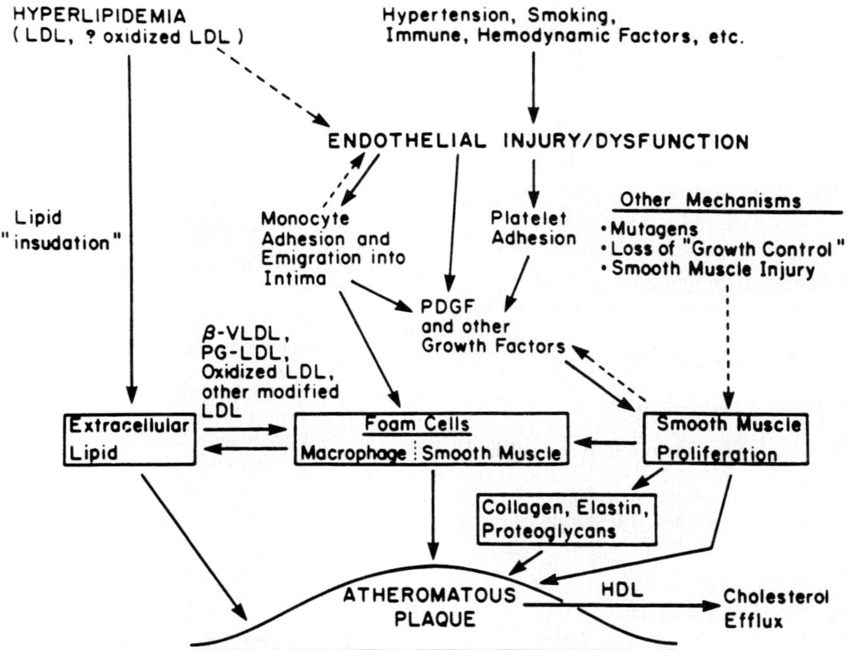

FIGURE 70–9 Diagram of postulated sequence of events and cellular interactions in atherogenesis. HDL, high-density lipoprotein; LDL, low-density lipoprotein; PG-LDL, proteoglycan–low-density protein. (From Cotran RS, Munro JM: Pathogenesis of atherosclerosis: recent concepts. *In* Grundy SM, Bearn AG [eds]: The Role of Cholesterol in Atherosclerosis: New Therapeutic Opportunities. p. 5. Philadelphia: Hanley & Belfus, 1988.)

TABLE 70–1 Cytokines, Hormones, and Chemical Mediators Potentially Operative in Cellular Responses in Injured Vessels

Endothelial cells	*Monocytes/macrophages (Continued)*
Prothrombotic factors (von Willebrand and others)	C5a (complement fragment C5a)
Antithrombotic factors (tissue-type plasminogen activator and others)	TGF-α (transforming growth factor-alpha)
IL-1 (interleukin-1) and other interleukins	TGF-β (transforming growth factor-beta)
TNF (tumor necrosis factor)	FGF (fibroblast growth factor)
MCAF (monocyte chemoattractant protein-1) and other monocyte factors	G M-CSF (granulocyte macrophage colony stimulating factor)
PGI_2 (prostacyclin)	*Platelets*
PAF (platelet-activating factor)	PDGF
PDGF (platelet-derived growth factor)	TXA_2 (thromboxane A_2)
EDRF (endothelium-derived relaxing factor)	Leukotrienes
EDHF (endothelium-derived hyperpolarizing factor)	Serotonin
EDCFs (endothelium-derived constricting factors, including endothelin)	*Smooth muscle cells*
Monocytes/macrophages	IL-1 and other interleukins
IL-1	TNF
TNF	MCAF and other monocyte factors
PAF	PDGF-like molecules
MDGF (macrophage-derived growth factor, i.e., PDGF-like molecule)	Prostaglandins

Modified from Buja LM, Murphree SS, Willerson JT: Pathobiology of arterial wall injury, atherosclerosis, and coronary angioplasty. *In* Black AJR, Anderson HV, Ellis S (eds): Complications of Coronary Angioplasty, pp. 11–33. New York: Marcel Dekker, 1989. By courtesy of Marcel Dekker, Inc.

event in the subsequent activation of physiologically important genes and gene products (Tables 70–5 and 70–6). NO production may be an important regulator of nuclear factor-κB activation.[58, 59] NO can inhibit the expression of adhesion molecules on the endothelial cell surface. Endothelial dysfunction can be determined by a decrease in endothelial NO activity, whereas endothelial activation is characterized by the expression of cellular adhesion molecules. Biomechanical forces generated by blood flow also act as important modulators of regional endothelial gene expression, phenotype, and function.[58–61]

Leukocyte-Endothelial Interactions

An important early event in lesion development is the adhesion of blood monocytes and platelets to the endothelial surface and the entry of monocytes into the intima.[3–8] Leukocyte recruitment involves the contributions of both adhesion and signaling molecules (Tables 70–7 and 70–8).[3–8, 55–71] Receptors called *selectins* mediate the transient adhesion of leukocytes to regionally activated endothelium. This is followed by activation of the loosely adherent leukocytes, with subsequent up-regulation of other molecules known as *integrins,* which increase adhesion and mediate emigration. The selectins are membrane proteins that interact with carbohydrate ligands on cell surfaces. E- and P-selectins are expressed on activated endothelium and bind the myeloid cells and subsets of lymphocytes. L-selectin is expressed on most leukocytes and binds to inducible ligands expressed on endothelium. However, firmer adhesion requires the interactions of leukocyte integrins with receptors on the endothelial cells, including intercellular adhesion molecule (ICAM)-1, ICAM-2, and vascular cell adhesion molecule-1. All leukocytes express

TABLE 70–2 Functions of Endothelial Cells

- Hemocompatibility
  - Anticoagulant, antithrombotic, profibrinolytic properties
  - Opposite properties—inducible
- Inflammatory and immune reactions
  - Leukocyte interactions
  - Expression of genes encoding for inflammatory mediators, including cytokines
  - Expression of histocompatibility or transplantation antigens
    - Class I (human leukocyte antigen-A, -B, and -C)—constitutive
    - Class II (HLA-DR, DP, and DQ)—inducible
- Production of growth regulatory factors
  - Platelet-derived and other growth factors
- Mechanical (flow and stretch)—biochemical coupling
- Regulation of vascular tone
  - Vasodilatation (nitric oxide)
  - Vasoconstriction (endothelins)

For a review, see Libby P, Schoen FJ: Vascular lesion formation. Cardiovasc Pathol 2(Suppl):43S–52S, 1993.

TABLE 70–3 Antithrombotic and Procoagulant Products of Endothelial Cells

Antithrombotic

- Plasminogen activators (tissue type, urokinase type)
- Prostacyclin
- Thrombomodulin
- Protein S
- Lipoprotein-associated coagulation inhibitor
- Glycosaminoglycans (heparan sulfate)

Procoagulant

- von Willebrand factor
- Factor V
- Plasminogen activator inhibitors 1 and 2

After In Vitro Stimulation

- Tissue factor
- Macrophage chemotaxin
- Macrophage adhesion receptors

From Tanaka K, Sueishi K: The coagulation and fibrinolysis systems and atherosclerosis. Lab Invest 69(1):5–18, 1993.

one or more of the three beta$_2$-integrins; mononuclear cells, eosinophils, and basophils also express the alpha$_4$ beta$_1$- or alpha$_4$ beta$_7$-integrins. Leukocyte activation increases the avidity of the immunoglobulin-like counterreceptors on the endothelial surface. Thus, leukocyte adhesion receptors implicated in recruitment include the β_2-integrins (leukocyte functional antigen-1, Mo-1/MAC-1, and p150,95), the β-integrin very late antigen-4, and L-selectin. The inducible endothelial adhesion receptors include the ICAMs, vascular cell adhesion molecule-1, and the two other members of the selectin family, E-selectin and P-selectin.[8, 66, 67]

Several chemical mediators are known to influence the expression of these molecules (see Tables 70–1 and 70–8).[3–8] Some agents, such as complement fragment 5a (C5a) and leukotriene B_4, act on leukocytes; others, including interleukin 1 and endotoxin, act on endothelial cells, and still others, such as tissue necrosis factor, act on both.[68, 69] Antibodies to leukocyte adhesion molecules can block the attachment and migration of monocytes and neutrophils in inflammatory states. It is possible that hypercholesterolemia heightens the expression of leukocyte adhesion molecules on monocytes, causes the expression of endothelial-leukocyte attachment molecules on endothelium, or both. The monocytes become macrophages that release growth factors that stimulate smooth muscle proliferation. It is also likely that hypercholesterolemia-induced alterations in vascular tone contribute to atherogenesis.[51–54]

PLAQUE GROWTH

The growth of atherosclerotic plaques involves the continued accumulation of macrophages and lymphocytes, proliferation of smooth muscle cells, and accumulation of lipid in the intima. Cytokines and growth factors mediate smooth muscle proliferation via paracrine and autocrine pathways (Table 70–9).[3–8] A key factor in local cellular lipid accumulation is the local formation of oxidized LDL and other forms of altered LDL.[41–46] This altered LDL can be taken up progressively via the scavenger receptor pathway into vascular cells. This pathway is not subject to feedback inhibition as is the LDL pathway. The intimal alterations are accompanied by progressive degeneration and weakening of the media and lymphocytic infiltration of the adventitia. Plaques develop a considerable content of collagen and glycosaminoglycans and some elastin. These matrix components are synthesized by smooth muscle cells. Repetitive endothelial injury, including patchy endothelial denudation, is important in the growth of plaques. This in turn leads to platelet aggregation and attachment with release of platelet-derived growth factor and other platelet products and further smooth muscle proliferation.[51–54, 70] Progressive intimal thickening leads to the development of hypoxia in the depths of the plaque in and around the intimal-medial junction. The hypoxia probably serves as an important initiating factor for necrosis of foam cells and release of their lipids and the vascularization of the plaques by the ingrowth of vessels from the vasa vasorum.[72] Local influence of vascular growth factors also is likely involved in

TABLE 70–4 Types of Endothelial Activation Programs

Stimulus	Response
Interleukin-1, tumor necrosis factor	Increase leukocyte adhesion molecules (~4 hours) Decrease blood compatibility Induce nitric oxide synthesis Decrease growth Increase cytokine, growth factor expression Increase prostanoid production
Thrombin	Increases PDGF, E-selectin gene expression
Platelet-activating factor	Increases P-selectin expression (minutes)
Interferon-gamma	Increases ICAM-1 expression (~24 hours) Induces nitric oxide synthesis Increases histocompatibility gene expression
Heparin-binding growth factors (acidic and basic FGF)	Stimulate proliferation
Shear	Activates an inward-rectifying K channel
Stretch	Activates a nonselective ion channel
Hypoxia	Increases PDGF gene expression Induces specific hypoxia-related genes of unknown function

Abbreviations: FGF, fibroblast growth factors; ICAM-1, intercellular adhesion molecule 1; PDGF, platelet-derived growth factor.
From Libby P, Schoen FJ: Vascular lesion formation. Cardiovasc Pathol 2(suppl):43S–52S, 1993. With permission from Elsevier Science.

TABLE 70–5 Genes Requiring Nuclear Factor-κB for Transactivation

Cellular adhesion molecules
- Intercellular adhesion molecule-1
- Vascular cell adhesion molecule-1
- Endothelial leukocyte adhesion molecule-1 (ELAM-1)

Inflammatory cytokines
- Interleukin-2, -6, and -8
- Tumor necrosis factor-α and -β
- Macrophage-colony stimulating factor (colony stimulating factor-1)
- Granulocyte colony stimulating factor
- Granulocyte macrophage-colony stimulating factor
- Interferon-β
- Tissue factor
- Macrophage chemotactic protein-1

Immunologic mediators
- Immunoglobulin (IgG) κ light chain
- T-cell receptor α and β chain
- Major histocompatibility complex class I
- Major histocompatibility complex class II invariant-chain (Ii)
- β_2-Microglobulin
- Type II inducible nitric oxide synthase

Viral enhancers
- Human immunodeficiency virus-1
- Cytomegalovirus
- Adenovirus
- Simian virus 40

Transcription factors
- IκB-α
- c-Rel
- NF-κB p105
- c-*myc*
- Interferon regulatory factor-1

Adapted from Liao JK, Libby P: Nitric oxide and gene transcription. *In* Rubanyi GM (ed): Pathophysiology and Clinical Applications of Nitric Oxide. Chur, Switzerland: Harwood Academic, 1999.

TABLE 70-6 **Factors That Activate Nuclear Factor-κB**

Inflammatory mediators	*Oxidants*
Tumor necrosis factor-α	Hydrogen peroxide
Interleukin-1 and -2	Ultraviolet light
Lymphotoxin	*Drugs*
Leukotriene B_4	Phorbolesters
Growth factors	Okadaic acid
Platelet-derived growth factor	Cycloheximide
Transforming growth factor-β_1	Anisomycin
Viral mediators	Pervanadate
Viral infection (human immunodeficiency virus, Epstein-Barr virus, cytomegalovirus, and so on)	*Physical stress*
Double-stranded RNA	Laminar shear stress
Epstein-Barr nuclear antigen-2	Stretch
Bacterial mediators	Cyclic strain
Lipopolysaccharide	
Muramyl proteins	
Exotoxin B	

Adapted from Liao JK, Libby P: Nitric oxide and gene transcription. *In* Rubanyi GM (ed): Pathophysiology and Clinical Applications of Nitric Oxide. Chur, Switzerland: Harwood Academic, 1999.

TABLE 70-7 **Some Molecules Involved in Endothelial-Leukocyte Adhesion**

Endothelial Surface	Leukocyte Surface
Selectins	
E-selectin	Sialyl-Lewis X, or Lewis X (CD15 glycoconjugate)
P-selectin	Sialyl-Lewis X, or Lewis X (CD15 glycoconjugate)
Immunoglobulin superfamily	
Intercellular adhesion molecule 1 (CD-1, CD54)	Leukocyte function antigen 1, (Mac 1 (CD11b/CD18) (CD11a/CD18, a β_2 integrin heterodimer)
Intercellular adhesion molecule 2	CD11a/CD18, a β_2 integrin heterodimer
Vascular cell adhesion molecule 1	Very late antigen 4 (CD 49d/CD 29) (a β_1 integrin)
Platelet-endothelial cell adhesion molecule-1 (CD31)	May bind to itself or other ligands

From Libby P, Schoen FJ: Vascular lesion formation. Cardiovasc Pathol 2(suppl):43S–52S, 1993. With permission from Elsevier Science.

TABLE 70-8 **Some Cytokines Produced by Vascular Endothelium and Smooth Muscle**

Cytokine	Typical Actions
Interleukin-1, tumor necrosis factor	Pyrogens Immunostimulators Endothelial and smooth muscle activators Induce nitric oxide synthesis
Interleukin 6	B- and T-lymphocyte activator
Interleukin 8	Neutrophil chemoattractant and activator Leukocyte adhesion inhibitor
Monocyte chemoattractant protein-1 (MCAF, JE [murine homolog])	Mononuclear phagocyte stimulator
Granulocyte monocyte-CSF	Hematopoietic growth factor
Monocyte-CSF (CSF-1)	Mononuclear phagocyte stimulator

Abbreviations: CSF, colony stimulating factor; MCAF, monocyte chemoattractant and stimulating factor.
From Libby P, Schoen FJ: Vascular lesion formation: Cardiovasc Pathol 2(suppl):43S–52S, 1993. With permission from Elsevier Science.

TABLE 70-9 Types of Smooth Muscle Activation Programs

Stimulus	Response
PDGF	Increases growth Stimulates migration Increases matrix synthesis
IL-1, tumor necrosis factor	Increases growth Increases cytokine, growth factor expression: (PDGF, basic FGF, IL-6, IL-8, MCAF, CSFs) Induce nitric oxide synthesis
Interferon-γ	Decreases growth Induces nitric oxide synthesis Increases histocompatibility gene expression
Heparin-binding growth factors (acidic and basic FGF)	Increases growth
Transforming growth factor-β	Increases interstitial collagen synthesis Variable effects on growth
Stretch	Increase matrix synthesis
Crush injury	Releases basic FGF

Abbreviations: CSF, colony stimulating factor; FGF, fibroblast growth factor; IL, interleukin; MCAF, monocyte chemoattractant and stimulating factor (MCP-1/JE); PDGF, platelet-derived growth factor.
From Libby P, Schoen FJ: Vascular lesion formation. Cardiovasc Pathol 2(suppl):43S–52S, 1993. With permission from Elsevier Science.

the vascularization of plaques.[73–75] Dystrophic calcification of the necrotic lipid frequently occurs. The vessels in the cores of the plaques are a source of petechial hemorrhages and leakage of plasma. These blood components contribute to lipid accumulation in the plaques. The major form of the intracellular lipid is esterified cholesterol, whereas the extracellular lipid is composed of free and esterified cholesterol and phospholipid, which is largely derived from necrosis of foam cells.

Disease progression results in atherosclerotic plaques that contain varying amounts of fibrous and lipid components. Hard plaque is composed predominantly of fibrous tissue, soft plaques, or atheromas and has a thin fibrous capsule that covers a core of necrotic, lipid-rich material. It is these atheromas that are susceptible to clinically important complications. Glagov and associates[33] have shown that as a result of medial weakening, there is significant remodeling and dilatation of coronary arteries as intimal lesions progress, such that the luminal diameter of the vessel is maintained until severe atherosclerotic involvement has occurred. However, the disease eventually leads to progressive encroachment on the luminal area.

The development of secondary changes (complications) in atherosclerotic lesions is directly linked to the development of clinical manifestations of atherosclerosis, including coronary artery disease. The most important complication is the development of major alterations of the surface of the plaque. These alterations are characterized by fissuring, ulceration, or rupture of the luminal surface of the plaque and are often associated with major hemorrhage into the plaque. The surface changes predispose to platelet aggregation and thrombosis, which are major mechanisms of induction of ischemic heart disease. The detailed relationships between complications of coronary atherosclerosis and ischemic heart disease are discussed in other chapters.

REFERENCES

1. Wissler RW, Vesselinovitch D, Getz GS: Abnormalities of the arterial wall and its metabolism in atherogenesis. Prog Cardiovasc Dis 18:341–369, 1976.
2. Willerson JT, Hillis LD, Buja LM: Pathogenesis and pathology of ischemic heart disease. *In* Ischemic Heart Disease: Clinical and Pathophysiological Aspects. pp. 7–83. New York: Raven, 1982.
3. Ross R: The pathogenesis of atherosclerosis—an update. N Engl J Med 314:488–500, 1986.
4. Ross R: The pathogenesis of atherosclerosis: a perspective for the 1990s. Nature 362:801–809, 1993.
5. Munro JM, Cotran RS: The pathogenesis of atherosclerosis: atherogenesis and inflammation. Lab Invest 58:249–261, 1988.
6. Cotran RS, Munro JM: Pathogenesis of atherosclerosis: recent concepts. *In* Grundy SM, Bearn AG (eds): The Role of Cholesterol in Atherosclerosis: New Therapeutic Opportunities. p. 5. Philadelphia: Hanley & Belfus, 1988.
7. Libby P, Schoen FJ: Vascular lesion formation. Cardiovasc Pathol 2(suppl):43S–52S, 1993.
8. Buja LM, Murphree SS, Willerson JT: Pathobiology of arterial wall injury, atherosclerosis, and coronary angioplasty. *In* Black AJR, Anderson HV, Ellis S (eds): Complications of Coronary Angioplasty. pp. 11–33. New York: Marcel Decker, 1989.
9. Haust MD: The morphogenesis and fate of potential and early atherosclerotic lesions in man. Hum Pathol 2:1–29, 1971.
10. Pearson TA, Kramer EC, Solez K, Heptinstall RH: The human atherosclerotic plaque. Am J Pathol 86:657–664, 1977.
11. Buja LM, Kovanen PT, Bilheimer DW: Cellular pathology of homozygous familial hypercholesterolemia. Am J Pathol 97:327–357, 1979.
12. Buja LM, Kita T, Goldstein JL, et al: Cellular pathology of progressive atherosclerosis in the WHHL rabbit, an animal model of familial hypercholesterolemia. Arteriosclerosis 3:87–101, 1983.
13. Buja LM, Clubb FJ Jr, Bilheimer DW, Willerson JT: Pathobiology of human familial hypercholesterolemia and a related animal model, the Watanabe heritable hyperlipidemic rabbit. Eur Heart J 11(suppl E):41–52, 1990.
14. Kannel WB: Contributions of the Framingham study to the conquest of coronary artery disease. Am J Cardiol 62:1109–1112, 1988.
15. Neaton JD, Wentworth D: Serum cholesterol, blood pressure, cigarette smoking and death from coronary heart disease: overall findings and differences by age for 316,099 white men. Arch Intern Med 152:56–64, 1992.
16. Malcom GT, Oalmann MC, Strong JP: Risk factors for atherosclerosis in young subjects: the PDAY study. Ann N Y Acad Sci 817:179–188, 1997.
17. Reddy KS, Yusuf S: Emerging epidemic of cardiovascular disease in developing countries. Circulation 97:569–601, 1998.
18. Goldstein JL, Brown MS: Atherosclerosis: the low-density lipoprotein receptor hypothesis. Metabolism 26:1257–1275, 1977.
19. Broze GJ Jr: Endothelial injury, coagulation and atherosclerosis. Coron Artery Dis 2:131–140, 1991.

20. Tanaka K, Sueishi K: The coagulation and fibrinolysis systems and atherosclerosis. Lab Invest 69:5–18, 1993.
21. McCully KS: Vascular pathology of homocysteinemia: implications for the pathogenesis of atherosclerosis. Am J Pathol 56:111–128, 1969.
22. Boushey CJ, Beresford SA, Omenn GS, Motulsky AG: A quantitative assessment of plasma homocysteine as a risk factor for vascular disease: probable benefits of increasing folic acid intakes. JAMA 274:1049–1057, 1995.
23. Graham IM, Daly LE, Refsum HM, et al: Plasma homocysteine as a risk factor for vascular disease: the European concerted action project. JAMA 277:1775–1781, 1997.
24. Hajjar DP: Viral pathogenesis of atherosclerosis: impact of molecular mimicry and viral genes. Am J Pathol 139:1195–1211, 1991.
25. Buja LM: Does atherosclerosis have an infectious etiology? [editorial]. Circulation 94:872–873, 1996.
26. Nieto FJ, Adam E, Sorlie P, et al: Cohort study of cytomegalovirus infection as a risk factor for carotid intimal-medial thickening, a measure of subclinical atherosclerosis. Circulation 94:922–927, 1996.
27. Davidson M, Kuo CC, Middaugh JP, et al: Confirmed previous infection with *Chlamydia pneumoniae* (TWAR) and its presence in early coronary atherosclerosis. Circulation 98:628–633, 1998.
28. Meier CR, Derby LE, Jick SS, et al: Antibiotics and risk of subsequent first-time acute myocardial infarction. JAMA 281:427–431, 1999.
29. Folsom AR: Antibiotics for prevention of myocardial infarction? Not yet! JAMA 281:461–462, 1999.
30. Bini A, Fenoglio JJ Jr, Mesa-Tejada R, et al: Identification and distribution of fibrinogen, fibrin, and fibrin(ogen) degradation products in atherosclerosis: use of monoclonal antibodies. Arteriosclerosis 9:109–121, 1989.
31. Casscells W, Hathorn B, David M, et al: Thermal detection of cellular infiltrates in living atherosclerotic plaques: possible implications for plaque rupture and thrombosis. Lancet 347:1447–1451, 1996.
32. Zand T, Nunnari JJ, Hoffman AH, et al: Endothelial adaptations in aortic stenosis: correlation with flow parameters. Am J Pathol 133:407–418, 1988.
33. Glagov S, Zarins C, Giddens DP, Ku DN: Hemodynamics and atherosclerosis: insight and perspectives gained from studies of human arteries. Arch Pathol Lab Med 112:1018–1031, 1988.
34. Benditt EP, Benditt JM: Evidence for a monoclonal origin of human atherosclerotic plaques. Proc Natl Acad Sci U S A 70:1753–1756, 1973.
35. Pearson TA, Wang A, Solez K, Heptinstall RH: Clonal characteristics of fibrous plaques and fatty streaks from human aortas. Am J Pathol 81:379–388, 1975.
36. Thomas WA, Reiner JM, Janakidevi K, et al: Population dynamics of arterial cells during atherogenesis, X: study of monotypism in atherosclerotic lesions of black women heterozygous for glucose-6-phosphate dehydrogenase (G-6-PD). Exp Mol Pathol 31:367–386, 1979.
37. Thomas WA, Kim DN: Atherosclerosis as a hyperplastic and/or neoplastic process. Lab Invest 48:245–255, 1983.
38. Parkes JL, Cardell RR, Hubbard FC Jr, et al: Cultured human atherosclerotic plaque smooth muscle cells retain transforming potential and display enhanced expression of the *myc* protooncogene. Am J Pathol 138:765–775, 1991.
39. Bondjers G, Glukhova M, Hansson GK, et al: Hypertension and atherosclerosis: cause and effect, or two effects with one unknown cause? Circulation 84(suppl VI):VI-2–VI-16, 1991.
40. Genest J Jr, Jenner JL, McNamara JR, et al: Prevalence of lipoprotein(a) [Lp(a)] excess in coronary artery disease. Am J Cardiol 67:1039–1145, 1991.
41. Steinberg D, Parthasarathy S, Carew TE, et al: Modifications of low-density lipoprotein that increase its artherogenicity. N Engl J Med 320:915–924, 1989.
42. Berliner JA, Navab M, Fogelman AM, et al: Atherosclerosis: basic mechanisms: oxidation, inflammation, and genetics. Circulation 91:2488–2496, 1995.
43. Navab M, Berliner JA, Watson AD, et al: The yin and yang of oxidation in the development of the fatty streak: a review based on the 1994 George Lyman Duff Memorial Lecture. Arterioscler Thromb Vasc Biol 16:831–842, 1996.
44. Sattar N, Petrie JR, Jaap AJ: The atherogenic lipoprotein phenotype and vascular endothelial dysfunction. Atherosclerosis 138:229–235, 1998.
45. Tardif JC, Coté G, Lespérance J, et al: Probucol and multivitamins in the prevention of restenosis after coronary angioplasty. N Engl J Med 337:365–372, 1997.
46. Diaz MN, Frei B, Vita JA, Keaney JF Jr: Antioxidants and atherosclerotic heart disease. N Engl J Med 337:408–416, 1997.
47. Tilney NL, Whitley WD, Diamond JR, et al: Chronic rejection: an undefined conundrum. Transplantation 52:389–398, 1991.
48. Hruban RH, Beschorner WE, Baumgartner WA, et al: Accelerated arteriosclerosis in heart transplant recipients is associated with a T-lymphocyte-mediated endothelialitis. Am J Pathol 137:871–882, 1990.
49. Salomon RN, Hughes CC, Schoen FJ, et al: Human coronary transplantation-associated arteriosclerosis: evidence for a chronic immune reaction to activated graft endothelial cells. Am J Pathol 138:791–798, 1991.
50. McDonald PC, Kenyon JA, McManus BM: The role of lipids in transplant vascular disease [minireview]. Lab Invest 78:1187–1201, 1998.
51. Hirsh PD, Campbell WB, Willerson JT, Hillis LD: Prostaglandins and ischemic heart disease. Am J Med 71:1009–1026, 1981.
52. Willerson JT, Golino P, Eidt J, et al: Specific platelet mediators and unstable coronary artery lesions: experimental evidence and potential clinical implications. Circulation 80:198–205, 1989.
53. Vanhoutte PM, Shimokawa H: Endothelium-derived relaxing factor and coronary vasospasm. Circulation 80:1–9, 1989.
54. Stein B, Fuster V, Israel DH, et al: Platelet inhibitor agents in cardiovascular disease: an update. J Am Coll Cardiol 14:813–836, 1989.
55. Collins T: Endothelial nuclear factor-κB and the initiation of the atherosclerotic lesion. Lab Invest 68:499–508, 1993.
56. Spiecker M, Peng HB, Liao JK: Inhibition of endothelial vascular cell adhesion molecule-1 expression by nitric oxide involves the induction and nuclear translocation of IκB-α. J Biol Chem 272:30969–30974, 1997.
57. Liao JK, Libby P: Nitric oxide and gene transcription. *In* Rubanyi GM (ed): Pathophysiology and Clinical Applications of Nitric Oxide. Chur, Switzerland: Harwood Academic, (in press).
58. Gimbrone MA Jr, Cybulsky MI, Kume N, et al: Vascular endothelium: an integrator of pathophysiological stimuli in atherogenesis. Ann N Y Acad Sci 748:122–131, 1995.
59. Gimbrone MA Jr, Nagel T, Topper JN: Biomechanical activation: an emerging paradigm in endothelial adhesion biology. J Clin Invest 99:1809–1813, 1997.
60. Davies PF: Flow-mediated endothelial mechanotransduction. Physiol Rev 75:519–560, 1995.
61. Topper JN, Cai J, Stavrakis G, et al: Human prostaglandin transporter gene (*h*PGT) is regulated by fluid mechanical stimuli in cultured endothelial cells and expressed in vascular endothelium in vivo. Circulation 98:2396–2403, 1998.
62. Harlan JM: Leukocyte-endothelial interactions. Blood 65:513–525, 1985.
63. Bevilacqua MP, Pober JS, Mendrick DL, et al: Identification of an inducible endothelial-leukocyte adhesion molecule, ELAM-1. Proc Natl Acad Sci U S A 84:9238–9242, 1987.
64. Cushing SD, Berliner JA, Valente AJ, et al: Minimally modified low-density lipoprotein induces monocyte chemotactic protein 1 in human endothelial cells and smooth muscle cells. Proc Natl Acad Sci U S A 87:5134–5138, 1990.
65. Yu X, Dluz S, Graves DT, et al: Elevated expression of monocyte chemoattractant protein 1 by vascular smooth muscle cells in hypercholesterolemic primates. Proc Natl Acad Sci U S A 89:6953–6957, 1992.
66. McEver RP: Misguided leukocyte adhesion. J Clin Invest 91:2340–2341, 1993.
67. Grober JS, Bowen BL, Ebling H, et al: Monocyte-endothelial adhesion in chronic rheumatoid arthritis: in situ detection of selectin and integrin-dependent interactions. J Clin Invest 91:2609–2619, 1993.
68. Williams SK: Regulation of intimal hyperplasia: do endothelial cells participate? Lab Invest 64:721–723, 1991.
69. Clinton SK, Fleet JC, Loppnow H, et al: Interleukin-1 gene expression in rabbit vascular tissue in vivo. Am J Pathol 138:1005–1014, 1991.
70. Jawien A, Bowen-Pope DF, Lindner V, et al: Platelet-derived growth

factor promotes smooth muscle migration and intimal thickening in a rat model of balloon angioplasty. J Clin Invest 89:507–511, 1992.

71. Jang Y, Lincoff AM, Plow EF, Topol EJ: Cell adhesion molecules in coronary artery disease. J Am Coll Cardiol 24:1591–1601, 1994.
72. Bennett MR, Boyle JJ: Apoptosis of vascular smooth muscle cells in atherosclerosis. Atherosclerosis 138:3–9, 1998.
73. Folkman J: Clinical applications of research on angiogenesis (Seminars in Medicine of the Beth Israel Hospital, Boston). N Engl J Med 333:1757–1763, 1995.
74. Folkman J, D'Amore PA: Blood vessel formation: what is its molecular basis? Cell 87:1153–1155, 1996.
75. Folkman J: Angiogenic therapy of the human heart. Circulation 97:628–629, 1998.

CHAPTER 71

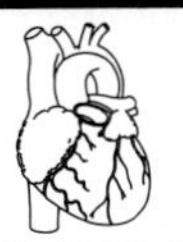

Atherosclerosis: Pathogenesis, Morphology, and Risk Factors

Antonio M. Gotto, Jr., and John Farmer

INTRODUCTION
PATHOGENESIS
Monoclonal Hypothesis
Infectious and Inflammatory Hypothesis
Lipid Hypothesis
Response to Injury
MORPHOLOGIC LESIONS
Type I Lesion
Type II Lesion
Type III Lesion
Type IV Lesion
Type V Lesion
Type VI Lesion
Type VII Lesion
Type VIII Lesion
RISK FACTORS
Major Risk Factors
Minor Risk Factors
CONCLUSION

Introduction

Despite an encouraging decline in age-adjusted morbidity and mortality, atherosclerosis remains the major cause of morbidity and mortality in the United States. The clinical manifestations of coronary atherosclerosis are gradually shifting to an older age group, and the absolute number of cardiovascular deaths in the United States is increasing. The complications of coronary, cerebral, and peripheral vascular disease account for approximately 50 percent of all-cause mortality in the United States and are associated with an economic burden of approximately $300 billion dollars per year when hospitalization, therapeutic intervention, and lost productivity are considered.[1]

Atherosclerosis is a syndrome with a multifactorial etiology, and a unifying hypothesis that explains all aspects of the process is lacking because the precise underlying mechanisms resulting in occlusive vascular disease remain unclear. The concept of risk factor identification and modification has been popularized in vascular medicine. Numerous modifiable risk factors have been identified that are associated with an increase in the statistical risk for the development of atherosclerosis. However, the identification of plausible risk factors and their statistical relation to risk for coronary heart disease does not necessarily prove a causal relation but may simply be a nonspecific marker of the pathophysiologic process that results in a specific condition. Criteria for determining whether a statistical association reflects causality include the strength of the association, as expressed by the relative risk of individuals exposed to a certain risk factor compared with individuals who have not been exposed; whether the association represents a dose-response relation, so that the relative risk is progressively increased at increasing levels of exposure to the factor; precedents of exposure to clinical onset of disease; consistency of results in different populations; independence of the association when other known risk factors are controlled for; predictivity of the disease incidence in different populations; and biologic plausibility.

A large body of epidemiologic and experimental evidence has identified an ever-expanding number of potential cardiac risk factors. Risk factors may be arbitrarily divided into major and minor or modifiable and nonmodifiable. The identification and stratification of the risk factor profile in an individual patient provide a method for identifying potential therapeutic interventions in an attempt to decrease risk for coronary heart disease and to improve quality and longevity of life.

Pathogenesis

Monoclonal Hypothesis

Benditt and Benditt[2] suggested that the origin of the smooth muscle cells within the atherosclerotic plaque is secondary to multiplication of a single clone of cells. Atherosclerosis may thus be similar to an unregulated neoplastic cellular growth rather than a response to vascular damage. Supporting evidence has come from numerous studies, including the finding of only one isozyme of glucose-6 phosphate dehydrogenase in atherosclerotic lesions from individuals with the genetic deficiency of this enzyme, which is compatible with the premise that the proliferation of one clone of cells is responsible for the cellular elements within the atherosclerotic plaque.

Infectious and Inflammatory Hypothesis

The concept of establishing the degree of cardiovascular risk by tabulation of the number and severity of conditions known to be statistically associated with increased rates for ischemic events has gained popularity in clinical medicine. However, a significant proportion of patients who have a documented acute myocardial infarction appear to be at relatively low risk when the commonly accepted modifiable risk factors are documented and stratified. The concept that infection and chronic inflammation may play a role in coronary disease has been popularized, although the concept is not new. Earlier histologic studies involving occlusive coronary artery lesions had demonstrated increased concentration of inflammatory cells, such as T lymphocytes and neutrophils within areas associated with plaque rupture.[3] Additionally, the early stages of atherosclerosis are characterized pathologically by an increased infiltration of inflammatory cellular elements into the involved area. Cytokines, which are associated with increased degrees of inflammation, aid in the migration of monocytes into the subendothelial space, which is also modulated by the production of a number of adhesion molecules that localize on the vascular endothelium and bind the circulating cellular elements associated with the early stages of atherosclerosis.[3]

Epidemiologic studies have attempted to correlate the presence and the degree of inflammatory markers with the severity of atherosclerosis. Large-scale epidemiologic trials are hampered by inability to control for potential confounding variables and frequently are designed as retrospective or case control studies, which are inherently limited as to the determination of causality. Considerable interest has been generated concerning the potential role of inflammation as correlated by the circulating level of C-reactive protein. The prospectively performed Physicians' Health Study evaluated the relationship between C-reactive protein and the risk of developing symptomatic coronary ischemia and stroke.[4] The Physicians' Health Study evaluated men who were clinically free of atherosclerosis and had no evidence of a prior myocardial infarction. Risk factor profiles were constructed, and the cohort was determined to be at relatively low risk by smoking rates and other demographic data. C-reactive protein level was determined, and the cohort was subsequently stratified into quartiles. Subjects whose C-reactive protein fell in the highest quartile had a doubling of the degree of risk for stroke and tripling of the risk for acute myocardial infarction, which were both statistically significant when compared with subjects in the lowest quartile for this nonspecific marker of systemic inflammation. The data from the Physicians' Health Study are in concordance with several epidemiologic trials that documented a higher level of C-reactive protein in patients with symptomatic coronary atherosclerosis. The Physicians' Health Study controlled for other risk factors and determined that the increased risk associated with increased levels of C-reactive protein was independent of lipid subfractions, fibrinogen, and smoking habits. The Physicians' Health Study, which was performed over an 8-year period, demonstrated that the increased prognostic significance of high levels of C-reactive protein was additive to the determination of cardiovascular risk by lipid levels. Subjects whose cholesterol and C-reactive proteins were both increased had a fivefold enhanced risk for future myocardial infarction. Although intriguing, the data from the Physicians' Health Study do not prove a definite cause and effect between increased inflammatory mediators and pathogenesis of atherosclerosis. Elevated C-reactive protein, fibrinogen, amyloid A, and other markers of acute phase reactants may represent an epiphenomenon, and the causal relation remains to be determined.

The role that infection potentially plays in atherosclerosis has been supported by several studies. *Helicobacter pylori,* cytomegalovirus, and chlamydia have all been postulated to be associated with increased risk for coronary atherosclerosis. Chlamydia are obligate intracellular bacteria which cannot replicate outside cells. *Chlamydia pneumoniae* has a global distribution, and infection most commonly occurs in children between the ages of 5 and 14 years.[5] Pathologic evidence has demonstrated the localization of the *C. pneumoniae* organism in specimens obtained from coronary atheroma. Chlamydia has also been observed by electron microscopy, immunocytochemical staining, and polymerase chain reaction. The presence of chronic chlamydia infection has also been correlated with serum lipid values in several clinical trials. The Helsinki Heart Study was a long-term primary prevention trial involving approximately 4000 dyslipidemic (as characterized by elevated non–high-density lipoprotein [HDL] cholesterol) men. Infection by *C. pneumoniae* was determined to be an independent risk factor for the development of coronary artery disease in a substudy of this trial.[6] Patients were stratified by the presence of immune complexes containing *C. pneumoniae* antigen or elevated immunoglobulin A titer against *C. pneumoniae* and were determined to be twice as likely to have an acute cardiac event that was independent of age, hypertension, and smoking.[7]

The epidemiologic studies involving serologic testing or epidemiologic analysis have generally been performed with a case-control design and not in a prospective manner. Epidemiologic studies of this type are difficult to interpret because of the potential for the presence of confounding factors. However, several treatment studies have been performed in survivors of acute myocardial infarction that provide further evidence of a potential role for infection in ischemic disease. Two hundred twenty male survivors of acute myocardial infarction were screened in a consecutive manner for the presence and magnitude of anti–*C. pneumoniae* antibodies.[8] Subjects were stratified into three groups on the basis of the detection and the level of circulating antibodies. Antibody titers were determined to be either absent, intermediate (1/8 to 1/32), and elevated (seropositive at > 1/64 dilution). Patients who had persisting seropositivity at a level of greater than 1/64 were subsequently randomly assigned to receive either oral azithromycin, 500 mg/day, or placebo. After 6 months of therapy, the anti–*C. pneumoniae* titer fell to less than 1/16 in 43 percent of patients receiving azithromycin, whereas only 10 percent who were randomly assigned to receive placebo were documented to have a decrease in antichlamydia titers. The azithromycin-treated group demonstrated a fivefold statistically significant reduction in cardiovascular events, with an odds ratio of 0.2. This was the first trial to assess the relation between elevated antichlamydia antibodies and clinical outcome after antibiotic treatment. The reduction in cardiovascular event rate was believed to be related possibly to alteration of the direct involvement of *C. pneumoniae* in atherogenesis. Chronic macrophage infection involving intracellular organisms has been postulated to contribute to an inflammatory process or to a procoagulant state via tissue factor expression.[8] The polysaccharide cell wall of chlamydia may also contribute to direct endothelial damage, and hypersensitivity to chlamydia may play a role in atherogenesis. Treatment with azithromycin was postulated to stabilize the vulnerable plaque lesion at least partially by altering inflammation or perhaps affecting other infections, such as *H. pylori.*

Roxithromycin was also studied in 202 patients who were randomly assigned to receive this drug, 150 mg/day, or placebo after the clinical diagnosis of unstable angina or non–Q wave infarction.[9] Antibiotic therapy was continued for 30 days, and patients were followed up for 6 months. The effect of roxithromycin was assessed on an intention-to-treat basis and cardiac ischemic death, myocardial infarction, and severe recurrent ischemia were used as a composite primary end point. Roxithromycin therapy was able to reduce the primary end point significantly, supporting again the potential role of antibiotic therapy in certain defined patient subsets in the treatment of atherosclerosis.

H. pylori has also been epidemiologically associated with coronary artery disease. Many studies have demonstrated a higher prevalence of *H. pylori* infections in patients with ischemic heart disease when compared with normal control subjects, although the results are often contradictory because of the inclusion of variable patient and control populations. Some studies have examined the potential role in atherosclerosis of the genetic polymorphisms of *H. pylori* that bear the cytotoxin-associated gene-A, which had been demonstrated to play a pathogenetic role in both gastric carcinoma and peptic ulcer disease.[10] A retrospective case-control study examined the prevalence of infection with *H. pylori* in 88 patients with ischemic heart disease and compared the prevalence of infection with that in a group of age- and sex-matched controls who were free of coronary artery disease. The prevalence of *H. pylori* infection was significantly elevated in patients with coronary artery disease when compared with control patients, and the virulence appeared to be mediated through cytotoxin-associated gene-A positivity. The genetically determined virulence factor may be associated with a greater inflammatory burden and was demonstrated to be significantly higher in patients with ischemic heart disease. However, no association between seropositivity and severity of angiographically defined coronary artery disease could be determined, although angiography has definite limitations in the assessment of coronary artery disease. The role of inflammation and infection in the possible pathogenesis of coronary heart disease is generating hypotheses and awaits further clinical trials.

Lipid Hypothesis

Dyslipidemia has been established as a major pathogenetic risk factor for the development of coronary artery disease by epidemiologic, genetic, pathologic, and controlled clinical trials.

Epidemiology

The Framingham Heart Study is a long-term epidemiologic trial that has evaluated the role of total cholesterol, low-density lipoprotein (LDL), HDL, very low density lipoprotein (VLDL), and apoproteins in the pathogenesis of atherosclerosis. The Framingham data, which linked dyslipidemia with the prevalence and the extent of coronary disease, are extensive and extend into the Framingham Offspring Study.[11] The Framingham Heart Study also documented a temporal change in the relation between dyslipidemia and acute myocardial infarction.[11] Elevated cholesterol was correlated with the incidence of acute myocardial infarction in the Framingham study in the decade encompassing the 1950s. During that time period, myocardial infarction was seen in relatively young individuals who were significantly dyslipidemic. The average age for both men and women who had symptomatic coronary artery disease was 48 years of age, with the cholesterol level in men approximating 246 mg/dl, compared with 281 mg/dl in women. The Framingham Study has subsequently demonstrated a gradual decline in the level of cholesterol that was associated with an acute myocardial infarction, coupled with the increasing age of the population at risk. In the decade encompassing the 1980s, the mean serum cholesterol associated with a myocardial infarction in men was 228 mg/dl and 248 mg/dl in women.

The Multiple Risk Factor Intervention Trial (MRFIT), although lacking the decades-long evaluation period of the Framingham Study, clearly demonstrated the curvilinear relation between total serum cholesterol level and coronary heart disease mortality in a large cohort consisting of 356,222 men who were initially free of documented atherosclerosis.[12] The 6-year, age-adjusted death rate from coronary artery disease demonstrated a continuous gradation that statistically linked the cholesterol levels and mortality rates, even after correction for smoking and elevated blood pressure in multivariate analysis. MRFIT did not demonstrate the threshold below which an excess risk could not be determined, although below a level of 200 mg/dl, the risk relation becomes less pronounced (Fig. 71–1). However, approximately 20 percent of acute myocardial infarctions occur in the range of cholesterol falling below 200 mg/dl, which is a level considered to be desirable by the National Cholesterol Education Program guidelines.

Genetics

The epidemiologic data in large-scale populations are strengthened by the close correlation between atherosclerotic complications and lipid concentration in numerous genetic syndromes involving lipid disorders. Genetic syndromes involving both overproduction of LDL and underproduction of HDL have been described, and the molecular genetics of these conditions have been elucidated. Familial hypercholesterolemia is the model for the consequences of increased circulating levels of LDL caused by reduced activity of the LDL receptor. The heterozygous form of familial hypercholesterolemia is associated with premature atherosclerosis, with males afflicted with this condition beginning to demonstrate increased risk for coronary disease in the fourth decade of life. Females are initially protected by their gender but also begin to demonstrate increased risk for vascular complications with a 10-year lag period compared with the male population.

Underproduction of HDL in familial hypoalphalipopro-

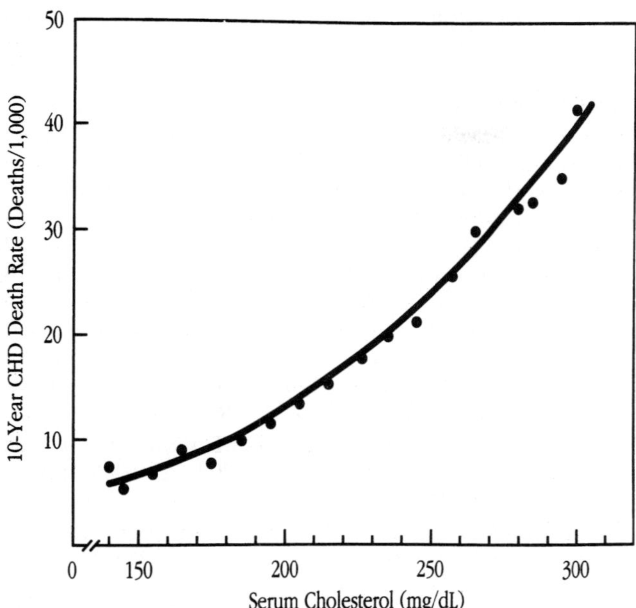

FIGURE 71–1 The relation between serum cholesterol concentration and coronary disease mortality. CHD, coronary heart disease. (Adapted from Neaton JD, Wentworth D: Serum cholesterol, blood pressure, cigarette smoking, and death from coronary heart disease: overall findings and differences by age for 316,099 white men. Arch Intern Med 152:56, 1992.)

teinemia is also associated with increased cardiovascular risk.

Clinical Trials Utilizing Statin Monotherapy

The most telling clinical evidence in support of the lipid hypothesis are the results of the statin trials. Earlier primary prevention trials, such as the Lipid Research Clinics Coronary Primary Prevention Trial and the Helsinki Heart Study, demonstrated benefit from the use of hypolipidemic interventions, but the absolute reductions in clinical end points were relatively modest.[13, 14] The advent of statin therapy has revolutionized the ability of the clinician to optimize the lipid profile. Statin monotherapy has been demonstrated to be clinically efficacious in both primary and secondary prevention trials that evaluated patients with either high or low cholesterol levels. Subset analysis of these trials has shown benefit across the patient population, with clinical improvement being documented in men, women, older patients, hypertensives, smokers, and diabetics.

Early studies testing the lipid hypothesis were fraught with problems resulting from poor design and relatively ineffective agents. Statin monotherapy has demonstrated effectiveness in angiographic plus primary and secondary prevention trials. Different statins have been demonstrated to be effective either clinically or angiographically, implying that the benefit is related to a hypolipidemic effect and is not solely the effect of a single pharmacologic agent or a class of agents. The fibric acid derivatives and bile acid sequestrants have also been demonstrated to be effective albeit at a decreased rate.

ANGIOGRAPHIC TRIALS

Angiographic trials utilizing statin monotherapy have clearly delineated the anatomic benefit attainable with statin therapy. The Multicenter Anti-Atheroma Study was a double-blind angiographic trial that evaluated 381 patients with documented coronary artery disease.[15] Subjects were randomly assigned to receive dietary therapy or simvastatin at a dose of 20 mg/day. Angiograms were quantitatively analyzed in a blinded fashion by use of computer-assisted cardiovascular angiographic analysis (CAAS), which determined mean lumen diameter, minimal lumen diameter, reference diameter, and percent diameter stenosis. Simvastatin therapy demonstrated beneficial effects on the lipid profile when compared with dietary therapy plus placebo: total cholesterol was reduced by 23 percent, LDL cholesterol was reduced by 31 percent, HDL cholesterol was increased by 9 percent, and triglycerides were reduced by 18 percent. Angiographic analysis demonstrated a decreased rate of progression of luminal stenosis in the group randomly assigned to receive simvastatin; this effect appeared to be more pronounced in subjects whose baseline lesion exceeded an initial 50 percent diameter reduction. Simvastatin therapy resulted in fewer new lesions or total occlusions than in the dietary group. The Multicenter Anti-Atheroma Study was not adequately powered to evaluate clinical end points, but a favorable trend was noted with simvastatin therapy: 20 percent of the simvastatin group had at least one major cardiac event, compared with 28 percent of the dietary group.

The Regression Growth Evaluation Statin Study (REGRESS) evaluated the use of pravastatin in a cohort of patients with documented coronary atherosclerosis but whose cholesterol levels were only moderately elevated.[16] The REGRESS trial was undertaken to establish the benefit of lipid reduction therapy by statins in a cohort that was more representative of the general population. Pravastatin therapy resulted in a 20 percent reduction in total cholesterol level, a 29 percent reduction in LDL cholesterol level, a 10 percent increase in HDL cholesterol level, and a 7 percent decrease in triglyceride levels. Pravastatin therapy was associated with decreased angiographic progression when compared with the control group, and the benefit was demonstrable in all LDL quartiles. Clinical events were also monitored, and 81 percent of the control group remained free of a cardiac event, compared with 89 percent of the group randomly assigned to receive pravastatin.

The Lipoprotein and Coronary Atherosclerosis Study (LCAS) evaluated the effect of fluvastatin on coronary atherosclerosis in patients with mild-to-moderate LDL cholesterol elevations.[17] Fluvastatin resulted in significant improvement in the lipid profile, with an 18 percent reduction in total cholesterol level, which was associated with a 26.5 percent reduction in LDL cholesterol level. HDL cholesterol was increased by 5.5 percent, and triglycerides were reduced by 10 percent. Fluvastatin therapy was associated with a considerable variability in patient response, with approximately 40 percent of the patients randomly assigned to receive fluvastatin demonstrating a 30 percent reduction in LDL cholesterol level. Fluvastatin therapy was associated with less angiographic progression, as demonstrated by a 0.028-mm decrease in minimum luminal diameter, compared with a 0.100-mm decrease with dietary therapy. Fluvastatin therapy was also associated with reduced progression of atherosclerosis, as determined by change in percent diameter, which was increased by 0.6 percent in fluvastatin patients, compared with 2.8 percent in placebo patients. Elevated levels of HDL cholesterol have been associated with reduced risk for the development of atherosclerosis in many epidemiologic studies.[18] The LCAS also analyzed the effect of baseline HDL cholesterol levels on subsequent angiographic production. Patients whose baseline HDL cholesterol level was less than 35 mg/dl had more progression when analyzed by decreases in minimum lumen diameter, but these patients also received the greatest angiographic benefit from fluvastatin therapy.[19] The implication of this subset analysis of the LCAS cohort suggests that statin therapy is beneficial not only to patients with elevated LDL cholesterol level but also to patients with relatively normal LDL cholesterol level and low levels of HDL cholesterol.

The Canadian Coronary Atherosclerosis Intervention Trial,[20] Pravastatin Limitation of Atherosclerosis in the Coronary Arteries,[21] the Monitored Atherosclerosis Regression Study,[22] and the Post Coronary Artery Bypass Graft Trial[23] have all demonstrated angiographic benefit. These trials of statin therapy clearly confirm and extend the epidemiologic and earlier trial evidence supporting the lipid hypothesis.

PRIMARY PREVENTION

Statin monotherapy has also been utilized in both primary prevention and secondary prevention trials that evaluated patients with normal or elevated cholesterol levels. The role of pharmacologic therapy in primary prevention has been controversial because of the presumed high cost associated with minimal-to-no clinical benefit and has been recommended only in extremely high-risk individuals or in patients with multiple risk factors. Statin therapy has been demonstrated to be effective in patients with elevated cholesterol levels in the West of Scotland Coronary Primary Prevention Study (WOSCOPS)[24] and in patients with average cholesterol levels in the Air Force Coronary Atherosclerosis Prevention Study (AFCAPS/TexCAPS).[25]

The WOSCOPS was a large-scale study involving 6595 men who had not had a documented myocardial infarction and were randomly assigned to receive 40 mg/day of either pravastatin or placebo to assess the efficacy of such treatment on subsequent development of symptomatic coronary atherosclerosis. WOSCOPS evaluated a relatively high-risk group whose average baseline cholesterol level was 272 mg/dl, and 78 percent were either current or exsmokers. Pravastatin therapy resulted in a reduction of total cholesterol level of 20 percent and LDL cholesterol level by 26 percent; HDL cholesterol level was increased by five percent, and triglyceride levels were reduced by twelve percent. Pravastatin therapy resulted in improvement in clinical events that correlated with a reduction in cholesterol. The primary end point of the WOSCOPS was the combination of nonfatal myocardial infarction and death from coronary heart disease, which was reduced by 31 percent. An increase in mortality from noncardiovascular causes was not demonstrated, and total mortality was reduced by 22 percent in the group randomly assigned to receive pravastatin.

The results of the West of Scotland Study were extended by AFCAPS/TexCAPS, which analyzed the effect of lovastatin in primary prevention targeted at a low-to-moderate risk cohort. The AFCAPS/TexCAPS trial was designed to evaluate a cohort that was similar to the general population, as determined by the National Health and Nutrition Examination Survey. Lovastatin was utilized in 6605 men and women without coronary disease at an initial dosage of 20 mg/day. Dosage was titrated to 40 mg/day if after 3 months participants had not reached the target goal of LDL cholesterol level of 110 mg/dl or lower. The primary end point of the AFCAPS/TexCAPS trial was the incidence of the first major coronary event, defined as unstable angina pectoris, fatal or nonfatal myocardial infarction, or sudden cardiac death. After a mean follow-up of 5.2 years, treated participants experienced a 37 percent reduction in the primary end point compared with placebo. The trial, originally intended to have a longer follow-up, was terminated early because of this demonstrated efficacy. Clinical improvement induced by lovastatin was consistent in subgroup analysis evaluating men, women, smokers, hypertensives, diabetics, and older patients.

SECONDARY PREVENTION

Secondary prevention is less controversial because of the strong evidence of benefit in high-risk patients who have had an acute myocardial infarction. The Scandinavian Simvastatin Survival Study (4S)[26] evaluated the effect of simvastatin therapy on total mortality in survivors of acute myocardial infarction with a mean average cholesterol level of 261 mg/dl. The primary end point of the 4S study was total mortality, and secondary end points included first major coronary event, coronary death, and definite silent myocardial infarction. Simvastatin therapy resulted in significant improvement in the lipid profile and resulted in a reduction in total cholesterol level of 28 percent, a reduction in LDL cholesterol of 38 percent, and an increase in HDL cholesterol level of 8 percent. Simvastatin therapy resulted in a statistically significant reduction of 30 percent in risk for death from all causes. No increase in noncardiovascular deaths was documented, and the improvement in survival was basically accounted for by a risk reduction of 42 percent for coronary mortality. Subgroup analysis demonstrated benefit of simvastatin therapy in patients older than 60 years, women, smokers, and hypertensive patients. The 4S trial is especially important because it is the first major statin trial to demonstrate the benefits of pharmacologic interventions on both total and coronary mortality.

Cholesterol lowering in secondary prevention has also been demonstrated to be effective in patients with relatively normal cholesterol levels. The Cholesterol and Recurrent Events (CARE) study[27] evaluated patients who had had an acute myocardial infarction that was associated with relatively normal cholesterol levels before randomization into the CARE trial. Participants were included who had a documented myocardial infarction and a total cholesterol level of less than 240 mg/dl. The average cholesterol level in the CARE cohort was 208 mg/dl. Participants were randomly assigned to receive either dietary therapy or pravastatin, 40 mg/day. Pravastatin therapy reduced LDL cholesterol by 32 percent and was associated with a reduction in LDL cholesterol level from 139 to 98 mg/dl. Pravastatin resulted in a 24 percent reduction in the incidence of the primary end point. The benefit of pravastatin therapy was documented across subgroups when it was analyzed for the presence of hypertension, diabetes, smoking, reduced ejection fraction, or sex. Retrospective subgroup analysis has questioned the benefit of pravastatin therapy in subjects whose baseline cholesterol level was less than 125 mg/dl. Pravastatin therapy in this group was not associated with clinical benefit and actually resulted in a 3 percent relative risk increase, which did not reach statistical significance. The clinical benefit of hypolipidemic therapy in patients with lower LDL cholesterol levels has been challenged even in secondary prevention. However, because the curvilinear relation between coronary artery disease and LDL cholesterol level becomes relatively flat below a level of 125 mg/dl, either larger numbers of patients or a longer duration of therapy may be required to detect a potential clinical difference.

The clinical trials involving statin therapy in both angiographic and clinical end point studies emphasize the increased risk associated with patients with dyslipidemia. The trials also support the lipid hypothesis in the demonstration of a reduction in cardiovascular morbidity and, in trials that were adequately powered, a reduction in total mortality.

Response to Injury

The response-to-injury hypothesis was advanced by Ross.[28] The response-to-injury hypothesis postulates that the origin and the progression of occlusive atherosclerotic coronary and peripheral vascular disease represent a nonspecific response incited by endothelial damage. The response-to-injury hypothesis emphasizes the concept of coronary artery disease as a syndrome with multiple potential underlying conditions that have as their unifying principle the potential for alteration of endothelial function. Endothelial function may be altered by metabolic abnormalities, such as dyslipidemia and diabetes, with resultant imbalance in clotting and vasoconstriction. Physical damage to the endothelium may occur with elevated blood pressure, immune-mediated injury, or toxic damage, as seen in exposure to tobacco inhalants. The endothelial response to damage is nonspecific and results in functional abnormalities followed by morphologic changes involving the deposition of lipid subfractions, calcium, and various types of connective tissue into the vessel wall.

Endothelial damage is associated with the involvement of numerous cell lines, which are characterized by their ability to accumulate lipid subfractions or generate growth factors, adhesion molecules, and chemoattractants. Early atherosclerosis is characterized by the movement into the endothelial space of monocytes, which subsequently transform into macrophages. Monocyte-derived macrophage cell lines have the ability to recognize, bind, and internalize lipoprotein subparticles, especially oxidized LDL. Macrophages thus act as localized tissue scavengers and have the ability to secrete growth factors and chemoattractants, such as platelet-derived growth factor.

Platelet-derived growth factor-beta enhances the proliferation and activation of smooth muscle cells and fibroblasts. Other growth factors, including transforming growth factor, are produced that interact in a complex manner with various cell lines and may alter the physicochemical composition of atherosclerotic plaque. Smooth muscle cells that have their origin in the vascular media are attracted into the area of potential atherosclerosis development and transform from the normal contractile to a synthetic phenotype, resulting in the production of growth factors, which modulate the localization of cellular elements and matrix formation. Smooth muscle cells have an autocrine function, which allows the production and local action of compounds such as platelet-derived growth factor, which stimulates the extensive extracellular connective tissue matrix and influences the activity of the expression of receptors that recognize lipid subforms. The response-to-injury theory has been extensively reviewed by Ross[28] and emphasizes the potential of atherosclerosis to evolve as a nonspecific response to numerous potentially noxious stimuli. That is, it emphasizes the concept of atherosclerosis as a syndrome with multiple potential predisposing factors and the difficulty of managing patients at risk for the development of coronary artery disease.

Morphologic Lesions

The classical concept of atherosclerosis is that of a gradual and progressive disease that begins in early life. A long subclinical exposure to the classic risk factors, such as dyslipidemia and hypertension, is believed to precede the development of anatomically identifiable lesions. Early pathologic studies described adaptive intimal thickening, which gradually progressed to a fatty streak that was visible on the surface of the involved vessels as a relatively flat or minimally raised lesion that was identifiable with staining utilizing Sudan exposure. The fatty streak is composed of macrophage- and smooth muscle cell–derived foam cells, which have accumulated oxidized LDL in droplet phase. The fatty streak was believed to progress to a lesion that was altered in its geometry and physiochemical composition and was termed the *fibrous plaque*. The fibrous plaque that had demonstrable collagen and lipid deposition was referred to as a *fibroatheroma*. The end-stage complex lesion resulted in significant impingement on the luminal dimensions and contained a lipid core of varying volume plus an increased deposition of calcium and collagen. Stary[29] reclassified the process of atherosclerosis into a more detailed pathologic schema and divided atherosclerotic lesions from type I through type VIII.

Type I Lesion

The type I lesion is the first atherosclerotic lesion that can be anatomically identified. The type I lesion is characterized by the presence in the intima of lipid-laden macrophages whose origin is secondary to an increased influx by elements of the circulating plasma monocyte cell line into the lesion. The macrophage density is increased in areas with intimal thickening. The macrophage cellular elements are also increased in density in areas known to be associated with an increased prevalence of clinical ischemic syndromes and are believed to represent progression-prone lesions.

Type II Lesion

The type II lesion represents an intensification of the pathologic process that is originally demonstrable in the type I lesion. Type II lesions are microscopically visible and may be stained with Sudan dyes, which react with lipid within the vessel and impart a red color to the involved lesion. The type II lesion has an increased density of lipid-laden cells that originated in the monocyte-derived macrophage line and also is associated with increased numbers of T lymphocytes and smooth muscle cells. Type I and type II lesions are generally clinically silent and are not associated with either a reduction of distal blood flow or an increased incidence of ischemic events. Type II lesions may progress to more advanced atherosclerotic involvement, which is especially more common in individuals with dyslipidemia and hypertension. Progression-prone lesions appear to be affected by mechanical and shearing forces, which are present at bifurcations and vascular branch points, and lesions in this area may progress rapidly in a coronary prone individual.

Type III Lesion

The type III lesion has been described as a bridge between minimal involvement of the intima and the more advanced atherosclerotic lesion. The type III lesion has also been termed the *intermediate* or *preatheromatous* stage of atherosclerosis and is characterized by the accumulation of an extracellular lipid deposition that is termed the *lipid core.* This core presumably forms by the confluence of droplet lipid that has been distributed in various areas of the lesion. Type III lesions are believed to progress to a more advanced state with the potential for an increased risk for developing an ischemic event.

Type IV Lesion

The type IV lesion is the first definite atheroma that may be determined pathologically and is considered to represent an advanced histologic stage. The type IV lesion is characterized by the presence of extracellular lipid, including the deposition of cholesterol crystals in the musculoelastic layer of the vessel, which has also been involved by adaptive intimal thickening. The accumulation of lipid in this area weakens the arterial wall as it displaces structural smooth muscle cells whose presence may yield stability to the involved area. Type IV lesions are frequently associated with thickening of the coronary artery opposite an anatomic bifurcation. Type IV lesions are generally crescent shaped and may be associated with mild luminal impingement. However, the type IV lesion may not be identifiable by coronary angiography. Mineral deposition may be identified microscopically and is frequently associated with cellular and lipid debris.

Type V Lesion

Type V lesions are defined pathologically by the demonstration of collagen deposition and are referred to as *fibroatheromas.* Type V lesions are associated with an increased risk for plaque rupture with the potential for generation of an obstructive thrombus. The fate of the mural thrombus is variable and may be progressive or incorporated into the lesion, with further diminution of luminal dimensions but no acute clinical sequelae. The collagen within the type V lesion is demonstrable between the lumen and the lipid core and is believed to replace proteoglycan matrix within the atherosclerotic lesion. The increased collagen is also associated with increased degrees of smooth muscle cell migration and lipid deposition.

Type VI Lesion

Coronary atherosclerosis mortality and morbidity are associated with the type VI lesion, which was referred to as the *complicated lesion* in prior classifications. The type VI lesion is associated with fissuring or disruption of the surface, which may be associated with the intravascular generation of thrombotic components. Fissures frequently develop at the margins of a lesion, which is characterized by an increased density of macrophages and foam cells. Fissuring may be enhanced by alterations of the shearing forces to which the lesion is exposed and reductions in the tensile strength of the plaque itself. Additionally, members of the metalloproteinase enzyme system (collagenase, gelatinase) generated by the macrophage cell line may weaken the plaque. Plaque fissuring may generate a thrombus on the surface of the lesion whose course is further influenced by thrombogenic risk factors, such as increased platelet aggregation, and high levels of fibrinogen and lipoprotein(a).

Type VII Lesion

Type VII, or advanced, atherosclerotic lesions are demonstrable frequently in older adults and are largely calcific. Calcium deposits are demonstrable in areas associated with remnants of extracellular lipid and dead lymphocytes, smooth muscle cells, and macrophages. The lipid core is minimal to nonexistent and is frequently entirely replaced by calcium. The deposition of calcium may add tensile strength to the vascular deformity.

Type VIII Lesion

Type VIII lesions are fibrotic and are also associated with minimal-to-no lipid involvement. The development of the fibrotic lesion is unknown from a pathogenetic standpoint. The absence of lipid implies that it may have been metabolized, reabsorbed, or not been deposited in the area. Fibrotic lesions may also represent organized thrombosis and have the potential to obstruct the lumen of medium-sized arteries.

RISK FACTORS

Major Risk Factors

Hypertension

Elevated systolic and diastolic blood pressure represent a major and potentially modifiable risk factor that has been statistically correlated with an increased incidence of both coronary artery and cerebrovascular disease. Epidemiologic studies in geographically and ethnically diverse populations have established a curvilinear relation between the incidence of acute coronary syndromes and both thrombotic and hemorrhagic stroke. Meta-analysis of major, prospective hypertension trials have demonstrated a graded and consistent relation between myocardial infarction and cerebrovascular disease. The epidemiologic data have been strengthened by clinical trials that clearly demonstrate reduction in the incidence of stroke and coronary artery disease after lowering of blood pressure. The decrease in coronary atherosclerosis resulting from antihypertensive treatment, although statistically significant, has been less than would be anticipated from the epidemiologic relation between blood pressure and acute ischemic events, despite plausibility from a mechanistic standpoint. The large-scale MRFIT study evaluated 356,222 middle-aged men in a 6-year follow-up study and evaluated the impact of hypertension on coronary atherosclerosis death rates. The MRFIT data established that approximately 32 percent of all acute ischemic coronary mortality could be related to increased diastolic blood pressure in excess of 80 mg/dl, and 42 percent of the mortality was due to systolic hypertension with elevations of blood pressure above 120 mm Hg.[30] Although many studies show a curvilinear relationship between elevated blood pressure and ischemic events, controversy has been generated over the potential of a J-shaped relationship between hypertension and acute coronary events, with an apparent increase in morbidity and mortality if blood pressure was lowered to less than 85 mm Hg. A J-shaped relation has not been definitely established, and an unequivocally increased incidence of morbidity and mortality below a certain level of blood pressure remains controversial.

The Hypertension Optimal Treatment (HOT) Trial addressed the potential adverse effects of overzealous lowering of blood pressure.[31] The HOT trial randomly assigned 18,790 subjects with documented hypertension in an international multicenter study. Subjects were randomly assigned to strategies designed to achieve a diastolic blood pressure of less than or equal to 90, 85, or 80 mm Hg. The dihydropyridine calcium channel blocker felodipine was administered as initial baseline therapy with the potential for addition of either an angiotensin-converting enzyme inhibitor or a beta-blocker. Titration of the agents was also allowed. All patients received either aspirin at 75 mg/day or placebo over a 3.8-year period. The mean diastolic blood pressure level after treatment was 85, 83, and 81 mm Hg, respectively, in the three target groups. Analysis of the HOT trial revealed a small reduction in the rate of myocardial infarction when the subjects with diastolic pressures of 85 and 80 mm Hg were compared with the group randomly assigned to a blood pressure of 90 mm Hg. The decrease in myocardial infarction was 25 and 28 percent, respectively, which, although representing a beneficial trend toward reduction of events in the lower blood pressure groups, did not reach statistical significance. Subgroup analysis of 1501 diabetics revealed that patients in the 80 mm Hg group had half the risk for major cardiovascular events compared with the group whose blood pressure target was 90 mm Hg. The HOT study did not demonstrate the J-curve phenomenon representing increased mortality at lower blood pressure levels and showed considerable improvement in diabetics.

A potential blunting of clinical benefit or even an adverse relation between antihypertensive therapy and cardiovascular disease has been attributed to overzealous reduction of blood pressure in patients with ostial or severe coronary lesions that may alter perfusion; severe diastolic abnormalities with resultant subendocardial ischemia due to inadequate perfusion of the innermost layers of the myocardium coupled with increased left ventricular end-diastolic pressure resulting in compression of the subendocardial blood flow; or the potential adverse metabolic effects of certain antihypertensive agents, including resultant dyslipidemia, electrolyte abnormalities, and abnormal glucose tolerance. Additionally, although left ventricular hypertrophy is clearly a risk factor for cardiovascular morbidity and is related to hypertension, not all antihypertensive agents result in a reduction in left ventricular mass. Pure arterial dilators, such as minoxidil, when utilized as monotherapy, may result in an increase in left ventricular mass as a result of activation of the sympathetic nervous system, which acts as a trophic factor for myocardial cell growth.

Tobacco

The use of tobacco products is recognized as a major modifiable risk factor for the development of atherosclerosis. The use of tobacco products has been epidemiologically associated with more than 170,000 cardiovascular deaths in the United States.[32] Cigarette smoking in the United States increased rapidly until the 1950s, when numerous government sponsored reports on the adverse health effects of cigarette smoking were published. Beginning in 1973, the consumption of cigarettes, when tabulated on a per capita basis, began a steady decline. In 1984, the consumption of tobacco products approximated the same level that was achieved in 1942. By 1993, approximately 25 percent of Americans older than 18 years were utilizing tobacco products.[33] The reduction in the use of tobacco products has been statistically accompanied by a significant parallel reduction in cardiovascular mortality, although the mechanism by which cigarette smoking is associated with increased risk is complex and multifactorial. Endothelial dysfunction, even without anatomically demonstrable lesions, is believed to be an initial step in atherosclerosis. The inhalation of tobacco smoke results in alterations in endothelial function, which may be modulated by oxidants, carbon monoxide, or nicotine.[34] Endothelial dysfunction results in alteration of the permeability barrier of the endothelium to lipoproteins and is associated with an imbalance between fibrinolysis and coagulation and with increased penetration of LDL into the subendothelial space. The increased oxidant stress associated with use of tobacco products results in an increased level of oxidized LDL.[35] Oxidized LDL is recognized, bound, and taken up by the scavenger receptor of the monocyte/macrophage system in an unregulated way and is associated with subsequent generation of the foam cell. Oxidized LDL may be immunogenic and may also alter the release of nitric oxide from the normally functioning endothelium, resulting in a tendency toward vasoconstriction.

The consumption of cigarette smoke also may play a role in hypercoagulable states secondary to alteration of normal endothelial function. Endothelial dysfunction is frequently associated with an imbalance between tissue plasminogen activators and tissue plasminogen inhibitors, resulting in a potential increase in hypercoagulability. Elevated fibrinogen levels have been positively correlated with risk for atherosclerosis in numerous epidemiologic trials. The use of tobacco products is one of the multitude of conditions associated with an increased level of fibrinogen, which may remain elevated for years, even after discontinuation of smoking.[36] The mechanism by which the inhalation of tobacco products is associated with increased fibrinogen levels has not been completely elucidated but may be secondary to increased hepatic synthesis, which occurs in response to enhanced interleukin-1 production after exposure to cigarette smoke. In addition to fibrinogen, factor VII coagulant activity is also increased in smokers with endothelial dysfunction.[37] Endothelial dysfunction in smokers is also associated with an increased level of plasminogen activator inhibitor, which blocks the generation of plasmin from plasminogen. Increased platelet aggregation is considered to be a major risk factor for the development of acute ischemic syndromes. Platelet aggregates form after the formation of plaque fissures and exposure to the thrombogenic intraplaque lipid core and has the potential to generate an occlusive intravascular thrombus. Smokers have decreased platelet survival time and increased platelet aggregation, which is associated with an increased production of thromboxane A_2, which causes further platelet aggregation and vasoconstriction.[38]

The use of tobacco products is a major atherosclerotic risk factor, even in populations with a low prevalence of coronary artery disease, such as China. Multivariate analysis of smokers in China demonstrates more than a threefold increased risk for the development of myocardial infarction in smokers.[39]

The Atherosclerosis Risk in Communities study examined the relation between cigarette smoking and progression of atherosclerosis in a longitudinal assessment over a 3-year period in 10,914 patients. Ultrasonographic measurement of intimal medial thickness of the carotid artery was the end point.[40] The current use of cigarette smoke was associated with a 50 percent increase in the progression of atherosclerosis over a 3-year period, and past smoking was associated with a 25 percent increase over the same time period. The rate of progression of intimal medial thickening was higher in hypertensive and diabetic subjects. The degree of pack years of smoking was associated with progression of atherosclerosis, although when subjects were analyzed for current versus past smoking, there was no significant relation with the degree of progression of carotid disease, suggesting that some adverse effects of smoking may be cumulative and irreversible. Because of the potential for permanent vascular damage, a concerted effort should be made to reduce the prevalence of smoking, which is a proven beneficial and highly cost-effective intervention in both primary and secondary prevention.

Diabetes

Type I and type II diabetic subjects have a significantly increased risk for coronary artery disease. Diabetes is a major cause of death in the United States, and vascular complications are common as the underlying cause of morbidity and mortality in these patients. Diabetics also have a significantly higher prevalence of obesity, hypertension, and dyslipidemia, which are frequently linked in risk factor clustering.

Approximately 16,000,000 Americans satisfy diagnostic criteria for diabetes, with the vast majority (> 90 percent) of afflicted individuals having type II diabetes. Hypertension is extremely common in the diabetic population; approximately 60 percent of diabetics have coexistent elevated blood pressure, which is approximately twice the prevalence documented in the general population.[41] Patients with type II diabetes may be hypertensive at the time of diagnosis, and elevated blood pressure may precede the development of the metabolic abnormalities generally attributed to diabetics.[42] The pathogenesis of hypertension in diabetic patients has not been clearly delineated and is multifactorial and may partially relate to abnormalities in ion transport, genetic factors, sympathetic nervous system activity, and hyperinsulinemia.

Hypertension has been related to abnormalities in the concentration and distribution of many intracellular electrolytes. The documented abnormalities may result from inability of the membrane ion transporter systems to regulate the movement and distribution of ions across cell membranes. Postulated enzyme systems with a potential role in hypertension include sodium-potassium adenosine triphosphatase, calcium hydrogen exchanger, the calcium adenosine triphosphatase and magnesium-sodium exchanger. Additionally, the sodium-lithium countertransporter and the sodium-hydrogen antiporter have been implicated to be important in the origin of elevated blood pressure in diabetic individuals because of the stimulatory effect of insulin in increasing sodium reabsorption. The causal relationship between abnormalities in the activity of these enzymes and hypertension is an area of active research. Additionally, type II diabetes is genetically transmitted, and data have implicated a potential heritable basis for elevated blood pressure in diabetic patients. However, a specific hypertensive gene has not been definitely elucidated, although mutations in the angiotensinogen gene have been correlated with elevated blood pressure in numerous studies in whites.[43]

Type II diabetes is frequently characterized by peripheral insulin resistance with increased circulating levels of insulin, despite the normal or minimally elevated glucose levels. Elevated insulin levels have been determined to be an independent cardiovascular risk factor and may also be involved in the pathogenesis of coexistent hypertension. Hyperinsulinemia is associated with increased sympathetic activity, vascular remodeling, and increased renal sodium reabsorption, which are all potential underlying mechanisms in hypertension. Additionally, hyperinsulinemia is also accompanied by increased sensitivity to pressors, such as angiotensin II.[44] Insulin resistance may result in significant dyslipidemia because of hepatic overproduction of triglyceride-rich lipoproteins and inadequate metabolism in the periphery caused by blunted activity of lipoprotein lipase.

The presence of diabetes mellitus is a significant independent risk factor for the development of cardiovascular disease. However, the role of intensive diabetic treatment in an attempt to decrease cardiovascular complications is controversial.[45] The University Diabetes Group and the Diabetes Control and Complications Trial had been the only available randomized intervention trials with long-term follow-up. However, the University Diabetes Group program was an inadequate trial that was not designed with sufficient power and in which separation of glycemic levels was not obtained. Additionally, the potential confounding use of tobacco products was not considered. The Diabetes Control and Complications Trial analyzed the incidence of cardiovascular events and other complications in a relatively young and presumably low-risk patient population with a short duration of the disease. The young age and risk factor profile of the patients resulted in an inadequate number of cardiovascular events for a definitive answer to the question of the benefits of intensive glycemic control.

In addition to the glycemic abnormalities, diabetics frequently have dyslipidemia that is amenable to therapy. The most characteristic abnormality found in diabetes is increased levels of circulating triglycerides, low levels of HDL cholesterol, and increased levels of small, dense LDL. Optimization of the glycemic abnormalities may improve but not necessarily normalize the associated dyslipidemia. Experts have recommended a more aggressive therapeutic approach to lipid disorders in the diabetic patient[46] to levels below that recommended by the National Cholesterol Education Program. The benefits of aggressive lipid lowering in diabetics have not been proved in prospective large scale clinical trials. However, subgroup analysis of the 4S study found a reduction in coronary events in diabetic patients and postulated that the improvement in diabetic subjects may be greater than in nondiabetic subjects.[47]

Despite the lack of definitive clinical trial data, most experts recommend a relatively rigorous control of the metabolic abnormalities in diabetic patients combined with optimization of blood pressure and dyslipidemia in an attempt to decrease cardiovascular risk.

Dyslipidemia

CHYLOMICRONS

Chylomicrons are large particles derived from dietary fat and composed predominantly of cholesteryl ester and exogenous triglycerides. The density of chylomicrons is less than 0.95 g/dl, and their diameter ranges from 800 to 5000 Å. Chylomicrons have essentially no electrophoretic mobility and remain at the origin during lipoprotein electrophoresis. Chylomicrons carry a number of apoproteins, including apo-AI, apo-AII, apo-AIV, apo-B48, apo-CI, apo-CII, apo-CIII, and apo-E. Chylomicrons are generally rapidly cleared from the plasma after a fatty meal and are elevated only in rare inherited lipid disorders. Chylomicrons are metabolized by lipoprotein lipase, and the genetically determined absence of this enzyme may result in massive accumulations of chylomicrons in plasma. Absence of lipoprotein lipase results in marked accumulation of circulating chylomicrons manifest by a milky white serum after overnight refrigeration. Hyperchylomicronemia is generally detected in childhood after recurrent bouts of pancreatitis. Hyperchylomicronemia is also characterized by the presence of a number of dermatologic manifestations, including cutaneous xanthomas. Lipoprotein lipase is physiologically activated by apo-CII on the surface of lipoproteins, and hyperchylomicronemia may also be secondary to the familial absence of this apoprotein, which occurs as a rare autosomal disorder, resulting in the impaired clearance of chylomicrons from the blood. Elevations in both chylomicrons and VLDL may be elevated, a condition that is clinically manifest as pancreatitis, presumably caused by vasocclusive crises. Inhibitors of the activation of lipoprotein lipase have been described in systemic lupus erythematosus, acute intermittent porphyria, and multiple myeloma with resultant chylomicronemia. Elevations of chylomicrons of a genetic basis are not associated with an increased risk for premature atherosclerosis.

VERY LOW DENSITY LIPOPROTEIN

VLDL is the major carrier of endogenously produced triglyceride and has a synthetic origin in the hepatocytes. VLDL carries numerous apoproteins, including apo-B100, apo-CI, apo-CII, apo-CIII, and apo-E. VLDL are large particles with a diameter ranging between 300 to 800 Å and a density of less than 1.006 g/ml. VLDLs demonstrate electrophoretic mobility in the pre-beta region. The evidence linking the elevation of LDL with increased risk for coronary artery disease is well established, whereas the triglyceride-rich lipoprotein relationship to atherosclerosis remains controversial. The potential link between elevated VLDL and coronary artery disease risk is difficult to assess because of the large intervariability and intravariability in triglyceride measurements coupled with the lack of precision in assays and a close metabolic interrelation with HDL. However, univariate analysis establishes a clear association between elevated triglyceride levels and atherosclerosis, although earlier epidemiologic studies demonstrate a weakening of the relationship in multivariate analysis and potential disappearance when HDL cholesterol is taken into consideration.[48] The role of triglyceride-rich lipoproteins as an independent cardiovascular risk factor is complicated by the fact that triglycerides circulate in various lipoproteins with variable impact on the prevalence of atherosclerosis. Chylomicrons are associated with extraordinarily elevated triglyceride levels but are not clearly associated with increased cardiovascular risk. Familial combined hyperlipidemia and dysbetalipoproteinemia are clearly associated with increased risk, which appears to be at least partially associated with small VLDL particles and especially the persistence in the circulation of VLDL and chylomicron remnants. Remnant particles are potentially cytotoxic and have been demonstrated to be associated with increased recognition, binding, and uptake by the macrophage, leading to the generation of foam cells. Additionally, triglyceride-rich lipoproteins are clearly a clinical marker of the presence of potentially atherogenic and prothrombotic conditions, including small, dense LDL; fibrinogen; plasminogen activator inhibitor type I; low HDL cholesterol level; insulin resistance; and hyperinsulinemia. Evaluation of hypertriglyceridemia is further complicated by the fact that triglyceride determinations are generally performed on a fasting sample to avoid measuring the presence of exogenously derived chylomicron remnants. Postprandial lipemia, defined as the inability to clear triglycerides after a fatty load, has been correlated with increased risk for coronary heart disease.[49] This relationship has persisted in multivariate analysis, implicating the inability of fasting triglyceride levels to accurately depict cardiovascular risk.

Epidemiologic and clinical trial evidence has supported the potential atherogenic role of triglyceride-rich lipoproteins. A meta-analysis of 16 population-based prospective studies involving both men and women established a positive relationship between elevated triglycerides and increased cardiovascular risk. The increased risk associated with hypertriglyceridemia persisted even after HDL cholesterol was adjusted for by use of multivariate analysis.[50]

The Prospective Cardiovascular Munster Study, which was a long-term epidemiologic trial, established the combination of elevated triglyceride levels (> 200 mg/dl) and an LDL-to-HDL cholesterol ratio of at least five as a subgroup that is at extremely high risk for coronary artery disease.[51]

The Copenhagen Male Study analyzed an 8-year follow-up evaluation of the relationship between triglycerides and ischemic heart disease.[52] The study consisted of 3387 men with a mean age of 63 years who participated in a continuation of the original Copenhagen Male Study. The study was stratified by HDL levels, and a clear gradient of the risk of developing ischemic heart disease was correlated with increasing triglyceride levels within each level of HDL cholesterol, even after other risk factors of ischemic heart disease were controlled for in multivariate analysis. The Copenhagen Male Study also controlled for the potential confounding effects of antihypertensive drugs, physical activity, social class, and alcohol use. An additional subgroup of hypertriglyceridemic individuals was also determined to be at increased risk for coronary artery disease, despite a potentially protective high level of circulating HDL cholesterol.

The Bezafibrate Coronary Atherosclerosis Intervention Trial was a 5-year angiographic study evaluating the potential benefits of bezafibrate or dietary intervention in dyslipidemic male survivors of an acute myocardial infarction who were younger than 45 years of age.[53] Angiographic analysis was performed in 81 subjects and demonstrated significantly less progression in the group randomly assigned to receive bezafibrate therapy. Bezafibrate resulted in a reduction of circulating triglycerides of 31 percent, which was coupled with an increase in HDL cholesterol of 9 percent. Bezafibrate administration resulted in essentially no significant alteration of circulating LDL. Fibrinogen levels were also decreased in concordance with the reduction in circulating triglycerides. The exact beneficial mechanisms associated with bezafibrate administration have not been completely determined. However, the results of this trial support the potential benefits of reductions in triglyceride rich lipoproteins.

The Cholesterol Lowering Atherosclerosis Study (CLAS) was also an angiographic regression trial utilizing the combination of colestipol and nicotinic acid in an attempt to determine the potential role of aggressive lipid lowering as a means to retard the progression of atherosclerosis.[54] Multivariate analysis of the CLAS population found that the primary predictor of atherosclerotic progression in subjects who were randomly assigned to receive combination therapy was the level of apo-CIII in HDL. Apo-C lipoproteins consist of apo-CI, apo-CII, and apo-CIII. Apo-CII is the physiologic activator of lipoprotein lipase, which is the key enzyme in the degradation of triglyceride-rich lipoproteins, such as VLDL. Apo-CIII, which is also found on VLDL, inhibits the activity of this enzyme. Apo-C particles can interchange between various circulating lipoprotein fractions, including HDL. Sequestration of apo-CIII into HDL would thus potentially enhance the degree of activation of lipoprotein lipase by unopposed apo-CII and thus increase the catabolic rate and clearance of VLDL, potentially reducing the exposure of the vascular endothelium to triglyceride-rich remnant particles.[55]

LOW-DENSITY LIPOPROTEIN

LDL is formed from the catabolism of intermediate-density lipoprotein and is strongly correlated with increased cardiovascular risk. LDL has a density of 1.019 to 1.063 g/ml and demonstrates electrophoretic mobility in the beta region. The particle is approximately 18 to 25 nm in diameter and has a molecular weight of 180 to 300 D and contains only one apoprotein (apo-B100). The prototype disease manifest by elevated LDL is familial hypercholesterolemia, which is a genetic disorder that occurs in the heterozygous state in approximately 1 in 500 individuals. Familial hypercholesterolemia may represent the underlying genetic defect in as many as 10 percent of premature myocardial infarctions. Familial hypercholesteremia is characterized by a decreased number or function of the apo-B/E receptor, which recognizes and internalizes circulating lipoproteins carrying these apoproteins on their surface. Heterozygous individuals have approximately a 50 percent reduction in the number or function of LDL receptors, which results in an approximate doubling of circulating LDL levels. Homozygous familial hypercholesterolemia is rare and occurs in approximately 1 in 1,000,000 individuals. Familial hypercholesterolemia in the homozygous form may be demonstrated at birth by use of cord blood analysis and is associated with severe, aggressive, premature atherosclerosis, with myocardial infarction being documented as early as 18 months of age.

Familial defective apo-B100 also results in an LDL cholesterol elevation that is secondary to reduced clearance of this lipoprotein in the presence of normally functioning LDL receptors. The LDL particle carries an amino acid substitution that renders the apo-B100 molecule to be structurally abnormal and results in reduced recognition and binding by the LDL receptor. The prevalence of this condition is approximately 1 in 700 in whites with circulating LDL cholesterol levels similar to those documented in heterozygous familial hypercholesterolemia.

Familial combined hyperlipidemia is due to hepatic overproduction of apo-B–containing particles and may present with different phenotypes, including elevated LDL cholesterol, elevated VLDL cholesterol, or elevated LDL and VLDL cholesterol levels. The clinical expression of this condition frequently occurs in adulthood and is associated with premature atherosclerosis.

LDL exists in several different subtypes, as determined by density ultracentrifugation, but for clinical purposes, it has been divided into patterns A (large, buoyant LDL) and B (small, dense LDL). Clinical trials have clearly demonstrated that pharmacologic therapy primarily directed at reduction of circulating LDL results in reduced cardiovascular morbidity and mortality and, in some cases, total mortality. However, despite significant reductions in circulating LDL levels, coronary atherosclerosis is often not reversed and frequently progresses, albeit at a reduced rate. This finding has directed clinical interest in the potential role of type A and type B LDL particles in the pathogenesis of atherosclerosis. The atherogenic lipoprotein profile has been characterized by a normal level of LDL cholesterol distributed in the LDL fraction but associated with increased numbers of small, dense LDL particles.[56] The atherogenic lipid profile is a genetic disorder and is also associated with elevated intermediate-density lipoprotein, apo-B100, and triglycerides. Reductions in HDL cholesterol and apo-A in combination with central obesity and subsequent insulin resistance are also frequently seen. The Friedewald equation, which calculates the amount of cholesterol distributed within the LDL fraction, is not adequate to determine the presence of the atherogenic lipoprotein profile.[57] The atherogenic lipid profile accounts for approximately 25 percent of subjects in the normal population but is demonstrated in 50 percent of patients who have had an acute myocardial infarction, demonstrating an overrepresentation within the subjects demonstrating overt atherosclerosis.[58] The atherogenic lipoprotein profile is genetically transmitted and has been variably linked to a position on the short arm of chromosome 19 and three other loci, including the apo-AI/CIII/AIV gene cluster on chromosome 11, which is associated with severe lipid abnormalities.

The presence of the atherogenic lipoprotein profile has been demonstrated to be associated with significant increased cardiovascular risk in epidemiologic and interventional trials. The Physicians' Health Study prospectively demonstrated a greater than threefold increased risk for atherosclerosis in the presence of this lipid profile that was independent of body mass index, HDL cholesterol, non-HDL cholesterol, and triglycerides.[59] The genetic and epidemiologic association of the atherogenic lipoprotein profile with coronary disease has been extended by subgroup analysis in the Helsinki Heart Study, which documented the beneficial response to gemfibrozil in a primary-prevention analysis of more than 4000 patients.[60] The bulk of clinical benefit (approximately 70 percent) was confined on retrospective analysis to the small (~10 percent) subgroup of patients whose triglyceride levels were in excess of 200 mg/dl and whose LDL/HDL ratio exceeded five. This lipid profile is compatible with the presence of the atherogenic lipoprotein phenotype and is similar to the high-risk subgroup in the PROCAM study.

The CLAS was retrospectively analyzed by evaluating clinical response relative to baseline triglyceride levels. Subjects with low triglyceride levels were presumed to have large, buoyant LDL, whereas patients with elevated triglyceride levels presumably had a higher prevalence of small, dense LDL. Clinical benefit appeared to be concentrated in the group with elevated triglycerides, despite the fact that subjects whose initial triglycerides were low achieved significant LDL reductions in response to nicotinic acid and colestipol. Additionally, CLAS demonstrated improved angiographic progression relative to markers of efficient triglyceride metabolism (apo-CIII levels in HDL).

HIGH-DENSITY LIPOPROTEIN

HDL is a major carrier of cholesteryl ester and is a relatively small particle ranging in diameter from 50 to 120 Å. The major circulating components of HDL are the HDL_2 and HDL_3 forms, which may carry apo-AI, apo-AII, apo-CI, apo-CII, apo-CIII, and apo-E. HDL has a density ranging between 1.125 and 1.063 g/ml and migrates with electrophoretic ability in the alpha region. HDL is synthesized and secreted as nascent HDL by the ileum and the liver. Nascent HDL is a discoid precursor particle consisting predominantly of phospholipid, cholesterol, and apo-A. Nascent HDL subsequently is transformed into a mature spheroidal particle by acquiring cholesterol via the enzymatic activity of lecithin: cholesterol acyltransferase. HDL_3 is converted into HDL_2, which is larger in diameter and has a higher cholesterol content. Women and participants in aerobic exercise have significantly higher levels of HDL_2.[61]

Elevated levels of HDL cholesterol are epidemiologically associated with a reduction in risk of ischemic events, and the National Cholesterol Education Program has designated an HDL cholesterol level above 60 mg/dl as a negative risk factor. However, the mechanism by which increased levels of HDL cholesterol confer a reduction in risk has not been totally elucidated and is multifactorial. HDL is believed to be the major particle involved in reverse cholesterol transport, which scavenges cholesterol from peripheral tissues with subsequent transfer to the liver, where it may be incorporated into the bile acid pool and excreted. HDL may have other potential mechanisms in reduction in risk, including enhanced endothelial repair, increased prostacyclin production, and antioxidant activity and may have a major metabolic role in the catabolism of triglyceride-rich lipoproteins. A low level of HDL cholesterol is associated with increased risk for coronary artery disease, and the National Cholesterol Education Program has designated an HDL cholesterol level of less than 35 mg/dl as a positive risk factor.[62]

However, certain genetic syndromes associated with extremely low HDL cholesterol levels may not exhibit increased risk for premature atherosclerosis. Tangier disease is a genetically determined lipid disorder associated with low total cholesterol level and marked reductions in HDL cholesterol levels, which frequently are below 20 mg/dl. Tangier disease is recognizable clinically by corneal arcus, hepatosplenomegaly, orange tonsils, and mild peripheral neuropathy. Despite the extremely low HDL cholesterol level, a significant increase in the incidence of premature atherosclerosis is not clinically documented, although there may be some mildly increased risk. Kinetic studies have demonstrated that the low plasma level in Tangier disease is secondary to markedly enhanced catabolism of HDL with facilitated cholesterol efflux from cellular elements, implying enhanced potential for reverse cholesterol transport.[63]

Familial hypoalphalipoproteinemia is more common and may be associated with up to 20 percent of all myocardial infarctions in the United States. Kindreds with this genetically determined condition have normal triglyceride levels, normal cholesterol level, normal LDL cholesterol level, and isolated low HDL cholesterol levels, which are associated with an increased risk of premature atherosclerosis.[64] Many rare syndromes, such as apo-AI/apo-CIII deficiency and apo-AI/apo-CIII/apo-AIV deficiency, are associated with severe, malignant, premature atherosclerosis. Isolated reductions in HDL cholesterol in the presence of other normal lipid subfractions are difficult to treat pharmacologically. Lifestyle alterations, such as exercise and smoking cessation, may result in increased HDL cholesterol levels. Fibric acid derivatives and nicotinic acid are the main pharmacologic agents utilized to elevate decreased HDL cholesterol levels.

LIPOPROTEIN(A)

An elevated circulating plasma level of lipoprotein(a) is an independent risk factor for the subsequent development of occlusive coronary, peripheral, and cerebrovascular disease. Lipoprotein(a) is a complex particle consisting of two major components—a large glycoprotein termed *apolipoprotein(a),* which demonstrates homology to plasminogen, is linked to an LDL particle via a disulfide bond interacting within the apo-B100 molecule. The major circulating lipoproteins in human plasma are distributed with a gaussian distribution. However, the levels of lipoprotein(a) are skewed, with most individuals having a circulating level of less than 10 mg/dl.[65]

Racial differences are found in the distribution of lipoprotein(a), and the median plasma level in Africans is approximately twofold to fourfold higher when compared with whites or Asians. The major circulating lipoprotein fractions have a limited variability in their plasma concentration, which is in contrast with lipoprotein(a), which may vary more than 1000-fold in different patients.[66] Lipoprotein(a) has been proposed as a major link between dyslipidemia, atherosclerosis, and thrombosis resulting from the presence of the LDL particle and the structural similarity of apo(a) and plasminogen. Plasminogen has five subunits termed *kringles,* which are defined in numerical order (K1 to K5). Kringles 1 to 3 are found in plasminogen but have not been determined to be present in apo(a), which is characterized by multiple repeating copies of kringle-4 of plasminogen. Despite the resultant structural similarity, lipoprotein(a) lacks serine protease activity and thus does not demonstrate the fibrinolytic activity of the product of the interaction between plasminogen (plasmin) and tissue plasminogen activators.

The circulating levels of lipoprotein(a) in humans are predominantly determined by genetic inheritance, and the role of environmental factors on circulating plasma levels has not been clearly delineated. The polymorphism of the apo(a) gene accounts for approximately 40 to 70 percent of the individual variation of circulating levels in whites.[67]

Lipoprotein(a) is synthesized in the liver and attaches to LDL particles either on the surface of the hepatocyte or after the migration of this particle into the circulation. After secretion of lipoprotein(a) into the circulation, the metabolic fate has not been clearly defined. The apo B/E receptor is not required for lipoprotein(a) catabolism, but has been demonstrated by in vitro studies to bind lipoprotein(a), although the affinity coefficients are significantly reduced compared with those for binding of LDL.[68] The circulating levels of lipoprotein(a) remain relatively constant throughout life, although many conditions may be associated with changes in plasma levels. Postmenopausal females have been documented to demonstrate a gradual increase in circulating levels of lipoprotein(a), and estrogen therapy may restore the level to normal. Anabolic steroids are also associated with a significant reduction in circulating levels of lipoprotein(a). Myxedema and acromegaly are also associated with high circulating levels of lipoprotein(a), and the administration of thyroid and growth hormone restores levels toward normal.

Pharmacologic therapy directed at reduction of lipoprotein(a) has been controversial, and commonly utilized agents, such as statins and bile acid sequestrants, are frequently ineffective. However, nicotinic acid, especially when utilized at high doses, can significantly reduce lipoprotein(a) level.[69] The mechanism by which nicotinic acid reduces lipoprotein(a) level has not been fully delineated but appears to be secondary to a reduction in the hepatic synthesis. The fibric acid derivatives are generally not associated with a reduction in lipoprotein(a) levels. However, in patients with combined hyperlipidemia, which is associated with elevations of both LDL and VLDL levels, fibric acids may be effective in the individual who also has elevated lipoprotein(a) levels.[70] LDL apheresis is an aggressive but effective method of reducing lipoprotein(a) levels. Lipoprotein(a) is clearly a risk factor for the development of atherosclerosis, but the potential beneficial role of altering the levels of this particle has not been determined.

Minor Risk Factors

Thrombosis

Increased tendency for coagulation has been recognized as a potential major modifiable risk factor for coronary atherosclerosis, and clinical interest has centered around the potential association and interrelation between endothelial dysfunction, hyperlipidemia, and hypercoagulability. Acute ischemic syndromes are believed to be related to the formation of an occlusive intravascular thrombus secondary to the fissuring of a vulnerable plaque. The local balance of procoagulant and fibrinolytic activity is a major determinant of the subsequent clinical course, which represents a complex interaction between levels of coagulation factors, platelet activation, tissue factor, and dyslipidemia. Dyslipidemia has been statistically correlated with various procoagulant markers, including elevated levels of fibrinogen, elevated levels of plasminogen activator inhibitor, and abnormal platelet binding and aggregation. Endothelial damage or dysfunction has been associated with increased levels of von Willebrand factor, which has been correlated with both increased platelet aggregation and the subsequent binding to the dysfunctional endothelium. The extent and the severity of atherosclerosis have been directly correlated with increased circulating levels of von Willebrand factor, implying a potential relation between the progression of vascular injury and a hypercoagulable state. Elevated levels of von Willebrand factor have also been documented in unstable angina, and an early rise of von Willebrand factor has also been determined to be an independent predictor of an adverse clinical outcome.[71] Circulating levels of von Willebrand factor have been demonstrated to be positively correlated with elevated levels of LDL and significantly reduced after successful treatment of dyslipidemia.[72] The mechanism involved has not been totally elucidated but presumably is at least partially related to the hypolipidemia-mediated restoration of normal endothelial function.

Cellular elements derived from the monocyte-macrophage line are a source of platelet-activating factor, which is generated at sites of inflammation within the intimal surface of the arterial beds. Activation of platelets results in the upregulation of thrombin receptors, which are localized on vascular smooth muscle and thus enhance the vasoconstrictor activity of thrombin. Dyslipidemia has been associated with increased platelet aggregation in addition to increased levels of beta-thromboglobulin and thromboxane A_2 and B_2. This finding is compatible with the concept that dyslipidemia is associated with both lipid peroxidation and resultant platelet activation.[73] Restoration of circulating lipid parameters to normal has been associated with improvement in platelet aggregation. Lovastatin therapy in dyslipidemic patients, as manifest by increased levels of LDL cholesterol, was demonstrated to reduce adenosine.[74] Platelet leukocyte adhesion and interactions have been modulated by the generation of P-selectin molecules expressed on the surface of platelets, which has been shown to be increased in patients with symptomatic coronary atherosclerosis.[75] Hypolipidemic therapy in the form of either the administration of statins or the utilization of LDL apheresis has been demonstrated to decrease the rate of platelet thrombosis and the activity of cellular adhesion molecules, which would have therapeutic implications. An arterial injury model that stimulates plaque rupture has been utilized in patients with atherosclerosis and demonstrated that the magnitude of platelet thrombus formation was correlated with the degree of dyslipidemia.[76] Pravastatin administration was demonstrated to reduce both the level of LDL cholesterol and the generation of platelet thrombus, which was not affected by the utilization of aspirin.

Tissue factor is a lipoprotein cofactor that increases the proteolytic activity of factor VII-A by acting on factor IX and factor X.[77] Tissue factor activity is associated with endothelial injury and has been demonstrated to be increased in numerous cellular processes associated with either inflammation or smooth muscle cell migration. Additionally, tissue factor has been reported to be up-regulated in human atherosclerotic lesions.[78] Dyslipidemia has been associated with increased tissue factor activity, as demonstrated by associated levels in human monocyte–derived macrophages after the exogenous administration of cholesterol.[79] Atherectomy specimens removed from human coronary artery obstructive lesions have also demonstrated an increased activity of tissue factor and have been correlated with unstable angina and acute myocardial infarction, which implies a potential role in the pathogenesis and clinical manifestations of atherosclerosis.

Epidemiologic studies have associated increased levels of fibrinogen with enhanced risk for atherosclerosis.[80] Elevated fibrinogen is a plausible risk factor because of its major role in both coagulation and blood viscosity. Fibrinogen also is a cofactor for platelet aggregation and is involved in growth factor activity, which may play a role in early stages of atherosclerosis.[81] Elevated levels of fibrinogen have also been correlated with other risk factors, including dyslipidemia. Statin therapy has been utilized as a possible therapeutic intervention to alter fibrinogen and has been evaluated in comparative trials with variable and contradictory results. Fibric acid derivatives, such as bezafibrate and fenofibrate, have been demonstrated to lower significantly circulating levels of fibrinogen, as opposed to gemfibrozil, which has been associated with an increase in fibrinogen, despite decreases in cardiac end points.[82] The potential role of statin therapy as a means to lower fibrinogen is controversial, and a consensus as to its benefit has not been reached.

Plasminogen activator inhibitor type I is increased in many conditions associated with increased cardiac risk, including hypertriglyceridemia, insulin resistance, and hypertension.[83] The endothelial-mediated balance between procoagulant and fibrinolytic activity is disturbed when the endothelium is dysfunctional and is associated with an increased production of plasminogen inhibitor type I coupled with a decrease in plasminogen activators. Plasminogen activator inhibitor type I interferes with the formation of plasmin from its precursors and thus contributes to a potential hypercoagulable state. Plasminogen activator inhibitor may be lowered by angiotensin-converting enzyme inhibitors, angiotensin-II receptor blockers, or various hypolipidemic agents, including fibric acid derivatives and statins.

Elevated levels of homocysteine have also been correlated with increased risk for hypercoagulability, myocardial infarction, and vascular disease.[84] Homocysteine is a metabolic intermediate that is generated during methionine metabolism. The rare genetic abnormality homocysteinuria is secondary to a deficiency of the enzyme cystathionine beta-synthase and results in markedly elevated levels of homocysteine due to incomplete catabolism. Homocysteinuria has been associated with vascular complications, and clinical research has indicated milder elevations of homocysteine as a potential risk factor for the development of coronary artery disease. Levels of homocysteine may be affected by both genetic and environmental factors.[85] Mutations in the structure of several of the genes associated with the production of enzymes involved in the metabolism of this essential sulfur–containing amino acid include the C677T mutation in the gene 45, 10-methylene tetrahydrofolic reductase. Cystathionine β-synthase has also been associated with mutations that result in elevated levels of homocysteine. The mechanism by which homocysteine is involved in vascular damage is complex and multifactorial, with endothelial function abnormalities thought to be an initial step.[86]

Obesity

Obesity is a highly prevalent condition in the United States, and the proportion of the population who exceeds ideal body weight is gradually increasing. Currently, approximately 20 percent of the United States population is obese if the definition of an increase in body weight exceeding 20 percent of ideal body weight is used.[87] Despite the frequent coexistence of obesity and coronary artery disease, the role of mild-to-moderately increased body weight as an independent risk factor remains controversial. Increased body weight is frequently associated with cardiovascular risk factors, including hypertension, dyslipidemia, diabetes, and physical inactivity, which raises the possibility that increased body weight may simply exist as a marker for other risk factors. However, the Framingham Study demonstrated an independent relation for obesity in cardiovascular illness, with the analysis controlling for other variables in multivariate analysis.[88] Obesity has been also correlated in numerous epidemiologic studies showing increased total and cardiovascular mortality. A meta-analysis analyzed 19 prospective studies that enrolled more than 600,000 subjects followed up over a 15-year period. The lowest mortality was documented in patients in the low range of body mass index. Patients whose body mass index was in the higher ranges had a concordant increase in all-cause cardiovascular mortality that was maintained in multivariate analysis.[89]

In addition to increased weight or body mass index, the localization of fat may also play a major role in the determination of cardiovascular risk. Truncal obesity, which is more common in male subjects, appears to increase the risk of coronary artery disease. Abdominal fat distribution can be determined by computed tomography or can be estimated by waist-to-hip circumference ratio. Men are considered to be at risk if the waist-to-hip ratio is greater than 0.95, and women demonstrate increased risk if the waist-to-hip ratio exceeds 0.8.[90] The distribution of body fat is associated with several metabolic abnormalities, especially as relates to glucose, insulin, and lipid metabolism. Truncal obesity is associated with insulin resistance and resultant hyperinsulinemia. Insulin resistance is associated with dyslipidemia secondary to overproduction of triglyceride-rich lipoproteins by the liver coupled with impaired activation of lipoprotein lipase resulting in elevated triglycerides; low HDL cholesterol; and small, dense LDL. Tumor necrosis factor may also have a direct role in the development of insulin resistance in obese subjects because of the impairment of insulin-stimulated glucose uptake in the periphery. Tumor necrosis factor may also decrease the activity of the insulin-responsive glucose transporter that regulates glucose uptake in the periphery independently of insulin level.

Obesity frequently coexists with hemostatic abnormalities that are compatible with a hypercoagulable state. Plasminogen activator inhibitor has been demonstrated to be increased in subjects with truncal obesity.[91] Plasminogen activator inhibitors may be lowered after dietary therapy. Obesity may also play a significant role in hypertension. Obese subjects have a higher prevalence (as high as 50 percent) of elevated blood pressure when compared with the general population. The degree of blood pressure elevation relates to the relative increase in body weight.[92] Importantly, obesity-related hypertension is potentially modifiable by increasing physical activity and losing weight, both of which also improve insulin resistance. Despite the complexities of establishing the independent relation of increased body weight and its distribution to coronary artery disease risk, patients should be encouraged to increase physical activity with a concerted effort to maintain ideal body weight.

Physical Activity

Physical inactivity is considered to be a modifiable risk factor, and the National Institutes of Health has established consensus guidelines on the relation between physical activity and cardiovascular health.[93] Physical inactivity is common in the United States, and approximately 60 percent of all adults describe no significant physical activity.[94] Additionally, approximately 50 percent of high school students are not enrolled in physical education courses. The role that physical activity plays in the development of cardiovascular disease is multifactorial, and increasing levels of exercise have been demonstrated to be associated with reductions in blood pressure, improvements in serum lipids, increased weight loss, and improvement of insulin resistance. Establishing and maintaining a regular physical activity pattern has been shown to reduce risk for cardiovascular events in several observational epidemiologic studies. A meta-analysis of studies that analyzed the physical activity in different occupations determined that the relative risk of death in sedentary occupations was 1.9 when compared with active occupations.[95] The Multiple Risk Factor Intervention Trial correlated cardiovascular risk and moderate physical activity and demonstrated that physically active subjects had an approximate 27 percent reduction in vascular complications compared with sedentary individuals.[96]

The impact of exercise on cardiovascular risk factors appears to be related to the intensity of physical activity. The level of physical activity determined by the kilometers run per week and the intensity in a 12-km run, as determined in kilometers/hour, were determined in 7059 male and 1837 female runners. The intensity of physical activity was correlated with lower blood pressure, triglyceride levels, ratio of total to HDL cholesterol, and body mass index. However, the effect on HDL cholesterol was more marked in long distance runners, as quantified by kilometers run per week, when compared with speed, as quantified by kilometers per hour.

Some studies have compared the impact on long distance runners (>80 km/wk) to runners who ran less than 16 km/wk. Long distance runners demonstrated a 2.5-fold increase in HDL cholesterol coupled with a 50 percent reduction in hypertension and medications used to control blood pressure and cholesterol levels.[97]

Physical activity can be considered to be generally inversely related to risk for coronary artery disease, although the specific shape of the dose-response curve is uncertain.[98] The greatest benefit may accrue from changing physical activity from a sedentary lifestyle to moderately active, and the degree of improvement may decrease at higher levels of exercise.[99]

Psychological Stress

The role of stress as a risk factor for coronary atherosclerosis remains controversial. The type A, or coronary-prone, behavior was described during the 1960s. A type A behavior pattern has been clinically characterized as being documented in individuals who displayed aggression, competitiveness, and time urgency. The prospective studies involving type A behavior and coronary atherosclerosis have met with mixed results.[100] Type A personality has been reported to be an independent risk factor in an 8-year study involving more than 3000 men who had no clinical evidence of coronary atherosclerosis on enrollment. However, the Framingham Heart Study showed no definite association between personality type and risk for either myocardial infarction or fatal events, despite an increase in angina.[101] The Multiple Risk Factor Intervention Trial did not demonstrate a statistical association between type A behavior and risk for first major coronary events when defined as coronary death or nonfatal myocardial infarction. Mental stress has been demonstrated to induce myocardial ischemia in patients with known coronary artery disease, which may act as a trigger for acute cardiac events.[102] The role of stress as a cardiovascular risk factor remains plausible but requires further delineation.

CONCLUSION

The age-related decline in cardiovascular morbidity and mortality is encouraging, but atherosclerosis remains a major clinical challenge in the United States. Increased recognition of the role of risk factors in the genesis of coronary, cerebral, and peripheral atherosclerosis has provided major therapeutic options for further clinical benefits in risk reduction.

REFERENCES

1. American Heart Association: Heart and Stroke Facts Statistical Update. Dallas, TX: American Heart Association, 2000.
2. Benditt EP, Benditt JM: Evidence for monoclonal origin of human atherosclerotic plaques. Proc Natl Acad Sci U S A 70:1773, 1993.
3. Ridker PM: Inflammation, infection, and cardiovascular risk: how good is the clinical evidence? Circulation 17:1671, 1997.
4. Ridker PM, Cushman M, Stampfer MJ, et al: Inflammation, aspirin and the risk of cardiovascular disease in apparently healthy men. N Engl J Med 336:973, 1997.
5. Leitinen K, Laurila A, Pyhala L, et al: *Chlamydia pneumoniae* infection induces inflammatory change in the aortas of rabbits. Infect Immun 65:4832, 1997.
6. Saikku P, Leinonen M, Tenkanen N: Chronic *Chlamydia pneumoniae* infection as a risk factor for coronary heart disease in the Helsinki Heart Study. Ann Intern Med 116:273, 1992.
7. Grayston JT: Antibiotic treatment of *Chlamydia pneumoniae* for secondary prevention of cardiovascular events. Circulation 97:1669, 1998.
8. Gupta S, Leatham EW, Carrington D, et al: Elevated *Chlamydia pneumoniae* antibodies, cardiovascular events and azithromycin in male survivors of myocardial infarction. Circulation 96:404, 1997.
9. Gurfinkel E, Bozovich G, Daroca A, et al: Randomized trial of roxithromycin in non–Q wave coronary syndromes: ROXIS pilot study. 350:404, Lancet 1997.
10. Pasceri V, Cammarota G, Patti G, et al: Association of virulent *Helicobacter pylori* strains with ischemic heart disease. Circulation 97:1675, 1998.
11. Kannel WB: Range of cholesterol values in the population developing coronary artery disease. Am J Cardiol 76:69C, 1995.
12. Stamler J, Wentworth D, Neaton JD: Is the relationship between serum cholesterol and risk of premature death from coronary heart disease continuous and graded? Findings in 356,222 primary screenees of the Multiple Risk Factor Intervention Trial. JAMA 256:2823, 1986.
13. Lipid Research Clinics Program: The Lipid Research Clinics Coronary Primary Prevention Trial results. I: reduction in incidence of coronary heart disease. JAMA 251:351, 1984.
14. Manninen V, Elo MO, Frick MH, et al: Lipid alterations and decline in the incidence of coronary heart disease in the Helsinki Heart Study. JAMA 260:641, 1988.
15. MAAS Investigators: Effect of simvastatin on coronary atheroma: the Multicentre Anti-Atheroma Study (MAAS). Lancet 344:633, 1994.
16. Jukema JW, Bruschke ADG, van Boven AJ, et al: Effects of lipid lowering by pravastatin on progression and regression of coronary artery disease in symptomatic men with normal to moderately elevated serum cholesterol levels: the Regression Growth Evaluation Statin Study (REGRESS). Circulation 91:2528, 1995.
17. Herd JA, Ballantyne CM, Farmer JA, et al: Effect of fluvastatin on coronary atherosclerosis in patients with mild to moderate cholesterol elevations (Lipoprotein in Coronary Atherosclerosis Study [LCAS]). Am J Cardiol 80:278, 1997.
18. Goldbourt U, Yaari S, Medalie JH: Isolated low HDL cholesterol as a risk factor for coronary heart disease mortality: a 21-year follow-up of 8000 men. Arterioscler Thromb Vasc Biol 17:107, 1997.
19. Ballantyne CM, Herd JA, West MS: Influence of low HDL cholesterol on progression of CAD in response to fluvastatin therapy. J Am Coll Cardiol 29:232A, 1997.
20. Waters D, Higginson L, Gladstone P, et al: Effects of monotherapy with an HMG CoA reductase inhibitor on the progression of coronary atherosclerosis as assessed by serial quantitative angiography: the Canadian Coronary Atherosclerosis Intervention Trial. Circulation 89:959, 1994.
21. Pitt B, Mancini JBJ, Ellis SG, et al: Pravastatin Limitation of Atherosclerosis in the Coronary Arteries (PLAC-1): reduction in atherosclerosis progression in clinical events. J Am Coll Cardiol 26:1133, 1995.
22. Blankenhorn DH, Azen SP, Kramsh DM, et al: Coronary angiographic changes with lovastatin therapy: the Monitored Atherosclerosis Regression Study (MARS). Ann Intern Med 119:969, 1993.
23. Post Coronary Artery Bypass Graft Trial Investigators: The effect of aggressive lipid lowering on low density lipoprotein cholesterol levels and low dose anticoagulation on obstructive changes and saphenous vein coronary artery bypass grafts. N Engl J Med 336:153, 1997.
24. Shepherd J, Cobbe SM, Ford I, et al: Prevention of coronary heart disease with pravastatin in men with hypercholesterolemia. N Engl J Med 333:1301, 1995.
25. Downs JR, Clearfield M, Weis S, et al: Primary prevention of acute coronary events with lovastatin in men and women with average cholesterol levels: results of AFCAPS/TexCAPS. JAMA 279:1615, 1998.
26. Scandinavian Simvastatin Survival Study Group: Randomized trial of cholesterol lowering in 4,444 patients with coronary artery disease: the Scandinavian Simvastatin Survival Study (4S). Lancet 344:1383, 1994.
27. Sacks FM, Pfeffer MA, Moye LA: The effect of pravastatin on coronary events after myocardial infarction in patients with normal cholesterol levels. N Engl J Med 335:1001, 1996.
28. Ross R: Cellular and molecular studies of atherogenesis. Atherosclerosis 131(suppl):S3, 1997.
29. Stary H: Composition and classification of human atherosclerotic lesions. Virchow Arch 421:277, 1992.
30. Stamler J: Epidemiology to establish risk factors in the primary prevention of coronary heart disease. *In* Parmley WW, Chatterjee K (eds): Cardiology. Vol. II. p. 1. Philadelphia: JB Lippincott, 1987.

31. Hansson L, Zanchetti A, Carruthers SG, et al: Effects of intensive blood pressure lowering and low dose aspirin in patients with hypertension: principal results of the Hypertension Optimal Treatment (HOT) randomized trial. Lancet 351:1755, 1998.
32. Centers for Disease Control: Cigarette smoking attribute to mortality and years of potential life lost, United States, 1990. MMWR Morb Mortal Wkly Rep 42:645, 1993.
33. Garfinkel L: Trends in cigarette smoking in the United States. Prev Med 26:447, 1997.
34. Pittilo RM: Cigarette Smoking and Endothelial Injury: A Review in Tobacco Smoking and Atherosclerosis. New York: Plenum, 1989.
35. Harats D: Cigarette smoking renders LDL susceptible to peroxidated modification and enhanced metabolism by macrophages. Atherosclerosis 79:245, 1989.
36. Meade TW, Imeson J, Stirling Y: Effects of changes in smoking and other characteristics on clotting factors and the risk of ischemic heart disease. Lancet 2:986, 1987.
37. Heinrich J: Fibrinogen and factor-VII in the prediction of coronary risk: results from the PROCAM and CAP study in healthy men. Arterioscler Thromb 14:54, 1994.
38. Schmidt KG, Rasmussen JW: Acute platelet activation induced by smoking. Thromb Haemost 51:279, 1994.
39. Lam TH, He Y, Li LS, et al: Mortality attributable to cigarette smoking in China. JAMA 278:1505, 1997.
40. Howard AG, Wagenknecht LE, Burke GL, et al: Cigarette smoking and the progression of atherosclerosis: the Atherosclerosis Risk in Communities (ARIC) study. JAMA 279:119, 1998.
41. Joint National Committee on Detection, Evaluation, and Treatment of High Blood Pressure: The sixth report of the Joint National Committee on Detection, Evaluation, and Treatment of High Blood Pressure. Arch Intern Med 157:2413, 1997.
42. Morales PA, Braxton DN, Valdez RA, et al: Incidence of NIDDM and impaired glucose tolerance in hypertensive subjects. Diabetes 42:154, 1993.
43. Caulfield M, Lavender P, Farrall M: Linkage of the angiotensinogen gene to essential hypertension. N Engl J Med 330:1629, 1994.
44. Stamler J, Vaccaro O, Neaton JD, et al: Diabetes, other risk factors, and 12-year cardiovascular mortality for men screened in the Multiple Risk Factor Intervention Trial. Diabetes Care 16:434, 1993.
45. Jenuth S. Exogenous insulin administration and cardiovascular risk in non-insulin dependent and insulin dependent diabetes. Ann Intern Med 124:104, 1996.
46. American Diabetes Association: Management of dyslipidemia in adults with diabetes. Diabetes Care 22(suppl S):S56, 1999.
47. Pyorala K, Pedersen TR, Kjekshus J, et al: Cholesterol lowering with simvastatin improves prognosis of diabetic patients with coronary heart disease: a subgroup analysis of the Scandinavian Simvastatin Survival Study (4S). Diabetes Care 20:614, 1997.
48. Gotto AM: Triglyceride: the forgotten risk factor. Circulation 97:1027, 1998.
49. Groot PHE, van Stiphout WAHJ, Crauss X: Postprandial lipoprotein metabolism in normal lipemic men with and without coronary artery disease. Arterioscler Thromb 11:653, 1991.
50. Hokanson JE, Austin MA: Triglyceride is a risk factor for coronary disease in men and women: a meta-analysis of population based prospective studies [abstract]. Circulation 88:I-510, 1993.
51. Assmann G, Schulte H: Role of triglycerides in coronary artery disease: lessons from the Prospective Cardiovascular Munster Study. Am J Cardiol 70:10H, 1992.
52. Jeppesen J, Hein HO, Suadicaini DD, et al: Triglyceride concentration and ischemic heart disease: an 8-year follow-up in the Copenhagen Male Study. Circulation 97:1029, 1998.
53. de-Faireu U, Ericsson CG, Grip L, et al: Secondary preventive potential of lipid lowering drugs: the Bezafibrate Coronary Atherosclerosis Intervention Trial. Eur Heart J 17(suppl F):37, 1996.
54. Blankenhorn DH, Sessim SA, Johnson RL: Beneficial effects of combined colestipol-niacin therapy on coronary atherosclerosis and coronary venous bypass grafts. JAMA 257:3233, 1987.
55. Blankenhorn DH, Alaupovic P, Wickham E: Prediction of angiographic change in human coronary arteries and aorto-coronary bypass grafts: lipid and nonlipid factors. Circulation 81:470, 1990.
56. Krauss RM: The tangled web of coronary risk factors. Am J Med 90(suppl 2A):2A, 1991.
57. Superko HR: What can we learn about dense low density lipoprotein and lipoprotein particles from clinical trials. Curr Opin Lipidol 7:363, 1996.
58. Austin MA, Breslow JL, Hennekens CH: Low density lipoprotein subclass patterns and risk of myocardial infarction. JAMA 260:1917, 1988.
59. Stampfer MJ, Krauss RM, Ma J, et al: A prospective study of triglyceride level, low-density lipoprotein particle diameter, and risk of myocardial infarction. JAMA 276:882, 1996.
60. Manninen D, Tenkanen L, Koskinen P, et al: Joint effects of serum triglyceride and LDL in HDL cholesterol concentrations on coronary heart disease risk in the Helsinki Heart Study. Circulation 85:37, 1992.
61. James RW, Pometta D: Immunofractionation of high density lipoprotein subclasses 2 and 3: similarities and differences of fractions isolated from male and female populations. Atherosclerosis 83:35, 1990.
62. National Cholesterol Education Program Expert Panel: Summary of the 2nd report of the National Cholesterol Education Program Expert Panel on detection, evaluation and treatment of high blood cholesterol in adults. JAMA 269:3015, 1993.
63. Serfaty-Lacrosniere C, Civeira F, Lanzberg A, et al: Homozygous Tangier disease and cardiovascular disease. Atherosclerosis 107:85, 1994.
64. Third JL, Montag J, Flynn M, et al: Primary and familial hypoalphalipoproteinemia. Metabolism 33:136, 1984.
65. Gabel BR, May LF, Marcovina SM, et al: Lipoprotein(a) assembly. Arterioscler Thromb Vasc Biol 16:1559, 1996.
66. Albers JJ, Hazzard WR: Immunochemical quantification of human plasma Lp (a) lipoprotein. Lipids 9:15, 1974.
67. Lakner C, Boerwinkle E, Leffert CC, et al: Molecular basis of apolipoprotein (a) isoform size heterogeneity as revealed by pulsed gel electrophoresis. J Clin Invest 87:2077, 1991.
68. Utermann G: Lipoprotein (a). *In* Scriver C, Baudet A, Sly W, Valle D (eds): The Metabolic and Molecular Bases of Inherited Disease. p. 1887. New York: McGraw-Hill, 1995.
69. Seed M, O'Conner B, Knight BL: The effect of nicotinic acid and acipimox on lipoprotein (a) concentration and turnover. Atherosclerosis 101:61, 1993.
70. Jones PH, Pownall HJ, Patsch W, et al: Effect of gemfibrozil on levels of lipoprotein (a) in type II hyperlipoproteinemic subjects. J Lipid Res 37:1298, 1996.
71. Montalescot G, Philippe F, Ankri A, et al: Early increase of von Willebrand factor predicts adverse outcome in unstable coronary artery disease: beneficial effects of enoxaparin. Circulation 98:294, 1998.
72. Bland AD, Davis A, Miller JP: von Willebrand factor and soluble E-selectin in hyperlipidemia: relationship to lipids and vascular disease. Am J Hematol 55:15, 1997.
73. Di Minno G, Silver MJ, Cerbone AM: Increased fibrinogen binding to platelets from patients with familial hypercholesterolemia. Arteriosclerosis 6:203, 1986.
74. Hochgraf E, Levy Y, Aviram M, et al: Lovastatin decreases plasma and platelet cholesterol levels and normalizes elevated platelet fluidity and aggregation in hypercholesterolemic patients. Metabolism 43:11, 1994.
75. Gawaz M, Reininger A, Neumann FJ: Platelet function and platelet leukocyte adhesion in symptomatic coronary heart disease. Thromb Res 83:341, 1996.
76. Lacoste L, Lamb JY, Hung J, et al: Hyperlipidemia in coronary artery disease: correction of the increased thrombogenic potential with cholesterol reduction. Circulation 92:3172, 1995.
77. Broze GJ: The tissue factor pathway of coagulation. *In* Loscalzo J, Schafer A (eds): Thrombosis and Hemorrhage. p. 57. Boston: Blackwell Scientific, 1994.
78. Sato Y, Asada Y, Marutsuka K: Tissue factor induces migration of cultured aortic smooth muscle cells. Thromb Haemost 75:389, 1996.
79. Lesnik P, Rouis M, Skarlatos S: Uptake of exogenous free cholesterol induces upregulation of tissue factor expression in human monocyte derived macrophages. Proc Natl Acad Sci U S A 89:10370, 1992.
80. Danesh J, Collins R, Appleby T, et al: Association of fibrinogen, C-reactive protein, albumin or leukocyte count with coronary heart disease. Meta-analysis of prospective studies. JAMA 279:1477, 1998.
81. Ernst E: Fibrinogen: its emerging role as a cardiac risk factor. Angiology 45:87, 1994.
82. Branchi A, Robelline A, Sommariva D: Effect of three fibrate

derivatives and of two HMG CoA reductase inhibitors on plasma fibrinogen level in patients with primary hypercholesterolemia. Thromb Haemost 70:241, 1993.
83. Holvoet P, Collen D: Thrombosis and atherosclerosis. Curr Opin Lipidol 8:320, 1997.
84. Kuller LH, Evans RW: Homocysteine, vitamins and cardiovascular disease. Circulation 98:196, 1998.
85. Verhoef P, Stampfer MJ, Rimm EB: Folate and coronary heart disease. Curr Opin Lipidol 9:17, 1998.
86. Mayer EL, Jacobson DW, Robinson KR: Homocysteine and coronary atherosclerosis. J Am Coll Cardiol 27:517, 1996.
87. National Institutes of Health Consensus Development Panel on the health implications of obesity. Ann Intern Med 103:1073, 1985.
88. Hubert HB, Feinleib M, McNamara PM, et al: Obesity as an independent risk factor for cardiovascular disease: a 26-year follow-up on participants in the Framingham Heart Study. Circulation 67:968, 1983.
89. Troino HP, Forngillo EAJ, Sobal J, et al: The relationship between body weight and mortality: a quantitative analysis of combined information from existing studies. Int J Obes Relat Metab Disord 20:63, 1996.
90. Bary GA: Pathophysiology of obesity. Am J Clin Nutr 55:448S, 1992.
91. Svendesen OL, Hassager C, Cristiansen C, et al: Plasminogen activator inhibitor type I, tissue type plasminogen activator and fibrinogen: effective dieting with or without exercise in overweight, postmenopausal females. Arterioscler Thromb Vasc Biol 16:381, 1996.
92. Bonora E, Targher G, Branzi P, et al: Cardiovascular risk profile in 38-year and 18-year old men: contribution of body fat content and regional fat distribution. Int J Obes Relat Metab Disord 20:28, 1996.
93. NIH Consensus Development Panel on Physical Activity in Cardiovascular Health. JAMA 270:3:241, 1996.
94. Prevalence of sedentary lifestyle-behavioral risk factor surveillance system, United States, 1991. MMWR Morb Mortal Wkly Rep 42:576, 1993.
95. Berlin JA, Colditz GA: A meta-analysis of physical activity in the prevention of coronary heart disease. Am J Epidemiol 132:612, 1991.
96. Leon AS, Connett J: Physical activity and 10.5-year mortality in the Multiple Risk Factor Intervention Trial. Int J Epidemiol 20:690, 1991.
97. Williams PT: The relationship of heart disease risk factors to exercise quantity and intensity. Arch Intern Med 158:237, 1998.
98. Blair SN, Cooper KH: Dose of exercise and health benefits. Arch Intern Med 157:153, 1997.
99. Pate RR, Pratt M, Blair SN: Physical activity and public health. JAMA 273:402, 1995.
100. Jonston DW: The current status of the coronary prone behavior pattern. J R Soc Med 86:406, 1993.
101. Eaker ED, Abbott RD, Kannel WB: Frequency of uncomplicated angina pectoris in type A compared to type B persons (the Framingham Study). Am J Cardiol 63:1042, 1989.
102. Jiang W, Babyak M, Krantz DS, et al: Mental stress–induced myocardial ischemia and cardiac events. JAMA 275:1651, 1996.

C H A P T E R **72**

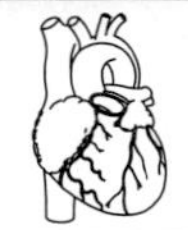

Diseases of the Aorta

James T. Willerson, Bharat Raval, Michael S. Sweeney, O. H. Frazier, Faisal Khan, David Ott, and Denton A. Cooley

ANATOMY AND NORMAL FUNCTION
PHYSIOLOGIC CONSIDERATIONS
PATHOPHYSIOLOGY
Coarctation of the Aorta
Pseudocoarctation
Thoracic Aortic Aneurysms
Abdominal Aortic Aneurysms
Aortic Dissection
Annuloaortic Ectasia
Arteritis Involving the Aorta
Aortic Trauma
Knife or Missile Wounds
Aortic Infections
Aortic Thromboembolic Disease
Thrombotic Occlusion of the Aorta
Embolization of Atherosclerotic Material
Aortic Tumors
Inflammatory Aortic Aneurysms

Anatomy and Normal Function

The ascending aorta lies just to the right of the midline of the pulmonary artery, which is positioned in front, and the left atrium, right pulmonary artery, and right main stem bronchus behind the aorta. The arch of the aorta gives rise to several vessels, including the innominate artery, the left common carotid artery, and the left subclavian artery (Fig. 72–1). The descending thoracic aorta is a continuation of the aorta beyond the arch, and it lies in the posterior mediastinum to the left of the vertebral column, occupying a position behind the esophagus. The aortic isthmus is the location at which the aortic arch and descending thoracic aorta join and is the usual location of coarctations of the aorta. It is also the point at which the aorta is most mobile and vulnerable to tear. The abdominal aorta is a continuation of the thoracic aorta, providing origin for the splanchnic arteries and ending in the aortic bifurcation at the approximate level of the fourth lumbar vertebra.

Physiologic Considerations

The aorta is responsible for the conductance of blood pumped into it with each cardiac systole. Its three layers include a thin, inner *intima*; a thicker middle layer, the *media*; and a thin outer layer, the *adventitia*. As blood is ejected into the aorta, it is propelled distally into the arterial bed at a speed of about 5 m/sec. The systolic pressure developed within the aorta is related to the volume of blood ejected into it, the compliance of the aorta, and the resistance to blood flow. Resistance is determined primarily by the tone in the peripheral muscular arteries and arterioles and, to a lesser extent, by the inertia of the static blood as systole begins. With aging, the aorta and its branches become stiffer, resulting in the typical increase in systolic blood pressure associated with aging.

Pathophysiology

Diseases of the aorta may be congenital or acquired (Tables 72–1 and 72–2).[1–10] Acquired diseases of the aorta result primarily from degenerative changes in the aortic wall. Contributing to degeneration of the aorta and acquired aortic diseases are arteriosclerosis, hypertension, aging, connective tissue diseases, inflammation, and infection. The rate of pressure rise and the blood pressure itself are important factors that contribute to the development of aortic dissection by their influence on shear stress. Familial aortic aneurysms have been described in some individuals with decreased ratios of type III collagen.[3] A study from Milewicz and associates[4] indicates that alterations in fibrillin content may also play a role. Hypertension causes structural aortic changes that may contribute to medial degeneration and decrease blood flow in the vasa vasorum, with resultant ischemia of the aortic wall leading to dissection, aneurysm development, or stiffening of the aortic wall, further perpetuating the development of systemic arterial hypertension. Selected diseases of the aorta as they manifest in the adult are discussed here.

Coarctation of the Aorta

The basic anatomic defect in coarctation of the aorta is a localized deformity of the media manifested by an in-

TABLE 72–1 **Congenital Defects of the Aorta**

Right-sided aortic arch	Cystic medial necrosis
Anomalous arterial branches	Coarctation
Double aortic arches	Pseudocoarctation

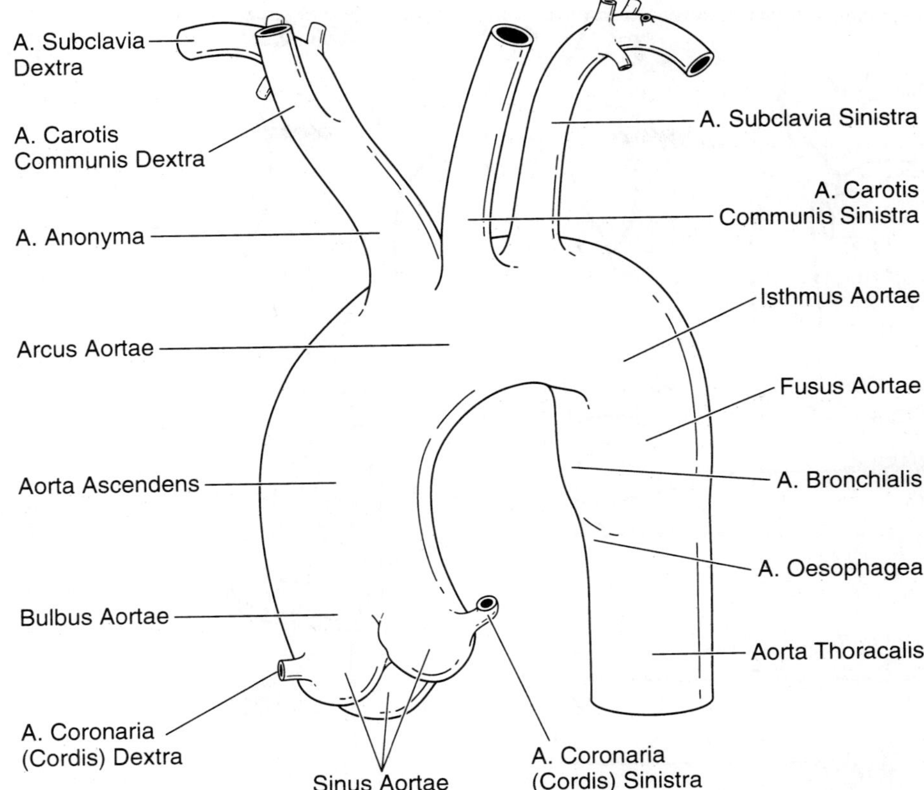

FIGURE 72–1 The aorta, its major branches, and the various anatomic locations of importance. (From Grossman, W: Cardiac Catheterization and Angiography. 3rd ed. Philadelphia: Lea & Febiger, 1985.)[139]

folding that concentrically narrows the aortic lumen (Fig. 72–2).[9, 10] The area of coarctation is characteristically located immediately beyond the origin of the left subclavian artery at or just distal to the insertion of the ligamentum arteriosum. However, the coarctation may take the form of a diffusely narrowed aortic segment that begins distal to the innominate artery and ends at a localized constriction just beyond the left subclavian artery. Occasionally, the area of coarctation is situated at or just proximal to the left subclavian artery so that the lumen of that vessel is compromised and the left radial pulse is reduced. On other occasions, the right subclavian artery arises anomalously below the zone of coarctation. In rare instances, the coarctation is located at sites remote from the aortic isthmus. Aortic coarctation can occur in the ascending aorta proximal to the innominate artery, in the descending thoracic aorta, or in the abdominal aorta above, below, or at the level of the renal arteries. Coarctation of the aorta is often associated with other cardiac malformations, of which the most common is the bicuspid aortic valve.[9, 11] The bicuspid valve may become stenotic, incompetent, or both. Occasionally, supravalvular or discrete subvalvular stenosis has been found in association with aortic coarctation.[12, 13] Moreover, coarctation of the aorta may coexist with patent ductus and aortic stenosis.

In patients with aortic coarctation, the ascending aorta is usually dilated. The dilatation may become aneurysmal and involve the ascending aorta and sinuses of Valsalva.[14, 15] Endocardial fibroelastosis may coexist with aortic coarctation.[16] Coarctation of the aorta occurs with mitral stenosis or incompetence, and the most important noncardiac anomaly in patients with coarctation is an *aneurysm of the circle of Willis*.[17] The most frequent shunt lesion associated with aortic coarctation is a *patent ductus arteriosus*. The most frequently encountered intracardiac shunt with coarctation of the aorta is *ventricular septal defect*.[18]

TABLE 72–2 Acquired Diseases of the Aorta

Atherosclerosis
Atherosclerotic aortic aneurysms
Syphilitic aortic aneurysms
Dissecting aortic aneurysms
Traumatic rupture
Arteritis such as Takayasu's and giant cell arteritis
Aortic embolism
Aortic bacterial infections
Aortic tumors

Natural History

Coarctation of the aorta occurs predominantly in males, but aortic coarctation in the abdomen is divided equally between the sexes. Familial coarctation has been reported, but the incidence is too low to be of clinical importance.

Coarctation of the aorta is particularly likely to produce significant symptoms at two times of life: the first period is in early infancy, and the second begins at age 20 to 30

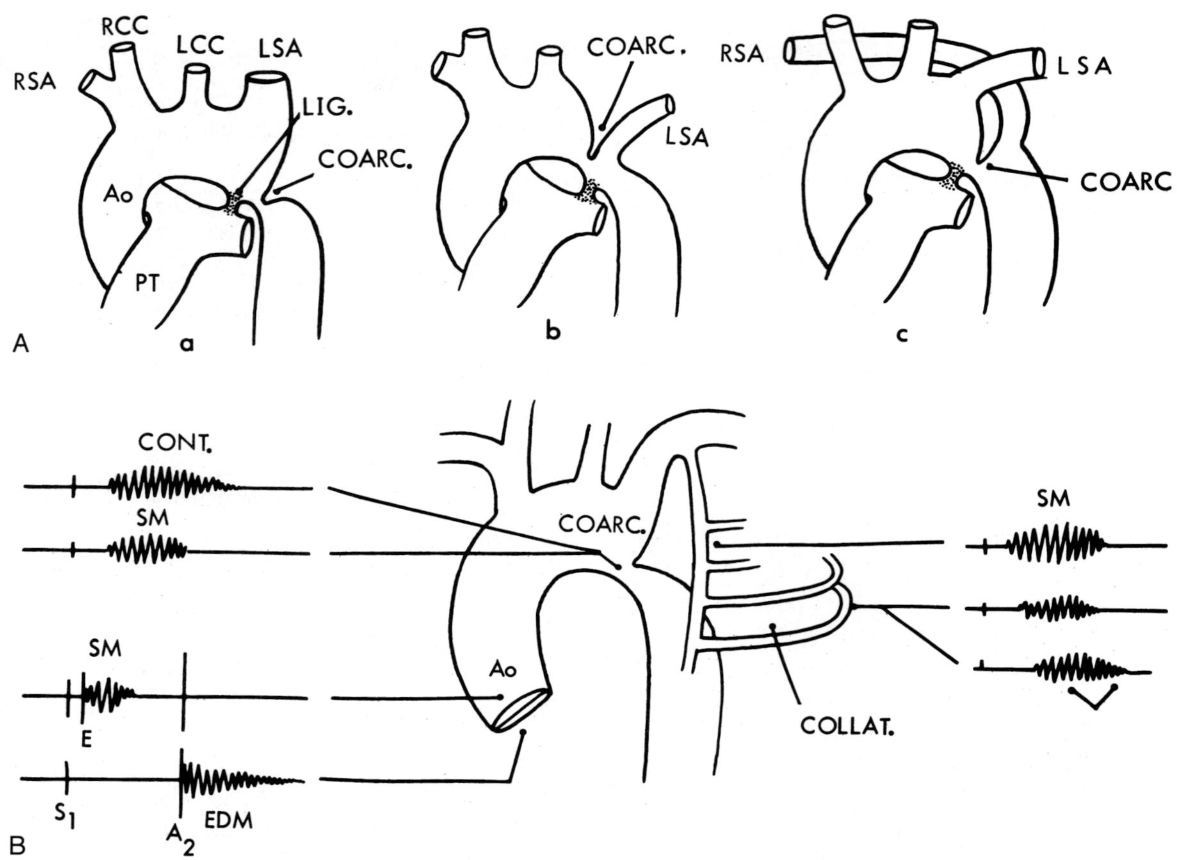

FIGURE 72–2 A, Schematic representation of the different kinds of coarctation (COARC.) of the aorta. *a,* In the usual variety, the area of coarctation is located immediately beyond the left subclavian artery (LSA), which is usually enlarged. The descending aorta is often dilated distal to the coarctation. Ao, ascending aorta; LIG., ligamentum arteriosum; PT, main pulmonary artery; RCC and LCC, right and left common carotid arteries; RSA, right subclavian artery. *b,* The site of coarctation proximal to the left subclavian artery; under these circumstances, the left subclavian artery is not dilated and blood pressure in the left arm is often reduced. *c,* The right subclavian artery (RSA) takes origin anomalously below the coarctation and may compress the esophagus in its unusual course, causing dysphagia. **B,** Diagrammatic illustration of the murmurs heard in patients with coarctation of the aorta (Ao). Bicuspid aortic valves often coexist with coarctation of the aorta, generating their own murmur. *Bottom left,* The typical ejection click (E) followed by a short systolic ejection murmur is demonstrated. In some patients, a diastolic murmur of aortic insufficiency (EDM) is also found. *Top left,* A continuous (CONT.) and a delayed (SM) systolic murmur are demonstrated, which are heard over the coarctation (COARC.) itself, particularly posteriorly over the thoracic spine. *Right,* Collateral (COLLAT.) arterial murmurs, which are often continuous or delayed systolic murmurs and often bilateral, being heard on both sides of the chest. (**A** and **B,** From Perloff, JM: The Clinical Recognition of Congenital Heart Disease. Philadelphia: WB Saunders, 1970.)

years. Most patients live to adulthood, but only a minority reach age 40, and only 10 percent live beyond age 50 if the coarctation is not corrected.[13, 19] However, survival to the age of 92 was recorded in one patient.[20]

Serious symptoms of aortic coarctation are uncommon before the age of 15 years, but it is uncommon for symptoms to be absent in patients beyond the age of 30 years. Systemic arterial hypertension is the most frequent finding in patients with aortic coarctation, and it may provide the initial suspicion of the presence of aortic coarctation. Headache, epistaxis, and leg fatigue are often described. Claudication of the legs is more common with abdominal coarctation. Dysphagia may occur when the right subclavian artery originates distal to the coarctation and passes behind the esophagus to reach the right arm.[21]

Congestive heart failure, dissection or rupture of the aorta, bacterial endarteritis or endocarditis, and cerebral hemorrhage may complicate aortic coarctations.[10, 13] Coarctation of the aorta is one of the most common causes of heart failure in the first few months of life, particularly in acyanotic infants without left-to-right shunts. Rupture of the aorta occurs either in the proximal ascending aorta or in a postcoarctation aneurysm.[19, 22, 23] Perforation of the aorta beyond the coarctation may result in bleeding into the esophagus. Recurrent episodes of hematemesis, melena, or both may be suggestive of severe bleeding from a ruptured postcoarctation aneurysm. Bacterial endocarditis is a complication of infection on the aortic valve or the coarctation itself. Fatal infections are more likely to occur during the first three decades of life, with the great majority occurring between ages 10 and 40 years. The bicuspid aortic valve is the usual site of endocarditis. Patients with aortic coarctation should receive antibiotic prophylaxis at the time of dental and surgical work.

Cerebral hemorrhage is a major complication of coarctation of the aorta; the hemorrhage is usually due to rupture of an aneurysm of the circle of Willis.[17] In pregnant women with coarctation, blood pressure fluctuations during gestation are similar in direction to those in uncomplicated pregnancy. Intracranial hemorrhage is not more likely to occur during pregnancy, and cardiac failure seldom develops. Pregnancy increases the risk of rupture of the aorta, especially during the end of the third trimester. Furthermore, the bacteremia that accompanies labor and delivery may cause endocarditis or endarteritis.[24]

CLINICAL RECOGNITION

Physical Examination. The physical appearance of patients with coarctation of the aorta may be normal, or the left arm may develop poorly when the coarctation compromises the origin of the left subclavian artery.[25] Differential cyanosis indicates reversed shunt through a coexisting patent ductus arteriosus distal to the coarctation.[26] In this entity, the feet are cyanosed, whereas the hands show little or no cyanosis.

In patients with *Turner's syndrome*, aortic coarctation may develop. The somatic features of Turner's syndrome include a female of short stature, webbing of the neck, absent or scanty pubic and axillary hair, wide-set nipples, low hairline, small chin, and wide carrying angle on the arms.[27, 28]

The characteristic physical finding in patients with aortic coarctation is markedly reduced or absent femoral artery pulses or marked lag between the radial artery impulse and a weak femoral artery impulse. In addition, the blood pressure in the legs is considerably lower than in the arms; this is a reverse of the normal finding, where systolic blood pressure in the legs is 10 mm Hg or more than in the arms.

Laboratory Examination. The radiograph provides considerable information regarding the presence of aortic coarctation (Fig. 72–3). Rib notching occurs on the inferior and undersurfaces of the ribs, presenting as irregular scalloped areas on the undersurfaces of the posterior ribs. Notching of the ribs seldom appears before the age of 7 years. When the area of coarctation is located just distal to the left subclavian artery, rib notching is bilateral and confined to the third to eighth posterior ribs.[10] However, rib notching is rarely found either above the third or below the ninth rib. Anatomic variation in coarctation of the aorta is accompanied by important variations in the patterns of notching. Collateral vessels depend on the patency of the origins of the subclavian arteries. When coarctation narrows the orifice of the left subclavian artery, collateral circulation fails to develop on the left side and unilateral notching develops in the right posterior ribs. When there is anomalous origin of the right subclavian artery distal to the coarctation, collateral circulation fails to develop in the right hemithorax and unilateral notching is confined to the left side. In the rare patient in whom coarctation occurs proximal to the innominate artery, rib notching is absent.[10] Rib notching is the most distinctive radiographic sign of aortic coarctation, but it may be caused by other clinical abnormalities as well.[29]

In patients with aortic coarctation, the ascending aorta may be inconspicuous, normal, or dilated. Aneurysms of the aortic sinuses have been described but are not usually seen on plain chest radiographs. The hypertensive ascending aorta is usually dilated and has a tendency to develop premature atherosclerosis. Aortic dilatation distal to the coarctation may produce a recognizable leftward convexity of the descending thoracic aorta. The barium-filled esophagus often demonstrates the mirror image impression, a reverse 3 or letter E. In the plain chest radiograph, the ascending aorta may form rightward convexity, a dilated left subclavian artery is seen above the coarctation, and the dilated descending aorta is seen below the silhouette in Figure 74–4.

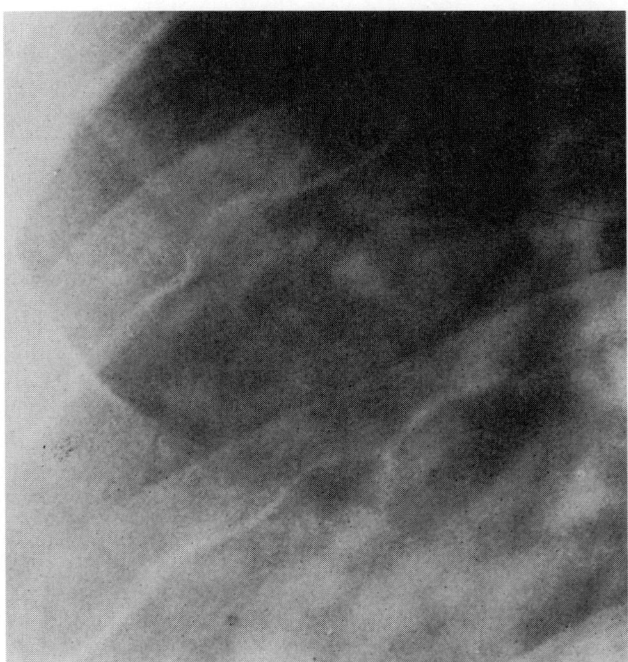

FIGURE 72–3 Rib notching of the inferior margins of the posterior ribs of a patient with a coarctation of the aorta. The notching varies from rib to rib and from patient to patient and may be single, multiple, shallow, deep, broad, or narrow. Rib notching occurs because of dilated intercostal arteries that are present in the costal grooves. Rib notching originates in the costal grooves. There are many causes of rib notching other than coarctation of the aorta. (From Perloff, JM: The Clinical Recognition of Congenital Heart Disease. Philadelphia: WB Saunders, 1970.)

Treatment of hypertension with inhibitors of the renin-angiotensin-aldosterone system (angiotensin-converting enzyme [ACE] inhibitors), angiotensin II type 1 receptor antagonists (AT_1) or aldosterone antagonists, a beta-blocker, or a centrally acting alpha-adrenergic agonist (i.e., clonidine) may control the predominantly elevated systolic blood pressure in the patient with aortic coarctation. If, on the other hand, the blood pressure elevation is severe and does not respond adequately to antihypertensive therapy, resection of the coarctation and replacement by a graft are usually indicated. However, this surgical correction is most effective in correcting systemic arterial hypertension when it is performed in early childhood. Alternatively, in some patients, it is possible to dilate the coarctation with a balloon device.

Pseudocoarctation

Pseudocoarctation of the aorta is a rare condition resulting from elongation of the aortic arch with redundancy and

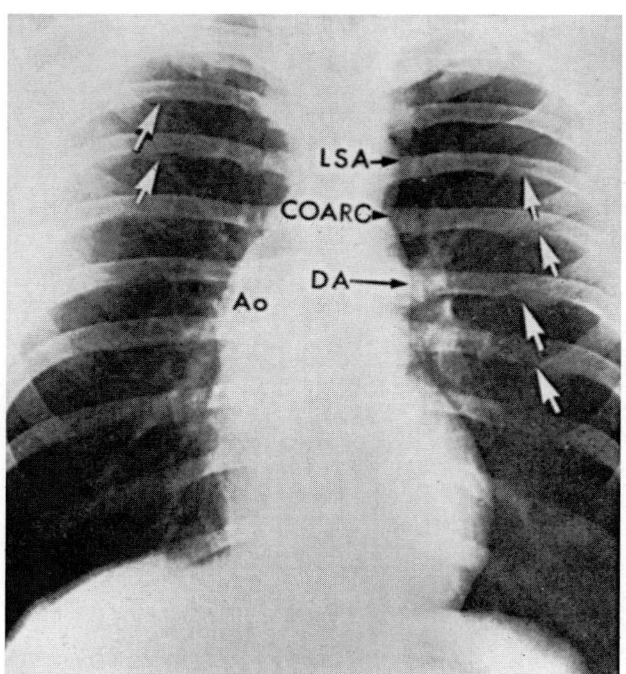

FIGURE 72–4 Chest radiograph from a man with coarctation (COARC) of the aorta. The *arrows* point to sites of notching on the undersurface of the ribs. The ascending aorta (Ao) forms a rightward convexity, and a dilated left subclavian artery (LSA) is demonstrated above the coarctation. The dilated descending aorta (DA) is shown below; together, these three shadows form the silhouette of a "figure 3." (From Perloff, JM: The Clinical Recognition of Congenital Heart Disease. Philadelphia: WB Saunders, 1970.)

kinking of the aorta just distal to the origin of the left subclavian artery at the level of the ligamentum arteriosum (Fig. 72–5).[30–34]

Etiology

The cause is thought to be a lack of compression and fusion of certain segments of the dorsal aortic root and fourth arch. As is the case for true coarctation of the aorta, associated abnormalities include bicuspid aortic valves, sinus of Valsalva aneurysms, and Turner's syndrome.

CLINICAL RECOGNITION

Physical Examination. Pseudocoarctation is differentiated from true coarctation of the aorta by the absence of a pressure gradient across the deformed area, the presence of normal lower extremity pulses, and a blood pressure in the legs that is higher than in the arms. A systolic murmur may be heard in the interscapular area.

Laboratory Examination. The laboratory examination is best performed with angiography, computed tomography (CT) scanning, or magnetic resonance imaging (MRI) with contrast agents. The pseudocoarctation may also be recognized from a chest radiograph as a double, rounded density in the left superior mediastinum (see Fig. 72–5), but the redundant aorta is sometimes mistaken for tumor or aneurysm, requiring angiography, CT with contrast agent, or MRI/magnetic resonance angiography (MRA) for precise delineation.

Treatment

Usually, no therapy is necessary for pseudocoarctation. Rarely, thrombus formation occurs with occlusion of the aorta or propagation or embolization of the thrombus, especially into the left subclavian artery. In these instances, therapy is necessary, including possible anticoagulation or surgical removal of the thrombus (or both) and repair of the pseudocoarctation. It seems wise to administer antibiotic prophylaxis for endocarditis before dental or surgical procedures, especially in patients who have a systolic murmur audible over the site of the pseudocoarctation.

Thoracic Aortic Aneurysms

Atherosclerosis may cause thoracic aortic aneurysms. Atherosclerotic thoracic aortic aneurysms most commonly involve the arch or descending portion of the aorta, whereas syphilitic aneurysms are located predominantly in the ascending aorta.

CLINICAL RECOGNITION

Physical Examination. Thoracic aortic aneurysms are often discovered accidentally on a chest radiograph or during another imaging procedure (Fig. 72–6). As they enlarge, they may impinge on adjacent structures, causing tracheal deviation, cough, dyspnea, stridor, or wheezing, or they may rupture into an adjacent bronchus, leading to hemoptysis.[35, 36] Their compression of adjacent bronchi can lead to recurrent pneumonia. The compression of the recurrent laryngeal nerve by thoracic aortic aneurysms may cause hoarseness, and compression of the esophagus may cause dysphagia. On occasion, a superior vena caval syndrome develops as a consequence of obstruction of venous return from the superior vena cava.

Compression of adjacent musculoskeletal structures or erosion of the aneurysm may lead to pain that is persistent and severe. Expansion of an ascending thoracic aortic aneurysm into the sternum or right thoracic cage may lead to pain anteriorly, whereas erosion of the vertebral column may result from expansion of a descending thoracic aortic aneurysm. Visible pulsatile masses are sometimes evident when aneurysms begin to erode through the chest wall. Rupture of the aneurysm is generally fatal, leading rapidly to hypotension, shock, and death associated with severe pain.

Laboratory Examination. Thoracic aortic aneurysms may be identified with chest fluoroscopy or radiography, CT scanning, MRI/MRA, digital subtraction angiography, or aortic angiography. CT scanning is performed in conjunction with the use of contrast media that more accurately allows detection of the extent and size of the aneurysms. Transesophageal echocardiography may also be used to image the thoracic aorta and detect atherosclerotic and dissecting aortic aneurysms (see Fig. 72–6).[35, 36]

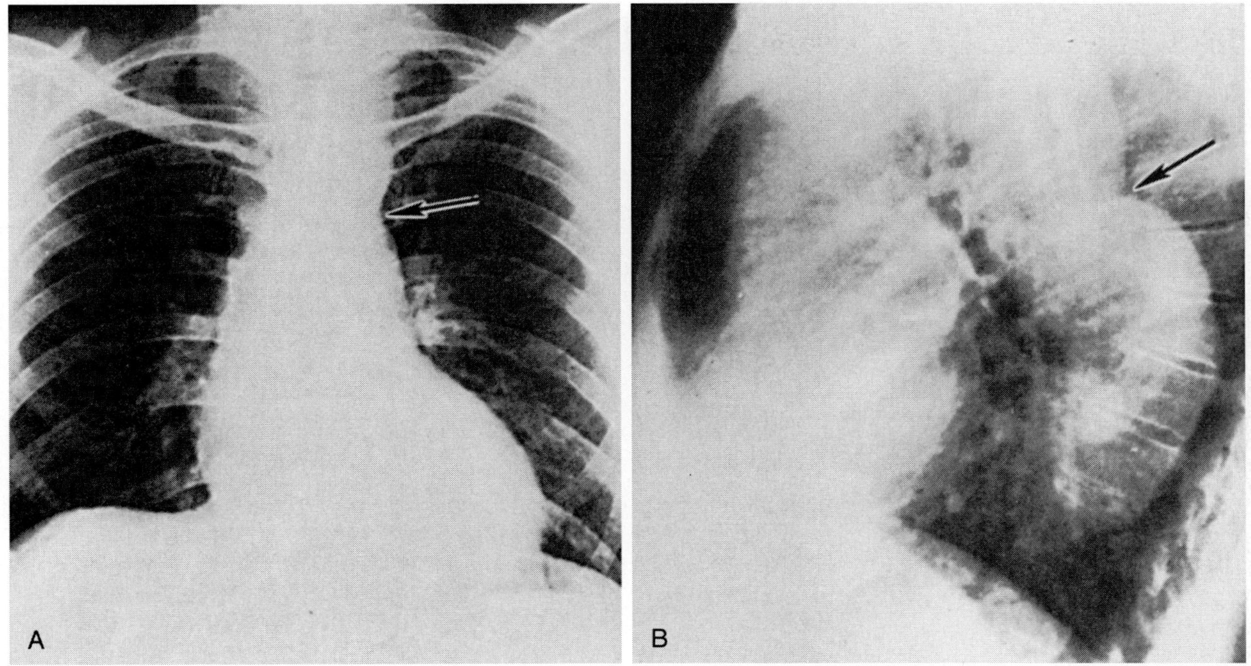

FIGURE 72–5 A and **B,** Chest radiographs from two patients with "pseudocoarctation" characterized by kinking of the aorta *(arrows)* at or just beyond the site of the ligamentum arteriosum. There is no real narrowing of the aortic lumen at the site of the kinking. **A,** Film from a man. **B,** Film from an elderly woman. (**A** and **B,** From Perloff, JM: The Clinical Recognition of Congenital Heart Disease. Philadelphia: WB Saunders, 1970.)

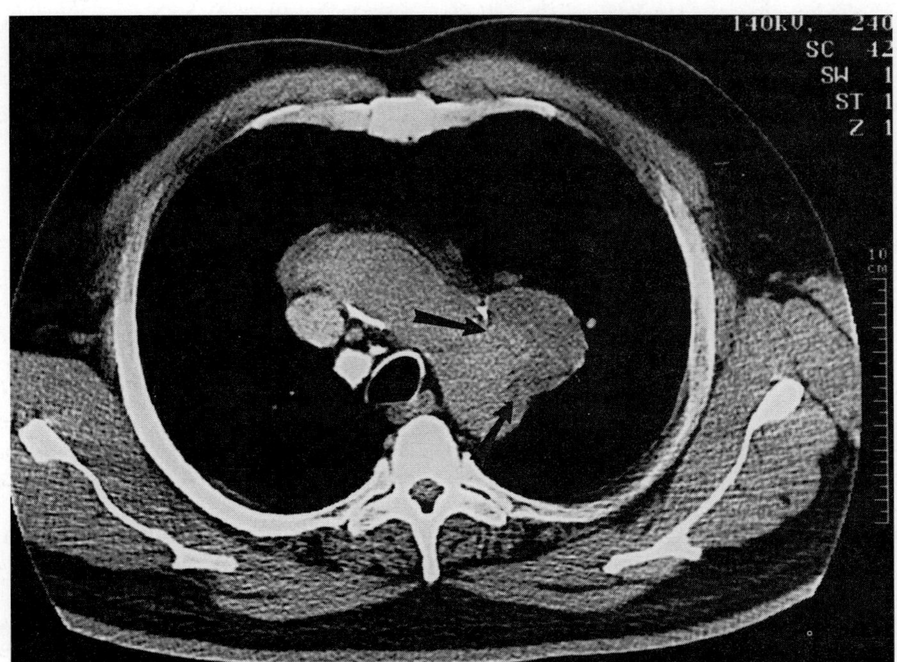

FIGURE 72–6 An aneurysm of the thoracic aorta at the level of the aortic arch is demonstrated with computed tomography. The majority of the aneurysm contains thrombus *(arrow).*

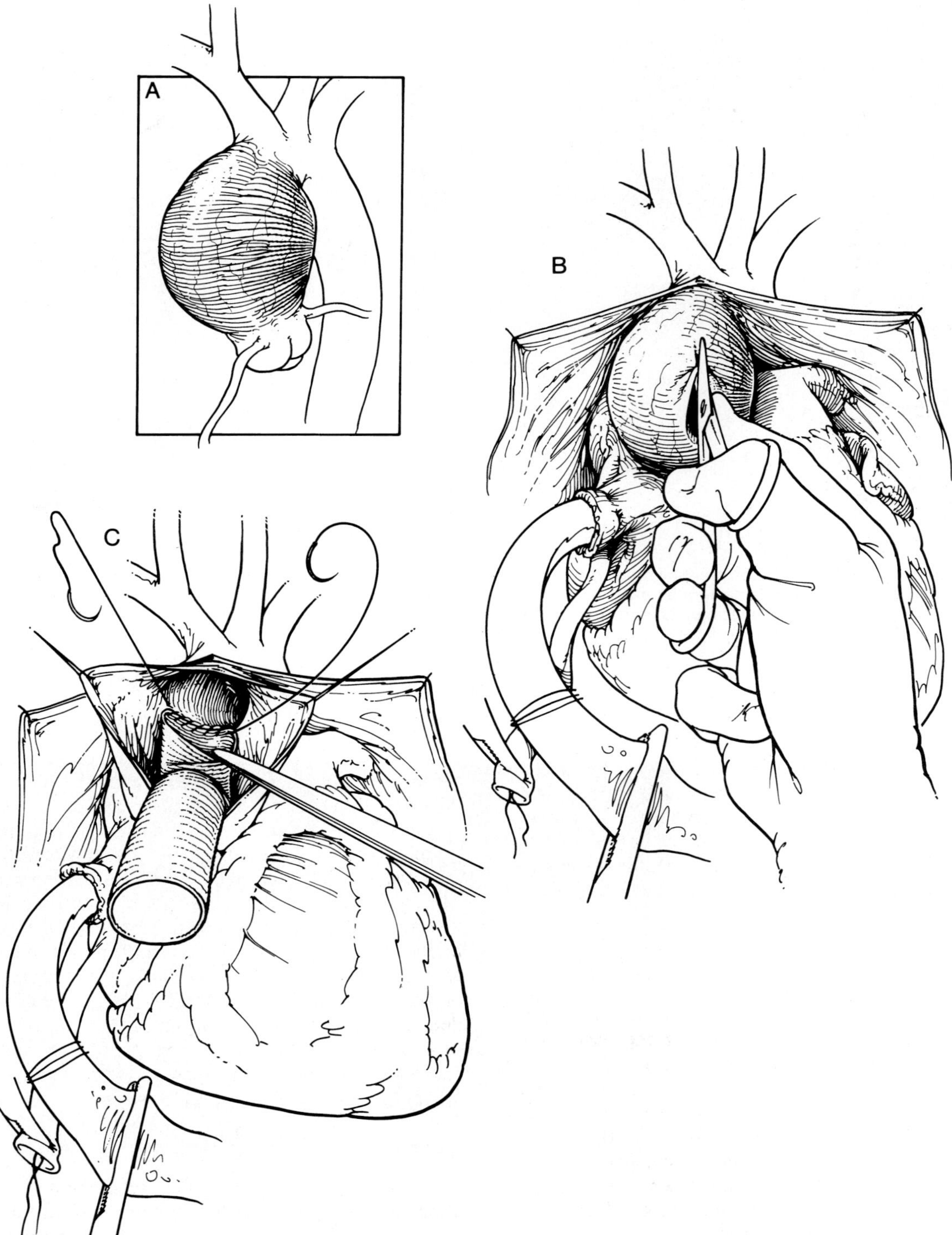

FIGURE 72–7 A–E, Aneurysm of the ascending aorta and proximal transverse arch. Open distal anastomosis is accomplished by reducing the patient's temperature to 18° to 20°C with an efficient heat exchanger in the extracorporeal circuit and by arresting the circulation. (**A–E,** From Cooley DA: Surgical Treatment of Aortic Aneurysms. Philadelphia: WB Saunders, 1986.)

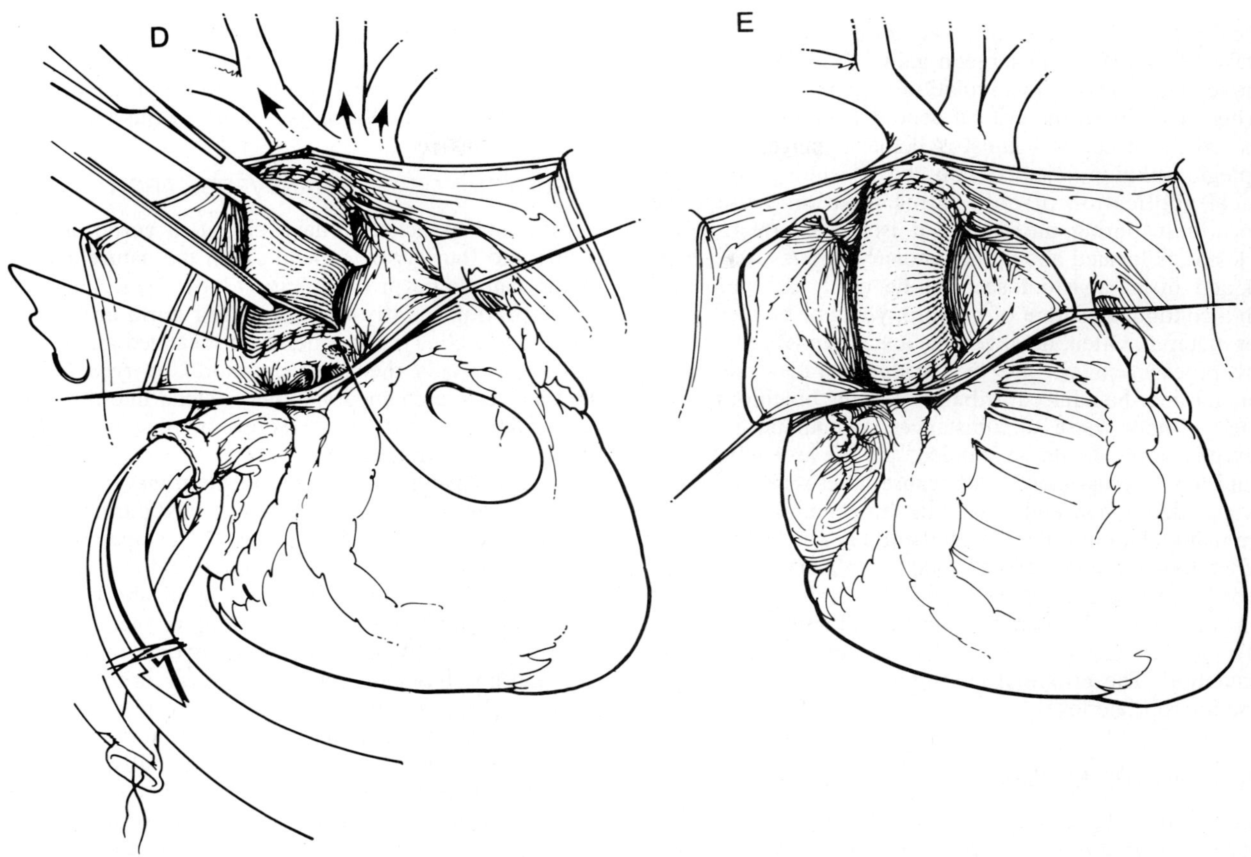

FIGURE 72–7 *Continued*

NATURAL HISTORY

Survival with thoracic aortic aneurysms is related directly to the size of the aneurysms. Thoracic aneurysms that are 6 to 7 cm in diameter are prone to rupture.[35, 36] Thoracic aortic aneurysms are often associated with atherosclerotic vascular disease elsewhere that may cause strokes or myocardial infarctions before the thoracic aortic aneurysm ruptures.

Surgical Treatment

Aneurysms of the thoracic aorta have long challenged the cardiovascular surgeon.[37, 38] Only during the past several decades has any effective treatment been developed. With the introduction of hypothermic circulatory arrest, surgeons were able to operate on aneurysms of the ascending aorta and arch in a dry, unobstructed operative field. By reducing basic metabolic requirements, hypothermic perfusion also provided protection for the brain and other vital organs. In addition, the development of graft materials reduced blood loss and improved surgical results.

We repair aortic aneurysms by replacing the aneurysm with a woven, low-porosity fabric graft that is placed in the aneurysmal bed. For ascending aortic and arch aneurysms, the operative field is rendered bloodless by circulatory arrest. After inducing hypothermia, the internal reconstruction is performed, and pulsatile circulation is thus restored to the patient's entire body. In addition, by leaving the wall of the aneurysm intact, anatomic structures such as the lung, phrenic and vagus nerves, duodenum, and left kidney (depending on the location of the lesion) are not disturbed. Limiting dissection also reduces blood loss.

Surgical treatment of aortic aneurysm depends on the morphology and, particularly, the anatomic location of the aneurysm, which may be anywhere from the aortic annulus and aortic valve to the distal thoracic aorta, including the visceral vessels in the abdomen. Therefore, aneurysms may be located in the aortic root, as in annuloaortic ectasia; the ascending aorta; the transverse arch; the descending aorta; or the thoracoabdominal aorta.[39] The surgeon must also determine whether the aneurysm is true and of a fusiform or sacciform type or, from a prognostic standpoint in surgical treatment, whether the operation is an elective repair or an emergency repair of an acute rupture.

ASCENDING AORTIC ANEURYSMS

When treating aneurysms of the ascending aorta, consideration must be given to the proximal and distal extent of the lesion and the involvement of the aortic valve. When the aortic valve is involved, it is replaced after the distal anastomosis is completed. We resect the aneurysm and line the ascending aorta with a low-porosity woven Dacron graft for almost all aneurysms in this location (Fig. 72–7).

In patients with lesions of the ascending aorta and proximal arch, hypothermic circulatory arrest using cardiopulmonary bypass has provided a practical solution to a critical problem. By reducing body temperature to approximately 18° to 20°C, the surgeon gains 30 to 45 minutes of relative safety while the circulation is completely arrested. During this period, the critical central nervous system tissues remain protected against ischemic damage. Cold cardioplegic solution injected into the ascending aorta and topical application of cold saline solution protect the myocardium during the period of ischemic arrest. When the lesion is located above the coronary orifices, the proximal and distal anastomoses can be easily accomplished with a continuous suture of polypropylene or braided polyester material. Often, however, the aneurysm and the pathologic process extend into the proximal transverse aortic arch and into the adjacent tributaries in the brachiocephalic vessels. Under these circumstances, cannulations in the transverse aorta should be avoided, and the ascending aorta should not be cross-clamped, because atherosclerotic particles and debris can embolize into the cerebral circulation from manipulation of the diseased aorta at this level. Induction of hypothermia permits total circulatory arrest with "open" repair distally.[40] Once the distal anastomosis has been accomplished, a clamp is placed on the woven Dacron graft, and circulation is restored from the femoral arterial cannulation. The proximal anastomosis is then performed at the appropriate level.

ANNULOAORTIC ECTASIA

Annuloaortic ectasia is usually related to an aortic pathology known as *Erdheim's cystic medial necrosis.* Often, Erdheim's cystic medial necrosis is associated with *Marfan's syndrome*, but it may also appear as an isolated lesion of the forme fruste type. In general, if the aneurysm is dilated and displaces the coronary artery ostia cephalad by 2 cm or more and if aortic insufficiency is present, the repair of Bentall and DeBono[41] with a composite graft is the standard of surgical treatment. The technique has been modified, however, especially the manner in which the coronary arteries are implanted, because restoration of coronary circulation is an important technical aspect in the repair of annuloaortic ectasia. Although others have advocated the interposition of grafts between the coronary orifices and the composite aortic graft, we have found this technique to be unnecessary.

We generally use a direct, conventional repair when the coronary ostia have maintained their normal relationship with the aortic annulus and the sinuses of Valsalva have not been grossly dilated. This method, first suggested by Groves and colleagues[42] and Wheat and colleagues,[43] involves the use of a supracoronary graft for the treatment of the aneurysm and conventional valve replacement. When the brachiocephalic vessels are involved, graft replacement of the stenotic or aneurysmal segment is performed from the aortic annulus to the distal extent of the aneurysm. This latter technique requires reimplantation of the coronary artery ostia for the reestablishment of coronary blood flow. When there is significant disease of the sinuses of Valsalva and aortic annulus, we use composite graft replacement for the repair (the Bentall technique), with direct coronary artery reimplantation and inclusion. When possible, we create a fistula between the perigraft space and the right atrium using the technique of Cabrol and colleagues,[44] which has helped control postoperative bleeding and formation of late false aneurysms at the coronary artery reimplantation sites.[45] Neither complications nor late persistence of the fistula has occurred as a result of this technique.

ANEURYSMS OF THE TRANSVERSE ARCH

Cooley and associates[39] have classified aortic arch aneurysms into four types, depending on the nature and extent of the pathologic process (Fig. 72–8). *Type A* lesions involve predominantly the ascending aorta and proximal transverse arch. *Type B* lesions are localized and sacciform and involve only the transverse aorta. In *type C* lesions, the transverse arch aneurysm may extend into the proximal descending aorta. *Type D* lesions involve predominantly the descending thoracic aorta.

To repair aneurysms located in the transverse arch, normal cerebral viability must be maintained during the period of circulatory interruption to avoid postoperative neurologic complications. Here we believe that the technique of hypothermic arrest has its greatest applicability. We use a method of core cooling with the pump oxygenator and heat exchanger. Usually, the aneurysms involve only the aortic wall and not the innominate, left carotid, or left subclavian arteries. As a result, reconstruction can be performed through reimplantation of the major tributaries as a unit into the new arch graft. This substantially reduces the possibility of postoperative bleeding or thrombosis in an arch vessel. In an occasional instance in which one of the vessels, particularly the left subclavian artery, has been occluded by the aneurysmal process, a separate graft may be placed from the fabric aortic graft to the side of the subclavian vessel (Fig. 72–9). In addition, the cerebral arteries need not be occluded during the period of circulatory arrest, because air embolism does not occur into these vessels.

ANEURYSMS OF THE DESCENDING THORACIC AORTA

Most aneurysms of the descending aorta are fusiform rather than sacciform in nature, involving almost the entire circumference of the aorta, and excision requires expeditious insertion of a fabric graft to restore circulatory continuity. The exact site of proximal occlusion depends on the extent of the aneurysm; the usual site is between the left common carotid and the left subclavian arteries.

In patients with aneurysms of the descending aorta, paraplegia is the most common and most feared complication. Thus, protection of the viability of the spinal cord is of prime importance in surgery on aneurysms in this location.[46, 47] The most common risk factors for paraplegia include location and extent of the lesion, duration of clamp time, intraoperative hypotension, elevated cerebral spinal fluid pressure, and variability of spinal cord blood supply.

Many measures to protect the spinal cord have been tried in the past, mostly to establish and maintain the distal circulation during the period of aortic cross-clamping. These methods have included shunts, pumps, pump oxygenators with femoral vein–to–femoral artery bypass, and others. After extensive experience with all of these modalities, we used a technique of exsanguination, or "open"

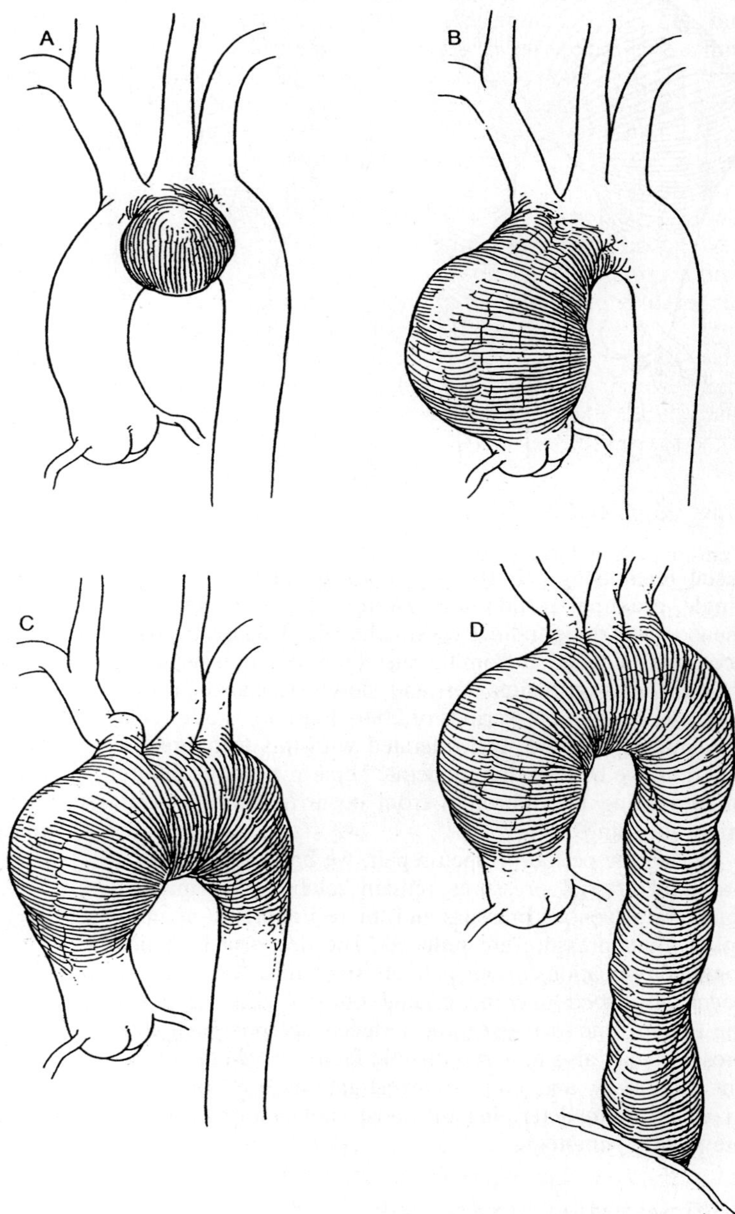

FIGURE 72–8 A–D, Classification for aneurysms of the transverse aorta according to location and extent. (**A–D,** From Cooley, DA: Surgical Treatment of Aortic Aneurysms. Philadelphia: WB Saunders, 1986.)

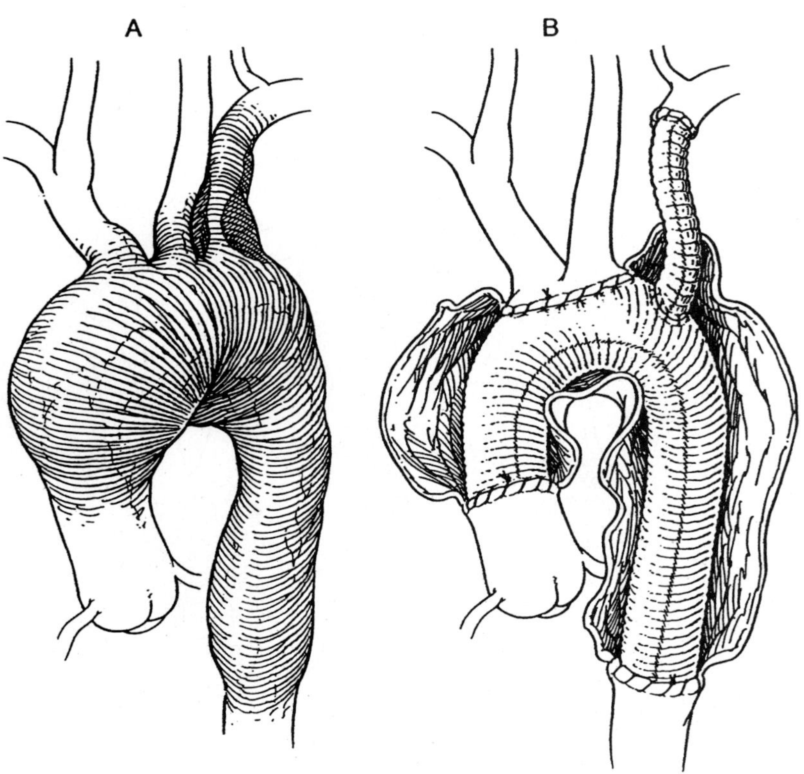

FIGURE 72–9 **A** and **B,** Repair of an aneurysm of the transverse aorta with involvement of the left subclavian artery through use of the technique of endoaneurysmorrhaphy. (**A** and **B,** From Cooley DA: Surgical Treatment of Aortic Aneurysms. Philadelphia: WB Saunders, 1986.)

distal repair (Fig. 72–10).[48] In open distal repair, only a single, proximal aortic clamp is applied. The aneurysm is then opened longitudinally, and the distal anastomosis is accomplished. Blood from the distal circulation is aspirated into an autotransfusion unit and slowly replaced into the systemic circulation. Periods of 20 to 30 minutes of circulatory interruption are well tolerated with this technique. In addition, we believe that moderate heparinization is helpful in preventing microthrombi from occurring during aortic cross-clamping.

During the period of open repair, we have noted that the proximal arterial pressures remain relatively normal but that central venous pressure and, more important, cerebrospinal fluid pressure are reduced. The decrease in neurologic complications in our patients since this technique has been introduced may be related only to the brevity of the clamp time; however, the reduced cerebrospinal fluid pressure may also be a responsible factor.[49, 50] Many different laboratory and clinical investigations are continuing in an effort to determine the most satisfactory means of preventing paraplegia.

POSTOPERATIVE MANAGEMENT

After surgery, optimal circulatory equilibrium must be maintained. Measurement of renal function and urinary output provides a good index of the general circulatory status. Because surgery to repair aortic aneurysms is extensive, these patients have a greater tendency to bleed than do those who have undergone many other cardiovascular procedures. As a result, blood volume, which can be determined by measuring central venous and systemic pressures, should be watched carefully, because patients who undergo these repairs may require blood replacement therapy.

When hypotension occurs, spinal cord ischemia may result. Neurologic deficits may also develop unexpectedly in the first 48 hours after surgery. Prolonged hypotension may lead to renal tubular necrosis and renal failure; therefore, personnel in the intensive care unit who care for these patients must be highly trained and instructed to watch for any symptoms that might portend such complications. Heavy sedation should be avoided. If blood pressure falls below normal, it should be immediately corrected by administering vasopressors and increasing blood volume.

RESULTS

We have achieved excellent results in repairing aneurysms of the thoracic aorta by carefully selecting the techniques used in the repair, based on the disease process in each patient. In the years since we began to repair ascending aortic aneurysms, the rate of early death has decreased significantly. In our practice, acute dissecting aneurysms compose 40 percent of the total repairs. We also see a large number of older patients (60 percent are 50 years of age or older), most of whom die from complications related to their heart disease. Although the repair of such dangerous aneurysms in older, sicker patients is difficult, the early mortality rate has averaged about 10 percent for all types of aortic aneurysms, including ruptured lesions. We attribute this improved mortality rate to our use of the techniques of hypothermic circulatory arrest and open aortic anastomosis.

The prognosis has changed for aneurysms of the aorta. Many patients who would have died in the early years of repair enjoy full lives as a result of progress in the treatment of these difficult lesions.

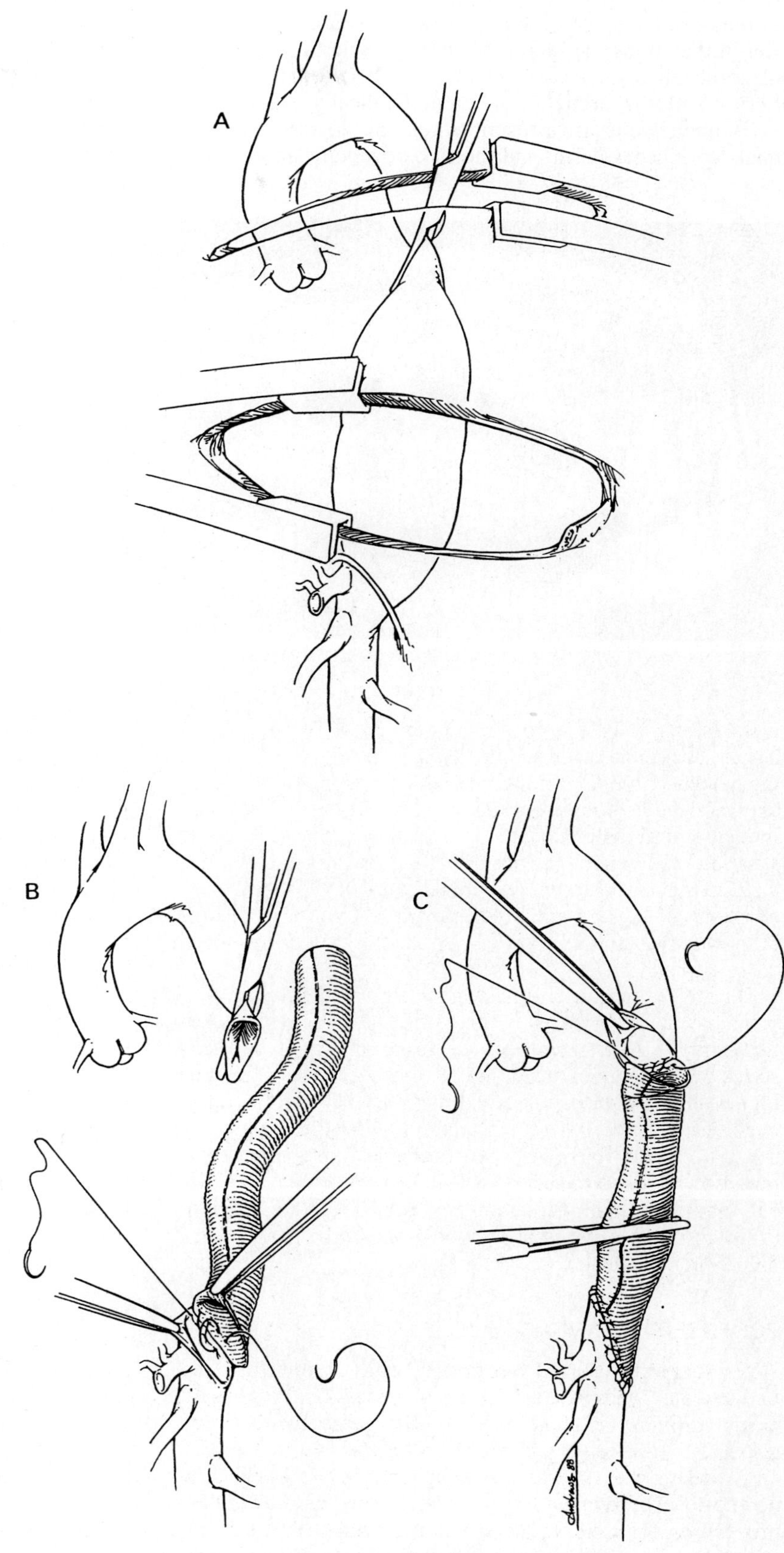

FIGURE 72–10 A–C, Resection of extensive fusiform aneurysm of the descending thoracic aorta, through use of the technique of "open" distal anastomosis and replacement with a fabric graft. Reinforcing tapes are placed around the aortic anastomoses, and the aneurysmal wall is sutured over the graft. (**A–C,** From Cooley DA: Surgical Treatment of Aortic Aneurysms. Philadelphia: WB Saunders, 1986.)

Abdominal Aortic Aneurysms

Aortic aneurysms caused by atherosclerosis are most common in the abdominal aorta. Most atherosclerotic abdominal aortic aneurysms arise in the area between the renal arteries and the aortic bifurcation. Clinically significant aortic aneurysms are present when the aorta diameter equals or exceeds 4 cm, and the risk of rupture of such an aneurysm increases with each degree of dilatation of the aorta, such that aneurysms that are 5 cm or larger have a substantial risk of rupture (Figs. 72–11 to 72–14).[51–56]

Atherosclerosis damages the aortic wall, leading to saccular dilatation. As the aorta widens, tension in the wall of the aorta increases (*Laplace's law*), promoting further enlargement of the aneurysm. Hypertension also contributes to dilatation of the aneurysm.

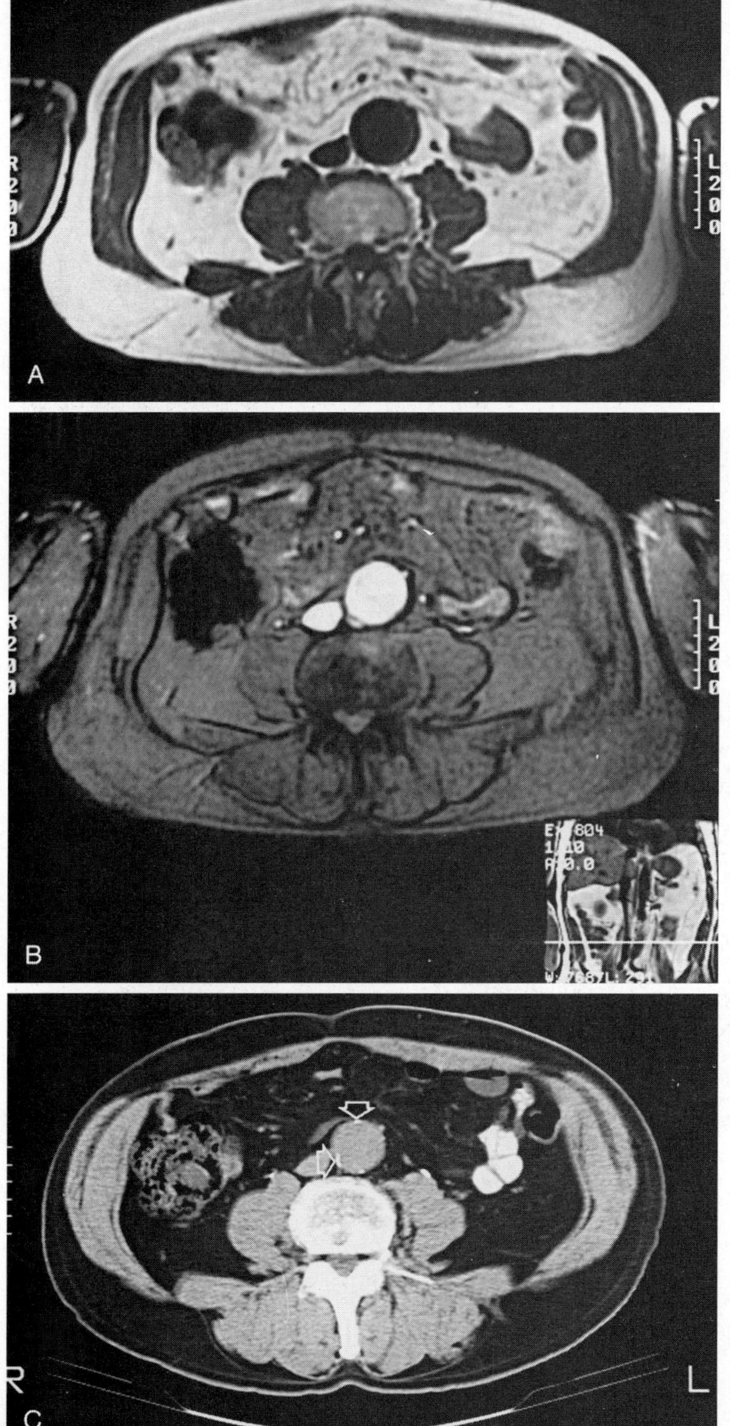

FIGURE 72–11 **A,** Spin-echo magnetic resonance image demonstrates black signal for flowing blood in an abdominal aorta aneurysm. **B,** Gradient-echo magnetic resonance image in the same patient reveals bright signal for blood in the aneurysm. **C,** An abdominal aorta aneurysm is demonstrated with computed tomography of the abdomen performed with intravenous contrast medium. A small amount of calcification is present in the wall.

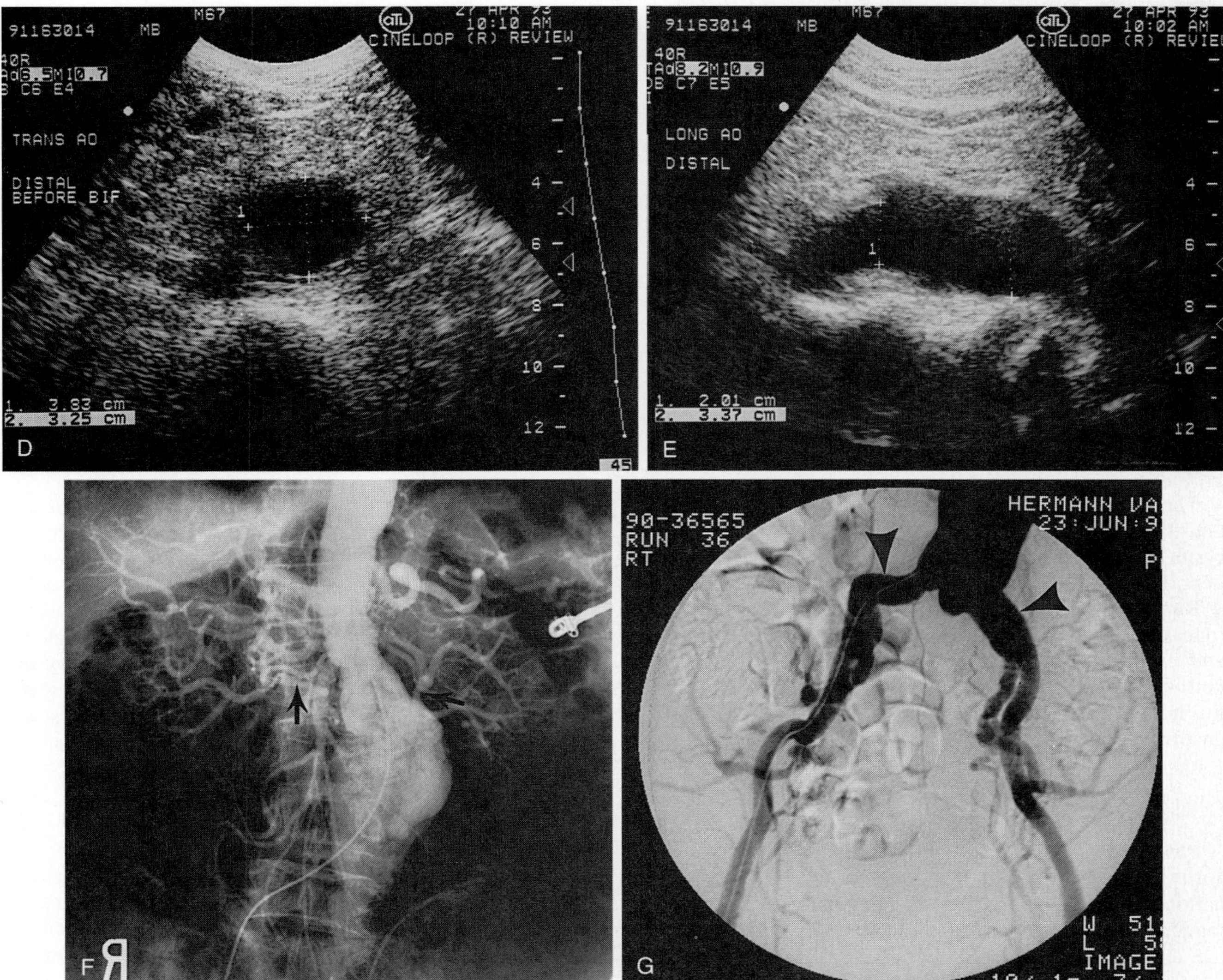

FIGURE 72–11 *Continued.* **D** and **E,** Transverse and longitudinal views of the abdominal aorta on an ultrasound examination permit an evaluation of the size of the aneurysm. Ultrasound can be used for serial follow-up. **F,** Aortogram demonstrates an abdominal aorta aneurysm that involves the origin of both renal arteries *(arrows).* **G,** Digital subtraction arteriogram obtained through the intra-arterial injection of contrast medium shows extension of an aortic aneurysm into both common iliac arteries.

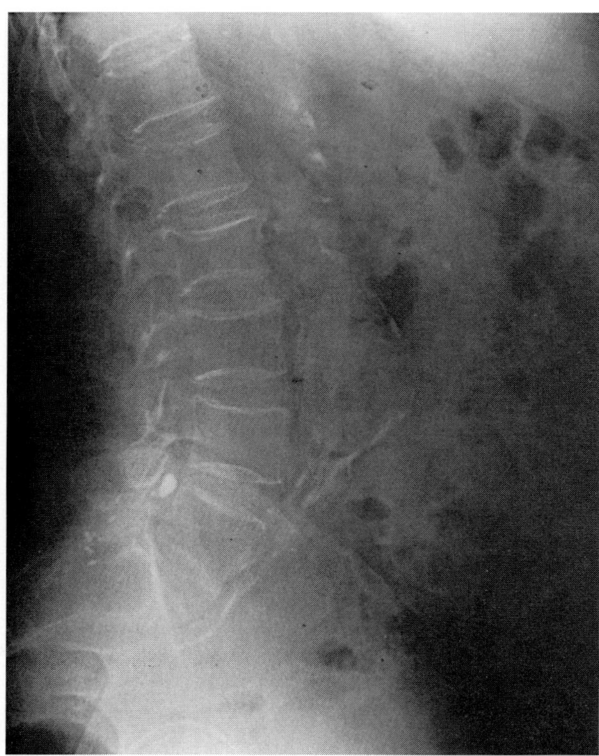

FIGURE 72–12 Lateral radiograph of the abdomen reveals an aortic aneurysm with extensive calcification in its wall *(arrows).*

Thrombotic material is usually present in the aneurysm, and it and cholesterol debris may embolize from the aneurysm into any organ, resulting in a cerebrovascular accident, loss of pulse in an extremity, or renal failure.

Rupture of abdominal aortic aneurysms occurs retroperitoneally in most cases, leading to hypotension, back pain, and circulatory collapse, but it may also occur into the peritoneal cavity or adjacent vessel or structure, including the inferior vena cava, iliac vein, or renal vein[57–59] or the gastrointestinal tract.[51–56, 59]

CLINICAL RECOGNITION

Physical and Laboratory Examinations. Most abdominal aortic aneurysms are discovered on routine physical examination or abdominal imaging procedure. When symptomatic, these aneurysms may cause a sense of fullness in the epigastrium or pain in the lower back. When pain develops, one is concerned about abrupt enlargement or rupture of the aneurysm. With rupture of the aneurysm, the discomfort is usually continuous, it may radiate into the back, and it is usually unaffected by movement, although it may be partially relieved by certain positions, such as assuming the fetal position with the legs drawn up. When rupture occurs, the pain is typically severe and radiates into the back or abdomen, and there is localized tenderness to palpation in the region of the aneurysm. With rupture, patients become hypotensive, and depending on the degree of rupture, they may quickly develop shock and die. Abdominal aortic aneurysms are the most difficult to detect by palpation in obese individuals and in those with marked organomegaly involving the liver or spleen. A pulsatile mass extending between the xiphoid process and the umbilicus that seems unduly wide usually represents an abdominal aortic aneurysm. Exact measurements of size are difficult on physical examination because of the presence of other organs in the same vicinity, and one is usually dependent on an imaging procedure for accurate measurement of the aneurysm size. The best of these measurements for the detection and sizing of thoracic aortic aneurysms are MRI, transesophageal echocardiography, and CT scanning.[60–64] For abdominal aortic aneurysms, MRI, CT scanning, and ultrasound are the noninvasive techniques,[60, 65] and aortography is an invasive technique (see Fig. 72–11).

An enlarged aortic aneurysm should be palpated cautiously and gently. A systolic murmur is often heard over the aneurysm.

Occasionally, an aneurysm may expand so as to obstruct the inferior vena cava or iliac vein or veins, resulting in edema and congestion in one or both legs. An arteriovenous fistula may result from spontaneous rupture of the aneurysm into the inferior vena cava, iliac vein, or renal vein, leading to acute high output heart failure and hemodynamic collapse.[57, 59, 66, 67]

Ruptured aortic aneurysms represent a surgical emergency, because patients may die rapidly after this occurrence. The patient quickly develops shock with hypotension, peripheral vasoconstriction, cool and clammy skin, diaphoresis, obtundation, oliguria, and, finally, cardiac arrest. Retroperitoneal hemorrhage may be identified by hematomas in the flanks and groin. Rupture into the abdominal cavity may cause abrupt abdominal distention, and rupture into the small bowel, especially the duodenum, may cause massive gastrointestinal bleeding.[57, 66, 67]

The surgical technique used to repair abdominal aortic aneurysms is shown in Figure 72–13.

Text continued on page 1374

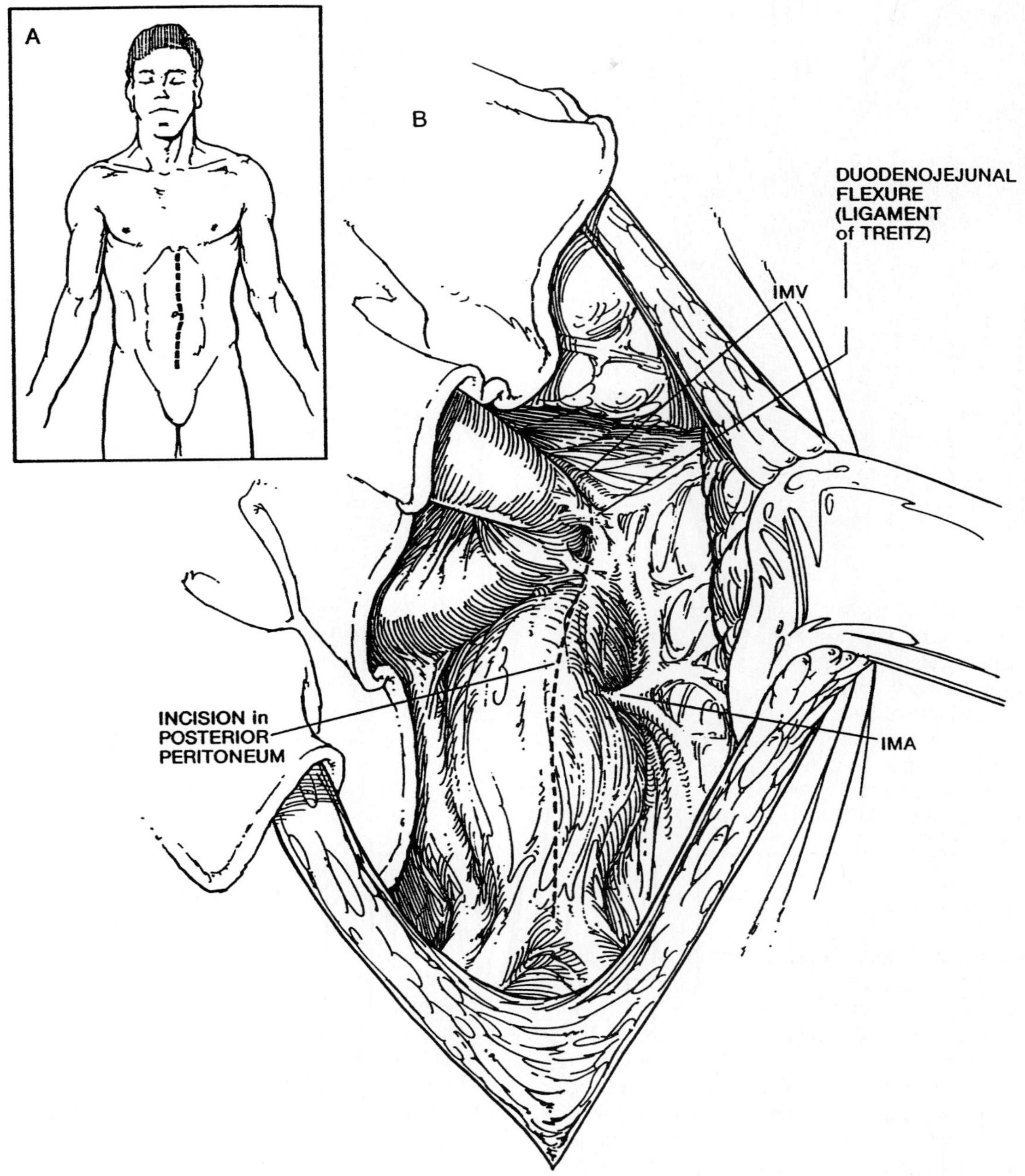

FIGURE 72–13 A–L, Technique used to repair an abdominal aorta aneurysm. In some instances, the aortic bifurcation may have to be replaced with a bifurcated graft **(J)**. See text for description. (**A–L,** From Cooley DA: Surgical Treatment of Aortic Aneurysms. Philadelphia: WB Saunders, 1986.)

Illustration continued on following page

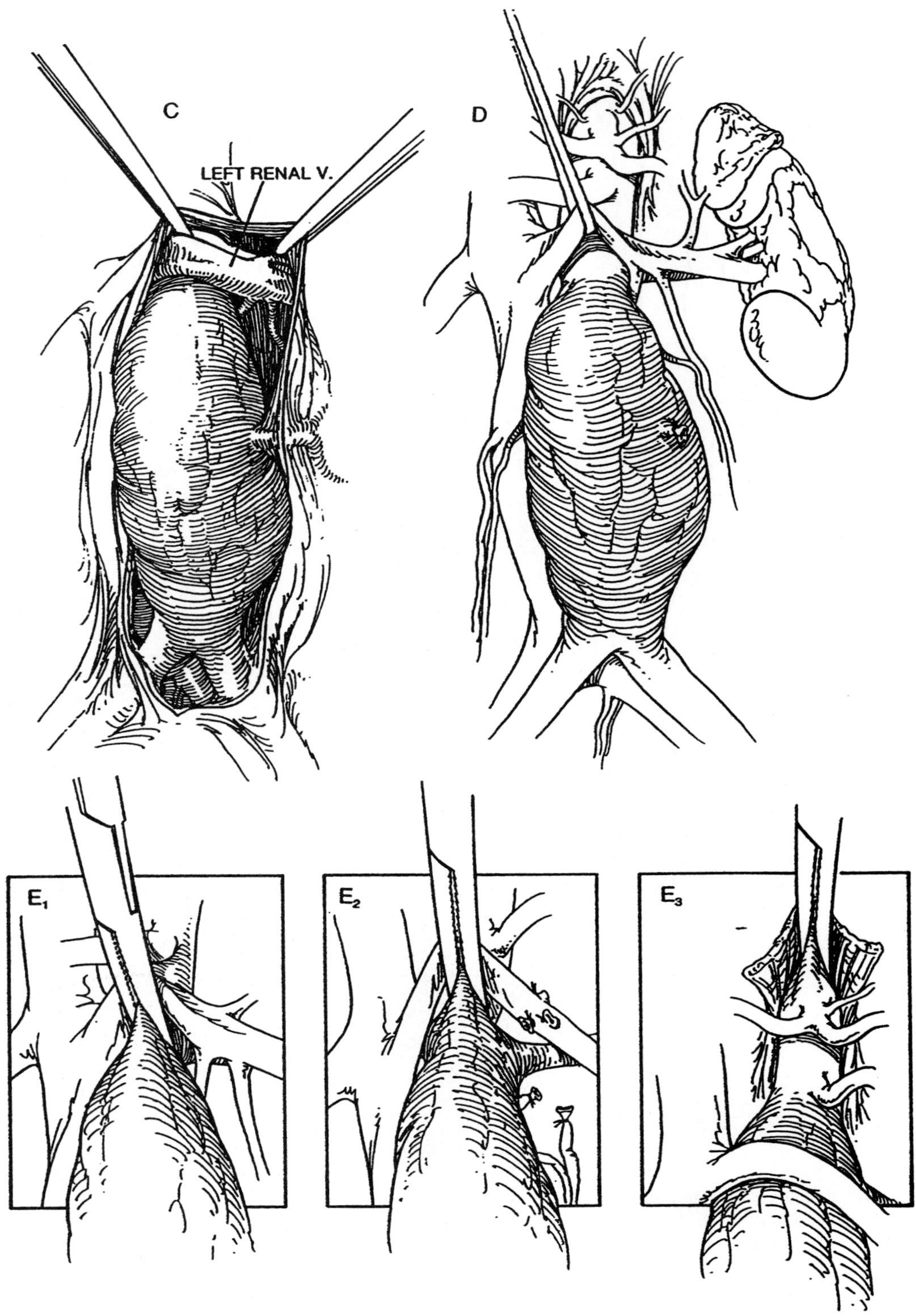

FIGURE 72–13C–E *Continued*

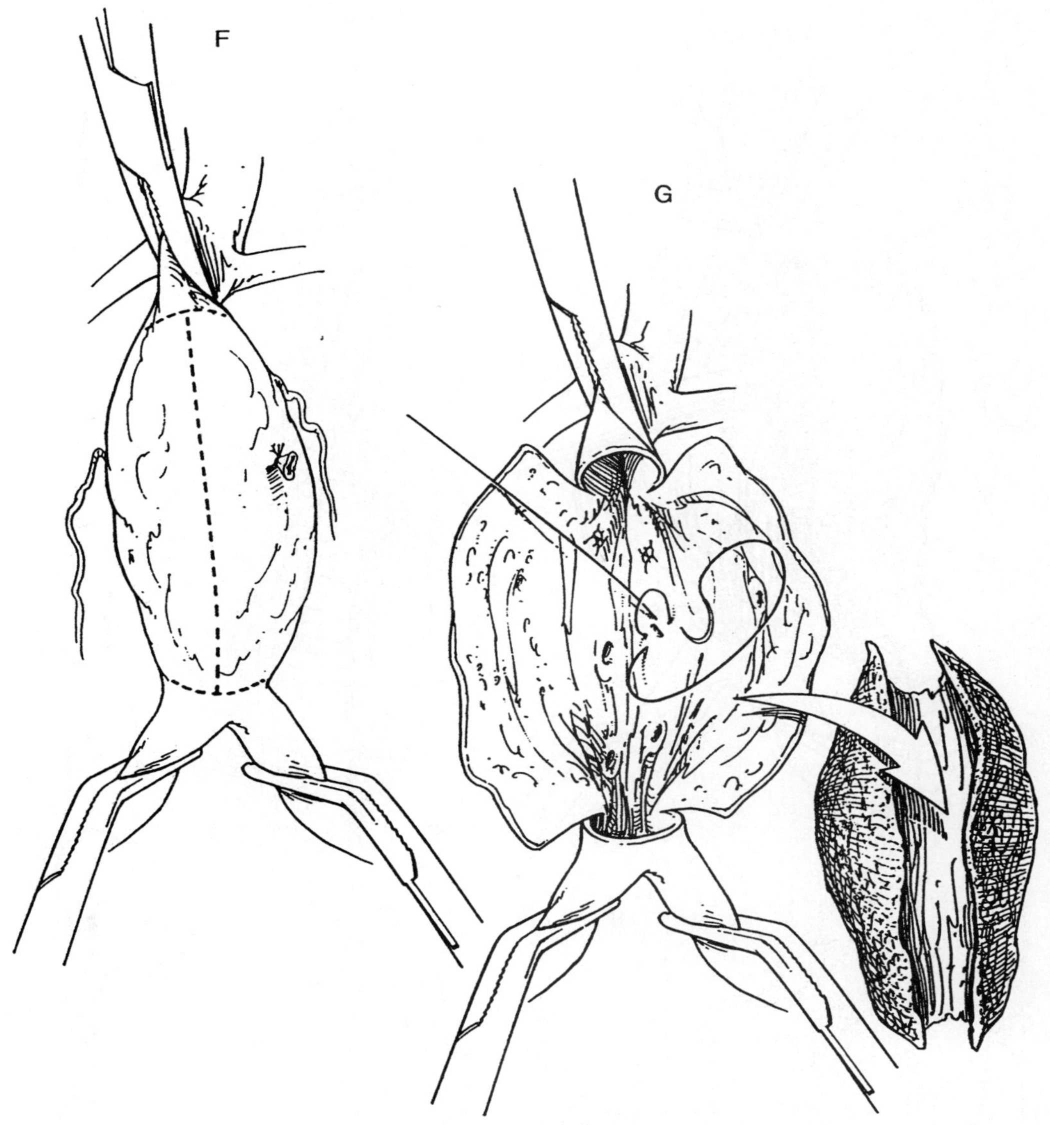

FIGURE 72–13F–G *Continued*

Illustration continued on following page

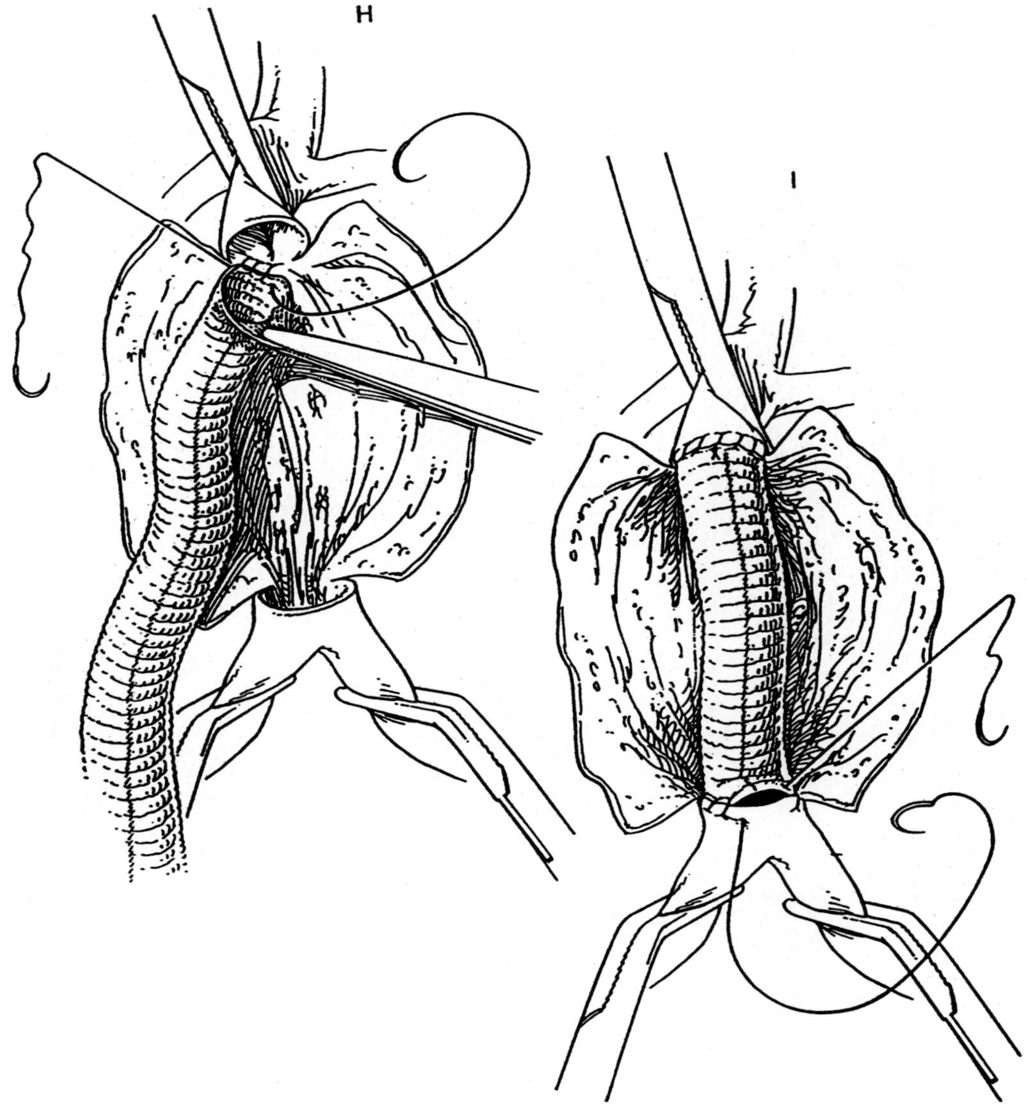

FIGURE 72–13H–I *Continued*

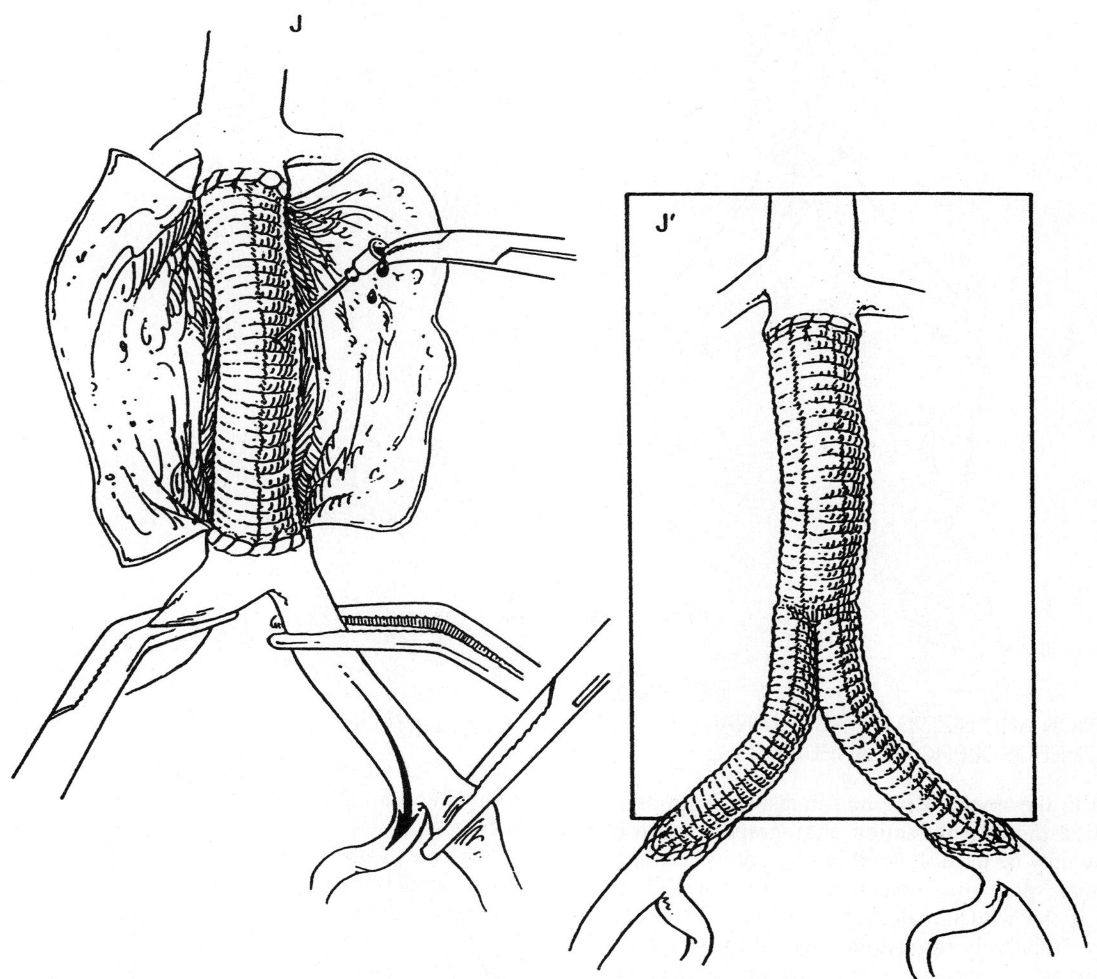

FIGURE 72–13J *Continued*

Illustration continued on following page

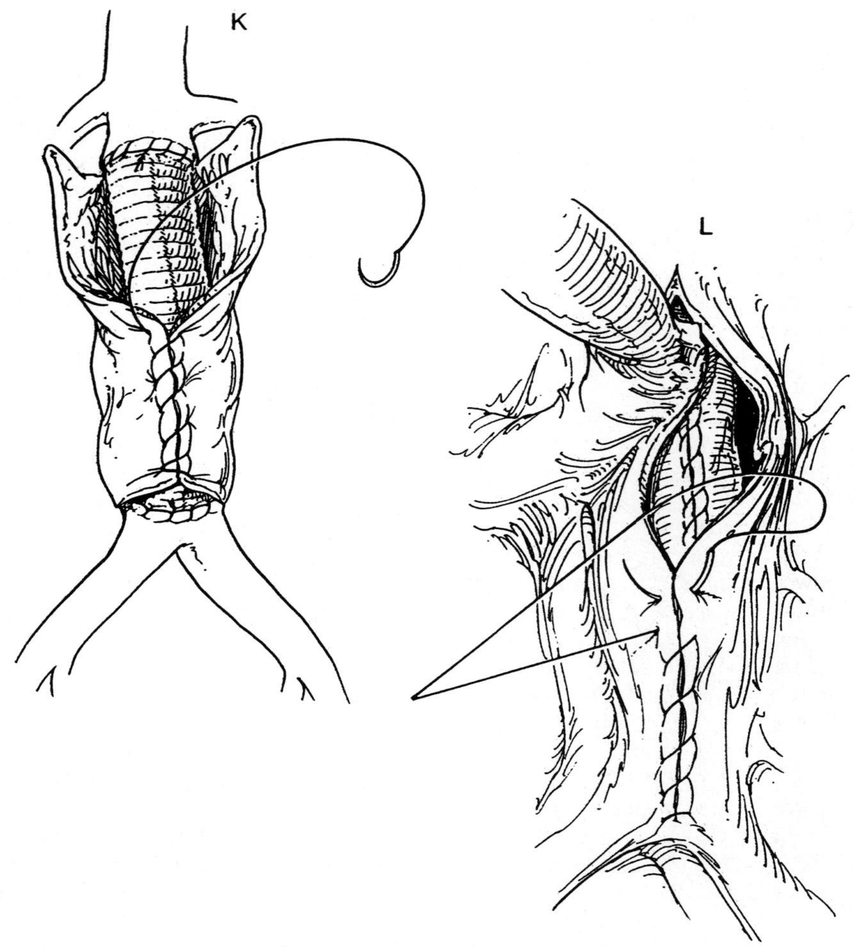

FIGURE 72–13K–L *Continued*

RECOGNITION AND SIZING OF ABDOMINAL AORTIC ATHEROSCLEROTIC ANEURYSMS

In addition to the noninvasive and invasive methods mentioned earlier, digital subtraction angiography and routine radiography may be used. Lateral radiographic examination of the lumbar spine may detect the outline of abdominal aneurysms if the wall is calcified (see Fig. 72–12). However, this is a relatively insensitive method for visualization of the aneurysm. Cross-sectional ultrasound is accurate in aneurysm detection and sizing and represents a simple way to detect most aneurysms (see Fig. 72–11). MRI and CT scanning of the abdomen provide excellent means for detecting and measuring the size of abdominal aortic aneurysms and for identifying the extent of these lesions, especially with the injection of contrast media or the use of MRA (see Fig. 72–11). Digital subtraction angiography allows the identification of aneurysms. Abdominal aortic angiography also allows the detection and sizing of aortic aneurysms,[68] but it carries a definite risk of complications, including aneurysm rupture, hematoma, localized dissection, infection, embolization, and the development of renal failure associated either with embolization of atherosclerotic debris into a renal artery or with the nephrotoxic effect of the contrast medium itself.

Natural History

The size of the aneurysm generally determines subsequent clinical abnormalities.[51–56] The rate of aneurysm expansion becomes greater as aneurysms become larger, and the risk of rupture of aneurysms becomes substantial when aneurysm diameter equals 5 cm or larger. As many as 50 percent of abdominal aortic aneurysms of more than 6 cm in diameter rupture within 1 year, but 20 percent or fewer of aneurysms less than 6 cm in size rupture within the same time period. With aneurysms measuring 4 to 7 cm, the rupture rate is 25 percent. An average aneurysm expansion rate is approximately 0.2 to 0.5 cm/yr.

Surgical Treatment

Elective surgery is advised for all abdominal aortic aneurysms 6 cm in diameter or larger.[51–56] In patients in good health otherwise, elective resection of aortic abdominal aneurysms of 5 cm in size is probably indicated. Patients with other serious medical problems must be evaluated and managed individually. Control of systemic arterial hypertension and reduction in serum cholesterol values seem logical in the management of these patients. In patients with other serious medical diseases, close follow-up of aortic aneurysms of 4 to 6 cm is indicated, with immediate surgery if the aneurysm expands or shows signs of early rupture.

Because small abdominal aortic aneurysms do rupture (23 percent of ruptured aneurysms were 4 to 5 cm in diameter in one study), and the operative mortality rate approaches 50 percent once rupture has occurred, all aortic abdominal aneurysms are potentially fatal lesions. The benefits of elective surgery must be weighed against the medical risks in advising patients toward proper therapy. There are several reports documenting mortality rates of less than 5 percent in octogenarians, so age alone should not be considered a major risk factor for elective aneurysm resection. A history of angina or congestive heart failure should prompt a thorough preoperative cardiac evaluation in patients of any age, and treatment of the underlying cause should be completed, if possible, before elective abdominal aortic aneurysm surgery. Patients with recent myocardial infarctions should be similarly evaluated, and elective surgery should be postponed for 4 to 6 months. Renal dysfunction, as manifested by low creatinine clearances or serum creatinine levels of more than 3 mg/dl, should be considered a major risk factor for aneurysm surgery. Similarly, chronic obstructive pulmonary disease, with a forced expiratory volume of less than 1 L/sec or simple dyspnea at rest, must be regarded as a very serious handicap in a patient's ability to have a successful operation and recovery.

The surgical approach to the abdominal aorta may be either through a midline laparotomy incision or through a left retroperitoneal incision (see Fig. 72–13A and B). The midline abdominal approach allows good exposure of the iliac arteries and veins and allows the surgeon the opportunity to perform a thorough exploratory laparotomy as well as associated surgical procedures. With the trends and successes associated with laparoscopic surgical technologies, this latter issue seems less important. In some patients, exposure of the proximal extent of the aneurysm may be difficult through the midline laparotomy incision. Moreover, one should expect both a prolonged ileus (from retraction of intestines during the operation) and some respiratory problems (from splinting of painful abdominal muscles) when midline incisions are used. In most cases, we prefer the extended left retroperitoneal approach to the aortic aneurysm. This incision, from near the umbilicus toward the left eleventh intercostal space, allows the peritoneal contents and left kidney to be easily mobilized and reflected medially. The resulting exposure of the aorta, its mesenteric branches, and the left renal artery is excellent (see Fig. 72–13C to E). Control of the proximal aorta is easily achieved, whether the neck of the aneurysm is above or below the renal arteries. The duodenum and intestines, which may be easily inspected if necessary, are not subjected to retraction or injury. Importantly, postoperative ileus and respiratory complications are minimized when the flank incision is used instead of the traditional midline approach.

Adequate proximal and distal control of the arteries is obviously essential. The proximal aorta should be clamped with a minimum of prior dissection and manipulation, so as to minimize the chances of embolization of atheromatous debris. For this reason, we do not advise encircling the aorta with tapes or ligatures before cross-clamping. If distal anastomoses are performed at the iliac artery level, these arteries should be dissected free from the iliac veins to avoid trauma to these fragile and inaccessible vessels. The infusion of mannitol (25 g) and furosemide (40 mg)15 to 20 minutes before aortic cross-clamping helps to promote a brisk diuresis and contributes to reducing the likelihood of postoperative renal dysfunction.

Once the aneurysm sac is opened, thrombus and debris are removed, and lumbar arteries are oversewn if they are backbleeding (see Fig. 72–13F and G). Great care should be used in examining the orifice of the inferior mesenteric artery (IMA). If either brisk backbleeding or no backbleeding is present, the IMA can be safely ligated. If there is a question about collateral flow into the IMA from the superior mesenteric artery (via the marginal artery of Drummond or other mesenteric vessels), a button of native aortic wall that includes the IMA orifice should be sewn into the body of the Dacron graft used in replacement of the aorta. It is important to note that there is no conclusive evidence that measurement of IMA stump pressures, as advocated by some, will prevent postoperative colon ischemia.

The aneurysm is replaced with an appropriately sized Dacron graft, either tube shaped or bifurcated in configuration (see Fig. 72–13). The proximal anastomosis is usually performed first and commonly involves a running end-to-end suture line of either 4-0 or 3-0 polypropylene material. The distal anastomoses are performed in either end-to-end (commonly for distal aorta or iliac arteries) or end-to-side (for femoral arteries) fashion, using a running 5-0 polypropylene suture. Before completing all anastomoses, the graft should be flushed of all debris to prevent distal embolization. The old aneurysm sac should then be loosely reclosed over the body of the graft.

In most large centers, the overall mortality rate for elective aortic aneurysm surgery ranges from 1 to 3 percent. Almost all postoperative deaths are due to either cardiac or renal causes, emphasizing again the importance of careful preoperative evaluation and treatment. Serious morbidity may occur in 10 to 15 percent of postoperative patients and may involve not only myocardial infarction and renal failure but also ischemic colitis, limb ischemia, or, less often, paraplegia. Moreover, sexual dysfunction is a well documented late complication and is likely related to either extraneous surgical dissection near the internal iliacs or postoperative lack of blood flow to the same area. Aortoenteric fistula formation is a rare but devastating late complication of abdominal aortic aneurysm surgery. If acute limb ischemia develops, it is an indication of either debris embolization or imperfect anastomoses, and immediate reexploration is advised. Fever, leukocytosis, and abdominal pain (in the absence of other causes) may alert one to the possibility of postoperative ischemic colitis. Multiple loose guaiac-positive stools may also suggest this complication, and endoscopy can be performed to aid in the diagnosis. In its severe forms, postoperative ischemic colitis carries with it mortality rates of 50 percent, despite aggressive treatment. Milder forms of the spectrum of this complication may respond to treatment with antibiotics and nasogastric suction, but if this regimen is prescribed, careful follow-up via repeat endoscopy is essential. Ischemic colitis may occur in up to 5 percent of postoperative patients. Paraplegia is a very rare complication, occurring in about 0.1 percent of patients after abdominal aortic aneurysm surgery. Although this incidence is fortunately very low, the complication is obviously devastating and seems to arise in a totally unpredictable fashion.

Aortic Dissection

Aortic dissections are usually caused by a tear in the intima of the aorta, leading to a dissecting hematoma in the aortic media. Indeed, the name is not an accurate description of the problem, and perhaps, as suggested by others, a better phrase to describe this catastrophic event is *dissecting hematoma*.[69–89] It is uncertain in every event whether the primary abnormality is a rupture of the intima with dissection of blood into the media or whether, on occasion, hemorrhage within a diseased media followed by disruption of the adjacent intima and subsequent propagation of the dissection through the intimal tear is the cause of the problem (Fig. 72–15).

A related entity that is considered to be clinically similar to dissecting aortic aneurysm by us and others is *intramural hematoma* (see Fig. 72–14B). This entity is characterized by the sudden development of severe pain and an aortic intramural hematoma with no identifiable intimal tear.[89a] The clinical prognosis for these patients is virtually identical to that of classic aortic dissection.[89a]

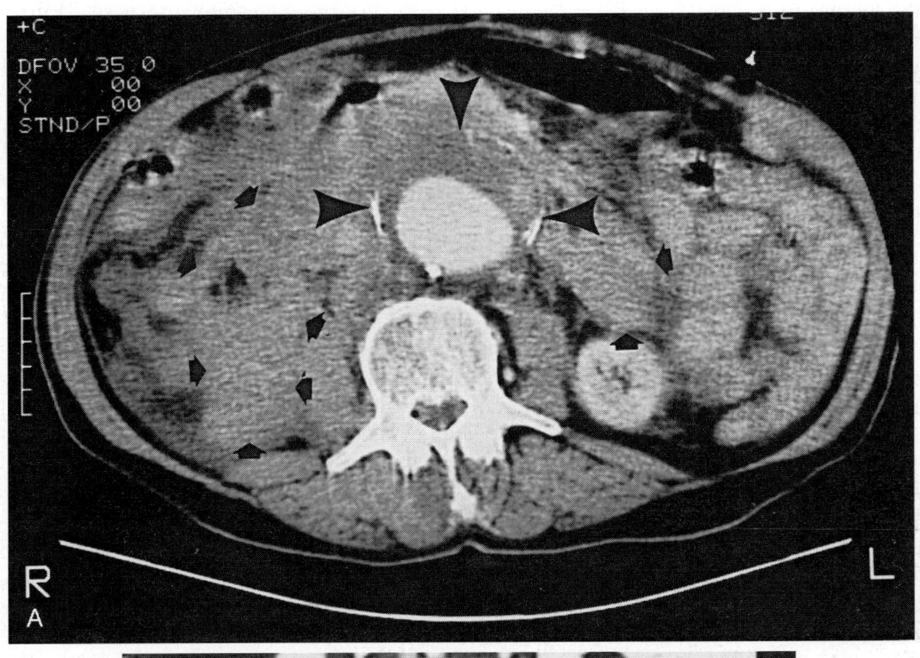

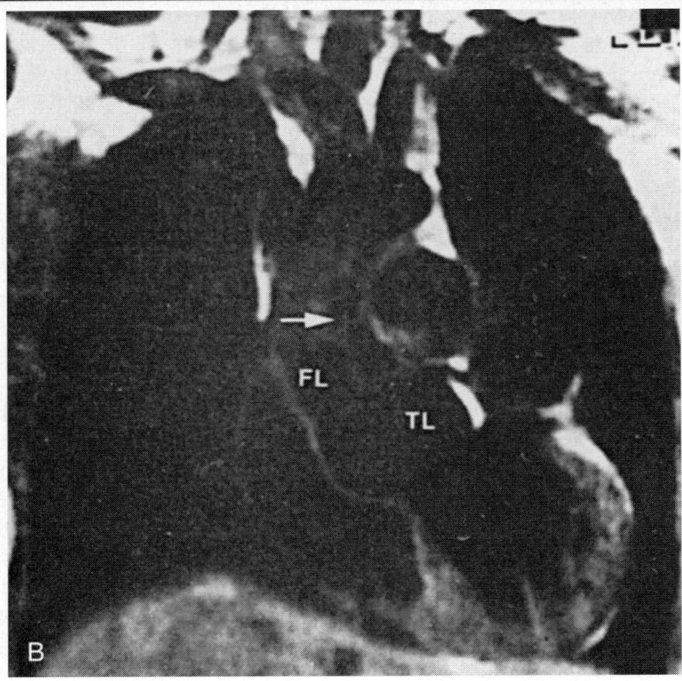

FIGURE 72–14 A, Computed tomography shows an aneurysm of the abdominal aorta *(arrowheads)* that has ruptured into the retroperitoneum *(arrows)*. These findings were confirmed at subsequent surgery. **B,** Magnetic resonance imaging study of an ascending aortic dissection *(arrow)*. FL, false lumen; TL, true lumen. (**A** and **B,** From Nienaber CA, von Kodolitsch Y, Nicolas V, et al: The diagnosis of thoracic aortic dissection by noninvasive imaging procedures. N Engl J Med 328:1, 1993. Copyright 1993, Massachusetts Medical Society. All rights reserved.)

Aortic dissections and intramural hematomas typically cause severe pain in a location suggesting either the origin or the path followed by the dissection. The circulation of any artery arising from the aorta may be compromised, resulting in vascular insufficiency, including the sudden development of a cerebrovascular accident, loss of arterial supply to a limb, the abrupt development of a myocardial infarction, mesenteric ischemia or infarction, or infarction of a kidney. The aortic dissection may rupture through the adventitia, resulting in immediate exsanguination, the development of pericardial tamponade with rupture into the pericardial space, a left pleural effusion with rupture into the left pleural cavity, or shock.

Types of Aortic Dissections

More than 90 percent of aortic dissections arise in one of two locations: the ascending aorta, within several centimeters of the aortic valve; or the descending aorta, ordinarily just beyond the origin of the left subclavian artery. DeBakey and colleagues[84, 85] have recognized three types of dissections, as shown in Figure 72–15. In types I and II, the intimal tear is in the ascending aorta. With *type I*, there is an extension beyond the ascending aorta and arch, whereas with *type II*, the dissection is confined to the ascending aorta. *Type III* dissections begin in the descending thoracic aorta and propagate proximally or distally for a variable distance. Type III dissections may be further subclassified into *type IIIa*, in which the process is limited to the thoracic aorta, and *type IIIb*, which indicates extension of the dissection below the diaphragm. Eagle and De Sanctis[2] simplified the classification of dissection, referring to *proximal* (DeBakey types I and II) and *distal* (DeBakey type III) dissections. Daily and associates[70] classified dissections into types A and B. *Type A* dissections include all proximal dissections and those distal dissections that extend retrograde to involve the arch and ascending aorta. *Type B* dissections include all other distal dissections without proximal extension.

On occasion, the site of origin of an aortic dissection is the aortic arch or the abdominal aorta. In addition, individual arteries may be the site of localized dissections, especially the coronary and carotid arteries in women in their last trimester of pregnancy or after delivery, in individuals

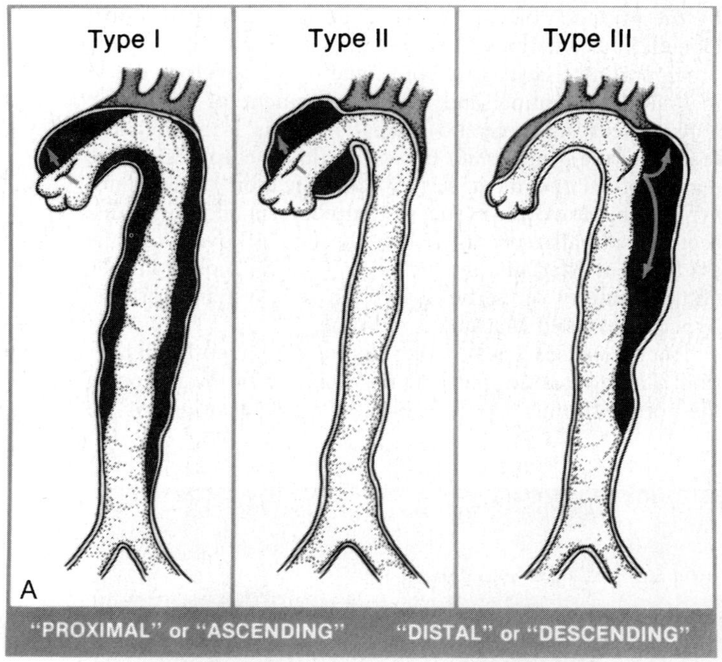

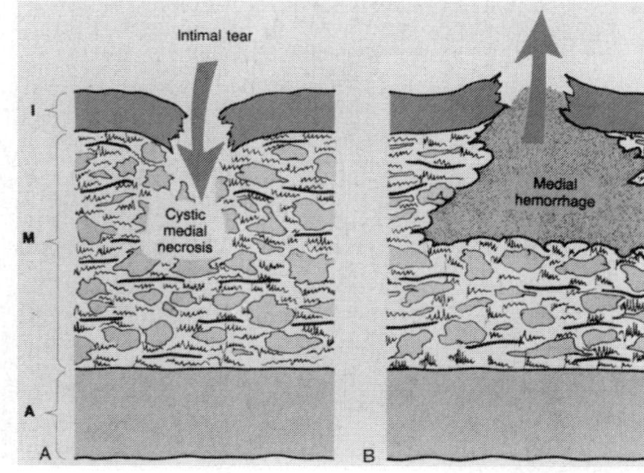

FIGURE 72–15 A, Classification scheme for aortic dissections as devised by DeBakey. **B,** A proposed mechanism for the initiation of aortic dissection. *Left,* An intimal tear is the initial event allowing blood to enter the media, resulting in a dissecting hematoma. *Right,* The initial event is the medial hemorrhage with rupture into the intima. I, intima; M, media; A, adventitia. (**A** and **B,** From Braunwald E [ed]: Heart Disease: A Textbook of Cardiovascular Medicine. 4th ed. Philadelphia: WB Saunders, 1992.)

TABLE 72–3 **Causes of Aortic Dissection**

Systemic arterial hypertension
Marfan's syndrome
Coarctation of the aorta and bicuspid aortic valve
Last trimester of pregnancy or soon after parturition
Atherosclerotic plaque
Ehlers-Danlos syndrome

with vasculitis in the same artery, and occasionally in association with intensive exercise.[71, 90, 91]

Etiology

Degeneration of the aortic media is thought to be the underlying lesion responsible for the development of an aortic dissection (Table 72–3).[2, 74, 82] Often, this results from deterioration of the collagen and elastic tissue with cystic change. Cystic medial necrosis can be the result of chronic stress against the aortic wall, such as may occur with severe and chronic hypertension. Medial degeneration appears to be part of the normal aging process in the aorta enhanced by the presence of chronic systemic arterial hypertension. Genetic abnormalities in the amount and type of collagen or supporting tissues may contribute to the development of medial degeneration and the development of dissecting aortic aneurysms.[4] Cystic medial necrosis is an intrinsic feature of the Marfan and Ehlers-Danlos syndromes. Aortic dissection is the most serious complication of Marfan's syndrome. However, cystic medial necrosis and aortic dissection can also occur in the absence of overt clinical evidence of Marfan's syndrome.[69, 72–74] The most common clinical causes of aortic dissection are systemic arterial hypertension and Marfan's syndrome.

Trauma causes a tear rather than a classic aortic dissection. These tears are particularly common in the region of the aortic isthmus, in close proximity to the origin of the left subclavian artery after sudden deceleration injury (Fig. 72–16).[92–98]

Clinical Findings

Aortic dissections occur most frequently in the sixth to seventh decades of life and are more common in men than in women. Severe chest pain is the most common clinical manifestation of aortic dissection. With dissections that are distal in location, the pain often begins in the back and may radiate in any direction. With other sites of origin of dissections, the pain may begin in other locations, especially in the left precordium or substernally. Typically, the pain is severe and unrelenting and sometimes described as tearing in nature. The chest pain is severe from the onset, and it migrates into the chest, abdomen, or back in accordance with the course of the aortic dissection. Associated symptoms, such as sweating, nausea, vomiting, and loss of consciousness sometimes occur, and when there is impairment of blood flow to other organs, the patient may experience the sudden development of a major neurologic event, including loss of consciousness or hemiparesis, pulse loss, a left pleural effusion, pericardial tamponade, a new murmur of aortic insufficiency, heart failure, severe hypertension with involvement of a renal artery, or limb ischemia. In the majority of patients, concomitant systemic arterial hypertension is present with the chest pain. Rarely, aortic dissection occurs without severe chest pain.

CLINICAL RECOGNITION

Physical Examination. The diagnosis can often be suspected from history and physical findings. Presentation with the typical chest or migrating abdominal or back pain described earlier in association with an absent left radial pulse or reduced blood pressure in the left arm and a widened ascending aortic silhouette is highly suggestive of aortic dissection. Other patients are peripherally vasocon-

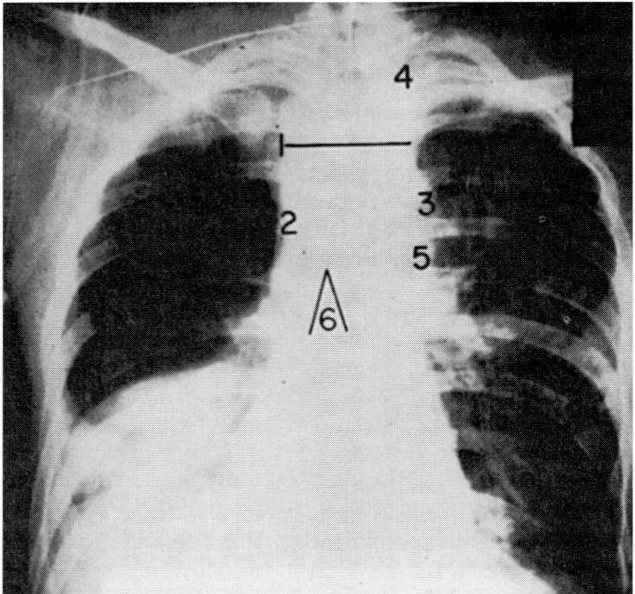

FIGURE 72–16 Demonstration of aortic trauma associated with sudden deceleration injury in which the aorta is torn, resulting in an increased mediastinal size. 1, Mediastinum diameter; 2, position of the trachea; 3, aortic outline; 4, upper lobe of left lung; 5, space between the aorta and the pulmonary artery; and 6, left main stem bronchus. (From Braunwald E [ed]: Heart Disease: A Textbook of Cardiovascular Medicine. 4th ed. Philadelphia: WB Saunders, 1992.)

stricted but have important systemic arterial hypertension. As noted earlier, hypotension or even shock may result from cardiac tamponade or intrapleural or intraperitoneal rupture. Severe heart failure usually develops when wide-open aortic insufficiency occurs. A new murmur of aortic insufficiency, especially one loudest in the second to third right intercostal spaces associated with the acute development of hypertension and chest pain, is suggestive of an acute aortic dissection. Pulse deficits in patients with aortic dissection may be transitory, tending to come and go depending on compression or decompression of the aorta or other vascular lumen by the hematoma, allowing distal reentry of blood flow into the true lumen or by movement of the intimal flap away from or toward the occluded orifice.

Aortic regurgitation occurs in the majority of patients with proximal aortic dissections. When the aortic insufficiency is severe, one expects bounding carotid and femoral pulses, a wide pulse pressure, enhanced capillary pulsations in the nail bed, and both a systolic ejection murmur and an aortic diastolic murmur. Severe aortic insufficiency is associated with a third heart sound and usually an apical low-frequency short diastolic rumble ("Austin Flint rumble") without an audible opening snap. Aortic regurgitation occurs in patients with proximal aortic dissections for one of three reasons:

1. Dilatation of the aortic root, widening the aortic annulus so that the aortic leaflets do not coapt normally during diastole
2. The dissecting hematoma depresses one or more leaflets below the line of closure of the remaining leaflets
3. Annular support of the leaflets may be weakened or interrupted, causing aortic valve incompetence

Neurologic deficits associated with aortic dissection include cerebrovascular accidents, ischemic peripheral neuropathy, ischemic paraparesis, and loss of consciousness. Each of these abnormalities is more common with proximal aortic dissection. *Horner's syndrome* due to compression of the superior cervical sympathetic ganglion, vocal cord paralysis and hoarseness from pressure against the left recurrent laryngeal nerve, superior mediastinal syndrome from superior vena cava compression,[99] pulsating neck masses, tracheal or bronchial compression with bronchospasm, hemorrhage into the tracheobronchial tree with hemoptysis as a consequence of the rupture of the dissection into the bronchus, hematemesis due to perforation into the esophagus, heart block from retrograde burrowing of the dissection into the atrial septum and atrioventricular node, a continuous murmur caused by rupture of the aortic dissection into the right atrium or right ventricle, pulsation of one of the sternoclavicular joints, or a combination is occasionally encountered.[70, 100–102] Infarction of the bowel, renal infarction with severe renovascular hypertension, and myocardial infarction are among the more serious associated clinical events.

DIFFERENTIAL DIAGNOSIS

Aortic dissections must be distinguished from myocardial ischemia and infarction, aneurysms of the thoracic and abdominal aorta that are not caused by dissection, mediastinal tumors, and pericarditis. The differential diagnosis is made more difficult when there are associated clinical conditions, such as aortic insufficiency, inequality of pulses or a left pleural effusion due to another cause, and presentation with chest pain suggesting aortic dissection.

None of the laboratory chemistries specifically differentiate aortic dissection, because it may coexist with acute myocardial infarction as occurs when a coronary artery is compromised by the aortic dissection. In this circumstance, creatine kinase, creatine kinase-MB, and troponins I and T are elevated. If the patient is actively bleeding as a consequence of the dissection, progressive anemia develops. In the absence of concomitant acute myocardial infarction or separate myocardial infarction, the electrocardiogram does not show specific changes indicative of aortic dissection.

LABORATORY EXAMINATION

Transesophageal echocardiography is especially useful in the detection of a proximal aortic dissection through identification of a widened aortic diameter and delineation of the dissecting aneurysm (Fig. 72–17 and Table 72–4).[103, 104] Doppler color flow imaging may allow sites of communication between the true and false lumen to be identified (see Fig. 72–17).

MRI/MRA is a noninvasive technique that is extremely useful in the anatomic evaluation of the aorta and the detection of dissecting aortic aneurysms (see Table 72–4).[62, 75, 104] Identification of an intimal flap is possible in most cases, as is identification of the extent of the dissection and involvement of branch vessels. In contrast to CT scanning, MRI/MRA does not require the administration of potentially toxic contrast material, nor does it involve ionizing radiation. It may be the most sensitive noninvasive imaging method for the detection of dissecting aortic aneurysms, but transesophageal echocardiography and CT scanning with contrast agent are also excellent noninvasive methods for the detection of aortic dissections (see Figs. 72–14 and 72–17).[102–104]

Aortic angiography is the most useful invasive study technique in the diagnosis of aortic dissection. It requires the injection of contrast media into the aorta, but it often allows one to make a definitive diagnosis, identify the site of origin of the dissection, and delineate the extent of the dissection and the arterial vessels that take origin from the true and false channels. There are some risks in contrast angiography, including (1) allergic responses, (2) introduction of infection, (3) causing transient worsening of renal function, (4) further extending the dissection, and (5) immediate rupture of the aortic aneurysm as a consequence of injecting contrast medium under pressure. In addition, angiography may fail to demonstrate a dissection if there is only faint or no opacification of the false lumen, a small and very localized dissection, or equal simultaneous opacification of both the true and the false channels. The noninvasive methods have largely replaced angiography in the detection of aortic dissections.

Chest radiographs generally reveal a widened aortic contour in patients with proximal aortic dissections. The major difficulty is in distinguishing aortic dilatation from aging, hypertension, atherosclerotic aneurysm, and combinations

TABLE 72-4 **Identification of Thoracic Aortic Dissection and Associated Findings, According to Imaging Procedure**

Finding	Sensitivity	Specificity	Accuracy (%)	Positive Predictive Value	Negative Predictive Value
Dissection					
Ascending Aorta					
TTE	78.1	86.7	84.1*	71.4	90.3
TEE	96.4†	85.7	90.0‡	81.8	97.3
CT	82.6	100§	94.9	100†	93.3
MRI	100†	98.7§	99.0	96.8†	100
Aortic Arch					
TTE	35.7	97.4	80.8	83.3	80.4
TEE	95.0¶	93.6	94.0	86.4	97.8
CT	89.5¶	96.7	94.9	89.5	96.7
MRI	96.1¶	100	99.0†	100	98.7
Descending Aorta					
TTE	31.3	100‖	66.0	100	59.8
TEE	97.1¶	94.4	95.7	94.3	97.1†
CT	90.2¶	86.8	88.6	88.1	89.2†
MRI	98.0¶	100§	99.0†	100	98.1†
Entry Location					
Ascending Aorta					
TTE	40.0	100	88.8	100	87.9
TEE	78.9†	100	94.1	100	92.5
CT	—	—	—	—	—
MRI	80.0†	100	86.2	100	95.5
Aortic Arch					
TTE	33.3	100	98.1	100	98.1
TEE	66.7	100	98.5	100	98.5
CT	—	—	—	—	—
MRI	100	100	100	100	100
Descending Aorta					
TTE	9.5	100	80.8	100	80.4
TEE	64.3*	100	92.6	100	91.5
CT	—	—	—	—	—
MRI	90.8*	100	98.1	100	97.6
Thrombosis					
Ascending Aorta					
TTE	0	100	93.6	0*	93.6
TEE	33.3	100	97.1	100	97.1
CT	83.2†	100	98.6	100	98.5
MRI	87.5†	100	99.0	100	98.8
Aortic Arch					
TTE	0	100	94.3	0	94.3
TEE	50	100	97.1	100	97.0
CT	100†	100	100	100	100
MRI	100†	98.0	98.0	75	100
Descending Aorta					
TTE	13.8	100	75.0	100	74.0
TEE	69.2†	100	94.1	100	93.2
CT	94.7**	98.1	97.2	94.6	98.1†
MRI	86.2**	100	96.2	100	95.0

Abbreviations: CT, computed tomography; MRI, magnetic resonance imaging; TEE, transesophageal echocardiography; TTE, transthoracic echocardiography.
Percentages were calculated on the basis of all assessable findings.
*$P < .01$ for the comparison with TEE, x-ray CT, and MRI.
†$P < .05$ for the comparison with TTE.
‡$P < .05$ for the comparison with MRI.
§$P < .05$ for the comparison with TTE and TEE.
¶$P < .005$ for the comparison with TTE.
‖$P < .05$ for the comparison with x-ray CT.
**$P < .01$ for the comparison with TTE.
From Nienaber CA, von Kodolitsch Y, Nicolas V, et al: The diagnosis of thoracic aortic dissection by noninvasive imaging procedures. N Engl J Med 328:1, 1993.

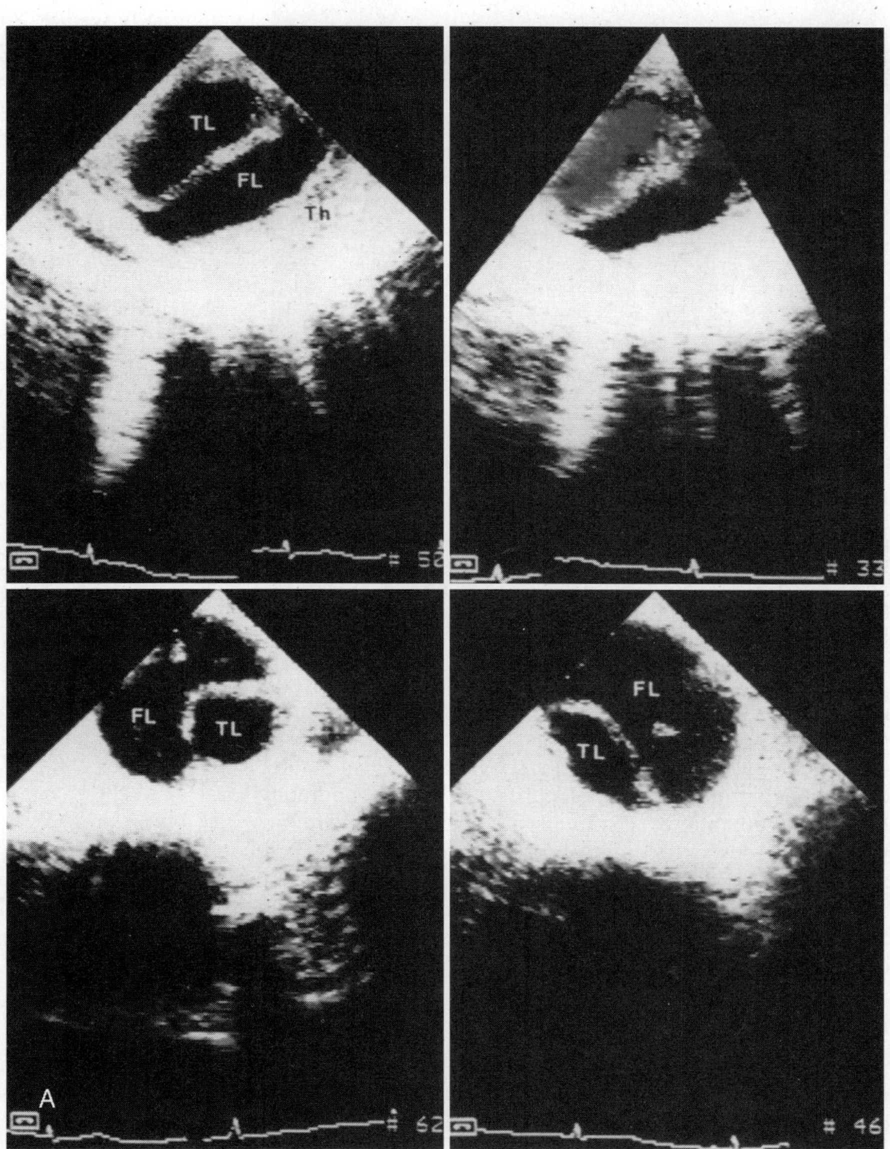

FIGURE 72–17. A, Transesophageal echocardiogram demonstrates an ascending aortic dissection. FL, false lumen; TL, true lumen.

Illustration continued on following page

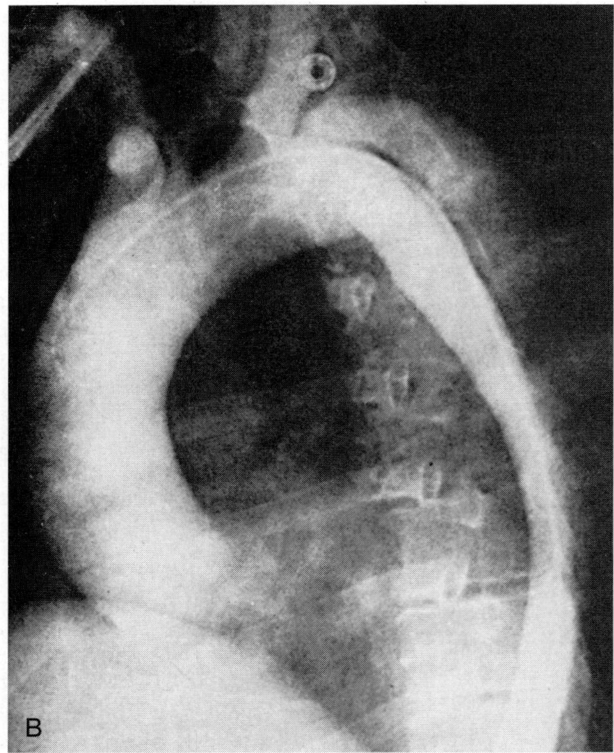

FIGURE 72–17 *Continued.* **B,** Aortogram demonstrates an aortic arch and descending aortic aneurysm with contrast medium in both the true and the false lumen. (**A,** From Nienaber CA, von Kodolitsch Y, Nicolas V, et al: The diagnosis of thoracic aortic dissection by noninvasive imaging procedures. N Engl J Med 328:1, 1993. Copyright 1993, Massachusetts Medical Society. All rights reserved.)

of these entities from that due to dissecting aortic aneurysm. Serial chest radiographs that allow comparisons with the recent past can be enormously helpful. Distal aortic dissections are difficult to identify on roentgenography. However, separation of intimal calcification from the adventitial border exceeding 1 cm, the "calcium sign," is suggestive of aortic dissection (Fig. 72–18).

Table 72–4 identifies the sensitivity, specificity, accuracy, and positive and negative predictive values for each of these imaging techniques for detection of aortic dissection.

Initial Evaluation of Patients With Aortic Dissections

All patients in whom there is a strong suspicion of aortic dissection should be admitted immediately to an intensive care unit, where blood pressure, heart rate and rhythm, and urine output can be closely monitored, and a general examination can be performed. An initial electrocardiogram followed by serial electrocardiograms with cardiac enzymes is also indicated in those patients with chest or back pain. On occasion, acute myocardial infarction develops as a consequence of compromise of the ostia of a major coronary artery by the dissection. The initial therapeutic goals are the reduction or elimination of pain and reduction in systolic blood pressure to the lowest levels compatible with adequate cerebral, renal, and cardiac perfusion.

For acute reduction of arterial pressure, the authors prefer a β-adrenergic antagonist or combined α/β-adrenergic antagonists administered intravenously.

Generally, a β-blocker, such as propranolol or a comparable β-blocker, is added in incremental doses of 1 mg IV every 5 minutes until there is evidence of satisfactory β-adrenergic blockade as indicated by a pulse rate of 60 to 80 beats/min and a reduction in systolic blood pressure. A test dose of 0.5 mg IV is usually administered initially. The maximal initial total dose should not exceed 0.15 mg/kg body weight. Additional propranolol should be administered intravenously every 4 to 6 hours to maintain a reduction in blood pressure and heart rate; usual subsequent doses are 2 to 6 mg. Subsequently, the patients are switched to oral β-blocker therapy, and for propranolol, this includes the administration of 20 to 40 mg every 6 hours with subsequent increases in dosage dependent on heart rate and systolic blood pressure. β-Blockers are contraindicated in patients with profound bradycardia, severe heart failure, bronchospasm/asthma, and labile and insulin-dependent diabetes mellitus. Atenolol or metoprolol, the more cardioselective β-blockers, may be used as alternatives to propranolol, especially in patients with chronic obstructive lung disease and those with labile diabetes. Labetalol is a combined α/β-adrenergic receptor blocker, and it is also useful in the treatment of patients with acute aortic dissections.

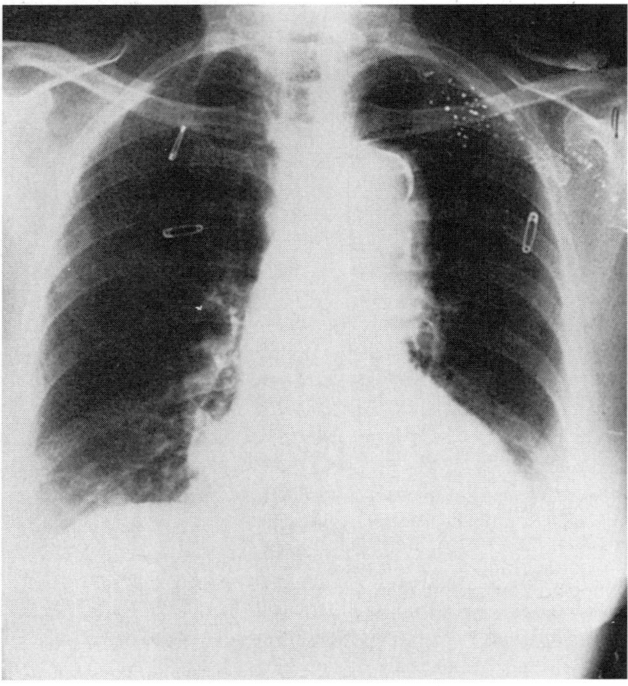

FIGURE 72–18 The "calcium sign" is demonstrated. Linear calcium is shown in the aortic arch and in the descending aorta. Calcium present in the descending or ascending aorta at least 1.0 cm from the outer border of the aortic silhouette is suggestive of aortic dissection. Calcium present in the aortic arch is not as useful in identifying the presence of a dissection because the curvature of the aorta at that point makes it difficult to obtain a reliable measurement that identifies calcium in the aortic wall from the outer border of the aorta and that is meaningful regarding the presence of a previous dissection. (From Braunwald E [ed]: Heart Disease: A Textbook of Cardiovascular Medicine. 4th ed. Philadelphia: WB Saunders, 1992.)

Labetalol is administered intravenously initially as 5 to 20 mg, and additional doses of 20 to 40 mg may be administered every 10 to 15 minutes until the blood pressure is controlled at the desired level or a total daily dose of 150 to 300 mg has been administered. One may give a continuous intravenous infusion of 0.5 mg/min to 2.0 mg/min. Subsequently, oral doses of 100 mg twice a day, with dose increases in 2 to 3 days up to 200 to 400 mg twice a day, to control systemic arterial hypertension may be used.

Sodium nitroprusside, administered parenterally as 15 to 100 mg in 500 ml of 5 percent dextrose and water and infused initially at a rate of 25 to 50 μg/min with subsequent dosages depending on blood pressure response, lowers blood pressure rapidly, but it does not depress the rate of propulsive force rise. One should not exceed 4 μg/kg/min in 3 hours to avoid cyanide intoxication. Indeed, it may actually increase it, which is an undesirable accompaniment of lowering blood pressure in the patient with aortic dissection. Nevertheless, it is sometimes necessary to add nitroprusside or nitroglycerin intravenously to gain control of blood pressure. When combined with a β-blocker or combined α/β-adrenergic antagonist, the unloading effect of nitroprusside is attenuated.

In the patient with occlusion of a renal artery as a consequence of the aortic dissection, severe and difficult to treat systemic arterial hypertension may develop. In this circumstance, the intravenous administration of an ACE inhibitor, such as enalapril or captopril, may be effective in dosages of 1 to 2 mg every 4 to 6 hours. The ACE inhibitor helps to control blood pressure, but it also increases the rate of propulsive force rise in the aorta, so it should be added only when absolutely necessary for blood pressure control, preferably in combination with a β-blocker that reduces the rate of propulsive force rise in the aorta. However, careful monitoring of renal function is necessary with this approach.

A calcium channel antagonist may also be used in the treatment of patients with acute aortic dissections, especially verapamil or diltiazem. Nifedipine is useful in treating systemic arterial hypertension, but like nitroprusside, it does not reduce the rate of propulsive force rise in the aorta and may actually increase it.

For longer-term therapy, control of blood pressure and the rate of propulsive force rise is important, so most patients remain on a β-adrenergic or combined α/β-adrenergic antagonist blocker with a calcium antagonist or ACE inhibitor and are followed closely with periodic MRI, CT scanning, or transesophageal echocardiography studies to evaluate possible progressive saccular enlargement of the aneurysm. Progressive saccular enlargement of an ascending aortic or descending aortic aneurysm to a maximal diameter of 5 cm or larger requires surgical resection and repair to reduce the risk of rupture. Progressive saccular enlargement of aortic dissections occurs more commonly in patients with ascending aortic dissections, even in those on medical therapy.

After medical therapy or combined medical and surgical therapy, it is important that the patient be monitored carefully for adequate blood pressure control and avoid excessive physical exercise, such as occurs in competitive athletics.

With the appropriate medical therapy, initial hospital survival rates of 80 percent or greater have been reported for patients with acute ascending aortic dissections treated surgically and for acute distal dissections treated medically. Hospital survival for patients with chronic aortic dissections, defined as presentations 2 weeks or more after the onset of dissection, who are treated either surgically or medically is usually 90 percent or greater.

Acute surgery in patients with aortic dissections is associated with greater difficulty in repair because of edema, bleeding, and fragility of the aortic wall. Improved survival in patients with chronic aortic dissections who subsequently undergo surgery probably results in part from the fact that some patients have selected themselves out as a group most likely to do well after surviving the initial high mortality rates. For patients with ascending aortic dissections who have other serious medical diseases or who refuse surgical therapy, medical therapy is used as described earlier.

Medical Treatment and Prognosis

The treatment of aortic dissections is directed initially at controlling blood pressure and reducing the rate of propulsive force rise in the aorta, because hypertension and increased rate of pressure rise in the aorta tend to expand the aneurysm and cause it to rupture. Without treatment, most patients with aortic dissections die relatively rapidly. In patients with aortic dissection, more than 25 percent are dead within 24 hours in the absence of any treatment, and more than half die within the first week. By 1 year, more than 90 percent of patients have died.

In patients with aortic dissection, medical therapy is started immediately, including medication to reduce systemic arterial blood pressure and the rate of propulsive force rise in the aorta. The goal of treatment is to lower blood pressure to the lowest level tolerated hemodynamically; ideally, systolic blood pressures of 90 to 100 mm Hg are achieved. One should intravenously administer antihypertensive medication without substantial afterload-reducing properties to lower blood pressure to the lowest level compatible with adequate cerebral, renal, and cardiac perfusion. As mentioned earlier, in the absence of a contraindication, a β-blocker or combined α/β-adrenergic blocker is generally administered intravenously originally and orally later, with the goal of reducing blood pressure and the rate of propulsive force rise. One attempts to avoid medications that substantially reduce afterload, because they may increase the rate of propulsive force rise even if they reduce systemic blood pressure.

Patients with ascending and aortic arch dissections (DeBakey types I and II) usually require surgery in combination with the medical therapy discussed earlier. Surgery may be performed acutely, or it may be deferred a few days. Modern surgical therapy for aortic dissections was developed by DeBakey and colleagues in the 1950s. The principles of surgical therapy are as follows:

1. To eliminate the intimal tear
2. To obliterate the false channel by oversewing aortic edges
3. To reconstitute the aorta with or without interposition of a synthetic graft

4. In the case of proximal dissection with valvular aortic insufficiency, to restore aortic valve competence through resuspension of the disrupted aortic leaflets or through prosthetic aortic valve replacement

Patients with distal or DeBakey type III dissections generally are as well treated with medical therapy as with surgery.

Aggressive medical therapy for patients with aortic dissection was first described by Wheat and colleagues.[87] The goals of pharmacologic therapy are to reduce systolic blood pressure to the lowest level compatible with adequate cerebral, renal, and cardiac perfusion and the rate of pressure rise in the aorta. This form of therapy is used as the primary treatment for patients with distal, or DeBakey type III, dissections, whereas surgical combined with medical therapy is the treatment of choice for acute proximal and aortic arch dissections (DeBakey types I and II). Table 72–5 lists the indications for surgical and medical therapy in patients with aortic dissections.

Surgical Treatment and Prognosis

The first successful management of aortic dissection was reported by DeBakey and colleagues in 1955,[85] and Wheat and colleagues described medical management in 1965.[87] Since then, considerable progress has been made in dealing with this problem, and there has also been controversy regarding the details of management. Aortic dissection is the most common catastrophic disease of the aorta, occurring two to three times more commonly than ruptured abdominal aneurysms. There are an estimated 2000 annual cases in the United States. The need for urgent diagnosis and treatment is obvious.

Once the diagnosis of an acute aortic dissection has been made, definitive therapy should begin. Types I and II dissections (or type A dissection, proximal to the left subclavian artery) have traditionally been treated with combined medical and surgical therapy, and the results have increasingly improved. Operative mortality rates of 7 to 10 percent have been reported, and even these results may be improving in medical centers with a particular interest in the treatment of acute aortic dissections. The goal of surgery is twofold. First, the aortic segment containing the original intimal tear is resected, with graft replacement of the ascending aorta redirecting blood into the true lumen (thereby obliterating the false lumen). Second, if severe aortic insufficiency is present, it should be corrected. Aortic insufficiency is typically due to downward displacement of the noncoronary cusp of the aortic valve into the left ventricle. Resuspension of the valve, if possible, is the preferred maneuver. If there is a question of valvular competence from simple resuspension, valve replacement can be performed, either as a separate prosthesis or as a combined valve-conduit. In the latter procedure, reimplantation of the coronary arteries may be required. With redirection of flow into the true lumen, obstruction or compromise of branch vessels will usually resolve. If it does not, selective revascularization of affected viscera or extremities may be indicated. Technical problems during the procedure may develop from the extreme friability of the acutely dissected aorta, which may not hold sutures well. Various techniques have been devised to deal with this problem. An intraluminal rigid prosthesis (a Dacron conduit with two rings at either end) may be placed in the affected aorta and the aorta secured around the rings at either end with a tape, proximal and distal to the site of origin of the dissection. Theoretically, this technique may eliminate bleeding from suture lines through friable tissue. Another helpful maneuver involves the use of woven Dacron grafts that have been preclotted with albumin or fresh frozen plasma and then baked in an autoclave. These grafts appear to bleed less than those not similarly treated. We prefer the "open" technique of operative repair shown in Figure 72–19. This maneuver uses a brief period of hypothermic circulatory arrest to effect a rapid, precise repair without the need for cannulae and clamps, which may obscure proper vision and tear the already friable vessel wall.

The only contraindication to repair of a type A dissection is the presence of a stroke in progress, because the occlusion of a carotid or vertebral artery will result in an ischemic infarction, and intraoperative heparinization with restoration of cerebral blood flow may result in a massive hemorrhagic cerebral infarction. Intimal tears that begin in the aortic arch (type II) are the most difficult to treat, and a variety of approaches have been devised. The best approach seems to involve deep hypothermia and create a circulatory arrest, because this allows a direct surgical approach in a tranquil, bloodless operative field. Although surgical results have been good, many continue to try to treat this condition medically.

The treatment of type III dissections (or type B, distal to the left subclavian artery) has generated more controversy. Traditionally, uncomplicated type B dissection has been treated medically, with results equal to or better than those obtained from surgical therapy. One group at the Massachusetts General Hospital reported an 80 percent in-hospital survival rate with medical management of such patients.[87a] Surgery has most often been reserved for those patients who develop complications from type III dissections, including unrelenting pain, occlusion of a major arterial trunk leading to visceral or limb ischemia, uncontrolled hypertension, or expansion of the aorta with threatened rupture. However, with improved preoperative, operative, and post-

TABLE 72–5 Indications for Surgical or Medical Therapy in Patients With Acute Aortic Dissection

Surgical Treatment

For patients with acute ascending aortic dissections
For acute aortic dissections complicated by any of the following:
- Occlusion of a major artery
- Leaking from the aneurysm
- Wide open valvular aortic insufficiency with congestive heart failure
- Pericardial tamponade
- Vital organ compromise
- Progressive enlargement of the saccular aneurysm with time

Medical Treatment

Treatment of choice for uncomplicated distal dissection (DeBakey type III dissections)
Used in combination with surgical therapy when surgical therapy is deemed most appropriate

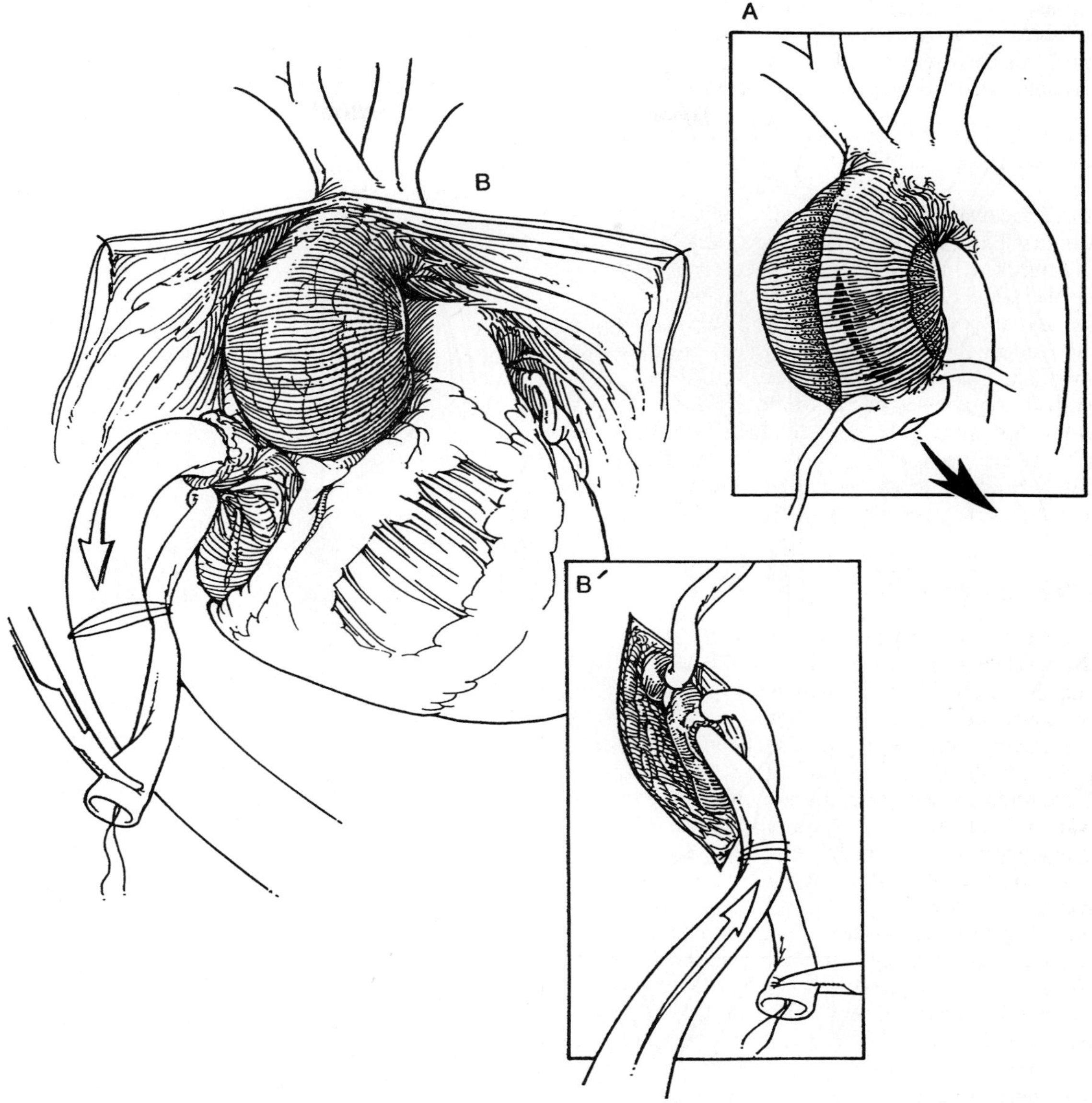

FIGURE 72–19 A–H, Technique used to repair acute and chronic dissection of the ascending aorta when aortic valve regurgitation is present. (**A–H,** From Cooley DA: Surgical Treatment of Aortic Aneurysms. Philadelphia: WB Saunders, 1986.)

Illustration continued on following page

operative management of these patients (as well as the fact that some patients with a chronic type III dissection will eventually require surgical intervention), the results of medical therapy are challenged by operative therapy. Surgeons at some medical centers report an operative mortality rate of 12 to 13 percent for repairs of acute type III dissections and recommend early surgical referral for patients with aortic dissection of any type. The major complication of surgery for type III dissections is spinal cord ischemia, and the incidence of paralysis appears to be directly related to cross-clamp time. Femorofemoral bypass, left aortofemoral bypass, shunts, and hypothermia have all been used in attempts to eliminate paraplegia, and opinion varies as to the advantages any or all may offer relative to a simple "clamp-and-sew" approach.

The impact of the use of a competent anesthesiologist on the results of surgical treatment of acute aortic dissection cannot be overestimated. Anesthesia for acute aortic dissection is similar to that for patients undergoing cardiopulmonary bypass. A pulmonary artery catheter is placed for the management of preload and afterload concerns, and a right radial artery line should be used in type III dissections where the left subclavian artery might be clamped. Anesthetic induction should be performed with the goal of avoiding hypertension. A double-lumen endotracheal tube should be used for type III repairs, allowing deflation of the left lung during some of the procedure. As with any surgery on the thoracic aorta, the most critical periods for anesthetic management are the times of clamping and unclamping the aorta. The anesthesiologist should have ready at all times a sodium nitroprusside drip, as well as the ability to rapidly replace major blood losses.

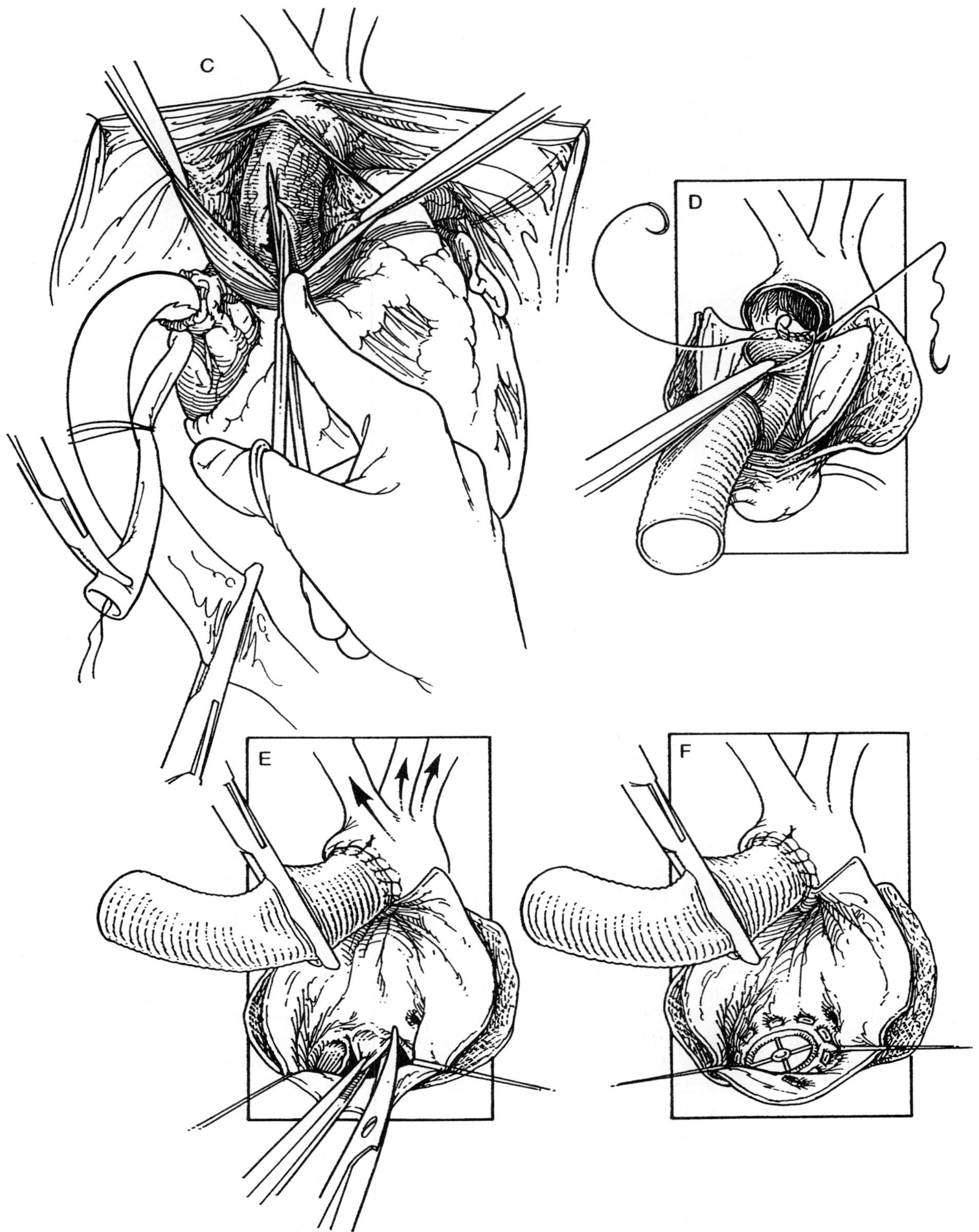

FIGURE 72–19C–F *Continued*

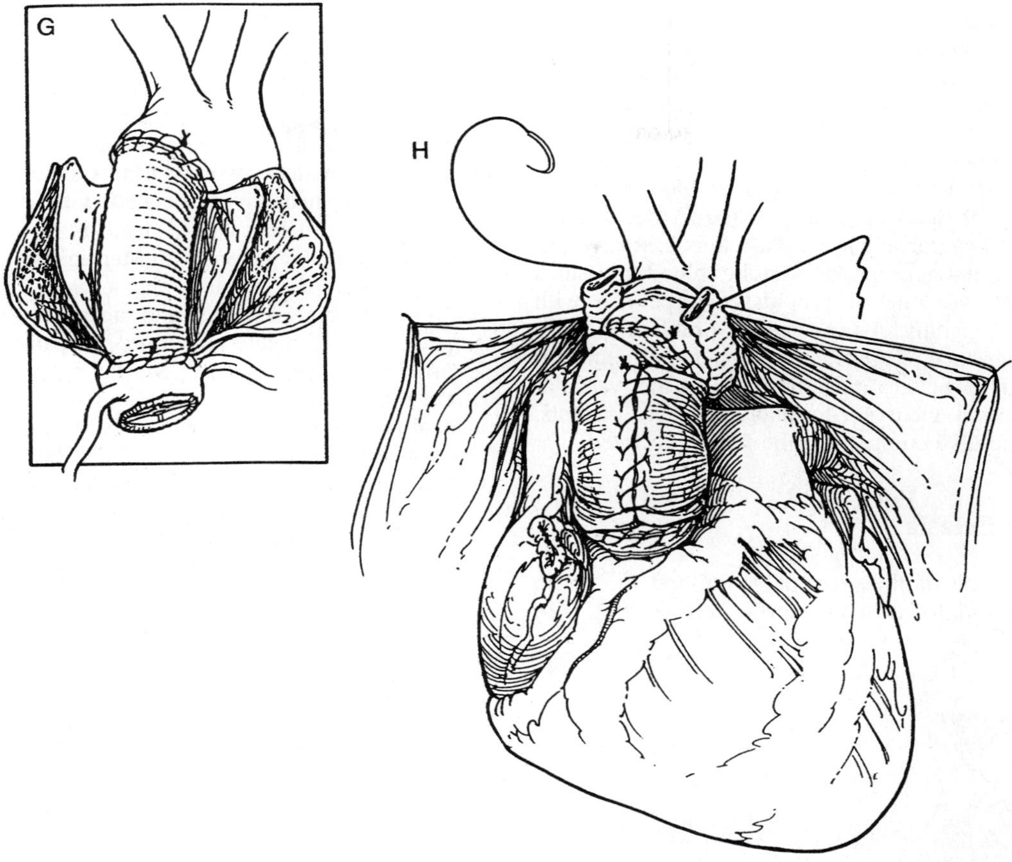

FIGURE 72–19G–H *Continued*

POSTOPERATIVE CARE

The most critical aspect of postoperative care (and with medical therapy generally) in the intensive care unit is the control of blood pressure. The use of β-adrenergic blockade, unloading therapy if necessary, attention to ongoing blood loss, correction of hypothermia, and treatment of coagulopathy are all of great importance. Heating blankets, convection shields, and warm blood products help to raise the patient's temperature and should all be used if necessary. The aggressive use of fresh frozen plasma, platelets, and fresh whole blood often helps to correct clotting abnormalities. As with any cardiovascular procedure, optimization of cardiac output with a thermodilution catheter, maintenance of adequate urine output, careful attention to respiratory function, and rapid weaning from the ventilator are performed. A careful postoperative neurologic examination should be performed, looking for evidence of cerebral or spinal cord ischemia.

RESULTS

The results of operative treatment for acute aortic dissection have improved, with many groups reporting operative mortality rates as low as 7 percent for types I and II repair and 12 to 13 percent for type III repairs. The predictors of operative death include renal dysfunction, tamponade, visceral ischemia, and pulmonary disease. Long-term results are surprisingly good, with actuarial survival rates of 82 percent at 5 years and 64 percent at 10 years. In one series, the incidence of dissection-related reoperation was 13 percent at 5 years and 23 percent at 10 years. Younger age, intimal tears in the aortic arch (type II), and the preoperative presence of cardiac tamponade made the need for reoperation more likely. Reoperation is usually required for aneurysm development, redissection, or onset of aortic insufficiency. In DeBakey's long-term follow-up series, ruptured aneurysms caused 29.3 percent of all late deaths.[84] The incidence and significance of late complications accent the importance of close follow-up of these patients, at least with frequent chest films and CT scans of the aorta. The appearance of any new problem warrants an aggressive evaluation and possible surgical correction. The nonoperative management of these patients on a long-term basis is similar to the strategy used for the acute problem, involving control of blood pressure and velocity of contractions. This is achieved with β-blockers, selected calcium channel blockers, and other standard antihypertensives. Labetalol, with its unique combination of α/β-adrenergic antagonism, or a separate β-blocker and α-adrenergic agonist in the central nervous system (clonidine) are helpful for the long-term care of the patient who has experienced an acute aortic dissection.

Patients With Marfan's Syndrome

Patients with Marfan's syndrome are particularly likely to develop aortic dissections. The indications for medical and surgical therapy are the same as those identified earlier. The avoidance of competitive exercise is important in these individuals. However, many of these patients are talented athletes. Nevertheless, the responsible physician should prevent patients with Marfan's syndrome from engaging in competitive athletics and strenuous exercise that will result in major increases in heart rate and systolic blood pressure. Close follow-up of these patients is required, because the risk of a new dissection always exists. It is critically important to maintain appropriate systolic blood pressures and to diminish the rate of propulsive force rise with selected medical therapy. A fundamental problem in these patients is the absence of a normal supporting structure for the aorta. With a better understanding of the vascular biology involved in aneurysm formation in these patients, the risk of aortic dissection should be further reduced.

Annuloaortic Ectasia

Idiopathic dilatation of the proximal aorta and the aortic annulus is referred to as annuloaortic ectasia (Fig. 72–20).[105–111]

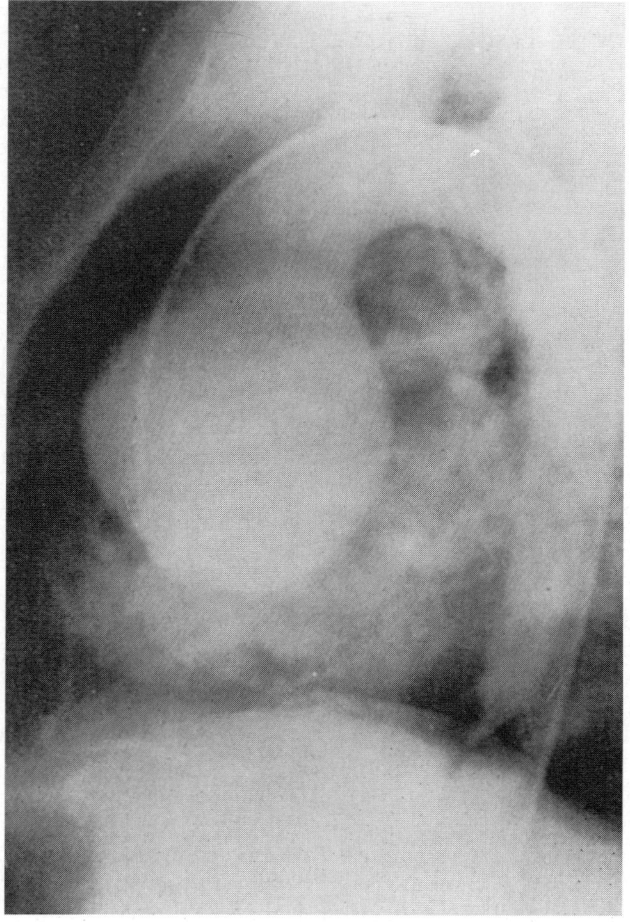

FIGURE 72–20 A patient with annuloaortic ectasia. Note the pear-shaped enlargement of the aorta immediately above the aortic valve and the associated aortic insufficiency. (From Braunwald E [ed]: Heart Disease: A Textbook of Cardiovascular Medicine. 4th ed. Philadelphia: WB Saunders, 1992.)

Etiology

Severe degenerative changes, often cystic medial necrosis, in the wall of the aorta lead to a pear-shaped enlargement of the aorta at the level of the aortic annulus. Patients with Marfan's syndrome may demonstrate annuloaortic ectasia; indeed, most patients with Marfan's syndrome have some cystic medial necrosis associated with dilatation of the proximal aorta. The cause of death is often aortic rupture or dissection in the patient with Marfan's syndrome; defects in the fibrillin gene appear to play a role in the development of cystic medial necrosis and aneurysm formation.[4] In general, approximately one third of patients with annuloaortic ectasia have classic Marfan's syndrome. In many of the remaining patients, the annuloaortic ectasia may be a localized expression of Marfan's syndrome without the other manifestations of the disease.[108] In the patients with this clinical problem, the aorta widens progressively; the annulus dilates, drawing apart the aortic leaflets; and in some patients, marked aortic insufficiency develops. Aortic dissection may also occur in the area of annuloaortic ectasia.

Clinical Recognition

Annuloaortic ectasia occurs more frequently in men than in women. The abnormality often becomes obvious in the fourth to sixth decades of life and may be announced initially by a new murmur of aortic insufficiency. Patients with Marfan's syndrome may be identified at an earlier age. Aortic root dissection with its associated pain is a common finding in patients with annuloaortic ectasia.[106] Patients with dissection and this clinical problem generally have severe chest pain, but some of these patients have recurrent episodes of chest pain without detectable aortic dissection.

The development of aortic regurgitation results in a diastolic decrescendo murmur, which may be heard best to the right of the sternum in the second to third intercostal spaces, as is true for other causes of aortic regurgitation resulting from aortic root disease. Moderately severe and severe aortic regurgitation results in an audible third heart sound, and severe aortic regurgitation causes a short apical diastolic rumble (the Austin Flint rumble).

Chest radiographs generally demonstrate a dilated aortic root. In patients with substantial aortic insufficiency, the left ventricle enlarges in relationship to the severity of aortic regurgitation and its chronicity. Often, proximal enlargement of the aorta is not apparent on chest radiography because it is at the level of the aortic annulus. Two-dimensional echocardiography, transesophageal echocardiography, MRI, or CT scanning are required to demonstrate the pear-shaped enlargement at the level of the aortic valve leaflets (see Fig. 72–8).

Aortic enlargement and the presence of aortic regurgitation are easily demonstrated angiographically. Most patients have pear-shaped enlargement of the aorta, but some demonstrate a diffuse symmetric dilatation, and in others the dilatation is limited to the sinuses of Valsalva. Aortic dissections occurring in the region of annuloaortic ectasia are characteristically small and confined to the ascending aorta; thus, they are not always easy to identify with any imaging technique.

Treatment

When the systemic blood pressure is elevated, it is controlled by appropriate medication. When the transaortic dilatation becomes 5 cm or larger, surgical correction is recommended; this includes resection of the aneurysmal aorta and replacement with a prosthetic graft. In patients with important aortic regurgitation, the prosthetic graft will contain an artificial aortic valve with reimplantation of the coronary arteries. Postoperatively, 5- and 10-year survival rates have been reported as 75 and 55 percent, respectively.[109, 110] Physicians at the Johns Hopkins Hospital have reported a 90-percent 8-year survival rate for 49 patients operated on for ascending aortic aneurysms associated with Marfan's syndrome.[107] These authors recommend elective repair of the aorta in patients with Marfan's syndrome and aortic root diameters equal to or larger than 6.0 cm.[107] Although there is some controversy over the precise degree of dilatation of the ascending aorta that should result in surgical repair, it is our feeling that aortic root dilatations of 5 to 6 cm should be repaired and those of 6 cm and larger must be repaired unless there is some compelling contraindication. It should be noted, however, that surgical repair of annuloaortic ectasia does not preclude later aortic dissection and sudden death.[109–111] In addition, repeat surgery for adjacent aneurysm formation or dissection has been necessary in at least one fourth of patients followed on a long-term basis.

Arteritis Involving the Aorta

See Table 72–6 for causes of arteritis involving the aorta.

Takayasu's Arteritis

The clinical features of Takayasu's arteritis are described in Table 72–7 and shown in Figure 72–21. Takayasu's arteritis was first noted by a Japanese ophthalmologist, M. Takayasu, who described a young woman with arteriovenous anastomoses surrounding the optic papillae and cataracts.[112] Subsequently, others called attention to two additional patients with similar ocular findings who also had absent radial pulses. This syndrome is also known as *pulseless disease* and *aortic arch syndrome*.[112–126]

ETIOLOGY

The majority of cases have been reported from Asia and Africa, and most large series consist of Asian women.[113] The anatomic alteration found is marked intimal proliferation with fibrosis, scarring, and degeneration of the elastic fibers of the media with mononuclear cell infiltration. Fibrosis predominates over inflammatory reaction. The intima and adventitia become thickened, and the vasa vasorum are injured. Proliferative changes lead to narrowing of the aorta and the origins of involved arteries. Localized aneurysm formation, poststenotic dilatation, and calcification in the aorta and involved arterial walls occur late in the process. Takayasu's arteritis primarily involves the arch of the aorta and its major branches. The changes that are most marked occur at the points of origin of the arteries from the aorta. The pulmonary artery may also be affected. In order of frequency, the most commonly involved arteries in patients studied in the United States are (1) a subclavian artery (90 percent), (2) a carotid artery (45 percent), (3) a vertebral artery (25 percent), and (4) a renal artery (20 percent).[114] However, the mesenteric arteries and abdominal aorta may also be involved.[116]

Ueno and associates[116] have divided Takayasu's arteritis into three types, depending on the arterial site of involvement (see Fig. 72–21). *Type I* arteritis involves the aortic arch and its branches; *type II* involves the thoracoabdominal aorta and its branches; and *type III* demonstrates involvement of both the aortic arch and the thoracoabdominal aorta and branches. A fourth category of arterial involvement has been suggested (*type IV*), in which pulmonary artery involvement occurs.[113]

The cause of Takayasu's arteritis is unknown. However, it is often preceded by an illness characterized by fever, malaise, weight loss, arthralgias, pleuritic pain, and fatigue. Giant cells may be found in some arterial specimens. The majority of the evidence suggests that it has an autoimmune cause. An association between Takayasu's arteritis and selected human leukocyte antigen types has been reported.[117, 118]

CLINICAL RECOGNITION

Takayasu's arteritis affects women more frequently than men, at a ratio of 8:1, with the disease expressing itself during teenage years. Often there is an initial systemic illness characterized by fever, anorexia, malaise, weight loss, night sweats, arthralgias, pleuritic pain, and fatigue. Localized pain and tenderness occur over affected arteries. Subsequently, signs and symptoms related to the narrowing of major blood vessels develop. Diminished or absent pulses, as well as bruits over the involved vessels, develop in the majority of patients. In some patients, systemic arterial hypertension develops, and occasionally heart failure occurs. Retinopathy described by Takayasu is found in only one fourth of patients, and it is usually associated with carotid arterial involvement. The ocular process may lead to blindness. Patients with types I and III Takayasu's arteritis demonstrate the most classic findings of the disease (i.e., absent or diminished upper body pulses and difficult-to-measure blood pressure in one or both arms). Patients with type II Takayasu's arteritis often develop hypertension because of the renal artery involvement, but it may be difficult to recognize because of the reduced pulses in the arms. Heart failure, when it occurs, generally does so in association with systemic arterial hypertension or aortic regurgitation. Ostial and proximal segments of coronary

TABLE 72–6 Arteritis Involving the Aorta

Arteritis Involving the Aorta
Takayasu's arteritis
Giant cell arteritis
Ankylosing spondylitis
Reiter's syndrome
Behçet's syndrome
Psoriatic arthritis
Relapsing polychondritis
Systemic lupus erythematosus

TABLE 72-7 **Proposed Criteria For The Clinical Diagnosis of Takayasu's Arteritis**

Criterion	Definition
Obligatory Criterion	
Age ≤ 40 yr	Age ≤ 40 yr at diagnosis or at onset of "characteristic signs and symptoms" of 1-mo duration in patient
Two Major Criteria	
1. Left midsubclavian artery lesion	The most severe stenosis or occlusion present in the midportion from the point 1 cm proximal to the left vertebral artery orifice to that 3 cm distal to the orifice determined by angiography
2. Right midsubclavian artery lesion	The most severe stenosis or occlusion present in the midportion from the right vertebral artery orifice to the point 3 cm distal to the orifice determined by angiography
Nine Minor Criteria	
1. High ESR	Unexplained persistent high ESR ≥ 20 mm/h (Westergren) at diagnosis or presence of the evidence in patient history
2. Carotid artery tenderness	Unilateral or bilateral tenderness of common carotid arteries by physician palpation: neck muscle tenderness is unacceptable
3. Hypertension	Persistent blood pressure ≥ 140/90 mm Hg brachial or ≥ 160/90 mm Hg popliteal at age ≤ 40 yr or presence of the history at age ≤ 40 yr
4. Aortic regurgitation	By auscultation or Doppler echocardiography or angiography
or	
Annuloaortic ectasia	By angiography or two-dimensional echocardiography
5. Pulmonary artery lesion	Lobar or segmental arterial occlusion or equivalent determined by angiography or perfusion scintigraphy; or presence of stenosis, aneurysm, luminal irregularity or any combination in pulmonary trunk or in unilateral or bilateral pulmonary arteries determined by angiography
6. Left mid common carotid lesion	Presence of the most severe stenosis or occlusion in the midportion of 5 cm in length from the point 2 cm distal to its orifice determined by angiography
7. Distal brachiocephalic trunk lesion	Presence of the most severe stenosis or occlusion in the distal third determined by angiography
8. Descending thoracic aorta lesion	Narrowing, dilatation or aneurysm, luminal irregularity, or any combination determined by angiography; tortuosity alone is unacceptable
9. Abdominal aorta lesion	Narrowing, dilatation or aneurysm, luminal irregularity, or any combination and absence of lesion in aortoiliac region consisting of 2 cm of terminal aorta and bilateral common iliac arteries determined by angiography; tortuosity alone is unacceptable

Abbreviation: ESR, erythrocyte sedimentation rate.

From Ishikawa K: Diagnostic approach and proposed criteria of the clinical diagnosis of Takayasu's arteriopathy. Am J Cardiol 12:964, 1988. With permission from Elsevier Science.

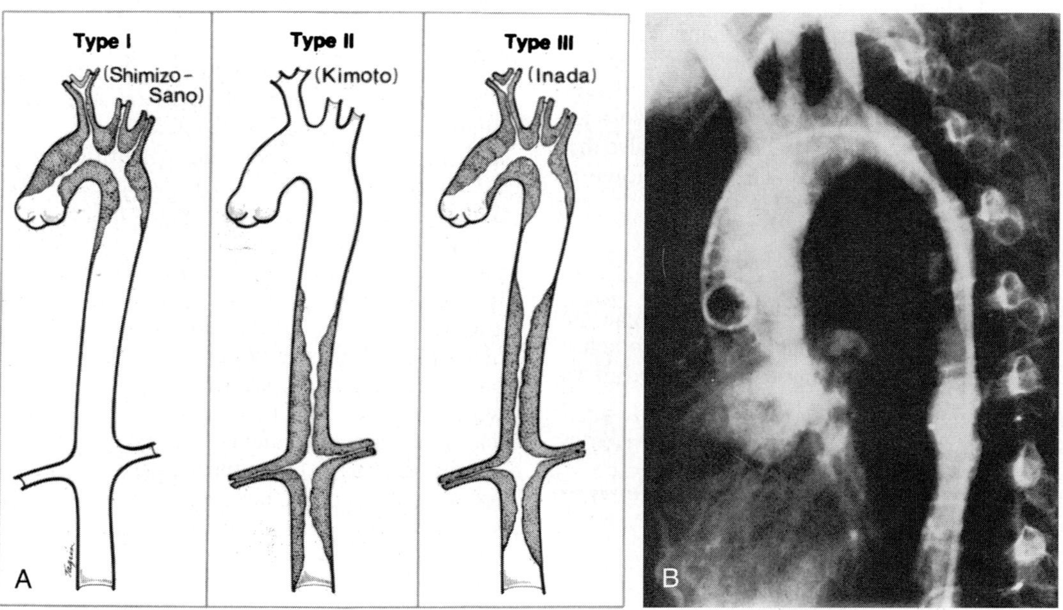

FIGURE 72–21 A, Various types of inflammatory involvement of the aorta in patients with Takayasu's arteritis. The figure also demonstrates the relative extent and involvement of branch vessels in types I, II, and III Takayasu's arteritis. **B,** Aortogram demonstrates narrowing of the descending thoracic aorta in a patient with Takayasu's arteritis. The rapid tapering of the descending aorta has been likened to a "rat's tail" appearance. (**A** and **B,** From Braunwald E [ed]: Heart Disease: A Textbook of Cardiovascular Medicine. 4th ed. Philadelphia: WB Saunders, 1992.)

arteries may be affected, leading to angina or myocardial infarction. Aneurysms of coronary arteries develop in some patients.[119–125]

Among laboratory abnormalities usually found in these individuals are an elevated sedimentation rate, mild anemia, increases in white blood cell counts, and elevations in the serum immunoglobulins IgG or IgM.

Chest radiographs often show enlargement of the heart in patients with hypertension, important coronary artery disease, or important aortic insufficiency. Arteriography demonstrates stenosis of the aorta or one of its major branches, saccular aneurysms, or complete occlusion of major branch arteries arising from the aorta (see Fig. 72–21). The thoracic aorta in these patients often demonstrates a "rat-tail" angiographic appearance (see Fig. 72–4).[125]

Most patients are relatively young at diagnosis. Table 72–7 lists the major criteria used to make a diagnosis of Takayasu's arteritis. For example, a young Asian woman less than 40 years of age with a preceding inflammatory illness who has reduced subclavian and radial artery pulses and blood pressure probably has Takayasu's arteritis.

TREATMENT

Adrenal steroids have been used to treat this entity; they reduce fever, malaise, fatigue, and the elevated sedimentation rate.[114, 115] Cyclophosphamide has also been used at a dosage of 2 mg/kg/day adjusted to maintain the white blood cell count above 3000/mm^2. More recently, immunoglobulin has been administered to patients with Takayasu's arteritis with apparent benefit, especially in more rapid resolution of the inflammatory process and in protection against the development of coronary artery aneurysms. Antiplatelet agents and anticoagulants, including Coumadin, aspirin, and dipyridamole, have been administered to treat ischemic symptoms, but their impact is uncertain. In the treatment of systemic arterial hypertension, ACE inhibitors may be effective. Occasional patients require a surgical procedure to reestablish blood flow, including bypass procedures for obstructed arteries, and excision and replacement of saccular aneurysms. Percutaneous transluminal angioplasty has also been used to relieve discrete stenotic lesions involving carotid, subclavian, renal, and mesenteric arteries.[115, 126]

NATURAL HISTORY

A slow progression of the occlusive disease over a period of months to years is the usual course. Morbidity and mortality rates depend on the presence or absence of critical narrowing of arteries in organs such as the heart, kidneys, and brain. Survival for 5 to 7 years has been reported as greater than 90 percent in patients without major complications but less than 60 percent in patients with complications such as those described earlier.[115, 126]

Giant Cell Arteritis

Giant cell arteritis involves medium-sized arteries[127–132]; the aorta and its major branches are involved in a minority of cases. Synonymous terms used to describe this entity are *granulomatous*, *cranial*, and *temporal arteritis*. Middle-aged and older patients complaining of diffuse muscle aching and stiffness and arthralgias have a connective tissue disease known as *polymyalgia rheumatica*.[128] Some of these patients have temporal arteritis and may be identified by having tender and swollen temporal arteries and a markedly elevated sedimentation rate, often greater than 70 mm/hr. These patients are at risk for loss of vision if not recognized and treated promptly with steroids.

PATHOPHYSIOLOGY

The characteristic histologic lesion distinguishing giant cell arteritis from the other arteritis syndromes is granulomatous inflammation of the medium-sized arteries, especially the arteries of the head and neck and, most particularly, the temporal arteries. An inflammatory infiltrate composed of plasma cells, eosinophils, and other mononuclear cells is usually found in the involved artery. On occasion, the inflammatory involvement of the artery may lead to obstruction. The aortic wall may be altered by the inflammatory process, leading to localized aneurysm formation, aortic annular dilatation, and aortic regurgitation.

CLINICAL RECOGNITION

Typically, giant cell arteritis involves women of 50 years of age and older and may be more common in black women.[130] Many of these patients also have polymyalgia rheumatica (i.e., diffuse muscle aching and arthralgias). The classic presentation consists of severe headaches, marked malaise, and fever in association with a markedly elevated sedimentation rate, often more than 60 mm/hr. The headaches are often intense and occur over the temporal artery and occipital regions. The temporal arteries are sensitive to pressure, and patients with this problem may complain of being unable to rest their head against a pillow, wear a hat, or comb their hair. Claudication in the jaw muscle while chewing occurs in a large number of patients and is suggestive of this diagnosis. Patients with temporal arteritis may develop sudden blindness from involvement of an ophthalmic artery, and it may be irreversible. Visual symptoms ranging from blurring of vision to diplopia and visual loss occur in some patients.

When the aorta and its major branches are involved, symptoms and signs are similar to those of Takayasu's arteritis. Symptoms include claudication of the upper extremities, paresthesias, Raynaud's phenomenon, myocardial ischemia, transient cerebral ischemic attacks, and, occasionally, ischemia of the lower extremities and abdominal angina. Rarely, aortic aneurysms, aortic regurgitation, and aortic dissection occur.[131] Renal artery involvement is rare in contrast with Takayasu's arteritis, where it is relatively common.

Fever is present in many patients with granulomatous arteritis. Involved arteries are thickened and tender. Pulses may be lost and bruits may occur over sites of arterial narrowing. A normocytic, normochromic anemia is often present.

DIAGNOSIS

The diagnosis of giant cell arteritis is made by biopsy of an involved artery, usually the temporal artery. Angiography may help to differentiate granulomatous arteritis from arteriosclerosis by demonstrating tapering stenoses alternating with segments of normal or even slightly increased arterial diameter; the absence of ulcerated atheromatous plaques; and the typical anatomic distribution of arteritis, including subclavian, axillary, and brachial arteries.[129]

TREATMENT

High-dose steroid therapy should be administered to patients with granulomatous arteritis, especially patients with temporal arteritis. The dosage of steroids is usually 60 to 80 mg/day prednisone, and one should attempt to give the steroids as single-dose therapy in the early morning. In patients with temporal arteritis, it is a relative emergency to begin steroid therapy to prevent blindness. The sedimentation rate may be used as a guide for the effectiveness of steroids and as an indication for when they may be reduced. In most patients after a period of high-dose steroid therapy, the steroids are reduced gradually to a maintenance dosage of 5 to 15 mg/day for 1 to 2 years. Most patients improve and eventually have complete resolution of their symptoms. In occasional patients, the disease does not respond adequately to steroids, and the administration of other immunosuppression therapy, such as Imuran or Cytoxan, may be necessary.

Aortic Trauma

Fatal automobile accidents are associated with rupture of the aorta in some individuals, especially with sudden deceleration.[94–98]

Etiology

The shear forces generated by sudden deceleration on impact may tear the aorta at sites where it is relatively mobile and joined to a fixed segment. Thus, sudden high-speed deceleration injuries resulting from motor vehicle accidents may tear the aorta. The aortic isthmus just distal to the origin of the left subclavian artery is the most frequent point of rupture of the aorta. The injury varies from a small tear to complete transection. A localized saccular aneurysm or pseudoaneurysm may develop at the site of the tear. Sudden deceleration trauma may injure the ascending aorta just above the aortic valve, the innominate artery, the aortic arch itself, the descending thoracic aorta, and the abdominal aorta.[96]

Clinical Findings

Tearing of the aorta without immediate exsanguination can lead to localized pressure from a hematoma and dyspnea or stridor from tracheal or bronchial compression, dysphagia from esophageal compression, or superior vena caval syndrome from compression of the superior vena cava. A localized hematoma or an aneurysm may cause hoarseness, cough, and dysphagia from compression of adjacent structures, including the recurrent laryngeal nerve, bronchus, and esophagus. The aorta itself may be obstructed, leading to the sudden development of upper extremity hypertension and reduced lower extremity pressures and pulses.

Clinical Recognition

One must have a high index of suspicion about the possibility of a tear in the aorta in any patient involved in sudden deceleration injury, especially in the patient with chest, cardiac, and abdominal injuries. The chest radiograph often provides the initial clue to the presence of an aortic tear by demonstrating one or more of the following[95]:

1. A mediastinum measuring more than 8 cm at the level of the aortic arch
2. A shift of the trachea toward the right
3. Blurring of the normally sharp outline of the aorta
4. Obliteration of the medial aspect of the apex of the upper lobe of the left lung
5. Opacification of the clear space between the aorta and the pulmonary artery
6. The depression of the left main stem bronchus below 40 degrees

Mediastinal widening of the aorta to a mean diameter of 9.4 cm or more is a sensitive marker of aortic injury.[96] Angiography, CT scanning with contrast injection, or MRI/MRA may provide the correct diagnosis.

Natural History

Most patients with aortic rupture die instantly from exsanguination. In those with a partial tear, death occurs within the first week from progressive hemorrhage. Alternatively, some patients develop a localized aneurysm or pseudoaneurysm over a period of months.

Treatment

Surgical repair is necessary for the treatment of aortic tears. Rupture of the aorta is usually treated by removing the torn segment and replacing it with a prosthetic graft. Prompt recognition and correction of a ruptured aorta have resulted in survival of most patients with this type of injury who reach the hospital alive.[97, 98] In patients with localized saccular aneurysms developing relatively late after the trauma, surgical correction is needed if the patient does not have other serious medical problems that prevent surgical repairs.

Knife or Missile Wounds

Perforation of the aorta from knife or missile wounds within the pericardial sac may cause pericardial tamponade. Perforation of the aorta elsewhere may cause massive hemorrhage and potential compression of surrounding structures or exsanguination. Penetration of both an adjacent artery and vein may lead to an arteriovenous fistula with the development of a continuous murmur over the site of the injury, wide pulse pressure, and increased cardiac output. Such injuries have followed surgical procedures, including cardiac catheterizations where an indwelling arterial cannula was placed.

Aortic Infections

Cardiovascular Syphilis

Linear calcification in the ascending aorta in patients younger than 40 years of age suggests that syphilitic aortitis may cause ascending aortic aneurysms, aortic regurgitation, and ostial narrowing of coronary arteries secondary to inflammation.[98a] In the patient with syphilitic aortitis and aneurysm or aortic insufficiency, there often is a history of syphilis, and other clinical manifestations of syphilis are found in up to one third of patients.[132] Some patients have negative routine serologic tests for syphilis, but a test such as the *Treponema pallidum* immobilization evaluation or the fluorescent treponemal antibody evaluation is almost always positive. In patients with large aortic aneurysms or important valvular aortic insufficiency in whom surgical correction is contemplated, it is important to obtain coronary arteriograms to evaluate the ostial portions of the major coronary arteries for evidence of the ostial inflammatory reaction that leads to severe narrowing of the major coronary arteries at their origins.

Patients with cardiovascular syphilis seen 1 year or more after the initial contact should receive penicillin (2.4 million U/wk IM benzathine penicillin G [Bicillin] for 3 weeks for a total of 7.2 million U). In patients allergic to penicillin, the recommended therapy is 200 mg doxycycline PO bid for 21 days. An alternate regimen is 500 mg erythromycin PO qid for 30 days. After therapy, repeated serologic measurements should be made, with the desired result being a fourfold reduction in titer within 1 to 2 years.

The indications for surgical repair of syphilitic aneurysms are similar to those for other thoracic aortic aneurysms. Specifically, when the aneurysm has reached a diameter of 6 cm or more or an aneurysm produces symptoms or is expanding rapidly, it must be surgically replaced. Where significant valvular aortic insufficiency is present, aortic valve replacement is indicated in association with the repair of an aortic aneurysm. Aortic valve replacement is also needed in the patient with symptoms related to moderately severe or severe valvular insufficiency with progressive decline in ventricular function at rest. In the patient with coronary disease resulting from inflammation at the coronary ostia, a localized endarterectomy may be feasible; if not, coronary artery bypass graft surgery is a good alternative.

Bacterial Infections

Bacterial infections may cause aneurysmal dilatation, including fusiform and saccular aneurysms. Rupture into the venous system may cause arteriovenous fistulas. Infection may also arise within preexisting aortic aneurysms.

Vascular infection may be caused by septic emboli from bacterial endocarditis or diffuse bacteremia; contiguous spread from adjacent sites of infection; and introduction from an external source with trauma, surgery, and so forth. *Salmonella* and *Staphylococcus aureus* are often the causes of bacterial infection of aortic aneurysms.[133, 134]

Patients with infected aortic aneurysms are usually febrile with shaking chills, and they have elevated white blood cell counts. They may have palpable and tender aneurysms. Blood cultures are usually positive. A tender and pulsatile mass in a febrile patient should be considered an infected aneurysm until proved otherwise. The femoral arteries and abdominal aorta account for most infected or mycotic aneurysms. Mycotic aneurysms expand progressively with a thinning of the aneurysm wall and eventual rupture. The treatment of such aneurysms is surgical excision in association with appropriate antibiotic, antituberculous, or antifungal therapy and replacement of the aneurysm with a prosthetic graft.

Aortic Thromboembolic Disease

Thrombotic material in the aorta may embolize and occlude branch vessels with subsequent manifestations of ischemia in the perfused organ. Thrombi from the left side of the heart, the left atrium, and the left ventricle may also embolize and obstruct branch vessels of the aorta. Arterial emboli that involve the aortic bifurcation into the iliac arteries are termed *saddle emboli*. Thrombus overlying an atherosclerotic plaque may embolize from within the aorta itself. Occasionally, paradoxical systemic embolism may originate in the venous circulation, especially the right atrium or right ventricle, and pass through a patent foramen ovale or atrial septal defect, leading to embolism into the aorta or its branches. Peripheral arterial embolism is most commonly associated with myocardial infarction from a mural thrombus or ventricular aneurysm. It also occurs from prosthetic heart valves on the left side of the heart, in patients with atrial fibrillation with enlarged left atria and dilated left ventricles, and in those with mitral valve disease or low output states. *Marantic endocarditis* occurs in an occasional chronically ill patient with neoplastic disease, and the sterile intracardiac thrombi may embolize to distal aortic or branch vessel sites. Left atrial myxomas and infectious lesions with vegetations on aortic or mitral valves may embolize into the aorta and its branch vessels. A classic presentation in cardiovascular medicine is the sudden occlusion of a femoral artery by embolic material in a relatively young person; in these individuals, the occlusion of an otherwise normal artery implies a large amount of embolic material, and this usually occurs in patients with a left atrial myxoma or fungal (*Candida*) endocarditis. Therefore, the embolic material removed from a femoral artery in such a patient must be examined microscopically and cultured to determine whether either myxoma or fungal endocarditis may be responsible. Women taking contraceptive pills and estrogens have an increased risk of thromboembolism, and so do patients with neoplastic diseases, especially those with carcinomas of the pancreas and kidney.

Clinical Presentation

Arterial embolization to a lower extremity, including saddle emboli, usually causes severe pain in one or both lower extremities. The pain usually progresses distally from the midthigh but can involve the buttocks. Numbness, paresthesias, and symmetric weakness of the legs may be present. Peripheral arterial emboli cause severe pain with cyanosis and a mottled, bluish appearance of the extremity.

These changes may progress to the blue-black color of gangrene. Pulses are absent or severely reduced below the abdominal aorta at the site or sites at which the embolization has occurred. If the ischemia persists for an extended period of time, there is a release of products from muscle breakdown into the blood stream, causing shock, hypotension, hyperkalemia, and myoglobinuria; systemic sepsis may also develop. Unless vascular perfusion is reestablished within a few hours, irreversible injury of the involved tissue occurs. With embolization into intracranial vessels or the carotid arteries, the clinical presentation is that of a cerebrovascular accident and neurologic deficits that represent the deficit lost through occlusion of a major cerebral blood vessel, including sudden hemiparesis, headaches, seizures, aphasia, loss of consciousness, or a combination. The differential diagnosis with the sudden occlusion of an artery includes in situ thrombosis, aortic dissection, and intense vasospasm. The correct diagnosis is generally made based on the clinical history and physical examination and confirmed with angiography. If the diagnosis of embolization is strongly suspected, prompt surgical intervention (or sometimes thrombolytic therapy or angioplasty) to restore blood flow is important to prevent irreversible damage to the perfused tissues.

Treatment

Many emboli may be removed with a Fogarty balloon-tipped catheter inserted through a transfemoral arterial approach under local anesthesia. If the embolus cannot be retrieved in this manner, removal through direct aortotomy becomes necessary. Anticoagulation with intravenous heparin should be begun on completion of the operation, and the heparin is administered in amounts to prolong the prothrombin time by 1.5 to 2 times normal values. Anticoagulation with intravenous heparin before the surgery is needed if the operation is to be delayed for any period of time. Long-term anticoagulation therapy with warfarin and sometimes antiplatelet therapy may be required. All removed embolic material should be examined histologically and cultured for routine organisms and fungi. Left atrial myxomas are sometimes recognized initially as a result of the histologic evaluation of the removed embolic specimen.

Thrombotic Occlusion of the Aorta

Thrombotic occlusion may occur because of a severe stenosis of a branch vessel of the aorta or of the distal aorta itself from atherosclerotic disease and, in rare patients, with antithrombin III deficiencies or other hypercoagulable states. Thrombolytic agents may be used to provide reperfusion, but in some patients surgical therapy is required.

Embolization of Atherosclerotic Material

Disruption of an atherosclerotic plaque in the aorta or a major branch vessel may occur after surgery or angiography in a patient with severe atherosclerosis of the aorta. Atherosclerotic embolism in the renal and the splanchnic arterial beds occurs after major abdominal vascular procedures, especially resection of abdominal aortic aneurysms. However, embolization of atherosclerotic plaque material may also occur as a complication of intra-arterial cannulation or angiography, cardiac catheterization, or cardiopulmonary bypass. Cholesterol embolization occurs from the aorta into any artery, especially the femoral and popliteal arteries. Embolization of cholesterol and atherosclerotic plaque debris often occurs repetitively and involves small arterial branches.

Cholesterol embolization after abdominal aortic surgery may cause pancreatitis or renal failure from diffuse microinfarction of the pancreas and kidneys. Gastrointestinal hemorrhage from microinfarction of abdominal viscera may also occur. In some patients, transient neurologic defects occur with embolization into the cerebral circulation. Cholesterol embolization of the lower extremities may cause purpuric and ecchymotic lesions in the lower legs, feet, and toes, and these may be paroxysmal and associated with skin necrosis and gangrene, especially in the toes. With this entity, arterial pulses of the lower extremities may be well preserved.

Aortic Tumors

Very rarely, primary aortic tumors develop, including fibrosarcomas, angiosarcomas, leiomyosarcomas, endotheliomas, fibromyxosarcomas, and malignant fibrous histiocytomas.[135, 136] Aortic tumors are more common in males than in females. The initial presentation often consists of abdominal or leg pain, proximal hypertension due to an acquired narrowing of the aorta by tumor with decreased femoral pulses, fever, or claudication.[137, 138] The correct diagnosis has been made in the past through the use of angiographic techniques, but presently, CT scanning with contrast medium, MRI/MRA, or, in selected circumstances, transesophageal echocardiography or intravascular ultrasound should be useful. Surgical exploration and biopsy are required to prove the presence of an aortic tumor. With a localized aortic tumor interfering with blood flow, local resection with graft replacement of that segment of the aorta is indicated.

Inflammatory Aortic Aneurysms

Inflammatory aortic aneurysms are also called porcelaneous aneurysms because of the shiny, pearly-white inflammatory process that surrounds the anterior, medial, and lateral walls of the aorta. The thickened inflammatory tissue does not usually involve the posterior wall. The back wall is thin and is often the point of rupture or vertebral erosion. Tissue planes are often obliterated, and inflammation involves the surrounding viscera and mesentery. The duodenum, small bowel, inferior vena cava, ureters, renal and iliac veins, and ascending and sigmoid colon are commonly fixed to the inflammatory process surrounding the aorta.

History

The first report of an inflammatory process involving the abdominal aorta was by James and colleagues in 1935.[141]

He described a patient dying of uremia secondary to obstruction of both ureters by an inflammatory process around a large abdominal aortic aneurysm. The first surgery was done by DeWeerd and associates in 1955 on a 45-year-old man with severe hydronephrosis, bilateral ureteral obstruction, and a large abdominal aortic aneurysm. He performed bilateral ureterolysis and placed bilateral nephrostomy tubes but did not resect the aneurysm. The patient survived the operation, and renal function returned to normal during a 15-month follow-up. Shumacker and Garrett did the first successful operative resection that same year, in which they replaced an aneurysm with a bifurcated graft made of fused nylon and polyethylene. They also performed bilateral ureterolysis. Walker and coworkers[142] in 1972 reported their experience in the treatment of 19 such patients, and they were the first to coin the term "inflammatory aneurysm." Since then, many groups have reported their experience in the treatment of such aneurysms.

Incidence

Inflammatory aneurysms constitute about 5 to 15 percent of total aortic aneurysms.[143] They are most common in males, females having only approximately 5 percent. They are mostly symptomatic (65 percent) as compared with atherosclerotic aneurysms (20 percent). The common age at presentation is in the seventh decade (62 to 68 years). Most of these patients have an elevated erythrocyte sedimentation rate (74 percent), suggestive of an inflammatory process, as compared with patients with atherosclerotic aneurysms who have an elevated erythrocyte sedimentation rate in only 33 percent of cases. The patients with inflammatory aneurysms typically have a smoking history and weight loss. The operative mortality for these aneurysms is 3 to 10 percent (7.9 percent) as compared with atherosclerotic aneurysms, which have operative mortality rates of 1 to 3 percent (2.4 percent).

Pathology

There is replacement of both tunica media and adventitia (Fig. 72–22)[144] with thick fibrous tissue and collagen deposition leading to medial destruction. There is also loss of smooth muscle cells and elastic fibers in the media. Endarteritis and phlebitis of adventitial vessels and the vessels within the perianeurysmal tissue are present. The inflammatory cells consist of lymphocytes, plasma cells, and multinucleated giant cells.

Pathogenesis

An inflammatory aneurysm is considered to be an exaggerated inflammatory response of an atherosclerotic aortic aneurysm; hence, all etiologic factors involved in the development of atherosclerotic aneurysms play a role in its pathogenesis.[145] In addition, there is a view that chronic blood leakage from atherosclerotic aneurysms produces an inflammatory process that spreads to involve the retroperitoneum and the peritoneal viscera. However, hemosiderin deposits have not been described, and immunologic techniques have failed to detect fibrinogen in the perianeurysmal tissue. Another theory is that sudden expansion of an atherosclerotic aneurysm or ischemia due to atheroemboli in vasa vasorum of the aorta leads to lymphatic obstruction, with leakage of lymph within the surrounding space, which causes an inflammatory reaction.[146] It has also been suggested that these aneurysms develop because of an autoimmune process similar to, but pathologically different from, retroperitoneal fibrosis.

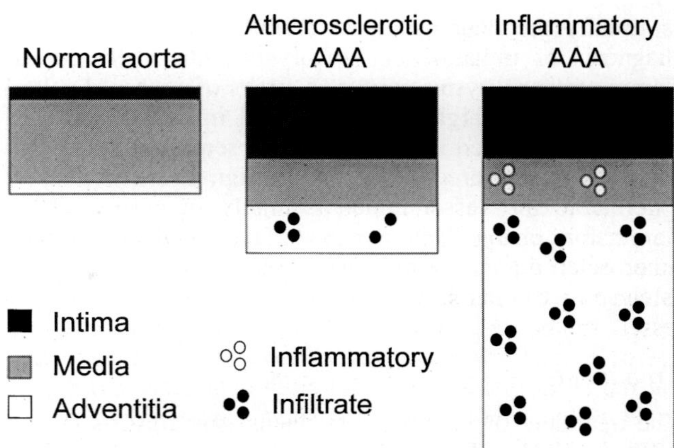

FIGURE 72–22 Histologic section of aortic wall depicting the three layers of aorta and showing the difference in diameter in layers between the normal, atherosclerotic, and inflammatory aorta. (From Pennell RC, Hollier LH, Lie JT, et al: Inflammatory abdominal aortic aneurysms: a thirty-year review. J Vasc Surg 2:859, 1985.)

Presentation

Most patients present with symptoms of either back or flank pain and, hence, are diagnosed as having either rupture or leakage of an atherosclerotic aortic aneurysm. These aneurysms are more easily palpable at the time of diagnosis. Thus, a classic patient with inflammatory aneurysm is a male in his early 60s, with a large abdominal aneurysm, pain on palpation, weight loss, and an elevated erythrocyte sedimentation rate.

Diagnosis

Preoperative diagnosis is possible in only 13 to 33 percent of cases. The diagnostic tests include ultrasound, CT scan, angiogram, excretory urogram, and MRI. Ultrasound shows an echogenic and thickened wall with a hypoechoic anterior and anterolateral rim around the aorta. CT scans show thickening and contrast enhancement of the aorta in the periadventitial region. Preoperative diagnostic accuracy of the CT scan is 50 to 70 percent. Angiograms fail to show any evidence of inflammatory aneurysm as only the lumen is enhanced, and the periaortic tissue is not included. In retrospective review, the diagnostic accuracy of angiograms is low. Excretory urograms are usually done in patients with abnormal renal function tests. In cases of inflammatory aneurysms, excretory urograms show medial deviation of the ureters due to their involvement in the inflammatory reaction, whereas in atherosclerotic aneurysms, one usually finds lateral displacement by the enlarged aneurysm. The diagnostic accuracy of urograms is 50 to 60 percent. MRI is usually the diagnostic test of choice for preoperative diagnosis of inflammatory aneurysms. On MRI, the inflammatory aneurysms appear as arrays of concentric alternating layers of high- and low-signal intensity, best seen on the T1-weighted images and STIR sequences. On MRI, the presence of three or more high–signal intensity layers external to the vessel lumen is highly suggestive of inflammatory change, whereas fewer layers indicate a simple atherosclerotic aneurysm. The diagnostic accuracy of MRI is close to 100 percent.

Treatment

The treatment of inflammatory aneurysms consists of steroids, surgical replacement, and endovascular grafting. Preoperative steroids may help reduce the inflammatory reaction.[147] However, steroids may mask the symptoms of rupture/leak and may contribute to sepsis; their discontinuation leads to recurrence of symptoms. Surgical replacement of the diseased aorta with a woven Dacron graft is the treatment of choice for inflammatory aneurysms. It not only treats the aneurysm, but the presence of synthetic material also decreases the extent of periaortic inflammatory process and separates the viscera involved in the reaction. The experience with endovascular grafting of inflammatory aneurysms is slowly increasing. The 5-year survival of patients after surgical replacement is approximately 80 percent.

REFERENCES

1. Aortic diseases. *In* Fowler NO (ed): Diagnosis of Heart Disease. p. 375. New York: Springer-Verlag, 1991.
2. Eagle KA, De Sanctis RW: Diseases of the aorta. *In* Braunwald E (ed): Heart Disease: A Textbook of Cardiovascular Medicine. pp. 1528–1557. Philadelphia: WB Saunders, 1992.
3. Powell JT, Greenhalgh RM: Cellular, enzymatic, and genetic factors in the pathogenesis of abdominal aortic aneurysms. J Vasc Surg 9:297, 1989.
4. Milewicz DM, Pyeritz RE, Crawford ES, Byers PH: Marfan syndrome: defective synthesis, secretion and extracellular matrix formation of fibrillin, a glycoprotein associated with elastic fibers. J Clin Invest 89:79, 1992.
5. Abbot ME: Coarctation of the aorta of adult type: statistical study and historical retrospect of 200 recorded cases with autopsy of stenoses or obliteration of descending arch in subjects above age of two years. Am Heart J 3:574, 1928.
6. Bahn RC, Edwards JE, DuShane JW: Coarctation of the aorta as a cause of death in early infancy. Pediatrics 8:192, 1951.
7. Cooley DA, McNamara DG, Latson JR: Aorticopulmonary septal defect: diagnosis and surgical treatment. Surgery 42:101, 1952.
8. Collett RW, Edwards JE: Persistent truncus arteriosus: classification according to anatomic types. Surg Clin North Am 29:1245, 1949.
9. Edwards JE, Carey LS, Newfeld HN, Lester RG: Congenital Heart Disease. Philadelphia: WB Saunders, 1965.
10. Perloff JM: The Clinical Recognition of Congenital Heart Disease. Philadelphia: WB Saunders, 1970.
11. Edwards JE: The congenital bicuspid aortic valve. Circulation 23:485, 1961.
12. Najafi H, Dye WS, Julian OC: Successful one-stage correction of both supravalvular aortic stenosis and typical coarctation of aorta in one patient. J Thorac Cardiovasc Surg 48:644, 1964.
13. Fontana RS, Edwards JE: Congenital Cardiac Disease. Philadelphia: WB Saunders, 1962.
14. Frederiksen T, Jagt T: Disease and congenital malformation at the aortic orifice complicating coarctation of the aorta. Acta Chir Scand 130:479, 1965.
15. Steinberg I, Stein JL, Goldberg HP: Aneurysms complicating the post-operative course of coarctation of the aorta: report of 3 cases. AJR 93:331, 1965.
16. Hallidie-Smith KA, Olsen EGJ: Endocardial fibroelastosis, mitral incompetence and coarctation of the abdominal aorta. Br Heart J 30:850, 1968.
17. Hodes HL, Steinfeld L, Blumenthal S: Congenital cerebral aneurysms and coarctation of the aorta. AMA Arch Pediatr 76:28, 1959.
18. Newcombe CR, Ongley PA, Edwards JE, Wood EH: Clinical, pathologic, and hemodynamic considerations in coarctation of the aorta associated with ventricular septal defects. Circulation 24:1356, 1961.
19. Campbell M, Baylis JH: Course and prognosis of coarctation of the aorta. Br Heart J 18:475, 1956.
20. Jarcho S: Coarctation of the aorta. Am J Cardiol 9:591, 1962.
21. Silander T: Anomalous origin of the right subclavian artery and its relation to coarctation of the aorta. Acta Chir Scand 124:412, 1962.
22. Reifenstein GH, Levine SA, Gross RE: Coarctation of the aorta: a review of 104 autopsied cases of the "adult-type," two years of age or older. Am Heart J 33:146, 1947.
23. Robiscek F, Taylor FH, Sanger PW: Spontaneous perforation of the aorta distal to the coarctation. Angiology 12:68, 1961.
24. Goodwin JF: Pregnancy and coarctation of the aorta. Clin Obstet Gynaecol 4:645, 1961.
25. Wood PH: Diseases of the Heart and Circulation. Philadelphia: JB Lippincott, 1956.
26. Burford TH, Ferguson TB, Goldring D, Behrer MR: Coarctation of the aorta in infants: a clinical and experimental study. J Thorac Cardiovasc Surg 39:47, 1960.
27. Albright F, Smith PH, Frase R: A syndrome characterized by primary ovarian insufficiency and decreased stature: report of 11 cases with a digression on hormonal control of axillary and pubic hair. Am J Med Sci 204:625, 1942.
28. Goldberg MB, Scully AL, Solomon IL, Steinbach HL: Gonadal dysgenesis in phenotypic female subjects. Am J Med 45:529, 1968.
29. Boone ML, Swenson BE, Felson G: Rib notching: its many causes. AJR 91:1075, 1964.
30. Lavin N, Mehta S, Liberson M, Pouget JM: Pseudocoarctation of the aorta. Am J Cardiol 24:584, 1969.
31. Steinberg I: Anomalies (pseudocoarctation) of the arch of the aorta—report of 8 new and review of 8 previously published cases. AJR 88:73, 1962.
32. Brinsfield DE, Shuford WM, Plauth WH Jr, Sybers RG: Congenital anomalies of the aorta. *In* Lindsay J Jr, Hurst JW (eds): The Aorta. p. 271. New York: Grune & Stratton, 1979.
33. Lajos TZ, Meckstroth CV, Klassen KP, Sherman NJ: Pseudocoarctation of the aorta: a variant or an entity? Chest 58:571, 1970.
34. Wolf WJ: Pseudocoarctation of the aortic arch in a patient with Turner's syndrome. Clin Cardiol 9:A5, 1986.
35. Collins JJ, Koster JK, Cohn LH, Van Devanter SH: Common aortic aneurysms: when to intervene. J Cardiovasc Med 8:245, 1983.
36. Joyce JW, Fairbairn JF, Kincaid OW, Jeurgens JL: Aneurysms of the thoracic aorta: clinical study with special reference to prognosis. Circulation 29:176, 1964.
37. Cooley DA, DeBakey ME: Surgical considerations of intrathoracic aneurysms of the aorta and great vessels. Ann Surg 135:660, 1952.
38. Cooley DA, DeBakey ME: Hypothermia in the surgical treatment of aortic aneurysms. Bull Soc Int Chir 15:206, 1956.
39. Cooley DA: Surgical Treatment of Aortic Aneurysms. Philadelphia: WB Saunders, 1986.
40. Livesay JJ, Cooley DA, Duncan JM, et al: Open aortic anastomosis: improved results in the treatment of aneurysms of the aortic arch. Circulation 66(suppl I):I-122, 1982.
41. Bentall H, DeBono A: A technique for complete replacement of the ascending aorta. Thorax 23:338, 1968.
42. Groves LK, Effler DB, Hawk WA, Gulati K: Aortic insufficiency secondary to aneurysmal changes in the ascending aorta: surgical management. J Thorac Cardiovasc Surg 48:362, 1964.
43. Wheat MW Jr, Wilson JR, Bartley TD: Successful replacement of the entire ascending aorta and aortic valve. JAMA 188:717, 1964.
44. Cabrol C, Pavie A, Mesnildrey P et al: Long-term results with total replacement of the ascending aorta and reimplantation of the coronary arteries. J Thorac Cardiovasc Surg 91:17, 1986.
45. Lewis CTP, Cooley DA, Murphy MP, et al: Surgical repair of aortic root aneurysms in 280 patients. Ann Thorac Surg 53:38, 1992.
46. Dommisse GF: The blood supply of the spinal cord. J Bone Joint Surg 56:225, 1974.

47. Berendes JN, Bredee JJ, Schipperheyn JJ, Mashour YAS: Mechanisms of spinal cord injury after cross-clamping of the descending thoracic aorta. Circulation 66(suppl I):I-112, 1982.
48. Cooley DA, Baldwin RT: Technique of open distal anastomosis for repair of descending thoracic aortic aneurysms. Ann Thorac Surg 54:932, 1992.
49. Blaisdell FW, Cooley DA: The mechanism of paraplegia after temporary thoracic aortic occlusion and its relationship to spinal fluid pressure. Surgery 51:351, 1962.
50. Colon R, Frazier OH, Cooley DA, McAllister HA: Hypothermic regional perfusion for protection of the spinal cord during periods of ischemia. Ann Thorac Surg 43:639, 1987.
51. Gliedman ML, Ayers WB, Vestal BL: Aneurysms of the abdominal aorta and its branches: a study of untreated patients. Ann Surg 217:1537, 1982.
52. Delin A, Ohlsen H, Swedenborg J: Growth rate of abdominal aortic aneurysms as measured by computed tomography. Br J Surg 72:530, 1985.
53. Bernstein EF, Chan EL: Abdominal aortic aneurysm in high risk patients. Ann Surg 200:255, 1985.
54. Nevitt MP, Ballard DJ, Hallett JW Jr: Prognosis of abdominal aortic aneurysms: a population-based study. N Engl J Med 321:1009, 1989.
55. Pasch AR, Ricotta JJ, May AG, et al: Abdominal aortic aneurysm: the case for elective resection. Circulation 70(suppl I):I-1, 1984.
56. Cooley DA, Carmichael MJ: Abdominal aortic aneurysm. Circulation 70(suppl I):I-5, 1984.
57. Darling RC: Ruptured arteriosclerotic abdominal aortic aneurysms. Am J Surg 119:397, 1970.
58. Rantakokko V, Havia T, Inberg MV, Vanttinen E: Abdominal aortic aneurysms: a clinical and autopsy study of 408 patients. Acta Chir Scand 149:151, 1983.
59. Astarita D, Filippone DR, Cohn JD: Spontaneous major intra-abdominal arteriovenous fistulas: a report of several cases. Angiology 36:656, 1985.
60. Valk PE, Hale JD, Kaufman L, et al: MR imaging of the aorta with three dimensional vessel reconstruction: validation by angiography. Radiology 157:721, 1985.
61. Glazer JS, Gutierrez FR, Levitt RE, et al: The thoracic aorta studied by MR imaging. Radiology 157:149, 1985.
62. Goldman AP, Kotler MN, Scanlon MH, et al: The complementary role of magnetic resonance imaging, Doppler echocardiography, and computer tomography in the diagnosis of dissecting thoracic aneurysms. Am Heart J 111:970, 1986.
63. Dinsmore RE, Liberthson RR, Wismer GL, et al: Magnetic resonance imaging of thoracic aortic aneurysms: comparison with other diagnostic techniques. AJR 146:309, 1986.
64. Taams MA, Gussenhoven WJ, Schippers LA, et al: The value of transesophageal echocardiography for diagnosis of thoracic aortic pathology. Eur Heart J 9:1308, 1988.
65. Gomes MN, Choyke PL: Preoperative evaluation of abdominal aortic aneurysms: ultrasound or computed tomography? J Card Surg 2:159, 1987.
66. Crew JR, Bashour TT, Ellerston D, et al: Ruptured abdominal aortic aneurysms: experience with 70 cases. Clin Cardiol 8:433, 1985.
67. Darling RC, Messina CR, Brewster DC, Ottinger LW: Autopsy study of unoperated abdominal aortic aneurysms: the case for early resection. Circulation 56(suppl II):II-161, 1977.
68. Brewster DC, Retana A, Waltman AC, Darling RC: Angiography in the management of aneurysms of the abdominal aorta: its value and safety. N Engl J Med 292:822, 1975.
69. Roberts WC: Aortic dissection: anatomy, consequences, and causes. Am Heart J 101:195, 1981.
70. Daily PO, Trueblood HW, Stinson EB, et al: Management of acute aortic dissection. Ann Thorac Surg 10:237, 1970.
71. Bulkley BH, Roberts WC: Dissecting aneurysm (hematoma) limited to coronary artery. Am J Med 55:747, 1973.
72. Cooke JP, Safford RE: Progress in the diagnosis and management of aortic dissection. Mayo Clin Proc 61:147, 1986.
73. Wheat MW Jr: Pathogenesis of aortic dissection. *In* Doroghazi RM, Slater EE (eds): Aortic Dissection. p. 55. New York: McGraw-Hill, 1983.
74. Dalen JR, Pape LA, Cohn LH, et al: Dissection of the aorta: pathogenesis, diagnosis, and treatment. Prog Cardiovasc Dis 23:237, 1980.
75. Amparo EG, Higgins CB, Hricak L, Solitto R: Aortic dissection: magnetic resonance imaging. Radiology 155:399, 1985.
76. Glower DD, Fann JI, Speier RH, et al: Comparison of medical and surgical therapy for uncomplicated descending aortic dissection. Circulation 80(suppl II):II-24, 1989.
77. Crawford ES, Svensson LG, Coselli JS, et al: Aortic dissection and dissecting aortic aneurysms. Ann Surg 208:254, 1988.
78. Cachera JP, Vouhe PR, Loisance DY, et al: Surgical management of acute dissections involving the ascending aorta. J Thorac Cardiovasc Surg 82:576, 1981.
79. Wheat MW Jr: Acute dissecting aneurysm of the aorta: diagnosis and treatment. Am Heart J 99:373, 1990.
80. Doroghazi RM, Slater EE: Aortic Dissection. New York: McGraw-Hill, 1983.
81. Slater EE, DeSanctis RW: The clinical recognition of dissecting aortic aneurysm. Am J Med 60:625, 1976.
82. Larson EW, Edwards WO: Risk factors of aortic dissection: a necropsy study of 161 cases. Am J Cardiol 53:849, 1984.
83. Pumprey CW, Fay T, Weir I: Aortic dissection during pregnancy. Br Heart J 1993.
84. DeBakey ME, McCollum CH, Crawford ES, et al: Dissection and dissecting aneurysms of the aorta: 20-year follow-up of 527 patients treated surgically. Surgery 92:1118, 1982.
85. DeBakey ME, Cooley DA, Creech O Jr: Surgical considerations of dissecting aneurysms of the aorta. Ann Surg 142:586, 1955.
86. Dinsmore RE, Willerson JT, Buckley MJ: Dissecting aneurysm of the aorta: aortographic features affecting prognosis. Diagn Radiol 105:567, 1972.
87. Wheat MW Jr, Palmer RF, Barley TD, Seelman RC: Treatment of dissecting aneurysms of the aorta without surgery. J Thorac Cardiovasc Surg 50:364, 1965.
87a. McFarland J, Willerson JT, Dinsmore RE, et al: The medical treatment of dissecting aortic aneurysms. N Engl J Med 286:115, 1972.
88. Anagnostopoulos CE, Prabhakar MJS, Kittle CF: Aortic dissections and dissecting aneurysms. Am J Cardiol 30:263, 1972.
89. Shuford WH, Sybers RG, Weens HS: Problems of the aortographic diagnosis of dissecting aneurysms of the aorta. N Engl J Med 280:225, 1969.
89a. Nienaber CA, von Kodolitsch Y, Petersen B, et al: Intramural hemorrhage of the thoracic aorta. Diagnostic and therapeutic implications. Circulation 92:1465, 1995.
90. Hochberg FH, Bean C, Fisher CM, Roberson GH: Stroke in a 15-year-old girl second to terminal carotid dissection. Neurology 25:725, 1980.
91. Demaio SJ Jr, Kinsella SH, Silverman ME: Clinical course and long-term prognosis of spontaneous coronary artery dissection. Am J Cardiol 64:471, 1989.
92. Greendyke RM: Traumatic rupture of aorta: special reference to automobile accidents. JAMA 195:527, 1966.
93. Parmley LF, Mattingly TW, Manion WC, Jahnke EJ: Nonpenetrating traumatic injury of the aorta. Circulation 17:1086, 1958.
94. Faro RS, Monson DO, Weinberg M, Javid H: Disruption of aortic arch branches due to nonpenetrating chest trauma. Arch Surg 118:1333, 1983.
95. March DG, Sturm JT: Traumatic aortic rupture: roentgenographic indications for angiography. Ann Thorac Surg 21:337, 1976.
96. Sturm JT, Olson FR, Cicero JJ: Chest roentgenographic findings in 26 patients with traumatic rupture of the thoracic aorta. Ann Emerg Med 12:598, 1983.
97. Atkins CW, Buckley MJ, Daggett W, et al: Acute traumatic disruption of the thoracic aorta: a ten-year experience. Ann Thorac Surg 31:305, 1981.
98. Stiles QR, Cohlmia GS, Smith JH, et al: Management of injuries of the thoracic and abdominal aorta. Am J Surg 150:132, 1985.
98a. Heggtveit HA: Syphilitic aortitis: a clinicopathologic autopsy study of 100 cases, 1950 to 1960. Circulation 29:346, 1964.
99. Riley DJ, Liv RT, Saxanoff S: Aortic dissection: a rare cause of the superior vena cava syndrome. J Med Soc NJ 78:187, 1981.
100. McCarthy C, Dickson GH, Besterman EMM, et al: Aortic dissection with rupture through ductus arteriosus into pulmonary artery. Br Heart J 34:284, 1972.
101. Thiene G, Rossi L, Beker AE: The atrioventricular conduction system in dissecting aneurysm of the aorta. Am Heart J 98:447, 1979.
102. Thorsen MD, San Dretto MA, Lawson TL, et al: Dissecting aortic aneurysms: accuracy of complete tomographic diagnosis. Radiology 148:773, 1983.

103. Perez JE: Noninvasive diagnosis: computed tomography and ultrasound. *In* Doroghazi RM, Slater EE (eds): Aortic Dissection. p. 133. New York: McGraw-Hill, 1983.
104. Savile N, Mathier D, Keitern K, et al: Computed tomography of thoracic aortic dissection: accuracy and pitfalls. J Comput Assist Tomogr 10:211, 1986.
105. Ellis PR, Cooley DA, DeBakey ME: Clinical consideration and surgical treatment of annulo-aortic ectasia. J Thorac Cardiovasc Surg 42:363, 1961.
106. Lemon DK, White CW: Annuloaortic ectasia: angiographic, hemodynamic and clinical comparison with aortic valve insufficiency. Am J Cardiol 41:482, 1978.
107. Gott VL, Pyeritz RE, Magovern GJ Jr, et al: Surgical treatment of aneurysms of the ascending aorta in the Marfan syndrome: results of composite-graft repair in 50 patients. N Engl J Med 314:1070, 1986.
108. Emanuel R, Ng RAL, Marcomichelakis J, et al: Formes frustes of Marfan's syndrome presenting with severe aortic regurgitation: clinicogenetic study of 18 families. Br Heart J 39:190, 1977.
109. Miller DC, Stinson EB, Oyer PE, et al: Concomitant resection of ascending aortic aneurysm and replacement of the aortic valve. J Thorac Cardiovasc Surg 79:388, 1980.
110. Svensson LG, Crawford S, Coselli JS, et al: Impact of cardiovascular operation on survival in the Marfan patient. Circulation 80(suppl I):I-233, 1989.
111. Crawford ES: Marfan's syndrome: broad spectral surgical treatment of cardiovascular manifestations. Ann Surg 198:487, 1983.
112. Takayasu M: Case with unusual changes of the central vessels in the retina. Acta Soc Ophthalmol Jpn 12:554, 1908.
113. Lupi-Herrera E, Sanchez-Torres G, Marcushamer J, et al: Takayasu's arteritis: clinical study of 107 cases. Am Heart J 93:94, 1977.
114. Shelhamer JH, Volkman DJ, Parillo JE, et al: Takayasu's arteritis and its therapy. Ann Intern Med 103:121, 1985.
115. Hall S, Barr W, Lie JT, et al: Takayasu arteritis. Medicine 64:89, 1985.
116. Ueno A, Awane G, Wakahayachi A: Successfully operated obliterative brachiocephalic arteritis (Takayasu) associated with the elongated coarctation. Jpn Heart J 8:538, 1967.
117. Volkman DJ, Mann DL, Fauci AS: Association between Takayasu's arteritis and a B-cell alloantigen in North Americans. N Engl J Med 306:464, 1982.
118. Numano F, Isohisa I, Egami M, et al: HLA-CR MT and MB antigens in Takayasu disease. Tissue Antigens 21:208, 1983.
119. Gronemeyer PS, deMello DE: Takayasu's disease with aneurysm of right common iliac artery and iliocaval fistula in a young infant: case report and review of the literature. Pediatrics 69:626, 1982.
120. Morooka S, Saito Y, Nonaka Y, et al: Clinical features of aortitis syndrome in Japanese women older than 40 years. Am J Cardiol 53:859, 1984.
121. Wu Y-JJ, Martin B, Ong K, et al: Takayasu's arteritis as a cause of fever of unknown origin. Am J Med 87:476, 1989.
122. Talwar KK, Chopra P, Narula J, et al: Myocardial involvement and its response to immuno-suppressive therapy in nonspecific aortoarteritis (Takayasu's disease): a study by endomyocardial biopsy. Int J Cardiol 23:323, 1988.
123. Cipriano PR, Silverman JF, Perlroth MG, et al: Coronary arterial narrowing in Takayasu's aortitis. Am J Cardiol 39:744, 1977.
124. Hashimoto Y, Numano F, Maruyama Y, et al: Thallium-201 stress scintigraphy in Takayasu arteritis. Am J Cardiol 67:879, 1991.
125. Lande A, Rossi P: The value of total aortography in the diagnosis of Takayasu's arteritis. Radiology 114:287, 1975.
126. Kakao K, Ikeda M, Kimata S, et al: Takayasu's arteritis: clinical report of 84 cases and immunological studies of 7 cases. Circulation 35:1141, 1967.
127. Klein RG, Hunder GG, Stanson AW, Sheps SG: Larger artery involvement in giant cell (temporal) arteritis. Ann Intern Med 83:806, 1975.
128. Alestig K, Uppsala MD, Barr J: Giant-cell arteritis, a biopsy study of polymyalgia rheumatica, including one case of Takayasu's disease. Lancet 1:1228, 1963.
129. Ghose MK, Shensa S, Lerner PI: Arteritis of the aged (giant cell arteritis) and fever of unexplained origin. Am J Med 60:429, 1976.
130. Gonzalez EB, Varner WT, Lisse JR, et al: Giant-cell arteritis in the southern United States: an 11-year retrospective study from the Texas Gulf Coast. Arch Intern Med 149:1561, 1989.
131. Salisbury RS, Hazleman BL: Successful treatment of dissecting aortic aneurysm due to giant cell arteritis. Ann Rheum Dis 40:507, 1981.
132. Healy LA, Wilske KR: Manifestations of giant cell arteritis. Med Clin North Am 61:261, 1977.
133. Brown SL, Busuttil RW, Baker JD, et al: Bacteriologic and surgical determinants of survival in patients with mycotic aneurysms. J Vasc Surg 1:541, 1984.
134. Jarrett F, Darling RC, Mundth ED, Austen WG: Experience with infected aneurysms of the abdominal aorta. Arch Surg 110:1281, 1975.
135. Schipper J, van Oostayen JA, den Hollander JC, van Seyen AJ: Aortic tumours: report of a case and review of the literature. Br J Radiol 62:35, 1989.
136. Schmid E, Port JS, Carroll RM, Friedman NB: Primary metastasizing aortic endothelioma. Cancer 54:1407, 1984.
137. Nienaber CA, von Kodolitsch Y, Nicolas V, et al: The diagnosis of thoracic aortic dissection by noninvasive imaging procedures. N Engl J Med 328:1, 1993.
138. Braunwald E (ed): Heart Disease: A Textbook of Cardiovascular Medicine. 4th ed. Philadelphia: WB Saunders, 1992.
139. Grossman W: Cardiac Catheterization and Angiography. 3rd ed. p. 232. Philadelphia: Lea & Febiger, 1985.
140. Ishikawa K: Diagnostic approach and proposed criteria of the clinical diagnosis of Takayasu's arteriopathy. Am J Cardiol 12:964, 1988.
141. Crawford JL, Stowe CL, Safi HJ, et al: Inflammatory aneurysms of the aorta. J Vasc Surg 2:113, 1985.
142. Walker DI, Bloor K, Williams G, et al: Inflammatory aneurysms of the abdominal aorta. Br J Surg 59:609, 1972.
143. Ernst CB, Stanley JC (eds): Current Therapy in Vascular Surgery. 3rd ed. St. Louis: Mosby, 1995.
144. Pennell RC, Hollier LH, Lie JT, et al: Inflammatory abdominal aortic aneurysms: a thirty-year review. J Vasc Surg 2:859, 1985.
145. Sterpetti AV, Hunter WJ, Feldhaus RJ, et al: Inflammatory aneurysms of the abdominal aorta: incidence, pathologic, and etiologic considerations. J Vasc Surg 9:643, 1989.
146. Rasmussen TE, Hallett JW: Inflammatory aortic aneurysms: a clinical review with new perspectives in pathogenesis. Ann Surg 225:155, 1997.
147. Shigeyuki S, Keishu Y, Kou T, et al: Inflammatory abdominal aortic aneurysms and atherosclerotic abdominal aortic aneurysms: comparisons of clinical features and long-term results. Jpn Circ J 61:231, 1997.

CHAPTER 73

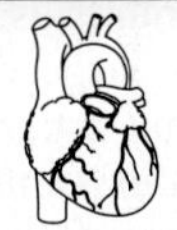

Peripheral Vascular Diseases

Alan T. Hirsch and Thom W. Rooke

PATHOLOGIC PROCESSES AFFECTING THE ARTERIAL SYSTEM
Atherosclerosis
Degenerative Diseases
Dysplastic Disease
Vascular Inflammation
Thrombosis
Embolic Disease
Vasospastic Disease
Other Arterial Diseases
CLINICAL MANIFESTATIONS OF ARTERIAL OCCLUSIVE DISEASES
Carotid Artery Disease
Renal Artery Disease
Peripheral Arterial Disease of the Lower Extremities

Peripheral vascular diseases are common and potentially serious, yet they often receive little clinical attention as distinct entities. Although the term *peripheral vascular disease* has been historically restricted to noncardiac arterial occlusive diseases, its correct definition encompasses a myriad of pathophysiologic syndromes affecting the arterial, venous, and lymphatic circulations, and it should include all vascular diseases altering end-organ perfusion. The *arterial diseases* include those disorders that cause either fixed obstruction or abnormal vascular reactivity of the arteries supplying a given tissue; the obstruction impairs blood delivery and can produce ischemia. *Venous diseases* occur in response to processes that impede normal venous function, including all noncardiac causes of venous hypertension. These disorders include venous valvular incompetence and venous hypertension, deep venous thrombosis, pulmonary embolism, postphlebitic syndrome, and varicose veins. *Lymphatic diseases* are a consequence of congenital or acquired processes that cause progressive destruction of the microvascular lymphatic networks; these disorders are often clinically manifested as lymphedema.

It has been proposed that the spectrum of vascular diseases be viewed as a single systemic biologic process because these diverse diseases share many common pathophysiologic processes that may alter endothelial function, vascular smooth muscle reactivity, and the propensity for local intravascular thrombosis and fibrinolysis. If permitted to progress without medical intervention, these processes may ultimately impede end-organ nutritive blood flow, eventually altering patient morbidity and mortality. The clinical implication of this systemic vascular paradigm has been the establishment of a growing clinical field known as vascular medicine.[1, 2] The conceptualization of vascular disorders as components of a single field of expertise has important implications for the provision of clinical vascular care. In lieu of vascular patients receiving care from multiple subspecialists (e.g., cardiologist, neurologist, nephrologist, lipid specialist, and vascular surgeon), it has been suggested that care be provided by a broadly trained vascular internist. Additionally, modern management of these complex disorders often requires a truly multidisciplinary collaboration between a cardiologist or a vascular internist, a vascular surgeon, and a radiologist to affect optimal care. The synergistic advances in both vascular biology and vascular medicine have come together in a clinical arena of tremendous depth, breadth, and rapid growth. Comprehensive coverage of this field is therefore far beyond the scope of this chapter. The discussion that follows focuses on the most common clinical disorders caused by arterial occlusive diseases of the carotid, renal, and lower extremity circulations.

Pathologic Processes Affecting the Arterial System

The arterial diseases include a wide range of pathologic processes that can affect anyone; however, specific diseases usually demonstrate specific patterns with regard to demographic factors (e.g., gender, age, race), certain risk factors (e.g., smoking, hypertension, hyperlipidemia), or the type and location of the vessels affected (e.g., large arteries versus medium arteries versus the microcirculation; elastic versus muscular arteries). Certain comorbid conditions (e.g., diabetes mellitus, limb trauma) are also associated with particular arterial diseases. The specific disease processes that affect arteries are pathologically diverse and are discussed in the following sections.

Atherosclerosis

The etiology, pathophysiology, and natural history of atherosclerosis have been previously described (see Ch. 70, Atherosclerosis: Pathologic Anatomy, and Ch. 71, Atherosclerosis: Pathogenesis and Risk Factors). Atherosclerosis is by far the most frequent arterial disease in industrialized countries, although its incidence in the general population is largely unknown. It is typically a generalized process that progresses to involve multiple arterial circulations, and coexistent clinical involvement of more than one organ system is common. The development of atherosclerosis is closely associated with several well-defined risk factors, including smoking, family history, male gender or postmenopausal state, diabetes, lipid abnormalities, hypertension, and homocysteinemia.[3]

Degenerative Diseases

Degenerative arteriopathies lead to a loss of the structural integrity and subsequent spontaneous dilatation of the arterial wall.[4] The pathophysiology of some specific progressive arterial degenerative diseases are relatively well understood (e.g., the collagen abnormalities that underlie Ehlers-Danlos syndrome), whereas the vascular defect responsible for other degenerative diseases remains elusive (e.g., Erdheim's cystic medial necrosis, Marfan's syndrome, spontaneous arteriomegaly, and most of the so-called idiopathic or atherosclerotic aneurysms). In these latter conditions, it is presumed that both atherosclerotic and hypertensive injury may contribute to the progression of these diseases. Arterial wall degeneration can lead to *aneurysm* formation and/or *dissection,* which may result in arterial rupture or occlusion.

Dysplastic Disease

Fibromuscular dysplasia is the most common dysplastic vascular condition and may affect many kinds of arteries.[5] Although the classic patient is a young female, this condition may occur in patients of either sex and at any age. Common clinical sequelae of fibromuscular dysplasia include arterial obstruction, occlusion, and aneurysm formation.

Vascular Inflammation

Vasculitis can affect most blood vessels, and the spectrum of clinical syndromes associated with vasculitis is broad.[6] *Large vessels* (the muscular aorta and its first and second-order branches) may be involved by giant cell arteritis (temporal arteritis or Takayasu's disease), Behcet's syndrome, relapsing polychondritis, and vasculitis associated with arthropathies. *Medium-sized vessels* (conduit muscular arteries and branches) are classically the target of polyarteritis nodosa, although Wegener's or lymphoid granulomatosis, Churg-Strauss syndrome, and Kawasaki's disease also affect vessels of this size. *Small-vessel* disease (arterioles and microvessels) is frequently seen in association with systemic disorders, such as rheumatoid arthritis, systemic lupus erythematosus, serum sickness, and other connective tissue or autoimmune diseases. *Buerger's disease* is an arterial obliterative process that almost exclusively occurs in smokers; it behaves like a vasculitis and can affect arteries of all sizes (small arteries more frequently than large ones) as well as veins.

Thrombosis

Prothrombotic states may be caused by (1) specific abnormalities in the clotting system (e.g., protein C, S, or antithrombin III deficiencies, factor V Leiden or prothrombin mutations),[7] (2) the presence of a lupus anticoagulant or anticardiolipin antibody,[8] (3) the procoagulant status caused by many cancers and inflammatory bowel disease,[9] and (4) a wide assortment of other disease states (e.g., atherosclerosis, trauma, aneurysms, and congestive heart failure).

Embolic Disease

Embolic vascular occlusive disease affects both large (*macroembolic*) and small (*microembolic*) vessels. Macroemboli usually originate from a cardiac source (e.g., an atrial clot associated with atrial fibrillation, ventricular thrombus secondary to either myocardial infarction or congestive heart failure), whereas microemboli may have either a cardiac source (typically a diseased native valve or a thrombogenic prosthetic valve) or a vascular source (most often a ruptured cholesterol-containing plaque producing distal *atheroembolization*).

Vasospastic Disease

Vasospasm refers to the pathologic vasoconstriction that may affect any muscular vessel in the body.[10] Migraine headache, cerebral vasospasm associated with intracranial bleeding, Prinzmetal's angina, Raynaud's phenomenon, and ergot toxicity are all well-recognized vasospastic syndromes. In the extremities, vasospasm may occur as a primary event (primary Raynaud's phenomenon), or it may occur secondary to an underlying disease process, such as scleroderma and systemic lupus erythematosus (secondary Raynaud's syndrome).

Other Arterial Diseases

The arterial diseases are characterized by pathophysiologic diversity. Additional disorders that alter normal peripheral arterial function include syndromes that cause extrinsic compression of the arteries, such as thoracic outlet syndrome and the popliteal entrapment syndrome; arterial remodeling caused by chronic hypertension; arterial calcification seen in association with diabetes mellitus (diabetic sclerosis) or with chronic renal failure, or as an isolated entity (Mönckeberg's calcific arterial sclerosis); various forms of penetrating and nonpenetrating trauma; congenital anomalies; and arteriovenous malformations.

Clinical Manifestations of Arterial Occlusive Diseases

The clinical manifestations of arterial disease depend on the vascular pathophysiology and the regional circulation that is affected. The occlusive diseases of the carotid arteries, the renal arteries, and the arteries to the lower extremities cause the most prevalent clinical disease and therefore serve as the focus of this chapter.

Carotid Artery Disease

Stroke is the third leading cause of death in the United States and is a major source of morbidity in the elderly. The annual worldwide incidence of stroke in middle-aged or older adults (greater than 75 years of age) is approximately 300 to 500/100,000,[11] although some data suggest that this incidence may be declining.[12] Most cases of stroke occur secondary to carotid atherosclerosis (Fig. 73–1), and therefore the demographic risk factor profile for patients with stroke is similar to that for patients with atherosclerosis in other circulations.[13] However, the vast array of other arterial pathologies outlined earlier (i.e., giant cell arteritis, emboli, dissection) can also affect the carotid and cerebral vessels; determining the underlying cause of carotid disease is often a challenging task for the clinician.

Diagnosis

The key to the diagnosis of carotid disease remains the history and physical examination. Even if neurologic episodes are transient, the responsible lesions can often be accurately localized on the basis of reported symptoms. It is imperative to document cervical or supraclavicular bruits, heart murmurs, retinal examination, and motor/sensory findings in patients with suspected or proven cerebrovascular disease. Specific diagnostic testing is an important adjunct in the assessment of neurovascular disease. Tests of particular importance include

1. *Oculoplethysmography.* This test measures ocular blood pressure, from which the adequacy of the anterior cerebral circulation can be inferred.[14] The oculoplethysmography is affected by collateral blood flow as well as flow through the major intracranial arteries; if collateral flow is well developed, the oculoplethysmography measurement may be normal despite high-grade stenotic disease (or complete occlusion) in the carotid system. The test is particularly useful for assessing the functional significance of carotid occlusive lesions.
2. *Duplex ultrasound.* A combination of two-dimensional real-time ultrasound imaging and pulsed-wave Doppler, this technique identifies, localizes, and determines the hemodynamic significance of particular carotid lesions.[15] Color-flow technology has helped to reduce the examination time and to expand the applicability of the examination.[16]
3. *Contrast angiography.* This remains the gold standard for the evaluation of cerebrovascular disease. Because it is invasive and carries a small but significant risk of complication,[17] it is best reserved for patients in whom revascularization surgery is being contemplated.
4. *Computed tomographic scanning.* Tomographic views of the brain are particularly useful for identifying and/or determining the location and extent of previous strokes. Computed tomographic scanning is generally indicated in patients with significant cerebrovascular disease, especially those preparing to undergo carotid artery surgery.[18]
5. *Magnetic resonance imaging.* Not only does magnetic resonance imaging offer an ability to image the brain (to localize acute infarction or intracerebral bleeds or other structural abnormalities) that is comparable to that of computed tomographic scanning, but new image acquisition, processing, and reconstruction modalities have transformed tomographic magnetic resonance imaging angiography into a useful clinical tool.[19]

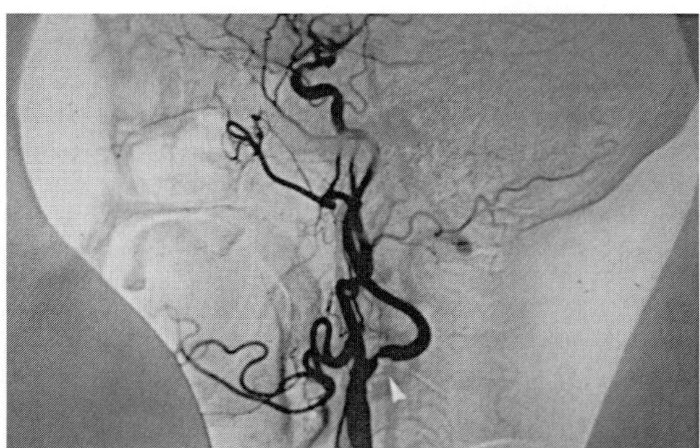

FIGURE 73–1 Cerebral angiogram demonstrates a high-grade proximal internal carotid artery atherosclerotic lesion (*arrow*).

Clinical Manifestations and Natural History

The usual clinical presentations of carotid disease include the asymptomatic carotid lesion (with or without bruit), transient ischemic attack (TIA), and stroke. The most common signs and symptoms of cerebrovascular disease are transient or fixed motor and sensory deficits, dysphasia, and visual abnormalities; when these occur, they may involve the anterior or posterior circulation and can be either hemispheric or nonhemispheric.

The natural history of the *asymptomatic* carotid lesion remains an area of clinical controversy, as new data continue to be accrued that may better define the role of carotid plaque morphology and ulceration to stroke risk, as well as the role of diagnostic methods to assess this risk.[20] Several clinical trials involving patients with asymptomatic disease have been completed and provide data that are helpful in assessing the relative risks and benefits of medical or surgical therapy in this large population of patients.[21–24] Asymptomatic carotid artery disease is a risk factor for stroke. More severe carotid arterial disease is associated with a greater likelihood of a subsequent neurologic event. Several studies confirm that patients with high-grade carotid artery lesions (>70 percent) have increased rates of subsequent TIA, stroke, or arterial occlusions; estimates of the yearly incidence for these outcomes range from 18 to 46 percent,[25–26] at least for the first year after diagnosis.

The natural history appears worse for patients with symptomatic carotid disease. Moore and associates[27] summarized the literature and suggest that patients with TIAs have a 12 to 13 percent risk of stroke (in the distribution of the TIA) during the ensuing year and a 5-year cumulative stroke risk of 30 to 35 percent after a TIA.

Treatment

Because the natural history of an asymptomatic carotid lesion is uncertain, selecting the proper therapy remains controversial. *Surgery* is a viable option provided that the perioperative morbidity and mortality rates remain less than 3 percent.[28] After successful surgery, patients with asymptomatic lesions generally have combined neurologic event rates (TIA and stroke) of less than 0.5 percent per year; the answer to whether this is truly better than the neurologic event rate for patients treated medically must await the outcomes of randomized clinical trials that are currently in progress. In the meantime, medical therapy should be considered for patients with relative or absolute contraindications to surgery, those with low-grade lesions (<70 percent stenosis), or those for whom surgery cannot be performed with an acceptable morbidity and mortality.

Patients with *symptomatic* carotid disease present a much stronger case for surgical intervention. If surgery can be performed with a morbidity and mortality of less than 5 percent in this group, then the rate of subsequent neurologic events can be significantly reduced by an operative procedure. In February 1991, the North American Symptomatic Carotid Endarterectomy Trial reported the 18-month follow-up for patients with symptomatic carotid lesions (70 to 99 percent stenosis) randomly assigned to surgical versus medical care. The morbidity and mortality in the surgical group (including perioperative events) was 7 percent, versus 24 percent in those treated medically.[29–30] Preliminary results from the European Carotid Surgery Trial suggest similar findings.[31]

For patients in whom surgery is contraindicated, antiplatelet agents may provide significant protection from stroke.[32] Ticlopidine or clopidogrel (adenosine diphosphate receptor antagonist antiplatelet agents)[33–35] and warfarin[36, 37] also appear to provide protection against neurologic events in certain patients with symptomatic disease.

Renal Artery Disease

The renal arteries are most commonly affected by atherosclerotic disease (Fig. 73–2), which accounts for 60 to 70 percent of renovascular lesions. Fibromuscular dysplasia is responsible for most of the remaining lesions,[38] although Takayasu's arteritis and other vasculitides, neurofibromatosis, and other rare conditions can also compromise renal arterial blood flow. Inadequate renal perfusion reduces the glomerular filtration rate and stimulates the renin-angiotensin-aldosterone system, leading to fluid retention and systemic vasoconstriction. Chronic hypoperfusion of the renal parenchyma may lead to permanent damage and renal atrophy. Clinical manifestations of renal artery disease include renovascular hypertension, renal failure, kidney infarction, and formation of renal artery aneurysms. It is difficult to estimate the incidence or the prevalence of renal artery disease in the general population, but certain high-risk groups have been studied. In a report of 395 patients with objective evidence of nonrenal atherosclerosis, the incidence of occult renal artery stenosis (defined as a lesion > 50 percent) was greater than 30 percent.[39] In patients with known hypertension, the incidence of a renovascular cause is typically 0.5 to 5.0 percent[38, 40]; the actual percentage depends on the subpopulation undergoing analysis. For example, in hypertensive children, the incidence of renovascular disease is estimated at 56 to 95 percent.[38] Similarly, the processes causing renovascular disease vary with the population studied. Atherosclerosis predominates in older patients with conventional risk factors, whereas younger patients (especially females) are more likely to have fibromuscular dysplasia.[38] The natural history of stenotic renal lesions appears variable. Studies with a mean follow-up time of 2 to 3 years[38] have shown a 44 percent progression rate in arteries with atherosclerosis (16 percent went on to occlusion) and a 33 percent progression in arteries with fibromuscular dysplasia (none of these went on to occlusion).

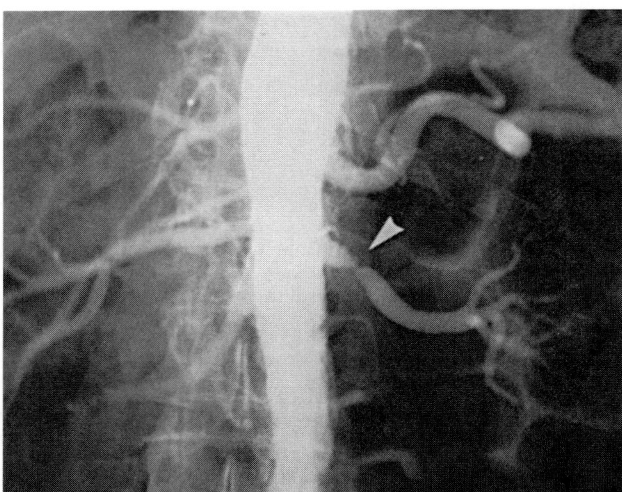

FIGURE 73–2 Aortic angiogram demonstrates high-grade focal left renal artery atherosclerotic lesion (*arrow*).

Diagnosis

The history and physical examination are notoriously unreliable methods for establishing the diagnosis of renal artery disease. Nevertheless, attention to historical details and aspects of the clinical examination provides clues that may raise suspicion to the astute clinician. Historical features suggesting renal artery disease include onset of hypertension or renal failure in the very young (<25 to 30 years of age) or older (>55 to 60 years of age) patient, hypertension that is difficult to control or demonstrates an accelerating pattern, or hypertension and renal failure in any patient with severe systemic atherosclerosis. A systolic or diastolic abdominal bruit is present in as many as 46 percent of patients with renovascular hypertension, as opposed to 9 percent of those with essential hypertension[41]; a higher incidence of bruits is generally noted in patients with fibromuscular dysplasia than in those with atherosclerosis.[42, 43] Other findings that can aid in the diagnosis include the presence of unilateral or bilateral renal atrophy on x-ray or ultrasound studies or the development of azotemia after initiation of therapy with converting enzyme inhibitors or angiotensin receptor antagonists.

Certain specific diagnostic tests may be useful in the evaluation of patients with suspected renal artery disease; these vary widely in terms of their sensitivity, specificity, cost, and relative invasiveness. The choice of diagnostic strategy may well be contingent on the experience and the reliability of the following techniques in the individual practice environment.

PLASMA RENIN ACTIVITY DETERMINATIONS

An isolated measurement of the plasma renin activity yields little diagnostic information regarding the presence of renal artery disease, primarily because plasma renin activity may be elevated in as many as 30 percent of patients with essential hypertension. Thus, in a survey of 540 patients, the plasma renin activity measurement was associated with a high false-negative (43 percent) and false-positive (34 percent) rate for the detection of renal artery disease.[44] Administration of an oral dose of captopril to stimulate renal renin release has been tried as a way of increasing the diagnostic discriminatory potential of plasma renin measurements; this technique has appeared promising in certain subgroups of patients[45] but has not proved universally reliable.[46]

Renal vein catheterization with selective renal vein sampling (with or without renin stimulation using captopril or furosemide) is another method that utilizes plasma renin activity to assess renal artery disease. A ratio of 1.4 to 1.5:1 in the relative venous renin concentrations between kidneys is predictive of renal vascular hypertension. Unfortunately, the reversibility of hypertension after renal revascularization cannot always be predicted on the basis of a lateralizing renin concentration.[47]

RAPID-SEQUENCE UROGRAPHY

The use of rapid, serial urograms after the intravenous administration of radio-opaque contrast has been used to screen for renovascular disease, but this technique is also associated with significant false-positive and false-negative rates.[48]

RADIONUCLIDE IMAGING/FLOW STUDIES

Pc-diethylenetriaminepentaacetic acid (DTPA),[42] ^{131}I-hippuran, ^{99m}Tc-mercaptoacetyltriglycine,[50] and other agents can be used to perform dynamic renography and renal scintigraphy (with or without the adjunctive use of captopril). Although these tests have definite diagnostic values, significant false-positive and false-negative rates are frequently reported.[49]

RENAL ARTERIAL DUPLEX SCANNING

Echo Doppler ultrasound scanning, especially when combined with color-flow technology, is generating considerable interest as a means of assessing the renal arteries. Although some authors report excellent results (95 percent sensitivity, 90 percent specificity) for the identification of renal artery stenosis,[51, 52] others have been less impressed, and the applicability and accuracy of the technique is not uniformly accepted.[53] These diagnostic limitations may be due to difficulty with the identification of the renal arteries, especially when multiple arteries are present, and to difficulty with the criteria used to judge the presence and the severity of renal artery stenosis.

MAGNETIC RESONANCE IMAGING

Magnetic resonance imaging is a very promising technique for assessing the renal arteries. In one study of 89 patients, the sensitivity and the specificity for detection of a stenosis greater than 60 percent were 90 percent and 86 percent, respectively.[54] It is likely that the use of magnetic resonance angiography scanning will continue to increase for this indication. As with all prior diagnostic techniques used to assess renal vascular disease, however, broader use of magnetic resonance angiography will be required to assess its relative limitations.

CONTRAST ANGIOGRAPHY

Angiography remains the gold standard for assessing renal artery disease. Both conventional and digital subtraction radiographic techniques (used to minimize contrast loads) yield excellent results. The role of intravenous digital angiography is less clear; the contrast load administered is often as great as that for standard renal angiography, and the image resolution is considerably poorer. However, for screening purposes, intravenous digital angiography may be adequate for detecting disease.[55–57]

Medical Treatment

The hypertension and azotemia associated with renal artery disease can often be adequately managed by use of conventional pharmacologic agents (e.g., diuretics, beta-blockers, calcium blockers, converting enzyme inhibitors, angiotensin receptor antagonists). Converting enzyme inhibitors, via their ability to inhibit the formation of angiotensin II, and angiotensin receptor antagonists have particular theoretical appeal in the treatment of renovascular disease.[58, 59] Administration of these classes of antihypertensive agents may be particularly efficacious in patients with unilateral renal artery disease. Whereas the high plasma renin and high circulating angiotensin II may be responsible for elevated blood pressure, this neurohormonal milieu may also sustain near-normal intrarenal hemodynamics. Therefore, reduction of the intrarenal hemodynamic effects of angiotensin II during treatment with a converting enzyme inhibitor or an angiotensin receptor antagonist may reduce efferent renal arteriolar vasomotor tone, cause a profound decline in the glomerular filtration rate, and potentially worsen renal function. This potential deleterious effect is especially problematic in patients with bilateral renal artery disease. In trials comparing the effects of converting enzyme inhibitors versus calcium blockers on glomerular filtration rate (in patients with renal artery transplants), only the converting enzyme inhibitor caused a reduction in glomerular filtration rate.[60]

Medical therapy is usually reserved for patients in whom (1) the renovascular disease is mild or easily controlled, (2) the arteries are not technically amenable to revascularization, or (3) the patient is not a good risk for invasive therapy. For patients with significant renal artery disease, the possibility of revascularization should be carefully considered.

Surgical Treatment

Surgical revascularization of the renal arteries remains the mainstay of invasive therapy. In experienced centers, these operations can be performed with reasonably low operative mortality (2 to 3 percent)[61, 62] and with excellent rates of cure or improvement (for hypertension or azotemia) ranging from 50 to 96 percent.[62, 63] Any kidney with occlusive disease and a pole-to-pole length greater than 8 to 10 cm has the potential for improved function after successful revascularization. Operations to restore blood flow include the aortorenal bypass, transaortic endarterectomy,[64] and splenorenal or hepatorenal bypass.

PERCUTANEOUS ANGIOPLASTY

Renal artery angioplasty is increasingly used in the treatment of renal artery disease, particularly in patients with fibromuscular dysplasia.[65–67] Results of angioplasty in atherosclerotic renal disease have been much less impressive; this is largely due to the high proportion of ostial renal artery lesions and the poor response of these lesions to dilatation.[68, 69] Restenosis remains a problem in approximately one third of successful dilatations,[66] especially for atherosclerotic lesions. The deployment of stents has improved the short- and long-term success of percutaneous renal revascularization.[70] However, when the cost of treating and retreating patients with restenosis is analyzed, it remains difficult to demonstrate any financial savings from the use of percutaneous transluminal angioplasty as opposed to initial surgery in the treatment of renal artery disease.[71, 72] Thus, the choice of percutaneous versus surgical renal revascularization is usually made on the basis of the clinical characteristics of the patient (e.g., the perioperative surgical risk and expected longevity) and the experience of the clinical center where care will be provided.

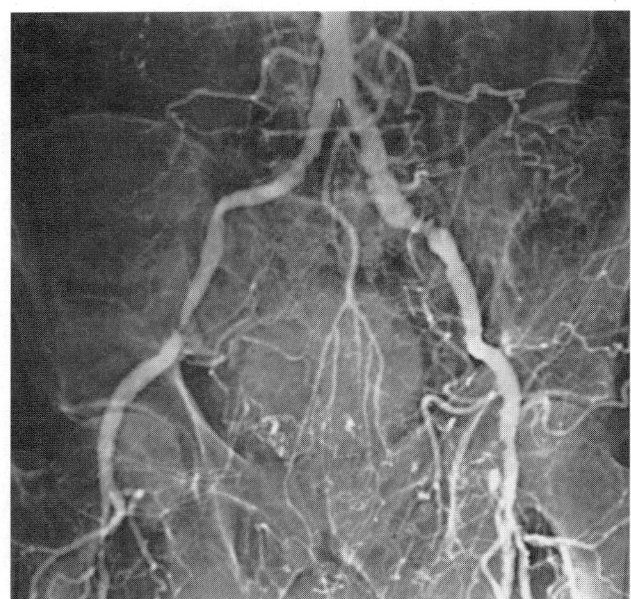

FIGURE 73–3 Arteriogram demonstrates diffuse bilateral aortoiliac and femoral artery atherosclerosis.

Peripheral Arterial Disease of the Lower Extremities

Peripheral arterial disease (PAD) of the lower extremities is an extremely prevalent disorder that causes significant disability and is associated with a very high rate of cardiovascular ischemic events. The most common cause of lower extremity arterial occlusive disease in Western societies remains atherosclerosis. Lower extremity atherosclerosis affects multiple anatomic sites in the distal abdominal aorta, iliac, femoral, and infrapopliteal arteries (Fig. 73–3). The incidence of atherosclerotic arterial disease of the legs increases synergistically in response to an individual's exposure to the common atherosclerosis risk factors.[73] Whereas many other disorders can duplicate the symptoms of lower extremity arterial insufficiency (e.g., thromboangiitis obliterans or other arteritides, arterial thromboemboli, intimal dissection, popliteal entrapment syndrome), these conditions account for only a small percentage of lower extremity arterial disease; however, recognition of the broad differential diagnosis of lower extremity arterial disease by the clinician is essential in order to permit specific therapies to be applied to individual patients. Progressive lower extremity arterial atherosclerosis may promote progressive focal stenoses or occlusion and may lead to arterial aneurysm formation. The clinical presentation (asymptomatic, mild-to-severe claudication, or a vascular emergency) depends on the rate of disease progression, the severity of the decrease in limb blood flow, and the propensity for development of collateral blood flow and/or sudden thrombosis. Thus, patients with anatomically comparable degrees of arterial occlusive disease may present with symptoms that range from mild claudication to rest pain to frank gangrene (Fig. 73–4).

The natural history of PAD has been carefully examined in the studies of Boyd,[74] Imparato and colleagues,[75] McAllister,[76] and others (Table 73–1).[73] Progression of disease may be slow, but in patients presenting with intermittent claudication, there is eventual symptomatic worsening in 15 to 30 percent over the 5 to 10 years after the diagnosis is established. Tissue necrosis and/or progression to rest pain requiring vascular surgery is needed in 2.7 to 5.0 percent of limbs with claudication annually, and amputation is ultimately required in 1 percent per year.[73] Whereas this amputation rate may appear small, when these events are summed over 5 to 10 years of follow-up, a 5 to 10 percent amputation rate for this prevalent disease is notable. An appropriate understanding of this natural history must encompass an appreciation of the complete atherosclerotic risk burden carried by the patient with PAD because the risk of fatal and nonfatal cardiovascular ischemic events is much higher (approximately 50 percent over

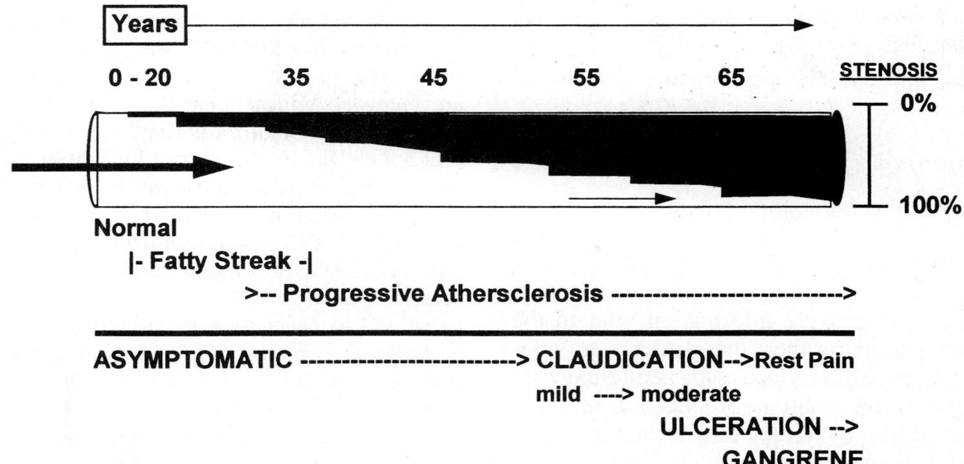

FIGURE 73–4 The natural history of atherosclerotic lower extremity arterial occlusive disease. As in other circulations, the course of atherosclerosis is slowly progressive. Clinical manifestations of disease usually occur late in the anatomic natural history. This provides a lengthy period of clinical opportunity to initiate preventive measures intended to decrease the incidence of claudication, rest pain, ischemic ulceration, or amputation.

5 years) than the risk of any clinical limb event (progressive claudication, requirement for revascularization, or amputation).[76, 77] New data demonstrate that risk factor modification and antiplatelet therapy can markedly lower the rate of cardiovascular ischemic events and disease progression in symptomatic individuals.

Diagnosis

HISTORY AND PHYSICAL EXAMINATION

The diagnosis of PAD can often be established with a high degree of certainty from the history and physical examination alone. Classic intermittent claudication is typically described as a reproducible aching, fatigue, or discomfort that occurs in the muscles of the legs on walking and resolves promptly (within 10 minutes) of rest. Stenoses in the aortoiliac arteries commonly elicit discomfort in the buttock or thigh, although symptoms may occasionally begin with distal foot and calf pain and then progress to involve the proximal leg musculature. Focal stenoses in the superficial femoral artery at Hunter's canal often present as calf claudication. Disease of the infrapopliteal vessels may present as foot claudication. Unfortunately, such typical lower extremity ischemic symptoms may be so insidious in onset that patients become quite disabled before the exercise intolerance is brought to the attention of the physician; exercise intolerance may be instead attributed to aging or to concomitant comorbid diseases (e.g., the arthritides, neuropathic syndromes). The exercise limitation is often noted by a spouse or other close family member rather than the patient. If exercise is also limited by orthopedic, neurologic, or other infirmities, or if the claudication history is atypical, then the optimal history may be best obtained during an exercise Doppler stress test.

Atherosclerosis is a systemic disease that progresses at variable rates in regional circulations. When patients are found to have lower extremity arterial occlusive disease, it is clinically appropriate to ascertain by physical examination whether coexistent coronary or carotid disease is present by assessing whether cardiac gallops or carotid bruits are present. In a large, well-known study by Hertzer and colleagues,[78] severe coronary artery disease was found angiographically in 36 percent of patients with an abdominal aortic aneurysm and in 28 percent of patients with lower extremity occlusive disease. In a separate report, Kramer and Hertzer[79] noted cervical bruits in 11 percent of patients with abdominal aortic aneurysm and 25 percent of patients with peripheral disease; a significant number of patients (44 percent) had high-grade (>75 percent) carotid stenoses or occlusions. Although disease of other arterial beds is common in patients with PAD, there are no data that can yet be used to support the cost-effectiveness of a deliberate screening search for other arterial disease by performance of surveillance duplex ultrasound examinations.

The femoral and popliteal pulses and both ankle pulses

TABLE 73–1 Selected Investigations of the Natural History of Lower Extremity Arterial Occlusive Disease

Author (yr)	n	Follow-Up (yr)	Stable or Improved (%)	Amputation (%)	Survival (%)
Boyd (1962)	1476	5	80	7.2	73
		10	6	12.0	38
Imparato (1975)	104	2.5	79	5.8	—
McAllister (1976)	100	6	78	7.0	89

can usually be readily assessed by palpation, and the signs of ischemia, such as discoloration, cool skin, chronic trophic skin changes, and skin breakdown, are evident on simple inspection.

THE NONINVASIVE VASCULAR LABORATORY

The noninvasive vascular laboratory provides a powerful set of tools that can objectively assess the status of lower extremity disease and thereby accelerate the delineation of a therapeutic plan. The combined use of physiologic data and imaging studies can provide information vital to the choice of interventional approaches; these studies are relatively inexpensive, can be performed with negligible risk, and provide prognostic information. Application of these tools to the lower extremity circulation is analogous to the use of electrocardiography and echocardiography for cardiac disease. When appropriately utilized, these noninvasive tools can either supplant or augment the data obtained by use of invasive angiographic methods. Noninvasive vascular laboratory examinations of the lower extremity arterial circulation should be performed: (1) to objectively establish the presence of arterial occlusive disease, (2) to quantitatively assess the severity of disease, (3) to localize lesions to specific arterial segments of the limb, and (4) to determine the temporal progression of disease or its response to specific therapy.[80] These tests are summarized in Table 73–2 and are reviewed in subsequent sections.

THE ANKLE-BRACHIAL INDEX

For most patients who present with asymptomatic or moderately symptomatic disease, the measurement of the ankle-brachial index (ABI) provides objective data that may predict limb survival, propensity for wound healing, and patient survival. The ABI can be utilized either as a screening tool for PAD or to follow the efficacy of therapeutic interventions. For this test, systolic blood pressure is recorded from both brachial arteries and from both the dorsal artery of the foot and the posterior tibial arteries while the patient is in the supine position. Optimal recordings are obtained by use of blood pressure cuffs that are appropriately sized to the patient's calves, and systolic pressures are recorded with a hand-held 5- or 10-mHz Doppler instrument. In normal individuals, there should be a minimal (<12 mm Hg) interarm systolic pressure gradient during a routine examination. Inasmuch as the incidence of atherosclerotic subclavian and axillary arterial occlusive disease is higher in this population, both arm pressures must be recorded. If the arm blood pressures are *not* equal, then the presence of a subclavian or axillary arterial stenosis is presumed to be present in the lower pressure arm and the higher blood pressure is used for subsequent blood pressure ratio calculations. Pulse wave reflection in healthy individuals causes the ankle pressure to be 10 to 15 mm Hg higher than the brachial arterial systolic pressure, and thus the normal ankle-arm systolic blood pressure ratio is greater than 1.0.

Abnormal ABI values represent a continuous variable less than 0.90. ABI values are often considered to be mildly diminished when they are between 0.80 and 0.90, moderately diminished when between 0.50 and 0.80, and severely decreased when less than 0.50. These relative categories have prognostic value. For example, the preservation of an ABI value greater than 0.50 (or an ankle pressure > 70 mm Hg) suggests that progression to critical leg ischemia is unlikely during the subsequent 6.5 years of follow-up.[81] In contrast, it is common for patients to experience ischemic rest pain when the ABI is less than 0.4; similarly, the low ankle systolic blood pressure in such individuals bodes poorly for the healing of ischemic wounds. The presence of a severely decreased ABI also identifies individuals who are at particularly high risk for the subsequent development of rest pain, ischemic ulceration, or gangrene.[82]

Despite its utility, the ABI may not be accurate in individuals in whom systolic blood pressure cannot be abolished by inflation of an air-filled blood pressure cuff. The incidence of noncompressible, calcified conduit arteries is highest in diabetics and elderly patients; in these individuals, it may be impossible to abolish the systolic pressure

TABLE 73–2 **Noninvasive Vascular Laboratory Testing Methods for Lower Extremity Arterial Occlusive Disease**

Anatomic Method	Quantitation of Disease Localization	Relative Severity	Cost	Benefits (Limitations)
Ankle-brachial indices	–	+ +	+	Ideal office screening tool[1] Predicts limb & patient survival
Segmental pressure analysis	+ +	+ +	+	Excellent arterial localization[1]
Pulse volume recordings	+	+	+	Objective qualitative data
Transcutaneous oximetry	+	+ + +	+ +	Assesses small-vessel disease Predicts wound healing
Doppler waveform analysis	+ + +	+ +	+ +	Accurate in all populations[2]
Arterial duplex	+ + +	+ +	+ + +	Excellent anatomic localization[2,3]
Exercise Doppler testing	–	+ + +	+ + +	Objective functional assessment Assesses exercise pain etiology Coronary ischemia assessment[4]

Limitations of Arterial Testing Methods

1. They may not be accurate in some elderly or diabetic patients.
2. They do not predict patient survival.
3. Duplex scanning may be time-consuming and costly and requires technical proficiency.
4. They have decreased sensitivity to assess exercise-induced ischemia in patients with claudication.

signal despite cuff inflation to pressures in excess of 200 mm Hg. Despite the artifactually "high" recorded systolic pressure, these individuals may have quite severe disease. It is also common for patients with either severely stenotic or totally occluded iliofemoral arteries to nevertheless have a normal ankle pressure if sufficient collaterals are present. If such patients have symptomatic evidence of arterial disease, the presence of a normal ABI should not be presumed to rule out significant arterial occlusive disease and an alternative diagnostic test (e.g., segmental pressure measurement, Doppler waveform analysis, pulse volume recording, and exercise Doppler test) should be performed.

Whereas this technique has served as an important diagnostic test for vascular physicians for many decades, its utility has been expanded by epidemiologic studies.[83–86] It has long been recognized that the presence of lower extremity atherosclerotic disease is predictive of the presence of coronary heart disease. The studies of Newman and coworkers[83] have confirmed the inverse relationship between the ABI and the presence of coronary artery disease risk factors, as well as with the presence of both cardiovascular and cerebrovascular disease. This relationship may be especially prominent in high-risk groups. For example, in a cohort of 1537 elderly men and women followed up in the Systolic Hypertension in the Elderly Program, the presence of a low ABI was predictive of total mortality and cardiovascular mortality (relative risk of cardiovascular mortality in the low ABI cohort was increased approximately threefold to fourfold).[84] It is notable that these findings are evident in subjects *without* lower extremity ischemic symptoms. Therefore, the increased mortality associated with a diminished ABI in symptomatic patients with claudication is not surprising. McKenna and colleagues[86] have documented 5-year mortalities of approximately 30 percent and 50 percent in patients with an ABI of 0.70 and 0.40, respectively. This prognostic information provides an index of survival similar to that obtained via use of the ejection fraction or the left ventricular end-diastolic diameter for patients with heart failure. Despite the increasing use of more sophisticated vascular diagnostic tests (e.g., arterial duplex), only the ABI yields such vital predictive cardiac event and survival data (Fig. 73–5).

Based on these data, it would seem prudent for the ABI test to be increasingly utilized in office practice in general, and in cardiovascular practices in particular, because this simple, cost-effective diagnostic test defines a cohort in whom both atherosclerosis risk-reduction interventions and PAD-specific interventions can potentially improve outcomes.[87] It has been proposed that the ABI be considered as a routine test for all patients who are at risk for PAD, especially those older than 70 years, or those who are 50 years of age and in whom other atherosclerosis risk factors would increase the PAD prevalence (especially tobacco use and diabetes).

SEGMENTAL PRESSURE MEASUREMENTS

Arterial pressures can also be measured by use of plethysmographic cuffs placed sequentially along the limb at various levels. In most vascular laboratories, these blood pressure cuffs are placed at the upper thigh, the lower thigh, the upper calf, and the lower calf above the ankle. The

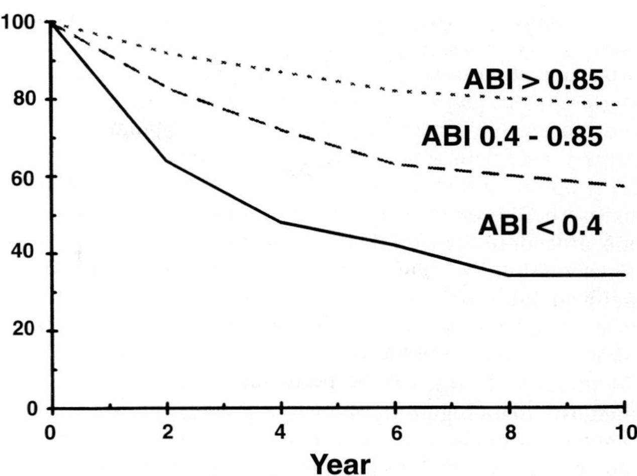

FIGURE 73–5 Prediction of patient survival by the ankle-brachial index (ABI). The magnitude of decrease in ankle blood pressure is an index of the systemic atherosclerotic disease burden and predicts patient survival. The primary causes of death of patients with lower extremity arterial occlusive disease are usually cardiac (myocardial infarction and heart failure). Thus, the ABI serves as a facile, noninvasive predictor of cardiac ischemic risk. (Modified from McKenna M, Wolfson S, Kuller L: The ratio of ankle and arm blood pressure as an independent risk factor of mortality. Atherosclerosis 87:119, 1991.)

systolic blood pressures obtained from the lower extremities can also be indexed relative to the brachial artery pressure, in a manner analogous to the simple ABI. These measurements provide a noninvasive corollary to intra-arterial pressure measurements, with the advantage that these determinations can be performed as a screening tool, can be repeated to assess disease natural history or to determine the efficacy of interventions, and can be performed at no risk to the patient. In contrast to ABI studies, the segmental pressure analysis is often able to accurately determine the location of individual arterial stenoses. For example, the presence of a prominent systolic pressure gradient between the brachial artery pressure and the upper thigh systolic pressure usually signifies the presence of an aortoiliac stenosis. A pressure gradient located between the upper and lower thigh cuffs would signify a lesion of the superficial femoral artery. Gradients between the lower thigh and upper calf cuffs would identify a distal superficial femoral or a popliteal arterial stenosis, and gradients between the upper and lower calf cuffs would identify infrapopliteal disease. In most laboratories, any gradient between adjacent sites of greater than 10 to 15 mm Hg may represent a physiologically important focal stenosis. Thus, segmental pressure measurements can identify the location and the magnitude of many arterial stenoses noninvasively. However, segmental pressure measurements may be artifactually elevated or uninterpretable in patients with calcified, noncompressible vessels, as is the case with simple ABI determinations. In such individuals, Doppler waveform analyses, arterial duplex studies, or transcutaneous oximetry studies may still be quite helpful.

EXERCISE DOPPLER STRESS TESTS

It is commonly taught that patients with PAD cannot be effectively evaluated by cardiovascular treadmill testing. It is true that standard exercise testing protocols may be inordinately arduous for many patients with claudication, with subjects less frequently reaching workloads adequate to provide optimal sensitivity to evaluate coronary ischemic symptoms. Nevertheless, treadmill testing may be extremely useful in objectively documenting the magnitude of symptom limitation in patients with mild-to-moderate disease before embarking on any aggressive revascularization procedure. Treadmill tests for patients with claudication should utilize less intense progressive workloads (e.g., the Naughton protocol) and should record the time of onset of specific leg symptoms, the presence of associated coronary ischemic symptoms, and the total walking time. Continuous electrocardiographic monitoring may provide diagnostic data regarding inducible myocardial ischemia in many individuals, even if the patient cannot achieve 85 percent of his or her age-predicted peak heart rate or workload. Such objective functional yardsticks may also be helpful in differentiating vascular from alternative, nonvascular causes of exercise-induced lower extremity discomfort.

The addition of a Doppler recording of the ankle systolic blood pressure at rest and after exercise yields objective data to grade the dynamic functional significance of an arterial stenosis. In normal individuals, the brachial and ankle blood pressures rise together and maintain their normal relationship with exertion. In contrast, the increased central blood pressure and the maximal exercise-induced ischemic vasodilatation in the claudicating limb cause a marked rise in the trans-stenosis blood pressure gradient. Thus, in the individual with true vasculogenic claudication, the postexercise ABI demonstrates a classical "paradoxical" fall from its baseline value. For example, in individuals with symptoms of thigh and buttock claudication caused by iliac arterial stenoses, the resting ABI may be normal. Measurement of a normal index at baseline with a subsequent diagnostic ABI fall immediately after exercise may reveal the functional significance of a high-grade stenosis that significantly limits ambulation. In contrast, the patient with pseudoclaudication resulting from spinal stenosis demonstrates a normal postexercise ABI, despite exercise limiting symptoms suggestive of arterial insufficiency.

PULSE VOLUME RECORDINGS

Additional objective data can be obtained to assess the adequacy of perfusion in patients via the use of simple plethysmographic techniques. Pulse volume recordings provide a method to evaluate the arterial pressure waveform profile via the use of either a pneumoplethysmograph or a mercury-in-Silastic strain gauge. Both of these devices can be applied in a segmental manner from the thigh to the ankle to assess the change in limb volume between diastole and systole. When such data are recorded on chart paper, the magnitude of the pulse volume provides an index of large-vessel patency and correlates with blood flow.

CONTINUOUS-WAVE DOPPLER WAVEFORM EXAMINATIONS

Continuous-wave Doppler waveform analysis can also provide important information that may establish arterial patency or localize arterial occlusive lesions. In many circumstances, a change in blood velocity and/or pulse waveform provides reasonably accurate information about the localization and the extent of specific lower extremity lesions. Doppler waveform analyses are reliable even in highly calcified vessels that are not amenable to pressure determinations.

DUPLEX SCANNING

Duplex scanning, utilizing dual imaging and Doppler waveform analysis, discussed earlier for both the carotid and the renal circulations, can also be used to assess PAD in the lower extremities. This technique can visualize and assess flow velocities in regions of arterial aneurysms or at sites of localized stenosis or occlusion. Duplex studies can assess plaque morphology and surgical graft patency and can establish the presence of arteriovenous fistulas. In most patients, diagnostic images can be easily obtained. However, this technique requires the presence of a technically proficient examiner, may require extensive time for a complete examination, and is significantly more expensive than most physiologic testing. Thus, despite the utility of these examinations, their use as a screening tool remains limited; duplex testing should be reserved for specific indications in which the precise anatomic information obtained by this technique is likely to be useful. Duplex techniques are particularly helpful in assessing proximal iliofemoral stenoses that may be amenable to angioplasty, in providing follow-up data to assess the continued patency of both native venous and prosthetic arterial grafts, and to evaluate the patency of prior angioplasty sites or intravascular stents.

TRANSCUTANEOUS OXIMETRY

In many clinical settings, the application of either physiologic or imaging measures of large-vessel perfusion (e.g., ABIs, Doppler waveform analysis, arterial duplex imaging) may demonstrate adequate blood flow to the ankle, yet the physical examination may suggest the presence of functionally important disease in the dorsal arterial arch or digital arteries. This may be particularly critical for the assessment of patients with ischemic ulcerations and/or impending gangrene. Thus, the measurement of the adequacy of both large- and small-vessel perfusion to the distal limb may be clinically valuable. Determination of the net delivery of oxygen to ischemic, but potentially salvageable, tissue may be accomplished by use of transcutaneous oximetry ($TcPo_2$) measurements using oxygen-sensing electrodes. These electrodes are usually attached to the skin in both a normally perfused region (e.g., the chest) and at calf or foot sites to directly measure the local cutaneous oxygen tension. $TcPo_2$ determinations provide a very sensitive means to assess the adequacy of skin perfusion, the severity of ischemic wounds, and the potential for cutaneous healing at specific sites.[88] Normal $TcPo_2$ values are usually greater than 50 to 60 mm Hg; in contrast, $TcPo_2$ values less than 20 to 30 mm Hg suggest severe local ischemia and bode poorly for future wound healing.[89] In summary, $TcPo_2$ studies provide an excellent method for the assessment of patients with concomitant large-vessel and microvascular disease, such as diabetic patients and patients with severe atheroembolic lesions.

CONTRAST ANGIOGRAPHY

Contrast studies remain the definitive means for examining the lower extremity circulation. As with angiography of other vascular regions, lower extremity arteriography should be undertaken only when the potential benefits exceed the foreseeable risks for a specific individual. Techniques utilizing intravenous, as opposed to arterial, contrast administration may reduce the risk of complications in some circumstances and still provide adequate imaging quality.[90] The advances in noninvasive vascular laboratory techniques during the past decade usually permit angiography to be restricted to the assessment of the patient before planned surgical or percutaneous revascularization.

Treatment

THE BENEFICIAL EFFECTS OF MEDICAL THERAPY FOR CLAUDICATION

Medical therapies can effectively both modify the natural history of atherosclerotic PAD and significantly blunt the accompanying morbidity of this disorder (Table 73–3). Effective medical therapy should be consistently prescribed to forestall the onset of limb-threatening events that might mandate interventional therapy. At the completion of successful revascularization procedures, atherosclerosis risk factor modification and antiplatelet therapies decrease the rate of cardiovascular ischemic events and have the potential to improve long-term patient survival.

Normalization of adverse atherosclerotic risk factors is critical in patients with PAD. It is often presumed that patients with claudication are more reluctant to become tobacco abstinent, or may be less successful at quitting, than other tobacco-using cohorts. This presumption ignores the intrinsic motivation to quit using tobacco that accompanies overt claudication, rest pain, an ischemic wound, or vascular reconstructive procedures. Even patients with stable, mild disease should be informed that continuation of tobacco use is likely to accelerate anatomic disease progression and cause progressive symptomatic worsening.[91] Jonason and Bergstrom[92] demonstrated that rest pain developed over the subsequent 5 years of observation in as many as 18 percent of patients with claudication who continued to smoke cigarettes; the advent of rest pain is a critical clinical landmark because this population is highly disabled, at high risk for gangrene, and often requires revascularization or amputation. In contrast, in patients who became tobacco abstinent, the development of rest pain was exceedingly rare. Successful tobacco cessation also has major effects on patient survival in this population.[93, 94] The 5-year mortality rates for patients with claudication who continue to smoke may be as high as 40 to 50 percent. In contrast, tobacco abstinence in this population is associated with markedly decreased rates of myocardial infarction and stroke, resulting in an impressive improvement in survival.[91]

Effective lipid management should also be considered a mandatory component of the medical therapy of patients with objective evidence of lower extremity arterial occlusive disease. This strategy has been sanctioned by the National Cholesterol Education Program recommendation that patients with evidence of atherosclerotic vascular disease (symptomatic or objective evidence, e.g., the ABI) be treated by diet and pharmacologic therapy to achieve a low-density lipoprotein cholesterol level of less than 100 mg/dl.[95] Such efforts should achieve a decreased rate of cardiovascular ischemic events in this fragile population. It is less well-recognized that lipid-lowering strategies have beneficial, although small, effects on the progression of atherosclerotic femoral arterial disease. The Cholesterol Lowering Atherosclerosis Study of Barndt and colleagues[96] assessed the rates of both coronary and femoral atherosclerosis disease progression in a cohort of 162 middle-aged, nonsmoking men in a double-blind, placebo-controlled study of dietary versus aggressive lipid-lowering drug treatment. Patients were either treated by combined dietary modification and colestipol and niacin therapy or by dietary management alone during a relatively brief 2-year study period. These data demonstrated that the rate of femoral arterial atherosclerotic disease progression, as assessed by paired quantitative angiography, was blunted and femoral arterial disease regression was greater in those subjects who achieved optimal effective lipid lowering by pharmacotherapy. These relatively short-term angiographic observations have been extended in the Program on the Surgical Control of the Hyperlipidemias study.[97] In these patients, lipid-lowering achieved by ileal bypass surgery extended the benefits of treatment throughout 10 years of follow-up. As in the Cholesterol Lowering Atherosclerosis Study, the rate of femoral arterial atherosclerosis disease progression was diminished; more impressively, the rate of development of symptomatic claudication was also reduced by 27 percent.

Whereas it has been demonstrated that optimal achievement of glucose control in diabetics is associated with an improved natural history of microvascular disease (e.g.,

TABLE 73–3 Treatment Goals for Patients With Peripheral Arterial Disease

Treatment Goal	Potential Therapeutic Strategies
Improve exercise capacity	Supervised exercise rehabilitation program Tobacco cessation Consider cilostazol or pentoxifylline therapy Consider revascularization (angioplasty or surgery)
Prevent amputation	Well-fitting footwear Foot hygiene (e.g., nail care, interdigital lamb's wool) Avoid trauma Prompt treatment of infection
Prevent MI, stroke, and cardiac death	Antiplatelet therapy (e.g., ASA, clopidogrel) Vigilance for cardiac ischemic symptoms Preoperative cardiac risk assessment
Blunt atherosclerosis disease progression	Tobacco cessation Effective lipid management Optimal diabetic control Optimal antihypertensive control

Abbreviations: ASA, aspirin; MI, myocardial infarction.

retinopathy and microalbuminuria), the effects of diabetic management on large-vessel arterial occlusive disease in this population have been less completely evaluated in controlled, prospective clinical trials, but current data suggest that ischemic events may be reduced.[98] Nevertheless, the potential beneficial impact of ideal glucose management in the diabetic population should not be discounted. Optimal diabetic management is presumed to improve the rate of lower extremity disease progression, the incidence of myocardial ischemic events, and the incidence of wound infection, gangrene, and amputation.

EXERCISE TRAINING AND REHABILITATION

As noted earlier, it is usual for patients with symptomatic lower extremity arterial occlusive disease, whether presenting with claudication, rest pain, or ischemic ulceration, to have restricted their activities of daily living before their presentation to the clinician. This profound deconditioning also contributes to the disability of the disease. Deconditioning may also be induced iatrogenically in the postoperative state after successful surgical revascularization. Prolonged periods of bed rest, as often prescribed for patients with ischemic foot wounds or new vein grafts, may thereby also delay functional recovery. Independent ambulation and freedom of mobility are the major "end-organ functions" of the lower extremities. Therefore, improved limb function assessed by walking distance (not simple angiographic or physiologic blood flow measures) may serve as the optimal "patient-focused" treatment goal. Exercise rehabilitation remains a critically important treatment modality and should be considered a mainstay of therapy for patients with lower extremity arterial disease.

The efficacy of claudication exercise training has been well-established by numerous investigators (Fig. 73–6).[99–106] Essentially all studies of the efficacy of exercise training have demonstrated an improvement in both the pain-free walking time (the intermittent claudication distance) and the maximal walking time (the absolute claudication distance). Using a constant-load treadmill protocol, these investigations have demonstrated improvements ranging from 50 to 300 percent. Similarly, exercise training may elicit improvements in maximal walking time of 25 to 200 percent. On average, patients can expect to double their intermittent claudication distance and absolute claudication distance. Exercise training has been postulated to improve performance in patients with claudication by directly augmenting limb blood or collateral flow, by improving blood viscosity, by promoting a change in walking techniques to more biomechanically efficient techniques, or by altering the ischemic pain threshold or tolerance.[103, 105] However, although improvements in these factors may be beneficial, the magnitude of functional benefit cannot be explained by these factors alone. Some studies have reported a pattern of abnormal skeletal muscle oxidative metabolism, with accumulation of acylcarnitines, denervation of muscle bundles (as documented by both electrophysiologic and histopathologic studies), and selective loss of type II myofibers in ischemic limbs.[100, 101] The exact mechanism underlying the impressive benefits of exercise training remain incompletely elucidated.

In order to achieve these clinical benefits, patients should receive rehabilitation in a structured claudication exercise rehabilitation program for at least three sessions weekly over at least 12 weeks.[99, 105, 106] Gardner and Poehlman[106] demonstrated that the greatest improvement in claudication pain distances during a structured exercise program can be achieved when individuals exercise to a moderate to near-maximal claudication pain end point, in programs that last at least 3 to 6 months, and when walking is the primary mode of exercise. Other factors that might underlie success include maintenance of exercise for greater than 30 minutes per session and an exercise frequency of at least three sessions per week. Despite the impressive documented efficacy of claudication rehabilitation programs, few patients now receive such therapeutic benefit, primarily because of the current lack of reimbursement for such care in established rehabilitation settings. Whereas there are perceived to be immediate functional benefits of surgical or percutaneous revascularization, few prospective, randomized trials have compared these invasive therapies directly with exercise training. Two such trials have con-

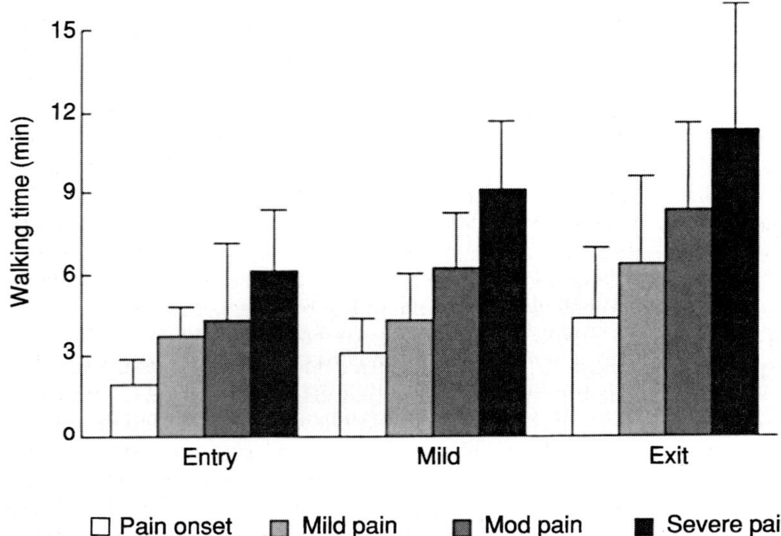

FIGURE 73–6 The beneficial effects of exercise training for functional status in patients with claudication. Patients with claudication typically experience an improvement in both the time of onset of claudication symptoms and the maximal treadmill walking time during a 12-week exercise rehabilitation program. In this study by Hiatt and associates, 10 subjects graded the time of onset and the severity of claudication at baseline, after 6 weeks of training, and at the 12-week time point. The sequential improvement in symptoms and doubling in maximal treadmill time are apparent. (Modified from Hiatt WR: Benefit of exercise conditioning for patients with peripheral arterial disease. Circulation 81:602, 1990. By permission of The American Heart Association.)

cluded that exercise training may be comparable or superior to revascularization in improving functional status in selected treatment groups.[107, 108] Clinical factors that might be presumed to impede the ability of patients to benefit from exercise rehabilitation have been assessed. For example, the presence of rest pain or associated coronary artery disease or the anatomic location of the lower extremity lesions do not preclude the achievement of functional benefit. Thus, when a patient presents with lifestyle-limiting claudication and is considered for referral to vascular specialists for possible revascularization, it is imperative that the patient and the physician ensure that the limitation is lifestyle limiting *after* prescription of an adequate exercise rehabilitation program. The structure of successful vascular rehabilitation programs usually involves a partnership of physicians and vascular nurses.[109]

OTHER SUPPORTIVE ASPECTS OF EFFECTIVE MEDICAL CARE

The relatively slow rate of progression of lower extremity arterial occlusive disease should provide many opportunities for primary prevention of the costly and morbid complications of the later disease stages. Certainly, optimal early supportive care should decrease the occurrence of refractory claudication, ischemic wounds, cellulitis, and amputation. The occurrence of these later symptoms is usually an indication for referral to a vascular specialist (vascular medicine, vascular surgery, or interventional radiology) for aggressive care (Table 73–4). In contrast, cardiovascular specialists and primary physicians should apply other effective preventive measures before these disease complications supervene. Patients in whom foot blood flow is diminished should be instructed to wear well-fitting, protective footwear to diminish the risk of accidental injury; this simple recommendation, although effective, remains an often neglected component of medical care. Instruction in foot care should be given to patients with diabetes, those with a history of an ischemic wound, and those with a severely diminished ABI ($\leq$ 0.30 to 0.40).

PHARMACOTHERAPIES FOR LOWER EXTREMITY ARTERIAL DISEASE

Pentoxifylline (Trental), an oral, well-tolerated methylxanthine derivative, was the first drug approved for use in the United States for the alleviation of the symptoms of claudication.[110–113] Pentoxifylline is presumed to improve limb perfusion by reducing red blood cell rigidity, blood viscosity, and platelet hyperreactivity. Numerous clinical investigations have demonstrated that when this agent is used in adequate dosages for an appropriate duration (400 mg three times daily for at least 3 months), treadmill walking distances significantly improve.[94] The results of these trials have been reviewed by Radack and Wyderski[111]; the reported 20 to 85 percent rates of improvement in pain-free walking time have been questioned inasmuch as few trials have been double-blind, placebo-controlled, and of an adequate sample size. Although pentoxifylline administration may yield therapeutic benefits, improvements in walking distances may be relatively mild, are difficult to predict in affected individuals, and have never been shown to improve patient-derived indices of quality of life.

With the approval of cilostazol (Pletal) for use in the United States, clinicians have a new pharmacologic treatment for claudication. Cilostazol inhibits platelet aggregation and promotes vasodilatation by blocking phosphodiesterase. This results in an increased concentration of cyclic adenosine monophosphate within both platelets and blood vessels. Cilostazol also is able to cause mild decreases in serum triglyceride levels and mild increases in high-density lipoprotein levels. In controlled clinical trials, cilostazol has been proved to increase absolute walking distance. In the study conducted by Money and colleagues,[114] 239 patients with claudication were randomly assigned to receive cilostazol (100 mg twice daily) or placebo for 16 weeks. Those patients who received cilostazol, compared with placebo, treatment demonstrated a significant increase in their maximal walking distance (47 percent versus 12.9 percent, $P < .001$). Cilostazol responses are uniform regardless of patient age, gender, or severity of claudication. Of note for cardiovascular practitioners, cilostazol use is absolutely contraindicated in patients with congestive heart failure. Inasmuch as patients with PAD have an increased frequency of myocardial ischemic events, patients who may be candidates for cilostazol use should be screened for heart failure by consideration of their clinical history, by physical examination, or by selective use of noninvasive assessments of left ventricular systolic function. Once therapy is initiated, patients should utilize this medication for a minimum period of 8 to 12 weeks to determine whether clinical benefit will be achieved.

An ideal claudication therapeutic plan might include a series of steps to be applied sequentially: (1) immediate efforts to stress the importance of prompt discontinuation of cigarette smoking, and (2) participation in a regular (and ideally supervised) exercise program, inclusive of broad efforts to normalize atherosclerosis risk factors. If the patient does not improve adequately with these interventions, then (3) a pharmacologic treatment trial (with either cilostazol or pentoxifylline) for 2 to 3 months may be indicated. Individuals who remain markedly symptomatic thereafter should undergo lower extremity arterial imaging studies and be considered candidates for (4) revascularization strategies, after completion of a clear discussion or relative risks, benefits, and durability of each procedure.

Vasodilator drugs have not been shown to improve symptoms in patients with claudication. Direct-acting vasodilators may have minimal effects at the focal atherosclerotic site, do not vasodilate lower extremity collateral vessels, and may elicit a fall in blood pressure (and thus limb perfusion pressure) if preferential vasodilatory effects occur in other nondiseased circulations.[115] Although β-blockers are widely believed to have detrimental clinical effects on

TABLE 73–4 Indications for Referral of Patients With Lower Extremity Arterial Occlusive Disease to a Vascular Specialist

Severe claudication (refractory to exercise rehabilitation and pharmacologic therapies)
Ischemic foot ulceration
Rest pain

claudication, well-controlled clinical trials have demonstrated a symptom-neutral effect of these agents in most patients.[116, 117] Inasmuch as β-blocker therapy may be efficacious for the treatment of associated coronary artery disease or myocardial infarction, these drugs need not be empirically withdrawn from the patient with claudication.

Antiplatelet therapy may alter the rate of atherosclerotic disease progression, the incidence of thrombotic events in the limb circulation, and the rate of adverse coronary and cerebrovascular ischemic events. Hess and coworkers[118] reported beneficial effects of aspirin and an aspirin/dipyridamole combination on quantitative angiographic rates of femoral arterial atherosclerosis disease progression in a small cohort of patients followed up over 2 years. In this study, the effects of antiplatelet therapy on claudication symptoms and ischemic event rates were not reported. Larger trials have generally corroborated beneficial effects of antiplatelet therapies in populations of subjects with documented arterial occlusive disease.[119, 120] Ticlopidine has been shown to blunt ischemic event rates, to perhaps improve claudication symptoms, and to improve patient survival, as documented in the Swedish Ticlopidine Multicentre Study and smaller trials in PAD patients.[121, 122]

The relative benefits of aspirin and clopidogrel (a new adenosine diphosphate receptor antagonist) on rates of myocardial infarction, stroke, and death have been reported from the prospective international evaluation studies in the Clopidogrel vs. Aspirin in Patients at Risk of Ischemic Events (CAPRIE) investigation.[123] CAPRIE was designed to recruit individuals with various manifestations of arterial atherosclerosis in the cerebrovascular, coronary arterial, or limb arterial circulations. This study was designed in this manner based on the observation that individuals who present with stroke, myocardial infarction, or claudication all experience the same systemic "atherothrombotic" disease and comparably high rates of heart attack, stroke, and vascular death. Thus, the CAPRIE investigators recruited 19,185 patients from these three eligible cohorts, and 6452 individuals with PAD were prospectively studied. For CAPRIE, PAD was defined as either (1) self-reported claudication with an ABI less than 0.85, or (2) the occurrence of prior lower extremity arterial revascularization procedures (either angioplasty or vascular surgery) or amputation. After a mean follow-up period of 1.91 years, there was an overall relative risk reduction of 8.7 percent over aspirin in the total study population (with a primary end point of decreased rates of ischemic stroke, myocardial infarction, or vascular death). Post hoc analysis demonstrated that patients with PAD had a significantly improved outcome, with a 23.8 percent risk reduction compared with aspirin alone. Overall, current clinical data therefore suggest that all patients with documented arterial occlusive disease of the limbs should receive antiplatelet therapy unless it is otherwise contraindicated. Warfarin may be beneficial in improving patency rates of lower extremity arterial grafts.[124]

The potential of certain medical therapies, such as iloprost (a stable prostaglandin analogue)[125, 126] and other novel vasodilators, appears promising, but their exact roles will await the results of ongoing clinical investigation. Chelation therapy using ethylenediaminetetraacetic acid does not appear to offer significant benefit for the claudicator.[127]

SURGICAL TREATMENT

Revascularization is indicated for all patients with severe debilitating claudication, ischemic rest pain, or tissue necrosis. In many medical centers, a surgical approach remains the commonest means of revascularization. Bypass operations (using autologous or synthetic grafts)[128–130] or endarterectomy[131] remain the procedures of choice.

Isolated proximal aortoiliac disease or multisegmental iliofemoral disease provides an anatomically favorable clinical scenario for surgical improvement of arterial inflow. The functional significance of proximal atherosclerosis can be determined by combined use of the noninvasively measured segmental pressures, intra-arterial pressures obtained during the angiographic study, and angiographic appearance of the involved vessels. Surgical approaches may include either local thromboendarterectomy or implantation of an aortoiliac Dacron vascular prosthesis. Five-year patency rates of 85 to 90 percent are typical for aortoiliac or femoral grafts.[132] Whereas such operations are generally long lasting, selected patients with concomitant coronary artery disease or other illnesses might not tolerate such an extensive vascular operative approach. For these individuals, unilateral iliac disease might be treated by either a femoral-femoral or an axillary-femoral bypass graft. Whereas these latter operative approaches may be less enduring, multiyear graft patency, effective limb salvage, and alleviation of symptoms may be an adequate clinical goal if long-term cardiac survival cannot be achieved or would be compromised by a more aggressive operative approach. Clearly, close consultation between medical caregivers, the vascular surgeon, and the patient is required to determine the optimal therapeutic revascularization approach.

The femoropopliteal and femorotibial segments may be successfully reconstructed by use of either native saphenous veins, prosthetic Dacron, or polytetrafluoroethylene grafts. As with all vascular procedures, the clinical success of the operative approach depends on the degree of impairment of arterial inflow, arterial outflow distal to the graft, choice of graft material, and other patient-related issues (e.g., successful tobacco abstinence, use of an antiplatelet agent). Careful review of the indications for distal lower extremity vascular reconstruction is required because the long-term patency rates in these sites have been less impressive than for more proximal disease. Establishment of above-the-knee femoropopliteal grafts by an experienced surgeon may result in 5-year patency rates of 70 to 80 percent. In contrast, below-knee saphenous vein femoropopliteal or femorotibial grafts usually achieve overall patency rates of only 40 to 50 percent.[133] The long-term patency rates for synthetic grafts placed below the knee are significantly less than those for autologous grafts.[134] Thus, whereas such operations are usually justified for patients with limb-threatening rest pain or ischemic ulceration, the reduced longevity of these procedures may make their use less beneficial for all but those with the most refractory claudication. The use of thrombolytic therapy in conjunction with surgery has become more widespread and appears to offer a distinct advantage in situations where relatively fresh thrombus (embolus or thrombosis in situ) complicates the intended revascularization.[135]

PERCUTANEOUS ANGIOPLASTY

The advent of catheter-based therapies has profoundly altered the treatment of lower extremity arterial occlusive disease, just as percutaneous transluminal coronary angioplasty has transformed care strategies for atherosclerotic disease in the coronary circulation. However, the relative benefits of such percutaneous approaches to limb arterial disease remain less well appreciated, despite the fact that these approaches offer less risk and greater long-term benefit in the limb than in the coronary circulation.[136] Angioplasty procedures using simple balloon dilatation, atherectomy, laser, and intravascular stent placements may offer an alternative to surgery in many clinical settings. As for any revascularization approach, simple angiographic success (the short- or long-term patency rate for the treated, diseased segment) cannot serve as the sole definition of success. The likelihood of achieving a clinical success (amelioration of symptoms without undue adverse procedural effects) is dependent on many individual features, such as the focality versus the extent of arterial disease and the relative functional limitations of the treated versus the untreated limb, in addition to the simple patency rate for the specific percutaneous procedure.

Percutaneous angioplasty may serve as the treatment of choice for many patients with aortoiliac disease. It is common to achieve initial success rates of greater than 80 percent for iliac artery angioplasty, and excellent 5-year patency rates are common (>65 to 85 percent).[137] Thus, percutaneous dilatation of diseased iliac arterial segments is the most successful site for angioplasty in the arterial circulation. Richter and coworkers[138] suggest that use of stents at these sites may further improve long-term angiographic patency at 4 years. For cases in which iliac disease coexists with stenoses of more distal arterial segments, initial treatment of the iliac lesion may sufficiently improve inflow so that the perfusion pressure beyond the residual lesions becomes adequate to achieve the clinical goals (to improve claudication or rest pain or to achieve wound healing). Additionally, a strategy of initial iliac angioplasty may improve the patency of a downstream vascular conduit and yield a more satisfactory operative approach. For example, a patient with high-grade bilateral iliac stenoses and femoropopliteal disease might require major aortoiliac bypass grafting with subsequent femoropopliteal bypass. A successful percutaneous approach to the iliac disease could avert the more demanding (and high-risk) intra-abdominal operation. This procedure may yield a satisfactory clinical result; if not, the patient may then subsequently undergo the distal bypass procedure. Thus, initial proximal limb arterial angioplasty can be used to lessen the magnitude of subsequent operative revascularization or to avert entirely an operative approach.

Short-term angiographic success for percutaneous treatment of disease in the superficial femoral and infrapopliteal arteries is common. However, long-term success decreases as the caliber of the more distal native artery diminishes. For example, whereas 60 to 90 percent success rates for above-the-knee femoropopliteal procedures are the rule, sustained clinical improvement may be achieved in only 40 to 80 percent of patients who undergo below-the-knee femorotibial angioplasty procedures.[139] The role of adjuvant measures, such as atherectomy and laser angioplasty, remains controversial.[136, 139, 140–142] Application of intravascular stents to the superficial femoral artery has not yielded results as favorable as in the iliac site because of a persistent high rate of restenosis.[143] As with surgery, thrombolysis is playing an increasing role as an aid to revascularization in limbs in which thrombus contributes to the vascular obstruction.[135] Although the long-term results of percutaneous procedures in the distal arterial sites remain somewhat problematic, the role of this approach can still be markedly beneficial for specific individuals. Distal arterial disease is less likely to be the cause of claudication, and such patients are more likely to require revascularization to treat a nonhealing ischemic wound. These patients are otherwise likely treated conservatively via methods that rely on months of bed rest (or non–weight-bearing ambulation), with associated risk of further wound infection, muscular deconditioning, bone demineralization, and venous thrombosis. Many of these individuals may achieve a satisfactory clinical result whose benefit, even if only short term, is strikingly favorable.

References

1. Shepherd JT, Bergan JJ, Cohen RA, et al: Report of the task force on vascular medicine. Circulation 89:532, 1994.
2. Cooke JP, Dzau VJ: The time has come for vascular medicine. Ann Intern Med 112:138, 1990.
3. Chisolm GM, DiCorleto PE, Ehrhart LA, et al: Pathogenesis of atherosclerosis. *In* Young JR, Graor RA, Olin JW, Bartholomew JR (eds): Peripheral Vascular Diseases. p. 137. St. Louis: Mosby–Year Book, 1991.
4. Rooke TW, Stanson AW: Acquired diseases of the aorta. *In* Guiliano ER, Fuster V, Gersh BJ, et al (eds): Cardiology: Fundamentals and Practice. 2nd ed. p. 1961. St. Louis: Mosby–Year Book, 1991.
5. Luscher TF, Lie JT, Stanson AW, et al: Arterial fibromuscular dysplasia. Mayo Clin Proc 62:931, 1987.
6. Conn DL: Update on systemic necrotizing vasculitis. Mayo Clin Proc 64:535, 1989.
7. Genton E: Primary hypercoagulable state. *In* Spittell JA Jr (ed): Contemporary Issues in Peripheral Vascular Disease. p. 19. Philadelphia: FA Davis, 1992.
8. Love PE, Santoro SA: Antiphospholipid antibodies: anticardiolipin and the lupus anticoagulant in systemic lupus erythematosus (SLE) and in non-SLE disorders. Ann Intern Med 112:682, 1990.
9. Lee JC, Spittell JA Jr, Sauer WG, et al: Hypercoagulability associated with chronic ulcerative colitis: changes in blood coagulation factors. Gastroenterology 68:245, 1975.
10. Coffman JD: Vasospastic diseases. *In* Young JR, Graor RA, Olin JW, Bartholomew JR (eds): Peripheral Vascular Diseases. p. 361. St. Louis: Mosby–Year Book, 1991.
11. Sudlow CL, Warlow CP: Comparable studies of the incidence of stroke and its pathological types: results from an international collaboration. Stroke 28:491, 1997.
12. Fogelholm R, Murros K, Rissanen A, Ilmavirta M: Decreasing incidence of stroke in central Finland, 1985–1993. Acta Neurol Scand 95:38, 1997.
13. Berger K, Schulte H, Stogbauer F, Assmann G: Incidence and risk factors for stroke in an occupational cohort: the PROCAM Study. Stroke 29:1562, 1998.
14. Eikelboom BC: Ocular pneumoplethysmography. *In* Bernstein EF (ed): Noninvasive Diagnostic Techniques in Vascular Disease. 3rd ed. p. 330. St. Louis: Mosby–Year Book, 1985.
15. Strandness DE Jr: Extracranial arterial disease. *In* Duplex Scanning in Vascular Disorders. p. 92. New York: Raven, 1990.

16. Strandness DE Jr: Color. *In* Duplex Scanning in Vascular Disorders. p. 185. New York: Raven, 1990.
17. Rooke TW: Vascular complications of interventional procedures. *In* Holmes DR Jr, Vlietstra RE (eds): Interventional Cardiology. p. 340. Philadelphia: FA Davis, 1989.
18. Whittemore AD: Carotid artery disease: surgical management. *In* Cooke JP, Frohlich ED (eds): Current Management of Hypertensive and Vascular Diseases. p. 142. St. Louis: Mosby–Year Book, 1992.
19. Levy RA, Maki JH: Three-dimensional contrast-enhanced MR angiography of the extracranial carotid arteries: two techniques. AJNR 19:688, 1998.
20. Kent KC, Kuntz KM, Patel MR, et al: Perioperative imaging strategies for carotid endarterectomy: an analysis of morbidity and cost-effectiveness in symptomatic patients. JAMA 274:888, 1995.
21. The Asymptomatic Carotid Artery Stenosis Study Group: Study design for randomized prospective trial of carotid endarterectomy for asymptomatic atherosclerosis. Stroke 20:844, 1989.
22. A Veterans Administration Cooperative Study: Role of carotid endarterectomy in asymptomatic carotid stenosis. Stroke 17:534, 1986.
23. The CASANOVA Study Group: Carotid surgery versus medical therapy in asymptomatic carotid stenosis. Stroke 22:1229, 1991.
24. Hobson RW II, Weiss DG, Fields WS, et al: Efficacy of carotid endarterectomy for asymptomatic carotid stenosis. N Engl J Med 328:221, 1993.
25. Chambers BR, Norris JW: Outcome in patients with asymptomatic neck bruits. N Engl J Med 315:860, 1986.
26. Roederer GO, Langlios YE, Jaeger KA, et al: The natural history of carotid arterial disease in asymptomatic patients with cervical bruits. Stroke 15:605, 1984.
27. Moore WS, Barnett HJM, Beebe HG, et al: Guidelines for carotid endarterectomy: a multidisciplinary consensus statement from the Ad Hoc Committee, American Heart Association. Circulation 91:566, 1995.
28. Beebe UG, Clagett CG, DeWeese JA, et al: Assessing risk associated with carotid endarterectomy. Stroke 20:314, 1989.
29. North American Symptomatic Carotid Endarterectomy Trial (NASCET) Investigators: Clinical alert: benefit of carotid endarterectomy for patients with high-grade stenosis of the internal carotid artery. Stroke 22:816, 1991.
30. North American Symptomatic Carotid Endarterectomy Trial Collaborators: Beneficial effect of carotid endarterectomy in symptomatic patients with high-grade carotid stenosis. N Engl J Med 325:445, 1991.
31. European Carotid Surgery Trialist's Collaborative Group: MRC European carotid surgery trial: interim results for symptomatic patients with severe (70–99%) or with mild (0–29%) carotid stenosis. Lancet 337:1235, 1991.
32. Sze PC, Reitman D, Pincus MM, et al: Antiplatelet agents in the secondary prevention of stroke: meta-analysis of the randomized control trials. Stroke 19:436, 1988.
33. Hass WK, Easton JD, Adams HP, et al: A randomized trial comparing ticlopidine hydrochloride with aspirin for the prevention of stroke in high risk patients. N Engl J Med 321:501, 1989.
34. Gent M, Blakely JA, Easton JD, et al: The Canadian American Ticlopidine Study (CATS) in thromboembolic stroke. Lancet 1:1215, 1989.
35. Diener HC: Antiplatelet drugs in secondary prevention of stroke: lessons from recent trials. Neurology 49(5 suppl 4):S75, 1997.
36. Whisnant JP, Matsumoto M, Elveback LR: The effect of anticoagulant therapy on the prognosis of patients with transient cerebral ischemic attacks in a community. Rochester, Minnesota 1965–1969. Mayo Clin Proc 48:844, 1973.
37. Jonas S: Anticoagulant therapy in cerebrovascular disease: review and meta-analysis. Stroke 19:1043, 1988.
38. Chiantella V, Dean RH: Basic data related to clinical decision making in renovascular hypertension. Ann Vasc Surg 2:92, 1988.
39. Olin JW, Melia M, Young JR, et al: Prevalence of atherosclerotic renal artery stenosis in patients with atherosclerosis elsewhere. Am J Med 88:46N, 1990.
40. Working Group on Renovascular Hypertension: Detection, evaluation and treatment of renovascular hypertension. Arch Intern Med 147:820, 1987.
41. Simon N, Franklin SS, Bleifer KH, Maxwell MH: Clinical characteristics of renovascular hypertension: cooperative study of renovascular hypertension. JAMA 220:1209, 1972.
42. Hunt JC, Sheps SG, Harrison EG Jr, et al: Renal and renovascular hypertension. Arch Intern Med 133:988, 1974.
43. Eipper DF, Gifford RW Jr, Stewart B, et al: Abdominal bruits in renovascular hypertension. Am J Cardiol 37:48, 1976.
44. Maxwell MH, Rudnick M, Waks AU: New approaches to the diagnosis of renovascular hypertension. Adv Nephrol Necker Hosp 14:285, 1985.
45. Muller FB, Sealey JE, Case DB, et al: The captopril test in identifying renovascular disease in hypertensive patients. Am J Med 80:633, 1986.
46. Materson BJ: Special uses for captopril. Am J Kidney Dis 10(1 suppl 1):88, 1987.
47. Hughes JS, Dove HG, Gifford RW Jr, Feinstein AR: Duration of blood pressure elevation in acutely predicting surgical cure of renovascular hypertension. Am Heart J 101:408, 1981.
48. Bookstein JJ, Abrams HL, Buenger RE, et al: Radiologic aspects of renovascular hypertension. The role of urography and unilateral renovascular disease: cooperative study of renovascular hypertension. JAMA 220:1225, 1972.
49. Kremer-Hovinga TK, de Jong PE, Piers DA, et al: Diagnostic use of angiotensin converting enzyme inhibitors in radioisotope evaluation of unilateral renal artery stenosis. J Nucl Med 30:605, 1989.
50. Dondi M, Monetti N, Fanti S, et al: Use of technetium-99m-MAG3 for renal scintigraphy after angiotensin-converting enzyme inhibition. J Nucl Med 32:424, 1991.
51. Hoffman U, Edwards JM, Carter S, et al: Role of duplex scanning for the detection of atherosclerotic renal artery disease. Kidney Int 39:1232, 1991.
52. Olin JW, Piedmonte MR, Young JR, et al: The utility of duplex ultrasound scanning of the renal arteries for diagnosing significant renal artery stenosis. Ann Intern Med 122:833, 1995.
53. Desberg AL, Paushter DM, Lammert GK, et al: Renal artery stenosis: evaluation with color Doppler flow imaging. Radiology 177:749, 1990.
54. Leung DA, Hoffman U, Pfammatter T, et al: Magnetic resonance angiography versus duplex sonography for diagnosing renovascular disease. Hypertension 33:726, 1999.
55. Dunnick NR, Svetkey LP, Cohan RH, et al: Intravenous digital subtraction renal angiography: use in screening for renovascular hypertension. Radiology 171:219, 1989.
56. Wilms GE, Baert AL, Staessen JA, Amery AK: Renal artery stenosis: evaluation with intravenous digital subtraction angiography. Radiology 160:713, 1986.
57. Harvey RJ, Krumlovsky F, del Greco F, Martin HG: Screening for renovascular hypertension: Is renal digital-subtraction angiography the preferred non-invasive test? JAMA 254:388, 1985.
58. Gavras I, Gavras H: Effects of eprosartan versus enalapril in hypertensive patients on the renin-angiotensin-aldosterone system and safety parameters: results from a 26-week, double-blind, multicentre study. Curr Med Res Opin 15:15, 1999.
59. Gradman AH, Gray J, Maggiacomo F, et al: Assessment of once-daily eprosartan, an angiotensin II antagonist, in patients with systemic hypertension. Clin Ther 21:442, 1999.
60. Mourad G, Ribstein J, Argiles A, et al: Contrasting effects of acute angiotensin converting enzyme inhibitors and calcium antagonists in transplant renal artery stenosis. Nephrol Dial Transplant 4:66, 1989.
61. Novick AC, Ziegelbaum M, Vidt DG, et al: Trends in surgical revascularization for renal artery disease: ten years experience. JAMA 257:498, 1987.
62. Stanley JC: David M. Hume memorial lecture: surgical treatment of renovascular hypertension. Am J Surg 174:102, 1997.
63. Olin JW, Novick AC: Renovascular disease. *In* Young JR, Graor RA, Olin JW, Bartholomew JR (eds): Peripheral Vascular Disease. p. 267. St. Louis: Mosby–Year Book, 1991.
64. Mason RA, Newton GB, Kvilekval K, et al: Transaortic endarterectomy of renal visceral artery lesions in association with infrarenal aortic surgery. J Vasc Surg 12:697, 1990.
65. Sos TA, Pickering TG, Phil D, et al: Percutaneous transluminal renal angioplasty in renovascular hypertension due to atheroma or fibromuscular dysplasia. N Engl J Med 309:274, 1983.
66. Beebe HG, Chesebro K, Merchant F, Bush W: Results of renal artery balloon angioplasty limit its indications. J Vasc Surg 8:300, 1988.
67. Hollenberg NK: The treatment of renovascular hypertension: surgery, angioplasty, and medical therapy with converting-enzyme inhibitors. Am J Kidney Dis 10(1 suppl 1):52, 1987.

68. Cicuto KP, McLean GK, Oleaga JA, et al: Renal artery stenosis: anatomic classification for percutaneous transluminal angioplasty. AJR 137:599, 1981.
69. Englund R, Brown MA: Renal angioplasty for renovascular disease: a reappraisal. J Cardiovasc Surg 32:76, 1991.
70. Van de Ven PJ, Kaatee R, Beutler JJ, et al: Arterial stenting and balloon angioplasty in ostial atherosclerotic renovascular disease: a randomised trial. Lancet 353:282, 1999.
71. Weibull H, Bergqvist D, Jendteg S, et al: Clinical outcome and health care costs in renal revascularization-percutaneous transluminal renal angioplasty versus reconstructive surgery. Br J Surg 78:620, 1991.
72. Xue F, Bettmann MA, Langdon DR, Wivell WA: Outcome and cost comparison of percutaneous transluminal renal angioplasty, renal arterial stent placement, and renal arterial bypass grafting. Radiology 212:378, 1999.
73. McDaniel MD, Cronenwett JL: Basic data related to the natural history of intermittent claudication. Ann Vasc Surg 3:273, 1989.
74. Boyd AM: The natural course of arteriosclerosis of the lower extremities. Proc R Soc Med 55:591, 1962.
75. Imparato AM, Kim GE, Davidson T, Crowley JG: Intermittent claudication: its natural course. Surgery 78:795, 1975.
76. McAllister FF: The fate of patients with intermittent claudication managed non-operatively. Am J Surg 132:593, 1976.
77. Weitz JI, Byrne J, Clagett P, et al: Diagnosis and treatment of chronic arterial insufficiency of the lower extremities: a critical review. Circulation 94:3026, 1996.
78. Hertzer NR, Beven EG, Young JR, et al: Coronary artery disease in peripheral vascular patients: a classification of 1000 coronary angiograms and results of surgical management. Ann Surg 199:223, 1984.
79. Kramer JR, Hertzer NR: Coronary atherosclerosis in patients undergoing elective abdominal aortic aneurysm resection. Cardiovasc Clin 12:143, 1981.
80. Rooke TW: Arterial disease: noninvasive assessment. *In* Cooke JP, Frohlich ED (eds): Current Management of Hypertensive and Vascular Diseases. p. 199. St. Louis: Mosby–Year Book, 1992.
81. Jelnes Gaardsting O, Jensen KH, Baekgaard Tonnesen KH: Fate in intermittent claudication: outcome and risk factors. BMJ 294:1137, 1986.
82. Yao JST: Hemodynamic studies in peripheral arterial disease. Br J Surg 57:761, 1970.
83. Newman AB, Siscovick DS, Manolio TA, et al, for the Cardiovascular Health Study (CHS) Collaborative Research Group: Ankle-arm index as a marker of atherosclerosis in the Cardiovascular Health Study. Circulation 88:837, 1993.
84. Newman AB, Sutton-Tyrrell K, Vogt MT, Kuller LH: Morbidity and mortality in hypertensive adults with a low ankle/arm blood pressure index. JAMA 270:487, 1993.
85. Vogt MT, Cauley JA, Newman AB, et al: Decreased ankle/arm blood pressure index and mortality in elderly women. JAMA 270:465, 1993.
86. McKenna M, Wolfson S, Kuller L: The ratio of ankle and arm blood pressure as an independent risk factor of mortality. Atherosclerosis 87:119, 1991.
87. Hirsch AT, Baker S, Treat-Jacobson D, et al: The Minnesota Regional Peripheral Arterial Disease Screening Program: toward a definition of community standards of care. Vasc Med (in press).
88. Bacharach JM, Rooke TW, Osmundson PJ, Gloviczki P: Predictive value of transcutaneous oxygen pressure and amputation success by use of supine and elevation measurements. J Vasc Surg 15:558, 1992.
89. Kram HB, Appel PL, Shoemaker WC: Multisensor transcutaneous oximetric mapping to predict below knee amputation wound healing: use of a critical Po_2. J Vasc Surg 9:796, 1989.
90. Harries S, Vaughan CJ, Torrie EP, Galland RB: An evaluation of intravenous digital subtraction angiography in assessing lower limb ischaemia. Eur J Vasc Surg 5:205, 1991.
91. Hirsch AT, Treat-Jacobson D, Lando HA, Hatsukami DK: The role of tobacco cessation, anti-platelet, and lipid-lowering therapies for the treatment of peripheral arterial disease. Vasc Med 2:243, 1997.
92. Jonason T, Bergstrom R: Cessation of smoking in patients with intermittent claudication: effects on the risk of peripheral vascular complications, myocardial infarction and mortality. Acta Med Scand 221:253, 1987.
93. Faulkner KW, House AK, Castleden WM: The effect of cessation of smoking on the accumulative survival rates of patients with symptomatic peripheral vascular disease. Med J Aust 1:217, 1983.
94. Lassila R, Lepantalo M: Cigarette smoking and the outcome after lower limb arterial surgery. Acta Chir Scand 154:635, 1988.
95. Expert Panel on Detection, Evaluation, and Treatment of High Blood Cholesterol in Adults: Summary of the second report of the National Cholesterol Education Program (NCEP) expert panel on detection, evaluation, and treatment of high blood cholesterol in adults (adult treatment panel II). JAMA 23:3015, 1993.
96. Barndt R, Blankenhorn DH, Crawford DW, Brooks SH: Regression and progression of early femoral atherosclerosis in treated hyperlipoproteinemic patients. Ann Intern Med 86:139, 1977.
97. Buchwald H, Varco RL, Matts JP, et al, and the POSCH Group: Effect of partial ileal bypass on mortality and morbidity from coronary heart disease in patients with hypercholesterolemia: report of the Program on the Surgical Control of the Hyperlipidemias. N Engl J Med 323:946, 1990.
98. UK Prospective Diabetes Study (UKPDS) Group: Effect of intensive blood-glucose control with metformin on complications in overweight patients with type 2 diabetes (UKPDS 34). Lancet 352:1557, 1998.
99. Hiatt WR, Regensteiner JG: Exercise rehabilitation in the treatment of patients with peripheral arterial disease. J Vasc Med Biol 2:163, 1990.
100. England JD, Regensteiner JG, Ringel SP, et al: Muscle denervation in peripheral arterial disease. Neurology 42:994, 1992.
101. Regensteiner JG, Wolfel EE, Brass EP, et al: Chronic changes in skeletal muscle histology and function in peripheral arterial disease. Circulation 87:413, 1993.
102. Dahloff A, Bjorntorp P, Holm J, Schersten T: Metabolic activity of skeletal muscle in patients with peripheral arterial insufficiency: effect of physical training. Eur J Clin Invest 4:9, 1974.
103. Dahloff A, Holm J, Schersten T, Sivertsson R: Peripheral arterial insufficiency: effect of physical training on walking tolerance, calf blood flow and blood flow resistance. Scand J Rehabil Med 8:18, 1976.
104. Hiatt WR, Nawaz D, Regenstein JG, et al: The valuation of exercise performance in patients with peripheral arterial disease. J Cardiopulm Rehabil 12:525, 1988.
105. Hiatt WR: Benefit of exercise conditioning for patients with peripheral arterial disease. Circulation 81:602, 1990.
106. Gardner AW, Poehlman ET: Exercise rehabilitation programs for the treatment of claudication pain. A meta-analysis. JAMA 274:975, 1995.
107. Lundgren F, Dahlloff A, Lundholm K, et al: Intermittent claudication—surgical reconstruction or physical training? A prospective randomized trial of treatment efficiency. Ann Surg 209:346, 1989.
108. Creasy TS, McMillan PJ, Fletcher EWL, et al: Is percutaneous transluminal angioplasty better than exercise for claudication? Preliminary results from a prospective randomized trial. Eur J Vasc Surg 4:135, 1990.
109. Hirsch AT, Ekers MA: A comprehensive vascular medical therapeutic approach to peripheral arterial disease: the foundation of effective vascular rehabilitation. *In* Fahey V (ed): Vascular Nursing. 3rd ed. Philadelphia: WB Saunders, 1999.
110. Dettelbach HR, Aviado DM: Clinical pharmacology of pentoxifylline with special reference to its hemorrheologic effect for the treatment of intermittent claudication. J Clin Pharmacol 25:8, 1985.
111. Radack K, Wyderski RJ: Conservative management of intermittent claudication. Ann Int Med 113:135, 1990.
112. Cameron HA, Waller PC, Ramsay LE: Drug treatment of intermittent claudication: a critical analysis of the methods and findings of published clinical trials, 1965–1985. Br J Clin Pharmacol 26:569, 1988.
113. Porter JM, Cutler BS, Lee BY, et al: Pentoxifylline efficacy in the treatment of intermittent claudication: multicenter controlled double-blind trial with objective assessment of chronic arterial occlusive disease patients. Am Heart J 104:66, 1982.
114. Money SR, Herd JA, Isaacsohn JL, et al: Effect of cilostazol on walking distances in patients with intermittent claudication caused by peripheral vascular disease. J Vasc Surg 27:267, 1998.
115. Coffman JD: Vasodilator drugs in peripheral vascular disease. N Engl J Med 300:713, 1979.

116. Radack K, Deck C: β-Adrenergic blocker therapy does not worsen intermittent claudication in subjects with peripheral arterial disease: a meta-analysis of randomized controlled trials. Arch Intern Med 151:1769, 1991.
117. Hiatt WR, Stoll S, Nies AS: Effect of beta-adrenergic blockers on the peripheral circulation in patients with peripheral arterial disease. Circulation 72:1226, 1985.
118. Hess H, Miewtaschik A, Deischsel G: Drug-induced inhibition of platelet function delays progression of peripheral occlusive arterial disease: a prospective, double-blind arteriographically controlled trial. Lancet 1:415, 1985.
119. Clagett GP, Genton E, Salzman EW: Antithrombotic therapy in peripheral vascular disease. Chest 95(suppl):128S, 1989.
120. Antiplatelet Trialists Collaboration: Collaborative overview of randomized trials of antiplatelet therapy. I: prevention of death, myocardial infarction, and stroke by prolonged antiplatelet therapy in various categories of patients. BMJ 308:81, 1994.
121. Janzon L, Bergquist D, Boberg J, et al: Prevention of myocardial infarction and stroke in patients with intermittent claudication: effects of ticlopidine. Results from STIMS, the Swedish Ticlopidine Multicentre Study. J Int Med 227:301, 1991.
122. Balsano F, Cocherri S, Libretti A, et al: Ticlopidine in the treatment of intermittent claudication: a 21-month double-blind trial. J Lab Clin Med 114:84, 1989.
123. CAPRIE Steering Committee: A randomised, blinded, trial of clopidogrel versus aspirin in patients at risk of ischaemic events (CAPRIE). Lancet 348:1329, 1996.
124. Arfvidsson B, Lundgren F, Drott C, et al: Influence of coumarin treatment on patency and limb salvage after peripheral arterial reconstructive surgery. Am J Surg 159:556, 1990.
125. Ylitalo P, Kaukinen S, Reinikainen P, et al: A randomized, double-blind, crossover comparison of iloprost with dextran in patients with peripheral arterial occlusive disease. Int J Clin Pharmacol Ther Toxicol 28:197, 1990.
126. Fiessinger JN, Schafer M: Trial of iloprost versus aspirin treatment for critical limb ischaemia of thromboangiitis obliterans: the TAO Study. Lancet 335:555, 1990.
127. Van Rij AM, Solomon C, Packer SG, Hopkins WG: Chelation therapy for intermittent claudication: a double-blind, randomized, controlled trial. Circulation 90:1194, 1994.
128. Bergmark C, Johansson G, Olofsson P, Swedenborg J: Femoropopliteal and femoro-distal bypass: a comparison between in situ and reversed technique. J Cardiovasc Surg 32:117, 1991.
129. Moore WS, Quinones-Baldrich WJ: An argument against all-autogenous tissue for vascular bypasses below the inguinal ligament. Adv Surg 24:91, 1991.
130. Rosenblatt MD, Quist WC, Sidaway AN, et al: Results of vein graft reconstruction of the lower extremity in diabetic and nondiabetic patients. Surg Gynecol Obstet 171:331, 1990.
131. Kalman PG, Johnston KW, Walker PM: The current role of isolated profundaplasty. J Cardiovasc Surg 31:107, 1990.
132. Brewster DC: Clinical and anatomical considerations for surgery in aortoiliac disease and results of surgical treatment. Circulation 83(suppl I):I-42, 1991.
133. Krajewski LP, Olin JW: Atherosclerosis of the aorta and lower extremity arteries. *In* Young JR, Graor RA, Olin JW, Bartholomew JR (eds): Peripheral Vascular Diseases. p. 179. St. Louis: Mosby–Year Book, 1991.
134. Hallett JW Jr: Trends in revascularization of the lower extremity. Mayo Clin Proc 61:369, 1986.
135. Comerota AJ, White JV, Grosh JD: Intraoperative intra-arterial thrombolytic therapy for salvage of limbs in patients with distal arterial thrombosis. Surg Gynecol Obstet 169:238, 1989.
136. Isner JM, Rosenfield K: Redefining the treatment of peripheral artery disease. Role of percutaneous revascularization. Circulation 88:1534, 1993.
137. Rooke TW, Stanson AW, Johnson CM, et al: Percutaneous transluminal angioplasty in the lower extremities: a 5-year experience. Mayo Clin Proc 62:85, 1987.
138. Richter GM, Roeren T, Noeledge G, et al: Prospective randomized trail: iliac stenting versus PTA [abstract]. Angiology 43:268, 1992.
139. Widlus DM, Osterman FA Jr: Evaluation and percutaneous management of atherosclerotic peripheral vascular disease. JAMA 261:3148, 1989.
140. Odink HF, de Valois HC, Eikelboom BC: Femoropopliteal arterial occlusions: laser-assisted versus conventional percutaneous transluminal angioplasty. Radiology 181:61, 1991.
141. Belli AM, Cumberland DC, Procter AE, Welsh CL: Total peripheral artery occlusions: conventional versus laser thermal recanalization with a hybrid probe in percutaneous angioplasty—results of a randomized trial. Radiology 181:57, 1991.
142. Rosenthal D, Pesa FA, Gottsegen WL, et al: Thermal laser-assisted balloon angioplasty of the superficial femoral artery: a multicenter "review" of 602 cases. J Vasc Surg 14:152, 1991.
143. Sapoval MR, Long AL, Raynaud AC, et al: Femoropopliteal stent placement: long-term results. Radiology 184:833, 1992.

CHAPTER 74

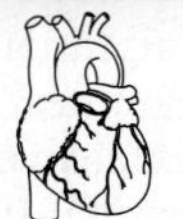

GENE THERAPY

Iris Baumgartner and Jeffrey M. Isner

VASCULAR DEVELOPMENT
THERAPEUTIC ANGIOGENESIS
VASCULAR ENDOTHELIAL GROWTH FACTOR
CLINICAL TRIALS IN PATIENTS WITH CRITICAL LIMB ISCHEMIA
ARTERIAL GENE THERAPY FOR INHIBITING RESTENOSIS
THERAPEUTIC ANGIOGENESIS FOR CORONARY ARTERY DISEASE

Angiogenic growth factors constitute a potentially novel form of therapy for patients with ischemic vascular disease. The feasibility of using recombinant formulations of angiogenic growth factors to augment collateral artery development through the stimulation of capillary growth in animal models of myocardial and hindlimb ischemia has been well established. This strategy for the treatment of vascular insufficiency, depicted schematically for peripheral vascular disease in Figure 74–1, has been termed *therapeutic angiogenesis.* Preclinical studies have suggested that at least five angiogenic growth factors, including acidic fibroblast growth factor, angiopoietin, basic fibroblast growth factor, hepatocyte growth factor, and vascular endothelial growth factor (VEGF), are sufficiently potent to merit further investigation. In the case of VEGF, a cytokine secreted from intact cells, bioavailability and meaningful angiogenic bioactivity were also shown to be achievable through intramuscular gene transfer, with a recent clinical phase I trial in patients with chronic critical limb ischemia cautiously interpreted to support both the strategy of somatic gene therapy and the concept of therapeutic angiogenesis.

VASCULAR DEVELOPMENT

Vascular development can be categorized into vasculogenesis, angiogenesis, and arteriogenesis. *Vasculogenesis* has been considered to be confined to embryogenesis and consists of the initial process of in situ differentiation of endothelial cells from mesodermal precursors (angioblasts) and their subsequent organization into a primary capillary plexus.[1] VEGF and its receptor, Flk-1/KDR, appear to modulate this developmental sequence, based on gene targeting studies performed in mice that showed that the deletion of either gene is lethal early in embryogenesis.[2, 3] More recent data indicate that vasculogenesis is not confined to fetal development and that bone marrow–derived circulating endothelial progenitor cells also contribute to postnatal neovascularization.[4] Proceeding from the primary vascular plexus, stationary endothelial cells can form new capillaries by sprouting from their vessel of origin, termed *angiogenesis.* This process, in which endothelial cells from a quiescent microvasculature with a turnover of thousands

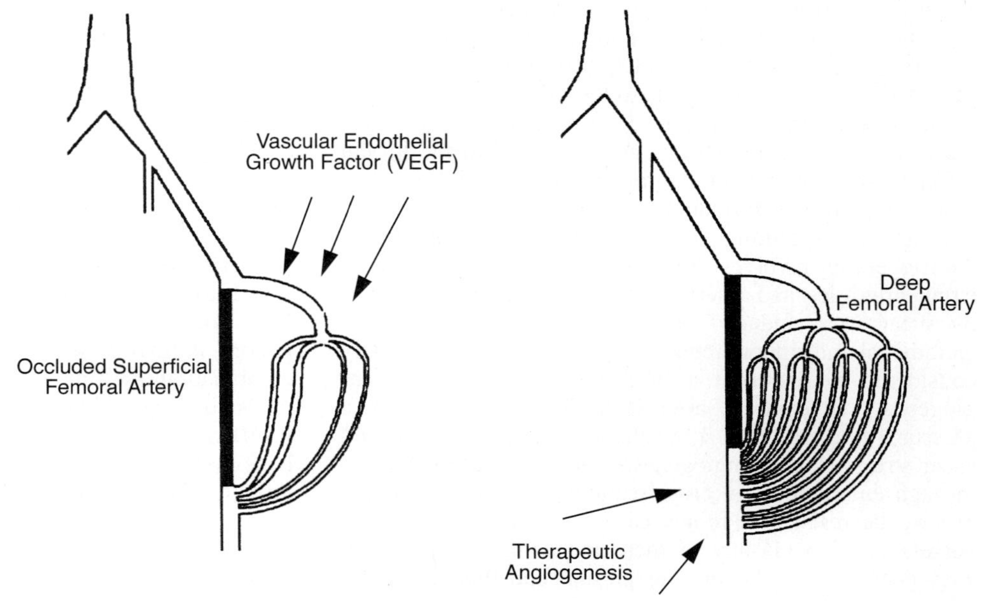

FIGURE 74–1 Schematic depiction of the strategy of therapeutic angiogenesis. **Left,** Before treatment, occlusion of the superficial femoral artery with the deep femoral artery reconstituting the popliteal artery. Stimulation of collateral vessel development by vascular endothelial growth factor (VEGF)–augmented therapeutic angiogenesis. **Right,** After treatment, collateral network has increased to accommodate greater volume of blood transport to distal limb.

of days are activated to undergo rapid proliferation and migration,[5] can be initiated by a variety of cytokines. The families of angiogenic growth factors investigated most extensively are VEGF and fibroblast growth factors.[6] Other cytokines in or near the blood vessel wall implicated in the process of angiogenesis include hepatocyte growth factor[7] and platelet-derived growth factor,[8] which each interact with specific receptors on endothelial or smooth muscle cells. Angiopoietin-1, which was first identified in 1996, is suggested to mediate vessel maturation conferred by recruitment and interaction of endothelial cells with periendothelial support cells.[9, 10] Angiopoietin-2, a natural antagonist of angiopoietin-1, was demonstrated to disrupt blood vessel formation in the mouse embryo with transgenic overexpression.[11]

The formation of new capillaries through sprouting from existing capillaries or venules occurs in a series of steps. Stationary, nonproliferative intimal endothelial cells are activated by cytokines, followed by the release of extracellular proteinases (plasminogen activators, metalloproteinases) required to degrade basement membrane and matrix constituents underlying the endothelium. Thereafter, endothelial cells actually migrate, reattach, and proliferate beyond the vessel of origin. The newly originated column of endothelial cells lengthens and forms a three-dimensional tubular structure (branch), and individual branches fuse to loops through which blood can flow. Loops generate new sprouts, and the process is repeated until a network of new capillaries is formed, which are capped and inactivated via reciprocal interaction with pericytes.[12] For vessels larger than capillaries, vascular smooth muscle cells must migrate as well. Pericytes and smooth muscle cells are attracted via chemotactic factors up-regulated in association with active capillary sprouting. Intraluminal and extraluminal factors are involved in further modification of blood vessels (*arteriogenesis*), which can mature or regress along with the demands of the tissue or organs they supply.

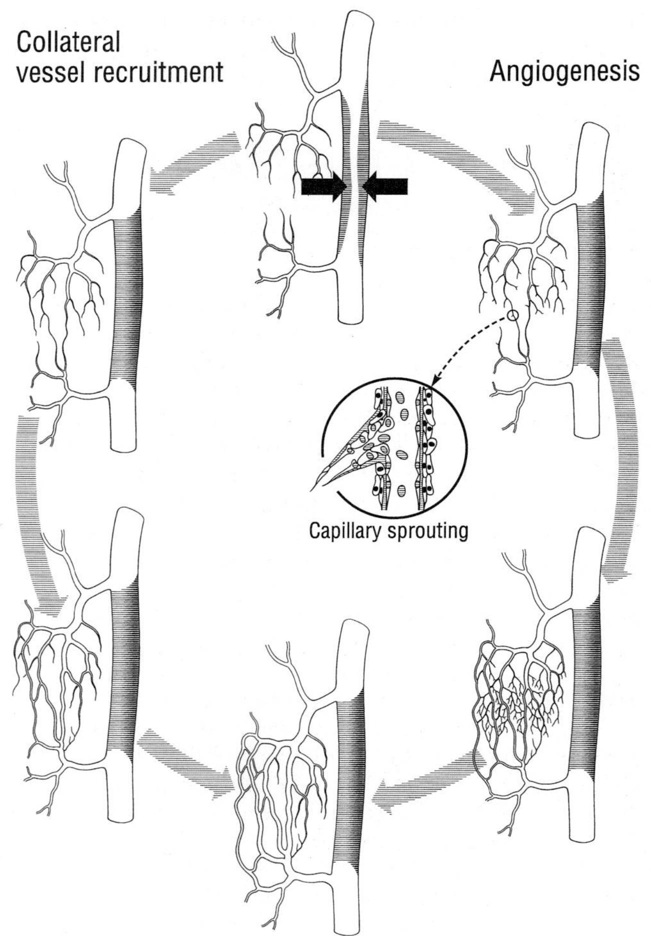

FIGURE 74–2 Schematic depiction of collateral vessel development. Three interconnected mechanisms are involved to partially adapt to regional tissue ischemia induced by an obstruction of the stem artery: recruitment of preexisting collateral vessels **(left),** capillary sprouting driven by angiogenic factors **(right),** and shear stress–induced in situ enlargement and remodeling of collateral vessels ultimately leading to new mature arterial networks **(below).** The figure within the *black circle* represents an enlarged graph of capillary sprouting. Stationary endothelial cells of the vascular intima are activated by cytokines, followed by the release of proteinases required to degrade basement membrane and matrix constituents underlying the endothelium. Then, activated endothelial cells and circulating bone marrow–derived endothelial progenitor cells migrate and proliferate beyond the vessel of origin to form new three-dimensional tubular structures.

THERAPEUTIC ANGIOGENESIS

Nature has created mechanisms for partial adaptation to regional ischemia through the compensatory development of a functional collateral circulation driven by angiogenic factors (Fig. 74–2). Analogous to the primary development of the vasculature, collateral vessel growth involves three principal mechanisms. *Vasculogenesis* refers to the in situ differentiation of endothelial progenitor cells.[4, 13] *Angiogenesis* refers to the formation of new capillary networks via capillary sprouting from existing parent vessels.[14, 15] Arteriogenesis involves the in situ enlargement of preexisting arterioles and arteries into larger muscular arteries by shear stress–induced proliferation and remodeling of endothelial and smooth muscle cells.[15] Hypoxia is generally considered to represent a fundamental stimulus for angiogenesis. In contrast, arteriogenesis is dependent on a pressure gradient with a resultant increase in flow and shear stress. Hence, angiogenesis can affect arteriogenesis through enlargement in cross-sectional area and reduction in vascular resistance. In any case, it is true that collateral vessels develop via any of these mechanisms only when angiogenic growth factors are present and their receptors are expressed. The adaptive development of collateral vessels, however, is rather slow and often unable to compensate fully for the effects of ischemia. Why the collateral flow does not usually increase to the point that it can restore normal flow is not clear; it may result from a combination of a time lag in collateral development in case of rapid progression of the occlusive process and either insufficient local generation of necessary cytokines or perhaps a decreased responsiveness of endothelial cells to growth factors involved in neovascularization. It therefore seems logical to supplement or replace angiogenic growth factors, which are not present in abundance. This novel strategy for the treatment of vascular insufficiency has been termed *therapeutic angiogenesis* and has been proved to be successful for recombinant formulations of acidic and basic growth factors and VEGF in animal models of myocardial and hindlimb ischemia, respectively.[16–19]

Vascular Endothelial Growth Factor

VEGF (or VEGF-A) was discovered in the early 1980s by Dvorak and coworkers[20] as a factor that made blood vessels leaky; hence, it was given the name *vascular permeability factor.*[20] In the late 1980s, three groups of researchers cloned and sequenced VEGF and showed that it could promote endothelial cell migration and replication.[21–23] VEGF differs from other angiogenic growth factors by several features. First, high-affinity binding sites (Flt-1, Flk-1/KDR) are nearly restricted to endothelial cells, so the action of VEGF is endothelial cell specific.[24] Second, in contrast to other angiogenic growth factors, the VEGF gene possesses a secretory signal sequence, so the protein is naturally secreted by intact cells.[25] Third, the expression of VEGF and its major receptor Flk-1/KDR are tightly regulated by hypoxia, providing a physiologic feedback mechanism to accommodate the angiogenic effect to tissue oxygenation. Analogous to other hypoxia-inducible genes, the VEGF gene has a hypoxia recognition site (hypoxia-inducible factor [HIF-1]) in its promoter.[26] Furthermore, mRNA stability is increased (post-transcriptional regulation),[27] and the Flk-1/KDR receptor may be up-regulated in response to factors released from hypoxic tissues.[28, 29] Fourth, VEGF promotes bone marrow–derived endothelial progenitor cell mobilization and exerts proliferatory and migratory effects on endothelial progenitor cells.[30]

Evidence that VEGF stimulates angiogenesis in vivo had been developed in experiments performed on rat and rabbit cornea and the chorioallantoic membrane and in the rabbit bone graft model. The concept that the angiogenic activity of VEGF is sufficiently potent to achieve augmented neovascularization in ischemic tissues was established with a rabbit ischemic hindlimb model (femoral artery, including inferior epigastric, deep femoral, lateral circumflex, and superficial epigastric arteries, ligated and completely excised).[19] In these experiments, physiologic evidence of an increased downstream perfusion was documented on serial measurements of the lower limb blood pressure ratio. The Doppler pressure ratio (ischemic/nonischemic limb) was significantly greater in animals receiving VEGF than in control animals (0.75 ± 0.14 versus 0.48 ± 0.19, $P < .05$), which is consistent with the development of more mature collateral vessels. Direct anatomic evidence of an augmented collateral circulation was apparent from the increased number of angiographically visible collateral vessels at 10 and 30 days after VEGF administration. Complementary flow studies (intra-arterial Doppler flow-wire measurements) documented an increase in maximum blood flow[31] and restored vasoreactivity.[32] Necropsy examination showed a significantly higher capillary density in ischemic muscles and an increased endothelial cell proliferative activity,[33] which is consistent with the classic definition of angiogenesis formulated by Klagsbrun and Folkman.[34] Despite the fact that the mitogenic effects of VEGF have been previously shown to be limited to endothelial cells, the proliferative activity of smooth muscle cells in small, so-called midzone collaterals was also increased. VEGF has been shown to interact with lower-affinity binding sites to induce mononuclear phagocyte chemotaxis[35] and to ligate Flt-1 expressed by smooth muscle cells.[36] Thus, one cannot exclude the possibility that increased smooth muscle cell proliferation observed in response to VEGF represents a direct effect of VEGF. Two indirect effects are also possible. The ability to induce vascular permeability is a well known feature of VEGF that is responsible for its alternate designation as vascular permeability factor.[20] It is possible that the extravasation of certain growth factors from circulating blood results in the activation of smooth muscle cell proliferation. Alternatively, endothelial cells stimulated by VEGF may secrete factors that promote smooth muscle proliferation.[37]

The fact that the VEGF gene encodes a secretory signal sequence was more recently exploited as part of a strategy designed to accomplish therapeutic angiogenesis via somatic gene transfer. Gene products that are secreted may have profound paracrine effects, even when the number of transduced cells remains low. In contrast to genes such as the fibroblast growth factors, which do not typically encode a secretory signal sequence, the transfection of a much larger cell population might be required for the intracellular gene product to express its biologic effects.[38] The first technique used to perform cardiovascular gene transfer in humans involved arterial gene transfer with naked plasmid DNA that encoded VEGF driven by a cytomegalovirus promoter ($phVEGF_{165}$).[39] For delivery, a hydrogel-coated standard angioplasty balloon was used.[40] The polymer surface of the balloon acts like a sponge onto which concentrated DNA can be applied ex vivo and subsequently delivered into the vessel wall at the time of balloon inflation (Fig. 74–3). Site-specific transfection of $phVEGF_{165}$ was confirmed through an analysis of transfected arteries with reverse-transcription polymerase chain reaction.[41] Wolff and coworkers[42] also demonstrated evidence of transgene expression with the direct intramuscular injection of nonviral, covalently closed plasmid DNA. Adapted to the rabbit hindlimb model, intramuscular injection of $phVEGF_{165}$ into ischemic muscles showed significantly augmented development of collateral vessels compared with control animals; this was documented by serial angiograms in vivo and increased capillary density at necropsy. Amelioration of the hemodynamic deficit in the ischemic limb was shown by improvement in the limb blood pressure ratio in VEGF-transfected animals (0.70 ± 0.08) versus control animals (0.50 ± 0.18, $P < .05$). With regard to the target of therapeutic use, it has been noted that VEGF-induced angiogenesis was not indiscriminate or widespread but instead restricted to sites of ischemia.[43]

At least four isoforms—$VEGF_{121}$, $VEGF_{165}$, $VEGF_{189}$, and $VEGF_{206}$—have been identified and shown to result from alternative splicing of the VEGF-A transcript. These isoforms all share the important biologic property of mitogenicity for endothelial cells but differ markedly in solubility: the longer the isoform and the more basic amino acid residues, the greater the avidity for cell-surface heparan sulfates and proteoglycans of the extracellular matrix.

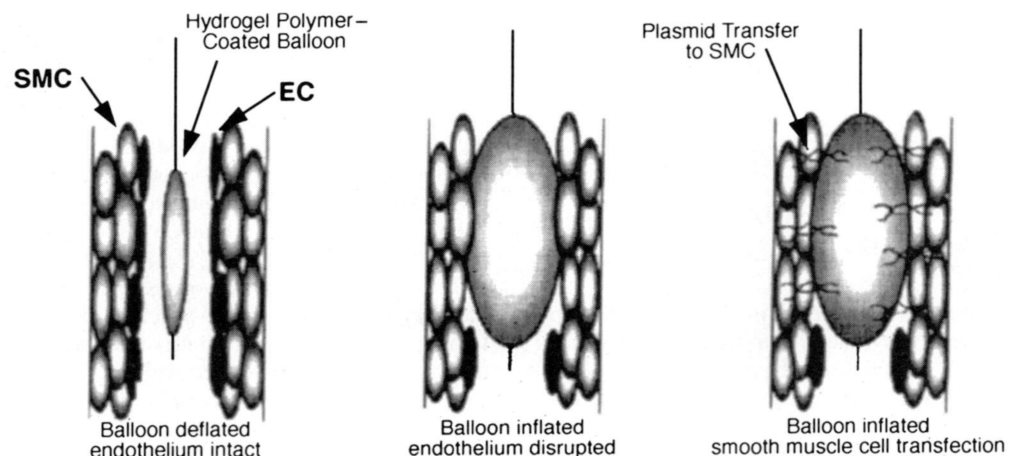

FIGURE 74–3 Schematic depiction of gene transfer with a hydrogel polymer–coated angioplasty balloon. EC, endothelial cell; SMC, smooth muscle cell.

Other VEGF-related genes have been identified: VEGF-B, VEGF-C, and placenta growth factor. VEGF-C was initially characterized for its lymphangiogenic potency induced by autophosphorylation of the tyrosine kinase receptor flk-4 (VEGFR-3) located on lymphatic cells. A VEGF-C signaling pathway via the endothelial cell specific receptor flk-1 was documented by Joukov and associates,[44] and stimulation of endothelial cell migration in vitro and augmented angiogenesis in the setting of tissue in vivo were shown by Witzenbichler and colleagues.[45]

CLINICAL TRIALS IN PATIENTS WITH CRITICAL LIMB ISCHEMIA

Striking advantages of VEGF gene transfer in particular are its confinement to the target organ, with minimal expression of the transgene in other organs, and an absent systemic effect due to its brief half-life of a few minutes in the circulation.[46] In December 1994, the first clinical trial of human gene therapy involving the percutaneous arterial gene transfer of phVEGF$_{165}$—a prospective, nonrandomized, open-label phase I trial for patients with critical limb ischemia[39]—was initiated. Although mechanical revascularization may be used to treat the majority of these patients, a considerable subset exists in whom the extent and distribution of arterial obstructions preclude revascularization. The situation is compounded by the lack of available medical therapy, so many of these patients face amputation.[47]

As tested in preclinical studies, plasmid DNA encoding VEGF$_{165}$ was applied to the hydrogel coating of a standard angioplasty balloon covered with a sheath to prevent the loss of genetic material. Under fluoroscopic guidance, the balloon was subsequently advanced and inflated within an artery supplying the critical ischemic limb. Dose-escalating treatment was initiated with 100 μg of phVEGF$_{165}$. Three patients presenting with rest pain and treated with 1000 μg were subsequently shown at 1-year follow-up to have improved blood flow to the ischemic limb and remained free of rest pain.[48] With the increase in dose of phVEGF$_{165}$ to 2000 μg, the first evidence of new blood vessel development became apparent.[49] One month after treatment, angiography revealed newly visible vessels at the calf level. Moreover, the patient developed three spider angiomas over the ankle and forefoot; however, unreliable transfection efficiency in atherosclerotic, calcified arteries and the potential risk of arterial injury at the site of transfection limited feasibility. In a second clinical trial, the same vector was delivered with an alternative delivery technique. Treatment was performed at the patient's bedside, with the DNA solution injected directly into ischemic muscles of the affected limb. For therapeutic use, four aliquots each consisting of 500 μg of naked plasmid DNA were injected with a 27-gauge needle (Fig. 74–4); the identical treatment was repeated 4 weeks later.[50] Gene expression at the protein level was documented as a transient peak of VEGF blood levels at 1 to 3 weeks after each treatment, measured with the use of an enzyme-linked immunosorbent assay. Ankle or toe brachial index increased from 0.33 at baseline to 0.48 at 12-week follow-up, and serial contrast angiograms at 4, 8, and 16 weeks showed newly visible, small (200–800 μm) collateral vessels in 70 percent of treated limbs (Fig. 74–5).

Several mechanisms may account for the angiogenic effect of VEGF seen in these patients. Because VEGF is mitogenic in vitro, the most obvious explanation is that the angiogenic effect in vivo was achieved via a similar mechanism, that is, from the proliferation and migration of endothelial cells followed by the formation of new blood vessels. Another possibility alone or in combination is the recruitment of preexisting collateral blood vessels. The importance of this distinction is further emphasized by the different stimuli that may be involved in the regulation of arteriogenesis and angiogenesis. Although proximal occlusion of an limb artery leads to ischemia distally, angiographically observed collateral vessels frequently develop or are visible in a region upstream from the ischemic territory that is not ischemic. A third possibility is that VEGF also improves the vasomotor function of large and small arteries of animals with chronic ischemia. In addition, there is evidence that VEGF may promote the mobilization of bone marrow–derived endothelial progenitor cells[30] and that such cells administered in vivo promote neovasculari-

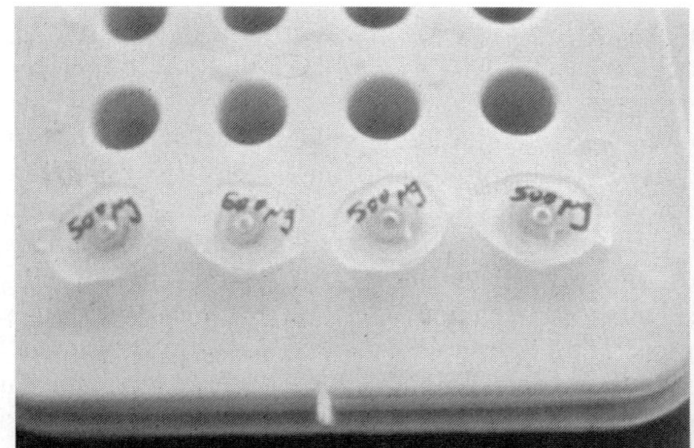
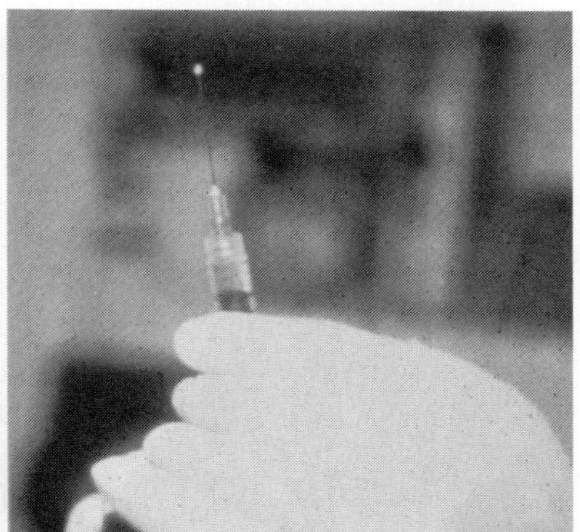

FIGURE 74–4 Elements of intramuscular gene transfer. Pure plasmid DNA is dissoluted in sterile 0.9 percent saline solution **(left)** and administered intramuscularly in a 5-ml syringe with a 27-gauge needle **(right).**

zation,[51] suggesting that vasculogenesis may have contributed. Promising hemodynamic and angiographic improvement were associated with profound clinical amelioration of symptoms. In a study of 19 limbs for which there was a mean follow-up period of 7 months after treatment, isolated rest pain resolved in 5 limbs, and gangrene healed or showed considerable improvement so that a major amputation could be prevented in 8 of 14 limbs. Despite below-the-knee amputation in six patients with intractable pain or infectious complications (32 percent), results were promising compared with historic controls.[52] Complications were limited to transient lower extremity edema, consistent with VEGF enhancement of vascular permeability, aggressively and successfully treated with diuretics. Although not found in any of the $phVEGF_{165}$-treated patients, all gene therapy designed to potentiate local angiogenesis carries the theoretical risk of potentiation of angiogenesis-driven diseases such as diabetic retinopathy[53] or tumor angiogenesis.[54] Data suggest that the former does not occur.[55] Concerning the latter, laboratory studies have established that VEGF expression did not lead to malignant proliferation or metastasis, a finding in agreement with the notion that the stimulation of angiogenesis is necessary but not sufficient for malignant growth.[56]

Arterial Gene Therapy for Inhibiting Restenosis

The term *restenosis* denotes recurrent narrowing of a blood vessel after successful revascularization procedure, such as percutaneous transluminal angioplasty (PTA). Despite the fact that PTA has been used widely to treat atherosclerotic obstructions in the coronary and peripheral vascular circulation for more than two decades, restenosis continues to be a vexing and expensive complication of this otherwise efficient intervention. Superficial femoral artery (SFA) stenosis represents one of the most common sites of peripheral

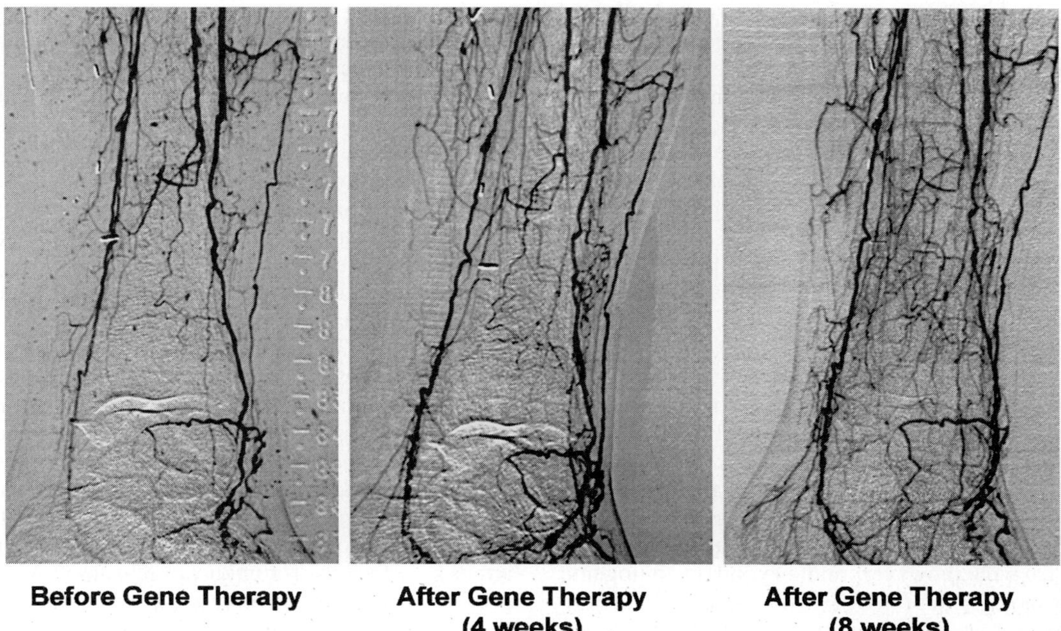

FIGURE 74–5 Serial digital subtraction angiograms in a patient before and 4 and 8 weeks after intramuscular vascular endothelial growth factor gene therapy. Newly visible collateral arteries, predominantly 200 to 800 μm in size, refill sparely vascularized areas around and above the ankle. The branching and regathering of the small collaterals are typical.

vascular obstruction. The acute procedural success rate for percutaneous revascularization of lesions in the SFA with the use of conventional guidewires and standard PTA is well in excess of 90 percent. On the other hand, as reported by Adar and associates,[57] who reviewed 12 selected clinical reports of SFA/popliteal PTA, the 3-year patency rate was 62 percent for patients presenting with intermittent claudication and 43 percent for patients undergoing revascularization for limb salvage, with the largest decline in patency occurring during the first 6 to 12 months. Multiple strategies have been used to inhibit recurrent intimal thickening (i.e., restenosis); these include antiproliferative strategies designed to interfere with smooth muscle cell proliferation, antiplatelet or anticoagulant therapy designed to prevent the development of a platelet-fibrin scaffold, anti-inflammatory drugs, spasmolytic drug therapy, and lipid-lowering agents. None of the clinical studies published to date have demonstrated significant reduction in restenosis, even for selected subgroups.

Previous studies in a variety of animal species demonstrated that extensive endothelial denudation of the arterial wall invariably leads to a proliferative response in smooth muscle cells.[58] These experimental studies have been cited to support the notion that certain functions of the endothelium, including its barrier function, antithrombogenicity, prevention of leukocyte adherence, and the production of growth-inhibitory molecules are critical to prevent luminal narrowing by neointimal thickening after vessel wall injury. The capability of certain cytokines to serve as mitogens for endothelial cells in vitro suggests that growth-stimulatory molecules might be exploited to accelerate *reendothelialization* after balloon injury. The first evidence that accelerated reendothelialization is indeed sufficiently potent to reduce intimal proliferation was shown by the direct application of VEGF recombinant protein to a balloon-denuded surface of a rat carotid artery.[59] The advantages and feasibility of direct arterial gene therapy using naked plasmid DNA encoding VEGF ($phVEGF_{165}$), as depicted schematically (see Fig. 74–4), were shown shortly thereafter. Experimentally, simultaneous balloon injury and $phVEGF_{165}$ transfection of the femoral artery in rabbits disclosed near-complete reendothelialization by 7 days, whereas the extent was less than 50 percent by day 7 and remained nearly 20 percent incomplete at 4 weeks in control animals transfected with a *LacZ* reporter gene. The impact on neointimal thickening was evaluated by light microscopic examination as the ratio of intimal area to medial area. *LacZ*-transfected arteries showed progressive neointimal thickening through 4 weeks (2-week ratio, 0.59 ± 0.04; 4-week ratio, 0.69 ± 0.10). In contrast, VEGF-transfected arteries disclosed significantly less intimal thickening, including the regression of intimal thickening between weeks 2 and 4 (2-week ratio, 0.20 ± 0.05; 4-week ratio, 0.14 ± 0.02, $P < .01$). In addition, $phVEGF_{165}$ transfection was associated with a concomitant reduction in proliferative activity in both the media and neointima.[60] Potentially contributory as well, however, and beyond its mitogenic effects, is the potential for VEGF to modulate qualitative aspects of endothelial cell function. Ku and colleagues[61] demonstrated that the direct application of VEGF to isolated segments of canine coronary arteries induces endothelium-dependent relaxation due to constitutive nitric oxide synthetase–mediated synthesis, release of endothelium-derived relaxing factor, or both.

In February 1994, the first clinical trial of human gene therapy involving the percutaneous arterial gene transfer of $phVEGF_{165}$—a nonrandomized, open-label phase I trial for patients with intermittent claudication due to femoropopliteal obstructions undergoing PTA[62]—was initiated. Gene transfer was made using a standard hydrogel-coated balloon angioplasty catheter to deliver a single application of $phVEGF_{165}$ (10 patients received 1000 μg and 9 patients received 2000 μg of plasmid DNA) to the site of balloon angioplasty. Clinical restenosis was defined by a subsequent fall in the ankle-brachial index by more than 0.15, a more than 50 percent stenosis on duplex, more than 50 percent luminal narrowing at the treatment site at angiography, and more than 75 percent narrowing in cross-sectional area with interventional ultrasonography. The average follow-up attained for the 19 patients was 9 months. No restenosis or only minimal intimal hyperplasia was observed in 14 (75 percent), and revascularization was required for clinical restenosis in only 4 (22 percent). These results may be cautiously interpreted to indicate that gene therapy, designed to accelerate reendothelialization at the site of PTA-induced endothelial disruption, represents a potentially useful strategy for the inhibition of restenosis in peripheral arterial disease.[63]

Therapeutic Angiogenesis for Coronary Artery Disease

Occlusions of one or more coronary arteries can occur unnoticed and may develop without overt myocardial infarction due to the development of collateral vessels. The time span necessary for collateral vascular growth in humans is, however, uncertain. Rentrop and associates[64] showed that there is a marked increase in the angiographic appearance of collateral vessels 10 to 14 days after persistent coronary occlusion in post-thrombolytic patients.[64] The functional importance of coronary collateral vessels is convincingly supported by a report from the Thrombolysis in Myocardial Infarction Phase 1 Trial.[65] In this study, patients were included only if coronary arteriography revealed absence of perfusion 90 minutes after the onset of thrombolytic therapy, thereby reducing the interference of antegrade flow in the limitation of myocardial damage. Under these conditions, collateral vascular supply reduced myocardial infarct size by 35 percent as assessed by enzymatic means and global ejection fraction, and by 12 percent at follow-up. Coronary collateral development has limitations: the time required for vascular growth and the incomplete nature of adaptation. The latter is particular significant because even under the best circumstances, collateral development usually remains incomplete; about 30 percent of the maximal blood flow capacity is restored, and collateral artery growth stops for unknown reasons.[66] Available therapeutic approaches to ischemic coronary artery disease have a goal of either relieving symptoms by reducing myocardial oxygen demand or restoring flow to a localized segment of the arterial tree by means of angioplasty or bypass surgery. However, a significant number of patients with ischemic heart disease are not candidates for these therapeutic strategies. At this stage, it is possible that the exogenous application of growth factors might be helpful, and studies in animals have conclusively shown improvement in myocardial perfusion by angiogenic growth factor administration.[18, 67, 68]

Schumacher and colleagues[69] reported the first angiogenic therapy of human coronary heart disease. In a randomized controlled clinical trial that included 20 patients with three-vessel coronary artery disease who underwent bypass surgery, recombinant human fibroblast growth factor-1 (FGF-1) was injected into the myocardium close to the left anterior descending coronary artery and distal to bypass anastomoses with the internal mammary artery. Follow-up angiography 12 weeks later showed coronary artery neovascularization extending from the area of FGF-1 injection. Meanwhile, the results of 20 patients treated in a phase I clinical trial of direct myocardial gene transfer of $phVEGF_{165}$ as the sole therapy in patients with medically intractable angina who were not candidates for further conventional revascularization procedures underscore the clinical benefit of therapeutic angiogenesis.[70, 71] The surgical procedure for direct intramyocardial gene delivery was performed under general anesthesia with a small anterior thoracotomy incision in the fourth or fifth intercostal space, exposing a 2 × 2-cm area of the left ventricle. The plasmid DNA was injected in 2-ml aliquots at four separate sites with a 3-ml syringe and a 25-gauge needle (Fig. 74–6). The first 10 patients received a total of 125 μg of $phVEGF_{165}$, whereas the second group of 10 patients received a total of 250 μg of $phVEGF_{165}$. All patients had experienced angina with minimal activity on a daily basis before gene therapy. By day 60, all patients had experienced a reduction in angina frequency, and 70 percent of patients followed up to 180 days were completely angina free. The use of nitroglycerin tablets decreased from a mean of 60 ± 5 per week before gene therapy to a mean of 7 ± 3 on day 60. Stress dobutamine or persantine single-photon emission computed tomography sestamibi studies provided evidence of an augmented collateral development with improvement between baseline and 60-day images in 13 of 17 patients analyzed (7 of 8 in the group with the 250-μg dose) (Plate 74–1). Angiographic collateral filling graded according to the Rentrop score (absent, 0; filling of side branches of the target occluded epicardial vessel without visualization of the vessel itself, +1; partial filling of the epicardial segment via collateral vessels, +2; complete filling of the epicardial segment of the occluded vessel, +3) at 60 days after gene transfer showed improvement in each of the 13 patients assessed.[64]

Therapeutic angiogenesis in patients with coronary artery disease is in its infancy, and it still must be clarified which cytokine and whether protein or gene therapy is preferred. In the case of VEGF, gene therapy is particular appealing because the VEGF gene encodes a signal sequence that permits the protein to be naturally secreted by intact cells. In addition, gene therapy could avoid systemic hypotension, which has been documented to occur with intracoronary administration of the VEGF protein.[72] For patients who are truly inoperable, gene transfer achieved percutaneously through a catheter-based system may ultimately be the most efficacious, and trials of such systems are under way. On the other hand, if additional studies confirm that angiogenic therapy is effective for the stimulation of collateral development, then its ultimate role will almost certainly include its use as an adjunctive revascularization strategy in patients undergoing bypass surgery who have a significant territory of ischemic myocardium that cannot be revascularized.

Theoretical concerns regarding growth factor therapy are that plaque angiogenesis might be exacerbated, that plaque progression is stimulated, and that plaque instability is induced.[73] In particular, it is suggested that VEGF-mediated enhancement of permeability adds an additional risk of plaque rupture. Nevertheless, there is little or no proof that therapeutic angiogenesis induced by VEGF is indeed dangerous with regard to plaque complications. First, there is no evidence from animal studies. Second, with regard to

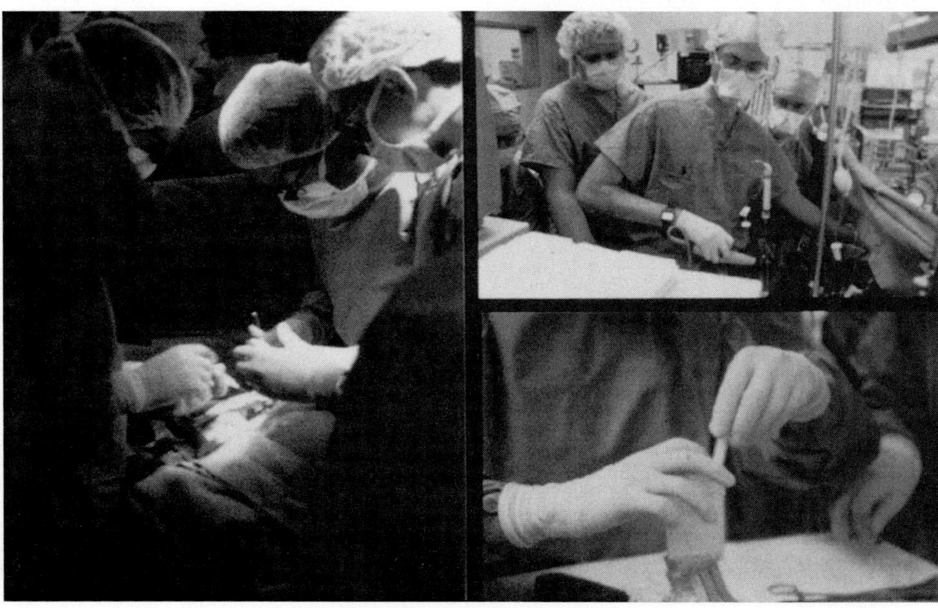

FIGURE 74–6 Exposure of the left ventricle via a small anterior thoracotomy incision in the fourth or fifth intercostal space and direct intramyocardial injection of plasmid DNA.

intramuscular plasmid or protein application, there is little or no circulating VEGF, a protein with a half-life of 3 minutes. Third, in patients with cancer who have high circulating levels of VEGF, there is no documentation of accelerated arteriosclerosis.[74] Fourth, more than 30 patients have undergone direct intra-arterial gene transfer of naked DNA encoding for VEGF (phVEGF$_{165}$) to a freshly injured arterial surface. In 12 patients, phVEGF$_{165}$ was administered to normal or moderately diseased arterial segments through the use of a hydrogel-coated angioplasty balloon to promote angiogenesis.[49] Follow-up angiography and intravascular ultrasonography showed no evidence of disease progression (J. M. Isner and colleagues, unpublished data). In an additional 20 patients, the same delivery strategy was used to accelerate reendothelialization after balloon angioplasty of femoral arteries. Follow-up examination up to 18 months after gene transfer[63] disclosed evidence of restenosis in only five patients (25 percent), approximately 50 percent of the anticipated incidence of restenosis predicted by historical controls.

REFERENCES

1. Risau W, Sariola H, Zerwes H-G, et al: Vasculogenesis and angiogenesis in embryonic stem cell–derived embryoid bodies. Development 102:471–478, 1988.
2. Shalaby F, Rossant J, Yamaguchi TP, et al: Failure of blood-island formation and vasculogenesis in Flk-1–deficient mice. Nature 376:62–66, 1995.
3. Ferrara N, Carver-Moore K, Chen H, et al: Heterozygous embryonic lethality induced by targeted inactivation of the VEGF gene. Nature 380:439–442, 1996.
4. Asahara T, Murohara T, Sullivan A, et al: Isolation of putative progenitor endothelial cells for angiogenesis. Science 275:964–967, 1997.
5. Schaper W, de Brabander M, Lewi P: DNA synthesis and mitoses in coronary collateral vessels of the dog. Circ Res 28:671–679, 1971.
6. Klagsbrun M, D'Amore PA: Regulators of angiogenesis. Annu Rev Physiol 53:217–239, 1991.
7. Van Belle E, Witzenbichler B, Chen D, et al: Potentiated angiogenic effect of scatter factor/hepatocyte growth factor via induction of vascular endothelial growth factor: the case for paracrine amplification of angiogenesis. Circulation 97:381–390, 1998.
8. Martins RN, Chleboun JO, Sellers P, et al: The role of PDGF-BB on the development of the collateral circulation after acute arterial occlusion. Growth Factors 10:299–306, 1994.
9. Suri C, Jones PF, Patan S, et al: Requisite role of angiopoietin-1, a ligand for the TIE2 receptor, during embryonic angiogenesis. Cell 87:1171–1180, 1996.
10. Kou-Gi S, Manor O, Magner M, et al: Direct intramuscular injection of plasmid DNA encoding angiopoietin-1 but not angiopoietin-2 augments revascularization in the rabbit ischemic hindlimb. Circulation 98:2081–2087, 1998.
11. Maisonpierre PC, Suri C, Jones PF, et al: Angiopoietin-2, a natural antagonist for Tie2 that disrupts in vivo angiogenesis. Science 277:55–60, 1997.
12. Sato Y, Rifkin DB: Inhibition of endothelial cell movement by pericytes and smooth muscle cells: activation of a latent transforming growth factor-beta 1–like molecule by plasmin during co-culture. J Cell Biol 109:309–315, 1989.
13. Risau W: Differentiation of endothelium. FASEB J 9:926–933, 1995.
14. D'Amore PA, Thompson RW: Mechanisms of angiogenesis. Annu Rev Physiol 49:453–464, 1987.
15. Schaper W, Ito WD: Molecular mechanisms of coronary collateral vessel growth. Circ Res 79:911–919, 1996.
16. Baffour R, Berman J, Garb JL, et al: Enhanced angiogenesis and growths of collaterals by in vivo administration of recombinant basic fibroblast growth factor in a rabbit model of acute lower limb ischemia: dose-response effect of basic fibroblast growth factor. J Vasc Surg 16:181–191, 1992.
17. Pu LQ, Sniderman AD, Brassard R, et al: Enhanced revascularization of the ischemic limb by means of angiogenic therapy. Circulation 88:208–215, 1993.
18. Banai S, Jaklitsch MT, Shou M, et al: Angiogenic-induced enhancement of collateral blood flow to ischemic myocardium by vascular endothelial growth factor in dogs. Circulation 89:2183–2189, 1994.
19. Takeshita S, Zheng LP, Brogi E, et al: Therapeutic angiogenesis: a single intra-arterial bolus of vascular endothelial growth factor augments revascularisation in a rabbit ischemic hindlimb model. J Clin Invest 93:662–670, 1994.
20. Dvorak HF, Brown LF, Detmar M, Dvorak AM: Vascular permeability factor/vascular endothelial growth factor, microvascular hyperpermeability, and angiogenesis. Am J Pathol 146:1029–1039, 1995.
21. Leung DW, Cachianes G, Kuang WJ, et al: Vascular endothelial growth factor is a secreted angiogenic mitogen. Science 246:1306–1309, 1989.
22. Plouet J, Shilling J, Gospodarowicz D: Isolation and characterization of a newly identified endothelial cell mitogen produced by AtT-20 cells. EMBO J 8:3801–3806, 1989.
23. Keck PJ, Hauser SD, Krivi G, et al: Vascular permeability factor, an endothelial cell mitogen related to PDGF. Science 246:1309–1312, 1989.
24. Klagsbrun M, D'Amore PA: Vascular endothelial growth factor and its receptors. Cytokine Growth Factor Rev 7:259–270, 1996.
25. Ferrara N, Houck K, Jakeman L, Leung DW: Molecular and biological properties of the vascular endothelial growth factor family of proteins. Endocr Rev 13:18–32, 1992.
26. Goldberg MA, Schneider TJ: Similarities between the oxygen-sensing mechanisms regulating the expression of vascular endothelial growth factor and erythropoietin. J Biol Chem 269:4355–4359, 1994.
27. Levy PL, Levy NS, Goldberg MA: Post-transcriptional regulation of vascular endothelial growth factor by hypoxia. J Biol Chem 271:2746–2753, 1996.
28. Brogi E, Schatteman G, Wu T, et al: Hypoxia-induced paracrine regulation of VEGF receptor expression. J Clin Invest 97:469–476, 1996.
29. Waltenberger, Mayr U, Pentz S, Hombach V: Functional upregulation of the vascular endothelial growth factor receptor KDR by hypoxia. Circulation 94:1647–1654, 1996.
30. Asahara T, Takahashi T, Kalka C, et al: A novel function for VEGF: mobilization of bone marrow–derived endothelial progenitor cells. Circulation 98(suppl I):I-605, 1998.
31. Bauters C, Asahara T, Zheng LP, et al: Physiological assessment of augmented vascularity induced by VEGF in ischemic rabbit hindlimb. Am J Physiol 267:H1263–H1271, 1994.
32. Bauters C, Asahara T, Zheng LP, et al: Recovery of disturbed endothelium-dependent flow in the collateral-perfused rabbit ischemic hindlimb after administration of vascular endothelial growth factor. Circulation 91:2802–2809, 1995.
33. Takeshita S, Kearney M, Loushin C, et al: In vivo evidence that vascular endothelial growth factor stimulates collateral formation by inducing arterial cell proliferation in a rabbit ischemic hindlimb. Am J Physiol 266:H1588–H1595, 1994.
34. Klagsbrun M, Folkman J: Angiogenesis. *In* Sporn MB, Roberts AB (eds): Peptide Growth Factors and Their Receptors. pp. 459–586. New York: Springer-Verlag, 1990.
35. Clauss M, Gerlach M, Gerlach H, et al: Vascular permeability factor: a tumor-derived polypeptide that induces endothelial cell and monocyte procoagulant activity, and promotes monocyte migration. J Exp Med 172:1535–1545, 1990.
36. Wang H, Keiser JA: Vascular endothelial growth factor upregulates the expression of matrix metalloproteinases in vascular smooth muscle cells: role of flt-1. Circ Res 83:832–840, 1998.
37. Folkman J, D'Amore PA: Blood vessel formation: what is its molecular basis? Cell 87:1153–1155, 1996.
38. Losordo DW, Pickering JG, Takeshita S, et al: Use of the rabbit ear artery to serially assess foreign protein secretion after site specific arterial gene transfer in vivo: evidence that anatomic identification of successful gene transfer may underestimate the potential magnitude of transgene expression. Circulation 89:785–792, 1994.
39. Isner JM, Walsh K, Symes JF, et al: Arterial gene therapy for therapeutic angiogenesis in patients with peripheral artery disease. Circulation 91:2687–2692, 1995.
40. Riessen R, Rahimizadeh H, Blessing E, et al: Arterial gene transfer using pure DNA applied directly to a hydrogel-coated angioplasty balloon. Hum Gene Ther 4:749–758, 1993.

41. Takashita S, Tsurumi Y, Couffinhal T, et al: Gene transfer of naked DNA encoding for three isoforms of vascular endothelial growth factor stimulates collateral development in vivo. Lab Invest 75:487–502, 1996.
42. Wolff JA, Malone RW, Williams P, et al: Direct gene transfer into mouse muscle in vivo. Science 247:1465–1468, 1990.
43. Tsurumi Y, Takeshita S, Chen D, et al: Direct intramuscular gene transfer of naked DNA encoding vascular endothelial growth factor augments collateral development and tissue perfusion. Circulation 94:3281–3290, 1996.
44. Joukov V, Pajusola K, Kaipainen A, et al: A novel vascular endothelial growth factor, VEGF-C, is a ligand for the Flt4 (VEGFR-3) and KDR (VEGFR-2) receptor tyrosine kinases. EMBO J 15:290–298, 1996.
45. Witzenbichler B, Asahara T, Murohara M, et al: Post-natal overexpression of vascular endothelial growth factor-C (VEGF-C/VEGF-2) promotes angiogenesis in the setting of tissue ischemia. Am J Pathol 153:381–394, 1998.
46. Isner JM: Therapeutic angiogenesis: a new frontier for vascular therapy. Vasc Med 1:79–87, 1996.
47. European Working Group on Critical Leg Ischemia: Second European consensus document on chronic critical leg ischemia. Circulation 84(suppl IV):IV-1–IV-26, 1991.
48. Isner JM: Arterial gene transfer of naked DNA for therapeutic angiogenesis: early clinical results. Adv Drug Delivery Rev 30:185–197, 1998.
49. Isner JM, Pieczek A, Schainfeld R, et al: Clinical evidence of angiogenesis following arterial gene transfer of phVEGF165 in a patient with ischemic limb. Lancet 348:370–374, 1996.
50. Baumgartner I, Pieczek A, Manor O, et al: Constitutive expression of phVEGF165 following intramuscular gene transfer promotes collateral vessel development in patients with critical limb ischemia. Circulation 97:1114–1123, 1998.
51. Kalka C, Masuda H, Takahashi T, et al: Administration of culture-expanded endothelial progenitor cells (EPC) augments therapeutic neovascularization. Circulation 98(suppl I):I-455, 1998.
52. Lepäntalo M, Mätzke S: Outcome of unreconstructed chronic critical leg ischaemia. Eur J Vasc Endovasc Surg 11:153, 1996.
53. Aiello LP, Avery RL, Arrigg PG, et al: Vascular endothelial growth factor in ocular fluids of patients with diabetic retinopathy and other retinal disorders. N Engl J Med 331:1480–1487, 1994.
54. Plate KH, Breier G, Weich HA, Risau W: Vascular endothelial growth factor is a potential tumor angiogenesis factor in vivo. Nature 359:845–847, 1992.
55. Vale PR, Rauh GF, Wuensch DI, et al: Influence of vascular endothelial growth factor on diabetic retinopathy. Circulation 98(suppl I):I-353, 1998.
56. Ferrara N, Winer J, Burton T, et al: Expression of vascular endothelial growth factor does not promote transformation but covers a growth advantage in vivo to Chinese hamster ovary cells. J Clin Invest 91:160–170, 1992.
57. Adar R, Critchfield GC, Eddy DM: A confidence profile analysis of the results of femoropopliteal percutaneous transluminal angioplasty in the treatment of lower-extremity ischemia. J Vasc Surg 10:57–67, 1989.
58. Scott-Burden T, Vanhoutte PM: The endothelium as a regulator of vascular smooth muscle proliferation. Circulation 87(suppl V):V-51–V-55, 1993.
59. Asahara T, Bauters C, Pastore CJ, et al: Local delivery of vascular endothelial growth factor accelerates reendothelialization and attenuates intimal hyperplasia in balloon-injured rat carotid artery. Circulation 91:2793–2801, 1995.
60. Asahara T, Chen D, Tsutumi Y, et al: Accelerated restitution of endothelial integrity and endothelium-dependent function following phVEGF165 gene transfer. Circulation 94:2892–2899, 1996.
61. Ku DD, Zaleski JK, Liu S, Brock TA: Vascular endothelial growth factor induces EDRF-dependent relaxation in coronary arteries. Am J Physiol 265:H586–H592, 1993.
62. Isner JM, Walsh K, Rosenfield K, et al: Arterial gene therapy for restenosis. Hum Gene Ther 7:989–1011, 1996.
63. Vale PR, Wuensch DI, Rauh GF, et al: Arterial gene therapy for inhibition restenosis in patients with claudication undergoing superficial femoral artery angioplasty. Circulation 98(suppl I):I-66, 1998.
64. Rentrop KP, Feit F, Sherman W, et al: Late thrombolytic therapy preserves left ventricular function in patients with collateralized total coronary occlusion: primary end-point findings of the 2nd Mount-Sinai New York University Reperfusion Trial. J Am Coll Cardiol 14:58–64, 1989.
65. Habib GB, Heibig J, Forman SA, et al: Influence of coronary collateral vessels on myocardial infarct size in humans: results of phase I Thrombolysis in Myocardial Infarction (TIMI) Trial. Circulation 83:739–746, 1991.
66. Schaper W, Piek JJ, Munoz-Chapuli R, et al: Collateral circulation of the heart. *In* Ware JA, Simons M (eds): Angiogenesis and Cardiovascular Disease. pp. 159–198. New York: Oxford University Press, 1999.
67. Pearlman JD, Hibberd MG, Chuang ML, et al: Magnetic resonance mapping demonstrates benefits of VEGF-induced myocardial angiogenesis. Nat Med 1:1085–1089, 1995.
68. Ware JA, Simons M: Angiogenesis in ischemic heart disease. Nat Med 3:158–164, 1997.
69. Schumacher B, Pecher P, von Specht BU, Stegmann T: Induction of neoangiogenesis in ischemic myocardium by human growth factors: first clinical results of a new treatment of coronary heart disease. Circulation 97:645–650, 1998.
70. Symes JF, Losordo DW, Vale PR, et al: Gene therapy with vascular endothelial growth factor for inoperable coronary artery disease: preliminary clinical results. Ann Thorac Surg 68(3):830–837, 1999.
71. Losordo DW, Vale PR, Symes JF, et al: Gene therapy for myocardial angiogenesis: initial clinical results with direct myocardial injection of phVEGF165 as sole therapy for myocardial ischemia. Circulation 98:2800–2804, 1998.
72. Lopez J, Laham R, Carrozza J, et al: Hemodynamic effects of intracoronary EGF delivery: evidence of tachyphylaxis and NO dependence of response. Am J Physiol 273:H1317–H1323, 1997.
73. Moulton KS, Heller E, Konerding MA, et al: Angiogenesis inhibitors endostatin or TNP-470 reduce intimal neovascularization and plaque growth in apolipoprotein E–deficient mice. Circulation 99:1726–1732, 1999.
74. Isner JM: Cancer and atherosclerosis. Circulation 99:1653–1655, 1999.

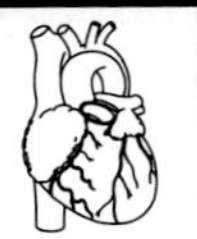

INTERVENTIONAL PROCEDURES FOR TREATMENT OF PERIPHERAL VASCULAR DISEASE

Zvonimir Krajcer

THE USE OF THROMBOLYTIC AGENTS FOR ARTERIAL OCCLUSIONS
Methods of Administration of Thrombolytic Agents
Doses of Infusion of Thrombolytic Agents
Predictors of Success of Thrombolysis
Patient Selection for Thrombolysis
Conclusion
RENOVASCULAR DISEASE
Prevalence and Natural History
Fibromuscular Dysplasia
Screening for Renovascular Hypertension
Renal Scintigraphy
Duplex Doppler
Magnetic Resonance Angiography
Renal Angiography
Indications for Revascularization
Surgical and Endovascular Revascularization for Renal Artery Stenosis
Percutaneous Transluminal Angioplasty and/or Stenting for Treatment of Atherosclerotic Renal Artery Stenosis
ABDOMINAL AORTIC ANEURYSMS
Epidemiology
Imaging Technology to Determine Patient Selection and/or Success of Treatment
Endovascular Treatment
CAROTID ARTERY DISEASE
Epidemiology
Carotid Endarterectomy
Carotid Angioplasty
Methods of Reducing the Incidence of Cerebral Emboli
Future Clinical Implications of Stent-Supported Carotid Angioplasty
ENDOLUMINAL TREATMENT OF TIBIOPERONEAL ATHEROSCLEROTIC DISEASE
Technique and Choice of Devices for Endoluminal Treatment
Results of Tibioperoneal Angioplasty
Thrombolytic Therapy for Tibioperoneal Occlusions
Atherectomy Devices
Stents
Laser Devices
Gene Therapy
Radiation Therapy
SUBCLAVIAN ARTERY OCCLUSIVE DISEASE
ENDOVASCULAR RADIATION THERAPY FOR TREATMENT OF PERIPHERAL ARTERIAL OCCLUSIVE DISEASE
Clinical Trials
Conclusions

THE USE OF THROMBOLYTIC AGENTS FOR ARTERIAL OCCLUSIONS

A principal goal of the treatment of acute limb ischemia is rapid restoration of blood flow to the ischemic region before irreversible changes occur. Surgical treatment of acute limb ischemia, because of comorbid illnesses, carries a 30-day mortality of between 15 and 25 percent.[1, 2]

Intravenous infusion of exogenous plasminogen activators, specifically streptokinase, was attempted about three decades ago for the treatment of peripheral arterial occlusion.[3] Several studies have shown that thrombolysis can be an effective initial treatment for many patients with acute arterial occlusions.[1–4] One of the advantages of thrombolysis over surgical intervention is that after thrombolysis, angiographic evaluation can uncover any underlying cause that played a role in thrombus formation.[1–4] After thrombolysis, when underlying lesions are identified, they can be treated either by transluminal balloon angioplasty or by elective surgical revascularization.[1, 2] The rationale for the use of thrombolytic therapy for arterial thrombotic disease includes:

1. Removal of thrombus and establishment of blood flow to ischemic limb
2. Identification of a hemodynamic cause of arterial or graft occlusion
3. Conversion of emergent into elective surgery
4. Removal of thrombus from the collateral circulation
5. Avoidance of the mechanical trauma of surgery to tibioperoneal vessels

Thrombolytic agents that have been used are streptokinase, urokinase, recombinant tissue plasminogen activator (rt-PA), acylated plasminogen streptokinase complex, and pro-urokinase. All these agents induce a systemic fibrinolytic state. In comparative studies on the treatment of arterial thrombosis, streptokinase, urokinase, rt-PA, and pro-urokinase were shown to be more effective than heparin alone in lysing the thrombus.[1–7] A retrospective study from Cleveland Clinic revealed that the clinical success rate was 60 percent for streptokinase, 95 percent for urokinase, and 91 percent for rt-PA.[5]

Previous studies in peripheral arterial occlusions revealed that urokinase has a greater success rate with fewer complications than streptokinase[3, 5, 7, 8] The early studies on the use of thrombolytic agents revealed that lysis was more likely to be successful if thrombosis was recent and involved proximal vessels.[1–3] McNamara and associates[6] demonstrated that the mean duration of infusion was also significantly shorter for urokinase than for streptokinase. Comparative studies of streptokinase, urokinase, and rt-PA have shown that rt-PA provides equal success in thrombolysis, but at a higher rate of major bleeding.[4, 5, 7] The use of streptokinase is limited because of the production of antibodies resulting from previous use of streptokinase or a recent streptococcal infection.

Methods of Administration of Thrombolytic Agents

Thrombolytic agents have been infused both systemically and locally. The *systemic* use of thrombolytic agents has been associated with significant bleeding complications.[3, 7] Conversely, several studies have revealed that the *local route (catheter-directed thrombolysis)* increases the concentration of the thrombolytic agent in the treatment area, which increases the chance of interaction with the thrombus and decreases the incidence of hemorrhagic side effects.[1, 2, 6, 7] Several investigators have shown the usefulness of the *guide wire traversal test* to assess the outcome of thrombolysis.[2–8] McNamara and coworkers[6] showed that before initiation of thrombolysis, if a guide wire can be easily advanced through the thrombus, the thrombus is likely to lyse; however, if the guide wire cannot be passed, the thrombolysis is less likely to be successful. A variety of multi–side-hole catheters and infusion wires are available for local administration of thrombolytic agents.[7] Coaxial systems of two catheters or a catheter and an infusion wire are commonly used to deliver thrombolytic agents throughout the length of a thrombotic occlusion.[6] This technique decreases the infusion time and requires less frequent angiographic monitoring because lysing is achieved throughout the length of thrombus and because catheter repositioning is usually not necessary. Some of the administration techniques that have been tried include *bolus lacing* (an initial bolus of agent is given over a short period of time throughout the length of the thrombus),[2, 6] *pulsed spray* (injection of a lytic agent through a multi–side-slit catheter by use of high-pressure intermittent pulses),[7] and *continuous infusion* of a thrombolytic agent over a longer period of time (hours to days).[2–8] Mechanical devices have been used to disrupt and macerate the freshly formed thrombus and subsequently remove it from the circulation.[9] It appears that these devices are of most value when combined with a lytic agent to lyse and then remove small thrombi of recent onset.[9]

Doses of Infusion of Thrombolytic Agents

The dosage and the length of infusion of thrombolytic agent depends on the *indication, agent used, route of administration, amount and age of thrombus, surface area, and degree of ischemia.* In general, the fresher the thrombus, the more effective the thrombolysis.[3, 5–7] In addition, the greater the amount of thrombus (thrombus burden), the longer the time to complete lysis.[6, 7] The higher the concentration of the thrombolytic agent in the area of thrombosis, the more rapid the lysis.[5–7] Several investigators have recommended the following dosage regimens for systemic infusion of a thrombolytic agent for the treatment of deep venous thrombosis and pulmonary emboli[3, 5–7]:

1. *Urokinase:* 4400 IU/kg intravenous bolus as a loading dose, followed by 4400 IU/kg/h for 12 to 24 hours
2. *Streptokinase:* 250,000 IU intravenous bolus (loading dose) over 30 minutes, followed by 100,000 IU/h for 24 to 72 hours
3. *rt-PA:* 100 mg as continuous intravenous infusion given over 2 hours for treatment of pulmonary embolism and 0.06 mg/kg/h for treatment of deep venous thrombosis

The dosage recommendations for local infusion of urokinase for treatment of deep venous thrombosis and arterial occlusions are as follows[5–7]:

1. *Low dose:* 60,000 IU/h, with or without bolus
2. *High dose:* 240,000 IU/h for 4 hours, then 120,000 IU/h for 12 to 24 hours, with or without bolus

The more severe the degree of ischemia, the more important it is to achieve rapid lysis. The rapidity of thrombolysis is increased with high-dose regimens; however, the complication rates may also be increased.[2–5, 7] The duration of therapy usually depends on the response to therapy, as determined by clinical and/or angiographic results. Several investigators have shown the benefit of concomitant anticoagulation with thrombolysis.[5–8] Concomitant anticoagulation with heparin reduces thrombus formation around the catheter and retards thrombus propagation and reocclusion of the treated vessel segment, particularly in a proximal vessel that has low blood flow above the occlusion. Conversely, heparin can increase the severity of a bleeding complication.

The end points of thrombolysis should be *restoration of antegrade flow, complete lysis of thrombus, failure to lyse residual thrombus, extension of thrombosis, and complications of therapy.*

Predictors of Success of Thrombolysis

The likelihood of success of thrombolysis depends on the factors listed in Table 75–1.

Patient Selection for Thrombolysis

The selection of patients for thrombolysis depends on the patient's presenting symptoms, history, physical findings, and objective laboratory test results. After the established diagnosis of thrombosis, it is essential to assess indications, contraindications, risk factors, and likelihood of success. If thrombolysis is a reasonable choice of therapy, after careful selection of the site of vascular access, angiography is performed. After the angiographic findings are evaluated

TABLE 75-1 Predictors of Successful Thrombolysis

Predictor	Likelihood of Success	
	High	*Low*
Guide wire traversal test	Successful	Unsuccessful
Duration of occlusion	Hours, <week	Weeks, months
Location of occlusion	Proximal	Distal
Distal vessel	Visualized	Not visualized
Doppler signal	Present	Absent
Relative contraindications	None	Present

and likelihood of success determined, the type of equipment and the dose of the thrombolytic agent are selected.

Before treatment with a thrombolytic agent is initiated, attention should be paid to possible hypercoagulable conditions:

- Anti–thrombin III deficiency
- Protein C and protein S deficiency
- Factor V Leiden level
- Anticardiolipin antibodies
- Antiphospholipid antibodies
- Malignancy

The presence of any of these conditions makes one even more thoughtful concerning the use of thrombolytic therapy, and clearly, alternative strategies need to be used, both short term and long term.

Conclusion

Accrued experience over the past decade has led to increased acceptance of selective intra-arterial thrombolytic therapy for peripheral arterial occlusions as an adjunct to definitive revascularization procedures. Although newer infusion techniques have significantly decreased treatment times, the times remain at about 24 hours for lower-extremity occlusions. Work continues on the optimization of infusion methods and new drugs and their dosing in order to shorten treatment times.

RENOVASCULAR DISEASE

Prevalence and Natural History

Renovascular hypertension is usually caused by partial or complete occlusion of one or both renal arteries. The overall incidence of hypertension due to renal artery stenosis (RAS) is less than 5 percent.[10] It is estimated, however, that 2 to 4 million people in the United States have renovascular disease. However, the prevalence of RAS in several autopsy series and among the older population is much higher and ranges from 27 to 62 percent.[11, 12] A notable feature in patients with renovascular disease is the high incidence of generalized vascular disease.[13] Harding and coworkers[13] found that only 15 percent of their patients who underwent routine cardiac catheterization did not have concomitant coronary artery or peripheral vascular disease. Arterial hypertension due to renovascular disease can be caused by many conditions, including *atherosclerotic disease, fibromuscular dysplasia (FMD), scleroderma, vasculitis, and atheroembolic disease.* However, atherosclerosis accounts for almost two thirds of the cases of renovascular hypertension, and fibromuscular dysplasia accounts for the remaining third.[13]

Atherosclerotic renovascular disease typically presents in patients older than 40 years and most commonly affects the renal ostium and/or the proximal third of the renal artery. This disease affects men twice as often as women.[13, 14]

Progression of Renal Atherosclerosis

The incidence of progression of renal artery disease in published studies varies between 29 and 71 percent, depending on the length of follow-up.[15, 16] Dean and coworkers[15] found in a prospective study that it was not possible to reliably quantify the rate of progression of the disease. Some of their patients remained stable for long periods, whereas others progressed rapidly. In United States, the incidence of end-stage renal disease due to hypertension has increased sharply over the past two decades, especially in elderly white dialysis patients.[16]

Fibromuscular Dysplasia

Fibromuscular dysplasia (FMD) is the most common type of nonatherosclerotic renal artery disease. It affects less than 1 percent of all patients undergoing renal angiography.[10, 13, 17] This disease primarily affects women between the third and sixth decade and has a marked predilection for whites.[16] The lesions are usually bilateral and, unlike those seen with atherosclerotic renovascular disease, affect the distal half of the renal artery.[17, 18]

The cause-and-effect relationship between RAS and a patient's hypertension is stronger for FMD than for atherosclerotic renal artery disease. There are three principal variants of this disease:[17, 18]

1. *Intimal dysplasia:* Fibrosis confined to intima
2. *Medial dysplasia:* Fibromuscular rings alternating with areas of thinning (most common variant affecting two thirds of cases)
   Subtypes: a. Medial hyperplasia
   b. Medial fibroplasia
   c. Perimedial fibroplasia
3. *Periadventitial dysplasia* (least common variant)

Differential diagnosis: the differential diagnosis should include atherosclerotic renal artery disease, Takayasu's arteritis, vascular lesions of neurofibromatosis, and inherited connective tissue disease (e.g., Ehlers-Danlos syndrome).[10–18]

Angiographic appearance: a. "String of beads" appearance
b. Unifocal or multifocal tubular stenoses
c. "Atypical"—diverticulum or saccular

Screening for Renovascular Hypertension

Several clinical variables are helpful in identifying patients with RAS[11, 14–18]:

- Severe or refractory hypertension after the age of 50 years ("late onset") or before the age of 20 years ("early onset")
- Accelerated hypertension in a patient who was previously normotensive or whose hypertension was well controlled with antihypertensive therapy
- Deterioration of renal function after initiation of an angiotensin-converting enzyme (ACE) inhibitor
- Malignant hypertension resistant to two or three antihypertensive medications
- Unexplained or progressive renal insufficiency
- Associated vascular disease
- A systolic-diastolic abdominal bruit
- Paradoxical worsening of hypertension on diuretic therapy
- Atrophic kidney or discrepancy in kidney size
- Recurrent "flash" pulmonary edema

Many noninvasive and invasive techniques are available to demonstrate the presence of renovascular disease:

- Duplex Doppler ultrasonography
- Intravenous pyelography
- ACE inhibitor radioisotope scans
- Renal vein renin measurements
- Magnetic resonance angiography

Plasma Renin Measurements

Because a hemodynamically significant lesion implies a renin-dependent basis for hypertension, the finding of a renal vein ratio of 1.5 or greater (affected-to-nonaffected side) suggests a hemodynamically significant lesion. The predictive value of this test regarding the reduction of blood pressure after intervention is high, with a sensitivity of 82 percent and a specificity of 62 percent.[19]

The use of ACE inhibitor before measuring renal vein renin level can enhance its predictive accuracy and increase its sensitivity to 90 percent in patients with unilateral renal artery disease. However, the renal vein renin levels may not accurately predict the blood pressure response after intervention in as many as 60 percent of patients who may improve after revascularization.[19]

Because of the cumbersome nature of this evaluation, the need to discontinue the medications that may affect renin secretion, and the high incidence of false-negative results, renal vein renin measurements are rarely used.

Intravenous Pyelography

Intravenous pyelography is now infrequently used as a screening test for renovascular hypertension because of its low sensitivity and specificity (both approximately 75 percent), the risk of contrast-induced nephrotoxicity, and the relatively high radiation dose required.[19]

Renal Scintigraphy

Renal scintigraphy using either ^{131}I-labeled *o*-iodohippurate or ^{99m}Tc-labeled diethylenetriamine pentaacetic acid, with an ACE inhibitor improves the predictive value as well as the sensitivity and specificity (90 to 95 percent for both) of the scan.[20] A test result is considered positive if it shows one or more of the following:

- Decreased uptake by the affected kidney
- Almost twice the usual time (5 minutes) to peak uptake of the isotope on the affected side
- Delayed washout of the radioisotope (>5 minutes) on the involved side when compared with the contralateral kidney

Although renal scintigraphy with an ACE inhibitor offers an excellent screening test, its use is limited in patients with bilateral renal artery stenosis and in patients whose creatinine clearance is less than 20 ml/min.

Duplex Doppler

Duplex Doppler ultrasonography provides anatomic and functional information and can detect renal artery stenosis of 60 percent or more. Olin and coworkers reported positive and negative predictive values of 99 percent and 97 percent respectively, and a sensitivity and specificity of 98 percent of duplex Doppler ultrasonography when compared with angiography.[21] They reported that peak systolic renal artery velocities higher than 200 cm/sec and a renal-aortic velocity ratio of 3.5 or higher reliably separated patients whose renal arteries have less than 60 percent stenosis from those with 60 percent or more stenosis. Duplex Doppler ultrasonography is a noninvasive test that does not require the discontinuation of medication and offers accurate results in patients with renal failure and bilateral RAS. It does not involve exposure to radiation or contrast material. This test is especially beneficial in detecting restenosis in patients who have undergone previous angioplasty, stenting, or vascular surgery (Plate 75–1). The greater use of this test is limited, however, because it is time consuming, operator dependent, and frequently difficult to perform in obese patients and in those with overlying intestinal gas.[21]

Magnetic Resonance Angiography

Magnetic resonance angiography is a useful noninvasive screening tool to evaluate patients with potential renovascular disease. This imaging technique eleminates the need for intravascular access and the use of potentially nephrotoxic radiocontrast material. Technical advances with the use of three-dimensional phase-contrast magnetic resonance angiography with cardiac synchronization have achieved a sensitivity of 100 percent and a specificity of 96 percent, for proximal lesions.[22] Unfortunately, the use of MRA is restricted because of its expense, its limited availability, and its contraindications in patients with metallic implants.

Renal Angiography

Renal angiographic techniques include

- Conventional renal angiography
- Intra-arterial digital subtraction angiography

- Intravenous digital subtraction angiography
- Spiral (helical) computed tomographic intravenous angiography
- Carbon dioxide digital angiography

Conventional renal angiography or intra-arterial digital subtraction angiography remains the diagnostic "gold standard" against which other imaging techniques are compared. Intravenous digital subtraction angiography is a less invasive technique than arterial angiography; however, the amount of radiocontrast material required is significantly greater (150 to 200 ml). The sensitivity and specificity of this technique are only 90 percent; this is significantly lower than the sensitivity and specificity of the arterial techniques.[19] Digital subtraction angiography, because of low contrast volume (25 to 50 ml), is a preferred procedure, especially in patients with impaired renal function.

Spiral computed tomography with intravenous administration of radiocontrast agent has been also used as a sensitive tool, with a sensitivity of 98 percent and a specificity of 94 percent.[19] Unfortunately, the sensitivity and specificity of this technique declines significantly in the presence of renal insufficiency. Another disadvantage of this technique is the risk of nephrotoxicity resulting from a large amount of contrast agent that is required to obtain adequate imaging.

Carbon dioxide digital angiography has been found to be of great benefit in patients with impaired renal function.[23] When used with digital subtraction, this technique offers quality and diagnostic accuracy similar to those of conventional renal angiography without exposing the patient to the potential risk of an allergic reaction and nephrotoxicity associated with the use of radiocontrast agents.[23] The disadvantages of carbon dioxide angiography is less than optimal visualization of distal renal artery, potential risk of air embolization, renal ischemia resulting from "vapor lock," and requirement for experienced technical support with electronic enhancement.[23]

Indications for Revascularization

The presence of RAS is not always associated with hypertension. Many patients with RAS have normal or mildly elevated blood pressure. Clinical features that are commonly present in patients with renovascular hypertension include

- Onset of diastolic hypertension after the age of 55
- Refractory hypertension
- Development of uncontrolled hypertension
- Malignant hypertension
- Rapid deterioration of renal function
- Recurrent flash pulmonary edema without readily explainable cause

Renal revascularization is indicated only in cases in which medical therapy offers suboptimal control of hypertension.[24] Although revascularization in atherosclerotic RAS is rarely curative, considerable improvement in blood pressure control is expected in most patients. Clinical predictors of cure with revascularization include duration of hypertension of less than 5 years, significant elevation of preprocedural diastolic blood pressure, and significant difference between renal vein renin levels.[25]

Surgical and Endovascular Revascularization for Renal Artery Stenosis

Revascularization for Fibromuscular Disease

The results of surgical and endovascular revascularization for severe FMD have been very rewarding[26] (Fig. 75–1). In the past decade, as a result of excellent results of percutaneous transluminal renal angioplasty (PTRA), the indications for surgical revascularization of FMD have declined significantly. PTRA for renal artery FMD is less invasive and less costly than surgery and is equally effective. The technical success rate of PTRA has been reported to be between 88 and 100 percent.[26–28] Klinge and coworkers[27] reported that initial clinical success rate (cure or significant improvement of hypertension) occurred in 87 percent of patients.[27] During 5 years of follow-up, only 6 percent of patients experienced recurrence.

Medial fibroplasia responds most favorably to PTRA.[29] Low inflation pressures usually result in a normal appearance on follow-up angiography. Intimal fibroplasia, medial hyperplasia, and adventitial fibroplasia cause eccentric stenosis, require higher inflation pressures and less commonly permit complete dilatation.[28]

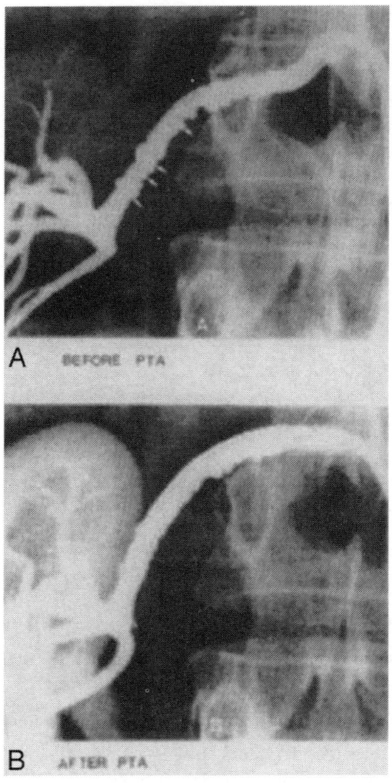

FIGURE 75–1 Cineangiographic frames of the right renal artery reveal typical features of fibromuscular dysplasia before percutaneous transluminal angioplasty (PTA) *(arrows)* **(A)** and improvement of renal artery luminal irregularities after PTA **(B)**.

Revascularization for Atherosclerotic Renal Artery Stenosis

There is now abundant evidence that revascularization by surgery or angioplasty can result in an improvement or stabilization of arterial hypertension and renal function. Hansen and coworkers[30] showed in 152 patients with atherosclerotic renovascular hypertension that 90 percent of patients demonstrated improvement in blood pressure control after surgical renal artery revascularization.

The surgical mortality rates range in reported studies from 3 to 17 percent, with an average of 6 percent.[31–33] However, Novick and coworkers[32] showed that surgical revascularization in patients with diffuse aortic atheromatosis can significantly worsen the outcome of the procedure. In their series of 241 patients, they reported that after a mean follow-up period of 39 months, thrombosis or restenosis occurred in 4.3 percent of operated arteries, and the mortality rate was 11.2 percent.[31] The average improvement in renal function occurred in 41 to 43 percent of patients.[31–33] The longevity of surgical repair procedures in the form of endarterectomy or bypass varies signifantly between the published reports. Several studies have revealed that patients in whom end-stage renal disease has recently developed may also benefit from revascularization.[30–33]

Based on the existing evidence in published studies, patients with progressive decline in renal function, accelerated hypertension, hypertension that is difficult to control, and/or congestive heart failure are likely to benefit from renal revascularization.

Percutaneous Transluminal Angioplasty and/or Stenting for Treatment of Atherosclerotic Renal Artery Stenosis

Since Gruentzig and coworkers'[34] original description in 1978 of successful renal artery balloon angioplasty, there has been ongoing controversy regarding the benefits of PTRA versus surgical revascularization. Unfortunately only one prospective randomized trial compared the results of these two revascularization alternatives.[35] In their randomized trial, Weibull and coworkers[35] reported that there was no statistically significant difference in acute outcomes between PTRA and surgical revascularization.[35] After 24 months of follow-up, the primary patency rates in the surgical group and in the PTRA group were 97 percent and 62 percent, respectively. The secondary patency rate in PTRA group was 90 percent after repeat PTRA or surgery. They also reported similar results between two groups regarding the cure or improvement in hypertension and complications. Their analysis also revealed that with the use of PTRA, 60 percent of patients would require additional treatment in the form of a repeat PTRA or surgery.

Several predictors of initial failure or restenosis after PTRA have been identified.[36–38] The most important predictor of restenosis after PTRA is lesion location.[36–38] PTRA of ostial stenosis, particularly when calcified, has offered disappointing results. The initial success rates range from 24 to 35 percent, and the rates of restenosis range from 15 to 42 percent.[36–38]

To overcome the problem of elastic recoil after angioplasty, several investigators have recommended the use of intravascular stents for the treatment of ostial renal artery stenosis.[36–38] These investigators have also demonstrated greater augmentation in luminal diameter and transstenotic pressure gradient after stent implantation compared with PTRA alone (Fig. 75–2). Several stents have been successfully used for renal artery revascularization.[36–38] We have shown a benefit of using a combination of a self-expandable stent and a balloon-expandable stent for the treatment of an iatrogenic renal artery dissection in a patient with atherosclerotic and FMD disease.[39]

In a prospective study of 68 patients who had not responded to PTRA for ostial renal artery stenosis, Blum and associates[40] reported a 100 percent initial technical success with Palmaz stent deployment. The restenosis rate in this study after 24 months of follow-up was 11 percent. Reintervention resulted in a secondary patency rate of 92 percent. Renal function remained stable, even in patients with abnormal baseline renal function. The improvement in arterial hypertension occurred in 62 percent of patients.

Dorros and associates[41] reported encouraging results of renal artery stenting in patients with normal baseline renal function. However, their results revealed a high mortality in patients with bilateral renal artery disease and a baseline serum creatinine concentration of 2.0 mg/dl or greater. They proposed that early diagnosis and revascularization

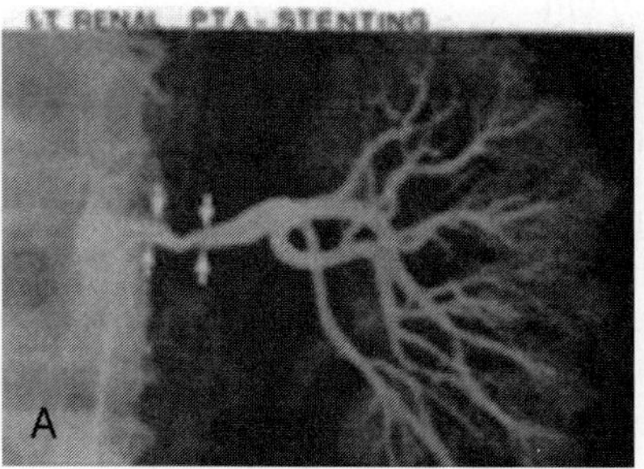

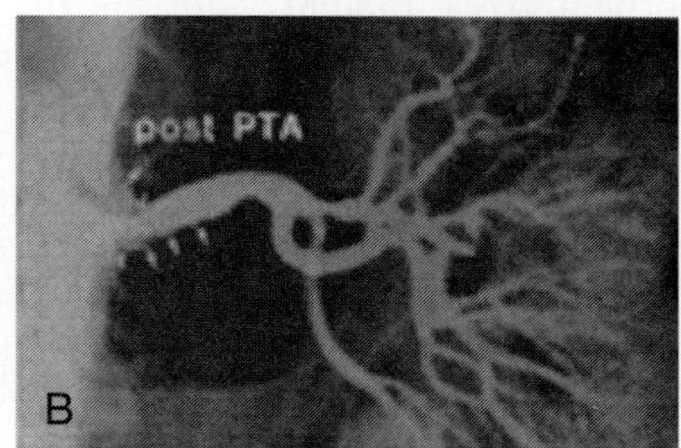

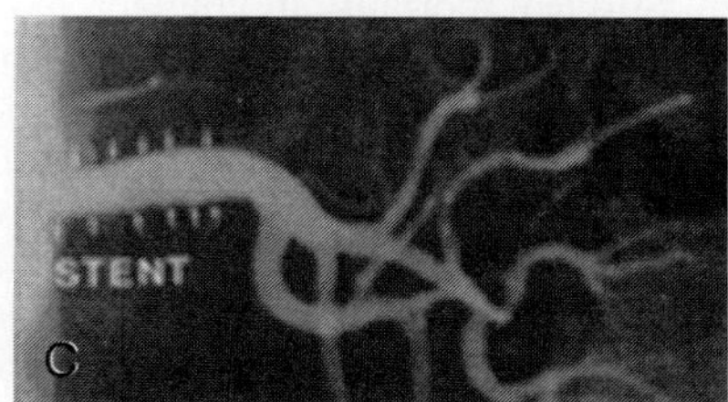

FIGURE 75–2 **A,** Seventy percent ostial stenosis of the left renal artery before the intervention. **B,** Reveals left renal artery dissection after percutaneous transluminal renal angioplasty. **C,** Excellent result after deployment of a Palmaz (P204) stent in the left renal artery *(arrows).*

before the onset of renal dysfunction could improve hypertension control, preserve or prevent deterioration of renal function, and improve patient survival. This hypothesis is currently being tested in several randomized trials between PTRA alone and stent-supported PTRA.

ABDOMINAL AORTIC ANEURYSMS

Epidemiology

Abdominal aortic aneurysm (AAA) is a serious vascular disorder characterized by a permanent dilatation of the abdominal aorta which has a diameter of at least 50 percent greater than normal. This disease predominantly affects men who are 60 years of age or older. Men are five times more frequently affected than women.[42, 43] More than 90 percent of these aneurysms are secondary to atherosclerosis, and 89 percent are located in the infrarenal aorta.[42, 43] The prevalence of AAAs that are 4 cm or larger in diameter in nonselected patients aged 65 to 80 years is 1.3 to 2.7 percent.[42, 43] The risk of rupture has been shown to be related to aneurysm size. Previous studies demonstrated that 25 percent of patients with AAA who did not undergo corrective surgery died of a ruptured aneurysm, and this percentage doubled when the diameter of the aneurysm exceeded 7.0 cm.[42, 43]

Abdominal aortic aneurysm is the 13th leading cause of death for patients 55 years of age and older and is responsible for approximately 15,000 deaths per year in the United States.[42] In the past 30 years, the incidence of AAA has increased threefold.[44] The generally accepted diameter of AAA at which repair is indicated is 5 cm.[42–44] This figure is based on historical information from the natural history and is at the crossover point where the risk of rupture exceeded the risk of open surgical repair.

There is a 90 percent mortality rate associated with an out-of-hospital AAA rupture, with the mortality rate decreasing to 50 percent for those who undergo emergency surgery.[42–44] To prevent this devastating event, more than 40,000 surgical repairs of AAA are currently being performed in the United States annually, making this the second most commonly performed vascular surgical procedure.[42] The current standard of treatment is replacement of the diseased aorta with the prosthetic graft. Surgical treatment requires opening of the aneurysmal sac and interposition of a synthetic graft, thereby excluding and bypassing the aneurysm. Surgical mortality in younger, asymptomatic patients undergoing elective resection is 3 to 5 percent.[42, 43] Because general anesthesia, laparotomy, aortic clamping, and blood transfusion are required, this procedure in an elderly population is associated with high morbidity. For patients who have undergone previous abdominal surgery or for those with severe pulmonary, cardiovascular, or renal disease, the risk of perioperative death may be between 20 and 60 percent, and they may often be denied surgery because the risks of surgery exceed the benefit.[42–45] The prognosis of these patients denied surgery is poor, with 72 percent dying within 2 years, 43 percent from aneurysm rupture.[45]

Imaging Technology to Determine Patient Selection and/or Success of Treatment

The simplest and most inexpensive noninvasive test available to confirm the presence of AAA is abdominal ultrasonography. This test has been shown to be a reliable method of evaluation before a surgical AAA repair is considered.[46] A spiral computed tomography with three-dimensional reconstruction with intravenous contrast injection has been an essential method of preprocedural and postprocedural evaluation after endovascular AAA repair.[46] This technique offers an accurate measurement of various segments of the abdominal aorta and iliac arteries, which is essential in selecting the appropriate diameter and the length of the endoprosthesis. This test also offers pertinent information regarding the presence or the absence of thrombus and calcifications in the abdominal aorta and the degree of tortuosity in the abdominal aorta and iliac arteries, which determine whether the patient is a candidate for endovascular repair. At the present time, abdominal aortography is also considered an essential component of preprocedural information for endovascular AAA repair. This evaluation is of great benefit to determine whether the iliac arteries are of adequate size to accommodate the endoprosthesis and whether any interventional procedures, such as percutaneous transluminal angioplasty (PTA) and stenting, are necessary before the endovascular repair. Angiography also accurately identifies aberrant renal arteries that originate in the landing zone of the endoprosthesis. Another benefit of angiography is the identification before the endovascular procedure of large abdominal aortic and iliac arterial branches, such as inferior mesenteric, lumbar, and internal iliac arteries, which, if they remain patent after the procedure, may continue to supply the blood flow to the aneurysm. Several views might be necessary to delineate the relationship of the aneurysm to these arteries and to determine the best approach and the type of the endoprosthesis to be used.

Endovascular Treatment

During the 1990s, no area of treatment of peripheral vascular disease has attracted more enthusiasm than the endovascular exclusion of AAA. This procedure has captured the interest of vascular surgeons, interventional radiologists, and interventional cardiologists. Whereas grafting had previously been the domain of the vascular surgeon, more recent developments in transcatheter delivery of vascular prostheses allowed nonsurgical specialties to use these devices for the treatment of a variety of vascular defects. The development of reliable noninvasive evaluation for the detection of AAA and the potential for a less invasive procedure for their repair should increase the number of endovascular AAA repairs, decrease the number of aneurysms that rupture, and thus decrease the overall mortality rate associated with aneurysmal disease.

The first endoluminal treatment of AAA in a clinical setting was introduced in 1990 and was reported on in 1991 by Parodi and colleagues.[44] Stent-mounted grafts have been introduced during the 1990s as a less invasive alternative to surgical AAA repair.

It is hoped that endoluminal grafts will help decrease morbidity and mortality associated with AAA repair, particularly in patients with comorbid illnesses. Initially, these devices were used in patients with comorbid illnesses or other conditions that increased the risk of conventional surgical procedure.[44] More recently, the use of endoluminal grafts has been proposed for patients without comorbid illnesses.[47–52] The purpose of this technique is to eliminate the risk of rupture of the aneurysm by excluding the aneurysm from the arterial circulation and the systemic arterial pressure. The first-generation endovascular endoluminal grafts were tubular grafts and, later, aorto-uni-iliac, one-piece, bifurcated construction (Figs. 75–3 and 75–4). The early prostheses were relatively inflexible and required 24 French internal diameter introducing the femoral sheath.[44] They are now available as tube grafts or bifurcated grafts[48–52] (Table 75–2). They are now more flexible and are available in smaller diameters.[50–52] Their structure is either completely stent supported (see Figs. 75–3 and 75–4)[50–52] or stented only at the level of attachment area.[48, 49] The original Parodi device consisted of a thin-walled, crimped, and knitted Dacron tube graft sutured to custom-made Palmaz-type stents at each end.[44] This device is mounted on an angioplasty catheter and introduced through

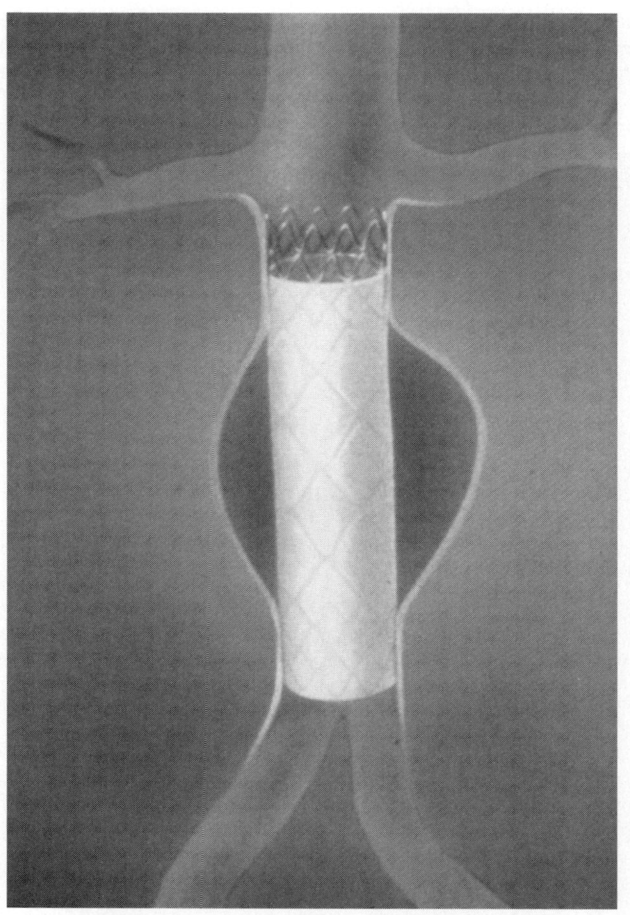

FIGURE 75–3 Artistic rendering of an aortoaortic (tubular stent) graft for endoluminal exclusion of abdominal aortic aneurysm. This illustration shows the infrarenal attachment of a stent graft by radial force (friction) of a fully supported Nitinol, self-expanding stent graft.

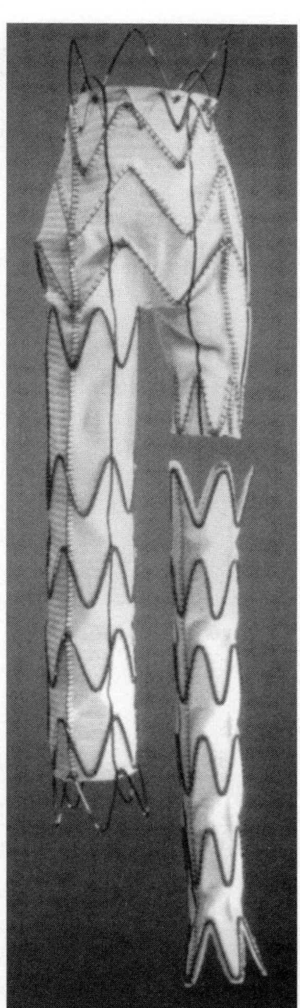

FIGURE 75–4 Modular design of a self-expanding stent graft that consists of a Nitinol stent and a thin-walled polyester graft material, which is sutured to the Nitinol frame. The stent graft consists of the bifurcated segment and the iliac segment, which are deployed separately by use of bilateral femoral artery percutaneous or direct surgical approach.

a 22 French sheath into a femoral artery through an arteriotomy. Balloon inflation at the proximal end is required to expand and deploy the proximal stent graft. The same procedure is then used to expand the distal stent graft in the distal abdominal aorta or ipsilateral iliac artery. The balloon-expandable stent was sutured to the Dacron graft at the level of infrarenal attachment, while the remaining segment of the graft was not supported.

These devices consist now of fabric grafts that are supported throughout their length by a self-expanding metal stent to minimize kinking and migration.[51] Stainless steel and Nitinol, which has thermal memory characteristics, are the most common materials used for stent designs[48–51] (see Table 75–2).

Endoluminal grafts have since undergone many modifications and improvements.[48–52] Many investigators believe that fully supported grafts offer higher degree of immediate and late success.[50–52] The stent may be placed on the outside of the graft material (exoskeleton)[50] or on the inside (endoskeleton).[52] The prosthetic wall is made of a polyethylene terephthalate textile in a woven or a knitted form,[50–52]

TABLE 75-2 **Stent Grafts for Abdominal Aortic Aneurysm Repair**

Company/Device	Stent Type	Deployment Mode	Graft Material	Means of Attachment	Special Features
Parodi/Barone Industries	316 L steel, slotted tube	Balloon expandable	Woven Dacron	Friction, radial force	Proximal & distal support, tubular
EVT/Guidant/Ancure	316 L steel spring	Self-expandable	Lightweight woven Dacron	Barbs, active fixation	Proximal & distal support, Y design
Cook/Zenith	Barbed Gianturco Z stent	Self-expandable	Woven, noncrimped Dacron	Barbs, active fixation	Fully supported
Medtronic/Talent	Nitinol spring	Self-expandable	Lightweight Dacron	Friction, radial force	Full support, modular
Corvita-BSC/CEG	Algiloy, braided tube	Self-expandable	Urethane-polycarbonate	Friction, radial force	Full support, modular
Meadox-BSC/Vanguard	Nitinol	Self-expandable	Thin-walled woven polyester	Friction, radial force	Full support, modular
Gore & Associates/ Excluder	Nitinol	Self-expandable	ePTFE	Friction, radial force	Full support, modular
Baxter/White-Yu	Algiloy wire	Self-expandable	Woven polyester	Friction, radial force	Partial support
Endologics/Bard/ PowerLink	Algiloy wire	Self-expandable	ePTFE	Friction, radial force	Full support, Y design

Abbreviation: ePTFE, expanded polytetrafluoroethylene.

urethane polycarbonate, or an expanded polytetrafluoroethylene material. The stent grafts are either *self-expandable*[50, 51] or *balloon expandable.*[44] The fixation of the stent graft can be achieved either by the radial force of the stent or by a specific attachment system that includes barbs or hooks.[49–51] The bifurcated prostheses are available in either a *one-piece*[49] or a *modular design.*[50–52] The modular design consists of introduction of the body and the ipsilateral limb of the prosthesis through the ipsilateral femoral access in a first step and insertion and attachment

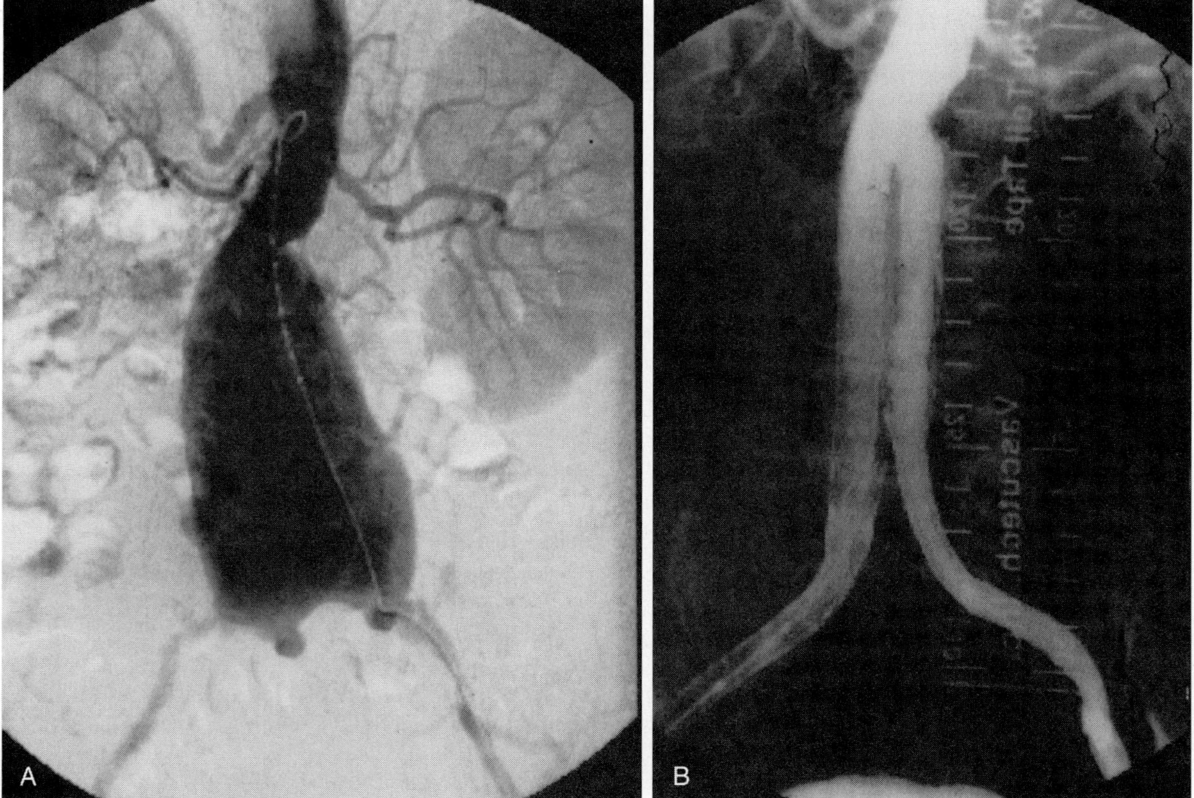

FIGURE 75–5 **A,** Preprocedural angiographic image of a patient with an 9-cm abdominal aortic aneurysm (AAA) in maximal diameter, revealing very tortuous iliac arteries. **B,** Postprocedural angiogram in the same patient as in **A** shows exclusion of AAA from the arterial flow after deployment of the AneuRx stent graft.

TABLE 75-3 **Stent Grafts for Abdominal Aortic Aneurysm Repair (1998)***

Company/ Product	Patients (n)	Technical Success (%)	Conversion to Surgery (%)	Endoleak (30-da) (%)	Mortality (30-da) (%)
Meadox/Vanguard	1500†	88.7	2.4	10.3	4.1
World Medical/Talent	2254†	92	1.8	3.9	1.8
Ancure/EVT/Guidant	300‡	91	8.5	23	3.3
Medtronic/AneuRx	250‡	91	0	9	NA
Corvita/BSC/CEG	200‡	90	4.8	4.0	1.0
Cook/Zenith	75‡	NA	3.5	3.5	NA
Baxter/White-Yu	60‡	81	5.6	14	3.1

Abbreviation: NA, not available.
*Numbers are approximate.
†World experience.
‡United States experience.
Adapted from World Medical Market Position 1997 & 1999: Endoluminal Stent Graft—Abdominal Aorta. World Medical Manufacturing Corporation, Sunrise, FL.

of the contralateral limb through the contralateral femoral access in a second step (Fig. 75-5; see also Table 75–2). Which of these materials and designs will ultimately produce superior long-term results remains to be seen when ongoing clinical studies are completed.

In 1998, more than 3000 endoluminal abdominal aneurysm repairs have been performed with various devices worldwide[53] (Table 75–3). Procedural success occurs in 90 percent of cases for most of the devices that have been used.[49–53] The need for surgical intervention because of device failure should be less than 8 percent.[49–53] The incidence of endoleak after 1 month has been less than 10 percent for most of the currently ongoing trials. The 1-month mortality was between 1 and 4 percent in one trial.[53] Even though significant improvements have been made in stent grafts since the original procedure described by Parodi and coworkers, further follow-up in currently ongoing trials will be necessary to determine the exact role of this procedure for the treatment of AAA.

Carotid Artery Disease

Epidemiology

Extracranial carotid artery occlusive disease causes 25 percent of the 500,000 cerebrovascular accidents (CVAs) that occur each year in the United States.[54] Stroke is the third most common cause of death in the United States. More than 2 million of CVA survivors have varying degrees of disability. One third of the patients who have ischemic stroke die, and another third remain permanently disabled.

Several studies revealed that patients with carotid artery stenosis greater than 75 percent have a 2 to 5 percent risk of having an ischemic CVA during the first year.[55, 56] After a transient ischemic attack, the risk of ischemic stroke is 12 to 13 percent in the first year and 30 to 37 percent in the 5 years after the initial event. For the patients who had a CVA, the risk of a subsequent CVA is 5 to 9 percent per year, and approximately 24 to 45 percent of these patients have another CVA within the next 5 years. The presence of an ulcerated lesion also increases the risk of an ischemic CVA.[57]

Carotid Endarterectomy

Carotid endarterectomy (CEA) was introduced in 1954 as a surgical therapy for the prevention of CVA in patients with extracranial carotid artery stenosis.[58] With the goal of minimizing mortality and morbidity, surgeons have refined CEA techniques over the past four decades, leading to acceptable perioperative complication rates for most patients.[59] The number of CEAs has dramatically increased in the United States from 15,000 in 1971 to 130,000 during the 1990s.[60, 61] However, medical therapy with antiplatelet agents remains as the standard of care for symptomatic patients with less than 50 percent stenosis.[55]

Prospective, randomized studies, such as North American Symptomatic Carotid Endarterectomy Trial (NASCET),[61] the European Carotid Surgery Trial (ECST),[62] and the Asymptomatic Carotid Atherosclerosis Study (ACAS),[63] have proved the superiority of CEA over medical therapy for a selected group of patients with symptomatic and asymptomatic extracranial carotid artery stenosis. In NASCET, for patients with 70 percent or greater carotid stenosis, the risk of ipsilateral stroke was reduced by 65 percent in surgical group.[61] In ACAS, for patients with 60 percent carotid stenosis, the risk of ipsilateral stroke was reduced by 53 percent.[63] In the NASCET and ACAS studies, a clear benefit from CEA was demonstrated, in spite of a perioperative stroke/death rate of 5.8 percent in symptomatic patients and 2.7 percent in asymptomatic patients.

Thus, the prospective randomized clinical trials have established that CEA performed by skilled surgeons who have low perioperative stroke rates is the gold standard for the treatment of patients with symptomatic and asymptomatic severe carotid artery stenosis.[64] However, CEA is not without its risks. There is a significant discrepancy in complications after CEA between reported studies. The clinical and anatomic diversity of patients with carotid disease could lead to differences in outcomes with CEA between different studies.

In a meta-analysis of 50 CEA studies, Rothwell and associates[64] reported the risk of CVA to be 7.7 percent in the studies followed up by a neurologist and 2.3 percent in the studies followed up only by surgeons.[64] The mortality and morbidity of CEA was particularly high (18 percent) for patients who also had significant coronary artery disease.

Other complications of CEA are cranial nerve palsies (7.6 to 27 percent), hematoma (5.5 to 11 percent) and restenosis (5 to 9 percent).[64] To determine the predictors of postoperative complications McCrory and colleagues[65] retrospectively analyzed the clinical data of 1160 patients who underwent CEA. They discovered that predictors of postoperative myocardial infarction, nonfatal strokes, and death were age greater than 75 years old, endarterectomy performed in preparation of bypass surgery, internal carotid artery thrombus, intracranial carotid artery disease, and perioperative neurologic instability.

Restenosis After Carotid Endarterectomy

Another complication of CEA is restenosis. Although studies with complete angiographic follow-up after CEA have not been performed, restenosis appears to occur in 8 to 19 percent of patients.[55, 59, 66, 67] Myointimal hyperplasia is a primary cause of restenosis within the first 24 months after CEA.[68] Progressive atherosclerosis plays a greater role in more delayed restenosis. Controversy remains as to whether vein or prosthetic patch repair results in a lower incidence of restenosis than does primary closure.[55, 58, 59, 66–68]

Endarterectomy for recurrent carotid artery stenosis after endarterectomy is more difficult because of scarring and carries a significantly higher complication rate than the original operation.[58, 66, 67] The scarring external to the artery lengthens the duration of the procedure and requires more manipulation of the carotid bifurcation that increases the risk of cerebral embolization and recurrent laryngeal nerve injury.[66–69]

In the two largest series, the major complication rate for repeat CEA ranged from 4.6 to 10.9 percent.[70] From previous studies, it is difficult to establish the frequency and the severity of symptoms leading to the second CEA. In a Cleveland Clinic series of carotid reoperations, 5.1 percent of the patients had neurologic symptoms leading to the operation.[68] In several retrospective studies, 22 to 90 percent of patients with restenosis had neurologic symptoms before their second CEA.[68, 69]

Carotid Angioplasty

PTA has become a standard treatment of occlusive atherosclerotic disease at different levels of the vascular system: coronary, renal, lower extremities, and others. For many years, PTA of atherosclerotic carotid stenosis was considered an unsuitable treatment because the atherosclerotic plaque is not removed by this method. Interventionists have been reluctant to use this technique because of the potential risks of dislodging the atherosclerotic debris, causing cerebral embolism and stroke.

Although Kerber and coworkers[70] first performed carotid artery PTA in 1980, this procedure is still debated and is controversial for the treatment of extracranial carotid artery stenosis. The European trial (Carotid and Vertebral Artery Transluminal Angioplasty Study [CAVATAS]) that compared CEA to PTA of the internal carotid artery in a prospectively randomized study showed no essential difference between the two methods in a period of more than 4 years.[71]

Stent-Supported Carotid Angioplasty

With technological advances in the endovascular treatment of peripheral vascular disease and the introduction of stents, several trials have been initiated for the treatment of extracranial carotid artery occlusive disease. The technique of stent-supported carotid angioplasty (SSCA) has expanded the indications and reduced the risk of neurologic complications. At the present time, the authors of several large studies propose on the basis of their experiences that carotid angioplasty not be performed without the use of stents.[72, 73] However, no randomized trial comparing SSCA and CEA has been completed to validate SSCA as a standard treatment of extracranial carotid artery disease.

However, several prospective nonrandomized SSCA trials have shown encouraging results. Roubin and associates[72] reported on a series of 238 SSCA procedures with a 6.3 percent incidence of neurologic complications. In their series of 110 patients (117 carotid arteries) treated with stent placement, Diethrich and colleagues[73] reported seven CVAs (6.4 percent) and 5 transient ischemic attacks (4.5 percent).[73] Woley and associates[74] reported on data from 114 procedures in which Palmaz stents were successfully placed in 108 carotid arteries. Their complications included two major CVAs, two minor CVAs, and five transient ischemic attacks, which occurred in only 61 symptomatic patients (8.2 percent). Yadev and colleagues[75] reported mean angiographic stenosis in 81 patients to be 18 $\pm$ 16 percent (range, 21 to 57 percent) at 6 months.

Wholey and coworkers[76] reported on the International Stent Supported Carotid Angioplasty experience on a total of 2591 procedures among 24 centers worldwide.[76] The overall technical success was 98.8 percent. Carotid stenting complication rates were 3.08 percent for minor strokes, 1.32 percent for major strokes, and 1.37 percent for periprocedural death. This revealed a combined periprocedural stroke and death rate of 5.77 percent. This rate varied from zero to 10 percent from the various centers. The restenosis rates in this survey were 4.80 percent at 6 months based on clinical and diagnostic studies. More detailed prospective randomized trials (Carotid Randomized Endarterectomy Stent Trial [CREST], Carotid Artery Stent Arterectomy Trial) are currently under way to answer these questions.

STENT-SUPPORTED EXTRACRANIAL CAROTID ARTERY ANGIOPLASTY TECHNIQUE

The technique of SSCA is rapidly changing with the advances in technology and the increasing experience of the interventionists.

Several factors are essential to achieve the optimal results of SSCA:

- Detailed preprocedural clinical, noninvasive, and angiographic cerebrovascular evaluation
- Appropriate choice of arterial access site
- Appropriate choice of guiding catheters, guide wires, PTA balloons

- Appropriate choice of stents (balloon expandable or self-expandable)
- Essential pharmacologic therapy
- Adequate knowledge or support in performing intracranial vascular rescue
- Adequate postprocedural neurologic, invasive, and noninvasive evaluation

The neurologic evaluation is essential to objectively assess the patient's condition before and after the interventional procedure. Carotid Duplex (Doppler and ultrasound) examination should be performed before the procedure and as a routine noninvasive follow-up. Aortic arch and selective cerebral angiography with intracranial images are necessary to identify the extent of the disease and possible associated intracranial lesions. The patients are usually given antiplatelet agents 8 days before the procedure.

The femoral access is the most commonly used access. The femoral artery access is obtained with a standard percutaneous technique. Cerebral angiography is then performed with a 5 French cerebral angiographic catheter. The patient is given 5000 U of heparin intravenously and the activated clotting time is maintained between 200 and 250 seconds. After the lesion is identified in multiple views, a 0.035-inch extra-support guide wire is advanced to the common or external carotid artery, and the diagnostic catheter is replaced with a 9 French guiding catheter or a 7 or 8 French, 90-cm-long sheath. At this point, the 0.035-inch wire is removed, and a coronary (0.014- or 0.018-inch) guide wire and a 4-mm × 20-mm coronary balloon are advanced through the lesion. The patient usually receives 0.5 to 1 mg of intravenous atropine just before the PTA to avoid severe bradyarrhythmia and hypotension. Very rarely, the patient might require the use of intravenous vasopressors or a temporary pacemaker for profound bradycardia and/or hypotension.

After PTA is completed, the balloon is removed, the self-expanding stent or the balloon-expandable stent is advanced to the lesion, and the stent is deployed. Various balloon-expandable and self-expandable stents have been successfully used for SSCA. It is usually necessary to perform PTA after deploying the self-expandable stent to achieve adequate apposition of the stent to the arterial wall. During the procedure, the patient's neurologic status is frequently evaluated to detect any possible complications. If there are no complications, the patient is given oral antiplatelet agents and is discharged from the hospital the following day. Before discharge, a neurologist evaluates the patient.

THE CHOICE OF STENT

The size of the internal carotid artery varies from 5 to 8 mm. The common carotid artery measures from 7 to 10 mm. When the stent is placed across the bifurcation of the common carotid artery, it must adapt itself to arteries of different diameters. The stent should be in close contact to the arterial wall to allow growth of neointima. Self-expandable stents, such as Wallstent (Schneider, Minneapolis, MN), Smart Stent (Cordis/Johnson & Johnson), and Integra stent (Medi-Tech), have varied radial expansion capabilities, flexibility, and compressibility. Their narrow meshwork is beneficial in preventing embolism during balloon dilatation. Some of the balloon-expandable stents, such as the Palmaz stent (Johnson & Johnson, Warren, NJ), offer more precise location, less metal, and more radial strength. The disadvantages of balloon-expandable stents are the risk of deformity and the tendency to collapse with external compression or trauma. This complication has been reported to occur at the rate of 4 to 15 percent.[77, 78] For this reason, most of the currently ongoing trials are using only self-expandable stents.

Even though many types of stents have been successfully used for SSCA, no ideal stent that has been specifically designed for this application is available at the present time. Several manufacturers are working on thermally expandable (Nitinol) stents, coated stents, and stent grafts, which should inhibit thrombus formation and myointimal proliferation. Covered stents are available outside of the United States; however, they will require several refinements to be of benefit for this application. It is possible that the covered stents will decrease the risk of embolization; however, the risk of occlusion of the external carotid artery should be taken into consideration. Based on several reports, it appears that the greatest benefit of SSCA is in patients with[73–77]:

- Postoperative recurrent carotid artery stenosis
- Nonatherosclerotic cause of carotid artery stenosis (FMD, Takayasu's arteritis, after radiation stenosis, after radical neck surgery stenosis)
- Increased operative risk because of comorbid illnesses

Methods of Reducing the Incidence of Cerebral Emboli

Cerebral embolization results from manipulation of the guide wires, balloons, and stents across the complex atherosclerotic carotid artery lesions. Echolucent plaques and lesions with greater than 90 percent stenosis have been shown to increase the risk of embolic particles.[77] Theron and coworkers[77] analyzed the aspirated blood after angioplasty under cerebral protection with the inflated balloon in the internal carotid artery and found cholesterol crystals ranging from 600 to 1300 μm in length in 17 of 21 cases.

Mathur and colleagues[78] reported that neurologic complications are significantly related to patient selection. Advanced age, severely stenosed lesions, and long and multiple stenosis are independent predictors of procedural CVA. In this study, there was no correlation with number of embolic particles, preprocedural symptoms, plaque ulceration, gender, diabetes mellitus, presence of coronary artery disease, hypercholesterolemia, prior CEA, history of smoking, contralateral carotid occlusion, or type of stent used. Several cerebral protection devices are currently being investigated in the United States and elsewhere:

- Cerebral protection techniques with occlusion balloon—Theron and coworkers'[77] technique
- Kachel's[79] reversing flow technique
- PercuSurge guide wire temporary occlusion and aspiration system[80]
- Medicorp Henry-Amor-Fried-Ruenacht (HAFR) device[80]
- Combined-techniques filters[80]

Theron and coworkers'[77] technique was originally described in 1990. It consists of the use of a triple-coaxial catheter that occludes the internal carotid artery beyond the stenosis with the use of a latex balloon. The angioplasty and stent placement are then performed under cerebral protection, thus avoiding distal embolization. The potential debris associated with the procedure can be then aspirated and/or flushed through the guiding catheter toward the external carotid artery. In their series of 259 carotid angioplasties, Theron and coworkers[77] reported that 136 were performed with their cerebral protection technique. They reported no neurologic events during the procedure and one event 6 hours after the procedure. Unfortunately, no other large study exists that has evaluated the benefit of this technique of cerebral protection. The limitations of this technique are the absence of a guide wire in the shaft of the protection balloon and the poor steerability of the catheter.

The PercuSurge guide wire (PercuSurge, Sunnyvale, CA) is a device that consists of a 0.014 or 0.018 angioplasty guide wire (190 and 300 cm in length) constructed of a hollow nitinol hypotube. Incorporated into the distal wire segment is an inflatable elastomeric balloon capable of occluding vessel flow.[80] The proximal end of the hypotube wire incorporates a Microseal, allowing inflation and deflation of the distal occlusion balloon by use of a Microseal adapter. On detachment of the Microseal adapter, the occlusion balloon remains inflated, during which time the angioplasty and stenting are performed. An aspiration catheter is then advanced over the wire into the vessel, and manual suction is applied to retrieve particulate debris. This device was studied experimentally in animal coronary vessels and then in human aortocoronary saphenous grafts. These studies revealed that this device is capable of capturing and retrieving atherosclerotic and thrombotic debris and that it may aid in the prevention of distal embolization in a vessel.

The MEDICORP device consists of a protection balloon, a dilatation balloon that can be used over a 0.014 coronary guide wire.[80] Although Henry and colleagues[80] have reported encouraging preliminary data, larger number of cases will be needed to determine the benefit of this cerebral protection device.

Kachel[79] reported on a cerebral protection technique that consists of occluding the upper part of the common carotid artery with a balloon attached to the distal end of the guiding catheter. The occlusion created by the balloon leads to the reversal of flow toward the external carotid artery. The angioplasty and the stenting are then performed through the guiding catheter. This technique seems easy to use; however, it does not offer sufficient safety against the risk of embolization. In his series, Kachel[79] reported a complication rate of 4.6 percent, which is not significantly different from complication rates reported in other series without cerebral protection.

The combined technique of occlusion of the internal carotid and the common carotid arteries could be entertained as another reasonable alternative. Occlusion of the internal carotid artery above the lesion and the common carotid artery below the lesion would create a dilatation zone, without a flow that could be easily aspirated and cleared of atherosclerotic debris. Filters are currently in the early experimental stages of investigation for cerebral protection. A filter could stop detached embolic particles without interrupting blood flow to the brain. This technique might be of benefit in patients with contralateral carotid occlusion or the incomplete circle of Willis that cannot tolerate prolonged interruption of ipsilateral carotid flow.

Future Clinical Implications of Stent-Supported Carotid Angioplasty

During the 1990s, significant achievements occurred in our understanding of the pathology and the treatment of extracranial carotid artery stenosis. CEA has proved to be superior to medical therapy for most patients with symptomatic carotid disease. SSCA is rapidly emerging as an alternative mode of treatment to CEA with encouraging preliminary results. Innovative stent designs that are adapted for SSCA are being evaluated worldwide. Cerebral protection devices are emerging as a useful tool to prevent cerebral embolization during SSCA. Further refinements in balloon, stent, and cerebral protection device technology will be needed to establish SSCA as the treatment of choice for extracranial carotid artery stenosis.

Endoluminal Treatment of Tibioperoneal Atherosclerotic Disease

Tibial and peroneal atherosclerosis usually occurs in patients with advanced and diffuse peripheral vascular disease in the presence of diabetes mellitus and generalized atherosclerosis.[81] Patients with this disease frequently present with severe symptoms of intermittent claudication and ischemia in the lower extremities. Until recently, most of the patients with infrapopliteal arterial disease were treated with various types of surgical procedures. It has been previously shown, however, that patients with infrapopliteal arterial disease have a periprocedural operative mortality between 2 and 6 percent.[81] Furthermore, it has also been reported that the 5-year survival of patients who underwent infrapopliteal surgical bypass was only 48 percent.[81] Endovascular interventions for treatment of tibioperoneal arterial disease have been reported shortly after Gruentzig's[82] original description of PTCA.

Technique and Choice of Devices for Endoluminal Treatment

If the patient's history, physical examination, and noninvasive testing results indicate that the patient might be a candidate for an interventional procedure, diagnostic angiography is performed. Numerous approaches can be used for endoluminal treatment of tibial and peroneal arterial disease. The usual approach for an interventional procedure of tibioperoneal vessels is ipsilateral antegrade puncture because this technique facilitates better catheter and guide wire control. For tibioperoneal angioplasty, it is usually sufficient to use 6 French sheaths. Many sheaths are available that are between 40 to 60 cm in length. Before the procedure, the patient is given an aspirin, and whenever possible, clopidogrel or ticlopidine.

During the interventional procedure, the patient should be anticoagulated with parenteral heparin to achieve an activated clotting time in the range of 200 to 300 seconds. During the procedure, if the run-off appears to be "sluggish" and/or persistent vasospasm is evident, it might be necessary to use small boluses of nitroglycerin or calcium antagonists intra-arterially. Various devices have been used successfully for the endoluminal treatment of tibioperoneal arterial disease (Table 75–4).

Results of Tibioperoneal Angioplasty

Balloon angioplasty has been the most established and the most commonly used infrapopliteal interventional technique.[82–85] Some publications have revealed that the use of low-profile angioplasty systems has allowed increased success and safety of this procedure.[82–84]

PTA of the tibioperoneal disease offers the highest technical success rate and long-term patency rates for the treatment of short, focal, and concentric atherosclerotic lesions.[83–85] When the disease is more diffuse and involves longer segments of multiple branches, surgery is generally recommended as a better choice for the treatment of lower-extremity ischemia.[83–85]

When balloon angioplasty is performed from the level of the tibioperoneal trunk to the mid-calf, one should use 3.5 to 4.5 French balloon catheters and 0.018-inch guide wires. For more distal lesions, it is common to use 2.5 to 3.5 French balloon catheters or coronary catheters and 0.014-inch guide wires. During the procedure, it is beneficial to use digital subtraction technique and road mapping to use less contrast and have better control of the guide wire and balloon catheters. Long lesions and occlusions can rarely be crossed with regular guide wires. In complex lesions, it is frequently necessary to use 0.0014- or 0.018-inch hydrophilically coated guide wires.

By life table analysis, Horvath and coworkers[83] calculated cumulative patency rates after balloon tibioperoneal angioplasty of 79.8 percent at 1 year and 75.3 percent at 3 years of follow-up. In a more recent publication on tibioperoneal angioplasty, Bull and coworkers[84] reported a cumulative clinical success rate of 83 percent at 3 years for angioplasty for single stenosis and a 76 percent clinical success rate for vessels treated with multilevel lesions. Their cumulative patency rate at 3 years, however, was only 44 percent when lytic therapy had been employed. They further reported that their cumulative patency rates at 3 years was only 36 percent for segmental occlusions and only 14 percent for anastomotic stenosis.[84] They concluded that factors that were statistically significant in predicting poor long-term patency included

1. A single patent artery
2. Anastomotic stenosis
3. Acute ischemia

Brown and associates[85] noted very unsatisfactory results with balloon angioplasty at or near distal bypass graft anastomosis (25 percent patency at 2½ months) and suggested that atherectomy may be preferable to a balloon angioplasty for these lesions.

Schwarten and Cutliff[86] reported significantly better results in 96 patients with 146 below-knee angioplasties who were followed up for 6 years. The primary success rate was 97 percent, and the 2-year limb salvage rate was 83 percent. On the basis of their findings, they suggested that the results of angioplasty are comparable to those of surgery in a selected group of patients. In their study, only 20 to 30 percent of patients who had isolated tibioperoneal disease and were suitable for PTA. They suggested that suitable lesions are five or fewer stenoses and occlusions 5 cm or less in length.[86]

Complications that occur with PTA of tibial and peroneal disease vary widely. Horvath and coworkers[83] reported an overall major complication rate of 4 percent and a minor complication rate of 26.4 percent. Bull and coworkers[84] reported that three of their 168 consecutive patients died from periprocedural complications.

TABLE 75–4 Devices and Techniques for Endoluminal Treatment of Tibial and Peroneal Arterial Disease

Balloon angioplasty	Laser angioplasty
Thrombolysis	Gene therapy
Atherectomy (directional, rotational)	Radiation therapy
Stents	

Thrombolytic Therapy for Tibioperoneal Occlusions

Thrombolytic agents have been successfully used for the treatment of acute and chronic tibial and peroneal occlusions.[87, 88] They are particularly beneficial for the treatment of acute embolism of native arteries and infrainguinal bypass thrombosis.[7, 87, 88] The choice of the thrombolytic agent and the technique vary with the circumstances; however, a contralateral femoral approach with a 5 or 6 French sheath is the preferred technique for most patients. The most effective method of thrombolysis is achieved with direct infusion of a thrombolytic agent at the site of thrombosis (catheter-directed technique). Various 0.038-inch infusion wires and 3 to 5 French infusion catheters are available for the catheter-directed infusion of a thrombolytic agent.[7, 87, 88] The infusion of a thrombolytic agent is given until there is evidence of improvement of arterial flow, as documented by relief of pain, appearance of arterial pulses, or angiographic evidence of arterial recanalization. The duration of infusion of a thrombolytic agent varies depending on the age of occlusion, the length of the occluded arterial segment, and the presence or absence of thrombus at the lesion. It is generally recommended that the infusion not be prolonged beyond 24 hours because the incidence of complications increases exponentially and the chances for success are small.[7, 87, 88] After successful recanalization of tibioperoneal vessels with a thrombolytic agent, it is frequently necessary to treat inflow or outflow disease, which is the culprit of thrombosis. The choice of an interventional or surgical technique should be determined on the basis of the anatomic findings and the patient's general condition. For instance, in patients with multiple previous surgical interventions, without suitable veins for bypass procedure, and failed distal tibioperoneal bypasses, it might be more advantageous to perform balloon angioplasty and/or stenting than a surgical procedure.

Atherectomy Devices

Atherectomy devices have been rarely used for the treatment of tibioperoneal atherosclerosis. Most investigators have reserved the use of rotational ablation devices for the treatment of short, focal, and calcific lesions. The rotational ablation device in this situation is used for debulking purposes and for facilitating subsequent balloon angioplasty (Fig. 75–6). Use of the rotational atherectomy device in total occlusions, long lesions, and multisegmented disease is not recommended because of the high risk of dissection, the potential risk of perforation, and the potential development of a compartment syndrome.[89, 90] Use of other atherectomy devices is even less beneficial, because they are large in profile and might not negotiate curvatures in the stenotic tibioperoneal vessels.[89, 90, 91]

Stents

Stents for treatment of tibioperoneal disease have not been adequately evaluated. Most of the reports refer to rare or occasional use of stents when no other alternatives were available to maintain the patency of a treated vessel.[90] Stents might be of benefit in treating flow-limiting dissection and threatened closure of the vessel after balloon angioplasty or rotational atherectomy. The stents have not been approved for use in the United States for tibioperoneal vessels. If absolutely necessary, it appears that self-expanding stents or stents that are not easily deformed by external compression might be the best choice.

Laser Devices

The use of laser devices for recanalization of total occlusions and treatment of long, diffusely diseased segments of small tibioperoneal vessels has been met with mixed reviews.[91, 92] Excimer laser has been used for these purposes by several investigators with satisfactory results in a small number of patients when no other alternatives appeared to be of benefit.[91, 92] Similar to its coronary applications, the use of lasers in this location is associated with high incidence of restenosis and the potential risk of perforation.[91, 92]

Gene Therapy

A large number of patients with critical limb ischemia are unsuitable for operative or percutaneous revascularization. No pharmacologic treatment has been shown to favorably affect the natural history of critical limb ischemia. Until recently, amputation was frequently the only available alternative in this subset of patients. Preclinical studies have indicated that angiogenic growth factors (vascular endothelial growth factor and basic fibroblast growth factor) can stimulate the development of collateral arteries in animal models of peripheral and myocardial ischemia, a concept called *therapeutic angiogenesis*.[93] In clinical studies, several authors have used a vascular endothelial growth factor, also known as vascular permeability factor, that has high affinity to bind to endothelial cells.[94] They have demonstrated angiographic and histologic evidence of angiogenesis after intra-arterial and intramuscular gene transfer of vascular endothelial growth factor in patients with critical limb ischemia.[94] Although the preliminary results are encouraging, further clinical studies of both recombinant protein and alternative dosing regimens will be required to define the relative risks and benefits of gene therapy.

Radiation Therapy

Radiation therapy for peripheral vascular disease is in its infancy. The preliminary data of radiation therapy for de novo and restenotic superficial and popliteal artery disease are encouraging.[95] No information is available regarding its

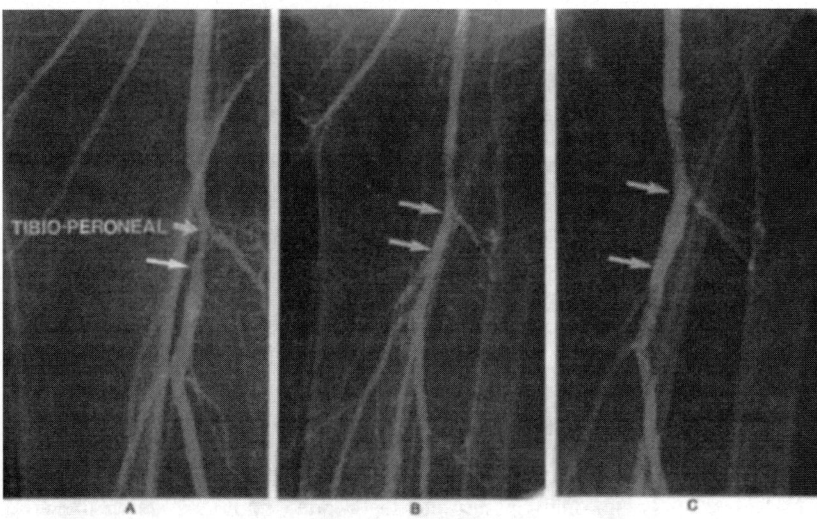

FIGURE 75–6 Selected cineangiographic frames of a patient with severe tibioperoneal atherosclerotic disease. **A,** Left tibioperoneal trunk angiogram reveals a severe, calcific lesion *(arrows)* at the origin of tibioperoneal trunk before intervention. **B,** Left tibioperoneal trunk angiogram reveals significant improvement of the stenosis *(arrows)* after rotablation with 2.5-mm burr. **C,** Left tibioperoneal angiogram of the same patient as in **A** and **B** after 6-month follow-up shows excellent result *(arrows)* of the interventional procedure.

application in the treatment of tibioperoneal disease. Because these vessels are of a small caliber and the disease is often manifested with long and calcified lesions, currently available radiation source delivery systems will require further refinement.

Subclavian Artery Occlusive Disease

The traditional treatment of subclavian arterial occlusive disease has been surgical bypass; however, morbidity ranges from 4 to 11 percent, and mortality risk can reach 5 percent.[96, 97] Since the original report of Bachman and Kim in 1980,[93] PTA for subclavian artery occlusive disease has gained significant popularity. This technique offers a safer and less invasive alternative to surgery.[99–101]

As in iliac artery angioplasty, the technical success rate of PTA for subclavian artery stenosis is achieved in 97 to 100 percent of patients.[100–102] On the other hand, several studies have revealed that the recanalization rate for subclavian artery occlusions is significantly lower than that for stenosis.[102] Henry and colleagues[102] reported only a 47 percent recanalization rate for occlusions. Hebrang and associates[103] reported an 80 percent patency at 4 years. Henry and colleagues[102] reported an 8-year secondary patency rate of 90 percent. For the less common innominate artery lesions, angioplasty results are similar to those obtained in the proximal left subclavian artery.[100–103] Although several studies confirmed the safety and efficacy of balloon angioplasty of the subclavian artery, potential complications and limitations continue to exist. Dissection has been reported to occur in 10 to 12 percent of cases, thrombosis in 2 to 8 percent, technical failures in 5 to 12 percent, and restenosis in 10 to 16 percent.[100–104]

Distal embolization of the plaque material into the vertebral artery was reported in 1 percent of the procedures, resulting in neurologic deficit.[102] It appears, however, that these neurologic ischemic events are mostly transient.[102–104]

Kumar and associates[101] originally proposed stent-supported balloon angioplasty to prevent intimal tears, abrupt vessel closure, and embolization by trapping atherosclerotic material between the stent and the atherosclerotic material. Several reports have revealed that initial success and short-term results of subclavian artery balloon angioplasty can be improved by adjunctive stenting[100–107] (Table 75–5).

However, to date, no randomized trial has been performed to compare the results of balloon angioplasty to those of subclavian artery stenting. The indications for angioplasty and/or stenting should be the same as for surgery.[96, 97, 102, 104] It is generally indicated for symptomatic patients with subclavian artery stenosis or occlusion with either neurologic signs of vertebrobasilar insufficiency and/or upper limb ischemia.[102–107] This procedure is also indicated in patients with subclavian steal syndrome and recurrent angina after internal mammary artery bypass[102–107] (Figs. 75–7 to 75–9).

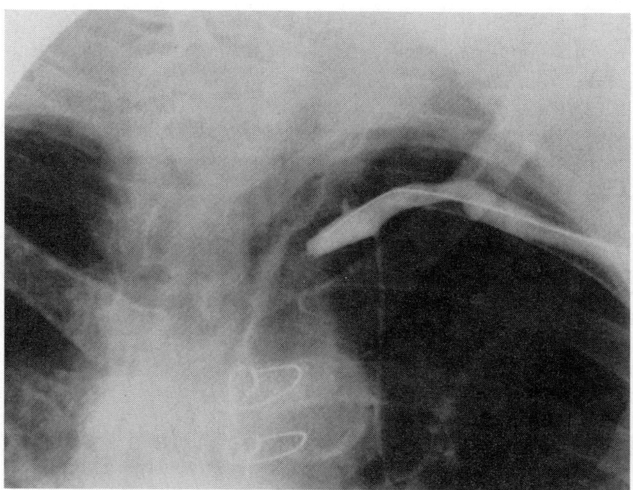

FIGURE 75–7 Cineangiographic frame of a left subclavian artery occlusion at the origin *(white arrow)* in a patient with angina pectoris. This patient recently underwent coronary artery bypass surgery utilizing the left internal mammary artery *(open arrow)*.

Many stents have been used for balloon-assisted angioplasty of the subclavian arteries. Even though none of the stents has been approved for this use in the United States, the Palmaz models P204, P294, and P394 (Johnson & Johnson, Warren, NJ) and the Wallstent (Schneider, Minneapolis, MN) have been used with encouraging immediate and long-term results.[102–107] The procedure is usually performed by femoral or ipsilateral brachial artery access. In the presence of an occlusion, the brachial site is useful, particularly if the occlusion begins at the origin of the subclavian artery.

Balloon angioplasty with or without stenting is safe and offers favorable immediate and late clinical outcomes for

TABLE 75-5 Review of Reports of Subclavian Artery Stenting

Author	Patients/Arteries (n)	Technical Success (%)	Restenosis Rate (%)	Mean Follow-Up (mo)
Mathias et al[100]	7/7	100	0	6
Kumar et al[101]	27/31	100	0	NR
Ansel et al[105]	37/37	97	5	NR
Bajwa et al[104]	29/29	100	10	NR
Pathan et al[106]	35/36	100	5	12
Henry et al[102]	113/113	91	15.5	108
Al-Mubarak et al[107]	38/38	92	6	20

Abbreviation: NR, not reported.

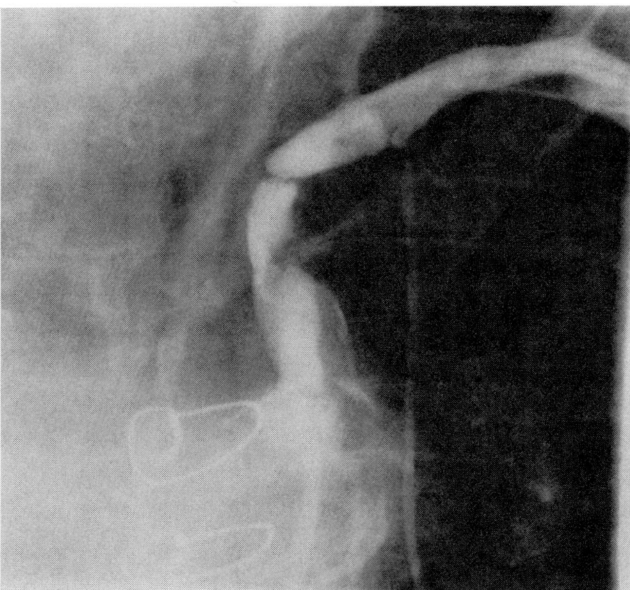

FIGURE 75–8 Cineangiographic frame of the same patient as in Figure 75–7 after left subclavian artery balloon angioplasty with utilization of brachial artery and femoral artery approaches. Note spiral dissection and recoil with significant residual stenosis of the recanalized subclavian artery *(arrows).*

most patients with subclavian artery stenosis. Recanalization of occlusions is more difficult to achieve and carries higher complication rates. Further randomized studies will be necessary to determine the particular benefit of stents in the treatment of these lesions.

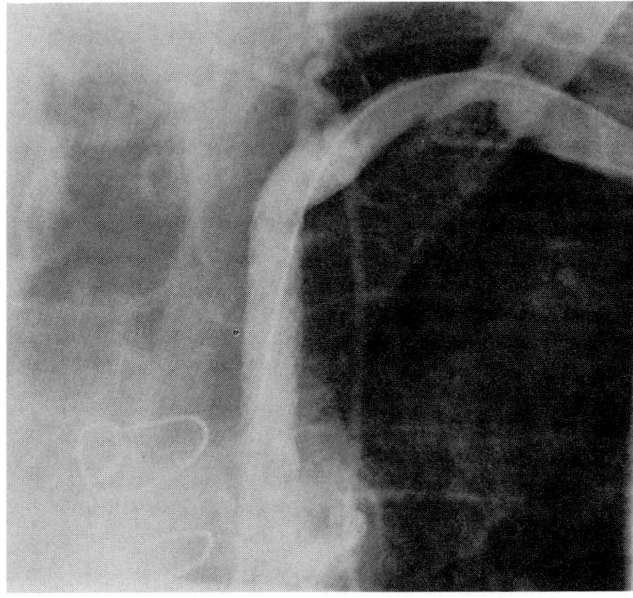

FIGURE 75–9 Cineangiographic frame of the same patient as in Figures 75–7 and 75–8 reveals excellent flow without residual stenosis after deployment of a balloon-expandable, Palmaz P294 stent *(arrows).*

Endovascular Radiation Therapy for Treatment of Peripheral Arterial Occlusive Disease

Despite improvements in long-term outcomes after PTA and stenting of the peripheral vessels, restenosis remains a significant problem, particularly in long lesions, vessels with smaller diameters, and restenotic lesions.[108] Therapeutic approaches have focused on atherectomy devices, stents, and stent grafts or pharmaceutical agents. None of these treatment options has been successful in resolving this problem.[108, 109] Vascular radiation therapy for the prevention of restenosis after PTA and stenting is a new frontier in the field of peripheral interventions. The first experience of in vivo endovascular radiation therapy was reported by Friedman and colleagues, in 1964.[110] The purpose of their study was to prevent the development of atherosclerosis.

Various radiation therapy platforms have been tried for the prevention of restenosis after angioplasty or stenting (Fig. 75–10). Nori and Parikh[111] tried external-beam radiation therapy in their pilot study using 8 to 12 Gy with encouraging preliminary results. However, no randomized trial with long-term follow-up after external-beam vascular radiation therapy is available to determine the long-term results and the potential consequences of radiation to the adjacent tissues.

Intravascular radiation therapy with various beta and gamma sources has been studied more extensively than external-beam radiation therapy.

The locally delivered ionizing radiation can inhibit vascular smooth muscle cell proliferation associated with restenosis. A large body of animal investigation and a more limited number of clinical trials have established that localized irradiation of the angioplasty site by intraluminal delivery of low-dose beta or gamma particles inhibits smooth muscle cell migration and proliferation in vitro and in vivo.[112]

Numerous isotopes have been tested for the treatment of coronary artery occlusive disease (Table 75–6).[113] Several of these have been proposed for the treatment of peripheral arterial disease. Previous studies have generally involved the use of high-activity gamma emitters. However, contro-

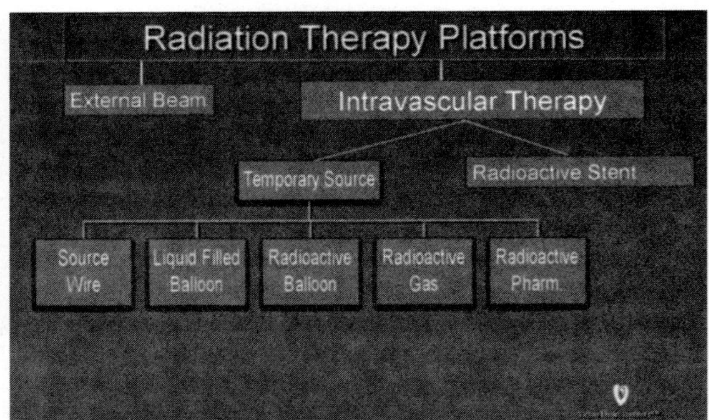

FIGURE 75–10 Radiation therapy platforms.

TABLE 75-6 Possible Isotopes for Endovascular Brachytherapy

Isotope	Emission	Half-Life	Activity Required
Ir 192	Gamma	74 da	1.0 Ci
I 125	X-ray	60 da	3.8 Ci
P 32	Beta	14 da	40 mCi
Sr/Y 90	Beta	28 yr	30 mCi
W/Re 188	Beta	69 da	35 mCi
V 48	Beta	16 da	1.0 μCi (stent)

versy regarding the choice of emitters still remains among the investigators. Two of the most controversial issues surrounding intravascular radiation therapy involve the preference of beta- or gamma-emitting radioisotope sources and the importance of the source centering in the arteries. The larger peripheral vessel diameters require higher energy sources than the coronary vessels. Eccentric atherosclerotic lesions frequently cause malcentering of the catheter in the vessel, and malcentering of the catheter-based solid source by as little as 0.5 mm could lead to as much as a fivefold error of dosing.[114, 115]

These errors are considerably worse for beta than for gamma emitters. However, because beta emitters deposit a large fraction of their energy locally, these isotopes have substantial safety advantages over the gamma emitters for both the operator and the patient.[115] Efforts to make use of beta radioisotopes in solution await the development of an appropriate compound with an adequate biodilution profile to deal with safety of the potential intravascular release of radioisotope-containing liquid.[114] Irradiated stents for the treatment of peripheral arterial occlusive disease await further advances in stent design and the most effective choice of the radioisotope.

Clinical Trials

The first clinical trial was started in 1990 by Liermann and associates[112] in an effort to reduce the restenosis rate after balloon angioplasty in superficial femoral-popliteal arteries. Their 6-year experience has been reported on by Schopohl.[113] In this study from 1990 to 1997, 29 patients with in-stent restenosis in the femoral-popliteal arteries were treated with another PTA or directional atherectomy followed by endovascular radiation with ^{192}Ir. The radiation was well tolerated, and the investigators reported a 5-year patency rate of 82 percent based on Doppler ultrasound. Restenosis occurred in 11 percent of patients, and 7 percent of patients experienced occlusion of the treated vessels. More recently, in a randomized trial between PTA and brachytherapy for superficial femoral artery lesions, Pokrajac and coworkers[114] reported a restenosis rate of 51.7 percent in PTA alone versus 25 percent for PTA plus brachytherapy.

The Peripheral Artery Radiation Investigational Study (PARIS) is currently evaluating the safety, feasibility, and efficacy of endovascular brachytherapy to prevent restenosis in the superficial femoral-popliteal arteries immediately after PTA without stenting.[115] Endovascular brachytherapy is administered through a balloon-centering catheter system using a ^{192}Ir source delivered to the target site by a remote afterloader. Twenty-seven patients completed phase II, 6-month angiographic follow-up. Their restenosis rate was 11 percent.

Conclusions

Brachytherapy for the treatment of peripheral arterial disease to prevent restenosis after an interventional procedure is still in the developmental stages. At the present time, various isotopes are being tested in an effort to reduce the radiation exposure to the patient and the operator and to reduce the dose delivery in near-field.[112–115] Centering balloons have been designed that center the catheter-based isotope within the lumen of the vessel, in spite of eccentric plaque. This improves the depth of dose delivery, especially for large vessels. Novel techniques, such as radioactive liquid–filled or gas-filled balloons that improve dose delivery, are currently under investigation.

Future potential brachytherapy sites include superficial femoral–popliteal arteries, tibioperoneal arteries, hepatic vascular system, arteriovenous dialysis grafts, renal arteries, and carotid arteries.

References

1. Yehear RA, Monta GL, Taylor LM, et al: Surgical management of severely acute lower extremity ischemia. J Vasc Surg 15:358–393, 1992.
2. Ouriel K, Veith FJ, Sasahara AA: A comparison of recombinant urokinase with vascular surgery as initial treatment for acute arterial occlusion of the legs. N Engl J Med 338:1105–1111, 1998.
3. McNicol GB, Reid W, Bain WH, Douglas AS: Treatment of peripheral arterial occlusions by streptokinase perfusion. BMJ 1:1508–1512, 1963.
4. Goldhaber SZ, Kessler CM, Heit JA, et al: Recombinant tissue-type plasminogen activator versus a novel dosing regimen of urokinase in acute pulmonary embolism: a randomized controlled multicenter trial. J Am Coll Cardiol 20:24–30, 1992.
5. Groar RA, Olin J, Bartholomew JR, et al: Efficacy and safety of intraarterial local infusion of streptokinase, urokinase, or tissue plasminogen activator for peripheral arterial occlusion: a retrospective review. J Vasc Med Biol 2:310–315, 1990.
6. McNamara TO, Fischer JR: Thrombolysis of peripheral arterial and graft occlusions: improved results using high dose urokinase. AJR 144:769–775, 1985.
7. Marder VJ, Sherry S: Thrombolytic therapy: current status (1) and (2). N Engl J Med 318:1512–1520, 1988.
8. Van Breda A, Katzen BT, Deutsch AS: Urokinase versus streptokinase in local thrombolysis. Radiology 165:109–111, 1987.
9. Dale WA: Differential management of acute peripheral arterial ischemia. J Vasc Surg 1:269–278, 1984.
10. Kaplan NM: Systemic hypertension: mechanisms and diagnosis. *In* Braunwald E (ed): Heart Disease: A Textbook of Cardiovascular Medicine. 3rd ed. pp. 819–861. Philadelphia: W B Saunders, 1988.
11. Holley KE, Hunt JC, Brown AL, et al: Renal artery stenosis: a clinical-pathologic study in normotensive and hypertensive patients. Am J Med 37:14–22, 1964.
12. Olin JW, Melia M, Young JR, et al: Prevalence of atherosclerotic RAS in patients with atherosclerosis elsewhere. Am J Med 88:46N–51N, 1990.
13. Harding MB, Smith LR, Himmelstein SI, et al: Renal artery stenosis: prevalence and associated risk factors in patients undergoing routine cardiac catheterization. J Am Soc Nephrol 2:1608–1616, 1992.
14. Ploth DW: Renovascular hypertension. *In* Jacobson HR, Striker GE, Klahr S (eds): The Principles and Practice of Nephrology. 2nd ed. pp. 379–386. St. Louis: Mosby, 1995.
15. Dean, RH, Kieffer RW, Smith BM, et al: Renovascular hypertension:

anatomic and renal function changes during drug therapy. Arch Surg 116:1408–1415, 1981.

16. Tollefson DF, Ernst CB: Natural history of atherosclerotic renal artery stenosis associated with aortic disease. J Vasc Surg 14:327–331, 1991.
17. Pohl MA, Novick AC: Natural history of atherosclerotic and fibrous renal artery disease: clinical implications. Am J Kidney Dis 5:A120–A130, 1985.
18. Harrison EG Jr, McCormack LJ: Pathologic classification of renal artery disease in neurovascular hypertension. Mayo Clin Proc 46:161, 1971.
19. Working Group on Renovascular Hypertension: Detection, evaluation and treatment of renovascular hypertension. Final report. Arch Intern Med 147:820–829, 1987.
20. Dondi M, Monetti N, Fanti S, et al: Use of technetium-99m-MAG_3 for renal scintigraphy after angiotensin converting enzyme inhibition. J Nucl Med 32:424–428, 1991.
21. Olin JW, Piedmonte MR, Young JR, et al: The utility of duplex ultrasound scanning of renal arteries for diagnosing renal artery stenosis. Ann Intern Med 122:833–838, 1995.
22. Klatzburg RW, Duomoulin CL, Buonocore MA, et al: Noninvasive measurement of renal hemodynamic function using gadolinium-enhanced magnetic resonance imaging. Invest Radiol 29:5123–5126, 1994.
23. Hawkins IF, Wilcox CS, Kerns SR, et al: CO_2 digital angiography: a safer contrast agent for renal vascular imaging. Am J Kidney Dis 24:685–694, 1994.
24. Diamond JR: Flash pulmonary edema and the diagnostic suspicion of occult RAS. Am J Kidney Dis 21:328–330, 1993.
25. Barri YM, Davidson RA, Senler S, et al: Prediction of cure of hypertension in atherosclerotic RAS. South Med J 89:679–683, 1996.
26. Novick AC, Ziegelboum M, Vidt DG, et al: Trends in surgical revascularization for renal artery disease: ten years' experience. JAMA 257:498–501, 1987.
27. Klinge J, Mali WPTM, Puijaelrt CBAJ, et al: Percutaneous transluminal renal angioplasty: Initial and long term results. Radiology 171:501–506, 1989.
28. Tegtmeyer CJ, Dyer R, Teates CD, et al: Percutaneous transluminal dilatation of renal the arteries. Radiology 135:589–599, 180.
29. Sos TA, Pickering TG, Phil D: Percutaneous renal angioplasty in renovascular hypertension due to atheroma or fibromuscular dysplasia. N Engl J Med 309:274–279, 1983.
30. Hansen KJ, Starr SM, Sands RE, et al: Contemporary surgical management of renovascular disease. J Vasc Surg 16:319–331, 1992.
31. Jamieson GG, Clarkson AR, Woodroff AJ, Faris I: Reconstructive renal vascular surgery for chronic renal failure. Br J Surg 71:338–340, 1984.
32. Novick AC, Textor SC, Bodie B, Khauli RB: Revascularization to preserve renal function in patients with atherosclerotic renovascular disease. Urol Clin North Am 11:477–490, 1984.
33. Libertino JA, Bosco PJ, Ying CY, et al: Renal revascularization to preserve and restore renal function. J Urol 147:1485–1487, 1992.
34. Gruntzig A, Kuhlmann U, Lutolf U, et al: Treatment of renovascular hypertension with percutaneous transluminal dilatation of a renal-artery stenosis. Lancet 1:801–802, 1978.
35. Weibull H, Berquist D, Bergantz SE, et al: Percutaneous transluminal renal angioplasty versus surgical reconstruction of atherosclerotic renal artery stenosis: a prospective randomized study. J Vasc Surg 18:841–852, 1993.
36. Martin LG, Cork RD, Kaufman SL: Long term results of angioplasty in 110 patients with renal artery stenosis. J Vasc Interv Radiol 3:619–626, 1992.
37. Rees CR, Palmaz JC, Becker GJ, et al: Palmaz stent in atherosclerotic stenoses involving the ostia of the renal arteries: preliminary report of a multicenter study. Radiology 181:507–514, 1991.
38. Eldrup-Jorgensen J, Harvey HR, Sampson LN, et al: Should transluminal renal angioplasty be applied to ostial artery atherosclerosis? J Vasc Surg 21:909–915, 1995.
39. Damaraju S, Krajcer Z: Successful Wallstent implantation for extensive iatrogenic renal artery dissection in a patient with fibromuscular dysplasia. J Endovasc Surg 6:297–300, 1999.
40. Blum U, Krumme B, Flügel P, Gabelmann A, et al: Treatment of ostial renal-artery stenosis with vascular endoprosthesis after unsuccessful balloon angioplasty. N Engl J Med 336:459–465, 1997.
41. Dorros G, Jaff M, Mathiak L, et al: Four-year follow-up of Palmaz-Schatz revascularization as treatment for atherosclerotic renal artery stenosis. Circulation 98:642–647, 1998.
42. Johnston WK: Multicenter prospective study of nonruptured abdominal aortic aneurysms. Part II: variables predicting morbidity and mortality. J Vasc Surg 9:437–447, 1989.
43. Chen JC, Hildebrand HD, Salvian AJ, et al: Predictors of death in ruptured and nonruptured abdominal aortic aneurysms. J Vasc Surg 24:614–620, 1996.
44. Parodi JC, Palmaz JC, Barone HD: Transfemoral intraluminal graft implantation for abdominal aortic aneurysms. Ann Vasc Surg 5:491–499, 1991.
45. Zarins CK, Haris EJ: Operative repair for aortic aneurysms: the gold standard. J Endovasc Surg 4:232–241, 1997.
46. Beebe HG: Imaging modalities for aortic endografting. J Endovasc Surg 4:111–123, 1997.
47. Balm R, Eikleboom BC, van Leewen MS, Noordzij J: Spiral CT-angiography of the aorta. Eur J Vasc Surg 8:544–551, 1994.
48. May J, White GH, Yu W, et al: Concurrent comparison of endoluminal repair versus no treatment for small abdominal aortic aneurysms. Eur J Vasc Endovasc Surg 13:472–426, 1997.
49. Moore WS, Rutherford RB: Transfemoral repair of abdominal aortic aneurysm: results of the North American EVT phase 1 trial. EVT investigators. J Vasc Surg 23:543–553, 1996.
50. Zarins CK, White RA, Schwarten D, et al: AneuRx stent graft versus open surgical repair of abdominal aortic aneurysms: multicenter prospective clinical trial. J Vasc Surg 29:292–305, 1999.
51. Taheri SA, Leonhardt HJ, Greenan T: The TALENT endoluminal graft placement system. *In* Yao JST, Pearce WH (eds): Techniques in Vascular Surgery. pp. 433–445. Stamford, CT: Appleton & Lange, 1998.
52. Beebe HG: The Meadox Vanguard Endovascular Graft. Presented at Techniques in Vascular and Endovascular Surgery Meeting, December 11, 1997, Chicago, IL.
53. Diethrich EB: Current status of endoluminal grafting for abdominal aortic aneurysms. Texas Heart Inst J 25:10–16, 1998.
54. McGovern PG, Burke GL, Sprafka JM, et al: Trends in mortality, morbidity, and risk factor levels for stroke from 1960 through 1990. JAMA 268:753–759, 1992.
55. Cohen M, Biller J, Saver JL: Advances in management of carotid disease. Curr Probl Cardiol 19:473–532, 1994.
56. Roederer GO, Langois YE, Jager KA, et al: The natural history of carotid artery disease in asymptomatic patients with cervical bruits. Stroke 15:605–613, 1984.
57. Autet A, Pourcelot L, Saudeau D, et al: Stroke risk in patients with carotid stenosis. Lancet 1:888–890, 1987.
58. De Bakey M: Carotid endarterectomy revisited. J Endovasc Surg 3:4, 1996.
59. Pokras R, Dyken ML: Dramatic changes in the performance of endarterectomy for diseases of the extracranial arteries of the head. Stroke 19:1289–1290, 1988.
60. Zarins CK: Carotid endarterectomy: the gold standard. J Endovasc Surg 3:10–15, 1996.
61. North American Symptomatic Carotid Endarterectomy Trial Collaborators: Beneficial effects of carotid endarterectomy in symptomatic patients with high grade carotid stenosis. N Engl J Med 325:445–453, 1991.
62. European Carotid Surgery Trialists' Collaborative Group: MRC European Carotid Surgery Trial: interim results of symptomatic patients with severe (70–99%) or with mild (0–29%) carotid stenosis. Lancet 337:1235–1243, 1991.
63. Executive Committee for the Asymptomatic Carotid Atherosclerotic Study: Endarterectomy for asymptomatic carotid artery stenosis. JAMA 273:1421–1428, 1995.
64. Rothwell PM, Slattery J, Warlow CP: A systemic review of the risks of stroke and death due to endarterectomy for symptomatic carotid stenosis. Stroke 27:260–265, 1996.
65. McCrory DC, Goldstein LB, Samsa GP, et al: Predicting complications of carotid endarterectomy. Stroke 24:1285–1291, 1993.
66. Edwards WH Jr, Edward WH Sr, Mulherin JL, et al: Recurrent carotid artery stenosis. Ann Surg 209:662–669, 1989.
67. Mattos MA, Hogson KJ, Londrey GL: Carotid endarterectomy: operative risks, recurrent stenosis, long term stroke rates in modern series. J Cardiovasc Surg 33:387–400, 1992.
68. Das MV, Hertzer NR, Ratcliffe NB, et al: Recurrent carotid stenosis: a five year series of 65 reoperations. Ann Surg 202:28–35, 1985.

69. Riccotta JJ, O'Brian MS, De Weesse JA: Natural history of reccurrent residual stenosis after carotid endarterectomy: implications for postoperative surveillance and surgical management. Surgery 112:656–663, 1992.
70. Kerber CW, Hornwell LD, Loehden OL: Catheter dilatation of proximal carotid artery stenosis during distal bifurcation endarterectomy. AJNR 1:348–349, 1980.
71. Sivaguru A, Venables GS, Beard JD, et al: European Carotid Angioplasty Trial. J Endovasc Surg 3:16–20, 1996.
72. Roubin GS, Yadev S, Iyer SS, et al: Carotid stent-supported angioplasty: a neurovascular intervention to prevent stroke. Am J Cardiol 78:8–12, 1996.
73. Diethrich EB, Ndiaye M, Reid DB: Stenting in the carotid artery: initial experience in 110 patients. J Endovasc Surg 3:42–62, 1996.
74. Wholey MH, Wholey M, Jarmolowski CR, et al: Endovascular stents for carotid occlusive disease. J Endovasc Surg 4:326–328, 1997.
75. Yadev JS, Roubin GS, Iyer S: Elective stenting of the extracranial carotid arteries: immediate and late outcome. Circulation 95:376–381, 1997.
76. Wholey MH, Wholey M, Bergeron P, et al: Current global status of carotid artery stent placement. Cathet Cardiovasc Diagn 44:1–6, 1998.
77. Theron J, Payelle G, Coskum O, et al: Carotid artery stenosis: treatment with protected balloon angioplasty and stent placement. Radiology 201:627–636, 1996.
78. Mathur A, Roubin GS, Iyer SS, et al: Predictors of stroke complicating carotid artery stenting. Circulation 97:1239–1245, 1998.
79. Kachel R: Results of balloon angioplasty in carotid arteries. J Endovasc Surg 3:22–30, 1996.
80. Henry M, Amor M, Masson I, et al: Angioplasty and stenting of the extracranial carotid arteries. J Endovasc Surg 5:293–304, 1998.
81. Rutherford RB, Becker GJ: Standards for evaluating and reporting the results of surgical and percutaneous therapy for peripheral arterial disease. J Vasc Interv Radiol 2:169–174, 1991.
82. Gruentzig A: Die perkutane rekanalisation chronischer arterialler verschlusse (Dotter-Prinzip) mit einem neuem dopplelumigen dilatationkatheter. Fortschr Geb Reontgenstr Nuklearmed 124:80–86, 1976.
83. Horvath W, Oertl M, Haidinger D: Percutaneous transluminal angioplasty of crural arteries. Radiology 177:565–569, 1990.
84. Bull PG, Mendel H, Hold M, et al: Distal popliteal and tibioperoneal transluminal angioplasty: long term follow-up. J Vasc Interv Radiol 3:522–532, 1992.
85. Brown RT, Moore ED, Getrajdman GI, Sadekni S: Infrapopliteal angioplasty: long term follow-up. J Vasc Interv Radiol 4:139, 1993.
86. Schwarten DE, Cutliff WC. Arterial occlusive disease below the knee: treatment with percutaneous transluminal angioplasty performed with low-profile catheters and steerable guide wires. Radiology 169:71–74, 1988.
87. McNamara TO, Fischer JR: Thrombolysis in peripheral arterial and graft occlusions: improved results using high dose urokinase. AJR 144:764–775, 1985.
88. Traughber PD, Cook PS, Micklos RJ, et al: Intraarterial fibrinolytic therapy for popliteal and tibial artery obstructions: comparison of streptokinase and urokinase. AJR 149:453–456, 1987.
89. Dorros G, Lyer S, Zaitoun R, et al: Acute angiographic and clinical outcome of high-speed percutaneous rotational atherectomy (Rotablator). Cathet Cardiovasc Diagn 22:157–166, 1991.
90. Dacca N, Rainier AE, Noon GP: Treatment of symptomatic peripheral atherosclerotic disease with a rotational atherectomy device. Am J Cardiol 63:77–80, 1989.
91. Diethrich EB: Laser angioplasty: development, current status and future. Angiology 41:757–767, 1990.
92. Litvack F, Grundfest WS, Adler L, et al: Percutaneous excimer-laser and excimer-laser-assisted angioplasty of the lower extremities: results of initial clinical trial. Radiology 172:331–335, 1998.
93. Baffour R, Berman J, Garb JL, et al: Enhanced angiogenesis and growth of collaterals by in vivo administration of recombinant basic fibroblast growth factor in a rabbit model of acute lower limb ischemia: dose-response effect of basic fibroblast growth factor. J Vasc Surg 16:181–191, 1992.
94. Baumgartner I, Pieczek A, Manor O, et al: Constitutive expression of phVEGF$_{165}$ after intramuscular gene transfer promotes collateral vessel development in patients with critical limb ischemia. Circulation 97:1114–1123, 1998.
95. Nori D, Parikh S, Moni J: Management of peripheral vascular disease: innovative approaches using radiation therapy. Int J Radiat Oncol Biol Phys 36:847–856, 1996.
96. Mingoli A, Feidhous RJ, Farina C, et al: Comparative results of carotid-subclavian artery bypass and axillo-axillary bypass in patients with symptomatic subclavian disease. Eur J Vasc Surg 6:26–30, 1992.
97. Thompson BW, Read RC, Campbell GC: Operative correction of proximal blocks of the subclavian or the innominate arteries. J Cardiovasc Surg 21:125–130, 1980.
98. Bachman DM, Kim RM: Transluminal dilatation of subclavian steal syndrome. AJR 135:995–996, 1980.
99. Dorros G, Ruben FL, Jamnadas P, Mathiak ML: Peripheral transluminal angioplasty of the subclavian and innominate arteries utilizing the brachial approach: acute outcome and follow-up. Cathet Cardiovasc Diagn 19:71–76, 1990.
100. Mathias DK, Leath I, Haarman P: Percutaneous transluminal angioplasty of proximal subclavian artery occlusions. Cardiovasc Interv Radiol 16:214–218, 1993.
101. Kumar K, Dorros G, Bates CM, et al: Primary stent deployment in occlusive subclavian artery disease. Cathet Cardiovasc Diagn 34:281–285, 1995.
102. Henry M, Amor M, Henry I, et al: Percutaneous transluminal angioplasty of subclavian arteries. J Endovasc Surg 6:33–41, 1999.
103. Hebrang A, Maskovic J, Berislav T: Percutaneous transluminal angioplasty of the subclavian arteries: long-term results in 52 patients. AJR 156:1091–1094, 1991.
104. Bajwa T, Shalev Y, Schmidt HD: Subclavian artery stenting for treatment of upper extremity claudication and subclavian steal syndrome: demonstration of long-term outcome. Circulation 94(suppl I):58, 1996.
105. Ansel GM, Barry SG, Yakabov JS: Primary stenting of symptomatic subclavian artery stenosis. Circulation 94(suppl I):58, 1996.
106. Pathan AS, Kenichi F, Ganim SM: Favorable long-term outcome of subclavian artery stenting. Circulation 94(suppl I):58, 1996.
107. Al-Mubarak N, Liu WM, Dean LS, et al: Immediate and late outcomes of subclavian artery stenting. Cathet Cardiovasc Diagn 46:169–172, 1999.
108. Johnston KW: Femoral and popliteal arteries: reanalysis of results of angioplasty. Radiology 183:767–771, 1992.
109. Martin EC, Katzen BT, Benenati JF, et al: Multicenter trial of the Wallstent in the iliac and femoral arteries. J Vasc Interv Radiol 6:843–849, 1995.
110. Friedman M, Felton L, Beyers S: The antiatherogenic effect of ^{192}Ir upon the cholesterol-fed rabbit. J Clin Invest 43:185–192, 1964.
111. Nori D, Parikh S, Moni J: Management of peripheral vascular disease: innovative approaches using radiation therapy. Int J Radiat Oncol Biol Phys 36:847–856, 1996.
112. Liermann D, Boettcher HD, Kollatch J: Prophylactic endovascular brachytherapy to prevent intimal hyperplasia after stent implantation in femoro-popliteal arteries. Cardiovasc Intervent Radiol 17:12–16, 1994.
113. Schopohl B: ^{192}Ir endovascular brachytherapy for avoidance of intimal hyperplasia after transluminal angioplasty and stent implantation in peripheral vessels: 6 years of experience. Int J Oncol Biol Phys 36:835–840, 1996.
114. Pokrajac B, Minar E, Knocke TH, et al: HDR-brachytherapy for prophylaxis of restenosis after femoropopliteal angioplasty: results from a randomized trial. Vienna 02. Presented at 1998 Endovascular Brachytherapy Workshop, Naples, Italy, May 10, 1998.
115. Waksman R, Laird JR, Benenati J, et al: Intravascular radiation for prevention of restenosis after angioplasty of narrowed femoral-popliteal arteries: preliminary six month results of a feasibility study. Circulation 98(suppl I):I-66, 1998.

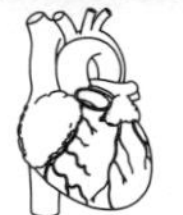

B-Mode Ultrasound: A Noninvasive Method for Assessing Atherosclerosis

John R. Crouse, Curt D. Furberg, Robert P. Byington, and Ward A. Riley

PRINCIPLES
REPRODUCIBILITY
VALIDITY
NORMAL AND ABNORMAL INTIMAL-MEDIAL THICKNESSES
Associations of Risk Factors With Intimal-Medial Thickness
Progression of Intimal-Medial Thickness
Influences of Risk Factors on Progression of Intimal-Medial Thickness in Clinical Trials
Associations of Intimal-Medial Thickness With Symptomatic Vascular Disease
Use of B-Mode Ultrasound to Define Arterial Dimensions
SUMMARY

Imaging of the extent and severity of arterial disease is an intuitively obvious approach for identifying individuals at high or low risk for the development of cardiovascular events. Invasive methods for imaging and quantifying arterial stenosis (coronary or peripheral angiography) have long been used with great benefit for this purpose in symptomatic patients (see Ch. 30, Coronary Angiography). However, the invasive nature of these methods has precluded their broad use in asymptomatic populations and stimulated investigators to develop noninvasive methods that might identify subclinical disease in larger healthy populations or those with minimal symptomatology. Furthermore, because it is recognized that stenosis is only the "tip of the iceberg" of atherosclerosis,[1] methods that directly image the degree of atherosclerosis would be desirable to identify disease before the occurrence of clinical events and thus permit intervention early in selected high-risk individuals. In addition, an individual might be more likely to comply with treatment if he knows he has the early stage of the disease. The identification of subclinical atherosclerosis would also enable investigators to accurately relate risk factors to atherosclerotic disease without the bias inherent in the study of symptomatic patients and to distinguish between underlying atherosclerosis and the development of symptoms.

Noninvasive methods for quantifying atherosclerosis of the coronary arteries are not yet available; the closest approximation is afforded by electron beam computed tomography, which has been used to quantify coronary calcification, an index of advanced atherosclerotic disease.[2] Because atherosclerosis is a generalized disease, other noninvasive (ultrasound) technology has focused on the extracranial carotid arteries. In the 1980s, studies with Doppler ultrasound demonstrated that asymptomatic individuals with extracranial carotid artery stenosis (>75 percent) had a 5.5- and 3-fold increased risk of incident stroke and coronary disease, respectively, compared with those with less than 50 percent stenosis.[3] Investigators have used surface B-mode ultrasound to quantify atherosclerosis of the extracranial carotid arteries. As a means of imaging chronic stable atherosclerotic vascular disease, B-mode ultrasound has many advantages, and it has been used to identify both traditional and new risk factors.[4–6] Investigators have also defined the rates of progression of extracranial carotid atherosclerosis[7, 8] and the effects of interventions (e.g., cholesterol lowering) on progression rates.[7–13] It is clear that atherosclerosis of the extracranial arteries is associated with prevalent coronary artery[14–16] and cerebrovascular[16, 17] disease. Extracranial carotid atherosclerosis has been related to incident coronary artery disease[18–22] and stroke,[22, 23] as well as all-cause mortality.[24]

This review summarizes new information with respect to B-mode ultrasound methodology and its reliability, validity, and relationships with "traditional" and "nontraditional" risk factors for coronary artery disease and associations of risk factor modification with progression of atherosclerosis. In addition, the association of extracranial carotid atherosclerosis with prevalent coronary artery and cerebrovascular disease and its ability to identify individuals at risk for incident coronary artery and cerebrovascular disease are reviewed.

Principles

Ultrasound B-mode imaging is based on the pulse-echo principle used in sonar from which measurements of the arrival times of echoes from a source of pulsed ultrasound are used to create a two-dimensional real-time display of the echo-producing structures. The positions of the structures relative to the source are computed using the arrival times and an assumed value for the speed of propagation of the ultrasound energy between the source and structures. The ultrasound instrumentation required for the noninvasive assessment of atherosclerosis in superficial vessels uses short (two or three cycle) pulses of 7.5 to 10 MHz ultrasound. This provides an axial resolution of approximately 0.1 to 0.2 mm. The distance between structures (e.g., arterial adventitia and lumen) initially separated by more than this resolution distance can be reliably measured, and changes in this distance over time can be ascertained with considerably greater precision, as determined by the changes in arrival times of the corresponding echoes.

To perform reproducible examinations on a specific arterial site, a highly standardized protocol is required that includes the definition of an anatomic landmark, identification of an initial interrogation plane defined relative to the patient's anatomy, and careful circumferential scanning of the segment to identify the maximum wall thickness. Figure 76–1 is a simplified diagram of the carotid artery that defines the segments of arterial walls examined with B-mode ultrasound in the Asymptomatic Carotid Artery Plaque Study (ACAPS).[25] This diagram shows the artery as imaged from the initial interrogation plane (in which the internal and external carotids divide) and shows the anatomic landmark (tip of flow divider) relative to the segments that are defined. The 12 segments of interest are the near and far walls of the common, bifurcation, and internal on the right and left sides of the neck. Different segments of the extracranial arteries have different potential for B-mode imaging: for example, in the Pravastatin, Lipids, and Atherosclerosis in the Carotid arteries (PLAC-II) study, the intimal-medial thickness (IMT) of the common carotid artery was visualized in 97 percent of segments, whereas the IMT of the internal carotid artery was visualized in only 50 percent of near wall sites and 75 percent of far wall sites. The IMT of the bifurcation was visualized to an intermediate degree in about 88 percent of segments.[26]

The extent of atherosclerosis can be quantified in a number of ways. Individual wall thicknesses can be examined, as well as a composite measure of global extracranial carotid arterial disease. A mean of multiple thickness measurements within a patient has the advantage of more broadly representing the total amount of disease. It also markedly reduces measurement variability. For these reasons, the primary atherosclerosis end point often selected for use in clinical trials has been the mean value of the maximum IMTs in each of the examined segments (common carotid, bifurcation, and/or internal carotid artery), the so-called mean maximum IMT.

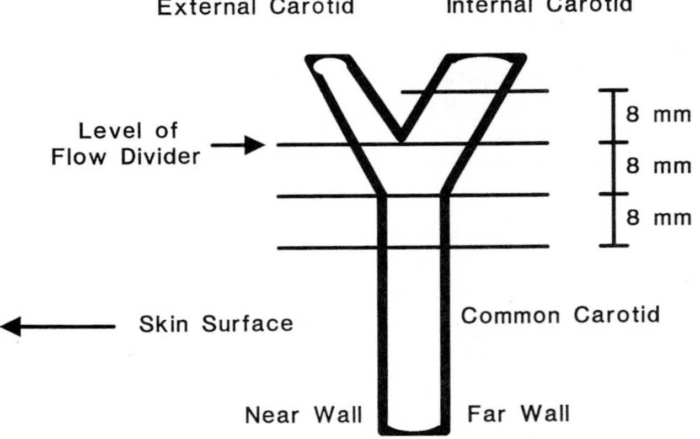

FIGURE 76–1 Simplified diagram of the carotid artery. (Adapted from Riley WA, Barnes RW, Applegate WB, et al: Reproducibility of noninvasive ultrasonic measurement of carotid atherosclerosis. Stroke 23:1062–1068, 1992.)

A standard training and certification program is a requirement for sonographers and readers and should preferably include instruction in ultrasound physics and instrumentation, the anatomy and pathology of atherosclerosis, B-mode image formation, and the visualization and identification of arterial wall boundaries. In our research projects, sonographers and readers submit 25 practice scans or readings that are reviewed and critiqued before they receive initial certification. An ongoing quality control program for both instrumentation and personnel should also be implemented; the latter involves annual recertification based on quantitative visualization and examination of reproducibility criteria.

Reproducibility

The measurement of IMTs in the carotid system is highly reproducible; this may in part reflect the chronic stable nature of this manifestation of arterial disease: IMT is unlikely to be affected by transient metabolic changes. Table 76–1 presents a portion of the reliability data obtained during the conduct of ACAPS.[25] Duplicate examinations, usually obtained within 1 month, were conducted on every participant at baseline and at the end of 3 years of follow-up. The average difference in the mean maximum IMT between the two baseline examinations was 0.01 mm, and the standard deviation of this difference was 0.14 mm. These values were almost identical at the end of the trial: 0.01 and 0.14 mm, respectively. With the standard deviation as a measure of variability, the within- and between-sonographer variabilities at baseline were comparable and low. Although the within-reader variability is half the between-reader variability (0.07 and 0.15 mm, respectively), both are fully acceptable. Although useful for identification of measurement error at baseline and follow-up, these replicability studies do not address the potential problem of equipment, sonographer, or reader drift over time. To address this, studies have incorporated contemporaneous repeat readings of baseline tapes throughout the study.

After conducting a literature review of a large number of protocols for measuring IMT, Kanters and colleagues[27] concluded that the variability of IMT measurements is lowest when determining the mean thickness in the common carotid artery from several different interrogation angles but that a consensus concerning the assessment of IMT is urgently needed so that results from studies in different laboratories can be accurately compared. Automated computerized edge-detection methods being evaluated in several laboratories have the potential to further improve reproducibility, as do harmonic imaging and other innovative techniques being developed and evaluated by ultrasound equipment manufacturers.

Validity

The in vitro and in vivo experiments of Pignoli and associates[28] focused on the aorta and common carotid arteries and indicated that IMT values obtained from B-mode im-

TABLE 76–1 **Reproducibility of Carotid Atherosclerosis Between Paired Examinations at Baseline and At 36 Months**

	Mean Maximum IMT (m) Values At Baseline					
	Overall at Baseline	***Within Sonographers***	***Between Sonographers***	***Within Readers***	***Between Readers***	**Overall at 36 Mo**
Exam 2 measurement						
Median	1.29*	1.30*	1.29*	1.32*	1.33*	1.31
Mean	1.32	1.31	1.32	1.32	1.32	1.32
SD	0.21	0.21	0.22	0.22	0.21	0.19
N	858	405	453	40	41	593
Difference, exam 2 − exam 1						
Median	−0.01	−0.02	0.00	−0.02	0.02	0.01
Mean	−0.01	−0.01	0.00	−0.04	0.05	0.00
SD	0.14	0.13	0.15	0.07	0.15	0.14
Pearson r between exam 1 and exam 2	0.77	0.79	0.75	0.95	0.73	0.73

Abbreviations: IMT, intimal-medial thickness; SD, standard deviation.
*Median, mean, and standard deviation for exam 2 value of paired exams.
From Riley WA, Barnes RW, Applegate WB, et al: Reproducibility of noninvasive ultrasonic measurement of carotid atherosclerosis. Stroke 23:1062–1068, 1992.

aging did not differ significantly from the IMT as measured on pathologic examination.[28] Wong and colleagues[29] performed similar measurements on carotid and femoral arteries and concluded that B-mode imaging of IMT on the far (deeper) wall did not provide significantly different results from those obtained by histology. Gamble and associates[30] described in vitro and in situ experiments in the common carotid arteries of cadavers; these studies indicated that B-mode imaging of the artery wall correlated best with the combined intimal-medial-adventitial thickness as measured from histologic sections but that increased wall thickness due to intimal atherosclerotic thickening still correlated well with the thickness obtained from B-mode images. Thickness measurements from the far (deeper) wall of a vessel are more clearly defined and valid than those from the near (shallower) wall, due to the basic physical principles used in the construction of B-mode images.[29, 31]

Normal and Abnormal Intimal-Medial Thicknesses

Data were reported on the distribution of IMTs from the Atherosclerosis Risk in Communities (ARIC) study, a probability sample of middle-aged men and women in four communities in the United States.[32] A portion of these data are presented in Table 76–2, which shows that the median IMT increases with age, is higher in men than in women, and is higher in the bifurcation than in the common and internal carotid arteries. A "normal" thickness may be represented by the median values of participants in their mid-40s (i.e., 0.60 mm for men and 0.54 mm for women in the common carotid artery).

As described in the review of Kanters and colleagues,[27] various investigators have used different protocols to characterize normal and abnormal arteries. Although it is attractive to use protocols that focus on the common carotid artery only (because imaging of other segments is sometimes difficult[26]), recent evidence suggests that imaging of the bifurcation or internal carotid artery may provide additional information regarding associations with disease.[5, 33, 34]

B-mode images of three common carotid artery far wall segments with increasing IMTs are shown in Figure 76–2. Figure 76–2A illustrates an IMT in the upper range of normal; Figure 76–2B shows an IMT slightly less than twice normal; and Figure 76–2C shows a protruding plaque with a maximum thickness that is four times that of normal.

Certain investigators have advocated the use of plaque rather than IMT as an index of disease because some increase in IMT may result from hyperplasia rather than atherosclerosis per se.[35] In theory, this approach has merit; however, in practice, different investigators have proposed different definitions of *plaque* (most characterize plaque as a lesion whose IMT is 50 percent greater than a normal-appearing nearby segment,[37] whereas others identify plaque as present if there is a localized irregular thickening of ≥ 1.5 mm[38]). Furthermore, plaque does not appear to add information about associations with risk factors or with prevalent or incident disease that is not available from the measurement of IMT alone.

Characterization of plaque composition from B-mode images has also been advocated by some investigators[38] because of the well described association of unstable plaque with acute events[39]; however, such characterization

TABLE 76–2 **Median Carotid Far Wall Intimal-Medial Thickness in Atherosclerosis Risk in Communities Study by Age and Gender**

	45 Yr	**55 Yr**	**65 Yr**
Left common			
White men	0.60	0.68	0.77
White women	0.54	0.62	0.71
Left bifurcation			
White men	0.68	0.83	0.96
White women	0.61	0.73	0.85
Left internal			
White men	0.56	0.66	0.74
White women	0.50	0.58	0.64

From Howard G, Sharrett AR, Heiss G, et al: Carotid artery intimal-medial thickness distribution in general populations as evaluated by B-mode ultrasound. Stroke 24:1297–1304, 1993.

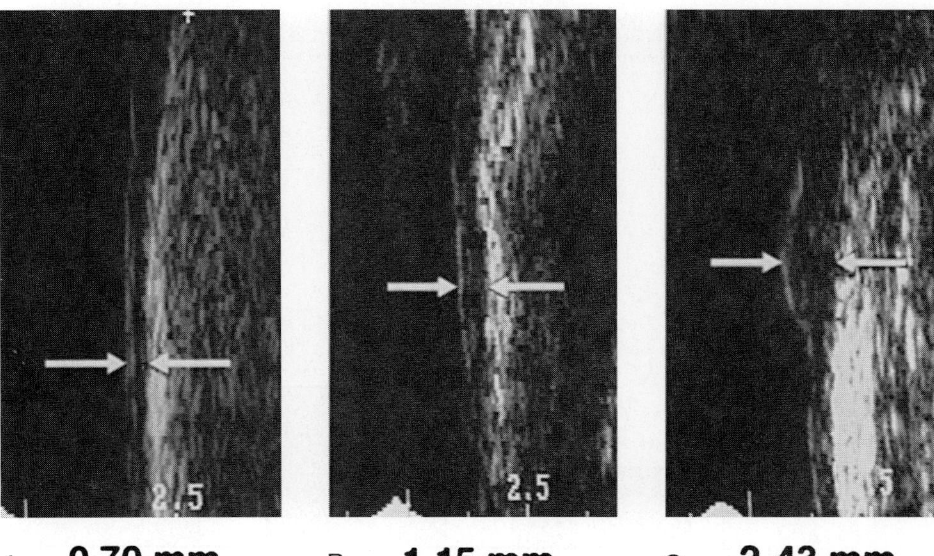

FIGURE 76–2 A–C, Three B-mode ultrasound images with different intimal-medial thicknesses *(arrows).*

is complex and difficult. The methods described earlier for the assessment of IMT evolved from validation studies on normal or near-normal arteries in which the lumen-intima and media-adventitia boundaries were clearly defined. When complex plaques are present, these boundaries may become less well defined and other boundaries may develop within the wall, which can significantly change the fundamental principles underlying the IMT measurement process and decrease the reproducibility. Investigations are under way to further explore the potential of ultrasonic B-mode imaging in the characterization of atherosclerotic plaque.

Associations of Risk Factors With Intimal-Medial Thickness

Because IMT is an index of chronic stable disease, associations with risk factors represent lifetime (more than current) exposure. Recent data from the Framingham Heart Study support this concept.[40] Well recognized risk factors for clinical manifestations of coronary artery disease include age, male gender, menopausal status, cigarette smoking, diabetes, hypertension, elevated low-density lipoprotein (LDL) cholesterol levels, and depressed high-density lipoprotein cholesterol levels; all of these have been shown to be related to increased IMT of the extracranial carotid arteries.[4–6, 36, 40] In addition, a number of risk factors of putative but hitherto unproved importance for clinical events have been associated with increased IMT; these include passive smoking,[41] elevated homocysteine levels,[42] dietary saturated fat intake,[43] factors related to thrombosis[44] and thrombolysis,[45] past *Chlamydia pneumoniae* infection,[46] elevated levels of E selectin and intercellular adhesion molecule-1,[47] psychosocial factors,[48] and insulin sensitivity.[49]

Progression of Intimal-Medial Thickness

Limited data are available on progression rates. The annual mean progression rate in the placebo group of the ACAPS study, a clinical trial of asymptomatic individuals, was approximately 0.01 mm.[8] On the other hand, the annual mean progression rate in the placebo group of the PLAC-II study, a clinical trial of symptomatic hypercholesterolemic patients, was 0.07 mm.[7] Within a group, certain individuals may show progression, whereas others have no noticeable change in IMT. The progression rate is typically higher in the bifurcation than in the common carotid artery. Data from a large population-based epidemiologic study in Finland found the following factors to be related to IMT progression: age, LDL cholesterol, pack-years, white blood cell count, and platelet aggregability, whereas systolic blood pressure and high-density lipoprotein were not related to progression.[50] Figure 76–3 depicts the annualized progression rate of IMT stratified by LDL level and smoking status. A stepwise relationship seems to exist, going from being a nonsmoker with low LDL levels to being a smoker with higher LDL levels. Other investigators have associated estrogen replacement with a slower progression of IMT in postmenopausal women[51]; passive smoking,[49] increases in dietary cholesterol, fiber, and body weight,[52] and hyperreactivity to psychologic stress[53] have been related to faster progression.

Influences of Risk Factors on Progression of Intimal-Medial Thickness in Clinical Trials

Clinical trials using B-mode ultrasound to quantify atherosclerosis have also related risk factor reduction with retardation of atherosclerosis progression. This has been evaluated most carefully in clinical trials with cholesterol-lowering agents; seven such trials are reviewed in Table 76–3. These trials have consistently shown that cholesterol lowering retards the rate of progression or, in three of these, is associated with net regression of atherosclerosis. Typically it takes 1 to 3 years to show differences in rates of progression of IMT between intervention and placebo groups. Effects of antihypertensive therapy on extracranial carotid IMT progression have also been evaluated.[54] How-

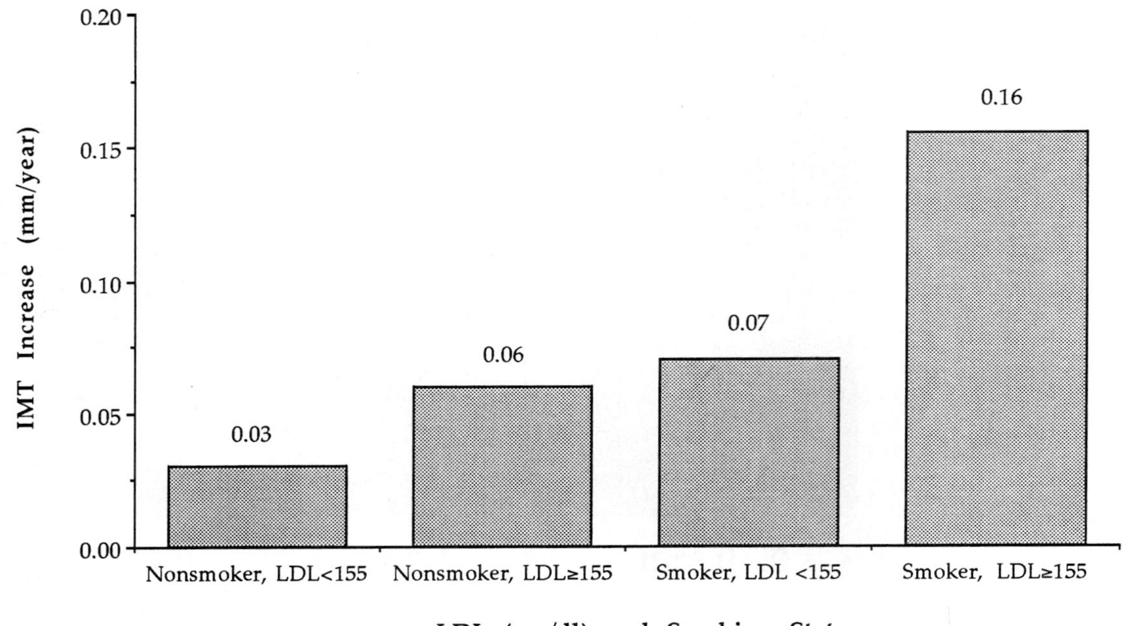

FIGURE 76–3 Annualized progression of intimal-medial thicknesses (IMT) by baseline low-density lipoprotein (LDL) and smoking status. (Adapted from Salonen R, Salonen JT: Progression of carotid atherosclerosis and its determinants: a population-based ultrasonography study. Atherosclerosis 81:33, 1990.)

ever, agents that influence intravascular volume (e.g., diuretics) may cause an artificial short-term apparent increase in IMT associated with a reduction in lumen diameter, thus confounding the interpretation of such studies.

Associations of Intimal-Medial Thickness With Symptomatic Vascular Disease

Extracranial carotid atherosclerosis has been independently associated with prevalent coronary artery[14–16, 56, 57] and cerebrovascular[15, 16, 55, 56] disease. The odds ratios for prevalent symptomatic coronary artery and cerebrovascular disease in the Cardiovascular Health Study were 2.84 and 2.56, respectively, when comparing the highest with the lowest quartile of internal carotid IMT.[16] Of interest, increased IMT has also been associated with cerebral white matter lesions,[57, 58] which have themselves been associated with neurologic abnormalities.[59]

Increased IMT as identified by B-mode ultrasound of the extracranial carotid arteries is also a predictor of incident coronary events[18–22] and stroke.[22, 23] During a mean follow-up of 5.2 years, 23 percent of incident coronary heart disease events were found in the population in the ARIC study with IMT of at least 1.0 mm (top 7 percent of population), and event rates were 1.17 percent per year for

TABLE 76-3 **Clinical Trials With Atherosclerosis Outcome**

	Clinical Features						IMT Progression Rate Difference			
Trial	N (Years of Follow-Up)	Symptom Status	Medication	Base LDL Level (mg/dl)	%Δ LDL	%Δ HDL	Common (mm/yr)	Bif (mm/yr)	Agg (mm/yr)	% Decrease
CLAS[9]	78 (4)*	CABG	C + N	170	↓ 43	↑ 37.0	−0.035			REG
MARS[10]	30 (2)*	CAD	L	155	↓ 45	↑ 8.5	−0.065			100
PLAC-II[7]	151 (3)	CAD	P	165	↓ 28	↑ 3.9	−0.016	−0.016	−0.008	30
LIPID[13]	522 (4)	CAD	P	153	↓ 27	↑ 4.0	−0.015			REG
ACAPS[8]†	461 (3)	None	L	157	↓ 28	↑ 5.0			−0.015	REG
KAPS[11]	447 (3)*	None	P	186	↓ 27	↑ 5.0	−0.019	−0.012		40
CAIUS[12]†	305 (3)	None	P	178	↓ 22	↑ 4.0	−0.011	−0.027	−0.013	REG

Abbreviations: ACAPS, Asymptomatic Carotid Artery Progression Study; Agg, aggregate IMT; Bif, bifurcation IMT; C, colestipol; CABG, coronary artery bypass graft surgery; CAD, coronary artery disease; CAIUS, Carotid Atherosclerosis Italian Ultrasound Study; CLAS, Cholesterol Lowering Atherosclerosis Study; Common, common carotid artery IMT; HDL, high-density lipoprotein; IMT, intimal-medial thickness; KAPS, Kuopio Atherosclerosis Prevention Study; L, lovastatin; LDL, low-density lipoprotein; LIPID, Long-term Intervention with Pravastatin in Ischemic Disease; MARS, Monitored Atherosclerosis Regression Study; N, niacin; P, pravastatin; PLAC-II, Pravastatin, Lipids, and Atherosclerosis in the Carotid Arteries; REG, net regression.

women and 1.29 percent per year for men in this subset with high IMT. By contrast, event rates for the entire population were 0.25 percent per year for women and 0.67 percent per year for men (Fig. 76–4). In the Cardiovascular Health Study, 14 percent of incident strokes occurred in the 6 percent of the population with the greatest carotid stenosis (>50 percent). A report has presented evidence for an independent association of IMT with all-cause mortality.[24]

Because IMT represents a chronic stable index of disease, changes in lifestyle or pharmacologic modification that might alter the risk of incident disease over weeks or months (e.g., lipid lowering) would not be rapidly reflected in changes in IMT. In this regard, it has been reported that the progression of extracranial carotid atherosclerosis is a stronger risk factor for incident coronary events than baseline coronary stenosis or progression of coronary stenosis.[60]

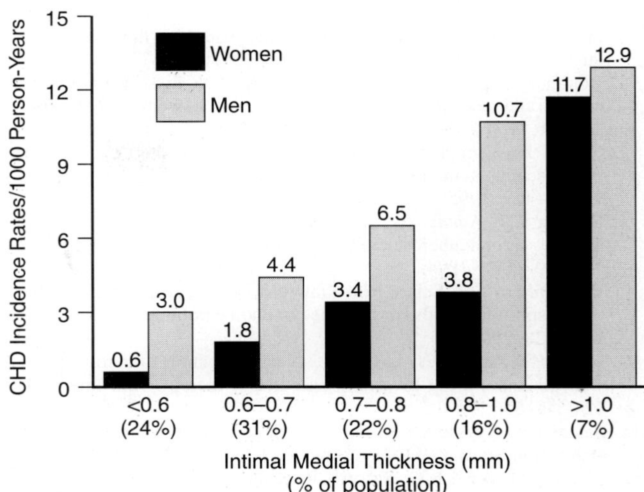

FIGURE 76–4 Age-, field center–, and race-adjusted coronary heart disease incidence rates (per 1000 person-years) in the Atherosclerosis Risk in Communities Study, 1987 to 1993. (Adapted from Chambless LE, Heiss G, Folsom AR, et al: Association of coronary heart disease incidence with carotid arterial wall thickness and major risk factors: the Atherosclerosis Risk in Communities [ARIC] Study, 1987–1993. Am J Epidemiol 146:483–494, 1997.)

Use of B-Mode Ultrasound to Define Arterial Dimensions

In addition to IMT, B-mode ultrasound is capable of defining arterial dimensions (lumen diameter and interadventitial diameter). Associations of risk factors with arterial dimensions are different from associations with atherosclerosis in the common carotid artery. Increased IMT of the common carotid is associated with increased lumen diameter,[61] and most risk factors that are associated with increased IMT (aging, male gender, cigarette smoking, hypertension, diabetes) are also associated with increased common carotid lumen diameter (LDL cholesterol is the exception; it is associated with smaller arterial lumens in the common carotid artery).[62–64] These noninvasively defined associations are consistent with remodeling of the artery due to atherosclerosis and are reminiscent of compensatory dilation observed in the coronary arteries.[1]

SUMMARY

The use of B-mode ultrasound to quantify and monitor the progression of IMT of the extracranial carotid arteries has provided important new insights about risk factors for arterial disease, as well as the risk of prevalent and incident coronary heart disease and stroke. Several controversies regarding its use are evident, including the use of characterization of "plaque" as opposed to IMT and of quantification of plaque characteristics. Because IMT and plaque identify structural aspects of arterial disease that may carry fundamentally different information regarding risk, this distinction may be important. Investigators differ in reliance on measurements of carotid disease from one segment (the common carotid artery) as opposed to multiple segments. In addition, the use of this technology in clinical trials of agents that may acutely increase or decrease arterial lumen diameter poses unique challenges.

The potential for B-mode ultrasound to identify individuals who stand to benefit most from lifestyle modification or pharmacologic intervention has not yet been fully realized. Extreme thickening of the intima-media complex identifies a small group of individuals whose risk of incident cardiac and cerebrovascular events is 2- to 5-fold greater than that of the parent population; however, because IMT changes slowly, it may not by itself precisely identify individuals at a short-term risk of incident disease. Furthermore, the underlying risk for otherwise healthy middle-aged populations is so low (<1 percent per year for cardiac events) that even those individuals with extreme thickening of the intima-media complex have a low risk rate, and in absolute terms, the vast majority of events occurs in the population with normal or only modestly increased IMT.

Conversely, the stability of IMT makes it an ideal marker for response of the arterial wall to long-term risk factor exposure. IMT is also ideally suited for identification of risk factors, and several new risk factors have been identified with this method. Furthermore, it is an excellent indicator of the long-term effects of risk factor change in clinical trials. It is likely that quantification of IMT in conjunction with risk factor measurements or other indices of vascular disease (e.g., indices of vascular function) that change more rapidly with behavior modification or pharmacologic intervention will allow investigators and clinicians to better predict individual risk in the future.

REFERENCES

1. Glagov S, Weisenberg E, Zarins CK, et al: Compensatory enlargement of human atherosclerotic coronary arteries. N Engl J Med 316:1371–1375, 1987.
2. Wexler L, Brundage B, Crouse J, et al: Coronary artery calcification: pathophysiology, epidemiology, imaging methods and clinical implications. Circulation 94:1175–1192, 1996.
3. Chambers BR, Norris JW: Outcome in patients with asymptomatic neck bruits. N Engl J Med 315:860–865, 1986.
4. Heiss G, Sharrett AR, Barnes R, et al, and the ARIC Investigators: Carotid atherosclerosis measured by B-mode ultrasound in populations: associations with cardiovascular risk factors in the ARIC study. Am J Epidemiol 134:250–256, 1991.

5. O'Leary DH, Polak JF, Kronmal RA, et al: Distribution and correlates of sonographically detected carotid artery disease in the Cardiovascular Health Study. Stroke 23:1752–1760, 1992.
6. Bonithon-Kopp C, Scarabin PY, Taquet A, et al: Risk factors for early carotid atherosclerosis in middle-aged French women. Arterioscler Thromb 11:966–972, 1991.
7. Crouse JR, Byington RP, Bond MG, et al: Pravastatin, Lipids, and Atherosclerosis in the Carotid Arteries (PLAC-II). Am J Cardiol 75:455–459, 1995.
8. Furberg CD, Adams HP, Applegate WB, et al: Effect of lovastatin on early carotid atherosclerosis and cardiovascular events. Circulation 90:1679–1687, 1994.
9. Blankenhorn DH, Selzer RH, Crawford DW, et al: Beneficial effects of colestipol-niacin therapy on the common carotid artery. Circulation 88:20–28, 1993.
10. Hodis HN, Mack WJ, LaBree L, et al: Reduction in carotid arterial wall thickness using lovastatin and dietary therapy. Ann Intern Med 124:549–556, 1996.
11. Salonen R, Nyyssonen K, Porkkala E, et al: Kuopio Atherosclerosis Prevention Study (KAPS). Circulation 92:1758–1764, 1995.
12. Mercuri M, Bond MG, Sirtori CR, et al: Pravastatin reduces carotid intima-media thickness progression in an asymptomatic hypercholesterolemic Mediterranean population: the Carotid Atherosclerosis Italian Ultrasound Study. Am J Med 101:627–634, 1996.
13. MacMahon S, Sharpe N, Gamble G, et al: Effects of lowering average or below-average cholesterol levels on the progression of carotid atherosclerosis: results of the LIPID atherosclerosis substudy. Circulation 98:1784–1790, 1998.
14. Craven TE, Ryu JE, Espeland MA, et al: Evaluation of the associations between carotid artery atherosclerosis and coronary artery stenosis: a case control study. Circulation 82:1230–1242, 1990.
15. Burke GL, Evans GW, Riley WA, et al: Arterial wall thickness is associated with prevalent cardiovascular disease in middle-aged adults: the Atherosclerosis Risk in Communities (ARIC) study. Stroke 26:386–391, 1995.
16. O'Leary DH, Polak JF, Kronmal RA, et al: Distribution and correlates of sonographically detected carotid artery disease in the Cardiovascular Health Study. Stroke 23:1752–1760, 1992.
17. Chambless LE, Shahar E, Sharrett AR, et al: Association of transient ischemic attack/stroke symptoms assessed by standardized questionnaire and algorithm with cerebrovascular risk factors and carotid artery wall thickness. Am J Epidemiol 144:857–866, 1996.
18. Salonen JT, Salonen R: Ultrasound B-mode imaging in observational studies of atherosclerotic progression. Circulation 87(suppl II):II-56–II-57, 1993.
19. Chambless LE, Heiss G, Folsom AR, et al: Association of coronary heart disease incidence with carotid arterial wall thickness and major risk factors: the Atherosclerosis Risk in Communities (ARIC) study, 1987–1993. Am J Epidemiol 146:483–494, 1997.
20. Kuller LH, Shemanski L, Psaty BM, et al: Subclinical disease as an independent risk factor for cardiovascular disease. Circulation 92:720–726, 1995.
21. Hodis HN, Mack WJ, LaBree L, et al: The role of carotid arterial intima-media thickness in predicting clinical coronary events. Ann Intern Med 128:262–269, 1998.
22. Bots ML, Hoes AW, Koudstaal PJ, et al: Common carotid intima-medial thickness and risk of stroke and myocardial infarction: the Rotterdam Study. Circulation 96:1432–1437, 1997.
23. Manolio TA, Kronmal RA, Burke GL, et al: Short-term predictors of incident stroke in older adults: the Cardiovascular Health Study. Stroke 27:1479–1486, 1996.
24. Fried LP, Kronmal RA, Newman AB, et al: Risk factors for 5-year mortality in older adults: the Cardiovascular Health Study. JAMA 279:585–592, 1998.
25. Riley WA, Barnes RW, Applegate WB, et al: Reproducibility of noninvasive ultrasonic measurement of carotid atherosclerosis. Stroke 23:1062–1068, 1992.
26. Crouse JR, Byington RP, Bond MG, et al: Pravastatin, Lipids, and Atherosclerosis in the Carotid Arteries: design features of a clinical trial with atherosclerosis outcome. Controlled Clin Trials 13:495–506, 1992.
27. Kanters SDJM, Algra A, van Leeuwen MS, Buanga J-D: Reproducibility of in vivo carotid intima-media thickness measurements: a review. Stroke 28:665, 1997.
28. Pignoli P, Tremoli E, Poli A, et al: Intimal plus medial thickness of the arterial wall: a direct measurement with ultrasound imaging. Circulation 74:1399–1406, 1986.
29. Wong M, Edelstein J, Wollman J, Bond MG: Ultrasonic-pathological comparison of the human arterial wall. Arterioscler Thromb 13:482–486, 1993.
30. Gamble G, Beaumont B, Smith H, et al: B-mode ultrasound images of the carotid artery wall: correlation of ultrasound with histological measurements. Atherosclerosis 102:163–173, 1993.
31. Atherosclerosis Risk in Communities Study Protocol, Manual 6: Ultrasound Assessment. Part B: Ultrasound B-Mode Image Reading. Chapel Hill, NC: ARIC Coordinating Center, Department of Biostatistics, University of North Carolina, 1987.
32. Howard G, Sharrett AR, Heiss G, et al: Carotid artery intimal-medial thickness distribution in general populations as evaluated by B-mode ultrasound. Stroke 24:1297–1304, 1993.
33. Crouse JR, Craven TE, Hagaman AP, Bond GM: Association of coronary disease with segment specific intimal medial thickening of the extracranial carotid artery. Circulation 92:1141–1147, 1995.
34. Hulthe J, Wikstrand J, Emanuelsson H, et al: Atherosclerotic changes in the carotid artery bulb as measured by B-mode ultrasound are associated with the extent of coronary atherosclerosis. Stroke 28:1189–1194, 1997.
35. Crouse JR: B-mode in clinical trials: answers and questions. Circulation 88:319–321, 1993.
36. Salonen R, Seppanen K, Rauramaa R, Salonen JT: Prevalence of carotid atherosclerosis and serum cholesterol levels in eastern Finland. Arteriosclerosis 8:788–792, 1988.
37. Veller MG, Fisher CM, Nicolaides AN, et al: Measurement of the ultrasonic intima-media complex thickness in normal subjects. J Vasc Surg 17:719–725, 1993.
38. El-Barghouty N, Nicolaides A, Behal V, et al: The identification of the high risk carotid plaque. Eur J Vasc Endovasc Surg 11:470–478, 1996.
39. Davies MJ: Stability and instability: two faces of coronary atherosclerosis: the Paul Dudley White Lecture 1995. Circulation 94:2013–2020, 1996.
40. Wilson PWF, Hoeg JM, D'Abostino RB, et al: Cumulative effects of high cholesterol levels, high blood pressure, and cigarette smoking on carotid stenosis. N Engl J Med 337:516–522, 1997.
41. Howard G, Wagenknecht LE, Burke GL, et al: Cigarette smoking and progression of atherosclerosis: the Atherosclerosis Risk in Communities (ARIC) study. JAMA 279:119–124, 1998.
42. Selhub J, Jacques PF, Bostom AG, et al: Association between plasma homocysteine concentrations and extracranial carotid-artery stenosis. N Engl J Med 332:286–291, 1995.
43. Tell GS, Evans GW, Folsom AR, et al: Dietary fat intake and carotid artery wall thickness: the Atherosclerosis Risk in Communities (ARIC) Study. Am J Epidemiol 139:979–989, 1994.
44. Tracy RP, Bovill EG, Yanez D, et al, for the Cardiovascular Health Study Investigators: Fibrinogen and factor VIII, but not factor VII, are associated with measures of subclinical cardiovascular disease in the elderly: results from the Cardiovascular Health Study. Arterioscler Thromb Vasc Biol 15:1269–1279, 1995.
45. Salomaa V, Stinson V, Kark JD, et al: Association of fibrinolytic parameters with early atherosclerosis: the ARIC Study. Circulation 15:1269–1279, 1995.
46. Melnick SL, Shahar E, Folsom AR, et al: Past infection by *Chlamydia pneumoniae* strain TWAR and asymptomatic carotid atherosclerosis. Am J Med 95:499–504, 1993.
47. Hwang S, Ballantyne CM, Sharrett AR, et al: Circulating adhesions molecules VCAM-1, ICAM-1 and E-selectin in carotid atherosclerosis and incident coronary heart disease cases: the Atherosclerosis Risk in Communities (ARIC) Study. Circulation 96:4219–4225, 1997.
48. Lynch J, Krause N, Kaplan G, et al: Workplace demands, economic reward and progression of carotid atherosclerosis. Circulation 96:302–307, 1997.
49. Howard G, O'Leary DH, Zaccaro D, et al, for the IRAS Investigators: Insulin sensitivity and atherosclerosis. Circulation 93:1809–1817, 1996.
50. Salonen R, Salonen JT: Progression of carotid atherosclerosis and its determinants: a population-based ultrasonography study. Atherosclerosis 81:33, 1990.
51. Espeland MA, Applegate W, Furberg CD, et al: Estrogen replacement therapy and progression of intimal-medial thickness in the carotid arteries of postmenopausal women. Am J Epidemiol 142:1011–1019, 1995.

52. Markus RA, Mack WJ, Azen SP, Hodis HN: Influence of lifestyle modification on atherosclerotic progression determined by ultrasonographic change in the common carotid intima-media thickness. Am J Clin Nutr 65:1000–1004, 1997.
53. Barnett PA, Spence JD, Manuck SB, Jennings JR: Psychological stress and the progression of carotid artery disease. J Hypertens 15:49–55, 1997.
54. Borhani NO, Mercuri M, Borhani PA, et al: Final outcome results of the Multicenter Isradipine Diuretic Atherosclerosis Study (MIDAS). JAMA 2765:785–791, 1996.
55. Bots ML, de Jong PTVM, Hofman A, Grobbee DE: Left, right, near or far wall common carotid intima-media thickness measurements: associations with cardiovascular disease and lower extremity arterial atherosclerosis. J Clin Epidemiol 50:801–807, 1997.
56. Salonen R, Tervahauta M, Salonen JT, et al: Ultrasonographic manifestations of common carotid atherosclerosis in elderly Eastern Finnish men. Arterioscler Thromb 14:1631–1640, 1994.
57. Bots ML, van Swieten JC, Breteler MMB, et al: Cerebral white matter lesions and atherosclerosis in the Rotterdam Study. Lancet 341:1232–1237, 1993.
58. Manolio TA, Kronmal RA, Burke GL, et al: Magnetic resonance abnormalities and cardiovascular disease in older adults. Stroke 25:318–327, 1994.
59. Price TR, Manolio TA, Kronmal RA, et al: Silent brain infarction on magnetic resonance imaging and neurological abnormalities in community-dwelling older adults. Stroke 28:1158–1164, 1997.
60. Hodis HN, Mack WJ, LaBree L, et al: The role of carotid arterial intima-media thickness in predicting clinical coronary events. Ann Intern Med 128:262–269, 1998.
61. Crouse JR III, Goldbourt U, Evans G, et al, for the ARIC Investigators: Arterial enlargement in the Atherosclerosis Risk in Communities (ARIC) cohort. Stroke 25:1354–1359, 1994.
62. Polak JF, Kronmal RA, Tell GS, et al: Compensatory increase in common carotid artery diameter. Stroke 27:2012–2015, 1996.
63. Bonithon-Kopp C, Touboul PJ, Berr C, et al: Factors of carotid arterial enlargement in a population aged 59 to 71 years: the EVA Study. Stroke 27:654–660, 1996.
64. Crouse JR III, Goldbourt U, Evans G, et al: Risk factors and segment specific carotid arterial enlargement in the Atherosclerosis Risk in Communities (ARIC) cohort. Stroke 27:69–75, 1996.

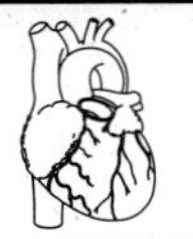

CHAPTER 77

Intravascular Ultrasound

Paul G. Yock and Peter J. Fitzgerald

BASIC FEATURES OF CATHETER ULTRASOUND TECHNOLOGY
INTERPRETATION OF THE IMAGES
IN VIVO ASSESSMENT OF PLAQUE MORPHOLOGY
CONCLUSIONS

There is a significant gap between our understanding of vascular pathophysiology, as outlined in the preceding chapters, and the concepts that clinicians actually use to treat a patient with vascular disease. The most influential test result in the evaluation of a patient with coronary atherosclerosis is the estimate of percent stenosis from the angiogram. The fact that a 50-percent, lipid-laden plaque may be more likely to rupture and occlude a coronary artery than a fibrotic, 90-percent lesion is an uncomfortable possibility that cannot be pursued clinically.

Intravascular ultrasound (IVUS) is a relatively new technology that may help address such issues by providing direct information about plaque composition and distribution. Ultrasound catheters generate a cross-sectional image of the vessel wall similar to a histologic section taken at the level of the catheter tip. The ability to image plaque in depth has opened the way to develop a much more detailed understanding of the clinical implications of atherosclerosis and the various modalities of treatment. This chapter briefly reviews (1) the basic design of the catheter systems and format of the images, (2) the potential and limitations of ultrasound for the assessment of plaque and vessel morphology, and (3) the early lessons regarding vessel structure and function that have been derived from clinical studies with IVUS. The clinical applications of IVUS imaging are addressed in more detail in a subsequent chapter.

Basic Features of Catheter Ultrasound Technology

The adaptation of ultrasound technology for catheter imaging has required not only extreme miniaturization of the transducers but also the development of catheters that can support the imaging electronics while remaining sufficiently flexible and trackable to access the coronary arteries. Two major design approaches have emerged on the basis of either solid state or mechanical catheter technology.[1] In the solid state approach, a cylindric array of transducer elements is positioned as a collar at the catheter tip.[2, 3] Depending on the configuration, 64 or more elements in the transducer are linked to a set of integrated circuits that are also contained in the catheter tip, with the resultant signals being sent along the length of the catheter over a small number of transmission lines. The image is rapidly assimilated by a computer, so an updated image can be presented at a rate of 20 to 30 frames per second. The solid-state approach in general has the advantage of having no moving parts within the catheter. Although for years the mechanical catheter systems generated better-quality images than the solid state catheters, the gap has narrowed substantially. The first solid state coronary catheter approved by the Food and Drug Administration was 3.2 French in caliber, and a 2.9 French catheter has been introduced.

In the mechanical approach to catheter imaging, a single transducer at the catheter tip is rotated by a flexible drive cable running the length of the catheter.[4–7] Advances in cable technology have provided very flexible catheters that are able to negotiate most coronary bends. In general, the dynamic range and resolution of the mechanical catheters are slightly superior to those of the solid state catheters for the same size catheter. The necessity to mechanically rotate the transducer in the mechanical system, however, leads to an image artifact that is not present in the solid state systems: nonuniform rotational distortion (NURD). This is a distortion of the image in the rotational (theta) dimension that is caused by drag on the drive cable during some portion of its rotation. Current mechanical coronary catheters range from 2.6 to 3.5 French in size. The mechanical catheters use a "rail"-style delivery system rather than an over-the-wire configuration, which some operators believe provides more convenient catheter exchange.

The images generated by all of the different catheters have the same basic format: a two-dimensional slice of the vessel is taken at the location of the transducer (Figs. 77–1A and 77–2). The catheter itself is seen at the center of the vessel within the lumen. At the higher frequencies used for catheter imaging (20 to 45 MHz), blood is visualized, with a finely speckled and dynamic appearance. At these high frequencies, penetration of the ultrasound signal is limited, typically to a radius of 0.5 to 1.0 cm, depending on the amount and composition of plaque within the vessel.

Interpretation of the Images

The strength of a reflected ultrasound signal depends on the acoustic impedance of the tissues being imaged. Among the tissue components present in a normal vessel wall, the

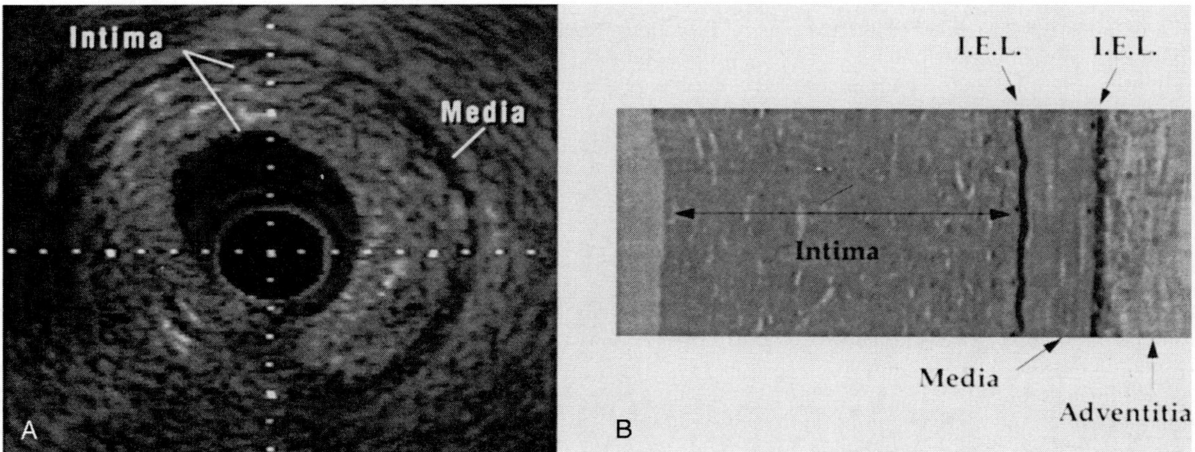

FIGURE 77–1 Example of a standard cross-sectional image of a coronary artery **(A)** and the corresponding histologic section **(B)**. The catheter is represented by the *black circle* in the center of the image; calibration marks are 0.5 mm. The guidewire artifact for this catheter is seen as a ray extending from the catheter in the 7 o'clock position which obscures the anatomy. IEL, EEL, internal and external elastic lamina.

media is weakly reflective of ultrasound compared with the other layers. The resultant image of a muscular artery (see Fig. 77–2), therefore, shows a relatively dark band corresponding to the medial layer. At the frequencies used for clinical imaging, resolution is not sufficiently fine to discriminate intima from internal elastic lamina, so these two layers merge to form a single, relatively bright inner layer on the image. Similarly, the external lamina, adventitia, and periadventitial tissue have acoustical properties that are sufficiently close to generally appear as a coherent band on the images. The resulting appearance of a muscular artery on the ultrasound scan, therefore, consists of three layers: a thin, darker medial layer sandwiched between the intima and adventitia.[4, 8]

Several factors may modify this basic three-layer pattern. In elastic arteries (e.g., the carotid arteries and aorta), the higher collagen and elastin contents of the media make this layer more highly reflective of ultrasound, and therefore the media does not stand out as clearly as a distinct layer.[9] Transitional arteries (e.g., the iliac arteries) are intermediate in this respect. In the coronary arteries, the intima and the internal elastic lamina in a normal segment of vessel may not have sufficient reflectivity to show up as a distinct layer (see Fig. 77–2). Both in vitro and in vivo studies have suggested that a certain degree of intimal thickening (~160 μm for a 30-MHz image) is necessary before the three-layer appearance can be resolved.[10] Another important point is that due to the properties of ultrasound passing through the arterial wall, the thickness of the media may be slightly underrepresented on the ultrasound scans.[11] As the beam passes from the more reflective intima and internal lamina to the media, there is "blooming," or setback of the apparent transition point into the media. The thickness of plaque is overrepresented by a corresponding amount. For this reason, most IVUS studies report the plaque-plus-media area measurement as a reproducible in-

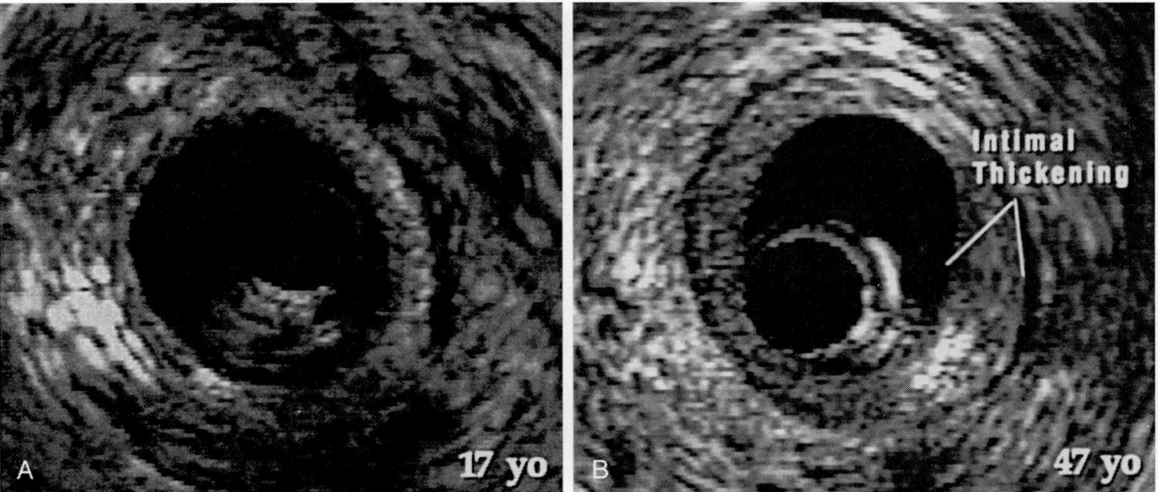

FIGURE 77–2 Intimal thickening and the three-layered appearance on ultrasound. **B,** A 47-year-old patient has significant intimal thickening, which gives rise to a clear three-layered appearance (the media is the dark band). **A,** In a 17-year-old patient, the intima is not sufficiently thickened to give a distinct three-layered appearance.

dex of the plaque area. Fortunately, for even a small plaque accumulation, the media contributes a very low proportion of the total plaque-plus-media area, so the use of this combined area as a surrogate for the plaque area measurement is an acceptable approximation.

Measurements of lumen area by IVUS are proving to be relatively accurate compared with other clinically applicable techniques. Theoretical calculations and in vitro calibration tests suggest that the errors involved in area measurements in the clinical setting may be in the range of 5 to 10 percent. Several studies have compared lumen area measurements made by ultrasound and histology in in vitro arterial specimens and have demonstrated good correlation.[3, 5, 7] Clinical studies that compare ultrasound lumen measurements with quantitative angiography have shown that the strength of correlation depends on the type of vessel segment being analyzed. Concentric plaques (as determined by ultrasound) yield a better correlation than do eccentric plaques, perhaps because the angiographic measurements of eccentric plaques depend on the projections chosen for analysis. There is a strikingly worse correlation for measurements in postangioplasty segments compared with measurements in noninstrumented arteries.[3] This has been attributed to the irregular contour of the segments after angioplasty, which is difficult to assess with angiography. In stented segments, the correlations between IVUS and angio are also weak.[12–14] This finding was initially surprising to investigators, given the assumption that the stent creates a round, regular lumen. In fact, often some portion of the stented segment is poorly expanded, typically in the area in which the plaque accumulation is the greatest. This area of incomplete expansion is usually very short (a few millimeters or less), so computerized, quantitative angiographic measurements miss this finding. In fact, these short stretches of incomplete expansion are usually very difficult to detect even with careful visual inspection of the angiogram.

The ability of ultrasound to penetrate below the surface of the lumen offers the possibility of identifying different plaque types in the clinical setting. Calcium or fibrocalcific deposits provide the most distinctive appearance on the ultrasound scan, as characterized by a bright image with shadowing of tissue structures deep to the calcium (Fig. 77–3).[6] Fibrous or fibrofatty plaques are intermediate in appearance, with a relatively fine speckled pattern and moderate brightness. Lipid "pools" within plaque are poorly reflective of ultrasound and therefore appear as a relatively dark region covered by the brighter reflections of the fibrous cap. In vitro studies suggest that the sensitivity and specificity for the detection of lipid accumulations by ultrasound are both relatively low.[14] Several other situations can mimic the appearance of a lipid pool, including attenuation of the beam by plaque or the presence of fibrocalcific deposits immediately adjacent to the imaging plane. Clinically, given the current generation of imaging catheters, the degree of confidence for identifying lipid accumulations is at best moderate. Another significant limitation with current catheter ultrasound technology is the difficulty in discriminating soft plaque from thrombus. These tissues are similar in the strength of reflectance of the ultrasound beam. In favorable cases, the motion of thrombus during the pulse cycle in the vessel is characteristic. Thrombus may also have a fairly distinctive "scintillating" appearance (reminiscent of amyloid in a cardiac echo) that is not seen with soft plaque.[15]

The difficulty in making subtle discriminations between different tissue types has prompted the development of enhanced "tissue characterization" methods based on further computer processing of the ultrasound signals used to make the images (Fig. 77–4).[16] These techniques take advantage of the fact that there are other parameters encoded in the ultrasound signals in addition to the strength of backscatter that can help to identify a target tissue. Preliminary work in this area has suggested that analysis of the radiofrequency signal can reliably help differentiate thrombus and soft plaque in vitro.

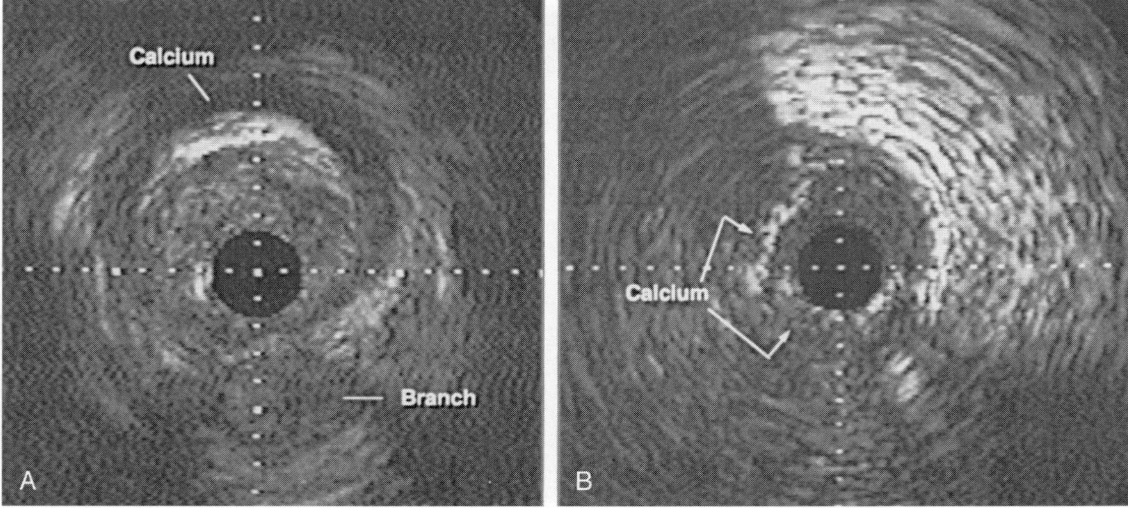

FIGURE 77–3 Examples of calcium deposits. **A,** There is a rim of calcium beneath an accumulation of softer plaque (the catheter is tightly intubated in the plaque). **B,** Calcium is deposited at the luminal border. Shadowing of the ultrasound signal beyond the calcium deposits is characteristic.

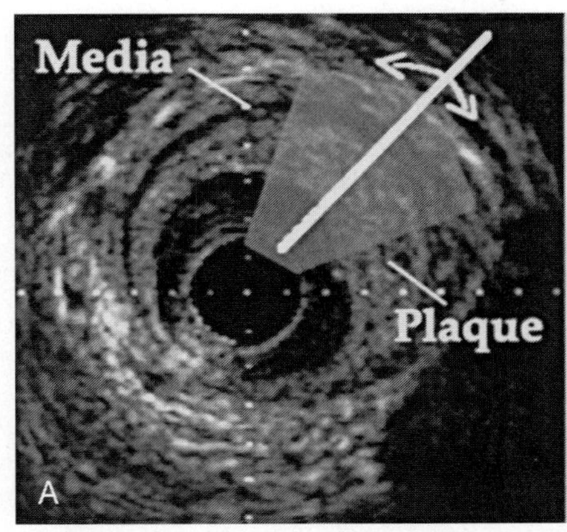

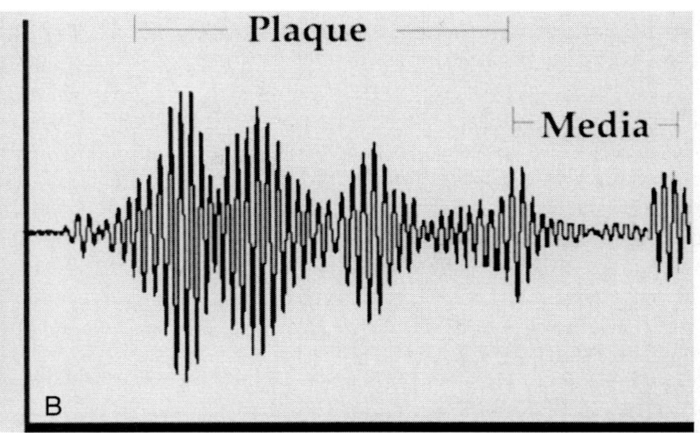

FIGURE 77–4 Example of the raw radiofrequency (RF) signal **(B)** used to generate the ultrasound signal. The RF signal for the line shown on the image **(A)** is displayed. This signal can be analyzed by computer-based statistical methods to more precisely identify the tissue characteristics of a region of interest.

IN VIVO ASSESSMENT OF PLAQUE MORPHOLOGY

As the technology of intravascular ultrasound has been refined, studies in coronary and peripheral vessels have begun to demonstrate features of plaque morphology that have not previously been appreciated in the clinical setting. Perhaps the most striking initial impression from an intracoronary ultrasound examination is the large amount of atheroma present, even in segments of vessel that appear to be normal on the angiogram. Quantitative catheter ultrasound studies have demonstrated, for example, that the proximal segment chosen as the "normal" reference site for the calculation of percent stenosis on angiography has an average of 30 to 40 percent of its cross-sectional area occupied by plaque.[3, 19] The phenomenon of remodeling (enlarging) of plaque segments in segments of disease, as first described by Glagov and colleagues,[20] is well illustrated with the use of IVUS.[21] In Figure 77–5, for example, two adjacent segments of a vessel have relatively similar lumen areas as determined by both angiography and ultrasound. The section shown in B, however, has a much larger deposit of plaque visualized by ultrasound than that in A. The total cross-sectional area of the vessel is correspondingly much larger at B, demonstrating the expansion of the media and adventitia at this point.

IVUS studies have revealed that the process of negative remodeling (shrinkage) has a major role in restenosis after angioplasty.[22, 23] In fact, studies have indicated that the loss in lumen area during the first 6 months after either percutaneous transluminal coronary angioplasty or directional coronary atherectomy is due primarily to negative remodeling of the treated segment and less to intimal proliferation.[24] During the first month after the procedure, an increase in plaque area is accompanied by positive remodeling, so net loss of lumen area is minimal. In the subsequent 1- to 6-month period, the rate of intimal proliferation slows—the plaque area may actually decrease. However, this favorable change is associated with a major shrinkage in overall vessel area (negative remodeling). This series of events has been compared with wound healing, in which there is early scar formation accompanied by late contracture.

Assessment of the eccentricity of plaque is another area in which ultrasound provides data that are discrepant with that from angiography in a large proportion of cases. Several studies have suggested that when a lesion is judged to be concentric by angiography, more likely than not the actual distribution of plaque is eccentric (as can be seen with IVUS).[25] This discrepancy has particular importance for therapeutic procedures that remove or ablate plaque, such as directional atherectomy. The angiogram can be highly misleading in the determination of whether a plaque is eccentric or concentric and in judging where to orient the device for the safest and most efficient removal of plaque.

The degree of calcification of plaque and the location of the calcium deposits within the plaque substance are also shown much more clearly on an ultrasound scan than on an angiogram. Clinical studies have suggested that calcium is demonstrated by ultrasound in 60 to 80 percent of severely stenotic lesions, in cases where the detection by fluoroscopy is 20 to 40 percent.[20, 21] The location of calcium within the plaque may be a critical parameter that influences the performance of different therapeutic devices. For example, if calcium is located at the luminal border (see Fig. 77–3), tissue retrieval by directional atherectomy will be inhibited due to tendency of the current cutter to glance off of hard materials.[27] Balloon dilatation or stenting of these lesions may also be difficult, because of the mechanical strength of these "napkin-ring" fibrocalcific stenoses. Luminal calcification is well suited, on the other hand, for treatment by high-speed rotational atherectomy. Deposits of calcium within the plaque substance or deep at the medial border cause plaque to respond in a different fashion. Directional atherectomy will remove plaque down to the fibrocalcific deposit. Balloon dilatation is effective, generally creating a tear associated with the localized calcium. Rotational ablation, on the other hand, may be less efficient because of the higher elasticity of the softer plaque.

The ability of ultrasound to image in depth is also leading to a better understanding of the process of dissection associated with balloon angioplasty (Fig. 77–6). Dissections are seen in 60 to 70 percent of coronary dilatations by ultrasound compared with 20 to 40 percent by angiography.[19, 28] In our experience, the rate of dissections

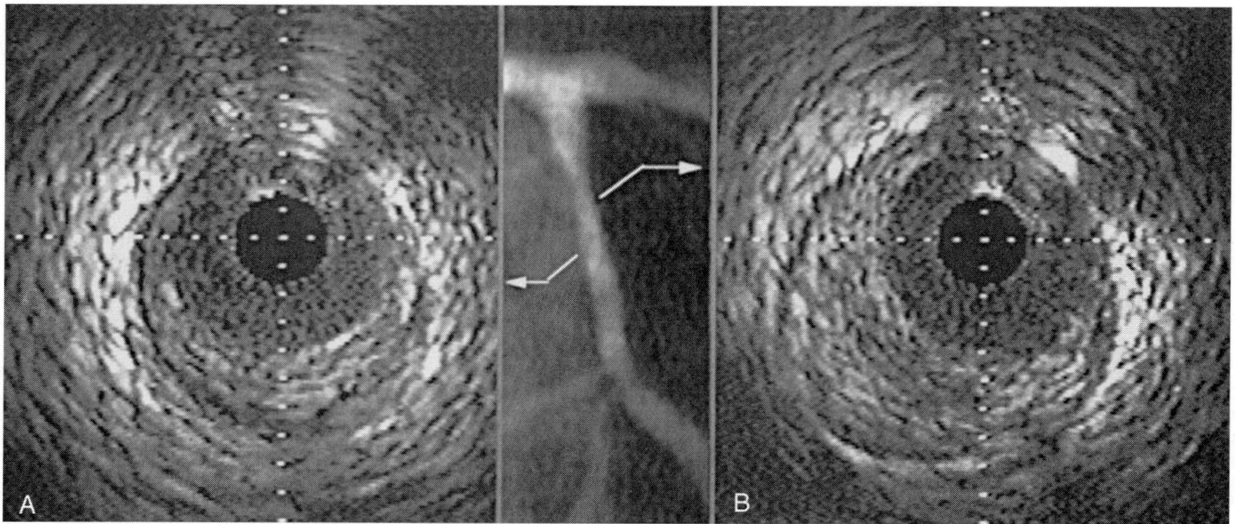

FIGURE 77–5 **A** and **B,** Deposits of soft plaque and the "remodeling" phenomenon. In these two adjacent segments of a left anterior descending coronary artery, the lumen dimensions are similar (~3.5 mm in diameter). However, there is a larger plaque deposit in **B**, and the entire cross-sectional area of the vessel (including plaque) is correspondingly much larger than in **A**. (**A** and **B,** From Hodgson J [ed]: Atlas of Intravascular Ultrasound. Raven, New York: 1993.)

detected by ultrasound is even higher in peripheral angioplasty, approaching 90 percent. The incidence of coronary dissections by ultrasound may be underestimated to some extent by the tendency of the imaging catheters to "prop up" the dissected tissue, so the tear is not as easily seen with ultrasound. The images of dissections have demonstrated that the tearing caused by the balloon follows some general patterns that would be predicted from the biomechanics of plaque and vessel wall. Tears often occur at the edge of an accumulation of plaque where the relatively rigid plaque meets more compliant vessel wall. Additional tears may be seen within the plaque substance. Tears within plaque are particularly common when there are localized fibrocalcific deposits in the plaque.[28] As a balloon is inflated in this type of lesion, the shear stresses are highest in the areas of interface between the hard deposits and the adjacent soft plaque.

Although by far the greatest use of IVUS is in coronary applications, transducer through the segment of interest.[33] Although three-dimensional reconstruction appears to be a feasible direction for image display, there are several practical limitations, including artifacts created by motion of the catheter relative to the artery during image acquisition.

The relative difficulty of discriminating thrombus from soft plaque with the use of IVUS has been mentioned previously. Although tissue characterization methods will probably provide better discrimination, from a practical standpoint it is likely that fiberoptic angioscopy will remain a superior technique for the direct visualization of thrombus.[34]

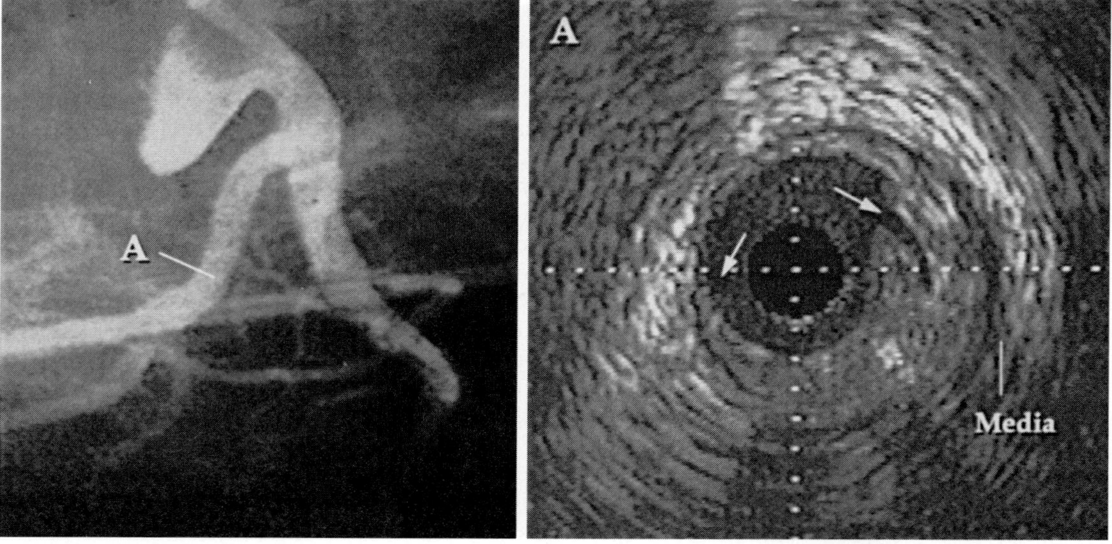

FIGURE 77–6 Dissections occurring after balloon angioplasty. **Right,** The ultrasound image shows two tears *(arrows)*. **Left,** The resolution of the angiogram is not sufficient to detect these tears.

Conclusions

IVUS has moved from the developmental arena into a clinically applicable technology for the assessment of plaque distribution and composition. Direct inspection of plaque with ultrasound is helping to refine clinical concepts of vascular disease that have previously been largely shaped with angiography. It is clear that knowledge regarding specific plaque morphology may be important in selecting a therapy for a given lesion and monitoring the results of that treatment.

References

1. Bom N, ten Hoff H, Lancee CT, et al: Early and recent intraluminal ultrasound devices. Int J Card Imaging 4:79, 1989.
2. Hodgson JM, Graham SD, Savakus AD, et al: Clinical percutaneous imaging of coronary anatomy using an over-the-wire ultrasound catheter system. J Card Imaging 4:1, 1989.
3. Nissen SE, Grimes CL, Gurley JC, et al: Application of a new phased-array ultrasound imaging catheter in the assessment of vascular dimensions. Circulation 81:2007, 1990.
4. Yock PG, Johnson EL, Linker DT: Intravascular ultrasound: development and clinical potential. Am J Card Imaging 2:185, 1988.
5. Mallery JA, Tobis JM, Griffith J, et al: Assessment of normal and atherosclerotic arterial wall thickness with an intravascular ultrasound imaging catheter. Am Heart J 119:1392, 1990.
6. Gussenhoven EJ, Essed CE, Lancee CR, et al: Arterial wall characteristics determined by intravascular ultrasound imaging: an in vitro study. J Am Coll Cardiol 14:957, 1989.
7. Pandian NG, Kreis A, Brockway B, et al: Ultrasound angioscopy: real-time, two-dimensional, intraluminal ultrasound imaging of blood vessels. Am J Cardiol 62:493, 1988.
8. Meyer CR, Chiang EH, Fechner KP, et al: Feasibility of high-resolution intravascular ultrasonic imaging catheters. Radiology 168:113, 1988.
9. Nishimura RA, Edwards WD, Warnes CA, et al: Intravascular ultrasound imaging: in vitro validation and pathologic correlation. J Am Coll Cardiol 16:145, 1990.
10. Fitzgerald PJ, St. Goar FG, Connolly AJ, et al: Intravascular ultrasound imaging of coronary arteries: is three layers the norm? Circulation 86:154, 1992.
11. Gussenhoven EJ, Frietman PA, The SH: Assessment of medial thinning in atherosclerosis by intravascular ultrasound. Am J Cardiol 68:1625, 1991.
12. Colombo A, Hall P, Nakamura S, et al: Intracoronary stenting without anticoagulation accomplished with intravascular ultrasound guidance. Circulation 91:1676, 1995.
13. Nakamura S, Colombo A, Gaglione A, et al: Intracoronary ultrasound observations during stent implantation. Circulation 89:2026, 1994.
14. Potkin BN, Bartorelli AL, Gessert JM, et al: Coronary artery imaging with intravascular high-frequency ultrasound. Circulation 81:1575, 1990.
15. Pandian NG, Kreis A, Brockway B: Detection of intraarterial thrombus by intravascular high frequency two-dimensional ultrasound imaging in vitro and in vivo studies. Am J Cardiol 15:1280, 1990.
16. Landini L, Samem R, Picano E, Salvadori M: Evaluation of frequency dependence of backscatter coefficient in normal and atherosclerotic aortic walls. Ultrasound Med Biol 12:397, 1986.
17. Barzilai B, Saffitz JE, Miller JG, Sobel BE: Quantitative ultrasonic characterization of the nature of atherosclerotic plaques in human aorta. Circ Res 60:459, 1987.
18. Linker DT, Kieven A, Gronningsaether A, et al: Tissue characterization with intra-arterial ultrasound: special promise and problems. Int J Card Imaging 6:255, 1991.
19. Tobis JM, Mallery JA, Gessert J, et al: Intravascular ultrasound cross-section imaging before and after balloon angioplasty in vitro. Circulation 80:873, 1989.
20. Glagov S, Weisenberg E, Zarins CK, et al: Compensatory enlargement of human atherosclerotic coronary arteries. N Engl J Med 316:1371, 1987.
21. Losordo DW, Rosenfield K, Kaufman J, et al: Focal compensatory enlargement of human arteries in response to progressive atherosclerosis: in vivo documentation using intravascular ultrasound. Circulation 89:2570, 1994.
22. Post MJ, Borst C, Kuntz RE: The relative importance of arterial remodeling compared with intimal hyperplasia in lumen renarrowing after balloon angioplasty. Circulation 89:2816, 1994.
23. Mintz GS, Popma JJ, Pichard AD, et al: Arterial remodeling after coronary angioplasty: a serial intravascular ultrasound study. Circulation 94:35, 1996.
24. Kimura T, Laburagi S, Tamura T, et al: Remodeling of human coronary arteries undergoing coronary angioplasty or atherectomy. Circulation 96:475, 1997.
25. Mintz GS, Popma JJ, Pichard AD, et al: Limitations of angiography in the assessment of plaque distribution in coronary artery disease: a systematic study of target lesion eccentricity in 1446 lesions. Circulation 93:924, 1996.
21. Mintz G, Douek P, Pichard AD, et al: Target lesion calcification in coronary artery disease: an intravascular ultrasound study. J Am Coll Cardiol 20:1149, 1992.
22. Matar FA, Mintz GS, Pinnow E, et al: Multivariate predictors of intravascular ultrasound end points after directional coronary atherectomy. J Am Coll Cardiol 25:318, 1995.
23. Fitzgerald PJ, Ports TA, Yock PG: Contribution of localized calcium deposits to dissection after angioplasty: an observational study using intravascular ultrasound. Circulation 86:64, 1992.
24. Crowley U, von Behren PL, Couvillon LA Jr, et al: Optimized ultrasound imaging catheters for use in the vascular system. Int J Card Imag 4:145, 1989.
25. Evans JL, Ng K-H, Vonesh MJ, et al: Arterial imaging utilizing a new forward viewing intravascular ultrasound catheter. Circulation 89:712, 1994.
26. Kitney RI, Moura L, Straughan K: 3-D visualization of arterial structures using ultrasound and Voxel modelling. Int J Card Imag 4:135, 1989.
27. Rosenfield K, Kauftnan J, Pieczek A, et al: Real-time three dimensional reconstruction of intravascular ultrasound images of iliac arteries. Am J Cardiol 70:412, 1992.
28. Gil R, von Birgelen C, Prati F, et al: Usefulness of three-dimensional reconstruction for interpretation and quantitative analysis of intracoronary ultrasound during stent deployment. Am J Cardiol 77:761, 1996.
29. Ramee SR, White CJ, Collins TJ, et al: Percutaneous angioscopy during coronary angioplasty using a steerable microangioscope. J Am Coll Cardiol 17:100, 1991.

CHAPTER 78

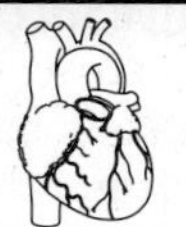

NEWER IMAGING MODALITIES: INTRAVASCULAR ULTRASOUND—CLINICAL APPLICATIONS

James J. Ferguson

INTRODUCTION
LIMITATIONS OF CONTRAST ANGIOGRAPHY
HISTORICAL DEVELOPMENT OF IVUS
EARLY VALIDATION STUDIES
CURRENT GUIDELINES FOR IMAGE ACQUISITION
CURRENT CLINICAL APPLICATIONS
Diagnostic Applications
Interventional Applications: Before Intervention, During Intervention
CLINICAL TRIALS
EMERGING AND FUTURE DIRECTIONS
Technical Advances
Expanded Clinical Applications
SUMMARY

INTRODUCTION

Intravascular ultrasound (IVUS) has emerged as a major new imaging modality for the evaluation of vascular pathology. It has taught us a great deal about the key mechanisms involved in restenosis following coronary intervention and has changed the way that we perform many of these procedures. In a few short years, it has moved beyond initial investigational applications to the mainstream of clinical practice. This chapter traces the historical development of IVUS, presents data from validation studies (both angiographic and pathologic), and discusses the modern-day clinical applicability of IVUS in detail.

LIMITATIONS OF CONTRAST ANGIOGRAPHY

There are clearly defined limitations to contrast angiography. Angiography is basically a two-dimensional representation of three-dimensional structures, a "shadow" projection on film of the lumen contour. Angiography does not visualize the wall itself or provide information about the structure or makeup of areas of obstruction. Visual interpretation of angiographic stenosis severity can be very inaccurate and subjective. Even modern quantitative techniques can have severe calibration errors and may not identify the true severity of diffuse atherosclerotic disease.

Angioscopy is an alternative imaging modality that directly visualizes the lumen interior, but it also has clear-cut limitations, including a requirement for a blood-free field, the need for flushing distally to clear blood from the field of view, and a limited steering capability. Moreover, angioscopy allows only visualization of the inner lining of the vessel wall and does not lend itself to quantification of vessel size or severity of obstruction.

HISTORICAL DEVELOPMENT OF IVUS

Since the 1970s, there has been a great deal of interest in the application of intraluminal imaging techniques as a means of providing cross-sectional imaging of blood vessels from the inside out. The obvious advantages of an intraluminal approach (as opposed to standard transcutaneous approaches) include close proximity of the transducer to the imaging target, higher frequency, shorter wavelength, small transducers, and better image resolution.[1] Cross-sectional imaging allows visualization of not only the lumen, but also the structure of the vessel wall.

Initial applications of intraluminal echocardiography focused on nonimaging echo transit-time measurements. Cieszynski was among the first to document such a use of intraluminal ultrasound in 1956.[2] He successfully obtained ultrasonic tissue reflections in both experimental models and dogs. In 1966, Kossoff described a catheter-mounted ultrasound device for intracardiac measurements of septal and ventricular wall thickness with an accuracy of up to 0.1 mm.[3] As technology evolved from single to multiple transducers, Peronneau utilized two transducers mounted on either side of the catheter,[4] and Carleton used a nondirectional cylindric transducer.[5] Hughes used a three-element, 10-MHz device in 1978 to measure aortic lumen diameter.[6]

In 1962, Omoto described one of the first intravascular imaging devices, which used a rotating probe with a fixed guide wire tip.[7] Eggleton utilized a four-element catheter to approximate cardiac cross-sectional images.[8] One of the major pioneers of true two-dimensional real-time intravascular ultrasound imaging was Klaas Bom, who as early as 1969 developed a 32-element phased-array device that operated at 5.6 MHz, had an outer diameter of 3.2 mm, and was mounted on a 9-French catheter.[9] Further refine-

ments of the technology evolved, including the very significant contributions of Paul Yock toward developing clinically applicable devices.

EARLY VALIDATION STUDIES

Early work in the field of IVUS was directed at validating measurements obtained from intravascular ultrasound images with angiographic and pathologic standards. St. Goar and colleagues examined 20 cardiac transplant patients with no angiographic coronary artery disease.[10] They compared quantitative angiography and ultrasound measurements of lumen diameter at 76 sites and found a close correlation when ultrasound diameter was compared to angiographic diameter (r = 0.86 for angiographic diameter perpendicular to the vessel; r = 0.88 for angiographic diameter perpendicular to the ultrasound catheter).

Davidson and coworkers compared angiography and ultrasound in 65 patients undergoing 70 interventional procedures.[11] They found a poor (r = 0.28) correlation between postprocedural angiography and ultrasound but concluded that for postintervention assessment, ultrasound was probably the more reliable and accurate of the two techniques. Vessel dissection was noted in 41 percent of segments by ultrasound but in only 20 percent of segments by angiography. In 10 of 11 atherectomy cases, residual atheroma was visible on ultrasound despite an angiographically adequate result.

Gussenhoven and associates reported the results of in vitro studies comparing histologic sections with ultrasound images in human arterial autopsy specimens.[12, 13] They observed a close relationship between plaque location, maximum plaque thickness, and circumferential extent of plaque involvement. Muscular arteries exhibited hypoechoic media in contrast to elastic arteries, in which the media were as echogenic as the intima and adventitia. Ultrasound could distinguish four basic components of atherosclerotic plaque: (1) hypoechoic lipid deposits, (2) moderately echoic fibromuscular tissue, (3) highly echoic fibrous tissue, and (4) highly echoic (with shadowing) calcium deposits.

Nissen and colleagues compared the ability of ultrasound and angiography to measure vascular dimensions in animals.[14] Anatomic deformations were created by external constriction and balloon dilation. There was a very close correlation between the two techniques for both diameter (r = 0.98) and area (r = 0.96) as well as percent diameter stenosis (r = 0.89). The correlation between angiography and ultrasound for vessel diameter and area before and after balloon dilation was somewhat stronger before dilation (diameter, r = 0.92; area, r = 0.88) than after dilation (diameter, r = 0.86; area, r = 0.81).

Nissen and coworkers also compared angiography and ultrasound images at 33 sites in 8 normal subjects and at 162 sites in 43 patients with coronary artery disease (CAD).[15] In normal subjects, there was an excellent correlation (r = 0.92) between the two techniques. In 90 concentric sites in CAD patients, the correlation was also excellent (r = 0.93), but in 72 eccentric sites, the correlation was not as good (r = 0.77). The authors attributed these differences in eccentric lesions to the inherent differences between tomographic and silhouette imaging techniques.

Tobis and associates performed in vivo clinical studies of IVUS and in vitro comparison studies with histology in human arterial specimens.[16] They concluded that intravascular images could provide accurate information about histologic characteristics of atherosclerotic plaques. Their studies showed relatively poor correlation between angiography and intravascular ultrasound, but they too concluded that intravascular ultrasound may be the more accurate of the two techniques—again, especially after interventional procedures.

Nishimura and colleagues comprehensively examined 130 segments of fresh peripheral arteries with intravascular ultrasound and compared the results with the corresponding histopathologic sections.[17] There was a strong correlation between ultrasound lumen area and calculated histologic area. Ultrasound demonstrated three vessel patterns: (1) a distinct media-adventitia interface; (2) an indistinct media-adventitial interface with different echo density layers; and (3) a diffuse homogeneous appearance, depending on the content, density, and location of elastin and smooth muscle in the vessel wall. They found that atherosclerotic plaque could be reliably detected but that its thickness and demarcation from the media could not always be determined.

Siegel and coworkers examined the sensitivity, specificity, and accuracy of IVUS and angioscopy in 70 postmortem human arterial segments.[18] Imaging sites were classified on the basis of density (normal, increased, or decreased) and lumen configuration (smooth or irregular). Using histologic analysis as a gold standard, they found ultrasound to be highly (>88 percent) sensitive, specific, and accurate for stable atheroma with results as good as, if not better than, those of angioscopy. For disrupted atheroma, the sensitivity of IVUS was 81 percent with specificity, accuracy, and predictive value all greater than 90 percent; angioscopy was slightly less sensitive and slightly more specific. For thrombus detection, IVUS was much less sensitive than angioscopy (57 percent versus 100 percent) because of false-negative interpretation of laminar clots in normal vessels and difficulty distinguishing thrombus from disrupted or stable atheroma. The specificity, accuracy, and predictive value of IVUS for the detection of thrombus were all greater than 93 percent.

Willard and associates studied 19 saphenous vein grafts (10 autopsy, 9 harvested at the time of bypass surgery) with IVUS, quantitative coronary angiography, and histologic analysis.[19] There was a strong correlation between lumen measurements obtained with IVUS and quantitative coronary angiography measurements (r = 0.91). There was a good correlation between ultrasound and histologic images in distinguishing normal intima, intimal hyperplasia, vessel wall fibrosis, and atheromatous plaque.

Fitzgerald and colleagues used IVUS to study 16 intact hearts at autopsy from patients without a history of CAD. They found intimal thickening (>178 μm) to be associated with a three-layer appearance. The nonlayered group also tended to be much younger than the three-layer group (27 ± versus 43 ± 9 years).[20]

Hodgson and coworkers compared plaque morphology (soft, fibrous, calcific, mixed plaque, concentric subintimal thickening) with angiographic morphologic features, proce-

TABLE 78–1 Ultrasound Lesion Characteristics Useful in Distinguishing Lesion Pathology

Characteristic	Normal	Stable Atheroma	Disrupted Atheroma	Thrombus
Calcium	Absent	Often present (with shadowing)	Often present (with shadowing)	Absent
Wall thickness	Normal	Increased	Increased	N/A
Lumen contour	Smooth, round, widely patent	Smooth, concentrically or eccentrically narrowed	Concentrically or eccentrically narrowed; disrupted (visible cracks, flaps, dissections, and ulcerations)	Intraluminal location; distinct borders
Apperarance	Usually three-layered; no layering may be present in young patients	Loss of layering	Loss of layering, cracks, splits	No layering; speckled, homogeneous
Media	Thin, hypoechoic	Thickened	Thickened; dissections may be present	N/A

dural results, and clinical angina patter (stable versus unstable) in 65 patients undergoing percutaneous transluminal coronary angioplasty (PTCA).[21] Unstable angina patients had more soft lesions, fewer calcified and mixed lesions, and less intralesional calcium. Ultrasound was more sensitive than angiography in identifying unstable lesions. There was a substantial amount of plaque in reference segments, and post-PTCA plaque burden remained high.

In summary, IVUS provides accurate images of the arterial lumen. It appears to be a good technique for defining lumen geometry and identifying wall pathology (Table 78–1). IVUS has the capability to document the normal three-layer appearance of healthy coronary arteries and to distinguish between muscular arteries (coronary arteries) and elastic arteries (aorta and pulmonary arteries). It can detect the presence of intimal thickening at an early stage, if it exceeds 150 to 200 μm. Additional issues of cardiac cycle variability, blood pressure effects, and study-to-study imaging reproducibility location have not been completely solved, although with modern-era devices, which are more user-friendly, these issues have dwindled in importance. There are obvious visible effects of blood pressure on arterial diameter, even in coronary arteries. These concerns notwithstanding, IVUS holds great promise for future studies that require precise measurements of arterial diameter. After interventions, such as PTCA, the correlation with angiography is generally less good, but this probably represents more of a limitation of angiographic techniques and the difficulties in tracking angiographic lumen boundaries after PTCA.

Current Guidelines for Image Acquisition

The European Society of Cardiology (the Study Group on Intracoronary Imaging of the Working Group of Coronary Circulation and the Subgroup on Intravascular Ultrasound of the Working Group of Echocardiography) set forth guidelines for image acquisition (Table 78–2).[22] They highlighted important features of IVUS image acquisition before, during, and after catheter insertion. Before catheter insertion, proper catheter preparation, intravenous heparin (5000–10,000 U), and intracoronary nitrates are important to ensure proper device function and patient safety. During insertion, standardized image orientation, advancement of the catheter beyond the lesion, optimized image quality, and video recording during automated pullback with voice annotation provide the best quality studies. After images are acquired, the device should be pulled into the guiding catheter lumen and the videotape reviewed (or the longitudinally reconstructed view examined, or both), the area and

TABLE 78–2 Guidelines for Image Acquisition

Before Insertion of the Intracoronary Ultrasound Catheter

Inject intracoronary nitroglycerin (0.1–0.3 mg) or isosorbide dinitrate (1–3 mg) to prevent spasm and induce maximal vasodilatation.

Inspect and prepare the catheter (flush carefully if mechanical); connect to ultrasound console or motor unit; test the catheter.

Subtract the ring-down artifact with catheter not in contact with the vessel wall (electronic transducers).

During Insertion of the Intracoronary Ultrasound Catheter

During insertion, set the rotation of the images to a predefined standard (i.e., place origin of the circumflex at 9 o'clock when imaging the left anterior descending).

Insert the catheter distal to the stenosis or the segment under investigation under fluoroscopy (attention must be paid to wire looping for short monorail catheters); for common sheath design, remove guide wire up to proximal marker and insert imaging cable.

Optimize image quality (gain and zoom setting).

Start recording on super-VHS videotape and check that the entire examination is recorded and that demographic and procedural data have been annotated.

Indicate when the pullback is started (written or voice annotation, possibly showing the position of the tip of the ultrasound catheter with fluoroscopy before starting the pullback).

Start the pullback, using a motorized pullback device operating at constant speed (0.25, 0.50 or 1.0 mm·s^{-1}).

Continue voice comment or annotate positions without interrupting the pullback until the ultrasound catheter is withdrawn into the guiding catheter.

After Insertion of the Intracoronary Ultrasound Catheter

Reassess the cross-sections of interest, reviewing the videotape or the longitudinal view generated after on-line three-dimensional reconstruction and perform area and diameter measurements of target stenosis and reference.

Reinsert the ultrasound probe only if doubts of the image interpretation remain (use contrast or saline to better delineate the lumen, if necessary).

Before new insertions, inspect and flush carefully the ultrasound catheter and test it again.

Adapted from DiMario C, Görge G, Peters R, et al: Clinical application and image interpretation in intracoronary ultrasound. Eur Heart J 19:207, 1998.

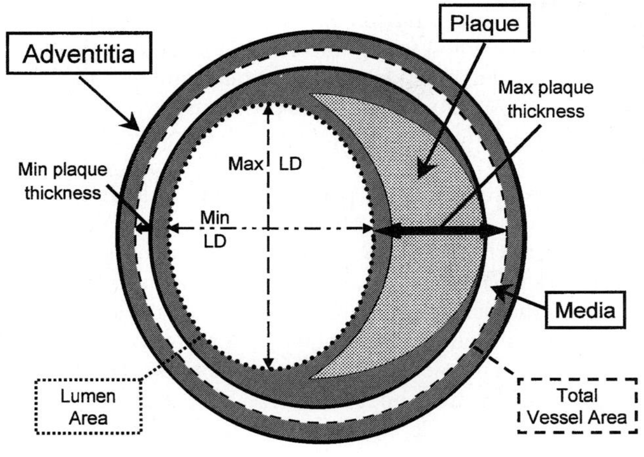

FIGURE 78–1

Measurement	Abbreviation/ Units of Measure	Comments
Plaque area (PA)	PA, mm^2	Vessel area (VA) minus lumen area (LA)
Percent PA	% PA, %	Percentage of VA occupied by plaque (VA − LA)/VA × 100
Mean lumen diameter (LD)	Mean LD, mm	Calculated as: $\left(\sqrt{(LA/\pi)}\right) \times 2$
Lumen symmetry index	Min D/max D	1 indicates circular lumen, <1 indicates increasing elliptical lumen shape
Plaque eccentric index	Min/max plaque thickness (min/max PT)	1 indicates concentric plaque, <1 indicates increasing plaque eccentricity

diameter measurements made of the reference vessel and target lesion, and the length of the target lesion assessed. Reinterrogation of the vessel should be necessary only in the case of unclear image interpretation or if contrast or saline is required to better define the exact borders of the lumen. Standardized measurements obtained from IVUS studies are given in Figure 78–1.

CURRENT CLINICAL APPLICATIONS

In its early years of clinical use, in the late 1980s and early 1990s, IVUS appeared to be a technology in search of an application. There was no question that IVUS provided unique image information, but it was less clear that the new information made any difference in patient management.

All that changed as the technique of stenting emerged as the dominant interventional technology in the later 1990s. In the early days of stenting, there was considerable uncertainty about what anticoagulant regimens should be employed and about how best to deliver stents. Although IVUS could not answer the former question, it taught operators a great deal about optimizing stent delivery and helped bring coronary stenting forward in a way that was not possible with any other catheterization laboratory imaging modality. In the modern-day world of invasive and interventional cardiology, the clinical application of IVUS falls into two general categories: diagnostic applications and interventional applications (Table 78–3).

Diagnostic Applications

There are three primary areas where IVUS provides clinically useful diagnostic information: for angiographically normal segments, for ambiguous lesions, and in patients following cardiac transplantation.

Patients undergoing angiography for suspected CAD may have "normal" coronary angiograms in approximately 10 to 15 percent of cases. However, as recently demonstrated by Erbel and associates,[23] almost one half of patients with ostensibly normal coronary angiograms will have atherosclerotic changes on IVUS. The superior sensitivity of IVUS in identifying atherosclerosis is not a new observation and was well documented in the early 1990s.[24] We have come to appreciate the importance of vessel remodeling in the progression of atherosclerotic disease, first described by Glagov in 1987.[25] As atherosclerotic lesions evolve over time, compensatory mechanisms within the vessel try to preserve lumen size, concealing early atherosclerotic lesions from angiographic disclosure. IVUS may also be useful in identifying other areas of vascular pathology, such as spontaneous coronary dissection,[26] myocardial bridging,[27] and clarifying of areas of inhomogeneous contrast distribution observed during angiography. Ultrasound is also able to detect the presence of significant atherosclerosis in what otherwise appears to be angiographically normal segments adjacent to stenotic segments.[23] St. Goar

TABLE 78–3 Clinical Applications of Intravascular Ultrasound

- Diagnostic applications
  - Angiographically inapparent disease
  - Angiographically ambiguous lesions
  - Postcardiac transplant
  - Identification of calcium
  - Identification of thrombus
  - Bypass grafts
- Therapeutic applications
  - Before procedure
    - Assessment of lesion length
    - Lesion localization
    - Device selection
  - During procedure
    - Balloon expandable stents
    - Self-expanding stents
    - Balloon angioplasty
    - Directional atherectomy
    - Rotational atherectomy
- Other applications
  - Intracardiac imaging
    - Pulmonary artery pathology
    - Chronic pulmonary thromboemboli
    - Restenosis trials
    - Venous structures
    - Vena caval filters
    - Arterial compliance and P-V relationships

Abbreviation: P-V, pressure-volume.

and colleagues have shown that IVUS can be used to detect early, angiographically inapparent CAD in young adults.[28] Ge and coworkers[29] performed IVUS studies in 55 patients with normal coronary angiograms and clinical symptoms of chest pain. Atherosclerotic plaque was identified in 25 of 55 patients (45%), occupying 28.8 ± 9.6 percent of the lumen area.

As previously mentioned, the limitations of contrast angiography in providing true measurements of lumen size or contour, particularly after interventional procedures or with complex lesions, are well recognized. Because of vessel overlap or difficulty in laying out the target vessel properly, there are circumstances where it is difficult (if not impossible) to angiographically determine whether or not there is a significant obstruction (Fig. 78–2). Ostial stenosis, diffuse lesions, highly eccentric lesions, and bifurcation lesions are all situations in which conventional contrast angiography can provide suboptimal or even inadequate or misleading diagnostic information. Furthermore, patient characteristics, such as extreme obesity, chest deformities, and emphysema, can severely limit the quality of angiographic imaging. IVUS, by providing precise tomographic visualization, allows precise characterization and localization of intralumen pathology.

Again, this is not a new observation; it has been recognized since the early 1990s.[30] However, two more recent studies further documented the utility of IVUS in defining the significance (or nonsignificance) of angiographically ambiguous lesions, although these studies did not use prespecified objective criteria for identifying "severe" disease requiring intervention.[31, 32] Particularly when coupled with other forms of physiologic assessment (such as poststenotic pressure measurements or intracoronary Doppler velocity measurements), IVUS provides a very powerful tool for more closely interrogating ambiguous lesions.

The single most important cause of morbidity and mortality in cardiac transplant patients after the first year is accelerated graft atherosclerosis.[33–35] Symptoms are not reliable in the denervated heart, and yearly coronary angiography is part of the routine follow-up of cardiac transplant patients, although it is significantly limited in how well it can identify disease progression.[36] The nature of the atherosclerotic involvement in transplant vasculopathy is concentric intimal proliferation throughout the vascular tree, progressing to obstruction, first in the smaller vessels ("pruning" of the vascular tree) and then more proximally.[37] Angiographically, transplant vascular disease appears to involve only the small arteries, with relative sparing of the major epicardial arteries. Coronary flow reserve has also been proposed as an alternative diagnostic means but is not readily applicable in clinical practice.

IVUS, on the other hand, provides a sensitive, accurate, reliable, and reproducible assessment of the extent of graft atherosclerosis (Fig. 78–3). The majority of patients will have IVUS evidence of angiographically silent intimal thickening a year or more after transplantation,[38–41] and IVUS provides a means for early detection of disease progression and even identification of focal lesions.[41, 42] In serial studies, IVUS detects changes in intimal thickness in approximately 40 percent of subjects,[43] usually within the first 2 years after transplant. A mean intimal thickness greater than or equal to 0.3 mm is an independent predictor of survival and freedom from retransplant.[44] Mills and associates have also documented posttransplant endothelial dysfunction using IVUS imaging and Doppler flow studies.[45]

Unfortunately, from the perspective of clinical outcome, identifying the presence of disease does not necessarily mean that anything can be done to alter its course. Nevertheless, IVUS has proved to be a very useful tool in exploring the pathogenetic mechanisms of accelerated atherosclerosis in cardiac transplant recipients. A number of immunologic and metabolic factors appear to correlate with the progression of intimal thickness, and the hope is that new mechanistic understandings will lead to improvements in clinical care.

Fluoroscopy is capable of detecting calcium, which occupies more than 180 degrees of the vessel circumference only 60 percent of the time, and is even less sensitive when less circumferential involvement is present. IVUS, on the other hand, can much more accurately identify the extent and depth of calcification. In an early study, Minz and colleagues reported a high incidence of ultrasound target lesion calcification in patients undergoing PTCA, which was poorly detected by fluoroscopy.[46] In a subsequent, much larger study,[47] they reported IVUS-identified calcium in 73 percent of 1155 coronary lesions compared with angiography that showed calcium in only 38 percent. The presence of calcium can have significant implications for the selection of interventional devices. Dissections are much more frequent if greater than 25 percent of the vessel circumference is involved. If subendothelial calcium is present, directional atherectomy is a much less attractive technique, and rotational atherectomy would be favored, particularly if more than 180 degrees of the circumference is involved.

The Washington Heart Center documented[32] that preintervention IVUS information resulted in a change in treatment strategy in 20 percent of cases. With increasing experience, operators tend to rely more and more on IVUS information to guide their therapy[31] when approaching a variety of lesion types. For instance, with restenotic lesions, particularly in patients with in-stent restenosis, IVUS provides very valuable information for guiding subsequent management. What kind of remodeling is present—intimal hyperplasia or vessel shrinkage? Is a previously implanted stent underdeployed, or is there a significant burden of in-stent neointimal hyperplasia? These types of questions become very important as one tries to apply the best technique for the clinical circumstance at hand. Another difficult clinical circumstance is degenerated saphenous vein grafts, with a much higher procedural risk of distal embolization and periprocedural myocardial infarction. Intragraft pathologic processes are not always well defined with angiography,[48] and appropriate choice of intervention (extraction atherectomy, stenting, PTCA, or referral for repeat coronary artery bypass graft) is possible with a better understanding of the extent of the disease and the true length of the involved segments.

An additional area where IVUS can provide valuable

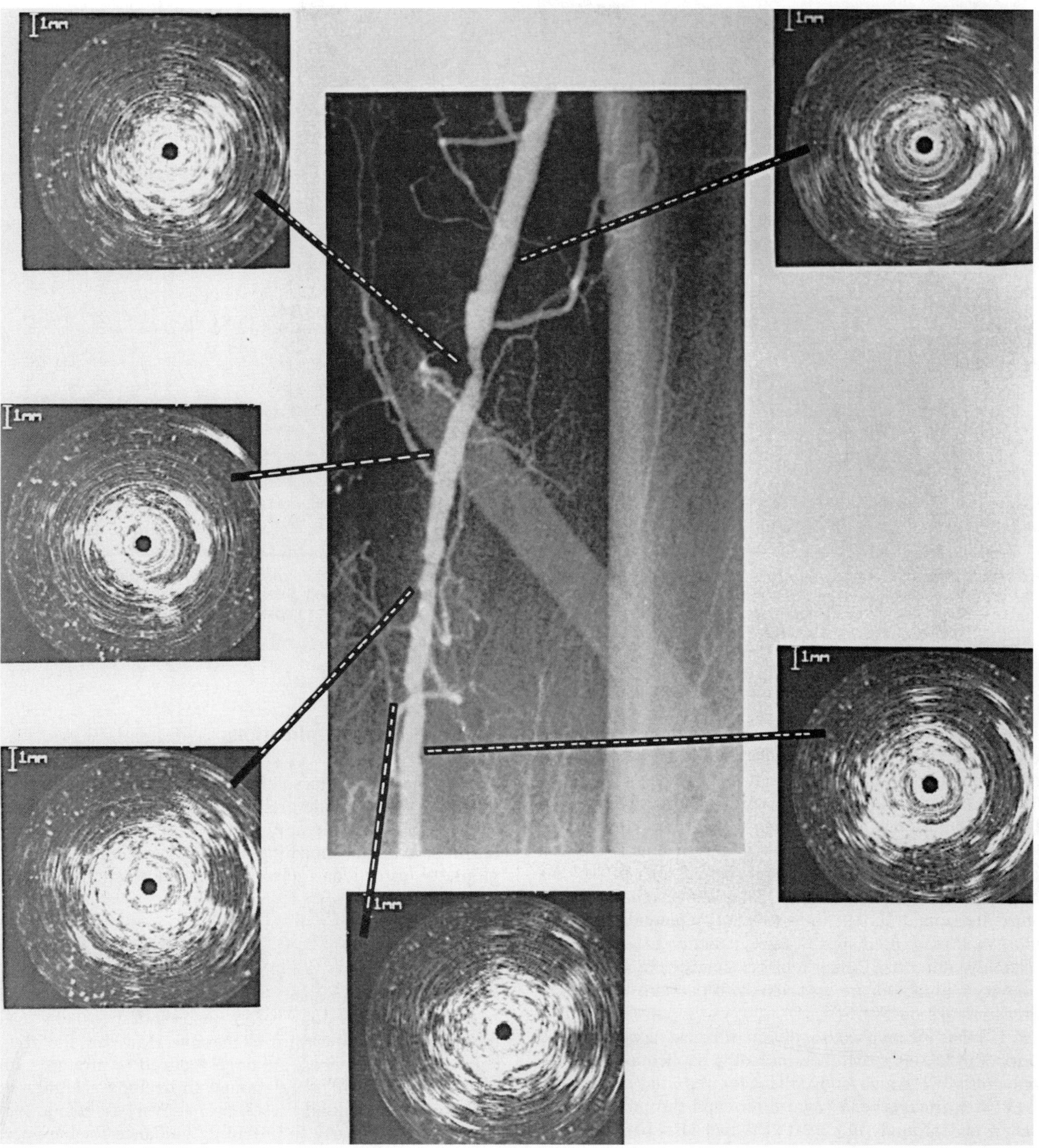

FIGURE 78–2 Intravascular ultrasound images from an angiographically ambiguous lesion in a superficial femoral artery. In the upper (distal) portion of the vessel is an obvious area of narrowing, with the corresponding ultrasound images. In the lower (proximal) portion of the vessel is an area with mild angiographic narrowing but severe narrowing on ultrasound.

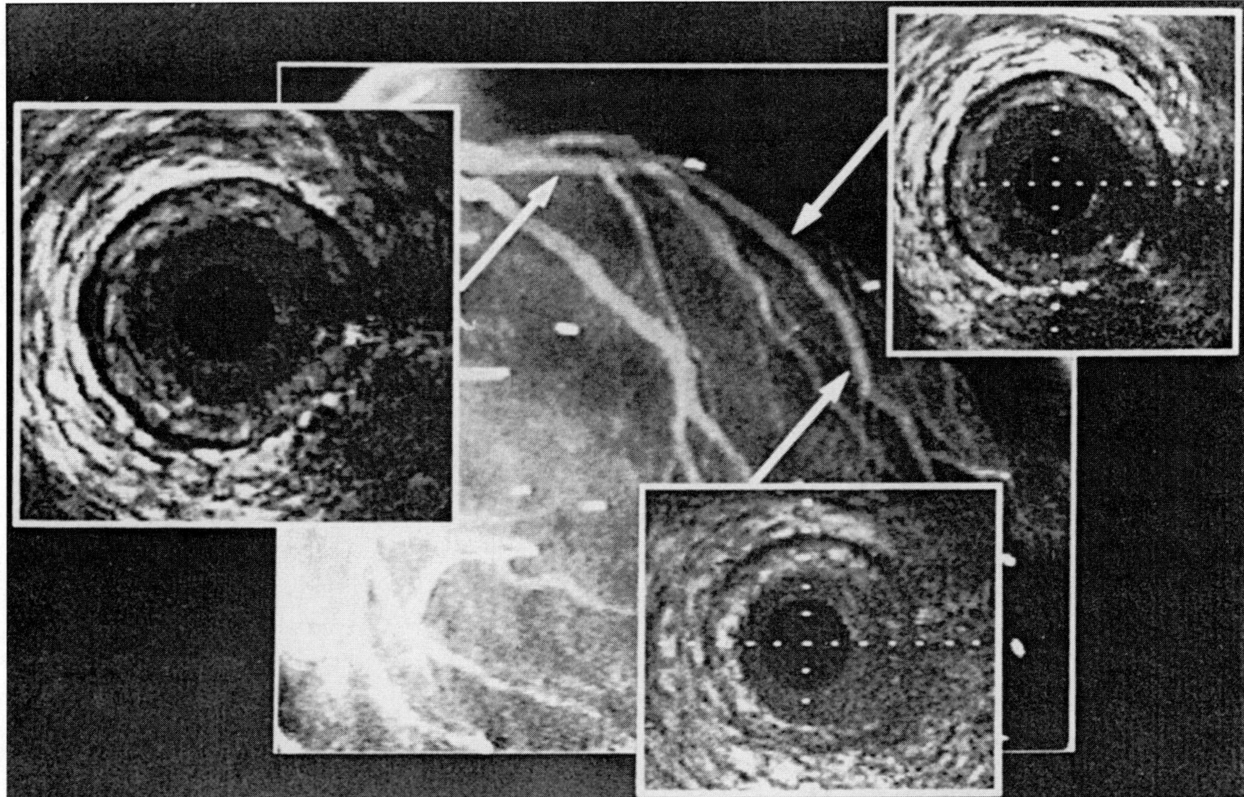

FIGURE 78–3 Angiogram and ultrasound images from a 37-year-old man 3 years after cardiac transplantation. Despite the normal angiogram, the ultrasound images show significant intimal thickening along the proximal/mid left anterior descending coronary artery. (From St. Goar FG, Pinto FJ, Alderman EL, et al: Intracoronary ultrasound in cardiac transplant recipients: In vivo evidence of angiographically silent" intimal thickening. Circulation 85:979, 1992.)

diagnostic information is in the identification of intraluminal thrombus. IVUS is not as sensitive as the more cumbersome technique of angioscopy, but it is clearly more sensitive than angiography in determining the presence or absence of thrombus (Fig. 78–4).[49–52]

Nissen and coworkers[53] have suggested that IVUS can be used to distinguish the type of plaque seen in patients with stable and unstable angina. They suggested that in the future ultrasound may be used to identify plaque characteristics that may predispose some patients to developing unstable syndromes. Zeiher and associates have shown that coronary risk factors are associated with certain vessel wall characteristics on IVUS.[54]

IVUS has been used to obtain images in central and peripheral venous structures, including saphenous vein bypass grafts.[55] Karnich and colleagues reported on the use of IVUS to image vena caval filters and thrombus formation in and around filters.[56] IVUS has also been used in experimental circumstances by some investigators to better define arterial pressure-area relationships and arterial compliance.[57–61] It can also be useful in providing a quantitative measure of vascular tone and has been used for finite element modeling of circumferential stress in atherosclerotic vessels[62] and for assessment of plaque distensibility,[63] as well as for assessment of endothelial function.[45]

Interventional Applications

As an adjunct to interventional therapy, potential applications of IVUS include preintervention assessment (to help select appropriate therapy) and specific assistance in guiding interventional modalities such as stenting, balloon angioplasty, directional atherectomy, and rotational atherectomy.

Before Intervention

As previously mentioned, IVUS is potentially a very useful tool to evaluate lesions before intervention to help select the most appropriate form of therapy. However, the physical size of the devices, although reduced to around 1 mm in diameter, is still large enough to occlude a highly stenotic lesion, potentially resulting in severe ischemia. Nevertheless, particularly in providing guidance for the necessity of using adjunctive debulking therapies with coronary stenting, IVUS may play a very valuable role. The most obvious circumstance, noted above, is in identifying the presence and extent of intralesion calcium. Highly calcified lesions are very resistant to dilation and may prevent full stent expansion. By identifying at-risk lesions and targeting them for debulking techniques such as rotational atherec-

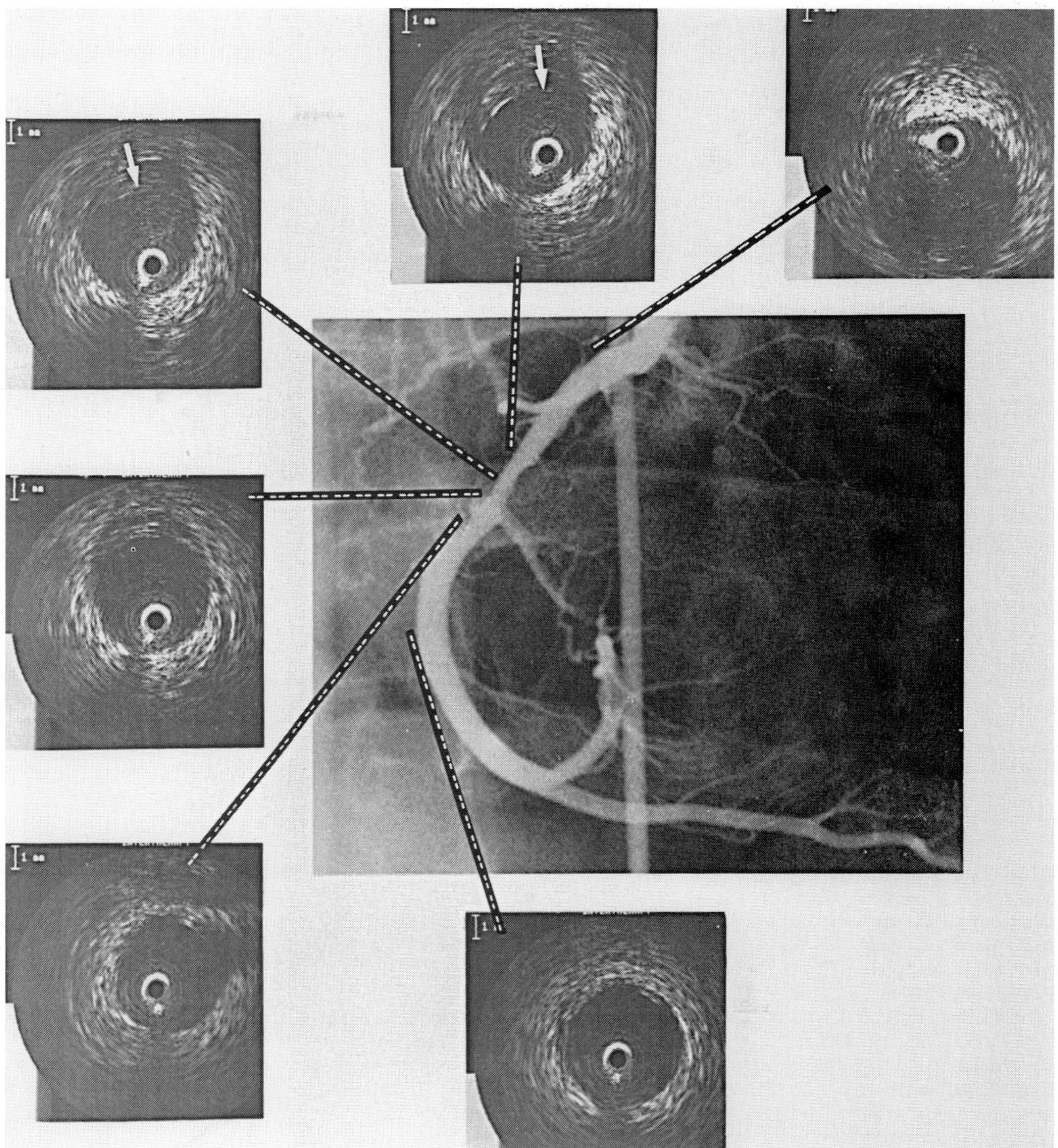

FIGURE 78–4 Intravascular ultrasound images of intracoronary thrombus in a right coronary artery. The thrombus *(arrows)* on ultrasound was a clearly defined intraluminal mass, but on angiography, it was seen as only an area of mild luminal narrowing.

tomy, there may be a much greater likelihood of final procedural success and avoidance of the clinical difficulties associated with underdeployed stents.

Overall, IVUS can be used to accurately assess lesion length (for selecting correct stent lengths or for defining the true treatment area), vessel diameter (to appropriately size devices), lesion eccentricity (for use in adjunctive therapy with directional atherectomy, for instance), and lesion composition (for identifying areas of calcium as noted above).

During Intervention

The specific area of coronary intervention where IVUS has had the most dramatic impact is in coronary stenting. IVUS played an essential role in improving the delivery of stents as they were initially employed in the coronary vasculature (Fig. 78–5). Early studies showed that incomplete apposition of stent to the vessel wall was still present in more than 80 percent of cases, despite a good angiographic result,[64] and that poor delivery techniques were associated

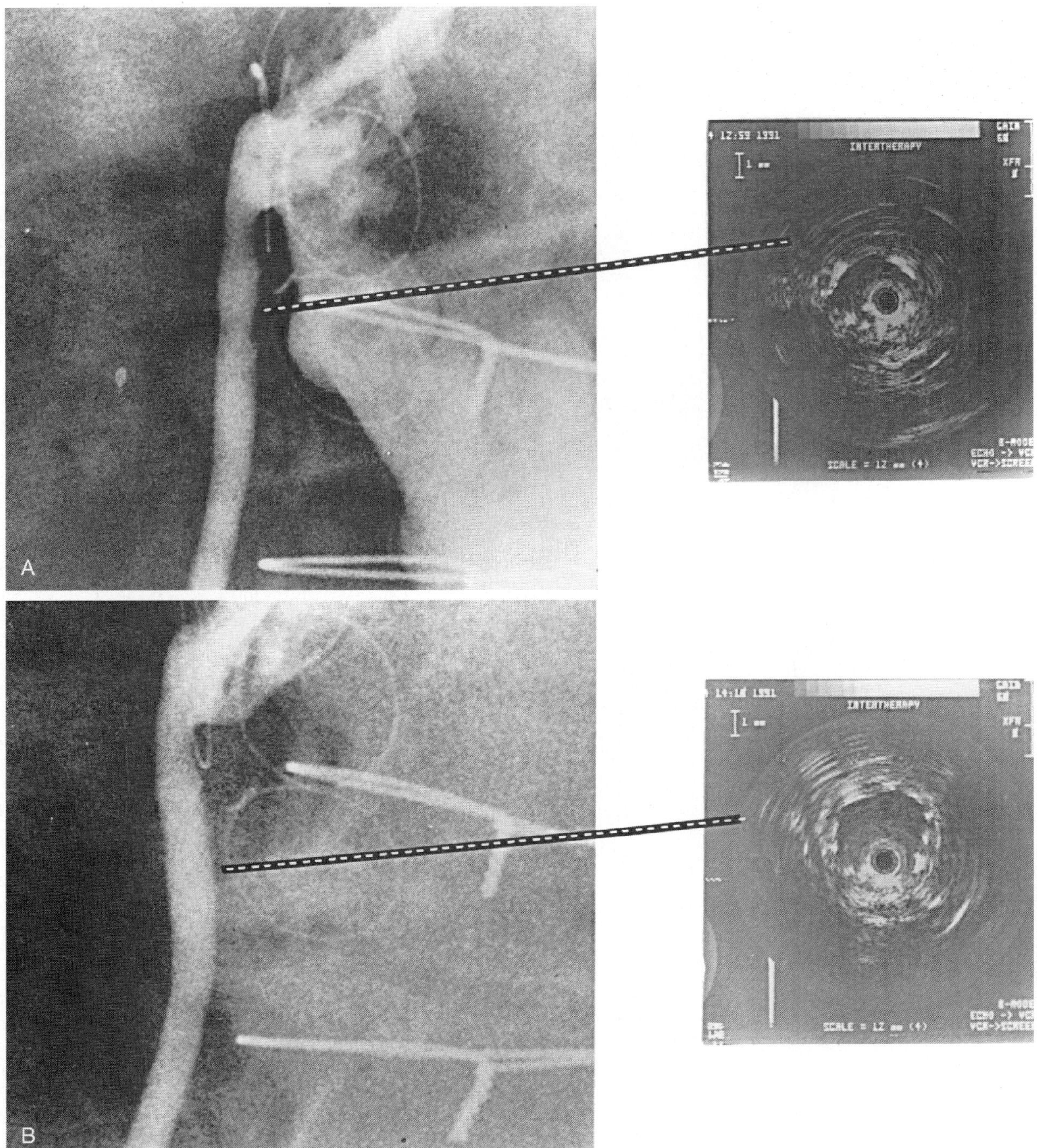

FIGURE 78–5 Intravascular ultrasound images during placement of a Johnson & Johnson Palmaz-Schatz balloon-expandable coronary stent in a saphenous vein graft. The stainless steel struts of the stent are readily visible for assessment of stent expansion. **A,** Angiogram and ultrasound after initial delivery. The stent is not fully expanded. **B,** Similar images after complete expansion of the stent.

with adverse outcomes. This led to the widespread adoption of high-pressure balloon dilation within the stent and a dramatic improvement in clinical outcomes.[65–68] Current guidelines for optimal stent expansion, as set forth by the MUSIC investigators, are listed in Table 78–4.

Because high-pressure balloon inflations have become widely applied, the question frequently arises as to whether IVUS is necessary for optimal stent delivery. Studies have suggested that angiography may provide a more accurate assessment of lumen dimensions after high-pressure inflation as opposed to low-pressure inflation.[69, 70] The subacute thrombosis rates for routine stent deployment without IVUS are still very low. A large-scale French registry reported an experience with 1156 patients without the use of IVUS[71] and documented a subacute thrombosis rate of 1.6 percent. Data from the MUST trial (a trial of aspirin and ticlopidine post stenting that did not use IVUS) showed successful stent deployment in 259 of 260 patients.[72] Dur-

TABLE 78-4 MUSIC Criteria for Optimal Stent Expansion

Complete apposition of the stent to the vessel wall along the entire length of the stents.
In-stent minimal lumen area is ≥90% of the average reference vessel area or ≥100% of the reference segment with the smallest lumen area.
If minimal lumen area inside the stent is >9.0 mm², criterion number 2 may be modified to ≥80% of the average reference vessel area of ≥90% of the reference segment with the smallest lumen area.
In-stent area of the proximal stent entrance is ≥90% of the proximal reference lumen area.
Symmetric stent expansion, with a maximal-minimal lumen diameter rate ≥0.7.

ing the hospital stay, there were no deaths, eight patients had a myocardial infarction (three Q wave and five non–Q wave), and four patients had repeat PTCA.

However, data from other groups routinely using IVUS for stent deployment (including the APLAUSE trial at Washington Heart Center,[73] the Milan group,[68] and the Cleveland Clinic[74]) suggest that subacute thrombosis rates can be reduced even further, significantly below 1 percent. A hybrid approach has also been advocated, strongly recommending IVUS for high-risk circumstances such as diffuse disease, bailout use of stents, acute coronary syndromes, multiple stents, and limited operator experience. Approaches to facilitate the applicability of IVUS to stent implantation, including combining the ultrasound probe and the balloon on the same catheter or using an IVUS imaging core within a conventional delivery balloon may help facilitate more routine IVUS use for stenting.

Concerns have also been raised about the vessel injury associated with high-pressure balloon inflation, and some operators have backed away from the very high pressures previously used. In these circumstances, there is a higher chance of inadequate stent expansion, and the use of IVUS to guide deployment becomes increasingly important as the deployment delivery pressure falls. Another important dilemma arises in saphenous vein grafts, when larger, self-expanding stents are employed, and the operator wishes to manipulate the vessel as little as possible to reduce the risk of embolization. In this circumstance, IVUS can tell the operator whether follow-up balloon inflations are really necessary and can reduce the risk of embolization that would accompany otherwise routine postdilation.

Given the dramatic reductions observed in the incidence of subacute stent thrombosis, more recent attention has turned to the vexing problem of in-stent restenosis. While, as yet, we do not know whether IVUS-guided stenting can significantly reduce restenosis, a number of trials, highlighted below, will help answer this question. Furthermore, as previously mentioned, the use of IVUS to select lesions that require debulking to optimize stent implantation (particularly in calcified, noncompliant vessels) would be expected to favorably influence restenosis. In the recent CRUISE trial (a subset of the STARS trial), the IVUS-guided stent group had a significant increase in within-stent cross-sectional area and a 40 percent reduction in target vessel revascularization.[75]

In much the same way that the benefits of (and need for) high-pressure balloon inflation were evident only on IVUS examination, IVUS also provides us with the only good mechanistic insights into restenosis (Fig. 78–6). Two processes appear to play complementary roles: (1) neointimal hyperplasia and (2) adverse vascular remodeling (pathologic shrinkage of the overall vessel size, perhaps as a consequence of adventiomedial scarring). In-stent restenosis within an optimally deployed stent is largely composed of neointimal hyperplasia. The future of clinical restenosis research lies with IVUS, as the only imaging technology to provide adequate anatomic detail. The ERASER trial[76] is a case in point, in which volumetric assessment of neointimal growth was the primary endpoint of the trial (which looked at whether the platelet GP IIb/IIIa antagonist abciximab could reduce restenosis). A similar IVUS subset is being investigated in the ongoing PRESTO trial of the antikeloid drug tranilast[77] and in other studies including ITALICS, ESSEX, TRAPIST, and BERT.

Although stenting has received the most attention and is the most obvious area in which IVUS can facilitate intervention, it may also be a useful adjunct to other forms of coronary intervention. For conventional balloon angioplasty, IVUS does allow better balloon sizing and a better delineation of the area requiring treatment. However, the *real* utility of IVUS for balloon angioplasty appears to be in assessing the adequacy of the results achieved.

Two primary factors limit modern-day angioplasty: abrupt closure and restenosis. The former represents an interaction between the injury done to the vessel and the thrombogenic milieu at the time of the procedure. Although platelet GP IIb/IIIa antagonists and the availability of stents have dramatically reduced the incidence of abrupt closure, the primary utility of stents in this circumstance comes in the setting of sealing post-PTCA dissections. Unfortunately, angiography is a poor tool for assessing the severity or extent of dissections; IVUS is much more sensitive in this regard.[78–80] The ultimate application of IVUS for this indication will probably involve three-dimensional reconstruction to fully appreciate the longitudinal and circumferential extent of dissection.[81]

With regard to restenosis, a number of trials are investigating whether IVUS can identify or reduce risk factors associated with restenosis. The small-scale PICTURE study showed no relationship between IVUS-identified dissections or lesion composition and outcome.[82] More recent data from the Washington Heart Center have suggested that residual plaque burden following intervention is a very powerful independent predictor of restenosis.[83] The ongoing GUIDE trial is examining on a larger scale the IVUS factors that predict restenosis following PTCA or directional coronary atherectomy (DCA).[84, 85] IVUS is certainly warranted in circumstances in which there is angiographic evidence of a suboptimal result (haziness, filling defects, etc.), but, in much the same way that IVUS taught us how to properly deliver stents, IVUS may also teach us that to optimize the long-term outcome of PTCA, we need to minimize the postprocedure plaque burden. The only way this will truly be feasible is with postprocedure IVUS examinations in more patients and with meticulous, large-scale prospective randomized studies.

For directional atherectomy, IVUS is useful in identifying highly eccentric lesions and in providing an assess-

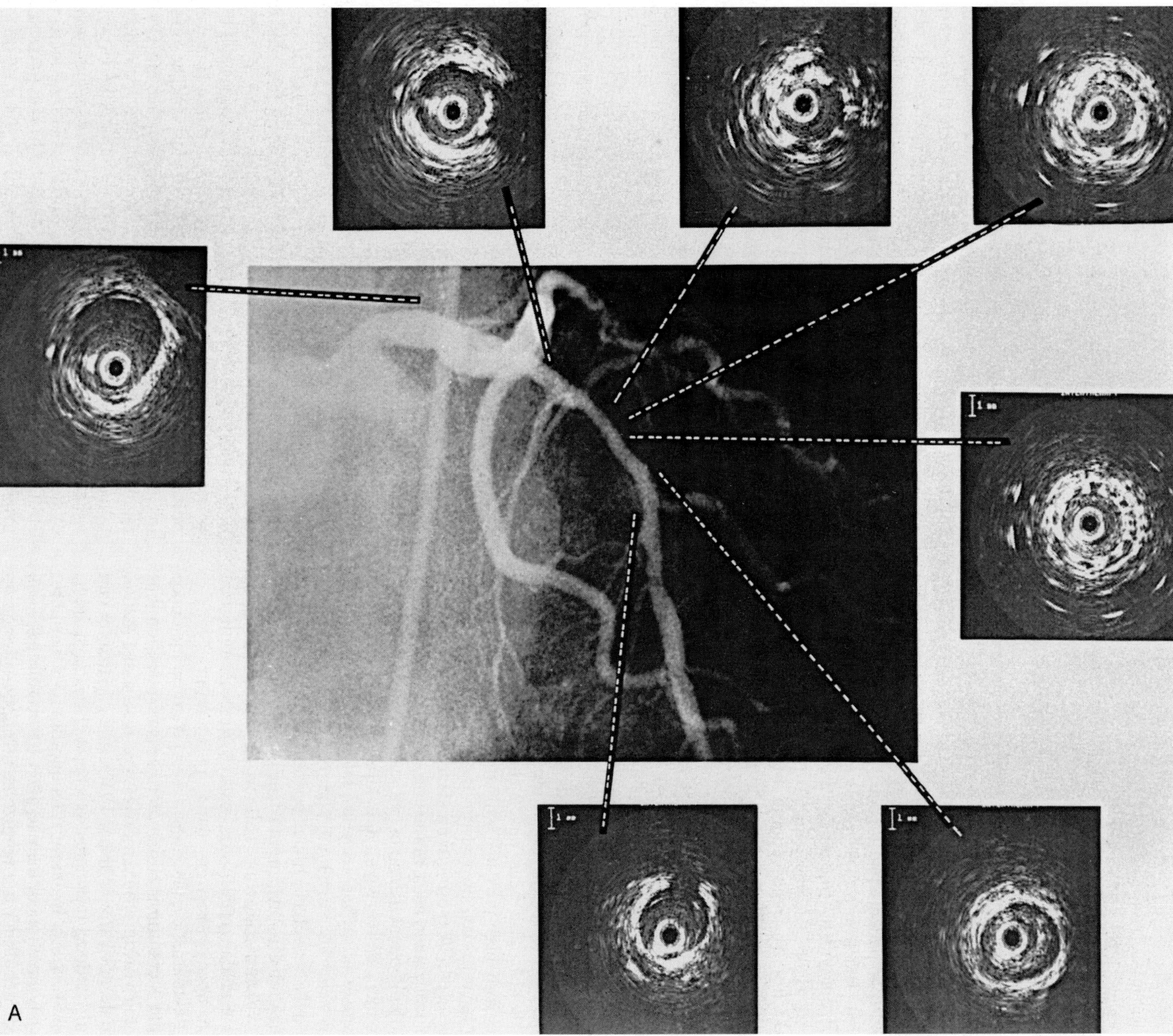

FIGURE 78–6 A, Intravascular ultrasound images in the left coronary tree of a patient 6 months after stent implantation. Note the presence of significant new atheroma within the stent. The atheroma extends beyond the distal border of the stent.

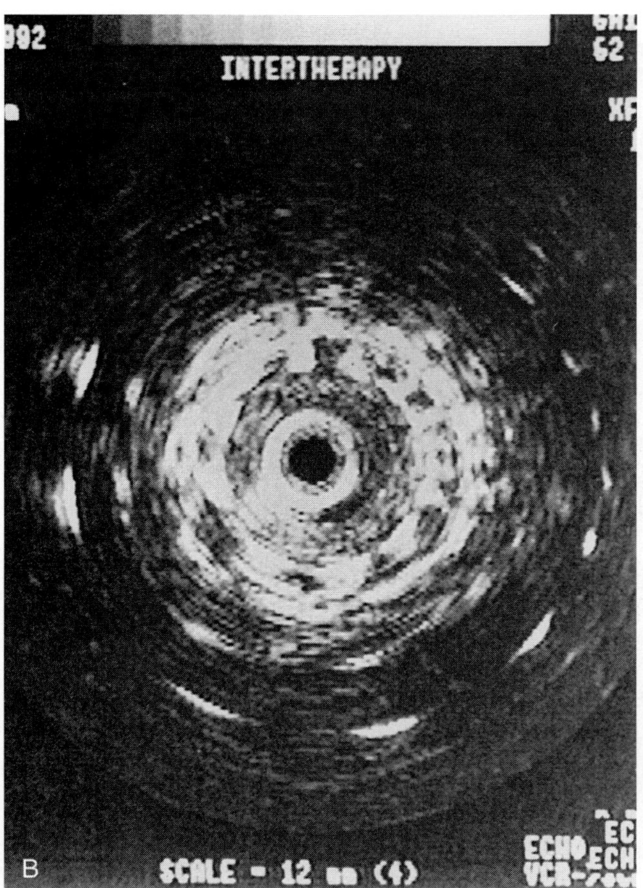

FIGURE 78–6 *Continued.* **B,** Close-up of atheroma within the stent.

ment of the adequacy of tissue removal (Fig. 78–7). Unfortunately, an interactive approach of sequential IVUS-DCA-IVUS-DCA is cumbersome, and combined ultrasound-atherectomy devices that take advantage of the rotating technology employed by both devices are in only experimental prototype stages. Also, circumferential anatomic localization usually depends on the identification of a landmark sidebranch for orientation.[86] Alternatively, a "reference cut" can be employed to guide orientation for tissue removal.[87] In addition, IVUS can provide valuable information about when *not* to use DCA, such as in the circumstance of extensive subendothelial calcification. Although the need for serial ultrasounds may seem onerous, in experienced hands it can be expeditiously accomplished. The OARS trial demonstrated the feasibility of aggressive ultrasound-guided directional atherectomy, with residual diameter stenosis of 8 ± 11 percent.[88] Disappointingly, the angiographic restenosis rate with aggressive atherectomy was still 29 percent. The more recent ABACAS trial, conducted in Japan, involved even more rigorous plaque removal (a residual plaque burden of 45 percent, in contrast to 57 percent in OARS) and demonstrated an angiographic restenosis rate of 21 percent.[89]

The primary utility of IVUS as an adjunct to rotational atherectomy, as described above, is in identifying lesions that would respond most favorably in this form of intervention—specifically, diffuse, concentric, calcific disease. Appropriate bur sizing is also possible with an accurate assessment of true vessel size.

Clinical Trials

Larger-scale clinical trials of IVUS are summarized in Table 78–5.

Emerging and Future Directions

Advances in IVUS will come both from a technical perspective and, as technology improves, in expanded clinical applications.

Technical Advances

Technical advancements can be anticipated in a number of areas. One major problem is device size. Despite the availability of devices in the 2.9- to 3.2-French (0.97–1.07 mm) range, potential ischemic problems are encountered in trying to get IVUS images of critical coronary lesions, particularly before intervention. The patients may develop ischemic changes, and there are always concerns of altering or damaging a complex plaque. Smaller-size devices, 2.6 French and even smaller, may be forthcoming in the near future. A high-frequency catheter from Boston Scientific (Mansfield, MA) has a removable imaging core that can be inserted into the guide wire lumen of a conven-

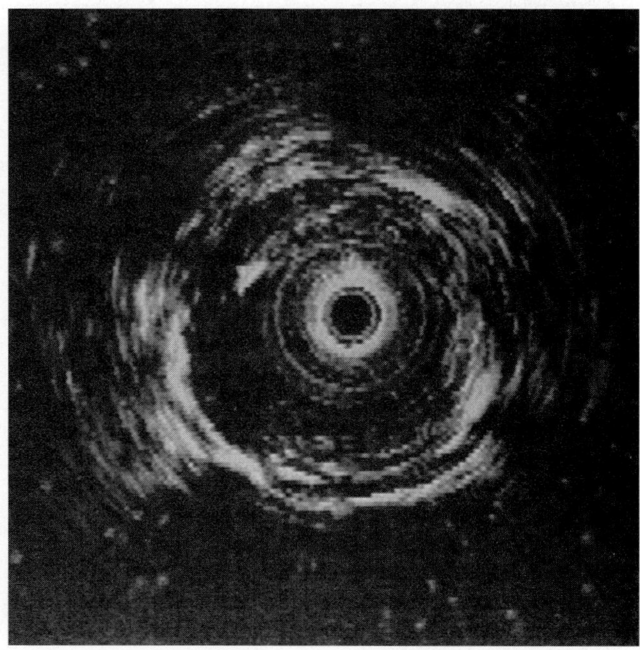

FIGURE 78–7 Intravascular ultrasound image of a coronary vessel after directional atherectomy with a DVI Simpson Atherocath. Note the focal area of atheroma removal.

TABLE 78–5 Recent Clinical Trials in Intravascular Ultrasound

Study	Intervention	Purpose	Findings
GUIDE (phase I) (n = 187)	PTCA/DCA	To compare IVUS and angiography	Discrepancies in evaluation of plaque morphology, composition, and distribution: Eccentric IVUS 77% Angio 38% Calcium IVUS 62% Angio 35% Dissection IVUS 49% Angio 22% Dissection leads to better lumen gain.
PICTURE (n = 200)	PTCA	IVUS predictors of restenosis	Positive predictors: Absence of dissection MLD Residual plaque burden Not predictive: Eccentricity Plaque composition
GUIDE (phase II) (n = 500)	PTCA/DCA	IVUS predictors of restenosis	Positive predictors: Residual plaque burden (strongest predictor) MLD (predicts death, MI, TVR)
CLOUT (pilot) (n = 102)	PTCA	IVUS-guided balloon upsizing (to midwall diameter)	Upsizing necessary in 73%. No complications of upsizing. 40% increase in IVUS lumen area. Residual DS—18%.
SIPS (n = 269)	PTCA/Stent	Angio versus IVUS guidance of balloon angioplasty	Procedural success ↓ Acute TVR in IVUS group (0.8% v. 4.6%) ↓ MACE in IVUS group (0.8% v. 6.1%) No difference once stented [Long-term results pending]
SURE (n = 100)	PTCA/DCA	To define time course of restenosis or remodeling	Reduction in total area (remodeling) occurs between 1 and 6 mo.
OARS (n = 200)	DCA	To define mechanism of acute lumen gain and restenosis	Tissue removal contributes 58% of ↑ lumen size. Remaining ↑ because of an increase in total vessel area (27% during DCA; 15% during adjunctive PTCA). Remodeling responsible for 85% of late lumen loss.
ABACAS (n = 200)	DCA	Aggressive IVUS-guided debulking	↓ Residual plaque burden reduced to 45%. 2.1% restenosis rate.
MUSIC (n = 160)	Stent	IVUS-optimized implantation, withdrawal of anticogulation	0.6% subacute thrombosis. 7% restenosis rate. 5.7% TLR.
OSTI (n = 89)	Stent	Relationship between balloon pressure and stent expansion	IVUS MLD increase with ↑ pressure. No increase in angio MLD. MUSIC criteria met in: 37% at 12 atm 61% at 15 atm 73% at 18 atm
STRUT (n = 111)	Stent	To define frequency of suboptimal stent expansion after high-pressure deployment	22% incomplete stent expansion (requiring additional balloon inflations, not detected angiographically). 12% marginal tears. Stent area expansion <90% in 68% of cases, <80% in 46% of cases, <70% in 28% of cases.
POST (n = 22)	Stent	Retrospective review of subacute stent thrombosis	Incomplete stent expansion—48% (not detectable angiographically). Marginal tears—18%.
CRUISE (n = 472)	Stent	(Substudy of STARS) Effect of IVUS guidance on TLR	15.3% TLR (IVUS documented). 8.5% TLR (IVUS guided).
AVID (n = 800)	Stent	Effect of IVUS guidance on TLR	Additional treatment: 1.5% in angiography-guided group; 41.6% in IVUS group. Postprocedure MLD greater in IVUS group. Total group TLR 12.4% in angiography-guided group; 8.4% in IVUS group. When protocol violators were excluded, TLR was lower in IVUS group (4.9% v. 10.8%). In SVG, TLR lower in IVUS group (5.1% v. 20.8%). IVUS-guided success criteria not met in 58%.
RESIST (n = 155)	Stent	Effect of IVUS guidance on restenosis	Postprocedure stent lumen greater with IVUS guidance (7.95 + 2.21 mm^2 v. 7.16 ± 2.48 mm^2 without IVUS). Nonsignificant trend toward lower restenosis (22.5% v. 28.8% without IVUS).
OPTICUS (n = 550)	Stent	Effect of IVUS on angiographic restenosis	[Pending]

Abbreviations: DCA, directional coronary atherectomy; DS, diameter stenosis; IVUS, intravascular ultrasound; MACE, major adverse cardiac events; MLD, minimal lesion disease; TLR, target lesion revascularization; TVR, target vessel revascularization; PTCA, percutaneous transluminal coronary angioplasty; SVG, saphenous vein graft.

tional balloon catheter; ultrasound imaging wires are also being explored.[90]

Currently, high-frequency (40 MHz) catheters are commercially available, which provide better imaging resolution[91] and can be combined with smaller catheter sizes. Some manufacturers have also been experimenting with lower-frequency (10 MHz and below) devices. Higher-frequency devices allow better spatial resolution and an enhanced ability to image small structures. Lower-frequency devices allow greater depth of field and extend the imaging window to allow better visualization of larger structures for aortic and intracardiac applications.

Intracardiac ultrasound is an extension of intraluminal imaging to include visualization of the structures of the heart from within.[92] A major driving force behind this application is the need for better guidance methods for catheter-based therapeutic techniques, such as balloon valvuloplasty, closure of atrial and ventricular septal defects, radiofrequency ablation of accessory conduction pathways and arrhythmia foci, and even transseptal catheterization or pericardiocentesis. Transthoracic and transesophageal ultrasound have been used to facilitate interventional procedures[93, 94] but are logistically cumbersome when performed simultaneously with catheterization laboratory procedures. As previously mentioned, the early development of intraluminal imaging involved intracardiac applications.[1–9] The technologic advances in catheter design have permitted the visualization of valves, cardiac chambers, and great vessels.[95–98] Experimental studies have also been performed using lower-frequency (5 MHz) transesophageal probes positioned in the inferior vena cava.[99–102] More recently, conventional ultrasound catheters have become available with lower-frequency devices.[102–105] As the frequency decreases, the depth of field increases, expanding the imaging window beyond the approximately 2-cm radius with 20-MHz systems.

Some commercially available systems permit three-dimensional image reconstruction.[106–108] The images presented include "stacked" images along a longitudinal view, or even rendered images of the vessel wall, and threshold-based rendered images of the lumen cast (Fig. 78–8). As computer processing speeds have increased, longitudinal views can essentially be constructed online as images are being acquired. This greatly facilitates visualization of things such as the exact area covered by a stent, the morphology and extent of a complex dissection, or the relationship of lesions to other landmarks such as side branches. "True" three-dimensional reconstructed images can also be reconstructed, maintaining the spatial curvature of the artery.[109, 110]

A major problem with imaging during manual pullbacks is that the pullback speed is not always uniform and that the catheter can jump across certain areas. Automatic pullback devices, which provide a uniform speed of pullback, are now routinely employed and are much more user-friendly than earlier versions. Automated pullback greatly enhances the accuracy of reconstructed three-dimensional images and subjectively provides a "smoother" view of the vessel during pullback. If three-dimensional reconstruction is used, automatic pullback is mandatory.[111, 112]

Significant advances have also taken place in the image-handling capabilities of IVUS equipment. With the widespread use of digital images and digital storage media, the user interface has become greatly streamlined, and sophisticated image stacking software and volumetric analyses are emerging as turn-key applications that can be routinely and effortlessly applied in clinical practice. Again, clinical utility, in terms of improving clinical outcomes, remains to be proven. However, in much the same way that catheterization laboratory imaging has leapt into the digital era, so too has IVUS capitalized on the rapid technical progress in digital imaging and archival technology. Further progress is also expected in the use of IVUS to provide more detailed tissue characterization and in more complex analyses of signals from the moving blood (as opposed to the relatively stationary vessel wall) that allow quantification of flow.

Expanded Clinical Applications

One obvious future application of IVUS is in closer combination with interventional techniques, such as balloon angioplasty or directional atherectomy. Several experimental catheters have been developed that are combination IVUS-angioplasty, IVUS-laser, or IVUS-atherectomy devices.[113–116] These allow imaging without the hindrance of changing catheters, and some can even image during balloon inflation or atherectomy cuts, although their ultimate utility also remains to be proven. Current quick-exchange monorail catheters have handling characteristics that are superior to more cumbersome combination devices, but the use of a removable imaging core that is deliverable down a conventional balloon catheter greatly enhances the likelihood of easily performed imaging studies that do not involve a lot of additional catheter exchanges. Ultrasound guidance of directional atherectomy has been talked about for many years but still falls short of clinical reality, perhaps partially as a consequence of the much less enthusiastic use of DCA with the widespread availability of stents.

The current clinical research experience with *intracardiac* ultrasound includes valvular interrogation, characterization of atrial septal defects,[117] detection of tumors,[104] detection of pericardial effusion and tamponade,[118] and even guidance for electrophysiologic procedures.[98] Interventional catheters have also been identified within the heart.[104] General areas of potential application include guidance during interventional procedures, intraoperative applications (similar to transesophageal echo), diagnostic uses, and monitoring ventricular function during interventional procedures.

Siegel and colleagues have also reported on the use of a simultaneous angioscopy–IVUS system that was felt to enhance the diagnostic information available from each technique alone.[119] Sudhir and coworkers have reported the use of transvenous coronary ultrasound imaging.[120] This novel approach to visualizing the coronary circulation involves passage of an ultrasound catheter into the cardiac venous system via the coronary sinus. There was a significant correlation between angiographic and ultrasound measurements in both animals and humans. This technique may allow for a less invasive visualization of coronary arteries that does not interfere with other interventions.

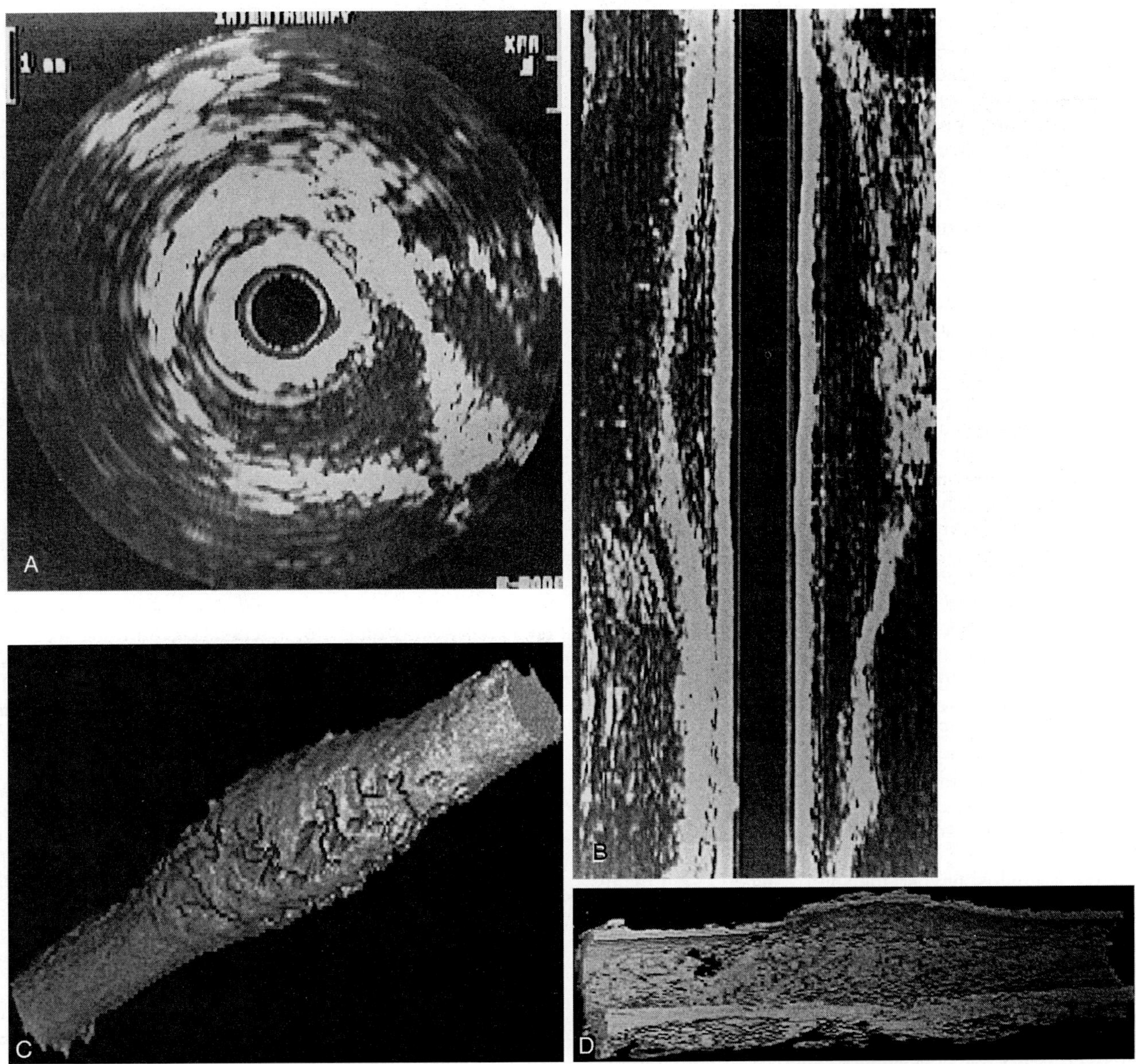

FIGURE 78–8 Three-dimensional reconstruction of intravascular ultrasound images. **A,** Cross-sectional two-dimensional image. **B,** "Stacked" images along a longitudinal view. **C,** Threshold-based reconstruction of the lumen cast. **D,** Reconstruction of the vessel wall.

SUMMARY

IVUS is an exciting new technique that provides unique information about intraluminal pathology and vessel wall structure. Enormous technical advances have made these devices much more user-friendly. IVUS has taught us a number of important lessons, including the necessity for high-pressure stent deployment, the recognition of the importance of pathologic vessel remodeling in restenosis, and the strong relationship that exists between residual plaque volume and subsequent risk of restenosis. In the very near future, we will have IVUS data that may lead to more refined strategies to reduce the risk of in-stent restenosis and to help determine when nonstent technologies may have provided "adequate results." In the 1990s, IVUS moved into the mainstream of interventional cardiology, and although the necessity of routine IVUS use for coronary intervention can be vigorously debated, there is no question that IVUS will be instrumental in providing the physiologic and mechanistic information that will serve as the basis for subsequent improvements in interventional technology.

REFERENCES

1. Bom N, ten Hoff H, Lancee CT, et al: Early and recent intraluminal ultrasound devices. Int J Cardiac Imaging 4:79, 1989.
2. Cieszynski T: Intracardiac method for the investigation of structure of the heart with the aid of ultrasonics. Arch Immun Ter Dow 8:551, 1960.
3. Kossoff G: Diagnostic applications of ultrasound in cardiology. Australas Radiol 10:101, 1966.
4. Peronneau P: Catheter with piezoelectric transducer. U.S. patent No. 3, 542, 014, 1970.

5. Carleton RA, Sessions RW, Graettinger JS: Diameter of heart measured by intracavitary ultrasound. Med Res Engng May/June:28, 1969.
6. Hughes DJ, Geddes LA, Bourland JD, Babbs CF: Dynamic imaging of the aorta in-vivo with 10 MHz ultrasound. *In* Metherell AF (ed): Acoustical Imaging 8. pp. 699–707. New York: Plenum, 1980.
7. Omoto R: Intracardiac scanning of the heart with the aid of ultrasonic intravenous probe. Jap Heart J 8:569, 1962.
8. Eggleton RC, Townsend C, Kossoff G, et al: Computerized ultrasonic visualization of dynamic ventricular configurations. 8th IC-MBE, Palmer House, Chicago, July 1969, Session 10-3.
9. Bom N, Lancee CT, Van Egmond FC: An ultrasonic intracardiac scanner. Ultrasonics 10:72–6, 1972 and U.S. patent no. 1, 402, 192, filed February 22, 1973.
10. St. Goar FG, Pinto FJ, Alderman EL, et al: Intravascular ultrasound imaging of angiographically normal coronary arteries: An in vivo comparison with quantitative angiography. J Am Coll Cardiol 18:952, 1991.
11. Davidson CJ, Sheikh KH, Kisslo KB, et al: Intracoronary ultrasound evaluation of interventional technologies. Am J Cardiol 68:1305, 1991.
12. Gussenhoven EJ, Essed CE, Frietman P, et al: Intravascular ultrasonic imaging: Histologic and echographic correlation. Eur J Vasc Surg 3:571, 1989.
13. Gussenhoven EJ, Essed CE, Lancee CT, et al: Arterial wall characteristics determined by intravascular ultrasound imaging: An in vitro study. J Am Coll Cardiol 14:947, 1989.
14. Nissen SE, Grines CL, Gurley JC, et al: Application of a new phased-array ultrasound imaging catheter in the assessment of vascular dimensions: In vivo comparison to cineangiography. Circulation 81:660, 1990.
15. Nissen SE, Gurley JC, Grines CL, et al: Intravascular ultrasound assessment of lumen size and wall morphology in normal subjects and patients with coronary artery disease. Circulation 84:1087, 1991.
16. Tobis JM, Mallery J, Mahon D, et al: Intravascular ultrasound imaging of human coronary arteries in vivo. Analysis of tissue characterizations with comparison to in vitro histological specimens. Circulation 83:913, 1991.
17. Nishimura RA, Edwards WD, Warnes CA, et al: Intravascular ultrasound imaging: In vitro validation and pathologic correlation. J Am Coll Cardiol 16:145, 1990.
18. Siegel RJ, Ariani M, Fishbein MC, et al: Histopathologic validation of angioscopy and intravascular ultrasound. Circulation 84:109, 1991.
19. Willard JE, Netto D, Demian SE, et al: Intravascular ultrasound imaging of saphenous vein grafts in vitro: comparison with histologic and quantitative angiographic findings. J Am Coll Cardiol 19:759, 1992.
20. Fitzgerald PJ, St. Goar FG, Connolly AJ, et al: Intravascular ultrasound imaging of coronary arteries: Is three layers the norm? Circulation 86:154, 1992.
21. Hodgson J McB, Reddy KG, Suneja R, et al: Intracoronary ultrasound imaging: Correlation of plaque morphology with angiography, clinical syndrome and procedural results in patients undergoing coronary angioplasty. J Am Coll Cardiol 21:35, 1993.
22. Di Mario C, Görge G, Peters R, et al on behalf of the Study Group on Intracoronary Imaging of the Working Group of Coronary Circulation and of the Subgroup on Intravascular Ultrasound of the Working Group of Echocardiography of the European Society of Cardiology: Clinical application and image interpretation in intracoronary ultrasound. Eur Heart J 19:207, 1998.
23. Erbel R, Ge J, Kearney P, et al: Value of intracoronary ultrasound and Doppler in the differentiation of angiographically normal coronary arteries: A prospective study in patients with angina pectoris. Eur Heart J 17:880, 1996.
24. Nissen SE, Gurley JC, Grines CL, et al: Intravascular ultrasound assessment of lumen size and wall morphology in normal subjects and coronary artery disease patients. Circulation 84:1087, 1991.
25. Glagov S, Weisenberg E, Zarnis CK, et al: Compensatory enlargement of human coronary arteries. N Engl J Med 316:1371, 1987.
26. Kearney P, Erbel R, Ge J, et al: Assessment of spontaneous coronary artery dissection by intravascular ultrasound in a patient with unstable angina. Cathet Cardiovasc Diagn 32:58, 1994.
27. Ge J, Erbel R, Rupprecht HJ, et al: Comparison of intravascular ultrasound and angiography in the assessment of myocardial bridging. Circulation 89:1725, 1994.
28. St. Goar FG, Pinto FJ, Alderman EL, et al: Intimal disease in young coronary arteries: Detection by intracoronary ultrasound [abstract]. Circulation 84:II, 1991.
29. Ge J, Erbel R, Gerber T, et al: Intravascular ultrasound imaging of angiographically normal arteries: A prospective study in vivo. Br Heart J 71:572, 1994.
30. White CJ, Ramee SR, Collin TJ, et al: Ambiguous coronary angiography: Clinical utility of intravascular ultrasound. Cathet Cardiovasc Diagn 26:200, 1992.
31. Lee DY, Nishioka T, Tabak SW, et al: Effect of intracoronary imaging on clinical decision making. Am Heart J 129:1084, 1995.
32. Mintz GS, Pichard AD, Kovach JA, et al: Impact of preintervention intravascular ultrasound imaging on transcatheter treatment strategies in coronary artery disease. Am J Cardiol 73:423, 1994.
33. Jamieson SW, Oyer PE, Baldwin J, et al: Heart transplantation in end-stage ischemic heart disease: The Stanford experience. Heart Transplantation 3:224, 1984.
34. Uretsky BF, Murali S, Reddy PS, et al: Development of coronary artery disease in cardiac transplant patients receiving immunosuppressive therapy with cyclosporine and prednisone. Circulation 76:827, 1987.
35. Gao S, Schroeder J, Hun S, Stinson E: Retransplantation for severe accelerated coronary artery disease in heart transplant recipients. Am J Cardiol 62:876, 1988.
36. Johnson DE, Alderman EL, Schroeder JS, et al: Transplant coronary artery disease: Histopathological correlations with angiographic morphology. J Am Coll Cardiol 17:449, 1991.
37. Gao SZ, Alderman EL, Schroeder JS, et al: Accelerated coronary vascular disease in heart transplant patients: Coronary arteriographic findings. J Am Coll Cardiol 12:334, 1988.
38. St. Goar FG, Pinto FJ, Alderman EL, et al: Intracoronary ultrasound in cardiac transplant recipients. In vivo evidence of angiographically "silent" intimal thickening. Circulation 85:979, 1992.
39. Rickenbacher PR, Pinto FJ, Chenzbraun A, et al: Incidence and severity of transplant coronary artery disease early and up to 15 years after transplantation as detected by intravascular ultrasound. J Am Coll Cardiol 25:171, 1995.
40. St. Goar FG, Pinto FJ, Alderman EL, et al: Detection of coronary atherosclerosis in young adult hearts using intravascular ultrasound. Circulation 86:756, 1992.
41. Tuzcu EM, De Franco AC, Goormastic M, et al: Dichotomous pattern of coronary atherosclerosis 1 to 9 years after transplantation: Insight from systematic intravascular ultrasound imaging. J Am Coll Cardiol 27:839, 1996.
42. Klauss V, Mudra H, Uberfuhr P, Theisen K: Intraindividual variability of cardiac allograft vasculopathy as assessed by intravascular ultrasound. Am J Cardiol 76:436, 1995.
43. Pinto FJ, Chenzbraun A, St. Goar FG, et al: Feasibility of serial intracoronary ultrasound imaging for assessment of progression of intimal proliferation in cardiac transplant recipients. Circulation 90:2348, 1994.
44. Rickenbacher PR, Pinto FJ, Lewis NP, et al: Prognostic importance of intimal thickness measured by intracoronary ultrasound after cardiac transplantation. Circulation 92:3445, 1995.
45. Mills RM Jr, Billett JM, Nichols WW: Endothelial dysfunction early after heart transplantation. Circulation 86:1171, 1992.
46. Mintz GS, Douek P, Pichard AD, et al: Target lesion calcification in coronary artery disease: An intravascular ultrasound study. J Am Coll Cardiol 20:1149, 1992.
47. Mintz GS, Popma JJ, Pichard AD, et al: Patterns of coronary artery calcification in coronary artery disease. A statistical analysis of intravascular ultrasound in 1155 lesions. Circulation 91:1959, 1995.
48. Mendelshon FO, Foster GP, Palacios IF, et al: In vivo assessment of enlargement in saphenous vein bypass grafts. Am J Cardiol 76:1066, 1995.
49. Pandian NG, Kreis A, Brockway B: Detection of intraarterial thrombus by intravascular high frequency two-dimensional ultrasound imaging in vitro and in vivo studies. Am J Cardiol 65:1280, 1990.
50. Ferguson JJ, Ober JC, Edelman SK, et al: Documentation of experimentally induced thrombus formation using intravascular ultrasound. Texas Heart Inst J 18:179, 1991.
51. Jain A, Paulsen DB, Milani RV: Ultrasonic characteristics of maturing intravascular thrombi: In vivo analysis [abstract]. Circulation 84:II-540, 1991.
52. Conness K, Fitzgerald PJ, Yock PG: Intracoronary ultrasound imaging of graft thrombosis. N Engl J Med 327:1691, 1992.

53. Nissen SE, Gurley JC, Booth DC, et al: Differences in intravascular ultrasound plaque morphology in stable and unstable patients [abstract]. Circulation 84:II-436, 1991.
54. Zeiher AM, Grove A, Bleile T, Fritz R: Intravascular ultrasound characteristics of coronary arterial wall architecture of early lesions relate to risk factors of coronary artery disease [abstract]. Circulation 84:II-676, 1991.
55. Jain SP, Roubin GS, Nanda NC, et al: Intravascular ultrasound imaging of saphenous vein graft stenosis. Am J Cardiol 69:133, 1992.
56. Karnik R, Winkler WB, Valentin A, et al: Intravascular ultrasound imaging of Guenter vena caval filters. Am J Cardiol 69:1504, 1992.
57. Gordon MR, Dick CD, Jarvis G, et al: Determination of regional arterial compliance by intravascular ultrasound [abstract]. Circulation 84:II-675, 1991.
58. Jeremy RW, Sinclair E, Brieger D, et al: Measurement of compliance of normal and diseased arteries by intravascular ultrasound [abstract]. Circulation 84:II-675, 1991.
59. Doerr R, Uebis R, Nase-Hueppmeier S, et al: The effect of aging on arterial compliance [abstract]. Circulation 84:II-675, 1991.
60. Doerr R, Heintz R, Krebs W, et al: Quantitative assessment of the elastic properties of human arteries by intravascular ultrasound: Pathological arterial stiffening in patients with hypertension [abstract]. Circulation 84:II-676, 1991.
61. Wilson R, Di Mario C, Krams R, et al: Changes in large artery compliance measured with intravascular ultrasound [abstract]. JACC 19:140A, 1992.
62. Lee RT, Loree HM, Stringfellow RG, Kamm RD: Finite element modeling of circumferential stress in atherosclerotic vessels: Implications for intravascular ultrasound [abstract]. JACC 19:300A, 1992.
63. Honye J, Mahon DJ, Tobis JM: Plaque distensibility of human coronary arteries documented by intravascular ultrasound imaging [abstract]. Circulation 84:II-437, 1991.
64. Nakamura S, Colombo A, Gaglione A, et al: Intracoronary ultrasound observations during stent implantation. Circulation 89:2026, 1994.
65. Goldberg SL, Colombo A, Nakamura S, et al: Benefit of intracoronary ultrasound in the deployment of Palmaz-Schatz stents. J Am Coll Cardiol 24:996, 1994.
66. Serruys PW, Di Marco C: Who was thrombogenic: The stent or the doctor? Circulation 91:1891, 1995.
67. Colombo A, Hall P, Nakamura S, et al: Intracoronary stenting without anticoagulation accomplished with intravascular ultrasound guidance. Circulation 91:1676, 1995.
68. Colombo A, Hall P, Itoh A, et al: The optimal pressure for stent implantation. *In* Sigwart (ed): Endoluminal Stenting. pp. 276–279. London: Saunders, 1996.
69. Blasini R, Schuhlen H, Mudra H, et al: Angiographic overestimation of lumen size after coronary stent placement: Impact of high pressure dilatation. Circulation 92(suppl I):I-223, 1995.
70. Gorge G, Haude M, Ge J, et al: Intravascular ultrasound after low and high inflation pressure coronary stent implantation. J Am Coll Cardiol 26:725, 1995.
71. Morice MC, Breton C, Bunouf P, et al: Coronary stenting without anticoagulation, without intravascular ultrasound. Results of the French registry. Circulation 92(suppl I):I-796, 1995.
72. Morice MC, Aubry P, Benveniste E, et al: The MUST trial: Acute results and six months' clinical follow-up. J Invas Cardiol 10:457, 1998.
73. Wong SC, Hong MK, Chuang YC, et al: The antiplatelet treatment after intravascular ultrasound guided optimal stent expansion (APLAUSE) trial. Circulation 92(suppl I):I-795, 1995.
74. Belli G, Whitlow PL, Gross L, et al: Intracoronary stenting without oral anticoagulation the Cleveland Clinic registry. Circulation 92(suppl I):I-796, 1995.
75. Metz JA, Fitzgerald PJ, Oshima A, et al: Impact of intravascular ultrasound guidance on stenting on the CRUISE substudy. Circulation Suppl I:1–199, 1996.
76. Ellis SG, Serruys PW, Popma JJ, et al: Can abciximab prevent neointimal proliferation in Palmaz-Schatz stents? The final ERASER results. Circulation 96(suppl I):I-87(abstr), 1997.
77. Holmes D, Fitzgerald P, Goldberg S, et al: The PRESTO (Prevention of Restenosis with Tranilast and its Outcomes) protocol: a double-blind, placebo-controlled trial. Am Heart J 139:23–31, 2000.
78. Honye J, Mahon DJ, White CJ, et al: Morphological effect of coronary balloon angioplasty in vivo assessed by intravascular ultrasound imaging. Circulation 85:1012, 1992.
79. Gerber TC, Erbel R, Gorge G, et al: Classification of morphologic effects of percutaneous transluminal coronary angioplasty assessed by intravascular ultrasound. Am J Cardiol 70:1546, 1992.
80. Yock PG, Fitzgerald PJ, Linker DT, et al: Intravascular ultrasound guidance for catheter-based coronary interventions. J Am Coll Cardiol 17(suppl B):39B, 1991.
81. Roelandt JRTC, Di Marco C, Pandian NG, et al: Three-dimensional reconstruction of intracoronary ultrasound images: Rationale, approaches, problems and directions. Circulation 90:1044, 1994.
82. Peters RJG, Kok WEM, Di Marco C, et al: Prediction of restenosis after coronary balloon angioplasty. Results of PICTURE (Post-intracoronary Treatment Ultrasound Result Evaluation). A prospective multicenter intracoronary ultrasound imaging study. Circulation 95:2254, 1997.
83. Mintz GS, Popma JJ, Pichard AD, et al: Intravascular ultrasound predictors of restenosis after percutaneous transcatheter coronary revascularization. J Am Coll Cardiol 27:1678, 1996.
84. GUIDE Trial Investigators. Discrepancies between angiographic and IVUS appearance of coronary lesions undergoing intervention: Report of phase I of the GUIDE trial. J Am Coll Cardiol 21(suppl A):118A (abstr), 1993.
85. GUIDE Trial Investigators. IVUS-determined predictors of restenosis in PTCA and DCA: Final report from the GUIDE trial, Phase II. J Am Coll Cardiol 29(suppl A):156A (abstr), 1996.
86. Kimura FJ, Fitzgerald PJ, Sudhir K, et al: Guidance of directional coronary atherectomy by intracoronary ultrasound imaging. Am Heart J 124:1385, 1992.
87. Bauman RP, Yock PG, Fitzgerald PJ, et al: Reference cut method of intracoronary ultrasound guided directional coronary atherectomy: Initial and six month results. Circulation 92(suppl I):I-546, 1995.
88. Simonton CA, Leon MB, Kuntz RE, et al: Acute and late clinical and angiographic results of directional atherectomy in the optimal atherectomy restenosis study (OARS). Circulation 92:I-545, 1995.
89. Sumitsuji, Suzuki T, Katoh O, et al for the ABACAS investigators: Restenosis mechanism after aggressive directional coronary atherectomy assessed by intravascular ultrasound in adjunctive balloon angioplasty following coronary atherectomy study (ABACAS) [abstract]. J Am Coll Cardiol 129A, 1997.
90. Tenaglia AN, Kisslo K, Kelly S, et al: Ultrasound guidewire directed stent deployment [abstract]. JACC 19:300A, 1992.
91. Foster FS, Knapik DA, Machado JC, et al: High-frequency intracoronary ultrasound imaging. Semin Interv Cardiol 2:33, 1997.
92. Pandian NG, Hsu T-L, Schwartz SL, Weintraub AR: Intracardiac ultrasound imaging: Rationale, current developments, and future directions *In* Tobis JM, Yock PG: Intravascular Ultrasound Imaging. pp. 231–246. New York: Churchill Livingstone, 1992.
93. Pandian NG, Isner JM, Hougen TJ: Percutaneous balloon valvuloplasty of mitral stenosis aided by cardiac ultrasound. Am J Cardiol 59:380, 1987.
94. Kronzon I, Tunick PA, Schwinger ME: Transesophageal echocardiography during percutaneous mitral valvuloplasty. J Am Soc Echocardiogr 2:380, 1989.
95. Pandian NG, Weintraub A, Kreis A, et al: Intracardiac, intravascular, two-dimensional, high-frequency ultrasound imaging of pulmonary artery and its branches in humans and animals. Circulation 80:2007, 1990.
96. Weintraub A, Pandian N, Salem D, et al: Realtime intracardiac two-dimensional echocardiography in the catheterization laboratory in humans [abstract]. J Am Coll Cardiol 15:16A, 1990.
97. Valdes-Cruz L, Sahn DJ, Yock P, et al: Experimental animal investigations of the potential for new approaches to diagnostic cardiac imaging in infants and small premature infants from intracardiac and transesophageal approaches using a 20 MHz real time ultrasound imaging catheter [abstract]. J Am Coll Cardiol 13:137A, 1989.
98. Berns E, Mitchel J, Mehran R, et al: Ablating catheter placement under direct visualization with the intravascular ultrasound probe: A potential aid to ablative therapy of arrhythmias [abstract]. J Am Coll Cardiol 15:19A, 1990.
99. Schwartz SL, Kusay BS, Pandian NG, et al: Utility of in vivo, intracardiac 2-dimensional echocardiography in the assessment of myocardial risk area and myocardial dyssynergy during coronary occlusion and reperfusion [abstract]. Circulation 80:II-374, 1989.
100. Schwartz S, Kusay B, Pandian N, et al: Intracardiac echocardio-

graphic guidance and monitoring during aortic and mitral balloon valvuloplasty: In vivo experimental studies, abstracted. J Am Coll Cardiol 15:104A, 1990.

101. Seward JB, Khandheria BK, McGregor CGA, et al: Transvascular and intracardiac two-dimensional echocardiography. Echocardiography 7:457, 1990.
102. Valdes-Cruz LM, Sideris E, Sahn DJ, et al: Transvascular intracardiac applications of a miniaturized phased-array ultrasonic endoscope: Initial experience with intracardiac imaging in piglets. Circulation 83:1023, 1991.
103. Pandian N, Katz S, Kumar R, et al: Enhanced depth of field in intracardiac 2-D echocardiography with a new prototype, low frequency (12 MHz, 9 French) ultrasound catheter [abstract]. Circulation 81(suppl III):III-442, 1990.
104. Schwartz SL, Gillam LD, Weintraub AR, et al: Intracardiac echocardiography in humans using a small-sized (6F), low frequency (12.5 MHz) ultrasound catheter. J Am Coll Cardiol 21:189, 1993.
105. Pandian NG, Kumar R, Katz S, et al: Real-time, intracardiac, two-dimensional echocardiography. Echocardiography 8:407, 1991.
106. DeJesus ST, Rosenfield K, Gal D, et al: 3-dimensional reconstruction of vascular lumen from images recorded during percutaneous 2-D intravascular ultrasound [abstract]. Clin Res 37:838A, 1989.
107. Kitney RI, Moura L, Straughan K: 3-D visualization of arterial structures using ultrasound and Voxel modeling. Int J Card Imaging 4:177, 1989.
108. Rosenfield K, Losordo DW, Ramaswamy K, et al: Three-dimensional reconstruction of human coronary and peripheral arteries from images recorded during two-dimensional intravascular ultrasound. Circulation 84:1938, 1991.
109. Slager CJ, Wentzel JJ, Oomen JS, et al: True reconstruction of vessel geometry from combined x-ray angiographic and intracoronary ultrasound data. Semin Interv Cardiol 2:43, 1997.
110. Evans JL, Ng KH, Wiet SG, et al: Accurate three-dimensional reconstruction of intravascular ultrasound data. Spatially correct three-dimensional reconstructions. Circulation 93:567, 1996.
111. Mintz GS, Leon MB, Eldredge SL, et al: A new comprehensive system for reliable three-dimensional intravascular ultrasound image acquisition, reconstruction, and analysis [abstract]. JACC 19:116A, 1992.
112. Rosenfield K, Kaufman J, Pieczek A, Isner JM: On-line three-dimensional reconstruction from 2D IVUS: Utility for guiding interventional procedures [abstract]. JACC 19:224A, 1992.
113. Isner JM, Rosenfield K, Losordo DW, et al: Combination balloon-ultrasound imaging catheter for percutaneous transluminal angioplasty. Validation of imaging, analysis of recoil, and identification of plaque fracture. Circulation 84:739, 1991.
114. Gregory KW, Martinelli MA, Aretz TH, Butterly JR: Intravascular ultrasound guided Holmium laser atherectomy [abstract]. Circulation 82(suppl III):III-2689, 1990.
115. Hsu T-L, Schwartz S, Cao Q-L, et al: Utility of combined intravascular ultrasound imaging and balloon dilatation device in the performance of balloon angioplasty of aortic coarctation and pulmonary artery branch stenosis—experimental studies [abstract]. JACC 19:299A, 1992.
116. Fitzgerald PJ, Sudir K, Gupta M, et al: Combined atherectomy/ultrasound imaging device reduces subintimal tissue injury [abstract]. JACC 19:223A, 1992.
117. Sanzobrino BW, Mitchel JF, Chameides L: Intracardiac two-dimensional ultrasonic assessment of atrial septal defects: Human studies [abstract]. Circulation 82:III-31, 1990.
118. Weintraub AR, Schwartz SL, Smith J, et al: Intracardiac two-dimensional echocardiography in patients with pericardial effusion and tamponade. J Am Soc Echocardiogr 4:571–576, 1991.
119. Siegel RJ, Ariani M, Maurer G: Development of a simultaneous intravascular ultrasound and angioscopy system to enhance diagnostic evaluation [abstract]. JACC 19:141A, 1992.
120. Sudhir K, Fitzgerald PJ, MacGregor JS, et al: Transvenous coronary ultrasound imaging: A novel approach to visualization of the coronary arteries. Circulation 84:1957, 1991.

C H A P T E R **79**

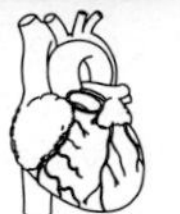

Arterial Compliance

Gary E. McVeigh, Alan J. Bank, and Jay N. Cohn

THE ARTERIAL CIRCULATION AND ARTERIAL COMPLIANCE
Physiology of the Arterial System
Compliance and the Arterial System
BLOOD VESSEL STRUCTURE
VASCULAR PRESSURE:VOLUME RELATIONSHIP
SMOOTH MUSCLE RELAXATION AND ARTERIAL COMPLIANCE
PRESSURE PULSE CONTOUR AND WAVE REFLECTION
TECHNIQUES FOR MEASURING ARTERIAL COMPLIANCE
Direct
Indirect
ABNORMALITIES OF VASCULAR COMPLIANCE IN AGING AND DISEASE STATES
Aging
Atherosclerosis
Hypertension
Diabetes Mellitus
Heart Failure
DEFINITIONS

The constituents of the walls of blood vessels make them compliant. Their compliance is demonstrated by the relationship between transmural pressure and vessel diameter. Arteries, in contrast to veins, exhibit a steep pressure:volume relationship indicative of less compliant vessels. The compliance characteristics of these vessels relate to their initial shape and to the components of the wall, including vascular smooth muscle, collagen, elastin, and other interstitial elements. The nonlinear relationship between volume and pressure is indicative of the physical properties of the components and of the heterogeneous nature of the wall. This nonlinearity means that no single number can be utilized to define the compliance characteristics of any blood vessel or any vascular bed.

Changes in vascular compliance can be induced by changes in the tone of vascular smooth muscle; by changes in the mass of the smooth muscle, collagen, or elastin components of the wall; by infiltration of the wall with cellular or interstitial elements; or by a change in tissue fluid in the wall. Since these changes in compliance may independently affect large arteries, small arteries, arterioles, and veins, a change in vascular compliance must be assessed separately in different segments of the vasculature.

The influence of vascular compliance on circulatory integrity is often not adequately emphasized. The conduit arterial system serves as a Windkessel that smooths out the pulsatile arterial flow and delivers it in a more continuous fashion into the capillary beds. This Windkessel effect is, in part, accomplished by compliance of the arterial system, which allows expansion of the arteries during systole and release of the stored blood in diastole to maintain diastolic flow. Changes in the compliance of these vessels can have important effects on systolic blood pressure, left ventricular load, and cardiac output. Compliance of the small arteries plays a role in the generation of reflected waves, which add an oscillatory component to the arterial pulse wave and are reflected backward toward the root of the aorta in late systole. These reflected waves may also affect left ventricular load.

This chapter reviews what is known about the factors affecting arterial compliance, the influence of disease processes on vascular structure and tone, techniques used to assess arterial compliance, and the possible impact of changes in arterial compliance on circulatory integrity.

The Arterial Circulation and Arterial Compliance

Physiology of the Arterial System

The arterial circulation is a branching system of conduits that conducts blood from the heart to the capillaries where an exchange of nutrients and waste products occurs between tissue cells and the blood. Since the arterial tree is distensible, it acts as an elastic reservoir that stores part of the energy of cardiac contraction, maintaining pressure and flow during diastole when the heart is not ejecting blood.[1] The smallest arteries and arterioles are the sites of greatest hemodynamic resistance and act in conjunction with the precapillary sphincters to form a variable resistance that controls the rate of blood flow through the tissues.[2] The arterioles also provide a step-down in the hydrostatic pressure within capillaries to prevent excessive loss of blood volume by transudation of fluid across capillary walls. An arterial system composed of elastic conduits and high-resistance terminals constitutes a hydraulic filter that converts the intermittent output from the heart into steady capillary flow.[3] For optimal function, this should be achieved with the least possible energy expenditure.[4] To minimize cardiac work during systole in this pulsatile system, the normal arterial bed provides a low-input impedance or opposition to left ventricular ejection.[5] This is accomplished in the periphery by desirable arterial elastic properties and geometric proportions. The heart has also adapted to the arterial system with its physiologic range of heart rates determined, in part, by arterial properties. Thus, a compromise is reached between the heart and the systemic circulation to provide optimal coupling so that the left ventricle can supply the amount of blood per unit time necessary for tissue metabolism at minimal energy cost and still be able to adapt quickly to increased metabolic demands.[6]

Compliance and the Arterial System

The pressure generated during left ventricular systole ejects a stroke volume that contributes to arterial distention and forward flow in the arterial circulation. The volume stored in the arteries is dependent on the arterial compliance. The forward flow is dependent on the perfusion pressure and the resistance in the smaller vessels. A normally compliant system can store a considerable volume of blood in the aorta and the large arteries during systole.[7] Compliance in young normal subjects has been measured at approximately 2 ml/mm Hg.[8] As the arterial system becomes less distensible, the storage capacity of the aorta and conduit arteries is diminished for any given pulse pressure. Under these circumstances, a larger fraction of the stroke volume must run off during systole or a greater rise in systolic pressure must occur to accommodate increased volume in the noncompliant arterial tree. If the arteries were totally nondistensible, capillary flow would be limited to systole and stroke volume would be dependent on systolic pressure and arteriolar resistance. The impact of these vascular changes on left ventricular function can be profound.[9] When the ventricle ejects into a compliant system, a slower rise in systolic pressure for any given stroke volume causes a lower wall stress and a lower oxygen consumption. Furthermore, the ventricle should eject more rapidly because of the lower impedance, and the greater rate of reduction in chamber size further reduces wall stress during ejection. Thus, changes in arterial compliance can alter the pulse contour, the dynamics of left ventricular ejection, and the ratio of systolic to diastolic flow into the capillary bed without necessarily affecting mean arterial pressure.[10]

Whereas it is recognized that the proximal aorta and its major branches are the most compliant portion of the arterial circulation,[11] the peripheral vasculature also contributes importantly to circulatory regulation. These vessels have a small storage capacity of their own and act as a major site for reflected waves that reverberate proximally and contribute to pressure phenomena in the arteries.[12] The waveform of pressure and flow transmitted to these vessels is more pulsatile if the proximal arteries are less compliant.[13] If the compliance of these smaller vessels were reduced, it would impair the mechanical damping of the pulse pressure, which has been shown to influence vessel structure and growth.[14] Little is known about the impact of pulsatile versus continuous flow into the precapillary and capillary vasculature, but physical materials are more susceptible to fatigue and fracture from intermittent changes in stress than from continuous stress.[15] Applying this observation to the arterial wall, it is possible that excessive pulsatile pressure in the small vessels could accelerate vascular damage.[16]

Clinically, *arterial compliance* has been defined as a change in area, diameter, or volume of an artery or arterial bed for a given change in pressure. Compliance is dependent on vessel geometry as well as the mechanical properties of the vessel wall.[17] Arterial wall properties are different in different vessels, in the same vessel at various distending pressures, and with activation of smooth muscle in the vessel wall. Although no single descriptor of arterial physical characteristics can completely describe the mechanical behavior of the vasculature, arterial compliance represents the best clinical index of the buffering function of the arterial system. Changes in the mechanical behavior of blood vessels, manifested by a reduced arterial compliance, can influence growth and remodeling of the left ventricle, large arteries, small arteries, and arterioles.[18] Clearly, arterial blood vessels can no longer be considered as passive conduits to deliver blood to peripheral tissues in response to metabolic demands. Instead, they should be viewed as biophysical sensors that respond to hemodynamic and neurohumoral stimuli that influence the tone and structure of the systemic circulation.[19]

Studies assessing the compliance characteristics of the arterial system have been hampered by the lack of a "gold standard," thus making comparison of results from different laboratories difficult if not impossible. Although an association between reduced arterial compliance and risk factors for vascular disease has been described previously, the results have not been uniformly consistent and may be critically dependent on the methodology used, the patient population under study, and the segment of the vasculature examined.[20] Furthermore, difficulties in drawing firm conclusions from published studies are compounded by confusion surrounding the terminology employed to describe the mechanical behavior of blood vessels, the lack of comparative studies using different techniques within the same patient, and the marked heterogeneity in the response of blood vessels to aging, disease, and therapeutic interventions.

Blood Vessel Structure

The arterial wall is composed of three concentric zones: the tunica intima, tunica media, and tunica adventitia. The *tunica intima* consists of the vascular endothelium and a thin layer of collagen and elastin fibers that anchor it to the internal elastic lamina. The *tunica adventitia* consists primarily of collagen that merges with the surrounding connective tissue.[21] The *tunica media* forms the largest part of the arterial wall and is the principal determinant of the vessel's mechanical properties. It is composed of the elastic materials collagen and elastin in addition to smooth muscle. The distribution of collagen and elastin differs strikingly between the central and the peripheral arteries.[22] In the proximal aorta, elastin is the dominant component, whereas collagen dominates in the more distal vessels.[23] Because the elastic modulus of collagen is much higher than that of elastin, the arteries are stiffer as the distance from the heart increases.[12, 24, 25]

Arterial blood vessels are, therefore, complex three-dimensional structures whose wall components differ in mechanical, biochemical, and physiologic characteristics. Traditionally, the mechanical strength of blood vessels has been viewed as residing in the media, with elastin fibers playing a major role at lower pressures and collagen fibers bearing most of the mechanical stress at higher pressures. The potential role of the endothelium in buffering pulsatile pressure in the arterial system has been emphasized.[26, 27] As a single monolayer of cells, the endothelium possesses little tensile strength but can profoundly alter the mechanical characteristics of blood vessels through the elaboration of vasoactive substances that influence vascular tone, structure, and growth.[28] Emerging data support the concept that the cardioprotective actions of drug interventions may, at least in part, be dependent on favorably influencing endothelial function and pulsatile arterial function.[29]

Vascular Pressure:Volume Relationship

The relationship between pressure and cross-sectional area or volume in a blood vessel is curvilinear. The slope of a tangent to the pressure volume curve (dV/dP) is defined as the *compliance*. As transmural pressure in an artery increases, the compliance decreases as a result of the more distensible elastin bearing a greater portion of the load at lower pressures than the less distensible collagen.[25, 30, 31] This elastic property of arterial walls demonstrates why the compliance of a vessel cannot be described by a single number but rather must be defined for a given distending pressure or volume.

A number of models of the arterial wall have been used to explain the relationships among the three main components of the wall and their contributions to arterial compliance.[32–35] A detailed description of these models is beyond the scope of this chapter; however, a brief description of one of these models follows. Figure 79–1 shows a modified Maxwell model of the arterial wall. In this model, smooth muscle is in parallel with collagen and elastin fibers, which combine to make up the parallel elastic component of the arterial wall. Collagen fibers are depicted as hooks that contribute little to arterial wall mechanics when not engaged, but that are quite stiff when recruited.[36] In addition, smooth muscle is in series with connective tissue components (collagen in this example) that compose the series elastic component. When pressure increases, the vessel is stretched and tension increases in the parallel collagen, the parallel elastin, and the combined smooth muscle–series elastic component. Additional collagen fibers are also recruited. When the vessel has little or no smooth muscle tone, the mechanical properties of the artery are almost entirely due to the parallel elastic component's mechanical properties.

Smooth Muscle Relaxation and Arterial Compliance

Whereas the effects of wall structure and distending pressure on vascular compliance are generally agreed on, the effects of smooth muscle tone on vascular compliance are controversial. Detailed reviews of this topic have previously been written.[37–41] In isolated vessel and intact animal studies, some investigators have claimed increases[37, 42, 43] and others decreases[24, 38, 44] in vessel compliance in response to smooth muscle contraction. Most in vivo studies in humans have demonstrated increases in arterial compliance in response to the systemic administration of vasodilator drugs.[45–48] However, in most studies, there are decreases in blood pressure following systemic drug administration owing to smooth muscle relaxation in resistance vessels. This indirect effect results in a leftward shift along a given compliance-pressure curve. This pressure effect alone improves arterial compliance and makes it difficult to determine the direct effects of the drug on the arterial wall.

In human subjects, several studies have been performed using intravascular ultrasound to assess the direct effects of smooth muscle relaxation on arterial wall mechanics.[49, 50] In these studies, the brachial artery transmural pressure was reduced by inflating a cuff surrounding the artery being imaged. Figure 79–2 shows the effects of smooth muscle relaxation with intra-arterial nitroglycerin on in vivo brachial artery area, compliance, and incremental elastic modulus in eight normal human subjects.[49] Intra-arterial

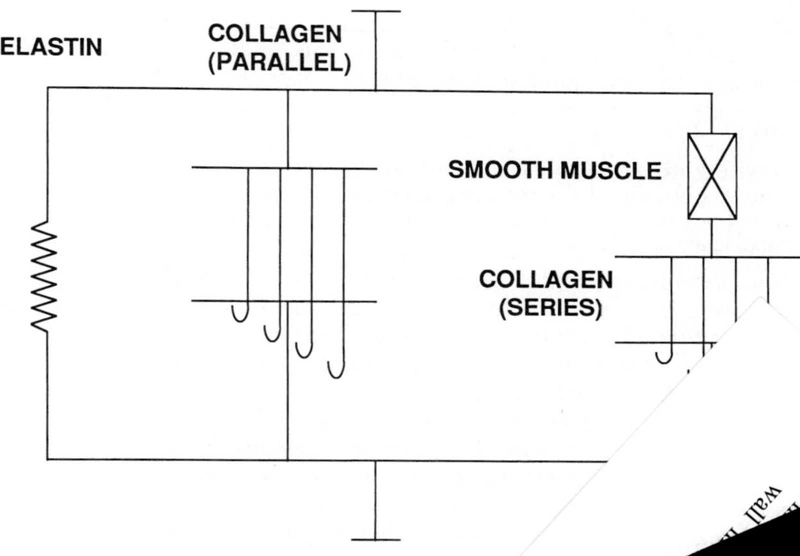

FIGURE 79–1 Modified Maxwell model of the arterial wall. Elastin and collagen (parallel) make up the parallel elastic component. Collagen is represented by stiff springs that are recruited as the arterial wall is stretched (parallel collagen) or as the smooth muscle contracts (series collagen).

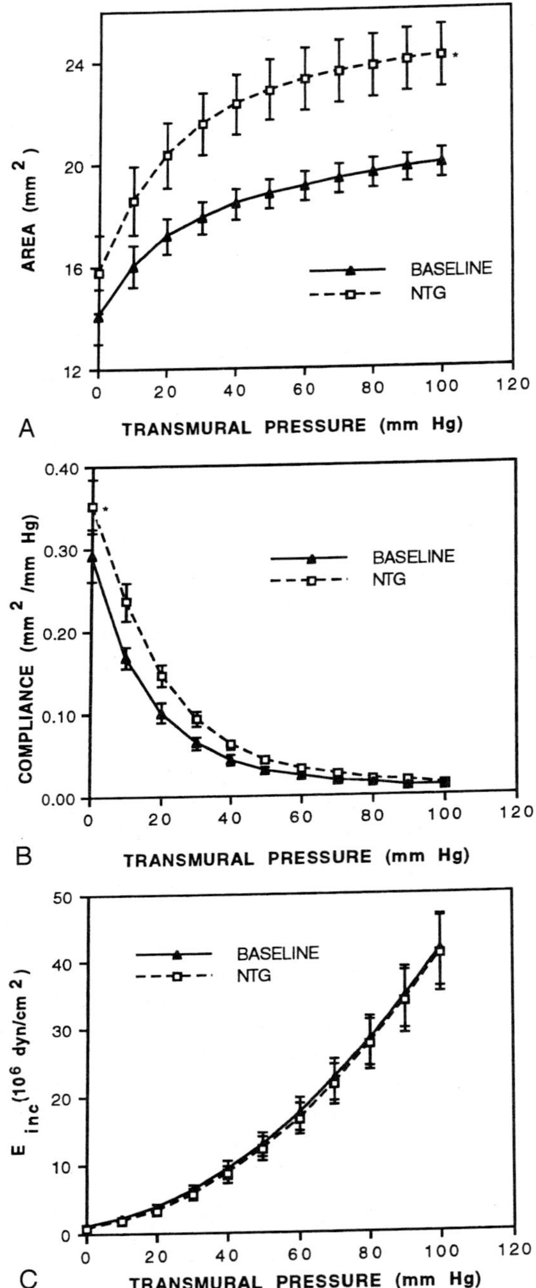

FIGURE 79–2 Effects of smooth muscle relaxation with intra-arterial nitroglycerin (NTG) (100 μg) on brachial artery area **(A)**, compliance **(B)**, and incremental elastic modulus **(C)** in eight normal human subjects. Nitroglycerin significantly increased isobaric brachial artery area and compliance without significantly changing incremental elastic modulus.

nitroglycerin shifted the pressure-area curve upward in a nonparallel fashion by approximately 22 percent. It also shifted the pressure-compliance curve upward by approximately 50 percent. There was no significant change in the incremental elastic modulus with nitroglycerin. These changes in arterial wall mechanics in response to smooth muscle relaxation can be explained based on the arterial model described previously. The compliance of a given artery at a given pressure (isobaric compliance) is dependent on two factors: the size of the vessel and the stiffness of the wall. Smooth muscle relaxation can alter both the size of the vessel and the functional stiffness of the wall. Table 79–1 shows the various factors that are altered with smooth muscle relaxation within the arterial wall and the mechanisms responsible for changes in arterial compliance as a result of these alterations. Smooth muscle relaxation decreases smooth muscle tone and thus decreases tension in both the smooth muscle and its associated series elastic component. It also increases vessel size, which alone is an important determinant of arterial compliance.[51] These geometric and stiffness changes increase arterial compliance. An increase in vessel size also results in increased stretch of parallel elastin and collagen fibers and increased recruitment of previously disengaged or coiled collagen fibers. These changes decrease arterial compliance. The direct effect of smooth muscle relaxation on arterial compliance is the net effect of these opposing factors. In the normal subjects described, arterial compliance increased because of an increase in arterial size (geometric effect) in conjunction with no change in arterial stiffness. The incremental elastic modulus, an intrinsic measure of wall stiffness, did not change because the decrease in stiffness owing to decreased smooth muscle–series elastic component tension was balanced by the increase in stiffness owing to increased parallel elastic component tension. Since the effects of a vasodilator drug on arterial compliance are complex and involve a number of competing mechanisms, it is not surprising that studies of arterial compliance in different species, different arteries, or different disease states have produced conflicting results.

PRESSURE PULSE CONTOUR AND WAVE REFLECTION

The arterial pressure waveform is derived from the complex interaction of the left ventricular stroke volume, the physical properties of the arterial tree, and the characteristics of the fluid in the system. During systole, only the proximal portion of the aorta becomes distended initially because the inertia of blood hinders the passage of the stroke volume to the periphery. The radial stretch of the

TABLE 79–1 Smooth Muscle Relaxation and Arterial Compliance

Factors That Increase Arterial Compliance	Mechanism
Decreased smooth muscle tone	Decreased tension in SM and SEC
Increased vessel size	Geometric effect
Factors That Decrease Arterial Compliance	
Increased stretch or recruitment of collagen	Increased tension in parallel collagen Recruitment of coiled or slack collagen
Increased stretch of parallel elastin	Increased tension in parallel elastin

Abbreviations: SEC, series elastic component; SM, smooth muscle.

ascending aorta brought about by left ventricular ejection initiates a pressure wave that is propagated down the aorta and its branches.[2] This pressure wave travels with a finite velocity that is considerably faster than the actual forward movement of the blood itself. There are marked changes in the shape of the arterial pulse wave as it is propagated peripherally[52] (Fig. 79–3). The distortion in the arterial waveform includes a delay in the time of onset of the initial pressure rise, damping of the high-frequency components of the pulse, and a narrowing and elevation of the systolic portions of the pressure wave.[53] In the proximal portion of the diastolic pressure waveform, a hump becomes more prominent as the pulse passes peripherally. These morphologic changes tend to diminish with age as the arteries become less compliant. The damping of the high-frequency components of the arterial pulse are largely due to the viscoelastic properties of the arterial walls. The mechanisms involved in the peaking of the pressure wave are not clearly defined.[54] Several factors appear to contribute, including wave reflections, geometric tapering, resonance, and pressure-dependent transmission velocity.

It is impossible to explain data on pressure wave transmission and changes in pulse pressure contour morphology without considering wave reflection and a type of damped resonance in the system.[55] Tapering and branching of the arteries alter the pulse contour because an incident wave will be reflected at branch points and the pressure wave becomes amplified as it progresses down a tapered tube. Furthermore, the arterial tree will resonate at certain frequencies while other frequencies are effectively damped.

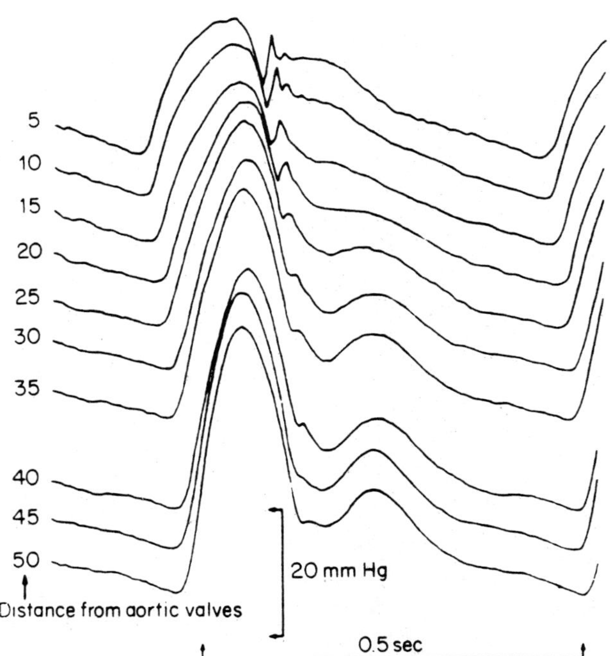

FIGURE 79–3 Pressure waves recorded sequentially at 5-cm intervals between the aortic arch (5 cm from the aortic valve) and the internal iliac artery (50 cm from the aortic valve) in a 16.5-kg wombat through a catheter inserted in the femoral artery. (From O'Rourke MF: Pressure and flow waves in systemic arteries and the anatomical design of the arterial system. J Appl Physiol 23:139, 1967.)

The transmission velocity varies inversely with arterial compliance that, in turn, varies inversely with pressure level. Thus, the peak of the pressure curve will tend to catch up with the "foot" of the same curve. Particularly in peripheral arteries, this phenomenon contributes to peaking and narrowing of the waveform. Reflection and resonance, in addition to influencing the peak of the pressure pulse contour, also contribute to the diastolic hump on the same peripheral waveforms.[56]

TECHNIQUES FOR MEASURING ARTERIAL COMPLIANCE

Table 79–2 depicts the various methods used for estimating arterial compliance along with the advantages and limitations of each technique. These methods are described in the following sections.

Direct

The most direct way to measure arterial compliance in vivo is by measuring simultaneous pulsatile pressure and diameter (or area) changes within an artery. Pulsatile changes in pressure can be measured either invasively or noninvasively using several techniques, including sphygmomanometry and applanation tonometry. It is critical, however, that the absolute pressure be measured at the same site as the caliber measurement. Accurate measurements of pulsatile changes in arterial diameter or cross-sectional area are more difficult to obtain. A number of techniques have been used in situ or in vivo to assess pulsatile changes in arterial diameter. In animals, ultrasound crystals,[57–60] differential transformers,[44] resistance strain-gauges,[61] and photoelectric gauges[62] are some of the techniques that have been utilized to measure arterial diameter. Whereas each of these techniques has its advantages, there are associated problems, including the effects of surgery, anesthesia, and hindrance produced by the device used, which can alter mechanical properties of the vessel wall.

In vivo studies of pulsatile arterial diameter changes in humans have been performed using a variety of techniques. Angiography,[63, 64] magnetic resonance imaging,[65] and transthoracic,[66] transesophageal echocardiography,[67] and intravascular wall motion detectors[68] have been used to assess aortic compliance. Studies of peripheral vascular compliance have utilized plethysmography[69, 70] and ultrasound techniques including Doppler velocimetry[71–73] and two-dimensional ultrasound.[74] Since the late 1980s, a number of laboratories have used noninvasive echo-tracking systems to measure arterial diameter as a function of time.[75–78] Figure 79–4A shows an example of the radiofrequency signal obtained from an A-mode image of a normal human brachial artery. The high-amplitude spikes represent the anterior and posterior arterial wall. Markers are placed over these spikes, and the movement of the arterial wall as a function of time is recorded with precision approaching 5 μm.[79] By using simultaneous noninvasive finger plethysmography or radial artery tonometry, pressure waveforms can be obtained simultaneously with the arterial diameter

TABLE 79-2 Methods Used to Estimate Arterial Compliance

Methods	Advantages	Limitations	Information
Direct			
Angiography	Evaluation of different aortic segments	Expensive, invasive, limited clinical application	Regional aortic compliance
Magnetic resonance imaging	Noninvasive, not limited by acoustic window, able to examine multiple segments, not overly operator dependent	Claustrophobia-inducing, expensive, limited availability, remote site of BP measurement	Regional aortic compliance
TTE/TEE	TTE noninvasive, reasonable availability	Expensive, TTE limited by acoustic window, operator-dependent techniques; TEE invasive, remote site of BP measurement	Regional aortic compliance
Transcutaneous ET/IVUS techniques	Transcutaneous technique noninvasive; both techniques reproducible	Operator dependent, IVUS invasive, remote site of BP measurement with ET, clinical research application	Regional compliance of peripheral arteries
Venous occlusion plethysmography	Noninvasive, reasonable availability	Remote site of BP measurement, clinical research application	Compliance of vascular bed under cuff
Indirect			
Stroke volume/pulse pressure ratio	Noninvasive, reasonable availability	Noninvasive estimate of stroke volume required brachial sphygmomanometer BP measurement	Total arterial compliance
Pulse wave velocity	Noninvasive reasonable availability, reproducible	Limited to larger arteries, errors estimating path length and waveform distortion with pulse propagation	Segmental arterial compliance
Fourier analysis of pressure and flow waveforms	Standard technique, reproducible	Expensive, invasive, limited to the clinical research arena	Total arterial compliance
Pulse contour analysis	Can be noninvasive, reproducible, potential for widespread clinical application	Measurement of stroke volume	Total arterial compliance

Abbreviations: BP, blood pressure; ET, echo-tracking; TEE, transesophageal echocardiography; TTE, transthoracic echocardiography; IVUS, intravascular ultrasound.

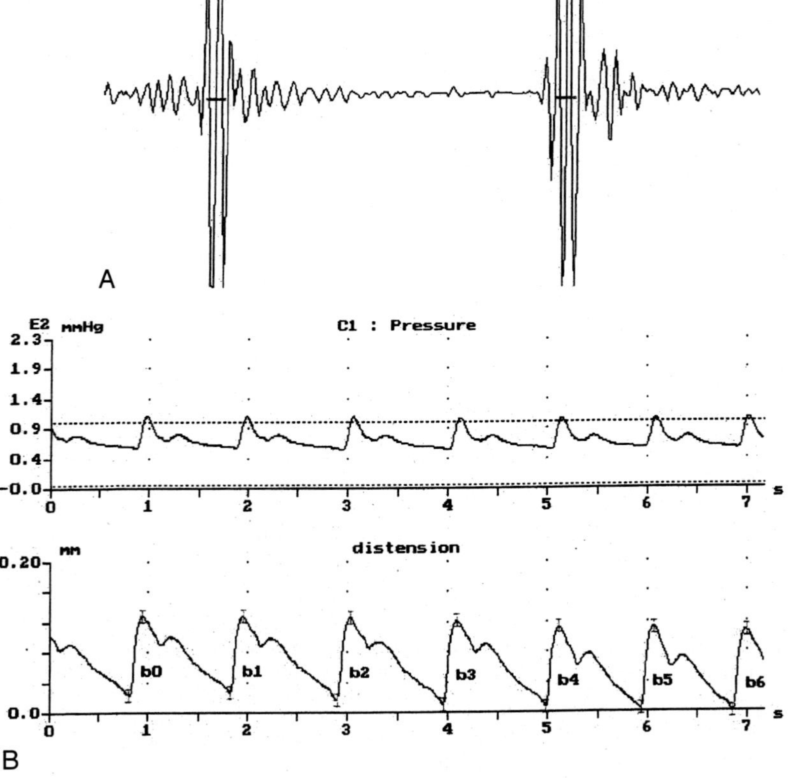

FIGURE 79–4 A, Radiofrequency signal of the brachial artery in a normal human subject. The first large spike represents the anterior wall of the brachial artery, and the second large spike represents the posterior wall of the artery. Motion of the brachial artery can be measured by tracking the movement of these signals. **B,** Simultaneous pressure *(above)* and diameter *(below)* waveforms from the brachial artery of a normal human subject. Arterial compliance can be determined by plotting instantaneous arterial pressure versus diameter and calculating the slope of the curve at any given pressure.

waveforms (see Fig. 79–4B) and calibrated based on cuff recordings of blood pressure. These noninvasive echo-tracking techniques are becoming refined and widely applied to the study of vascular physiology and pathophysiology in human subjects in vivo. Finally, intravascular ultrasound is an invasive technique that has been used to assess human pulmonary,[80] aortic,[81] coronary,[82–85] and brachial[49, 50] artery compliance.

Indirect

A number of indirect techniques for measuring arterial compliance have been utilized by physiologists and clinical investigators. It is well recognized that a pressure pulse wave is transmitted more slowly in distensible than in rigid tubes. The method most commonly employed in humans to measure pulse wave velocity has estimated the time of travel of the foot of the waveform over a known distance.[86] The *foot* is defined as the point at the end of diastole when the steep rise of the wavefront begins. Mathematical equations have been proposed by Moens and Korteweg[87] and Bramwell and Hill[88] to quantitatively express the relation between pulse wave velocity and elastic modulus. These formulas assume that the pulse wave velocity depends only on vessel diameter, blood density, and local arterial wall properties. However, pulse wave velocity is also sensitive to changes in heart rate, blood pressure, and wave reflections in the system.[89] The increase in pulse wave velocity with increased stiffness of the arteries does not strictly represent a measure of *compliance of the arteries,* which is defined as an increment in volume produced by an increment in pressure. The use of the Bramwell and Hill formula also assumes that pulse wave reflections are negligible in the system. Although reflections are small for high frequencies corresponding to the wavefoot, it has previously been demonstrated that the propagation coefficients can be modified by reflected waves.[90, 91] Neglecting the viscous properties of the blood also introduces small errors in relating pulse wave velocity to arterial compliance. Inconsistencies in the literature also arise from the variable methods employed to define the foot of the pulse contour and accurately describe the distance between the pressure or the flow probes. Finally, pulse wave velocity is proportional to the square root of arterial wall stiffness and, therefore, is not particularly sensitive to changes in intrinsic wall properties that influence large vessel compliance. Finally, although pulse wave velocity remains an accepted index of arterial elastic properties, small changes may not be detected because the data generated can often show considerable scatter.[92]

Generalized changes in the physical characteristics of the arterial circulation will influence the impedance to left ventricular ejection. Information about the static and pulsatile elements of the impedance load can be quantified by analyzing the altered pressure and flow relationships and pulse contour parameters produced through the effects of disease on the structural and functional components of the arterial system.[93] In the frequency domain analysis of pressure and flow waveforms, characteristic impedance defines a relationship between pressure and flow in an artery when pressure and flow waves are not influenced by wave reflections (Figs. 79–5 and 79–6). It is measured by averaging moduli of high-frequency values of impedance when fluctuations caused by wave reflections are negligible and provides an indirect measure of compliance distal to a site of measurement.[94] However, the values of moduli used are often close to the noise level of the recording instruments. Therefore, characteristic impedance, which is not a standardized parameter, can be difficult to calculate and interpret.[95] Clearly, the aortic impedance spectrum contains a great deal of information about the physical state of the arterial circulation, and although it is considered the gold standard for studying the opposition to left ventricular ejection, the utility of the technique is limited by the invasive nature of the procedures involved.

There is a growing interest in the quantitative and descriptive analysis of the arterial pressure pulse waveform in the time domain. During systole, the heart imparts energy into the arterial circulation, producing changing values of pressure and flow at all points in the system. A minor part of the stroke volume is dissipated as forward capillary

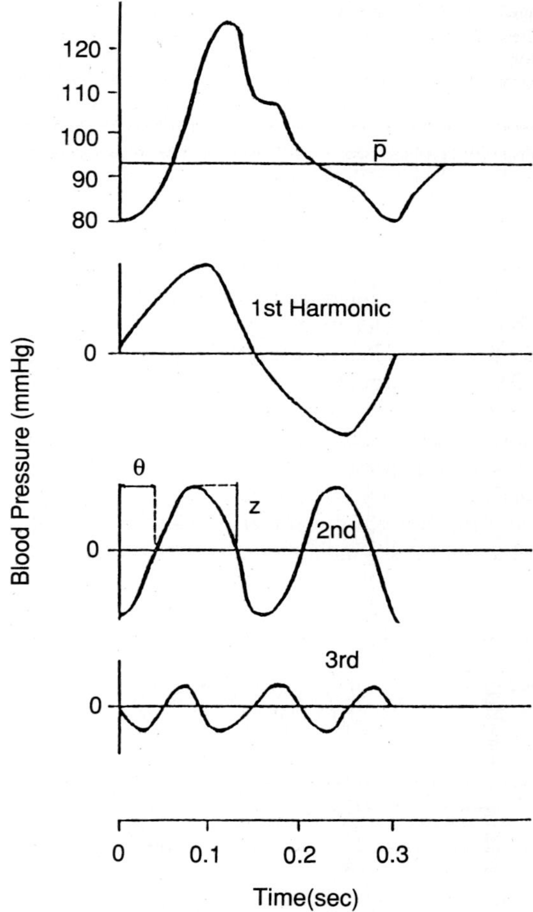

FIGURE 79–5 The Fourier series of the pressure waveform consists of the mean pressure (p̄) and a series of sinusoidal waves or harmonics. The first harmonic is at the frequency of the heart rate, the second is twice that frequency, and so on. The amplitude of each harmonic is termed the *modulus* (z), and the timing of each sinusoidal wave in relation to others is called its *phase angle* (θ). The sum of all terms in the Fourier series approaches the original wave in configuration as additional harmonics are computed.

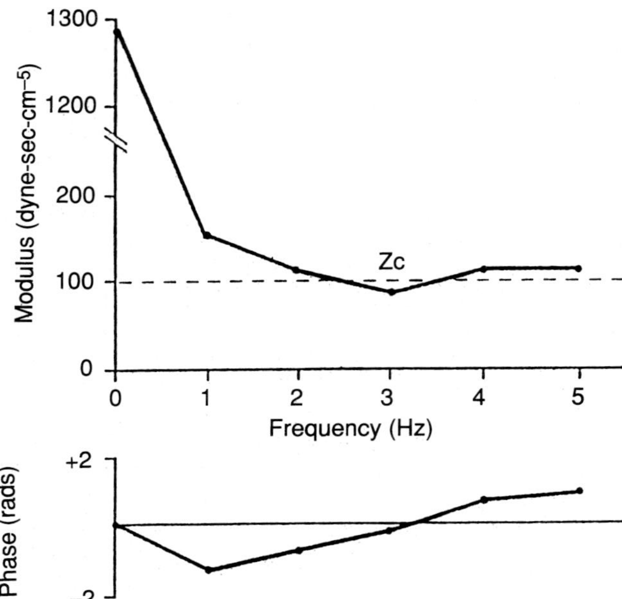

FIGURE 79–6 Hypothetical aortic input impedance spectrum. The impedance modulus values decline from a high value of 0 Hz (i.e., resistance) to a minimum usually between 2 and 4 Hz. This is approximately the same frequency that phase crosses the zero line. Negative phase angles denote that flow leads pressure. Impedance moduli oscillate due to wave reflections around the characteristic impedance, Zc (average of moduli > 2 Hz) that is approximately 10 percent of the resistance.

flow during systole. The remainder is retained by the distensible arteries as potential energy.[96] Closure of the aortic valve prevents further transfer of energy from the heart to the blood vessels. During diastole, this stored energy will passively decay through the arterial tree, and the shape of the end result (the diastolic waveform) will be reflected in the interaction between the input (stroke volume) and the arterial wall properties. Using the technique of pulse contour analysis, arterial compliance values can be estimated by analyzing diastolic arterial pressure decay and employing a modified Windkessel model to interpret the decay of the pressure pulse wave in terms of compliance, inertance, and resistance[97, 98] (Fig. 79–7).

It has been recognized for many years that qualitatively consistent changes in the arterial pulse contour occur in many disease states and with physiologic and pharmacologic interventions.[99] The pulse contour technique quantifies these changes to provide additional information about arterial wall properties and the load imposed on the heart. The Windkessel, as popularized by Frank,[100] represents a nonpropagative model of the arterial circulation that views the peripheral vasculature as a lumped capacitance in parallel with a terminal resistance. This and other closely related models have been employed to simulate the load on the heart or interpret this load in terms of the mechanical properties of the arterial circulation. Estimates of compliance, like estimates of pulse wave velocity, are sensitive to changes in heart rate and blood pressure.[101] The derived values are also sensitive to wave reflections in the system, and different estimation methods applied to the same data can yield different results. For example, methods that integrate pressure with respect to time during the diastolic interval (area method) specifically minimize the effects of wave reflections in distorting the diastolic pressure decay from a monoexponential form. Conversely, the pulse contour technique is exquisitely sensitive in quantifying the impact of wave reflections in distorting the pressure pulse decay in diastole.

A number of techniques have been described in an attempt to determine central aortic pressure from peripheral arterial waveforms.[102–104] A feature of the central aortic waveform is a late systolic pressure peak that is assumed to represent a reflection from more distal sites.[102] This late systolic peak can, therefore, provide insight into the magnitude of the reflection and its transit time from the reflecting site back to the aortic root. A late systolic peak that surpasses the peak pressure of the incident wave in early systole is characteristic of vasoconstricted states, such as hypertension, and of aging. This augmented pressure in late systole is, therefore, suggestive of an increase in pulse wave velocity or a decrease in distensibility or compliance of the smaller arteries where reflections emanate. Thus, the so-called augmentation index utilizes changes in the pres-

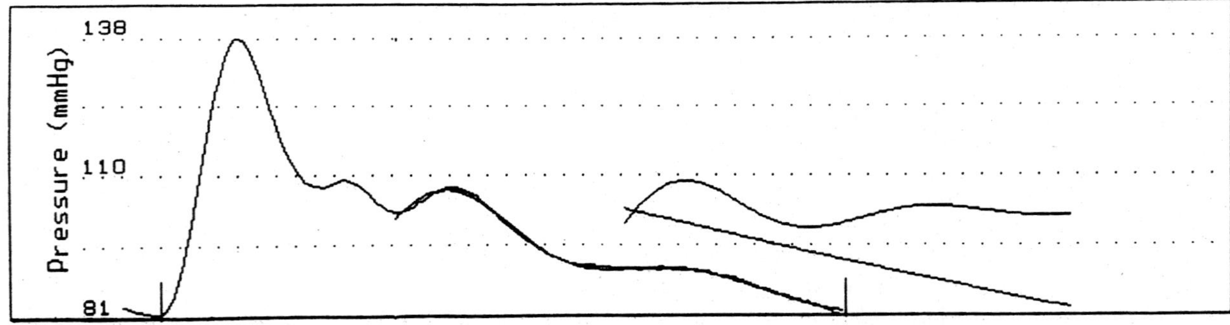

FIGURE 79–7 The passive transient response of the arterial vasculature to the initial loading conditions produced during systole during left ventricular ejection is determined by analyzing the diastolic portion of the pressure pulse waveform. A curve-fit software program utilizes a third-order equation $[A_1e^{-A_2t} + A_3e^{-A_4t}\cos(A_5t + A_6)]$ to represent the time course of the diastolic pressure decay and produce a set of A constants that describe an average waveform that accurately fits each marked pressure pulse contour. The first term in the equation fits to the exponential decay of pressure in diastole and the second term to the oscillatory dicrotic waveform as depicted here. Elements in the modified Windkessel model[153] are calculated from the systemic resistance and the six A constants by equating the A constants with comparable coefficients from the solution to the circuit equations.

sure waveform during systole in an attempt to provide a quantitative measure of the incremental increase in arterial pressure attributed to pulse wave reflections. However, its utility is limited to analysis of waveforms obtained from the more central arteries, and in elderly patients, an inflection point on the systolic upstroke can be difficult to identify.[105] Furthermore, morphologic changes in the pulse contour have been well described before significant augmentation of the systolic peak becomes apparent. The earliest change in the arterial pulse contour morphology with aging and disease involves a diminution in the amplitude and duration of the pressure waveform that interrupts the monoexponential pressure decay owing to wave reflections in the system.

Abnormalities of Vascular Compliance in Aging and Disease States

Aging

An understanding of age-related physiologic changes occurring in the vascular system is crucial in order to appreciate the influence of age on the development of cardiovascular disease and its response to treatment. Although it is recognized that the interindividual variability and the severity of the age-related vascular disease can be substantial,[106] a major problem in studying the effects of age on the cardiovascular system relates to separating age-related from disease-related changes.[107] Adaptations in the arterial vasculature play a critical role in influencing the rise in blood pressure and the left ventricular afterload that accompany advancing age.[108] These changes also contribute to alterations in regional blood flow,[109] atherosclerosis,[110] and the microvascular abnormalities[111] that occur during senescence. The age-related changes in the properties of the arterial system are both structural and functional in nature.

Aging effects involve the arterial intima but are most marked in the media, where there is loss of the orderly arrangement of elastic fibers, which display thinning, fraying, and fragmentation.[112] Elastic degeneration is associated with an increase in collagenous material, often with the deposition of calcium in the degenerating media. The progressive arterial stiffening with aging is more rapid in the central than in the peripheral vessels,[113] so that in the elderly, the aorta and larger arteries exhibit similar stiffness. Studies by Learoyd and Taylor[25] showed that the viscoelastic properties of human arterial walls are altered with age. These authors performed static and dynamic stress-strain studies on arteries removed at autopsy. They concluded that Young's modulus of elasticity increased progressively with increasing distance from the heart and that older vessels (age $>$ 35 years) had a higher modulus than young vessels (age $<$ 35 years). These findings and those of other investigators demonstrate that aging changes do not simply develop in the elderly but are progressive throughout life and are well developed by early adulthood.[114]

Measurement of pulse wave velocity has been the indirect method most commonly employed to evaluate age-related compliance changes in large artery segments.[113, 115–117] Although it has not been extensively studied, functional changes in the properties of the arterial system could influence the compliance characteristics of the blood vessels. The well-recognized reduction in beta-mediated adrenergic function with age may make a significant contribution to changes in vascular tone, vasodilating capacity, and vascular compliance in senescence.[118] Age-related changes in the intima of the arterial blood vessels may also contribute to altered smooth muscle tone by influencing the release of endothelium-derived relaxing factors.[119] The clinical implication of the reduction in compliance may reside in a diminished vasodilator reserve and an inability to respond to increased metabolic demands. A decrease in compliance will also increase the impedance load opposing left ventricular ejection. Although the results of previous studies are not entirely consistent, it would appear that characteristic impedance increases with age, signifying an increased opposition to pulsatile flow.[120–122] This senescent increase in vascular impedance could provide a stimulus for the increase in left ventricular mass in the aged population. Cardiac morphology studied at autopsy[123] and by echocardiography[124] shows a modest degree of myocardial hypertrophy in advanced years. This adaptive left ventricular hypertrophy is associated with an increased risk of cardiovascular morbidity and mortality and, therefore, cannot be dismissed as an unimportant manifestation of the aging process.[125, 126]

Age-related changes in the vasculature are not confined to the large arteries but involve the small arteries and arterioles as well.[111, 127] Peripheral vascular resistance has been employed to estimate hemodynamic adaptations in arterial resistance vessels in previous studies, and a modest increase with aging has usually been documented.[128] This measurement represents a steady-state situation based on continuously fixed pressure and a constant flow model of the circulation in which resistance is calculated from mean arterial pressure and cardiac output. This model ignores pressure fluctuations occurring in the circulation, where the compliance characteristics of the arterial vasculature provide the vital buffering function required to smooth pulsatile outflow from the heart. In these smaller vessels, atherosclerotic changes are much less prevalent and medial arteriosclerotic change is predominant.[129] Furthermore, as the increase in systemic resistance is attributed to medial degenerative changes that rarely produce significant vascular narrowing,[111, 127, 129] measurement of the compliance characteristics of these vessels may provide important information about senescent changes that are not reflected in flow resistance.

Whereas it is generally accepted that the structural and functional changes associated with aging impair the buffering function of the arterial circulation, most studies have been confined to the large conduit arteries and have emphasized that changes in pulsatile function do not progress in a uniform or consistent manner.[130, 131] Prior studies employing pulse wave velocity to estimate the stiffness of arterial segments indicate that the aorta stiffens progressively at an accelerated rate compared with other arterial segments. Echo-tracking technology has revealed that age-related changes in pulsatile function are inhomogeneous within localized arterial segments of elastic and muscular arteries and that the compliance characteristics of the radial artery may paradoxically increase with age. In contrast to the marked heterogeneity in the physical characteristics of localized arterial segments with aging, consistent and predictable changes occur in the arterial pulse contour, regardless of the site of measurement.

We[132] have recently examined the effects of aging on the compliance characteristics of the arterial circulation, applying the pulse contour analysis technique to waveforms recorded invasively and noninvasively from the brachial and radial arteries, respectively. Consistent age-related reductions in arterial compliance estimates were found regardless of measurement site or method employed. The decline in small artery compliance with aging was significantly greater than estimates recorded for large arteries. As the smaller arterial vessels are generally free from atheroma and the decline in small artery compliance with aging was independent of changes in blood pressure, this estimate may reflect the effects of the degenerative aging process per se in altering pulsatile arterial function. One plausible explanation for our findings may reside in impaired endothelial function, which is known to accompany advancing age and may negatively affect pulsatile arterial function.

Atherosclerosis

Atherosclerosis and the increase in mean arterial pressure that occurs with advancing age could account, at least in part, for a decrease in arterial compliance estimates. Changes in arterial compliance have been documented with atherosclerosis, but the findings have not been consistent. Farrar and coworkers[133, 134] in experimental atherosclerosis in the rhesus monkey, demonstrated the loss of aortic distensibility by pulse wave velocity with the development of atherosclerosis and the improvement of aortic distensibility with regression of atherosclerosis. By contrast, in vitro studies of human aortas failed to show any difference in distensibility attributable to atherosclerosis when comparing atheroma-filled and atheroma-free specimens.[135] Similarly, studies of pulse wave velocity change in populations with a high and low prevalence of atherosclerosis failed to show any differences between groups,[114] and studies in patients with and without coronary artery disease revealed no difference in arterial wall characteristics.[136] More recent studies employing ultrasound techniques to investigate changes in the physical characteristics of the coronary arteries in the immediate vicinity of plaque found a decrease in wall distensibility that appeared related to the presence, size, and intrinsic characteristics of the plaque.[137] Other investigators[27] reported decreased distensibility of peripheral arteries in patients with known atherosclerotic disease in remote vascular beds and implicated the generalized effects of atherosclerosis on the endothelium to explain the changes in pulsatile arterial function. Whereas it is probable that atherogenesis does play a role in reducing arterial compliance or distensibility, the changes may be too small to be detected by the crude methods employed and may be lost in the wide scatter of values taken from persons of the same age and blood pressure. The strong positive effect of age could be clearly distinguished from the effects of a modest increase in mean arterial pressure in increasing pulse wave velocity and decreasing arterial compliance estimates in previous studies.[113]

Some authorities have hypothesized that atherosclerotic disease in the aorta progressively stiffens the vessel and that the accompanying increase in aortic pulse wave velocity may be used as a surrogate marker for subclinical atherosclerosis.[138] They further postulate that the measure may predict future coronary events, given the close correlation between aortic and coronary atherosclerosis. However, assuming a close linear correlation does exist between the severity of atherosclerosis and the changes in pulse wave velocity,[139] the recognition that most coronary events occur in patients with only mild-to-moderate disease will severely limit the usefulness of this clinical application.

Hypertension

Hypertension is a vascular disease characterized by structural and functional changes in the cardiovascular system. Left ventricular hypertrophy and arterial wall thickening of the blood vessels have been well documented in chronic hypertension, both in experimental animals and in human subjects at autopsy.[140, 141] Therapeutic trials in hypertension have suggested a dissociation between blood pressure control and prevention of cardiovascular complications of hypertension.[142, 143] Thus, coronary events[144, 145] and left ventricular hypertrophy[146, 147] are not necessarily prevented by drugs that lower blood pressure. These observations raise the possibility that blood pressure itself may not be the primary determinant of these cardiovascular events.[148] To some extent, the cardiovascular structural alterations are natural physiologic responses to the high blood pressure and are protective. However, it is suggested increasingly that effective antihypertensive treatment requires normalization not only of the blood pressure but also of cardiovascular structure.[149]

An increased peripheral vascular resistance is regarded as a hemodynamic hallmark of sustained hypertension.[150] Folkow[151] demonstrated quantitatively that the observed increases in vascular resistance could be fully explained in terms of an alteration in vascular wall architecture without any need to postulate a change in excitation-contraction coupling in hypertension. Thus, the increased vascular resistance can be explained by alterations in vascular structure if there is encroachment of the tunica media into the lumen, thus decreasing the lumen diameter and increasing the media thickness:lumen diameter ratio. Evidence would suggest that the altered vascular architecture described in the small arteries may in large part be due to a remodeling process rather than growth.[149, 152] The fact that remodeling rather than growth may be primarily responsible for the abnormal small artery structure may explain why antihypertensive therapy rarely normalizes vascular architecture in essential hypertensive patients.[153, 154] Intuitively, changes in small artery structure and growth would be expected to alter the compliance characteristics of these vessels in addition to increasing resistance to blood flow in the tissues.

With regard to the large arteries, hypertension can be viewed as an accelerated form of aging. The pathologic changes in the aortic wall and the associated aortic dilatation occur at an earlier age if blood pressure is elevated.[141] Arterial compliance will decrease as the blood pressure increases, owing to the nonlinear distensible characteristics of the arteries. The decrease in arterial compliance will increase the pulse pressure. This has been demonstrated in closed-chest anesthetized dogs, in which a stiff tube was inserted around the ascending aorta.[10] This maneuver produced an increase in systolic and a decrease in diastolic blood pressure without influencing mean arterial pressure or systemic resistance. A reduced large artery compliance is a well-accepted finding in hypertension, whatever the site and method of measurement.[155–157] Because the elevated blood pressure itself will induce a decrease in arterial compliance, it remains a matter of debate whether the reduction in compliance represents an alteration of wall properties or is merely a consequence of elevated pressure.

Several tentative observations would suggest that a decreased large artery compliance in essential hypertension is not solely a mechanical consequence of an elevated blood pressure. In patients with isolated systolic and borderline essential hypertension, the observed decrease in arterial compliance may not be fully accounted for by the marginal increase in mean arterial pressure.[157, 158] In established hypertension, compliance estimates appear reduced to the same extent regardless of the degree of blood pressure elevation.[159] In addition, different drugs exhibit disparate effects on arterial compliance despite similar reductions in blood pressure.[160] Armentano and associates[161] used a nonlinear mathematical model to represent diameter-pressure relationships in the brachial artery to permit comparison of data in hypertensive and normotensive subjects under isobaric conditions from pressure-diameter and pressure-compliance curves in the artery. These authors[161] concluded that the reduced compliance estimates found in hypertensive patients could not be attributed solely to the stretching effect of elevated blood pressure. In summary, these indirect observations suggest that factors in addition to the level of blood pressure, either structural or functional in nature, participate in the mechanisms influencing arterial compliance.[162]

A reduced arterial compliance in hypertensive patients has not been a universal finding. With blood pressure controlled as a confounding variable, no difference in forearm arterial compliance between hypertensive and normotensive subjects has been reported in prior studies.[92, 163] More recent observations appear to confirm these earlier findings and suggest that a decreased arterial compliance in muscular conduit arteries may not be a prominent feature of hypertension.[75] As emphasized by the authors, observations recorded from the muscular radial artery cannot be extrapolated to the more elastic central arteries. The lumen diameter of the radial artery was not increased in hypertensive patients, a finding that has been observed in the carotid and femoral vessels as well.[164] That carotid and femoral wall thicknesses were increased in hypertensive subjects despite a normal lumen diameter provides strong evidence for large artery growth in these subjects.[164, 165] Changes involving alterations in the proportion and mechanical characteristics of wall components would intuitively be expected to influence the arterial compliance estimates. As emphasized by Mulvany,[166, 167] however, this may not always be the case. A reduction in the elastic modulus (an intrinsic measure of stiffness of the vascular wall materials) would serve to normalize arterial compliance estimates despite an increase in wall thickness.

A decrease in the elastic modulus of the wall materials has been described in small arteries in experimental hypertension and may serve as a means whereby the vasculature can functionally maintain its distensibility characteristics despite the relatively increased wall thickness required by the increased intravascular pressure. However, the extent to which the altered structure measured under in vitro conditions reflects the in vivo situation remains to be determined. Other caveats include sampling issues, the representative nature of the vascular bed under study, the experimental model of hypertension employed, and the role of the arterial smooth muscle in altering the mechanical properties of the vessel wall. Although speculative, it may be that individuals who do not normalize compliance under isobaric conditions and expose the vessel wall to high pulsatile stress are destined to experience early cardiovascular complications.

Changes in arterial smooth muscle cell phenotype can occur during hypertension.[168] A well-differentiated phenotype is predominant in resistance vessels that contract in response to chemical or mechanical stimuli. The dedifferentiation toward a more immature phenotype in hypertensive states may be associated with a partial loss of contractile properties of the smooth muscle cells. The decreased capacity of the arterial wall to withstand high systolic pressures may, in turn, favor an increase in vascular events. It is of interest that the administration of diuretic therapy has been reported to prevent smooth muscle cell phenotype modification and fibrinoid necrosis in blood vessels, independent of effects on blood pressure and vascular medial hypertrophy.

The small arteries and arterioles appear to be the most important dysfunctional segment of the vasculature in hypertension.[169] Pulse contour analysis has identified a striking change in the oscillatory component of the diastolic waveform consistent with an alteration in the compliance characteristics of the smaller arteries that serve as a site of pulse wave reflections in the arterial system.[155] In addition to altered structural properties of the vessel wall, functional modifications in the endothelium or in responses to vasoactive substances elaborated by the endothelium can influence arteriolar tone in hypertensive vascular disease.[170]

It has been suggested that prevention of hypertensive-related cardiovascular events requires the prescription of drug therapy that lowers blood pressure and affects vascular and cardiac structure. Left ventricular hypertrophy is recognized as an independent predictor of future cardiovascular events. The low correlation between left ventricular hypertrophy and blood pressure as well as the incomplete regression of left ventricular hypertrophy with blood pressure lowering suggests that left ventricular hypertrophy is not solely a pressure-related phenomenon. It is also apparent that antihypertensive drugs exert different effects on vascular and cardiac structure. In health, optimal coupling between the heart and the peripheral vasculature produces a characteristic waveform that changes predictably with aging, disease, and drug interventions. Although unproved, it would appear intuitively appealing to restore this situation by prescribing drugs that lower arterial pressure by influencing both compliance and resistance to reproduce the waveform morphology that identifies optimal matching between the heart and the circulation.

Diabetes Mellitus

The altered metabolism associated with diabetes mellitus produces structural and functional changes in the arterial vasculature and accounts for the increased cardiovascular morbidity and mortality found in diabetic subjects.[171, 172] Large vessel disease represents a major threat to health in patients with diabetes.[173] Although the pathogenesis remains unresolved, it is generally considered to be of atherosclerotic origin.[174] Angiographic[175] and autopsy studies[176] have demonstrated that diabetic patients have more severe and diffuse atheromatous disease than do age-matched controls. However, it is now recognized that a specific vascular process can occur in diabetic patients to produce large vessel damage. In contrast to the distribution of atherosclerosis, which is often confined to particular vessels and territories, diabetic macroangiopathy represents a constellation of changes that affect the entire arterial system.[177] The histologic findings include the accumulation of periodic acid–Schiff–positive substance, connective tissue membrane components such as fibronectin, and type IV collagen, as well as deposition of calcium in the arterial media.[178] The term *diabetic microangiopathy* usually includes arteriolosclerosis and thickening of capillary walls. *Arteriolosclerosis* refers to concentric hyaline thickening of the arteriolar walls and is recognized as a generalized change in diabetes mellitus.[179] The development of microangiopathy involves capillary basement membrane thickening,[172] nonenzymatic glycation of long-lived tissue proteins, abnormalities of endothelial cells and platelets, and perhaps, increased blood vessel damage by free radicals.[180] The functional consequences of these changes involve an increased permeability of capillary networks and, eventually, acellular capillaries, resulting in a decreased microvascular density.[181] These changes in the vessel wall will affect vessel elasticity.[182] With such widespread changes occurring in both large and small arterial vessels, one would expect these changes to influence the arterial compliance characteristics in diabetic subjects.

Pulse wave velocity has been the method most commonly employed in prior studies to examine the effects of carbohydrate intolerance on arterial stiffness in diabetic subjects.[183–187] However, there is little consensus in the literature regarding a change in pulse wave velocity, used as an index of the arterial wall stiffness, in subjects with diabetes mellitus. Although a majority of reports indicate increased stiffness of arterial segments in diabetic subjects versus controls, the results are not uniform and, in many cases, have been influenced by confounding variables. Monnier and colleagues[183] found an increase in patients with a long-standing insulin-dependent diabetes versus nondiabetic controls only if they had retinopathy. However, this measurement reflects a stiffness of the large artery segments, and the higher blood pressures recorded in the diabetic subjects with retinopathy could have accounted for their findings. Scarpello and coworkers[185] reported an increase in pulse wave velocity in the popliteal to posterior tibial arteries only in diabetic subjects with neuropathy and active or healed foot ulceration. In the upper limbs, pulse wave velocity was similar for all groups. It would appear that the combination of severe degenerative atherosclerotic changes and possible medial arterial calcification was required to stiffen the vessel sufficiently to detect an increase in foot-to-foot wave velocity. Using echo-tracking technology, a number of investigators examined the mechanical behavior of the arterial wall in different arterial territories in diabetes mellitus. In insulin-dependent diabetes mellitus, a decreased arterial distensibility has been reported but appears dependent on the arterial territory studied.[188] In type 2 diabetes mellitus, increased stiffness of the common carotid artery was evident in the Atherosclerosis Risk in Communities (ARIC) Study[189] and was positively correlated with fasting glucose levels. By contrast, consistent abnormalities in the arterial pressure pulse contour have been recognized for many years in diabetic subjects.[187, 190, 191] The principal change in arterial wave shape, found in both the smaller digital and the larger conduit arteries, consists of the shortening and damping of the oscillatory diastolic wave. Similar abnormalities in pulse wave contour are found with aging and hypertension and have been shown to reflect the loss of vessel wall distensibility.[99, 192, 193]

The arterial diastolic waveform was able to separate patients with non–insulin-dependent diabetes mellitus from age- and sex-matched controls.[194] Using the pulse contour analysis methodology, quantitative changes in the arterial waveform, reflected by a reduced oscillatory compliance estimate, were identified in patients with diabetes. This change acts as a measure of oscillation in the arterial system reflecting altered compliance characteristics of the more peripheral vessels.[155, 195] No differences were found in large artery compliance estimates or in peripheral vascular resistance. The reduced oscillatory compliance values were found in diabetic subjects, regardless of whether they exhibited one or more complications of the disease detected during the initial screening procedures. These findings suggested that this estimate may represent a sensitive marker for early vascular abnormalities that occur in diabetes. It may also indicate that the ability of a vessel to distend in response to pressure is more sensitive than its basal caliber in identifying abnormal structure and tone.

In a series of follow-up studies using a crossover design with the diabetic subjects as their own controls, we found that the administration of fish oil improved arterial compliance estimates compared with responses recorded after the ingestion of olive oil.[196] Significantly improved forearm dilator responses to the infusion of acetylcholine were also apparent after dietary fish oil supplementation. We postulated that the improved compliance characteristics of the vasculature observed with fish oil administration probably resulted from its direct effect on improving endothelial function.

Heart Failure

The failing heart is exquisitely sensitive to arterial loading conditions.[197, 198] Although many studies have demonstrated the importance of altering the nonpulsatile left ventricular load (systemic vascular resistance), there is less information on the pulsatile load faced by the failing heart. Determinations of ascending aortic impedance using high-fidelity pressure and flow measurements have shown both reduced[199] and normal[200, 201] impedance in patients with heart failure. Radial[202] and carotid[203] artery compliance is impaired in patients with heart failure. Brachial artery compliance is decreased and brachial-radial pulse wave velocity is increased in patients with heart failure.[204] These abnormalities correlate with New York Heart Association class. Although Ramsey and associates[205] did not find differences in baseline pulse wave velocity or distensibility in patients with idiopathic dilated cardiomyopathy, they demonstrated that improvements in arterial elastic properties in response to endothelium-dependent stimuli were impaired. Pulse contour analysis studies in heart failure have demonstrated abnormalities of oscillatory but not proximal arterial compliance.[206] Although the mechanisms of abnormal arterial compliance have not been extensively investigated, possible etiologies include increased vessel smooth muscle tone as a result of neurohumoral activation, increased sodium or water content of blood vessels, and structural abnormalities of the vessel wall. Of note, abnormalities in arterial elastic properties occur at early stages of left ventricular dysfunction or heart failure in some animal models,[207, 208] and these abnormalities may precede increases in peripheral vascular resistance.[207]

Acute drug administration has been demonstrated to alter pulsatile loading conditions in patients with heart failure. Both nitroprusside[209] and dobutamine[210] can decrease aortic characteristic impedance in patients with heart failure, although the effects of nitroprusside on characteristic impedance are not uniform. There is general agreement, however, that nitroprusside decreases the frequency of the first harmonic of the impedance spectrum, probably as a result of decreased wave reflection.[211, 212] Chronic angiotensin-converting enzyme inhibition improves radial artery compliance in patients with heart failure.[202] Studies of drug effects on arterial elastic properties in patients with heart failure have involved systemic administration of drugs. These drugs can have a number of effects, including decreases in blood pressure, changes in autonomic reflexes, and changes in heart rate. It is thus difficult to separate the *indirect* effects of the drug (e.g., improved compliance due solely to decreased blood pressure) from the direct effects on the arterial wall.

DEFINITIONS

A number of different definitions have been used in the literature for the terms describing vascular elastic properties. The following is a summary of these terms and their definitions. Definitions are given using cross-sectional area (A) as the parameter describing vascular dimension; however, blood vessel diameter or volume can be used interchangeably.

Compliance (C): the change in cross-sectional area (ΔA) for a given change in pressure (ΔP). The compliance of an artery can be determined as the slope of a tangent to the pressure-area curve (dA/dP) for that blood vessel.

Distensibility (D): the fractional change in area (ΔA/A) for a given change in intravascular pressure (ΔP). Distensibility is, thus, the quotient of compliance (ΔA/ΔP) and area (A). This term refers to the relative extensibility of a vessel and serves to facilitate comparison between blood vessels of different sizes.

Wall tension (T): the circumferential force in the vessel wall per unit of vessel length. The relationship between tension and radius (R) for a thin-walled vessel is often referred to as the law of Laplace: T = PR.

Pulse wave velocity: the distance traveled by a pressure or flow wave divided by the time required to travel that distance. Pulse wave velocity is inversely related to vascular compliance because wave travel is slower along compliant vessels.

Impedance: the total opposition to flow offered by the arterial system.

Input impedance: the ratio of pressure and flow at a given site, which is considered the input to the vascular tree distal to that site.

Characteristic impedance: the ratio of pressure and flow in an artery when pressure and flow waves are not influenced by wave reflection.

Stress (σ): the force per unit area that produces a change in arterial cross-sectional area. Stress is, therefore, wall tension (T) divided by wall thickness (h) or PR/h.

Strain (ϵ): the ratio of change in area (ΔA) to the *initial* area (A).

Elastic modulus: the change in stress (Δσ) for a given change in strain (Δϵ). Because the relationship between stress and strain in an artery is nonlinear, the term *incremental elastic modulus* is used and is defined as the slope of a tangent to the stress-strain curve ($d\sigma/d\epsilon$). A single incremental elastic modulus cannot be determined for a blood vessel, but rather, the value must be reported at a specific distending pressure or cross-sectional area. Unlike compliance, the incremental elastic modulus is an intrinsic characteristic of the vessel wall materials and independent of vessel geometry.

REFERENCES

1. Pepine CJ, Nichols WW: Aortic impedance in cardiovascular disease. Prog Cardiovasc Dis 24:307–318, 1982.
2. Guyton AL: Vascular distensibility and functions of the arterial and venous systems. *In* Guyton AL (ed): Textbook of Medical Physiology. 8th ed. pp. 159–167. Philadelphia: WB Saunders, 1991.
3. Noble MIM: Left ventricular load, arterial impedance and their interrelationship. Cardiovasc Res 13:183–198, 1979.
4. Piene H: Impedance matching between ventricle and load. Ann Biomed Eng 12:191–207, 1984.
5. Nichols WW, Pepine CJ, Geiser EA, Conti R: Vascular load defined by the aortic input impedance spectrum. Fed Proc 39:196–201, 1980.
6. O'Rourke MF, Avolio AP, Nichols WW: Left ventricular–systemic arterial coupling in humans and strategies to improve coupling in disease states. *In* Yin FCP (ed): Ventricular/Vascular Coupling. pp. 3–19. New York: Springer-Verlag, 1987.
7. Arndt JO, Stegall HF, Wicke HJ: Mechanics of the aorta in vivo. Circ Res 28:693–704, 1971.
8. Simon AC, Safar ME, Levenson JA, et al: An evaluation of large arteries compliance in man. Am J Physiol 237:H550–H554, 1979.
9. Covell JW, Pouleur H, Ross J Jr: Left ventricular wall stress and aortic input impedance. Fed Proc 39:202–207, 1980.
10. Randall OS, Van den Bos GC, Westerhof N: Systemic compliance: does it play a role in the genesis of essential hypertension? Cardiovasc Res 18:455–462, 1984.
11. Westerhof N, Bosman R, DeFries CJ, Noordergraaf A: Analog

studies of the human systemic arterial tree. J Biomech 2:121–143, 1969.
12. Latham RD, Westerhof N, Sipkema P, et al: Regional wave travel and reflections along the human aorta: a study with six simultaneous micromanometric pressures. Circulation 72:1257–1269, 1985.
13. Safar M: Therapeutic trials and large arteries in hypertension. Am Heart J 115:702–710, 1988.
14. Christensen KL: Reducing pulse pressure in hypertension may normalize small artery structure. Hypertension 18:722–727, 1991.
15. O'Rourke MF, Yaginuma T, Avolio AP: Physiological and pathophysiological implications of ventricular:vascular coupling. Ann Biomed Eng 12:119–134, 1984.
16. Milnor WR: Pulsatile blood flow. N Engl J Med 287:27–34, 1972.
17. Lee RT, Kamm RD: Vascular mechanics for the cardiologist. J Am Coll Cardiol 23:1289–1295, 1994.
18. Safar ME, Frohlich ED: The arterial system in hypertension. A prospective view. Hypertension 26:10–14, 1995.
19. Dzau VJ, Gibbons GH, Cooke JP, et al: Vascular biology and medicine in the 1990s: scope, concepts, potentials and perspectives. Circulation 87:705–719, 1993.
20. Glasser SP, Arnett DK, McVeigh GE, et al: Vascular compliance and cardiovascular disease. A risk factor or a marker? Am J Hypertens 10:1175–1189, 1997.
21. Caro CCT, Pedley TJ, Schroter RC, Seed WA: The Mechanics of the Circulation. pp. 243–346. Oxford: Oxford University Press, 1978.
22. Fischer GM, Llaurado JG: Collagen and elastin content in canine arteries selected from functionally different vascular beds. Circ Res 19:394–399, 1966.
23. Harkness MLR, Harkness RD, McDonald DA: The collagen and elastin content of the arterial wall in the dog. Proc R Soc Lond 146B:541–551, 1957.
24. Nichols WW, McDonald DA: Wave-velocity in the proximal aorta. Med Biol Eng 10:327–335, 1972.
25. Learoyd BM, Taylor MG: Alterations with age in the visco-elastic properties of human arterial walls. Circ Res 18:278–292, 1966.
26. McVeigh GE, Morgan DJ, Finkelstein SM, et al: Vascular abnormalities associated with long-term cigarette smoking identified by arterial waveform analysis. Am J Med 102:227–231, 1997.
27. Heintz B, Dorr R, Gillessen T, et al: Do arterial endothelin 1 levels affect local arterial stiffness? Am Heart J 26:987–989, 1993.
28. Glasser SP, Selwyn A, Ganz P: Atherosclerosis, risk factors and the vascular endothelium. Am Heart J 131:379–384, 1996.
29. Simon A, Megnien JL, Levenson J: Detection of preclinical atherosclerosis may optimize the management of hypertension. Am J Hypertens 10:813–824, 1997.
30. Roach MR, Burton AC: The effect of age on the elasticity of human iliac arteries. Can J Biochem Physiol 37:557–570, 1959.
31. Bergel DH: The static elastic properties of the arterial wall. J Physiol (Lond) 156:445–457, 1961.
32. Sonnenblick EH: Series elastic and contractile elements in heart muscle: changes in muscle length. Am J Physiol 207:1330–1338, 1964.
33. Pringle JWS: Models of muscle. Symp Soc Exp Biol 14:41–68, 1960.
34. Cox RH: Passive mechanics and connective tissue composition of canine arteries. Am J Physiol 234:H533–H541, 1978.
35. Dobrin P, Canfield T: Identification of smooth muscle series elastic component in intact carotid artery. Am J Physiol 232:H122–H130, 1977.
36. Wiederhielm CA: Distensibility characteristics of small blood vessels. Fed Proc 24:1075–1084, 1965.
37. Gow BS: Circulatory correlates: vascular impedance, resistance and capacity. *In* Shepherd JT, Abboud FM (eds): American Physiological Society Handbook of Physiology. Sect. 2. The Cardiovascular System. Vol. 2. pp. 353–408. Bethesda, MD: American Physiological Society, 1983.
38. Cox RH: Mechanics of canine iliac artery smooth muscle in vitro. Am J Physiol 230:462–470, 1976.
39. Dobrin PB: Mechanical properties of arteries. Physiol Rev 58:397–460, 1978.
40. Nichols WW, O'Rourke MF: Properties of the arterial wall. *In* Nichols WW, O'Rourke MF (eds): McDonald's Blood Flow in Arteries. 3rd ed. pp. 99–102. London: Edward Arnold, 1990.
41. Bank AJ: Physiologic aspects of drug therapy and large artery elastic properties. Vasc Med 2:44–50, 1997.
42. Wiggers CJ, Wegria R: Active changes in size and distensibility of the aorta during acute hypertension. Am J Physiol 124:603, 1938.
43. Alexander RS: The influence of constrictor drugs on the distensibility of the splanchnic venous system, analyzed on the basis of an aortic model. Circ Res 2:140–147, 1954.
44. Peterson LH, Jensen RE, Parnell J: Mechanical properties of arteries in vivo. Circ Res 8:622–639, 1960.
45. Safar ME, London GM, Bouthier JA, et al: Brachial artery cross-sectional area and distensibility before and after arteriolar vasodilation in men with sustained hypertension. J Cardiovasc Pharmacol 9:734–742, 1987.
46. Safar ME, Laurent S, Bouthier JA, London GM: Comparative effects of captopril and isosorbide dinitrate on the arterial wall of hypertensive human brachial arteries. J Cardiovasc Pharmacol 8:1257–1261, 1986.
47. Fitchett DH: Forearm arterial compliance: a new measure of arterial compliance. Cardiovasc Res 18:651–656, 1984.
48. Westling H, Jansson L, Jonson B, Nilsen R: Vasoactive drugs and elastic properties of human arteries in vivo, with special reference to the action of nitroglycerine. Eur Heart J 5:609–616, 1984.
49. Bank AJ, Wilson RF, Kubo SH, et al: Direct effects of smooth muscle relaxation and contraction on in vivo brachial artery elastic properties. Circ Res 77:1008–1016, 1995.
50. Bank AJ, Wang H, Holte J, et al: The contribution of collagen, elastin and smooth muscle to in vivo human brachial artery wall stress and elastic modulus. Circulation 94:3263–3270, 1996.
51. Bank AJ, Kaiser DR: Smooth muscle relaxation: effects on arterial compliance, distensibility, elastic modulus and pulse wave velocity. Hypertension 32:356–359, 1998.
52. Murgo JP, Westerhof N, Giolima JP, Altobelli SA: Effects of exercise on aortic input impedance and pressure waveforms in normal humans. Circ Res 48:334–343, 1981.
53. Remington JW, Wood EH: Formation of the peripheral pulse contour in man. J Appl Physiol 9:433–442, 1956.
54. Berne RM, Levy MW: *In* Berne RM, Levy MW (eds): Physiology. 2nd ed. pp. 486–495. St. Louis: CV Mosby, 1988.
55. Nichols WW, O'Rourke MF: Contours of pressure and flow waves in arteries. *In* Nichols WW, O'Rourke MF (eds): McDonald's Blood Flow in Arteries. 3rd ed. pp. 216–245. London: Edward Arnold, 1990.
56. Little RC, Little WC: Physiology of the Heart and Circulation. 4th ed. pp. 236–243. Chicago: Year Book Medical, 1989.
57. Gross DR, Hunter JF, Allert JA, et al: Pressure-diameter relationship in the coronary artery of intact, awake calves. J Biomech 14:613–620, 1981.
58. Pagani M, Gaig H, Sherman A, et al: Measurement of multiple simultaneous small dimensions and study of arterial pressure-diameter relation in conscious animals. Am J Physiol 229:286–290, 1975.
59. Vatner SF, Hintze TH: Effects of calcium-channel antagonist on large and small coronary arteries in conscious dogs. Circulation 66:579–588, 1982.
60. Barra JG, Armentano RL, Levenson J, et al: Assessment of smooth muscle contribution to descending thoracic aortic elastic mechanics in conscious dogs. Circ Res 73:1040–1050, 1993.
61. Patel DJ, Mallos AJ, Fry DL: Aortic mechanics in the living dog. J Appl Physiol 16:293–299, 1961.
62. Wetterer E, Bauer RD, Busse R: New ways of determining the propagation coefficient and the visco-elastic behavior of arteries in situ. *In* Bauer RD, Busse R (eds): The Arterial System. pp. 35–47. New York: Springer-Verlag, 1978.
63. Merillon JP, Motte G, Fruchand J, et al: Evaluation of the elasticity and characteristic impedance of the ascending aorta in man. Cardiovasc Res 12:401–406, 1978.
64. Stefanadis C, Wooley CF, Bush CA, et al: Aortic distensibility abnormalities in coronary artery disease. Am J Cardiol 59:1300–1304, 1987.
65. Mohiaddin RH, Underwood SR, Bogren HG, et al: Regional aortic compliance studied by magnetic resonance imaging: the effects of age, training, and coronary artery disease. Br Heart J 62:90–96, 1989.
66. Dart AM, LaLombe F, Yeoh JK, et al: Aortic distensibility in patients with isolated hypercholesterolaemia, coronary artery disease or cardiac transplant. Lancet 338:270–273, 1991.
67. Mugge A, Daniel WG, Niedermeyer J, et al: Usefulness of a new automated boundary detection system (acoustic quantification) for

assessing stiffness of the descending thoracic aorta by transesophageal echocardiography. Am J Cardiol 70:1629–1631, 1992.
68. Stefanadis C, Dernellis J, Vlachopoulos C, et al: Aortic function in arterial hypertension determined by pressure-diameter relation: effects of diltiazem. Circulation 96:1853–1858, 1996.
69. Dahn I, Jonson B, Nilsen R: Plethysmographic in vivo determination of elastic properties of arteries in man. J Appl Physiol 28:328–332, 1970.
70. Fitchett DH: Forearm arterial compliance: a new measure of arterial compliance. Cardiovasc Res 18:651–656, 1984.
71. Safar ME, Peronneau PA, Levenson JA, et al: Pulsed Doppler: diameter, velocity and flow of the brachial artery in sustained essential hypertension. Circulation 63:393–400, 1981.
72. Levenson JA, Peronneau PA, Simon A, Safar ME: Pulsed Doppler: determination of diameter, blood flow velocity and volumic flow of brachial artery in man. Cardiovasc Res 15:164–170, 1981.
73. Laurent S, Juillerat L, London GM, et al: Increased response of brachial artery diameter to norepinephrine in hypertensive patients. Am J Physiol 255:H36–H43, 1988.
74. Buntin CM, Silver FH: Noninvasive assessment of mechanical properties of peripheral arteries. Ann Biomed Eng 18:549–566, 1990.
75. Hayoz D, Rutschmann B, Perret F, et al: Conduit artery compliance and distensibility are not necessarily reduced in hypertension. Hypertension 20:1–6, 1992.
76. Boutouyrie P, Lacolley P, Girerd XJ, et al: Sympathetic activation decreases medium-sized arterial compliance in humans. Am J Physiol 267:H1368–H1376, 1994.
77. Joannides R, Richard V, Haefeli WE, et al: Role of basal and stimulated release of nitric oxide in the regulation of radial artery caliber in humans. Hypertension 26:327–331, 1995.
78. Van Merode TP, Hick PJJ, Hoeks APG, et al: Carotid artery wall properties in normotensive and borderline hypertensive subjects of various ages. Ultrasound Med Biol 14:563–569, 1988.
79. Hoeks APG, Brands PJ, Smeets FAM, Reneman RS: Assessment of the distensibility of superficial arteries. Ultrasound Med Biol 16:121–128, 1990.
80. Porter TR, Taylor D, Pandian NG, et al: Pulmonary arterial dynamics in congestive heart failure in humans: significance of pulmonary arterial stiffness. J Vasc Med Biol 4:105–114, 1993.
81. Xu J, Shiota T, Omota R, et al: Intravascular ultrasound assessment of regional aortic wall stiffness, distensibility, and compliance in patients with coarctation of the aorta. Am Heart J 134:93–98, 1997.
82. Reddy KG, Suneja R, Nair RN, et al: Measurement by intracoronary ultrasound of in vivo arterial distensibility within atherosclerotic lesions. Am J Cardiol 72:1232–1237, 1993.
83. Kerber S, Heinemann-Vechtel O, Gunther F, et al: Coronary compliance in patients following orthotopic heart transplantation. An intravascular ultrasound study. Eur Heart J 17:1891–1897, 1996.
84. Alfonso F, Macaya C, Goicolea J, et al: Determinants of coronary compliance in patients with coronary artery disease: an intravascular ultrasound study. J Am Coll Cardiol 23:879–884, 1994.
85. Nakatani S, Yamagishi M, Tamai J, et al: Assessment of coronary artery distensibility by intravascular ultrasound: application of simultaneous measurements of luminal area and pressure. Circulation 91:2904–2910, 1995.
86. McDonald DA: Regional pulse-wave velocity in the arterial tree. J Appl Physiol 24:73–78, 1968.
87. Moens AI: Die Pulskurve. p. 90. Leiden, The Netherlands: EJ Brill, 1878.
88. Bramwell JC, Hill AV: The velocity of the pulse wave in man. Proc R Soc Lond 93B:298–306, 1922.
89. Mitchell GF, Pfeffer MA, Finn PV, Pfeffer JM: Comparison of techniques for measuring pulse-wave velocity in the rat. J Appl Physiol 82:203–207, 1997.
90. Milnor WR: Wave reflection. *In* Milnor WR (ed): Hemodynamics. pp. 192–210. Baltimore: Williams & Wilkins, 1982.
91. Wright JS, Cruickshank JK, Kontis S, et al: Aortic compliance measured by non-invasive Doppler ultrasound: description of a method and its reproducibility. Clin Sci 78:463–468, 1990.
92. Smulyan H, Vardan S, Griffiths A, Gribbin B: Forearm arterial distensibility in systolic hypertension. J Am Coll Cardiol 3:387–393, 1984.
93. Finkelstein SM, Collins VR: Vascular hemodynamic impedance measurement. Prog Cardiovasc Dis 24:401–418, 1982.
94. Chang K-C, Hsieh K-S, Kuo T-S, Chen HI: Effects of nifedipine on systemic hydraulic vascular load in patients with hypertension. Cardiovasc Res 24:719–726, 1990.
95. Fitchett DH, Simkus GJ, Beaudry JP, Marpole DGF: Reflected pressure waves in the ascending aorta: effect of glyceryl trinitrate. Cardiovasc Res 22:494–500, 1988.
96. McVeigh GE, Finkelstein SM, Cohn JN: Assessment of arterial compliance in hypertension. Curr Opin Nephrol Hypertens 2:82–86, 1993.
97. Goldwyn RM, Watt TB Jr: Arterial pressure pulse contour analysis via a mathematical model for the clinical quantification of human vascular properties. IEEE Trans Biomed Eng 14:11–17, 1967.
98. Watt TB Jr, Burrus CS: Arterial pressure contour analysis for estimating human vascular properties. J Appl Physiol 40:171–176, 1976.
99. Freis ED, Heath WC, Luchsinger PC, Snell AE: Changes in the carotid pulse which occur with age and hypertension. Am Heart J 71:757–765, 1966.
100. Frank O: Die Grundform des arteriellen Pulses. Z Biol 37:483–526, 1899.
101. Quick CM, Berger DS, Noordergraaf A: Apparent arterial compliance. Am J Physiol 274: H1393–H1403, 1998.
102. O'Rourke MF, Kelly RP: Wave reflection in the systemic circulation and its implications in ventricular function. J Hypertens 11:327–337, 1993.
103. Roman MJ, Saba S, Pini R, et al: Parallel cardiac and vascular adaptation in hypertension. Circulation 86:1909–1918, 1992.
104. Sharir T, Marmor A, Ting CT, et al: Validation of a method for non-invasive measurement of central arterial pressure. Hypertension 21:74–82, 1993.
105. Nichols WW, Avolio AP, Kelly RP, O'Rourke MF: Effects of age and of hypertension on wave travel and reflections. *In* O'Rourke MF, Safar ME, Dzau VJ (eds): Arterial Vasodilation. Mechanisms and Therapy. pp. 23–40. Philadelphia: Lea & Febiger, 1993.
106. Shock NW: Aging of physiological systems. J Chronic Dis 36:137–142, 1983.
107. Fleg JL: Alterations in cardiovascular structure and function with advancing age. Am J Cardiol 57:33C–44C, 1986.
108. Salisbury PF, Cross CE, Rieben PA: Ventricular performance modified by elastic properties of outflow system. Circ Res 11:319–328, 1962.
109. Leithe ME, Hermiller JB, Magorien RD, et al: The effect of age on central and regional hemodynamics. Gerontology 30:240–246, 1984.
110. Stout RW: Aging and atherosclerosis. Age Aging 16:65–72, 1987.
111. Auerbach O, Hammond EC, Garfinkel L: Thickening of walls of arterioles and small arteries in relation to age and smoking habits. N Engl J Med 278:980–984, 1968.
112. Gerrity RG, Cliff WJ: The aortic tunica media of the developing rat, Part I. Quantitative stereologic and biochemical analysis. Lab Invest 32:585–600, 1975.
113. Schimmler W: Correlation between the pulse wave velocity in the aortic-iliac vessel and age, sex and blood pressure. Angiology 17:314–322, 1966.
114. Avolio AP, Chen S-G, Wang R-P, et al: Effects of aging on changing arterial compliance and left ventricular load in a Northern Chinese urban community. Circulation 68:50–58, 1983.
115. Simonson E, Nakagawa K: Effect of age on pulse wave velocity and aortic ejection time in healthy men and in men with coronary artery disease. Circulation 22:126–129, 1960.
116. Smulyan H, Csermely TJ, Mookherjee S, Warner RA: Effect of age on distensibility in asymptomatic humans. Arteriosclerosis 3:199–205, 1983.
117. Avolio AP, Deng F-Q, Li W-Q, et al: Effects of aging on arterial distensibility in populations with high and low prevalence of hypertension: comparison between urban and rural communities in China. Circulation 71:202–210, 1985.
118. Walsh RA: Cardiovascular effects of the aging process. Am J Med 82(suppl 1B):34–40, 1987.
119. Shirasaki Y, Su C, Lee TJ-F, et al: Endothelial modulation of vascular relaxation to nitrovasodilators in aging and hypertension. J Pharmacol Exp Ther 239:861–866, 1986.
120. Yin FCP, Weisfeldt ML, Milnor WR: Role of aortic input impedance in the decreased cardiovascular response to exercise with aging dogs. J Clin Invest 68:28–38, 1981.
121. Gundel W, Cherry G, Rajagopalan B, et al: Aortic input impedance in man: acute response to vasodilator drugs. Circulation 63:1305–1314, 1981.

122. Nichols WW, O'Rourke MF, Avolio AP, et al: Effects of age on ventricular-vascular coupling. Am J Cardiol 55:1179–1184, 1985.
123. Linzbach AJ, Akuamoa-Boateng E: Die alternsveranderungen des menschlichen herzens. I. Das Herzgewicht im alter. Klin Wochenschr 52:156–163, 1973.
124. Gerstenblith G, Frederiksen J, Yin FCP, et al: Echocardiographic assessment of a normal adult aging population. Circulation 56:273–278, 1977.
125. Capasso JM, Sonnenblick EH: Myocardial hypertrophy and diastolic heart failure in the aging heart. Heart Failure 3:219–227, 1986.
126. Lakatta EG: Cardiovascular system aging. *In* Kent B, Butler R (eds): Human Aging Research: Concepts and Techniques. pp. 199–219. New York: Raven, 1988.
127. Rosenthal J: Aging and the cardiovascular system. Gerontology 33(suppl 1):3–8, 1987.
128. Landowne M, Brandfonbrener M, Shock NW: The relation of age to certain measures of performance of the heart and circulation. Circulation 12:567–576, 1955.
129. Wallace AG: Pathophysiology of cardiovascular disease. *In* Smith LH Jr, Thier SO (eds): Pathophysiology: The Biological Principles of Disease. pp. 1162–1167. Philadelphia: WB Saunders, 1981.
130. Van Merode T, Brands PJ, Hoeks APG, Reneman RS: Different effects of ageing on elastic and muscular arterial bifurcations in men. J Vasc Res 33:47–52, 1996.
131. Khder Y, Bray Des Boscs L, Aliot E, Zannad F: Endothelial, viscoelastic and sympathetic factors contributing to the arterial wall changes during aging. Cardiol Elderly 4:161–165, 1996.
132. McVeigh GE, Bratteli CW, Morgan DJ, et al: Age-related abnormalities in arterial compliance identified by pressure pulse contour analysis. Hypertension 33:1392–1398, 1999.
133. Farrar DJ, Green HD, Bond MG, et al: Aortic pulse wave velocity, elasticity and composition in a non-human primate model of atherosclerosis. Circ Res 43:52–62, 1978.
134. Farrar DJ, Green HD, Wagner WD, Bond MG: Reduction in pulse wave velocity and improvement of aortic distensibility accompanying regression of atherosclerosis in the rhesus monkey. Circ Res 47:425–432, 1980.
135. Nakashima T, Tanikawa J: A study of human aortic distensibility with relation to atherosclerosis and aging. Angiology 22:477–490, 1971.
136. Hickler RB: Aortic and large artery stiffness: current methodology and clinical correlations. Clin Cardiol 13:317–322, 1990.
137. El-Tamimi H, Mansour M, Wargovich TJ, et al: Constrictor and dilator responses in intracoronary acetylcholine in adjacent segments of the same coronary artery in patients with coronary disease. Circulation 89:45–51, 1994.
138. Lehmann ED: Elastic properties of the aorta. Lancet 342:1417, 1993.
139. Vonesh MJ, Cheol-Hyung C, Pinto JV Jr, et al: Regional vascular mechanical properties by 3-D intravascular ultrasound with finite-element analysis. Am J Physiol 272:H425–H437, 1997.
140. Folkow B: Physiological aspects of primary hypertension. Physiol Rev 62:347–504, 1982.
141. Wolinsky H: Long-term effects of hypertension on rat aortic wall and their relation to concurrent aging changes: morphological and chemical studies. Circ Res 30:301–309, 1972.
142. Medical Research Council Working Party: MRC trial of treatment of mild hypertension. BMJ 29:97–104, 1985.
143. Helgeland A: Treatment of mild hypertension: a 5-year controlled drug trial, The Oslo Study. Am J Med 69:725–732, 1980.
144. Hodge JV, Smirk FH: The effect of drug treatment of hypertension on the distribution of deaths from various causes. Am Heart J 73:441–452, 1967.
145. Chobanian AV: The influence of hypertension and other hemodynamic factors in atherogenesis. Prog Cardiovasc Dis 26:177–196, 1983.
146. Devereux RB, Savage DD, Sachs I, Laragh JH: Relation of hemodynamic load to left ventricular hypertrophy and performance in hypertension. Am J Cardiol 51:171–176, 1983.
147. Leenen FHH: Left ventricular hypertrophy in hypertensive patients. Am J Med 86(suppl IB):63–65, 1989.
148. Cohn JN: Arteries, myocardium, blood pressure and cardiovascular risk: towards a revised definition of hypertension. J Hypertens 16:2117–2124, 1998.
149. Heagerty AM, Aalkjaer C, Bund SJ, et al: Small artery structure in hypertension. Dual process of remodeling and growth. Hypertension 21:391–397, 1993.
150. Lund-Johansson P: Hemodynamics in essential hypertension. Clin Sci 59:343–354, 1980.
151. Folkow B: The Fourth Volhard Lecture. Cardiovascular structural adaptation: its role in the initiation and maintenance of primary hypertension. Clin Sci Mol Med 55(suppl):2s–22s, 1978.
152. Baumbach GL, Heistad DD: Remodeling of cerebral arterioles in chronic hypertension. Hypertension 13:968–972, 1989.
153. Jennings GL, Esler MD, Korner PI: Effect of prolonged treatment on haemodynamics of essential hypertension before and after autonomic block. Lancet 2:166–169, 1980.
154. Hartford M, Wendelhag I, Berglund G, et al: Cardiovascular and renal effect of long-term antihypertensive treatment. JAMA 259:2553–2557, 1988.
155. McVeigh GE, Burns DE, Finkelstein SM, et al: Reduced vascular compliance as a marker for essential hypertension. Am J Hypertens 4:245–257, 1991.
156. Liu Z, Ting C-T, Zhu S, Yin FCP: Aortic compliance in human hypertension. Hypertension 14:129–136, 1989.
157. Simon A, Levenson J: Use of arterial compliance for evaluation of hypertension. Am J Hypertens 4:97–105, 1991.
158. Ventura H, Messerli FH, Oigman W, et al: Impaired systemic arterial compliance in borderline hypertension. Am Heart J 108:132–136, 1984.
159. Simon ACH, Laurent S, Levenson JA, et al: Estimation of forearm arterial compliance in normal and hypertensive men from simultaneous pressure and flow measurements in the brachial artery, using a pulsed Doppler device and a first-order arterial model during diastole. Cardiovasc Res 17:331–338, 1983.
160. Levenson J, Simon A: Heterogeneity of response of peripheral arteries to antihypertensive drugs in essential hypertension. Basic effects and functional consequences. Drugs 35(suppl 5):34–39, 1988.
161. Armentano R, Simon A, Levenson J, et al: Mechanical pressure versus intrinsic effects of hypertension on large arteries in humans. Hypertension 18:657–666, 1991.
162. Dzau VJ, Safar ME: Large conduit arteries in hypertension: role of the vascular renin-angiotensin system. Circulation 77:947–954, 1988.
163. Gribben B, Pickering TG, Sleight P: Arterial distensibility in normal and hypertensive man. Clin Sci 56:413–417, 1979.
164. Gariepy J, Massonneau M, Levenson J, et al: Evidence for in vivo carotid and femoral wall thickening in human hypertension. Hypertension 22:111–118, 1993.
165. Lever AF, Harrup SB: Essential hypertension: a disorder of growth with origins in childhood. J Hypertens 10:101–120, 1992.
166. Mulvany MJ: A reduced elastic modulus of vascular wall components in hypertension? Hypertension 20:7–9, 1992.
167. Mulvany MJ: Biophysical aspects of resistance vessels studied in spontaneous and renal hypertensive rats. Acta Physiol Scand 133(suppl 571):129–135, 1988.
168. Contard F, Abbelkarim S, Glukhova M, et al: Arterial smooth muscle cell phenotype in stroke-prone spontaneously hypertensive rats. Hypertension 22:665–676, 1993.
169. Bohlen HG: Localization of vascular resistance changes during hypertension. Hypertension 8:181–183, 1986.
170. Falloon BJ, Bund SJ, Tulip JR, Heagerty AM: In vitro perfusion studies of resistance artery function in genetic hypertension. Hypertension 22:486–495, 1993.
171. Colwell JA, Lopes-Virella MF: A review of the development of large vessel disease in diabetes mellitus. Am J Med 85(suppl 5A):113–118, 1988.
172. Siperstein MD: Diabetic microangiopathy, genetics, environment and treatment. Am J Med (suppl 5A):119–130, 1988.
173. Garcia MJ, McNamara PM, Gordon T, Kannel WB: Morbidity and mortality in diabetics in the Framingham population. Sixteen year follow-up study. Diabetes 23:105–111, 1974.
174. Ruderman NB, Haudenschild C: Diabetes as an atherogenic factor. Prog Cardiovasc Dis 26:373–408, 1984.
175. Freedman DS, Gruchow HW, Bamrah VS, et al: Diabetes mellitus and arteriographically-documented coronary artery disease. J Clin Epidemiol 41:659–668, 1988.
176. Waller BF, Palumbo PJ, Lie JT, Roberts WC: Status of the coronary arteries at necropsy in diabetes mellitus with onset after age 30 years. Analysis of 229 diabetic patients with and without clinical evidence of coronary heart disease and comparison to 183 control subjects. Am J Med 69:498–506, 1980.

177. Ledet T, Heickendorff L, Rasmussen LM: Pathology of macrovascular disease. *In* Nattrass M, Hale PJ (eds): Bailliere's Clinical Endocrinology and Metabolism. Vol. 2, No. 2. Non-Insulin Dependent Diabetes. pp. 391–405. Eastbourne, England: Bailliere Tindall, 1988.
178. Ledet T: Diabetic macroangiopathy and growth hormone. Diabetes 30(suppl):14–17, 1981.
179. Legg MA, Harawi SJ: *In* Marble A, Krall LP, Bradley RF, et al (eds): Joslin's Diabetes Mellitus. 12th ed. pp. 298–331. Philadelphia: Lea & Febiger, 1975.
180. Barnett AH: Pathogenesis of diabetic microangiopathy. An overview. Am J Med 90(suppl 6A):67S–73S, 1991.
181. Lorenzi M, Cagliero E: Pathobiology of endothelial and other vascular cells in diabetes mellitus. Diabetes 40:653–659, 1991.
182. Merimee TJ: Diabetic retinopathy. A synthesis of perspectives. N Engl J Med 322:978–983, 1990.
183. Monnier VM, Vishwanath V, Frank KE, et al: Relation between complications of type 1 diabetes mellitus and collagen-linked fluorescence. N Engl J Med 314:403–408, 1986.
184. Woolham GL, Schnur PL, Vallbona C, Hoff HE: The pulse wave velocity as an early indicator of atherosclerosis in diabetic subjects. Circulation 25:533–539, 1962.
185. Scarpello JHB, Martin TRP, Ward JD: Ultrasound measurements of pulse-wave velocity in the peripheral arteries of diabetic subjects. Clin Sci 58:53–57, 1980.
186. Wahlqvist ML, Lo CS, Myers KA: Fish intake and arterial wall characteristics in healthy people and diabetic subjects. Lancet 2:944–946, 1989.
187. Pillsbury HC, Hung W, Kyle MC, Fries ED: Arterial pulse waves and velocity and systolic time intervals in diabetic children. Am Heart J 87:783–790, 1973.
188. Kool MJ, Lambert J, Stehouwer CD, et al: Vessel wall properties of large arteries in uncomplicated IDDM. Diabetes Care 18:618–624, 1995.
189. Salomaa V, Riley W, Kark JD, et al: Non-insulin dependent diabetes mellitus and fasting glucose and insulin concentrations are associated with arterial stiffness indexes. Circulation 91:1432–1443, 1995.
190. Lax H, Feinburg AW: Abnormalities of the arterial pulse wave in young diabetic subjects. Circulation 20:1106–1110, 1959.
191. Feinburg AW, Lax H: Vascular abnormalities in children with diabetes mellitus. JAMA 201:515–518, 1967.
192. Freis ED, Kyle ML: Computer analysis of carotid and brachial pulse waves. Effects of age in normal subjects. Am J Cardiol 22:691–695, 1968.
193. Kelly R, Hayward C, Avolio A, O'Rourke M: Non-invasive determination of age-related changes in the human arterial pulse. Circulation 80:1652–1659, 1989.
194. McVeigh G, Brennan G, Hayes R, et al: Vascular abnormalities in non–insulin-dependent diabetes mellitus identified by arterial waveform analysis. Am J Med 95:424–430, 1993.
195. McVeigh GE: Pulse contour and impedance parameters derived from analysis of arterial waveforms. Automedica 13:141–148, 1991.
196. McVeigh GE, Brennan GM, Cohn JN, et al: Fish oil improves arterial compliance in non–insulin-dependent diabetes mellitus. Arterioscler Thromb 14:1425–1429, 1994.
197. Ross J: Afterload mismatch and preload reserve: a conceptual framework for the analysis of ventricular function. Prog Cardiovasc Dis 18:255–264, 1976.
198. Weber KT, Janicki JS, Hunter WC, et al: The contractile behavior of the heart and its functional coupling to the circulation. Prog Cardiovasc Dis 24:375–400, 1982.
199. Pepine CJ, Nichols WW, Conti CR: Aortic input impedance in heart failure. Circulation 58:460–465, 1978.
200. Laskey WK, Kussmaul WG, Martin JL, et al: Characteristics of vascular hydraulic load in patients with heart failure. Circulation 72:61–67, 1985.
201. Merillon JP, Fontenier G, Leralluit JF, et al: Aortic input impedance in heart failure: comparison with normal subjects and its changes during vasodilator therapy. Eur Heart J 5:447–455, 1984.
202. Giannattasio C, Failla M, Stella ML, et al: Alterations of radial artery compliance in patients with congestive heart failure. Am J Cardiol 76:381–385, 1995.
203. Lage SG, Kopel L, Monachini MC, et al: Carotid arterial compliance in patients with congestive heart failure secondary to idiopathic dilated cardiomyopathy. Am J Cardiol 74:691–695, 1994.
204. Arnold JMO, Marchiori GE, Emrie JR, et al: Large artery function in patients with chronic heart failure. Circulation 84:2418–2425, 1991.
205. Ramsey MW, Goodfellow J, Jones CJH, et al: Endothelial control of arterial distensibility is impaired in chronic heart failure. Circulation 92:3212–3219, 1995.
206. Finkelstein SM, Cohn JN, Collins VR, et al: Vascular hemodynamic impedance in congestive heart failure. Am J Cardiol 55:423–427, 1985.
207. Eaton GM, Cody RJ, Binkley PF: Increased aortic impedance precedes peripheral vasoconstriction at the early stage of ventricular failure in the paced canine model. Circulation 88:2714–2721, 1993.
208. Gaballa MA, Raya RE, Goldman S: Large artery remodeling after myocardial infarction. Am J Physiol 268:H2092–H2103, 1995.
209. Pepine CJ, Nichols WW, Curry Jr RC, Conte CR: Aortic input impedance during nitroprusside infusion. J Clin Invest 64:643–654, 1979.
210. Binkley PF, Van Fossen DB, Nunziata E, et al: Influence of positive inotropic therapy on pulsatile hydraulic load and ventricular-vascular coupling in congestive heart failure. J Am Coll Cardiol 15:1127–1135, 1990.
211. Yin FCP, Guzman PA, Brin KP, et al: Effect of nitroprusside on hydraulic vascular loads on the right and left ventricle of patients with heart failure. Circulation 67:1330–1339, 1983.
212. Laskey WK, Kussmaul WG: Arterial wave reflection in heart failure. Circulation 75:711–722, 1987.

CHAPTER 80

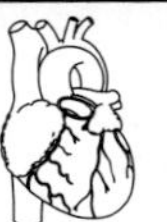

HYPERTENSION

Bernard Waeber, Hans R. Brunner, Michel Burnier, and Jay N. Cohn

PATHOPHYSIOLOGY
Monogenic Forms of Hypertension
Essential Hypertension
Secondary Forms of Hypertension
CLINICAL RECOGNITION
History
Physical Examination
Measurement of Blood Pressure
Workup of the Hypertensive Patient
The Search for Secondary Hypertension
NATURAL HISTORY
Pathologic Consequences of Hypertension
Prevention of Cardiovascular Diseases by Antihypertensive Treatment
Definition of Hypertension
Hypertension in Childhood and Adolescence
Hypertension in Pregnancy
Malignant Hypertension
TREATMENT
Nonpharmacologic Control of Hypertension
Pharmacologic Treatment
Sequential Monotherapy
Combination Therapy
Associated Diseases
Special Considerations
CONCLUSIONS

Hypertension is a common disorder that contributes importantly to the high cardiovascular morbidity and mortality observed in industrialized countries. The proper diagnosis and management of this condition afford considerable reduction of the risk of developing cardiac, cerebral, and renal complications. Approximately 95 percent of patients with high blood pressure exhibit a so-called essential, or primary, form of hypertension. Various mechanisms are involved in the pathogenesis of this type of hypertension. This heterogeneity accounts for the diverse therapeutic approaches that have been utilized and for the rationale for individualizing treatment programs. In a small fraction of patients, the elevation of blood pressure is due to a specific cause (secondary hypertension). The recognition of such patients has improved markedly in recent years. This is relevant because secondary hypertension can often be cured by appropriate interventions.

The diagnosis of hypertension has been based entirely on the demonstration of a measured blood pressure above the normal range of values. Although this measurement clearly identifies individuals at an increased risk of developing morbid cardiovascular events, the disease is not the blood pressure but is rather the vascular abnormality that results in these morbid events.[1] Indeed, morbid vascular events occur in many individuals whose blood pressure is within the normal range, and many individuals with frankly elevated blood pressures do not experience morbid events. Consequently, there is a growing sense that measured blood pressure is not, by itself, an adequate marker for the presence of the vascular disease that requires aggressive treatment. Efforts to develop methods to more specifically assess the blood vessels that are the site of abnormality in hypertension are still too preliminary to advocate their widespread clinical use at the present time. Therefore, in this section, we focus our attention on the magnitude of elevation of the blood pressure, with full recognition that the disease represents a blood vessel abnormality and its treatment is aimed at preventing vascular events, not merely lowering an elevated pressure.

PATHOPHYSIOLOGY

Monogenic Forms of Hypertension

The genetic and molecular basis of several mendelian, single-gene forms of hypertension has been identified.[2] A better understanding of the pathways involved in the pathogenesis of these rare forms of hypertension may help in the future to recognize new mechanisms involved in the pathogenesis of essential hypertension. The well-defined monogenic forms of hypertension are glucocorticoid-remediable aldosteronism, the syndrome of apparent mineralocorticoid excess, and Liddle's syndrome. Some characteristics of these diseases are given in Table 80–1.

Patients with glucocorticoid-remediable aldosteronism have a chimeric gene encoding both aldosterone synthase and 11β-hydroxylase in the adrenal fasciculata.[3] In normal individuals, aldosterone synthase is found only in the adrenal fasciculata, and the expression and the activity of this enzyme is not controlled by adrenocorticotropic hormone (ACTH). In patients with glucocorticoid-remediable aldosteronism, aldosterone secretion becomes dependent on ACTH because of the presence of an ACTH-sensitive regulatory element in the chimeric gene (this regulatory element is physiologically present in the 11β-hydroxylase gene). In this form of hypertension, dexamethasone treatment suppresses ACTH secretion and, by this means, aldosterone secretion.

In patients with the syndrome of apparent mineralocorticoid excess, the activity of 11β-hydroxysteroid dehydrogenase is decreased.[4] This enzyme normally metabolizes cortisol (by activating the mineralocorticoid receptor) to

TABLE 80–1 **Principal Characteristics of Monogenic Forms of Hypertension**

Form	Transmission	Gene Abnormality	Pathophysiologic Mechanism
GRA	Autosomal dominant	Chimeric gene encoding aldosterone synthase and 11β-hydroxylase	Increased ACTH-dependent secretion of aldosterone → salt and water retention
AME	Autosomal recessive	11β-hydroxysteroid dehydrogenase deficiency	Decreased metabolism of cortisol, increased activation of the mineralocorticoid receptor → salt and water retention
LS	Autosomal dominant	Mutations in genes encoding either the β or the γ subunits of the ENaC	Increased activity of the ENaC → salt and water retention

Abbreviations: ACTH, adrenocorticotropic hormone; AME, syndrome of apparent mineralocorticoid excess; ENaC, amiloride-sensitive epithelial Na^+ channel; GRA, glucocorticoid-remediable aldosteronism; LS, Liddle's syndrome.

cortisone (devoid of mineralocorticoid activity). The impaired degradation of cortisol leads, therefore, to an increased activation of the mineralocorticoid receptor.

The amiloride-sensitive epithelial Na^+ channel (ENaC) is a rate-limiting step of sodium reabsorption regulated by aldosterone. This channel is composed of 3 subunits (α, β, and γ). Patients with Liddle's syndrome have mutations in genes encoding either the β or the γ subunits, with an ensuing hyperactivity of the channel.[5]

Patients with glucocorticoid-remediable aldosteronism, the syndrome of apparent mineralocorticoid excess, or Liddle's syndrome are all retaining excessive sodium and water in the renal distal tubule, where mineralocorticoid receptors are located. The mineralocorticoid effect is associated with a loss of potassium and a suppression of renin secretion owing to the plasma volume expansion.

Essential Hypertension

Cardiovascular homeostasis is normally maintained by a close interplay among various mechanisms. In patients with essential hypertension, one or more of these mechanisms may be dysregulated, the imbalance manifesting by an increase in blood pressure (Fig. 80–1).

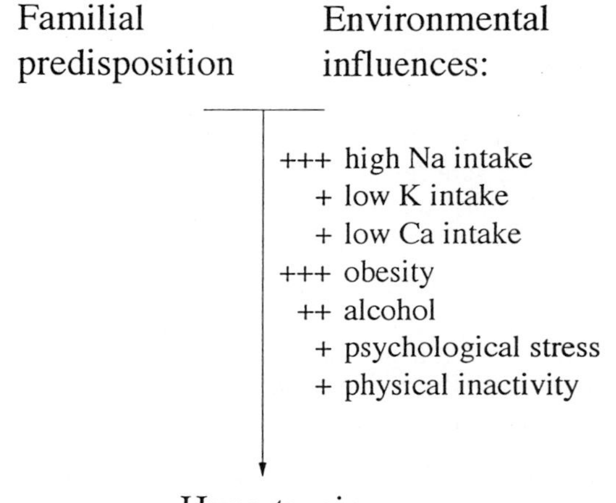

FIGURE 80–1 Interaction between genetic (familial) and environmental factors in the pathogenesis of hypertension. The clinical relevance of the different environmental factors is rated from minor (+) to major (+ + +).

Familial Predisposition

There exists a clear familial aggregation of blood pressure. Newborns of hypertensive parents have higher blood pressures than those of normotensive parents, the difference becoming prominent in adolescence. Also, blood pressure correlates better between monozygotic than dizygotic twins. Finally, subjects with a positive family history of hypertension are particularly prone to develop hypertension.[6] In most patients, hypertension seems to be polygenic. Most likely, specific genes interact with environmental factors to determine the expression of hypertension. This view is compatible with the heterogeneous character of hypertension. The expression of some genes can be detected with the aid of specific biochemical markers. For instance, several membrane cation flux abnormalities are present in a fraction of prehypertensives and hypertensives as well as in their first-degree relatives (see Membrane Abnormalities). Another example is a low urinary kallikrein excretion in hypertension-prone families (see Decreased Activity of Vasodilating Systems). Also well established is a genetic influence on salt sensitivity of blood pressure (see Environmental Influences). Recently, an inherited form of hypertension has been recognized in patients presenting with high blood pressure, obesity, insulin resistance, and dyslipidemia (see Hyperinsulinemia). In this subset of patients, a genetic component is clearly apparent. Several criteria may be clinically useful to identify normotensive persons genetically prone to develop future hypertension. These criteria include an excessive blood pressure increase in response to physical exercise or mental arithmetic.[7, 8] Searching for the expression of candidate genes for hypertension may help to detect persons susceptible to become hypertensive and to initiate early preventive treatment.[9] Conceivably, it may also provide better insight into the mechanisms responsible for the blood pressure elevation and allow for more rational therapeutics.

Specific mutations of several candidate genes seem to be positively related to essential hypertension. They include genes encoding angiotensinogen,[10, 11] aldosterone synthase,[12] endothelial nitric oxide synthase,[13] and alpha-adducin, a cytoskeleton protein involved in cell membrane ion transport.[14]

Noteworthy, there exists in humans a polymorphism of angiotensin-converting enzyme (ACE) consisting of either the absence (deletion, D) or the presence (insertion, I) of a 287 base-pair DNA fragment inside intron 16.[15] The DD and DI genotypes have been claimed to be associated with a higher risk of hypertension, but whether this is true remains controversial.[16] There is, however, good evidence that the D allele, which is linked with increased circulating levels of ACE, behaves as a marker of atherosclerotic and renal microvascular complications. A polymorphism in the gene encoding the angiotensin II type 1 (AT_1) receptor has also been described, but it is still unclear whether mutations in this gene are linked with high blood pressure.[17, 18] Finally, the ENaC gene was also studied in patients with essential hypertension. So far, no cosegregation between mutations of this channel and high blood pressure has been found in hypertensive patients.[19]

Environmental Influences

SODIUM INTAKE

Among environmental factors known to influence blood pressure, salt intake holds a predominant position. Salt consumption can be assessed best by measuring 24-hour urinary sodium excretion. Numerous epidemiologic studies have pointed to a positive association between dietary sodium chloride overload and the prevalence of hypertension.[20] This is particularly apparent in between-population studies, when comparing low-salt–consuming with high-salt–consuming ethnic groups. A striking feature is the lack of blood pressure elevation with aging in nonindustrialized civilizations accustomed to eating less than 30 mmol/da of sodium. Migration studies have also suggested a blood pressure–raising effect of the sodium ion. Such studies are of great interest because migrant and nonmigrant communities have a similar genetic background. In contrast to between-population and migration studies, most within-population studies have not found any close relationship between blood pressure and sodium intake. Only a 2.2 mm Hg difference in systolic blood pressure can be expected for a difference of 100 mmol/da of sodium.[21] The susceptibility to increase blood pressure in response to sodium loading is highly variable. The salt sensitivity of blood pressure has a familial character and can be evidenced already in the prehypertensive state.[22] Low birth weight has been associated with elevated blood pressure in children and with hypertension in adults.[23] This association may be due to an inborn deficit in nephron number and an ensuing increased renal retention of sodium. In Western societies, sodium intake is generally between 150 and 250 mmol/da. Individuals becoming hypertensive on such a diet presumably represent salt-sensitive persons.

POTASSIUM INTAKE

The day-to-day variation in potassium intake is larger than that in sodium intake. Potassium consumption can be evaluated either by performing a 24-hour dietary recall or by measuring 24-hour urinary electrolyte excretion. Migration as well as between-population and within-population studies have shown an inverse relationship between potassium intake and the prevalence of hypertension.[24] Black subjects ingest less potassium than do white subjects. This could explain, in part, the tendency for more severe hypertension observed in blacks.

CALCIUM INTAKE

The prevalence of hypertension is higher in geographic areas supplied with "soft" water (i.e., water containing only a limited amount of calcium). Population data indicate that the lower the dietary calcium intake, the greater the likelihood of becoming hypertensive.[25]

OBESITY

There is a strong positive correlation between body fat and blood pressure levels. This relationship is seen within the whole range of body fat distribution. The prevalence of hypertension is greater in persons with central, abdominal obesity, as reflected by a high waist:hip ratio, than in those with peripheral, gluteal fat and a low waist:hip ratio.[26] Hypertension in the obese with fat accumulation in the upper body segments is often associated with insulin resistance and hyperlipidemia (see Hyperinsulinemia).

ALCOHOL

Regular consumption of more than 30 g/da ethanol is linked with an increased prevalence of hypertension.[27] It is, however, still unclear whether smaller amounts exert a pressor effect.

PSYCHOLOGICAL STRESS

Behavioral factors are often believed to play a pathogenic role in the development of hypertension.[28] Mental stress can undoubtedly elicit pressor responses. The blood pressure reactivity to environmental stimuli seems to be related to personality traits, being exaggerated, for instance, in type A individuals—that is, patients who display a high degree of competitiveness, aggressiveness, impatience, and a striving for achievement.[29] Basal blood pressure of type A people is most often not abnormally elevated. It remains, therefore, uncertain whether intermittent elevations in blood pressure resulting from repeated exposure to psychological stressors can lead to sustained elevations of blood pressure.

PHYSICAL INACTIVITY

A number of epidemiologic studies have demonstrated an inverse relationship between estimates of physical activity and blood pressure levels.[30] Unfortunately, it is difficult to ascertain whether these observations are independent of body fat. This is because physically fit people are usually less obese than persons not exposed to regular physical activity.

Increased Activity of Vasoconstrictor Systems

SYMPATHETIC NERVOUS SYSTEM

The sympathetic nervous system plays a pivotal role in the regulation of vascular tone.[31] It modulates the cardiac output and peripheral vascular resistance, the two determinants of blood pressure. Norepinephrine released by adrenergic nerve endings causes an arterial and venous constriction via activation of postsynaptic $alpha_1$-receptors and α_2-receptors

(Fig. 80–2). The resulting increase in arteriolar tone is responsible for a blood pressure elevation. Beta$_2$-adrenergic receptors are also found postsynaptically, and their activation leads to vasorelaxation. Cardiac output may be augmented in response to sympathetic stimulation because of an increased venous return and β-adrenergic receptor–mediated direct inotropic and chronotropic effects. Sympathetic effects are mediated by epinephrine, predominantly released from the adrenal medulla, and norepinephrine, released into the synaptic cleft from sympathetic nerve endings. Epinephrine, therefore, largely circulates as a hormone, whereas the circulating norepinephrine represents the overflow of a local hormone whose site of action is largely on receptors exposed to the synaptic cleft. Presynaptic activation of β_2-receptors facilitates the neurotransmitter release, whereas this process is inhibited by activation of prejunctional α_2-adrenergic receptors. The activity of the sympathetic nervous system is under the control of brain areas involved in cardiovascular homeostasis—for example, brain stem centers governing reflex responses. These cardiovascular centers receive afferent neurons from peripheral cardiopulmonary and arterial baroreceptors and actively adjust the sympathoadrenal outflow.

Clinical evaluation of the neurogenic component of hypertension is difficult. Plasma norepinephrine concentrations are elevated in only a fraction of patients with high blood pressure.[32] Increased levels are observed mainly in younger patients with borderline hypertension, a "hyperkinetic" form of hypertension associated with a high cardiac output.[33] The norepinephrine concentration in the circulation, however, does not necessarily reflect the actual concentration prevailing in the vicinity of prejunctional and postjunctional adrenergic receptors.[34] Moreover, sympathetic outflow is organ specific. Direct evidence for a neurogenic hyperactivity in hypertensive patients has been provided by recording peripheral sympathetic drive.[35] Also, spectral analysis of the heart rate variability has suggested enhanced sympathetic and reduced vagal activities in hypertensive patients.[36] In older patients with established hypertension, cardiac output is no longer elevated and there is generally no evidence for a causal sympathetic component, at least as assessed by plasma norepinephrine determination. In fact, an age-dependent increase in plasma norepinephrine occurs in normotensive individuals, but not in hypertensive patients. Nevertheless, neurogenic factors may contribute to the enhanced peripheral vascular resistance in patients with sustained hypertension, perhaps because of an increased arteriolar responsiveness to α-adrenergic receptor stimulation.[37]

Several dysfunctions of the sympathetic nervous system have been described in hypertensive patients.[37–39] As already pointed out (see Environmental Influences), some patients have a genetically linked hyper-responsiveness to ordinary daily psychosocial stimuli or to exaggerated salt intake. Centrally mediated reinforcement of sympathetic nerve activity may contribute to the elevation of blood pressure seen in these patients. Another abnormality involving the central nervous system seems to be an impaired baroreceptor reflex sensitivity, which might be accompanied in hypertensive patients by an enhanced blood pressure variability. Hypertension might also be associated with alterations of β-adrenergic receptors. Young patients with borderline or mild hypertension frequently present with increased heart rate, cardiac output, and forearm blood flow, which points to an enhanced involvement of β-adrenergic receptors. This could be attributed to a heightened density of β-adrenergic receptors or to a hyper-responsiveness of these receptors. Speculatively, as hypertension becomes established, a functional uncoupling of the β-adrenergic receptor activation from the cellular response could occur, which might be manifest by a greater α-adrenergic receptor–mediated vasoconstriction. Epinephrine is also a vasoconstrictor potentially contributing to the genesis of hypertension.[40] Plasma levels of this catecholamine are often elevated in patients with borderline or mild hypertension. Epinephrine may act principally by stimulating presynaptic β_2-adrenergic receptors and thereby augmenting the discharge of norepinephrine.

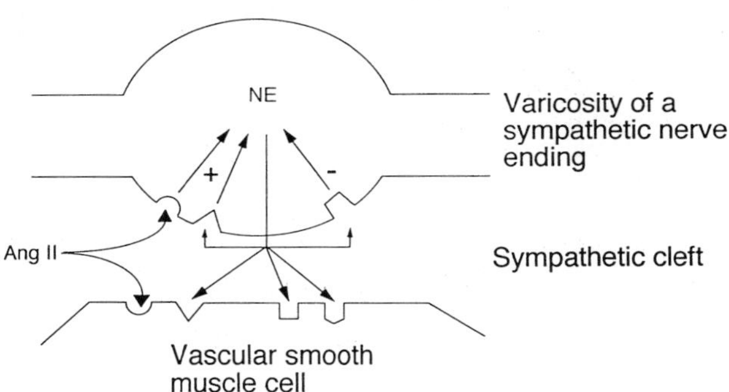

FIGURE 80–2 Presynaptic regulation of norepinephrine release. A positive feedback is exerted by the stimulation of β_2-adrenergic receptors and angiotensin II (Ang II) receptors and a negative feedback by activation of α_2-adrenergic receptors. Postsynaptically, the stimulation of α_1, α_2, and Ang II receptors causes a vasoconstriction; that of β_2-receptors, a vasodilatation.

RENIN-ANGIOTENSIN SYSTEM

Activation of the renin-angiotensin system starts with renin secretion from the kidney and culminates in the formation of angiotensin II (Fig. 80–3). Renin is a proteolytic enzyme cleaving off the decapeptide angiotensin I from angiotensinogen, a protein substrate synthesized by the liver and circulating in the blood. Angiotensin I is devoid of any vasoactive effect; a converting enzyme splits it into two fragments, of which the larger, an octapeptide, represents the final hormone angiotensin II.[41] The ACE is also called kininase II because it is one of the enzymes physiologically involved in breaking down bradykinin, a vasodilating peptide (see Decreased Activity of Vasodilating Systems). Most of the angiotensin I is converted to angiotensin II during its passage through the pulmonary circulation, but the ACE is ubiquitously present at the surface of endothelial cells.[42] Moreover, the enzyme is found in the circulation. Renin may, therefore, generate angiotensin II within all vascular beds. In addition, there seems to exist in the vascular wall all the components required for the genera-

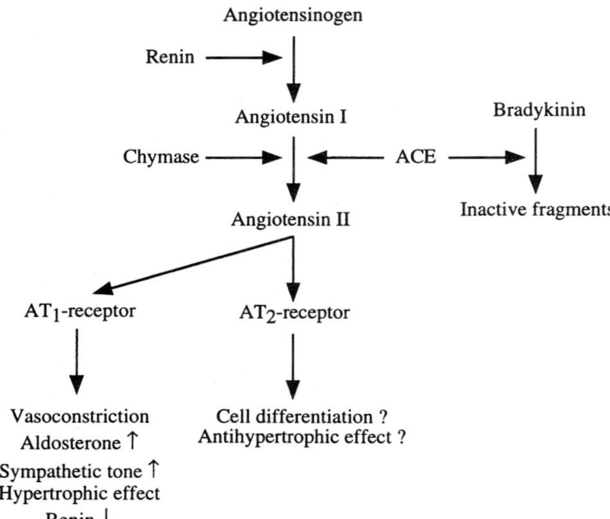

FIGURE 80–3 Biochemical cascade of the renin-angiotensin system. ACE, angiotensin-converting enzyme; AT_1, AT_2, subtypes of angiotensin II receptors.

tion of angiotensin II.[43] Whether renin and angiotensinogen found in vascular smooth muscle cells are originating from the circulation or are produced locally is, however, still debated. Noteworthy, non–ACE-dependent pathways can also transform angiotensin I into angiotensin II. This can be done, for example, by chymase, a chymotrypsin-like proteinase present in the heart and blood vessels.[44]

Two functionally different angiotensin II receptors have been characterized in humans, the AT_1 and AT_2 receptors.[45] Stimulation of the AT_1 receptor is responsible for all known physiologic effects of angiotensin II. The AT_1 receptor has been cloned and sequenced. It is G-protein–coupled and contains 359 amino acids. Angiotensin II can increase blood pressure by several mechanisms. It is a potent vasoconstrictor, stimulates aldosterone release from the adrenal glomerulosa (see Renin Sodium Retention), and reinforces the neurogenic-controlled vascular tone. Angiotensin II interacts with the peripheral sympathetic nervous system by activating receptors located on sympathetic nerve endings to facilitate norepinephrine release.[46] Postsynaptically, it may enhance the contractile response to α-adrenergic receptor stimulation. Circulating angiotensin II may also reach brain stem cardiovascular centers through areas devoid of a tight blood-brain barrier, thereby increasing sympathetic efferent activity.[46] Other effects of AT_1 receptor stimulation are an activation of vascular and cardiac growth and a suppression of renin release. The role of the AT_2 receptors has not yet been identified with certainty. Stimulation of this receptor might be involved in cell differentiation and exert an antihypertrophic action.

In a majority of patients with essential hypertension, renin secretion, for a given state of sodium balance, is within the same limits as those established in normotensive subjects. In approximately 15 percent of the patients, however, plasma renin activity is higher than normal, whereas in roughly 25 percent, renin release seems to be reduced.[47] Renin secretion is increased by sodium depletion and suppressed by sodium loading. In a given hypertensive patient, the contribution of angiotensin II to the maintenance of high blood pressure is thus augmented by shifting from a high-sodium to a low-sodium diet.[48] Activation of β-adrenergic receptors triggers the release of renin from juxtaglomerular cells.[49] In the early phase of hypertension, the high renin levels may be secondary to an increased autonomic nervous activity.[50] Renin secretion decreases with age, in both normotensive and hypertensive people, reflecting presumably a sodium retention associated with a progressive decline in functional nephrons.[51]

Decreased Activity of Vasodilating Systems

KALLIKREIN-KININ SYSTEM

The basic elements of the kallikrein-kinin system consist of proteases (kallikreins) that release kinins from precursor proteins (kininogen).[52] There exist two kinds of kallikrein, namely, plasma and tissue, also called glandular kallikrein (Fig. 80–4). Plasma kallikrein produces the nonapeptide bradykinin from a high-molecular-weight kininogen, whereas renal kallikrein cleaves both low-molecular-weight and high-molecular-weight kininogen to generate the decapeptide kallidin, the latter then being processed to bradykinin. The stimulation of bradykinin receptors situated on the endothelium causes the release of the vasodilator endothelium-derived relaxing factor (nitric oxide [NO]; see Endothelial Dysfunction) and prostacyclin. In the kidney, kinins have a diuretic and a natriuretic effect. Part of this effect might be due to a bradykinin-induced stimulation of prostaglandin synthesis. Of note is that mineralocorticoids, prostaglandins, and a high-sodium intake are known to increase urinary kallikrein excretion. The plasma kallikrein-kinin system is involved mainly in the local regulation of vascu-

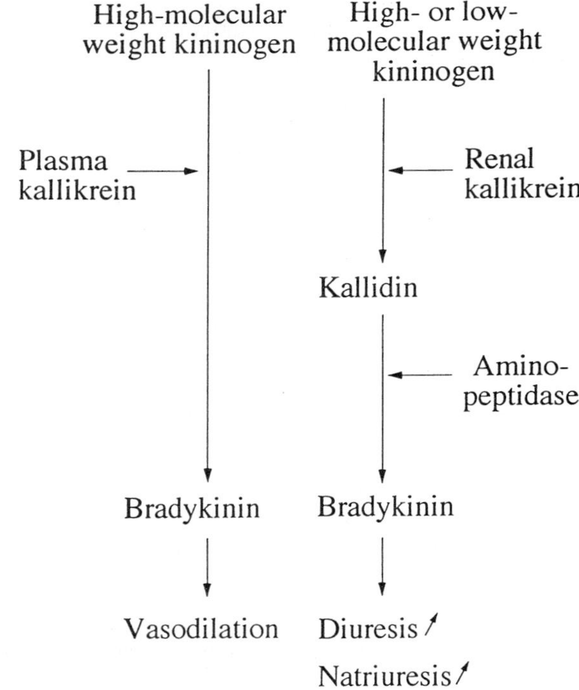

FIGURE 80–4 Components and actions of the kallikrein-kinin system.

lar tone and blood flow. During infusion of bradykinin in hypertensive patients, extremely high concentrations of the peptide must be reached to reduce systemic blood pressure.[53] An abnormality in the activity of the renal kallikrein-kinin system is, however, possible in hypertension. Urinary kallikrein excretion is often lessened in hypertensive patients, but a causal relationship between a decreased intrarenal formation of kinins and the abnormal elevation of blood pressure has not yet been proved. As already mentioned in this chapter (see Familial Predisposition), a deficiency in urinary kallikrein has been recognized as a strong marker of a genetic component of essential hypertension.

ATRIAL NATRIURETIC FACTOR

Atrial natriuretic factor (ANF) is a 28-amino acid residue that is released into the circulation by cardiac atria.[54, 55] ANF possesses diuretic, natriuretic, and vasodilatory properties (Fig. 80–5). It also exerts an inhibitory action on aldosterone and renin release. Moreover, this peptide produces a shift of fluid from the vascular space to the extravascular compartment. ANF is secreted mainly as a result of atrial stretching. Raised plasma levels of ANF have been described in a fraction of patients with essential hypertension, but a role for atrial distention in the genesis of the elevated levels has not been fully established. Blood volume is generally not expanded in such patients, but it is possible that, owing to a greater venous return, a shift of blood to the thorax occurs, with an ensuing increase in central blood volume. Evidence for an enhanced venous tone in essential hypertensive patients has been presented.[56] Furthermore, enlarged atria have been demonstrated by echocardiography in hypertensive persons with elevated plasma ANF levels, and this can be taken as an argument in favor of atrial distention as a major stimulus for ANF release.[57] This finding is also compatible with the increased central venous pressures measured in some hypertensive patients.[58] Plasma ANF levels have repeatedly been shown to increase in response to sodium loading, in both normotensive and hypertensive persons. The propensity of ANF to increase during exposure to a high dietary intake appears to be blunted in normotensive individuals with a family history of hypertension, suggesting a link between this hereditary disturbance and the predisposition to future hypertension.[59]

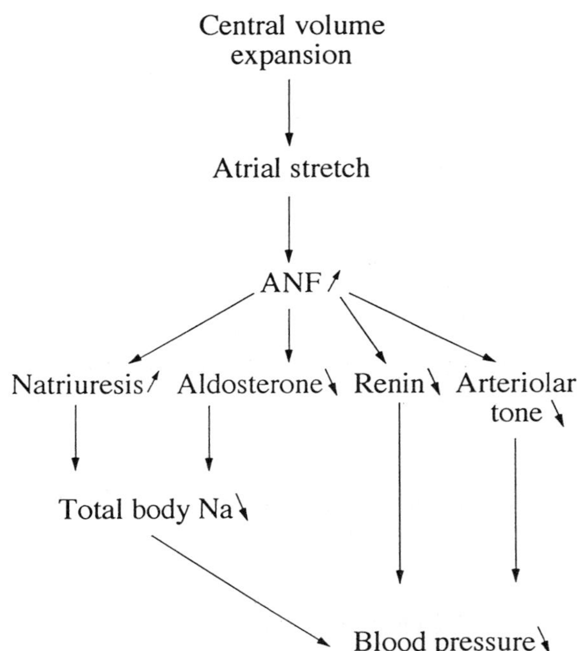

FIGURE 80–5 Atrial natriuretic factor (ANF) is secreted into the circulation in response to atrial stretch. This hormone then acts on target organs to lower blood pressure.

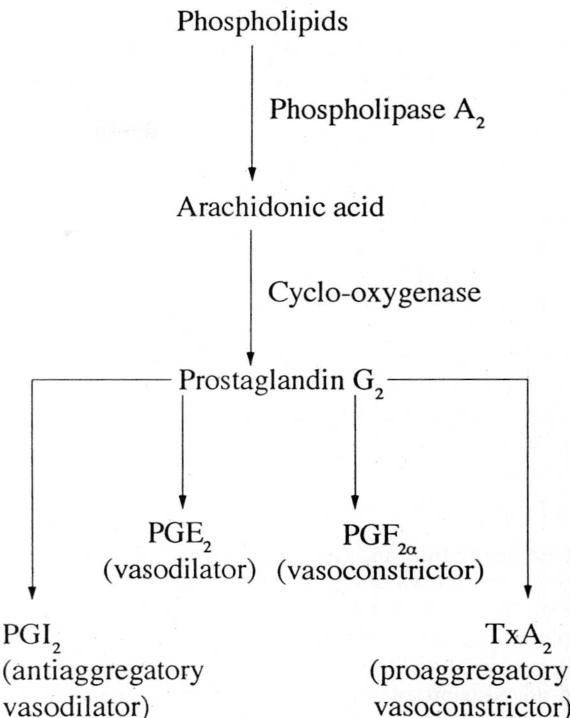

FIGURE 80–6 Steps in prostaglandin (PG) synthesis. TxA_2, thromboxane A_2.

PROSTAGLANDINS

Arachidonic acid, the precursor of prostaglandins, is released from phospholipids contained in cell membranes under the action of phospholipase A_2 (Fig. 80–6). Activation of this enzyme may result from a variety of stimuli, including angiotensin II, norepinephrine, and bradykinin. Arachidonic acid is converted to prostaglandin E_2 (PGE_2, a vasodilator), prostaglandin F_2 (PGF_2, a vasoconstrictor), thromboxane A_2 (TxA_2, a proaggregatory vasoconstrictor), or prostacyclin (PGI_2, an antiaggregatory vasodilator).[60] Prostaglandins are rapidly destroyed by local metabolism, and it is therefore unlikely that these substances play a major role away from the site of their synthesis. Vasodilatory prostaglandins not only possess direct relaxant properties but also attenuate the vasoconstrictor effect of angiotensin II and norepinephrine. PGI_2 and PGE_2, via a presynaptic effect, diminish the release of norepinephrine induced by sympathetic nerve stimulation. These two prostaglandins are also known to stimulate renin secretion. In the kidneys, prostaglandin-related mechanisms seem to participate in the regulation of renal perfusion and blood flow distribution. PGE_2 is believed to be the main prostaglandin synthesized in the kidney. It can promote water and sodium excretion and might mediate, at least in part, the renal effects of kinins. A deficiency in vasodilatory prostaglandins may exist in patients with essential hypertension.[61] This is suggested by the finding of a reduced urinary excretion of PGE_2 and 6-keto-PGF_1 (the stable metabolite of PGI_2) in some hypertensive patients. On the other hand, there is evidence for an increased production of TxA_2 in essential hypertension.[62] These observations point therefore to an imbalance between antihypertensive and prohypertensive prostaglandins as a possible pathogenic factor in hypertension.

Renal Sodium Retention

Salt accumulation in the body is one of the principal mechanisms contributing to the development of essential hypertension. As already discussed, all major determinants of blood pressure control can, in one way or another, influence renal sodium handling, serving mainly for short-term adjustments of sodium balance. This is the case, for instance, for the sympathetic nervous system and the renin-angiotensin-aldosterone system, which both induce sodium retention. The kidneys also have a key role in controlling the long-term arterial pressure level because of their intrinsic ability to respond to an elevation in blood pressure by an increase in fluid excretion.[63] The so-called pressure diuresis-natriuresis encourages the return of high blood pressure to normal. Any dysfunction in this renal volume mechanism for blood pressure homeostasis could lead to hypertension. In fact, this mechanism is still operating in hypertensive patients, but at higher blood pressure values and in the presence of a volume overload.

During the initial phase of hypertension, cardiac output is usually high, perhaps as a consequence of a subtle increase in blood volume and venous return (Fig. 80–7). With time, the "high cardiac output" hypertension might be converted to a "high peripheral resistance" hypertension, a process that could be accounted for by so-called whole body autoregulation.[63] This process implies that blood vessels progressively adapt to protect against a high cardiac output–associated local hyperperfusion. The mechanism of this autoregulation includes increased vascular tone, as well as structural changes, which might include a reduction in the lumen diameter or a decrease in tissue vascularity. At this late stage, the high blood pressure is due primarily to an increase in total peripheral resistance, the cardiac output being generally normal again because of nervous reflex responses. The pressure diuresis-natriuresis mechanism is still operating, but with a higher blood pressure for a given urinary sodium and water excretion. About half of patients with essential hypertension increase their blood pressure during the shift from a low-sodium to a high-sodium intake.[64] These salt-sensitive patients with a difficulty in handling sodium often have a positive family history for hypertension. They are also known as *nonmodulators,* as they seem unable to respond adequately to a sodium overload–induced suppression in angiotensin II formation with an increase in renal blood flow and a decrease in aldosterone secretion.

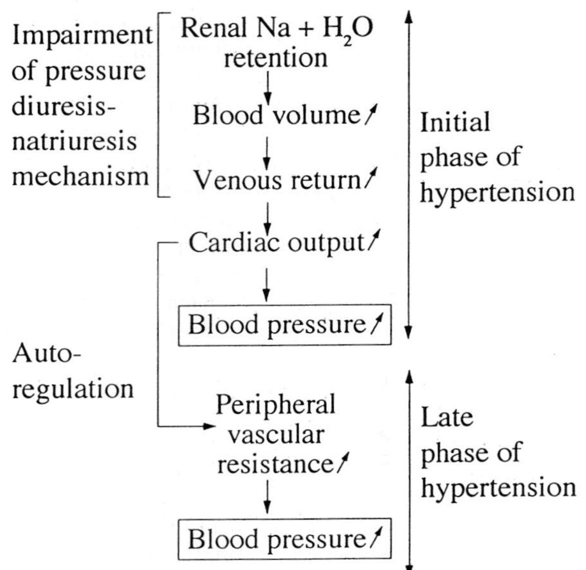

FIGURE 80–7 Sequence of events leading from a high cardiac output to a high vascular resistance hypertension.

Hyperinsulinemia

Hypertension, obesity (increased waist:hip ratio), hyperlipidemia, and glucose intolerance represent a cluster of cardiovascular risk factors that are often associated (known as *syndrome X*).[65] These different disorders not only might coexist incidentally but also could be the direct consequence of a common disturbance. In this respect, resistance of peripheral tissues to the action of insulin may play a pivotal role. Hypertensive patients often exhibit some degree of hyperinsulinemia. The excessive production of insulin may by itself lead to an increase in blood pressure. Insulin causes a renal sodium reabsorption, has a stimulatory effect on the sympathetic nervous system, and constitutes a growth factor (see Vascular Structural Changes). The hyperinsulinemia-associated hypertension has a strong genetic component.

Endothelial Dysfunction

The endothelium has a strategic position in the cardiovascular system, being located between the blood and the vasculature, and produces a variety of vasoactive factors.[66, 67] One of the most important of them is NO, known as endothelium-derived relaxing factor, which possesses potent vasorelaxant properties. NO is released from the endothelial cell in response to physical stimuli (shear stress, hypoxia), as well as to the activation of endothelial receptors (Fig. 80–8). Thus, acetylcholine and bradykinin exert their vasodilatory action via the NO pathway. Endothelium-derived relaxing factor may also attenuate vasoconstrictor responses—for example, that induced by α-adrenergic receptor or vasopressin stimulation. The crucial role of NO is illustrated by the fact that acetylcholine, in the absence

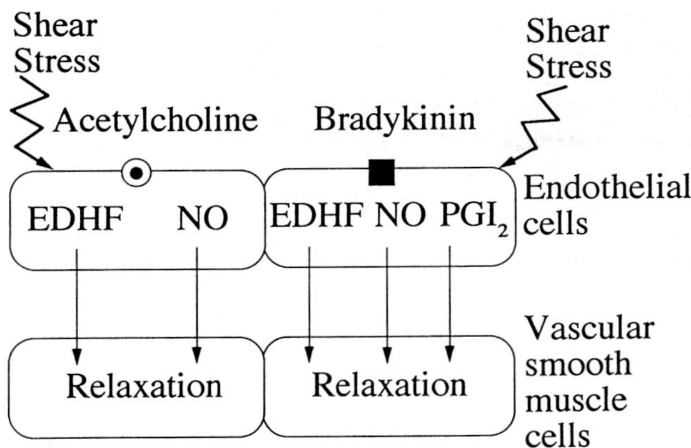

FIGURE 80–8 Vasorelaxing factors released by the endothelium. EDHF, endothelium-derived hyperpolarizing factor; NO, nitric oxide; PGI_2, prostaglandin I_2.

of endothelium, is a vasoconstrictor rather than a vasodilator. NO is synthesized from L-arginine by a nitric oxide synthase, an enzyme present constitutively in endothelial cells. NO is emerging also as a factor that might suppress renin release while having a natriuretic effect.[68] Vasorelaxant factors other than NO can be formed by the endothelium, in particular PGI_2 and the endothelium-derived hyperpolarizing factor.[67] The vasorelaxing effect of NO can be counteracted by oxidation at the tissue level. A role for angiotensin II in inducing oxidative stress has led to the concept that vascular tone may represent a balance between angiotensin II and NO at the vascular wall.[69]

The endothelium also produces the most potent endogenous vasoconstrictor known so far, a 21-amino acid peptide called *endothelin* (Fig. 80–9).[70] This peptide comes from a precursor (big endothelin) on the action of an endothelin-converting enzyme. Stimuli of endothelin release include the shear stress, thrombin, angiotensin II, vasopressin, and catecholamines. Stimulation of endothelin receptors located on the endothelium (ET_B receptors) causes the release of NO and PGI_2. The vasoconstrictor effect of endothelin is due to the activation of ET_A and ET_B receptors present in the vasculature. The contractile response to endothelin is markedly blunted by NO but is considerably enhanced by other vasoconstrictors.

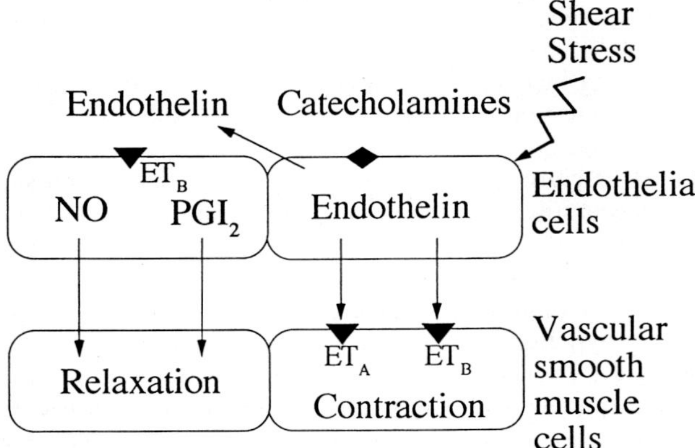

FIGURE 80–9 Effects of endothelin. ET_A and ET_B, subtypes of endothelin receptors; NO, nitric oxide; PGI_2, prostaglandin I_2.

There might exist an endothelium dysfunction in hypertensive humans. This is suggested by the demonstration in these patients of an impaired vasodilatory response to acetylcholine.[71] Endothelial dysfunction seems to be frequently present in hypertensive patients with the DD polymorphism of ACE gene.[72] Regarding circulating levels of endothelin, consistent augmentations have been reported only in patients with severe hypertension, but plasma endothelin levels do not necessarily reflect the local concentrations achieved at the surface of vascular smooth muscle cells.[73]

Abnormalities in Signal Transduction

The tone of vascular smooth muscle cells increases in response to a rise in cytosolic free calcium.[74] The calcium ion can enter into the cell through either voltage-operated or receptor-regulated calcium channels. The former respond to the depolarization of the cell membrane, and the latter to the ligand-receptor interaction. The principal agonists thought to play a role in the pathogenesis of hypertension are coupled to G-protein receptors (α-adrenergic receptor stimulants, angiotensin II, endothelin, vasopressin, TxA_2).[75, 76] The cytosolic part of these receptors is connected through a G-protein to phospholipase C. On stimulation with the ligand—for instance, the AT_1 receptor with angiotensin II—phospholipase C becomes activated, leading to the hydrolysis of phosphatidylinositol 4,5-biphosphate into diacid glycerol and inositol 1,4,5-triphosphate ($InsP_3$) (Fig. 80–10). Diacid glycerol activates protein kinase C within the membrane, thereby facilitating a number of cellular functions. Regarding $InsP_3$, it diffuses into the cytosol and activates specific receptors from endoplasmic reticulum, causing the release of calcium necessary for the mediation of the angiotensin II effects. The rapid calcium mobilization by this pathway then stimulates a sustained entry of calcium through the plasma membrane.

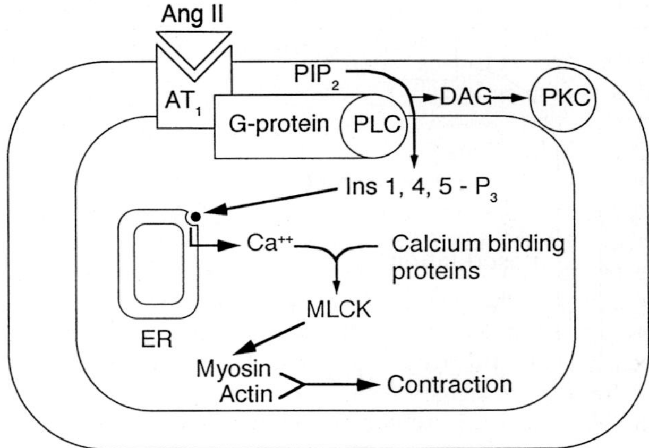

FIGURE 80–10 Mode of action of angiotensin II (Ang II) in vascular smooth muscle cells. AT_1, AT_2, subtypes of Ang II receptors; DAG, 1,2-diacylglycerol; ER, endoplasmic reticulum; Ins 1,4,5-P_3, inositol 1,4,5-triphosphate; MLCK, myosin light chain kinase; PIP_2, phosphatidylinositol 4,5-biphosphate; PKC, protein kinase C; PLC, phospholipase C.

In the vascular smooth muscle cell, the calcium ion bonds to calcium-binding proteins. The resulting complex activates a myosin light chain kinase, and the myosin filaments are phosphorylated and interact with actin filaments to generate a contraction. Whether alterations in this second messenger system contribute to the pathogenesis of hypertension remains to be elucidated. This is conceivable considering the fact that the basal and agonist-stimulated intracellular free calcium concentration is increased in platelets from hypertensive patients.[77]

The vasorelaxation resulting from β-adrenergic receptor stimulation is mediated by the intracellular formation of cyclic adenosine monophosphate (cAMP) (Fig. 80–11). The ligand-receptor interaction activates a stimulatory G-protein. During this process, the guanosine triphosphatase activity of a G-protein subunit is modified, permitting the replacement of the bound guanosine diphosphate by guanosine triphosphate. This leads to the activation of adenylate cyclase and thereby to the generation of cAMP from adenosine triphosphate. This second messenger activates specific protein kinase, with subsequent dephosphorylation of myosin light chain kinase and reduction of myosin phosphorylation, which in turn causes vasodilatation. The β-receptor–stimulated adenylate cyclase activity is reduced in lymphocytes of hypertensive patients.[78] Interestingly, this abnormality can be corrected by a low-sodium diet. On the other hand, a cAMP hyper-responsiveness has been found in platelets of hypertensive patients.[79] It remains uncertain, therefore, whether alterations in the cAMP signaling pathway modulate in essential hypertensive patients the vascular response to β-adrenergic receptor activation.

ANF and NO exert their vasodilatory action by increasing the generation of cyclic guanosine monophosphate (cGMP). ANF activates a particulate, membrane-bound guanylate cyclase, leading to the transformation of guanosine triphosphate to cGMP. This latter nucleotide activates specific kinases, with a reduction in intracellular free calcium as the ultimate consequence. cGMP can eventually

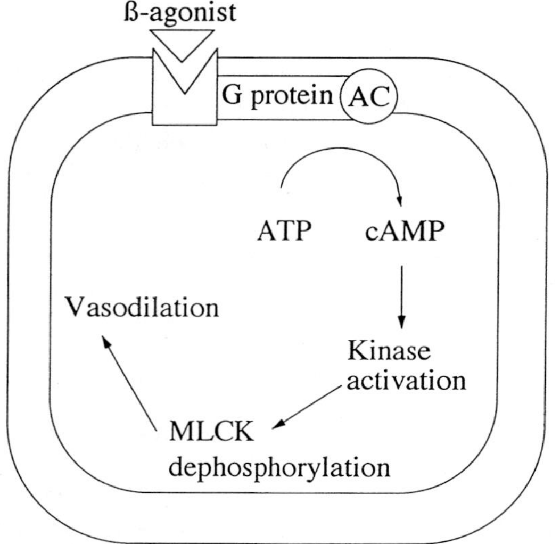

FIGURE 80–11 Cellular mechanisms involved in the β-adrenergic receptor–induced vasodilatation. AC, adenylate cyclase; ATP, adenosine triphosphate; cAMP, cyclic adenosine monophosphate; MLCK, myosin light chain kinase.

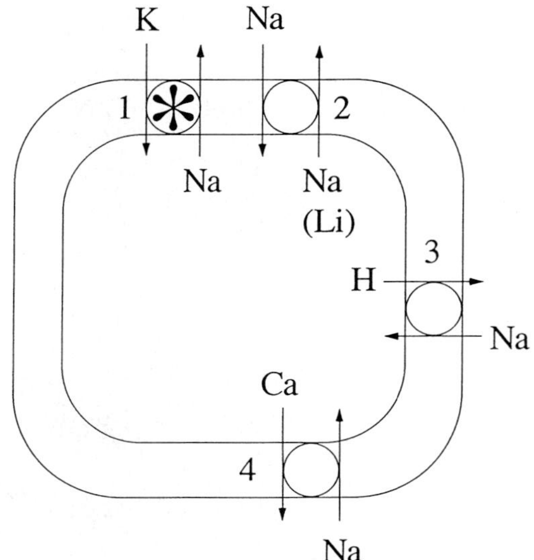

1 Sodium-potassium ATPase
2 Sodium-lithium countertransport
3 Sodium-hydrogen antiport
4 Sodium-calcium exchanger

FIGURE 80–12 Electrolyte transport systems that function abnormally in essential hypertension. ATPase, adenosine triphosphatase.

egress through the cellular membrane. Both the circulating concentration and the urinary excretion of cGMP are, on average, similar in patients with essential hypertension and in normotensive subjects.[80, 81] With regard to NO, it acts on a soluble, cytosolic guanylate cyclase.

Membrane Abnormalities

Sodium metabolism has been extensively examined in erythrocytes, leukocytes, and platelets of hypertensive patients, the assumption being that the ionic membrane transport of these blood cells is identical with that of vascular smooth muscle cells. Only the main abnormalities are described here.[82] The ouabain-sensitive, sodium-potassium adenosine triphosphatase is inhibited in many patients with essential hypertension (Fig. 80–12). This defect may be due to the presence in the circulation of a factor able to block this pump and appears to have an inherited character. The pathogenesis of essential hypertension has been hypothetically linked to the inhibition of the sodium pump and the ensuing increase in intracellular sodium, which reduces the concentration gradient between extracellular and intracellular sodium. As a consequence, the activity of the sodium-calcium exchanger might be increased and result in an accumulation of intracellular calcium and vasoconstriction.[74]

The activity of the erythrocyte sodium-lithium countertransport is abnormally increased in some patients with primary hypertension. In the absence of lithium, this system allows the exchange of sodium between the extracellular and the intracellular compartment. The physiologic role of this transport system is not yet understood. Intriguingly, essential hypertensive patients with insulin resistance often exhibit an increased activity of this countertransport.[83] A third ionic perturbation present in essential hypertension is linked to the sodium-hydrogen antiport. This system allows the extrusion of intracellular protons in exchange for extracellular sodium and plays a role in the regulation of cytosolic pH. The activity of this sodium-hydrogen antiport is increased in platelets of essential hypertensives. Diacid glycerol, formed together with $InsP_3$ on activation of phospholipase C, stimulates protein kinase C and can enhance the activity of the sodium-hydrogen antiport.

Vascular Structural Changes

When exposed to high blood pressure, resistance blood vessels undergo an adaptive hypertrophy that makes it possible to keep the wall stress constant but that amplifies considerably the vascular responsiveness to all constrictors.[84] The increase in media:lumen ratio found in small arteries of hypertensive patients seems to be due more to a rearrangement of the material normally present in the wall (remodeling) than to a real growth.[85] Vascular hypertrophy may also be promoted by growth factors such as angiotensin II, catecholamines, and endothelin. The raised intracellular free calcium and activation of protein kinase C mediated by these vasoconstrictors induces the expression of proto-oncogenes (*c-fos, c-myc, c-jun*), which in turn stimulate cell growth.[86] The enhanced sodium-proton exchange activity observed in patients with essential hypertension seems to be associated with vascular hypertrophy, but it is still unknown whether this abnormality represents a causal factor for structural changes.[87]

Hypertensive patients tend to have an increased arterial stiffness compared with normotensive individuals.[88, 89] A change in the viscoelastic properties of the wall of the large conduit arteries is due, in part, to an increased collagen content and leads to an acceleration of pulsed-wave velocity. As a consequence, reflected pressure waves return early to the root of the aorta, thus resulting in a late systolic amplification of aortic systolic pressure. Increased stiffness of the smaller arteries, at the site of wave reflections from the peripheral arterial tree, alters the cushioning function of the arteries and affects the frequency and damping of reflected waves observed in diastole.[90] This alteration can be identified by diastolic pulsed-wave analysis utilizing a modified Windkessel model of the circulation.[91] Abnormal stiffness of these reflecting sites is characteristic of hypertension, diabetes, and other conditions associated with endothelial dysfunction. These changes may be functional, structural, or more likely, a combination of both.

Vascular structural changes in hypertension may result from genetic, hemodynamic, or hormonal influences. A genetic contribution has been implicated on the basis of AT_1 receptor gene polymorphism.[92] Regardless of cause, increased stiffness of the large conduit arteries is a major contributor to a rise in systolic blood pressure and to the widened pulse pressure that has been identified as a risk factor for cardiovascular morbid events.[93, 94]

Secondary Forms of Hypertension

Renal Diseases

Renal diseases are observed in 3 to 4 percent of hypertensive adults.[95] The kidney has a pivotal position in hypertensive disorders. On the one hand, it may cause or accelerate hypertension. On the other hand, the kidney is a target, high blood pressure being a major determinant of renal function deterioration. All forms of renal parenchymal disease may be associated with hypertension, including glomerulonephritis, interstitial nephritis, diabetic nephropathy, polycystic kidney disease, and reflux nephropathy. The prevalence of hypertension in these disorders ranges, depending on the series, from 25 to 80 percent. At the stage of terminal renal failure, 80 to 90 percent of patients have hypertension. Unilateral renal diseases can also be involved in the pathogenesis of hypertension. To be mentioned are hydronephrosis, radiation nephritis, and renal tumors or cysts. A hallmark of chronic renal failure is salt and water retention, resulting in increased plasma and extracellular fluid volumes. The activity of the renin-angiotensin systems may be not adequately suppressed in the face of the volume overload. Increased intraglomerular pressure and hyperfiltration are thought to play critical roles in the deterioration of renal function, especially in diabetic nephropathy and nephrotic syndrome. Angiotensin II seems to have a deleterious effect in this respect because it acts preferentially at the efferent arteriole. The renin-angiotensin system contributes to the maintenance of high blood pressure in many patients with polycystic kidney disease. In patients with hydronephrosis, large tumors, or cysts, localized renal ischemia with stimulation of renin release may occur. Furthermore, some tumors can secrete renin. This is typically the case for benign juxtaglomerular cell tumors, but some nephroblastomas and renal cell carcinomas may also be a source of renin.

Renovascular Hypertension

Renovascular hypertension is the prototype of renin-dependent hypertension. Any obstructing lesion located on the renal arterial tree may cause, beyond a critical degree of stenosis, a pressure gradient and a blood flow reduction, thereby triggering the release of renin from the ischemic kidney.[96] Not every stenotic lesion is functionally significant, so the diagnosis of renovascular hypertension should not be based exclusively on the documentation of an anatomic obstruction. In the population of hypertensive patients, the prevalence of this form of hypertension has been estimated at about 5 percent, but it may be much higher, at around 30 percent among severely hypertensive patients.[97] The main causes of renovascular hypertension are atherosclerosis, fibromuscular dysplasia, renal artery stenosis on a transplant kidney, and dissection of the aorta involving renal arteries. Atherosclerotic lesions (stenosis, occlusion, and aneurysm) are most frequent in middle-aged and older patients, especially in men having a generalized vascular disease. In patients with long-standing hypertension, the presence of a renal artery stenosis may aggravate the severity of hypertension. Most patients exhibit other risk factors for cardiovascular disease. The kidney function is often impaired owing to concurrent nephroangiosclerosis, and bilateral lesions are frequent. Fibromuscular dysplasia involves primarily medium-sized arteries in the renal and cerebral vascular bed.[98] The cause of this disease is unknown, but genetic factors, female sex hormones, and ischemia of the arterial wall may play a role. Patients with fibromuscular dysplasia are often young women. Progression of stenotic lesions is slower in patients with fibromuscular dysplasia than in those with atherosclerotic lesions. Rare causes of renovascular hypertension are renal atheroembolism, which may be precipitated by catheterization of the aorta, Takayasu's arteritis, and hereditary connective tissue disorders (Ehlers-Danlos syndrome, Marfan's syndrome, and neurofibromatosis).

Coarctation of the Aorta

Hypertension developing during childhood or early adulthood might be due to a narrowing (coarctation) of the aorta just below the origin of the left subclavian artery. Typically, blood pressure is much higher in the upper than in the lower part of the body. The renin-angiotensin system may be activated in some patients with coarctation, contributing to the elevation of blood pressure, which, however, seems to result primarily from the mechanical obstruction.[99]

Pheochromocytoma

Pheochromocytomas are potentially lethal, catecholamine-secreting tumors.[100, 101] They consist of chromaffin cells (i.e., cells of neuroectodermal origin that become black when exposed to chromium salts). These tumors are localized predominantly in the adrenal medulla, either unilaterally or bilaterally. They can also occur in extra-adrenal sites, the chromaffin cells being associated with sympathetic ganglia (para-aortic, urinary bladder, chest, neck, rectum). About 10 percent of patients with pheochromocytoma harbor multicentric lesions. A familial character is found in approximately 10 percent of pheochromocytomas, and some of them may be associated with other endocrine tumors (multiple endocrine neoplasia). The prevalence of pheochromocytoma among hypertensive patients is estimated at less than 0.1 percent. In about half of the patients, the discharge of catecholamines from the tumor causes only paroxysmal hypertension. Malignant pheochromocytomas are rare. Pheochromocytoma cells may secrete norepinephrine, epinephrine, and dopamine, with usually a prominence of norepinephrine over the other catecholamines. Some pheochromocytomas may also release vasoactive peptides, for instance, the vasoconstrictor neuropeptide Y. Catecholamines are metabolized more or less rapidly within the tumor, so that the amount of catecholamines reaching the circulation can greatly vary.

Primary Aldosteronism

Primary aldosteronism is a syndrome characterized by hypertension with excessive production of aldosterone, potassium loss, sodium retention, and suppressed renin secretion.[102, 103] The prevalence rate of this disorder has traditionally been thought to be very low, about 0.1 percent among unselected hypertensives. However, some have suggested that more subtle degrees of aldosteronism, including genetic forms, may be more common if detected by the ratio of aldosterone levels:renin activity.[104] The increased aldosterone secretion may be due to the presence of a unilateral adrenocortical adenoma (known as Conn's syndrome). Very seldom is the tumor an aldosterone-secreting carcinoma. Ectopic aldosterone-producing tumors have been described in the ovaries. In about a third of patients with primary aldosteronism, no tumor can be identified. In this subset of patients, the increased production of aldosterone is associated with a diffuse or focal hyperplasia of the adrenal zona glomerulosa. These changes are bilateral, and the glands usually bear multiple nodules (idiopathic aldosteronism). Deoxycorticosterone is a precursor in aldosterone formation and also possesses salt-retaining properties. Hypertension with suppression of both renin and aldosterone secretion can therefore also result from excessive synthesis of deoxycorticosterone, either by an adrenal tumor (benign or malignant) or by adrenal hyperplasia.

Cushing's Syndrome

Hypertension may be due to an overproduction of cortisol from the adrenal, a condition known as Cushing's syndrome. The excessive secretion of cortisol may be due to an increased release of ACTH (pituitary Cushing's syndrome) caused by the corticotropin-releasing factor originating from the hypothalamus.[105] This idiopathic form of glucocorticoid excess is associated with bilateral adrenal hyperplasia and accounts for about 70 percent of all cases of Cushing's syndrome. In some patients, ACTH or ACTH-like peptides are produced by nonendocrine malignant tumors. Hypersecretion of cortisol, and sometimes also of other steroids, may arise from adrenal neoplasms, either benign or malignant (adrenal Cushing's syndrome). Cortisol has a weak mineralocorticoid activity. At high plasma concentrations, this steroid may, however, lead to some sodium retention. Glucocorticoids increase the hepatic synthesis of angiotensinogen, perhaps enhancing the generation of angiotensin II. The major mechanism involved in the pathogenesis of hypertension in Cushing's syndrome seems to be a vascular hyper-reactivity to angiotensin II and norepinephrine, possibly as a result of reduced synthesis of prostacyclin.

Congenital Adrenal Hyperplasia

Inborn errors of corticosteroid biosynthesis are rare causes of hypertension.[106] Figure 80–13 illustrates the steps of aldosterone and cortisol synthesis, with the position of two key enzymes, the 17-hydroxylases and the 11-hydroxylases. The deficiency of these enzymes may be more or less complete. In both cases, the production of cortisol is impaired, preventing the feedback inhibition of ACTH release. Consequently, steroids proximal to the biosynthetic impediment accumulate. Subjects with 17-hydroxylase deficiency have a marked elevation in plasma 11-deoxycorticosterone, a steroid with potent mineralocorticoid properties, whereas androgens and estrogens cannot be formed normally (primary amenorrhea and sexual infantilism in females and pseudohermaphroditism in males). Reduced 11-hydroxylation leads to an increase in 11-deoxycorticosterone, 11-deoxycortisol, and androgen levels (virilization and pseudohermaphroditism).

Thyroid Disease

Thyroid hormone is implicated in cardiovascular regulation.[107] It mediates a decrease in peripheral vascular resis-

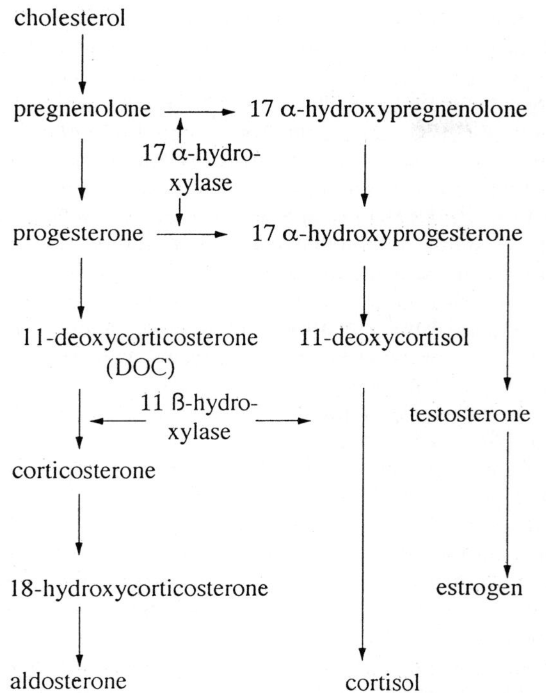

FIGURE 80–13 Steps in aldosterone and cortisol synthesis.

tance, an increase in blood volume, cardiac contractility, and chronotropy, as well as cardiac output. ANF is released by thyroid hormone and might, therefore, be implicated in the regulation of blood volume in hyperthyroidism and hypothyroidism.[108] In hyperthyroidism, the pulse pressure is usually widened and high systolic pressure can be seen together with normal or even low diastolic pressures. In patients with hypothyroidism, the prevalence of hypertension is high, at around 20 percent, and the elevation of blood pressure is mainly diastolic.

Hyperparathyroidism

The incidence of hypertension is increased among patients with primary hyperparathyroidism.[109] Several factors might contribute to this association, such as hypercalcemia, an activation of the renin-angiotensin system, or a vascular hyper-responsiveness to vasoconstrictors. Evidence has also been provided for the release of a hypertensive factor in the circulation of hypertensive patients with primary hyperparathyroidism.[110] This parathyroid hypertensive factor can actually increase calcium uptake in vascular smooth muscle and potentiate the contractile response to norepinephrine and angiotensin II.

Acromegaly

Patients with acromegaly produce an excess of growth hormone in the anterior lobe of the pituitary and commonly exhibit an elevated blood pressure. Vascular hypertrophy may have a role in the pathogenesis of acromegalic hypertension. Another potential mechanism is an increase in intracellular calcium owing to the presence in the circulation of a substance with an inhibitory activity on the sodium-potassium adenosine triphosphatase.[111]

Pregnancy

Pre-eclampsia is a form of hypertension developing most often in nulliparous women, usually during the third trimester of gestation, and accompanied by proteinuria, edema, and possibly also microangiopathic hemolytic anemia and liver function disturbances.[112] Pre-eclampsia may progress to eclampsia, a condition characterized by life-threatening convulsions. Pre-eclampsia can be seen early during the course of pregnancy in women with chronic, pre-existing hypertension. Pregnant women are normally highly resistant to the action of pressor agonists—for instance, to that of angiotensin II. In contrast, the sensitivity to vasoconstrictors is markedly increased in women with pre-eclampsia, accounting, at least in part, for the raised vascular peripheral resistance. The abnormal reactivity of the vasculature may be caused by an imbalance in the production of vasodilating and vasoconstricting prostaglandins. It may also reflect to some extent an endothelial dysfunction, with a deficiency in NO synthesis[113] and an increased endothelin formation.[114] Blood pressure typically normalizes within a few days during the postpartum period.

Obstructive Sleep Apnea

Patients with obstructive sleep apnea (OSA) experience repetitive apneic periods during sleep.[115] These patients have a high prevalence of hypertension. OSA is especially common in obese middle-aged men. Snoring and alcohol abuse may contribute to the pathogenesis of this disease. During cessation of air flow, arterial oxygen content decreases and arterial carbon dioxide levels increase. Hypoxia and hypercapnia, acting via the chemoreflexes, activate the sympathetic nervous system and, thereby, increase blood pressure during sleep.[116] The elevation of blood pressure may carry over to the daytime and cause sustained hypertension. OSA is often associated with an exaggerated cardiovascular risk, an excessive daytime sleepiness, and impaired cognitive and sexual functions.

Oral Contraceptives

Oral contraceptives tend to increase blood pressure in the majority of women, but true hypertension develops in less than 5 percent of pill users.[117] The estrogenic component is the main determinant of the blood pressure elevation.[118] Progestagens alone generally have no blood pressure effect.[119, 120] Estrogen-containing contraceptive pills stimulate the hepatic synthesis of angiotensinogen, but this, however, does not result in consistent raised plasma angiotensin II levels,[121] even if increased angiotensin II concentrations have been measured.[122] Estrogens and synthetic gestagens may induce some fluid retention in susceptible persons, whereas natural progesterone has the opposite effect on sodium metabolism.[123] The precise mechanisms responsible for this type of hypertension, therefore, remain unclear. The blood pressure effect of oral contraceptives is dose dependent, thus encouraging prescription of preparations with low estrogen-progesterone content. After withdrawal of oral contraceptives, several months are sometimes needed for recovery of normal blood pressure values.

Iatrogenic Hypertension

A number of medications can be responsible for a sustained elevation of blood pressure.[123] They include substances with glucocorticoid or mineralocorticoid activities. Chronic excessive ingestion of licorice may cause a form of hypertension mimicking primary aldosteronism. This is because the licorice extract contains a substance, glycyrrhizic acid, that inhibits 11β-hydroxysteroid dehydrogenase activity, thus leading to increased plasma cortisol levels, a steroid possessing mineralocorticoid activities. A derivative of glycyrrhizic acid is found in carbenoxolone, an obsolete drug used to heal gastric ulcers. Some drugs may increase blood pressure by enhancing, via a direct or an indirect effect, α-adrenoceptor stimulation. Phenylephrine as well as other α-adrenergic receptor agonists, including alkaloids related to ergotamine, produce vasoconstriction by activating postsynaptic adrenergic receptors. Cocaine, like amphetamine, augments the discharge of norepinephrine from terminal nerve endings while simultaneously preventing the catecholamine neuronal reuptake. This may lead to severe hypertension, tachycardia, and seizures.[124] Monoamine oxidase (MAO) inhibitors can also precipitate hypertensive crisis when patients ingest tyramine contained, for instance, in cheese or fermented foods. Tyramine taken up by sympathetic terminals is normally oxidized by MAO and thus accumulates during inhibition of the enzyme activity. Tyramine triggers the release of stored norepinephrine, and this catecholamine, having its metabolism impaired under MAO inhibition, reaches pressor concentrations in the synaptic cleft.

Cyclosporine has a hypertensive effect, depending on the dosage and duration of treatment.[125] Exposure to cyclosporine is associated with a predominantly renal afferent vasoconstriction, sodium retention, and augmented vasoconstrictive responses to pressor peptides and catecholamines. Sympathetic nerve stimulation as well as enhanced TxA_2 and endothelin release might be involved in the cyclosporine-induced vasoconstriction, which is reversible after discontinuation of the drug. There is now available a recombinant human erythropoietin that can be used to correct anemia in patients on chronic hemodialysis. Striking increments in blood pressure can be seen in patients receiving erythropoietin, the overall prevalence of erythropoietin-induced hypertension being about 30 percent.[126] The hormone may increase blood pressure via a direct effect or indirectly by heightening the vascular responsiveness to angiotensin II. The erythropoietin-induced rise in hematocrit and blood viscosity is also a potential cause of increased peripheral resistance. Nonsteroidal anti-inflammatory drugs raise blood pressure only modestly in individuals not on antihypertensive treatment. These drugs, by inhibiting cyclooxygenase and thereby prostaglandin synthesis, may, however, attenuate the blood pressure–lowering effect of practically all antihypertensive agents.[127]

Clinical Recognition

History

Each patient should be questioned regarding family history of hypertension, diabetes, hyperlipidemia, ischemic heart disease, and stroke.[128, 129] Information should also be obtained about the personal history of cardiovascular, cerebrovascular, and renal symptoms or diseases, as well as about the existence of associated risk factors or any clinically relevant disorder. Attention must be paid to the dietary habits, with special reference to sodium intake, to alcohol consumption and smoking, to weight gain, and to physical activities. Psychosocial and environmental factors (e.g., lifestyle, family situation, working conditions, educational level) should be detailed. It is essential to get a history of the patient's hypertension, including the known duration of the blood pressure elevation, the efficacy and tolerability of previous antihypertensive therapy, as well as the presence of symptoms suggesting a secondary form of hypertension, such as symptomatic hypertensive attacks (hypertension is paroxysmal in 25 percent of patients with pheochromocytoma, and headache, sweating, and tachycardia are encountered in 95 percent of them). Palpitations, anxiety, and tremulousness are suggestive of pheochromocytoma producing predominantly epinephrine.[100, 101] Symptoms are unusual in patients with uncomplicated essential hypertension, the most common consisting of early morning, usually occipital headache, tinnitus, blurred vision, and dizziness. All prescribed and over-the-counter medications taken by the patient should be known.

Physical Examination

A complete physical examination, including weight and height measurements, is mandatory in each patient.[128, 129] Particularly pertinent for the evaluation of hypertension is auscultation of the abdomen (a bruit is present in about 40 percent of patients with renal artery stenosis) and the main large arteries. The diminution or the absence of peripheral arterial pulsation may point to a generalized arteriopathy. Reduced and delayed femoral pulses with preserved pulses in the upper extremities may be a clue for the diagnosis of the coarctation of the aorta, especially if a systolic murmur is audible in the back. An abnormal aortic pulsation may reveal the presence of an aneurysm. Funduscopic examination must be performed, with pupil dilatation if necessary. Hypertensive retinopathy can be classified in four grades according to the severity of the retinal changes (grade I, arteriolar narrowing; grade II, narrowing and arteriovenous nicking; grade III, narrowing, nicking, and retinal hemorrhages and/or exudates; grade IV, papilledema).

Inspection of the skin may reveal "café-au-lait" spots and widespread subcutaneous neuromas characteristic of neurofibromatosis, a condition frequently associated with pheochromocytoma. Patients with pheochromocytoma are often pale during catecholamine surge. Truncal striae and central obesity along with atrophy of the skin may be due to hypercortisolism. Patients with advanced renal failure exhibit a urochrome pigmentation. The presence of tophi points to the diagnosis of gout. Hyperlipidemic patients may have xanthelasmas, xanthomas, or a corneal arcus. The acromegalic patient has typical appearance, with enlarged hands and feet and coarsening of the facial features (broad nose, prominent lips, thickened skin). Patients with hypothyroidism may present with thin, brittle nails, thinning of hair, hard pitting edema, and delayed return of deep tendon reflexes, whereas those with hyperthyroidism often show a goiter, a tremor, and an exophthalmos that is at times associated with a pretibial, hard, and nonpitting swelling.

Cardiac examination may be a sensitive means of identifying left ventricular hypertrophy. The apical impulse felt with the patient lying in the left lateral decubitus position exhibits a sustained outward thrust often occupying an area larger than 2 cm in diameter in patients with hypertrophy. A diffuse apical heave is indicative of left ventricular dilatation. An early diastolic murmur of aortic regurgitation along the left sternal border may be observed in severe hypertension and often disappears when the blood pressure is lowered.

Measurement of Blood Pressure

Obtaining correct blood pressure readings is critical for the diagnosis of hypertension.[130] This implies the use of accurate equipment and an appropriate technique of measurement. The cuff bladder should transmit the pressure evenly to the underlying brachial artery. To be adequate, a bladder should have a length and a width corresponding to 100 and 40 percent of the patient's arm circumference, respectively. A standard-sized bladder (12 × 23 cm) is suitable for most adults. For those with large obese or muscular arms, a special bladder (18 × 36 to 50 cm) is required. A bladder adapted to the arm circumference is also necessary in children. The manometer (mercury, aneroid, or electronic device) should be checked regularly. The patient should rest for at least 5 minutes, in the seated posture preferably for routine measurements, with the arm fully relaxed at the level of the heart. When pressure is taken for the first time, the cuff should be inflated and deflated rapidly and the systolic blood pressure approximated by disappearance and reappearance of the radial pulse. Subsequent readings can then be made by inflating the cuff to 20 to 30 mm Hg above this value. In this way, it is possible to avoid errors in the determination of systolic blood pressure owing to an auscultatory gap. Deflation of the cuff should be performed at a rate of about 2 mm/s. The *systolic* pressure is defined as the first appearance of a Korotkoff sound, and the *diastolic* by the disappearance of the Korotkoff sound (phase 5). In some subjects (mainly in young subjects and in pregnant women), sounds can be detected until nearly zero. In this case, the diastolic pressure represents the level at which a muffling of the Korotkoff sounds becomes apparent (phase 4). A blood pressure reading should also be performed with the patient standing for 2 minutes. Blood pressure should be measured to the nearest 2 mm Hg in order not to give preference to 0 and 5 as terminal digits.

Workup of the Hypertensive Patient

The goal of the initial workup of the hypertensive patient is to assess whether there is damage of target organs, to look for coexisting risk factors, and to judge whether additional investigations are needed for the diagnosis of a potentially curable form of secondary hypertension.[128, 129] Table 80–2 summarizes the proposed laboratory tests and complementary investigations. Urinalysis should be performed on a fresh, if possible first-morning, specimen. Dipstick tests can be used in everyday practice for the detection of glucose and protein in the urine. The measurement of microalbuminuria (defined as a urinary albumin excretion of 30 to 300 mg/24 hr) is increasingly advocated.[131] Getting an electrocardiogram is a necessity. Although not very sensitive as an indicator of cardiac hypertrophy, this test gives useful information on conduction disturbances and ischemic heart disease. Echocardiography is not recommended in every patient, but it is superior to the electrocardiogram in assessing left ventricular mass[132] and it also allows evaluation of the systolic and diastolic function of the myocardium. The chest x-ray may identify cardiomegaly, pulmonary congestion, and unfolding of the thoracic aorta, suggestive of aortic aneurysm. Moreover, erosion of the ribs secondary to the dilatation of intercostal arteries can be seen in patients with coarctation of the aorta. Physician-measured blood pressures may not be representative of blood pressures prevailing when patients undergo their usual daily activities outside the medical setting.[133, 134] It seems, therefore, appealing to try to learn more about the behavior of blood pressure in the patient's environment, either by self-measurement at home or by noninvasive ambulatory blood pressure monitoring (see Definition of Hypertension, later).

TABLE 80–2 Routine Workup of the Hypertensive Patient

Blood

Hemoglobinemia
Hematocrit
Serum concentration of
  Creatinine
  Sodium
  Potassium
  Calcium
  Uric acid
  Glucose (fasting)
  Total cholesterol, HDL cholesterol, and triglycerides (fasting) in patients with abnormally high concentrations of total cholesterol
  Self blood pressure measurement at home (optional)
  Ambulatory blood pressure monitoring (optional)

Urine

Examination for the presence of
  Cells
  Casts
  Glucose
  Protein
Microalbuminuria (optional)

Electrocardiogram

Posteroanterior Chest X-Ray (Optional)

Echocardiography (Optional)

Abbreviation: HDL, high-density lipoprotein.

The Search for Secondary Hypertension

Renovascular Hypertension

Identification of patients with renovascular hypertension is an important task because this form of hypertension is potentially curable. Special examinations for detecting renal artery stenosis cannot, however, be performed in every individual with hypertension.[135] The diagnostic tests should be limited to patients with increased likelihood of disease. Such patients are those presenting with an abrupt onset of hypertension, a severe or malignant hypertension, a treatment-resistant hypertension, a known occlusive arterial disease, an unexplained elevation of serum creatinine, or a deterioration of renal function reversibly induced by an ACE inhibitor (see Renovascular Hypertension). A history of smoking heightens the suspicion of renovascular disease. Table 80–3 lists the most common procedures used to detect and confirm the presence of a renal artery stenosis.

Measurement of plasma renin activity is of no help in the screening for renovascular hypertension, as renin secretion is not necessarily elevated in this condition and can be high even in patients with essential hypertension. Measurement of plasma renin activity at peak ACE inhibition—for instance, 90 minutes after oral administration of 25 mg of captopril (captopril test)—helps to discriminate between patients with renovascular stenosis and those with essential hypertension, the reactive hyperreninemia (owing to the lack of angiotensin II to exert a feedback inhibitory action on renin secretion) being clearly more pronounced in the former than in the latter. This test must be performed after discontinuation of all antihypertensive medications. Demonstration that renal arterial stenosis is sufficient to have functional consequences requires determination of renin levels bilaterally in the renal veins to confirm lateralization of renin secretion. In this case, the afflicted kidney constitutes the source of circulating renin levels while renin release is suppressed in the contralateral kidney. The difference in renal vein renins can be amplified by prior stimulation of renin secretion using either a diuretic or an ACE inhibitor.

TABLE 80–3 Diagnostic Procedures for Renovascular Hypertension, Primary Aldosteronism, and Pheochromocytoma

Renovascular Hypertension
Plasma renin activity
Captopril test
Renal vein renins
Renal scintigram during angiotensin-converting enzyme inhibition
Intravenous pyelogram
Intravenous or intra-arterial digital subtraction angiography
Duplex ultrasound
Primary Aldosteronism
Plasma renin activity
Plasma and/or urinary aldosterone
Computed tomography scan
Magnetic resonance imaging
Adrenal scintillation scanning with radioiodinated cholesterol
Adrenal vein sampling and adrenal venography
Pheochromocytoma
Urinary catecholamine, metanephrine, and/or vanillylmandelic acid
Plasma catecholamines
Clonidine test
Computed tomography scan
Magnetic resonance imaging
Scintigraphy with radioiodinated metaiodobenzylguanidine
Vena cava blood sampling

A convenient, noninvasive screening test is the renal scintigram. The value of this test is considerably increased by comparing renograms obtained before and after a single dose of captopril. It may be adequate to perform only one scintigraphy, but at peak ACE inhibition. In the affected kidney, the inhibition of angiotensin II synthesis produces a dilatation of the efferent arteriole, with a consequent fall in glomerular filtration and delay in renal excretion of the radioactive tracer. An asymmetry of uptake (suggestive of a severe lesion), excretion, or both, can be seen. A major advantage of renal scintigraphy coupled with captopril challenge is its predictive value in terms of detecting patients who are most likely to benefit from revascularization of renal artery stenosis.

The use of intravenous pyelography in diagnosing renovascular hypertension is declining because bilateral or branch stenoses are regularly missed by this examination. Intravenous digital subtraction angiography is a much better alternative, but its resolution is not as good as that obtained by intra-arterial injection of the dye. The invasive route may, therefore, be preferable, except in patients with severe atherosclerotic disease who are at higher risk to develop complications such as hemorrhage, thrombosis, and cholesterol embolization. The experience with Doppler flow studies is still inadequate to position this technique in the screening of renovascular hypertension. A major concern is the skill of the sonographer, which greatly influences the value of the ultrasound investigation.

Primary Aldosteronism

Classically, patients with primary aldosteronism present with hypokalemia.[102] Serum potassium concentration may occasionally be normal. This is mostly the case when dietary sodium intake is low, so that only a small amount of sodium is available at the distal tubule to be exchanged with potassium. An underlying primary aldosteronism should also be suspected when patients develop marked hypokalemia in response to diuretic therapy. The diagnosis of primary aldosteronism is based on the demonstration of a suppressed plasma renin activity together with elevated plasma aldosterone concentrations and/or increased urinary aldosterone excretion (see Table 80–3). There is no functional test to differentiate with certainty adenoma and hyperplasia. The highly efficient imaging techniques (computed tomography and magnetic resonance imaging) may be unable to detect small adrenal tumors. In some cases, adrenal scintillation scanning using radioionated cholesterol may be useful. Other investigations such as adrenal vein sampling, for separately exploring aldosterone secretion from each gland, and adrenal venography are no longer recommended.

Pheochromocytoma

Pheochromocytoma should be suspected in all patients with a suggestive history, with or without associated hypertension (approximately 15 percent of patients are normotensive).[100, 101] Patients with a family history of pheochromocytoma should also be systematically screened for the presence of a catecholamine-secreting tumor. The first diagnostic step is the demonstration of an excessive release of catecholamines. This can be done either by measuring 24-hour urinary excretion of free (i.e., unconjugated) catecholamines or their metabolites (metanephrines, vanillylmandelic acid) or by determining plasma catecholamine concentrations (see Table 80–3). In most patients, the urinary determinations are adequate for establishing the diagnosis. The assays of catecholamines and metanephrines should be performed preferentially by high-performance liquid chromatography and electrochemical detection or radioenzymatic techniques to avoid interference with a number of medications. The false-negative rate for urinary vanillylmandelic acid is very high (around 30 percent), which strongly limits its diagnostic value. In principle, large tumors tend to release mainly metabolized catecholamines into the circulation, giving high concentrations of metabolites relative to free catecholamines in the urine, the converse being true for small pheochromocytomas.

In some patients with only slightly elevated plasma catecholamines, a clonidine suppression test may be helpful. Clonidine is an α_2-adrenergic receptor stimulant lowering blood pressure via a centrally mediated decrease in sympathetic activity and, in the periphery, by a presynaptic inhibition of norepinephrine release. This agent is, therefore, expected to decrease the plasma concentration of norepinephrine in patients with essential hypertension, but not that of patients with pheochromocytoma, in whom the regulation of catecholamine release is autonomous. Computed tomographic scanning is a convenient and efficient way to localize pheochromocytomas anywhere in the body. Magnetic resonance imaging is excellent in visualizing tumors located in the adrenal and can be used safely in pregnant women. Another way to locate adrenal and extra-adrenal pheochromocytomas is scintigraphy with radioiodinated metaiodobenzylguanidine (MIBG). This substance is taken up by chromaffin tissues by the catecholamine pump. The MIBG scintigraphy can be very useful in locating metastatic tumors. Selective blood sampling along the vena cava for catecholamine determination is rarely required for the localization of the tumor.

Others

Renal ultrasound examination, intravenous pyelogram, and biopsy are the principal methods used for diagnosing kidney diseases. In patients with primary hyperparathyroidism, serum calcium levels (corrected for serum albumin) and serum ionized calcium levels are raised, whereas serum inorganic phosphorus concentration is low. The diagnosis is confirmed by the measurement of elevated levels of parathyroid hormone–like protein in the plasma. Hypothyroidism is characterized by low free serum thyroxine values in the face of increased serum concentrations of thyroid-stimulating hormone, the opposite being true for hyperthyroidism. The diagnosis of Cushing's syndrome is highly suspected based on the measurement of an increase in plasma cortisol concentration or 24-hour urinary free cortisol excretion, but should be confirmed by a dexamethasone suppression test. Elevated fasting serum growth hormone levels and nonsuppression of growth hormone secretion after an oral glucose tolerance test are typical diagnostic features in patients with acromegaly. Polysomnography is helpful to assess whether patients have OSA.[115]

Natural History

Pathologic Consequences of Hypertension

Hypertension is a strong and independent risk factor for cardiovascular diseases.[136–138] There is a consistent and graded relation between both systolic and diastolic blood pressure and various cardiovascular complications, including stroke, coronary heart disease, cardiac hypertrophy, and congestive heart failure. The likelihood of developing renal disease,[139] peripheral arterial disease, and aneurysm of the aorta is also augmented by hypertension. The relative risk for stroke and heart attack as a function of diastolic blood pressure is illustrated in Figure 80–14.[140] A continuum obviously exists between the level of diastolic pressure and the expectation of a cardiovascular event. The implication is that hypertension is more a quantitative than a qualitative disorder and that there is no threshold blood pressure below which full protection against cardiovascular events is ensured. An increased pulse pressure is also an independent predictor of cardiovascular risk, especially for cardiac complications.[93, 94]

The epidemiologic association of blood pressure and cardiovascular risk does not necessarily imply that it is the blood pressure itself that produces the risk. An elevated blood pressure may be a marker for endothelial dysfunction that renders the vasculature sensitive to structural changes that may eventuate in atherosclerosis (Fig. 80–15). Thus, an elevated blood pressure may, in part, identify individuals "at risk," and the greater the elevation, the more likely is

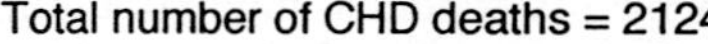

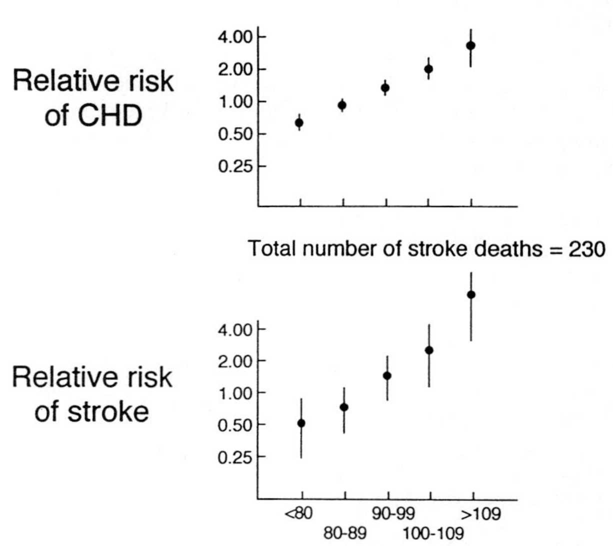

FIGURE 80–14 Relative risks and approximate 95 percent confidence limits for deaths from stroke and from coronary heart disease (CHD) during 6 years of follow-up, stratified by diastolic blood pressure (DBP) at baseline. The results are reported for 350,977 men without previous history of myocardial infarction who were screened for the Multiple Risk Factor Intervention Trial. (From MacMahon S, Cutler JA, Stamler J: Antihypertensive drug treatment. Potential, expected, and observed effects on stroke and coronary heart disease. Hypertension 13[suppl I]:45, 1989.)

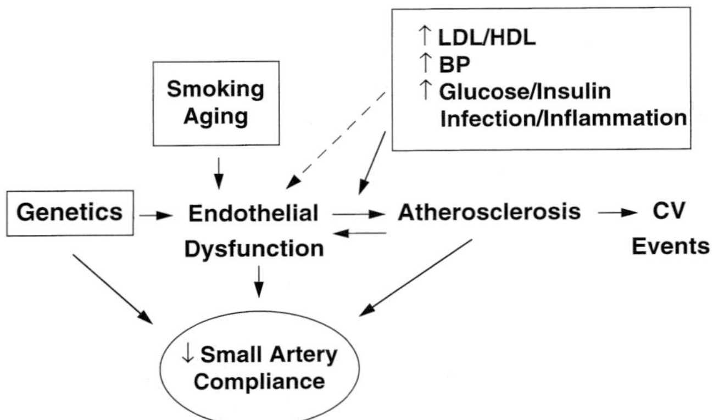

FIGURE 80–15 Proposed sequence of events in progressive atherosclerosis. Endothelial dysfunction, whether resulting from genetic factors, aging, or smoking, sensitizes the blood vessel to the damaging effects of increased cholesterol, high blood pressure (BP), or insulin resistance that accelerate the atherosclerotic process. A decrease in small artery compliance, or elasticity, may be an early marker for the endothelial dysfunction. CV, cardiovascular; LDL/HDL, low-density lipoprotein/high-density lipoprotein ratio.

the individual to be at risk because of endothelial dysfunction. A number of other factors can contribute to or be associated with increased event rates. Traditional risk factors for cardiovascular events include, in addition to age, gender (the risk is greater in men than in women), family history of coronary artery disease or stroke, hypercholesterolemia, smoking, and diabetes.[141] Novel risk factors have now been recognized, such as left ventricular hypertrophy, hypertriglyceridemia, microalbuminuria, male-type obesity, insulin resistance (syndrome X), and hyperhomocysteinemia.[65, 141, 142] Noteworthy, left ventricular hypertrophy is a major cause of cardiac systolic and diastolic dysfunction, inadequate coronary blood flow, and increased incidence of life-threatening cardiac arrhythmia.[132] A key point is that the coexistence of several risk factors amplifies drastically the likelihood of developing cardiovascular events, the final risk being much greater than the sum of the individual risks. It is, therefore, necessary to take into account all risk factors in caring for hypertensive patients. This approach provides an estimate of absolute risk in an individual patient with a goal for intervention targeted to reduce that risk.[143]

Prevention of Cardiovascular Diseases by Antihypertensive Treatment

There is now ample evidence that cardiovascular morbidity and mortality can be effectively reduced by antihypertensive therapy.[140, 144, 145] Beneficial effects have been observed not only in patients with severe hypertension but also in those with modestly elevated blood pressures (diastolic ≥ 90 mm Hg). In a meta-analysis of 14 randomized intervention studies of antihypertensive treatment,[144] the morbidity and mortality from stroke and coronary heart disease were both significantly reduced, the protecting effect being manifestly more pronounced for the cerebrovascular than the coronary heart diseases (Fig. 80–16). In adults, for a drug-induced 6 mm Hg decrease in diastolic pressure, a 42 percent reduction in the incidence of stroke can be anticipated over a 2- to 3-year period, compared with 12 percent for the incidence of heart attacks. When considering elderly hypertensives, almost the same figures are true. The combined results of five randomized trials of antihypertensive treatment in patients older than 60 years have shown a 34 percent and a 19 percent reduction in the incidence of stroke and coronary heart disease, respectively.[146] This protecting effect was observed over an average follow-up of nearly 5 years and for a blood pressure reduction of 15 mm Hg for systolic and 6 mm Hg for diastolic. Even elderly patients with isolated systolic hypertension, as defined by a systolic pressure of 160 mm Hg or higher and a diastolic pressure of 90 mm Hg or less, exhibit a benefit from antihypertensive therapy. Over a 5-year treatment

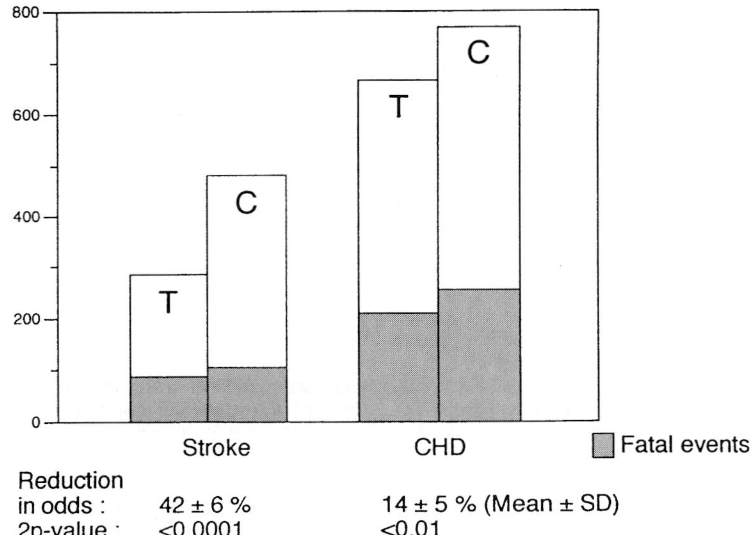

FIGURE 80–16 Effects of blood pressure reduction on stroke and coronary heart disease (CHD). The results represent a compilation of 14 randomized intervention studies of antihypertensive treatment. C, control group; T, treatment group. (From Collins R, Peto R, MacMahon S, et al: Blood pressure, stroke and coronary heart disease. Part 2. Short-term reductions in blood pressure: overview of randomized drug trials in their epidemiological context. Lancet 335:827, 1990.)

period, a 36 percent reduction in stroke incidence and a 27 percent reduction in coronary heart disease have been observed.

A major area of uncertainty remains the limited effectiveness of antihypertensive drugs in preventing myocardial infarction relative to the marked beneficial impact on stroke incidence. Several reasons have been advanced in an attempt to explain this phenomenon. The development of coronary heart disease depends (probably more than that of stroke) on risk factors commonly associated with hypertension. Unfortunately, trials aimed to evaluate antihypertensive therapy were not directed to correct simultaneously in each patient the whole constellation of risk factors. Possibly a treatment-induced slowing of the progression of coronary lesions may have passed unnoticed because of a too short follow-up. Furthermore, some antihypertensive agents may have a deleterious effect on lipid or glucose metabolism. This might conceptually attenuate the coronary protection otherwise provided by the blood pressure reduction. The absence of a tight link between blood pressure reduction and coronary disease events adds further credence to the view that blood pressure is a marker for but not necessarily the major causative factor in coronary artery disease.

The suboptimal results of antihypertensive therapy, with regard to coronary heart disease, could also result from too aggressive treatment, especially in patients with pre-existing ischemic heart disease. In these patients, lowering diastolic blood pressure below a critical level might conceivably impair myocardial perfusion and precipitate myocardial infarction.[147] A large trial aimed to assess the optimal diastolic blood pressure to reach during antihypertensive treatment has been completed recently.[148] Almost 19,000 patients aged 50 to 80 years were randomly allocated to a target diastolic blood pressure of either 90 mm Hg or less, 85 mm Hg or less, or 80 mm Hg or less. The treatment was initiated in all patients with the calcium antagonist felodipine, with the possibility of adding other drugs (β-blocker, ACE inhibitor) or increasing the doses according to a predetermined schedule when needed. The average follow-up was 3.8 years. No difference was found among the three target groups with regard to the cardiovascular morbidity and mortality (Table 80–4). The lowest incidence of major cardiovascular events, however, occurred at a mean achieved diastolic blood pressure of 82.6 mm Hg, and the lowest risk of cardiovascular mortality at a mean diastolic blood pressure of 86.5 mm Hg. Further reductions of diastolic blood pressures below these values were safe, indicating that the warning against an intensive lowering of diastolic blood pressure in hypertensive patients is not justified. It has also to be pointed out that an intervention directed to optimally control all risk factors in hypertensive patients on antihypertensive therapy allows the attainment of a further reduction of cardiovascular mortality.[149] With respect to congestive heart failure and chronic renal insufficiency, consistent beneficial effects can be expected from antihypertensive therapy.[150, 151]

Definition of Hypertension

Blood pressure is normally distributed within the population, with no natural cut-off point allowing discrimination between normotensive and hypertensive individuals. Moreover, the tendency for blood pressure to rise with age makes it difficult to uniformly apply any criteria of normal blood pressure. The definition of hypertension is in some way arbitrary. By choosing specific blood pressure levels as upper limits of normal, it is meant that the cardiovascular risk becomes high enough to warrant an intervention. Most so-called hypertensive individuals have only slightly elevated blood pressures. Small blood pressure reductions in this large fraction of hypertensive people may be associated with a substantial percentage reduction in cardiovascular risk, but the majority of patients who will not experience an event do not derive any benefit from the blood pressure reduction. On the other hand, most patients with severe hypertension who are at higher risk to have an event are likely to benefit from the blood pressure lowering.[128, 129] Table 80–5 proposes a new way of defining normotension and classifying hypertension.[129] The definitive diagnosis of

TABLE 80–4 Events in Relation to Target Blood Pressure Groups

	Events/1000 Patient-Years	*P* for Trend
All Myocardial Infarction, Including Silent Cases		
≤90 mm Hg	5.4	
≤85 mm Hg	4.6	
≤80 mm Hg	4.6	0.19 (NS)
All Stroke		
≤90 mm Hg	4.0	
≤85 mm Hg	4.7	
≤80 mm Hg	3.8	0.74 (NS)
Cardiovascular Mortality		
≤90 mm Hg	3.7	
≤85 mm Hg	3.8	
≤80 mm Hg	4.1	0.49 (NS)

Abbreviation: NS, not significant.

From Hansson L, Zanchetti A, Carruthers SG, et al: Effects of intensive blood-pressure lowering and low-dose aspirin in patients with hypertension: principal results of the Hypertension Optimal Treatment (HOT) randomized trial. Lancet 351:1755, 1998.

TABLE 80–5 Definition of Normotension and Classification of Hypertension by Blood Pressure Level

Category	Systolic (mm Hg)		Diastolic (mm Hg)
Optimal BP	<120	and	<80
Normal BP	<130	and	<85
High-normal	130–139	or	85–89
Hypertension*			
Stage 1	140–159	or	90–99
Stage 2	160–179	or	100–109
Stage 3	≥180	or	≥110

Abbreviation: BP, blood pressure.

*When systolic and diastolic BPs fall into different categories, the higher category should be selected to classify the individual's BP status. Isolated systolic hypertension is defined as systolic BP of 140 mm Hg or greater and diastolic BP below 90 mm Hg and staged appropriately.

From The Sixth Report of the Joint National Committee on Prevention, Detection, Evaluation, and Treatment of High Blood Pressure. NIH Publication No. 98-4080. Bethesda, MD: National Institutes of Health, National High Blood Pressure Educational Program. 1997.

TABLE 80–6 Recommendations for Follow-Up Based on Initial Blood Pressure Measurements in Adults

Initial BP (mm Hg)		
Systolic	**Diastolic**	**Follow-Up Recommendations***
<130	<85	Recheck in 2 yr
130–139	85–89	Recheck in 1 yr†
149–159	90–99	Confirm within 2 mo†
160–179	100–109	Evaluate or refer to source of care within 1 mo
≥180	≥110	Evaluate or refer to source of care immediately or within 1 wk, depending on clinical situation

Abbreviation: BP, blood pressure.
*Modify the scheduling of follow-up according to reliable information about past BP measurements, other cardiovascular risk factors, or target organ disease.
†Provide advice about lifestyle modifications.
From the Sixth Report of the Joint National Committee on Prevention, Detection, Evaluation, and Treatment of High Blood Pressure. NIH Publication No. 98-4080. Bethesda, MD: National Institutes of Health, National High Blood Pressure Educational Program. 1997.

hypertension should be based on repeated blood pressure measurements on different occasions. The practical approach is exemplified in Table 80–6. The goal of treatment is to lower blood pressure below 140/90 mm Hg, while simultaneously controlling other coexisting cardiovascular risk factors.[128, 129] Decreasing blood pressure further, if antihypertensive treatment is well tolerated, may be desirable.[148]

Blood pressure readings obtained by a doctor may greatly differ from those determined away from the clinical setting. Indeed, the magnitude of the blood pressure increase that may be elicited by the presence of the doctor is totally unpredictable.[152] Increasing evidence suggests that blood pressures recorded during everyday activities better predict the long-term prognosis of the patient than blood pressure measured conventionally in the doctor's office.[133] This is particularly true for cardiac hypertrophy, which is more closely related to ambulatory recorded pressures than to office blood pressures.[153] Nocturnal blood pressure is normally lower than daytime blood pressure. An interesting feature is that patients whose amplitude of nocturnal fall in blood pressure exceeds 10 percent of the average daytime blood pressure values are less prone to develop cardiac hypertrophy than patients lowering blood pressure by less than 10 percent relative to daytime values.[154] The lack of a normal nocturnal decline in blood pressure may be seen in patients with essential hypertension, but this is observed particularly in patients with secondary forms of hypertension, in pre-eclampsic women, in patients with OSA, as well as in patients with congestive heart failure or with peripheral neuropathy due, for example, to diabetes.

There is still no firm consensus on the use of noninvasive ambulatory blood pressure monitoring, but this technique may help to recognize patients whose blood pressure is abnormally elevated even in their familiar environment (i.e., the patients who are expected to derive the greatest benefit from antihypertensive therapy).[155] The same considerations apply to blood pressure self-measured at home.[156] One should, however, be cautious in interpreting ambulatory blood pressure recordings and home blood pressure measurements because normal blood pressure for these techniques have not yet been established in prospective studies. Also to be considered is the fact that many patients with white-coat hypertension may develop sustained hypertension over a few years.[157] Patients with white-coat hypertension should therefore not be lost to follow-up.

Hypertension in Childhood and Adolescence

The prevalence of hypertension in the young is much lower than in adults. The blood pressure elevation is generally mild when it is an early expression of essential hypertension, and severe hypertension mandates a screen for secondary forms of hypertension.[158] Guidelines for upper limits of blood pressure normalcy in children and adolescents are given in Table 80–7.[159]

Hypertension in Pregnancy

Blood pressure during pregnancy should not exceed 140/90 mm Hg, and lower values are desirable.[160] Women with

TABLE 80–7 Classification of Hypertension in the Young by Age Group

		High-Normal	Significant Hypertension	Severe Hypertension
Percentile		≥90th	≥95th	≥99th
Infants (≥2 yr)	SBP	≥104	≥112	≥118
	DBP	≥70	≥74	≥82
Children (3–5 yr)	SBP	≥108	≥116	≥124
	DBP	≥70	≥76	≥84
Children (6–9 yr)	SBP	≥114	≥122	≥130
	DBP	≥74	≥78	≥86
Children (10–12 yr)	SBP	≥122	≥126	≥134
	DBP	≥78	≥82	≥90
Adolescents (13–15 yr)	SBP	≥130	≥136	≥144
	DBP	≥80	≥86	≥92
Adolescents (16–18 yr)	SBP	≥136	≥142	≥150
	DBP	≥84	≥92	≥98

Abbreviations: DBP, diastolic blood pressure (mm Hg); SBP, systolic blood pressure (mm Hg).
From Task Force on Blood Pressure Control in Children: Report of the Second Task Force on Blood Pressure Control in Children, 1987. Reproduced with permission from Pediatrics 79:1, 1988.

a diastolic pressure greater than 75 mm Hg and 85 mm Hg during, respectively, the second and third trimesters must be followed carefully.

Malignant Hypertension

Malignant hypertension is a form of hypertension progressing rapidly to terminal renal failure if untreated.[161] This condition is characterized by a severe hypertension, grade IV retinopathy, and impaired renal function owing to thrombotic microangiopathy. All types of hypertension may progress to this fulminating disease, but the risk is particularly prominent in patients with underlying renal disease. The incidence of malignant hypertension has declined, probably because of early diagnosis and improved management of hypertension in recent years.

TREATMENT

Nonpharmacologic Control of Hypertension

Environmental factors may contribute importantly to the blood pressure elevation observed in hypertensive patients. By changing lifestyle, it is possible to lower blood pressure in a large portion of patients with established hypertension as well as to prevent the development of hypertension in many persons at risk to develop high blood pressure. Various nonpharmacologic therapies are now advocated as first-line intervention in patients diagnosed as hypertensive. This approach is safe and may be enough to normalize blood pressure, mainly in patients with slightly increased blood pressure. Moreover, nondrug therapy may enhance the efficacy of antihypertensive therapy, allowing a reduction of medication requirements.[128, 129, 162] Table 80–8 summarizes the risk stratification and its implication on the therapeutic approach using lifestyle modifications and antihypertensive drugs in the management of hypertensive patients.[129] It is important to recognize, however, that no data are available or studies in progress to address whether nonpharmacologic blood pressure reduction will reduce the risk of cardiovascular events.

Sodium Restriction

Long-term adherence to rigid sodium restriction, especially for asymptomatic hypertensive patients, is difficult. It is therefore reasonable to only modestly restrict dietary sodium intake, to about 100 mmol/da. That the dietary manipulation is really effective in lowering blood pressure is exemplified in Figure 80–17, which relates the changes in diastolic pressure to those in 24-hour urinary sodium excretion observed in 16 studies.[163] For a 100 mmol/da reduction in sodium intake, systolic pressure may be expected to decrease by 5.4 mm Hg and diastolic pressure by 6.5 mm Hg. Not every patient responds to the change in sodium balance with a blood pressure fall, however. Moderate salt restriction also has a demonstrable blood pressure–lowering effect as an adjuvant to antihypertensive therapy.

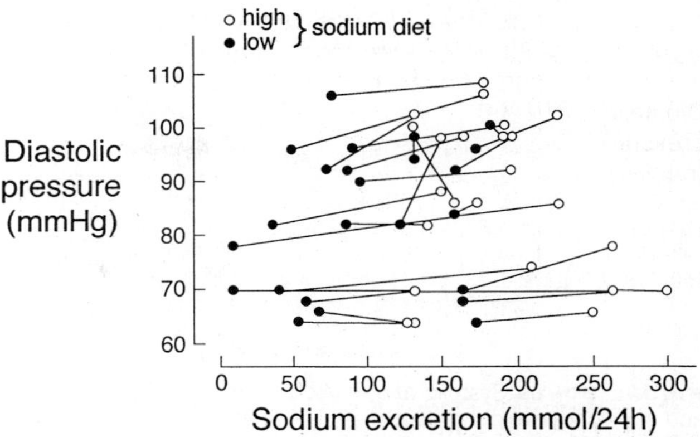

FIGURE 80–17 Systolic and diastolic blood pressures on a high-sodium and a low-sodium intake in 16 studies published from 1973 to 1987. (From Staessen J, Fagard R, Lijnen P, Amery A: Body weight, sodium intake and blood pressure. J Hypertens 7[suppl 1]:S19–S23, 1989.)

Weight Reduction

Weight reduction in obese patients is associated with a well-documented reduction of blood pressure. This is illustrated in Figure 80–18, which is taken from an analysis of 11 published trials.[163] For each 1-kg fall in body weight, systolic and diastolic pressures are anticipated to decrease by 1.6 mm Hg and 1.3 mm Hg, respectively. Part of the blood pressure–lowering effect of low calorie diets may be due to a concomitant reduction in sodium intake.

Alcohol Restriction

Reduction of alcohol consumption has a significant blood pressure–lowering effect. Moderating alcohol intake to no

TABLE 80–8 Risk Stratification and Treatment

Blood Pressure Stages (mm Hg)	Risk Group A (No risk factors: no TOD/CCD)	Risk Group B (At least 1 risk factor, not including diabetes; no TOD/CCD)	Risk Group C (TOD/CCD and/or diabetes, with or without other risk factors)
High-normal (130–139/80–89)	Lifestyle modifications	Lifestyle modifications	Drug therapy
Hypertension Stage 1 (140–159/90–99)	Lifestyle modifications (up to 12 mo) Drug therapy	Lifestyle modifications (up to 6 mo) Drug therapy	Drug therapy
Stages 2 and 3 (≥160/≥100)	Drug therapy	Drug therapy	Drug therapy

Abbreviations: CCD, cardiovascular disease; TOD, target organ disease.

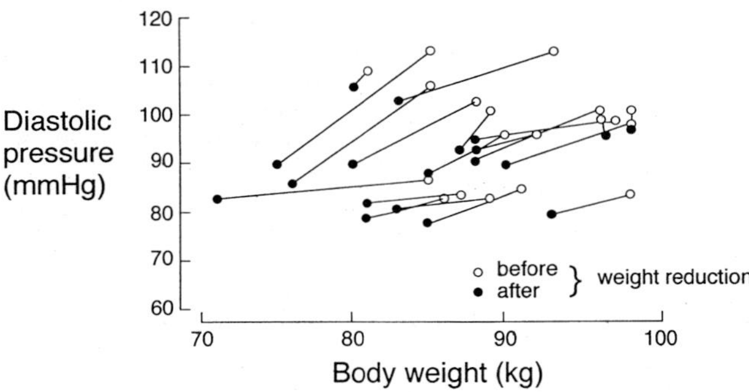

FIGURE 80–18 Systolic and diastolic blood pressures before and after body weight reduction in 11 studies published from 1954 to 1985. (From Staessen J, Fagard R, Lijnen P, Amery A: Body weight, sodium intake and blood pressure. J Hypertens 7[suppl 1]:S19–S23, 1989.)

more than 2 standard drinks a day (20 g equivalent absolute ethanol) seems to be wise advice, particularly because alcohol consumption in this range may have a protective effect against cardiovascular disease.[164]

Physical Exercise

Regular physical exercise not only has a lowering effect on blood pressure but also favorably influences other risk factors by increasing high-density lipoprotein (HDL) cholesterol and by helping to maintain normal body weight and to discourage smoking.[165] The physical training need not be strenuous to be efficacious. Dynamic, predominantly isotonic exercise (walking, jogging, running, bicycling, swimming) should be preferred to static, isotonic exercise (weight lifting), the latter inducing considerable elevations of blood pressure during the effort.

Pharmacologic Treatment

Since the late 1970s, the treatment of hypertension has improved considerably. Several new well-tolerated antihypertensive drugs have become available that have enhanced the therapeutic possibilities at the expense of other compounds such as the centrally acting sympatholytic agents.[166] In most industrialized countries, six classes of antihypertensive agents are recommended for first-line therapy (diuretics, β-blockers, ACE inhibitors, angiotensin II antagonists, calcium antagonists, and α_1-blockers; Fig. 80–19).[128] All these drugs have the advantage of lowering blood pressure by different mechanisms. This is very important because hypertension is a highly heterogeneous disease. In addition, these drugs can be combined when required. Table 80–9 gives a list of specific antihypertensive agents and their recommended doses.

Diuretics

Diuretics are still a cornerstone in the management of hypertension.[167, 168] These medications inhibit renal sodium reabsorption in the early distal convoluted tubule (thiazides, metolazone, indapamide), in the thick ascending limb of the loop of Henle (furosemide, bumetanide, ethacrynic acid), or in the late distal convoluted tubule and the collecting duct (spironolactone, triamterene, amiloride). Thiazides (hydrochlorothiazide, chlorothiazide, chlortalidone, bendrofluazide) become ineffective when glomerular filtration rate is below 30 to 40 ml/min. In patients with impaired renal function, the natriuretic action of metolazone and, even more, that of loop diuretics, is preserved. Thiazides, metolazone, and loop diuretics increase urinary potassium excretion and tend to decrease body potassium stores, which may result in hypokalemia. On the contrary, spironolactone (which competes with aldosterone for receptor sites), amiloride, and triamterene are potassium sparing. The dose-response curve of thiazides, in terms of natriuresis, is quite flat. The occurrence of side effects such as hypokalemia, hyponatremia, hyperuricemia, hyperglycemia, and hypercholesterolemia has a clear-cut dose-dependent character, so that there is an advantage to using only low doses of thiazides. With regard to loop diuretics, increments in doses, even if considerable, are still associated with an enhanced natriuretic response. A disadvantage of these diuretics is a rapid onset and a short duration of action, whereas the other types of diuretics have a smoother and more prolonged action, allowing once-a-day administration. Diuretics with potassium-retaining properties should not be used in patients with renal failure, as the risk of developing a life-threatening hyperkalemia exists. Combinations of thiazide with potassium-sparing diuretics are very popular. Triamterene and amiloride have only a limited natriuretic activity, but their antikaliuretic effect is sufficient to prevent the thiazide-induced hypokalemia in most patients.

The mechanisms involved in the blood pressure–lowering action of diuretics are not yet fully understood. At initiation of therapy, the plasma volume is reduced, but this effect does not persist after a few weeks of treatment, despite a persistent decrease in total body sodium, as manifested by a weight gain after drug withdrawal. The long-term antihypertensive effect of diuretics may be due to an attenuation of the vascular responsiveness to pressor stimuli, perhaps as a consequence of a decreased vascular wall thickness and content in sodium, the latter being expected

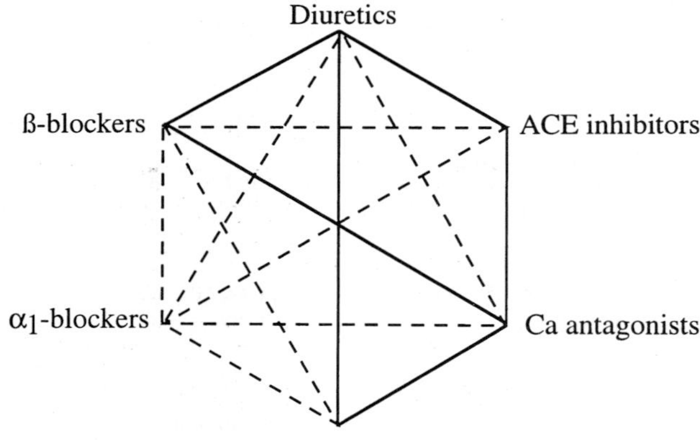

FIGURE 80–19 Six classes of drugs that may be used for monotherapy for hypertension. As noted, their combination provides additive and sometimes synergistic effects on blood pressure. ACE, angiotensin-converting enzyme.

TABLE 80-9 Individual Antihypertensive Drugs and Recommendations for Dosage

Type of Drug	Usual Dosage* Range (total mg/day)	Frequency (times/day)
Diuretics		
Thiazides and Related Agents		
Bendroflumethiazide	2.5–5	1
Benzthiazide	12.5–50	1
Chlorothiazide	125–500	2
Chlorthalidone	12.5–50	1
Cyclothiazide	1–2	1
Hydrochlorothiazide	12.5–50	1
Hydroflumethiazide	12.5–50	1
Indapamide	2.5–5	1
Methyclothiazide	2.5–5	1
Metolazone	0.5–5	1
Polythiazide	1–4	1
Quinethazone	25–100	1
Trichlormethiazide	1–4	1
Loop Diuretics		
Bumetanide	0.5–5	1–3
Ethacrynic acid	25–100	1–3
Furosemide	20–320	2–3
Furosemide (slow release)	30–120	1–3
Potassium-Sparing Diuretics		
Amiloride	5–10	1
Spironolactone	25–100	1
Triamterene	50–150	1
Adrenergic Inhibitors		
β_1-Blockers		
Atenolol	25–100†	1
Betaxolol	5–40	1
Bisoprolol	5–20	1
Metoprolol	50–200	1 or 2
Metoprolol (extended release)	50–200	1
β_1- + β_2-Blockers		
Nadolol	20–240†	1
Propranolol	40–240	2
Propranolol (slow release)	60–240	1
Sotalol†	160–320	1
Timolol	20–40	2
β-Blockers With ISA		
Acebutolol	200–1200†	2
Bopindolol	0.5–1	1
Carteolol	2.5–10†	1
Oxprenolol	80–160	1
Penbutolol	20–80†	1
Pindolol	10–60†	2
α + β-Blocker		
Carvedilol	12.5–50	2
Labetalol	20–1200	2–3
β_1-Blocker + β_2-Agonist		
Celiprolol	100–400	1–2
α_1-Blockers		
Doxazosin	1–16	1
Prazosin	1–20	2–3
Terazosin	1–20	1
ACE Inhibitors		
Benazepril	10–40†	1–2
Captopril	12.5–150†	2
Cilazapril	2.5–5	1–2
Enalapril	2.5–40†	1–2
Fosinopril	10–40	1–2
Lisinopril	5–40†	1–2
Perindopril	1–16†	1–2
Quinapril	5–80†	1–2
Ramipril	12.5–20†	1–2
Spirapril	12.5–50	1–2
Angiotensin II Receptor Blockers		
Candesartan	8–16	1
Irbesartan	150–300	1
Losartan	25–100	1–2
Valsartan	80–160	1
Calcium Antagonists		
Diltiazem	90–360	3
Diltiazem (slow release)	120–360	2
Diltiazem (extended release)	180–360	1
Verapamil	80–480	2
Verapamil (slow release)	120–480	1–2
Dihydropyridines		
Amlodipine	2.5–10	1
Felodipine	5–20	1–2
Isradipine	2.5–10	2
Isradipine (slow release)	5–10	1–2
Nicardipine	60–120	3
Nifedipine	30–60	3
Nifedipine (slow release)	20–60	2–3
Nifedipine (GITS)	30–90	1
Centrally Acting α_2-Agonists		
Clonidine	0.1–1.2	2
Guanabenz	4–64	2
Guanfacine	1–3	1
Methyldopa	250–750	1–3
Rauwolfia Alkaloid		
Reserpine	0.05–0.25	1
Direct Vasodilators		
Hydralazine	50–300	2–4
Minoxidil	2.5–80	1–2

Abbreviations: ACE, angiotensin-converting enzyme; GITS, gastrointestinal therapeutic system; ISA, intrinsic sympathomimetic activity.
*This usual dosage range may differ slightly from that recommended in the package insert.
†A drug that is excreted by the kidney and requires dosage reduction in the presence of renal impairment (serum creatine $\geq$ 221/μmol/L $\geq$ 2.5 mg/dl).
Adapted from the Sixth Report of the Joint National Committee on Prevention, Detection, Evaluation, and Treatment of High Blood Pressure. NIH Publication No. 98-4080. Bethesda, MD: National Institutes of Health, National High Blood Pressure Educational Program. 1997.

to reduce free intracellular calcium.[74] A key limiting determinant of the blood pressure–lowering effect of diuretics is the hyperreninemia triggered by the salt depletion.

A major source of concern for the widespread use of thiazides is the development of hypokalemia (and hypomagnesemia), which may be linked to an enhanced risk of ventricular arrhythmia and the existence of unfavorable effects on carbohydrate and lipid metabolism. Diuretics can increase insulin resistance, precipitate overt diabetes in susceptible patients, and increase cholesterol and triglyceride levels. The same concern is valid for the use of metolazone and loop diuretics, whereas indapamide and spironolactone seem to be more neutral with regard to the glucose and lipid profiles. As already stressed, potassium depletion is rarely a problem when thiazides are prescribed at a low dosage. Moreover, with the doses currently recommended (e.g., 6.25 to 25 mg/da for hydrochlorothiazide), there is generally no sustained metabolic alteration. Finally, diuretics have proven beneficial effects in the prevention of cardiovascular diseases. There is, therefore, no sound reason to discard these nonexpensive agents, if used at appropriate doses, as first-choice medications for the treatment of hypertension. Nonsteroidal anti-inflammatory drugs importantly blunt the natriuretic potency of diuretics and may lead to deterioration of renal function. Of note are that spironolactone, mainly at doses exceeding 50 mg/day, can occasionally cause a gynecomastia and that rapid intravenous administration of loop diuretics at high doses is potentially ototoxic.

β-*Blockers*

A large number of β-blockers are now registered worldwide. All of them compete with catecholamines for β-adrenergic receptors. Some agents bind selectively to β_1-adrenergic receptors that are confined, in the cardiovascular system, to cardiac muscle and conductive system (atenolol, betaxolol, bisoprolol, metoprolol), whereas others (nadolol, propranolol, sotalol, timolol) block at the same time β_1-adrenergic and β_2-adrenergic receptors, the latter being located presynaptically and postsynaptically at the level of sympathetic endings innervating blood vessels as well as on the bronchial smooth muscle. Several agents have an intrinsic sympathomimetic activity (acebutolol, bopindolol, carteolol, oxprenolol, pindolol). Labetolol is a mixture of stereoisomers, one being β-blocker and another α_1-blocker. Carvedilol has also at the same time β-blocking and α-blocking properties. Some β-blockers are hydrophilic (acebutolol, atenolol, sotalol) and do not easily pass the blood-brain barrier. Sotalol possesses a class III, amiodarone-like antiarrhythmic activity. Celiprolol has some β_2-agonistic activity.

The various ancillary properties of β-blockers may not be relevant for long-term antihypertensive efficacy,[169] but they may be more important for the safety profile. Cardioselective agents may be preferred in diabetics on insulin therapy because β_2-stimulation helps to restore normal glucose in patients with hypoglycemia. It appears also rational to use a β_1-selective agent in patients with peripheral artery disease as well as in those at risk of pulmonary decompensation, because bronchial spasm could be more easily reversed by a β_2-agonist. The intrinsic sympathomimetic activity can influence the hemodynamic response. Agents with such an activity decrease heart rate and cardiac output only slightly at rest. β-Blockers tend to reduce HDL cholesterol. This is, however, probably less the case for compounds with intrinsic sympathomimetic or β_1-selective effects. β-Blockers having poor access to the brain may have fewer central side effects. During chronic administration, all β-blockers can be given once a day or at most twice daily. The mechanisms of action of β-blockers are still not fully elucidated. The contribution of a centrally mediated decrease in sympathetic nerve activity cannot be ruled out. Acutely, the fall in blood pressure induced by β_1-adrenergic and β_2-adrenergic receptor blockade is associated with an increase in peripheral vascular resistance, but a progressive decline in peripheral resistance is observed with prolonged treatment. One possible explanation is a presynaptic inhibition by the β-blocker of the positive feedback normally exerted by catecholamines on the release of norepinephrine (see Fig. 80–2). Also to be considered is an autoregulatory dilatation of resistance vessels in response to the β-blocker–induced reduction in cardiac output and tissue perfusion. Still another factor is an inhibition of renin release, mainly with agents lacking any sympathomimetic activity.

A disadvantage of β-blockers is the diminution of exercise capacity. The occurrence of side effects is dose related (asthenia, vivid dreams, sexual dysfunction, cold extremities). β-Blockers have negative inotropic and chronotropic effects and may precipitate heart block or congestive heart failure, especially in older patients remaining severely hypertensive during treatment. Asthma may develop in predisposed patients. There is a large body of evidence to suggest a "cardioprotective" effect of β-blockers.[170] Such an effect is well documented in postinfarction patients using agents with no intrinsic sympathomimetic activity. β-Blockers were also part of the treatment of the major recent trials that have demonstrated a beneficial effect of antihypertensive therapy in the primary prevention of cardiovascular complications.[144–146] Undoubtedly, these agents represent a valuable first-line modality for treating hypertensive patients.

ACE Inhibitors

ACE inhibitors have acquired a wide acceptance as first-line antihypertensive drugs.[171, 172] These agents are generally well tolerated when lowering blood pressure, and the patient's well-being and quality of life do not deteriorate during treatment. Captopril and lisinopril are effective without bioactivation after oral ingestion and absorption, whereas all other ACE inhibitors are administered as prodrugs (benazepril, cilazapril, enalapril, fosinopril, perindopril, quinapril, ramipril, spirapril) and require de-esterification in the liver to form the active metabolite. Captopril has a rapid onset of action and may decrease blood pressure within minutes, whereas the antihypertensive action of the other inhibitors starts with a few (usually 1 to 3) hours' delay. The inhibitory effect of captopril on ACE activity is short lasting, and even high doses of this agent are not sufficient to block the angiotensin I–processing enzyme around the clock when given once a day. The other compounds have a more or less longer duration of action. Noteworthy during prolonged therapy, effective control of blood pressure can be maintained even if converting enzyme intermittently recovers enough activity to generate angiotensin II.[173] The discrepancy between the profile of ACE inhibition and that of the blood pressure fall is particularly striking for captopril, as this compound can often be used successfully in one dose per day. The dosage of most ACE inhibitors should be reduced in patients with impaired renal function. This is less a problem for benazepril, fosinopril, quinapril, and spirapril because these agents have a dual excretion by the kidney and the liver.

The ACE inhibitor–induced blood pressure fall is due primarily to the disappearance of angiotensin II from the circulation. Typically, ACE inhibitors cause a dilatation not only of arterioles and large arteries but also of the capacitive system. This might partly explain the lack of reflex increase in heart rate even in the face of a blood pressure drop. Another potential reason is that angiotensin II may reinforce the contribution of the sympathetic nervous system to blood pressure maintenance. Whether ACE inhibitors act to some extent by blocking the generation of angiotensin II within vascular smooth muscle cells is still debated. Also to be considered is the local accumulation, in response to ACE inhibition, of bradykinin. This peptide could trigger the release of both NO and prostacyclin from the endothelium. Aldosterone secretion tends to decrease during ACE inhibition, an effect that may help to counteract the antinatriuretic effect of the blood pressure fall. Angiotensin I levels increase during ACE inhibition. This leads to an increased production of angiotensin-(1–7) by the action of endopeptidases that are not blocked by ACE inhibitors. Interesting, angiotensin-(1–7) might function as a vasodilator hormone.[174]

ACE inhibitors are effective in lowering blood pressure in all forms of hypertension. Their efficacy is on the average better in patients with high renin levels than in those with normal or low renin levels, but blockade of angiotensin II synthesis normalizes blood pressure even in a substantial number of patients with suppressed renin activity. Therefore, renin profiling cannot serve as a reliable indicator of the blood pressure response to ACE inhibition in the individual patient. ACE inhibitors show equivalent efficacy in all age classes of the population.[175] As monotherapy, these agents are more likely to control blood pressure in white than in black individuals. The mechanism for this racial difference is not fully understood, although differential activation of the renin-angiotensin system may play a role.

ACE inhibitors have few side effects. By far the most common is a dry cough, which may be related to the accumulation of kinins, substance P, or prostaglandins.[176] Angioedema is a rare but potentially serious reaction to this type of drug. Its mechanisms may again involve kinins, together with an activation of the complement system.[177] The risk of a dangerous increase in serum potassium is small during ACE inhibition unless the drug is combined with a potassium-sparing diuretic, the patient takes oral potassium supplementation, or the renal function is impaired. Skin rashes and dysgeusia were seen quite often during the early years of experience with captopril, when very high doses of this agent were commonly administered. ACE inhibitors may cause a deterioration of renal function in patients with renal impairment and in those with renal artery stenosis, especially if bilateral. This adverse effect of ACE inhibition relates to the dependence in these patients of glomerular filtration pressure on an angiotensin II–mediated contraction of the efferent arteriole (Fig. 80–20).[178] ACE inhibitors seem very attractive in view of the lack of adverse effects on carbohydrate and lipid metabolism. A consistent finding during ACE inhibition is an increased sensitivity to insulin. Furthermore, ACE inhibitors have no detrimental effects on serum lipids, and beneficial alterations have even been reported.

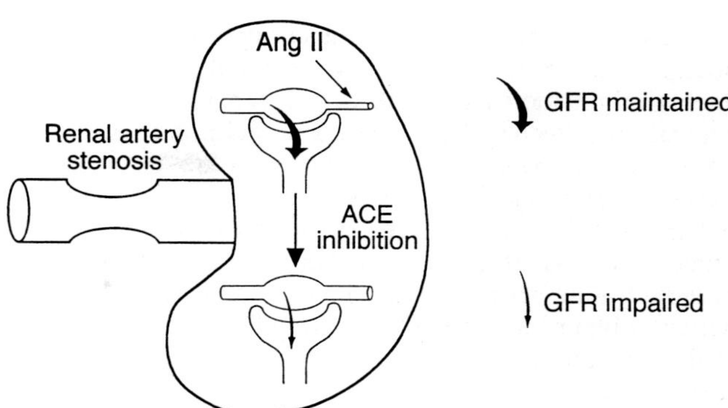

FIGURE 80–20 Effect of angiotensin-converting enzyme (ACE) inhibition on glomerular filtration rate (GFR) in a kidney irrigated by a stenotic renal artery. Ang II, angiotensin II.

Calcium Antagonists

There exist three major classes of calcium antagonists, the phenylalkylamines (verapamil), the dihydropyridines (amlodipine, felodipine, isradipine, nicardipine, nifedipine, nimodipine, nisoldipine, nitrendipine), and the benzothiazepines (diltiazem).[179, 180] These agents cause vasodilatation by blocking the entry of calcium ions from the extracellular space into the cytoplasm of the cell through voltage-dependent calcium channels. The various types of calcium antagonists can be more or less selective for the heart and the vasculature. Verapamil has the greatest chronotropic and inotropic depressant actions, whereas the dihydropyridines exert more effect on vascular smooth muscle cells. Diltiazem has an intermediate position—less potent than verapamil in the heart and less potent than dihydropyridines in blood vessels.

The blood pressure–lowering effect of calcium antagonists is clearly dose dependent, and the duration of action is related both to the drug and to the form of administration. Slow-release preparations have now been developed for most calcium antagonists, often making it possible to administer the medication in a single daily dose. Calcium antagonists are highly metabolized by the liver. The vasodilatation induced by dihydropyridines is frequently accompanied by a reflex increase in sympathetic nerve activity. This counter-regulatory mechanism may oppose the fall in blood pressure and tends to be most pronounced at initiation of treatment and to resolve thereafter, perhaps by resetting of the baroreceptor reflex at a lower blood pressure. The most common side effects of calcium antagonists, mainly of the dihydropyridines, are due to the vasodilatation (headache, palpitations, flushing, edema). These effects are dose dependent, and their incidence can be reduced by using controlled-release forms that tend to prevent large fluctuations in the concentration of the active drug in the blood. The edema is not due to sodium retention because calcium antagonists possess a natriuretic action, but likely reflects an increased capillary pressure due to arteriolar dilatation. For verapamil, constipation may become a problem when high doses are used. With this medication, atrioventricular block may occasionally occur. Diltiazem is usually well tolerated. Calcium antagonists are neutral in terms of carbohydrate and lipid metabolism and, in preclinical studies, have been noted to impede the development of atherosclerosis. However, definitive evidence for an antiatherosclerotic effect in hypertensive patients is still lacking.

There has been a controversy about the safety of calcium antagonists.[181–183] The concerns were that these vasodilating agents might increase the risk of coronary heart disease, cancer, and bleeding. The experience accumulated so far with calcium blockers has been reviewed in detail by experts. The conclusions were that long-acting calcium antagonists have no adverse impact on the cardiovascular outcome of hypertensive patients.[184] Preference should be given to long-acting compounds because, unlike short-acting calcium antagonists, they usually do not trigger a reflex activation of the sympathetic nervous system when lowering blood pressure. Calcium antagonists also appeared not to be harmful with regard to the risk of cancer and bleeding.[184] This view is supported by the results of a placebo-controlled prevention trial involving elderly patients with isolated systolic hypertension.[185] In this study, the long-acting dihydropyridine nitrendipine importantly decreased the incidence of stroke, and the beneficial effect observed on the incidence of myocardial infarction was very close to achieving statistical significance.

α_1-Blockers

Selective α_1-adrenergic receptor blockade lowers blood pressure by preventing catecholamine-induced vasoconstriction.[186] Norepinephrine released by sympathetic terminals can still exert an inhibitory action on catecholamine discharge, as presynaptic receptors belong to the α_2-subtype. This probably explains the greater long-term efficacy of pure α_1-blockers relative to nonselective α_1-blockers and α_2-blockers, as well as the lack of tachycardia. Prazosin was the first α_1-blocker available for clinical use. This drug's effect is short lasting, and it has to be given at rather high doses three times a day to be effective. Early experience with this agent has revealed a high incidence of orthostatic hypotension. Moreover, syncopal episodes can occur during initiation of treatment unless a very small dose is used. Slow-release preparations of prazosin now exist in some countries and provide a smoother delivery of the drug. With these formulations, orthostatic hypotension and first-dose collapse have become infrequent. The newer long-acting α_1-blockers (terazosin, doxazosin) have a slow onset of action and are well tolerated. Doxazosin can be administered once daily. α_1-Blockers also have the advantage of no adverse effect on carbohydrate and lipid metabolism. These agents improve insulin sensitivity and HDL cholesterol while reducing modestly total cholesterol, low-density lipoprotein cholesterol, and triglycerides.[187, 188] The hypothesis that α_1-blockers offer, in virtue of their favorable metabolic effects, a heightened protection against atherosclerosis remains to be demonstrated, however.

Angiotensin II Antagonists

A specific approach to block the renin-angiotensin system is to prevent the binding of angiotensin II at its receptor. This can be done using orally active competitive antagonists of angiotensin II.[189–191] Those available for clinical use selectively block the AT_1 subtype of angiotensin II (i.e., the receptor responsible for all well established actions of angiotensin II). The largest experience has been accumulated with losartan potassium. After oral administration, this compound is rapidly and extensively transformed to its long-acting metabolite, whereas the parent compound has, in addition to a short-lasting blocking effect on the AT_1 receptor, an uricosuric effect that results in a slight decrease in uricemia. Other angiotensin II antagonists (candesartan, irbesartan, valsartan) have been developed. These agents do not need any transformation to block AT_1 receptor. The comparative antihypertensive efficacy of angiotensin II antagonists and ACE inhibitors is a key issue. Although the two types of blockers of the renin-angiotensin system seem to provide equivalent blood pressure results, this cannot be assumed to mean that the drugs act through a similar mechanism. ACE inhibitors enhance the action of bradykinin, whereas angiotensin receptor blockers more effectively inhibit the effects of angiotensin II. Indeed, data suggest that the drugs have an additive effect on blood pressure reduction.[192, 193]

Angiotensin II antagonists typically have a flat dose-response curve with regard to the incidence of adverse events. Usually, with these drugs, the rate of adverse effects is comparable with that of placebo. Unlike ACE inhibitors, angiotensin II antagonists do not cause cough. During AT_1 receptor blockade, the negative feedback on renin secretion normally exerted by angiotensin II is prevented, so that a reactive hyperreninemia develops. AT_1 receptor antagonists leave the other angiotensin II receptors, notably the AT_2 receptor, unopposed. During AT_1 blockade, there is therefore an increased stimulation of AT_2 receptors. Whether this is clinically relevant remains unknown. Until now, there is no evidence for any problem related to a hyperstimulation of AT_2 receptors.

Others

Second-choice antihypertensive agents include a number of medications that are still widely used in some areas of the world but that are being increasingly replaced by modern drugs with greater patient acceptability. Reserpine acts by depleting norepinephrine stores in sympathetic nerve endings. Common complaints are drowsiness, sedation, and nasal congestion. A major drawback of this medication is depression, which may develop insidiously. α-Methyldopa is metabolized to α-methylnorepinephrine, which stimulates α_2-adrenergic receptors located at strategic sites in the brain stem, resulting in an inhibition of sympathetic outflow. α-Methyldopa–associated side effects are sedation, dizziness, dry mouth, orthostatic hypotension, and impotence. The direct antiglobulin test (Coombs test) may be positive, and hemolytic anemia is sometimes observed. Rebound hypertension on withdrawal of treatment might occur. Clonidine is an α_2-adrenergic receptor agonist readily crossing the blood-brain barrier and decreasing sympathetic nerve activity via a central mechanism. This agent frequently causes sedation, dry mouth, constipation, and impotence. Clonidine treatment should not be stopped abruptly in order to avoid the occurrence of rebound hypertension. Moxonidine is a centrally acting imidazoline receptor agonist that exerts a similar antihypertensive action by inhibiting sympathetic activity.

Hydralazine, dihydralazine, and minoxidil are pure dilators of the arterial bed. Their long-term antihypertensive efficacy is limited by reflexly mediated counter-regulatory mechanisms (increase in heart rate and myocardial contractility, sodium retention). The most common side effects are in conjunction with the vasodilatation (headache, tachycardia, palpitations). Hydralazine and dihydralazine might cause a systemic lupus erythematosus–like syndrome. Minoxidil has the most potent vasodilatory activity. It has to be given with large doses of diuretics to avoid sodium and water retention, and a β-blocker should be systematically coadministered to prevent heart rate acceleration. The minoxidil-induced vasodilatation is associated with a marked hirsutism, which represents a major problem in children and women. These vasodilator drugs are potent when added to other drugs in patients with resistant hypertension.

Sequential Monotherapy

For many years, hypertensive patients have been treated according to the classic stepped-care approach, a second drug being added to the first-line therapy whenever the latter is insufficient to normalize blood pressure.[194] The concept of sequential monotherapy has now emerged.[195] It is derived directly from the inability to predict the blood pressure response to antihypertensive drugs in an individual patient. The purpose of this approach is to establish for each patient the most adequate drug that will control blood pressure when administered as monotherapy (Fig. 80–21). The concept is based on the following observation: most antihypertensive agents of the different therapeutic classes exhibit similar response rates, of approximately 40 to 60 percent. However, not every drug normalizes blood pressure in exactly the same 40 to 60 percent of patients. If one assumes that the fraction of a hypertensive population that responds to a given drug shifts by 20 percent from one drug to another, it follows that if two compounds were tested sequentially as monotherapy, an overall response rate of 60 to 70 percent could be expected. This does not mean, however, that every patient should receive consecutively a diuretic, a β-blocker, a calcium antagonist, an ACE inhibitor, and an α_1-blocker. The presence of associated diseases may preclude the administration of some classes of drug. In some patients, agents may be avoided in order to preserve the patient's lifestyle. For example, β-blockers might not be chosen for a young patient involved in heavy athletic activities. One important aspect of sequential monotherapy is that drugs must be administered for several weeks in order to appropriately evaluate their efficacy. Thus, antihypertensive therapy should ideally not be modified at intervals of less than 4 to 6 weeks. In general, this does not represent a major limitation in patients with moderate uncomplicated hypertension. What is the attitude if the successive monotherapies remain unsuccessful in controlling blood pressure? In fact, most patients respond to antihypertensive therapy at relatively low doses. Increasing the dosage allows blood pressure to be controlled in more patients, but often at the expense of a higher incidence of side effects.

Combination Therapy

When monotherapy is insufficient to control blood pressure, it is wiser to use a low-dose combination therapy than to increase the dose of a given drug used as monotherapy.[196, 197] The six major therapeutic classes act via different mechanisms and can therefore be combined successfully (see Fig. 80–19). Diuretics are very useful when associated with any other class of agents. The combination of an ACE inhibitor or an angiotensin II antagonist with a diuretic is particularly efficacious. Indeed, after blockade of the renin-angiotensin system, blood pressure maintenance depends very much on total body sodium. Commonly, small doses of diuretics are sufficient when combined with a blocker of the renin-angiotensin system. In some cases, however, more potent diuretics such as loop diuretics must be used and titrated to obtain an optimal blood pressure response. In general, it is safer to introduce the ACE inhibitor or the angiotensin II antagonist first and the diuretic in a second step. In this way, the occurrence of acute hypotension on initiation of ACE inhibitor therapy is prevented. In patients

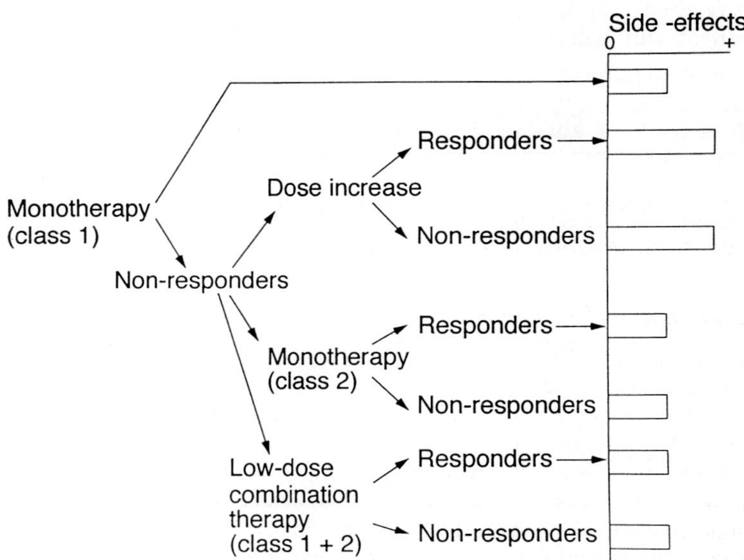

FIGURE 80–21 In nonresponders to a drug acting by a given mechanism, it is preferable to switch to another type of antihypertensive agent than to increase the dose. If required, small doses of antihypertensive agents may be combined.

already being treated with diuretics, the introduction of a blocker of the renin-angiotensin system should be done cautiously, and it may be wise to interrupt diuretic therapy for 2 or 3 days before adding the blocker. Aldosterone secretion is decreased during ACE inhibition and angiotensin II blockade and may cause serum potassium levels to increase. Nevertheless, potassium-sparing diuretics may be safely combined with ACE inhibitors or angiotensin II antagonists as long as renal function is normal.[198] Diuretics also potentiate the antihypertensive efficacy of calcium channel blockers and of β-blockers. An efficacious and logical combination is the association of a calcium antagonist and a β-blocker. The vasodilatation induced by dihydropyridine-type calcium antagonists is generally better tolerated after blockade of β-adrenergic receptors.

The association of a β-blocker with verapamil, a calcium channel blocker with negative inotropic and chronotropic properties, is not recommended because of the increased likelihood of heart block. ACE inhibitors and angiotensin II antagonists may be combined successfully with a β-blocker or a calcium antagonist and β-blockers with all types of agents. The principal goal of combination therapy is to maximize therapeutic efficacy while minimizing side effects. This is usually possible because low doses of the drugs are often adequate. The treatment can sometimes gain considerably in simplicity and acceptance from the patients by using well-balanced fixed-dose combinations. Such combinations may even become valuable options to initiate antihypertensive therapy.[129]

Associated Diseases

Hypertensive patients often present with concomitant diseases that must be taken into account when initiating antihypertensive therapy. The individualization of treatment is therefore aimed at finding an efficacious and well-tolerated drug that possibly improves or at least does not worsen the course of associated diseases (Table 80–10).

Congestive Heart Failure

Any drug that lowers blood pressure in a hypertensive patient will reduce the risk of heart failure. Once heart failure has developed and blood pressure is normalized, however, drug therapy needs to be more selective. ACE inhibitors and β-blockers have emerged as important classes of agents to be used for this indication.[199–202] Given alone or in combination with diuretics, ACE inhibitors are effective in treating moderate or severe congestive heart failure. β-Blockers exert additive effect on slowing the progression of the cardiac dysfunction in heart failure. Angiotensin receptor blockers may also be useful in patients with congestive heart failure, but the benefit observed in a preliminary study[203] has not been confirmed in a large-scale mortality trial recently completed.

Coronary Artery Disease

β-Blockers and calcium antagonists belong to the first-line therapy of coronary insufficiency in normotensive patients. In patients with coronary artery disease, ACE inhibitors (as well as probably angiotensin II antagonists) may also be beneficial because they lower blood pressure and may reduce the incidence of ischemic events.[201, 204] These drugs are, therefore, appropriate agents as monotherapy or combined therapy in hypertensive patients with coronary artery disease.

Left Ventricular Hypertrophy

Cardiac hypertrophy usually regresses if a sustained reduction in blood pressure is achieved. This is indeed the case for patients treated with all classes of antihypertensive agents used as first-line therapy.[205] In a meta-analysis, the beneficial effect was less pronounced for diuretics and most prominent for ACE inhibitors.[206]

Renal Failure

Diuretics have an important role in the management of hypertensive patients with renal failure, and their administration is generally necessary to adequately control blood pressure. ACE inhibitors may be particularly effective in reducing the rate of progression of chronic renal failure,[151] perhaps by preferentially vasodilating the efferent arteriole, thus decreasing the intraglomerular capillary pressure and the proteinuria. Alterations in pore size selectivity owing

TABLE 80–10 **Suggested Use of Antihypertensive Drugs in Patients With Hypertension and Associated Diseases**

Disease	Diuretics	β-Blockers	ACE Inhibitors	Angiotensin II Antagonists	Calcium Antagonists	α-Blockers
Congestive heart failure	+ + +	+ +	+ + +	(+)	+	+
Coronary artery disease	+	+ + +	+ +	(+)	+ + +	+
Left ventricular hypertrophy	+ +	+ + +	+ + +	(+)	+ + +	+ + +
Renal failure	+ + +	+ +	+ +	(+)	+ +	+ +
Peripheral artery disease	+ +	+	+ +	(+)	+ + +	+ + +
Pulmonary obstructive disease or asthma	+ + +	−	+ + +	+ + +	+ + +	+ + +
Diabetes mellitus	+ +	+ +	+ + +	(+)	+ +	+ + +
Hyperlipidemia	+	+	+ + +	+ + +	+ + +	+ + +
Hypertension during pregnancy	−	+ + +	−	−	(+)	(+)

Abbreviation: ACE, angiotensin-converting enzyme.
Key: −, contraindicated; +, + +, + + +, little to strongly indicated; (+), encouraging preliminary experience.

to a fall in plasma angiotensin II levels may also contribute to the antiproteinuric effect of ACE inhibitors. The renal effects of ACE inhibitors seem to favorably influence the natural history of kidney disease.[207]

Peripheral Vascular Diseases

ACE inhibitors, calcium antagonists, and β-blockers are safe first-line therapies in hypertensive patients suffering from peripheral vascular disease. In contrast, β-blockers are not usually recommended because they may aggravate claudication. However, a meta-analysis of 11 controlled studies suggested that the effect of β-blockers on intermittent claudication is minor.[208]

Bronchial Asthma and Chronic Obstructive Pulmonary Disease

Diuretics, ACE inhibitors, and calcium channel blockers can usually be administered safely in patients with bronchial asthma or chronic obstructive pulmonary disease. In contrast, β-blockers can worsen respiratory function in these patients. An agent with β_2-agonistic activity such as celiprolol might be safer if the administration of a β-blocker is mandatory.[209]

Diabetes Mellitus

The most important task in treating diabetics with hypertension is to normalize blood pressure, whatever the drugs used to achieve this goal. This is crucial because lowering blood pressure decreases proteinuria and reduces the rate of decline in renal function. In the Hypertension Optimal Treatment (HOT) study, patients with diabetes mellitus had half the major cardiovascular events in the target group of 80 mm Hg or less compared with the target group of 90 mm Hg or less.[148] In diabetics, blood pressure should not exceed 130/85 mm Hg. ACE inhibitors appear particularly beneficial in hypertensive diabetics. These agents can indeed delay the progression of the nephropathy to the end-stage more effectively than blood pressure control alone.[210] The mechanisms underlying the antiproteinuric effect of ACE inhibitors have already been discussed. Calcium antagonists are also effective antihypertensive drugs in hypertensive diabetics, but in contrast to ACE inhibitors, nifedipine appears to increase rather than decrease proteinuria in patients with diabetic nephropathy.[211] However, this does not appear to be the case for long-acting dihydropyridines. Studies have demonstrated that diltiazem, verapamil, and ACE inhibitors have similar effects on proteinuria in diabetic nephropathy.[211]

Hyperlipidemia

As already mentioned, thiazides and β-blockers may adversely alter lipid metabolism, whereas β-blockers might have a favorable effect.[188, 212] During prolonged therapy with the various classes of first-choice antihypertensive agents, however, no significant change in total cholesterol and HDL cholesterol was demonstrated.[205]

Cerebrovascular Diseases

There is no evidence that some medications are more appropriate than others in the primary prevention of stroke. Elevations in blood pressure are commonly seen in patients with acute stroke, whether they were previously hypertensive or not.[213] In such patients, lowering blood pressure too rapidly and too drastically may reduce cerebral perfusion below the autoregulatory limit, which is generally shifted at a higher level of systemic pressure in ischemic brain areas. Overtreatment after an acute cerebrovascular event may, therefore, aggravate the brain damage. In patients with extreme hypertension, it seems nevertheless justified to lower blood pressure cautiously to about 170/100 mm Hg within a few hours.

Special Considerations

Elderly Patients

Diuretics and calcium antagonists have been claimed to be the most effective in patients with low renin levels, as is often the case in older people, the converse being true for β-blockers and ACE inhibitors.[214] This view has received little support from most trials.[215] Indeed, any drug may normalize blood pressure in a given patient whatever her or his age.

Pregnant Women

Nonpharmacologic therapy is particularly attractive for women with pregnancy-induced hypertension.[216] It may be particularly tempting to restrict salt intake, as the elevation of blood pressure is often accompanied by an excessive gain in body weight and edema. On the other hand, preeclampsic women generally have a decreased intravascular volume and salt depletion may worsen this condition, leading to an additional reduction in placental and renal function. Severe salt restriction is not currently recommended during pregnancy. The best nonpharmacologic measure is bed rest, which helps to shift interstitial fluid to the intravascular compartment and which improves uterine and renal blood flow. Hospitalization is unfortunately most often required. Practically, it is more convenient to prescribe antihypertensive drugs and to propose bed rest if blood pressure cannot be satisfactorily controlled. Hydralazine and methyldopa have long been used as first-choice medications in pregnancy.[217] β-Blockers now appear to be preferable. Diuretics should not be used because they may cause an inappropriate contraction of blood volume. ACE inhibitors are contraindicated, as they increase the risk of oligohydramnios, fetal anuria, and stillbirth when administered late during pregnancy. The experience with calcium antagonists is still limited but promising.[218] α_1-Blockers might also be useful, particularly when combined with a β-blocker.

Refractory Hypertension

There is no general consensus regarding the definition of refractory hypertension.[219] Patients resistant to a combination of three medications acting by different mechanisms represent a minority. In those patients, it is imperative to search for secondary forms of hypertension and to eliminate a problem of noncompliance with the prescribed drug regimen. It may also be wise to make sure that the patient is really hypertensive outside the medical setting.[220] Furthermore, blood pressure measured noninvasively may overestimate the true intra-arterial pressure of patients with rigid arteries.[221] There is unfortunately no easy, reliable test to recognize patients with such a pseudohypertension component. Frequently, blood pressure control can be improved by intensifying diuretic therapy, mainly when given on top of a blocker of the renin-angiotensin system. If needed, the dosage of calcium antagonist (preferably of the dihydropyridine class) or α_1-blockers can be increased. The potent vasodilator minoxidil may be useful, but it should be coadministered with a loop diuretic and a β-blocker to prevent the occurrence of sodium retention and reflex tachycardia. Noteworthy, poor compliance with treatment still represents a leading cause of unsatisfactory blood pressure control.

Hypertensive Crisis

Alarming conditions necessitating a normalization of blood pressure within a few minutes are exceptional.[222] They consist mainly of hypertensive encephalopathy, a severe form of hypertension accompanied by neurologic manifestations (headache, alterations of mental status, seizures), and of hypertension associated with pulmonary edema, acute myocardial infarction, dissecting aortic aneurysm, eclampsia, and sudden blood pressure elevations due to a surge of catecholamines (pheochromocytoma, rebound hypertension after clonidine withdrawal, acute blood pressure increase during treatment with an MAO inhibitor). The most appropriate drug for the treatment of true hypertensive emergency is sodium nitroprusside, an arterial and venous vasodilator acting as a donor of NO inside the vascular smooth muscle cell. This parenterally active drug can be titrated very precisely according to the blood pressure response and usually does not cause a troublesome reflex heart rate acceleration. Accumulation of thiocyanate may occur if treatment is prolonged for several days. Thiocyanate toxicity may be manifested by blurred vision, tinnitus, confusion, and seizures. Labetolol can be used if needed as small bolus or by continuous infusion even outside an intensive care unit (unlike sodium nitroprusside). This combination of α- and β-blockade is particularly appropriate for the treatment of hyperadrenergic states. In patients with pheochromocytoma, intravenous administration of the α_1- and α_2-adrenergic receptor blocker phentolamine is effective, but a β-blocker has generally to be added to prevent tachycardia. Nitrates may be helpful to lower blood pressure in patients with pulmonary edema or acute myocardial infarction.

Except in the situations described previously, it is safer to try to lower blood pressure progressively within a few hours (hypertensive crisis). This is even true in patients with poststroke hypertension (see Cerebrovascular Diseases). Abrupt and marked drops in blood pressure may be hazardous for both the cerebral and the coronary circulation.[223, 224] Nifedipine has become very popular for nonparenteral treatment of hypertensive crisis.[225] When given sublingually or after chewing, this agent can bring blood pressure down within a few minutes. A slow-release formulation of nifedipine maintains more stable blood pressure control. Oral captopril may also be useful, but hypotension may occur in salt-depleted subjects.[226]

Renovascular Hypertension

As expected, ACE inhibitors are often very effective in patients with renovascular hypertension, especially if the renal artery stenosis is unilateral. With other types of medications, multiple combinations are often needed to achieve a satisfactory blood pressure control. As pointed out earlier (in ACE Inhibitors), the disappearance of angiotensin II under ACE inhibition might be detrimental for renal function. Glomerular filtration may be strikingly reduced because of the dependence on angiotensin II for the maintenance of an adequate filtration pressure. Cessation of glomerular filtration rate may pass unnoticed in cases of unilateral renal artery stenosis, as the contralateral kidney can still function normally. The experience available to date suggests that the impairment of renal function induced by ACE inhibition is reversible after withdrawal of the drug. ACE inhibitors are not strictly contraindicated in patients with renovascular hypertension. They may represent the only way to normalize blood pressure in some patients in whom a correction of the stenosis cannot be performed. Low doses of ACE inhibitors are advocated in such instances, so that the intermittent generation of angiotensin II can restore glomerular filtration for a few hours during the day. It is relevant in this context that a recent randomized trial has shown similar effects of antihypertensive treatment and angioplasty on blood pressure control in patients with atherosclerotic renal artery stenosis.[227]

CONCLUSIONS

Hypertension is a heterogeneous disorder associated with an increased cardiovascular risk. The early diagnosis and management of this disease is imperative in order to derive the maximum of benefit from blood pressure–lowering interventions. A large number of antihypertensive drugs acting by various mechanisms are now available. Administered alone or in association, these medications make it possible to normalize blood pressure in nearly all hypertensive persons. Effects should be directed to find a drug regimen that is efficacious and well tolerated for each patient. The evidence is now available that blood pressure can be normalized in almost all patients without adversely altering the quality of life.[228]

REFERENCES

1. Cohn JN: Arteries, myocardium, blood pressure and cardiovascular risk: towards a revised definition of hypertension. J Hypertens 16:2117, 1998.
2. Lifton RP: Molecular genetics of human blood pressure variation. Science 272:676, 1996.
3. Mune T, Rogerson FM, Nikkila H, et al: Human hypertension caused by mutations in the kidney isozyme of 11β-hydroxysteroid dehydrogenase. Nat Genet 10:394, 1995.

4. Lifton RP, Dluhy RG, Powers M, et al: A chimaeric 11β-hydroxylase/aldosterone synthase gene causes glycocorticoid-remediable aldosteronism and human hypertension. Nature 355:262, 1992.
5. Schimkets RA, Warnock D, Bositis CM, et al: Liddle's syndrome: heritable human hypertension caused by mutations in the β subunit of the epithelial sodium channel. Cell 79:407, 1994.
6. Williams RR, Hunt SC, Hasstedt SJ, et al: Are there interactions and relations between genetic and environmental factors predisposing to high blood pressure? Hypertension 18(suppl I):29, 1991.
7. Hunt SC, Hasstedt SJ, Kuida H, et al: Genetic heritability and common environmental components of resting and stressed blood pressures, lipids, and body mass index in Utah pedigrees and twins. Am J Epidemiol 129:625, 1989.
8. Smith TW, Turner CW, Ford MH, et al: Blood pressure reactivity in adult male twins. Health Psychol 6:209, 1987.
9. Hamet P, Pausova Z, Adarichev V, et al: Hypertension: genes and environment. J Hypertens 16:397, 1998.
10. Jeunemaître X, Soubrier F, Kotelevtsev YV, et al: Molecular basis of human hypertension: role of angiotensinogen. Cell 71:169, 1992.
11. Caulfield M, Lavender P, Farral M, et al: Linkage of the angiotensinogen gene to essential hypertension. N Engl J Med 330:1629, 1994.
12. Brand E, Chatelain N, Mulatero P: Structural analysis and evaluation of the aldosterone synthase gene in hypertension. Hypertension 32:198, 1998.
13. Miyamoto Y, Saito Y, Kajiyama N, et al: Endothelial nitric oxide synthase gene is positively associated with essential hypertension. Hypertension 32:3, 1998.
14. Tripodi G, Valtorta F, Torielli K, et al: Hypertension-associated point mutations in the adducin alpha and beta subunits affect actin cytoskeleton and ion transport. J Clin Invest 97:2815, 1996.
15. Rigat B, Hubert C, Alhenc-Gelas F, et al: An insertion/deletion polymorphism in the angiotensin I–converting enzyme gene accounting for half the variance of serum enzyme levels. J Clin Invest 86:1343, 1990.
16. Staessen JA, Wang JG, Ginocchio G, et al: The deletion/insertion polymorphism of the angiotensin converting enzyme gene and cardiovascular-renal risk. J Hypertens 15:1579, 1997.
17. Bonnardeaux A, Davies E, Jeunemaître X, et al: Angiotensin II type 1 receptor gene polymorphisms in human essential hypertension. Hypertension 24:63, 1994.
18. Schmidt S, Beige J, Walla-Friedel M, et al: A polymorphism in the gene for the angiotensin II type 1 receptor is not associated with hypertension. J Hypertens 15:1385, 1997.
19. Persu A, Barbry P, Bassilana F, et al: Genetic analysis of the β subunit of the epithelial Na^+ channel in essential hypertension. Hypertension 32:129, 1998.
20. Muntzel M, Drucke T: A comprehensive review of the salt and blood pressure relationship. Am J Hypertens 5:1S, 1992.
21. Stamler J, Rose G, Elliot P, et al: Findings of the international cooperative INTERSALT study. Hypertension 17(suppl I):9, 1991.
22. Luft FC, Miller JZ, Weinberger MH, et al: Genetic influences on the response to dietary salt reduction, acute salt loading or salt depletion in humans. J Cardiovasc Pharmacol 12(suppl 3):49, 1988.
23. Chertow GM, Brenner BM: Low birth weight as a risk factor for juvenile and adult hypertension. *In* Laragh JH, Brenner BM (eds): Hypertension: Pathophysiology, Diagnostic, and Management. 2nd ed. pp. 89–97. New York: Raven, 1995.
24. Langford HG: Dietary potassium and hypertension: epidemiologic data. Ann Intern Med 98:770, 1985.
25. Campese VM: Calcium, parathyroid hormone and blood pressure. Am J Hypertens 2:34S, 1989.
26. Reisin E: Sodium and obesity in the pathogenesis of hypertension. Am J Hypertens 3:164, 1990.
27. MacMahon SW, Norton RN: Alcohol and hypertension: implications for prevention and treatment. Ann Intern Med 105:124, 1986.
28. Henry JP, Grim CE: Psychosocial mechanisms of primary hypertension. J Hypertens 8:783, 1990.
29. Contrada RJ, Krantz DS: Stress, reactivity, and type A behavior: current status and future directions. Ann Behav Med 10:64, 1988.
30. Maiorano G, Contursi V, Saracino E, Ricapito M: Physical exercise and hypertension. New insights and clinical applications. Am J Hypertens 2:60S, 1989.
31. Izzo JL: Sympathoadrenal activity, catecholamines, and the pathogenesis of vasculopathic hypertensive target-organ damage. Am J Hypertens 2:305S, 1989.
32. Goldstein DS: Plasma catecholamines and essential hypertension: an analytical review. Hypertension 5:86, 1983.
33. Julius S: The blood pressure seeking properties of the central nervous system. J Hypertens 6:177, 1988.
34. Esler MD, Jennings GL, Korner P, et al: Assessment of human sympathetic nervous system activity from measurements of norepinephrine turnover. Hypertension 11:3, 1988.
35. Floras JS, Hara K: Sympathoneural and haemodynamic characteristics of young subjects with mild essential hypertension. J Hypertens 11:647, 1993.
36. Malliani A, Pagani M, Lombardi F, et al: Spectral analysis to assess increased sympathetic tone in arterial hypertension. Hypertension 17(suppl III):36, 1993.
37. Folkow B: Sympathetic nervous control of blood pressure. Role in primary hypertension. Am J Hypertens 2:103S, 1989.
38. Ferrario CM, Averill DB: Do primary dysfunctions in neural control of arterial pressure contribute to hypertension? Hypertension 18(suppl I):38, 1991.
39. Rosendorff C, Susanni E, Hurwitz ML, Ross FP: Adrenergic receptors in hypertension: radioligand binding studies. J Hypertens 3:571, 1985.
40. Floras JS: Epinephrine and the genesis of hypertension. Hypertension 19:1, 1992.
41. Oparil S, Haber E: The renin-angiotensin system. N Engl J Med 291:389, 1974.
42. Erdös EG: Angiotensin I converting enzyme and the changes in our concepts through the years. Hypertension 16:363, 1990.
43. Swales JD, Heagerty AM: Vascular renin-angiotensin system: the unanswered questions. J Hypertens 5(suppl 2):1, 1987.
44. Urata H, Nishimura H, Ganten D, et al: Angiotensin-converting enzyme–independent pathways of angiotensin II formation in human tissues and cardiovascular diseases. Blood Press 5(suppl 2):22, 1996.
45. Chung O, Stoll M, Unger T: Physiologic and pharmacologic implications of AT_1 versus AT_2 receptors. Blood Press 5(suppl 2):47, 1996.
46. Zimmerman BG, Sybert EG, Wong PC: Interaction between sympathetic and renin-angiotensin system. J Hypertens 2:581, 1984.
47. Brunner HR, Laragh JH, Baer L, et al: Essential hypertension: renin and aldosterone, heart attack and stroke. N Engl J Med 286:441, 1972.
48. Brunner HR, Gavras H: Clinical implications of renin in the hypertensive patient. JAMA 233:1091, 1975.
49. Churchill PC, Churchill MC, McDonald FD: Evidence that beta-adrenoceptor activation mediates isoproterenol stimulated renin secretion in the rat. Endocrinology 113:687, 1983.
50. Julius S: Interaction between renin and the autonomic nervous system in hypertension. Am Heart J 116:611, 1988.
51. Weidmann PS, De Muyttenaere-Bursztein S, Maxwell MH, Lima JD: Effect of aging on plasma renin and aldosterone in normal man. Kidney Int 8:325, 1975.
52. Carretero OA, Scicli AG: Local hormonal factors (intracrine, autocrine, and paracrine) in hypertension. Hypertension 18(suppl I):58, 1991.
53. Bönner G, Preis S, Schunk U, et al: Hemodynamic effects of bradykinin on systemic and pulmonary circulation in healthy and hypertensive humans. J Cardiovasc Pharmacol 15(suppl 6):46, 1990.
54. Cantin M, Genest J: The heart and the atrial natriuretic factor. Endocrine Rev 6:107, 1985.
55. Laragh JH: Atrial natriuretic hormone, the renin-aldosterone axis and blood pressure electrolyte homeostasis. N Engl J Med 313:1330, 1985.
56. Safar ME, London GM: Venous system in essential hypertension. Clin Sci 69:497, 1985.
57. Ganau A, Devereux RB, Atlas SA, et al: Plasma atrial factor in essential hypertension: relation to cardiac size, function and systemic hemodynamics. J Am Coll Cardiol 14:715, 1989.
58. Fioventini C, Barbier P, Galli C: Pulmonary vascular overreactivity in systemic hypertension: a pathophysiological link between the greater and the lesser circulation. Hypertension 7:995, 1985.
59. Ferrari P, Weidmann P, Ferrier CI, et al: Dysregulation of atrial natriuretic factor in hypertension-prone man. J Clin Endocrinol Metab 71:944, 1990.
60. McGiff JC, Carroll MA, Escalante B: Arachidonate metabolites and kinins in blood pressure regulation. Hypertension 18(suppl III):150, 1991.
61. Cinotti GA, Pugliese F: Prostaglandins and hypertension. Am J Hypertens 2:10S, 1989.

62. Hornych A, Safar M, Bariety J, et al: Thromboxane A_2 in borderline and essential hypertensive patients. Prostaglandins Leukot Med 10:145, 1983.
63. Guyton AC: Dominant role of the kidneys and accessory role of whole-body autoregulation in the pathogenesis of hypertension. Am J Hypertens 2:575, 1989.
64. Hollenberg NK, Williams GH: Sodium-sensitive hypertension. Implications of pathogenesis for therapy. Am J Hypertens 2:809, 1989.
65. De Fronzo RA: Insulin resistance, hyperinsulinemia, and coronary artery disease: a complex metabolic web. J Cardiovasc Pharmacol 20(suppl 11):1, 1992.
66. Moncada S, Palmer RMJ, Higgs EA: Nitric oxide: physiology, pathophysiology and pharmacology. Pharmacol Rev 43:109, 1991.
67. Vanhoutte PM: Other endothelium-derived vasoactive factors. Circulation 87(suppl V):9, 1993.
68. Raij L: Nitric oxide and the kidney. Circulation 87(suppl V):26, 1993.
69. Gibbons GH, Dzau VJ: Mechanism of disease: the emerging concept of vascular remodeling. N Engl J Med 330:1431, 1994.
70. Luscher TF, Bong-Gwan S, Buhler FR: Potential role of endothelin in hypertension. Controversy on endothelin in hypertension. Hypertension 21:752, 1993.
71. Panza JA, Quiyyumi AA, Brush JE Jr, Eastein SE: Abnormal endothelium-dependent vascular relaxation in patients with essential hypertension. N Engl J Med 323:22, 1990.
72. Perticone F, Ceravolo R, Maio R, et al: Angiotensin-converting enzyme polymorphism is associated with endothelium-dependent vasodilation in never treated hypertensive patients. Hypertension 31:900, 1998.
73. Widimsky J Jr, Horky K, Dvorakova J: Plasma endothelin-1,2 levels in mild and severe hypertension. J Hypertens 9:194s, 1991.
74. Blaustein MP: Sodium ions, calcium ions, blood pressure regulation and hypertension: a reassessment of a hypothesis. Am J Physiol 232:165, 1977.
75. Tonyz RM, Schiffrin EL: Signal transduction in hypertension: part I. Curr Opin Nephrol Hypertens 2:5, 16, 1993.
76. Tonyz RM, Schiffrin EL: Signal transduction in hypertension: part II. Curr Opin Nephrol Hypertens 2:17, 1993.
77. Haller H, Lindschau C, Quass P, Distler A: Protein phosphorylation and intracellular free calcium in platelets of patients with essential hypertension. Am J Hypertens 5:117, 1992.
78. Feldman RD, Lawton WJ, McArdle WL: A low sodium diet corrects the defect in lymphocyte beta-adrenergic receptors in hypertensive subjects. J Clin Invest 79:290, 1987.
79. Resink TJ, Burgisser E, Buhler FR: Enhanced platelet cyclic AMP response to prostaglandin E_1 in essential hypertension. Hypertension 8:662, 1986.
80. Muller FB, Bolli P, Kiowski W, et al: Atrial natriuretic peptide is elevated in low-renin essential hypertension. J Hypertens 4(suppl 6):489, 1986.
81. Sagnella GA, Singer DR, Markandu ND, et al: Is atrial natriuretic peptide 3′,5′ cyclic monophosphate coupling a determinant of urinary sodium excretion in essential hypertension? J Hypertens 10:349, 1992.
82. Aviv A, Lasker N: Defects in membrane transport of ions as possible pathogenic factors in hypertension. Curr Opin Nephrol Hypertens 1:68, 1992
83. Doria A, Fioretto P, Avogaro A, et al: Insulin resistance is associated with high sodium-lithium counter-transport in essential hypertension. Am J Physiol 261:E684, 1991
84. Folkow B: Physiological aspects of primary hypertension. Physiol Rev 62:347, 1982.
85. Mulvany MJ: Remodeling of resistance vessel structure in essential hypertension. Curr Opin Nephrol Hypertens 2:77, 1993.
86. Diez J: Cardiovascular growth associated with arterial hypertension. J Cardiovasc Pharmacol 20(suppl B):1, 1992.
87. Rosskopf D, Dusing R, Siffert W: Membrane sodium-proton exchange and primary hypertension. Hypertension 21:607, 1993.
88. Glasser SP, Arnett DK, McVeigh GE, et al: Vascular compliance and cardiovascular disease. A risk factor or a marker? Am J Hypertens 10:1175, 1997.
89. Safar E, London GM, Asmar R, et al: Recent advances on large arteries in hypertension. Hypertension 32:156, 1998.
90. Finkelstein SM, Cohn JN: First- and third-order models for determining arterial compliance. J Hypertens 10(suppl):11, 1992.
91. Cohn JN, Finkelstein SM: Abnormalities of vascular compliance in hypertension, aging and heart failure. J Hypertens 10:S61, 1992.
92. Benetos A, Gauthier S, Richard S, et al: Influence of angiotensin-converting enzyme and angiotensin II type I receptor gene polymorphisms on aortic stiffness in normotensive and hypertensive patients. Circulation 94:698, 1996.
93. Verdecchia P, Schillaci G, Borgioni C, et al: Ambulatory pulse pressure. A potent predictor of total cardiovascular risk in hypertension. Hypertension 32:983, 1998.
94. O'Rourke M, Frohlich ED: Pulse pressure. Is this a clinically useful risk factor? Hypertension 34:372, 1999.
95. Brown MA, Whitworth A: Hypertension in human renal disease. J Hypertens 10:701, 1992.
96. Vaughan DE: Renovascular hypertension. Kidney Int 27:811, 1985.
97. Davis BA, Crook JE, Vestal RE, Oates JA: Prevalence of renovascular hypertension in patients with grade III or IV hypertensive retinopathy. N Engl J Med 301:1273, 1979.
98. Luscher TF, Lie JT, Stanson AW, et al: Arterial fibromuscular dysplasia. Mayo Clin Proc 63:931, 1987.
99. Alpert BS, Bain HH, Balfe JW, et al: Role of the renin-angiotensin-aldosterone system in hypertensive children with coarctation of the aorta. Am J Cardiol 43:828, 1979.
100. Manger WM, Gifford RW, Hoffmann B: Pheochromocytoma: a clinical and experimental overview. Curr Probl Cancer 9:1, 1985.
101. Bravo EL: Pheochromocytoma: new concepts and future trends. Kidney Int 40:544, 1991.
102. Noth RH, Biglieri EG: Primary aldosteronism. Med Clin North Am 72:1117, 1988.
103. Biglieri EG: The mineralocorticoid hormones in human hypertension. Am J Hypertens 1:313, 1988.
104. Stowasser M, Bachmann AW, Jonsson JR, et al: Clinical, biochemical and genetic approaches to the detection of familial hyperaldosteronism type I. J Hypertens 13:1610, 1995.
105. Kaye TB, Crapo L: The Cushing's syndrome: an update on diagnostic tests. Ann Intern Med 112:434, 1990.
106. Connel JMC, Fraser R: Adrenal corticoid synthesis and hypertension. J Hypertens 9:97, 1991.
107. Polikar R, Burger AG, Scherrer U, Nicod P: The thyroid and the heart. Circulation 87:1435, 1993.
108. Gardner DG, Gertz BJ, Hane S: Thyroid hormone increases rat atrial natriuretic peptide messenger ribonucleic acid accumulation in vivo and in vitro. Mol Endocrinol 1:260, 1987.
109. Hellstrom J, Birke G, Edvall CA: Hypertension in hyperparathyroidism. Br J Urol 30:13, 1988.
110. Lewanczuk KZ, Pang PKT: Expression of parathyroid hypertensive factor in hypertensive primary hyperparathyroid patients. Blood Press 2:22, 1993.
111. Deray G, Rieu M, Devynck MA, et al: Evidence of an endogenous digitalis-like factor in the plasma of patients with acromegaly. N Engl J Med 316:575, 1987.
112. Cunningham FG, Lindheimer MD: Hypertension in pregnancy. N Engl J Med 326:927, 1992.
113. Pinto A, Sorrentino R, Sorrentino P, et al: Endothelial-derived relaxing factor released by endothelial cells of human umbilical vessels and its impairment in pregnancy-induced hypertension. Am J Obstet Gynecol 164:507, 1991.
114. Clark BA, Halvorson L, Sachs B, Epstein FH: Plasma endothelin levels in preeclampsia: elevation and correlation with uric acid levels and renal impairment. Am J Obstet Gynecol 166:962, 1992.
115. Silverberg DS, Oksenberg A, Iaina A: Sleep related breathing disorders are common contributing factors to the production of essential hypertension but are neglected, underdiagnosed, and undertreated. Am J Hypertens 10:1319, 1997.
116. Narkiewics K, Somers VK: The sympathetic nervous system and obstructive sleep apnea: implications for hypertension. J Hypertens 15:1613, 1997.
117. Woods JW: Oral contraceptives and hypertension. Hypertension 11(suppl II):11, 1988.
118. Khaw K, Peart WS: Blood pressure and contraceptive use. BMJ 285:402, 1982.
119. Mackay EV, Khoo SH, Adam R: Contraception with a six monthly injection of progestagen. Effects on blood pressure, body weight, and uterine bleeding pattern, side effects, efficacy and acceptability. Aust N Z J Obst Gynaecol 11:148, 1971.
120. Hawkins DF, Benster B: A comparative study of three low dose

progestagens, chlormadinone acetate, megestrol acetate and norethisterone, as oral contraceptives. Br J Obstet Gynaecol 84:708, 1977.
121. Weir RJ, Davies DL, Fraser R, et al: Contraceptive steroids and hypertension. J Steroid Biochem 6:961, 1975.
122. Cain MD, Walters WA, Catt KJ: Effects of oral contraceptive therapy on the renin-angiotensin system. J Clin Endocrinol Metab 33:671, 1971.
123. Crane MG: Iatrogenic hypertension and contraceptive pills. *In* Genest J, Koiw E, Kuchel O (eds): Hypertension. pp. 855–866. New York: McGraw-Hill, 1977.
124. Gawin FH, Ellinwood EH: Cocaine and other stimulants: actions, abuse, and treatment. N Engl J Med 318:1173, 1988.
125. Luke RG: Mechanism of cyclosporine-induced hypertension. Am J Hypertens 4:468, 1991.
126. Ad Hoc Committee for the National Kidney Foundation: Statement on the clinical use of recombinant erythropoietin in anemia of end-stage renal disease. Am J Kidney Dis 14:163, 1989.
127. Swartz SL: The role of prostaglandins in mediating the effects of angiotensin converting enzyme inhibitors and other antihypertensive drugs. Cardiovasc Drugs Ther 1:39, 1987.
128. 1999 World Health Organization–International Society of Hypertension: Guidelines for the management of hypertension. J Hypertens 77:151, 1999.
129. The Sixth Report of the Joint National Committee on Prevention, Detection, Evaluation, and Treatment of High Blood Pressure. NIH Publication No 98–4080. Bethesda, MD: National Institutes of Health, National High Blood Pressure Educational Program, 1997.
130. American Society of Hypertension: Recommendations for routine blood pressure measurement by indirect cuff sphygmomanometry. Am J Hypertens 5:207, 1992.
131. Ljungman S: Microalbuminuria in essential hypertension. Am J Hypertens 3:956, 1990.
132. Frohlich ED, Apstein C, Chobanian AV, et al: The heart in hypertension. N Engl J Med 327:998, 1992.
133. Pickering TG: Ambulatory monitoring and the definition of hypertension. J Hypertens 10:401, 1992.
134. Appel LJ, Stason WB: Ambulatory blood pressure monitoring and blood pressure self-measurement in the diagnosis and management of hypertension. Ann Intern Med 118:867, 1993.
135. Mann SJ, Pickering TG: Detection of renovascular hypertension. State of the art. Ann Intern Med 117:845, 1992.
136. Kannel WB, Neaton JD, Wentworth P, et al, for the MRFIT Research Group: Overall and coronary health disease mortality rates in relation to major risk factors in 325,348 men screened for the MRFIT. Am Heart J 112:825, 1986.
137. Stokes J, Kannel WB, Wolf PA, et al: The relative importance of selected risk factors for various manifestations of cardiovascular disease among men and women from 35 to 64 years old: 30 years of follow-up in the Framingham Study. Circulation 75(suppl V):65, 1987.
138. MacMahon S, Peto R, Cutler J, et al: Blood pressure, stroke, and coronary heart disease. Part I. Prolonged differences in blood pressure: prospective observational studies corrected for the regression, dilution bias. Lancet 335:765, 1990.
139. Whelton PK, Klag MJ: Hypertension as a risk factor for renal disease. Review of clinical and epidemiological evidence. Hypertension 13(suppl I):19, 1989.
140. MacMahon S, Cutler JA, Stamler J: Antihypertensive drug treatment. Potential, expected, and observed effects on stroke and coronary heart disease. Hypertension 13(suppl I):45, 1989.
141. Hansson L: The key issues in preventive cardiology. Blood Press 1(suppl 4):7, 1992.
142. Dennis VW, Nurko S, Robinson K: Hyperhomocysteinemia: detection, risk assessment, and treatment. Curr Opin Nephrol Hypertens 6:483, 1997.
143. Alderman MH: Blood pressure management: individualized treatment based on absolute risk and the potential for benefit. Ann Intern Med 119:329, 1993.
144. Collins R, Peto R, MacMahon S, et al: Blood pressure, stroke and coronary heart disease. Part 2. Short-term reductions in blood pressure: overview of randomized drug trials in their epidemiological context. Lancet 335:827, 1990.
145. Cutler JA, MacMahon SW, Furberg CD: Controlled clinical trials of drug treatment for hypertension. A review. Hypertension 13(suppl I):36, 1989.
146. MacMahon S, Rodgers A: The effects of blood pressure reduction in older patients: an overview of five randomized controlled trials in elderly hypertensives. Clin Exp Hypertens 15:967, 1993.
147. Cruickshank JM: Coronary flow reserve and the J curve relation between diastolic blood pressure and myocardial infarction. BMJ 297:726, 1988.
148. Hansson L, Zanchetti A, Carruthers SG, et al: Effects of intensive blood-pressure lowering and low-dose aspirin in patients with hypertension: principal results of the Hypertension Optimal Treatment (HOT) randomized trial. Lancet 351:1755, 1998.
149. Fagerberg B, Wilkstrand J, Berglund G, et al: Mortality rates in treated hypertensive men with additional risk factors are high but can be reduced. A randomized intervention study. Am J Hypertens 11:14, 1998.
150. Furberg CD, Yusuf S: Effect of drug therapy on survival in chronic heart failure. Adv Cardiol 34:124, 1986.
151. Mimran A, Ribstein J: Antihypertensive therapy in renal disease and transplantation. J Hypertens 10(suppl 5):79, 1992.
152. Waeber B, Rutschmann B, Nussberger J, Brunner HR: Evaluation of antihypertensive therapy: discrepancies between office and ambulatory recorded blood pressure. J Hypertens 9(suppl 3):53, 1991.
153. Devereux RB, Pickering TG: Relationship between ambulatory or exercise blood pressure and left ventricular structure: prognostic implications. J Hypertens 8(suppl 6):125, 1990.
154. Verdecchia P, Schillacci G, Guerrieri M, et al: Circadian blood pressure changes and left ventricular hypertrophy in essential hypertension. Circulation 81:528, 1990.
155. The Scientific Committee: Consensus document on non-invasive ambulatory blood pressure monitoring. J Hypertens 8(suppl 6):135, 1990.
156. World Hypertension League: Self-measurement of blood pressure: a statement by the World Hypertension League. J Hypertens 6:257, 1988.
157. Bildingmeyer I, Burnier M, Bildingmeyer M, et al: Isolated office hypertension: a prehypertensive state? J Hypertens 14:327, 1996.
158. Falkner B: Hypertension in childhood and adolescence. Clin Exp Hypertens 15:1315, 1993.
159. Task Force on Blood Pressure Control in Children: Report of the Second Task Force on Blood Pressure Control in Children, 1987. Pediatrics 79:1, 1988.
160. National High Blood Pressure Education Program: Working Group Report on High Blood Pressure in Pregnancy. Am J Obstet Gynecol 163:1689, 1990.
161. Kincaid-Smith P: Malignant hypertension. J Hypertens 9:893, 1991.
162. Kaplan NM: Long-term effectiveness of non pharmacological treatment of hypertension. Hypertension 18(suppl I):153, 1991.
163. Staessen J, Fagard R, Lijnen P, Amery A: Body weight, sodium intake and blood pressure. J Hypertens 7(suppl 1):19, 1989.
164. Marmot M, Brunner E: Alcohol and cardiovascular disease: the status of the U shaped curve. BMJ 303:565, 1991.
165. Arakawa K: Hypertension and exercise. Clin Exp Hypertens 15:1171, 1993.
166. Van Zwieten PA: Development and trends in the drug treatment of essential hypertension. J Hypertens 10(suppl 7):1, 1992.
167. Gifford RW, Borazanian RA: Traditional first-line therapy. Overview of medical benefits and side effects. Hypertension 13(suppl I):119, 1989.
168. Johnston CI: The place of diuretics in the treatment of hypertension in 1993: can we do better? Clin Exp Hypertens 15:1239, 1993.
169. Man in't Veld AJ, van den Meiracker A, Schalekamp MADH: The effect of beta-blockers on total peripheral resistance. J Cardiovasc Pharmacol 8(suppl 4):49, 1986.
170. Cruickshank JM: The case for beta-blockers as first-line antihypertensive therapy. J Hypertens 10(suppl 3):21, 1992.
171. Brunner HR, Waeber B, Nussberger J: Treatment of hypertension with ACE inhibition as first step: pharmacologic and clinical considerations. J Cardiovasc Pharmacol 10(suppl 7):36, 1987.
172. Williams GH: Converting-enzyme inhibitors in the treatment of hypertension. N Engl J Med 319:1517, 1989.
173. Waeber B, Nussberger J, Juillerat L, Brunner HR: Angiotensin converting enzyme inhibition: discrepancy between antihypertensive effect and suppression of enzyme activity. J Cardiovasc Pharmacol 14(suppl 4):53, 1989.
174. Iyer SN, Ferrario CM, Chappell MC: Angiotensin-(1–7) contributes to the antihypertensive effects of blockade of the renin angiotensin system. Hypertension 31:356, 1998.

175. Ball SG: Age-related effects of converting enzyme inhibitors: a commentary. J Cardiovasc Pharmacol 12(suppl 8):105, 1988.
176. McEwan JR, Fuller RW: Angiotensin converting enzyme inhibitors and cough. J Cardiovasc Pharmacol 13(suppl 3):67, 1989.
177. Nussberger J, Cugno M, Amstutz C, et al: Plasma bradykinin in angio-oedema. Lancet 351:1693, 1998.
178. Levenson DJ, Dzau VJ: Effects of angiotensin-converting enzyme inhibition on renal hemodynamics in renal artery stenosis. Kidney Int 31(suppl 20):173, 1987.
179. Dustan HP: Calcium channel blockers. Potential medical benefits and side effects. Hypertension 13(suppl I):37, 1989.
180. Luft FC, Haller H: Calcium channel blockers in current medical practice: an update for 1993. Clin Exp Hypertens 15:1263, 1993.
181. Psaty B, Heckbert S, Koepsell T, et al: The risk of myocardial infarction associated with antihypertensive drug therapies. JAMA 274:620, 1995.
182. Pahor M, Guralnik J, Furberg C, et al: Risk of gastrointestinal haemorrhage with calcium antagonists in hypertensive persons over 67 years old. Lancet 347:1061, 1996.
183. Pahor M, Guralnik J, Ferruci L, et al: Calcium-channel blockade and incidence of cancer in aged populations. Lancet 348:493, 1996.
184. Ad Hoc Subcommittee of the Liaison Committee of the World Health Organization and the International Society of Hypertension: Effects of calcium antagonists on the risks of coronary heart disease, cancer and bleeding. J Hypertens 15:105, 1997.
185. Staessen JA, Fagard R, Thijs L, et al: Morbidity and mortality in the European trial on isolated systolic hypertension in the elderly. Lancet 350:757, 1997.
186. Grimm RH: Alpha-antagonists in the treatment of hypertension. Hypertension 13(suppl I):131, 1989.
187. Pollare T, Lithell H, Selinus I, Berne C: Application of prazosin is associated with an increase in insulin sensitivity in obese patients with hypertension. Diabetologica 31:415, 1988.
188. Lithell HOL: Effect of antihypertensive drugs on insulin, glucose and lipid metabolism. Diabetes Care 14:203, 1991.
189. Waeber B, Brunner HR: Angiotensin II antagonists: a new class of antihypertensive agent. Br J Clin Pract 50:265, 1996.
190. Bauer JH, Reams GP: The angiotensin II type 1 receptor antagonists. A new class of antihypertensive agents. Arch Intern Med 155:1361, 1995.
191. Csajka C, Buclin T, Brunner HR, et al: Pharmacokinetic-pharmacodynamic profile of angiotensin II receptor antagonists. Clin Pharmacokinet 32:1, 1997.
192. Azizi M, Chatellier G, Guyene T-T, et al: Additive effects of combined angiotensin-converting enzyme inhibition and angiotensin II antagonism on blood pressure and renin release in sodium-depleted normotensives. Circulation 92:825–834, 1995.
193. Baruch L, Anand I, Cohen IS, et al: Augmented short- and long-term hemodynamic and hormonal effects of an angiotensin receptor blocker added to angiotensin converting enzyme inhibitor therapy in patients with heart failure. Circulation 99:2658–2664, 1999.
194. Zanchetti A: A re-examination of "stepped care": a retrospective and a prospective. J Cardiovasc Pharmacol 7(suppl 1):126, 1985.
195. Brunner HR, Menard J, Waeber B, et al: Treating the individual hypertensive patient: considerations on dose, sequential monotherapy and fixed-dose combinations. J Hypertens 8:3, 1990.
196. Chalmers J: The place of combination therapy in the treatment of hypertension in 1993. Clin Exp Hypertens 15:1299, 1993.
197. Waeber B, Brunner HR: Low-dose combinations versus monotherapies in the treatment of hypertension. J Hypertens 15(suppl 2):17, 1997.
198. Schohn DC, Spiesser R, Wehrlen M, et al: Aldactazine/captopril combination, safe and effective in mild to moderate systemic hypertension: report on a multicenter study of 967 patients. Am J Cardiol 65(suppl K):4, 1990.
199. Deedwania PC: Angiotensin-converting enzyme inhibitors in congestive heart failure. Arch Intern Med 150:1798, 1990.
200. Cohn JN: Physiological variables as markers for symptoms, risk, and interventions in heart failure. Circulation 87(suppl VII):110, 1993.
201. Gavras H, Gavras I: Cardioprotective potential of angiotensin converting enzyme inhibitors. Hypertension 9:385, 1991.
202. CIBIS-II Investigators and Committees: The Cardiac Insufficiency Bisoprolol Study II (CIBIS-II): a randomized trial. Lancet 353:9, 1999.
203. Pitt B, Segal R, Martinez FA, et al: Randomised trial of losartan versus captopril in patients over 65 with heart failure. Evaluation of Losartan in the Elderly Study, ELITE. Lancet 349:747, 1997.
204. Yusuf S, Pepine CJ, Garces C, et al: Effect of enalapril on myocardial infarction and unstable angina in patients with low ejection fractions. Lancet 340:1173, 1992.
205. Neaton JD, Grimm RH, Prineas RJ, et al: Treatment of Mild Hypertension Study. Final results. JAMA 270:713, 1993.
206. Dahlof B, Pennert K, Hansson L: Reversal of left ventricular hypertrophy in hypertensive patients: a meta-analysis of 109 treatment studies. Am J Hypertens 5:95, 1992.
207. Maschio M, Alberti D, Janin G, et al: Effect of the angiotensin-converting-enzyme inhibitor benazepril on the progression of chronic renal insufficiency. N Engl J Med 334:939, 1996.
208. Radack K, Deck C: Beta-adrenergic blocker therapy does not worsen intermittent claudication in subjects with peripheral arterial disease. A meta-analysis of randomized controlled trials. Arch Intern Med 151:1769, 1991.
209. Weber MA: Hypertension with concomitant conditions: the changing role of beta-adrenoceptor blockade. Am Heart J 121:716, 1991.
210. Lewis EJ, Hunsicker LG, Pain RP, Rohde RD: The effect of angiotensin-converting-enzyme inhibition on diabetic nephropathy. N Engl J Med 329:1456, 1993.
211. Demarie BK, Bakris GL: Effects of different calcium antagonists on proteinuria associated with diabetes mellitus. Ann Intern Med 113:987, 1990.
212. Weidmann P, Uehlinger DE, Gerber A: Antihypertensive treatment and serum lipoproteins. J Hypertens 3:297, 1985.
213. Powers WJ: Acute hypertension after stroke: the scientific basis for treatment decisions. Neurology 43:461, 1993.
214. Buhler FR, Bolli P, Kiowski W, et al: Renin profiling to select antihypertensive baseline drugs. Renin inhibitors for high-renin and calcium-entry blockers for low-renin patients. Am J Med 77(suppl 2A):36, 1984.
215. Kaplan NM: Critical comments on recent literature. Age and the response to antihypertensive drugs. Am J Hypertens 2:213, 1989.
216. Brown MA: Non-pharmacological management of pregnancy-induced hypertension. J Hypertens 8:295, 1990.
217. Lowe SA, Rubin PC: The pharmacological management of hypertension in pregnancy. J Hypertens 10:201, 1992.
218. Fenakel K, Fenakel G, Appelman Z, et al: Nifedipine in the treatment of severe preeclampsia. Obstet Gynecol 77:331, 1991.
219. Setaro JF, Black HR: Current concepts: refractory hypertension. N Engl J Med 327:543, 1992.
220. Waeber B, Scherrer U, Petrillo A, et al: Are some hypertensive patients overtreated? Results of a prospective study of ambulatory blood pressure recordings. Lancet 2:732, 1998.
221. Zweifler AJ, Shahab ST: Pseudohypertension: a new assessment. J Hypertens 11:1, 1993.
222. Gifford RW: Management of hypertensive crises. JAMA 266:829, 1991.
223. Strandgaard S: Autoregulation of cerebral blood flow in hypertensive patients. Circulation 53:720, 1976.
224. Cruickshank JM, Thorp JM, Zacharias FJ: Benefits and potential harm of lowering high blood pressure. Lancet 1:581, 1987
225. Schillinger DS: Nifedipine in hypertensive emergencies: a prospective study. J Emerg Med 5:463, 1987.
226. Biollaz J, Waeber B, Brunner HR: Hypertensive crisis treated with orally administered captopril. Eur J Clin Pharmacol 25:145, 1983.
227. Plouin PF, Chatellier G, Darné B, et al: Blood pressure outcome of angioplasty in atherosclerotic renal artery stenosis. A randomized trial. Hypertension 31:823, 1998.
228. Wirklund I, Halling K, Ryden-Bergsten T, et al: Does lowering the blood pressure improve the mood? Quality-of-life results from the Hypertension Optimal Treatment (HOT) Study. Blood Press 6:357, 1997.

CHAPTER 81

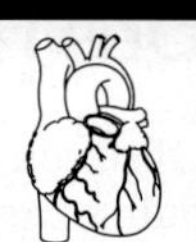

Shock

Henry S. Loeb and Jay N. Cohn

VOLUME DEPLETION
SEPTIC SHOCK
OBSTRUCTIVE SHOCK
CARDIOGENIC SHOCK
Predictors, Incidence, and Mortality
Clinical Recognition
Treatment

Shock is a syndrome in which an acute deficiency of vital tissue perfusion due to hemodynamic dysfunction leads to progressive metabolic and functional deterioration that, if not reversed, will lead to death. The common feature of shock is that cardiac output is inadequate to perfuse all the organs with sufficient blood to maintain tissue integrity. This inadequacy of perfusion is usually but not always accompanied by hypotension and intense regional vasoconstriction. The perfusion deficit may result in a cascade of further complications, such as the release of vasodilator factors that increase capillary permeability and may further lower blood pressure, leading ultimately to cardiac dysrhythmias and death. Shock can result from both cardiovascular and noncardiovascular illnesses (Table 81–1). Cardiac causes are the focus of concern for the cardiologist, and it is critical to exclude noncardiac causes before launching into aggressive cardiovascular therapy.

TABLE 81–1 Causes of Shock

Hypovolemic shock	Hemorrhage
	Trauma
	Burns
	Dehydration
	Diuresis
	Plasma volume loss
Vasodilatation shock	Drugs
	Pyrexia
	Endogenous vasodilatation
Cardiogenic shock	Acute myocardial infarction
	Myocarditis
	Arrhythmias
	Impaired filling
	Pericardial, valvular
	Pulmonary, vascular
	Obstructed emptying
	Aortic valve
Septic shock	Gram-negative and gram-positive infections

Volume Depletion

The most common and most easily treated form of shock is that due to functional hypovolemia. Whether caused by hemorrhage, severe intravascular plasma volume depletion, or an increased capacitance of the vascular system, inadequate cardiac filling and a fall in cardiac output are hallmarks of the syndrome. Recognition of the problem and prompt restoration of volume are generally curative unless the perfusion deficit has persisted long enough to activate tissue-damaging local and circulating toxins.

Recognition of volume depletion as the cause of shock generally is simple when the patient has sustained hemorrhage or trauma. More subtle inadequacies of venous return may occur with dehydration, infections, malnutrition, and some edematous states.[1] A low blood pressure, a narrow pulse pressure, and a low jugular venous pressure are hallmarks of hypovolemia. A challenge with intravenous infusion of fluids is the most effective way to diagnose and treat the syndrome. When pulmonary symptoms cloud the picture and there is concern about volume loading in an individual who may have pulmonary edema, a bedside right heart catheterization may be necessary to clarify the hemodynamic abnormality.

Septic Shock

The mechanisms responsible for septic shock continue to be an area of considerable research. The role of factors such as nitric oxide from the endothelium and the monokines and eicosanoids from macrophages continues to be pursued, and the use of arginine analogues and monoclonal antibodies in endotoxic shock has been a potential therapeutic advance. A role for endogenous opioids has been proposed, and the ability in some situations of the opioid antagonist naloxone to reverse endotoxic shock has been partly supportive.

Double-blind, randomized controlled trials have included a monoclonal antibody to tumor necrosis factor-alpha,[2] antithrombin III replacement,[3] low-dose corticosteroids,[4] pentoxifylline,[5] antioxidants,[6] human interleukin-1 receptor antagonist,[7] and p55 tumor necrosis factor receptor fusion protein.[8] Although the results of some of these trials have been encouraging, there is at present no established regimen for the treatment of septic shock beyond the prompt and effective eradication of infection coupled with appropriate supportive measures based on accurate and frequent physiologic and clinical assessment.

Obstructive Shock

Obstruction of blood flow through the lungs due to massive pulmonary embolism or tension pneumothorax will reduce left heart filling and impair cardiac output. Similarly, obstruction of blood flow into the left ventricle because of pericardial tamponade or valvular or intracardiac obstruction may result in an acute reduction in cardiac output that demands aggressive specific intervention. These conditions are considered further in the discussion of cardiogenic shock.

Cardiogenic Shock

The most common cause of cardiogenic shock is acute *myocardial infarction* or *ischemia* resulting in a deficit of regional or global myocardial contraction. Several conditions can mimic cardiogenic shock due to acute myocardial infarction. *Pericardial tamponade* should be considered whenever a paradoxical pulse is detected or in patients with malignancy, renal failure, chest trauma, anticoagulant therapy, aortic dissection, or postinfarction free wall rupture. Bedside echocardiography can be used to confirm the diagnosis and is a useful guide during emergency pericardiocentesis. *Massive pulmonary embolization* must be considered in postoperative patients or in patients with other known risk factors. Emergency cardiopulmonary bypass followed by embolectomy or, in less critical patients, the administration of thrombolytic agents is indicated. *Tension pneumothorax* can impair ventricular filling, resulting in shock, and thus should be excluded particularly when shock develops in patients undergoing mechanical ventilation. In patients with mechanical heart valves, shock may develop as the result of *acute thrombi* that are occluding the valve orifice or preventing the valve from opening adequately. The treatment of this condition requires prompt surgical intervention or, for nonsurgical candidates, the administration of thrombolytic agents.

Patients who develop shock soon after an acute myocardial infarction usually have marked impairment of left ventricular contractile function. In a minority of patients, however, there is a mechanical abnormality that contributes to the development or persistence of shock and that may be amenable to surgical correction. *Rupture of the intraventricular septum with a resultant left-to-right shunt* places an excessive volume load on the already damaged left ventricle and has a nearly 100 percent mortality rate if not surgically corrected. Similarly, *severe acute mitral insufficiency from necrosis and rupture of a papillary muscle* or its head may lead to pulmonary edema and shock even in patients with relatively small infarctions. Finally, *partial free wall rupture with a progressively enlarging left ventricular pseudoaneurysm* can, in addition to sudden rupture, severely compromise cardiac function and lead to cardiogenic shock. Although these mechanical complications might be suspected in the presence of typical physical findings and hemodynamic abnormalities, the availability of high-resolution two-dimensional and Doppler echocardiography that is performed at the bedside has made it relatively easy to identify patients who may require immediate surgery to repair mechanical complications. The decision as to whether to perform coronary angiography and, on occasion, angioplasty before taking such patients to the operating room will depend on the patient's stability, the availability of a catheterization laboratory, and the preferences of the surgeon and cardiologist.

The first physiologic studies on acute myocardial infarction by Gilbert and associates[9] in 1951 were followed by studies in which more sophisticated equipment was used to define the hemodynamics of shock.[10] Procedures to obtain hemodynamic data in the acutely ill patient that were once difficult are now routine with the use of flotation catheters, intra-arterial pressure measurements, and bedside thermodilution cardiac output measurements. Initial studies demonstrated that cardiac output was markedly reduced in the face of high ventricular filling pressures.[9, 10] Systemic vascular resistance, however, was not increased in proportion to the fall in cardiac output. This was unexpected because the patients appeared to be markedly vasoconstricted. Animal shock models, usually as the result of hemorrhage, indicated marked vasoconstriction of the systemic vasculature, and it was expected that similar responses would pertain to shock in acute myocardial infarction. As various receptors were isolated in the experimental models, it became apparent that vascular resistance in acute myocardial infarction was being determined by conflicting afferent signals.[11–13] The aortic and carotid baroreceptors signaled systemic vasoconstriction. Chemoreceptors in the carotid arteries activated by hypoxemia and low pH produced differential vasoconstriction, with a shift of flow away from skeletal muscles and the splanchnic bed to the coronary and cerebral circulation. On the other hand, left ventricular chemoreceptors or stretch receptors were activated by ischemia or stretch and presented afferent signals that called for a decrease in vascular resistance. The integration of these afferent signals in the medullary centers is responsible for the level of efferent sympathetic outflow and differential vasoconstriction to various vascular beds.[13] Thus, patients with shock in myocardial infarction are not maximally vasoconstricted, and alpha-adrenergic receptor agonists can be administered to elevate central arterial pressure by increasing systemic vascular resistance.

In shock after an acute myocardial infarction, there usually is severe left ventricular dysfunction, and two autopsy studies established the association with loss of 40 percent or more of left ventricular myocardium.[14, 15] These investigations also noted the high incidence of recent coronary thrombosis in 18 of 20[14] and 16 of 22[15] patients, with almost universal evidence of fresh marginal extension and focal areas of necrosis scattered throughout the remaining myocardium. The syndrome of *right ventricular infarction* as a cause of shock has also been recognized[16]; this is usually associated with right coronary occlusion and extensive right ventricular free wall and septal infarction that impair left ventricular filling and systemic blood flow.

Predictors, Incidence, and Mortality

The Multicenter Investigation of the Limitation of Infarct Size (MILIS) Study Group[17] attempted to define the predictors of in-hospital development of cardiogenic shock after myocardial infarction to identify likely patients and improve therapy. Of their 845 patients who presented with acute myocardial infarction, 60 (7.1 percent) developed cardiogenic shock. One half developed shock within 24 hours of hospital admission. Multivariate analysis indicated that the independent predictors of in-hospital development of cardiogenic shock were age above 65 years, left ventricular ejection fraction on admission below 0.35, large infarcts as estimated from enzyme determinations, a history of diabetes mellitus, and a previous myocardial infarction.

Goldberg and colleagues[18] reviewed the experience of a community hospital to define the incidence of and mortality rates for shock after acute myocardial infarction. Those who developed shock were more likely to have very proximal occlusion of the left anterior descending coronary artery and to lack adequate collateral vessels. They were likely to have had one or more previous myocardial infarcts and severe multivessel coronary disease and to develop a left bundle branch block during the course of the acute infarction. The incidence of cardiogenic shock of 7.5 percent was consistent with that of several studies.[17, 18] Patients who developed cardiogenic shock often had a faster heart rate, lower arterial pressure, neck vein distention, and pulmonary rales. Evidence of infarct extension occurred in 23 percent, and in two thirds of the patients this occurred before or at the time of onset of cardiogenic shock. Patients also had more frequent conduction defects, cardiac arrhythmias, and episodes of cardiac arrest before the development of cardiogenic shock.

In addition to these patients, some develop cardiogenic shock later, in the 7 to 10 days after an acute myocardial infarction. They develop a low output state, arrhythmias, and then cardiogenic shock. The pathology is characterized by the softening of a large infarct that becomes aneurysmal and absorbs the energy of the remaining myocardium. It also absorbs the volume necessary to lengthen the normal myocardial fibers in diastole, so the normal myocardium functions less effectively on the Frank-Starling curve.[19] Because of the aneurysmal infarct, ventricular arrhythmias are more frequent and difficult to reverse. It is often difficult to separate the relative contribution of pump failure and arrhythmias to the hemodynamic difficulty.

Patients with cardiogenic shock often have multivessel disease, and thus noninfarcted areas of the myocardium become ischemic at central aortic pressures that are adequate if the coronary vasculature were normal.[10] Vessels leading to noninfarcted areas may be sufficiently narrow that the pressure drop across the partial obstruction leaves the myocardium supplied by these vessels pressure dependent and unable to autoregulate to improve myocardial blood flow. Therefore, in addition to the large area of infarction that is noncontractile, remaining segments of the myocardium may be hypocontractile on the basis of ischemia secondary to the low arterial pressure.[14]

Clinical Recognition

Shock is defined clinically as inadequate perfusion of the vital organs manifested by obtundation, cyanosis, cold extremities, thready pulse, and oliguria. It should be distinguished from the low-blood-pressure, normal-output states sometimes seen in acute myocardial infarction associated with increased vagal tone. These latter patients are not obtunded, they continue to excrete urine adequately, and they have warm extremities, even though their systolic blood pressure may be less than 100 mm Hg. They usually require no treatment—only observation.

Patients in cardiogenic shock frequently have a slightly elevated venous pressure. With right ventricular infarction, however, the neck veins may be quite distended. There is clinical evidence of pulmonary edema ranging from a few rales to pulmonary edema. The heart is quiet, and the heart tones are distant. The first sound is soft; the second sound may be single or paradoxically split, and the third and fourth sounds are usually present, but at the heart rates associated with cardiogenic shock they frequently fuse to form a summation gallop. There may be a subtle parasternal systolic lift, particularly in the presence of an anteroseptal infarct. A new systolic murmur from mitral insufficiency may arise. At the time of presentation in cardiogenic shock, there usually is no evidence of peripheral edema or hepatic congestion.

Useful hemodynamic information can be derived from the placement of a flotation catheter to measure left ventricular filling pressure, right atrial pressure, and cardiac output. If patients are hypotensive, a catheter should be placed into the central arterial system for measurement of arterial pressure. Large discrepancies of arterial pressure between cuff pressures and central aorta have been described in patients in shock with acute myocardial infarction.[20] There may even be a significant gradient from brachial to radial arteries because of arterial vasoconstriction.

Treatment

Pharmacologic

Early attempts at treatment included the use of pure pressor agents to elevate arterial pressure without increasing myocardial contractility, which was considered myocardial oxygen wasting. Methoxamine was used as a peripheral vasoconstrictor, but this therapy was not successful.[10] Norepinephrine was then tried and was able to increase the cardiac output as well as elevate arterial pressure. As long as the arterial pressure was not raised above 110 mm Hg systolic, cardiac output tended to increase incrementally. This use of norepinephrine provides $beta_1$ cardiac inotropic stimulation as well as modest peripheral vasoconstriction, thus elevating the arterial pressure while improving perfusion.[10, 21]

In an attempt to unload the ventricle at the same time that arterial pressure would be sustained by increased cardiac output, isoproterenol was used. However, the differential flow to skeletal muscle and the inability to raise arterial pressure sufficiently, as well as the chronotropic effects of this agent, gave it a short-lived prominence.[22]

Dopamine was developed to increase cardiac output, elevate arterial pressure, and act as a moderate vasoconstrictor.[23] At low doses, it tends to vasodilate, but as the infusion rate is raised, the alpha-vasoconstrictor activity increases. At high infusion dose rates, the hemodynamic effects are similar to those of norepinephrine except for greater chronotropic activity, and this becomes a limiting feature.

To further enhance the inotropic effects of adrenergic stimulation, dobutamine was synthesized. It has only minimal peripheral vascular effects, and through its β-adrenergic receptor effects, it increases myocardial contractility.[24] The decrease in ventricular volume offsets the oxygen costs of increased contractility. In acute myocardial infarction, it has minimal adverse effects on oxygen demand. It is not, however, an effective agent for increasing arterial pressure.

Chatterjee and Parmley[25] and Cohn[26] developed the clinical concept of unloading the left ventricle in congestive heart failure and applied this to acute myocardial infarction and cardiogenic shock. Thus, they broadened the definition of shock to include patients who were clinically in shock and had low cuff pressures but preserved intra-arterial pressures. This expansion of the definition through a spectrum of shock-pump failure was useful because ventricular unloading is effective in increasing cardiac output, decreasing myocardial oxygen demand, and alleviating the shock syndrome if arterial blood pressure can be preserved. In some, particularly when mitral insufficiency is present, systemic arterial pressure has increased as cardiac pump function improved with this type of therapy.

Finally, the definition of right ventricular infarction, which can produce an entirely different therapeutic dilemma, made it imperative that there be hemodynamic classification of patients in shock-pump failure due to acute myocardial infarction.[27]

ACUTE MYOCARDIAL INFARCTION WITH HYPOVOLEMIC SHOCK

Hypovolemic shock may occur in patients with acute myocardial infarction and must be recognized because this necessitates volume repletion rather than pressor therapy. Such patients are clinically similar to patients with cardiogenic shock, except for absent neck vein distention and third heart sounds. Causes of hypovolemia include the overjudicious use of diuretics, third space redistribution of intravascular volume after cardiac arrest, the prolonged use of pressor agents, unrecognized sepsis or bleeding, and vomiting or profuse diaphoresis, which can occur early in the course of a myocardial infarction.[28] These patients have filling pressures of less than 15 mm Hg and require rapid fluid repletion to bring left ventricular filling pressure to 18 mm Hg before redefining the patient as undergoing cardiogenic shock or pump failure if the low output persists.

PHARMACOLOGIC AND LEFT VENTRICULAR ASSIST THERAPY

The management of the patient who exhibits shock from left ventricular failure in the setting of an acute myocardial infarction varies depending on its severity and hemodynamic profile.[27] Because persistent myocardial ischemia and stunned myocardium may play a critical role in the impaired contractile force, consideration must always be given to the balance between myocardial perfusion and oxygen consumption. In general, all therapies that augment contractile force through a positive inotropic effect will increase myocardial oxygen consumption. When aortic diastolic pressure is low, however, coronary perfusion may be critically impaired, especially in areas subserved by stenotic coronary arteries. Thus, a rise in aortic pressure may increase oxygen consumption but might also augment blood flow to improve myocardial ischemia. Vasodilator therapy, on the other hand, by lowering impedance to left ventricular ejection, can improve left ventricular emptying while reducing myocardial oxygen consumption. The net effect on ischemia will depend on the change in aortic diastolic pressure and its effect on myocardial perfusion. These considerations make clear the physiologic rationale for counterpulsation, which reduces aortic systolic pressure and augments aortic diastolic pressure.

Because blood pressure is difficult to obtain accurately through noninvasive means in patients with intense peripheral vasoconstriction, it is critical to monitor pressure intra-arterially with a transducer in this clinical setting. When pressure is not critically reduced (>90/60 mm Hg), cardiac filling pressure (jugular venous pressure or pulmonary capillary wedge pressure) is elevated, and peripheral perfusion is impaired (reduced urine output, cool extremities, disturbed mentation, metabolic acidosis), the cautious administration of a vasodilator drug is indicated. In the early postinfarct period, the agent of choice is nitroglycerin in escalating doses until perfusion is improved or unacceptable hypotension develops. When the shock state has developed more than 12 hours after the acute infarction and regional myocardial perfusion is therefore less tenuous, sodium nitroprusside in gradually escalating doses may be more effective.

If blood pressure is critically reduced or if it falls during vasodilator therapy, a positive inotropic drug is mandated. Dobutamine, dopamine, or norepinephrine is appropriate depending on the severity of the hypotension and its contribution to the clinical state. Dobutamine will produce the greatest augmentation in output but is least reliable in raising blood pressure. Norepinephrine will reliably raise blood pressure but often at the expense of regional perfusion, including that of the kidney. The use of phosphodiesterase inhibitors such as milrinone in the setting of cardiogenic shock is more unpredictable because the balance of inotropic and vasodilator effects cannot be individually titrated as is possible with, for example, the infusion of dobutamine and nitroprusside.

If the syndrome is not quickly corrected or the arterial pressure is profoundly reduced, intra-aortic balloon counterpulsation should be instituted as quickly as possible. Proper timing of this counterpulsation should result in adequate diastolic pressure to maintain perfusion of the heart and brain and often will augment renal and peripheral perfusion as well (Fig. 81–1). Only norepinephrine and intra-aortic balloon counterpulsation have been shown through direct measurement of lactate metabolism to improve myocardial metabolism in the hypotensive shock patient with acute myocardial infarction.[29]

Overall pharmacologic management of the circulatory deficiency in cardiogenic shock also requires close attention to urine output (high-dose loop diuretics when indicated) and to ventricular arrhythmias that may contribute

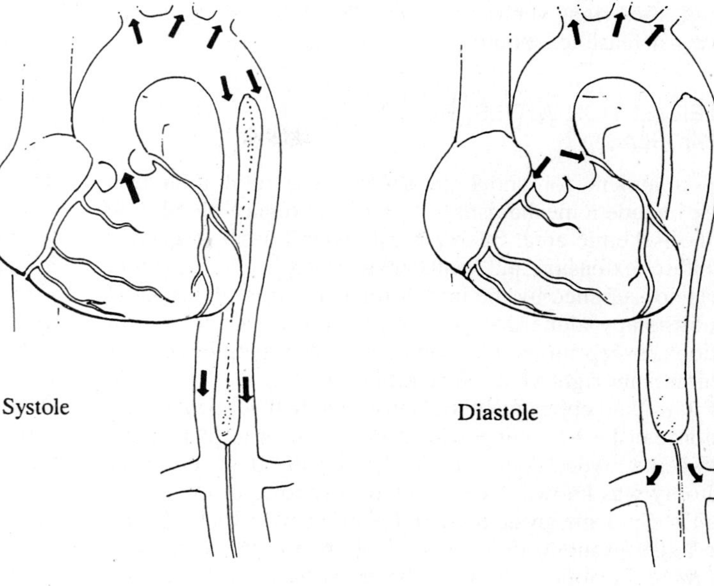

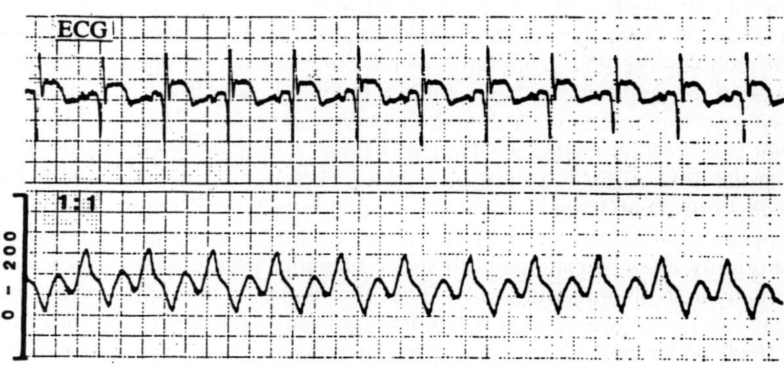

FIGURE 81–1 Top, Diagram of collapsed aortic balloon in systole and distended balloon in diastole augmenting perfusion to coronary arteries and aortic branches. **Bottom,** Electrocardiogram (ECG) is accompanied by a pressure recording showing proper timing of balloon inflation to produce prominent diastolic augmentation and low end-diastolic pressure to facilitate left ventricular systolic ejection. (Modified from Pierpont GL: Mechanical support of the failing circulation in acute coronary insufficiency and myocardial infarction. *In* Francis GS, Alpert JS [Eds]: Coronary Care, 2nd ed. pp. 261–288. Boston: Little, Brown, 1995.)

to the reduced cardiac output. The judicious use of drugs and devices may be critical to the patient's survival.

The use of emergency cardiopulmonary bypass was investigated in 109 patients with cardiogenic shock by Overlie and associates,[30] who reported a 50 percent 1-year survival rate in 52 patients who subsequently underwent surgery versus 37 percent in 57 patients who were treated medically. The use of left ventricular assist devices as a temporary circulatory support or a bridge to transplantation in patients whose cardiac function does not recover is a rational therapeutic option that has not yet been subjected to controlled study.

RIGHT VENTRICULAR INFARCTION

The presence of right ventricular infarction presents a therapeutic dilemma different from that presented by pump failure due to left ventricular damage. Right atrial and right ventricular diastolic pressures are elevated, whereas the cardiac index and arterial pressure are low. Left ventricular filling pressures can be elevated or normal. Unless left ventricular filling pressure is also elevated, the primary therapy is to increase right ventricular output by elevating right ventricular filling pressure while monitoring left ventricular filling pressure so the wedge pressure does not exceed 20 mm Hg. Venodilators, particularly nitroglycerin, are contraindicated, and diuretics should not be administered unless there is pulmonary congestion.[31–33]

Because patients with right ventricular infarction usually have occlusion of the right (or a dominant left circumflex) coronary artery, bradyarrhythmias or atrioventricular conduction abnormalities are common and may cause an inadequate cardiac output and hypotension. Under these circumstances, temporary pacing should be instituted promptly.

Fluid infusion should be administered as a challenge because even slow infusion may not exceed loss from intravascular space and leads to diffuse edema, including pulmonary edema, without effectively raising the filling pressure. Furthermore, left ventricular damage may be masked by the right heart failure[33] and only manifest after right ventricular filling pressures have been increased. The pressor agent of choice is dobutamine because dopamine and norepinephrine increase pulmonary vascular resistance.[34] There is a good response to intra-aortic balloon counterpulsation in these patients, and many improve remarkably after several days of counterpulsation without more aggressive intervention.[33, 35] Nevertheless, because mortality rates remain high in patients with cardiogenic shock after right ventricular infarction, emergency angioplasty, if feasible, should be considered.[36]

INTERVENTION WITH SURGERY AND ANGIOPLASTY

The treatment for shock in acute myocardial infarction must include a mechanism to improve coronary blood flow to the ischemic area. Such patients have a high frequency of infarct extension and spotty myocardial necrosis even in areas not supplied by the infarct-related artery.[14] Pharmacologic therapy alone does not improve a dismal long-term outlook, except in patients with associated hypovolemia or predominant right ventricular infarction.[35]

Pifarre and colleagues[37] demonstrated that surgical reperfusion can be lifesaving with a good outcome in patients with acute myocardial infarction, especially if the coronary anatomy was known and the infarct occurred in the hospital. The Spokane group showed the efficacy of such therapy in a larger group of patients in a community that organized for rapid identification of, catheterization of, and surgery in patients with chest pain. DeWood and associates[38] reviewed the Spokane data and demonstrated the importance of reducing the time from onset of pain to reperfusion. The advent of angioplasty has enabled coronary reperfusion without thoracotomy. Although primary angioplasty has not been recommended as standard therapy for acute myocardial infarction, it is the therapy of choice in patients with shock and acute Q wave myocardial infarction.[27] This apparent dichotomy makes sense in the context of the high mortality rates of patients with shock or pump failure who are treated pharmacologically. The improvement in such patients with reperfusion far outweighs any deleterious effects of the procedure. Thus, the large amount of myocardium in jeopardy and frequently nonfunctioning is improved much more quickly with angioplasty reperfusion than with thrombolytic therapy.[39] Improved outcome with thrombolytic therapy has not been as definitively demonstrated in these patients,[40] and therefore, reperfusion should be performed when possible through primary angioplasty. If angioplasty is unavailable, there may be a role for thrombolytic therapy in conjunction with intra-aortic balloon support[41] while transfer is being made to a center for invasive treatment. O'Neill and colleagues[39] compared the use of thrombolysis with that of angioplasty and showed similar rates of reperfusion. However, in the patients who underwent angioplasty, there was significant improvement in wall motion, unlike with in those who received thrombolytic therapy alone. The residual stenosis was much greater in the thrombolytic than in the angioplasty group.

O'Neill and colleagues[42] proposed the use of angioplasty for the treatment of shock in acute myocardial infarction, and their reported experience demonstrated improved survival rates in this group of patients. Using historical controls, they showed a 50 percent survival rate at 30 days in patients treated with angioplasty and a 17 percent survival rate at 30 days in those treated with conventional therapy without angioplasty. In patients with successful reperfusion, there was a 77 percent survival rate at 30 days.[43]

In a multicenter registry arising out of experience in Michigan and reported by Lee and colleagues,[44] there were 69 patients who were treated with attempted angioplasty for shock in acute myocardial infarction. The procedure was unsuccessful in 20 patients who were, in all respects, similar to the 49 patients who had successful angioplasty. These two groups were then compared. The immediate survival rate in the two groups was 69 percent for those with successful angioplasty and 20 percent for those with unsuccessful angioplasty. The survival rate at 24 months was 54 percent for the successful angioplasty group and 11 percent for the unsuccessful group. A more recent report from Henry Ford Hospital confirms the efficacy of revascularization with either angioplasty or bypass surgery, with a 56 percent survival rate in the revascularized group and an 8 percent survival rate in the nonrevascularized group (Fig. 81–2).[45]

Consistent with these results is a report on experience with primary angioplasty. Thirty-three patients with more than one diseased vessel had shock,[46] and 36 patients with one diseased vessel had shock.[47] The survival rates were

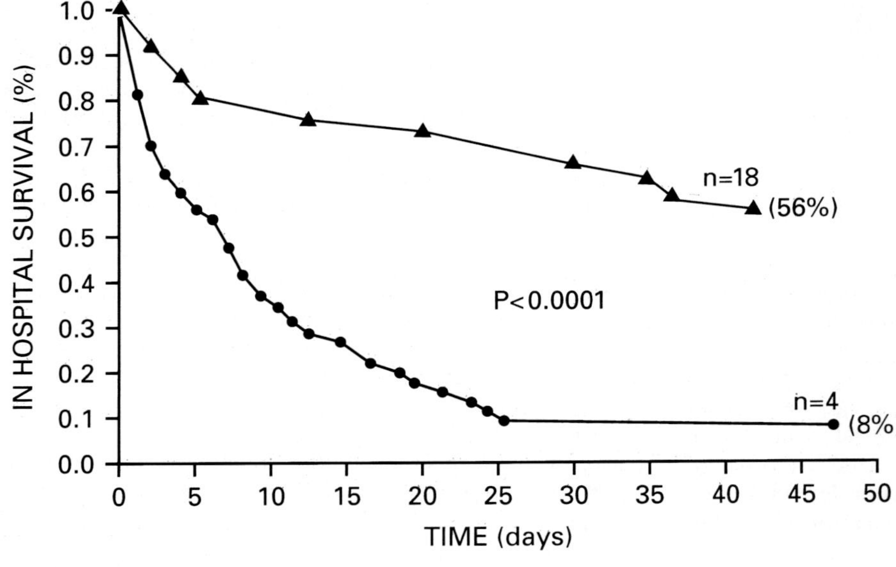

FIGURE 81–2 Comparison of in-hospital cumulative survival rates for 32 patients with (*triangles*) and 49 patients without (*circles*) revascularization. At 42 days, there were 18 surviving patients (56 percent) in the group with revascularization and 4 (8 percent) in the group without revascularization. (Reprinted with permission from the American College of Cardiology *[Journal of the American College of Cardiology]* 19:907, 1992.)

55 percent in the multivessel group and 59 percent in the one-vessel group. The treatment consisted of placement of an intra-aortic balloon pump, movement of the patient to the catheterization laboratory for angiography, and angioplasty where indicated. The long-term survival rate was excellent compared with pharmacologic therapy. Overall, the patients were treated within less than 6 hours of the onset of their chest pain. Rothbaum and colleagues[48] also reported the use of primary angioplasty for acute myocardial infarction; shock was present in 18 of their patients. There were seven deaths, resulting in a survival rate of 61 percent.

Berger and colleagues[49] reported the effects of early angiography and revascularization strategy in 2200 patients with cardiogenic shock who were entered into the Global Utilization of Streptokinase and Tissue Plasminogen Activator for Occluded Coronary Arteries trial. The 30-day survival rate was 62 percent among 406 patients who underwent early angiography (within 24 hours) versus a 30-day survival rate of only 38 percent in the 1794 patients who did not undergo early angiography. When these two groups were compared, however, it was found that patients undergoing early angiography tended to be younger, to have less prior infarction, and to have received thrombolytic therapy earlier. Among the 406 patients who underwent early angiography, 233 patients underwent early revascularization with angioplasty, bypass surgery, or both; the 30-day survival rate in these patients was 60 percent. In 173 of these patients, early revascularization was not performed after angiography, and the 30-day survival rate was 65 percent. Although these data suggest a favorable effect of early angiography in patients with cardiogenic shock after acute myocardial infarction, it is unclear how much of this benefit is due to selection bias versus early revascularization for patients found at angiography to be suitable candidates.

Experience with primary angioplasty in patients with acute myocardial infarction, including those with cardiogenic shock,[50] has demonstrated the feasibility of coronary stenting coupled with antiplatelet therapy, including blockers of the platelet IIa/IIIb receptor, to achieve an optimal angiographic result. It is anticipated that the wider use of early revascularization with improved techniques will continue to have a favorable impact on the outcome of patients who develop cardiogenic shock after acute myocardial infarction.

SUMMARY OF THERAPEUTIC STRATEGY

The treatment of patients in shock with myocardial infarction for which the cause is pump failure should be to stabilize the patient with pharmacologic therapy according to a regimen based on the hemodynamic disorder. Patients with shock syndrome should have an intra-aortic balloon pump placed and be taken to the cardiac catheterization laboratory as quickly as possible, the anatomy should be defined, and reperfusion with either angioplasty or surgery should be undertaken. The attempt should be made to have this completed within the first 6 hours from the onset of the chest pain. The earlier such reperfusion is established, the better the outcome, although patients presenting within 24 hours of the onset of myocardial infarction have been treated in this manner with results improved over pharmacologic therapy. Whether thrombolysis should be used either intravenously at the onset of this process or intracoronarily during the attempt at angioplasty is still not settled, but if there are delays in mechanical reperfusion, thrombolysis may be a reasonable part of initial therapy.

REFERENCES

1. Cohn JN, Luria MH, Daddario RC, Tristani FE: Studies in clinical shock and hypotension, V: hemodynamic effects of dextran. Circulation 35:316–326, 1967.
2. Anzueto AE, Gutierrez G, Tessler S, et al: Double-blind randomised controlled trial of monoclonal antibody to human tumour necrosis factor in the treatment of septic shock. Lancet 351:929–933, 1998.
3. Baudo F, Caimi D, de Cataldo F, et al: Antithrombin III replacement therapy in patients with sepsis and/or post surgical complications: a controlled double-blind, randomised, multicenter study. Intens Care Med 24:336–342, 1998.
4. Bollaert PE, Charpentier C, Levy B, et al: Reversal of late septic shock with supraphysiologic doses of hydrocortisone. Crit Care Med 26:645–650, 1998.
5. Staubach KH, Schroder J, Stuber F, et al: Effect of pentoxifylline in severe sepsis: results of a randomised double-blind, placebo-controlled study. Arch Surg 133:94–100, 1998.
6. Gally HF, Howdle PD, Walker BE, Webster NR: The effects of intravenous antioxidants in patients with septic shock. Free Radic Biol Med 23:768–774, 1997.
7. Opal, SM, Fisher CJ, Dhainaut JF, et al: Confirmatory interleukin-1 receptor antagonist trial in severe sepsis: a phase III, randomised, double-blind, placebo-controlled, multicenter trial. Crit Care Med 25:1115–1124, 1997.
8. Abraham E, Glauser MP, Butler T, et al: p55 tumor necrosis factor receptor fusion protein in the treatment of patients with severe sepsis and septic shock: a randomised controlled multicenter trial. JAMA 277:1531–1538, 1997.
9. Gilbert RP, Aldrich SL, Anderson L: Cardiac output in acute myocardial infarction. J Clin Invest 30:640, 1951.
10. Gunnar RM, Cruz A, Boswell J, et al: Myocardial infarction with shock: hemodynamic studies and results of therapy. Circulation 33:753, 1966.
11. Sleight P, Widdicombe JG: Action potential in fibers from receptors in the epicardium and myocardium of the dog's left ventricle. J Physiol 181:235, 1966.
12. Brown AM: Excitation of afferent cardiac sympathetic nerve fibers during myocardial ischemia. J Physiol 190:35, 1967.
13. Abboud FM: Integration of reflex responses in the control of blood pressure and vascular resistance. Am J Cardiol 44:903, 1979.
14. Page DL, Caulfield JB, Kastor JA, et al: Myocardial changes associated with cardiogenic shock. N Engl J Med 285:133, 1971.
15. Alonso DR, Scheidt S, Post M, Killip T: Pathophysiology of cardiogenic shock: quantification of myocardial necrosis, clinical, pathologic and electrocardiographic correlations. Circulation 48:588, 1973.
16. Cohn JN, Guiha NH, Broder MI, Limas CJ: Right ventricular infarction: clinical and hemodynamic features. Am J Cardiol 33:209–214, 1974.
17. Hands ME, Rutherford JD, Muller JE, et al: The in-hospital development of cardiogenic shock after myocardial infarction: incidence, predictors of occurrence, outcome and prognostic factors. J Am Coll Cardiol 14:40, 1989.
18. Goldberg RJ, Gore JM, Alpert JS, et al: Cardiogenic shock after acute myocardial infarction—incidence and mortality from a community-wide perspective, 1975 to 1988. N Engl J Med 325:1117, 1991.
19. Swan HJC: Functional Basis of the Hemodynamic Spectrum Associated With Myocardial Infarction in Shock in Myocardial Infarction. New York: Grune & Stratton, 1974.
20. Cohn NJ: Blood pressure measurement in shock. JAMA 199:972, 1967.
21. Gunnar RM, Loeb HS, Pietras RJ, Tobin JR Jr: Hemodynamic measurements in a coronary care unit. Prog Cardiovasc Dis 11:29, 1968.
22. Gunnar RM, Loeb HS, Pietras RJ, Tobin JR Jr: Ineffectiveness of isoproterenol in the treatment of shock due to acute myocardial infarction. JAMA 202:1124, 1967.

23. Goldberg LI, Talley RC, McNay JL: The potential role of dopamine in the treatment of shock. Prog Cardiovasc Dis 12:40, 1969.
24. Tuttle RR, Mills J: Dobutamine: development of a new catecholamine to selectively increase cardiac contractility. Circ Res 38:185, 1975.
25. Chatterjee K, Parmley WW: The role of vasodilator therapy in heart failure. Prog Cardiovasc Dis 19:301, 1977.
26. Cohn JN: Vasodilator therapy for heart failure: the influence of impedance on left ventricular performance. Circulation 48:5, 1973.
27. Gunnar RM, Bourdillon PDV, Dixon DW, et al: Guidelines for the early management of patients with acute myocardial infarction: a report of the American College of Cardiology/American Heart Association Task Force on Assessment of Diagnostic and Therapeutic Cardiovascular Procedures (Subcommittee to Develop Guidelines for the Early Management of Patients with Acute Myocardial Infarction). J Am Coll Cardiol 16:249, 1990.
28. Loeb HS, Pietras RJ, Tobin JR Jr, Gunnar RM: Hypovolemia in shock due to acute myocardial infarction. Circulation 40:653, 1969.
29. Mueller H, Ayres SM, Giannelli S Jr, et al: Effect of isoproterenol, *l*-norepinephrine and intra-aortic counter pulsation on hemodynamics and myocardial metabolism in shock following acute myocardial infarction. Circulation 45:335, 1972.
30. Overlie PA, Shawl FA, George EM, et al: Cardiogenic shock: survival rates from the National Registry for Emergency Cardiopulmonary Bypass Investigators. J Am Coll Cardiol 29:398A, 1997.
31. Cohn JN: Right ventricular infarction revisited. Am J Cardiol 43:666, 1979.
32. Dell'Italia LJ, Starling MR, Blumhardt R, et al: Comparative effects of volume loading, dobutamine, and nitroprusside in patients with predominant right ventricular infarction. Circulation 72:1327, 1985.
33. Creamer JE, Edwards JD, Nightingale P: Mechanism of shock associated with right ventricular infarction. Br Heart J 65:63, 1991.
34. Loeb HS, Bredakis J, Gunnar RM: Superiority of dobutamine over dopamine for augmentation of cardiac output in patients with chronic low output cardiac failure. Circulation 55:375, 1977.
35. Johnson SA, Scanlon PJ, Loeb HS, et al: Treatment of cardiogenic shock in myocardial infarction by intra-aortic balloon counterpulsation and surgery. Am J Med 62:687, 1977.
36. Bier JD, Cohen JS, Sleeper L, et al: Characteristics and outcome of patients with cardiogenic shock due to right ventricular dysfunction: a report from SHOCK trial registry. J Am Coll Cardiol 29:460A, 1997.
37. Pifarre R, Spinazzola A, Nemickas R, et al: Emergency aortocoronary bypass for acute myocardial infarction. Arch Surg 103:525, 1971.
38. DeWood MA, Notske RN, Hensley GR, et al: Intra-aortic balloon counterpulsation with and without reperfusion for myocardial infarction shock. Circulation 61:1105, 1980.
39. O'Neill W, Timmis GC, Bourdillon PD, et al: A prospective randomized clinical trial of intracoronary streptokinase versus coronary angioplasty for acute myocardial infarction. N Engl J Med 314:812, 1986.
40. Mueller HS, Cohen LS, Braunwald E, et al: Predictors of early morbidity and mortality after thrombolytic therapy of acute myocardial infarction: analyses of patient subgroups in the Thrombolysis in Myocardial Infarction (TIMI) trial, phase II. Circulation 85:1254, 1992.
41. Kovack PJ, Rasak MA, Bates ER, et al: Thrombolysis plus aortic counterpulsation: improved survival in patients who present to community hospitals with cardiogenic shock. J Am Coll Cardiol 29:1454–1458, 1997.
42. O'Neill W, Erbel R, Laufer M, et al: Coronary angioplasty therapy of cardiogenic shock complicating acute myocardial infarction. Circulation 72(suppl III):III-309, 1985.
43. Lee L, Bates ER, Pitt B, et al: Percutaneous transluminal coronary angioplasty improves survival in acute myocardial infarction complicated by cardiogenic shock. Circulation 78:1345, 1988.
44. Lee L, Erbel R, Brown TM, et al: Multicenter registry of angioplasty therapy of cardiogenic shock: initial and long-term survival. J Am Coll Cardiol 17:599, 1991.
45. Moosvi AR, Khaja F, Villanueva L, et al: Early revascularization improves survival in cardiogenic shock complicating acute myocardial infarction. J Am Coll Cardiol 19:907, 1992.
46. Kahn JK, Rutherford BD, McConahay DR, et al: Results of primary angioplasty for acute myocardial infarction in patients with multivessel coronary artery disease. J Am Coll Cardiol 16:1089, 1990.
47. Stone GW, Rutherford BD, McConahay DR, et al: Direct coronary angioplasty in acute myocardial infarction: outcome in patients with single vessel disease. J Am Coll Cardiol 15:534, 1990.
48. Rothbaum DA, Linnemeier TJ, Landin RJ, et al: Emergency percutaneous transluminal coronary angioplasty in acute myocardial infarction: a 3-year experience. J Am Coll Cardiol 10:264, 1987.
49. Berger PB, Holmes DR, Stebbins AL, et al: Impact on an aggressive invasive catheterization and revascularization strategy on mortality in patients with cardiogenic shock in Global Utilization of Streptokinase and Tissue Plasminogen Activator for Occluded Coronary Arteries (GUSTO-I) trial. Circulation 96:122–127, 1997.
50. Antoniucci D, Valenti R, Santoro GM, et al: Systematic direct angioplasty and stent-supported direct angioplasty therapy for cardiogenic shock complicating acute myocardial infarction: in-hospital and long-term survival. J Am Coll Cardiol 31:294–300, 1998.

CHAPTER 82

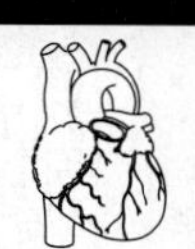

Autonomic Dysfunction and Hypotension

Christopher J. Mathias

CLASSIFICATION OF AUTONOMIC DISORDERS
CLINICAL MANIFESTATIONS
Cardiovascular Features
Noncardiovascular Features
INVESTIGATION OF AUTONOMIC DYSFUNCTION
Cardiovascular System
DESCRIPTION OF KEY AUTONOMIC DISORDERS
Localized Autonomic Disorders
Primary Autonomic Failure Syndromes
Secondary Autonomic Disorders
Neurally Mediated Syncope
Postural Tachycardia Syndrome (Orthostatic Intolerance)
Drugs, Poisons, and Toxins
MANAGEMENT OF POSTURAL HYPOTENSION
Nonpharmacologic Measures
Pharmacologic Measures
Therapy in Specific Disorders

The autonomic nervous system, especially through the cranial parasympathetic and lumbosacral sympathetic outflow, is closely involved in the beat-to-beat control of systemic blood pressure, heart rate, and the regional blood supply to skeletal muscle and vital organs. It is of major importance in ensuring adequate tissue perfusion, in maintaining supplies of oxygen and nutrients, and in transporting metabolic end-products in response to the demands of varying situations. It accomplishes these actions through a complex system of pathways that involves the brain and spinal cord, preganglionic and postganglionic pathways, and synapses at the target organ (Fig. 82–1). The immense flexibility and capability of the autonomic nervous system are dependent on intricate pathways that may be damaged in a variety of conditions that affect one or more sites. This chapter provides an outline classification of autonomic disorders that affect the cardiovascular system, followed by a description of the main clinical manifestations, an investigation of autonomic dysfunction, and a brief description of some of the major autonomic disorders. There is an emphasis on postural (orthostatic) hypotension, as it is a cardinal feature of many autonomic disorders. It is now recognized that a number of factors in daily life, such as food ingestion and exercise, can cause hypotension and worsen postural hypotension in patients with autonomic dysfunction, and these factors are described.

Classification of Autonomic Disorders

Autonomic disorders may result in localized or generalized dysfunction (Table 82–1).[1] Examples of *localized dysfunction* include cardiac transplantation. Examples of *generalized dysfunction* include primary disorders where there is no clear etiologic factor (e.g., multiple system atrophy, synonymous with the Shy-Drager syndrome) and secondary disorders associated with a clearly defined lesion (e.g., spinal cord transection), disease (e.g., diabetes mellitus), or a specific biochemical deficit (e.g., dopamine beta-hydroxylase deficiency). A separate category includes *neurally mediated syncope*, in which there is an intermittent autonomic abnormality, often associated with specific events. The *postural tachycardia syndrome* is a disorder in which there is orthostatic intolerance usually without orthostatic hypotension. A wide variety of drugs, toxins, and chemicals either directly or indirectly result in cardiovascular autonomic dysfunction (Table 82–2). Autonomic dysfunction often results in diminished activity, leading to hypotension and bradycardia; the reverse, overactivity, also may occur causing hypertension and tachycardia. In some disorders, such as neurally mediated syncope, both overactivity and underactivity may occur simultaneously.

Clinical Manifestations

Cardiovascular Features

Autonomic dysfunction can affect the regulation of blood pressure and heart rate and may impair regional vascular control mechanisms.

Hypotension

Postural (orthostatic) hypotension is a cardinal feature of sympathetic vasoconstrictor failure (Fig. 82–2). It may provide the first clue to an underlying diagnosis of an autonomic disorder. Postural hypotension is defined as a fall in systolic blood pressure of more than 20 mm Hg (or diastolic blood pressure of more than 10 mm Hg) on either standing upright or head-up tilt for 3 minutes; normally, there is no fall in blood pressure on head-up postural

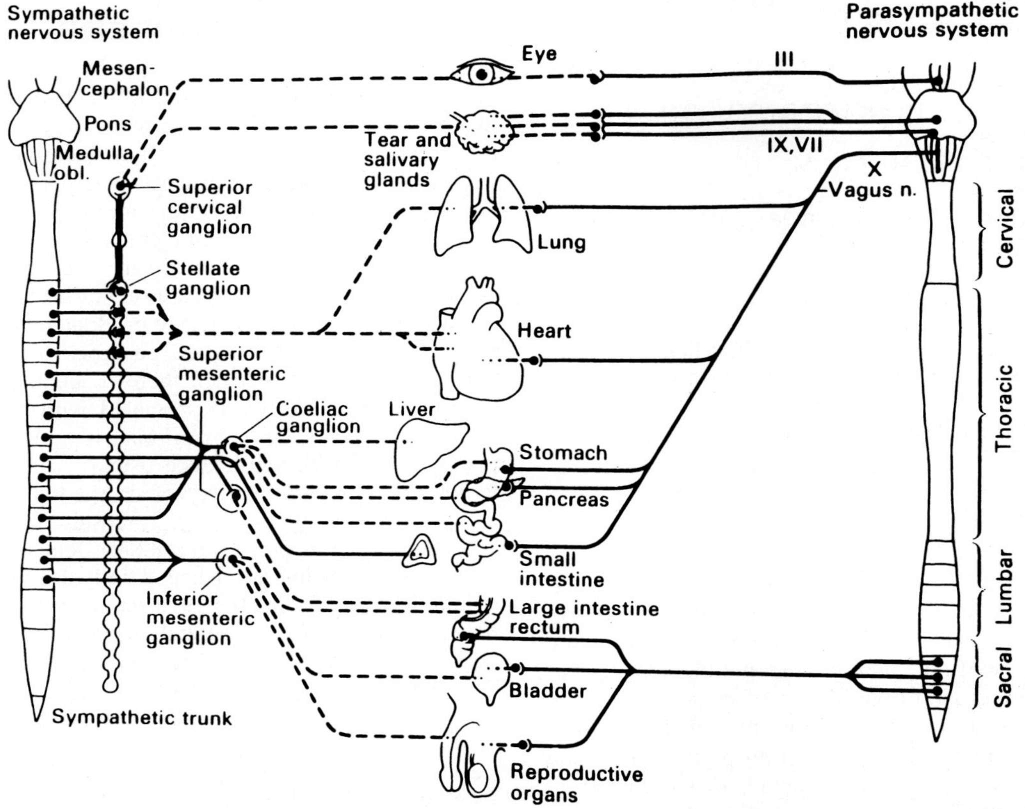

FIGURE 82–1 Peripheral autonomic nervous system. The sympathetic innervation of vessels, sweat glands, and piloerector muscles is not shown. *Solid lines,* preganglionic axons; *dashed lines,* postganglionic axons. (From Janig W: Autonomic nervous system. *In* Schmidt RF, Thews G [eds]: Human Physiology. 2nd ed. pp. 333–370. New York: Springer-Verlag, 1987.)

TABLE 82-1 Outline Classification and Examples of Disorders That Cause Cardiovascular Autonomic Dysfunction

Primary

Acute/Subacute Dysautonomias

Pure cholinergic dysautonomia
Pure pandysautonomia
Pandysautonomia with neurologic features

Chronic Autonomic Failure Syndromes

Pure autonomic failure
Multiple system atrophy (Shy-Drager syndrome)
Autonomic failure with Parkinson's disease

Secondary

Congenital

Nerve growth factor deficiency

Hereditary

Autosomal dominant trait
  Familial amyloid neuropathy
  Porphyria
Autosomal recessive trait
  Familial dysautonomia (Riley-Day syndrome)
  Dopamine beta-hydroxylase deficiency
  Friedreich's ataxia

Metabolic Diseases

Diabetes mellitus
Chronic renal failure
Chronic liver disease
Thyroid disease (thyrotoxicosis and myxedema)
Vitamin B_{12} deficiency
Alcohol induced

Inflammatory Diseases

Guillain-Barré syndrome
Transverse myelitis

Infections

Bacterial: tetanus
Viral: human immunodeficiency virus infection
Parasitic: *Trypanosomiasis cruzi*; Chagas' disease
Prion: fatal familial insomnia

Neoplasia

Brain tumors, especially of the third ventricle or posterior fossa
Paraneoplastic, to include adenocarcinomas of lung and pancreas and Lambert-Eaton syndrome

Surgery

Organ transplantation: heart, kidney
Vagotomy and drainage procedures: "dumping syndrome"
Regional sympathectomy: splanchnic

Trauma

Spinal cord transection

Miscellaneous Neurologic Disorders

Subarachnoid hemorrhage
Epilepsy
Narcolepsy
Reflex sympathetic dystrophy

Neurally Mediated Syncope

Vasovagal syncope
Carotid sinus hypersensitivity
Micturition syncope
Cough syncope
Swallow syncope
Associated with glossopharyngeal neuralgia

Postural Tachycardia Syndrome

Drugs

See Table 82–2

Adapted from Mathias CJ: Disorders of the autonomic nervous system. *In* Bradley WG, Daroff RB, Fenichel GM, Marsden CD (eds): Neurology in Clinical Practice. 3rd ed. pp. 2131–2165. Boston: Butterworth-Heinemann, 2000.

TABLE 82-2 Examples of Drugs, Chemicals, Poisons, and Toxins That May Alter Cardiovascular Autonomic Activity; Many Are Used Therapeutically

Decreasing Sympathetic Activity

Centrally Acting

Clonidine
Methyldopa
Moxonidine
Reserpine
Barbiturates
Anesthetics

Peripherally Acting

Sympathetic nerve ending (guanethidine, bethanidine)
Alpha-adrenoceptor blockade (phenoxybenzamine)
Beta-adrenoceptor blockade (propranolol)

Increasing Sympathetic Activity

Amphetamines
Releasing noradrenaline (tyramine)
Uptake blockers (imipramine)
Monoamine oxidase inhibitors (tranylcypromine)
Beta-adrenoceptor stimulants (isoprenaline)

Decreasing Parasympathetic Activity

Antidepressants (imipramine)
Tranquillizers (phenothiazines)
Antidysrhythmics (disopyramide)
Anticholinergics (atropine, probanthine, benzotropine)
Toxins (botulinum)

Increasing Parasympathetic Activity

Cholinomimetics (carbachol, bethanechol, pilocarpine, mushroom poisoning)
Anticholinesterases
  Reversible carbamate inhibitors (pyridostigmine, neostigmine)
  Organophosphorus inhibitors (parathion, sarin)

Miscellaneous

Alcohol, thiamine (vitamin B_1 deficiency)
Mercury poisoning ("pink" disease)
Ciguatera toxicity
Jellyfish and marine animal venoms
First dose of certain drugs (captopril, prazosin)

Adapted from Mathias CJ: Disorders of the autonomic nervous system. *In* Bradley WG, Daroff RB, Fenichel GM, Marsden CD (eds): Neurology in Clinical Practice. 3rd ed. pp. 2131–2165. Boston: Butterworth-Heinemann, 2000.

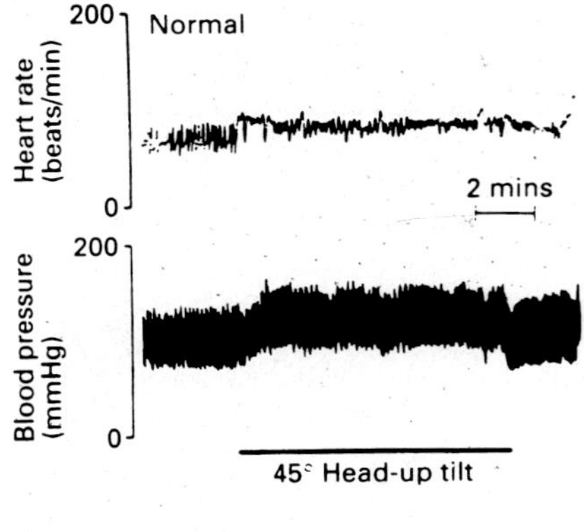

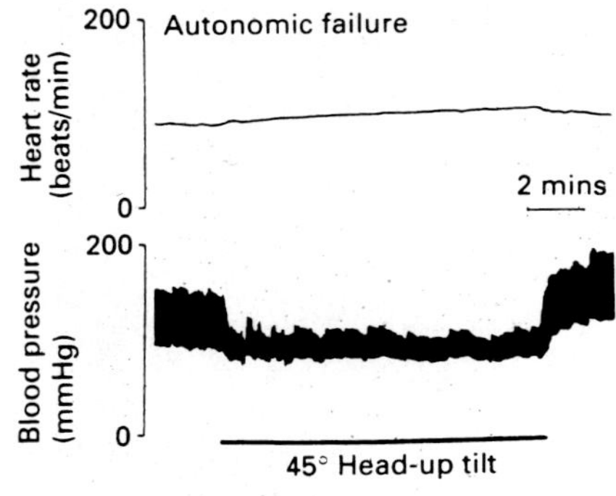

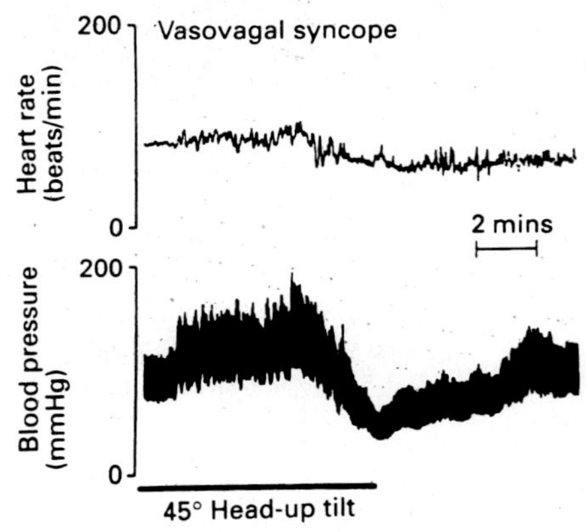

FIGURE 82–2 Blood pressure and heart rate before, during, and after head-up tilt in a normal subject **(top),** a patient with autonomic failure **(middle)**, and a patient with vasovagal syncope **(bottom)**. In the normal subject, there was no fall in blood pressure during head-up tilt. In the patient with autonomic failure, blood pressure fell promptly and remained low, with a blood pressure overshoot on return to the horizontal position. In addition, there was only a minimal change in heart rate despite the marked blood pressure fall. In the patient with vasovagal syncope, there initially was no fall in blood pressure during head-up tilt; in the latter part of tilt, as indicated in the record, blood pressure initially rose and then markedly fell, to extremely low levels, so the patient had to be returned to the horizontal position. Heart rate also fell. In each case, continuous blood pressure and heart rate were recorded with the Portapress II. (From Mathias CJ, Bannister R: Investigation of autonomic disorders. *In* Mathias CJ, Bannister R [eds]: Autonomic Failure: A Textbook of Clinical Disorders of the Autonomic Nervous System. 4th ed. pp. 169–195. Oxford: Oxford University Press, 1999.)

change.[2, 3] A fall of this magnitude usually is associated with symptoms of hypoperfusion to various organs, in particular to the brain (Table 82–3). Symptoms arising from cerebral hypoperfusion are often the reason for requesting medical advice.[4] They are precipitated by sitting or standing and are relieved by lying flat; they may vary in the same individual at different times. Their magnitude may be independent of the fall in blood pressure. With time, symptoms of cerebral hypoperfusion often are reduced, probably due to improved cerebrovascular autoregulation.

Common symptoms of cerebral hypoperfusion include dizziness and visual disturbances; these usually, but not necessarily, precede loss of consciousness (syncope, fainting). Symptoms of postural hypotension often are worse when getting out of bed in the morning and may be enhanced by a variety of stimuli in daily life, ranging from food ingestion and even modest amounts of alcohol, to mild exercise and a raised environmental temperature (Table 82–4). Straining during micturition and bowel movements, which commonly are affected in autonomic disorders, may induce symptoms; these stimuli presumably raise intrathoracic pressure and result in a Valsalva-like maneuver, thus lowering blood pressure. Many patients recognize the association between postural change and symptoms of cerebral hypoperfusion and sit down, lie flat, or assume postures such as squatting or stooping.[5] Syncope may occur rapidly if the blood pressure falls precipitously, and this may be similar to a drop attack. Syncope may result in injury. Seizures occasionally occur, especially if cerebral hypoxia is prolonged. A number of drugs, ranging from sublingual glyceryl trinitrate to those with minimal cardiovascular effects such as levodopa (for parkinsonism), may unmask or aggravate postural hypotension. In diabetics with autonomic neuropathy, insulin may enhance postural hypotension through its effects in causing vasodilatation or a reduction in blood volume.[6] Occasionally, symptoms may occur even with a small postural fall in blood pressure, when perfusion is compounded by impairment of the vas-

TABLE 82–3 Some of the Symptoms Resulting from Postural Hypotension and Impaired Perfusion of Various Organs

Cerebral Hypoperfusion

Dizziness
Visual disturbances
  Blurred
  Tunnel
  Scotoma
  Graying out
  Blacking out
  Color defects
Loss of consciousness
Impaired cognition

Muscle Hypoperfusion

Paracervical and suboccipital "coathanger" ache
Lower back/buttock ache
Calf claudication

Cardiac Hypoperfusion

Angina pectoris

Renal Hypoperfusion

Oliguria

Nonspecific

Weakness, lethargy, fatigue

Adapted from Mathias CJ: Orthostatic hypotension: causes, mechanisms and influencing factors. Reproduced with permission from Advanstar Communications Inc. as adapted from Neurology®, 1995, Vol. 45, Suppl. 5, pp. S6–S11. Neurology® is a registered trademark of the American Academy of Neurology.

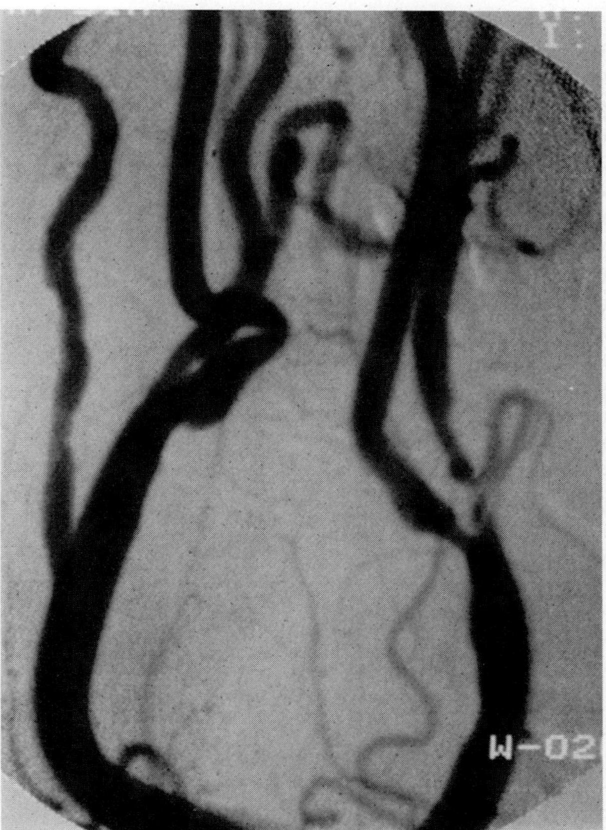

FIGURE 82–3 Intravenous digital subtraction angiogram of the carotid vessels in a patient with hypertension and widespread atherosclerosis. She had symptoms of cerebral ischemia associated with postural change, which occurred despite a small blood pressure fall of approximately 10 mm Hg. In the presence of left carotid artery stenosis, as demonstrated, this was sufficient to induce symptoms. She benefited from a reduction in her antihypertensive therapy, which abolished the small orthostatic fall in blood pressure. (From Mathias CJ: Autonomic disorders. *In* Bogousslavsky J, Fisher M [eds]: Textbook of Neurology. pp. 519–545. Boston: Butterworth-Heinemann, 1998.)

cular supply of the organ. An example is carotid artery stenosis, in which symptoms of cerebral hypoperfusion may be difficult to distinguish from transient ischemic attacks caused by thromboembolism (Fig. 82–3).

Hypoperfusion of organs other than the brain may result in a variety of symptoms. Suboccipital and paracervical pain in a "coathanger" distribution is probably due to reduced perfusion of head and neck muscles that tonically must be kept active.[7] Symptoms suggestive of angina pectoris may occur even in young subjects with apparently normal coronary arteries.[8] Oliguria while upright probably results from renal hypoperfusion, with the reverse occurring during recumbency.[9]

In neurally mediated syncope, hypotension often is associated with, but may be independent of, head-up posture. In the young, a common cause is vasovagal syncope, which often has an emotional cause; there may be a family history, especially in those presenting before the age of 20.[10] There have been numerous variants of emotionally induced cardiovascular syndromes described over the years, including Da Costa's syndrome (soldier's heart, neurocirculatory asthenia), in which dizziness and syncope on effort are accompanied by exhaustion, dyspnea, headache, palpitations, and pain over the heart.[11] Orthostatic intolerance and syncope may occur in chronic fatigue syndrome.[12] These disorders differ from carotid sinus hypersensitivity, where bradycardia and hypotension may be associated with neck movements, and it is more frequently recognized in the elderly with recurrent unexplained falls.[13] A variety of other stimuli, ranging from coughing, micturition, and even laughing, can induce syncope, probably via similar mechanisms.

An increasingly recognized disorder is *orthostatic intolerance with tachycardia* (*postural tachycardia syndrome*), often without a postural fall in blood pressure.[14] It is more common in young women.

TABLE 82–4 Factors That May Influence Postural Hypotension

Speed of postional change
Time of day (worse in the morning)
Prolonged recumbency
Warm environment (hot weather, central heating, hot bath)
Raising intrathoracic pressure: micturition, defecation, or coughing
Food and alcohol ingestion
Physical exertion
Maneuvers and positions (bending forward, abdominal compression, leg crossing, squatting, activating calf muscle pump)*
Drugs with vasoactive properties (including dopaminergic agents and nitroglycerin)

*These maneuvers usually reduce the postural fall in blood pressure, unlike the others.
From Mathias CJ, Bannister R: Investigation of autonomic disorders. *In* Mathias CJ, Bannister R (eds): Autonomic Failure: A Textbook of Clinical Disorders of the Autonomic Nervous System. 4th ed. p. 174. Oxford: Oxford University Press, 1998.

Hypertension

Supine hypertension (in addition to postural hypotension) may occur in primary chronic autonomic failure. The mechanisms are not clear and include impaired baroreflex activity, adrenoceptor supersensitivity, an increase in central blood volume due to a shift from the periphery, and the continuing effects of drugs used to prevent postural hypotension.[15] Supine hypertension may cause headache; there have been reports, albeit rarely, of papilledema, cerebral hemorrhage, aortic dissection, myocardial ischemia, and heart failure. Hypertension may occur in cerebral tumors, especially when in the posterior fossa.[16] Paroxysmal hypertension may occur in bulbar poliomyelitis, tetanus, the Guillain-Barré syndrome, and porphyria with rapid fluctuations in cardiovascular autonomic activity; in some, as reported in tetanus and the Guillain-Barré syndrome, episodes of hypotension and bradycardia may complicate management. In high spinal cord lesions, hypertension is a major component of autonomic dysreflexia and can cause a throbbing headache and occasionally result in neurologic complications such as epileptic seizures or cerebral hemorrhage (Fig. 82–4). In subarachnoid hemorrhage, severe hypertension may occur, along with electrocardiographic abnormalities due to increased sympathetic activity.[17] Hypertension, often paroxysmal, is a common feature of pheochromocytoma and may occur with other symptoms, such as sweating and palpitations.[18] Increased sympathetic nervous activity may initiate or maintain hypertension in organ transplantees receiving cyclosporin as immunosuppressant therapy,[19] in renovascular disease such as renal artery stenosis,[20] and in preeclamptic toxemia.[21]

Cardiac Dysrhythmias

Tachycardia may occur due to increased sympathetic neural discharge in the Guillain-Barré syndrome and tetanus. In pheochromocytoma, it is due to catecholamine release and beta-adrenoceptor stimulation. Tachycardia may result from cardiac parasympathetic denervation, as in diabetes mellitus; it may be an early sign of cardiovascular autonomic dysfunction in familial amyloid polyneuropathy.

Bradycardia due to abnormal vasovagal reflex activity may complicate tracheal suction in tetraplegics on artificial respirators.[22] Bradycardia due to increased cardiac parasympathetic activity may be a key feature in carotid sinus hypersensitivity and other forms of neurally mediated syncope. The rapid rise in pressure in a pheochromocytoma may result in bradycardia with escape rhythms and atrioventricular dissociation. Bradycardia in high spinal injuries also may occur during autonomic dysreflexia in response to the rise in blood pressure.

Vascular Effects

FACIAL VASCULATURE

In autonomic failure, facial pallor often occurs as the blood pressure falls, with prompt restoration when the blood pressure rises. Facial pallor due to vasoconstriction may accompany other features of excessive sympathoadrenal activation during an attack in pheochromocytoma. Facial vasodilatation accompanied by nasal congestion (the Guttmann sign) may occur in high spinal cord lesions in the acute phase when in spinal shock; it also is seen in patients receiving alpha-adrenoceptor blockers and sympatholytics, such as phenoxybenzamine, guanethidine, and reserpine. In

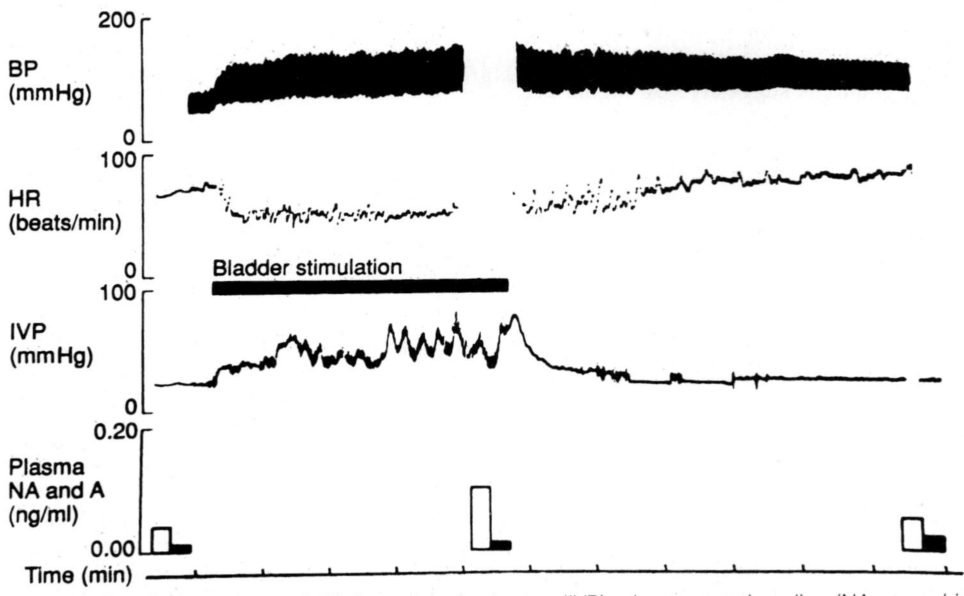

FIGURE 82–4 Blood pressure (BP), heart rate (HR), intravesical pressure (IVP), plasma noradrenaline (NA, *open histograms*), and adrenaline (A, *filled histograms*) levels in a tetraplegic patient before, during, and after bladder stimulation induced by suprapubic percussion of the anterior abdominal wall. The rise in BP is accompanied by a fall in HR as a result of increased vagal activity in response to the rise in BP. Plasma NA, but not A, levels rose, suggesting an increase in sympathetic neural activity independent of adrenomedullary activation (From Mathias CJ, Frankel H: Autonomic disturbances in spinal cord lesions. *In* Mathias CJ, Bannister R [eds]: Autonomic Failure: A Textbook of Clinical Disorders of the Autonomic Nervous System. 4th ed. pp. 494–513. Oxford: Oxford University Press, 1999.)

TABLE 82–5 Some of the Clinical Manifestations and Possible Presentations in Primary Chronic Autonomic Failure Syndromes

Cardiovascular	Orthostatic hypotension
Sudomotor	Anhidrosis, heat intolerance
Gastrointestinal	Constipation, occasionally diarrhea, dysphagia
Renal and urinary bladder	Nocturia, frequency, urgency, incontinence, retention
Sexual	Erectile and ejaculatory failure in the male
Ocular	Aniscoria, Horner's syndrome
Respiratory	Stridor, inspiratory gasps, apneic episodes
Other neurologic deficits	Parkinsonian and cerebellar/ pyramidal features

Certain features, such as oropharyngeal dysphagia and respiratory abnormalities (including those resulting from laryngeal cord paresis), occur in multiple system atrophy, rather than in pure autonomic failure.

From Mathias CJ: Autonomic disorders and their recognition, N Engl J Med 10:721–724, 1997.

chronic high spinal lesions, hypertension during autonomic dysreflexia is often accompanied by flushing and sweating over the face and neck; the mechanisms are unclear. In Horner's syndrome, facial vasodilatation and anhidrosis with pupillary constriction may result from lesions to sympathetic neural pathways within the brain, spinal cord, or periphery.

LIMB VASCULATURE

Raynaud's phenomenon, due to cold hypersensitivity, may occur in both hands and feet in primary chronic autonomic failure (pure autonomic failure and multiple system atrophy).[23] The blue, violaceous phase often persists. Abnormal vascular changes, with sweating and pain, occur in reflex sympathetic dystrophy,[24] for reasons that are unclear and could include sympathetic denervation and the cardiovascular autonomic effects of neuropeptides such as substance P and calcitonin gene–related peptide.

SKELETAL MUSCLE AND ORGAN VASCULATURE

The regional vascular control of skeletal muscle and various organs may be affected in autonomic failure and account for various manifestations. Thus, abnormal peripheral vascular and splanchnic control may contribute to postprandial hypotension,[25] and renal oligemia while upright to oliguria. Hypoperfusion of specific areas within the brain, or their increased sensitivity to ischemia, may be of relevance to symptoms of postural hypotension; thus, hypoperfusion of the brain stem may account for dizziness, and reduced blood supply to the retina and occipital lobes may result in visual disturbances.

Noncardiovascular Features

The function of virtually every organ is influenced by the autonomic nervous system, and a wide variety of features occur in the generalized autonomic disorders (Table 82–5).[26]

INVESTIGATION OF AUTONOMIC DYSFUNCTION

The key aims of investigation of autonomic dysfunction are as follows:

1. To determine whether autonomic function is normal or abnormal; screening investigations to evaluate cardiovascular autonomic function are highlighted in Table 82–6.
2. If an abnormality has been observed, to assess the degree of autonomic dysfunction with an emphasis on the site of the lesion and the functional deficit

TABLE 82–6 Outline of Investigations in Autonomic Failure

Cardiovascular	
Physiologic	Head-up tilt (45 degrees)*; standing*; Valsalva maneuver*
	Pressor stimuli*: isometric exercise,* cold pressor,* mental arithmetic*
	Heart rate responses: deep breathing,* hyperventilation,* standing,* head-up tilt,* 30:15 ratio
	Liquid meal challenge
	Exercise testing
	Carotid sinus massage
Biochemical	Plasma norepinephrine: supine and head-up tilt or standing; urinary catecholamines; plasma renin activity and aldosterone
Pharmacologic	Norepinephrine: alpha-adrenoceptors, vascular
	Isoprenaline: beta-adrenoceptors, vascular and cardiac
	Tyramine: pressor and norepinephrine response
	Edrophonium: norepinephrine response
	Atropine: parasympathetic cardiac blockade
Sudomotor	Central regulation: thermoregulatory sweat test
	Sweat gland response: intradermal acetylcholine quantitative sudomotor axon reflex test (Q-SART), localized sweat test
	Sympathetic skin response
Gastrointestinal	Barium studies, video cine fluoroscopy, endoscopy, gastric emptying studies
Renal Function and Urinary Tract	Day and night urine volumes and sodium/ potassium excretion
	Urodynamic studies, intravenous urography, ultrasound examination, sphincter electromyography
Sexual Function	Penile plethysmography
	Intracavernosal papaverine
Respiratory	Laryngoscopy
	Sleep studies to assess apnea and oxygen desaturation
Eye	Schirmer's test
	Pupil function: pharmacologic and physiologic

Screening cardiovascular autonomic investigations used in our laboratory are indicated by an asterisk.

From Mathias CJ, Bannister R: Investigation of autonomic disorders. *In* Mathias CJ, Bannister R (eds): Autonomic Failure: A Textbook of Clinical Disorders of the Autonomic Nervous System. 4th ed. pp. 169–195. Oxford: Oxford University Press, 1999.

3. To determine whether the abnormality is of the primary or secondary variety, as the need for further investigation, along with prognosis and management, is dependent on the diagnosis; in some, investigation of various systems may be required.[2]

Cardiovascular System

Postural hypotension is a cardinal and often disabling feature of autonomic failure, and investigations are designed to confirm its presence and evaluate exacerbating factors in daily life, so as to guide treatment strategies. In our laboratories, screening investigations to determine whether there is a neurogenic cause include measuring the blood pressure to both head-up tilt and standing and a variety of tests to assess sympathetic vasoconstrictor and cardiac parasympathetic function. It is important that non-neurogenic causes of postural hypotension are considered (Table 82–7); these also may worsen hypotension resulting from neurogenic failure.

Blood pressure and heart rate can be accurately measured with automated noninvasive techniques. Investigation on a tilt table is advantageous when patients have severe postural hypotension or neurologic deficits, as they can be returned rapidly to the horizontal, especially if they are near syncope or have lost consciousness. Prolonged head-up tilt is of value in the investigation of neurally mediated syncope. Carotid sinus massage should be performed during head-up tilt,[27] especially in the vasodepressor forms, because in the head-up position there is greater dependence on sympathetic neural activity and its withdrawal, after massage, can have substantial effects.

The cardiovascular responses to the Valsalva maneuver, during which intrathoracic pressure is raised, also tests the integrity of the entire baroreflex pathway (Fig. 82–5); changes in heart rate alone, even in the absence of continuous blood pressure recordings, provide a useful guide.

TABLE 82–7 Non-Neurogenic Causes of Postural Hypotension

Low Intravascular Volume	
Blood/plasma loss	Hemorrhage, burns, hemodialysis
Fluid/electrolyte	Inadequate intake: anorexia nervosa
	Fluid loss: vomiting, diarrhea, losses from ileostomy
	Renal endocrine: salt-losing nepropathy, adrenal insufficiency (Addison's disease), diabetes insipidus, diuretics
Vasodilatation	Drugs: glyceryl trinitrate
	Alcohol
	Heat, pyrexia
	Hyperbradykinism
	Systemic mastocytosis
	Extensive varicose veins
Cardiac Impairment	
Myocardial	Myocarditis
Impaired ventricular filling	Atrial myxoma, constrictive pericarditis
Impaired output	Aortic stenosis

From Mathias CJ, Bannister R: Investigation of autonomic disorders. *In* Mathias CJ, Bannister R (eds): Autonomic Failure: A Textbook of Clinical Disorders of the Autonomic Nervous System. 4th ed. pp. 169–195. Oxford: Oxford University Press, 1999.

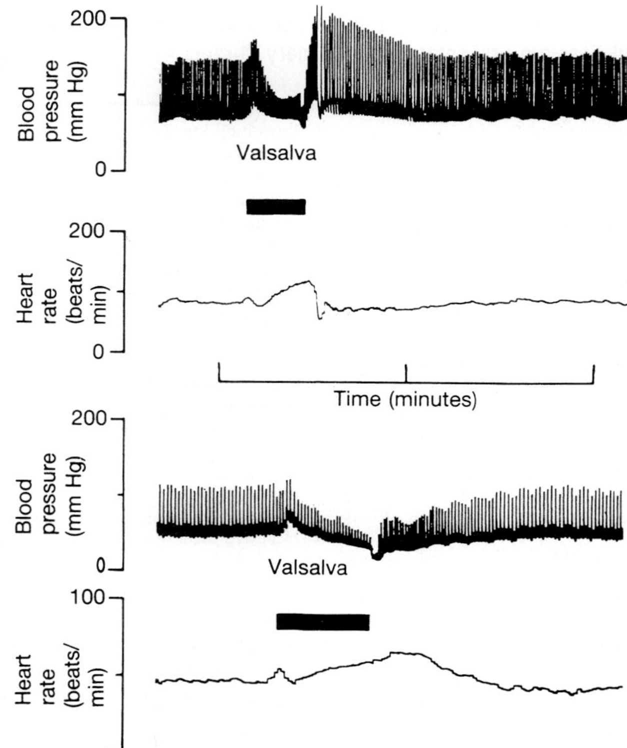

FIGURE 82–5 Blood pressure (BP) and heart rate (HR) before and during a Valsalva maneuver. **Top,** Expiratory pressure is maintained at 40 mm Hg in a subject with intact sympathetic reflexes. The fall in BP is accompanied by a rise in HR. The fall in BP is due to the reduction in venous return, which then stimulates sympathetic activity. BP then partially recovers. After the release of intrathoracic pressure, there is a BP overshoot, and the HR falls below the pre-Valsalva level. **Bottom,** In a patient with impaired autonomic function, raising intrathoracic pressure lowered BP substantially, with no BP recovery. Note that the HR scale differs from that of the normal subject. After the release of intrathoracic pressure, there was no BP overshoot or an immediate fall in HR below basal levels. There was a slow return of BP to pre-Valsalva levels. (From Mathias CJ, Bannister R: Investigation of autonomic disorders. *In* Mathias CJ, Bannister R [eds]: Autonomic Failure: A Textbook of Clinical Disorders of the Autonomic Nervous System. 4th ed. pp. 169–195. Oxford: Oxford University Press, 1999.)

Some patients, however, may have raised intraoral pressure without raised intrathoracic pressure. This can result in a falsely abnormal response; in such situations, continuous blood pressure measurements are of particular value. Stimuli that raise blood pressure, such as isometric exercise (by sustained handgrip for 3 minutes), cutaneous cold (the cold pressor test, by immersing the hand in ice slush for 90 seconds), and mental arithmetic (using serial 7s or subtraction of 17), activate different afferent or central pathways, which then stimulate the sympathetic efferent outflow. The heart rate responses to postural change, deep breathing (sinus arrhythmia) (Fig. 82–6), and hyperventilation assess the integrity of cardiac parasympathetic efferent pathways.

The 24-hour noninvasive ambulatory measurement of blood pressure and heart rate (with a suitably modified protocol as used in our laboratory) records responses to key stimuli such as posture, food, and exercise. It also provides information on whether there is a diurnal fall in

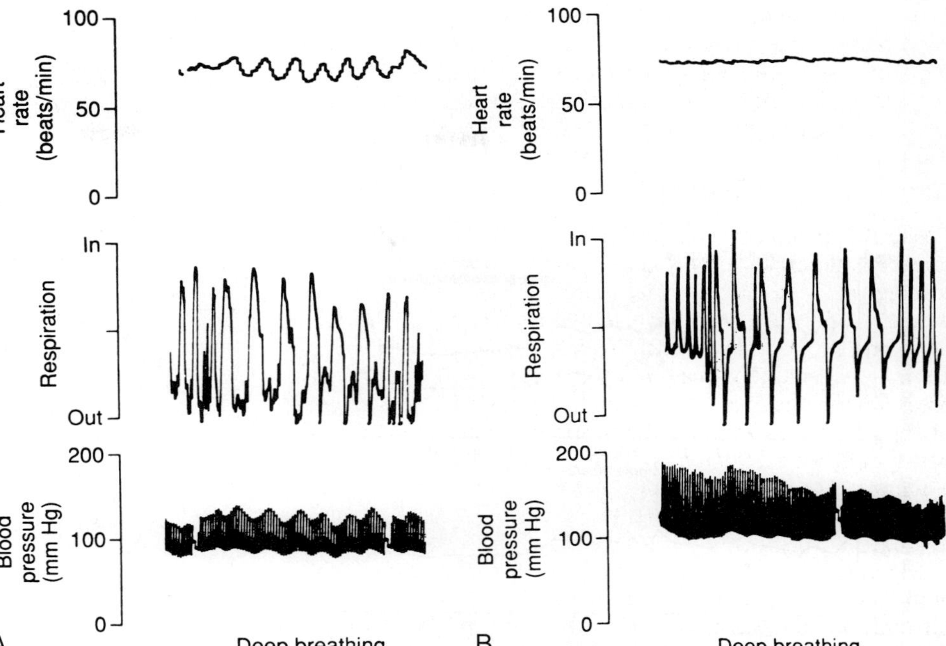

FIGURE 82–6 The effect of deep breathing on heart rate ***(upper panel)*** and blood pressure ***(lowest panel)*** in a normal subject **(A)** and a patient with autonomic failure **(B)**. There is no sinus arrhythmia in the patient despite a fall in blood pressure. Respiratory changes are indicated in the ***middle panel***. (**A** and **B,** From Mathias CJ, Bannister R: Investigation of autonomic disorders. *In* Mathias CJ, Bannister R [eds]: Autonomic Failure: A Textbook of Clinical Disorders of the Autonomic Nervous System. 4th ed. pp 169–195. Oxford: Oxford University Press, 1999.)

blood pressure at night (as occurs normally) and on the presence and severity of supine or paroxysmal hypertension (Fig. 82–7). It is useful in the evaluation of therapy.[15] In some patients, additional investigations may be needed to further determine the factors causing or contributing to postural hypotension and syncope. Thus, there are established laboratory protocols to determine the responses to food ingestion[28] (Fig. 82–8) and exercise[29] (Fig. 82–9), that are major stimuli in daily life and must be therapeutically targeted in some patients. In neurally mediated syncope, prolonged tilt may be needed; some laboratories also use drugs such as isoprenaline[30] to induce an episode, but this carries potential dangers and does not provide a physiologic evaluation of the problem. Others use a combination of head-up tilt and lower body negative pressure.[31] Carotid sinus massage should be performed in suspected carotid sinus hypersensitivity while horizontal and also during head-up tilt (Fig. 82–10)[27]; it is important that carotid artery stenosis is excluded and that due precautions are taken.

The measurement of plasma catecholamines may further determine the neurogenic component to postural hypotension. Basal norepinephrine levels often are normal in multiple system atrophy (where the autonomic lesion is predominantly central), and low in pure autonomic failure (where the lesion is peripheral). With head-up tilt or standing, plasma norepinephrine levels do not rise in autonomic failure, as they do normally (Fig. 82–11). Catecholamine measurements may lead to a diagnosis of dopamine beta-hydroxylase deficiency, as basal plasma norepinephrine and epinephrine levels are undetectable, whereas dopamine levels are elevated.[8] In high spinal cord lesions, paroxysmal hypertension during autonomic dysreflexia may be mistaken for a pheochromocytoma. However, in the former, the basal plasma norepinephrine levels are low, and although they rise during autonomic dysreflexia, the levels often are no higher than basal levels in normal humans; this is in contrast to the grossly elevated plasma catecholamine levels that are often observed in pheochromocytoma. The neurohormonal responses to the predominantly centrally acting sympatholytic agent clonidine are of value in diagnosis. In pheochromocytoma, with autonomous catecholamine secretion, plasma norepinephrine and epinephrine levels are not suppressed after clonidine, unlike in normal subjects and essential hypertensives (Fig. 82–12). In multiple system atrophy with central autonomic failure, there is no clonidine-induced rise in levels of serum growth hormone that is dependent on α_2-adrenoceptor–mediated hypothalamic release of growth hormone–releasing hormone; this differs from the rise in growth hormone levels caused by clonidine in normal subjects and autonomic failure due to peripheral causes (Fig. 82–13).[32]

The measurement of plasma renin activity and plasma aldosterone may be helpful. In diabetes mellitus, there may be hyporeninemia and hypoaldosteronism, which contribute to hyperkalemia. Plasma cortisol levels before and after synthetic adrenocorticotropic hormone administration help exclude Addison's disease, an endocrine cause of postural hypotension.

A number of approaches, especially in research laboratories, are contributing substantially to our understanding of the pathophysiologic processes in autonomic disorders. An example is the measurement of muscle or skin sympathetic nerve activity using the percutaneous insertion of a tungsten microelectrode into the peroneal or median nerve.[33] Sympathetic microneurography has enabled further understanding of the mechanisms in disorders where there is a reduction (vasovagal syncope) or an increase (cyclosporin-induced hypertension and preeclamptic toxemia) in sympathetic neural activity (Fig. 82–14). Other invasive techniques include the measurement of total body and regional norepinephrine spillover to the heart, splanchnic region, kidney, and brain.[34, 35] A variety of noninvasive computer-assisted approaches, using spectral analyses, can determine the sympathetic and parasympathetic contribu-

Text continued on page 1550

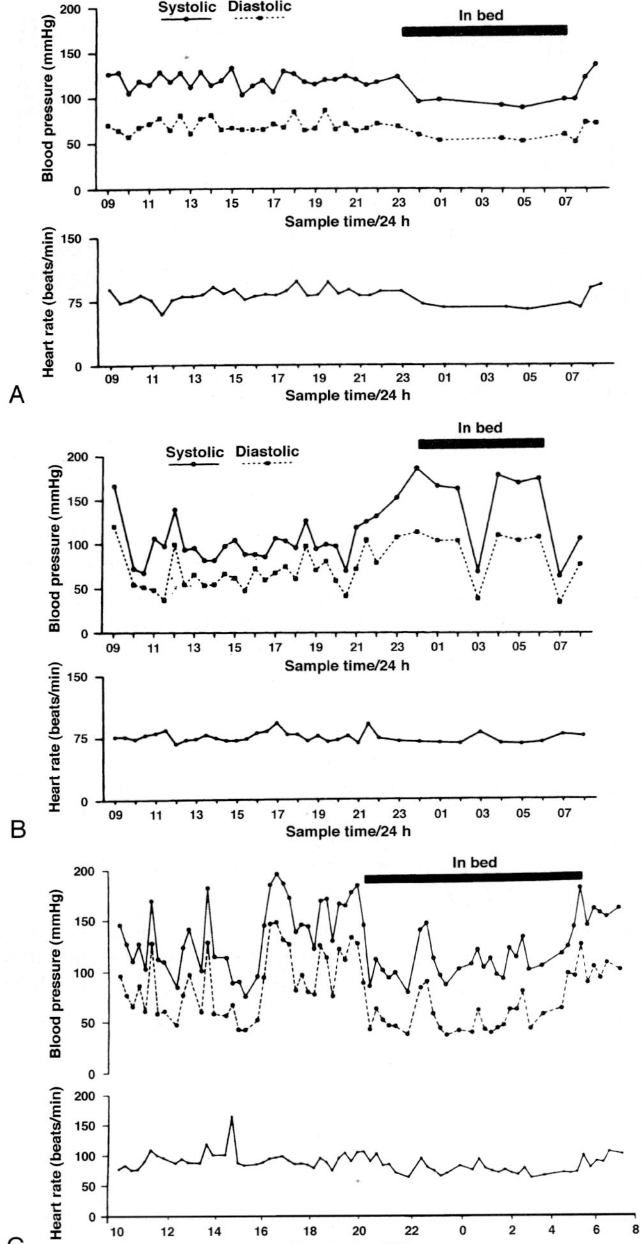

FIGURE 82–7 Twenty-four-hour noninvasive, ambulatory blood pressure profiles showing systolic *(circles)* and diastolic *(squares)* blood pressure and heart rate at intervals through the day and night. **A,** Changes in a normal subject with no postural fall in blood pressure; there was a fall in blood pressure at night while asleep, with a rise in blood pressure on wakening. **B,** Marked fluctuations in blood pressure in a patient with pure autonomic failure. The marked falls in blood pressure are usually the result of postural changes, either sitting or standing. Supine blood pressure, particularly at night, is elevated. Getting up to micturate causes a marked fall in blood pressure (at 3 AM). There is a reversal of the diurnal changes in blood pressure. There are relatively small changes in heart rate considering the marked changes in blood pressure. **C,** A 24-hour profile in a patient with Riley-Day syndrome (familial dysautonomia). The recording shows marked variability in blood pressure with both hypotension and extreme hypertension. (**A** and **B,** From Mathias CJ, Bannister R: Investigation of autonomic disorders. *In* Mathias CJ, Bannister R [eds]: Autonomic Failure: A Textbook of Clinical Disorders of the Autonomic Nervous System. 4th ed. pp. 169–195. Oxford: Oxford University Press, 1999. **C,** From Mathias CJ: Disorders of the autonomic nervous system in childhood. *In* Berg BO [ed]: Principles of Child Neurology. pp. 413–436. New York: McGraw-Hill, 1996. Reproduced with permission of The McGraw-Hill Companies.)

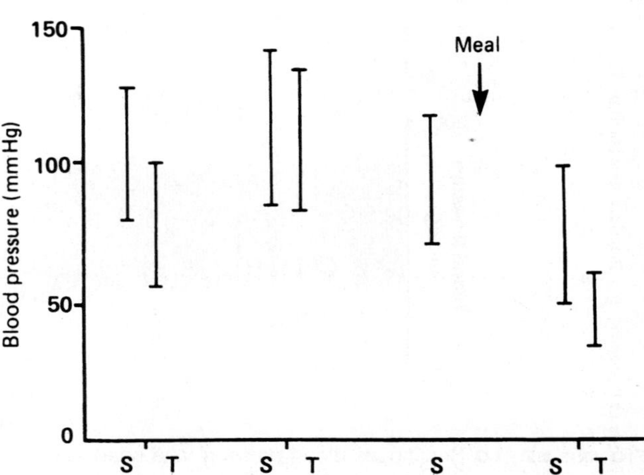

FIGURE 82–8 Systolic and diastolic blood pressure in a patient with multiple system atrophy while supine (S) and after 45-degree head-up tilt (T) on three occasions. On the first two occasions, food intake was not controlled. The patient, however, had not eaten on the second occasion when the postural blood pressure fall was negligible. On the third occasion, supine blood pressure was measured while fasting and 45 minutes after the meal. Postprandial tilt caused a considerable fall in blood pressure, and the patient had to be returned to the horizontal position within 3 minutes. (From Mathias CJ, Holly E, Armstrong E, et al: The influence of food on postural hypotension in three groups with chronic autonomic failure; clinical and therapeutic implications. J Neurol Neurosurg Psychiatry 54:726–730, 1991.)

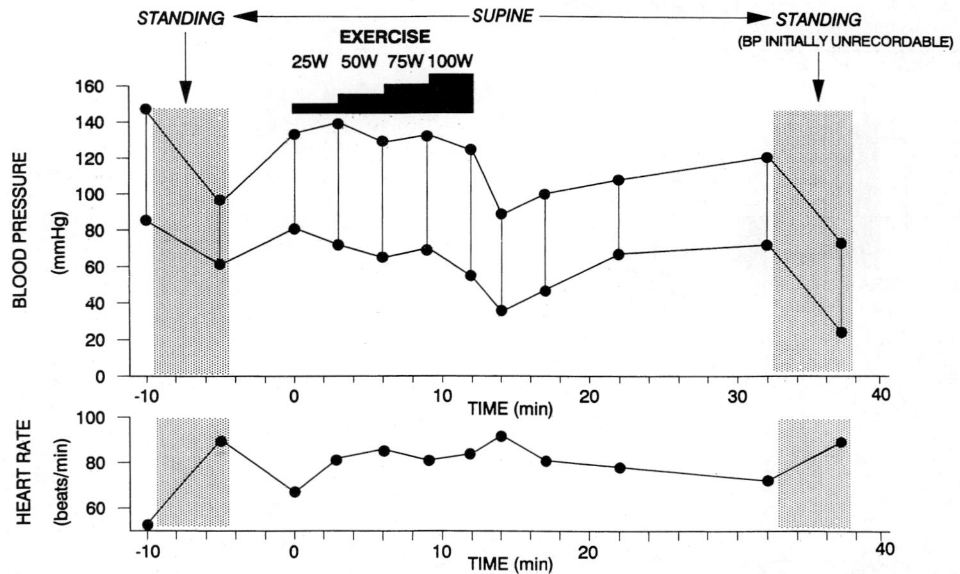

FIGURE 82–9 Blood pressure (BP) and heart rate responses in a patient with autonomic failure while lying and standing, before and after exercise. The *stippled areas* were during standing when there was a fall in BP. Exercise was performed on a bicycle erogometer in the supine position, and unlike normal subjects, in whom there is a rise in BP, there was little or no change. On stopping exercise, BP fell even while the patient was supine; after standing 20 minutes later, the BP was initially unrecordable and the patient was near syncope. The observations were consistent with the patient's symptoms because he did not feel faint during exercise but did on stopping exercise. (From Smith GDP, Bannister R, Mathias CJ: Post-exercise dizziness as the sole presenting symptom of autonomic failure. Br Heart J 69:359–361, 1993.)

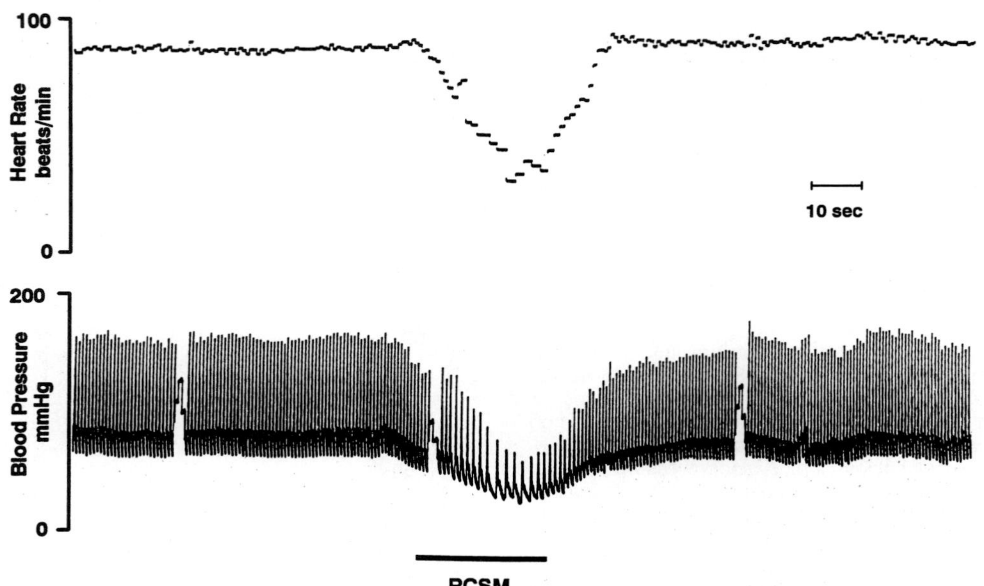

FIGURE 82–10 Continuous blood pressure and heart rate measured noninvasively (by Finapres) in a patient with falls of unknown cause. Right carotid sinus massage (RCSM) caused a fall in both heart rate and blood pressure. The findings indicate the mixed (cardioinhibitory and vasodepressor) form of carotid sinus hypersensitivity. (From Mathias CJ: Autonomic dysfunction and the elderly. *In* Grimley-Evans J, Williams TF, Beattie BL, et al [eds]: Oxford Textbook of Geriatric Medicine. 2nd ed. Oxford: Oxford University Press, 2000.)

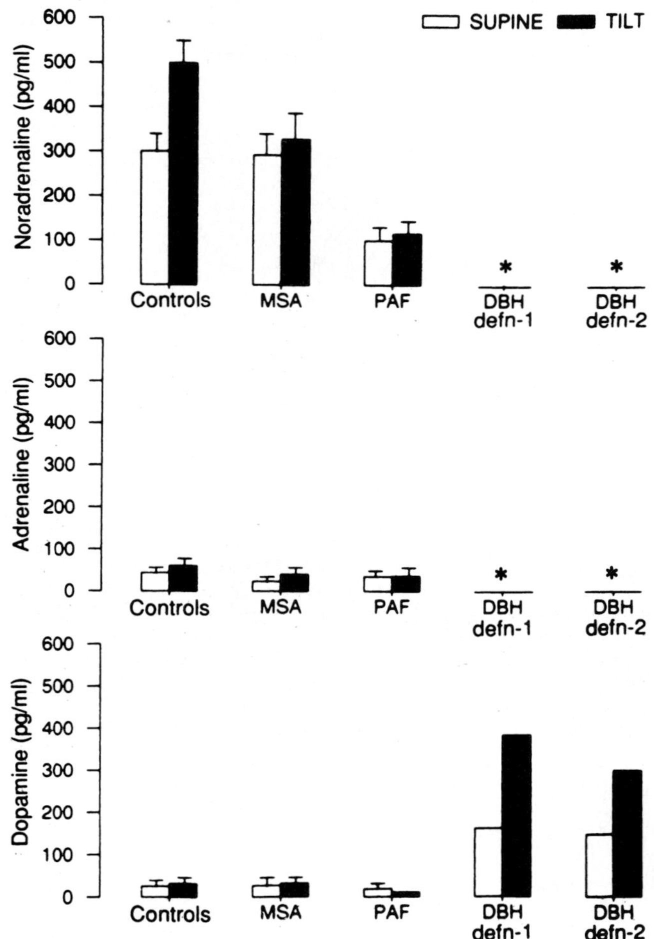

FIGURE 82–11 Plasma noradrenaline (norepinephrine), adrenaline (epinephrine), and dopamine levels (measured with high-pressure liquid chromatography) in normal subjects (controls), patients with multiple system atrophy (MSA), patients with pure autonomic failure (PAF), and two patients with dopamine beta-hydroxylase (DBH) deficiency while supine and after head-up tilt to 45 degrees for 10 minutes. The *asterisk* indicates levels below the detection limits for the assay, which are less than 5 pg/ml for noradrenaline and adrenaline and less than 20 pg/ml for dopamine. *Bars* indicate ± SEM values. (From Mathias CJ, Bannister R: Investigation of autonomic disorders. *In* Mathias CJ, Bannister R [eds]: Autonomic Failure: A Textbook of Clinical Disorders of the Autonomic Nervous System. 4th ed. pp. 169–195. Oxford, Oxford University Press, 1999.)

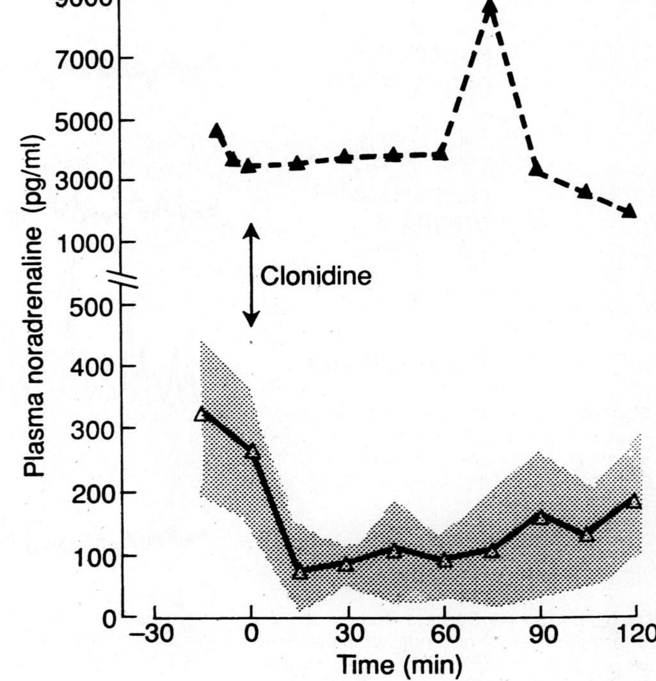

FIGURE 82–12 Plasma noradrenaline (norepinephrine) levels in a patient with a pheochromocytoma (▲----▲) and in a group of patients with essential hypertension (△———△) before and after intravenous clonidine *(arrow)* (2 μg/kg over 10 minutes). Plasma noradrenaline levels fall rapidly in the essential hypertensives after clonidine and remain low during the period of observation. *Stippled area,* ± SEM values. Plasma noradrenaline levels are considerably higher in the patient with pheochromocytoma and are not affected by clonidine. (From Mathias CJ, Bannister R: Investigation of autonomic disorders. *In* Mathias CJ, Bannister R [eds]: Autonomic Failure: A Textbook of Clinical Disorders of the Autonomic Nervous System. 4th ed. pp. 169–195. Oxford: Oxford University Press, 1999.)

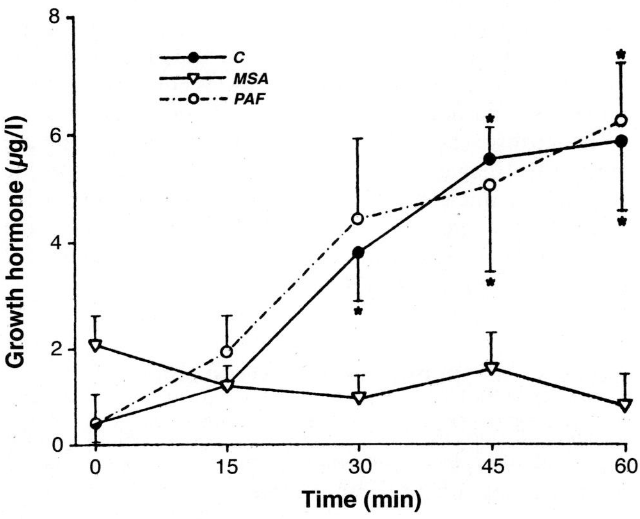

FIGURE 82–13 Serum growth hormone concentrations before (0) and at 15-minute intervals for 60 minutes after clonidine (2 μg/kg per minute) in normal subjects (control [C]) and in patients with pure autonomic failure (PAF) and multiple system atrophy (MSA). Growth hormone concentrations rise in control subjects and in patients with PAF with a peripheral lesion; there is no rise in patients with MSA with a central lesion. (From Thomaides TN, Ray Chaudhuri K, Maule S, et al: Growth hormone response to clonidine in central and peripheral primary autonomic failure. Lancet 340[8814]:263–266, 1992. © by The Lancet Ltd, 1992.)

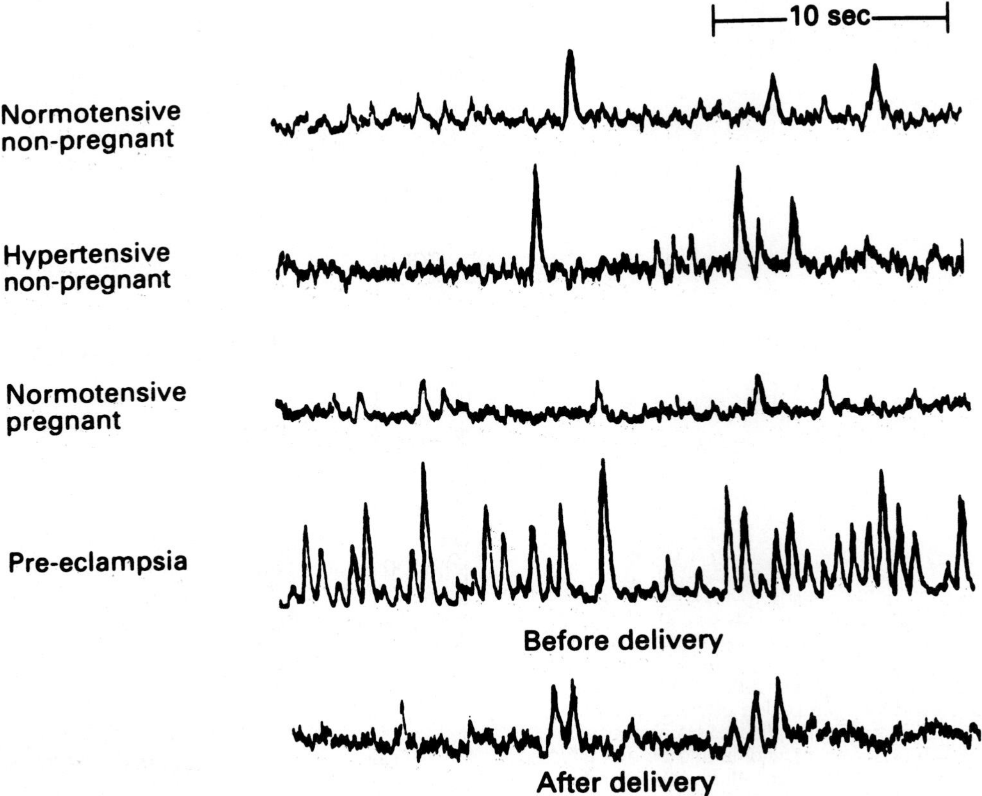

FIGURE 82–14 Representative recordings of sympathetic nerve activity in a normotensive nonpregnant woman, a hypertensive nonpregnant woman, a normotensive pregnant woman, and a woman with preeclampsia (before and after delivery). The rates of sympathetic nerve discharge were similar in the two nonpregnant women and the normotensive pregnant woman, but the rate was much higher in the patient with preeclampsia. After delivery, blood pressure and sympathetic activity returned to normal levels in this patient. (From Schobel HP, Thorsten-Fischer MD, Heuszer K, et al: Pre-eclampsia: a state of sympathetic overactivity. N Engl J Med 335:1480–1485, 1996. Copyright © 1996 Massachusetts Medical Society. All rights reserved.)

tion to heart rate and blood pressure control.[36] Other relatively noninvasive techniques include scintigraphy (metaiodobenzyl guanidine) and positron emission tomography (6-[^{18}F]fluorodopamine), which visualize sympathetic innervation of the heart.[37]

Description of Key Autonomic Disorders

Localized Autonomic Disorders

After heart transplantation, the cardiac parasympathetic and sympathetic pathways are severed, and the heart is incapable of responding to stimuli depending on these extrinsic pathways. There are abnormal cardiac rate changes to head-up postural change and respiratory stimuli such as the Valsalva maneuver, deep breathing, and hyperventilation. Up-regulation of cardiac adrenoreceptors may result in enhanced responses to adrenoceptor agonists such as isoprenaline[38] (Fig. 82–15). Endogenous stimuli, such as exercise, that elevate plasma norepinephrine and epinephrine levels, raise heart rate in cardiac transplantees; the responses in patients with heterotopic cardiac transplantation (with both donor and recipient atria and their sinoatrial nodes) enable further dissection of responses. Mild exercise results in a similar rise in heart rate in both denervated donor and innervated recipient atria; in the former, the rise is slower because of dependence on elevation of circulating catecholamines, rather than reflex neural activity.[39] The reverse, a slower return to baseline levels follows cessation of exercise and occurs in the denervated donor heart.

The intrinsic cholinergic plexuses to the heart and gut are affected in Chagas' disease. The reasons for such specific targeting are unclear and include the effects of neurotoxins released from parasites or an immunologic process that selects intrinsic cholinergic plexuses.[40] Abnormalities of conduction, with bradycardia, may occur.

Primary Autonomic Failure Syndromes

Primary autonomic failure syndromes include the rarer acute and subacute dysautonomias and the more common chronic autonomic failure syndromes.

Acute and Subacute Dysautonomias

In pure pandysautonomia, both sympathetic and parasympathetic pathways are involved, without additional neurologic involvement. Thus, there is postural hypotension with impairment of cardiac parasympathetic responses to stim-

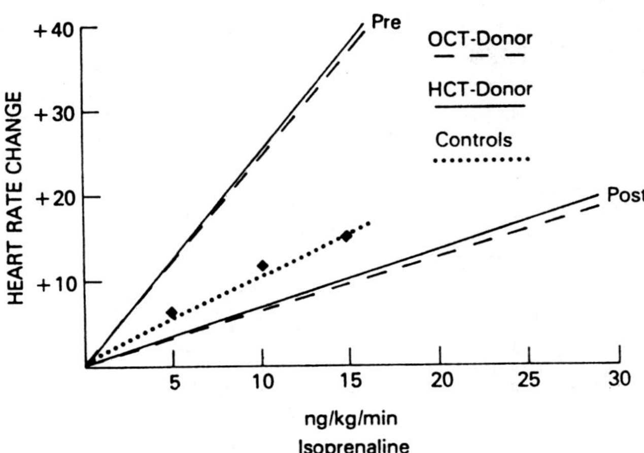

FIGURE 82–15 Changes in heart rate during infusion of isoprenaline in the donor hearts of patients with heterotopic (HCT) and orthotopic (OCT) heart transplants before (pre) and after (post) beta-adrenoceptor blockade. The response in 10 normal subjects (Controls) is also plotted. There is a greater response in both HCT and OCT heart transplant recipients before β-blockade. (From Yusuf S, Theodropoulos S, Mathias CJ, et al: Increased sensitivity of the denervated transplanted human heart to isoprenaline both before and after beta-adrenergic blockade. Circulation 75[4]:696–704, 1987.)

uli. When only the cholinergic nervous system is targeted, the term *pure cholinergic dysautonomia* has been favored, as it involves not only the parasympathetic nervous system but also sympathetic cholinergic fibers to sweat glands; the lesion appears to be presynaptic, as cholinergic receptors are responsive to cholinomimetic agents. Postural hypotension does not occur, but the cardiac parasympathetic pathways are affected, resulting in a raised heart rate. Investigation may indicate preservation of cardiac sympathetic pathways; thus, during head-up postural change, the heart rate may rise modestly, as it may during various pressor tests that affect sympathetic efferent pathways, but the heart rate changes during the Valsalva maneuver usually are impaired, and sinus arrhythmia is not present. In a third group, there is additional neurologic involvement, usually manifesting in a peripheral neuropathy.

The cause of acute dysautonomias is not known. An immunologic basis has been suggested as there have been two cases in whom intravenous immunoglobulin apparently reversed the autonomic features.

Chronic Autonomic Failure Syndromes

There are three groups, in each of which the cause is unknown (Fig. 82–16).[26] In *pure autonomic failure*, the lesions are peripheral, as based on a series of detailed physiologic and biochemical investigation, although with limited postmortem data; there is no additional neurologic involvement. The prognosis in this condition is favorable and thus differs from the more frequently encountered multiple system atrophy (synonymous with the Shy-Drager syndrome).[41] In the majority of these patients, parkinsonian features occur at some stage of the disease. *Multiple system atrophy* is considered to account for about 20 percent of patients initially diagnosed as having Parkinson's disease. It is a sporadic and progressive disorder, with the clinical features occurring and advancing in an unpredictable manner.[26, 41, 42] There is a less common group of patients with drug-responsive Parkinson's disease who later develop autonomic failure that appears to be *peripheral* in nature, as distinct from the central involvement in multiple system atrophy. When postural hypotension and genitourinary disturbances occur in a patient with parkinsonian features, especially if the patient is poorly responsive to levodopa therapy, multiple system atrophy should be considered.

Secondary Autonomic Disorders

Familial Dysautonomia (Riley-Day Syndrome)

This is a disorder that usually is diagnosed at birth.[43] It is transmitted as an autosomal recessive disorder, mainly in Ashkenazi Jews. The genotype has been identified. The cardiovascular system can be affected variably, with hypotension during postural change and exercise, and hypertension especially in response to stress (see Fig. 82–7C). Management therefore is difficult. Cardiovascular disturbances may contribute to renal failure, which in the past was one of the major factors resulting in increased mortality rates.

Diabetes Mellitus

In this common metabolic disorder, a peripheral neuropathy often accompanies the autonomic neuropathy, which ini-

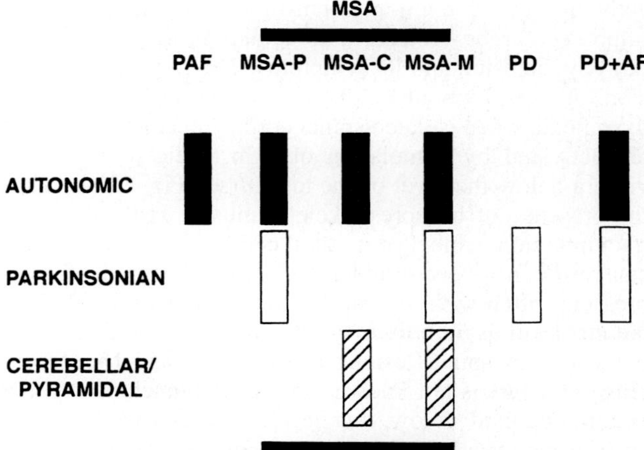

FIGURE 82–16 Schematic representation indicates the major clinical features in patients with primary chronic autonomic failure syndromes, including pure autonomic failure (PAF) and the three major neurologic forms of multiple system atrophy (MSA): the parkinsonian form (MSA-P; synonymous with striatonigral degeneration), the cerebellar form (MSA-C; the olivopontocerebellar degeneration form), and the multiple/mixed form (MSA-M; with both features). Also included are Parkinson's disease (PD) and the rarer subgroup with Parkinson's disease and autonomic failure (PD+AF). (Adapted from Mathias CJ: Autonomic disorders and their recognition. N Engl J Med 1997, 10:721–724, 1997. Copyright © 1997 Massachusetts Medical Society. All rights reserved.)

tially involves the cardiac parasympathetic pathways, with a resting tachycardia and lack of response to stimuli that normally influence heart rate. Sympathetic vasoconstrictor failure may occur later. Patients with diabetes are prone to coronary artery disease and myocardial ischemia, and it is unclear whether the altered cardiac autonomic balance (with preservation of increased sympathetic activity) may predispose them to cardiac dysrhythmias and thus contribute to sudden death.

Familial Amyloid Polyneuropathy

This disorder is due to a genetic abnormality involving the transthyretin protein, which is mainly produced in the liver.[44] It is an autosomal dominant disorder that affects people mainly over the age of 20, and it relentlessly damages peripheral somatic and autonomic nerves. The involvement of cardiac parasympathetic function is an early autonomic feature. Cardiac dysrhythmias may occur along with postural hypotension. The only means to halt the disease appears to be through liver transplantation, which prevents abnormal hepatic transthyretin production.

High Spinal Cord Lesions

In cervical and high thoracic spinal cord lesions, the majority of autonomic pathways to the heart and blood vessels are separated from cerebral control.[45] The baroreceptor afferents, however, are preserved, and the cardiac parasympathetic efferents to the heart remain intact and functional. Thus, hypotension occurs during postural change because of the inability of the brain to activate peripheral sympathetic efferent pathways, and heart rate rises because of baroreceptor activation and withdrawal of cardiac vagal tone. With time, compensatory mechanisms, which include activation of the renin-angiotensin-aldosterone system and improved cerebrovascular autoregulation, help reduce postural hypotension and its symptoms. The reverse, hypertension followed by bradycardia, may occur during autonomic dysreflexia when isolated spinal cord sympathetic pathways are activated by stimulation of skin, skeletal muscle, or viscera below the level of the lesion (see Fig. 82–4). Thus, the presence of bedsores, skeletal muscle spasms, urinary tract infection, a blocked urethral catheter, or an anal fissure can result in a severe and paroxysmal elevation of blood pressure, often with a compensatory bradycardia. The segmental level is important as autonomic dysreflexia does not occur in spinal lesions below level T5. The precise reason for this is not known; the large splanchnic vascular bed is supplied below this level, and this may provide an explanation. A key component in the management of autonomic dysreflexia is identifying the cause and alleviating it; drugs acting on various components of the reflex may be used (Table 82–8).

Patients with high cervical lesions (above the diaphragmatic innervation at the fourth and fifth cervical segments) require artificial respiration. They are prone to severe bradycardia and cardiac arrest, especially in the early phases after injury, when they are in a state of "spinal shock" (Fig. 82–17A). In this phase, isolated spinal cord sympathetic reflexes often are absent, and therefore autonomic dysreflexia does not occur. Disconnection of the respirator and tracheal suction, as for intermittent tracheal toilette, activates vagal afferents that increase vagal efferent activity (Table 82–9). This is not opposed by sympathetic nerves, as would occur normally. The cardiac effects of the vagus cannot be reversed by the inflation "reflex" because of respiratory paralysis. Furthermore, the vagi also may be increasingly sensitive because of hypoxia that could be secondary to a variety of reasons, from respiratory infections to pulmonary emboli. Thus, activation of vagal afferents can result rapidly in severe bradycardia and hypotension with potentially disastrous sequelae. The importance of the final efferent pathway is emphasized by the effectiveness of the muscarinic cholinergic blocker atropine in preventing bradycardia and cardiac arrest (see Fig. 82–17B).

A key factor in preventing excessive vagovagal reflex activity is adequate oxygenation. If bradycardia occurs, intravenous atropine may be necessary. The cholinomimetics neostigmine and carbachol, which may be used to reverse urinary bladder and bowel paralysis in spinal shock, should be avoided or used with caution. The β_2-adrenocep-

TABLE 82–8 Drugs Used in Autonomic Dysreflexia With Their Major Site of Action

Afferent	Topical lignocaine
Spinal cord	Clonidine
	Reserpine
	Spinal anesthetics
Sympathetic efferent	Ganglia: hexamethonium
	Nerve terminals: guanethidine
	Alpha-adrenoceptors: phenoxybenzamine
Target organ	
Blood vessels	Glyceryl trinitrate, nifedipine
Sweat glands	Probanthine

Note: Drugs such as clonidine may act at multiple sites. Some drugs must be administered at specific sites, such as lignocaine into the bladder, if this is the source of the stimulus causing autonomic dysreflexia.

From Mathias CJ, Frankel HL: Autonomic disturbances in spinal cord lesions. *In* Mathias CJ, Bannister R (eds): Autonomic Failure: A Textbook of Clinical Disorders of the Autonomic Nervous System. 4th ed. pp. 494–513. Oxford: Oxford University Press, 1999.

TABLE 82–9 The Major Mechanisms Contributing to Bradycardia and Cardiac Arrest in Recently Injured Tetraplegics in Spinal Shock During Tracheal Suction and Hypoxia

	Tracheal Suction	Hypoxia
Normal	Increased sympathetic nervous activity causes tachycardia and raises blood pressure	Bradycardia is the primary response opposed by the pulmonary (inflation) vagal reflex, resulting in tachycardia
Tetraplegics	There is no increase in sympathetic nervous activity, so there is no rise in heart rate or blood pressure. Vagal afferent stimulation may lead to unopposed vagal efferent activity	The primary response, bradycardia, is not opposed by the pulmonary (inflation) vagal reflex, because of disconnection from respirator or "fixed" respiratory rate

↘ ↙

Increased vagal cardiac tone

↓

Bradycardia and cardiac arrest

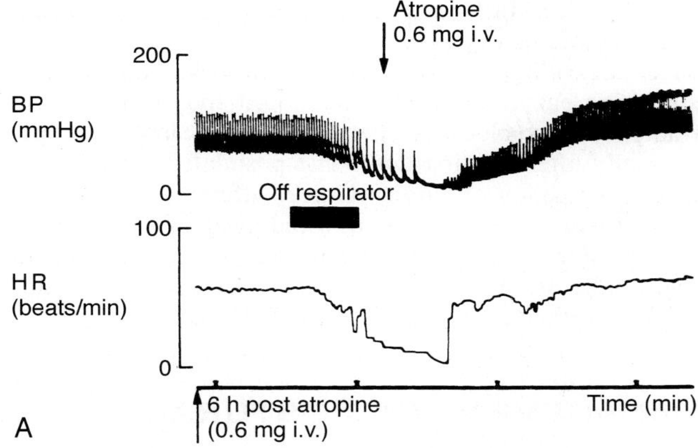

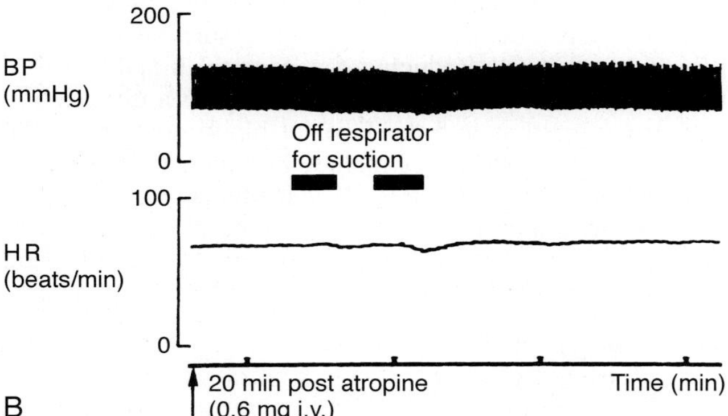

FIGURE 82–17 **A,** Effect of disconnecting the respirator (as required for aspiration of the airways) on the blood pressure (BP) and heart rate (HR) of a recently injured tetraplegic patient (C4-5 lesion) in spinal shock 6 hours after the last dose of intravenous atropine. Sinus bradycardia and cardiac arrest (also observed on the electrocardiogram) were reversed with reconnection, intravenous atropine, and external cardiac massage. **B,** Effect of tracheal suction 20 minutes after atropine. Disconnection from the respirator and tracheal suction did not lower either heart rate or blood pressure. (**A,** From Frankel HL, Mathias CJ, Spalding JMK: Mechanisms of reflex cardiac arrest in tetraplegic patients. Lancet 2:1183–1185, 1975. © 1975 by The Lancet Ltd. **B,** From Mathias CJ: Bradycardia and cardiac arrest during tracheal suction—mechanisms in tetraplegic patients. Eur J Int Care Med 2:147–156, 1976.)

tor agonist isoprenaline may be used to raise heart rate, but it can reduce blood pressure because of enhanced vasodilatation due to vascular β_2-adrenoceptor stimulation. Temporary cardiac demand pacemakers may be of value. Similar problems may occur in chronic tetraplegics undergoing general anesthesia when vagal afferents are stimulated during intubation, especially when there is inadequate cardiac vagal blockade. Such patients should be administered atropine, ideally intravenously, before intubation.

In patients with incomplete spinal cord lesions at different levels, various forms of cardiovascular autonomic dysfunction may occur depending on the degree of disruption to sympathetic pathways.

Neurally Mediated Syncope

In neurally mediated syncope disorders, there is an intermittent abnormality of the autonomic nervous system resulting in a rapid fall in heart rate due to increased cardiac vagal activity and hypotension due to withdrawal of sympathetic neural tone. In the young, the most common cause is vasovagal syncope, often with a family history.[10] Precipitating stimuli are often emotional and include venipuncture, exposure to a needle, or even discussion of venipuncture. In others, painful stimuli induce an attack. The overall prognosis is good, but attacks may be disruptive. In some, convulsions and seizures may lead to an erroneous diagnosis of epilepsy. The management initially consists of making an accurate diagnosis, identifying precipitating factors, and dealing with them. This may necessitate behavioral psychotherapy and even the use of selective serotonin reuptake inhibitors. Increased salt intake and regular exercise should be advised. In some, further measures are needed and include sympathomimetic agents. The insertion of a cardiac pacemaker alone to prevent bradycardia may not prevent syncope, emphasizing the importance of withdrawal of sympathetic nerve activity in the causation of hypotension.

In carotid sinus hypersensitivity, the stimulation of glossopharyngeal afferents induces syncope. There may be a classic history of attacks induced by neck movements or fastening of the collar. In the elderly, however, in whom this condition is increasingly recognized,[13] this history may not be elicited, and the diagnosis should be actively sought where there is no other cause for recurrent falls. There are three major forms: (1) the cardioinhibitory form with marked bradycardia, (2) the rarer vasodepressor form with hypotension but without bradycardia, and (3) the common mixed form with a combination of hypotension and bradycardia, which accounts for the majority of cases (see Fig. 82–10). When bradycardia occurs, often there is a response to a cardiac demand pacemaker. When hypotension occurs, vasopressor drugs may be needed, although there may be potential dangers in their use, especially in the elderly. In some, carotid sinus denervation may be needed.

Neurally mediated syncope may have other rarer causes, ranging from coughing and laughing to swallowing and the onset of glossopharyngeal neuralgia. It may be difficult to distinguish from other causes of syncope, including epilepsy. A precise diagnosis is of importance, together with delineation of the mechanisms (Fig. 82–18), as this is of crucial importance in planning treatment.

Postural Tachycardia Syndrome (Orthostatic Intolerance)

Postural tachycardia syndrome (orthostatic intolerance) is increasingly recognized in women between the ages of 15 and 50 in whom there is orthostatic intolerance with tachycardia (of $\geq$ 30 bpm on head-up postural tilt), often without postural hypotension. There are associations with mitral valve prolapse, chronic fatigue syndrome, and panic attacks. The pathophysiologic basis may include partial autonomic denervation, adrenoceptor changes, hypovolemia, and hyperventilation. The various descriptions suggest that it is a heterogeneous disorder.[46] The symptoms usually diminish with time. There often is a favorable response to β-adrenoceptor blockers such as propranolol.

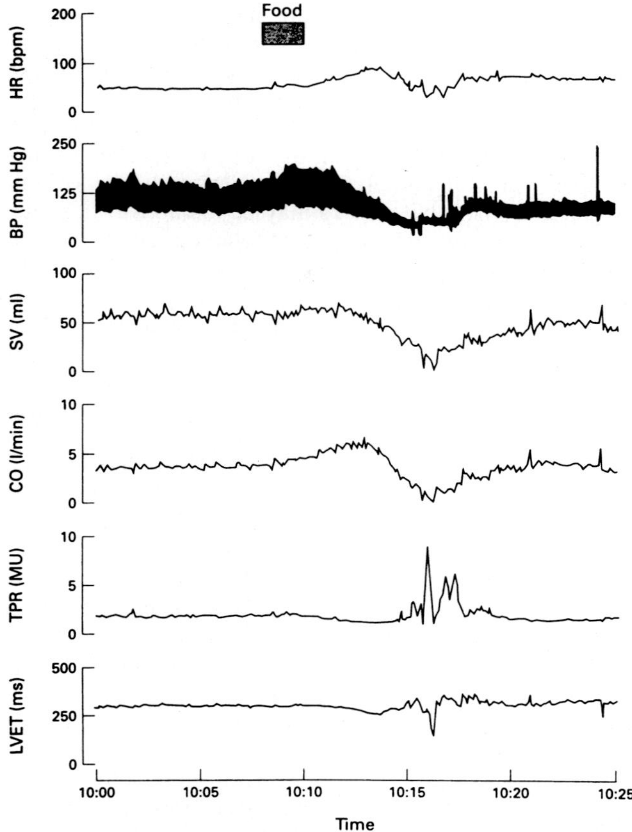

FIGURE 82–18 Continuous measurement of heart rate (HR), blood pressure (BP), stroke volume (SV), cardiac output (CO), and total peripheral vascular resistance (TPR) and left ventricular ejection time (LVET) before, during, and after a solid meal, eaten after an overnight fast. After completion of the food, there is a fall in blood pressure, stroke volume, and cardiac output and then a fall in heart rate. The patient collapsed at this point, hence the change in the record. On recovery from syncope, while lying flat, heart rate recovered, but stroke volume, cardiac output, and blood pressure remained low. A cardiac pacemaker was avoided. (From Deguchi K, Mathias CJ: Continuous haemodynamic monitoring in an unusual case of swallow-induced syncope. J Neurol Neurosurg Psychiatry 67:220–222, 1999.)

Drugs, Poisons, and Toxins

These may impair cardiovascular function either by a direct action on neural pathways and receptors or by causing an autonomic neuropathy (see Table 82–2). Included are drugs successfully used in the therapy of hypertension that act centrally (e.g., clonidine, methyldopa, and the newer imidazoline agonist moxonidine) or peripherally (e.g., β-adrenoceptor blockers). They occasionally may cause marked bradycardia and hypotension even when used locally; examples are xylometazoline hydrochloride used intranasally as a decongestant and timoptolol used intraocularly for glaucoma. Drugs may raise heart rate either through increasing sympathetic activity (e.g., amphetamines), or by reducing cardiac parasympathetic activity (e.g., botulinum toxin). Cholinomimetics and anticholinesterases (e.g., pyridostigmine) increase parasympathetic activity and can lower heart rate. Reef fish containing ciguatera toxin may cause bradycardia through increased vagal tone, which can be reversed by atropine. Alcohol and perhexiline maleate may affect cardiovascular autonomic function by causing an autonomic neuropathy.

Certain antihypertensive agents such as the angiotensin-converting enzyme inhibitors (captopril and enalapril) and α-adrenoceptor blockers (prazosin) may cause syncope, especially after the first dose. The postulated mechanisms include activation of cardiac C-fiber afferents, an increase in cholinergic activity, and a withdrawal of sympathetic activity, similar to the Bezold-Jarisch reflex, resulting in bradycardia and vasodilatation. These are probably examples of drug-induced neurally mediated syncope.

Management of Postural Hypotension

The key aims in management are to provide low-risk therapy, ensure appropriate mobility and function, prevent falls and associated trauma, and maintain a suitable quality of life (Table 82–10). Reducing the postural blood pressure fall is not the singular aim, as there may be a dissociation between symptoms and the level of blood pressure.[47] The main therapeutic strategies include both nonpharmacologic and pharmacologic measures. Patient education is of importance because appropriate implementation of nonpharmacologic approaches, in particular, is especially dependent on the cooperation of the patient and his or her caregivers.

Nonpharmacologic Measures

Nonpharmacologic measures can be divided into measures that should be avoided, introduced, and considered (Table 82–11). Simple explanations often suffice in enabling motivated patients to avoid stimuli that worsen postural hypotension. However, the reasons for some of the measures to be introduced may not be obvious and require further explanation. Head-up tilt, especially at night, probably acts by reducing renal perfusion pressure and activating nonneural mechanisms such as the renin-angiotensin-aldosterone system, which then reduce recumbency-induced diuresis and help maintain blood pressure. Determining the appropriate degree and type of exercise (Fig. 82–19) is important, and the advice requires individual tailoring. Exercising in a more horizontal position, such as swimming or the use of a rowing machine, may be less likely to lower blood pressure. The use of various body positions and appropriate aids, such as lightweight portable chairs, can be of value (Fig. 82–20).[48]

Antigravity suits have virtually no role; they often are difficult to apply, having been designed mainly for the physically able, and are of limited value as the compensatory mechanisms that must be recruited to reduce postural hypotension are not activated when the suit is not is use.

TABLE 82–10 Key Aims of Treatment

Low-risk therapy
Ensuring appropriate mobility and function
Preventing falls and associated trauma
Maintaining a suitable quality of life

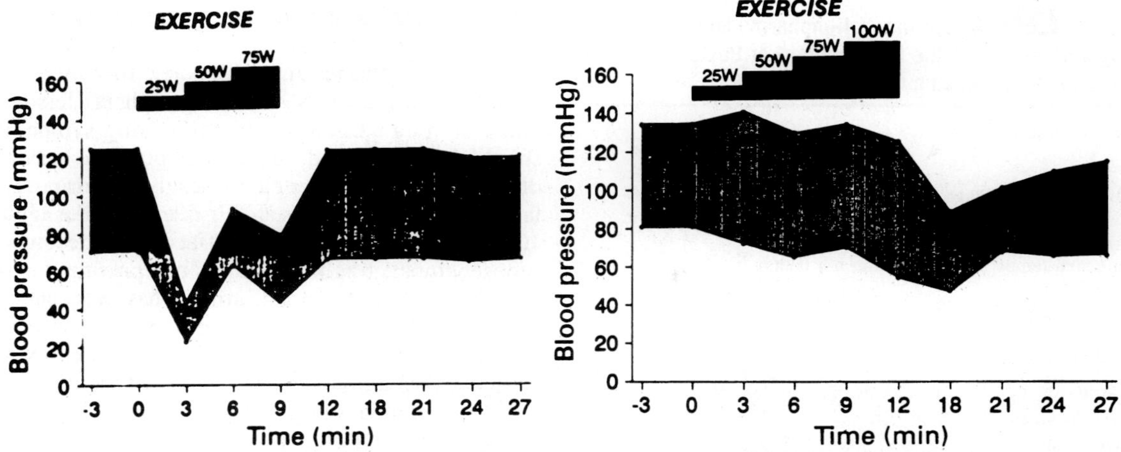

FIGURE 82–19 Systolic and diastolic blood pressure **(top)** in two patients with primary autonomic failure before, during, and after bicycle exercise performed in the supine position at different workloads, ranging from 25 to 100 W. **Left,** In this patient, there was a marked fall in blood pressure on initiation of exercise; she had to crawl upstairs because of severe exercise-induced hypotension. **Right,** In this patient, there were minor changes in blood pressure during exercise but a marked decrease soon after stopping exercise. This patient was usually asymptomatic while walking but developed postural symptoms when he stopped walking and stood still. Postexercise hypotension probably was due to vasodilatation in exercising skeletal muscle, not opposed by the calf muscle pump. (Adapted from Mathias CJ, Williams AC: The Shy-Drager syndrome [and multiple system atrophy]. *In* Calne DB [ed]: Neurodegenerative Diseases. 1st ed. pp. 743–768. Philadelphia: WB Saunders, 1994.)

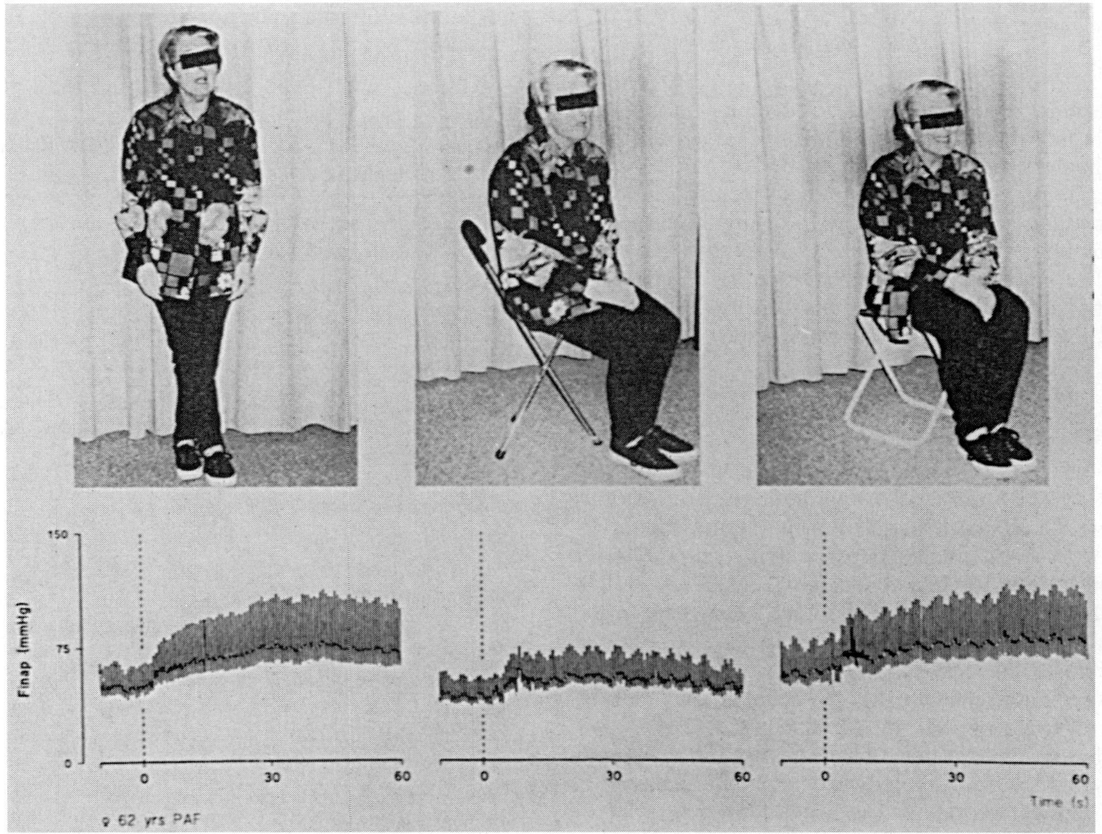

FIGURE 82–20 Effects on finger arterial blood pressure of standing in the crossed-leg position with leg muscle contraction **(left)** and of sitting on a derby **(middle)** and on a fishing chair **(right)** in a patient with autonomic failure. Orthostatic symptoms were present while standing and disappeared while crossing legs and sitting on the fishing chair. Sitting on a derby chair caused the least blood pressure rise and did not completely relieve the patient's symptoms. (From Smit AA, Hardjowijono MA, Wieling W: Are portable folding chairs useful to combat orthostatic hypotension? Ann Neurol 42[6]:975–978, 1997.)

TABLE 82–11 Outline of Nonpharmacologic and Pharmacologic Measures in the Management of Postural Hypotension Due to Neurogenic Failure

Nonpharmacologic Measures

To Be Avoided

Sudden head-up postural change (especially on waking)
Prolonged recumbency
Straining during micturition and defecation
High environmental temperature (including hot baths)
"Severe" exertion
Large meals (especially with refined carbohydrates)
Alcohol
Drugs with vasodepressor properties

To Be Introduced

Head-up tilt during sleep
Small, frequent meals
High-salt intake
Judicious exercise (including swimming)
Body positions and maneuvers

To Be Considered

Elastic stockings
Abdominal binders

Pharmacologic Measures

Starter drug:	fludrocortisone
Sympathomimetics:	ephedrine or midodrine
Specific targeting:	octreotide, desmopressin, or erythropoietin

It should be emphasized that non-neurogenic factors, such as fluid loss due to vomiting or diarrhea (Table 82–7), may substantially worsen postural hypotension.
From Mathias CJ, Kimber JR: Treatment of postural hypotension. J Neurol Neurosurg Psychiatry 65:285–289, 1998.

Cardiac pacemakers usually have no place in the management of chronic neurogenic postural hypotension; in such patients, the lack of sympathetic vasoconstriction causes peripheral pooling and reduces venous return and thus ventricular filling and cardiac output. Raising the heart rate neither affects the underlying defect nor provides benefit. In certain forms of neurally mediated syncope, and especially in the cardioinhibitory form of carotid sinus hypersensitivity, a cardiac demand pacemaker is of value.

Pharmacologic Measures

Drugs are needed when nonpharmacologic approaches are unsuccessful. They may raise blood pressure in various ways (Table 82–12). The starter drug is the mineralocorticoid fludrocortisone, which acts by reducing salt and water loss and may increase α-adrenoceptor sensitivity. A low dose of 100 to 200 μg is used at night, when there is the greatest natriuresis and diuresis. Side effects are minimal with these doses. In higher doses, hypokalemia and excessive fluid retention may occur. Its benefits may not be realized until it is stopped.

Drugs that mimic the deficient neurotransmitter norepinephrine should be considered next. Ephedrine has both direct and indirect actions and is of value in central autonomic disorders such as multiple system atrophy at dosages of 15 to 45 mg twice daily. It is best taken on waking up, with further doses before lunch and dinner. It is not recommended at night, when its pressor effects are not needed and when it may cause insomnia. Other side effects, especially with higher doses, include tremulousness, a reduction in appetite, and urinary retention in males due to its effects on the urethral sphincter. In patients refractory to ephedrine, as in those with peripheral lesions such as pure autonomic failure, a directly acting sympathomimetic should be introduced. An example is the prodrug midodrine, which is converted to desglymidodrine and stimulates α_1-adrenoreceptors.[49, 50] It is used in dosages of 2.5 to 10 mg twice daily. Its side effects include cutis anserina (goosebumps); tingling of the skin; pruritus, especially of the scalp; and in the male, urinary hesitancy and retention.

Sympathomimetics should be avoided or used with caution in patients with coexisting ischemic heart disease, cardiac dysrhythmias, and peripheral vascular disease.

If the combination of fludrocortisone and a sympathomimetic does not produce the desired effect, selective targeting is needed, depending on the underlying pathophysiologic abnormalities. Octreotide, a somatostatin analogue, reduces postprandial hypotension,[51] presumably because it inhibits the release of vasodilatatory/gastrointestinal peptides[52]; importantly, it does not enhance nocturnal hypertension.[15] It may reduce postural and exercise-induced hypotension.[53, 54] A dose of 25 to 50 μg subcutaneously 30 minutes before a meal reduces postprandial hypotension and may influence postural and exercise-induced hypotension. Side effects include nausea and abdominal colic. Desmopressin, a vasopressin analogue, acts on renal tubular vasopressin-2 receptors to reduce nocturnal polyuria and improve morning postural hypotension.[55] It is used as a nasal spray (10 to 40 μg) or orally in tablet form (100

TABLE 82–12 Major Actions by Which a Variety of Drugs May Reduce Postural Hypotension

Reducing Salt Loss/Plasma Volume Expansion

Mineralocorticoids (fludrocortisone)

Reducing Nocturnal Polyuria

Vasopressin-2 receptor agonists (desmopressin)

Vasoconstriction: Sympathetic

Directly on resistance vessels (phenylephrine, norepinephrine, clonidine) and on capacitance vessels (dihydroergotamine)
Indirectly (ephedrine, tyramine with monoamine oxidase inhibitors, yohimbine)
Prodrug (midodrine, L-threo-dihydroxyphenylserine)

Vasoconstriction: Nonsympathetic

Vasopressin-1 receptor agents: terlipressin

Preventing Vasodilatation

Prostaglandin synthetase inhibitors (indomethacin, flurbiprofen)
Dopamine receptor blockade (metoclopramide, domperidone)
$Beta_2$-2 adrenoceptor blockade (propranolol)

Preventing Postprandial Hypotension

Adenosine receptor blockade (caffeine)
Peptide release inhibitors (somatostatin analogue: octreotide)

Increasing Cardiac Output

Beta-blockers with intrinsic sympathetic activity (pindolol, xamoterol)
Dopamine agonists (ibopamine)

Increasing Red Cell Mass

Recombinant erythropoietin

From Mathias CJ, Kimber JR: Treatment of postural hypotension. J Neurol Neurosurg Psychiatry 65:285–289, 1998.

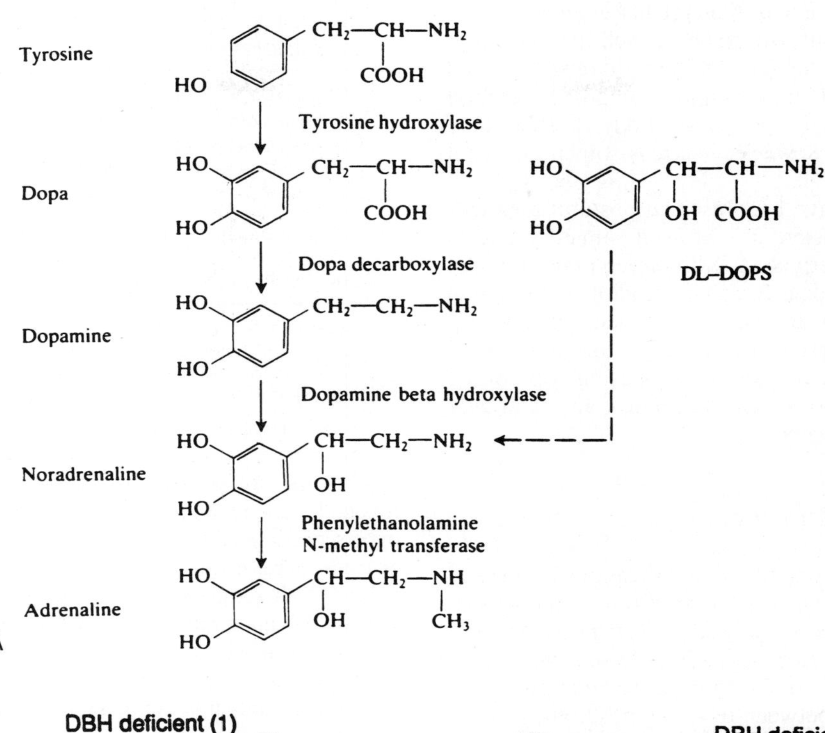

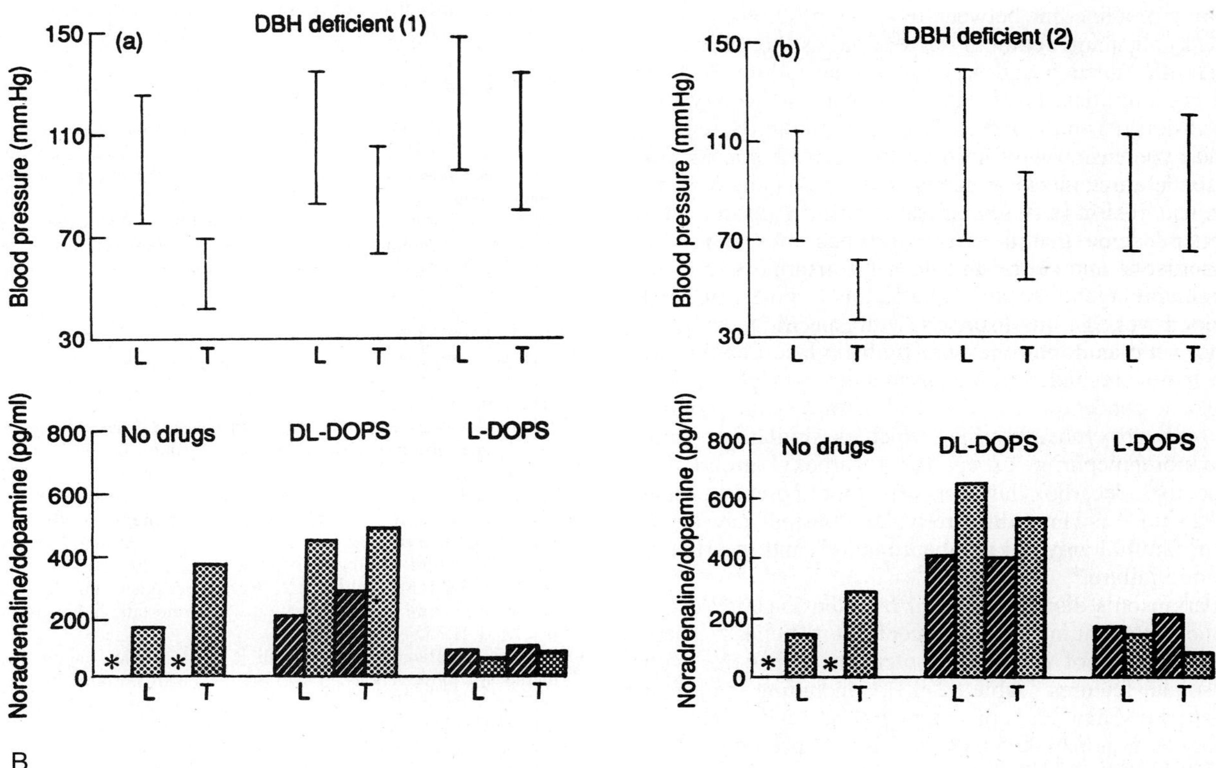

FIGURE 82–21 **A,** Biosynthetic pathway for noradrenaline synthesis and the structure of DL-threo-3,4-dihydroxyphenylserine (DL-DOPS) alongside. The enzyme dopa-decarboxylase, which is present both intraneuronally and extraneuronally, converts it to noradrenaline thus bypassing the hydroxylation step, which depends on dopamine beta-hydroxylase. **B,** Blood pressure (systolic and diastolic) while lying (L) and during head-up tilt (T) in two patients with dopamine beta-hydroxylase (DBH) deficiency (1 and 2, respectively, in figures), before and during treatment with DL-DOPS (racemic mixture; DOPS, dihydroxyphenylserine) and L-DOPS (laevoform). (**A** and **B,** From Mathias CJ, Bannister R: Dopamine beta-hydroxylase deficiency and other genetically determined autonomic disorders. *In* Mathias CJ, Bannister R [eds]: Autonomic Failure: A Textbook of Clinical Disorders of the Autonomic Nervous System. 4th ed. pp. 387–401. Oxford: Oxford University Press, 1999.)

to 400 μg) nocturnally. Side effects include hyponatremia and water intoxication. Erythropoietin is beneficial[56, 57] in anemic patients, especially in diabetes mellitus and amyloidosis with complicating renal failure. It raises the red cell mass and hematocrit and presumably improves cerebral oxygenation. A dosage of 50 μg/kg body weight three times a week for 6 to 8 weeks is used, sometimes with oral iron.

A variety of drugs have been used in postural hypotension, ranging from nonsteroidal anti-inflammatory agents (indomethacin), ergot derivatives (dihydroergotamine), and drugs that stimulate cardiac function (pindolol) (see Table 82–11). It is important in the management of postural hypotension that appropriate trials are performed in adequate numbers of clearly defined patients using appropriate therapeutic end points to ensure that their value and side effects are clearly delineated.

Therapy in Specific Disorders

In secondary autonomic disorders, modifications to therapy often are needed to encompass the different pathophysiologic processes, the effects of the underlying disease, and the specific treatment of these disorders. In diabetes mellitus, insulin therapy itself may lower blood pressure; also, there may be a fine line between reducing postural hypotension and enhancing supine hypertension, as the latter may impair renal function and accelerate renal failure. In high spinal cord injuries, the balance between the paroxysmal hypertension that may occur during autonomic dysreflexia and the hypotension with head-up tilt must be considered. In systemic amyloidosis, excessive proteinuria and hypoalbuminuria result in a low intravascular volume, with peripheral edema that is often worsened by the use of fludrocortisone and compounded by refractoriness to sympathomimetic agents because of amyloid deposits in heart and blood vessels. In disorders with specific enzymatic defects, such as dopamine-beta-hydroxylase deficiency, where there are undetectable plasma norepinephrine and epinephrine concentrations, the ideal therapy is the prodrug L-threo-dihydroxyphenylserine, which is similar in structure to norepinephrine except for a carboxyl group; the enzyme dopa-decarboxylase converts it into norepinephrine (Fig. 82–21).[58] L-Threo-dihydroxyphenylserine may be of value in familial amyloid polyneuropathy[59] and in primary autonomic failure.[60]

In Parkinson's disease, postural hypotension may occur in a substantial number (58 percent) of patients.[61] There are many causes of postural hypotension in patients with parkinsonian features (Table 82–13),[42] including the effect of anti-parkinsonian and coincidental drugs, and an erroneous diagnosis, as parkinsonism may be the presenting feature of the primary autonomic failure syndrome multiple system atrophy. There are particular problems in the elderly and patients with dementia to which multiple factors contribute[62, 63]; lack of adherence to advice and poor drug compliance are additional factors that complicate their management. In neurally mediated syncope with an emotional or a central component, treatment may require a combination of behavioral and psychotherapeutic approaches along with inhibitors of serotonin reuptake.[64]

TABLE 82–13 Possible Causes of Orthostatic Hypotension and Autonomic Dysfunction in a Patient With Parkinsonian Features

Multiple system atrophy
Parkinson's disease with autonomic failure
Side effects of antiparkinsonian therapy
To include L-DOPA and selegiline
Coincidental disease causing autonomic dysfunction such as diabetes mellitus
Concomitant administration of drugs for an allied condition
Antihypertensives (for hypertension)
Alpha-adrenoceptor blockers (for benign prostatic hyperplasia)

From Mathias CJ, Polinsky RJ: Separating the primary autonomic failure syndromes, multiple system atrophy and pure autonomic failure from Parkinson's disease. *In* Stern G (ed): Advances in Neurology. pp. 353–361. Philadelphia: Lippincott Williams & Wilkins, 1999.

In some disorders, the prevention of progression, or reversal, of the underlying pathophysiologic mechanisms may reduce postural hypotension. Thus, in acute dysautonomia, intravenous gamma-immunoglobulin may be of value.[65, 66] It remains to be determined whether transplantation of the pancreas in diabetes mellitus[67] and of the liver in familial amyloid polyneuropathy,[68] which appear to improve somatic and probably halt autonomic nerve damage, will reduce postural hypotension in these conditions.

References

1. Mathias CJ: Disorders of the autonomic nervous system. *In* Bradley WG, Daroff RB, Fenichel GM, Marsden CD (eds): Neurology in Clinical Practice. 3rd ed. pp. 2131–2165. Boston: Butterworth-Heinemann, 2000.
2. Mathias CJ, Bannister R: Investigation of autonomic disorders. *In* Bannister R, Mathias CJ (eds): Autonomic Failure: A Textbook of Clinical Disorders of the Autonomic Nervous System. 4th ed. pp. 169–195. Oxford: Oxford University Press, 1999.
3. Schatz IJ, Bannister R, Freeman RL, et al: Consensus statement on the definition of orthostatic hypotension, pure autonomic failure and multiple system atrophy. Clin Auton Res 6:125–126, 1996.
4. Mathias CJ: Orthostatic hypotension—causes, mechanisms and influencing factors. Neurology 45(suppl 5):s6–s11, 1995.
5. Wieling W, van Lieshout JJ, van Leeuwen AM: Physical manoeuvres that reduce postural hypotension in autonomic failure. Clin Auton Res 3:57–65, 1993.
6. Watkins PJ, Edmonds ME: Diabetic autonomic neuropathy. *In* Mathias CJ, Bannister R (eds): Autonomic Failure: A Textbook of Clinical Disorders of the Autonomic Nervous System. 4th ed. pp. 378–386. Oxford: Oxford University Press, 1999.
7. Bleasdale-Barr K, Mathias CJ: Neck and other muscle pains in autonomic failure: their association with orthostatic hypotension. J R Soc Med 91:355–359, 1998.
8. Mathias CJ, Bannister R, Cortelli P, et al: Clinical autonomic and therapeutic observations in two siblings with postural hypotension and sympathetic failure due to an inability to synthesize noradrenaline from dopamine because of a deficiency of dopamine beta hydroxylase. Q J Med N Ser 75 278:617–633, 1990.
9. Kooner JS, da Costa DF, Frankel HL, et al: Recumbency induces hypertension, diuresis and natriuresis in autonomic failure but diuresis alone in tetraplegia. J Hypertens 5(suppl 5):327–329, 1987.
10. Mathias CJ, Deguchi K, Bleasdale-Barr K, et al: Frequency of family history in vasovagal syncope. Lancet 352:33–34, 1998.
11. Da Costa JM: An irritable heart: a clinical study of a form of function cardiac disorder and its consequences. Am J Med Sci 61:71, 1871.
12. De Lorenzo F, Hargreaves J, Kakkar VV: Pathogenesis and management of delayed orthostatic hypotension in patients with chronic fatigue syndrome. Clin Auton Res 7:185–190, 1997.
13. McIntosh SJ, Lawson J, Kenny RA: Clinical characteristics of vaso-

depressor, cardioinhibitory and mixed carotid sinus syndrome in the elderly. Am J Med 95:203–208, 1993.
14. Schondorf, R, Low PA: Idiopathic postural orthostatic tachycardia syndrome (POTS): an attenuated form of acute pandysautonomia. Neurology 43:132–137, 1993.
15. Alam M, Smith GDP, Bleasdale-Barr K, et al: Effects of the peptide release inhibitor, octreotide, on daytime hypotension and on nocturnal hypertension in primary autonomic failure. J Hypertens 13:1664–1669, 1995.
16. Mathias CJ: Role of the central nervous system in human secondary hypertension. J Cardiovasc Pharmacol 10(suppl 12):593–599, 1987.
17. Cruickshank JM, Neil-Dwyer G, Lane J: The effect of oral propranolol upon the ECG changes occurring in subarachnoid haemorrhage. J Neurol Neurosurg Psychiatry 37:755–759, 1974.
18. Manger WM, Gifford RW: Clinical and Experimental Phaeochromocytoma. 2nd ed. Cambridge, MA: Blackwell Science, 1996.
19. Scherrer U, Vissing SF, Morgan BJ, et al: Cyclosporine-induced sympathetic activation and hypertension after heart transplantation. N Engl J Med 323:693–699, 1990.
20. Kooner JS, Peart WS, Mathias CJ: The sympathetic nervous system in hypertension due to unilateral renal artery stenosis in man. Clin Auton Res 1:195–204, 1991.
21. Schobel HP, Fischer T, Heuszer K, et al: Pre-eclampsia—a state of sympathetic overactivity. N Engl J Med 335:1480–1485, 1996,
22. Mathias CJ: Bradycardia and cardiac arrest during tracheal suction—mechanisms in tetraplegic patients. Eur J Int Care Med 2:147–156, 1976.
23. Mallipedi R, Mathias CJ: Raynaud's phenomenon after sympathetic denervation in patients with primary autonomic failure: questionnaire survey. BMJ 316:438–439, 1998.
24. Schott GD: Pain and the sympathetic nervous system. *In* Mathias CJ, Bannister R (eds): Autonomic Failure: A Textbook of Clinical Disorders of the Autonomic Nervous System. 4th ed. pp. 520–526. Oxford: Oxford University Press, 1999.
25. Mathias CJ, Bannister R: Postcibal hypotension in autonomic disorders. *In* Mathias CJ, Bannister R (eds): Autonomic Failure: A Textbook of Clinical Disorders of the Autonomic Nervous System. 4th ed. pp. 283–295. Oxford: Oxford University Press, 1999.
26. Mathias CJ: Autonomic disorders and their recognition. N Engl J Med 10:721–724, 1997.
27. Mathias CJ, Armstrong E, et al: Value of non-invasive continuous blood pressure monitoring in the detection of carotid sinus hypersensitivity. Clin Auton Res 2:157–159, 1991.
28. Mathias CJ, Holly E, Armstrong E, et al: The influence of food on postural hypotension in three groups with chronic autonomic failure: clinical and therapeutic implications. J Neurol Neurosurg Psychiatry 54:726–730, 1991.
29. Smith GDP, Mathias CJ: Postural hypotension enhanced by exercise in patients with chronic autonomic failure. Q J Med 88:251–256, 1995.
30. Almquist A, Goldenberg IF, Milstein S, et al: Provocation of bradycardia and hypotension by isoproterenol and upright posture in patients with unexplained syncope. N Engl J Med 320:346, 1989.
31. El-Badawi KM, Hainsworth R: Combined head-up tilt and lower body suction: a test of orthostatic tolerance. Clin Auton Res 4:41–47, 1994.
32. Kimber JR, Watson L, Mathias CJ: Distinction of idiopathic Parkinson's disease from multiple system atrophy by stimulation of growth hormone release with clonidine. Lancet 349:1877–1881, 1997.
33. Wallin BG: *In* Mathias CJ, Bannister R (eds): Autonomic Failure: A Textbook of Clinical Disorders of the Autonomic Nervous System. 4th ed. pp. 224–231. Oxford: Oxford University Press, 1999.
34. Esler M: Clinical application of noradrenaline spillover methodology: delineation of regional human sympathetic nervous responses. Pharmacol Toxicol 75:243–253, 1993.
35. Lambert GW, Thompson JM, Turner AG, et al: Cerebral noradrenaline spillover and its relation to muscle sympathetic nervous activity in healthy human subjects. J Auton Nerv Syst 64:57–64, 1997.
36. Omboni S, Parati G, Di Rienzo M, et al: Blood pressure and heart rate variability in autonomic disorders: a critical review. Clin Auton Res 6:171–182, 1996.
37. Goldstein DS, Holmes C, Stuhlmuller, et al: 6-[^{18}F]Fluorodopamine positron emission scanning in the assessment of cardiac sympathoneural function—studies in humans. Clin Auton Res 7:17–29, 1997.
38. Yusuf S, Theodropoulos S, Mathias CJ, et al: Increased sensitivity of the denervated transplanted human heart to isoprenaline both before and after beta-adrenergic blockade. Circulation 75:696–704, 1987.
39. Yusuf S, Theodoropoulos S, Dhalla N, et al: Influence of beta blockade on exercise capacity and heart rate response after human orthotopic and heterotopic cardiac transplantation. Am J Cardiol 64:636–641, 1989.
40. Fernandez A, Hontebeyrie M, Said G: Autonomic neuropathy and immunological abnormalities in Chagas disease. Clin Auton Res 2:409–412, 1992,
41. Mathias CJ, Williams AC: The Shy-Drager syndrome (and multiple system atrophy). *In* Calne DB (ed): Neurodegenerative Diseases. 1st ed. pp. 743–768. Philadelphia: WB Saunders, 1994.
42. Mathias CJ, Polinsky RJ: Separating the primary autonomic failure syndromes, multiple system atrophy and pure autonomic failure from Parkinson's disease. *In* G Stern (ed): Advances in Neurology. pp. 353–361. Philadelphia: Lippincott Williams & Wilkins, 1999.
43. Axelrod FB: Familial dysautonomia. *In* Mathias CJ, Bannister R (eds): Autonomic Failure: A Textbook of Clinical Disorders of the Autonomic Nervous System. 4th ed. pp. 402–409. Oxford: Oxford University Press, 1999.
44. Reilly MM, Thomas PK: Amyloid polyneuropathy. *In* Mathias CJ, Bannister R (eds): Autonomic Failure: A Textbook of Clinical Disorders of the Autonomic Nervous System. 4th ed. pp. 410–418. Oxford: Oxford University Press, 1999.
45. Mathias CJ, Frankel HL: Autonomic disturbances in spinal cord lesions. *In* Mathias CJ, Bannister R (eds): Autonomic Failure: A Textbook of Clinical Disorders of the Autonomic Nervous System. 4th ed. pp. 494–513. Oxford: Oxford University Press, 1999.
46. Khurana RK: Orthostatic intolerance and orthostatic tachycardia: a heterogeneous disorder. Clin Auton Res 5:12–18, 1995.
47. Mathias CJ, Kimber JR: Treatment of postural hypotension. J Neurol Neurosurg Psychiatry 65:285–289, 1998.
48. Smit AAJ, Hardjowijono MA, Wieling W: Are portable folding chairs useful to combat orthostatic hypotension? Ann Neurol 42:975–978, 1997.
49. Jankovic J, Gilden JLD, Heine BC, et al: Neurogenic orthostatic hypotension: a double blind, placebo controlled study with midodrine. Am J Med 95:38–48, 1993.
50. Low PA, Gilden JL, Freeman R, et al: Efficacy of midodrine vs placebo in neurogenic orthostatic hypotension: a randomized, double-blind multicenter study. JAMA 277:1046–1051, 1997.
51. Hoeldtke RD, Horvath GG, Bryner KD, Hobbs GR: Treatment of orthostatic hypotension with midodrine and octreotide. J Clin Endocrinol Metab 83:339–343, 1998.
52. Raimbach SJ, Cortelli P, Kooner JS, et al: Prevention of glucose-induced hypotension by the somatostatin analogue, octreotide (SMS 201-995) in chronic autonomic failure—haemodynamic and hormonal changes. Clin Sci 77:623–628, 1989.
53. Armstrong E, Mathias CJ: The effects of the somatostatin analogue, octreotide, on postural hypotension, before and after food ingestion in primary autonomic failure. Clin Auton Res 2:135–140, 1991.
54. Smith GDP, Alam M, Watson LP, et al: Effects of the somatostatin analogue, octreotide, on exercise induced hypotension in human subjects with chronic sympathetic failure. Clin Sci 89:367–373, 1995.
55. Mathias CJ, Fosbraey P, da Costa DF, et al: The effect of desmopressin on nocturnal polyuria, overnight weight loss and morning postural hypotension in patients with autonomic failure. BMJ 293:353–354, 1986.
56. Hoeldtke RD, Streeten DH: Treatment of orthostatic hypotension with erythropoietin. N Engl J Med 329:611–615, 1993.
57. Perera R, Isola L, Kaufmann H: Effect of recombinant erythropoietin on anemia and orthostatic hypotension in primary autonomic failure. Clin Auton Res 5:211–214, 1995.
58. Mathias CJ, Bannister R: Dopamine beta-hydroxylase deficiency and other genetically determined autonomic disorders. *In* Mathias CJ, Bannister R (eds): Autonomic Failure: A Textbook of Clinical Disorders of the Autonomic Nervous System. 4th ed. pp. 387–401. Oxford: Oxford University Press, 1999.
59. Suzuki S, Higa S, Tsuga I, et al: Effects of infused L-threo-3,4-dihydroxyphenylserine in patients with familial amyloid polyneuropathy. Eur J Clin Pharmacol 17:429–435, 1980.
60. Freeman R, Young J, Landsbert L, Lipsitz L: The treatment of postprandial hypotension in autonomic failure with 3,4-DL-threo dihydroxyphenylserine. Neurology 47:1414–1420, 1996.

61. Senard JM, Rai S, Lapeyre-Mestre M, et al: Prevalence of orthostatic hypotension in Parkinson's disease. J Neurol Neurosurg Psychiatry 63:584–589, 1997.
62. Ooi WL, Hossain S, Keeley-Gagnon N, Lipsitz LA: Patterns of orthostatic blood pressure change and their clinical correlates in a frail elderly population. JAMA 277:1299–1304, 1997.
63. Passant U, Warkentin S, Gustafson L: Orthostatic hypotension and low blood pressure in organic dementia: a study of prevalence and related clinical characteristics. Int J Geriatr Psychiatry 12:395–403, 1997.
64. Samoil D, Grubb BP: Neurally mediated syncope and serotonin reuptake inhibitors. Clin Auton Res 5:251–255, 1995.
65. Heafield MT, Gammage MD, Nightingale S, et al: Idiopathic dysautonomia treated with intravenous gammaglobulin. Lancet 347:28–29, 1996.
66. Smit AAJ, Vermeulen M, Koelman JHTM, et al: Unusual recovery from acute panautonomic neuropathy after immunoglobulin therapy. Mayo Clin Proc 72:333–335, 1995.
67. Kennedy WR, Navarro X, Goetz FL, et al: Effects of pancreatic transplantation on diabetic neuropathy. N Engl J Med 322:1031–1037, 1990.
68. Suhr OB, Holmgren G, Steen L, et al: Liver transplantation in familial amyloidotic polyneuropathy: follow-up of the first 20 Swedish patients. Transplantation 60:933–938, 1995.

SECTION IX

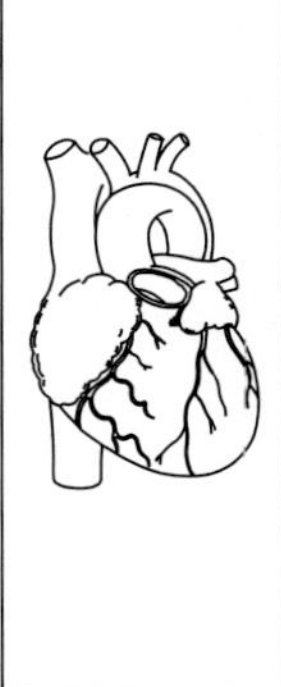

ELECTRICAL DISTURBANCES OF THE HEART

Recognition and Physiologic Treatment of Cardiac Arrhythmias and Conduction Disturbances

Sinus Node Dysfunction

Atrioventricular Nodal and Subnodal Conduction Disturbances

Supraventricular Tachycardias

Preexcitation

Atrial Fibrillation/Flutter

Transesophageal Echocardiography for Patients With Atrial Fibrillation

Long QT Syndromes

Arrhythmogenic Right Ventricular Dysplasia

The Importance of Atrioventricular Dissociation

Syncope

Sudden Cardiac Death

Antiarrhythmic Drugs

Pacing and Defibrillation

Radiofrequency Catheter Ablation of Supraventricular and Ventricular Arrhythmias

Surgical Treatment of Arrhythmias

CHAPTER 83

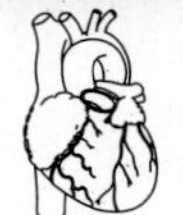

Recognition and Physiologic Treatment of Cardiac Arrhythmias and Conduction Disturbances

Gerald V. Naccarelli, C. Gunnar Blomqvist, and James T. Willerson

SINUS NODE RHYTHM DISTURBANCES
Sinus Arrhythmia
Sinus Bradycardia
Sinus Tachycardia
Sinus Pause or Sinus Arrest
ATRIAL ECTOPIC RHYTHM DISTURBANCES
Atrial Premature Beats
Paroxysmal Supraventricular Tachycardia
Atrial Flutter
Atrial Fibrillation
Multifocal Atrial Tachycardia
ATRIOVENTRICULAR JUNCTIONAL ECTOPIC RHYTHMS
Accelerated Atrioventricular Junctional Rhythm
VENTRICULAR RHYTHM DISTURBANCES
Ventricular Extrasystoles
Ventricular Tachycardia
Idioventricular Tachycardia
Polymorphic Ventricular Tachycardia ("Torsades de Pointes")
Bedside Evaluation
Atrioventricular Block

The mechanisms of tachycardia have been classified as those caused by disorders of impulse formation and those caused by disorders of impulse propagation. An example of a disorder of impulse formation is enhanced normal automaticity. In this situation, natural pacemaker cells, such as those existing in the sinus node or the atrioventricular (AV) junction, may undergo enhancement of their "normal automaticity" by an external stimulus, such as sympathetic stimulation. The sinus node has natural inherent pacemaker activity, which exhibits a phasic, spontaneous depolarization during diastole. This phase IV depolarization results in generation of an action potential and a threshold potential under normal conditions.

Sympathetic stimulation may accelerate the rate of rise of phase IV depolarization and therefore the number of action potentials that reach threshold over a period of time, thus increasing the heart rate under appropriate circumstances. Natural pacemaker cells, such as those in the sinus and AV nodes, depolarize more rapidly than other cardiac tissue; the remaining tissue remains dormant, owing to overdrive suppression of these subsidiary pacemakers. In both the sinus node and the AV node, the action potentials are secondary to "slow" inward calcium channel-dependent action potentials, which exhibit a rapid rise of phase IV depolarization (Fig. 83–1).

The remainder of the cardiac tissue normally remains at a high negative resting membrane potential, in the range of 90 mV. These tissues depolarize only when stimulated. The action potentials of these tissues are predominantly dependent on the "fast" inward sodium channel (Fig. 83–2). Phase 0 of the "fast" action potential is caused by a rapid influx of sodium. During phase I, outward potassium current begins. In phase II there is a plateau of the action potential owing to a balance of inward calcium (also a small amount of inward sodium) and outward potassium current. During phase III (repolarization), the outward potassium current predominates. Finally, in phase IV (diastole) the resting membrane potential returns to about 90 mV, with an ionic balance maintained by the sodium-potassium pump. Under certain pathologic circumstances, this action potential can be transformed into one with a reduced membrane potential, exhibiting spontaneous phase IV depolarization and triggering an arrhythmia secondary to abnormal automaticity. Clinical examples of arrhythmia secondary to abnormal automaticity include ectopic atrial and ventricular tachycardias.

Another disorder of impulse formation is secondary to triggered activity. Triggered activity can be defined as pacemaker activity that requires at least one preceding impulse or action potential. Triggered activity is caused by after-depolarizations. These after-depolarizations occur either early (EAD) or late or delayed (DAD) during depolarization. When one of these subthreshold depolarizations reaches threshold activation of tissue, an arrhythmia can be induced. Early after-depolarizations can be induced by hypoxia, ischemia, hypokalemia, cesium, catecholamines, and by anti-arrhythmic drugs, such as quinidine and sotalol. EADs are initiated under conditions associated with bradycardia and long action potential durations, and may be suppressed by pacing at more rapid rates. Because of this latter association, it is believed that EADs may be a mechanism for pause-dependent torsades de pointes. Delayed after-depolarizations have been implicated as the cause of

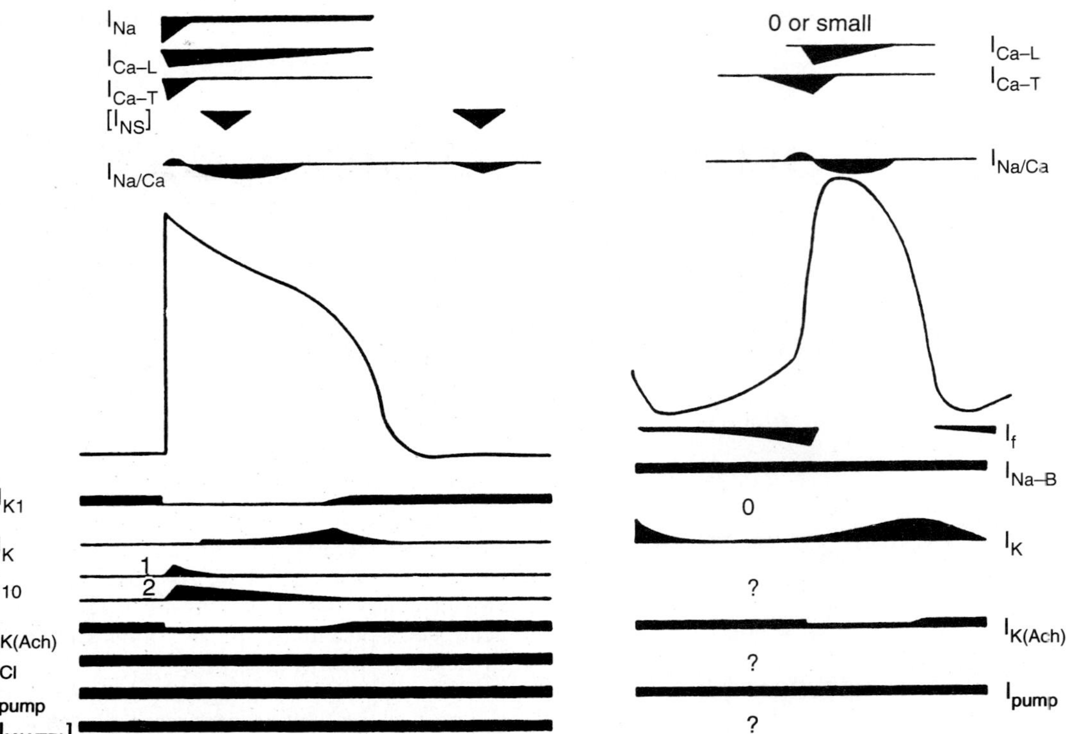

FIGURE 83–1 Currents and channels involved in generating the resting and action potentials. The time course of a stylized action potential of atrial and ventricular cells is shown on the left and of sinoatrial node cells on the right. Above and below are the various channels and pumps that contribute the currents underlying the electrical events. (From Task Force of the Working Group on Arrhythmias of the European Society of Cardiology: the Sicilian Gambit. Cardiology 84:1831, 1991.)

some clinical arrhythmias associated with digitalis toxicity (nonparoxysmal junctional tachycardia) and idiopathic ventricular tachycardia.

Disorders of impulse propagation include re-entry and reflection. Re-entry is the more common mechanism for clinical arrhythmias. Classic re-entry requires unidirectional block of a propagated impulse, followed by slow conduction of the impulse in an alternate pathway, with return of that impulse to the original pathway after this tissue has recovered excitability. The barrier that separates these two pathways can be anatomic, as in reciprocating orthodromic supraventricular tachycardia in patients with Wolff-Parkinson-White (WPW) syndrome, or it can be functional, as in some ischemia-induced re-entrant ventricular tachycardias. Arrhythmias that are thought to be secondary to re-entry include intra-atrial re-entrant tachycardias, AV nodal re-entrant tachycardias, AV re-entrant tachycardias in patients with WPW syndrome, bundle branch re-entrant tachycardia, many sustained ischemic ventricular tachycardias, atrial flutter, and atrial fibrillation.

This chapter discusses the various cardiac arrhythmias.[1] Extensive discussion of the specific clinical entities are reviewed in other chapters in this section. For purposes of the present discussion, we will divide the various cardiac arrhythmias into those concerned with sinus node responses, atrial ectopic rhythm disturbances, AV junctional (AV nodal) ectopic rhythms, and ventricular rhythm disturbances.

SINUS NODE RHYTHM DISTURBANCES

Sinoatrial (SA node) rhythm disturbances of importance are sinus arrhythmia, sinus bradycardia, sinus tachycardia, and sinus pause or arrest.

Sinus Arrhythmia

Sinus arrhythmia is defined as a slight variation in the cycling of the sinus rhythm, usually one that exceeds 0.12 second between the longest and the shortest cycles. Sinus arrhythmia is a normal finding in children and young adults and tends to diminish or disappear with age. Sinus arrhythmia is often somewhat more prominent with fluctuations in the respiratory cycle because heart rate accelerates with inspiration and slows with expiration. The alternating acceleration and deceleration of heart rate with respiration are mainly the result of fluctuations in vagal tone. Sinus arrhythmia may be aggravated by any factor that increases vagal tone.

Sinus Bradycardia

Sinus bradycardia is defined as a rate of less than 60 beats per minute (bpm), with the origin of the pacemaker being in the SA node. In adulthood, under basal conditions, sinus

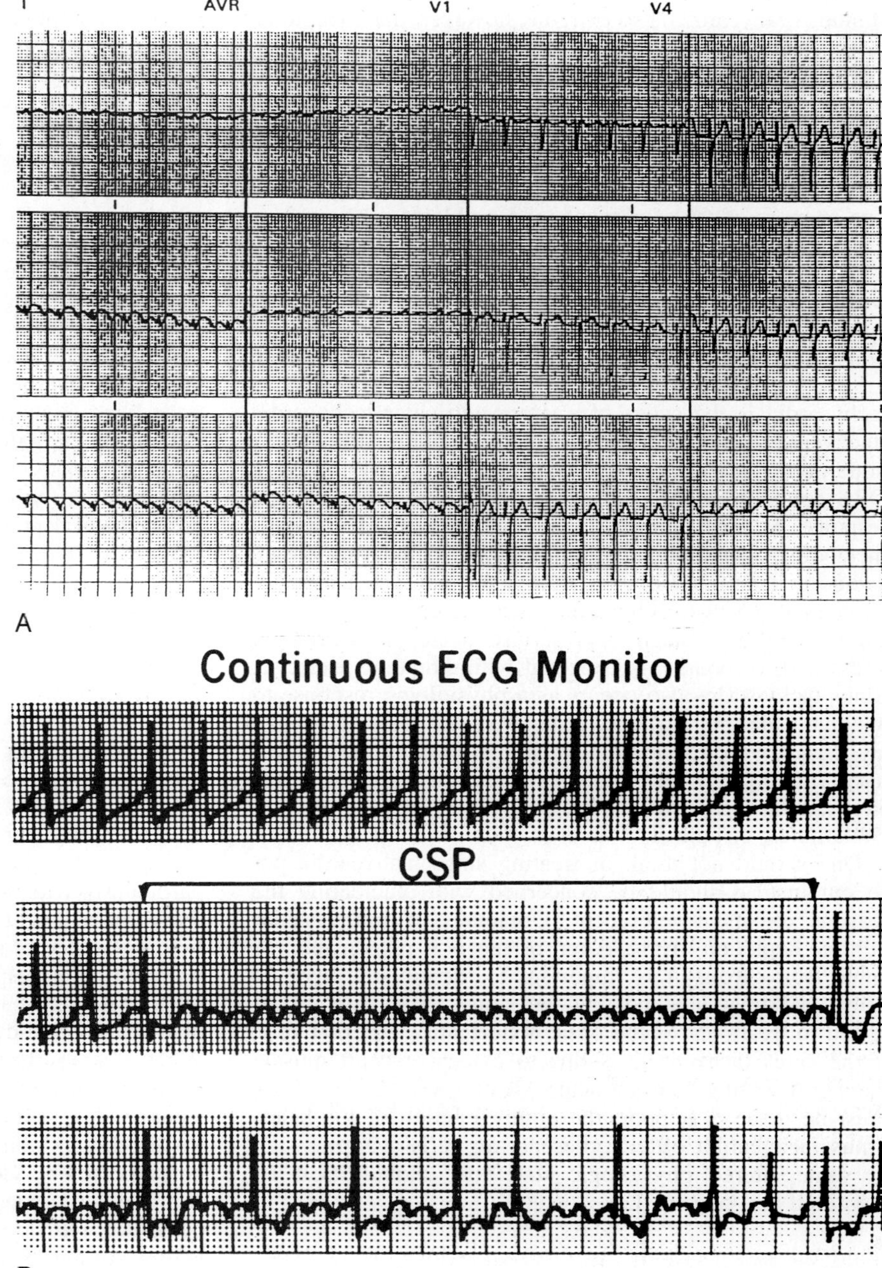

FIGURE 83–2 A, Atrial flutter with 2:1 conduction. Atrial rate 3000, ventricular rate 150 bpm. The atrial activity (F waves) is clearly seen in leads II, III, aVF, and V_1. The vertical leads show the characteristic sawtoothed pattern. **B,** Atrial flutter shown in the top panel with a ventricular rate of 150 bpm without clear P waves. With the application of carotid sinus pressure (CSP), the flutter waves are brought out, and a high-grade atrioventricular block is produced. In the bottom panel with termination of CSP, atrial flutter is evident with an irregular ventricular response. ECG, electrocardiogram.

bradycardia is encountered much more often than sinus tachycardia. Sinus bradycardia may be present in otherwise normal individuals and is common in well-trained athletes (particularly in long-distance runners) and in most persons during deep sleep. It is part of the normal reaction to vagal stimulation and is expected with carotid sinus pressure, with eyeball compression, during the Valsalva maneuver, during facial immersion in cold water (the so-called diving reflex), and sometimes during periods of pain or anticipated pain, such as with venipuncture, severe injury, or organic disease associated with pain. Certain drugs, including verapamil, diltiazem, and propranolol, may produce sinus bradycardia. Sinus bradycardia may also occur during the vagal stimulation produced by vomiting and in certain infectious diseases (particularly typhoid fever) and may be associated with metabolic abnormalities, including hypothermia and myxedema. In addition, nonvagally mediated sinus bradycardia may occur as a manifestation of organic heart disease, including ischemic heart disease, particularly when the SA node is damaged, as with certain types of acute myocardial infarction (MI) (particularly during acute inferior and/or true posterior MIs) and with severe chest pain of acute MI. Sinus bradycardia may also be a complication of myocardial disease in which the SA node is damaged by scarring or infiltrative processes or may simply be a reflection of the wear and tear associated with aging as part of a degenerative conduction system process.

Asymptomatic sinus bradycardia requires no treatment.

If sinus bradycardia is so extreme, however, that symptoms result, including syncope, congestive heart failure (CHF), angina pectoris, and hypotension, or if it leads to ventricular ectopic beats (slow sinus rates predispose to reentry mechanisms), then it should be treated. In some instances, temporary and even permanent ventricular pacing is necessary to ensure an adequate ventricular rate and to relieve one or more of the aforementioned problems.

Sinus Tachycardia

Sinus tachycardia is defined as sinus rhythm with a rate greater than 100 bpm. In order to be certain that sinus tachycardia is the cause of a supraventricular tachycardia (tachycardia with its origin in the AV junction, atria, or SA node), one must identify a constant single P wave for every QRS complex. Sinus tachycardia represents a physiologic response to fever, intravascular volume depletion, hypermetabolism, anxiety, and administration of pharmacologic agents that dramatically increase sinus rate, such as catecholamines. Sinus tachycardia is an integral part of the "fight or flight" adaptive response to severe emotional stress and, of course, is expected with strenuous exercise. Sinus tachycardia also occurs as a physiologic response to anemia, CHF, hemorrhage, extensive heart muscle damage associated with a reduction in cardiac output, and pulmonary embolism. Physiologically, sinus tachycardia results from either vagal withdrawal, endogenous release of catecholamines, or both.

One should not think of treating sinus tachycardia per se but instead should be concerned with elucidating the reasons for its development. Obviously, if intravascular volume depletion, fright, fever, or sepsis is responsible for sinus tachycardia, it is important to identify the specific cause and treat it, expecting the sinus tachycardia to respond to treatment of the basic abnormality. Alternatively, if the sinus tachycardia is due to extensive heart muscle damage resulting from an acute MI or severe CHF, efforts must be made to support the pump function of the heart. Sinus tachycardia often represents an early warning sign of some altered physiologic state that should itself be identified and corrected.

Sinus Pause or Sinus Arrest

In sinus arrest, the automaticity of the SA node ceases for a few seconds or longer. No sinus impulses are formed, and no P waves are generated on the electrocardiogram (ECG). A pause follows, which is usually interrupted by an AV junctional or ventricular escape beat and which, in the event of prolonged sinus arrest, may result in a sustained AV junctional or ventricular pacemaker rhythm. This is an uncommon rhythm disturbance but is occasionally noted in elderly patients, in those with ischemic heart disease (particularly with acute inferior or true posterior MI), in some patients with myocardial disease, and sometimes in those with digitalis toxicity. The development of an AV junctional or ventricular escape rhythm implies that the firing rate of the SA node is slower than that of the AV junction (or the ectopic ventricular pacemaker) and may even be completely absent, thus reflecting sinus pause or sinus arrest. This is particularly true if the AV junctional pacemaker (or the ectopic ventricular pacemaker) is not accelerated but instead exhibits its expected relatively slow firing rate.

The treatment of SA pause or arrest ordinarily includes administration of atropine or temporary or permanent ventricular pacing. Reasons to pace sinus pause or sinus arrest include the development of an AV junctional or ectopic ventricular pacemaker that is slow enough to result in syncope, CHF, angina, or frequent ventricular ectopic beats. If the escape AV junctional or ectopic ventricular pacemaker is rapid enough, particularly if the pacemaker is an AV junctional one, it may not be necessary to treat the underlying sinus pause or arrest except to ensure that it is not due to digitalis toxicity and, when possible, to determine its cause. If this rhythm disturbance is associated with bradyarrhythmias or tachyarrhythmias and appears to be an integral part of the sick sinus syndrome, pacemaker therapy is indicated. Pacemaker therapy is also indicated when any of the aforementioned signs or symptoms are a consequence of the slower AV junctional ectopic pacemaker.

SA Block

Distinction of SA block from SA pause or arrest is not usually easy, but SA block generally demonstrates a pause equal to two or more basic P-P intervals. Persistent absence of SA activity suggests the presence of either SA block or SA arrest. Intermittent failure of sinus P waves to occur, particularly with some recurring regularity, is also suggestive of intermittent SA block. SA block would be suspected by the absence of an expected sinus P wave. In this event, no ventricular response may occur, so that the entire P-QRS-T sequence is missing unless the sinus cycle is replaced by an escape AV junctional or ventricular beat. When a sinus beat is absent and the mechanism is SA block, the resulting pause is equal to almost exactly two sinus cycles; if an existing sinus rate exactly halves, 2:1, SA block can be identified. SA Wenckebach's block might be suspected by identifying periodic failure of P and QRS complexes to appear and recognizing that within any group cycle of P-QRS complexes, there is P-P interval shortening before the pause. SA block is relatively uncommon. Most instances of SA block are caused by structural disease or drug toxicity. Digitalis toxicity may cause SA block, especially that producing Wenckebach's periods. SA block may also result from ischemia, infarction, infectious processes (e.g., diphtheria), infiltrative myocardial disease, and structural degenerative conduction system disease.

Treatment of SA block is largely dependent on its cause and its complications. If an adequate lower escape pacemaker is present and its rate is sufficient to maintain normal blood supply to the various organs, and if angina, syncope, frequent ventricular premature beats, or CHF is not present, no specific therapy is necessary. Obviously, if drug toxicity is responsible for the SA block, the medication involved should be withdrawn and reinstituted later in lower doses. If symptoms related to a slow heart rate occur (syncope, CHF, angina, and/or frequent ventricular premature beats), ventricular pacing becomes necessary.

In theory, sinus arrest cannot be distinguished from complete SA block. In both conditions, there is an absence of P waves. However, in patients with complete SA block, the block is frequently associated with atrial or AV junctional escape rhythms, whereas sinus arrest or pause is usually associated with depression of other potential atrial pacemakers, so that atrial escape is infrequent.

ATRIAL ECTOPIC RHYTHM DISTURBANCES

Atrial Premature Beats

Atrial premature beats are common. They may or may not be conducted to the ventricle, depending on their prematurity and the status of AV and intraventricular conduction. Frequent atrial premature beats occur in some normal persons. It has been empirically noted that excess alcohol intake, fatigue, cigarettes, fever, anxiety, and infectious diseases of all sorts may result in atrial premature beats, and elimination of these factors may correct the disorder. Atrial premature beats also occur in some patients with CHF and in some with myocardial ischemia. They may also be noted in patients with underlying myocardial disease, in those with pulmonary disease and systemic hypoxia, and in those with hemodynamically important mitral valve disease.

Atrial extrasystoles or premature beats are usually perceived by patients as "palpitations" and sometimes are of concern to patients who notice "skipped" beats or "fluttering" that are frightening. Often, atrial premature beats cause no symptoms and are not recognized by the patient. Atrial premature beats require no specific therapy. If they are a source of aggravation or concern to the patient and one of the aforementioned factors can be identified and easily corrected, this measure should be taken.

The hallmark of atrial premature beats on the ECG is a premature and abnormal P wave morphology as compared with the sinus P wave activity. The premature P wave may be obvious on the ECG or it may be buried in the T wave, which makes it more difficult, although not impossible, to recognize, particularly if one seeks to establish whether T-wave morphology is somewhat variable on the ECG. The premature P wave may or may not be conducted and, when conducted, would be followed by a QRS that often has a normal duration but sometimes is prolonged as a consequence of aberrant conduction, usually with a right bundle branch block configuration. Most atrial premature beats are conducted in the ventricles, with a QRS configuration quite similar to that of normally conducted sinus beats. Conventional means by which atrial beats are recognized include the determination that the pause after a conducted atrial premature beat is usually less than a fully compensatory one. Nonconducted atrial premature beats may be followed by prolonged pauses; indeed, the most common reason for a pause on the ECG is a blocked or nonconducted atrial premature beat. In addition, atrial premature beats usually produce cannon A waves in the neck if they are premature enough to occur before the opening of the tricuspid valve.

When suppression of frequent atrial premature beats seems desirable, type IA or IC drugs may be utilized. Often, however, simple sedation and withdrawal of some of the precipitating factors are quite effective.

Paroxysmal Supraventricular Tachycardia

Paroxysmal supraventricular tachycardia (PSVT) is a supraventricular tachycardia with an atrial rate of 150 to 250 bpm, typically 150 to 180 bpm. Mechanisms for the development of PSVT have been discussed elsewhere. The rhythm disturbance typically has a sudden onset and termination and is characterized by a series of premature and morphologically bizarre P waves. The simplest definition of PSVT is a series of three or more consecutive atrial systoles. PSVT may be conducted on a 1:1 basis into the ventricles, producing similar atrial and ventricular rates or second-degree AV block. Regular or irregular conduction ratios may occur, or phasic aberrant ventricular conduction may be noted, leading to a series of bizarre QRS complexes.

The rhythm disturbance appears to be most common in women but may occur in either sex. It is frequently observed in anxious young people and in those who are physically fatigued; consuming large amounts of coffee, tea, or alcohol; or smoking in excess. It is also noted occasionally (but is uncommon) with myocardial ischemia and in the setting of acute MI. PSVT occurs in some patients with myocardial diseases during systemic arterial hypoxia and in some patients with serious mitral valve disease. PSVT most commonly occurs secondary to AV nodal re-entrant tachycardia or macro–re-entry in patients with Wolff-Parkinson-White syndrome.

The presence of intermittent PSVT may not necessitate treatment, although some patients experience angina, shortness of breath, and/or syncope during the rapid supraventricular tachycardia. Others are concerned by the "palpitations," and these concerns may constitute an indication for suppression of the arrhythmia in some patients. Pharmacologic interventions used to suppress PSVT are discussed elsewhere. Certain maneuvers that produce vagal stimulation may convert these tachycardias to sinus rhythm. In particular, carotid sinus massage, pressure on the eyeballs, the Valsalva maneuver, and/or the diving reflex may convert PSVT to sinus rhythm. Sedation and withdrawal from excesses of coffee, tobacco, alcohol, and fatigue may also be corrective. If the rhythm disturbance occurs in association with the Wolff-Parkinson-White syndrome, pharmacologic intervention or catheter ablation may be necessary to control the recurrent episodes of PSVT.

Atrial Flutter

Atrial flutter is a supraventricular tachycardia with an atrial rate of 250 to 350 bpm (see Fig. 83–2). F waves tend to be negatively oriented in the inferior leads, and the baseline tends to have a sawtoothed or picket-fence appearance. The sawtoothed appearance is most frequently noted in standard leads 2, 3, and AVF. Atrial flutter is frequently associated with second-degree AV block, usually a 2:1 AV block. This results in a characteristic ventricular rate of 140 to 160 ventricular beats per minute. In some instances, F-wave activity may not be obvious on the standard ECG, but instead, a regular ventricular rate of 140 to 160 bpm may be noted. It is wise to be cautious in analyzing ventricular rates of 140 to 160 bpm that are regular when no obvious P wave activity is noted because this phenomenon may represent atrial flutter (or AV junctional tachycardia). In some instances, carotid sinus massage may elicit the underlying atrial flutter waves so that the true nature of the supraventricular tachycardia can be recognized (see Fig. 83–2).

Atrial flutter with a rapid ventricular response may also be associated with angina, dyspnea, or syncope. Some patients perceive this as "palpitations," which may be annoying and of concern. Pharmacologic means of treating atrial flutter are described elsewhere, but although carotid sinus massage can sometimes convert atrial flutter to sinus rhythm, it often does not interrupt the atrial flutter. Atrial pacing at a rapid rate more often converts atrial flutter to sinus rhythm, as does cardioversion. Indeed, low energy levels of 10 to 20 W/s often convert atrial flutter to sinus rhythm. Whether the patient remains in sinus rhythm after being cardioverted depends on the initial cause of the supraventricular tachycardia, on whether the left atrium is markedly enlarged, on the duration of atrial flutter before conversion, and on whether the stimulus for its development (e.g., thyrotoxicosis, serious myocardial damage, acute MI with extensive myocardial damage, and severe mitral valve disease) persists. In the latter situation, one can expect the atrial flutter to recur or to be unable to convert the patient to sinus rhythm with cardioversion. Some patients with intrinsic AV junctional disease experience much slower ventricular rates with atrial flutter than would otherwise be expected (i.e., 60 to 100 bpm). In this event, there is no compelling reason to convert atrial flutter to sinus rhythm, but one should realize that the slow ventricular response is a complication of existing AV junctional disease. It has been said that the presence of atrial flutter indicates intrinsic cardiac disease and that this rhythm disturbance does not commonly occur in individuals who have no disease-related abnormality, particularly organic heart disease. Atrial flutter is usually encountered in patients with severe mitral valve disease, those with thyrotoxicosis, those with primary myocardial disease, those with pericardial disease, some patients with acute MIs, those with chronic obstructive pulmonary disease and systemic arterial hypoxia, and sometimes patients after open heart surgery.

Atrial Fibrillation

Atrial fibrillation is characterized by irregular, chaotic fibrillation waves of variable rate and amplitude, which distort the baseline and result in an irregular ventricular response (Fig. 83–3). The atrial rate of this supraventricular tachycardia is in excess of 350 bpm, but there is no discrete and forceful atrial contraction and no discrete atrial relaxation. The arrhythmia can be either paroxysmal or sustained. It is sometimes preceded by, and possibly is the result of, frequent atrial extrasystoles, particularly multifocal atrial premature beats. It leads to ineffective atrial transport and loss of the atrial contribution to cardiac output. The very rapid atrial rate also produces a large number of stimuli for the AV junction and causes irregular conduction of the impulses through the AV junction, producing the irregular ventricular response. Atrial fibrillation also renders individual patients at risk for development of an atrial thrombus and systemic arterial embolism. The risk for systemic arterial embolization is dependent on the cause of the atrial fibrillation and the associated cardiac findings, but it has been estimated that approximately 30 percent of all persons with long-standing atrial fibrillation experience at least one embolic episode during the course of the atrial fibrillation. Patients with atrial fibrillation who also have significant mitral stenosis, those with severe myocardial disease and generalized cardiomegaly, and those with the sick sinus syndrome and paroxysmal atrial fibrillation appear to be at the greatest risk for systemic arterial emboli.

Atrial fibrillation is a relatively common supraventricular

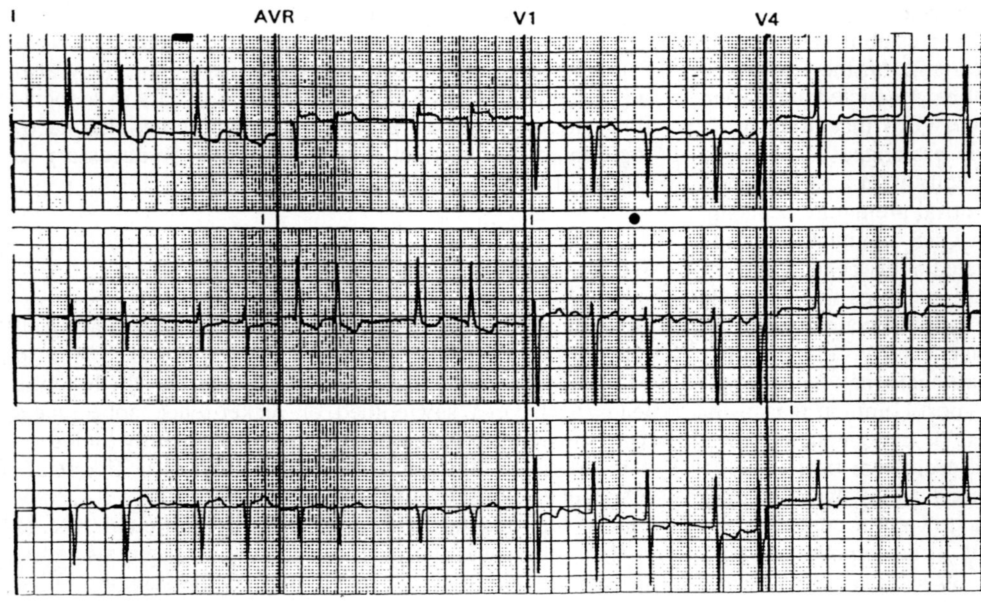

FIGURE 83–3 Coarse atrial fibrillation. Note random variations of the R-R interval. The atrial activity, F waves of variable amplitude, shape, and duration are best seen in leads II, III, aVF, and V_{1-2}. The ECG also demonstrates left axis deviation and left ventricular hypertrophy and strain.

tachycardia, more so than either atrial tachycardia or atrial flutter. Causes of atrial fibrillation include hemodynamically important mitral valve disease (mitral regurgitation, mitral stenosis, and mixed mitral valve disease); thyrotoxicosis; myocardial diseases, including those due to infiltrative processes, infection, and/or coronary artery disease; acute MI with extensive heart muscle damage (or with atrial infarction); pericarditis; hypoxia; and atrial septal defect. Atrial fibrillation may also occur in otherwise apparently healthy persons (particularly during periods of stress, fatigue and with excessive use of coffee, alcohol, or cigarettes). Atrial fibrillation may be either a paroxysmal rhythm disturbance or a sustained one, not only in patients with some of the abnormalities listed earlier but also in apparently otherwise healthy individuals for no apparent reason. In this latter circumstance, it is often referred to as *lone atrial fibrillation*.

Clinical problems related to atrial fibrillation include palpitations, CHF, angina, or syncope as a complication of the rapid ventricular response and/or loss of atrial contribution to cardiac output, and systemic arterial emboli, presenting as either a loss of pulse in an upper or lower extremity or a cerebrovascular accident. Patients with hypertrophic obstructive cardiomyopathy tolerate the development of atrial fibrillation particularly poorly, and many experience shock and severe CHF with the onset of this rhythm disturbance. Therefore, recognition and prompt treatment of atrial fibrillation in these individuals are absolutely necessary. Patients with significant mitral obstruction who experience atrial fibrillation may abruptly develop marked worsening of their CHF as inadequate left ventricular filling time occurs. For patients with rheumatic heart disease and severe mitral stenosis and those with mitral prosthetic valves, control of the ventricular rate and/or conversion to sinus rhythm may be an immediate necessity to prevent cardiovascular collapse.

Atrial fibrillation is recognizable on the ECG by the irregularly irregular ventricular responses and the absence of single discrete P-wave activity. Occasional QRS complexes are aberrantly conducted with atrial fibrillation, known as *Ashman's phenomenon*. Ashman's beats can be determined by the presence of the aberrancy in the short cycle after a longer pause ("long cycle–short cycle" rule). Ashman's beats can often be distinguished from premature ventricular contractions by determining the length of the pause after the beat (QRS) in question. The longer the pause after the QRS complex, the more likely the beat is to be a ventricular premature one. Ashman's beats are often conducted with a right bundle branch block configuration.

Wide fluctuations in peripheral arterial pressure can also be expected with rapid and irregular atrial fibrillation, depending on when blood pressure is recorded with respect to variations in heart rate and cycling. In the neck veins, one does not expect to see a discrete A wave in the jugular venous pulse but instead a fused CV wave. The presence of atrial fibrillation also precludes detection of an atrial sound (S_4) by auscultation because of the absence of discrete atrial contractions.

Atrial fibrillation with a well-controlled ventricular response may need no treatment. Acute and chronic management of atrial fibrillation are extensively reviewed in the section on atrial fibrillation.

Multifocal Atrial Tachycardia

Multifocal atrial tachycardia is defined as three or more ectopic sites of atrial activity and a ventricular rate of 100 or greater (Fig. 83–4). The different ectopic atrial foci are recognizable by distinguishing three or more distinct P-wave morphologies in the same ECG or lead. This rhythm disturbance has also been referred to as *chaotic atrial rhythm*. It occurs primarily during severe systemic hypoxia, especially in patients with severe chronic lung disease but also in those who experience severe hypoxia regardless of the cause. As noted earlier, multifocal atrial tachycardia is a precursor of atrial fibrillation and on physical examination may actually be confused with atrial fibrillation because an irregular ventricular response is noted. The treatment of this disorder is correction of the severe hypoxia when possible. Pharmacologic approaches to the treatment of this arrhythmia can include the use of drugs to suppress the ectopic atrial focus in conjunction with correction of the systemic arterial hypoxia. Rate-controlling drugs, such as verapamil and diltiazem, have some use in the treatment of this arrhythmia. This rhythm disturbance is not a manifestation of digitalis toxicity in most patients, although some individuals have digoxin serum levels at the upper limit of normal.

Atrioventricular Junctional Ectopic Rhythms

AV junctional (AV nodal) ectopic rhythms develop either as a consequence of default of upper sinus pacemakers (as

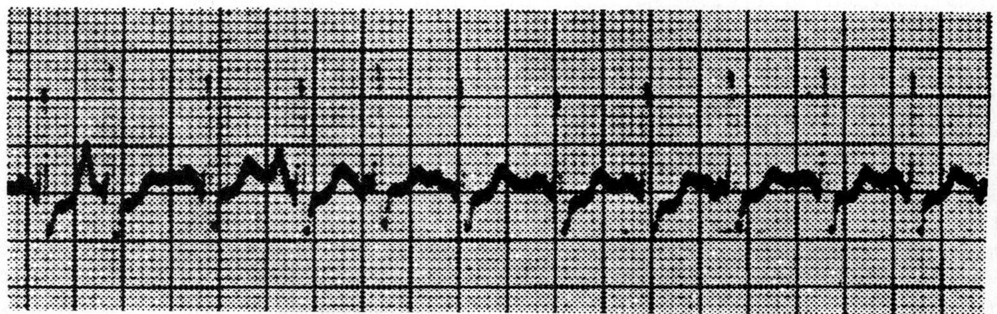

FIGURE 83–4 Multifocal atrial tachycardia (MAT) is shown. One may identify at least three different P-wave morphologies and a heart rate of more than 100 (beats per minute). This rhythm occurs in patients with hypoxia.

with sinus pause or arrest or SA block) or because of acceleration of the basic rate of impulse formation in the AV junction as a so-called AV junctional tachycardia. An escape AV junctional rhythm is expected with prolonged periods in which sinus SA node activity does not occur. The expected AV junctional pacemaker rate is 50 to 60 bpm. The term *AV junctional rhythm* is preferred over AV nodal rhythm because it has been difficult to determine whether or not pacemaking cells exist in the AV node proper, although they are found at its junction with the common bundle and in the bundle of His itself. For this reason, it is perhaps best to refer to AV junctional tissue or rhythms rather than to AV node or AV nodal rhythms.

AV junctional premature beats are much less common than either atrial or ventricular premature beats. The presence of AV junctional premature beats can be demonstrated by premature beats without preceding P waves or with a PR interval that is too short to represent conduction through the AV junction and into the ventricle with a narrow QRS complex. Aberrant conduction of premature AV junctional beats does occur and results in broad bizarre QRS complexes; aberrant conduction of AV junctional impulses can be extremely difficult and are often impossible to distinguish from premature ventricular contractions. Physical signs related to the development of premature AV junctional beats depend on the relationship of atrial to ventricular contraction.

Impulses arising in the AV junction spread simultaneously upward to the atria and downward to the ventricles in many instances. Depending on the rate of spread in each direction, atria may be activated before, simultaneously with, or after the ventricles. If the atria are activated first, the AV sequence is relatively normal, and the physical signs are similar to those resulting from atrial premature beats. However, if the atrium contracts on a closed tricuspid valve with an abnormally short PR interval (interval between atrial and ventricular contractions), a cannon A wave in the jugular venous pulse and an abnormally loud first heart sound result. If atrial contraction occurs simultaneously with ventricular contraction, a cannon A wave in the jugular venous pulse would be expected, but the first sound is not increased in intensity. If ventricular activation occurs before atrial activation, a cannon A wave follows ventricular contraction, and the first sound is soft. The pause after premature AV junctional beats is usually less than compensatory (a compensatory pause is one that does not disturb the underlying sinus mechanism).

On the ECG, P waves resulting from retrograde activation of the atria by the AV junctional pacemaker may be inverted in standard lead 1 and are usually inverted in leads 2, 3, and aVF. The P waves may precede, may occur simultaneously with, or may follow the QRS complex. When the P waves precede the QRS complex, the PR interval should be short (i.e., < 0.12 second, implying the unlikely possibility of AV conduction).

No treatment is usually required for premature AV junctional beats unless their frequency is such that one is concerned about preventing a sustained AV junctional rhythm. In such a case, the physiologic and pharmacologic approaches to the treatment are the same as those for the treatment of atrial premature beats.

Accelerated Atrioventricular Junctional Rhythm

Accelerated AV junctional rhythm (AV nodal tachycardia) consists of three or more AV junctional premature beats in a row. The rate is somewhat accelerated over the usual pacemaker rate of the AV junction and is characteristically in the range of 70 to 150 bpm. The ECG morphology of the QRS complex is similar to that of the AV junctional premature beats, usually narrow and similar to the QRS morphology of conducted sinus P waves. As already noted, however, occasionally aberrant conduction occurs with both premature AV junctional beats and with AV junctional tachycardia. In these instances, distinction from ventricular tachycardia or ventricular premature beats is difficult.

This particular rhythm disturbance usually occurs in the setting of organic heart disease or as a result of drug intoxication. AV junctional tachycardia may be particularly associated with acute MI (either inferior or anterior) and usually implies, when recurrent, a poor prognosis. In addition, AV junctional tachycardia may occur with digitalis toxicity, occasionally with serious myocardial disease, sometimes with infectious myocarditis, and sometimes with acute rheumatic fever or after open heart surgery.

If the rate is hemodynamically tolerated, there is no strong indication for the treatment of AV junctional tachycardia. Of course, if digitalis excess is responsible for the rhythm disturbance, the medication should be discontinued. This should be suspected as a possibility in any patient receiving a cardiac glycoside, usually digoxin, who develops this rhythm disturbance. It should also be appreciated that AV tachycardia may be a manifestation of extensive heart muscle damage after acute MI.

VENTRICULAR RHYTHM DISTURBANCES

Ventricular Extrasystoles

A ventricular premature beat, or extrasystole, is an impulse that arises from an ectopic ventricular focus that is premature with respect to the prevailing sinus rhythm. In general, ventricular premature beats are recognized by a premature beat with a broad, bizarre QRS morphology compared with the dominant conducted QRS morphology. In addition, the ventricular premature beat is usually followed by a full compensatory pause. At the bedside, one expects to find evidence of AV dissociation with isolated ventricular premature beats and with sustained ventricular rhythm disturbances, including cannon A waves in the jugular venous pulse and a first sound that varies in intensity. Premature ventricular contractions result in pulse irregularity, which may be noted by the patient and described as palpitations and may be detected by the physician by feeling the pulse at the wrist. Premature ventricular contractions have a fixed coupling interval to the preceding QRS complex unless they are multifocal in origin, in which case they have different QRS morphologies within the same ECG lead and do not necessarily possess a fixed coupling interval. Recognition of a fixed coupling interval of premature ventricular contractions helps to distinguish this form of ventricular ectopic beat from a parasystolic ventricular focus, in which the coupling interval is not fixed and there is a zone of surrounding protection with regard to the penetration of descending impulses from above.

There are many causes of premature ventricular contractions, including anxiety, fever, volume depletion, infection, drug excesses of all types (in particular, digitalis toxicity), and acute myocardial ischemia or infarction. Premature ventricular contractions also occur in association with myocardial disease, as a complication of hypokalemia or hypercalcemia, and after excess alcohol intake. Ventricular premature beats that occur every second beat, so that there is coupling of a normal QRS followed by a premature ventricular contraction on a repetitive basis, are termed *bigeminal rhythm*.

Certain types of ventricular premature beats are of particular concern to the physician because of their potential to degenerate or warn of more serious arrhythmias. Ventricular premature beats that occur with a frequency of greater than 10 bpm (some clinicians believe > 5 to 7 bpm), those on or close to the apex of the T wave (this represents a period of vulnerability during repolarization), multiform ventricular premature beats, and ventricular premature beats that occur in pairs or triplets sometimes represent dangerous ventricular premature beats. Some studies have suggested that these types of ventricular premature beats can be associated with an increased likelihood for development of ventricular tachycardia or ventricular fibrillation, especially in the patient with severe coronary artery disease or dilated or hypertrophied myocardium. Three or more ventricular premature beats in a row constitute the simplest definition of ventricular tachycardia. The apex of the T wave represents a time interval during ventricular repolarization in which a single ectopic impulse of even rather low energy may produce ventricular fibrillation. From a practical point of view, this is most likely to occur in the setting of digitalis toxicity or during acute myocardial ischemia or infarction.

If warranted, acute suppression of ventricular premature beats can be achieved with intravenous lidocaine or procainamide, and long-term suppression can be achieved by various class I, II, or III antiarrhythmic drugs.

Ventricular Tachycardia

There are four basic types of ventricular tachycardia. One represents a sustained ventricular ectopic rhythm disturbance ordinarily manifested by a regular rate of 150 bpm. Regularity is recognized by defining variation in RR intervals less than or equal to 0.08 second. The second variety of ventricular tachycardia is *slow ventricular tachycardia*, *accelerated ventricular rhythm*, or *idioventricular tachycardia*; the three terms are used synonymously to describe an ectopic ventricular rhythm disturbance with a rate of 100 bpm or less that occurs at a regular rate (Fig. 83–5). The third variety of ventricular tachycardia is known as *parasystolic ventricular tachycardia*. This form of ventricular tachycardia is generated by a "protected ectopic focus." It discharges continuously, activating the ventricles when they are not rendered refractory by a conducted supraventricular impulse. At the same time, the ectopic focus itself is not depolarized by these supraventricular impulses. It therefore maintains its own rhythmicity over long periods of time. The interval between bizarre QRS complexes can be calculated as a multiple of the basic cycle length. Fusion beats are common. At times, the abnormal QRS does not appear when expected because of the presence of so-called exit block from the ectopic focus. This variety of ventricular tachycardia is not commonly recognized, and the remainder of this discussion focuses on two more common varieties of ventricular tachycardia.

Sustained ventricular tachycardia is basically a continuous string of ventricular extrasystoles. Each paroxysm begins with a ventricular premature impulse linked to the preceding, normally conducted QRS complex by a fixed coupling interval. This particular rhythm disturbance is usually not well tolerated by patients, and one expects to find decreased blood pressure, disturbed sensorium, and increasing CHF in most patients with ventricular tachycardia. In an occasional patient, however, the rhythm disturbance is surprisingly well tolerated, allowing time to attempt to suppress the disorder by pharmacologic means. If this variety of ventricular tachycardia is not being hemodynamically tolerated, which is typical, cardioversion is performed as an emergency procedure. Usually, several hundred watt/seconds are required for conversion to sinus rhythm. Occasionally, this rhythm disturbance converts to sinus rhythm after a sharp blow to the chest. There are many different causes of extrasystolic ventricular tachycardia, but acute myocardial ischemia and infarction, digitalis toxicity, severe hypoxia and/or acidosis, hypokalemia, hypercalcemia, hyperkalemia, systemic infection, viral myocarditis, and hypotension are the most common. Occasionally, this rhythm disturbance occurs in apparently normal individuals; the reason for this is not known.

Idioventricular Tachycardia

The two major reasons for the development of idioventricular tachycardia ("slow VT") are digitalis toxicity and acute MI (see Fig. 83–5). This rhythm is common in acute MI and is usually benign. It may be present in as many as 30 to 40 percent of patients with acute MI and is usually so

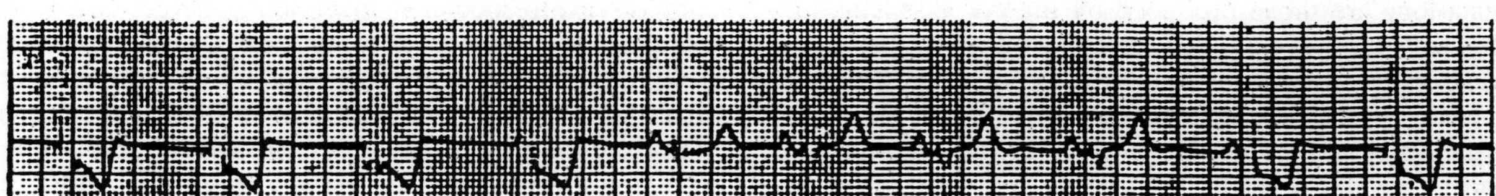

FIGURE 83–5 Idioventricular tachycardia ("slow ventricular tachycardia," "accelerated idioventricular rhythm") at a rate of 62 bpm. The "slow VT" is interrupted by a short run of regular sinus rhythm at a rate of 75 bpm.

benign that it goes unnoticed by the patient, nurse, and physician. Even when discovered, it usually requires no treatment if the patient is hemodynamically well compensated and there are no other foci of ventricular ectopic activity and no bursts of more rapid ventricular tachycardia, as described earlier. When this rhythm disturbance is caused by digitalis toxicity, the medication should be discontinued. This possibility should be suspected in any patient receiving digitalis who experiences the rhythm disturbance. This rhythm is also encountered in patients with acute MI with reperfusion. When pharmacologic treatment is necessary, atropine is preferred. Administration of atropine is based on the recognition that this rhythm disturbance generally occurs by default (i.e., the accelerated ventricular rhythm usurps pacemaker control from a slower sinus or AV junctional pacemaker). However, almost always, no treatment of this rhythm disturbance is required.

Polymorphic Ventricular Tachycardia ("Torsades de Pointes")

The fourth type of ventricular tachycardia is called *polymorphic ventricular tachycardia* or *torsades de pointes* (twisting about a point) to describe a rapid, regular ventricular tachycardia whose QRS morphology is frequently changing so that it appears that its QRS vector alternates around an imaginary point. This rhythm disturbance occurs congenitally in children with long QT intervals, and it may be acquired with electrolyte abnormalities, especially hypokalemia, hypocalcemia, and hypomagnesemia if they prolong the QT interval, and with several other cardiac abnormalities, including acute myocardial ischemia and infarction if they prolong the QT interval. Torsades de pointes often develops in patients with preceding bradycardia, and its medical treatment includes increasing heart rate with isoproterenol or pacing and using antiarrhythmic drugs that do not increase the QT interval further, including lidocaine and lidocaine-like drugs, and long-term treatment with beta-blockers, especially in children with this abnormality. One should never give a patient with a long QT interval procainamide, disopyramide phosphate (Norpace), or quinidine, because these medications further prolong the QT interval, and they may cause torsades de pointes even with their initial dose. Rapid torsades de pointes that is not tolerated hemodynamically should be cardioverted immediately. The long QT syndromes are discussed in detail in another chapter in this book.

Bedside Evaluation

Bedside examination of the patient may be very helpful in correctly identifying ventricular tachycardia. Clinical manifestations are those produced by the AV dissociation. The physical findings include cannon A waves in the jugular venous pulse, varying intensity of the first heart sound, and variations in systemic peak systolic blood pressure. Atrial gallops, ventricular filling gallops, and summation gallops of constant or variable intensity may also occur as a manifestation of the AV dissociation. Wide splitting of the first and second heart sounds is also frequently noted. Another helpful clue to AV dissociation can be obtained from the ECG itself if one can identify the presence of Dressler's or fusion beats, which represent a "hybrid beat" between a partially conducted supraventricular impulse and a ventricular ectopic beat. The presence of fusion beats identifies independent supraventricular and ventricular pacemakers and, in our opinion, helps to prove the presence of ventricular ectopy. Occasionally, AV junctional tachycardia may also be characterized by AV dissociation and may demonstrate the same clinical signs, but this phenomenon is uncommon. As a practical point, the presence at the bedside of signs of AV dissociation in conjunction with a rapid regular tachycardia and bizarre QRS complexes indicates the presence of ventricular tachycardia.

Atrioventricular Block

The different types of AV block are usually classified into three degrees. In first-degree AV block, there is a delay in AV conduction manifested by a prolonged PR interval on the ECG (usually $>$ 0.20 second), but each atrial impulse is conducted into the ventricles. In second-degree heart block, some atrial impulses are not conducted into the ventricles. In third-degree heart block, there is a complete inability to conduct atrial impulses into the ventricles, with the existence of a totally independent ventricular pacemaker. Third-degree heart block must be differentiated from complete AV dissociation, in which independent atrial and/or AV junctional and ventricular pacemakers do exist but only for temporary periods, because the mechanism of the AV dissociation is an accelerated AV junctional or idioventricular pacemaker with, for example, slowing of the sinus rate, digitalis toxicity, and ischemia. Third-degree heart block implies complete inability to conduct supraventricular impulses into the ventricles, and complete AV dissociation suggests that conduction would be possible if physiologic circumstances were appropriate.

First-Degree Heart Block

As previously discussed, first-degree heart block is identified by a prolonged PR interval on the resting ECG. In both normal and diseased hearts, atropine, exercise, and catecholamines tend to shorten PR intervals. In addition, in normal hearts, physiologic increases in heart rate tend to shorten PR intervals, although in diseased hearts, physiologic and artificial increases in heart rate may lead to PR prolongation. Prolonged PR intervals in first-degree heart block can be caused by vagal stimulation; pharmacologic interventions, including digitalis (toxicity); and disease processes, such as ischemic heart disease, infiltrative myocardial diseases, acute MI (especially acute inferior or diaphragmatic MI), myocarditis, Addison's disease, congenital heart disease (especially atrial septal defect and Ebstein's anomaly), rheumatic fever, and streptococcal infections. Prolonged PR intervals are occasionally found in otherwise apparently normal subjects and in well-trained athletes.

The presence of first-degree heart block usually does not necessitate any particular therapy. In children, first-degree heart block may represent digitalis toxicity, and cardiologists usually decrease the amount of digitalis a child is receiving after development of first-degree heart block. In adults, the development of first-degree heart block in association with digitalis administration is not necessarily an indication for either withdrawal or reduction of the amount of digitalis. First-degree heart block in association with the acute development of left bundle branch block after acute MI does constitute an indication for temporary pacing, because in two thirds of the cases, the combination of first-degree heart block and left bundle branch block developing during MI represents bilateral bundle branch block.

Second-Degree Heart Block

The two types of second-degree heart block are Mobitz I (Wenckebach's) AV block and Mobitz II block.

MOBITZ I (WENCKEBACH'S) AV BLOCK

The Mobitz I AV block is characterized by progressive PR prolongation, culminating in a nonconducted P wave followed by a pause and then either an escape AV junctional or idioventricular beat or resumption of the same cycle with progressively longer PR intervals until a P wave is again not conducted. The block is usually located in the AV junction but sometimes is located subjunctionally in a bundle branch. The physiologic mechanism for the AV block is thought to be AV junctional fatigue. Typically, QRS morphology is normal (i.e., there is no delay in intraventricular conduction), and this serves as a helpful distinction from Mobitz II block, in which prolonged QRS duration is the rule. If a bundle branch abnormality exists concomitantly with Wenckebach's block, QRS prolongation can be expected. In case of Mobitz I block in which the site of the conduction delay is in a bundle branch, QRS prolongation can also be expected. There are several different causes of Mobitz I block, including digitalis toxicity, acute myocardial ischemia or infarction (particularly acute inferior MI), rheumatic fever, myocardial disease, calcium deposition in conduction tissue (either as a complication of calcific aortic valve disease or as a manifestation of an increased calcium-phosphorus serum product in some patients with severe renal insufficiency), and myocarditis (e.g., diphtheria, virus). It may occasionally be a manifestation of congenital or degenerative conduction system disease. Vagal stimulation may also produce Mobitz I block, and it is also occasionally found in well-trained athletes. In some patients with chronic Wenckebach's heart block, the cause of the delay in AV conduction is not apparent. Presumably, arteriosclerotic heart disease, degenerative conduction system disease, or myocardial disease is the correct explanation.

Digitalis intoxication should be suspected as the cause of this form of heart block in any patient receiving digitalis at the time that it develops, and the drug should be discontinued to assess the effect. In general, temporary or permanent pacing is not necessary for patients with Wenckebach's heart block if the ventricular rate is fast enough that problems do not develop. However, if the ventricular response is so slow that the patient experiences angina, CHF, syncope, and/or frequent ventricular premature beats, then temporary and sometimes permanent pacing is necessary to ensure a rapid enough ventricular rate that these complications are not encountered. Wenckebach's heart block is relatively common in acute inferior MI. In this circumstance, it may progress to complete heart block, but this usually resolves within 5 or 6 days (although sometimes as long as 2 weeks). Permanent pacing is not usually necessary for complete heart block that develops after acute inferior MI.

MOBITZ II HEART BLOCK

In contrast to Wenckebach's block, Mobitz II heart block represents an intraventricular form of block and is associated with QRS prolongation on the ECG. This entity is characterized by a constant PR interval in the conducted SA beats and multiple P waves for every QRS complex. When only a 2:1 heart block exists, it may be difficult to distinguish Mobitz I from Mobitz II heart block, but if one pays attention to whether first-degree heart block exists in the conducted beats and whether QRS prolongation is present, one can generally distinguish Mobitz I from Mobitz II block. The distinction is an important one because some of the causes and the treatments for the two forms of heart block are different. Specifically, digitalis toxicity is almost never the cause of Mobitz II heart block. More common explanations for its development are degenerative conduction system disease, acute MI, calcium deposition in the conduction tissue (either as an extension of calcific aortic stenosis or as a complication of severe renal insufficiency), myocarditis, myocardial disease, and chronic ischemic heart disease. This particular form of heart block is treacherous and unpredictable, and most clinicians believe that it should be paced as soon as it is discovered. Temporary ventricular pacing is usually provided initially, and this is followed when convenient by permanent cardiac pacing. This approach to the treatment of Mobitz II heart block has reduced the incidence of complete heart block, cardiac asystole, and sudden death.

Complete Heart Block

As indicated earlier, in this situation of complete heart block, there is a totally independent ectopic ventricular pacemaker. In general, the ventricular rate is 30 to 40 bpm, and it should not be possible to identify conduction of any SA impulses. Physical examination usually documents various cardiac signs of complete heart AV dissociation as long as supraventricular electrical activity exists. In particular, one expects to find intermittent cannon A waves in the jugular venous pulse and a first heart sound that varies in intensity. A systolic ejection murmur is also present, and the heart rate is obviously slow. The causes of complete heart block are numerous, but some of the following are the most common: digitalis or potassium intoxication, acute MI, chronic ischemic heart disease, myocarditis, myocardial disease, tumors involving the heart, collagen disease involving the heart (particularly rheumatoid arthritis with rheumatoid nodules positioned in the conduction system), calcium deposition in the AV junction, and trauma (e.g., as a complication of surgical closure of ventricular septal defects). When complete heart block develops as a complication of an acute inferior MI, it tends to be tempo-

TABLE 83–1 Electrocardiographic Manifestations That May Represent Bilateral Bundle Branch Block

Left axis deviation and right bundle branch block
Right axis deviation and right bundle branch block
First-degree heart block and left bundle branch block
Alternating left and right bundle branch block within the same lead of an electrocardiogram
Left bundle branch block in the extremity leads and right bundle branch block in the precordial leads or vice versa

rary, but when it occurs as a complication of an acute anterior MI, it is usually permanent, and the prognosis is worse. Complete heart block should be paced, at least temporarily. In most clinical settings, the insertion of a temporary demand ventricular pacemaker followed by the placement of a permanent ventricular demand pacemaker, if the complete heart block does not resolve, is indicated.

Bilateral Bundle Branch Block

Several ECG patterns suggest the presence of bilateral bundle branch block (Table 83–1), and development of this conduction abnormality has prognostic and therapeutic significance. Left axis deviation and right bundle branch block represent block of the anterior fascicle of the left bundle and delay in conduction in the right bundle branch, thus signifying bilateral bundle branch disease. Right axis deviation and right bundle branch block sometimes represent a delay in conduction in the posterior fascicle of the left bundle and in the right bundle branch. In this entity, however, congenital heart disease, right ventricular failure, recurrent pulmonary emboli, and/or severe lung disease may also produce the same ECG pattern and do not necessarily reflect bilateral bundle branch block. First-degree heart block and left bundle branch block represent bilateral bundle branch block in two thirds of patients and represent delay in conduction in the left bundle and through the AV junction in the remaining one third of patients. The recognition of these patterns is important because when they develop in a setting of acute MI and are clearly new and persistent, they suggest the need for temporary ventricular pacing and also represent a very poor prognostic sign. In particular, the risk for development of complete heart block is increased in patients who experience acute bilateral bundle branch block, and, in addition, the development of bilateral bundle branch block in this setting identifies a large infarct; subsequent death as a complication of "power failure" is relatively common. These patients frequently experience cardiogenic shock, severe and medically refractory heart failure, or severe and medically refractory ventricular arrhythmias as a complication of their large infarct, and even those that survive their hospitalization are usually severely limited in later exercise performance.

One reservation about these patterns must be mentioned. If the bilateral bundle branch block precedes (i.e., is a chronic pattern occurring before the acute MI), the same cautions do not necessarily exist. Therefore, in this setting, it is not so clear that there is a significant risk for development of complete heart block, and there is much less evidence for poor prognostic expectations regarding the conduction pattern that represents a large infarct and a forerunner of the development of, for example, cardiogenic shock and severe CHF. Temporary and then often permanent ventricular pacemaker insertion is usually indicated in patients who experience bilateral bundle branch block with acute infarcts who survive their infarct. However, as noted earlier, many die in hospital of complications of "power

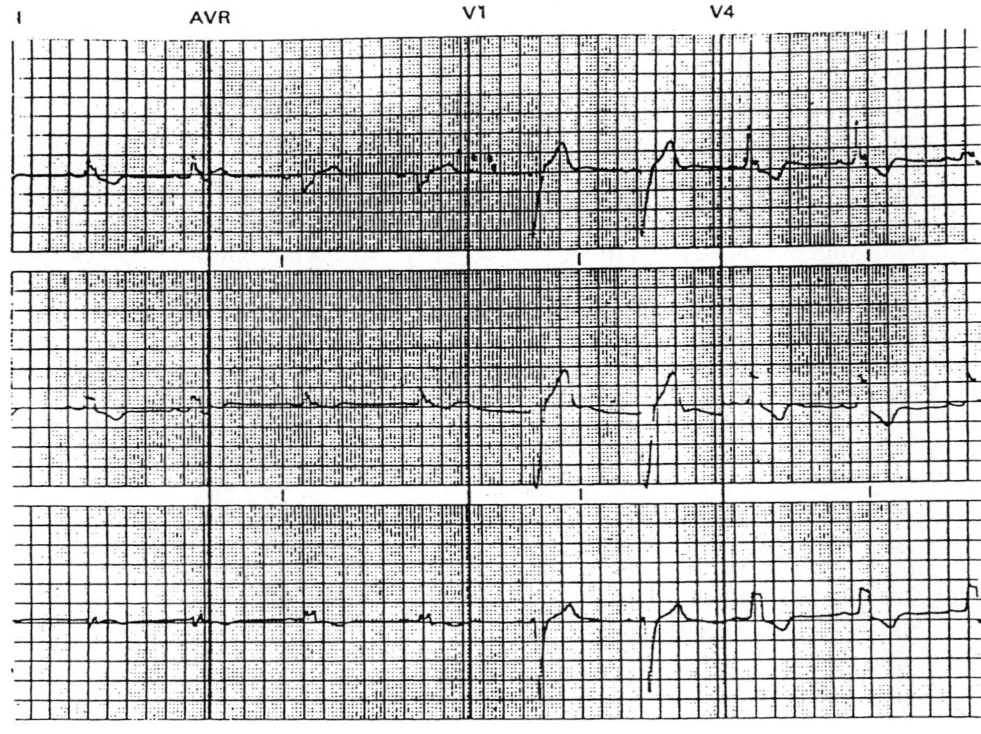

FIGURE 83–6 Complete left bundle branch block (LBBB). QRS duration is 0.14 second with typical distribution of QRS voltages and secondary STT wave change of LBBB.

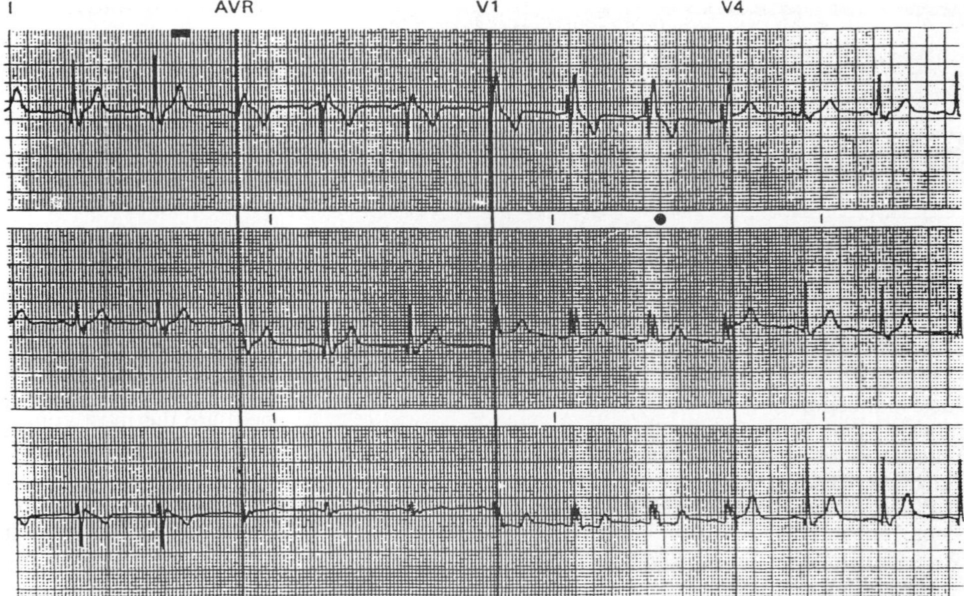

FIGURE 83–7 Complete right bundle branch block, QRS duration 0.14 second. Note the wide S wave on leads I, II, aVL, and V_{4-6} and tall R′ in V_{1-3}. Secondary ST-T wave changes are also present in lead V_1.

failure" of the left ventricle. Table 83–1 lists the ECG manifestations that may represent bilateral bundle branch block.

The chronic development of bilateral bundle branch block has different therapeutic implications. There is a risk of complete heart block in individuals with chronic bilateral bundle branch block, but the present best estimate of the frequency with which this occurs is 3 to 5 percent of patients per year. Therefore, ventricular pacing is not believed to be necessary in patients with chronic bilateral bundle branch block unless they are admitted to the hospital with syncopal spells that might well represent temporary complete AV block or ventricular arrhythmias associated with the conduction problem. In such instances, ventricular pacing may be important. Otherwise, most clinicians believe that these patients should be carefully followed and a pacemaker inserted when it is clearly indicated to do so.

Intraventricular Conduction Defects

LEFT BUNDLE BRANCH BLOCK

Left bundle branch block is characterized by QRS prolongation and the ECG pattern mentioned in the chapter on electrocardiography (Fig. 83–6). Rarely, normal individuals have the abnormality, but it more commonly reflects the presence of acute or chronic myocardial ischemia and develops with an acute MI (particularly anterior MI), myocarditis, myocardial disease, collagen disease, or calcium deposition in the conduction system. If it develops as a chronic abnormality, there is no specific indication for treatment. If it develops as a new event after acute MI, there is controversy about the appropriate treatment. It is clear, however, that there is a significant risk of complete heart block in patients who acquire left bundle branch block with acute MI, and it is our opinion that the entity should probably be ventricularly paced, at least temporarily. In addition, the acquisition of complete left bundle branch block with an acute anterior MI ordinarily occurs with relatively large infarcts and is itself a poor prognostic sign and often a precursor of the subsequent development of severe CHF or cardiogenic shock.

RIGHT BUNDLE BRANCH BLOCK

Right bundle branch block (Fig. 83–7) is described in the chapter on electrocardiography. It occurs in some individuals who have no other evidence of heart disease. It may also occur with various types of heart disease, including congenital heart disease, especially atrial septal defects; with myocardial ischemia, acute MI, and myocarditis; as a complication of pulmonary hypertension, right ventricular volume or pressure overload, and calcium deposition in conduction tissue; or as a manifestation of degenerative conduction system disease. When this form of intraventricular conduction defect is an isolated entity, it requires no additional treatment.

REFERENCES

1. Task Force on the Working Group on Arrhythmias of the European Society of Cardiology: the Sicilian gambit. Cardiology 84:1831, 1991.

CHAPTER 84

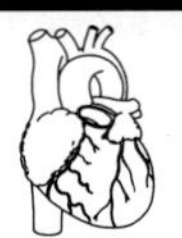

Sinus Node Dysfunction

David G. Benditt

PATHOPHYSIOLOGY
Basic Concepts
Intrinsic Sinus Node Dysfunction
Extrinsic Sinus Node Dysfunction
CLINICAL RECOGNITION
SPECTRUM OF ARRHYTHMIAS
Sinus Tachycardia
Sinus Bradycardia, Sinus Pause/Sinus Arrest, and Sinoatrial Exit Block
Bradycardia-Tachycardia Syndrome
Atrial Fibrillation
Prolonged Asystolic Pause or Failure to Restore Sinus Rhythm After Cardioversion
Sinus Node Reentrant Tachycardia
DIAGNOSTIC TECHNIQUES
Electrocardiographic Recordings and Ambulatory Monitoring
Exercise Testing
Clinical Studies of Sinus Node Autonomic Control
Invasive Electrophysiologic Testing
NATURAL HISTORY
Mortality Rates
Conduction System Disturbances
Arrhythmia Progression
Thromboembolic Complications
TREATMENT OF SINUS NODE DYSFUNCTION
Drug Therapy in Sinus Node Dysfunction
Pacing Therapy
Innovative Atrial Pacing Methods and Atrial Defibrillation Techniques
Percutaneous Transcatheter Cardiac Tissue Ablation
CONCLUSION

Sinus node dysfunction (also termed *sick sinus syndrome* or *sinoatrial disease*) encompasses an array of sinus node or atrial rhythm disturbances that result in persistent or intermittent periods of inappropriate slow or fast heart beating or inadequate heart rate responsiveness to physical exertion or emotional stress (so-called chronotropic incompetence).[1–5] Any or all of these may occur in the same patient at various times. The most common bradyarrhythmias are severe sinus bradycardia and sinus pauses. However, atrial fibrillation with an excessively slow ventricular response, sinoatrial exit block, or chronotropic incompetence may also contribute to symptoms. The most frequent tachyarrhythmia observed in these patients tends to be paroxysmal atrial fibrillation; atrial flutter or other primary atrial tachycardias are also relatively frequent. Inappropriate sinus tachycardia has become more widely appreciated as a troublesome arrhythmia and can be reasonably considered to be a manifestation of sinus node dysfunction.

Symptoms arising as a direct result of arrhythmia (e.g., palpitations, fatigue, dizziness/syncope, exertional intolerance) are the most common reason for patients with sinus node dysfunction to seek medical advice; however, it is the potential for thromboembolic complications that is usually the greatest concern. In fact, to the extent that patients with sinus node dysfunction exhibit greater morbidity and mortality rates than an age-matched cohort, embolic events are principally responsible. Furthermore, repeated subclinical embolism is suspected of contributing to gradual diminution of mental acuity in many older individuals with subtle forms of sinoatrial disease (presumably via small strokes).

Sinus node dysfunction most frequently occurs in older individuals. In some instances, aging is the only apparent "cause." More often, however, coronary artery disease, hypertensive heart disease, or cardiomyopathy is present and is thought to be contributory. In younger age groups, sinus node dysfunction may be observed in the newborn or child on a familial basis, but more frequently, it occurs somewhat later as a consequence of cardiac surgery (particularly if it involves the atria) or acquired cardiac disease. Heart transplantation surgery is an increasingly important addition to the list of cardiac operations with a propensity for initiating sinus node disturbances. In all age groups, cardioactive drugs and abnormalities of the autonomic nervous system can also produce or exacerbate arrhythmias characteristic of sinus node dysfunction.

The treatment of sick sinus syndrome is primarily directed toward the relief of symptoms stemming from paroxysmal or chronic bradyarrhythmias or tachyarrhythmias. The tachycardias are for the most part treated with one or more of the many available antiarrhythmic drugs. Bradycardias, when not the result of a reversible cause (e.g., drug effects, myocardial ischemia), are best treated with implanted cardiac pacemakers. Finally, every effort should be made to prevent thromboembolic complications through the use of anticoagulation; this is especially necessary in the older individual or those exhibiting recognized risk factors (e.g., structural heart disease, diabetes, hypertension).

The prevention of the development of sinus node disturbances is not possible in the vast majority of cases if reversible drug-induced disturbances are excluded; however, in the segment of the population in whom the condition is due to surgical trauma, careful surgical technique may reduce the frequency of severity of atrial dysrhythmias.

This chapter provides a summary of the origins and principal clinical manifestations of sinus node dysfunction.

Numerous detailed treatments of the cellular electrophysiology of the sinus node region are available in the literature; some sources[5–11] are suggested as a first step.

PATHOPHYSIOLOGY

Disturbances in sinus node function encompass abnormalities of the generation of the sinus node impulse, its subsequent emergence into the atria, or both; abnormal impulse transmission within the atria and specialized cardiac conduction system; failure of physiologic subsidiary pacemaker function; and increased susceptibility to paroxysmal or chronic atrial tachycardias.[1–5, 7] Disorders of sinus node function may be caused by processes that directly alter the anatomy and functional integrity of the sinus node or the surrounding atrium (intrinsic disturbances) or by factors that impair sinus node function without evidence of structural sinoatrial injury (extrinsic disturbances).[5, 7] The latter may be the result of disturbances of autonomic neural control,[5, 12, 13] the effects of cardioactive drugs (e.g., sympatholytic agents, antiarrhythmic drugs),[5, 14–17] or both.

Basic Concepts

Initial activation of each heartbeat in the normal heart arises from spontaneously depolarizing pacemaker cells within an anatomic region that lies laterally in the epicardial groove of the sulcus terminalis.[6–10] This sinus node region is far more diffuse than previously thought and consists of nests of potential pacemaker cells. The identification and characterization of the specific cells responsible for cardiac activation at a given point in time are exceedingly difficult tasks and one that complicates the study of sinus node cellular electrophysiology.

The principal pacemaker cells of the heart exhibit both relatively low resting potentials and the important property of spontaneous diastolic depolarization (phase 4 depolarization) leading to the generation of another action potential (Fig. 84–1). The rate of depolarization (i.e., the firing rate of the cell) is influenced by a number of factors, including autonomic tone, chemical milieu, and drug effects. As a rule, from an autonomic nervous system perspective, the healthy sinus node in the resting individual is predominantly influenced by parasympathetic (vagal) input.[7] Increases in heart rate due to physical exertion or emotional stress are mediated first by parasympathetic withdrawal in conjunction with increased sympathetic neural activity. Circulating catecholamines may contribute to further heart rate increments if the exertion or stress is sustained for a sufficiently prolonged period of time.

Apart from principal pacemaker cells, the sinus node is composed of a variety of comparable pacemaker cell nests that may exhibit somewhat slower intrinsic firing rates and consequently are considered to be backup or subsidiary pacemakers. These backup pacemaker cells or cell groups may be called on to take over under a variety of physiologic and pathologic conditions (e.g., vagal stimulation, sympathetic stimulation, electrolyte disturbances, atrial arrhythmias). The result is an apparent shift in the principal pacemaker site within the sinus node region.[9–11] In essence, therefore, the sinus node is a pacemaker complex in which periodic shifts of the principal pacemaker site complicate electrophysiologic assessment of sinus node function and may even result in alterations of P-wave morphology.[11]

Conduction of electrical impulses within the elements of the sinus node is very slow (2 to 5 cm/s).[13] Therefore, the potential for intranodal conduction failure is quite high, even in the normal situation.[5, 6, 10, 18–22] Any additional adverse impact on direct cell-to-cell transmission by disease or autonomic nervous system (particularly parasympathetic) disturbance can cause intranodal conduction block leading to sinus pauses or sinus arrest (Fig. 84–2). Alternatively, fibrosis due to disease (or possibly as a result of the aging process alone) in the sinoatrial region may establish the functional substrate needed for reentry to occur[23]; the outcome in some patients is a paroxysmal reentrant tachycardia with P-wave morphology similar to that present during sinus rhythm in that same individual (i.e., sinoatrial reentry tachycardia).[5]

Factors extrinsic to the sinus node itself play an important role not only as modulators of normal sinus node function but also as contributors to sinus node dysfunction. Both parasympathetic and sympathetic mediators (i.e., acetylcholine, norepinephrine, epinephrine) alter spontaneous

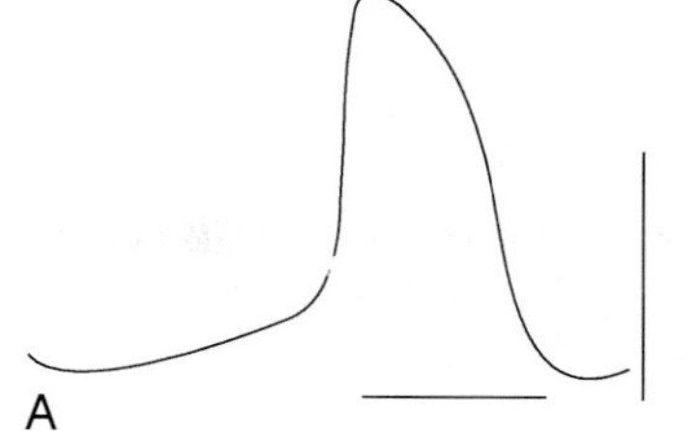

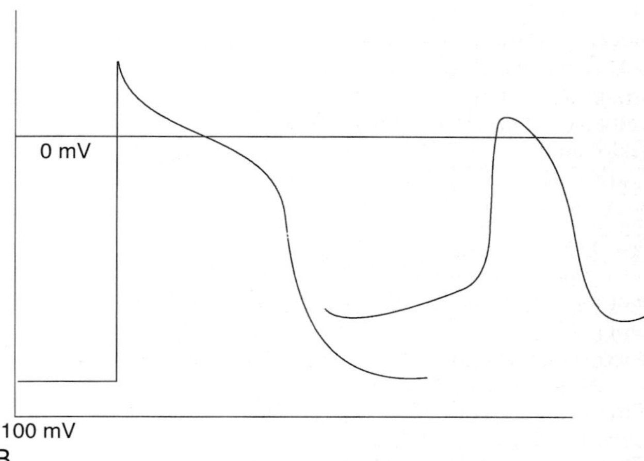

FIGURE 84–1 Transmembrane action potential recordings contrasting sinus node and His-Purkinje action potentials. **A,** Illustration of a sinus node pacemaker cell transmembrane action potential. The spontaneous diastolic depolarization accounts for the spontaneous generation of new action potentials and therefore the normal heart rate. Variation in the rate of diastolic depolarization largely accounts for changes in heart rate. **B,** Illustration of His-Purkinje and sinus node action potentials. Note that the sinus node potential has a lower amplitude and a slower rate of rise (phase 0).

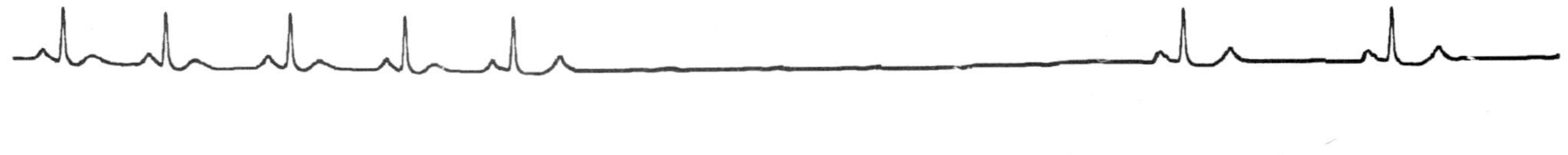

FIGURE 84–2 Electrocardiographic rhythm strip illustrates sinus pause/sinus arrest.

depolarization rates of sinus node cells and may also influence the site of the principal pacemaker within the node.[9, 11] Acetylcholine released from parasympathetic nerve endings reduces pacemaker firing rate, prolongs refractoriness of sinus node cells, and further slows intranodal conduction velocity.[20] On the other hand, norepinephrine released from sympathetic nerves and circulating epinephrine increases both sinus rate and intranodal conduction velocity. In vivo, parasympathetic influences usually predominate in the sinus node. However, excessive parasympathetic influence may result in marked sinus bradycardia or even lengthy pauses in the rhythm due to sinus arrest or sinoatrial exit block.[20–22, 24, 25] Cartoid sinus syndrome and vasovagal syncope are examples of clinical conditions in which these electrocardiographic abnormalities may occur.

Intrinsic Sinus Node Dysfunction

Certain pathologic states have been associated with the presence of sinus node dysfunction in adult patients and are presumed to have contributed to its development; coronary atherosclerosis has been most prominent among these.[26, 27] However, a causal relationship between coronary atherosclerosis and sinoatrial disease remains controversial; both tend to occur in older individuals, and the concordance may therefore be coincidental. The sinus node artery has also been reported to be subject to embolic events as well as to occlusive and inflammatory diseases. Again, however, the significance of such findings in the broad range of sinus node dysfunction patients remains uncertain. Indeed, a number of reports that have examined this issue have tended to emphasize the patency of the sinus node artery in patients with sinus node dysfunction.[26–30] For example, Shaw and associates[30] used postmortem angiography to investigate sinus node blood supply in 25 patients with sinus node disease and compared these findings with those for 54 individuals who died from heart block but in whom sinoatrial function was believed to be normal. Despite the frequent presence of extensive coronary artery disease in patients with sinus node dysfunction, more than 50 percent stenosis of the sinus node artery was observed in only 7 of 25 cases. On the other hand, sinoatrial artery disease was not present in any of the 54 patients with heart block. These findings may be interpreted to suggest that ischemia due to coronary artery disease affecting the sinus node artery (the principal blood supply to the central sinus node region) contributes to the development of sinus node disease in perhaps one third of affected adult patients.

Replacement or displacement of normal sinus node cells by fibrous tissue, with loss of functional components or alteration of regional architecture, has been the most common observation in the pathologic examination of cardiac tissues from patients with sinus node dysfunction.[28, 29, 31] Apart from ischemic heart disease, other potential causes include cardiomyopathy, surgical trauma, or inflammation (e.g., pericardial disease, rheumatic heart disease, viral myocarditis, collagen vascular diseases). In some instances, the condition appears to be familial in origin.[32–34] In most instances, however, the cause of the intrinsic sinus node dysfunction is not evident, and the structural changes in the sinoatrial region may not be measurably different from the normal increase in fibrous tissue that accompanies aging.[23, 35, 36]

In children and young adults, intrinsic sinoatrial disease has been most commonly associated with presumed direct sinus node damage (e.g., hemorrhage, necrosis, suture injury) due to previous atrial surgery, such as closure of atrial septal defects, and, most importantly, after atrial redirection procedures (Mustard/Senning operation) for transposition of the great arteries.[37–43] However, sinus node dysfunction has also been observed in patients with unoperated congenital heart disease (including relatively benign conditions such as persistent left superior vena cava, as well as lesions of potential hemodynamic significance) and even in ostensibly normal children and adolescents.[44–48] Again, in some of these patients, a familial disturbance of sinoatrial function may have been the cause, but in most instances, the origin is unknown. Patients undergoing heart transplantation have been recognized as exhibiting sinus node dysfunction of the donor heart.[49] Presumably, proximity of the atrial suture lines to the donor sinus node complex may account for this problem, although the role of rejection or inflammation cannot be disregarded. Most often, problems occur in the immediate postoperative period and tend to be transient. However, cardiac pacing has been necessary in approximately 5 percent of these patients. Future evolution of surgical technique may ameliorate this cause of sinoatrial disease.

Extrinsic Sinus Node Dysfunction

Of the extracardiac factors that affect sinus node function without inducing evident structural changes, the most important are cardioactive drugs and autonomic nervous system influences. Electrolyte (e.g., hyperkalemia, hypocalcemia) and endocrine (e.g., hyperthyroidism) disturbances may also play a role in individual cases, but these seem to occur only rarely.

Drugs may alter sinus node function directly, as a result of their pharmacologic action on nodal cells (e.g., membrane-active antiarrhythmics), or indirectly via neurally mediated effects (e.g., cardiac glycosides, beta-adrenergic blockers). Potential drug effects include new-onset or aggravation of preexisting sinus bradycardia, sinus pauses, sinoatrial exit block, or chronotropic incompetence. In addition, although not widely recognized, antiarrhythmic drugs may exert proarrhythmic effects in the atrium, with the outcome being more frequent episodes of atrial ectopy or runs of tachycardia. The latter effects are, however, difficult to recognize; more often than not, the drug is just assumed to have been ineffective and its use is discontinued.

The drugs that have been most often implicated in extrinsic sinus node dysfunction include β-adrenoceptor blockers, calcium channel blockers, and "membrane-active" antiarrhythmics.[14–17, 50–55] In the past, sympatholytic antihypertensive agents were among the most common offenders.[14–17] These latter agents are far less important, having in large part been replaced by more effective and better tolerated antihypertensive agents. Among the other drugs known to affect sinus node function (although less commonly encountered in clinical practice) are lithium carbonate, cimetidine, amitriptyline, and phenothiazines.[5, 16, 17, 56–58] Cardiac glycosides have also been implicated in the provocation of sinus node dysfunction; however, given the frequency with which they are used in older patients, glycosides are only rarely associated with clinically significant problems in this regard.

As noted earlier, disturbances in sinus node autonomic control (particularly enhanced parasympathetic activity) can be responsible for electrocardiographic (ECG) findings of sinus node disease.[20, 22, 24, 59–64] In this regard, marked sinus bradycardia, sinus pauses, sinoatrial exit block, and slow ventricular responses in atrial fibrillation may, in some cases, be primarily the result of marked hypervagatonia. In the extreme case, autonomically induced asystole may result in sudden cardiac death syndrome. The mechanism of the event appears to be the result of exaggerated neurally mediated bradycardia in conjuction with peripheral vasodepressor effects. Conversely, although not widely recognized as a manifestation of sinus node disease, persistent or inappropriate sinus tachycardia may reflect unbalanced or excessive sympathetic activity.

In summary, sinus node dysfunction may result from disease states that directly alter the anatomy and function of the pacemaker complex or from external, often reversible, factors (e.g., drugs). Distinguishing these two major pathophysiologic groups has obvious prognostic and therapeutic implications.

Clinical Recognition

As noted earlier, *sinus node dysfunction*, *sick sinus syndrome*, and *sinoatrial disease* or *dysfunction* are synonymous terms that encompass a clinical syndrome characterized by the presence of any of a wide variety of bradydysrhythmias or tachydysrhythmias and conduction disturbances.[1–5] In addition, disturbances of chronotropic responsiveness, as well as certain intraventricular conduction system disturbances (when present in conjuction with other manifestations of sinoatrial disease), are often considered to be an integral part of the global picture.[65]

As a rule, symptoms alone are not sufficiently specific to permit the establishment of a diagnosis of sinus node dysfunction based on medical history alone. Many individuals are essentially asymptomatic despite apparent ECG abnormalities. Others manifest various complaints due to inappropriate bradyarrhythmias, paroxysmal tachycardias, or exertional intolerance. Thus, the clinical picture may include syncope, dizziness, shortness of breath, palpitations, fatigue, and lethargy. Other disturbances, some of which may be very subtle, particularly in older patients, consist of personality changes, memory loss, and gastrointestinal disturbances.[3–5, 31, 66–68] In this regard, it is thought that multiple "minor" embolic episodes may be responsible for premature cerebral dysfunction as the principal clinical abnormality in some patients with sinus node dysfunction. Finally, systemic embolism is common and can be a devastating complication of sinus node disease. Embolism is particularly important in patients with bradycardia-tachycardia syndrome, with the risk appearing to be greatest within 24 hours of spontaneous or medically initiated termination of atrial tachyarrhythmias (particularly atrial fibrillation).[69]

It is often difficult to obtain unequivocal documentation of the relationship between symptomatology and dysrhythmia in patients with sinus node dysfunction. First, the ECG manifestations of sinus node dysfunction are often transient and therefore difficult to "capture." Second, the symptoms associated with sinus node dysfunction are sufficiently nonspecific in most instances (e.g., fatigue, changes in mental acuity, dizziness) that they overlap with many other medical conditions, especially in older patients. Consequently, symptoms noted during ambulatory ECG monitoring might not be associated with any arrhythmia at that moment. Third, even after thorough instruction, many older or infirm patients (i.e., those comprising the bulk of patients with sinus node dysfunction) do not understand or comply well with the need to maintain a detailed symptom diary during outpatient monitoring of their heart rhythm. Finally, the range of normal ECG findings and heart rate variations observed in health complicate the identification of sinus node dysfunction. For example, minor alterations in P-wave morphology are common in normal healthy subjects and may reflect physiologic variation in sinus node and atrial activation with changes in rate, site of principal pacemaker cells, or autonomic tone.[11] Similarly, impressive degrees of sinus bradycardia may occur in normal individuals (especially during sleep) and are not necessarily indicative of sinus node disease. For example, rates as slow as 35 to 40 beats/min may be observed in healthy resting individuals.[70, 71] In addition, sinus arrhythmia, a heart rate variation most often associated with respiratory cycles (rate increases with inspiration and decreases with expiration), is common in healthy individuals and must be differentiated from pathologic sinus pauses. The criteria for the normal range of sinus arrhythmia vary, but P-P interval variations less than 120 or 160 ms or 10 percent or less of the basic cycle length are most widely accepted.

Spectrum of Arrhythmias

Sinus Tachycardia

As a rule, maximum achievable heart rates decline with age (the most common calculation used is maximum heart rate [beats/min] = 220 − age [years]). However, the most commonly used heart rates through the day (i.e., activity of daily living rates) are very similar across all age ranges. Therefore, a single definition for sinus tachycardia is appropriate, at least beginning in older childhood and extending throughout the adult years.

Sinus tachycardia (generally defined as a sinus rate of > 100 beats/min) is usually a normal response to physiologic demands (e.g., exercise, anxiety) and pathologic conditions (e.g., fever, anemia, hyperthyroidism). Typically, heart rates of more than 180 beats/min are only rarely the result of sinus tachycardia in the adult (other than very athletic individuals), and rates above 140 beats/min are usually associated only with vigorous exercise or severe stress (e.g., hemorrhage). In general, sinus tachycardia occurring in response to an appropriate stimulus (e.g., exercise, fright) exhibits a rapid (but not abrupt) onset. After removal of the instigating factor or event, the rate slows gradually (in the case of exercise, this slow recovery is important to permit thermoregulation to be restored to normal levels). To some extent, these onset and offset features (along with the setting in which the rhythm is noted) help to distinguish sinus tachycardia from most other paroxysmal supraventricular tachycardias.

From time to time, it may be difficult to differentiate sinus tachycardia from pathologic rhythm disturbances, particularly atrial ectopic tachycardias (including so-called sinus node reentry; see later). Maneuvers such as carotid sinus massage or the Valsalva maneuver may be useful in helping to make a distinction. Similarly, the response to certain pharmacologic interventions (e.g., adenosine, β-adrenergic blockers, or calcium channel blockers) may be helpful.

In some cases, intractable idiopathic nonphysiologic sinus tachycardia proves to be a perplexing and troublesome clinical problem. This finding has been attributed to abnormal enhanced sinus node automaticity in some instances,[65, 72–74] but for the most part, its origin is usually unclear. The propensity for this arrhythmia to occur after radiofrequency ablation in the vicinity of the atrioventricular junction has raised the possibility that disturbances of local neutral reflexes play a role. In other cases, inflammation may account for the rapid rate (although this would not be expected to result in the often long-lasting sinus tachycardia occurring in many patients). Certainly, it is crucial to exclude other causative factors, such as hyperthyroidism, drug effects, infection, anemia, postoperative state, and restrictive cardiomyopathy, before attributing symptoms to idiopathic sinus tachycardia (especially if radiofrequency modification of the sinus node region is contemplated).

Sinus Bradycardia, Sinus Pause/Sinus Arrest, and Sinoatrial Exit Block

Sinus bradycardia is common in healthy (and especially in athletic) individuals. Sinus rates as low as 35 to 40 beats/min are compatible with normal sinus node function.[70, 71] On the other hand, slow heart rates can be responsible for many symptoms, especially in the elderly patient. Clinical correlation of bradycardia with symptoms is often difficult but is nevertheless essential for proper evaluation of these individuals.

Sinus pause and *sinus arrest* are synonymous terms, implying failure of the principal pacemaker cells of the sinus node to discharge, with a consequent absence of an expected atrial activation of sinus node origin (see Fig. 84–2). The duration of pause necessary to qualify as a sinus pause or sinus arrest has yet to be clearly defined, in part due to the fact that it depends on the magnitude of underlying sinus arrhythmia (i.e., normal variation of cardiac cycle length). Asymptomatic sinus pauses of more than 2 seconds' duration have been reported to occur in a substantial number of patients undergoing ambulatory monitoring, especially in trained athletes. These findings, in conjunction with reports indicating that pauses of up to 1.75 seconds are common in healthy young subjects, suggest that these durations are not typically considered abnormal.[70, 71, 75, 76] On the other hand, several reports have noted that sinus pauses of more than 3 seconds were rare during ambulatory ECG monitoring (2.4 and 0.8 percent of patients, respectively).[77, 78] However, even these studies differed in the significance of these longer pauses. Ector and colleagues[77] indicated that pauses of this duration were commonly associated with symptoms (85 percent of instances) and concluded that such pauses may be an indication of pacemaker implantation. Conversely, Hilgard and associates[78] found symptoms to be uncommon during such pauses. Therefore, it is probably reasonable to conclude that asymptomatic sinus pauses of up to 3 seconds are relatively common and without clear-cut adverse prognostic implications. Pauses of more than 3 seconds should trigger further clinical assessment; specifically, further attempts should be made to detect symptomatic correlations, other evidence of sinus node dysfunction, or both before consideration of therapeutic intervention. Ambulatory ECG monitoring would be most appropriate. However, in selected cases, invasive electrophysiologic testing may be preferrable for obtaining additional support for a diagnosis of sinus node dysfunction.

Sinoatrial Exit Block

Sinoatrial exit block implies that the transmission of a normally generated sinus node pacemaker impulse from the sinus node region to the atrium is either delayed (first-degree sinoatrial exit block) or blocked entirely (second- and third-degree sinoatrial exit block). The site of block is probably most often within the node itself, because conduction within this region is exceedingly slow, even under normal conditions. As indicated, sinoatrial exit block is usually classified in a manner analogous to that of atrioventricular (AV) blocks:[79–82]

1. First-degree sinoatrial block implies a prolonged conduction time for each impulse leaving the sinus node. This conduction delay cannot be observed on the surface electrocardiogram but can be identified through either direct recording or indirect estimation of sinoatrial conduction time (SACT) during electrophysiologic study.
2. Second-degree sinoatrial exit block, in a fashion anal-

ogous to that of second-degree AV block, indicates periodic failure of a sinus impulse to exit the sinus node and activate the atria. In some cases, a Wenckebach-type periodicity of this block may be inferred from surface ECG tracings by recognition of progressive P-P interval shortening preceding a pause in the atrial rhythm (a "dropped" P wave). In higher grades of second-degree sinoatrial exit block, abrupt failure of sinus impulses to exit the node may result in periodic absence of one or more normally generated atrial activations. The ECG hallmark of the interruption in the atrial rhythm in high-grade sinoatrial block is that the duration of the pause is an "exact" whole-number multiple of the immediately preceding P-P interval. However, it should be obvious that some leeway in measurement must be allowed to account for normal variations of sinus rhythm (i.e., sinus arrhythmia), as well as for autonomically induced variations that may occur secondary to the hemodynamic effects of the bradyarrhythmia itself.

3. Third-degree or complete sinoatrial exit block cannot readily be distinguished from a prolonged sinus pause or sinus arrest, other than if the pause is a whole-number multiple of the basic sinus cycle, or through direct recordings of sinus node pacemaker activity during electrophysiologic study. As a rule, high-grade block (in the absence of autonomic disturbance or drug toxicity) implies severe sinoatrial dysfunction and is usually associated with bradycardia-related symptoms.

Bradycardia-Tachycardia Syndrome

The occurrence of intermittent bradyarrhythmias and tachyarrhythmias of sinoatrial origin is an important and relatively common manifestation of sinus node dysfunction[5, 7, 31, 83, 84] (Fig. 84–3). This aspect of sinoatrial disease is often characterized as a syndrome of its own (i.e., bradycardia-tachycardia syndrome). It most commonly consists of the association in the same patient of sinus bradycardia with paroxysmal atrial fibrillation, although atrial flutter or other primary atrial tachycardias may also occur. In any case, it is important to document the tachyarrhythmia and verify the diagnosis before embarking on a treatment program. It is important to bear in mind that in these often older patients, ventricular tachyarrhythmias may be the cause of palpitations. In addition, such patients may be more susceptible to proarrhythmic effects of antiarrhythmic drug treatments.

Symptoms in patients with bradycardia-tachycardia syndrome may occur as a result of bradycardic periods, episodic tachycardia, or both. Furthermore, therapeutic interventions (particularly drugs) designed to achieve tachyarrhythmia control may exacerbate the tendency to bradycardia, thereby aggravating those symptoms due to slow heart rates. In addition, drug-induced tachyarrhythmias (proarrhythmia) may be more of a concern in patients with a predisposition to bradycardia. For both of these latter situations, cardiac pacing may become a necessity and is considered appropriately indicated if drug therapy is essential.

An important further concern in patients with bradycardia-tachycardia syndrome is their susceptibility to systemic embolism.[84] A wide range of symptoms may result from this complications. Consequently, anticoagulation is often an important part of the overall treatment strategy in these patients.

Atrial Fibrillation

Atrial fibrillation is usually considered to be part of the spectrum of sinus node disease when it is associated with

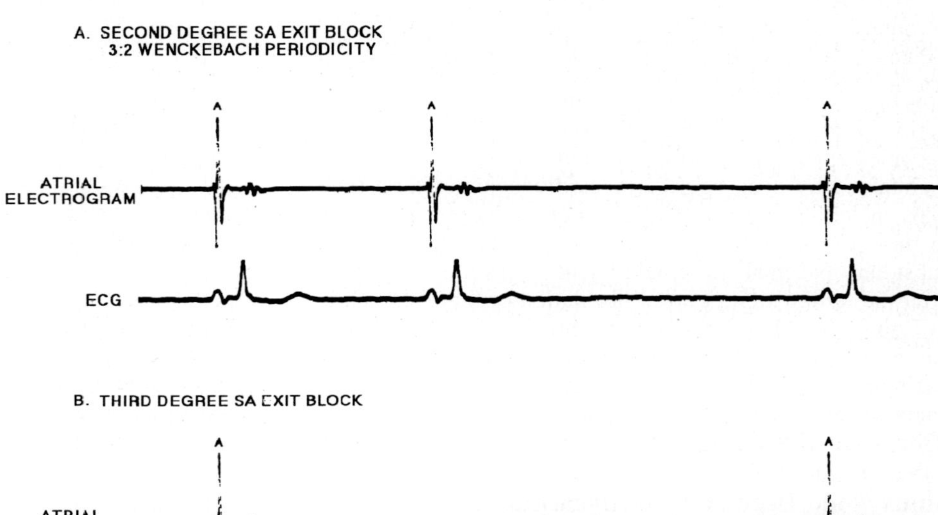

FIGURE 84–3 A and **B,** Electrocardiographic (ECG) tracing and atrial electrograms illustrate two forms of sinoatrial (SA) exit block. **B,** The pause was three times the basic sinus cycle in duration.

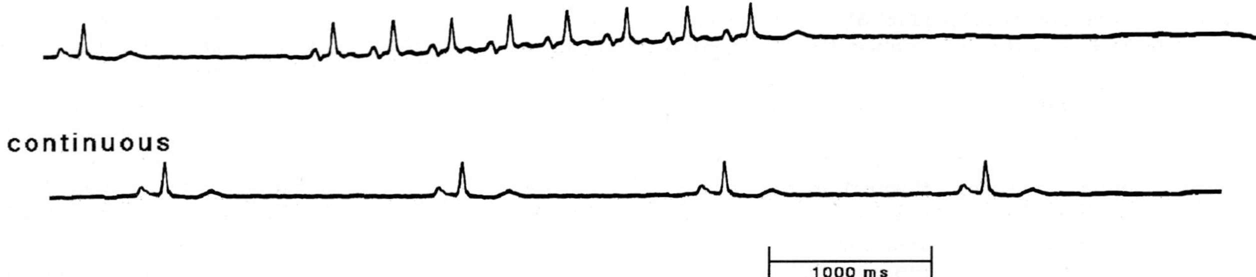

FIGURE 84–4 Electrocardiographic tracing illustrates an example of a record obtained from a patient with "bradycardia-tachycardia" syndrome.

a relatively slow ventricular response (in the absence of drugs). Presumably, concomitant disease of the atrioventricular conduction system or the inadequacy of subsidiary cardiac pacemakers accounts for this picture. However, it is not unreasonable to similarly categorize all atrial fibrillation within the sinus node dysfunction rubric (excluding perhaps transient postoperative events or those clearly the result of an associated illness or endocrine/metabolic disorder). The rationale lies in the apparent defect in sinoatrial electrophysiology that must be present to permit atrial fibrillation to occur. Furthermore, insisting on a "slow" ventricular response is inappropriate because many patients with sinus node dysfunction manifest surprisingly rapid ventricular rates during atrial tachycardias (Fig. 84–4). Not infrequently, it is these rapid rates that may be the primary cause of symptoms. Consequently, the presence of a slow ventricular response is not a necessary aspect of the diagnosis of sinus node dysfunction.

Prolonged Asystolic Pause or Failure to Restore Sinus Rhythm After Cardioversion

Prolonged pauses or severe bradycardia is common after cardioversion of tachyarrhythmias in patients with underlying sinoatrial disease. In some patients, sinus node dysfunction first becomes clinically evident when a long asystolic period occurs after a cardioversion procedure or when it becomes apparent that sinus rhythm cannot be restored or maintained by even aggressive cardioversion efforts (perhaps including internal cardioversion at centers proficient in the technique).[85, 86] In instances in which the atria and subsidiary pacemakers remain silent or severely depressed after the termination of atrial fibrillation or flutter (a condition that should be particularly anticipated if the patient has been taking antiarrhythmic drugs), immediate cardiac pacing may become essential. Ready access to transthoracic pacing is a prudent preparatory step in such cases.

Sinus Node Reentrant Tachycardia

The inherently slow conduction properties of the sinus node region provide fertile substrate for local reentry (presumably of the leading circle type, with a functional refractory center). Surgical trauma (e.g., postoperative cardiac surgical states, especially after a Mustard or Senning procedure) or fibrosis secondary to aging or disease can also be expected to add the potential for reentry around a structural obstacle. Thus, reentry within the vicinity of the sinoatrial node is an expected possibility (albeit relatively uncommon) in patients with sinoatrial disease.[87–89]

The ECG and electrophysiologic characteristics associated with atrial rhythms thought to be due to reentry within the sinus node region can be summarized as follows:

1. The morphology of the P waves generated by the reentrant cycles is essentially identical to those of sinus beats in that patient.
2. The sequence of atrial activation of reentrant cycles is identical to that of sinus impulses when studied in the clinical electrophysiology laboratory.
3. Induction of the reentry phenomenon is reproducible with atrial extrastimulus testing.
4. The tachycardia is usually relatively slow (i.e., < 150 beats/min) but exhibits wide rate fluctuations.[87, 88]

DIAGNOSTIC TECHNIQUES

A variety of diagnostic tools is available for the evaluation of patients with suspected sinus node dysfunction. Among the methods of long standing are conventional ambulatory ECG recordings (Holter-type and "event" recorders), exercise testing, pharmacologic assessment of sinus node autonomic neural control, and invasive clinical electrophysiologic testing. The introduction of atrial signal-averaged electrocardiography *(P-wave signal averaging)* may provide an additional useful screening tool, although further assessment is still needed.[90, 91] In addition, implantable long-term event monitors (*implantable loop* recorders) provide a powerful tool for identifying even very infrequent arrhythmias.[92] As a rule, however, one or another form of ambulatory ECG monitoring is the usual first step in the assessment of suspected sinus node dysfunction. Conventional invasive electrophysiologic studies have tended to become less widely used than had been the case in the 1980s. Nevertheless, such testing remains useful in selected cases. In essence, the diagnostic strategy must vary from patient to patient depending on the relative frequency with which symptoms occur, their severity, and the ability of the patient to manage some of the diagnostic tools (especially portable event recorders).

Electrocardiographic Recordings and Ambulatory Monitoring

The documentation of cardiac arrhythmia occurring in conjuction with spontaneous symptoms is the most specific diagnostic observation in any patient with cardiac arrhythmia and, depending on the circumstance, may essentially eliminate the need for additional diagnostic studies.[93–95] An obvious situation in which this would not be the case is when the same arrhythmia is recorded at other times in the absence of symptoms. In any case, establishing a diagnosis via this approach entails the exposure of patients to the recurrence of potentially serious rhythm disturbances and often is both time consuming and expensive. Therefore, although ambulatory monitoring with conventional 24- or 48-hour magnetic tape recording systems continues to be widely used as an initial diagnostic procedure, usually repeated recordings over a relatively long period of time may be needed to establish the diagnosis. For example, among 44 symptomatic patients evaluated with this technique, Stern and colleagues[93] apparently obtained satisfactory ECG correlates in 48 percent. However, an average of 5.8 recording days was required.

In many patients with suspected sinus node disease, symptoms are relatively infrequent. Consequently, long-term ECG event recorders with memory retention capability and 24-hour central monitoring and recording stations accessible by telephone transmission may be more helpful than conventional magnetic tape recording systems. If necessary, these event recorder systems can be used in the continuous-loop mode for patients in whom the duration of symptomatic episodes is too brief to permit a recording to be obtained in the conventional manner. This diagnostic strategy has been enhanced by the introduction of a patient-interactive, telemetry addressable, miniature implantable event recorder system with memory.[92] Future developments may include fully automatic implantable systems with microprocessor-based arrhythmia recognition techniques.

Exercise Testing

Exercise testing is not particularly useful in the diagnostic assessment of suspected sinus node dysfunction. Although abnormal heart rate responses during exercise have been reported in such patients,[96–100] the sensitivity and specificity of these observations remain unaddressed. Furthermore, exercise heart rate response in patients with suspected sinus node dysfunction often lacked reproducibility, suggesting that a single "negative" test (i.e., absence of evident chronotropic disturbance) did not exclude sinus node dysfunction. Despite these limitations, however, exercise testing may be useful in the management of individual patients. For example, exercise testing may permit distinguishing patients with resting sinus bradycardia but essentially normal exercise heart rate responses from those with more severe degrees of chronotropic incompetence. Furthermore, exercise testing may be helpful in identifying the potential benefits of sensor-triggered, rate-adaptive pacing in patients who exhibit sluggish heart rate responses at the onset of exercise or who manifest excessively rapid heart rate deceleration after exercise.[101, 102] In this context, it should be emphasized that although many patients with sinus node disease may achieve peak heart rates comparable to those expected of control subjects, the temporal course of heart rate acceleration might be abnormal. The latter, if slow or erratic, may limit activities of daily living and provide a basis for diminished exercise tolerance.

A number of exercise protocols are used for the assessment of sinus node function. These tend to be more gradual in their demands than are the more conventional exercise protocols used for the diagnosis of ischemic heart disease (e.g., the Bruce protocol). The best known of the heart rate response exercise assessments is the Chronotropic Assessment Exercise Protocol (CAEP).[103] Another assessment is the Minnesota Pacemaker Response Exercise Protocol (M-PREP).[104, 105] From a theoretical point of view, however, the assessment of heart rate responses during activities that mimic those of everyday activities (activities of daily living) would be a more desirable method for these patients. Unfortunately, although such methods are available, they are not widely accessible and diagnostic standards remain in evolution.

Clinical Studies of Sinus Node Autonomic Control

Disturbances in sinus node autonomic control, either alone or in conjunction with structural sinoatrial disease, can result in the clinical and ECG features of sinus node dysfunction ("extrinsic" sinus node disease discussed earlier). The potential role of the central nervous system in causing or exacerbating apparent disturbances of sinus node function may be evaluated through assessment of the following:

1. The nature of the bradycardic responses to carotid sinus massage, Valsalva maneuver, cough, or pharmacologically induced hypertension (e.g., phenylephrine administration)
2. The appropriateness of the tachycardic response to upright tilt or pharmacologically induced hypotension (e.g., amyl nitrite or nitroprusside administration)
3. The heart rate response to pharmacologic interventions such as β-adrenergic blockade, β-adrenergic stimulation, parasympathetic muscarinic blockade (atropine infusion), or parasympathetic enhancement (i.e., parenteral edrophonium).

Through the use of these various physical and pharmacologic interventions, one can attempt to determine, at least qualitatively, whether sinus node responsiveness is appropriate. Unfortunately, for many of these tests, the normal response is poorly defined. Consequently, such studies have not gained widespread clinical use. Nevertheless, they may be useful to assess the basis of sinus node dysfunction in specific patients. In this regard, the assessment of intrinsic heart rate (IHR; sinus node rate in the absence of neural control) by pharmacologic autonomic blockade has become relatively widely used.

The measurement of IHR was introduced for sinus node evaluation in the late 1970s by Jordan and associates.[12] Propranolol (0.2 mg/kg is slowly administered intravenously (~1 mg/min), after which 0.04 mg/kg atropine is similarly infused slowly. The subsequent observed sinus rate becomes temporarily independent of autonomic parasympathetic-muscarinic and β-adrenergic influences. The resulting rate is then characterized as the observed IHR (IHR_o). Normal values for IHR are predicted (IHR_p) from the linear regression obtained by Jose and Collison[106]:

$$IHR_p = 118.1 - (0.57 \times \text{age [in years]})$$

with a 95 percent confidence limit of ±14 percent for patients younger than 45 years and ±18 percent for patients older than 45 years.

A comparison of IHR_o to IHR_p provides an estimation of the contribution of autonomic influences to heart rate at a given time[5] and has been used as a relatively noninvasive stand-alone assessment of sinus node function.[61, 64, 107–109]

Invasive Electrophysiologic Testing

A number of invasive electrophysiologic techniques have been developed with the objective of identifying sinus node dysfunction in symptomatic patients. However, despite years of development and study, the use of invasive electrophysiologic testing as either a diagnostic tool or a means for predicting the need for treatment in patients with sinus node dysfunction remains limited.[5, 110, 111]

Overdrive Atrial Pacing Studies

The phenomenon of overdrive suppression of cardiac pacemakers has been recognized for more than 100 years. In the early 1970s, Mandel and associates[112] proposed that the assessment of the magnitude of overdrive suppression could be useful in distinguishing abnormal from healthy sinus node function. In essence, the time taken for sinus node activity to return after the termination of a period of rapid "overdrive" atrial pacing could be used as a means of assessing sinus node function (i.e., the sinus node recovery time [SNRT]). This procedure has been the subject of considerable clinical study, and despite its limitations, the overdrive atrial pacing technique remains the most widely used invasive assessment of sinus node function (Fig. 84–5).

Several factors affect the SNRT measurement. First, the degree of sinus node suppression achieved by an overdrive atrial pacing train depends not only on the intrinsic automaticity of the principal sinus node pacemaker cells (the subject of most clinical interest) but also on the number of pacing impulses entering and depolarizing the node, the relative effects of stimulation on local acetylcholine and norepinephrine release, and the overall hemodynamic impact of a prolonged period of atrial pacing (i.e., baroreceptor effects, influence of circulating catecholamines). Furthermore, the SNRT measurement itself includes two principal conduction intervals: the time required for the atrial impulse to enter the "sinus node" region and depolarize the active pacemaker site, and the time taken by the recovering sinus impulse to leave the node and become apparent in the atrium (recall that activity within the sinus node cannot be readily recorded and consequently is assessed by inference). In addition, SNRT is dependent on the patient's sinus cycle length at time of study and on the magnitude of sinus arrhythmia present.[113]

To establish normal values and permit interpatient com-

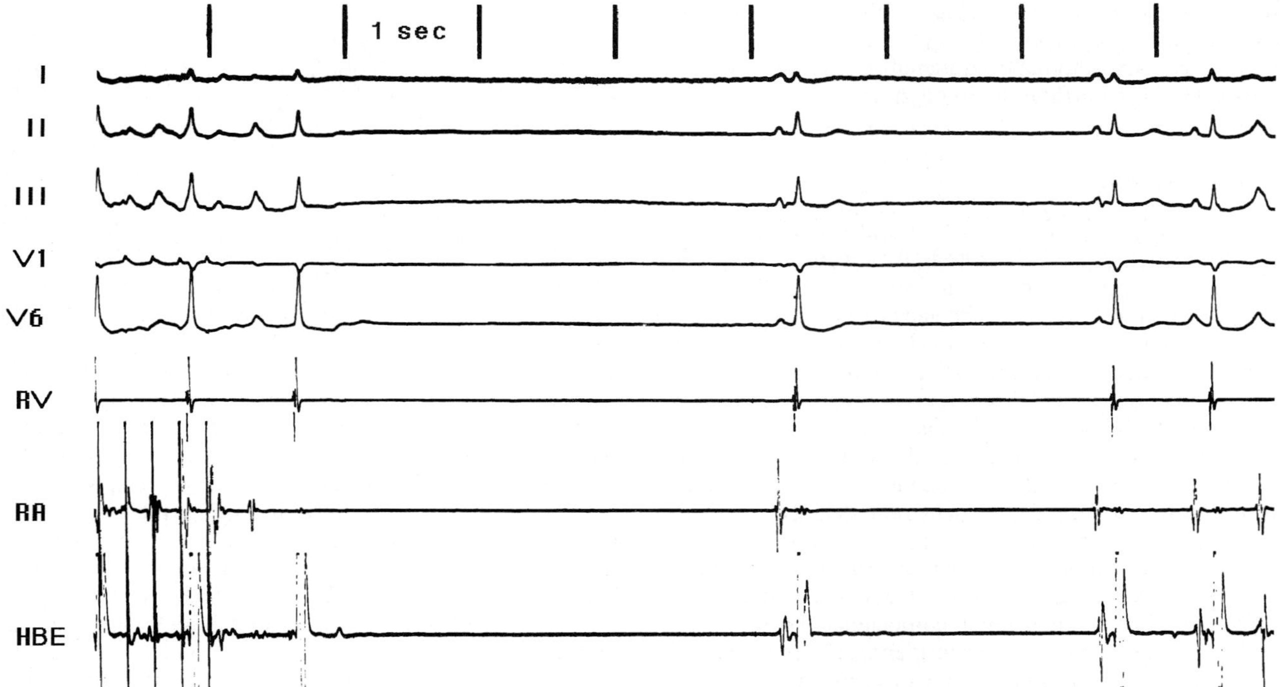

FIGURE 84–5 Electrocardiographic and intracardiac tracings illustrate a prolonged pause after the termination of a period of overdrive atrial pacing (i.e., measurement of the sinus node recovery time). A "secondary" pause is present in the second recovery cycle. HBE, His bundle electrogram; RA, right atrium; RV, right ventricle.

parisons, several approaches have been suggested to "correct" SNRT (corrected SNRT [CSRT]) and thus to take into account some of the many variables at play, especially baseline sinus cycle length (SCL) and degree of sinus arrhythmia. Most commonly, SCL correction is obtained by subtracting the baseline SCL from SNRT:[114]

$$\text{CSRT} = \text{SNRT} - \text{SCL baseline}$$

where normal CSRT is less than 525 ms (several "normal" values may be found in the literature, but this is the value most often used in clinical studies).

An alternative "correction" method entails the expression of SNRT as a ratio of the spontaneous sinus cycle length. Thus, Benditt and colleagues[113] determined the upper limit of normal SNRT to be 1.61 times the baseline SCL for patients with an SCL of less than 800 milliseconds and 1.83 times the baseline SCL for patients with an SCL of more than 800 milliseconds. In addition, the latter study provided a technique, albeit somewhat cumbersome, for incorporating a correction to account for sinus arrhythmia.

Although infrequently used in clinical practice, the technique of direct sinus node electrogram recording with the use of conventional intracavitary electrode catheters has provided additional insight into SNRT/CSRT measurements. Gomes and associates[115] observed that SNRT values determined with direct sinus node electrogram recordings tended to be shorter than those obtained through the conventional measurement of atrial signals (direct $SNRT_{max}$, 989 ± 304 ms; indirect $SNRT_{max}$, 1309 ± 356 ms). Moreover, conduction time out of the node of the first recovery beat was longer than that for control sinus beats, and more than 80 percent of patients manifested evidence of either sinus node suppression (56 percent) or sinus node acceleration (26 percent) as a result of the pacing train. In addition, Asseman and colleagues[116] demonstrated the occurrence of "nonconducted" sinus node electrograms during postpacing atrial pauses (i.e., undetected sinoatrial exit block may confound interpretation of SNRT recordings). Therefore, SNRT/CSRT as determined in most laboratories must be viewed as a composite assessment of sinus node automaticity, pacemaker site shifts, and sinoatrial conduction. In disease states, disturbances of any or all of these electrophysiologic characteristics of the sinus node pacemaker complex may account for a prolonged postpacing recovery time.

Secondary Pauses After Rapid Atrial Pacing

In addition to the duration of the first recovery cycle after the termination of rapid atrial pacing, unexpected prolongation of subsequent postpacing cycles has proved to be a highly specific indicator of sinus node dysfunction (see Fig. 84–5). Benditt and associates[113] developed diagnostic criteria for the identification of abnormal prolongation of the second through tenth postpacing cycles (secondary pauses). This technique increases the value of atrial overdrive pacing by permitting the identification of abnormal responses after the termination of rapid atrial pacing in individuals in whom the first postpacing cycle (SNRT) is normal. However, again, the method is cumbersome and is used infrequently.

Sinoatrial Conduction Time

An assessment of the time taken for an impulse arising in the principal pacemaker cells of the sinus node region to exit the sinus node region and activate the atrium (thereby becoming manifest to conventional recording techniques) has been proposed as a marker for sinus node disease (i.e., SACT). Several indirect and direct techniques have been developed to characterize SACT during clinical electrophysiologic studies.[18, 79, 80, 117, 118]

The atrial extrastimulus method was the first systematic approach to the estimation of SACT and remains the most widely used. This technique uses timed premature extrastimuli (A1–A2) introduced near the sinus node region during sinus rhythm (A1–A1). With the insertion of A2, the sequence of sinoatrial activation is reversed for one cycle. Ignoring the adverse effect of the retrogradely conducted premature impulse on the suppression of intrinsic sinus node automaticity, the return cycle (A2–A3) will be equal to A1–A1 plus an interval equal to the time required for A2 to enter the node plus the time taken for the next sinus impulse to exit the node and result in A3. Therefore, the total conduction time into and out of the sinus node region can be estimated as:

$$\text{SACT a} + \text{r} = (\text{A2–A3 interval}) - (\text{A1–A1 interval})$$

where a is antegrade direction (sinus node to atrium), and r is retrograde direction (atrium to sinus node).

In practice, responses to multiple atrial extrastimuli scanning the atrial (A1–A1) cycle (usually inserted every 8 to 10 sinus cycles) are examined and averaged to calculate the SACT a + r values. The initial extrastimulus coupling interval is set just shorter than the basic SCL and is progressively reduced to 10- and 20-ms decrements until the cardiac cycle has been scanned and atrial refractoriness has been reached. The A2–A3 responses are "normalized" with respect to the immediately preceding A1–A1 interval to account for SCL variation and are plotted (on the ordinate) against the normalized atrial extrastimulus coupling interval (A1–A2/A1–A1) (Fig. 84–6).

An alternative approach to the indirect estimation of SACT involves the analysis of the sinus return cycle after the termination of relatively brief atrial pacing trains (usually 8 to 16 beats) at rates preferably no more than 5 or 10 beats/min faster than the intrinsic sinus rate.[117] The interval between the last paced atrial electrogram and the next atrial activation of sinus node origin is assumed to compose the sum of the basic SCL and SACT a + r. An average of three to five estimations is usually made to calculate SACT a + r.

A relatively close correlation between SACTs determined with the constant atrial pacing technique and those estimated with the premature atrial extrastimulus method has been reported by Narula and colleagues,[117] whereas others have noted discrepancies.[118] In any event, although the constant atrial pacing technique offers the advantage of simplicity, its limitations and those of the atrial extrastimulus method are essentially the same[119]: the methods are indirect, pacing (either single extrastimulus or train) may fail to capture the principal pacemaker site, pacing may suppress sinus node automaticity or shift the principal pacemaker site (or both), and the measurements are critically dependent on the regularity of the basic SCL.

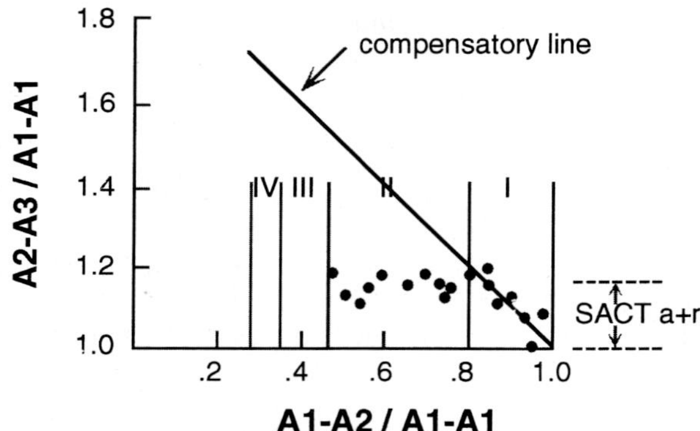

SACT a+r = sinoatrial conduction time into and out of the sinus node

FIGURE 84–6 Graphic representation illustrates the manner in which the atrial extrastimulus technique is used to estimate (indirectly) the sinoatrial conduction time (SACT). SACT a+r is generally calculated by taking an average of the points in the plateau phase (in this case averaging approximately 1.18) and multiplying this number by the average A1-A1 cycle length.

Techniques for in vivo sinus node electrogram recording, and thereby direct measurement of SACT, have been devised.[120–122] However, measurement may be difficult to obtain in the presence of rapid heart rates (e.g., in children[123] or when preceding T waves merge with the P wave of interest (e.g., prolonged repolarization, marked first-degree heart block). In addition, the procedure is time consuming, with success rates ranging from 50 percent in early studies to perhaps 80 percent as experience develops with the method. Nevertheless, although direct SACT measurements tend to be longer than indirect measurements, the two methods tend to correlate well.

Sinus Node Effective Refractory Period

Estimation of refractoriness of sinus node cells or sinoatrial junctional tissue has been proposed as a clinically useful test to assess sinus node function during electrophysiologic testing. However, an assessment of the refractoriness of these tissues cannot be carried out in a conventional manner because techniques for reliable direct stimulation and recording of sinus node pacemaker sites in human subjects have yet to be developed. As a result, an indirect sinus node effective refractory period (SNERP) measurement made with an extrastimulus technique has been evaluated as a clinical tool.

The SNERP method takes advantage of certain aspects of atrial extrastimulus testing discussed above. Specifically, relatively late atrial extrastimuli induced during electrophysiologic testing can enter the sinus node and reset it, whereas very early atrial extrastimuli may be blocked in sinoatrial tissues and the subsequent expected sinus beat emerges on time. This zone of interpolation occurs when the entering atrial impulse encroaches on the refractory period of the preceding sinus beat.[124, 125] Consequently, an estimate of SNERP can be obtained.

Initial studies of the clinical usefulness of SNERP measurements indicated a potentially useful difference between SNERP values in patients with and without known sinus node dysfunction.[126, 127] However, the method has not proved to be particularly popular in clinical electrophysiology laboratories and is mainly used in research.

Clinical Usefulness of Electrophysiologic Testing in Assessment of Sinus Node Function

The ability of electrophysiologic testing to confirm the presence of sinus node disease in patients in whom electrocardiographic documentation is already available has yielded variable results. Pooling findings from various studies suggest that the sensitivity (test positives/true positives) and specificity (test negatives/true negatives) of a combined testing procedure (i.e., incorporating both $CSRT_{max}$ and SACT) to be 70 and 90 percent, respectively.[125, 128–131] Therefore, the most commonly used electrophysiologic tests of "sinus node function" lack the necessary sensitivity to serve as adequate screening tools but, on the other hand, are relatively specific.

Equal in importance to the detection of sinus node disease during electrophysiologic testing is the determination of whether it is the cause of the patient's symptoms. Unfortunately, the use of electrophysiologic testing in this regard can be inferred only indirectly by examining the frequency with which symptoms have been suppressed in patients in whom therapy was directed on the basis of the findings of abnormal sinus node function test results. To date, combined findings from studies in patients with syncope indicate that when test results suggest sinus node dysfunction, the therapy selected was appropriate in 40 to 50 percent of cases.[132, 133] However, certain limitations must be considered in interpreting these results. First, symptom status in patients with syncope and dizziness is notoriously variable. Second, methodologic differences among studies bring into question the validity of pooling observations. Finally, results from comparable asymptomatic control groups are not available.

A third desirable attribute of sinus node function studies would be the capacity to predict whether cardiac pacing would be beneficial in symptomatic patients experiencing dizziness, syncope, or both. In the classic report by Gann and associates,[134] 30 of 68 symptomatic patients had prolonged $CSRT_{max}$ values, and 25 of 26 of these patients who agreed to pacemaker implantation obtained symptomatic relief. Of the 38 symptomatic patients with normal $CSTR_{max}$, pacemakers were eventually placed in 16 (of whom symptoms were suppressed in 12 of 16), and spontaneous resolution of symptoms occurred in 17 patients; 5 patients remained undiagnosed. Therefore, although an abnormal $CSRT_{max}$ value in a symptomatic patient tended to suggest that cardiac pacing would be beneficial, a normal $CSRT_{max}$ value did not exclude this possibility. Furthermore, although this may be the most important study to address the predictive value of sinus node function testing, it did not provide direct evidence that it was the pacemaker that provided the "cure."

The value of atrium-based pacing therapy for both optimizing hemodynamics and reducing susceptibility to atrial tachyarrhythmias has become increasingly accepted. Where possible, atrial pacing alone offers this benefit at lesser cost (although care must be taken to avoid excessive PR interval prolongation with atrial single chamber pacing). If atrial pacing is being considered, the stability of intact AV conduction over the long term becomes an important concern. In this regard, the new onset of clinically significant concomitant AV conduction system disturbance probably is not nearly as common a problem as was previously believed.[135–140] Nevertheless, characterization of AV conduction during electrophysiologic testing may help to facilitate appropriate selection of pacing mode (i.e., single-chamber atrial [AAI/AAIR] versus dual-chamber [DDD/DDDR]). Electrophysiologic assessment documenting a normal H-V interval and 1:1 AV conduction to heart rates in the range of 140 beats/min suggests that atrial pacing (usually AAIR mode) may be safe, physiologic, and cost effective in a given patient (again, bearing in mind potentially undesirable excessive PR interval prolongation). In the absence of normal AV conduction, dual-chamber pacing (DDD or DDDR modes) is a better choice. Finally, evaluation of the status of ventriculoatrial conduction may be useful in programming dual-chamber pacing systems. Specifically, the absence of ventriculoatrial conduction permits the maintenance of a relatively short atrial refractory period and thereby avoids limiting upper rate operation of dual-chamber pacemakers in these patients.

NATURAL HISTORY

An understanding of the natural history of sinus node dysfunction has important implications in regard to lifestyle concerns, potential complications, and treatment strategy. For example, recognition of the importance of embolic complications in patients with sinus node dysfunction is crucial to patient education and provides the justification for treatment programs encompassing both stabilization of the atrial rhythm and anticoagulant prophylaxis.

Mortality Rates

Five- to 10-year survival statistics appear to be similar both in patients with sinus node dysfunction and in patients with other severe conduction system disease.[141–145] Thus, when mortality statistics in patients with sinus node dysfunction were compared with those in otherwise well age- and sex-matched control subjects, Skagen and Hansen[144] concluded that patients with sinus node disease exhibit a 4 to 5 percent excess annual mortality rate in the first 5 years of follow-up. However, among patients with sinus node dysfunction who had no other coexisting disease at the time of initial diagnosis, mortality rates did not differ significantly from those observed in control subjects. The findings of Shaw and colleagues[145] were similar. On the other hand, among other patients with sinus node dysfunction who had a variety of concomitant illness (primarily acute and chronic cardiovascular disease), mortality rates were markedly higher; the latter group exhibited a 4-year survival rate of 40 percent versus a rate of 85 percent for patients with sinus node dysfunction who had no coexisting disease and 91 percent for control subjects.

Sutton and Kenny[135] calculated overall survival statistics for patients with sinus node dysfunction of 85 to 92 percent at 1 year, 62 to 65 percent at 5 years, and 52 percent at 7 years. However, certain forms of sinus node dysfunction appear to have a worse prognosis than others.[74] Sinus bradycardia is reported to be more benign than sinus pauses/arrest, whereas bradycardia-tachycardia syndrome has a more disconcerting outlook.

Differences in natural history among the various forms of sinus node dysfunction may in large part reflect the relative risk for thromboembolic complications. Although concomitant cardiac and renal disease importantly affect mortality rates in patients with sinus node dysfunction, systemic embolism is the most frequent and potentially preventable cause of death. Embolic events (primarily cerebrovascular embolism) are reported to account for 30 to 50 percent of deaths in these patients,[84, 146–148] a finding that may diminish given the increasingly widespread use of long-term anticoagulant therapy and greater attention to atrium-based pacing systems when the use of cardiac pacemakers is indicated.[149]

Conduction System Disturbances

The presence of clinically significant concomitant AV block at the time of diagnosis of sinus node dysfunction and the incomplete understanding of the propensity for conduction system disease to develop or worsen over time in such patients have been the subjects of considerable concern. Sutton and Kenny[135] used the presence of one or more of the following criteria as indicative of conduction system involvement: P-R interval of more than 0.24 second, complete bundle branch block, development of Mobitz I second-degree AV block during atrial pacing at heart rates of 120 beats/min or higher, H-V interval prolongation, or spontaneous appearance of second- or third-degree AV block. Among the more than 1800 patients included in the studies that the authors reviewed, approximately 17 percent manifested conduction system disease based on these broad criteria at time of diagnosis of sinus node dysfunction. However, high-grade AV block was reported in only 5 to 10 percent of cases. Importantly, in studies in which follow-up was available, only approximately 8 percent of patients developed new conduction system disturbances during a mean follow-up time of 34.2 months (approximately 2.7 percent per year).

These statistics indicate that the frequency with which AV conduction system disease develops during follow-up in sinus node dysfunction patients is low but not zero. However, in interpretation of the clinical implications of even this low progression rate, the acuteness with which such disturbances develop and the possibility of predicting their occurrence are important considerations. Findings such as those of Rosenqvist and associates[150] and Stangl and associates[147] suggest that the rate with which conduction system involvement progresses is usually both slow and detectable by careful periodic clinical and electrocardiographic follow-up. In the former report,[150] only 1 of 30 patients with sinus node disease followed over a 5-year period developed high-grade AV block (i.e., less than 1 percent incidence of progression per year), and that patient had marked H-V interval prolongation on entry into the study. Similarly, Stangl and colleagues[147] found that only 6 of 110 patients followed for 52 ± 28 months exhibited conduction disease progression. In most cases, the progression was minor (third-degree AV block, 0 patients; Mobitz II second-degree AV block, 1 patient; first-degree AV block, 5 patients). Furthermore, it appears that susceptibility to subsequent conduction system involvement is essentially independent of the features of sinus node dysfunction.[129] Thus, only 1 of 17 patients with primarily bradycardia developed high-grade AV block during 36-month follow up (~2 percent per year) compared with 3 of 22 patients with bradycardia-tachycardia who were followed for 53 months (~3.1 percent per year). Van Mechelen and associates[151] noted that the deterioration of AV conduction system performance in sinus node dysfunction patients (as assessed by serial estimation of the atrial paced rate at which Mobitz type I second-degree AV block was observed) appeared to correlate closely with the use of antiarrhythmic drugs. Finally, in an important prospective study of atrial versus ventricular pacing, Andersen and colleagues[138, 139] estimated the annual risk of AV block to be approximately 0.6 percent.

In summary, single-chamber atrial pacing can be safe and highly effective for the treatment of patients with sinus node dysfunction. Catastrophic bradycardia does not appear to be an issue even among those individuals who develop significant AV conduction disturbances. The exclusion of patients with baseline H-V interval prolongation, diligent electrocardiographic follow-up, and careful control of exposure of patients to antiarrhythmic drugs may substantially diminish the risk for untoward conduction system complications and facilitate the safe use of atrial pacing techniques in patients in whom cardiac pacing is indicated.[149] On the other hand, the disadvantages of atrial pacing must be kept in mind when weighing single- versus dual-chamber modes. Most important, excessive P-R interval prolongation may occur as the atrial pacing rate increases (i.e., during sensor-driven increased atrial rate). This may lead to a form of "pacemaker syndrome" as atrial contraction impinges on the still-closed AV valves from the previous heart beat.

Arrhythmia Progression

Relatively little is known about the natural history of progression of arrhythmic states in patients with sinus node disease. Vardas and colleagues[152] indicated that among patients with resting sinus bradycardia and normal CSRT, chronotropic responsiveness was well preserved during an approximate 4-year follow-up. On the other hand, the deterioration of chronotropic response was common in patients with sinus bradycardia and very abnormal CSRT (>1000 ms). Comparable studies of the tendency for sinus bradycardia to progress to sinus pauses or bradycardia-tachycardia syndrome would be of interest. In this regard, however, the report by Gann and associates[134] provides some insight. These investigators followed the clinical course of 103 patients with persistent sinus bradycardia during a mean duration of 4.6 years. All patients had corrected sinus node recovery time measurements (CSRT) made at entry into the study. Thirty-five patients were initially asymptomatic, and of these individuals, the CSRT was normal in 24 and abnormal in 11. During follow-up, 14 of the 35 patients (40 percent) ultimately required pacemaker implantation (7 of 24 with normal initial CSRT and 7 of 11 with abnormal CSRT). Therefore, it appears that bradyarrhythmias progress in severity in a substantial proportion of patients with sinus node dysfunction, and CSRT measurements may help to define a high-risk subset.

In 21 studies reviewed by Sutton and Kenny,[135] atrial fibrillation was present at the time sinus node disease was diagnosed in 79 of 958 patients (8.2 percent). During a mean follow-up of 38.2 months, the new onset of atrial fibrillation was 15.8 percent overall (~5.2 percent/year). However, during approximately the same follow-up duration, the onset of atrial tachyarrhythmias occurred in only 3.9 percent in atrially paced patients compared with 22.3 percent in ventricularly paced patients.

Thromboembolic Complications

Thromboembolic complications are a major concern in patients with sinoatrial disease, particularly among those with bradycardia-tachycardia syndrome. The modern era of a more aggressive use of systemic anticoagulation in high-risk patient populations should substantially reduce this propensity with only a slightly increased chance of bleeding problems. Rubenstein and associates[3] reported eight thromboembolic events among 33 such patients followed for an average of 9 years (incidence of ~2.7 percent/year). Similarly, Fairfax and colleagues[84] noted a prevalence rate of thromboembolism of 16 percent among 100 patients with sinoatrial disease (annual incidence of ~1.6 percent) compared with 1.3 percent among 712 age-matched control subjects (~0.13 percent/year). Finally, Sutton and Kenny[135] reported a 15.2 percent overall incidence of thromboembolism among unpaced patients with sinus node dysfunction. Moreover, this incidence was not particularly affected by conventional single-chamber ventricular pacing (~13 percent) but appeared to be markedly diminished in atrially paced patients (1.6 percent). In the Danish prospective pacing trial, the protective effects of atrium-based pacing were clearly confirmed in the population with sinus node dysfunction.[138, 139] During an approximately 8-year follow-up, thromboembolic events were approximately half as frequent in the atrially paced patients (relative risk, 0.47 [0.24–0.92 confidence interval], $P = .023$) compared with patients with ventricular pacing alone.

In summary, the natural history of sinus node dysfunction is relatively well understood in terms of mortality and morbidity but is poorly understood in terms of arrhythmia progression. Essentially, mortality rates in patients with sick sinus syndrome are somewhat greater than those in control subjects of a comparable age. However, if attention is paid to the control of atrial tachyarrhythmias and prevention of thromboembolic complications, much of the difference may be eliminated. Anticoagulation and atrially based pacing are important tools in diminishing morbidity and mortality risk in these patients.

Treatment of Sinus Node Dysfunction

The treatment of patients with sinus node dysfunction must be individualized. In many instances, the electrocardiographic disturbances are an incidental finding and are unassociated with symptoms. In such cases, no therapy is needed. On the other hand, when symptoms do occur, they may be due to either bradyarrhythmias, tachyarrhythmias, or both. Drug or pacemaker therapy, or both, may be warranted. However, treatment must also focus on the avoidance of agents believed to exacerbate arrhythmia in this setting (e.g., alcohol, caffeine, stimulants) and on the control of medical conditions that may aggravate arrhythmia susceptibility (e.g., chronic pulmonary disease, congestive heart failure, hypertension). Finally, the management of patients with sinus node dysfunction must incorporate the prevention of serious complications known to be prevalent in these patients, particularly thromboembolic events.

Drug Therapy in Sinus Node Dysfunction

Drugs are not used to any extent to prevent bradycardia in sinus node dysfunction. Theophylline has been advocated from time to time but is only rarely used for this indication.[153] Similarly, at times, new drugs with positive chronotropic propensities undergo study, but none have proved to be appealing enough to replace cardiac pacing. On the other hand, patients with sinus node disease are commonly exposed to a wide range of agents that may aggravate bradycardia-related symptoms.[5, 14–17, 50–58] For example, cardiac glycosides, β-adrenergic blockers, calcium channel blockers, and membrane-active antiarrhythmic agents used to treat tachyarrhythmias in patients with sinoatrial dysfunction may exacerbate susceptibility to bradycardia.[14–17, 50–55] Similarly, sympatholytic antihypertensives have been shown to accentuate bradyarrhythmias in patients with sinus node dysfunction.[14–17] Finally, certain infrequently used agents, such as radiography contrast materials, lithium carbonate, cimetidine, and adenosine, are known to depress sinus node function, at least transiently.[5, 16, 17, 56–58]

The potential impact of membrane-active antiarrhythmic drugs on sinus node function is particularly important because of the frequency with which older patients are treated with such agents. It should be expected that these drugs will depress both sinus node and subsidiary pacemaker function. However, the severity of antiarrhythmic drug effects on sinus node function is quite variable. For example, quinidine, disopyramide, and, to a lesser extent, procainamide exhibit vagolytic actions that may minimize their direct depressant effects on sinus node tissues. Nevertheless, in patients with sinus node dysfunction, quinidine has been shown to prolong sinus node recovery times and to induce marked bradycardia and asystolic pauses. Similar findings have been reported with disopyramide and procainamide.[154–161] Finally, the so-called type 3 antiarrhythmics (e.g., amiodarone, sotalol, dofetilide) exhibit potent direct depressant membrane actions and, in some cases, antisympathetic effects as well.[162] Amiodarone, in particular, has proved extremely useful for controlling refractory, disabling atrial tachyarrhythmias in sinus node dysfunction patients with bradycardia-tachycardia syndrome. However, many of these patients ultimately exhibit chronotropic incompetence (presumably in part as a result of drug effects on sinus rode function), and cardiac pacing then becomes indicated.

Pacing Therapy

Since the 1960s, pacemakers have progressively evolved into small, sophisticated devices with multiple programmable features and increasingly physiologic operating characteristics. In addition, the overall strategy of cardiac pacing has advanced to incorporate the important concepts of rate adaption, preservation of atrial electrical stability, and maintenance of a normal AV relationship.[101, 135, 138, 139, 149, 150, 163, 164] In addition, the frontier is rapidly progressing to incorporate multiple and selective-site pacing as a means of furthering atrial stabilization.[165–167] In this regard, pacing at several atrial sites either simultaneously or with programmable delays (designed to mimic normal intra-atrial conduction delays) appears to be a promising technique for preventing atrial tachyarrhythmias (particularly atrial fibrillation).

Table 84–1 summarizes current nomenclature for cardiac pacing systems. The earliest pulse generators were designed to pace the ventricles at a fixed rate. This was a life-saving device, and there was no capability to sense native heartbeats (VOO mode). Subsequently, sensing was added, and the device could "inhibit" its output if a native heartbeat occurred (VVI mode). The latter devices could also be used in the atrial position (AOO, AAI), although this did not prove particularly popular due to the inadequacy of atrial leads and the fact that in most cases AV conduction system disease was the primary indication for pacing. Subsequently, dual-chamber pacemakers were developed. These devices were initially large, provided fixed-rate pacing (DVI mode), and continued to lack easily positioned and reliable atrial pacing leads. Device improvements have resulted in sensor-triggered, rate-adaptive single-chamber pacemakers for ventricular or atrial locations (VVIR, AAIR), as well as sophisticated dual-chamber systems that can track native atrial electrical activity (DDD mode) and, when necessary, provide additional sensor-triggered rate adaption (DDDR mode). In addition, the development of pacemaker lead technology has substantially improved the reliability of pacing systems for both atrial and ventricular positions. Furthermore, improvements in pacing algorithms provide options for the device to deal automatically with atrial arrhythmic events (mode switching) or even try to prevent such events (consistent atrial pacing technique, dynamic atrial overdrive).

Among the many advances that have occurred in pacing therapy, the two that have had the greatest impact on the treatment of patients with sinus node dysfunction have been the introduction of increasingly sophisticated rate adaptive capabilities and atrium-based pacing techniques (including multisite atrial pacing). In regard to the former, pacing systems with on-board sensors (often more than one) responsive to physical exertion or other markers of increased metabolic demand have provided a crucial avenue to "normalize" chronotropic responsiveness in patients in whom atrial tracking cannot provide an appropriate paced rate.[101, 163, 164] The importance of atrially based pacing was alluded to earlier. Although most available studies are retrospective in nature, atrially based pacing systems appear to improve overall cardiovascular hemodynamics through the maintenance of a normal AV relationship. The outcome has translated into improved feelings of well-

TABLE 84-1 Pacemaker Function Code (Simplified From NASPE/BPEG Code)

First Letter: Chamber Paced	Second Letter: Chamber Sensed	Third Letter: Response Mode	Fourth Letter*: Sensor Triggered, Rate Responsive	Fifth Letter*: Tachycardia Treatment
V = ventricle A = atrium D = dual (both chambers) S = single (may be O = none; used to indicate either chamber)	V = ventricle A = atrium D = dual	I = inhibited T = triggered D = dual (both I and T) O = none	R = sensor triggered	P = pacing S = shock D = both

Abbreviations: BPEG, British Pacing and Electrophysiology Group; NASPE, North American Society of Pacing and Electrophysiology.
*In detailed NASPE/BPEG versions of this code, there are a number of letters indicated for positions 4 and 5. However, except for R in the fourth position when appropriate, these fourth and fifth letters are rarely used in practice. A separate code has been developed for implantable cardioverter-defibrillators.

being,[164] a reduced incidence of congestive heart failure, and diminished mortality rates[135, 138, 139, 150, 168] compared with ventricular single-chamber pacing. In addition, atrially based pacing appears to diminish the incidence of atrial fibrillation and its attendant thromboembolic complications, as attested to by both retrospective analysis and the prospective Danish study.[138, 139] A recent prospective U.S. study provided a less glowing conclusion regarding the clinical benefits of dual-chamber pacing; however, the findings in that study are colored by the fact that a large crossover (>25 percent) occurred from single-chamber to dual-chamber pacing, and this was not considered fairly when the data were reported.[169]

Optimization of pacemaker therapy is an ongoing process that continues throughout the follow-up period. Therefore, device follow-up must be designed not only to provide safe and reliable pacing by ensuring the adequacy of pacemaker capture and identifying "end-of-life indicators" (i.e., predetermined changes in operating characteristics or telemetered values that indicate impending need for pulse generator/lead replacement) or other system problems but also to evaluate pacing mode and to identify opportunities to adjust programmable parameters to account for evolving clinical circumstances. In many respects, modern pacing systems are beginning to incorporate automatic systems to assist with these important functions.

Indications for Cardiac Pacing in Sinus Node Dysfunction

Guidelines for the implantation of cardiac pacemakers are periodically reviewed and summarized by the American College of Cardiology/American Heart Association Task Force on Assessment of Diagnostic and Therapeutic Cardiovascular Procedures.[170, 171] Indications for pacemaker therapy have been divided into three categories. Class I consists of conditions for which there is general agreement that a cardiac pacemaker should be implanted. Class II incorporates conditions for which pacemakers are frequently used but there may be a divergence of opinion with regard to necessity. Class III consists of conditions for which there is general agreement that a pacemaker is not needed. In the most recent modification of these guidelines, the task force subdivided the class II indications into IIa, where the "weight of evidence/opinion is in favor of usefulness/efficacy," and IIb, where "usefulness/efficacy is less well established by evidence/opinion."

In general, symptomatic bradycardia is the principal indication for cardiac pacemaker implantation. The task force defined "symptomatic bradycardia" as encompassing those "clinical manifestations that are directly attributable to the slow heart rate; transient dizziness, lightheadedness, near syncope or frank syncope as manifestations of transient cerebral ischemia, and more generalized symptoms such as marked exercise intolerance or frank congestive heart failure."[171]

Sinoatrial dysfunction (sick sinus syndrome) is the most commonly cited diagnosis for cardiac pacing in the United States, Canada, and many other Western countries. AV conduction disease is second. Under these circumstances, it is clear that in many candidates for cardiac pacemakers, the tracking of native atrial rates may not provide optimal physiologic chronotropic response due to intrinsic sinoatrial disease. In these individuals, physiologic sensors designed to adjust pacing rate appropriately with physical exertion offer valuable backup. In addition, as noted earlier, there has been a growing appreciation of the importance of providing the paced patient, whenever possible, an atrial pacing component in an attempt to stabilize atrial rhythm and to maintain and normalize the AV relationship. Both of these features can be provided in some patients through the use of single-chamber, sensor-triggered, rate-adaptive pacemakers with a single atrial lead (AAIR mode). Alternatively, in individuals in whom AV conduction is suspect, dual-chamber pacing systems are usually prescribed (DDDR mode).

Innovative Atrial Pacing Methods and Atrial Defibrillation Techniques

Atrial tachyarrhythmias, particularly atrial fibrillation, remain a vexing problem in the treatment of patients with sinus node dysfunction. The combination of pharmacologic and cardiac pacing techniques, when chosen appropriately, appears to reduce susceptibility. However, complete success has yet to be achieved. Potentially, pacing the atrium at multiple sites (e.g., right atrial free wall, right atrial appendage, left atrium) either simultaneously or with programmable delays,[165-167] may further enhance atrial fibrillation prevention by reducing intra-atrial conduction delays. The addition of specialized pacing algorithms, such as "consistent atrial pacing" or "dynamic atrial overdrive," may also diminish tachyarrhythmia susceptibility. Should these methods prove inadequate, however, there has been renewed interest in the development of low-energy implantable atrial defibrillators that may operate in conjunction with conventional or innovative pacing techniques to both diminish risk of atrial fibrillation and treat breakthrough episodes promptly[172–175]

Percutaneous Transcatheter Cardiac Tissue Ablation

Percutaneous transcatheter cardiac tissue ablative techniques have begun to play an important role in tachyarrhythmia control in patients with sinus node dysfunction. His bundle ablation is the most widely accepted of these techniques. Ablation of the bundle of His by electrode catheter technique with the placement of a cardiac pacemaker (so-called ablate-and-pace technique) has proved useful in certain patients with primary atrial tachyarrhythmias refractory to or intolerant of drug therapy.[176] This approach, although perhaps still best reserved for the most difficult to treat patient, has nevertheless been associated with marked amelioration of tachycardia-induced symptoms. In some cases, improvement of left ventricular function (by reversal of tachycardia-induced cardiomyopathic changes) has also been observed. Of course, because His bundle ablation does not eliminate the atrial tachyarrhythmia (usually atrial fibrillation) itself, anticoagulation remains a necessity.

Permanent elimination of arrhythmia susceptibility is the ultimate objective of ablation. In patients with typical atrial flutter, ablation of the isthmus region between the inferior vena cava orifice and the tricuspid valve annulus has been very effective in curing the patient by permanently blocking a segment of atrial tissue critical for the macroreentrant rhythm to sustain itself.[177, 178] Success rates for cure of atrial flutter exceed 90 percent in most centers (although some of these same patients may still be susceptible to atrial fibrillation). Based on the pioneering surgical experience for treatment of atrial fibrillation,[179, 180] development of techniques for transcatheter ablation of atrial fibrillation itself has been of increasing interest. Focal ablation, particularly to critical sites in the pulmonary veins, has been effective in some cases, whereas linear ablation lines causing segmentation of the atria have eliminated atrial fibrillation in other cases (so-called catheter maze procedure).[181–183] However, more investigative work remains to be done before ablation of atrial fibrillation can be claimed to be a standard approach to the treatment of this arrhythmia.

In summary, percutaneous transcatheter ablation of the bundle of His (primarily using radiofrequency energy) followed by permanent cardiac pacing remains the most valuable ablation tool for achieving symptomatic relief in patients with refractory primary atrial tachyarrhythmias. In such cases, the placement of a rate-adaptive pacing system provides a controlled heart rate capable of the appropriate adjustment for level of physical activity. Anticoagulation remains essential for the prevention of thromboembolic complications.

CONCLUSION

Sinus node dysfunction is a very common and multifaceted syndrome. Its origins may be multifactorial and usually are not readily identified in individual patients. The diagnosis is established as a result of the electrocardiographic manifestations. Electrophysiologic testing in the clinical laboratory has specific but limited utility in most cases. Treatment strategy is largely dictated by symptoms and electrocardiographic findings. However, an important focus is that of reducing thromboembolic complications by preserving organized atrial electrical activation in conjunction with anticoagulation. The anticoagulation strategy is well supported in the literature. The importance and feasibility of maintaining atrial electrical stability are the subject of large trials (e.g., AFFIRM), as well as smaller, more defined studies.[184] Treatment should place a high priority on diminishing symptoms of exertional intolerance by providing appropriate chronotropic support when indicated and enhancing survivorship using the principles of physiologic pacing therapy in conjunction with prudent concomitant pharmacologic interventions.

REFERENCES

1. Ferrer MI: The sick sinus syndrome in atrial disease. JAMA 206:645, 1968.
2. Ferrer MI: The sick sinus syndrome. Circulation 47:635, 1973.
3. Rubenstein JJ, Schulman CL, Yurchak PM, DeSanctis RW: Clinical spectrum of the sick sinus syndrome. Circulation 46:5, 1972.
4. Bigger JT Jr, Reiffel JA: Sick sinus syndrome. Annu Rev Med 30:91, 1979.
5. Benditt DG, Milstein S, Goldstein MA, et al: Sinus node dysfunction: pathophysiology, clinical features, evaluation, and treatment. *In* Zipes DP, Jalife J (eds): Cardiac Electrophysiology: From Cell to Bedside. pp. 708–734. Philadelphia: WB Saunders, 1990.
6. Brooks CM, Lu H-H: The Sinoatrial Pacemaker of the Heart. Springfield, IL: Charles C Thomas, 1972.
7. Strauss HC, Prystowsky EN, Scheinman MM: Sino-atrial and atrial electrogenesis. Prog Cardiovasc Dis 19:385, 1977.
8. Anderson RH, Yen HS, Becker AE, Gosling JA: The development of the sinoatrial node. *In* Bonke FM (ed): The Sinus Node: Structure, Function and Clinical Relevance. pp. 166–182. The Hague: Martinus Nijhoff, 1978.
9. Bouman LN, Mackaay AJC, Bleeker WK, Becker AE: Pacemaker shifts in the sinus node: effects of vagal stimulation, temperature and reduction of extracellular calcium. *In* Bonke FIM (ed): The Sinus Node: Structure, Function and Clinical Relevance. pp. 245–257. The Hague: Martinus Nijhoff, 1978.
10. Bonke FIM, Kirchhoff CJHJ, Allessie MA, Wit AL: Impulse propagation from the S-A node to the ventricles. Experientia 43:1044, 1987.
11. Boineau JP, Canavan TE, Schuessler RB, et al: Demonstration of a widely distributed atrial pacemaker complex in the human heart. Circulation 77:1221, 1988.
12. Jordan JL, Yamaguchi I, Mandel WJ: Studies on the mechanism of sinus node dysfunction in the sick sinus syndrome. Circulation 57:217, 1978.
13. Desai JM, Scheinman MM, Strauss HC, et al: Electrophysiologic effects of combined autonomic blockade in patients with sinus node disease. Circulation 63:953, 1981.
14. Scheinman MM, Strauss HC, Evans GT, et al: Adverse effects of sympatholytic agents in patients with hypertension and sinus node dysfunction. Am J Med 64:1013, 1978.
15. Seipel L, Both A, Breithardt G, et al: Action of antiarrhythmic drugs on His bundle electrogram and sinus node function. Acta Cardiol 18(suppl):251, 1974.
16. Benditt DG, Benson DW Jr, Dunnigan A, et al: Drug therapy in sinus node dysfunction. *In* Rapaport E (ed): Cardiology Update-1984. pp. 79–101. New York: Elsevier, 1984.

17. Strauss HC, Scheinman MM, LaBarre A, et al: Review of the significance of the drugs in the sick sinus syndrome. *In* Bonke FM (ed): The Sinus Node: Structure, Function and Clinical Relevance. pp. 103–111. The Hague: Martinus Nijhoff, 1978.
18. Strauss HC, Bigger JT Jr, Saroff AL, Giardina EGV: Electrophysiologic evaluation of sinus node function in patients with sinus node dysfunction. Circulation 53:763, 1976.
19. Miller HC, Strauss HC: Measurement of sinoatrial conduction time by premature atrial stimulation in the rabbit heart by constant atrial pacing technique. Circulation 60:597, 1979.
20. Prystowsky EN, Grant AO, Wallace AG, Strauss HC: An analysis of the effects of acetylcholine on conduction and refractoriness in the rabbit sinus node. Circ Res 44:112, 1979.
21. Thormann J, Schwarz F, Ensslen R, Sesto M: Rolle des Vagotonus bei der symptomatischen Sinusknotendysfunktion. Z Kardiol 67:323, 1978.
22. Santinelli V, Chiariello M, Clarizia M, Condorelli M: Sick sinus syndrome: the role of hypervagatonia. Int J Cardiol 5:532, 1984.
23. Davies MJ, Pomerance A: Quantitative study of ageing changes in the human sinoatrial node and internodal tract. Br Heart J 34:150, 1972.
24. Strasberg B, Sclarovsky S, Arditti A, et al: Deep inspiration induced sinus arrest: an unusual manifestation in a patient with the sick sinus syndrome. J Electrocardiol 19:91, 1986.
25. Jordan J, Yamaguchi J, Mandel WJ: Characteristics of sinoatrial conduction in patients with coronary artery disease. Circulation 55:569, 1977.
26. Engel TR, Meister SG, Feitosa GS, et al: Appraisal of sinus node artery disease. Circulation 52:286, 1975.
27. Evans R, Shaw DB: Pathological studies in sinoatrial disorder (sick sinus syndrome). Br Heart J 39:778, 1977.
28. Demoulin J-C, Kubertus HE: Pathological correlates of atrial arrhythmias. *In* Kulbertus HE (ed): Reentrant Arrhythmias: Mechanisms and Treatment. pp. 99–113. Lancaster, England: MTP, 1977.
29. Demoulin J-C, Kulbertus HE: Histopathological correlates of sinoatrial disease. Br Heart J 40:1384 ,1978.
30. Shaw DB, Linker NJ, Heaver PA, Evans R: Chronic sinoatrial disorder (sick sinus syndrome): a possible result of cardiac ischemia. Br Heart J 58:598, 1987.
31. Kaplan BM, Langendorf R, Lev M, Pick A: Tachycardia-bradycardia syndrome (so-called "sick sinus syndrome"). Am J Cardiol 26:497, 1973.
32. Rasmussen K: Chronic sinus node disease: natural course and indications for pacing. Eur Heart J 2:455, 1981.
33. Barak M, Herschkowitz S, Shapiro I, Roguin N: Familial combined sinus node and atrioventricular conduction dysfunction. Int J Cardiol 15:231, 1987.
34. Mehta AV, Chidambaram B, Garrett A: Familial symptomatic sinus bradycardia: autosomal dominant inheritance. Pediatr Cardiol 16:231–234, 1995.
35. Lev M: Aging changes in the human sinoatrial node. Gerontology 9:1, 1954.
36. Becker AE: General comments. *In* Bonke FM (ed): The Sinus Node: Structure, Function, and Clinical Relevance. pp. 212–222. The Hague: Martinus Nijhoff, 1978.
37. Sasaki R, Theilen EO, January LE, Ehrenhaft JL: Cardiac arrhythmias associated with the repair of atrial and ventricular septal defects. Circulation 18:909, 1958.
38. Young D: Later results of closure of secundum atrial septal defect in children. Am J Cardiol 31:14, 1973.
39. Greenwood RD, Rosenthal A, Sloss LJ, et al: Sick sinus syndrome after surgery for congenital heart disease. Circulation 52:208, 1975.
40. Gillette PC, Kugler JD, Garson AT Jr, et al: Mechanisms of cardiac arrhythmias after Mustard operation for transposition of the greater arteries. Am J Cardiol 45:1225, 1980.
41. Driscoll DJ, Offord KP, Feldt RH, et al: Five to fifteen year follow-up after Fontan operation. Circulation 85:469–496, 1992.
42. Paridon SM, Humes RA, Pinsky WW: The role of chronotropic impairment during exercise after the Mustard operation. J Am Coll Cardiol 17:729–732 1991.
43. Kanter RJ, Garson A Jr: Atrial arrhythmias during chronic follow-up of surgery for complex congenital heart disease. Pacing Clin Electrophysiol 20:502–511, 1997.
44. Yabek YM, Jarmakani JM: Sinus node dysfunction in children, adolescents, and young adults. Pediatrics 61:593, 1978.
45. James TN, Marshall TK, Edwards JE: Cardiac electrical instability in the presence of a left superior vena cava. Circulation 54:689, 1977.
46. Scott O, Macartney FJ, Deverall PB: Sick sinus syndrome in children. Arch Dis Child 51:100, 1976.
47. Beder SD, Gillette PC, Garson A Jr, et al: Symptomatic sick sinus syndrome in children and adolescents as the only manifestation of cardiac abnormality or associated with unoperated congenital heart disease. Am J Cardiol 51:1133, 1983.
48. Yabek SM, Dillion T, Berman W, Niland CJ: Symptomatic sinus node dysfunction in children without structural heart disease. Pediatrics 69:590, 1982.
49. Heinz G, Kratochwill C, Schmid S, et al: G. Sinus node dysfunction after orthotopic heart transplantation: the Vienna experience 1987–1993. Pacing Clin Electrophysiol 17:2057–2063, 1994.
50. Falk RH: Proarrhythmia in patients treated for atrial fibrillation or flutter. Ann Intern Med 117:141, 1992.
51. Margolis JR, Strauss HC, Miller HC, et al: Digitalis and the sick sinus syndrome: clinical and electrophysiologic documentation of a severe toxic effect on sinus node function. Circulation 52:162, 1975.
52. Engel TR, Schaal SF: Digitalis in the sick sinus syndrome: the effect of digitalis on sinoatrial automaticity and atrioventricular conduction. Circulation 43:1201, 1973.
53. Narula OS, Vasquez M, Shantha N, et al: Effect of propranolol on normal and abnormal sinus node function. *In* Bonke FIM (ed): The Sinus Node: Structure, Function and Clinical Relevance. pp. 113–128. The Hague: Martinus Nijhoff, 1978.
54. Motte G, Bellanger P, Vogel M, et al: Asystole suivie de choc cardiogenique après injection intraveineuse de verapamil. Ann Cardiol Angeiol 24:157, 1975.
55. Andrivet P, Beasley V, Kiger JP, vu Gnoc C: Complete sinus arrest during diltiazem therapy: clinical correlates and efficacy of intravemous calcium. Eur Heart J 15:350–354, 1994.
56. Montalescot G, Levy Y, Farge D, et al: Lithium causing a serious sinus-node dysfunction at therapeutic doses. Clin Cardiol 7:617, 1984.
57. Wellens HJJ, Cats V, Duren DR: Symptomatic sinus node abnormalities following lithium carbonate therapy. Am J Med 59:285, 1975.
58. Steckler TL: Lithium and carbamazepine-associated sinus node dysfunction: nine year experience in a psychiatric hospital. J Clin Psychopharmacol 14:336–339, 1994.
59. Talano JV, Euler D, Randall WC, et al: Sinus node function: an overview with emphasis on autonomic and pharmacologic consideration. Am J Med 64:773, 1978.
60. Dighton DG: Sinus bradycardia: autonomic influences and clinic assessment. Br Heart J 36:791, 1974.
61. de Marneffe M, Jacobs P, Haardt R, Englert M: Variations of normal sinus node function in relation to age: role of autonomic influence. Eur Heart J 7:662, 1986.
62. Milstein S, Buetikofer J, Lesser et al: Cardiac asystole: a manifestation of neurally-mediated hypotension-bradycardia. J Am Coll Cardiol 14:1626, 1989.
63. Kollai M, Jokkel G, Bonyhay I, et al: Relation between tonic sympathetic and vagal control of human sinus node function. J Auto Nerv Syst 46:273–280, 1994.
64. de Marneffe M, Gregoire JM, Waterschoot P, Kestemont MP: The sinus node and the autonomic nervous system in normals and sick sinus patients. Acta Cardiol 50:291–308, 1995.
65. Yee R, Guiraudon GM, Gardner MJ, et al: Refractory paroxysmal sinus tachycardia: management by subtotal right atrial exclusion. J Am Coll Cardiol 3:400, 1984.
66. Chung EK: Sick sinus syndrome: currert views. Mod Concept Cardiovasc Dis 49:61, 1980.
67. Marmor BM, Black MM: Unusual manifestations of severe sick sinus syndrome. Am Heart J 100:95, 1980.
68. Fowler NO, Fenton JC, Conway GF: Syncope and cerebral dysfunction caused by bradycardia without atrioventricular block. Am Heart J 80:303, 1970.
69. Atrial Fibrillation Investigators: Risk factors for stroke and efficacy of antithrombotic therapy in atrial fibrillation. Arch Intern Med 154:1449–1457, 1994.
70. Brodsky M, Wu D, Denes P, et al: Arrhythmias documented by 24 hour continuous electrocardiographic monitoring in 50 male medical students without apparent heart disease. Am J Cardiol 39:390, 1997.
71. Romano M, Clariia M, Onofrio E, et al: Heart rate, PR, and QT intervals in normal children: a 24-hour Holter monitoring study. Clin Cardiol 11:839, 1988.

72. Bauernfeind RA, Amat-y-Leon F, Dhingra RC, et al: Chronic paroxysmal sinus tachycardia in otherwise healthy persons. Ann Intern Med 91:702, 1979.
73. Pappone C, Stabile G, Oreto G, et al: Inappropriate sinus tachycardia after radiofrequency ablation of para-Hisian accessory pathways. J Cardiovasc Electrophysiol 8:1357–1365, 1997.
74. Cossu SF, Steinberg JS: Supraventricular tachyarrhythmias involving the sinus node: clinical and electrophysiological characteristics. Prog Cardiovasc Dis 41:51–63, 1998.
75. Viitasalo MT, Kala R, Eisalo A: Ambulatory electrocardiographic recording in endurance athletes. Br Heart J 47:213, 1982.
76. Hattori M, Toyama J, Ito A, et al: Comparative evaluation of depressed automaticity in sick sinus syndrome by Holter monitoring and overdrive suppression test. Am Heart J 105:587, 1983.
77. Ector H, Rolies L, De Geest H: Dynamic electrocardiography and ventricular pauses of 3 seconds and more: etiology and therapeutic implications. Pacing Clin Electrophysiol 6:548, 1983.
78. Hilgard J, Ezri MD, Denes P: Significance of ventricular pauses of three seconds or more detected on twenty-four hour Holter recordings. Am J Cardiol 55:1005, 1985.
79. Strauss HC, Grant AO, Scheinman MM, Wallace AG: The use of cardiac stimulation techniques to evaluate sinus node dysfunction. *In* Little RC (ed): Physiology of Atrial Pacemakers. pp. 339–365. Mt. Kisco, NY: Futura, 1980.
80. Strauss HC, Saroff AL, Bigger JT Jr, Giardina EGV: Premature atrial stimulation as a key to the understanding of sinoatrial conduction in man. Circulation 47:86, 1973.
81. Engel TR, Bond RC, Schaal SF: First degree sinoatrial heart block: sinoatrial block in the sick sinus syndrome. Am Heart J 91:303, 1976.
82. Benditt DG, Remole S. Sick sinus syndrome. *In* Kastor J (ed): Arrhythmias. pp. 225–249. Philadelphia: WB Saunders, 1994.
83. Short DS: The syndrome of alternating bradycardia and tachycardia. Br Heart J 16:208–214, 1954.
84. Fairfax AJ, Lambert CD, Leatham A: Systemic embolism in chronic sinoatrial disorder. N Engl J Med 295:190, 1976.
85. Levy S, Lacombe P, Cointe R, Bru P: High energy transcatheter cardioversion of chronic atrial fibrillation. J Am Coll Cardiol 12:514–518, 1988.
86. Levy S, Lauribe P, Dolla E, et al: A randomized comparison of external and internal cardioversion of chronic atrial fibrillation. Circulation 86:1415–1420, 1992.
87. Narula OS: Sinus node re-entry: a mechanism for supraventricular tachycardia. Circulation 50:1114, 1974.
88. Curry PVL, Krikler DM: Paroxysmal reciprocating sinus tachycardia. *In* Kulbertus HE (ed): Re-entrant Arrhythmias: Mechanisms and Treatment. pp. 39–62. Lancaster, England: MTP, 1977.
89. Gomes JAC, Hariman RI, Chowdry IA: New application of direct sinus node recordings in man: assessment of sinus node recovery time. Circulation 70:663, 1984.
90. Yamada T, Fukunami M, Ohmori M, et al: Characteristics of frequency content of atrial signal-averaged electrocardiograms during sinus rhythm in patients with paroxysmal atrial fibrillation. J Am Coll Cardiol 19:559–563, 1992.
91. Sasaki R, Sugisawa K, Tani H, et al: Correlation between initial potentials on a signal-averaged P-wave and indices of electrophysiologic measurements in the right atrium. Jpn Circ J 62:279–283, 1998.
92. Krahn AD, Klein GJ, Norris C, et al: The etiology of syncope in patients with negative tilt table and electrophysiologic testing. Circulation 91:1819–1824, 1995.
93. Stern S, Ben-Shachar G, Tzivoni D, Braun K: Detection of transient arrhythmias by continuous long-term recording of electrocardiograms of active subjects. Israel J Med Sci 6:103, 1970.
94. Crook BRM, Cashman PMM, Stott FD, Raftery EB: Tape monitoring of the electrocardiogram in ambulant patients, with sinoatrial disease. Br Heart J 35:1009, 1973.
95. Johansson BW: Long-term ECG in ambulatory clinical practice. Eur J Cardiol 5:39, 1977.
96. Holden W, McAnulty JW, Rahimtoola SN: Characterization of heart rate response to exercise in the sick sinus syndrome. Br Heart J 40:923, 1978.
97. Valin HO, Edhag KO: Heart rate responses in patients with sinus node disease compared to controls: physiological implications and diagnostic possibilities. Clin Cardiol 3:391, 1980.
98. Chin C-F, Messenger JC, Greenberg PS, Ellestad MH: Chronotropic incompetence in exercise testing. Clin Cardiol 2:12, 1979.
99. Johnston FA, Robinson JF, Fyfe T: Exercise testing in the diagnosis of sick sinus syndrome in the elderly: implications for treatment. 10:831, 1987.
100. Abbott JA, Hirschfeld DS, Kunkel FW, Scheinman MM: Graded exercise testing in patients with sinus node dysfunction. Am J Med 62:330, 1977.
101. Benditt DG, Milstein S, Gornick CC, et al: Sensor-triggered rate-variable cardiac pacing: current technologies and clinical implications. Ann Intern Med 107:714, 1987.
102. Kay GN, Bubien RS, Epstein AE, Plumb VJ: Rate-modulated cardiac pacing based on transthoracic measurements of minute ventilation: correlation with gas exchange. J Am Coll Cardiol 14:1283–1289, 1989.
103. Wilkoff B, Corey J, Blackburn G: Mathematical model of the cardiac chronotropic response to exercise. J Electrophysiol 3:176, 1989.
104. Mianulli MJ: Exercise physiology: relation to physiologic pacing. *In* Benditt DG (ed): Rate-Adaptive Pacing. pp. 69–82. London: Blackwell Scientific, 1993.
105. Mianulli M, Crossley G, Wilkoff B, Benditt DG: The utility and stability of a new automatic rate response algorithm to achieve desired rate behaviour [abstract]. Arch Mal Coeur 91:146, 1998.
106. Jose AD, Collison D: The normal range and the determinants of the intrinsic heart rate in man. Cardiovasc Res 4:160, 1970.
107. Szatmary LJ: Autonomic blockade and sick sinus syndrome: new concepts in the interpretation of electrophysiological and Holter data. Eur Heart J 5:637, 1984.
108. Bhandari S, Talwar KK, Kaul U, Bhatia ML: Value of physical and pharmacological tests in predicting intrinsic and extrinsic sick sinus syndrome. Int J Cardiol 12:203, 1986.
109. Jordan JL, Yamaguchi I, Mandel MJ: Function and dysfunction of the sinus node: clinical studies in the evaluation of sinus node function. *In* Bonke FIM (ed): The Sinus Node: Structure, Function, and Clinical Relevance. pp. 3–22. The Hague: Martinus Nijhoff, 1978.
110. Benditt DG, Gornick CC, Dunbar D, et al: Indications for electrophysiologic testing in the diagnosis and assessment of sinus node dysfunction. Circulation 75(suppl III):III-93, 1987.
111. Rahimtoola SH, Zipes DP, Akhtar M, et al: Consensus statement of the conference on the state of the art of electrophysiologic testing in the diagnosis and treatment of patients with cardiac arrhythmias. Circulation 75(suppl III):III-3, 1987.
112. Mandel WJ, Hayakawa H, Allen HN, et al: Assessment of sinus node function in patients with sick sinus syndrome. Circulation 46:761, 1972.
113. Benditt DG, Strauss HC, Scheinman MM, et al: Analysis of secondary pauses following termination of rapid atrial pacing in man Circulation 54:436, 1976.
114. Narula OS, Samet P, Javier R: Significance of the sinus node recovery time. Circulation 45:140, 1972.
115. Gomes JAC, Kang PS, El-Sherif N: The sinus node electrogram in patients with and without sick sinus syndrome: techniques and correlation between directly measured and indirectly estimated sinoatrial conduction time. Circulation 66:864, 1982.
116. Asseman P, Berzin B, Desry D, et al: Persistent sinus nodal electrograms during abnormally prolonged postpacing atrial pauses in sick sinus syndrome in humans: sinoatrial block versus overdrive suppression. Circulation 68:33–41, 1983.
117. Narula OS, Shanttha N, Vasquez M, et al: A new method for measurement of sinoatrial conduction time. Circulation 58:706, 1978.
118. Breithardt G, Seipel L: Comparative study of two methods of estimating sinoatrial conduction time in man. Am J Cardiol 42:965, 1978.
119. Grant AO, Kirkorian G, Benditt DG, Strauss HC: The estimation of sinoatrial conduction time in rabbit heart by the constant atrial pacing technique. Circulation 60:597, 1979.
120. Reiffel JA, Gang E, Gliklich J, et al: The human sinus node electrogram: transvenous catheter technique and a comparison of directly measured and indirectly estimated sinoatrial conduction time in adults. Circulation 62:1324, 1980.
121. Reiffel JA, Kuehnert MJ: Electrophysiological testing of sinus node function: diagnostic and prognostic application—including updated information from sinus node electrograms. Pacing Clin Electrophysiol 17:349–365, 1994.
122. Juillard A, Guillerm F, Chuong HV, et al: Sinus node electrogram

recording in 59 patients: comparison with simulation. Br Heart J 50:75, 1983.

123. Yabek SM: Electrophysiologic evaluation. *In* Yabek SM, Gillette PC, Kugler JD (eds): The Sinus Node in Pediatrics. pp. 48–88. Edinburgh: Churchill Livingstone, 1984.
124. Langendorf R, Lesser ME, Plotkin P. Levin BD: Atrial parasystole with interpolation: observations on prolonged sinoatrial conduction. Am Heart J 63:649, 1962.
125. Dhingra RC, Wyndham C, Amat-y-Leon F, et al: Sinus nodal responses to atrial extrastimuli in patients without apparent sinus node disease. Am J Cardiol 36:445, 1975.
126. Kerr CR, Strauss HC: The measurement of sinus node refractoriness in man. Circulation 68:1231, 1984.
127. Kerr CR: Effect of pacing cycle length and autonomic blockade on sinus node refractoriness. Am J Cardiol 62:1192, 1988.
128. Gupta PK, Lichstein E, Chadda KD, Badui E: Appraisal of sinus nodal recovery time in patients with sick sinus syndrome. Am J Cardiol 34:265, 1974.
129. Pop T, Fleischmann D: Measurement of sinus node recovery time after atrial pacing. *In* Bonke FM (ed): The Sinus Node: Structure, Function, and Clinical Relevance. pp. 23–35. The Hague: Martinus Nijhoff, 1978.
130. Luderitz B, Steinbeck G, Naumann d'Alnoncourt C, Rosenberger W: Relevance of diagnostic atrial stimulation for pacemaker treatment in sinoatrial disease. *In* Bonke FM (ed): The Sinus Node: Structure, Function and Clinical Relevance. pp. 77–88. The Hague: Martinus Nijhoff, 1978.
131. Seipel L, Breithardt G, Leuner C: Programmed atrial stimulation used for the calculation of sinoatrial conduction time (SACT) in man *In* Bonke FM (ed): The Sinus Node: Structure, Function, and Clinical Relevance. pp. 36–45. The Hague: Martinus Nijhoff, 1978.
132. Hess DS, Morady F, Scheinman MM: Electrophysiologic testing in the evaluation of patients with syncope of undetermined origin. Am J Cardiol 50:1309, 1982.
133. Akhtar M, Shenasa M, Denker S, et al: Role of cardiac electrophysiologic studies in patients with unexplained recurrent syncope. Pacing Clin Electrophysiol 6:192, 1983.
134. Gann D, Tolentino R, Samet P: Electrophysiologic evaluation of elderly patients with sinus bradycardia. Ann Intern Med 90:24, 1979.
135. Sutton R, Kenny RA: The natural history of sick sinus syndrome. Pacing Clin Electrophysiol 9:1110, 1986.
136. Brandt J, Anderson H, Fahreaus T, Schuller H: Natural history of sinus node disease treated with atrial pacing in 213 patients: implications for selection of stimulation mode. J Am Coll Cardiol 20:633–639, 1992.
137. Elshot SRE, El Gamal MIH, Tielen van Gelder BM: Incidence of atrioventricular block and chronic atrial flutter/fibrillation after implantation of atrial pacemakers: follow-up of more than ten years. Int J Cardiol 38:303–308, 1993.
138. Andersen HR, Thuesen L Bagger JP, et al: Prospective randomised trial of atrial versus ventricular pacing in sick-sinus syndrome. Lancet 344:1523–1528, 1994.
139. Andersen HR, Nielsen JC, Thomsen PE, et al: Long-term follow-up of patients from a randomised trial of atrial versus ventricular pacing for sick-sinus syndrome. Lancet 350:1210–1216, 1997.
140. Zanini R, Facchinetti AI, Gallo G, et al: Morbidity and mortality of patients with sinus node disease: comparison of atrial and ventricular pacing. Pacing Clin Electrophysiol 13:2076, 1990.
141. Santini M, Alexidou G, Ansalone G, et al: Relation of prognosis in sick sinus syndrome to age, conduction defects and modes of permanent cardiac pacing. Am J Cardiol 65:729, 1990.
142. Alt E, Volker R, Wirtzfeld A, Ulm K: Survival and follow-up after pacemaker implantation: a comparison of patients with sick sinus syndrome, complete heart block and atrial fibrillation. Pacing Clin Electrophysiol 8:849, 1985.
143. Fisher JD, Furman S, Escher DJW: Pacing in the sick sinus syndrome: profile and prognosis. *In* Feruglio G (ed): Cardiac Pacing, Electrophysiology and Pacemaker Technology. pp. 519–520. Padova: Piccin, 1982.
144. Skagen K, Hansen JF: The long-term prognosis for patients with sinoatrial block treated with permanent pacemaker. Acta Med Scand 199:13, 1975.
145. Shaw DB, Holman RR, Gowers JI: Survival in sinoatrial disorder (sick-sinus syndrome). Br Med J 290:139, 1980.
146. Mond H: The bradyarrhythmias: current indications for permanent pacing: part II. Pacing Clin Electrophysiol 4:538, 1981.
147. Stangl K, Wirtzfeld A, Seitz K, et al: Atrial stimulation (AAI): long-term follow-up of 110 patients. *In* Belhassen B, Feldman S, Copperman Y (eds): Cardiac Pacing and Electrophysiology. Proceedings of the VIIIth World Symposium on Cardiac Pacing and Electrophysiology. Jerusalem: R & L Creative Communications, pp. 283–285, 1987.
148. Hartel G, Talvensaari T: Treatment of sinoatrial syndrome with permanent cardiac pacing in 90 patients. Acta Med Scand 198:341, 1975.
149. Sutton R: Pacing in atrial arrhythmias. Pacing Clin Electrophysiol 13:1823, 1990.
150. Rosenqvist M, Brandt J, Schuller H: Atrial versus ventricular pacing in sinus node disease: a treatment comparison study. Am Heart J 111:292, 1986.
151. van Mechelen R, Segers A, Hagemeijer F: Serial electrophysiologic studies after single chamber atrial pacemaker implantation in patients with symptomatic sinus node dysfunction. Eur Heart J 5:628, 1984.
152. Vardas PE, Fitzpatrick A, Ingram A, et al: Natural history of sinus node chronotropy in paced patients. Pacing Clin Electrophysiol 14:155, 1991.
153. Alboni P, Menozzi C, Brigole M, et al: Effects of permanent pacemaker and oral theophylline in sick sinus syndrome: the THEOPACE study: a randomized controlled study. Circulation 96:260–266, 1997.
154. Strauss HC, Gilbert M, Svenson RH, et al: Electrophysiologic effects of propranolol on sinus node function in patients with sinus node dysfunction. Circulation 54:452 1976.
155. Qi A, Tuna IC, Gornick CC, et al: Potentiation of cardiac electrophysiologic effects of verapamil following autonomic blockade or cardiac transplantation. Circulation 75:888, 1987.
156. Seipel L, Breithardt G: Medical treatment of sinus node disease: antiarrhythmic drugs and sinoatrial conduction *In* Bayes A, Cosin J (eds): Diagnosis and Treatment of Cardiac Arrhythmias. pp. 636–647. New York: Pergamon, 1980.
157. Adams DF, Paulin S: Effect of radiographic contrast media in selective injections into the sinus node artery. Radiology 91:719, 1968.
158. Mason JW, Winkle RA, Rider AK, et al: The electrophysiologic effects of quinidine in the transplanted human heart. J Clin Invest 59:481, 1977.
159. Jeresaty RM, Kahn AH, Landry AB Jr: Sinoatrial arrest in a patient receiving quinidine. Chest 61:683, 1972.
160. Seipel L, Breithardt G: Sinus recovery time after disopyramide phosphate. Am J Cardiol 37:1118, 1976.
161. Josephson ME, Caracta AR, Lau SH, et al: Electrophysiologic properties of procainamide in man. Am J Cardiol 33:596, 1974.
162. Hoffmann A, Kappenberger L, Jost M, Burckhardt D: Effect of amiodarone on sinus node function in patients with sick sinus syndrome. Clin Cardiol 10:451, 1987.
163. Fearnot NE, Smith HJ, Geddes LA: A review of pacemakers that physiologically increase rate: the DDD and rate-responsive pacemakers. Prog Cardiovasc Dis 29:145, 1986.
164. Sulke N, Dritsas A, Bostock J, et al: "Subclinical" pacemaker syndrome: a randomised study of symptom free patients with ventricular demand (VVI) pacemakers upgraded to dual chamber devices. Br Heart J 67:57, 1992.
165. Daubert C, Mabo P, LeClercq C: Physiologic pacing systems for patients with sick sinus syndrome. *In* Benditt DG (ed): Rate-Adaptive Pacing. pp. 151–171. London: Blackwell, 1993.
166. Saksena S, Prakash A, Hill M, et al: Prevention of recurrent atrial fibrillation with chronic dual-site right atrial pacing. J Am Coll Cardiol 28:687–694, 1996.
167. Daubert JC, Pavin D, Victor F, Mabo P: Cardiac pacing for terminating and preventing atrial flutter and fibrillation. *In* Saoudi N, Schoels W, El-Sherif N (eds): Atrial Flutter and Fibrillation: From Basic to Clinical Applications. pp. 293–315. Armonk, NY: Futura, 1998.
168. Hesselson AB, Parsonnet V, Bernstein AD, Bonavita GJ: Deleterious effects of long-term single-chamber ventricular pacing in patients with sick sinus syndrome: the hidden benfits of dual-chamber pacing. J Am Coll Cardiol 19:1542–1549, 1992.
169. Lamas GA, Orav EJ, Stambler BS, et al: Quality of life and clinical outcomes in elderly patients treated with ventricular pacing as com-

pared with dual-chamber pacing. N Engl J Med 338:1097–1104, 1998.
170. Gregoratos G, Cheitlin MD, Conill A, et al: ACC/AHA guidelines for implantation of cardiac pacemakers and antiarrhythmia devices: a report of the American College/American Heart Association Task Force on Practice Guidelines. J Am Coll Cardiol 31:1175–1209, 1998.
171. Dreifus LS, Fisch C, Griffin JC, et al: Guidelines for implantation of cardiac pacemakers and antiarrhythmia devices: a report of the American College of Cardiology/American Heart Association Task Force. Circulation 84:455, 1991.
172. Dunbar DN, Tobler HG, Fetter J, et al: Intracavitary electrode catheter cardioversion of atrial tachyarrhythmias in the dog. J Am Coll Cardiol 7:1015–1027, 1986.
173. Benditt DG, Kriett JM, Tobler HG, et al: Cardioversion of atrial tachyarrhythmias by low energy transvenous technique. *In* Steinbach K (ed): Cardiac Pacing: Proceedings of the VIIth World Symposium on Cardiac Pacing. p. 845. Darmstadt: Steinkopff, 1982.
174. Mirowski M, Mower MM: An automatic implantable defibrillator for recurrent atrial tachyarrhythmias. *In* Touboul P, Waldo AL (ed): Atrial Arrhythmias: Current Concepts and Management. p. 419. St. Louis: Mosby–Year Book, 1990.
175. Cooper RAS, Alferness CA, Smith WM, Ideker RE: Internal cardioversion of atrial fibrillation in sheep. Circulation 87:1673–1676, 1993.
176. Scheinman MM, Evans GT: Catheter electrical ablation of cardiac arrhythmias: a summary report of the percutaneous cardiac mapping and ablation registry. *In* Brugada P, Wellens HJJ (eds): Cardiac Arrhythmias: Where to Go From Here. pp. 529–538. Mt. Kisco, NY: Futura, 1995.
177. Kay GN, Chong F, Epstein AE, et al: Radiofrequency ablation for treatment of primary atrial tachycardias J Am Coll Cardiol 21:901–909, 1993.
178. Lesh MD, Van Hare GF, Epstein LM, et al: Radiofrequency catheter ablation of atrial arrhythmias: Results and mechanisms. Circulation 89:1074–1089, 1994.
179. Cox JL: The surgical treatment of atrial fibrillation, IV: surgical technique. J Thorac Cardiovasc Surg 101:584–592, 1991.
180. Guiraudon G, Klein GJ, Guiraudon CM, Yee R: Surgical treatment of atria fibrillation: what's new. *In* Saoudi N, Schoels W, El-Sherif N (eds): Atrial Flutter and Fibrillation: From Basic to Clinical Applications. pp. 349–360. Armonk, NY: Futura, 1998.
181. Haissaguerre M, Jais P, Shah D, et al: Right and left radiofrequencey catheter therapy of paroxysmal atrial fibrillation. J Cardiovasc Electrophysiol 7:1132–1144, 1996.
182. Gaita F, Riccardi R, Calo L, et al: Atrial mapping and radiofrequency catheter ablation in patients with idiopathic atrial fibrillation: electrophysiological findings and ablation results. Circulation 97:2136–2145, 1998.
183. Haissaguerre M, Jais P, Shah D, et al: Spontaneous initiation of atrial fibrillation by ectopic beats originating in the pulmonary veins. N Engl J Med 339:659–666, 1998.
184. Friedman PA, Hill MRS, Hammill SC, et al: Randomized prospective pilot study of long-term dual-site atrial pacing for prevention of atrial fibrillation. Mayo Clin Proc 73:848–854, 1998.

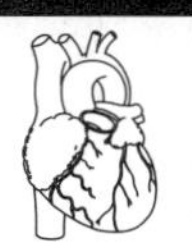

CHAPTER 85

Atrioventricular Nodal and Subnodal Conduction Disturbances

Hein J. J. Wellens

THE ELECTROCARDIOGRAM IN ATRIOVENTRICULAR CONDUCTION DISTURBANCES
NONINVASIVE METHODS TO DETERMINE THE SITE OF ATRIOVENTRICULAR BLOCK
BUNDLE BRANCH BLOCK
Bundle Branch Block in Acute Myocardial Infarction
Chronic Bundle Branch Block

After its origin in the sinus node region, the cardiac impulse is conducted from atrium to ventricle over the atrioventricular (AV) node, the bundle of His, and the bundle branches.

Abnormalities in conduction may occur at any of these levels, alone or in combination.[1] These abnormalities can be the result of developmental anomalies (congenital heart disease), reversible or irreversible interruption of blood supply to the conduction system (Fig. 85–1), inflammatory or infiltrative disease, calcified aortic valve disease, calcified mitral annulus, cardiomyopathy, space-occupying lesions, drug toxicity, abnormalities in electrolyte levels, trauma (also during open heart surgery), and fibrotic changes that occur with aging.[2] Abnormalities in conduction are common in acute myocardial infarction (MI). They are usually transient (not requiring long-term ventricular pacing) and have prognostic implications as to hospital mortality. Their site in the AV conduction system is related to the location of the MI. As shown in Figure 85–1, a branch from the right coronary artery perfuses the AV node. Therefore, AV nodal block may occur in inferoposterior MI caused by an occlusion of the right coronary artery. AV nodal block is a common complication of occlusion of the proximal right coronary artery. As described elsewhere, the location of the obstruction in the coronary artery leading to inferoposterior MI can easily be derived from the additional recording of right precordial leads (Fig. 85–2).[3] In contrast, conduction abnormalities distal to the AV node may occur after a proximal occlusion of the left anterior descending coronary artery. As shown in Table 85–1, both AV nodal and subnodal conduction disturbances in acute MI increase mortality.

A common cause of abnormalities in the AV conduction system is fibrosis of the intraventricular conduction system. The incidence increases with age.[3] This may lead to a primary conduction system disorder and may involve the AV node, the bundle of His, the right bundle branch, and the common part and the fascicles of the left bundle branch.[4]

The ability to record the electrical activity of the bundle

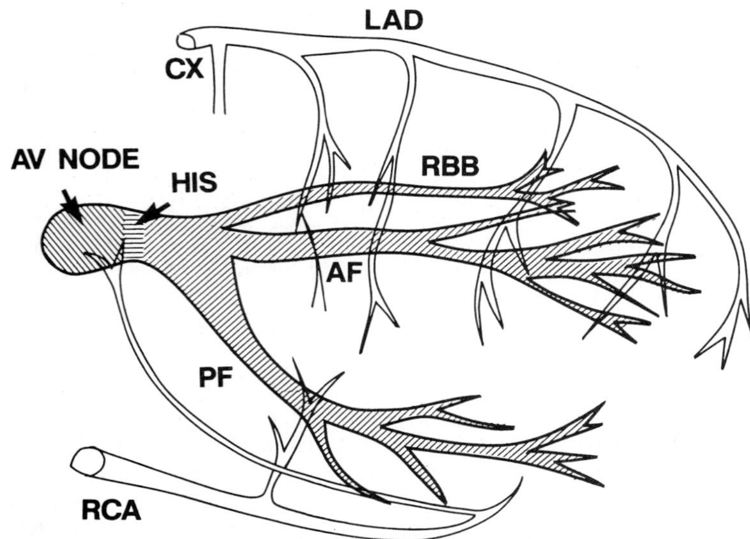

FIGURE 85–1 The components of the atrioventricular (AV) conduction system and the coronary arteries responsible for their blood supply. The AV node is perfused by a branch from the right coronary artery (RCA). The right bundle branch (RBB) and the anterior fascicle (AF) of the left bundle branch are perfused by the left anterior descending (LAD) coronary artery and are therefore vulnerable in anteroseptal myocardial infarction. The posterior fascicle (PF) of the left bundle branch is supplied by both the LAD and the RCA. CX, circumflex.

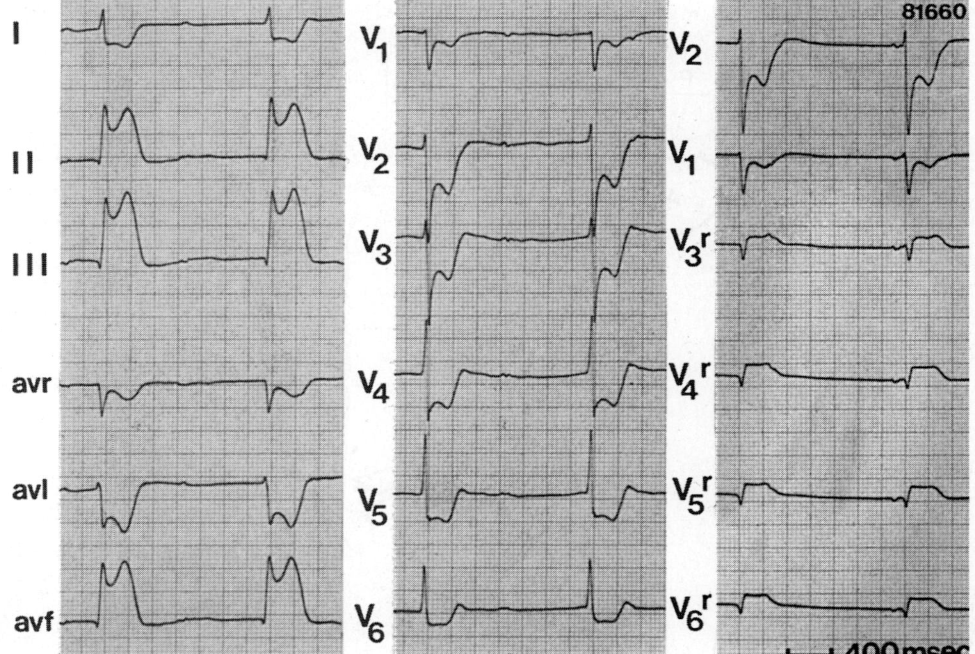

FIGURE 85–2 Example of complete AV nodal block in a patient with an acute inferoposterior myocardial infarction and right ventricular involvement. Right ventricular involvement is indicated by the ST-segment elevation in the right precordial leads. (From Braat SH, Gorgels APM, Bar TW, Wellens HJJ: Value of the ST-T segment in lead V4R in inferior wall acute myocardial infarction to predict the site of coronary artery occlusion. Am J Cardiol 62:140, 1988. With permission from Elsevier Science.)

of His makes it possible to identify the area of block or impaired conduction (Fig. 85–3). As indicated in Figure 85–3, block at the different levels of the AV conduction system is traditionally divided into first-, second-, and third-degree types. First-degree block is characterized by prolonged conduction; each impulse is conducted, but with a longer conduction time than normal. Second-degree block is divided into type 1, characterized by a series of impulses showing progressive lengthening in conduction time, terminated by one blocked impulse; type 2, in which impulses are conducted with a normal or slightly prolonged conduction time until one of the impulses is suddenly blocked; and 2:1 or 3:1 block, in which only every second or third impulse is conducted over the conduction system. In third-degree or complete block, each impulse fails to be conducted through the conduction system. Second-degree type 2 and third-degree or complete heart block are treated with a pacemaker.

TABLE 85-1 Features of Atrioventricular Conduction Disturbances Complicating Acute Myocardial Infarction

Feature	Inferior MI	Anterior MI
Site of block	AV node	Bundle branches
Artery involved	RCA	LAD
Escape rhythm	Narrow QRS Rate 40–60/min Dependable	Wide QRS Rate < 40/min Undependable
Duration of block	Transient	Transient
Increase in hospital mortality (compared with same infarction location block)	2.5 times	4 times

Abbreviations: AV, atrioventricular; LAD, left anterior descending coronary artery; MI, myocardial infarction; RCA, right coronary artery.

Table 85–2 illustrates how common or uncommon these different forms of conduction disturbances are in relation to the different components of the AV conduction system.

THE ELECTROCARDIOGRAM IN ATRIOVENTRICULAR CONDUCTION DISTURBANCES

Figure 85–4 shows an example of type 1 second-degree AV block (Wenckebach's type). The narrow QRS places the conduction abnormality in the AV node. Figure 85–5 gives an example of type 2 second-degree AV block. The QRS complex shows left bundle branch block (LBBB), indicating that the AV block occurred in the right bundle branch. Figure 85–6 shows a 2:1 AV block with a sudden change to complete AV block. The QRS complex on the left reveals complete block in the right bundle branch and the posterior fascicle of the left bundle branch. Two-to-one conduction in the anterior fascicle of the left bundle branch changes into complete block.

NONINVASIVE METHODS TO DETERMINE THE SITE OF ATRIOVENTRICULAR BLOCK

As pointed out, AV block may be located in the AV node, bundle of His, bundle branches, or any combination of these locations (see Fig. 85–2). Because AV nodal block has a better prognosis and treatment differs from that of subnodal block, determination of the location and type of block is important. In this regard, much can be learned on the surface electrocardiogram from the PR interval, the QRS duration, and the response of the block to noninvasive

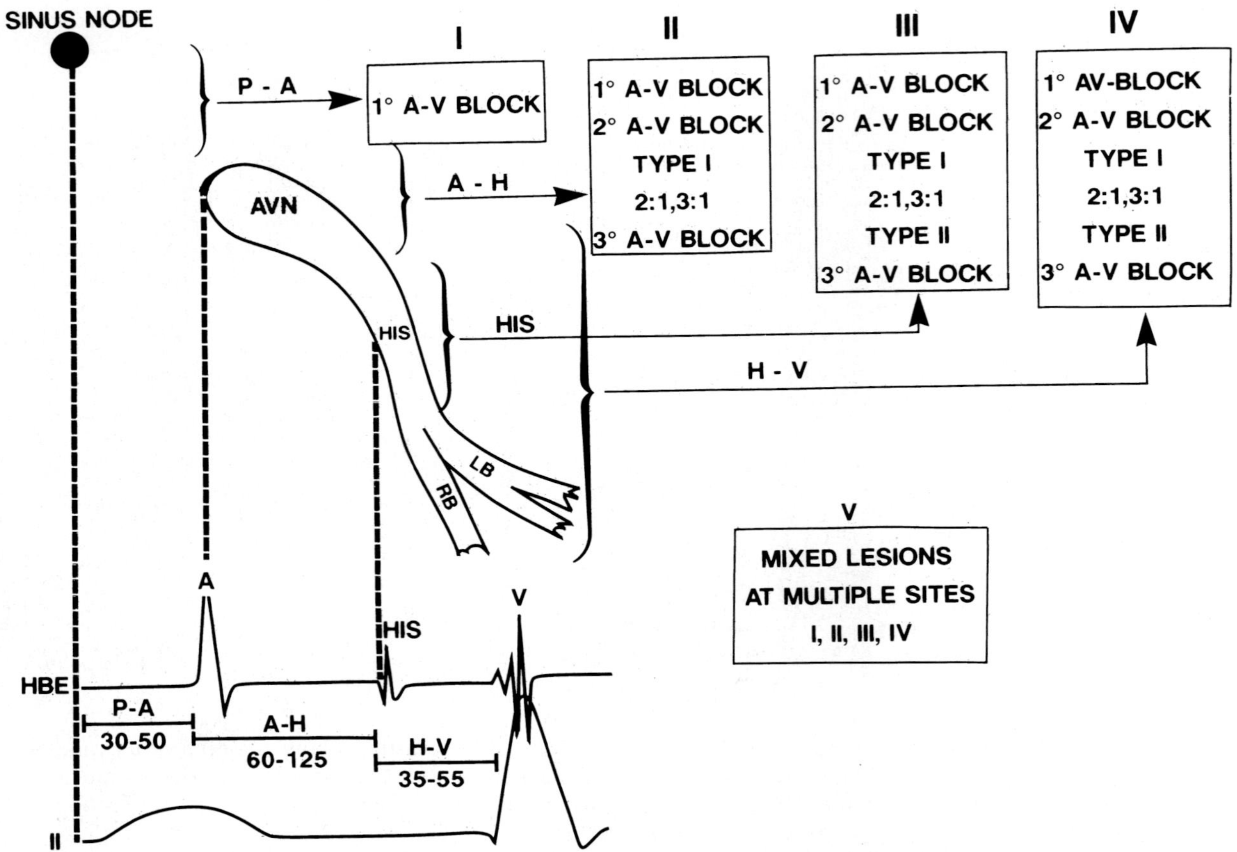

FIGURE 85–3 Location and types of block from the sinus node area to the ventricles and the corresponding measurements in the His bundle electrogram (HBE). In the *left lower portion* of the figure, a His bundle electrogram (ECG) and lead II tracing are schematically shown. The intervals noted are P-A, A-H, and H-V; normal values are shown in milliseconds. P-A interval, from the beginning of the P wave in the ECG to the atrial deflection (A) in the His bundle electrogram; A-H interval, from the atrial deflection to the first deflection of the His bundle (corresponds to A-V nodal transmission time); H-V interval, from the onset of the His bundle deflection to the onset of the ventricular deflection in the His bundle electrogram, indicating the time required to travel from the bundle of His to the ventricles over the bundle branch system. A-V, atrioventricular. (Modified from Narula DS, Scherlag BJ, Samet P, et al: Atrioventricular block localization and classification by His bundle recordings. Am J Med 50:146, 1971.)

interventions, such as atropine, exercise, catecholamines, and vagal maneuvers (Table 85–3).

Interventions that slow AV conduction, such as vagal maneuvers, worsen AV nodal block, but because the number of impulses passing through the AV node declines, such maneuvers improve subnodal block (Fig. 85–7). On the other hand, interventions such as atropine and exercise improve AV nodal conduction, but because of the increase in number of impulses conducted through the AV node, they worsen subnodal conduction. Thus, carotid sinus massage worsens AV nodal block and improves subnodal block; atropine, exercise, and catecholamines improve AV nodal block and worsen subnodal block.

TABLE 85–2 Prevalence of the Different Forms of Conduction Disturbances at Different Sites of the Atrioventricular Conduction System

	First	Second			Third
		Type 1	*Type 2*	*2:1*	
AVN	C	C	N	C	C
His	C	U	C	C	C
Bundle branches	C	U	C	C	C

Abbreviations: AVN, atrioventricular node; C, common; N, virtually never; U, uncommon.

BUNDLE BRANCH BLOCK

There are two major areas of clinical interest in the discussion of prognosis and treatment of bundle branch block: (1) bundle branch block in association with acute MI and (2) chronic bundle branch block in patients with or without symptoms of transient neurologic impairment.

Bundle Branch Block in Acute Myocardial Infarction

As pointed out by Lie and associates[5] in cases of MI, the prognosis depends on whether the bundle branch block is the consequence of the MI or was present before the

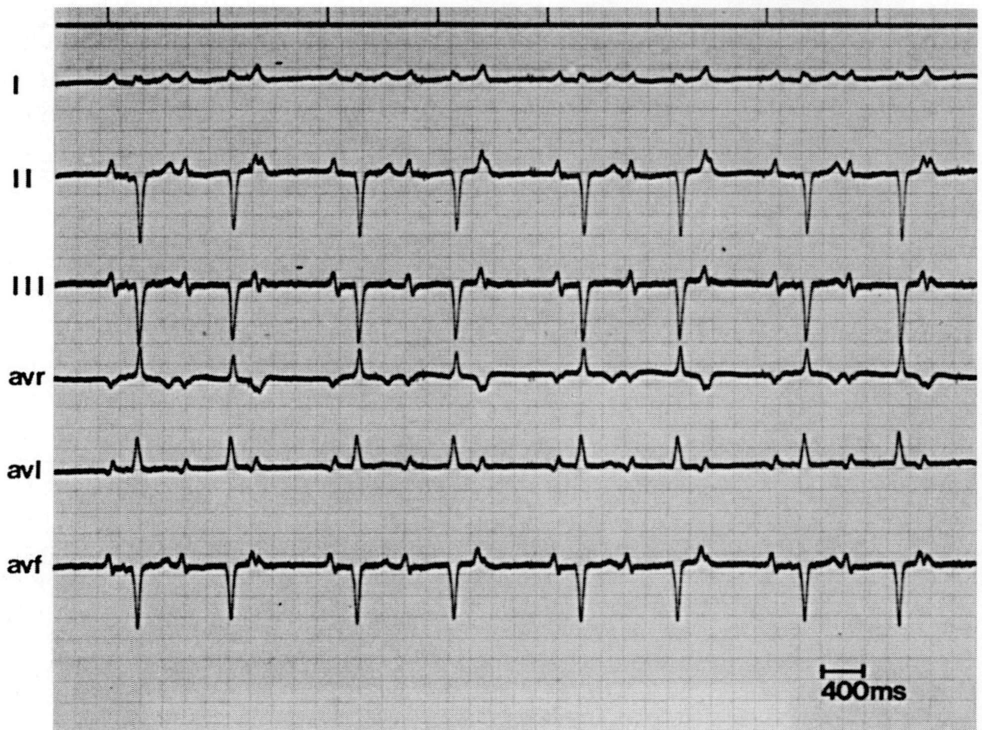

FIGURE 85–4 Type 1 second-degree AV block (Wenckebach's type). After progressive P-R prolongation of the first and second P wave, the third P wave fails to be conducted to the ventricle.

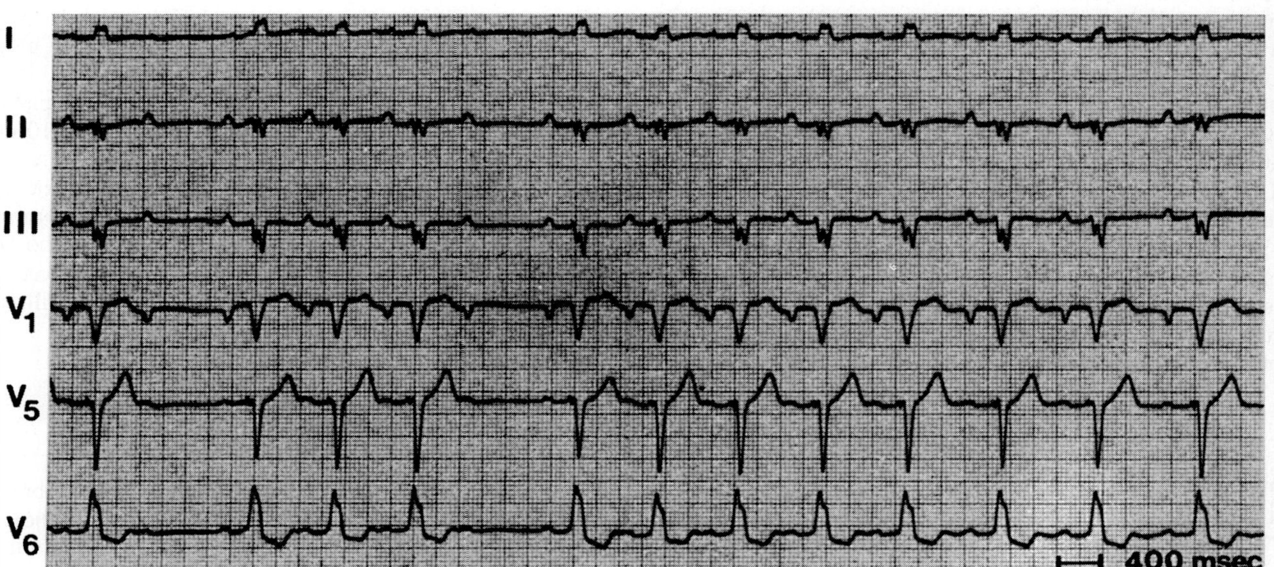

FIGURE 85–5 Type 2 second-degree AV block (Mobitz II). The PR intervals, although prolonged, stay the same before and after the nonconducted P wave. The QRS has a typical left bundle branch block configuration, indicating that the Mobitz II block is located in the right bundle branch.

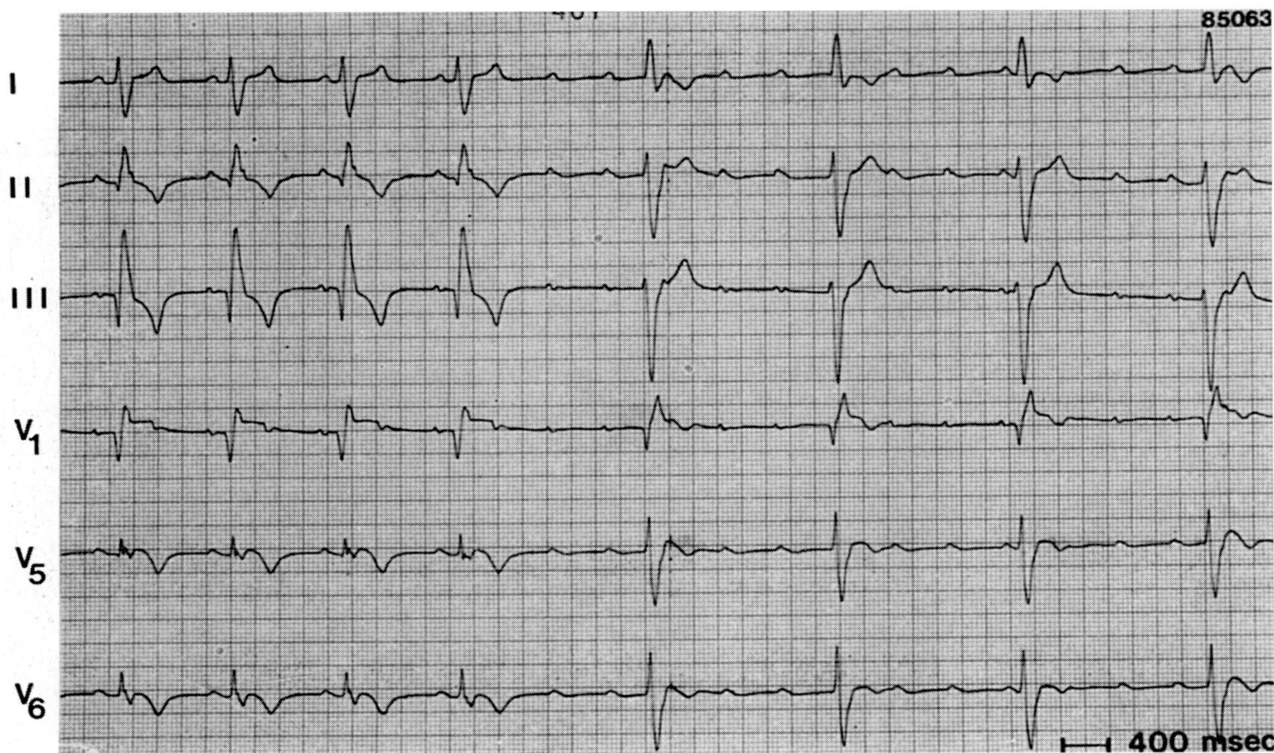

FIGURE 85–6 On the *left,* 2:1 AV block with a QRS configuration, indicating block in the right bundle branch and the posterior fascicle of the left bundle branch. This suddenly changes into complete AV block, with an escape rhythm arising in the left posterior fascicle.

MI. Acquired right bundle branch block (RBBB) is more common in anterior wall MI, and LBBB in inferior wall MI (see Fig. 85–1). The risk of progression to high-degree AV block is lower in old (preexistent) versus new (acquired) bundle branch block.[5] It would be helpful, therefore, to be able to distinguish old from new bundle branch block if bundle branch block is already present on admission. Lie and colleagues[5] pointed out that age greater than 70 years and an rSR rather than a QR pattern in lead V_1 favor preexistent rather than new RBBB (Fig. 85–8). In anterior wall MI, acquired RBBB carries a higher in-hospital mortality than preexistent RBBB.[5] In inferior wall MI, preexistent RBBB does not affect hospital mortality.[5]

The significance of preexistent versus acquired LBBB in association with an acute MI is less clear.[6] LBBB is often a sign of more generalized left ventricular disease and, as such, has more ominous significance than RBBB. If it is not possible to determine a relation between acute MI and bundle branch block, it is useful, especially in patients with anterior MI and bifascicular block (RBBB with anterior or posterior left fascicular block), to make a His bundle recording.[5] In patients with a prolonged HV interval, there is a high risk for development of complete subnodal block, in contrast to patients with a normal HV interval. In patients with acute MI and acquired bundle branch block, hospital mortality is high and is mainly due to failure of pump function.[7, 8] In the absence of prophylactic pacing, complete heart block contributes to approximately 10 percent of the short-term mortality, usually within the first few days.[8] Complete heart block in patients with anterior wall MI is associated with a high mortality, even with prophylactic pacing.[9–11] Patients with this complication who survive pump failure in the acute phase frequently experience sustained ventricular tachycardia and ventricular fibrillation in the first to third week after the onset of MI.[12–14]

TABLE 85–3 Noninvasive Interventions to Determine Site of Atrioventricular Block: Effects on Atrioventricular Conduction

Intervention	AV Nodal Conduction	Subnodal Conduction
Atropine	Improves	Worsens
Exercise or catecholamines	Improves	Worsens
Carotid sinus massage	Worsens	Improves

Abbreviation: AV, atrioventricular.

Treatment of Bundle Branch Block Associated With Acute Myocardial Infarction

The data on the significance of acquired bundle branch block after an MI were obtained in the prethrombolysis and pre–percutaneous transluminal coronary angioplasty period. Development of RBBB signifies a proximal occlusion in the left anterior descending coronary artery and the presence of an extensive anterior wall MI. Reperfusion of that region should therefore be attempted. If thrombolytic therapy fails or is contraindicated, one should try to reopen the coronary vessel by emergency angioplasty. If RBBB with anterior or posterior left fascicular block persists after

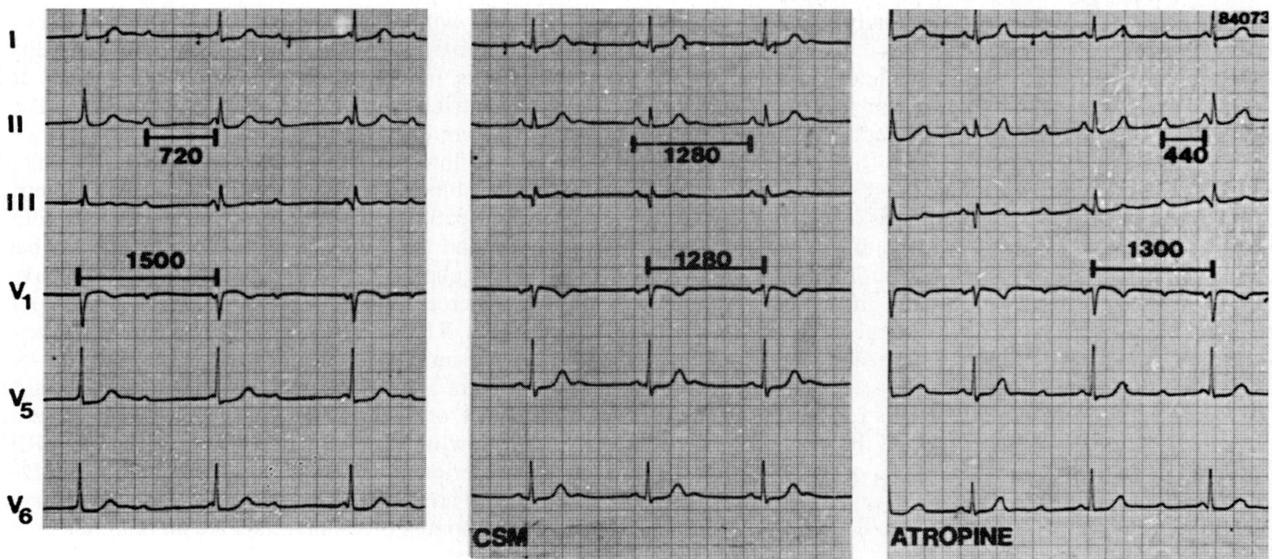

FIGURE 85–7 Example of the value of carotid sinus massage (CSM) and atropine administration in locating the site of block in a patient with complete AV block with a narrow QRS. As shown, slowing of the sinus node by CSM improves AV conduction, whereas atropine worsens conduction. This indicates a sub–AV-nodal location of the block in the bundle of His.

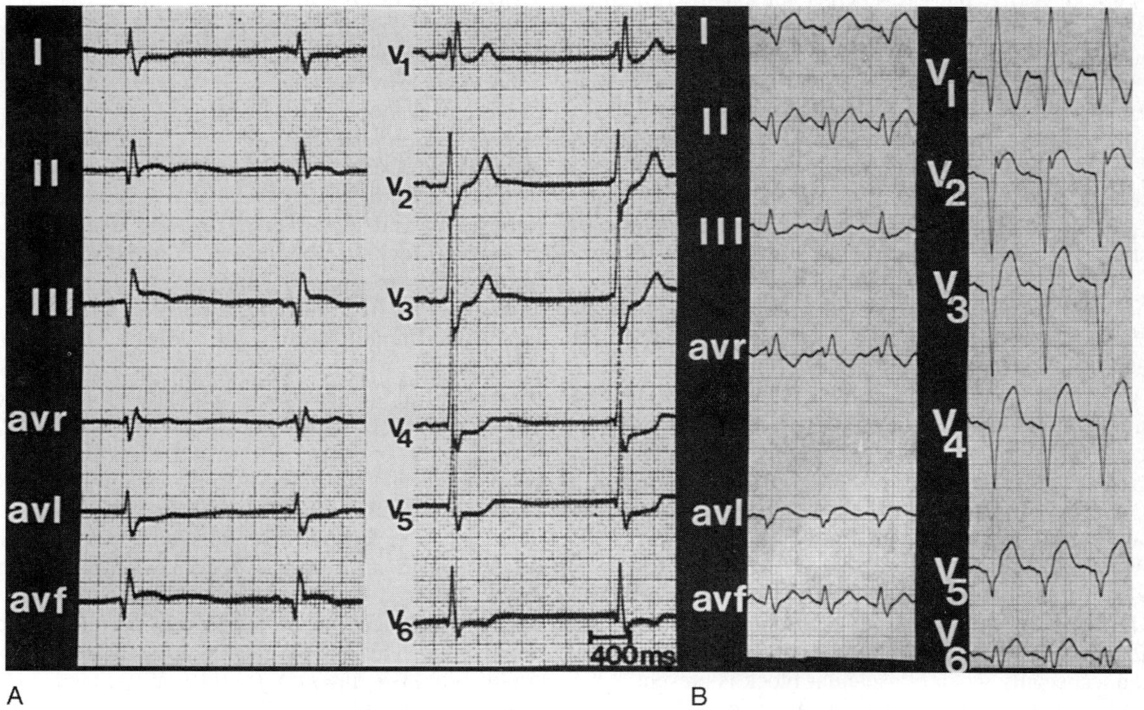

FIGURE 85–8 **A,** Right bundle branch block not caused by myocardial infarction. Note the classic rSR′ pattern in lead V_1 and the qRS pattern in V_6. The patient has an inferior wall infarction. **B,** Right bundle branch block caused by anteroseptal myocardial infarction. Note qR pattern in lead V_1.

reperfusion, temporary prophylactic pacing is recommended. Prophylactic pacing enables a smooth transition to a paced rhythm when complete heart block occurs and avoids the need for cardiopulmonary resuscitation associated with the low ventricular rates usually seen in complete block with anterior infarction.

As pointed out elsewhere, if complete AV block develops, it is usually transient.[5] Permanent pacing should be reserved for patients who have persistent or recurrent high-degree AV block.

A special problem is the patient presenting with acute chest pain and LBBB. First, LBBB masks the characteristic electrocardiographic changes that are diagnostic for acute MI, hampering the use of the electrocardiogram in decision making as to myocardial reperfusion measures. Although occasionally ST-segment changes suggestive of acute MI are present,[15] administration of reperfusion therapy should be based on the clinical impression.[16]

Second, pacing in MI with LBBB is required only if MI occurs in the setting of high-degree AV block. Prophylactic cardiac pacing is not required if LBBB occurs with 1:1 AV conduction.

Chronic Bundle Branch Block

Bundle branch block is a common finding, and the incidence increases with age.[17] With the exception of LBBB, males are more frequently affected than females.[18] The prognostic significance varies in relation to the type of patient studied, and it increases when the chance finding of bundle branch block in the community is compared with that in the asymptomatic and symptomatic hospital patient.[19] In general, prognosis is determined by the overall cardiac status of the patient rather than by bundle branch block alone. In treating a patient with chronic bundle branch block, several questions should be answered.

Frequently, bundle branch block is accompanied by significant pathologic changes in the intraventricular conduction system.[4] Widespread fibrosis is often present, especially if there is an associated hemiblock.[3] Many diseases can cause chronic impairment of intraventricular conduction, including coronary artery disease, hypertension, aortic valve disease, idiopathic degenerative diseases of the conduction system, and cardiomyopathy. In the young population, bundle branch block is rare, especially LBBB. The presence of the latter should raise the suspicion for underlying heart disease. RBBB may occur in congenital cardiac disease, such as atrial septal defect, but is frequently not accompanied by associated heart disease and in such cases has an excellent prognosis.

In older patients with RBBB, clinical cardiovascular disease is present in 50 percent, according to a general population survey,[17] rising to about 80 percent in a hospital population, especially when bifascicular block is present.[20, 21] LBBB has an even higher incidence of associated cardiac disease.[17, 22] The prognosis for patients with chronic bundle branch block is primarily determined by the presence and the type of associated cardiovascular disease. McAnulty and colleagues[20] reported a cumulative mortality after 3 years of 56 percent and 20 percent, respectively, in hospitalized patients with coronary artery disease with or without a previous MI. The same authors[20] found a 3-year cumulative mortality of 26 percent in patients with valvular heart disease and bundle branch block. In community surveys, a lower mortality rate is found than in the hospital inpatient or outpatient population.[17, 23, 24]

In patients with bundle branch block, death occurs suddenly in approximately 50 percent of the total mortality. In those patients in whom the terminal rhythm was documented, ventricular tachyarrhythmias were found more commonly than complete block with asystole.[20, 25]

There is a low incidence of progression to documented complete AV block, and it is therefore difficult to determine such risk in patients with bundle branch block in relation to the type and the cause of their conduction disturbance. In a general population study, Kulbertus and coworkers[18] found a 2 percent incidence of complete heart block in patients with RBBB and left anterior hemiblock after a mean follow-up period of 3 years. In a hospital-based series, Dhingra and colleagues[21] found a 7 percent cumulative incidence of documented complete heart block after 5 years of follow-up in patients with bifasciular block (RBBB with left anterior or left posterior hemiblock and LBBB). Rarely, there are electrocardiographic findings in patients with bundle branch block that indicate an ominous prognosis, such as alternating bundle branch block (Fig. 85–9) and paroxysmal AV block.[26]

The hope that information on the AV conduction system obtained by using His bundle recordings and atrial pacing would help in predicting risk for complete block in the asymptomatic patient with bundle branch block, with or without accompanying hemiblock, has not been fulfilled. Most studies did not find a correlation between a prolonged HV interval and the development of complete block.[20, 27] Only patients with documented transient AV block or syncope in whom ventricular tachyarrhythmias and noncardiac causes of syncope can be excluded have a high incidence of progression to complete block in cases of prolonged HV interval.[28–31] Occasionally, electrophysiologic study can be useful in asymptomatic patients with bundle branch block. Scheinman and coworkers[32] reported a high incidence of complete block in patients with an H-V interval of 100 milliseconds or greater. Dhingra and colleagues[33] pointed to the prognostic value of the development of block distal to the His bundle during 1:1 AV nodal conduction with atrial pacing at rates less than 140 beats/min. Rarely, it is possible to induce complete subnodal block by electrically inducing atrial or ventricular premature beats (Fig. 85–10).

A special problem is the patient with bundle branch block and syncope but no documentation of bradycardia. In these patients, other causes for syncope must be excluded.[31] After this has been done and prolonged electrocardiographic monitoring has not revealed bradyarrhythmias, an electrophysiologic study should be performed. If high-degree AV block can be induced, a permanent pacemaker is indicated. This should also be done in case of a markedly prolonged H-V interval (>100 milliseconds). If no AV block is inducible and the H-V interval is not severely prolonged, programmed stimulation should be performed in the ventricle to exclude sustained ventricular tachycardia as the cause of syncope.

The patient with paroxysmal AV block presents a diagnostic challenge. Characteristically, these patients experience periods of asystole on reaching a critical duration of the P-P interval; this may occur after a premature (atrial,

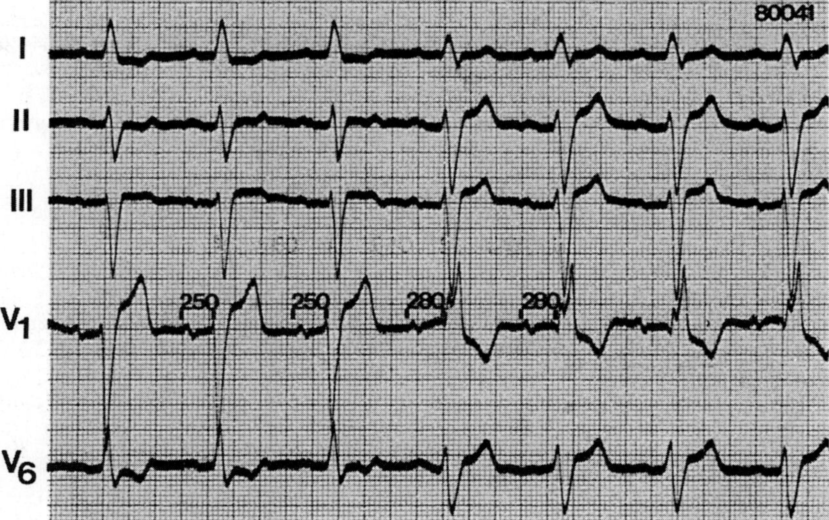

FIGURE 85–9 Example of alternating bundle branch block. The left part of the figure shows sinus rhythm with left bundle branch block and a PR interval of 250 msec. This suddenly changes into right bundle branch block with a PR interval of 280 msec.

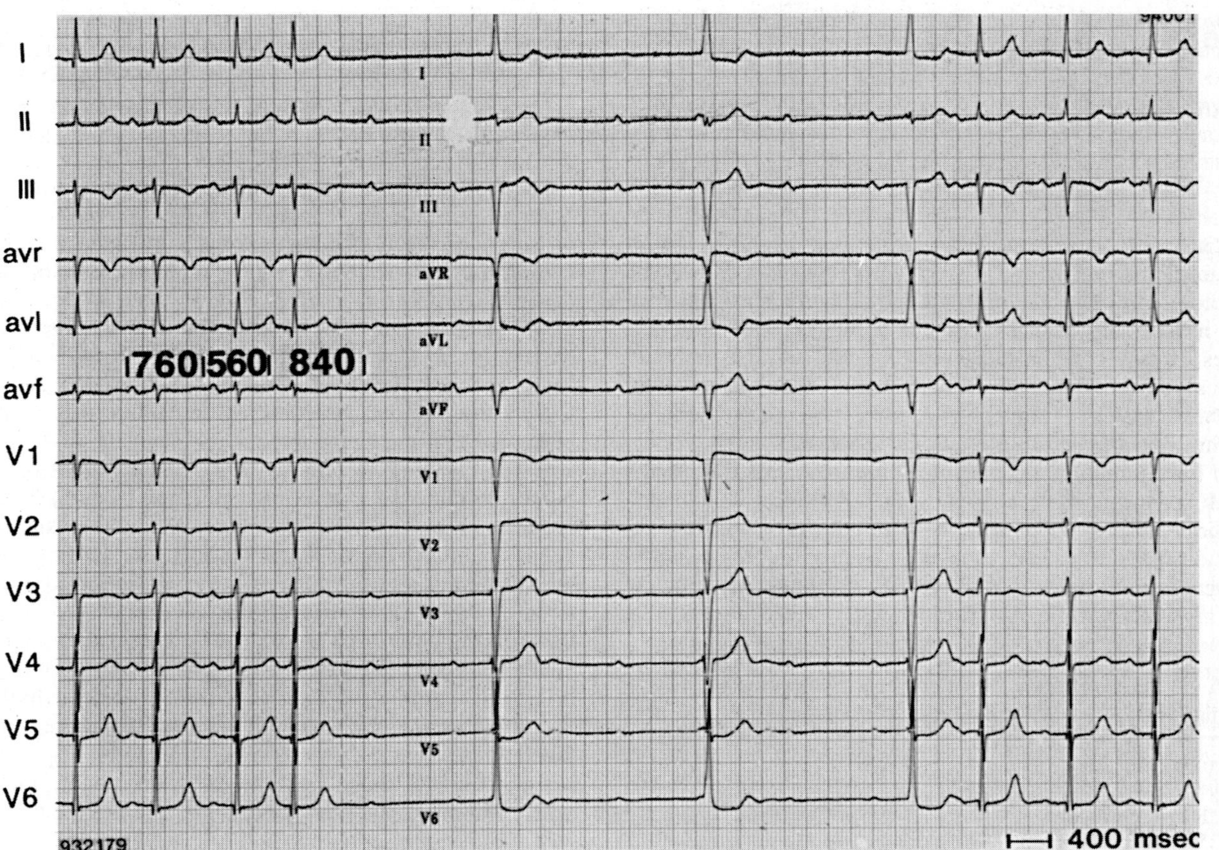

FIGURE 85–10 Paroxysmal complete AV block after a conducted atrial premature beat (occurring after 560 msec during sinus rhythm) is followed by an interval to the next sinus P wave of 840 msec. This P-P interval is sufficiently long to induce local phase 4 depolarization in the bundle of His, resulting in complete AV block for subsequent atrial impulses. The escape rhythm shows a narrow QRS complex, indicating an origin high in the specific AV conduction system.

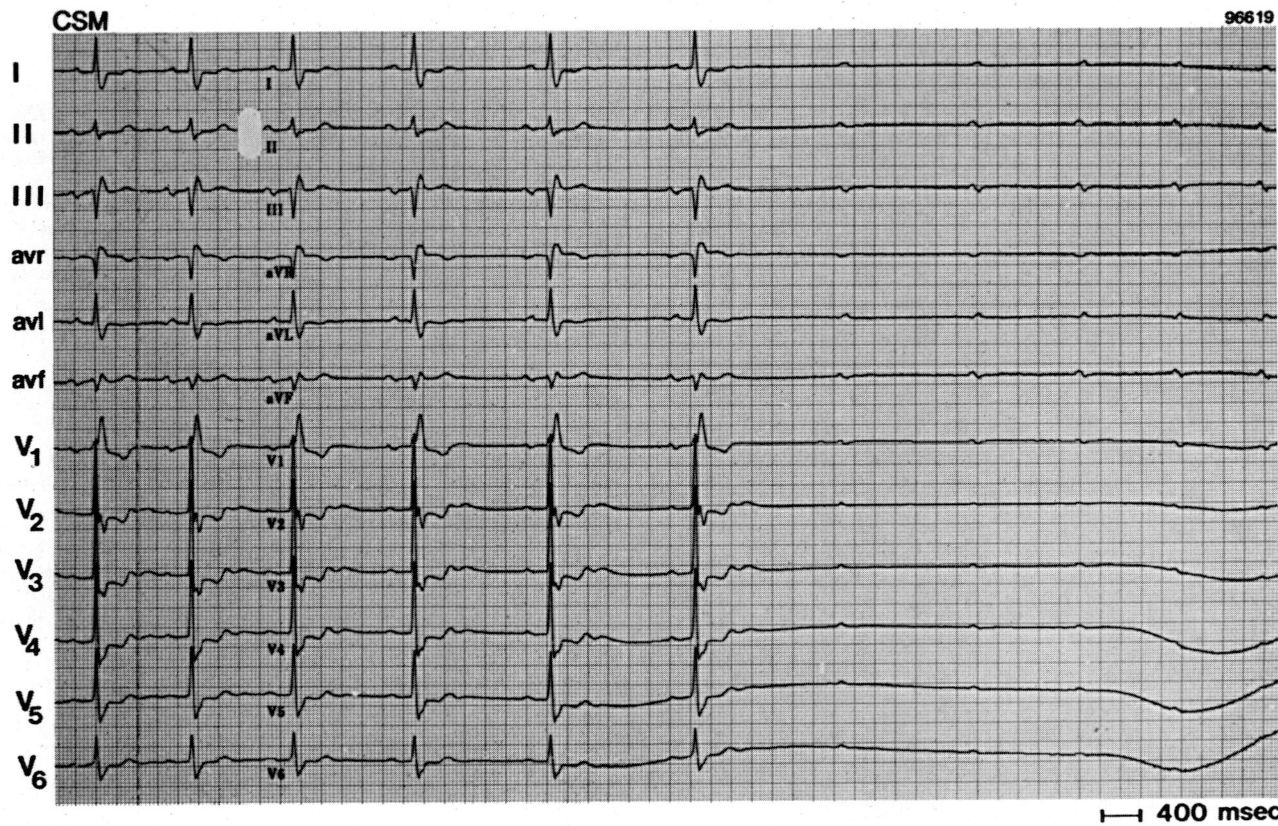

FIGURE 85–11 Paroxysmal complete AV block on reaching a critical length of the P-P interval during carotid sinus massage. Note that there is no change in PR interval up to the moment of complete AV block, indicating that the block is not in the AV node. Local phase 4 depolarization in the left bundle branch is responsible for this type of AV block.

AV junctional or ventricular) beat (see Fig. 85–10) or carotid sinus massage (Fig. 85–11). The mechanism is the development of local phase 4 depolarization in the subnodal (intrahissal or bundle branch) tissue.[26] Outside the episodes of asystole, the electrocardiogram may be perfectly normal or showing only bundle branch block. Especially in these patients, Holter monitoring or other forms of rhythm documentation are particularly useful.

In the asymptomatic patient with chronic bundle branch block, electrophysiologic study is not indicated unless a systemic disease is present with rapidly progressive conduction system disease, such as in dystrophia myotonica.[34]

Occasionally, the question arises of prophylactic acute or long-term pacing in asymptomatic patients with bundle branch block in situations such as general anesthesia, cardiac catheterization, cardiac surgery, and use of His-Purkinje system–depressant antiarrhythmic drugs. Prophylactic pacing during general anesthesia is not recommended, because the risk for progression to high-degree AV block is very low.[35] Electrocardiographic monitoring should be performed during the procedure. Placement of temporary epicardial pacing electrodes is indicated in patients with bundle branch block who are undergoing cardiac surgical procedures in the vicinity of the conduction system. In general, antiarrhythmic drugs that depress the His-Purkinje system, such as quinidine, procainamide, and disopyramide, can be used safely in patients without symptoms that are suggestive of paroxysmal distal heart block.[36–38] When in doubt, especially when high dosages of these drugs are required to control ventricular tachyarrhythmias, the effect of the drug should be tested during an electrophysiologic study.

Table 85–4 summarizes the questions to be addressed when treating a patient with chronic bundle branch block.

TABLE 85–4 Questions to Be Addressed in Treating the Patient With Chronic Bundle Branch Block

Underlying pathology
Prognosis of the patient
Risk of progression to complete heart block
Value of electrophysiologic studies
Management of patients with bundle branch block and syncope but no documentation of bradycardia
Role of permanent pacing in the asymptomatic patient with bundle branch block
Management of the patient with bundle branch block under circumstances such as general anesthesia, open heart surgery, and use of His-Purkinje system–depressant drugs

REFERENCES

1. Narula OS: Atrioventricular block. *In* Narula OS (ed): Cradiac Arrhythmias: Electrophysiology, Diagnosis and Management. p. 113. Baltimore: Williams & Wilkins, 1979.
2. Lev M, Bharati S: Atrioventricular and intraventricular conduction disease. Arch Intern Med 135:405, 1975.

3. Braat SH, Gorgels APM, Bar FW, Wellens HJJ: Value of the ST-T segment in lead V4R in inferior wall acute myocardial infarction to predict the site of coronary artery occlusion. Am J Cardiol 62:140, 1988.
4. Kulbertus HE, Demoulin JC: Pathological basis of concept of left hemiblock. *In* Wellens HJJ, Lie KI, Janse MJ (eds): The Conduction System of the Heart: Structure, Function and Clinical Implications. p. 287. The Hague: Martinus Nijhoff, 1976.
5. Lie KI, Wellens HJJ, Schuilenburg RM: Bundle branch block and acute myocardial infarction. *In* Wellens HJJ, Lie KI, Janse MJ (eds): The Conduction System of the Heart: Structure, Function and Clinical Implications. p. 662. The Hague: Martinus Nijhoff, 1976.
6. Rosenbaum MB, Elizari MV, Lazzari JO: The Hemiblocks: New Concepts of Intraventricular Conduction Based on Human Anatomical, Physiological and Clinical Studies. Oldsmare, FL: Tampa Tracings, 1970.
7. Roos JC, Dunning AJ: Bundle branch block in acute myocardial infarction. Eur J Cardiol 6:403, 1978.
8. Hindman MC, Wagner GS, JaRo M, et al: The clinical significance of bundle branch block complicating acute myocardial infarction. 1: clinical characteristics, hospital mortality, and one-year follow-up. Circulation 58:679, 1978.
9. Godman MJ, Lassers BW, Julian DG: Complete bundle branch block complicating acute myocardial infarction. N Engl J Med 282:237, 1970.
10. Fenig S, Lichstein E: Incomplete bilateral bundle branch block and AV block complicating acute myocardial infarction. Am Heart J 84:38, 1972.
11. Norris RM, Mercer CJ, Croxon MS: Conduction disturbances due to anteroseptal myocardial infarction and their treatment by endocardial pacing. Am Heart J 84:560, 1972.
12. Wellens HJJ, Bar FWHM, Vanagt EJDM, Brugada P: Medical treatment of ventricular tachycardia: considerations in the selection of patients for surgical treatment. Am J Cardiol 49:186, 1982.
13. Lie KOI, Liem KL, Schuilenburg RM, et al: Early identification of patients developing late in-hospital ventricular fibrillation after discharge from the coronary care unit: a 5½ year retrospective and prospective study of 1,897 patients. Am J Cardiol 41:674, 1978.
14. Hauer R, Lie KI, Liem KL, Durrer D: Long-term prognosis in patients with bundle branch block complicating acute anteroseptal infarction. Am J Cardiol 49:1581, 1982.
15. Sgarbossa EB, Pinski SL, Barbagelata A, et al: Electrocardiographic diagnosis of evolving acute myocardial infarction in the presence of left bundle branch block. N Engl J Med 334:481, 1996.
16. Wellens HJJ: Acute myocardial infarction and left bundle branch block: can we lift the veil? N Engl J Med 334:528, 1996.
17. Siegman-Igra Y, Yahini JH, Goldbourt U, Neufeld HN: Intraventricular conduction disturbances: a review of prevalence, etiology, and progression for 10 years within a stable population of Israeli adult males. Am Heart J 96:669, 1978.
18. Kulbertus HE, De Laval-Rutten F, Dubois M, Petit JM: Prognostic significance of left anterior hemiblock with right bundle branch block in mass screening. Am J Cardiol 41:385, 1978.
19. Ross DL: Approach to the patient with bundle branch block. *In* Wellens HJJ, Kulbertus HE (eds): What's New in Electrocardiography. p. 111. Hague: Martinus Nijhoff, 1981.
20. McAnulty JH, Rahimtoola SH, Murphy ES, et al: A prospective study of sudden death in "high risk" bundle branch block. N Engl J Med 299:209, 1978.
21. Dhingra RC, Wyndham CR, Amat-y-Leon F, et al: Incidence and site of atrioventricular block in patients with chronic bifascicular block. Circulation 59:238, 1979.
22. Dhingra RC, Amat-y-Leon, Wyndham C, et al: Significance of left axis deviation in patients with chronic left bundle branch block. Am J Cardiol 43:551, 1978.
23. Schneider JF, Thomas HE, Kreger BE, et al: Newly acquired left bundle branch block: the Framingham study. Ann Intern Med 90:303, 1979.
24. Schneider JF, Thomas HE, Kreger BE, et al: Newly acquired right bundle branch block: the Framingham study. Ann Intern Med 92:37, 1980.
25. Denes P, Dhingra RC, Wu D, et al: Sudden death in patients with chronic bifascicular block. Arch Intern Med 137:1005, 1977.
26. Rosenbaum MB, Elizari MV, Levi RJ, et al: Paroxysmal atrioventricular block related to hypopolarization and spontaneous diastolic depolarization. Chest 63:678, 1973.
27. Dhingra RC, Denes P, Wu D, et al: Prospective observations in patients with chronic bundle branch block and marked H-V prolongation. Circulation 53:600, 1976.
28. Scheinman M, Weiss A, Kunkel F: His bundle recordings in patients with bundle branch block and transient neurologic symptoms. Circulation 48:322, 1973.
29. Narula OS, Gann D, Samet P: Prognostic value of H-V intervals. *In* Narula OS (ed): His Bundle Electrocardiography and Clinical Electrophysiology. p. 437. Philadelphia: FA Davis, 1975.
30. Vera Z, Mason DT, Fletcher RD, et al: Prolonged His-Q interval in chronic bifascicular block: relation to impending complete heart block. Circulation 53:46, 1976.
31. Altschuler H, Fisher JD, Furman S: Significance of isolated H-V interval prolongation in symptomatic patients without documented heart block. Am Heart J 97:19, 1979.
32. Scheinman MM, Peters RW, Modin G, et al: Prognostic value of infranodal conduction time in patients with chronic bundle branch block. Circulation 56:240, 1977.
33. Dhingra RC, Wyndham C, Bauernfeind R, et al: Significance of block distal to the His bundle induced by atrial pacing in patients with chronic bifascicular block. Circulation 60:1455, 1979.
34. Prystowsky EN, Pritchett ELC, Roses AD, Gallagher J: The natural history of conduction system disease in myotonic muscular dystrophy as determined by serial electrophysiologic studies. Circulation 60:1360, 1979.
35. Pastore JO, Yurchak PM, Janis KM, et al: The risk of advanced heart block in surgical patients with right bundle branch block and left axis deviation. Circulation 57:677, 1978.
36. Scheinman MM, Weiss AN, Benowitz N, Rowland M: Electrophysiologic effects of procainamide in patients with intraventricular conduction delay. Circulation 49:522, 1974.
37. Hirschfield DS, Ueda CT, Rowland M, Scheinman MM: Clinical and electrophysiological effects of intravenous quinidine in man. Br Heart J 39:309, 1977.
38. Desai JM, Scheinman M, Peters RW, O'Young J: Electrophysiological effects of disopyramide in patients with bundle branch block. Circulation 59:215, 1979.
39. Narula OS, Scherlag BJ, Samet P, et al: Atrioventricular block localization and classification by His bundle recordings. Am J Med 50:146, 1971.

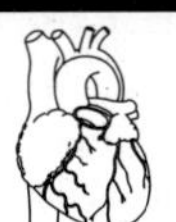

CHAPTER 86

SUPRAVENTRICULAR TACHYCARDIAS

Hein J. J. Wellens

CLASSIFICATION OF SUPRAVENTRICULAR TACHYCARDIAS
Atrial Tachycardia
Atrial Flutter
Atrial Fibrillation
Atrioventricular Nodal Tachycardia
Accelerated Atrioventricular Junctional Rhythm
Circus Movement Tachycardia
FINDINGS AND MANEUVERS HELPFUL IN MAKING THE DISTINCTION BETWEEN THE DIFFERENT TYPES OF SUPRAVENTRICULAR TACHYCARDIA
Electrical Alternans of the QRS Complex
Slowing in Heart Rate During Tachycardia When Bundle Branch Block Develops
Mode of Initiation
Mode of Termination
The Practical Approach

CLASSIFICATION OF SUPRAVENTRICULAR TACHYCARDIAS

The outcomes of programmed electrical stimulation of the heart and excitation mapping, the effect of antiarrhythmic drugs, the knowledge from experiments using the tissue bath and the intact animal, and the outcome of catheter ablation using radiofrequency energy have led to a much better understanding of the site of origin and the mechanism of supraventricular tachycardias.[1–4] This has led to the classification shown in Table 86–1. Each of these different types of supraventricular tachycardias has its own characteristic electrocardiographic features.[5–7] Knowledge of these features is essential to recognize those types that are curable by catheter ablation therapy.

Atrial Tachycardia

As shown in Table 86–1, different forms of atrial tachycardia need to be recognized. Typically, during atrial tachycardia, the electrocardiogram shows that the P wave precedes the QRS complex (Fig. 86–1). The polarity of the P wave, the PR interval, and the ratio between P waves and QRS complexes depend on the site of origin in the atrium, the rate of abnormal impulse formation, and the atrioventricular (AV) nodal transmission characteristics. The paroxysmal form is the most common type of atrial tachycardia and is characterized by a sudden onset and cessation of the arrhythmia (Fig. 86–2). The behavior of this arrhythmia during programmed electrical stimulation of the heart and its response to different antiarrhythmic drugs suggest that paroxysmal atrial tachycardia is based either on reentry (80 percent of cases) or on triggered activity (20 percent). Triggered activity is an arrhythmogenic mechanism resulting from delayed after-depolarization.[1, 8, 9] However, it is not always possible to identify the exact mechanism of paroxysmal atrial tachycardia.

A relatively rare but serious arrhythmia is the incessant (or permanent) form of atrial tachycardia (Fig. 86–3). In patients with this rhythm disturbance, the arrhythmia is present for more than 50 percent of the day. The rate of atrial impulse formation, which is most likely caused by abnormal automaticity, increases during exercise. The persistent nature of the tachycardia and the inability to control the ventricular rate by failure to prevent rate increase of the arrhythmia and 1:1 AV conduction may result in a dilated (tachycardia-induced) cardiomyopathy.[10] Recognition that the arrhythmia is the cause rather than the conse-

TABLE 86–1 Classification of Supraventricular Tachycardia According to Site of Origin and Mechanism

	Reentry	DAD	Abn Auto
Atrial tachycardia			
Paroxysmal	+	+	
Incessant			+
Atrial flutter	+		
Atrial fibrillation	+ (mult. circ.)		
AV nodal tachycardia			
Common form (slow-fast)	+		
Uncommon form (fast-slow)		+	
AV junctional accelerated rhythm			
Digitalis induced		?	
Post cardiac surgery			+
Infectious			+
Ischemic			+
AV junctional circus movement tachycardia			
Paroxysmal: VA conduction over a rapidly conducting AP	+		
Nonparoxysmal: VA conduction over a slowly conducting AP	+		

Abbreviations: Abn, abnormal; AP, accessory pathway; Auto, automaticity; AV, atrioventricular; DAD, delayed after-depolarization; multi. circ., multiple circuits; VA, ventriculoatrial.

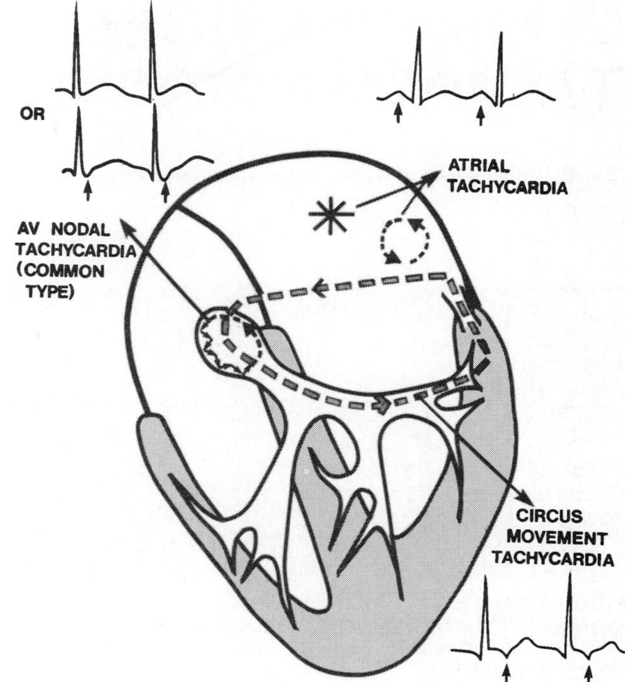

FIGURE 86–1 Three types of supraventricular tachycardia and the relation between QRS and P wave during tachycardia. Note that in atrial tachycardia, P precedes QRS; P occurs simultaneously with QRS in the common type of atrioventricular (AV) nodal tachycardia and follows QRS in circus movement tachycardia using a fast-conducting accessory AV pathway.

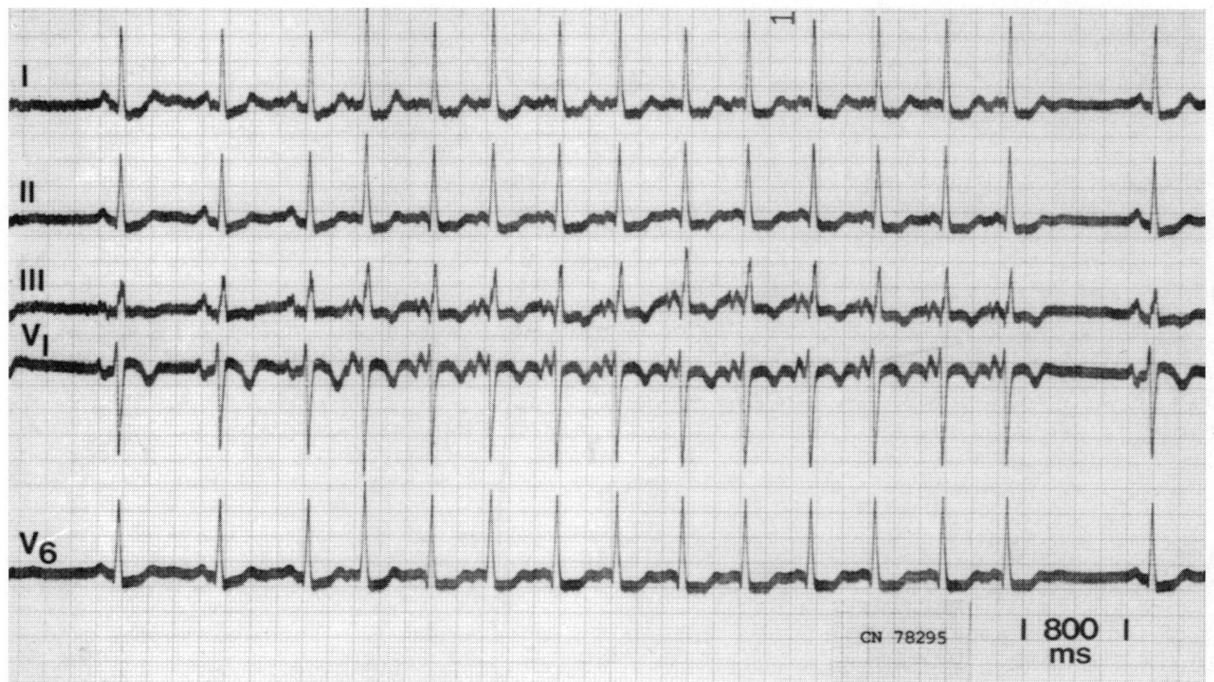

FIGURE 86–2 Example of a paroxysmal atrial tachycardia. Note the onset of the arrhythmia after three conducted sinus beats with a P wave that precedes the QRS complex but has a different configuration from the sinus P waves.

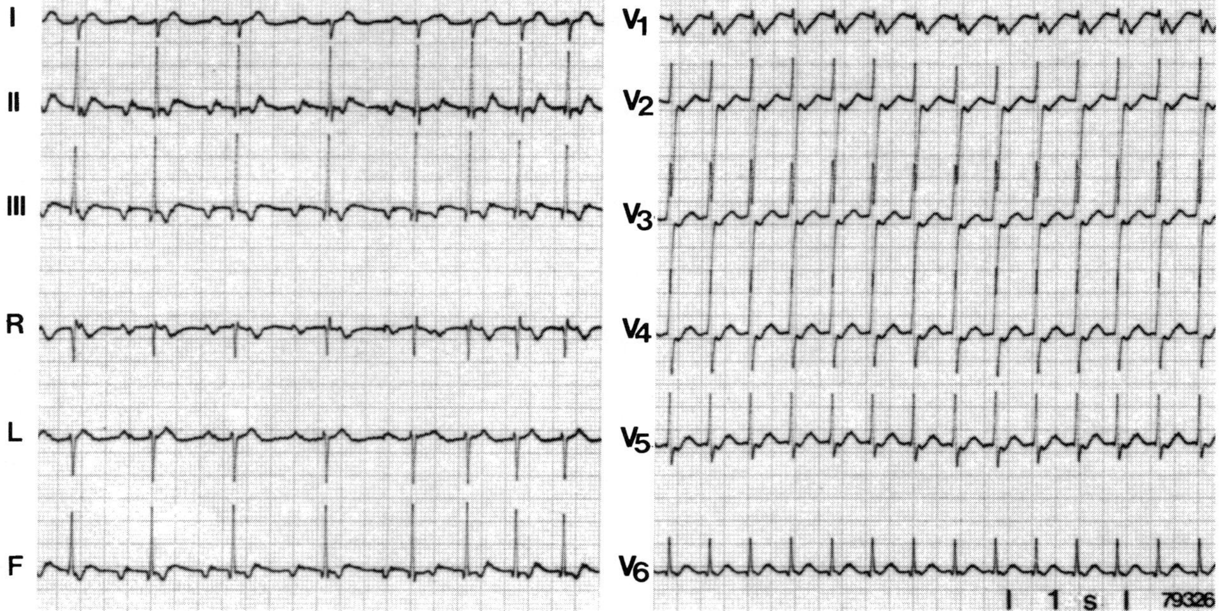

FIGURE 86–3 Example of an incessant atrial tachycardia. This patient, initially showing 2:1 and later 1:1 AV conduction, has been continuously in tachycardia for 12 years and presented with the picture of dilated cardiomyopathy.

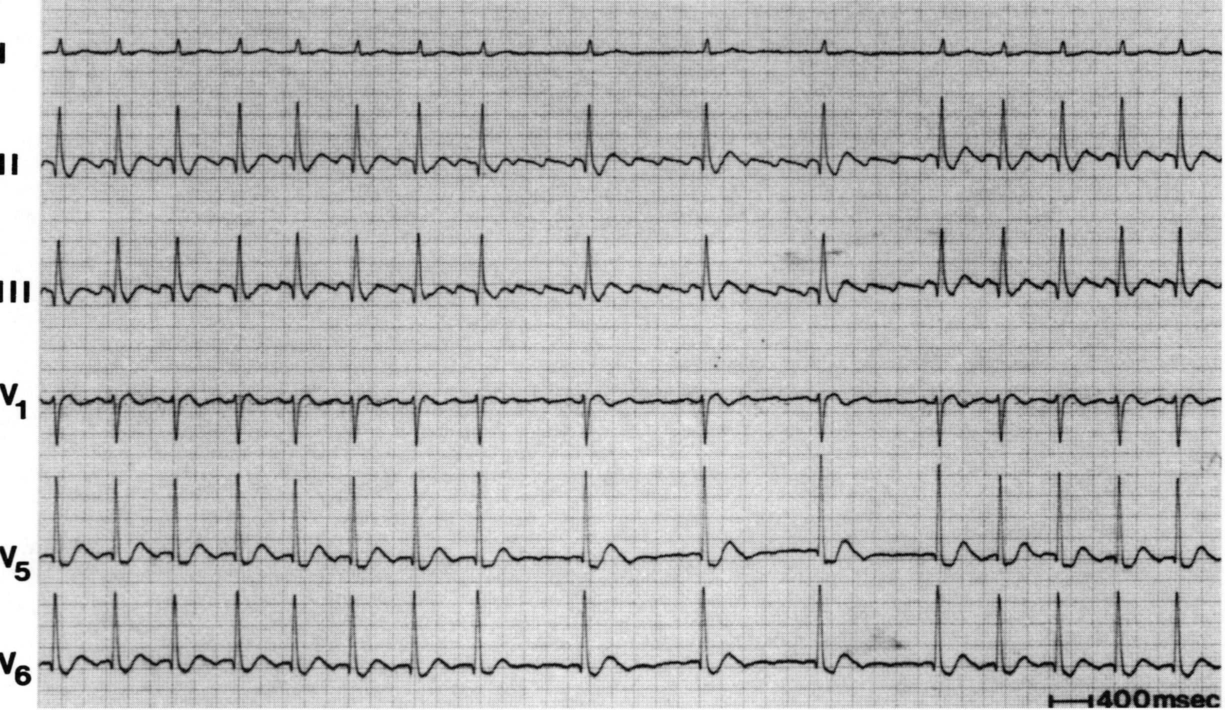

FIGURE 86–4 Carotid sinus massage reveals that atrial flutter is the underlying rhythm at the atrial level.

quence of the cardiomyopathy is important. Destruction of the atrial area of abnormal impulse formation by radiofrequency catheter ablation leads to cure of the arrhythmia and improvement in pump function.

Atrial Flutter

Observations both in the tissue bath and in patients[1, 11–14] suggest macro–reentry in the right atrium as the mechanism for atrial flutter. The classical sawtoothed pattern of atrial activity is the electrocardiographic hallmark of the arrhythmia. Carotid sinus massage–induced AV block facilitates recognition of the arrhythmia (Fig. 86–4).

Atrial Fibrillation

Experimental work in animals and mapping studies during surgery and in the catheterization laboratory suggest that different mechanisms like focal firing in, or close to, the pulmonic veins or multiple reentrant wavelets in the atria are the basis for atrial fibrillation.[15–17]

It is important to be aware of two types of paroxysmal atrial fibrillation that can occur in patients without apparent heart disease. As emphasized by Coumel and associates,[18] one should recognize the so-called vagally induced and the catecholamine-sensitive type. Characteristically, the former arrhythmia is found in middle-aged men and begins at night, during rest, or after a meal. Catecholamine-sensitive atrial fibrillation is less commonly encountered in clinical practice. The arrhythmia is most often observed in young women. It is related to stress and exercise and can be provoked by caffeine or alcohol.[18] Infusion of catecholamines or stress provocation testing is capable of reproducing the arrhythmia more easily than exercise testing. Holter recordings show the occurrence of the arrhythmia in the daytime, usually in the morning, and preceded by an increase in sinus rate.

Atrioventricular Nodal Tachycardia

The reproducible initiation and termination of paroxysmal AV nodal tachycardia by programmed stimulation of the heart suggest reentry as the underlying mechanism. This is supported by the finding of "dual" AV nodal conduction in many of these patients.[19] The common type of paroxysmal AV nodal tachycardia typically shows simultaneous activation of the atrium and the ventricle during the arrhythmia. Anterograde conduction in the AV node during tachycardia is considered to occur over a slowly conducting pathway, and retrograde conduction, over a rapidly conducting pathway. During tachycardia, this results in an electrocardiogram with the P wave either completely hidden in the QRS complex or distorting the terminal portion of the QRS complex. This pattern is graphically represented in Figure 86–1, and an electrocardiogram of the arrhythmia is shown in Figure 86–5. The common type of AV nodal tachycardia occurs twice as often in women as in men.

The uncommon type of paroxysmal AV nodal tachycardia is characterized by a P wave that follows the QRS complex, the mechanism being anterograde AV nodal conduction over a rapid pathway and retrograde conduction over a slow pathway. The RP interval is long, and the P wave becomes located in front of the next QRS complex. This is a rare arrhythmia that is seldom sustained and must

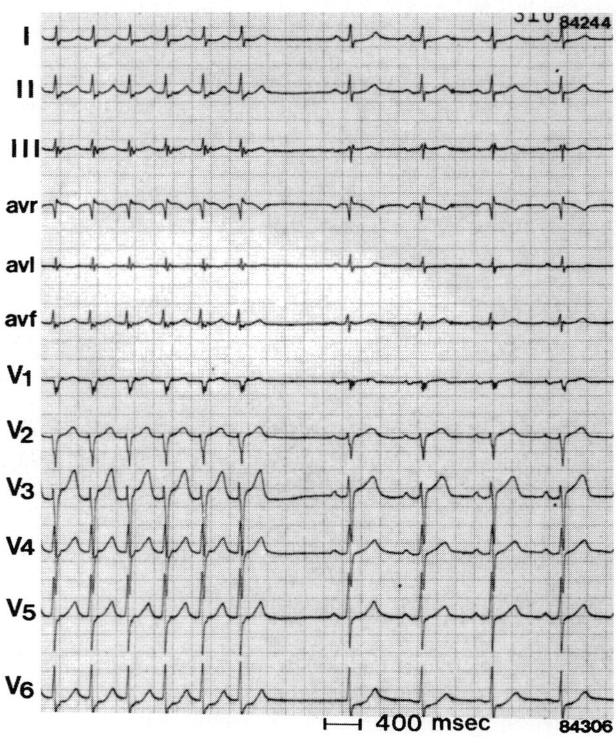

FIGURE 86–5 Example of the common form of AV nodal tachycardia. Note the pseudo-S wave in leads II and III and the pseudo incomplete right bundle branch block pattern in lead V_1, caused by the P wave during tachycardia.

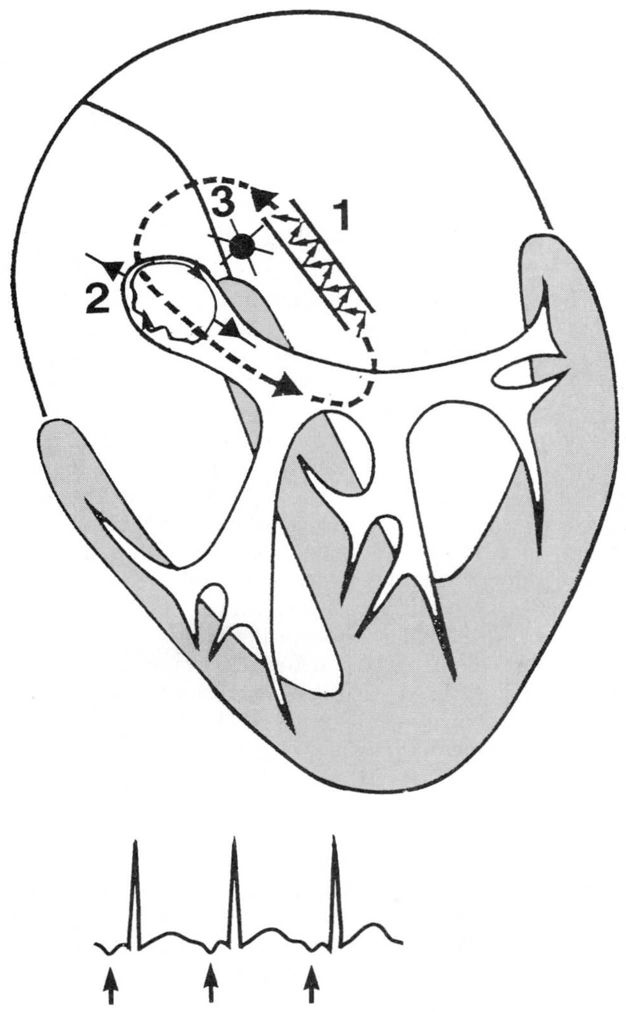

FIGURE 86–6 The three types of supraventricular tachycardia resulting in an electrocardiogram during tachycardia show a negative P wave in front of the QRS complex on lead II. Statistically most likely is a circus movement tachycardia with atrioventricular conduction over the AV node and ventriculoatrial conduction over a slowly conducting accessory pathway **(1)**. The other two possibilities are an AV nodal tachycardia of the unusual (fast-slow) form **(2)** or a low atrial tachycardia in the vicinity of the AV node **(3)**.

be differentiated from a low atrial tachycardia and a circus movement tachycardia using a slowly conducting accessory pathway for ventriculoatrial conduction (Fig. 86–6).

Accelerated Atrioventricular Junctional Rhythm

Accelerated AV junctional impulse formation (of a nonparoxysmal type) may occur in ischemia, with inflammation, after cardiac surgery, and in digitalis intoxication. The exact site of origin in the AV junction (bundle of His?) is not known. It is likely, however, as shown in Table 86–1, that the enhanced impulse formation is based on delayed after-depolarizations (digitalis intoxication) or abnormal automaticity.

Circus Movement Tachycardia

Epicardial mapping and electrophysiologic investigations have shown that accessory connections between atrium and ventricle frequently participate in tachycardia circuits.[1, 20–22] Intracardiac stimulation techniques and recordings are required for demonstration of the location and participation of these extra connections.

An interesting subgroup of patients with supraventricular tachycardia are those with a so-called concealed accessory pathway.[23, 24] These connections conduct the impulse in only a ventriculoatrial direction. They are often present in patients referred for evaluation of their supraventricular tachycardia. There are two groups of concealed accessory pathways (Figs. 86–7 and 86–8). The group using a slowly conducting accessory pathway is small, and most of the patients are women. Atrial activation typically follows the QRS complex, with an RP interval that is longer than the PR interval. This type of supraventricular tachycardia must be differentiated from a low atrial tachycardia and an AV nodal tachycardia of the uncommon type (see Fig. 86–6).

Circus movement tachycardia using a rapidly conducting accessory atrioventricular pathway is twice as common in men than in women. Concealed accessory pathways are about half as common as overt anterogradely conducting accessory pathways (ventricular preexcitation). The mean age at onset of the first attack of tachycardia in patients with accessory pathways is 10 years younger than that in patients with AV nodal tachycardia.[25]

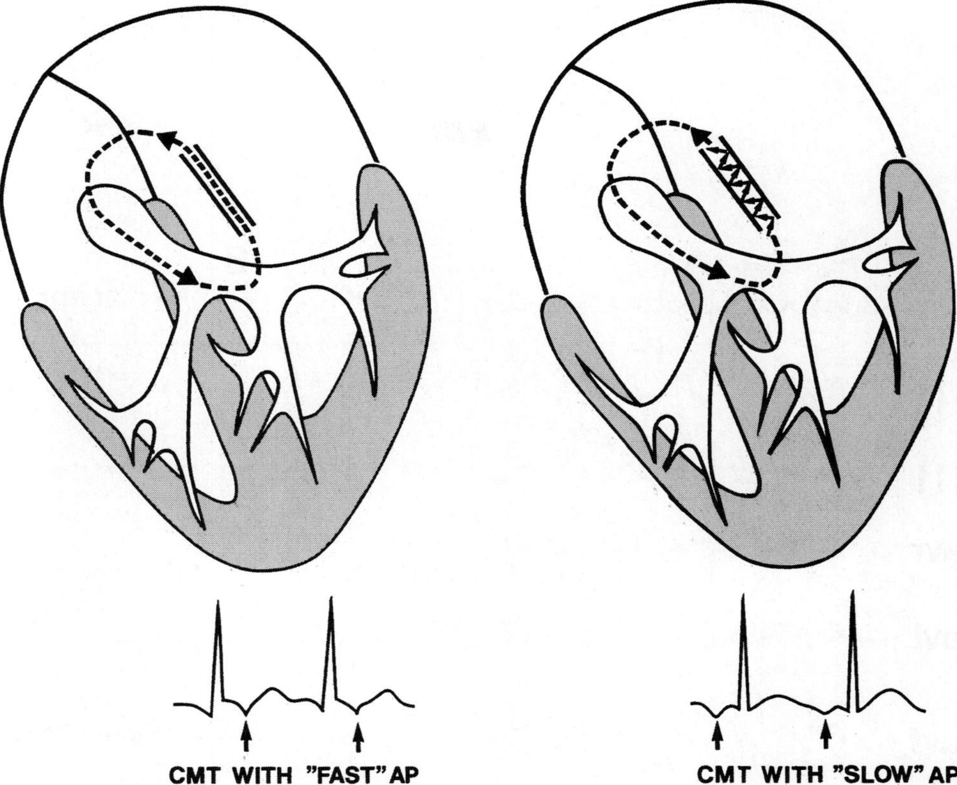

FIGURE 86–7 Schematic representation of a circus movement tachycardia using a "concealed" fast-conducting **(A)** or slow-conducting **(B)** accessory atrioventricular pathway. The corresponding electrocardiograms during tachycardia with their characteristic RP/PR ratio are shown in Figure 86–8.

Findings and Maneuvers Helpful in Making the Distinction Between the Different Types of Supraventricular Tachycardia

Findings on both physical examination and spontaneously occurring or carotid sinus massage–induced changes in the electrocardiogram during tachycardia can be helpful in differentiating between the different types of supraventricular tachycardia. Table 86–2 shows how findings on physical examination, such as characteristics of the radial pulse, jugular venous pulsations, behavior of blood pressure, and loudness of the first heart sound, can be used to make this distinction. Table 86–3 indicates the value of carotid massage in unraveling the different types of tachycardia.

Electrical Alternans of the QRS Complex

Alternating changes in the QRS complex during a narrow QRS tachycardia are highly suggestive of a circus movement tachycardia using an accessory pathway for ventriculoatrial conduction.[26] QRS alternation as a clue to a circus movement tachycardia can be used only when it is present more than 5 seconds after the start of tachycardia. Changes in QRS configuration are common at the start of supraventricular tachycardia because the sudden acceleration in ventricular rate leads to different degrees of changes in refractoriness and conduction velocity in the conduction system. In patients with circus movement tachycardia and a narrow QRS, the incidence of electrical alternans increases with increasing heart rate during tachycardia. An example of electrical alternans is shown in Figure 86–9.

Slowing in Heart Rate During Tachycardia When Bundle Branch Block Develops

Figures 86–10 and 86–11 illustrate the importance of careful measurements of rate of tachycardia when bundle branch block develops and disappears during supraventricular tachycardia. As shown in Figure 86–11, a slowing in tachycardia rate during bundle branch block indicates the presence of a circus movement tachycardia using an accessory AV pathway for ventriculoatrial conduction inserting into the free wall of the ventricle on the same side as the blocked bundle branch.

Mode of Initiation

Initiation of a supraventricular tachycardia by a single atrial premature beat during sinus rhythm after marked prolongation of the PR interval suggests the presence of dual AV nodal pathways and AV nodal reentrant tachycardia as the mechanism of the arrhythmia (Figs. 86–12 and 86–13). In contrast, initiation of a supraventricular tachycardia during sinus rhythm without prolongation of the PR interval suggests a circus movement tachycardia using an

Text continued on page 1618

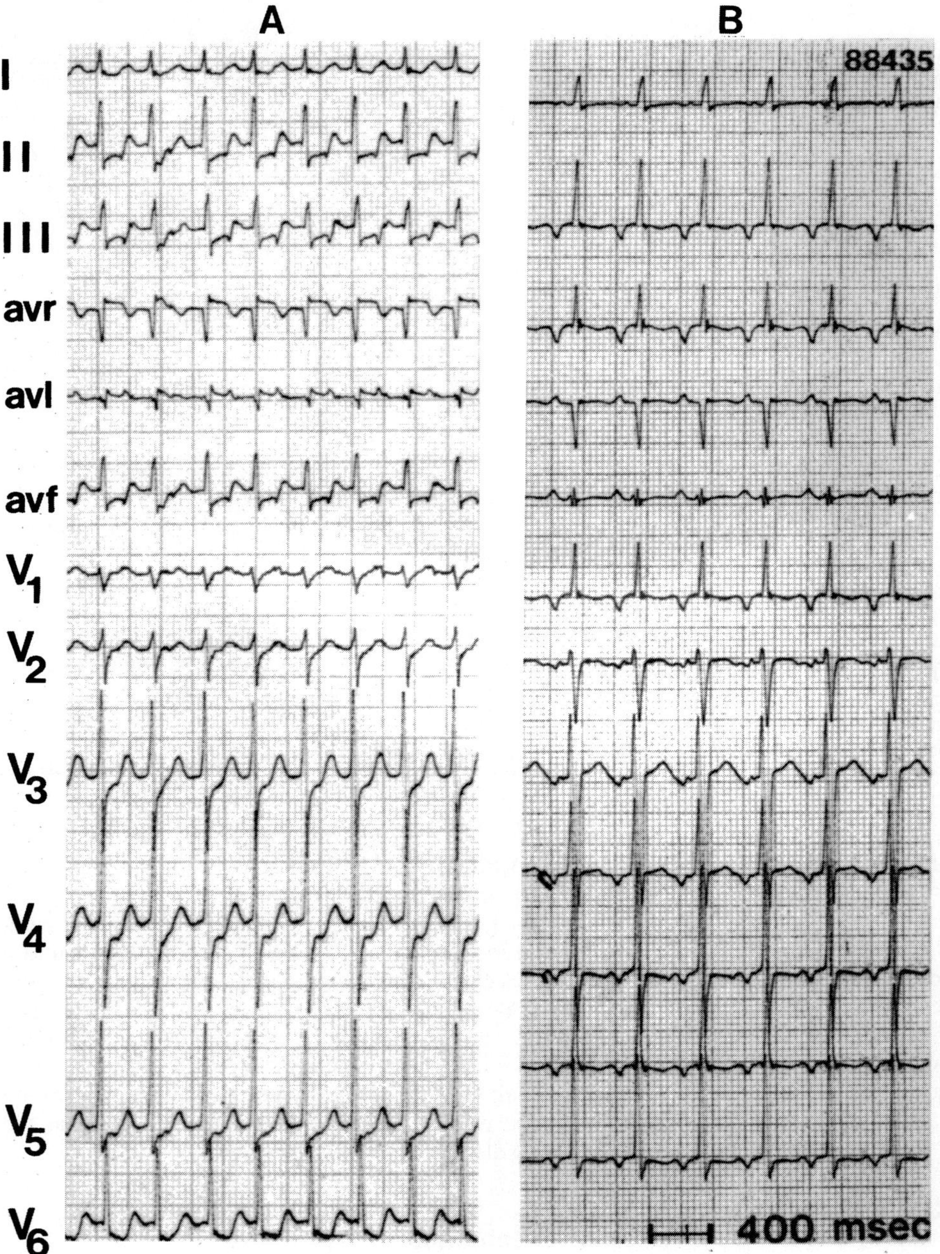

FIGURE 86–8 Two types of circus movement tachycardias. Circus movement tachycardia due to a rapid- **(A)** and slow-conducting **(B)** accessory pathway (AP). The rapidly conducting AP **(A)** is associated with a short RP, the slow-conducting AP **(B)** with a long RP. The P waves are relatively narrow, inverted in the inferior leads, and isoelectric in lead I, suggesting a septal or paraseptal location.

TABLE 86–2 Clinical Findings and Blood Pressure Measurements in Different Types of Supraventricular Tachycardia

Tachycardia	Pulse	Neck Veins	Blood Pressure	Loudness of First Heart Sound
Sinus tachycardia	Regular	No abn.	Constant	Constant
Atrial tachycardia	Regular	No abn.	Constant	Constant
Atrial flutter	Regular during 2:1 AV conduction	Flutter waves	Constant during regular pulse	Constant
	Irregular during changing AV conduction		Changing	Changing
Atrial fibrillation	Irregular	Irregular pulsations	Changing	Changing
AV nodal tachycardia	Regular	"Frog" sign	Constant	Changing
Circus movement tachycardia (using concealed accessory pathway)	Regular	"Frog" sign	Constant	Changing

Abbreviation: AV, atrioventricular.

TABLE 86–3 Findings on Carotid Sinus Massage in Different Types of Tachycardia

Tachycardia	Effect of Carotid Sinus Massage
Sinus tachycardia	Gradual and temporary slowing in heart rate
Atrial tachycardia	
Paroxysmal form	Cessation of tachycardia
	No effect
Incessant form	Temporary slowing because of increase in AV block
	No effect
Atrial flutter	Temporary slowing because of increase in AV block
	Transformation into atrial fibrillation
	No effect
Atrial fibrillation	Temporary slowing because of increase in AV block
	No effect
AV nodal tachycardia	Cessation of tachycardia
	No effect
Circus movement tachycardia (using overt or concealed accessory pathway)	Cessation of tachycardia
	No effect

Abbreviation: AV, atrioventricular.

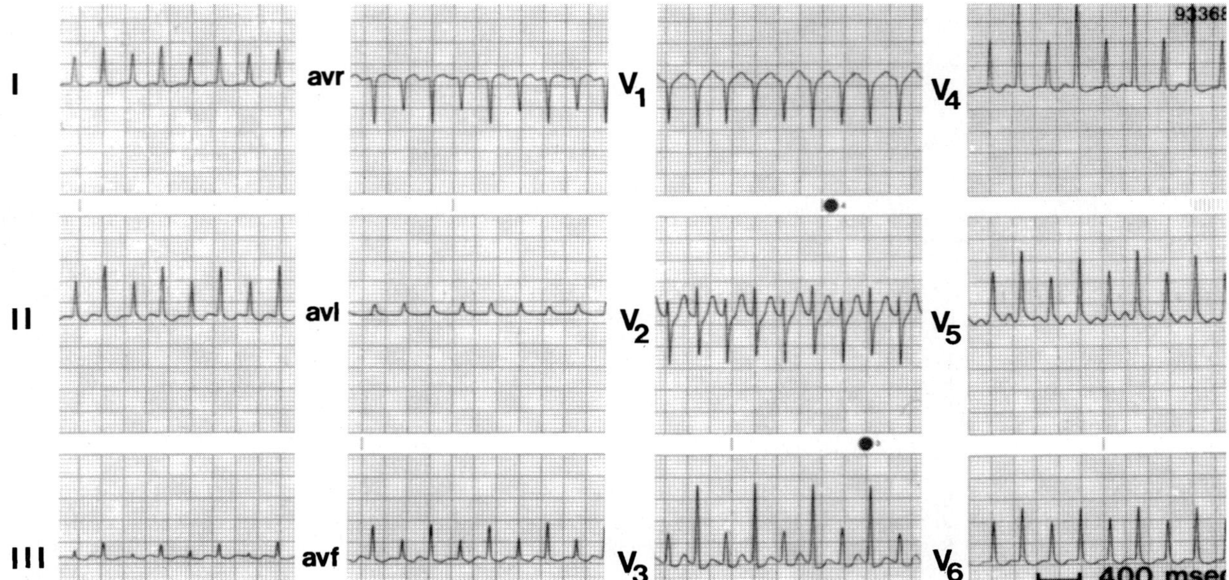

FIGURE 86–9 Example of electrical alternans of the QRS complex during a circus movement tachycardia using a "concealed" accessory AV pathway. Note that QRS alternation is best seen in leads II, V_3, and V_4.

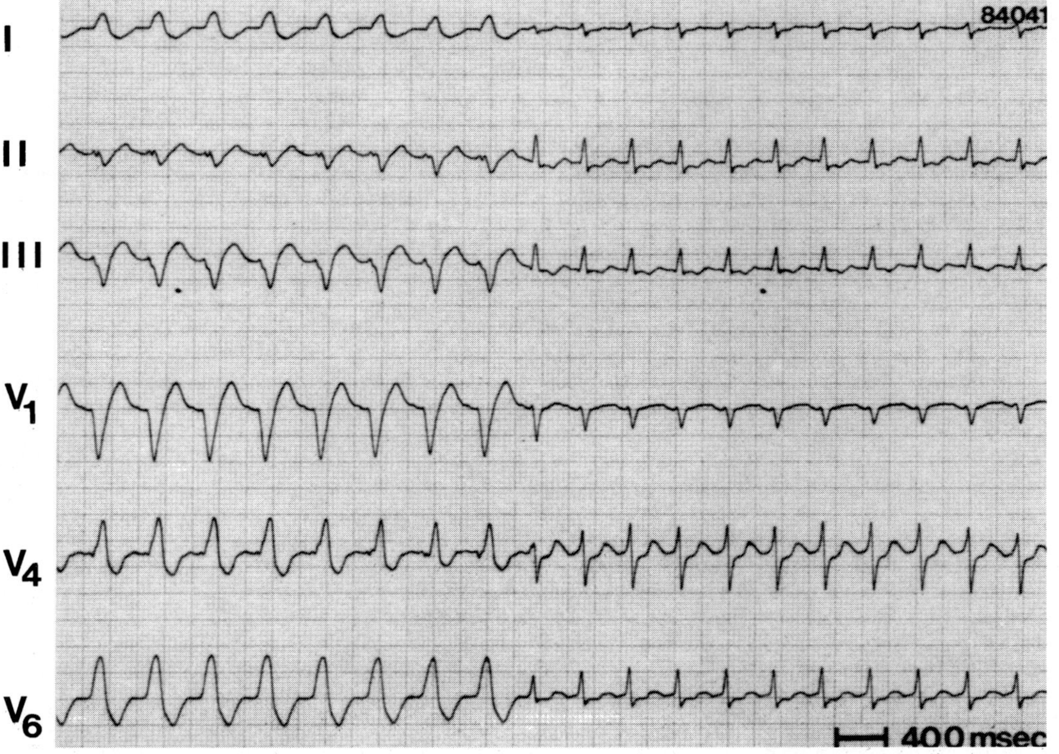

FIGURE 86–10 The presence of a slower heart rate during supraventricular tachycardia in a case of left bundle branch block. As explained in Figure 86–11, this indicates a circus movement tachycardia using an accessory AV pathway on the same side as the blocked bundle branch. In this example, therefore, the accessory pathway is between the left atrium and the left ventricle.

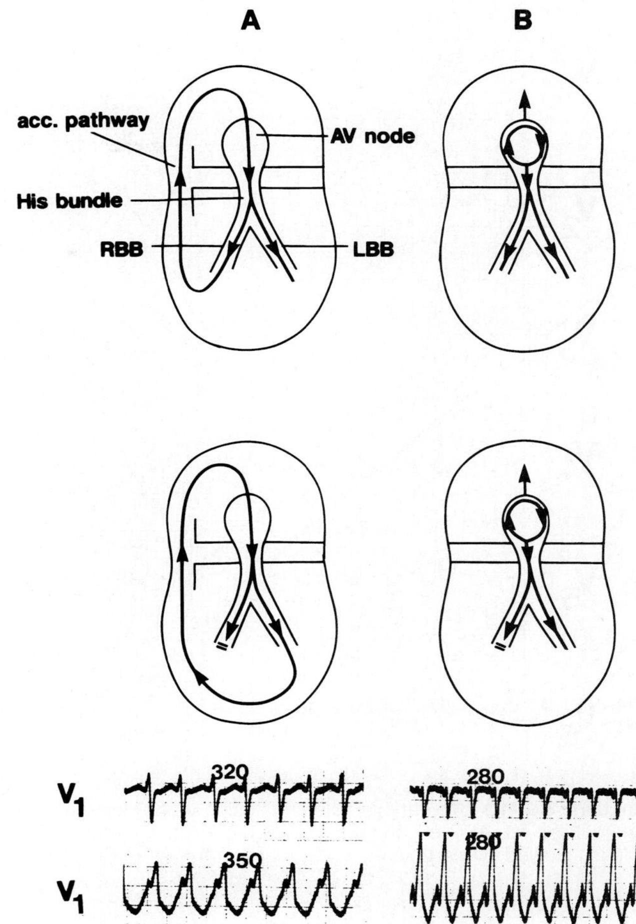

FIGURE 86–11 Increase in the length of the re-entry circuit when bundle branch block develops during circus movement tachycardia using an accessory pathway that is on the same side as the bundle branch block. **A,** There is a right-sided accessory pathway. **B,** The tachycardia circuit is confined to the AV node. When right bundle branch block develops in the patient with a right-sided accessory pathway, the circuit becomes longer and the tachycardia rate slows (compare V_1 before and after right bundle branch block on the left). In contrast **(B)**, nothing happens to the tachycardia rate when bundle branch block develops during AV nodal re-entrant tachycardia (measurements are in milliseconds).

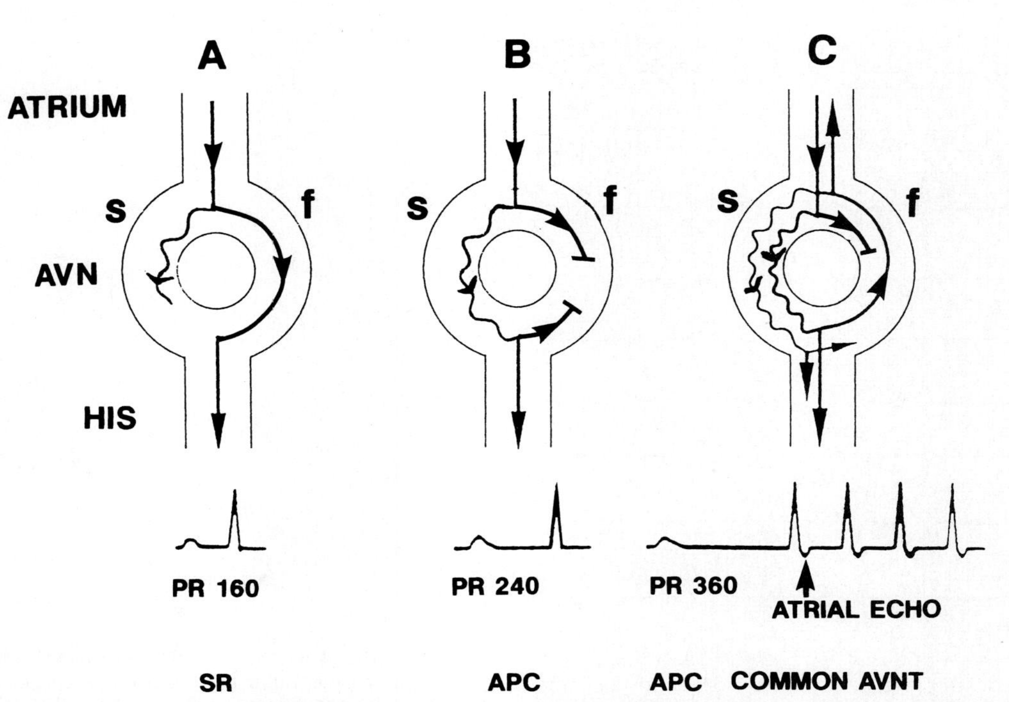

FIGURE 86–12 Initiation of an AV nodal tachycardia by an atrial premature complex (APC) during sinus rhythm (SR). **A**, During sinus rhythm, the atrial impulse reaches the bundle of His by way of the most rapidly conducting (the fast f) pathway. **B**, An APC is conducted to the bundle of His over the slow (s) pathway because of block in the fast (f) pathway. This results in sudden prolongation of the PR interval compared with sinus rhythm. **C**, An even earlier APC with slower conduction in the slow pathway is able to re-enter the fast pathway and to initiate the common form of AV nodal tachycardia.

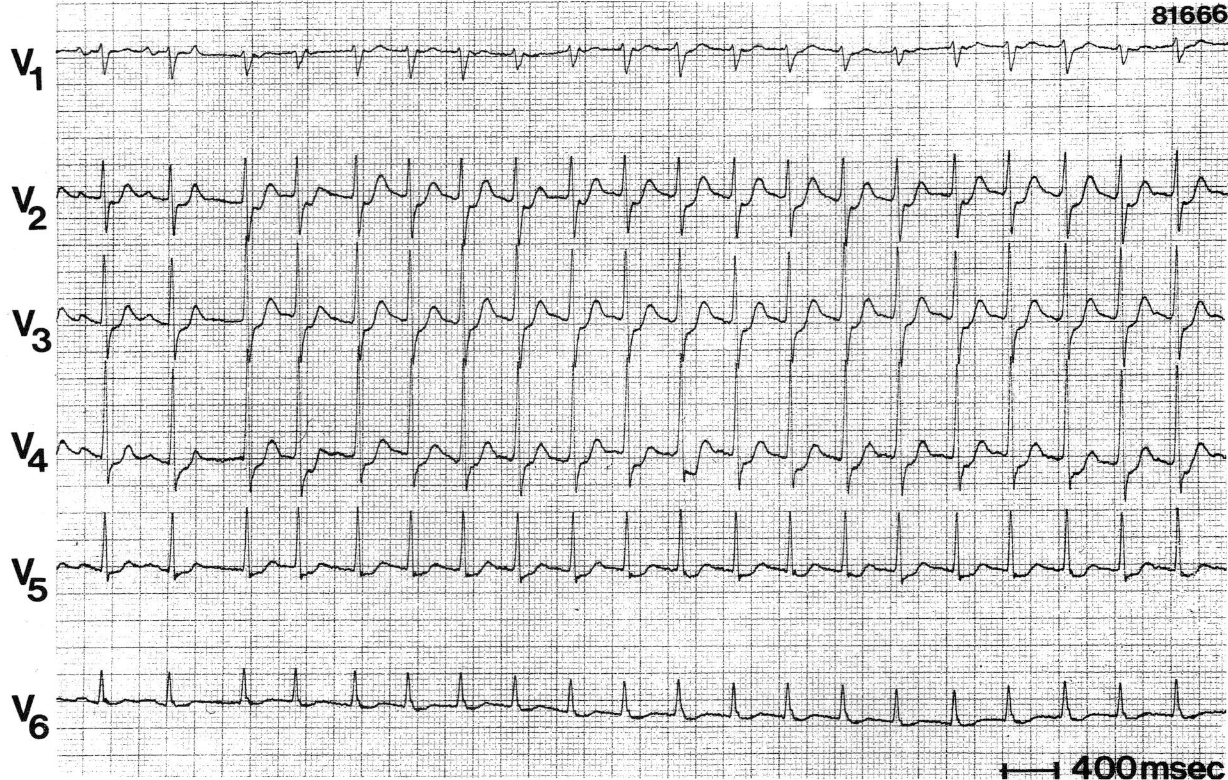

FIGURE 86–13 Clinical example of initiation of the common form of AV nodal tachycardia. After two sinus beats that are conducted to the ventricle, an APC is conducted to the ventricle, with marked PR prolongation indicating conduction over the slow AV nodal pathway. This is followed by perpetuation of re-entry in the AV node and AV nodal tachycardia. Six precordial leads were recorded simultaneously.

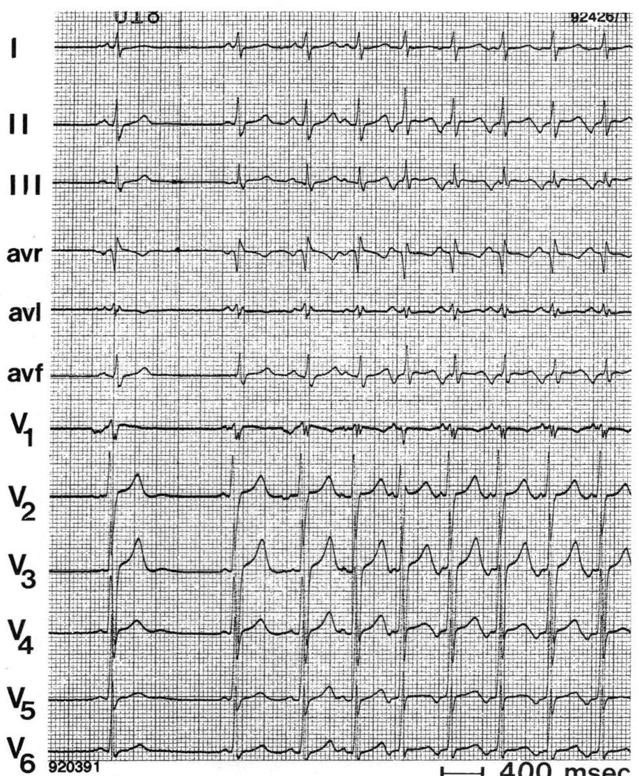

FIGURE 86–14 Initiation of a supraventricular tachycardia during sinus rhythm. Note that an acceleration in rate during sinus rhythm is followed by a tachycardia with a narrow QRS complex. The RP interval exceeds the PR interval during tachycardia, with negative P waves in leads II, III, V_3, and V_6. These findings indicate the presence of a circus movement tachycardia using a slowly conducting accessory pathway for ventriculoatrial conduction.

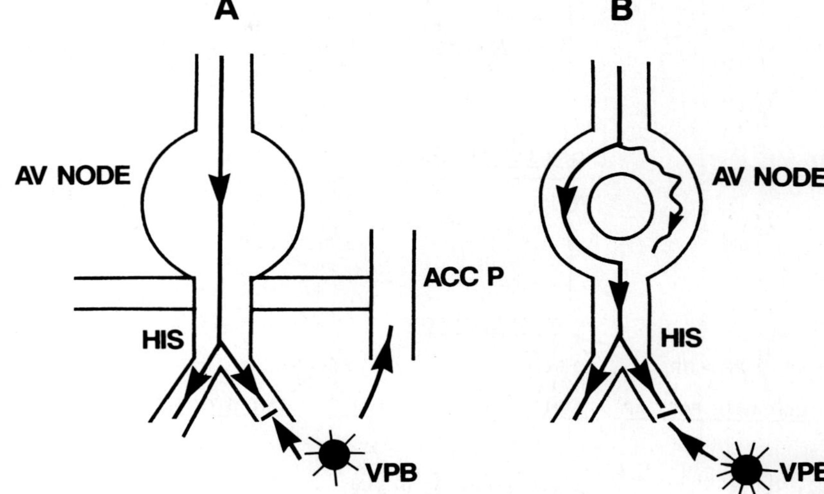

FIGURE 86–15 **A**, During sinus rhythm a circus movement tachycardia using an accessory AV pathway can easily be initiated by a single ventricular premature beat (VPB) because the VPB finds the distal conduction system refractory and is retrogradely conducted to the atrium over the accessory pathway (ACC P). **B**, In contrast, because of refractoriness of the distal conduction system, a VPB cannot get to the AV node to initiate AV nodal reentry.

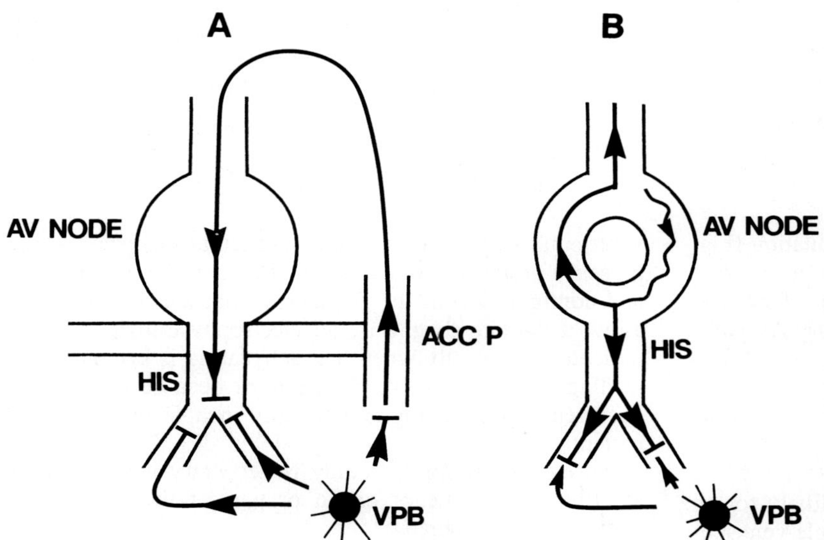

FIGURE 86–16 Differences for a ventricular premature beat (VPB) to get into the tachycardia circuit (and to terminate tachycardia) in AV nodal tachycardia and in a circus movement tachycardia using an accessory pathway for ventriculoatrial conduction. The VPB in AV nodal tachycardia will be blocked distal to the reentry circuit **(B)**, whereas the VPB easily invades the reentry circuit during circus movement tachycardia **(A)**.

STEPS IN DIAGNOSIS OF NARROW QRS TACHYCARDIA (QRS< 0,12 SEC)

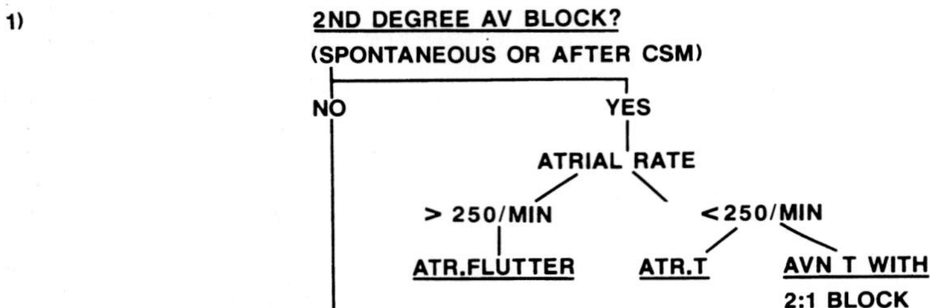

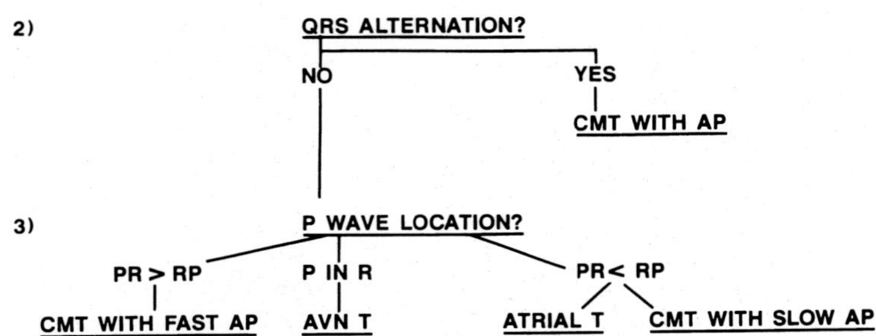

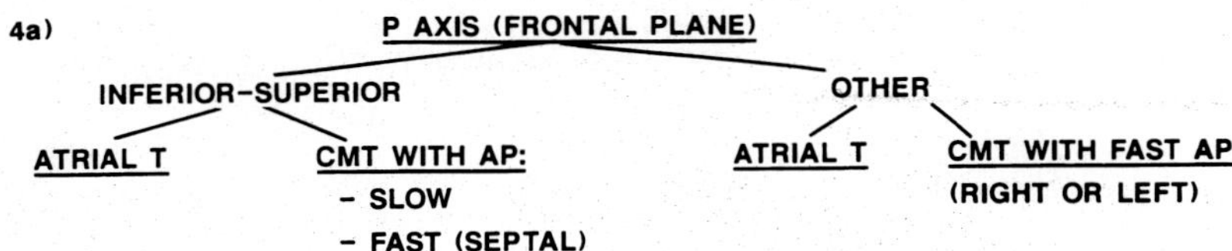

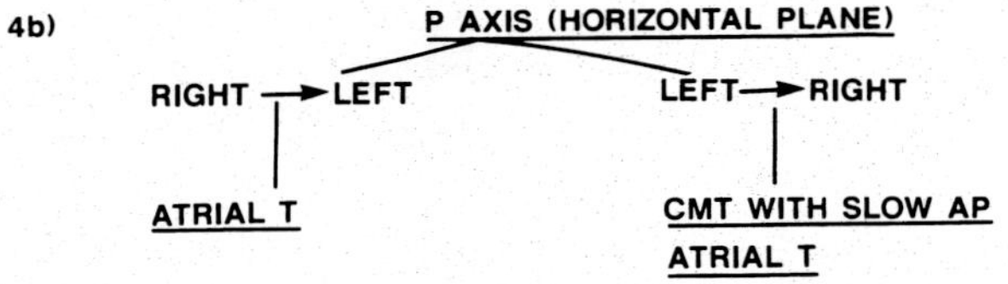

FIGURE 86–17 Four steps to be taken when analyzing the 12-lead ECG of a regular supraventricular tachycardia. As shown, information should be obtained about the relation between atrial and ventricular events during supraventricular tachycardia (spontaneously and after carotid sinus massage [CSM]) followed by a look for electrical alternans of the QRS complex. Thereafter, the location of the P wave in relation to the QRS complex and the polarity of the P wave in the frontal and horizontal plane should be studied.

accessory AV pathway for ventriculoatrial conduction (Fig. 86–14). Initiation of a supraventricular tachycardia by a single ventricular premature beat argues in favor of a circus movement tachycardia incorporating an accessory AV pathway (Fig. 86–15).

Mode of Termination

As shown in Figure 86–16, it is extremely unlikely for an AV nodal tachycardia to be terminated by a single ventricular premature beat. However, this is quite common in a circus movement tachycardia using an accessory AV pathway for ventriculoatrial conduction.

The Practical Approach

A stepwise approach is advised for analyzing the 12-lead electrocardiogram during supraventricular tachycardia (Fig. 86–17). The steps include the relation between atrial and ventricular events during supraventricular tachycardia, the presence or absence of electrical alternans, and the location and configuration of the P wave. If that analysis does not allow a definite diagnosis, an electrophysiologic study is indicated, especially when the tachycardia is symptomatic, leading to myocardial dysfunction, or because its frequent occurrence is annoying and socially incapacitating for the patient.

An electrophysiologic study is necessary when catheter ablation of the site of origin or part of the tachycardia pathway is considered.

REFERENCES

1. Wellens HJJ: Electrical Stimulation of the Heart in the Study and Treatment of Tachycardias. Baltimore: University Park Press, 1971.
2. Rosen MR: The links between basic and clinical cardiac electrophysiology. Circulation 77:251, 1988.
3. Zipes DP: Cardiac electrophysiology: promises and contributions. J Am Coll Cardiol 13:1329, 1989.
4. Wellens HJJ, Brugada P: Treatment of cardiac arrhythmias: when, how and where? J Am Coll Cardiol 14:1417, 1989.
5. Wellens HJJ: Differential diagnosis of narrow QRS tachycardia. *In*

Fisch C, Surawicz S (eds): Cardiac Electrophysiology and Arrhythmias. pp. 164–175. New York: Elsevier, 1991.
6. Josephson ME, Wellens HJJ: Differential diagnosis of supraventricular tachycardia. Cardiol Clin 8:411, 1990.
7. Wellens HJJ, Conover MB: The ECG in Emergency Decision Making. Philadelphia: WB Saunders, 1992.
8. Wellens HJJ, Brugada P: Mechanisms of supraventricular tachycardia. Am J Cardiol 62:10, 1988.
9. Wellens HJJ, Brugada P, Vanagt E, et al: New studies with triggered automaticity. *In* Harrison DC (ed): Cardiac Arrhythmias. A Decade of Progress. pp. 601–610. Boston: GK Hall, 1981.
10. Wellens HJJ: The electrocardiogram in digitalis intoxication. *In* Yu PN, Goodwin JF (eds): Progress in Cardiology. Vol. 5. pp. 271–290. Philadelphia: Lea & Febiger, 1976.
11. Puech P, Latour M, Grolleau R: Le flutter et ses limites. Arch Mal Coeur 63:116, 1970.
12. Boineau JP, Mooney CR, Hudson RD, et al: Observations on reentrant excitation pathway and refractory period distributions in spontaneous and experimental atrial flutter in the dog. *In* Kulbertus HE (ed): Re-entrant Arrhythmias: Mechanisms and Treatment. pp. 72–98. Baltimore: University Park Press, 1977.
13. Waldo AL, Maclean WAH, Karp RB, et al: Entrainment and interruption of atrial flutter with atrial pacing: studies in man following open heart surgery. Circulation 56:737, 1977.
14. Allessie MA, Bonke FIM, Schopman FJG: Circus movement in rabbit atrial muscle as a mechanism of tachycardia III. The "leading circle" concept: a new model of circus movement in cardiac tissue without the involvement of an anatomic obstacle. Circ Res 41:9, 1977.
15. Allessie MA, Lammers WJEP, Bonke FIM, Hollen J: Experimental evaluation of Moe's multiple wavelet hypothesis of atrial fibrillation. *In* Zipes DP, Jalife J (eds): Cardiac Arrhythmias. pp. 265–276. New York: Grune & Stratton, 1985.
16. Falk RH, Podrid PJ: Atrial Fibrillation: Mechanism and Management. New York: Raven Press, 1991.
17. Haissaguerre M, Jais P, Shah DC, et al: Spontaneous initiation of atrial fibrillation by ectopic beats originating in the pulmonary veins. N Engl J Med 339:659, 1998.
18. Coumel P, Attuel P, Leclercq JF: Arhythmies auriculaires d'origine vagale ou catecholergique: effects compares du traitment beta-bloqueur et phenomenes d'echappement. Arch Mal Coeur 75:373, 1982.
19. Denes P, Wu D, Dhingra RC, et al: Demonstration of dual AV nodal pathways in patients with paroxysmal supraventricular tachycardia. Circulation 48:549, 1973.
20. Wellens HJJ, Durrer D: The role of an accessory pathway in reciprocal tachycardia. Circulation 52:58, 1975.
21. Durrer D, Roos JP: Epicardial excitation of the ventricles in a patient with Wolff-Parkinson-White syndrome (type B). Circulation 35:15, 1967.
22. Durrer D, Schoo L, Schuilenburg RM, Wellens HJJ: The role of premature beats in the initiation and termination of supraventricular tachycardia in the Wolff-Parkinson-White syndrome. Circulation 36:644, 1967.
23. Wellens HJJ, Brugada P, Farre J, et al: Diagnosis and treatment of concealed accessory pathways in patients suffering from paroxysmal AV junctional tachycardia. *In* Rosenbaum MB, Elizari MV (eds): Frontiers of Cardiac Electrophysiology. pp. 773–797. The Hague: Martinus Nijhoff, 1983.
24. Coumel Ph, Attuel P: Reciprocating tachycardia in overt and latent pre-excitation: influence of functional bundle branch block on the rate of tachycardia. Eur J Cardiol 1:423, 1974.
25. Rodriguez LM, De Chillou C, Schlapfer J, et al: Age at onset and gender of patients with different types of supraventricular tachycardias. Am J Cardiol 70:1213, 1992.
26. Green M, Heddle B, Dassen W, et al: The value of QRS alternation in diagnosing the site of origin of narrow QRS supraventricular tachycardia. Circulation 68:368, 1983.

CHAPTER 87

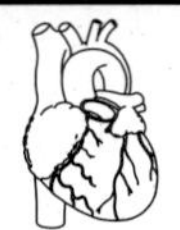

PREEXCITATION

Hein J. J. Wellens

UNDERSTANDING THE ELECTROCARDIOGRAM
INCIDENCE OF PREEXCITATION
ARRHYTHMIAS
Circus Movement Tachycardia
Atrial Fibrillation
NONINVASIVE TESTS TO RECOGNIZE THE LOW-RISK PATIENT
TREATMENT
Drugs
Surgery and Electrical Ablation
PRACTICAL APPROACH TO THE PATIENT
The Patient With an Arrhythmia
The Patient Without an Arrhythmia

In 1930, Wolff, Parkinson, and White[1] described patients with electrocardiograms (ECGs) showing a short PR interval, a delta wave, and a wide QRS complex. In 1933, Wolferth and Wood[2] postulated the presence of an accessory atrioventricular (AV) pathway to explain the peculiar ECG and the frequently occurring tachycardias in these patients.

Subsequently, electrophysiologic investigations, epicardial mapping, surgical findings, and anatomic studies have shown that there are several pathways by which a part of or the whole ventricle can be activated earlier than expected[3–10] (Fig. 87–1). The old and new nomenclature is given in Table 87–1. By far the most common type of extra connection leading to ventricular preexcitation is an accessory AV pathway or Kent bundle. The other connections are rare and require sophisticated intracardiac stimulation techniques and recordings to be demonstrated. Emphasis in this section is therefore focused on the recognition, consequences, and treatment of patients who have an accessory AV pathway.

UNDERSTANDING THE ELECTROCARDIOGRAM

Essential to our understanding of the electrocardiographic findings in ventricular preexcitation is the awareness that in activation of the ventricles over two pathways, a fusion QRS complex results whose configuration depends on the contribution of each of the two activation fronts. As shown in Figures 87–2 and 87–3, a left-sided accessory AV pathway is present. In Figures 87–2A and 87–3A, because of the time required to conduct the impulse from the sinus node to the ventricle over the two AV pathways, an important part of the ventricle is preexcited, leading to a short PR interval, a delta wave (representing activation of the left ventricular free wall), and a widened QRS complex. In Figures 87–2B and 87–3B, contribution to ventricular activation over the accessory AV pathway is minor and therefore the PR interval is longer, the delta wave small, and the QRS complex relatively narrow.

The conclusion is that an ECG showing a classic Wolff-Parkinson-White (WPW) syndrome (PR interval less than 0.12 second) is not always present. The form of the ECG depends on the amount of ventricular muscle activated over the accessory AV pathway. Several factors may play a role here, such as location of the accessory pathway, the site of atrial impulse formation in relation to the location of the accessory pathway, the size of the atria, and the transmission characteristics of the AV node and of the accessory AV pathway. These considerations should be kept in mind

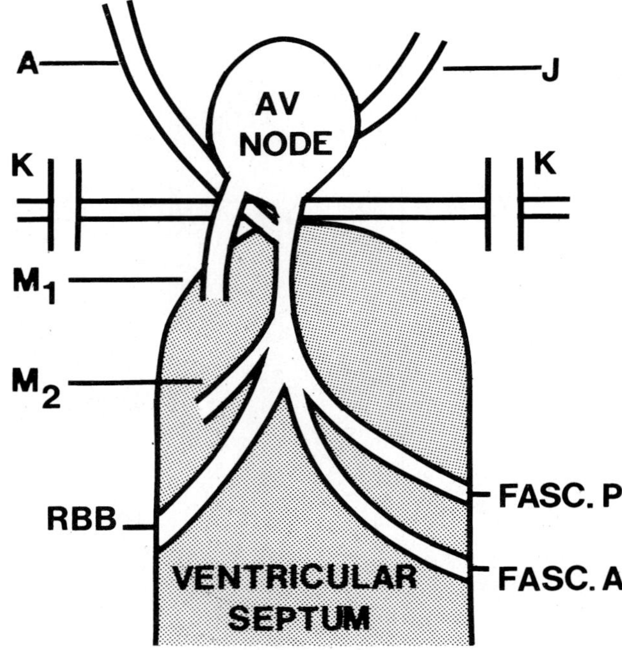

FIGURE 87–1 Schematic of the atrioventricular (AV) conduction system and the possible accessory connection(s) partially or totally bypassing that system. A, atriofascicular bypass tract; Fasc. A, fasciculus anticus of left bundle branch; Fasc. P, fasciculus posticus of left bundle branch; J, intranodal bypass tract; K, accessory AV pathway; M_1, nodoventricular pathway; M_2, fasciculoventricular pathway; RBB, right bundle branch. See also Table 87–1. (From Anderson RH, Becker AE, Brechenmacher C, et al: Ventricular pre-excitation: a proposed nomenclature for its substrates. Eur J Cardiol 3:27, 1975.)

TABLE 87–1 Old and New Nomenclature of Accessory Connections

Old	Symbol In Figure 87–1	New	Connections
Kent's bundle	K	Accessory atrioventricular pathway	Atrium to ventricle
Mahaim fiber	M_1	Nodoventricular pathway*	Atrioventricular node to ventricle
Mahaim fiber	M_2	Fasciculoventricular pathway	His bundle or bundle branch to ventricle
Atrio-Hissian fiber	A	Atriofascicular bypass tract	Atrium to His bundle
James fiber	J	Intranodal bypass tract	Atrium to atrioventricular node

*The fiber may insert into the bundle branch and is then called a *nodofascicular fiber.*

From Anderson RH, Becker AE, Brechenmacher C, et al: Ventricular pre-excitation: a proposed nomenclature for its substrates. Eur J Cardiol 3:27, 1975.

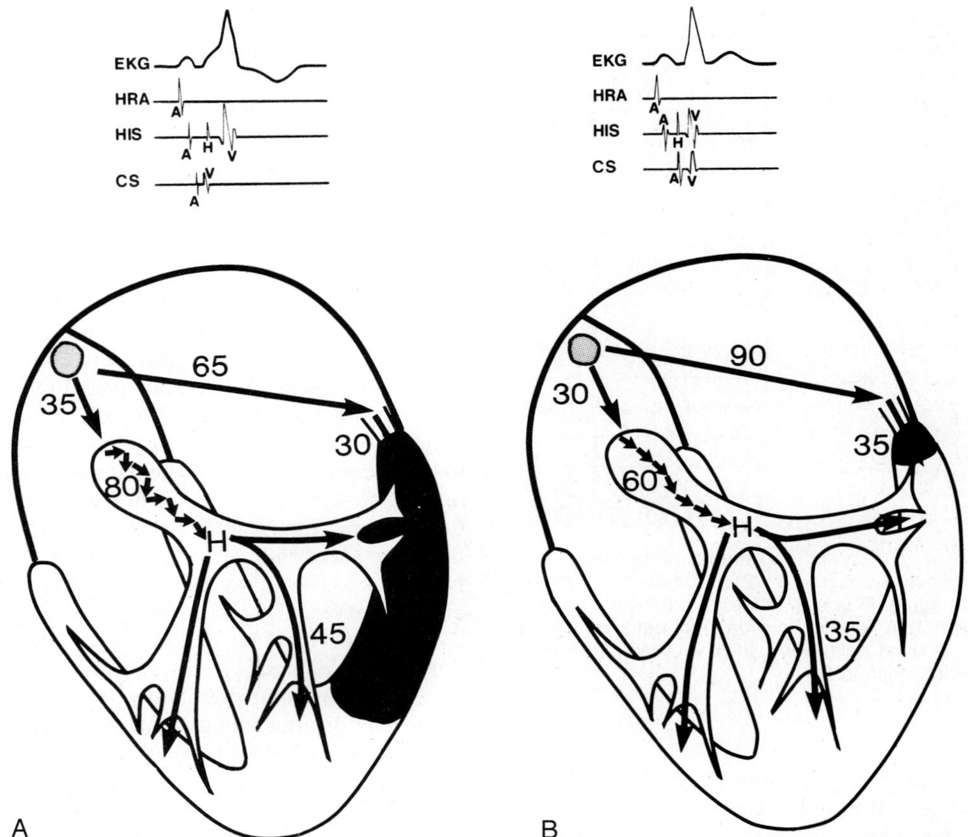

FIGURE 87–2 Factors determining the degree of preexcitation in a left-sided accessory atrioventricular (AV) pathway during sinus rhythm. **A,** Because of a shorter conduction time from the sinus node to the ventricle over the accessory pathway (65 + 30 = 95 ms versus 35 + 80 + 45 = 160 ms over the normal AV conduction system), an important part of the ventricle is preexcited, resulting in an electrocardiogram (ECG) with a short PR interval, a clear delta wave, and a widened QRS complex (**A,** *top*). This is in contrast with **B,** where activation of the ventricle starts simultaneously over the normal AV conduction system (30 + 60 + 35 = 125 ms) and accessory pathway (90 + 35 = 125 ms). This leads to an EKG with a longer PR interval, hardly any delta wave, and a more narrow QRS complex (**B,** *top*). CS, carotid sinus; HIS, His bundle; HRA, high right atrium.

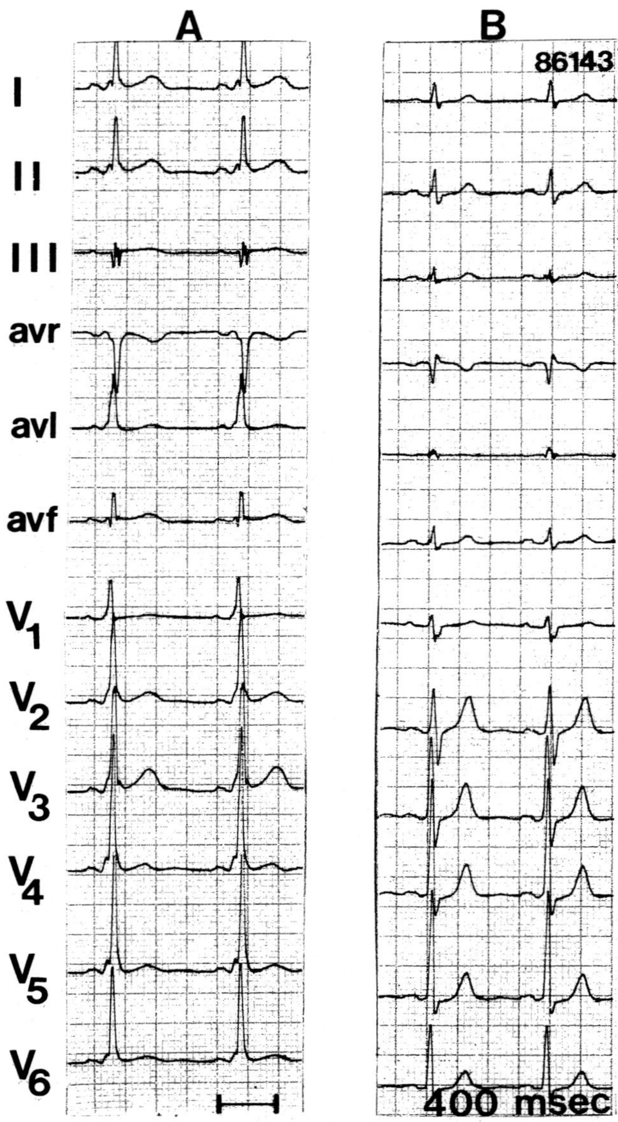

FIGURE 87–3 Electrocardiographic examples of the two schematic drawings shown in Figure 87–2. **A** and **B** correspond to the left and right sides of Figure 87–2. Note that the electrocardiogram (ECG) in **A** shows a prominent delta wave, and the ECG in **B** shows a small delta wave. In **A,** a much larger area of ventricle is preexcited than in **B.**

when one tries to locate the accessory pathway on the 12-lead ECG. Only when an important amount of ventricular preexcitation (a clear delta wave) is present can dependable predictions be made.

Incidence of Preexcitation

The true incidence of preexcitation is unknown; the reported figures vary from 0.1 to 3/1000 ECGs.[11] The WPW syndrome is undoubtedly underdiagnosed because, as pointed out, the contribution to ventricular activation over the accessory pathway may vary.

Arrhythmias

Pathways leading to ventricular preexcitation can be classified as shown in Figure 87–1. These pathways may be incorporated into several different types of reentry circuits (Fig. 87–4). Again, it should be stressed that from a practical point of view, a direct connection between the atrium and the ventricle, a true accessory AV pathway, or a Kent bundle is most commonly involved in the tachycardia mechanism. The incidence of tachyarrhythmias in the WPW syndrome is unknown. The reported figures range from 12 to 80 percent.[12, 13]

Although any type of arrhythmia, such as atrial, AV nodal, or ventricular tachycardia, may occur in the presence of an accessory connection, the clinically most common types of arrhythmia in patients with preexcitation are circus movement tachycardia and atrial fibrillation.

Circus Movement Tachycardia

Programmed electrical stimulation of the heart has made it possible to demonstrate and understand how a circus movement tachycardia can be initiated and terminated in a patient having two connections between atrium and ventricle instead of one.[4] As shown in Figure 87–5, a critically timed atrial premature beat that finds the accessory pathway refractory is conducted from atrium to ventricle over the AV node–His pathway only and returns from the ventricle to the atrium over the accessory pathway. Perpetuation of this type of conduction results in a circus movement tachycardia. A circus movement tachycardia with AV conduction over the AV node and ventriculoatrial conduction over the accessory AV pathway is called an *orthodromic* circus movement tachycardia (see Figs. 87–4A and 87–5A). A tachycardia running in the reverse direction (AV conduction over the accessory AV pathway and ventriculoatrial conduction over the His–AV node) is called an *antidromic* circus movement tachycardia (see Fig. 87–4B). Orthodromic tachycardia is 10 to 15 times more common than the antidromic type. Programmed stimulation of the heart has shown that there are many ways to initiate a circus movement tachycardia.[7] However, they all have in common the creation of a unidirectional block in one of the two AV pathways. This can occur by a critically timed atrial or ventricular premature beat, by reaching a critical sinus rate, or after administration of a drug.[7]

Intracardiac recordings during circus movement tachycardia, findings on epicardial mapping preceding surgery, and observations during radiofrequency energy catheter ablation have shown that the most common location of an accessory AV pathway is the one connecting the left atrium with the left ventricle (50 percent).[14] A posteroseptal, right ventricular, or anteroseptal insertion of the AV pathway is found in approximately 30 percent, 13 percent, and 7 percent of patients, respectively.

Circus movement tachycardia is the most common type of tachycardia in the patient with preexcitation. Intracardiac recordings during supraventricular tachycardia have shown that an accessory AV pathway that can conduct only retrogradely, a so-called concealed accessory AV pathway, is often incorporated into the tachycardia circuit. These pa-

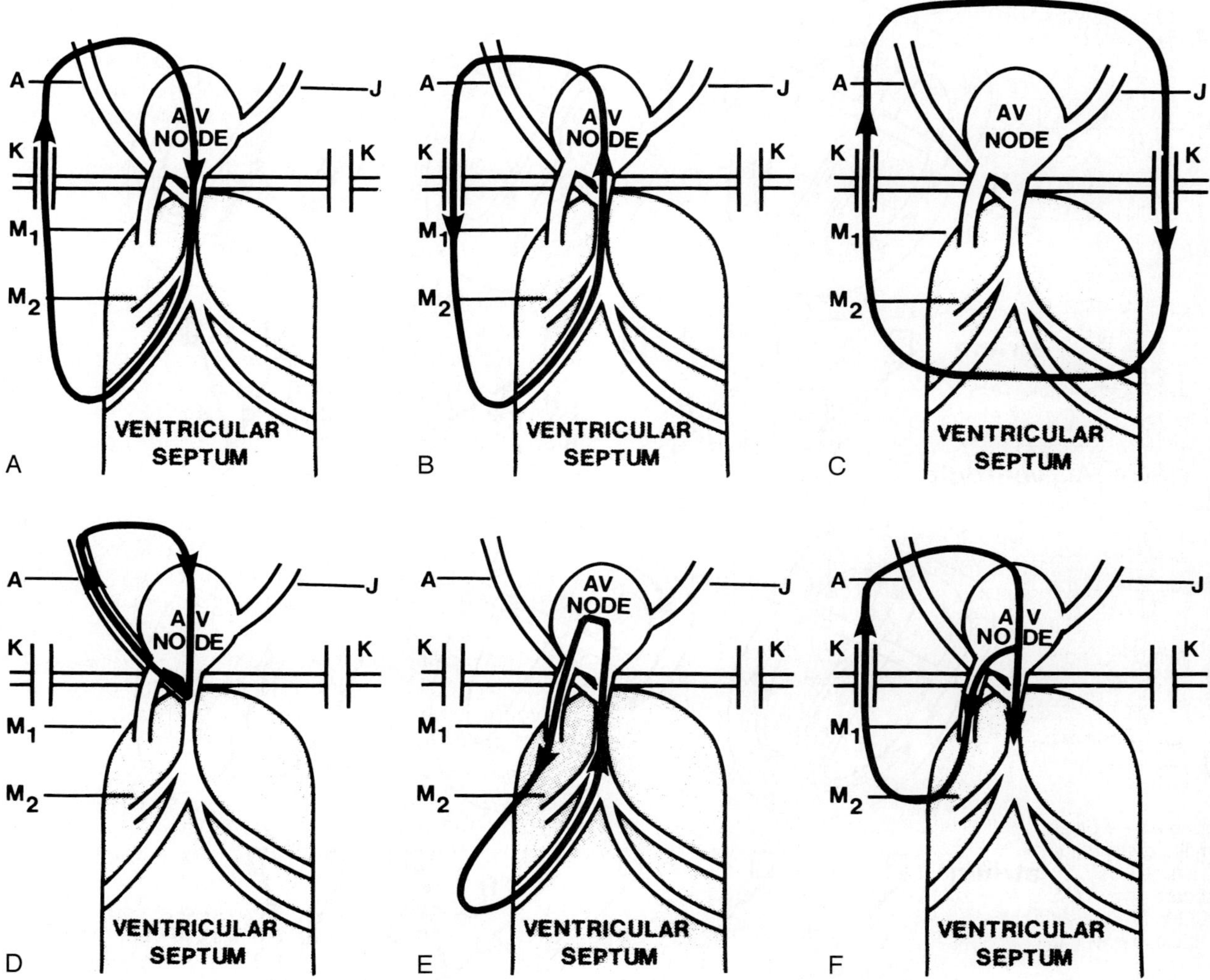

FIGURE 87–4 Some examples of possible reentry circuits in patients with accessory connections. **A,** Classic orthodromic circus movement tachycardia using an atrioventricular (AV) node–His pathway in anterograde and an accessory pathway in retrograde direction. **B,** Antidromic circus movement tachycardia shows reversed direction of tachycardia shown in **A**. **C,** Tachycardia circuit using one accessory AV pathway for anterograde and another accessory AV pathway for retrograde conduction. **D,** Circuit using AV node and atriofascicular bypass tract. **E,** Tachycardia circuit with anterograde conduction over nodoventricular fiber and retrograde conduction over bundle branch–His system. **F,** Circus movement tachycardia with anterograde conduction over nodoventricular fiber and retrograde conduction over accessory AV pathway. Abbreviations as in Figure 87–1.

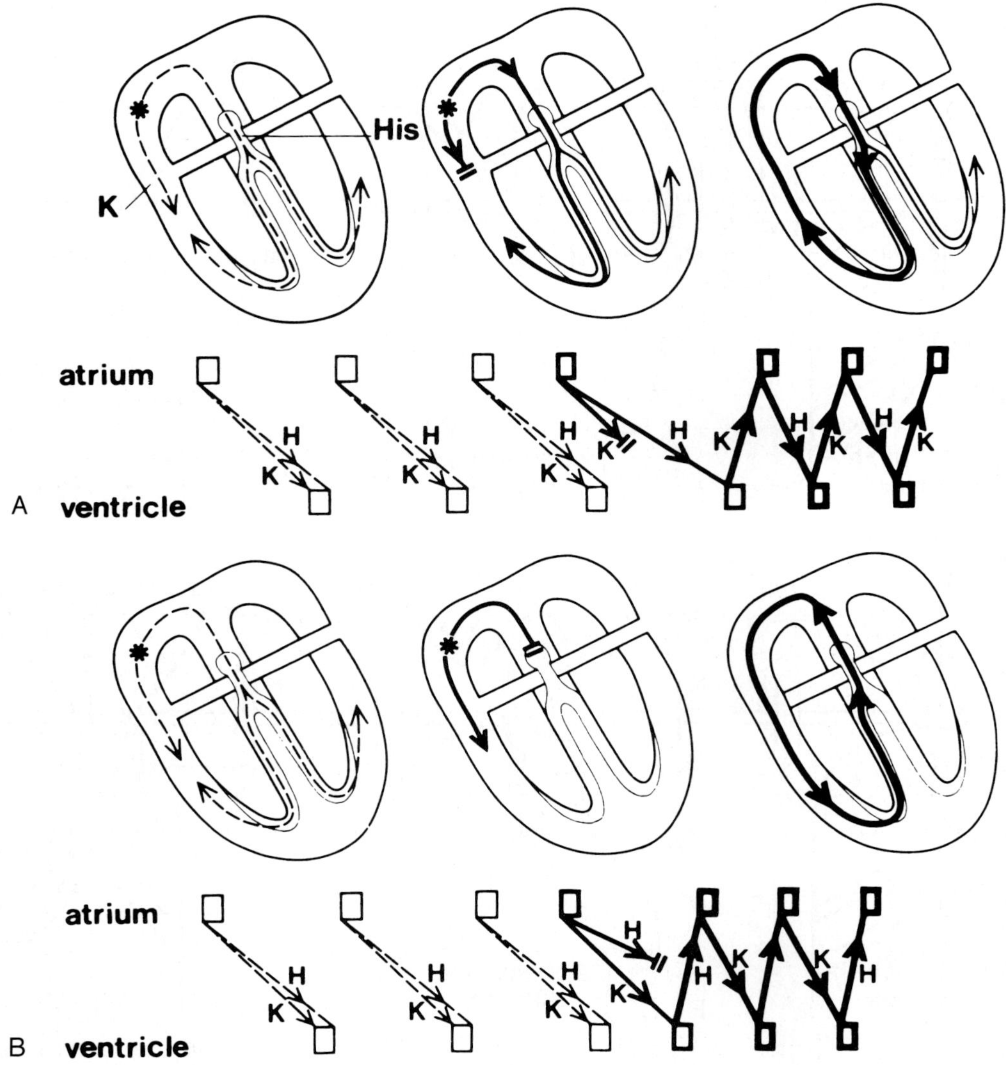

FIGURE 87–5 Mode of initiation of circus movement tachycardia by atrial premature beat. **A,** Critically timed atrial premature beat during atrial pacing leads to unidirectional block in the accessory pathway. AV conduction over the AV node–His pathway is followed by an orthodromic circus movement tachycardia. **B,** Initiation of reversed (antidromic) type of circus movement tachycardia. The ECG during orthodromic circus movement tachycardia will show disappearance of the delta wave, whereas the delta wave will become more prominent during an antidromic circus movement tachycardia. H, His bundle; K, accessory pathway.

tients never show ventricular preexcitation during sinus rhythm but do have an accessory connection between the atrium and the ventricle that plays an essential role in the tachycardia mechanism.

Atrial Fibrillation

In the human heart, the ventricles are protected by the refractory period of the AV node against a high ventricular rate during a rapid atrial rhythm. In patients having an accessory pathway or an atriofascicular bypass tract, atrial fibrillation can be an extremely dangerous arrhythmia if the accessory connection has a short anterograde refractory period (Fig. 87–6B). In that situation, the occurrence of ventricular fibrillation has been documented.[6] An example is shown in Figure 87–7. In patients with WPW syndrome, the ventricular rate during atrial fibrillation is determined not only by the duration of the refractory period of the accessory pathway in anterograde direction but also by factors such as the length of the refractory period of the AV node and ventricle and concealed anterograde and retrograde penetration into the accessory pathway and into the AV node.[15]

The duration of the anterograde refractory period of the accessory pathway is influenced by the autonomic nervous system. Sympathetic discharge induced by the fall in blood pressure and the anxiety that accompany atrial fibrillation may lead to abbreviation of the refractory period of the accessory pathway and an increase in ventricular rate.[16]

Noninvasive Tests to Recognize the Low-Risk Patient

As pointed out, the presence of an accessory AV pathway with a short anterograde refractory period may lead to life-threatening high ventricular rates if atrial fibrillation supervenes. Is it possible to identify such risk when a patient has an ECG showing preexcitation? We have previously reported[17] that three noninvasive techniques can give an idea about the approximate length of the refractory period of the accessory pathway in an anterograde direction. First, the finding of intermittent preexcitation (Fig. 87–8) indicates a long anterograde refractory period of the accessory pathway. Second, as first shown by Levy and coworkers,[18] disappearance of preexcitation during exercise points to a long anterograde refractory period of the accessory pathway (Fig. 87–9). One should be careful in interpretation, however, because sympathetic stimulation during exercise will speed up trans-AV nodal conduction and might thereby diminish the area of the ventricles preexcited over the accessory pathway. Several electrocardiographic leads should therefore be taken simultaneously, and special

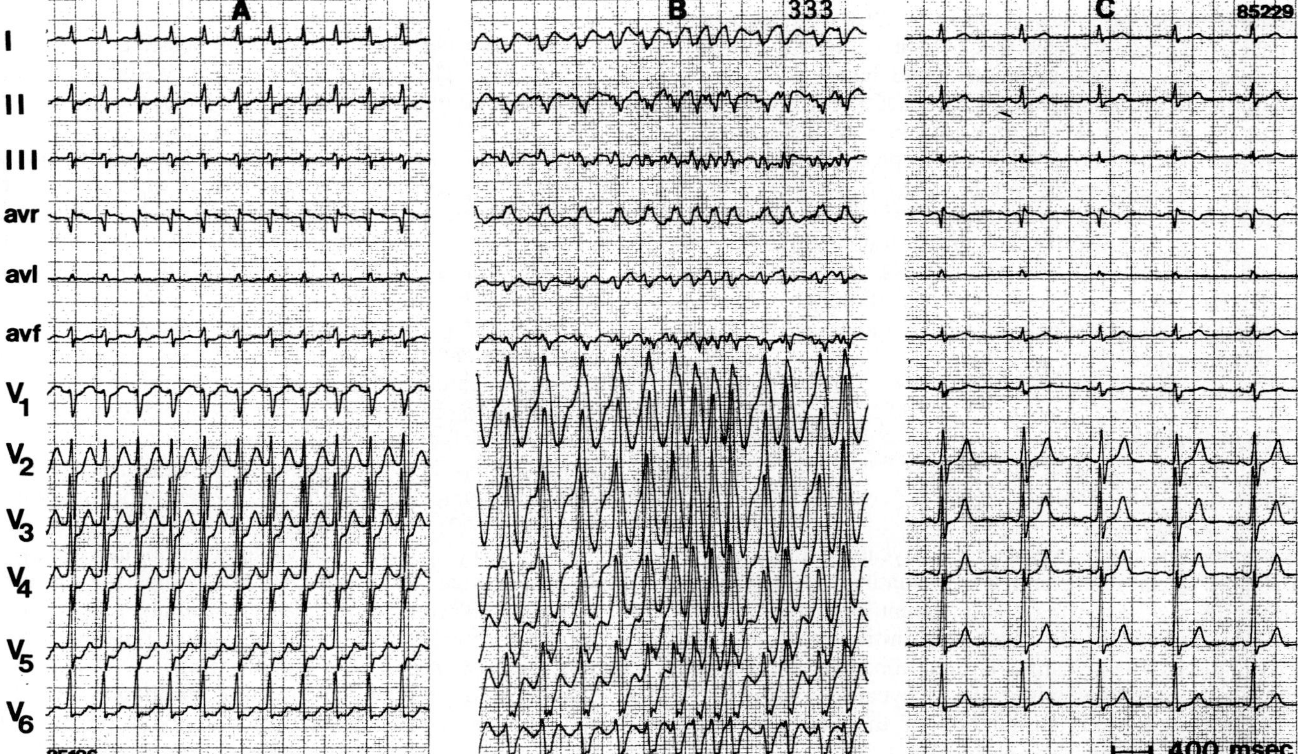

FIGURE 87–6 Two most common types of tachycardia in the Wolff-Parkinson-White syndrome. **A,** An orthodromic circus movement tachycardia with AV conduction over the AV node–His pathway and ventriculoatrial conduction over the accessory pathway. **B,** Atrial fibrillation with a shortest RR interval of 200 ms. Both arrhythmias were recorded in a patient with an ECG, shown in **C,** during sinus rhythm. This is the same patient as in Figure 87–3B. This example is chosen to stress that maximal preexcitation and high ventricular rates can occur during atrial fibrillation in patients showing little ventricular preexcitation during sinus rhythm.

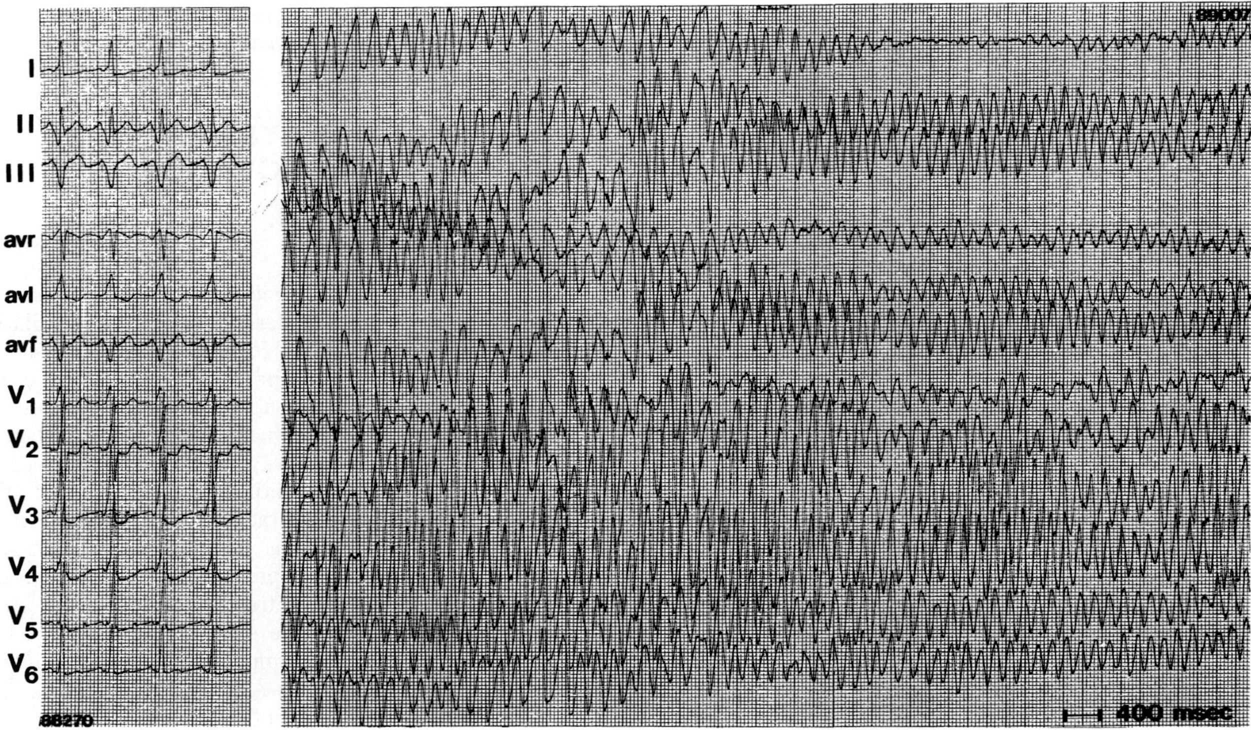

FIGURE 87–7 Example of deterioration of atrial fibrillation into ventricular fibrillation in a patient with the Wolff-Parkinson-White syndrome. Twelve electrocardiographic leads were recorded simultaneously. The *left panel* shows the ECG during sinus rhythm.

attention should be given to the ECG *after* exercise when, in case of exercise-induced block in the accessory pathway, a sudden marked change in the ECG takes place on resumption of AV conduction over the accessory connection. Third, failure to produce complete block in the accessory pathway by intravenous injection of procainamide hydrochloride (10 mg/kg body weight over a 5-minute period)[19] strongly suggests a short anterograde refractory period of the accessory pathway (<270 milliseconds) (Fig. 87–10). Because procainamide also prolongs the refractory period of the His-Purkinje system, the test should be done in surroundings in which complete heart block can be appropriately managed.

TREATMENT

Drugs

As pointed out, circus movement tachycardias in preexcitation have an initiating and a perpetuating mechanism. A premature beat exposing the different properties of the two AV connections is usually the initiating mechanism. Perpetuation of tachycardia is determined by the electrophysiologic properties within the tachycardia circuit.

Using programmed stimulation of the heart, we have learned how different drugs affect the properties of the AV node–His pathway and the accessory AV pathway (Fig. 87–11). Before discussing the choice of a drug for treatment of a circus movement tachycardia, emphasis should be placed on the effectiveness of the vagal maneuvers that block conduction in the AV node in the patient with a circus movement tachycardia (Table 87–2). These maneuvers should be performed as soon as possible after onset of tachycardia. The longer the physician waits, the higher the sympathetic tone and the less likely that the maneuvers will be successful. Note that eyeball pressure is disliked by most patients, carries the risk of retinal detachment, and in our experience, rarely proves effective. If vagal maneuvers are unsuccessful, the intravenous injection of a drug that suddenly prolongs the refractory period of the AV node (e.g., verapamil hydrochloride or adenosine phosphate) or produces lengthening of the refractory period of the accessory AV pathway (e.g., procainamide) usually breaks the circus movement tachycardia (Table 87–3). Pacing or cardioversion is rarely required to interrupt circus movement tachycardia. To prevent circus movement tachycardia, amiodarone hydrochloride in small doses (100 to 200 mg/day) or drugs such as the class IC agents propafenone, flecainide acetate, or sotalol hydrochloride, a beta-blocking agent with class III effects, are usually effective. There is also still a place for "classic" drugs such as quinidine sulfate and procainamide. Controlled studies comparing the efficacy of the different drugs are not available. It is clear, however, that there is no "magic" drug. The physician should therefore prescribe a familiar drug.

Choice of drug treatment of atrial fibrillation is influenced by the ventricular rate and hemodynamic consequences of the arrhythmia. Cardioversion should be done immediately if a rapid ventricular rhythm during atrial fibrillation leads to severe circulatory impairment. If the arrhythmia is better tolerated, drugs that prolong the anterograde refractory period of the accessory pathway should be given.

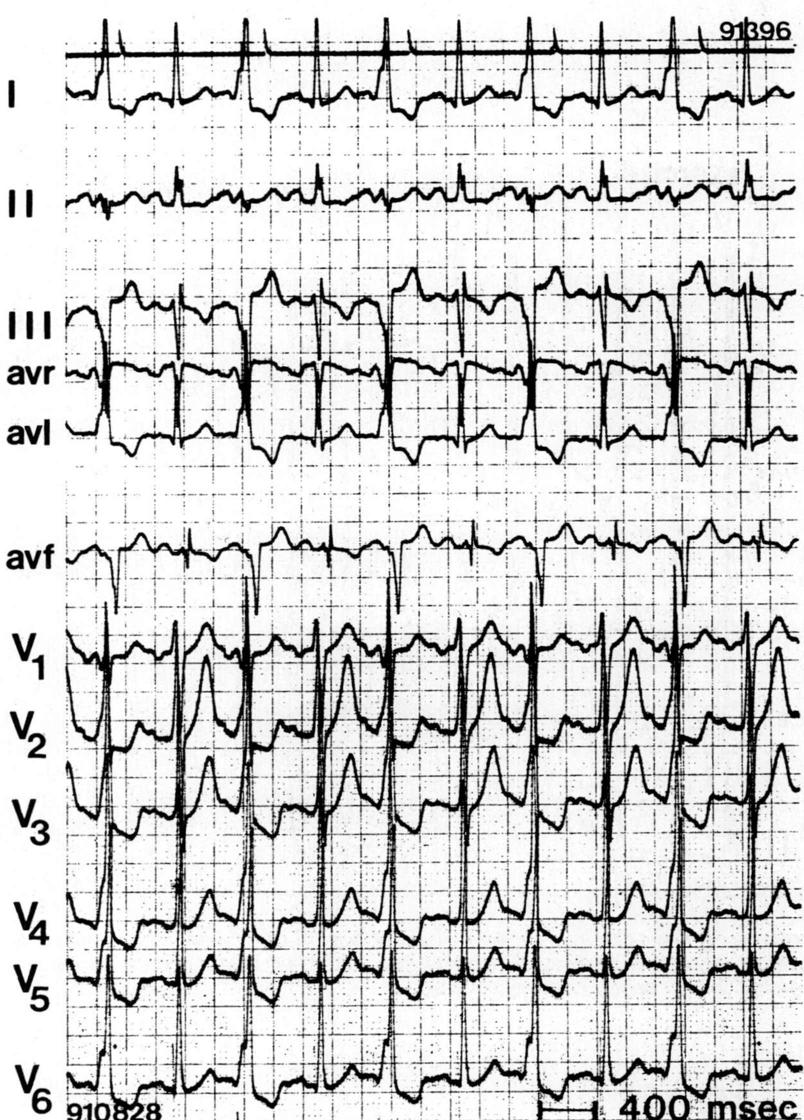

FIGURE 87–8 Intermittent preexcitation. The ECG shows alternating conduction over both the accessory pathway and the AV node and AV conduction over the AV node only.

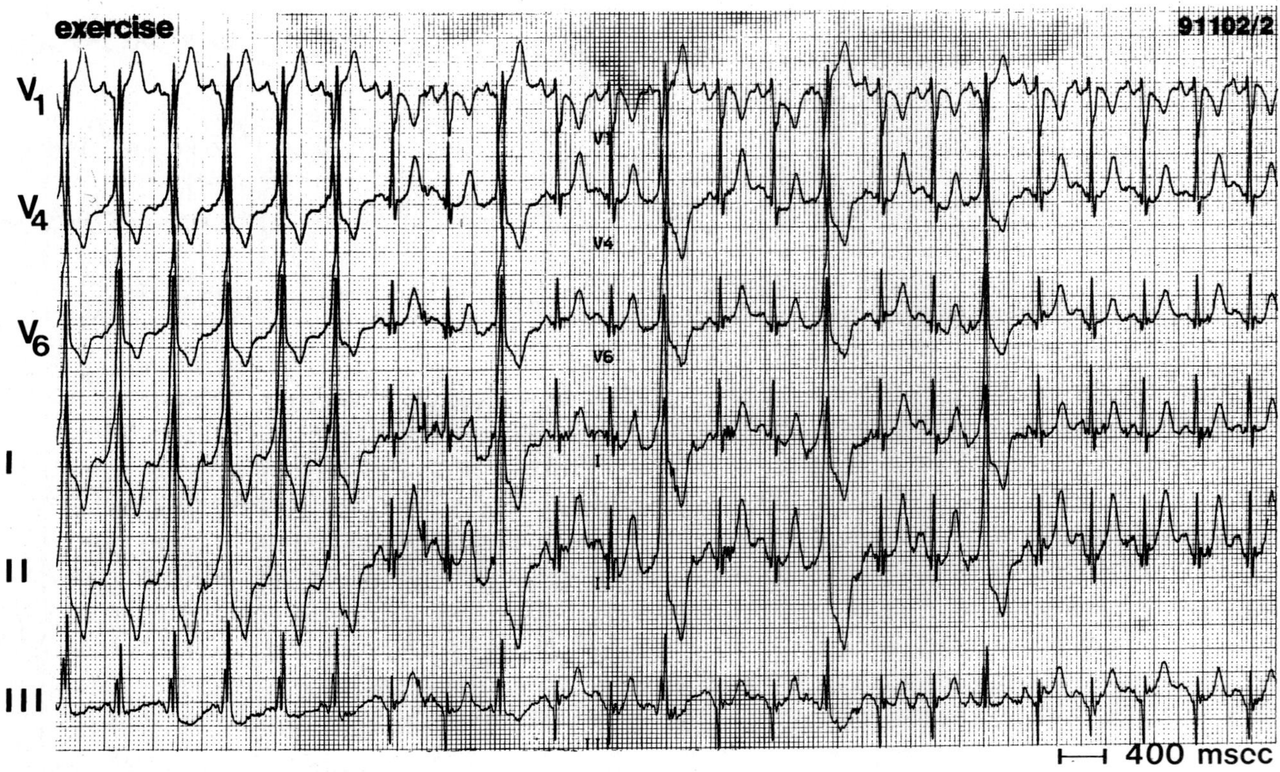

FIGURE 87–9 Effect of exercise in a patient with the Wolff-Parkinson-White syndrome. On reaching a critical sinus rate 1:1, conduction over the accessory pathway disappears. Thereafter, only every third sinus beat is conducted over the accessory pathway until complete block in the accessory pathway occurs.

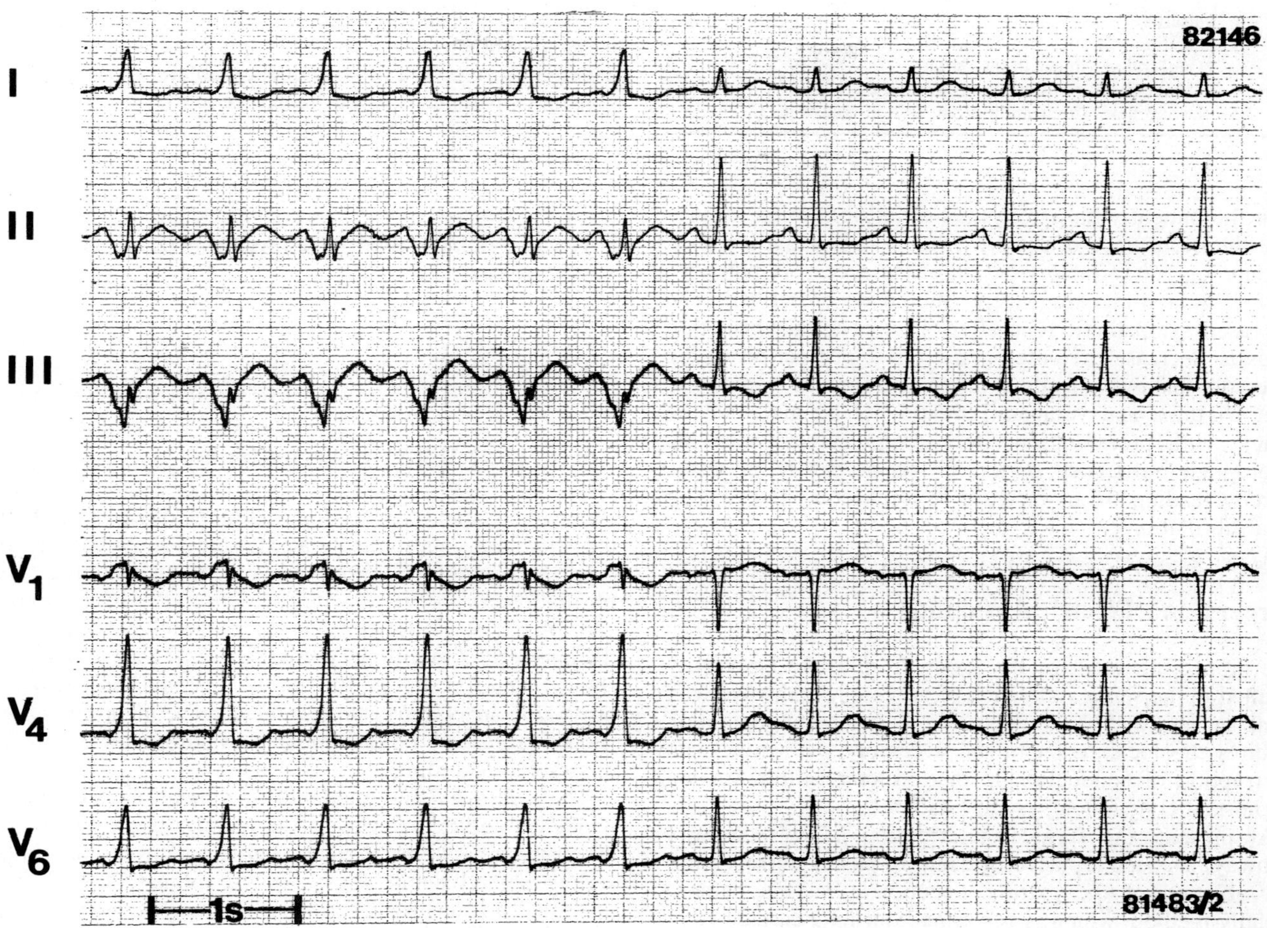

FIGURE 87–10 Example of the occurrence of complete block in the accessory AV pathway after the IV administration of procainamide (600 mg). This indicates a long anterograde refractory period of the accessory pathway.

VAGAL STIMULATION
β-BLOCKING AGENT
VERAPAMIL
DILTIAZEM
ADENOSINE PHOSPHATE
DIGITALIS

ATRIUM

QUINIDINE
PROCAINAMIDE
DISOPYRAMIDE
AJMALINE

VENTRICLE

FLECAINIDE
ENCAINIDE
PROPAFENONE
SOTALOL
AMIODARONE

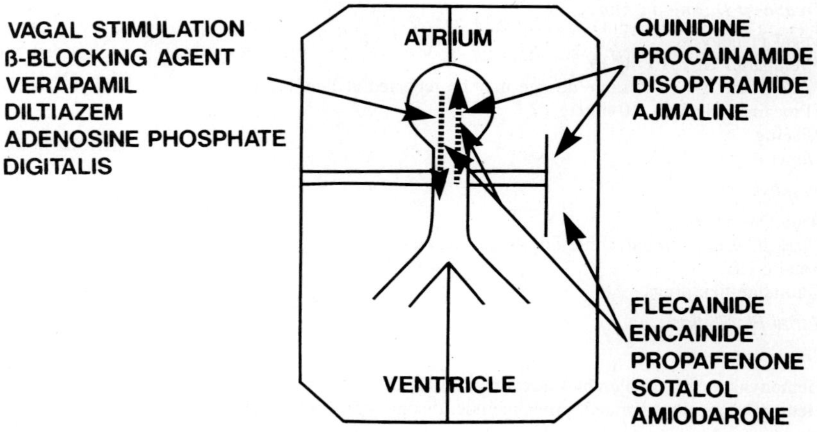

FIGURE 87–11 Site of prolongation of refractory period in AV nodal–His pathway and accessory AV pathway by different drugs. Note that several drugs have effects on both pathways. Note also that some drugs (e.g., quinidine sulfate) lengthen the refractory period of the accessory pathway in anterograde and retrograde direction and the refractory period of the His–AV nodal pathway in retrograde direction only.

TABLE 87-2 Maneuvers Used to Interrupt a Supraventricular Tachycardia

Valsalva
Squatting (Valsalva maneuver)
"Gag" reflex (finger in the throat)
"Upside-down position" (legs against the wall)
"Dive reflex" (immersion of the face in cold water)

In the patient with paroxysmal atrial fibrillation, to prevent the occurrence of the arrhythmia, drugs that lengthen the anterograde refractory period of the accessory pathway, as well as a β-blocking agent, should be prescribed. The increased sympathetic tone after onset of atrial fibrillation tends to decrease the anterograde refractory period of the accessory pathway, leading to an increase in ventricular rate. Digitalis and verapamil should not be given to the patient with preexcitation. Both drugs may shorten the anterograde refractory period of an accessory pathway, thereby leading to an increase in ventricular rate during atrial fibrillation.

Surgery and Electrical Ablation

The pioneering work of the group from Duke University resulted in the surgical division of accessory pathways with great success and at low risk.[8, 14] A successful operation requires the localization of the accessory pathways, with interruption of conduction in that structure while leaving the normal conduction system intact.

At present, the surgical interruption of an accessory pathway has been replaced by radiofrequency current catheter ablation of the extra connection.[20, 21] This patient-friendly method, which is performed during a cardiac catheterization, is associated with a low risk and a high success rate.[22] The indication for radiofrequency current ablation has been medical refractoriness of a disabling arrhythmia, intolerance to drug therapy, detrimental side effects of antiarrhythmic agents, and poor patient compliance. The excellent results of a radiofrequency ablation make it likely that more patients will be treated (even on a prophylactic basis in case of a short anterograde refractory period of the accessory pathway) by this approach.

TABLE 87-3 Treatment of Tachycardia in Patients with Pre-Excitation

Circus Movement Tachycardia

Treatment During an Attack

Vagal maneuvers
*Verapamil HCl, 10 mg IV
*Adenosine 6 mg IV; same dosage may be repeated at 1-min intervals
*Procainamide HCl, 10 mg/kg IV
*Pacing
Direct-current shock

Prophylaxis

Amiodarone HCl
Class IC drugs: propafenone, flecainide acetate
Sotalol HCl
Quinidine-like drugs

Atrial Fibrillation

Treatment

Hemodynamically intolerable: direct-current shock
Hemodynamically tolerated: procainamide, disopyramide, phosphate

Prophylaxis

Amiodarone
Sotalol

*Quinidine-like drugs plus a beta-blocking agent.

PRACTICAL APPROACH TO THE PATIENT

As always in medicine, treatment of the patient with preexcitation should be individualized.

The Patient With an Arrhythmia

When the patient comes for treatment of an arrhythmia, the important questions relate to the following: (1) the type of arrhythmia (circus movement tachycardia, atrial fibrillation, or both); (2) its incidence; (3) its symptoms and tolerance; (4) its tachycardia-initiating events; and (5) the presence of additional cardiac disease. Careful attention should therefore be paid to the history and circumstances provoking arrhythmias, so that they can be identified. These should preferably be documented by long-term electrocardiographic recordings.

The necessity and mode of treatment depend on the incidence and/or severity of the attacks of tachycardia. If the problem is a rare circus movement tachycardia without serious hemodynamic consequences, the patient should try the vagal maneuvers described previously. If they fail, the patient should take medication by mouth, such as quinidine or disopyramide phosphate, and wait for the arrhythmia to subside. This "cocktail" approach is preferred in the patient with rare, well-tolerated tachycardia. We have already discussed the steps to be taken when a persistent arrhythmia occurs or when a recurrent arrhythmia must be prevented.

The Patient Without an Arrhythmia

Although this is still a controversial matter, we believe that patients with an ECG showing ventricular preexcitation should be evaluated to identify those at risk for sudden death if atrial fibrillation occurs. As we have discussed, noninvasive means can be of help in obtaining this information.

Considerable interest exists in the appropriate management of the asymptomatic patient discovered to have a WPW pattern on a routine ECG.[23, 24] In general, our policy is to withhold antiarrhythmic drug therapy in patients who show the WPW ECG without a history of arrhythmias but who have a short anterograde refractory period of the accessory pathway on noninvasive and invasive testing. We agree with Leitch and associates[23] and Beckman and colleagues[24] that these patients have a good prognosis.

However, in selected asymptomatic patients with a short anterograde refractory period of the accessory pathway, we have interrupted conduction over that structure by surgical or radiofrequency current ablation for occupational reasons (e.g., for a patient to be licensed to fly a commercial airliner or to be insured as a professional football player).

REFERENCES

1. Wolff L, Parkinson J, White PD: Bundle branch block with short PR interval in healthy young people prone to paroxysmal tachycardia. Am Heart J 5:685, 1930.
2. Wolferth LC, Wood FC: The mechanism of production of short PR intervals and prolonged QRS complexes in patients with presumably undamaged hearts. Hypothesis of an accessory pathway of atrioventricular conduction (bundle of Kent). Am Heart J 8:297, 1933.
3. Durrer D, Schuilenburg RM, Wellens HJJ: Preexcitation revisited. Am J Cardiol 25:690, 1970.
4. Durrer D, Schoo L, Schuilenburg RM, et al: The role of premature beats in the initiation and termination of supraventricular tachycardia in the Wolff-Parkinson-White syndrome. Circulation 36:644, 1967.
5. Durrer D, Roos JP: Epicardial excitation of the ventricles in a patient with Wolff-Parkinson-White syndrome (type B). Circulation 35:15, 1967.
6. Gallagher JJ, Pritchett ELC, Sealy WC, et al: The pre-excitation syndromes. Prog Cardiovasc Dis 20:285, 1978.
7. Wellens HJJ, Brugada P: Value of programmed stimulation of the heart in patients with the Wolff-Parkinson-White syndrome. *In* Josephson ME, Wellens HJJ (eds): Tachycardias. pp. 199–222. Philadelphia: Lea & Febiger, 1984.
8. Sealy WC, Gallagher JJ, Pritchett ELC: The surgical anatomy of Kent bundles on electrophysiologic mapping and surgical exploration. J Thorac Cardiovasc Surg 76:804, 1978.
9. Becker AE, Anderson RH, Durrer D, Wellens HJJ: The anatomical substrates of Wolff-Parkinson-White syndrome. A clinicopathologic correlation in seven patients. Circulation 57:870, 1978.
10. Anderson RH, Becker AE, Brechenmacher C, et al: Ventricular preexcitation: a proposed nomenclature for its substrates. Eur J Cardiol 3:27, 1975.
11. Chung KY, Walsh TJ, Massie E: Wolff-Parkinson-White syndrome. Am Heart J 69:1, 1965.
12. Bellet S: Clinical Disorders of the Heart Beat. 2nd ed. Philadelphia: Lea & Febiger, 1971.
13. Averill KM, Fosmoe RJ, Lamb LE: Electrocardiographic findings in 67,375 asymptomatic subjects. IV. Wolff-Parkinson-White syndrome. Am J Cardiol 6:108, 1960.
14. Gallagher JJ, Sealy WC, Cox JL, et al: Results of surgery for preexcitation caused by accessory atrioventricular pathways in 267 consecutive cases. *In* Josephson ME, Wellens HJJ (eds): Tachycardias. pp. 259–269. Philadelphia: Lea & Febiger, 1984.
15. Wellens HJJ, Durrer D: Relation between refractory period of the accessory pathway and ventricular frequency during atrial fibrillation in patients with the Wolff-Parkinson-White syndrome. Am J Cardiol 34:777, 1974.
16. Wellens HJJ, Brugada P, Roy D, et al: Effect of isoproterenol on the antegrade refractory period of the accessory pathway in patients with the Wolff-Parkinson-White syndrome. Am J Cardiol 50:180, 1982.
17. Wellens HJJ: Wolff-Parkinson-White syndrome. Part I. Mod Concepts Cardiovasc Dis 52:53, 1983.
18. Levy S, Bronstet JP, Clemency J: Syndrome de Wolff-Parkinson-White. Corrélations entre l'exploration électrophysiologique et l'effet de l'épreuve d'effort sur l'aspect électrocardiographique de pre-excitation. Arch Mal Coeur 72:634, 1979.
19. Wellens HJJ, Braat SH, Brugada P, et al: Use of procainamide in patients with the Wolff-Parkinson-White syndrome to disclose a short refractory period of the accessory pathway. Am J Cardiol 50:921, 1982.
20. Jackman W, Wang X, Friday KJ, et al: Catheter ablation of accessory atrioventricular pathways (Wolff-Parkinson-White syndrome) by radiofrequency current. N Engl J Med 324:1605, 1991.
21. Calkins H, Sousa J, El-Atassi R, et al: Diagnosis and cure of the Wolff-Parkinson-White syndrome or paroxysmal supraventricular tachycardia during a single electrophysiologic test. N Engl J Med 324:1612, 1991.
22. Calkins H, Yong P, Miller JM, et al: Catheter ablation of accessory pathways, atrioventricular nodal reentrant tachycardia and the atrioventricular junction: final results of a prospective, multicenter clinical trial. The Atakr Multicenter Investigators Group. Circulation 99:262, 1999.
23. Leitch JW, Klein GJ, Yee R, Murdock C: Prognostic value of electrophysiologic testing in asymptomatic patients with Wolff-Parkinson-White pattern. Circulation 82:1718, 1990.
24. Beckman KJ, Gallastegui JL, Bauman JL, Hariman RJ: The predictive value of electrophysiologic studies in untreated patients with Wolff-Parkinson-White syndrome. J Am Coll Cardiol 15:640, 1990.

CHAPTER 88

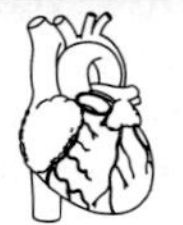

ATRIAL FIBRILLATION/FLUTTER

Gerald V. Naccarelli

EPIDEMIOLOGY AND NATURAL HISTORY
ETIOLOGY
MECHANISM
ATRIAL REMODELING
DEFINITIONS
DIAGNOSIS AND ELECTROCARDIOGRAPHIC FEATURES
EVALUATION
TREATMENT
Acute Treatment
Chronic Treatment
ATRIAL FIBRILLATION AND WOLFF-PARKINSON-WHITE SYNDROME
RISKS OF ANTIARRHYTHMIC THERAPY FOR ATRIAL FIBRILLATION
CHOOSING AN ORAL AGENT FOR MAINTENANCE OF SINUS RHYTHM
POST-THORACOTOMY ATRIAL FIBRILLATION
PRIMARY PREVENTION OF ATRIAL FIBRILLATION
EMBOLIC RISK AND ANTICOAGULATION ISSUES
ANTICOAGULATION FOR CARDIOVERSION
NONPHARMACOLOGIC THERAPIES FOR ATRIAL FIBRILLATION

EPIDEMIOLOGY AND NATURAL HISTORY

Atrial fibrillation is the most common tachyarrhythmia encountered in clinical practice. Several million Americans are affected by this disorder. According to the Framingham Heart Study,[1, 2] atrial fibrillation has a prevalence of 4 percent in the adult population. Feinberg and colleagues[3] reported that the absolute numbers of men and women with atrial fibrillation are equal; however, in patients older than 75 years old, more women than men had atrial fibrillation given the fact that more women are alive in this elderly age group. Atrial fibrillation is a disease of aging; only 0.05 percent of 25- to 30-year-olds and more than 5 percent of patients older than 69 years have this disorder.[1, 4] Independent risk factors for atrial fibrillation include advancing age, diabetes, hypertension, congestive heart failure, and myocardial infarction.[2]

Prognostically, the presence of atrial fibrillation is associated with a fivefold increase in morbidity risk and a twofold increase in mortality risk.[2, 5] Most complications and deaths associated with atrial fibrillation are due to complications associated with cerebrovascular embolic events. Atrial fibrillation accounts for 75,000 strokes per year in the United States. In patients with valvular heart disease, there is a 17-fold increase in the incidence of cerebrovascular embolic accidents. Even in patients without valvular disease, the annual cerebrovascular accident risk averages 3 to 5 percent per year.[6–10] Patients without identifiable heart disease ("lone" atrial fibrillators) have minimal complications associated with their condition.[11, 12] In the Mayo Clinic experience,[11] the cumulative incidence of stroke was only 1.3 percent in 15 years of follow-up.

Patients with previous episodes of paroxysmal atrial fibrillation are at a higher risk for recurrence and the development of chronic atrial fibrillation. Acute conversion and maintenance of sinus rhythm may depend on the duration of atrial fibrillation and atrial size.[13–16]

ETIOLOGY

A large left atrium predisposes toward the development of atrial fibrillation regardless of the type of underlying heart disease. Table 88–1 lists diseases that are commonly associated with atrial fibrillation. Hypertensive cardiovascular disease is the most frequent cause of atrial fibrillation.[1] Other common causes include coronary artery disease, cardiomyopathy, and sick sinus syndrome. Women are more likely to have atrial fibrillation due to congestive heart failure or valvular heart disease, and men are more likely to have atrial fibrillation due to a previous myocardial infarction.[17] From 10 to 28 percent of cases of atrial fibrillation[10, 11, 18] have idiopathic or "lone" atrial fibrillation with no discernible cause identified even after extensive evaluation. Increased parasympathetic tone may predispose patients with otherwise normal hearts to develop vagally mediated atrial fibrillation.[19] Antibodies against myosin

TABLE 88-1 **Causes of Atrial Fibrillations**

Hypertensive cardiovascular disease
Coronary artery disease
Rheumatic mitral valve disease with mitral stenosis or regurgitation
Dilated or hypertrophic cardiomyopathy
Congestive heart failure
Tachycardia-bradycardia syndrome
Post-thoracotomy
Hyperthyroidism
Pericarditis
Congenital heart disease
Idiopathic
Wolff-Parkinson-White syndrome
Alcohol/toxins
Pulmonary embolism

have been noted in one group of patients with atrial fibrillation, suggesting an immune-related cause.[20] A genetic locus for a rare form of familial atrial fibrillation has been identified.[21]

Mechanism

The electrophysiologic mechanisms of atrial arrhythmias are not completely defined. Ectopic atrial arrhythmias appear to arise from disorders of impulse generation either by abnormal automaticity through enhancement of normal ion mechanisms or by triggered activity during or after repolarization (*afterdepolarization*). This may explain why some of these arrhythmias occur with stress, exercise, or digitalis toxicity. Some atrial tachyarrhythmias, such as intra-atrial reentrant tachycardia, are probably caused by micro-reentry.

Reentry is the most widely accepted mechanism used to explain atrial fibrillation and atrial flutter.[22] Heterogeneity of atrial refractoriness creates the milieu for the initiation of atrial fibrillation. Anatomic or physiologic conditions provide the necessary substrate to sustain reentry within atrial tissue. Processes that increase atrial size provide a greater surface area for the development of multiple reentrant wavelets; when refractory atrial tissue is encountered, the reentrant wavelet extinguishes. Slow intra-atrial conduction allows the atrial tissue to electrically recover before another reentrant wavelet passes through the tissue, Shortened refractory periods allow the atria to recover faster and thus allow atrial fibrillation to perpetuate. Thus, antiarrhythmic drugs that prolong atrial refractoriness may help terminate and prevent atrial fibrillation. Atrial stretch, by heterogeneously prolonging atrial refractoriness, may make the initiation of atrial fibrillation more likely.[22] Electrical remodeling, thyrotoxicosis, and increased vagal and sympathetic tone may decrease atrial refractory periods. Decreased conduction velocity may occur secondary to ischemia, fibrosis, or electrolyte abnormalities.

Premature beats frequently act as a trigger to initiate any atrial tachyarrhythmia. Some patients with atrial fibrillation may have triggering activity in the pulmonary veins. In such patients, catheter ablation of the arrhythmogenic focus may prevent further episodes of atrial fibrillation.[23]

In atrial flutter, a single organized right atrial circuit usually propagates in a caudal-cranial direction at a particular cycle length, thereby determining the rate of tachycardia. On the other hand, multiple reentrant wavelets with irregular and rapid propagation patterns appear to cause atrial fibrillation. For both atrial flutter and fibrillation, speeding up conduction velocity of the reentrant wavelets may result in the wavelets encountering refractory tissue and thus terminate the arrhythmia.

Atrial Remodeling

Atrial fibrillation appears to cause an electrical remodeling in the atria. Wijffels and colleagues[24] demonstrated in an instrumented caprine model that the repeated induction of atrial fibrillation results in prolonged episodes of atrial fibrillation by shortening atrial refractoriness. This has popularized the concept that "atrial fibrillation begets atrial fibrillation." Marked changes in atrial myocyte substructure have been noted secondary to this remodeling. Experimental[25] and clinical[26–28] data suggest that this electrical remodeling is mediated by changes in calcium current flux. Verapamil has been shown to attenuate the shortening of atrial refractoriness[25–28] and to shorten the postatrial fibrillation recovery of atrial refractoriness back to baseline. The use of verapamil before cardioversion has also been associated with a higher incidence of postcardioversion maintenance of sinus rhythm.[29] Other drugs, such as propranolol, procainamide, propafenone, and amiodarone, have not demonstrated any beneficial effect on atrial remodeling.[27] Stretch, ischemia, autonomic tone, and atrial natiuretic factor do not appear to be mechanistically associated with electrical remodeling.[28]

Definitions

Atrial fibrillation can occur paroxysmally (intermittently) or in its chronic form. Paroxysmal atrial fibrillation has been defined as recurrent spells that self-terminate within 48 hours. Persistent atrial fibrillation has been defined as spells that last longer than 48 hours and may require medical intervention to revert back to sinus rhythm. Permanent atrial fibrillation is a form of chronic atrial fibrillation that is resistant to cardioversion.[30]

Diagnosis and Electrocardiographic Features

Patients presenting with atrial arrhythmias may be asymptomatic or complain of palpitations, shortness of breath, or dizziness. Hypotension, syncope, and congestive heart failure will often be a function of ventricular rate, degree of underlying ventricular dysfunction, and dependence on the atrial contribution for left ventricular filling and cardiac output. It is difficult to discern one atrial arrhythmia from another through physical examination. An irregularly irregular pulse most commonly occurs with atrial fibrillation; however, atrial flutter and atrial tachycardia with variable atrioventricular (AV) block will cause similar pulse irregularities. A variable intensity of the first heart sound is consistent with atrial fibrillation.

Electrocardiographically, atrial fibrillation is recognized on the basis of irregular baseline undulations or discrete atrial activity of variable amplitude at rates of 350 to 600 beats/min. These atrial deflections are best seen in the inferior leads or precordial lead V_1 (Fig. 88–1). In either case, the ventricular response is usually irregular, ranging from 100 to 180 beats/min in untreated patients.

Atrial flutter rates range from 250 to 350 beats/min. With drug-treated atrial flutter, the atrial rate may be slower (Fig. 88–2). The P wave is usually negative in the inferior or precordial leads, and there is no isoelectric segment between P waves. This results in the characteristic sawtooth pattern. The ventricular response is usually regular and half the atrial rate, most commonly 150 beats/min.

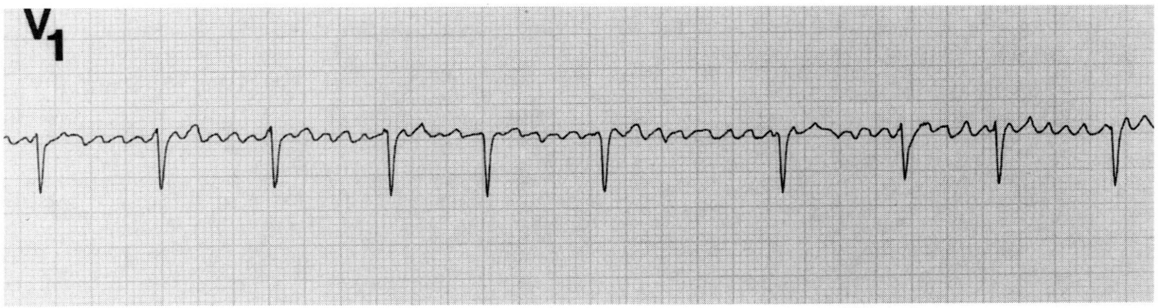

FIGURE 88–1 Lead V_1 rhythm strip demonstrates typical electrocardiographic features of atrial fibrillation.

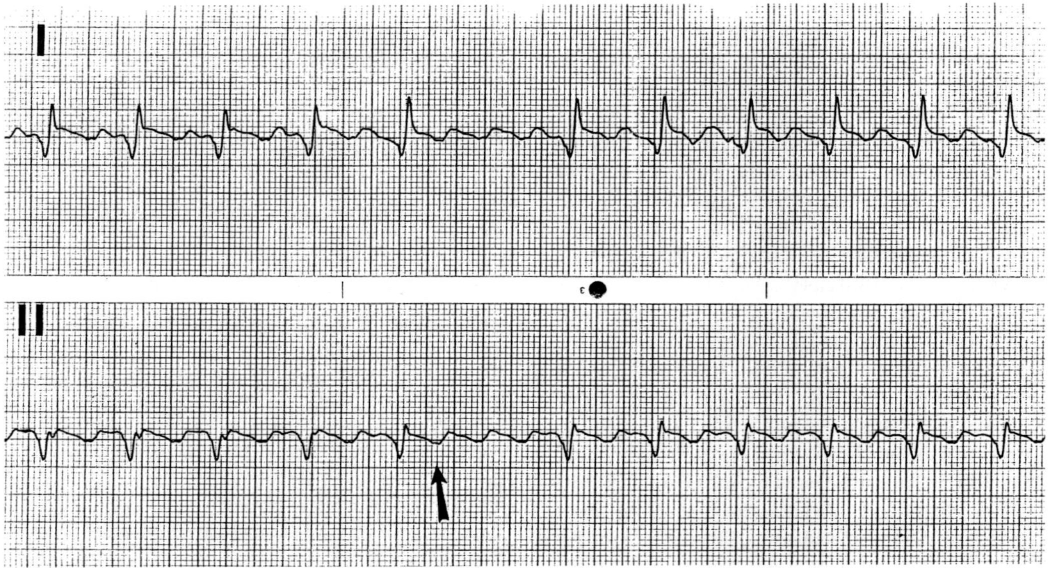

FIGURE 88–2 Electrocardiographic leads I and II demonstrate drug-treated atrial flutter with predominantly 2:1 and transient 4:1 atrioventricular conduction *(arrow).*

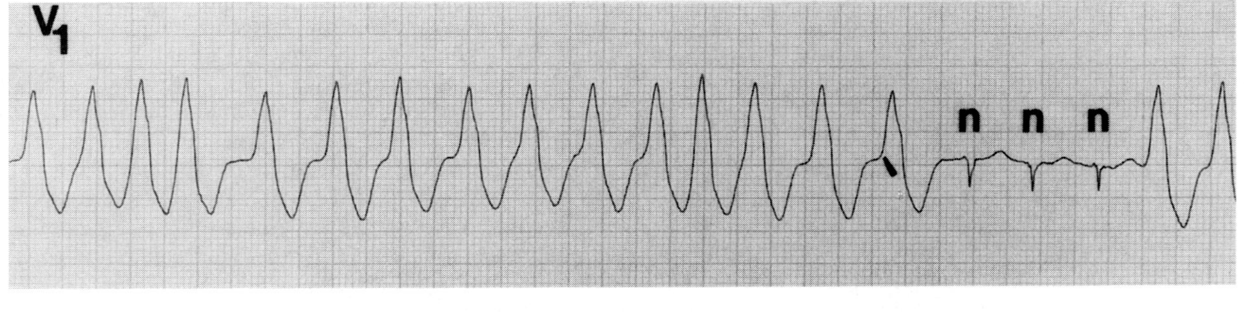

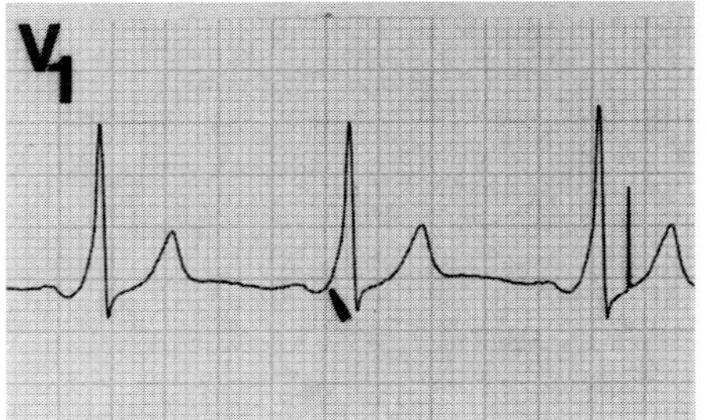

FIGURE 88–3 Electrocardiographic lead V_1 demonstrates atrial fibrillation with wide QRS conduction secondary to antegrade conduction down a left free wall accessory pathway. **Bottom,** in sinus rhythm, there is a similarity of the preexcited QRS complexes. *Arrow,* delta wave; n, conduction down atrioventricular node. (From Berns E, Naccarelli GV: Diagnosis and management of patients with primary atrial arrhythmias. *In* Naccarelli GV [ed]: Cardiac Arrhythmias: A Practical Approach. pp. 177–198. Mt Kisco, NY: Futura, 1991.)

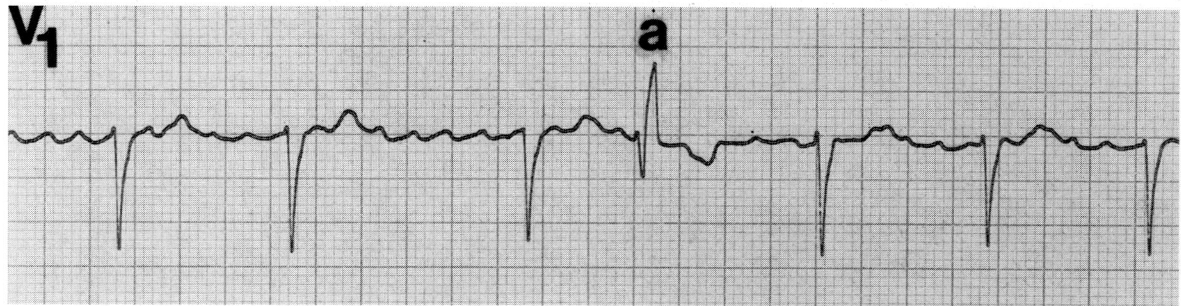

FIGURE 88–4 Lead V_1 demonstrates atrial fibrillation with periods of right bundle branch aberrancy (Ashman phenomenon).

Patients with the Wolff-Parkinson-White syndrome who present with an atrial dysrhythmia associated with an antegrade conducting accessory pathway will have a wide and bizarre-appearing QRS complex secondary to overt preexcitation (Fig. 88–3); intermittent narrow QRS complexes with conduction down the AV node may be present. Aberrant conduction usually occurs when a short RR interval follows a long RR interval (*Ashman's phenomenon*) with the ensuing wide beats frequently assuming a right bundle branch block configuration (Fig. 88–4), although left bundle branch block can also be noted.

EVALUATION

History and physical examination may help diagnose an associated condition that is responsible for the arrhythmia. Echocardiography is useful to confirm the presence or absence of valvular heart disease, pericardial effusion, ventricular hypertrophy, or wall motion abnormalities. In addition, cardiac chamber size can be assessed. Transesophageal echocardiography is useful to screen for risk factors of embolic events, such as aortic placquing, atrial thrombus, and atrial "smoke."[31–43]

Correlation of symptoms with the presence of arrhythmia is important before treatment is undertaken to confirm the diagnosis and to use symptoms as a guide to therapeutic efficacy.[44, 45] An electrocardiogram may confirm the diagnosis of the rhythm and screen for hypertrophy, intraventricular conduction disturbances, previous myocardial infarction, coexisting ischemia, or ventricular arrhythmias. Although chronic arrhythmias are easily documented by electrocardiography, paroxysmal arrhythmias can be difficult to record. Continuous electrocardiographic monitoring (Holter monitoring) for 24 to 48 hours rarely captures infrequent symptomatic episodes but may record nonsustained asymptomatic runs that may represent an electrical instability and predisposition for a sustained event. Holter recordings can also document concomitant ventricular arrhythmias and bradycardias that might influence therapy (Fig. 88–5). When a patient's history suggests exertion as an initiating factor, exercise treadmill testing may be useful

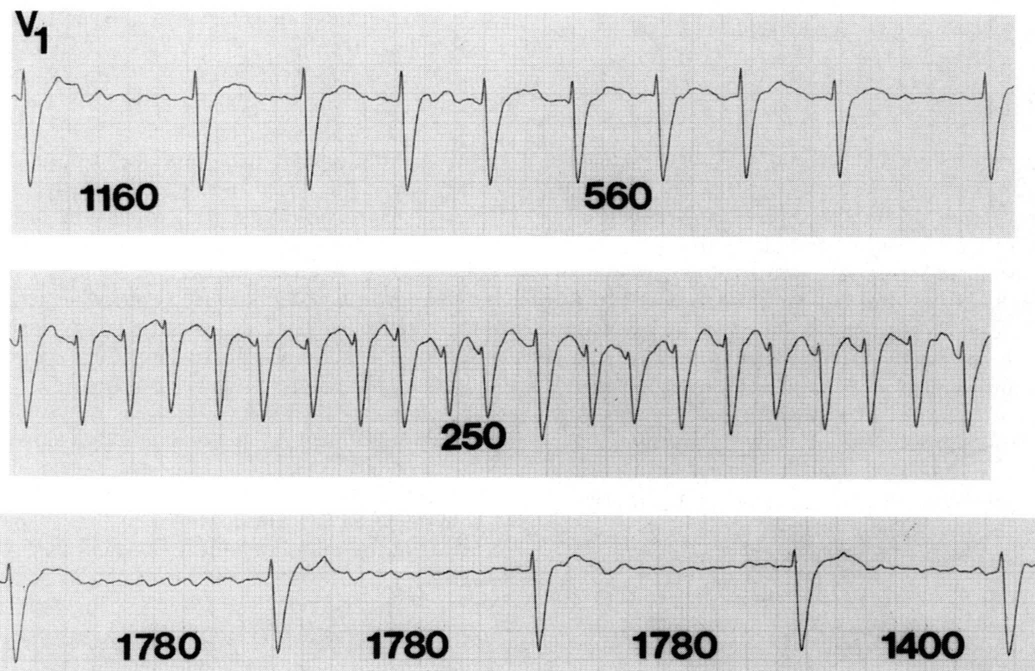

FIGURE 88–5 Holter lead V_1 demonstrates a well-controlled ventricular response **(top)**, a rapid ventricular response (240 beats/min; cycle length, 250 ms) **(middle)**, and a junctional escape rhythm of 34 beats/min (cycle length, 1780 ms) **(bottom)**. All occurred in a patient on digoxin therapy alone during a 24-hour period.

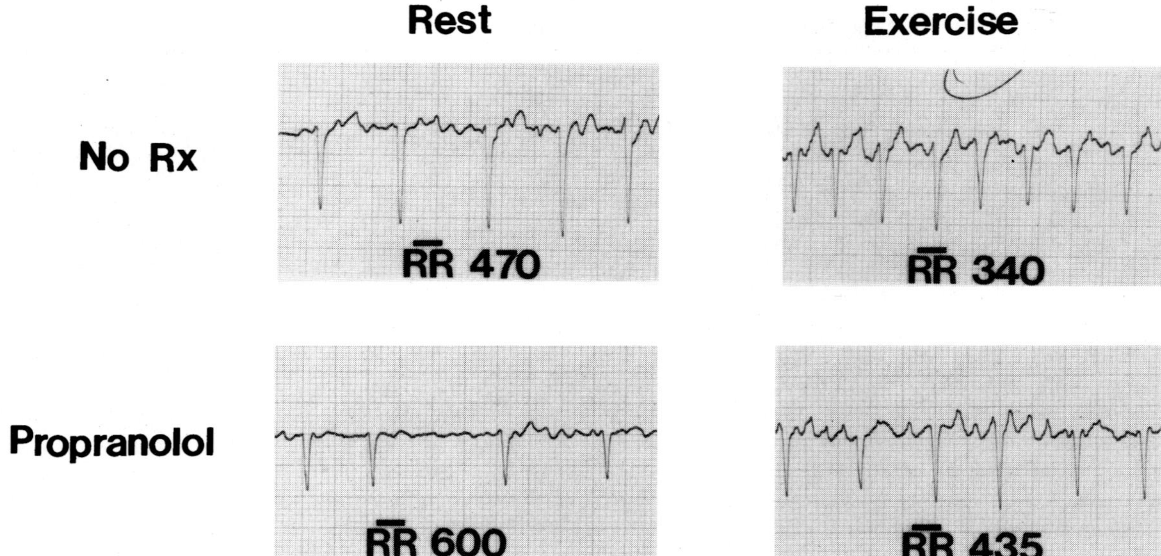

FIGURE 88–6 Electrocardiogram demonstrates better control of ventricular response at rest and during exercise with a combination of propranolol plus digoxin compared with monotherapy with digoxin.

to initiate atrial fibrillation.[46] Stress testing may also be useful to assess the effect of drugs on the ventricular response during exercise (Fig. 88–6). Finally, patient-activated transtelephonic event recorders can record paroxysmal symptomatic occurrences of arrhythmia and define the type of arrhythmia. Once diagnosed, Holter monitoring or transtelephonic recordings may confirm symptomatic recurrence and determine whether the frequency of asymptomatic runs has been decreased with therapy. Patients with persistent atrial arrhythmias in whom the major therapeutic goal is to control the ventricular response under a variety of physiologic conditions should have their heart rates recorded with Holter monitoring and during treadmill testing to assess the heart rate at rest and during exercise.

TREATMENT

In all patients, reversible causes, such as thyrotoxicosis, should be screened for and treated. Major goals of therapy include the prevention of embolic events and reduction in symptoms. There are two general antiarrhythmic treatment strategies for atrial arrhythmias: control of ventricular response or restoration and/or maintenance of sinus rhythm.[47, 48] Except for patients with overt preexcitation, the ventricular response to an atrial arrhythmia is usually dependent on propagation of impulses through the AV node. Table 88–2 outlines pharmacologic agents used to control the ventricular response by slowing AV nodal conduction and prolonging AV nodal refractoriness; the table also lists antiarrhythmic drugs with active electrophysiologic effects in the atria. These drugs are useful to pharmacologically convert atrial fibrillation and maintain sinus rhythm.

Acute Treatment

Figure 88–7 depicts an algorithm for the acute management of atrial fibrillation.[49] The route of drug administration depends on the urgency of the clinical situation. Digitalization is often used to control the ventricular response.[50, 51] Although safe, digitalization often takes hours and is less useful when there is an acute need to quickly slow the ventricular response. During loading, one should observe for signs of digitalis toxicity, such as significant slowing of the ventricular response, accelerated junctional rhythm, junctional escape rhythm, or an increase in ventricular ectopic activity.

Intravenous β-blockers or calcium channel blockers are faster and more effective than digitalis for controlling the ventricular rate. When verapamil is administered over a 1- to 2-minute period, the maximal effect on the AV node is achieved within 2 to 3 minutes, and the duration of action lasts about 30 minutes.[52, 53] Verapamil should be used cautiously in patients with a history of left ventricular dysfunction, tachycardia-bradycardia syndrome, or concurrent use of β-blockers. In addition, intravenous verapamil is a potent vasodilator and may produce profound hypotension, especially if the blood pressure is already low. Because of these concerns, diltiazem (0.25 mg/kg IV bolus) has gained popularity for acute use in slowing the ventricular response.[54, 55] After an intravenous bolus of diltiazem, a 25 to 35 percent reduction in ventricular response usually occurs within 3 to 7 minutes and may last for hours. If necessary, continuous infusions of diltiazem can be used to help control the ventricular response.

Intravenous β-blockers, such as propranolol, may also achieve significant AV node conduction slowing, especially when a rapid ventricular response is due to a heightened adrenergic state. Esmolol is an intravenous β-blocker with an acute onset of action similar to that of propranolol but a rapid termination half-life of 9 minutes.[56] Because of its short half-life, esmolol may provide an added element of safety if adverse reactions should occur. Studies with esmolol, propranolol, and verapamil demonstrate that they are equally effective for controlling ventricular rates and have a similar incidence of drug-induced hypotension.[57–59] Due to its extremely short half-life, adenosine has no role in the management of this heart disturbance.

TABLE 88-2 **Pharmacologic Therapies of Atrial Arrhythmias**

Drug	Loading Dose	Maintenance Dose
Intravenous and Oral Agents to Control Ventricular Response		
Digoxin	0.75–1.0 mg IV 0.75–1.5 mg PO	0.125–0.25 mg qod–qd PO or IV
Propranolol	0.15–0.20 mg/kg IV	20–80 mg q6h PO or IV
Esmolol	500 μg/kg/min IV loading doses	50–300 μg/kg/min IV
Verapamil	5–10 mg IV	80–160 mg q6–8h PO 0.005 mg/kg/min IV
Diltiazem	0.25 mg/kg IV	30–90 mg q8h PO 5–15 mg/h IV
Amiodarone*	1100 mg IV over 24 h	1 mg/min IV
Agents to Restore and Maintain Sinus Rhythm		
Ibutilide	1 mg IV (may repeat ×1)	NA
Procainamide*	10–15 mg/kg IV	2–4 mg/min IV 500–1000 mg q6h PO (SR)†
Quinidine		200–600 mg q6h PO
Disopyramide*		100–200 mg q6h PO†
Flecainide	300 mg PO × 1 dose	100–150 mg bid PO
Propafenone	600 mg PO × 1 dose	150–300 mg tid PO
Sotalol		80–160 mg bid PO
Amiodarone*	800–1600 mg/da tapered to 400 mg/da by 2–6 wk	200–400 mg qd PO
Dofetilide		250–500 μg bid
Azimilide‡		100–125 mg qd

Abbreviations: NA, not applicable; SR, sustained release.
*Not approved by the U.S. Food and Drug Administration for this indication.
†Same daily dose split bid with controlled-release forms.
‡Investigational.

Digitalis, verapamil, diltiazem, propranolol, and esmolol rarely terminate atrial arrhythmias. Two studies have noted no difference in the reversion of atrial fibrillation acutely in digitalized versus nondigitalized patients.[50, 51] Most reversions after the administration of AV nodal blocking agents are due to spontaneous conversion. Several studies have demonstrated that spontaneous conversion rates are as high as 50 to 70 percent during the first 24 hours after presentation with symptoms.[60, 61] Patients with symptomatic atrial fibrillation of less than 24 to 48 hours have the highest spontaneous reversion rates.[60, 61] If a patient with atrial fibrillation is admitted to the hospital from the emergency department, the mean length of stay is 3.9 days with average hospital costs of $6,692.[61] Given the fact that there are more than 1 million hospital admissions per year in the United States, more cost-effective and efficient treatment strategies are needed. Rate control with spontaneous conversion to sinus rhythm may represent the most cost-effective approach to patients who present with recent-onset atrial fibrillation. Patients who do not revert spontaneously within a short period of time are good candidates for medical or direct current (DC) cardioversion.

Although DC cardioversion is effective in reverting about 85 percent of patients to sinus rhythm,[62] intravenous drugs, such as ibutilide and procainamide, and oral class IA, IC, and III agents, including bolus oral class IC, are commonly used for medical cardioversion of both atrial fibrillation and atrial flutter. The ability to acutely terminate and chronically maintain sinus rhythm may be enhanced when oral pharmacologic therapy is instituted before electrical cardioversion and then continued after sinus rhythm is restored. Drug-refractory atrial flutter usually requires either pacing or DC shock for the restoration of sinus rhythm.

Because embolic risk of cardioversion increases if symptoms exists for longer than 48 hours,[65] an efficient decision process is necessary. If patients present with atrial fibrillation of longer than 48 hours, several weeks of rate control with warfarin is required. The role of transesophageal echocardiography–guided cardioversion is under investigation.[66] Although the risk of embolic events is lower for the cardioversion of atrial flutter, the persistence of atrial stunning[63, 64] suggests that similar antiembolic strategies, used for the cardioversion of atrial fibrillation, should be considered.

Intravenous procainamide can acutely terminate atrial fibrillation in about 20 percent of cases.[67] The main side effects of intravenous procainamide include hypotension, QRS and QT interval prolongation, and drug-induced torsades de pointes.

Ibutilide is more effective than procainamide and can revert 35 to 40 percent of patients to sinus rhythm within 1 hour of administration.[67–69] Ibutilide is administered in a dose of 1 mg IV over 10 minutes. Up to 70 percent of all conversions occur within 20 minutes of infusion. If the first dose is ineffective, a second may be administered before alternative strategies are considered. Atrial flutter is even more likely to convert with intravenous ibutilide.[69] The side effects of ibutilide include significant QT prolongation with sustained polymorphc ventricular tachycardia (torsades de pointes) in 1.7 percent of patients and nonsustained polymorphic ventricular tachycardia in 2.6 percent of patients.[68] Essentially all ibutilide-induced proarrhythmias occur within 1 hour; however, given the short half-life of the drug, a 4-hour observation period is recommended before discharging patients.

Oral quinidine also may be used for the acute termination of atrial fibrillation. The conversion rate is reported to be up to 60 percent and is noted to be more effective than

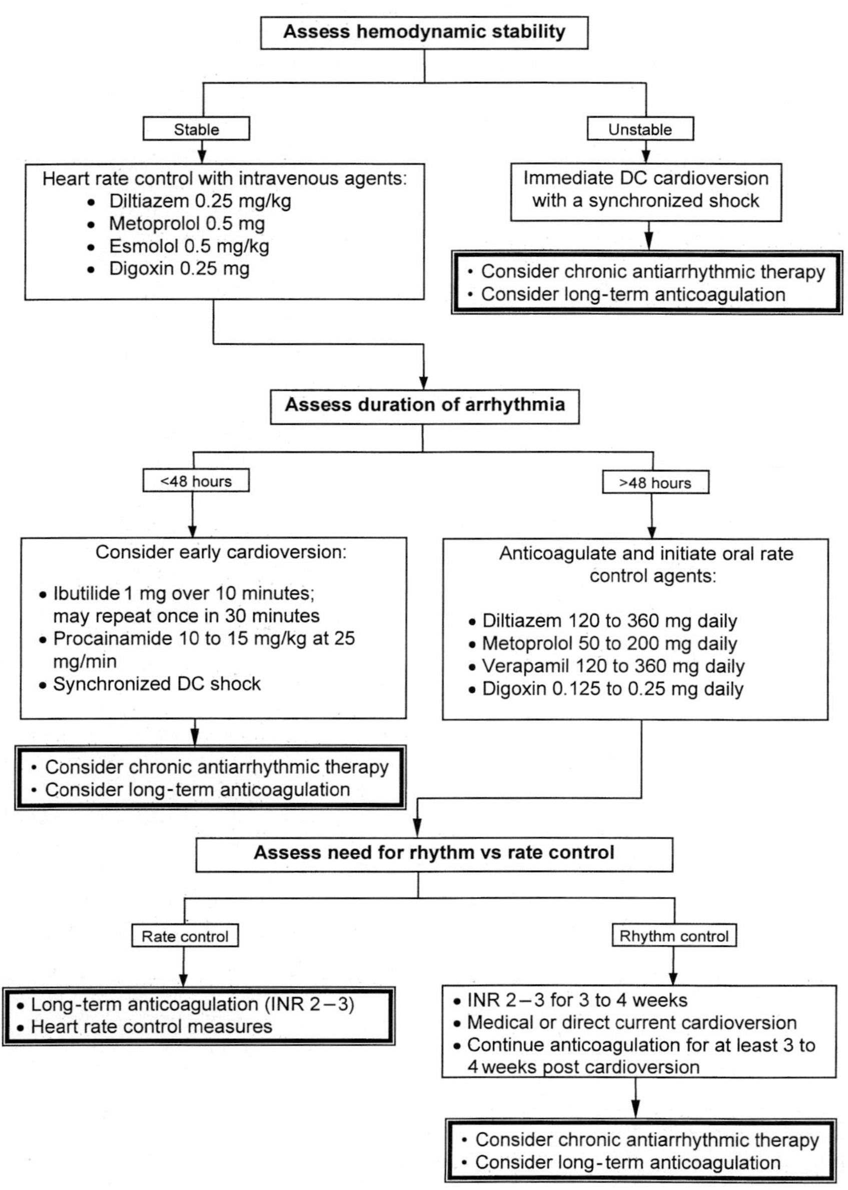

FIGURE 88–7 Algorithm for the acute management of atrial fibrillation.

oral sotalol.[70, 71] Torsades de pointes is a major side effect in patients who undergo therapy with quinidine. This proarrhythmia is most likely to occur after reversion to sinus rhythm,[70, 71] when postectopic pauses may prolong the QT interval the most.

A single high-bolus dose of oral flecainide (300 mg) will convert 60 to 70 percent of recent-onset atrial fibrillation to sinus rhythm within 3 hours and up to 91 percent within 8 hours of administration.[72] A high-bolus dose (600 mg) of oral propafenone has also been shown to be effective for reversion of recent-onset atrial fibrillation, with conversion rates of up to 76 percent within 8 hours of administration.[72, 73] Efficacy rates are similar for patients with and without structural heart disease.[74] Studies in patients with persistent atrial fibrillation are not available.

Intravenous amiodarone has little effect in atrial tissue but acutely slows AV nodal conduction and prolongs AV nodal refractoriness through its calcium-blocking and sympatholytic properties.[75] Although intravenous amiodarone is useful in controlling the ventricular response, a placebo-controlled study demonstrated that amiodarone (68 percent conversion rate) was no more effective ($P = .5$) than placebo (60 percent conversion rate) for the acute conversion of atrial fibrillation to sinus rhythm.[76] The most common side effects of intravenous amiodarone include hypotension and bradyarrhythmias. On the other hand, oral amiodarone, which prolongs atrial refractoriness, may be effective in cardioversion, either alone or as an adjunct to DC cardioversion.[77] However, due to the long half-life of amiodarone, it is not useful for acute cardioversion.

Patients who have severe hypotension, congestive heart failure, or angina associated with their arrhythmia should have immediate electrical cardioversion to sinus rhythm with a synchronized DC countershock. Electrical cardioversion has a success rate of 85 to 90 percent. Atrial flutter is frequently terminated with as little as 10 to 50 J. Atrial fibrillation usually requires a minimum of 50 to 100 J and up to 400 J to restore sinus rhythm.

Chronic Treatment

Chronic treatment strategies include rate control, maintenance of sinus rhythm, and antiembolic measures.[18, 44, 47, 48, 78] Three multicenter randomized trials are ongoing to compare the risks and benefits of rate control with those of rhythm control therapy. These three trials include Atrial Fibrillation Follow-up Investigation of Rhythm Management (AFFIRM), Pharmacologic Intervention in Atrial Fibrillation (PIAF), and Rate Control versus Electrical Cardioversion (RACE).[78, 79] The results of these trials will determine the appropriate role of the two treatment strategies in the future.

On a chronic basis, the same drugs, useful for acute rate control, are often used orally to control the ventricular response in chronic or recurring paroxysmal atrial fibrillation. Although digoxin is quite popular, its efficacy as monotherapy is limited because it may not be effective in rate control during acute paroxysms of atrial fibrillation or during exercise[80–82] (see Fig. 88–6). Because of these limitations, once-a-day β-blockers verapamil and diltiazem have gained popularity either as monotherapy or in combination with digoxin. The added benefit of calcium blockers may be the attenuation of atrial fibrillation–induced atrial remodeling; however, in one study, the addition of atenolol to digoxin appeared to control the ventricular response better than digoxin plus diltiazem.[82] Due to their negative inotropic potential, β-blockers and calcium blockers must be used cautiously in patients with congestive heart failure. Obviously, chronic rate control does not eliminate the risk of peripheral embolization, and concomitant antiembolic therapy should be used when appropriate.

Restoration and maintenance of sinus rhythm may improve symptoms and hemodynamics. Class IA, IC, and III antiarrhythmic drugs often restore sinus rhythm. Oral procainamide, disopyramide, flecainide, propafenone, and sotalol are as effective as quinidine for the prevention of atrial fibrillation.[83–92] Several comparative trials have compared the efficacy of these agents in maintaining sinus rhythm. On the average, about 50 percent of patients will maintain sinus rhythm at 1 year with the use of these agents.[83, 85, 92] Dofetilide and azimilide, new class III agents, appear to have similar efficacy.[93, 94] Even if a type IA agent has failed previously, one half to two thirds of patients treated with a type IC agent or with sotalol will be maintained in sinus rhythm with fewer side effects compared with patients taking the more conventional type IA agents.[87, 89]

Amiodarone appears to be the most effective agent available for drug refractory, symptomatic, recurrent atrial fibrillation.[95–101] A small trial has demonstrated that it is more effective than sotalol,[102] and larger randomized trials are attempting to verify this finding.[103] Nearly two thirds of patients treated remained in sinus rhythm for up to 1 year. Most patients with persistent atrial fibrillation will require DC cardioversion after a 4- to 6- week loading period with oral amiodarone because medical cardioversion will occur in fewer than 50 percent of patients. However, once converted, amiodarone is effective in maintaining sinus rhythm in more than 50 percent of patients. The use of low-dose amiodarone (≤200 mg/da) limits its potentially severe and life-threatening side effects.[104]

Regardless of the antiarrhythmic used, about 50 percent of patients will have recurrence of their arrhythmia during the first year. The recurrence rates in patients with longstanding atrial fibrillation, a large left atrial size, or multiple previous drug failures will be even higher. Concomitant rate control therapy with oral digoxin, diltiazem, verapamil, or a β-blocker should be considered along with appropriate oral antiembolic therapy. Although recurrence of atrial fibrillation is common, antiarrhythmic drugs are often effective in decreasing the frequency of atrial fibrillation as measured by the time to first recurrence and the arrhythmia-free interval.[91, 98] Complete abolition of symptoms is rare. An acceptable therapeutic end point is a marked reduction in symptomatic episodes.

Atrial Fibrillation and Wolff-Parkinson-White Syndrome

Patients presenting with antegrade conduction over an accessory pathway during atrial fibrillation or flutter (Fig. 88–3) are often hemodynamically unstable, and emergency electrical cardioversion is the treatment of choice. These patients represent the subgroup with supraventricular tachyarrhythmias who are at risk for sudden cardiac death if their ventricular response is rapid.[105] These patients should not receive AV node–blocking agents such as digitalis, β-blockers, or calcium channel–blocking agents because the ventricular rate is rarely slowed and frequently enhanced down the accessory pathway, resulting in hypotension or the precipitation of a ventricular tachyarrhythmia.[106, 107]

In patients whose blood pressure is stable, the intravenous administration of procainamide may slow conduction over the accessory pathway and terminate the atrial arrhythmia. Intravenous lidocaine should not be used because it is ineffective and may rarely enhance conduction over the accessory pathway.

Individuals presenting with atrial arrhythmias and overt preexcitation should be stabilized and undergo electrophysiologic evaluation to determine whether pharmacologic therapy with a type IA or IC agent to maintain sinus rhythm will also slow or prevent antegrade accessory pathway conduction should there be a recurrence. Radiofrequency catheter ablation of the accessory pathway remains a frontline therapy to eliminate accessory pathway conduction and often eliminates atrial fibrillation that may have been triggered by atrioventricular reentrant supraventricular tachycardia.

Risks of Antiarrhythmic Therapy for Atrial Fibrillation

It is assumed that antiarrhythmic therapy will reduce the recurrence of atrial fibrillation and thus complications, such as stroke, associated with these recurrences. This hypothesis has not been well tested. Asymptomatic recurrences of atrial fibrillation episodes appear to be common.[108] It is not known whether these asymptomatic recurrences are associated with an increased risk for stroke.

Data suggest that the use of membrane-active antiarrhythmic drugs may be associated with increased mortality risk secondary to drug-induced ventricular proarrhythmia. A meta-analysis[83] reported that quinidine use was associated with a 2.9 percent mortality rate compared with only 0.9 percent in patients not treated with quinidine ($P <$ .05). In the Stroke Prevention in Atrial Fibrillation (SPAF) trial,[109] an enhanced mortality rate was noted in atrial fibrillation patients with associated heart failure who were treated with drugs such as quinidine and procainamide. In patients with congestive heart failure, only amiodarone and dofetilide have been shown to have no adverse effects on survival.[110–113] The safety of the use of azimilide in the post–myocardial infarction setting is being studied.[114] Due to the results of the Cardiac Arrhythmia Suppression Trial (CAST), flecainide should be avoided in the post–myocardial infarction setting.[115] However, Pritchett and colleagues[116] reported that the use of flecainide and encainide was not associated with any enhanced mortality rates in a cohort of patients with supraventricular tachycardia who did not have significant structural heart disease. In post–myocardial infarction patients, amiodarone, sotalol, and dofetilide have demonstrated no adverse effects on survival rates.[112, 113, 117–119] Other class I antiarrhythmic agents have not been well studied in the post–myocardial infarction setting and should be used with caution.

Because of its vagolytic effect and resultant rapid ventricular response, quinidine should not be given without prior administration of agents to slow AV nodal conduction. Type IA and IC agents occasionally slow the atrial rate, allowing for more impulses to be conducted and resulting in a faster ventricular rate. The occurrence of wide QRS tachycardias in patients with atrial fibrillation treated with class IC agents is most often secondary atrial flutter with 1:1 AV nodal conduction and QRS widening.[120, 121] This situation can be misdiagnosed as ventricular tachycardia (Fig. 88–8). This is commonly prevented or treated by the addition of agents that slow AV node conduction, such as β-blockers and calcium channel blockers. Occasionally, treatment of patients with antiarrhythmic drugs may worsen sinus node function or AV node or His-Purkinje conduction, resulting in symptomatic bradyarrhythmias that require pacemaker support.

Quinidine syncope is due to a drug-induced arrhythmia—torsades de pointes.[122–124] This is a rapid, polymorphic ventricular tachycardia commonly associated with the use of class IA and III agents and frequently seen in patients with left ventricular dysfunction, hypokalemia, prolonged QT interval, or atrial fibrillation (Fig. 88–9). It is our practice to initiate antiarrhythmic drugs, with the potential to cause torsades de pointes, in the hospital under electrocardiographic monitoring for about 72 to 96 hours. This is the usual time for drugs to reach a steady state and to detect most early proarrhythmic events.[125–127] The initiation of antiarrhythmic therapy under inpatient monitoring has been shown to be a cost-effective strategy in selected patients.[127]

Class IC agents may precipitate a ventricular proarrhythmia in patients with left ventricular dysfunction, a left ventricular scar, or coexisting ventricular arrhythmias.[128] However, in patients with idiopathic atrial fibrillation and no evidence of structural heart disease, the incidence of IC-induced ventricular proarrhythmia is very low. In this latter low-risk patient group, we usually initiate flecainide and propafenone therapy on an outpatient basis.

The development of incessant atrial arrhythmias or atrial arrhythmia not previously documented is a rare but well described atrial proarrhythmic response.[129] These arrhythmias are frequently resistant to pharmacologic or electrical cardioversion with spontaneous conversion occurring after the drug is metabolized. Because it is difficult to predict the hemodynamic and ventricular responses to an incessant atrial proarrhythmia after the drug is discontinued, treatment is most safely done in the hospital with telemetry monitoring.

Finally, the risk of antiarrhythmia-induced subjective and end-organ toxicity must be considered before initiating

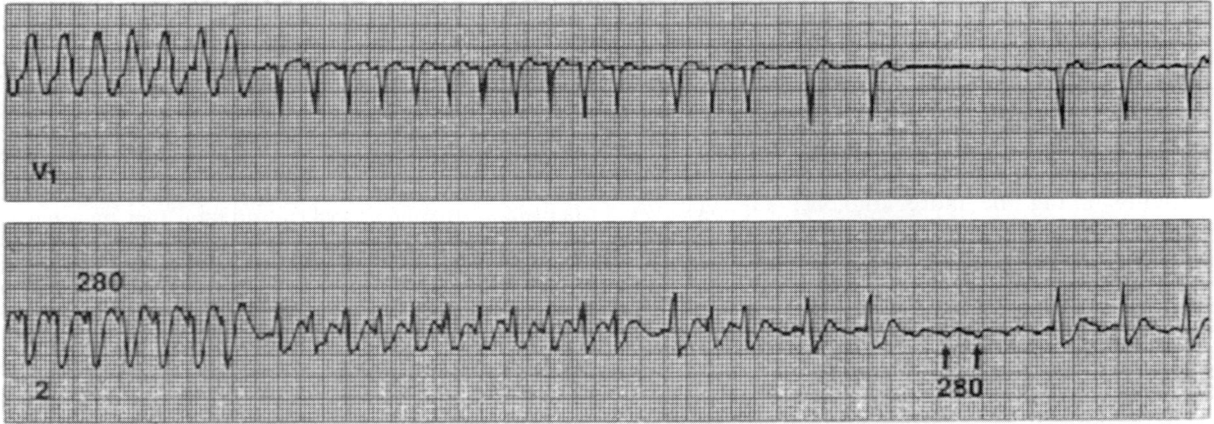

FIGURE 88–8 Wide QRS tachycardia secondary to flecainide-treated atrial flutter and 1:1 atrioventricular conduction in an atrial fibrillation patient occurring during the recovery phase of a stress test. After several seconds of recovery, normalization of the QRS complex occurs, followed by atrioventricular block with the atrial flutter cycle length of 280 msec, being identical to the R-to-R cycle length during 1:1 conduction.

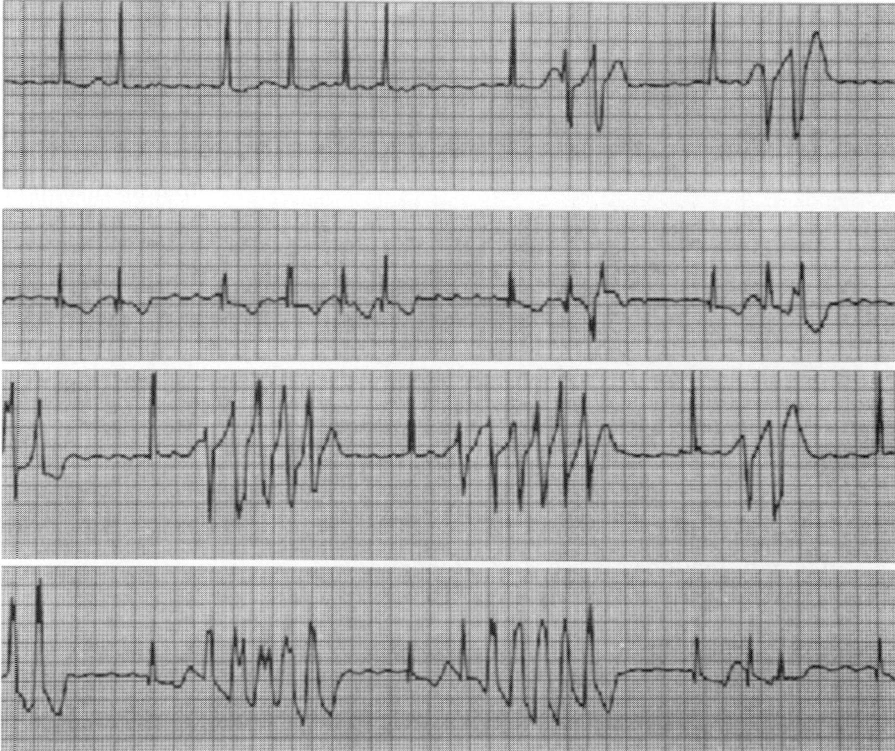

FIGURE 88–9 Simultaneous Holter, V_5, and V_1 leads of a patient with atrial fibrillation treated with quinidine. **Bottom,** the occurrence of pause-dependent, nonsustained polymorphic ventricular tachycardia (torsades de pointes).

therapy for atrial fibrillation. Lethal examples of drug-induced end-organ toxicity include drug-induced neutropenia, thrombocytopenia, and pulmonary fibrosis.

Choosing an Oral Agent for Maintenance of Sinus Rhythm

All of the class IA, IC, and III agents are chronically useful in maintaining sinus rhythm and have 1-year efficacy rates of about 5 percent. Thus, atrial fibrillation recurrences are common after the initiation of these oral drugs. Because the complete abolition of recurrences may be unrealistic, a reasonable end point of therapy is to markedly reduce the frequency and duration of any recurrences. Because these drugs have similar efficacy, drugs are usually chosen based on their lack of end-organ, cardiac, subjective toxicity. The frequency and type of proarrhythmic potential of the drug are key factors in the front-line use of these drugs. Front-line choices vary depending on the presence (Fig. 88–10) or absence (Fig. 88–11) of structural heart disease. In idiopathic atrial fibrillation (Fig. 88–12), flecainide and propafenone are first drugs of choice given their safety record,[116] lack of end-organ toxicity, low incidence of subjective toxicity, and low ventricular proarrhythmic risk in this patient population. In patients after myocardial infarction (see Fig. 88–11), sotalol, dofetilide, and amiodarone are preferred due to their neutral survival effects on this population.[112, 113, 117–119] In patients with congestive heart failure, dofetilide and amiodarone are the only drugs with studies demonstrating neutral survival[110–113] and therefore are used as front-line agents in this population.

Post-Thoracotomy Atrial Fibrillation

Postoperative atrial arrhythmias are commonly seen after thoracic surgery, especially pneumonectomy and open-heart surgery.[128, 129] More than 30 percent of post-thoracotomy patients may develop postoperative atrial fibrillation. Acute treatment to restore sinus rhythm is often ineffective or associated with early recurrence. However, most patients who develop postoperative atrial fibrillation will have sinus rhythm restored either spontaneously or with pharmacologic therapy within 1 week of surgery, and only 15 percent will require long-term treatment. Hemodynamic and embolic complications from postoperative paroxysmal atrial

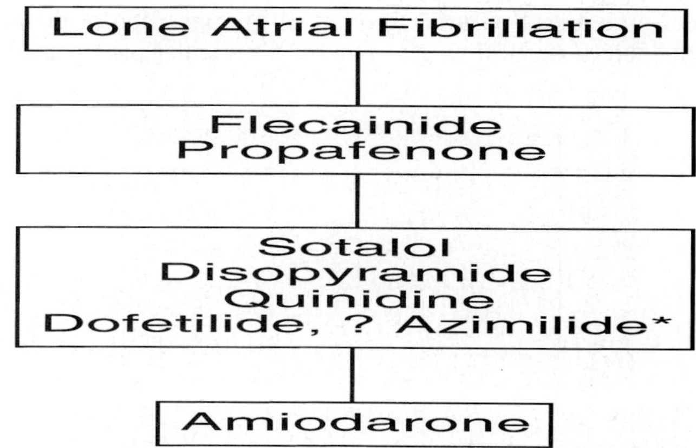

FIGURE 88–10 Algorithm for choosing oral antiarrhythmic drug for idiopathic atrial fibrillation.

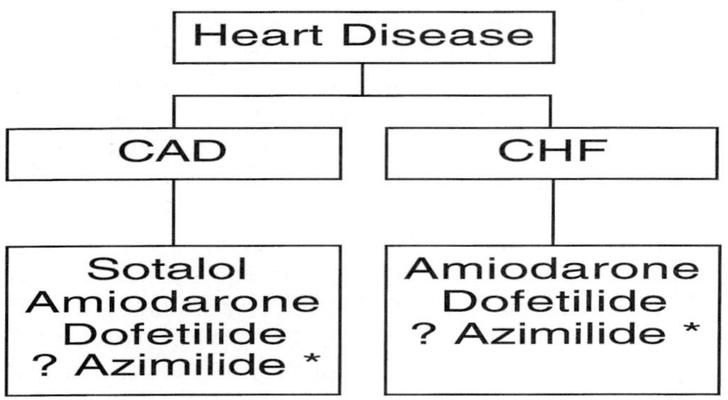

FIGURE 88–11 Algorithm for choosing oral antiarrhythmic drug for treatment of atrial fibrillation associated with significant structural heart disease. CAD, coronary artery disease; CHF, congestive heart failure.

fibrillation are rare. Multiple studies have shown that prophylaxis with low-dose β-blockers preoperatively frequently prevent the acute episodes.[130] Randomized studies with digoxin are less conclusive although in a meta-analysis report, digoxin added to β-blockers was more effective than β-blockers alone in maintaining sinus rhythm.[131] Intravenous procainamide has not been shown to be of prophylactic use.[132] Although preoperative oral[133] and postoperative intravenous amiodarone[134] appears to prevent post-thoracotomy atrial fibrillation, amiodarone may have little to offer over the use of preoperative β-blockers. Rate control and antiembolic therapy may be a cost-effective strategy to expedite hospital discharge.[135] Within 6 weeks of surgery, more than 85 percent of patients will have resolvement of their atrial fibrillation and will not require chronic suppressive therapy. Patients treated in the short term with antiarrhythmic agents to suppress atrial fibrillation should be reassessed to determine their need for ongoing antiarrhythmic treatment.

PRIMARY PREVENTION OF ATRIAL FIBRILLATION

Primary prevention of atrial fibrillation has not been well studied. However, control of hypertension and treatment of coronary artery disease and congestive heart failure may delay the onset of atrial fibrillation. The insertion of dual-chamber instead of single-chamber ventricular pacemakers has lowered the incidence of patients developing atrial fibrillation.[136–138] As noted, the prophylactic use of β-blockers before open heart surgery has been shown to decrease the incidence of post-thoracotomy atrial fibrillation. Finally, ablation of accessory pathways in patients with the Wolff-Parkinson-White syndrome will eliminate the recurrence of atrial fibrillation in 80 percent of patients.[139, 140]

EMBOLIC RISK AND ANTICOAGULATION ISSUES

Many studies have demonstrated a 1 to 5 percent annual risk of peripheral embolization even in patients with nonvalvular atrial fibrillation. The risk of systemic embolism and ischemic stroke in patients with nonrheumatic, chronic atrial fibrillation is five to seven times higher than that for similar patients in sinus rhythm, particularly during the first year after the onset.[4–10] Trials[6–10] have provided information suggesting that oral anticoagulation is significantly beneficial in reducing system embolization in patients with nonvalvular atrial fibrillation (Table 88–3). More than 2000 patients in these trials were randomized to receive placebo versus warfarin. Except for the Canadian trial (CAFA), which was prematurely terminated due to the beneficial findings of SPAF and AFASAK, all trials demonstrated a statistical reduction in stroke and systemic embolism with warfarin compared with placebo. Warfarin, with International Normalized Ratio (INR) ranges of 1.8 to 2.4, decreased the average annual embolic rate by 68 percent and the rate of death by 33 percent. Most embolic events in these trials occurred in patients with an INR of less than 2.0, and most hemorrhagic events occurred in patients with an INR of more than 4.0. Thus, careful monitoring of INR levels is mandatory. The incremental risk of serious bleeding was less than 1 percent per year among patients on anticoagulation who were selected to participate in these clinical trials and followed carefully on protocols. Low-intensity anticoagulation (INR, 2.0 to 3.0) clearly confers antiembolic benefit[141] with little risk of hemorrhagic sequelae.

The safety of long-term anticoagulation has been less clear in elderly patients (>75 years old), the age group encompassing perhaps half of atrial fibrillation–associated stroke patients. A placebo-controlled trial involving atrial fibrillation patients with a mean age of 75 years reported a 38 percent withdrawal rate from anticoagulation after 1

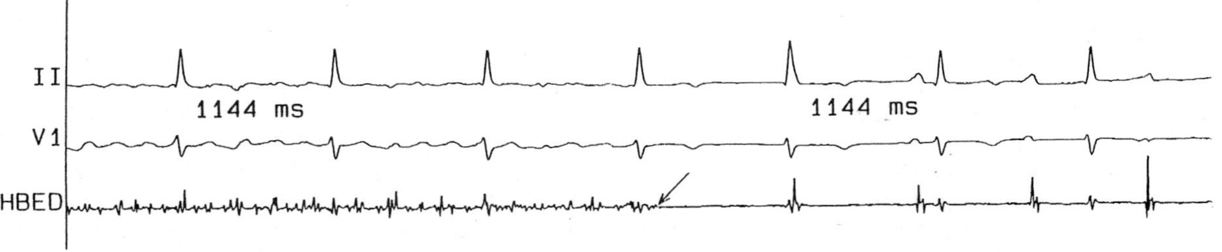

FIGURE 88–12 Leads II and V_1 and atrial and ventricular recordings near the atrioventricular junction demonstrate junctional escape rhythm after successful radiofrequency catheter ablation of atrioventricular junction in a patient with atrial fibrillation and a rapid ventricular response not controlled by antiarrhythmics. Note persistent junctional escape rhythm at cycle length of 1144 ms, with complete atrioventricular block during and after spontaneous termination of atrial fibrillation *(arrow)* to sinus rhythm.

TABLE 88-3 Results of Anticoagulation Trials in Nonvalvular Atrial Fibrillation

Study	Annual Incidence of Embolic Events (%)		
	Placebo	*Aspirin*	*Warfarin*
Copenhagen Atrial Fibrillation, Aspirin, Anticoagulation Study[9]	5.5	5.5	2.0*
Stroke Prevention in Atrial Fibrillation Study[10]	6.3	3.6*	ND
	7.4	ND	2.3*
Boston Area Anticoagulation Trial for Atrial Fibrillation[6]	3.0†	ND	0.4*
Canadian Atrial Fibrillation Anticoagulation Study[7]	5.2	ND	3.5
Stroke Prevention in Nonrheumatic Atrial Fibrillation Study[8]	4.3	ND	0.9*

Abbreviation: ND, no data.
*$P < .05$ compared with placebo.
†46% of control group took aspirin.

year.[142] A recent clinical trial comparing anticoagulation in atrial fibrillation patients younger and older than 75 years found that risk of major hemorrhage during anticoagulation (INR range, 2.0 to 4.5; mean INR, 2.7) was substantially increased in the patients older than 75 years.[143] In contrast, pooled data from five atrial fibrillation trials demonstrated only one intracranial hemorrhage in 223 patients older than 75 years receiving warfarin.[144] Furthermore, in the European Atrial Fibrillation Trial,[145] 63 percent of patients were more than 70 years old, and no intracranial hemorrhages occurred during warfarin therapy (mean INR, 2.9). In SPAF II, the yearly incidence of major bleeding complications was significantly higher during warfarin treatment versus control (2.8% versus 0.07 percent).[141] INR levels should be closely monitored when warfarin is used in the elderly.

The efficacy of aspirin, an antiplatelet agent, for stroke prevention in atrial fibrillation patients is less clear. Aspirin in doses between 75 and 325 mg/da has been assessed in three randomized, placebo-controlled clinical trials. Pooled data demonstrate statistically significant risk reduction of about 25 percent (range, 14 to 44 percent) in aspirin-treated patients.[146] However, aspirin was significantly less effective than anticoagulation in two of these clinical trials and also on secondary on-therapy analysis of the third trial. Aspirin has some degree of efficacy for preventing atrial fibrillation–associated stroke but clearly less than the benefits of warfarin. In the AFASAK study (median age, 75 years old),[9] 75 mg/da aspirin had no effect compared with placebo in reducing embolic events. In SPAF,[10] 325 mg/da of aspirin decreased the annual risk of stroke from 6.3 to 3.6 percent ($P < .05$). Several studies are ongoing to compare aspirin with warfarin in this group of patients. SPAF II[141] demonstrated that in patients less than 75 years old, the risk of stroke was less than 2 percent in patients treated with either aspirin (1.9 percent) or warfarin (1.3 percent). In patients more than 75 years old, warfarin was more effective than aspirin in preventing thrombotic stroke. However, the rate of thrombotic stroke plus intracranial hemorrhage was not different in the two groups. In SPAF III,[147] INR-regulated warfarin in patients older than 80 years had a lower incidence (risk reduction, 74 percent) of embolic events (1.9 percent) than low-dose warfarin in combination with aspirin (7.9 percent).

Episodes of "lone" atrial fibrillation, especially in patients less than 40 years old, may not carry the same risk of thromboembolism as for other patients with nonvalvular atrial fibrillation. Patients with nonvalvular atrial fibrillation and no risk factors for stroke appear to be at low risk for embolic events, averaging about 1 percent per year.[31, 148] This embolic risk is no higher than that for other low-risk patients taking warfarin. Low-risk patients who are younger than 65 years and have idiopathic atrial fibrillation may be given 325 mg/da aspirin to prevent stroke unless high-risk criteria develop.

Major risk factors for thromboembolic events include age of more than 65 years, recent stroke or thromboembolic event, congestive heart failure, diabetes, hypertension, left ventricular hypertrophy, left atrial dilatation, left atrial thrombus or "smoke," intracardiac thrombus, aortic plaques, and valvular heart disease. In patients with nonvalvular atrial fibrillation and one risk factor, warfarin therapy costs only $8000 per quality-adjusted life year saved. In elderly patients (>75 years old), close surveillance of INR levels is recommended because of the greater likelihood of bleeding complications. Chronic anticoagulation benefits must be weighed against the risk of major hemorrhagic complications, which occur at a rate of up to 3 percent per year. The risk of major bleeding increases with duration of therapy, INR of more than 4.0, and age of more than 75 years.

Patients with atrial fibrillation who cannot safely receive anticoagulation should be given aspirin. The value of other antiplatelet agents, such as ticlopidine and clopidogrel, and low-dose heparin preparations have not been assessed in patients with atrial fibrillation.

Anticoagulation for Cardioversion

The risk of thromboembolic events after cardioversion of atrial fibrillation ranges from 1 to 5 percent in nonanticoagulated patients to about 1 percent in those anticoagulated.[149] Arnold and colleagues[63] noted embolic events in 6 of 179 cardioversions for atrial fibrillation lasting 48 hours or longer compared with 0 of 153 when anticoagulation therapy was used. Although thromboembolic events after cardioversion from atrial flutter are rare, due to postcardioversion atrial stunning, prophylactic anticoagulation is probably warranted. Systemic embolism is a complication of electrical and pharmacologic cardioversion of atrial fibrillation to sinus rhythm. Prior anticoagulation appears to decrease the embolic risk, although randomized prospective trials to evaluate the effectiveness of anticoagulation in this setting have not been performed. Patients who have atrial fibrillation of unknown duration or more than 48 hours should be given warfarin for approximately 3 weeks before and 4 weeks after cardioversion because mechanical atrial systole may not return for up to 1 month after restoration of sinus rhythm. Because pharmacological cardioversion may lead to systemic emboli, antiarrhythmic agents to restore sinus rhythm should be withheld until anticoagulation has been achieved. The rationale for the recommendations to anticoagulate before and after cardioversion are based largely on theory and have never been rigorously proved in controlled clinical trials. Patients presenting with paroxysmal atrial fibrillation, of less than 2 days' duration can undergo chemical or electrical cardioversion without delay so as to enhance the possibility of restoring sinus rhythm. Patients requiring emergency electrical cardioversion have rarely been in atrial fibrillation for a long period of time and should not have the procedure delayed to be anticoagulated.

An alternative approach using transesophageal echocardiography (TEE) has been suggested for in-hospital patients with atrial fibrillation lasting for more than 2 days[34–42, 66] This strategy avoids delaying cardioversion for several weeks until adequate anticoagulation has been achieved. Theoretically, this strategy could minimize atrial remodeling. TEE offers better visualization of the left atrium and its appendage than conventional transthoracic echocardiography. When TEE is used, left atrial appendage thrombi and spontaneous echogenic densities ("smoke"), possibly indicative of stasis, and aortic plaques are more often found in patients with atrial fibrillation who develop a thromboembolic event. Stoddard and associates[38] used TEE to evaluate the frequency of left atrial thrombus in 143 patients with atrial fibrillation of less than 3 days' duration. Twenty patients (14 percent) had left atrial thrombus and 56 (39 percent) had spontaneous echocardiographic contrast. A recent systemic embolus occurred in 24 patients, of whom 5 had documented left atrial thrombus. Although thromboembolic events are more likely to occur in patients with these findings noted on TEE, thromboembolic complications can occur after cardioversion in patients without evidence of atrial thrombus on precardioversion TEE.[33, 35, 43] The predictive value of TEE findings for subsequent stroke has yet to be validated by adequate clinical studies. Thus, data are insufficient to recommend the routine use of TEE to stratify thromboembolic potential in atrial fibrillation patients; the results of the ACUTE trial[63] may clarify the routine use of TEE in this setting.

Although most ischemic strokes associated with atrial fibrillation are due to embolism of stasis-induced thrombi forming in the left atrium, other risk factors for stroke exist. Up to 25 percent of atrial fibrillation–associated stroke is due to associated intrinsic cerebrovascular diseases, other cardiac sources of embolism, or aortic arch atheroma[33, 150] About half of elderly patients with atrial fibrillation also have chronic hypertension, another major risk factor for stroke. Although about 12 percent of elderly patients have carotid artery stenoses, the frequency of carotid disease is not substantially greater in atrial fibrillation patients with stroke. Thus, carotid artery stenoses appears to be a minor contributor to atrial fibrillation–associated stroke.[148]

Nonpharmacologic Therapies for Atrial Fibrillation

In some patients with atrial tachyarrhythmias, rate control or suppression of the arrhythmia cannot be achieved with antiarrhythmic drugs. Rate control may be a problem in patients with depressed ejection fractions who cannot tolerate the negative inotropy of high doses of β-blockers or calcium channel blockers.

There are surgical and catheter ablative techniques for the treatment of atrial arrhythmias that are acceptable alternatives to drug therapy. Surgical or radiofrequency catheter ablation of accessory pathways is the most effective therapy for the Wolff-Parkinson-White syndrome, frequently obviating the need for drug therapy and removing the stimulus for future episodes of paroxysmal atrial fibrillation.[151, 152]

Patients refractory to drug therapy, either because of inefficacy or adverse reactions, may be symptomatically improved by percutaneous radiofrequency catheter ablation of the AV nodal junction.[153–156] This technique creates complete heart block and a junctional escape rhythm in up to 99 percent of patients (see Fig. 88–12). Even though the patient continues to have recurrence of the atrial tachyarrhythmia, the complete AV block ensures that there is no transmission of the atrial impulse to the ventricle, with resultant rate control without the need for antiarrhythmic drugs. Despite the need for a permanent pacemaker, quality of life and left ventricular systolic function are significantly improved.[155] Rate control after catheter ablation has been associated with an improvement in left ventricular hemodynamics secondary to reversal of a tachycardia-induced cardiomyopathy.[157–161] In a comparative study[156] with pharmacologic rate control, ablation and insertion of a VVIR pacemaker were superior to drug therapy in controlling symptoms in 66 patients with chronic atrial fibrillation, heart rates of more than 90 beats/min, concomitant heart failure. Attempt to modify and slow AV node conduction, without the need for a pacemaker,[162, 163] has not had widespread acceptance due to the recurrence of rapid rates, the need for repeated procedures, and the rare risk of complete AV block. Comparative studies have not shown any clinical benefit of modification versus creating complete heart block, although both groups have improved left ventricular systolic function in patients when these procedures were performed in patients with rapid rates and depressed ejection fractions.[164] Complete AV junction ablation has been demonstrated to be superior to AV nodal modification with respect to quality-of-life indicators and reduction in the frequency of major symptomatic attacks.[164] Rare sudden cardiac deaths have been noted after radiofrequency catheter ablation of the AV junction. Whether these deaths are secondary to the procedure or expected sudden deaths in a high-risk population with left ventricular dysfunction is not known.

Atrial pacing may prevent the onset of atrial fibrillation by suppressing triggers or by decreasing the dispersion of atrial refractoriness. Atrium-based pacing, along with concomitant antiarrhythmic drugs, appears to be more effective than ventricular pacing in decreasing the frequency of atrial fibrillation occurrences.[136–138] Pacing techniques may be most useful in patients with pause-dependent (e.g., sick sinus syndrome) atrial fibrillation. Creative pacing techniques such as dual-site or coronary sinus pacing may be superior to single-site atrial pacing in preventing atrial fibrillation.[165, 166] Multiple prospective trials are ongoing to assess the benefit of atrial pacing in suppressing atrial fibrillation.[79]

Patients with infrequent episodes of paroxysmal atrial flutter, without the Wolff-Parkinson-White syndrome, in whom medication is ineffective, not indicated, or not desirable, may have acute episodes terminated by the implantation of a permanent antitachycardia pacemaker. Patients with refractory atrial flutter may also undergo a catheter ablation procedure to ablate the atrial flutter circuit. This technique has been successful in up to 90 percent of patients.[167, 168]

Implantable atrial defibrillators may be used to terminate recurrences of atrial fibrillation.[169] Terminating spells within minutes should minimize the need for antiembolic measures. Theoretically, synchronized transvenous atrial defibrillating shocks might cause a proarrhythmic effect with initiation of ventricular fibrillation.[170] To date, no clinical reports of this complication exist; however, due to this concern, a dual-chamber defibrillator is undergoing clinical study. Unfortunately, patient discomfort from the low-energy (1 to 3 J) shocks limits widespread clinical acceptance of such a device.[171]

The Maze operation[172] has been extensively studied for the prevention of refractory atrial fibrillation. This operation has had a high success rate but has been reserved for refractory patients due to the risk of surgery and frequent need of permanent pacing after the procedure. Catheter ablation of patients with pulmonary vein atrial ectopic triggers has been successful[23] in preventing future recurrences of atrial fibrillation. In one study,[23] 28 of 45 (62 percent) patients had no recurrence of atrial fibrillation after radiofrequency catheter ablation of an initiating focus 2 to 4 cm inside the os of the pulmonary veins. Although curative, only a small number of patients are candidates for this procedure. Attempts to simulate the Maze procedure with radiofrequency catheter ablation techniques have only had limited success despite repeat procedures and the frequent need for concomitant antiarrhythmic drugs. Thus, catheter Maze procedures should be reserved for drug-refractory patients until further advances demonstrate more acceptable efficacy and safety.[173]

References

1. Kannel WB, Abbot RD, Savage DD, McNamara PM: Epidemiologic features of chronic atrial fibrillation. N Engl J Med 306:1018–1022, 1982.
2. Benjamin EJ, Levy D, Vaziri SM, et al: Independent risk factors for atrial fibrillation in a population-based cohort: the Framingham Study. JAMA 271:840–844, 1994.
3. Feinberg WM, Blackshear JL, Laupacis A, et al: Prevalence, age distribution, and gender of patients with atrial fibrillation. Arch Intern Med 155:469–473, 1995.
4. Wolf PA, Abbott RD, Kannel WB: Atrial fibrillation as an independent risk factor for stroke: the Framingham Study. Stroke 22:983–988, 1991.
5. Alpert JS, Petersen P, Godtfredsen J: Atrial fibrillation: natural history, complications and management. Annu Rev Med 39:41–52, 1988.
6. The Boston Area Anticoagulation Trial for Atrial Fibrillation Investigators: The effect of low-dose warfarin on the risk of stroke in patients with nonrheumatic atrial fibrillation. N Engl J Med 323:1505–1511, 1990.
7. Connolly SJ, Laupacis A, Gent M, et al: Canadian Atrial Fibrillation Anticoagulation (CAFA) Study. J Am Coll Cardiol 18:349–355, 1991.
8. Ezekowitz MD, Bridgers SL, James KE, et al: Warfarin in the prevention of stroke associated with nonrheumatic atrial fibrillation: Veterans Affairs Stroke Prevention in Nonrheumatic Atrial Fibrillation Investigators. N Engl J Med 327:1406–1412, 1992.
9. Petersen P, Boysen G, Godtfredsen J, et al: Placebo-controlled, randomized trial of warfarin and aspirin for prevention of thromboembolic complications in chronic atrial fibrillation: the Copenhagen AFASAK study. Lancet 1:175–179, 1989.
10. Stroke Prevention in Atrial Fibrillation Investigators: Stroke Prevention in Atrial Fibrillation Study: final results. Circulation 84:527–539, 1991.
11. Brand FN, Abbott RD, Kannel WB: Characteristics and prognosis of lone atrial fibrillation: 30-year follow-up on the Framingham Study. JAMA 254:3449–3453, 1985.
12. Kopecky SL, Jersh BJ, McGoon MD, et al: The natural history of lone atrial fibrillation: a population based study over three decades. N Engl J Med 317:669–674, 1987.
13. Ravelli F, Allessie M: Effects of atrial dilatation on refractory period and vulnerability to atrial fibrillation in the isolated Langendorff-perfused rabbit heart. Circulation 96:1686–1695, 1997.
14. Henry WL, Morganroth J, Pearlman AS, et al: Relation between echocardiographically determined left atrial size and atrial fibrillation. Circulation 53:273–279, 1976.
15. Dittrich HC, Ericson JS, Schneiderman T, et al: Echocardiographic and clinical predictors for outcome of elective cardioversion of atrial fibrillation. Am J Cardiol 63:193–197, 1989.
16. Brodsky MA, Allen BJ, Capparelli EV, et al: Factors determining maintenance of sinus rhythm after chronic atrial fibrillation with left atrial dilatation. Am J Cardiol 63:1065–1068, 1989.
17. Benjamin EJ, Wolf PA, D'Agostino RB, et al: Impact of atrial fibrillation on the risk of death: the Framingham Heart Study. Circulation 98:946–952, 1998.
18. Prystowsky EN, Benson DW Jr, Fuster V, et al: Management of patients with atrial fibrillation: a statement for healthcare professionals: the Subcommittee on Electrocardiography and Electrophysiology, American Heart Association. Circulation 93:1262–1277, 1996.
19. Coumel P: Neurogenic and humoral influences of the autonomic nervous system in the determination of paroxysmal atrial fibrillation. *In* Atteul P, Coumel P, Janse MJ (eds): The Atrium in Health and Disease. pp. 213–232. Mount Kisco, NY: Futura, 1989.
20. Maixent JM, Paganelli F, Scaglione J, Lévy D: Antibodies against myosin in sera of patients with idiopathic parosysmal atrial fibrillation. J Cardiovasc Electrophysiol 9:612–617, 1998.
21. Brugada R, Tapscott T, Czernuszewicz GZ, et al: Identification of a genetic locus for familial atrial fibrillation. N Engl J Med 336:905, 1997.
22. Zipes DP: Atrial fibrillation: from cell to bedside. J Cardiovasc Electrophysiol 8:927–938, 1997.
23. Haissaguerre M, Jais P, Shah DC, et al: Spontaneous initiation of atrial fibrillation by ectopic beats originating in the pulmonary veins. N Engl J Med 339:659–666, 1998.
24. Wijffels MCEF, Kirchhof CJHJ, Dorland R. Allessie MA: Atrial fibrillations begets atrial fibrillation: a study in awake chronically instrumented goats. Circulation 92:1954–1968, 1995.
25. Tieleman RG, DeLangen CDH, Van Gelder IC, et al: Verapamil reduces tachycardia-induced electrical remodeling of the atria. Circulation 95:1945–1953, 1997.
26. Yu WC, Chen SA, Lee SH, et al: Tachycardia-induced change of atrial refractory period in humans: rate dependency and effects of antiarrhythmic drugs. Circulation 97:2331–2337, 1998.
27. Daoud EG, Knight BP, Wiess R, et al: Effect of verapamil and procainamide on atrial fibrillation–induced electrical remodeling in humans. Circulation 96:1542–1550, 1997.
28. Tieleman RG, Van Gelder IC, Crijns HJGM, et al: Early recurrences of atrial fibrillation after electrical cardioversion: a result of fibrillation induced electrical remodeling in man? J Am Coll Cardiol 31:167–173, 1998.
29. Wijffels MCEF, Kirchhof CJHJ, Dorland R, et al: Electrical remodeling due to atrial fibrillation in chronically instrumented conscious goats: roles of neurohumoral changes, ischemia, atrial stretch, and high rate of electrical activation. Circulation 96:3710–3720, 1997.
30. Levy S: Epidemiology and classification of atrial fibrillation. J Cardiovasc Electrophysiol 9:S78–S82, 1998.
31. The Stroke Prevention in Atrial Fibrillation Investigators: Predictors of thromboembolism in atrial fibrillation, 1: clinical features of patients at risk. Ann Intern Med 116:1–5, 1992.

32. Albers GW, Atwood EW, Hirsh J, et al: Stroke prevention in nonvalvular atrial fibrillation. Ann Intern Med 115:727–736, 1991.
33. The Stroke Prevention in Atrial Fibrillation Investigators Committee on Echocardiography: Transesophageal echocardiographic correlates of thromboembolism in high-risk patients with nonvalvular atrial fibrillation. Ann Intern Med 128:639–647, 1998.
34. Manning WJ, Silverman DI, Gordon SPF, et al: Cardioversion from atrial fibrillation without prolonged anticoagulation with use of transesophageal echocardiography to exclude the presence of atrial thrombi. N Engl J Med 328:750–756, 1993.
35. Fatkin I, Kuchar DL, Thorburn CW, Feneley MP: Transesophageal echocardiography before and during direct current cardioversion of atrial fibrillation: evidence for "atrial stunning" as a mechanism of thromboembolic complications. J Am Coll Cardiol 23:307–316, 1994.
36. Grimm RA, Stewart WJ, Black IW, et al: Should all patients undergo transesophageal echocardiography before electrical cardioversion of atrial fibrillation? J Am Coll Cardiol 23:533–541, 1994.
37. Chimowitz MI, DeGeorgia MA, Poole RM, et al: Left atrial spontaneous echo contrast is highly associated with previous stroke in patients with atrial fibrillation or mitral stenosis. Stroke 24:1015–1019, 1993.
38. Stoddard MF, Dawkins PR, Prince CR, Ammash NM: Left atrial appendage thrombus is not uncommon in patients with acute atrial fibrillation and a recent embolic event: a transesophageal echocardiographic study. J Am Coll Cardiol 25:452–459, 1995.
39. Manning WJ, Leeman DE, Gotch PJ, et al: Pulsed Doppler evaluation of atrial mechanical function after electrical cardioversion of atrial fibrillation. J Am Coll Cardiol 13:617–623, 1989.
40. Manning WJ, Silverman DI, Keighley CS, et al: Transesophageal echocardiography facilitated early cardioversion from atrial fibrillation using short-term anticoagulation: final results of a prospective 4.5-year study. J Am Coll Cardiol 25:1354–1361, 1995.
41. Stöllberger C, Chnupa P, Kronik G, et al, for the ELAT Study Group: Transesophageal echocardiography to assess embolic risk in patients with atrial fibrillation. Ann Intern Med 128:630–638, 1998.
42. Manning WJ: Role of transesophageal echocardiography in the management of thromboembolic stroke. Am J Cardiol 80:19D–28D, 1997.
43. Black IW, Fatkin D, Sagar KB, et al: Exclusion of atrial thrombus by transesophageal echocardiography does not preclude embolism after cardioversion of atrial fibrillation: a multicenter study. Circulation 89:2509–2513, 1994.
44. Pritchett EL: Management of atrial fibrillation. N Engl J Med 326:1264–1271, 1992.
45. Naccarelli GV, Dougherty AH, Berns E, et al: Assessment of antiarrhythmic drug efficacy in the treatment of supraventricular arrhythmias. Am J Cardiol 58:31C–36C, 1986.
46. Yeh SJ, Lin FC, Wu D: The mechanism of exercise provocation of supraventricular tachycardia. Am Heart J 117:1041–1049, 1989.
47. Pritchett ELC, Anderson JL: Antiarrhythmic strategies for the chronic management of supraventricular tachycardias. Am J Cardiol 62:1D–2D, 1988.
48. Sopher SM, Camm AJ: Atrial fibrillation: maintenance of sinus rhythm versus rate control. Am J Cardiol 77:24A–37A, 1996.
49. Dell'Orfano JT, Luck JC, Wolbrette DW, et al: Drugs for conversion of atrial fibrillation. Am Fam Phys 58:471–480, 1998.
50. Falk RH, Knowlton AA, Bernard SA, et al: Digoxin for converting recent-onset atrial fibrillation to sinus rhythm. Ann Intern Med 106:503–506, 1987.
51. The Digitalis in Acute Atrial Fibrillation (DAAF) Trial Group: Intravenous digoxin in acute atrial fibrillation: results of a randomized, placebo-controlled multicentre trial in 239 patients. Eur Heart J 18:649–654, 1997.
52. Rinkenberger RL, Prystowsky EN, Heger JJ, et al: Effects of intravenous and chronic oral verapamil administration in patients with supraventricular tachyarrhythmias. Circulation 62:996–1010, 1980.
53. Waxman HL, Myerburg RJ, Appel R. Sung RJ: Verapamil for control of ventricular rate in paroxysmal supraventricular tachycardia and atrial fibrillation or flutter: a double-blind randomized crossover study. Ann Intern Med 94:1–6, 1981.
54. Ellenbogen KA, Dias VC, Plumb VJ, et al: A placebo-controlled trial of continuous intravenous diltiazem infusion for 24-hour heart rate control during atrial fibrillation and atrial flutter: a multicenter study. J Am Coll Cardiol 18:891–897, 1991.
55. Salerno DM, Dias VC, Kleiger RE, et al: Efficacy and safety of intravenous diltiazem for treatment of atrial fibrillation and atrial flutter: the Diltiazem-Atrial Fibrillation/Flutter Study Group. Am J Cardiol 63:1046–1051, 1989.
56. Turlapaty P, Laddu A, Murphy VS, et al: Esmolol: short-acting intravenous beta blocker for an acute critical care setting. Am Heart J 114:866–885, 1987.
57. Esmolol Multicenter Study Research Group: Efficacy and safety of esmolol vs. propranolol in the treatment of supraventricular tachyarrhythmias: a multicenter double-blind clinical trial. Am Heart J 110:913–922, 1985.
58. Platia EV, Michelson EL, Porterfield JK, et al: Esmolol vs. verapamil in the acute treatment of atrial fibrillation or atrial flutter. Am J Cardiol 63:925–929, 1989.
59. Anderson S, Blanski L, Byrd RC, et al: Comparison of the efficacy and safety of esmolol, a short-acting beta blocker, with placebo in the treatment of supraventricular tachyarrhythmias. Am Heart J 111:42–48, 1986.
60. Dainias PG, Caulfield TA, Weigner MJ, et al: Likelihood of spontaneous conversion of atrial fibrillation to sinus rhythm. J Am Coll Cardiol 31:558–592, 1998.
61. Dell'Orfano JT, Luck JC, Wolbrette DW, et al: Acute treatment of atrial fibrillation: spontaneous conversion rates and cost of care. Am J Cardiol 83:788–790, 1999.
62. Mancini DGB, Goldberger AL: Cardioversion of atrial fibrillation: consideration of embolization, anticoagulation, prophylactic pacemaker and long-term success. Am Heart J 104:617–621, 1982.
63. Arnold AZ, Mick MJ, Mazurek RP, et al: Role of prophylactic anticoagulation for direct current cardioversion in patients with atrial fibrillation or atrial flutter. J Am Coll Cardiol 19:851–855, 1992.
64. Irani WN, Grayburn PA, Afridi I: Prevalence of thrombus, spontaneous echo contrast, and atrial stunning in patients undergoing cardioversion of atrial flutter. Circulation 95:962–966, 1997.
65. Weigner MJ, Caulfield TA, Danias PG, et al: Risk for clinical thromboembolism associated with conversion to sinus rhythm in patients with atrial fibrillation lasting less than 48 hours. Ann Intern Med 126:615–620, 1997.
66. Klein AL, Grimm, RA, Black IW, et al: Cardioversion guided by transesophageal echocardiography: the ACUTE pilot study: a randomized, controlled trial. Ann Intern Med 126:200–209, 1997.
67. Volgman AS, Carberry PA, Stambler B, et al: Conversion efficacy and safety of intravenous ibutilide compared with intravenous procainamide in patients with atrial flutter or fibrillation. J Am Coll Cardiol 31:1414–1419, 1998.
68. Naccarelli GV, Lee KS, Gibson JK, VanderLugt J: Electrophysiology and pharmacology of ibutilide. Am J Cardiol 78:12, 1996.
69. Ellenbogen KA, Stambler BS, Wood MA, et al: Efficacy of intravenous ibutilide for rapid termination of atrial fibrillation and atrial flutter: a dose-response study. J Am Coll Cardiol 28:130–136, 1996.
70. Halinen MO, Huttunen M, Paakkinen S, Tarssanen L: Comparison of sotalol with digoxin-quinidine for conversion of acute atrial fibrillation to sinus rhythm (the Sotalol-Digoxin-Quinidine Trial). Am J Cardiol 76:495–498, 1995.
71. Hohnloser SH, van de Loo A, Baedeker F: Efficacy and proarrhythmic hazards of pharmacologic conversion of atrial fibrillation: prospective comparison of sotalol versus quinidine. J Am Coll Cardiol 26:852–858, 1995.
72. Capucci A, Boriani G, Luca Botto G, et al: Conversion of recent-onset atrial fibrillation by a single oral loading dose of propafenone or flecainide. Am J Cardiol 74:503–505, 1994.
73. Capucci A, Lenzi T, Boriani G, et al: Effectiveness of loading oral flecainide for converting recent-onset atrial fibrillation to sinus rhythm in patients without organic heart disease or with only systemic hypertension. Am J Cardiol 70:69–72, 1992.
74. Boriani G, Biffi M, Capucci A, et al: Oral propafenone to convert recent-onset atrial fibrillation in patients with and without underlying heart disease: a randomized, controlled trial. Ann Intern Med 126:621–625, 1997.
75. Clemo HF, Wood MA, Giligan DM, Ellenbogen KA: Intravenous amiodarone for acute heart rate control in the critically ill patient with atrial tachyarrhythmias. Am J Cardiol 81:594–598, 1998.
76. Galve E, Rius T, Ballester R, et al: Intravenous amiodarone in treatment of recent-onset atrial fibrillation: results of a randomized, controlled study. J Am Coll Cardiol 27:1079–1082, 1996.
77. Tieleman RG, Gosselink AT, Crijins HJ, et al: Efficacy, safety, and

determinants of conversion of atrial fibrillation and flutter with oral amiodarone. Am J Cardiol 79:53–57, 1997.
78. The Planning and Steering Committees of the AFFIRM Study for the NHLBI AFFIRM Investigators: Atrial fibrillation follow-up investigation of rhythm management—the AFFIRM study design. Am J Cardiol 79:1198–1202, 1997.
79. Sopher SM, Camm AJ: New trials in atrial fibrillation. J Cardiovasc Electrophysiol 9:S211–S215, 1998.
80. Klein HO, Kaplinsky E: Digitalis and verapamil in atrial fibrillation and flutter: is verapamil now the preferred agent? Drugs 31:185–197, 1986.
81. David D, Segni ED, Klein HO, Kaplisky E: Inefficacy of digitalis in the control of heart rate in patients with chronic atrial fibrillation: beneficial effect of an added beta adrenergic blocking agent. Am J Cardiol 44:1378–1382, 1979.
82. Farshi R, Kistner D, Sarma JSM, et al: Ventricular rate control in chronic atrial fibrillation during daily activity and programmed exercise: a crossover open-label study of five drugs regimens. J Am Coll Cardiol 33:304–310, 1999.
83. Coplen SE. Antman EM, Berlin JA, et al: Efficacy and safety of quinidine therapy for maintenance of sinus rhythm after cardioversion: a meta-analysis of randomized control trials. Circulation 82:1106–1116, 1990.
84. Karlson BW, Torstensson I, Abjorn C, et al: Disopyramide in the maintenance of sinus rhythm after electroconversion of atrial fibrillation: a placebo-controlled one-year follow-up study. Eur Heart J 9:284–290, 1988.
85. Juul-Moller S, Edvardsson N, Rehnqvist-Ahlberg N: Sotalol versus quinidine for the maintenance of sinus rhythm after direct current conversion of atrial fibrillation. Circulation 82:1932–1939, 1990.
86. Naccarelli GV, Dorian P, Hohnsloser SH, Coumel P, for the Flecainide Multicenter Atrial Fibrillation Study Group: Prospective comparison of flecainide versus quinidine for the treatment of paroxysmal atrial fibrillation. Am J Cardiol 77:53A–59A, 1996.
87. Anderson JL, Gilbert EM, Alpert BL, et al: Prevention of symptomatic recurrences of paroxysmal atrial fibrillation in patients initially tolerating antiarrhythmic therapy: a multicenter, double-blind, crossover study of flecainide and placebo with transtelephonic monitoring. Circulation 80:1557–1570, 1989.
88. Pritchett ELC, DaTorre SD, Platt ML, et al: Flecainide acetate treatment of paroxysmal supraventricular tachycardia and paroxysmal atrial fibrillation: dose-response studies. J Am Coll Cardiol 17:297–303, 1991.
89. Antman EM, Beamer AD, Cantillon C, et al: Long-term oral propafenone therapy for suppression of refractory symptomatic atrial fibrillation and atrial flutter. J Am Coll Cardiol 12:1005–1011, 1989.
90. Connolly SJ, Hoffert DL: Usefulness of propafenone for recurrent paroxysmal atrial fibrillation. Am J Cardiol 63:817–819, 1989.
91. Pritchett ELC, McCarthy EA, Wilkinson WE: Propafenone treatment of symptomatic paroxysmal supraventricular arrhythmias: a randomized, placebo-controlled, crossover trial in patients tolerating oral therapy. Ann Intern Med 114:539–544, 1991.
92. Reimold SC, Cantillon CO, Friedman PL, Antman EM: Propafenone versus sotalol for suppression of recurrent symptomatic atrial fibrillation. Am J Cardiol 71:558–563, 1993.
93. Greenbaum Ra, Campbell TJ, Channer KS, et al: Conversion of atrial fibrillation and maintenance of sinus rhythm by dofetilide: the EMERALD (European and Australian Multicenter Evaluative Research on Atrial Fibrillation Dofetilide) study [abstract]. Circulation 98(suppl I):I-633, 1998.
94. Pritchett E, Page R, Connolly S, et al: Azimilide treatment of atrial fibrillation [abstract]. Circulation 98(suppl I):I-633, 1998.
95. Horowitz LN, Spielman SR, Greenspan AM, et al: Use of amiodarone in the treatment of persistent and paroxysmal atrial fibrillation resistant to quinidine therapy. J Am Coll Cardiol 6:1402–1407, 1985.
96. Brodsky MA, Allen BJ, Walker CJ, et al: Amiodarone for maintenance of sinus rhythm after conversion of atrial fibrillation in the setting of a dilated left atrium. Am J Cardiol 60:572–574, 1987.
97. Gosselink AT, Crijns HJ, Van Gelder IC, et al: Low-dose amiodarone for maintenance of sinus rhythm after cardioversion of atrial fibrillation or flutter. JAMA 267:3289–3293, 1992.
98. Disch DL, Greenberg ML, Holzberger PT, et al: Managing chronic atrial fibrillation: a Markov decision analysis comparing warfarin, quinidine, and low-dose amiodarone. Ann Intern Med 120:449–457, 1994.
99. Van Gelder IC, Crijns HJGM, Tieleman RG, et al: Chronic atrial fibrillation: success of serial cardioversion therapy and safety of oral anticoagulation. Arch Intern Med 156:2585–2592, 1996.
100. Levy S, Lauribe P, Dolla E, et al: A randomized comparison of external and internal cardioversion of chronic atrial fibrillation. Circulation 86:1415–1420, 1992.
101. Zehender M, Hohnloser S, Muller B, et al: Effects of amiodarone versus quinidine and verapamil in patients with chronic atrial fibrillation: results of a comparative study and a 2-year follow-up. J Am Coll Cardiol 19:1054–1059, 1992.
102. Kochiadakis GE, Igoumenidis NE, Marketou ME, et al: Low-dose amiodarone versus sotalol for suppression of recurrent symptomatic atrial fibrillation. Am J Cardiol 81:995–998, 1998.
103. Roy D, Talajic M, Thibault B, et al, and the CTAF Investigators: Pilot study and protocol of the Canadian Trial of Atrial Fibrillation (CTAF). Am J Cardiol 80:464–468, 1997.
104. Vorperian CR, Havighhurst TC, Miller S, January CT: Adverse effects of low dose amiodarone: a meta-analysis. J Am Coll Cardiol 30:791–798, 1997.
105. Klein GJ, Bashore TM, Sellers TD, et al: Ventricular fibrillation in the Wolff-Parkinson-White syndrome. N Engl J Med 301:1080–1085, 1979.
106. McGovern B, Garan H, Ruskin JM: Precipitation of cardiac arrest by verapamil in patients with Wolff-Parkinson-White syndrome. Ann Intern Med 104:791–794, 1986.
107. Gulamhusein S, Ko P, Klein GJ: Ventricular fibrillation following verapamil in the Wolff-Parkinson-White syndrome. Am Heart J 106:145–147, 1983.
108. Page RL, Wilkinson WE, Clair WK et al: Asymptomatic arrhythmias in patients with symptomatic paroxysmal atrial fibrillation and paroxysmal supraventricular tachycardia. Circulation 89:224–227, 1994.
109. Flaker GC, Blackshear JL, McBride R, et al: Antiarrhythmic drug therapy and cardiac mortality in atrial fibrillation: the Stroke Prevention in Atrial Fibrillation Investigators. J Am Coll Cardiol 20:527–532, 1992.
110. Doval HC, Nul DR, Grancelli HO, et al: Randomized trial of low-dose amiodarone in severe congestive heart failure: Grupo de Estudio de la Sobrevida en la Insuficiencia Cardiaca en Argentina (GESICA). Lancet 344:493–498, 1994.
111. Singh SN, Fletcher RD, Fisher SG, et al: Amiodarone in patients with congestive heart failure and asymptomatic ventricular arrhythmia: Survival Trial of Antiarrhythmic Therapy in Congestive Heart Failure. N Engl J Med 333:77–82, 1995.
112. The DIAMOND Study Group: Dofetilide in patients with left ventricular dysfunction and either heart failure or acute myocardial infarction: rationale, design, and patient characteristics of the DIAMOND studies. Clin Cardiol 20:704–710, 1997.
113. Naccarelli GV, Wolbrette DL, Dell'Orfano JT, et al: A decade of clinical trial developments in post-myocardial infarction, congestive heart failure and sustained ventricular tachyarrhythmia patients: from CAST to AVID and beyond. J Cardiovasc Electrophysiol 9:864–889, 1998.
114. Camm AJ, Karam R, Pratt C: The azimilide post-infarct survival evaluation (ALIVE) trial. Am J Cardiol 81:35D–39D, 1998.
115. Echt DS, Liebson PR, Mitchell LB, et al: Mortality and morbidity in patients receiving encainide, flecainide, or placebo. N Engl J Med 324:781–788, 1991.
116. Pritchett ELC, Wilkinson WE: Mortality in patients treated with flecainide and encainide for supraventricular arrhythmias. Am J Cardiol 67:976–980, 1991.
117. Julian DG, Camm AJ, Frangin G, et al, for the European Myocardial Infarct Amiodarone Trial Investigators: Randomized trial of effect of amiodarone on mortality in patients with left-ventricular dysfunction after recent myocardial infarction: EMIAT. Lancet 349:667–674, 1997.
118. Cairns, JA, Connolly SJ, Roberts R, Gent M, for the Canadian Amiodarone Myocardial Infarction Arrhythmia Trial Investigators: Randomized trial of outcome after myocardial infarction in patients with frequent or repetitive ventricular premature depolarisations: CAMIAT. Lancet 349:675–682, 1997.
119. Julian DG, Prescott RJ, Jackson FS, Szekely P: Controlled trial of sotalol for one year after myocardial infarction. Lancet 1:1142–1147, 1982.
120. Crijns HJ, van Gelder IC, Lie KI: Supraventricular tachycardia mimicking ventricular tachycardia during flecainide treatment. Am J Cardiol 62:1303–1306, 1988.

121. Feld GK, Chen P-S, Nicod P, et al: Possible atrial proarrhythmic effects of class IC antiarrhythmic drugs. Am J Cardiol 66:378–383, 1990.
122. Selzer A, Wray HW: Quinidine syncope: paroxysmal ventricular fibrillation occurring during treatent of chronic atrial arrhythmias. Circulation 30:17–26, 1964.
123. Roden DM. Woosley RL, Primm RK: Incidence and clinical features of the quinidine-associated long QT syndrome: implications for patient care. Am Heart J 111:1088–1093, 1986.
124. Jackman WM, Friday KJ, Anderson JL, et al: The long QT syndromes: a critical review, new clinical observations and a unifying hypothesis. Prog Cardiovasc Dis 31:115–172, 1988.
125. Chung MK, Schweikert RA, Wilkoff BL, et al: Is hospital admission for initiation of antiarrhythmic therapy with sotalol for atrial arrhythmias required? Yield of in-hospital monitoring and prediction of risk for significant arrhythmia complications. J Am Coll Cardiol 32:169–176, 1998.
126. Maisel WH, Kuntz KM, Reimold SC, et al: Risk of initiating antiarrhythmic drug therapy for atrial fibrillation in patients admitted to a university hospital. Ann Intern Med 127:281–284, 1997.
127. Simons GR, Eisenstein El, Shaw LJ, et al: Cost effectiveness of inpatient initiation of antiarrhythmic therapy for supraventricular tachycardias. Am J Cardiol 80:1551–1557, 1997.
128. Rinkenberger RL, Naccarelli GV, Berns E, et al: Efficacy and safety of class IC antiarrhythmic agents for the treatment of coexisting supraventricular and ventricular tachycardia. Am J Cardiol 62:44D–55D, 1988.
129. Lauer MS, Eagle KA, Buckley MJ, DeSanctis RW: Atrial fibrillation following coronary artery bypass surgery. Prog Cardiovasc Dis 31:367–378, 1989.
130. Aranki SF, Shaw DP, Adams DH, et al: Predictors of atrial fibrillation after coronary artery surgery: current trends and impact on hospital resources. Circulation 94:390–397, 1996.
131. Kowey PR, Taylor JE, Rials SJ, Marinchak RA: Meta-analysis of the effectiveness of prophylactic drug therapy in preventing supraventricular arrhythmias early after coronary artery bypass grafting. Am J Cardiol 69:963–965, 1992.
132. Gold MR, O'Gara PT, Buckley MJ, DeSanctis RW: Efficacy and safety of procainamide in preventing arrhythmias after coronary artery bypass surgery. Am J Cardiol 78:975–979, 1996.
133. Daoud EG, Strickberger SA, Ching Man K, et al: Preoperative amiodarone as prophylaxis against atrial fibrillation after heart surgery. N Engl J Med 337:1785–1791, 1997.
134. Guarnieri T: Amiodarone reduces CABG hospitalization (ARCH). American College of Cardiology presentation, 1998.
135. Solomon AJ, Kouretas PC, Hopkins RA, et al: Early discharge of patients with new-onset atrial fibrillation after cardiovascular surgery. Am Heart J 135:557–563, 1998.
136. Sgarbossa EB, Pinski S, Maloney JD, et al: Chronic atrial fibrillation and stroke in paced patients with sick sinus syndrome: relevance of clinical characteristics and pacing modalities. Circulation 88:1045–1053, 1993.
137. Barold SS, Wyndham CRC, Kappenberger LL, et al: Implanted atrial pacemakers for paroxysmal atrial flutter. Ann Intern Med 107:144–149, 1987.
138. Feuer JM, Shandling AH, Messenger JC: Influence of cardiac pacing mode on the long-term development of atrial fibrillation. Am J Cardiol 64:1376–1379, 1989.
139. Sharma AD, Klein GJ, Guiraudon GM, et al: Atrial fibrillation in patients with Wolff-Parkinson-White syndrome: incidence after surgical ablation of the accessory pathway. Circulation 72:161–169, 1985.
140. Prystowsky EN: Tachycardia-induced tachycardia: a mechanism of initiation of atrial fibrillation. *In* DiMarco JP, Prystowsky EN (eds): Atrial Arrhythmias: State of the Art. pp. 81–95. Armonk, NY: Futura, 1995.
141. Stroke Prevention in Atrial Fibrillation Investigators: Warfarin versus aspirin for prevention of thromboembolism in atrial fibrillation: Stroke Prevention in Atrial Fibrillation II Study. Lancet 343:687–691, 1994.
142. European Atrial Fibrillation Study Group: Secondary prevention in non-rheumatic atrial fibrillation after transient ischaemic attack or minor stroke: EAFT (European Atrial Fibrillation Study Group Trial). Lancet 342:1255–1262, 1993.
143. Miller VT, Pearce LA, Feinberg WM, et al, for the Stroke Prevention in Atrial Fibrillation Investigators: Differential effect of aspirin versus warfarin on clinical stroke types in patients with atrial fibrillation. Neurology 46:238–240, 1996.
144. Singer DE, Hughes RA, Gress DR, et al, for the BAATAF Investigators: The effect of aspirin on the risk of stroke in patients with nonrheumatic atrial fibrillation: the BAATAF study. Am Heart J 124:1567–1573, 1992.
145. The European Atrial Fibrillation Trial Study Group: Optimal oral anticoagulant therapy in patients with nonrheumatic atrial fibrillation and recent cerebral ischemia. N Engl J Med 333:5–10, 1995.
146. The National Heart, Lung and Blood Institute Working Group on Atrial Fibrillation: Atrial fibrillation: current understandings and research imperatives. J Am Coll Cardiol 22:1830–1834, 1993.
147. SPAF III: Adjusted-dose warfarin versus low-intensity, fixed-dose warfarin plus aspirin for high-risk patients with atrial fibrillation: Stroke Prevention in Atrial Fibrillation III randomised clinical trial. Lancet 348:633–638, 1996.
148. Risk factors for stroke and efficacy of antithrombotic therapy in atrial fibrillation: analysis of pooled data from five randomized controlled trials. Arch Intern Med 154:1449–1457, 1994.
149. Shapiro EP, Effron MB, Lima S, et al: Transient atrial dysfunction after conversion of chronic atrial fibrillation to sinus rhythm. Am J Cardiol 62:1202–1207, 1988.
150. The Stroke Prevention in Atrial Fibrillation Investigators: Predictors of thromboembolism in atrial fibrillation, II: echocardiographic features of patients at risk. Ann Intern Med 116:6–12, 1992.
151. Jackman WM, Wang X, Friday KJ, et al: Catheter ablation of accessory atrioventricular pathways (Wolff-Parkinson-White syndrome) by radiofrequency current. N Engl J Med 324:1612–1618, 1991.
152. Calkins H, Langberg JJ, Sousa J, et al: Radiofrequency catheter ablation of accessory atrioventricular connections in 250 patients: abbreviated therapeutic approach to Wolff-Parkinson-White syndrome. Circulation 85:1337–1346, 1992.
153. Langberg JJ, Chin MC, Rosenqvist M, et al: Catheter ablation of the atrioventricular junction with radiofrequency energy. Circulation 80:1527–1535, 1989.
154. Jackman WM, Wang X, Friday KJ, et al: Catheter ablation of the atrioventricular junction using radiofrequency current in seventeen patients: comparison of standard and large-tip catheter electrodes. Circulation 83:1562–1576, 1991.
155. Kay GN, Ellenbogen KA, Giudici M, et al, and the APT Investigators: The Ablate and Pace Trial: a prospective study of catheter ablation of the AV conduction system and permanent pacemaker implantation for treatment of atrial fibrillation. J Intervent Card Electrophysiol 2:121–135, 1998.
156. Brignole M, Menozzi C, Gianfranchi L, et al: Assessment of atrioventricular junction ablation and VVIR pacemaker versus pharmacologic treatment in patients with heart failure and chronic atrial fibrillation. Circulation 98:953–960, 1998.
157. Gallagher MM, Obel OA, Camm AJ: Tachycardia-induced atrial myopathy: an important mechanism in the pathophysiology of atrial fibrillation? J Cardiovasc Electrophysiol 8:1065–1074, 1997.
158. Kieny JR, Sacrez A, Facello A, et al: Increase in radionuclide left ventricular ejection fraction after cardioversion of chronic atrial fibrillation in idiopathic dilated cardiomyopathy. Eur Heart J 13:1290–1295, 1992.
159. Packer DL, Brady GH, Worley SJ, et al: Tachycardia-induced cardiomyopathy: a reversible form of left ventricular dysfunction. Am J Cardiol 57:563–570, 1986.
160. Grogan M, Smith HC, Gersh BJ, Wood DL: Left ventricular dysfunction due to atrial fibrillation in patients initially believed to have idiopathic dilated cardiomyopathy. Am J Cardiol 69:1570–1573, 1992.
161. Rodriguez LM, Smeets JLRM, Xie B, et al: Improvement in left ventricular function by ablation of atrioventricular nodal conduction in selected patients with lone atrial fibrillation. Am J Cardiol 72:1137–1141, 1993.
162. Williamson BD, Man KC, Daoud E, et al: Radiofrequency catheter modification of atrioventricular conduction to control the ventricular rate during atrial fibrillation. N Engl J Med 331:910–917, 1994.
163. Feld GK, Fleck RP, Fujimura O, et al: Control of rapid ventricular response by radiofrequency catheter modification of the atrioventric-

ular node in patients with medically refractory atrial fibrillation. Circulation 90:2299–2307, 1994.
164. Lee SH, Chen SA, Tai CT, et al: Comparison of quality of life and cardiac performance after complete atrioventricular junction ablation and atrioventricular junction modification in patients with medically refractory atrial fibrillation. J Am Coll Cardiol 31:637–644, 1998.
165. Saksena S, Prakash A, Hill M, et al: Prevention of recurrent atrial fibrillation with chronic dual-site right atrial pacing. J Am Coll Cardiol 28:687–694, 1996.
166. Papageorgiou P, et al: Coronary sinus pacing prevents induction of atrial fibrillation. Circulation 96:1893–1898, 1997.
167. Feld GK, Fleck RP, Chen PS, et al: Radiofrequency catheter ablation for the treatment of human type I atrial flutter: identification of a critical zone in the reentrant circuit by endocardial mapping techniques. Circulation 86:1233–1340, 1992.
168. Lesh, MD, VanHare GF, Epstein LM, et al: Radiofrequency catheter ablation of atrial arrhythmias: results and mechanisms. Circulation 89:1074–1089, 1994.
169. Powell AC, Garan H, McGovern BA, et al: Low energy conversion of atrial fibrillation in the sheep. J Am Coll Cardiol 20:707–711, 1992.
170. Lau CP, Tse HF, Lok NS, et al: Initial clinical experience with an implantable human atrial defibrillator. Pacing Clin Electrophysiol 20:220–225, 1997.
171. Heisel A, Jung J: The atrial defibrillator: a stand-alone device or part of a combined dual-chamber system? Am J Cardiol 83:218D–226D, 1999.
172. Cox JL Scheussler RB, Lappas DG: An 8½ year clinical experience with surgery for atrial fibrillation. Ann Surg 224:267–275, 1996.
173. Haissaguerre M, Jais P, Shah D, et al: Right and left atrial radiofrequency catheter therapy for paroxysmal atrial fibrillation. J Cardiovasc Electrophysiol 7:1132–1144, 1996.

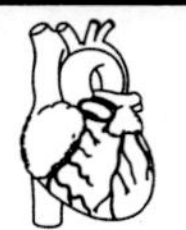

TRANSESOPHAGEAL ECHOCARDIOGRAPHY FOR PATIENTS WITH ATRIAL FIBRILLATION

Warren J. Manning

EFFICACY OF WARFARIN BEFORE ELECTIVE CARDIOVERSION
CARDIOVERSION WITH TRANSESOPHAGEAL ECHOCARDIOGRAPHY
Transesophageal Echocardiography–Guided Cardioversion in Concert With Heparin/Warfarin Anticoagulation
Transesophageal Echocardiography Cardioversion Without Anticoagulation
Cost Effectiveness of Transesophageal Echocardiography–Guided Cardioversion
Role of Transesophageal Echocardiography for Patients With Atrial Fibrillation of Less Than 48 Hours

Atrial fibrillation is the most common sustained arrhythmia. It is characterized by a lack of organized atrial electric and mechanical activity. The loss of orderly atrial systolic contraction leads to impaired left ventricular filling with resultant depressed cardiac output and symptoms of dyspnea and fatigue. In addition, the consequent stasis of blood with enhanced platelet aggregation and coagulation[1] predisposes to the formation of atrial thrombi and subsequent clinical thromboembolism.[1, 2]

For patients presenting with their first episode of atrial fibrillation, transthoracic (surface) echocardiography is often helpful for initial evaluation and management. Many cardiac disorders associated with atrial fibrillation, including mitral valve disease, hypertensive heart disease (left ventricular hypertrophy), or ischemic heart disease (focal left ventricular systolic dysfunction), are readily diagnosed with the use of transthoracic echocardiography. Information regarding left ventricular systolic function is of assistance in guiding the choice of ventricular rate–controlling agent. Finally, the absence of both clinical risk factors and structural heart disease on transthoracic echocardiography identifies patients for whom chronic therapy with aspirin (versus warfarin) may be preferred.[3] Because of the frequent inability to adequately image the left atrial appendage, however, surface echocardiography is not advocated for the identification or exclusion of atrial thrombi.

Although inadequate for the visualization of atrial thrombi, transthoracic echocardiography is an excellent technique for the assessment of left atrial size. Left atrial enlargement is common among patients with atrial fibrillation.[4] Sustained (chronic) atrial fibrillation is associated with progressive biatrial enlargement.[5] Cardioversion and maintenance of sinus rhythm may reverse this process.[6–8] Data are conflicting on the relationship between mild or moderate left atrial enlargement and long-term maintenance of sinus rhythm.[9–12] Because of this uncertainty, left atrial enlargement alone should not be used as a criterion to forego an attempt at cardioversion. We generally attempt cardioversion for almost all patients who present with their first episode of atrial fibrillation (assuming the duration of atrial fibrillation is brief and reversible causes of atrial fibrillation have been treated). Patients with prolonged (>1 year) atrial fibrillation, rheumatic mitral valve disease, and those with a left atrial dimension of more than 6.0 cm are less likely to have long-term maintenance of sinus rhythm. Repeated echocardiographic studies are generally not indicated for those with recurrent or chronic atrial fibrillation (unless there is a change in their clinical status, such as new heart failure).

EFFICACY OF WARFARIN BEFORE ELECTIVE CARDIOVERSION

Cardioversion of atrial fibrillation is often advocated to improve cardiac function, relieve symptoms, and decrease the risk of thrombus formation.[2] Unfortunately, successful cardioversion may be associated with clinical thromboembolism, usually occurring within the first 10 days after conversion. Patients with atrial fibrillation for at least 2 days are at a 6 percent risk for cardioversion-related clinical thromboembolism if cardioversion is not preceded by several weeks of warfarin (Table 89–1).[13–16] The use of 3 to 4 weeks of prophylactic warfarin (INR 2.0 to 3.0) reduces this risk to less than 1 percent (Table 89–2).[13–15, 17, 18]

Although warfarin prophylaxis offers the advantage of a reduction in postcardioversion thromboembolism, this approach delays cardioversion for the vast majority of patients who might otherwise undergo early cardioversion without complication. This delay exposes most patients to prolonged precardioversion warfarin therapy (with associated risk of

TABLE 89–1 Risk of Cardioversion-Related Thromboembolism Without 3 to 4 Weeks of Warfarin Therapy Before Elective Cardioversion

Study	Patients (n)	Incidence of Thromboembolism
Bjerkelund and Orning[13]	162	6.8%
Weinberg and Mancini[14]	28	7.1%
Arnold et al[15]	115*	6.3%
Roy et al[16]	42	4.8%

*Excludes post-thoracotomy patients with atrial fibrillation.

hemorrhagic complications) and also serves to prolong the duration of atrial fibrillation before cardioversion.

Among patients receiving warfarin in preparation for elective cardioversion, hemorrhagic complications requiring hospitalization, blood transfusion, or urgent surgery are reported in 1 to 2 percent of patients.[14, 17] For these patients, warfarin is often fully reversed to minimize further complications, yet if the event occurs before elective cardioversion, the patient remains unprotected and in atrial fibrillation. Minor complications (e.g., epistaxis, hematuria, menorrhagia) have been reported in an additional 6 to 18 percent of patients.[14, 17] For such patients, the clinician is faced with the difficult choice of reducing the intensity of anticoagulation, often to a subtherapeutic range (with the patient remaining in atrial fibrillation), or continuing warfarin at the risk of continued or worsening hemorrhage.

Finally, although 3 to 4 weeks of warfarin therapy are recommended before elective cardioversion, many patients are not treated in this manner. In one study, at least 25 percent of warfarin-eligible patients did not receive 1 month of prophylactic warfarin before cardioversion.[19] The proportion of elderly patients who do not receive 1 month of prophylactic warfarin may exceed 50 percent.[20] Even among patients for whom 1 month of warfarin is intended, transient subtherapeutic prothrombin times are common.[17] For these patients, a strategy of increasing the warfarin dose and restarting the "1-month clock" is generally followed.

Cardioversion With Transesophageal Echocardiography

A diagnostic imaging technique that provides the accurate assessment of atrial thrombi would allow for early and safe cardioversion for patients without thrombi. Such an approach is available; transesophageal echocardiography (TEE), a moderately invasive but well-tolerated procedure,[21] provides high-resolution imaging of the body of the atrium and the left atrial appendage. Comparative intraoperative series have demonstrated the excellent sensitivity and predictive accuracy of TEE for the identification and exclusion of left atrial thrombi (Fig. 89–1).[22–26] Achieving this level of diagnostic accuracy demands a systematic and careful examination of the atria and appendages[25] by an experienced operator with the use of multiplane (or biplane) transesophageal echocardiographic probes. Although TEE validation data for right atrial appendage thrombi are unreported, isolated right atrial thrombi appear to be quite rare.[17, 27–30]

In addition to reduced anticoagulation risk, several physiologic arguments can be made for abbreviating the duration of atrial fibrillation before cardioversion. Long-term maintenance of sinus rhythm is inversely related to the duration of atrial fibrillation before cardioversion.[31, 32] Preliminary data suggest that those with atrial fibrillation of less than 3 weeks before conversion have a decreased likelihood of atrial fibrillation recurrence and an enhanced likelihood of sinus rhythm at 1 year.[30] In addition, the recovery of atrial mechanical function has been shown to be inversely related to the duration of atrial fibrillation before cardioversion.[33] Patients with atrial fibrillation for less than 2 weeks before cardioversion demonstrate near-complete return of atrial mechanical function within 24 hours of cardioversion, whereas those with atrial fibrillation for more than 6 weeks require 3 weeks or longer for full recovery of atrial mechanical function.[33]

Transesophageal Echocardiography–Guided Cardioversion in Concert With Heparin/Warfarin Anticoagulation

We[27, 28, 30] and others[17, 29, 34] have advocated the use of TEE to guide early cardioversion in concert with therapeutic

TABLE 89–2 Risk of Cardioversion-Related Thromboembolism With Use of 3 to 4 Weeks of Prophylactic Warfarin Before Cardioversion

Study	Patients (n)	Incidence of Thromboembolism
Bjerkelund and Orning[13]	186	1.1%
Weinberg and Mancini[14]	51	0.0%
Arnold et al[15]	52*	0.0%
Klein et al[17]	64	1.6%
Seidl et al[18]	357	0.8%

*Excludes post-thoracotomy patients with atrial fibrillation.

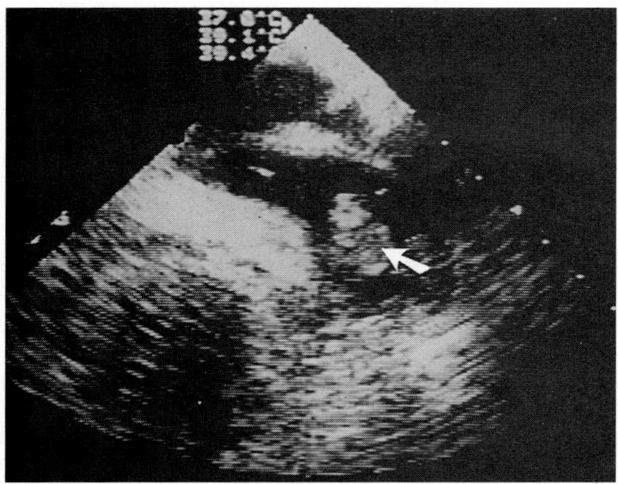

FIGURE 89–1 Transesophageal echocardiogram in vertical (90 degrees) imaging plane demonstrating a 1.5-cm thrombus *(white arrow)* within the left atrial appendage. (From Silverman DI, Manning WJ: Role of echocardiography in patients undergoing elective cardioversion of atrial fibrillations. Circulation 98[5]:479–486, 1998.)

anticoagulation (with heparin or warfarin) beginning at the time of TEE and extending to 1 month after cardioversion (Fig. 89–2). The rationale for this strategy is based on two assumptions: (1) TEE will detect clinically relevant thrombi and (2) heparin/warfarin anticoagulation will prevent the formation of new, clinically relevant thrombi during the interval between TEE and cardioversion and during the postcardioversion period. Regardless of the method (including spontaneous), conversion to sinus rhythm has been shown to be associated with relatively depressed left atrial and left atrial appendage mechanical function[29, 35–37] and, therefore, increased risk for postcardioversion thrombus formation.[29] The use of systemic anticoagulation for 1 month after cardioversion serves to inhibit the formation of new thrombi during recovery of atrial function and for prophylaxis should the patient revert to atrial fibrillation.

At least four independent trials[17, 27–30, 34, 38] have prospectively reported on the safety of a TEE-guided approach to early cardioversion among patients presenting with atrial fibrillation of at least 48 hours' duration (Table 89–3). These studies demonstrate that approximately 13 percent of patients presenting with atrial fibrillation will have atrial thrombi on initial TEE (see Table 89–3). The apparent discrepancy between the 13 percent prevalence rate of atrial thrombi and the 6 percent historical rate of clinical thromboembolism for nonanticoagulated patients is likely explained by (1) the imperfect specificity of TEE (especially among patients with extensive spontaneous echocardiographic contrast), (2) the likelihood that not all thrombi migrate after cardioversion, and (3) the fact that thrombi that do migrate may not always cause clinical events.[39] Predictors of atrial thrombi have included atrial spontaneous echocardiographic contrast,[27–29] depressed left ventricular systolic function,[17, 27, 28] and initial presentation with clinical thromboembolism.[27] Mitral regurgitation does not appear to be protective against thrombus formation in this group.[17, 27, 28]

With the use of the anticoagulation strategy described (see Fig. 89–2), early cardioversion in patients without transesophageal echocardiographic evidence of thrombi has resulted in only one systemic thromboembolic complication[30] among more than 1000 prospectively followed patients (0.1 percent; see Table 89–3). Safety data from a pilot prospective study that directly compared the conventional treatment of atrial fibrillation (4 weeks of warfarin before cardioversion) with the TEE-guided approach[17] also appears favorable for the transesophageal echocardiographic strategy with regard to safety and anticoagulation management and complications but not for the short-term maintenance of sinus rhythm. Data from the much larger (>3000 subjects), multicenter Assessment of Cardioversion Using Transesophageal Echocardiography study are not expected

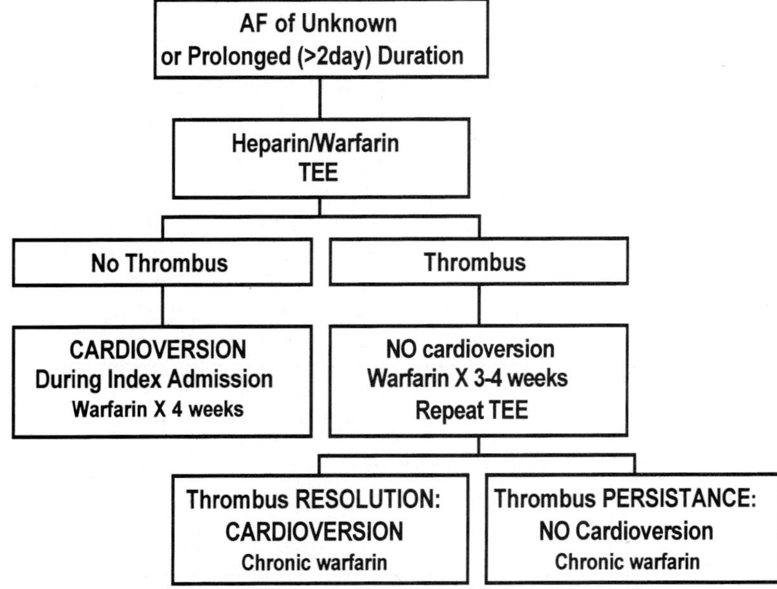

FIGURE 89–2 Schematic of transesophageal echocardiography–guided early cardioversion protocol for patient in whom cardioversion is desired. Decision analytic models demonstrate equal effectiveness with cost benefit if the transthoracic echocardiogram is omitted. AF, atrial fibrillation; TEE, transesophageal echocardiography.

TABLE 89-3 Incidence of Thrombi and Safety of Early Cardioversion Among Patients Referred for Transesophageal Echocardiography–Guided Cardioversion

Study	Number of Patients (n)	Number of Patients with Left Atrial Thrombi	Postcardioversion Thromboembolism*
Manning et al[27, 28, 30]	501†	64 (13%)	1 (0.25%)
Stoddard et al[29]	206‡	37 (18%)	0 (0%)
Klein et al[17]	62§	7 (13%)	0 (0%)
Grimm et al[38]	417	28 (7%)	0 (0%)
Corrado et al[34]	112	12 (10%)	0 (0%)

*Of patients without atrial thrombi.
†Five (1%) patients could not complete transesophageal echocardiography.
‡Forty-six received short-term anticoagulation.
§Six patients did not undergo transesophageal echocardiography.

for several years. Until the final randomized study data are published, the TEE-guided approach to cardioversion should be considered as having a safety profile similar to, but not safer, than that of conventional therapy. Patients ideally suited for the TEE-guided approach include patients at an increased risk for complications due to warfarin and those with a relatively short (<1 month) duration of atrial fibrillation at presentation. Patients with transesophageal echocardiographic evidence of atrial thrombi[40] or those in whom the left atrial appendage cannot be adequately visualized should not undergo early cardioversion but should be conservatively treated with 4 weeks of warfarin therapy.

As might be anticipated, the presence of an atrial thrombus on TEE confers an adverse prognosis. In our experience, despite the maintenance of systemic anticoagulation and the avoidance of cardioversion, 10 percent of these patients die during their index admission.[27, 28, 30] Of survivors with nonvalvular atrial fibrillation, the majority (>75 percent) of thrombi resolve during the subsequent month of warfarin anticoagulation.[17, 34, 41] Although there are no randomized data to support the use of a second TEE before cardioversion, this is our recommendation, and cost-effectiveness data support this second transesophageal echocardiographic approach.[40] We also advocate the long-term use of warfarin for these patients regardless of rhythm (see Fig. 89–2). We generally do not perform cardioversion until thrombus has completely resolved, and we treat patients with persistent thrombi with long-term warfarin and the avoidance of cardioversion.

Transesophageal Echocardiography Cardioversion Without Anticoagulation

Adverse events have been documented among patients with a "negative" TEE who have undergone early cardioversion *without* systemic anticoagulation.[42] Thromboembolism in these reports has uniformly occurred in patients who have not received therapeutic anticoagulation before TEE and extending 3 to 4 weeks after cardioversion. Many underwent electric cardioversion several days or weeks after TEE with no anticoagulation during this interval.[42] For these patients, it is impossible to exclude the possibility that atrial thrombi formed either between the TEE and cardioversion or after cardioversion. Impaired atrial mechanical function,[33, 35] new left atrial spontaneous echo contrast,[29, 35, 37] and even thrombus formation[29] have all been documented after successful cardioversion.

Cost Effectiveness of Transesophageal Echocardiography–Guided Cardioversion

In the health care environment, the cost effectiveness of novel treatment strategies must be considered in addition to its therapeutic benefits. The cost-benefit considerations of a TEE-guided approach to cardioversion must include (1) the complications of TEE, (2) the cost of performing the TEE, and (3) health care costs for patients who experience thromboembolism after a negative transesophageal echocardiogram. For conventional therapy, the costs are (1) the additional risk of hemorrhagic complications and (2) health care costs for patients who experience thromboembolism after 4 weeks of warfarin therapy. The cost effectiveness of the TEE-guided approach has been examined using decision analytic models.[43, 44] Using hospital *costs* (not *charges*), the TEE-guided approach has been identified as being more cost effective for hospitalized patients with atrial fibrillation but only when the initial transthoracic (surface) echocardiogram is eliminated[43]; this is because the use of transthoracic echocardiography cannot adequately exclude atrial thrombi. We therefore do not perform transthoracic echocardiography for patients in whom a TEE-guided approach is planned (see Fig. 89–2). In addition, it is important to proceed with expeditious TEE for hospitalized patients. Any cost savings are attenuated (or even reversed) if TEE is delayed and the hospital stay is prolonged. We advocate the use of therapeutic heparin and the initiation of oral warfarin at time of presentation to the emergency department. TEE should be performed within 24 hours of admission, with pharmacologic (or electric) cardioversion immediately after TEE or the next morning. The patient is then ready for discharge when the prothrombin time is therapeutic.

Role of Transesophageal Echocardiography for Patients With Atrial Fibrillation of Less Than 48 Hours

The general teaching (and clinical impression) that the incidence of atrial thrombi among patients with a relatively brief (<2 days) duration of atrial fibrillation came under closer scrutiny when Stoddard and associates[45] reported left atrial thrombi in 14 percent of patients with atrial fibrillation of less than 3 days' duration. These provocative data prompted an examination of the incidence of thromboembolism among patients presenting with atrial fibrillation of less than 48 hours' duration. In a consecutive series of more than 350 hospitalized patients with nonvalvular atrial fibrillation of less than 48 hours' duration, we found that more than 95 percent of patients converted (spontaneously or actively) to sinus rhythm during the index admission. None had a screening TEE. The incidence of cardioversion-related thromboembolism was 0.8 percent, and all events occurred in patients who had spontaneously converted to sinus rhythm.[46] This incidence of thromboembolism is similar to the expected incidence of thromboembolism had this entire group been treated with 1 month of warfarin before cardioversion. Preliminary data from Mitchell and colleagues[47] are also consistent with these patients being at a very low risk of postcardioversion thromboembolism. Accordingly, we do not advocate a screening TEE or prolonged warfarin therapy before cardioversion for patients with nonvalvular atrial fibrillation of less than 48 hours' duration, except for patients at high risk for thromboembolism (history of prior or recent thromboembolism, rheumatic valvular disease, severe left ventricular systolic dysfunction). Although the benefit has not been proved, we do recommend that patients presenting with atrial fibrillation of less than 48 hours' duration be anticoagulated with heparin at the time of presentation so as to minimize the likelihood that a thrombus will develop while they are undergoing management and so they are "protected" during the periconversion period of atrial and atrial appendage dysfunction.

REFERENCES

1. Sohara H, Amitani S, Kurose M, Miyahara K: Atrial fibrillation activates platelets and coagulation in a time-dependent manner: a study in patients with paroxysmal atrial fibrillation. J Am Coll Cardiol 29:106, 1997.
2. Pritchett E: Management of atrial fibrillation. N Engl J Med 326:1264, 1992.
3. The Stroke Prevention in Atrial Fibrillation Investigators: Predictors of thromboembolism in atrial fibrillation, II: echocardiographic features of patients at risk. Ann Intern Med 116:6, 1992.
4. Vaziri SM, Larson MG, Benjamin EJ, Levy D: Echocardiographic predictors of nonrheumatic atrial fibrillation: the Framingham Heart Study. Circulation 89:724, 1994.
5. Sanfillippo AJ, Abascal VM, Sheehan M, et al: Atrial enlargement as a consequence of atrial fibrillation: a prospective echocardiographic study. Circulation 82:792, 1990.
6. Manning WJ, Leeman DE, Gotch PJ, Come PC: Pulsed Doppler evaluation of atrial mechanical function after electrical cardioversion of atrial fibrillation. J Am Coll Cardiol 13:617, 1989.
7. Gosselink ATM, Crijns HJGM, Hamer HPM, et al: Changes in left and right atrial size after cardioversion of atrial fibrillation: role of mitral valve disease. J Am Coll Cardiol 22:1666, 1993.
8. Van Gelder IC, Crijns HJ, Van Gilst WH, et al: Decrease of right and left atrial sizes after direct current electrical cardioversion in chronic atrial fibrillation. Am J Cardiol 67:93, 1991.
9. Hoglund C, Rosenhamer G: Echocardiographic left atrial dimension as a predictor of maintaining sinus rhythm after conversion of atrial fibrillation. Acta Med Scand 217:411, 1985.
10. Dittrich HC, Erickson JS, Schneiderman T, et al: Echocardiographic and clinical predictors for outcome of elective cardioversion of atrial fibrillation. Am J Cardiol 63:193, 1989.
11. Volgman AS, Iftikhar F, Soble JS, et al: Effect of left atrial size on recurrence of atrial fibrillation after electrical cardioversion: atrial dimension versus volume. Am J Card Imaging 10:261, 1996.
12. Arnar DO, Danielsen R: Factors predicting maintenance of sinus rhythm after direct current cardioversion of atrial fibrillation and flutter: a reanalysis with recently acquired data. Cardiology 87:181, 1996.
13. Bjerkelund C, Orning OM: The efficacy of anticoagulant therapy in preventing embolism related to DC electrical conversion of atrial fibrillation. Am J Cardiol 23:208, 1969.
14. Weinberg DM, Mancini GBJ: Anticoagulation for cardioversion of atrial fibrillation. Am J Cardiol 63:745, 1989.
15. Arnold AZ, Mick MJ, Mazurek RP, et al: Role of prophylactic anticoagulation for direct cardioversion in patients with atrial fibrillation or atrial flutter. J Am Coll Cardiol 19:851, 1992.
16. Roy D, Marchand E, Gagné P, et al: Usefulness of anticoagulant therapy in the prevention of embolic complications of atrial fibrillation. Am Heart J 112:1039, 1986.
17. Klein AL, Grimm RA, Black IW, et al, for the ACUTE Investigators: Cardioversion guided by transesophageal echocardiography: the ACUTE pilot study: a randomized, controlled trial. Ann Intern Med 126:200, 1997.
18. Seidl K, Hauer B, Schwacke H, Droegemueller A: Intrahospital stroke rates after acute electrical cardioversion in atrial fibrillation and atrial flutter despite effective anticoagulation: a prospective study [abstract]. Circulation 98(suppl I):I-298, 1998.
19. Schlicht JR, Davis RC, Naqi K, et al: Physician practices regarding anticoagulation and cardioversion of atrial fibrillation. Arch Intern Med 156:290, 1996.
20. Carlsson J, Tebbe U, Rox J, et al, for the ALKK Study Group: Cardioversion of atrial fibrillation in the elderly. Am J Cardiol 78:1380, 1996.
21. Daniel WG, Erbel R, Kasper W, et al: Safety of transesophageal echocardiography: a multicenter survey of 10,419 examinations. Circulation 83:817, 1991.
22. Mügge A, Daniel WG, Hausmann D, et al: Diagnosis of left atrial appendage thrombi by transesophageal echocardiography: clinical implications and follow-up. Am J Card Imaging 4:173, 1990.
23. Olson JD, Goldenberg IF, Pedersen W, et al: Exclusion of atrial thrombus by transesophageal echocardiography. J Am Soc Echocardiogr 5:52, 1992.
24. Hwang JJ, Chen JJ, Lin SC, et al: Diagnostic accuracy of transesophageal echocardiography for detecting left atrial thrombi in patients with rheumatic heart disease having undergone mitral valve operations. Am J Cardiol 72:677, 1993.
25. Manning WJ, Weintraub RM, Waksmonski CA, et al: Accuracy of transesophageal echocardiography for identifying left atrial thrombi: a prospective, intraoperative study. Ann Intern Med 123:817 1995.
26. Fatkin D, Scalia G, Jacobs N, et al: Accuracy of biplane transesophageal echocardiography in detecting left atrial thrombus. Am J Cardiol 77:321, 1996.
27. Manning WJ, Silverman DI, Keighley CS, et al: Transesophageal echocardiographically facilitated early cardioversion from atrial fibrillation using short term anticoagulation: final results of a prospective 4.5-year study. J Am Coll Cardiol 25:1354, 1995.
28. Manning WJ, Silverman DI, Gordon SPF, et al: Cardioversion from atrial fibrillation without prolonged anticoagulation with the use of transesophageal echocardiography to exclude the presence of atrial thrombi. N Engl J Med 328:750, 1993.
29. Stoddard MF, Dawkins P, Prince CR, Longaker RA: Transesophageal echocardiographic guidance of cardioversion in patients with atrial fibrillation. Am Heart J 129:1204, 1995.
30. Weigner MJ, Silverman DI, Patel U, et al: Transesophageal echocardiography facilitated cardioversion from atrial fibrillation: safety and one year follow-up [abstract]. Circulation 98(suppl I):I-849, 1998.
31. Dittrich HC, Erickson JS, Schneiderman T, et al: Echocardiographic and clinical predictors for outcome of elective cardioversion of atrial fibrillation. Am J Cardiol 63:193, 1989.
32. Flaker GC, Fletcher KA, Rothbart RM, et al: Clinical and echocardiographic features of intermittent atrial fibrillation that predict recurrent atrial fibrillation. Am J Cardiol 76:355, 1995.
33. Manning WJ, Silverman DI, Katz SE, et al: Impaired left atrial mechanical function after cardioversion: relationship to the duration of atrial fibrillation. J Am Coll Cardiol 23:1535, 1994.
34. Corrado G, Tadeo G, Beretta S, et al: Atrial thrombus resolution after

prolonged anticoagulation in patients with atrial fibrillation. Chest 115:140, 1999.

35. Grimm RA, Leung DY, Black IW, et al: Left atrial appendage "stunning" after spontaneous conversion of atrial fibrillation demonstrated by transesophageal Doppler echocardiography. Am Heart J 130:174, 1995.
36. Manning WJ, Silverman DI, Katz SE, et al: Temporal dependence of the return of atrial mechanical function on the mode of cardioversion of atrial fibrillation to sinus rhythm. Am J Cardiol 75:624, 1995.
37. Grimm RA, Stewart WJ, Maloney JD, et al: Impact of electrical cardioversion of atrial fibrillation on left atrial appendage function and spontaneous echo contrast: characterization by simultaneous transesophageal echocardiography. J Am Coll Cardiol 22:1359, 1993.
38. Grimm RA, Agler DA, Vaughn SE, et al: TEE-guided anticoagulation in patients undergoing electrical cardioversion of atrial fibrillation: results from the ACUTE registry [abstract]. J Am Coll Cardiol 31:353A, 1998.
39. Ezekowitz MD, James KE, Nazarian SM, Davenport J, et al: Silent cerebral infarction in patients with nonrheumatic atrial fibrillation: the Veterans Affairs Stroke Prevention in Nonrheumatic Atrial Fibrillation Investigators. Circulation 92:2178, 1995.
40. Seto TB, Taira DA, Manning WJ: Cardioversion in patients with nonvalvular atrial fibrillation and left atrial thrombi on initial TEE: should TEE be repeated prior to elective cardioversion? J Am Soc Echocardiogr 12:508, 1999.
41. Collins LJ, Silverman DI, Douglas PS, Manning WJ: Cardioversion of non-rheumatic atrial fibrillation: reduced thromboembolic complications with 4 weeks of pre-cardioversion anticoagulation are related to atrial thrombus resolution. Circulation 92:160, 1995.
42. Black IW, Fatkin D, Sagar KB, et al: Exclusion of atrial thrombus by transesophageal echocardiography does not preclude embolism after cardioversion of atrial fibrillation: a multicenter study. Circulation 89:2509, 1994.
43. Seto TB, Taira DA, Tsevat J, Manning WJ: Cost-effectiveness of transesophageal echocardiography-guided cardioversion for hospitalized patients with atrial fibrillation. J Am Coll Cardiol 29:122, 1997.
44. Klein AL, Grimm RA, Black IW, et al: Cost effectiveness of TEE-guided cardioversion with anticoagulation compared to conventional therapy in patients with atrial fibrillation [abstract]. J Am Coll Cardiol 23:128A, 1994.
45. Stoddard MF, Dawkins PR, Prince CR, Ammash NM: Left atrial appendage thrombus is not uncommon in patients with acute atrial fibrillation and a recent embolic event: a transesophageal echocardiographic study. J Am Coll Cardiol 25:452, 1995.
46. Weigner MJ, Caulfield TA, Danias PG, et al: Risk for clinical thromboembolism associated with conversion to sinus rhythm in patients with atrial fibrillation of less than 48 hours' duration. Ann Intern Med 126:615, 1997.
47. Mitchell MA, Hughes GS, Ellenbogen KA, et al: Cardioversion-related stroke rates in atrial fibrillation and atrial flutter [abstract]. Circulation 96(suppl I):I-453, 1997.

CHAPTER **90**

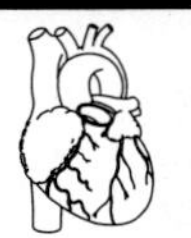

Long QT Syndromes

Steven J. Compton and Jay W. Mason

PATHOPHYSIOLOGY
Historical
Competing Hypotheses
New Gene and Ion Channel Findings
Acquired (Drug-Induced) Long QT Syndrome
Jervell and Lange-Nielsen Syndrome: Homozygous Carriers
New Models of Torsades de Pointes
PHYSICAL EXAMINATION
NATURAL HISTORY
TREATMENT
SUMMARY

The inherited long QT syndrome (LQTS) is characterized by QT interval prolongation, syncope and sudden death due to polymorphic ventricular tachycardia (torsades de pointes), and ventricular fibrillation. Although the syndrome was first described about four decades ago,[1–4] descriptions of the abnormal cellular electrophysiology have only emerged since 1996. Powerful molecular genetic techniques (linkage analyses, positional cloning, and candidate gene analyses) have identified mutations responsible for disease in most affected families. This work was immediately followed by study of the biophysics of the mutant ion channels causing LQTS, which has led to an understanding of the disease sufficient to permit development of new treatments of affected patients. The rapid application of benchside genetic discoveries to treatment powerfully illustrates the clinical utility of molecular genetics.

Pathophysiology

Historical

Jervell and Lange-Nielsen[1] first described the familial occurrence of QT interval prolongation and sudden death associated with congenital deafness in 1957. This syndrome was typically associated with consanguinuity, and thus an autosomal recessive pattern of genetic transmission seemed apparent. An autosomal dominant form of the disease was later described by Romano and coworkers[2] and Ward[3, 4]; this form was not associated with congenital deafness and was later found to be far more common. Syncope in these patients was found to be caused by torsades de pointes, a pause-dependent ventricular tachycardia characterized by a gradual oscillation of the QRS axis. Sudden death is caused by degeneration of this rhythm into ventricular fibrillation. The incidence of both syncope and sudden death varies among families, and these events are often associated with sudden changes in adrenergic tone. Triggers for syncope and sudden death include sudden loud noises, fear, anger, exertion, and distress. Sudden death may also occur during both sleep and rest.

Several therapies have been used to prevent ventricular arrhythmia. These include beta-adrenergic blocking drugs, left cardiac sympathetic denervation (LCSD), and permanent pacing. The effectiveness of these treatments has never been tested in randomized trials, but reductions in event rates have been reported.[5–7] Refractory cases have been treated with implantable cardioverter-defibrillators (ICDS)[8] or cardiac transplantation.

Competing Hypotheses

Two competing hypotheses have been proposed to explain the clinical features of LQTS. James[9] noted the frequent initiation of arrhythmias by adrenergic fluctuations, and Moss and McDonald[10] suggested that a right-left imbalance of cardiac sympathetic innervation was responsible. This concept, promoted by Schwartz[11] as the *sympathetic imbalance* hypothesis, was supported by the observations that left stellate ganglion stimulation or right stellectomy prolonged the QT interval,[12] reproduced T wave alternans,[13] and increased ventricular arrhythmias[14] in animals. Based on the hypothesis that patients with LQTS have lower than normal right cardiac sympathetic activity, with reflex hyperactivity of the left cardiac sympathetic nerves, LCSD was first attempted as therapy for LQTS in 1971.[10] Although LCSD did not shorten the QT interval in all patients, the procedure eventually gained favor as a nonspecific protective therapy based on increases in ventricular fibrillation thresholds.[13]

The second hypothesis explaining LQTS was the *myocyte abnormality* hypothesis, which holds that an intrinsic myocellular abnormality, rather than an extrinsic neuroadrenergic mechanism, is the cause of LQTS. This hypothesis was favored by the observation that QT prolongation and torsades de pointes can be observed in normal hearts exposed to class III antiarrhythmics, cesium, hypocalcemia, or hypokalemia. All of these conditions reduce repolarizing potassium currents, prolonging action potential duration and, therefore, QT interval duration. In the familial LQTS, mutations of genes coding for repolarizing cardiac ion channels could cause prolongation of repolarization.

New Gene and Ion Channel Findings

Since 1996, the myocyte abnormality hypothesis has been proved to account for most cases of familial LQTS. Over 90 percent of genotyped families suffer from mutations of any of four different genes coding for ion channel proteins (Table 90–1).

Cardiac ion channels are proteins that span the bilipid membrane of the cardiac myocyte, controlling inflow and outflow of charged ions. Selective movement of ions across the membrane results in measurable changes in transmembrane voltages. Cardiac ion channel activity determines the magnitude and duration of voltage changes across the myocyte membrane. In any vertebrate, movements of sodium, calcium, and potassium ions are largely responsible for generation of the ventricular action potential, measured indirectly on the body surface as the QRST complex. The normal ventricular action potential is shown in the first panel of Figure 90–1, together with the principal currents. The resting cell potential is about −90 mV relative to the outside of the cell. Depolarization occurs when inward flow of positive ions (sodium, followed by calcium) abruptly raises the cellular membrane potential. Later, outward flow of positively charged potassium ions results in repolarization of the cell membrane. Augmentation of the depolarizing currents, or reduction of the repolarizing currents, prolongs the action potential duration, thereby prolonging the QT interval (see Fig. 90–1).

Augmented Sodium Current

In a small proportion of LQTS families, a genetic defect on chromosome 3 was discovered.[15] This defect is due to mutations in the *SCN5A* gene coding for a protein domain involved in the inactivation of the cardiac sodium channel. When *Xenopus* oocytes (frog eggs) are injected with cRNA corresponding to these mutations and allowed to incubate, sodium channel proteins are formed and transported to the oocyte surface. Whole cell and patch-clamp studies then allow characterization of the abnormal channels. Normally, the SCN5A channel opens briefly at the beginning of the action potential, allowing rapid depolarization by an inward sodium current. In the *Xenopus* system, the mutant channels open briefly under voltage clamp, but then intermittently reopen during prolonged membrane depolarization (simulating the plateau phase of the action potential). Thus, there is a sustained sodium current that prolongs action potential duration.[16, 17]

Strikingly similar pathology has been described in inherited disorders of the skeletal muscle counterpart of this channel, SCN4A. Mutations affecting inactivation of this channel cause myotonia, hyperkalemic periodic paralysis, and paramyotonia congenita.[18]

The effect of the sodium channel blocker mexiletine has now been investigated in the *Xenopus* system, a ventricular myocyte model,[19] and humans affected by this form of LQTS. Mexiletine appears to block the intermittent reopening of the mutant sodium channels,[17] and a small clinical study has demonstrated QT interval shortening in patients with this form of LQTS.[20] Finally, mutations causing *diminished* function of this channel have been associated with idiopathic ventricular fibrillation.[21]

Diminished Potassium Current

Repolarization of cardiac myocytes is accomplished by opening of potassium channels, allowing outward flow of potassium ions and restoration of the negative resting membrane potential. One repolarizing potassium current, I_K, is subdivided into rapid and slow components: I_{Kr} and I_{Ks}.[22] Abnormalities of three different genes have been found to result in diminished function of these two channels. Predictably, reduction of these currents results in prolongation of the action potential and QT interval.

Mutations of I_{Ks} channels are responsible for disease in over half of LQTS families (Fig. 90–2). The I_{Ks} channel is a very slowly activating, slowly deactivating channel that is variably present in mammalian ventricular tissue.[23] Each action potential activates a small fraction of I_{Ks} channels, but with faster rates, the number of activated channels accumulates, resulting in gradual increases of this repolarizing current. The accumulation of activated I_{Ks} channels

TABLE 90–1 **Characteristics of Inherited Long QT Syndromes**

LQT Type	Chromosome	Gene	Gene Product	Current	Clinical Characteristics/? Possible Gene-Specific Treatment
LQT1	11p15.5	*KVLQT1*	KvLQT1 (I_{Ks} α-subunit)	I_{Ks}	Adrenergic onset/β-blockers
LQT2	7q35-36	*HERG*	HERG α-subunit	I_{Kr}	? Potassium therapy
LQT3	3p21-24	*SCN5A*	SCN5A	I_{Na}	Onset at rest/? mexiletine
LQT4	4q25-257	?	?	?	One large French family
LQT5	21q22.1-22.2	*KCNE1*	minK (I_{Ks} β-subunit)	I_{Ks}	Rare; ? similar to LQT1
LQT6	21q22.1-22.2	*KCNE2*	MiRP1 (minK-related peptide)	I_{Kr}	Rare. MiRP1 is an ion channel subunit that affects I_{Kr}
LQT7	?	?	?	?	Certain LQTS families do not have any of the mutations listed above
LQT8	?	?	?	?	LQTS with syndactyly
JLN1	11p15.5	*KVLQT1*	KvLQT1 (I_{Ks} α-subunit)	I_{Ks}	Autosomal recessive, congenital hearing loss, high sudden death risk
JLN2	21q22.1-22.2	*KCNE1*	minK (I_{Ks} β-subunit)	I_{Ks}	Autosomal recessive, congenital hearing loss, high sudden death risk

Abbreviations: JLN[n], variants of the autosomal dominant Jervell and Lange-Nielsen syndrome; LQT[n], variants of the autosomal recessive Romano-Ward syndrome; LQTS, long QT syndrome.

is due to their slow deactivation kinetics. This property may explain aspects of normal repolarization physiology, such as QT interval shortening at faster heart rates, as well as the observation that changes in QT interval with abrupt heart rate changes are not instantaneous. Finally, I_{Ks} is increased by β-adrenergic stimulation, a property that may have important clinical implications.[24] Among the various LQTS subtypes, patients with I_{Ks} channel mutations are most likely to have clinical events triggered by adrenergic stress.[25–27] Retrospective analysis of patients with I_{Ks} mutations showed a marked reduction in event rates when these patients were treated with beta-blockers.[28]

It now appears that each I_{Ks} channel is composed of coassembled subunits, which are coded for by two separate genes,[29, 30] *KCNE1* and *KVLQT1*. *KCNE1* encodes the minK subunit; *KVLQT1* encodes the KvLQT1 subunit. The smaller subunit, minK, does not form functional channels when expressed alone in *Xenopus* oocytes. When expressed with the second subunit, KvLQT1, functional potassium channels form. It is likely that I_{Ks} channels are formed by two minK subunits coassembling with four KvLQT1 subunits. In most families, I_{Ks} abnormalities are due to *KVLQT1* mutations. The finding that minK is an I_{Ks} subunit resulted in an immediate search for LQTS families with mutations of this protein.[31] Although the minK protein also modifies I_{Kr} function,[32] this property may not be physiologically relevant. A related gene, *KCNE2*, codes for a minK-related peptide (MiRP1). The MiRP1 subunit coassembles with *HERG*; *KCNE2* mutations have been associated with diminished I_{Kr} current and LQTS.[33]

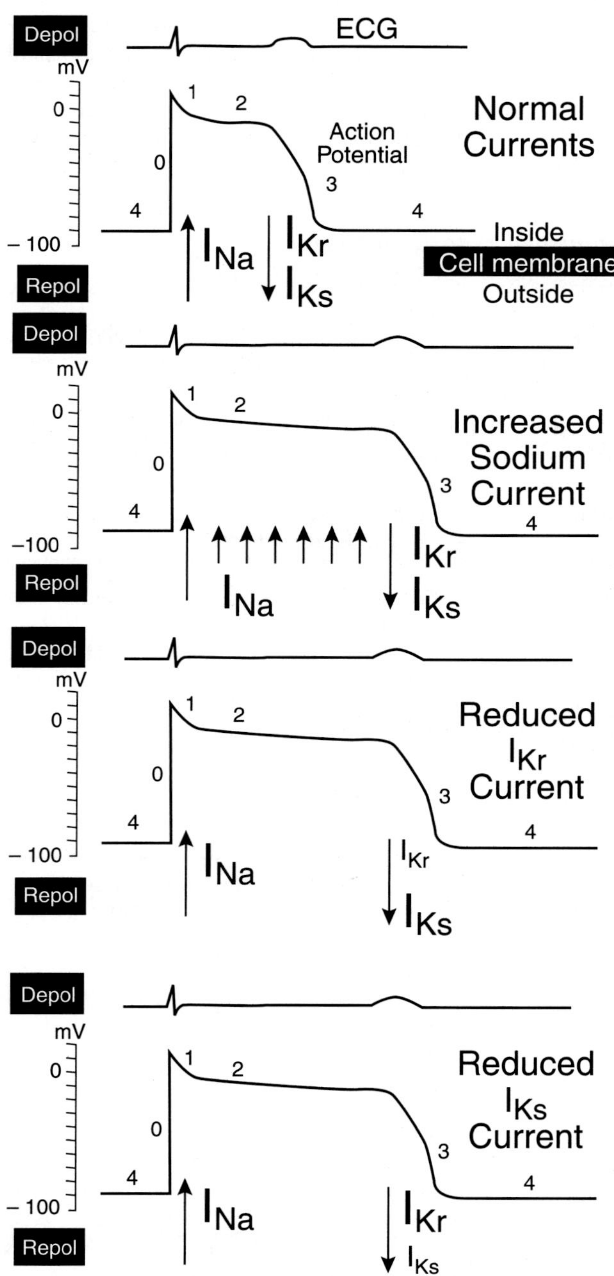

FIGURE 90–1 Action potential and currents. ECG, electrocardiogram.

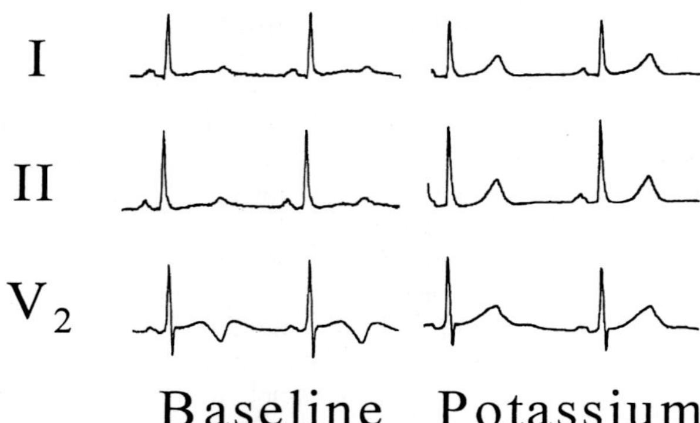

FIGURE 90–2 Effect of potassium on resting QT morphology. These recordings were taken from a patient with a *HERG* mutation causing diminished I_{Kr} channel function. After infusion of potassium, the QT interval shortens and the biphasic T wave in lead V_2 becomes more normal.

Although specific I_{Ks}-agonist drugs are not clinically available, nicorandil has been used in a group of LQTS patients with inherited KVLQT1 defects.[34] Nicorandil is an agonist affecting the adenosine triphosphate (ATP)–sensitive potassium channel, K_{ATP}. In this study, epinephrine prolonged action potential duration and QT interval, and these effects were partly reversed by intravenous nicorandil. Shimizu and colleagues[34] concluded that the shortening of repolarization was likely through activation of K_{ATP} channels. There is a single case report of successful clinical use of this drug.[35]

The other component of I_K is the *rapid* delayed rectifier current, I_{Kr}. As the name implies, the activation kinetics are fast compared with those of I_{Ks}. This channel is not directly modified by β-adrenergic stimulation, and unlike with I_{Ks}, accumulation does not occur with faster heart rates. Where I_{Kr} and I_{Ks} coexist, I_{Kr} contributes more to repolarization at slow heart rates, and I_{Ks} plays more of a role at fast heart rates.

Inherited mutations of I_{Kr} are now thought to be the second most prevalent cause of LQTS. The gene *HERG*, located on chromosome 7, codes for the protein forming an alpha-subunit of the human I_{Kr} channel.[36] Each single I_{Kr} channel is normally composed of four identical α-subunits. Patients who are heterozygous carriers of the mutant *HERG* gene will express both normal and mutant α-subunits, possibly in equal proportions. When mutant and normal subunits are allowed to randomly coassemble in the *Xenopus* expression system, diminished channel function is observed. As with the I_{Ks} defect, reduction of repolarizing current leads to prolongation of action potential and QT duration. Patients with the I_{Kr} form of LQTS have an exaggerated reduction in QT interval with faster heart rates,[37, 38] presumably related to a greater reliance on the I_{Ks} channel for repolarization. This is in contrast to patients with the I_{Ks} defect, who show a blunted QT reduction with faster heart rates compared with those of normals.[39]

Since intracellular potassium concentration is lower than extracellular potassium ($[K^+]_o$) one would expect that raising $[K^+]_o$ would *decrease* the potassium current by reducing the transmembrane chemical gradient. In myocytes and HERG channels expressed in *Xenopus* oocytes, the opposite effect is seen, because I_{Kr} is directly modulated by $[K^+]_o$.[36, 40] In LQTS patients with the I_{Kr} defect, acute elevation of serum potassium levels reduced QT intervals and QT dispersion and improved baseline T wave abnormalities (see Fig. 90–2).[37]

Acquired (Drug-Induced) Long QT Syndrome

Acquired LQTS is much more common than the congenital form, and it is most commonly related to exposure of a normal heart to medications, such as quinidine or sotalol, that block I_{Kr}. With these and other medications, toxicity may manifest as QT interval prolongation, with syncope or sudden death associated with pause-dependent torsades de pointes. A physiologic connection to inherited LQTS had long been suspected, but was not proved until 1995, when the I_{Kr} defect in LQTS was described. The physiologic manifestations of I_{Kr}-blocking drugs are identical to those of patients with inherited I_{Kr} dysfunction. As in the inherited I_{Kr} defect, acute elevation of serum potassium has now been shown to decrease QT intervals and QT dispersion and improve baseline T wave abnormalities in acquired QT prolongation due to quinidine use.[41] This is consistent with clinical observations that hypokalemia is a risk factor for torsades de pointes[42] and with experimental work in which increased $[K^+]_o$ inhibits I_{Kr} blockade by quinidine.[43]

The identification of I_{Kr} blockade as a risk factor for sudden death has led to closer scrutiny of I_{Kr}-blocking drugs. Terfenadine (Seldane) was highly prescribed after receiving U.S. Food and Drug Administration approval in 1982 as a nonsedating antihistamine. After market release, QT prolongation and sudden death were noted in patients receiving terfenadine in the setting of hepatic failure or concomitant use of medications blocking the hepatic metabolism of terfenadine.[44] Terfenadine proved to be a weak I_{Kr} blocker[45] and was ultimately replaced in the North American market by fexofenadine, a metabolite found to block histamine receptors but without significant effects on I_{Kr}. A similar drug, astemizole (Hismanal), is also metabolized to an I_{Kr} blocker,[46] but this has remained on the market. A list of commonly prescribed medications with proven or suspected I_{Kr}-blocking properties is given in Table 90–2. Although several groups have reported cases of drug-induced QT prolongation secondary to subclinical LQTS mutations,[47] it is not yet known whether this is the general case.

Jervell and Lange-Nielsen Syndrome: Homozygous Carriers

As predicted by family pedigree data showing autosomal dominant transmission, patients with the Romano-Ward syndrome are heterozygous carriers of these gene mutations. The autosomal recessive inheritance pattern of the more severe Jervell and Lange-Nielsen (JLN) syndrome raised the possibility that JLN patients might be homozygous carriers of the same mutations. This proved to be true when JLN was associated with homozygous mutations of both the *KVLQT1*[48, 49] and the *KCNE1*[50] genes. Since both of these genes code for I_K subunits, these patients have markedly reduced I_{Ks} cardiac currents. Congenital deafness in these patients has been explained by the requirement of I_{Ks} for endolymph production in the inner ear.[49]

New Models of Torsades de Pointes

Torsades de pointes is a distinctive form of polymorphic ventricular tachycardia[51] that is associated with both inherited and acquired QT prolongation. QT interval prolongation represents the surface manifestation of ventricular action potential prolongation, which is linked to development

TABLE 90–2 I_{Kr}-Blocking Agents

Class Ia antiarrhythmics with class III effects
Quinidine
Procainamide
Disopyramide
Class III antiarrhythmics
Sotalol
Dofetilide
Bretylium
Ibutilide
Antiarrhythmic drug metabolites
N-Acetylprocainamide
Desethylamiodarone
Antibiotics
Erythromycin
Azithromycin
Trimethoprim-sulfamethoxazole
Chloroquine
Pentamidine
Antidepressants
Tricyclics: amitriptyline, imipramine, desipramine
Tetracyclics
Antifungals
Itraconazole
Ketoconazole
Antihistamines
Diphenhydramine
Terfenadine
Astemizole
Antireflux
Cisapride
Neuroleptics
Phenothiazines: haloperidol, thioridazine

of early afterdepolarizations (EADs) in Purkinje (conduction system) tissue. EADs are oscillations in membrane voltage during the plateau or recovery phase of the action potential. When the EADs are of sufficient magnitude, they give rise to triggered action potentials. The upstroke of the triggered potential is most likely due to abnormal reactivation of L-type calcium channels, but sodium channels may also be involved. The observation that both EADs and torsades de pointes follow pauses has raised the possibility that torsades de pointes is initiated by a triggered depolarization.

The generation of torsades de pointes rhythm has been poorly understood, and two hypotheses have been advanced. In the first, advanced by Dessertenne[51] in his original description of torsades de pointes, fused beats from multiple foci may result in the distinctive electrocardiographic findings. In fact, a rhythm resembling torsades de pointes can be generated by simultaneously pacing different ventricular sites at slightly different rates. In the second hypothesis, functional block occurs within the ventricle after a triggered beat, and intraventricular reentry ensues. This hypothesis has been supported by computer simulations[52] and by the observation that dispersion of refractoriness appears to be a prerequisite for torsades de pointes.[53–55]

After initial descriptions of the channel abnormalities in congenital LQTS, several laboratories have developed animal models of this disease.[19, 54, 55] Anthopleurin-A is a polypeptide poison that prolongs the QT interval by slowing sodium channel inactivation,[56] similar to that seen in the SCN5A form of LQTS described previously. In dogs exposed to this toxin, El-Sherif's group[57] mapped the three-dimensional activation sequence during torsades de pointes and demonstrated functional reentry.[57] Consistent findings have been demonstrated in epicardial optical mapping studies of isolated rabbit hearts.[58] In this model, torsades de pointes is a triggered arrhythmia that is sustained through functional reentry in the ventricle. Sudden death is likely caused by degeneration to ventricular fibrillation.

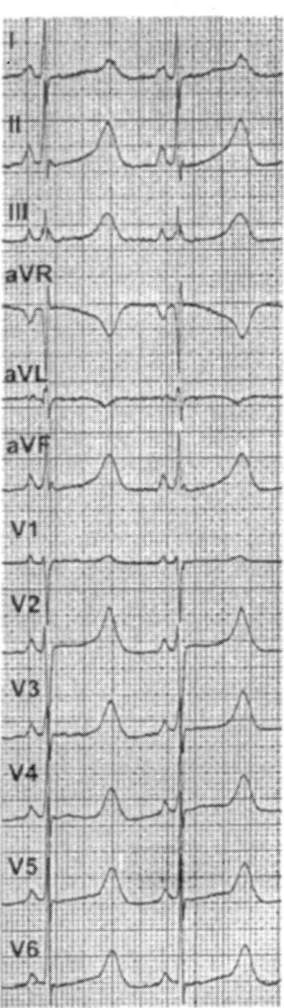

FIGURE 90–3 Typical electrocardiographic findings in long QT syndrome. This recording was taken from a patient with a *KVLQT1* mutation causing diminished I_{Ks} channel function.

PHYSICAL EXAMINATION

There are no physical examination findings diagnostic of LQTS. Associated physical findings include slow pulse secondary to sinus bradycardia or 2:1 atrioventricular block (generally seen in infants). Congenital deafness may be seen in patients with homozygous mutations affecting I_{Ks}, and QT prolongation may be more common among the congenitally deaf population.[59] Rarely, congenital syndactyly has been described in infants with severe congenital LQTS.[60] Electrocardiographic screening (Fig. 90–3) is warranted in patients with physical findings of unexplained bradycardia, congenital deafness, or syndactyly.

NATURAL HISTORY

The prevalence of LQTS in the general population is unknown. LQTS has been described in virtually every population group worldwide, and it has been implicated in the sudden infant death syndrome.[61] Mortality risk in LQTS is somewhat difficult to define and may vary with the specific ion channel defect.[62, 63] There are often marked differences in measured QT intervals and symptoms between affected individuals within a family.[64, 65] Not surprisingly, the proband (first diagnosed case within a family) carries a higher sudden death risk than affected family members.[66] Published mortality data are confounded by the inclusion of both treated and untreated LQTS patients. In an initial case review with a 5-year follow-up, Schwartz and Stone[14] estimated an alarming 5 percent annual sudden death risk in untreated LQTS. This study included a large number of high-risk patients (congenital deafness, untreated probands), and subsequent studies have yielded lower mortality estimates. The most recent LQTS registry update reported annual sudden death risks of 0.9 percent in probands and 0.2 percent in affected relatives of probands.[66] Cardiac arrest (rather than syncope) may be the initial symptom in 6 to 22 percent of patients.[67, 68]

Numerous risk factors have been demonstrated using prospective registry data. These include congenital deafness, history of syncope, documented ventricular arrhythmias,[69] and QT_c duration.[66] Retrospective studies have also identified certain T wave morphologies,[70] QT dispersion,[71, 72] history of asthma,[73] and postpartum state,[74] as risk factors for syncope or sudden death. Males appear to be at greater risk until puberty, and females are at greater risk during adulthood.[75] The specific LQTS genotype has also been shown to influence the clinical course. Defects of I_{Kr} and I_{Ks} appear to confer significantly higher risk of cardiac events (syncope, aborted cardiac arrest, sudden death) than do sodium channel defects.[62] Although their overall clinical risk was lower, the patients with sodium channel mutations were more likely to have fatal events.

Updated clinical diagnostic criteria have been proposed by Schwartz and coworkers.[76] As shown in Table 90–3, these authors have proposed a point-based system for estimation of clinical risk. This system recognizes the marked variability in QT intervals and symptoms among LQTS patients. It is important to note that depending on the upper QT limit used, 20 to 40 percent of LQTS gene carriers will have normal or borderline QT intervals.[64] In the international registry, "unaffected" family members, with QTc less than 440 milliseconds, carried a 5 percent risk of syncope or cardiac arrest.[77] The diagnosis can now be more confidently made on the basis of genotyping studies, if a specific known channel disorder can be defined. As of this writing, routine clinical genotyping is not yet available, and this time-consuming procedure is being performed only in research protocols.

Once clinical genotyping becomes widely available, new clinical problems will have to be addressed. There are currently no methods for extrapolating clinical risk from knowledge of a specific mutation. It is possible that different forms of LQTS will vary in their response to β-blockade and other standard treatments. Now that LQTS patients are being split into subgroups, rather than lumped together, reanalysis of risk and treatment efficacy will be required based on genotype. Until better data are available, counseling of certain patient subgroups will remain fairly speculative. These groups will include asymptomatic genotype-proven LQTS patients with minimal QT prolongation and families with newly characterized mutations.

TABLE 90–3 1993 Diagnostic Criteria for Long QT Syndrome

Criteria	Points
ECG Findings	
QT_c >480 ms	3
460–470 ms	2
450 ms (male)	1
Documented torsades de pointes	2
T wave alternans	1
Notched T wave in three leads	1
Resting HR below second percentile for age (children only)	½
Clinical History	
Syncope	
With stress	2
Without stress	1
Congenital deafness	½
Family History	
Family members with definite LQTS (i.e., score > 4 points)	1
Unexplained sudden cardiac death below age 30 yr among immediate family	½
Scoring of Total Points	
<1 point	Low probability of LQTS
2–3 points	Intermediate probability of LQTS
>4 points	High probability of LQTS

Notes: The ECG must be obtained in the absence of medications or conditions known to affect these electrocardiographic measurements, such as hypokalemia. QT_c is calculated by Bazett's formula:

$$QT_c = \frac{QT}{\sqrt{RR}}$$

Abbreviations: ECG, electrocardiogram; HR, heart rate; LQTS, long QT syndrome.
From Schwartz PJ, Moss AJ, Vincent GM, et al: Diagnostic criteria for the long QT syndrome: an update. Circulation 88:782, 1993.

TREATMENT

Traditionally, treatment options for LQTS have included β-blocker therapy, left cardiac sympathetic denervation, and permanent pacing. The implantable cardioverter-defibrillator (ICD) has been reserved for patients with refractory arrhythmias. The advent of small, transvenous ICDs has lowered the threshold to prophylactic ICD implantation.

β-Blockade remains the most firmly established medical therapy for LQTS. There are no placebo-controlled studies demonstrating efficacy, but multivariate analysis of prospectively collected registry data suggested treatment benefits of both β-blockade and left cardiac sympathetic denervation.[69] The utility of β-blockade is also supported by acute studies of repolarization in LQTS patients. Intravenous β-agonists have been shown to lengthen QT intervals[24, 78] and induce EADs.[78] These effects were reversed by intravenous propranolol.

Permanent pacing has been proposed as a therapy, based on the observation that repolarization abnormalities and torsades de pointes are often bradycardia- or pause-dependent.[79] After early positive findings, Eldar and colleagues[80] paced 21 symptomatic LQTS patients treated with β-blockers, most of whom had had symptoms refractory to β-blockade and left cardiac sympathetic denervation. Using paced rates between 70 and 125 beats/min, these authors demonstrated significant reductions in symptoms and QT intervals. Over a 55-month follow-up period, 2 patients (10 percent) had recurrent syncope and 1 patient died suddenly after discontinuing β-blockers. In a study by Moss and associates,[81] 30 patients from the international LQTS registry received permanent pacemakers. Although QTc and cardiac event rates were significantly reduced after pacemaker implantation, 1 patient died suddenly and another suffered an aborted cardiac arrest.

The published pacing data are uncontrolled observational studies that do not allow conclusions to be drawn concerning absolute risk reduction. Since sudden death risk in LQTS appears to decrease with advancing age, this reduction may be a source of bias in any interventional study that monitors event rates. Furthermore, the published studies do not permit conclusions to be drawn about optimal programmed pacing modes and rates. Both single-chamber and dual-chamber pacemakers have been employed, with rates up to 125 beats/min. Although faster paced rates are more likely to eliminate torsades de pointes, tachycardia-induced cardiomyopathy may result.[82] Finally, ventricular pacing rates may be limited by the prolonged ventricular refractory periods seen in these patients.

Left cardiac sympathetic denervation has also been referred to as left stellectomy in various reports. As noted previously, this procedure evolved from animal models in which LQTS could be mimicked by imbalances of sympathetic cardiac innervation. In 1970, Moss and McDonald[10] first attempted left sympathetic denervation in a LQTS patient, based on the presumption that the underlying abnormality was a congenital imbalance of sympathetic cardiac innervation. Although LCSD did not shorten QT intervals in most patients, a subsequent series[7] demonstrated reductions in event rates after surgery in 84 LQTS registry patients with symptoms refractory to β-blocking medications. In this study, 5-year survival was 94 percent, with 7 sudden deaths reported during the follow-up period. The surgical techniques varied somewhat in this multicenter study, and these uncontrolled data are subject to the same bias mentioned in the discussion of pacing therapy.

The ICD may be an appropriate treatment option for high-risk, medically refractory patients. The threshold for implantation has dropped in recent years, owing to the development of nonthoracotomy lead systems and smaller pulse generators. In patients with frequent, self-terminating episodes of torsades de pointes, extension of the ICD's programmed detection times may reduce the risk of frequent recurrent shocks. Additionally, the painful stimulation of an ICD shock may result in adrenergic stimulation, precipitating repetitive runs of torsades de pointes and repetitive shocks.[8] Finally, the cumulative lifetime risks of lead fracture and device infection are higher in this young population. Since current generation ICDs are also capable of dual-chamber pacing, multimodal therapy is now available for LQTS using a single device.

With the discovery of the genetic and channel defects responsible for LQTS, new gene-based therapies are being investigated. These have been discussed more fully in the pathophysiology section of this chapter, and are briefly summarized in Table 90–1. At the time of this writing, clinical trials are under way, using potassium and mexiletine for patients with I_{Kr} and I_{Na} channel mutations, respectively.

Treatment of asymptomatic individuals with LQTS is controversial, owing to the lack of controlled treatment data. These patients are often diagnosed through family investigations or when electrocardiograms are obtained for other purposes. Although event rates are relatively low (~1 percent/yr), most authorities are currently offering β-blockade to such patients. The most compelling rationale for treatment is that in the absence of therapy, as many as 22 percent of these patients suffer sudden death as their initial clinical presentation.[19]

SUMMARY

Recent genetic findings in LQTS have accelerated the pace of research in this field. As a result, the *myocyte abnormality* hypothesis of LQTS has been confirmed; three human cardiac ion channels have been cloned, expressed, and studied; the mechanism of acquired LQTS has been explained; and the pathogenesis of torsades de pointes has been clarified. Early clinical work has raised the possibility of gene-specific therapies for the different channel defects.

This explosion of findings in a 3-year period is remarkable, considering that the disease was first described in the late 1950s and remained unexplained until now. The congenital LQTS is an excellent example of rapid translation of bench research to bedside understanding.

REFERENCES

1. Jervell A, Lange-Nielsen F: Congenital deaf mutism, functional heart disease with prolongation of the Q-T interval and sudden death. Am Heart J 54:59–68, 1957.
2. Romano C, Genrme G, Pongiglione R: Aritmie cardiache rare dell'eta pediatrica. II. Assessi sincopali per fibrillozione ventricolare parossistics. (Presentazione del primo case della letteratura pediatrica Italiana.) Clin Paediatr 45:656, 1963.
3. Ward O: Report to the Council for the Royal Academy of Medicine in Ireland, 1963.
4. Ward O: A new familial cardiac syndrome in children. J Ir Med Assoc 54:103, 1964.
5. Schwartz PJ, Locati E: The idiopathic long QT syndrome. Pathogenetic mechanisms and therapy. Eur Heart J 6(suppl D):103, 1985.
6. Eldar M, Griffin JC, VanHare GE, et al: Combined use of beta-adrenergic blocking agents and long-term cardiac pacing in patients with the long QT syndrome. J Am Coll Cardiol 20:830–837, 1992.
7. Schwartz PJ, Locati EH, Moss AJ, et al: Left cardiac sympathetic denervation in the therapy of congenital long QT syndrome: a worldwide report. Circulation 84:503–511, 1991.
8. Groh WJ, Silka MJ, Oliver RP, et al: Use of implantable cardioverter-defibrillators in the congenital long QT syndrome. Am J Cardiol 78:703–706, 1996.
9. James TN: QT prolongation and sudden death. Mod Concepts Cardiovasc Dis 38:35–38, 1969.
10. Moss AJ, McDonald J: Unilateral cervicothoracic ganglionectomy for the treatment of long QT interval syndrome. N Engl J Med 285:903–904, 1971.
11. Schwartz PJ: Idiopathic long QT syndrome: progress and questions. Am Heart J 109:399–411, 1985.
12. Yanowitz R, Preston JB, Abildskov JA: Functional distribution of right and left stellate innervation of the ventricles: production of neurogenic electrocardiographic changes by unilateral alternation of sympathetic tone. Circ Res 18:416, 1966.
13. Schwartz PJ, Periti M, Malliani A: The long QT syndrome. Am Heart J 89:378–390, 1975.
14. Schwartz PJ, Stone HL: Effects of unilateral stellectomy upon cardiac performance during exercise in dogs. Circ Res 44:637, 1979.
15. Wang Q, Shen J, Splawski I, et al: *SCN5A* mutations associated with an inherited cardiac arrhythmia, long QT syndrome. Cell 80:805–811, 1995.
16. Bennett PB, Yazawa K, Makita N, George AL Jr: Molecular mechanism for an inherited cardiac arrhythmia. Nature 376:683–685, 1995.
17. Dumaine R, Wang Q, Keating MT, et al: Multiple mechanisms of Na^+ channel–linked long-QT syndrome. Circ Res 78:916–924, 1996.
18. Hudson AJ, Ebers GD, Bulman DE: The skeletal muscle sodium and chloride channel diseases. Brain 118:547–563, 1995.
19. Priori SG, Napolitano C, Cantu F, et al: Differential response to Na^+ channel blockade, beta-adrenergic stimulation, and rapid pacing in a cellular model mimicking the *SCN5A* and *HERG* defects present in the long-QT syndrome. Circ Res 78:1009–1115, 1996.
20. Schwartz PJ, Priori SG, Locati EH, et al: Long QT syndrome patients with mutations of the *SCN5A* and *HERG* genes have differential responses to Na^+ channel blockade and to increases in heart rate. Implications for gene-specific therapy. Circulation 92:3381–3386, 1995.
21. Chen Q, Kirsch GE, Zhang D, et al: Genetic basis and molecular mechanism for idiopathic ventricular fibrillation. Nature 392:293–296, 1998.
22. Sanguinetti MC, Jurkiewicz NK: Delayed rectifier outward K^+ cur-

rent is composed of two currents in guinea pig atrial cells. Am J Physiol 260:H393–H399, 1991.
23. Kass RS: Delayed potassium channels in the heart: cellular, molecular, and regulatory properties. *In* Zipes DP, Jalife J (eds): Cardiac Electrophysiology: From Cell to Bedside. 2nd ed. pp. 74–82 Philadelphia: WB Saunders, 1995.
24. Compton SJ, Zhang L, Vincent GM, et al: Adrenergic Ca^{++} and K^{+} currents in patients with KVLQT1 mutations [abstract]. Circulation 98:I-776, 1998.
25. Timothy KW, Zhang L, Meyer KJ, Vincent GM: Differences in precipators of cardiac arrest and sudden death in chromosome 11 versus 7 genotype long QT syndrome patients [abstract]. Circulation 94:I-204, 1996.
26. Ali RH, Zareba W, Rosero SZ, et al: Adrenergic triggers and nonadrenergic factors associated with cardiac events in long QT syndrome patients [abstract]. Pacing Clin Electrophysiol 20:1072, 1997.
27. Schwartz PJ, Moss AJ, Priori SG, et al: Gene-specific influence on the triggers for cardiac arrest in the long QT syndrome [abstract]. Circulation 96:I-212, 1997.
28. Vincent GM, Fox J, Zhang L, Timothy KW: Beta-blockers markedly reduce risk and syncope in KVLQT1 long QT patients [abstract]. Circulation 94:I-204, 1995.
29. Sanguinetti MC, Curran ME, Zou A, et al: Coassembly of KvLQT1 and minK (IsK) proteins to form cardiac I_{Ks} potassium channel. Nature 384:80–83, 1996.
30. Barhanin J, Lesage F, Guillemare E, et al: KvLQT1 and IsK (minK) proteins associate to form the I_{Ks} cardiac potassium current. Nature 384:78–80, 1996.
31. Splawski I, Tristani-Firouzi M, Lehmann MH, et al: Mutations in the hminK gene cause long QT syndrome and suppress I_{Ks} function. Nat Genet 17:338–340, 1997.
32. McDonald TV, Yu Z, Ming Z, et al: A minK-HERG complex regulates the cardiac potassium current I_{Kr}. Nature 388:289–292, 1997.
33. Abbott GW, Sesti F, Splawski I, et al: MiRP1 forms I_{Kr} potassium channels with HERG and is associated with cardiac arrhythmia. Cell 97:175–187, 1999.
34. Shimizu W, Kurita T, Matsuo K, et al: Improvement of repolarization abnormalities by a K^{+} channel opener in the LQT1 form of congenital long-QT syndrome. Circulation 97:1581–1588, 1988.
35. Sato T, Hata Y, Yamamoto M, et al: Early afterdepolarization abolished by potassium channel opener in a patient with idiopathic long QT syndrome. J Cardiovasc Electrophysiol 6:279–282, 1995.
36. Sanguinetti MC, Jiang C, Curran ME, Keating MT: A mechanistic link between an inherited and an acquired cardiac arrhythmia: HERG encodes the I_{Kr} potassium channel. Cell 81:299–307, 1995.
37. Compton SJ, Lux RL, Ramsey MR, et al: Genetically defined therapy of inherited long-QT syndrome: correction of abnormal repolarization by potassium. Circulation 94:1018–1022, 1996.
38. Compton SJ: Genetically defined therapy of inherited long QT syndrome [letter]. Circulation 95:1675–1676, 1997.
39. Vincent GM, Jaiswal D, Timothy KW: Effects of exercise on heart rate, QT, QTc, and QT/QS2 in the Romano-Ward inherited long QT syndrome. Am J Cardiol 68:498–503, 1991.
40. Sanguinetti MC, Jurkiewicz NK: Role of external Ca^{2+} and K^{+} in gating of cardiac delayed rectifier K^{+} currents. Pflugers Arch 420:180–186, 1992.
41. Choy AM, Lang CC, Chomsky DM, et al: Normalization of acquired QT prolongation in humans by intravenous potassium. Circulation 96:2149–2154, 1997.
42. Bauman JL, Bauman JL, Bauernfeind RA, et al: Torsades de pointes due to quinidine: observation in 31 patients. Am Heart J 107:425–430, 1984.
43. Yang T, Roden DM: Extracellular potassium modulation of drug block I_{Kr}: implications for torsades de pointes and reverse use-dependence. Circulation 93:407–411, 1996.
44. Woosley RL, Chen Y, Freiman JP, Gillis RA: Mechanism of the cardiotoxic actions of terfenadine. JAMA 269:1532–1536, 1993.
45. Roy M, Dumaine R, Brown AM: HERG, a primary human ventricular target of the nonsedating antihistamine terfenadine. Circulation 94:817–823, 1996.
46. Vorperian VR, Zhou Z, Mohammad S, et al: Torsades de pointes with an antihistamine metabolite: potassium channel blockade with desmethylastemizole. J Am Coll Cardiol 28:1556–1561, 1996.
47. Donger C, Denjoy I, Berthet M, et al: KVLQT1 C-terminal missense mutation causes a forme fruste long-QT syndrome. Circulation 96:2778–2781, 1997.
48. Splawski I, Timothy KW, Vincent GM, et al: Molecular basis of the long-QT syndrome associated with deafness. N Engl J Med 336:1562–1567, 1997.
49. Neyroud N, Tesson F, Denjoy I, et al: A novel mutation in the potassium channel gene KVLQT1 causes the Jervell and Lange-Nielsen cardioauditory syndrome. Nat Genet 15:186–189, 1997.
50. Schulze-Bahr E, Wang Q, Wedekind H, et al: KCNE1 mutations cause Jervell and Lange-Nielsen syndrome. Nat Genet 17:267–268, 1997.
51. Dessertenne F: La tachycardie ventriculaire a deux foyers opposes variables. Arch Mal Coeur 59:263–272, 1966.
52. Abildskov JA, Lux RI: Mechanisms in adrenergic dependent onset of torsades de pointes. Pacing Clin Electrophysiol 20:88–94, 1997.
53. Hii JT, Wyse DG, Gillis AM, et al: Precordial QT interval dispersion as a marker of torsades de pointes. Disparate effects of class Ia antiarrhythmic drugs and amiodarone. Circulation 86:1376–1382, 1992.
54. Volders PG, Sipido KR, Vos MA, et al: Cellular basis of biventricular hypertrophy and arrhythmogenesis in dogs with chronic complete atrioventricular block and acquired torsades de pointes. Circulation 98:1136–1147, 1998.
55. Verduyn SC, Vos MA, van der Zande J, et al: Further observations to elucidate the role of interventricular dispersion of repolarization and early afterdepolarizations in the genesis of acquired torsades de pointes arrhythmias: a comparison between almokalant and D-sotalol using the dog as its own control. J Am Coll Cardiol 30:1575–1584, 1997.
56. El-Sherif N, Caref EB, Yin H, Restivo M: The electrophysiological mechanism of ventricular arrhythmias in the long QT syndrome. Tridimensional mapping of activation and recovery patterns. Circ Res 79:474–492, 1996.
57. El-Sherif N, Chinushi M, Caref EB, Restivo M: Electrophysiological mechanism of the characteristic electrocardiographic morphology of torsades de pointes tachyarrhythmias in the long-QT syndrome: detailed analysis of ventricular tridimensional activation patterns. Circulation 96:4392–4399, 1997.
58. Asano Y, Davidenko JM, Baxter WT, et al: Optical mapping of drug-induced polymorphic arrhythmias and torsades de pointes in the isolated rabbit heart. J Am Coll Cardiol 29:831–842, 1997.
59. Habbal MH, Wait TD, Mahony CO: QTc in congenital sensory-neural hearing loss [abstract]. Circulation 98:I-777, 1998.
60. Marks ML, Trippel DL, Keating MT: Long QT syndrome associated with syndactyly identified in females. Am J Cardiol 25:59–64, 1995.
61. Schwartz PJ, Stramba-Badiale M, Segantini A, et al: Prolongation of the QT interval and the sudden infant death syndrome. N Engl J Med 338:1709–1714, 1998.
62. Zareba W, Moss AJ, Schwartz PJ, et al: Influence of genotype on the clinical course of the long-QT syndrome. N Engl J Med 339:960–965, 1998.
63. Vincent GM: Heterogeneity in the inherited long QT syndrome. J Cardiovasc Electrophysiol 6:137–146, 1995.
64. Vincent GM, Timothy KW, Leppert M, Keating M: The spectrum of symptoms and QT intervals in carriers of the gene for the long QT syndrome. N Engl J Med 327:846–852, 1992.
65. Ackerman MJ: The long QT syndrome: ion channel diseases of the heart. Mayo Clin Proc 73:250–269, 1998.
66. Moss AJ, Schwartz PJ, Crampton RS, et al: The long QT syndrome: prospective longitudinal study of 328 families. Circulation 84:1136–1144, 1991.
67. Garson AJ Jr, Dick MI II, Fournier A, et al: The long QT syndrome in children: an international study of 287 patients. Circulation 87:1855–1872, 1993.
68. Priori SG, Maugeri FS, Napolitano C, et al: The risk of sudden death as first cardiac event in asymptomatic patients with the long QT syndrome [abstract]. Circulation 98:I-777, 1998.
69. Moss AJ, Schwartz PJ, Crampton RS, et al: The long QT syndrome: a prospective international study. Circulation 71:17–21, 1985.
70. Malfatto G, Beria G, Sala S, et al: Quantitative analysis of T wave abnormalities and their prognostic implications in the idiopathic long QT syndrome. J Am Coll Cardiol 23:296–301, 1994.
71. Day CP, McComb JM, Campbell RWF: QT dispersion: an indication of arrhythmia risk in patients with long QT intervals. Br Heart J 63:342–344, 1990.
72. Priori SG, Napolitano C, Dieh L, Schwartz PJ: Dispersion of the QT interval: a marker of therapeutic efficacy in the idiopathic long QT syndrome. Circulation 89:1681–1689, 1994.

73. Rosero SZ, Zareba W, Ali RHH, et al: Asthma in the long QT syndrome: a modifier of cardiac morbidity [abstract]. 96:I-212, 1997.
74. Rashba EJ, Zareba W, Moss AJ, et al: Influence of pregnancy on the risk for cardiac events in patients with hereditary long QT syndrome. LQTS Investigators. Circulation 97:451–456, 1998.
75. Locati EH, Zareba W, Moss AJ, et al: Age- and sex-related differences in clinical manifestations in patients with congenital long-QT syndrome. Circulation 97:2237–2244, 1998.
76. Schwartz PJ, Moss AJ, Vincent GM, et al: Diagnostic criteria for the long QT syndrome: an update. Circulation 88:782, 1993.
77. Schwartz PJ, Locati EH, Napolitano C, Priori SG: The long QT syndrome. *In* Zipes DP, Jalife J (eds): Cardiac Electrophysiology: From Cell to Bedside. 2nd ed. pp. 788–811 Philadelphia: WB Saunders, 1995.
78. Shimizu W, Ohe T, Kurita T, et al: Effects of verapamil and propranolol on early after depolarizations and ventricular arrhythmias induced by epinephrine in congenital long QT syndrome. J Am Coll Cardiol 26:1299–1309, 1994.
79. Jackman WM, Friday KJ, Anderson JL, et al: The long QT syndromes: a critical review, new clinical observations and a unifying hypothesis. Prog Cardiov Dis 31:115–172, 1988.
80. Eldar M, Griffin JC, Abbott JA, et al: Permanent cardiac pacing in patients with the long QT syndrome. J Am Coll Cardiol 10:600–607, 1987.
81. Moss AJ, Lieu JE, Gottlieb S, et al: Efficacy of permanent pacing in the management of high-risk patients with long QT syndrome. Circulation 84:1524–1529, 1991.
82. Klein HO, Levi A, Kaplinsky E, et al: Congenital long QT syndrome: deleterious effect of long-term high-rate ventricular pacing and definitive treatment by cardiac transplantation. Am Heart J 132:1079–1081, 1996.

CHAPTER 91

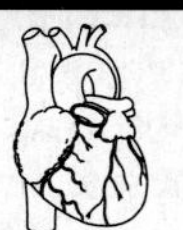

Arrhythmogenic Right Ventricular Dysplasia

G. Fontaine, F. Fontaliran, J. L. Hebert, D. Chemla, O. Zenati, Y. LeCarpentier, and R. Frank

SYMPTOMS
Palpitations
Dyspnea and Asthenia
Chest Pain
ELECTROCARDIOGRAM DURING VENTRICULAR ARRHYTHMIAS
ELECTROCARDIOGRAM IN SINUS RHYTHM
Repolarization and Depolarization Abnormalities
Epsilon Waves
SIGNAL-AVERAGING TECHNIQUE
M-MODE AND TWO-DIMENSIONAL ECHOCARDIOGRAPHY
CONTRAST ECHOCARDIOGRAPHY
TRANSESOPHAGEAL AND THREE-DIMENSIONAL ECHOCARDIOGRAPHY
CHEST X-RAYS
NUCLEAR ANGIOGRAPHY
NUCLEAR MAGNETIC RESONANCE
CONTRAST ANGIOGRAPHY
Right Ventricular Angiography
Left Ventricular Abnormalities in ARVD
Normal Coronary Arteries
ENDOMYOCARDIAL BIOPSY
ELECTROPHYSIOLOGIC STUDY
ANATOMY AND PATHOLOGY OF ARVD
Gross Pathology
Basic Histology
Histologic Basis of Ventricular Arrhythmias (New Concepts)
ARVD AND SUDDEN DEATH IN YOUNG ADULTS
FAMILIAL OCCURRENCE OF ARVD
PATHOGENESIS
CLINICAL FORMS
Dysplasia With Major Left Ventricular Involvement
Right Precordial ST-Segment Elevation
Right Ventricular Outflow Tract Tachycardia
Uhl's Anomaly
ANTIARRHYTHMIC DRUG TREATMENT
IMPLANTABLE DEFIBRILLATOR
RADIOFREQUENCY AND REDUCED ENERGY DIRECT-CURRENT ABLATION
HEART TRANSPLANTATION
RISK STRATIFICATION
CONCLUSIONS

Arrhythmogenic right ventricular dysplasia (ARVD) is an underdiagnosed clinical entity characterized by ventricular arrhythmias originating in the right ventricle and a specific pathology. This pathology mostly consists of massive replacement of right ventricular (RV) myocardium by fat occupied by surviving strands of cardiomyocytes bordered by or embedded in, fibrosis.[1] The term arrythmogenic right ventricular dysplasia was proposed in 1977 to describe sustained ventricular tachycardia (VT) in patients who did not have overt heart disease and were resistant to antiarrhythmic medications. The term *arrhythmogenic right ventricular cardiomyopathy,* introduced by the World Health Organization in 1996, encompasses a wide spectrum of diseases that have in common VTs of RV origin and have the similar basic histologic structure, but different presentations and outcome (Table 91–1).[2]

Symptoms

Palpitations

Palpitations are the most common symptom and might be related to ventricular arrhythmias ranging from symptomatic extrasystoles to sustained poorly tolerated VT showing a left bundle branch block pattern. Rapid VT or ventricular fibrillation observed in patients who present with

TABLE 91–1 Classification of Arrhythmogenic Right Ventricular Cardiomyopathies

Arrhythmogenic right ventricular dysplasia (ARVD):
  Typical form of description
  Primitive form of ARVD
  Occult form of ARVD
Clinical forms of ARVD with major left ventricular involvement
  Pure biventricular dysplasia
  Dysplasia complicated by myocarditis
    Superacute
    Acute-subacute
    Chronic
    Chronic active (autoimmune)
Naxos disease
Venetian cardiomyopathy
Noncoronary ST-segment elevation*
Right ventricular outflow tract tachycardia*
Mitral valve prolapse*
Benign extrasystoles
Uhl's anomaly

*Only a limited number of these cases suggests ARVD.
Data from Fontaine G, Fontaliran F, Frank R: Arrhythmogenic right ventricular cardiomyopathies: clinical forms and main differential diagnoses [editorial]. Circulation 65:384–399, 1982.

syncopal episodes may occur during competitive sports and strenuous exercise. However, sudden death has been also observed at rest or even during sleep. Sudden death could be the first presenting symptom of the disease. This situation may be observed in young individuals, mostly male, with no evidence of heart disease at physical examination. However, supraventricular arrhythmias, including atrial extrasystoles, flutter, or fibrillation, may also be the initial marker of the disease.[3] Therefore, palpitation is not necessarily the marker of ventricular arrhythmias.

Dyspnea and Asthenia

Because of minor involvement of the left ventricle, left ventricular (LV) failure is not present, and VT may be relatively well tolerated. However, in some cases, RV failure could be the result of progression of the original dysplastic phenomenon in this ventricle. In the complicated forms resulting from a superimposed myocarditis or in cases of biventricular dysplasia, symptoms suggesting progression toward congestive heart failure may be observed. This situation accounts for an additional mortality of 1 percent per year.[4]

Chest Pain

Chest pain is a new marker of the disease that was previously overlooked because of the rarity of atheromatous coronary artery disease studied by contrast angiography. However, identification of the increased thickness of the media in distal coronary arteries suggested that the mechanism of atypical chest pain may be the result of a small-vessel disease.[5]

Electrocardiogram During Ventricular Arrhythmias

The electrocardiogram (ECG) during ventricular arrhythmias shows a left bundle branch block pattern consistent with delayed activation of the LV chamber. The QRS axis is normal or shifted to the right when the arrhythmia originates in the pulmonary infundibulum; it may show extreme left-axis deviation when arising from the diaphragmatic wall or the apex of the right ventricle.[1] These two areas of origin of VT may be present in the same patient.

Electrocardiogram in Sinus Rhythm

Repolarization and Depolarization Abnormalities

Repolarization abnormalities in terms of T-wave inversion in leads beyond V_1 are generally the first sign that attracts attention. It is observed in roughly half of the cases. Extension of T-wave inversion in left precordial leads has a positive correlation with RV end-diastolic index.[6, 7]

Variable degrees of delayed RV activation from complete (15 percent) or, more frequently, incomplete right bundle branch block pattern (18 percent) with low voltage of the rapid-phase potentials may also be observed. Correlation of surface ECGs and epicardial mapping have suggested that these patterns may be due to a parietal block without distinct alteration of conduction in the bundle branches.[8]

Selective prolongation of the QRS complex duration in lead V_1, V_2, or V_3 of more than 25 milliseconds above the QRS duration in lead V_6 in the presence of right bundle branch block is another diagnostic marker of the disease[9] (Figs. 91–1 and 91–2). However, involvement of the conduction system by apoptotic phenomena[10] or myocarditis has also been described in the complicated forms of ARVD.[11]

Increased QT dispersion on the 12-lead ECG and changes in ST-segment elevation in the precordial leads over the right ventricle may identify the patient at risk[12] (see Fig. 91–2).

Epsilon Waves

In 30 percent of cases, more specific changes, such as ventricular postexcitation waves, may be recorded.[13] These are potentials of small amplitude that are termed *epsilon waves* (see Fig. 91–1). They occur after the QRS complex at the beginning of the ST segment.[14] They reflect the presence of delayed activation of some RV muscle on the surface ECG. The recording of epsilon waves may also be enhanced by increasing the sensitivity of the recording two or three times.

The vertical bipolar lead FI, which has the same orientation as VF, seems to be the most sensitive to record epsilon waves. It also magnifies atrial potentials and may be useful in documenting atrioventricular dissociation during VT as well as in studying atrial rhythms when the P wave is of too small amplitude in other leads.[15]

In many instances, the shape of epsilon waves is different from the usual pattern of small potentials at the beginning of the ST segment. When a smaller number of myocardial fibers is activated after the end of the QRS complex, the epsilon wave may look like a smooth potential forming an atypical prolonged R′ wave in leads V_1 through V_3. Therefore, any potential in V_1 through V_3 that is more than 25 milliseconds longer than the QRS duration in lead V_6 should be considered an epsilon wave representing the late excitation of some myocardial fibers (see Fig. 91–2). These postexcitation waves are the surface counterpart of "delayed" or "late" potentials detected during endocardial or epicardial mapping or with signal-averaged ECG.[14]

Signal-Averaging Technique

This is another technique to increase the gain without the distortion induced by the exceedingly large noise produced by muscle potentials. These postexcitation waves are frequently observed in patients with documented episodes of VT.[16, 17] Using a band pass of 25 Hz instead of 40 Hz increases the sensitivity of this technique in patients with

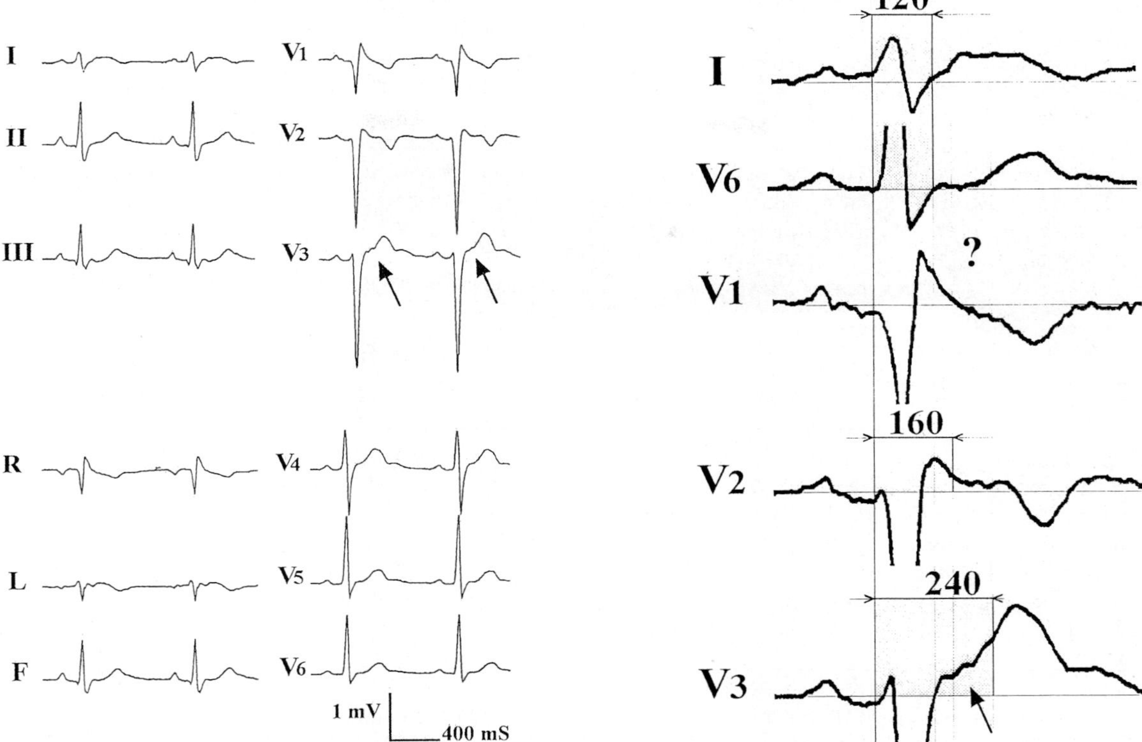

FIGURE 91–1 Right bundle branch block pattern, with a QRS complex duration in lead V_1, V_2, or V_3 larger than that in V_6. Epsilon waves are indicated by arrows. QRS complex duration is difficult to analyze in lead V_1.

ARVD.[18] The use of frequency domain in addition to time domain also increases the sensitivity of ARVD detection.[19]

M-Mode and Two-Dimensional Echocardiography

Echocardiographic studies may show localized abnormalities or dilation of the right heart cavities, especially of the right ventricle with an increased RV/LV ratio.[20, 21] However, in patients with minimal abnormalities, the echocardiogram may be normal.

The structural abnormalities of most cases of ARVD are moderate, and therefore, they may be overlooked when a routine study is performed. ARVD is recognized only if it is looked for systematically, especially by making measurements of diameters at several strategic points of the right ventricle. The echocardiographic signs of the disease are (1) dilatation of the right ventricle, (2) presence of aneurysms during diastole, and (3) dyskinetic areas in the inferobasal region (these are especially specific when they are observed below the tricuspid valve).

It is also possible to find hypertrophy of the moderator band and/or isolated dilatation of the outflow tract. The apical region has to be carefully evaluated for dyskinesia as well as hypertrophied trabeculations.

In addition to the standard echographic examination, we believe that right parasternal views with the patient lying in the right lateral position should be obtained routinely when ARVD is suspected.

With the subcostal approach, it is possible to see the free wall of the right ventricle both in the two-dimensional mode and also on time motion. By rotating the probe 90 degrees, it is possible to visualize the long axis of the right ventricle, which is useful for studying the infundibulum and the pulmonary artery.

Attention has to be paid to evaluate the presence of tricuspid valve prolapse and regurgitation in the severe forms of the disease as well as to look for mitral valve prolapse, which has been recognized as being associated with ARVD.[22]

Contrast Echocardiography

Contrast echocardiography using injections of saline may help to evaluate RV, regional, or global function.[23] Contrast echocardiography may better outline the right ventricle to permit measurement of RV volume analysis, as proposed by Levine and colleagues.[24]

Transesophageal and Three-Dimensional Echocardiography

Transesophageal echocardiography may be more sensitive than a transthoracic approach in detecting wall motion abnormalities.[25, 26] Three-dimensional echocardiography,

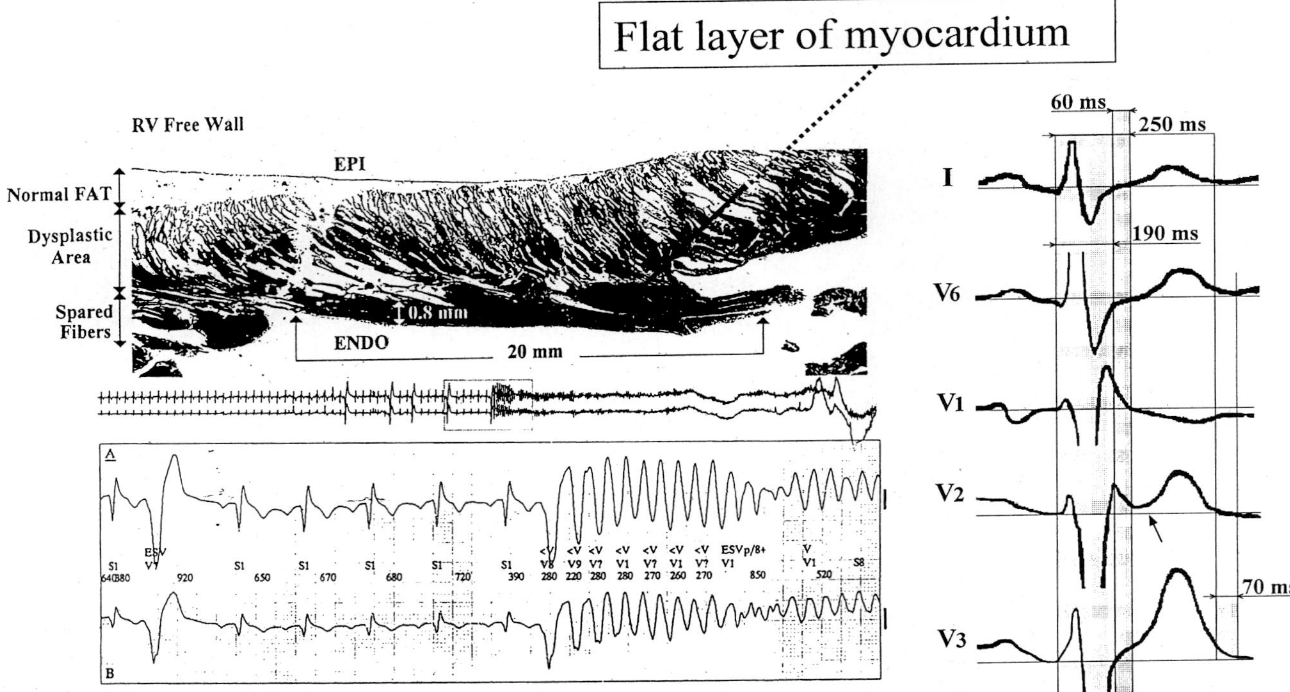

FIGURE 91–2 Upper left, Panoramic view of the right ventricular (RV) free wall showing that most of the myocardium is replaced by fat, which is dissociating surviving myocardium. There is, however, a compact layer of myocardium remaining in the subendocardial area. This structure may explain the mechanism of reentrant tachycardia, drifting on this part of myocardium. **Lower left,** Mechanism of torsades de pointes–like ventricular tachycardia recorded on Holter monitor in the same patient who died suddenly at night. The low-speed recording located in the middle shows presence of isolated extrasystoles leading to the arrhythmia. The electrocardiogram (ECG) recorded a few days before death shows a QRS complex duration of 60 msec larger in leads V_1 and V_2 than in V_6 (parietal block, also called *more than complete right bundle branch block*). Note also the presence of a saddle-back ST-segment elevation in lead V_2 and dispersion of repolarization of 70 msec between V_3 and V_6 as compared with lead I. EPI, epicardium; ENDO, endocardium. (Modified from Fontaine G, Aouate P, Fontaliran F: Dysplasie ventriculaire droite arhythmogene, torsades de pointes et mort subite: nouveaux concepts. Ann Cardiol Angeiol 46:531–538, 1997; Fontaine G, Aouate P, Fontaliran F: Repolarization and the genesis of cardiac arrhythmias: role of body surface mapping [editorial]. Circulation 12:2600–2602, 1997. By permission of the American Heart Association, Inc.)

particularly combined with the transesophageal approach, is being investigated to enhance the diagnostic accuracy of this technique.[27, 28]

Chest X-Rays

Chest x-rays may show a moderate cardiac enlargement with a convexity between the aortic knob and the left ventricle without pulmonary vascular redistribution. The cardiothoracic index is less than 0.6 in most cases. However, a wide spectrum from a completely normal cardiac silhouette to a definitely enlarged heart may be observed.[29, 30] In the young athletic adult, this relative cardiomegaly may be wrongly attributed to training only.

Nuclear Angiography

This examination provides data concerning the size and the function of the ventricles, their contraction pattern, and possibly the site of origin of VT. It is also an elegant form of studying both left and right ejection fractions.[31, 32] Specific isotopic markers have demonstrated the abnormality of regional sympathetic dysinnervation.[33, 34]

Nuclear Magnetic Resonance

This new and promising technique can be used to analyze the dimensions and the dynamic behavior of the cardiac chambers, as well as to identify abnormal amount of distribution of adipose tissue within ventricular myocardium[35–41] (Fig. 91–3).

Magnetic resonance imaging can be an effective noninvasive examination to detect patients with *fatty* infiltration of the myocardium. However, because fat is a normal component of the right ventricle in human, it is necessary to incorporate all these dynamic and morphologic parameters to increase both the sensitivity and the specificity of this examination.[42]

Contrast Angiography

Right Ventricular Angiography

RV cineangiography remains the gold standard for the diagnosis of ARVD (Fig. 91–4). The broad spectrum of angiographic patterns is based on the presence of segmental

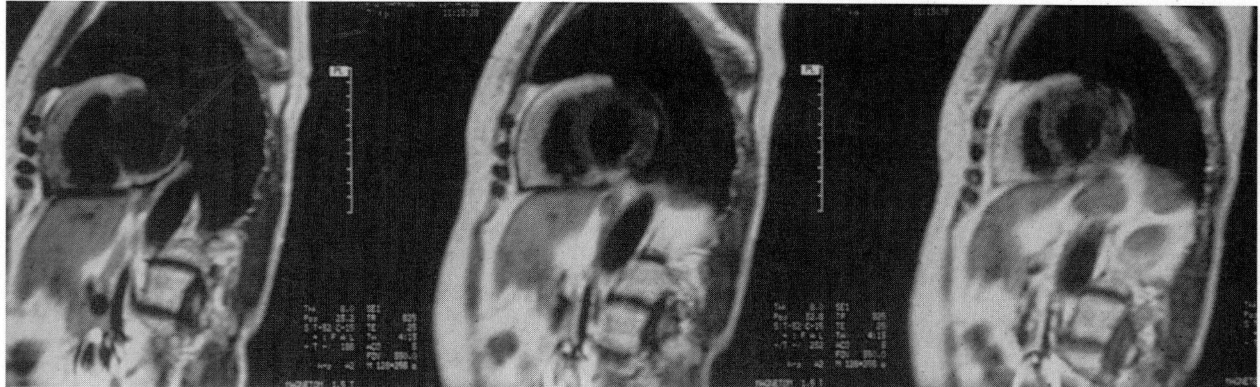

FIGURE 91–3 Magnetic resonance imaging of an asymptomatic 68-year-old woman who had dilatation of the right ventricle detected by systematic two-dimensional echocardiography. Inhomogeneous right ventricular free wall, which is almost totally replaced by fat. (Courtesy of Pr Kunze, Germany.)

morphologic abnormalities and wall motion abnormalities. Localized lesions should be sought specifically in three RV regions: the pulmonary infundibulum, the anterior RV free wall (including the apex), and the inferior wall (including the subtricuspid area). These regions are named the *triangle of dysplasia.*[1]

Several abnormalities can be observed in the right anterior oblique projection, including (1) infundibular aneurysm; (2) hypertrophic trabeculae thicker than 4 mm, the so-called deep fissures; (3) areas of negative contrast in the trabecular zone and/or the moderator band; (4) fissures and/or bulgings at the apex or inferior area; (5) multiple outpouchings in the inferior wall; (6) diastolic bulging of the subtricuspid area; and (7) tricuspid valve prolapse, usually associated with mild tricuspid insufficiency.[43] The RV free wall is usually normal and the septum is vertical in the left anterior oblique projection. Patients who have diffuse RV myocardial involvement due to ARVD may have global dilatation[44, 45] with reduced contractility.

Slow evacuation of dye in an otherwise normal heart by physical examination is an excellent sign that can be observed along the inferior wall, in fissures and aneurysms, and in poor contractile areas, where the contrast medium may stagnate for more than 20 beats.[45–47]

Left Ventricular Abnormalities in ARVD

Usually, the LV end-diastolic volume is normal, and the LV ejection fraction is either preserved or moderately decreased.[43, 46] However, segmental LV contraction abnormalities, increased LV volumes, and reduced LV ejection fraction have been reported in 20 to 50 percent of ARVD patients.[29, 43, 45, 46, 48] LV dysfunction can also be primarily due to pathologic abnormalities of the left ventricle. Contrary to fibrofatty changes of the right ventricle, LV lesions are predominantly fibrotic. LV volumes are generally increased in these patients, LV ejection fraction is reduced, and LV hemodynamic function progressively deteriorates. In the right anterior oblique projection, akinetic areas may be observed on the upper anterolateral wall, on the mid-inferior wall, or on the apex of the LV.[46, 49]

Normal Coronary Arteries

An increased right atrial *a* wave has been reported, together with normal RV and pulmonary artery systolic pressures.[1, 50] This suggests a prominent contribution of right atrial contraction to RV filling. Interestingly, LV end-diastolic pressure is preserved in ARVD patients with depressed LV systolic function.[49, 51] This could explain the absence of pulmonary artery hypertension in ARVD.

Endomyocardial Biopsy

The confirmation of the diagnosis of ARVD by endocardial biopsy lacks sensitivity because the typical pathologic changes are not consistently seen in the septum, the usual site of biopsy. The RV free wall does not usually undergo biopsy because of possible myocardial perforation. Only the disposable King's College bioptome (manufactured by Cordis Corp) should be used. On a practical basis, however, myocardial biopsy cannot be routinely recommended to confirm the diagnosis of ARVD.[52]

Electrophysiologic Study

Electrophysiologic investigations should be carried out to detect late potentials, which are tiny waves occurring after the QRS complex in addition to the normal synchronous potential. Their dynamic behavior exhibits time-dependent properties that could be significant for intramyocardial reentrant phenomena.[53] In addition, it is sometimes possible to observe a delay of more than 80 milliseconds between stimuli and ventricular activation that also may show time-dependent properties.[53]

An elevated pacing threshold is frequently seen in the abnormal area.[54] Programmed stimulation or bursts of rapid ventricular stimulation usually induce and terminate VT.[1, 14, 55, 56] In some cases, however, it can be difficult to induce VT, and many attempts may be necessary to induce the first attack. Pacing should be carried out in several places of the right ventricle using different basic cycle lengths, introducing several extra stimuli, and even burst pacing or

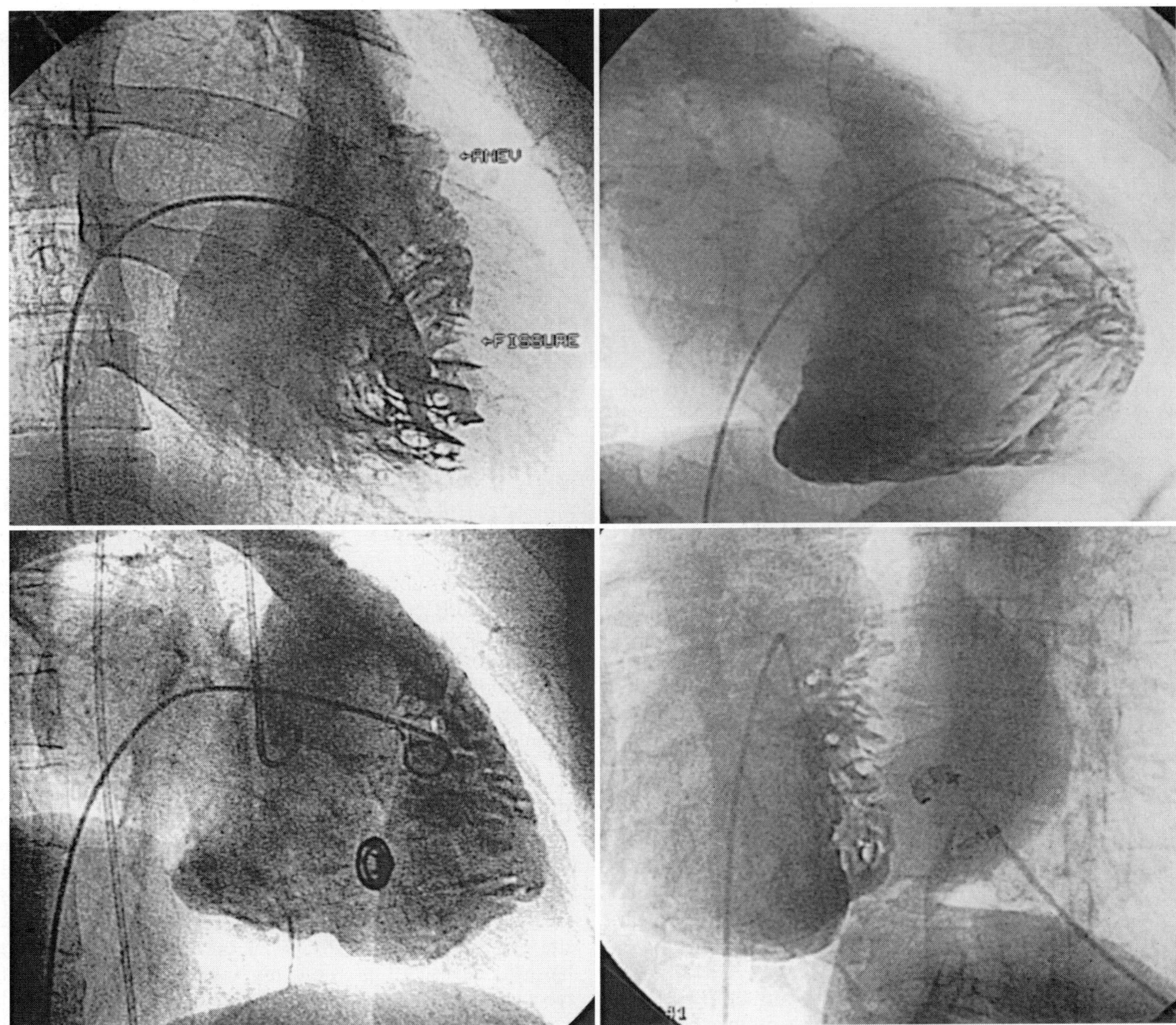

FIGURE 91–4 Upper left, Male, 27 years old (right anterior oblique [RAO] 45-degree projection). Typical aspect of limited ARVD: presence of a small aneurysm (ANEV) at the upper anterior junction of true infundibulum with trabecular zone. Deep fissuring (FISSURE) and polycyclic images of the anteroapical zone. **Lower left,** Female, 48 years old (RAO 45-degree projection). More diffuse form including deep fissuring of the anteroapical zone and large inferoapical bulging. **Upper right,** Male, 56 years old (RAO 45-degree projection). Right ventricular global dilation. Diffuse fissuring of the anterior wall and typical diastolic bulging of the subtricuspid zone with late stagnation. **Lower right,** Male, 56 years old (left anterior oblique 45-degree projection). Right ventricular transversal dilation. Major disarrangement of the trabecular zone with polycyclic images and clifflike right ventricular septal zone.

a more premature stimulus at the end of the burst. In contrast, when the initial episode of VT has been induced, reinitiation is easier. These maneuvers may induce spontaneous or undocumented episodes of VT. The axis of VT is generally consistent with the area involved. Isoproterenol infusion may be used during electrophysiologic study to increase its sensitivity. Finally, programmed stimulation may be used to evaluate the induction of supraventricular tachycardia.[57]

Endocardial mapping in sinus rhythm may demonstrate fragmented and/or delayed activation of the right ventricular free wall that is globally consistent with parietal block seen on the surface ECG. Epicardial mapping during surgery has demonstrated the bunching of the isochrones that is always observed over the dysplastic areas. The amplitude of RV endocardial as well as epicardial potentials is generally markedly reduced. They could be part of the substrate for the development of reentry phenomena, provided that delayed activity could reactivate adjacent normal myocardium. Epicardial maps show delayed activation of the right ventricle, even if the activation of the free wall is within the normal range, suggesting in these particular cases a preserved conduction system.[8]

Anatomy and Pathology of ARVD

ARVD has been probably overlooked as a cause of sudden unexpected death in the population at large. In a study reporting systematic autopsy examination in such cases, a prevalence of 5 percent was observed in patients younger than 65 years.[58]

Gross Pathology

Gross pathology confirms dilatation of the right ventricle, covered by fat. After the RV free wall is cut through, the thinness of the remaining endocardial layer is striking. This explains why it can be transilluminated. In most cases, endocardium appears to be normal, but in some cases, plaques of thick fibrosis have been observed. This may be due to the organization of a mural thrombus, as suggested by histologic and some echocardiographic studies.[59–62]

Basic Histology

The typical histologic pattern of ARVD consists of the presence of an exceedingly large amount of fat and fibrosis occupying the RV myocardium and, to a much lesser extent, the left myocardium (Fig. 91–5). Fibrosis bordering or embedding strands or sheets of cardiomyocytes may provide a basis for slow conduction (delayed potentials) and reentry.[63]

Histologic Basis of Ventricular Arrhythmias (New Concepts)

Vortex-Like Reentrant Mechanism, Torsades de pointes, and Sudden Death at Rest

The histologic structure of ARVD suggests that the onset of the arrhythmia may be due to a vortex-like reentrant mechanism drifting in the right ventricle.[64] If the subepicardial and midzonal layers are modified and/or destroyed by a pathologic process, the thickness of remaining tissue creates a bidimensional structure that could support spirals drifting on the sheet of remaining endocardial layers (see Fig. 91–2). It is probable that ventricular fibrillation is induced when the adjacent three-dimensional structure of myocardium is attained.

Activation of Neutrophils and Early After-Depolarization

We have previously stressed the role played by myocarditis in the histology of ARVD (see Fig. 91–5). One report has suggested the possible role of neutrophil activation in arrhythmogenesis. This is due to the platelet aggregating factor, which becomes operative by the creation of early after-depolarization.[65] This new concept may explain the genesis of arrhythmias in ARVD not only as a unique parameter involved in arrhythmogenesis but also as a potential trigger of sustained reentrant arrhythmias in a latent arrhythmogenic substrate.

ARVD and Sudden Death in Young Adults

ARVD has been recognized as a rare but important cause of sudden death in competitive athletes. In our own series, we know four patients who died suddenly. In two, sudden death was observed during sports or major exercise. In two cases, syncope or near-syncope was present before death. In a systematic study of the risk of sudden death in competitive athletes in which a series of 1642 Italian competitive athletes were screened, 136 of whom were of champion levels, 60 percent of sudden deaths were related to ARVD, and the same proportion was observed in champion level as compared with common athletes. In patients who experienced cardiac arrest or sudden death in Italian athletes, one fourth were due to ARVD.[66] However, this result is different from the reports published in the United States.[67]

Familial Occurrence of ARVD

Familial forms of RV dysplasia as well as arrhythmogenic RV dysplasia have been reported.[1, 68–74] Penetrance of the disease based on the identification of clinical signs in family members is 15 to 25 percent.[75] This figure will probably increase if sophisticated techniques of identification are performed that lead to the identification of form fruste.[76] Risk stratification of these healthy carriers is difficult to assess.

Pathogenesis

ARVD appears to be the result of an abnormality in myocardial development. This reasoning is based on the fact that ARVD has been observed in members of the same family (siblings or father), suggesting some genetic factor.[1, 73] A 27-week-old fetus that was arrhythmogenic in utero was brought to our attention after routine echography, it demonstrated bulging of the lateral RV free wall. Spontaneous abortion led to the demonstration of histologic picture compatible with ARVD without signs of inflammation or fibrosis.[2]

Therefore, the genetically determined abnormality becomes apparent with time, with an increasing number of myocardial fibers replaced by fatty tissue. This occurs mainly in the medial and/or subepicardial layers. When this process is advanced, only the subendocardial layers demonstrate normal myocardial tissue, and the remaining part of the wall consists of fatty tissue[29] (see Fig. 91–5). Dysplasia is also believed to be complicated by an acquired myocardial damage produced by an inflammatory or infectious process superimposed on the genetic background of RVD (see Fig. 91–5). It could explain why arrhythmogenicity is not frequently observed in the pediatric age group.[77–80]

The abnormality of development observed early in life, possibly even in the embryo, is the possible result of an anomaly in the genetic program of cardiomyocytic genesis.[81]

It is likely that an ongoing process is present, modifying the structure of the heart with the creation of the arrhythmogenic substrate. Apoptosis, adipogenesis, fibrogenesis not related to inflammatory reaction, and environmental factors are responsible for remodeling the myocardial structure over time.[82–85]

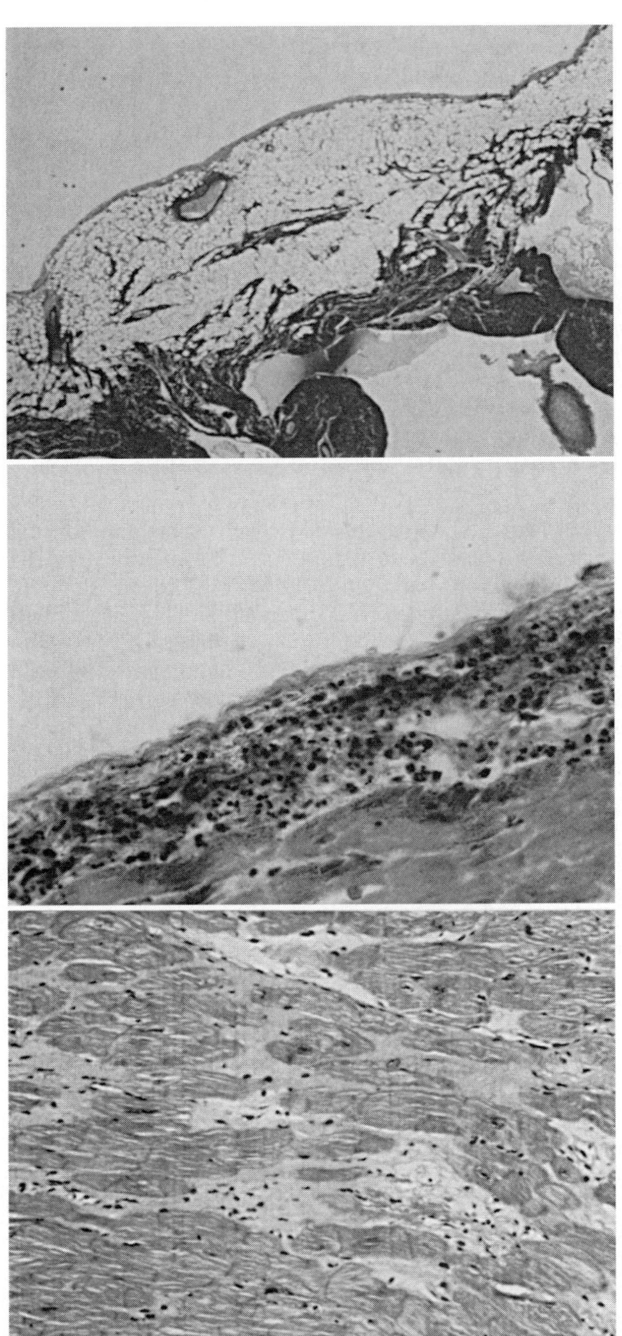

FIGURE 91–5 Top, Anterior wall of the right ventricle in a typical pattern of dysplasia. The epicardium is thicker than normal, and the endocardium is also thin but shows hypertrophic trabeculations. Most of the myocardium is replaced by a thick layer of fat. The black areas inside the fat indicate the presence of surviving strands of cardiomyocytes. **Middle,** This patient died of congestive cardiac failure 9 years after successful antiarrhythmic surgery. Signs of acute epicarditis in a different patient with a typical pattern of dysplasia. **Bottom,** Cardiomyocytes interspersed with zones of fibrosis showing the presence of lymphocytes or lymphoplasmocytes bordering necrotic myocardial cells, suggesting an ongoing process of myocardial destruction. (H&E, ×10).

CLINICAL FORMS

Dysplasia With Major Left Ventricular Involvement

Biventricular Dysplasia

The same disease process involving the left ventricle as the right ventricle[86] characterizes this unusual form. Biventricular dysplasia can lead to cardiac insufficiency because of excessive loss of LV myocardial tissue and may be wrongly diagnosed as idiopathic dilated cardiomyopathy.[87] However, magnetic resonance identification of infiltration of the left ventricle by fat should lead to the correct diagnosis.[88]

Dysplasia Complicated by Myocarditis

In a small percentage of cases, dysplasia may also be complicated by a large amount of inflammatory reaction. In this case, both ventricles are generally involved, and the prognosis is poor.[48] Because only a small number of patients with ARVD have no inflammatory infiltrates, it may be deduced that myocarditis is probably superimposed on the genetically determined structural background of ARVD. A striking demonstration of this concept is the study of identical twins with completely different evolution, suggesting both familial and environmental factors.[89] Another is the presence of old hyaline fibrosis bordering strands of cardiomyocytes within fat in cases presenting with hyperacute myocarditis.[90]

The term *myocarditis* is used to indicate a histologic picture consistent with acute inflammation. This inflammatory process may be the result of multiple causes (viral, bacterial, fungal, toxic, or autoimmune). It may be localized or diffuse and may be observed at different stages of evolution.[91, 92] It may also be associated with a wide spectrum of clinical manifestations ranging from absence of symptoms, apparent complete resolution, sudden death, or even death due to acute congestive heart failure within a few days.[49, 93]

When myocarditis involves both ventricles, congestive heart failure can occur. At a late stage of the disease, it is difficult to distinguish ARVD from an advanced form of idiopathic dilated cardiomyopathy.[94] The diagnosis of ARVD is even more difficult in cases of myocarditis complicating the nonarrhythmogenic form. Therefore, these patients could present a clinical overt or concealed myocarditis and a clinical evolution consistent with idiopathic dilated cardiomyopathy. The microscopic histologic examination of the RV free wall shows the pattern of dysplasia. However, this diagnosis could be obscured by the signs of myocarditis and may escape attention if it is not specifically looked for.[94]

Right Precordial ST-Segment Elevation

This syndrome (also called the Brugada's syndrome) has been observed in young adults who have a risk of sudden death during rest or sleep.[95] It has been reported with an increased prevalence in South East Asia.[96] Some cases with the typical electrocardiographic findings of this condition have clinically or histologically proven ARVD.[97, 98]

Right Ventricular Outflow Tract Tachycardia

Some patients with RV outflow tract tachycardia studied by magnetic resonance imaging show signs of structural heart disease. This was confirmed in some cases by contrast angiography strongly suggesting the presence of ARVD localized to the infundibular area.[99, 100] The *benign extrasystoles* have a pattern suggesting an infundibular origin similar to patients with outflow tract VT. Therefore, it is not surprising that some patients who have premature ventricular contractions of this morphology may have ARVD.

Uhl's Anomaly

This rare anomaly[101–103] does not represent a late form of ARVD. This disease falls into two age groups and has a clearly distinctive clinical as well as pathologic presentation. Uhl's anomaly generally leads to congestive cardiac failure at an early age and death after few weeks or months. In the adult age group, death is the result of congestive heart failure and/or cardiac arrhythmias.[104] Uhl's disease shows the unmistakable pattern of a huge and transparent RV free wall that is easily diagnosed by magnetic resonance imaging. This is the result of apposition of the endocardium with the epicardium with some fatty tissue but without intervening myocardium (paper-thin right ventricle or parchment heart).

Antiarrhythmic Drug Treatment

Drug treatment is the first and most frequently used therapy.[105] If, as is generally the case, LV function is preserved, class I antiarrhythmic drugs may be used safely, provided that the arrhythmia is not severe and the patient is observed carefully at the beginning of treatment. If the LV function is depressed, amiodarone therapy is the treatment of choice. Combination therapy, including amiodarone plus beta-blocking agents, have been used.[106] Because of the incidence of the long-term side effects of amiodarone, sotalol seems to be a reasonable alternative.[107] Because of the excellent results of programmed pacing to guide antiarrhythmic drug therapy in ARVD, this technique is appropriate to predict arrhythmia control.[108] Nevertheless, some reports have stressed the limitations of drug treatment, including sotalol therapy, to prevent sudden death.[109, 110]

Implantable Defibrillator

This therapy is being used more and more frequently in this disease[111] because of the small size and longevity of currently available equipment as well as the transvenous mode of implantation.[108] In addition, the automatic implantable cardioverter/defibrillator may be used to evaluate the efficacy of drug therapy using noninvasive programmed pacing, as well as to evaluate the result of pacing or shock events in the treatment of ventricular arrhythmias observed despite drug therapy. However, the low amplitude of endocardial signals related to the particular structure of the RV myocardium in ARVD may make it more difficult to sense and pace appropriately.[112]

Radiofrequency and Reduced Energy Direct-Current Ablation

Radiofrequency ablation may be used to treat VT that is resistant to drug therapy or in patients who have unacceptable side effects or are not compliant. Reduced-energy direct-current ablation is still used in resistant cases. VT with multiple morphologies are not a deterrent to ablation. It has been commonly observed that a single zone of application of current may lead to the ablation of more than one morphology of VT. It is also critical to pay attention to all the technical aspects for identification of the zone of slow conduction.[113, 114] Reassessment of drug therapy could prove effective after an apparent ineffective ablation session. Failure of a first session is generally followed by a successful repeat session.[115]

Heart Transplantation

This treatment has been used in cases with extreme forms of RV or biventricular involvement.[116] Until now, all our cases with cardiac arrhythmias were amenable to treatment by ablation.

Risk Stratification

This is probably the most difficult problem in ARVD management. The fruste forms are not exempt from the risk of sudden death. The only protection is based on the implantable defibrillator after explanation of the possible complications of this form of therapy. Periodic re-evaluation of drug effectiveness by programmed pacing (eventually using noninvasive techniques in patients with the implantable defibrillator) is advisable. An international registry including a large number of cases is necessary to learn more about the long-term follow-up.

Conclusions

ARVD may be suspected in the presence of ventricular arrhythmias with left bundle branch block pattern as well as supraventricular arrhythmias. ARVD may show a spectrum of RV abnormalities that are emerging as an important cause of sudden death in young, otherwise healthy persons as well as a cause of congestive heart failure. In some cases, it could be the cause of temporary incapacitation with potential catastrophic consequences. It seems probable that ECG with specific criteria may be used as a screening tool able to identify most of these individuals before the first symptom appears. Magnetic resonance imaging is the only noninvasive tool available to analyze the size and the function of both ventricles and to detect the presence of fat in the heart. Echocardiography needs special expertise. Contrast angiography remains the gold standard to ascertain the diagnosis.

The wide clinical spectrum of ARVD appears to be the result of a genetically determined replacement of myocardium by fat and susceptibility to environmental factors. These features could be a contributing component in many causes of death. The incidence of this disease in the population at large is difficult to evaluate. Current treatment modalities include drug therapy, catheter ablative techniques, and modern treatment of congestive heart failure. Heart transplantation is performed in exceptional cases. Implantable defibrillator, used alone or in combination with drug therapy, is playing an increasing role in the treatment of this condition.

Acknowledgments

We gratefully acknowledge the technical assistance of Mrs. Françoise Moreau-Raillecove from the Association Claude Bernard and of Mrs. Nicole Proust for the manuscript preparation and the support of the Fondation Gustave Prevot (Geneva, Switzerland).

References

1. Marcus FI, Fontaine G, Guiraudon G, et al: Right ventricular dysplasia: a report of 24 cases. Circulation 65:384–399, 1982.
2. Fontaine G, Fontaliran F, Frank R: Arrhythmogenic right ventricular cardiomyopathies: clinical forms and main differential diagnoses [editorial]. Circulation 97:1532–1535, 1998.
3. Tonet J, Castro Miranda R, Iwa T, et al: Frequency of supraventricular tachyarrhythmias in arrhythmogenic right ventricular dysplasia. Am J Cardiol 67:1153, 1991.
4. Fontaine G, Fontaliran F, Iwa T, et al: Arrhythmogenic right ventricular dysplasia: definition and mechanism of sudden death. *In* Akhtar M, Myerburg RJ, Ruskin JN (eds): Sudden Cardiac Death. Prevalence, Mechanisms, and Approaches to Diagnosis and Management. pp. 226–237. Malvern: Williams & Wilkins, 1994.
5. Gutierrez PS: Arrhythmogenic right ventricular dysplasia. Br Heart J 70:294, 1993.
6. Corrado D, Basso C, Thiene G, et al: Spectrum of clinico-pathologic manifestations of arrhythmogenic right ventricular cardiomyopathy/dysplasia: a multicenter study. J Am Coll Cardiol 30:1512–1520, 1997.
7. Wada J, Kasanuki H, Ohnishi S, Hosoda S: Left ventricular lesions in arrhythmogenic right ventricular dysplasia and 12-lead electrocardiographic findings. J Cardiol 28:337–344, 1996.
8. Fontaine G, Frank R, Guiraudon G, et al: Signification des troubles de conduction intraventriculaires observes dans la dysplasie ventriculaire droite arythmogene. Arch Mal Coeur 77:872–879, 1984.
9. Fontaine G, Sohal PS, Piot O, et al: Parietal block superimposed on right bundle branch block: a new ECG marker of right ventricular dysplasia [abstract]. J Am Coll Cardiol 29(suppl 2):110A, 1997.
10. James TN, Nichols MM, Sapire DW, et al: Complete heart block and fatal right ventricular failure in an infant. Circulation 93:1588–1600, 1996.
11. Bharati S, Feld AW, Bauernfeind RA, et al: Hypoplasia of the right ventricular myocardium with ventricular tachycardia. Arch Pathol Lab Med 107:249–253, 1983.
12. Fontaine G, Aouate P, Fontaliran F: Dysplasie ventriculaire droite arythmogene, torsades de pointes et mort subite: nouveaux concepts. Ann Cardiol Angeiol (Paris) 46:531–538, 1997.
13. Fontaine G, Guiraudon G, Frank R: Intramyocardial conduction defects in patients prone to ventricular tachycardia. I: the postexcitation syndrome in sinus rhythm. *In* Sandoe E, Julian DG, Bell JW (eds): Management of Ventricular Tachycardia. Role of Mexiletine. pp. 39–55. Amsterdam: Excerpta Medica, 1978.
14. Fontaine G, Guiraudon G, Frank R, et al: Stimulation studies and epicardial mapping in ventricular tachycardia: study of mechanisms and selection for surgery. *In* Kulbertus HE (ed): Reentrant Arrhythmias. pp. 334–350. Lancaster, England: MTP, 1977.
15. Hurst JW: Naming of the waves in the ECG, with a brief account to their genesis. Circulation 98:1837–1942, 1998.
16. Iwa T, Lascault G, Frank R, et al: Value of the signal-averaged electrocardiogram in identifying patients with arrhythmogenic right ventricular dysplasia [abstract]. Eur Heart J 12(suppl):192, 1991.
17. Leclercq JF, Coumel Ph: Late potentials in arrhythmogenic right ventricular dysplasia: prevalence, diagnostic and prognostic values. Eur Heart J 14(suppl E):80–83, 1993.
18. Kinoshita O, Fontaine G, Rosas Andrade F, et al: Optimal high-pass filter settings of the signal-averaged electrocardiogram in patients with arrhythmogenic right ventricular dysplasia. Am J Cardiol 15:1074–1075, 1994.
19. Kinoshita O, Fontaine G, Rosas Andrade F, et al: Time- and frequency-domain analyses of the signal-averaged ECG in patients with arrhythmogenic right ventricular dysplasia. Circulation 91:715–721, 1995.
20. Laurenceau JL, Dumesnil JG: Right and left ventricular dimensions as determinants of ventricular septal motion. Chest 69:388–393, 1976.
21. Scognamiglio R, Fasoli G, Nava A, et al: Relevance of subtle echocardiographic findings in early diagnosis of the concealed form of right ventricular dysplasia. Eur Heart J 10(suppl D):27–28, 1989.

22. Corrado D, Basso C, Angelini A, Thiene G: Sudden death in young people with apparently isolated mitral valve prolapse [abstract]. Pacing Clin Electrophysiol 20(Pt II):1120, 1997.
23. Beckman-Suurkula M, Johansson M, Gustavsson T, Blomstrom-Lundqvist C: Regional right ventricular function in patients with arrhythmogenic right ventricular dysplasia and healthy controls assessed by contrast echocardiography and videodensitometry [abstract]. 1st International Symposium on Arrhythmogenic Right Ventricular Cardiomyopathy-Dysplasia, Paris, June 1996.
24. Levine RA, Gibson TC, Aretz HT, et al: Echocardiographic measurement of right ventricular volume. Circulation 69:497–505, 1984.
25. De Piccoli B, Rigo F, Caprioglio F, et al: The usefulness of transesophageal echocardiography in the diagnosis of arrhythmogenic right ventricular cardiomyopathy. G Ital Cardiol 23:247–259, 1993.
26. Monducci I, Tomasi AM, Bacchi M, Menozzi C: Usefulness of biplanar transesophageal echocardiography in arrhythmogenic right ventricular dysplasia: clinical experience with seven cases. Echocardiography 13:1–8, 1996.
27. King DL, Gopal AS, King DL Jr: 3-Dimensional echocardiography: a method for right ventricular volume and endocardial surface area computation in vivo by polyhedral surface reconstruction [abstract]. J Am Coll Cardiol 23:333A, 1994.
28. Zachara E, Greco C, Salustri A, et al: Three-dimensional echocardiography in right ventricular dysplasia [abstract]. 1st International Symposium on Arrhythmogenic Right Ventricular Cardiomyopathy-Dysplasia, Paris, June 1996.
29. Fontaine G, Guiraudon G, Frank R, et al: Dysplasie ventriculaire droite arythmogene et maladie de Uhl. Arch Mal Coeur 75:361–372, 1982.
30. Uhl HS: A previously undescribed congenital malformation of the heart: almost total absence of the myocardium of the right ventricle. Bull John Hopkins Hosp 91:197–205, 1952.
31. Le Guludec D, Slama M, Frank R, et al: Fourier analysis of gated blood pool studies in the detection of arrhythmogenic right ventricular dysplasia [abstract]. Circulation 80(suppl II):155, 1989.
32. Le Guludec D, Slama M, Frank R, et al: Evaluation of radionuclide angiography in diagnosis of arrhythmogenic right ventricular cardiomyopathy. J Am Coll Cardiol 26:1476–1483, 1995.
33. Wichter T, Hindrinks G, Lerch H, et al: Regional myocardial sympathetic dysinnervation in arrhythmogenic right ventricular cardiomyopathy: an analysis using 1231-meta-iodobenzylguaninidine scintigraphy. Circulation 89:667–683, 1994.
34. Takahashi M, Ishida Y, Maeno M, et al: Significance of 123I-metaiodobenzylguanidine SPECT for detecting left ventricular involvement in patients with arrhythmogenic right ventricular dysplasia. Kaku Igaku 33:57–67, 1996.
35. Fontaine G, Fontaliran F, Frank R, et al: La dysplasie ventriculaire: nosologie et mort subite. Ann Cardiol Angeiol (Paris) 37:347–355, 1988.
36. Klersy C, Raisaro A, Salerno JA, et al: Arrhythmogenic right and left ventricular disease: evaluation by computed tomography and nuclear magnetic resonance imaging. Eur Heart J 10(suppl D):33–36, 1989.
37. Wolf JE, Rose-Pittet L, Page E, et al: Mise en evidence par l'IRM des lesions parietales au cours de dysplasies arythmogenes du ventricule droit. Arch Mal Coeur 82:1711–1717, 1989.
38. Midiri M, Finazzo M, Brancato M, et al: Arrhythmogenic right ventricular dysplasia: MR features. Eur Radiol 7:307–312, 1997.
39. Ricci C, Longo R, Pagnan L, et al: Magnetic resonance imaging in right ventricular dysplasia. Am J Cardiol 70:1589–1595, 1992.
40. Menghetti L, Basso C, Nava A, et al: Spin-echo nuclear magnetic resonance for tissue characterisation in arrhythmogenic right ventricular cardiomyopathy. Heart 76:467–470, 1996.
41. Molinari G, Sardanelli F, Gaita F, et al: Right ventricular dysplasia as a generalized cardiomyopathy? Findings on magnetic resonance imaging. Eur Heart J 16:1619–1624, 1995.
42. Fontaliran F, Fontaine G, Fillette F, et al: Frontieres nosologiques de la dysplasie arythmogene: variations quantitatives du tissu adipeux ventriculaire droit normal. Arch Mal Coeur 84:33–38, 1991.
43. Daliento L, Rizzoli G, Thiene G, et al: Diagnostic accuracy of right ventriculography in arrhythmogenic right ventricular cardiomyopathy. Am J Cardiol 66:741–745, 1990.
44. Blomstrom-Lundqvist C, Selin K, Jonsson R, et al: Cardioangiographic finding in patients with arrhythmogenic right ventricular dysplasia. Br Heart J 59:556–563, 1988.
45. Drobinski G, Verdiere C, Fontaine G, et al: Diagnostic angiocardiographique des dysplasies ventriculaires droites. Arch Mal Coeur 78:544–551, 1985.
46. Daubert JC, Descaves C, Foulgoc JL, et al: Critical analysis of cineangiographic criteria for diagnosis of arrhythmogenic right ventricular dysplasia. Am Heart J 115:448–459, 1988.
47. Pietras RJ, Lam W, Bauernfeind RA: Chronic recurrent right ventricular tachycardia in patients without ischemic heart disease: clinical hemodynamic and angiographic findings. Am Heart J 105:357–366, 1983.
48. Fontaine G, Fontaliran F, Rosas Andrade F, et al: The arrhythmogenic right ventricle: dysplasia versus cardiomyopathy. Heart Vessels 10:227–235, 1995.
49. Pinamonti B, Sinagra G, Salvi A, et al: Left ventricular involvement in right ventricular dysplasia. Am Heart J 123:711–724, 1992.
50. Hebert JL, Chemla D, Zenati O, et al: Right ventricular function in arrhythmogenic right ventricular dysplasia: an hemodynamic study [abstract]. Cardiostim 1996.
51. Hebert JL, Chemla D, Coirault C, et al: Left ventricular function hemodynamics in arrhythmogenic right ventricular dysplasia. Cardiostim 1996.
52. Peters S, Davies MJ, McKenna WJ: Diagnostic value of endomyocardial biopsies of the right ventricular septum in arrhythmias originating from the right ventricle. Jpn Heart J 37:195–202, 1996.
53. Fontaine G, Guiraudon G, Frank R: Intramyocardial conduction defects in patients prone to ventricular tachycardia. II: a Dynamic Study of the Post-Excitation Syndrome. *In* Sandoe E, Julian DG, Bell JW (eds): Management of Ventricular Tachycardia. Role of Mexiletine. pp. 56–66. Amsterdam: Excerpta Medica, 1978.
54. Bharati S, Ciraulo DA, Bilitch M, et al: Inexcitable right ventricle and bilateral bundle branch block in Uhl's disease. Circulation 57:636–644, 1978.
55. Frank R, Fontaine G, Vedel J, et al: Electrocardiologie de quatre cas de dysplasie ventriculaire droite arythmogene. Arch Mal Coeur 71:963–972, 1978.
56. Belhassen B, Webb CR, Shapira I, et al: Unusual features of ventricular tachycardia during respiration and exercises in arrhythmogenic right ventricular dysplasia. Am J Cardiol 54:1280, 1984.
57. Brembilla-Perrot B, Terrier de la Chaise A, Beurrier D, et al: Incidence du déclenchement des tachyarythmies supraventriculaires dans la dysplasie du ventricule droit. Arch Mal Coeur 86:203–207, 1993.
58. Loire R, Tabib A: Mort subite cardiaque inattendue. Bilan de 1000 autopsies. Arch Mal Coeur 1:13–18, 1996.
59. Calvo JR, Duran RM, Vazquez de Prada JA: Resolution of relapsing thrombus by heparin therapy in right ventricular dysplasia. Int J Cardiol 26:238–239, 1990.
60. Wlodarska EK, Rydlewska-Sadowska W, Konka M, et al: Thrombotic complications in arrhythmogenic right ventricular dysplasia/cardiomyopathy [abstract]. *In* The 4th International Symposium on Cardiomyopathy and Myocarditis. Tokyo: Japan Research Promotion Society for Cardiovascular Diseases, 1997.
61. Kesoi I, Gojak I, Enyezdi J, Deak G: Arrhythmogenic right ventricular cardiomyopathy associated with multiple right atrial thrombi. Orv Hetil 138:3185–3188, 1997.
62. Schionning JD, Frederiksen P, Kristensen IB: Arrhythmogenic right ventricular dysplasia as a cause of sudden death. Am J Forensic Med Pathol 18:345–348, 1997.
63. Fontaine G, Guiraudon G, Frank R, et al: The pathophysiology of chronic disturbances of ventricular rhythm. *In* Masoni A, Alboni P (ed): Cardiac Electrophysiology Today. pp. 251–271. London: Academic, 1982.
64. Fontaine G, Aoute P, Fontaliran F: Repolarization and the genesis of cardiac arrhythmias: role of body surface mapping [editorial]. Circulation 12:2600–2602, 1997.
65. Hoffman BF, Feinmark SJ, Guo SD: Electrophysiologic effects of interactions between activated canine neutrophils and cardiac myocytes. J Cardiovasc Electrophysiol 8:679–687, 1997.
66. Furlanello F, Bertoldi A, Dallago M, et al: Cardiac arrest and sudden death in competitive athletes with arrhythmogenic right ventricular dysplasia. Pacing Clin Electrophysiol 21:331–335, 1998.
67. Maron BJ, Shirani J, Poliac LC, et al: Sudden death in young competitive athletes: clinical, demographic, and pathological profiles. JAMA 276:199–204, 1996.
68. Thiene G, Nava A, Corrado D, et al: Right ventricular cardiomyopathy and sudden death in young people. N Engl J Med 318:129–133, 1988.

69. Rakovec P, Rossi L, Fontaine G, et al: Familial arrhythmogenic right ventricular disease. Am J Cardiol 58:377–378, 1986.
70. Diggelmann U, Baur HR: Familial Uhl's anomaly in the adult. Am J Cardiol 53:1402–1403, 1984.
71. Nava A, Scognamiglio R, Thiene G, et al: A polymorphic form of familial arrhythmogenic right ventricular dysplasia. Am J Cardiol 59:1405–1409, 1987.
72. Waynberger M, Courtadon M, Peltier JM, et al: Tachycardie ventriculaire familiale: a propos de 7 cas. Nouv Presse Med 3:1857–1860, 1974.
73. Blomstrom-Lundqvist C, Enestrom S, Edvardsson N, Olsson SB: Arrhythmogenic right ventricular dysplasia presenting with ventricular tachycardia in a father and a son. Clin Cardiol 10:277–283, 1987.
74. Ruder MA, Winston SA, Davis JC, et al: Arrhythmogenic right ventricular dysplasia in a family. Am J Cardiol 56:799–800, 1985.
75. Lascault G, Laplaud O, Frank R, et al: Ventricular tachycardia features in right ventricular dysplasia [abstract]. Circulation 78 (suppl II):300, 1988.
76. Hermida JS, Minassian A, Jarry G, et al: Familial incidence of late ventricular potentials and electrocardiographic abnormalities in arrhythmogenic right ventricular dysplasia. Am J Cardiol 79:1375–1380, 1997.
77. Dallavolta S: Arrhythmogenic cardiomyopathy of the right ventricle: thoughts on aetiology. Eur Heart J 10(suppl D):2–6, 1989.
78. Pawel BR, Donner RM: Sudden death in childhood due to right ventricular dysplasia: report of two cases. Pediatr Pathol 14:987–995, 1994.
79. Makanda A, Tremouroux-Wattiez M, Stijns-Cailteux M, et al: Dysplasie arythmogene du ventricule droit chez un enfant de 16 mois. Arch Mal Coeur 82:811–814, 1989.
80. Atalay S, Imamoglu A, Gumus H, et al: Value of the echocardiographic findings of arrhythmogenic right ventricular involvement in a child. Pediatr Cardiol 17:40–42, 1996.
81. James TN: Normal and abnormal consequences of apoptosis in the human heart: from postnatal morphogenesis to paroxysmal arrythmias. Circulation 90:556–573, 1994.
82. Abou Jaoude S, Leclercq JF, Coumel Ph: Progressive ECG changes in arrhythmogenic right ventricular disease: evidence for an evolutive disease. Eur Heart J 17:1717–1722, 1996.
83. Fontaine G, Fontaliran F: Arrhythmogenic right ventricular disease, dysplasia and cardiomyopathy [editorial]. Eur Heart J 17:1613–1614, 1996.
84. McKenna WJ, Thiene G, Nava A, et al: Diagnosis of arrhythmogenic right ventricular dysplasia/cardiomyopathy. Br Heart J 71:215–218, 1994.
85. Baraka M, Fontaliran F, Frank R, Fontaine G: Value of task force criteria in the diagnosis of arrhythmogenic right ventricular dysplasia-cardiomyopathy. Herzschr Elektrophys 9:1–6, 1998.
86. Letac B, Tayot J, Barthes P: Infiltration graisseuse du coeur et maladie de Uhl. (A propos d'une observation de lipomatose cardiaque). Arch Mal Coeur 70:107–113, 1977.
87. Gallo P, D'Amati G, Pelliccia F: Pathologic evidence of extensive left ventricular involvement in arrhythmogenic right ventricular cardiomyopathy. Hum Pathol 23:948–952, 1992.
88. Pinamonti B, Pagnan L, Bussani R, et al: Right ventricular dysplasia with biventricular involvement. Circulation 98:1943–1945, 1998.
89. Buja G, Nava A, Daliento L, et al: Right ventricular cardiomyopathy in identical and nonidentical young twins. Am Heart J 126:1187–1193, 1993.
90. Fontaine G, Brestescher C, Fontaliran F, et al: Modalites evolutives de la dysplasie ventriculaire droite arythmogene: a propos de 4 observations. Arch Mal Coeur 88:973–980, 1995.
91. Martino TA, Liu P, Petric M, Sole MJ: Enteroviral myocarditis and dilated cardiomyopathy: a review of clinical and experimental studies. *In* Rotbart HA (ed): Human Enterovirus Infections. pp. 291–351. Washington, DC: American Society of Microbiology, 1995.
92. Wesslen L, Pahlson C, Lindquist O, et al: An increase in sudden unexpected cardiac deaths among young Swedish orienteers during 1979–1992. Eur Heart J 17:902–910, 1996.
93. Fontaliran F, Fontaine G, Brestescher C, et al: Signification des infiltrats lymphoplasmocytaires dans la dysplasie ventriculaire droite arythmogene. Arch Mal Coeur 88:1021–1028, 1995.
94. Girard F, Fontaine G, Fontaliran F, et al: Catastrophic global heart failure in a case of non arrhythmogenic right ventricular dysplasia. Heart Vessels 12:152–154, 1997.
95. Brugada P, Brugada J: Right bundle branch block, persistent ST segment elevation and sudden cardiac death: a distinct clinical and electrocardiographic syndrome. J Am Coll Cardiol 20:1391–1396, 1992.
96. Nademanee K, Veerakul G, Nimmannit S, et al: Arrhythmogenic marker for the sudden unexplained death syndrome in Thai men. Circulation 96:2595–2600, 1997.
97. Corrado D, Nava A, Buja G, et al: Familial cardiomyopathy underlies syndrome of right bundle branch block, ST segment elevation and sudden death. J Am Coll Cardiol 27:443–448, 1996.
98. Fontaine G, Piot O, Sohal PS, et al: Sus-decalage du segment ST en dérivations precordiales droites et mort subite. Relation avec la dysplasie ventriculaire droite arythmogene. Arch Mal Coeur 89:1323–1329, 1996.
99. Carlson MD, White RD, Trohman RG, et al: Right ventricular outflow tract ventricular tachycardia: detection of previously unrecognized anatomic abnormalities using cine magnetic resonance imaging. J Am Coll Cardiol 24:720–727, 1994.
100. Proclemer A, Basadonna PT, Slavich GA, et al: Cardiac magnetic resonance imaging findings in patients with right ventricular outflow tract premature contractions. Eur Heart J 18:2002–2010, 1997.
101. Caglar NM, Pamir G, Kural T: Right ventricular cardiomyopathy similar to Uhl's anomaly with atrial flutter and complete AV block. Int J Cardiol 38:199–201, 1993.
102. Gerlis LM, Schmidt-Ott SC, Ho SY, Anderson RH: Dysplastic conditions of the right ventricular myocardium: Uhl's anomaly versus arrhythmogenic right ventricular dysplasia. Br Heart J 69:142–150, 1993.
103. Gaffney FA, Nicod P, Lin JC, Rude RE: Noninvasive recognition of the parchment right ventricle (Uhl's anomaly, arrhythmogenic right ventricular dysplasia) syndrome. Clin Cardiol 6:235–242, 1983.
104. Vedel J, Frank R, Fontaine G, et al: Tachycardies ventriculaires recidivantes et ventricule droit papyrace de l'adulte. (A propos de deux observations anatomo-cliniques). Arch Mal Coeur 71:973–981, 1978.
105. Leclercq JF, Coumel Ph: Characteristics, prognosis and treatment of the ventricular arrhythmias of right ventricular dysplasia. Eur Heart J 10(suppl D):61–67, 1989.
106. Fontaine G: Amiodarone drug interactions: potential beneficial and adverse effects. Clin Cardiol 10:I-17–I-20, 1987.
107. Wichter T, Borggrefe M, Haverkamp W, et al: Efficacy of antiarrhythmic drugs in patients with arrhythmogenic right ventricular disease: results in patients with inducible and noninducible ventricular tachycardia. Circulation 86:29–37, 1992.
108. Wichter T, Martinez-Rubio A, Kottkamp H, et al: Reproducibility of programmed ventricular stimulation in arrhythmogenic right ventricular dysplasia/cardiomyopathy [abstract]. Circulation 94(suppl I):626, 1996.
109. Haverkamp W, Martinez-Rubio A, Hief C, et al: Efficacy and safety of d,l-sotalol in patients with ventricular tachycardia and in survivors of cardiac arrest. J Am Coll Cardiol 30:487–495, 1997.
110. Constantin L, Martins JB: Autonomic control of ventricular tachycardia: direct effects of beta-adrenergic blockade in 24 hour old canine myocardial infarction. J Am Coll Cardiol 9:366–373, 1987.
111. Link MS, Wang PJ, Haugh CJ, et al: Arrhythmogenic right ventricular dysplasia: clinical results with implantable cardioverter defibrillators. J Intervent Card Electrophysiol 1:41–48, 1997.
112. Fontaine G: Implantable defibrillator in arrhythmogenic right ventricular dysplasia [letter to the editor]. J Intervent Card Electrophysiol 1:329, 1997.
113. Fontaine G, Frank R, Tonet J, Grosgogeat Y: Identification of a zone of slow conduction appropriate for VT ablation: theoretical and practical considerations. Pacing Clin Electrophysiol 12(Pt II):262–267, 1989.
114. Yamabe H, Okumura K, Tsuchiya T, Yasue H: Demonstration of Entrainment and presence of slow conduction during ventricular tachycardia in arrhythmogenic right ventricular dysplasia. Pacing Clin Electrophysiol 17:172–178, 1994.
115. Fontaine G, Zenati O, Tonet J, et al: The role of electrophysiological stimulation in the treatment of life-threatening ventricular tachycardia. *In* Caturelli G (ed): Cura Intensiva Cardiologica 1995. pp. 482–494. Milano: Librex, 1995.
116. Oteo JF, Alonso-Pulpon L, Cavero MA, et al: Right ventricular arrhythmogenic dysplasia: the role of heart transplantation in its management. Rev Esp Cardiol 47:839–842, 1994.

CHAPTER 92

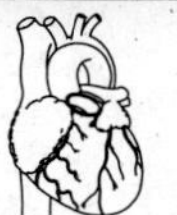

The Importance of Atrioventricular Dissociation

Hein J. J. Wellens

THE IMPORTANCE OF ATRIOVENTRICULAR DISSOCIATION
The Jugular Pulse
Varying Intensity of the First Heart Sound
Changes in Systolic Blood Pressure
MECHANISMS OF WIDENED QRS DURING SUPRAVENTRICULAR TACHYCARDIA
Phase 3 Block
Concealed Retrograde Conduction
ELECTROCARDIOGRAPHIC DIAGNOSIS OF WIDE QRS TACHYCARDIA
Atrioventricular Dissociation
Width of the QRS Complex
The QRS Axis in the Frontal Plane
Configurational Characteristics of the QRS Complex
THE PRACTICAL APPROACH

Because a drug given for the treatment of supraventricular tachycardia (SVT) may be deleterious to a patient with a ventricular tachycardia (VT),[1,2] the differential diagnosis in broad-QRS tachycardia is critical. Errors are made because physicians wrongly consider VT unlikely if the patient is hemodynamically stable,[3] and they are often unaware that certain findings on physical examination and on the electrocardiogram (ECG) may quickly and accurately lead to the correct diagnosis.

The possible causes of wide QRS tachycardia are as follows (Fig. 92–1):

1. SVT with preexisting or functional bundle branch block (BBB). This includes sinus tachycardia, atrial tachycardia, atrial flutter, atrial fibrillation, and atrioventricular (AV) nodal reentry tachycardia.
2. Orthodromic circus movement tachycardia using the AV node in the anterograde direction and an accessory pathway in the retrograde direction with preexisting or functional BBB.
3. SVT with conduction over an accessory pathway.
4. Antidromic circus movement tachycardia using an accessory pathway in the anterograde direction and the AV node or another accessory pathway in the retrograde direction.
5. AV reentry tachycardia using a nodoventricular fiber in the anterograde direction and the bundle of His or another accessory pathway in the retrograde direction.
6. Ventricular tachycardia.

The Importance of Atrioventricular Dissociation

In addition to careful evaluation of the ECG, examination of the patient should include a search for physical signs of AV dissociation. AV dissociation is present in approximately 50 percent of all VTs. The other 50 percent show some form of retrograde conduction to the atria.[4] Therefore, the finding of AV dissociation is an important diagnostic clue.

The physical signs of AV dissociation are as follows[5]:

1. Irregular cannon A waves in the jugular pulse
2. Varying intensity of the first heart sound
3. Beat-to-beat changes in systolic blood pressure

Any one of these three clues indicates AV dissociation. However, in the absence of such clues, VT cannot be ruled out; there remains the possibility of coexistent atrial fibrillation or ventriculoatrial conduction, in which case none of the signs of AV dissociation would be present. In theory, it is also possible for an AV junctional tachycardia with retrograde block to have AV dissociation; however, in view of the rarity of such a rhythm, AV dissociation remains a valuable diagnostic clue for VT.

The Jugular Pulse

In VT with independent beating of atria and ventricles, the atria occasionally beat against closed AV valves, resulting in retrograde blood flow into the jugular vein, producing the so-called cannon A wave. Inspection of the jugular vein reveals the characteristic occasional expansive pulsation.

Varying Intensity of the First Heart Sound

The first heart sound marks the onset of ventricular systole and is caused by the closing of the mitral and tricuspid valves. During AV dissociation, there is a beat-to-beat change in the loudness of the first heart sound, owing to the varying position of the AV valves at the time of ventricular contraction. Therefore, the first heart sound varies in inten-

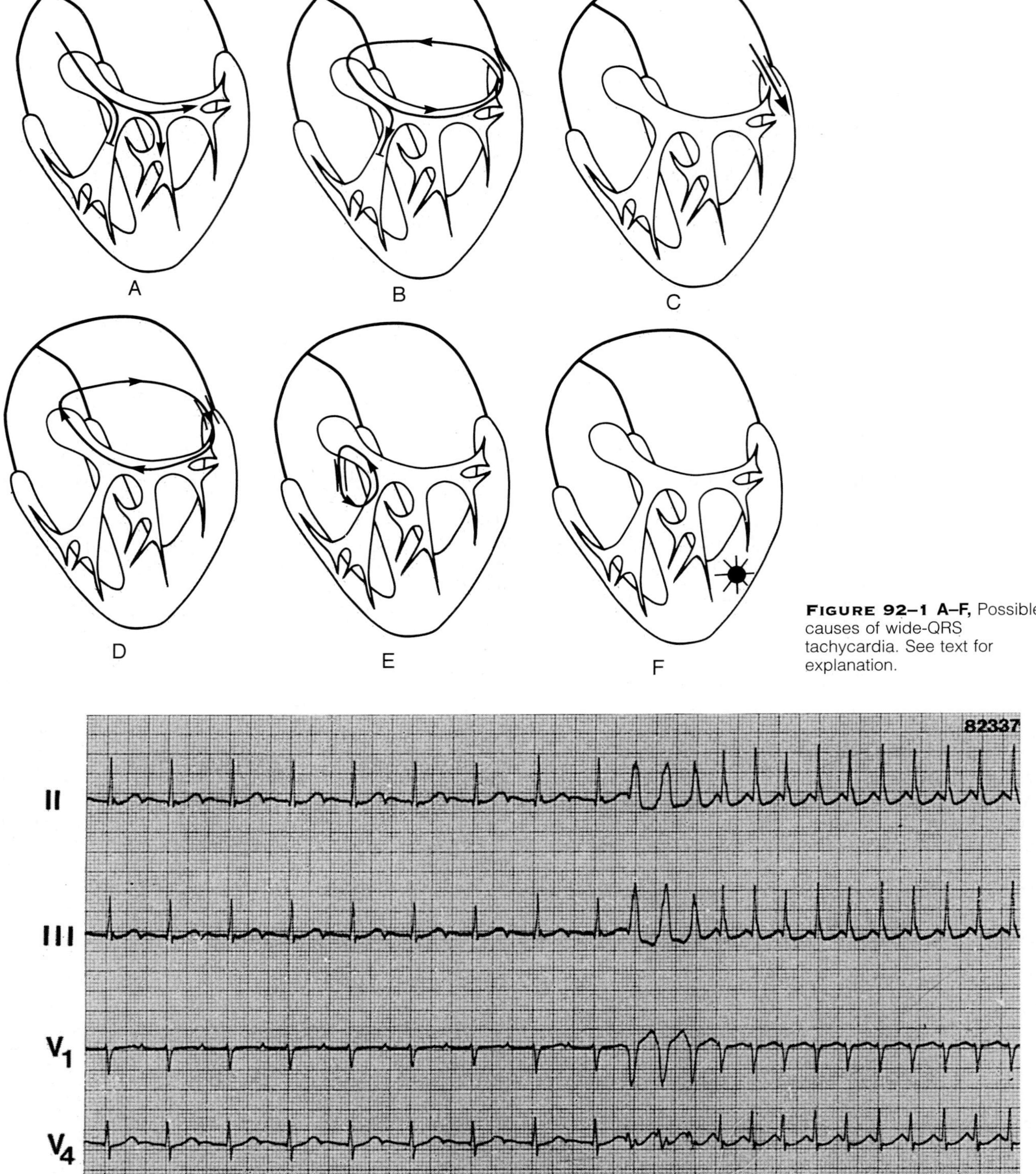

FIGURE 92–1 A–F, Possible causes of wide-QRS tachycardia. See text for explanation.

FIGURE 92–2 Phase 3 aberration. In a patient with supraventricular tachycardia and 2:1 atrioventricular (AV) conduction *(left)*, there is a sudden change in 1:1 AV conduction. This sudden increase in ventricular rate is accompanied by widening of the first three QRS complexes (left bundle branch block). Note that the third QRS shows less widening than the first and second QRS complexes. This sequence is typical of phase 3 aberration.

sity during VT and in complete heart block, as well as during AV Wenckebach's and atrial fibrillation.

Changes in Systolic Blood Pressure

During AV dissociation, ventricular filling from the atria varies, depending on the time interval between atrial and ventricular contraction. These differences in ventricular filling lead to a beat-to-beat change in systolic stroke volume into the aorta, which in turn causes beat-to-beat changes in systolic blood pressure. This sign of AV dissociation can easily be detected at the bedside by use of the blood pressure recorder. Thus, a typical finding in VT with AV dissociation is that the rhythm is regular, whereas the systolic blood pressure differs from beat to beat.

Mechanisms of Widened QRS During Supraventricular Tachycardia

As shown in Figure 92–1, BBB may be one of the causes of a wide QRS tachycardia. This block may be preexistent (also present during sinus rhythm) or functional. Functional BBB during SVT may occur because of phase 3 block or retrograde invasion into the bundle branch.

Phase 3 Block

Phase 3 (tachycardia-dependent) aberration usually occurs in the right bundle branch because that bundle commonly has the longest refractory period.[6–9] Left bundle branch block (LBBB) aberration accounts for approximately one third of cases of aberrant ventricular conduction. It may occur in normal fibers if the impulse is premature enough to reach the cell when the membrane has not fully repolarized. This is the form of aberration commonly observed at the beginning of paroxysmal SVT (Fig. 92–2). Phase 3 aberration is promoted by a long-short cycle sequence because the refractory period of the bundle branch of the beat following the long cycle is prolonged.

Concealed Retrograde Conduction

Although the mechanism of QRS widening at the onset of SVT commonly is phase 3 aberration, the sustaining mechanism is often concealed retrograde conduction up one of the bundle branches. Figure 92–3 is a schematic representation of how, during sinus rhythm, LBBB aberration is initiated by the premature atrial beat that also initiates SVT. This phase 3 block of the left bundle is followed by conduction over the right bundle and retrograde invasion into the left bundle branch. This makes the left bundle branch refractory when the next supraventricular impulse passes through the AV node. The impulse is conducted down the right bundle branch and then in a retrograde direction again up the left bundle branch. This mechanism is responsible for continuation of LBBB during SVT. Retrograde invasion into the left bundle branch continues until it is disrupted by a ventricular premature beat. Figure 92–4 gives a clinical example of the latter mechanism during SVT with right BBB.

Retrograde concealed conduction into one of the bundle branches is a common mechanism of perpetuation of aberration during SVT.[8]

Electrocardiographic Diagnosis of Wide QRS Tachycardia

A 12-lead ECG is required for the correct diagnosis of wide QRS tachycardia on the basis of morphology. The physician should examine the ECG systematically, looking for the presence of AV dissociation and analyzing QRS characteristics, such as width, axis, and configuration.

Atrioventricular Dissociation

Traditionally (and correctly), dissociation between atrial and ventricular activity during tachycardia has been considered a hallmark of VT. As pointed out previously, however,[4] some form of ventriculoatrial conduction is frequently present during VT. Identification of atrial activity during VT can be difficult or impossible on the 12-lead ECG. Recognition of the P wave in a wide QRS tachycardia is important, however, because of the diagnostic value of AV dissociation. It is extremely rare for an AV nodal tachycardia to show a widened QRS complex and AV dissociation. This may occur in the presence of an accelerated AV junctional rhythm (as in digitalis intoxication or after cardiac surgery) in the patient with preexistent BBB. Independent beating of atria and ventricles during a VT can result in "capture" or "fusion" complexes (Fig. 92–5). This occurs when the ventricular rate during VT is such that appropriately timed atrial impulse is able to traverse the AV node to depolarize the ventricles completely (capture) or partially (fusion). In the latter situation, fusion occurs because of concomitant ventricular activation from the VT focus (see Fig. 92–5). The occurrence of a narrower-QRS VT is not always the result of a conducted supraventricular beat; it may also result from fusion with a ventricular premature depolarization arising in the ventricle contralateral to the ventricle in which the tachycardia originates or fuses with a ventricular echo beat when a retrogradely conducted impulse during VT travels to the AV node and reenters the ventricle.[9]

Width of the QRS Complex

When we compared the width of the QRS complex in 100 cases of VT and 100 cases of SVT with aberrant conduction, we found that all cases of SVT with aberrant conduction had a QRS width of less than or equal to 0.14 second, whereas 59 percent of cases of VT had a QRS width of more than 0.14 second. These findings indicate that a QRS width of more than 0.14 second is highly suggestive of a ventricular origin of the tachycardia. The cause of VT plays a role in the width of the QRS complex. As reported

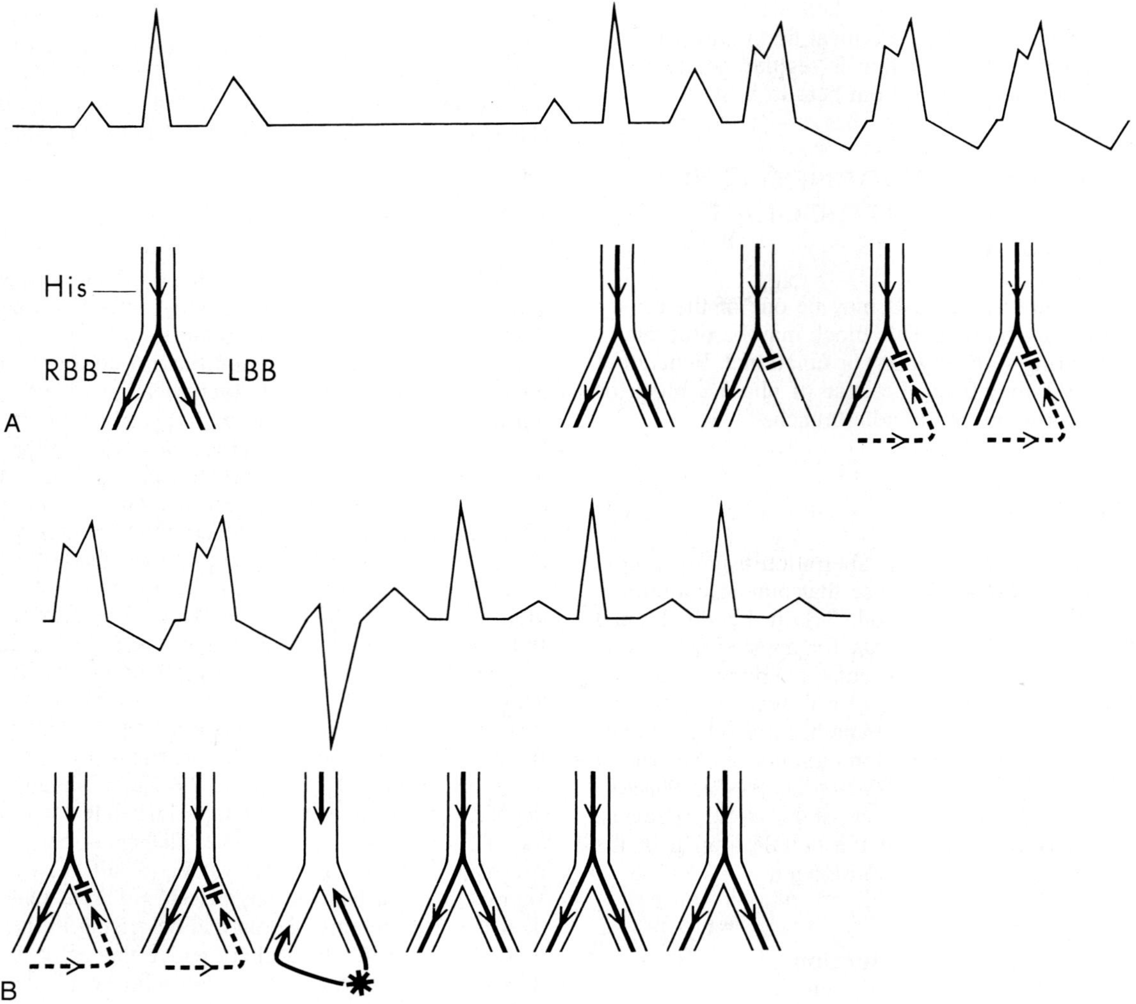

FIGURE 92–3 A and **B,** Schematic representation of initiation of left bundle branch (LBB) block aberration (see text).

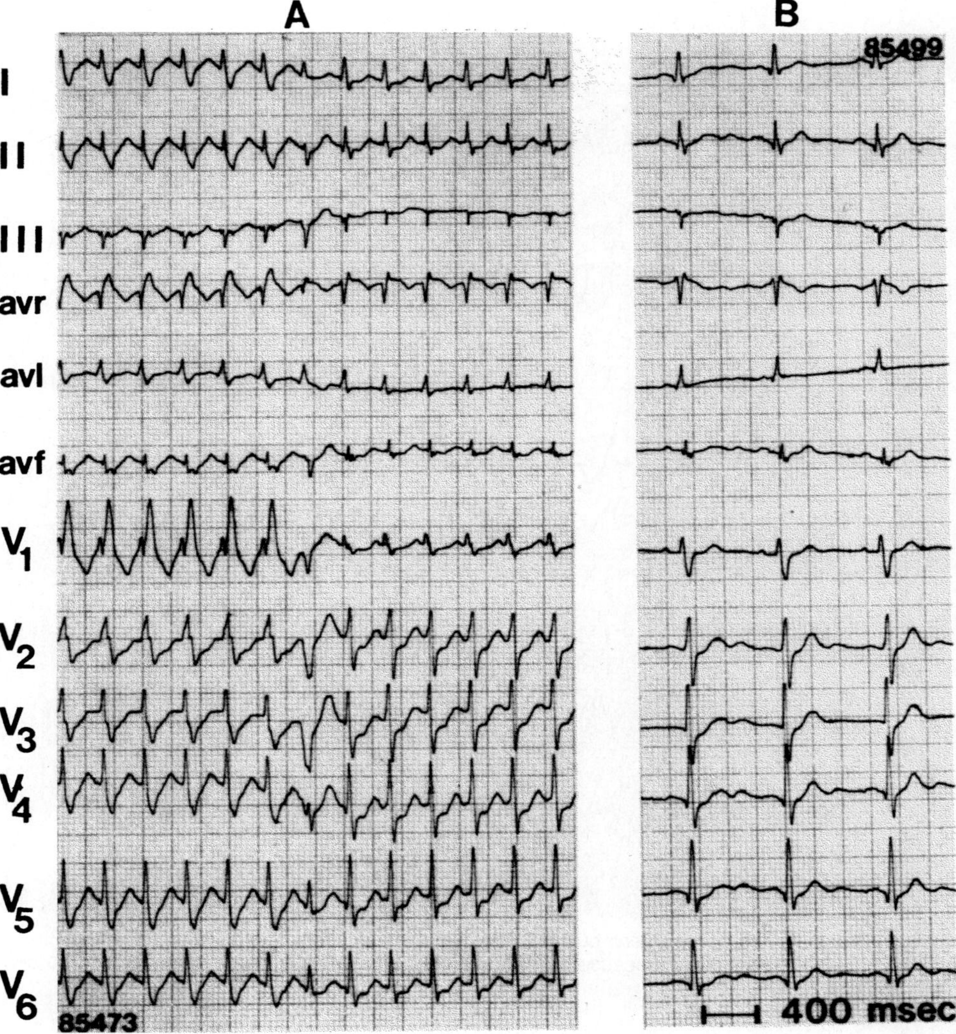

FIGURE 92–4 A, Example of widening of the QRS complex during tachycardia by retrograde invasion into the right bundle branch. The critical time relations required for perpetuation of retrograde invasion into the right bundle branch are disrupted by a right-sided ventricular premature beat. **B,** Same patient during sinus rhythm.

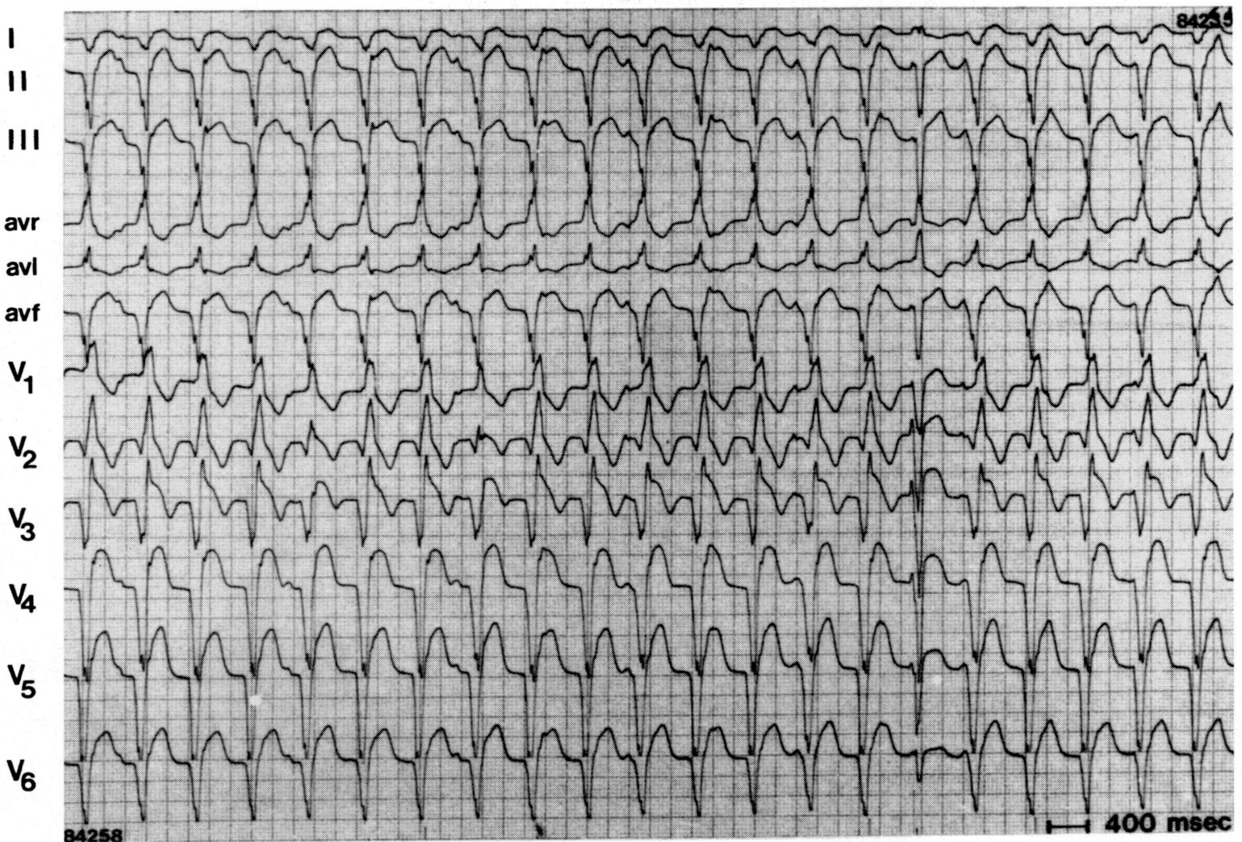

FIGURE 92–5 An example of ventricular tachycardia with ventricular fusion beats. The 5th, 8th, and 16th QRS complexes are narrower than the other QRS complexes because of fusion between a ventricular ectopic complex and a conducted supraventricular beat.

by Coumel and associates,[10] in coronary artery disease, the average QRS complex is wider during VT than the QRS complex of the patient with idiopathic VT (171 10 milliseconds versus 135 11 milliseconds; *P* .001). There are three situations in which an SVT can have a QRS width of more than 0.14 second. The first occurs when the patient has an SVT in the presence of preexistent BBB. The second involves an SVT with AV conduction over an accessory pathway. The third is marked QRS widening during SVT because of the use of antiarrhythmic drugs that prolong intraventricular conduction.

The QRS Axis in the Frontal Plane

Most patients with VT secondary to a previous myocardial infarction have a markedly abnormal QRS axis in the frontal plane. Especially in the right bundle branch block (RBBB)–like VT, the axis usually points superiorly, in contrast to SVT with RBBB, in which the axis is to the right. Patients with idiopathic VT can have a normal QRS axis in the frontal plane, but the two most common types of idiopathic VT may have marked left-axis or right-axis deviation (Fig. 92–6). In fact, an LBBB-shaped tachycardia with a vertical-axis or a right-axis deviation is very likely to be VT. In discussing the importance of the axis in the frontal plane in the differential diagnosis of wide QRS tachycardia, it is important to realize that a markedly abnormal axis can occur in patients with preexistent BBB during SVT and in patients who, during tachycardia, have AV conduction over an accessory pathway. In the latter situation, marked left-axis deviation can be found during anterograde conduction over a right-sided or posteroseptal accessory bundle and marked right-axis deviation in case of a left lateral accessory pathway.

Configurational Characteristics of the QRS Complex

The Concordant Pattern in the Precordial Leads

When ventricular activation starts in the posterobasal region of the left ventricle, the precordial leads from V_1 to V_6 show a positive QRS complex. A "concordant" positive QRS complex in the precordial leads is therefore found not only in a VT originating in the posterobasal left ventricle (Fig. 92–7) but also in a tachycardia with AV conduction over accessory pathway inserting into the posterobasal left ventricle. A concordant negative QRS pattern in the precordial leads is typical of VT originating in the anteroapical left ventricle.

Bundle Branch Block–Shaped QRS Complexes

SVT with RBBB aberration is recognized because of a triphasic rSR pattern in lead V_1 and a triphasic QRS pattern in lead V_6.[4, 11] In lead V_1, the initial R wave reflects normal septal activation, the S wave reflects left ventricular activation, and the R wave reflects late activation of the right ventricle. Lead V_6 shows a narrow little Q wave as

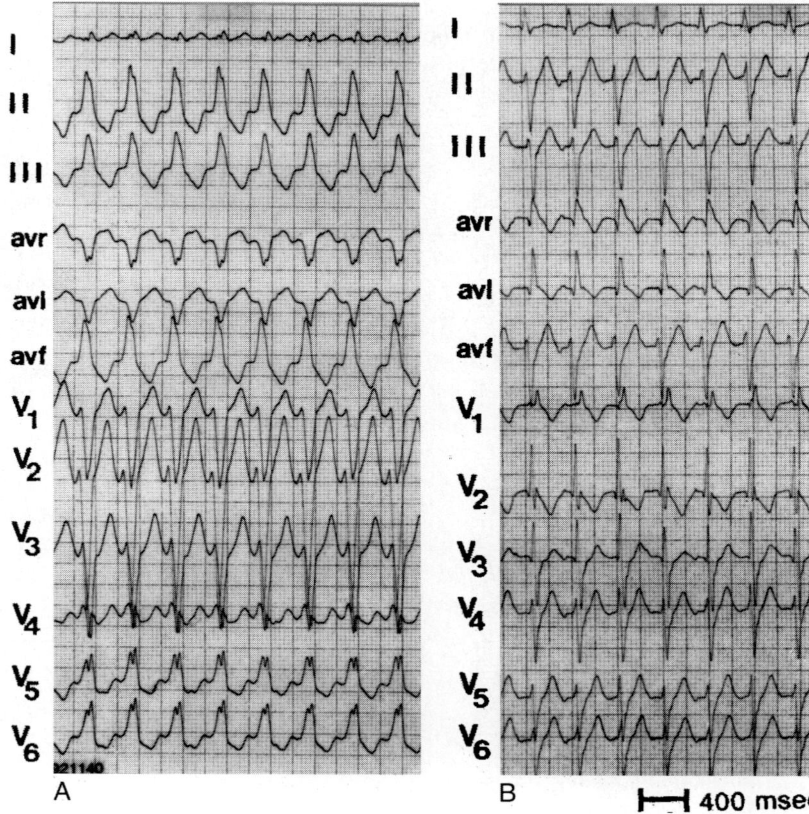

FIGURE 92–6 The two most common forms of idiopathic ventricular tachycardia. **A,** The origin is in the outflow tract of the right ventricle. The QRS shows a left bundle block–shaped QRS and a vertical axis. **B,** The origin is in the inferoseptal portion of the left ventricle. The QRS shows a right bundle branch block shape and left-axis deviation.

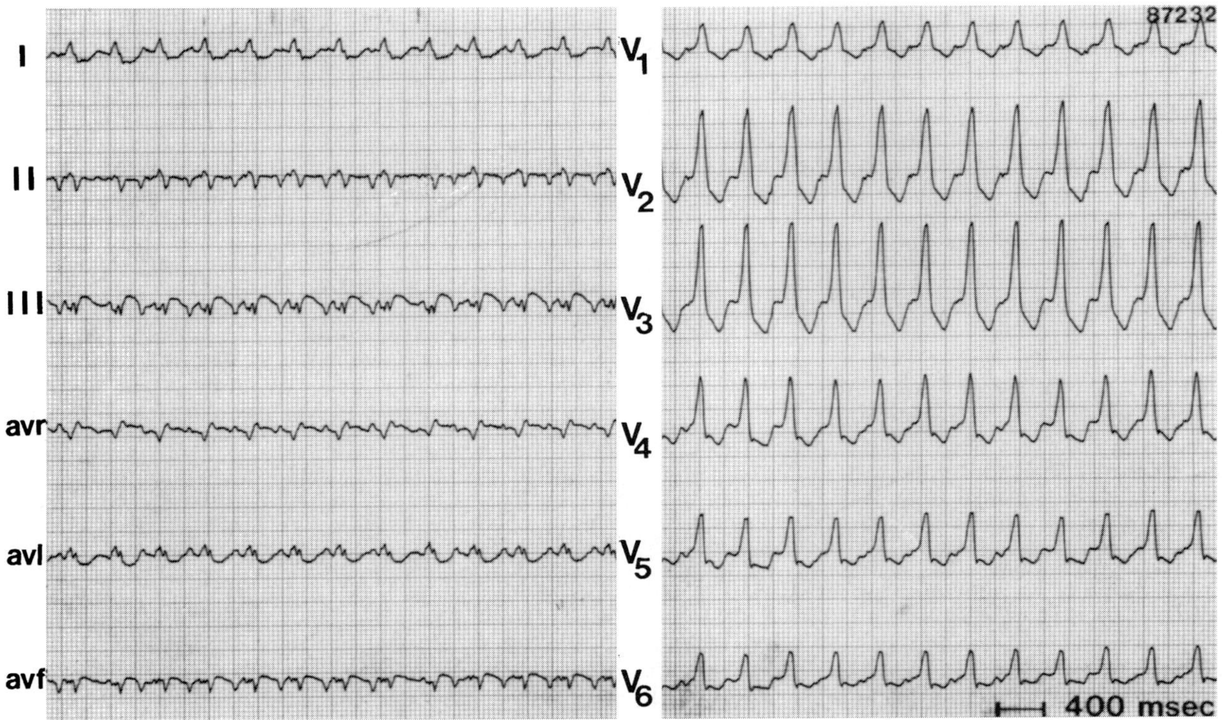

FIGURE 92–7 Positive concordant pattern in the precordial leads in a patient with an old inferior myocardial infarction and a ventricular tachycardia originating in the posteroinferior region. Ventriculoatrial conduction showing a Wenckebach type of conduction can be seen in the limb leads.

the result of normal septal activation and an R/S ratio of more than 1. A typical example of RBBB aberration during SVT is shown in Figure 92–8. In VT with an RBBB-like QRS contour, lead V_1 usually shows a monophasic or biphasic R wave. The presence of a deep S wave in lead V_6 (R/S ratio < 1) supports a diagnosis of VT. An R/S ratio of less than 1 in lead V_6 is more common when left-axis deviation is present (Fig. 92–9).

The differential diagnosis of an LBBB-shaped VT and SVT with LBBB aberration is made in leads V_1 and V_2 and in lead V_6. If an R wave is present in either lead V_1 or V_2, it is narrow (< 0.04 second) in LBBB aberration,

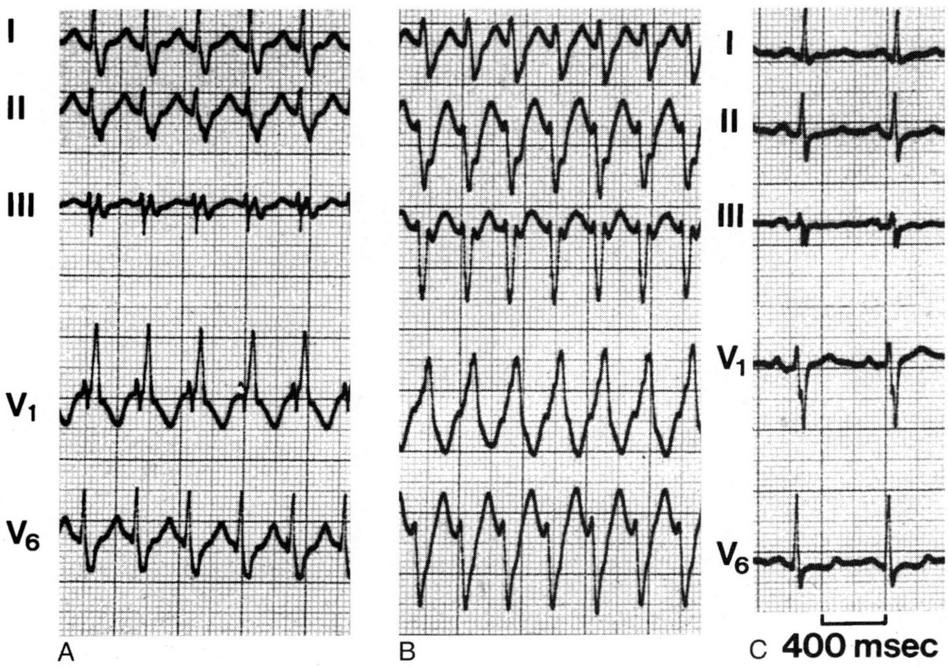

FIGURE 92–8 A, A supraventricular tachycardia with right bundle branch block. **B,** A ventricular tachycardia. **C,** Same patient as in **A** and **B** but during sinus rhythm (see text).

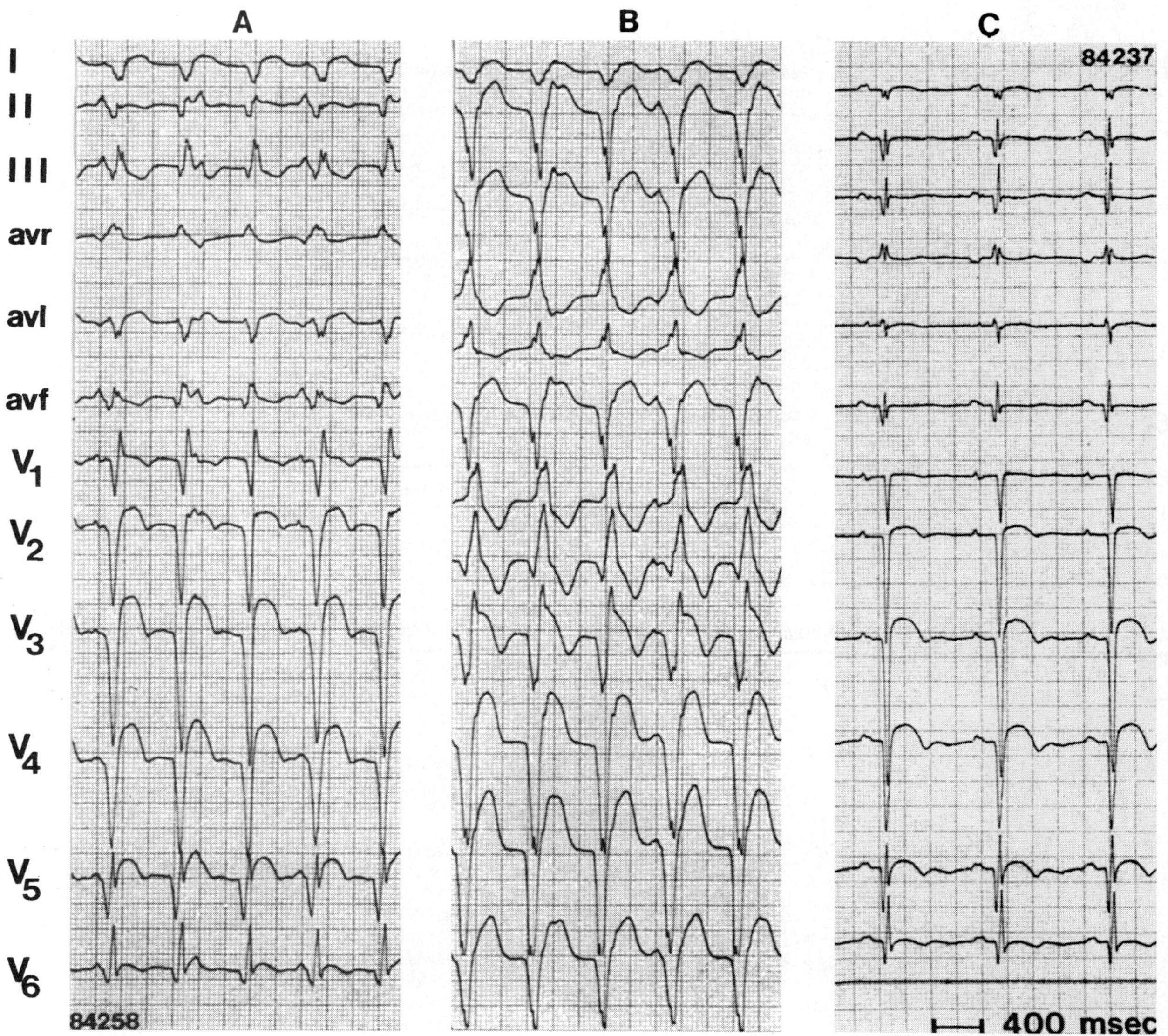

FIGURE 92–9 Two examples of ventricular tachycardia with a right bundle branch block–shaped ventricular tachycardia in the same patient. Note left-axis deviation and an R/S ratio of less than 1 in V_6 **(B)**. **A,** An R/S ratio of more than 1 in V_6 in the presence of right-axis deviation in the frontal plane. **C,** Same patient during sinus rhythm.

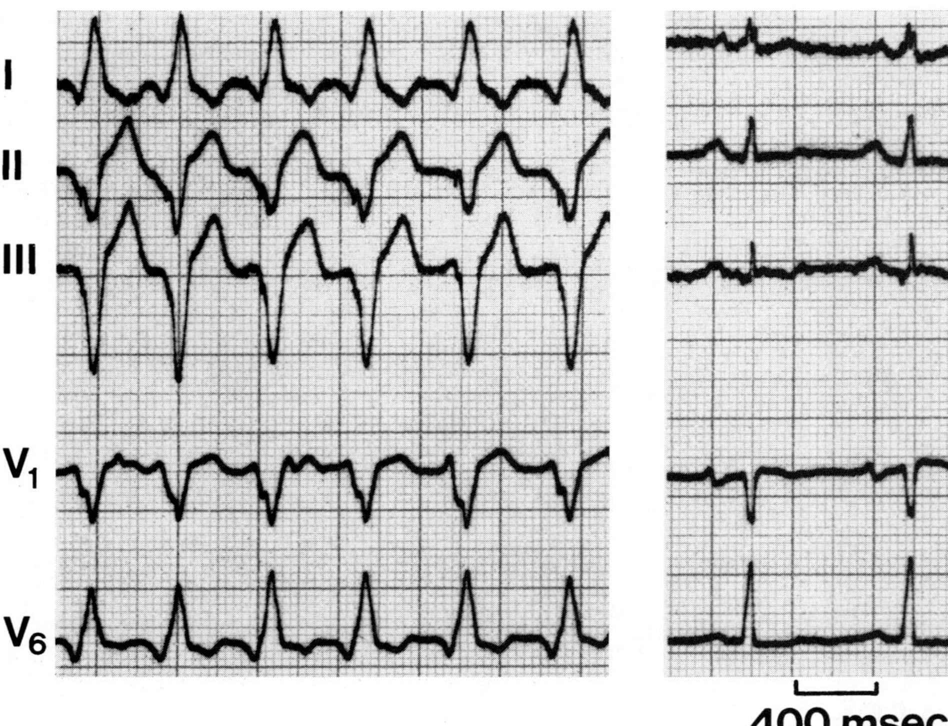

FIGURE 92–10 Ventricular tachycardia with a left bundle branch block–shaped QRS complex. Note AV dissociation and the characteristic QRS changes in leads V_1 and V_6 (see text).

TABLE 92-1 Limitations of Electrocardiographic Signs Suggestive of a Ventricular Origin for a Wide QRS Tachycardia

Sign	Limitations
AV dissociation	VA conduction may occur during VT AV junctional rhythm with BBB and AV dissociation
QRS width > 0.14 s	Preexistent BBB (especially LBBB) SVT with AV conduction over an accessory pathway Use of drugs slowing intraventricular conduction (class IA, IC, amiodarone)
Left-axis deviation (to the left of −30°)	Not helpful in LBBB-shaped QRS SVT with AV conduction over a right-sided or posteroseptal accessory AV pathway SVT during use of class IC drugs
Right-axis deviation (to the right of +90°)	Not helpful in RBBB-shaped QRS
Presence of q(Q)R complexes in leads other than AVR	Only in VT with localized myocardial scarring or infiltration (MI, sarcoidosis, amyloidosis)
Concordant pattern in precordial leads	Positive concordancy may occur during SVT with AV conduction over a left posterior accessory AV pathway
R-nadir S ⩾ 100 ms in one or more precordial leads	SVT on drugs showing intraventricular conduction SVT with AV conduction over an accessory AV pathway Preexistent BBB (especially LBBB)
Presence of a supraventricular impulse able to depolarize the ventricles completely ("capture beat") or partially (fusion complex)	Occurs only at relatively slow VT rates R/O fusion with a contralateral VPC during VT R/O fusion with a ventricular echo beat
Presence of premature beats during sinus rhythm with the same QRS configuration as during wide QRS tachycardia	Requires availability of ECG during sinus rhythm R/O atrial premature beat with aberrant conduction

Abbreviations: AV, atrioventricular; BBB, bundle branch block; ECG, electrocardiogram; LBBB, left bundle branch block; MI, myocardial infarction; R/O, rule out; SVT, supraventricular tachycardia; VA, ventriculoatrial; VPC, ventricular premature complex; VT, ventricular tachycardia.

and the downstroke of the S wave is clean and swift (no slurs or notches). Because of the narrow R wave and/or the clean downstroke, the distance from the beginning of the QRS to the nadir of the S wave is 0.06 second or less. In contrast, an R wave of more than 0.04 second, with a slurred downstroke and a delayed S nadir in V_1 and/or V_2, supports a diagnosis of VT. A Q wave in lead V_6 confirms VT (Fig. 92–10).

Presence of Q Waves During Tachycardia

Coumel and associates[10] demonstrated the value of QR complexes during a wide QRS tachycardia as pointing to a ventricular origin for the arrhythmia. This is the case in VT in patients with a localized ventricular scar, as in previous myocardial infarction or localized infiltrative or inflammatory myocardial disease.

Duration of the Onset of R to Nadir of S in Precordial Leads

This distance is increased in VT. As pointed out by Brugada and colleagues,[12] the presence of an RS interval of more than 100 milliseconds in one or more precordial leads is highly suggestive of VT. However, such a duration may occur in SVT with AV conduction over an accessory pathway, in SVT during the administration of drugs that slow intraventricular conduction, and in SVT with preexistent BBB (especially LBBB).

Ventricular Premature Beats With the Same QRS Configuration as During Wide QRS Tachycardia

In the patient with a wide QRS tachycardia, the finding of ventricular premature beats with the same QRS during sinus rhythm points to a ventricular origin for the tachycardia. One has to be careful, however, to rule out aberrant conduction of supraventricular premature beats as the cause of the widened QRS complex during sinus rhythm!

Table 92–1 lists all the limitations of these different electrocardiographic findings.

THE PRACTICAL APPROACH

It is important not to panic when one is confronted with a wide QRS tachycardia. The patient should be examined for clinical signs of AV dissociation, and the 12-lead ECG should be systematically evaluated. This usually leads to the correct diagnosis of SVT versus VT. Statistically, VT is much more common in the regular wide QRS tachycardia than SVT. In addition, patients can tolerate VT well hemodynamically (they can walk into the hospital). If the diagnosis is in doubt, the patient should not be treated with verapamil; procainamide should be used instead.

REFERENCES

1. Stewart RB, Bardy GH, Greene HL: Wide complex tachycardia: misdiagnosis and outcome after emergent therapy. Ann Intern Med 104:766, 1986.
2. Buxton AE, Marchlinski FE, Doherty JU: Hazards of intravenous verapamil for sustained ventricular tachycardia. Am J Cardiol 59:1107, 1987.
3. Dancy M, Camm AJ, Ward D: Misdiagnosis of chronic recurrent ventricular tachycardia. Lancet 2:320, 1985.
4. Wellens HJJ, Bar FWHM, Lie KI: The value of the electrocardiogram in the differential diagnosis of a tachycardia with a widened QRS complex. Am J Med 64:27, 1978.
5. Harvey WP, Ronan JA: Bedside diagnosis of arrhythmias. Prog Cardivasc Dis 8:419, 1966.
6. Moe GK, Mendez C, Han J: Aberrant AV impulse propagation in the dog heart: a study of functional bundle branch block. Circ Res 16:261, 1965.
7. Cohen SI, Lau SH, Stein E, et al: Variations of aberrant ventricular conduction in man: evidence of isolated and combined block within the specialized conduction system. Circulation 38:899, 1968.
8. Wellens HJJ, Ross DL, Farre J, Brugada P: Functional bundle branch block during supraventricular tachycardia in man: observations on mechanisms and their incidence. *In* Zipes D, Jalife J (eds): Cardiac Electrophysiology and Arrhythmias. pp. 435–441. New York: Grune & Stratton, 1985.
9. Vermeulen A, Wellens HJJ: Paroxysmal ventricular tachycardias showing fusion with reciprocal ventricular beats. Br Heart J 33:320, 1971.
10. Coumel P, Leclercq JF, Attuel P, Slama R: The QRS morphology in postmyocardial infarction ventricular tachycardia: a study in 100 tracings compared with 70 cases of idiopathic ventricular tachycardia. Eur Heart J 5:792, 1984.
11. Marriott HJL: Differential diagnosis of supraventricular and ventricular tachycardia. Geriatrics 25:91, 1970.
12. Brugada P, Brugada J, Mont L, et al: A new approach to the differential diagnosis of a regular tachycardia with a wide QRS complex. Circulation 83:1649, 1991.

CHAPTER 93

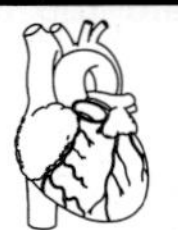

SYNCOPE

David G Benditt, William Fabian, and Scott Sakaguchi

PHYSIOLOGY OF THE CEREBRAL CIRCULATION
CLINICAL PATHOPHYSIOLOGY OF SYNCOPE
Cardiovascular Causes of Syncope
Noncardiovascular Causes of Syncope
DIAGNOSTIC STRATEGY
Initial Evaluation
Noninvasive Cardiovascular Studies
Invasive Electrophysiologic Testing
Autonomic Function Testing
Combined Electrophysiologic and Tilt-Table Studies in Syncope
Neurologic Studies
NATURAL HISTORY AND EPIDEMIOLOGY
General Considerations
Specific Conditions
TREATMENT
Neurally Mediated Syncopal Syndromes
Orthostatic and Dysautonomic Disturbances of Blood Pressure Control
Primary Cardiac Arrhythmias
LQTS Diagnostic Criteria and Treatment
Structural Cardiovascular or Cardiopulmonary Disease
Cerebrovascular, Neurologic, and Psychiatric Diseases
Miscellaneous Disturbances
ECONOMIC ASPECTS
CONCLUSION

Syncope is defined clinically as a relatively abrupt loss of both consciousness and postural tone, with subsequent prompt spontaneous recovery. For the medical practitioner, the first challenge when confronted by a patient who has apparently experienced a "syncopal spell" is to distinguish true syncope from other disturbances of consciousness and/or postural tone that may mimic a syncopal event (e.g., seizures, "drop attacks," sleep disorders, inadvertent falls). The next challenge is to define the basis for the event. Only after a reasonably certain etiology is established, can the prevention of further episodes be approached in a rational manner.

The potential causes of syncope are numerous (Table 93–1). However, in the vast majority of cases, the principal physiologic disturbance is transient diminution of cerebral blood flow owing to a self-limited period of systemic arterial hypotension. In this regard, conditions that affect the stability of the cardiovascular system either directly (e.g., arrhythmias, drug effects, gravity) or indirectly (e.g., autonomic disturbances of heart rate or vascular tone) are by far the most frequent causes of syncopal symptoms. On rare occasion, local disturbances of cerebral blood flow (e.g., cerebrovascular spasm) or abnormalities of the composition of cerebral nutrient flow (e.g., hypoxia, and hypercapnia) may be responsible for syncopal spells. Metabolic abnormalities and primary neurologic diseases are infrequent causes of syncope.

This chapter provides a brief review of the physiology of the cerebral circulation as it relates to the pathophysiology of syncope. The principal causes of syncopal spells are examined and classified in terms of their relative frequency of occurrence. Finally, diagnostic and treatment strategies are addressed.

PHYSIOLOGY OF THE CEREBRAL CIRCULATION

Normally, the brain receives blood flow of 50 to 60 ml/min/100 g tissue, or approximately 10 to 15 percent of resting cardiac output. As a rule, total cerebral blood flow is relatively constant, although regional variations in flow occur in response to local metabolic requirements.[1]

Control of cerebral blood vessels is largely the result of local metabolic and chemical factors. Sympathetic adrenergic innervation is present (although not uniformly distributed), but it appears capable of causing only relatively minor changes in blood flow. These nerves may play a protective constrictor role when the cerebral circulation is faced with an abrupt rise in central blood pressure. Parasympathetic nerve fibers are also present; however, their role in blood flow control is uncertain. In terms of metabolic mediators of cerebral blood flow, the partial pressures of carbon dioxide (P_{CO_2}), pH, and hypoxia are probably the most influential. Thus, over a certain range, increased P_{CO_2} may be associated with marked increases in cerebral blood flow, with the response being diminished at the extremes of P_{CO_2} (Fig. 93–1A). The effect is primarily attributed to alteration of cerebrospinal fluid pH, since CO_2 is able to cross the blood-brain barrier rapidly and react with water to form H^+ and HCO_3. Given the modest buffering capacity of the cerebrospinal fluid, abrupt pH changes may occur, and it is the altered H^+ concentration that is responsible for vasodilatation. Of note, systemic metabolic acidosis may not affect the cerebrospinal fluid to the same extent as respiratory acidosis, since the H^+ ion does not readily cross the blood-brain barrier.

Severe hypoxia is associated with increased cerebral blood flow, an effect probably mediated by local metabolites (see Fig. 93–1B). However, to the extent that hypoxia is often associated with hyperventilation, the vasoconstrictor action of reduced P_{CO_2} may tend to offset the cerebral

TABLE 93–1 Syncope: Diagnostic Classification

Neurally Mediated Reflex Disturbances of Blood Pressure Control

Vasovagal faint
Carotid sinus syncope
Cough syncope and related disorders
Gastrointestinal, pelvic, or urologic origin (swallowing, defecation, postmicturition)
Airway stimulation

Orthostatic and Dysautonomic Disturbances of Blood Pressure Control

Primary autonomic failure
Multisystem atrophy
Diabetic neuropathy
Drug-induced orthostasis

Primary Cardiac Arrhythmias

Sinus node dysfunction (including bradycardia/tachycardia syndrome)
Atrioventricular conduction system disease
Paroxysmal supraventricular tachycardias
Paroxysmal ventricular tachycardia (including torsades de pointes)
Implanted pacing system malfunction, pacemaker-mediated tachycardia, "pacemaker syndrome"

Structural Cardiovascular or Cardiopulmonary Disease

Cardiac valvular disease/ischemia
Acute myocardial infarction
Obstructive cardiomyopathy
Subclavian steal syndrome
Pericardial disease/tamponade
Pulmonary embolus
Primary pulmonary hypertension

Cerebrovascular, Neurologic, and Psychiatric Diseases

Obstructive Vascular Disease

Intracerebral steal

Central Nervous System Substrates

Seizure disorders
Subarachnoid hemorrhage
Narcolepsy
Hydrocephalus

Psychiatric Disorders

Panic attacks
Hysteria

Miscellaneous Causes of Syncope

Metabolic/Endocrine Disturbances

Hyperventilation (hypocapnia)
Hypoglycemia
Volume depletion (Addison's disease, pheochromocytoma)
Hypoxemia

blood flow effects of hypoxia. Operating together, these factors result in a special form of cerebral blood flow "autoregulation" in the setting of hypoxia.

The more traditional so-called autoregulatory capacity of the cerebral vascular bed is one of its most distinctive features (see Fig. 93–1C); in essence, cerebral blood flow tends to be well maintained over a relatively wide range of mean arterial pressures. Outside this range, marked rises in flow occur at higher pressures, whereas dramatic declines are observed at lower pressures. Once again, local metabolic effects are likely the key operative factors.

It has been estimated that maintenance of consciousness requires cerebral oxygen (O_2) delivery of at least 3.5 ml O_2/100 g of tissue each minute.[2, 3] Diminution of cerebral O_2 delivery below minimal requirements for 10 seconds or longer may be expected to be functionally deleterious, and depending on a number of factors (e.g., the individual's posture at the time), loss of both consciousness and postural tone may occur. Briefer periods of cerebral hypoperfusion may initiate a transient premonitory sensation of imminent loss of consciousness (often-termed *presyncope* or *near-syncope*).[4] Regional blood flow disturbances also contribute to the clinical picture. Thus, for example, since the visual cortex is highly vulnerable in terms of greatest gravitational risk (i.e., high up and remote from the central circulation), it is understandable that visual loss ("gray-out") is often an early symptom in an evolving complete or nearly complete faint.

In the healthy young to middle-aged individual, assuming absence of severe hypoxemia, cerebral O_2 requirements are easily met under almost all circumstances. Specifically, maintenance of blood flow is achieved over a relatively wide range of perfusion pressures owing to the health of the "autoregulatory" features of the cerebrovascular bed.[5] Furthermore, in health, since the various local and systemic control mechanisms discussed previously are intact, and usually efficient, the central vascular baroreceptor system provides additional protection for cerebral perfusion by altering heart rate, and adjusting systemic vascular resistance, to accommodate for hypotensive states. Finally, under normal conditions, vascular volume is protected by normal renal function (usually unimpeded by drugs in young healthy individuals) acting in conjunction with hormonal influences, particularly those attributable to the renin-angiotensin-aldosterone system and vasopressin. Nevertheless, even healthy individuals exposed to extreme conditions of cardiovascular stress (e.g., dehydration, excessive tachycardia or bradycardia, or marked peripheral vascular dilatation) may experience transient diminution of cerebral blood flow. Given the brain's minimal nutrient storage capacity, syncope may occur.

With increasing age, especially given the greater predilection for concomitant disease in older individuals, many of the compensatory and protective mechanisms associated with the more youthful healthy cerebrovascular bed may become compromised. Aging alone has been associated with diminution of cerebral blood flow by up to 25 percent between ages 20 and 70 years.[6, 7] In one report,[8] cerebral blood flow was found to average 50 ml/min/100 g tissue in healthy individuals over 75 years of age, but fell to the 40 ml/min range in elderly hospitalized patients with hypertension or atherosclerotic disease. Consequently, the usual wide safety factor for cerebral O_2 delivery is compromised in many older patients, and it may be even further undermined in the presence of hypertension, diminished cardiac output, concomitant anemia, and/or hypoxia.

Hypertension, a common accompaniment of the aging process, is associated with a shift of the autoregulatory curve to higher pressures (i.e., placing adequacy of blood flow at greater risk should a transient drop in systemic pressure occur). Additionally, coexisting diseases (including drug treatments employed to deal with them) may contribute to a less effective compensatory response. Thus, diabetes alters the chemoresponsiveness of the cerebrovascular bed.[9] Furthermore, normal protective reflexes become less reliable. For instance, the carotid baroreceptors become less sensitive to phenylephrine-induced blood pressure in-

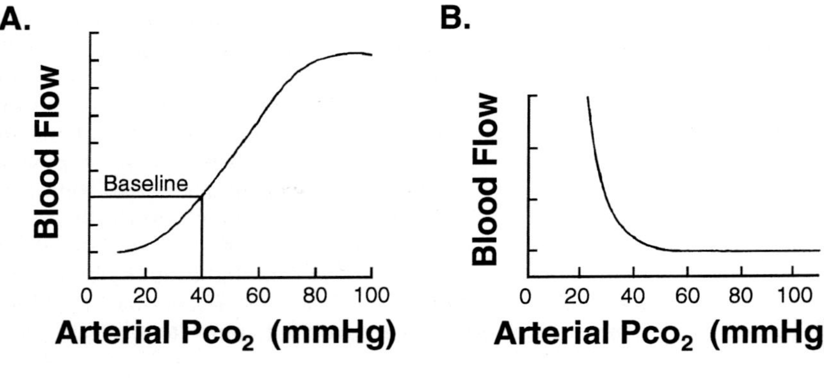

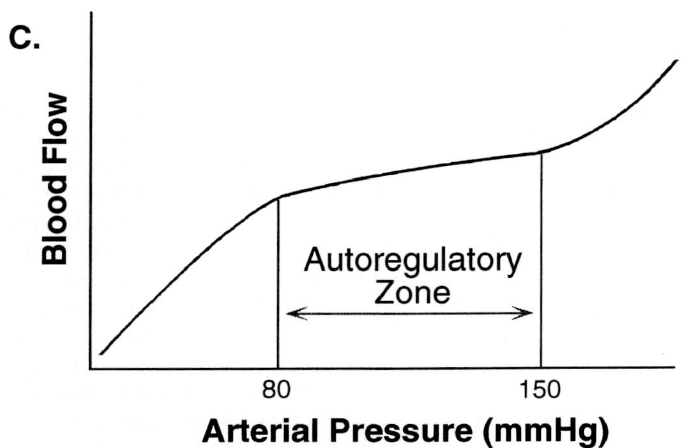

FIGURE 93–1 Changes in cerebral blood flow as a function of alterations of arterial P_{CO_2} **(A),** arterial P_{O_2} **(B),** and mean arterial pressure **(C).**

creases or drug-induced hypotension in the elderly. Consequently, compensatory heart rate and vascular changes may be inadequate to adjust for even such relatively transient disturbances as postural change, cough, straining, or dehydration, let alone more serious problems such as arrhythmias or hemorrhage. On the other hand, from time to time, it seems that certain reflex responses become overactive in the older individual.[10–13] By way of example, the carotid baroreceptors appear to become "hypersensitive" in some older patients (carotid sinus hypersensitivity) and to contribute to transient neurologic disturbances (carotid sinus syndrome). Although the latter may, in fact, be less a problem with baroreceptor sensitivity than with the concordance of various head and neck neural afferent signals to the brain stem,[10] the outcome is greater susceptibility to syncope in older patients.

CLINICAL PATHOPHYSIOLOGY OF SYNCOPE

Causes of syncope may be broadly classified as being either cardiovascular or noncardiovascular in origin. However, a more detailed classification is helpful (see Table 93–1). Cardiovascular causes include syncope owing to neurally mediated reflex disturbances of blood pressure control, effects of cardiovascular drugs, cardiac and pulmonary disease, and peripheral and/or cerebrovascular disease. The noncardiovascular etiologies encompass primarily conditions that more often than not produce "syncope mimics" (e.g., seizure disorders, metabolic and endocrine disturbances, and psychiatric disorders). As a rule, cardiovascular disturbances are by far the more common causes of true syncope.

Cardiovascular Causes of Syncope

Neurally Mediated Syncopal Syndromes

The neurally mediated syncopal syndromes (Table 93–2) are the most common causes of syncope in all age groups. Of these conditions, the *emotional* or vasovagal faint and

TABLE 93–2 Neurally Mediated Syncopal Syndromes

Emotional syncope (common or "vasovagal" faint, "malignant" vasovagal faint)
Carotid sinus syncope
Gastrointestinal stimulation
Swallow syncope, defecation syncope
Micturition syncope
Cough syncope
Sneeze syncope
Glossopharyngeal neuralgia
Airway stimulation
Raised intrathoracic pressure
Playing a brass wind instrument, lifting weights

carotid sinus hypersensitivity are the best known, and these account for the vast majority of all syncopal events. Certain others, such as postmicturition syncope, cough syncope, and the postexercise variant of neurally mediated syncope are also encountered relatively frequently in general medical practice. The remaining neurally mediated syncopal syndromes tend to be far less common, but they may be encountered in specific circumstances (e.g., syncope accompanying gastrointestinal or genitourinary tract instrumentation in medical clinic environments).

Although each of the various neurally mediated syncopal syndromes appear to be distinct entities owing to differences in the source of the "trigger" for the syncopal episodes (e.g., pain, carotid sinus stimulation, cough, and micturition), they are nevertheless pathophysiologically closely related. In regard to the initiation of these syncopal events, the presumed triggering neural signals may arise within the central nervous system itself (e.g., syncope associated with fear or anxiety) or from any of a number of peripheral "receptors" that respond to various stimuli (e.g., mechanical, chemical, and pain). The nature of these receptors is clearest in carotid sinus syncope and postmicturition syncope, although even in these cases, much remains to be learned. Specifically, the interaction of the afferent neural signals with signals coming from other sources may be both important and complex.[10] For instance, in the case of carotid sinus syndrome, the triggering signals are initiated by stimulation of autonomic receptors in the cervical region.[14–18] However, Tea and associates[10] pointed out the potential importance of parallel afferent inputs from the sternocleidomastoid muscles. When these signals are not concordant, susceptibility to carotid sinus syndrome is greater. In postmicturition syncope, the status of wakefulness seems to play an important role in terms of an individual patient's susceptibility to an event. In typical vasovagal syncope, on the other hand, the location and nature of the trigger sites are less certain. In particular, the proposed role of cardiac and other central cardiopulmonary mechanoreceptors remains controversial.[14–17] The concept that such receptors play a role in the syncopal event is consistent with the fact that diminution of central circulatory volume (volume depletion, hemorrhage, or adoption of the erect posture) tends to enhance the risk of syncope.

The afferent neural signals in neurally mediated syncope initiate a little understood series of events within the medullary cardiovascular control areas, ultimately resulting in the efferent bradycardic and vasodilatory response. The efferent reflex pathways comprise two principal elements: (1) increased vagus nerve activity inducing bradycardia and (2) reduced sympathetic neural activity causing dilatation of skeletal muscle arterioles[19–21] and splanchnic venules (i.e., the vasodepressor component).[22, 23] The relative impact of these two elements may differ substantially among patients (and perhaps even within patients at various times); thus, systemic hypotension in some syncopal events may be characterized primarily by bradycardia (i.e., cardioinhibitory syncope), whereas others are principally due to vasodilatation (i.e., vasodepressor syncope). In most cases, both mechanisms are operative (i.e., a mixed response).

Paradoxic cerebrovascular arteriolar vasoconstriction may be an additional contributor to some forms of neurally mediated syncope.[24, 25] In this regard, Grubb and colleagues[24] studied 30 patients with recurrent unexplained syncope undergoing head-up tilt-table testing using transcranial Doppler sonography to assess middle cerebral artery blood flow. Syncope occurred during testing in 20 of the 30 patients (67 percent). At the time of development of hypotension and bradycardia, there was a mean 73 percent increase in resistance index, suggesting an unexpected vasoconstriction in the face of increasing systemic hypotension. Thus, the possibility exists that cerebral hypoperfusion with loss of consciousness and postural tone may occur in some cases in the absence of systemic hypotension. In the past, such a finding was thought (perhaps mistakenly) to imply syncope of psychiatric origin (e.g., hysteria).

Orthostatic and Dysautonomic Causes of Syncope

Symptomatic hypotension associated with movement to the upright posture (orthostatic hypotension) may be the consequence of transient or chronic diminution of intravascular volume and/or abnormal vasomotor compensatory mechanisms. The former is among the most frequent causes of syncope and dizziness. Iatrogenic factors such as excessive diuresis or aggressive use of antihypertensive and vasodilator agents are particularly common contributors. Environmental factors (e.g., excessive heat), diminished mobility, and/or a reduced appetite may be important aggravating factors, especially in the elderly or physically impaired patient. Additionally, complications associated with any number of medical conditions (e.g., hemorrhage, anemia, and third space fluid loss) or the disease processes themselves (e.g., adrenal insufficiency, diabetes insipidus, and hyperglycemia) may provoke syncopal episodes. Primary autonomic dysfunction resulting in abnormal vasomotor control as a cause of syncope may occur in the absence of other neurologic disturbances or in association with multiple system involvement (Shy-Drager syndrome) (Table 93–3). More commonly, however, the disturbance of the autonomic nervous system is secondary to drugs or other diseases (see Table 93–3). In regard to drugs, the most common ones at fault are antihypertensives, diuretics, nitrates, and beta-adrenergic blockers. However, a wide range of commonly used vasoactive drugs or sedatives may impair neural reflex compensation. Among the common disease states to be concerned about in this setting, neuropathies of alcohol or diabetic origin, spinal cord lesions, and paraneoplastic syndromes are relatively common. However, even prolonged periods of physical inactivity such as occur during hospitalization for any reason may be responsible.

Cardiac Causes of Syncope

RHYTHM DISTURBANCES

Cardiac rhythm disturbances are among the most frequent and potentially hazardous causes of syncope and dizziness. Bradyarrhythmias due to sinus node dysfunction and/or conduction system disease are important considerations, especially in the older patient. However, ventricular tachyarrhythmias may be even more frequent, and they may have even greater adverse prognostic importance.

TABLE 93-3 Orthostasis and Dysautonomias: A Classification of Causes of Autonomic Failure

Primary
Progressive primary AF
Progressive AF with multiple-system atrophy (Shy-Drager syndrome)
Progressive AF with Parkinson's disease
Secondary
Various medical disorders (e.g., diabetes)
Autoimmune acute and subacute dysautonomias (e.g., Guillain-Barré syndrome, myasthenia gravis)
Autonomic neuropathy associated with malignancies
Metabolic diseases (e.g., porphyria, Fabry's disease)
CNS infections (e.g., syphilis, Chagas' disease)
Hypothalamic and midbrain lesions/tumors (e.g., craniopharyngioma)
Familial dysautonomia
Spinal cord lesions/tumors
Drug/Toxin-Induced
Alcohol
Sedatives/tranquilizers: phenothiazines, barbiturates
Vasodilators (e.g., peripheral and central sympatholytic agents)
ACE inhibitors
Tricyclic antidepressants

Abbreviations: ACE, angiotensin-converting enzyme; AF, autonomic failure; CNS, central nervous system.

Modified from Bannister R (ed): Autonomic Failure. A Textbook of Clinical Disorders of the Autonomic Nervous System. Oxford: Oxford University Press, 1988, by permission of Oxford University Press.

Sinus Node Dysfunction. Disturbances of sinus node function encompass a variety of sinoatrial, atrial, and at times, atrioventricular (AV) electrophysiologic abnormalities.[26–30] Thus, electrocardiographic (ECG) manifestations of sinus node dysfunction may include severe sinus bradycardia, sinus pauses or sinus arrest, sinoatrial exit block, chronic atrial tachyarrhythmias, and alternating periods of atrial bradyarrhythmias and tachyarrhythmias. Additionally, increasing recognition of exertional symptoms due to abnormal heart rate responses during physical exercise or emotional stress (so-called chronotropic incompetence) provides another facet to sinoatrial disease.[30–32] Any of these abnormal rhythms could occur with sufficient severity to result in persistent or intermittent diminution of blood flow to critical organ systems, particularly the brain. In the case of bradyarrhythmias, a finding of a 3-second or greater asystolic pause or a persistent heart rate of 40 beats/min or less in a symptomatic patient (i.e., with a history of syncope) is usually considered sufficient to warrant treatment with a pacemaker.[30] On the other hand, the evaluation of tachycardias is more difficult unless spontaneous symptoms and arrhythmia are correlated during ECG monitoring (e.g., event recorder, Holter monitor). Electrophysiologic testing may prove helpful, although interpretation of the findings must be undertaken with care and in the light of other coexisting information in a given patient.

Unfortunately, the propensity of sinus node dysfunction patients to develop thromboembolic complications adds another facet to their potential for manifesting neurologic disturbances. Thus, transient loss of consciousness with subsequent residual neurologic deficit raises the possibility of embolic stroke as the underlying cause. Greater recent attention to prophylactic anticoagulation in high-risk subsets of this population will likely diminish the frequency with which this potentially devastating scenario is seen in the future.

Cardiac Conduction Disease. Cardiac conduction system disease is common in patients with underlying structural heart disease. Structural disturbances of the cardiac conduction system may be the result of acute ischemic syndromes as well as the effects of long-standing atherosclerotic disease, cardiomyopathy, hypertension, and valvular heart disease. However, not infrequently, the etiology cannot be specified and a chronic degenerative process is assumed. In any event, ECG findings indicative of cardiac conduction system disease (unless correlated with patient symptoms) should not lead to immediate assumption that transient AV block is the cause of syncope. In such cases, the same disease substrate may be responsible for more subtle but potentially important abnormalities, particularly sinus node dysfunction and ventricular tachyarrhythmias.

Persistent or episodic AV block may result in diminution of cardiac output and cerebrovascular flow sufficient to cause loss of consciousness. Since the impact of the hemodynamic disturbance is greatest with upright posture, the patient may recover when supine only to faint once again when she or he tries to get up. The recording of AV block in association with such symptoms is the most powerful diagnostic evidence, but this is difficult to obtain in many cases and searching for it may expose patients to excessive hazard. Electrophysiologic evidence of an excessively prolonged His-ventricle (HV $>$ 100 ms) interval may be taken to imply worrisome conduction system disease.[33] Similarly, documentation of infra-His block (Mobitz type 1 or type 2) during atrial pacing at moderate rates is also considered indicative of the potential for undocumented higher-grade block being responsible for syncope. In such cases, pacemaker therapy is probably warranted. However, in all such cases, it must be kept in mind that susceptibility to ventricular tachyarrhythmias is also common in patients with conduction system disease. Thus, among 30 patients with chronic bifascicular block and syncope, Dhingra and coworkers[34] found that ventricular tachyarrhythmias were the most likely cause of symptoms in 9 cases (30 percent). The remaining patients evidenced various other causes, with a full 30 percent remaining undiagnosed. Consequently, careful assessment of this possibility is a necessary feature of the electrophysiologic assessment of all syncope patients with conduction system disease.

Tachyarrhythmias. The abrupt onset of tachyarrhythmias (either ventricular or supraventricular) may be accompanied by hypotension with consequent dizziness or syncope, particularly if the onset of arrhythmia occurs when the patient is in the upright posture. This is especially the case in older patients, in the individual with coexisting cardiac or vascular disease. However, even in the apparently healthy patient, the occurrence of tachycardia in the face of upright posture (i.e., gravitational stress) can lead to dizziness or syncope, especially if the patient is volume depleted owing to a hot environment or after physical exertion. As a rule, supraventricular tachyarrhythmias (SVT) are less often implicated as causes of syncope among patients referred for electrophysiologic assessment than are ventricular tachyarrhythmias.[35] In either case, however, programmed electrical stimulation of the heart during electrophysiologic testing has proved highly effective for eliciting susceptibility to tachyarrhythmias and directing therapy. In particular, the feasibility in many patients of eliminating arrhythmia susceptibility by radiofrequency ablation, or reducing risk by implantation of a pacemaker or implantable cardioverter-defibrillator (ICD) during the same procedure, provides further incentive for recommending electrophysiologic testing in syncope patients.

Although electrophysiologic studies are effective for eliciting susceptibility to symptomatic ventricular tachyarrhythmias in patients with some forms of ischemic heart disease (particularly ischemic disease), the method has important limitations. For example, torsades de pointes ventricular tachycardia is not easily provoked (see Long QT Syndromes, later), even with exogenous catecholamine provocation and long-short stimulation sequences. Conversely, the initiation of nonsustained ventricular tachycardia during studies (especially if polymorphous) has uncertain diagnostic implications.

Long QT Syndromes. The long QT syndromes (LQTSs) may not be among the most common causes of syncope, but they must always be kept in mind.[35–38] As a rule, they are most often iatrogenic, always life-threatening, and usually treatable if recognized promptly (Table 93–4). Syncope is primarily due to tachyarrhythmia (specifically torsades de pointes ventricular tachycardia). Torsades de pointes is a form of polymorphous ventricular tachycardia characterized by an undulating ECG waveform produced by a shifting QRS axis in the setting of QT interval prolongation (acquired or congenital in origin) (Fig. 93–2).

Acquired LQTS. The acquired form of LQTS is by far the more common, and it is most frequently the result of drugs that prolong the QT interval. Torsades de pointes in this setting is most often seen during periods of bradycardia (e.g., sleep) or after pauses in the cardiac rhythm (e.g., after premature ventricular contractions) that accentuate the QT interval. Some of the best known offending drugs are listed in Table 93–5. The majority of these act by antagonizing outward (i.e., repolarizing) potassium currents (e.g., class 1A and class 3 antiarrhythmic drugs). Other agents in this list are reported to interfere with the metabolism of drugs that directly prolong the QT interval. In general, the risk of torsades de pointes increases in proportion to the duration of the QT. However, although amiodarone may cause torsades de pointes, it does so less frequently than might be expected for the degree of QT interval lengthening it induces.[36]

Hypokalemia or hypomagnesemia may cause QT interval prolongation and torsades de pointes. On the other hand, although hypocalcemia prolongs the QT interval, torsades de pointes is rare. Other causes of QT interval prolongation and torsades de pointes include organophosphate insecticides, arsenic poisoning, intracranial disease (e.g., subarachnoid hemorrhage), extreme bradycardia, and liquid protein modified fast diets.[36]

Congenital LQTS. Congenital, idiopathic, or familial LQTS is caused by mutations in cardiac ion channels that contribute to the action potential repolarization process. Congenital LQTS is a very infrequent cause of syncope, but its identification can be life-saving. Affected individuals have QT prolongation and a high risk of recurrent syncope and sudden cardiac death owing to torsades de pointes. An international registry for LQTS was established in 1979.[37] Among 235 probands reported in a 1991 report,[37] the annual rates of recurrent syncope and probable LQTS-related death were 5 percent and 0.9 percent, respectively. Syncope and sudden death in this setting are frequently associated with emotional or physical arousal such as may be triggered by fear, loud noises, or exertion.[37, 38] Heterogeneity in clinical presentation exists, however, so that in other individuals torsades de pointes occurs owing to bradycardia or during sleep in conjunction with rate-dependent QT interval prolongation.[39]

The ECG hallmark of congenital LQTS is demonstration of abnormal ventricular repolarization (characterized by QT interval prolongation as well as by notched T waves or T wave alternans), potentially leading to torsades de pointes, in the absence of drugs or other disorders (e.g., acute neurologic injury) known to cause these ECG features. The abnormally long QT interval on the electrocardiogram results from lengthening of the cardiac action potential as a consequence of either prolongation of the depolarizing transmembrane currents (e.g., inward sodium current) or slowing of repolarizing currents (e.g., one of many outward potassium currents). Congenital LQTS has been shown to be caused by mutations in cardiac ion channels that contribute to the repolarization process. Prolongation of cellular repolarization allows the development of afterdepolarizations: depolarizing, subthreshold oscillations in transmembrane potential during or after the plateau phase of the action potential. Afterdepolarizations may reach threshold potential and thereby generate new premature action potentials (so-called triggered activity).[40] The

TABLE 93–4 1993 Long QT Syndrome Diagnostic Criteria

Criteria	Points*
ECG Findings†	
QT_c‡	
≥480 ms$^{1/2}$	3
460–470 ms$^{1/2}$	2
450 ms$^{1/2}$ (in males)	1
Torsades de pointes§	2
T wave alternans	1
Notched T wave in three leads	1
Low heart rate for age‖	0.5
Clinical History	
Syncope§	
With stress	2
Without stress	1
Congenital deafness	0.5
Family History	
Family members with definite LQTS**	1
Unexplained sudden cardiac death below age 30 among immediate family members	0.5

Abbreviations: ECG, electrocardiographic; LQTS, long QT syndrome.

**Scoring*: 1 point, low probability of LQTS; 2–3 points, intermediate probability of LQTS; 4 points, high probability of LQTS.

†In the absence of medications or disorders known to affect these ECG features.

‡QT_c calculated by Bazett's formula, where $QT_c = QT/(RR)^{1/2}$.

§Mutually exclusive.

‖Resting heart rate below the second percentile for age.

¶The same family member cannot be counted in both subcriteria.

**Definite LQTS is defined by an LQTS score 4.

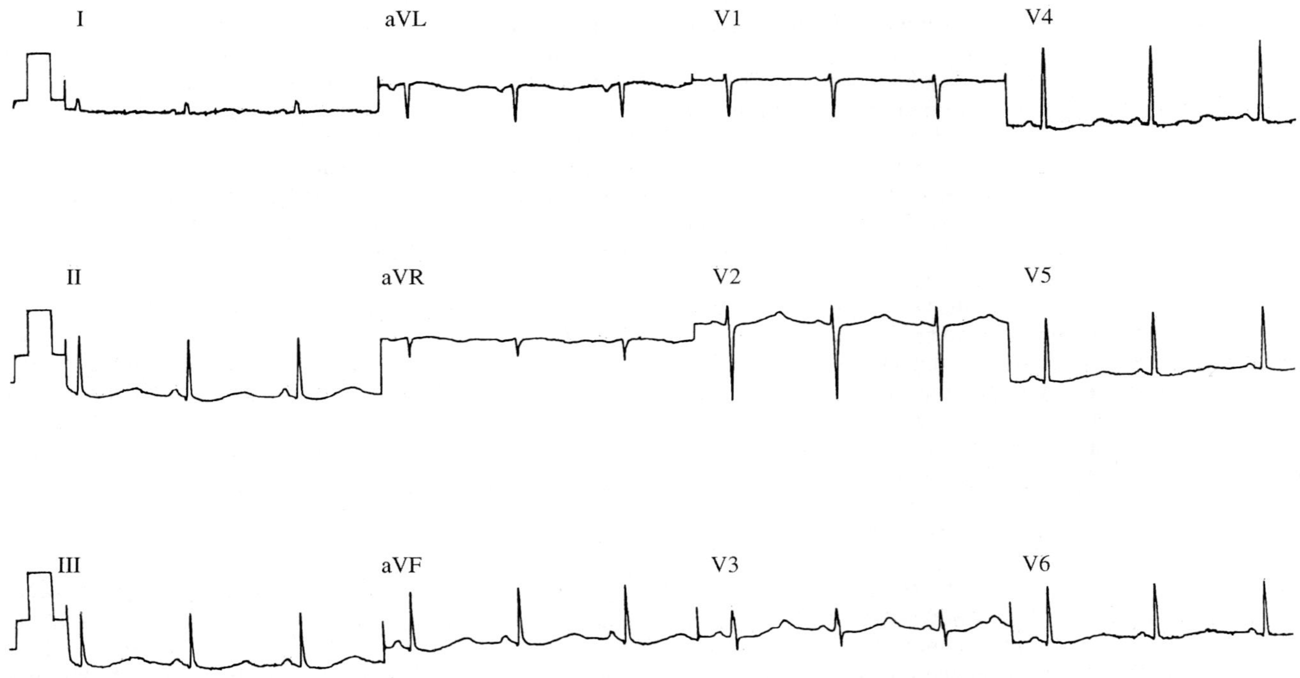

FIGURE 93–2 A 12-lead ECG from a young woman with a history of recurrent syncope. A prolonged QT interval is evident. Analysis of blood samples revealed her to exhibit a mutation in *KVLQT1* as the cause of the long QT interval.

current concept is that these afterdepolarizations and triggered activity are responsible for torsades de pointes.[36]

Molecular Biology of LQTS. The 1990s have witnessed extraordinary developments in the understanding of the molecular basis of LQTS. At the time of this writing, mutations causing LQTS have been identified in genes coding four specific cardiac ion channel proteins. A fifth LQTS locus has been identified on chromosome 4 (locus LQT4) but the associated gene remains to be identified.[40]

LQT1 was the first association reported between LQTS and a specific chromosome. A large family was found with autosomal dominant LQTS in which the genetic abnormality appeared on chromosome 11 and was in very close physical proximity to an oncogene known as HRAS.[41]

TABLE 93–5 Drugs Frequently Implicated in QT Prolongation and Torsades de Pointes

Antiarrhythmic Agents	*Tricyclic Antidepressants*
Class IA	Amitriptyline
Quinidine	Imipramine
Procainamide	*Antibiotics*
Disopyramide	Erythromycin
Class III	Pentamidine
Sotalol	Fluconazole
Ibutilide	*Nonsedating Antihistamines*
Amiodarone	Terfenadine
N-Acetylprocainamide (NAPA)	Astemizole
Antianginal Agents	*Others*
Bepridil	Cisapride
Psychoactive Agents	
Phenothiazines	
Thioridazine	

Initial speculation that HRAS might, in fact, be the *LQTS* gene in this family was ultimately rejected, but further study identified a gene labeled *KVLQT1* in which a mutation was clearly responsible for LQTS (see Fig. 93–2).[42] Expression of *KVLQT1* produces a protein that conducts potassium current unlike any previously seen. It was subsequently shown that the KVLQT1 protein coassembled with another protein known as minimal potassium channel subunit (minK) to form a slowly activating potassium current analogous to I_{Ks} (see later) described in guinea pig heart.[43, 44]

Before this understanding of the molecular basis of LQTS, two eponymous syndromes were frequently cited. The Jervell-Lange-Nielsen syndrome consists of congenital sensory deafness, prolonged QT interval, frequent syncope, and sudden death; the mode of inheritance is autosomal recessive.[45] In contrast, the more common Romano-Ward syndrome is not associated with deafness, and affected persons generally have milder symptoms. Its mode of inheritance is autosomal dominant.[46, 47] It has now been shown that a heterozygous mutation of *KVLQT1* can cause LQTS with normal hearing, whereas a homozygous mutation will also produce deafness and the Jervell-Lange-Nielsen syndrome.[48] Another form of LQTS (LQT5) has been demonstrated in patients with mutations in the *KCNE1* gene on chromosome 21 that produce an abnormal minK protein.[48] Conceivably, mutations in minK would also produce the Jervell-Lange-Nielsen syndrome. The Romano-Ward syndrome is presumably a heterogeneous group of patients in which a family may have mutations in any of the genes responsible for cardiac repolarization.

The LQT2 locus has been identified in humans on chromosome 7 where one of the major potassium channels is coded by a gene labeled *HERG*.[49] Multiple outward potassium currents are responsible for repolarization in myocardium. Two major components were originally described in guinea pig heart and named I_{Kr} and I_{Ks} for rapidly and slowly activating components, respectively.[50] The name *HERG,* human eag-related gene, derives from a distant *Drosophila* mutant termed *ether-a-go-go* (eag), in which a mutant potassium channel produced a distinctive "dance" in the fruit flies. The gene product of *HERG* is a potassium channel that appears analogous to I_{Kr} described in guinea pig.[51] Mutations in *HERG* have been identified in certain families with LQTS.[52] Several different mutations have subsequently been identified, ranging from simple amino acid substitutions to large deletions in families with LQTS linked to chromosome 7. Of particular importance, I_{Kr} and/or the *HERG* product is blocked by many drugs known to produce QT prolongation and torsades de pointes, including sotalol,[50] ibutilide,[53] terfenadine,[54] and erythromycin.[55] Thus, many forms of acquired QT prolongation and torsades de pointes are functionally similar to patients with LQTS2.

The LQT3 locus was mapped to chromosome 3 in several families with LQTS.[56] Mutations were subsequently found in the gene *SCN5A* on this chromosome that encodes for the sodium channel.[57] The mutations described do not allow normal inactivation of the sodium channel, resulting in prolonged sodium entry during repolarization.

Currently, only a few laboratories provide the capability to identify the variants of congenital LQTS. However, inasmuch as the variations have therapeutic implications, the availability of ready access to diagnostic testing should evolve. Ultimately, many more forms of LQTS will probably come to light.

MECHANICAL DISTURBANCES (OBSTRUCTION/INADEQUATE FLOW)

Syncope, occurring as a result of diminished cardiac output secondary to structural heart disease, is far less common than that due to disturbances of the heart's rhythm. Nevertheless, structural disturbances can contribute to syncopal symptoms both directly (i.e., reduced blood flow) and indirectly (i.e., disturbances of autonomic vascular control).

Perhaps the most common basis for syncope in association with structural heart disease is in conjunction with acute myocardial ischemia or infarction.[58, 59] In this setting, however, the mechanism of the faint may be multifactorial. Transient reduction of cardiac output, neural reflex mechanisms, cardiac arrhythmias, or a combination of these may be operative in a given patient. In the setting of obstruction to left ventricular outflow (e.g., aortic stenosis, hypertrophic obstructive cardiomyopathy), syncope has a grave prognostic significance, and may be contributed to both by the mechanical obstruction and by ventricular mechanoreceptor-mediated bradycardia and vasodilatation.[60, 61] The former mechanism may predominate during abrupt change in posture (e.g., sitting to standing) or in the presence of increased metabolic demand (e.g., fever), when fixed outflow limitation precludes an appropriate increase in forward flow. In the case of hypertrophic obstructive cardiomyopathy in particular, spontaneous occurrence of tachyarrhythmias, particularly atrial fibrillation but also ventricular tachycardia, may markedly impair forward flow and directly contribute to a syncopal event. Less commonly, left ventricular inflow obstruction may cause syncope on exertion in patients with mitral stenosis or at unpredictable times in patients with atrial myxoma. Other causes of syncope falling in this category (although the mechanisms are again multifactorial) include pulmonary hypertension, acute pulmonary embolism, and severe pericardial disease (see Table 93–1).

Noncardiovascular Causes of Syncope

Excluding seizure disorders and psychiatric disturbances, both of which tend to mimic rather than cause syncope, the most important contributors to the so-called noncardiovascular etiologies are cerebrovascular disease and metabolic and endocrine disturbances.

Cerebrovascular Disease

Cerebrovascular disease is only infrequently a primary cause of syncope. Nevertheless, its presence may increase susceptibility to syncope in patients who develop transient hypotensive periods (e.g., orthostatic drops in systemic pressure or otherwise benign arrhythmias). On rare occasion, transient ischemic attacks, especially those involving the vertebrobasilar system, may be associated with syncope. In cases in which a vertebrobasilar etiology seems likely, the cause may be atherosclerotic narrowings or extrinsic mechanical compression of the vertebral arteries (e.g., cervical spondylosis, cervical osteoarthritis, and cervical rib). Mechanical disturbances should receive particular consideration if attacks are associated with positional changes of the head, particularly extension or lateral rotation. However, in general terms, a vertebrobasilar etiology for symptoms is unlikely in the absence of residual focal neurologic findings.

Subclavian steal syndrome or severe carotid artery disease (e.g., atherosclerotic disease, Takayasu's disease) may be associated with syncope in some patients. In subclavian steal syndrome, narrowing of the subclavian artery at its origin results in syncope or dizziness in conjunction with upper extremity exercise as blood is shunted from the brain to the exercising limb via the vertebral artery system. Usually a bruit can be detected over the affected subclavian artery, along with diminution of ipsilateral brachial artery pressure.

Metabolic and Endocrine Disturbances

Metabolic and endocrine disturbances are rarely causes of syncope; they are more often responsible for confusional states or behavioral disturbances. In the older patient, it is not uncommon for several metabolic and/or endocrine conditions to interact, resulting in diminished cerebral nutrient or oxygen supply. Thus, hypoxemia due to heart failure, pneumonia, or pulmonary embolism may compound a chronic anemia in older individuals. Similarly, hypoglycemia or excessive hyperglycemia could similarly contribute to altered state of consciousness. In general, though, these conditions are not transient and do not reverse spontaneously. Consequently, disturbances of consciousness induced by metabolic and endocrine abnormalities are usually distinguishable from true syncopal events.

Symptoms virtually indistinguishable from true syncope may occur in association with anxiety attacks or hysteria.[62, 63] These cases tend to be more common in young patients, and in some cases, alcohol or drug abuse may be contributory. Hyperventilation may also contribute to symptoms in such patients. Whether cerebrovascular spasm in the absence of systemic hypotension accounts for a portion of patients currently categorized as manifesting *hysterical* faints remains to be determined.

Miscellaneous Conditions

Drop attacks are often incorporated along with considerations of syncope. However, they differ from true syncope by virtue of the fact that the patient retains consciousness despite abrupt loss of postural tone. The mechanism is not understood. However, selective, albeit transient, cerebral or spinal column ischemia could be at fault. In any event, the long-term prognosis seems to be favorable,[64] but further study is needed.

In summary, the essential pathophysiologic mechanism of syncope in the vast majority of cases is transient diminution of global cerebral nutrient flow. Although many disease states may contribute to susceptibility to syncope, cardiovascular disorders (including neurally mediated syncopal syndromes) are most frequently at fault.

DIAGNOSTIC STRATEGY

Although, as has been noted earlier, other conditions (e.g., seizures, sleep disorders, and accidents) may be misinterpreted as syncopal spells, in most instances it is not difficult to determine that the patient has suffered a syncopal spell. The greater challenge usually lies in identifying the specific cause of the faint. In this regard, Kapoor[65] provided important insight (from the perspective of the general internist or cardiologist) into the origins of syncope and its appropriate evaluation. Among 433 syncope patients assessed over an approximately 3-year period, a cause for symptoms was assigned in 254 (59 percent). The most common causes identified were cardiovascular: neurally mediated syncope in 71 patients, ventricular tachycardia in 49, orthostatic hypotension in 43, and drug-induced syncope in 9. Vascular disease compromising cerebrovascular blood flow accounted for 10 cases (4 percent of those assigned a diagnosis), with transient ischemic attacks occurring in 8 patients and subclavian steal in 2. Importantly, neurologic studies had an exceedingly low diagnostic yield, and despite the skill and experience of the investigator, 41 percent of cases remained unknown.

As a rule, a tentative basis for the cause of a syncopal event can often be established after careful assessment of the medical history (especially the history surrounding the symptomatic events, including eyewitness accounts), physical examination, and noninvasive cardiovascular studies (particularly 12-lead electrocardiogram and echocardiogram). However, diagnoses based on these findings alone are rarely definitive (ECG identification of congenital LQTS discussed earlier may be an exception, as would echocardiographic evidence of a large left atrial myxoma). Additional effort is usually necessary to establish the etiology with sufficient certainty to confidently begin therapy. For example, in a patient with pre-excitation syndrome, there is a tendency to assume that syncope is related to the predisposition to tachyarrhythmia. However, in so doing, one may overlook the actual cause of the problem. Similar judgment errors will occur if one assumes that frequent premature ventricular contractions mean that syncope was due to ventricular arrhythmia or that the presence of bifascicular conduction system disease signals AV block as the cause. Establishing a secure diagnosis usually demands further studies (e.g., long-term ECG monitoring, autonomic function testing, and electrophysiologic studies).

Initial Evaluation

The assessment of a syncopal episode requires careful questioning of the patient and witnesses. Circumstances surrounding the event, prodromal symptoms, the rapidity with which loss of consciousness occurred, duration of the event, and speed of recovery should be noted. As a rule, cardiac tachyarrhythmias and paroxysmal AV block result in rapid onset and prompt resolution of symptoms. Premonitory symptoms are variable, and palpitations may or may not be noted. Neurally mediated syncope may be suggested by association with characteristic scenarios or trigger events (e.g., medical procedures, pain, emotional upset, voiding, and cough), and this is often accompanied by a prodrome of sweating, nausea, pallor, and slow loss of vision and hearing. Recovery may be prompt, but a prolonged period of fatigue lasting hours to days after the event is relatively common.

An approach to the diagnostic evaluation of syncope is depicted in Figure 93–3. As a rule, routine unselected screening tests have a low diagnostic yield in the evaluation of syncopal spells and should be avoided. Additionally, as emphasized by Kapoor's experience,[65] neurologic testing (i.e., electroencephalogram, head computed tomography, or magnetic resonance imaging) is not often helpful in the early stages of the syncope assessment, and these studies are discouraged unless specific abnormal neurologic symptoms or signs are detected by history or during physical examination.

The choice of initial diagnostic studies is far more cost effective if based on careful consideration of the medical history, with the more common causes of syncope (i.e., neurally mediated and orthostatic—particularly drug-induced) being evaluated first. Thus, in the patient with hypertension or heart failure, the role of diuretics, angiotensin-converting enzyme inhibitors, and/or nitrates in causing syncope merits early consideration. In individuals with a history suggestive of acute or chronic gastrointestinal bleeding, the identification of anemia or blood in the stool may be the crucial test. In a known diabetic, appropriate biochemical studies may be directed to assess blood sugars and volume status. However, in the syncopal patient without history of other medical conditions and not taking suspect drugs, the focus should be to identify and characterize the severity of underlying structural heart disease. In the absence of clinically remarkable structural heart disease

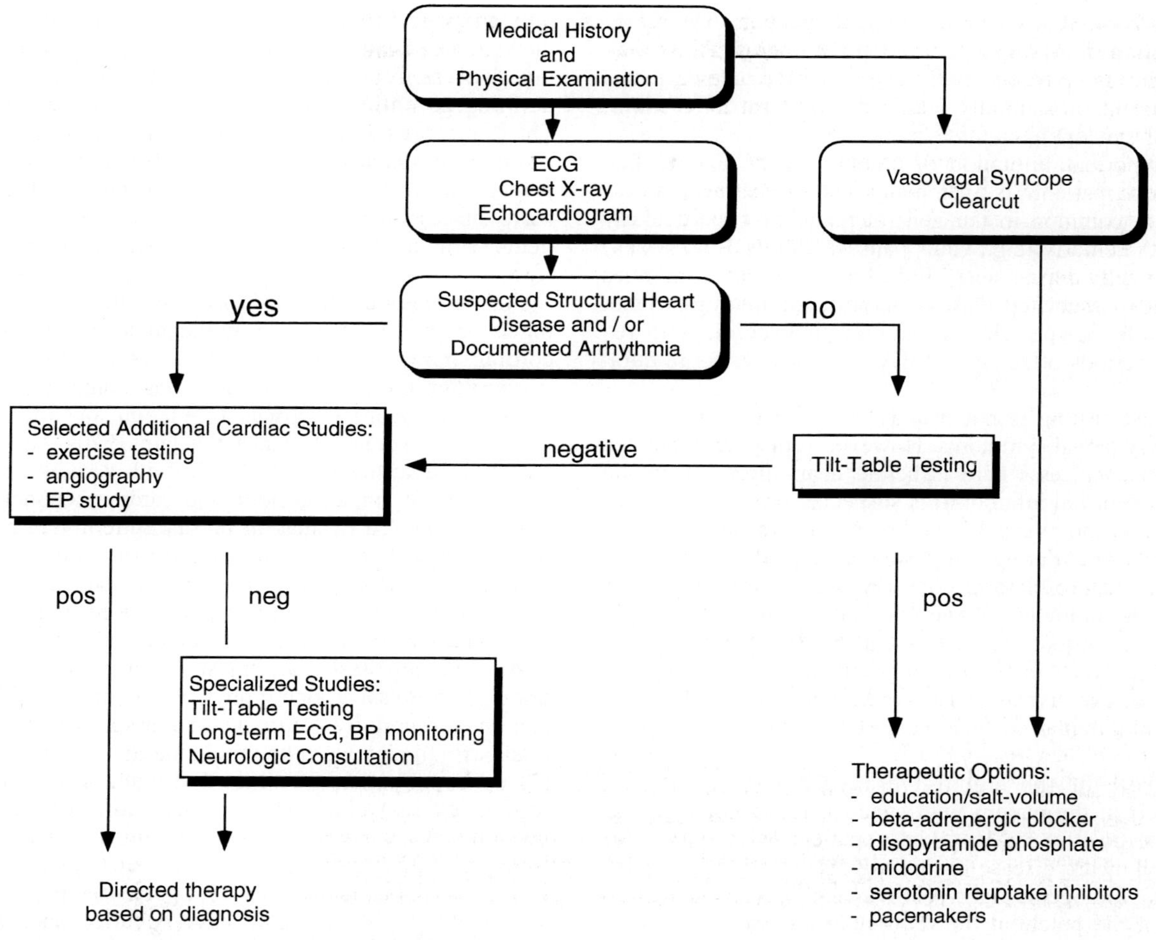

FIGURE 93–3 A strategy for selection of diagnostic studies for patients with syncope. BP, blood pressure; ECG, electrocardiogram; EP, electrophysiologic.

(as assessed by history, physical examination, electrocardiography, and echocardiography), autonomic system evaluation (particularly tilt-table testing) is the most effective place to start the syncope diagnostic evaluation. In addition, in the presence of significant structural heart disease, invasive cardiovascular studies (angiography, intracardiac pressure measurements) and electrophysiologic testing would seem prudent first steps. In individuals in whom these techniques prove to be unrewarding (or the outcomes are unconvincing), long-term ECG monitoring (including the use of an implantable loop recorder if necessary[66]) may be helpful.

Noninvasive Cardiovascular Studies

The 12-lead electrocardiogram and echocardiogram (and, to a lesser extent, the chest x-ray) are of particular value in the initial search for underlying cardiovascular disease. In the sense that the recognition of cardiovascular disease has important diagnostic implications in the syncope patient (see earlier), these studies are important. However, apart from a few cases in which unsuspected complete AV block, severe aortic valvular stenosis, or a left atrial myxoma is identified, they only rarely provide a complete explanation for syncopal symptoms.

Among patients with evident cardiovascular disease, cardiac arrhythmias are a particularly important cause of syncope (in terms of both frequency and prognostic significance). Consequently, vigorous attempts to correlate symptoms with rhythm disturbances are a common feature of the diagnostic evaluation of many syncope patients. In this regard, long-term outpatient ECG recordings are extremely valuable if symptoms occur during the recording session. However, conventional 24- or 48-hour Holter-type magnetic tape recordings are usually of inadequate duration unless the patient is experiencing very frequent symptoms. Event recorders, which can be used for much longer periods of time, are a more effective approach, and their effectiveness can be further enhanced by use of the continuous-loop mode. In this operating mode, the device is always monitoring the heart rhythm. However, only when the patient feels symptoms is a portion of the record saved (usually starting from some moments before the record button is pressed and continuing on for some time thereafter). Unfortunately, conventional continuous-loop event recorders require the patient to replace ECG electrodes on the skin each day (or sometimes several times each day);

this task is often too onerous for many patients. The recent introduction of an implantable loop recorder (ILR, Reveal, Medtronic Inc., Minneapolis, MN) should alleviate this problem and substantially facilitate long-term ECG monitoring of syncope patients.[66]

An important limitation of ambulatory ECG recording in syncope patients is that many "abnormalities" are in fact quite common in the general population, particularly among the elderly (e.g., sinus pauses, Mobitz 1 AV block) and especially during sleep. Therefore, unless abnormalities are clearly associated with symptoms, the findings cannot be considered specific. Persistence is crucial, with recording periods often several days to many weeks in duration.

Exercise testing is not usually of value in defining the basis of syncopal symptoms. However, it may be warranted in those instances where ischemic heart disease (but not acute myocardial infarction) is suspected or where exercise precipitated the event. In such cases, marked drop of systemic pressure during exertion may signal the presence of severe atherosclerotic coronary artery disease or even congenital anomalies of the coronary circulation in some cases. In addition, rate-dependent AV block or exercise-induced neurally mediated hypotension may be reproduced. Of course, exercise testing is contraindicated in the setting of critical valvular or dynamic aortic outflow tract obstruction.

The role of the signal-averaged electrocardiogram (SAECG) in the patient with syncope is incompletely defined. A positive SAECG in a patient with underlying structural heart disease (especially ischemic disease, but also arrhythmogenic right ventricular dysplasia) raises suspicion of the potential for ventricular tachyarrhythmias as the cause of syncope. However, the positive predictive accuracy of the SAECG is only moderate in this setting, and further invasive electrophysiologic testing would be warranted. On the other hand, a negative SAECG in a patient with ischemic heart disease is a valuable finding, as it largely eliminates the likelihood that ventricular tachyarrhythmia was at fault.[67, 68]

Certain new noninvasive tools have begun to become more widely available. Of these, the cine magnetic resonance imaging study is perhaps the most effective tool to evaluate patients for evidence of arrhythmogenic right ventricular dysplasia. However, its applicability should be restricted to those syncope patients in whom the diagnosis is being seriously considered. The roles of the P wave–averaged electrocardiogram for diagnosing sinus node dysfunction and of T wave dispersion for assessing arrhythmia risk in ischemic heart disease have yet to be determined in the syncope population.

Invasive Electrophysiologic Testing

Although noninvasive studies are often sufficient to identify and to some extent assess the severity of underlying structural heart disease in the syncope patient, invasive hemodynamic evaluation and angiography are often required as well in order to define treatment direction. Most often, though, the presence of structural heart disease implies susceptibility to arrhythmia (tachycardia or bradycardia), and it is arrhythmia that is most often responsible for the syncopal symptoms. In general, it is in these cases that invasive electrophysiologic testing has proved useful for defining potential arrhythmic causes of syncope.[35, 69–72] Thus, in a review by Camm and Lau,[35] electrophysiologic testing was deemed to have provided a diagnosis in 56 percent of all patients. However, the testing was clearly more successful in patients with (71 percent) than in patients without (36 percent) apparent structural cardiac disease.

For purposes of this discussion, electrophysiologic testing is deemed to comprise multichannel surface ECG recording, intracardiac electrogram recording (generally from two or three sites, including the cardiac conduction system–His bundle region), electrical stimulation, and arterial blood pressure measurement. Since the late 1970s, such testing has evolved sufficiently to permit (with variable precision) assessment of sinoatrial node and cardiac conduction system function and evaluation of susceptibility to many supraventricular and ventricular tachyarrhythmias (the latter usually determined using programmed electrical stimulation techniques). Tilt-table testing and related studies of autonomic system function are considered separately later.

As with any test, care must be taken in interpreting findings of invasive electrophysiologic studies. For example, in a report by Fujimura and associates,[73] in which bradyarrhythmias were known to be the cause of syncope (21 syncopal patients with known symptomatic AV block or sinus pauses), electrophysiologic testing correctly identified only 3 of 8 patients with documented sinus pauses (sensitivity 37.5 percent) and 2 of 13 patients with documented AV block (sensitivity 15.4 percent). However, other abnormalities not known to have occurred spontaneously in these individuals were often induced during electrophysiologic study. Consequently, one must be alert to false-positive results, especially in patients with structural heart disease. Conversely, false-negative studies may occur owing to failure to elicit certain fastidious rhythm disturbances during testing. Nevertheless, certain findings, such as Mobitz type 2 AV block, an atrio-His interval greater than 100 ms, infra-His type 1 (Wenckebach) AV block during moderate rate atrial pacing, or inducible monomorphic sustained supraventricular or ventricular tachycardia, are probably of diagnostic significance in the syncope patient. Other findings, including abnormal sinus node recovery times, drug-induced His-ventricular interval prolongation, and inducible polymorphous ventricular tachycardia, are often suggestive of a diagnosis but are of less certain significance.

Autonomic Function Testing

The role played by the autonomic nervous system function in triggering symptomatic hypotension has become increasingly appreciated in recent years, and it appears to be particularly important when syncope occurs in individuals who otherwise seem to be in good health (e.g., exhibit no evidence of structural cardiovascular or neurologic disease). At the present time, head-up tilt-table testing and carotid sinus massage are the most widely applied tests used in this setting. However, other procedures such as response to Valsalva maneuver, assessment of baroreceptor sensitivity, response to cough, and evaluation of intrinsic heart rate may provide additional insight in specific patients.

In regard to the role of tilt-table testing for evaluation of syncope patients, a number of observations support the notion that symptomatic hypotension-bradycardia associated with a positive head-up tilt test is comparable to the spontaneous neurally mediated vasovagal syncope.[74–78] First, both induced and spontaneous syncopal episodes tend to be associated with similar premonitory symptoms (e.g., nausea, diaphoresis) and signs (e.g., marked pallor, loss of postural tone). Second, the temporal sequence of blood pressure and heart rate changes during tilt-induced syncopal spells parallel those reported for spontaneous episodes. Finally, plasma catecholamines measured before and during spontaneous and tilt-induced syncope exhibit important similarities. In particular, premonitory increases in circulating catecholamines appear to characterize both the spontaneous vasovagal faint and the tilt-induced hypotension-bradycardia.

Tilt-table testing, especially when undertaken in the absence of provocative pharmacologic agents, appears to discriminate quite well between symptomatic patients and asymptomatic control subjects. de Mey and Enterling[79] reported only 8 instances of hypotension-bradycardia among 40 apparently normal subjects (20 percent). Fitzpatrick and colleagues[80, 81] indicated that 60-degree upright tilt for 45 minutes was accompanied by development of syncope in only 7 percent of 27 subjects without a history of syncope (mean time to syncope, 35 ± 5 minutes). Similarly, during a 45-minute drug-free tilt at 60 degrees, Raviele and coworkers[82] noted that among 35 control subjects, none developed syncope. Grubb and associates[83, 84] also observed a relatively low false-positive rate associated with tilt-testing in both elderly and young patients. Finally, in regard to the potential impact of pharmacologic agents on specificity of tilt testing, Natale and colleagues[85] examined the outcome of tilt-testing at various angles and with various doses of isoproterenol provocation in 150 volunteers with no prior history of syncope or presyncope. They found tilt-table testing at 60, 70, and 80 degrees to exhibit specificities of 92 percent, 92 percent, and 80 percent, respectively, when low doses of isoproterenol were used. In summary, most studies suggest that tilt-table testing at angles of 60 to 70 degrees, in the absence of pharmacologic provocation, exhibits a specificity of approximately 90 percent. In the presence of pharmacologic provocation, test specificity may be reduced, although the magnitude of this reduction is unclear. Recent experience, however, suggests that in the case of isoproterenol provocation, an infusion rate of 1 μg/min is associated with test specificity not much diminished from a drug-free tilt.

The response to upright tilt-table testing in patients with suspected neurally mediated syncope differs from that observed in syncope patients in whom other diagnostic studies have provided a firm basis for symptoms. In an early report advocating the use of upright posture during conventional electrophysiologic testing to assess the hemodynamic impact of observed arrhythmias, Hammill and coworkers[86] noted that only the 6 patients with histories most compatible with vasovagal syncope developed hypotension-bradycardia–related syncopal symptoms during head-up tilt. Similarly, Fitzpatrick and colleagues[81] found that a 60-degree upright tilt reproduced symptoms in 53 of 71 patients (75 percent) with unexplained syncope; 40 exhibited both hypotension and bradycardia, whereas 13 manifested primarily a vasodepressor response.

The methodology for tilt-table testing has been the subject of some debate for a number of years. Although differences remain, the American College of Cardiology Expert Task Force report provides a useful starting point for most laboratories.[87] As a rule, tilt-testing should be undertaken in a quiet environment, using an angle of 70 to 80 degrees for 45 minutes in the absence of pharmacologic provocation. Thereafter, various agents have been used to enhance test sensitivity (although with some inevitable loss of specificity). Isoproterenol, edrophonium, and nitroglycerin are currently the most widely used provocative agents.

Carotid sinus stimulation provides a means of directly initiating afferent neural activity from at least one set of mechanoreceptors known to be capable of inducing a neurally mediated hypotensive bradycardic response. However, false-positive observations are a concern, especially among older men and patients with atherosclerotic disease (so-called carotid sinus hypersensitivity). True carotid sinus syncope is much less common, but not rare. In fact, carotid sinus syndrome may be responsible for more falls in older patients than has previously been recognized.[88] An induced pause of 5 seconds or longer is probably of clinical relevance, and even shorter pauses may be suggestive if the medical history is compatible (e.g., syncope with neck/head movement, prior head/neck irradiation or surgery).[89–92]

The Valsalva maneuver and the blood pressure response to cough may be useful diagnostic tests in certain forms of neurally mediated syncope such as the mess trick or cough syncope. However, the range of normal values for these tests remains uncertain, and the positive predictive value of a presumably abnormal test result is as yet unstudied.

Combined Electrophysiologic and Tilt-Table Studies in Syncope

The addition of tilt-table testing to electrophysiologic testing has substantially enhanced diagnostic capabilities in syncope patients. For example, Sra and associates[71] reported results of electrophysiologic testing in conjunction with head-up tilt testing in 86 consecutive patients referred for evaluation of unexplained syncope. Electrophysiologic testing was abnormal in 29 patients (34 percent), with the majority of these (21 patients) being inducible sustained monomorphic ventricular tachycardia. The remainder comprised inducible supraventricular tachycardias (5 patients), sinoatrial dysfunction (1 patient), and conduction system disease (2 patients). Among the remaining patients, head-up tilt-testing proved positive in 34 cases (40 percent), and 23 patients (26 percent) remained undiagnosed. In general, patients exhibiting positive electrophysiologic findings were older, more frequently male, and exhibited lower ventricular ejection fractions and higher frequency of evident heart disease than was the case in patients with positive head-up tilt-table tests or patients in whom no diagnosis was determined. During follow-up, syncope recurrence occurred in approximately 13 percent of patients. Importantly, however, syncope recurrence in patients in whom treatment was directed by electrophysiologic testing or tilt-table testing seemed to be highly associated with discontinuation of recommended therapies.

A further evaluation of the combined use of electrophysiologic testing and head-up tilt-table testing in the assessment of syncope is provided in the report by Fitzpatrick and coworkers.[81] Among 322 syncope patients evaluated between 1984 and 1988, conventional electrophysiologic testing provided a basis for syncope in 229 of 322 cases (71 percent), with 93 patients having a normal electrophysiologic study. Among the patients with abnormal electrophysiologic findings, AV conduction disease was diagnosed in 34 percent, sinus node dysfunction in 21 percent, carotid sinus syndrome in 10 percent, and an inducible sustained tachyarrhythmia in 6 percent. As noted previously, in the 93 patients with normal conventional electrophysiologic studies, tilt-table testing was undertaken in 71 cases and reproduced syncope, consistent with a vasovagal mechanism, in 53 of the 71 patients (75 percent). Overall, a diagnosis of neurally mediated vasovagal syncope was made in 16 percent of the entire patient population, a percentage that largely reflects the selected nature of the study population, and is therefore lower than would be expected in a broader range of syncope patients (e.g., those presenting to emergency rooms or general medical clinics).

Neurologic Studies

In general, conventional neurologic laboratory studies (electroencephalogram, head computed tomography, and magnetic resonance imaging) have relatively low diagnostic yield in the syncope patient. However, given the importance of orthostatic and dysautonomic causes of syncope, tilt-table testing and other tests of autonomic function have (always used with and interpreted in the light of a careful medical history) an increasingly important role to play. Tilt-table testing has been dealt with in some detail earlier. However, in addition to the tilt-table's utility in diagnosing susceptibility to the vasovagal faint, assessment of the heart rate and blood pressure response during head-up tilt may also be helpful in identifying patients with a propensity for orthostatic hypotension and/or postural orthostatic tachycardia syndrome.

NATURAL HISTORY AND EPIDEMIOLOGY

General Considerations

Syncope may be a presenting feature of a wide range of disorders. In terms of natural history, the ultimate clinical outcome depends primarily on the nature and severity of the underlying disease process. Thus, in the case of acquired complete AV block, the onset of which is often accompanied by syncope, untreated mortality risk is quite high. Similarly, syncope associated with valvular aortic stenosis or occurring during exertion in patients with severe coronary artery disease has a worrisome prognostic implication. On the other hand, the natural history of neurally mediated syncope (especially vasovagal syncope) is less certain, but available evidence suggests that the mortality risk is low (although the risk of syncope recurrences is high).

The Framingham study provides the best overview of the epidemiologic aspects of syncope in a large free-living population.[93] More than 2300 men and 2800 women were examined every 2 years from entry into the study (1948 to 1952). After 13 biennial (26-year) follow-ups, 27 subjects (15 men, 12 women) with a known history of cardiac or neurologic disease reported syncopal symptoms. So-called isolated syncope (e.g., syncope in the absence of evident cardiovascular or neurologic disease) occurred in 56 men and 89 women. Thus, during this 26-year period, 3 percent of men and 3.5 percent of women experienced a syncopal episode. Further, among the isolated syncope cohort, approximately 30 percent reported syncope recurrences.

The age-specific incidence of isolated syncope increased with age for both men and women. By way of example, for men in the 35- to 44-year age group, the incidence was 7 per 1000 person examinations, compared with 56 per 1000 in those patients aged 75 years and older. Findings were comparable in women. In terms of subsequent morbidity and mortality, isolated syncope did not seem to predispose individuals to increased likelihood of stroke, myocardial infarction, or cardiovascular mortality. However, concern remains that syncope recurrences could increase the possibility of nonfatal accidents and consequent increased medical costs.

The outcome of patients with syncope associated with cardiovascular disease seems to be much more alarming than is the case for isolated syncope. In an early report, Kapoor and associates[94] provided patient outcome during follow-up based on categorization of the syncopal event as being more or less likely to be due to a cardiovascular versus a noncardiovascular disturbance (neurally mediated events were considered noncardiovascular in this case). Among the 204 patients included in the study, 53 were classified as having cardiovascular syncope, 54 as noncardiovascular, and the remainder as unknown. The findings, although subject to substantial limitation owing to the inadequate diagnostic tools at the time, indicated a 12-month mortality rate of 30 percent among patients with a cardiovascular cause compared with 12 percent among patients with noncardiovascular syncope and 6.4 percent in the unknown group. The incidence of sudden death was particularly worrisome (24 percent in the cardiovascular group versus 4 percent and 3 percent in the other two groups, respectively).

In more recent years, electrophysiologic testing was added to the diagnostic armamentarium. Using this tool, Bass and colleagues[95] from Kapoor's laboratory reassessed outcomes in syncope patients. Tilt-table testing was not undertaken. Among 70 patients included in the study, an apparent basis for syncope was obtained by electrophysiologic testing in 37 cases (electrophysiology positive). Compared with the electrophysiology-negative patients, the electrophysiology-positive subgroup (not unexpectedly) had a higher incidence of previous myocardial infarction (43 percent versus 21 percent), bundle branch block (38 percent versus 15 percent), and Holter monitor evidence of ventricular tachycardia (>3 beats: 57 percent versus 27 percent). These latter patients also tended more often to be male and to exhibit a higher frequency of congestive heart failure, stroke, valvular heart disease, and premature ventricular contractions. On the other hand, multiple syncopal episodes tended to be more common in the electrophysiology-negative group (possibly indicating that these patients were exhibiting a more benign form of syncope from a mortality perspective).

The observations by Bass and colleagues[95] do not address natural history, but they nevertheless provide valuable insight into outcomes in syncope patients risk-stratified by electrophysiologic testing. The 3-year actuarial rate of recurrent syncope was 28 percent among all patients (32 percent in electrophysiology-positive versus 24 percent in the negative patients). In addition, there was a substantial difference between the groups with respect to sudden death and total mortality. At 3 years, the group with positive electrophysiologic findings exhibited a 48 percent sudden death rate and a 61 percent total mortality. This finding is consistent with a high prevalence of ventricular tachycardia diagnoses (31 of 37 patients) in this group (and possibly the lack of ready availability of ICD therapy at the time). By contrast, the electrophysiology-negative group had a 9 percent sudden death rate and a 15 percent total mortality.

As noted earlier, the Kapoor and Bass studies[94, 95] do not give a clear picture of the natural history of syncope. The patients were treated according to the therapeutic principles of the time. Such treatment may have masked potential morbidity and mortality in some cases, although it is just as likely that the unrecognized proarrhythmic effects of certain treatments may have biased the outcomes adversely in many other instances (especially patients with ventricular tachyarrhythmias treated with conventional antiarrhythmic agents).

A pure natural history study can no longer be justified in syncope patients with significant underlying structural heart disease, given our current understanding of the risk associated with delaying therapy. Indirect information may, however, still be obtainable in certain patient subgroups that receive pacemakers and/or implantable cardioverter defibrillators. These devices are capable of logging arrhythmic events quite accurately in a prospective manner. On the other hand, studies designed to obtain greater understanding of the natural history of neurally mediated syncope remain defensible. In fact, important progress has already been reported by Sheldon and coworkers.[96, 97] In essence, these investigators have been able to show that the risk of syncope recurrence is greatest in those patients with vasovagal syncope having already experienced a large number of prior syncopal episodes, and in whom the preceding duration of syncopal symptom history is relatively long.

Specific Conditions

Neurally Mediated Syncopal Syndromes

The natural history of vasovagal syncope has been alluded to earlier. Of the other neurally mediated syncopal syndromes, only carotid sinus syndrome has been studied in sufficient detail to provide some insight into untreated patient outcomes.

In a relatively early report, Sugrue and associates[98] assessed outcomes in 56 patients with syncope and carotid sinus hypersensitivity. During 6 to 120 months of follow-up, syncope recurred in 3 of 13 patients who received no treatment, compared with 2 of 23 who received single-chamber pacemakers. Based on these findings, the authors concluded that therapeutic intervention was not crucial. However, their findings may be criticized as not having been based on what would now be considered adequate diagnostic testing. In this regard, Brignole and colleagues[99] provided a more recent examination of this issue. During an 8-month follow-up in their patients with well-documented carotid sinus syndrome, 47 percent of patients on no therapy exhibited syncope recurrences and 68 percent experienced at least some symptoms. By the 16th month of follow-up, only 36 percent of patients remained syncope free. Thus, carotid sinus syndrome patients are at risk for recurrences of syncope, and prompt treatment (usually with a cardiac pacemaker) is warranted once the diagnosis is established.

Cardiac Causes of Syncope

The risks associated with syncope caused by cardiac arrhythmias have been discussed in some detail earlier. As pointed out, a true natural history outcome cannot be readily derived, but the risks seem to be worrisome. The same can be said for syncope associated with acquired AV block.

In regard to syncope accompanying valvular heart disease, those patients with left ventricular outflow obstruction are clearly at gravest risk. Patients with syncope associated with aortic stenosis have been reported to have an average survival of only 3 years. Of course, these patients now tend to undergo prosthetic valve replacement, and the natural history of the condition has thereby been entirely changed. Syncope is also a worrisome symptom in hypertrophic obstructive cardiomyopathy patients.[100–103] For example, in one follow-up study incorporating 37 young patients, Romeo and coworkers[100] reported 9 sudden deaths (24 percent) at an average follow-up of 9 years (3 percent per year). Syncope was among the most important adverse prognostic risk factors.

Syncope Associated With Congenital and Acquired Repolarization Disorders (LQTSs)

The basis of LQTSs has been considered at length earlier. In brief, the congenital forms are associated with a high frequency of syncope and a very grave prognosis untreated. For instance, among the four deaf siblings reported by Jervell and Lange-Nielsen,[45] three died before age 10 years. Similarly, among 235 probands reported in the previously noted international LQTS registry, the annual rate of recurrent syncope and probable LQTS-related death was 5 percent and 0.9 percent, respectively.[37] The same level of risk probably applies in acquired LQTSs, although in these cases, prompt recognition of the problem and removal of the offending agent(s) provides a ready solution to the problem.

TREATMENT

Neurally Mediated Syncopal Syndromes

In the case of neurally mediated syncopal syndromes, treatment strategies remain in evolution. Specific treatment should, when possible, be directed at relieving apparent trigger factors. Examples include alleviating the cause of cough in cough syncope or treating esophageal abnormalities in swallow syncope. However, in conditions such as carotid sinus syncope and vasovagal syncope, this type of direct approach is not usually available. Therefore, in the former case, cardiac pacing has become a primary treatment modality (recognizing that in many instances additional consideration must be given the concomitant vasodepressor element of the syndrome). In the case of vasovagal syncope, the mainstay in treatment is explanation and reassurance, followed, if necessary, by drugs and, on rare occasion, by cardiac pacing. Education alone proves most effective when there is a prodrome of sufficient duration to permit the patient to take suitable evasive action. Patients whose symptoms demand more aggressive approaches to therapy than education and reassurance are those whose attacks have minimal or no prodrome (especially if they have had resulting injury), those who cannot be taught to abort attacks, and those whose attacks are complicated by seizure-like activity or incontinence. Additionally, patients with high-risk occupations or avocations in which syncope might lead to injury to themselves or others present a concern (e.g., pilots, commercial drivers, window-washers, and swimmers).

Among patients with vasovagal syncope in whom conservative treatment measures are either ineffective or not applicable, a variety of pharmacologic approaches have been the subject of recent attention. In this regard, β-adrenergic blocking drugs, disopyramide, and to a lesser extent, vasoconstrictor agents (e.g., midrodine, ergotamine preparations, and ephedrine) are the principal agents utilized in treatment of patients with recurrent vasovagal syncope. Volume expanders (e.g., fludrocortisone and salt tablets) continue to find application, particularly in pediatric and young adult patients. Vagolytic agents (e.g., scopolamine), on the other hand, are less popular owing to uncertain efficacy and frequent annoying side effects (e.g., dry mouth, constipation, and urinary retention). Another group of drugs that appears to be useful in selected cases is the serotonin-reuptake inhibitors. However, only a very small experience currently exists regarding their effectiveness.

Despite the existence of a substantial literature on the pharmacologic treatment of vasovagal syncope, the efficacy of any of the proposed agents is uncertain.[104–107] Most of the published reports are uncontrolled studies. The few small controlled studies that have been reported (atenolol, Caffedrine, disopyramide, scopolamine, and etilefrine) all have methodologic problems. Nonetheless, only one of these (β-adrenergic blocker, atenolol) has shown a drug benefit over a 1 month follow-up.[108] One report suggests that the magnitude of sinus tachycardia present before syncope offers a clue to the potential benefit of β-adrenergic blockade therapy.

Cardiac pacing has proved highly successful in carotid sinus syndrome when bradycardia has been documented.[109] Currently, pacing is acknowledged to be the treatment of choice in all but the mildest forms of carotid sinus syndrome. Debate exists only concerning the mode of pacing (e.g., single-chamber versus dual-chamber ventricular pacing). In general, dual-chamber pacing with an abrupt rate-drop recognition feature and rapid pacing rate hysteresis response is desirable. The VVI or VVIR pacing mode should be chosen only if there is clear absence of both susceptibility to ventricular pacing effect (e.g., a drop in systemic pressure as a result of ventricular pacing alone) and a substantial concomitant vasodepressor element.[99, 109, 110] Single-chamber atrial pacing (AAI or AAIR) is contraindicated in carotid sinus syndrome (and other forms of neurally mediated syncope) owing to the propensity for these patients to exhibit paroxysmal high-grade AV block during the episodes. Incidentally, the presence of AV block may be "masked" by marked sinus bradycardia or asystole, but it becomes immediately evident when the atrium is paced.

In contrast to carotid sinus syndrome, experience with pacing in vasovagal syncope other forms of neurally mediated syncope has been much more limited, although seemingly favorable.[111–113] In the case of vasovagal syncope, pacing may play a useful role when reserved for severe cases in which recurring periods of cardioinhibitor appear to be responsible for symptoms. In other cases, currently available pacing techniques may be expected to prolong the prodrome. Ultimately, if evasive action is not taken, syncope will occur in most cases. Nevertheless, a delay in onset of syncope, which permits the patient to recognize what is transpiring, may prove beneficial in avoiding injury and accidents. Again, atrial pacing alone (e.g., AAI or AAIR modes) is contraindicated owing to the potential for paroxysmal AV block. Similarly, single-chamber ventricular pacing (VVI or VVIR modes) is not likely to be effective. Further, as was true for carotid sinus syncope, it is essential that the pacing system be capable of detecting imminent neurally mediated syncopal events and providing a form of rate hysteresis in order to pace sufficiently rapidly when necessary. Currently, an abrupt change in heart rate is used to trigger the vasovagal treatment response. Ultimately, other sensor systems may prove helpful for improving the specificity and timeliness of the response.

Orthostatic and Dysautonomic Disturbances of Blood Pressure Control

Although the recognition of patients with some form of symptomatic autonomic disturbance has increased in recent years, treatment remains unsatisfactory. Indeed, apart from perhaps placement of greater emphasis on physical maneuvers (e.g., counterpressure clothing, leg crossing, and sleeping with the head of the bed elevated),[114, 115] the treatment of orthostatic and dysautonomic causes of syncope is in many respects similar to that of the neurally mediated syncopal syndromes. Unfortunately, unlike most neurally mediated syncopal syndromes, many autonomic disturbances tend to be persistent over very long periods of time (an exception being those resulting directly from prolonged bed rest or similar inactivity or exposure to weightlessness) and relatively unresponsive to most available pharmacologic therapies.

The mainstay of treatment has been attempted chronic expansion of central circulating volume. To this end, certain pharmacologic approaches are well accepted; specifically, administration of increased salt in the diet and use of salt-retaining steroids (e.g., principally fludrocortisone, which may in addition provide some vasoconstrictor action) are usually the first steps. Additional benefit has been reported with the use of agents, such as erythropoietin, that increase blood volume. A second element in the treatment strategy is reduction of the tendency for central volume to be displaced to the lower extremities with upright posture. To this end, both directly and indirectly acting vasoconstrictors have been employed, although with limited success owing to the tendency for tachyphylaxis to develop. Thus, ephedrine has limited efficacy. Clonidine has been reported to be helpful,[116] but there appears to be little ongoing enthusiasm for its use. Serotonin reuptake inhibitors may also be helpful, but clinical experience is limited to date. Of greatest current interest is midrodine, an agent that has prominent venoconstrictor properties and that has proved to be well tolerated.[117] Physical maneuvers such as the use of counterpressure clothing (e.g., fitted stockings and abdominal compression devices) can be helpful, but these are uncomfortable (especially in hot climates) and expose the patient to even worse symptoms when removed.

Physical rehabilitation (gentle progressive increments of exercise), with enforced periods of increasing exposure to upright posture, is generally an advisable ancillary therapeutic approach.[114, 115, 118, 119] Another option, cardiac tachypacing, may prove valuable in certain selected cases, but this has yet to be adequately tested in large numbers of individuals.[120–122]

Primary Cardiac Arrhythmias

The appropriate treatment of patients in whom bradyarrhythmias or tachyarrhythmias are the cause of syncope is relatively well understood and is not dealt with in detail here. Suffice it to say that patients in whom there is a well-defined correlation between documented bradyarrhythmias and symptoms of syncope or dizziness do very well with cardiac pacemaker therapy.[123, 124] However, other factors are often important contributors to the decision process. For instance, in the case of individuals with sinus node dysfunction, optimal selection of treatment necessitates consideration of not only the culprit arrhythmic disturbance but also the effects of drugs on sinus node and AV conduction properties and on ventricular function and proarrhythmic tendency. Additionally, current indications for and available modes of cardiac pacing and the role of anticoagulation must be incorporated in the overall treatment strategy. Finally, the currently evolving role of transcatheter or surgical ablation for atrial arrhythmia control warrants examination. In regard to ablation, only a relatively small proportion of sinus node dysfunction patients undergo such procedures currently. In the majority of these cases, His bundle ablation is used to facilitate control of ventricular rate.[125] On occasion, modification of the sinus node region has been advocated for cases of symptomatic inappropriate sinus tachycardia (a condition that seems to be frequently associated with syncope, although probably most often neurally mediated in origin).[126, 127] The longer-term success of the latter approach has been quite variable. Transcatheter ablation for control of atrial flutter, on the other hand, has been highly successful (reported success rates of 80 to 90 percent). It is best reserved for those patients in whom atrial flutter is the solitary primary atrial tachycardia, but it may be beneficial in a broader array of individuals in whom atrial flutter either is the most symptomatic arrhythmia or is thought to initiate other arrhythmias such as atrial fibrillation.

Transcatheter techniques for altering atrial electrophysiologic milieu and reducing susceptibility to atrial fibrillation have evolved rapidly in the past few years. The potential for such procedures to be of benefit to patients with recurrent syncope owing to the abrupt onset of atrial fibrillation is now a real possibility.[128–130] Surgical methods for direct treatment of atrial fibrillation are currently confined to a selected small number of patients who are undergoing surgery for other cardiac problems (e.g., mitral valve repair or replacement) and are routinely undertaken at relatively few surgical centers.[131]

In general, cardiac pacemaker therapy has proved highly effective in preventing symptom recurrences in patients with syncope owing to bradyarrhythmias, whether due to sinus node dysfunction or to AV conduction disturbances. For the most part, modern pacing practice is moving away from use of single-chamber ventricular pacing (VVI, VVIR modes), unless persistent atrial fibrillation precludes atrial pacing. Pacing techniques that endeavor to maintain a normal AV relationship not only offer better hemodynamic responses but also eliminate symptoms commonly associated with pacemaker syndrome and tend to diminish the likelihood of later development of atrial fibrillation and its consequent risk of thromboembolism.[132–137] However, stroke risk reduction by anticoagulation is an important element in the treatment of individuals with paroxysmal or persistent atrial fibrillation. In this regard, there is solid evidence supporting the use of warfarin therapy (for review, see Laupacis and accosiates[138]). Further, while the merits of full-dose (325 mg) aspirin therapy remain to be resolved, warfarin is clearly superior to minidose aspirin (75 mg) and is probably the most effective drug available for thromboembolic prophylaxis. In brief, long-term oral anticoagulant therapy should be considered for all older patients (usually characterized as older than 65 years) and for younger patients with the following risk factors: a previous transient ischemic attack or stroke, hypertension, heart failure, diabetes, clinical coronary artery disease, mitral stenosis, prosthetic heart valve, or thyrotoxicosis.[138]

In large measure, paroxysmal supraventricular tachyarrhythmias can be adequately controlled by conventional antiarrhythmic drug treatment. β-Adrenergic blockers or calcium channel blockers may be effective alone or, if necessary, in combination with class 1 antiarrhythmics (particularly class 1C drugs such as flecainide and propafenone). Class 3 drugs such as sotalol or dofetilide may also be used effectively, although there is greater concern regarding QT interval prolongation and its potential proarrhythmic consequences. However, long-term drug treatment is not readily maintained in many paroxysmal supraventricular tachyarrhythmia patients owing to side effects, issues of compliance, and occasionally, expense. Transcatheter ablation (currently primarily undertaken using radiofrequency heating [e.g., radiofrequency ablation]) has become a highly effective and very safe treatment option.[139, 140] In the case of paroxysmal re-entrant supraventricular tachyarrhythmia associated with syncope, transcatheter ablation is probably the treatment of choice because a successful ablation is the most secure method for eliminating the potential for symptomatic arrhythmia recurrence. At the same time, the risks of drug-related side effects or proarrhythmia are averted.

In the case of syncope due to ventricular tachycardia, underlying heart disease (especially left ventricular dysfunction) of varying degrees of severity is usually present. The latter increases the proarrhythmic risk associated with antiarrhythmic drug therapy, especially with class 1 agents. Consequently, pharmacologic therapeutic strategies often involve early consideration of class 3 agents (principally sotalol or amiodarone at the present time). However, given the difficulty of ensuring effective prophylaxis in this apparently high-risk patient population, the use of ICDs has become an important element of the overall treatment plan in many cases.[141–146] In regard to the latter, prospective evaluation of ICD efficacy in syncope patients with poor left ventricular function is needed before concrete recommendations can be made. However, reports examining this issue retrospectively provide strong support for the ICD option. Specifically, Middlekauff and colleagues[147] noted that among patients with severe left ventricular dysfunction, the presence of a history of syncope was accompanied by a significantly higher 1-year mortality (65 percent versus 25 percent in comparable patients without syncope) and a greater tendency toward sudden death (45 percent of deaths versus 12 percent in comparable patients).

Currently, ablation techniques are appropriate first choices in patients with right ventricular outflow tract tachycardia and bundle branch re-entry tachycardia. The future may bring more extensive use of such techniques in a broader range of ventricular tachycardia patients.[148–150]

LQTS Diagnostic Criteria and Treatment

Diagnosis of LQTS may be straightforward in patients with marked QT prolongation in the absence of drugs and with stress-induced syncope or documented ventricular arrhythmias. Clinical diagnosis is more difficult, however, in patients with borderline QT prolongation, particularly in the absence of symptoms. Even among subjects with a genetically identified mutation of a LQTS gene, there is a wide variation of QT intervals that includes normal values.[151] For clinical diagnosis, a set of diagnostic criteria was proposed in 1985 and updated in 1993 (see Table 93–4).[152] The new criteria incorporate gender differences in normal QT intervals, broaden the ECG criteria for repolarization abnormalities, and generally expand non-ECG criteria in an attempt to overcome the limitations of QT measurements. A few centers are capable of genetic identification of LQTS and currently accept blood from patients for evaluation, but this work is costly and time consuming and, at this time, is performed as part of ongoing research rather than as a clinical tool.

The goal of therapy in LQTS is to prevent recurrent syncope and sudden cardiac death. There are currently four treatment modalities: β-adrenergic antagonists, permanent pacing, left cervicothoracic sympathetic ganglionectomy, and implanted defibrillators. β-Adrenergic antagonists are the foundation of therapy and appear to reduce the incidence of cardiac events.[151, 153] The dose is maximized to ensure adequate beta-blockade as judged by the heart rate response to exercise: an exercise heart rate of less than 130 beats/min has been suggested.[154] β-Blockers may antagonize the sudden surges in sympathetic activity that often trigger arrhythmias in LQTS patients. Evidence suggests that the left cardiac sympathetic nerves (see later) mediate these influences. On a cellular level, efficacy of β-adrenergic blockade may be due to antagonism of afterdepolarizations.[155] These benefits may be countered by the pause-dependent nature of torsades de pointes in many patients. β-Blockade may worsen arrhythmias in these patients. Permanent cardiac pacing appears to reduce the rate of recurrent syncope in high-risk LQTS patients.[37, 156] Cardiac pacing may be beneficial by preventing pauses that prolong the QT interval and may allow higher doses of β-blockers. Because of the high association of cardiac events with exertion, patients should avoid competitive athletics. High-risk patients may be treated with implanted defibrillators; newer defibrillators with sophisticated bradycardia pacing capabilities may be particularly applicable. Treatment plans must be individualized because an accurate assessment of risk in an individual patient or family member of a patient remains difficult. Electrophysiologic testing as currently performed is of minimal value in diagnosis or management of LQTS (with the possible exception of catecholamine provocation for assessing susceptibility to torsades de pointes).

The efficacy of left cervicothoracic sympathetic ganglionectomy is controversial. The treatment is based on animal models: right stellectomy shortened ventricular refractoriness and increased the incidence of ventricular arrhythmias, whereas left stellectomy had the opposite effects.[157] In patients with LQTS, left cardiac sympathetic denervation has been shown in one study to produce a highly significant reduction in syncope,[38] but similar efficacy has not been found in other reports.[158] At present, the procedure is reserved for patients with recurrent symptoms in spite of maximal β-blockade and pacing. The procedure should probably be reserved for centers with significant experience in this surgery.

Future Directions

Currently, β-adrenergic blockers are the primary therapy for LQTS. In the future, treatment may become tailored to the identified genotype. Gene replacement therapy may ultimately be the ideal treatment for LQTS, and this possibility is already being addressed. Meanwhile, the sodium channel blocker mexiletine significantly shortened the QT interval in six patients with LQT3 (e.g., impaired sodium channel inactivation) but not in seven patients with LQT2 (e.g., abnormalities in I_{Kr}).[159] In patients with LQT1, LQT2, or LQT5, repolarization may be rendered more normal by a new class of antiarrhythmic agents (potassium channel openers) not yet widely available.[160] Increases in extracellular potassium will paradoxically increase current through I_{Kr}, even though the electrochemical gradient for potassium is diminished. In seven patients with LQT2, acute administration of potassium decreased QT interval and normalized T wave morphology and QT dispersion.[161]

Structural Cardiovascular or Cardiopulmonary Disease

In these cases, syncope is often only one of several types of symptoms being experienced by the patient. In such cases, treatment is almost best directed at amelioration of the specific structural lesion or its consequences. Thus, in syncope associated with myocardial ischemia, pharmacologic therapy and/or revascularization is clearly the appropriate strategy in most cases. If successful, syncope susceptibility (whether the result of tachyarrhythmias or bradyarrhythmias or neural reflex effects) will be reduced. Of course, of perhaps greater importance is the potential improvement in overall function and prognosis. Similarly, when syncope is closely associated with surgically addressable lesions (e.g., valvular aortic stenosis, pericardial disease, atrial myxoma, and congenital cardiac anomaly), a direct corrective approach is often feasible. On the other hand, when syncope is caused by certain difficult-to-treat conditions such as primary pulmonary hypertension or restrictive cardiomyopathy, it is often impossible to ameliorate the underlying problem adequately. Even modifying outflow gradients in hypertrophic obstructive cardiomyopathy is not readily achieved surgically. In the latter condition, the effectiveness of standard pharmacologic therapies remains uncertain; and consequently, despite ongoing controversy, recent success with cardiac pacing techniques offers considerable promise to symptomatic individuals.[103, 162, 163]

Cerebrovascular, Neurologic, and Psychiatric Diseases

Treatment of the conditions in this group are critically dependent on an accurate diagnosis. For example, arterial entrapment in conjunction with cervical spine disease is correctable but so rare as to be almost never considered. Migraine is far more common, and although it is an infrequent cause of syncope, pharmacologic treatment is highly effective.

Recognition of temporal lobe seizures or akinetic seizures and drop attacks requires considerable clinical acumen and appropriate laboratory testing. The first two are controllable with antiepileptic medications, whereas the latter has proved difficult to control. Similarly, syncope accompanying anxiety attacks and hysteria can prove to be a chronically recurring problem, since the underlying psychiatric condition is often refractory to long-term control.

Miscellaneous Disturbances

Syncope (more often syncope-like states) occurring in the setting of conditions such as diabetic coma or severe hypoxia or hypercapnia obviously requires addressing the underlying problem. Perhaps syncope owing to psychogenic hyperventilation is the most difficult of these to reverse, and this is likely to require psychiatric assistance. Pharmacotherapy, counseling, and biofeedback may be needed in combination.

ECONOMIC ASPECTS

Syncope is a relatively common symptom, and consequently, the cost of its evaluation is substantial. Furthermore, syncopal spells may result in loss of mobility and occupational opportunity, resulting in a loss of productivity that needs to be considered along with medical costs when evaluating the overall economic impact.

In 1982, Kapoor and coworkers[164] identified a need for a more cost-effective approach to the syncope evaluation. At that time, the average cost for evaluating syncope patients was estimated to be $2600 in United States dollars. However, since the actual etiology was determined in only relatively few cases, the real cost was far greater (approximately U.S. $24,000 per specific diagnosis). Given inflation, and the more widespread proliferation of diagnostic imaging procedures, conventional electrophysiologic testing, and tilt-table testing, it is reasonable to assume that the per-patient expenditure has increased substantially during the 1990s.[165] However, given the marked improvement in the frequency with which a specific diagnosis is now obtained, the cost-per-specific diagnosis is probably considerably lower than was the case in 1982.

CONCLUSION

Syncope has many possible causes. In the setting of underlying structural cardiovascular disease, syncopal symptoms are associated with worrisome prognostic implications. In the otherwise healthy patient, syncope tends to be more benign, but nonetheless, it can have important effects on lifestyle and occupational status. Furthermore, in all patients, syncope tends to recur. Consequently, aggressive pursuit of the cause is well warranted.

The principal diagnostic step in syncope evaluation is differentiation of those individuals with normal cardiovascular status from those with evident structural disease. In the former, assuming that the medical history or physical examination has not identified another system problem, autonomic function studies including tilt-table testing should be undertaken. In the latter group, a functional assessment of the suspected structural disturbance (e.g., hemodynamic, angiographic, and electrophysiologic studies as appropriate) and evaluation of susceptibility to tachyarrhythmias and bradyarrhythmias by conventional electrophysiologic testing are appropriate at an early stage. Tilt-table testing should follow if the diagnosis remains in doubt. In only a few instances should special neurologic studies be selected as an initial step. In all cases, the ultimate objective is obtaining a sufficiently strong correlation between the syncopal symptoms and the detected abnormalities to permit both an accurate assessment of prognosis and an initiation of an appropriate treatment plan.

References

1. Heistad DD, Kontos HA: Cerebral circulation. *In* Shepherd JT, Abboud FM (eds): Handbook of Physiology. Vol. III: The Cardiovascular System. Part I: Peripheral Circulation and Blood Flow. pp. 137–182. Bethesda, MD: The American Physiological Society, 1983.
2. Gibson GE, Pulsinelli W, Blass JP, et al: Brain dysfunction in mild to moderate hypoxia. Am J Med 70:1247–1254, 1981.
3. McHenry LC, Fazekas JF, Sullivan JF: Cerebral hemodynamics of syncope. Am J Med Sci 214:173–178, 1961.
4. Wood E: Hydrostatic homeostatic effects during changing force environments. Aviat Space Environ Med 61:366–373, 1990.
5. Rowell LB: Human Circulation. Regulation During Physical Stress. New York: Oxford University Press, 1986.
6. Cook P, James I: Cerebral vasodilators. N Engl J Med 305:1508–1513, 1981.
7. Scheinberg P, Blackburn I, Rich M, et al: Effects of aging on cerebral circulation and metabolism. Arch Neurol Psychiatry 70:77–85, 1953.
8. Lipsitz LA: Syncope in the elderly. Ann Intern Med 99:92–105, 1983.
9. Dandona P, James IM, Newbury PA, et al: Cerebral blood flow in diabetes mellitus: evidence of abnormal cerebral vascular reactivity. BMJ 2:325–326, 1978.
10. Tea SH, Mansourati J, L'Heveder G, et al: New insights into the pathophysiology of carotid sinus syndrome. Circulation 93:1411–1416, 1996.
11. Nathanson MH: Hyperactive cardioinhibitory carotid sinus reflex. Arch Intern Med 77:491–502, 1946.
12. Thomas JE: Hyperactive carotid sinus reflex and carotid sinus syncope. Mayo Clin Proc 44:127–139, 1969.
13. Almquist A, Gornick C, Benson DW Jr, et al: Carotid sinus hypersensitivity: evaluation of the vasodepressor component. Circulation 71:927–936, 1985.
14. Benditt DG, Goldstein MA, Adler S, et al: Neurally mediated syncopal syndromes: pathophysiology and clinical evaluation. *In* Mandel WJ (ed): Cardiac Arrhythmias. 3rd ed. pp. 879–906. Philadelphia: JB Lippincott, 1995.
15. Morley CA, Sutton R: Carotid sinus syncope. Int J Cardiol 6:287–293, 1984.
16. Sharpey-Schafer EP, Hayter CJ, Barlow ED: Mechanism of acute hypotension from fear and nausea. BMJ 2:878–880, 1958.
17. Thoren P: Role of cardiac C fibres in cardiovascular control. Rev Physiol Biochem Pharmacol 86:1–94, 1979.
18. Oberg B, Thoren P: Increased activity in left ventricular receptors during hemorrhage or occlusion of caval veins in the cat. A possible cause of the vaso-vagal reaction. Acta Physiol Scand 85:164–173, 1972.
19. Barcroft H, Edholm OG: On the vasodilatation in human skeletal muscle during posthemorrhagic fainting. J Physiol [Lond] 104:161–175, 1945.
20. Vallin BG, Sundlof G: Sympathetic outflow to muscles during vasovagal syncope. J Auton Nerv Syst 6:287–291, 1982.
21. Robinson BJ, Johnson RH: Why does vasodilatation occur during syncope? Clin Sci 74:347–350, 1988.
22. Van Lieshout JJ, Wieling W, Karemaker JM, et al: The vasovagal response. Clin Sci 81:575–586, 1991.
23. Bearn AG, Billing B, Edholm OG, et al: Hepatic blood flow and carbohydrate changes in man during fainting. J Physiol [Lond] 115:442–445, 1951.
24. Grubb BP, Gerard G, Rouish K, et al: Cerebral vasoconstriction during head-upright tilt-induced vasovagal syncope: a paradoxic and unexpected response. Circulation 84:1157–1164, 1991.
25. Njemanze PC: Cerebral circulation dysfunction and hemodynamic abnormalities in syncope during upright tilt test. Can J Cardiol 9:238–24,2 1993.
26. Ferrer MI: The sinus syndrome in atrial disease. JAMA 206:645–646, 1968.
27. Ferrer MI: The sick sinus syndrome. Circulation 47:635–641, 1973.
28. Strauss HC, Prystowsky EN, Scheinman MM: Sino-atrial and atrial electrogenesis. Prog Cardiovasc Dis 19:385–404, 1977.
29. Scheinman MM, Strauss HC, Abbott JA: Electrophysiologic testing for patients with sinus node dysfunction. J Electrocardiol 12:211–216, 1979.
30. Benditt DG, Milstein S, Goldstein MA, et al: Sinus node dysfunction: pathophysiology, clinical features, evaluation and treatment. *In* Zipes DP, Jalife J (eds): Cardiac Electrophysiology: From Cell to Bedside. pp. 708–734. Philadelphia: WB Saunders, 1990.
31. Chin C-F, Messenger JC, Greenberg PS, Ellestad MH: Chronotropic incompetence in exercise testing. Clin Cardiol 2:12–18, 1979.
32. Buetikofer J, Fetter J, Milstein S, et al: Variability of sinoatrial rate-response during exercise: impact on assessment of chronotropic competence in sinus node dysfunction [abstract]. Pacing Clin Electrophysiol 11:531, 1988.
33. Morady F, Shen E, Schwartz A, et al: Long-term follow-up of patients with recurrent unexplained syncope evaluated by electrophysiologic testing. J Am Coll Cardiol 2:1053–1059, 1983.
34. Dhingra RC, Denes P, Wu D, et al: Syncope in patients with chronic bifascicular block. Ann Intern Med 81:302–306, 1974.
35. Camm AJ, Lau CP: Syncope of undetermined origin: diagnosis and management. Prog Cardiol 1:139–156, 1988.
36. Jackman WM, Friday KJ, Anderson JL, et al: The long QT syndromes: a critical review, new clinical observations and a unifying hypothesis. Prog Cardiovasc Dis 31:115–172, 1988.
37. Moss AJ, Schwartz PJ, Crampton RS, et al: The long QT syndrome: prospective longitudinal study of 328 families. Circulation 84:1136–1144, 1991.
38. Schwartz PJ, Zaza A, Locati E, et al: Stress and sudden death: the case of the long QT syndrome. Circulation 83(suppl II):71–80, 1991.
39. Tobe TJ, de Langen CD, Bink-Boelkens MT, et al: Late potentials in bradycardia-dependent long QT syndrome associated with sudden death during sleep. J Am Coll Cardiol 19:541–549, 1992.
40. Schott J-J, Charpentier F, Peltier S, et al: Mapping of a gene for long QT syndrome to chromosome d4qf25-27. Am J Hum Genet 57:1114–1122, 1995.
41. Keating M, Atkinson D, Dunn C, et al: Linkage of a cardiac arrhythmia, the long QT syndrome, and the Harvey ras-1 gene. Science 252:704–706, 1991.
42. Wang Q, Curran ME, Splawski I, et al: Positional cloning of a novel potassium channel gene: KVLQT1 mutations cause cardiac arrhythmias. Nat Genet 12:17–23, 1996.
43. Barhanin J, Lesage F, Guillemare E, et al: K(V)LQT1 and 1sK (minK) proteins associate to form the I(Ks) cardiac potassium current. Nature 384:78–80, 1996.
44. Sanguinetti MC, Curran ME, Zou A, et al: Coassembly of KvLQT1 and minK (IsK) proteins to form cardiac I(Ks) potassium channel. Nature 384:78–80, 1996.
45. Jervell A, Lange-Nielsen F: Congenital deaf-mutism, functional heart disease with prolongation of the QT interval and sudden death. Am Heart J 54:59–68, 1957.
46. Romano C, Gemme G, Pongiglione R: Aritime cardiach rare deell-eta'pediatrica: Accessi sincopali per fibrillazione ventriculare parossistica. Clinica Pediatrica [Parma], 1963.
47. Ward OC: A new familial cardiac syndrome in children. J Ir Med Assoc 54:103–106, 1964.
48. Splawski I, Tristani-Firouzi M, Lehmann M, et al: Mutations in the hminK gene cause long QT syndrome and suppress IKs function. Nat Genet 17:338–340, 1997.
49. Warmke JW, Ganetzky B: A family of potassium channel genes related to eag in *Drosophila* and mammals. Proc Nat Acad Sci U S A 91:3438–3442, 1994.
50. Sanguinetti MC, Jurkiewicz NK: Two components of cardiac delayed rectifier K+ current: differential sensitivity to block by class III antiarrhythmic agents. J Gen Physiol 96:195–215, 1990.
51. Sanguinetti MC, Jiang C, Curran ME, et al: A mechanistic link between an inherited and an acquired cardiac arrhythmia: HERG encodes the IKr potassium channel. Cell 82:299–307, 1995.
52. Curran ME, Splawski I, Timothy KW, et al: A molecular basis for cardiac arrhythmias. HERG mutations cause long QT syndrome. Cell 80:795–803, 1995.
53. Yang T, Snyders DJ, Roden DM: Ibutilide, a methylsulfonanilide antiarrhythmic, is a potent blocker of the rapidly activating delayed rectifier K+ current (IKr) in AT-1 cells. Circulation 91:1799–1806, 1995.

54. Berul CI, Morad M: Regulation of potassium channels by nonsedating antihistamines. Circulation 91:1799–1806, 1995.
55. Daleau P, Lessard E, Groleau MF, et al: Erythromycin blocks the rapid component of the delayed rectifier potassium current and lengthens repolarization of guinea pig myocytes. Circulation 91:3010–3016, 1995.
56. Jiang C, Atkinson D, Towbin JA, et al: Two long QT loci map to chromosomes 3 and 7 with evidence of further heterogeneity. Nat Genet 8:141–147, 1994.
57. Wang Q, Shen J, Splawski I, et al: SCN5A mutations associated with an inherited cardiac arrhythmia, long QT syndrome. Cell 80:805–811, 1995.
58. Pathy MS: Clinical presentations of myocardial infarction in the elderly. Br Heart J 29:190–199, 1967.
59. Dixon MS, Thomas P, Sheridon DJ: Syncope is the presentation of unstable angina. Int J Cardiol 19:125–129, 1988.
60. Lombard JT, Selzer A: Valvular aortic stenosis. Ann Intern Med 106:292–298, 1987.
61. Atwood JE, Kawanishi S, Myers J, et al: Exercise testing in patients with aortic stenosis. Chest 93:1083–1087, 1988.
62. Linzer M, Varia I, Pontinen M, et al: Medically unexplained syncope: relationship to psychiatric illness. Am J Med 92:18–25, 1992.
63. Grubb BP, Gerard G, Wolfe DA, et al: Syncope and seizures of psychogenic origin: identification with head-upright tilt table testing. Clin Cardiol 15:839–842, 1992.
64. Ross RT: Syncope. London: WB Saunders, 1988.
65. Kapoor W: Evaluation and outcome of patients with syncope. Medicine 69:160–175, 1990.
66. Krahn AD, Klein GJ, Norris C, et al: The etiology of syncope in patients with negative tilt table and electrophysiologic testing. Circulation 92:1819–1824, 1995.
67. Simson MB: Signal-averaged electrocardiography. *In* Zipes DP, Jalife J (eds): Cardiac Electrophysiology: From Cell to Bedside. 2nd ed. pp. 1038–1048. Philadelphia: WB Saunders, 1995.
68. Kuchar DL, Thorburn CW, Sammel NL: Signal-averaged electrocardiogram for evaluation of recurrent syncope. Am J Cardiol 58:949–953, 1986.
69. Kudenchuk PJ, McAnulty JH: Syncope: evaluation and treatment. Mod Concepts Cardiovasc Dis 54:25–29, 1985.
70. Benditt DG, Remole S, Milstein S, et al: Syncope: causes, clinical evaluation, and current therapy. Annu Rev Med 43:283–300, 1992.
71. Sra JS, Anderson AJ, Sheikh SH, et al: Unexplained syncope evaluated by electrophysiologic studies and head-up tilt testing. Ann Intern Med 114:1013–1019, 1991.
72. DiMarco JB, Garan H, Hawthorne WJ, et al: Intracardiac electrophysiologic techniques in recurrent syncope of unknown cause. Ann Intern Med 95:542–548, 1981.
73. Fujimura O, Yee R, Klein GJ, et al: The diagnostic sensitivity of electrophysiologic testing in patients with syncope caused by bradycardia. N Engl J Med 321:1703–1707, 1989.
74. Chosy JJ, Graham DT: Catecholamines in vasovagal fainting. J Psychosom Res 9:189–194, 1965.
75. Sander-Jensen K, Secher NH, Astrup A, et al: Hypotension induced by passive head-up tilt: endocrine and circulatory mechanisms. Am J Physiol 251:R743–R749, 1986.
76. van Lieshout JJ, Wieling W, Karemaker JM, Eckberg DL: The vasovagal response. Clin Sci 81:575–586, 1991.
77. Fitzpatrick A, Williams T, Ahmed R, et al: Echocardiographic and endocrine changes during vasovagal syncope induced by prolonged head-up tilt. Eur J Cardiac Pacing Electrophysiol 2:121–128, 1992.
78. Benditt DG, Lurie KG, Adler SW, Sakaguchi SW: Rationale and methodology of head-up tilt table testing for evaluation of neurally mediated (cardioneurogenic) syncope. *In* Zipes DP, Jalife J (eds): Cardiac Electrophysiology: From Cell to Bedside. 2nd ed. pp. 1115–1128. Philadelphia: WB Saunders, 1995.
79. de Mey C, Enterling D: Assessment of the hemodynamic responses to single passive head-up tilt by non-invasive methods in normotensive subjects. Methods Find Exp Clin Pharmacol 8:449–457, 1986.
80. Fitzpatrick A, Theodorakis G, Vardas P, et al: Methodology of head-up tilt testing in patients with unexplained syncope. J Am Coll Cardiol 17:125–130, 1991.
81. Fitzpatrick A, Theodorakis G, Vardas P, et al: The incidence of malignant vasovagal syndrome in patients with recurrent syncope. Eur Heart J 12:389–394, 1991.
82. Raviele A, Gasparini G, DiPede F, et al: Usefulness of head-up tilt test in evaluating patients with syncope of unknown origin and negative electrophysiologic study. Am J Cardiol 65:1322–1327, 1990.
83. Grubb BP, Temesy-Armos P, Hahn H, et al: Utility of upright tilt table testing in the evaluation and management of syncope of unknown origin. Am J Med 90:6–10, 1991.
84. Grubb BP, Wolfe D, Samoil D, et al: Recurrent unexplained syncope in the elderly: the use of head-upright tilt table testing in evaluation and management. J Am Geriatr Soc 40:1123–1128, 1992.
85. Natale A, Akhtar M, Jazayeri M, et al: Provocation of hypotension during head-up tilt testing in subjects with no history of syncope or presyncope. Circulation 92:54–58, 1995.
86. Hammill SC, Holmes DR, Wood DL, et al: Electrophysiologic testing in the upright position: improved evaluation of patients with rhythm disturbances using a tilt table. J Am Coll Cardiol 4:65–71, 1984.
87. Benditt DG, Ferguson DW, Grubb BP, et al: Tilt-table testing for assessing syncope. An American College of Cardiology expert consensus document. J Am Coll Cardiol 28:263–275, 1996.
88. Richardson DA, Bexton R, Shaw FE, et al: Prevalence of cardioinhibitory carotid sinus hypersensitivity in patients 50 years or over presenting to the accident and emergency department with "unexplained" or "recurrent" falls. Pacing Clin Electrophysiol 20:820–823, 1997.
89. Weiss S, Baker JP: The carotid sinus reflex in health and disease. Its role in the causation of fainting and convulsions. Medicine 12:297–354, 1933.
90. Nathanson MH: Hyperactive cardioinhibitory carotid sinus reflex. Arch Intern Med 77:491–502, 1946.
91. Thomas JE: Hyperactive carotid sinus reflex and carotid sinus syncope. Mayo Clin Proc 44:127–139, 1969.
92. Almquist A, Gornick C, Benson DW Jr, et al: Carotid sinus hypersensitivity: evaluation of the vasodepressor component. Circulation 71:927–936, 1985.
93. Savage DD, Corwin L, McGee DL, et al: Epidemiologic features of isolated syncope: the Framingham study. Stroke 16:626–629, 1985.
94. Kapoor WN, Karpf M, Wieand S, et al: A prospective evaluation and follow-up of patients with syncope. N Engl J Med 309:197–204, 1983.
95. Bass EB, Elson JJ, Fogoros RN, et al: Long-term prognosis of patients undergoing electrophysiologic studies for syncope of unknown origin. Am J Cardiol 62:1186–1191, 1988.
96. Sheldon R, Rose S, Flanagan P, et al: Risk factors for syncope recurrence after a positive tilt table test in patients with syncope. Circulation 93:973–981, 1996.
97. Malik P, Koshman ML, Sheldon RS: Timing of first syncope recurrence predicts syncope frequency following a positive tilt table test. J Am Coll Cardiol 29:1284–1289, 1997.
98. Sugrue DD, Gersh BJ, Holmes DR, et al: Symptomatic "isolated" carotid sinus hypersensitivity: natural history and results of treatment with anticholinergic drugs or pacemaker. J Am Coll Cardiol 7:158–162, 1986.
99. Brignole M, Menozzi C, Lolli G, et al: Long-term outcome of paced and nonpaced patients with severe carotid sinus syndrome. Am J Cardiol 69:1039–1043, 1992.
100. Romeo F, Cianfrocca C, Pelliccia F, et al: Long-term prognosis in children with hypertrophic cardiomyopathy: an analysis of 37 patients aged 14 years at diagnosis. Clin Cardiol 13:101, 1990.
101. McKenna WJ, Deanfield J, Faruqui A, et al: Prognosis in hypertrophic cardiomyopathy: role of age and clinical electrocardiographic and hemodynamic features. Am J Cardiol 47:532–538, 1981.
102. Maron BJ, Roberts WC, Epstein SE: Sudden death in hypertrophic cardiomyopathy: a profile of 78 patients. Circulation 65:1388–1394, 1982.
103. McAreavey D, Epstein ND, Fananapazir L: Dual chamber pacing is effective therapy for hypertrophic cardiomyopathy patients with provocable LV outflow tract obstruction and symptoms refractory to medical therapy [abstract]. J Am Coll Cardiol 23:11, 1994.
104. Fitzpatrick AP, Ahmed R, Williams S, et al: A randomized trial of medical therapy in malignant vasovagal syndrome or neurally-mediated bradycardia/hypotension syndrome. Eur J Cardiac Pacing Electrophysiol 1:991–202, 1991.
105. Brignole M, Menozzi C, Gianfranchi L, et al: A controlled trial of acute and long-term medical therapy in tilt-induced neurally mediated syncope. Am J Cardiol 70:339–342, 1992.

106. Morillo CA, Leitch JU, Yee R, et al: A placebo-controlled trial of intravenous and oral disopyramide for prevention of neurally mediated syncope induced by head-up tilt. J Am Coll Cardiol 22:1843–1848, 1993.
107. Moya A, Permanyer-Miralda G, Sagrista-Sauleda J, et al: Limitations of head-up tilt test for evaluating the efficacy of therapeutic interventions in patients with vasovagal syncope: results of a controlled study of etilefrine versus placebo. J Am Coll Cardiol 25:65–69, 1995.
108. Mahanonda N, Bhuripanyo K, Kangkagate C, et al: Randomized double-blind placebo-controlled trial of oral atenolol in patients with unexplained syncope and positive upright tilt table results. Am Heart J 130:1250–1253, 1995.
109. Benditt DG, Remole S, Asso A, et al: Cardiac pacing for carotid sinus syndrome and vasovagal syncope. *In* Barold S, Mugica J (eds): New Perspectives in Cardiac Pacing. Vol. 3. pp. 15–28. Mount Kisco, NY: Futura, 1993.
110. Sutton R: Pacing in atrial arrhythmias. Pacing Clin Electrophysiol 13:1823, 1990.
111. Benditt DG, Peterson M, Lurie K, et al: Cardiac pacing for prevention of recurrent vasovagal syncope. Ann Intern Med 122:204–209, 1995.
112. Petersen MEV, Chamberlain-Webber R, Fitzpatrick AP, et al: Permanent pacing for cardioinhibitory malignant vasovagal syndrome. Br Heart J 71:274–281, 1994.
113. Connolly SJ, Sheldon R, Roberts RS, et al, for the Vasovagal Pacemaker Study Investigators: The North American Vasovagal Pacemaker Study (VPS): a randomized trial of permanent cardiac pacing for the prevention of vasovagal syncope. J Am Coll Cardiol 33:16–20, 1999.
114. Ten Harkel ADJ, van Lieshout JJ, Wieling W: Treatment of orthostatic hypotension with sleeping in the head-up tilt position, alone and in combination with fludrocortisone. J Int Med 232:139–145, 1992.
115. Weiling W, van Lieshout JJ, van Leeuwen AM: Physical maneuvers that reduce postural hypotension in autonomic failure. Clin Auton Res 3:57–65, 1993.
116. Robertson D, Goldberg M, Hollister AS, et al: Clonidine raises blood pressure in severe orthostatic hypotension. Am J Med 74:193–200, 1983.
117. Sra J, Maglio C, Biehl M, et al: Efficacy of midodrine hydrochloride in neurocardiogenic syncope refractory to standard therapy. J Cardiovasc Electrophysiol 8:42–46, 1997.
118. Bannister R, Mathias C: Management of postural hypotension. *In* Bannister R (ed): Autonomic Failure. A Textbook of Clinical Disorders of the Autonomic Nervous System. pp. 569–595. Oxford: Oxford University Press, 1988.
119. Ector H, Reybrouck T, Heidbuchel F, et al: Tilt training: a new treatment for neurocardiogenic syncope [abstract]. Arch Mal Coeur 91(III):32, 1998.
120. Moss AJ, Glasser W, Topol E: Atrial tachypacing in the treatment of a patient with primary orthostatic hypotension. N Engl J Med 302:1465–1467, 1980.
121. Weissmann P, Chin MT, Moss AJ: Cardiac tachypacing for severe refractory orthostatic hypotension. Ann Intern Med 116:650–651, 1992.
122. Grubb BP, Wolfe D, Samoil D, et al: Adaptive rate pacing controlled by right ventricular pre-ejection interval for severe refractory orthostatic hypotension. Pacing Clin Electrophysiol 16:801–805, 1993.
123. Parsonnet V, Bernstein AD, Galasso D: Cardiac pacing practices in the US in 1985. Am J Cardiol 62:71, 1988.
124. Rattes MF, Klein GJ, Sharma AD, et al: Efficacy of empirical cardiac pacing in syncope of unknown cause. Can Med Assoc J 140:381–385, 1989.
125. Scheinman MM, Evans-Bell T, and the Executive Committee of the Percutaneous Cardiac Mapping and Ablation Registry: Catheter ablation of the atrioventricular junction: a report of the Percutaneous Mapping and Ablation Registry. Circulation 70:1024–1029, 1984.
126. Lee RJ, Kalman JM, Fitzpatrick AP, et al: Radiofrequency catheter modification of the sinus node for "inappropriate" sinus tachycardia. Circulation 92:2919–2928, 1995.
127. Kalman JM, Lee RJ, Fischer WG, et al: Radiofrequency catheter modification of the sinus pacemaker function guided by intracardiac echocardiography. Circulation 92:3070–3081, 1995.
128. Haissaguerre M, Gencel L, Fischer B, et al: Successful catheter ablation of atrial fibrillation. J Cardiovasc Electrophysiol 5:1045–1052, 1994.
129. Gaita F, Riccardi R, Calo L, et al: Atrial mapping and radiofrequency catheter ablation in patients with idiopathic atrial fibrillation. Electrophysiological findings and ablation results. Circulation 97:2136–2145, 1998.
130. Haissaguerre M, Jais P, Shah D, et al; Spontaneous initiation of atrial fibrillation by ectopic beats originating in the pulmonary veins. N Engl J Med 339:659–666, 1998.
131. Cox JL, Boineau JP, Schuessler RB, et al: Modifications of the MAZE procedure for atrial flutter and atrial fibrillation: I—rationale and surgical results. J Thorac Cardiovasc Surg 110:473–484, 1995.
132. Rosenqvist M, Brandt J, Schuller H: Atrial versus ventricular pacing in sinus node disease: A treatment comparison study. Am Heart J 111:292–297, 1986.
133. Stangl K, Wirtzfeld A, Seitz K, et al: Atrial stimulation (AAI): long-term follow-up of 110 patients. *In* Belhassen B, Feldman S, Copperman Y (eds): Cardiac Pacing and Electrophysiology. pp. 283–285. Proceedings of the VIIIth World Symposium on Cardiac Pacing and Electrophysiology. Jerusalem: R & L Creative Communications, 1987.
134. Sutton R, Bourgeois I: The Foundations of Cardiac Pacing. Part 1. p. 131. Mt. Kisco, NY: Futura, 1991.
135. Rosenqvist M, Brandt J, Schuller H: Long-term pacing in sick sinus node disease: effects of stimulation mode on cardiovascular morbidity and mortality. Am Heart J 116:16–22, 1988.
136. Andersen HR, Thuesen L, Bagger JP, et al: Prospective randomised trial of atrial versus ventricular pacing in sick-sinus syndrome. Lancet 344:1523–1528, 1994.
137. Andersen HR, Nielsen JC, Thomsen PEB, et al: Long-term follow-up of patients from a randomised trial of atrial versus ventricular pacing for sick sinus syndrome. Lancet 350:1210–1216, 1997.
138. Laupacis A, Albers G, Dalen J, et al: Antithrombotic therapy in atrial fibrillation. Chest 108:352S–359S, 1995.
139. Jackman WM, Wang W, Friday K, et al: Catheter ablation of accessory atrioventricular pathways (Wolff-Parkinson-White syndrome) by radiofrequency current. N Engl J Med 324:1605–1611, 1991.
140. Naccarelli GV, Dougherty AH, Jalal S, et al: Paroxysmal supraventricular tachycardia: comparative role of therapeutic methods—drugs, devices, and ablation. *In* Saksena S, Luderitz B (eds): Interventional Electrophysiology. A Textbook. 2nd ed. pp. 461–470. Armonk, NY: Futura, 1996.
141. Saksena S, Madan N, Lewis C: Implantable cardioverter-defibrillators are preferable to drugs as primary therapy in sustained ventricular arrhythmias. Prog Cardiovasc Dis 38:445–454, 1996.
142. The AVID Investigators: A comparison of antiarrhythmic-drug therapy with implantable defibrillators in patients resuscitated from near-fatal ventricular arrhythmias. N Engl J Med 337:1576–1583, 1997.
143. Moss AJ, Hall WJ, Cannom DS, et al: Improved survival with an implanted defibrillator in patients with coronary artery disease at high risk for ventricular arrhythmias. N Engl J Med 335:1933–1940, 1996.
144. Bigger JT Jr: Prophylactic use of implanted cardiac defibrillators in patients at high risk for ventricular arrhythmias after coronary artery bypass graft surgery. N Engl J Med 337:1569–1575, 1997.
145. Connolly S: Non-pharmacologic therapy for sustained ventricular tachycardia and ventricular fibrillation. *In* Yusuf S, Cairns J, Camm J, et al (eds): Evidence Based Cardiology. pp. 586–595. London: BMJ Books, 1998.
146. Gregoratos G, Cheitlin MD, Conill A, et al: ACC/AHA guidelines for implantation of cardiac pacemakers and antiarrhythmia devices: a report of the American College/American Heart Association Task Force on Practice Guidelines. J Am Coll Cardiol 31:1175–1209, 1998.
147. Middelkauff HR, Stevenson WG, Stevenson LW, Saxon LA: Syncope in advanced heart failure: high risk of sudden death regardless of origin of syncope. J Am Coll Cardiol 21:110–116, 1993.
148. Morady F, Harvey M, Kalbfleisch SJ, et al: Radiofrequency catheter ablation of ventricular tachycardia in patients with coronary artery disease. Circulation 87:363–372, 1993.
149. Stevenson WG, Khan H, Sager P, et al: Identification of reentry circuit sites during catheter mapping and radiofrequency ablation of ventricular tachycardia late after myocardial infarction. Circulation 88:1647–1670, 1993.

150. Borgreffe M, Chen X, Hindricks G, et al: Catheter ablation of ventricular tachycardia in patients with heart disease. *In* Zipes DP (ed): Catheter Ablation of Arrhythmias. pp. 277–308. Armonk, NY: Futura, 1994.
151. Zareba W, Moss AJ, Schwartz PJ, et al: Influence of the genotype on the clinical course of the long-QT syndrome. N Engl J Med 339:960–965, 1998.
152. Schwartz PJ, Moss AJ, Vincent GM: Diagnostic criteria for the long QT syndrome: an update. Circulation 88:782–784, 1993.
153. Moss AJ, Schwartz PJ, Crampton RS, et al: The long QT syndrome: a prospective international study. Circulation 71:17–21, 1985.
154. Moss AJ, Zareba W, Robinson JL: The long QT syndrome. Cardiol Rev 3:79–85, 1995.
155. Priori SG, Mantica M, Schwartz PJ: Mechanisms underlying early and delayed afterdepolarizations induced by catecholamines. Am J Physiol 258:H1796–H1805, 1990.
156. Eldar M, Griffin JC, Van Hare GF, et al: Combined use of beta-adrenergic blocking agents and long-term cardiac pacing for patients with the long QT syndrome. J Am Coll Cardiol 20:830–837, 1992.
157. Schwartz PJ: Idiopathic long QT syndrome: progress and questions. Am Heart J 109:399–411, 1985.
158. Bhandari AK, Scheinman MM, Morady F, et al: Efficacy of left cardiac sympathectomy in the treatment of patients with the long QT syndrome. Circulation 70:1018–1023, 1984.
159. Schwartz PJ, Priori SG, Locati EH, et al: Long QT syndrome patients with mutations of the SCN5A and HERG genes have differential responses to Na+ channel blockade and to increases in heart rate: implications for gene-specific therapy. Circulation 92:3381–3386, 1995.
160. Sato T, Hata Y, Yamamoto M, et al: Early afterdepolarizations abolished by potassium channel opener in a patient with idiopathic long QT syndrome. J Cardiovasc Electrophysiol 6:279–282, 1995.
161. Compton SJ, Lux RL, Ramsey MR, et al: Genetically defined therapy of inherited long-QT syndrome: correction of abnormal repolarization by potassium. Circulation 94:1018–1022, 1996.
162. Fananapazir L, Cannon R, Tripodi D, et al: Impact of dual-chamber pacing in patients with obstructive hypertrophic cardiomyopathy with symptoms refractory to verapamil and beta-adrenergic blocker therapy. Circulation 85:2149–2161, 1992.
163. Gadler F, Linde C, Juhlin-Dannfelt A, et al: Influence of right ventricular pacing site on left ventricular obstruction in patients with hypertrophic obstructive cardiomyopathy. J Am Coll Cardiol 27:1219–1224, 1996.
164. Kapoor W, Karpf M, Maher Y, et al: Syncope of unknown origin: the need for a more cost-effective approach to its evaluation. JAMA 247:2687–2691, 1982.
165. Calkins H, Byrne M, El-Atassi R, et al: The economic burden of unrecognized vasodepressor syncope. Am J Med 95:473–479, 1993.

CHAPTER 94

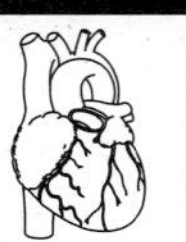

SUDDEN CARDIAC DEATH

Abdi Rasekh, Munir Zaqqa, and Ali Massumi

DEFINITION
EPIDEMIOLOGY
POPULATION DYNAMICS
TIME DEPENDENCE OF RISK
RISK FACTORS
Influence of Age, Race, and Gender
Activity
Psychological Factors
Risk Factors for Coronary Artery Disease and Ischemic Heart Disease
TRANSIENT RISK FACTORS
Transient Ischemia and Reperfusion Arrhythmias
Systemic Factors
Autonomic Variation
Toxins and Drugs
UNDERLYING DISEASES
Coronary Artery Disease and Acute Myocardial Infarction
Coronary Artery Abnormalities
Hypertrophic Obstructive Cardiomyopathy
Arrhythmogenic Right Ventricular Dysplasia
Valvular Heart Disease
Dilated Cardiomyopathy
Primary Electrophysiologic Abnormalities
PATHOLOGY AND PATHOPHYSIOLOGY
EVALUATION AND RISK STRATIFICATION
PREVENTION
Primary Prevention
Secondary Prevention

DEFINITION

Sudden cardiac death (SCD) is defined as an unexpected natural death from a cardiac cause that occurs instantaneously or within 1 hour from the onset of an abrupt change in clinical status in a person without a prior condition that would appear to be fatal.[1, 2]

The classification of death based on clinical circumstances is difficult because as many as 40 percent of sudden deaths are unwitnessed,[3] and only monitoring of the patient at the time of sudden death provides a clear answer.

Prodromal symptoms, which are defined as relatively abrupt changes that begin during an arbitrarily defined period of up to 24 hours before the cardiac arrest, are often nonspecific. Symptoms such as chest pain, palpitations, and dyspnea can only be considered suggestive of certain causes.

EPIDEMIOLOGY

SCD accounts for more than 300,000 deaths in the United States each year,[1, 2, 4–6] which corresponds to about 50 percent of all cardiac deaths in the United States and other developed countries.

The incidence of SCD ranges from 36 to 128 per 100,000 inhabitants per year in different studies.[7–9] However, only victims of SCD resuscitated by emergency medical services personnel were included in these studies. Rates of SCD in other industrialized countries are quite consistent with those in the United States. In developing countries, the rates of SCD are considerably lower, paralleling the rates of ischemic heart disease.

A review of data from several population-based studies that reported time trends showed a 15- to 19-percent decline in the incidence of SCD. This decline has paralleled the decline in death from ischemic heart disease that began more than 20 years ago (Fig. 94–1).[2, 10, 11]

POPULATION DYNAMICS

The epidemiological data from the Framingham Heart Study, a 26-year follow-up of 5209 men and women who were 30 to 59 years old and free of identified heart disease at baseline, showed that SCD accounted for 46 percent of deaths due to coronary artery disease (CAD) among men and for 34 percent among women.[12] The incidence of SCD increased with age. However, the proportion of deaths from CAD that were sudden and unexpected was greater in the younger age groups.

The 300,000 SCDs that occur annually in the United States can be expressed as a fraction among an unselected adult population; the overall incidence, therefore, is 0.1 to 0.2 percent per year. When the high-risk subgroups are identified and removed from this population base, the calculated incidence for the remainder of the population decreases and the identification of individuals at risk becomes more difficult (Fig. 94–2). Based on these estimates, any preventive measure must be applied to the 999 of 1000 individuals who will not have an event during the course of 1 year to potentially influence the outcome in 1 of 1000. The costs of such a low-yield intervention are obviously prohibitive, and therefore the identification of more specific markers of high risk is needed. The present risk factors generally identify the risk of developing structural heart disease rather than the proximate precipitator of the SCD event.

TIME DEPENDENCE OF RISK

The risk of death after a major change in cardiovascular status is not linear over time for most clinical

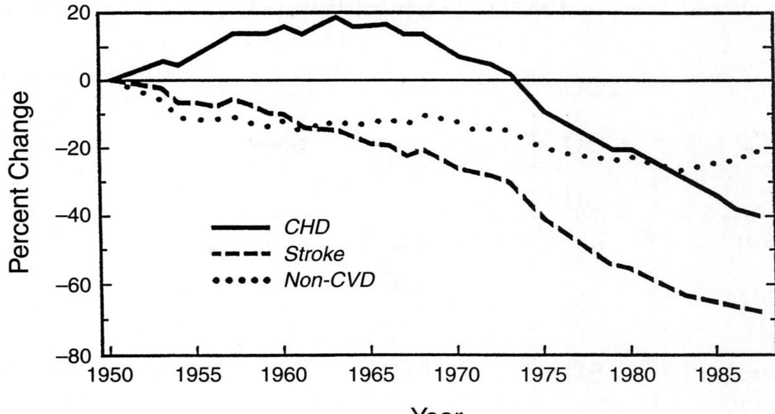

FIGURE 94–1 Percent change in age-adjusted death rates since 1950. CHD, coronary heart disease; non-CVD, total mortality rate minus cardiovascular disease. (From Morbidity and Mortality Chartbook on Cardiovascular, Lung, and Blood Disease. Washington, DC: National Heart, Lung, and Blood Institute, U.S. Department of Health and Human Services; 1990.)

circumstances.[13, 14] The highest secondary death rates occur during the first 6 to 18 months after a major index event such as myocardial infarction (MI). The slope of survival curves approach that of a similar population who have remained free of an interposed major event at 18 to 24 months (Fig. 94–3).[1, 13]

RISK FACTORS

In a study by Gillum[5] of persons between the ages of 35 and 74 years in 40 states, the epidemiology of SCD parallels that of CAD. The annual incidence of SCD was 1.91:1000 for white and nonwhite men, 0.57:1000 for white women, and 0.90:1000 for nonwhite women (Fig. 94–4).

In patients with ischemic heart disease, 60 percent of deaths in men and 50 percent in women occurred out of hospital.

Influence of Age, Race, and Gender

Age

The incidence of SCD increases with age in men and women, both white and nonwhite, as the prevalence of ischemic heart disease increases with age.

The peak incidences of SCD are between birth and 6 months, as a result of sudden infant death syndrome, and between 45 and 75 years, as a result of CAD. However, the proportion of SCD caused by CAD decreases with age, from approximately 75 percent at ages 35 to 44 to approximately 50 percent at ages 75 to 84.

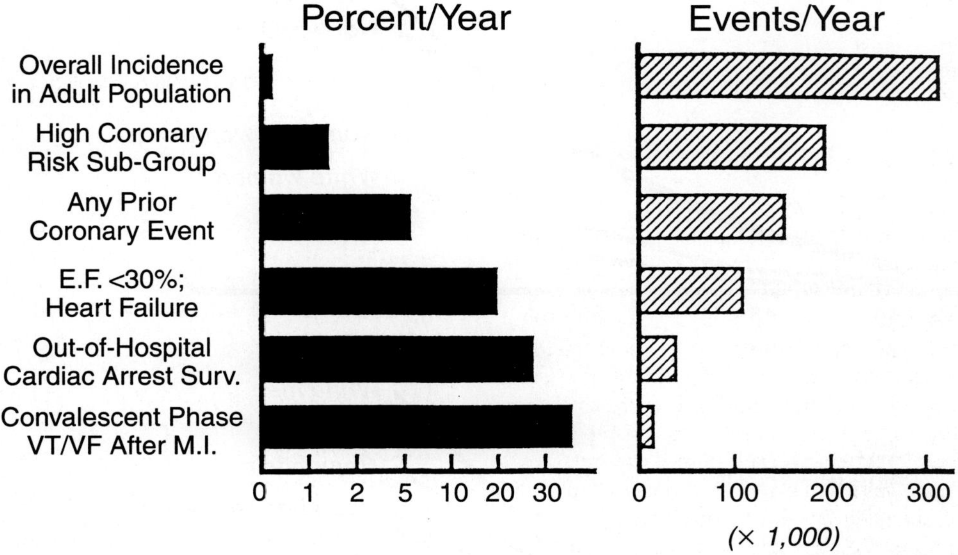

FIGURE 94–2 Sudden cardiac deaths among population subgroups. Estimates of incidence (percent per year) and total number of sudden cardiac deaths per year are shown for the overall adult population in the United States and for higher-risk subgroups. The overall estimated incidence is 0.1–0.2% per year, accounting for more than 300,000 deaths per year. Within subgroups identified by increasingly powerful risk factors, the increasing incidence is accompanied by progressively decreasing total numbers. Practical interventions for the larger subgroups will require identification of specific markers to increase their ability to identify patients who will have a future event. EF, ejection fraction; MI, myocardial infarction; VT/VF: ventricular tachycardia–ventricular fibrillation. (From Myerburg RJ, Kessler KM, Castellanos A: Sudden cardiac death. Structure, function, and time-dependence of risk. Circulation 85[1 suppl]:I2–I10, 1992.)

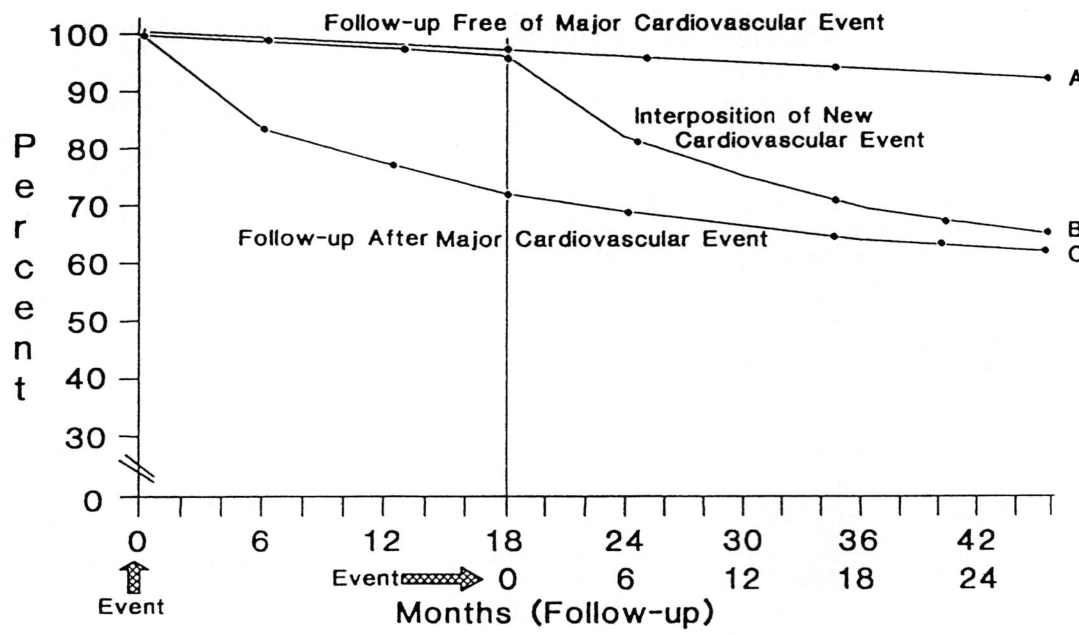

FIGURE 94–3 Time dependence of risk after cardiovascular events. Survival curves for hypothetical patients with known cardiovascular disease free of major index event (*curve A*) and for patients surviving major cardiovascular events (*curve C*). Attrition is accelerated during the initial 6–24 months after the event. *Curve B* shows the dynamics of risk over time in low-risk patients with an interposed major event that is normalized to a time point (e.g., 18 mo). The subsequent attrition is accelerated for 6–24 mo. (From Myerburg RJ, Kessler KM, Castellanos A: Sudden cardiac death. Structure, function, and time-dependence of risk. Circulation 85[1 suppl]:I2–I10, 1992.)

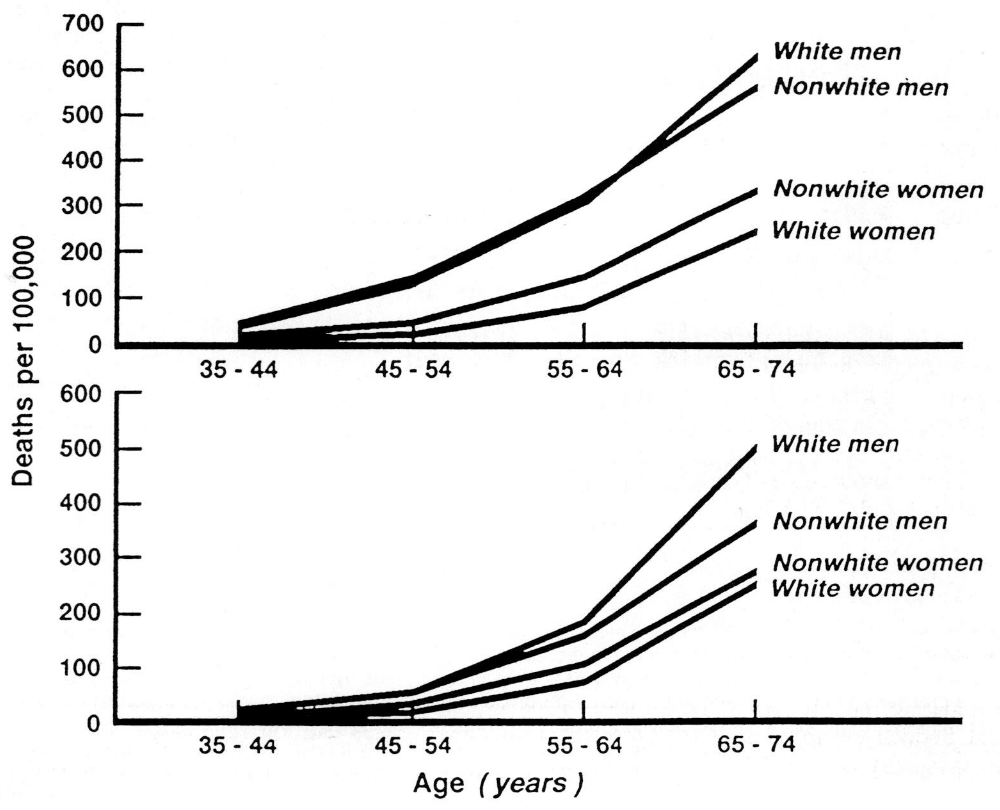

FIGURE 94–4 Mortality rates for ischemic heart disease occurring out of hospital or in emergency departments *(top)* and occurring in hospital *(bottom)* by age, gender, and race in 40 states during 1985. (From Gillum RF: Sudden coronary death in the United States: 1980–1985. Circulation 79:756–765, 1989.)

Race

Data on racial differences in sudden death suggest that blacks are more likely than whites to experience sudden death in excess of their risk of death from ischemic heart disease.[4, 15, 16] However, the data are conflicting, and the interpretation of data is complicated by several factors, as follows[16]:

1. A younger age distribution of the black population, so crude rates give the impression of lower rates of CAD in blacks although age-specific rates are similar
2. Frequent failure to report data for nonwhites separately from those for whites and to distinguish minorities (who have varying rates of ischemic heart disease) from each other (e.g., blacks, Hispanics, Asians, American Indians, and so on)

A large study in Chicago concluded that the incidence of cardiac arrest was significantly higher for blacks than for whites in every age group.[17] The survival rate after cardiac arrest was 2.6 percent in whites compared with 0.8 percent in blacks. Blacks were significantly less likely to have a witnessed cardiac arrest, bystander-initiated cardiopulmonary resuscitation, or a "favorable" initial rhythm on admittance to the hospital. When they were admitted, blacks were half as likely to survive.

Gender

The annual incidence of SCD is three to four times higher in men than in women; approximately 75 percent of SCDs occur in men. This difference can be explained by the difference in the incidence of CAD and the protection that women have from atherosclerosis before menopause.

At 20 years of follow-up in the Framingham Heart Study, there was a 3.8-fold excess incidence of SCD in men compared with that in women. The excess risk in men peaked at 6.75:1 in the 55- to 64-year-old age group and then fell to 2.17:1 in the 65- to 74-year-old age group.[12]

Activity

The impact of physical activity on SCD remains controversial. Although heavy exercise can trigger the onset of an acute MI, particularly in persons who are habitually sedentary, this correlation has not yet been shown with SCD.[18] It has been suggested that vigorous exercise increases platelet adhesiveness and aggregability, whereas moderate physical activity may be beneficial by decreasing platelet adhesiveness and aggregability.[19]

Cardiac arrests occur at a rate of 1:12,000 to 15,000 during rehabilitation programs, whereas during stress testing cardiac arrest occurs at a rate of 1:2000. This is at least six times greater than the incidence of SCD for patients known to have heart disease.[2]

Other data indicate that the impact of activity on SCD may be small. In the Maastricht Sudden Death study, 67 percent of SCD victims were physically inactive at the time of the event.

Psychological Factors

Psychological factors appear to influence the risk of SCD. Psychological factors such as a recent life change have been associated with an increased risk of SCD.[20] Rahe and associates[20] reported a correlation between an increased life change score in the preceding 6 months and the risk of coronary events. This association was particularly notable for victims of SCD.

A study of SCDs in women showed an increased risk for women who were not married, who had none or fewer children, and who had a greater difference in educational level compared with their spouse.[21] Other risk factors in this group included prior psychiatric treatment, greater alcohol consumption, and cigarette smoking.[21]

In a large study of 2320 men who survived MI, social isolation and high life stress were associated with an increased risk of SCD. Both of these factors were directly associated with low educational levels.[22]

Type A personality has also been associated with an increased incidence of CAD and with manifestations of CAD, including SCD.[23] However, the validity of this risk factor remains somewhat controversial.[23]

Risk Factors for Coronary Artery Disease and Ischemic Heart Disease

The risk factors of SCD parallel those of CAD, which is the most common cause of SCD in developing countries. The investigators of the Albany-Framingham study considered age, smoking, hypertension, hypercholesterolemia, and left ventricular hypertrophy in a combined fashion to produce a multivariate model of the probability of SCD. In their study of 4120 men, they showed a 16-fold gradation in the incidence of sudden death from the lowest to the highest decile of this risk score[24] (Table 94–1).

A prior history of CAD is a powerful risk factor for

TABLE 94–1 Incidence of Sudden Death According to Decile of Multivariate Risk: Framingham-Albany Combined Analysis

Decile of Multivariate Risk	Sudden Deaths (n)			
		Prior CHD?		
	Total	Yes	No	*2-Yr Incidence of SCD/1000*
1	2	1	1	0.89
2	2	2	0	0.89
3	2	0	2	0.89
4	6	3	3	2.69
5	8	2	6	3.58
6	6	1	5	2.69
7	12	5	7	5.37
8	10	4	6	4.48
9	17	6	11	7.61
10	32	13	19	14.32
Total	97	37	60	4.34

Abbreviations: CHD, coronary heart disease; SCD, sudden cardiac death.

From Kannel WB, Doyle JT, McNamara PM, et al: Precursors of sudden coronary death. Factors related to the incidence of sudden death. Circulation 51:606–613, 1975.

SCD. In a review of SCD in the Framingham study, the risk of SCD was 3 to 12 times higher among those with clinical manifestation of CAD than among the general population of the same age. In men, the risk was on average 6.7 times that of persons without a CAD event. The risk of SCD was higher in persons with an MI than in those who had angina pectoris. However, even angina carried an almost 5-fold increased risk.[25] In those without interim CAD, virtually all of the major risk factors were related to the incidence of SCD. After the onset of ischemic heart disease, none of the major modifiable risk factors were predictive of sudden death in men. In women, diabetes was the only significant predisposing factor, and cigarette smoking had a sizable standardized logistic coefficient.[25]

In persons with established ischemic heart disease, factors that reflect ischemic myocardial damage were the chief predictors of sudden death. Electrocardiographic abnormalities indicating old MI, left ventricular hypertrophy, interventricular conduction delay, or repolarization abnormality were significant predictors of SCD. Ventricular ectopy was a risk factor for SCD in men[25] (Fig. 94–5). In the Finnish cohort study, smoking appeared to be a more important predictor of SCDs than of non-SCDs, whereas other coronary risk factors seemed to equally predict SCDs and non-SCDs.[26] Kuller and associates[27] also found that smoking probably is the most important risk factor for SCD.

In patients with known ischemic heart disease, left ventricular dysfunction is the most powerful predictor of risk of subsequent SCD. The mortality rate due to SCD increases when the left ventricular ejection fraction (LVEF) is less than 0.50; however, the rise in probability of SCD is particularly remarkable in the group with an LVEF of 0.30 to 0.39 (a rise from 0.10 in the former to 0.30 in the latter group).[28] An LVEF of 0.30 or less is the most powerful predicator of SCD. However, it has a low specificity. There also is a suggestion that an LVEF of less than 0.30 is a better predictor of early death (<6 months), whereas the presence of ventricular arrhythmia was a better predictor of late death (>6 months).

Several studies suggested that the presence of three or more premature ventricular contractions (PVCs) is a powerful predictor of SCD.[28, 29] High-risk forms of ventricular ectopy also include multifocal PVCs, bigeminy, short coupling intervals with risk of R-on-T phenomenon, and three or more consecutive ectopic beats.[30]

Certain electrocardiographic findings also could be helpful in identifying patients with an increased risk of SCD, including the presence of interventricular conduction delays, QT prolongation, an increase in resting heart rate of more than 90 beats/min, and an increased QT dispersion in survivors of out-of-hospital cardiac arrest.[2] However, a study by Zabel and colleagues[31] failed to support the usefulness of QT dispersion in survivors of out-of-hospital cardiac arrest. In survivors of cardiac arrest who have an LVEF of less than 0.30 and in whom the cause of arrest is obscure, the risk of SCD exceeds 30 percent if they do not have inducible ventricular tachycardia (VT) by programmed extrastimulation over a period of 1 to 3 years.[2, 32–34] In those who have inducible VT, the risk of recurrent arrest ranges from 15 to 50 percent over a 2- to 3-year period despite therapy that suppresses inducible arrhythmias or with amiodarone.[32, 34–36]

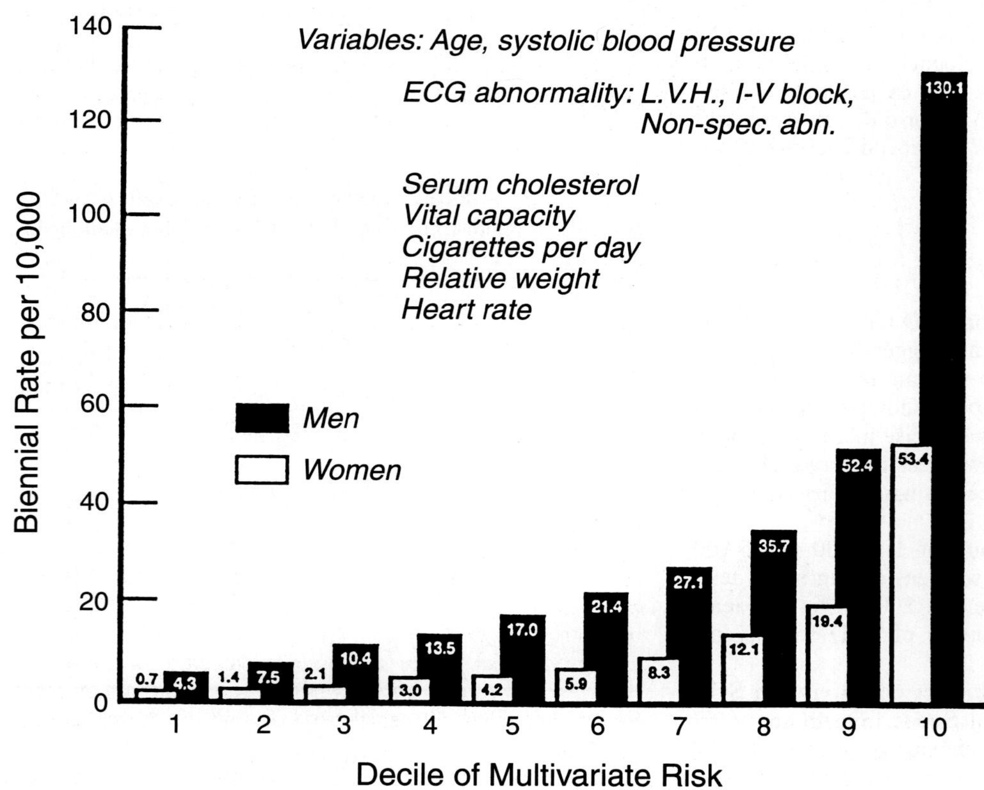

FIGURE 94–5 Risk of sudden cardiac death by decile of multivariate risk: 28-yr follow-up, Framingham Study. ECG, electrocardiographic; I-V, interventricular; LVH, left ventricular hypertrophy; non-spec. abn., nonspecific abnormality. (From Kannel WB, Schatzkin A: Sudden death: lessons from subsets in population studies. J Am Coll Cardiol 5[6 suppl]:141B–149B, 1985.)

Transient Risk Factors

Transient risk indicates a time-limited and unpredictable event or state that has the potential to initiate or allow the initiation of an unstable electrophysiologic (EP) condition. It increases the probability of transition from normal to benign cardiac rhythm to VT or ventricular fibrillation (VF).[1] Unfortunately, due to the transient nature of these risk factors, they lack sufficient sensitivity, specificity, and predictive values to be used for a specific preventive or therapeutic intervention before an actual event.

Transient Ischemia and Reperfusion Arrhythmias

Ischemia has a clear clinical correlation with potentially fatal ventricular arrhythmias during the early phase of an acute MI. However, approximately 80 percent of SCDs caused by CAD are not associated with an acute MI. It is assumed that transient acute ischemia is one of the major triggering factors of SCD.[37]

A study in an experimental model demonstrated that smaller decreases in blood flow are required to induce VT or VF in the presence of prior MI compared with controlled subjects without a prior infarction.[38] Reperfusion can also induce electrical instability via reentrant[39] or triggered activity[40] mechanisms.

Systemic Factors

Reversible systemic abnormalities could contribute to the life-threatening arrhythmias. Electrolyte imbalances, such as hypokalemia and hypomagnesemia, hypoxemia, and acidosis, may influence EP stability and cause VT/VF and SCD. Recognition and correction of these factors are the only required interventions.

Hemodynamic dysfunction in patients with an abnormal heart can result in cardiac arrest. In an experimental model, volume loading of isolated perfused canine left ventricles shortened refractory periods,[1, 41] and regional disparity in hearts with prior MI has been demonstrated.[1, 41]

Autonomic Variation

Alteration of heart rate variability has been suggested as a marker for SCD among survivors of MI[42] and survivors of out-of-hospital cardiac arrest.[43] A blunted baroreceptor response to phenylephrine has also been suggested as a marker for the risk of VT or SCD after MI.[1, 44]

Clinically, the induction of sustained VT by the use of isoproterenol among survivors of cardiac arrest and its prevention by the use of beta-blockers suggest a role for autonomic influence in the genesis of ventricular arrhythmias.

Huikuri and associates[45] studied the sinus node rate, as an estimate of cardiac autonomic tone, immediately after the onset of VT. Sinus node rate during ventriculoatrial dissociation increases progressively during the first 30 seconds of VT in patients with stable VT, whereas in patients with unstable VT, the sinus node rate increases more rapidly during the first 5 seconds and then abruptly decreases.[1, 45]

All of these observations support the role of abnormal autonomic function as a risk factor for VT/VF and SCD.

Toxins and Drugs

The risk of VF during anesthesia with chloroform was the first recognized and published report of a drug that caused a potentially fatal arrhythmia.[1, 46] Subsequently, the risk of arrhythmic death by torsade de pointes was reported during the treatment of chronic atrial arrhythmias with quinidine.

It is well recognized that class IA antiarrhythmic agents can cause torsade de pointes. The Cardiac Arrhythmia Suppression Trial (CAST) also showed an increased risk of death with class IC agents in an ischemic context.[47] Death in this population treated with class IC agents may have resulted from an interaction among the substrate of CAD, the transient risk factor of ischemia, and the exacerbation of ischemia-induced slowing in conduction by drugs with negative dromotropic actions, such as encainide or flecainide.[2, 48] Class III antiarrhythmic drugs also can cause QT prolongation and torsade de pointes.

There are an emerging number of medications that are not antiarrhythmic drugs but can be responsible for similar proarrhythmic responses. Drug interaction during therapy by apparently innocuous medications could be dangerous. Diverse categories of medications, such as erythromycin, ketoconazole, cisipride, and psychotropic agents, can cause prolonged QT interval. Other agents, such as terfenadine and cocaine, cause prolonged QT interval through an effect on repolarizing currents such as delayed potassium current rectifier, I_{ks}.[49, 50]

Phosphodiesterase inhibitors and other positive inotropic agents can increase intracellular calcium loading, which has also been demonstrated to exert proarrhythmic actions and to increase the risk of SCD.[2]

Hypokalemia caused by potassium-wasting diuretics and hypomagnesemia can cause QT prolongation and trigger ventricular arrhythmia and SCD. However, it is sometimes difficult to determine whether the arrhythmia was the result of hypokalemia or whether the serum concentration of potassium was decreased as a result of catecholamine release after cardiac arrest and the resuscitation effort.

Underlying Diseases

Coronary Artery Disease and Acute Myocardial Infarction

As discussed earlier, CAD is the most common cause of SCD in Western countries. Approximately 80 percent of patients who experience SCD have CAD. Death in this population may occur in the acute ischemic phase or at a time remote from a previous MI. In the Framingham Heart Study, more than 50 percent of coronary death was related to SCD.[51]

In survivors of SCD, CAD with more than 75 percent

cross-sectional stenosis is found in approximately 40 to 86 percent of patients, depending on the age and gender of the population studied.[2]

Autopsy studies have reported that a recent occlusive coronary thrombus was found in 15 to 64 percent of victims of SCD caused by ischemic heart disease. A study by Roberts and associates[52] found intraluminal thrombi in 29 percent of victims of SCD. However, the thrombus was nonocclusive in more than 80 percent of this group.

There is evidence of MI on the basis of elevated cardiac enzymes in fewer than 50 percent of patients with VF and fewer than 25 percent have Q wave MI.[2]

Many factors can play a role in the process of SCD in patients with CAD or a history of previous MI. Three main factors are ischemia, left ventricular dysfunction, and electrical instability.[4]

Healed MIs are present in 50 percent or more of SCD victims.[2] Observation during the ambulatory monitoring of victims of SCD who had a history of a previous MI showed that the most common mode of death was either VF or VT deteriorating to VF.

Mapping of ventricular activation during VT[53] showed the presence of fragmented, repetitive, low-voltage electrical activity in the area of abnormal impulse formation covering most of the interval between two successive tachycardia beats. This was initially interpreted as an indication of reentry circuit with a zone of slow conduction.[54] However, it was subsequently demonstrated that although the cells incorporated in the circuit may have a normal intracellular structure with normal electrical properties, they have lost lateral intercellular connections that led to a very long maze-type circuit, which gives the impression of marked slowing of conduction velocity in the circuit.[55, 56]

Sudden death due to VF is most common in the 6-month period after MI. It is independently predicted by LVEF,[28, 57] extent of CAD, premature ventricular beats,[28, 58] evidence of ischemia during post-MI exercise testing,[59] late potentials,[60] and decreased heart rate variability.[61]

Approximately one third of SCD survivors were not inducible during EP testing despite aggressive programmed stimulation.[62, 63] This may represent a population in whom ischemia is important as a trigger or to facilitate the induction of reentrant arrhythmias through modulation of the underlying EP substrate.[4]

Coronary Artery Abnormalities

A higher incidence of coronary anomalies has been consistently observed in young victims of sudden death than in adults undergoing routine autopsy (4 to 15 percent in the former group versus 1 percent in the latter group).[64]

In patients with an anomalous origin of the left main coronary artery from the right (anterior) sinus of Valsalva, with passage of the left main coronary artery between the aorta and the pulmonary trunk, there is an increased risk of SCD. About 75 percent of the patients reported with this malformation die before age 20, usually during or soon after vigorous exertion.[65]

The "mirror image" coronary anomaly in which the right coronary artery originates from the left sinus of Valsalva has also been associated with an increased risk for SCD, although the risk is not as high as the former congenital anomaly.[66]

Other unusual variants of coronary artery anomalies, including hypoplasia of the right coronary and left circumflex arteries,[67] the left or right coronary artery originating from the pulmonary trunk, and coronary arterial intussusception that causes coronary lumen occlusion,[68] could be rarely associated with SCD.

Myocardial bridges have also been associated with SCD during exercise in healthy individuals.[69] It has been suggested that dynamic mechanical obstruction may cause myocardial ischemia. However, evidence that myocardial bridges are responsible for sudden death remains controversial.[70]

Coronary dissection with or without aortic dissection occurs in patients with Marfan's syndrome.[71] Among other rare mechanical causes of SCD is rupture of the sinus of Valsalva aneurysm with the involvement of coronary arteries.[72] Prolapse of myxomatous polyps from aortic valve into coronary arteries has also been reported as a rare cause of SCD.[73]

Coronary spasm can cause ischemia and SCD.[74] Coronary arteritis as seen in polyarteritis nodosa can be associated with SCD.[75] Kawasaki's disease can cause SCD through involvement of the coronary arteries.[76]

Hypertrophic Obstructive Cardiomyopathy

The incidence of SCD associated with hypertrophic cardiomyopathy has been reported to be 2 to 4 percent per year in adults.[2, 77] Other studies reported an overall annual mortality rate of less than 1 percent.[78, 79] The authors attributed previous reported excess mortality rates to selection and referral bias.[80]

The incidence of SCD is higher in younger patients than in elderly patients with hypertrophic cardiomyopathy. It is the most common cause of sudden death in young competitive athletes younger than 35 years[81] (Fig. 94–6).

Despite intense investigation, the identification of patients at high risk remains a challenge. The multiplicity of mechanisms that can result in SCD and their interrelation represent different aspects of the same phenomenon. The variables that seem to identify patients at an increased risk include a history of aborted SCD or sustained VT, family history of sudden death, identification of a high-risk genotype, multiple repetitive nonsustained VT (NSVT) on ambulatory monitoring, recurrent syncope, and massive left ventricular hypertrophy.[82, 83] Although it was initially thought that the magnitude of the left ventricular outflow gradient is a risk for sudden death, data have not shown an association.[84]

There is no convincing evidence that EP testing has an important role in identifying patients with hypertrophic cardiomyopathy who are at a high risk for sudden death.[82]

Available data on genetic markers of SCD in patients with hypertrophic cardiomyopathy suggest that β-myosin heavy chain mutations may account for 30 to 40 percent of cases of familial hypertrophic cardiomyopathy.[85–87] The prognosis for patients with different myosin mutations varies considerably. Genotype-phenotype correlation studies have shown that mutations carry prognostic significance.

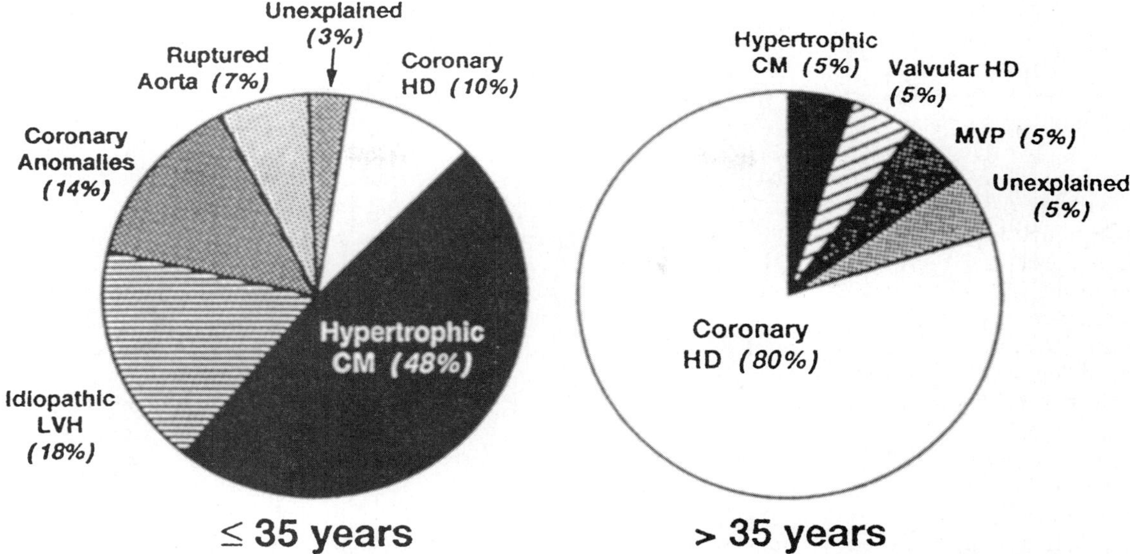

FIGURE 94–6 Causes of sudden death in competitive athletes. Estimated prevalences of disease responsible for death are compared in young (≤35 yr) and older (>35 yr) athletes. CM, cardiomyopathy; HD, heart disease; LVH, left ventricular hypertrophy; MVP, mitral valve prolapse. (From Maron BJ, Epstein SE, Roberts WC: Causes of sudden death in competitive athletes. J Am Coll Cardiol 7:204–214, 1986.)

The Arg403Gln, Arg719Trp, and Arg453Cys mutations in the β-myosin heavy chain are associated with a high incidence of SCD. Mutations in cardiac troponin T are also associated with a high incidence of SCD, although there is a mild degree of hypertrophy.[88]

Arrhythmogenic Right Ventricular Dysplasia

Arrhythmogenic right ventricular dysplasia (ARVD) is characterized by ventricular arrhythmias and a specific right ventricular cardiomyopathy that shows fatty infiltration of the right ventricle.[89] The term *arrhythmogenic right ventricular dysplasia* was first proposed in 1977 by Fontaine and colleagues[89] in a report of six patients with sustained VT who were resistant to medical therapy and did not have overt heart disease. In the three patients who underwent surgery, the right ventricle was dilated and had paradoxical wall motion.

ARVD should be considered as a possible differential diagnosis in patients with frequent premature ventricular beats or VT, particularly if the ventricular arrhythmias have a left bundle branch block morphology.[90] It is a rare but important cause of sudden death in young, otherwise healthy populations and a subtle cause of congestive heart failure.[91]

Typically, ARVD occurs in young adults; there is a predominance for males. In a review of a series of 52 patients,[92] there was an 80 percent predominance of males. At least 80 percent of the cases were diagnosed before the age of 40 years.

The disease seems to be common in northern Italy (prevalence, 1:1000), with an autosomal dominant inheritance (30 percent). An autosomal recessive variant of ARVD, which is associated with wooly hair and palmoplantar keratoderma, has been reported from Naxos Island in Greece.[93, 94]

The most common form of presentation includes ventricular arrhythmias, ranging from symptomatic or asymptomatic isolated ventricular extrasystoles to sustained poorly tolerated VT with left bundle branch morphology. Sudden unexpected death could be the first presentation of the disease.[95] VF and SCD may be observed during competitive sports and strenuous exercise,[96] but they can also occur at rest or even during sleep.[97]

During VT, the electrocardiogram (ECG) shows a left bundle branch block pattern, suggesting delayed activation of the left ventricle. The QRS axis is normal or shifted to the right when the tachycardia originates in the pulmonary infundibulum. There may be extreme left-axis deviation when tachycardia arises from the diaphragmatic wall or near the apex of the right ventricle.[98]

The ECG in sinus rhythm may show changes compatible with right-sided abnormality. Repolarization abnormalities in term of T wave inversion in precordial leads beyond V_1, which are observed in 54 percent of cases, are the first sign that attracts medical attention.[91] Extension of T wave inversion in all precordial leads had a positive correlation with left ventricular involvement.[99]

In patients with suspected ARVD, a QRS duration of more than 110 milliseconds in lead V_1 has a sensitivity of 55 percent and a specificity of 100 percent for this condition.[100] Another diagnostic marker of the disease is the selective prolongation of the QRS complex duration in lead V_1, V_2, or V_3 of more than 25 milliseconds compared with the QRS duration in lead V_6 in the presence of right bundle branch block.[101]

In 30 percent of cases, a more specific change with the presence of a discrete wave just beyond the QRS complex at the beginning of the ST segment can be observed; this has been named the *epsilon* wave (Fig. 94–7). These waves represent potentials of small amplitude, suggesting delayed ventricular activation of some portion of the right ventricle.

Patients with ARVD who have clinical VT may have an

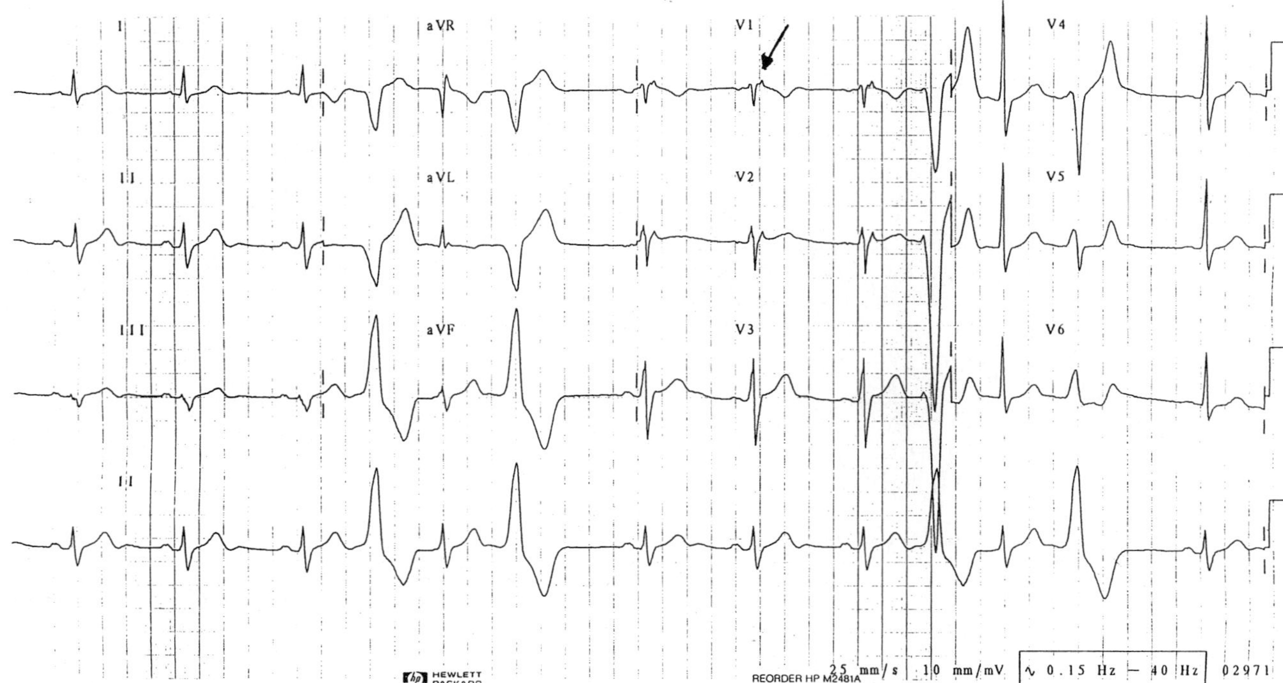

FIGURE 94–7 The presence of the epsilon wave (*arrow*).

abnormal signal-averaged ECG.[102] However, if the disease is localized, the signal-averaged ECG may be normal.

Echocardiography may show localized abnormalities of the right ventricle, but structural abnormalities are usually moderate. They would be recognized only if systematically sought. These abnormalities include dilatation of the right ventricle, presence of aneurysmal areas in the infundibulum during diastole, and dyskinetic areas in the inferobasal region.

Magnetic resonance imaging (MRI) could be the most effective noninvasive test to locate and localize increased adipose tissue within the ventricular myocardium. The diagnostic value of MRI was evaluated by Auffermann and associates[103] in 36 consecutive patients with biopsy-proved ARVD. They concluded that this method can replace angiography and possibly biopsy for the diagnosis of ARVD. MRI in combination with signal-averaged ECG may help in the differential diagnosis of ARVD as opposed to idiopathic right ventricular outflow tract VT.[104]

Right ventriculography remains the reference imaging method for the diagnosis of ARVD.[71] A broad spectrum of different ventriculography patterns can be observed in ARVD. The diagnosis is based on segmental wall motion and morphologic abnormalities.

Valvular Heart Disease

Aortic stenosis was one of the most common noncoronary causes of SCD in the pre–valvular surgery era. However, asymptomatic aortic stenosis is associated with a low risk of SCD. Both ventricular tachyarrhythmias and bradyarrhythmias have been associated with SCD in this population.

The primary cause of ventricular arrhythmia in this population is believed to be subendocardial ischemia due to left ventricular hypertrophy and high end-diastolic intracavitary pressure. Bradyarrhythmia may be due to atrioventricular block caused by calcium penetration in the conduction system or neurocardiogenic mechanism. Patients with aortic valve replacement remain at some risk for SCD caused by arrhythmias, prosthetic valve dysfunction, or coexistent CAD.[105] SCD has been reported to be the second most common mode of death after valve replacement surgery, with an incidence of 2 to 4 percent over a follow-up period of 7 years, accounting for 21 percent of postoperative deaths. The incidence peaked 3 weeks after surgery and then plateaued after 8 months.[106]

It is not clear whether mitral valve prolapse can cause SCD. Its prevalence is so high that its presence may be just a coincidental finding in victims of SCD.[2] Severe mitral regurgitation, left ventricular dysfunction, and myxomatous degeneration of the valve can be the markers for the patients with a higher risk of complication such as endocarditis, cerebroembolic events, and SCD.[2]

It has been shown that patients who have valvular heart disease may develop bundle branch reentrant tachycardia, particularly after valvular replacement.[107, 108] This arrhythmia usually occurs in the immediate postoperative period and can result in either cardiac arrest or syncope.[108] Almost all VTs occurred within 4 weeks after surgery (median, 10 days). Due to the proximity of the His-Purkinje system, valvular surgery may result in His-Purkinje system conduction abnormalities that facilitate bundle branch reentry.

Dilated Cardiomyopathy

Approximately 10 percent of SCDs in the adult population occur in patients with dilated cardiomyopathy (DCM).[109]

Overall survival rates after clinical diagnosis is estimated to be 70 percent at 1 year and 50 percent at 2 years.[110, 111] Mortality rates among patients with DCM are high, reaching 10 to 50 percent annually, depending on the severity of disease.[112]

In an overview of 14 studies that included a total of 1432 patients with DCM, the mortality rate was 42 percent at 4 years, and 28 percent of the deaths were classified as sudden.[112] SCD in this population is attributed to ventricular tachyarrhythmias because of the high frequency of complex ventricular ectopic activity in this population.[113] However, the terminal event can be asystole or electromechanical dissociation, especially in patients with advanced left ventricular dysfunction.[114]

In this population, syncope is another variable that may identify patients at high risk for SCD. In a study by Middlekauff and associates,[115] the probability of SCD was 45 percent among patients with New York Heart Association (NYHA) functional class III or IV who had unexplained syncope in 1 year.

Primary Electrophysiologic Abnormalities

These are the conditions in which an EP abnormality predisposes the patient to VT/VF in the absence of structural heart disease. Electrocardiographic findings may provide a clue to diagnosis.

Congenital Long QT Syndrome

The idiopathic long QT syndrome (LQTS) is a congenital disease with frequent familial transmission, characterized primarily by prolongation of the QT interval and by the occurrence of life-threatening tachyarrhythmias, particularly in association with emotional or physical stress.[116] It is caused by the prolongation of repolarization due to abnormal inward movement of sodium or outward movement of potassium from cardiac myocytes, creating prolonged periods of intracellular positivity.[117] Such prolongation of repolarization could cause the development of early afterdepolarizations. Early afterdepolarizations trigger torsade de pointes in patients with congenital or acquired LQTS.

The diagnosis of LQTS is reasonably certain when the corrected QT (QT_c) interval is unequivocally prolonged ($QT_c \geq 0.480$ millisecond) in the absence of secondary causes or if the QT_c is borderline prolonged with either an abnormal configuration of the T wave or a history of unexplained syncope.[118]

Schwartz and colleagues[116] developed LQTS diagnostic criteria with a score system ranging from a minimum value of 0 to a maximum value of 9. The patients who have a score 4 or higher have a high probability of LQTS (Table 94–2). Congenital LQTS includes a group of genetic disorders that affect cardiac ion channels.

One form of LQTS that was originally described in 1957 by Jervell and Lange-Nielsen[119] was associated with deafness and was thought to be an autosomal recessive disorder. A similar condition without deafness but with autosomal dominant transmission was subsequently reported in 1963 by Romano and colleagues[120] and in 1964 by Ward.[121] Four specific mutant LQT genes (*LQT1, LQT2, LQT3,* and *LQT5*) have been identified. The mutant gene for *LQT4* has not yet been identified.

TABLE 94–2 Long QT Syndrome Diagnostic Criteria

	Points*
ECG Findings†	
QT_c‡	
≥480 ms	3
460–470 ms	2
450 ms (in males)	1
Torsades de pointes§	2
T wave alternans	1
Notched T wave in three leads	1
Low heart rate for age‖	.5
Clinical History	
Syncope	
With stress	2
Without stress	1
Congenital deafness	.5
Family History¶	
Family members with definite LQTS**	1
Unexplained sudden cardiac death below age 30 yr among immediate family members	.5

Abbreviations: ECG, electrocardiographic; LQTS, long QT syndrome.
**Scoring:* ≤1 point, low probability of LQTS; 2–3 points, intermediate probability of LQTS; ≥4 points, high probability of LQTS.
†In the absence of medications or disorders known to affect these ECG features.
‡QT_c calculated by Bazzett's formula, where $QT_c = QT/RR^2$.
§Mutually exclusive.
‖Resting heart rate below the second percentile for age.
¶The same family member cannot be counted in either of the following criteria.
**Definite LQTS is defined by LQTS score ≥4.
From Schwartz PJ, Moss AJ, Vincent GM, Crampton RS: Diagnostic criteria for the long QT syndrome. An update. Circulation 88:782–784, 1993.

The four specific mutant cardiac ion channel genes that encode abnormal channel proteins include the following:

1. *LQT1:* A mutant *KvLQT1* gene on chromosome 11 encodes an abnormal potassium channel protein (α-subunit). Patients with Jervell-Lange-Nielsen syndrome, dominant for the long QT manifestation but recessive for associated deafness, were found to have a homozygous mutation of *KvLQT1*. When expressed with minK protein (β-subunit), the α-subunit produces a negative effect in the slowly activating delayed rectifier potassium current (I_{ks}).[118, 122]
2. *LQT2:* A mutant *HERG* gene on chromosome 7 encodes an abnormal potassium channel protein that produces a dominant negative effect in rapidly activating delayed rectifier potassium current (I_{kr}).[117, 123]
3. *LQT3:* A mutant *SCN5A* gene on chromosome 3 encodes an abnormal sodium channel protein, resulting in a continued leakage of sodium current I_{Na} into the cell with prolongation of repolarization.[118, 124]
4. *LQT4:* The *KCNE1* gene on chromosome 21 encodes β-subunit (minK protein) that coassembles with *KvLQT1* α-subunits to form I_{ks} and complex with *HERG* to regulate I_{kr}. Mutations in *KCNE1* gene cause LQTS and suppress I_{ks}.[117, 125]

The four mutant ionic channel genes account for an estimated 50 percent of known families with LQTS, so additional mutant genes surely exist.[118]

The incidence of cardiac events is higher in *LQT1* and *LQT2* than in *LQT3,* whereas the lethality of cardiac events is higher in *LQT3* than *LQT1* and *LQT2* patients.[117]

An international, prospective, longitudinal study of patients with congenital LQTS was initiated in 1979.[126] The registry shows that mean age at enrollment was 21 ± 15 years, and the mean age at the first cardiac event was 14 ± 12 years. Eighty-five percent had a family member with a QT_c of more than 0.44 second, and 69 percent were women. The frequency of syncope was 5 percent per year, and the cardiac mortality rate was 0.9 percent per year. Syncope occurred in association with intense emotion, vigorous physical activity, or arousal by auditory stimuli. In this study, the risk of syncope or sudden death was related to the length of the QT_c, a history of prior cardiac events, and an elevated heart rate.[107, 127]

Acquired Long QT Syndrome

Antiarrhythmic drugs have long been recognized as a possible cause of ventricular tachyarrhythmias, torsade de pointes, and SCD. Class IA agents such as quinidine can cause torsade de pointes by prolongation of QT interval. The reported incidence of torsade de pointes from quinidine ranges from 0.5 to 8.8 percent. Quinidine at low plasma concentrations blocks potassium channels, whereas at higher plasma concentrations it also blocks sodium channels. Therefore, QT prolongation and torsade de pointes can be observed even at subtherapeutic doses.

Sotalol, a class III drug that blocks potassium channels and therefore lengthens repolarization, can be responsible for QT prolongation and torsade de pointes. Prolonged QT is dose related, with increasing incidence at higher doses.

Ibutilide is another class III drug that prolongs repolarization by activating the slow inward sodium current during the plateau phase. Polymorphic VT has been reported after the infusion of ibutilide. Almost all of these episodes occurred within a few hours after ibutilide infusion.

We discussed earlier in detail the role of a number of nonantiarrhythmic drugs in the genesis of ventricular arrhythmias caused by QT prolongation. Table 94–3 summarizes the causes of acquired LQTS.

TABLE 94–3 Causes of Acquired Long QT Syndrome

Antiarrhythmic agents
- Class IA: Quinidine, procainamide, disopyramide, *N*-acetylprocainamide
- Class III: sotalol, bretylium, ibutilide, amiodarone (low risk for torsades de pointes)
- Class IV: bepridil, mibefradil

Antihistamines
- Astemizole, terfenadine

Antimicrobials
- Erythromycin, clarithromycin, azithromycin
- Trimethoprim-sulfamethoxazole
- Ketoconazole, cotrimoxazole
- Pentamidine
- Chloroquine

Serotonin antagonists
- Ketanserin, zindeline

Lipid-lowering agents
- Probucol

Gastrointestinal agents
- Cisapride, liquid protein diets

Psychotropic agents
- Tricyclic and tetracyclic antidepressants
- Phenothiazines
- Haloperidol
- Risperidone

Other drugs
- Chloral hydrate amantidine
- Anthracyclines
- Diuretics (reduced K^+, Mg^{2+})
- Vasopressin (severe bradycardia)

Organophosphorus
- Insecticides

Electrolyte abnormalities
- Hypokalemia
- Hyponatremia
- Hypocalcemia

Bradyarrhythmias

Anorexia nervosa and altered nutritional states

Cerebrovascular diseases
- Intracranial and subarachnoid hemorrhage

Intracranial trauma

Wolff-Parkinson-White Syndrome

Sudden death in the Wolff-Parkinson-White (WPW) syndrome is rare. The estimated prevalence of WPW varies from 0.1 to 0.3 percent of the population.[126, 128, 129] SCD in the majority of the patients with WPW occurs during atrial fibrillation. In these patients, antegrade conduction via the accessory pathway is very rapid. This rapid ventricular response causes hemodynamic dysfunction, and disorganization of the ventricular rhythm leads to VF and SCD. The estimated incidence of SCD in WPW has been suggested to be from 0 to 0.4 percent.[130, 131] The most pessimistic estimate would be no more than 1 per 100 patient-years.[132]

A review of retrospective data from patients resuscitated from VF and found to have the WPW pattern showed that the most important risk factor was a rapid ventricular response over the accessory pathway during atrial fibrillation. The shortest RR interval during atrial fibrillation was less than 250 milliseconds.[133, 134] Although this criterion identifies virtually 100 percent of patients at risk for developing VF, its specificity is low. Other risk factors include the presence of multiple accessory pathways,[135] presence of symptoms (particularly a history of both reciprocating tachycardia and atrial fibrillation), and the use of digitalis and intravenous verapamil. Patients with Ebstein's anomaly are probably also at a greater risk of developing VF.[136] The propensity to develop this complication can be accurately assessed with EPS.

Brugada's Syndrome

In 1992, Brugada and Brugada[137] described eight patients with a history of aborted SCD who had a distinct electrocardiographic pattern of right bundle branch block with ST-segment elevation in precordial leads (V_1, V_2, and V_3) and a normal QT interval without any demonstrable structural heart disease. The entity is increasingly recognized. To date, 108 symptomatic and 66 asymptomatic patients with a characteristic electrocardiographic pattern have been described.[138] There is a male preponderance (an 8:1 to 10:1 ratio of males to females).[139, 140] Although age at presentation varied from 2 to 77 years, there was a peak around the fourth decade.[140] The risk of recurrent syncope or SCD was high. During a mean follow-up of 34 ± 32 months, an arrhythmic event occurred in 34 percent of previously symptomatic patients and 27 percent of patients without any prior event.

The administration of the class I antiarrhythmic drug ajmaline or procainamide reproduces the abnormal ECG in patients with transient normalized ECGs and in family members of affected individuals with a normal ECG.

Although the underlying pathogenesis of electrocardiographic changes remains unclear, it has been suggested that heterogeneity of repolarization across the wall of the right ventricular outflow tract contributes to the electrocardiographic patterns and the genesis of arrhythmias in Brugada's syndrome.[139]

In contrast to endocardial cells, action potentials (APs) of epicardial cells display a pronounced phase 1 referred to as *spike-and-dome morphology.* The transient outward current, I_{to}, which is present in epicardial cells and virtually absent in endocardial cells, underlines the difference between the AP configurations.[140] The loss of AP dome in epicardial cells but not endocardial cells may cause transmural heterogeneity and ST-segment elevation as a result of transmural current flow from the endocardium to the epicardium.[140]

It is unclear whether this entity can have any correlation or may be responsible for the sudden unexplained nocturnal death that occurs in young healthy males of southeast Asia that has several names, such as *lai-lai* ("sleep death"; Laos), *pokkuri* ("sudden death at night"), and *bangugut* ("moaning and dying during sleep"; Philippines).

Idiopathic Ventricular Tachycardia

Idiopathic VTs with monomorphic morphology that occur in patients with structurally normal hearts include paroxysmal and repetitive forms that may originate from the following:

1. Right ventricular outflow tract: they have left bundle branch block morphology and inferior axis and terminate with vagal maneuvers such as adenosine infusion.[141]
2. Left posterior septum: Also called *fascicular tachycardia* because it is often preceded by a fascicular potential, it has a right bundle branch block morphology with left-axis deviation. Calcium channel blockers usually suppress this arrhythmia.

SCD is extremely rare in patients with idiopathic VT.

Catecholamine-Sensitive Polymorphic Ventricular Tachycardia

These VTs are associated with less favorable outcome than idiopathic monomorphic VTs. In 1994, Leenhardt and colleagues[142] reported this variant. In this series, VTs were typically triggered by emotion or physical activity and could be reproduced by exercise or infusion of isoproterenol. The mean age at the onset of symptoms was 7.8 ± 4 years. A family history of syncope or sudden death was noted in 30 percent of the patients. During a 7-year follow-up period, there were 5 deaths of the initial 21 patients, and four of the five deaths were sudden. A typical sequence of events was noted during exercise. Although baseline rhythm was normal, sinus tachycardia would lead to a junctional tachycardia during exercise. Isolated monomorphic premature ventricular beats gradually increased in frequency and became polymorphic, followed by bursts of monomorphic and bidirectional salvos. If activity persisted, polymorphic VT and VF eventually occurred.

Idiopathic Ventricular Fibrillation

An estimated 1 to 5 percent of SCDs are due to idiopathic VF without apparent evidence of structural heart disease.[143, 144] The mean age is the mid 30s to early 40s, and the ratio of men to women is approximately 2:1. Preliminary data suggest that these patients have a 30 percent recurrence rate of VF, syncope, and cardiac arrest. The use of implantable cardioverter-defibrillators (ICDs) could be particularly useful in this population.

Specialized Conduction System Abnormalities

Primary fibrosis (Lenegre's disease)[145] or secondary mechanical injury (Lev's disease)[146] of the His-Purkinje system can be the cause of intraventricular conduction abnormalities and symptomatic atrioventricular block. However, these entities are less commonly associated with SCD.

Pathology and Pathophysiology

There is no uniform hypothesis regarding the pathophysiology of SCD. A combination of multiple triggering factors in a susceptible myocardium results in the sudden cessation of cardiac output, leading to hypotension, hypoperfusion of the organs of the body, and death. Factors that can trigger SCD include circulating catecholamines, autonomic sympathetic input, electrolyte abnormalities, antiarrhythmic drugs, and myocardial ischemia.[147] Although more than half of patients with SCD have no previous history of CAD,[148] significant coronary stenosis is the most commonly encountered factor in 75 to 94 percent of SCD victims.[149–151] Direct pathologic evidence that links CAD to SCD through the documentation of recent thrombotic occlusion of a major coronary vessel can be found in 4 to 64 percent[152] of these patients. Even in the absence of total occlusion, ischemia may be due to sudden plaque fissuring and rupture[153] or to vasospasm.[154] Experimental animal models suggest that vulnerability to arrhythmia during coronary occlusion is increased in the early period of occlusion (0 to 30 minutes), peaking at 5 to 6 minutes and again at 12 to 30 minutes and during reperfusion.[155, 156] Acute ischemia results in acidosis and the accumulation of extracellular potassium and intracellular calcium, as well as various metabolites of fatty acid and glycolysis that result in sarcolemmal and gap junction dysfunction.[157–159] The EP consequences of these changes are an increased spontaneous impulse formation, a decreased myocyte refractoriness, and slowing of conduction through the myocardium.[160] These changes lead to electrical inhomogenicity in the myocardium, which predisposes to arrhythmia.[2] When a PVC is coupled to the underlying rhythm by a critical period, a reentrant circuit is created.[161] The wave of activation from the PVC blocks in the ischemic area, while the surrounding normal tissue continues to activate to the area distal to the ischemia; the impulse then moves back slowly through the ischemic zone to create a circuit. *Reentry* is the major mechanism by which an arrhythmia is created and maintained, although other mechanisms, such as increased automaticity and triggered activity, are also important.

For 6 to 8 hours and for 2 to 3 days after an acute MI, the myocardium is vulnerable to arrhythmias to a lesser degree, mainly as a result of increased automaticity of the Purkinje fibers in the infarcted area.[162] Chronically, after an acute MI, areas of scar tissue can lead to a reentry circuit and predispose to tachyarrhythmias.[163]

The most common ultimately lethal arrhythmia in patients with cardiac arrest is VF.[164] Acute ischemia in experimental animals can lead to VT, which can degenerate into VF in 1 to 5 minutes.[165] The transition from VT to VF appears to be due to acceleration of the tachycardia in both the subendocardium and the subepicardium. VF is then maintained by multiple disorganized reentrant circuits that follow constantly changing pathways, with the rapid recovery of excitability.[166] Tachyarrhythmias are frequently encountered in acute coronary syndromes. In hearts with severe chronic diffuse disease, however, bradyarrhythmia or pulseless electrical activity more commonly occurs as a terminal event.[32]

Atherosclerosis resulting in ischemia is the disease process seen in most patients with SCD. In the remainder of patients, a wide spectrum of congenital and acquired diseases can be found. In some of these cases, the heart may show macroscopic changes such as hypertrophy (in aortic stenosis and hypertrophic cardiomyopathy) and focal fatty or fibrous fatty infiltrates (in arrhythmogenic right ventricular dysplasia). If the heart is normal at the gross and microscopic levels, careful examination of the conduction system may reveal pathologic changes related to SCD; these changes include fibrosis, degeneration, inflammation, and abnormal conduction pathways in the sinoatrial node, atrioventricular node, and bundle branches. Conduction system disorders can result in abnormal impulse formation or propagation and can predispose to reentrant arrhythmias.[167] Advances in molecular biology are revealing new causes of SCD at the cellular level, such as LQTS, several forms of distinctive tachycardias, idiopathic VF, and diseases of the sinoatrial and atrioventricular nodes.[168]

EVALUATION AND RISK STRATIFICATION

Although during the past two decades multiple diagnostic tests have been used to evaluate different cardiac and noncardiac factors that play a role in occurrence of SCD, the relatively low positive predictive accuracy of these tests affects their usefulness.[169] Our understanding of these risk factors is incomplete. When screening a patient for the presence of risk factors for SCD, one should first evaluate the underlying cardiac pathology as well as the presence of possible comorbid noncardiac conditions. The first step would be a complete history and physical examination, which can provide clues regarding the risk of SCD.

Because CAD is the most common underlying factor in SCD, particular attention should be directed towards a history of chest discomfort or recent exertional intolerance. Because left ventricular dysfunction is a major risk factor for SCD, potential symptoms of congestive heart disease (CHF) should be carefully evaluated. A prior history of cardiac arrest is the most significant risk factor recurrent cardiac arrest.[170] In patients with structural heart disease, particular attention should be paid to history of unexplained syncope that puts this population at higher risk for SCD.[169] In the setting of unexplained syncope in patients with structural heart disease or in patients who survived SCD, the interrogation of those who witnessed the event can provide crucial information. Documentation of all rhythm strips recorded during the event is also paramount. Any current use of cardiac or noncardiac drugs, whether prescribed or over-the-counter medications, must be carefully determined because of the possibility of QT prolongation. Interrogation of the patient should include any family history of hypertrophic cardiomyopathy, Marfan's syndrome, and sudden or unexplained death.

A careful physical examination also provides further insight into the presence of underlying structural heart disease and other comorbid conditions. Various noninvasive methods are used to evaluate the underlying cardiac pathology and help the risk stratification process.

Electrocardiography. An ECG is helpful in the diagnosis of underlying CAD and MI. Furthermore, it provides other helpful markers such as prolonged QT interval (in acquired and congenital LQTS), delta waves (a clue to WPW syndrome), epsilon wave (in ARVD), and right bundle branch block and ST-segment elevation in V_1 to V_3 (in Brugada's syndrome). An ECG is also a specific but insensitive tool with which to evaluate left ventricular hypertrophy.

Echocardiography. Echocardiography provides information regarding LVEF, which is one of the most powerful predictors of recurrent cardiac arrest.[171] LVEF is an independent predictor of death. An EF of less than 0.40 indicates an increased risk of death by at least 3- to 4-fold.[172] When left ventricular dysfunction is associated with ventricular arrhythmia, the risk for SCD increases further. The presence of LV dysfunction precludes the use of certain antiarrhythmic agents that can produce a negative inotropic effect or a proarrhythmic event.

Echocardiography can also be used to evaluate segmental wall motion abnormalities associated with CAD, significant valvular dysfunction, evidence of hypertrophic cardiomyopathy, pericardial disease, intracardiac tumors, and congenital heart disease.

Exercise Stress Testing. Exercise stress testing is a recognized prognostic test in survivors of acute MI. Several studies have shown that the presence of ST-segment changes, the occurrence of exercise-induced angina, inappropriate blood pressure response, and exercise-induced ventricular arrhythmia in post-MI patients during submaximal predischarge stress testing is a predictor of recurrent ischemic events, need for revascularization, and overall cardiac mortality rates. Certain authors found that these findings are predictive of ventricular arrhythmia and sudden death.[173–175] However, other investigators have not found exercise test results to specifically predict the risk of SCD.[59, 176, 177]

Exercise testing is also useful in the identification of patients with exercise-induced or exercise-aggravated ventricular tachycardia.[178–180]

Stress testing is most commonly used as a noninvasive test to evaluate the presence of CAD in patients with chest pain. The sensitivity and specificity of stress test improve when it is combined with nuclear methods.

Radionuclide Imaging. Radionuclide angiography is another noninvasive method that can be used to quantitatively assess left ventricular function. It can also provide information regarding regional left ventricular performance.

Ambulatory Electrocardiographic Monitoring. The role of Holter monitoring in the evaluation of patients with arrhythmias has been the subject of multiple studies, particularly in post-MI patients. Several studies confirmed the prognostic significance of frequent premature ventricular complexes and NSVT in post-MI patients.[181, 182] However, the specificity of spontaneous ventricular ectopy is limited.[183] Mortality rates are not influenced by the frequency, duration, or rate of NSVT.[181, 182]

The presence of frequent ventricular ectopy in asymptomatic patients without structural heart disease and normal left ventricular function has little, if any, prognostic significance.

Signal-Averaged Electrocardiography. Low-amplitude, fragmented, and delayed electrical activity can be recorded from areas bordering the infarction in an experimental model of MI. The signal-averaged ECG records this delayed fractionated activity from the body surface. A number of studies have evaluated the prognostic significance of the signal-averaged ECG alone or in combination with Holter monitoring or LVEF in the post-MI population.[60, 184, 185] In these studies, the sensitivity during a follow-up period of 6 to 24 months in patients who experienced sustained VT or SCD was between 50 and 90 percent. Its primary benefit was its excellent negative predictive value, which has been reported to be about 95 percent. However, the positive predictive value of signal-averaged ECG (the risk of arrhythmia in a patient with positive results) has been lower, averaging 20 percent in these studies. Kuchar and colleagues[185] risk-stratified patients after an acute MI by using signal-averaged ECG, Holter monitoring, and radionuclide ventriculography. Patients were followed for a median of 14 months for an arrhythmic event that was defined as sudden death or sustained VT. The results of each of these three tests were independently predictive of arrhythmic events. An LVEF of less than 0.40 was the most powerful predictor of an arrhythmic event. The addition of a positive signal-averaged ECG to the LVEF further increased the probability of predicting an event (from 4 percent for LVEF of less than 0.40 alone to 34 percent with LVEF of less than 0.40 plus a positive signal-averaged ECG). A signal-averaged ECG is most predictive of arrhythmic events in inferior infarctions and is less useful in anterior infarctions. This difference is probably due to the fact that peri-infarct tissue in anterior infarction is activated relatively early in the sequence of ventricular activation. This makes it more difficult to detect late potentials.

Heart Rate Variability. Heart rate variability is a measure of beat-to-beat variations of sinus-initiated RR intervals. It has been evaluated as an indicator of decreased parasympathetic tone, which is associated with poor prognosis in post-MI patients. Schneider and Costiloe[186] evaluated the relationship between sinus arrhythmia and prognosis after MI and concluded that sinus arrhythmia decreases in normal patients with age, that sinus arrhythmia is less evident after MI, and that patients with the least evidence of sinus arrhythmia had the worst prognosis during follow-up.

Kleiger and colleagues demonstrated the relation between increased mortality rates and decreased heart rate variability in a study of 808 post-MI patients. They showed that heart rate variability has a significant relation with other prognostic indicators, relating directly to LVEF and exercise capacity. However, the heart rate variability correlated to a much lower degree with ventricular ectopy, suggesting that these two factors acted independently.

Farrell and associates[187] observed that the sensitivity of heart rate variability in the prediction of arrhythmic events (sudden death and sustained VT) was higher than that of other risk factors, including exercise testing, LVEF, ventricular ectopy, and signal-averaged ECG. In the analysis of a combination of risk factors, the combination of a decrease in heart rate variability and the presence of late potentials in signal-averaged electrocardiography was more predictive of arrhythmic events than other combinations.

The decrease in heart rate variability suggests a relative decrease in parasympathetic tone.[188] Another possible explanation is that increased vagal tone protects against VF in the presence of ischemia.

Cardiac Catheterization. Cardiac catheterization should be performed in almost all survivors of SCD to establish the presence, extent, and severity of CAD. It can also exclude congenital coronary vessel anomalies in younger SCD survivors. Cardiac catheterization can confirm the results of noninvasive studies for evaluation of left ventricular function, wall motion abnormalities, and valvular disease.

Electrophysiologic Testing. Wellens and colleagues[163] demonstrated that programmed stimulation could safely and reproducibly initiate VT in the majority of the patients who experienced sustained VT.

Subsequent studies confirmed this observation. From 60 to 90 percent of patients who survived sudden death unassociated with acute MI are inducible during EP study.[163, 189–192] Sustained monomorphic VT can be induced during EP study in 50 to 60 percent of cardiac arrest survivors, and polymorphic VT or VF can be induced in an additional 10 to 20 percent.[193–195] Ventricular arrhythmia is inducible in more than 90 percent of patients who had a prior MI and clinical VT.

The difference in the incidence of induced ventricular arrhythmias among studies depends on the extent of left ventricular dysfunction, the clinical arrhythmia, and the aggressiveness of stimulation protocol. Considerable controversy still exists regarding the optimal EP protocol for the evaluation of sudden death survivors. The optimal protocol achieves a high rate of inducibility but minimizes the induction of poorly reproducible and clinically irrelevant arrhythmias. The studies that used stimulation protocols limited to two or fewer ventricular extrastimuli with a follow-up period of less than 1 year have reported low sensitivity and low positive predictive values for inducible VT.[196, 197] Studies that used stimulation protocols with three or more extrastimuli and a follow-up period of at least 1 year reported 25 to 36 percent arrhythmic events in patients with inducible VT.[198, 199] The group in Sydney who evaluated more than 1200 patients and followed them for at least 2 years[199] has shown that the patients who had inducible polymorphic VT or VF in the EP laboratory were not at any higher risk of arrhythmic events than were patients who were not inducible. Like several other reports, they showed that programmed stimulation has an excellent negative predictive value (~98 percent).[200]

The prognostic value of a number of tests in the same population was evaluated, and it was concluded that EP testing had the highest positive predictive value (~30 percent)[176] and was the only test that specifically identified patients at risk for SCD. Programmed stimulation has also been evaluated for risk stratification in patients with CAD and NSVT.[201–205] These studies have shown inducible VT in 21 to 45 percent of the patients. If we consider only the protocols that used three ventricular extrastimuli, the rate of inducibility increases to 40 to 45 percent. These studies also confirm the excellent negative predictive value of EP testing. However, the positive predictive value of EP testing in these studies was poor, with a range of 12.5 to 23 percent.

The relatively low positive accuracy of these tests, which at best, alone or on combination, reaches 30 percent, is a major problem considering the cost of adequate protective therapy.

PREVENTION

The majority of SCD victims have no symptoms and are not identified as being at high risk before the event.[146] Therefore, in addition to the secondary prevention of SCD (prevention of recurrent cardiac arrest), primary prevention is a major therapeutic goal.

As discussed earlier, patients with the highest risk factor profile constitute a small percentage of the total number of people at risk for SCD. Furthermore, when the high-risk subgroups are identified and removed from this population base, the calculated incidence for the remainder of the population decreases and the identification of individuals at high risk becomes more difficult.

During the past decade, multiple trials have been conducted regarding the primary prevention of SCD in patients with heart disease who are at high risk and the secondary prevention of SCD in patients who have been successfully resuscitated. Here, we summarize pertinent data from the extensive literature that is available, but it is beyond the scope of this chapter to review the extensive data from numerous trials.

Primary Prevention

Pharmacologic Studies

β-BLOCKER THERAPY

Available data from several prospective double-blind studies revealed that β-blockers reduce the overall mortality and SCD rates after acute MI. In the Beta-Blocker Heart Attack Trial (BHAT),[206] propranolol (180 to 240 mg/da) decreased the total mortality rate over an average follow-up period of 25 months by 26.5 percent (from 9.8 percent in the placebo group to 7.2 percent in the propranolol group). The benefit was remarkable in high-risk patients. Propranolol reduced the risk of death in this group by 43 percent ($P < .001$).[207] Propranolol decreased the incidence of SCD by 47 percent in patients who had previous heart failure versus 13 percent in the patients who did not, with a 35 percent reduction in adjusted mortality rate (Fig. 94–8).

In the Norwegian Multicenter Study on Timolol after Acute Myocardial Infarction,[208] timolol reduced total mortality by 38 percent. SCD was decreased by 45 percent from 13.9 percent in the placebo group to 7.7 percent in the timolol group ($P = .0001$). The beneficial results persisted for up to 72 months.[209] In the Acebutolol Post-Infarction Trial (Acebutolol et Prevention Secondaire de l'Infarctus [APSI]),[210] acebutolol reduced mortality rates by 48 percent and cardiovascular death by 58 percent compared with placebo. The benefit was maintained after several years of follow-up.[211]

In the Goteborg trial,[212] metoprolol (intravenous infusion followed by 200 mg/da PO) reduced mortality rates by 36 percent from 8.9 to 5.7 percent. In the Metoprolol in Acute Myocardial Infarction (MIAMI) study,[213] the metoprolol group had a statistically insignificant 13 percent reduction in mortality rates. However, retrospective analysis showed that the treatment was beneficial in high-risk patients and reduced mortality rates from 8.5 to 6 percent ($P = .03$). Metoprolol was also used in the Thrombolysis in Myocardial Infarction (TIMI) II-B study[214] as an adjunct to intravenous tissue plasminogen activator. The patients were randomly assigned to receive immediate intravenous metoprolol followed by oral therapy or to deferred therapy with metoprolol starting on day 6 after the MI. There was a lower rate of recurrent ischemia and nonfatal MI in the group that received immediate therapy. In a meta-analysis of 26 trials by Yusuf and associates,[215] therapy with β-

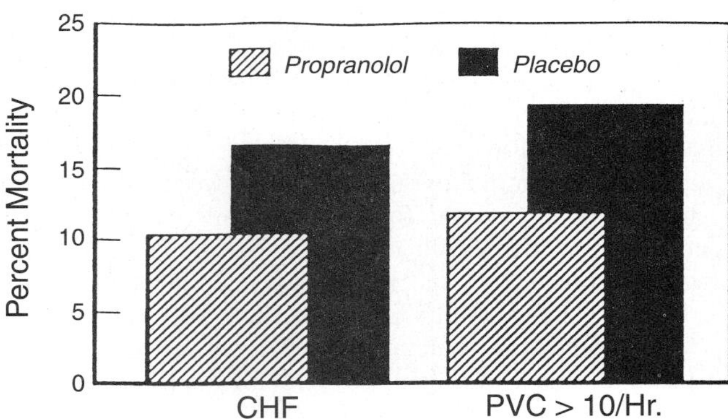

FIGURE 94–8 Mortality rates in two high-risk subgroups in the Beta-Blocker Heart Attack Trial demonstrate a substantial survival benefit associated with β-blockers *(hatched bars)* relative to placebo *(solid bars)*. CHF, congestive heart failure; PVC, premature ventricular contraction. (From Wilber DJ, Kall JG, Kapp DE: What can we expect from prophylactic implantable defibrillators? Am J Cardiol 80:20F–27F, 1997.)

blockers resulted in a 23 percent reduction in mortality rates.

The mechanism of beneficial effect of β-blockers is unclear. The survival benefits appear to be mediated by a reduction in arrhythmia-related deaths and recurrent MI.

β-Blockers reduce the threshold for VF, most likely through their antisympathetic effect. β-Blockers also reduce hypokalemia by blocking the catecholamine-induced influx of potassium into cells.[216]

Patients with depressed left ventricular function and a history of congestive heart failure show the greatest survival benefit. β-Blockers may improve survival in patients with congestive heart failure by reducing myocardial oxygen demand, improving diastolic relaxation, reducing sympathetic-mediated vasoconstriction and tachycardia, or reducing catecholamine-induced myocardial damage or by their antiarrhythmic effect.[216]

The Metoprolol in Dilated Cardiomyopathy (MDC) Trial decreased the risk of death or need of heart transplantation by 35 percent. It also caused a significant improvement in cardiac function and exercise capacity.

Bisoprolol was noted to be beneficial in the Cardiac Insufficiency Bisoprolol Study (CIBIS).[218] Although there was no overall benefit in survival, there was a 57 percent reduction in mortality rate in patients without previous MI. In the CIBIS-II study,[219] bisoprolol showed a significant mortality benefit. In this multicenter, double-blinded, randomized, placebo-controlled trial, all enrolled patients were in NYHA functional class III or IV with an LVEF of less than 0.35. The all-cause mortality rate was significantly lower with bisoprolol (11.8 percent versus 17.3 percent in the placebo group, $P < .0001$). Furthermore, the incidence of SCD decreased by 44 percent among patients receiving bisoprolol (3.6 percent versus 6.3 percent in placebo group, $P = .0011$).

In the Mortality Effect of Metoprolol in Patients with Heart Failure (MERIT-HF) trial,[220] treatment with metoprolol CR/XL was associated with a 34 percent decrease in all-cause mortality rates, a 38 percent decrease in cardiovascular mortality rates, a 41 percent decrease in SCD, and a 49 percent decrease in death due to progressive heart failure. Carvedilol, a nonselective β-receptor agonist with some α_1-receptor antagonist activity, improved survival rates in patients with CHF in a U.S. multicenter study.[221] There was a 65 percent reduction in mortality rates. The findings of this study have been criticized because four U.S. trials were combined to achieve these values, and the primary objective was to rule out excess mortality by the drug. However, the result of this trial was supported by another trial from Australia/New Zealand,[222] which showed a 26 percent decrease in death or hospital admission in patients with ischemic cardiomyopathy.

ANGIOTENSIN-CONVERTING ENZYME INHIBITORS AND THE ANGIOTENSIN II RECEPTOR ANTAGONISTS

The beneficial effect of angiotensin-converting enzyme (ACE) inhibitors appears to be a class effect that is mediated by a reduction in ventricular size, reinfarction, the appearance of CHF, and a new ischemic event.

There has been a 6 to 22 percent reduction in mortality rate in several studies. Despite the beneficial effect on total mortality rate, the precise role of these agents in reducing SCD is still not clear.

In the Veterans Administration Cooperative II Study (V-HeFT II),[223] there was a 28 percent reduction in mortality rate in the enalapril group from reduced incidence of SCD compared with the hydralazine-isosorbide group.

In the Trandolapril Cardiac Evaluation[224] (TRACE) study, trandolapril reduced mortality rates by 22 percent and SCD rates by 24 percent ($P = .03$) in post-MI patients with evidence of left ventricular dysfunction. However, other studies did not show any significant reduction in the SCD rate. In the Survival and Ventricular Enlargement (SAVE) trial,[225] although captopril reduced total mortality rates by 19 percent in survivors of MI with asymptomatic left ventricular dysfunction (LVEF $\leq$ 40 percent), there was no statistical difference in the SCD rate. In the Studies on Left Ventricular Dysfunction (SOLVD) prevention trial,[226] captopril did not reduce significantly total mortality and SCD rates in asymptomatic (NYHA functional class I or II) patients with an LVEF of 0.35 or less.

Losartan is an angiotensin II receptor antagonist that blocks the receptor without increasing bradykinin levels. Because angiotensin II can be produced through alternate pathways, this class of drugs may have an advantage over ACE inhibitors.

In the Evaluation of Losartan in the Elderly (ELITE) trial,[227] the mortality rate was 46 percent lower in the losartan group than in the captopril group. The precise role of this new class of medication in reducing SCD needs to be further evaluated in larger studies.

ANTIARRHYTHMIC DRUG THERAPY

Class I Antiarrhythmic Drugs. Frequent and complex ventricular activities in survivors of MI have been demonstrated to be a risk marker for subsequent SCD. The objective of the CAST Trials I and II[228, 229] was to test the hypothesis that the suppression of ventricular ectopy after an MI would reduce the incidence of SCD.

In the CAST I study,[228] patients who had asymptomatic PVCs after MI suppressed by encainide or flecainide were randomly assigned to receive long-term drug therapy or placebo. After an average of 9.7 months, the total mortality rate was 7.7 percent in the type IC group versus 3 percent in the placebo group (relative risk, 2.5; $P = .0001$). Arrhythmic death was more common in the class IC group (4.5 percent versus 1.2 percent in the placebo group). The relative risk of death or resuscitated cardiac arrest was 2.38 (Fig. 94–9). Further analysis showed that the adverse event rate was highest in patients with the lowest LVEF. The presence of an LVEF of more than 0.30 was associated with improved survival rates. In a subgroup analysis, patients who were treated with β-blockers in addition to class IC antiarrhythmic agents had lower mortality rates than the group of patients who were treated with class IC agents alone. This observation suggests a protective effect of β-blockers.[230]

The results of the CAST trial disproved the hypothesis that suppression of ventricular arrhythmia improves mortality rates. Furthermore, meta-analysis of other class I agent trials showed a significantly higher mortality rate for antiar-

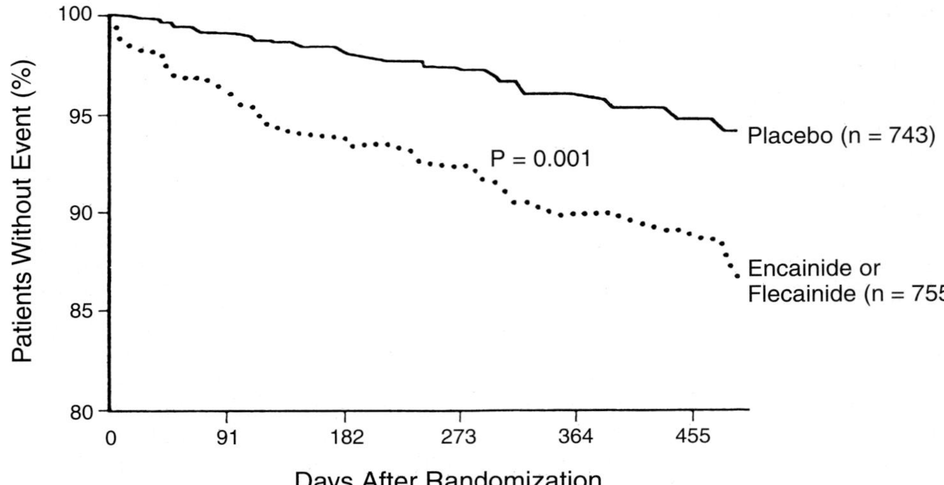

FIGURE 94–9 Actuarial probabilities of freedom from death or cardiac arrest from arrhythmias in 1498 patients receiving encainide, flecainide, or corresponding placebo. (From Echt DS, Liebson PR, Mitchell LB, et al: Mortality and morbidity in patients receiving encainide, flecainide, or placebo. The Cardiac Arrhythmia Suppression Trial. N Engl J Med 324:781–788, 1991.

rhythmic agent–treated patients compared with placebo-treated patients.[231]

A third drug, moracizine, was subsequently studied in the CAST II trial.[229] The overall mortality rate was similar for patients treated with moracizine and those treated with placebo. However, there was a significantly higher mortality rate among patients treated with moracizine during the initial 2 weeks of therapy (2.3 percent versus 0.3 percent). The cause of this proarrhythmic response is unknown. The unexpectedly low placebo mortality rate suggests that a low-risk population was chosen for the trial, which exposed the patients to all the risks of active therapy without much hope of benefit.

Class III Antiarrhythmic Drugs. Amiodarone is a unique antiarrhythmic drug with class I, II, III, and IV effects. The effect of amiodarone in the prevention of SCD was extensively studied in post-MI patients. In the Basel Antiarrhythmic Study of Infarct Survival (BASIS) trial,[232] there was 61 percent reduction in mortality rate with amiodarone. Amiodarone also decreased VF or SCD compared with control group (P = .024). The beneficial effect of amiodarone persisted several years after drug discontinuation.

The Polish Amiodarone Trial (PAT)[233] showed a reduction in cardiac death rates from 10.7 percent in the placebo group to 6.9 percent in the amiodarone arm of study.

The goal of the European Myocardial Infarct Amiodarone Trial (EMIAT)[234] was to assess the efficacy of amiodarone in reducing mortality rates in patients with depressed left ventricular function after an MI. This study enrolled 1486 patients with an LVEF of 0.40 or less within 5 to 21 days of MI. The median follow-up period was 21 months. Patients were randomly assigned to treatment with amiodarone or placebo. The primary end point was all-cause mortality, and secondary end points were cardiac death, arrhythmic death, and the combination of arrhythmic death and resuscitated cardiac arrest.

Amiodarone reduced arrhythmic death by 35 percent (P = .05) and arrhythmic death and resuscitated cardiac arrest by 32 percent (P = .05). However, amiodarone did not show any beneficial or detrimental effect on all-cause mortality rates.

The Canadian Amiodarone Myocardial Infarction Trial (CAMIAT)[235] evaluated the hypothesis that amiodarone could reduce arrhythmic death among post-MI patients (6 to 45 days after MI) who had frequent PVCs (≥10 PVCs per hour) or any run of VT on baseline Holter recording. The primary end point was arrhythmic death or resuscitated VF. Secondary end points were arrhythmic death, cardiac death, and all-cause mortality. In the efficacy analysis, resuscitated VF or arrhythmic death occurred in 6 percent of patients in the placebo group and 3.3 percent of patients in the amiodarone group. Amiodarone reduced the relative risk by 48.5 percent. Intention-to-treat analysis showed 38.2 percent risk reduction in the amiodarone group compared with the placebo group (from 6.9 percent in the placebo group to 4.5 percent in the amiodarone group, P = .029). The absolute risk reduction was greatest among patients with CHF or a history of MI. Although amiodarone reduced all-cause mortality by 18 percent, the difference was not statistically significant.

In EMIAT and CAMIAT, there was a significant reduction in arrhythmic death among patients. However, these two trials did not show any benefit in total mortality rates. CAMIAT was not powered to predict the overall survival benefit.

Sim and associates[236] showed a 21 percent reduction in overall mortality rates in a meta-analysis of eight post-MI trials in patients who received amiodarone.

Two other studies investigated the effect of amiodarone in patients with CHF. The Grupo de Estudio de la Sobrevida en la Insuficiencia Cardiaca en Argentina (GESICA) trial[237] studied the effect of amiodarone in patients with severe CHF who did not have any symptomatic ventricular arrhythmia. In this multicenter prospective study, 516 patients with LVEF of less than 0.35 were randomized to receive optimal medical therapy with or without amiodarone. Thirty-nine percent of patients had a prior history of MI; the remainder of the patients had nonischemic dilated cardiomyopathy or Chagas' disease. The mortality rate was 33.5 percent in the amiodarone-treated group and 41.4 percent in the control group. The primary end point was total mortality, and there was 28 percent risk reduction (P = .024), which was observed after 90 to 120 days of therapy and persisted to the end of the study. The reduction in mortality rates reflected improved rates of SCD and deaths due to worsening of heart failure. However, these trends were not statistically significant. Further subsequent analysis showed that 2-year SCD rate increased from 8.7 percent in patients without NSVT to 23.7 percent in patients with NSVT ($P < .001$). Therefore, the presence of NSVT was an independent risk marker for SCD.[238] However, these results were not reproducible in the Survival Trial of Antiarrhythmic Therapy in Congestive Heart Failure (CHF-STAT) trial,[239] which examined the use of amiodarone in patients with CHF with an LVEF of less than 0.40 and asymptomatic ventricular arrhythmias (>10 PVCs per hour). This was a multicenter, double-blind, placebo-controlled study that was performed to determine whether amiodarone could reduce overall mortality rates. Six hundred seventy-four patients were randomly assigned to treatment with either amiodarone or a placebo. There was no significant difference in the rates of overall mortality or sudden death between the two groups, despite the improved left ventricular function and suppressed ventricular arrhythmia in the amiodarone-treated group.

However, amiodarone tended to improve survival rates in the nonischemic heart disease group ($P = .07$). The difference in the results between the GESICA study and the CHF-STAT trial can be attributed to the much higher percentage of patients with nonischemic cardiomyopathy in the GESICA study.[240]

Sotalol is another class III antiarrhythmic medication with β-blocking properties that was studied in post-MI patients. In a double-blind randomized trial, Julian and associates[241] studied 1465 patients 5 to 14 days after MI. The patients were randomized to receive 320 mg/d *dl*-sotalol or placebo. The *dl*-sotalol group had an 18 percent improvement in survival rates. However, the total mortality rate was not significantly different at 1 year (8.4 percent for placebo versus 7.3 percent for *dl*-sotalol). Reinfarction rates were 41 percent lower ($P < .05$) in the *dl*-sotalol–treated group. *d*-sotalol was developed as a "pure" type III antiarrhythmic medication without β-blocking properties, as an alternative to *dl*-sotalol.

The Survival With Oral d-Sotalol (SWORD) trial[242] studied the effect of *d*-sotalol, a racemic isomer of *dl*-sotalol, in survivors of acute MI to evaluate reduction in all-cause mortality rates. There were 3121 patients who were randomized to receive *d*-sotalol or placebo. Entry criteria included history of MI 6 to 42 days before entry and an LVEF of less than 0.40. In addition, patients who had an MI more than 42 days earlier could be enrolled if they had symptomatic NYHA functional class II or III CHF. The study was prematurely terminated due to excess death rates in the *d*-sotalol arm (5 percent versus 3.1 percent in the placebo arm). The majority of excess death appeared to be secondary to enhanced arrhythmic death ($P = .008$).

Newer class III agents, such as azmilide and dofetilide, are under investigation.

Implantable Converter-Defibrillator Trials for Primary Prevention

The efficacy of defibrillators in the termination of ventricular arrhythmias is well established.[243, 244] Several recent or ongoing primary prevention trials have focused on the role of prophylactic ICDs in patients at a high risk of SCD (Table 94–4).

MULTICENTER AUTOMATIC DEFIBRILLATOR IMPLANTATION TRIAL

The presence of NSVT in patients with depressed left ventricular function, CAD, and inducible nonsuppressible VT on EP study is a predictor of poor prognosis with a 2-year mortality rate of 30 percent. The Multicenter Automatic Defibrillator Implantation Trial (MADIT)[245] was designed to evaluate the possible benefit of prophylactic ICD implantation in these patients. One hundred ninety-six patients from 32 centers in the United States and Europe were enrolled in this trial. The enrollment criteria included history of Q wave MI (≥3 weeks before entrance in study), LVEF of 0.35 or less, documented NSVT, inducible sustained VT not suppressed by antiarrhythmic drug on EP study, and NYHA functional class I to III. The average LVEF among MADIT patients was 26 percent and half of the patients had evidence of CHF. There were 101 patients in the drug therapy arm, including 80 receiving amiodarone and 95 receiving ICD therapy. MADIT was terminated early by the safety monitoring committee due to significant improvement in survival rates in the ICD group. There were 39 deaths (38.6 percent) in the antiarrhythmic group compared with 15 (12 percent) in the ICD group (hazard ratio, 0.46; 95 percent confidence interval, 0.26 to 0.82; $P = .009$). Death from cardiac causes was reduced by 57 percent in the ICD group (Fig. 94–10). Subanalysis from the MADIT database revealed a 2-year mortality rate of 8 percent in MADIT noninducible patients, 20 percent in MADIT inducible and suppressible patients, and 25 percent in inducible nonsuppressible patients who refused randomization into the study.[246] The investigators concluded that in a high-risk population with LV dysfunction and CAD, ICD therapy improved survival rates.

Critics of the MADIT study raised several issues regarding the study. A large number of patients in the antiarrhythmic arm were not taking any antiarrhythmic drug at the time of death (~23 percent), and approximately 30 percent of the patients who initially received amiodarone therapy discontinued it. On the other hand, 25 percent of patients assigned to the ICD group were taking amiodarone by the end of the study. β-Blockers, which are known to improve survival in post-MI patients, were administered more frequently in the ICD group.

Thus, critics have argued that MADIT demonstrates that an ICD in combination with an antiarrhythmic agent was better than no antiarrhythmic agent at all. The MADIT investigators believe that the reduction in overall mortality rate cannot be attributed to the more frequent use of β-blockers in the ICD arm and cite the BHAT trial,[206] which reported just a 2.5 percent difference in mortality rates between the placebo arm and the propranolol arm over an average follow-up period of 25 months.

Despite these concerns, the MADIT trial was the first randomized study that suggested that the prophylactic use of an ICD not only can save lives in a selected group of patients with LV dysfunction but also might save more lives than amiodarone therapy.

TABLE 94–4 **Prospective Multicenter Intracardiac Defibrillator Prevention Trials**

Study	Patient Inclusion Criteria	Endpoint(s)	Treatment Arms	Key Results
MADIT[245]	Q wave MI ≥ 3 wk Asymptomatic NSVT LVEF ≤ 0.35 Inducible, nonsuppressible VT on EPS with procainamide NYHA classes I–III	Overall mortality Costs and cost effectiveness	ICD (n = 95) Conventional therapy (n = 101)	ICD reduced overall mortality by 54% ICDs cost $16,900 per life-year saved versus conventional therapy
CABG Patch[247]	Scheduled for elective CABG surgery LVEF < 0.36 Abnormal SAECG	Overall mortality	ICD (n = 446) Standard treatment (n = 454)	Survival was not improved by prophylactic implantation of ICD at time of elective CABG
MUSTT[249–251]	CAD EF ≤ 0.40 NSVT Inducible VT or VF	Sudden arrhythmic death or spontaneous sustained VT	ICD in nonsuppressible group Antiarrhythmic drug therapy in suppressible group No therapy	EP-guided therapy is useful in reducing sudden arrhythmic death or VT with benefit seeming to be arising mainly from ICD use
SCD HeFT	Ischemic or nonischemic dilated cardiomyopathy NYHA classes II–III EF ≤ 0.35	Total mortality Arrhythmic mortality Costs Quality of life	ICD Amiodarone Placebo	Ongoing
Cardiomyopathy Study	Dilated nonischemic cardiomyopathy LVEF ≤ 0.30 NYHA classes II–III	Total mortality Sudden death Serious arrhythmia	ICD Standard treatment	Ongoing
DEFIBRILLAT	CHF patients awaiting heart transplantation	Total mortality Serious arrhythmia	ICD Standard treatment	Ongoing

Abbreviations: CABG, coronary artery bypass graft; CAD, coronary artery disease; CHF, congestive heart failure; EF, ejection fraction; EP, electrophysiologic; EPS, electrophysiologic study; ICD, implantable cardioverter-defibrillator; LVEF, left ventricular ejection fraction; MADIT, Multicenter Automatic Defibrillator Implantation Trial; MI, myocardial infarction; MUSTT, Multicenter Unsustained Tachycardia Trial; NSVT, nonsustained ventricular tachycardia; NYHA, New York Heart Association; SAECG, signal-averaged electrocardiogram; SCD HeFT, Sudden Cardiac Death in Heart Failure Trial; VF, ventricular fibrillation; VT, ventricular tachycardia.
From Khoshnevis GR, Massumi A: Ventricular arrhythmias in congestive heart failure: clinical significance and management. Tex Heart Inst J 26:42–59, 1999.

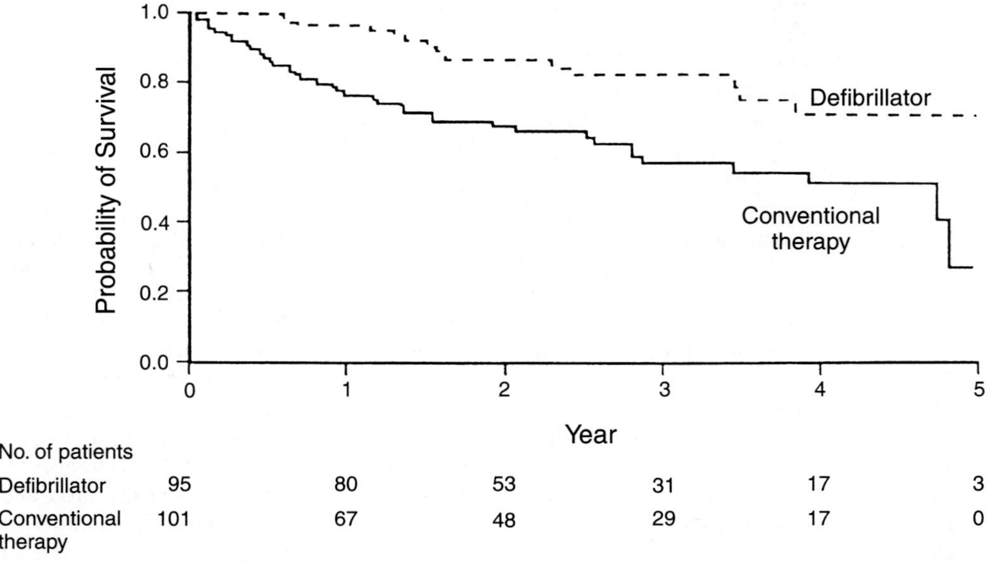

FIGURE 94–10 Kaplan-Meier analysis of probability of death according to assigned treatment. The difference in mortality rates between two treatment groups was significant (P = .009). (From Moss AJ, Hall WJ, Cannon DS, et al: Improved survival with an implanted defibrillator in patients with coronary disease at high risk for ventricular arrhythmia. Multicenter Automatic Defibrillator Implantation Trial Investigators. N Engl J Med 335:1933–1940, 1996.)

CORONARY ARTERY BYPASS GRAFT PATCH TRIAL

In the Coronary Artery Bypass Graft (CABG)-Patch trial,[247] the prophylactic use of ICDs was evaluated in a high-risk population with established CAD, depressed LV function, and an abnormal signal-averaged ECG. The trial was based on evidence that the 2-year mortality rate of patients who undergo bypass graft surgery with a baseline LVEF of less than 0.36 is 27.5 percent,[248] and approximately 40 percent of these patients died suddenly. Pilot data also suggested that a positive signal-averaged ECG increased the mortality risk. The prestudy hypothesis was that an ICD would reduce the 3-year total mortality rate by 26 percent.

Nine hundred patients younger than 80 years with an LVEF of less than 0.36 and a positive signal-averaged ECG were randomized to undergo elective coronary artery bypass graft surgery alone (n = 454) or to undergo prophylactic implantation of an ICD during elective coronary artery bypass graft surgery (n = 446). The primary end point was overall mortality. During an average follow-up period of 32 ± 16 months, there were 101 deaths in the ICD group (71 from cardiac causes) and 95 deaths in the control group (72 from cardiac causes) by intention-to-treat analysis.[247] The hazard ratio overall mortality rate was 1.07 (95 percent confidence interval, 0.81 to 1.42; $P = .64$). The CABG-Patch trial demonstrated no benefit from the prophylactic ICD implantation in patients with depressed LVEF and ischemia who underwent revascularization.

NSVT was present in only 30 percent of the CABG-Patch trial patients (based on an average of 16 hours of Holter monitoring) but was present in 100 percent of the MADIT trial patients. Signal-averaged ECG was abnormal in 100 percent of the CABG-Patch trial patients compared with 60 percent of the MADIT trial patients. All of the patients in the CABG-Patch trial had been revascularized compared with only two thirds of the MADIT patients, Only 90 patients (10 percent of enrolled patients) in the CABG-Patch trial had EP study during enrollment, but inducibility is estimated to be about 22 percent using mathematical models. Considering these facts, the different results of MADIT and CABG-Patch trials could be explained in two ways. A positive signal-averaged ECG seems to be a poor risk stratifier in this subset of patients. As demonstrated in the MADIT trial, inducible sustained VT during EP study may be a better risk stratifier for subsequent arrhythmic event.

Furthermore, this study provides additional evidence that revascularization may have reduced the number of arrhythmic deaths by preventing the ischemic trigger and led to subsequent preservation and even improvement of LVEF.

THE MULTICENTER UNSUSTAINED TACHYCARDIA TRIAL

The Multicenter Unsustained Tachycardia Trial (MUSTT)[249–251] is not a direct study of the efficacy of ICD, but the inclusion of device therapy in one arm of the trial offers an opportunity to evaluate the usefulness of ICD therapy. The hypothesis was that EP study–guided antiarrhythmic or ICD therapy, or both, would reduce the risk of arrhythmic death or cardiac arrest in patients with nonsustained VT and left ventricular dysfunction. The inclusion criteria for this study were LVEF of 0.40 or less, history of MI preceding entrance to study for at least 1 week, and nonsustained VT. A total of 704 patients were randomly assigned to EP-guided therapy with different antiarrhythmic medications or an ICD if the patient had persistent inducible VT, or no antiarrhythmic therapy. All of these patients had inducible sustained VT, VF, or both on programmed electrical stimulation. The primary end point of the trial was arrhythmic death or cardiac arrest. The secondary end point was total or cardiovascular death. There was no difference between the two groups in average age, gender, LVEF, history of prior MI, prior CABG and use of β-blockers or ACE inhibitors.

The mean duration of follow-up was 39 months. The incidence of arrhythmic death or cardiac arrest at 2 years was 18 percent in patients randomized to no antiarrhythmic therapy and 12 percent in the EP-guided therapy group. At 5 years, the incidence of primary end point was 32 percent in the former group and 25 percent in the EP-guided group. A total of 46 percent of patients in the EP-guided therapy group underwent defibrillator implantation after failing EP-guided drug testing. Primary end point events in the EP-guided group patients who received an ICD were reduced by more than 50 percent compared with the patients who did not receive an ICD in this group,[251] whereas EP-guided pharmacologic therapy alone did not seem to convey a survival benefit.

The investigators concluded that in high-risk patients with CAD, depressed LV function, and inducible sustained VT, EP-guided therapy is useful in reducing the risk of arrhythmic death and cardiac arrest. The benefit seems to arise from the use of ICDs. These preliminary results, which were presented at the American College of Cardiology meeting in 1999, were consistent with MADIT trial results.

There are several ongoing trials that consider the role of intracardiac defibrillators in the primary prevention of SCD (see Table 94–4).

MADIT II TRIAL

This trial has been designed to expand and simplify the inclusion criteria of the MADIT trial by eliminating risk stratification by programmed extrastimulation. In this trial, post-MI patients with an LVEF of less than 30 percent will be randomly assigned to receive either ICD or conventional therapy.

CABG-PATCH II TRIAL

In the CABG-Patch II trial, all survivors of the CABG-Patch trial will undergo EP study. If the inducibility rate of survivors is far beyond the mathematical estimation of 22 percent, then it will support the protective effect of revascularization against arrhythmic death by preventing the ischemic triggering.

SUDDEN CARDIAC DEATH IN HEART FAILURE

This is a prospective primary prevention trial in patients with LV dysfunction. The hypothesis in this trial is that

SCD might be preventable in as many as 50 percent of patients with moderate heart failure by the use of prophylactic amiodarone or defibrillator therapy, or both. The plan is to enroll 2500 patients with symptomatic heart failure (NYHA functional class II or III) of at least 3 months' duration with an LVEF of 0.35 or less.

All patients will be treated maximally with ACE inhibitors, vasodilators, or both. The study population would be randomized into three different treatment arms. The first arm of the study is the control arm; the patients will receive conventional heart failure therapy and placebo. The second arm combines conventional heart failure therapy and amiodarone. In these two arms of study, amiodarone and placebo are delivered in a double-blind fashion.

The patients randomized to the third arm of study will receive conventional therapy and implantation of a single-lead pectoral ICD.

Patients with NYHA functional class I and IV heart failure, a life expectancy of less than 1 year, or restrictive, hypertrophic, or infiltrative cardiomyopathy are excluded.

The primary end point of the study is all-cause mortality. Complications, economics, and quality of life will be evaluated separately as secondary end points.

Secondary Prevention

In patients with a history of sustained VT/VF, aborted SCD, or both, antiarrhythmic drugs have been the cornerstone of therapy for several years. Different studies were performed to determine the best method to guide antiarrhythmic therapy.[252–256] Several studies have been performed to determine whether antiarrhythmic drugs or ICDs are the therapy of choice to prolong survival.[257–262]

Role of Antiarrhythmic Drugs

The debate on whether antiarrhythmic therapy is best guided by Holter monitoring or invasive EP study led to prospective trials.

CALGARY STUDY[252]

This small study randomized patients with a history of sustained VT to receive antiarrhythmic therapy guided by Holter monitoring or EP study. By intention-to-treat analysis, the recurrence of symptomatic sustained VT/VF or sudden death was 19 percent in the invasive arm and 47 percent in the noninvasive arm ($P = .02$). It showed the superiority of the invasive approach in decreasing the frequency of recurrent VT/VF.

THE ELECTROPHYSIOLOGIC STUDY VERSUS ELECTROCARDIOGRAPHIC MONITORING TRIAL

The Electrophysiologic Study Versus Electrocardiographic Monitoring (ESVEM) study[254, 255] was performed to compare whether Holter monitoring or EP drug testing is superior in predicting long-term efficacy of different antiarrhythmic drugs. A total of 486 patients with sustained VT/VF who were inducible during EP study and had more than 10 PVCs per hour during 48-hour Holter monitoring were randomized to EP drug testing or ambulatory electrocardiographic monitoring while on antiarrhythmic therapy.

Drug efficacy was defined in the Holter arm as 100 percent suppression of VT runs of more than 15 beats, 80 percent suppression of pairs, and 70 percent suppression of PVCs. EP study efficacy was defined as suppression of inducible VT (no inducible VT of >15 beats in duration).

The primary end point was recurrence of arrhythmia in a patient receiving a drug that was predicted to be more effective by serial testing. Secondary end points were death from any cause, death from cardiac cause, and death from arrhythmia. Forty-five percent of patients in the EP arm (108 of 242 were included in this limb of study) and 77 percent (187 of 244) in the Holter monitoring arm achieved efficacy. There was no statistical difference between the two methods in predicting arrhythmia recurrence, which was 58 percent at 2 years.[255]

Patients received up to six drugs in a random order; amiodarone was not used in this study. Sotalol was found to be more effective than other drugs tested and statistically had a lower recurrence rate of arrhythmia ($P < .001$), all-cause mortality ($P < .004$), cardiac death ($P < .02$), and arrhythmic death ($P = .04$).[263] ESVEM investigators therefore concluded that Holter monitoring was equally predictive of arrhythmia recurrence as EP testing.

CARDIAC ARREST STUDY IN SEATTLE: CONVENTIONAL VERSUS AMIODARONE DRUG EVALUATION TRIAL

In the Cardiac Arrest Study in Seattle: Conventional versus Amiodarone Drug Evaluation (CASCADE) study,[264] 228 cardiac arrest survivors (out-of-hospital VF not associated with a Q wave MI) were randomly assigned to receive empirical amiodarone or a conventional class I antiarrhythmic drug guided by EP studies or Holter monitoring. Patients were included in this study if they had 10 PVCs or more per hour on Holter monitoring and had inducible sustained VT or VF. The primary end point was cardiac survival, which was defined as being free of syncope/ICD shock, resuscitated cardiac arrest, and/or cardiac death.

During a follow-up of 6 years, the rate of cardiac survival was 30 percent. The patients treated with amiodarone had a better outcome (amiodarone, 41 percent survival rate; conventional class I agent, 20 percent survival rate; $P < .001$). There was no significant difference in outcomes between conventionally treated patients whose inducible arrhythmias were or were not suppressed.

Based on findings of ESVEM, CASCADE, and CAST trials as we discussed earlier, it should be concluded that therapy with class I antiarrhythmic drugs for VT/VF was either ineffective or caused more harm. Although class III agents, sotalol in the ESVEM trial, and amiodarone in the CASCADE trial were more effective than class I agents, the chance of long-term event-free survival (no cardiac death or sustained ventricular arrhythmia) was less than 50 percent during follow-up. Therefore, ICD therapy was considered as an alternative for the secondary prevention of SCD. Several studies evaluated the role of ICDs for secondary prevention.

Role of ICD Therapy

ANTIARRHYTHMIC VERSUS IMPLANTABLE DEFIBRILLATOR TRIAL

The Antiarrhythmic Versus Implantable Defibrillator (AVID) trial[258, 259] was designed to determine whether best antiarrhythmic drug (empiric amiodarone or guided sotalol) or ICD therapy is superior in reducing mortality rates in patients with a history of sustained VT/VF. Secondary objectives of the study considered the cost effectiveness of the two arms and quality of life assessment (Table 94–5).

The study enrolled 1016 patients who had either been resuscitated from VF (45 percent) or undergone cardioversion from sustained VT (55 percent). The patients who had VT also had syncope or other serious cardiac symptoms and LVEF of 0.40 or less. The patients were randomized to either class III antiarrhythmic drugs, primarily amiodarone, or ICD implantation.

The study was terminated prematurely in April 1997 after data analysis and safety monitoring revealed a significant survival advantage in the ICD group.[201] The survival rates in the ICD group were 89.3, 81.6, and 75.4 percent at 1, 2, and 3 years, respectively. The survival rate in the drug group was 82.3, 74.4, and 64.1 percent at 1, 2, and 3 years. The corresponding reductions in mortality rates in the ICD group were 39 percent at 1 year, 27 percent at 2 years, and 31 percent at 3 years (Fig. 94–11). The majority of ICD benefit occurred in the first 9 months. ICD survival benefit was most prominent in patients with an LVEF of less than 0.35. No significant statistical benefit of the ICD was noted with an LVEF of more than 0.35.

CARDIAC ARREST STUDY HAMBURG TRIAL

The Cardiac Arrest Study Hamburg (CASH) trial[257] was initiated in 1987 and designed to compare the efficacy of empiric antiarrhythmic therapy with amiodarone, propafenone, or metoprolol compared with an ICD in survivors of SCD not related to MI. The primary end point was total mortality. The secondary end points were hemodynamically unstable VT and incidence of drug withdrawal. The mean LVEF was 0.46, and approximately 75 percent of the patients had CAD. The main exclusion criterion was MI within 72 hours of SCD.

In July 1992, an interim analysis showed an excessive mortality rate in the propafenone arm compared with the ICD group, and the propafenone arm was dropped. The other three arms of trial continued, and follow-up evaluation was conducted for a minimum of 2 years after the randomization of 349 patients. The analysis revealed that ICD implantation significantly decreased overall mortality rates in the first year of follow-up (63 percent decrease in overall mortality rates). The 2-year mortality rate was 12.1 percent in the ICD group and 19.6 percent in the combined drug therapy group (37 percent reduction in 2-year overall mortality rates, $P = .047$). There was no significant differ-

TABLE 94–5 Prospective Multicenter Intracardiac Defibrillator Secondary Prevention Trials

Study	Patient Inclusion Criteria	End Point(s)	Treatment Arms	Key Results
AVID[258, 259]	VF or Sustained VT with syncope or Sustained VT without syncope and LVEF ≤ 0.40 and SBP < 80 mm Hg, chest pain, or near-syncope	Overall mortality Quality of life Cost and cost effectiveness	ICD therapy (n = 29) EP or Holter-guided sotalol or empiric amiodarone	ICD reduced total mortality 39% after 1 yr, 27% after 2 yr, and 31% after 3 yr compared with antiarrhythmic drugs
CASH[257]	Survivors of sudden cardiac death documented to be associated with VF or Hemodynamically significant sustained VT	Total mortality Recurrence of sudden cardiac death Arrhythmic mortality	ICD Propafenone Metoprolol Amiodarone	Propafenone arm was associated with excess mortality and was discontinued No significant mortality difference between amiodarone and metoprolol ICD decreased total mortality by 63% in 1 yr and 37% in 2 yr compared with combination arms of amiodarone and metoprolol
CIDS[260]	Survivors of sudden cardiac death documented to be associated with VF or VT with syncope or Sustained VT and LVEF ≤ 0.35 Syncope of unknown cause and inducible VT in EPS and LVEF < 0.35	All-cause mortality Arrhythmic death	ICD Amiodarone	ICD decreased all-cause mortality slightly but not significantly Results were consistent with AVID and CASH

Abbreviations: AVID, Antiarrhythmic Versus Implantable Defibrillator; CASH, Cardiac Arrest Study Hamburg; CIDS, Canadian Implantable Defibrillator Study; EP, electrophysiologic; EPS, electrophysiologic study; ICD, implantable converter-defibrillator; LVEF, left ventricular ejection fraction; SBP, systolic blood pressure; VF, ventricular fibrillation; VT, ventricular tachycardia.

From Khoshnevis GR, Massumi A: Ventricular arrhythmias in congestive heart failure: clinical significance and management. Tex Heart Inst J 26:42–59, 1999.

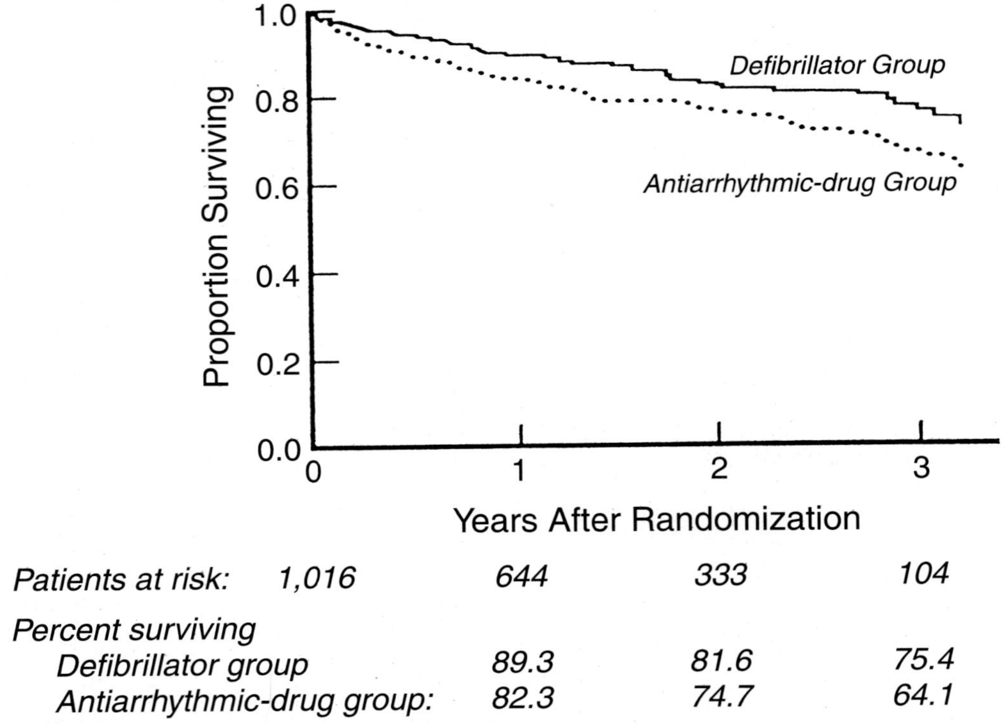

FIGURE 94–11 Difference in mortality rates between two treatment groups was significant at 1, 2, and 3 years after randomization. (From The Antiarrhythmics Versus Implantable Defibrillators (AVID) Investigators: A comparison of antiarrhythmic-drug therapy with implantable defibrillators in patients resuscitated from near-fatal ventricular arrhythmias. N Engl J Med 337:1576–1583, 1997.)

ence in mortality rate between the amiodarone and metoprolol groups.

The results of this trial were consistent with the results of the AVID trial.

CANADIAN IMPLANTABLE DEFIBRILLATOR STUDY

The Canadian Implantable Defibrillator Study (CIDS) trial[260] randomized 659 patients with prior history of cardiac arrest or hemodynamically unstable VT to receive either ICD therapy (n = 328) or amiodarone (n = 331). The inclusion criteria included documented VF, out-of-hospital cardiac arrest requiring defibrillation, documented sustained VT at a rate of 150 beats/min or greater causing presyncope or angina in a patient with an LVEF of 0.35 or less, syncope with documented spontaneous VT of 10 seconds or greater duration or inducible sustained VT in EP laboratory.

The study end point was all-cause mortality in a comparison of the two therapeutic options. The study also considered arrhythmic death. By the end of 5 years after enrollment, 22 percent of patients in the amiodarone group received an ICD and 30 percent of the ICD patients had been started on amiodarone.

ICD therapy trended toward overall improvement in survival. Overall mortality rate was approximately 27 percent at 4 years with ICD versus approximately 33 percent with amiodarone (P = .07).

The trial showed a modest, but not statistically significant, reduction in mortality rates with ICD. These results are consistent with AVID and CASH results that showed a beneficial effect of ICD therapy for the secondary prevention of SCD.

Although insight into the mechanism and circumstances of SCD is increasing, the majority of victims of SCD are not identified as high risk before the event. A search for more effective methods must continue to identify patients at risk of SCD and to predict the efficacy of our preventive measures as SCD remains a major health care issue.

REFERENCES

1. Dunbar SB, Ellenbogen K, Epstein AE: *In* Sudden Cardiac Death: Past, Present, and Future. Armonk, NY: Futura, 1997.
2. Zipes DP, Wellens HJ: Sudden cardiac death. Circulation 98:2334–2351, 1998.
3. de Vreede-Swagemakers JJ, Gorgels AP, Dubois-Arbouw WI, et al: Out-of-hospital cardiac arrest in the 1990's: a population-based study in the Maastricht area on incidence, characteristics and survival. J Am Coll Cardiol 30:1500–1505, 1997.
4. Akhtar M, Myerburg RJ, Ruskin JN: Sudden Cardiac Death. Malvern, PA: 1994.
5. Gillum RF: Sudden coronary death in the United States: 1980–1985. Circulation 79:756–765, 1989.
6. DiMarco JP, Haines DE: Sudden cardiac death. Curr Probl Cardiol 15:183–232, 1990.
7. Becker LB, Smith DW, Rhodes KV: Incidence of cardiac arrest: a neglected factor in evaluating survival rates. Ann Emerg Med 22:86–91, 1993.
8. Vertesi L: The paramedic ambulance: a Canadian experience. Can Med Assoc J 119:25–29, 1978.
9. Bachman JW, McDonald GS, O'Brien PC: A study of out-of-hospital cardiac arrests in northeastern Minnesota. JAMA 256:477–483, 1986.
10. Gillum RF, Folsom A, Luepker RV, et al: Sudden death and acute

myocardial infarction in a metropolitan area, 1970–1980: the Minnesota Heart Survey. N Engl J Med 309:1353–1358, 1983.
11. Goldberg RJ, Gore JM, Alpert JS, Dalen JE: Incidence and case fatality rates of acute myocardial infarction (1975–1984): the Worcester Heart Attack Study. Am Heart J 115:761–776, 1988.
12. Kannel WB, Thomas HE Jr: Sudden coronary death: the Framingham Study. Ann N Y Acad Sci 382:3–21, 1982.
13. Myerburg RJ, Kessler KM, Castellanos A: Sudden cardiac death. Structure, function, and time-dependence of risk. Circulation 85(suppl I):I-2–I-10, 1992.
14. Furukawa T, Rozanski JJ, Nogami A, et al: Time-dependent risk of and predictors for cardiac arrest recurrence in survivors of out-of-hospital cardiac arrest with chronic coronary artery disease. Circulation 80:599–608, 1989.
15. Gillum RF: Coronary heart disease in black populations. I. Mortality and morbidity. Am Heart J 104(4 pt 1):839–851, 1982.
16. Gillum RF, Liu KC: Coronary heart disease mortality in United States blacks, 1940–1978: trends and unanswered questions. Am Heart J 108(3 pt 2):728–732, 1984.
17. Becker LB, Han BH, Meyer PM, et al: Racial differences in the incidence of cardiac arrest and subsequent survival: the CPR Chicago Project. N Engl J Med 329:600–660, 1993.
18. Mittleman MA, Maclure M, Tofler GH, et al: Triggering of acute myocardial infarction by heavy physical exertion: protection against triggering by regular exertion: Determinants of Myocardial Infarction Onset Study Investigators. N Engl J Med 329:1677–1683, 1993.
19. Wang JS, Jen CJ, Kung HC, et al: Different effects of strenuous exercise and moderate exercise on platelet function in men. Circulation 90:2877–2885, 1994.
20. Rahe RH, Romo M, Bennett L, Siltanen P: Recent life changes, myocardial infarction, and abrupt coronary death: studies in Helsinki. Arch Intern Med 133:221–228, 1974.
21. Talbott E, Kuller LH, Detre K, Perper J: Biologic and psychosocial risk factors of sudden death from coronary disease in white women. Am J Cardiol 39:858–864, 1977.
22. Ruberman W, Weinblatt E, Goldberg JD, Chaudhary BS: Psychosocial influences on mortality after myocardial infarction. N Engl J Med 311:552–559, 1984.
23. Weinblatt E, Ruberman W, Goldberg JD, et al: Relation of education to sudden death after myocardial infarction. N Engl J Med 299:60–65, 1978.
24. Kannel WB, Doyle JT, McNamara PM, et al: Precursors of sudden coronary death: factors related to the incidence of sudden death. Circulation 51:606–613, 1975.
25. Kannel WB, Cupples LA, D'Agostino RB: Sudden death risk in overt coronary heart disease: the Framingham Study. Am Heart J 113:799–804, 1987.
26. Suhonen O, Reunanen A, Knekt P, Aromaa A: Risk factors for sudden and non-sudden coronary death. Acta Med Scand 223:19–25, 1988.
27. Kuller LH, Perper JA, Dai WS, et al: Sudden death and the decline in coronary heart disease mortality. J Chron Dis 39:1001–1019, 1986.
28. Bigger JT Jr, Fleiss JL, Kleiger R, et al: The relationships among ventricular arrhythmias, left ventricular dysfunction, and mortality in the 2 years after myocardial infarction. Circulation 69:250–258, 1984.
29. Ruberman W, Weinblatt E, Goldberg JD, et al: Ventricular premature complexes and sudden death after myocardial infarction. Circulation 64:297–305, 1981.
30. Myerburg RJ, Kessler KM, Luceri RM, et al: Classification of ventricular arrhythmias based on parallel hierarchies of frequency and form. Am J Cardiol 54:1355–1358, 1984.
31. Zabel M, Klingenheben T, Franz MR, Hohnloser SH: Assessment of QT dispersion for prediction of mortality or arrhythmic events after myocardial infarction: results of a prospective, long-term follow-up study. Circulation 97:2543–2550, 1998.
32. Stevenson WG, Stevenson LW, Middlekauff HR, Saxon LA: Sudden death prevention in patients with advanced ventricular dysfunction. Circulation 88:2953–2961, 1993.
33. Wilber DJ, Garan H, Finkelstein D, et al: Out-of-hospital cardiac arrest. Use of electrophysiologic testing in the prediction of long-term outcome. N Engl J Med 318:19–24, 1988.
34. Sager PT, Choudhary R, Leon C, et al: The long-term prognosis of patients with out-of-hospital cardiac arrest but no inducible ventricular tachycardia. Am Heart J 120(6 pt 1):1334–1342, 1990.
35. Weinberg BA, Miles WM, Klein LS, et al: Five-year follow-up of 589 patients treated with amiodarone. Am Heart J 125:109–120, 1993.
36. Herre JM, Sauve MJ, Malone P, et al: Long-term results of amiodarone therapy in patients with recurrent sustained ventricular tachycardia or ventricular fibrillation. J Am Coll Cardiol 13:442–449, 1989.
37. Myerburg RJ, Kessler KM, Zaman L, et al: Survivors of prehospital cardiac arrest. JAMA 247:1485–1490, 1982.
38. Furukawa T, Moroe K, Mayrovitz HN, et al: Arrhythmogenic effects of graded coronary blood flow reductions superimposed on prior myocardial infarction in dogs. Circulation 84:368–377, 1991.
39. Coronel R, Wilms-Schopman FJ, Opthof T, et al: Reperfusion arrhythmias in isolated perfused pig hearts: inhomogeneities in extracellular potassium, ST and TQ potentials, and transmembrane action potentials. Circ Res 71:1131–1142, 1992.
40. Furukawa T, Bassett AL, Furukawa N, et al: The ionic mechanism of reperfusion-induced early afterdepolarizations in feline left ventricular hypertrophy. J Clin Invest 91:1521–1531, 1993.
41. Calkins H, Maughan WL, Weisman HF, et al: Effect of acute volume load on refractoriness and arrhythmia development in isolated, chronically infarcted canine hearts. Circulation 79:687–697, 1989.
42. Kleiger RE, Miller JP, Bigger JT Jr, Moss AJ: Decreased heart rate variability and its association with increased mortality after acute myocardial infarction. Am J Cardiol 59:256–262, 1987.
43. Huikuri HV, Linnaluoto MK, Seppanen T, et al: Circadian rhythm of heart rate variability in survivors of cardiac arrest. Am J Cardiol 70:610–615, 1992.
44. La Rovere MT, Specchia G, Mortara A, Schwartz PJ: Baroreflex sensitivity, clinical correlates, and cardiovascular mortality among patients with a first myocardial infarction: a prospective study. Circulation 78:816–824, 1988.
45. Huikuri HV, Zaman L, Castellanos A, et al: Changes in spontaneous sinus node rate as an estimate of cardiac autonomic tone during stable and unstable ventricular tachycardia. J Am Coll Cardiol 13:646–652, 1989.
46. Hill IGW: Cardiac irregularities during chloroform anesthesia. Lancet 1:1139–1142, 1932.
47. Goldstein S, Brooks MM, Ledingham R, et al: Association between ease of suppression of ventricular arrhythmia and survival. Circulation 91:79–83, 1995.
48. Greenberg HM, Dwyer EM, Hochman JS, et al: Interaction of ischemia and encainide/flecainide treatment: a proposed mechanism for the increased mortality in CAST I. Br Heart J 74:631–655, 1995.
49. Woosley RL, Chen Y, Freiman JP, Gillis RA: Mechanism of the cardiotoxic actions of terfenadine. JAMA 269:1532–1536, 1993.
50. Kimura S, Bassett AL, Xi H, Myerburg RJ: Early afterdepolarizations and triggered activity induced by cocaine: a possible mechanism of cocaine arrhythmogenesis. Circulation 85:2227–2235, 1992.
51. Josephson ME, Horowitz LN, Farshidi A, et al: Recurrent sustained ventricular tachycardia. 2. Endocardial mapping. Circulation 57:440–447, 1978.
52. Roberts WC, Kragel AH, Gertz SD, Roberts CS: Coronary arteries in unstable angina pectoris, acute myocardial infarction, and sudden coronary death. Am Heart J 127:1588–1593, 1994.
53. Kleber AG, Janse MJ, Wilms-Schopmann FJ, et al: Changes in conduction velocity during acute ischemia in ventricular myocardium of the isolated porcine heart. Circulation 73:189–198, 1986.
54. Josephson ME, Horowitz LN, Farshidi LN, Farshidi A, Kastor JA: Recurrent sustained ventricular tachycardia. 1. Mechanisms. Circulation 57:431–440, 1978.
55. Rohr S, Kucera JP, Kleber AG: Slow conduction in cardiac tissue, I: effects of a reduction of excitability versus a reduction of electrical coupling on microconduction. Circ Res 83:781–794, 1998.
56. Spach MS, Josephson ME: Initiating reentry: the role of nonuniform anisotropy in small circuits. J Cardiovasc Electrophysiol 5:182–209, 1994.
57. Lampert S, Lown B, Graboys TB, et al: Determinants of survival in patients with malignant ventricular arrhythmia associated with coronary artery disease. Am J Cardiol 61:791–797, 1988.
58. Moss AJ, Davis HT, DeCamilla J, Bayer LW: Ventricular ectopic beats and their relation to sudden and nonsudden cardiac death after myocardial infarction. Circulation 60:998–1003, 1979.

59. Fioretti P, Brower RW, Simoons ML, et al: Prediction of mortality during the first year after acute myocardial infarction from clinical variables and stress test at hospital discharge. Am J Cardiol 55:1313–1318, 1985.
60. Breithardt G, Schwarzmaier J, Borggrefe M, et al: Prognostic significance of late ventricular potentials after acute myocardial infarction. Eur Heart J 4:487–495, 1983.
61. Bigger JT, Fleiss JL, Rolnitzky LM, Steinman RC: The ability of several short-term measures of RR variability to predict mortality after myocardial infarction. Circulation 88:927–934, 1993.
62. Eldar M, Sauve MJ, Scheinman MM: Electrophysiologic testing and follow-up of patients with aborted sudden death. J Am Coll Cardiol 10:291–298, 1987.
63. Swerdlow CD, Bardy GH, McAnulty J, et al: Determinants of induced sustained arrhythmias in survivors of out-of-hospital ventricular fibrillation. Circulation 76:1053–1060, 1987.
64. Angelini P: Coronary Artery Anomalies. pp. 27–78. Baltimore, MD: Lippincott Williams & Wilkins, 1999.
65. Maron BJ, Roberts WC: *In*: Sudden Cardiac Death: Prevalence, Mechanism, and Approaches to Diagnosis and Management. pp. 238–257. Malvern, PA: 1994.
66. Roberts WC, Kragel AH: Anomalous origin of either the right or left main coronary artery from the aorta without coursing of the anomalistically arising artery between aorta and pulmonary trunk. Am J Cardiol 62:1263–1267, 1988.
67. Menke DM, Waller BF, Pless JE: Hypoplastic coronary arteries and high takeoff position of the right coronary ostium: a fatal combination of congenital coronary artery anomalies in an amateur athlete. Chest 88:299–301, 1985.
68. Roberts WC, Silver MA, Sapala JC: Intussusception of a coronary artery associated with sudden death in a college football player. Am J Cardiol 57:179–180, 1986.
69. Faruqui AM, Maloy WC, Felner JM, et al: Symptomatic myocardial bridging of coronary artery. Am J Cardiol 41:1305–1310, 1978.
70. Roberts WC, Dicicco BS, Waller BF, et al: Origin of the left main from the right coronary artery or from the right aortic sinus with intramyocardial tunneling to the left side of the heart via the ventricular septum: the case against clinical significance of myocardial bridge or coronary tunnel. Am Heart J 104:303–305, 1982.
71. Roberts WC, Honig HS: The spectrum of cardiovascular disease in the Marfan syndrome: a clinico-morphologic study of 18 necropsy patients and comparison to 151 previously reported necropsy patients. Am Heart J 104:115–135, 1982.
72. Roberts WC: Pathology of arterial aneurysms. *In* Bergan JJ, Yao ST (eds): Aneurysms: Diagnosis and Treatment. pp. 17–43: New York: Grune & Stratton, 1982.
73. Harris LS, Adelson L: Fatal coronary embolism from myxomatous polyp of the aortic valve: an unusual cause of sudden death. Am J Clin Pathol 43:61–66, 1965.
74. Nakamura M, Takeshita A, Nose Y: Clinical characteristics associated with myocardial infarction, arrhythmias, and sudden death in patients with vasospastic angina. Circulation 75:1110–1116, 1987.
75. Thiene G, Valente M, Rossi L: Involvement of the cardiac conducting system in panarteritis nodosa. Am Heart J 95:716–724, 1978.
76. Kegel SM, Dorsey TJ, Rowen M, Taylor WF: Cardiac death in mucocutaneous lymph node syndrome. Am J Cardiol 40:282–286, 1977.
77. Shah PM, Adelman AG, Wigle ED, et al: The natural (and unnatural) history of hypertrophic obstructive cardiomyopathy. Circ Res 35(suppl II):179–195, 1974.
78. Hada Y, Sakamoto T, Amano K, et al: Prevalence of hypertrophic cardiomyopathy in a population of adult Japanese workers as detected by echocardiographic screening. Am J Cardiol 59:183–184, 1987.
79. Savage DD, Castelli WP, Abbott RD, et al: Hypertrophic cardiomyopathy and its markers in the general population: the great masquerader revisited: the Framingham study. J Cardiovasc Ultrasonogr 2:41–47, 1983.
80. Cannan CR, Reeder GS, Bailey KR, et al: Natural history of hypertrophic cardiomyopathy: a population-based study, 1976 through 1990. Circulation 92:2488–2495, 1995.
81. Maron BJ, Epstein SE, Roberts WC: Causes of sudden death in competitive athletes. J Am Coll Cardiol 7:204–214, 1986.
82. Spirito P, Seidman CE, McKenna WJ, Maron BJ: The management of hypertrophic cardiomyopathy. N Engl J Med 336:775–785, 1997.
83. Maron BJ: Hypertrophic cardiomyopathy. Lancet 350:127–133, 1997.
84. Maron BJ: Heart disease and other causes of sudden death in young athletes. Curr Probl Cardiol 23:477–529, 1998.
85. Watkins H, Rosenzweig A, Hwang DS, et al: Characteristics and prognostic implications of myosin missense mutations in familial hypertrophic cardiomyopathy. N Engl J Med 326:1108–1114, 1992.
86. Schwartz K, Carrier L, Guicheney P, Komajda M: Molecular basis of familial cardiomyopathies. Circulation 91:532–540, 1995.
87. Marian AJ, Roberts R: Recent advances in the molecular genetics of hypertrophic cardiomyopathy. Circulation 92:1336–1347, 1995.
88. Marian AJ, Roberts R: Molecular genetic basis of hypertrophic cardiomyopathy: genetic markers for sudden cardiac death. J Cardiovasc Electrophysiol 9:88–99, 1998.
89. Fontaine G, Guiraudon G, Frank R, et al: Stimulation studies and epicardial mapping in ventricular tachycardia: study of mechanisms and selection for surgery. Re-entrant Arrhythmias September 29, 1977, pp. 334–350.
90. Marcus FI, Fontaine G: Arrhythmogenic right ventricular dysplasia/cardiomyopathy: a review. Pacing Clin Electrophysiol 18:1298–1314, 1995.
91. Fontaine G, Fontaliran F, Hebert JL, et al: Arrhythmogenic right ventricular dysplasia. Annu Rev Med 50:17–35, 1999.
92. Lascault G, Laplaud O, Frank R, et al: Ventricular tachycardia features in right ventricular dysplasia. Circulation 78(suppl II):300, 1988. Abstract.
93. Priori SG, Barhanin J, Hauer RN, et al: Genetic and molecular basis of cardiac arrhythmias: impact on clinical management parts I and II. Circulation 99:518–528, 1999.
94. Coonar AS, Protonotarios N, Tsatsopoulou A, et al: Gene for arrhythmogenic right ventricular cardiomyopathy with diffuse non-epidermolytic palmoplantar keratoderma and woolly hair (Naxos disease) maps to 17q21. Circulation 97:2049–2058, 1998.
95. Thiene G, Nava A, Corrado D, et al: Right ventricular cardiomyopathy and sudden death in young people. N Engl J Med 318:129–133, 1988.
96. Furlanello F, Bertoldi A, Dallago M, et al: Cardiac arrest and sudden death in competitive athletes with arrhythmogenic right ventricular dysplasia. Pacing Clin Electrophysiol 21(1 pt 2):331–335, 1998.
97. Aouate P, Fontaliran F, Fontaine G, et al: [Holter and sudden death: value in a case of arrhythmogenic right ventricular dysplasia]. Arch Mal Coeur Vaiss 86:363–367, 1993.
98. Marcus FI, Fontaine GH, Guiraudon G, et al: Right ventricular dysplasia: a report of 24 adult cases. Circulation 65:384–398, 1982.
99. Corrado D, Basso C, Thiene G, et al: Spectrum of clinicopathologic manifestations of arrhythmogenic right ventricular cardiomyopathy/dysplasia: a multicenter study. J Am Coll Cardiol 30:1512–1520, 1997.
100. Fontaine G, Umemura J, Di Donna P, et al: [Duration of QRS complexes in arrhythmogenic right ventricular dysplasia: a new non-invasive diagnostic marker]. Ann Cardiol Angeiol (Paris) 42:399–405, 1993.
101. Fontaine G, Sohal PS, Piot O et al: Parietal block super imposed on right bundle branch block: a new ECG marker of right ventricular dysplasia [abstract]. J Am Coll Cardiol 29:110A, 1997.
102. Blomstrom-Lundqvist C, Hirsch I, Olsson SB, Edvardsson N: Quantitative analysis of the signal-averaged QRS in patients with arrhythmogenic right ventricular dysplasia. Eur Heart J 9:301–312, 1988.
103. Auffermann W, Wichter T, Breithardt G, Joachimsen K, Peters PE: Arrhythmogenic right ventricular disease: MR imaging vs. Angiography. AJR 161:549–555, 1993.
104. Grimm W, List-Hellwig E, Hoffmann J, Menz V, Hahn-Rinn R, Klose KJ, Maisch B: Magnetic resonance imaging and signal-averaged electrocardiography in patients with repetitive monomorphic ventricular tachycardia and otherwise normal electrocardiogram. Pacing Clin Electrophysiol 20:1826–1833, 1997.
105. Rahimtoola SH: Valvular heart disease: a perspective. J Am Coll Cardiol 1:199–215, 1983.
106. Blackstone EH, Kirklin JW: Death and other time-related events after valve replacement. Circulation 72:753–767, 1985.
107. Sra J, Dhala A, Blanck Z, Deshpande S, Cooley R, Akhtar M: Sudden cardiac death. Curr Probl Cardiol 24:461–538, 1999.
108. Narasimhan C, Jazayeri MR, Sra J, DhalaA, Deshpande S, Biehl M, Akhtar M, Blanck Z: Ventricular tachycardia in valvular heart disease: facilitation of sustained bundle-branch reentry by valve surgery. Circulation 96:4307–4313, 1997.

109. Khoshnevis GR, Massumi A: Ventricular arrhythmias in congestive heart failure; clinical significance and management. Tex Heart Instj 26:42–59, 1999.
110. Fuster V, Gersh BJ, Giuliani ER, et al: The natural history of idiopathic dilated cardiomyopathy. Am J Cardiol 47:525–531, 1981.
111. Unverferth DV, Magorien RD, Moeschberger ML, et al: Factors influencing the one-year mortality of dilated cardiomyopathy. Am J Cardiol 54:147–152, 1984.
112. Tamburro P, Wilber D: Sudden death in idiopathic dilated cardiomyopathy. Am Heart J 124:1035–1045, 1992.
113. Larsen L, Markham J, Haffajee CI: Sudden death in idiopathic dilated cardiomyopathy: role of ventricular arrhythmias. Pacing Clin Electrophysiol 16:1051–1059, 1993.
114. Luu M, Stevenson WG, Stevenson LW, et al: Diverse mechanisms of unexpected cardiac arrest in advanced heart failure. Circulation 80:1675–1680, 1989.
115. Middlekauff HR, Stevenson WG, Stevenson LW, Saxon LA: Syncope in advanced heart failure: high risk of sudden death regardless of origin of syncope. J Am Coll Cardiol 21:110–116, 1993.
116. Schwartz PJ, Moss AJ, Vincent GM, Crampton RS: Diagnostic criteria for the long QT syndrome. An update. Circulation 88:782–784, 1993.
117. Schwartz PJ, Priori SG, Napolitano C: Long QT syndrome. *In* Zipes DP, Jalife J (eds): Cardiac Electrophysiology: From Cell to Bedside. Orlando, FL: WB Saunders, 1999.
118. Moss AJ: Management of patients with the hereditary long QT syndrome. J Cardiovasc Electrophysiol 9:668–674, 1998.
119. Jervell A, Lange-Nielsen F: Congenital deaf-mutism, functional heart disease with prolongation of the Q-T interval and sudden death. Am Heart J 54:59–68, 1957.
120. Romano C, Gemme G, Pongiglione R: Aritmie cardiache rare dell'eta pediatrica: II accessi sincopali per fibrillazione ventricolare parossistica. Clin Pediatr (Bologna) 45:656–683, 1963.
121. Ward OC: A new familial cardiac syndrome in children. J Ir Med Assoc 54:103–106, 1964.
122. Wang Q, Curran ME, Splawski I, et al: Positional cloning of a novel potassium channel gene: KVLQT1 mutations cause cardiac arrhythmias. Nat Genet 12:17–23, 1996.
123. Curran ME, Splawski I, Timothy KW, et al: A molecular basis for cardiac arrhythmia: HERG mutations cause long QT syndrome: Cell 80:795–803, 1995.
124. Wang Q, Shen J, Splawski I, et al: SCN5A mutations associated with an inherited cardiac arrhythmia, long QT syndrome. Cell 80:805–118, 1995.
125. Splawski I, Tristani-Firouzi M, Lehmann MH, et al: Mutations in the hminK gene cause long QT syndrome and suppress IKs function. Nat Genet 17:338–340, 1997.
126. Moss AJ, Schwartz PJ, Crampton RS, et al: The long QT syndrome: prospective longitudinal study of 328 families. Circulation 84:1136–1144, 1991.
127. Guize L, Soria R, Chaouat JC, et al: [Prevalence and course of Wolff-Parkinson-White syndrome in a population of 138,048 subjects]. [In French] Ann Med Interne (Paris) 136:474–478, 1985.
128. Vidaillet HJ Jr, Pressley JC, Henke E, et al: Familial occurrence of accessory atrioventricular pathways (preexcitation syndrome). N Engl J Med 317:65–69, 1987.
129. Wellens HJ, Durrer D: Wolff-Parkinson-White syndrome and atrial fibrillation: relation between refractory period of accessory pathway and ventricular rate during atrial fibrillation. Am J Cardiol 34:777–782, 1974.
130. Cosio FG, Benson DW Jr, Anderson RW, et al: Onset of atrial fibrillation during antidromic tachycardia: association with sudden cardiac arrest and ventricular fibrillation in a patient with Wolff-Parkinson-White syndrome. Am J Cardiol 50:353–359, 1982.
131. Papa LA, Saia JA, Chung EK: Ventricular fibrillation in Wolff-Parkinson-White syndrome, type A. Heart Lung 7:1015–1019, 1978.
132. Bromberg BI, Lindsay BD, Cain ME, Cox JL. Impact of clinical history and electrophysiologic characterization of accessory pathways on management strategies to reduce sudden death among children with Wolff-Parkinson-White syndrome. J Am Coll Cardiol 27:690–695, 1996.
133. Klein GJ, Bashore TM, Sellers TD, et al: Ventricular fibrillation in the Wolff-Parkinson-White syndrome. N Engl J Med 301:1080–1085, 1979.
134. Montoya PT. Ventricular fibrillation in the Wolff-Parkinson-White syndrome. Circulation 78(suppl II):II-22, 1998.
135. Teo WS, Klein GJ, Guiraudon GM, et al: Multiple accessory pathways in the Wolff-Parkinson-White syndrome as a risk factor for ventricular fibrillation. Am J Cardiol 67:889–891, 1991.
136. Smith WM, Gallagher JJ, Kerr CR, et al: Ebstein's anomaly of the tricuspid valve. Am J Cardiol 49:1223–1234, 1982.
137. Brugada P, Brugada J: Right bundle branch block, persistent ST segment elevation and sudden cardiac death: a distinct clinical and electrocardiographic syndrome: a multicenter report. J Am Coll Cardiol 20:1391–1396, 1992.
138. Alings M, Wilde A: "Brugada" syndrome: clinical data and suggested pathophysiological mechanism. Circulation 99:666–673, 1999.
139. Brugada J, Brugada P: Further characterization of the syndrome of right bundle branch block, ST segment elevation, and sudden cardiac death. J Cardiovasc Electrophysiol 8:325–331, 1997.
140. Brugada J, Brugada R, Brugada P: Right bundle-branch block and ST-segment elevation in leads V1 through V3: a marker for sudden death in patients without demonstrable structural heart disease. Circulation 97:457–460, 1998.
141. Buxton AE, Waxman HL, Marchlinski FE, et al: Right ventricular tachycardia: clinical and electrophysiologic characteristics. Circulation 68:917–927, 1983.
142. Leenhardt A, Glaser E, Burguera M, et al: Short-coupled variant of torsade de pointes: a new electrocardiographic entity in the spectrum of idiopathic ventricular tachyarrhythmias. Circulation 89:206–215, 1994.
143. Viskin S, Lesh MD, Eldar M, et al: Mode of onset of malignant ventricular arrhythmias in idiopathic ventricular fibrillation. J Cardiovasc Electrophysiol 8:1115–1120, 1997.
144. Belhassen B, Viskin S: Idiopathic ventricular tachycardia and fibrillation. J Cardiovasc Electrophysiol 4:356–368, 1993.
145. Lenegre J: The pathology of complete atrioventricular block. Prog Cardiovasc Dis 6:317–324, 1964.
146. Bharati S, Lev M: The Cardiac Conduction System in Unexplained Sudden Death. Mt Kisco, NY: Futura, 1990.
147. Gilman JK, Naccarelli GV: Sudden cardiac death. Curr Prob Cardiol 17:693–778, 1992.
148. Kannel WB, Schatzkin A: Sudden death: lessons from subsets in population studies. J Am Coll Cardiol 5(6 suppl):141B–149B, 1985.
149. Spain DM, Bradess VA: Relationship of coronary thrombosis to coronary atherosclerosis and ischemic heart disease (a necropsy study covering a period of 25 years). Am J Med Sci 240:701, 1960.
150. Baroldi G, Falzi G, Mariani F: Sudden coronary death: a postmortem study in 208 selected cases compared to 97 "control" subjects. Am Heart J 98:20–31, 1979.
151. Liberthson RR, Nagel EL, Hirschman JC, et al: Pathophysiologic observations in prehospital ventricular fibrillation and sudden cardiac death. Circulation 49:790–798, 1974.
152. Davies, MJ: Pathological view of sudden cardiac death. Br Heart J 45:88–96, 1981.
153. Davies MJ, Thomas A: Thrombosis and acute coronary artery lesion in sudden cardiac ischemic death. N Engl J Med 310:1137–1140, 1984.
154. Myerburg RJ, Kessler KM, Mallon SM, et al: Life-threatening ventricular arrhythmias in patients with silent myocardial ischemia due to coronary artery spasm. N Engl J Med 326:1451–1455, 1991.
155. Battle WE, Naimi S, Avitall B, et al: Distinctive time course of ventricular vulnerability to fibrillation during and after release of coronary ligation. Am J Cardiol 34:42–47, 1974.
156. Kaplinsky E, Ogawa S, Balke C, Dreifus L: Two periods of early ventricular arrhythmia in the canine acute myocardial infarction model. Circulation 60:397–403, 1979.
157. Corr PB, Gross RW, Sobel BE: Amphipathic metabolites and membrane dysfunction in ischemic myocardium. Circ Res 55:135–154, 1984.
158. Downer E, Janse MJ, Durrer D: The effect of "ischemic" blood on transmembrane potentials of normal porcine ventricular myocardium. Circulation 55:455–462, 1977.
159. Owens LM, Fralix TA, Murphy E, et al: Correlation of ischemia-induced extracellular and intracellular ion changes to cell-to-cell electrical uncoupling in isolated blood perfusion rabbit hearts. Circulation 94:10–13, 1996.
160. Zipes DP: Electrophysiological mechanisms involved in ventricular fibrillation. Circulation 52(suppl I):I-120–I-130, 1975.
161. Pogwizd SM, Corr PB: Reentrant and nonreentrant mechanisms

contribute to arrhythmogenesis during early myocardial ischemia: results using three-dimensional mapping. Circ Res 61:352–371, 1987.

162. Wit AL, Friedman PL: Basis for ventricular arrhythmias accompanying myocardial infarction: alterations in electrical activity of ventricular muscle and Purkinje fibers after coronary artery occlusion. Arch Intern Med 135:459–472, 1975.
163. Wellens HJJ, Schuilenburg RM, Durrer D: Electrical stimulation of the heart in patients with ventricular tachycardia. Circulation 46:216–226, 1972.
164. Eisenberg MS, Hallstrom A, Bergner L: Long term survival after out-of-hospital cardiac arrest. N Engl J Med 306:1340, 1982.
165. Pogwizd SM, Corr PB: Mechanism underlying the development of ventricular fibrillation during early myocardial ischemia. Circ Res 66:672–695, 1990.
166. Pogwizd SM, Corr PB: Electrophysiologic mechanisms underlying arrhythmias due to reperfusion of ischemic myocardium. Circulation 76:404–426, 1987.
167. Bharati S, Lev M: The conduction system findings in sudden cardiac death. J Cardiovasc Electrophysiol 5:356–366, 1994.
168. Brugada R, Roberts R: The molecular genetics of arrhythmias and sudden death. Clin Cardiol 21:553–560, 1998.
169. Kapoor WN, Karpf M, Wieand S, et al: A prospective evaluation and follow-up of patients with syncope. N Engl J Med 309:197–204, 1983.
170. Cobb LA, Baum RS, Alvarez H 3d, Schaffer WA: Resuscitation from out-of-hospital ventricular fibrillation: 4 years follow-up. Circulation 52(suppl III):III-223–III-35, 1975.
171. Swerdlow CD, Winkle RA, Mason JW: Determinants of survival in patients with ventricular tachyarrhythmias. N Engl J Med 308:1436–1442, 1983.
172. Volpi A, De Vita C, Franzosi MG, et al: Determinants of 6-month mortality in survivors of myocardial infarction after thrombolysis: results of the GISSI-2 data base: The Ad hoc Working Group of the Gruppo Italiano per lo Studio della Sopravvivenza nell'Infarto Miocardico (GISSI)-2 data base. Circulation 88:416–429, 1993.
173. Jansson K, Dahlstrom U, Karlsson E, et al: The value of exercise test, Holter monitoring, and programmed electrical stimulation in detection of ventricular arrhythmias in patients with hypertrophic cardiomyopathy. Pacing Clin Electrophysiol 13:1261–1267, 1990.
174. Dilsizian V, Bonow RO, Epstein SE, Fananapazir L: Myocardial ischemia detected by thallium scintigraphy is frequently related to cardiac arrest and syncope in young patients with hypertrophic cardiomyopathy. J Am Coll Cardiol 22:796–804, 1993.
175. Maron BJ, Savage DD, Wolfson JK, Epstein SE: Prognostic significance of 24 hour ambulatory electrocardiographic monitoring in patients with hypertrophic cardiomyopathy: a prospective study. Am J Cardiol 48:252–257, 1981.
176. Waters DD, Bosch X, Bouchard A, et al: Comparison of clinical variables and variables derived from a limited predischarge exercise test as predictors of early and late mortality after myocardial infarction. J Am Coll Cardiol 5:1–8, 1985.
177. Starling MR, Crawford MH, Kennedy GT, O'Rourke RA: Exercise testing early after myocardial infarction: predictive value for subsequent unstable angina and death. Am J Cardiol 46:909–914, 1980.
178. Palileo EV, Ashley WW, Swiryn S, et al: Exercise provocable right ventricular outflow tract tachycardia. Am Heart J 104(2 pt 1):185–193, 1982.
179. Savage DD, Seides SF, Maron BJ, et al: Prevalence of arrhythmias during 24-hour electrocardiographic monitoring and exercise testing in patients with obstructive and nonobstructive hypertrophic cardiomyopathy. Circulation 59:866–875, 1979.
180. McKenna WJ, Chetty S, Oakley CM, Goodwin JF: Arrhythmia in hypertrophic cardiomyopathy: exercise and 48 hour ambulatory electrocardiographic assessment with and without beta adrenergic blocking therapy. Am J Cardiol 45:1–5, 1980.
181. Anderson KP, DeCamilla J, Moss AJ: Clinical significance of ventricular tachycardia (3 beats or longer) detected during ambulatory monitoring after myocardial infarction. Circulation 57:890–897, 1978.
182. Bigger JT Jr, Weld FM, Rolnitzky LM: Prevalence, characteristics and significance of ventricular tachycardia (three or more complexes) detected with ambulatory electrocardiographic recording in the late hospital phase of acute myocardial infarction. Am J Cardiol 48:815–823, 1981.
183. Maggioni AP, Zuanetti G, Franzosi MG, et al: Prevalence and prognostic significance of ventricular arrhythmias after acute myocardial infarction in the fibrinolytic era: GISSI-2 results. Circulation 87:312–322, 1993.
184. Gomes JA, Winters SL, Stewart D, et al: A new noninvasive index to predict sustained ventricular tachycardia and sudden death in the first year after myocardial infarction: based on signal-averaged electrocardiogram, radionuclide ejection fraction and Holter monitoring. J Am Coll Cardiol 10:349–357, 1987.
185. Kuchar DL, Thorburn CW, Sammel NL: Prediction of serious arrhythmic events after myocardial infarction: signal-averaged electrocardiogram, Holter monitoring and radionuclide ventriculography. J Am Coll Cardiol 9:531–538, 1987.
186. Schneider RA, Costiloe JP: Relationship of sinus arrhythmia to age and its prognostic significance in ischemic heart disease (abstract). Clin Res 13:219, 1965.
187. Farrell TG, Bashir Y, Cripps T, et al: Risk stratification for arrhythmic events in postinfarction patients based on heart rate variability, ambulatory electrocardiographic variables and the signal-averaged electrocardiogram. J Am Coll Cardiol 18:687–697, 1991.
188. Zipes DP. Influence of myocardial ischemia and infarction on autonomic innervation of the heart. Circulation 82:1095, 1990.
189. Schaffer WA, Cobb LA: Recurrent ventricular fibrillation and modes of death in survivors of out-of-hospital ventricular fibrillation. N Engl J Med 293:259–262, 1975.
190. Cain ME, Anderson JL, Arnsdorf MF, et al: Signal-averaged electrocardiography. J Am Coll Cardiol 27:238–249, 1996.
191. Richards DA, Byth K, Ross DL, Uther JB. What is the best predictor of spontaneous ventricular tachycardia and sudden death after myocardial infarction? Circulation 83:756–763, 1991.
192. Ohnishi Y, Inoue T, Fukuzaki H: Value of the signal-averaged electrocardiogram as a predictor of sudden death in myocardial infarction and dilated cardiomyopathy. Jpn Circ J 54:127–136, 1990.
193. Schoenfeld MH, McGovern B, Garan H, et al: Determinants of the outcome of electrophysiologic study in patients with ventricular tachyarrhythmias. J Am Coll Cardiol 6:298–306, 1985.
194. Roy D, Waxman HL, Kienzle MG, et al: Clinical characteristics and long-term follow-up in 119 survivors of cardiac arrest: relation to inducibility at electrophysiologic testing. Am J Cardiol 52:969–974, 1983.
195. Kelly P, Ruskin JN, Vlahakes GJ, et al: Surgical coronary revascularization in survivors of prehospital cardiac arrest: its effect on inducible ventricular arrhythmias and long-term survival. J Am Coll Cardiol 15:267–273, 1990.
196. Bhandari AK, Rose JS, Kotlewski A, et al: Frequency and significance of induced sustained ventricular tachycardia or fibrillation two weeks after acute myocardial infarction. Am J Cardiol 56:737–742, 1985.
197. Roy D, Marchand E, Theroux P, et al: Long-term reproducibility and significance of provokable ventricular arrhythmias after myocardial infarction. J Am Coll Cardiol 8:32–39, 1986.
198. Iesaka Y, Nogami A, Aonuma K, et al: Prognostic significance of sustained monomorphic ventricular tachycardia induced by programmed ventricular stimulation using up to triple extrastimuli in survivors of acute myocardial infarction. Am J Cardiol 65:1057–1063, 1990.
199. Bourke JP, Richards DA, Ross DL, et al: Routine programmed electrical stimulation in survivors of acute myocardial infarction for prediction of spontaneous ventricular tachyarrhythmias during follow-up: results, optimal stimulation protocol and cost-effective screening. J Am Coll Cardiol 18:780–788, 1991.
200. Bourke JP, Richards DA, Ross DL, et al: Does the induction of ventricular flutter or fibrillation at electrophysiologic testing after myocardial infarction have any prognostic significance? Am J Cardiol 75:431–435, 1995.
201. Gomes JA, Hariman RI, Kang PS, et al: Programmed electrical stimulation in patients with high-grade ventricular ectopy: electrophysiologic findings and prognosis for survival. Circulation 70:43–51, 1984.
202. Buxton AE, Marchlinski FE, Flores BT, et al: Nonsustained ventricular tachycardia in patients with coronary artery disease: role of electrophysiologic study. Circulation 75:1178–1185, 1987.
203. Klein RC, Machell C: Use of electrophysiologic testing in patients with nonsustained ventricular tachycardia: prognostic and therapeutic implications. J Am Coll Cardiol 14:155–161, 1989; discussion 162–163.

204. Manolis AS, Estes NA 3d: Value of programmed ventricular stimulation in the evaluation and management of patients with nonsustained ventricular tachycardia associated with coronary artery disease. Am J Cardiol 65:201–205, 1990.
205. Wilber DJ, Olshansky B, Moran JF, Scanlon PJ: Electrophysiological testing and nonsustained ventricular tachycardia: use and limitations in patients with coronary artery disease and impaired ventricular function. Circulation 82:350–358, 1990.
206. Beta-Blocker Heart Attack Trial Research Group. A randomized trial of propranolol in patients with acute myocardial infarction. I. Mortality results. JAMA 247:1707–1714, 1982.
207. Viscoli CM, Horwitz RI, Singer BH: Beta-blockers after myocardial infarction: influence of first-year clinical course on long-term effectiveness. Ann Intern Med 118:99–105, 1993.
208. The Norwegian Multicenter Study Group. Timolol-induced reduction in mortality and reinfarction in patients surviving acute myocardial infarction. N Engl J Med 304:801–807, 1981.
209. Pedersen TR: Six-year follow-up of the Norwegian Multicenter Study on Timolol after Acute Myocardial Infarction. N Engl J Med 313:1055–1058, 1985.
210. Boissel JP, Leizorovicz A, Picolet H, Ducruet T: Efficacy of acebutolol after acute myocardial infarction (the APSI trial): the APSI Investigators. Am J Cardiol 66:24C–31C, 1990.
211. Cucherat M, Boissel JP, Leizorovicz A: Persistent reduction of mortality for five years after one year of acebutolol treatment initiated during acute myocardial infarction: the APSI Investigators: Acebutolol et Prevention Secondaire de l'Infarctus. Am J Cardiol 79:587–589, 1997.
212. Hjalmarson A, Elmfeldt D, Herlitz J, et al: Effect on mortality of metoprolol in acute myocardial infarction: a double-blind randomised trial. Lancet 2:823–827, 1981.
213. The MIAMI Trial Research Group. Metoprolol in Acute Myocardial Infarction (MIAMI): a randomised placebo-controlled international trial: the MIAMI Trial Research Group. Eur Heart J 6:199–226, 1985.
214. Roberts R, Rogers WJ, Mueller HS, et al: Immediate versus deferred beta-blockade following thrombolytic therapy in patients with acute myocardial infarction: results of the Thrombolysis in Myocardial Infarction (TIMI) II-B Study. Circulation 83:422–437, 1991.
215. Yusuf S, Wittes J, Friedman L: Overview of results of randomized clinical trials in heart disease. I. Treatments following myocardial infarction. JAMA 260:2088–2093, 1988.
216. Brown MJ, Brown DC, Murphy MB: Hypokalemia from beta2-receptor stimulation by circulating epinephrine. N Engl J Med 309:1414–1419, 1983.
217. Waagstein F, Bristow MR, Swedberg K, et al: Beneficial effects of metoprolol in idiopathic dilated cardiomyopathy: Metoprolol in Dilated Cardiomyopathy (MDC) Trial Study Group. Lancet 342:1441–1446, 1993.
218. CIBIS Investigators and Committees. A randomized trial of beta-blockade in heart failure: the Cardiac Insufficiency Bisoprolol Study (CIBIS). Circulation 90:1765–1773, 1994.
219. The Cardiac Insufficiency Bisoprolol Study Investigators. The Cardiac Insufficiency Bisoprolol Study II (CIBIS-II): a randomised trial. Lancet 353:9–13, 1999.
220. Goldstein S, Hjalmarson A: The mortality effect of metoprolol CR/XL in patients with heart failure: results of the MERIT-HF Trial. Clin Cardiol 22(suppl 5):V30–V35, 1999.
221. Packer M, Bristow MR, Cohn JN, et al: The effect of carvedilol on morbidity and mortality in patients with chronic heart failure. N Engl J Med 334:1349–1355, 1996.
222. Australia/New Zealand Heart Failure Research Collaborative Group. Randomised, placebo-controlled trial of carvedilol in patients with congestive heart failure due to ischaemic heart disease. Lancet 349:375–380, 1997.
223. Cohn JN, Johnson G, Ziesche S, et al: A comparison of enalapril with hydralazine-isosorbide dinitrate in the treatment of chronic congestive heart failure. N Engl J Med 325:303–310, 1991.
224. Kober L, Torp-Pedersen C, Carlsen JE, et al: A clinical trial of the angiotensin-converting-enzyme inhibitor trandolapril in patients with left ventricular dysfunction after myocardial infarction: Trandolapril Cardiac Evaluation (TRACE) Study Group. N Engl J Med 333:1670–1676, 1995.
225. Pfeffer MA, Braunwald E, Moye LA, et al: Effect of captopril on mortality and morbidity in patients with left ventricular dysfunction after myocardial infarction: results of the survival and ventricular enlargement trial. The SAVE Investigators. N Engl J Med 327:669–677, 1992.
226. The SOLVD Investigators. Effect of enalapril on mortality and the development of heart failure in asymptomatic patients with reduced left ventricular ejection fractions. N Engl J Med 327:685–691, 1992.
227. Pitt B, Segal R, Martinez FA, et al: Randomised trial of losartan versus captopril in patients over 65 with heart failure. Lancet Mar 15;349(9054):747–752, 1997.
228. Echt DS, Liebson PR, Mitchell LB, et al: Mortality and morbidity in patients receiving encainide, flecainide, or placebo: the Cardiac Arrhythmia Suppression Trial. N Engl J Med 324:781–788, 1991.
229. The Cardiac Arrhythmia Suppression Trial II Investigators. Effect of the antiarrhythmic agent moricizine on survival after myocardial infarction. N Engl J Med 327:227–233, 1992.
230. Kennedy HL, Brooks MM, Barker AH, et al: Beta-blocker therapy in the Cardiac Arrhythmia Suppression Trial: CAST Investigators. Am J Cardiol 74:674–680, 1994.
231. Hennekens CH, Albert CM, Godfried SL, et al: Adjunctive drug therapy of acute myocardial infarction—evidence from clinical trials. N Engl J Med 335:1660–1667, 1996.
232. Smith GD, Egger M: Who benefits from medical interventions? BMJ 308:72–74, 1994.
233. Burkart F, Pfisterer M, Kiowski W, et al: Effect of antiarrhythmic therapy on mortality in survivors of myocardial infarction with asymptomatic complex ventricular arrhythmias: Basel Antiarrhythmic Study of Infarct Survival. J Am Coll Cardiol 16:1711–1718, 1990.
234. Julian DG, Camm AJ, Frangin G, et al: Randomised trial of effect of amiodarone on mortality in patients with left-ventricular dysfunction after recent myocardial infarction: EMIAT: European Myocardial Infarct Amiodarone Trial Investigators. Lancet 349:667–674, 1997.
235. Cairns JA, Connolly SJ, Roberts R, Gent M: Randomised trial of outcome after myocardial infarction in patients with frequent or repetitive ventricular premature depolarisations: CAMIAT: Canadian Amiodarone Myocardial Infarction Arrhythmia Trial Investigators. Lancet 349:675–682, 1997.
236. Sim I, McDonald KM, Lavori PW, et al: Quantitative overview of randomized trials of amiodarone to prevent sudden cardiac death. Circulation 96:2823–2829, 1997.
237. Doval HC, Nul DR, Grancelli HO, et al: Randomised trial of low-dose amiodarone in severe congestive heart failure: Grupo de Estudio de la Sobrevida en la Insuficiencia Cardiaca en Argentina. Lancet 344:493–498, 1994.
238. Doval HC, Nul DR, Grancelli HO, et al: Nonsustained ventricular tachycardia in severe heart failure: independent marker of increased mortality due to sudden death: GESICA-GEMA Investigators. Circulation 94:3198–3203, 1996.
239. Singh SN, Fletcher RD, Fisher SG, et al: Amiodarone in patients with congestive heart failure and asymptomatic ventricular arrhythmia: Survival Trial of Antiarrhythmic Therapy in Congestive Heart Failure. N Engl J Med 333:77–82, 1995.
240. Massie BM, Fisher SG, Radford M, et al: Effect of amiodarone on clinical status and left ventricular function in patients with congestive heart failure: CHF-STAT Investigators. Circulation 93:2128–2134, 1996.
241. Julian DG, Prescott RJ, Jackson FS, Szekely P: Controlled trial of sotalol for one year after myocardial infarction. Lancet 1:1142–1147, 1982.
242. Waldo AL, Camm AJ, deRuyter H, et al: Effect of d-sotalol on mortality in patients with left ventricular dysfunction after recent and remote myocardial infarction: the SWORD Investigators: Survival With Oral d-Sotalol. Lancet 348:7–12, 1996.
243. Zipes DP, Roberts D: Results of the International Study of the Implantable Pacemaker Cardioverter-Defibrillator: a comparison of epicardial and endocardial lead systems: the Pacemaker-Cardioverter-Defibrillator Investigators. Circulation 92:59–65, 1995.
244. Fogoros RN, Elson JJ, Bonnet CA, et al: Efficacy of the automatic implantable cardioverter-defibrillator in prolonging survival in patients with severe underlying cardiac disease. J Am Coll Cardiol 16:381–386, 1990.
245. Moss AJ, Hall WJ, Cannom DS, et al: Improved survival with an implanted defibrillator in patients with coronary disease at high risk for ventricular arrhythmia: Multicenter Automatic Defibrillator

Implantation Trial Investigators. N Engl J Med 335:1933–1940, 1996.

246. Naccarelli GV, Wolbrette DL, Dell'Orfano JT, et al: A decade of clinical trial developments in postmyocardial infarction, congestive heart failure, and sustained ventricular tachyarrhythmia patients: from CAST to AVID and beyond: Cardiac Arrhythmic Suppression Trial: Antiarrhythmic Versus Implantable Defibrillators. J Cardiovasc Electrophysiol 9:864–891, 1998.

247. Bigger JT Jr: Prophylactic use of implanted cardiac defibrillators in patients at high risk for ventricular arrhythmias after coronary-artery bypass graft surgery: Coronary Artery Bypass Graft (CABG) Patch Trial Investigators. N Engl J Med 337:1569–1575, 1997.

248. The CABG Patch Trial Investigators and Coordinators. The Coronary Artery Bypass Graft (CABG) Patch Trial. Prog Cardiovasc Dis 36:97–114, 1993.

249. Buxton AE, Fisher JD, Josephson ME, et al: Prevention of sudden death in patients with coronary artery disease: the Multicenter Unsustained Tachycardia Trial (MUSTT). Prog Cardiovasc Dis 36:215–226, 1993.

250. Buxton AE, Lee KL, DiCarlo L, et al: Nonsustained ventricular tachycardia in coronary artery disease: relation to inducible sustained ventricular tachycardia: MUSTT Investigators. Ann Intern Med 125:35–39, 1996.

251. Ferguson JJ: Meeting highlights of the 48th Scientific Sessions of the American College of Cardiology. Circulation 100:570–575, 1999.

252. Mitchell LB, Duff HJ, Manyari DE, Wyse DG: A randomized clinical trial of the noninvasive and invasive approaches to drug therapy of ventricular tachycardia. N Engl J Med 317:1681–1687, 1987.

253. Mitchell LB, Duff HJ, Gillis AM, et al: A randomized clinical trial of the noninvasive and invasive approaches to drug therapy for ventricular tachycardia: long-term follow-up of the Calgary trial. Prog Cardiovasc Dis 38:377–384, 1996.

254. The ESVEM Investigators. The ESVEM trial: Electrophysiologic Study Versus Electrocardiographic Monitoring for selection of antiarrhythmic therapy of ventricular tachyarrhythmias. Circulation 79:1354–1360, 1989.

255. Mason JW: A comparison of electrophysiologic testing with Holter monitoring to predict antiarrhythmic-drug efficacy for ventricular tachyarrhythmias: Electrophysiologic Study versus Electrocardiographic Monitoring Investigators. N Engl J Med 329:445–451, 1993.

256. Reiffel JA, Hahn E, Hartz V, Reiter MJ: Sotalol for ventricular tachyarrhythmias: beta-blocking and class III contributions, and relative efficacy versus class I drugs after prior drug failure: ESVEM Investigators: Electrophysiologic Study Versus Electrocardiographic Monitoring. Am J Cardiol 79:1048–1053, 1997.

257. Siebels J, Cappato R, Ruppel R, et al: Preliminary results of the Cardiac Arrest Study Hamburg (CASH): CASH Investigators. Am J Cardiol 72:109F–113F, 1993.

258. The Antiarrhythmics versus Implantable Defibrillators (AVID) Investigators. Antiarrhythmics Versus Implantable Defibrillators (AVID)—rationale, design, and methods. Am J Cardiol 75:470–475, 1995.

259. The Antiarrhythmics Versus Implantable Defibrillators (AVID) Investigators: A comparison of antiarrhythmic-drug therapy with implantable defibrillators in patients resuscitated from near-fatal ventricular arrhythmias. N Engl J Med 337:1576–1583, 1997.

260. Connolly SJ, Gent M, Roberts RS, et al: Canadian Implantable Defibrillator Study (CIDS): study design and organization. CIDS Co-Investigators. Am J Cardiol 72:103F–108F, 1993.

261. Curtis AB, Hallstrom AP, Klein RC, et al: Influence of patient characteristics in the selection of patients for defibrillator implantation (the AVID Registry): Antiarrhythmics Versus Implantable Defibrillators. Am J Cardiol 79:1185–1189, 1997.

262. Kim SG, Hallstrom A, Love JC, et al: Comparison of clinical characteristics and frequency of implantable defibrillator use between randomized patients in the Antiarrhythmics Vs Implantable Defibrillators (AVID) trial and nonrandomized registry patients. Am J Cardiol 80:454–457, 1997.

263. Mason JW: A comparison of seven antiarrhythmic drugs in patients with ventricular tachyarrhythmias: Electrophysiologic Study versus Electrocardiographic Monitoring Investigators. N Engl J Med 329:452–458, 1993.

264. The CASCADE Investigators. Randomized antiarrhythmic drug therapy in survivors of cardiac arrest (the CASCADE Study). Am J Cardiol 72:280–287, 1993.

265. Wilber DJ, Kall JG, Kapp DE: What can we expect from prophylactic implantable defibrillators? Am J Cardiol 80:20F–27F, 1997.

CHAPTER 95

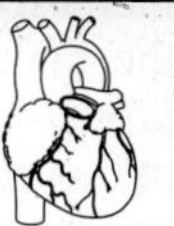

Antiarrhythmic Drugs

Gerald V. Naccarelli

PHARMACOKINETIC AND PHARMACODYNAMIC PRINCIPLES OF ANTIARRHYTHMIC AGENTS
ANTIARRHYTHMIC CLASSIFICATION
Quinidine (Quinidex, Quinaglute, Cardioquin)
Procainamide (Procan SR, Pronestyl-SR, Procanbid)
Disopyramide (Norpace, Norpace CR)
Lidocaine Hydrochloride (Xylocaine)
Tocainide (Tonocard)
Mexiletine (Mexitil)
Flecainide (Tambocor)
Propafenone (Rythmol)
Moricizine (Ethmozine)
Propranolol (Inderal, Inderal LA)
Acebutolol (Sectral)
Esmolol Hydrochloride (Brevibloc)
Amiodarone (Cordarone)
Bretylium (Bretylol)
Sotalol (Betapace)
Ibutilide (Corvert)
Dofetilide (Tikosyn)
Azimilide (Stedicor)
Verapamil (Calan, Isoptin)
Diltiazem (Cardizem)
Adenosine (Adenocard)
Digoxin (Lanoxin, Lanoxicaps); Digitoxin (Crystodigin)

Parenteral and oral antiarrhythmic agents remain front-line therapy for acute and chronic arrhythmias. The purpose of this chapter is to review the electrophysiology, pharmacokinetic properties, antiarrhythmic efficacy, and adverse reaction profiles of currently available antiarrhythmic agents.

Pharmacokinetic and Pharmacodynamic Principles of Antiarrhythmic Agents

Plasma concentrations of an antiarrhythmic drug are affected by its absorption, distribution, metabolism, and excretion. The therapeutic range of a specific drug is based on studies that have provided information regarding the plasma concentrations associated with the desired pharmacologic outcome or toxic effects of the drug. Several factors may affect the plasma drug concentration in an individual patient. Disease states can affect the rate or the extent of absorption. Distribution is often affected by alterations in protein binding, such as increased quinidine binding after a myocardial infarction (MI), saturated binding sites by high disopyramide levels, and fewer available binding sites with the digoxin-quinidine interaction. Changes in renal and hepatic function may prolong the time it takes to remove a drug from the body. Drug concentration of parent compounds and metabolites is often genetically predetermined by inherited phenotypes determining the amount of enzyme available to metabolize drugs. Finally, other drugs that the patient is taking can interact with any of the aforementioned four phases.[1]

Drug absorption is usually a fairly rapid process; however, the rate and the extent of absorption are subject to change. Absorption may be affected by gastric and bowel pH, bowel bacterial flora, concomitant food intake, bowel motility, or other drugs.

Bioavailability is the percentage of drug that reaches the systemic circulation after absorption and first-pass clearance. Bioavailability may be affected by the formulation of the drug, such as sustained-release preparations.

The systemic circulation distributes the drug to the various compartments. The volume of distribution indicates the extent that a drug distributes into body fluids and tissues. The volume of distribution is thus a function of the lipid-versus-water solubility and the plasma and tissue protein binding properties of the drug. In most cases, the drug behaves as though there are two or more compartments. The first compartment is a rapidly equilibrating volume, usually made up of blood and highly perfused organs. The time it takes to get one half of the drug distributed in this initial compartment is referred to as the alpha (α) half-life. The second compartment equilibrates with the drug in the initial compartment over a longer period of time.

Another important pharmacokinetic parameter is clearance, which is the ability of the body to remove drug from the blood. Clearance represents the volume of blood from which the drug is removed over a specific period of time. Body surface area, plasma protein binding, extraction ratio, renal function, hepatic function, and cardiac output are factors that alter clearance. A drug's clearance and volume of distribution determine the rate of removal from the body. First-pass clearance may be affected by congestive heart failure (CHF) with decreased perfusion of the liver, cirrhosis, inherited metabolism phenotype, and drug interactions that alter metabolism.

Enzymatic metabolism of a drug is genetically determined.[2] Several antiarrhythmic drugs undergo biotransformation by hepatic oxidative metabolism through the cytochrome P450 system. Cimetidine and amiodarone inhibit the P450 enzymes, causing an increased concentration of certain drugs when they are used concomitantly. Phenytoin and phenobarbital induce the P450 system, resulting in increased metabolism of some antiarrhythmics. P450D6 is the major enzyme system responsible for biotransforming propafenone, flecainide, acebutolol, metoprolol, and propranolol. Most patients are "extensive metabolizers." Five to 10 percent of the population, who have reduced amounts of the P450D6 enzyme, are labeled as "poor metabolizers." Low doses of quinidine can inhibit P450D6, thus increasing the peak and steady state plasma concentrations and half-life of parent compounds, such as propafenone.

The cytochrome P450A4 system is responsible for the metabolism of lidocaine, quinidine, and certain antihistamines. This system is inhibited by erythromycin and ketoconazole, thus increasing the concentrations of drugs such as quinidine when used concomitantly, and thereby increasing the risk of torsades de pointes.

Certain drugs, such as procainamide, are metabolized by *N*-acetyltransferase. About 50 percent of blacks and whites and 90 percent of Asians are rapid acetylators.

Many drugs have active metabolites. The time to reach steady state is determined by the half-life of the active metabolite if it has a longer half-life than the parent compound. This is typical for drugs such as propafenone and acebutolol.

Drugs are assumed to enter and leave the body from the initial or central compartment. Most drugs follow a first-order elimination process. First-order elimination kinetics refers to a process in which the amount of drug in the body diminishes logarithmically over time. This means that the fraction of a drug in the body eliminated over a period of time remains constant. The time it takes to get 50 percent of the drug eliminated from this initial compartment is referred to as the beta (β) half-life. One would expect the serum drug concentration to decline by one half over this period; this is known as the *elimination half-life*. After a drug is discontinued, approximately five half-lives pass before it is completely removed from the body. With drugs that follow first-order elimination, if the dose given is doubled, the serum drug concentrations also double. Some drugs are said to follow nonlinear or dose-dependent pharmacokinetics. In this situation, doubling the dose may increase serum concentrations by much more than a factor of two, thus leading to toxicity. In cases of toxicity, peritoneal dialysis is not effective in clearing antiarrhythmic drugs. However, hemodialysis may be effective in clearing procainamide, disopyramide, tocainide, and sotalol.

As successive doses of a drug are given, the drug begins to accumulate in the body. Steady state means that the rate of drug administered equals the rate of drug eliminated. For drugs that follow first-order elimination, the time to reach a steady state equilibrium is dependent on the drug's elimination half-life. It takes five half-lives to reach more than 96 percent of the steady state concentration. Thus, the five half-lives rule can be used to estimate the time necessary to reach steady state. Each time the maintenance dose is changed, another five half-lives must pass before the new steady state level is reached.

In CHF, the volume of distribution may be decreased by as much as 40 percent, and drug clearances may be diminished as a result of decreased renal or hepatic blood flow and reduced hepatic enzyme activity.[3] The aforementioned changes may prolong elimination half-life and require a reduction in dosage to avoid toxicity.

TABLE 95–1 Vaughn Williams Antiarrhythmic Drug Classification

Class	Action	Drug
I	Sodium channel blockers	
IA	Moderate phase 0 depression	Quinidine
	Moderate conduction slowing	Procainamide
	Prolongs repolarization	Disopyramide
IB	Minimal phase 0 depression	Lidocaine
	Shortens repolarization	Tocainide
		Mexiletine
IC	Marked phase 0 depression	Flecainide
	Marked conduction slowing	Propafenone
	Slight effect on repolarization	Moricizine
II	Beta-blockers	Propranolol
		Acebutolol
		Esmolol
III	Prolongs repolarization	Bretylium
		Amiodarone
		Sotalol
		Ibutilide
		Dofetilide*
		Azimilide*
IV	Calcium channel blockers	Verapamil
		Diltiazem
	Purine agonist	Adenosine
	Digitalis glycosides	Digoxin
		Digitoxin

*Investigational.

TABLE 95–2 Offset/Onset Kinetics of Class I Antiarrhythmic Drugs

Group I: fast onset/fast offset	Procainamide
Lidocaine	Flecainide
Tocainide	Group III: fast onset/slow offset
Mexiletine	Disopyramide
Group II: slow onset/slow offset	Propafenone
Quinidine	Moricizine

ANTIARRHYTHMIC CLASSIFICATION

Table 95–1 lists a classification of antiarrhythmic drugs as proposed by Vaughn Williams.[4] This classification has been modified over the years. The largest group of antiarrhythmic drugs are the sodium channel blockers. Because of the size of this class, these drugs have been subclassified into

TABLE 95–3 Principal States Blocked by Specific Drugs

Open-state blockers	Procainamide
Quinidine	Lidocaine
Disopyramide	Tocainide
Flecainide	Mexiletine
Propafenone	Moricizine
Inactivated-state blockers	Amiodarone
Disopyramide	

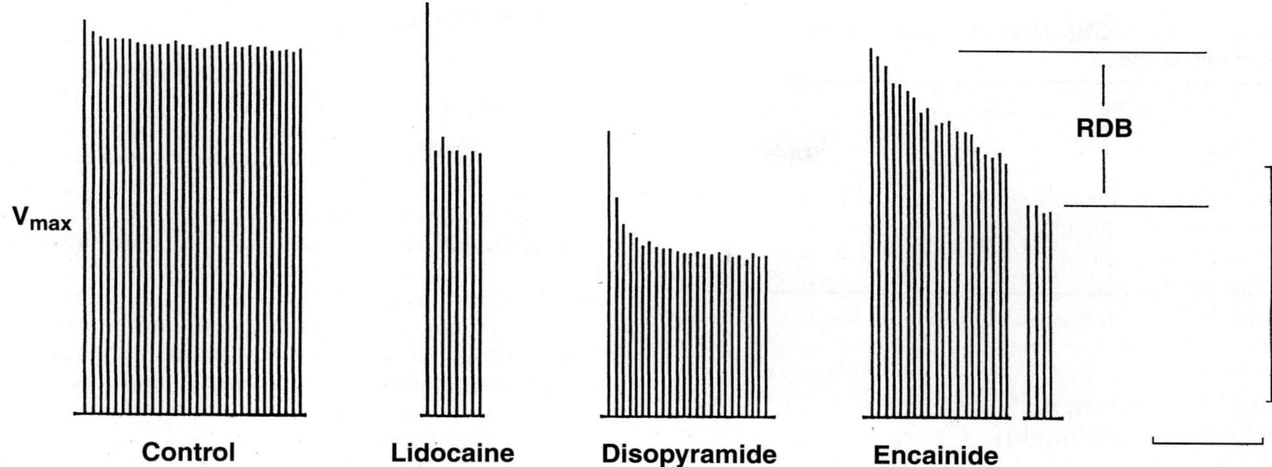

FIGURE 95–1 Rate-dependent block (RDB) demonstrated fast use dependence by lidocaine, intermediate use dependence by disopyramide, and slow use-dependent block by encainide. V_{max}, maximum flow per unit of time. (From Campbell TJ: Kinetics of onset of rate-dependent effects of class I antiarrhythmic drugs are important in determining effects on refractoriness in guinea pig ventricle, and provide a theoretical basis for their subclassification. Cardiovasc Res 17:344–352, 1983. With permission from Elsevier Science.)

IA, IB, and IC groups on the basis of their electrophysiologic actions. This simplified classification scheme is limited in its usefulness in that it does not characterize drugs by basic electrophysiologic differences, such as onset-offset kinetics (Table 95–2),[5–7] use dependency (Fig. 95–1), and whether drugs block open or inactivated states (Table 95–3).[8] In addition, autonomic and unique features of these drugs are not used as part of this classification. These characteristics as listed in the paper describing the Sicilian Gambit[9] are listed in Table 95–4. Table 95–5 lists the expected electrocardiographic effects of the antiarrhythmic agents.

In the remainder of this chapter, I individually review the electrophysiology, pharmacokinetics, efficacy, and adverse effect profile of the older and newer antiarrhythmic agents. Comparative pharmacokinetic data (Tables 95–6 and 95–7), drug interactions (Table 95–8), and hemodynamics (Table 95–9) are listed.

TABLE 95-4 **Sicilian Gambit Classification of Antiarrhythmic Drugs**

	Channel Blockers					Receptors			
	Na								
Drug	Fast	Medium	Slow	*Ca*	*K*	α	β	M_2	*P*
Lidocaine	L								
Mexiletine	L								
Tocainide	L								
Moricizine	H, I								
Procainamide		H, A			M				
Disopyramide		H, A			M			L	
Quinidine		H, A			M			L	
Propafenone		H, A					L		
Flecainide			H, A		L				
Verapamil	L			H		M			
Diltiazem				M					
Bretylium					H	Ag/Ant	Ag/Ant		
Sotalol					H				
Amiodarone	L			L	H	M	M		
Ibutilide*					L				
Dofetilide					H				
Azimilide					H				
Propranolol	L						H		
Acebutolol							H		
Esmolol							H		
Adenosine							H		Ag

Abbreviations: A, activated; Ag, agonist; Ant, antagonist; H, high; L, low; M, medium; M2, muscarinic; O, open, P, purine.
*Ibutilide enhances sodium (Na) flow into the cell during the plateau phase of the action potential.

TABLE 95–5 Electrocardiographic Effects of Antiarrhythmic Agents

	PR	QRS	QT	JT
IA	↑	↑	↑↑	↑↑
IB	—	—	—↓	—↓
IC	↑↑	↑↑	↑	—
II	↑	—	—	—
III	↑	↑	↑↑	↑↑
IV	↑	—	—	—

Abbreviations: ↑↑, markedly increase; ↑, increase; ↓, decrease; —, no change.

Quinidine (Quinidex, Quinaglute, Cardioquin)

Quinidine is a type IA antiarrhythmic agent (see Table 95–1). It is manufactured as a sulfate salt (82.8 percent quinidine base) with long-acting trade name formulations (Quinidex) and also as polygalacturonate (Cardioquin) and gluconate salts (62 percent quinidine base) (Quinaglute).

Electrophysiology. Basic experiments demonstrate that quinidine reduces automaticity by raising the threshold potential and decreasing the rate of rise of phase 4 depolarization. Quinidine decreases the rate of rise of phase 0 of the action potential by blocking sodium influx predominantly in the activated state, thus slowing conduction. This action of quinidine is frequency dependent, with depression of V_{max} being greater at faster heart rates.[5, 6] Quinidine prolongs action potential duration (APD), primarily by blocking the potassium channel (see Table 95–9). Quinidine also prolongs the effective refractory period (ERP) and the ERP/APD ratio.

Quinidine has vagolytic effects that can increase sinus heart rate, enhance atrioventricular (AV) nodal conduction, and shorten AV node refractory periods. Quinidine mildly blocks alpha and muscarinic subtype 2 receptors[9] (see Table 95–9). Because of conduction slowing and competitive vagolytic properties, the PR and AH intervals may not increase. Quinidine increases the ERP of the atria, His-Purkinje system, ventricles, and accessory pathways. Quinidine increases the HV, QT, and QRS intervals.[10]

Pharmacokinetics. Because quinidine comes in different preparations, pharmacokinetics vary. With quinidine sulfate, 95 percent is absorbed orally, bioavailability is about 70 to 90 percent, and peak levels occur 1 to 3 hours after ingestion. Twenty to 50 percent is excreted unchanged by the kidneys. Otherwise, quinidine is metabolized by hydroxylation in the liver. 3-Hydroxyquinidine and 2′-oxoquinidine appear to have some antiarrhythmic activity. The half-life of quinidine sulfate is 5 to 7 hours, and thus the drug takes about 24 to 36 hours to reach steady state. Therapeutic plasma levels are 2 to 7 μg/ml. Extended release preparations release about one third of the dose immediately, with the remainder time released over 6 to 10 hours.

Dosing. Dosage of the quinidine sulfate is usually 200 to 600 mg qid, depending on levels, efficacy, and intolerance. Quinidex is given at the same total daily dose using a bid or tid schedule. Quinaglute doses range from 324 to 972 mg bid or tid.

Efficacy. Quinidine is effective in suppressing premature atrial contractions and ectopic atrial tachycardias. Quinidine has been useful in the chemical cardioversion and maintenance of patients with atrial flutter and fibrillation. About 50 percent of atrial fibrillation patients treated with quinidine remain in sinus rhythm 1 year after cardioversion.[11]

By suppressing premature atrial contractions and premature ventricular contractions (PVCs) and by slowing conduction and prolonging refractoriness of accessory path-

TABLE 95–6 Antiarrhythmic Drugs: Pharmacokinetic Summary

Drug	Route of Administration	Oral Bioavailability (%)	Protein Bindings (%)	Half-Life* (h)
Quinidine	po, IM, IV	80	75–95	6
Procainamide	po, IV	85	15	3
Disopyramide	po	80	40–81	7
Lidocaine	IV	35	70	1.7
Phenytoin	po, IV	90	—	22
Tocainide	po	95	15	13–15
Mexiletine	po	85	70	10–12
Moricizine	po	38	95	2–5 (9 long-term)
Flecainide	po	90	40	20
Propafenone	po	<25	95	4–6
Propranolol	po, IV	10	—	3–6 (po)
Acebutolol	po	40	25	3–4
Esmolol	IV	NA	56	9 min
Bretylium	IV	NA	—	8
Amiodarone	po, IV	50	90	53 da
Sotalol	po, IV	90	50	7–15
Verapamil	po, IV	16	90	5 (po)
Diltiazem	po, IV	40	75	3.5
Digoxin	po, IV	70	25	36–48
Digitoxin	po	95	90	7–9 da

Abbreviation: NA, not applicable.
*Parent compound.

TABLE 95-7 **Antiarrhythmic Drugs: Pharmacokinetic Summary**

	Principal Route of Elimination	Active Metabolites	Half-Life (hr) Active Metabolites	Steady State (da*)	Therapeutic Range (μg/ml)	Usual Maintenance Dose (mg)
Quinidine	Hepatic	3-hydroxy-quinidine	NA	1–2	2–7	200–400 qid
Procainamide	Hepatic + renal	*N*-acetylprocainamide	9–10	1–2	4–10	500–1500 qid
Disopyramide	Renal + hepatic	*N*-monodeakyl disopyramide	NA	2	2–8	100–200 qid
Licocaine	Hepatic	MEGX	NA	NA	1.5–6.0	1–4 mg/min
Phenytoin	Hepatic	No	NA	3	10–20	200–600 qd
Tocainide	Hepatic + renal	No	NA	2–3	4–10	300–600 tid
Mexiletine	Hepatic	No	NA	2–3	0.5–2	150–300 tid
Moricizine	Hepatic	No	NA	2	NE	200–300 tid
Flecainide	Hepatic + renal	No	NA	4	0.4–1	100–150 bid
Propafenone	Hepatic	OH-propafenone	6–12	3	NE	150–300 tid
Propranolol	Hepatic	No	NA	2	100–150	10–40 qid
Acebutolol	Hepatic + renal	Diacetolol	8–13	3	NE	200–400 qd
Esmolol	Hepatic	No	NA	NA	NE	500 μg/kg (load)
Bretylium	Renal	No	NA	NA	NE	1–4
Amiodarone	Hepatic	Desethylamiodarone	months	months	1.5–2.5	200–400 qd
Sotalol	Renal	No	NA	2–3	NE	80–320 bid
Verapamil	Hepatic	No	NA	1	0.1–0.4	0.1 mg/kg IV (80–160 po tid)
Diltiazem	Hepatic	No	NA	1	NE	30–90 po tid
Adenosine	Cellular	No	NA	NA	NE	6–12 mg IV
Digoxin	Renal	No	NA	10	0.1–2.0	0.25 mg qd
Digitoxin	Hepatic	No	NA	30	10–20	0.15 mg qd

Abbreviations: MEGX, monoethylglycinexylidide; NA, not applicable; NE, not established.
*Takes into account active metabolites.

TABLE 95–8 Important Antiarrhythmic Drug Interactions

Drug	Interacts With	Results
Quinidine	Digoxin	Doubling of digoxin levels
Propafenone	Digoxin	Doubling of digoxin levels
Amiodarone	Digoxin	Doubling of digoxin levels
	Quinidine Procainamide Disopyramide Flecainide	15–35% increase in Na channel blocker levels
	Warfarin	2–3× increase in prothrombin times
Disopyramide	Phenytoin	Decreases disopyramide levels
Verapamil	Digoxin	Increase in digoxin levels
Moricizine	Theophylline	Decreases theophylline levels

ways and the retrograde limb of the AV node, quinidine has been effective in treating paroxysmal supraventricular tachycardia (PSVT) secondary to AV nodal reentrant tachycardia and AV reentrant tachycardia. Similar to procainamide, quinidine rarely completely blocks conduction in accessory pathways with refractory periods of 270 ms or less.[12]

Quinidine is effective for the long-term suppression of ventricular ectopic activity. Holter monitoring shows that quinidine effectively suppresses PVCs, couplets, and nonsustained ventricular tachycardia (VT) in about 60 percent of patients.[13, 13a–13c, 14] In patients with sustained VT/ventricular fibrillation (VF), efficacy rates, as determined by programmed stimulation, are 20 to 25 percent.[10, 14] Patients with ejection fractions greater than 30 percent appear to have higher efficacy rates in the latter group.

Combination therapy with tocainide or mexiletine using lower maintenance doses of both drugs achieves added efficacy and lower toxicity.[15] Quinidine can also be used in conjunction with amiodarone although, because of a drug interaction, quinidine doses need to be lowered by about one third.[16]

Adverse Effects. Subjective toxicity with quinidine is common. Ten to 35 percent of patients experience nausea, vomiting, anorexia, or diarrhea. Some of these adverse reactions are dose related. Fever, rash, and tinnitus can rarely occur. End-organ toxicity includes a rare drug-induced thrombocytopenia and granulomatous hepatitis.

TABLE 95–9 Antiarrhythmic Drugs: Inotropic Potential

Positive/neutral Digitalis Ibutilide Dofetilide Azimilide Mild negative Quinidine Procainamide Lidocaine Tocainide Mexiletine Moricizine Bretylium Amiodarone	Moderate negative Flecainide Propafenone D,L-Sotalol Diltiazem Most negative Disopyramide Beta-blockers Verapamil

Quinidine has mild negative inotropic activity (see Table 95–9), but its overall effect on cardiac output appears to be minimal. Some of its direct negative inotropic activity may be counterbalanced by its peripheral vasodilatory effects, mediated partially by alpha-blockade. Rarely, the vasodilatory properties of quinidine can lead to orthostatic hypotension.

Importantly, quinidine interacts with digoxin (see Table 95–8), increasing digoxin levels by a factor of two.[16, 17] This occurs secondary to quinidine's displacing digoxin from the tissues and by its reducing renal clearance rates of digoxin. When used in combination, digoxin doses should be halved. As noted earlier, amiodarone also interacts with quinidine.

Because of its vagolytic effects, quinidine may cause an increase in ventricular response when it is used to treat patients for atrial fibrillation or flutter. Also, by slowing the atrial rate and decreasing concealed AV nodal block in the AV node, atrial flutter with 1:1 conduction can occur. Prophylactic digitalization may minimize the occurrence of this phenomenon.

Quinidine may worsen infranodal block. By slowing conduction, quinidine can be proarrhythmic with the development of new-onset monomorphic VT. Of more concern, quinidine may prolong the QT interval and cause drug-aggravated torsades de pointes in up to 5 percent of patients.[18, 19] There are no large controlled trials defining the safety of the use of quinidine in patients who have had an MI or in those with CHF. One small study suggested that quinidine increases mortality in patients with CHF.[20]

Procainamide (Procan SR, Pronestyl-SR, Procanbid)

Procainamide is a type IA antiarrhythmic agent that is useful in both atrial and ventricular arrhythmias. It is available intravenously and in oral shorter acting and sustained-release preparations. Procan SR is delivered via an early-release wax matrix and Pronestyl-SR as an early-release inner core.

Electrophysiology. Procainamide has electrophysiologic properties similar to those of quinidine (see Tables 95–1 and 95–4) but has fewer vagolytic effects.

Pharmacokinetics. Procainamide is 95 percent absorbed in the small intestine, with peak levels occurring 15 minutes to 2 hours after oral administration. Bioavailability is about 85 percent. Procainamide is acetylated in the liver by *N*-acetyltransferase to an active metabolite, *N*-acetylprocainamide (NAPA). The rate of acetylation depends on a genetically determined acetylation phenotype. In rapid acetylators, NAPA levels usually exceed levels of the parent compound. NAPA is an active metabolite with 70 percent of the antiarrhythmic activity of the parent compound. Thirty to 60 percent of the drug is excreted unchanged in the urine, and the remainder is excreted as

NAPA. Orally, the half-life of procainamide is only 3 to 4 hours; thus, steady state is achieved within 24 hours. NAPA has a half-life of 6 hours. Therapeutic procainamide levels are in the 4- to 8-μg/ml range with NAPA levels of 8 to 16 μg/ml, and combined levels in excess of 16 to 20 μg/ml are commonly associated with toxicity.

Dosing. Procainamide is usually initiated at about 50 mg/kg/da. Doses are titrated according to efficacy, toxicity, and blood levels. IV procainamide requires loading doses of 10 to 15 mg/kg given over 25 to 50 mg/min, depending on blood pressure. This can be followed by a 1- to 4-mg/min IV drip.

Efficacy. Both IV and oral procainamide may be used to chemically convert and treat patients with ectopic atrial tachycardia, atrial flutter, atrial fibrillation, and PSVT. In hemodynamically tolerated atrial fibrillation with overt preexcitation, IV procainamide is the treatment of choice to slow antegrade accessory pathway conduction and thus the ventricular response. Procainamide is about 60 percent effective in suppressing PVCs, couplets, and nonsustained VT, as assessed by Holter monitoring.[13, 13a–13c, 14] Procainamide is effective in about 20 to 25 percent of cases of sustained VT, as assessed by programmed stimulation.[13, 13a–13c, 14, 21] Added efficacy is achieved when procainamide is used in combination with mexiletine. The response to IV procainamide in the electrophysiology laboratory appears to predict an acceptable electrophysiologic response to oral procainamide and other antiarrhythmic agents.[22] IV procainamide is one of the parenteral treatments of choice for ventricular tachyarrhythmias and is more likely to terminate VT than lidocaine.[23]

Adverse Effects. Procainamide may cause nausea, anorexia, vomiting, and rash. End-organ toxicity of concern is a rare agranulocytosis that usually occurs during the first 3 months of treatment.

The major limiting adverse reaction to procainamide has been the development of a systemic lupus–like reaction in 10 to 20 percent of patients. This is more likely to occur in slow acetylators (50 percent of the population). More than 70 percent of patients have a positive antinuclear antibody titer within a year. This laboratory abnormality alone does not warrant discontinuation of therapy.

Procainamide has a negative inotropic effect that is mild and may be less than that of quinidine (see Table 95–9). In a 21-patient comparative study, procainamide caused less hemodynamic compromise than tocainide or encainide.[24] Procainamide can cause high-degree AV block and ventricular proarrhythmia, including the new onset of sustained, monomorphic VT or torsades de pointes. In renal failure, patients may have significantly increased levels of both procainamide and NAPA with the development of torsades de pointes. Similar to quinidine, procainamide has been associated with increased mortality when used in CHF patients.[20] No safety data exist in the post-MI setting.

Disopyramide (Norpace, Norpace CR)

Disopyramide is a type IA antiarrhythmic agent that was approved by the United States Food and Drug Administration (FDA) in 1977 for the treatment of ventricular arrhythmias.

Electrophysiology. In basic animal and human experiments, disopyramide has electrophysiologic and vagal effects similar to those of quinidine and procainamide (see Tables 95–1 and 95–4).

Pharmacokinetics. Ninety percent of an oral dose of disopyramide is orally absorbed, and its bioavailability is 70 to 85 percent. Peak levels occur within 2 hours. Fifty-five percent of a dose is recovered unchanged in the urine after renal excretion, and 25 percent is recovered as the active *N*-monodealkylated metabolite. Disopyramide has nonlinear pharmacokinetics, with decreasing plasma protein binding as serum concentrations increase.

The half-life varies from 4 to 10 hours (average, 6 to 7 hours), and steady state is achieved within 40 hours. In patients with renal failure and CHF, elimination half-life is significantly increased. Usually, therapeutic levels are in the 2- to 5-μg/ml range.

Dosing. Dosing ranges from 100, 150 to 200 mg orally qd. The controlled-release formulation is effective with a bid dosing schedule.

Efficacy. Disopyramide is very effective in treating patients with ectopic atrial tachycardia, atrial flutter, atrial fibrillation, and PSVT associated with and not associated with the Wolff-Parkinson-White syndrome. Disopyramide is as effective as procainamide and quinidine in suppressing PVCs, ventricular couplets, and nonsustained runs of VT, as assessed by Holter monitoring, and in suppressing sustained VT, as assessed by programmed stimulation.[13, 13a–13c, 14, 25] Because of disopyramide's anticholinergic properties, it is often used to treat patients with neurocardiogenic syncope.

Adverse Effects. Disopyramide's subjective toxicity is primarily secondary to its anticholinergic activity and include dry mouth, blurred vision, urinary retention, constipation, and worsening of glaucoma. These reactions require discontinuation in about 10 percent of patients. No significant end-organ toxicity has been noted with disopyramide.

Disopyramide's most important adverse reaction is a worsening of CHF secondary to its significant negative inotropic activity and an increase of peripheral vascular resistance. CHF occurs in 50 percent of patients with a prior history of CHF and in only 5 percent of other patients.[26] No well-controlled data exist to determine the safety of the use of disopyramide in CHF or post-MI patients.

Disopyramide, by slowing conduction, can cause complete AV block and bundle branch block. Slowing of conduction and prolongation of the QT interval can cause proarrhythmias, such as monomorphic sustained VT and torsades de pointes.

Lidocaine Hydrochloride (Xylocaine)

Lidocaine hydrochloride, used intravenously, is a short-acting type IB antiarrhythmic agent (see Tables 95–1 and 95–4).

Electrophysiology. Electrophysiologically, lidocaine minimally blocks the sodium channels and thus minimally slows conduction in the His-Purkinje system and the myocardium. Lidocaine has more conduction-slowing properties in ischemic tissue. Lidocaine has little to no effect on atrial, AV nodal, or accessory pathway tissue; thus, it is ineffective in treating supraventricular arrhythmias. Lidocaine depresses automaticity in Purkinje fibers and thus would be predicted to be efficacious in suppressing irritable ventricular foci. Its ability to slow conduction in cardiac tissue and to cause a net increase in the ERP/APD ratio may help prevent reentrant ventricular arrhythmias.

Pharmacokinetics. Lidocaine has poor oral absorption, and 90 percent of an administered dose is rapidly metabolized in the liver into two major metabolites—monoethylglycinexylidide (MEG) and glycinexylidide.[27] Monoethylglycinexylidide is 80 percent and glycinexylidide is 10 percent as potent as the parent compound. Because of its rapid first-pass metabolism, lidocaine is not useful orally and must be administered parenterally for therapeutic blood levels to be achieved.

Lidocaine administered as an intravenous bolus is distributed rapidly into the intravascular compartment (half-life, 8 minutes) and then diffuses quickly into the peripheral compartment. Lidocaine has a half-life of 1½ to 2 hours in the second pass of redistribution, with extensive metabolism occurring hepatically. Because of this, if an infusion is started without a bolus loading dose, it takes from 20 to 60 minutes to attain therapeutic levels.

Dosing. Recommended dosing includes a loading bolus infusion of 75 mg IV, followed by a 1- to 4-mg/min maintenance infusion. Within 15 minutes of the first bolus, a second bolus can be given to maintain levels. If maintenance infusions at higher doses are needed, patients should receive a 50- to 75-mg IV bolus before the rate of the maintenance infusion is increased, in order to avoid delays in attaining higher blood levels.[28]

In patients with severe heart failure, there is decreased hepatic blood flow and metabolism of lidocaine. In this situation, lower doses need to be used to avoid toxicity.[29] Elderly patients are more sensitive to the toxic effects of lidocaine. In older patients, lower loading and maintenance doses should be used.

Efficacy. Lidocaine is used as a drug of choice for the rapid suppression of PVCs, warning arrhythmias, and prophylaxis in the post-MI setting.[30] A meta-analysis suggests that lidocaine should not be routinely used as a post-MI prophylactic antiarrhythmic against the occurrence of VT/VF.[31] It is not as effective as procainamide for slowing or terminating sustained VT.[23]

Adverse Effects. Lidocaine has dose-related neurologic and gastrointestinal adverse effects. Neurologic side effects include numbness, tingling, seizures, tremors, paresthesias, disorientation, dulled sensorium, tinnitus, and drowsiness. Gastrointestinal side effects include nausea and vomiting. Lidocaine is well tolerated hemodynamically. Lidocaine only minimally slows conduction in the His-Purkinje system. Therapeutic blood levels are in the 1- to 5-μg/ml range.

Tocainide (Tonocard)

Tocainide is an orally useful primary amine analogue of lidocaine with class IB effects (see Tables 95–1 and 95–4).

Electrophysiology. Its electrophysiologic effects in vitro are similar to those of lidocaine and mexiletine.

Pharmacokinetics. Tocainide has excellent oral absorption and bioavailability that exceed 95 percent. Tocainide is eliminated by both the renal and the hepatic routes. No major active metabolites exist. Its onset of action is 1½ hours, and its half-life averages 11 to 19 hours. Therapeutic levels of tocainide are between 4 and 10 μg/ml.[32]

Dosing. Oral dosing with tocainide is usually initiated at 300 to 400 mg bid or tid. Rarely, doses as high as 600 mg tid are required.

Efficacy. Tocainide has been found to be an effective suppresser of premature ventricular beats. An effective response to lidocaine seems to be predictive of tocainide response. As measured by programmed stimulation, tocainide is effective in less than 15 percent of patients with sustained ventricular tachyarrhythmias.[13, 13a–13c, 14, 32–34] Combination therapy of tocainide with a type IA agent has demonstrated an added efficacy of 15 to 35 percent in patients with ventricular arrhythmias compared with either agent alone.

Adverse Effects. Similar to lidocaine and mexiletine, tocainide's side effects are primarily gastrointestinal and neurologic. Gastrointestinal side effects include anorexia, nausea, vomiting, abdominal pain, and constipation. Neurologic side effects include tremors, nervousness, dizziness, paresthesias, and confusion. Because of subjective intolerance, which is often dose related, tocainide has to be discontinued in 15 to 30 percent of patients. Subjective side effects can often be minimized by lowering the dose or taking the medication after meals. Up to 8 percent of patients who take tocainide get a drug-induced rash, which resolves on discontinuation of the drug. Of significant concern are the rare occurrences of pulmonary fibrosis or agranulocytosis (0.2 percent) with tocainide use. These end-organ toxicities have limited the use of this drug. From a cardiac viewpoint, tocainide is well tolerated. The incidence of drug-aggravated heart failure or arrhythmia is less than 4 percent. No major drug interaction problems have been reported. No post-MI or CHF safety data exist for tocainide.

Mexiletine (Mexitil)

Mexiletine is a class IB oral agent that resembles lidocaine and tocainide in structure.

Electrophysiology. Its electrophysiologic and electrocardiographic effects are similar to those of lidocaine and tocainide (see Tables 95–1 and 95–4).

Pharmacokinetics. Mexiletine is well absorbed orally and has an 85 percent bioavailability. Hepatic metabolism is the major route of elimination, and only 10 to 15 percent of the parent drug is excreted unchanged in the urine. The onset of action occurs within 1 to 2 hours, and the elimination half-life averages 10 to 12 hours. Mexiletine is 70 percent protein bound. No important drug interactions have been identified with mexiletine.[35]

Dosing. Mexiletine dosing is usually initiated at 200 mg tid. Maintenance doses vary between 150 and 300 mg tid. In some patients, bid dosing may be effective.

Efficacy. Similar to tocainide, mexiletine has been effective in approximately 50 percent of patients with potentially lethal ventricular arrhythmias studied by a Holter monitor model.[13, 13a–13c, 14] In the Electrophysiologic Study Versus Electrocardiographic Monitoring (ESVEM) study, more than 60 percent of patients had suppression of their ventricular arrhythmia, as assessed by Holter monitoring.[36] Mexiletine has been shown to be comparable to quinidine in suppressing ventricular ectopic activity. Adding a type IA antiarrhythmic agent to mexiletine is associated with added efficacy and decreased toxicity.[15, 37] Mexiletine was not found to reduce mortality in a post-MI population IMPACT study, although it significantly reduced the frequency of PVCs.[38] Mexiletine's effects on survival in CHF patients have not been studied. In patients with recurrent sustained VT studied in the electrophysiology laboratory, mexiletine appears to be effective in 10 to 15 percent of patients.[14] Efficacy rates of 20 to 30 percent have been demonstrated in patients with VF who survived an out-of-hospital cardiac arrest.[39, 40] Combination therapy with type IA agents in patients with sustained ventricular tachyarrhythmias may increase the efficacy rates by an additional 15 to 30 percent.[15, 37] Mexiletine is very effective in treating children who have ventricular arrhythmias after surgery for tetralogy of Fallot. Mexiletine, by shortening the QT interval, is effective in treating some patients with the prolonged QT syndrome.

Adverse Effects. Similar to lidocaine and tocainide, mexiletine has dose-related central nervous system and gastrointestinal side effects. Central nervous system toxicity includes tremors, dizziness, blurred vision, and confusion. The primary gastrointestinal side effect is nausea, although vomiting and heartburn also occur. Subjective side effects can be minimized by giving the drug with meals.

Mexiletine is relatively free of end-organ toxicity. Only rare cases of a possible drug-induced hepatitis have been reported.

Hemodynamically, mexiletine is well tolerated. No change in left ventricular ejection fraction has been noted during mexiletine therapy when compared with baseline. Mexiletine has minimal proarrhythmic effects. Because mexiletine shortens the QT interval, torsades de pointes does not occur.

Flecainide (Tambocor)

Flecainide was the first type IC antiarrhythmic agent approved by the FDA (see Tables 95–1 and 95–4).

Electrophysiology. Flecainide is a type IC antiarrhythmic agent that prolongs refractoriness and slows conduction in the atria, AV node, His-Purkinje system, ventricles, and accessory pathways.[41, 42]

Pharmacokinetics. Flecainide has a bioavailability of 90 to 95 percent and a half-life averaging between 12 and 27 hours (mean, 20 hours). Although flecainide is metabolized mainly (70 percent) in the liver, 30 percent is excreted by the kidney. Peak blood levels are achieved within 2 to 4 hours.[43] Because of its long half-life, flecainide is effective with a bid dosing schedule. Its only significant drug interaction is with amiodarone. When used in combination with amiodarone, flecainide levels may increase 15 to 30 percent.

Dosing. Flecainide is available as 100-mg tablets. I usually initiate therapy at 100 mg bid, and then after steady state has been achieved, increase the dose to 150 mg bid as necessary. Rarely, higher doses (200 mg bid) are required. Therapeutic levels are 0.2 to 1.0 μg/ml. Prolongation of the PR and QRS intervals occurs when therapeutic plasma levels are achieved.

Efficacy. Flecainide has been shown to be extremely effective (>70 percent) in decreasing the frequency of PVCs in patients with frequent ventricular ectopy.[13, 13a–13c, 14, 44, 45] In comparative trials with quinidine and disopyramide, flecainide has been shown to be statistically superior in the suppression of PVCs, ventricular couplets, and runs of nonsustained VT. In patients with symptomatic ventricular arrhythmias in the post-MI period, the Cardiac Arrhythmia Suppression Trial (CAST) demonstrated that both encainide and flecainide enhanced mortality compared with placebo, despite effective PVC suppression.[46] In patients with sustained VT, the efficacy of flecainide (20 percent) has been comparable with that of type IA antiarrhythmic agents.[14, 47, 48] Efficacy rates are higher in patients with preserved left ventricular function and ejection fractions greater than 30 percent.[49]

Flecainide has been demonstrated to be a very effective agent in the treatment of reentrant supraventricular arrhythmias,[42] atrial origin arrhythmias,[48] and atrial fibrillation.[42] A prospective study demonstrated that flecainide was equally effective as quinidine in treating atrial fibrillation and was associated with less toxicity.[50] Flecainide has been approved by the FDA for the treatment of supraventricular tachyarrhythmias without concomitant organic heart disease.

Adverse Effects. Subjectively, flecainide is very well tolerated. Noncardiac side effects that are dose related include dizziness, visual disturbances, and headache. Cardiovascular adverse reactions of concern include depression of left ventricular function and aggravation of CHF in some patients[41, 42] (see Table 95–9).

Of major concern is flecainide's proarrhythmic potential. In patients with PVCs and nonsustained VT that do not occur in the post-MI period, the incidence of ventricular proarrhythmia appears to be less than 3 percent. In the CAST study, mortality was increased compared with placebo in patients treated for asymptomatic ventricular arrhythmias after MI.[46] In patients without significant structural heart disease and supraventricular tachycardia (SVT), there is no risk of worsening survival.[51] In patients with sustained ventricular tachyarrhythmias, the incidence of proarrhythmia, including the development of incessant VT, averages between 7 and 17 percent,[41, 47, 49] the higher incidence being noted in patients with severe organic heart disease and left ventricular dysfunction. Flecainide may worsen pre-existing sinus node dysfunction and, because of its potent effects on slowing His-Purkinje conduction, it may aggravate pre-existing conduction disturbances and precipitate the development of advanced AV block. Flecainide has caused acute and chronic elevation of permanent pacemaker thresholds. Flecainide may slightly increase digoxin levels.

Propafenone (Rythmol)

Propafenone is a new type IC–like antiarrhythmic agent with weak associated beta-blocking characteristics.[52, 53]

Electrophysiology. Besides having type IC electrophysiologic effects (see Tables 95–1 and 95–4), propafenone also has strong membrane-stabilizing activity and weak β-blocking effects (and a structure similar to that of propranolol). Its onset-offset kinetics are more similar to those of disopyramide than those of flecainide[7] (see Table 95–2).

Pharmacokinetics. Propafenone is totally absorbed, then undergoes first-pass hepatic elimination via a saturable oxidative pathway. Metabolism of propafenone is genetically determined by use of the P450D6 enzyme system.[54, 55] Ten percent of patients are "poor metabolizers" and experience a prolonged half-life of the parent compound. The half-life of the parent compound ranges from 2 to 12 hours (mean, 6 hours). Poor metabolizers often have half-lives in the 10- to 12-hour range. The major metabolites of propafenone are 5-hydroxy propafenone (active) and *N*-debutyl propafenone. Although the half-life of the parent compound is only 6 hours, steady state is not usually reached for 72 hours because of the active metabolite's half-life.

Dosing. The recommended starting dose of propafenone is 150 mg tid. Doses may be increased up to 300 mg tid if necessary. I often used 225 mg as an intermediate dose.

Efficacy. In patients with potentially lethal ventricular arrhythmias, propafenone has been effective in controlling PVCs, couplets, and nonsustained VT in more than 65 percent of patients.[13, 13a–13c, 14, 36, 53] Studies have demonstrated at least equal and, in some cases, greater efficacy than quinidine, mexiletine, and disopyramide.[56] In patients with a history of sustained VT/VF, programmed stimulation studies have demonstrated propafenone to be effective in suppressing inducible VT in about 20 percent of patients.[14, 36, 57] Similar to other type IC agents, it can profoundly slow the rate of induced and recurrent VT.

Propafenone prolongs refractoriness and slows conduction in the atria, AV node, and accessory AV connections.[58] Propafenone is effective in treating more than 50 percent of patients with reentrant SVT and paroxysmal atrial fibrillation.[53]

Adverse Effects. Subjective adverse effects with propafenone include a bitter metallic taste, nausea, vomiting, constipation, and dizziness. A drug-induced rash has been induced in about 3 percent of patients. End-organ toxicity, such as neutropenia and a positive antinuclear antibody titer with a drug-induced lupus syndrome, is rarely caused by propafenone. Because of its β-blocking activity, it can accentuate AV nodal block. Because of its type IC effects, it can aggravate His-Purkinje block. Propafenone has some negative inotropic activity and should be used cautiously in patients with left ventricular dysfunction. Proarrhythmia occurs in about 3 percent of patients treated for benign or potentially lethal ventricular arrhythmias and in 10 percent of patients with a prior history of sustained VT or VF.

Propafenone interacts with digoxin and can raise digoxin levels by 40 to 60 percent. Propafenone also appears to increase the plasma concentration of warfarin and can significantly increase prothrombin times. No post-MI or CHF safety data exist for propafenone.

Moricizine (Ethmozine)

Moricizine hydrochloride is a phenothiazine derivative developed in the Soviet Union that is useful in the treatment of ventricular arrhythmias.[59, 60]

Electrophysiology. Moricizine has membrane-stabilizing activity and local anesthetic activity, and it moderately inhibits the sodium channels in phase 0 of the action potential. It primarily blocks the fast sodium channel in the inactivated state (see Table 95–3). Moricizine's electrophysiologic effects do not clearly define this agent into any of the subclasses as defined by Vaughn Williams. Its electrophysiologic actions are similar to those of a mild class IC agent. In isolated dog Purkinje fibers, moricizine shortens phase II and III repolarization and causes a dose-related decrease in V_{max}. In the canine model, no significant effects have been observed in the sinus node or atria. In humans, moricizine decreases conduction velocity through the AV node and increases the AH interval. It also slows conduction in the ventricular myocardium and prolongs the HV, PR, and QRS intervals. There is little change in the JT interval, suggesting that the drug does not prolong ventricular repolarization or block potassium channels. Intracardiac studies have shown that moricizine slows AV node conduction without prolonging VERP.[61] Retrograde AV node and accessory pathway conduction is also slowed.

Pharmacokinetics. Moricizine is the ethyl ester hydrochloride of 10-(3-morpholinoproprinonyl) phenothiazine-2-carbonic acid. It is well absorbed by the gastrointestinal tract. However, because of significant first-pass metabolism, bioavailability is only 38 percent. Peak blood levels are reached 0.5 to 2 hours after oral administration. Moricizine is highly plasma bound to protein (95 percent). The mean elimination half-life is 6 hours. With long-term dosing, the half-life may increase to 12 hours. Moricizine is extensively metabolized (at least 26 metabolites), with significant first-pass metabolism occurring. Two active metabolites probably have little importance because they represent less than 1 percent of the administered parent drug dose. About 56 percent of moricizine is excreted in the feces and 39 percent in the urine.

Dosing. Moricizine is available as 200-, 250-, and 300-mg tablets. The typical daily oral dosing is 200 to 400 mg tid. I usually initiate therapy at 200 mg tid, then increase by 150-mg/da at 3-day intervals.

Efficacy. In non–life-threatening ventricular arrhythmias, moricizine is usually effective in 50 to 65 percent of patients, as assessed by Holter monitoring, regardless of ejection fraction.[14, 45] In comparative studies, moricizine has been demonstrated to be equally effective as propranolol, quinidine, and disopyramide. In CAST II, moricizine was shown to have an early (first 14 days) enhanced mortality ($P = .02$) when compared with placebo in post-MI ventricular arrhythmia patients. Over long-term follow-up, no statistical difference in mortality was noted.[62] These results have limited the use of this drug. In refractory sustained VT, as assessed by programmed stimulation, the response rate is less than 20 percent, although moricizine usually slows the VT rate in patients who remain inducible. The efficacy of moricizine in treating various supraventricular tachyarrhythmias has not been well established. It has been shown to suppress retrograde AV nodal and accessory pathway conduction and to have some efficacy in suppressing atrial fibrillation.

Adverse Effects. Moricizine can cause proarrhythmia in about 3 to 4 percent of patients, with potentially lethal ventricular arrhythmias. In CAST II, some early post-MI mortality secondary to moricizine is believed to be secondary to enhanced proarrhythmic potential in the ischemic setting.[62] In patients with depressed ejection fractions and lethal arrhythmias, the proarrhythmic rate exceeds 10 percent. The most common adverse reactions include dry mouth, paresthesias, vertigo, dizziness (15 percent), nausea, headache, fatigue, dyspnea, palpitations, dyspepsia, nausea, diarrhea, vomiting, and sweating. Dizziness appears to be dose related. Rarely, moricizine can cause a drug fever and elevation of liver function test results. No other significant end-organ toxicity has been reported. Moricizine has minimal negative inotropic activity. Moricizine worsened heart failure in 2.8 percent of 374 patients with a prior history of heart failure and only 0.1 percent of 545 patients without a history of heart failure. There is no known significant interaction with digoxin or warfarin. Cimetidine raises moricizine levels by 40 percent, and moricizine improves the clearance and shortens the half-life of theophylline derivatives.

Propranolol (Inderal, Inderal-LA)

Propranolol is β-blocker that has had FDA approval for treating supraventricular and ventricular arrhythmias since 1973. Propranolol is noncardioselective and has no intrinsic sympathomimetic activity, but it does have membrane stabilizing activity. It is available as a short-acting and long-acting (Inderal-LA) oral preparation and also as a parenteral preparation.

Pharmacokinetics. Propranolol is almost completely absorbed orally, but bioavailability is markedly reduced because of first-pass metabolic breakdown via the P450D6 enzyme system in the liver. With long-term administration, there is saturation of the hepatic system with an increase in bioavailability from 10 to 50 percent. The major metabolite is 4-OH-propranolol. The half-life of propranolol is 3 to 6 hours, and steady state is achieved within 30 hours. Inderal-LA has a duration of action exceeding 24 hours. Intravenously, propranolol has an initial half-life of 10 minutes followed by a β half-life of 2 to 3 hours. Therefore, after intravenous administration of propranolol, systemic effects may last for hours.

Dosing. Oral dosing varies from 40 to 640 mg daily. Because of first-pass metabolism, only about 10 percent of an IV dose is given (1 to 10 mg). Complete sympathetic blockade requires 0.15 to 0.2 mg/kg of IV propranolol.

Electrophysiology. Propranolol has membrane-stabilizing effects with mild sodium channel blocking effects. Propranolol inhibits many of the effects of beta-receptor stimulation, such as blocking enhanced automaticity and adrenergic improvement in conduction velocities and shortening of refractory periods. Propranolol also blocks adrenergic activation of calcium channels. Propranolol decreases resting heart rate, prolongs sinus node recovery times, increases PR and AH intervals, and may decrease the QT interval. Propranolol prolongs refractoriness in the AV node with little effect in refractoriness of other cardiac tissues.

Efficacy. Propranolol is effective in slowing the ventricular response (especially during exercise) but rarely terminates or prevents the occurrence of atrial flutter, fibrillation, and PSVT. Propranolol is also effective in slowing sinus heart rate in patients with inappropriate symptomatic sinus tachycardia. In ventricular arrhythmias, propranolol suppresses PVCs, ventricular couplets, and nonsustained VT in 45 to 50 percent of patients. In the electrophysiology laboratory, propranolol is effective in fewer than 5 percent of patients with inducible sustained VT. Propranolol is the drug of choice in exercise-aggravated or exercise-induced arrhythmias and in patients with the prolonged QT syndrome. Propranolol is effective as adjunct therapy in combination with a sodium channel blocker for both SVT and VT. Adrenergic reversal of sodium channel blockers can be blunted by propranolol. Intravenously, propranolol can be emergently used to slow the ventricular response or treat arrhythmia patients in the critical care setting. Similar to timolol, metoprolol, and acebutolol, propranolol has been shown to significantly reduce mortality in the post-MI period.[63, 64]

Adverse Effects. Propranolol can aggravate sinus node dysfunction and AV block, and it can slow heart rate. Because propranolol is not cardioselective, it can cause bronchospasm or mask the sympathetic-mediated warning signs of hypoglycemia in insulin-dependent diabetics. Because of its significant negative inotropy, dose-related worsening of CHF is common. Subjective side effects include fatigue and mental blunting.

Acebutolol (Sectral)

Acebutolol is a β-blocker that has been approved for the management of ventricular arrhythmias. Acebutolol differs from propranolol in that it is more cardioselective, has intrinsic sympathomimetic activity, and is more hydrophilic. Similar to propranolol, it has membrane-stabilizing activity at higher doses.

Electrophysiology. Acebutolol has electrophysiologic effects similar to those of other β-blockers except that, because of intrinsic sympathomimetic activity, it causes less reduction in heart rate than propranolol.

Pharmacokinetics. Acebutolol is well-absorbed from the gastrointestinal tract and is subject to extensive first-pass hepatic metabolism via the P450D6 enzyme system into the pharmacologically active *N*-acetyl metabolite, diacetolol. Although the half-life of acebutolol is only 3 to 4 hours, the half-life of diacetolol is longer (8 to 13 hours), making twice-daily dosing an option. The drug is partially excreted in the urine.

Dosing. I usually initiate therapy with 200 mg bid and increase to 400 mg bid if necessary.

Efficacy. Acebutolol has efficacy rates similar to those of propranolol in suppressing ventricular ectopic activity.[65] Acebutolol is effective in controlling about 45 to 50 percent of benign and potentially lethal ventricular arrhythmias, as defined by Holter monitoring.[66] In one study, efficacy rates were similar to those of quinidine. In patients with sustained VT, acebutolol has been effective in less than 5 percent of patients. Acebutolol reduced mortality by 48 percent in one high-risk post-MI study,[67] and there was long-term maintenance of this protective effect.

Adverse Effects. The most common adverse reactions from acebutolol are those typically associated with β-blockers, such as depression and fatigue. Because of its intrinsic sympathomimetic activity, symptomatic bradycardia is less common than with propranolol. Although acebutolol is relatively cardioselective, asthma and other bronchospastic lung disease can be exacerbated. Worsening of AV block and aggravation of heart failure as a result of negative inotropy may occur. Rare cases of reversible hepatic toxicity represent the only known end-organ toxicity.

Esmolol Hydrochloride (Brevibloc)

Esmolol is an intravenously available β-blocking agent that is relatively cardioselective, has no intrinsic sympathomimetic activity or membrane stabilizing activity, and is weakly lipid soluble.

Electrophysiology. After an intravenous infusion of esmolol, electrophysiologic effects, as determined by a slowing in sinus cycle length and a prolongation of sinus node recovery times, occur within 5 minutes. Esmolol also slows AV nodal conduction. No direct effect on atrial or ventricular refractoriness or HV interval has been noted.

Pharmacokinetics. Esmolol is an ultra–short-acting intravenous β-blocker (about 1⁄40th the blocking potency of propranolol). Within 24 hours of termination, up to 88 percent of the drug is accounted for in the urine as the clinically inactive acid metabolites. Esmolol given IV has a distribution half-life of 2 minutes and an elimination half-life of 9 minutes. After a loading infusion, steady state blood levels can be reached within 5 minutes. After discontinuation, blood levels deplete rapidly within 10 minutes and are negligibly present within 30 minutes.

Dosing. Esmolol is usually given as a 500-mg/kg loading dose IV over 1 minute. This is usually followed by a 4-minute infusion at 50 μg/kg/min. The infusion can be increased up to 30 μg/kg/min if necessary.

Efficacy. In patients with SVT and atrial fibrillation, a slowing of mean ventricular rate is quickly achieved. In a 63-patient study, esmolol produced a therapeutic response in 72 percent of patients with various SVTs, compared with 6 percent receiving placebo. In a comparative study, a therapeutic response was noted in 72 percent of patients taking esmolol, compared with 69 percent taking intravenous propranolol.[68]

Adverse Effects. Esmolol exhibits effects of heart rate slowing equal to those of propranolol, with more rapid reversal of β-blockade on discontinuation. Esmolol, similar to other β-blockers, has significant negative inotropic activity. Decreases in hemodynamics are similar to those seen after 4 mg of intravenous propranolol. Dose-related hypotension is the most common adverse effect.

Amiodarone (Cordarone)

Amiodarone is an iodinated benzofuran derivative that is commercially available intravenously and orally.

Electrophysiology. Amiodarone has been subclassified as a class III antiarrhythmic agent. However, amiodarone has class I, II, III, and IV actions[9, 16] (see Table 95–4). Because the sodium channels are depressed in phase 0 in a use-dependent fashion, amiodarone's effects become more pronounced at faster heart rates. Amiodarone also has some sympatholytic properties. In vivo, amiodarone prolongs refractoriness and slows conduction in the atria, AV node, His-Purkinje system, ventricles, and accessory pathways. Both in vitro and in vivo, amiodarone slows sinus node automaticity and thus heart rate. Prolongation of APD is secondary to potassium channel blocking effects.

Intravenously, amiodarone slows heart rate and prolongs AV nodal refractoriness. IV amiodarone has few short-term effects on atrial or ventricular refractoriness.[69] Intravenous amiodarone is not associated with any significant prolongation of APD or use-dependent sodium channel blockade. Its short-term effects may be partially explained by its sympatholytic and calcium channel blocking effects.

Pharmacokinetics. The clinical pharmacology of oral amiodarone is not well understood, although it is best represented by a three-compartment model.[16] Amiodarone has a large volume of distribution (500 L) and a long half-life (average, 53 days), requiring months for blood levels to reach equilibrium. The bioavailability of amiodarone averages 30 to 50 percent. Excretion is minimal by both hepatic and fecal routes. Because of high lipophilicity, amiodarone and its metabolites are extensively distributed into fat, muscle, liver, lung, and spleen. Amiodarone is extensively metabolized to desethylamiodarone. Amiodarone has biphasic elimination, with a decrease in levels over the first 10 days after cessation of therapy, followed by an increase in drug concentration that is believed to be from elimination of parent compound from poorly perfused tissues. Because of the drug's long half-life, plasma levels of amiodarone and desethylamiodarone can be measured as long as 9 months after cessation of therapy.

Intravenous amiodarone has complex pharmacokinetics. Peak serum concentrations range from 5 to 41 mg/L after a 15-minute infusion. Because of the rapid distribution of the drug, serum concentrations decrease to 19 percent of peak values within 30 to 45 minutes of discontinuation of an infusion. Although parent compound plasma levels are high with intravenous use, desethylamiodarone levels are quite low.

Dosing. Amiodarone requires an oral loading dose of 800 to 1400 mg/da for several weeks. By 4 weeks of therapy, doses average abut 600 mg/da. By 4 months, most of our patients are taking 400 mg/da. In an attempt to minimize toxicity, maintenance doses ranging from 200 mg every other day to 400 mg/da are preferred. Therapeutic blood levels are in the 1.0- to 2.5-μg/ml range. Blood levels, along with a clinical judgment of efficacy and toxicity, are used to titrate the dose downward. Low doses of 200 mg qod to qd can be used in patients with atrial fibrillation.

Intravenous dosing starts with a 150-mg bolus injection given over 10 minutes, followed by a slow loading infusion of 360 mg given over 6 hours at 1 mg/min and 540 mg given at 0.5 mg/min over the remaining 18 hours. Supplemental infusions of 150 mg given over 10 minutes can be given for breakthrough arrhythmias.

Efficacy. Amiodarone has been approved for the treatment of life-threatening ventricular arrhythmias. Amiodarone is effective in more than 60 percent of patients with refractory sustained VT/VF.[70, 70a, 70b, 71] Although empirical therapy with amiodarone has been demonstrated to be more effective than guided therapy with more conventional antiarrhythmics,[72] several trials have demonstrated that the implantable-cardioverter defibrillator is more effective in improving survival in patients with sustained ventricular tachyarrhythmias.[64, 73–75] Although not approved for use in patients with potentially lethal ventricular arrhythmias, amiodarone is a very effective (>70 percent) suppresser of ventricular ectopic activity, as assessed by Holter monitoring. In the Multicenter Automatic Defibrillator Implantation Trial (MADIT), there was a 54 percent improvement in survival in patients treated with an ICD compared with amiodarone or other antiarrhythmics in a post-MI population with a depressed ejection fraction, nonsustained VT, and inducible sustained VT that was not suppressed by IV procainamide.[76] Although the Grupo de Estudio de la Sobrevida en la Insuficiencia Cardiaca en Argentina (GESICA) trial[77] demonstrated an improvement in survival in patients with CHF who were taking amiodarone (most with concomitant ventricular arrhythmias), the Survival Trial of Antiarrhythmic Therapy in Congestive Heart Failure (CHF-STAT)[78] demonstrated a neutral effect on survival, even in patients whose ventricular arrhythmia was suppressed. In the Canadian Amiodarone Myocardial Infarction Arrhythmia Trial (CAMIAT),[79] post-MI patients with concomitant ventricular arrhythmias had decreased arrhythmic death but no statistical improvement in total survival when treated with amiodarone. In the European Myocardial Infarct Amiodarone Trial (EMIAT),[80] amiodarone was used to treat post-MI patients with depressed ejection fractions. In EMIAT, similar to CAMIAT, arrhythmic death was statistically reduced, but there was no statistical improvement in overall survival.

Oral amiodarone, even at low doses, can be effective in controlling two thirds of the patients with otherwise drug-refractory atrial fibrillation or PSVT.

Intravenous amiodarone has been demonstrated to control life-threatening ventricular tachyarrhythmias with an efficacy comparable to that of bretylium.[81] Intravenous amiodarone is also effective in slowing AV nodal conduction in patients with rapid atrial tachyarrhythmias in the critical care setting. Because it has little effect on atrial ERP, intravenous amiodarone is no more effective than placebo in terminating atrial fibrillation.[82]

Adverse Effects. Adverse effects during amiodarone therapy are common.[16, 83, 84] Minor side effects seldom requiring drug discontinuation include corneal microdeposits, asymptomatic transient elevation of hepatic enzyme levels, photosensitivity of the skin, bluish-gray skin discoloration, and subjective gastrointestinal side effects. Amiodarone-induced hypothyroidism occurs in about 8 percent of my patients and requires the addition of thyroid replacement therapy. Drug-induced hyperthyroidism (2 percent) may require discontinuation of therapy. Other serious end-organ toxicities that may require discontinuation of amiodarone include interstitial pneumonitis (3 to 7 percent) and drug-induced hepatitis (2 percent). Neurologic side effects include a peripheral neuropathy and myopathy that usually resolve on lowering the dose. Drug-induced bradycardia may require backup permanent pacing in up to 2 percent of patients. Low-dose amiodarone may minimize the frequency of the aforementioned adverse effects.[83] Venous sclerosis can be minimized if intravenous amiodarone is given through a central venous line.

Amiodarone is well tolerated hemodynamically, with minimal negative inotropic effects. Amiodarone's vasodilating properties partially compensate for its negative inotropy. The predominant adverse effect of intravenous amiodarone is drug-induced hypotension.[69] Fewer than 4 percent of orally treated patients have worsening of CHF.

Although amiodarone prolongs APD, amiodarone-induced torsades de pointes is rare, and the development of incessant sustained VT occurs in less than 4 percent of patients.

Amiodarone has been shown to interact with digoxin, warfarin, quinidine, procainamide, and flecainide[16, 84] (see Table 95–8). Digoxin levels double, type I antiarrhythmic levels increase 15 to 35 percent, and prothrombin times double or triple. Concomitant use of these drugs requires lower doses and close monitoring.

Bretylium (Bretylol)

Bretylium is an intravenous class III agent that is useful in the emergent treatment of sustained ventricular tachyarrhythmias.

Electrophysiology. Bretylium affects the heart through direct action on the membrane and indirectly through sympathetic denervation of the heart. Bretylium prolongs the APD and the ERP of Purkinje fibers in ventricular muscle through a direct effect without altering the ERP/APD ratio. However, this prolongation seems to be more significant in normal tissue than in ischemic tissue. Thus, bretylium may raise the VF threshold by reducing the disparity of ventricular refractoriness between ischemic and nonischemic tissue.

Pharmacokinetics. Intravenous bretylium has a rapid onset of action that occurs within minutes. It is primarily excreted by the kidneys, with 80 to 90 percent of the parent compound being recovered unchanged in the urine. The half-life is 4 to 17 hours, and the therapeutic blood levels are in the range of 1 μg/ml.

Dosage. The initial recommended dosage of bretylium is 5 to 10 mg/kg given intravenously. The maintenance dosage schedule is 1 to 2 mg/min as a continuous intravenous infusion.

Efficacy. Bretylium is a unique antiarrhythmic agent. In addition to its antiarrhythmic properties, the drug has excellent antifibrillatory properties. Several studies have shown that defibrillation is possible with bretylium alone or with bretylium and cardioversion when lidocaine alone or cardioversion alone have failed to revert the patient to sinus rhythm.[85] IV bretylium has been demonstrated to be as effective as IV amiodarone[81] in suppressing VT/VF recurrences in patients with sustained ventricular tachyarrhythmias. In addition to its use as an antiarrhythmic agent in the emergent treatment of VT and VF, bretylium has been found to be as efficacious as lidocaine in the treatment of out-of-hospital VF.[86]

Adverse Effects. Bretylium has no significant negative inotropic effects on the myocardium. Clinical studies have shown that bretylium may improve myocardial function directly by increasing the amount of calcium available for myocardial contraction from intracellular stores, and indirectly by its effect in the sympathetic nervous system.

Because of the release of norepinephrine caused by bretylium, there may be a transient increase in blood pressure and heart rate, and there may be a transient increase in blood pressure, heart rate, and PVCs during the initial 20 minutes. Later, because of some antiadrenergic effects after a dose, postural hypotension and, less frequently, supine hypotension may occur. Rarely, some nausea and vomiting occur during administration of bretylium.

Sotalol (Betapace)

Sotalol is a unique, noncardioselective β-blocker with type III properties[14, 87] (see Table 95–4). The commercially available drug is a racemic mixture of D- and L-sotalol. Sotalol has one third the β-blocking potency of propranolol. It exhibits no intrinsic sympathomimetic or local anesthetic activity.

Electrophysiology. Sotalol prolongs repolarization in a concentration-dependent fashion, resulting in increases in the QT interval and the APD, as determined by basic electrophysiologic measurements and monophasic action potential recordings in humans. Action potential lengthening is predominantly caused by a reduction in the delayed rectifier potassium current in addition to a decrease in the inward rectifier current. In high concentrations, sotalol inhibits the inward sodium, but no calcium, currents. Sotalol slows sinus node cycle length and lengthens AV nodal conduction time (AH interval) and ERPs of the atria, AV node, ventricle, and accessory pathway. Sotalol demonstrates reverse use dependence in the atria and has less electrophysiologic effects at faster heart rates. No effect on the HV interval has been noted. Electrocardiographically, sotalol prolongs the PR and JTc intervals and causes no significant change in the QRS duration (see Table 95–5). Sotalol's β-blocking properties predominate at lower doses, and its type III effects predominate at higher doses.[14, 87]

Pharmacokinetics. Sotalol is nearly completely absorbed (>90 percent) and excreted via the kidney with minimal metabolic breakdown.[88] Bioavailability approaches 100 percent. Peak blood levels are noted 2 hours after a dose, and the elimination half-life varies from 7 to 15 hours. The β-adrenergic antagonism effects of sotalol are longer than the elimination half-life.

Dosing. Oral sotalol is initiated at 80 mg bid. Doses are increased to 120 mg to 160 mg bid as needed.

Efficacy. Because of sotalol's effects on atrial, AV node, and accessory pathway refractoriness, it is effective in converting and maintaining sinus rhythm in patients with atrial fibrillation. Rate control at the level of the AV node is also achieved in these patients. Sotalol is also effective in the treatment of PSVT and atrial fibrillation and has efficacy rates similar to those of quinidine and propafenone.

Sotalol appears to be effective in suppressing ventricular ectopic activity, as assessed by Holter monitoring, in 50 to 60 percent of patients. In the ESVEM trial, sotalol was as effective as quinidine, procainamide, mexiletine, and propafenone in achieving suppression of ventricular arrhythmias, as assessed by serial Holter monitoring.[36] In a post-MI study, sotalol reduced mortality by 18 percent (*P* not significant compared with placebo) and reduced reinfarction rate by 41 percent ($P < .05$) during the year after infarction.[89]

In sustained VT, as assessed by programmed stimulation, sotalol has been demonstrated to be effective in suppressing VT induction in 30 percent of patients in numerous trials, including ESVEM.[36]

Adverse Effects. Because of its β-blocking properties, sotalol has some negative inotropic potential; however, this is minimal compared with other β-blocking agents because lengthening of APD may enhance cardiac contractility. Noncardiac side effects are those typically noted of the other β-blockers. Cardiac side effects of sotalol include hypotension, symptomatic bradycardia, and AV nodal conduction abnormalities. Torsades de pointes is the most common proarrhythmia caused by sotalol, with a frequency similar to that of quinidine. This side effect is minimized to less than 2 percent if the total daily dose is no more than 320 mg/da and the QTc is 525 ms or less. Given its post-MI safety, sotalol is commonly used to treat symptomatic arrhythmias in this setting.

Ibutilide (Corvert)

Ibutilide is a class III intravenous antiarrhythmic agent with a novel mechanism of action. It is useful for the pharmacologic conversion of atrial fibrillation and atrial flutter.

Electrophysiology. Ibutilide prolongs APD and thus the QT interval by enhancing sodium flow into the cell during the plateau phase of the action potential.[90] Some of its effects may be secondary to blocking of the delayed rectifier potassium channel. Ibutilide prolongs atrial refractoriness. It has no evidence of reverse use dependence and has equal effects on atrial refractoriness at both slow and fast heart rates. It has negligible effects on heart rate and AV nodal conduction and refractoriness. Ibutilide prolongs ventricular ERPs and lowers the defibrillation threshold.[90, 91]

Pharmacokinetics. The pharmacokinetics of ibutilide are linear, with rapid extravascular distribution and hepatic metabolism, and it has a half-life of 3 to 6 hours. Ibutilide is 41 percent plasma protein bound and is rapidly metabolized to eight inactive metabolites.[90, 91]

Dosing. The usual dosing is 1 mg IV over 10 minutes, followed by a second dose if the first is ineffective.

Efficacy. Ibutilide is effective in terminating atrial fibrillation within 1 hour in about 35 percent of patients, compared with 3 percent efficacy in placebo patients and 18 percent efficacy with intravenous procainamide.[92] It is even more effective in terminating atrial flutter, with efficacy rates averaging 60 percent. Similar efficacy rates for both atrial fibrillation and flutter have been reported in the post–coronary artery bypass grafting setting.

Adverse Effects. Ibutilide's main toxicity is secondary to its ability to prolong APD and thus the QT interval. Nonsustained drug-induced torsades de pointes occurs in about 2 percent of patients, with sustained polymorphic VT occurring in an additional 2 percent of patients. All drug-induced proarrhythmia has occurred within 40 minutes of drug administration.

Dofetilide (Tikosyn)

Dofetilide is a class III antiarrhythmic that is being evaluated by the FDA for the treatment of atrial fibrillation.

Electrophysiology. Dofetilide is a methanesulfonanilide derivative with a structure that is similar to that of the non–β-blocking moiety of sotalol. Dofetilide prolongs APD in a dose-dependent manner. Dofetilide selectively inhibits Ikr channels without major effects on other potassium channels.[93] Dofetilide prolongs the atrial and ventricular ERP and the QT interval without affecting other conduction parameters. Reverse use dependence of these changes have been reported. Dofetilide displays little affinity for adrenergic, adenosine, dopamine, or muscarinic receptors.

Pharmacokinetics. Dofetilide is well-absorbed and has a systemic bioavailability of greater than 90 percent. The peak plasma concentrations are achieved at about 2 hours, and the elimination half-life averages 9.5 hours. Steady state is achieved in about 2 days. More than 60 percent of the drug is excreted unchanged in the urine, and the remainder is metabolized in the liver.

Dosing. Dosing under telemetry conditions is based on baseline creatinine clearance as a result of the drug's predominant renal excretion. In patients with normal renal function, the dose is 500 μg bid, and in those with abnormal renal function, 250 μg bid.

Efficacy. Although effective in suppressing ventricular ectopy, dofetilide has been primarily studied in the suppression of atrial fibrillation, with efficacy rates averaging about 50 percent.

Adverse Effects. Subjectively, dofetilide is well tolerated. Its predominant adverse effect that causes concern is a 1.3 percent rate of torsades de pointes. Hemodynamically, the drug is well tolerated and, by prolonging APD, is a positive inotropic agent. Dofetilide has been used safely in post-MI and CHF patients in the DIAMOND trial[94] with neutral effects on overall survival. No known drug interactions with dofetilide exist.

Azimilide (Stedicor)

Azimilide is a class III antiarrhythmic that is currently undergoing study to assess its efficacy and safety in treating atrial fibrillation.

Electrophysiology. Azimilide prolongs APD in a dose-dependent manner. It selectively inhibits both Ikr and Iks.[95] At higher doses, it blocks the L-type calcium, and also sodium, channels. It prolongs the atrial and ventricular ERP and the QT interval without any other significant conduction interval changes. These effects occur at varying heart rates with no evidence of reverse use dependence. No significant adrenergic or muscarinic blocking properties have been demonstrated.

Pharmacokinetics. Azimilide is almost completely absorbed and has high bioavailability. The elimination half-life is long (about 115 hours)[96]; thus, the drug takes weeks to reach steady state. The drug is predominantly hepatically metabolized, and only 10 percent clearance is via the kidney.

Dosing. Dosing is still being tested. A dose of 100 to 125 mg bid appears to be safe and effective.

Efficacy. Azimilide is effective in suppressing atrial fibrillation in about 50 percent of patients.

Adverse Effects. Similar to other drugs that prolong APD, there is about a 1 percent risk of torsades de pointes. Other subjective adverse effects are uncommon. Hemodynamically, the drug is well tolerated because it is a positive inotropic agent. Azimilide's safety in a post-MI population is being tested in the Azimilide Post-Infarct Survival Evaluation (ALIVE) trial.[97]

Verapamil (Calan, Isoptin)

Verapamil is a papaverine derivation that is classified as a type IV antiarrhythmic agent. Intravenous verapamil is available for the emergent treatment of SVT. Oral verapamil is available in a short-acting and controlled-release formulation and has some usefulness in controlling the ventricular response in atrial fibrillation and in treating reentrant PSVT.

Electrophysiology. As a calcium L-channel antagonist, verapamil inhibits the slow channels by blocking the inward calcium current. Verapamil slows sinus rate, although this direct suppressant effect may be counteracted by its vasodilatory properties, and it prolongs the AH interval and the AV nodal ERP and AV nodal functional refractory period. Verapamil has been noted to shorten the refractory period of accessory pathway tissue.

Pharmacokinetics. Although 90 percent of verapamil is absorbed, only 10 to 20 percent is bioavailable as a result of first-pass hepatic metabolism. Only 7 percent of the drug is excreted unchanged in the urine. Orally, peak levels occur within 2 hours, and the half-life is 3 to 7 hours.

Dosing. When the drug is given intravenously, effects occur within 3 to 5 minutes and last 20 to 30 minutes. Intravenously, I usually administer a dose of 0.1 mg/kg as a bolus. If continuous infusions are needed, I maintain patients at 0.005 mg/kg/min. Orally, the total daily dose ranges from 160 to 720 mg/da.

Efficacy. Intravenous verapamil has been the drug of choice for the emergent termination of reentrant PSVT utilizing the AV node. Efficacy rates of 80 to 95 percent for reversion to sinus rhythm are comparable with those of intravenous adenosine. IV verapamil can also be used to emergently slow the ventricular response in patients with SVTs, including atrial fibrillation and flutter.[98–100] Intravenous verapamil should not be used in wide QRS tachycardias of undetermined cause because most of these tachycardias are VTs and verapamil may cause further hemodynamic compromise.[101] Continuous infusions (0.1 mg/kg/h) of verapamil may be useful for temporary rate control of multifocal atrial tachycardia and atrial fibrillation in the critical care setting.

Oral verapamil is useful in the control of the ventricular response in patients with atrial fibrillation and flutter. Oral verapamil may rarely be effective in preventing the recurrence of PSVT. Rarely, verapamil is effective in treating certain types of VT in patients with normal hearts.

Adverse Effects. Verapamil can cause symptomatic bradycardia and sinus arrest and may worsen AV nodal block. Because of significant negative inotropy, verapamil can depress left ventricular function and cause or worsen CHF (see Table 95–9). IV verapamil can accelerate the pre-excited ventricular response in patients with atrial fibrillation and Wolff-Parkinson-White syndrome.[102] Subjective toxicity includes nausea, dizziness, and constipation. Verapamil may increase the serum digoxin level during concomitant administration. Several trials suggest that verapamil has neutral effects on survival when used in the post-MI setting.[64, 103]

Diltiazem (Cardizem)

Diltiazem is a L-channel calcium blocker with electrophysiologic effects similar to those of verapamil. Orally, it is approved for the treatment of angina and hypertension, although it is frequently used as adjunct therapy in rate control of atrial fibrillation. Intravenously, diltiazem has proved to be an effective drug for emergently terminating PSVT[104] (efficacy rates similar to those of verapamil) and for controlling the ventricular response with rapid atrial arrhythmias.[105]

Dosing. Oral diltiazem is used at total daily doses of 90 to 360 mg. Intravenously, the dose is 0.25 mg/kg. Continuous IV infusions can be used at a dose of 0.15 mg/kg/hr.

Electrophysiology. Diltiazem has electrophysiologic effects similar to those of verapamil. Because it causes less peripheral vasodilatation than verapamil, reflex changes are not as common. Because of this, diltiazem more consistently slows heart rate. Diltiazem slows conduction (AH) in the AV node and prolongs antegrade AV nodal refractoriness. It has no effect on accessory pathway tissue.

Efficacy. After an intravenous bolus, diltiazem slows the ventricular response by about 25 percent within 3 to 7 minutes in patients with atrial tachyarrhythmias and a rapid ventricular response. Continuous intravenous infusion of diltiazem maintains a greater than 20 percent decrease in heart rate in patients in atrial flutter/fibrillation.[105] Intravenous diltiazem has been effective in terminating SVT in more than 80 percent of cases within 3 minutes.[104] Oral diltiazem is very effective in controlling the ventricular response in patients with rapid atrial fibrillation/flutter.

Adverse Effects. Intravenous diltiazem may cause heart rate slowing, AV block, and hypotension. Compared with verapamil, hemodynamic compromise is less likely to occur. Oral diltiazem is safe to use in the post-MI setting, except in patients with pulmonary congestion.[64, 106, 107]

Adenosine (Adenocard)

Adenosine is a purine agonist that is effective in terminating PSVT. The effects of adenosine are mediated by extracellular purinergic receptors.

Electrophysiology. Adenosine has negative chronotropic and dromotropic effects on the sinoatrial and AV node. No effects on His-Purkinje conduction or ventricular refractoriness have been noted.

Pharmacokinetics. After injection, adenosine is rapidly cleared from the circulation by cellular uptake and metabolism. Adenosine enters the blood pool and metabolizes to inosine and adenosine monophosphate. It has an elimination half-life of less than 10 seconds. Onset of action is about 15 to 30 seconds after injection. Aminophylline counteracts the effects of adenosine. Dipyridamole, which is a potent adenosine uptake inhibitor, may potentiate the effect of adenosine.[108, 109]

Dosing. Adenosine is available in 6-mg vials and more than 90 percent of patients with PSVT revert to sinus rhythm with a dose of 50 mg/kg (<10 mg). The current recommended dose is 6 mg IV push, followed by a 12-mg IV dose, if necessary.

Efficacy. Adenosine given at doses of 12 mg IV is effective in terminating PSVT in 91 percent of cases.[108, 109] Conversion to sinus rhythm usually occurs in less than 1 minute. Adenosine terminates SVT quicker than verapamil (median, 30 versus 170 seconds). Adenosine has been found to be effective in terminating certain types of sustained VT in normal hearts that are calcium influx sensitive. Because adenosine rarely affects VT and has a short half-life, it has been used as a diagnostic test in wide QRS tachycardia of undetermined cause.[110] In patients with structural heart disease and hypotensive wide QRS tachycardia, adenosine should be avoided.

Adverse Effects. Dyspnea and flushing are the most common adverse effects that may occur transiently. Cardiac side effects include transient but significant sinus bradycardia, sinus tachycardia, sinus pauses, and AV block. At high doses, a transient decrease in blood pressure has been noted.

Digoxin (Lanoxin, Lanoxicaps); Digitoxin (Crystodigin)

Digoxin and digitoxin are cardiac glycosides, often grouped in the digitalis glycoside family. These drugs are useful in controlling the ventricular response in atrial tachyarrhythmias and also as positive inotropic agents in patients with systolic dysfunction.[111]

Pharmacokinetics. Digoxin is 60 to 80 percent absorbed. After drug administration, a 6- to 8-hour distribution phase occurs. The volume of distribution is large. Twenty to 25 percent of digoxin is bound to protein. The time to onset effect is ½ to 2 hours and peak effect occurs at 2 to 6 hours. Elimination of digoxin follows first-order kinetics. Because digoxin is primarily renally excreted, excretion may be diminished in patients with abnormal renal function. The elimination half-life in patients with normal renal function is 1.5 to 2 days. This may be extended to 6 days in patients with significant renal dysfunction.

Digitoxin differs from digoxin in having a longer elimination half-life of 7 to 9 days and is primarily metabolized in the liver.

Electrophysiology. Digitalis glycosides cause some indirect action that is mediated by the autonomic nervous system secondary to vagal action. Thus, digitalis may slow sinus node automaticity and slow AV node conduction, prolonging AV node refractoriness. Directly, digoxin may increase the force velocity of myocardial systolic contractions.

Dosing. The usual maintenance dose of digoxin is 0.125 to 0.25 mg/da. The dose should be decreased in patients who are taking concomitant quinidine, propafenone, or amiodarone. It also should be decreased in patients with renal dysfunction. Because of the long elimination half-life, it may take more than a week for digoxin to reach steady state. Orally or intravenously, patients could be more rapidly digitalized with loading doses of 8 to 12 μg/kg.

For digitoxin, digitalization can occur with 0.2 mg bid for 4 days, followed by maintenance doses of 0.05 to 0.3 mg daily, with the most common dose being 0.1, 0.15, or 0.2 mg daily. In patients who experience life-threatening digitalis toxicity, Digibind can be given in an attempt to reverse some direct effects of digoxin emergently.

Efficacy. There is little proof in the literature that digoxin has significant benefit in treating ventricular arrhythmias. However, there are some minimal reports and indirect evidence that in patients with systolic dysfunction, optimizing hemodynamics may have a beneficial antiarrhythmic effect.[112] Digoxin is primarily used to control the ventricular rate in patients with atrial fibrillation, atrial flutter, and atrial tachycardia. Although digitalis is a useful drug for slowing conduction through the AV node and prolonging AV node refractoriness, β-blockers and calcium blockers are more effective. Although rapid digitalization is often used in patients who present with new-onset atrial fibrillation, placebo-controlled studies have demonstrated that the conversion rates are similar to those of placebo.[113, 114] In patients with vagally induced atrial fibrillation, digitalis may make atrial fibrillation more likely to recur. Digitalis, by slowing conduction antegrade in the AV node, may be useful in slowing the ventricular response of patients with reentrant PSVTs. In rare circumstances, this effect on AV nodal conduction may be beneficial in preventing recurrence of PSVT.

Adverse Effects. Noncardiac toxic manifestations of digitalis excess include anorexia, nausea, vomiting, headache, visual scotomas, and changes in color perception. Cardiac toxicity includes AV junctional escape rhythms, ventricular ectopic beats and bigeminy, VT, nonparoxysmal functional tachycardias, atrial tachycardia with block, and Mobitz type I AV block.[115] In patients with heart failure, digitalis has been shown to have neutral effects on long-term survival.[116]

References

1. Woosley RL, Shand DG: Pharmacokinetics of antiarrhythmic drugs. Am J Cardiol 41:986–995, 1978.
2. Siddoway LA, Thompson EA, McAllister CB, et al: Polymorphism propafenone metabolism and disposition in man: clinical and pharmacokinetic consequences. Circulation 75:785–791, 1987.
3. Woosley RL, Echt DS, Roden DM: Effects of congestive heart failure on the pharmacokinetics and pharmacodynamics of antiarrhythmic agents. Am J Cardiol 57:25B–33B, 1986.
4. Vaughn Williams EM: A classification of antiarrhythmic actions reassessed after a decade of new drugs. J Clin Pharmacol 24:129–147, 1984.
5. Campbell TJ: Kinetics of onset of rate-dependent effects of class I antiarrhythmic drugs are important in determining effects on refractoriness in guinea pig ventricle, and provide a theoretical basis for their subclassification. Cardiovasc Res 17:344–352, 1983.
6. Grant AO, Wendt DJ: Blockade of ion channels by antiarrhythmic drugs. J Cardiovasc Electrophysiol 2:5153–5158, 1991.
7. Weirich J, Antoni H: Differential analysis of the frequency-dependent effects of class I antiarrhythmic drugs according to periodic ligand binding: implications for antiarrhythmic and proarrhythmic efficacy. J Cardiovasc Pharmacol 15:998–1003, 1990.
8. Hondegehem LM, Katzung BG: Antiarrhythmic agents: modulated receptor applications. Circulation 75:514–520, 1987.
9. Task Force of the Working Group on Arrhythmias of the European Society of Cardiology: The Sicilian Gambit: a new approach to the classification of antiarrhythmic drugs based on their actions on arrhythmogenic mechanisms. Circulation 84:1831–1851, 1991.
10. DiMarco JP, Garan H, Ruskin JN: Quinidine for ventricular arrhythmias: value of electrophysiologic testing. Am J Cardiol 51:90–95, 1983.
11. Coplen SE, Antman EM, Berlin JA, et al: Efficacy and safety of quinidine therapy for maintenance of sinus rhythm after cardioversion: a meta-analysis of randomized controlled trials. Circulation 82:1106–1116, 1990.
12. Wellens HJJ, Bar F, Dassen WRM, et al: Effect of drugs in the Wolff-Parkinson-White syndrome: importance of initial length of the effective refractory period of the accessory pathway. Am J Cardiol 46:665–669, 1980.
13. Salerno DM: Review: antiarrhythmic drugs; 1987. Electrophysiology l(pts I–J):217, 1987.

13a. Salerno DM: Review: antiarrhythmic drugs. Electrophysiology 1(pt II):300–319, 1987.

13b. Salerno DM: Review: antiarrhythmic drugs. Electrophysiology 1(pt III):435–465, 1987.

13c. Salerno DM: Review: antiarrhythmic drugs. Electrophysiology 2(pt IV):55–87, 1988.

14. Singh BN: Electrophysiologic basis for the antiarrhythmic actions of sotalol and comparison with other agents. Am J Cardiol 72:8A–18A, 1993.
15. Duff HJ, Mitchell LB, Manuari D, Wyse DG: Mexiletine-quinidine combination: electrophysiologic correlates of a favorable antiarrhythmic interaction in humans. J Am Coll Cardiol 10:1149–1156, 1987.
16. Naccarelli GV, Rinkenberger RL, Dougherty AH, Giebel RA: Amiodarone: pharmacology and antiarrhythmic and adverse effects. Pharmacotherapy 5:298–313, 1985.
17. Mungall DR, Robichaux RP, Perry W, et al: Effects of quinidine on serum digoxin concentration: a prospective study. Ann Intern Med 93:689–693, 1980.
18. Selzer A, Wray HW: Quinidine syncope: paroxysmal ventricular fibrillation occurring during treatment of chronic atrial arrhythmias. Circulation 30:17, 1964.
19. Roden DM, Woosley RL, Primm K: Incidence and clinical features of the quinidine-associated long QT syndrome: implications for patient care. Am Heart J 111:1088–1093, 1986.
20. Flaker GC, Blackshear JL, McBride R, et al: Antiarrhythmic drug therapy and cardiac mortality in atrial fibrillation. J Am Coll Cardiol 20:527–532, 1992.
21. Greenspan AM, Horowitz LN, Spielman SR, Josephson ME: Large-dose procainamide therapy for ventricular tachyarrhythmia. Am J Cardiol 46:453–462, 1980.
22. Waxman HL, Buxton AE, Sadowski LM, Josephson ME: Response to procainamide during electrophysiologic study for sustained ventricular tachycardia predicts response to other drugs. Circulation 67:30–37, 1982.
23. Gorgels APM, van den Dool A, Hofs A, et al: Comparison of procainamide and lidocaine in terminating sustained monomorphic ventricular tachycardia. Am J Cardiol 78:43–46, 1996.
24. Gottlieb SS, Kukin ML, Medina N, et al: Comparative hemodynamic effects of procainamide, tocainide and encainide in severe chronic heart failure. Circulation 81:860–864, 1991.
25. Lermann BB, Waxman HL, Buxton AE, Josephson ME: Disopyramide: evaluation of electrophysiologic effects and clinical efficacy in patients with sustained ventricular tachycardia or ventricular fibrillation. Am J Cardiol 51:759–764, 1983.
26. Podrid PJ, Schoeneberger A, Lown B: Congestive heart failure caused by oral disopyramide. N Engl J Med 302:614–617, 1980.
27. Collingsworth KA, Kalman SN, Harrison DC: The clinical pharmacology of lidocaine as an antiarrhythmic drug. Circulation 50:1217–1230, 1974.
28. Harrison DC: Practical guidelines for the use of lidocaine: prevention and treatment of cardiac arrhythmias. JAMA 233:1202–1204, 1975.
29. Thompson PD, Melmon KL, Richardson JA, et al: Lidocaine pharmacokinetics in advanced heart failure, liver disease and renal failure in humans. Ann Intern Med 78:499–508, 1973.

30. Lie KI, Wellens HJJ, VanCapelle FJ, Durrer D: Lidocaine in the prevention of ventricular fibrillation. N Engl J Med 291:1324–1326, 1974.
31. Hine LK, Laird N, Hewitt P, et al: Meta-analytic evidence against prophylactic use of lidocaine in acute myocardial infarction. Arch Intern Med 149:2694–2698, 1989.
32. Kutalek SP, Morganroth J, Horowitz LN: Tocainide: a new oral antiarrhythmic agent. Ann Intern Med 103:387–391, 1985.
33. Morganroth J, Nestico FF, Horowitz LN: A review of the uses and limitations of tocainide: a class IB antiarrhythmic agent. Am Heart J 110:856–863, 1985.
34. Podrid PJ, Lown B: Tocainide for refractory symptomatic ventricular arrhythmias. Am J Cardiol 49:1279, 1982.
35. Campbell RWF: Mexiletine. N Engl J Med 316:29–34, 1987.
36. Mason JW and the ESVEM Investigators: A comparison of seven antiarrhythmic drugs in patients with ventricular tachyarrhythmias. N Engl J Med 329:452–458, 1993.
37. Duff HJ, Kolodgie FD, Roden DM, Woosley RL: Electropharmacologic synergism with mexiletine and quinidine. J Cardiovasc Pharmacol 8:840–846, 1986.
38. Impact Research Group: International mexiletine and placebo antiarrhythmic coronary trial. I: report on arrhythmia and other findings. J Am Coll Cardiol 4:1148–1163, 1984.
39. DiMarco JP, Garan H, Ruskin JN: Mexiletine for refractory ventricular arrhythmias: results using serial electrophysiologic testing. Am J Cardiol 47:131, 1981.
40. Berns E, Naccarelli GV, Dougherty AH, et al: Mexiletine: lack of predictors of clinical response in patients treated for life-threatening tachyarrhythmias. J Electrophysiol 2:201–206, 1988.
41. Roden DM, Woosley RL: Drug therapy: flecainide. N Engl J Med 315:36–41, 1986.
42. Anderson JL, Pritchett ELC (eds): International Symposium on Supraventricular Arrhythmias: focus on flecainide. Am J Cardiol 62:1D–67D, 1988.
43. Nappi JM, Anderson JL: Flecainide: a new prototype antiarrhythmic agent. Pharmacotherapy 5:209–221, 1985.
44. Lal R, Chapman PD, Naccarelli GV, et al: Flecainide in the treatment of nonsustained ventricular tachycardia. Ann Intern Med 105:493–498, 1986.
45. The Cardiac Arrhythmia Pilot Study (CAPS) Investigators: Effects of encainide, flecainide, imipramine and moricizine on ventricular arrhythmias during the year after myocardial infarction: the CAPS. Am J Cardiol 61:501–509, 1988.
46. The Cardiac Arrhythmia Suppression Trial Investigators: Preliminary report: effect of encainide and flecainide on mortality in a randomized trial of arrhythmia suppression after myocardial infarction. N Engl J Med 321:406–412, 1989.
47. Lal, R, Chapman PD, Naccarelli GV, et al: Short- and long-term experience with flecainide acetate in the management of refractory life-threatening ventricular arrhythmias. J Am Coll Cardiol 6:772, 1985.
48. Berns E, Rinkenberger RL, Jeang M, et al: Clinical efficacy and safety of flecainide acetate in the treatment of primary atrial tachycardias. Am J Cardiol 59:1337–1341, 1987.
49. Flecainide Ventricular Tachycardia Study Group: Treatment of resistant ventricular tachycardia with flecainide acetate. Am J Cardiol 57:1299–1304, 1986.
50. Naccarelli GV, Dorian P, Hohsloser SH, Coumel P, for the Flecainide Multicenter Atrial Fibrillation Group: Prospective comparison of flecainide versus quinidine for the treatment of paroxysmal atrial fibrillation/flutter. Am J Cardiol 77:53A–59A, 1996.
51. Pritchett ELC, Wilkinson WE, Clair WK, et al: Comparison of mortality in patients treated with propafenone to those treated with a variety of antiarrhythmic drugs for supraventricular arrhythmias. Am J Cardiol 72:108–110, 1993.
52. Podrid PJ, Lown B: Propafenone: a new agent for ventricular arrhythmias. J Am Coll Cardiol 4:117–125, 1984.
53. Podrid PJ (ed): Symposium on propafenone. J Electrophysiol 1:517–590, 1989.
54. Connally SJ, Kates RE, Lebsack CS, et al: Clinical pharmacology of propafenone. Circulation 68:589–596, 1983.
55. Siddoway LA, Thompson EA, McAllister CB, et al: Polymorphism propafenone metabolism and disposition in man: clinical and pharmacokinetic consequences. Circulation 75:785–791, 1987.
56. Naccarella F, Bracchetti D, Palmieri M, et al: Comparison of propafenone and disopyramide for treatment of chronic ventricular arrhythmias: placebo-controlled, double-blind, randomized crossover study. Am Heart J 109:833–839, 1985.
57. Chilson DA, Heger JJ, Zipes DP, et al: Electrophysiologic effects and clinical efficacy of oral propafenone therapy in patients with ventricular tachycardia. J Am Coll Cardiol 5:1407, 1985.
58. Ludmer PL, McGowan NE, Antman EM, Friedman PL: Efficacy of propafenone in Wolff-Parkinson-White syndrome: electrophysiologic findings and long-term followup. J Am Coll Cardiol 9:1357–1363, 1987.
59. Podrid PJ, Lyakishev A, Lown B, et al: Ethmozine, a new antiarrhythmic drug for suppressing ventricular premature complexes. Circulation 61:450–457, 1980.
60. Ruggio JM, Somberg JC: New therapy focus: Ethmozine. Cardiovasc Rev Rep 5:738–741, 1984.
61. Mann DE, Luck JC, Herre JM, et al: Electrophysiologic effects of Ethmozine in patients with ventricular tachycardia. Am Heart J 107:674, 1984.
62. The Cardiac Arrhythmia Suppression Trial II Investigators: Effect of the antiarrhythmic agent moricizine on survival after myocardial infarction. N Engl J Med 327:227–233, 1992.
63. Beta Blocker Heart Attack Trial Research Group: A randomized trial of propranolol in patients with acute myocardial infarction. I: mortality results. JAMA 247:1707–1714, 1982.
64. Naccarelli GV, Wolbrette DL, Dell'Orfano JT, et al: A decade of clinical trial developments in postmyocardial infarction, congestive heart failure, and sustained ventricular tachyarrhythmia patients: from CAST to AVID and beyond. J Cardiovasc Electrophysiol 9:864–891, 1998.
65. Singh SN, DiBianco R, Davidson ME, et al: Comparison of acebutolol and propranolol for treatment of chronic ventricular arrhythmia: a placebo-controlled, double-blind, randomized crossover study. Circulation 65:1356–1364, 1982.
66. DeSoyza N, Shapiro W, Chandraratna PAN, et al: Acebutolol therapy for ventricular arrhythmias: a randomized, placebo-controlled double-blind multicenter study. Circulation 65:1129–1133, 1982.
67. Boissel JP, Leizorowitc A, Picolet H, Ducruet T, for the ASPI Investigators: Efficacy of acebutolol after acute myocardial infarction (the ASPI trial). Am J Cardiol 66:24C–31C, 1990.
68. Anderson S, Blanski L, Byrd RC, et al: Comparison of the efficacy and safety of esmolol, a short-acting beta blocker with placebo in the treatment of supraventricular arrhythmias. Am Heart J 111:429–438, 1986.
69. Desai AD, Chun S, Sung RJ: The role of intravenous amiodarone in the management of cardiac arrhythmias. Ann Intern Med 127:294–303, 1997.
70. Kehoe RF, Zheutlein T (eds): Amiodarone I. Prog Cardiovasc Dis 31:249–294, 1989.
70a. Kehoe RF, Zheutlein T (eds): Amiodarone II. Prog Cardiovasc Dis 31:319–366, 1989.
70b. Kehoe RF, Zheutlein T (eds): Amiodarone III. Prog Cardiovasc Dis 31:393–453, 1989.
71. Herre JM, Sauve MJ, Malone P, et al: Long-term results of amiodarone therapy in patients with recurrent sustained ventricular tachycardia or ventricular fibrillation. J Am Coll Cardiol 13:442–449, 1989.
72. The CASCADE Investigators: Randomized antiarrhythmic drug therapy in survivors of cardiac arrest (the CASCADE study). Am J Cardiol 72:280–287, 1993.
73. Siebels J, Cappato R, Ruppel R, et al, and the CASH Investigators: Preliminary Results of the Cardiac Arrest Study Hamburg (CASH). Am J Cardiol 72:109F–113F, 1993.
74. The Antiarrhythmics Versus Implantable Defibrillators (AVID) Investigators: A comparison of antiarrhythmic drug therapy with implantable defibrillators in patients resuscitated from near fatal ventricular arrhythmias. N Engl J Med 337:1576–1583, 1997.
75. Connolly S, Gent M, Roberts R, et al: Canadian Implantable Defibrillator Study (CIDS): study design and organization. Am J Cardiol 72:103F–108F, 1993.
76. Moss AJ, Hall WJ, Cannom DS, et al, for the Multicenter Automatic Defibrillator Implantation Trial Investigators: Improved survival with an implanted defibrillator in patients with coronary disease at high risk for ventricular arrhythmia. N Engl J Med 335:1933–1940, 1996.
77. Doval HC, Nul DR, Grancelli HO, et al, for Grupo de Estudio de

la Sobrevida en la Insuficiencia Cardiaca en Argentina (GESICA): Randomized trial of low-dose amiodarone in severe congestive heart failure: Grupo de Estudio de la Sobrevida en la Insuficiencia Cardiaca en Argentina (GESICA). Lancet 344:493–498, 1994.

78. Singh SN, Fletcher RD, Fisher SG, et al, for the Survival Trial of Antiarrhythmic Therapy in Congestive Heart Failure (CHF-STAT): Amiodarone in patients with congestive heart failure and asymptomatic ventricular arrhythmia (CHF-STAT). N Engl J Med 333:77–82, 1995.
79. Cairns, JA, Connolly SJ, Roberts R, et al, for the Canadian Amiodarone Myocardial Infarction Arrhythmia Trial Investigators: Randomized trial of outcome after myocardial infarction in patients with frequent or repetitive ventricular premature depolarisations: CAMIAT. Lancet 349:675–682, 1997.
80. Julian DG, Camm AJ, Franglin G, et al, for the European Myocardial Infarct Amiodarone Trial Investigators: Randomized trial of effect of amiodarone on mortality in patients with left-ventricular dysfunction after recent myocardial infarction: EMIAT. Lancet 349:667–674, 1997.
81. Kowey PR, Levine JH, Herre JM, et al: Randomized, double-blind comparison of intravenous amiodarone and bretylium in the treatment of patients with recurrent, hemodynamically destabilizing ventricular tachycardia or fibrillation. Circulation 92:3255–3263, 1995.
82. Galve E, Rius T, Ballester R, et al: Intravenous amiodarone in treatment of recent-onset atrial fibrillation: results of a randomized, controlled study. J Am Coll Cardiol 27:1079–1082, 1996.
83. Vorperian VR, Havighurst TC, Milleer S, January CT: Adverse effects of low dose amiodarone: a meta-analysis. J Am Coll Cardiol 30:791–798, 1997.
84. Podrid PJ: Amiodarone: reevaluation of an old drug. Ann Intern Med 122:689–700, 1995.
85. Kerber RE, Pandian NG, Jensen SR, et al: Effect of lidocaine and bretylium on energy requirements for transthoracic defibrillation: experimental studies. J Am Coll Cardiol 7:397–405, 1986.
86. Haynes RE, Chinn TL, Capass MK, Cobb LA: Comparison of bretylium tosylate and lidocaine in management of out-of-hospital ventricular fibrillation: a randomized clinical trial. Am J Cardiol 48:353–356, 1981.
87. Singh BN (ed): A symposium: controlling cardiac arrhythmias with sotalol, a broad spectrum antiarrhythmic with beta-blocking effects and class III activity. Am J Cardiol 65:IA–88A, 1990.
88. Hanyok JJ: Clinical pharmacokinetics of sotalol. Am J Cardiol 72:19A–26A, 1993.
89. Julian DG, Jackson FS, Prescott RJ, Szekely P: Controlled trial of sotalol for one year after myocardial infarction. Lancet 1:1142–1147, 1982.
90. Naccarelli GV, Lee KS, Gibson JK, VanderLugt J: Electrophysiology and pharmacology of ibutilide. Am J Cardiol 78:12–16, 1996.
91. Murray KT: Ibutilide. Circulation 97:493–497, 1998.
92. Volgman AS, Carberry PA, Stambler B, et al: Conversion efficacy and safety of intravenous ibutilide compared with intravenous procainamide in patients with atrial flutter or fibrillation. J Am Coll Cardiol 31:1414–1419, 1998.
93. Ward KJ, Gill JS: Dofetilide: first of a new generation of class III agents. Exp Opin Invest Drugs 6:1269–1281, 1997.
94. The DIAMOND Study Group: Dofetilide in patients with left ventricular dysfunction and either heart failure of acute myocardial infarction: rationale, design, and patient characteristics of the DIAMOND studies. Clin Cardiol 20:704–710, 1997.
95. Fermini B, Jurkiewicz NK, Jow B, et al: Use-dependent effects of the class III antiarrhythmic agent NE-10064 (azimilide) on cardiac repolarization: block of delayed rectifier potassium and L-type calcium currents. J Cardiovasc Pharmacol 26:259–271, 1995.
96. Corey A, Agnew J, Bao J, et al: Effect of age and gender on azimilide pharmacokinetics after a single oral dose of azimilide dihydrochloride. J Clin Pharmacol 37:946–953, 1997.
97. Camm AJ, Karam R, Pratt C: The azimilide post-infarct survival evaluation (ALIVE) trial. Am J Cardiol 81:35D–39D, 1998.
98. Rinkenberger RL, Prystowsky EN, Heger JJ, et al: Effects of intravenous and chronic oral verapamil administration in patients with supraventricular tachyarrhythmias. Circulation 62:996–1010, 1980.
99. Sung RJ, Elser B, McAllister RG Jr: Intravenous verapamil for termination of reentrant supraventricular tachycardias: intracardiac studies correlated with plasma verapamil concentrations. Ann Intern Med 93:682–689, 1980.
100. Waxman HL, Myerburg RJ, Appel R, Sung RJ: Verapamil for control of ventricular rate in paroxysmal supraventricular tachycardia and atrial fibrillation or flutter: a double-blind randomized cross-over study. Ann Intern Med 94:1–6, 1981.
101. Buxton AE, Marchlinski FE, Doherty JW, et al: Hazards of intravenous verapamil for sustained ventricular tachycardia. Am J Cardiol 59:1107–1110, 1987.
102. Gulamhusein S, Ko P, Carruthers SG, Klein GJ: Acceleration of the ventricular response during atrial fibrillation in the Wolff-Parkinson-White syndrome after verapamil. Circulation 65:348–354, 1982.
103. The Danish Study Group on Verapamil in Myocardial Infarction: Effect of verapamil on mortality and major events after acute myocardial infarction (the Danish Verapamil Infarction Trial II—DAVIT II). Am J Cardiol 66:779–785, 1990.
104. Dougherty AH, Jackman WM, Naccarelli GV, et al, the IV Diltiazem Study Group: Acute conversion of paroxysmal supraventricular tachycardia with intravenous diltiazem: a multicenter dose response study. Am J Cardiol 70:587–592, 1992.
105. Salerno DM, Dias VC, Kleiger RE, et al: Efficacy and safety of intravenous diltiazem for treatment of atrial fibrillation and atrial flutter. Am J Cardiol 63:1046–1051, 1989.
106. The Multicenter Diltiazem Postinfarction Trial Research Group: The effect of diltiazem on mortality and reinfarction after myocardial infarction. N Engl J Med 319:385–392, 1988.
107. Gibson RS, Boden WE, Theroux P, et al: Diltiazem and reinfarction in patients with non Q-wave infarction. N Engl J Med 315:423–429, 1986.
108. DiMarco JP, Sellers TD, Lerman BB, et al: Diagnostic and therapeutic use of adenosine in patients with supraventricular tachyarrhythmias. J Am Coll Cardiol 6:417–425, 1985.
109. DiMarco, Sellers TD, Berne RM, et al: Adenosine: Electrophysiologic effects and therapeutic use for terminating paroxysmal supraventricular tachycardia. Circulation 68:1254–1263, 1983.
110. Griffith MJ, Linker NJ, Ward DE, Camm A: Adenosine in the diagnosis of broad complex tachycardia. Lancet 1:672–675, 1988.
111. Smith TW: Digitalis: mechanisms of action and clinical use. N Engl J Med 318:358–365, 1988.
112. Lown B, Graboys TB, Podrid PJ, et al: Effect of a digitalis drug on ventricular premature beats. N Engl J Med 296:301–306, 1977.
113. Falk RH, Knowlton AA, Bernard SA, et al: Digoxin for converting recent-onset atrial fibrillation to sinus rhythm: a randomized, double-blind trial. Ann Intern Med 106:503–506, 1987.
114. The Digitalis in Acute Atrial Fibrillation (DAAF) Trial Group: Intravenous digoxin in acute atrial fibrillation: results of a randomized, placebo-controlled multicentre trial in 239 patients. Eur Heart J 18:649–654, 1997.
115. Pick A: Digitalis and the electrocardiogram. Circulation 15:603–608, 1957.
116. Garg R, Gorlin R, Smith T, Yusuf S, for the Digitalis Investigation Group: The effect of digoxin on mortality and morbidity in patients with heart failure. N Engl J Med 336:525–533, 1997.

CHAPTER 96

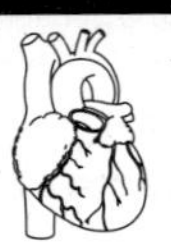

Pacing and Defibrillation

PERMANENT CARDIAC PACING
Michael H. Gollob, Michael F. Lenis, and John J. Seger
NASPE/BPEG Generic Pacemaker Code
Indications for Permanent Cardiac Pacing
Pacing System Components
Pacing and Sensing Thresholds
Pacemaker Timing Intervals
Pacemaker Modes and Clinical Application
Pacemaker Syndrome
Special Pacemaker Features
Use of Pacemaker Diagnostics
Procedure-Related Pacemaker Complications
Pacemaker Malfunction
Pacemaker Follow-Up
THE IMPLANTABLE CARDIOVERTER-DEFIBRILLATOR
Michael H. Gollob and John J. Seger
Evolution of the ICD
The Modern ICD
Defibrillation Threshold
The Magnet Response and Electromagnetic Interference
Evaluation of ICD Malfunction
Clinical Trials of the ICD
Cost-Effectiveness
Future Developments

Permanent Cardiac Pacing

Michael H. Gollob, Michael F. Lenis, and John J. Seger

Cardiac pacing had its origins in the 1920s, when Dr. Mark Lidwill successfully paced and resuscitated a stillborn infant.[1] Little is known about the equipment used, although it did involve a skin electrode and a needle electrode percutaneously advanced into the ventricle. In the early 1950s, Zoll demonstrated transthoracic pacing with high-voltage plate electrodes strapped to the chest wall.[2] In the late 1950s, Lillehei paced patients at the time of cardiac surgery with epicardial leads, and shortly thereafter, Fuhrman and Schwedel developed a transvenous pacing electrode.[2] The development of the transistor allowed for small, self-contained, battery-operated pulse generators (PGs) and led to the first pacemaker implantation by Senning and Elmquist in 1958.[2]

Since Senning's initial pacemaker implant, cardiac pacing has developed from a novelty into a significant part of modern cardiovascular therapeutics. Pacing technology advances have led to the pacemaker's evolving from a simple asynchronous pacing device to a sophisticated computerized pacing system. Indications for permanent pacemaker therapy continue to evolve.

NASPE/BPEG Generic Pacemaker Code

Pacemaker terminology has been standardized by a joint effort of the North American Society of Pacing and Electrophysiology (NASPE) and the British Pacing and Electrophysiology Group (BPEG).[3] This NASPE/BPEG coding standard allows for the communication of device type and capability.

In the NASPE/BPEG coding standard, pacemaker function and modality are expressed in a five-position lettering system (Table 96–1). Although the NASPE/BPEG standard allows for five positions, it is customary for most pacemakers to be described in an abbreviated three- or four-position form. The fifth position describes antitachycardia functions, including antitachycardia pacing and cardioversion-defibrillation. It is therefore possible to describe implantable cardioverter-defibrillators (ICDs) with the NASPE/BPEG coding system, although this rarely occurs in clinical practice.

Each letter position is filled according to the established NASPE/BPEG standard lettering system. The first letter position denotes the chamber paced and the second refers to the chamber sensed. Both are abbreviated with the standard *A,* representing the atrial chamber, and *V,* the ventricular chamber. *D* represents dual chamber, and *O,* off. The third letter position, which refers to a pacemaker's response to a sensed event, is denoted *I* for inhibited or *T* for triggering a paced event after a programmable interval, or by *D,* designating either inhibited or triggered, depending on the chamber sensed. *O,* again, denotes the absence of either triggering or inhibition. The fourth position denotes

TABLE 96–1 The NASPE-BPEG Pacemaker Code

I *Chambers Paced*	II *Chambers Sensed*	III *Response to Sensing*	IV *Programmability, Rate Response*	V *Antitachycardia Functions*
O—none	O—none	O—none	O—none	O—none
A—atrium	A—atrium	T—triggered	P—simple programmable	P—pacing (antitachycardias)
V—ventricle	V—ventricle	I—inhibited	M—multiprogrammable	S—shock
D—dual (A + V)	D—dual (A + D)	D—dual (T + I)	C—communicating	D—dual (P + S)
S—single	S—single		R—rate modulation	

Abbreviations: BPEG, British Pacing and Electrophysiology Group; NASPE, North American Society of Pacing and Electrophysiology.

programmability and rate response, using the letter abbreviations *O, P, M, C,* and *R*. These letters represent nonprogrammable, simple programmable, multiprogrammable, communicating, and rate-adaptive programmability.

Indications for Permanent Cardiac Pacing

The most recent consensus statement from the American College of Cardiology (ACC) and the American Heart Association (AHA) was issued in 1998 (Table 96–2).[4] This is the third set of guidelines after the initial publication in 1984 and the second publication in 1991. These guidelines are subdivided into three classifications on the basis of the level of general agreement for the specific indication (Table 96–3). The current guidelines have a new feature: a level of evidence designation for the pacing indication.[4]

Sinus Node Dysfunction

Sinus node dysfunction is the most common indication for permanent pacing in the United States, accounting for up to 50 percent of primary pacemaker implantations.[5] The spectrum of arrhythmias in sinus node dysfunction includes sinus bradycardia, sinus arrest, chronotropic incompetence, and the tachy-brady syndrome with alternating tachycardia and bradycardia events. Significant bradycardia seen in sinus node dysfunction may be caused by drug therapy required for the prevention of rapid recurrent paroxysms of atrial tachycardia, flutter, or fibrillation. Up to 50 percent of patients with sinus node dysfunction have episodes of paroxysmal atrial fibrillation, which carries with it an increased risk of arterial thromboembolism.[6]

The current guidelines include as a class IIB indication for permanent pacing an absolute heart rate of less than 30 beats per minute (bpm) in awake patients who are minimally symptomatic.[7] This is, however, uncommon, and symptoms correlated with bradycardia remain the primary indication for pacing in sinus node dysfunction.

It is well recognized that cardiac pacing is effective in abolishing bradycardia-related symptoms in patients with sinus node dysfunction. A randomized trial compared the efficacy of permanent cardiac pacing with theophylline in the treatment of patients with symptomatic sinus node dysfunction.[8] Patients were randomly assigned to DDDR pacing, theophylline, or no therapy and were followed up for a mean of 19 months. Although both treatment arms were associated with a lower incidence of heart failure, permanent pacing markedly reduced the incidence of syncope when compared with the theophylline (P = .07) and the no-therapy (P = .02) groups. This study further confirms the absence of acceptable pharmacologic alternatives and reaffirms pacing as the treatment of choice for patients with symptomatic sinus node dysfunction. The appropriate pacing mode in sinus node dysfunction remains controversial and, as is discussed, is the focus of ongoing clinical trials.

Chronotropic Incompetence

Symptomatic chronotropic incompetence is now a class I indication for permanent pacing in the new ACC/AHA guidelines. The ability to accelerate the heart rate with exercise is the most important factor in increasing cardiac output with physical exertion. The ability to increase stroke volume is limited, whereas heart rate can be increased more than threefold from resting rates.[9] Chronotropic incompetence may therefore lead to a significant decrease in functional capacity. In addition, there is evidence that chronotropic incompetence may be a risk factor for coronary artery disease and total mortality.[10]

The initial definition of chronotropic incompetence was the inability to increase the heart rate to a level of 100 bpm in response to an exercise test.[11] This definition may be arbitrary and does not take into account differing patient subgroups with markedly different predicted maximal heart rates. Modifications for defining chronotropic incompetence have been proposed and are evolving. Future criteria will likely include failure to achieve 75 percent of the age-predicted maximal heart rate along with a modification of heart rate to work rate ratio.[12]

Acquired AV Block

Acquired atrioventricular (AV) block may be subdivided into complete AV block, second-degree AV block types I and II, first-degree AV block, and finally, chronic bifascicular and trifascicular block. The indications for pacing for these entities are discussed separately.

COMPLETE AV BLOCK

Complete AV block at any anatomic level associated with symptoms is a class I indication for permanent pacing. Studies dating to the 1970s have demonstrated improved survival for patients with third-degree AV block treated with permanent pacemakers.[13] The current guidelines designate asymptomatic complete AV block to be a class I indication for pacing only if the escape rhythm is less than 40 bpm or an asystolic pause greater than 3 seconds is documented. These cut-off rates are arbitrary and may not predict rate stability. Patients with irreversible acquired complete AV block should probably have permanent pacemakers implanted, regardless of the escape rate.[14]

SECOND-DEGREE AV BLOCK

Second-degree AV block is divided into type I and type II. Type I AV block is of the Wenckebach type and is presumed to be at the level of the AV node, whereas type II block is presumed to be infranodal. However, it is known that up to 30 percent of type I second-degree AV blocks in the setting of chronic bundle branch block occur in the His-Purkinje system.[15] Conversely, type II second-degree AV block can occur at the level of the AV node, particularly when there is slowing of the PP interval before AV block.[16]

The 1998 ACC/AHA guidelines designate second-degree block of either type with symptomatic bradycardia as a class I indication for permanent pacing. In asymptomatic patients with second-degree AV block, cardiac pacing may be necessary if the level of block is infranodal because it is known that progression to complete heart block is common.[17, 18] In the setting of type I second-degree AV block with chronic bundle branch block, electrophysiologic docu-

TABLE 96–2 ACC/AHA Guidelines for Pacemaker Implantation

	Class I	Class II-A	Class II-B	Class III
Acquired AV block	1. Third-degree AV block at any anatomic level associated with any of the following conditions:	1. Asymptomatic third-degree AV block at any anatomic site with associated ventricular rates of 40 beats/min	Marked first-degree AV block of greater than 300 msec in patients with LV dysfunction and CHF in whom a shorter AV interval results in improved hemodynamics	1. Asymptomatic first-degree AV block
	A. Bradycardia with symptoms presumed secondary to AV block B. Arrhythmias and other medical conditions requiring medications that result in symptomatic bradycardia	2. Asymptomatic type II second-degree block 3. Asymptomatic type I AV block at intrahisian or infrahisian levels		2. Asymptomatic type I second-degree AV block 3. Temporary AV block
	C. Documented periods of asystole greater than 3 seconds or any escape rhythm of <40 beats/min in an awake asymptomatic patient D. Post AV nodal ablation E. Permanent postoperative AV block F. Neuromuscular disorders with AV block 2. Second-degree AV block with associated symptomatic bradycardia	4. First-degree AV block with symptoms consistent with pacemaker syndrome and documented improvement with temporary pacing		
Pacing in sinus node dysfunction	1. Sinus node dysfunction with documented symptomatic bradycardia, including frequent sinus pauses that produce symptoms. This may be iatrogenic secondary to required medications.	1. Sinus node dysfunction occurring spontaneously or as a result of necessary drug therapy, with heart rate <40 beats/min when a clear association between significant symptoms consistent with bradycardia and the actual presence of bradycardia has not been documented	In minimally symptomatic patients, chronic heart rate less than 30 beats/min	1. Sinus node dysfunction in asymptomatic patients, including those in whom substantial sinus bradycardia, <40 beats/min, is a consequence of long-term drug treatment
	2. Symptomatic chronotropic incompetence.			2. Sinus node dysfunction in patients with symptoms suggestive of bradycardia that are clearly documented as not associated with a slow heart rate 3. Sinus node dysfunction with symptomatic bradycardia due to nonessential drug therapy

Chronic bifascicular and trifascicular block	1. Intermittent third-degree AV block. 2. Type II second-degree heart block.	1. Syncope not proved to be due to AV block when other causes have been excluded, including VT 2. Incidental finding of markedly prolonged HV interval (>100 msec) at EPS 3. Incidental finding of pacing induced nonphysiologic infrahisian block	None	1. Fascicular block without AV block or symptoms 2. Fascicular block with first-degree AV block without symptoms
AV block with acute myocardial infarction	1. Persistent second-degree AV block in the His-Purkinje system with bilateral branch block or third-degree AV block within or below the His-Purkinje system 2. Transient advanced (second- or third-degree) infranodal block and associated bundle branch block; if site of block uncertain, EPS may be necessary 3. Persistent and symptomatic second- or third-degree AV block	None	Persistent second- or third-degree AV block at the AV node	1. Transient AV block in the absence of intraventricular conduction defects 2. Transient AV block in the presence of an isolated left anterior hemiblock 3. Acquired left anterior hemiblock in the absence of AV block 4. Persistent first-degree AV block in the presence of chronic or indeterminate age bundle branch block
Hypersensitive carotid sinus syndrome	Recurrent syncope caused by carotid sinus stimulation; minimal carotid sinus pressure induces ventricular asystole of >3 seconds duration in the absence of any medication that depresses the sinus node or AV conduction	1. Recurrent syncope without clear, provocative events and with a hypersensitive cardioinhibitory response 2. Syncope of unexplained origin when major abnormalities of sinus node dysfunction or AV conduction are discovered or provoked in EPSs	Neurally mediated syncope with significant bradycardia reproduced by a head-up tilt with or without isoproterenol or other provocative maneuvers	1. A hyperactive cardioinhibitory response to carotid sinus massage in the absence of symptoms 2. A hyperactive cardioinhibitory response to carotid sinus stimulation in the presence of vague symptoms, e.g., dizziness, light-headedness, or both 3. Situational vasovagal syncope in which avoidance behavior is effective

Abbreviations: ACC, American College of Cardiology; AHA, American Heart Association; AV, atrioventricular; CHF, congestive heart failure; EPS, electrophysiologic study; LV, left ventricular; VT, ventricular tachycardia.

TABLE 96-3 **Classification of Pacemaker Indications**

Class I	Conditions for which there is general agreement and evidence that permanent pacing is beneficial
Class II	Conditions for which there is conflicting opinion and evidence regarding whether a pacemaker should be implanted
	A. Weight of evidence in favor of efficacy
	B. Efficacy less well established
Class III	Conditions for which there is general agreement and evidence that permanent pacing is not beneficial or harmful

mentation of an infranodal location of the block may be required. Finally, with 2:1 AV block, the level of block may be impossible to determine on the surface electrocardiogram. In patients with bundle branch block and 2:1 AV block, the level of block is usually but not invariably infranodal, and pacing may be required.[15]

CHRONIC BIFASCICULAR AND TRIFASCICULAR BLOCK

Bifascicular block refers to right bundle branch block and left anterior hemiblock, right bundle branch block and left posterior hemiblock, or left bundle branch block. The addition of first-degree AV block to this phenomenon is frequently referred to as *trifascicular block*, although this is not strictly correct, because the site of AV block causing the first-degree AV block may be in either the AV node or the His-Purkinje system.[19] True trifascicular block during 1:1 conduction is diagnosed in the presence of alternating right bundle branch block and left bundle branch block or fixed right bundle branch block and alternating left anterior hemiblock and left posterior hemiblock.[20] These patients may require permanent pacing.[19]

Bifascicular block or bifascicular block with first-degree AV block defines disease in the infranodal conduction system. However, in asymptomatic patients, this does not represent an indication for pacemaker implantation, because the risk of progression to complete AV block is known to be low.[21] The ACC/AHA guidelines designate bifascicular block with intermittent complete heart block and symptoms as a class I indication. Bifascicular block with type II second-degree AV block is also a class I indication for permanent pacing. Patients with syncope and electrocardiographic evidence of bifascicular block without AV block should undergo electrophysiologic study (EPS), particularly in the presence of structural heart disease. This allows assessment for ventricular tachycardia (VT) and assessment of the infrahisian conduction system. In the absence of a diagnostic EPS, pacing is a class IIA indication by the current guidelines. Finally, the identification of an HV interval of greater than 100 ms or pacing-induced infrahisian block, regardless of symptoms, is a class IIA indication for permanent pacemaker implantation.[4]

EXERCISE-INDUCED AV BLOCK

Exercise-induced AV block is almost invariably infranodal and is associated with a poor prognosis.[22, 23] Permanent pacing is usually required. Ischemia and neurocardiogenic syndromes are treatable causes of exertional AV block that may not require permanent pacing.[24]

FIRST-DEGREE AV BLOCK

Asymptomatic first-degree AV block is common and does not require permanent pacing.[25] In the setting of marked PR interval prolongation, however, atrial contraction may occur against closed AV valves, producing symptoms of pacemaker syndrome. If a temporary AV pacing study confirms improved hemodynamics, permanent pacing is a class IIA indication. In patients with a long PR interval in the setting of dilated cardiomyopathy and congestive heart failure, permanent pacing is a class IIB indication after demonstration of hemodynamic benefit.[4] The requirement for a pacing study is controversial, however, because it is not clear that a dual-chamber temporary study will predict long-term benefit.[26]

Congenital AV Block

Congenital complete heart block usually presents with relatively asymptomatic AV block with a narrow QRS escape. Congenital AV block has been associated with life-threatening complications, including recurrent syncope and sudden cardiac death (SCD).[26–28] Patient characteristics associated with higher risk include marked bradycardia for age, chamber enlargement or ventricular dysfunction, mitral regurgitation, prolonged corrected QT interval, and ventricular ectopy. In addition, some studies have suggested that even patients without risk factors may have significant bradycardia complications.[29] Congenital complete heart block is a class IIA indication in the current guidelines in the asymptomatic neonate, child, or adolescent, regardless of risk factors.

Post–Myocardial Infarction Permanent Pacing

Bradyarrhythmias and conduction disturbances are frequently observed in acute myocardial infarction. Significant sinus bradycardia is seen after both anterior and inferior myocardial infarctions and may occur in up to 25 percent of patients. Presumably on the basis of increased vagal tone, bradycardia is more common in inferior myocardial infarction.[30] Permanent pacemakers are rarely required for postinfarction symptomatic bradycardia.

The incidence of AV conduction disturbances in acute myocardial infarction is approximately 20 percent, with more than half of these being first-degree AV block. Second-degree block and third-degree AV block occur in 5 and 3 percent, respectively. AV conduction disturbances in the setting of inferior infarction are usually caused by reversible ischemia of the AV node, and these patients tend to have less extensive infarctions.[31] Although conduction disturbances in inferior infarctions have been noted to last for up to 16 days, they are typically reversible, and pacemakers are infrequently needed.[32] The incidence of AV block complicating inferior infarction in the prethrombolytic era appears similar to that in the post-thrombolytic era.[33] However, early reperfusion does appear to be associated with a shorter duration of AV block.[33]

In contrast, AV conduction disturbances in anterior myocardial infarction are often caused by more extensive myocardial necrosis with involvement of the infranodal conduction system and congestive heart failure, leading to a poor prognosis.[34, 35] The prevalence of right bundle branch block or left bundle branch block complicating a myocardial infarction is approximately 6 percent for each entity.[34] The development of these conduction defects is associated with a higher short- and long-term mortality, particularly with persistence of the bundle branch block.[35] However, it has not been established that mortality is a result of progression to complete AV block.

Identifying patients who would benefit from permanent pacing after myocardial infarction is often difficult. Only three class I indications exist; these are listed in Table 96–2. These class I indications require documentation of extensive infranodal conduction system disease or symptomatic AV block.

Neurally Mediated Syncope and Carotid Sinus Hypersensitivity

Neurally mediated syncope is a syndrome of episodic loss of consciousness caused by an exaggerated autonomic nervous system reflex with depression of blood pressure and heart rate to various degrees.[36] Carotid sinus hypersensitivity is a subset of neurally mediated syncope in which the abnormal cardioinhibitory or vasodepressor responses occur with carotid sinus massage. This subset is distinct in that it tends to occur in elderly individuals who have a more prominent cardioinhibitory component.[36, 37] In addition, considerable literature demonstrates the effectiveness of pacing in patients with documented carotid sinus hypersensitivity.[38–42] The diagnosis of carotid sinus hypersensitivity is confirmed with a history consistent with spontaneous recurrent syncopal events provoked by maneuvers that would potentially evoke carotid sinus stimulation (turning one's head, looking up, "barber chair" syncope). A carotid sinus massage–induced asystolic pause of greater than 3 seconds in the absence of medications that depress sinus or AV nodal function is required for a class I indication. Dual-chamber pacing is generally preferred because of improved hemodynamics with AV sequential pacing.[42–46] Carotid sinus hypersensitivity is relatively common in patients without a history of recurrent syncope.[36] Therefore, patients with vague symptoms of dizziness who respond abnormally to carotid sinus massage do not in general meet indications for permanent pacemaker implantation.

Pacing in other neurally mediated syndromes is controversial. These patients tend to be younger and have a more prominent vasodepressor component.[36] However, the North American Vasovagal Pacemaker Study did indicate that in a selected group of medically refractory patients with recurrent neurally mediated syncope and bradycardia during tilt table testing, permanent pacemaker implantation is beneficial.[47] These dual-chamber devices had a specific algorithm providing an interventional pacing rate for precipitous bradycardic events. During follow-up, 19 of the 27 patients randomly assigned to standard therapy had recurrent syncope, whereas only 6 of 27 patients in the pacemaker group experienced recurrent syncopal events. The study was planned for 284 patients but was terminated early after the enrollment of only 54 patients because of a significant treatment effect. Although these results are promising, the study has limitations, including potential significant placebo benefit, the variable pattern of recurrent syncopal events, and the relatively small numbers in the trial at the time of its termination.[48] In addition, these were highly symptomatic, medically refractory patients. These factors require serious consideration before a permanent pacemaker is implanted in a generally young and otherwise healthy patient.

Hypertrophic Cardiomyopathy

The potential for hemodynamic benefit from permanent pacing in hypertrophic obstructive cardiomyopathy was postulated nearly 25 years ago.[49] More recently, enthusiasm for the role of pacing in hypertrophic cardiomyopathy has increased with the reporting of observational studies demonstrating an improvement in left ventricular outflow tract gradient, symptoms, and exercise capacity.[50–53] The precise mechanism of these effects, although not completely clear, includes a right ventricular apical "preexcitation" with paradoxical septal motion and an increase in the left ventricular outflow tract diameter that leads to a decrease in the outflow tract gradient. Another potential mechanism is a primary negative inotropic effect from right ventricular apical pacing and dyssynchronous left ventricular contraction. Short AV delays are typically required to allow complete apical capture from the pacing stimulus and reduce the contribution of native AV conduction.[54, 55]

The initial enthusiasm for pacing has been tempered after three randomized crossover trials involving 150 patients: the Mayo Clinic Trial, the European Pacing and Cardiomyopathy Trial, and the Multi-center Pacing Therapy for Hypertrophic Cardiomyopathy Trial.[56–58] Although these trials have shown a 40 to 50 percent reduction in left ventricular outflow tract gradient, no change in exercise capacity was demonstrated. Permanent pacing remains an option in selected medically refractory patients. Surgery and the emerging therapy of alcohol septal ablation are other therapeutic considerations.[59]

Pacing for Atrial Fibrillation Prevention

Retrospective studies in patients who have received permanent pacemakers for sinus node dysfunction have demonstrated a lower incidence of atrial fibrillation with AAI or DDD pacing than with VVI pacing.[60] The first prospective study was published in 1994 by Andersen and colleagues[61]; this study compared AAI with VVI pacing in patients with sinus node dysfunction. This study demonstrated a statistically lower incidence of atrial fibrillation and thromboembolism at just over three years. When the study group was reassessed at 5½ years, statistical significance had been achieved for atrial fibrillation, thromboembolic events, heart failure, and total mortality.[6, 61] Subsequent prospective randomized trials have been less compelling and have shown mixed results. The Pacemaker Selection Elderly Trial compared VVIR with DDDR pacing in 407 patients 65 years of age or older who received permanent pacemakers for standard indications. Although not statistically significant, a strong trend showing a reduced incidence of stroke, death, and atrial fibrillation was seen in the sinus node dysfunction subgroup.[62] In the Pacemaker Atrial Tachycardia Trial, 198 patients with tachy-brady syndrome were randomly assigned to DDDR or VVIR pacing.[63] At 2-year follow-up, there was no statistical difference in recurrence of atrial fibrillation, which was the primary end point of the study. However, there was a statistically significant increase in mortality in the VVIR group (6.8 percent versus 3.2 percent, $P = .007$). In the Canadian Trial of Physiologic Pacing, more than 2500 patients requiring a permanent pacemaker were randomly assigned to either VVI or DDD pacing.[64, 65] At 3-year follow-up, there was no statistically significant difference in cardiovascular death or stroke. There was a statistically significant difference in the incidence of atrial fibrillation, with a 19 percent risk reduction at 2 years.[65] Further trials are ongoing.[66, 67]

Multisite atrial pacing has been reported to reduce the occurrence of atrial fibrillation.[68, 69] Multisite pacing was originally described as a means of resynchronizing atrial contraction for patients with intra-atrial conduction defects in an attempt to improve hemodynamics.[70, 71] Preliminary studies utilizing multisite atrial pacing from the right atrial appendage and the ostium of the coronary sinus indicate a significant increase in arrhythmia-free intervals.[68, 69]

Permanent Pacing for Dilated Cardiomyopathy

The benefits of cardiac pacing in dilated cardiomyopathy and congestive heart failure are the focus of interest and investigation. The potential long-term efficacy of dual-chamber pacing in end-stage cardiomyopathy was initially reported by Hochleitner and associates.[72] An improvement in left ventricular ejection fraction and functional class was reported with dual-chamber pacing and a short AV delay. Echocardiographic studies suggested that the improvement was limited to patients with diastolic mitral regurgitation or first-degree AV block.[73] Subsequent controlled studies have not demonstrated consistent benefits.[74, 75] In addition, it had previously been shown that right ventricular apical pacing had a potential negative effect on hemodynamics.[76, 77] Nonetheless, some patients with marked first-degree AV block and diastolic mitral regurgitation may benefit from this pacing therapy.

More recently, interest has shifted to biventricular pacing in patients with dilated cardiomyopathies and intraventricular conduction delays, particularly of the left bundle branch block type. The goal of biventricular pacing is to "re-synchronize" ventricular contraction. Small observational studies have demonstrated hemodynamic benefit.[78] The mechanism is not entirely clear but may relate to improved ventricular filling times.[79]

Pacing System Components

Pulse Generators

The pacemaker pulse generator (PG) consists of the pacemaker casing, header, power source, and internal circuitry. Most currently available PGs weigh between 20 and 35 g.

PACEMAKER CASING AND HEADER

The pacemaker casing in currently manufactured devices is hermetically sealed and made of titanium. Allergies to pacemaker casings have been reported and have been managed by coating the device with an inert biocompatible polymer or gold.[80, 81] Some unipolar pacing systems, which utilize the pacemaker casing as the anode in the pacing circuit, use an inert polymer coating on the back and sides of the device to aid in the prevention of muscle stimulation. Most pacemaker headers are made of polyurethane. This serves as the interface between the lead and the PG. In currently manufactured devices, the headers and lead pins are of standardized sizing, permitting interchanging of different manufacturers' products without the need for cumbersome adapters.

PULSE GENERATOR POWER SOURCE

The initial power source for cardiac pacemakers was the zinc-mercury battery. The average battery half-life for these chemical batteries was only 2 to 4 years, and decay characteristics were not predictable, with sudden failure being a common difficulty. Nuclear batteries were reliable and had projected longevity of up to 20 years.[82] However, because of expense, radiation concerns, and strict nuclear controls, their use was limited.

The first lithium-iodine powered pacemaker was implanted in 1972.[83] These batteries gained rapid popularity because of high energy densities, low self-discharge, and voltage/impedance characteristics that allowed smaller size and good longevity characteristics. A lithium-iodine battery has a beginning-of-life voltage of approximately 2.8 V, an end-of-life voltage at 90 percent depletion of approximately 1.8 V, and predictable decay characteristics.[84] Because of these factors and its proven reliability, the lithium-iodine battery is the most common PG battery used today.[84]

PULSE GENERATOR CIRCUITRY

PG circuitry includes the pacing/timing circuitry, telemetry and diagnostic circuitry. With the development of microprocessor technology, pacemaker electronics have become smaller, more energy efficient, reliable, and capable of more complex functions.

The pacing/timing circuitry provides the basic functions of pacing and sensing for the device. This includes the algorithms for the different pacing modes and timing intervals. Signals of sensed cardiac events are received from sensing amplifiers, while pacing output signals are emitted to output amplifiers based on the algorithms for the specific mode and timing intervals programmed.

The output amplifiers and sense amplifiers are the interface between the myocardium and the pacing/timing circuitry. Output pulses in modern pacemakers are generally constant voltage. Constant current waveforms are frequently used in temporary external pacing systems. The sensing amplifier system amplifies input signals approximately 100-fold. Band pass filters allow passage of signals within a certain frequency range and are used to filter out noncardiac signals and environmental noise.[85] As is discussed later, blanking periods during which sensing does not occur and refractory intervals during which the device does not react to sensed signals also help eliminate sensing of unwanted nonphysiologic or inappropriate signals.

The diagnostics circuitry is generally a memory circuit where PG data are stored and where pacing and sensing observational data, such as from rate histograms and intracardiac electrograms (EGMs), are stored. The telemetry circuitry controls the interaction between the PG and the pacemaker programmer, delivering commands to the pacing/timing circuitry and diagnostic data to the programmer.

Pacemaker Leads

The pacemaker lead both conducts intracardiac signals to the sensing amplifiers and delivers the PG waveform from the output amplifiers to the myocardium. The currently manufactured transvenous pacemaker lead includes the connector pins, conductor material, insulation material, fixation system, and electrode or electrodes. Epicardial leads are relatively rare in modern cardiac pacing, with the exception of the pediatric population, in which they are commonly used in children younger than 5 years.

LEAD POLARITY

Pacemaker lead configurations are either unipolar or bipolar. A unipolar lead has only one distal tip electrode. This represents the cathode of the circuit, and the PG casing is the anode. In bipolar pacing, the lead has two electrodes, one on the distal tip and the other a short distance proximally. As in unipolar pacing, the distal electrode is the cathode.

The preferred lead configuration has been the subject of controversy for many years.[86] The primary disadvantage of unipolar pacing is oversensing. Because of the large interelectrode spacing, unipolar systems are much more sensitive to extracardiac potentials, including skeletal myopotentials, far-field sensing, and cross-talk. Unipolar pacing configurations are also prone to skeletal muscle stimulation because the anode in the PG casing is close to skeletal muscle.

The larger size of the unipolar pacemaker stimulus artifact is an advantage during pacemaker testing. However, the primary advantage of unipolar systems has been the simplicity of the lead design, which has resulted in reliable longevity.[87] The original bipolar leads were bulky and had a more complex lead design and, not surprisingly, a higher failure rate. One of the main reasons for these high failure rates was insulation defects associated with specific polyurethane-insulated lead systems.[88] Modern bipolar leads are now similar to unipolar leads in size and, with changes in conductor configuration and insulation, it is anticipated that their longevity will approach that of unipolar leads. There is, therefore, a growing trend for the use of bipolar leads, although long-term reliability data demonstrating equality with unipolar pacing systems have not been confirmed.

Pacing Electrodes

Pacing electrode materials have included platinum-iridium, iridium oxide, activated carbon, and Elgiloy.[89, 90] Electrode material should be biologically inert and resistant to chemical degradation and corrosion, thereby reducing the inflammatory response at the tissue-electrode interface.

ELECTRODE SIZE, COMPOSITION, AND POLARIZATION

Early electrodes were large with relatively low current density and high stimulation thresholds. This resulted in large current drains and shortened battery life. High current densities were achieved by reducing the electrode surface area, thereby lowering stimulation thresholds.[91] Modern pacing electrodes have small surface areas and higher impedances, which result in lower stimulation thresholds and increased battery longevity.

The reduction in electrode size also leads to energy loss from high electrode polarization following stimulus delivery. Increasing the electrode surface area can significantly diminish polarization. Current density remains high because of the small electrode radius. Modern pacing electrode designs are therefore porous in order to increase surface area and diminish polarization, while maintaining a small electrode radius.[92] The electrode material also affects the polarization properties of the electrode.

STEROID-ELUTING ELECTRODES

After implantation, stimulation thresholds may rise up to 10 times the implant threshold because of acute inflammation at the electrode-myocardial interface.[93] The threshold rise usually peaks within 4 weeks and typically returns to two to three times the implant threshold within the first few months. The use of a steroid-eluting electrode may virtually eliminate this postimplant threshold rise.[94, 95] Steroid-eluting electrodes are available as both passive and active fixation electrodes.

LEAD-INSULATING MATERIAL

The predominant lead-insulating materials have been silicone rubber and polyurethane. Initial leads insulated with silicone required thick insulation because of low tear strength properties. This led to the development of thinner polyurethane insulation in the 1970s. Although this did result in improved handling characteristics, follow-up confirmed a high incidence of surface cracking and insulation failure.[88] Not surprisingly, these failures were more commonly seen in bipolar leads, with loss of integrity between the inner and outer coils. New varieties of polyurethane, which are stiffer and harder, have demonstrated improved performance. In addition, silicone rubber hybrids have been developed that are thinner and stronger (NovusR, Medtronic). Finally, combination polyurethane silicone leads have been developed. Although long-term data are lacking, it is anticipated that lead longevity will continue to improve. For currently implanted leads, maximal longevities are estimated to be about 15 years and possibly slightly longer for unipolar lead systems.

LEAD FIXATION DEVICES

Pacemaker leads are either active fixation or passive fixation. Most active fixation transvenous devices are a screw helix, which is either extendable-retractable or exposed. With a clockwise motion, these leads are screwed into the myocardium. Many exposed screw helices are imbedded in a soluble material (e.g., mannitol), which dissolves in the blood pool within a short interval. This facilitates introduction of the lead through the sheath and venous system. Passive fixation devices are most commonly tines or fins, which are umbrella-like extensions of the insulation material and facilitate entrapment in right atrial or right ventricular trabeculated myocardium (Fig. 96–1). Passive fixation leads are less traumatic to the myocardium and generally have lower acute thresholds. Their use is generally limited to the standard implant sites of the right atrial appendage and the right ventricular apex, where there are consistent trabeculations for fixation. Right atrial passive fixation leads have a preformed J shape, which holds the lead in place. The tines are rapidly covered with fibrous tissue, which may render removal of chronic leads more difficult, although it does not appear to affect overall extraction success rates.[97, 98]

Active fixation leads are frequently favored in younger patients, in whom the potential need for subsequent lead extraction is greater, in patients in whom nonstandard sites for lead implantation are anticipated, and in patients with large right ventricles, pulmonary hypertension, or significant tricuspid regurgitation, in whom dislodgment may occur.

SPECIAL USE LEADS

Single-pass leads have been developed and released for dual-chamber systems. These leads incorporate atrial and ventricular electrodes on the same lead body. At present, these systems do not provide atrial pacing. Atrial sensing with ventricular tracking allows for AV synchrony. Atrial sensing problems have been reported and may be dependent on body position because this sensing electrode is not fixed to atrial tissue.[99, 100] This lead system is limited for use in patients with normal sinus node function and AV block. Because of increased lead complexity, there is concern regarding lead longevity and reliability, although long-term data are lacking.

The impetus to develop coronary sinus leads has grown from both multisite atrial and multisite ventricular pacing studies, as described previously. Angulated leads, which allow wedging of these leads in the coronary sinus veins, have been developed.[101] In addition, over-the-wire coronary sinus leads are under investigation.[102]

Pacing and Sensing Thresholds

The two basic functions inherent in all cardiac pacemakers are pacing and sensing. Many factors influence the ability of the pacing system to deliver an adequate pacing stimulus and appropriately sense cardiac electrical activity. This includes hardware issues, such as electrode design, active versus passive fixation leads, and steroid-eluting electrodes. The electrode-tissue interface is crucial for pacing and sensing and may be affected by acute infarction, postimplant inflammation, and chronic fibrosis. Electrolyte abnormalities and antiarrhythmic drugs may affect pacing thresholds.[103, 104] Pacing and sensing functions are therefore continually evolving throughout the life of the pacemaker system.

Pacing

Myocardial stimulation requires the delivery of an electrical impulse of adequate intensity to produce a propagating wavefront throughout the atrial and ventricular myocardium. This pacing threshold is defined as the minimal energy required to consistently generate a depolarizing wavefront. The energy delivered is a function of both the intensity (voltage) and the duration (pulse width) of the electrical stimulus. The relationship between the voltage and the pulse width for myocardial stimulation is exponential and is represented by the strength-duration curve (Fig. 96–2). As can be seen from this relationship, at short pulse widths, there is a steep and marked change in threshold voltage required for successful stimulation, whereas at longer pulse widths, there is little change in threshold voltage for large changes in pulse width duration. This flat portion of the curve at longer pulse durations is referred to as the *rheobase* and represents the lowest voltage that depolarizes the myocardium at any pulse width. By convention, this value is generally taken at a pulse width of 2.0 ms. The *chronaxy* is defined as the pulse width threshold that corresponds to twice the rheobase voltage. An understanding of the strength-duration curve is important for proper programming of the voltage and the pulse width, allowing for adequate safety margin and optimal energy consumption. Because the steep portion of the strength-duration curve occurs at very narrow pulse widths, programming the pulse width less than 0.3 ms is not recommended, because a small shift in the strength-duration curve may potentially lead to a marked increase in the voltage threshold. Additionally, little is gained from

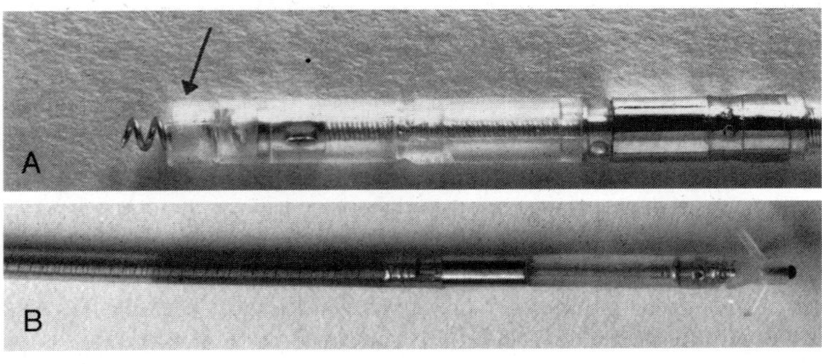

FIGURE 96–1 Active and passive fixation leads. **A,** The top lead illustrates an active fixation lead with an extendable/retractable helix, which is electrically active. A steroid collar is indicated by an *arrow.* **B,** The bottom lead is a passive fixation tine lead.

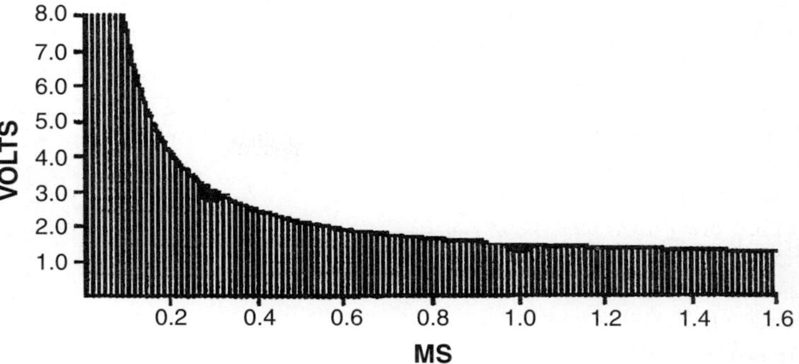

FIGURE 96–2 Strength-duration curve relates voltage and pulse width at capture threshold. Values above the curve capture the heart, whereas values below in the *shaded area* do not. As pulse width is extended beyond 1 ms, little is gained in voltage threshold. The curve is steep at narrow pulse widths, where small changes in pulse width duration may result in large changes in voltage threshold.

markedly prolonged pulse durations because the curve becomes flat.

The recommended safety margin for a stable pacing threshold has traditionally been three times the *energy* threshold. Because

$$\text{Energy} = [\text{Volts}^2 \times \text{Pulse Duration}] \div \text{Impedance},$$

this can be achieved by increasing the voltage 1.7 to 2 times the voltage threshold at a given pulse width or tripling the pulse width threshold at a given voltage. Some currently available devices incorporate algorithms that automatically measure thresholds at programmable intervals and self-adjust the pacing output. In addition, devices are available that identify optimal settings for battery longevity on the basis of a measured strength-duration curve.

Sensing

Sensing of the intracardiac EGM is essential for the proper function of a permanent pacemaker. The sensing circuits must allow appropriate detection of atrial and ventricular EGMs while rejecting unwanted noncardiac signals and inappropriate cardiac signals, such as T waves.

The intracardiac EGM is typically biphasic, and predominantly negative or positive deflections are less frequently seen. The transition between predominantly upright to predominantly downgoing is known as the *intrinsic deflection* and is believed to reflect the movement of the myocardial activation wavefront across the region of the recording electrode. The intracardiac EGM is filtered by the sensing circuits, with the least sensitive setting at which sensing occurs reflecting the sensing threshold. The slew rate is defined as the change in voltage over time (dV/dt) of the EGM. The larger the value of the slew rate, the "sharper" the EGM, and the more easily sensed.[105]

Unipolar pacing systems, because of greater interelectrode spacing, have considerable differences in sensing characteristics. The interelectrode spacing on a typical transvenous bipolar lead is generally less than 3 cm. A unipolar lead, which utilizes the generator casing as one of the electrodes, may have an interelectrode spacing of up to 40 to 50 cm. As discussed previously, far-field sensing is therefore much more common in unipolar systems and represents the major disadvantage of this configuration. At the time of implant, it is recommended that a larger atrial EGM amplitude be achieved with unipolar systems than with bipolar systems because of this increased risk of oversensing. With bipolar systems, reasonable sensing thresholds are 1.5 mV or greater and, in unipolar systems, ideally should be 2 mV or greater. Ventricular EGMs are significantly larger because of mass differences. Acceptable ventricular EGMs are 5 mV or greater, although they are in general readily obtainable in the 10- to 20-mV range.

Pacemaker Timing Intervals

An understanding of pacemaker timing intervals is required to fully understand pacemaker function and interpret pacemaker electrocardiograms. The timing intervals are discussed as they relate to single- and dual-chamber pacing. Timing intervals by convention are expressed in milliseconds.

Timing Intervals in Single-Chamber Pacing

The *lower rate interval* of a single-chamber pacemaker defines the lowest rate at which the pacemaker will pace. The *refractory period* is an interval initiated by a paced or sensed event. The device ignores any sensed event that occurs during this interval. It is designed to prevent inhibition by inappropriate cardiac or noncardiac signals. The *blanking period* is the first portion of the refractory period. During this interval, the pacemaker is blind to any events. In the single-chamber device, the blanking period is designed to prevent oversensing of the pacing stimulus. In single-chamber devices with rate-adaptive capability, the *upper sensor rate interval* defines the shortest interval the pacemaker can pace as dictated by an activity sensor. Single-chamber timing intervals are illustrated in Figure 96–3.

Timing Intervals in Dual-Chamber Pacing

The four possible expressions of dual-chamber pacing are a sensed or paced atrial event in combination with a sensed or paced ventricular event. The lower rate interval in dual-chamber pacing refers to the lowest rate the pacemaker will pace the atrium in the absence of intrinsic atrial activity. The *AV interval* is defined as the interval initiated by a paced or sensed atrial event and terminates with a ventricular paced or sensed event. The AV interval in most current devices may be separately programmed for a sensed AV interval and a paced AV interval. The paced AV interval by definition initiates with the pacing stimulus, which is followed by atrial depolarization. The sensed AV interval

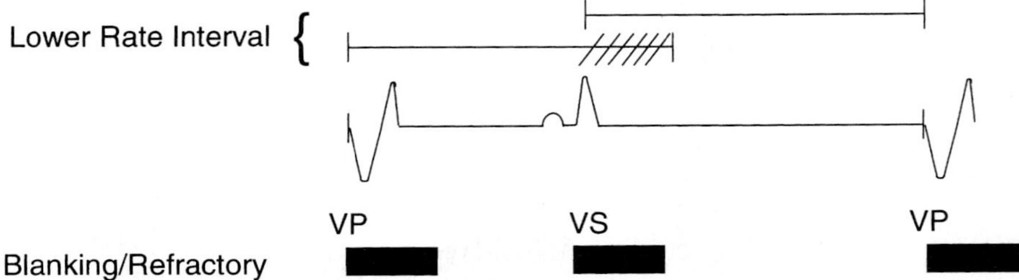

FIGURE 96–3 Single-chamber (VVI) timing. A ventricular-paced event (VP) is followed by a blanking period and a refractory period, preventing oversensing of pacing stimuli, paced complexes, and T waves. A ventricular-sensed (VS) event occurs before the end of the lower rate interval (LRI). The LRI is reset and, in the absence of another VS event, results in a VP event.

is programmed shorter because atrial sensed events occur after the initiation of the P wave (Fig. 96–4). The *atrial escape interval* or *VA interval* is the interval initiated by a sensed or paced ventricular event and terminates with the next atrial paced event. The programmed lower rate interval is equal to the paced AV interval plus the VA interval. The *upper or maximal tracking rate* (MTR) in dual-chamber systems represents the maximal rate the ventricle can be paced in response to sensed atrial events. The *ventricular refractory period* is similar to that in single-chamber systems and is intended to prevent oversensing of the evoked potential or T waves. The *postventricular atrial refractory period* (PVARP) is an atrial refractory interval initiated by a ventricular paced or sensed event and is intended primarily to prevent atrial sensing of retrograde P waves that could initiate pacemaker-mediated tachycardia (PMT). In addition, the atrium is refractory to sensed events during the AV interval. The *total atrial refractory period* then is equal to the sum of the AV interval and the PVARP. Blanking periods on the atrial channel of the dual-chamber device occur at the time of an atrial paced event (*atrial blanking period*) and after ventricular paced events (*post-ventricular atrial blanking period*). Similarly, ventricular blanking periods occur after atrial depolarization (*post-atrial ventricular blanking*) and after ventricular paced events (*ventricular blanking period*). The atrial blanking period on the atrial channel and the ventricular blanking period on the ventricular channel are generally nonprogrammable. As with single-chamber devices, these blanking periods are designed to prevent oversensing of pacing stimuli in either chamber. Dual-chamber timing intervals are illustrated in Figure 96–5.

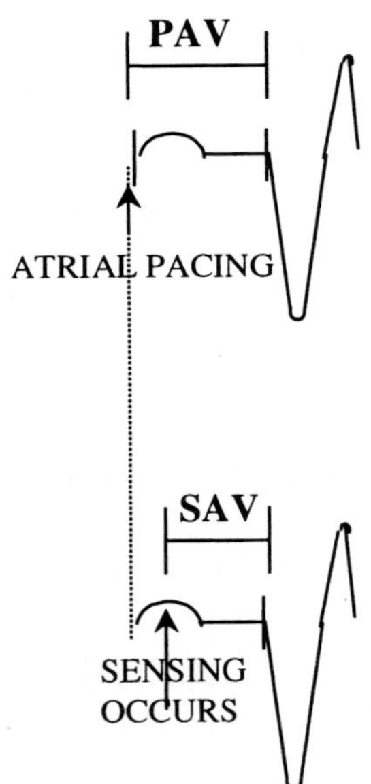

FIGURE 96–4 Relationship between sensed atrioventricular (SAV) and paced atrioventricular (PAV) intervals. **Top,** An atrial pacing stimulus initiates the PAV interval. **Bottom,** The SAV interval is programmed shorter than the PAV interval because atrial-sensed events occur after the beginning of the P wave.

Dual-chamber pacemaker system timing intervals are either atrial based or ventricular based (Fig. 96–6). With atrium-based timing, the *AA interval* is held constant. The AA interval is the lower rate interval and is equal to the AV interval plus the VA, or atrial escape interval. The effective ventricular rate in dual-chamber devices with atrium-based timing may vary because the AV interval may shorten from the programmed value as a result of intrinsic conduction, which in turn may lead to variations in the VV interval. In ventricular-based timing, the VA interval is held constant. The lower rate interval is again equal to the VA interval plus the AV interval. Because neither the AA interval nor the VV interval is held constant, the ventricular rate and the atrial rate may vary with intrinsic conduction and shortening of the AV interval from the programmed value. During atrium-based timing, therefore, the atrial rate is held constant and the ventricular rate may vary slightly, depending on native AV conduction. During ventricular-based timing, atrial and ventricular rates may vary slightly, again on the basis of intrinsic AV nodal conduction.

Upper-Rate Behavior

The total atrial refractory period is defined by the AV interval and the PVARP. This interval defines the maximal upper tracking limit of a dual-chamber pacemaker. If the sinus cycle length shortens to less than the total atrial refractory period, every other P wave falls within the postventricular atrial refractory period and is not sensed. This results in an abrupt fixed rate block. In patients who have AV block and require these faster physiologic rates, the abrupt development of 2:1 AV block may be poorly tolerated.

Decreasing the programmed AV interval or the postventricular atrial refractory period will allow a higher rate before 2:1 AV block occurs. In addition, several features have been developed to prevent or delay the development of 2:1 block. Wenckebach upper-rate behavior can occur if the total atrial refractory period is shorter than the programmed upper tracking rate. The difference between these intervals is the "Wenckebach interval." A P wave sensed during this interval does not initiate an AV interval until the end of the upper tracking rate interval. This effectively progressively prolongs the PR interval until the P wave

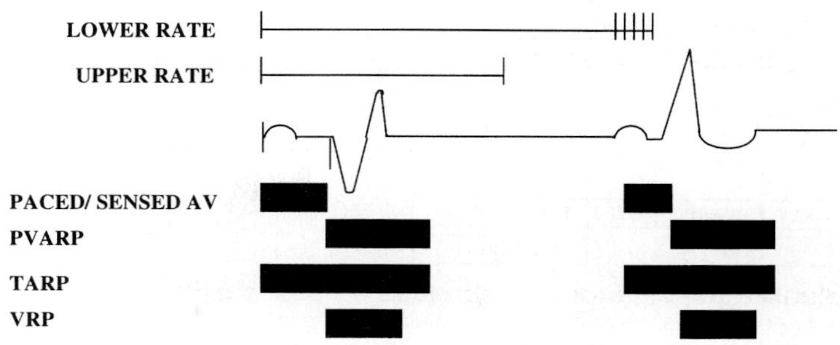

FIGURE 96–5 Dual-chamber timing. After a paced atrial event, a paced atrioventricular (PAV) interval is initiated. A sensed ventricular event does not occur within the programmed PAV interval, and a paced ventricular (VP) event occurs, followed by the postventricular atrial refractory period (PVARP) and the ventricular refractory period (VRP). After the end of the total atrial refractory period (TARP) and before the end of the lower rate interval (LRI), an atrial sensed event occurs. A sensed atrioventricular interval is triggered, and the LRI is reset. A ventricular-sensed event occurs and inhibits a VP event.

falls within the end of the total atrial refractory period, which results in a nonconducted beat (Fig. 96–7). Abrupt 2:1 AV block still occurs when the atrial cycle length drops below the total atrial refractory period.

Other features designed to modulate upper-rate behavior include rate-adaptive AV delay. This feature shortens the AV delay at faster atrial rates as occurs in normal physiology. In addition, the total atrial refractory period is shortened, allowing for tracking of faster rates. If, for example, the programmed AV delay shortens by 50 ms at faster atrial rates, the total atrial refractory period shortens by 50 ms. If the total atrial refractory period is 450 ms and therefore shortens to 400 ms, the upper tracking rate may be increased to a heart rate of 150 bpm from 133 bpm. Rates greater than 150 bpm would still result in 2:1 block. Rate smoothing is a programmable feature that may be used to prevent abrupt fixed rate block. This feature prevents abrupt changes in cycle length by limiting the maximal change between consecutively paced beats to a programmed value. At rates exceeding the upper tracking rate, the ventricular rate falls gradually to the 2:1 block rate or to the sensor rate if rate responsiveness is programmed on. Although rate smoothing may occur at the expense of AV synchrony, this may be less important at rates exceeding 100 bpm.[106]

Pacemaker Modes and Clinical Application

An understanding of the operational characteristics of pacemaker modes is essential to ensure optimal mode settings for specific conduction disturbances. Table 96–4 reviews a general consensus of appropriate modes for various pacing indications.

Single-Chamber Modes

VVI

The VVI mode, or "ventricular demand" pacing, prevents the ventricular rate from decreasing below a programmed lower rate limit (LRL). The ventricle is paced and sensed, and pacemaker output is inhibited when an intrinsic QRS occurs. The clinical use of VVI pacing is most appropriate in the setting of chronic atrial fibrillation and AV block.[60, 107, 108] VVI pacing is not recommended for patients who have normal atrial function, paroxysmal atrial fibrillation, or sick sinus syndrome.[61] In such patients, it is preferred to maintain AV synchrony by use of other pacing modes to optimize hemodynamics, avoid the symptoms of pacemaker syndrome, and decrease the future development of atrial fibrillation.[6] For patients with a short life expectancy or individuals are incapacitated because of severe illness, VVI pacing is acceptable.

VVT

The VVT mode is primarily reserved for diagnostic applications. In this mode, sensing of an intrinsic QRS complex immediately triggers a pacemaker stimulus. If no intrinsic rhythm is present, the device essentially operates identically to the VVI mode and paces at the programmed LRL.

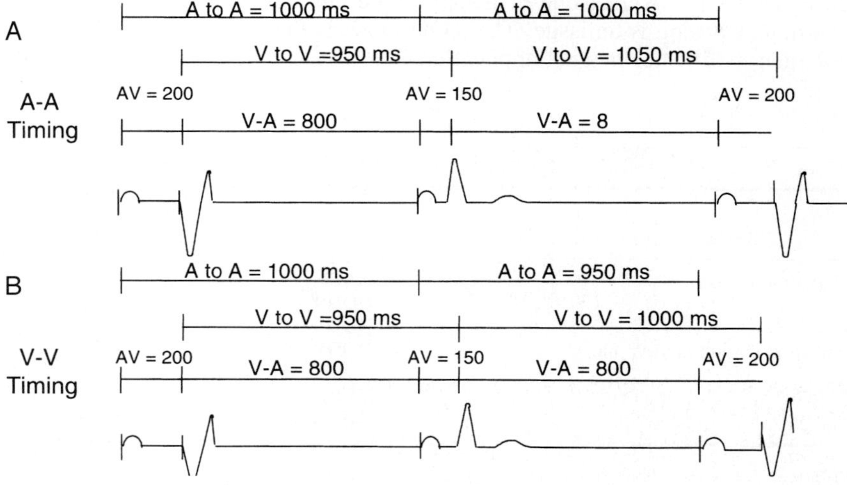

FIGURE 96–6 Atrial- and ventricular-based timing. **A,** In atrial-based timing, the AA interval is fixed, in this example at 1000 ms. The first and last complexes have paced atrioventricular (AV) intervals at the programmed value of 200 ms. The middle complex has a shortened AV interval of 150 ms because of native AV conduction. This results in a first VV interval of 950 ms and a second VV interval lengthened to 1050 ms. **B,** In ventricular-based timing, the ventriculoatrial (VA) interval is fixed, in this case at 800 ms. Shortening of the middle AV interval to 150 ms because of native conduction results in variation of both the AA and the VV intervals.

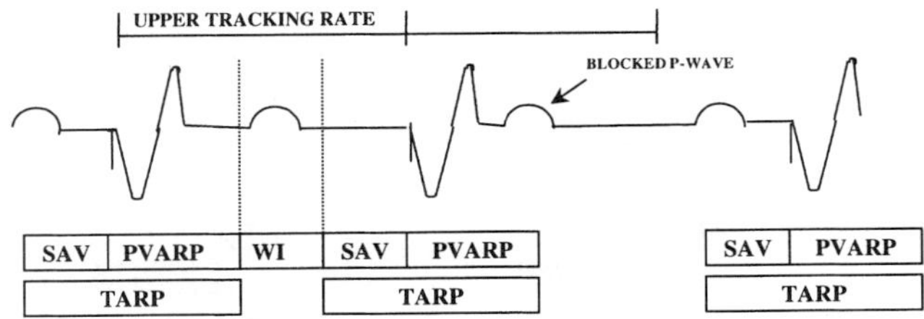

FIGURE 96–7 Wenckebach upper-rate behavior. The first atrial-sensed event is tracked, and ventricular pacing occurs at the sensed atrioventricular (SAV) interval. The second atrial event occurs after the postventricular atrial refractory period (PVARP) and is therefore sensed. Triggering of an SAV interval at this point would result in a paced event at a rate faster than the upper tracking rate (UTR). The SAV interval is thus extended by the Wenckebach interval (WI) such that the resultant VV interval occurs at the UTR. The third atrial event occurs within the PVARP and is not tracked, resulting in a blocked P wave. The fourth atrial event is sensed and an SAV interval is triggered as the UTR interval has ended. The cycle may then be repeated, resulting in a 3:2 Wenckebach pattern. TARP, total atrial refractory period.

The VVT mode may be used to pace terminate hemodynamically stable monomorphic VT. By applying external electrical stimuli to the chest wall that are sensed by the device, pacing stimuli are triggered. In this way, rapid external stimuli may be applied, giving rise to rapid ventricular pacing. Similarly, this technique may be utilized to perform a noninvasive EPS. These procedures are not necessary with current pacemaker models, which have noninvasive programmed stimulation capability. At the bedside, the VVT mode may be useful in assessing for oversensing. While telemetry is being observed, triggering of ventricular pacing would be noted to occur by nonspecific sensed events.

VOO

In the VOO mode, ventricular pacing occurs at a fixed rate with no relationship to the underlying, spontaneous heart rhythm. The earliest pacemakers functioned in this mode only. The risk of "R on T" induction of a malignant ventricular arrhythmia is a concern, although it has been observed rarely.[109] The clinical use of VOO pacing is limited. It may be considered in patients who are pacemaker dependent when oversensing or inappropriate inhibition of ventricular pacing is an issue. The VOO mode is the most common mode after magnet application.

AAI

The AAI mode is the atrial correlate of VVI. The atrium is paced, sensed, and inhibited by P waves. An atrial refractory period is longer than the corresponding ventricular refractory period in order to avoid far-field sensing of ventricular EGMs. The use of AAI pacing is far more common in Europe than in the United States. In sick sinus syndrome with normal AV conduction, the superiority of AAI pacing over VVI pacing in reducing the incidence of atrial fibrillation has been suggested by numerous studies.[6, 110]

Many physicians still opt for dual-chamber pacing in the setting of sinoatrial disease with normal AV conduction because of the concern of future AV block. However, in patients with a normal PR interval, no bundle branch block, and demonstrable 1:1 AV conduction at atrial rates of greater than 120 beats per minute, the annual incidence of second- or third-degree AV block is less than 1 percent per year.[111] It is estimated that AAI pacing could safely be used in approximately 40 percent of patients with sick sinus syndrome.[99]

AAT and *AOO* modes are seldom used but may serve functions similar to those described for the corresponding ventricular modes.

Dual-Chamber Modes

DDD

The DDD mode provides dual-chamber pacing, sensing, and dual mode of response. Four electrocardiographic patterns may be observed while the device is programmed in a DDD mode. Atrial sensing followed by ventricular pacing (AS-VP) occurs when the intrinsic atrial rate exceeds the LRL, and native AV conduction is either not present or longer than the programmed AV interval. This pattern illustrates ventricular "tracking" of the intrinsic atrial rhythm. When the intrinsic atrial rate is slower than the LRL and the AV interval duration completes before a native QRS does, atrial pacing and ventricular pacing (AP-VP) ensues. Should native AV conduction be faster than the programmed AV interval, a ventricular paced stimulus will not occur (AP-VS). Lastly, when the intrinsic atrial rate exceeds the LRL and native AV conduction is faster than the programmed AV interval, no pacing occurs (AS-VS).

The value of dual-chamber pacing over single-chamber pacing is the maintenance of AV synchrony, providing optimal hemodynamics in AV block. A diminished risk

TABLE 96–4 Recommended Pacing Modes and Programmable Features

Clinical Diagnosis	Pacing Mode and Programmable Feature(s)	Inappropriate Pacing Mode
Sinoatrial disease	AAIR DDDR	VVI
AV block	DDD	DDI, VVI
Sinoatrial disease and AV block	DDDR and automatic mode switching if a history of paroxysmal atrial fibrillation	VVI
Chronic atrial fibrillation and AV block	VVIR	DDD
Malignant vasovagal syncope	DDD with rate-drop response	VVI

Abbreviation: AV, atrioventricular.

of atrial fibrillation and mortality have been reported in subgroups.[63, 65] DDD pacing may also be successfully used in patients with cardioinhibitory syncope when combined with the rate-drop feature, as is discussed later. Prior to the development of automatic mode switching, a disadvantage of the DDD mode was ventricular tracking of rapid atrial tachyarrhythmias.

DDI

The DDI mode differs from the DDD mode in that no ventricular tracking of intrinsic atrial activity can occur. The device paces the atrium if the atrial rate is slower than the programmed LRL. At atrial rates exceeding the LRL, atrial pacing is inhibited, and the ventricle is paced as if in the VVI mode. This prevents tracking of atrial tachyarrhythmias. DDI pacing is often the conversion mode of automatic mode switching algorithms when an atrial tachyarrhythmia is detected in the DDD mode. The availability of automatic mode switching has made the need for DDI programming infrequent.

DVI

The DVI mode is similar to the DDI mode, except only the ventricle is sensed. Nonsensing of atrial activity gives rise to asynchronous atrial pacing and may increase the risk of atrial fibrillation. The DVI mode is rarely used. It may be seen functionally if sensing failure of the atrial lead occurs.

VDD

In the VDD mode, the atrium is sensed but not paced. In the setting of complete heart block and normal sinus node function, ventricular tracking and AV synchrony are maintained. The VDD mode may be accomplished with the use of a single tripolar lead with a sensing electrode within the atrial chamber. The disadvantage of the VDD mode is the loss of AV synchrony should the intrinsic atrial rate fall below the LRL.

Magnet Mode

All pacemakers contain a magnetic reed switch within the PG, which is activated by magnet application. The application of this switch disables all pacemaker sensing, leading to asynchronous pacing in either the VOO or the DOO mode. Dual-chamber devices programmed DDD may be converted to either the VOO or the DOO mode, depending on the model of the device. Removal of the magnet returns the device to its original mode. Some devices may have the magnet response programmed off and are not affected by magnet application.

Magnet application can provide valuable information. Depending on the pacemaker model, each device paces at specific rates relative to the battery status. Asynchronous pacing rates with magnet application identify batteries of normal status, those requiring elective replacement, and those at end of life. Patients observed to have inappropriate pauses on telemetry may be assessed for oversensing with magnet application at the bedside. If the pauses are eliminated in the asynchronous mode, oversensing, as opposed to failed pacemaker output, is confirmed. In the presence of ventricular tracking of atrial tachyarrhythmia, magnet application may help diagnose the atrial rhythm, for example, by uncovering atrial flutter waves during asynchronous ventricular pacing.

Pacemaker Syndrome

The pacemaker syndrome refers to a variety of symptoms classically associated with VVI pacing in patients with normal sinus activity. The mechanism is attributed to retrograde VA conduction during ventricular systole with subsequent atrial contraction against closed AV valves. Clinical signs may include the presence of "cannon A waves" on examination of the jugular venous pressure waveform. Symptoms may range from mild shortness of breath, fatigue, and neck pulsations to overt congestive heart failure and syncope.[112, 113] It is now recognized that the hemodynamic perturbations caused by the loss of AV synchrony alone are enough to cause symptoms of the pacemaker syndrome, and these perturbations may be seen in any pacing mode. The adverse consequences of the loss of atrial kick are particularly manifest in conditions with diastolic dysfunction in which the additional preload contributed by atrial systole significantly improves cardiac output and maintains hemodynamic stability.[114]

Chronic loss of AV synchrony has been shown to correlate with neurohormonal changes that may also contribute to persistent hypotension and risk of syncope.[115] Levels of atrial natriuretic peptide have been shown to be higher in patients with normal sinus activity paced in VVI mode as compared with DDD mode.[115] Elevated levels of atrial natriuretic peptide have been demonstrated to have well-defined vasodilator properties, contributing to lower blood pressure levels in patients with pacemaker syndrome.[116]

Definitive management of patients with pacemaker syndrome is restoration of AV synchrony. In some patients, symptoms may be diminished by decreasing the LRL and using the hysteresis feature to lengthen the interval before the first paced beat, thereby allowing a longer time for sinus rhythm to emerge.

Special Pacemaker Features

Rate-Adaptive Pacing

Cardiac output is defined as the product of stroke volume and heart rate. During exercise, a normally contracting ventricle consumes its stroke volume reserve before achieving 50 percent of maximal exertional activity.[117] Peak cardiac output may be achieved only by an appropriate increase in heart rate. In patients with poorly contracting ventricles, maximizing cardiac output is further dependent on increasing heart rate because stroke volume may be fixed.[118] The need for hemodynamic support in patients with chronotropic incompetence or atrial fibrillation with AV block has led to the development of artificial sensors to provide rate responsiveness. In addition, physiologic AV coupling may now be achieved by a programmable feature that allows AV shortening in response to increasing heart rate.

Artificial sensor designs have been based on *activity detection* via body movements or monitoring of *physiologic parameters* associated with exercise. The first activity sensor that was approved utilized a *piezoelectric crystal* attached to the inner case of the PG.[119] In response to *vibration*, the piezoelectric crystal generates an electrical output that signals the PG microprocessor of an increased activity level. Rate-responsiveness is triggered according to physician-selected parameters defining the signal threshold, acceleration (deceleration) slope of heart rate, and maximal upper sensor rate. The electrical signal of the sensor is proportional to the strength of its vibration. Thus, running generates a greater rate response than walking. Difficulties with the vibration sensor are encountered during certain activities, such as swimming and bicycling, that lack significant vibration. Additionally, inappropriate rate response may occur as a result of vibration transmitted from extraneous sources, such as bumpy roads and loud music. The *accelerometer* is a variation of the vibration system. This design removes the piezoelectric crystal from the inner PG case, diminishing the influence of body vibration.[120] The piezoelectric crystal is suspended within the PG and emits its signals in response to changes in body movements beyond those ordinarily occurring with running and walking. This allows for improved response to activities such as swimming and bicycling. Although the accelerometer is more sensitive to a variety of activities, it may still fail to provide adequate rate response when body movements may decline during increased strain, as in bicycling uphill. Spurious rate-responsiveness may be diminished with the accelerometer.

Physiologic sensors were designed in the hope of providing rate responsiveness that is more proportional to physiologic demand. These sensors are based on the premise that metabolic demand may be predicted by a monitored change in a physiologic parameter. *Minute ventilation* sensing is achieved by detecting changes in chest wall impedance and in respiratory rate. Chest wall impedance changes because of fluctuations in inspiratory/expiratory effort.[121] The advantage of this technique is the known linear relationship of O_2 uptake and workload. This sensor parameter responds well to various physical and emotional demands by virtue of its accurate estimation of true minute volume. *Central venous temperature* sensing relies on measurement of right ventricular temperature via a thermistor in the pacemaker lead and is based on the assumption that increased muscular activity generates heat and warms the blood.[122] Temperature elevation due to fever or hot baths increases heart rate. *Evoked QT interval* rate responsiveness takes advantage of the electrocardiographic QT interval response to sympathetic tone, which is independent of the observed QT shortening seen with increasing heart rate.[123] An individual with chronotropic incompetence exhibits QT shortening in response to catecholamines alone, which is detected from the paced stimulus to the end of the T wave. The degree of shortening generates a rate response. This algorithm depends on the presence of pacing and requires the documentation of adequate T-wave sensing. Numerous other physiologic sensors have been investigated or are under development, including sensors monitoring blood pH, stroke volume, and mixed venous O_2 saturation.[119]

Some newer devices are now incorporating a combination of an activity sensor and a physiologic sensor.[124, 125] This dual-sensor technique aims to overcome the relative strengths and limitations of each method alone. Sophisticated PG circuitry allows for dual sensors to reach a consensus on the ideal rate-responsive needs during exercise and thereby enhances the specificity of rate adaptation. The clinical benefit of this method awaits further testing.

Hysteresis

Hysteresis is a feature that is designed to promote optimal hemodynamics and preserve battery life. The hysteresis rate is a separate escape rate that follows sensed events and is programmed lower than the LRL. The hysteresis rate comes into effect anytime a native beat is sensed and is maintained if intrinsic complexes continue. This allows extra time for sinus rhythm to emerge before the onset of pacing. After paced events, the escape rate is at the LRL. Observation of the electrocardiogram indicates two escape intervals, the LRL following paced events and the hysteresis rate interval following sensed events (Fig. 96–8).

Hysteresis can be applied to the AV interval in patients with variable AV conduction. In a DDD mode, the ability to achieve intrinsic AV conduction is "searched" on an intermittent basis by adding an additional time duration (e.g., 50 ms) to the programmed AV interval for one cycle. If a sensed QRS occurs during this added time, the device maintains this AV interval. When a native QRS fails to occur during this new interval, ventricular pacing resumes at the programmed AV interval. Conversely, AV interval hysteresis may be applied in order to ensure that ventricular pacing is maintained. In hypertrophic obstructive cardiomyopathy, it has been suggested that left bundle branch block induced by pacing minimizes outflow tract obstruction. In this context, a "reverse" AV interval hysteresis may be programmed to intermittently search for a sensed QRS. If a sensed QRS is detected, the programmed AV

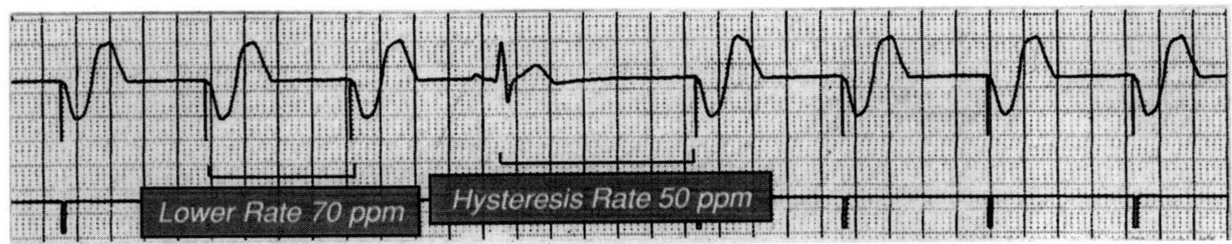

FIGURE 96–8 Hysteresis. The pacemaker paces at the programmed lower rate interval of 70 beats/min. When a sensed beat occurs, pacing does not resume until the heart falls to the hysteresis rate of 50 pulses per minute (ppm).

interval is shortened. The new AV interval persists if ventricular pacing ensues.

Automatic Mode Switching

The introduction of automatic mode switching in the early 1990s was a significant advancement for the management of intermittent atrial tachyarrhythmias in dual-chamber systems. In the DDD or VDD modes, the presence of an atrial arrhythmia leads to ventricular tracking to the MTR. Although this may be prevented by DDI or DVI programming, these modes are not appropriate in patients with predominant normal sinus activity and AV block. Clinical evaluation of the use of mode switching algorithms in dual-chamber systems has confirmed a significant improvement in quality of life for most patients.[126, 127]

Most devices manufactured in the United States use a similar algorithm in their approach to automatic mode switching. A programmable atrial detection rate is selected with which all AA intervals are compared. When a specified number of AA intervals exceed the detection rate and continue to do so over a programmable time duration, mode switching occurs. The ventricular response to atrial-sensed events is changed from a tracking to nontracking mode. Depending on the initially programmed mode and the manufacturer model, the mode may change to DDI(R), VVI(R), or VDI(R). Additional features of mode switching prevent an abrupt decline in heart rate. A programmable or automatic *fallback time duration* allows a gradual decrease in heart rate to the LRL or sensor-indicated rate (if a rate-responsive mode is on). AA intervals continue to be monitored, and when they decline to less than the detection rate on a consistent basis, reversion to the originally programmed mode occurs.

Rate-Drop Response

The rate-drop response algorithm was designed for patients with neurally mediated syncope and a cardioinhibitory response alone or combined with a vasodepressor component.[128] A detection bradycardia rate zone is programmed with a specified slope of heart rate change needed to trigger the rate-drop response. Should the heart rate enter this detection zone precipitously and exceed the acceptable slope of heart rate change, the pacemaker intervenes with "overshoot" DDD pacing in an attempt to compensate for any vasodepressor component. The intervention pacing rate and duration are programmable. Episodes are stored in the device diagnostics and may be reviewed at routine follow-up.

The effect of the rate-drop response was evaluated in the North American Vasovagal Pacemaker Study.[47] As discussed previously, patients with frequent neurally mediated syncope (greater than six episodes) and documented bradycardia on tilt-table testing were randomly assigned to standard medical therapy or to pacemaker implantation with rate-drop therapy at an intervention pacing rate of 100 bpm. The trial was terminated early because of a large benefit in favor of the pacemaker group. Further studies are needed to clarify the role of pacing and optimal rate-drop algorithm programming.

Use of Pacemaker Diagnostics

Diagnosis of Tachyarrhythmias

Although the vast majority of patients receive permanent pacemakers for symptomatic bradycardia, co-existing paroxysmal tachyarrhythmias are common. Most current pacemakers provide the option for storage of detected atrial and/or ventricular episodes exceeding a programmable rate. An atrial high rate episode is detected when *four of seven* PP intervals exceed the programmed rate. Detection of a high-rate ventricular episode occurs when a programmed number of *consecutive* RR intervals exceed the selected detection rate. Details indicating the number of episodes, date/time, duration, and maximal chamber heart rate are displayed during pacemaker interrogation (Fig. 96–9). In patients with nonspecific symptoms possibly related to tachyarrhythmia events, patient-triggered recording of heart rhythm during an episode may be accomplished by use of a hand-held remote. EGMs from both chambers are stored, thereby facilitating diagnosis (Fig. 96–10). The use of these diagnostics may eliminate the need for Holter monitoring

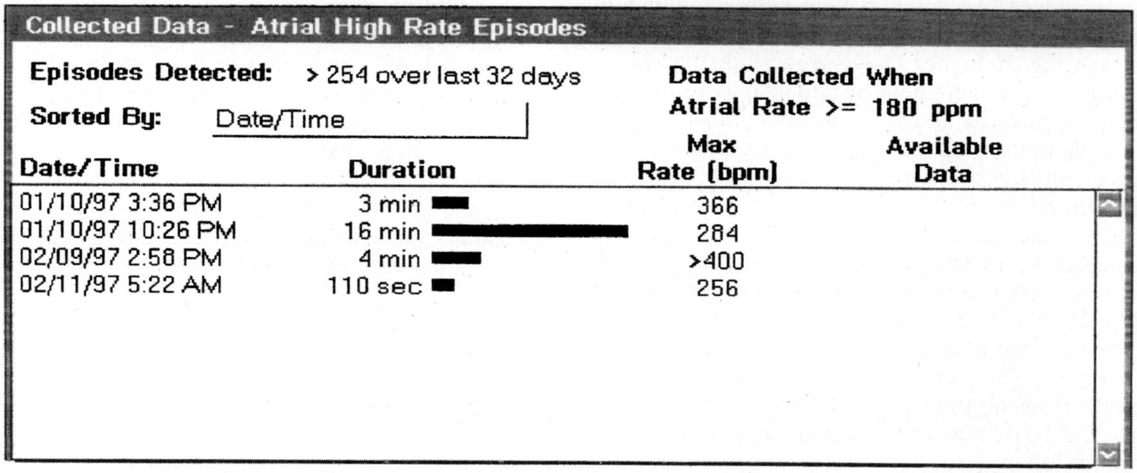

Collected Data - Atrial High Rate Episodes

Episodes Detected: > 254 over last 32 days

Sorted By: Date/Time

Data Collected When Atrial Rate >= 180 ppm

Date/Time	Duration	Max Rate (bpm)	Available Data
01/10/97 3:36 PM	3 min	366	
01/10/97 10:26 PM	16 min	284	
02/09/97 2:58 PM	4 min	>400	
02/11/97 5:22 AM	110 sec	256	

FIGURE 96–9 Diagnostic data of high-rate atrial episodes since last pacemaker interrogation are displayed.

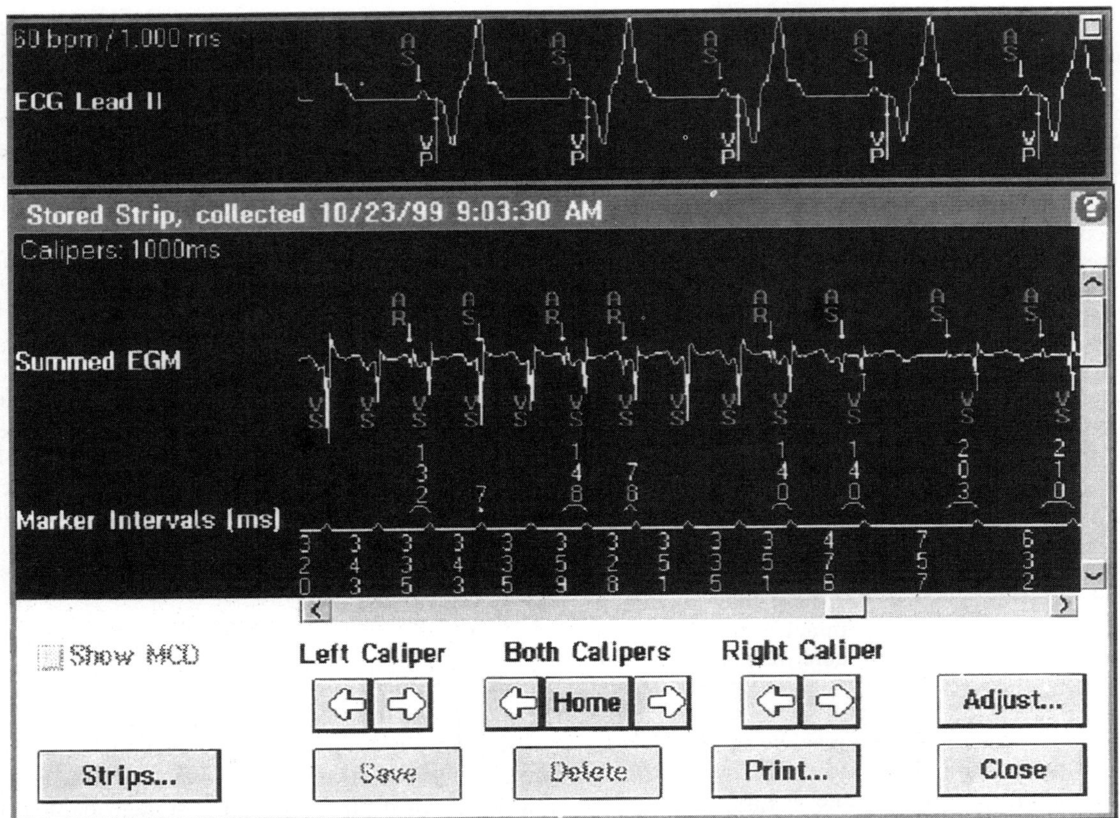

FIGURE 96–10 Stored electrograms (EGMs) of a high-rate ventricular episode. Analysis of the summed atrial and ventricular EGMs shows nonsustained ventricular tachycardia with atrial-sensed (AS) events dissociated from ventricular-sensed (VS) events. The last two beats are normal sinus rhythm. The electrocardiogram (ECG) strip at the top is the rhythm during device interrogation. AR, atrial-sensed event during total atrial refractory period; MCD, marker channel diagram (this is a "hidden" command on the screen and is rarely shown/used).

and provides the opportunity to objectively monitor the efficacy of medical therapy for arrhythmia suppression.

Optimal Device Programming

Counter and *histogram* storage provides information on the number of paced and sensed events at specific heart rates. These data allow assessment of the appropriateness of programmed rate-adaptive pacing in patients with chronotropic incompetence. An active patient with symptoms of fatigue at peak exercise may show evidence of minimal pacing or sensing at higher rates, suggesting inadequate rate responsiveness. As a guide to rate-adaptive programming, most pacemakers allow for a programmer-directed exercise test that may be performed during a routine office visit. The patient is asked to perform an activity, such as a brisk walk. Based on the rate-adaptive setting, the device plots the heart rate versus time. Should the rate response appear inadequate, an alternative setting is programmed, and the device plots the expected rate response at the new setting (Fig. 96–11). Some devices now allow evaluation of the programmed rate-adaptive setting during the patient's specific activities. The patient may activate the device just before exercise, which triggers heart rate collection for up to 1 hour. The heart rate response during this activity is reviewed on a follow-up visit.

Counter and *histogram* data may also be useful in determining the appropriateness of the programmed AV interval in patients with sinoatrial disease and normal AV conduction. In this clinical context, it is preferable for native AV conduction rather than pacing to occur. This preserves battery life and maintains optimal hemodynamics. A high percentage of AP-VP counters suggests that prolonging the AV interval may be beneficial, depending on underlying AV conduction.

Some devices provide AV conduction histograms indicating the heart rates at which ventricular pacing events occur. Figure 96–12 shows that the pacemaker is preempting normal AV conduction at higher rates. This typically occurs because dynamic or rate-adaptive AV intervals are programmed shorter than native AV conduction at these heart rates. The patient may have native AV conduction measured during moderate exercise in the clinic. Programming the minimal dynamic AV interval longer than the measured value or programming on AV search hysteresis may allow native AV conduction at higher rates.

Monitoring System Function

The ability to automatically monitor trends in lead impedance and capture/sensing thresholds is now available in some devices. Automatic lead impedance measurements are performed daily at a consistent pacing amplitude and pulse width. Measurements are displayed in graphic form, indicating values at specific time intervals. This information may allow early detection of potential lead failure before such problems jeopardize patient safety. A gradual decline in lead impedance may be a sign of an insulation break, whereas an abrupt jump may suggest coil fracture. Some newer pacemakers provide a programmable option for periodic capture threshold measurements, which may be viewed on follow-up. In addition, automatic adjusting of pacing outputs to a selected safety margin may be enabled. This feature maintains patient safety while minimizing battery drain. Similarly, P- and R-wave amplitudes may be monitored and sensitivity thresholds adjusted automatically to ensure reliable sensing. Battery status is readily available on initial device interrogation, and the need for elective or urgent replacement is displayed.

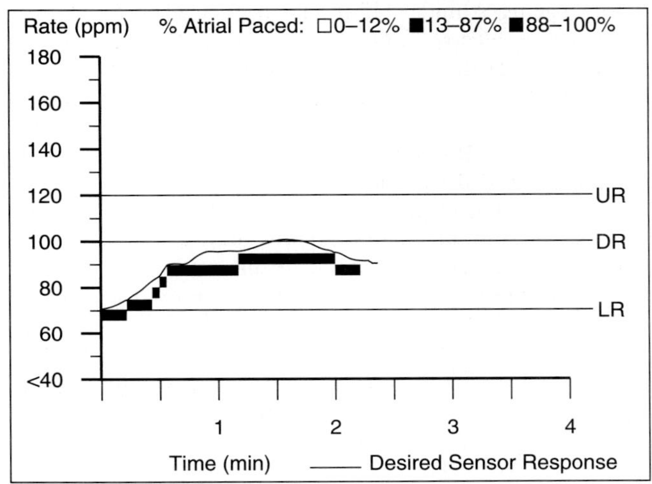

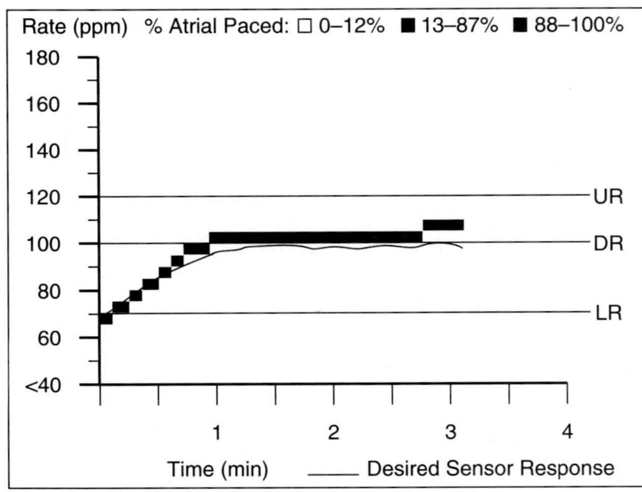

FIGURE 96–11 Plots of heart rate versus time for optimal rate-adaptive programming. The *narrow line* depicts the desired sensor rate for the activity, whereas the *heavy line* is the actual sensor-indicated rate. **Top,** An inadequate rate response during moderate activity is shown. **Bottom,** After reprogramming to an increased rate-adaptive threshold, the device plots the expected rate response for the same amount of activity and more closely approximates the desired sensor response. This assessment is performed during a clinic visit.

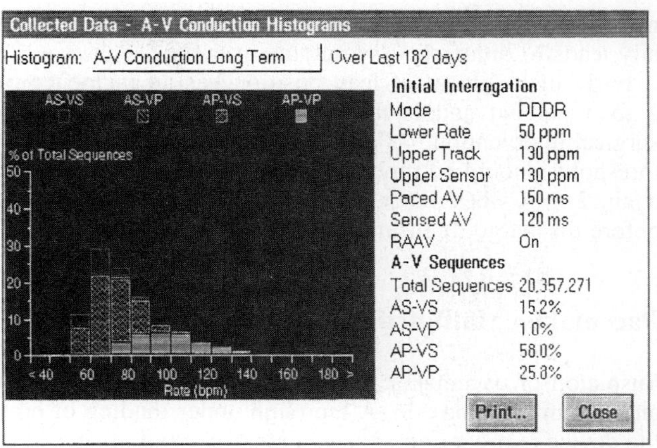

FIGURE 96–12 Atrioventricular (AV) conduction histogram indicates a high percentage of ventricular pacing (25.8%) in a patient with intact AV conduction. Appropriate programming of AV intervals and AV search hysteresis may promote native AV conduction.
AP-VP, atrial-paced event followed by ventricular-paced event; AP-VS, atrial-paced event followed by ventricular-sensed event; AS-VP, atrial-sensed event followed by ventricular-paced event; AS-VS, atrial-sensed event followed by ventricular-sensed event.

Procedure-Related Pacemaker Complications

Procedural-related complications are principally related to venous access, lead placement, and pocket healing. Inadvertent lung puncture during attempted venous access may lead to pneumothorax. This occurs in approximately 2 percent of patients and is related to operator experience.[129] During lead placement, care must be taken to avoid air suction through the venous sheath, causing air embolus, which may prove fatal.[130] Myocardial perforation by the pacing lead occurs rarely and may be unrecognized because of the frequent absence of symptoms. Evidence of a right bundle branch pacing pattern suggests pericardial or left ventricular lead position. After the procedure, a friction rub may be audible. Development of cardiac tamponade is unusual, but if it occurs, it typically does so within 24 hours.[131]

Pacemaker pocket infections may present with local erythema, abscess formation, or fever of unknown cause. Patients at increased risk include diabetics, corticosteroid users, and those with a temporary pacing wire in place.[132] Early infection is most commonly caused by *Staphylococcus aureus*, whereas late infection is usually caused by *Staphylococcus epidermidis*. Late infections may be associated with wound dehiscence or device erosion.[133] Evidence of pacemaker infection generally mandates removal of the entire system because lead involvement is common.[134] The use of prophylactic antibiotics has been shown to significantly reduce the risk of infection.[135] Various durations and timings of antibiotic therapy are reported.[136] In general, antistaphylococcal antibiotics are administered 2 hours before the procedure and maintained for 24 hours.

Symptomatic venous occlusion occurs infrequently despite evidence on contrast venography of significant subclavian vein obstruction in up to 40 percent of patients.[137] In the event of symptoms or notable edema, conservative management with short-term anticoagulation is recommended.[137, 138] The development of venous collaterals usually leads to diminished symptoms over time.

Early dislodgment of lead position has an incidence of 2 to 5 percent and is the most common cause of early surgical intervention.[139] For this reason, capture and sensing thresholds should be repeated on postprocedural day 1 and again 2 to 4 weeks later. A chest x-ray should be viewed before discharge to ensure appropriate lead position.

Pacemaker Malfunction

Suspicion of pacemaker malfunction requires a thoughtful and organized approach. A thorough understanding of how the device is programmed is essential to avoid misinterpretation of normal pacemaker behavior. Special features, such as automatic mode switch, hysteresis, and rate-drop behavior, may lead to the false conclusion of erratic pacemaker activity. Once the physician is comfortable with the programmed features and the nature of their response, he or she may undertake a stepwise approach.

Failure to Pace

A first approach to suspected failure to pace is to observe the *presence* or *absence of the pacing stimulus* (Fig. 96–13). In situations where the pacing stimulus is present without capture, the appropriateness of the timed stimulus should be determined on the basis of the programmed settings. An appropriately timed stimulus that fails to capture may indicate elevation of pacing thresholds and may reflect a problem at the electrode-tissue interface. After adequate pacemaker output settings are confirmed, consideration of drug effect or metabolic abnormalities is warranted. Type 1A and 1C antiarrhythmic agents have been noted to adversely effect pacing thresholds.[140, 141] Hyperkalemia may also increase pacemaker output requirements as well as pose a risk of malignant arrhythmias.[141] Myocardial infarction may lead to scarring in the vicinity of the electrode. Lead insulation defects or coil fracture may attenuate the pacemaker output. A common site of lead damage is at the junction of the first rib and clavicle, where chronic forces on the lead may precipitate damage. A thorough assessment of failure to pace with an appropriately timed stimulus should include a test of capture thresholds and lead impedance, a chest x-ray for lead assessment, a relevant history, and a routine metabolic profile.

The presence of an apparently inappropriately timed pacing stimulus without capture may reflect normal pacemaker function. Electrode sensing of an intrinsic QRS complex occurring very near the programmed escape interval may not occur until after some degree of surface electrocardiographic deflection. The resulting QRS is a fusion of the native QRS and paced QRS with an interposed pacing stimulus. If the intrinsic QRS deflection on the surface electrocardiogram is completed before it is sensed, a pacing stimulus occurs on the latter part of the QRS complex without apparent capture. This phenomenon is referred to as *pseudofusion* (Fig. 96–14). Fusion and pseudofusion QRS complexes give the impression of inappropriately timed and failed pacing stimuli but actually do occur according to programmed settings. True inappropriate pacing stimuli without capture may occur because of *undersensing*. Lack of capture in this setting results from pacing during the refractory period of the myocardium.

Failure to pace early after implant (less than 30 days) without evidence of a pacing stimulus usually reflects lead dislodgment or loose connectors. Later development raises the concern of *oversensing*. Oversensing may have many causes, including myopotential sensing, "electrical chatter" from lead defects, atrial/ventricular cross-talk, and T-wave sensing. Myopotential sensing is more common with unipolar systems and is often induced by arm movements. Electrical chatter may be secondary to lead fracture, an

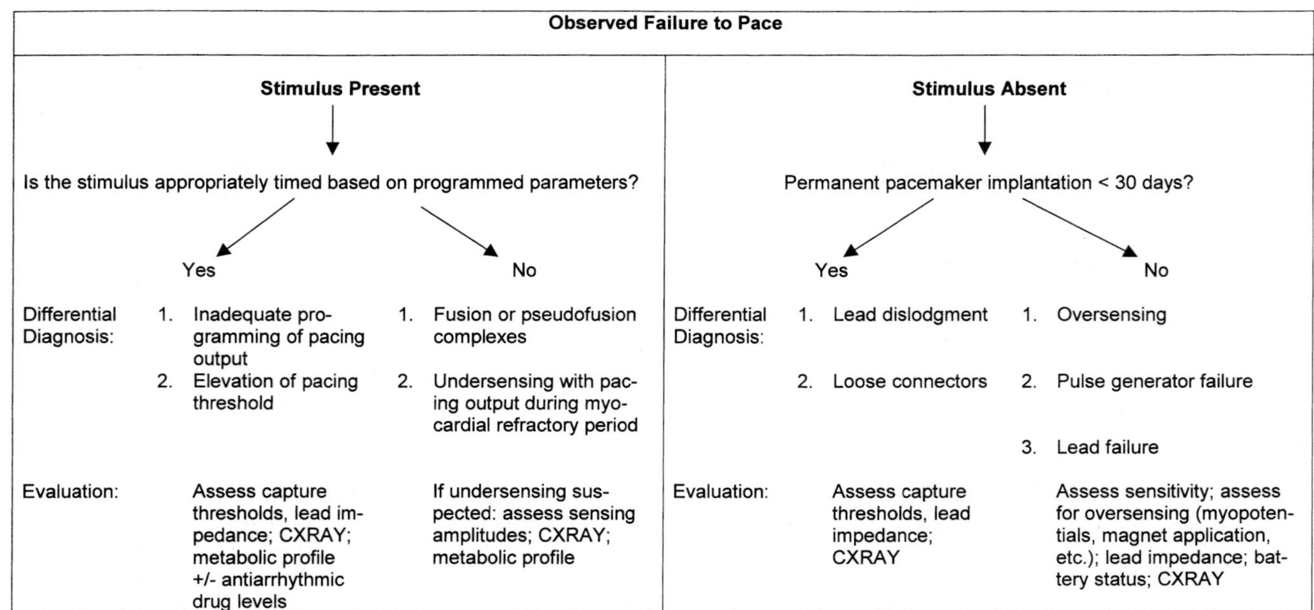

FIGURE 96–13 An approach to pacemaker failure to pace. CXRAY, chest x-ray.

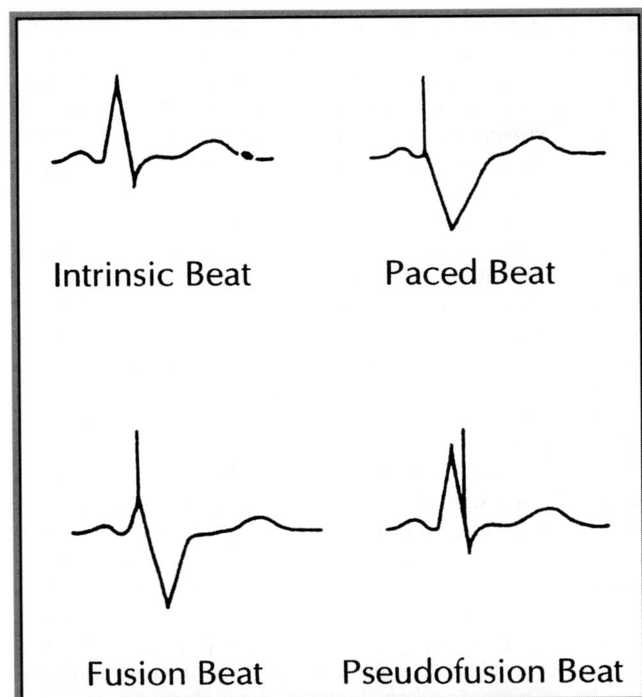

FIGURE 96–14 Fusion and pseudofusion complexes. The fusion complex is a composite of intrinsic and paced beats. A pseudofusion complex has the QRS morphology of the intrinsic beat with an interposed pacing stimulus. These complexes may be seen in normal pacemaker function.

insulation defect, or loose connectors. Pacemaker cross-talk occurs when the ventricular sensing amplifier interprets the atrial pacing stimulus as an intrinsic ventricular beat. The ventricular output is then inhibited, and only atrial pacing proceeds. Current dual-chamber pacemaker systems avoid this problem with blanking periods and a programmable "safety pacing" feature. If a ventricular sensed event occurs within a short interval after an atrial pacing stimulus is delivered, a ventricular paced event is delivered with a short AV delay. If this sensed event is a premature ventricular contraction, the short AV delay prevents R on T pacing. Safety pacing does not prevent cross-talk but will prevent asystole. The presence of safety pacing must be recognized and appropriate steps taken to correct cross-talk. This may involve decreasing atrial output and ventricular sensitivity or, infrequently, new lead positioning.

Magnet application may confirm the presence of oversensing by disabling sensing and allowing the return of regular pacing. If pacing does not resume, lead failure or primary PG failure is suspected. Management of oversensing includes decreasing device sensitivity and assessing for myopotentials through physical arm movements while observing telemetry. Suspected lead failure requires evaluation of lead impedance and chest x-ray. T-wave oversensing is resolved by prolonging the ventricular refractory period.

Failure of Pacing Inhibition

Failure of pacemaker inhibition is recognized by the presence of paced complexes at inappropriately short intervals. With the exception of the normal function of safety pacing, this is invariably caused by undersensing. Attenuation of sensing signals may be the result of a lead insulation defect or a coil fracture. EGM signals may be diminished as a result of altered tissue substrate in the setting of hyperkalemia, class IA/IC antiarrhythmic drug use, or myocardial scar formation.[141] Assessment of undersensing necessitates evaluation of R- and P-wave amplitude and increasing sensitivity as required. Lead impedance measurements and chest x-ray should be reviewed. A metabolic profile and antiarrhythmic drug review may be required.

Pacemaker-Mediated Tachycardia

PMT, also known as endless loop tachycardia, is unique to dual-chamber systems. PMT may develop when a premature ventricular contraction results in VA conduction. The retrograde P wave triggers an AV interval and a ventricular paced beat, which may again conduct retrograde and perpetuate the cycle.[142] PMT is analogous to antidromic AV reentry tachycardia with the accessory AV connection mediated by the pacemaker. PMT is most often initiated by a premature ventricular contraction. Transient loss of atrial capture, sensing, or myopotential ventricular tracking may also result in VA conduction and PMT.[142] There are two prerequisites for the initiation of PMT. First, retrograde VA conduction, which is present in up to 50 percent of patients receiving dual-chamber devices for standard indications, must be intact.[142] Second, a retrograde P wave must occur outside of the programmed PVARP in order for triggering of the AV interval and ventricular pacing to occur. PMT typically persists at the programmed MTR. As with other reentry tachycardias involving the AV node, PMT may be terminated by vagal maneuvers or adenosine. More commonly, magnet application quickly resolves the tachycardia by disabling sensing and initiating asynchronous pacing (VOO or DOO).

PMT may be avoided by assessing for VA conduction while in VVI mode. Should retrograde conduction be present, the PVARP can be programmed to exceed the VA conduction time. However, in cases of a prolonged VA conduction time, too long a PVARP (and therefore total atrial refractory period) leads to unwanted restrictions on the programmable MTR. Most devices now employ one of several algorithms to prevent or terminate PMT. One method automatically extends the PVARP for one cycle when a ventricular sensed event not preceded by an atrial event is detected, returning to the programmed PVARP thereafter. Another algorithm turns off atrial sensing after an isolated ventricular sensed event, adapting a DVI mode for a single cycle and preventing PMT. Automatic PMT termination algorithms in many devices insert a single long PVARP whenever tracking at the MTR is detected. If the tachycardia represents PMT, it is terminated.

"Runaway pacemaker" is a rare malfunction caused by PG circuit failure. Paced rates exceeding the MTR may occur and are unaffected by magnet application. PG circuit failure leading to runaway pacemaker has been reported secondary to electrocautery and radiation therapy.[143, 144] Treatment requires surgical removal of the device.

Pacemaker Interference

Pacemakers with a unipolar sensing configuration are more prone to high-energy electrical interference than are those with bipolar sensing configurations.[145] As previously discussed, this reflects the greater area encompassed by the sensing circuit and therefore the increased potential of sensing external electrical signals. Various pacemaker malfunctions may be observed as a result of electrical interference, most commonly inappropriate pacemaker inhibition or ventricular tracking.[146, 147] Modern devices are equipped with a "noise reversion mode." When electrical noise is consistently detected during a noise sampling period, the device paces asynchronously. Periodic noise sampling similarly detects the absence of the external noise and returns the pacemaker to its original mode.

In the hospital setting, electrocautery is the most common source of electrical interference.[148] Electrocautery used in close proximity to the PG or leads may precipitate noise sensing. Before the automatic noise reversion mode, devices were routinely programmed asynchronously before performing procedures using electrocautery. Magnetic resonance imaging is generally contraindicated in patients with devices, although there are multiple reports of magnetic resonance imaging being safely used in patients with pacemakers or implantable defibrillators.[146, 149] Although no permanent component damage has been reported, inhibition of pacing and inappropriate tracking have been observed.[150]

In the home environment, there are no reports of normally functioning domestic appliances causing any significant malfunction of modern pacemakers. Microwave ovens, electric shavers, portable telephones, or personal computers have not been linked to interference with modern pacemakers.

Theoretical complications from exposure to arc-welding, combustion engines, or power generators have traditionally led to advising against occupations involving contact with these sources. On brief exposure, metal detectors may induce transient single-beat inhibition or asynchronous pacing, which is of minimal clinical significance.[146] Electronic article surveillance systems utilizing acoustomagnetic equipment have been reported to induce inappropriate pacemaker inhibition and ventricular tracking on persistent device exposure.[147] Patients are recommended to walk briskly through such equipment. Cellular telephones have received much attention because of their increasing use. Preliminary studies indicated significant electromagnetic interference from cellular telephones.[146] Subsequently, a large multicenter study testing cellular phones produced by various manufacturers showed no clinically significant interference when telephones were tested during normal use.[151] Cellular phones of the digital variety have been observed to provoke intermittent pacemaker malfunction to a greater extent than analog cell telephones.[152] Because of the potential interference from cellular telephones, patients are advised to restrict usage to the opposite ear and not store the telephones inside inner coat pockets over the device.

Pacemaker Follow-Up

Approximately 500,000 patients in the United States have permanent pacemakers.[5] Most of the patients are older than 65 years and survive approximately 9 years after implantation.[153] This is approaching the expected life span of current PGs and emphasizes the need for efficient programming to extend battery life. In addition, despite the reliability of current pacemaker systems, up to 38 percent have complications or require specific intervention within the first year.[154] Dual-chamber systems are twice as likely as single-chamber systems to malfunction.[155] Although most can be corrected by reprogramming, up to 20 percent may go unrecognized.[156]

Pacemaker follow-up includes both office visits and trans-telephonic monitoring. Medicare and NASPE have published follow-up guidelines for both office and telephone surveillance.[157] The Medicare standards were set in 1984 and are in need of revision for current modern pacemaker systems. The NASPE guidelines that were issued in 1994 are listed in Table 96–5.[158] In both guidelines, follow-up is more frequent at the beginning and end of a pacemakers life span, reflecting the higher early need for intervention and the need for closer surveillance as the battery and the lead system age. Outpatient evaluations are best performed in specialized pacemaker clinics, which are more likely to identify pacing system problems.[156] Pacemaker clinics also allow for prompt identification and notification of patients when device or lead alerts occur.

The outpatient evaluation should consist of a relevant history and physical examination. Symptoms suggestive of pacemaker malfunction, pacemaker syndrome, or inappropriate programming, including dizziness or syncope, palpitations, muscle stimulation, shortness of breath, and exertional intolerance, should be noted. Fluctuations in systolic blood pressure and orthostatic changes may suggest pacemaker syndrome. The PG site should be examined for evidence of infection, erosion, "twiddler's syndrome," and muscle stimulation. For pectoral implants, evidence of sub-

TABLE 96–5 1994 NASPE Guidelines for Pacemaker Follow-Up

- Before discharge
  - Full clinic evaluation
  - CXR (PA + LAT), ECG
  - TTM transmitter education
- Discharge through 2 months
  - Full clinic evaluation
  - Program chronic settings as appropriate
  - Education reinforcement
  - No routine TTM
- Early surveillance (3–5 months)
  - One clinic or TTM evaluation
- Maintenance period (beginning at 6 months)
  - One full clinic evaluation yearly
  - Clinic evaluation or TTM with interview every 3 months
- Intensified follow-up period*
  - One full clinic evaluation yearly
  - Monthly clinic evaluation or TTM with interview every 4 weeks

Abbreviations: CXR, chest x-ray study; ECG, electrocardiogram; LAT, lateral; NASPE, North American Society of Pacing and Electrophysiology; PA, posteroanterior; TTM, transtelephonic monitoring.

*Begins at a time based on Medicare guidelines. For pacemakers with > 90% longevity at 5 years, whose output voltages decrease < 50% over 3 months and magnet rate decreases < 20% or 5 pulses over 3 months, this period begins at 73 months for single-chamber and 49 months for dual-chamber devices. For devices that do not meet the criteria, intensified surveillance begins at 37 months for single- and dual-chamber devices.

clavian vein thrombosis or rarely superior vena cava syndrome should be noted, and the jugular venous pulse should be examined for evidence of AV dyssynchrony. During cardiac auscultation a "pacemaker sound" may be heard infrequently after pacing and may be due to diaphragmatic or intercostal muscle stimulation.[159] Clicks and musical murmurs, possibly related to whipping of the lead on the tricuspid valve and movement of the lead within the right ventricle, have been described.[160, 161] A pericardial friction rub early after implantation may indicate perforation. A thorough history and examination may indicate specific programmed parameters that require special attention or evaluation.

The baseline interrogation assesses battery voltage and impedance, lead integrity, sensing and pacing thresholds, and stored diagnostic data. Determination of pacing and sensing thresholds is an integral part of the clinic visit. Pacing thresholds frequently change over the life of the pacing system, with one study demonstrating only approximately 40 percent of patients with stable long-term thresholds and 20 percent with rising thresholds.[162] When stable pacing thresholds allow, reducing the pacing output may significantly increase battery life. With appropriate reprogramming, battery life may be safely extended up to 4 to 5 years.[163] Nevertheless, up to 30 percent of pacing systems are left at manufacturer settings.[5] Sensing thresholds are measured in many ways, and some devices are capable of automatic measurements. In pacemaker-dependent patients without an adequate underlying escape rhythm, sensing assessment is not performed.

Transtelephonic monitoring is an important adjunct to the pacemaker clinic for pacing system follow-up. Typically, bracelet electrodes are attached to a transmitter, and, via a telephone adapter, rhythm strips are transmitted to the pacemaker clinic. A baseline strip and a strip during magnet application are routinely transmitted, allowing assessment of the baseline rhythm and magnet rate. Artifact sometimes limits interpretation, and dual-chamber undersensing and noncapture are less frequently identified than at a pacemaker clinic visit, but a partial assessment of pacing and/or sensing function is almost invariably obtainable.[164] Telephonic monitoring is very useful for battery decay monitoring and for acute rhythm assessment in patients with symptoms suggesting arrhythmias.

THE IMPLANTABLE CARDIOVERTER-DEFIBRILLATOR

Michael H. Gollob and John J. Seger

The ICD was first conceptualized by Dr. Michael Mirowski in the late 1960s after the death of a close colleague. While at the Sinai Hospital in Baltimore in 1969, Dr. Mirowski and colleagues successfully tested a prototype ICD in dogs.[165] This experimental model employed a right ventricular pressure sensor to detect ventricular fibrillation (VF). A modified pacing catheter electrode was inserted in the right ventricle, and an additional electrode implanted in the anterior chest wall completed the defibrillation circuit.

Since these early beginnings, the impetus for more sophisticated engineering of the ICD has grown. It is recognized that sudden cardiac death (SCD) accounts for an estimated 350,000 deaths annually in the United States alone.[166] Most of these events occur out of hospital and are associated with consequential delays in implementing external defibrillation. The ability of the ICD to provide therapy within 5 to 15 seconds of arrhythmia detection allows for defibrillation success rates approaching 100 percent.

The first human ICD implant occurred in 1980.[167] Approval for general use by the United States Food and Drug Administration was granted in 1985. The ICD has now become the treatment of choice for survivors of SCD and symptomatic sustained ventricular arrhythmias (AHA/ACC guidelines).[168] To date, roughly 200,000 patients around the world have received an ICD (personal communication, Medtronics).

Evolution of the ICD

System Function

The early ICDs of the 1980s had limited features. These devices were ordered by the physician specifying a detection heart rate and were delivered by the manufacturer to perform defibrillation-aggressive therapy should the ventricular rate exceed this value. Detection rates were not programmable, and the device could merely be turned on or off. These devices had obvious limitations. First, should initiation of an antiarrhythmic agent be required, VT rates could be slowed below preset detection rates. Subsequent advances have allowed programming of several detection zones, with the alternative of less aggressive therapy for termination of slower, hemodynamically stable VT. A second major limitation of early devices was the lack of rhythm discrimination capabilities. Sinus tachycardia or other supraventricular rhythms with rapid ventricular rates within a detection zone could not be discerned from ventricular-based rhythms, leading to a high incidence of inappropriate shocks. Analysis of stored EGMs and RR intervals in later device models confirmed a rate of inappropriate shocks ranging from 25 to 40 percent.[169–172] The development of sophisticated rhythm discrimination algorithms in the 1990s has resulted in the decline of the inappropriate shock rate to less than 5 percent.[173, 174]

The modern ICD may be equipped to perform routine dual-chamber pacing for bradycardia, obviating a separate procedure should a pacemaker be required. In addition, the risk of device cross-talk between the ICD and the pacemaker, leading to spurious shocks or failure to sense VF, is avoided. Cross-talk occurs when unipolar pacemakers and some bipolar pacemakers have their pacing pulses sensed by the ICD, leading to double or triple counting of a given heart rate in VVI or DDD pacing, respectively. Pacemaker pulses may also be detected as QRS complexes when VF truly exists, resulting in failure to deliver appropriate therapy.[175, 176]

Implantation

Although the Mirowski ICD prototype demonstrated successful defibrillation in dogs by use of a transvenous system, the high defibrillation energy requirements could not be consistently met in these early models.[177] Further studies in dogs indicated that the use of patch electrodes placed directly on the heart or pericardium, and thus covering a larger surface area of myocardial tissue, reliably achieved defibrillation at lower energy levels.[178] The first ICD in humans adopted this design, requiring a thoracotomy to surgically place two wire mesh patches directly on the heart (Fig. 96–15). Epicardial screw-in leads were also placed for rate sensing. The large size of PGs, primarily resulting from bulky capacitors needed to store sufficient defibrillation energy (750 to 800 V), necessitated an abdominal pocket. These procedures required general anesthesia, were associated with longer hospital stays, and had a perioperative mortality rate of about 4 percent.[180]

Two major technological advances led to successful transvenous pectoral ICD system implants in 1993. The first development involved the design of integrated lead systems incorporating both sensing and shocking elements (Fig. 96–16). High-energy coils situated on the lead and located within the superior vena cava and right ventricle formed an efficient defibrillation circuit. In the early use of these leads, additional hardware in the form of a subcutaneous patch or array was occasionally required to ensure effective therapy. PG size remained too large for pectoral implantation. Therefore, extensive tunneling was needed from the abdominal pocket site of the PG to the subclavian vein insertion site of the lead.

The second major advancement was the observation that a biphasic defibrillation waveform significantly lowered the amount of energy necessary to restore sinus rhythm as compared with a monophasic waveform.[180, 181] The biphasic waveform delivers energy with a biphasic pulse whereby the initial direction of current is reversed (Fig. 96–17). Initial defibrillation circuits consisted of a combination of high-energy coils and/or subcutaneous patch. Today's ICDS utilize an "active" PG casing that acts as a shocking surface in the defibrillation circuit (Fig. 96–18). These developments significantly lowered the defibrillation threshold (DFT) and, coupled with newer capacitor designs, allowed for the development of smaller capacitors and PGs for pectoral implantation without jeopardizing defibrillation efficacy (Fig. 96–19). Perioperative mortality with implantation of current ICD systems is less than 1 percent.[182]

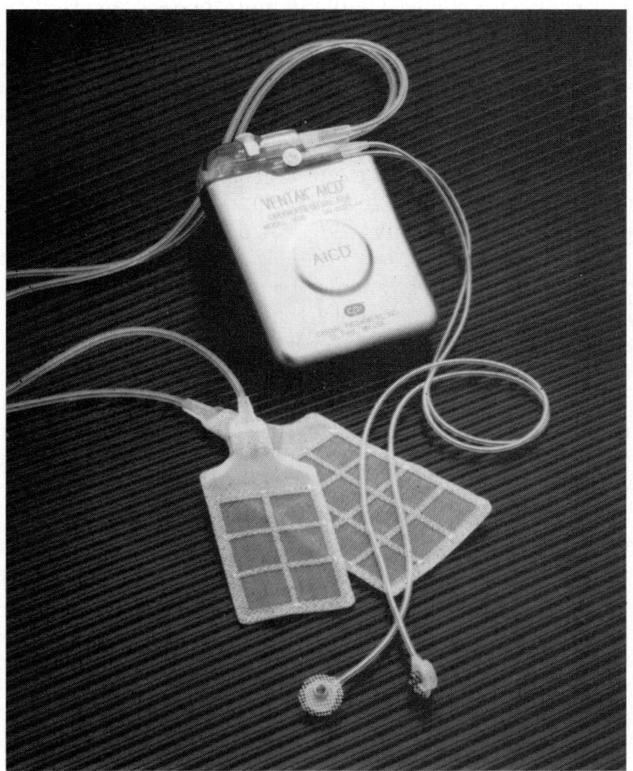

FIGURE 96–15 An early implantable cardioverter-defibrillator (ICD) system shows the epicardial patch electrodes used for defibrillation and epicardial screw-in leads for rate sensing. The large pulse generator was placed in the abdominal wall.

The Modern ICD

Device Components

Except for size, the PG of an ICD and that of a pacemaker appear quite similar. Unique to the ICD is the energy-storing capacitor and battery requirements. Capacitors must be charged fully at regular intervals to avoid age-related current leakage and therefore inefficient energy storage and delivery. Intermittent charging, or "reforming," of the capacitor repairs any electrochemical imperfections developed while the device is not in use. Early devices required visits by patients every several months in order to perform this procedure. Modern ICDs perform the procedure automatically.

The battery within the ICD PG must have the ability to deliver a large amount of current quickly in order to charge the defibrillation capacitors. This cannot be achieved by a lithium iodine battery, the power source for pacemakers. ICDs utilize the chemistry of silver vanadium pentoxide. Although this battery type is capable of rapid current delivery, the chemistry shelf life is inadequate for long-term pacing. Thus, newer ICDs with dual-chamber pacing capabilities employ two batteries, one to power pacing and the other to charge the capacitors.

The covering of the PG is made of titanium and provides an electrically active surface for use in the defibrillation circuit. An epoxy header is attached with two to four connectors for rate sensing, pacing, and shocking leads.

Sensing

Accurate sensing of the ventricular rate is essential because this is the first step in determining whether a ventricular arrhythmia is present. Two possible lead configurations are used to sense ventricular EGMs. True bipolar sensing uses the same methodology as that used in pacing, with sensing between a distal tip cathode and a proximal ring anode. Integrated bipolar sensing occurs between the distal tip cathode and the right ventricular shocking coil as the anode. Although this configuration has the advantages of simplicity and ability to incorporate two shocking coils in a single lead, there is potential undersensing immediately after a shock is delivered. Indeed, delayed redetection of

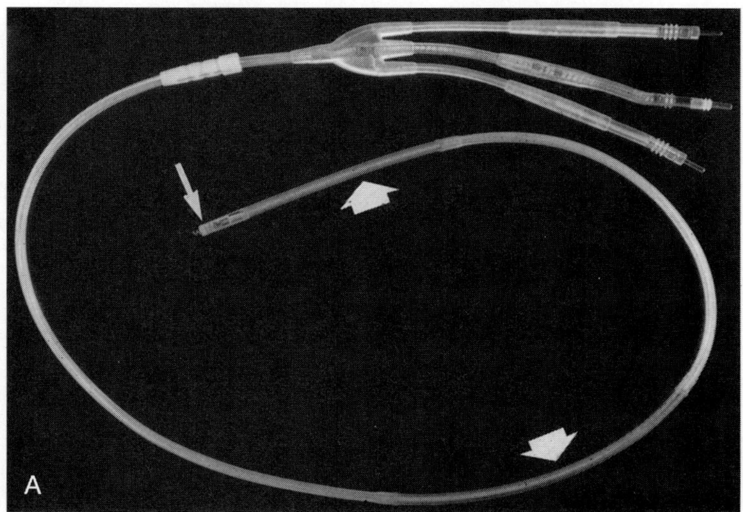

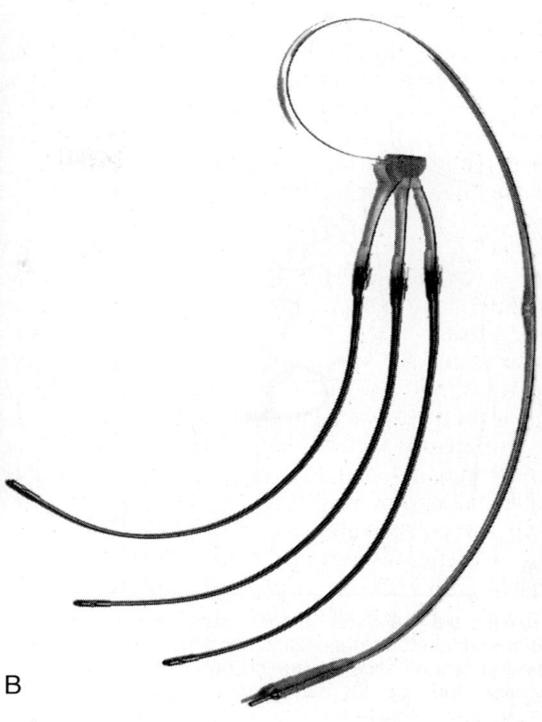

FIGURE 96–16 A, A transvenous implantable cardioverter-defibrillator (ICD) lead. Proximal (superior vena cava [SVC]) and distal (right ventricular [RV]) shocking coils are indicated *(large arrows).* The distal RV coil is involved in the sensing circuit (integrated bipolar) with the distal electrode *(thin arrow).* The lead's fixating screw is exposed. **B,** A subcutaneous array may be added to the defibrillation circuit, although this is rarely required. The array is placed in the axilla and radiates posteriorly.

VF relative to true bipolar sensing has been demonstrated, although normal sensing rapidly resumes.[183]

The size of intracardiac EGM signals may decrease significantly during VF. Programming a fixed sensitivity threshold low enough to detect small-amplitude VF EGM signals runs the risk of oversensing. Therefore, ICDs must use a continuously adjusting sensitivity to adapt to wide beat-to-beat variations in EGM amplitude. Two basic techniques are used to accomplish this task (Fig. 96–20). The first, automatic gain control (CPI, Ventritex), employs a fixed sensing threshold and increases the amplifier gain as necessary to sense low-amplitude fibrillatory EGMs. The second technique is autoadjusting sensitivity (Medtronics, Angeion), whereby the sensing threshold is reset to 75 percent of the amplitude of each successive EGM and becomes increasingly more sensitive until the following EGM is sensed.

Detection

Detection refers to the processing of sensed ventricular EGMs for the purpose of detecting the presence of a

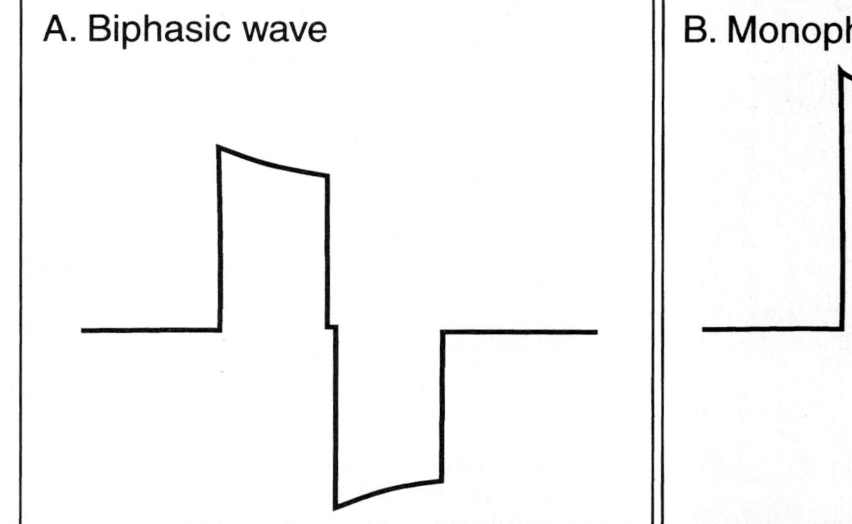

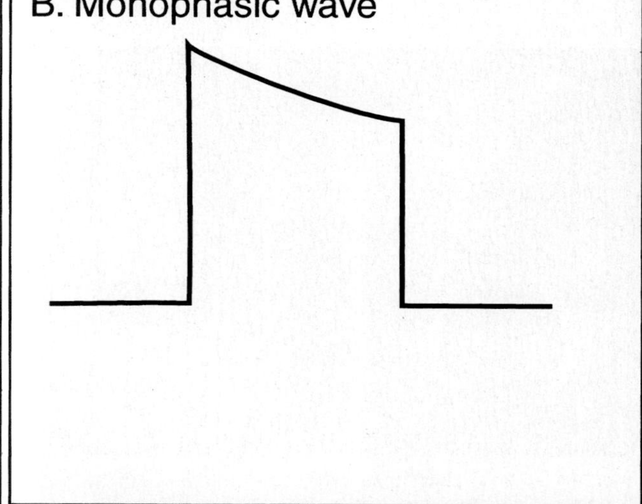

FIGURE 96–17 A, The biphasic waveform illustrates reversal of the pulsed energy current during defibrillation. **B,** The monophasic waveform requires a relatively higher energy for consistent defibrillation.

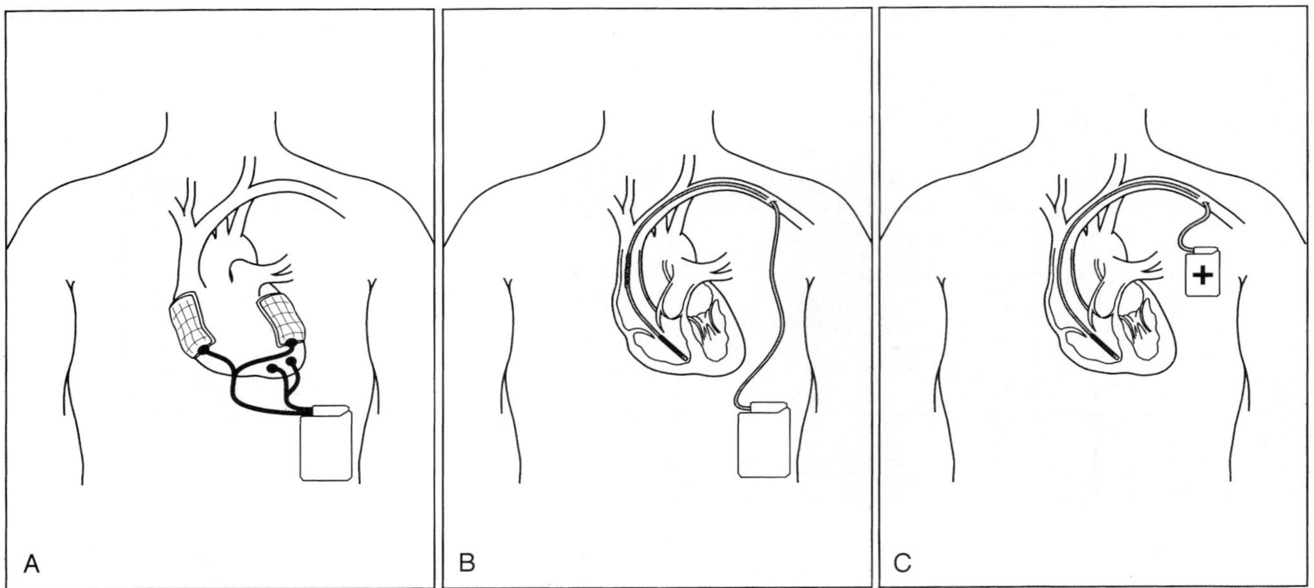

FIGURE 96–18 Evolving implantable cardioverter-defibrillator (ICD) systems. **A,** The earliest ICD system illustrates epicardial patch electrodes used for defibrillation and epicardial leads for rate sensing. This system required thoracotomy for implantation. **B,** The development of leads integrating both sensing and shocking elements allowed for nonthoracotomy implants. Pulse generator size remained too large for routine pectoral implant. **C,** The modern ICD utilizes the pulse generator as an "active can" in the defibrillation circuit and is of sufficiently small size for pectoral implant.

tachyarrhythmia. A continuous spectrum of RR intervals is generated and compared with programmable rate zone limits. Devices in use today allow for the programming of at least three tachyarrhythmia zones. Typically, the highest rate zone (defined by the shortest cycle length) is referred to as the *VF zone*. A fast ventricular tachycardia and a slower VT zone (VT-1) may be programmed to comprise three tachycardia zones with specific detection and therapy options.

VF Zone Detection. Because of the risk of sudden hemodynamic collapse or death during rapid ventricular arrhythmias, 100 percent sensitivity in detection is mandated. This is achieved by use of rate criteria alone as the method of detecting VF. In the VF zone, an X/Y algorithm is employed, requiring a certain proportion of the preceding cycle lengths to be within the programmed zone (e.g., 12/16) for initial detection. If cycle lengths continue to satisfy VF detection over a programmed duration of time, capacitor charging ensues. During this phase, most devices utilize a reconfirmation algorithm using a similar X/Y strategy. Should detection criteria not be met during reconfirmation, the defibrillation shock is aborted, averting unnecessary therapy for a self-terminating arrhythmia. If the arrhythmia is re-detected within 30 seconds of diverting a shock, defibrillation therapy becomes "committed" without an option for reconfirmation. The feature of committed or noncommitted first shocks is programmable and has been shown to prevent unnecessary therapy in 37 percent of patients over an average of 10 months of follow-up.[184]

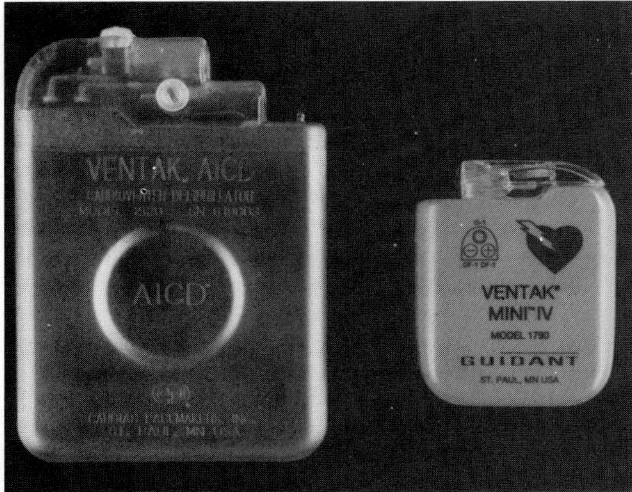

FIGURE 96–19 An early implantable cardioverter-defibrillator (ICD) model *(left)* and a current ICD model *(right).*

VT Zone Detection. Detection within VT zones may use an X/Y algorithm such as that used by VF. More commonly, a required minimal number of consecutive RR intervals within the detection heart rate zone is used, avoiding detection of short, nonsustained VT runs. However, rate criteria as the sole method for detection in VT zones results in a significant number (25 to 40 percent) of inappropriate shocks.[169–172] Most unnecessary therapies result from sinus tachycardia or atrial fibrillation with ventricular rates overlapping the programmed VT zones.[179, 180, 185–188] Therefore, enhanced detection algorithms to provide rhythm discrimination and increase detection specificity for VT have been developed. Unfortunately, increasing specificity occurs at the expense of sensitivity. Thus, all detection enhancers are programmable only for the presumed more hemodynamically stable, slower VT zones.

The first detection enhancement algorithms developed and still in use are *onset* and *stability. Onset* algorithms are intended to inhibit therapy precipitated by sinus tachycardia rates that overlap in the slow VT zone. When a change in heart rate is gradual, as is the case in sinus tachycardia,

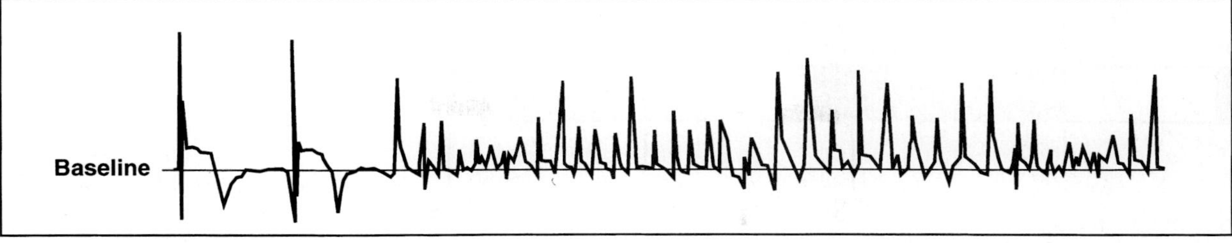

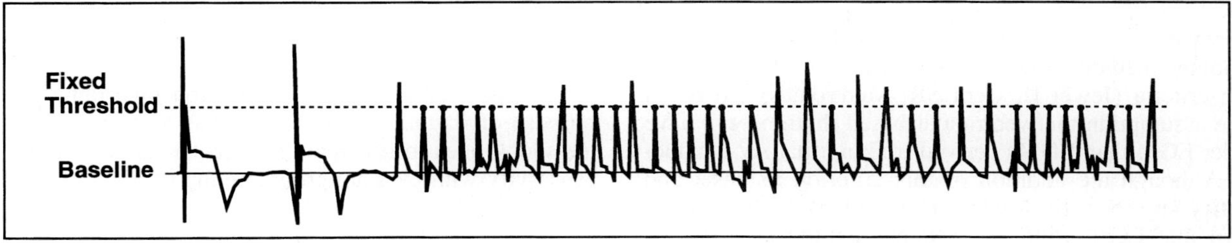

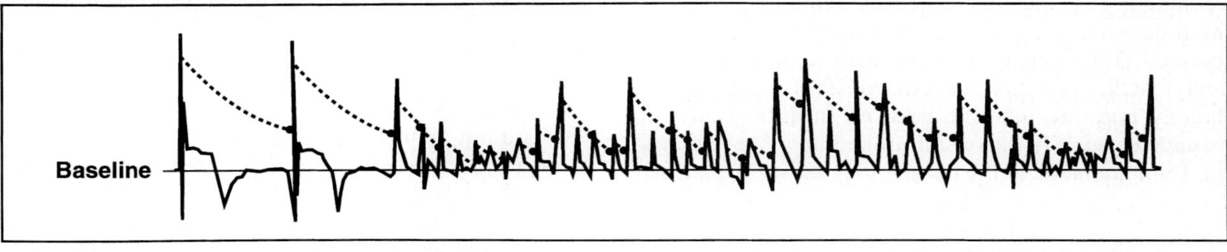

FIGURE 96–20 **A,** Unfiltered ventricular electrograms illustrate low-amplitude signals during ventricular fibrillation. **B,** Automatic gain control. Low-amplitude electrogram signals during ventricular fibrillation are amplified to the programmed sensing threshold. Amplifier gain increases when previously stable electrograms are not sensed. **C,** Automatic adjusting threshold control. Sensing threshold adjusts to 75 percent of the current electrogram signal and decreases until the next electrogram signal is sensed, resetting or adjusting the sensing threshold from beat to beat.

therapy is inhibited. Conversely, a sudden change in RR interval over a programmable value (e.g., 50 ms) is detected as VT. The limitation of this feature is the failure to detect VT that arises during exercise and lacks an abrupt onset. Similarly, some VTs may initiate with highly variable RR intervals and may not satisfy the programmed parameter value. The *onset* criterion has been reported to underdetect 5 to 13 percent of VTs.[189–191] *Stability* refers to the RR interval variability of the detected tachycardia. Ventricular rates caused by atrial fibrillation would be expected to show a wide range of RR intervals, as opposed to a more regular RR interval range in monomorphic VT. A programmable RR stability algorithm would detect as VT any rhythm with RR intervals varying less than the programmed value, for example, 40 ms. A potential difficulty is polymorphic VT, although this rhythm tends to be faster and to occur in higher detection zones.

Despite the limitations of onset and stability, the use of ICDs has decreased the incidence of inappropriate shocks to the range of 10 percent.[190] A programmable safety feature known as *sustained rate duration* (SRD) can apply therapy if the heart rate remains in the VT zone over a set period of time, thereby returning sensitivity for VT to near 100 percent.[190]

The availability of dual-chamber ICD systems with the capability of atrioventricular (AV) sequential pacing has allowed the design of newer enhancement detection algorithms. Sensing of atrial EGMs permits atrial fibrillation rate detection by use of X/Y criteria identical to that used for the VF zone. Comparison of V and A rates for evidence of dissociation is also programmable (Ventak AV II/III DR, CPI). PR Logic (Gem DR, Medtronics) is a more complex rhythm discrimination algorithm that integrates information about A-V patterns and regularity during tachycardia. A-V patterns representing 1:1 supraventricular tachycardias (SVTs), such as AV nodal reentry, may be differentiated as a result of an observed A-V pattern of near-simultaneous depolarization (Fig. 96–21).

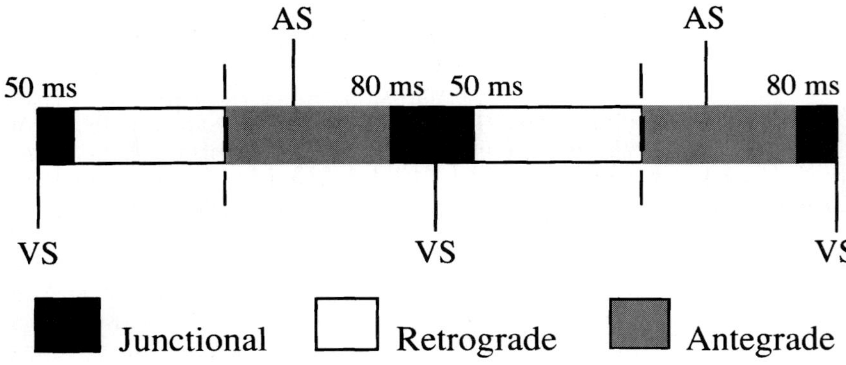

FIGURE 96–21 PR Logic (Medtronics) A-V pattern recognition. Atrial-sensed (AS) events occurring at intervals relative to a ventricular-sensed (VS) event are classified as representing a junctional, antegrade A-V, or retrograde A-V rhythm pattern.

Assessment of ventricular EGMs has been incorporated as another method to differentiate VTs from SVTs. EGM width criteria (Jewel II, Gem SR, Medtronics) are based on the assumption that ventricular-based rhythms will have a wider EGM than EGMs derived from normal AV conduction. Although the addition of this criterion to onset and stability significantly lowers inappropriate shocks, it is known that EGM width can change significantly at high sinus rates and over time.[192] Morphology discrimination (MD, Ventritex) is a novel algorithm whereby the device stores a template of the baseline (sinus) ventricular EGM morphology (Fig. 96–22). During tachycardia detection, each complex is compared with the template, and the algorithm determines the percent match. Should the tachyarrhythmia EGM complex be less than a programmable "percent match," therapy is initiated. The use of EGM morphology may preclude the need of an atrial lead and reduce undetected VTs due to unfulfilled *onset* or *stability* criteria. Limitations of EGM morphology exist for patients with underlying bundle branch block or rate-related bundle branch block.

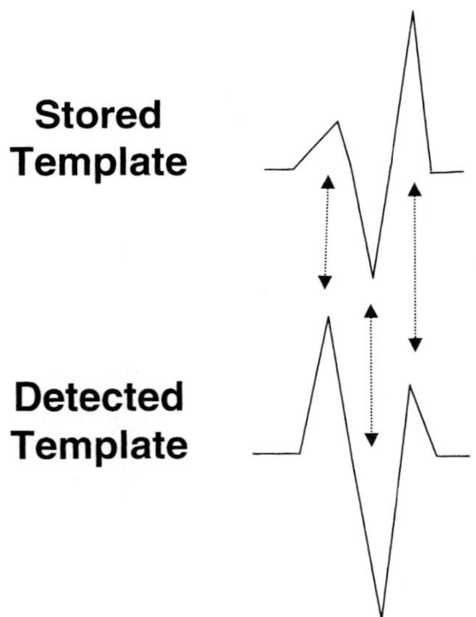

FIGURE 96–22 Morphology discrimination (Ventritex). A stored ventricular electrogram is compared with the detected ventricular electrogram with alignment of the three largest contiguous peaks. A morphology score or "percent match" is calculated. The tachycardia is assumed to be ventricular in origin if the percent match is less than a programmable value or if initial complex alignment is not possible.

The addition of enhanced detection algorithms for the purpose of rhythm discrimination has lowered inappropriate shock rates to less than 5 percent without jeopardizing sensitivity with back-up programming of SRD.[173, 174]

Therapy

VF. All ICDs utilize electrical defibrillation as the only therapeutic option for heart rates detected in the VF zone. As opposed to the small amount of tissue needed for successful capture in pacing, defibrillation requires recruitment of a wide area of myocardium. Therefore, the high-voltage coils and "active can" are separated by several centimeters in order to depolarize as much intervening myocardium as possible. Defibrillation circuits usually involve the active can of the PG and the right ventricular coil with or without a superior vena cava coil. Energy is always delivered in the biphasic waveform.

VT. Multiple, or "tiered," therapeutic options are available for VT detection zones. A sequence of therapy is programmable and followed as needed until an episode is terminated. These programmable options include antitachycardic pacing (ATP), low-energy synchronized cardioversion, and defibrillation.

The objective of ATP is to terminate monomorphic VT promptly with little discomfort to the patient. Delivery of ATP is applied in successive paced beats at a rate faster than the tachycardia cycle length. Intervals may be fixed (burst) or progressively shorter between each pulse (ramp) and are fully programmable. The mechanism of termination of reentry VT depends on the entry of a depolarizing wavefront into the circuit, creating a collision of wavefronts and cessation of reentry.

ATP therapy successfully terminates approximately 90 percent of spontaneous VTs.[178, 193] In addition, the use of this therapy is associated with a statistically significant 36 to 28 percent reduction of first ICD shocks over a 2-year follow-up.[194] The risk of this therapy is the potential for accelerating VT to VF, which may occur in up to 10 percent of attempts.[195] Therefore, tiered therapy must always include programming of back-up defibrillation. Most successful terminations by ATP occur within the first three attempts and therefore should be the programmed limit of sequences.[196] An option of low-energy synchronized cardioversion is programmable for VT zones. This therapy appears to have an efficacy similar to that of ATP.[197]

Pacing

It is estimated that 20 to 30 percent of ICD patients require permanent pacing for sinoatrial and AV conduction disturbances.[198, 199] All devices currently in use provide VVI pacing for primary rate support and/or postshock pacing. To offset the significant impact that pacing would have on device longevity, separate batteries are used for pacing requirements and capacitor charging. The preservation of AV synchrony in patients with depressed left ventricular function may optimize hemodynamic requirements and prevent atrial fibrillation.[200, 201] ICDs with dual-chamber pacemaker capabilities are now available (GemDR, Medtronics, Ventak AV II/III DR, CPI). These devices provide many of the essential features of stand-alone pacemakers, including rate-adaptive pacing and mode-switching. Presently, a dual-chamber device incorporating both atrial and ventricular cardioversion/defibrillation is under clinical investigation.

Diagnostic Storage

Early ICDs provided little information, noting only the number of device discharges. Current devices store and display extensive data. An updated therapy history is provided on each interrogation. A large number of episodes may be stored and their details viewed individually (Fig. 96–23). Specifics regarding the date/time, therapy delivered, detection zone, criteria satisfied, and total length of the episode are displayed. Additional details, such as onset and stability of the episode, may be displayed, even if these features were not programmed for rhythm detection. This allows the physician to decide which settings on these features would be most appropriate. Intracardiac EGMs of episodes requiring therapy are retrievable, including the onset segment (Fig. 96–24). Marker annotations indicating RR intervals and the device's interpretation of the ongoing rhythm are displayed. Simultaneous EGMs from atrial and ventricular leads may be viewed, thereby assisting the physician in determining the appropriateness of applied therapy. Lead impedance is measured in the event of a shock, which may give valuable information for assessing the integrity of the lead system and excluding the presence of lead fracture.

Defibrillation Threshold

There is no specific defibrillation energy level above which all applied shocks are guaranteed to succeed. Rather, the DFT for a patient is represented by a probability curve describing the probable success rate of a given defibrillation energy level. Developing a probability curve would require far too many VF inductions and defibrillations at various energy levels, subjecting the patient to excessive risk.

An acceptable approach at the time of implantation is to demonstrate two or three successful VF conversions without failure at a given energy level. Testing should be attempted at least 10 joules below the maximal output of the device to ensure the ability to program an adequate safety margin. Alternatively, energy levels during testing

```
Episode  80

Elapsed Time      Date            Time        Type
                  11-NOV-99       14:36       Spontaneous

                  Initial Detection           VT-1 Zone
                   Pre-Attempt Avg A Rate            47 bpm
                   Pre-Attempt Avg V Rate           150 bpm
                   Measured Onset             34 %, 309 ms
                   Measured Stability                 4 ms
                   A Fib                            OFF
                   V Rate > A Rate                  OFF

00:02  -   00:02  Attempt 1          VT-1 ATP1 Ramp/Scan
                   Therapy Delivered           1 Burst
                   Post-Attempt Avg A Rate              bpm
                   Post-Attempt Avg V Rate          312 bpm

                  Redetection                 VF Zone
                   Pre-Attempt Avg A Rate               bpm
                   Pre-Attempt Avg V Rate           329 bpm
                   Measured Stability                33 ms
                   A Fib                            OFF
                   V Rate > A Rate                  OFF

     00:07        Attempt 2  VF Shock 1
                   Therapy Delivered         31 J, Biphasic
                    Charge Time                    7.1 sec
                    Shocking Impedance                  Ω
                   Post-Attempt Avg A Rate              bpm
                   Post-Attempt Avg V Rate           71 bpm

     00:45        End of Episode
```

FIGURE 96–23 An episode detail retrieved from stored diagnostics. This episode describes ventricular tachycardia (VT) detection (rate, 150 beats per minute [bpm]) with attempted antitachycardia pacing (ATP) for termination. The ATP resulted in degeneration of VT to ventricular fibrillation (VF), requiring defibrillation therapy. A Fib, atrial fibrillation. A rate, atrial rate; V rate, ventricular rate.

A

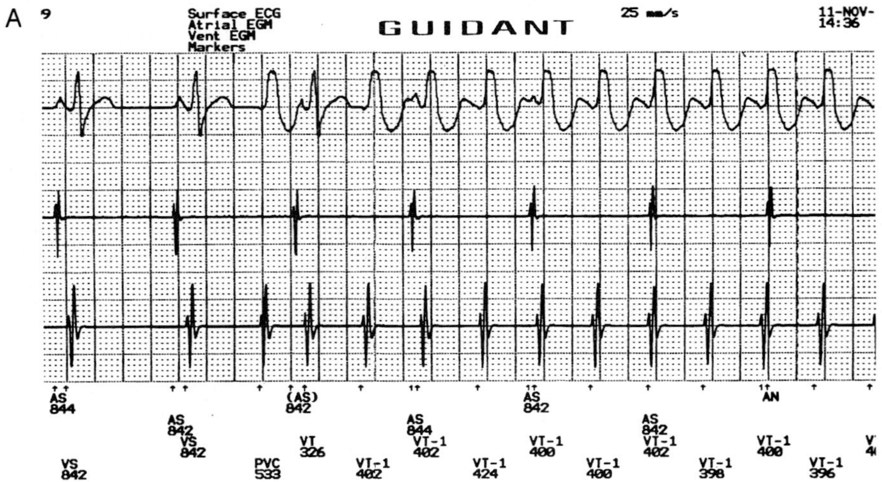

B

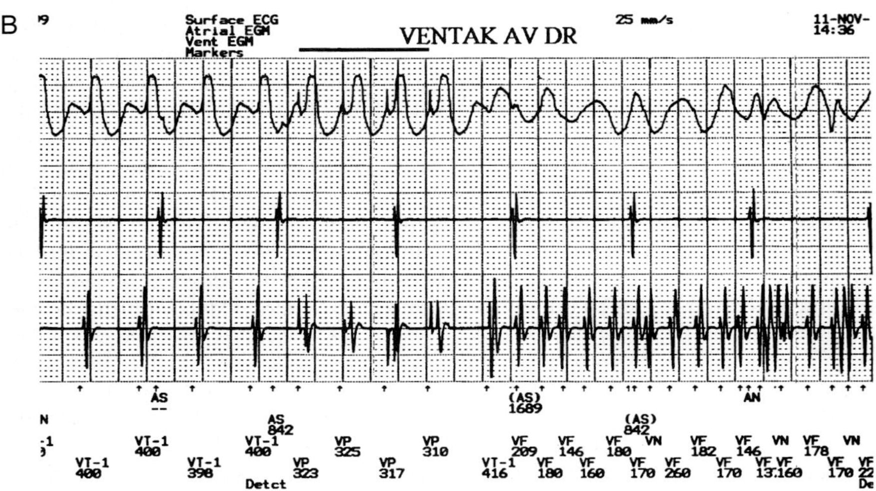

C

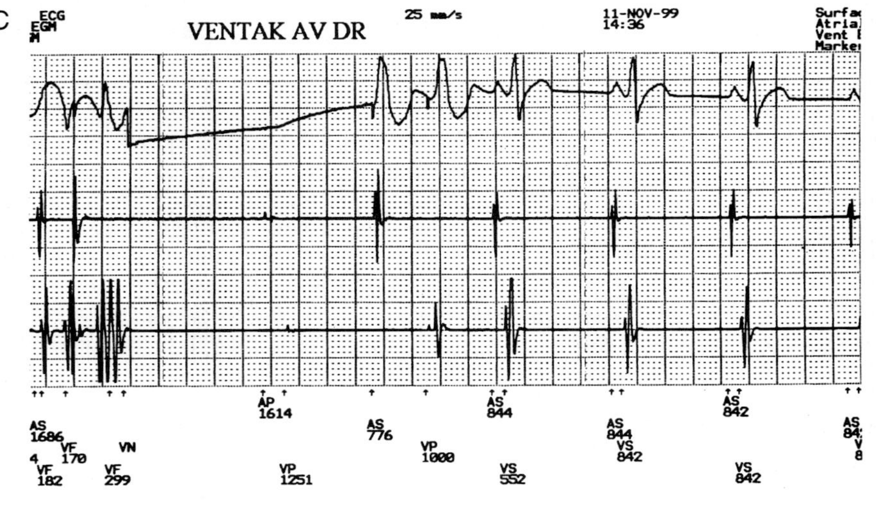

FIGURE 96–24 Intracardiac electrograms from Figure 96–9. **A,** Onset of monomorphic ventricular tachycardia (VT) from normal sinus rhythm after a premature ventricular contraction (PVC). **B,** Four-beat burst of antitachycardia pacing (ATP) therapy (*black bar*), which resulted in degeneration of VT to ventricular fibrillation (VF). VN, ventricular noise (VN marker occurs at RR intervals < 135 ms); VP, ventricular-paced event. **C,** Successful defibrillation and return to normal sinus rhythm. Marker annotations at the bottom of the tracings indicate the detected rhythm and the RR cycle length. AS, atrial-sensed event; ECG, electrocardiogram; EGM, electrogram; VS, ventricular-sensed event.

may be decreased in successive shocks until the shock fails to defibrillate. The lowest shock strength to successfully terminate VF is referred to as the DFT. Programming 10 to 15 joules above the DFT provides the necessary safety margin to compensate for potential increases in the DFT. DFTs may be increased by the addition of antiarrhythmic drugs, particularly amiodarone.[202, 203] Increased fibrosis in the region of the shocking elements caused by progressive disease or myocardial infarction may also adversely effect DFTs.[204] Strickberger and colleagues[205] demonstrated a 96 percent probability of successful first-shock defibrillation if a safety margin of 7 joules was added to the determined DFT. In the event an adequate safety margin cannot be programmed because of limitations of the maximal energy output of the device, addition of a subcutaneous patch or array may suffice. As a last resort, surgical placement of epicardial patches via thoracotomy may be required.

The Magnet Response and Electromagnetic Interference

ICDs and pacemakers have very different responses to magnet application. Additionally, ICD models may differ in their magnet response. However, a feature common to all ICDs is the suspension of tachycardia therapy on magnet application. This may be useful in a patient receiving repetitive inappropriate shocks. A concern is the inadvertent programming of the device to "off" in some ICDs. This may occur on exposure of the device to a magnet for 30 seconds, for example, when stereo speakers are carried close to the chest. Certain devices resume detection and therapy once the magnet is removed, regardless of the duration of exposure. Some devices now allow a programmable magnet response, providing the option to ignore the effect of magnet application. Although therapy responses may be affected by magnet application, required pacing is not, ensuring that asystole does not occur.

Electromagnetic interference may prevent arrhythmia detection or cause the device to falsely detect tachycardia and deliver inappropriate therapy. Patients should be advised to avoid the strong magnetic fields of electronic theft surveillance systems and, if they cannot be avoided, to walk through them without pausing. Similarly, caution is needed in the use of cellular telephones. When used, the telephone should be held on the side opposite the device. Avoidance of close contact of cellular phones with the PG and lead system is recommended, and therefore, telephones should not be placed in nearby pockets.[206, 207] Airport security systems may also pose a risk. Patients are advised to present their device identification card and avoid prolonged device exposure to hand-held metal detectors. Finally, the use of electrocautery in surgery may cause "electrical chatter" and oversensing. The ICD is best turned off in this setting with appropriate monitoring and external defibrillator nearby. In addition, electrocautery in close proximity to the device should be avoided to prevent the risk of damage to internal circuitry.

Evaluation of ICD Malfunction

Because modern ICDs provide pacing capabilities, problems similar to those with stand-alone pacemakers may be seen. These were discussed previously. Major issues specific to ICD malfunction include inappropriate delivery of therapy, failure to deliver therapy, and unsuccessful conversion of arrhythmia after therapy.

In assessing a patient with a recent defibrillation discharge, the first issue is determining whether therapy was appropriate. Despite sophisticated rhythm discrimination algorithms in current use, rapid atrial fibrillation remains the most common cause of inappropriate shocks.[185, 186] The main reason for this is atrial fibrillation ventricular rates that meet VF zone criteria where enhanced detection algorithms are not in effect. Preventative options include increasing VF detection rate, administering AV nodal blocking agents, or considering AV nodal ablation. Sensing of electrical chatter that falsely detects an arrhythmia occurs less frequently. This develops in the presence of lead fractures or insulation breaks or may result from a loose connection to the header device.[208–210] These problems may be evident on analysis of stored EGMs, where nonphysiologic RR intervals (<150 ms) may be observed. Lead problems should be suspected on device interrogation when marked variation of R-wave sensing, pacing thresholds, and impedance measurements exists. Occasionally, having the patient perform physical maneuvers, such as straining and arm movements, may reproduce electrical chatter that can be seen on ICD telemetry. An overpenetrated chest x-ray may localize a lead fracture. Issues related to lead failure or loose connections require surgical intervention.

Failure to deliver therapy occurs rarely. Most commonly, this phenomenon involves undersensing of EGMs and is associated with lead failure. Should this complication arise early after implantation (<30 days), lead malposition, dislodgment, or myocardial perforation is of concern. Lead fractures or insulation breaks leading to signal dropout typically require a duration of time to evolve. Undersensing may also occur as a result of a change in tissue substrate in the vicinity of the sensing electrodes. This may be seen after myocardial infarction with resultant weak EGM signals caused by myocyte loss. Lastly, failure to deliver therapy may be due to programming of too high a detection rate. Addition of antiarrhythmic agents, such as amiodarone and sotalol, may lower the rate of previously observed ventricular arrhythmias. Differentiating the cause of failure to deliver therapy requires a chest x-ray and thorough device interrogation.

Failure of therapy to convert an arrhythmia may have dire consequences. Again, lead failure or malposition may be a culprit, resulting in insufficient energy delivery. Altered tissue substrate may render ATP unsuccessful as a result of failure to adequately capture. DFTs may be increased because of amiodarone initiation or severe electrolyte/acid-base abnormalities. Increasing programming shock energy level may suffice, but a thorough device evaluation is required.

Clinical Trials of the ICD

Secondary Prevention of Sudden Cardiac Death

It is noteworthy that 12 years passed after Food and Drug Administration approval in 1985 before definitive mortality data on the ICD were available. The impact of the ICD on survival in patients with a history of life-threatening arrhythmias has now been assessed in three trials (Table 96–6).

The Anti-arrhythmics Versus Implantable Defibrillator (AVID) trial compared the effect of ICD or antiarrhythmic drug therapy with empiric amiodarone or EPS/Holter-guided sotalol therapy in survivors of SCD, syncopal VT, and an ejection fraction of less than 40 percent.[211] The study was terminated early after the enrollment of 1016 patients. At 3-year follow-up, survival was 75 percent for the ICD group, versus 61 percent for the antiarrhythmic group. More than 90 percent of patients in the antiarrhythmic group were receiving amiodarone. Although β-blocker use was more prevalent in the ICD group, adjusting for this imbalance did not alter the mortality reduction attributable to the ICD.

The Canadian Implantable Defibrillator Study randomized a patient population similar to that in the AVID trial to therapy with an ICD or empiric amiodarone. The primary end point was a composite of all-cause mortality at 3 years after randomization. At 5 year follow-up, a strong trend in favor of reduced mortality secondary to arrhythmic death in the ICD arm was observed: 25 percent versus 30 percent with amiodarone (P = 3.0/4.5 .072).[212]

The Cardiac Arrest Study—Hamburg randomly assigned survivors of cardiac arrest to ICD therapy or treatment with propafenone, metoprolol, or amiodarone. The propafenone arm was withdrawn early because of an observed excess mortality. All-cause mortality was 12.1 percent in the ICD arm versus 19.6 percent in the combined arms of amiodarone and metoprolol at 2-year follow-up, a statistically significant reduction. Interestingly, no difference was observed between the amiodarone and metoprolol arms.[213]

Treatment with an ICD is a class I indication for secondary prevention in survivors of cardiac arrest without a reversible cause, for patients with syncope of unknown cause and inducible VT/VF, and for spontaneous, sustained VT (Table 96–7).[168]

TABLE 96–6 Randomized Clinical Trials of the Implantable Cardioverter-Defibrillator

Trial	Patient Population	Control	Result
Primary Prevention			
Multicenter Automatic Implantable Defibrillator Trial (MADIT)	Prior myocardial infarction *and* left ventricular ejection fraction ≤ 35% *and* nonsustained VT *and* inducible VT *and not* suppressible with IV procainamide	Medical therapy	Significant reduction in total mortality in the ICD group
Coronary Artery Bypass Graft–Implantable Cardioverter Defibrillator Study (CABG-PATCH)	Coronary artery bypass grafting *and* left ventricular ejection fraction ≤ 35% *and* positive signal-averaged ECG	Medical therapy	No difference in total mortality
Multicenter Unsustained Tachycardia Trial (MUSTT)	Coronary artery disease *and* left ventricular ejection fraction ≤ 40% *and* nonsustained VT *and* inducible VT	Medical therapy or EPS-guided antiarrhythmic therapy	Significant reduction in sudden cardiac death and/or resuscitated cardiac arrest in the ICD group
Second Multicenter Automatic Implantable Defibrillator Trial (MADIT II)	Prior myocardial infarction *and* left ventricular ejection fraction ≤ 30% *without* arrhythmia entry criteria	Medical therapy	Ongoing
Sudden Cardiac Death in Heart Failure Trial (SCD-HeFT)	NYHA class II or III congestive heart failure *and* left ventricular ejection fraction < 35%	Placebo or amiodarone	Ongoing
Defibrillator in Acute Myocardial Infarction Trial (DINAMIT)	Acute myocardial infarction (< 30 da) *and* left ventricular ejection fraction < 35% *and* depressed heart rate variability *or* mean 24-hour heart rate > 80 beats/min	Medical therapy	Ongoing
Defibrillator in Nonischemic Cardiomyopathy Treatment Evaluation (DEFINITE)	Nonischemic cardiomyopathy *and* left ventricular ejection fraction < 35% *and* nonsustained VT *or* > 10 PVCs/h	Beta-blocker and conventional heart failure therapy	Ongoing
Secondary Prevention			
Antiarrhythmics Versus Implantable Defibrillator Trial (AVID)	Left ventricular ejection fraction ≤ 40% *and* cardiac arrest *or* syncopal VT *or* symptomatic sustained VT	Amiodarone or sotalol	Significant reduction in total mortality in the ICD group
Cardiac Arrest Study—Hamburg (CASH)	Resuscitated cardiac arrest	Propafenone or metoprolol or amiodarone	Significant reduction in total mortality in the ICD group
Canadian Implantable Defibrillator Study (CIDS)	Resuscitated cardiac arrest *or* syncopal VT or symptomatic sustained VT with left ventricular ejection fraction ≤ 35% *or* syncope and inducible VT	Amiodarone	Nonsignificant reduction in total mortality in the ICD group

Abbreviations: ECG, electrocardiogram; EPS, electrophysiologic study; ICD, implantable cardioverter-defibrillator; NYHA, New York Heart Association; PVC, premature ventricular contraction; VT, ventricular tachycardia.

TABLE 96-7 Clinical Indication for ICD Implantation (AHA/ACC Guidelines)

Class I

1. Cardiac arrest due to VF or VT, not due to a transient or a reversible cause
2. Spontaneous sustained VT
3. Syncope of undetermined origin with clinically relevant, hemodynamically significant sustained VT or VF induced at electrophysiologic study when drug therapy is ineffective, not tolerated, or not preferred
4. Nonsustained VT with coronary disease, prior MI, LV dysfunction, and inducible VF or sustained VT and electrophysiologic study that is not suppressible by a class I antiarrhythmic drug

Class IIa

None

Class IIb

1. Cardiac arrest presumed to be due to VF when electrophysiologic testing is precluded by other medical conditions
2. Severe symptoms attributable to sustained ventricular tachyarrhythmias while awaiting cardiac transplantation
3. Familial or inherited condition with a high risk for life-threatening ventricular tachyarrhythmias, such as long QT syndrome and hypertrophic cardiomyopathy
4. Nonsustained VT with coronary artery disease, prior MI, and LV dysfunction and inducible sustained VT or VF at electrophysiologic study
5. Recurrent syncope of undetermined cause in the presence of ventricular dysfunction and inducible ventricular arrhythmias at electrophysiologic study when other causes of syncope have been excluded

Class III

1. Syncope of undetermined cause in a patient without inducible ventricular tachyarrhythmias
2. Incessant VT or VF
3. VF or VT resulting from arrhythmias amenable to surgical or catheter ablation, e.g., atrial arrhythmias associated with the Wolff-Parkinson-White syndrome, right ventricular outflow tract VT, idiopathic left ventricular tachycardia, and fascicular VT
4. Ventricular tachyarrythmias due to a transient or reversible disorder (e.g., AMI, electrolyte imbalance, drugs, trauma)
5. Significant psychiatric illnesses that may be aggravated by device implantation or may preclude systematic follow-up
6. Terminal illnesses with projected life expectancy ≤ 6 months
7. Patients with coronary artery disease with LV dysfunction and prolonged QRS duration in the absence of spontaneous or inducible sustained or nonsustained VT who are undergoing coronary bypass surgery
8. NYHA class IV drug-refractory congestive heart failure in patients who are not candidates for cardiac transplantation

Abbreviations: ACC, American College of Cardiology; AHA, American Heart Association; AMI, acute myocardial infarction; ICD, implantable cardioverter-defibrillator; LV, left ventricular; MI, myocardial infarction; NYHA, New York Heart Association; VF, ventricular fibrillation; VT, ventricular tachycardia.

Primary Prevention of Sudden Cardiac Death

The ability to identify patients at high risk for SCD by invasive and noninvasive testing is well established. Thus, clinical trial designs for primary prevention have sought to identify high-risk groups that are most likely to benefit from ICD implantation.

The Multicenter Automatic Defibrillator Trial (MADIT) was the first prospective, randomized trial assessing the value of the ICD. Patients with prior myocardial infarction, left ventricular ejection fraction of less than 35 percent, evidence of documented nonsustained VT, and inducible VT not suppressed by intravenous procainamide, randomly received an ICD or "conventional therapy." A statistically significant difference in total mortality was observed: 15 percent in the ICD group and 39 percent in the conventional therapy group over an average follow-up of 2.5 years. Although a striking benefit for the ICD was present, the trial was criticized for lack of a unified approach to drug therapy in the conventional-treatment group. At last patient contact, only 5 percent of patients in the conventional group were receiving β-blocker therapy, versus 27 percent in the ICD group. Angiotensin-converting enzyme inhibitors and amiodarone use were 51 percent and 45 percent in the conventional group, respectively.[214]

The Multicenter Unsustained Tachycardia Trial randomized a patient population similar to that in MADIT. Patients with inducible VT received medical therapy alone (excluding antiarrhythmics) or an EPS-guided approach. Patients in the EPS-guided group with inducible VT/VF not suppressible with at least one trial of antiarrhythmic therapy received an ICD. At 5-year follow-up, a statistically significant benefit in the EPS-guided group was evident with respect to the primary end point of SCD or resuscitated cardiac arrest: 25 percent in the EPS-guided group versus 32 percent in the medical therapy group. Further analyses indicated that the benefit seen with the EPS-guided approach was due solely to the ICD subgroup. EPS-guided antiarrhythmic therapy did not show improved outcomes over medical treatment that did not include antiarrhythmic therapy.[215] Patients enrolled in this trial who were not inducible at EPS were followed up in a registry. Interestingly, this patient population had a higher mortality at 2 years than those in the ICD arm of the trial.

The Coronary Artery Bypass Graft–Implantable Cardioverter-Defibrillator (CABG-Patch) study randomly assigned patients with ejection fractions of less than 35 percent and positive signal-averaged electrocardiogram before coronary surgery to an ICD or a control group. No difference in overall mortality was observed.[216] The study did not require nonsustained VT or inducible VT for trial enrollment. Some investigators have suggested that patients with a similar degree of LV dysfunction but without inducible VT may be at a lower risk for SCD.[217, 218] In addition, revascularization may have decreased the risk for ischemia-induced arrhythmias in this patient population. These factors may help explain the much lower mortality rate in the CABG-Patch control arm (18 percent) as compared with the MADIT control group (39 percent).

The ongoing Sudden Cardiac Death in Heart Failure Trial will present the most stringent control intervention thus far versus the ICD. Patients with symptomatic (New York Heart Association classes II and III) ischemic or nonischemic cardiomyopathy and ejection fractions of less than 35 percent are being randomly assigned to ICD, amiodarone, or placebo. A key component of this trial is the strong encouragement for β-blocker use, targeting 70 percent of the patient population. The relevance of this is highlighted by trials that indicate a significant reduction in all-cause and sudden death mortality in congestive heart failure patients randomly assigned to β-blockers.[219, 220] Furthermore, the combination of β-blocker and amiodarone has been suggested in post hoc analyses to have a significant impact on reducing arrhythmic death.[221] Additional ongoing trials in primary prevention are listed in Table 96–6. Presently, patients fulfilling the MADIT criteria have a class I indication for ICD implantation in the primary prevention of SCD.[168]

Cost-Effectiveness

The cost associated with ICD implantation has declined in recent years, primarily as a result of the transition to the nonthoracotomy, pectoral approach. Vorperian and coworkers[222] compared the costs for ICD replacement procedures requiring an operating room setting versus an EPS laboratory. Total costs were significantly less in the EPS laboratory ($4,541) than in the operating room ($9,431). This lower cost was attributable to lower physician fees, lower hospital charges, and shorter postprocedural convalescence.

Present data analyzing the cost-effectiveness of the ICD relative to conventional medical therapy are obscured, given the rapid technological advances of the ICD. Owens and associates[223] provided an economic model estimating that a 30 percent reduction in mortality by the ICD relative to amiodarone would satisfy current standards of cost-effectiveness (< $50,000 per life-year gained). This estimate compares favorably with the observed risk reduction of 31 percent at 3 years in AVID and a 59 percent risk reduction at 2 years in MADIT.

Prior clinical information regarding the cost-effectiveness of ICDs has been limited by small patient numbers and trial design.[224, 225] Completion of the MADIT study in 1996 has allowed for an adequate duration of patient follow-up to assess the costs accumulated by each treatment group.[226] The expenses of recurrent hospitalizations, physician visits, medications, laboratory tests, and procedures were analyzed. In view of the significant mortality reduction in MADIT, the resulting cost-effectiveness ratio was $27,000 per life-year gained. In patients who received nonthoracotomy procedures, this ratio was reduced to $23,000 per life-year gained.

Advances in ICD technology will reduce the cost of this therapeutic strategy further. Improved batteries are increasing device longevity, better diagnostic features avoid in-patient or ambulatory Holter monitoring, and dual-chamber pacing capabilities prevent the need for separate pacemaker implantation when required.

Future Developments

The evolution of ICD technology moved rapidly during the 1990s. Continued improvements in shock waveforms and battery and capacitor technology will lead to even smaller devices. It is feasible that unique and sophisticated algorithms will make possible the monitoring of additional clinical parameters, allowing device intervention before arrhythmia onset. Detection of repolarization alternans, heart rate variability, long-short RR intervals, or hemodynamic changes may be treated by novel therapies.[227–231] Such programmable therapies may include intermittent antiarrhythmic drug infusion, pacing to avoid long-short coupling, and multisite pacing to improve hemodynamics. Undoubtedly, the role of the ICD will continue to evolve in the primary and secondary prevention of SCD.

References

1. Mond HG, Sloman JG, Edwards RH: The first pacemaker. Pacing Clin Electrophysiol 5:278–282, 1982.
2. Schecter D: Background of clinical cardiac electrico-stimulation. VII: modern era of artifical pacemakers. NY State J Med 72:1666, 1972.
3. Bernstein AD, et al: The NASPE/BPEG generic pacemaker code for antibradyarrhythmia and adaptive-rate pacing and antitachyarrhythmia devices. Pacing Clin Electrophysiol 10:794–799, 1987.
4. Gregoratos G, et al: ACC/AHA Guidelines for Implantation of Cardiac Pacemakers and Antiarrhythmia Devices: Executive Summary—a report of the American College of Cardiology/American Heart Association Task Force on Practice Guidelines (Committee on Pacemaker Implantation). Circulation 97:1325–1335, 1998.
5. Bernstein AD, Parsonnet V: Survey of cardiac pacing and defibrillation in the United States in 1993. Am J Cardiol 78:187–196, 1996.
6. Andersen HR, et al: Long-term follow-up of patients from a randomised trial of atrial versus ventricular pacing for sick-sinus syndrome [see comments]. Lancet 350:1210–1216, 1997.
7. Kay R, Estioko M, Weiner I, et al: Primary sick sinus syndrome as an indication for chronic pacemaker therapy in young adults: incidence, clinical features, and long term evaluation. Am Heart J 103:338–342, 1982.
8. Alboni P, et al: Effects of permanent pacemaker and oral theophylline in sick sinus syndrome—the THEOPACE study: a randomized controlled trial. Circulation 96:260–266, 1997.
9. Wilkoff BL, Blackburn G: Analytic techniques in the assessment of chronotropic response to exercise. Pacing Clin Electrophysiol 11:530, 1988.
10. Lauer MS, et al: Impaired heart rate response to graded exercise: prognostic implications of chronotropic incompetence in the Framingham Heart Study [see comments]. Circulation 93:1520–1526, 1996.
11. Dreifus LS, et al: Guidelines for implantation of cardiac pacemakers and antiarrhythmia devices: a report of the American College of Cardiology/American Heart Association Task Force on Assessment of Diagnostic and Therapeutic Cardiovascular Procedures (Committee on Pacemaker Implantation). Circulation 84:455–467, 1991.
12. Lewalter T, et al: Heart rate to work rate relation throughout peak exercise in normal subjects as a guideline for rate-adaptive pacemaker programming. Am J Cardiol 76:812–816, 1995.
13. Donmoyer TL, DeSanctis RW, Austen WG: Experience with implantable pacemakers using myocardial electrodes in the management of heart block. Ann Thorac Surg 3:218–227, 1967.
14. Hayes DL, et al: Evolving indications for permanent cardiac pacing: an appraisal of the 1998 American College of Cardiology/American Heart Association Guidelines [editorial]. Am J Cardiol 82:1082–1086, A6, 1998.
15. Denes P: Atrioventricular and intraventricular block. Circulation 75:III-19–III-25, 1987.
16. Rardon DT, Mitrani RD: Atrioventricular block and dissociation. *In* Zipes D, Jalife J (eds): Cardiac Electrophysiology: From Cell to Bedside. pp. 935–942. Philadelphia: WB Saunders, 1995.
17. Ranganathan N, et al: His bundle electrogram in bundle-branch block. Circulation 45:282–294, 1972.
18. Dhingra RC, et al: The significance of second degree atrioventricular block and bundle branch block: observations regarding site and type of block. Circulation 49:638–646, 1974.
19. Barold SS: ACC/AHA guidelines for implantation of cardiac pacemakers: how accurate are the definitions of atrioventricular and intraventricular conduction blocks? [editorial]. Pacing Clin Electrophysiol 16:1221–1226, 1993.
20. Rosenbaum N, DR, Phillips JH, Wigle ED: Syndrome of right bundle branch block and intermittent left anterior hemiblock and left posterior hemiblock. *In* Castellanos A (ed): The Hemiblocks. pp. 55–69. Oldsmar, FL: Tampa Tracings, 1970.
21. McAnulty JH, et al: Natural history of "high-risk" bundle-branch block: final report of a prospective study. N Engl J Med 307:137–143, 1982.

22. Luscure M, Lagorge T: Blocs auriculoventriculaires d'effort. Ann Cardiol Angeiol 44:486–492, 1995.
23. Sumiyoshi M, et al: Clinical and electrophysiologic features of exercise-induced atrioventricular block. Am Heart J 132:1277–1281, 1996.
24. Barold SS, et al: Exercise-induced second-degree AV block: is it type I or type II? J Cardiovasc Electrophysiol 8:1084–1086, 1997.
25. Sakaguchi S, et al: Syncope associated with exercise, a manifestation of neurally mediated syncope. Am J Cardiol 75:476–481, 1995.
26. Freedman RA: Standard indications and contraindications for pacemaker implantation. Cardiac Electrophysiol Rev 2:353–357, 1999.
27. Pinsky WW, et al: Diagnosis, management, and long-term results of patients with congenital complete atrioventricular block. Pediatrics 69:728–733, 1982.
28. Michaelsson M, Engle MA: Congenital complete heart block: an international study of the natural history. Cardiovasc Clin 4:85–101, 1972.
29. Michaelsson M, Jonzon A, Riesenfeld T: Isolated congenital complete atrioventricular block in adult life: a prospective study [see comments]. Circulation 92:442–449, 1995.
30. Chadda KD, et al: Effects of atropine in patients with bradyarrhythmia complicating myocardial infarction: usefulness of an optimum dose for overdrive. Am J Med 63:503–510, 1977.
31. De Guzman M, Kawanishi DT, Rahimtoola SH: AV node–His–Purkinje system disease. *In* Ellenbogen K, Kay GN, Wilkoff BL (eds): Clinical Cardiac Pacing. pp. 321–331. Philadelphia: WB Saunders, 1995.
32. Barold SS: American College of Cardiology/American Heart Association guidelines for pacemaker implantation after acute myocardial infarction: what is persistent advanced block at the atrioventricular node? [editorial]. Am J Cardiol 80:770–774, 1997.
33. Sgarbossa EB, et al: Acute myocardial infarction and complete bundle branch block at hospital admission: clinical characteristics and outcome in the thrombolytic era. GUSTO-I Investigators. Global Utilization of Streptokinase and t-PA [tissue-type plasminogen activator] for Occluded Coronary Arteries. J Am Coll Cardiol 31:105–110, 1998.
34. Go AS, et al: Bundle-branch block and in-hospital mortality in acute myocardial infarction: National Registry of Myocardial Infarction 2 Investigators. Ann Intern Med 129:690–697, 1998.
35. Zipes D: Anatomy of the cardiac conduction system. *In* Braunwald E (ed): Heart Disease: A Textbook of Cardiovascular Medicine. pp. 548–550. Philadelphia: WB Saunders, 1997.
36. Jaeger F, Fouad-Tarazi FM, Castle LW: Carotid sinus hypersensitivity and neurally mediated syncope. *In* Ellenbogen KA (ed): Clinical Cardiac Pacing. pp. 332–352. Philadelphia: WB Saunders, 1995.
37. Clemmensen P, et al: Complete atrioventricular block complicating inferior wall acute myocardial infarction treated with reperfusion therapy. TAMI Study Group. Am J Cardiol 67:225–230, 1991.
38. Strasberg B, et al: Carotid sinus hypersensitivity and the carotid sinus syndrome. Prog Cardiovasc Dis 31:379–391, 1989.
39. Almquist A, et al: Carotid sinus hypersensitivity: evaluation of the vasodepressor component. Circulation 71:927–936, 1985.
40. Sugrue DD, et al: Symptomatic "isolated" carotid sinus hypersensitivity: natural history and results of treatment with anticholinergic drugs or pacemaker. J Am Coll Cardiol 7:158–162, 1986.
41. Morley CA, et al: Carotid sinus syncope treated by pacing: analysis of persistent symptoms and role of atrioventricular sequential pacing. Br Heart J 47:411–418, 1982.
42. Morley C, Perrins EJ: Long term comparison of DVI and VVI pacing in carotid sinus syndrome. *In* 7th World Symposium on Cardiac Pacing. Darmstadt, Germany: Steinkopff, 1983.
43. Brignole M, et al: Natural and unnatural history of patients with severe carotid sinus hypersensitivity: a preliminary study. Pacing Clin Electrophysiol 11:1628–1635, 1988.
44. Brignole M, et al: Ventricular and dual chamber pacing for treatment of carotid sinus syndrome. Pacing Clin Electrophysiol 12:582–590, 1989.
45. Brignole M, et al: Pacing for carotid sinus syndrome and sick sinus syndrome. Pacing Clin Electrophysiol 13:2071–2075, 1990.
46. Benditt DG, et al: Tilt table testing for assessing syncope. American College of Cardiology. J Am Coll Cardiol 28:263–275, 1996.
47. Connolly SJ, et al: The North American Vasovagal Pacemaker Study (VPS): a randomized trial of permanent cardiac pacing for the prevention of vasovagal syncope [see comments]. J Am Coll Cardiol 33:16–20, 1999.
48. Barlow M, Krahn AD: The role of cardiac pacing in neurocardiogenic syncope. Cardiol Electrophysiol Rev 4:369–372, 1999.
49. Hassenstein P, Storch HH, Schmitz W: Results of electrical pacing in patients with hypertrophic obstruction cardiomyopathy [author's translation]. Thoraxchir Vask Chir 23:496–468, 1975.
50. Slade AK, et al: DDD pacing in hypertrophic cardiomyopathy: a multicentre clinical experience. Heart 75:44–49, 1996.
51. Gadler F, et al: Long-term effects of dual chamber pacing in patients with hypertrophic cardiomyopathy without outflow tract obstruction at rest. Eur Heart J 18:636–642, 1997.
52. Fananapazir L, et al: Long-term results of dual-chamber (DDD) pacing in obstructive hypertrophic cardiomyopathy: evidence for progressive symptomatic and hemodynamic improvement and reduction of left ventricular hypertrophy [see comments]. Circulation 90:2731–2742, 1994.
53. Jeanrenaud X, Kappenberger L: Regional wall motion during pacing for hypertrophic obstructive cardiomyopathy. Pacing Clin Electrophysiol 20:1673–1681, 1997.
54. Pak PH, et al: Mechanism of acute mechanical benefit from VDD pacing in hypertrophied heart: similarity of responses in hypertrophic cardiomyopathy and hypertensive heart disease. Circulation 98:242–248, 1998.
55. Gottfridsson C, et al: Full ventricular capture indicated by the QT interval function. Pacing Clin Electrophysiol 21:2171–2177, 1998.
56. Nishimura RA, et al: Dual-chamber pacing for hypertrophic cardiomyopathy: a randomized, double-blind, crossover trial. J Am Coll Cardiol 29:435–441, 1997.
57. Kappenberger L, et al: Pacing in hypertrophic obstructive cardiomyopathy: a randomized crossover study. PIC Study Group [see comments]. Eur Heart J 18:1249–1256, 1997.
58. Maron BJ, et al: Assessment of permanent dual-chamber pacing as a treatment for drug-refractory symptomatic patients with obstructive hypertrophic cardiomyopathy: a randomized, double-blind, crossover study (M-PATHY). Circulation 99:2927–2933, 1999.
59. Lakkis NM, et al: Echocardiography-guided ethanol septal reduction for hypertrophic obstructive cardiomyopathy. Circulation 98:1750–1755, 1998.
60. Sgarbossa EB, et al: Chronic atrial fibrillation and stroke in paced patients with sick sinus syndrome: relevance of clinical characteristics and pacing modalities. Circulation 88:1045–1053, 1993.
61. Andersen HR, et al: Prospective randomised trial of atrial versus ventricular pacing in sick-sinus syndrome [see comments]. Lancet 344:1523–1528, 1994.
62. Lamas GA, et al: Quality of life and clinical outcomes in elderly patients treated with ventricular pacing as compared with dual-chamber pacing. Pacemaker Selection in the Elderly Investigators [see comments]. N Engl J Med 338:1097–1104, 1998.
63. Wharton J, Sorrentino RA, Campbell P, et al, the PAC-A Tach Investigators: Effect of pacing modality on atrial tachyarrhythmia recurrence in the tachycardia-bradycardia syndrome: preliminary results of the pacemaker atrial tachycardia trial. Circulation 98:I-494, 1998.
64. Connolly SJ, et al: Dual-chamber versus ventricular pacing: critical appraisal of current data [see comments]. Circulation 94:578–583, 1996.
65. Sami M, Abdollah S, Connolly L: Profile of cardiovascular mortality in the CTOPP Study. Pacing Clin Electrophysiol 22:A195, 1999.
66. Lamas GA: Pacemaker mode selection and survival: a plea to apply the principles of evidence based medicine to cardiac pacing practice. Heart 78:218–220, 1997.
67. Andersen HR, Nielsen JC: Pacing in sick sinus syndrome: need for a prospective, randomized trial comparing atrial with dual chamber pacing [editorial]. Pacing Clin Electrophysiol 21:1175–1179, 1998.
68. Saksena S, et al: Prevention of recurrent atrial fibrillation with chronic dual-site right atrial pacing. J Am Coll Cardiol 28:687–694, 1996.
69. Defaut P, et al: Long-term outcome of patients with drug-refractory atrial flutter and fibrillation after single- and dual-site right atrial pacing for arrhythmia prevention. J Am Coll Cardiol 32:1900–1908, 1998.
70. Levy S, et al: Atrial fibrillation: current knowledge and recommendations for management. Working Group on Arrhythmias of the European Society of Cardiology. Eur Heart J 19:1294–1320, 1998.

71. Barold SS, et al: Permanent multisite cardiac pacing [editorial]. Pacing Clin Electrophysiol 20:2725–2729, 1997.
72. Hochleitner M, et al: Long-term efficacy of physiologic dual-chamber pacing in the treatment of end-stage idiopathic dilated cardiomyopathy. Am J Cardiol 70:1320–1325, 1992.
73. Nishimura RA, et al: Mechanism of hemodynamic improvement by dual-chamber pacing for severe left ventricular dysfunction: an acute Doppler and catheterization hemodynamic study. J Am Coll Cardiol 25:281–288, 1995.
74. Innes D, Leitch JW, Fletcher PJ: VDD pacing at short atrioventricular intervals does not improve cardiac output in patients with dilated heart failure. Pacing Clin Electrophysiol 17:959–965, 1994.
75. Linde C, et al: Results of atrioventricular synchronous pacing with optimized delay in patients with severe congestive heart failure. Am J Cardiol 75:919–923, 1995.
76. Rosenqvist M, et al: Relative importance of activation sequence compared to atrioventricular synchrony in left ventricular function. Am J Cardiol 67:148–156, 1991.
77. Burkhoff D, Oikawa RY, Sagawa K: Influence of pacing site on canine left ventricular contraction. Am J Physiol 251:H428–435, 1986.
78. Leclercq C, et al: Acute hemodynamic effects of biventricular DDD pacing in patients with end-stage heart failure. J Am Coll Cardiol 32:1825–1831, 1998.
79. Ansalone G, et al: Multisite stimulation in refractory heart failure. G Ital Cardiol 29:451–459, 1999.
80. Abdallah HI, Balsara RK, O'Riordan AC: Pacemaker contact sensitivity: clinical recognition and management. Ann Thorac Surg 57:1017–1018, 1994.
81. Looks like a million works like a charm [editorial]. *In* Medtronic Pulse. p. 3. New York: Plenum, 1985.
82. Purdy D: Nuclear batteries for implantable applications. *In* Owens B (ed): Batteries for Implantable Biomedical Devices. New York: Plenum, 1986.
83. Greatbatch W, Holmes CF: The lithium/iodine battery: a historical perspective. Pacing Clin Electrophysiol 15:2034–2036, 1992.
84. Utereker DF, Shepard RB: Power sources for implantable pacemakers. *In* Ellenbogen KA (ed): Clinical Cardiac Pacing. pp. 91–111. Philadelphia: WB Saunders, 1995.
85. Ireland J, Kay GN: Pulse generator circuitry. *In* Ellenbogen KA (ed): Clinical Cardiac Pacing. pp.112–126. Philadelphia: WB Saunders, 1995.
86. Mond HG: Unipolar versus bipolar pacing: poles apart. Pacing Clin Electrophysiol 14:1411–1424, 1991.
87. Medtronic Inc.: Product Performance Report, March 1999. Minneapolis: Medtronic, 1999.
88. Timmis GC, et al: The significance of surface changes on explanted polyurethane pacemaker leads. Pacing Clin Electrophysiol 6:845–857, 1983.
89. Ripart A, Mugica J: Electrode-heart interface: definition of the ideal electrode. Pacing Clin Electrophysiol 6:410–421, 1983.
90. Elmqvist H, Schueller H, Richter G: The carbon tip electrode. Pacing Clin Electrophysiol 6:436–439, 1983.
91. Schuchert A, Kuck KH: Influence of internal current and pacing current on pacemaker longevity. Pacing Clin Electrophysiol 17:13–16, 1994.
92. Amundson DC, McArthur W, Mosharrafa M: The porous endocardial electrode. Pacing Clin Electrophysiol 2:40–50, 1979.
93. Furman S: Basic concepts. *In* Furman S (ed): A Practice of Cardiac Pacing. pp. 27–73. Mt. Kisco, NY: Futura, 1986.
94. Kruse IM, Terpstra B: Acute and long-term atrial and ventricular stimulation thresholds with a steroid-eluting electrode. Pacing Clin Electrophysiol 8:45–49, 1985.
95. Pirzada FA, Moschitto LJ, Diorio D: Clinical experience with steroid-eluting unipolar electrodes. Pacing Clin Electrophysiol 11:1739–1744, 1988.
96. Medtronic, Inc.: NovusR Leads. Minneapolis: Medtronic.
97. Amitani S, et al: Tensile force of pacing lead extraction: a comparison between tined type and screw-in type. Jpn Heart J 37:495–501, 1996.
98. Byrd CL, Wilkoff BL: Clinical Cardiac Pacing and Defibrillation. Philadelphia: WB Saunders, 1999.
99. Toivonen L, Lommi J: Dependence of atrial sensing function on posture in a single-lead atrial triggered ventricular (VDD) pacemaker. Pacing Clin Electrophysiol 19:309–313, 1996.
100. Crick JC: European multicenter prospective follow-up study of 1,002 implants of a single lead VDD pacing system. The European Multicenter Study Group. Pacing Clin Electrophysiol 14:1742–1744, 1991.
101. Daubert C, et al: Permanent left atrial pacing with a specifically designed coronary sinus lead. Pacing Clin Electrophysiol 20:2755–2764, 1997.
102. Auricchio A, et al: Transvenous biventricular pacing for heart failure: can the obstacles be overcome? Am J Cardiol 83:136D–142D, 1999.
103. O'Reilly MV, Murnaghan DP, Williams MB: Transvenous pacemaker failure induced by hyperkalemia. JAMA 228:336–337, 1974.
104. Hellestrand KJ, et al: Effect of the antiarrhythmic agent flecainide acetate on acute and chronic pacing thresholds. Pacing Clin Electrophysiol 6:892–899, 1983.
105. Kay GN, Ellenbogen KA: Sensing. *In* Ellenbogen KA, Kay GN (eds): Clinical Cardiac Pacing. pp. 38–68. Philadelphia: WB Saunders, 1985.
106. Higano ST, Hayes DL, Eisinger G: Sensor-driven rate smoothing in a DDDR pacemaker. Pacing Clin Electrophysiol 12:922–929, 1989.
107. Sutton R, Bourgeois I: Cost benefit analysis of single and dual chamber pacing for sick sinus syndrome and atrioventricular block: an economic sensitivity analysis of the literature [see comments]. Eur Heart J 17:574–582, 1996.
108. Hesselson AB, et al: Deleterious effects of long-term single-chamber ventricular pacing in patients with sick sinus syndrome: the hidden benefits of dual-chamber pacing. J Am Coll Cardiol 19:1542–1549, 1992.
109. Santini M, et al: Relation of prognosis in sick sinus syndrome to age, conduction defects and modes of permanent cardiac pacing. Am J Cardiol 65:729–735, 1990.
110. Mattioli AV, Vivoli D, Mattioli G: Influence of pacing modalities on the incidence of atrial fibrillation in patients without prior atrial fibrillation: a prospective study. Eur Heart J 19:282–286, 1998.
111. Brandt J, Schuller H: Conisideration for the selection of rate adaptive single lead atrial pacing. *In* Barold S (ed): New Perspectives in Cardiac Pacing. pp. 74–80. Mt. Kisco, NY: Futura, 1993.
112. Ausubel K, Furman S: The pacemaker syndrome. Ann Intern Med 103:420–429, 1985.
113. Alicandri C, et al: Three cases of hypotension and syncope with ventricular pacing: possible role of atrial reflexes. Am J Cardiol 42:137–142, 1978.
114. Gaasch WH, et al: Left ventricular compliance: mechanisms and clinical implications. Am J Cardiol 38:645–653, 1976.
115. Vardas PE, et al: Effect of dual chamber pacing on raised plasma atrial natriuretic peptide concentrations in complete atrioventricular block. BMJ 296:94, 1988.
116. Stangl K, et al: Influence of AV synchrony on the plasma levels of atrial natriuretic peptide (ANP) in patients with total AV block. Pacing Clin Electrophysiol 11:1176–1181, 1988.
117. MacGregor DC, et al: Relations between afterload, stroke volume, and descending limb of Starling's curve. Am J Physiol 227:884–890, 1974.
118. Katz AM: The descending limb of the Starling curve and the failing heart. Circulation 32:871–875, 1965.
119. Lau CP: The RAN sensors and algorithms used in rate adaptive cardiac pacing. Pacing Clin Electrophysiol 15:1177–1211, 1992.
120. Lau CP, et al: Clinical experience with an activity sensing DDDR pacemaker using an accelerometer sensor. Pacing Clin Electrophysiol 15:334–343, 1992.
121. Lau CP, et al: Initial clinical experience with a minute ventilation sensing rate modulated pacemaker: improvements in exercise capacity and symptomatology. Pacing Clin Electrophysiol 11:1815–1822, 1988.
122. Alt E, et al: Rate control of physiologic pacemakers by central venous blood temperature. Circulation 73:1206–1212, 1986.
123. Rickards AF, Donaldson RM, Thalen HJ: The use of QT interval to determine pacing rate: early clinical experience. Pacing Clin Electrophysiol 6:346–356, 1983.
124. Cowell R, et al: Are we being driven to two sensors? Clinical benefits of sensor cross-checking. Pacing Clin Electrophysiol 16:1441–1444, 1993.
125. Leung SK, Lau CP, Tang MO: Cardiac output is a sensitive indicator of difference in exercise performance between single and dual sensor pacemakers. Pacing Clin Electrophysiol 21:35–41, 1998.

126. Kamalvand K, et al: Is mode switching beneficial? A randomized study in patients with paroxysmal atrial tachyarrhythmias. J Am Coll Cardiol 30:496–504, 1997.
127. Brignole M, et al: Assessment of atrioventricular junction ablation and DDDR mode-switching pacemaker versus pharmacological treatment in patients with severely symptomatic paroxysmal atrial fibrillation: a randomized controlled study. Circulation 96:2617–2624, 1997.
128. Sheldon R, et al: Effect of dual-chamber pacing with automatic rate-drop sensing on recurrent neurally mediated syncope. Am J Cardiol 81:158–162, 1998.
129. Parsonnet V, Bernstein AD, Lindsay B: Pacemaker-implantation complication rates: an analysis of some contributing factors. J Am Coll Cardiol 13:917–921, 1989.
130. Zeft HJ: Pulmonary air embolism during insertion of a permanent transvenous cardiac pacemaker. Circulation 36:456–459, 1967.
131. Rubenfire M, et al: Clinical evaluation of myocardial perforation as a complication of permanent transvenous pacemakers. Chest 63:185–188, 1973.
132. Lewis AB, et al: Update on infections involving permanent pacemakers: characterization and management. J Thorac Cardiovasc Surg 89:758–763, 1985.
133. Choo MH, et al: Permanent pacemaker infections: characterization and management. Am J Cardiol 48:559–564, 1981.
134. Smith HJ, et al: Five-years experience with intravascular lead extraction. U.S. Lead Extraction Database. Pacing Clin Electrophysiol 17:2016–2020, 1994.
135. Da Costa A, et al: Antibiotic prophylaxis for permanent pacemaker implantation: a meta-analysis. Circulation 97:1796–1801, 1998.
136. Classen DC, et al: The timing of prophylactic administration of antibiotics and the risk of surgical-wound infection [see comments]. N Engl J Med 326:281–286, 1992.
137. Spittell PC, Hayes DL: Venous complications after insertion of a transvenous pacemaker. Mayo Clin Proc 67:258–265, 1992.
138. Mazzetti H, et al: Superior vena cava occlusion and/or syndrome related to pacemaker leads. Am Heart J 125:831–837, 1993.
139. Morley-Davies A, Cobbe SM: Cardiac pacing [see comments]. Lancet 349:41–46, 1997.
140. Salel AF, Seagren SC, Pool PE: Effects of encainide on the function of implanted pacemakers. Pacing Clin Electrophysiol 12:1439–1444, 1989.
141. Dohrmann ML, Goldschlager NF: Myocardial stimulation threshold in patients with cardiac pacemakers: effect of physiologic variables, pharmacologic agents, and lead electrodes. Cardiol Clin 3:527–537, 1985.
142. Barold SS: Timing cycles and operational characteristics of pacemakers. *In* Ellenbogen KA, Kay GN, Wilkoff BL (eds): Clinical Cardiac Pacing. pp. 567–572. Philadelphia: WB Saunders, 1995.
143. Heller LI: Surgical electrocautery and the runaway pacemaker syndrome. Pacing Clin Electrophysiol 13:1084–1085, 1990.
144. Raitt MH, et al: Runaway pacemaker during high-energy neutron radiation therapy. Chest 106:955–957, 1994.
145. Marco D, Eisinger G, Hayes DL: Testing of work environments for electromagnetic interference. Pacing Clin Electrophysiol 15:2016–2022, 1992.
146. Hayes DL, et al: State of the science: pacemaker and defibrillator interference from wireless communication devices [see comments]. Pacing Clin Electrophysiol 19:1419–1430, 1996.
147. McIvor ME, et al: Study of Pacemaker and Implantable Cardioverter Defibrillator Triggering by Electronic Article Surveillance Devices (SPICED TEAS) [see comments]. Pacing Clin Electrophysiol 21:1847–1861, 1998.
148. van Gelder BM, Bracke FA, el Gamal MI: Upper rate pacing after radiofrequency catheter ablation in a minute ventilation rate adaptive DDD pacemaker. Pacing Clin Electrophysiol 17:1437–1440, 1994.
149. Gimbel JR, et al: Safe performance of magnetic resonance imaging on five patients with permanent cardiac pacemakers. Pacing Clin Electrophysiol 19:913–919, 1996.
150. Lauck G, et al: Effects of nuclear magnetic resonance imaging on cardiac pacemakers. Pacing Clin Electrophysiol 18:1549–1555, 1995.
151. Hayes DL, et al: Interference with cardiac pacemakers by cellular telephones [see comments]. N Engl J Med 336:1473–1479, 1997.
152. Naegeli B, et al: Intermittent pacemaker dysfunction caused by digital mobile telephones. J Am Coll Cardiol 27:1471–1477, 1996.
153. Gillis AM: The impact of pulse generator longevity on the long-term costs of cardiac pacing [see comments]. Pacing Clin Electrophysiol 19:1459–1468, 1996.
154. Neglia D, Parsonnett V, Berstein AD: An analysis of clinical events in routine follow-up of pacemaker patients. Pacing Clin Electrophysiol 14:655, 1991.
155. Sweesy MW, et al: Analysis of the effectiveness of in-office and transtelephonic follow-up in terms of pacemaker system complications. Pacing Clin Electrophysiol 17:2001–2003, 1994.
156. Roelke M, Krauser DG, Rubinstein VJ, Parsonnet V: Improved follow up in a specialized pacemaker center as compared to physicians not specifically trained in pacemaker patient care. Pacing Clin Electrophysiol 20:1108, 1997.
157. Medicare: Cardiac pacemaker evaluation services. HCFA Publication, No. 6, Section 50–1. Washington, DC: HCFA, 1984.
158. Bernstein AD, et al: Report of the NASPE Policy Conference on antibradycardia pacemaker follow-up: effectiveness, needs, and resources. North American Society of Pacing and Electrophysiology. Pacing Clin Electrophysiol 17:1714–1729, 1994.
159. Korn M, et al: The pacemaker sound. Am J Med 49:451–458, 1970.
160. Shirato C, Ishikawa K: Newly developed systolic murmur in patients with a transvenous pacemaker. Am Heart J 99:722–726, 1980.
161. Cheng TO, Ertem G, Vera Z: Heart sounds in patients with cardiac pacemakers. Chest 62:66–70, 1972.
162. Toivonen L, Heikkola E: Comparison of pacing threshold development in membrane coated and steroid eluting electrodes. Pacing Clin Electrophysiol 19:610, 1996.
163. Crossley GH, et al: Reprogramming pacemakers enhances longevity and is cost-effective. Circulation 94(9 suppl):II-245–II-247, 1996.
164. Vallario LE, et al: Pacemaker follow-up and adequacy of Medicare guidelines. Am Heart J 116:11–15, 1988.
165. Mirowski M, et al: Standby automatic defibrillator: an approach to prevention of sudden coronary death. Arch Intern Med 126:158–161, 1970.
166. Gillum RF: Sudden coronary death in the United States: 1980–1985. Circulation 79:756–765, 1989.
167. Mirowski M, Mower MM, Reid PR: The automatic implantable defibrillator. Am Heart J 100:1089–1092, 1980.
168. Gregoratos G, et al: ACC/AHA Guidelines for Implantation of Cardiac Pacemakers and Antiarrhythmia Devices: Executive Summary—a report of the American College of Cardiology/American Heart Association Task Force on Practice Guidelines (Committee on Pacemaker Implantation). Circulation 97:1325–1335, 1998.
169. Grimm W, Flores BF, Marchlinski FE: Electrocardiographically documented unnecessary, spontaneous shocks in 241 patients with implantable cardioverter defibrillators. Pacing Clin Electrophysiol 15:1667–1673, 1992.
170. Neuzner J, Pitschner HF, Schlepper M: Programmable VT detection enhancements in implantable cardioverter defibrillator therapy. Pacing Clin Electrophysiol 18:539–547, 1995.
171. Marchlinski FE, et al: Benefits and lessons learned from stored electrogram information in implantable defibrillators. J Cardiovasc Electrophysiol 6:832–851, 1995.
172. Reiter MJ, Mann DE: Sensing and tachyarrhythmia detection problems in implantable cardioverter defibrillators. J Cardiovasc Electrophysiol 7:542–558, 1996.
173. Schaumann A, et al: Enhanced detection criteria in implantable cardioverter-defibrillators to avoid inappropriate therapy. Am J Cardiol 78:42–50, 1996.
174. Trappe HJ, et al: Single-chamber versus dual-chamber implantable cardioverter defibrillators: indications and clinical results. Am J Cardiol 83:8D–16D, 1999.
175. Calkins H, et al: Clinical interactions between pacemakers and automatic implantable cardioverter-defibrillators. J Am Coll Cardiol 16:666–673, 1990.
176. Lampert R, et al: Inappropriate sensing of atrial stimuli in patients with third-generation defibrillators and DDD pacemakers. Pacing Clin Electrophysiol 21:1225–1229, 1998.
177. Kastor JA: Michel Mirowski and the automatic implantable defibrillator. Am J Cardiol 63:1121–1126, 1989.
178. Mower MM: Automatic implantable cardioverter-defibrillator: history and future developments. Z Kardiol 84(suppl 2):123–126, 1995.
179. Clinical outcome of patients with malignant ventricular tachyarrhythmias and a multiprogrammable implantable cardioverter-defi-

brillator implanted with or without thoracotomy: an international multicenter study. PCD Investigator Group. J Am Coll Cardiol 23:1521–1530, 1994.
180. Neuzner J: Clinical experience with a new cardioverter defibrillator capable of biphasic waveform pulse and enhanced data storage: results of a prospective multicenter study. European Ventak P2 Investigator Group. Pacing Clin Electrophysiol 17:1243–1255, 1994.
181. Block M, et al: A prospective randomized cross-over comparison of mono- and biphasic defibrillation using nonthoracotomy lead configurations in humans. J Cardiovasc Electrophysiol 5:581–590, 1994.
182. Bardy GH, Yee R, Jung W: Multicenter experience with a pectoral unipolar implantable cardioverter-defibrillator. Active Can Investigators. J Am Coll Cardiol 28:400–410, 1996.
183. Cooklin M, et al: Comparison of bipolar and integrated sensing for redetection of ventricular fibrillation. Am Heart J 138:133–136, 1999.
184. Hurwitz JL, et al: Importance of abortive shock capability with electrogram storage in cardioverter-defibrillator devices. J Am Coll Cardiol 21:895–900, 1993.
185. Schaumann A: Managing atrial tachyarrhythmias in patients with implantable cardioverter defibrillators. Am J Cardiol 83:214D–217D, 1999.
186. Anderson MH, et al: Performance of basic ventricular tachycardia detection algorithms in implantable cardioverter defibrillators: implications for device programming. Pacing Clin Electrophysiol 20:2975–2983, 1997.
187. Wood MA, et al: Lessons learned from data logging in a multicenter clinical trial using a late-generation implantable cardioverter-defibrillator. The Guardian ATP 4210 Multicenter Investigators Group. J Am Coll Cardiol 24:1692–1699, 1994.
188. Nunain SO, et al: Limitations and late complications of third-generation automatic cardioverter-defibrillators. Circulation 91:2204–2213, 1995.
189. Swerdlow CD, et al: Underdetection of ventricular tachycardia by algorithms to enhance specificity in a tiered-therapy cardioverter-defibrillator. J Am Coll Cardiol 24:416–424, 1994.
190. Weber M, et al: Efficacy and safety of the initial use of stability and onset criteria in implantable cardioverter defibrillators. J Cardiovasc Electrophysiol 10:145–153, 1999.
191. Brugada J: Is inappropriate therapy a resolved issue with current implantable cardioverter defibrillators? Am J Cardiol 83:40D–44D, 1999.
192. Barold HS, et al: Prospective evaluation of new and old criteria to discriminate between supraventricular and ventricular tachycardia in implantable defibrillators. Pacing Clin Electrophysiol 21:1347–1355, 1998.
193. Porterfield JG, et al: Conversion rates of induced versus spontaneous ventricular tachycardia by a third generation cardioverter defibrillator. The VENTAK PRx Phase I Investigators. Pacing Clin Electrophysiol 16:170–173, 1993.
194. Gross JN, et al: The antitachycardia pacing ICD: impact on patient selection and outcome. Pacing Clin Electrophysiol 16:165–169, 1993.
195. Rosenqvist M: Antitachycardia pacing: which patients and which methods? Am J Cardiol 78:92–97, 1996.
196. Newman D, Dorian P, Hardy J: Randomized controlled comparison of antitachycardia pacing algorithms for termination of ventricular tachycardia. J Am Coll Cardiol 21:1413–1418, 1993.
197. Bardy GH, et al: A prospective randomized repeat-crossover comparison of antitachycardia pacing with low-energy cardioversion. Circulation 87:1889–1896, 1993.
198. Geelen P, et al: The value of DDD pacing in patients with an implantable cardioverter defibrillator. Pacing Clin Electrophysiol 20:177–181, 1997.
199. Higgins SL, et al: Indications for implantation of a dual-chamber pacemaker combined with an implantable cardioverter-defibrillator. Am J Cardiol 81:1360–1362, 1998.
200. Santini M, et al: Indications for dual-chamber (DDD) pacing in implantable cardioverter-defibrillator patients. Am J Cardiol 78:116–118, 1996.
201. Hesselson AB, et al: Deleterious effects of long-term single-chamber ventricular pacing in patients with sick sinus syndrome: the hidden benefits of dual-chamber pacing. J Am Coll Cardiol 19:1542–1549, 1992.
202. Zhou L, et al: Effects of amiodarone and its active metabolite desethylamidarone on the ventricular defibrillation threshold. J Am Coll Cardiol 31:1672–1678, 1998.
203. Jung W, et al: Effects of chronic amiodarone therapy on defibrillation threshold. Am J Cardiol 70:1023–1027, 1992.
204. Venditti FJ Jr, et al: Rise in chronic defibrillation thresholds in nonthoracotomy implantable defibrillator. Circulation 89:216–223, 1994.
205. Strickberger SA, et al: Probability of successful defibrillation at multiples of the defibrillation energy requirement in patients with an implantable defibrillator. Circulation 96:1217–1223, 1997.
206. Occhetta E, et al: Implantable cardioverter defibrillators and cellular telephones: is there any interference? [see comments]. Pacing Clin Electrophysiol 22:983–989, 1999.
207. Barbaro V, et al: Electromagnetic interference of digital and analog cellular telephones with implantable cardioverter defibrillators: in vitro and in vivo studies. Pacing Clin Electrophysiol 22:626–634, 1999.
208. Lawton JS, et al: Sensing lead-related complications in patients with transvenous implantable cardioverter-defibrillators. Am J Cardiol 78:647–651, 1996.
209. Daoud EG, et al: Incidence, presentation, diagnosis, and management of malfunctioning implantable cardioverter-defibrillator rate-sensing leads. Am Heart J 128:892–895, 1994.
210. Roelke M, et al: Subclavian crush syndrome complicating transvenous cardioverter defibrillator systems [see comments]. Pacing Clin Electrophysiol 18:973–979, 1995.
211. A comparison of antiarrhythmic-drug therapy with implantable defibrillators in patients resuscitated from near-fatal ventricular arrhythmias. The Antiarrhythmics versus Implantable Defibrillators (AVID) Investigators [see comments]. N Engl J Med 337:1576–1583, 1997.
212. Connolly S: Results of the Canadian Implantable Defibrillator Study (CIDS). Presented at the 20th Annual Scientific Session of the North American Society of Pacing and Electrophysiology, 1999.
213. Kuck K: Results of the Cardiac Arrest Study-Hamburg (CASH). Presented at the 47th Annual Scientific Session of the American College of Cardiology. 1998.
214. Moss AJ, et al: Improved survival with an implanted defibrillator in patients with coronary disease at high risk for ventricular arrhythmia. Multicenter Automatic Defibrillator Implantation Trial Investigators [see comments]. N Engl J Med 335:1933–1940, 1996.
215. Buxton A, Leek L, Fisher JD, et al: A randomized study of the prevention of sudden death in patients with coronary artery disease. Multicenter Unsustained Tachycardia Trial Investigators. N Engl J Med 341:1882–1890, 1999.
216. Bigger JT Jr: Prophylactic use of implanted cardiac defibrillators in patients at high risk for ventricular arrhythmias after coronary-artery bypass graft surgery. Coronary Artery Bypass Graft (CABG) Patch Trial Investigators [see comments]. N Engl J Med 337:1569–1575, 1997.
217. Wilber DJ, et al: Electrophysiological testing and nonsustained ventricular tachycardia. Use and limitations in patients with coronary artery disease and impaired ventricular function [see comments]. Circulation 82:350–358, 1990.
218. Bhandari AK, et al: Prognostic significance of programmed ventricular stimulation in patients surviving complicated acute myocardial infarction: a prospective study. Am Heart J 124:87–96, 1992.
219. The Cardiac Insufficiency Bisoprolol Study II (CIBIS-II): a randomised trial [see comments]. Lancet 353:9–13, 1999.
220. Effect of metoprolol CR/XL in chronic heart failure: Metoprolol CR/XL Randomised Intervention Trial in Congestive Heart Failure (MERIT-HF) [see comments]. Lancet 353:2001–2007, 1999.
221. Boutitie F, et al: Amiodarone interaction with beta-blockers: analysis of the merged EMIAT (European Myocardial Infarct Amiodarone Trial) and CAMIAT (Canadian Amiodarone Myocardial Infarction Trial) databases. The EMIAT and CAMIAT Investigators. Circulation 99:2268–2275, 1999.
222. Vorperian VR, Lawrence S, Chlebowski K: Replacing abdominally implanted defibrillators: effect of procedure setting on cost. Pacing Clin Electrophysiol 22:698–705, 1999.
223. Owens DK, et al: Cost-effectiveness of implantable cardioverter defibrillators relative to amiodarone for prevention of sudden cardiac

death [see comments]. Ann Intern Med 126:1–12, 1997.
224. Larsen GC, et al: Cost-effectiveness of the implantable cardioverter-defibrillator: effect of improved battery life and comparison with amiodarone therapy. J Am Coll Cardiol 19:1323–1334, 1992.
225. Wever EF, et al: Cost-effectiveness of implantable defibrillator as first-choice therapy versus electrophysiologically guided, tiered strategy in postinfarct sudden death survivors: a randomized study [see comments]. Circulation 93:489–496, 1996.
226. Mushlin AI, et al: The cost-effectiveness of automatic implantable cardiac defibrillators: results from MADIT. Multicenter Automatic Defibrillator Implantation Trial. Circulation 97:2129–2135, 1998.
227. Nearing BD, Huang AH, Verrier RL: Dynamic tracking of cardiac vulnerability by complex demodulation of the T wave. Science 252:437–440, 1991.
228. Zehender M, et al: Continuous monitoring of acute myocardial ischemia by the implantable cardioverter defibrillator. Am Heart J 127:1057–1063, 1994.
229. Steinhaus DM, et al: Initial experience with an implantable hemodynamic monitor. Circulation 93:745–752, 1996.
230. Daubert J: The Compensatory Pause Prevention Algorithm: Preliminary Results at the Ventricular Level. New York: Futura, 1997.
231. Pinski SL, Fahy GL: Implantable cardioverter-defibrillators. Am J Med 106:446–458, 1999.

CHAPTER 97

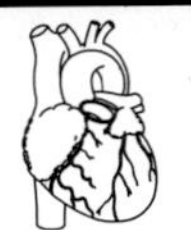

Radiofrequency Catheter Ablation of Supraventricular and Ventricular Arrhythmias

Luz Maria Rodriguez, Carl Timmermans, and Hein J. J. Wellens

HISTORICAL ASPECTS
INDICATIONS FOR RADIOFREQUENCY CATHETER ABLATION OF TACHYCARDIAS
Supraventricular Tachycardia
Ventricular Tachycardia
SUMMARY

Historical Aspects

In 1967, programmed electrical stimulation of the heart was introduced into clinical cardiology independently by Durrer and coworkers[1] in Amsterdam and by Coumel and associates[2] in Paris. Programmed electrical stimulation of the heart has revolutionized our methods of diagnosis and treatment of cardiac arrhythmias.[3] It resulted not only in the ability to localize the site of origin of the arrhythmia but also in a better understanding of arrhythmia mechanisms, better interpretation of the arrhythmia electrocardiogram (ECG), and the development of new treatment modalities such as antitachycardia pacing[4] and surgical[5] or catheter[6, 7] ablation of the tachycardia focus or pathway.

In 1986, the first successful clinical arrhythmia ablation with radiofrequency (RF) current was reported.[8] Early experience in the ablation of supraventricular arrhythmias had variable results. With evolving understanding of the anatomy of the heart and the introduction of a new RF ablation catheter with a large (4-mm) distal electrode, the success rate improved dramatically.[9, 10] To date, radiofrequency catheter ablation (RFCA) has become the first truly curative treatment for many supraventricular and some ventricular tachycardias (VTs).[11]

The RF ablation procedure should be preceded by a careful analysis of the 12-lead arrhythmia ECG and an electrophysiologic study. The electrophysiologic study should consist of a systematic analysis of the arrhythmia by recording and measuring a variety of electrophysiologic parameters during the basal state and by evaluating the response to programmed electrical stimulation. Programmed electrical stimulation of the heart not only gives important information about the electrophysiologic properties of the atrioventricular (AV) node, the His-Purkinje system, the atria, and the ventricles but also allows the study of the mechanism and localization of the site of origin or pathway of an arrhythmia. How the electrophysiologic study and the subsequent RF procedure should be conducted depends on the specific arrhythmia of the patient.

Indications for Radiofrequency Catheter Ablation of Tachycardias

The efficacy and the safety profile of RFCA resulted in the indications shown in Table 97–1. The approaches to the different types of supraventricular tachycardias and VTs are discussed separately.

Supraventricular Tachycardia

Accessory Pathways

LOCALIZATION

As also discussed in Chapter 87, Preexcitation, an accessory AV pathway is a connection between the atrium and

TABLE 97–1 Indications for Radiofrequency Catheter Ablation of Arrhythmias

Life threatening arrhythmias: Wolff-Parkinson-White patients with a short anterograde refractory period of their accessory atrioventricular pathway and patients with ventricular tachycardias, poorly tolerated hemodynamically
Arrhythmias leading to pump failure: Incessant atrial tachycardia; circus movement tachycardia using a slowly conducting accessory pathway in ventriculoatrial direction; atrial fibrillation
Symptomatic tachycardias, not controlled by antiarrhythmic drugs or because of patient preference: Paroxysmal atrial tachycardia; atrial flutter; atrioventricular nodal reentrant tachycardia; tachycardias using an accessory pathway; ventricular tachycardias
Prophylactic: Asymptomatic patients with an accessory pathway with a short anterograde refractory period resulting in an occupational hazard (pilots, professional athletes, and so on)

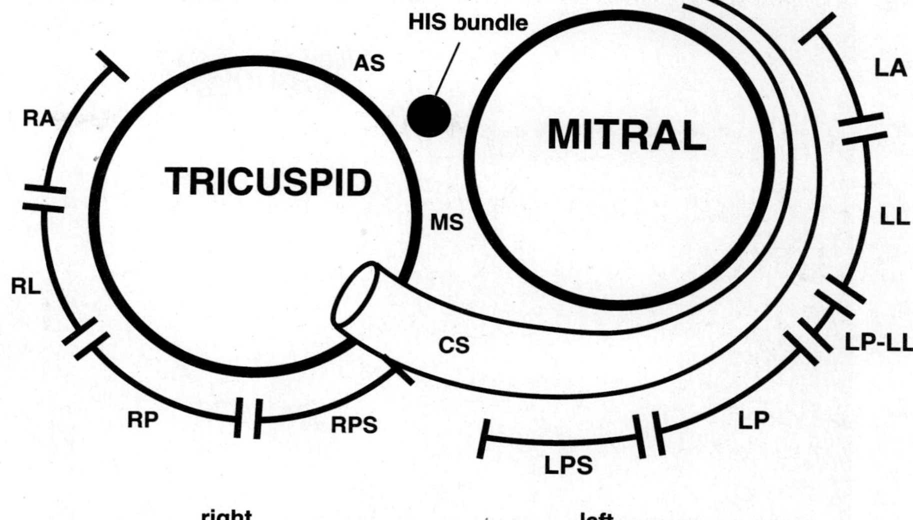

FIGURE 97–1 Localization of the different accessory pathways along the atrioventricular groove on the left and right sides. AS, anteroseptal; CS, coronary sinus; LA, left anterior, LL, left lateral; LP, left posterior; LPS, left posteroseptal; MS, midseptal; RA, right anterior; RL, right lateral; RP, right posterior; RPS, right posteroseptal.

the ventricle crossing the AV groove on the left or right side of the heart. Originally, accessory AV connections were divided into those located on the right or left free wall and the posteroseptal, anteroseptal, and midseptal regions. The use of RF catheter ablation requires a more precise localization of the accessory pathways in the AV groove (Fig. 97–1). Free wall accessory pathways are subdivided in a posterior, lateral, and anterior localization. Posteroseptal accessory pathways may also be found in the wall of the coronary sinus and in some cases in the middle cardiac vein.[12] Anteroseptal accessory pathways are those pathways located above the His bundle, and midseptal accessory pathways are those located in the midseptal area.[13, 14] The midseptum is the region located superior to the ostium of the coronary sinus but below the His bundle (Fig. 97–2). It is important to stress that accessory pathways may be conducting in both directions (anterogradely and retrogradely), only anterogradely, or only retrogradely. The latter pathway is called a *concealed* pathway. Concealed pathways are of two types: the rapidly and the slowly conducting one.

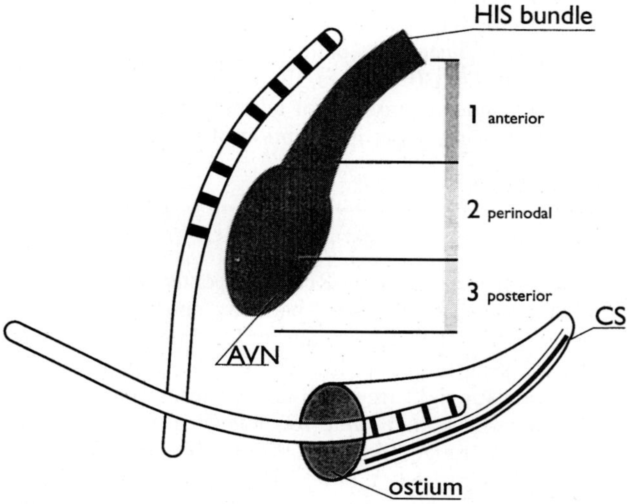

FIGURE 97–2 Localization of the three types of midseptal accessory pathways (anterior, perinodal, posterior) in the space between the ostium of the coronary sinus (CS) inferiorly and the His bundle superiorly. AVN, atrioventricular node.

PROCEDURE

To perform a RF ablation procedure, catheters are inserted through both femoral veins, the subclavian vein, or both and positioned in the heart under fluoroscopy. A quadripolar catheter is placed in the high right atrium, the His bundle, and the right ventricular apex. A multipolar catheter is placed in the coronary sinus. Finally, an RF catheter is positioned at the site of the accessory pathway as determined during the electrophysiologic study. In general, two fluoroscopic views—the left anterior oblique and the right anterior oblique projections—are used to position the RF ablation catheter in the accessory pathway region. In patients with a left-sided accessory pathway, the usual approach is to insert the RF catheter into the femoral artery retrogradely advance the catheter across the aortic valve, followed by positioning under the mitral annulus (Fig. 97–3). Mapping of the left AV groove to obtain specific electrograms, indicating the exact localization of the accessory pathway, is performed before attempting RF ablation. This requires a careful manipulation of the RF catheter under the mitral annulus and a good understanding and interpretation of the recorded electrograms. This approach is used when the ventricular insertion of the accessory pathway is the target of the RF ablation. If the atrial insertion of the accessory pathway must be ablated, the RF catheter should be positioned on the mitral annulus. Some centers prefer a transseptal catheterization to ablate left-sided accessory pathways, and in those patients, RF energy is delivered at the atrial insertion of the accessory pathway. The catheter inserted in the coronary sinus anatomically marks the AV groove and helps in mapping left-sided accessory pathways.

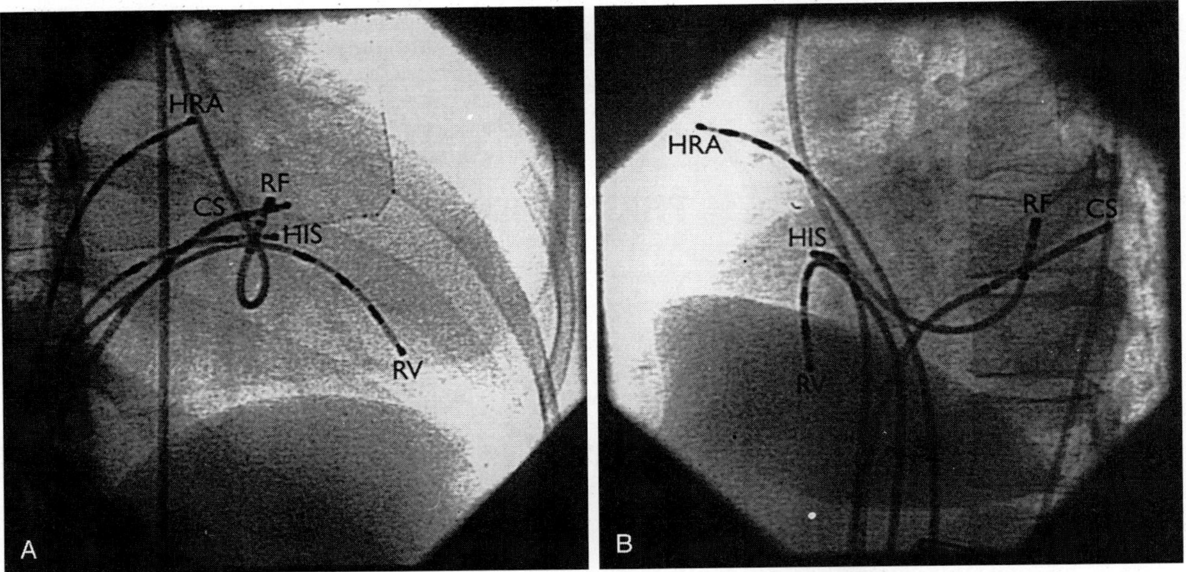

FIGURE 97–3 **A,** Right anterior oblique projection of catheters positioned in the coronary sinus (CS), high right atrium (HRA), His bundle (HIS), and right ventricle (RV). The tip of the radiofrequency ablation catheter (RF) is located under the mitral valve in the left lateral region. **B,** The same catheters in the left anterior oblique projection.

In patients with right-sided accessory pathways, the procedure is performed using either the femoral or subclavian approach. The RF catheter is carefully advanced most of the time over and sometimes under the tricuspid annulus to obtain the optimal electrograms indicating the exact location of the accessory pathway. Posteroseptal accessory pathways are located in the posteroseptal space (right and left) just outside and below the coronary sinus ostium. Some accessory pathways can also be located within the coronary sinus or in one of its branches (e.g., middle cardiac vein); therefore, mapping of the posteroseptal space should also include the first centimeters of the coronary sinus and its posterior branches.[12] Anteroseptal accessory pathways are pathways located above the His bundle, and midseptal accessory pathways are located in the midseptal region. Because of the vicinity of the conduction system (right bundle for anteroseptal accessory pathways; His bundle and AV node for midseptal accessory pathways), mapping of these regions should carefully and precisely be performed before delivering RF energy to avoid complications such as right bundle branch block or complete AV block, which may require permanent pacemaker implantation.

OPTIMAL SITE

Several electrophysiologic criteria are used to localize the optimal site to deliver RF energy.[15–18] During preexcited rhythms, the following parameters are used to localize the ventricular insertion of an accessory pathway: the local AV interval, the earliest ventricular activation compared with the delta wave, and the recording of an accessory pathway potential (Fig. 97–4). Certain morphologies of the unipolar electrogram and an early intrinsic deflection of the unipolar recording relative to the delta wave onset may also indicate an optimal ablation site.[17] The atrial insertion of an accessory pathway is usually localized by the site of the shortest ventriculoatrial (VA) interval during ventricular pacing or during circus movement tachycardia or by recording an accessory pathway potential. In general, the following criteria are considered to identify the optimal site for delivering RF energy in preexcited rhythms: the presence of an accessory pathway potential, the onset of a local ventriculogram preceding the delta wave by 5 to 20 milliseconds, a local AV interval of less than 40 milliseconds, and a PQS morphology in the unipolar recordings.[17, 18] In patients with a concealed accessory pathway, the ablation site of the atrial insertion is indicated by the shortest VA interval. [19] If the RF catheter has good tissue contact and the previously mentioned criteria are present, loss of preexcitation, retrograde conduction, or both should occur within seconds after the delivery of RF energy. Disappearance of preexcitation within 10 seconds after the delivery of RF energy is a good predictor for long-term success (Fig. 97–5). After the interruption of accessory pathway conduction and after a waiting period of 30 minutes, the electrophysiologic study is repeated under isoproterenol administration (1 to 3 μg/kg) to ensure permanent interruption of the accessory pathway.

SUCCESS RATE

The long-term success of RFCA depends on the correct localization of the accessory pathway and the experience of the operator. The success rate for left free wall accessory pathways is currently as high as 95 to 99 percent.[6] The success rate for right free wall and posteroseptal accessory pathways is less than that for left free wall accessory pathways and ranges between 90 and 93 percent. This is due to less catheter stability (right free wall accessory pathways) and to the complexity of the posteroseptal space (posteroseptal accessory pathways) where the accessory pathways may have an anatomic epicardial insertion with widespread branching, making complete ablation difficult.

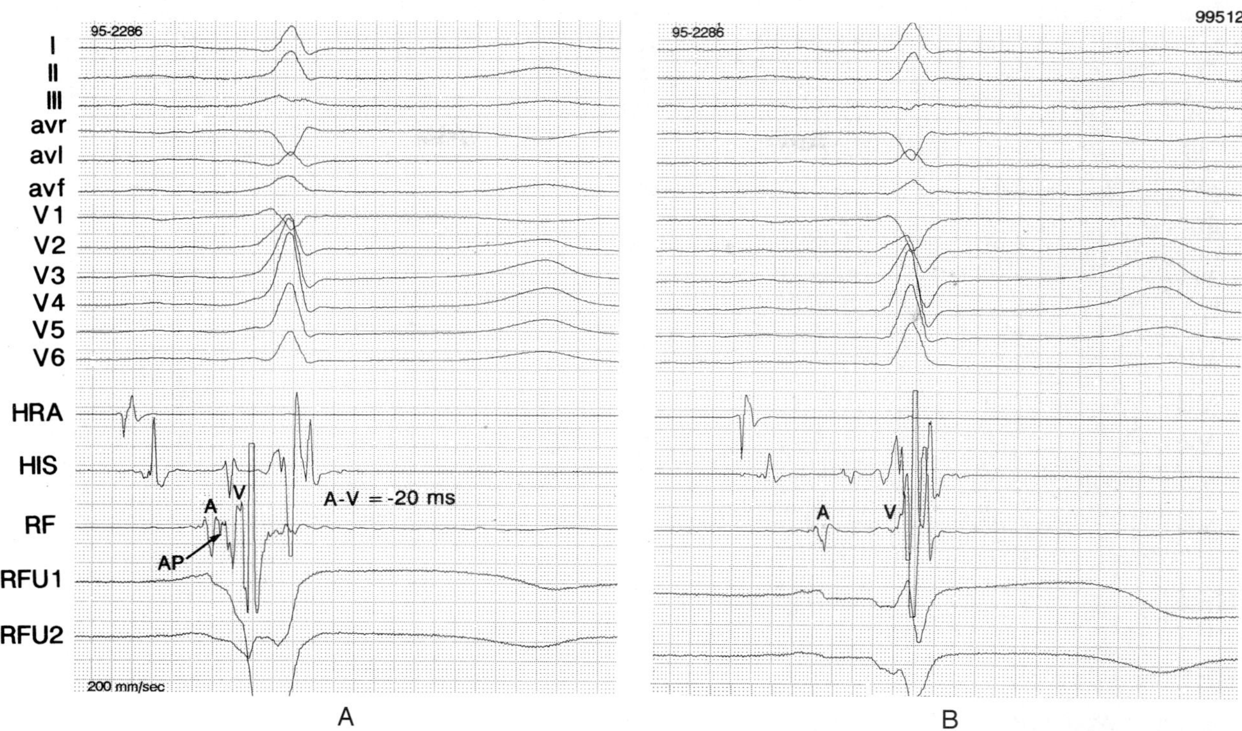

FIGURE 97–4 **A,** A 12-lead electrocardiogram (ECG) in a patient with a left lateral accessory pathway **(top)** and endocardial recordings recorded from the high right atrium (HRA), His bundle (HIS), and the tip of the radiofrequency ablation catheter with the bipolar (RF) and corresponding unipolar recordings (RFU1, RFU2) **(bottom)**. Note that the bipolar electrogram of the radiofrequency catheter located at the successful ablation site shows an accessory pathway potential (AP) and an atrioventricular interval of 20 ms. Furthermore, the unipolar RFU1 shows a PQS pattern. **B,** After successful ablation, pre-excitation and the AP potential have disappeared, and the atrioventricular interval recorded from the tip of the radiofrequency catheter ablation has lengthened to 100 ms.

The success rate for anteroseptal and midseptal accessory pathways ranges between 95 and 100 percent, but the risk of creating complete AV block in patients with midseptal accessory pathway is not negligible. The success rate for a Mahaim-type accessory pathway (a slowly conducting pathway inserting into the right ventricle) has also been reported to be as high as 90 to 100 percent.[20] Recording of a Mahaim potential on the tricuspid annulus is a good indicator for a successful ablation (Fig. 97–6). Finally, in patients with circus movement tachycardias using a slowly conducting accessory pathway for VA conduction, the success rate is as high as 95 to 100 percent. [21]

RECURRENCE OF CONDUCTION

In our institution, the incidence of reappearance of conduction through an accessory pathway after RFCA is around 8 percent. The time of recurrence of accessory pathway conduction ranged from 3 hours to 3 months.[22] These figures are in agreement with other studies reporting a recurrence rate of 8 to 12 percent after a time delay of 4 to 7 months.[23] Several variables have been reported to be predictors for recurrence of conduction over an accessory pathway: the presence of multiple accessory pathways, a high number of RF applications, young age,[23] and a right-sided location.[22] In general, the overall recurrence rate is low, and if necessary, the patient can be reablated with a high success rate. Based on this information, patients should be followed for 6 months after ablation.

COMPLICATIONS

The risk of RFCA is related to the location of the accessory pathway. As previously mentioned, ablation of a midseptal accessory pathway carries the risk of complete AV block. In posteroseptal epicardially located accessory pathways, where the ablation has to be performed from the coronary sinus, there is a risk of damage to the coronary artery or perforation of the venous system leading to cardiac tamponade.[12] A Multicenter European Survey[24] reported on the complications of RFCA in 2222 patients with accessory pathways. Fourteen patients (0.63 percent) developed complete AV block, 16 patients (0.72 percent) had a cardiac perforation with or without tamponade, and 12 patients developed a clinically significant pericardial effusion. In 3 patients, death was thought to be related to the procedure. However, it is important to mention that this study analyzed retrospective data from an early period (1987 to 1992) of RFCA. Calkins and associates[25] in a prospective study found a similar incidence of the same complications in the period of 1992 to 1995. In children and adolescents, the American Society of Pediatric Electrophysiology[26] reported 3.2 percent of complications after RFCA of supraventricular tachycardias in 4135 patients. The complications were complete AV block, cardiac perforation, pericardial effusion, cerebral emboli, and pneumothorax. A multivariate analysis showed three independent factors for recognizing patients with a high probability to develop a complication: the experience of the operator, the presence of right-sided

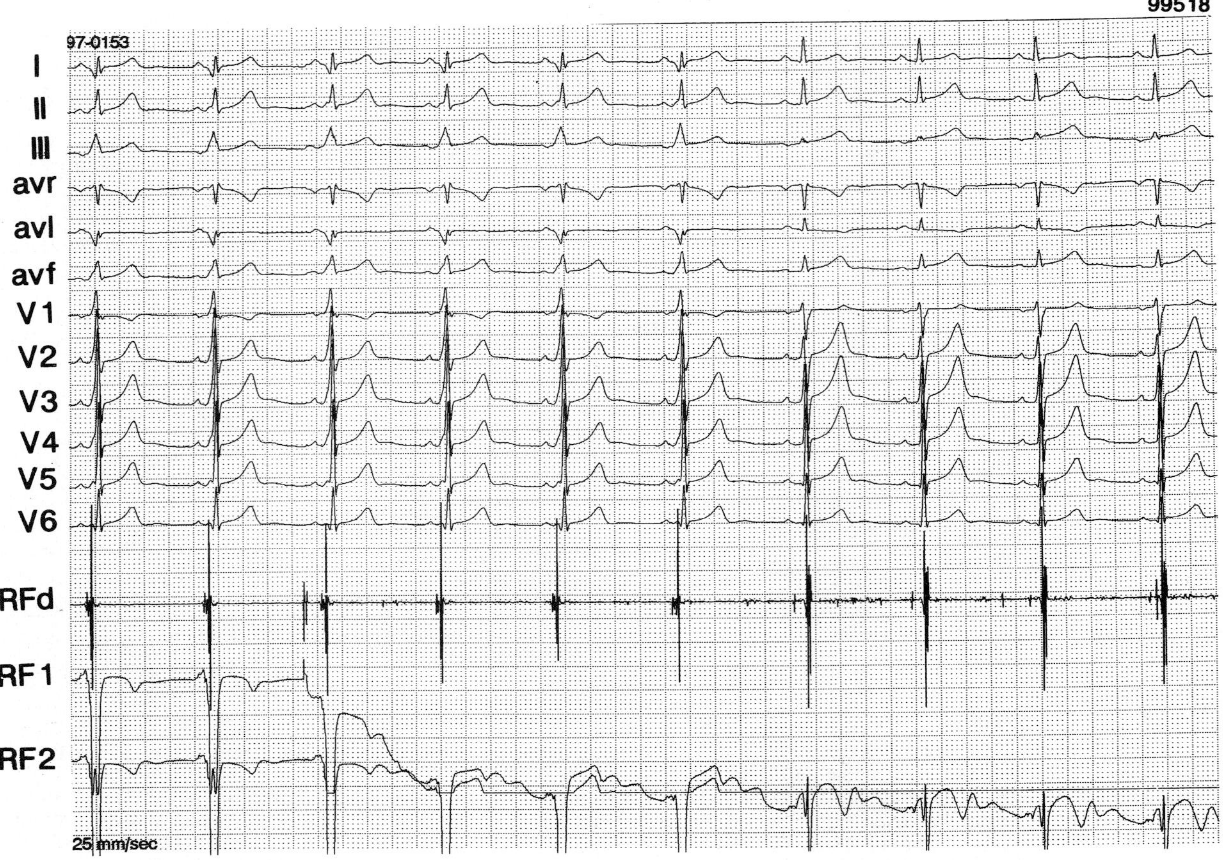

FIGURE 97–5 A 12-lead ECG and the bipolar (RFd) and unipolar (RF 1, RF 2) electrograms during radiofrequency ablation in a patient with an anterograde-conducting left lateral accessory pathway. Note the disappearance of pre-excitation immediately after radiofrequency energy application.

accessory pathways, and a body weight of less than 15 kg. Also in this survey, four deaths (0.11 percent) were reported. In the early days of RFCA, the fluoroscopy time was an important concern for eventual complications. To date, with more experience, procedure and fluoroscopy times have shortened, thereby reducing the risk of complications due to radiation.

Atrioventricular Nodal Reentrant Tachycardia

RFCA in patients with AV nodal reentrant tachycardia (AVNRT) has been quite successful in curing patients.[27–31] It has become the treatment of choice when the patient is symptomatic with this arrhythmia, not responding to or not willing to take antiarrhythmic medication. In the early days of RFCA, two approaches were suggested: the anterior approach to interrupt the fast and the posterior approach to block the slow pathway. These approaches were called anterior and posterior based on the location of the fast and slow pathways in the triangle of Koch. The fast pathway is located close to the His bundle, in the anterior part of the triangle of Koch, and the slow pathway is situated in the posterior part of this triangle (Fig. 97–7). Fast pathway ablation is seldom used in view of the high risk of complete AV block (5 to 10 percent) because of the proximity of the ablation site to the compact AV node and proximal His bundle.[32, 33]

SLOW PATHWAY ABLATION PROCEDURE

Two techniques have been used to ablate the slow pathway: the anatomic technique[29, 33] and the electrophysiologic technique.[27, 28] In the anatomic technique, fluoroscopic landmarks are used to guide the positioning of the ablation catheter. Using the posterior approach, the RF catheter is positioned in the posterior third of Koch's triangle (Fig. 97–8). An AV ratio of 0.5 or less than 1 in the ECG recorded with the tip of the RF catheter is required before the delivery of RF energy. A successful RF application is frequently associated with the appearance of a short episode of an accelerated junctional rhythm. After each RF application, conduction over the slow pathway and inducibility of AVNRT should be assessed. If this posterior approach is unsuccessful, the catheter is carefully moved to the midseptal region, where RF energy is again delivered. When using the electrophysiologic technique, RF ablation is performed based on specific electrograms representing slow pathway conduction. Two distinct morphologies of slow pathway potentials have been described. Jackman and colleagues[27] described a sharp spike-like potential preceded by a lower-frequency, lower-amplitude atrial potential during sinus rhythm. The slow pathway potential usually follows the atrial potential after 10 to 40 milliseconds. The slow pathway potential is recorded in the vicinity of the coronary sinus ostium, near the tricuspid annulus.

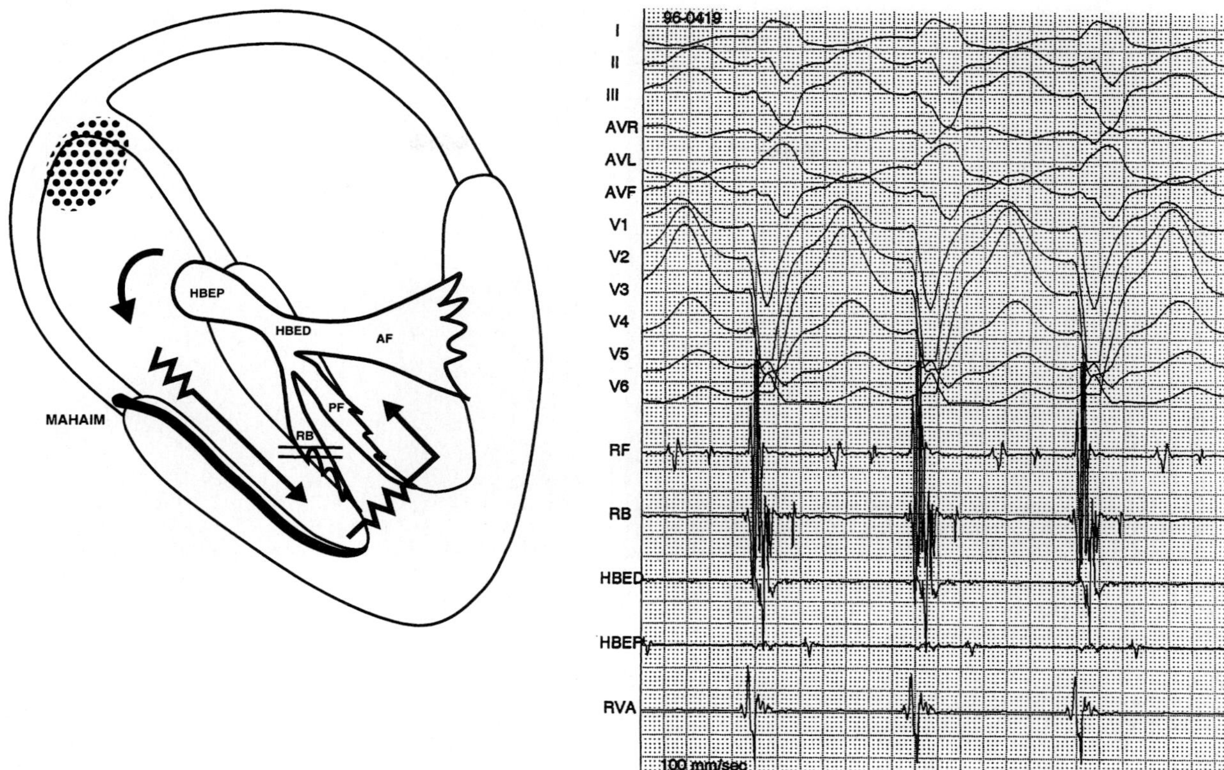

FIGURE 97–6 An electrophysiologic study in a patient with pre-excited tachycardia with atrioventricular conduction over a Mahaim fiber and ventriculoatrial conduction over the His–atrioventricular node pathway. Note the presence of a Mahaim potential recorded with the tip of the radiofrequency (RF) catheter where successful ablation was performed. AF, anterior fascicle; PF, posterior fascicle; RB, right bundle; HBED, His bundle electrogram distal; HBEP, His bundle electrogram proximal; RVA, right ventricular apex.

Another type of slow pathway potential was described by Haissaguerre and associates.[28] This is a low-amplitude, low-frequency signal and follows the atrial electrogram and is recorded in the midseptal area. Acute success of AVNRT ablation ranges from 90 to 100 percent.[27, 31] Few patients (1 percent in our laboratory) experience a recurrence of the arrhythmia and require a second procedure. The risk of AV block using the posterior approach is low (1 percent) compared with the anterior approach (5 to 10 percent).[25, 32] Other complications, like venous thrombosis and pericardial effusion, can occur, but in general, the risk of the procedure is low because no arterial catheterization is required.

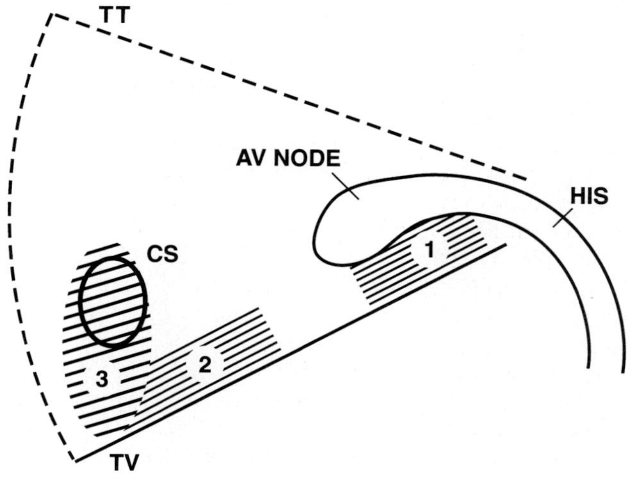

FIGURE 97–7 This figure depicts the triangle of Koch composed by the tendon of Todaro (TT) superiorly and the tricuspid valve (TV) inferiorly. The coronary sinus (CS) ostium forms the base, and the His bundle forms the apical portion. The numbers in the triangle represent the three approaches to perform radiofrequency ablation of atrioventricular (AV) nodal reentrant tachycardia: 1, anterior; 2, midseptal; and 3, posterior.

Right Atrial Common Flutter

The most frequent form of atrial flutter, the so-called common or typical atrial flutter, occurs in the right atrium and may rotate in a counterclockwise (CCW) or clockwise (CW) manner.[33, 34] Nonfluoroscopic mapping[35] and the use of multiple endocardial electrograms[36] have identified the circuit of the right atrial common flutter. The CCW atrial flutter is a broad band of peritricuspid activation that enters the isthmus (the atrial tissue between the inferior vena cava [IVC] orifice and the tricuspid annulus [TA]), slows in its medial part, ascends up the atrial septum, reaches the root of the superior vena cava, usually crosses anteriorly, and rarely fuses around it to descend down the free wall. The CW atrial flutter, although running in the opposite direction, shares the same circuit with the same endocardial borders as the CCW atrial flutter. On the 12-lead ECG, the common atrial flutter shows the "saw-tooth" appearance.

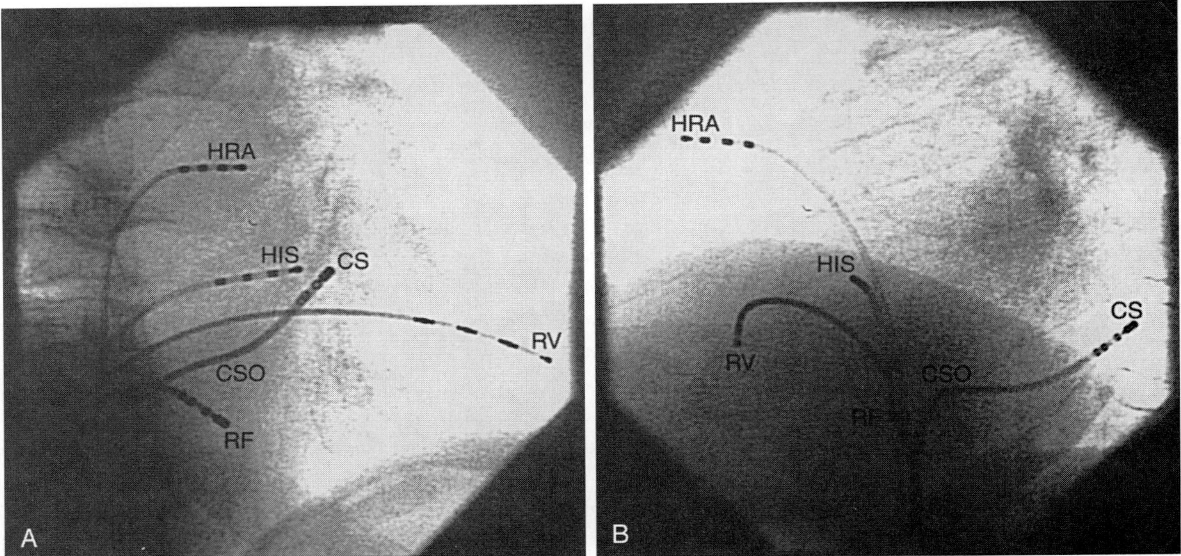

FIGURE 97–8 The catheter position used for ablation of atrioventricular nodal reentrant tachycardia in two fluoroscopic views: the right anterior oblique view **(A)** and the left anterior oblique view **(B)**. CS, coronary sinus; CSO, coronary sinus ostium; HRA, high right atrium; RF, radiofrequency catheter; RV, right ventricle.

PROCEDURE

An atrial flutter ablation procedure usually requires the insertion of the following catheters. A duodecapolar catheter is used for detailed mapping of the lateral right atrial wall and the IVC-TA isthmus, and multipolar catheters are used to record the activation of the coronary sinus ostium–TA isthmus, the His bundle, and the coronary sinus. During the electrophysiologic study, the atrial flutter is induced, and the type of isthmus conduction is evaluated.[37] Thereafter, an RF ablation catheter is positioned in the right atrial isthmus. The left and right anterior oblique fluoroscopic projections are used to guide the ablation (Fig. 97–9). Two approaches have been described to ablate common atrial flutter: the anatomic approach[38–41] and the electrophysiologic approach.[42] The first approach uses fluoroscopic landmarks to localize the right atrial isthmus, and the electrophysiologic approach targets areas with critical isthmus conduction determined on the basis of concealed entrainment or the presence of double potentials.[42] Two

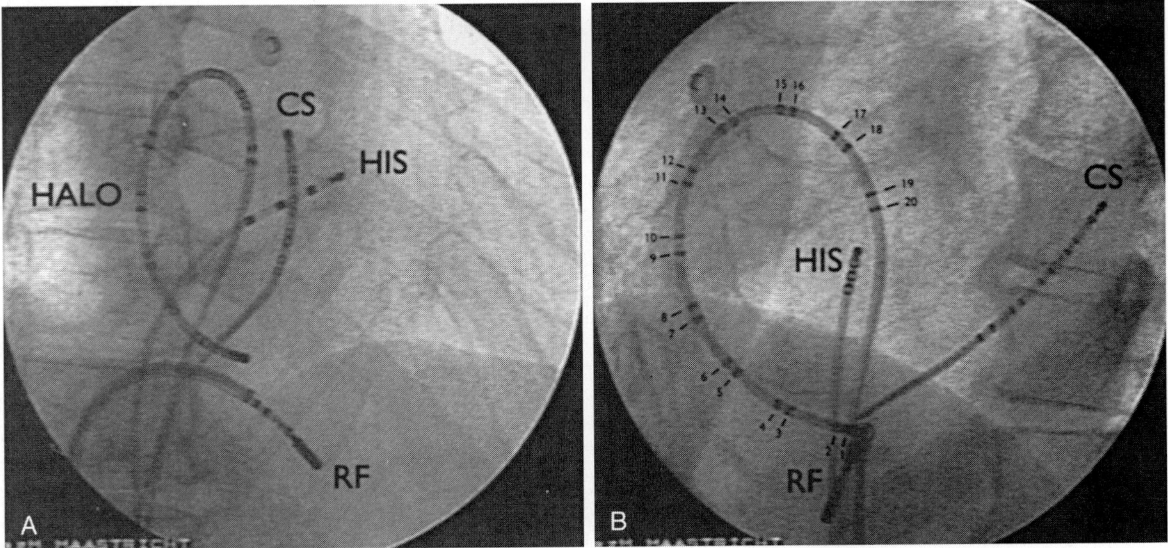

FIGURE 97–9 The catheter positions for radiofrequency (RF) ablation of a common atrial flutter in the right anterior oblique view **(A)** and the left anterior oblique view **(B)**. A duodecapolar catheter (HALO) is positioned around the tricuspid annulus in such a way that the proximal poles (bipolar 20 to 19 and 18 to 17) are septally located and the distal portion (bipolar 1 to 2 and 3 to 4) covers the posterior isthmus region. The remainder of the catheter covers the lateral wall of the right atrium. The radiofrequency ablation catheter is positioned in the posterior isthmus. A quadripolar catheter is located in the His bundle region, and a decapolar catheter inserted in the coronary sinus (CS) records left atrial activation.

isthmi have been described[37]: the posterior isthmus (IVC-TA), which includes the space between the IVC and the TA (IVC-TA), and the septal (TA-CS) isthmus, which is the space between the TA (at the level of the posterior margin of the coronary sinus ostium) to the posteroapical margin of the coronary sinus ostium (CS) or to the Eustachian ridge. In patients without atrial conduction between the coronary sinus ostium and the Eustachian ridge, ablation of the septal isthmus produces complete conduction block from the TA to the coronary sinus ostium and to the IVC, eliminating both CCW and CW atrial flutter.[37] A linear ablation is performed in one of the previously mentioned isthmi, either by applying point-by-point RF energy or by dragging the catheter during the RF application. Regardless of the approach used, the end point for successful RF ablation is the noninducibility of atrial flutter after completion of the RF line and the demonstration of a bidirectional isthmus conduction block.[40] Before RF ablation, pacing from the ostium of the coronary sinus results in the propagation of the atrial impulse in a CW direction to the IVC-TA isthmus and the lateral right atrium and in a CCW direction to the septum and the high right atrium. This pacing maneuver creates a collision of the atrial wavefronts in the lateral right atrium (Fig. 97–10A). In contrast, during pacing from the right lateral wall, the atrial impulse propagates in CCW direction along the ICV-TA isthmus and in a CW direction to the high right atrium and septum (see Fig. 97–10B). After completion of the ablation during bidirectional isthmus block, pacing from the coronary sinus ostium results in a single atrial wavefront descending along the lateral right atrium (see Fig. 97–10C). Pacing from the right lateral wall results in a single atrial wavefront ascending the high right atrium and descending through the atrial septum (see Fig. 97–10D). Finally, pacing is repeated under isoproterenol perfusion[43] to confirm noninducibility of atrial flutter and bidirectional isthmus conduction block. With this methodology, the acute success rate of RFCA for common atrial flutter ranges between 65 and 98 percent.[37–42]

In a number of patients with atrial fibrillation, the arrhythmia may organize into atrial flutter during the treatment of these patients with class III[44] or class IC[45, 46] antiarrhythmic drugs. RF ablation of the right atrial isthmus may significantly reduce the incidence of atrial fibrillation in these patients.[44–46] After RF ablation, these patients should continue to take the medication that changed atrial fibrillation into atrial flutter.

RF ablation of the septal isthmus has a (small) risk of complete AV block. Other complications are similar to those reported for right-sided RFCA procedures.

RECURRENCES

A high recurrence rate (10 to 55 percent) has been reported if noninducibility of atrial flutter alone is used as criterion for successful RF ablation.[39, 47, 48] The recurrence rate is lower (6 to 9 percent) in patients with bidirectional isthmus conduction block than in patients with unidirectional isthmus conduction block or bidirectional isthmus conduction delay at the end of the procedure.[49] In our laboratory,

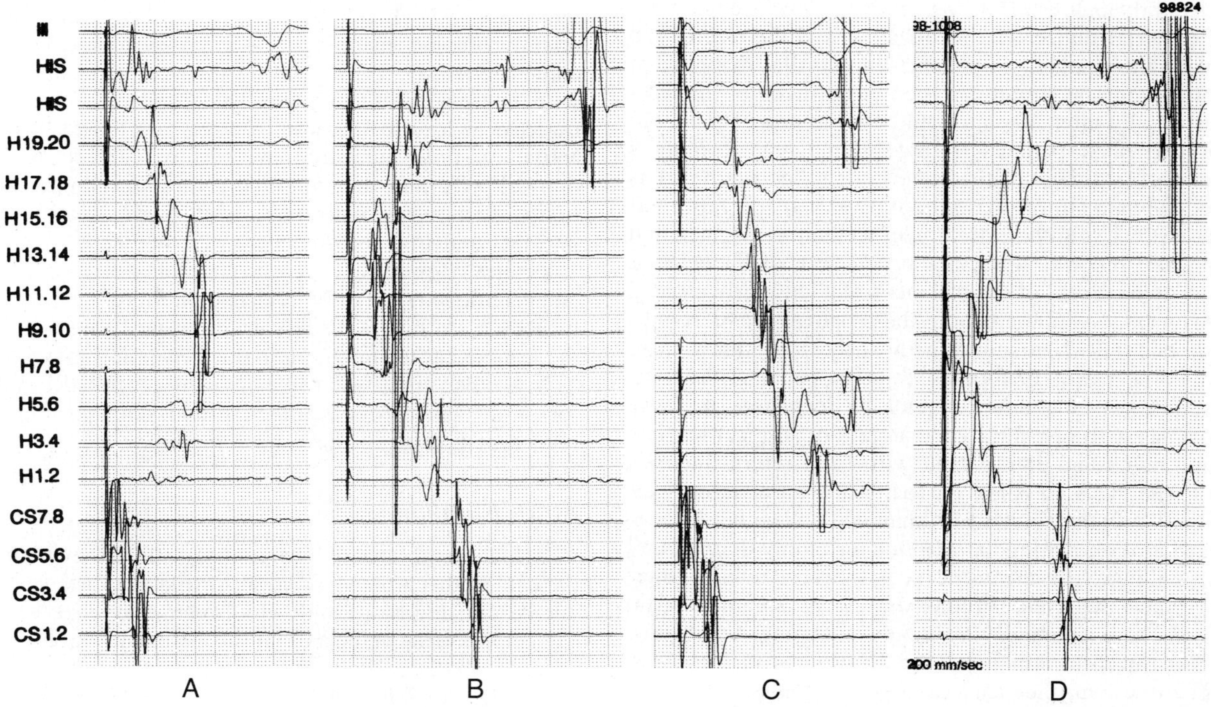

FIGURE 97–10 Pacing at the coronary sinus ostium **(A)** and at the low lateral right atrium **(B)** shows atrial pacing during sinus rhythm before ablation. Note a dual wavefront of right atrial activation with bidirectional conduction that collides in H9.10 acting at the coronary sinus ostium **(C)** and at the low lateral right atrium **(D)** shows bidirectional conduction block. Surface ECG lead III is shown. Intracardiac electrograms are recorded from the His bundle area. H1.2 to H19.20 indicate 10 bipoles of the duodecapolar (HALO) catheter positioned around the tricuspid annulus, and CS1.2 to CS7.8 represent 4 bipoles of a decapolar catheter placed in the coronary sinus (CS).

isoproterenol is used to evaluate resumption of conduction after right atrial isthmus ablation.[43] In some patients, isoproterenol infusion can unmask an apparent bidirectional isthmus conduction block, necessitating a new ablative procedure in the isthmus to create complete isthmus block.

Left Atrial Flutter

Although rare, atrial flutter may be caused by a left atrial reentrant circuit.[50] Using the conventional catheter positions, endocardial recordings show atrial activation in the coronary sinus that proceeds from the left to the right atrium or from the mid coronary sinus in both right and left directions. Pacing from the right atrium shows a long local return interval, with return cycles equal to the flutter cycle length recorded in the coronary sinus.[51] There is no standard approach for mapping and ablation of left atrial flutter, and the present experience is very limited.

"Incisional Tachycardia"

Atrial arrhythmias are a frequent clinical problem after surgical correction of congenital heart disease. Hemodynamic impairment and pressure overload together with the presence of surgical scars and prosthetic material may result in an arrhythmogenic combination of fixed artificial obstacles and electrophysiologic abnormalities that cause scar flutters, or "incisional tachycardia."[52] These tachycardias can occur after the correction of atrial or ventricular septal defects and after corrective surgery for complex anomalies, such as the Mustard, Senning, or Fontan procedures. The electrocardiographic pattern of these scar flutters, or incisional tachycardia, is variable, with the rate often slightly below the lower limit usually accepted for common atrial flutter. The localization and the size of the scar vary from patient to patient. Endocardial mapping of the entire reentrant circuit is sometimes difficult or impossible (especially after Mustard and Senning procedures). RF ablation in these patients is targeted to areas forming a critical part (isthmus) of the circuit, identified on the basis of electrogram timing, fragmentation,[53] or entrainment techniques.[52] Using the entrainment technique, Kalman and colleagues[52] reported an acute success rate of 83 percent. Seventy-two percent of the patients had a long-term clinical improvement, and 50 percent of these patients were asymptomatic and did not required medical therapy after a mean follow-up period of 17 months. In some patients, the critical isthmus of conduction cannot be localized. In these cases, areas with proximity to anatomic or surgical barriers showing concealed entrainment with local return intervals equal to the cycle length of the tachycardia are targeted for ablation.[51–54] In the study of Kalman and colleagues,[52] reentry was more often found around the atriotomy than around the septal patch of the atrial septal defect repair. Other authors have reported isthmus dependent common atrial flutter in these patients.[56] With new mapping techniques, like the three-dimensional, nonfluoroscopic mapping (CARTO) system, the scar can be more precisely located, and the RF ablation site can be better directed and verified.

Atrial Tachycardia

Atrial tachycardia can be classified according to its mechanism into automatic, triggered activity, and reentry. As pointed out in Chapter 86, Supraventricular Tachycardias, they may be paroxysmal or incessant. Results from a meta-analysis study show that the clinical and electrophysiologic characteristics of atrial tachycardia may vary among age groups.[57] This study demonstrated that pediatric patients more often have automatic and incessant forms, whereas adult patients more often present with the nonautomatic forms with a paroxysmal pattern.[57] Furthermore, right-sided atrial tachycardia and multifocal atrial tachycardia were more common in adults. It is important to know that in patients with incessant atrial tachycardia, the inability to control the ventricular rate may result in a dilated (tachycardia-induced) cardiomyopathy. In these patients, RFCA of the site of abnormal impulse formation leads to cure of the arrhythmia and regression of pump failure.[58, 59] Atrial tachycardia can originate in the right or left atrium. The localization in the right atrium includes the crista terminalis, the right atrial appendage, the intra-atrial septum, and the coronary sinus ostium. In a few patients, the site of origin of the atrial tachycardia can be localized in the sinus node (sinoatrial node reentrant). Atrial tachycardia originating from the left atrium is more commonly located in the ostia of the pulmonary veins and less frequent in the free wall and the atrial appendage.

As shown in Chapter 86, Supraventricular Tachycardias, the p wave morphology can be very helpful in localizing the site of origin of atrial tachycardia.

PROCEDURE

Two techniques are used to localize the site of origin of atrial tachycardia: the technique with multielectrode catheters (Figs. 97–11 and 97–12) and the three-dimensional, nonfluoroscopic mapping (CARTO) system (Fig. 97–13 and Plate 97–1). The left atrial tachycardia is approached with the transseptal technique. The electrophysiologic criteria used to localize the site of origin are the earliest atrial activation time preceding the surface ECG p wave, an optimal pace map, and concealed entrainment. RFCA ablation of focal atrial tachycardia has a high success rate (99 percent) and low recurrence rate (4 percent).[60] Chen and associates[60] found that the presence of a right-sided atrial tachycardia was the only independent predictor of successful RFCA. Although the left atrium is easily accessed using the transseptal technique, left-sided mapping may be more difficult than right-sided mapping. In general, RF ablation for atrial tachycardia is effective and safe; no procedure-related complications have been reported.

Atrial Fibrillation

RF ablation of atrial fibrillation is still in evolution. In patients with paroxysmal atrial fibrillation, the paroxysms can be initiated by a single atrial premature beat. RFCA of the ectopic beat or beats may be beneficial in controlling atrial fibrillation. The triggering ectopic beat may originate in the right or left atrium. In a study by Haissaguerre and associates,[61] the majority of the atrial premature beats that initiated atrial fibrillation originated from the pulmonary veins. In the 45 patients studied, a single focus of atrial ectopy was identified in 29 patients, two foci were identified in 9 patients, and three or four foci were identified in

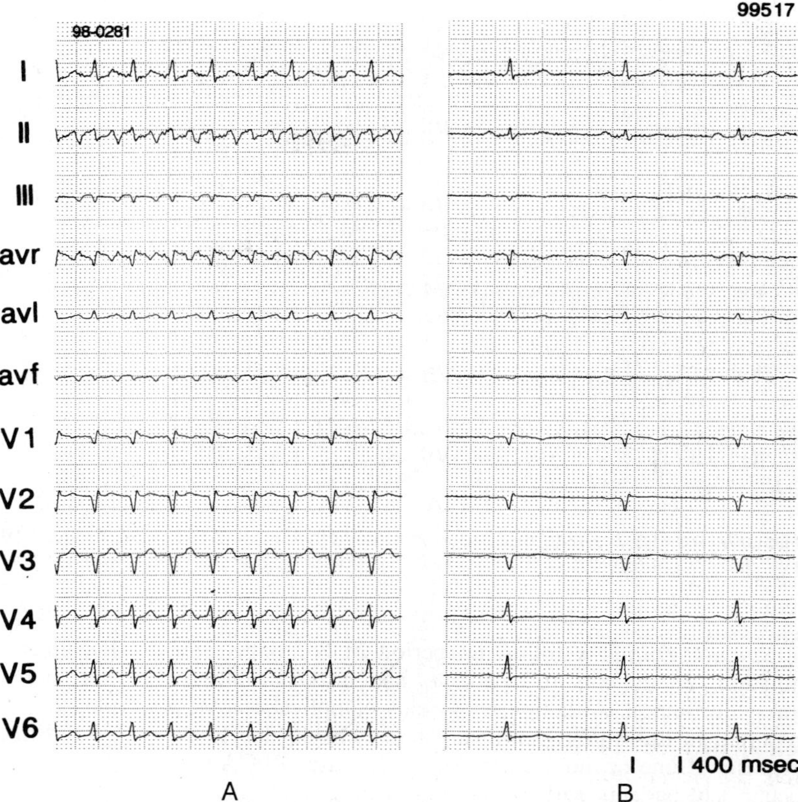

FIGURE 97–11 A 12-lead ECG during atrial tachycardia **(A)** and sinus rhythm **(B)**. Note that the P waves are negative in leads II, III, and aVF and positive in leads I and aVL, indicating an inferior origin in the right atrium.

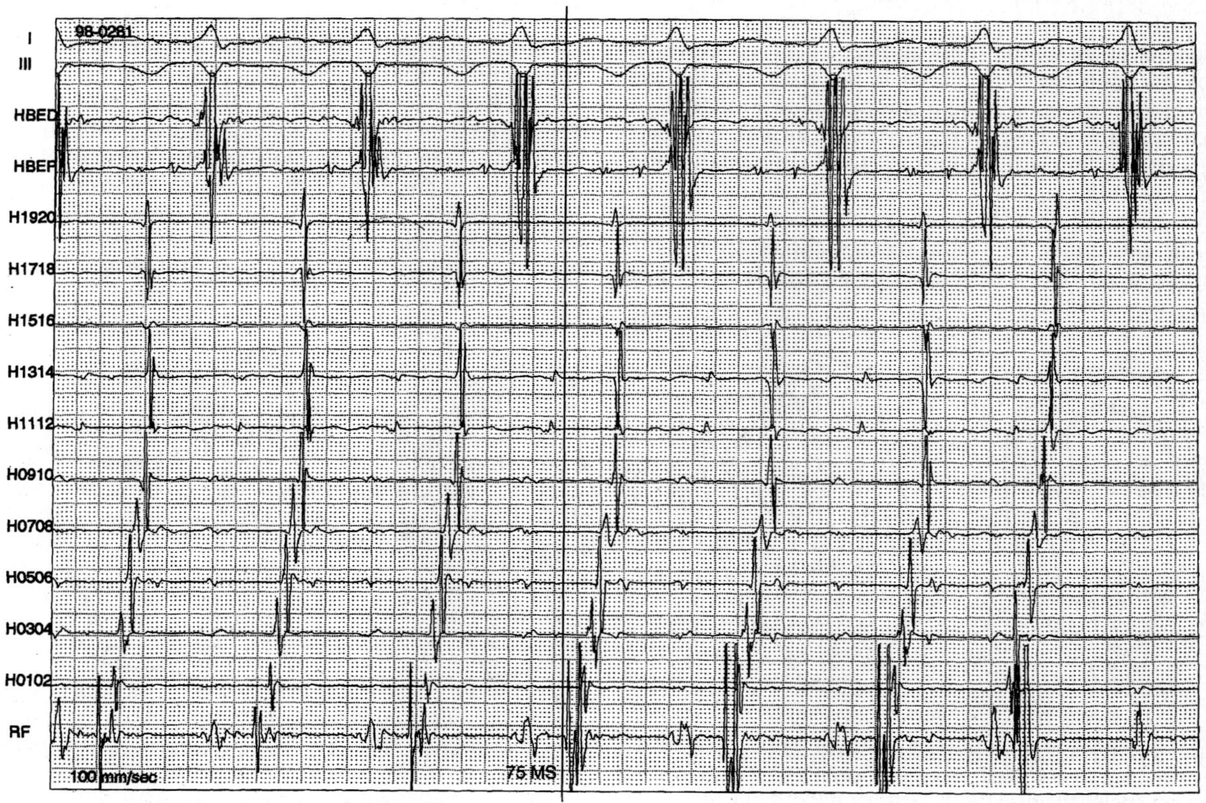

FIGURE 97–12 Endocardial recordings during tachycardia in the patient represented in Figure 97–11. Recordings were obtained using a multipolar catheter located in the right atrium (H0102 to H1920) and in the His bundle region (HBED, His bundle electrogram distal; HBEP, His bundle electrogram proximal). The earliest atrial endocardial activation (−75 ms) was found in the right inferoposterior region. At this site, the atrial tachycardia was successfully terminated with one radiofrequency (RF) application. Surface ECG leads I and III are shown.

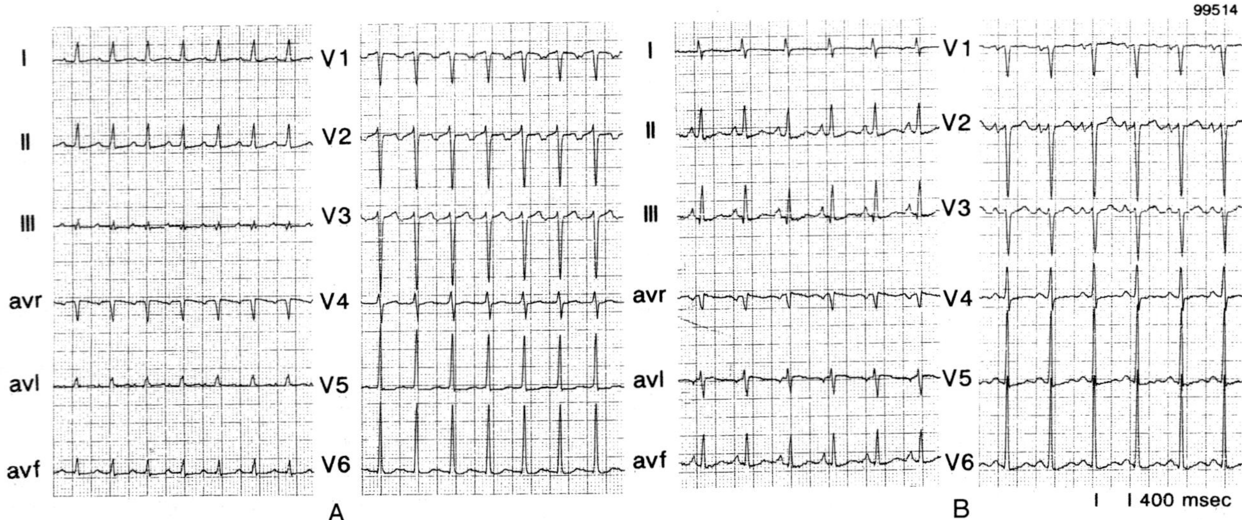

FIGURE 97–13 A 12-lead ECG during atrial tachycardia **(A)** and sinus rhythm **(B)**. Note that the P waves are positive in leads I, II, III, aVF, and aVL and negative in leads V_1 to V_3, indicating a high anterior origin in the right atrium.

7 patients. During a follow-up period of 8 months after ablation, 28 patients (62 percent) had no recurrence of atrial fibrillation. Although no serious complications were reported in this study, pulmonary hypertension due to the stenosis of one or more pulmonary veins after RFCA may occur.[62] In patients with chronic atrial fibrillation, the aim of RFCA is to divide both atria with linear ablations distributed in a systematic manner. The rationale of this technique is based on the surgical maze operation in which multiple incision lines are placed in the right and the left atrium.[63] The reasoning behind the operation is that atrial fibrillation is due to random reentry in the atrium, a perpetuating self-sustaining mechanism.[63] Compartmentalization of the atria with linear RF ablations will prevent random reentry.[65] The RF ablation lines have to be connected to avoid the possibility of a new reentry circuit around the RF line (Fig. 97–14). The long-term success is low when RF lines are placed only in the right atrium: the success rate increases to 50 percent when the RF lines are also placed in the left atrium.[66] With the available technology, a solid linear line is still difficult to achieve and to verify.

Atrioventricular Junction

AV junctional ablation followed by pacemaker implantation is limited to patients in whom RF ablation cannot cure the supraventricular arrhythmia (e.g., left atrial flutter, multifocal atrial tachycardia, and atrial fibrillation). It is an accepted treatment for symptomatic patients with atrial fibrillation in whom the arrhythmia and the ventricular response cannot be controlled by the treatment modalities such as antiarrhythmic drugs, external or internal cardioversion, and the implantable atrial defibrillator.[67] AV junctional ablation results in complete heart block and requires chronic

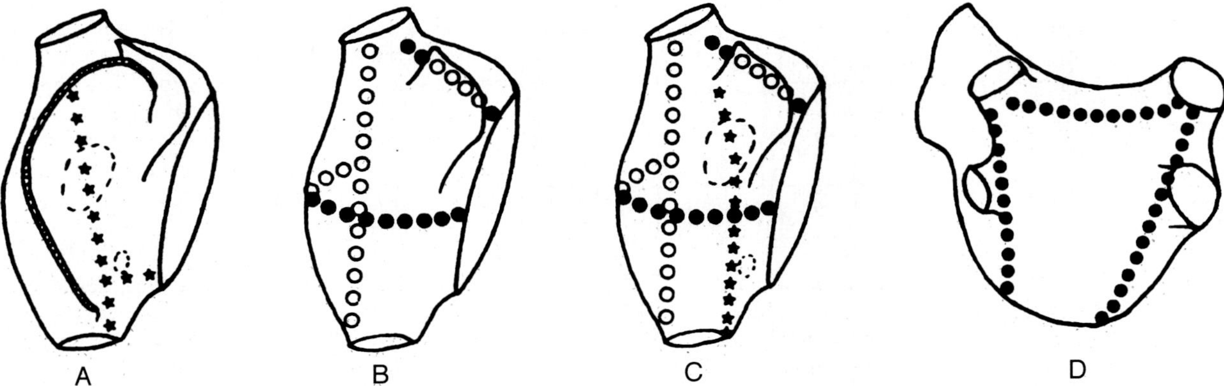

FIGURE 97–14 Ablation lines used for atrial fibrillation in the right (**A–C,** anterior view) and left atrium (**D,** posterior view). **A,** Single posterior line from the superior cava vein via the fossa ovalis and the coronary sinus ostium. **B,** Three lines are shown—one is longitudinal posteriorly between the inferior and the superior venae cavae, and one is between the superior vena cava and anterior to the tricuspid annulus. The third line is drawn transversely in the free wall from the anterolateral tricuspid annulus to the posterior line across the lateral free wall. **C,** Four lines are shown—the three previously mentioned ones and a fourth in the atrial septum. **D,** Ablation lines vertically from the two superior pulmonary veins to the posterior mitral annulus, including the inferior pulmonary veins; another horizontal line connects the superior point of the vertical lines. (**A–D,** Modified from Haissaguerre M, Jaïs P, Shah DC, et al: Right and left atrial radiofrequency catheter therapy of paroxysmal atrial fibrillation. J Cardiovasc Electrophysiol 7:1132–1144, 1996.)

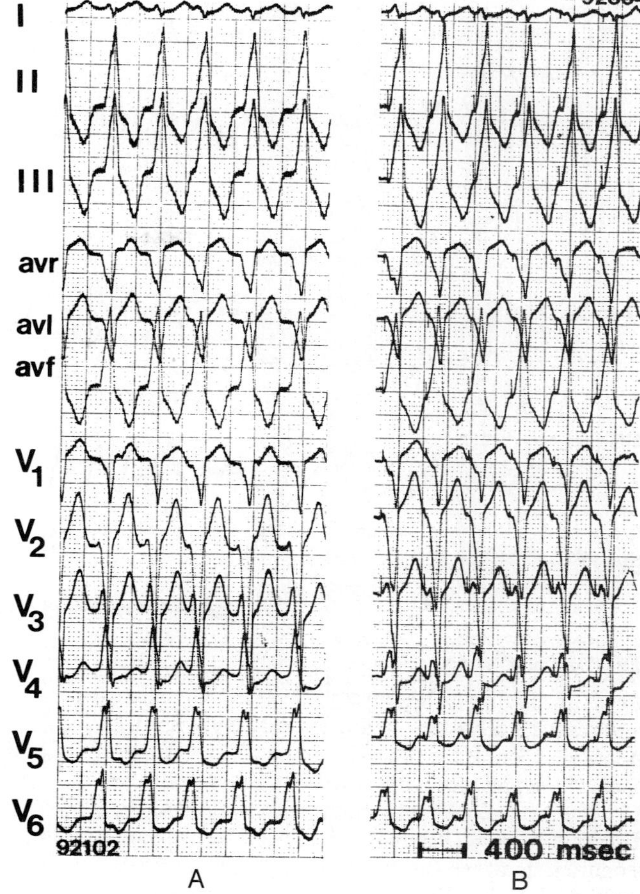

FIGURE 97–15 A typical example of an idiopathic right ventricular outflow tract tachycardia. **A,** Note the vertical axis and the left bundle branch block–like shape of the QRS complex. **B,** An optimal match between the clinically recorded 12-lead ECG and the ECG recorded during pacing on the septal site of the right ventricular outflow tract.

pacing. For successful ablation, the RF catheter is positioned across the tricuspid valve to record a high atrial, small His bundle and small ventricular deflection. The success rate of this technique is close to 100 percent. On rare occasions, interruption of conduction over the AV node–His–Purkinje system cannot be achieved from the right side, and a left-sided approach is necessary. Modification or partial, instead of complete, AV nodal conduction[68] has a moderate long-term success rate; therefore, complete interruption of the AV junction and pacemaker implantation is preferred in patients with rapid, uncontrollable ventricular rates.

Ventricular Tachycardia

In 75 percent of cases, sustained monomorphic VT is associated with ischemic heart disease. In the remaining patients, cardiomyopathy (dilated or hypertrophied), valvular heart disease, and right ventricular dysplasia are among the underlying cardiac causes. Sustained monomorphic VT may also occur in the absence of any other cardiac abnormality and is then called idiopathic. The 12-lead ECG during VT may be of great help to identify the cause; therefore, an effort should always be made to obtain a 12-lead ECG during VT.[69] An electrophysiologic study is performed to analyze the number of VTs, their morphology, their site of origin (using mapping and entrainment techniques), and (in ischemic VT) the critical zone of slow conduction in the reentry circuit.

In comparison with the outcome of RFCA in the patients with supraventricular tachycardias, the success rate of RFCA in treating patients with VT is more modest.

Idiopathic Ventricular Tachycardia

Idiopathic VT may originate from the right ventricular outflow tract or from the left ventricle. In the left ventricle, the majority of the VTs are localized in the inferoposterior aspect of the septum close to or in the left posterior fascicle.[70] Rarely, VTs are localized close to or in the anterior fascicle.[71] VTs originating in the right ventricular outflow tract typically have a left bundle branch block–like configuration with an intermediate or a vertical QRS axis in the extremity leads (Fig. 97–15). The mechanism of this VT is considered to be triggered activity. These VTs are frequently exercise related and catecholamine sensitive and can be terminated by intravenous adenosine or beta-blocker administration. VTs originating in the inferoposterior aspect of the septum of the left ventricle have a right bundle branch block–like configuration and a left or northwest QRS axis (Fig. 97–16). These VTs can frequently be initiated by programmed electrical stimulation and terminated by intravenous verapamil.[70] The mechanism of these VTs is probably micro-reentry in the left posterior fascicle. Mapping of either VT consists of localizing the earliest

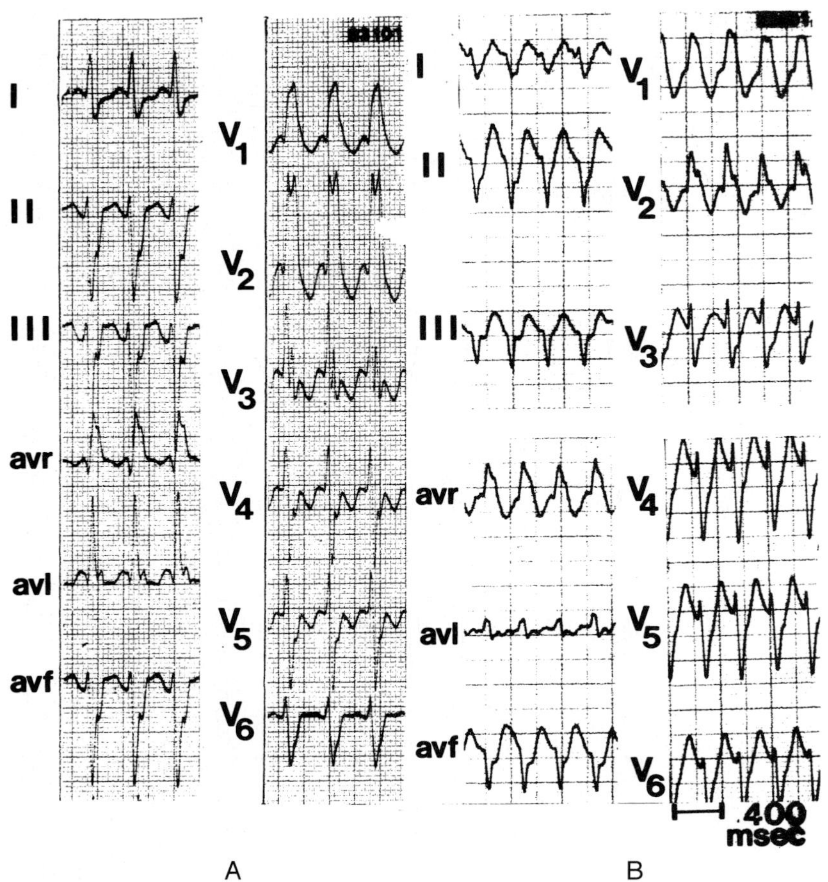

FIGURE 97–16 A, A 12-lead ECG of a patient with an idiopathic ventricular tachycardia originating in the left ventricle in the inferoposterior aspect of the septum close to the posterior fascicle. Note that the ventricular tachycardia has a right bundle branch block–like configuration and a left-axis deviation. **B,** A 12-lead ECG of an idiopathic ventricular tachycardia originating more anteriorly in the apicoseptal aspect of the left ventricle. That ventricular tachycardia shows a right bundle branch block–like configuration and a northwest axis.

ventricular endocardial activation during VT (Fig. 97–17). Additionally, an optimal pace map (with the 12-lead ECG showing an identical QRS morphology during ventricular pacing as the QRS during spontaneous VT; see Fig. 97–15) is required. Furthermore, recording of a fascicular potential can be useful in selecting successful sites in idiopathic VT originating from the inferoposterior aspect of the left ventricle (Fig. 97–18).[72] In our experience,[73] RF catheter ablation of the right ventricular outflow tract VT successfully eliminated the arrhythmia in 29 of 35 patients (83 percent) and in 12 of 13 VTs (92 percent) from the left ventricle. After a mean follow-up period of 30 months, there were four recurrences (14 percent) in patients with right ventricular outflow tract VT and none in patients with left ventricular VT. In our patients, unsuccessful ablation for right and left VT was characterized by more than one VT morphology, the presence of a delta wave–like beginning of the QRS (see Fig. 97–18), and a pace map showing a correlation in fewer than 11 of the 12 ECG leads. Other series of right ventricular outflow tract and left ventricular VT have shown similar success rate and rare complications.[74, 75] In idiopathic VT, RFCA is a curative technique and therefore should be offered early in the treatment of symptomatic patients.

Postinfarction Ventricular Tachycardia

Monomorphic VT due to the presence of scar tissue, most often after myocardial infarction, is commonly due to reentry.[11] Interruption of the reentry circuit by RFCA requires identification of an essential part of the reentry circuit. A reentry circuit varies in size, configuration, and location (subendocardial, midmyocardial, or subepicardial). The region where the wavefront emerges from the circuit is termed the *exit site*. The region proximal to the exit consists of a central and a proximal part (Fig. 97–19). After the wavefront emerges from the exit, it propagates through a loop, back to the proximal region of the circuit. The outer loop is a broad pathway along the margin of the scar.[11] Identification of the central part of the reentry circuit, which in general exhibits slow conduction is of importance to obtain successful RF ablation. If the zone of slow conduction is not too broad, a single RF ablation may terminate the VT. However, in some cases a broad portion of the reentry circuit has to be interrupted by a series of RF applications in a manner similar to that used for RF ablation for atrial flutter.[76] Stevenson and colleagues[11] proposed criteria to identify the central part (slow conduction zone) of the reentry circuit; these criteria include the presence of a mid-diastolic potential and the demonstration of concealed entrainment (Fig. 97–20). The strategy in these patients varies from center to center. Some centers advocate to ablate all inducible stable VTs.[11, 77, 78] Other groups[79, 80] prefer to target only the clinical stable one. In our institution, we prefer to target only the clinical VTs. Fifty-two patients underwent RFCA in our institution. After a mean follow-up period of 25 months, 10 patients had a VT recurrence (26 percent) and 9 patients died (17 percent; 3

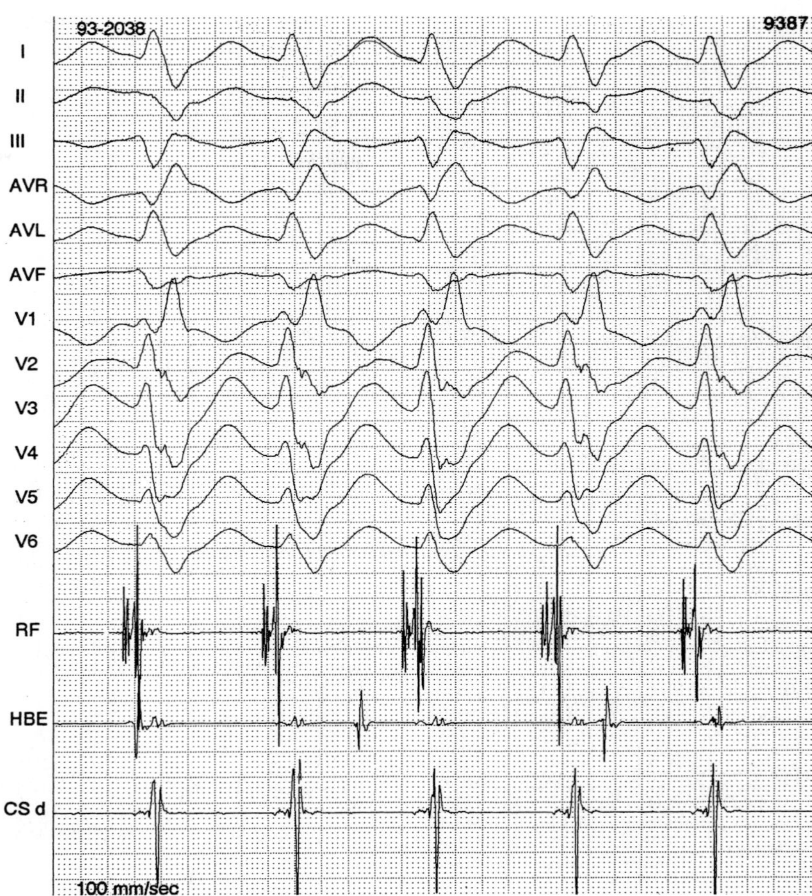

FIGURE 97–17 A 12-lead ECG of an idiopathic left ventricular tachycardia with a right bundle branch block–like morphology and left axis. Note the very sharp potential (the posterior fascicle) preceding the QRS complex in the endocardial recording from the radiofrequency ablation catheter. CS d, distal coronary sinus; HBE, His bundle electrogram.

patients from pump failure and 6 from sudden cardiac death). Our results are comparable to those reported by Stevenson and colleagues.[81] In their population, all inducible stable VTs were targeted. Ten patients died (10 of 52 patients, 17 percent) and 16 patients (16 of 52, 31 percent) had VT recurrences. In general, the long-term success rate ranges from 45 to 75 percent.[77–81] In the majority of the patients reported in those studies and in our patients, antiarrhythmic drugs were continued. The incidence of sudden death during follow-up raises the question of the necessity of additional implantation of a defibrillator in these patients. RFCA is usually not possible in those patients presenting with multiple unstable VT morphologies and with calcified and fibrotic scars, for which RF energy cannot penetrate deep in these areas. The success rate in postinfarction VT may be improved by the development of new mapping systems, which will allow better localization of the reentry circuits, not only for stable VT but also for unstable ones. Furthermore, new catheter designs (irrigated tip catheter) and the development of new ablative sources (cryotechnology) that can produce deeper lesions in scar tissue are needed to improve results. RFCA in postinfarction VT provides excellent palliation for many patients who have repeated episodes of spontaneous well tolerated VT.

Another uncommon form of VT that can be cured by RF ablation is the so-called bundle branch reentry VT.[82] These VTs are observed in patients with conduction disturbances in the bundle branches and in the interventricular septum (e.g., patients with ischemic or dilated cardiomyopathy after aortic valve replacement, myotonic dystrophy, and after chest trauma). The reentrant circuit in this type of VT may use one bundle branch as the anterograde limb of the circuit with transseptal retrograde conduction over the other bundle branch. These VTs therefore may show a left or right bundle branch block–like morphology.[83] They can be cured by ablation of one of the bundle branches. Another possibility is that the reentry circuit uses the anterior and posterior fascicles of the left bundle branch; this is called *interfascicular* VT. In the latter situation, the VT shows a right bundle branch block–like configuration with right- or left-axis deviation.[84] RF ablation is one of the fascicles that can cure this type of VT.

The results of RF ablation of VT in patients with right ventricular dysplasia are frequently disappointing because of the progressive nature of the disease. Only a limited number of cases of VT ablation in patients with hypertrophic[85] and dilated cardiomyopathy have been reported.

SUMMARY

In the past 12 years, RFCA has developed into an effective and safe curative treatment for patients with different types of supraventricular arrhythmias. This is also the case in a high number of patients with idiopathic VT and patients

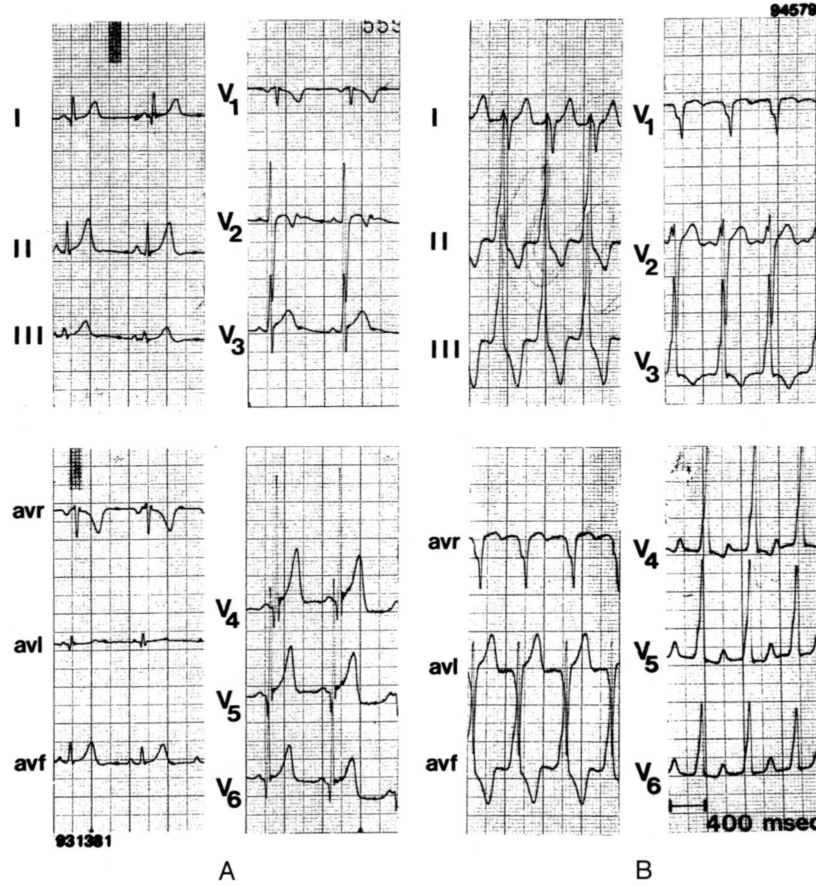

FIGURE 97–18 Example of a patient in whom radiofrequency catheter ablation failed. **A,** A 12-lead ECG during sinus rhythm. **B,** A 12-lead ECG during ventricular tachycardia with a left bundle branch block–like morphology and right axis. Note the slow, delta wave–like beginning of the QRS complex.

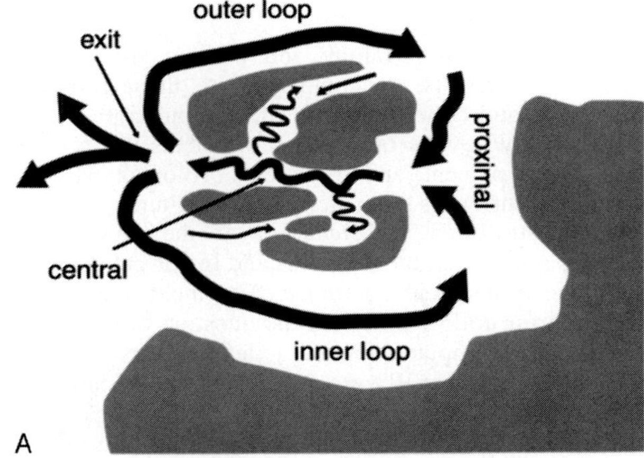

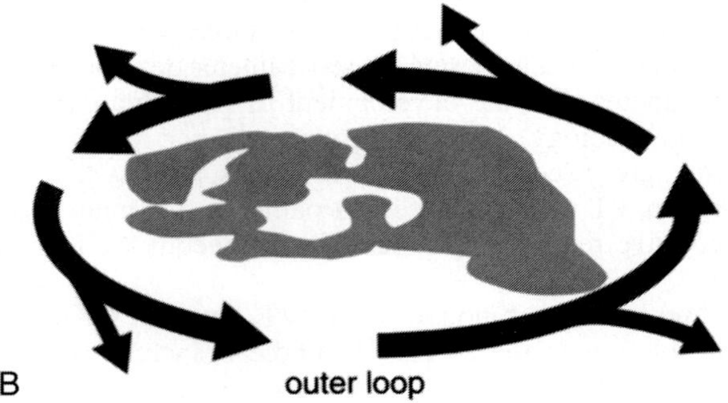

FIGURE 97–19 Parts of a re-entry circuit with an inner loop **(A)** and a broad outer loop **(B)** in scarred myocardium. (**A** and **B,** Modified from Stevenson WG, Delacretaz E, Friedman PL, Ellison K: Identification and ablation of macroreentrant ventricular tachycardia with the CARTO electroanatomical mapping system. Pacing Clin Electrophysiol 21:1448–1456, 1998.)

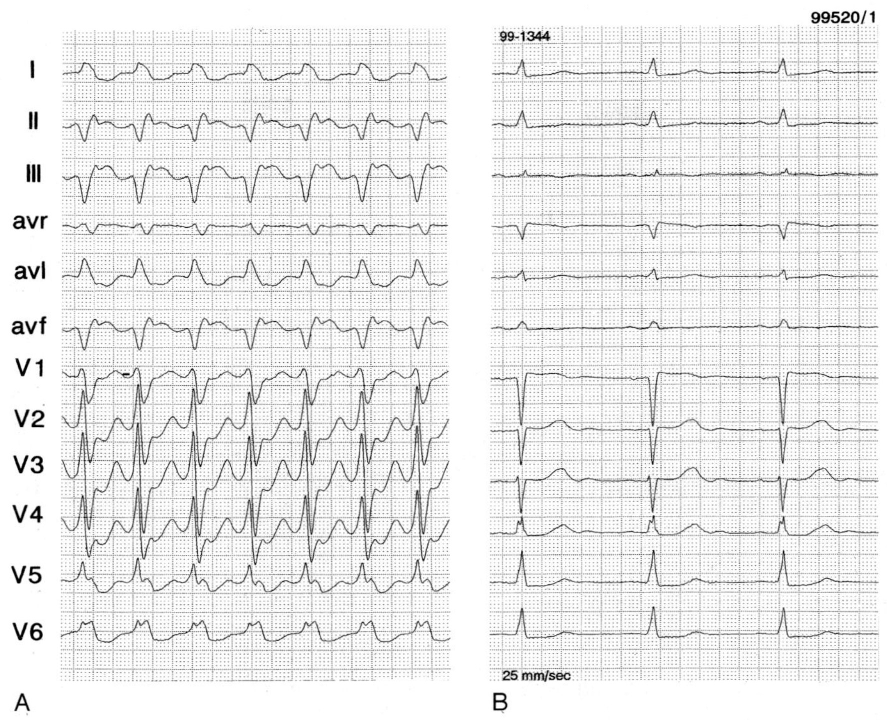

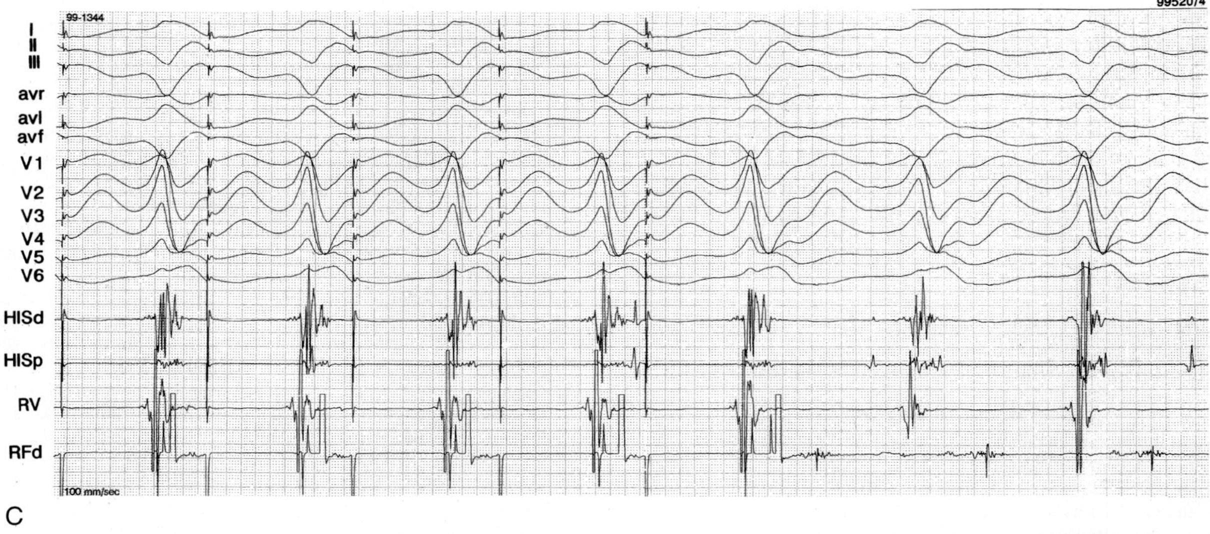

FIGURE 97–20 **A,** A 12-lead ECG during ventricular tachycardia in a patient with an old inferoposterior infarction. The ventricular tachycardia shows a left bundle branch block–like morphology with QR complexes in lead II, III, and aVF. **B,** Sinus rhythm with incomplete left bundle branch block. **C,** Ventricular pacing in the infarcted area by way of the radiofrequency ablation catheter. Pacing is performed 60 ms faster that the ventricular tachycardia rate (first four QRS complexes). Note that the morphology of the QRS during ventricular pacing is identical to that during ventricular tachycardia, indicating concealed entrainment. This suggests that the radiofrequency catheter is located in the zone of slow conduction (central part). Note that the endocardial recording obtained from the radiofrequency catheter (RFd) (last three nonpaced QRS) registers mid-diastolic potentials preceding the QRS complex by 260 ms. This is exactly the same interval as from the pacing spike to the QRS complex during pacing. HISd, His distal; HISp, His proximal; RV, right ventricle.

Illustration continued on following page

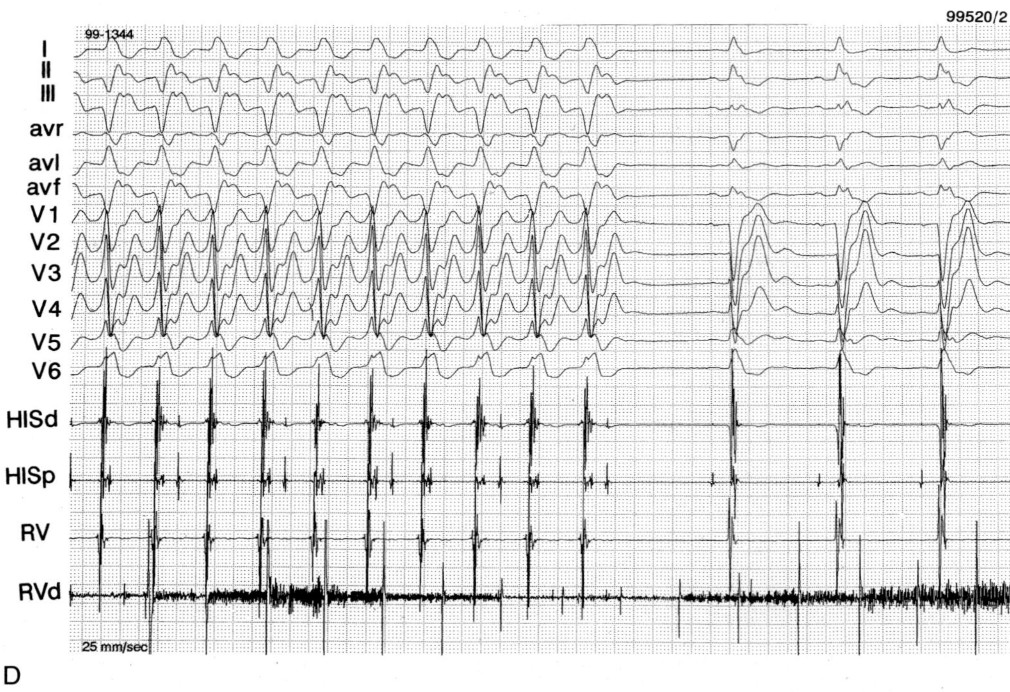

FIGURE 97–20 *Continued.* **D,** Radiofrequency ablation at the site shown in **C** terminates the ventricular tachycardia within 3 seconds.

with bundle branch reentrant VT. The technique should therefore be considered early in the therapy of the above-mentioned arrhythmias. RF ablation provides palliative treatment in patients with recurrent episodes of spontaneous, well-tolerated postinfarction VT. In the future, results may be improved by the use of new catheter designs and new ways to make deeper legions (in VT) and more solid ablation lines (in atrial fibrillation). RFCA should be performed only in centers in which the clinical electrophysiologist has sufficient experience to perform these sometimes complicated and time-consuming procedures.

REFERENCES

1. Durrer D, Schoo L, Schuilenburg RM, Wellens HJJ: The role of premature beats in the initiation and termination of supraventricular tachycardia in the Wolff-Parkinson-White syndrome. Circulation 36:644–662, 1967.
2. Coumel PH, Carbrol C, Fabiato A, et al: Tachycardie permanente par rhythm réciproque en dehors du syndrome de Wolff-Parkinson-White. Arch Mal Coeur 60:1830–1837, 1967.
3. Wellens HJJ: Electrical Stimulation of the Heart in the Study and Treatment of Tachycardias. Baltimore: University Park Press, 1971.
4. den Dulk K, Bartholet M, Brugada P, et al: A versatile pacemaker system for termination of tachycardias. Am J Cardiol 52:731–738, 1983.
5. Cobb FR, Blumenschein SD, Sealy WC, et al: Successful surgical interruption of the bundle of Kent in a patient with the Wolff-Parkinson-White syndrome. Circulation 38:1018–1025, 1968.
6. Gallagher JJ, Svenson R, Kasell JH, et al: Catheter technique for closed-chest ablation of the atrioventricular conduction system: a therapeutic alternative for the treatment of refractory supraventricular tachycardia. N Engl J Med 306:194–200, 1982.
7. Scheinman MM, Morady F, Hess DS, et al: Catheter induced ablation of the atrioventricular junction to control refractory supraventricular arrhythmias. JAMA 248:851–857, 1982.
8. Borggrefe M, Budde T, Podczeck A, Breithardt G: High frequency alternating current ablation of an accessory pathway in humans. J Am Coll Cardiol 10:576–582, 1987.
9. Jackman W, Wang X, Friday KLJ, et al: Catheter ablation of accessory atrioventricular pathways (Wolff-Parkinson-White syndrome) by radiofrequency current. N Engl J Med 324:1605–1611, 1991.
10. Kuck KH, Schlutter M, Geiger M, et al: Radiofrequency current catheter ablation of accessory atrioventricular pathways. Lancet 337:1557–1561, 1991.
11. Stevenson WG, Khan H, Sager P, et al: Identification of the reentry circuit sites during catheter mapping and radiofrequency ablation of ventricular tachycardia. Circulation 88:1647–1670, 1993.
12. Arruda M, Nakagawa H, Chandresekaran K, et al: Radiofrequency ablation in the coronary venous system is associated with risk of coronary artery injury which may be prevented by use of intravascular ultrasound. J Am Coll Cardiol 27(suppl II):160A, 1996.
13. Scheinman MM, Wang YS, Van Hare GF, Lesh MD: Electrocardiographic and electrophysiologic characteristics of anterior-midseptal and right anterior free wall accessory pathways. J Am Coll Cardiol 20:120–129, 1992.
14. Rodriguez LM, Smeets JLRM, de Chillou C, et al: The 12-lead ECG in mid-septal, anteroseptal, posteroseptal and right free wall accessory pathways. Am J Cardiol 72:1274–1280, 1993.
15. Chen X, Borgrefe M, Shenasa M, et al: Characteristics of local electrogram predicting successful transcatheter radiofrequency ablation of left sided accessory pathways. J Am Coll Cardiol 20:656–665, 1992.
16. Calkins H, Kim YN, Schmaltz S, et al: Electrogram criteria for identification of appropriate target sites for radiofrequency catheter ablation of accessory atrioventricular connections. Circulation 85:565–573, 1992.
17. Haissaguere M, Dartigues JF, Warin JF: Electrogram pattern predictive of successful catheter ablation of accessory pathways: value of unipolar recordings. Circulation 84:188–202, 1991.
18. Silka M, Kron J, Halperin B, et al: Analysis of local electrogram characteristics correlated with successful radiofrequency catheter of accessory atrioventricular pathway. Pacing Clin Electrophysiol 15:1000–1007, 1992.
19. Villacastin J, Almendral J, Medina O, et al: "Pseudodisappearance" of atrial electrogram during orthodromic tachycardia: new criteria for successful ablation of concealed left-sided accessory pathway. J Am Coll Cardiol 27:853–859, 1996.
20. Klein LS, Hacket FK, Zipes DP, Miles WM: Radiofrequency catheter ablation of Mahaim fibers at the tricuspid annulus. Circulation 87:738, 1993.

21. Shih HT, Miles WM, Klein LS, et al: Multiple accessory pathways in the permanent form of junctional reciprocating tachycardia. J Am Coll Cardiol 73:361–36, 1994.
22. Timmermans C, Smeets J, Rodriguez LM, et al: Recurrence rate after accessory pathway ablation. Br Heart J 72:571–574, 1994.
23. Langberg JJ, Calkins H, Kim YN, et al: Recurrences of conduction in accessory atrioventricular connections after initially successful radiofrequency catheter ablation. J Am Coll Cardiol 19:1588–1592, 1992.
24. Hendricks G: Complications of radiofrequency catheter ablation of arrhythmias. Eur Heart J 14:1644–1653, 1993.
25. Calkins H, Yong P, Miller JM, et al: Catheter ablation of accessory pathways, atrioventricular modal reentrant tachycardia and the atrioventricular junction: final results of a prospective multicenter clinical trial. Circulation 98:262–270, 1998.
26. Kugler JD, Danford DA, Houston K, et al: Radiofrequency catheter ablation for paroxysmal supraventricular tachycardia in children and adolescents without structural heart disease. Am J Cardiol 80:1438–1443, 1997.
27. Jackman WM, Beckman KJ, McClelland JH, et al: Treatment of supraventricular tachycardia due to atrioventricular nodal reentry by radiofrequency catheter ablation of slow pathway conduction. N Engl J Med 327:313–317, 1992.
28. Haissaguerre M, Gaita F, Fischer B, et al: Elimination of atrioventricular nodal reentrant tachycardia using discrete slow potentials to guide application of radiofrequency energy. Circulation 85:2162–2165, 1992.
29. Jazayeri MR, Hempe SL, Sra JS, et al: Selective transcatheter ablation of the fast and slow pathways using radiofrequency energy in patients with atrioventricular nodal reentry tachycardia. Circulation 85:1318–1328, 1992.
30. Langberg JJ, Leon A, Borganelli M, et al: A randomized prospective comparison of anterior and posterior approaches to radiofrequency catheter ablation of atrioventricular nodal reentry tachycardia. Circulation 87:1551–1556, 1993.
31. Kay GN, Epstein AE, Dailey SM, et al: Selective radiofrequency ablation of the slow pathway for the treatment of AV reentrant tachycardia: evidence of involvement of perinodal myocardium within the reentrant circuit. Circulation 85:1675–1688, 1992.
32. Langberg JJ, Harvey M, Calkins H, et al: Titration of power output during radiofrequency catheter ablation of atrioventricular nodal reentrant tachycardia. Pacing Clin Electrophysiol 16:465–470, 1993.
33. Olgin JE, Kalman JM, Firzpatrick AP, Lesh MD: Role of the right atrial endocardial structures as barriers to conduction during human type I atrial flutter: activation and entrainment mapping guided by intracardiac echocardiography. Circulation 92:1939–1848, 1995.
34. Kalman J, Olgin J, Lee R, et al: Activation and entrainment mapping defines the tricuspid annulus as the anterior barrier in typical atrial flutter. Circulation 94:398–406, 1996.
35. Shah DC, Jais P, Haissaguerre M, Chouairi S, et al: Three-dimensional mapping of the common atrial flutter circuit in the right atrium. Circulation 96:3904–3912, 1997.
36. Arribas F, Lopez-Gill M, Cosio F, et al: The upper link of human common atrial flutter circuit: definition by multiple endocardial recordings during entrainment. Pacing Clin Electrophysiol 20:2924–2929, 1997.
37. Nakagawa H, Lazarra R, Khastigir T, et al: Role of the tricuspid annulus and eustachian valve/ridge on atrial flutter: relevance to catheter ablation of the septal isthmus and a new technique for rapid identification of ablation success. Circulation 94:407–424, 1996.
38. Kirkorian G, Moncada E, Chevalier P, et al: Radiofrequency ablation of atrial flutter: efficacy of an anatomical guided approach. Circulation 90:2804–2814, 1994.
39. Philippon F, Plumb VI, Epstein A, et al: The risk of atrial fibrillation following radiofrequency catheter ablation of atrial flutter. Circulation 92:430–435, 1995.
40. Poty H, Soudi N, Nair M, et al: Radiofrequency catheter ablation of type I atrial flutter: predictors of late success by electrophysiological criteria. Circulation 92:1389–1392, 1995.
41. Nabar A, Rodriguez LM, Timmermans C, et al: Effect of the right atrial isthmus ablation on the occurrence of atrial fibrillation: observations in four patients groups having type I atrial flutter with or without associated atrial fibrillation. Circulation 99:1441–1445, 1999.
42. Kalman JM, Olgin JE, Saxon LA, et al: Electrocardiographic and electrophysiologic characteristic of atypical atrial flutter in man: use of activation and entrainment mapping and implications for catheter ablation. J Cardiovasc Electrophysiol 8:121–144, 1997.
43. Nabar A, Rodriguez LM, Timmermans C, et al: Isoproterenol to evaluate resumption of conduction after right atrial isthmus ablation in type I atrial flutter. Circulation 99:3286–3291, 1999.
44. Huang DT, Monahan KM, Zimetbaum P, et al: Hybrid pharmacologic and ablative therapy: a novel and effective approach for management of atrial fibrillation. J Cardiovasc Electrophysiol 9:462–469, 1998.
45. Nabar A, Rodriguez LM, Timmermans C, et al: Radiofrequency ablation of "class Ic atrial flutter" in patients with resistant atrial fibrillation. Am J Cardiol 83:785–787, 1999.
46. Schumacher B, Jung W, Lewalter T, et al: Radiofrequency ablation of atrial flutter due to administration of class Ic antiarrhythmic drugs for atrial fibrillation. Am J Cardiol 83:710–713, 1999.
47. Cosio FG, Lopez-Gil M, Goicoles A, et al: Radiofrequency ablation of the inferior vena cava-tricuspid valve isthmus in common atrial flutter. Am J Cardiol 71:705–709, 1993.
48. Fisher B, Haissaguerre M, Garrigues S, et al: Radiofrequency catheter ablation of common atrial flutter in 80 patients. J Am Coll Cardiol 25:1365–1372, 1995.
49. Schumacher B, Pfeiffer D, Tebbenjohanns J, et al: Acute and long-term effects of consecutive radiofrequency applications on conduction properties on the subeustachian isthmus in type I atrial flutter. J Cardiovasc Electrophysiol 9:152–163, 1998.
50. Cosio FG, Goicoles A, Lopez-Gil M, et al: Atrial endocardial mapping in the rare forms of atrial flutter. Am J Cardiol 66:715–720, 1990.
51. Cosio FG, Arribas F, Lopez-Gil M, et al: Atrial flutter mapping and ablation, I: studying atrial flutter mechanisms by mapping and entrainment. Pacing Clin Electrophysiol 19:841–853, 1996.
52. Kalman JM, Van Hare GF, Olgin JE, et al: Ablation of "incisional" re-entrant atrial tachycardia complicating surgery for congenital heart disease: use of entrainment to define a critical isthmus of conduction. Circulation 93:502–512, 1996.
53. Triedman, JK, Saul P, Weindling SN, et al: Radiofrequency ablation of intra-atrial reentrant tachycardia after surgical palliation of congenital heart disease. Circulation 91:707–714, 1995.
54. Olgin JE, Kalman JM, Lesh MD: Conduction barriers in human atrial flutter: correlation of electrophysiology and anatomy. J Cardiovasc Electrophysiol 7:1112–1126, 1996.
55. Baker SM, Cain ME: Catheter ablation of clinical intra-atrial reentrant tachycardias resulting from previous atrial surgery: localizing and transecting the critical isthmus. J Am Coll Cardiol 28:411–417, 1996.
56. Arribas F, Lopez-Gil M, Cosio FG: Atrial flutter ablation: role of endocardial mapping. *In* Farre J, Moro C (eds): Ten Years of Radiofrequency Catheter Ablation. pp. 339–359. Armonk, NY: Futura, 1998.
57. Chen SA, Tai CT, Chiang CE, et al: Focal atrial tachycardia: Reanalysis of the clinical and electrophysiologic characteristics and prediction of successful radiofrequency ablation. J Cardiovasc Electrophysiol 9:355–365, 1998.
58. Packer DL, Bardy GH, Worly SJ, et al: Tachycardia induced cardiomyopathy: a reversible form of left ventricular dysfunction. Am J Cardiol 57:563–570, 1986.
59. Wellens HJJ, Rodriguez LM, Smeets JLRM, et al: Tachycardiomyopathy in patients with supraventricular tachycardia with emphasis on atrial fibrillation. *In* Olsson SB, Allessie MA, Campbell RWF (eds): Atrial Fibrillation: Mechanisms and Therapeutic Strategies. pp. 333–342. Armonk, NY: Futura, 1994.
60. Chen SA, Chiang CE, Yang CJ, et al: Sustained atrial tachycardia in adults patients: electrophysiological characteristics, pharmacological response, possible mechanisms, and effects of radiofrequency ablation. Circulation 90:1262–1278, 1994.
61. Haissaguerre M, Jais P, Shah DC, et al: Spontaneous initiations of atrial fibrillation by beats originating in the pulmonary veins. N Engl J Med 339:659–666, 1998.
62. Robbens IV, Colvin EV, Doyle TP, et al: Pulmonary vein stenosis after catheter ablation of atrial fibrillation. Circulation 98:1769–1775, 1998.
63. Cox JL: Evolving application of the maze procedure for atrial fibrillation. Ann Thorac Surg 55:578–580, 1993.
64. Allessie MA. Reentrant mechanisms underlying atrial fibrillation. *In* Zipes DP, Jalife J (eds): Cardiac Electrophysiology: From Cell to Bedside. 2nd ed. pp. 562–566. Philadelphia: WB Saunders, 1995.
65. Guiraudon GM, Guiraudon C, Klein GJ, Yee R: Atrial fibrillation:

functional anatomy and surgery rationales. *In* Farre J, Moro C (eds): Ten Years of Radiofrequency Catheter Ablation. pp. 289–310. Armonk, NY: Futura, 1998.

66. Haissaguerre M, Jais P, Shah D, Clementy J: Radiofrequency catheter ablation for paroxysmal atrial fibrillation in humans: elaboration of a procedure based on electrophysiological data. *In* Murgatroyd FD, Camm AJ (eds): Nonpharmacological Management of Atrial Fibrillation. pp. 257–279. Armonk, NY: Futura, 1997.
67. Wellens HJJ, Lau CP, Lüderitz B, et al: Atrioverter: an implantable device for the treatment of atrial fibrillation. Circulation 98:1651–1656, 1998.
68. Della Bella P, Carbucicchо C, Tondo C, et al: Modification of atrioventricular conduction by ablation of the "slow" atrioventricular node pathway in patients with drug-refractory atrial fibrillation or flutter. J Am Coll Cardiol 25:39–46, 1995.
69. Wellens HJJ, Smeets JLRM, Rodriguez LM, Timmermans C: Clinical and electrocardiographic profiles of patients with ventricular tachycardia. *In* Farre J, Moro C (eds): Ten Years of Radiofrequency Catheter Ablation. pp. 205–217. Armonk, NY: Futura, 1998.
70. Belhassen B, Shapira I, Pelleg A: Idiopathic recurrent sustained ventricular tachycardia responsive to verapamil: an ECG-electrophysiologic entity. Am Heart J 108:1034–1037, 1984.
71. Rodriguez LM, Smeets JLRM, Timmermans C, et al: Radiofrequency catheter ablation of idiopathic ventricular tachycardia originating in the anterior fascicle of the left bundle branch. J Cardiovasc Electrophysiol 7:1211–1216, 1996.
72. Nagakawa H, Beckman KL, McClelland HJ, et al: Radiofrequency catheter ablation of left ventricular tachycardia guided by a Purkinje potential. Circulation 88:2607–2617, 1993.
73. Rodriguez LM, Smeets JLRM, Timmermans C, Wellens HJJ: Predictors for successful ablation of right and left-sided idiopathic ventricular tachycardia. Am J Cardiol 79:309–314, 1997.
74. Klein LS, Shih HT, Hackett K, et al: Radiofrequency catheter ablation of ventricular tachycardia in patients without structural heart disease. Circulation 85:1666–1674, 1992.
75. Coggins DL, Lee RJ, Sweeney J, et al: Radiofrequency catheter ablation as a cure for idiopathic tachycardia of both right and left ventricular origin. J Am Coll Cardiol 23:1333–1341, 1994.
76. Ellison K, Stevenson WG, Couper GS, et al: Ablation of ventricular tachycardia due to post-infarct ventricular septal defect: identification and insertion of a broad reentry loop. J Cardiovasc Electrophysiol 8:1163–1166, 1997.
77. Morady F, Harvey M, Kalbfleisch SJ, et al: Radiofrequency catheter ablation of ventricular tachycardia in patients with coronary artery disease. Circulation 87:363–372, 1993.
78. Rothman SA, Hsia HH, Cossu SF, et al: Radiofrequency catheter ablation of postinfarction ventricular tachycardia: long-term success and the significance of inducible nonclinical arrhythmias. Circulation 96:3499–3508, 1997.
79. Gonska DB, Cao K, Schaumman A, Dorszewski A, et al: Catheter ablation of ventricular tachycardia in 136 patients with coronary artery disease. Circulation 87:363–372, 1993.
80. Kim YH, Sosa-Suarez G, Troutont TG, et al: Treatment of ventricular tachycardia by transcatheter radiofrequency ablation in patients with ischemic heart disease. Circulation 89:1094–1102, 1994.
81. Stevenson WG, Friedman P, Kosovic D, et al: Radiofrequency catheter ablation of ventricular tachycardia after myocardial infarction. Circulation 98:308–314, 1998.
82. Tchou P, Jazayeri M, Denker S, et al: Transcatheter electrical ablation of the right bundle branch: a method of treating macroreentrant ventricular tachycardia attributed to bundle branch reentry. Circulation 78:246–250, 1988.
83. Oretto G, Smeets J, Rodriguez LM, et al: Wide QRS complex tachycardia with AV dissociation and QRS morphology identical to that of sinus rhythm: a manifestation of bundle branch re-entry. Heart 76:541–547, 1996.
84. Crijns HJGM, Smeets JLRM, Rodriguez LM, et al: Cure of interfascicular reentrant ventricular tachycardia by ablation of the anterior fascicle of the left bundle branch. J Cardiovasc Electrophysiol 6:486–492, 1995.
85. Rodriguez LM, Smeets J, Timmermans C, et al: Radiofrequency ablation of sustained monomorphic ventricular tachycardia in a patient with hypertrophic cardiomyopathy. J Cardiovasc Electrophysiol 8:803–806, 1997.

CHAPTER 98

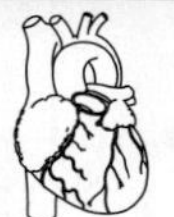

SURGICAL TREATMENT OF ARRHYTHMIAS

James L. Cox

ATRIAL FIBRILLATION
Historical Aspects
Anatomic-Electrophysiologic Basis
Surgical Indications and Contraindications
Preoperative Electrophysiologic Evaluation
Surgical Technique
Surgical Results
WOLFF-PARKINSON-WHITE SYNDROME
Surgical Technique
Associated Abnormalities
Surgical Results
PAROXYSMAL SUPRAVENTRICULAR TACHYCARDIA
Concealed Accessory Pathway
ATRIOVENTRICULAR NODE REENTRY TACHYCARDIA
Historical Aspects
AUTOMATIC ATRIAL TACHYCARDIAS
SUPRAVENTRICULAR ARRHYTHMIAS DUE TO MAHAIM FIBERS
IDIOPATHIC VENTRICULAR TACHYCARDIA
NONISCHEMIC CARDIOMYOPATHY
ARRHYTHMOGENIC RIGHT VENTRICULAR DYSPLASIA
UHL'S SYNDROME
LONG QT SYNDROME
ISCHEMIC VENTRICULAR TACHYCARDIA
Historical Aspects

The therapy for cardiac arrhythmias, including antiarrhythmic drugs, catheter ablation, and surgery, is capable of curing essentially all supraventricular and ventricular tachyarrhythmias. When these therapeutic interventions fail or when surgery is contraindicated, antitachycardia pacemaker cardioverter-defibrillators may provide substantial benefit. Although the indications for surgical intervention have narrowed, surgery remains an important treatment of cardiac arrhythmias, especially for the most common of all arrhythmias—atrial fibrillation.

ATRIAL FIBRILLATION

Atrial fibrillation is present in 0.4 to 2.0 percent of the general population[1–5] and in approximately 10% of the population older than 60 years,[6–9] making it the most common of all sustained cardiac arrhythmias. Although atrial fibrillation is frequently considered to be an innocuous arrhythmia, it is associated with significant morbidity and mortality rates because of its three detrimental sequelae:

1. An irregularly irregular heartbeat, which causes patient discomfort and anxiety
2. Loss of synchronous atrioventricular (AV) contraction, which compromises cardiac hemodynamics, resulting in varying levels of congestive heart failure
3. Stasis of blood flow in the left atrium, which increases the vulnerability to thromboembolism

Historical Aspects

Because medical therapy frequently fails to control atrial fibrillation, several previous surgical techniques have been designed to either ablate the arrhythmia or ameliorate its attendant detrimental sequelae. In 1980, we[10] described the *left atrial isolation procedure* (Fig. 98–1), which is capable of confining atrial fibrillation to the left atrium while leaving the remainder of the heart in normal sinus rhythm (Fig. 98–2). This procedure was successful in restoring a regular ventricular rhythm without the need for a permanent pacemaker; unexpectedly, it also restored normal cardiac hemodynamics. The reason for the latter is that the right atrium and right ventricle beat in synchrony after the procedure. This provides normal right-sided cardiac output that is then delivered to the left side of the heart. Despite the fact that the left atrium is isolated, and therefore cannot beat in synchrony with the left ventricle, the left ventricle adapts instantaneously to the normal right-sided output and delivers a normal forward cardiac output (Fig. 98–3). Thus, the left atrial isolation procedure alleviates two of the three detrimental sequelae of atrial fibrillation, namely, the irregular heartbeat and the compromised hemodynamics. Unfortunately, because the left atrium may continue to fibrillate, the vulnerability to systemic thromboembolism is unchanged after this procedure.

In 1982, Scheinman and colleagues[11] introduced *catheter fulguration of the His bundle* as a means of controlling the irregular cardiac rhythm associated with atrial fibrillation and other refractory supraventricular arrhythmias. During the 1990s, elective His bundle ablation has been accomplished through radiofrequency catheter ablation. Regardless of how His bundle conduction is interrupted, the procedure functions as a type of isolation procedure in that it isolates the supraventricular arrhythmia to the atria and away from the ventricles. Elective His bundle ablation dictates the implantation of a permanent ventricular pacemaker, which restores a normal ventricular rhythm. However, the atria continue to fibrillate after His bundle abla-

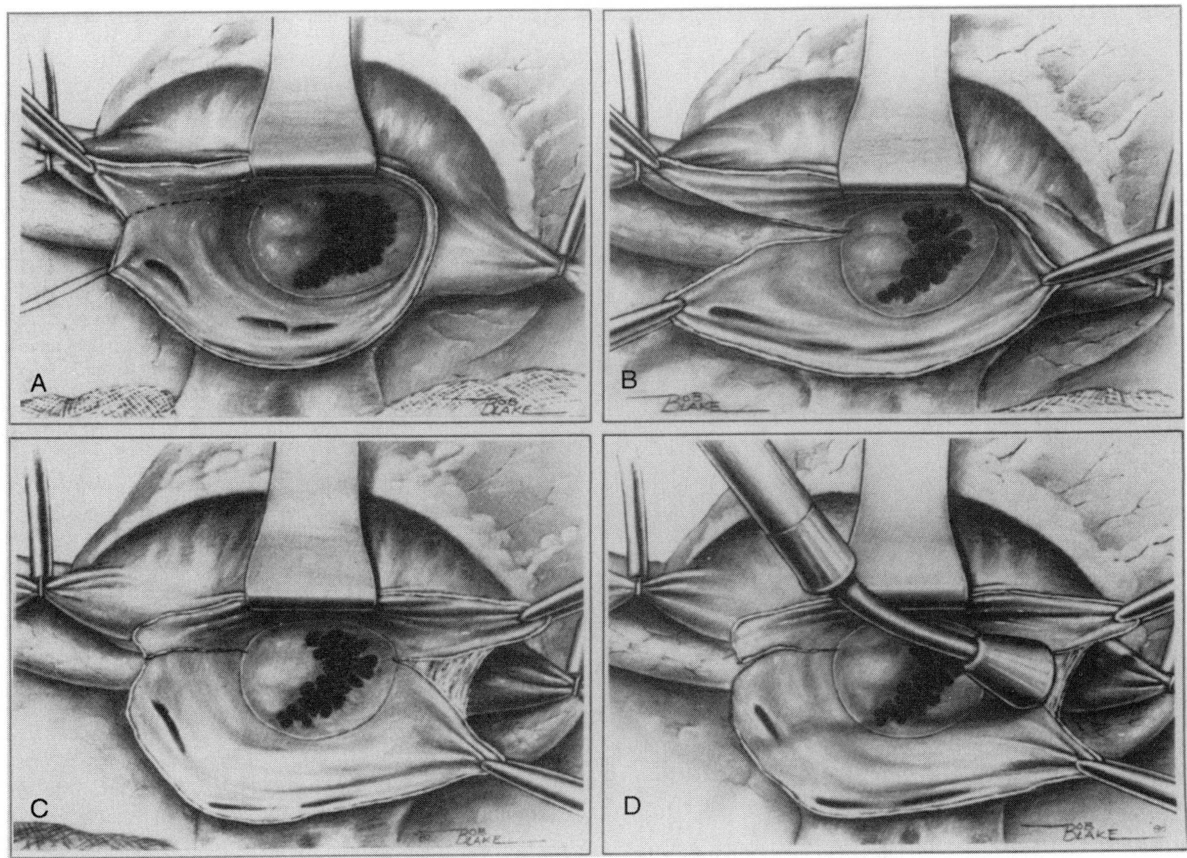

FIGURE 98–1 Left atrial isolation procedure. **A,** After a standard left atriotomy incision, the interatrial septum is retracted gently, and the atriotomy is extended anteriorly *(dashed line)* across Bachmann bundle to the level of the mitral valve annulus just to the left of the right fibrous trigone. **B,** The anterior extension of the standard left atriotomy has been completed. The base of the aorta and its juxtaposition with the anterior leaflet of the mitral valve are demonstrated. Note that the anterior atriotomy extends across the mitral valve annulus. The main body of the left atrium has been separated anteriorly from the remainder of the heart. **C,** The transmural left atriotomy is extended posteriorly to the level of the coronary sinus. The remaining portion of the incision is made through the endocardium and extends across the mitral valve annulus posteriorly just to the left of the interatrial septum. At this point, electrical activity continues to be propagated in a 1:1 fashion between the right and left atria because of the presence of interatrial muscular connections accompanying the coronary sinus. **D,** A cryoprobe is positioned over the endocardial aspect of the posterior atriotomy, and its temperature is decreased to −60°C for 2 minutes. This cryolesion ablates the endocardial interatrial fibers accompanying the coronary sinus. A similar cryolesion is created on the epicardial aspect of the atrioventricular groove on the opposite side of the coronary sinus to ablate all remaining interatrial epicardial connections. The left atriotomy is closed with a continuous 4-0 nonabsorbable suture. (**A–D,** From Williams JM, Ungerleider RM, Lofland GK, Cox JL: Left atrial isolation: new technique for the treatment of supraventricular arrhythmias. J Thorac Cardiovasc Surg 80:373, 1980.)

tion, and therefore, this technique alleviates only one of the detrimental sequelae of atrial fibrillation: the irregular heartbeat. The hemodynamic compromise due to loss of AV synchrony and the vulnerability to thromboembolism are unaffected by His bundle ablation.

In 1985, Guiraudon and associates[12] described the *corridor procedure* for the treatment of atrial fibrillation, an open-heart technique that does not always require a permanent pacemaker.[13, 14] The corridor procedure isolates a strip of atrial septum (the "corridor") harboring both the sinoatrial (SA) node and the AV node, thereby allowing the SA node to drive the ventricles. This procedure corrects the irregular heartbeat associated with atrial fibrillation, but both atria may continue to fibrillate postoperatively because they are totally isolated from the septal corridor. In addition, both atria are isolated from their respective ventricles, thereby precluding the possibility of AV synchrony on either side of the heart. Therefore, neither the hemodynamic compromise nor the vulnerability to thromboembolism associated with atrial fibrillation is alleviated by the corridor procedure. Indeed, this procedure accomplishes the same physiologic result as elective His bundle ablation, a procedure that can be performed without the need for open-heart surgery.

In assessing the results of such procedures, one should pay particular attention to the terminology used to describe "success." When speaking of a "cure" for atrial fibrillation, it is essential to take into account all of the detrimental sequelae of the arrhythmia and the status of the heart once the arrhythmia has been abolished. The described nonpharmacologic therapies for atrial fibrillation have been deemed successful, but they have been so only in terms of their limited goals. For example, the success rate of catheter ablation of the His bundle for atrial fibrillation is reported as being more than 90 percent.[15] However, this simply means that *permanent heart block* can be accom-

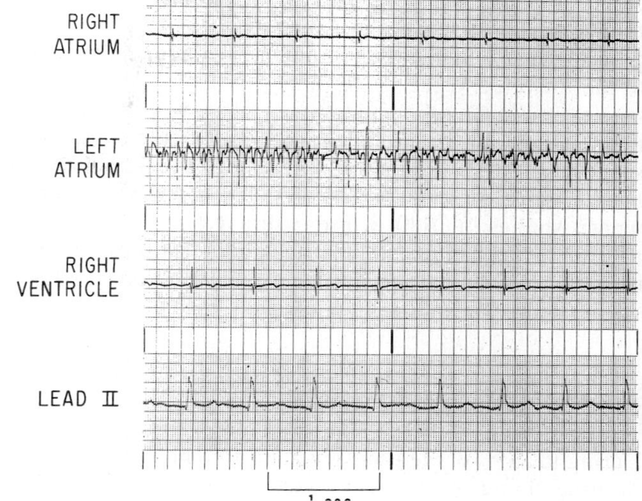

FIGURE 98–2 After the left atrial isolation procedure, atrial fibrillation is confined to the left atrium while the remainder of the heart is in normal sinus rhythm. Note that the right atrium and the right ventricle are beating in synchrony. The P waves are inconspicuous on the lead II electrocardiogram because of the loss of synchronous contraction of the left atrial mass. (From Williams JM, Ungerleider RM, Lofland GK, Cox JL: Left atrial isolation: new technique for the treatment of supraventricular arrhythmias. J Thorac Cardiovasc Surg 80:373, 1980.)

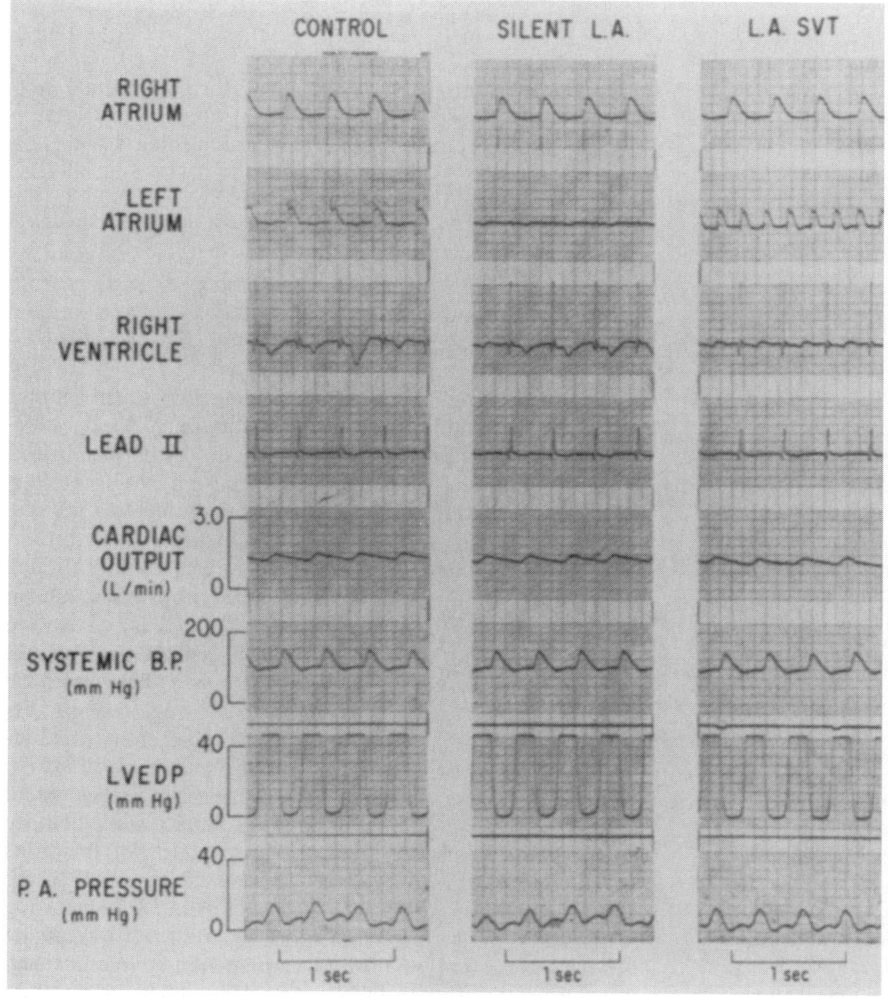

FIGURE 98–3 Postoperative electrograms of the right atrium, left atrium (L.A.), right ventricle, and lead II electrocardiogram are recorded during simultaneous monitoring of the cardiac output (aortic flow), systemic arterial blood pressure (B.P.), left ventricular end-diastolic pressure (LVEDP), and pulmonary artery (P.A.) pressure. In the control tracings, the right and left atria are both paced, but the pacing stimulus to the left atrium is delayed 30 ms to simulate the exact activation pattern that existed preoperatively during normal sinus rhythm. The pacing stimulus to the left atrium is then abruptly discontinued (silent L.A.). No alterations in normal atrioventricular conduction occur, and there is no change noted in left ventricular preload, afterload, or cardiac output. The left atrium is then paced at a rate of 300 pulses per minute (L.A. SVT) with no alteration in normal atrioventricular conduction, preload, afterload, or cardiac output. (From Williams JM, Ungerleider RM, Lofland GK, Cox JL: Left atrial isolation: new technique for the treatment of supraventricular arrhythmias. J Thorac Cardiovasc Surg 80:373, 1980.)

plished by the catheter technique in more than 90 percent of cases. The atrial fibrillation in those patients is never cured, although the ventricular response rate can be controlled with a permanent pacemaker.

In summary, each of these nonpharmacologic approaches to the treatment of atrial fibrillation provides some advantage over allowing the patient to continue with the arrhythmia, but none of them alleviates all three of the detrimental sequelae of atrial fibrillation. Because of the limitations of these surgical procedures, we initiated a series of experimental studies in 1980 with the ultimate aim of achieving a better understanding of the anatomic-electrophysiologic basis of atrial flutter and fibrillation and then developing a surgical cure for both arrhythmias.

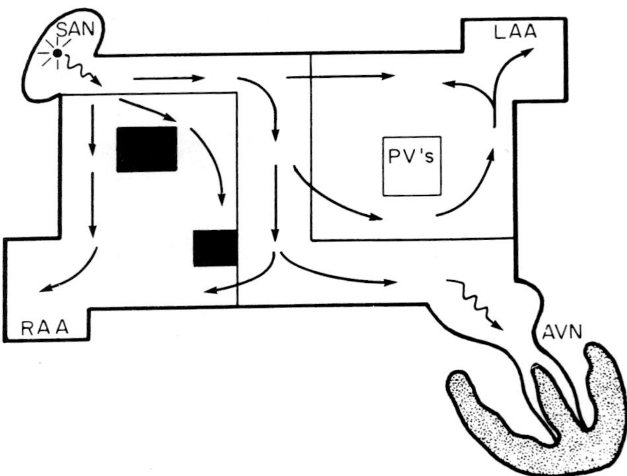

FIGURE 98–5 Normal atrial activation. During normal sinus rhythm, the electrical impulse is generated within the sinoatrial node and propagates across the right and left atria and the atrial septum to the atrioventricular node and then to the ventricles. Same anatomic schema and abbreviations as in Figure 98–4. (From Cox JL, Canavan TE, Schuessler RB, et al: The surgical treatment of atrial fibrillation, II: intraoperative electrophysiologic mapping and description of the electrophysiologic basis of atrial flutter and atrial fibrillation. J Thorac Cardiovasc Surg 101:406–426, 1991.)

Anatomic-Electrophysiologic Basis

During the 1980s, we used several different animal models of atrial flutter and atrial fibrillation in combination with computerized mapping in patients with atrial fibrillation to develop a comprehensive and inclusive concept of the anatomic-electrophysiologic basis of these arrhythmias.[16–24] These studies documented that there are three interacting components in atrial flutter and atrial fibrillation that determine the findings on the peripheral electrocardiogram (ECG) and, therefore, dictate the clinical diagnosis: (1) a macro-reentrant circuit or circuits, (2) passive atrial conduction in that portion of the atrium not involved in the macro-reentrant circuit, and (3) AV conduction. The electrophysiologic characteristics of these three components define a *spectrum* of atrial arrhythmias, extending from simple atrial flutter through several types of transitional arrhythmias to complex atrial fibrillation (Figs. 98–4 to 98–7).

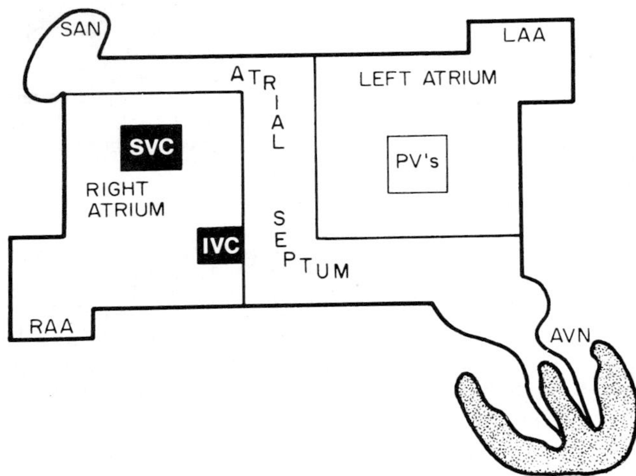

FIGURE 98–4 Atrial anatomy pertinent to atrial electrophysiology and the surgical treatment of atrial arrhythmias. The entire atrial myocardium, including the atrial septum, is depicted as a two-dimensional rectangle, with the atrial septum separating the right atrium from the left atrium. The left atrial appendage (LAA) and right atrial appendage (RAA) are depicted as contiguous with their respective atria. The superior vena cava (SVC) and the inferior vena cava (IVC) are depicted as black boxes within the right atrium, indicating that there are two large anatomic "holes" (i.e., the orifices of these two vessels) around which electrical activity must propagate. The orifices of the pulmonary veins (PVs) are also indicated schematically, but because electrical activity can conduct between the orifices of each of these veins, they are illustrated with the same background as that of the left atrium. Finally, the sinoatrial node (SAN) is located at the top of the atrial septum near its junction with the right atrium, and the atrioventricular node (AVN) is depicted at the bottom of the atrial septum. (From Cox JL, Canavan TE, Schuessler RB, et al: The surgical treatment of atrial fibrillation, II: intraoperative electrophysiologic mapping and description of the electrophysiologic basis of atrial flutter and atrial fibrillation. J Thorac Cardiovasc Surg 101:406–426, 1991.)

In addition to elucidating the mechanism of atrial flutter and atrial fibrillation, these experimental and clinical electrophysiologic studies also documented that our initial hopes of obtaining computerized electrophysiologic maps of atrial fibrillation and using them to guide the specific surgical technique, as we had done in other arrhythmias, were not feasible. Because the macro-reentrant circuits responsible for atrial flutter and atrial fibrillation are so fleeting in nature, it would be impossible to use activation maps to guide surgery even with on-line maps. As a result, we sought to develop a surgical technique that would be capable of interrupting any and all macro-reentrant circuits that might potentially develop in the atria, thereby precluding the ability of the atrium to flutter or fibrillate. In addition, it was recognized that the surgical incisions would have to be placed so that the SA node could resume activity postoperatively and "direct" the propagation of the sinus impulse throughout both atria. This would allow all of the atrial myocardium to be activated postoperatively, resulting in preservation of atrial transport function, a prerequisite for the restoration of normal cardiac hemodynamics and the prevention of stasis of blood flow in the left atrium with the resultant potential for thromboembolism. The surgical procedure that was conceived to accomplish these goals is

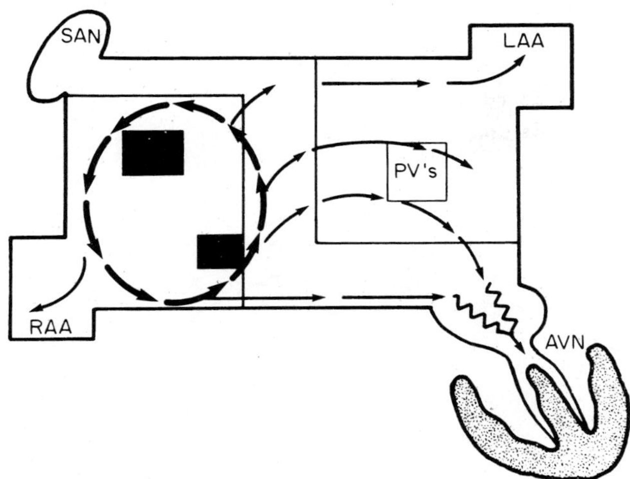

FIGURE 98–6 Single macro-reentrant circuit. Electrophysiologic basis of the standard electrocardiographic findings in the simplest type of atrial flutter. Same anatomic schema and abbreviations as in Figure 98–4. (From Cox JL, Canavan TE, Schuessler RB, et al: The surgical treatment of atrial fibrillation, II: intraoperative electrophysiologic mapping and description of the electrophysiologic basis of atrial flutter and atrial fibrillation. J Thorac Cardiovasc Surg 101:406–426, 1991.)

based on the concept of a maze[19, 25] and as a result was named the Maze procedure (Figs. 98–8 to 98–10).

Surgical Indications and Contraindications

The major indication for surgery is intolerance of the arrhythmia. In many respects, patients with paroxysmal atrial flutter/fibrillation are more symptomatic than are those with chronic atrial fibrillation. Major symptoms in the paroxysmal group include dyspnea on exertion, easy fatigability, lethargy, malaise, and a general sense of impending doom during the periods of atrial flutter/fibrillation. The patients with chronic atrial fibrillation are usually better adapted to the sensation of an irregular heartbeat, but the majority complain of exercise limitations, dypsnea on exertion, and easy fatigability. In addition, they frequently express concern over the possibility of having a stroke.

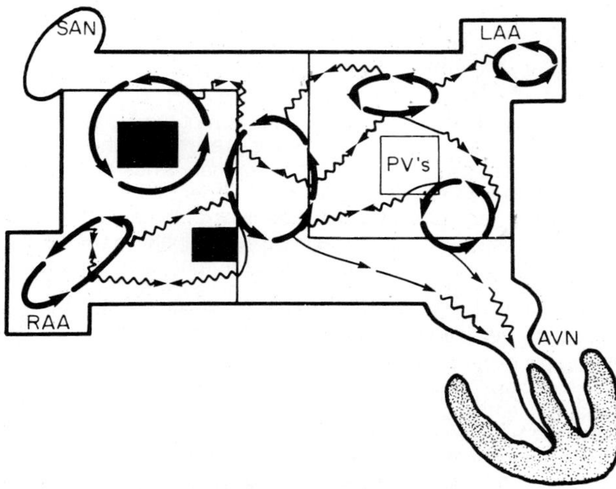

FIGURE 98–7 Multiple macrore-entrant circuit. Electrophysiologic basis of the standard electrocardiographic findings in the most complex type of atrial fibrillation. Same anatomic schema and abbreviations as in Figure 98–4. (From Cox JL, Canavan TE, Schuessler RB, et al: The surgical treatment of atrial fibrillation, II: intraoperative electrophysiologic mapping and description of the electrophysiologic basis of atrial flutter and atrial fibrillation. J Thorac Cardiovasc Surg 101:406–426, 1991.)

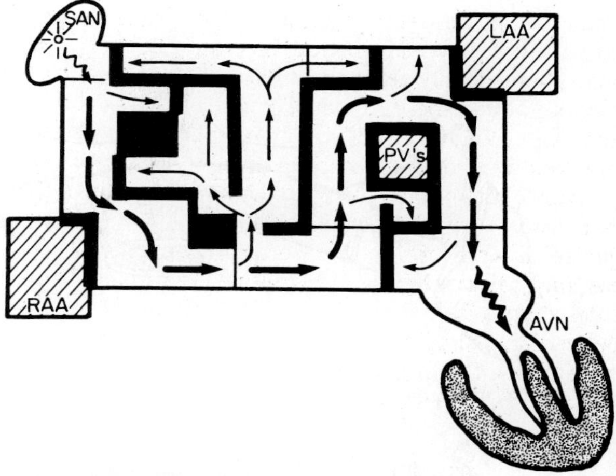

FIGURE 98–8 Conceptual diagram of the Maze procedure for atrial fibrillation. Because atrial fibrillation is characterized by the presence of multiple macro-reentrant circuits that are fleeting in nature and can occur anywhere in the atria, a surgical procedure based on the principle of a maze was developed. Both atrial appendages are excised, and the pulmonary veins are isolated. Appropriately placed atrial incisions not only interrupt the conduction routes of the most common reentrant circuits but also direct the sinus impulse from the sinoatrial node to the atrioventricular node along a specified route. The entire atrial myocardium (except for the atrial appendages and pulmonary veins) is electrically activated by providing for multiple blind alleys off the main conduction route between the sinoatrial node and the atrioventricular node, thereby preserving atrial transport function postoperatively. Same anatomic schema and abbreviations as in Figure 98–4. (From Cox JL, Canavan TE, Schuessler RB, et al: The surgical treatment of atrial fibrillation, II: intraoperative electrophysiologic mapping and description of the electrophysiologic basis of atrial flutter and atrial fibrillation. J Thorac Cardiovasc Surg 101:406–426, 1991.)

To be considered for surgery, the maximum amount of tolerable drug therapy must have been unsuccessful for a patient preoperatively. In addition, 19 percent of the patients in our series had experienced at least one episode of cerebral thromboembolism that resulted in significant temporary or permanent neurologic deficit.

Contraindications to the Maze procedure include the presence of significant left ventricular dysfunction not attributable to the arrhythmia itself and concomitant cardiac or noncardiac disease that constitutes an excessive surgical risk.

Preoperative Electrophysiologic Evaluation

For several years, a preoperative endocardial catheter electrophysiologic study was required in all patients with atrial flutter and in patients with *paroxysmal* atrial fibrillation.

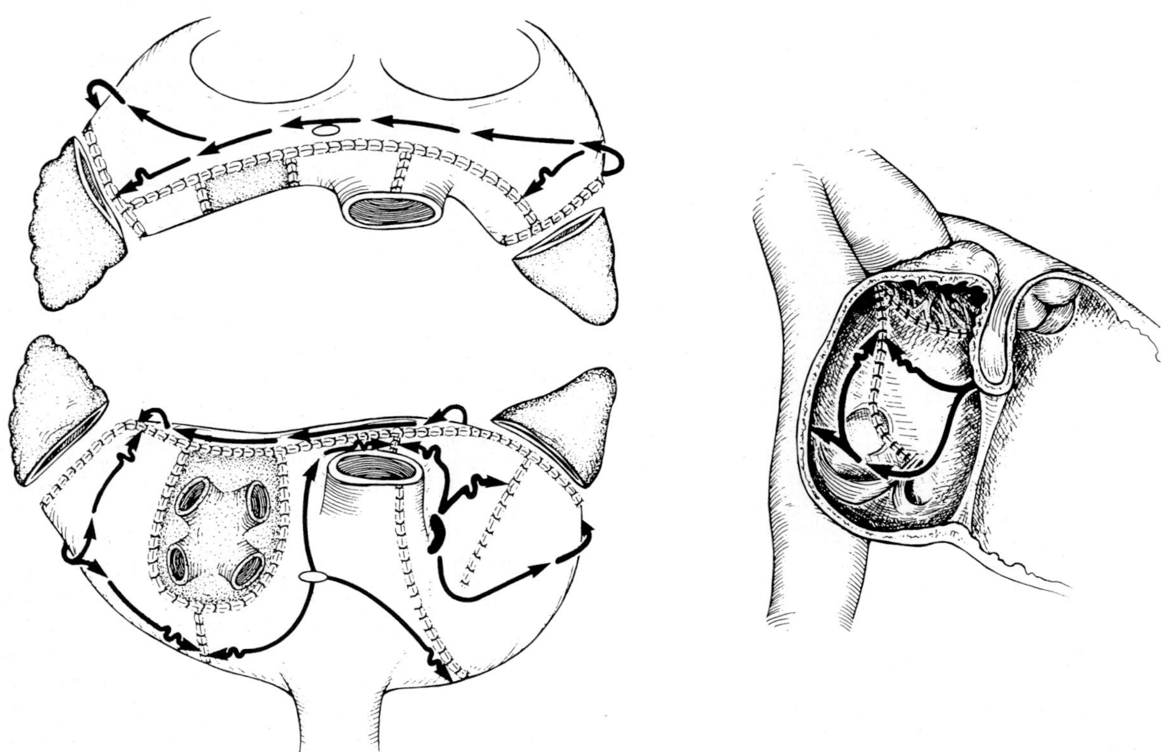

FIGURE 98–9 Two-dimensional drawing of the incisions made in the Maze I procedure. (From Cox JL, Schuessler RB, D'Agostino HJ Jr, et al: The surgical treatment of atrial fibrillation, III: development of a definite surgical procedure. J Thorac Cardiovasc Surg 101:569–583, 1991.)

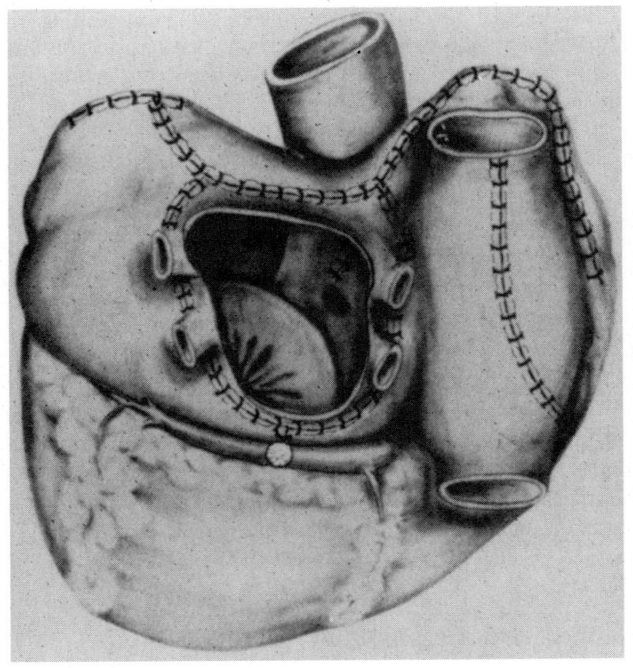

FIGURE 98–10 Three-dimensional depiction of the incisions used to perform the Maze I procedure. Note the presence of the transmural cryolesions *(white dot)* of the coronary sinus at the site of the posteroinferior left atriotomy. Both atrial appendages have been excised. The only completely isolated portions of the atrium are the orifices of the pulmonary veins. The impulse originates from the region of the sinoatrial node and can escape from that region only by passing inferiorly and anteriorly around the base of the right atrium. The impulse continues to propagate around the anterior right atrium onto the top of the interatrial septum. There, it bifurcates into two wavefronts—one passing through the septum in an anterior-to-posterior direction to activate the posteromedial right and left atria, and the other continuing around the base of the excised left atrial appendage to activate the posterolateral left atrial wall. In this manner, all atrial myocardium, except the pulmonary vein orifices, is activated. The activation of this atrial myocardium is fundamental to the preservation of atrial transport function postoperatively. (From Cox JL, Schuessler RB, D'Agostino HJ Jr, et al: The surgical treatment of atrial fibrillation, III: development of a definite surgical procedure. J Thorac Cardiovasc Surg 101:569–583, 1991.)

The primary purpose of this study was to (1) determine SA node function, (2) localize the site of the reentrant circuit in patients with atrial flutter, and (3) try to detect any underlying electrophysiologic abnormality that might be triggering the atrial fibrillation, such as an automatic atrial focus, an accessory atrioventricular connection, or AV node reentry. These electrophysiologic studies have proved to be a bit superfluous, so we no longer require that a patient undergo a formal study before surgery. We have never thought it wise to try to perform electrophysiologic studies in patients with *chronic* atrial fibrillation because the SA node cannot be evaluated without electric cardioversion, which would introduce too great a risk of thromboembolism.

Surgical Technique

The original surgical technique, the Maze I procedure (see Fig. 98–9),[25] was modified to become the Maze II procedure (Fig. 98–11) because of late chronotropic problems with the SA node and intra-atrial conduction delays that resulted in decreased left atrial contraction. However, the Maze II procedure proved to be exceedingly difficult technically, and as a result, it was modified again to become the Maze III procedure (Fig. 98–12).[26, 27] The Maze III procedure is considered to be the surgical technique of choice for the treatment of medically refractory atrial flutter and atrial fibrillation. Most of the incisions originally performed as a part of the Maze III procedure have been replaced by cryolesions so the procedure can be performed with minimally invasive techniques. In addition, the new minimally invasive technique avoids the removal of the left atrial appendage. The orifice of the appendage is now cryoablated circumferentially and then closed from inside the left atrium.

Surgical Results

Between September 25, 1987, and March 25, 1999, 32 patients had the Maze I procedure, 15 patients had the Maze II procedure, and 259 patients had the Maze III procedure for the treatment of atrial flutter/fibrillation. Forty-two percent of all patients experienced temporary perioperative atrial fibrillation within the first 3 months after surgery. These early postoperative arrhythmias invariably disappeared and had no correlation with long-term results of the surgery. Once the atrium healed from surgery (3 months), the recurrent arrhythmia rate was less than 5 percent for the entire group and 2 percent for the Maze III group. The recurrent arrhythmias have been easily controlled with medical therapy in those patients, despite the fact that an average of five drugs were unsuccessful postoperatively. Thus, for the past 7 years, 98 percent of patients have been cured of atrial fibrillation with the surgery alone and the other 2 percent of patients have been cured with a

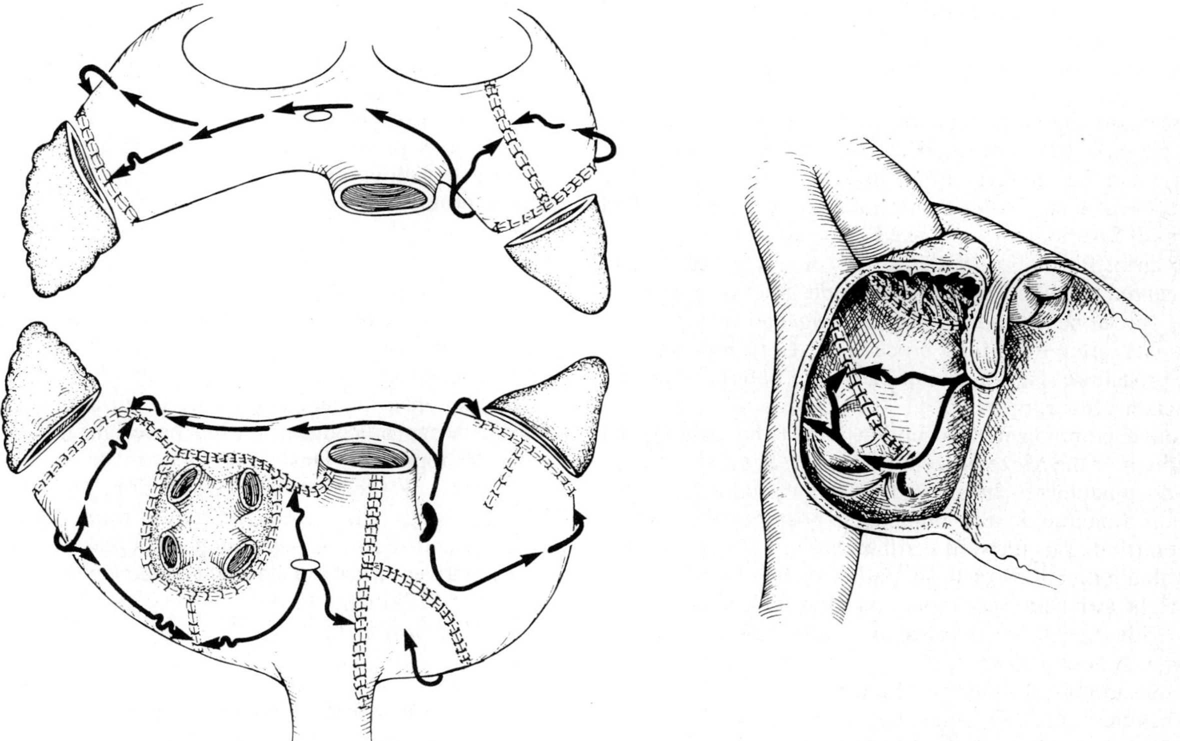

FIGURE 98–11 Maze II procedure. Same view as in Figure 98–9. The previous incision through the "sinus tachycardia" area has been deleted and the transverse atriotomy across the dome of the left atrium has been moved posteriorly to allow better intra-atrial conduction. The major problem with this modification of the Maze procedure is that it was necessary to completely transsect the superior vena cava to gain exposure of the left atrium. (From Cox JL, Boineau JP, Schuessler RB, Lappas DG: Modification of the maze procedure for atrial flutter and atrial fibrillation, I: rationale and surgical results. J Thorac Cardiovasc Surg 110:473–484, 1995.)

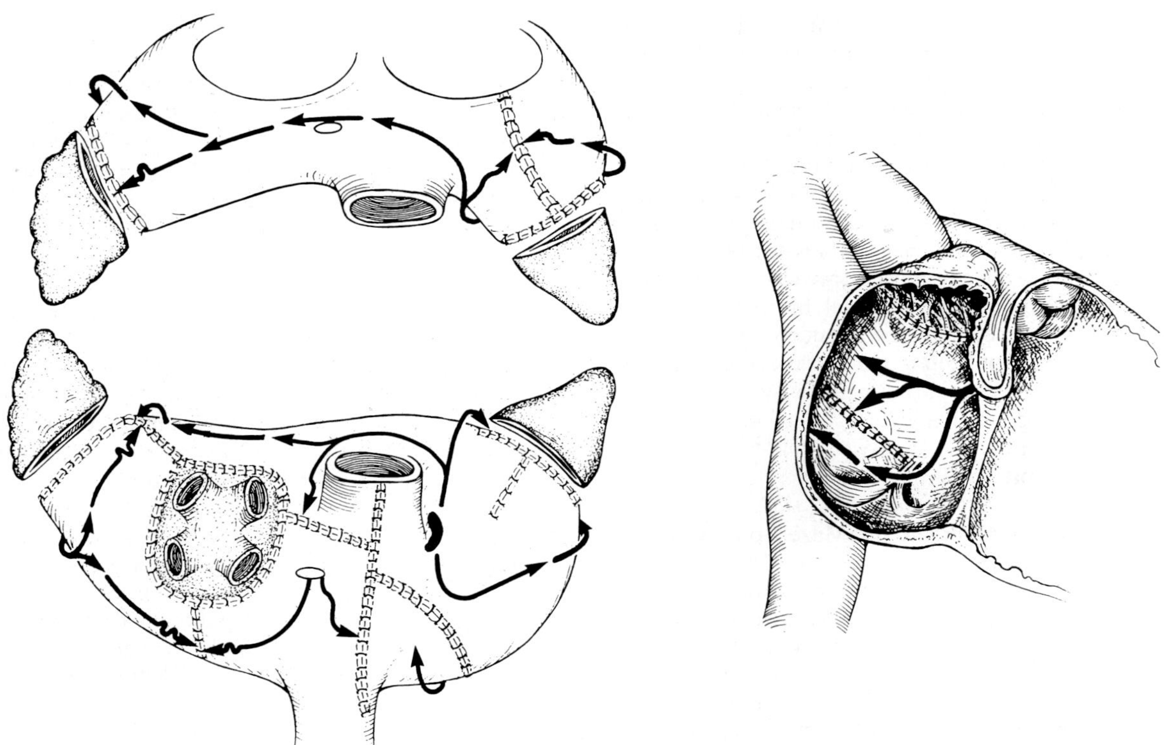

FIGURE 98–12 Maze III procedure: Same view as in Figure 98–9. By placing the septal incision posterior to the orifice of the superior vena cava, the exposure of the left atrium is excellent. (From Cox JL, Boineau JP, Schuessler RB, Lappas DG: Modification of the maze procedure for atrial flutter and atrial fibrillation, I: rationale and surgical results. J Thorac Cardiovasc Surg 110:473–484, 1995.)

combination of surgery and postoperative medicine, for an overall postoperative cure rate of 100 percent.

One of the commonly repeated misconceptions regarding the Maze procedure is that it causes patients to need pacemakers postoperatively. Overall, 19 percent of all postoperative patients have pacemakers, but all of them either already had pacemakers implanted before surgery, were known to have sick sinus syndrome preoperatively, or had abnormal SA nodes "unmasked" by abolishing the patient's atrial fibrillation. Indeed, 123 of our patients were documented to have normal sinus node function preoperatively, and none of those patients have had a permanent pacemaker after the Maze procedure. It is clear that the Maze procedure itself does not cause the patient to need a pacemaker after surgery.

Another common misconception is that the atria do not function after the Maze procedure. In our series, all patients were documented to have both right atrial and left atrial transport function in the immediate postoperative period that contributed to forward cardiac output. On late follow-up evaluation, 98 percent of patients have continued to have right atrial transport function, and 93 percent of patients with the Maze III procedure have had documented left atrial function as well.

We documented that the Maze procedure essentially abolishes the threat of stroke associated with atrial fibrillation. Fifty-eight of our patients (19 percent) had experienced a thromboembolic episode before surgery. There were 40 patients with a history of frank stroke and 18 patients with a history of at least one significant transient ischemic attack. Because of the presence of atrial fibrillation per se, the remainder of our patients were also at a higher-than-normal risk for thromboembolism than the normal population, although not as high a risk as that for the 58 patients. Despite the inherently high risk of stroke in these patients, there have been only two perioperative strokes (0.7 percent) and only one minor stroke during long-term follow-up (11.5 years; mean 3.9 ± 2.7 years). The long-term stroke rate after the Maze procedure is 0.1 percent per year. Although the long-term stroke rate for lone atrial fibrillation is 10 times that rate, we do not use the threat of stroke as an indication for the Maze procedure in patients with lone atrial fibrillation.

As mentioned, we have developed a minimally invasive Maze procedure that we perform routinely in the majority of our patients. Indeed, 76 percent of all patients undergoing the Maze procedure in 1999 have had this minimally invasive approach. This newer, less invasive surgical approach has resulted in earlier extubation, shorter intensive care unit stays, shorter hospitalization times, quicker recuperation and return to work, and a decreased incidence of perioperative atrial fibrillation (22 percent). In addition, only 1 of 51 patients (2 percent) has required a permanent pacemaker postoperatively.

Wolff-Parkinson-White Syndrome

The introduction of endocardial catheter techniques with the use of radiofrequency energy has had its most dramatic impact on the treatment of supraventricular arrhythmias due to the Wolff-Parkinson-White (WPW) syndrome.[28] Before October 1990, we performed nearly 100 WPW operations per year. Although we now see relatively few cases of failed radiofrequency catheter ablation (RFCA) of the accessory pathways, we have performed WPW surgery on a total of 25 such patients during the "catheter ablation era" since 1990. These patients represent a relatively large group in terms of patients who have undergone surgery only after failed RFCA, and they are instructive in terms of how interventional electrophysiologists should consider dealing with difficult-to-ablate cases.

At the time of surgery in these patients, we noted that the vast majority had some type of anatomic abnormality capable of making RFCA either more difficult or totally impossible to accomplish. These anatomic abnormalities or extreme variations in normal anatomy included anomalous coronary sinuses, Ebstein's anomaly, cardiac hypertrophy, mitral regurgitation, coronary artery disease, previous catheter perforation of the right ventricle, or a small heart due to age.

Several patients were noted to have severe scarring in the dissection planes of the AV groove, making surgical dissection both difficult and hazardous. The patients with Ebstein's anomaly frequently demonstrated a heavy muscle layer encompassing the coronary sinus that extended directly down to the posterior ventricular septum as a thick (6 to 8 mm) band of muscle fibers, representing the *accessory pathway.* It would have been technically impossible in these patients to ablate the accessory pathway with current RFCA technology.

This surgical experience with failed RFCA suggests that if one cannot ablate an accessory pathway in a reasonable period of time, it is highly probable that some type of anatomic abnormality exists that precludes one from doing so. Thus, electrophysiologists should exercise common sense in knowing when to terminate their attempts at RFCA because too much local radiofrequency trauma and injury can render a patient surgically incurable.

All patients who are now subjected to surgery for the WPW syndrome have undergone an endocardial catheter electrophysiologic study in association with their failed attempt at radiofrequency catheter ablation. The most important information for the surgeon to know before surgery is the location of the accessory pathway, the technique and number of ablative attempts used by the electrophysiologist during the attempted RFCA, and the associated (if any) anatomic abnormalities to be encountered during surgery.

Surgical Technique

Two surgical approaches are commonly used to divide accessory AV connections. The endocardial technique is designed to divide the ventricular end of the accessory pathway, and the epicardial technique is directed toward division of the atrial end of the pathway. Excellent results were obtained with both techniques during the pre-RFCA era,[29–31] but the specific operations for the WPW syndrome are usually more difficult because of the above-mentioned anatomic anomalies and the presence of scarring from previous RFCA attempts.

Associated Abnormalities

Certain types of congenital heart abnormalities are frequently associated with the WPW syndrome; the most common is Ebstein's anomaly, in which the septal leaflet, and occasionally the posterior leaflet, of the tricuspid valve is displaced downward into the right ventricle.[32] The position of the AV node and conduction bundles in patients with Ebstein's anomaly is normal, although the right bundle branch may be compressed by thickened endocardium. In our experience, there is a distinct association between patients with Ebstein's anomaly and the specific location of the accessory pathways. Most commonly, patients with this anomaly have posterior septal accessory pathways. However, in our series, a majority of patients with Ebstein's anomaly have also had a combination of right free wall and posterior septal accessory pathways.[30]

Standard endocardial techniques are used to interrupt these accessory pathways. If valve replacement or the placement of an annuloplasty ring is necessary to correct severe Ebstein's anomaly, the valve or annuloplasty ring should be placed below the coronary sinus with sutures placed through the true tricuspid annulus. Plication of the atrialized ventricle may or may not be necessary.

Surgical Results

The incidence of successful surgical correction of the WPW syndrome is nearly 100 percent with an operative mortality rate for elective, uncomplicated cases that ranges from 0 to 0.5 percent.[30, 31] There have been no early or late recurrences after surgery with the endocardial technique in our own series,[30] and the recurrence rate after the epicardial technique is low.[31] Moreover, the inadvertent creation of heart block is no longer a problem.

Paroxysmal Supraventricular Tachycardia

Paroxysmal supraventricular tachycardia is a clinical condition in which supraventricular tachycardia occurs suddenly in a patient who otherwise has a normal ECG. There are two abnormalities that account for essentially all paroxysmal supraventricular tachycardias: (1) a concealed accessory AV connection, and (2) AV node reentry.

Concealed Accessory Pathway

Accessory AV connections may be *manifest* or *concealed.* If an accessory pathway is capable of conducting in the antegrade (atrial-to-ventricular) direction, thereby causing a delta wave on the standard ECG, it is said to be manifest, (i.e., its presence is apparent electrocardiographically). The retrograde (ventricular-to-atrial) conduction characteristics of such a pathway determine the heart rate and frequency of occurrence of the associated reciprocating tachycardia. Some patients harbor accessory AV connections that are capable of conducting in the retrograde direction only. Because antegrade conduction across the accessory pathway does not occur, the ventricles are activated only through the normal AV node–His bundle complex and the standard ECG is normal. Therefore, such accessory pathways are said to be concealed. Because these accessory pathways are capable of conducting in the retrograde direction, however, reciprocating tachycardia can occur just as it does in the classic WPW syndrome. Thus, from a clinical standpoint, the only difference between patients with manifest accessory pathways and those with concealed accessory pathways is the appearance of the standard ECG during normal sinus rhythm. The former have ECGs characteristic of the WPW syndrome, and the latter have normal ECGs.

In patients with a concealed accessory pathway, the absence of antegrade conduction across the pathway precludes the necessity of performing antegrade ventricular mapping intraoperatively. Thus, only retrograde atrial mapping is performed, and these maps are recorded during ventricular pacing or during induced reciprocating tachycardia. The surgical technique used to divide concealed accessory pathways is the same as that for patients with the classic WPW syndrome.

Atrioventricular Node Reentry Tachycardia

Historical Aspects

In 1980, we began a series of experiments in dogs that were designed to gradually encroach on the anatomic AV node with a 2-mm cryoprobe in the hope of being able to modify AV node conduction without creating complete heart block.[33–35] During the course of these experiments, three dogs were discovered to have naturally occurring dual AV node pathways. This *discrete cryosurgical ablation* of the tissues around the AV node resulted in the abolition of the slow pathway of conduction while leaving the fast pathway intact, thereby preserving normal atrioventricular conduction through the AV node. These experiments led directly to the first clinical success in the treatment of AV node reentry tachycardia in August 1982.[36, 37] This discrete cryosurgical approach proved to be uniformly successful without creating heart block in any patients. Thereafter, other surgical techniques[38] were developed that were similarly effective and gained widespread use until the introduction of radiofrequency catheter ablation replaced them in the mid-1980s. It is no longer necessary to perform such procedures surgically because of the virtually uniform success of the catheter techniques.

Automatic Atrial Tachycardias

Clinical data suggest that derangements in automaticity, and not reentry, underlie the genesis of these arrhythmias. These tachycardias appear to have a focal origin and usually originate from the body of the right atrium or left atrium, although they may occasionally arise from the interatrial septum. Accurate preoperative localization is particularly important for patients with automatic atrial tachycardias if surgical ablation of the ectopic focus is contemplated. These tachycardias are frequently suppressed with general anesthesia, and as a result, intraoperative mapping to localize their site of origin may not be possible. In addition, automatic tachycardias are not inducible by standard programmed stimulation techniques. Without accurate intraoperative localization, elective His bundle ablation was once the only surgical alternative. However, alternative surgical techniques that leave the normal atrioventricular conduction intact while isolating the arrhythmogenic atrial myocardium from the remainder of the heart have been developed. If the site of origin of an automatic atrial tachycardia can be localized precisely through intraoperative mapping, the arrhythmogenic focus may be either excised or cryoablated.[39] Automatic foci located in the free wall of the left atrium or in either of the atrial appendages are ideal for excision or cryoablation. Automatic atrial tachycardias arising near the orifices of the pulmonary veins are best treated with pulmonary vein isolation or left atrial isolation (see Fig. 98–1).[10]

Theoretically, if intraoperative mapping properly localizes automatic foci in the free wall of the body of the right atrium, those foci can be either excised or cryoablated. However, automatic right atrial tachycardias are frequently multifocal in origin, and the ablation or excision of one automatic focus may be followed by the appearance of another at a later date. Thus, the recurrence rate after local excision or cryoablation of automatic right atrial tachycardias is unacceptably high. As a result, we prefer to perform a right atrial isolation procedure (Fig. 98–13),[40, 41] even though the site of origin of the tachycardia may be well defined with intraoperative computerized mapping.

Supraventricular Arrhythmias Due to Mahaim Fibers

Nodofascicular and fasciculoventricular connections, as described by Mahaim, occur between the nodal and fascicular components of the AV node–His bundle complex and the ventricular septum. Classically, these fibers have been depicted as originating from the atrioventricular node or its penetrating (His) bundle and then perforating the central fibrous body to insert into the ventricular myocardium. However, the appropriateness of depicting these accessory pathways as nodoventricular has been questioned. Tchou and associates[42] have suggested that such pathways represent atriofascicular connections with decremental conduction properties without direct anatomic connection to the AV nodal tissue, and Klein and colleagues[43] suggested that "typical" nodoventricular connections may be atypical accessory pathways with decremental conduction properties and a distal right ventricular insertion site. Regardless of the exact substrate, from a surgical point of view, Mahaim fibers may connect the His bundle to the ventricular septum by traversing the posterior septal space or the anterior septal space, in which case the Mahaim fiber is anterior to the His bundle. In addition, right free wall

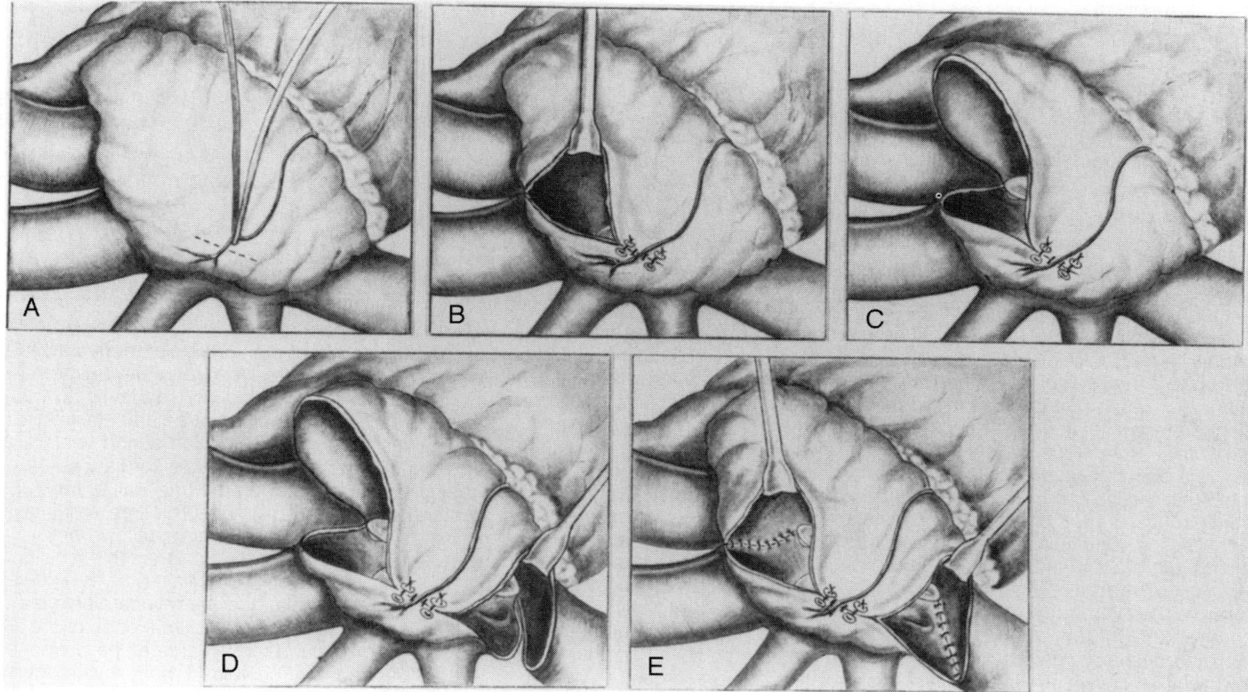

FIGURE 98–13 Right atrial isolation. **A,** Initially, the sinoatrial node artery is dissected free from the atrial tissue 5 mm anterior to the crista terminalis. A 2-cm incision parallel to the crista terminalis is placed beneath the artery. **B,** The incision beneath the sinoatrial node artery is closed with a continuous nonabsorbable 5-0 suture, with care taken to not damage the artery. The small pledgets are used above and below the artery to reinforce the incision. The right atriotomy is then extended to a point anterior to the junction of the superior vena cava and the base of the right atrial appendage. **C,** The atriotomy is extended along the anterior limbus of the fossa ovalis to the anteromedial tricuspid valve annulus, just anterior to the membranous interatrial septum. **D,** Caudad extension of the right atriotomy around the posterior right atrial–inferior vena cava junction to the posterolateral tricuspid valve annulus. A cryolesion (−60°C for 2 minutes) is placed at the end of the incision to ensure complete interruption of connecting atrial muscle fibers between the body of the right atrium and the remainder of the heart. **E,** The atriotomy is closed with a continuous 4-0 nonabsorbable suture. (From Harada A, D'Agostino HJ Jr, Boineau JP, Cox JL: Right atrial isolation: a new surgical treatment for supraventricular tachycardia. I. surgical technique and electrophysiological effects. J Thorac Cardiovasc Surg 95:643, 1988; and Harada A, D'Agostino HJ Jr, Boineau JP, Cox JL: Right atrial isolation: a new surgical treatment for supraventricular tachycardia. II. hemodynamic effects. J Thorac Cardiovasc Surg 95:651, 1988.)

accessory pathways with typical "Mahaim-like" characteristics have been reported,[43] and left-sided nodoventricular connections have been described as well.[44]

Depending on the spatial separation of the Mahaim fiber and the His bundle, these accessory connections can be interrupted with standard endocardial surgical dissection techniques that are used for the WPW syndrome in combination with cryosurgery. The precise surgical approach depends on the location of the accessory pathway as determined with preoperative and intraoperative electrophysiologic mapping. When the posterior septal space is involved, a combination of discrete cryosurgery[37] and a posterior septal space dissection is required in some patients, whereas in others, cryosurgery alone is sufficient to interrupt the pathway. In other patients, a combination of cryosurgery with both anterior and posterior septal dissections is necessary. Finally, a subset of patients have what should be classified as "para-Hisian" connections because despite all maneuvers, the accessory connection is so closely juxtaposed to the His bundle that it cannot be separated surgically. Simultaneous cryosurgical ablation of the His bundle and accessory pathway is the only therapeutic alternative in such cases.

Idiopathic Ventricular Tachycardia

This term refers to an arrhythmia in patients in whom the only clinical manifestation of cardiac disease is the ventricular arrhythmia. Both the macroscopic appearance of the heart at surgery and the pathologic data acquired at the time of autopsy in such patients fail to show any evidence of primary cardiac disease. The only abnormality noted has been global dilatation of the heart secondary to functional post-tachycardia heart failure. If these patients require surgery, they first undergo intraoperative electrophysiologic mapping during ventricular tachycardia in an effort to localize the apparent site of origin of the arrhythmia. Initial surgical approaches included simple ventriculotomy, exclusion procedures, and cryoablation, but the results were poor, primarily because many of these arrhythmias arise within the ventricular septum.[45] Our approach has been to use local isolation procedures (Fig. 98–14) if the site of origin is in the right ventricular free wall[36, 46] and multipoint map-guided cryoablation if it is in the septum.

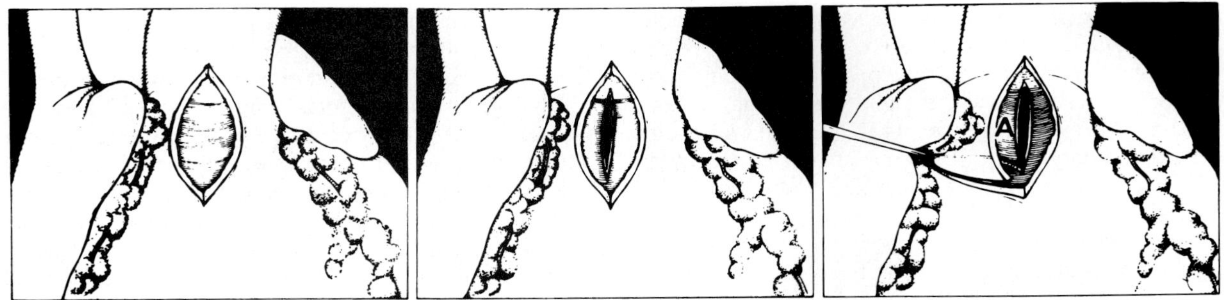

FIGURE 98–14 Surgical treatment of recurrent ventricular tachycardia in a 16-year-old girl with nonischemic cardiomyopathy secondary to coxsackievirus myocarditis. Initial intraoperative electrophysiologic mapping indicated that the ventricular tachycardia arose from the free wall of the pulmonary outflow tract near the atrioventricular groove and just proximal to the level of the pulmonic valve annulus (A). An intramural needle electrode was inserted at that epicardial site and was passed transmurally so that its tip was positioned in the interventricular septum between the crista supraventricularis and the pulmonic valve annulus. Intramural electrograms were recorded from electrode contacts located every millimeter along the needle shaft. Earliest ventricular activation during ventricular tachycardia occurred at the electrode contact point at the tip of the needle shaft, indicating that the ventricular tachycardia was originating in the supracristal portion of the interventricular septum. **Left,** A longitudinal incision was made on the free wall of the pulmonary outflow tract, beginning just distal to the level of the pulmonic valve annulus and extending proximally. This free wall incision did not alter the ventricular tachycardia. **Middle,** A counterincision was made on the posterior wall of the pulmonary outflow tract beginning just distal to the pulmonic valve annulus and extending proximally to the level of the crista supraventricularis. This incision was transmural, and the aortic root could be visualized through this posterior incision. This counterincision did not alter the ventricular tachycardia. A cryoprobe was positioned over the site of earliest activation during ventricular tachycardia, and the myocardium was frozen at −60°C for 2 minutes. This cryolesion resulted in cessation of the ventricular tachycardia. **Right,** The proximal ends of the anterior and posterior ventriculotomies were then connected by a transmural semicircular incision around the left side of the pulmonary outflow tract, as shown. This resulted in total isolation of the segment of the pulmonary outflow tract that contained the arrhythmogenic myocardium. The incisions were closed with a continuous 3-0 nonabsorbable suture, as shown. The patient has remained free of ventricular tachycardia for 20 years after this surgical procedure. (From Cox JL, Bardy GH, Damiano RJ, et al: Right ventricular isolation procedures for nonischemic ventricular tachycardia. J Thorac Cardiovasc Surg 90:212, 1985.)

Nonischemic Cardiomyopathy

A small group of patients has been shown to have ventricular tachycardia due to cardiomyopathy unassociated with ischemic heart disease. This group consists of patients with angiographic and catheter data indicating some type of abnormal myocardial contractility associated with recurrent ventricular tachycardia. These patients usually show a diffuse dilatation of both ventricles with widespread patchy myocardial fibrosis. These tachyarrhythmias frequently arise in the right ventricle, and our approach to such patients has been to use a combination of surgical isolation and cryoablation of the apparent site of origin of the arrhythmia.

Arrhythmogenic Right Ventricular Dysplasia

Fontaine and associates[47] described a previously unrecognized form of cardiomyopathy localized to the right ventricle that they termed *arrhythmogenic right ventricular dysplasia*. This syndrome is a congenital cardiomyopathy characterized by transmural infiltration of adipose tissue resulting in weakness and aneurysmal bulging of the infundibulum, apex, or posterior basilar region of the right ventricle, or a combination. The syndrome is characterized clinically by intractable ventricular tachycardia originating from one or all of the three pathologic areas of the right ventricle (Fig. 98–15). Because the origin of the tachycardia is in the right ventricle, the standard ECG shows a pattern consistent with left bundle branch block during the tachycardia. Right ventricular angiography should be performed in all patients who exhibit ventricular tachycardia with a left bundle branch block pattern. In patients with arrhythmogenic right ventricular dysplasia, the right ventricle appears enlarged; ventricular bulges or frank aneurysms are seen in the infundibulum, the apex, or the basal portion of the inferior wall; and right ventricular

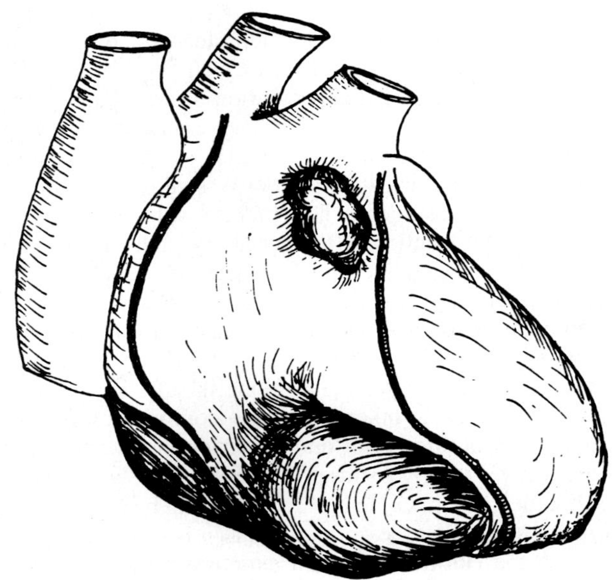

FIGURE 98–15 Sketch of the three areas of pathologic involvement in arrhythmogenic right ventricular dysplasia. (Courtesy of Dr. G. Fontaine.)

contractility is usually markedly decreased. Hypertrophic muscular bands in the infundibulum and anterior right ventricular wall result in apparent pseudodiverticula, the "feathering" appearance of the right ventricular outflow tract. Our approach to such patients is a transmural encircling ventriculotomy that effectively isolates the arrhythmogenic myocardium from the remainder of the heart (Fig. 98–16).[46]

Although Fontaine's original description of arrhythmogenic right ventricular dysplasia suggested that the cardiomyopathy was confined to three discrete areas of the right ventricle, intraoperative mapping of these patients has suggested that the entire right ventricular free wall may be arrhythmogenic in certain cases. In our experience, there may be as many as seven different sites of origin of tachycardia in these patients, with each site giving rise to a different morphologic type of ventricular tachycardia. Computerized intraoperative mapping systems are able to localize these tachycardias only if each of them can be induced at the time of surgery, which is an unrealistic expectation. As a result of these problems, we have had to resort to surgical isolation of the entire right ventricular free wall (Fig. 98–17) on occasion to relieve the life-threatening sequelae of arrhythmogenic dysplasia.[36] Although the follow-up of these patients documents excellent control of their tachycardia (Fig. 98–18), the right ventricle may undergo progressive dilatation postoperatively. Nevertheless, the patients in whom we performed this procedure have remained in excellent functional status for more than 17 years.

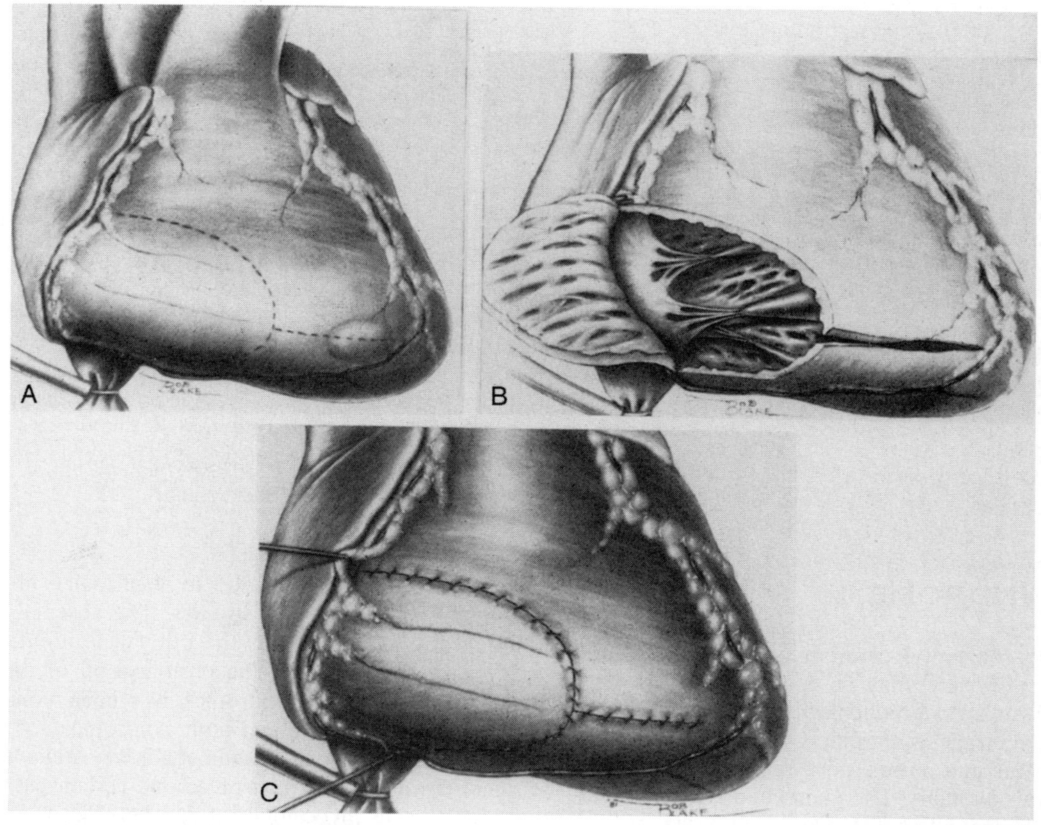

FIGURE 98–16 A, Appearance of the right ventricle in a patient with arrhythmogenic right ventricular dysplasia. Note the three coronary arteries coursing from the atrioventricular groove across the surface of the right ventricle. The acute margin of the right ventricle corresponded to the location of the middle coronary artery shown in this drawing. An area approximately 2 × 3 cm near the upper coronary artery was electrically silent. Epicardial mapping during ventricular tachycardia showed the earliest site of activation to be located near the lower edge of this electrically silent region just below the midsegment of the middle coronary region on the posterior basilar region of the right ventricle. A transmural ventriculotomy was placed around the electrically silent area and included the apparent site of origin of the ventricular tachycardia on the posterior basilar region of the heart *(broken line)*. The two ends of this incision were based at the atrioventricular groove, where cryolesions were applied to ensure isolation of the arrhythmogenic region of myocardium from the remainder of the heart. In addition, a second transmural incision was made from the apex of the semicircular incision to the apex of the right ventricle to include the small saccular aneurysm in that region. **B,** The isolated pedicle of right ventricular myocardium containing the electrically silent area and the apparent site of origin of the ventricular tachycardia has been reflected to show the internal anatomy of the right ventricle. Note the extension of the incision to the right ventricular apex to open the small aneurysm located in that region. **C,** The transmural encircling ventriculotomy around the arrhythmogenic region of the right ventricle and the simple ventriculotomy through the right ventricular apical aneurysm have been closed with a continuous 3-0 nonabsorbable suture. After completion of this procedure for arrhythmogenic right ventricular dysplasia, the isolated pedicle was paced at a rapid rate, but the paced impulses were not conducted to the remainder of the heart. In addition, the remainder of the right ventricle was then paced rapidly, but those paced impulses were not conducted into the isolated pedicle, confirming total isolation of the arrhythmogenic right ventricular myocardium from the remainder of the heart. (From Cox JL: Surgery for cardiac arrhythmias. *In* Current Problems in Cardiology. Vol. VIII, No. 4. Chicago: Year Book Medical, 1983.)

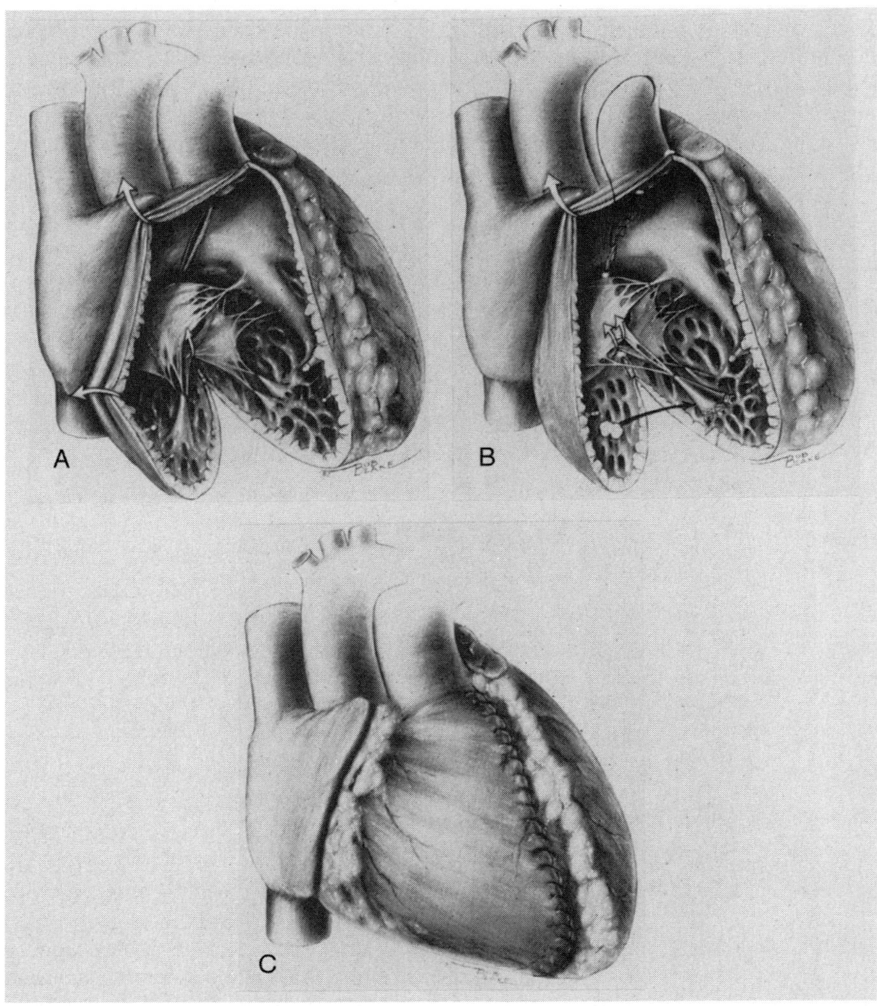

FIGURE 98–17 Right ventricular disconnection procedure. **A,** A transmural right ventriculotomy is placed parallel to and 5 mm from the interventricular septum extending from just across the pulmonic valve annulus anteriorly to the tricuspid valve posteriorly. It is necessary to divide several large infundibular muscular bundles and to divide the moderator band of the right ventricle. Although the entire incision is transmural, special care must be taken to avoid injury to the right coronary artery lying in the atrioventricular groove at the posterior extent of this incision. After identification of the location of the His bundle and right bundle branch, a second transmural incision is placed from the posterior pulmonic valve annulus to the anterior medial tricuspid valve annulus, exposing the underlying aortic root. If the tricuspid portion of this incision is placed too far anteriorly, the bundle of His may be inadvertently divided. **B,** After completion of the two transmural incisions, the papillary muscle attached to the anterior leaflet of the tricuspid valve is divided at its base and reimplanted on the lower ventricular septum using interrupted 3-0 pledgeted Prolene suture. Cryolesions are placed at each end of the anteroposterior ventriculotomy and at each end of the ventriculotomy between the posterior pulmonic valve annulus and the anterior medial suture, followed by closure of the long free wall ventriculotomy with continuous 3-0 nonabsorbable suture **(C)**. (From Cox JL: Surgery for cardiac arrhythmias. *In* Current Problems in Cardiology. Vol. VIII, No. 4. Chicago: Year Book Medical, 1983.)

UHL'S SYNDROME

This is a rare congenital cardiomyopathy that, from the anatomic point of view, may be considered to be a more complete form of arrhythmogenic right ventricular dysplasia. The right ventricle is extremely dilated, but the tricuspid valve remains in a normal position, thus differentiating it from Ebstein's anomaly. The main characteristic of Uhl's syndrome is the complete absence of myocardium in the right ventricular free wall, resulting in the endocardial and epicardial layers being in direct contact without interposition of myocardial fibers. Since Uhl's description of this cardiomyopathy in 1952,[48] the descriptive term *parchment heart* has been applied to the abnormality. Although Uhl's syndrome usually leads to rapid cardiac failure in the first month or years of life, an adult form of this condition occurs in which associated ventricular tachycardia is the dominant feature.

LONG QT SYNDROME

In 1957, Jervell and Lange-Nielsen[49] described a clinical entity consisting of a long QT interval, congenital deafness, and syncopal attacks due to ventricular fibrillation after emotional or physical stresses. The absence of congenital deafness characterizes the otherwise identical Romano-Ward syndrome.[50, 51] The prolongation of the QT interval in both of these syndromes has been considered to be congenital in orgin, and both syndromes are recognized to contribute to sudden death in children.[52, 53] However, Schwartz and coworkers[53] demonstrated that certain patients who sustained acute myocardial infarctions subsequently developed QT interval prolongation and thereafter experienced a significantly higher rate of sudden death. Although the pathogenesis of the long QT syndrome is poorly understood, James and associates[54] demonstrated the presence of focal neuritis and neural degeneration within the specialized conduction system and the ventricular myocardium. They suggested the possibility that a chronic viral infection or some noninfectious degenerative process of the cardiac nerves might be responsible for the prolongation of the QT interval and the associated fatal ventricular arrhythmias.

Ventricular tachycardia that occurs in association with the long QT syndrome is frequently of a distinct type called *torsades de pointes*.[55] This term is derived from the appearance of the ventricular tachycardia on a standard ECG, on which the polarity of the tachcardia is inconstant.

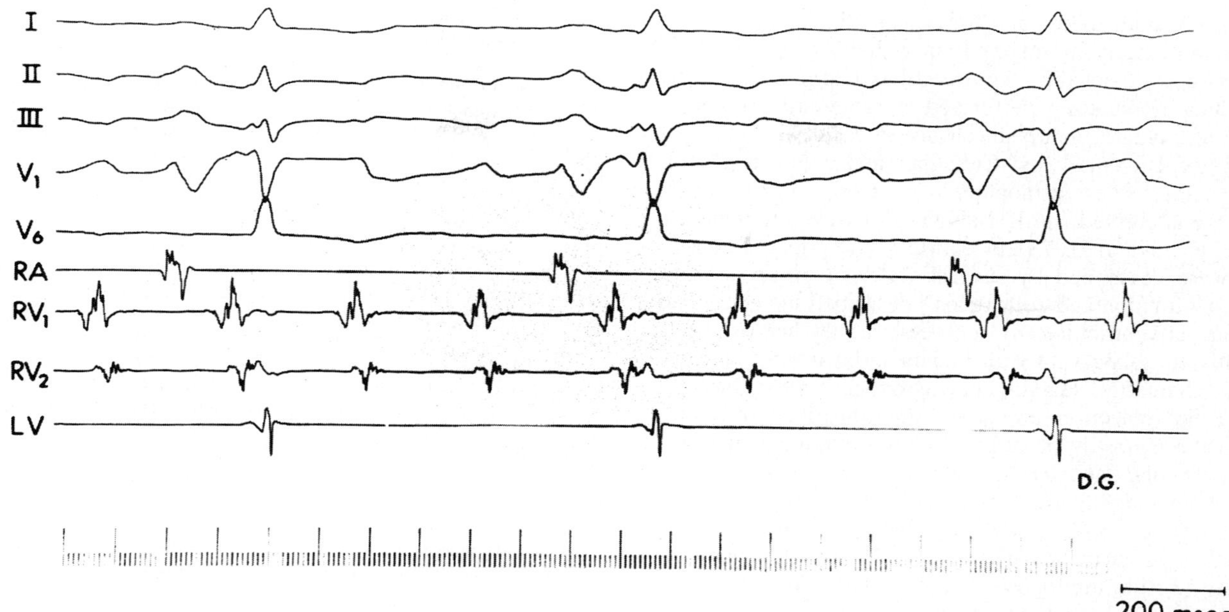

FIGURE 98–18 Surface recordings and intracardiac electrograms in a 16-year-old boy during an episode of right ventricular (RV) tachycardia after the right ventricular isolation procedure. The limb-lead (I-III) and precordial lead (V1 and V6) electrograms demonstrated normal sinus rhythm in the remainder of the heart documented by right atrial (RA) activity preceding each left ventricular (LV) complex. (From Cox JL, Bardy GH, Damiano RJ, et al: Right ventricular isolation procedures for nonischemic ventricular tachycardia. J Thorac Cardiovasc Surg 90:212, 1985.)

One of the most frequent causes of torsades de pointes is the administration of medications that prolong ventricular repolarization, particularly quinidine.[56]

These observations support the concept that torsades de pointes represents an abnormality in myocardial *repolarization*, as opposed to most other types of ventricular tachycardia, which are thought to be abnormalities in myocardial *depolarization*. As a result, the surgical treatment of recurrent ventricular tachycardia associated with long QT syndrome initially centered around efforts to modify cardiac innervation. Left stellate ganglion resection was reported to abolish symptoms in many patients with the long QT syndrome.[53, 57–59] However, our experience[60] and that of others[61] was characterized by early success and late failure. If medical therapy fails, the majority of these patients are treated with implantable cardioverter-defibrillator devices.

Ischemic Ventricular Tachycardia

Historical Aspects

Sir Thomas Lewis apparently was the first to recognize the relationship between ventricular aneurysm and ventricular tachycardia in 1909, when he suggested the need for a controlled method of inducing tachycardia so it could be studied in a systematic fashion.[62] In the absence of such a technique even 50 years later, Couch and associates[63] performed a simple aneurysmectomy specifically for the treatment of intractable ventricular tachycardia. In 1967, Dirk Durrer and Hein Wellens and colleagues of Amsterdam[64] and Phillipe Coumel and coworkers of Paris[65] described the technique of programmed electric stimulation, precisely the tool desired by Lewis to induce and terminate tachycardia in a reproducible manner for the purposes of diagnosis and evaluation of interventional therapy.

Experimental studies in the mid- and late 1960s documented the heterogeneity of tissue injury in acute myocardial infarction,[66] and the reentrant basis of ischemic ventricular tachyarrhythmias was confirmed.[67–72] Thus, with the advent of coronary artery bypass graft surgery in the late 1960s, it seemed that ischemic ventricular tachycardia would be easily corrected with this new procedure, because the basis for the arrhythmia (myocardial ischemia) could be alleviated by myocardial revascularization. During the 1970s, however, it became apparent that neither revascularization nor resection of the injured myocardium resulted in acceptable cure rates; in addition, the operative mortality rates reported when these procedures were performed primarily for ventricular tachycardia control were prohibitively high.[73] Although the demonstration that ischemic ventricular tachyarrhythmias occurred on a reentrant basis improved our concept of the arrhythmia, there remained a profound ignorance of the uncharted interplay among the autonomic nervous system, endogenous humoral stimulants, intracellular electrophysiology, extracellular electrophysiology, the specialized conduction system, coronary artery disease, myocardial ischemia and infarction, and normal myocardial conduction, all of which undoubtedly play a role in the genesis and perpetuation of ischemic ventricular tachyarrhythmias.

Because of the lack of efficacy of myocardial revascularization or resection in controlling ischemic ventricular tachycardia, several groups began to approach the problem in a more direct surgical manner. In 1969, Daniel and associates[74] and Kaiser and associates[75] independently reported intraoperative mapping in patients with ischemic heart disease to localize the area of ischemic injury. Fontaine and associates[76] performed intraoperative mapping before a standard aneurysmectomy in 1974, but in 1975, Wittig and Boineau[77] and Gallagher and colleagues[78] first reported the use of intraoperative mapping specifically to guide the attempted surgical ablation of ischemic ventricular tachycardia. In 1978, an entirely new group of operations were developed by several different groups of surgeons. Guiraudon and colleagues[79] described the encircling endocardial ventriculotomy, a procedure they had used successfully to ablate ventricular tachycardia in five patients. Shortly thereafter, Harken and associates[80] described the endocardial resection procedure, modifications of which remain the mainstay of surgery for the treatment of ischemic ventricular tachycardia. Jatene[81] and Dor and associates[82] independently described surgical techniques for repairing left ventricular aneurysms that have the unexpected side effect of curing most associated ventricular tachycardias. As a result, intraoperative electrophysiologic mapping in such patients is no longer necessary. In reality, however, the surgeon rarely sees such patients because they are usually treated with radiofrequency catheter ablation, implantable cardioverter-defibrillators, or both.

References

1. Savage DD, Garrison RJ, Castelli WP, et al: Prevalence of submitral (anular) calcium and its correlates in a general population-based sample (the Framingham study). Am J Cardiol 51:1375–1378, 1983.
2. Diamantopoulos EJ, Anthopoulos L, Nanas S, et al: Detection of arrhythmias in a representative sample of the Athens population. Eur Heart J 8(suppl D):17–19, 1987.
3. Onundarson PT, Thorgeirsson G, Jonmundsson E, et al: Chronic atrial fibrillation: epidemiologic features and 14 year follow-up: a case control study. Eur Heart J 8:521–527, 1987.
4. Hirosawa K, Sekiguchi M, Kasanuki R, et al: Natural history of atrial fibrillation. Heart Vessels 2(suppl):14–23, 1987.
5. Cameron A, Schwartz MJ, Kronmal RA, Kosinski AS: Prevalence and significance of atrial fibrillation in coronary artery disease (CASS Registry).: Am J cardiol 61:714–717, 1988.
6. Tammaro AE, Ronzoni D, Bonaccorso O, et al: Le aritmie nell'anziano. Minerva Med 74:1313–1318, 1983.
7. Cobler JL, Williams ME, Greenland P: Thyrotoxicosis in institutionalized elderly patients with atrial fibrillation. Arch Inter Med 144:1758–1760, 1984.
8. Martin A, Benbow LJ, Butrous GS, et al: Five-year follow-up of 101 elderly subjects by means of long-term ambulatory cardiac monitoring. Eur Heart J 5:592–596, 1984.
9. Treseder AS, Sastry BS, Thomas TP, et al: Atrial fibrillation and stroke in elderly hospitalized patients. Age Aging 15:89–92, 1986.
10. Williams JM, Ungerleider RM, Lofland GK, Cox JL: Left atrial isolation: new technique for the treatment of supraventricular arrhythmias. J Thorac Cardiovasc Surg 80:373, 1980.
11. Scheinman MM, Morady F, Hess DS, Gonzalez R: Catheter-induced ablation of the atrioventricular junction to control refractory supraventricular arrhythmias. JAMA 248:851, 1982.
12. Guiraudon GM, Campbell CS, Jones DL, et al: Combined sino-atrial node atrio-ventricular node isolation: a surgical alternative to His bundle ablation in patients with atrial fibrillation. Circulation 72 (suppl 3):220, 1985.
13. Cox JL: Surgical therapy of paroxysmal atrial fibrillation with the "corridor" operation. Ann Thorac Surg 53:571, 1992.
14. Cox JL: Surgical treatment of atrial fibrillation [letter reply]. J Thorac Cardiovas Surg 104:1492–1494, 1992.
15. Scheinman MM, Evans-Bell T: Catheter ablation of the atrioventricular junction: a report of the Percutaneous Mapping and Ablation Registry. Circulation 70:1024–1029, 1984.
16. Smith PK, Holman WL, Cox JL: Surgical treatment of supraventricular tachyarrhythmias. Surg Clin North Am 65:553–570, 1985.
17. Boineau JP, Mooney C, Hudson R, et al: Observations on re-entrant excitation pathways and refractory period distribution in spontaneous and experimental atrial flutter in the dog. *In* Kulbertus HE (ed): Reentrant Arrhythmias. pp. 79–98. Baltimore, MD: University Park, 1977.
18. Boineau JP, Schuessler RB, Mooney CR, et al: Natural and evoked atrial flutter due to circus movement in dogs. Am J Cardiol 45:1167, 1980.
19. Cox JL, Schuessler RB, D'Agostino HJ Jr, et al: The surgical treatment of atrial fibrillation, III: development of a definite surgical procedure. J Thorac Cardiovasc Surg 101:569–583, 1991.
20. D'Agostino HJ Jr, Harada A, Schuessler RB, et al: Global epicardial mapping of atrial fibrillation in a canine model of chronic mitral regurgitation. Circulation 76(suppl IV):IV-165, 1987.
21. Yamauchi S, Sato S, Schuessler RB, et al: Induced atrial arrhythmias in a canine model of left atrial enlargement. Pacing Clin Electrophysiol 13:556, 1990.
22. Canavan TE, Schuessler RB, Boineau JP, et al: Computerized global electrophysiological mapping of the atrium in patients with Wolff-Parkinson-White syndrome. Ann Thorac Surg 46:223–231, 1988.
23. Canavan TE, Schuessler RB, Cain ME, et al: Computerized global electrophysiological mapping of the atrium in a patient with multiple supraventricular tachyarrhythmias. Ann Thorac Surg 46:232–235, 1988.
24. Cox JL, Canavan TE, Schuessler RB, et al: The surgical treatment of atrial fibrillation, II: intraoperative electrophysiologic mapping and description of the electrophysiologic basis of atrial flutter and atrial fibrillation. J Thorac Cardiovasc Surg 101:406–426, 1991.
25. Cox JL: The surgical treatment of atrial fibrillation, IV: surgical technique. J Thorac Cardivasc Surg 101:584–592, 1991.
26. Cox JL, Boineau JP, Schuessler RB, Lappas DG: Modification of the maze procedure for atrial flutter and atrial fibrillation, I: rationale and surgical results. J Thorac Cardiovasc Surg 110:473–484, 1995.
27. Cox JL, Jaquiss RD, Schuessler RB, Boineau JP: Modification of the maze procedure for atrial flutter and atrial fibrillation, II: surgical technique of the maze III procedure. J Thorac Cardiovasc Surg 110:485–495, 1995.
28. Jackman WM, Wang XZ, Friday KJ, et al: Catheter ablation of accessory atriventricular pathways (Wolff-Parkinson-White syndrome) by radiofrequency current. N Engl J Med 324:1605–1611, 1991.
29. Klein GJ, Guiraudon GM, Perkins DG, et al: Surgical correction of the Wolff-Parkinson-White syndrome in the closed heart using cryosurgery: a simplified approach. J Am Coll Cardiol 3:405–409, 1984.
30. Cox JL, Gallagher JJ, Cain ME: Experience with 118 consecutive patients undergoing surgery for the Wolff-Parkinson-White syndrome. J Thorac Cardiovasc Surg 90:490–501, 1985.
31. Guiraudon GM, Klein GJ, Sharma AD, et al: Closed-heart technique for Wolff-Parkinson-White syndrome: further experience and potential limitations. Ann Thorac Surg 42:651–657, 1986.
32. Lev M, Liberthson RR, Joseph RH, et al: The pathologic anatomy of Ebstein's disease. Arch Pathol, 90:334, 1970.
33. Holman W, Ikeshita M, Lease J, et al: Elective prolongation of atrioventricular conduction by multiple discrete cryolesions: a new technique for the treatment of the paroxysmal supraventricular tachycardia. J Thorac Cardiovasc Surg 84:554, 1982.
34. Holman WL, Ikeshita M, Lease JG, et al: Alteration of antegrade atrioventricular conduction by cryoablation of peri-atrioventricular nodal tissue. J Thorac Cardiovasc Surg 88:67–75, 1984.
35. Holman WL, Ikeshita M, Lease JG, et al: Cryosurgical modification of retrograde atrioventricular conduction: implications for the surgical treatment of atrioventricular node reentry tachycardia. J Thorac Cardiovasc Surg 91:826–834, 1986.
36. Cox JL: Surgery for cardiac arrhythmias. *In* Current Problems in Cardiology Vol. VIII, No. 4. Chicago: Year–Book Medical, 1983.
37. Cox JL, Holman WL, Cain ME: Cryosurgical treatment of atrioventricular node reentry tachycardia. Circulation 76:1329–1336, 1987.
38. Ross DL, Johnson DC, Denniss AR, et al: Curative surgery for atrioventricular junctional ("A-V nodal") reentrant tachycardia. J Am Coll Cardiol 6:1383, 1985.
39. Gallagher JJ, Cox JL, German LD, Kasell JH: Nonpharmacologic treatment of supraventricular tachycardia. *In* Josephson ME, Wellens

HJJ (eds): Tachycardias: Mechanisms, Diagnosis, and Treatment. pp. 271–285. Philadelphia: Lea & Febiger, 1984.
40. Harada A, D'Agostino HJ Jr, Boineau JP, Cox JL: Right atrial isolation: a new surgical treatment for supraventricular tachycardia, I: surgical technique and electrophysiologic effects. J Thorac Cardiovasc Surg 95:643, 1988.
41. Harada A, D'Agostino HJ Jr, Boineau JP, Cox JL: Right atrial isolation: a new surgical treatment for supraventricular tachycardia, II: hemodynamic effects. J Thorac Cardiovasc Surg 95:651, 1988.
42. Tchou P, Lehmann MJ, Jazayeri M, Akhtar M: Atriofascicular connection or a nodoventricular Mahaim fiber? Electrophysiologic elucidation of the pathway and associated reentrant circuit. Circulation 44:837–848, 1988.
43. Klein GJ, Guiraudon GM, Kerr CR, et al: "Nodoventricular" accessory pathway: evidence for a distinct accessory atrioventricular pathway with atrioventricular node-like properties. J Am Coll Cardiol 11:1035–1040, 1988.
44. Abbott JA, Scheinman MM, Morady F, et al: Coexistent Mahaim and Kent accessory connections: diagnostic and therapeutic implications. J Am Coll Cardiol 10:364–372, 1987.
45. Guiraudon G, Fontaine G, Frank R, et al: Surgical treatment of ventricular tachycardia guided by ventricular mapping in 23 patients without coronary artery disease. Presented at the 17th Annual Meeting of the Society of Thoracic Surgery, January 1981.
46. Cox JL, Bardy, GH, Damiano RJ, et al: Right ventricular isolation procedures for non-ischemic ventricular tachycardia. J Thorac Cardiovasc Surg 90:212, 1985.
47. Fontaine G, Guiraudon G, Frank R: Management of chronic ventricular tachycardia. *In* Narula OS (ed): Innovations in Diagnosis and Management of Cardiac Arrhythmias. Baltimore, MD: Williams & Wilkins, 1979.
48. Uhl HS: A previously undescribed malformation of the heart: almost total absence of the myocardium of the right ventricle. Bull Johns Hopkins Hosp 91:197, 1952.
49. Jervell A, Lange-Nielsen F: Congenital deaf-mutism, functional heart disease with prolongation of the Q-T interval, and sudden death. Am Heart J 54:59, 1957.
50. Romano C, Gemme G, Pongiglione R: Aritmie cardiacherare dell'eta pediatrica. Clin Pediatr 45:656, 1963.
51. Ward OC: New familial cardiac syndrome in children. J Irish Med Assoc 54:103, 1964.
52. Fraser GR, Froggatt P: Unexpected cot deaths. Lancet 2:56, 1966.
53. Schwartz PJ, Periti M, Malliani A: The long Q-T syndrome. Fund am Clin Cardiol 89:378, 1975.
54. James TN, Froggatt P, Atkinson WJ Jr, et al: De subitaneis mortibus XXX: observations on the pathophysiology of the long Q-T syndromes with special reference to the neuropathology of the heart. Circulation 57:1221, 1978.
55. Kulbertus HE, La torsades de pointes. Rev Med Liege 33:63, 1978.
56. Kulbertus HE: The arrhythmogenic effects of anti-arrhythmicagents. *In* Befeler B (ed): Selected Topics in Cardiac Arrhythmias. p. 113. Mount Kisco, NY: Futura, 1980.
57. Moss AJ, McDonald J: Unilateral cervicothoracic sympathetic ganglionectomy for the treatment of long Q-T interval syndrome. N Engl J Med 285:903, 1971.
58. Smith W, Gallagher JJ: Q-T prolongation syndromes. Pract Cardiol 5:118, 1979.
59. Malliani A, Schwartz PJ, Zanchetti A: Neuralmechanisms and life-threatening arrhythmias. Am Heart J 100:705, 1980.
60. Benson DW Jr, Cox JL: Surgical treatment of cardiac arrhythmias. *In* Roberts NK, Gelband H (eds): Cardiac Arrhythmias in the Neonate, Infant and Child. 2nd ed. pp. 341–366. New York: Appleton-Century-Crofts, 1982.
61. Bhandari AK, Scheinman MM, Morady F, et al: Efficacy of left cardiac sympathectomy in the treatment of patients with the long QT syndrome. Circulation 70:1018–1023, 1984.
62. Lewis T: The experimental production of paroxysmal tachycardia and the effects of ligation of the coronary arteries. Heart, 1:98, 1909.
63. Couch OA Jr: Cardiac aneurysm with ventricular tachycardia and subsequent excision of aneurysm. Circulation 20:251, 1959.
64. Durrer D, Schoo L, Schuilenburg RM, Wellens HJJ: The role of premature beats in the initiation and the termination of supraventricular tachycardia in the Wolff-Parkinson-White syndrome. Circulation 36:644, 1967.
65. Coumel P, Cabarol C, Fabiato A, et al: Tachycardia permanente par rythme reçiproque. Arch Mal Coeur 60:1830, 1967.
66. Cox JL, McLaughline VW, Flowers NC, Horan LG: The ischemic zone surrounding acute myocardial infarction: Its morphology as detected by dehydrogenase staining. Am Heart J 76:650, 1968.
67. Cox JL, Daniel TM, Sabiston DC Jr, Boineau JP: De-synchronized activation in myocardial infarction—a re-entry basis for ventricular arrhythmias. Circulation 40:III-63, 1969.
68. Boineau JP, Cox JL: Slow ventricular activation in acute myocardial infarction: a source of re-entrant premature ventricular contractions. Circulation 48:702, 1973.
69. Han J, Gael BG, Hansen CS: Re-entrant beats induced in the ventricle during coronary occlusion. Am Heart J 80:778, 1970.
70. Durrer D, van Dam RT, Freud GE, Janse MJ: Re-entry and ventricular arrhythmias in local ischemia and infarction of the intact dog heart. Proc K Ned Akad Wet (Biol Med) 74:321, 1971.
71. Waldo AL, Kaiser GA: A study of ventricular arrhythmias associated with acute myocardial infarction in the canine heart. Circulation 47:1222, 1973.
72. El-Sherif N, Scherlag BJ, Lazzara R, Hopen RR: Re-entrant ventricular arrhythmias in the late myocardial infarction period, I: conduction characteristics of the infarction zone. Circulation 55:686, 1977.
73. Boineau JP, Cox JL: Rationale for a direct surgical approach to control ventricular arrhythmias. Am J Cardiol 49:381, 1982.
74. Daniel TM, Cox JL, Sabiston DC Jr, Boineau JP: Epicardial and intramural mapping activation of the human heart: a technique for localizing infarction and ischemia of the myocardium [abstract]. Circulation 40(suppl III):III-66, 1969.
75. Kaiser GA, Waldo AL, Harris PD, et al: New method to delineate myocardial damage at surgery. Circulation 39(suppl 1):83, 1969.
76. Fontaine G, Frank R, Guiraudon G: Surgical treatment of resistant re-entrant ventricular tachycardia by ventriculotomy: a new application of epicardial mapping [abstract]. Circulation 50(suppl III):III-82, 1974.
77. Wittig JH, Boineau JP: Surgical treatment of ventricular arrhythmias using epicardial transmural and endocardial mapping. Ann Thorac Surg 20:117, 1975.
78. Gallagher JJ, Oldham HN Jr, Wallace AG, et al: Ventricular aneurysm with ventricular tachycardia: report of a case with epicardial mapping and successful resection. Am J Cardiol 35:696, 1975.
79. Guiraudon G, Fontaine G, Frank R, et al: Encircling endocardial ventriculotomy: A new surgical treatment of life-threatening ventricular tachycardias resistant to medical treatment following myocardial infarction. Ann Thorac Surg 26:438, 1978.
80. Josephson ME, Harken AH, Horowitz LN: Endocardial excision—a new surgical technique for the treatment of recurrent ventricular tachycardia. Circulation 60:1430, 1979.
81. Jatene AD: Left ventricular aneurysmectomy: resection or reconstruction: J Thorac Cardiovasc Surg 89:321–331, 1985.
82. Dor V, Saab M, Coste P, et al: Left ventricular aneurysm: a new surgical approach. Thorac Cardiovasc Surg 37:11, 1989.

SECTION X

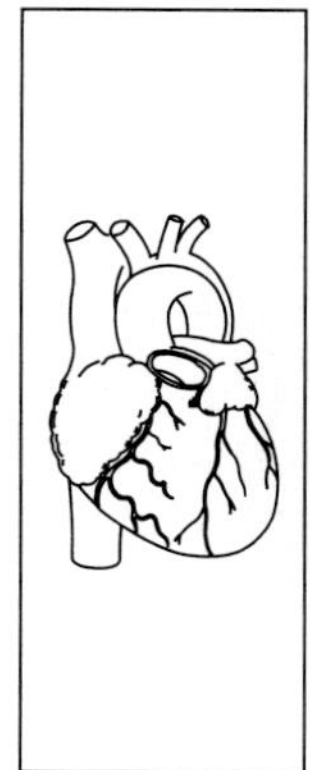

CARDIAC EFFECTS OF SYSTEMIC DISORDERS, PREGNANCY, AGING, AND ENVIRONMENTAL CHANGE

Pulmonary Thromboembolism

Pulmonary Hypertension

Chronic Obstructive Pulmonary Disease

Tumors of the Heart

Endocrine Disorders and the Heart

Connective Tissue Diseases and the Heart

Substance Abuse and the Heart

Cardiovascular Involvement in AIDS

Neuromuscular Disorders and Heart Disease

Hematologic Disease and Heart Disease

Aging and the Cardiovascular System

Pregnancy and the Heart

Cardiovascular Changes Associated With Space Flight

CHAPTER 99

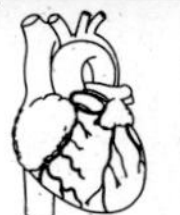

Pulmonary Thromboembolism

Herbert L. Fred and Ramesh Hariharan

PREDISPOSING FACTORS
SOURCES OF EMBOLI
CLINICAL FEATURES
PTE Without Infarction
PTE With Infarction
RADIOGRAPHIC FINDINGS
ELECTROCARDIOGRAPHIC FINDINGS
MISCELLANEOUS LABORATORY FINDINGS
DIAGNOSIS
DIFFERENTIAL DIAGNOSIS
Parenchymatous Respiratory Disorders
Pleural and Congenital Respiratory Disorders
Cardiovascular Disorders
Neurologic Disorders
Psychiatric Disorders
Abdominal Disorders
Infectious Disorders
Pulmonary-Renal Disorders
Hematologic Disorders
Metabolic Disorders
Particulate Matter Disorders
TREATMENT
COURSE AND PROGNOSIS
In Brief

Each year in the United States, an estimated 5,000,000 people suffer an episode of venous thrombosis,[1] 650,000 experience a pulmonary embolic event,[2] and as many as 200,000 die.[3] Although pulmonary thromboembolism (PTE)* occurs in all age groups, most victims are middle-aged or older.[4] A concurrent illness usually is present, but PTE can strike seemingly healthy, active persons,[5] including children[6] and adolescents.[7] Factors such as race, gender,[2] and season of the year have no significant influence on the incidence of the disease.

Predisposing Factors

PTE characteristically occurs in a setting of congestive heart failure, trauma (especially to the lower extremities and pelvis), immobility (resulting from medical illness, surgical procedures, or prolonged sitting), venous disease in the legs, or any combination thereof. In up to 50 percent of patients with deep vein thrombosis, the syndrome of activated protein C resistance may be responsible.[8–11] This syndrome results primarily from a point mutation in factor V (factor V Leiden) that involves the binding site of protein C.[12, 13] Other predisposing factors include obesity; pregnancy; polycythemia; malignancy; antiphospholipid antibodies[14]; hyperhomocysteinemia[15, 16]; use of oral contraceptives; deficiencies of protein C, S, or antithrombin III; and mutations in the prothrombin gene.[17, 17a]

Sources of Emboli

For several reasons, statistics vary as to the sites from which pulmonary emboli originate. The mere presence of thrombi in peripheral veins, right atrium, or right ventricle does not prove that these sites are the source of such emboli. Indeed, thrombi sometimes exist in these areas when no pulmonary emboli are evident. And once a clot becomes detached from a vein, that vessel may be empty when examined by imaging techniques or at autopsy.

These points aside, most pulmonary emboli arise from veins in the lower extremities[18] or pelvis.[19] Occasionally, the heart is the source[20] (Fig. 99–1C; see also Plate 99–1C), particularly in patients with septic pulmonary emboli from right-sided endocarditis.[21] Other sites of origin at times are the inferior vena cava, veins in the upper extremities,[22] prostatic venous plexus,[23] renal veins,[24] and veins of the cerebral sinuses and nasopharynx.[6]

Clinical Features

Manifestations of PTE depend on the number and size of emboli, presence or absence of infarction, duration of the thromboembolic process, and type and severity of associated disease(s). The clinical picture, therefore, varies considerably. Moreover, one cannot consistently judge the seriousness of PTE by the nature of its presentation. A large embolus, for example, may be clinically silent, whereas a small embolus may produce an alarming set of findings. We believe that the best way to understand and remember the protean expressions of PTE is to divide them into two groups: those occurring before and those appearing after pulmonary infarction develops.

**Pulmonary thromboembolism* (PTE) as used here refers to acute or subacute pulmonary thromboembolism with or without resultant infarction of the lung. The term does not include septic pulmonary embolism or chronic major vessel pulmonary hypertension.

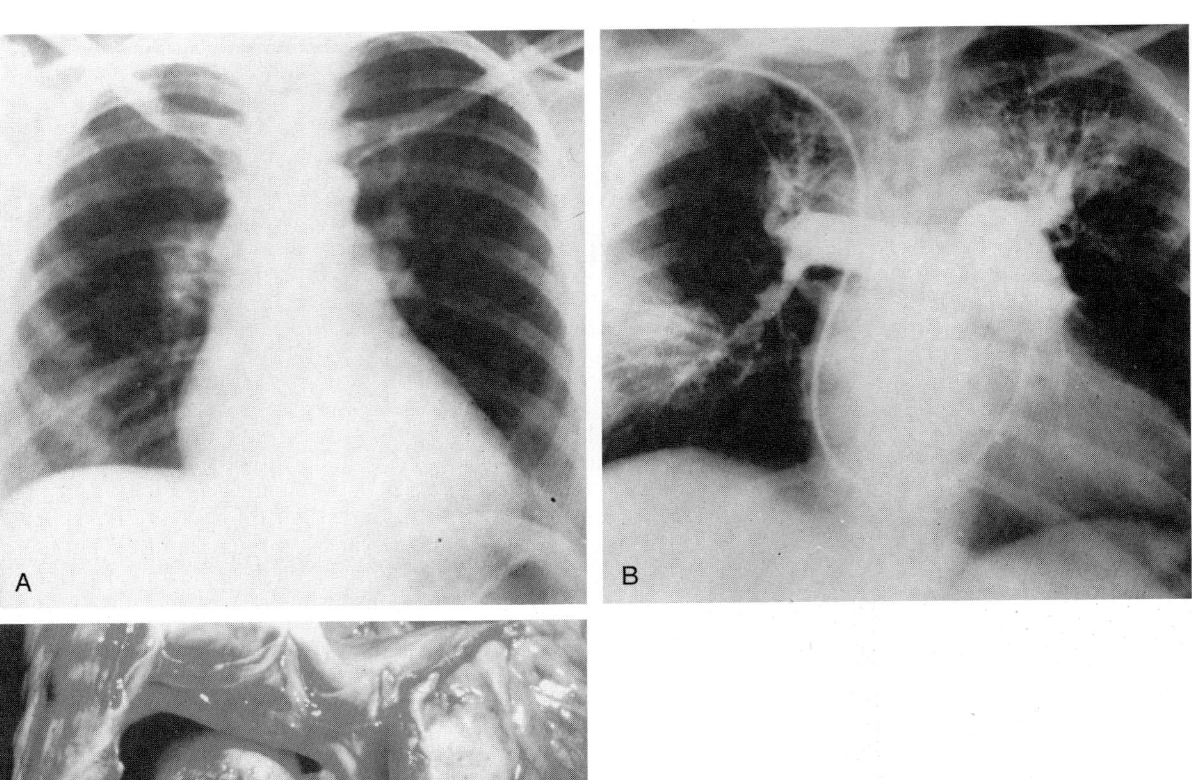

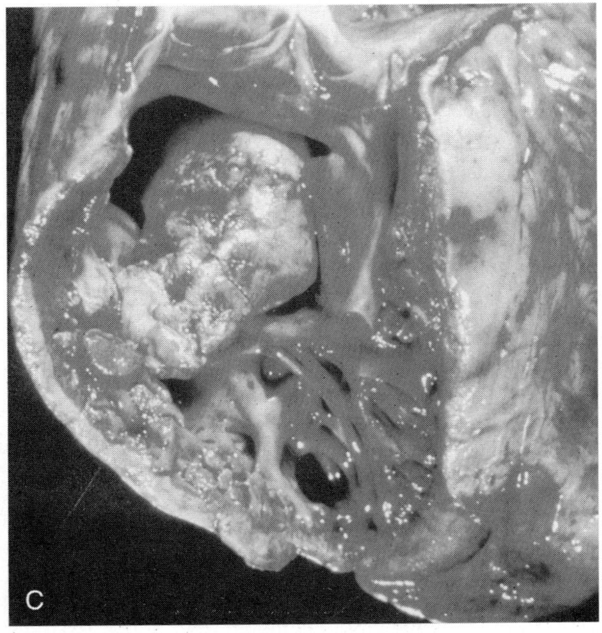

FIGURE 99–1 A 47-year-old woman with unexplained shortness of breath had a referring diagnosis of Munchausen's syndrome. **A,** Chest radiograph shows mild cardiomegaly, prominent central pulmonary arteries, and distal oligemia bilaterally. **B,** Pulmonary arteriogram demonstrates obstructed blood flow to both lungs, especially the lower lobes. **C,** Autopsy view of a large thrombus in the right ventricle. Numerous old and new thromboemboli were present throughout the pulmonary arterial tree. (See also Plate 99–1C.)

PTE Without Infarction

Dyspnea without orthopnea is the most common and important symptom.[4] It is often sudden in onset, progressing at times to gasping respirations. Frequently, however, the dyspnea is mild and fleeting. *Chest pain* is rare; when present, it is typically dull and retrosternal and usually reflects occlusion of major pulmonary arteries.[25] *Wheezing respirations,* ordinarily transient and occasionally recurrent, can be a heralding feature.[26] *Neurologic abnormalities* such as syncope, convulsions, restlessness, anxiety, stupor, coma, and weakness or paralysis of limbs predominate in about 5 percent of the cases and may be the first, the most prominent, or the only manifestation.[27] Unexplained *apprehension* and *a sense of impending doom* are common.[28] Rarely, the patient experiences a sudden strong urge to defecate or may faint or die during defecation.[29]

Tachycardia[28] and *tachypnea*[30] are frequent and often disproportionately severe. *Signs of venous thrombosis in the legs,* such as pain, heat, discoloration, or enlargement, develop in less than half of the patients and may not appear for days or even months after the onset of pulmonary symptoms.[31] *Cyanosis* may appear when embolism is massive or there is coexisting cardiopulmonary disease, shock, or both. *Hypotension* is relatively uncommon. Characteristically, it is of short duration, but if persistent, it indicates that the diagnosis is wrong or that embolism is massive. In some cases, sudden, profound, or prolonged shock is the *only* indication of PTE. *Acute cor pulmonale* can result from massive PTE and may be accompanied by an accentuated pulmonic valve closure sound, right ventricular gallop rhythm, or increased jugular venous pressure.

One point merits special attention. Signs of PTE without infarction may regress spontaneously just as dramatically as they appear. In these cases, the patient seems well one minute and moribund the next, only to recover rapidly.

PTE With Infarction

Less than 10 percent of pulmonary thromboemboli lead to infarction of the lung.[32] *Pleuritic pain* emerges in only half of these patients and may be sudden or gradual in onset and mild or severe.[33] *Hemoptysis* occurs in about one third of these patients.[4] At first it is bright red; it then appears as dark clots, and finally as dark brown, semiliquid material. *Fever* of varying duration and pattern is common.[34, 35] Temperatures usually range between 100° and 103°F but can reach 105°F in the absence of demonstrable infection (Fig. 99–2). *Cough* is uncommon and, when present, is intermittent and mild.[36] *Pleural friction rub,* audible in only about one fourth of these patients,[33] sometimes precedes radiographic evidence of pulmonary infarction. *Rales* and *signs of pleural effusion* are common, but classic signs of consolidation are distinctly rare. *Jaundice* can develop when the infarction is extensive or when congestive heart failure, hepatic disease, or both are present.[37]

Radiographic Findings

The radiographic patterns of PTE depend on the size, number, and distribution of the thromboemboli, the preexisting anatomic and functional status of the heart and lungs, and the frequency with which chest radiographs are obtained. *Before frank infarction develops,* the chest radiograph typically shows no abnormality. This is true even when one suspects PTE and searches specifically for its signs. In some cases, however, one or both main pulmonary arteries become enlarged (Figs. 99–3A and 99–4; see also Fig. 99–1A), with decreased peripheral vascular markings in the affected portions of lung (oligemia) and engorged vessels in the nonaffected areas (pleonemia) (see Fig. 99–4). The hemidiaphragm on the involved side may be elevated consequent to atelectasis.

After infarction develops, the chest radiograph almost always shows some abnormality, typically within 24 hours (Fig. 99–5). Rarely, it takes up to 5 days for an abnormality to appear.[38] Any segment of lung may be involved, but the lower lobes, especially the right, are the usual sites.[39] Atelectasis and small pleural effusions are common, but large pleural effusions may also occur. Parenchymal densities range in size from mere visibility to that of an opacified lobe (see Fig. 99–2). Their patterns are so diverse that no shape necessarily suggests or excludes pulmonary infarction. Traditional teaching that the typical radiographic appearance of a pulmonary infarct is that of a "wedge-shaped" shadow has served more to confuse than to facilitate the diagnosis of pulmonary infarction.

The radiographic findings of pulmonary infarction can mimic those of many diseases, especially pulmonary infection.[35] Sometimes it simulates cancer[40] (Fig. 99–6A; see also Plate 99–6C), and if cavitation occurs, the lesion can be mistaken for pulmonary abscess (see Fig. 99–2). Infarction involving an upper lobe occasionally masquerades as pulmonary tuberculosis. Septic pulmonary embolism—an infectious rather than an obstructive process—typically appears as many small, patchy lesions (frequently cavitary) scattered throughout the lungs, often mimicking metastases or tuberculosis.[21]

Chronic major vessel thromboembolic pulmonary hypertension usually results in clear lung fields. In some patients, however, the right atrium and right ventricle are dilated with enlargement or asymmetry of the central pulmonary arteries.[41]

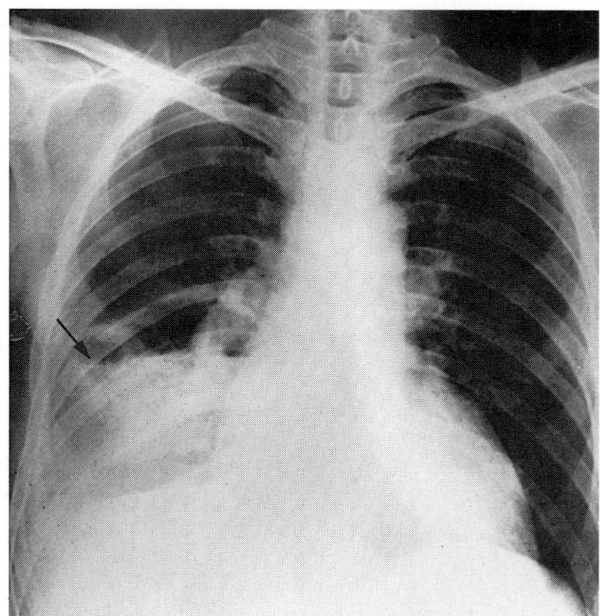

FIGURE 99–2 Chest radiograph of a 61-year-old man with chronic heart failure, hemoptysis, fever of 105°F, and a total leukocyte count of 40,000/mm³. Note the cardiomegaly, opacified right lower lobe with an air-fluid level *(arrow)*, and enlarged right pulmonary artery. Autopsy the next day showed a large thromboembolus occluding the right pulmonary artery with extensive infarction and cavitation of the right lower lobe. There was no evidence of pulmonary infection.

Electrocardiographic Findings

Electrocardiographic abnormalities are commonly absent and always nonspecific. Moreover, preexisting cardiac or pulmonary disease can modify or prevent the changes that might otherwise suggest PTE. When abnormalities do appear (Table 99–1), they are often fleeting and may go undetected unless multiple tracings are made within a short time. The transient nature of these alterations is characteristic, however, and serves as an important clue to PTE. Sinus or supraventricular tachycardias, ST-segment and T wave changes in the right precordial leads, and right bundle branch block are the most frequent electrocardiographic abnormalities (Figs. 99–7A and 99–8A; see also Fig. 99–3B). But even when the embolism is acute and massive, the electrocardiogram may show no signs of right ventricular strain.[42]

In patients with obliterative pulmonary hypertension from recurrent small pulmonary emboli[43] or from chronic

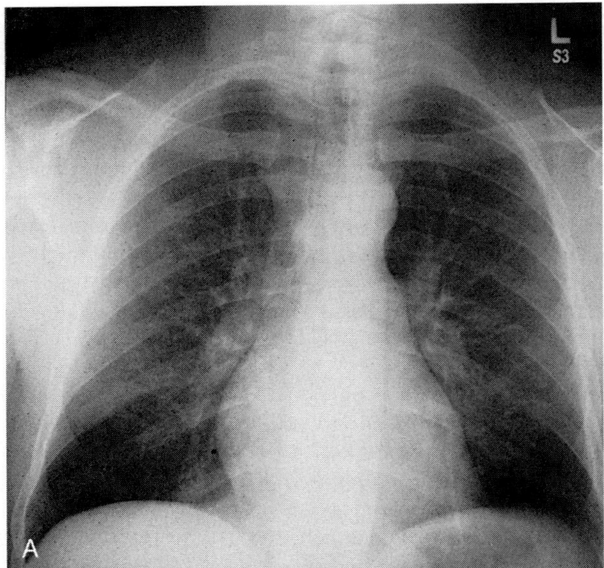

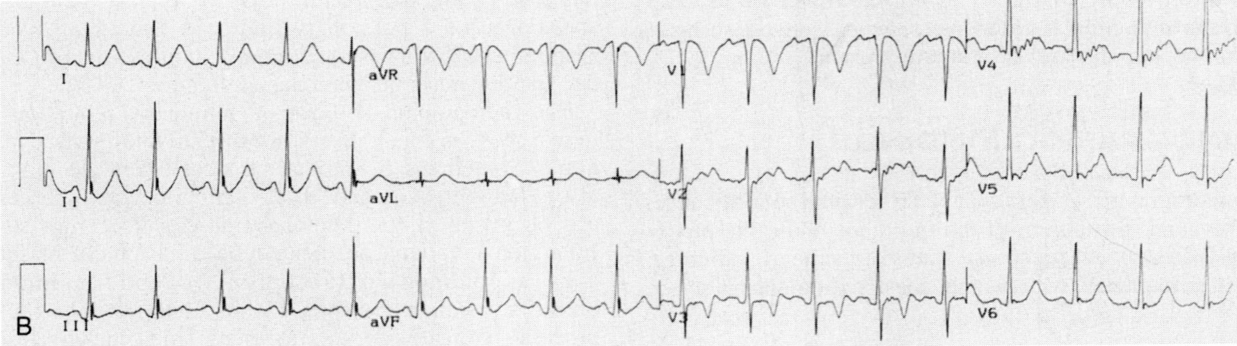

FIGURE 99–3 A previously healthy 37-year-old man had a sudden syncopal episode followed by persistent dyspnea. Six hours later, he died. **A,** Chest radiograph shows prominence of the central pulmonary arteries with abrupt tapering of the lower lobe branches and possible enlargement of the pulmonary outflow tract and right atrium. **B,** Electrocardiogram demonstrates sinus tachycardia, prolonged QT interval, and anterior T wave changes consistent with ischemia or acute right heart strain. Autopsy disclosed a saddle embolus at the bifurcation of the pulmonary arterial trunk extending into and obstructing the right and left main pulmonary arteries.

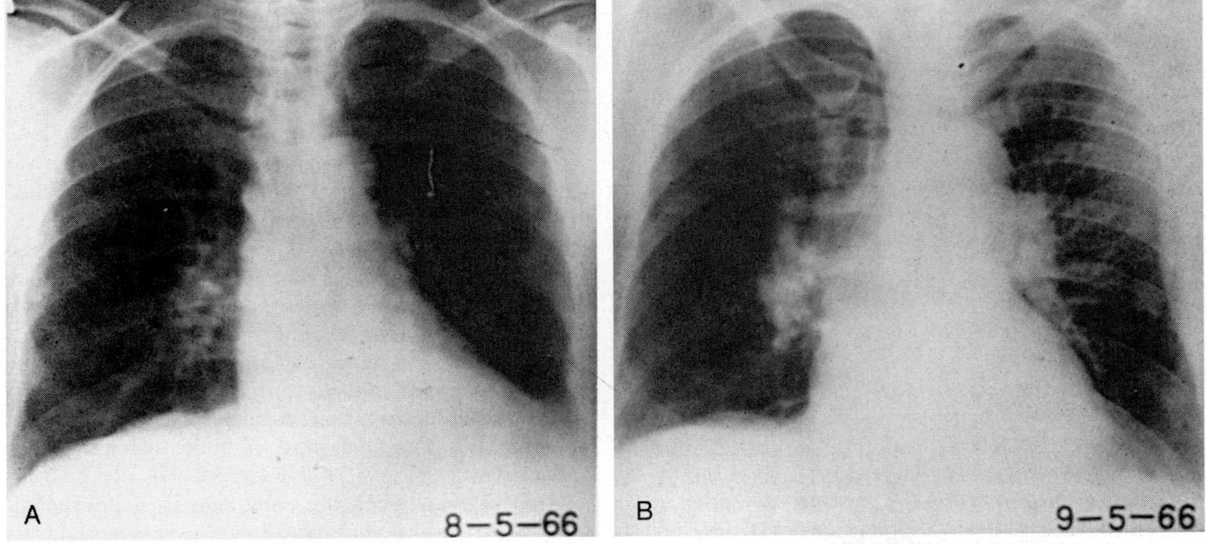

FIGURE 99–4 A 66-year-old woman had rapidly progressive shortness of breath initially attributed to cardiac failure. **A,** Chest radiograph at the onset of symptoms showed slight prominence of the right hilar vessels. **B,** Repeat study 1 month later demonstrated marked enlargement of the central pulmonary arteries, oligemia of the right lung, and relative pleonemia of the left lung. At autopsy, large thromboemboli completely occluded the right pulmonary artery and severely obstructed the left pulmonary artery.

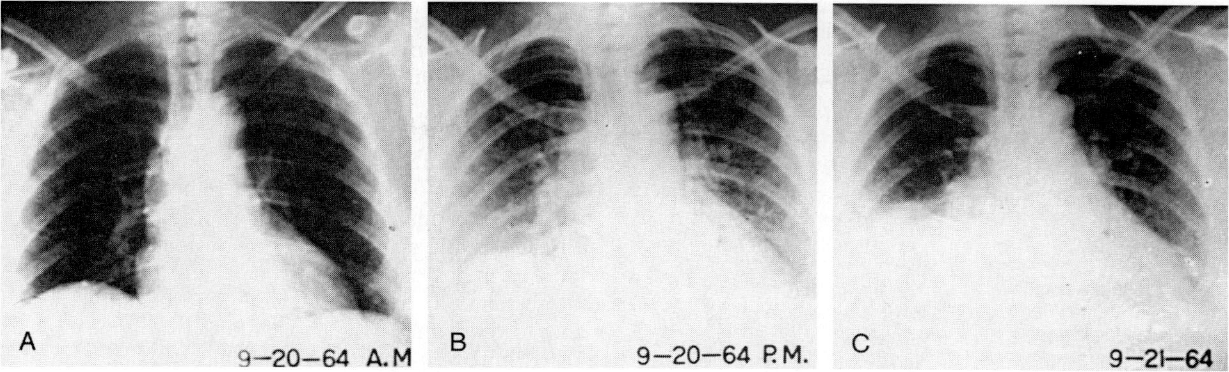

FIGURE 99–5 Serial chest radiographs of a 33-year-old woman who complained of severe right upper quadrant pain 3 weeks after undergoing a hysterectomy. The admitting diagnosis was acute cholecystitis. On the second hospital day, pulmonary arteriography showed complete obstruction of the arteries supplying the right middle and lower lobes.

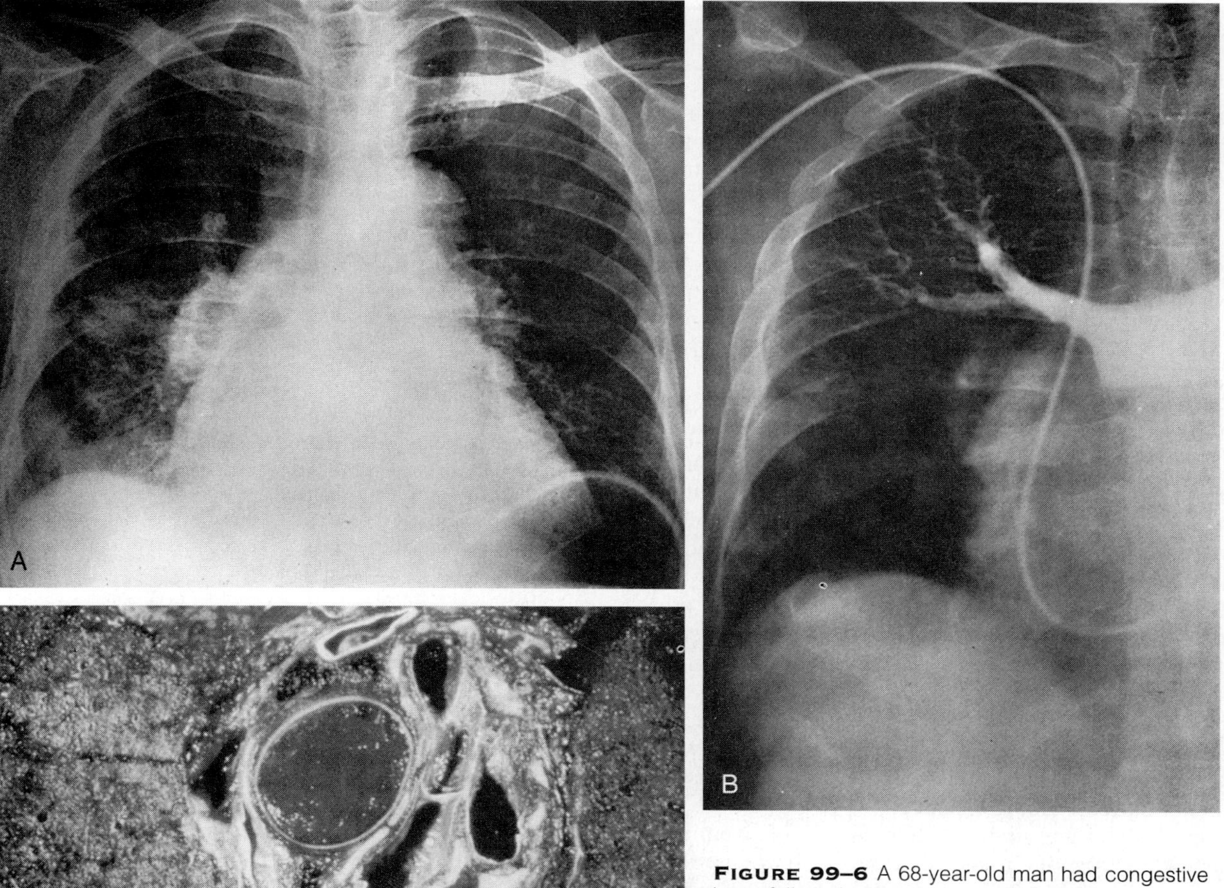

FIGURE 99–6 A 68-year-old man had congestive heart failure, hemoptysis, and a right hilar mass thought to represent bronchogenic carcinoma. **A,** Chest radiograph shows cardiomegaly, density in the right hilar region, and patchy infiltrates in the right lower lobe. **B,** Selective pulmonary arteriogram demonstrates complete obstruction of the arteries to the middle and lower lobes. **C,** Sagittal section of the right lung shows an organized thrombus extending 8 cm from the hilum, totally occluding the right middle and lower lobe arteries, and accounting for the hilar mass seen on the chest radiograph. (See also Plate 99–6C.)

TABLE 99–1 Electrocardiographic Findings in Pulmonary Thromboembolism*

No change at all
Sinus tachycardia
S_1–Q_3 pattern
S_1, S_2, S_3 pattern
Appearance of right-axis deviation and change to a vertical heart position
ST-segment depression in leads II, III, aVF, and occasionally, in I and left precordial leads
Flat or inverted T waves in leads II, III, aVF, and occasionally, in I and left precordial leads
Peaked P waves in leads II, III, and aVF
Development of extreme clockwise rotation of the heart
Appearance of right bundle branch block or right ventricular enlargement patterns
Inverted T waves with ST-segment deviations in the right precordial leads
Development of various types of transient supraventricular and, rarely, ventricular tachycardias
Combinations of these

*Not listed in order of frequency or importance.

major vessel pulmonary thromboemboli,[41] the electrocardiogram may be normal or may show right-axis deviation, P pulmonale, or a pattern of right ventricular hypertrophy and strain.

Miscellaneous Laboratory Findings

Results of routine laboratory tests in patients with PTE are nonspecific. The total leukocyte count usually is normal or slightly elevated,[43a] but in the presence of massive, bland necrosis of pulmonary tissue, it may reach 40,000/mm^3 (see Fig. 99–2). The sputum, if examined soon after infarction develops, commonly shows many erythrocytes but few leukocytes or organisms. Pleural fluid, when present, is bloody in 50 percent[33] to 65 percent[44] of the cases and may be a transudate or exudate.[44]

Plasma levels of D-dimer, a degradation product of cross-linked fibrin, are nearly always increased,[45] but because of poor specificity, such increase has limited diagnostic usefulness. Conversely, a *normal* plasma level of D-dimer is strong evidence against PTE.[45–47, 47a] Nevertheless, until D-dimer testing becomes standardized and more widely validated in prospective outcome studies, its widespread use is not currently recommended.[48]

Arterial blood gas analysis often shows hypoxemia, hypocarbia, respiratory alkalosis, and an increase in the $P(A - a)O_2$ gradient.[49–51] Yet up to a fourth of patients with documented PTE do not have hypoxemia while breathing room air,[50–52] and an increase in the $P(A - a)O_2$ gradient can occur in conditions other than PTE.[51, 52] Hence, a normal blood gas analysis does not exclude PTE,[53] and abnormal results, in and of themselves, do not appreciably increase the likelihood of PTE.[54]

Diagnosis

Constant awareness of PTE is the key to early diagnosis. If one waits for hemoptysis, pleural friction rub, signs of venous disease in the legs, pulmonary parenchymal infiltrates, or abnormal electrocardiographic patterns to develop, most cases will escape recognition. By contrast, the diagnosis never should be doubted or rejected simply because of high fever, leukocytosis, normal jugular venous pressure, "atypical" pulmonary lesions, or failure to detect the source of emboli or because the arterial blood gas analysis is normal.

Findings that should alert the physician to the possibility of PTE are fever of unknown origin and fever that does not respond to antibiotic therapy (especially in patients who have congestive heart failure or in those who are postpartum or postsurgical), congestive heart failure that increases rapidly in severity or is unresponsive to the usual therapeutic measures, wheezing of unknown cause, paroxysmal arrhythmias, unexplained sinus tachycardia, appearance of an "abscess" on a chest radiograph, bloody pleural effusion, and sudden, profound, or prolonged shock.

The *ventilation/perfusion* ($\dot{V}/\dot{Q}$) *lung scan* is a rapid, safe, and easy way to screen for PTE[55–60] and to follow its course. Perfusion scans image the distribution of intravenously injected macroaggregates of albumin labeled with ^{99m}Tc. Because these radioactive particles are 10 to 100 μm in diameter, even the smallest has a cross-sectional area larger than that of the average pulmonary capillary. Consequently, most of these particles become trapped at the precapillary level during their transit through the lungs. Distribution of macroaggregated albumin in a segment of lung is proportional to the relative pulmonary blood flow to that segment. Thus, the radioactivity recorded from different regions of the lung is an index of the relative amounts of capillary perfusion in those sites.

Ventilation scans involve the inhalation and washout of a tracer, usually ^{133}Xe gas. This technique determines regional pulmonary ventilation and, when done in association with the perfusion scan, may enhance recognition of PTE. Ventilation without perfusion points to pulmonary vascular obstruction,[61] whereas reduction of both ventilation and perfusion generally implies parenchymal or bronchial disease.[62]

Abnormal scans show high, intermediate, or low probability for PTE.[56, 58, 59, 61, 62] High-probability scans typically demonstrate large segmental perfusion defects without corresponding ventilatory or radiographic abnormalities. Low-probability scans demonstrate small segmental or nonsegmental perfusion defects with matching ventilatory and radiographic abnormalities. Intermediate scans fit neither of these patterns and are indeterminate.

The literature on lung scanning is extensive,[55–68, 68a] but the Prospective Investigation of Pulmonary Embolism Diagnosis (PIOPED)[59] is particularly noteworthy. It compared $\dot{V}/\dot{Q}$ scanning with pulmonary arteriography. Of 755 patients studied, 251 had PTE by arteriography but only 102 of them (41 percent) had a *high*-probability lung scan. Other smaller studies have shown similar results.[63, 64] Moreover, from 15 to 30 percent of patients with *low*-probability lung scans do, in fact, have PTE.[59, 61–63, 66] These findings show that both high-probability and low-probability lung scans have distinct limitations in predicting the presence or absence of pulmonary thromboemboli. On the other hand, a normal lung scan is as reliable as a normal pulmonary arteriogram in ruling out PTE.[57, 65, 66]

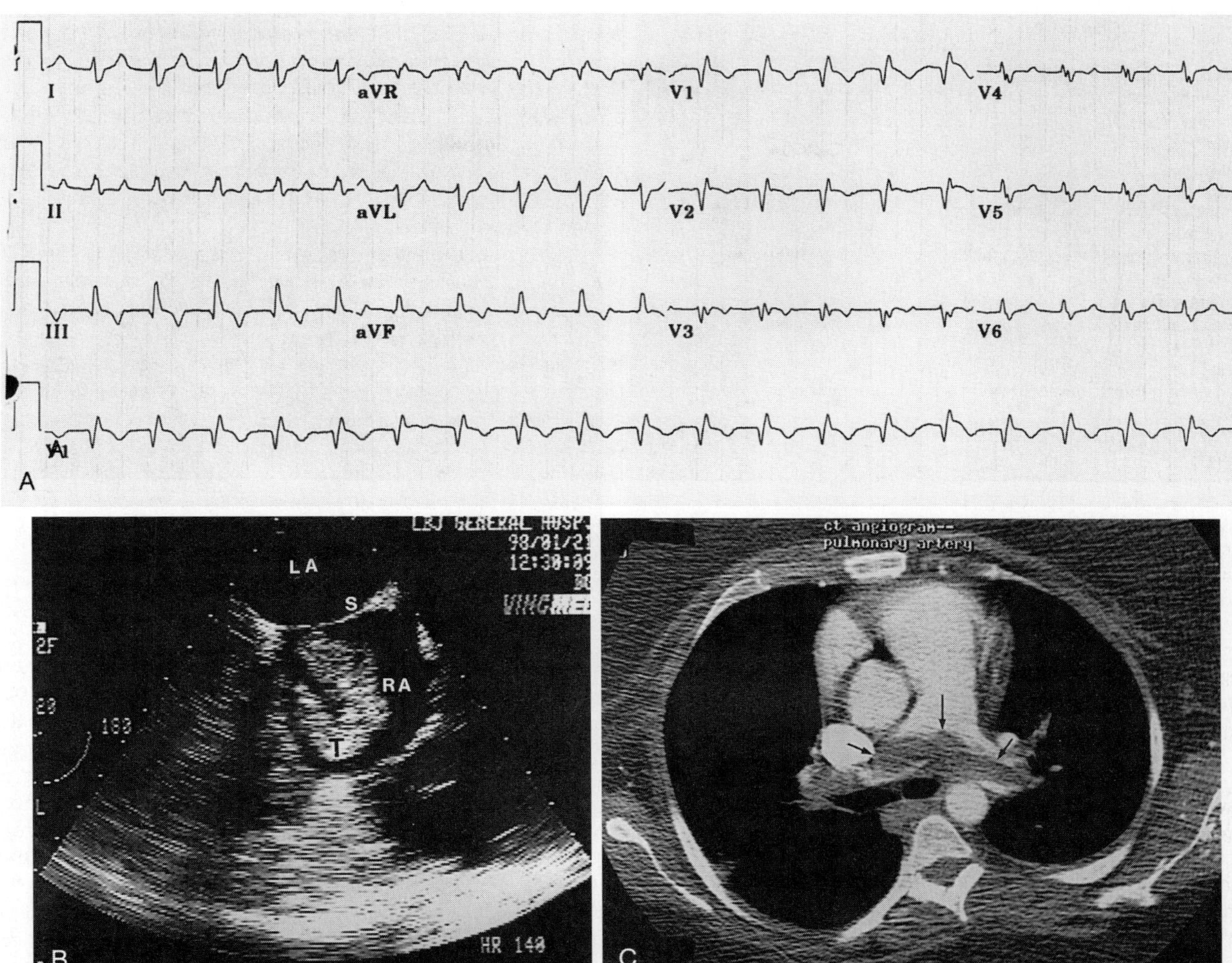

FIGURE 99–7 A 31-year-old diabetic woman with a painful, swollen right leg suddenly became dyspneic. $\dot{V}/\dot{Q}$ lung scan showed intermediate probability for pulmonary thromboembolism. Ultrasonography demonstrated clots in the right common femoral and popliteal veins. **A,** Electrocardiogram shows accelerated nodal tachycardia with retrograde P waves, right bundle branch block, pathologic anteroseptal Q waves, and an S_1-Q_3-T_3 pattern—findings consistent with severe pulmonary hypertension. **B,** Transesophageal echocardiogram, short-axis view (20 degrees), shows a large, lobulated opacity in the right atrium (RA) suggestive of a thrombus (T). LA, left atrium; S, atrial septum. **C,** Contrast-enhanced spiral computed tomographic study shows a large filling defect *(arrows)* in the bifurcation of the pulmonary arterial trunk. The patient died just as thrombolytic therapy was being initiated.

Pulmonary arteriography remains the most reliable means of establishing the presence of pulmonary thromboemboli and of determining their location and extent.[59, 61, 64] In experienced hands, it is relatively safe.[61, 67, 69] The arteriographic findings diagnostic of PTE are completely obstructed pulmonary arteries (Fig. 99–9; see also Figs. 99–1B and 99–6B) and intra-arterial filling defects (see Fig. 99–9).[67, 70, 71] Decrease in volume of affected lung segments (see Fig. 99–9) and changes in arterial caliber proximal or distal to the embolus may also appear. Intra-arterial webs, pouchlike filling defects, or intimal irregularities suggest previous thromboemboli.[72, 73]

Echocardiography is valuable in detecting right ventricular dysfunction, particularly when the systemic arterial pressure remains normal.[74–76] Such testing is important because right ventricular dysfunction in patients with PTE correlates with increased mortality.[77, 78] In addition, because such dysfunction is not always clinically apparent, the echocardiogram becomes an excellent means of monitoring therapeutic efficacy.[79, 80, 80a] It can also identify diseases that masquerade as PTE.

The echocardiographic signs of PTE include dilated right atrium, dilated hypokinetic right ventricle, flattening or paradoxical motion of the interventricular septum, and Doppler evidence of tricuspid or pulmonary regurgitation.[80–83] Regional right ventricular dysfunction with normal motion of the apical wall is another strong clue.[84] In addition, the echocardiogram may show clots in the right atrium (see Fig. 99–7B) or right ventricle[84a] and, occasionally, in the central pulmonary arteries.[83, 85]

Contrast-enhanced *spiral* or *electron-beam computed tomography* (CT) images the pulmonary vessels directly. Emboli appear as filling defects within the opacified arteries (see Fig. 99–7C). Compared with pulmonary arteriography, this technique has a mean sensitivity and specificity of about 90 percent for detecting emboli in the segmental and larger pulmonary arteries.[86–88] It has the advantage of being minimally invasive and of demonstrating chest dis-

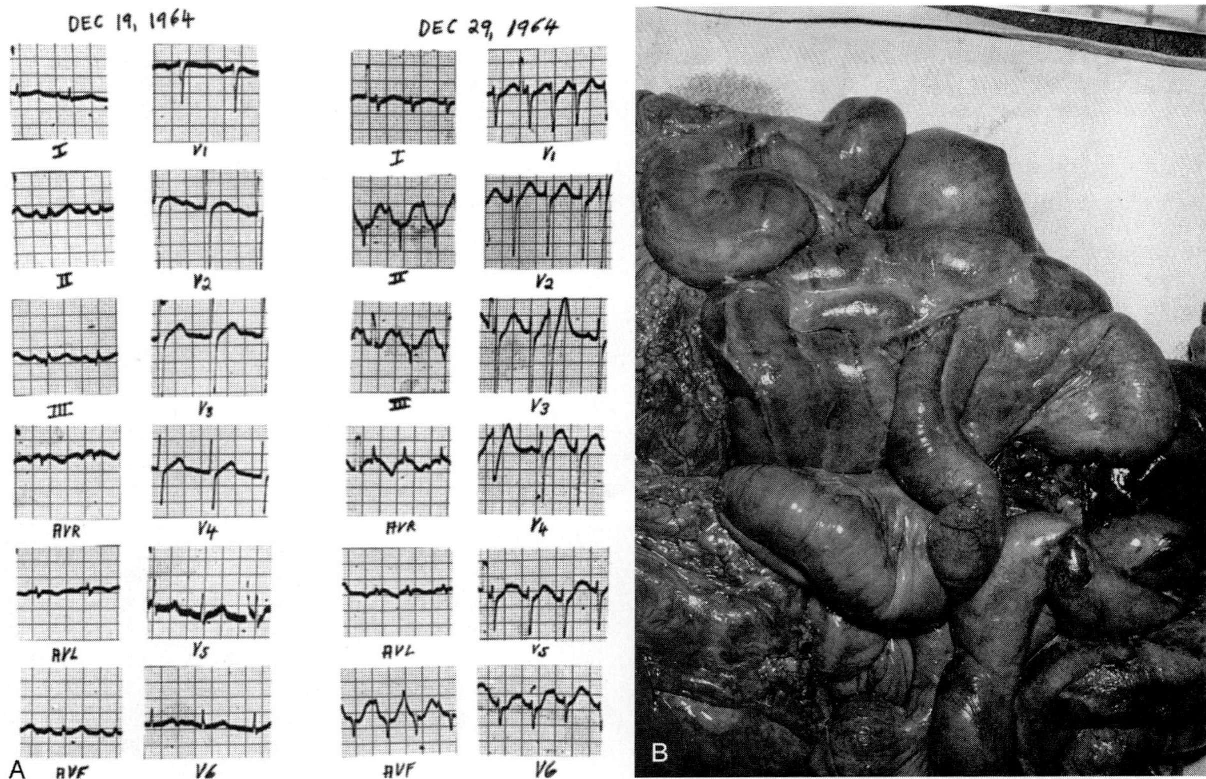

FIGURE 99–8 A, Electrocardiograms of a 55-year-old man who underwent surgical correction of sigmoid volvulus. **Left,** The preoperative tracing was within normal limits. On the ninth postoperative day, the patient abruptly became dyspneic, tachypneic, cyanotic, and hypotensive. **Right,** A tracing made at that time showed a marked shift in the QRS electrical axis to the right. These clinical and electrocardiographic changes prompted an erroneous diagnosis of massive pulmonary thromboembolism. Several hours later, the patient died. **B,** Autopsy view of the patient's intestines shows purulent peritonitis that resulted from disruption of the colon at the site of operative repair. There were no pulmonary thromboemboli. (See also Plate 99–8B.)

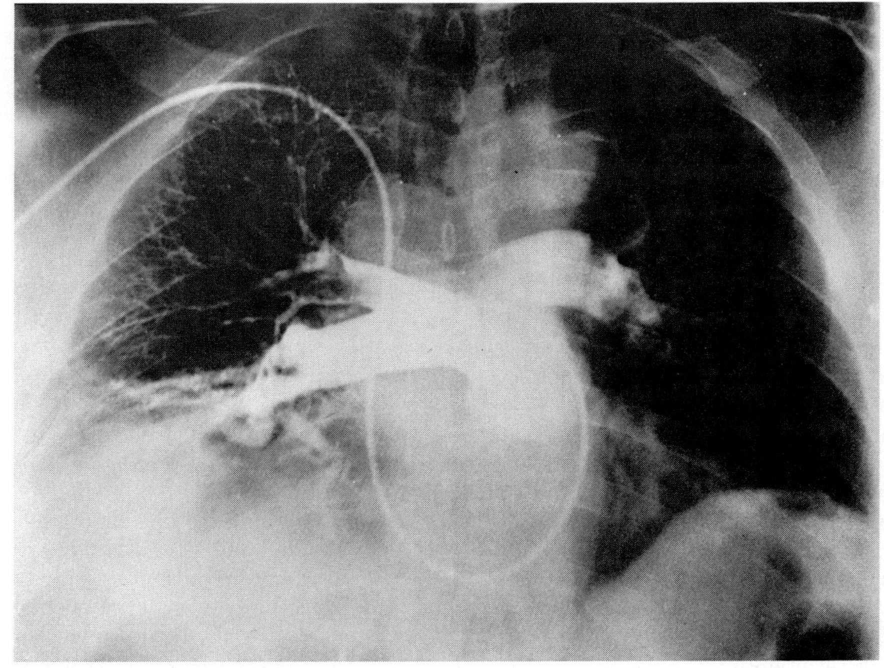

FIGURE 99–9 Pulmonary arteriogram obtained 24 hours after the onset of dyspnea and right pleuritic pain in a 71-year-old man. Note the large filling defect in the right upper lobe artery, collapse of the right middle and lower lobes, and multiple occlusive lesions in the lobar and segmental arteries of the left lung. Autopsy confirmed the arteriographic findings.

ease that can masquerade clinically as PTE.[89, 89a] In addition, it provides an excellent means of monitoring the resolution of centrally located emboli.[87] Some investigators believe that this technique should replace $\dot{V}/\dot{Q}$ scans as the initial investigation for PTE,[90] particularly in patients with underlying cardiorespiratory disorders.[91, 92] Others say that it could replace pulmonary arteriography in most patients whose $\dot{V}/\dot{Q}$ scans have intermediate probability for PTE and whose legs show no evidence of deep vein thrombosis.[89]

Certain disadvantages of CT deserve mention. The spiral type requires a 24-second breath-hold, which poses difficulty for the tachypneic patient.[86] It also exposes the patient to a relatively high dose of radiation.[93] Furthermore, neither the spiral nor the electron-beam type can detect clots in the periphery of the lung. In patients with renal insufficiency and high probability of PTE, exposure to contrast material can be minimized by foregoing CT and proceeding directly to conventional pulmonary arteriography.[94] Clearly, further studies are necessary to delineate the precise role of spiral and electron-beam CT in the diagnosis of acute PTE.

Gadolinium-enhanced *magnetic resonance angiography* can also identify large thromboemboli in the central pulmonary arteries but is not reliable in detecting clots in arteries beyond the segmental level.[95, 95a] Although its sensitivity is slightly lower than that of spiral CT, its specificity is the same.[96, 97] Moreover, it is a valid means of documenting venous thrombosis in the pelvis and lower limbs.[48, 97, 97a]

Venous ultrasonography,[98–102] *impedance plethysmography,*[103] and *contrast venography*[104–106] are standard means of establishing the diagnosis of deep vein thrombosis. Based on the concept that pulmonary embolism and lower extremity deep vein thrombosis are manifestations of the same disease process, these investigations, when positive, are frequently used as surrogate evidence of PTE.[60, 61, 107, 108] Venous ultrasonography using compression is the most accurate noninvasive means of diagnosing the first episode of symptomatic proximal deep vein thrombosis.[102] When negative, however, this study is not conclusive and should be repeated 5 to 7 days later before excluding deep vein thrombosis.[101, 102] Venous ultrasonography and impedance plethysmography are especially useful screening tests in pregnant women suspected of having PTE.[102, 109]

Contrast venography remains the "gold standard" for diagnosing deep vein thrombosis. Although invasive and associated with risks from the use of contrast media, this technique may become necessary in situations in which noninvasive studies typically yield inconclusive results.[102] These situations include asymptomatic postoperative patients suspected of having proximal deep vein thrombosis, those thought to have calf vein thrombosis, and those suspected of having recurrent deep vein thrombosis.[102, 105, 110]

Angioscopy[111–113] and *intravascular ultrasound*[114] have not been adequately tested as methods for diagnosing PTE. Nevertheless, angioscopy may prove useful in assessing the resolution of pulmonary thromboemboli.

DIFFERENTIAL DIAGNOSIS

The manifestations of PTE are so protean that even experienced clinicians occasionally mistake the illness for some other disorder. In addition, many other disorders often masquerade as PTE (Table 99–2). In this section, we show how confusion in diagnosis comes about and mention, when possible, simple means of resolving the issue. We also indicate when specialized diagnostic procedures are indispensable for proper management.

Parenchymatous Respiratory Disorders

Pneumonia

Both pulmonary infarction and bacterial pneumonia can cause dyspnea, tachypnea, cough, pleuritic pain, fever, hemoptysis, leukocytosis, and similar abnormalities on chest radiograph.[35] To minimize diagnostic error, physicians should consider both disorders whenever they make a tentative diagnosis of either, particularly when the process involves the lower lobes, especially the right. Accurate clinical differentiation of pulmonary infarction from pneumonia often takes several days and may be impossible without pulmonary arteriography. Therefore, as long as the diagnosis is uncertain, we favor treatment for both conditions.

Certain features are useful in distinguishing between these two illnesses. Patients with pneumonia frequently experience gradually increasing malaise followed by shaking chills and a cough productive of purulent sputum.

TABLE 99–2 Differential Diagnosis of Pulmonary Thromboembolism

Respiratory Disorders	*Abdominal Disorders*
Parenchymatous	Acute cholecystitis
Pneumonia	Subdiaphragmatic abscess
Pyogenic abscess	Ruptured viscus
Neoplasm	Pancreatitis
Granulomatous infection	Splenic infarction
Amebiasis	*Infectious Disorders*
Obstructive pulmonary disease	Bacteremia
Atelectasis	Peritonitis
Asthma	*Pulmonary-Renal Disorders*
Pleural	Goodpasture's syndrome
Viral (coxsackie)	Wegener's granulomatosis
Tuberculosis	Uremia
Neoplasm	*Hematologic Disorders*
Systemic lupus erythematosus	*Acute Blood Loss*
Congenital	Intraintestinal
Agenesis of pulmonary artery	Intrathoracic
Cardiovascular Disorders	Intraperitoneal and/or retroperitoneal
Myocardial infarction	*Sickle Cell Disease*
Congestive heart failure	*Disseminated Intravascular Coagulation*
Pericarditis	*Metabolic Disorders*
Acute cardiac tamponade	Pheochromocytoma
Dissecting hematoma of aorta	Lactic acidosis
Right-sided intracavitary cardiac lesions	*Particulate Matter Disorders*
Neurologic Disorders	Fat
Disturbances of consciousness	Amniotic fluid
Convulsive disorders	Tumor
Cerebrovascular disease	Air
Psychiatric Disorders	
Anxiety states	
Munchausen's syndrome	

Physical signs of consolidation are common. By contrast, patients with pulmonary infarction often become ill with dramatic suddenness, seldom have a troublesome cough, never experience true shaking chills (unless the emboli are septic), and almost never show physical signs of consolidation. Parenchymal infiltrates that appear first in one lung and then the other, or "pneumonia" unresponsive to therapy, suggests pulmonary infarction.

A pleural friction rub is of no value in differentiating pneumonia from pulmonary infarction, unless it occurs in the absence of parenchymal infiltrates on chest radiograph. In such cases, pneumonia is unlikely, and the prime considerations would be pulmonary infarction, fractured rib, viral pleuritis, and subdiaphragmatic inflammation.

Sputum examination is particularly helpful in differentiating pneumonia from pulmonary infarction. In pneumonia, the sputum classically is purulent, is occasionally foul smelling, and may contain bright red flecks of blood. Gram stain typically shows many bacteria. Conversely, early in the course of pulmonary infarction, sputum (when present) usually is frankly bloody with few bacteria or inflammatory cells. Blood cultures often yield the causative microorganism in patients with bacterial pneumonia but show no growth in patients with PTE.

The total leukocyte count may be normal or high in either disorder. Therefore, this test does not differentiate PTE from pneumonia.

Pleural fluid in PTE is often sanguineous and characteristically sterile. In pneumonia, however, it rarely is frankly bloody and often harbors the causative microorganism. The specific gravity and protein concentration of the pleural fluid are not distinctive for either disorder.

Pulmonary arteriography is the most specific means of differentiating bacterial pneumonia from pulmonary infarction. The pulmonary arteries in pneumonia—in contrast to those in PTE—show no filling defects or obstruction.[35]

Pyogenic Abscess, Neoplasm, Granulomatous Infection, and Amebiasis

These disorders, like PTE, can manifest fever, cough, dyspnea, hemoptysis, and pleuritic pain. In addition, like PTE, their radiographic features may include any combination of enlarged hilum, "mass lesion," parenchymal infiltrate, cavity (with or without an air-fluid level),[115, 116] and pleural effusion. Correct diagnosis, therefore, often requires bronchoscopy, pulmonary arteriography, pleural biopsy, or thoracotomy.

Obstructive Pulmonary Disease

Like PTE, obstructive pulmonary disease, especially when complicated by acute bronchitis, may cause wheezing, breathlessness, cough, hemoptysis, fever, and cyanosis. The chest radiograph in either disorder may show prominence of one or both main pulmonary arteries, together with localized or diffuse zones of increased radiolucency in which the peripheral vascular markings are diminished or absent. Moreover, either disorder may manifest electrocardiographic evidence of supraventricular arrhythmias, right-axis deviation, or a pattern suggesting right ventricular overload. In such instances, purulent sputum and hypercapnia suggest obstructive pulmonary disease, whereas hypocapnia favors PTE. Because perfusion defects occur in both conditions, lung scanning has limited usefulness, and spiral CT[91, 92] or pulmonary arteriography may become necessary.

Atelectasis

Both atelectasis and PTE may appear in bedridden and postoperative patients and cause dyspnea, tachypnea, and cyanosis, together with rales and decreased breath sounds over the involved areas of lung. These disorders may also cause similar radiographic changes, such as segmental collapse. Marked radiographic improvement after tracheobronchial suction or bronchoscopy indicates atelectasis.

Asthma

Common to both PTE and bronchial asthma are recurrent attacks of wheezing, dyspnea, and anxiety, associated with either a normal-appearing chest radiograph or scattered pulmonary parenchymal infiltrates, cyanosis, and signs of rapidly developing pulmonary hypertension. Ordinarily, these illnesses are easy to separate on clinical grounds. A long-standing history of atopy, elevated blood eosinophil count, tenacious and occasionally purulent sputum, or prompt therapeutic response to bronchodilators favors bronchial asthma. If, however, the patient is acutely ill, the diagnosis is in doubt, and precise differentiation is mandatory, pulmonary arteriography may become necessary.

Pleural and Congenital Respiratory Disorders

Coxsackievirus

Epidemic pleurodynia and early pulmonary infarction may have in common pleuritic pain, pleural friction rub, tenderness of intercostal muscles, and normal chest radiograph. Development of bloody sputum or parenchymal infiltrates, or both, points strongly toward pulmonary infarction and weighs heavily against pleurodynia. However, a cluster of cases of pleurisy in the community suggests pleurodynia.

Tuberculosis and Neoplasm

These illnesses, like PTE, can present with pleuritic pain, pleural friction rub, and grossly bloody pleural effusion. Definitive diagnosis rests on bacteriologic and histologic examination of the pleura and associated effusion.

Systemic Lupus Erythematosus

Patients known to have systemic lupus erythematosus occasionally exhibit sudden breathlessness, tachypnea, hyperpnea, tachycardia, cyanosis, pleuritic pain, pleural friction rub, and pleural effusion, accompanied at times by pulmonary parenchymal infiltrates and hemoptysis. In this circumstance, there is no consistent clinical means of distinguishing between systemic lupus erythematosus per se and concomitant PTE. Therefore, we sometimes resort to pulmonary arteriography for guidance in managing these patients.

Agenesis of the Pulmonary Artery

Congenital absence of a main branch of the pulmonary artery (usually the left) can lead to recurrent hemoptysis and dyspnea simulating PTE. In almost all cases, however, findings on conventional chest radiograph are sufficiently characteristic to permit recognition of this syndrome.[117] The findings consist of decreased volume of the affected lung with ipsilateral shift of the heart and mediastinal structures, absence of normal hilar shadow on the involved side, and plethora of the contralateral lung. Exact diagnosis requires pulmonary arteriography.

Cardiovascular Disorders

Myocardial Infarction

PTE often mimics myocardial infarction (MI), particularly in the first few hours after the embolic episode and before distinct clinical or radiographic signs of pulmonary infarction develop. To complicate matters, PTE occasionally is a sequel of MI,[118] and MI occasionally results from the systemic hypotension and pulmonary hypertension brought about by PTE. Certain features, however, are helpful in distinguishing between these two entities.

One good way of differentiating these disorders is to correlate the patient's blood pressure with the electrocardiogram. If hypotension develops concomitant with or after the onset of chest pain, and the accompanying electrocardiogram does not show definite or strongly suggestive evidence of acute MI, cardiac necrosis is most unlikely. In contrast, when PTE causes hypotension, the electrocardiogram typically shows only sinus tachycardia and nonspecific T wave changes or, sometimes, right-heart strain.

The duration of hypotension is another important diagnostic clue. Hypotension from MI ordinarily persists and usually requires vasopressor therapy. By contrast, hypotension from PTE ordinarily is transient, disappearing within minutes to a few hours, and often without the aid of vasopressors. If prolonged, it indicates massive obstruction to pulmonary blood flow with consequent decrease in cardiac output.

Finally, two contrasting features of PTE and MI deserve emphasis. Patients with PTE characteristically have dyspnea out of proportion to the degree of pain, hypotension, cyanosis, or radiographic changes. They may also appear moribund one minute and nearly well the next. Conversely, in patients with acute MI, dyspnea frequently is absent and, when present, usually reflects the degree of associated pulmonary vascular congestion. And once patients with MI appear moribund, they rarely recover spontaneously or rapidly.

Congestive Heart Failure

Among features common to both congestive heart failure and PTE are dyspnea, wheezing, apprehension, cyanosis, tachycardia, rales in the lung, hypotension, pleural effusion, bright red sputum, elevated jugular venous pressure, hepatomegaly, and peripheral edema.

To complicate the picture, congestive heart failure predisposes to PTE, and PTE sometimes precipitates and is responsible for the persistence of congestive heart failure.

Although clinical differentiation of these two disorders may be quite difficult, points favoring PTE are distinct *clots* of blood in the sputum, a normal heart size, and no pulmonary congestion on chest radiograph. Echocardiographic demonstration of contractile dysfunction predominantly of or limited to the left ventricle will usually establish a cardiac cause. Occasionally, pulmonary arteriography or direct measurement of pulmonary capillary pressure, or both, may be necessary for exact diagnosis.

Pericarditis

When infarction of the lung develops contiguous with the pericardium, a pleuropericardial friction rub or electrocardiographic signs of pericarditis, or both, may appear. A pericardial-like rub may also become audible in the area overlying a main pulmonary artery distended by massive thromboemboli.[25, 119] In our experience, the pericarditis induced by PTE is not associated with demonstrable pericardial effusion.

Acute Cardiac Tamponade

When acute cardiac tamponade presents with abrupt onset of dyspnea, tachypnea, tachycardia, cyanosis, distended neck veins, hepatomegaly, hypotension, and occasionally chest pain, it closely simulates massive PTE. Pulsus paradoxus, inspiratory distention of neck veins (Kussmaul sign), and distant heart sounds may also occur in either disorder. Because small amounts of pericardial fluid accumulated rapidly can lead to significant hemodynamic alteration without significant cardiomegaly, chest radiographs may not be useful in separating these two processes. Correct diagnosis may require echocardiography, CT, magnetic resonance angiography, cardiac catheterization, or pulmonary arteriography.

Dissecting Hematoma of the Aorta

Chest pain, usually severe and occasionally pleuritic, together with dyspnea, tachypnea, hypotension, neurologic manifestations, and even hemoptysis are features of dissecting hematoma of the aorta that simulate PTE. Additional difficulty in diagnosis can develop if the hematoma ruptures into the pericardial sac, causing cardiac tamponade, or into the pleural space (usually the left), resulting in hemothorax. A hematocrit value of the pleural fluid approaching that of peripheral blood is evidence of a ruptured vessel and weighs heavily against pulmonary infarction. Widening of the aorta, mediastinum, or both, on chest radiograph is another sign of dissecting hematoma. Precise diagnosis ordinarily requires CT, magnetic resonance imaging, echocardiography, pulmonary arteriography, or combinations thereof.

Right-Sided Intracavitary Cardiac Lesions

When the ball-valve action of a right-sided cardiac thrombus or neoplasm impedes orderly flow of blood into the lungs, the patient may exhibit intermittent dyspnea, syncope, tachycardia, cyanosis, chest pain, arrhythmias, or various cardiac murmurs. But unlike the findings in PTE, these signs and symptoms may change as the patient's position changes. If the lesion abuts the pulmonic valve, the pulmonic component of the second heart sound may be muffled. If the lesion becomes calcified, it may be evident on chest radiograph. Echocardiography, however, is the most sensitive and reliable means of detecting right-sided intracavitary masses.

Neurologic Disorders

Because the neurologic manifestations of PTE are usually abrupt in onset and often transient and recurrent, they commonly masquerade as cerebrovascular disease.[27] Conversely, cerebrovascular disease, such as hemorrhagic infarction and subdural hematoma, may be associated with labored respirations, pulmonary parenchymal infiltrates,[120] and electrocardiographic changes.[121] Therefore, differentiation of these two conditions can be difficult. Findings suggestive of PTE are cardiorespiratory abnormalities or signs of phlebitis that occur in association with sudden, transient, or recurrent neurologic dysfunction. Another clue to PTE is syncope at rest in the elderly, bedridden, or cardiac patient.

Psychiatric Disorders

It is easy to mistake PTE for a functional disorder when tachypnea, diaphoresis, apprehension, and feelings of suffocation are the major clinical features. Conversely, functional disorders can mimic PTE, particularly when spurious hemoptysis is part of the clinical picture. We have seen this diagnostic dilemma over a full spectrum, from fatal PTE masquerading as Munchausen's syndrome* (see Fig. 99–1) to true Munchausen's syndrome prompting vena caval ligation for suspected PTE. Differentiation depends primarily on thorough probing of the patient's complaints and credibility and use of tests appropriate for the given situation.

Abdominal Disorders

Acute cholecystitis and other diseases involving upper abdominal structures share with pulmonary infarction the capacity to cause abdominal discomfort and muscle guarding, chest pain on movement, tachycardia, frequent shallow and sometimes painful respirations, and radiographic changes at the base of one or both lungs. Early correct diagnosis is particularly difficult when the initial chest radiograph is normal and imaging studies of the abdomen are negative. In such cases, serial chest radiographs will point to PTE (see Fig. 99–5).

*A label applied to persons "who, in the absence of appropriate medical or surgical need, have made hospitalization a primary way of life."[122]

Infectious Disorders

Bacteremia

When bacteremia presents with breathlessness, hyperpnea, tachypnea, tachycardia, peripheral cyanosis, and hypotension, the clinical picture closely mimics that of PTE. Hints of bacteremia are high fever, shaking chills, warm dry skin, and an obvious source of infection. If the diagnosis remains unsettled and the chest radiograph shows no parenchymal disease, a normal lung scan excludes PTE.

Peritonitis

Postoperative peritonitis (see Fig. 99–8B; see also Plate 99–8B) can simulate PTE when it causes sudden circulatory collapse, rapid respirations, cyanosis, and pleural friction rub without causing the usual signs of peritoneal inflammation. Moreover, concomitant electrocardiograms may show changes consistent with those of massive PTE (see Fig. 99–8A). Clues to peritonitis in such cases are a progressive rise in the hematocrit value (indicating sequestration of fluid in the peritoneal cavity), a low central venous pressure, or a purulent peritoneal aspirate.

Pulmonary-Renal Disorders

Goodpasture's Syndrome

Recurrent dyspnea, hemoptysis, and transient pulmonary infiltrates are features of Goodpasture's syndrome that mimic PTE. Despite such similarities, clinical separation of these two entities ordinarily is easy. Patients with Goodpasture's syndrome characteristically are young and previously healthy and have iron-deficiency anemia along with iron-filled macrophages in their sputum. They may also exhibit proteinuria, hematuria, and cylindruria. During the acute stages of hemoptysis, their chest radiographs commonly show ill-defined, bilateral nodular densities, usually in a perihilar distribution sparing the apices and bases. Between bouts of hemoptysis, a finely granular, reticular pattern of increased interstitial markings may develop throughout the lungs.

Wegener's Granulomatosis

Wegener's granulomatosis, like PTE, may give rise to breathlessness, pleuritic pain, hemoptysis, pleural friction rub, pleural effusion, and cavities in the lung. Ultimately, most of these patients show evidence of widespread, multisystem disease, especially nephritis. Definitive diagnosis requires histologic demonstration of granulomatous disease of the respiratory tract, necrotizing vasculitis, and focal glomerulitis.

Uremia

We and others[123] have observed patients with advanced uremia who exhibit apprehension, tachypnea, hyperpnea, wheezing, pleuritic pain, pleural friction rub, progressive cyanosis, and occasionally, hemoptysis and hypotension. When these manifestations develop abruptly, and demise is rapid, the similarity to PTE is remarkable. Our experience indicates that differentiating these entities may not be possible without an autopsy.

Hematologic Disorders

Acute Blood Loss

When internal blood loss is sudden and severe, it may present as syncope associated with air hunger, tachycardia, peripheral cyanosis, and hypotension. These same features may also herald massive PTE. Because both disorders can be fatal if not treated promptly and appropriately, early correct diagnosis is essential. In that regard, a low central venous pressure favors hypovolemia whereas an elevated central venous pressure with an accentuated pulmonic valve closure sound points to massive PTE.

Sickle Cell Disease

Patients with sickle cell disease often experience acute chest pain accompanied at times by fever, dyspnea, tachypnea, hypoxemia, pulmonary parenchymal infiltrates, and small pleural effusions. This so-called acute chest syndrome[124] presumably results from pulmonary infection or in situ pulmonary microthromboses. Whatever the cause, the clinical picture closely mimics that of PTE.

Differentiating these two illnesses is important, particularly from the standpoint of therapy. In sicklers, anticoagulation is relatively ineffectual and inferior vena caval interruption potentially deleterious. Moreover, pulmonary arteriography is generally contraindicated because the hypertonic radiographic contrast material might precipitate further sickling and aggravate the condition. Thus, initial management of these patients should be conservative—pain control, hydration, supplemental oxygen, and if necessary, empirical antibiotics and partial exchange transfusion.

Disseminated Intravascular Coagulation

Like PTE, disseminated intravascular coagulation can cause fulminant dyspnea, cyanosis, neurologic abnormalities, and hypotension. In addition, like PTE, it tends to occur in obstetric and postsurgical patients. It may even be the presenting manifestation of unrecognized PTE.[125] Unlike PTE, however, disseminated intravascular coagulation commonly leads to purpuric skin lesions, proteinuria, hematuria, fragmented erythrocytes on peripheral blood film, thrombocytopenia, and depletion of plasma coagulation factors.

Metabolic Disorders

Pheochromocytoma

This tumor can cause paroxysms of *hypo*tension, tachycardia, tachypnea, sweating, peripheral cyanosis, cardiac murmur, fever, and leukocytosis. The patient may also seem well one minute, desperately ill the next, and then recover spontaneously and rapidly. So similar are these findings to those of PTE that the true nature of the illness can be totally overlooked while lung scanning,[126] pulmonary arteriography, right heart catheterization, and even ligation of the inferior vena cava are carried out.[127] Clues to pheochromocytoma in such instances are hyperglycemia, signs of hypermetabolism, a history of *hypo*tension, a pronounced sensitivity to the hypotensive effects of phenothiazines, or discovery of an abdominal mass.

Lactic Acidosis

Rarely, lactic acidosis leads to acute and increasingly severe signs of pulmonary hypertension simulating massive PTE. In one case, clinical evidence of PTE was so convincing that the surgeon did an emergency pulmonary arteriotomy but found no pulmonary emboli.[128] Any process responsible for decreased oxygenation of peripheral tissues coupled with low serum carbon dioxide content should alert the physician to the possibility of lactic acidosis. Demonstration of an extremely low arterial pH in association with excess blood lactate confirms the diagnosis.

Particulate Matter Disorders

Fat Embolism

In a patient with recent fracture of the long bones, sudden development of respiratory disability, pulmonary parenchymal infiltrates, central nervous system abnormalities, or combinations thereof suggests fat embolism as well as PTE. The best clue to fat embolism in such cases is the appearance of a petechial rash over the anterior part of the shoulders, the anterosuperior portion of the chest, the base of the neck, the axillae and conjunctivae, or occasionally, the abdomen and thighs.[129] When present, the petechiae typically emerge 24 to 36 hours after the injury, persist for 3 to 4 days, and then fade rapidly. Additional points favoring fat embolism are onset of symptoms within hours to a few days after the injury; diffuse, bilateral, "snowstorm-like" densities on chest radiograph simulating pulmonary edema but without pleural effusion or cardiomegaly; sharp drop in the hematocrit value consequent to intrapulmonary hemorrhage; increased erythrocyte aggregation and hemolysis; thrombocytopenia resulting from platelet aggregation; and demonstration of fat globules in the retinal arterioles, in the cerebrospinal fluid, or on the surface of the urine.

More typical of PTE are symptoms beginning 1 to 3 weeks after the accident; localized and larger pulmonary parenchymal lesions, often with pleural effusion; pleural friction rub; and signs of venous thrombosis.

Clinical differentiation of fat embolism from PTE can be difficult and, sometimes, impossible. In such cases, pulmonary arteriography is the best means of resolving the problem.

Amniotic Fluid Embolism

Precipitous hypotension, often accompanied by cardiorespiratory embarrassment, is characteristic of amniotic fluid embolism and is not uncommon in PTE. Accurate premortem distinction between these two types of embolism may be impossible. Guides to amniotic fluid embolism are multiparity; maternal age over 30 years; onset of symptoms late in labor, during delivery, or in the immediate postpartum period; difficult or prolonged labor; overweight or stillborn infant; radiographic signs of pulmonary edema; or coagulation defects such as thrombocytopenia, hypoprothrombinemia, and hypofibrinogenemia. By contrast, frank hemoptysis, pleural friction rub, signs of venous thrombosis, and oligemic lung fields suggest PTE.

Tumor Embolism

Pulmonary arterial tumor emboli can cause a clinical picture just like that of PTE. Knowledge that the patient has a malignancy offers little diagnostic help, because PTE is frequent in persons with cancer. Although cytologic examination of blood obtained from the pulmonary artery may show malignant cells,[130, 131] lung biopsy provides the best means of establishing the diagnosis. Recognizing a surgically curable lesion such as myxoma of the right atrium or right ventricle is particularly important; in that regard, echocardiography is indispensable.

Venous Air Embolism

Accidental introduction of air into a systemic vein may result from a variety of diagnostic, therapeutic, or surgical procedures.[132] The gas characteristically collects in the right ventricular outflow tract or occasionally in the pulmonary arterial tree and, if sufficient in amount, provokes gasping respirations, cyanosis, chest pain, tachycardia, convulsions, and hypotension. In most cases, death or total recovery ensues within an hour after onset of symptoms. A unique but inconstant diagnostic sign is a precordial "mill-wheel" murmur, a churning and splashing noise that masks the heart sounds. Palpation of air in the jugular veins or radiographic demonstration of air in the right ventricle provides additional diagnostic aid.

TREATMENT

The ideal treatment of PTE is *prevention* of the initial thrombus formation.[133–135] Such measures—used singly or in various combinations—include early full ambulation (especially for postoperative and postpartum patients), elastic stockings or intermittent pneumatic compression for bedridden persons and those undergoing major operative procedures,[136] and anticoagulant medication for patients at particular risk for PTE. Current options for preventing deep vein thrombosis in hospitalized patients,[134, 137–169] in patients discharged after lower extremity arthroplasty,[153, 154] and in pregnant women[109, 170] appear in Table 99–3.

Once PTE has occurred, the type of therapy depends on the severity of the illness, the nature of any associated disease(s), the skill and experience of the physician, and the available facilities. Even considering these factors, it may be difficult, at times, to decide on a fixed course of treatment, primarily because one cannot accurately predict in a given patient whether or when another embolus will occur, whether it will be clinically detectable, or how extensive it may be.

In addition to supportive measures, *immediate anticoagulation* with unfractionated heparin is standard (barring obvious contraindications). Heparin acts largely by binding to antithrombin III.[171] The resultant heparin–antithrombin III complex inactivates both thrombin and activated factor X. Because of the heterogeneous nature of unfractionated heparin, the response to therapy with this agent varies considerably.[172] Hence, frequent monitoring of the activated partial thromboplastin time (APTT) is necessary.

It is important to achieve a therapeutic threshold rapidly (i.e., an APTT ratio 1.5 times the control).[173–175] Failure to do so is associated with a high incidence of recurrent PTE.[176] We favor an intravenous bolus of 5000 to 10,000 U of heparin followed by a continuous infusion of 1200 to 1500 U/h. Based on the APTT value, the dose is adjusted at intervals of 4 to 6 hours, and the infusion is continued for at least 5 days.[177]

Pregnant women with PTE should receive heparin intravenously for 10 days followed by heparin subcutaneously throughout gestation.[109] The intravenous regimen is the same as that mentioned previously. The subcutaneous regimen consists of approximately 20,000 U every 12 hours, adjusted to maintain the APTT at 1.5 times the control. For patients in labor, heparin therapy should be discontinued at the onset of regular uterine contractions.

Some reports[155, 178–183, 183a] indicate that low-molecular-weight heparin offers several therapeutic advantages over unfractionated heparin: longer half-life, more predictable anticoagulant activity, no need for laboratory monitoring, and lower incidence of thrombocytopenia. It is also effective when administered subcutaneously. But since low-molecular-weight heparins are distinct compounds with different pharmacokinetic profiles and dosage regimens, the results with one preparation cannot be extended to that of another. Nevertheless, these agents are safe and effective in the treatment of proximal deep vein thrombosis[155, 179, 180] and may become the best option for treating PTE.[48, 182, 184–186]

The cornerstone of *long-term anticoagulation* is warfarin sodium.[187] This drug inhibits the enzyme vitamin K epoxide reductase. As a consequence, body stores of vitamin K become depleted, the synthesis of coagulation factors II, VII, IX, and X impaired, and the prothrombin time prolonged.

Warfarin can be administered along with, or shortly after, the institution of heparin therapy.[177, 188, 189] The usual recommended therapeutic range is an international normalized ratio (INR) of 2.0 to 3.0.[190] But in patients with the antiphospholipid antibody syndrome, the target INR is 3.5.[191] Because warfarin readily crosses the placenta, its use during pregnancy is contraindicated.

Levels of coagulation factor VII decrease within hours after the initiation of warfarin therapy. But it takes about 5 days for levels of the other coagulation factors to decrease.[187, 192] Therefore, heparin therapy should be continued for at least 2 to 3 days after the target INR has been reached.

The duration of anticoagulation varies.[193, 194] Two months may suffice in patients with a definable and reversible cause of PTE (e.g., fractured pelvis, postoperative state, or postpartum). When the cause cannot be identified, therapy should be continued for at least 6 months.[190, 194a, 194b] For patients with recurrent PTE and for those with the antiphospholipid antibody syndrome, lifelong anticoagulation is probably necessary. In patients with other underlying

TABLE 99-3 **Prophylaxis of Venous Thromboembolism***

Indication	Prophylaxis
Medical inpatients	Unfractionated heparin 5000 U twice daily[134, 137] (with or without GCS, IPC, or aspirin†[138, 139]) **or** Low-molecular-weight heparin Enoxaparin 40 mg daily[139a]
Intensive care unit	Same as Medical inpatients[140–142]
General surgery	Unfractionated heparin 5000 U twice daily[143–146] **or** Low-molecular-weight heparin[146, 147] Enoxaparin 40 mg daily **or** Dalteparin 2500 to 5000 U daily[148, 149] **or** Nadroparin‡ 3100 U daily **or** Tinzaparin‡ 3500 U daily (Each of the above with or without GCS, IPC, or aspirin)
Cardiothoracic surgery	Same as Medical inpatients[150]
Hip replacement	Low-molecular-weight heparin Enoxaparin 30 mg twice daily[151–154] **or** Heparinoid Danaparoid 750 U twice daily[155] **or** Recombinant hirudin Desirudin‡ 15 U twice daily[156, 157] **or** Adjusted-dose unfractionated heparin to maintain APTT ratio 1.5 times that of the control value[158] **or** Adjusted-dose warfarin (target INR 2.5)[159] (Each of the above with or without GCS[160] and IPC[161])
Knee replacement	Low-molecular-weight heparin Enoxaparin 30 mg twice daily[153, 154, 162] **or** Ardeparin 50 U/kg twice daily[163] (Each of the above with or without IPC)
Radical prostatectomy	Adjusted-dose warfarin (target INR 2.5) with or without GCS and IPC[164]
Neurosurgery	GCS and IPC[165] **or** GCS with low-molecular-weight heparin Enoxaparin 40 mg daily[166]
Spinal surgery	GCS with or without IPC[167]
Trauma (excluding brain)	GCS and IPC With or without Low-molecular-weight heparin Enoxaparin 30 mg twice daily[168] **or** Adjusted-dose unfractionated heparin to maintain APTT ratio 1.5 times that of the control value[169]
Pregnancy	Adjusted-dose unfractionated heparin to maintain APTT ratio 1.5 times that of the control value[169] **or** Low-molecular-weight heparin Dalteparin 5000 U daily[170] **or** Enoxaparin 40 mg daily[169]

Abbreviations: APTT, activated partial thromboplastin time; GCS, graduated compression stockings; INR, international normalized ratio; IPC, intermittent pneumatic compression.
*All listed medications except aspirin and warfarin are administered subcutaneously.
†Dose varies from 80 to 325 mg daily.
‡Not approved by U.S. Food and Drug Administration.

thrombophilic conditions, the duration of therapy remains unclear.[94, 192, 194]

Thrombolytic therapy deserves immediate consideration in patients who are hemodynamically unstable from massive PTE. Such treatment promotes dissolution of clots much faster than that achieved with anticoagulants alone.[69, 79, 195–198] The resultant decrease in clot burden relieves strain on the right ventricle, allowing cardiac function to improve.[79, 82, 198a, 199] This therapy may also reduce the rate of recurrent PTE by dissolving the initiating thrombi. Proof of such an effect, however, is lacking.[200]

Some patients with massive PTE are hemodynamically

stable but have echocardiographic evidence of right ventricular dysfunction. Experience to date, albeit observational, suggests that these patients may also benefit from thrombolytic therapy.[75, 76, 78] Although randomized clinical trials of thrombolytic therapy in PTE demonstrate no reduction in mortality, the scintigraphic, echocardiographic, and angiographic findings do improve.[200–203]

One additional point deserves emphasis. If the patient is in shock and the clinical evidence points strongly to PTE, thrombolytics can be lifesaving and should be administered without seeking absolute diagnostic confirmation. The potential benefit of thrombolytics in such cases far outweighs the risk of significant hemorrhage.[198a, 203a] In this setting, bedside transthoracic echocardiography can be invaluable in demonstrating right ventricular pressure overload while excluding other diagnostic considerations such as cardiac tamponade, left ventricular failure, and aortic dissection.[75, 198a]

Whereas the window for thrombolytic therapy in MI is but a few hours,[204–206] it is days to weeks in PTE.[79, 207] The U.S. Food and Drug Administration has approved three thrombolytic treatment protocols for PTE (Table 99–4). All three lyse clots effectively, but recombinant tissue-plasminogen activator acts most rapidly and produces the fewest systemic reactions. No laboratory monitoring or dose adjustment is necessary, and heparin is not used during the infusion. Anticoagulation is mandatory, however, on completion of thrombolytic therapy.

Contraindications to thrombolytic therapy ordinarily include active internal bleeding, pregnancy, multiple trauma, and intracranial hemorrhage.[69] All contraindications become relative, however, when the patient is dying from massive PTE.

Interruption of blood flow through the inferior vena cava, either totally (by ligation) or partially (by use of filters or various suturing techniques), merits serious consideration when anticoagulant therapy is contraindicated or when PTE recurs despite optimal anticoagulation.[42, 208, 209] Caval interruption is mandatory after pulmonary embolectomy. Moreover, in patients with suppurative pelvic thrombophlebitis and septic pulmonary emboli unresponsive to antibiotic or anticoagulant therapy, ligation of the inferior vena cava and both ovarian or spermatic veins may be lifesaving.

Six caval filters are currently available in this country[209–212]—three types of Greenfield filters, the Bird's-nest filter, the Simon nitinol filter, and the Vena Tech filter. In some European centers, caval filters specifically designed for temporary use are also available.[213–216] All of these devices are being used prophylactically with increasing frequency in a wide variety of clinical circumstances.[209, 217–222] In some cases, however, thrombi proximal to a filter, especially thrombi in the heart, can obviate the filter's potential advantages.[223]

The role of *pulmonary embolectomy* remains controversial. Some authors suggest that this procedure should be considered more often,[224] even in patients with no hemodynamic compromise.[225] Others argue that the successful completion of pulmonary arteriography virtually precludes the need for embolectomy.[226] Still others say that there are no indications for pulmonary embolectomy.[227] We favor this operation when thrombolytic therapy is contraindicated or has failed and the patient is either moribund or shows steady deterioration despite vigorous medical management.[228] Arteriography is still the best means of establishing the presence and precise location of surgically accessible pulmonary thromboemboli.

Transvenous pulmonary embolectomy with catheter suction is another method of treating massive PTE.[229, 230] Its in-hospital mortality rate of about 30 percent is similar to that of open embolectomy.[231] Catheter embolectomy, however, is limited in its ability to remove thrombi that have already become adherent to the wall of the pulmonary artery. More recent catheter-based techniques attempt mechanical fragmentation of the clot with high-velocity jets of saline solution.[232, 233] These various techniques offer promise for patients who, from old age and coexisting disease, are particularly poor surgical risks, do not have access to cardiopulmonary bypass facilities, or have contraindications to heparin and thrombolytic therapy.

Pulmonary artery thromboendarterectomy is currently the only effective therapy for patients with chronic major vessel thromboembolic pulmonary hypertension.[234, 235]

TABLE 99–4 Thrombolytic Treatment Protocols for Pulmonary Thromboembolism

Agent	Loading Dose	Maintenance Dose
Streptokinase	250,000 U over 30 min	100,000 U/h for 24 h
Urokinase	4400 IU/kg over 10 min	4400 IU/kg/h for 12–24 h
Recombinant tissue-type plasminogen activator	None	50 mg/h for 2 h

COURSE AND PROGNOSIS

Pulmonary arteriograms performed serially have shown that major clots can resolve spontaneously and completely within 7[236] to 14[237] days. In one case, an embolus to a lobar artery resolved almost completely within 30 hours.[238] These observations help explain why most patients with PTE survive the initial episode, irrespective of the type of treatment.

Deaths from PTE usually occur in the first 2 weeks after diagnosis.[239] About 75 percent of the patients with fatal PTE die within the first hour.[240] Most of them have serious underlying disease such as heart failure or cancer.

Recurrence is uncommon in patients who are properly diagnosed and treated.[200, 241] In a prospective study comprising 399 cases of PTE diagnosed by lung scanning and arteriography, 33 patients (8.3 percent) had clinically apparent recurrence.[239] Other prospective therapeutic trials have shown rates of recurrence ranging from 4 to 19 percent.[195, 196]

The long-term outlook for patients with PTE depends largely on the nature and severity of any underlying disease. For those without preexisting heart disease, prognosis is good.[242] During a 9-year follow-up, 12 of 72 patients who had survived massive PTE died; in no case, however, did death result from chronic pulmonary hypertension or from definite recurrence of PTE.[243] Chronic cor pulmonale from PTE is relatively rare[242] but may arise in patients with repeated embolic episodes that go unrecognized and therefore untreated.

In Brief

Although some battles have been won, the war against venous thrombosis and pulmonary embolism is far from over. This disease continues to pose problems for both patient and doctor. Its etiology is still unclear, its true incidence in doubt, its diagnosis often questionable, and its treatment unsettled.

> Few conditions in medicine have been subjected to so much analysis with so little elucidation.
>
> Michael E. De Bakey[244]

Written in 1954, those words remain true today.

References

1. Moser KM: Venous thromboembolism. Am Rev Respir Dis 141:235, 1990.
2. Bell WR, Simon TL: Current status of pulmonary thromboembolic disease: pathophysiology, diagnosis, prevention, and treatment. Am Heart J 103:239, 1982.
3. Lilienfeld DE, Chan E, Ehland J, et al: Mortality from pulmonary embolism in the United States: 1962 to 1984. Chest 98:1067, 1990.
4. Goyette EM: The diagnosis and management of pulmonary embolism and infarction. Dis Chest 25:15, 1954.
5. Rexrode WO: Massive pulmonary embolism in an otherwise healthy young patient. Respir Care 31:803, 1986.
6. Emery JL: Pulmonary embolism in children. Arch Dis Child 37:591, 1962.
7. Ramirez LM: Thromboembolic disease in adolescence. JAMA 170:1808, 1959.
8. Dahlback B, Carlsson M, Svensson PJ: Familial thrombophilia due to a previously unrecognized mechanism characterized by poor anticoagulant response to activated protein C: prediction of a cofactor to activated protein C. Proc Natl Acad Sci U S A 90:1004, 1993.
9. Zoller B, Svensson PJ, He X, et al: Identification of the same factor V mutation in 47 out of 50 thrombosis prone families with inherited resistance to activated protein C. J Clin Invest 94:2521, 1994.
10. Svensson PJ, Dahlback B: Resistance to activated protein C as a basis for venous thrombosis. N Engl J Med 330:517, 1994.
11. Hooper WC, Evatt BL: The role of activated protein C resistance in the pathogenesis of venous thrombosis. Am J Med Sci 316:120, 1998.
12. Bertina RM, Koeleman BPC, Koster T, et al: Mutation in factor V associated with resistance to activated protein C. Nature 369:64, 1994.
13. Greengard JS, Sun X, Xu X, et al: Activated protein C resistance caused by Arg506Gln mutation in factor Va. Lancet 343:1361, 1994.
14. Hughes GRV: The antiphospholipid antibody syndrome: ten years on. Lancet 342:341, 1993.
15. den Heijer M, Koster T, Blom HJ, et al: Hyperhomocysteinemia as a risk factor for deep-vein thrombosis. N Engl J Med 334:759, 1996.
16. Selhub J, D'Angelo A: Relationship between homocysteine and thrombotic disease. Am J Med Sci 316:129, 1998.
17. Margaglione M, Brancaccio V, Giuliani N, et al: Increased risk for venous thrombosis in carriers of the Prothrombin G $\rightarrow$ A[20210] gene variant. Ann Intern Med 129:89, 1998.

17a. DeStefano V, Martinelli I, Mannucci PM, et al: The risk of recurrent deep venous thrombosis among heterozygous carriers of both factor V Leiden and the G20210A prothrombin mutation. N Engl J Med 341:801, 1999.

18. Gore I, Tanaka K: Phlebothrombosis, pulmonary embolization and pulmonary hypertension. Am J Med Sci 244:351, 1962.
19. Sevitt S, Gallagher N: Venous thrombosis and pulmonary embolism: a clinicopathological study in injured and burned patients. Br J Surg 48:475, 1961.
20. Chakko S, Richards F III: Right-sided cardiac thrombi and pulmonary embolism. Am J Cardiol 59:195, 1987.
21. Fred HL, Harle TS: Septic pulmonary embolism. Dis Chest 55:483, 1969.
22. Harley DP, White RA, Nelson RJ, et al: Pulmonary embolism secondary to venous thrombosis of the arm. Am J Surg 147:221, 1984.
23. Moran TJ: Pulmonary embolism in nonsurgical patients with prostatic thrombosis. Am J Clin Pathol 17:205, 1947.
24. Marks J, Truscott BM, Withycombe JFR: Treatment of venous thrombosis with anticoagulants: review of 1,135 cases. Lancet 2:787, 1954.
25. Gorham LW: A study of pulmonary embolism. Arch Intern Med 108:8, 189, 418, 1961.
26. Olázabal FJ Jr, Román-Irizarry LA, Oms JD, et al: Pulmonary emboli masquerading as asthma. N Engl J Med 278:999, 1968.
27. Fred HL, Yang M: Sudden loss of consciousness, dyspnea, and hypoxemia in a previously healthy young man. Circulation 91:3017, 1995.
28. Miller R, Berry JB: Pulmonary infarction: a frequently missed diagnosis. Am J Med Sci 222:197, 1951.
29. Kollef MH, Schacter DT: Acute pulmonary embolism triggered by the act of defecation. Chest 99:373, 1991.
30. Sagall EL, Bornstein J, Wolff L: Clinical syndrome in patients with pulmonary embolism. Arch Intern Med 76:234, 1945.
31. Stevens AE: The late appearance of leg symptoms in pulmonary embolus. Lancet 2:1005, 1961.
32. Smith GT, Dammin GJ, Dexter L: Postmortem arteriographic studies of the human lung in pulmonary embolization. JAMA 188:143, 1964.
33. Israel HL, Goldstein F: The varied clinical manifestations of pulmonary embolism. Ann Intern Med 47:202, 1957.
34. Murray HW, Ellis GC, Blumenthal DS, et al: Fever and pulmonary thromboembolism. Am J Med 67:232, 1979.
35. Fred HL: Bacterial pneumonia or pulmonary infarction? Dis Chest 55:422, 1969.
36. Parker BM, Smith JR: Pulmonary embolism and infarction: a review of the physiologic consequences of pulmonary arterial obstruction. Am J Med 24:402, 1958.
37. Kugel MA, Lichtman SS: Factors causing clinical jaundice in heart disease. Arch Intern Med 52:16, 1933.
38. Fleischner FG: Pulmonary embolism. Clin Radiol [Lond] 13:169, 1962.
39. Smith MJ: Roentgenographic aspects of complete and incomplete pulmonary infarction. Dis Chest 23:532, 1953.
40. Perkins RB, Bradshaw HH: Pulmonary infarction mistaken for bronchogenic carcinoma. JAMA 151:545, 1953.
41. Moser KM, Auger WR, Fedullo PF: Chronic major-vessel thromboembolic pulmonary hypertension. Circulation 81:1735, 1990.
42. Beall AC Jr, Fred HL, Cooley DA: Pulmonary embolism: cause, consequences, prevention and treatment. Curr Probl Surg, February, 1964.
43. Goodwin JF, Harrison CV, Wilcken DEL: Obliterative pulmonary hypertension and thromboembolism. BMJ 701:777, 1963.

43a. Afzal A, Noor HA, Gill SA, et al: Leukocytosis in acute pulmonary embolism. Chest 115:1329, 1999.

44. Bynum LJ, Wison JE III: Characteristics of pleural effusions associated with pulmonary embolism. Arch Intern Med 136:159, 1976.
45. Perrier A, Desmarais S, Goehring C, et al: D-Dimer testing for suspected pulmonary embolism in outpatients. Am J Respir Crit Care Med 156:492, 1997.
46. Oger E, Leroyer C, Bressollette L, et al: Evaluation of a new, rapid, and quantitative D-dimer test in patients with suspected pulmonary embolism. Am J Respir Crit Care Med 158:65, 1998.
47. Perrier A: Noninvasive diagnosis of pulmonary embolism. Hosp Pract 33:47, 1998.

47a. Ginsberg JS, Wells PS, Kearon C, et al: Sensitivity and specificity of a rapid whole-blood assay for D-dimer in the diagnosis of pulmonary embolism. Ann Intern Med 129:1006, 1998.

48. ACCP Consensus Committee on Pulmonary Embolism: Opinions regarding the diagnosis and management of venous thromboembolic disease. Chest 113:499, 1998.
49. Dantzker DR, Bower JS: Clinical significance of pulmonary function

tests: alterations in gas exchange following pulmonary thromboembolism. Chest 81:495, 1982.
50. Cvitanic O, Marino PL: Improved use of arterial blood gas analysis in suspected pulmonary embolism. Chest 95:48, 1989.
51. Stein PD, Goldhaber SZ, Henry JW, et al: Arterial blood gas analysis in the assessment of suspected acute pulmonary embolism. Chest 109:78, 1996.
52. Stein PD, Terrin ML, Hales CA, et al: Clinical, laboratory, roentgenographic and electrocardiographic findings in patients with acute pulmonary embolism and no pre-existing cardiac or pulmonary disease. Chest 100:598, 1991.
53. Stein PD, Goldhaber SZ, Henry JW: Alveolar-arterial oxygen gradient in the assessment of acute pulmonary embolism. Chest 107:139, 1995.
54. Ely EW, Smith JM, Haponik EF: Pulmonary embolism and normal oxygenation: application of PIOPED-derived likelihood ratios. Am J Med 103:541, 1997.
55. Hull RD, Hirsch J, Carter CJ, et al: Diagnostic value of ventilation-perfusion lung scanning in patients with suspected pulmonary embolism. Circulation 88:819, 1985.
56. Alderson PO, Martin EC: Pulmonary embolism: diagnosis with multiple imaging modalities. Radiology 164:297, 1987.
57. Hull RD, Raskob GE, Coates G, et al: Clinical validity of a normal perfusion lung scan in patients with suspected pulmonary embolism. Chest 97:23, 1990.
58. Webber MM, Gomes AS, Roe D, et al: Comparison of Biello, McNeil, and PIOPED criteria for the diagnosis of pulmonary emboli on lung scans. AJR 154:975, 1990.
59. Value of the ventilation/perfusion scan in acute pulmonary embolism: results of the Prospective Investigation of Pulmonary Embolism Diagnosis (PIOPED). JAMA 263:2753, 1990.
60. Moser KM, Fedullo PF, Littlejohn JK, et al: Frequent asymptomatic pulmonary embolism in patients with deep venous thrombosis. JAMA 271:223, 1994.
61. Hull RD, Hirsch J, Carter CJ, et al: Pulmonary angiography, ventilation lung scanning, and venography for clinically suspected pulmonary embolism with abnormal perfusion lung scan. Ann Intern Med 98:891, 1983.
62. McNiel BJ: Ventilation-perfusion studies and the diagnosis of pulmonary embolism: concise communication. J Nucl Med 21:319, 1980.
63. Alderson PO, Rujanevech N, Seckler-Walker RH, et al: The role of Xe-133 ventilation studies in the radionuclide detection of pulmonary embolism. Radiology 120:633, 1976.
64. Cheeley R, McCartney WH, Perry JR: The role of noninvasive tests versus pulmonary angiography in the diagnosis of pulmonary embolism. Am J Med 70:17, 1981.
65. Kipper MS, Moser KM, Kortman KE, et al: Long-term follow-up of patients with suspected pulmonary embolism and a normal lung scan. Chest 82:411, 1982.
66. Kelley MA, Carson JL, Palevsky HI, et al: Diagnosing pulmonary embolism: new facts and strategies. Ann Intern Med 114:300, 1991.
67. Alexander JK, Gonzalez DA, Fred HL: Angiographic studies in cardiorespiratory diseases. JAMA 198:575, 1966.
68. Stein PD, Gottschalk A: Critical review of ventilation-perfusion lung scans in acute pulmonary embolism. Prog Cardiovasc Dis 37:13, 1994.
68a. Meyerovitz MF, Mannting F, Polak JF, et al: Frequency of pulmonary embolism in patients with low-probability lung scan and negative lower extremity venous ultrasound. Chest 115:980, 1999.
69. Stein PD, Hull R, Raskob G: Risks for major bleeding from thrombolytic therapy in patients with acute pulmonary embolism: consideration of noninvasive management. Ann Intern Med 121:313, 1994.
70. Ferris EJ, Stanzler RM, Rourke JA, et al: Pulmonary angiography in pulmonary embolic disease. Am J Roentgenol Rad Ther Nucl Med 100:355, 1967.
71. Lowman RM, Reardon J, Hipona FA, et al: The role of pulmonary angiography in pulmonary embolism. Angiology 18:291, 1967.
72. Peterson KL, Fred HL, Alexander JK: Pulmonary arterial webs: a new angiographic sign of previous thromboembolism. N Engl J Med 277:33, 1967.
73. Auger WR, Fedullo PF, Moser KM, et al: Chronic major-vessel thromboembolic pulmonary artery obstruction: appearance at angiography. Radiology 182:393, 1992.
74. Wolfe MW, Lee RT, Feldstein ML, et al: Prognostic significance of right ventricular hypokinesis and perfusion defects in pulmonary embolism. Am Heart J 127:1371, 1994.
75. Kasper W, Konstantinides S, Geibel A, et al: Management strategies and determinants of outcome in acute major pulmonary embolism: results of a multicenter registry. J Am Coll Cardiol 30:1165, 1997.
76. Goldhaber SZ: Pulmonary embolism thrombolysis: broadening the paradigm for its administration. Circulation 96:716, 1997.
77. Ribeiro A, Lindmarker P, Juhlin-Dannfelt A, et al: Echocardiography Doppler in pulmonary embolism: right ventricular dysfunction as a predictor of mortality rate. Am Heart J 134:479, 1997.
78. Konstantinides S, Geibel A, Olschewski M, et al: Impact of thrombolytic treatment on the prognosis of hemodynamically stable patients with major pulmonary embolism: results of a multicenter registry. Circulation 96:882, 1997.
79. Goldhaber SZ, Haire WD, Feldstein ML, et al: Alteplase versus heparin in acute pulmonary embolism: randomized trial assessing right ventricular function and pulmonary perfusion. Lancet 341:507, 1993.
80. Goldhaber SZ: Pulmonary embolism for cardiologists. J Am Coll Cardiol 30:1172, 1997.
80a. Ribeiro A, Lindmarker P, Johnsson H, et al: Pulmonary embolism: one-year follow-up with echocardiography Doppler and five-year survival analysis. Circulation 99:1325, 1999.
81. Kasper W, Meinertz T, Henkel B, et al: Echocardiographic findings in patients with proved pulmonary embolism. Am Heart J 112:1284, 1986.
82. Come PC: Echocardiographic evaluation of pulmonary embolism and its response to therapeutic interventions. Chest 101:151, 1992.
83. Ritoo D, Sutherland GR, Samuel L, et al: Role of transesophageal echocardiography in diagnosis and management of central pulmonary artery thromboembolism. Am J Cardiol 71:1115, 1993.
84. McConnell MV, Solomon SD, Rayan ME, et al: Regional right ventricular dysfunction detected by echocardiography in acute pulmonary embolism. Am J Cardiol 78:469, 1996.
84a. Chartier L, Béra J, Delomez M, et al: Free-floating thrombi in the right heart: diagnosis, management, and prognostic indexes in 38 consecutive patients. Circulation 99:2779, 1999.
85. Pruszczyk P, Torbicki A, Pacho R, et al: Noninvasive diagnosis of suspected severe pulmonary embolism: transesophageal echocardiography vs spiral CT. Chest 112:722, 1997.
86. Teigen CL, Maus TP, Sheedy PF II, et al: Pulmonary embolism: diagnosis with contrast-enhanced electron-beam CT and comparison with pulmonary angiography. Radiology 194:313, 1995.
87. Remy-Jardin M, Remy J, Wattinne L, et al: Central pulmonary thromboembolism: diagnosis with spiral volumetric CT with the single-breath-hold technique—comparison with pulmonary angiography. Radiology 185:381, 1992.
88. Remy-Jardin M, Remy J, Deschildre F, et al: Diagnosis of pulmonary embolism with spiral CT: comparison with pulmonary angiography and scintigraphy. Radiology 200:699, 1996.
89. Ferretti GR, Bosson J-L, Buffaz P-D, et al: Acute pulmonary embolism: role of helical CT in 164 patients with intermediate probability at ventilation-perfusion scintigraphy and normal results at duplex US of the legs. Radiology 205:453, 1997.
89a. Garg K, Welsh CH, Feyerabend AJ, et al: Pulmonary embolism: diagnosis with spiral CT and ventilation-perfusion scanning—correlation with pulmonary angiographic results or clinical outcome. Radiology 208:201, 1998.
90. Goodman LR, Lipchik RJ: Diagnosis of acute pulmonary embolism: time for a new approach. Radiology 199:25, 1996.
91. Mayo JR, Remy-Jardin M, Müller NL, et al: Pulmonary embolism: prospective comparison of spiral CT with ventilation-perfusion scintigraphy. Radiology 205:447, 1997.
92. Cross JJL, Kemp PM, Walsh CG, et al: A randomized trial of spiral CT and ventilation perfusion scintigraphy for the diagnosis of pulmonary embolism. Clin Radiol 53:177, 1998.
93. Hansell DM, Flower CDR: Imaging pulmonary embolism: a new look with spiral computed tomography. BMJ 316:490, 1998.
94. Goldhaber SZ: Pulmonary embolism. N Engl J Med 339:93, 1998.
95. White RD, Winkler ML, Higgins CB: MR imaging of pulmonary arterial hypertension and pulmonary emboli. AJR 149:15, 1987.
95a. Gupta A, Frazer CK, Ferguson JM, et al: Acute pulmonary embolism: diagnosis with MR angiography. Radiology 210:353, 1999.
96. Meaney JFM, Weg JG, Chenevert TL, et al: Diagnosis of pulmonary embolism with magnetic resonance angiography. N Engl J Med 336:1422, 1997.

97. Ellis D: Acute pulmonary embolism: advances in imaging. Br J Hosp Med 58:303, 1997.
97a. Evans AJ, Sostman HD, Witty LA, et al: Detection of deep venous thrombosis: prospective comparison of MR imaging and sonography. J Magn Reson Imaging 6:44, 1996.
98. Cronan JJ: Venous thromboembolic disease: the role of US. Radiology 186:619, 1993.
99. Turkstra F, Kuijer PMM, van Beek EJR, et al: Diagnostic utility of ultrasonography of leg veins in patients suspected of having pulmonary embolism. Ann Intern Med 126:775, 1997.
100. Lensing AWA, Doris CI, McGrath FP, et al: A comparison of compression ultrasound with color Doppler ultrasound for the diagnosis of symptomless postoperative deep vein thrombosis. Arch Intern Med 157:765, 1997.
101. Birdwell BG, Raskob GE, Whitsett TL, et al: The clinical validity of normal compression ultrasonography in outpatients suspected of having deep venous thrombosis. Ann Intern Med 128:1, 1998.
102. Kearon C, Julian JA, Math M, et al: Noninvasive diagnosis of deep venous thrombosis. Ann Intern Med 128:663, 1998.
103. Hull RD, Hirsch J, Carter CJ, et al: Diagnostic efficacy of impedance plethysmography for clinically suspected deep-vein thrombosis. Ann Intern Med 102:21, 1985.
104. Weinmann EE, Salzman EW: Deep-vein thrombosis. N Engl J Med 331:1630, 1994.
105. Hull R, Hirsh J, Sackett DL, et al: Clinical validity of a negative venogram in patients with clinically suspected venous thrombosis. Circulation 64:622, 1981.
106. Agnelli G, Ranucci V, Veschi F, et al: Clinical outcome of orthopedic patients with negative lower limb venography at discharge. Thromb Haemost 74:1042, 1995.
107. Bone RC: Ventilation/perfusion scan in pulmonary embolism: the emperor is incompletely attired. JAMA 263:2794, 1990.
108. Stein PD, Dalen JE, Goldhaber SZ, et al: Opinions regarding the diagnosis and management of venous thromboembolic disease. Chest 109:233, 1996.
109. Toglia MR, Weg JG: Venous thromboembolism during pregnancy. N Engl J Med 335:108, 1996.
110. Anderson D, Gross M, Robinson S, et al: Ultrasonography screening for deep vein thrombosis following arthroplasty fails to reduce posthospital thromboembolic complications: the Postarthroplasty Screening Study (PASS). Chest 114:119S, 1998.
111. Moser KM, Shure D, Harrell JH, et al: Angioscopic visualization of pulmonary emboli. Chest 2:198, 1980.
112. Beckman D, Solmos B, Herod G, et al: Intraoperative pulmonary angioscopy using the flexible fiberoptic choledochoscope. Ann Thorac Surg 41:563, 1986.
113. Uchida Y, Oshima T, Hirose J, et al: Angioscopic detection of residual pulmonary thrombi in the differential diagnosis of pulmonary embolism. Am Heart J 130:854, 1995.
114. Sagar KB, Rhyne TL, Greenfield LJ: Intravascular ultrasound. Circulation 67:365, 1983.
115. Good CA, Holman CB: Cavitary carcinoma of the lung: roentgenographic features in 19 cases. Dis Chest 37:289, 1960.
116. Dodd GD, Boyle JJ: Excavating pulmonary metastases. AJR 85:277, 1961.
117. Sherrick DW, Kincaid OW, DuShane JW: Agenesis of a main branch of the pulmonary artery. AJR 87:917, 1962.
118. Ahdout DJ, Damani P, Ultan LB: Recurrent acute pulmonary emboli in association with acute myocardial infarction. Chest 96:682, 1989.
119. Barritt DW, Jordan SC: Clinical features of pulmonary embolism. Lancet 1:729, 1961.
120. Richards P: Pulmonary oedema and intracranial lesions. BMJ 2:83, 1963.
121. Surawicz B: Electrocardiographic pattern of cerebrovascular accident. JAMA 197:913, 1966.
122. Ireland P, Sapira JD, Templeton B: Munchausen's syndrome: review and report of an additional case. Am J Med 43:579, 1967.
123. Bluemie LWJ: Acute tubular necrosis: analysis of one hundred cases with respect to mortality, complications, and treatment with and without dialysis. Arch Intern Med 104:180, 1959.
124. Krachman SL, Lodato RF, D'Alonzo GE: Managing the acute chest syndrome in sickle cell patients. J Crit Illness 9:375, 1994.
125. Stahl RL, Javid JP, Lackner H: Unrecognized pulmonary embolism presenting as disseminated intravascular coagulation. Am J Med 76:772, 1984.
126. Fred HL, Allred DP, Garber HE, et al: Pheochromocytoma masquerading as overwhelming infection. Am Heart J 73:149, 1967.
127. Richmond J, Frazer SC, Millar DR: Paroxysmal hypotension due to an adrenaline-secreting phaeochromocytoma. Lancet 2:904, 1961.
128. Sproule BJ, Phillipson EA, Couves CM, et al: Acute pulmonary hypertension in idiopathic lactic acidosis. Can Med Assoc J 94:141, 1966.
129. Stephens JH, Fred HL: Petechiae associated with systemic fat embolism. Arch Dermatol 86:515, 1962.
130. Masson RG, Ruggieri J: Pulmonary microvascular cytology: a new diagnostic application of the pulmonary artery catheter. Chest 88:908, 1985.
131. Babar SI, Sobonya RE, Snyder LS: Pulmonary microvascular cytology for the diagnosis of pulmonary tumor embolism. West J Med 168:47, 1998.
132. Bailey H: Air embolism. J Int Coll Surg 25:675, 1956.
133. Hirsh J: Antithrombotic therapy in deep vein thrombosis and pulmonary embolism. Am Heart J 123:1115, 1992.
134. Clagett GP, Anderson FA, Heit J, et al: Prevention of venous thromboembolism. Chest 108:312, 1995.
135. Prevention of venous thromboembolism: international consensus statement (guidelines according to scientific evidence). Int Angiol 16:3, 1997.
136. Morehead RS, Tzouanakis AE, Berger R: Preventing VTE: a guide to nonpharmacologic therapies. J Crit Illness 13:486, 1998.
137. Halkin H, Goldberg J, Modan M, et al: Reduction of mortality in general medical in-patients by low-dose heparin prophylaxis. Ann Intern Med 96:561, 1982.
138. Collaborative overview of randomized trials of antiplatelet therapy—III: reduction in venous thrombosis and pulmonary embolism by antiplatelet prophylaxis among surgical and medical patients. BMJ 308:235, 1994.
139. Cohen AT, Skinner JA, Kakkar VV: Antiplatelet treatment for thromboprophylaxis: a step forward or backwards? BMJ 308:1213, 1994.
139a. Samama MM, Cohen AT, Darmon JY, et al: A comparison of enoxaparin with placebo for the prevention of venous thromboembolism in acutely ill medical patients. N Engl J Med 341:793, 1999.
140. Hirsch DR, Ingenito EP, Goldhaber SZ: Prevalence of deep venous thrombosis among patients in medical intensive care. JAMA 274:335, 1995.
141. Ryskamp RP, Trottier SJ: Utilization of venous thromboembolism prophylaxis in a medical-surgical ICU. Chest 113:162, 1998.
142. Goldhaber SZ: Venous thromboembolism in the intensive care unit: the last frontier for prophylaxis. Chest 113:5, 1998.
143. Abernathy EA, Hartsuck JM: Postoperative pulmonary embolism: a prospective study utilizing low dose heparin. Am J Surg 128:739, 1974.
144. Prevention of fatal postoperative pulmonary embolism by low doses of heparin: an international multicenter trial. Lancet 2:45, 1975.
145. Collins R, Scrimgeour A, Yusuf S, et al: Reduction in fatal pulmonary embolism and venous thrombosis by perioperative administration of subcutaneous heparin: overview of results of randomized trials in general, orthopedic, and urologic surgery. N Engl J Med 318:1162, 1988.
146. Nurmohamed MT, Rosendaal FR, Büller HR, et al: Low-molecular-weight heparin versus standard heparin in general and orthopaedic surgery: a meta-analysis. Lancet 340:152, 1992.
147. Jørgensen LN, Wille-Jørgensen, Hauch O: Prophylaxis of postoperative thromboembolism with low molecular weight heparins. Br J Surg 80:689, 1993.
148. Bergqvist D, Matzch T, Burmark US, et al: Low molecular weight heparin given the evening before surgery compared with conventional low-dose heparin in prevention of thrombosis. Br J Surg 75:888, 1988.
149. Caen JP: A randomized double-blind study between a low molecular weight heparin Kabi 2165 and standard heparin in the prevention of deep vein thrombosis in general surgery: a French multicenter trial. Thromb Haemost 59:216, 1988.
150. Ramos R, Salem BI, De Pawlikowski MP, et al: The efficacy of pneumatic compression stockings in the prevention of pulmonary embolism after cardiac surgery. Chest 109:82, 1996.
151. Turpie AGG, Levine MN, Hirsch J, et al: A randomized controlled trial of a low-molecular-weight heparin (enoxaparin) to prevent deep-vein thrombosis in patients undergoing elective hip surgery. N Engl J Med 315:925, 1986.

152. Mohr DN, Silverstein MD, Murtaugh PA, et al: Prophylactic agents for venous thrombosis in elective hip surgery: meta-analysis of studies using venographic assessment. Arch Intern Med 153:2221, 1993.
153. Leclerc JR, Gent M, Hirsh J, et al: The incidence of symptomatic venous thromboembolism during and after prophylaxis with enoxaparin: a multi-institutional cohort study of patients who underwent hip or knee arthroplasty. Arch Intern Med 158:873, 1998.
154. Hirsh J: Evidence for the needs of out-of-hospital thrombosis prophylaxis: introduction. Chest 114:113S, 1998.
155. de Valk HW, Banga JD, Wester JWJ, et al: Comparing subcutaneous danaparoid with intravenous unfractionated heparin for the treatment of venous thromboembolism: a randomized controlled trial. Ann Intern Med 123:1, 1995.
156. Eriksson BI, Ekman S, Kälebo P, et al: Prevention of deep-vein thrombosis after total hip replacement: direct thrombin inhibition with recombinant hirudin, CGP 39393. Lancet 347:635, 1996.
157. Eriksson BI, Wille-Jørgensen P, Kälebo P, et al: A comparison of recombinant hirudin with a low-molecular-weight heparin to prevent thromboembolic complications after total hip replacement. N Engl J Med 337:1329, 1997.
158. Leyvraz PF, Richard J, Bachman F, et al: Adjusted- versus fixed-dose subcutaneous heparin in the prevention of deep vein thrombosis after total hip replacement. N Engl J Med 309:954, 1983.
159. Hamilton HW, Crawford JS, Gardiner JH, et al: Venous thrombosis in patients with fracture of the upper end of the femur. J Bone Joint Surg Br 52:268, 1970.
160. Imperiale TF, Speroff T: A meta-analysis of methods to prevent venous thromboembolism following total hip replacement. JAMA 271:1780, 1994.
161. Hull RD, Raskob GE, Gent M, et al: Effectiveness of intermittent pneumatic leg compression for preventing deep vein thrombosis after total hip replacement. JAMA 263:2313, 1990.
162. Leclerc JR, Geerts WH, Desjardins L, et al: Prevention of venous thromboembolism after knee arthroplasty: a randomized, double-blind trial comparing enoxaparin with warfarin. Ann Intern Med 124:619, 1996.
163. Levine MN, Gent M, Hirsh J, et al: Ardeparin (low-molecular-weight heparin) vs graduated compression stockings for the prevention of venous thromboembolism: a randomized trial in patients undergoing knee surgery. Arch Intern Med 156:851, 1996.
164. Chandhoke PS, Gooding GAW, Narayan P: Prospective randomized trial of warfarin and intermittent pneumatic leg compression as prophylaxis for postoperative deep venous thrombosis in major urological surgery. J Urol 147:1056, 1992.
165. Turpie AGG, Hirsh J, Gent M, et al: Prevention of deep vein thrombosis in potential neurosurgical patients: a randomized trial comparing graduated compression stockings alone or graduated compression stockings plus intermittent pneumatic compression with control. Arch Intern Med 149:679, 1989.
166. Agnelli G, Piovella F, Buoncristiani P, et al: Enoxaparin plus compression stockings compared with compression stockings alone in the prevention of venous thromboembolism after elective neurosurgery. N Engl J Med 339:80, 1998.
167. Catre MG: Anticoagulation in spinal surgery: a critical review of the literature. Can J Surg 40:413, 1997.
168. Geerts WH, Jay RM, Code KI, et al: A comparison of low-dose heparin with low-molecular-weight heparin as prophylaxis against venous thromboembolism after major trauma. N Engl J Med 335:701, 1996.
169. Green D, Lee MY, Ito VY, et al: Fixed- vs adjusted-dose heparin in the prophylaxis of thromboembolism in spinal cord injury. JAMA 260:1255, 1988.
170. Hunt BJ, Doughty HA, Majumdar G, et al: Thromboprophylaxis with low molecular weight heparin (Fragmin) in high risk pregnancies. Thromb Haemost 77:39, 1997.
171. Hirsh J, Dalen JE, Deykin D, et al: Heparin: mechanism of action, pharmacokinetics, dosing considerations, monitoring, efficacy, and safety. Chest 102:337S, 1992.
172. Brill-Edwards P, Ginsberg S, Johnston M, et al: Establishing a therapeutic range for heparin therapy. Ann Intern Med 119:104, 1993.
173. Hull RD, Raskob GE, Hirsh J, et al: Continuous intravenous heparin compared with intermittent subcutaneous heparin in the initial treatment of proximal-vein thrombosis. N Engl J Med 315:1109, 1986.
174. Cruickshank MK, Levine MN, Hirsh J, et al: A standard heparin nomogram for the management of heparin therapy. Arch Intern Med 151:333, 1991.
175. Raschke RA, Reilly BM, Guidry JR, et al: The weight-based heparin dosing nomogram compared with a "standard care" nomogram: a randomized controlled trial. Ann Intern Med 119:874, 1993.
176. Hull RD, Raskob GE, Brant RF, et al: Relation between the time to achieve the lower limit of the APTT therapeutic range and recurrent venous thromboembolism during heparin treatment for deep vein thrombosis. Arch Intern Med 157:2562, 1997.
177. Hull RD, Raskob GE, Rosenbloom D, et al: Heparin for 5 days as compared with 10 days in the initial treatment of proximal venous thrombosis. N Engl J Med 322:1260, 1990.
178. Tapson VF, Hull RD: Management of venous thromboembolic disease: the impact of low-molecular-weight heparin. Clin Chest Med 16:281, 1995.
179. Levine M, Gent M, Hirsh J, et al: A comparison of low-molecular-weight heparin administered primarily at home with unfractionated heparin administered in the hospital for proximal deep-vein thrombosis. N Engl J Med 334:677, 1996.
180. Koopman MMW, Prandoni P, Piovella F, et al: Treatment of venous thrombosis with intravenous unfractionated heparin administered in the hospital as compared with subcutaneous low-molecular-weight heparin administered at home. N Engl J Med 334:682, 1996.
181. Weitz JI: Low-molecular-weight heparins. N Engl J Med 337:688, 1997.
182. Koopman MMW, Büller HR: Low-molecular-weight heparins in the treatment of venous thromboembolism. Ann Intern Med 128:1037, 1998.
183. Antman EM, Handin R: Low-molecular-weight heparins: an intriguing new twist with profound implications. Circulation 98:287, 1998.
183a. Aguilar D, Goldhaber SZ: Clinical uses of low-molecular-weight heparins. Chest 115:1418, 1999.
184. Schafer AI: Low-molecular weight heparin: an opportunity for home treatment of venous thrombosis. N Engl J Med 334:724, 1996.
185. Simonneau G, Sors H, Charbonnier B, et al: A comparison of low-molecular-weight heparin with unfractionated heparin for acute pulmonary embolism. N Engl J Med 337:663, 1997.
186. The Columbus Investigators: Low-molecular-weight heparin in the treatment of patients with venous thromboembolism. N Engl J Med 337:657, 1997.
187. Hirsh J, Dalen JE, Deykin D, et al: Oral anticoagulants: mechanism of action, clinical effectiveness, and optimal therapeutic range. Chest 102:312S, 1992.
188. Gallus A, Tillett H, Jackaman J, et al: Safety and efficacy of warfarin started early after submassive venous thrombosis or pulmonary embolism. Lancet 2:1293, 1986.
189. Rosiello RA, Chan CK, Tencza F, et al: Timing of oral anticoagulation therapy in the treatment of angiographically proven acute pulmonary embolism. Arch Intern Med 147:1469, 1987.
190. Schulman S, Rhedin A-S, Lindmarker P, et al: A comparison of six weeks with six months of oral anticoagulant therapy after a first episode of venous thromboembolism. N Engl J Med 332:1661, 1995.
191. Khamashta MA, Cuadrado MJ, Mujic F, et al: The management of thrombosis in the antiphospholipid-antibody syndrome. N Engl J Med 332:993, 1995.
192. Hull RD, Pineo GF: Current concepts of anticoagulation therapy. Clin Chest Med 16:269, 1995.
193. Research Committee of the British Thoracic Society: Optimum duration of anticoagulation for deep-vein thrombosis and pulmonary embolism. Lancet 340:873, 1992.
194. Hirsh J: The optimal duration of anticoagulant therapy for venous thrombosis. N Engl J Med 332:1710, 1995.
194a. Kearon C, Gent M, Hirsh J, et al: A comparison of three months of anticoagulation with extended anticoagulation for a first episode of idopathic venous thromboembolism. N Engl J Med 340:901, 1999.
194b. Schafer AI: Venous thrombosis as a chronic disease. N Engl J Med 340:955, 1999.
195. Urokinase Pulmonary Embolism Trial: phase I results. JAMA 214:2163, 1970.
196. Urokinase-Streptokinase Embolism Trial: phase 2 results. JAMA 16:1606, 1974.
197. Goldhaber SZ, Kessler CM, Heit J, et al: A randomized controlled

trial of recombinant tissue-type plasminogen activator versus urokinase in the treatment of acute pulmonary embolism. Lancet 2:293, 1988.

198. Meyer G, Sors H, Charbonnier B, et al: Effects of intravenous urokinase versus alteplase on total pulmonary resistance in acute massive pulmonary embolism: a European multicenter double-blind trial. J Am Coll Cardiol 19:239, 1992.

198a. Arcasoy SM, Kreit JW: Thrombolytic therapy of pulmonary embolism: a comprehensive review of current evidence. Chest 115:1695, 1999.

199. Come PC, Kim D, Parker JA, et al: Early reversal of right ventricular dysfunction in patients with acute pulmonary embolism after treatment with intravenous tissue plasminogen activator. J Am Coll Cardiol 10:971, 1987.

200. Dalen JE, Alpert JS, Hirsh J: Thrombolytic therapy for pulmonary embolism: is it effective? is it safe? when is it indicated? Arch Intern Med 157:2550, 1997.

201. Levine M, Hirsh J, Weitz J, et al: A randomized trial of a single bolus dosage regimen of recombinant tissue plasminogen activator in patients with acute pulmonary embolism. Chest 98:1473, 1990.

202. PIOPED Investigators: Tissue plasminogen activator for the treatment of acute pulmonary embolism. Chest 97:528, 1990.

203. Dalla-Volta S, Palla A, Santolicandro A, et al: PAIMS 2: alteplase combined with heparin versus heparin in the treatment of acute pulmonary embolism. Plasminogen Activator Italian Multicenter Study 2. J Am Coll Cardiol 20:520, 1992.

203a. Ahearn GS, Hadjiliadis D, Tapson VF, et al: Thrombolytic therapy with tissue plasminogen activator (TPA) in the first trimester of pregnancy after massive pulmonary embolism (PE). Chest 116:405S, 1999.

204. Gruppo Italiano Per Lo Studio Della Streptochinasi Nell'infarto Miocardio (GISSI): Effectiveness of intravenous thrombolytic treatment in acute myocardial infarction. Lancet 1:397, 1986.

205. Randomized trial of intravenous streptokinase, oral aspirin, both, or neither among 17,187 cases of suspected acute myocardial infarction: ISIS-2. Lancet 2:349, 1988.

206. Bobbio M, Bergerone S, Maggioni AP, et al: Administration of thrombolytic therapy to 17944 patients with acute myocardial infarction: the GISSI-3 database. Am Heart J 135:443, 1998.

207. Daniels LB, Parker JA, Patel SR, et al: Relation of duration of symptoms with response to thrombolytic therapy in pulmonary embolism. Am J Cardiol 80:184, 1997.

208. Bomalski JS, Martin GJ, Hughes RL, et al: Inferior vena cava interruption in the management of pulmonary embolism. Chest 82:767, 1982.

209. Greenfield LJ, Proctor MC: Current indications for caval interruption: should they be liberalized in view of improving technology? Semin Vasc Surg 9:50, 1996.

210. Dorfman G: Percutaneous inferior vena caval filters. Radiology 174:987, 1990.

211. Grassi CJ: Inferior vena caval filters: analysis of five currently available devices. AJR 156:813, 1991.

212. Whitehill TA: Caval interruption methods: comparison of options. Semin Vasc Surg 9:59, 1996.

213. Bovyn G, Gory P, Reynaud P, et al: The Tempofilter: a multicenter study of a new temporary caval filter implantable for up to six weeks. Ann Vasc Surg 11:520, 1997.

214. Neill AM, Appleton DS, Richards P: Retrievable inferior vena caval filter for thromboembolic disease in pregnancy. Br J Obstet Gynaecol 104:1416, 1997.

215. Vos LD, Tielbeek AV, Bom EP, et al: The Gunther temporary inferior vena cava filter for short-term protection against pulmonary embolism. Cardiovasc Intervent Radiol 20:91, 1997.

216. Neuerburg JM, Gunther RW, Vorwerk D, et al: Results of a multicenter study of the retrievable Tulip vena cava filter: early clinical experience. Cardiovasc Intervent Radiol 20:10, 1997.

217. Mansour M, Chang AE, Sindelar WF: Interruption of the inferior vena cava for the prevention of recurrent pulmonary embolism. Am Surg 51:375, 1985.

218. Cohen JR, Tenenbaum N, Citron M: Greenfield filter as primary therapy for deep venous thrombosis and/or pulmonary embolism in patients with cancer. Surgery 109:12, 1991.

219. Arnold TE, Karabinis VD, Mehta V, et al: Potential for overuse of the inferior vena cava filter. Surg Gynecol Obstet 177:463, 1993.

220. Decousus H, Leizorovicz A, Parent F, et al: A clinical trial of vena caval filters in the prevention of pulmonary embolism in patients with proximal deep-vein thrombosis. N Engl J Med 338:409, 1998.

221. Rogers FB, Strindberg G, Shackford SR, et al: Five-year follow-up of prophylactic vena cava filters in high-risk trauma patients. Arch Surg 133:406, 1998.

222. Haire WD: Vena caval filters for the prevention of pulmonary embolism. N Engl J Med 338:463, 1998.

223. Alberts WM, Tonner JA, Goldman AL: Echocardiography in planned interruption of the inferior vena cava. South Med J 82:772, 1989.

224. Stoschitzky K, Stark G, Dacar D: Massive pulmonary embolism. N Engl J Med 337:1561, 1997.

225. Glassford DJ Jr, Alford WC Jr, Burrus GR, et al: Pulmonary embolectomy. Ann Thorac Surg 32:28, 1981.

226. Crane C, Hartsuck J, Birtch A, et al: The management of major pulmonary embolism. Surg Gynecol Obstet 128:27, 1969.

227. Sautter RD, Myers WO, Ray JF III, et al: Pulmonary embolectomy: review and current status. Prog Cardiovasc Dis 17:371, 1975.

228. Fred HL, Natelson EA: Selection of patients for pulmonary embolectomy. Dis Chest 56:139, 1969.

229. Timsit J-F, Reynaud P, Meyer G, et al: Pulmonary embolectomy by catheter device in massive pulmonary embolism. Chest 100:655, 1991.

230. Greenfield LJ, Proctor MC, Williams DM, et al: Long-term experience with transvenous catheter pulmonary embolectomy. J Vasc Surg 18:450, 1993.

231. Gray HH, Miller GAH, Paneth M: Pulmonary embolectomy: its place in the management of pulmonary embolism. Lancet 1:1441, 1988.

232. Koning R, Cribier AC, Gerber L, et al: A new treatment for severe pulmonary embolism: percutaneous rheolytic thrombectomy. Circulation 96:2498, 1997.

233. Fava M, Loyola S, Flores P, et al: Mechanical fragmentation and pharmacologic thrombolysis in massive pulmonary embolism. J Vasc Interv Radiol 8:261, 1997.

234. Moser KM, Auger WR, Fedullo PF, et al: Chronic thromboembolic pulmonary hypertension: clinical picture and surgical treatment. Eur Respir J 5:334, 1992.

235. Jamieson SW: Pulmonary thromboendarterectomy. Heart 79:118, 1998.

236. Fred HL, Axelrad MA, Lewis J, et al: Rapid resolution of pulmonary thromboemboli in man: an angiographic study. JAMA 196:1137, 1966.

237. Dalen JE, Banas JSJ, Brooks HL, et al: Resolution rate of acute pulmonary emboli in man. N Engl J Med 280:1194, 1969.

238. Sautter RD, Fletcher FW, Ousley JL, et al: Extremely rapid resolution of a pulmonary embolus: report of a case. Dis Chest 52:825, 1967.

239. Carson JL, Kelley MA, Duff A, et al: The clinical course of pulmonary embolism. N Engl J Med 326:1240, 1992.

240. Donaldson GA, Williams C, Scannell JG, et al: A reappraisal of the application of the Trendelenberg operation to massive fatal embolism: report of a successful pulmonary-artery thrombectomy using a cardiopulmonary bypass. N Engl J Med 268:171, 1963.

241. Douketis JD, Kearon C, Bates S, et al: Risk of fatal pulmonary embolism in patients with treated venous thromboembolism. JAMA 279:458, 1998.

242. Paraskos JA, Adelstein SJ, Smith RE, et al: Late prognosis of acute pulmonary embolism. N Engl J Med 289:55, 1973.

243. Hall RJC, Sutton GC, Kerr IH: Long-term prognosis of treated acute massive pulmonary embolism. Br Heart J 39:1128, 1977.

244. De Bakey ME: A critical evaluation of the problem of thromboembolism. Surg Gynecol Obstet 98:1, 1954.

CHAPTER 100

PULMONARY HYPERTENSION

E. Kenneth Weir, Evangelos D. Michelakis, Stephen L. Archer, and Lewis J. Rubin

DEFINITION
PREVALENCE
PATHOPHYSIOLOGY OF PULMONARY HYPERTENSION
Elevated Left Heart Filling Pressures
Hyperkinetic Pulmonary Hypertension
Obstructive and Obliterative Pulmonary Hypertension
CLINICAL RECOGNITION
Historical Assessment of Pulmonary Hypertension
Review of Systems
Physical Examination
Use of Laboratory Tests to Assess Pulmonary Hypertension
NONINVASIVE ASSESSMENT OF THE PULMONARY CIRCULATION
Electrocardiography
Chest Radiography
Echocardiography
Magnetic Resonance Imaging
Computed Tomography
Exercise Testing
CARDIAC CATHETERIZATION
Technical Considerations
Risks
NUCLEAR MEDICINE
Ventilation/Perfusion Scans
Thallium Scintigraphy
PULMONARY ANGIOGRAPHY
Technique
Complications
LUNG BIOPSY
MANAGEMENT OF PULMONARY HYPERTENSION
General Measures
Specific Measures
Medical Management
Surgical Management
PROGNOSIS AND NATURAL HISTORY

DEFINITION

Pulmonary hypertension is a syndrome, not a disease. The elevation of pulmonary arterial pressure (PAP) can be a complication of many diseases. Even primary pulmonary hypertension (PPH) is not a single entity, and it is hoped in the near future that the etiologic mechanisms responsible for the several forms of PPH will be understood. The decision as to what level of PAP constitutes pulmonary hypertension is somewhat arbitrary. In the case of the PPH Registry initiated by the National Heart, Lung, and Blood Institute in 1981, pulmonary hypertension was defined as a mean PAP greater than 25 mm Hg at rest or 30 mm Hg on exercise. However, PAP varies with age, and the range of normal values provides a more precise indication of what should be considered to be pulmonary hypertension. Between days 1 and 3 of neonatal life, the mean PAP falls to 26 ± 4 (SD) mm Hg.[1] From 6 to 45 years of age, it remains constant at approximately 14 ± 3 mm Hg, increasing to 16 ± 3 mm Hg between 60 and 83 years. Consequently, the mean +2 SDs provides an upper limit of normal of 20 mm Hg from childhood to approximately 60 years of age. The upper limit for the pulmonary vascular resistance (PVR) index (PAP − wedge pressure/cardiac index) in normal subjects increases from approximately 2.8 mm Hg/L/min/m^2 (6 to 10 years) to 3.2 (32 to 45 years) to 4.6 (60 to 83 years).

During exercise, both PAP and wedge pressures are elevated. In normal young men and women, PAP increases from 14 ± 3 mm Hg at rest to 29 ± 5 mm Hg on heavy exertion, whereas wedge pressure rises from 8 ± 3 to 16 ± 5 mm Hg.[2] Thus, mean PAP on exercise in normal young subjects can exceed the cutoff point of 30 mm Hg used by the PPH Registry to define pulmonary hypertension. In healthy older men (61 to 83 years), the mean PAP can be more than 40 mm Hg during exercise. Because of the increase in wedge pressure and cardiac output, PVR does not increase on exertion in normal subjects.[2] It is important to consider age, level of exercise, and normal values before a diagnosis of pulmonary hypertension is made on the basis of PAP measurements obtained during exercise.

PREVALENCE

What is the prevalence of pulmonary hypertension in the general population? Based on a measurement of the diameter of the right descending pulmonary artery, it has been suggested that a mean PAP above 20 mm Hg is present in about 13 percent of men between 35 and 44 years of age and that this percentage doubles by the age of 65 to 74 years (28 percent).[3] If the criterion for pulmonary hypertension is raised to 25 mm Hg, the prevalence becomes 10 and 25 percent, respectively, for these two age groups. Although this level of pulmonary hypertension may seem relatively insignificant, it can provide important prognostic information. In a study of survival in patients with chronic obstructive pulmonary disease (COPD), 87 percent of those whose mean PAP was less than 20 mm Hg survived for 4 years. Only half as many lived for 4 years when the mean PAP was between 21 and 30 mm Hg.[4]

PATHOPHYSIOLOGY OF PULMONARY HYPERTENSION

In mechanistic terms, the subdivisions of pulmonary hypertension described by Paul Wood in the 1950s remain a useful conceptual framework.[5] These subdivisions are as follows:

1. Passive, usually related to elevated left heart filling pressures
2. Hyperkinetic, usually secondary to high blood flow through the lungs
3. Obstructive or obliterative, usually associated with either intravascular obstruction, such as emboli, or loss of vessels, as in emphysema or pulmonary fibrosis
4. Vasoconstrictive, a mechanism that rarely occurs in isolation (perhaps in acute hypoxia) but may provide a "reactive" element superimposed on the other causes

Elevated Left Heart Filling Pressures

An increase in PAP directly related to an increase in left atrial (LA) pressure is relatively easy to understand. Dilatation and medial hypertrophy of the pulmonary veins and eccentric intimal fibrosis are seen in patients with elevated LA pressures (Table 100–1). Capillary congestion may be present, and thickening of the capillary basement membrane occurs when pulmonary venous pressure is chronically elevated.[6] Hemosiderin deposition is the result of rupture of bronchial veins[7] or capillary stress failure.[8]

When pulmonary capillary wedge pressure exceeds 20 mm Hg, there usually is an additional rise in mean PAP,[9] the "reactive" component of pulmonary hypertension mentioned by Wood.[5] This is caused by constriction of the small pulmonary arteries, which can be attenuated in an experimental model by the use of an alpha-adrenergic blocker such as phentolamine.[10] In patients with mitral stenosis, acetylcholine often transiently reduces the vasoconstriction.[11] Pulmonary hypertension secondary to elevated left heart filling pressures has three components: a passive rise in pressure, reactive vasoconstriction, and structural remodeling of the pulmonary arterial and venous beds. Alleviation of the high downstream pressure usually results in a rapid return toward normal PAPs as the passive and reactive components are reversed.[12]

TABLE 100–1 Passive Pulmonary Hypertension: Elevated Left Heart Filling Pressures

Left ventricular increased diastolic pressure
Atherosclerotic heart disease
Hypertensive cardiovascular disease
Aortic valve disease, coarctation of the aorta
Cardiomyopathy
Mitral regurgitation
Constrictive pericarditis
Left atrial hypertension
Mitral stenosis
Left atrial tumor or thrombosis
Cor triatriatum, supravalvar mitral ring
Pulmonary venous obstruction
Mediastinal fibrosis and tumors
Congenital pulmonary vein stenosis
Anomalous pulmonary venous drainage with obstruction

Hyperkinetic Pulmonary Hypertension

When normal subjects exercise so that pulmonary flow reaches 23 L/min, the mean PAP is approximately 31 mm Hg, whereas PVR is normal at 0.6 mm Hg/L/min.[2] Similarly, when pulmonary blood flow is increased as a result of a left-to-right shunt at the atrial level, pulmonary hypertension may reflect only high flow rather than vasoconstriction or remodeling. However, if the high flow is the result of a nonrestrictive ventricular septal defect or a patent ductus arteriosus, the pulmonary circulation is directly exposed to the pressure generated by the left ventricle, in addition to the effect of the increased flow. Under these circumstances, the histologic changes induced by high flow and pressure may be superimposed on a failure of the remodeling of the small pulmonary arteries that usually occurs in the neonate. The normal involution of the thick arterial media, present in the fetus, fails to occur in the presence of pressure/flow overload.

The histologic changes in the pulmonary vasculature associated with high-flow shunts have been well described.[13, 14] The earlier forms include medial hypertrophy; the extension of smooth muscle into small, usually nonmuscular pulmonary arteries; intimal proliferation; and concentric intimal fibrosis. If the intimal fibrosis is mild, the histologic changes may regress after the shunt is closed.[15] Other arterial lesions associated with irreversible pulmonary hypertension include plexiform lesions, dilatation lesions, and necrotizing arteritis. A plexiform lesion from a 40-year-old man with Eisenmenger's syndrome due to a ventricular septal defect is shown in Figure 100–1. Scanning electron microscopy shows the endothelial surface to have deep twisted ridges.[16] It is interesting to note that intimal proliferation of myofibroblasts is also frequently observed in the pulmonary veins.[17]

The exact sequence of pathophysiologic events that results in Eisenmenger's syndrome is not known. However, it is likely that the high pressure and flow give rise to increased shear forces that cause endothelial dysfunction. This dysfunction can be manifest as a loss of response to endothelium-dependent dilators.[18]

Platelet deposition is enhanced at high shear rates.[19] Consequently, the production of thromboxane A_2 and 5-hydroxytryptamine can cause vasoconstriction, and platelet-derived growth factor (PDGF) release from the platelets may contribute to intimal proliferation. The production of chemotactic and growth factors by the endothelium is further evidence of endothelial dysfunction. The generation of factors that promote or inhibit migration and proliferation is normally tightly controlled.[20] The pathologic proliferation in the intima as described is due to the abnormal migration of smooth muscle cells from the media through the internal elastic lamina, to lie beneath the endothelium.[21] Proliferation of these cells and the laying down of collagen result in encroachment on the lumen of the small pulmonary arteries. Thrombosis occurs probably due to loss of

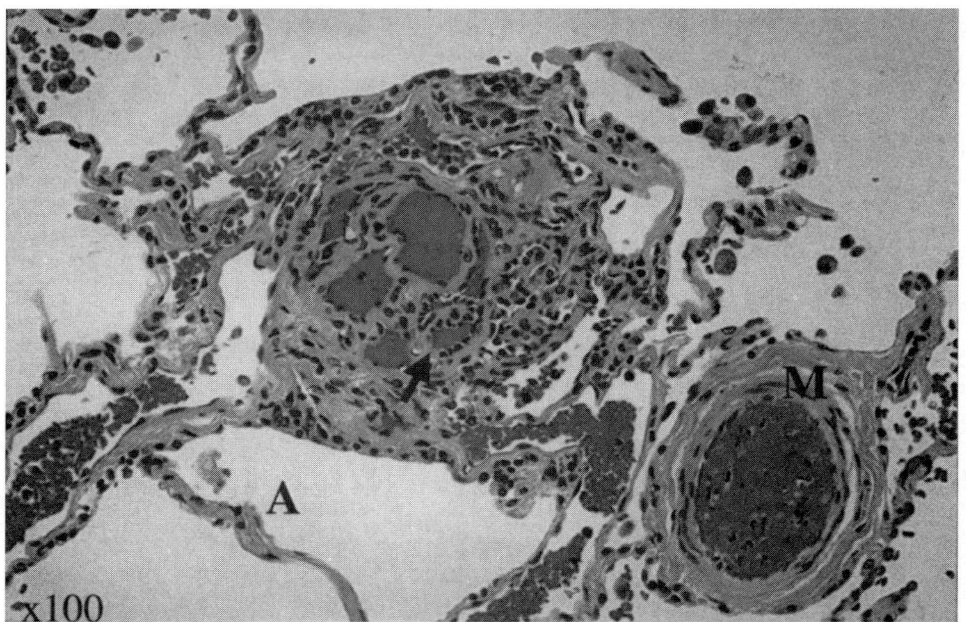

FIGURE 100–1 Plexogenic lesion from a 40-year-old man with Eisenmenger's syndrome due to a ventricular septal defect (H&E stain) shows a mass of proliferating endothelial cells obliterating the lumen *(arrow).* A, alveoli; M, media. (×100 magnification.)

the antithrombotic properties of the endothelium, such as prostacyclin and endothelium-derived relaxing factor (EDRF) production. Remodeling and thrombosis may lead to the loss of vessels, but this theory is controversial.[22]

Obstructive and Obliterative Pulmonary Hypertension

Vascular obstruction is common to many forms of pulmonary hypertension and may be primary (as in thromboembolic pulmonary hypertension) or may result from vascular remodeling. A condition such as thromboembolism of the major pulmonary arteries is the paradigm for the category of obstructive pulmonary hypertension. However, most causes fall under the "obstructive" heading. Pulmonary fibrosis as a cause of pulmonary hypertension comes under the "obliterative" heading, along with several other conditions. In the case of the left-to-right shunts associated with congenital heart disease, discussed earlier, pulmonary hypertension is induced via several mechanisms: the high-flow (*hyperkinetic*) mechanism, the vasoconstriction (*reactive*) mechanism, and the remodeling (*obstructive*) mechanism. The overlap in terms of responsible mechanisms is emphasized by the fact that vasoconstriction is an important secondary factor in many forms of pulmonary hypertension, in addition to obstruction or obliteration (Tables 100–2 to 100–4).

The histopathologic findings described in the pulmonary hypertension associated with intracardiac shunts are not specific. With minor variations, the pattern of plexogenic pulmonary arteriopathy can also be seen in pulmonary hypertension induced by toxic oil syndrome,[23] infection with human immunodeficiency virus,[24] familial platelet storage pool disease,[25] and schistosomiasis,[15] or associated with portal hypertension,[26] ingestion of anorectic drugs such as aminorex[27] or the fenfluramines,[28] and PPH.[14]

The cell proliferation, vasoconstriction, and thrombosis that characterize the plexogenic lesion can result from abnormalities in endothelial cells, smooth muscle cells, and

TABLE 100–2 Pulmonary Hypertension Secondary to Pulmonary Vascular Disease

Recurrent or massive pulmonary emboli
Tumor "microemboli"
Sickle cell disease
Schistosomiasis
Congenital heart disease with left-to-right shunt leading to Eisenmenger's syndrome
Peripheral pulmonary arterial stenoses
Vasculitis (scleroderma, mixed connective tissue disease, lupus erythematosus)
Granulomatous pulmonary arteritis (e.g., intravenous drug abuse)
Behçet's syndrome
Pulmonary vascular amyloidosis
Familial platelet storage pool disease
Toxic oil syndrome
Human immunodeficiency virus infection
Eosinophilia-myalgia syndrome
Pulmonary tuberous sclerosis?
Pulmonary lymphangiomyomatosis
Diet- or drug-induced pulmonary hypertension (e.g., aminorex, cocaine)
Primary pulmonary hypertension (PPH)
Portal hypertension associated with PPH

TABLE 100–3 Pulmonary Hypertension Secondary to Pulmonary Airway and Parenchymal Disease

Chronic obstructive pulmonary disease
Cystic fibrosis
Severe pulmonary fibrosis
  Sarcoidosis and other granulomatous lung diseases
  Diffuse interstitial fibrosis (e.g., radiation, Hamman-Rich syndrome, idiopathic)
  Pneumoconiosis
Adult respiratory distress syndrome
Pneumonectomy

TABLE 100–4 Pulmonary Hypertension Secondary to Hypoxia and/or Hypercapnia

High-altitude residence
Upper airway obstruction (e.g., enlarged tonsils, pharyngeal obstruction during sleep)
Primary hypoventilation
  Sleep-induced disorders of breathing
  Obesity-hypoventilation syndrome
  Primary alveolar hypoventilation
Neuromuscular disorders
  Myasthenia gravis
  Polio
  Mechanical hypoventilation (e.g., kyphoscoliosis)

platelets. The particular element that predominates in a given histologic picture may depend on several factors, such as the age and sex of the patient, the presence of coagulation or fibrinolytic defects, and the degree of vascular or platelet reactivity. This concept is illustrated in Figure 100–2 and has previously been discussed in more detail.[28] There is evidence implicating all three cell types in the pathogenesis of plexogenic arteriopathy and PPH.

The Endothelial Cell

Endothelium-dependent vasodilation is impaired in patients with PPH[29] and in the pulmonary arteries of those with end-stage COPD.[30] This impaired endothelial function is characterized by decreased production of vasodilation/antiproliferative factors as well as increased production of vasoconstriction/proliferation factors. In both the primary and several secondary forms of pulmonary hypertension, the urinary excretion of 6-keto-prostaglandin F_1 (a stable metabolite of prostacyclin) is diminished.[31] The expression of prostacyclin synthase has been found to be decreased in patients with severe pulmonary hypertension.[32] In addition, the expression of endothelial nitric oxide (NO) synthase is decreased in the lungs of patients with either primary or secondary pulmonary hypertension.[33] Given these observations on the underlying pathophysiology, it is logical that the "replacement" of endogenous EDRF by inhaled NO (a putative EDRF) or the infusion of prostacyclin should reduce pulmonary hypertension.[34, 36]

In contrast, increased expression[37] and circulating levels of the peptide endothelin-1 have been noted in patients with both PPH and some secondary forms of pulmonary hypertension.[38] Apart from its mainly vasoconstrictive effects, endothelin-1 also enhances smooth muscle proliferation.

What Is the Molecular Basis of the Endothelial Cell Dysfunction? Although injury of the endothelial cell frequently occurs in secondary pulmonary hypertension (e.g., due to the pressure overload and high flow in patients with Eisenmenger's syndrome), the cause of endothelial cell dysfunction in PPH is unclear.

The recognition that a viral illness can be associated with the histologic appearance of plexogenic pulmonary arteriopathy[24] raises the possibility that a viral infection might initiate PPH in some patients. Several viruses are capable of infecting vascular endothelial cells in culture.[39] Herpes simplex virus type 1 can inhibit proteoglycan synthesis by human vascular endothelial cells.[40] Proteoglycans are important in maintaining a nonthrombogenic surface and in inhibiting smooth muscle proliferation. Therefore, viral inhibition of proteoglycan synthesis could, in theory, explain the intimal proliferation and thrombosis seen in PPH. A viral etiology has been advanced for the rare form of PPH known as *pulmonary veno-occlusive disease.*[41]

Elegant studies have shown that the proliferating endothelial cells in primary, but not secondary, pulmonary hypertension are monoclonal. Using a microdissection technique, Lee and colleagues[42] selectively dissected

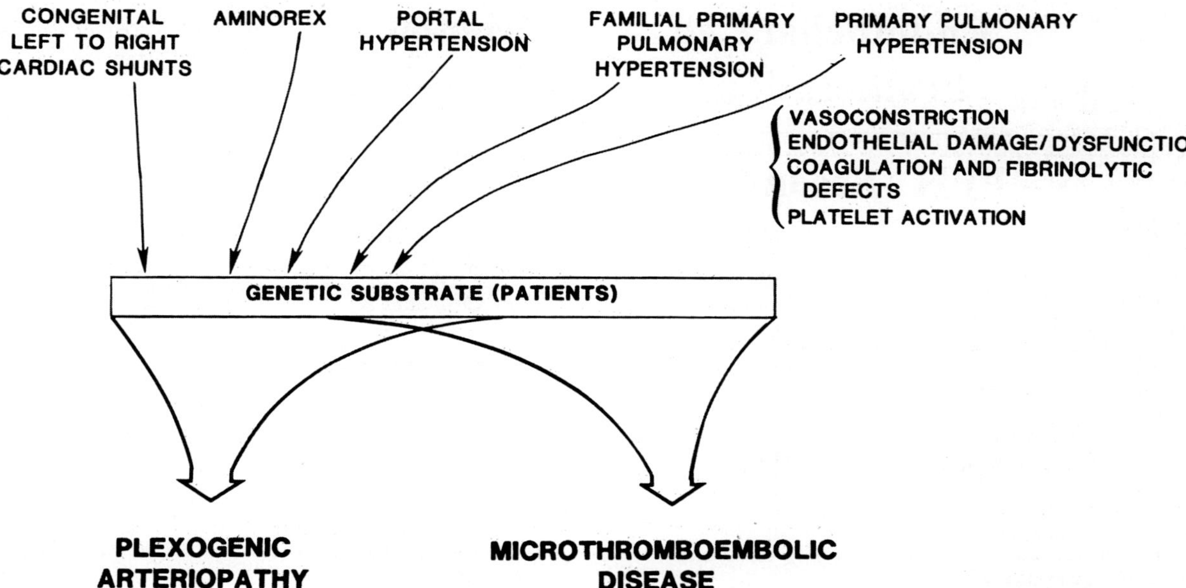

FIGURE 100–2 Common final pathways in some forms of pulmonary hypertension. A variety of stimuli may result in either plexogenic arteriopathy or microthromboembolic disease, or a combination of both, depending on factors such as the age and gender of the patient, genetic susceptibility, and others.

endothelial cells from plexogenic lesions from patients with primary or secondary pulmonary hypertension (Fig. 100–3). By assessing the methylation pattern of the human androgen receptor gene (HUMARA) with the use of polymerase chain reaction, they showed that endothelial cells from patients with PPH were monoclonal, whereas those from patients with secondary or no pulmonary hypertension were polyclonal (Fig. 100–3).[42]

These findings suggest that a somatic genetic alteration, similar to that present in neoplastic processes, may be responsible for the pathogenesis of PPH. They also provide a marker for the distinction between primary and secondary hypertension, an often difficult task for the pathologist.

The Smooth Muscle Cell

There is evidence of abnormalities intrinsic to the pulmonary arterial smooth muscle cells of patients with PPH. Yuan and associates[43] have shown that at least one voltage-gated potassium (K^+) channel (Kv) is downregulated in smooth muscle cells in PPH but not in secondary pulmonary hypertension.

What Is the Role of K^+ Channels in Vascular Smooth Muscle? K^+ channels are transmembrane proteins with a pore-forming unit that allows the selective efflux of K^+ ions from the cytoplasm. Based on pharmacologic and molecular criteria, K^+ channels in the vasculature are separated into three families: Kv, Calcium (Ca^{2+}) activated (K_{Ca}), and inward rectifier (Kir). When K^+ channels open, there is an efflux of K^+ ions from the cells down a concentration gradient (intracellular/extracellular K^+ concentration = 140/5 mEq), and the interior of the cell becomes more negatively charged (*hyperpolarization*). In contrast, when K^+ channels close, the cell becomes depolarized. Depolarization beyond a certain level, due to failure of the K^+ channels to open (whether because they are pharmacologically inhibited, mutated, or downregulated) causes opening of the voltage-gated L-type Ca^{2+} channels, influx of Ca^{2+}, activation of the actin-myosin complex, and contraction.[44]

In blood vessels, K^+ channel openers are vasodilators and K^+ channel inhibitors are vasconstrictors. For example, NO causes vasodilatation in part by opening the K_{Ca} channels.[45] In contrast, hypoxia causes pulmonary artery vaso-

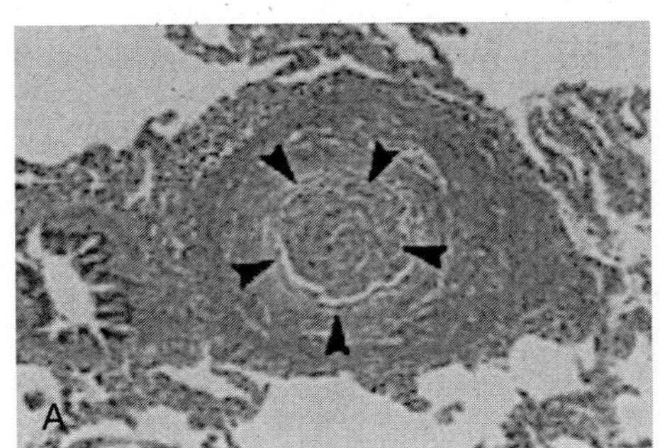

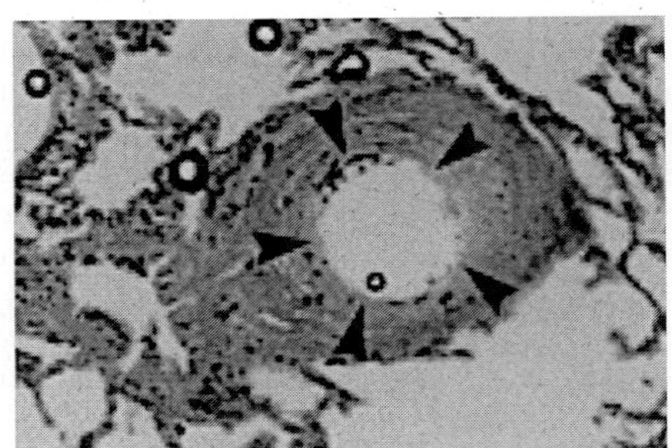

B

Endothelial Cell Proliferation

Medial hypertrophy

PPH Secondary PH

CLONALITY RATIO

1.0

0.75

0.5

0.25

0

FIGURE 100–3 **A,** In this plexiform lesion *(left)*, the investigators selectively harvested *(right)* the proliferating endothelial cells for subsequent polymerase chain reaction analysis *(arrowheads)* (H&E stain, 200×). **B,** Summary of clonality analysis with the human androgen receptor gene of endothelial cells and of hyperplastic smooth muscle cells from plexiform lesions. A clonality ratio of less than 0.25 is considered an index of monoclonality. In contrast to the endothelial cells from a patient with secondary pulmonary hypertension or the smooth muscle cells from a patient with primary or secondary hypertension, the endothelial cells of most primary pulmonary hypertension (PPH) lesions had very low clonality ratios (monoclonal). *Open squares,* small allele; *solid squares,* larger allele; *gray squares,* congenital heart disease (left-to-right shunt); *gray crosses,* CREST (*c*alcinosis cutis, *R*aynaud's phenomenon, *e*sophageal dysfunction, *s*clerodactyly, and *t*elangiectasia) syndrome; *Open circles,* smooth muscle cells from PPH lesions; *open triangles,* smooth muscle cells from secondary hypertension lesions. (**A** and **B,** Republished with permission of J Clin Invest from Lee SD, Shroyer KR, Markham NE, et al: Monoclonal endothelial cell proliferation is present in primary but not secondary pulmonary hypertension. J Clin Invest 101:927, 1998; permission conveyed through Copyright Clearance Center, Inc.)

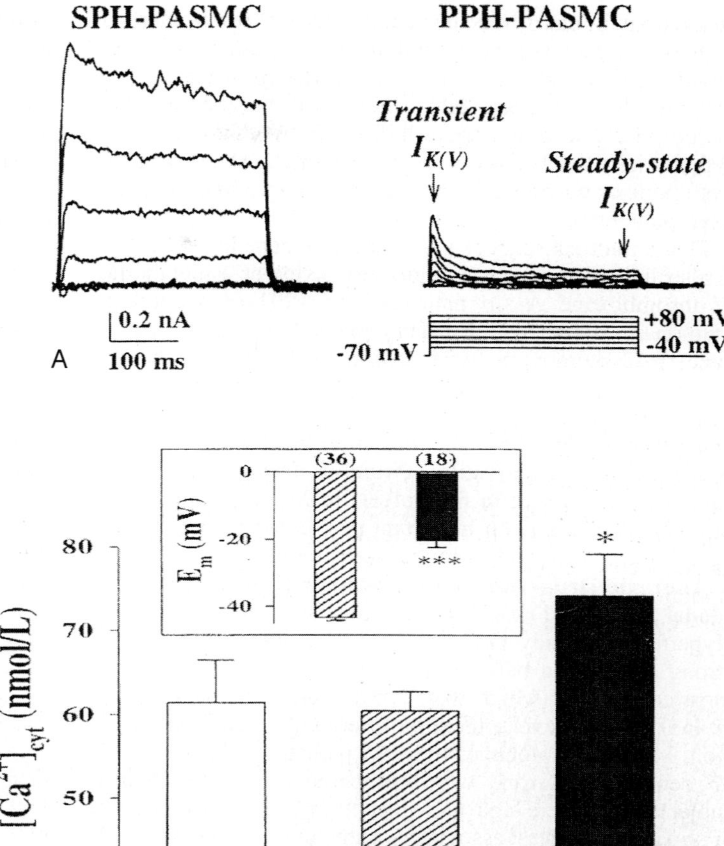

FIGURE 100–4 Cellular electrophysiology and intracellular Ca^{2+} imaging from isolated pulmonary artery smooth muscle cells (PASMCs) from patients with secondary pulmonary hypertension (SPH), primary pulmonary hypertension (PPH), or no pulmonary hypertension (NPH). **A,** Standard whole-cell patch-clamping: the membrane potential of the cell is held at −70 mV and with current injections depolarized to +80 mV (20-mV steps). With each current injection, the outward K^+ current is recorded (the more positive the potential, the higher the current). The PASMCs from patients with PPH have a significantly decreased outward K^+ current compared with those from patients with SPH. Based on standard pharmacology (not shown), this current was found to be due to open Kv channels. In another study, these investigators have shown that there is a selective decrease in the mRNA levels of a specific Kv channel (Kv1.5) in PPH PASMCs. **B** *(Inset)*, Using the same patch-clamping technique, the resting membrane potential of these cells can be measured. Cells from patients with PPH are more depolarized, as expected from the decrease in the outward K^+ current. Fluorescence microscopy shows higher intracellular Ca^{2+} levels in PASMCs from patients with PPH compared with those from patients with NPH or SPH. Depolarization due to the down-regulation of Kv channels causes the opening of L-type voltage-gated Ca^{2+} channels and the influx of extracellular Ca^{2+}. $*P < .05$, $***P < .001$ for PPH versus SPH. (**A** and **B,** From Yuan XJ, Wang J, Juhaszova M, et al: Attenuated K^+ channel gene transcription in primary pulmonary hypertension. Lancet 351[9104]:726–727, © by The Lancet Ltd, 1998.)

constriction via the inhibition of Kv channels, thus initiating hypoxic pulmonary vasoconstriction (HPV).[46–48]

In the carotid body type 1 cell, hypoxia inhibits an outward K^+ current and thus causes depolarization of the cell membrane,[49–51] suggesting that K^+ channel inhibition might be a well preserved mechanism, mediating the tissue response to hypoxia. In pulmonary artery smooth muscle cells, certain subfamilies of Kv channels (Kv1.2, 1.5, 2.1, and 9.3) have been shown to be oxygen-sensitive channels, the inhibition of which initiates hypoxic pulmonary vasoconstriction (HPV).[52, 53] Interestingly, it is the Kv1.5 channel that Yuan and associates[54] found to be selectively downregulated in PPH. As expected, the pulmonary artery smooth muscle cells from patients with PPH were found to be more depolarized and had higher concentrations of intracellular Ca^{2+} than cells from patients with secondary pulmonary hypertension and similar levels of PAP (Fig. 100–4).

These important findings suggest that K^+ channel abnormalities, which could be genetically controlled, might contribute to the pathogenesis of the vasoconstrictive component of PPH. These observations may help to explain the efficacy of drugs that open K_{Ca} or K_{ATP} channels in causing pulmonary vasodilatation, presumably by hyperpolarizing the cell membrane.[55–57] Ca^{2+} channel blockers act one step further down the sequence of HPV.[31, 58] It is possible that this mechanism, studied in HPV, is also involved in the vasoconstriction present in other types of pulmonary hypertension. In a recent study of the use of Ca^{2+} channel blockers in patients with PPH, a convincing acute vasodilator effect could be demonstrated in 26 percent of patients.[59] Similar observations were made in the National Institutes of Health (NIH) Primary Pulmonary Hypertension Registry[60] and in a literature review.[61]

Platelets and the Fibrinolytic System

Thrombosis is frequently observed in the small muscular pulmonary arteries of patients who die as a result of severe pulmonary hypertension. Whether endothelial dysfunction is primary or secondary, it is not surprising that thrombosis might ensue or that fibrinolytic mechanisms might be depressed. In PPH, thrombin activity may be increased, as demonstated by elevated levels of fibrinopeptide A in the plasma[62] and a decrease in the half-life of fibrinogen.[63] On the other hand, fibrinolytic activity was reported to be reduced in seven members of a family with PPH.[64] The presence of a high level of plasminogen activator inhibitor in as many as 70 percent of patients in one PPH series also suggests diminished fibrinolytic activity.[62]

The von Willebrand factor, which is present in platelets and endothelial cells,[65] plays an important role in the adhesion of platelets to a damaged vessel wall and in the aggregation of one platelet to another.[66] In patients with pulmonary hypertension secondary to congenital heart disease, the pulmonary vascular endothelium shows a marked increase in the intensity of immunostaining for von Willebrand factor antigen.[67] This implies a change secondary to the high-flow situation. Abnormalities of von Willebrand factor have also been noted in PPH.[68] These changes in von Willebrand factor activity and antigen suggest endothelial dysfunction and possibly the release of α-granule contents from platelets.

Platelet activation secondary to pulmonary hypertension is also indicated by elevated urinary levels of a metabolite of thromboxane A_2 in patients with PPH or secondary pulmonary hypertension.[32] This platelet activation could exacerbate pulmonary hypertension by leading to the release of substances that cause vasoconstriction, such as 5-hydroxytryptamine and thromboxane A_2, and substances that stimulate cell proliferation, such as PDGF. The evidence of platelet activation, thrombus formation, and, in some cases, a defect in fibrinolysis makes it apparent that thrombosis can play an important part in the pathophysiology of many forms of pulmonary hypertension.

Anorexic Drug–Induced Pulmonary Hypertension—A Model for PPH? In 1996, the International Pulmonary Hypertension Study Group published evidence showing a strong association between the use of anorexic drugs (the most common of which were dexfenfluramine and fenfluramine) and the development of severe pulmonary hypertension. In this case-control study, 95 patients with PPH from 35 centers in Europe were compared with 355 control subjects who were age and gender matched. The use of anorexic drugs was associated with an increased risk of PPH (odds ratio with any anorexic drug use, 6.3; 95% confidence interval, 3.0 to 13.2). For the use of anorexic agents in the preceding year, the odds ratio was 10.1 (95% confidence interval, 3.4 to 29.9). When anorexic drugs were used for more than 3 months, the odds ratio was 23.1 (95% confidence interval, 6.9 to 77.7).[69] This epidemic was reminiscent of the outbreak of pulmonary hypertension in several European countries in the late 1960s, which resulted from the use of another anoretic agent with a very similar structure, aminorex. The U.S. Food and Drug Administration withdrew the fenfluramines from the market in late 1997 when it was shown that a significant percentage of the patients using these drugs had developed "carcinoid-like" valvular insufficiency, often requiring valve replacement.

Several animal and human studies showed that the pathogenesis of anorexic drug–induced pulmonary hypertension and PPH involves similar mechanisms i.e., Kv channel inhibition, 5-hydroxytryptamine, and endothelial dysfunction). Because the plexogenic arteriopathy resulting from anorexic drug use is indistinguishable from that in PPH, it is possible that anorexic drug–induced pulmonary hypertension might prove to be a good model for PPH.

Aminorex and the fenfluramines have been shown to inhibit Kv channels in rat pulmonary artery smooth muscle as well as in cellular expression systems (Fig. 100–5).[70, 71] This Kv channel inhibition is associated with cell depolarization and an increase in intracellular Ca^{2+} in isolated pulmonary artery smooth muscle cells.[72] Fenfluramine was later shown to also inhibit Kv channels in human pulmonary artery smooth muscle cells.[73]

The fenfluramines are known to suppress appetite through an increase in 5-hydroxytryptamine levels in the nervous system. Increased plasma 5-hydroxytryptamine levels have been shown in patients with PPH.[74] Furthermore, these drugs have been shown to cause an increase in the PVR in rat isolated perfused lungs, especially if NO synthase is inhibited (see Fig. 100–5).[70] These data in the rat suggest that endothelial dysfunction could be a predisposing factor in the pathogenesis of anorexic drug–induced pulmonary hypertension. The results of studies in humans suggested that this might be true. In a prospective case-control study, Archer and colleagues[75] studied lung NO production in patients with anorexic drug–induced pulmonary hypertension and other forms of PPH. Lung NO production was lower in patients with anorexic drug–induced pulmonary hypertension than in control subjects and patients with PPH and correlated well with pulmonary vascular resistance (Fig. 100–6). These patients had a relative NO deficiency years after discontinuation of the anorexic drugs, perhaps accounting for their original susceptibility.[75]

Interestingly, the endothelial cells in patients with anorexic drug–induced pulmonary hypertension, similar to PPH and in contrast to secondary pulmonary hypertension, have also been found to be monoclonal.[76]

Preliminary experiments have shown that the fenfluramines inhibit Kv channels in megakaryocytes, the precursors of platelets, in the rabbit.[77] This could suggest a primary mechanism of platelet activation rather than a secondary mechanism of endothelial dysfunction. Thus, the pathogenesis of anorexic drug–induced pulmonary hypertension involves the endothelial and smooth muscle cells, as well as the platelets. It also suggests that one or more predisposing factors might be required for the development of PPH. This might explain why in several diseases known to also cause pulmonary hypertension, only a small percentage of the population at risk is affected. Such conditions include exposure to denatured repeseed oil,[23] eosinophilia myalgia syndrome,[23, 78, 79] systemic amyloidosis,[29] Behçet's syndrome,[29, 30, 80] pulmonary tuberous sclerosis,[81] pulmonary lymphangiomyomatosis,[82] and infection with human immunodeficiency virus.[24, 83]

CLINICAL RECOGNITION

Historical Assessment of Pulmonary Hypertension

Pulmonary hypertension is an uncommon condition and its symptoms are nonspecific, so patients often have symptoms for months or years before a correct diagnosis is made.[38, 84–86] In the national NIH PPH Registry, the average time from the onset of symptoms to the diagnosis of pulmonary hypertension was 2 ± 5 years.[87] Although symptoms of pulmonary hypertension do not directly reflect PAP, patients usually remain asymptomatic until PAP has doubled.[1]

The earliest and most common symptom of pulmonary hypertension is *dyspnea,* the subjective assessment by the patient of inadequate or difficult respiration.[84, 92] In the NIH Registry, 60 percent of the patients had dyspnea as a presenting symptom, although 98 percent had dyspnea by

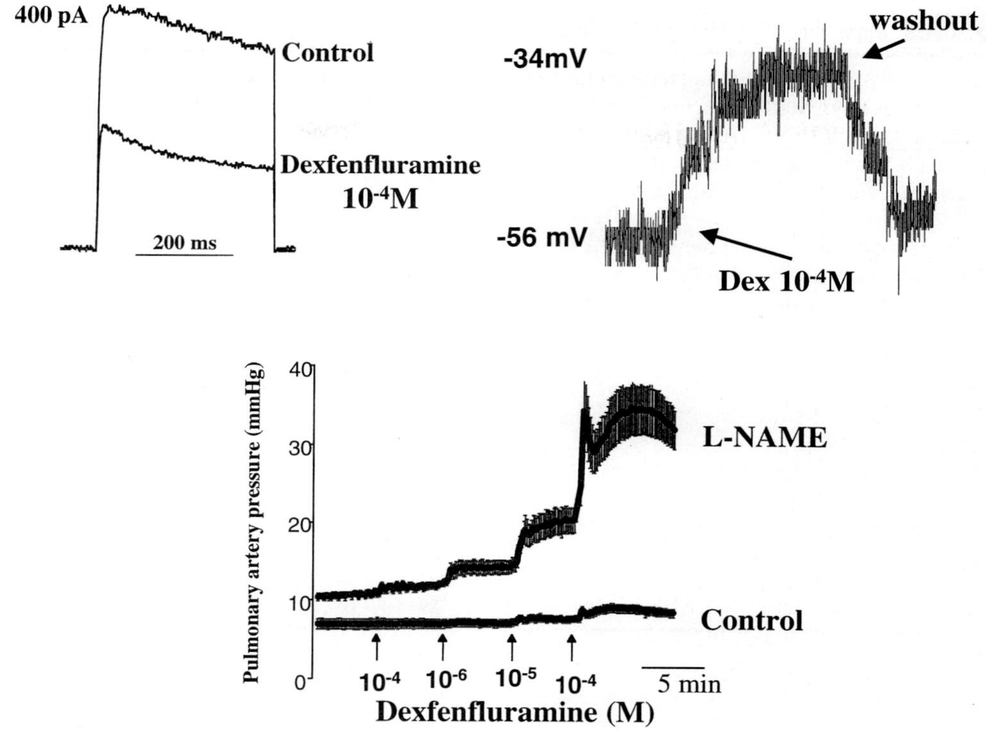

FIGURE 100–5 Top, Standard whole-cell patch-clamping on a resistance pulmonary artery smooth muscle cell from the rat. A protocol similar to that discussed in Figure 100–4 was used. The current elicited from a depolarization from −70 to +70 mV (control) is significantly inhibited on superfusion with dexfenfluramine (Dex) *(left).* This K^+ current inhibition (which was shown to be Kv current with standard pharmacology) causes significant depolarization *(right).* **Bottom,** Pulmonary artery recordings in the isolated perfused rat lung model. In this model, the perfusion through the pulmonary circulation is kept constant with a pump; therefore, changes in the recorded pressure reflect changes in the pulmonary vascular resistance. A dose-response to dexfenfluramine is shown with and without N^G-nitro-L-arginine methyl ester (L-NAME), an inhibitor of nitric oxide synthase. Note that in the presence of L-NAME, dexfenfluramine causes an increase even at the low dose of 10^{-6} M, which is similar to the steady-state drug levels achieved in treated humans. (From Weir EK, Reeve HL, Huang JM, et al: Anorexic agents aminorex, fenfluramine, and dexfenfluramine inhibit potassium current in rat pulmonary vascular smooth muscle and cause pulmonary vasoconstriction. Circulation 94:2216, 1996.)

the time they were enrolled in the registry (Table 100–5).[87] The causes of dyspnea in pulmonary hypertension are diverse, varying somewhat according to the cause of the syndrome. Dyspnea is found in the majority of pulmonary hypertensive syndromes, with the notable exception of sleep apnea. In most cases, dyspnea appears to relate more to altered lung mechanics and reflex activation than to hypoxemia. In PPH, there is often a respiratory alkalosis with mild hypoxemia. In these patients, dyspnea may relate to increased J receptor activity, possibly a result of altered

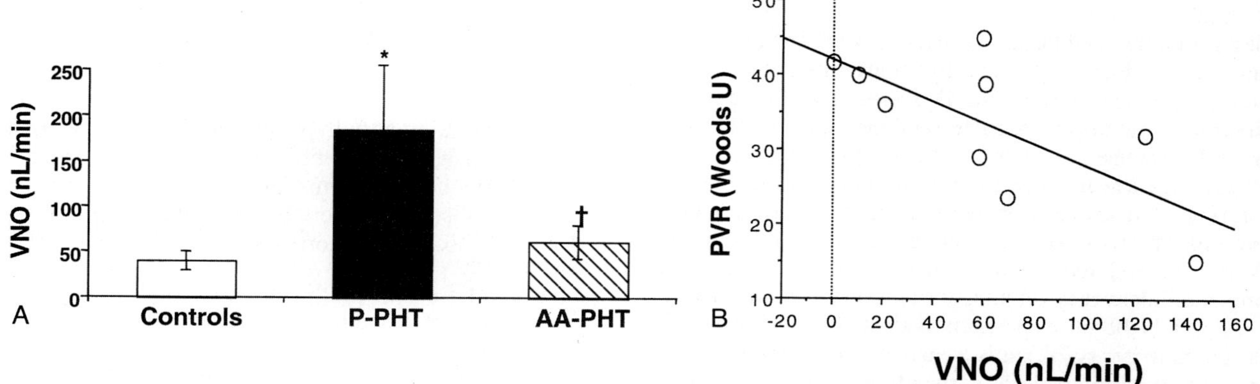

FIGURE 100–6 A, Lung nitric oxide production (VNO) measured by a chemiluminescence technique is reduced in patients with anorexia-induced pulmonary hypertension (AA-PHT) compared with patients with primary pulmonary hypertension (P-PHT). Values were obtained with patients at rest, while breathing medical air. $^*P < .05$ value differs from all other groups. $^\dagger P < .05$ value differs from P-PHT group. **B,** Invasively measured pulmonary vascular resistance (PVR) is inversely proportional to VNO in patients with AA-PHT. (**A** and **B,** From Archer SL, Djaballah K, Humbert M, et al: Nitric oxide deficiency in fenfluramine-induced pulmonary hypertension. Am J Respir Crit Care Med 158:1061, 1998.)

TABLE 100–5 **Signs and Symptoms of Pulmonary Hypertension**

	NIH PPH Registry (ref. 87)	Thromboembolic PHT (ref. 85)	PPH (ref. 89)	Thromboembolic PHT (ref. 89)	PPH (ref. 84)	Thromboembolic PHT (ref. 84)
Sample size	187	15	36	16	17	8
History						
Age (years)	36 ± 15	21–67	N/A	N/A	36 ± 15	39 ± 13
Female/male	1.7/1	0.4/1	1/1	1/1	7.5/1	1/1
Positive family history (%)	6	0	9	0	6	0
Symptoms (%)						
Dyspnea	60	100	88	93	>90	88
Fatigue	73	N/A	N/A	N/A	71	50
Syncope	36	33	N/A	N/A	24	13
Chest pain	47	60	N/A	N/A	77	75
Raynaud's phenomenon	10	N/A	24	0	12	0
Signs (%)						
Venous stasis/DVT	N/A	40	N/A	>than in PPH	12	12
Loud P2	93	47	N/A	N/A	100	88
Right-sided S3	23	2	N/A	N/A	12	25
Tricuspid regurgitation	40	40	N/A	N/A	71	50
Laboratory (%)						
Right-axis deviation	79	53	94	69	100	50
RVH	87	40	73	38	88	50
Enlarged PA on CXR	90	20%	89	89	94	38

Abbreviations: CXR, chest radiograph; DVT, deep vein thrombosis; N/A, information not available; PA, pulmonary artery; PHT, pulmonary hypertension; PPH, primary pulmonary hypertension; RVH, right ventricular hypertension.

vascular and, therefore, lung compliance. Hypoxemia may also lead to dyspnea in patients with pulmonary hypertension due to intracardiac shunting (e.g., Eisenmenger's syndrome). Interstitial lung disease, with reduced lung compliance and hypoxemia, is another cause of dyspnea in patients with pulmonary hypertension and is a prevalent symptom in patients with certain connective tissue diseases (e.g., mixed connective tissue disease, scleroderma, CREST [*c*alcinosis cutis, *R*aynaud's phenomenon, *e*sophageal dysfunction, *s*clerodactyly, and *t*elangiectasia] syndrome). In patients with mitral stenosis or left ventricular (LV) failure, the elevation of pulmonary capillary pressure and infiltration of fluid into the perivascular space stimulate the J receptors and thus promotes dyspnea.

Like dyspnea, fatigue is a common and nonspecific symptom in these patients (see Table 100–5). Fatigue may reflect reduced cardiac output and impaired oxygen delivery to the tissues. In addition, PVR increases dramatically with exercise in patients with pulmonary hypertension, unlike normal individuals. The rises in PAP and PVR that occur with exercise undoubtedly contribute to impaired exercise tolerance and fatigue. Dyspnea and fatigue occur with similar frequency regardless of the cause of the pulmonary hypertension.[84, 88, 89]

Syncope and near-syncope are common in some, but not all, forms of pulmonary hypertension. Although syncope occurs in roughly one third of patients with PPH (see Table 100–5), it is relatively uncommon in patients with cor pulmonale unless they have coexistent cough-induced syncope, possibly because the pulmonary hypertension is seldom severe in cor pulmonale. Syncope may occur at rest or with exercise. During exercise, the obstructed or obliterated pulmonary vascular bed may be unable to accommodate adequate increases in cardiac output, culminating in reduced cerebral blood flow and syncope.

Chest pain is not unusual in pulmonary hypertension and may be described by the patient as sharp and pleuritic or as a dull ache. Pleuritic chest pain is equally common in patients with primary or thromboembolic pulmonary hypertension. The dull chest ache noted by some patients with pulmonary hypertension is suggestive of angina. The mechanism of this angina-like pain is unclear. Potential mechanisms for chest pain in pulmonary hypertension include right ventricular (RV) ischemia and distention of the pulmonary arteries.

A somewhat unusual symptom of pulmonary hypertension is hoarseness (Ortner's syndrome). Hoarseness results when the left recurrent laryngeal nerve, which passes between the aorta and the pulmonary artery,[88, 90] is compressed by an enlarged pulmonary artery.[1, 90] Ortner's syndrome had been described in 6 to 8 percent of patients with severe chronic pulmonary hypertension but has been reported less frequently in recent series.[84, 86, 87]

Hemoptysis also occurs in many types of pulmonary hypertension. Moser and associates[85] noted a history of hemoptysis in 53 percent of patients undergoing thromboendarterectomy for thromboembolic pulmonary hypertension. It has been reported that in the capillary bed of patients with pulmonary hypertension there are microaneurysms that may be susceptible to rupture, resulting in hemoptysis.[1] In certain forms of pulmonary hypertension, such as mitral stenosis, there is elevated capillary pressure, which predisposes to hemorrhage.

Review of Systems

Certain screening questions can help to define the severity and cause of the pulmonary hypertension syndrome; these should be asked of each patient.

Family History

A history of familial pulmonary hypertension is present in approximately 6 percent of patients with PPH (see Table 100–5). The familial form of the disease appears to have clinical and prognostic features similar to the sporadic form of the syndrome. Genetic transmission of PPH behaves in autosomal dominant fashion with variable penetrance and displays a disturbing ability to skip generations.[91]

Thromboembolic Disease

Patients with thromboembolic pulmonary hypertension may have had a prior history of deep venous thrombosis or pleuritic chest pain.[92] Although the incidence of clinically recognized thromboembolism before the diagnosis of thromboembolic pulmonary hypertension is low,[85] more than one half of these patients have had an episode that in retrospect is consistent with prior venous thrombosis or acute pulmonary embolism.[92] Screening questions for trauma, immobility, pleurisy, hemoptysis, or "pneumonia" may be useful.

Environmental Factors

Sporadic cases of diet-induced pulmonary hypertension have been reported, including those after the ingestion of L-tryptophan. Aminorex, a weight loss medication used in Europe in the 1960s, was associated with an outbreak of pulmonary hypertension that histologically resembled PPH.[93] When the drug was withdrawn, the epidemic subsided.

Another epidemic of pulmonary hypertension occurred as a result of the ingestion of adulterated industrial rapeseed oil, sold illegally as cooking oil.[94] The industrial oil, recognizable by its aniline dye, became contaminated with oleoanilides when distributors attempted to extract the aniline dye to disguise its industrial origins.[95] These examples illustrate the potential for medications and dietary factors to cause pulmonary hypertension.

Connective Tissue Disease and Raynaud's Phenomenon

Pulmonary hypertension is relatively common in scleroderma,[96] systemic lupus erythematosus,[97] and mixed connective tissue disease,[98] and has been noted on rare occasions in patients with rheumatoid arthritis.[99] Ungerer and colleagues[96] found definite pulmonary hypertension in 16 percent of patients with progressive systemic sclerosis, with borderline pulmonary hypertension in an additional 16 percent.[96] Therefore, the clinician should elicit a history of arthritis, pleuritis, skin rashes, and dysphagia. Raynaud's syndrome is common in patients with connective tissue disease, in the absence of pulmonary hypertension, but it was also present in 24 percent of patients with PPH in the NIH registry. Raynaud's phenomenon does not occur with increased frequency in high-flow pulmonary hypertension, cor pulmonale, or thromboembolic pulmonary hypertension.[89] A history of Raynaud's phenomenon in a patient with pulmonary hypertension strongly suggests a diagnosis of primary or connective tissue disease–related pulmonary hypertension.

Pulmonary Disease

Pulmonary hypertension is usually a late manifestation of parenchymal pulmonary disease, and therefore a history of asthma, bronchitis, or recurrent pneumonia is usually present. Pulmonary fibrosis is more likely to cause significant pulmonary hypertension than COPD, and a history of pulmonary fibrosis or exposure to toxins that may cause fibrosis (e.g., beryllium and asbestos) should be sought. Sleep apnea, one of the more treatable causes of pulmonary hypertension, should be actively investigated. We routinely inquire about daytime hypersomnolence and nocturnal apnea.

Cardiac Disease

The most common cause of pulmonary hypertension is passive pulmonary hypertension due to LV dysfunction or mitral valve disease. A history of ischemic cardiac disease or heart murmur should be sought in each patient.

Liver Disease

Patients with cirrhosis have an increased frequency of pulmonary hypertension, which fits into the general category of PPH. McDonnell and associates[100] found that the incidence of pulmonary hypertension among cirrhotics in one autopsy study was higher than that among patients without cirrhosis (0.73 and 0.13 percent, respectively). The review of systems should document a patient's history of alcohol intake, cirrhosis, or jaundice.

Physical Examination

Like the history, the findings on physical examination in pulmonary hypertension are often nonspecific. A number of patients with pulmonary hypertension will have an entirely normal physical examination. Furthermore, the physical examination rarely allows quantification of the severity of pulmonary hypertension until the terminal stages of the disease, when right heart failure appears. The physical findings of pulmonary hypertension reflect the presence of an enlarged, noncompliant right ventricle and insufficiency of the tricuspid or pulmonic valves. Characteristic findings include the following (see also Table 100–5):

1. Elevation of a jugular venous pulse with prominent A or V waves
2. Right side fourth heart sound.
3. Enhanced intensity of the pulmonic component of the second heart sound (occasionally palpable)
4. Prominent left parasternal lift or heave
5. The murmurs of tricuspid or pulmonic regurgitation

Although a loud pulmonic component of the second heart sound is common in patients with pulmonary hypertension, as the hypertension becomes more severe, the interval between closure of the aortic and pulmonic valves may decrease so that the valves close almost simultaneously, eliminating the value of this sign.

Pulmonary Insufficiency

The so-called Graham-Steele murmur of pulmonary insufficiency occasionally accompanies severe pulmonary hypertension. This diastolic murmur is usually best heard in the second or third inner space near the sternum. Pulmonary insufficiency may be distinguished from aortic insufficiency by observing the response to the Valsalva maneuver. The pulmonary regurgitation murmur usually returns to pre-Valsalva intensity within several beats, whereas the aortic regurgitation murmur usually takes a somewhat longer time to return to its intensity. The time delay occurs because the blood excluded from the thorax by the Valsalva maneuver must first traverse the pulmonary circulation before reaching the aorta and augmenting the murmur.

Tricuspid Regurgitation

Although echocardiographic evidence of mild tricuspid and pulmonic regurgitation is prevalent even in normal individuals, audible or hemodynamically significant insufficiency is rare. The blowing systolic murmur of tricuspid regurgitation is best heard over the lower right sternal border and may briefly enhance with inspiration (Carvallo's sign). The right side third heart sound occurs primarily once the right ventricle has decompensated from chronic pressure overload and is usually accompanied by a murmur of tricuspid regurgitation.

There is one sign of pulmonary hypertension that has a degree of specificity for a single cause. A flow murmur over the lung fields has been noted in some patients with thromboembolic pulmonary hypertension.[85, 101] This sign may also be present in patients with stenosis of peripheral pulmonary arteries, as may occur in the rubella syndrome or with Takayasu's disease.

Use of Laboratory Tests to Assess Pulmonary Hypertension

Diagnostic testing in pulmonary hypertension may serve three purposes: (1) to document and quantify pulmonary hypertension, (2) to define the cause, and (3) to assess the prognosis.

Our approach to the patient with presumed pulmonary hypertension is to establish its presence, preferably with a noninvasive test, such as Doppler echocardiography. If the pressure is elevated or cannot be accurately measured, then a right heart catheterization is performed.

Once a diagnosis of pulmonary hypertension is established, the next goal is to determine the cause. This requires integration of the history, physical examination, and laboratory test results. A particular emphasis of the diagnostic assessment is the identification of causes of pulmonary hypertension that are reversible, such as mitral stenosis, thromboembolic pulmonary hypertension, intracardiac shunting, and sleep apnea. Unfortunately, most pulmonary hypertension can be palliated but not cured. In patients such as those with severe lung disease, PPH, or passive pulmonary hypertension due to LV dysfunction, the purpose of testing is to establish a diagnosis and to monitor therapy. In patients with cor pulmonale, for example, the response to oxygen therapy can be documented. In patients with PPH, one can determine whether vasodilator therapy is safe and effective. We obtain the following tests on a routine basis in virtually all patients in whom the cause of pulmonary hypertension is not evident: electrocardiography, chest radiography, arterial blood gases, pulmonary function tests (forced expiratory volume in 1 second [FEV_1], forced vital capacity [FVC], diffusing capacity [DLCO]), serology for rheumatic diseases (e.g., fluorescent antinuclear antibody [FANA]), ventilation perfusion scan, and echocardiography with contrast study. This relatively inexpensive and safe battery of tests can detect patients with chronic lung disease, mitral stenosis, most intracardiac shunts, thromboembolic pulmonary hypertension, passive pulmonary hypertension due to LV dysfunction, and connective tissue disease. The patients who remain undiagnosed and therefore most often require catheterization or other studies are those with pulmonary fibrosis, sleep apnea, or PPH. Because PPH is a diagnosis of exclusion, we routinely perform right heart catheterizations in these patients.

Laboratory Tests

BLOOD TESTS

Patients with PPH often have a positive FANA test.[87] A positive FANA result in PPH usually occurs without evidence of rheumatologic diseases (arthritis, pleuritis, skin rash). However, patients with CREST syndrome,[102] systemic lupus erythematosus, or, to a lesser extent, rheumatoid arthritis are at an increased risk for the development of pulmonary hypertension.[99] The FANA and other markers of autoimmunity provide a tantalizing clue to the cause of some cases of PPH.

Patients with thromboembolic pulmonary hypertension may have recognizable procoagulant abnormalities. Approximately 10 percent of patients with thromboembolic hypertension have lupus "anticoagulant" without clinical evidence of systemic lupus erythematosus.[92] The other known procoagulant abnormalities (protein C, protein S, or antithrombin III deficiency) occur in fewer than 1 percent of patients with thromboembolic pulmonary hypertension.

The finding of polycythemia is compatible with but not diagnostic of pulmonary hypertension in patients with chronic lung disease. It is also important to determine the hemoglobin level as a measure of blood viscosity. Excessive elevations of hemoglobin increase PVR, and phlebotomy may be beneficial in selected patients. The pulmonary hypertensive patient with cyanotic heart disease often has thrombocytopenia as well as polycythemia.

ARTERIAL BLOOD GASES

Arterial blood gases are usually abnormal in patients with pulmonary hypertension (Table 100–6). In COPD, a Po_2 of less than 60 mm Hg and a Pco_2 of more than 40 mm Hg are thought to be threshold values for the development of pulmonary hypertension.[103] Milder hypoxemia is typically present in PPH as well, but it is almost always associated with hypocapnia (see Table 100–2).[87]

TABLE 100–6 **Comparison of Invasive and Noninvasive Tests in Three Forms of Pulmonary Hypertension**

	NIH Primary PHT Registry (ref. 87)	Primary PHT (ref. 84)	Thromboembolic PHT (ref. 84)	Thromboembolic PHT (refs. 85, 86)	Cor Pulmonale (ref. 103)
Pulmonary function (% predicted)					
FEV_1	83 ± 17	79 ± 8	75 ± 9	N/A	33 ± 14
TLC	89	87 ± 12	96 ± 12	N/A	105 ± 15
DLCO	82	59 ± 22	60 ± 19	75–107	
Arterial blood gases (mm Hg)					
Po_2	70 ± 2	65 ± 12	62 ± 8	<80 in 80%	59 ± 8
Pco_2	30 ± 6	31 ± 5	32 ± 5	24–37	46 ± 8
Right heart catheterization (mm Hg)					
Mean PAP	61 ± 20	57 ± 15	48 ± 16	49 ± 9	24 ± 5
Wedge pressure	9 ± 4	7 ± 4	7 ± 4	9 ± 3	9 ± 3
Ventilation/perfusion scans					
Low probability or normal	97%	100%	0%	0%	N/A
High probability	0.6%	0%	100%	100%	N/A
Pulmonary angiography (%)					
Positive for proximal thrombi	0	0	100	100	N/A
Deaths from angiography	0	0	0	0	N/A

Abbreviations: N/A, not applicable; PAP, pulmonary artery pressure; PHT, pulmonary hypertension.
Values are expressed as mean ± SD if available.

PULMONARY FUNCTION TESTS

Pulmonary function tests are often abnormal in patients with pulmonary hypertension (see Table 100–6). The abnormality of lung function may be the cause of the pulmonary hypertension, as in cor pulmonale, or vice versa. For example, patients with thromboembolic and primary pulmonary hypertension often have mild restrictive or obstructive patterns noted on spirometry. Pulmonary hypertensive patients with collagen vascular disease tend to have more severe lung disease than a cohort with primary pulmonary hypertension: DLCO of 11.9 ± 1.5 and 17.6 ± 0.6 ml/min/mm Hg, respectively; FEV_1 of 1.9 ± 0.1 and 2.6 ± 0.1 L/sec, respectively; and FVC of 2.4 ± 0.1 and 3.3 ± 0.1 L, respectively.[104]

NONINVASIVE ASSESSMENT OF THE PULMONARY CIRCULATION

Electrocardiography

Electrocardiography is a specific but nonsensitive means of diagnosing RV hypertrophy (Fig. 100–7). Lehtonen and colleagues[105] compared four sets of electrocardiographic criteria for the diagnosis of RV hypertrophy in patients whose RV thickness was measured at autopsy. Hearts were considered normal if the total weight was less than 250 g, the right ventricle was less than 65 g, and the combined left ventricle plus septum weight was less than 190 g (ratio of [left ventricle + septum]/right ventricle, 2.3 to 3.3). In the patients with RV hypertrophy in this series, a common cause of death was respiratory failure. By combining aspects of the four sets of electrocardiographic criteria, the authors achieved a diagnostic sensitivity of 63 percent and a specificity of 96 percent. These combined criteria included right-axis deviation of more than 110 degrees, R or R′ wave equal to or greater than the S wave (in V_1 or V_2), R wave equal to or less than the S wave in lead V_6, and the calculated value of A + R − PL = 0.7 (where A is maximum R wave amplitude in lead V_1 or V_2, R is maximal S wave amplitude in lead I or V_6, and PL is minimal S wave amplitude in lead I or V_6). This set of criteria was quite specific, despite the presence of LV hypertrophy and myocardial infarction in the study population.

The electrocardiographic criteria for RV hypertrophy (Table 100–7) become less specific in the presence of right bundle branch block, posterior myocardial infarction, left posterior hemiblock, and Wolff-Parkinson-White syndrome with a posteroseptal accessory pathway. These conditions may cause right-axis deviation or a predominant R in lead V_1, similar to the findings in RV hypertrophy. Fortunately, there often are clues that permit differentiation of RV hypertrophy from these conditions. Posterior infarction usually involves associated inferior infarction. One should be cautious in making a diagnosis of RV hypertrophy in patients with inferior Q waves and dominant R waves in lead V_1. Furthermore, patients with RV hypertrophy typically have RA hypertrophy, with the diagnosis based on the presence of asymmetric peaked P waves of more than 2.5 mm in amplitude in any lead. Therefore, in attempting to distinguish between a posterior hemiblock and RV hypertrophy, the presence of atrial hypertrophy would militate in favor of the diagnosis of hypertrophy.

Because RV hypertrophy is usually associated with pulmonary hypertension, the electrocardiogram (ECG) remains a reasonable screening test for pulmonary hypertension. The ECG also correlates with pulmonary hemodynamics. In one study, the ECG was a sensitive and specific predictor of PAP and cardiac index in patients with severe pulmonary hypertension (see Table 100–7). Nevertheless, a normal ECG does not exclude mild or moderate degrees of pulmonary hypertension.

Chest Radiography

The chest radiograph, like the ECG, is a convenient and widely available screening test for pulmonary hypertension.

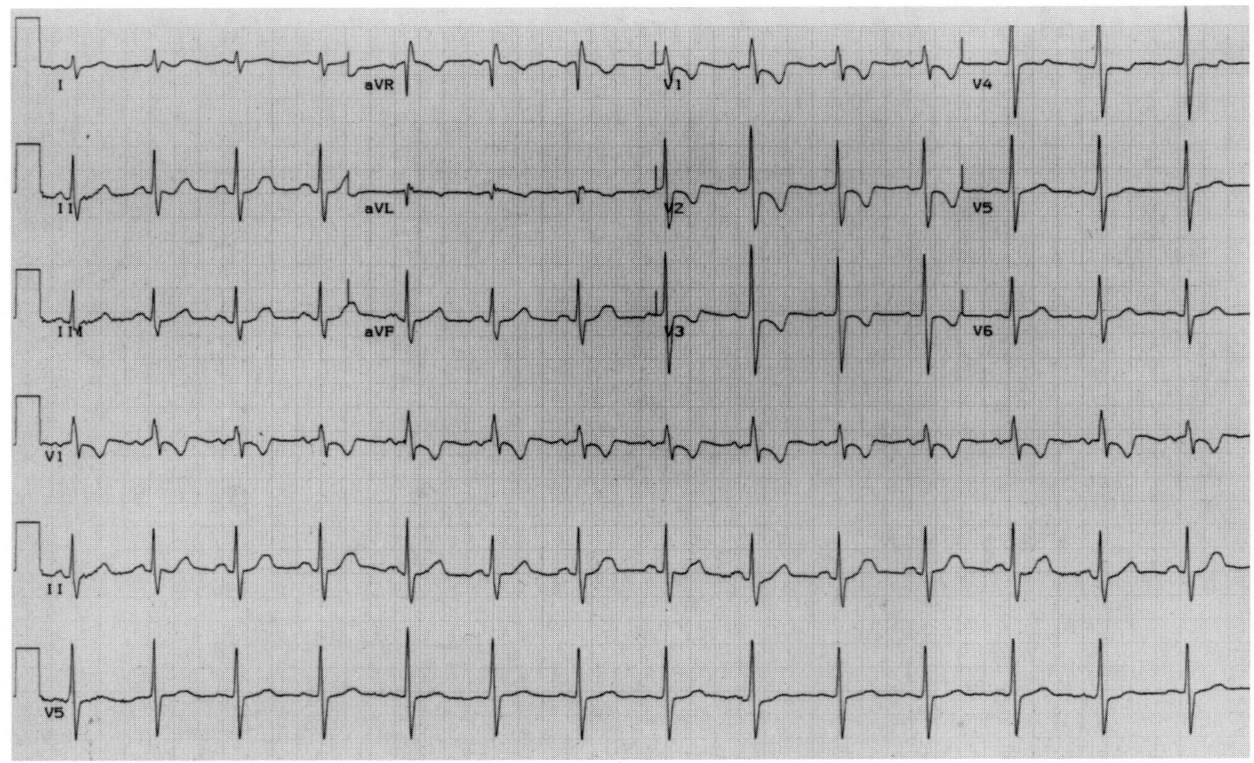

FIGURE 100–7 Electrocardiogram (ECG) of a patient with primary pulmonary hypertension. This 12-lead ECG reveals a number of typical findings in patients with pulmonary hypertension and right ventricular hypertrophy, including right-axis deviation and RS wave amplitude in lead V_1. The depression of the ST-T segments in leads V_1 to V_3 is a right ventricular strain pattern. This ECG has a specificity of 90 percent for right ventricular hypertrophy, but these findings are often absent in patients with pulmonary hypertension.

Although many criteria have been suggested to screen for the presence of pulmonary hypertension, the following three measurements are the most widely used radiographic criteria for the diagnosis of pulmonary hypertension[106–108]:

1. Descending right pulmonary artery (normal width, 12.1 ± 1.2 mm)
2. Hilar width percent (hilar width ÷ ½ the transverse thoracic diameter; normal value, 28 ± 5 percent)
3. Hilar/thoracic index percent (total hilar width ± total transverse diameter of the thorax; normal value, 34 ± 4 percent)[1]

TABLE 100–7 Specificity and Sensitivity of ECG in Diagnosis of Right Ventricular Hypertrophy

Criteria	Sensitivity	Specificity	Reference
QRS axis (limb leads) > 110°	19	96	1
$S_1S_2S_3$	24	87	
R/S V_6 < 1	16	93	
R/S V_1 > 1	6	98	
Prediction of pulmonary hypertension (pressure >90 mm Hg) by ECG			
R V_1 >1.2 mm	94	47	89
Prediction of reduced cardiac index (<2.8 l/min/m²) by ECG			
QRS axis (limb leads) > 100° + R/S V_6 < 2	84	100	89

Abbreviations: ECG, electrocardiography; R/S, ratio of the amplitude of the R wave to that of the S wave on standard 12-lead ECG.

In populations with a high pretest probability of pulmonary hypertension, the chest radiograph appears to be quite sensitive. In clinical practice, where pulmonary hypertension is uncommon, the positive and negative predictive values for the chest radiograph are less impressive.

Echocardiography

There are a number of excellent articles and chapters that review the use of echocardiography in the detection and quantification of pulmonary hypertension.[109, 110] Although the echocardiogram can be "normal" in patients with severe pulmonary hypertension,[85, 111] this is rare.[85] If the image quality is adequate and anatomic data (RV chamber size and thickness, mitral valve anatomy), physiologic measurements (Doppler measurement of valve insufficiency and shunts), and a few simple calculations of PAP are integrated, the echocardiogram is a reliable test to suggest the presence of pulmonary hypertension (Table 100–8). The likelihood of finding and estimating the severity of pulmonary hypertension is directly proportional to the diligence of the sonographer and the experience of the physician who interprets the study.

M-Mode Echocardiography

Although the M-mode echocardiogram is less widely used since the advent of two-dimensional echocardiography, it

TABLE 100–8 **Useful Formulas for Assessment of Pulmonary Hypertension**

Pulmonary/systemic flow	$\frac{PBF}{SBF} = \frac{\text{Systemic A} - \text{V } O_2 \text{ difference}}{\text{Pulmonary A} - \text{V } O_2 \text{ difference}}$
Pulmonary blood flow (Fick)	$PBF = \frac{O_2 \text{ consumption}}{\text{Pulmonary A} - \text{V } O_2 \text{ difference}}$
O_2 content of blood	O_2 content (volume%) = (1.34 × hemoglobin) × O_2 saturation Multiply by 10 to permit flow calculations in L/min
Pulmonary vascular resistance (PVR)	$\text{PVR (Wood Units)} = \left[\frac{PAP_{mean} - P_{wedge}}{\text{Cardiac output}}\right]$ $\text{PVR (dyne/s/cm}^{-5}) = \left[\frac{PAP_{mean} - P_{wedge}}{\text{Cardiac output}}\right] \times 80$
Total pulmonary resistance (TPR)	$\text{TPR (Wood Units)} = \left[\frac{PAP_{mean}}{\text{Cardiac output}}\right]$
PAP mean (acceleration time) PAP systolic (modified Bernoulli's equation)	PAP mean = 79 − (0.45 × AT) PAP systolic = $4 \times V^2_{TR}$

Abbreviations: AT, acceleration time; P, pressure; PAP, pulmonary artery pressure; PBF, pulmonary blood flow; SBF, systolic blood flow.

is occasionally a useful modality in the diagnosis of pulmonary hypertension. The M-mode signs of pulmonary hypertension are indirect measurements that predominantly reflect the rigid, noncompliant nature of the diseased pulmonary vasculature. Unlike Doppler techniques, the M-mode signs of pulmonary hypertension are unable to reliably measure PAP and are used as evidence for or against the presence of pulmonary hypertension. A characteristic sign of pulmonary hypertension is the absence of an A dip on the M-mode of the pulmonic valve.[112, 113] The A dip, which occurs when atrial systole causes a bulging or partial opening of the pulmonic valve, is present only in patients in sinus rhythm. The sensitivity and specificity of this sign are relatively low.[114]

A second sign of pulmonary hypertension is the transient midsystolic closure of the pulmonic valve. The reasons for the premature closure of the pulmonic valve in pulmonary hypertension include the reduced capacitance of the pulmonary vascular bed and a prominent flow reversal within the hypertensive pulmonary artery.[115] Reflection of the systolic wave front may be enhanced in the hypertensive pulmonary vasculature, resulting in deceleration of midsystolic flow.[116] This M-mode sign of pulmonary hypertension is related to the finding on pulsed Doppler of a transient, early systolic pulmonary arterial flow deceleration. The notched morphology on M-mode is fairly specific but is insensitive as a test for pulmonary hypertension and has been reported in patients with normal PAP who have idiopathic dilatation of the pulmonary artery.[117]

Two-Dimensional Echocardiography

The right ventricle has a complex geometric shape. Unlike the somewhat ellipsoid configuration of the left ventricle, the right ventricle is crescentic and is not readily described with simple geometric equations. Even the measurement of wall thickness is difficult due to the trabeculation, which can result in significant variations in wall thickness within a relatively small sample volume. Levine and associates[118] evaluated whether echocardiography could be used to measure the volume of the right ventricle using molded latex casts of the postmortem human heart. Goerke and Carlsson[119] have previously shown that Simpson's rule can be used to calculate volumes of ventricular casts in a similar model. Starling and colleagues[120] showed that RV volume could be calculated as area multiplied by length of the right ventricle, but the appropriate subcostal views could be obtained in only 64 percent of patients. Levine and associates[118] demonstrated that the volume of human RV casts could be accurately assessed by combining the single-plane RV area (from the apical four-chamber view) and chamber length (RV outflow tract view) in the following equation:

$$2A \times L2 \div 3$$

where A is area and L is length. This mathematical construct, based on the formula for a simple pyramid, reflects the fact that the human right ventricle is somewhat larger than the formula for a simple pyramid would dictate.

Right Ventricular Hypertrophy

RV hypertrophy can be measured with the M-mode echocardiogram or the electronic calipers on the two-dimensional image. Measurements are typically made in either the long-axis parasternal or subcostal acoustic windows with the cursor positioned at the level of the tips of the tricuspid valve leaflets. Care must be take to ensure that the M-mode cursor avoids the papillary muscles and the RV muscular bands. The right ventricle can be measured from many acoustic windows, but it is optimally measured from a medially angulated parasternal or subcostal window, using a 5-MHz transducer.[121] With this technique, Gottdiener and colleagues[122] found that normal subjects have an RV wall thickness of 4 mm. It is important to remember that RV hypertrophy is not specific for pulmonary vascular disease. Patients with aortic stenosis or systemic hypertension who have LV hypertrophy often have mild RV hypertrophy.[122] Tsuda and colleagues[121] reported normal RV thickness of 2.4 ± 0.5 mm. Patients with pulmonary hypertension in this study had an increased thickness (2.5 to 16 mm), and the degree of hypertrophy was related directly to the PAP.[121]

Miscellaneous Echocardiographic Findings in Pulmonary Hypertension

The end-systolic configuration of the ventricular septum is a useful indirect measurement of the relative pressures in the left and right ventricles.[123] As RV systolic pressure increases, there is a gradual change in septal configuration from convex (bulging toward the right ventricle) to flat and finally to concave (indented toward the left ventricle).

Pericardial effusion is a common but nonspecific finding in chronic severe pulmonary hypertension. In one study, in large part composed of patients with thromboembolic pulmonary hypertension, 41 percent of patients had small or medium-sized effusions; none of the patients were symptomatic. The likelihood of effusion was increased in the patients with the highest right atrial (RA) pressure or PAP.[116]

Pulsed Doppler

The normal pulmonary artery flow velocity is 81 ± 17 cm/sec and occurs with an acceleration time of 121 ± 27 seconds.[124] In pulmonary hypertension, there usually is a more rapid acceleration of the pulmonary flow velocity with or without early systolic deceleration. A typical Doppler signal in patients with pulmonary hypertension is often triangular rather than the normal broad shield shape seen in normotensive patients.[125] Kitabatake and associates[125] have shown that the acceleration time is shortened in patients with pulmonary hypertension. In pediatric patients, an acceleration time of less than 106 ms predicts an elevated PAP with a sensitivity of 79 percent and a specificity of 100 percent.[126] Although there is a fair correlation between acceleration time and systolic PAP, Mahan and colleagues[127] found a better correlation between acceleration time and mean PAP. They used a regression equation to develop the following formula predictive of mean PAP:

$$\text{PAP} = 79 - 0.45 \times \text{AT}$$

where AT is acceleration time. This technique is somewhat heart rate dependent but correlates well with mean PAP in patients with heart rates between 60 and 100.[128]

Continuous-Wave Doppler

Although M-mode and pulsed Doppler techniques can help to determine whether pulmonary artery hypertension is present or absent, they are suboptimal for the quantification of PAP. The recent development of continuous-wave Doppler imaging has greatly advanced the noninvasive measurement of systolic and diastolic PAP. Even normal individuals have tricuspid regurgitation velocities that exceed the Nyquist limit for pulsed-Doppler measurement. Consequently, these jets must be measured by continuous-wave Doppler. Tricuspid regurgitation is extremely common and increases in prevalence and severity as PAP increases.[129, 130] Berger and associates[129] found tricuspid regurgitation in approximately 39 of 49 patients with systolic pressures of less than 35 mm Hg and in 26 of 27 patients with pressures of more than 50 mm Hg.[21] They noted an excellent correlation between Doppler and catheter estimates of systolic PAP (r = 0.97; See, 4.9 mm Hg).[21] Morrison and colleagues[131] used contrast ventriculography and noted tricuspid regurgitation in 12 of 48 normal control subjects and 22 of 36 patients with a PAP of 20 to 30 mm Hg.

With the use of steerable continuous-wave Doppler, guided by color flow Doppler to a position roughly parallel to the regurgitant jet, it is usually possible to measure peak tricuspid regurgitation velocity (Fig. 100–8). The modified Bernoulli principle states that if there is no pulmonary stenosis, RV pressure and systolic PAP can be estimated by measuring the systolic pressure gradient across the tricuspid valve (Table 100–8) and adding to this the RA pressure (the pressure into which the tricuspid regurgitation is injected). Yock and Popp[132] used the modified Bernoulli equation to estimate RV systolic pressures in patients with clinical signs of pulmonary hypertension. In their study, tricuspid regurgitation velocity could be measured in 54 of 62 patients. There was a good correlation between the pressures obtained by catheter and by Doppler. The use of the tricuspid regurgitation jet in the evaluation of systolic PAP has been validated by a number of authors.[128, 133, 134]

Diastolic Pulmonary Artery Pressure

The same modified Bernoulli principle can be used to determine the diastolic PAP. Assuming that there is no RV pressure gradient, diastolic PAP can be determined with the following equation:

$$(PI_{EDV})^2 \times 4 + \text{mean right atrial pressure}$$

where PI_{EDV} is the end-diastolic velocity of the pulmonic insufficiency jet. The principle underlying this measurement is that the diastolic PAP is the pressure gradient across the pulmonic valve in diastole plus the RV end-diastolic pressure. Because RV end-diastolic pressure is not clinically available in most patients, the RA pressure is usually added to the pulmonic diastolic gradient to obtain the diastolic PAP. RA pressure must be either measured by catheter or estimated by echocardiography, as described later. Masuyama and colleagues[135] used continuous-wave Doppler to estimate diastolic PAP and showed a useful correlation between the Doppler- and catheter-determined pressures in both hypertensive and normotensive patients.

Estimation of Right Atrial Pressure

It is apparent that accurate estimation of PAP relies on knowledge of the RA pressure. A number of authors have advocated adding an arbitrary value for atrial pressure to the pressure determined with the Bernoulli equation,[135] but this practice is suboptimal. RA pressure can be estimated at the bedside by measuring the jugular venous pulse (JVP). Unfortunately, in many patients it is considerably difficult to accurately measure the jugular venous distention. The RA pressure is approximated by the perpendicular height of the JVP above the manubriosternal angle plus the estimated distance from the RA to the manubriosternal angle. This estimated atrial pressure (in cm H_2O) can be converted to millimeters of mercury by dividing by 1.3.

Because Yock and Popp[132] found only a modest correlation between estimates of RA pressure based on JVP and

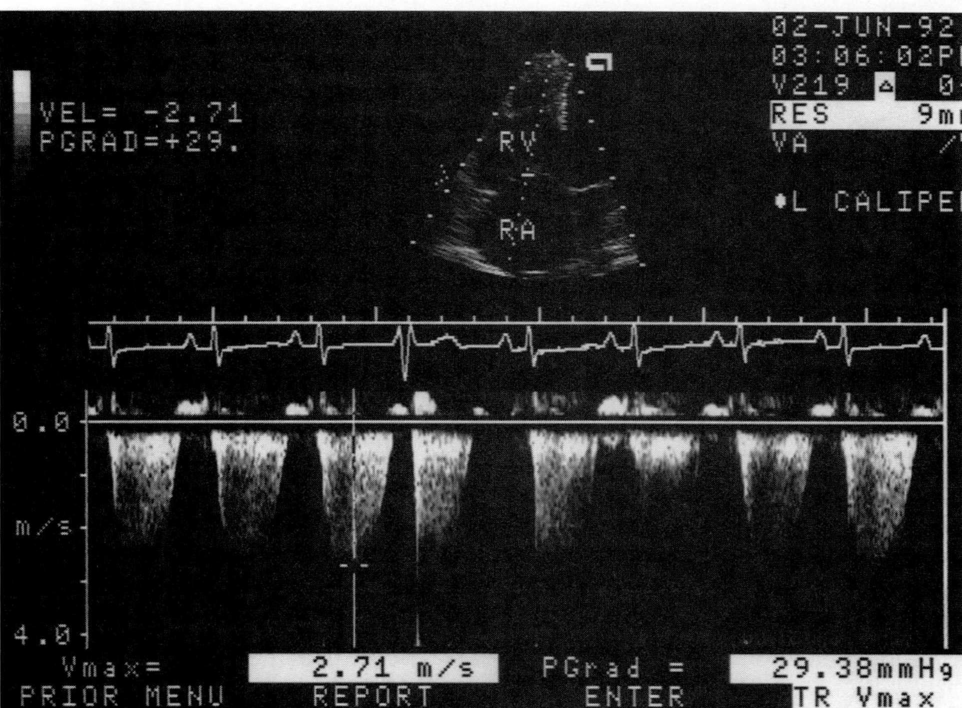

FIGURE 100–8 Noninvasive determination of pulmonary artery systolic pressure: tricuspid regurgitation velocity and the modified Bernoulli equation. The steerable continuous-wave Doppler is placed across the tricuspid valve and guided by color flow Doppler (color not seen in this figure). The systolic Doppler envelope of tricuspid regurgitation is seen below the baseline, consistent with the jet moving from the right ventricle (RV) toward the right atrium (RA). The peak velocity is 2.7 m/s. The pulmonary artery systolic pressure is calculated as $4\ (2.7)^2$ right atrial pressure (or 29 mm Hg right atrial pressure). The right atrial pressure can be measured clinically or estimated by observing the size and respiratory motion of the inferior vena cava, as in Figure 100–9.

the measured RA pressure, even in the hands of experienced examiners, it would be ideal to have a more accurate method of measuring atrial pressure. There is good correlation between the behavior of the proximal inferior vena cava and the RA pressure. Kircher and colleagues[136] showed that the normal response of the vena cava to inspiration is a decrease in size. A 50 percent reduction in caval dimension occurs with inspiratory pressures of 0 to 5 mm Hg. Much higher inspiratory pressures are required to achieve the same degree of collapse in patients with elevated RA pressure. Although there is a good correlation between the inspiratory pressure at which 85 percent of the maximal caval collapse occurs and RA pressure, there is an even better relationship between RA pressure and the inspiratory pressure required to alter caval size. Measurement of the inspiratory pressure required to alter the caval size requires the use of sonospirometry.[109] Although our method is imperfect, we use the diameter of the vena cava, measured 2 cm proximal to the junction with the right atrium, and the change in caval diameter with respiratory maneuvers, such as a sniff, to estimate RA pressure (Fig. 100–9).[137] As a rule, an inferior vena cava that is more than 2.5 cm in diameter and that collapses by less than 50 percent when the patient sniffs is "plethoric" and usually has a pressure in excess of 10 mm Hg. Conversely, cavae that are less than 1.5 cm and collapse by more than 50 percent with spontaneous respiration tend to have atrial pressures in the normal range (0 to 6 mm Hg).

TABLE 100–8 Useful Formulas for Assessment of Pulmonary Hypertension

Pulmonary/systemic flow	$\frac{PBF}{SBF} = \frac{\text{Systemic A} - \text{V } O_2 \text{ difference}}{\text{Pulmonary A} - \text{V } O_2 \text{ difference}}$
Pulmonary blood flow (Fick)	$PBF = \frac{O_2 \text{ consumption}}{\text{Pulmonary A} - \text{V } O_2 \text{ difference}}$
O_2 content of blood	O_2 content (volume%) = (1.34 × hemoglobin) × O_2 saturation Multiply by 10 to permit flow calculations in L/min
Pulmonary vascular resistance (PVR)	$\text{PVR (Wood Units)} = \left[\frac{PAP_{mean} - P_{wedge}}{\text{Cardiac output}}\right]$ $\text{PVR (dyne/s/cm}^{-5}) = \left[\frac{PAP_{mean} - P_{wedge}}{\text{Cardiac output}}\right] \times 80$
Total pulmonary resistance (TPR)	$\text{TPR (Wood Units)} = \left[\frac{PAP_{mean}}{\text{Cardiac output}}\right]$
PAP mean (acceleration time)	PAP mean = 79 − (0.45 × AT)
PAP systolic (modified Bernoulli's equation)	PAP systolic = $4 \times V^2_{TR}$

Abbreviations: AT, acceleration time; P, pressure; PAP, pulmonary artery pressure; PBF, pulmonary blood flow; SBF, systolic blood flow.

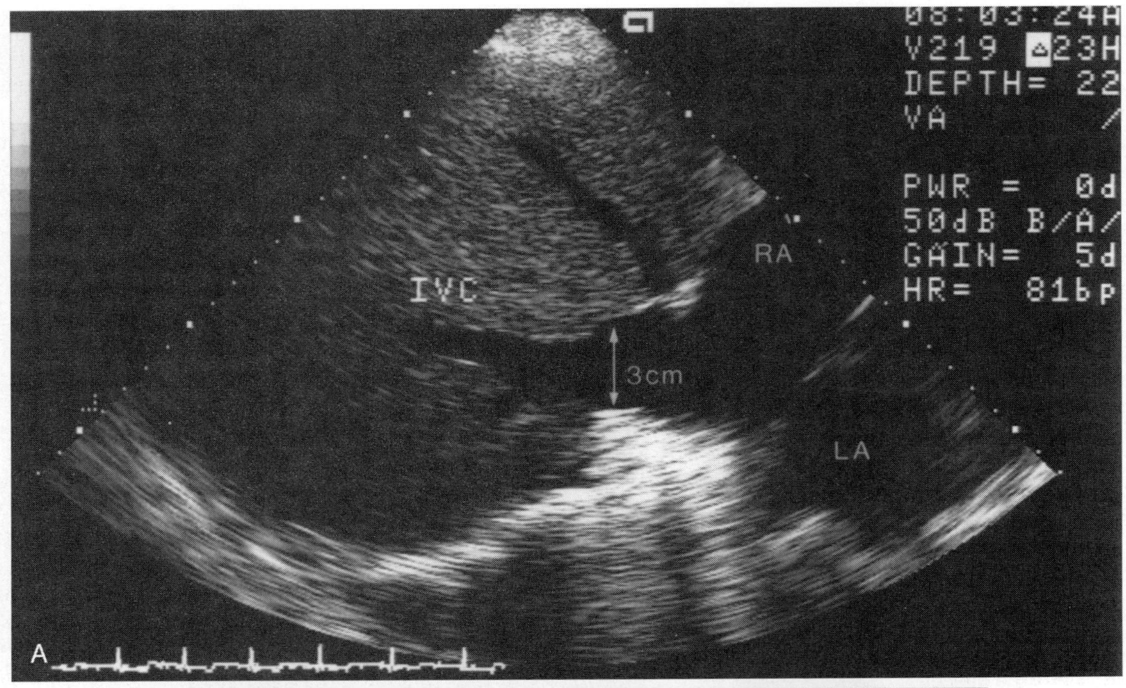

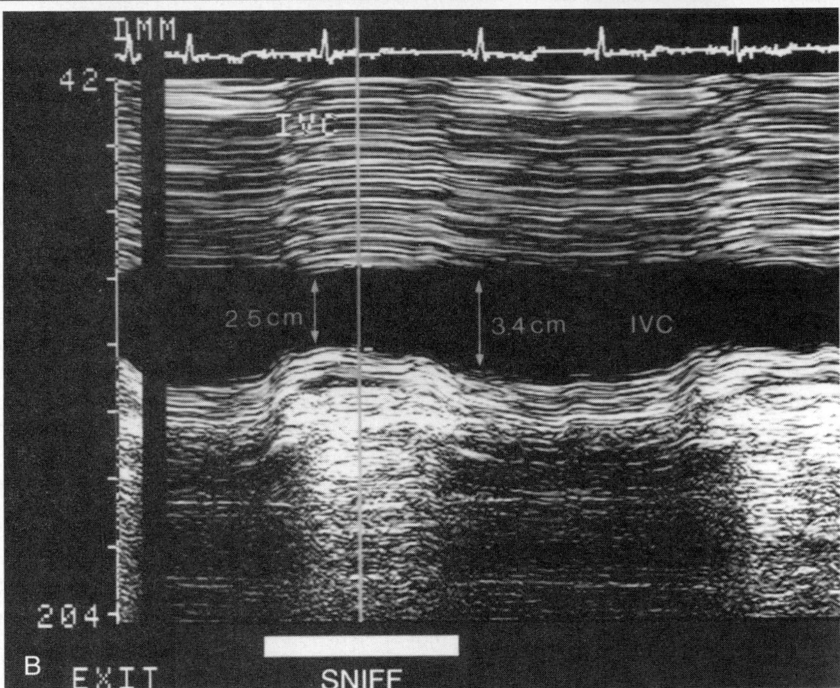

FIGURE 100–9 Estimation of right atrial pressure using the dimensions of the inferior vena cava (IVC). **A,** Subcostal view on a two-dimensional echocardiogram shows a plethoric IVC of approximately 3 cm. **B,** M-mode echocardiogram of the same view shows a dilated IVC (3.4 cm) that decreased to 2.5 cm when the patient sniffed. This is consistent with IVC plethora and indicates elevated right atrial pressure. LA, left atrium; RV, right ventricle.

Magnetic Resonance Imaging

Magnetic resonance imaging (MRI) permits volumetric flow measurement in the major pulmonary arteries. Bogren and associates[138] used this technique to evaluate compliance in the arteries of normal subjects and patients with pulmonary hypertension. They defined compliance, a measure of vascular distensibility, as the change in pulmonary artery volume resulting from a change in pressure.[138] Although this study included only four patients with pulmonary hypertension, it showed that the systolic change in volume in the main pulmonary arteries was considerably less in the hypertensive group (8 percent) than in control subjects (23 percent). Furthermore, although normal subjects had a small (2 percent), late reversal of pulmonary flow, patients with pulmonary hypertension had a larger volume (26 percent) of retrograde flow, accounting for the partial early closure of the valve in the latter group. Pulmonary flow velocity was slower in hypertensive patients than in control subjects, but the acceleration time was reduced, as noted in Doppler studies. The potential for MRI to define pathology in the pulmonary arteries and to measure PAP has not been systematically explored.

MRI also permits the accurate, noninvasive measurement of RV volume.[139] Boxt and colleagues[139] compared ventricular volumes in normal and pulmonary hypertensive patients by using Simpson's rule. The end-diastolic and end-systolic volume indices in patients with pulmonary hypertension (121 ± 45 and 70 ± 42 ml/m^2, respectively) were greater than those in normal individuals (68 ± 13 and 28 ± 8 ml/m^2, respectively).[139] In addition to the dilatation of the right heart and pulmonary arterial tree, there are other characteristic signs of pulmonary hypertension on MRI, including a reduced RV ejection fraction (patients with pulmonary hypertension, 0.43 ± 0.21; control subjects, 0.59 ± 0.9)[139] and an increase in the MRI signal intensity throughout the cardiac cycle.

Computed Tomography

The computed tomography (CT) scan can be used to measure pulmonary artery size, to rule out proximal pulmonary artery thrombi, and to evaluate the possibility of occult interstitial lung disease.[140, 141] Intuitively, one would expect that the CT scan, which provides a more accurate measure of pulmonary artery size, should be superior to the chest radiograph in the estimation of PAP. Moore and associates[142] evaluated the relationship between pulmonary artery size and pressure by the use of CT. They studied 6 patients with cor pulmonale and 18 with pulmonary vascular hypertension (primary or thromboembolic). In the patients with pulmonary vascular hypertension, pulmonary artery size correlated directly with PVR and inversely with cardiac output but did not correlate with PAP.[142] They speculated that the reduced compliance of the pulmonary arteries in pulmonary vascular hypertension might account for the lack of correlation between vessel size and pressure. Compliance is reduced in pulmonary arteries in patients with pulmonary vascular hypertension[143] but normal in patients with pulmonary hypertension associated with lung disease (cor pulmonale).[144] In cor pulmonale, a condition in which muscular hypertrophy of the media predominates, there was a trend toward a direct correlation between pulmonary artery size and pressure.[142] Although this small study lacked control subjects with normal pressures, it suggests that main pulmonary artery size, measured with CT, reflects PVR, an important prognostic factor. The diameter of the main pulmonary artery corrected for body surface area in patients with pulmonary hypertension (pressure, 65 ± 10 mm Hg) was 36 ± 6 mm.

CT has also been used to differentiate thromboembolic from primary pulmonary hypertension.[145] In addition to avoiding the need for catheterization, the CT scan allows characterization of tissue density. The tomographic assessment of tissue density enables a blood clot to be distinguished from the vessel wall. The CT scan may be helpful in the crucial assessment of whether the origins of the thrombi are sufficiently proximal to permit thromboendarterectomy.[145]

Patients with interstitial fibrosis may have entirely normal chest radiographs, and for these patients (10 percent of those with biopsy-proved interstitial fibrosis[140]), CT scans are a more sensitive technique. The use of ultrathin-slice CT scanning has enhanced our ability to diagnose the small group of patients with interstitial fibrosis who would otherwise be misdiagnosed as having "primary" pulmonary hypertension.

Exercise Testing

There are two major reasons to perform exercise testing in patients with pulmonary hypertension. The first is to evaluate the patient's functional capacity. Rhodes and colleagues[146] showed that patients with PPH who performed poorly at low work levels had a poor prognosis. In this small study, patients who exercised to greater than 75 percent of predicted capacity had positive responses to vasodilator therapy, whereas three patients who could exercise only to less than 10 percent of predicted levels died during diagnostic catheterization.[146] Larger studies are required to evaluate the true prognostic value of exercise capacity in patients with pulmonary hypertension.

The second reason to exercise the pulmonary hypertensive patient is to expose occult pulmonary hypertension. In normal individuals, exercise causes a proportionate increase in PAP and cardiac output. Consequently, PVR does not increase.[147, 148] In contrast, patients with mild or moderate pulmonary vascular disease may have minimal elevations of vascular resistance at rest but may develop marked elevations of pressure and resistance with exercise. The rise in PVR with exercise may account for symptoms such as exertional dyspnea and fatigue.

CARDIAC CATHETERIZATION

Catheterization of the pulmonary artery remains the "gold standard" for the determination of PAP and, despite a plethora of available noninvasive techniques, is usually required to firmly establish a diagnosis of pulmonary hypertension. The goals of right heart catheterization include the measurement of pressure, flow, and resistance. In addition, the catheter is used to establish the type of pulmonary hypertension.

The normal mean PAP compiled from the literature is 14 ± 3 (SD) mm Hg. Pulmonary hypertension is defined as a mean pressure of more than 18 mm Hg.[1] However, pressure alone is a crude measurement of the status of the pulmonary vascular bed. In normal adults, PVR, a calculated value that integrates flow and pressure drop across the circuit, is approximately 2 ± 1 Wood Units.[1] The normal cardiac index is 3.2 ± 0.5 L/min/m^2.

Pulmonary hypertension can generally be considered the result of vascular obstruction, as in thromboembolic and primary pulmonary hypertension, or a passive response to elevated LV end-diastolic pressure, as in congestive cardiomyopathy (Fig. 100–10). In patients with pulmonary vascular hypertension, there is a large gradient between the

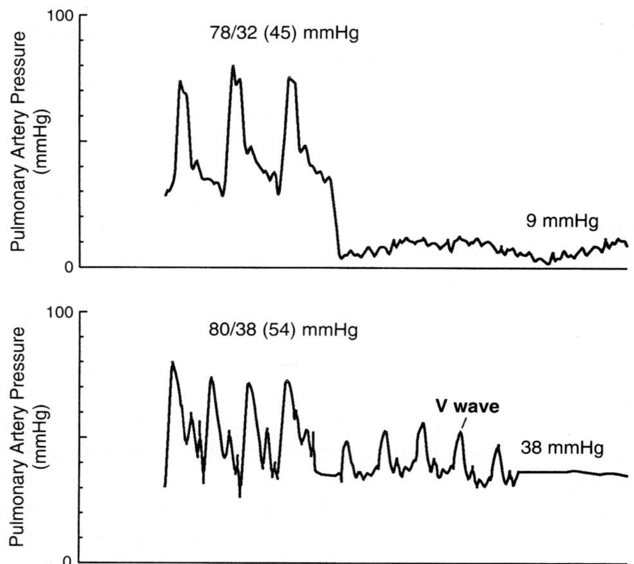

FIGURE 100–10 Comparison of the hemodynamic characteristics of passive and pulmonary vascular hypertension. These patient tracings were obtained with a balloon flotation catheter. **Top,** This patient has pulmonary vascular hypertension characterized by the large gradient between the pulmonary artery diastolic pressure (32 mm Hg) and the wedge pressure (9 mm Hg). This pattern indicates obstruction within the pulmonary vasculature and may be seen with primary or thromboembolic pulmonary hypertension. **Bottom,** This patient has "passive," or secondary, pulmonary hypertension due to elevated left atrial pressure, the result of severe left ventricular damage by a myocardial infarction. Note that there is no difference between the pulmonary artery diastolic pressure and the wedge pressure (both 38 mm Hg). This pattern indicates the cause of the pulmonary hypertension distal to the pulmonary vasculature. Such a pattern may be seen with valvular heart disease and various cardiomyopathies. Note the elevated wedge pressure with V waves, resulting from mitral regurgitation.

pulmonary diastolic pressure and the wedge pressure. This may be due to fixed vascular obstruction in a narrowed and partially obliterated vascular bed or may be due in part to increased pulmonary vascular tone. Based on studies of vasodilator therapy in patients with PPH, which consistently show only one third of patients responding to vasodilators, one can speculate that the majority of patients have fixed anatomic vascular disease as the proximate cause of the gradient between their diastolic pulmonary artery and wedge pressure. Consequently, PVR (calculated as mean PAP − wedge pressure divided by cardiac output) is elevated (see Fig. 100–10). In normoxic individuals, the normal difference between the pulmonary artery mean and wedge pressures is 5 to 9 mm Hg.[1]

In patients with LV failure, pulmonary artery diastolic and wedge pressures are similar (see Fig. 100–10). In these patients, the total pulmonary resistance, which does not take into account LA pressure, may be elevated, but PVR is not increased. Right heart catheterization readily distinguishes these forms of hypertension and thus aids in achieving a specific mechanistic diagnosis.

Technical Considerations

The goal of right heart catheterization in the assessment of a patient with unexplained pulmonary hypertension is to measure the pressure in all chambers, estimate LA pressure by obtaining a wedge pressure, and measure cardiac output. Additional studies may be necessary if there a suspicion of intracardiac shunting or valvular disease. In any patient with a question of shunting, we perform oximetry in all right heart chambers and use indocyanine green "dye curves" to localize and quantify the shunt.

We perform right heart catheterization via a femoral vein approach under fluoroscopic guidance. Most right heart catheterizations are performed with a balloon flotation catheter. Although this catheter is convenient and has a port for measurement of cardiac output using a thermodilution technique, the fidelity of the recording is poor. The small lumen and flexible walls ensure poor frequency response and significant catheter "whip." In patients with hypertension and large pulmonary arteries, it may be difficult to "float" the catheter into the artery. In this case, the use of a 0.018-inch wire within the catheter may adequately increase its stiffness to allow success. Alternatively, there are more rigid flotation catheters that may be useful. In general, it is a good policy to minimize the number of wedge measurements in patients with pulmonary hypertension and to monitor the catheter's position during attempted wedging. These practices minimize the risk of pulmonary artery rupture.

The use of a rigid catheter, such as a Goodale-Lubin catheter, provides better hemodynamic traces and allows more controlled manipulation, which is useful in an attempt to cross an atrial septal defect. These nonfloatation catheters have a higher risk of causing dysrhythmias, right bundle branch block, or myocardial perforation and therefore must be handled cautiously.

Risks

Right heart catheterization carries increased risks in patients with pulmonary hypertension. The risks of right heart catheterization can be divided into three categories:

1. Risks related to obtaining vascular access (e.g., vasovagal reactions)
2. Risks of having a catheter in the heart (pulmonary artery rupture, arrhythmia)
3. Risks of administering medications (e.g., negative inotropic effects, systemic vasodilatation with hypotension)

Pulmonary hypertensive patients may be intolerant to vasovagal reactions that may occur during attempted vascular access. When systemic vasodilatation occurs, whether due to a drug or reflex, the dysfunctional RV and obstructed pulmonary vascular bed may not support the normal increase in left heart output that accompanies systemic vasodilatation. Therefore, a simple vasovagal reaction may lead to a fatal cycle of bradycardia, hypotension, acidosis, and death. Rhodes and associates[146] reported a 19 percent mortality rate related to catheterization in a study of 16 consecutive patients with PPH. All of the deaths in this small study occurred in patients with poor exercise tolerance, and the authors advocated that catheterization be avoided in patients who were intolerant to low-level exercise (less than 10 percent of predicted exercise tolerated). In an accompanying editorial, Brundage[149] pointed out the need for meticulous attention to the prevention of pain and vasovagal reactions in the patient with pulmonary hypertension. It is noteworthy that there were no deaths during diagnostic catheterization in the NIH registry study, in which 187 patients, mostly of class III or IV, underwent right heart catheterization.[150]

NUCLEAR MEDICINE

Ventilation/Perfusion Scans

Ventilation/perfusion ($\dot{V}/Q$) scans are widely used in the assessment of patients with pulmonary hypertension to exclude a thromboembolic cause. Hull and associates[151] compared the relative roles of $\dot{V}/Q$ scans, objective testing for venous thrombosis, and pulmonary angiography in 305 consecutive patients with suspected pulmonary embolism. Patients underwent pulmonary angiography unless they had "prolonged life-threatening, known cardiac or respiratory disorders" (18 percent of eligible patients). This classic study proved that the common clinical practice of excluding pulmonary embolism when $\dot{V}/Q$ scans were abnormal in the same area, the so-called "matched defect," was incorrect. Although a segmental or larger, unmatched perfusion defect was associated with an 86 percent frequency of pulmonary embolism, segmental and subsegmental matched "low probability" $\dot{V}/Q$ abnormalities were associated with a 36 and 25 percent incidence of angiographically confirmed embolism, respectively. Fortunately for the diagnostician, virtually all patients with thromboembolic pulmonary hypertension have one or more high-probability defects (Fig. 100–11; see Table 100–2).

Risks

The major risk of $\dot{V}/Q$ scans in pulmonary hypertension is misdiagnosis. Patients with PPH often have diffuse, inhomogeneous perfusion scans that are interpreted as being "low probability" (see Fig. 100–11). This may lead to unnecessary angiography. There have been a handful of reports of death within minutes of injection of the albumin macroaggregates, which are the small particles (75 mm) that are labeled with technetium.[152] These complications have usually occurred in patients with severe pulmonary hypertension and may represent the inability of a severely obstructed vascular bed to deal with a shower of microemboli. Nevertheless, a $\dot{V}/Q$ scan should be included in the evaluation of every patient with unexplained pulmonary hypertension.

Thallium Scintigraphy

Although ^{201}Tl scintigraphy is used clinically for the diagnosis of LV ischemia, thallium may occasionally be evident in the wall of the right ventricle.[153] Khaja and colleagues[154] noted ^{201}Tl uptake in the right ventricle of 33 patients with RV hypertrophy or pulmonary hypertension. RV systolic

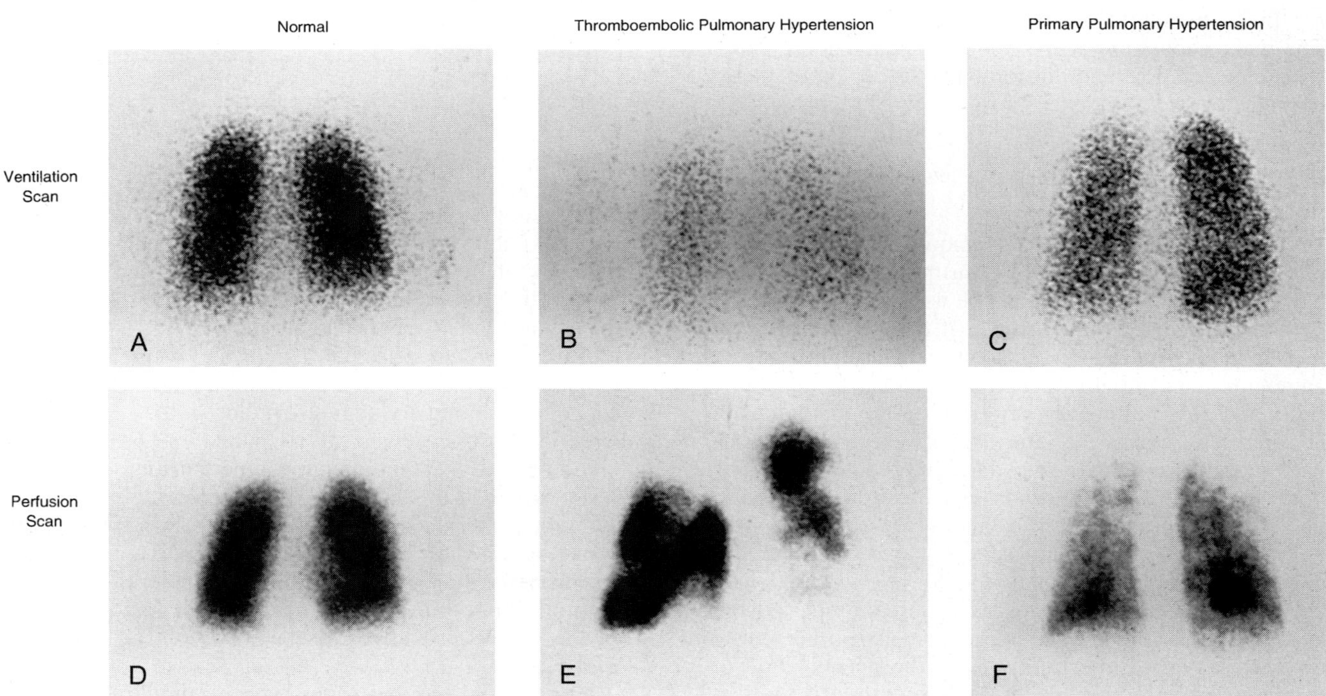

FIGURE 100–11 Comparison of ventilation/perfusion scans in normal individuals and patients with primary and thromboembolic pulmonary hypertension. **A–C,** Ventilation scans from patients with no lung disease, thromboembolic pulmonary hypertension, primary pulmonary hypertension. **D–F,** These perfusion scans were taken from the same patients as in **A–C** (no lung disease, thromboembolic pulmonary hypertension, and primary pulmonary hypertension). **E,** Note the segmental defects in the perfusion scan, which are typical of thromboembolic pulmonary hypertension. **F,** This contrasts with the mottled appearance of the perfusion scan from the patient with primary pulmonary hypertension.

hypertension (greater than 30 mm Hg) was present in 85 percent of the cases, and 9 percent had left-to-right intracardiac shunts with right heart enlargement. A group of patients whose right ventricles were not seen on thallium scintigraphy had normal PAPs.[154] These authors found thallium scintigraphy to be more sensitive for RV pressure-volume overload than the ECG, chest roentgenogram, or echocardiogram. Although thallium is not a routine part of our evaluation of the patient with pulmonary hypertension, it is important that the clinician realizes the potential significance of RV thallium uptake, because these patients periodically undergo thallium tests when their chest pain is mistaken for coronary artery stenosis–induced angina.

Pulmonary Angiography

Pulmonary angiography is primarily used to evaluate the possibility that the pulmonary hypertensive patient has chronic pulmonary emboli. Angiography is also a useful test to diagnose peripheral pulmonary artery stenoses, arteriovenous fistulas, and obliterative pulmonary vascular disease. The technique typically involves the placement of a catheter in the pulmonary artery via the Seldinger technique. Unless the femoral veins and inferior vena cava are shown to be free of thrombus, it is best to use an antecubital or internal jugular route for vascular access to avoid embolization. Although pulmonary angiography often is not attempted in pulmonary hypertension due to the perceived risk, it nevertheless is a safe procedure, with minimal morbidity and mortality risks. The incremental risk of the injection of contrast material beyond the risk of placing a catheter merely to measure pressures is relatively small. The main population at risk for complications are patients with elevated RV end-diastolic pressures (more than 20 mm Hg) or overt evidence of right heart failure.

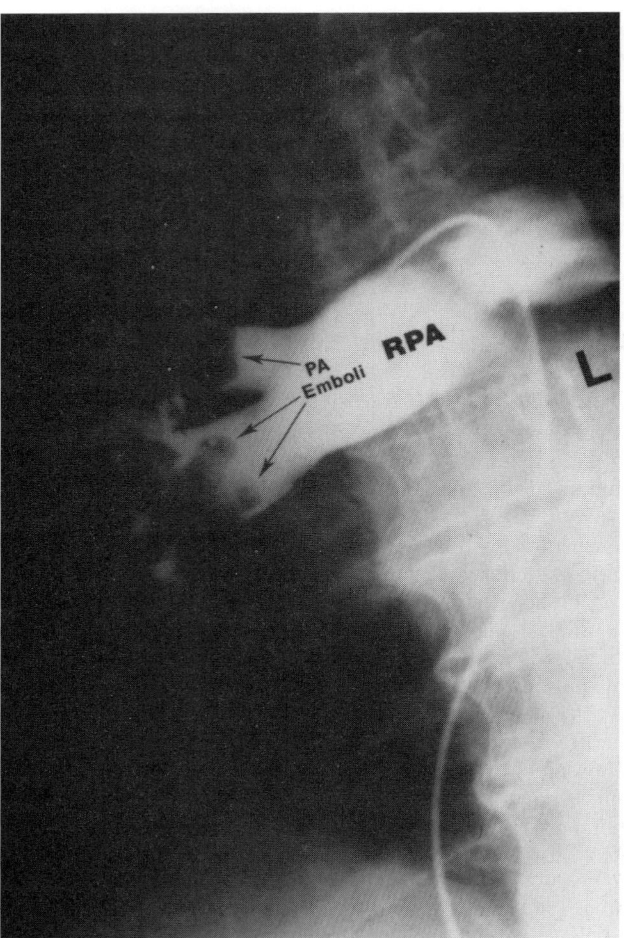

FIGURE 100–12 Selective right pulmonary angiogram (RPA) from a patient with chronic thromboembolic pulmonary hypertension shows multiple filling defects in the right lobar arteries and cutoff of distal vessels. PA, pulmonary artery.

Technique

V̇/Q scans underestimate the amount of thrombi in the patient with thromboembolic pulmonary hypertension. Nevertheless, the V̇/Q scan can be used to guide the angiographic procedure. For example, if a high-probability defect is noted in the lower lobe of the right lung, the angiogram can initially focus on this lobe. In general, the right and left pulmonary arteries, or their subdivisions, are injected selectively. The use of selective pulmonary angiography minimizes dye dilution, reduces overlap of opacified vessels, and ensures opacification of embolized vessels.[155] Although many catheters are available, 7 and 8 French NIH or Berman catheters are widely used for angiography. Hemodynamics should be measured before angiography. Biplanar images are acquired (anteroposterior and 30-degree left anterior oblique) using either cut-film or cine. A typical injection rate for the opacification of a single pulmonary artery is 3510 ml at a rate of 184 ml/s.[156] An acute embolism is present when there is either an intraluminal filling defect or an abrupt cutoff of a vessel (Fig. 100–12). However, in chronic thromboembolic pulmonary hypertension, the embolus often has become incorporated into the vessel wall, and the angiographic signs may be subtle. Shure and colleagues[157] studied patients with unexplained pulmonary hypertension and equivocal pulmonary angiograms with the use of intravascular angioscopy. They found that patients with chronic thromboembolism have pitted masses, scalloping of the vessel wall with intimal irregularities, and bands and webs (consistent with partial revascularization). These findings often are not evident on a pulmonary angiogram, and in the small series, fiberoptic angioscopy led to a change in the diagnosis in four patients with pulmonary hypertension.[157] Unusual diseases that can be diagnosed with CT or angioscopy but may mimic thromboembolic pulmonary hypertension on angiography include congenital absence of a pulmonary artery and fibrosing mediastinitis. Many patients with PPH have undergone pulmonary angiography, which usually shows a dilated proximal vessel with "pruning" of distal vessels.

Although conventional angiography is used to image the large vessels, an alternative angiographic technique called *wedge angiography* can be used to study the microvasculature. This technique is primarily used to assess the anatomy of the small vessels and capillary bed. Small amounts of contrast material are injected distal to the inflated balloon while the catheter is "wedged," and magnified angiograms are obtained. In normal subjects, the subsegmental vessel is plump and smooth, and there is a distal "blush" produced by the microcirculation. Narrowing of the vessel or reduction in the size of the microvascular bed occurs with progressive pulmonary vascular disease.[158] Findings on wedge angiography correlate fairly well with histologic assessment of the pulmonary vasculature obtained at lung biopsy.[159]

Complications

The literature contains many reports of deaths caused by pulmonary angiography, especially in patients with pulmonary hypertension. Advances in catheter design, the use of nonionic contrast agents, and the advent of selective angiography have all contributed to improved safety (see Table 100–2). Nicod and associates[138] analyzed the safety of pulmonary angiography in 67 patients with moderate to severe PPH or thromboembolic pulmonary hypertension. These authors observed no significant complications but noted occasional transient episodes of hypotension, cough, and flushing. The use of supplemental oxygen to avoid hypoxemia and careful attention to analgesia are critical for safe pulmonary angiography. The Prospective Investigation of Pulmonary Embolism Diagnosis (PIOPED) multicenter cooperative trial recently reported on the safety and use of pulmonary angiography in patients with acute pulmonary embolism.[160] The 1111 pulmonary angiograms were performed with ionic contrast injected at a rate of 20 to 35 ml/s for a total volume of 40 to 50 ml. The mortality rate from pulmonary angiography was 0.5 percent, with major, nonfatal complications occurring in 1 percent and minor complications occurring in 5 percent of patients.[160] Mean PAP did not differ in those with major (22 ± 14 mm Hg), minor (19 ± 9 mm Hg), or no (23 ± 11 mm Hg) complications. A review of the complications of pulmonary angiography revealed several incidents of cardiac perforation, which were attributed to the use of older, rigid catheters; therefore, the use of these should be avoided.

Lung Biopsy

Biopsy of the lung parenchyma, either transbronchially via the fiberoptic bronchoscope or by open thoracotomy, is a critically important diagnostic tool in the approach to patients with a variety of diffuse lung diseases. However, lung biopsy plays a less important role in the diagnosis of pulmonary hypertension in most clinical settings. A clinical diagnosis of PPH can be established with reasonable certainty when the criteria for this disease established by the NIH PPH registry are used. Indeed, pathology data from the PPH registry demonstrated that no other diagnosis was made pathologically in patients entered into the registry when lung tissue became available for review. In cases where the cause is less certain, such as patients with significant elevations in PAP associated with moderately abnormal lung function tests or evidence of interstitial disease on chest radiography or high-resolution CT scans of the chest, or patients with serologic abnormalities or other clinical signs that are suggestive of a vasculitis, lung biopsy may be highly useful in establishing a diagnosis and guiding therapy.

Transbronchial lung biopsy is not advocated in patients with pulmonary hypertension, because the small size of the specimen generally precludes the establishment of a definitive diagnosis, and the risk of hemorrhage from hypertensive pulmonary vessels is increased. Open lung biopsy via a standard thoracotomy had been considered the approach of choice, but the risks of this procedure are increased in patients with pulmonary vascular disease, who tolerate anesthesia and surgical interventions poorly. Thoracoscopic lung biopsy, which is less invasive and provides adequate tissue for diagnosis, is the preferred approach when a histologic diagnosis is deemed necessary.

There is marked variability in the extent and type of vascular lesions observed histologically in the lungs of patients with pulmonary hypertension due to primary vascular disease. This often makes a definitive diagnosis difficult, even by experienced pulmonary pathologists. It is even more difficult, therefore, to establish a prognosis or to reliably predict responsiveness to therapy based on pathologic findings. It has been suggested that patients with the greatest extent of medial hypertrophy are more likely to be responsive to vasodilators, presumably because these changes represent an earlier and more vasoreactive stage of the disease.

Although extensive prior thoracic surgery or chemical pleurodesis may preclude consideration for lung or heart-lung transplantation for technical reasons, prior lung biopsy, particularly if performed using a thoracoscope, does not constitute a contraindication for transplantation because the degree of scarring in the thorax is usually minor.

Management of Pulmonary Hypertension

General Measures

Regardless of the cause, pulmonary hypertension is a serious and often life-threatening illness that requires meticulous attention on the part of the patient and the treating physician. Conditions that can exacerbate the pathophysiologic process, such as pregnancy, high altitude, and air travel in nonpressurized aircraft, should be avoided if at all possible. Similarly, medications that can potentiate pulmonary vasoconstriction, such as sympathomimetics used for allergic symptoms or vasoconstrictor prostaglandins used as abortifacients, should not be used. Because oral contraceptives may exacerbate pulmonary hypertension in susceptible patients by increasing their risk for a thromboembolic event, other methods of birth control should be used.

Specific Measures

The guiding principle for the management of pulmonary hypertension is to treat the underlying cause, if one can be identified. Patients with pulmonary hypertension secondary to parenchymal lung disease often manifest significant improvement when a regimen directed at optimization of lung function and gas exchange is implemented. Such an approach usually consists of the maximization of airflow in patients with COPD with bronchodilators and mucolytics and the use of corticosteroids or other immunosuppressive agents to reduce the degree of inflammation and fibrosis in the setting of interstitial lung disease. Patients with cor pulmonale due to sleep apnea syndrome may show dramatic improvement when nocturnal hypoxemia and hypercapnia are corrected with, for example, the use of continuous positive airway pressure or supplemental oxygen therapy.[161, 162]

Medical Management

Oxygen Therapy

Supplemental oxygen therapy is indicated in the management of hypoxemic pulmonary vascular disease. In addition to maximizing oxygen delivery, supplemental oxygen therapy reduces the component of pulmonary hypertension that is due to active hypoxic pulmonary vasoconstriction. Patients with an arterial Po_2 of less than 55 mm Hg at rest or an arterial oxygen saturation of less than 90 percent with ambulation, measured while breathing ambient air, should be considered candidates for supplemental oxygen therapy.[163] Oxygen is most effective in this setting when it is used continuously. The British Medical Research Council[164] and the United States Nocturnal Oxygen Therapy Trial (NOTT)[163] studies demonstrated that the greatest benefit from supplemental oxygen was achieved in the patients who used it for the most time per day. However, although supplemental oxygen therapy prolongs life in patients with hypoxemic chronic respiratory disease, its effect on pulmonary hemodynamics is often variable and incomplete.[165] Patients with nonhypoxemic pulmonary vascular disease do not usually manifest hemodynamic improvement with supplemental oxygen therapy. Arterial oxygenation does not usually improve with supplemental oxygen when hypoxemia is due to right-to-left shunting, although patients may experience some symptomatic relief with its use.

Diuretics

Diuretics are useful for the treatment of right heart failure secondary to pulmonary vascular disease, but aggressive diuresis should be avoided because it can compromise right heart function by excessively reducing preload. Furosemide in doses of 40 to 160 mg/d is usually sufficient for patients with mild to moderate degrees of right heart failure. Patients refractory to furosemide may require the addition of more potent diuretics, such as metolazone or bumetanide. Serum potassium and magnesium levels should be monitored frequently when these agents are used.

Cardiac Glycosides

Cardiac glycosides appear to be most useful in patients whose right heart failure is accompanied by LV dysfunction.[166] These drugs should be used cautiously in patients with chronic lung disease, because the risk of digitalis toxicity is enhanced in this setting.[167]

Vasodilators

The rationale for the use of vasodilators to treat pulmonary hypertension is based on the premise that pulmonary vasoconstriction is a significant contributor to the vascular disease and that even small reductions in afterload will result in a substantial improvement in RV function. Although pulmonary vasoconstriction is present to varying degrees in some forms of pulmonary hypertension, others are characterized by vascular obstruction or obliteration. In the latter setting, it is unlikely that vasodilators will be of benefit, and they may produce serious adverse effects. Therefore, consideration of the use of vasodilators should be based on establishment of the cause of pulmonary vascular disease and assessment of the potential for reversible vasoreactivity in each patient.

Approximately one fourth of patients with PPH manifest substantial reductions in PAP and increases in cardiac output in response to vasodilator administration,[59] and approximately 50 percent of patients experience an increase in cardiac output with a minimal decrease or no change in PAP.[60] In the remainder of patients, vasodilators either have no substantial hemodynamic effect or produce deleterious effects. Mild adverse events occur in approximately 10 percent of patients during acute vasodilator trials when they are performed by experienced physicians. In the NIH registry, two deaths occurred in more than 400 patients who underwent acute testing, and right heart failure appeared to be the most significant risk factor for the development of severe hypotension or death.[60]

The Ca^{2+} channel–blocking agents nifedipine and diltiazem are the orally active vasodilators that are most widely used to treat pulmonary hypertension. In general, verapamil is not useful, in part because it possesses the greatest tendency to produce negative inotropic effects. The doses required to produce the optimal effects are variable, although it appears that responsive patients require higher doses than they do of agents that are conventionally used to treat systemic hypertension or angina pectoris. Some authors have advocated acute challenges in patients with serial doses of these agents under hemodynamic monitoring to identify patients who are likely to benefit from chronic therapy (Figs. 100–13 and 100–14).[59] Although this approach has the advantage of testing patients with the agents that are most likely to be used for chronic therapy, it has the disadvantage of using drugs that are long acting and not titratable.

The major adverse effect of vasodilator therapy is systemic hypotension, which occurs when the systemic effects of these agents predominate. Similarly, severe hypoxemia can develop in this setting if a preexistent right-to-left shunt, such as a patent foramen ovale, is present. Patients with pulmonary hypertension due to parenchymal lung disease may also experience a deterioration in gas exchange as perfusion increases to poorly ventilated lung units owing to the suppression of hypoxic pulmonary vasoconstriction. Peripheral edema can also complicate Ca^{2+} channel blocker therapy. This may be due to the salt and water retention

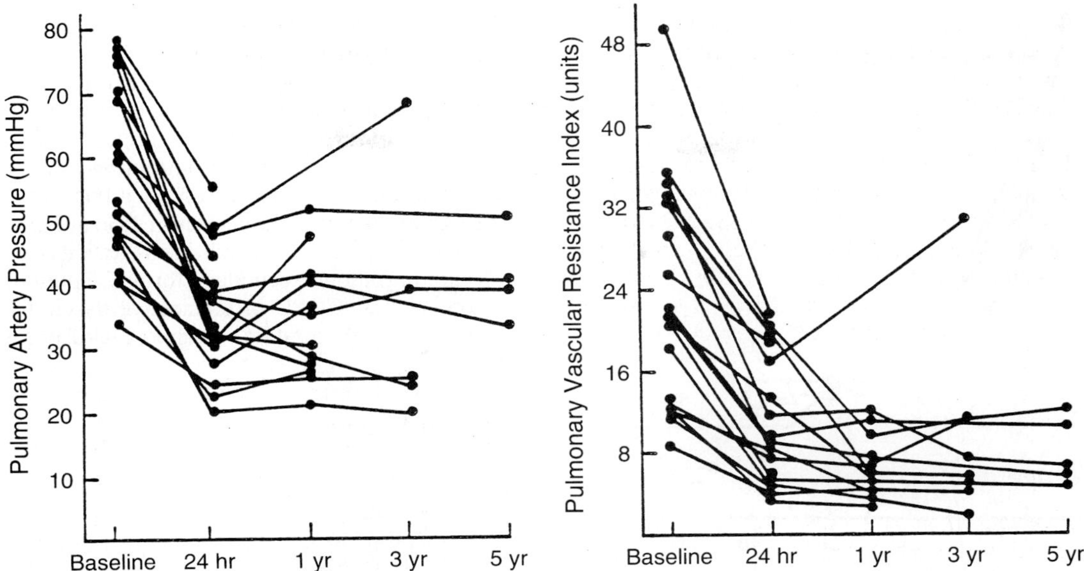

FIGURE 100–13 Mean pulmonary artery **(A)** pressure and **(B)** resistance in patients with primary pulmonary hypertension who responded to high-dose calcium channel blockers. Responders (26 percent of those tested) were defined as having an acute decrease of more than 20 percent in both pulmonary artery pressure and resistance. (**A** and **B,** From Rich S, Kaufmann E, Levy P: The effect of high doses of calcium channel blockers on survival in primary pulmonary hypertension. N Engl J Med 327:76, 1992. Copyright 1992 Massachusetts Medical Society. All rights reserved.)

properties of these agents or to the negative inotropic effects that are occasionally observed with their use.

Several other orally or topically active vasodilators have been used to treat pulmonary hypertension, including hydralazine, diazoxide, nitrates, and angiotensin-converting enzyme inhibitors, with mixed results.[169] Prostaglandins E_1 and I_2 (prostacyclin) are potent, titratable intravenous vasodilators that have been used acutely to evaluate vasoreactivity,[170, 171] although only prostaglandin$_1$ is commercially available. Intravenous adenosine has also been used as an acute test of pulmonary vasoreactivity in patients with pulmonary hypertension and shares with the prostaglandins the safety of a short half-life.[172] In general, responses to these agents are predictive of the responses to orally acting agents, although the magnitude of the response may differ.[173, 174] Side effects of prostaglandin infusions include headache, flushing, nausea, and hypotension: these are usually reversible within 15 minutes after discontinuation of the infusion. In our experience, more than 75 percent of patients manifest a decrease in PAP, an increase in cardiac output, or both in response to prostacyclin infused acutely in incremental doses. In addition, the continuous intravenous infusion of prostacyclin (epoprostenol, Flolan) has been approved by the U.S. Food and Drug Administration to treat patients with severe (New York Heart Association functional classes III and V) PPH and may be particularly useful as a bridge to transplantation in patients who are refractory to other forms of medical treatment.[36] Most patients with PPH who receive continuous-infusion prostacyclin therapy have manifested hemodynamic and symptomatic improvement, with follow-up in several patients on therapy for as long as 10 years.

Very recent data on the long-term effects of epoprostenol therapy have challenged the traditional view that the only patients responding to acute vasodilator challenges will benefit from long-term vasodilator treatment. McLaughlin and associates[175] have shown that the long-term hemodynamic effects of epoprostenol exceed the short-term pulmonary vasodilator response to adenosine. Long-term treatment with epoprostenol decreased PVR even in patients who had no response to adenosine (Fig. 100–15). These important findings suggest that epoprostenol, in addition to vasoactive effects, might improve and even reverse vascular remodeling.

A major limitation to the use of vasodilators to treat pulmonary hypertension is the lack of selectivity of the available agents for the pulmonary circulation. Therefore, some degree of systemic vasodilation occurs in all patients and may limit the use of these drugs. Preliminary experience with inhaled NO suggests that this agent may exert selective pulmonary vasodilation when administered via this route, due to its rapid inactivation.[34] However, this mode of administration is not practical for long-term administration, and the safety and efficacy of NO therapy have not been addressed to date.

Anticoagulants

The role of anticoagulants in nonthromboembolic pulmonary hypertension is controversial. Patients with pulmonary vascular disease appear to be at an increased risk for thromboembolic events because of their physical inactivity, right heart dilatation, and sluggish pulmonary blood flow. Sudden death, often due to pulmonary thromboembolism, occurs frequently in this setting. In both a retrospective[168] and a prospective[59] study, survival was significantly enhanced in patients with PPH who received anticoagulant therapy. The prospective study showed that the patients

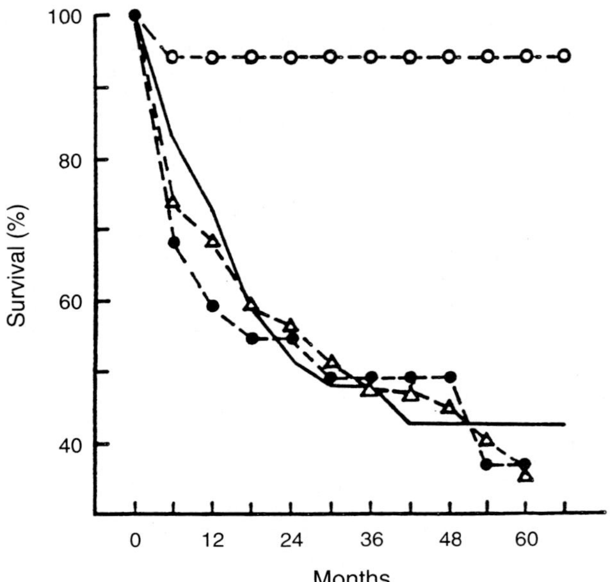

FIGURE 100–14 Significance of a response to high-dose calcium channel blockers in terms of survival. Kaplan-Meier estimates of survival among patients who responded to treatment *(open circles)* and those who did not respond *(solid line)*, patients enrolled in the National Institutes of Health Registry who were treated at the University of Illinois *(solid circles)*, and the National Institutes of Health Registry Cohort *(open triangles)*. Responders are defined in the legend to Figure 100–13. The percentages were calculated every 6 months for 5.5 years. The rate of survival was significantly better in the patients who responded (P = .003) than in the other groups. (From Rich S, Kaufmann E, Levy P: The effect of high doses of calcium channel blockers on survival in primary pulmonary hypertension. N Engl J Med 327:76, 1992. Copyright 1992 Massachusetts Medical Society. All rights reserved.)

who benefit the most from warfarin are those who do not respond to Ca^{2+} channel blockers. However, this study was not designed to assess the effects of anticoagulation, and results must be interpreted with caution. Warfarin was recommended only in the presence of an abnormal lung scan, and it is therefore possible that these patients had simply a higher likelihood of survival.

The adjustment of anticoagulant medications may be particularly difficult in patients prone to altered drug metabolism due to hepatic congestion, and bleeding complications can occur even in the face of therapeutic degrees of anticoagulation. Warfarin is the preferred drug, with the dose adjusted to achieve a prothrombin time of 1.5 to 2.0 times control. In our practice, we advise anticoagulation with warfarin in all patients with PPH, unless clearly contraindicated. We do not routinely anticoagulate patients with nonthrombotic secondary forms of pulmonary hypertension, such as COPD or connective tissue diseases, inasmuch as there are no data to support its use in this setting.

Surgical Management

Patients with pulmonary hypertension due to chronic thrombotic obstruction should be evaluated for thromboendarterectomy, because this procedure has the potential to restore both the integrity of pulmonary circulation and the function of the right heart.[86] Unfortunately, only patients with proximal large-vessel thrombosis, as determined on pulmonary angiography or angioscopy, are suitable candidates for this procedure. Surgical results are excellent; most patients experience a dramatic hemodynamic improvement, with an overall mortality rate of less than 10 percent in experienced hands.

Patients with severe pulmonary hypertension may be considered for either combined heart-lung or lung transplantation. Although there is no consensus regarding the preferred procedure for most patients with pulmonary vascular disease, patients with pulmonary hypertension due to complex congenital heart disease should undergo combined heart-lung transplantation, and the procedure of choice for patients with cor pulmonale due to cystic fibrosis is double lung transplantation because of the chronic lung infection that is often present in this condition. Single lung transplantation has been performed successfully in patients with PPH and pulmonary hypertension due to COPD and fibrotic lung disease.[176] The major complications of transplantation surgery for pulmonary vascular disease are organ rejection and opportunistic infection. Bronchiolitis obliterans occurs

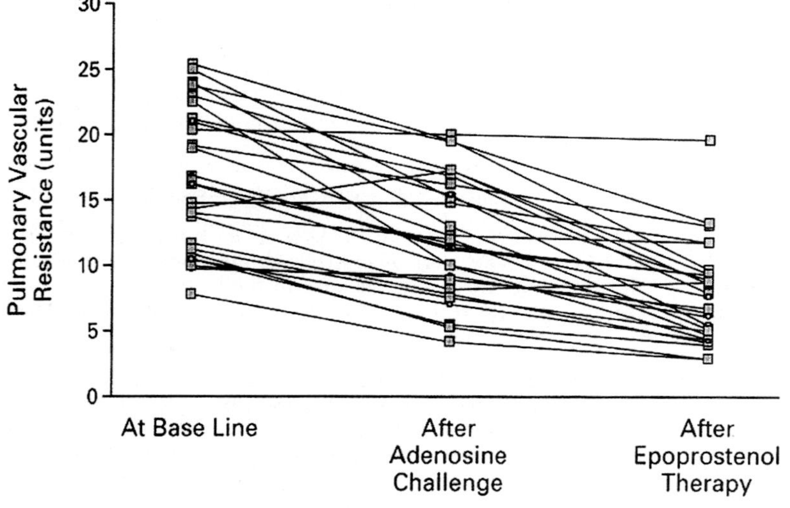

FIGURE 100–15 Pulmonary vascular resistance at baseline, after the administration of intravenous adenosine to test pulmonary vasoreactivity, and after long-term epoprostenol therapy. In all except one patient, the long-term effects of epoprostenol in lowering pulmonary vascular resistance exceeded the short-term pulmonary vasodilator response to adenosine. (From McLaughlin VV, Genthner DE, Panella MM, et al: Reduction in pulmonary vascular resistance with long term epoprostenol therapy in primary pulmonary hypertension. N Engl J Med 338:273, 1998. Copyright 1998 Massachusetts Medical Society. All rights reserved.)

in 25 to 40 percent of transplant patients and may result in serious respiratory embarrassment or death.

Prognosis and Natural History

The course of PPH is variable. Some patients survive for many years, whereas others experience an inexorable course leading to death within months of the diagnosis. Survival appears to be related to the state of function of the right heart, as indicated by functional class, cardiac output, and RA pressure. Patients with severe activity limitations (New York Heart Association functional class IV) and signs of right heart failure usually survive for less than 1 year.[150] To date, no form of therapy for this disease has been shown to alter survival rates, although large-scale prospective studies have not been performed.

The presence of concomitant pulmonary vascular disease in the setting of chronic lung disease has a significant impact on mortality rates, although most patients die within several years of progressive respiratory embarrassment rather than of RV failure.[177] Supplemental oxygen therapy is the only form of treatment that has been shown to improve survival rates in patients in this setting.[163]

References

1. Reeves JT, Groves BM: Approach to the patient with pulmonary hypertension. *In* Weir EK, Reeves JT (eds): Pulmonary Hypertension. pp. 1–44. Mount Kisco, NY: Futura, 1984.
2. Reeves J, Dempsey J, Grover R: Pulmonary circulation during exercise. *In* Weir EK, Reeves JT (eds): Pulmonary Vascular Physiology and Pathophysiology. pp. 107–133. Mount Kisco, NY: Futura, 1989.
3. Rich S, Chomka E, Hasara L, et al: The prevalence of pulmonary hypertension in the United States. Chest 96:236, 1989.
4. Jandova R, Widinsky J, Nikodymova L: Long-term prognosis in pulmonary hypertension in chronic lung disease. Prog Respir Res 20:157, 1985.
5. Wood P: Diseases of the Heart and Circulation. London: Eyre & Spottiswoode, 1962.
6. Lee Y-S: Electron microscopic studies of the alveolarcapillary barrier in the patients of chronic pulmonary edema. Jpn Circ J 43:945, 1979.
7. Ohmichi M, Tagaki S, Nomura N, et al: Endobronchial changes in chronic pulmonary venous hypertension. Chest 94:1127, 1988.
8. West J: Strength and failure of pulmonary capillaries. *In* Wagner W, Weir EK (eds): The Pulmonary Circulation and Gas Exchange. Mount Kisco, NY: Futura, 1994.
9. Dexter L: Pulmonary vascular disease in acquired heart disease. *In* Moser K (ed): Pulmonary Vascular Diseases. pp. 427–480. New York: Marcel Dekker, 1979.
10. Shirai M, Ninomiya I, Sada K: Constrictor response of small pulmonary arteries to acute pulmonary hypertension during left atrial pressure elevation. Jpn J Physiol 41:129, 1991.
11. Wood P, Besterman E, Towers M, McIlroy M: The effect of acetylcholine on pulmonary vascular resistance and left atrial pressure in mitral stenosis. Br Heart J 19:279, 1957.
12. Foltz B, Hessel E, Ivey T: The early course of pulmonary hypertension in patients undergoing mitral valve replacement with cardioplegic arrest. J Thorac Cardiovasc Surg 88:238, 1984.
13. Heath D, Edwards J: The pathology of hypertensive pulmonary vascular disease. Circulation 18:533, 1958.
14. Edwards W: Pathology of pulmonary hypertension. Cardiovasc Clin 18:321, 1988.
15. Wagenvoort C: Lung biopsies and pulmonary vascular disease. *In* Weir EK, Reeves JT (eds): Pulmonary Hypertension. pp. 393–437. Mount Kisco, NY: Futura, 1984.
16. Rabinovitch M: Problems of pulmonary hypertension in children with congenital cardiac defects. Chest 93:119S, 1988.
17. Caslin A, Heath D, Madden B, et al: The histopathology of 36 cases of plexogenic pulmonary arteriopathy. Histopathology 16:9, 1990.
18. Dinh-Xuan A, Higenbottam T, Clelland C, et al: Impairment of pulmonary endothelium-dependent relaxation in patients with Eisenmenger's syndrome. Br J Pharmacol 99:9, 1990.
19. Inauen W, Baumgartner H, Bombeli T, et al: Dose and shear rate-dependent effects of heparin on thrombogenesis induced by rabbit aorta subendothelium exposed to flowing human blood. Arteriosclerosis 10:607, 1990.
20. Reid L, Davies P: Control of cell proliferation in pulmonary hypertension. *In* Weir EK, Reeves JT (eds): Pulmonary Vascular Physiology and Pathophysiology. pp. 541–611. Mount Kisco, NY: Futura, 1989.
21. Berger M, Haimowitz A, Van Tosh A, et al: Quantitative assessment of pulmonary hypertension in patients with tricuspid regurgitation using continuous wave Doppler ultrasound. J Am Coll Cardiol 6:359, 1985.
22. Takahashi T, Wagenvoort C: Density of muscularized arteries in the lung: its role in congenital heart disease and its clinical significance. Arch Pathol Lab Med 107:23, 1983.
23. Gomez-Sanchez M, Mestre de Juan M, Gomez-Pajuelo C, et al: Pulmonary hypertension secondary to toxic oil syndrome: a clinicopathologic study. Chest 95:325, 1989.
24. Copland N, Shimony R, Ioachin H, et al: Primary pulmonary hypertension associated with human immunodeficiency viral infection. Am J Med 89:96, 1990.
25. Herve P, Drouet L, Dosquet C, et al: Primary pulmonary hypertension in a patient with a familial platelet storage pool disease: role of serotonin. Am J Med 89:117, 1990.
26. Edwards B, Weir E, Edwards W, et al: Coexistent pulmonary and portal hypertension: Morphologic and clinical features. J Am Coll Cardiol 10:1233, 1987.
27. Gurtner H: Pulmonary hypertension, "plexogenic pulmonary arteriopathy" and the appetite depressant drug aminorex: post or propter. Bull Eur Physiopathol Res 15:897, 1979.
28. Mark EJ, Patalas ED, Chang HT, et al: Fatal pulmonary hypertension associated with short-term use of fenfluramine and phentermine. N Engl J Med 337:602, 1997.
29. Johnson W, Lie J: Pulmonary hypertension and familial Mediterranean fever: a previously unrecognized association. Mayo Clin Proc 66:919, 1991.
30. Efthimiou J, Johnston C, Spiro S, Turner-Warwick M: Pulmonary disease in Behçet's syndrome. Q J Med 227:259, 1986.
31. Young T, Lundquist L, Chesler E, Weir E: Comparative effects of nifedipine, verapamil, and diltiazem on experimental pulmonary hypertension. Am J Cardiol 51:195, 1983.
32. Tuder RM, Cool CD, Geraci MW, et al: Prostacyclin synthase expression is decreased in lungs from patients with severe pulmonary hypertension. Am Rev Respir Crit Care Med 159:1925, 1999.
33. Giaid A, Saleh D: Reduced expression of endothelial nitric oxide synthase in the lungs of patients with pulmonary hypertension. N Engl J Med 333:214, 1995.
34. Pepka-Zaba J, Higenbottam T, Dinh-Xuan A, Wallwork J: Inhaled nitric oxide as a cause of selective pulmonary vasodilatation in pulmonary hypertension. Lancet 338:1173, 1991.
35. Jones K, Higenbottam T, Wallwork J: Pulmonary vasodilation with prostacyclin in primary and secondary pulmonary hypertension. Chest 96:784, 1989.
36. Rubin L, Mendoza J, Hood M, et al: Treatment of primary pulmonary hypertension with continuous intravenous prostacyclin (epoprostenol). Ann Intern Med 112:485, 1990.
37. Giaid A, Yanagisawa M, Langleben D, et al: Expression of endothelin-1 in the lungs of patients with pulmonary hypertension. N Engl J Med 328:1732, 1993.
38. Stewart D, Levy R, Cernacek P, Langlehben D: Increased plasma endothelin-1 in pulmonary hypertension: marker or mediator of disease? Ann Intern Med 114:464, 1991.
39. Friedman H, Macarak E, MacGregor R, et al: Virus infection of endothelial cells. J Infect Dis 143:266, 1981.
40. Kaner R, Iozzo R, Ziaie Z, Kefalides N: Inhibition of proteoglycan synthesis in human endothelial cells after infection with herpes simplex virus type 1 in vitro. Am J Respir Cell Mol Biol 2:423, 1990.

41. McDonnell P, Sumner W, Hutchins G: Pulmonary venoocclusive disease: morphologic changes suggesting a viral cause. JAMA 246:667, 1981.
42. Lee SD, Shroyer KR, Markham NE, et al: Monoclonal endothelial cell proliferation is present in primary but not secondary pulmonary hypertension. J Clin Invest 101:927, 1998.
43. Yuan XJ, Wang J, Juhaszova M, et al: Attenuated K^+ channel gene transcription in primary pulmonary hypertension. Lancet 351:726, 1998.
44. Nelson MT, Quayle JM: Physiological roles and properties of potassium channels in arterial smooth muscle. Am J Physiol 268:C799, 1995.
45. Archer SL, Huang JMC, Hampl V, et al: Nitric oxide and cGMP cause vasorelaxation by activation of charybdotoxin-sensitive K^+ channel by cGMP-dependent protein kinase. Proc Natl Acad Sci U S A 91:7583, 1994.
46. Yuan X-J, Goldman W, Tod M, et al: Hypoxia reduces potassium currents in cultured rat pulmonary but not mesenteric arterial myocytes. Am J Physiol 264:L116, 1993.
47. Archer SL, Huang JMC, Reeve HL, et al: Differential distribution of electrophysiologically distinct myocytes in conduit and resistance arteries determines their response to nitric oxide and hypoxia. Circ Res 78:431, 1996.
48. Yuan XJ, Wang J, Juhaszova M, et al: Molecular basis and function of voltage-gated K^+ channels in pulmonary arterial smooth muscle cells. Am J Physiol 274:L621, 1998.
49. Lopez-Barneo J, Lopez-Lopez J, Urena J, Gonzalez C: Chemotransduction in the carotid body: K current modulated by PO_2 in type I chemoreceptor cells. Science 242:580, 1988.
50. Delpiano M, Hescheler J: Evidence for a PO_2-sensitive K channel in the type-I cell of the rabbit carotid body. FEBS Lett 249:195, 1989.
51. Peers C: Hypoxic suppression of K currents in type I carotid body cells: selective effect on the Ca^2-activated K current. Neurosci Lett 119:253, 1990.
52. Archer SL, Couil E, Dinh-Xuan AT, et al: Molecular identification of the role of voltage-gated K^+ channels, kv1.5 and kv2.1, in hypoxic pulmonary vasoconstriction and control of resting membrane potential in rat pulmonary artery myocytes. J Clin Invest 101:2319, 1998.
53. Hulme JT, Coppock EA, Felipe A, et al: Oxygen sensitivity of cloned voltage-gated K^+ channels expressed in the pulmonary vasculature. Circ Res 85:489, 1999.
54. Yuan JX, Aldinger AM, Juhaszova M, et al: Dysfunctional voltage-gated K^+ channels in pulmonary artery smooth muscle cells of patients with primary pulmonary hypertension. Circulation 14:1400, 1998.
55. Weir E, Chidsey C, Weil J: Minoxidil reduces pulmonary vascular resistance in dogs and cattle. J Lab Clin Med 88:885, 1976.
56. Hasunuma K, Rodman D, McMurtry I: Effects of K channel blockers on vascular tone in the perfused rat lung. Am Rev Respir Dis 144:884, 1991.
57. Chan N, McLay J, Kenmore A: Reversibility of primary pulmonary hypertension during six years of treatment with oral diazoxide. Br Heart J 57:207, 1987.
58. McMurtry I, Davidson B, Reeves J, Grover R: Inhibition of hypoxic pulmonary vasoconstriction by calcium antagonists in isolated rat lungs. Circ Res 38:99, 1976.
59. Rich S, Kaufmann E, Levy P: The effect of high doses of calcium channel blockers on survival in primary pulmonary hypertension. N Engl J Med 327:76, 1992.
60. Weir E, Rubin L, Ayres S: The acute administration of vasodilators in primary pulmonary hypertension. Am Rev Respir Dis 140:1623, 1989.
61. Reeves J, Groves B, Turkevich D: The case for treatment of selected patients with primary pulmonary hypertension. Am Rev Respir Dis 134:342, 1986.
62. Eisenberg P, Lucore C, Kaufman L, et al: Fibrinopeptide A levels indicative of pulmonary vascular thrombosis in patients with primary pulmonary hypertension. Circulation 82:841, 1990.
63. Langleben D, Moroz L, McGregor M, Lisbona R: Decreased half-life of fibrinogen in primary pulmonary hypertension. Thromb Res 40:577, 1985.
64. Inglesby T, Singer J: Abnormal fibrinolysis in familial pulmonary hypertension. Am J Med 55:5, 1973.
65. Sadler JE, Mancuso DJ, Randi AM, et al: Molecular biology of von Willebrand factor. Ann N Y Acad Sci 614:114, 1991.
66. Weiss H: von Willebrand factor and platelet function. Ann N Y Acad Sci 614:125, 1991.
67. Rabinovitch M, Andrew M, Thom H, et al: Abnormal endothelial factor VIII associated with pulmonary hypertension and congenital heart defects. Circulation 76:1043, 1987.
68. Geggel R, Carvalho A, Hover L, Reid L: von Willebrand factor abnormalities in primary pulmonary hypertension. Am Rev Respir Dis 135:294, 1987.
69. Abenhaim L, Moride Y, Brenot F, et al: Appetite-suppressant drugs and the risk of primary pulmonary hypertension: International Primary Pulmonary Hypertension Study Group. N Engl J Med 33:609, 1996.
70. Weir EK, Reeve HL, Huang JM, et al: Anorexic agents aminorex, fenfluramine, and dexfenfluramine inhibit potassium current in rat pulmonary vascular smooth muscle and cause pulmonary vasoconstriction. Circulation 94:2216, 1996.
71. Patel AJ, Lazdunski M, Horore E: Kv2.1/Kv9.3, a novel ATP-dependent delayed-rectifier K^+ channel in oxygen-sensitive pulmonary artery myocytes. EMBO J 16:6615, 1997.
72. Reeve HL, Archer SL, Soper M, Weir EK: Dexfenfluramine increases pulmonary artery smooth muscle intracellular Ca^{++}, independent of membrane potential. Am J Physiol 277:L662, 1999.
73. Wang J, Juhaszova M, Conte JV Jr, et al: Action of fenfluramine on voltage-gated K^+ channels in human pulmonary-artery smooth-muscle cells. Lancet 352:290, 1998.
74. Herve P, Launay JM, Scrobohaci ML, et al: Increased plasma serotonin in primary pulmonary hypertension. Am J Med 99:249, 1995.
75. Archer SL, Djaballah K, Humbert M, et al: Nitric oxide deficiency in fenfluramine- and dexfenfluramine-induced pulmonary hypertension. Am J Respir Crit Care Med 158:1061, 1998.
76. Tuder RM, Radisavljevic Z, Shroyer KR, et al: Monoclonal endothelial cells in appetite suppressant-associated pulmonary hypertension. Am J Respir Crit Care Med 158:1999, 1998.
77. Weir EK, Reeve HL, Johnson G, et al: A role for potassium channels in smooth muscle cells and platelets in the etiology of primary pulmonary hypertension. Chest 114:200S, 1998.
78. Tazelaar H, Myers J, Drage C, et al: Pulmonary disease associated with L-tryptophan–induced eosinophilic myalgia syndrome. Clinical and pathologic features. Chest 97:1032, 1990.
79. Yakovlevitch M, Siegel M, Hoch D, Rutlen D: Pulmonary hypertension in a patient with tryptophan-induced eosinophilia-myalgia syndrome. Am J Med 90:272, 1991.
80. Erkan F, Cavdar T: Pulmonary vasculitis in Behçet's disease. Am Rev Respir Dis 146:232, 1992.
81. Wagner O, Roncoroni A, Barcat J: Severe pulmonary hypertension with diffuse smooth muscle proliferation of the lungs. Chest 95:234, 1989.
82. Kawahara Y, Taniguchi T, Kadou T, et al: Elevated pulmonary arterial pressure in pulmonary lymphangiomyomatosis. Jpn J Med 28:520, 1989.
83. Mette S, Palevsky H, Pietra G, et al: Primary pulmonary hypertension in association with human immunodeficiency virus infection. Am Rev Respir Dis 145:1196, 1992.
84. D'Alonzo GE, Bower JS, Dantzker DR: Differentiation of patients with primary and thromboembolic pulmonary hypertension. Chest 85:457, 1984.
85. Moser K, Spragg R, Utley J, Daily P: Chronic thrombotic obstruction of major pulmonary arteries. Ann Intern Med 99:299, 1983.
86. Moser KM, Daily PO, Peterson K, et al: Thromboendarterectomy for chronic, major-vessel thromboembolic pulmonary hypertension. Ann Intern Med 107:560, 1987.
87. Rich S, Dantzker DR, Ayres SM, et al: Primary pulmonary hypertension: a national prospective study. Ann Intern Med 107:216, 1987.
88. Voekel NF, Reeves JT: Primary pulmonary hypertension. *In* Lenfont F, Moser K (eds): Pulmonary Vascular Disease. pp. 573–628. New York: Marcel Dekker, 1979.
89. Chapman P, Bateman E, Benatar S: Primary pulmonary hypertension and thromboembolic pulmonary hypertension: similarities and differences. Respir Med 84:485, 1990.
90. Wood P: Disease of the Heart and Circulation. 2nd ed. Philadelphia: JB Lippincott, 1956.
91. Newman JH, Loyd JE: Familial pulmonary hypertension. *In* Fishman AP (ed): Pulmonary Circulation: Normal and Abnormal. pp. 301–313. Philadelphia: University of Pennsylvania Press, 1990.
92. Moser KM, Fedullo PF, Auger WR: Results of pulmonary thrombo-

endarterectomy for chronic, major-vessel thromboembolic pulmonary hypertension. *In* Weir EK, Archer SL, Reeves JT (eds): The Diagnosis and Treatment of Pulmonary Hypertension. pp. 311–329. Mount Kisco, NY: Futura, 1992.

93. Gurtner HP: Aminorex pulmonary hypertension. *In* Fishman AP (ed): The Pulmonary Circulation: Normal and Abnormal. pp. 397–411. Philadelphia: University of Pennsylvania Press, 1990.
94. Garcia-Dorado D, Miller DD, Garcia EJ, et al: An epidemic of pulmonary hypertension after toxic rapeseed oil ingestion in Spain. J Am Coll Cardiol 1:1216, 1983.
95. Lopez-Sendon J, Gomez Sanchez MA, Mestre de Juan MJ, Coma-Canella I: Pulmonary hypertension in the toxic oil syndrome. *In* Fishman AP (ed): Pulmonary Circulation: Normal and Abnormal. pp. 385–395. Philadelphia: University of Pennsylvania Press, 1990.
96. Ungerer RG, Tashkin DP, Furst D, et al: Prevalence and clinical correlates of pulmonary arterial hypertension in progressive systemic sclerosis. Am J Med 75:65, 1983.
97. Santini D, Fox D, Kloner RA, et al: Pulmonary hypertension in systemic lupus erythematosus: hemodynamics and effects of vasodilator therapy. Clin Cardiol 3:406, 1980.
98. Weiner-Kronish JP, Solinger AM, Warnock ML, et al: Severe pulmonary involvement in mixed connective tissue disease. Am Rev Respir Dis 124:499, 1981.
99. Young I, Ford S, Ford P: The association of pulmonary hypertension with rheumatoid arthritis. J Rheumatol 16:1266, 1989.
100. McDonnell PJ, Toye PA, Hutchins GM: Primary pulmonary hypertension and cirrhosis: are they related? Am Rev Respir Dis 127:437, 1983.
101. Auger WR, Moser KM: Pulmonary flow murmurs: a distinctive physical sign found in chronic pulmonary thromboembolic disease [abstract]. Clin Res 37:145A, 1989.
102. LeRoy E: Pulmonary hypertension: the bete noire of the diffuse connective tissue diseases. Am J Med 90:539, 1991.
103. Keller CA, Shepard JW, Chun DS, et al: Pulmonary hypertension in obstructive pulmonary disease: multivariate analysis. Chest 90:185, 1986.
104. Brundage B: Pulmonary hypertension in collagen vascular disease. *In* Fishman AP (ed): The Pulmonary Circulation: Normal and Abnormal. pp. 353–358. Philadelphia: University of Pennsylvania Press, 1990.
105. Lehtonen J, Sutinen S: Electrocardiographic criteria for the diagnosis of right ventricular hypertrophy verified at autopsy. Chest 93:839, 1988.
106. Viamonte M, Parks RE, Barrera F: Roentgenographic prediction of pulmonary hypertension in mitral stenosis. AJR 87:936, 1962.
107. Kanemoto N, Furuya H, Etoh T, et al: Chest roentgenograms in primary pulmonary hypertension. Chest 76:45, 1979.
108. Change CH: The normal roentgenographic measurement of the right descending pulmonary artery in 1085 cases. AJR 87:929, 1962.
109. Schiller NB, Sahn DJ: Pulmonary pressure measurement by Doppler and two-dimensional echocardiography in adult and pediatric populations. *In* Weir EK, Archer SL, Reeves JT (eds): The Diagnosis and Treatment of Pulmonary Hypertension. pp. 41–59. Mount Kisco, NY: Futura, 1992.
110. Missri J: Evaluation of pulmonary hypertension by Doppler echocardiography. J Cardiovasc Ultrasound 7:277, 1988.
111. Salvaterra CG, Brundage BH, Rubin LJ: Is the early diagnosis of pulmonary hypertension possible, useful, and cost-effective? *In* Weir EK, Archer SL, Reeves JT (eds): The Diagnosis and Treatment of Pulmonary Hypertension. pp. 3–12. Mount Kisco, NY: Futura, 1992.
112. Nanda N, Gramiak R, Robinson T, Shah P: Echocardiographic evaluation of pulmonary hypertension. Circulation 50:575, 1974.
113. Lew W, Karliner J: Assessment of pulmonary valve echogram in normal subjects and in patients with pulmonary arterial hypertension. Br Heart J 42:147, 1979.
114. Acquatella H, Schiller N, Sharpe D, Chatterjee K: Lack of correlation between echocardiographic pulmonary valve morphology and simultaneous pulmonary arterial pressure. Am J Cardiol 43:946, 1979.
115. Okamoto M, Miyatake K, Kinoshite N, et al: Analysis of blood flow in pulmonary hypertension with the pulsed Doppler flowmeter combined with cross-sectional echocardiography. Br Heart J 51:407, 1984.
116. Park B, Dittrich H, Polikar R, Olson L: Echocardiographic evidence of pericardial effusion in severe chronic pulmonary hypertension. Am J Cardiol 63:143, 1989.
117. Bauman W, Wann L, Childress R, et al: Mid systolic notching of the pulmonary valve in the absence of pulmonary hypertension. Am J Cardiol 43:1049, 1979.
118. Levine R, Gibson T, Aretz T, et al: Echocardiographic measurement of right ventricular volume. Circulation 69:497, 1984.
119. Goerke RJ, Carlsson E: Calculation of left and right ventricular volumes: methods using standard computer equipment and biplane angiograms. Invest Radiol 2:360, 1967.
120. Starling MR, Crawford MH, Sorenson SG, O'Rourke RA: A new two-dimensional echocardiographic technique for evaluating right ventricular size and performance in patients with obstructive lung disease. Circulation 66:612, 1982.
121. Tsuda T, Sawayama T, Kawai N, et al: Echocardiographic measurement of right ventricular wall thickness in adults by anterior approach. Br Heart J 44:55, 1980.
122. Gottdiener J, Gay J, Maron B, Fletcher R: Increased right ventricular wall thickness in left ventricular pressure overload: echocardiographic determination of hypertrophic response of the "nonstressed" ventricle. J Am Coll Cardiol 6:550, 1985.
123. Schimada R, Takeshita A, Nakamura M: Noninvasive assessment of right ventricular systolic pressure in atrial septal defect: analysis of the end-systolic configuration of the ventricular septum by two-dimensional echocardiography. Am J Cardiol 53:1117, 1984.
124. Wilson N, Goldberg SJ, Dickinson DF: Normal intracardiac and great artery blood velocity measurements by pulsed Doppler echocardiography. Br Heart J 53:451, 1985.
125. Kitabatake A, Inoue M, Asao M, et al: Noninvasive evaluation of pulmonary hypertension by a pulsed Doppler technique. Circulation 68:302, 1984.
126. Kosturakis D, Goldberg S, Allen H, Loeber C: Doppler echocardiographic prediction of pulmonary arterial hypertension in congenital heart disease. Am J Cardiol 53:1110, 1984.
127. Mahan G, Dabestani A, Gardin J, et al: Estimation of pulmonary artery pressure by pulsed Doppler echocardiography [abstract]. Circulation 68(suppl III):III-367, 1983.
128. Chan K, Currie P, Seward J, et al: Comparison of three Doppler ultrasound methods in the prediction of pulmonary artery pressure. J Am Coll Cardiol 9:549, 1987.
129. Berger M, Hect S, Van Tosh A, et al: Pulsed and continuous wave Doppler echocardiographic assessment of valvular regurgitation in normal subjects. J Am Coll Cardiol 13:1540, 1989.
130. Choong C, Abascal V, Weyman J, et al: Prevalence of valvular regurgitation by Doppler echocardiography in patients with structurally normal hearts by two-dimensional echocardiography. Am Heart J 117:636, 1989.
131. Morrison D, Ovitt T, Hammermeister K, Stovall J: Functional tricuspid regurgitation and right ventricular dysfunction in pulmonary hypertension. Am J Cardiol 62:108, 1988.
132. Yock P, Popp R: Noninvasive estimation of right ventricular systolic pressure by Doppler ultrasound in patients with tricuspid regurgitation. Circulation 70:657, 1984.
133. Currie P, Seward J, Chan K-L: Continuous wave Doppler determination of right ventricular pressure: a simultaneous Doppler-catheterization study in 127 patients. J Am Coll Cardiol 6:750, 1985.
134. Saal A, Otto C, Janko C, et al: Measurement of pulmonary systolic pressure in adults with tricuspid regurgitation using high pulse repetition frequency Doppler [abstract]. Circulation 70(suppl II):II-117, 1984.
135. Masuyama T, Kodama K, Kitabatake A, et al: Continuous-wave Doppler echocardiographic detection of pulmonary regurgitation and its application to noninvasive estimation of pulmonary artery pressure. Circulation 74:484, 1986.
136. Kircher B, Himelman R, Schiller N: Right atrial pressure estimation from respiratory behavior of the inferior vena cava. Circulation 78:2196, 1988.
137. Simonson J, Schiller N: Sonospirometry: a new method for noninvasive estimation of mean right atrial pressure based on two-dimensional echographic measurements of the inferior vena cava during measured inspiration. J Am Coll Cardiol 11:557, 1988.
138. Bogren H, Klipstein R, Mohiaddin R, et al: Pulmonary artery distensibility and blood flow patterns: a magnetic resonance study of normal subjects and of patients with pulmonary arterial hypertension. Am Heart J 118:990, 1989.
139. Boxt LM, Katz J, Kolb T, et al: Direct quantitation of right and left ventricular volumes with nuclear magnetic resonance imaging in

patients with primary pulmonary hypertension. J Am Coll Cardiol 19:1508, 1992.
140. Epler GR, McLoud TC, Gaensler EA, et al: Normal chest roentgenograms in chronic diffuse infiltrative lung disease. N Engl J Med 298:934, 1978.
141. Muller NL, Miller RR: Computed tomography of chronic diffuse infiltrative lung disease. Am Rev Respir Dis 142:1206, 1990.
142. Moore N, Scott J, Flower C, Higenbottam T: The relationship between pulmonary artery pressure and pulmonary artery diameter in pulmonary hypertension. Clin Radiol 39:486, 1988.
143. Reuben SR, Butler J, Lee GJ: Pulmonary arterial compliance in health and disease. Br Heart J 33:147, 1971.
144. Enson Y, Schmidt DH, Ferrer MI, Harvey RM: The effect of acutely induced hypervolemia on resistance to pulmonary blood flow and pulmonary arterial compliance in patients with chronic obstructive lung disease. Am J Med 57:395, 1974.
145. Kereiakes D, Herfkens R, Brundage B, et al: Computerized tomography in chronic thromboembolic pulmonary hypertension. Am Heart J 106:1432, 1983.
146. Rhodes J, Barst R, Garafano R, et al: Hemodynamic correlates of exercise function in patients with primary pulmonary hypertension. J Am Coll Cardiol 18:1738, 1991.
147. Stanek V, Jebavy P, Horych J, Widimsky J: Central hemodynamics during supine exercise and pulmonary artery occlusion in normal subjects. Bull Physiol Pathol Respir 9:1203, 1973.
148. Harris P, Segal N, Bishop JM: The relationship between pressure and flow in the pulmonary circulation in normal subjects and in patients with chronic bronchitis and mitral stenosis. Cardiovasc Res 2:73, 1968.
149. Brundage B: Exercise testing in primary pulmonary hypertension: a valuable diagnostic tool. J Am Coll Cardiol 18:1745, 1991.
150. D'Alonzo GE, Barst R, Ayres S: Survival in patients with primary pulmonary hypertension: results from a national prospective registry. Ann Intern Med 115:343, 1991.
151. Hull RD, Hirsh J, Carter C, et al: Diagnostic value of ventilation-perfusion lung scanning in patients with suspected pulmonary embolism. Chest 88:819, 1985.
152. Child J, Wolfe J, Tashkin D, Nakano F: Fatal lung scan in a case of pulmonary hypertension due to obliterative pulmonary vascular disease. Chest 67:308, 1975.
153. Cohen HA, Baird MG, Ronleau JR, et al: Thallium-201 myocardial imaging in patients with pulmonary hypertension. Circulation 54:790, 1976.
154. Khaja F, Alam M, Goldstein S, et al: Diagnostic value of visualization of the right ventricle using thallium-201 myocardial imaging. Circulation 59:182, 1979.
155. Bookstein JJ: Segmental arteriography in pulmonary embolism. Radiology 93:1007, 1969.
156. Nicod P, Peterson K, Levine M, et al: Pulmonary angiography in severe chronic pulmonary hypertension. Ann Intern Med 107:565, 1987.
157. Shure D, Gregoratos G, Moser KM: Fiberoptic angioscopy: role in the diagnosis of chronic pulmonary arterial obstruction. Ann Intern Med 103:844, 1985.
158. Schrijen F, Jezek V: Hemodynamic and pulmonary wedge angiography findings in chronic bronchopulmonary disease. Scand J Respir Dis 58:151, 1977.
159. Rabinovitch M, Keane JF, Fellows KE, et al: Quantitative analysis of the pulmonary wedge angiogram in congenital heart defects: correlation with hemodynamic data and morphometric findings in lung biopsy tissue. Circulation 63:152, 1981.
160. Stein P, Athanasoulis C, Alavi A, et al: Complications and validity of pulmonary angiography in acute pulmonary embolism. Circulation 85:462, 1992.
161. Hoffstein V, Slutsky A: Central sleep apnea reversed by continuous positive airway pressure. Am Rev Respir Dis 135:1210, 1987.
162. Motta J, Guilleminault C: Effects of oxygen administration in sleep-induced apneas. *In* Guilleminault C, Dement W (eds): Sleep Apnea Syndromes. pp. 137–144. New York: Alan R. Liss, 1978.
163. Nocturnal Oxygen Therapy Trial Group: Continuous or nocturnal oxygen therapy in hypoxemic chronic obstructive lung disease. Ann Intern Med 93:391, 1980.
164. Party MRCW: Long-term domiciliary oxygen therapy in chronic hypoxic cor pulmonale complicating bronchitis and emphysema. Lancet 1:681, 1981.
165. Timms R, Khaja F, Williams G: Hemodynamic response to oxygen therapy in chronic obstructive pulmonary disease. Ann Intern Med 102:29, 1985.
166. Mathur P, Powles R, Pugsley S, et al: Effect of digoxin on right ventricular function in severe chronic airflow obstruction. Ann Intern Med 95:283, 1981.
167. Green L, Smith T: The use of digitalis in patients with pulmonary disease. Ann Intern Med 87:459, 1977.
168. Fuster V, Steele P, Edwards W: Primary pulmonary hypertension: natural history and the importance of thrombosis. Circulation 70:580, 1984.
169. Brown G: Pharmacologic treatment of primary and secondary pulmonary hypertension. Pharmacotherapy 11:137, 1991.
170. Halpern S, Shah P, Lehrman S, et al: Prostaglandin E_1 as a screening vasodilator in primary pulmonary hypertension. Chest 92:686, 1987.
171. Rubin L, Groves B, Reeves J, et al: Prostacyclin-induced acute pulmonary vasodilation in primary pulmonary hypertension. Circulation 66:334, 1982.
172. Morgan JM, McCormack DG, Griffiths MB, et al: Adenosine as a vasodilator in primary pulmonary hypertension. Circulation 84:1145, 1991.
173. Barst R: Pharmacologically induced pulmonary vasodilation in children and young adults with primary pulmonary hypertension. Chest 89:497, 1986.
174. Groves B, Rubin L, Frosolono M, et al: A comparison of the acute hemodynamic effects of prostacyclin and hydralazine in primary pulmonary hypertension. Am Heart J 110:1200, 1985.
175. McLaughlin VV, Genthner DE, Panella MM, et al: Reduction in pulmonary vascular resistance with long term epoprostenol therapy in primary pulmonary hypertension. N Engl J Med 338:273, 1998.
176. Pasque M, Trulock E, Kaiser L, Cooper J: Single-lung transplantation for pulmonary hypertension. Circulation 84:2275, 1991.
177. Traver G, Cline M, Burrows B: Predictors of mortality in chronic obstructive pulmonary disease. Am Rev Respir Dis 119:895, 1979.

CHAPTER 101

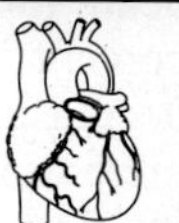

Chronic Obstructive Pulmonary Disease

Steven D. Brown and Rosa Maria Estrada y Martin

DEFINITIONS
PREVALENCE
RISK FACTORS
α_1-ANTIPROTEASE DEFICIENCY (α_1-ANTITRYPSIN DEFICIENCY)
PATHOPHYSIOLOGY AND PATHOGENESIS
CLINICAL PRESENTATION
Medical History
Physical Examination
Testing
DIFFERENTIAL DIAGNOSIS
NONSURGICAL TREATMENT
Smoking Cessation
Vaccination
Inhaled Bronchodilators
Theophylline
Corticosteroids
Antibiotics
α_1-Antiprotease Deficiency
Oxygen Therapy
Assisted Ventilation
Other Considerations
SURGICAL TREATMENT
PROGNOSIS

Definitions

Emphysema was first described by Laennec in the 1800s, so *chronic obstructive pulmonary disease* (COPD) has been recognized for many years but remains difficult to define. Since the 1940s, many authors have attempted to reach an acceptable definition.[1–4] Three disorders are included in COPD: emphysema, peripheral airway disease, and chronic bronchitis (Fig. 101–1).[1, 5] COPD is a disorder characterized by abnormal expiratory flows that do not change markedly over several months of observation. The airflow obstruction may be structural, as in emphysema, or functional, as in chronic bronchitis.[1] Bronchial hyperreactivity may be present and can be partially reversible.[1, 5] Bronchiectasis, cystic fibrosis, and asthma are excluded from the definition of COPD.

Emphysema is characterized by abnormal permanent enlargement of the airspaces distal to the terminal bronchiole, accompanied by destruction of the walls and pulmonary capillary beds without obvious fibrosis.[1] Physiologically, the consequence is a decrease in the elastic recoil of the lungs with outward displacement of the chest wall and flattening of the diaphragm, hyperinflation of the lung, and increased resistance to airflow due to circumferential narrowing of the airways. The hyperinflation increases respiratory muscle work with subsequent increase in oxygen consumption and cardiac output devoted to respiratory muscles.

Chronic bronchitis is a condition in which excessive mucus secretion and sputum production are chronic or recurrent. *Chronic* is defined as sputum production occurring on most days for at least 3 months of the year for at least 2 successive years; that should not be related to any other disease.[1]

Peripheral airway disease results from inflammation of the terminal and respiratory bronchioles, fibrosis with narrowing of airway walls, and goblet cell metaplasia of the bronchiolar epithelium. These changes may represent "an early or preclinical" COPD.[1]

Prevalence

In the United States, COPD affects at least 16 million people and is the fourth leading cause of death.[6] The

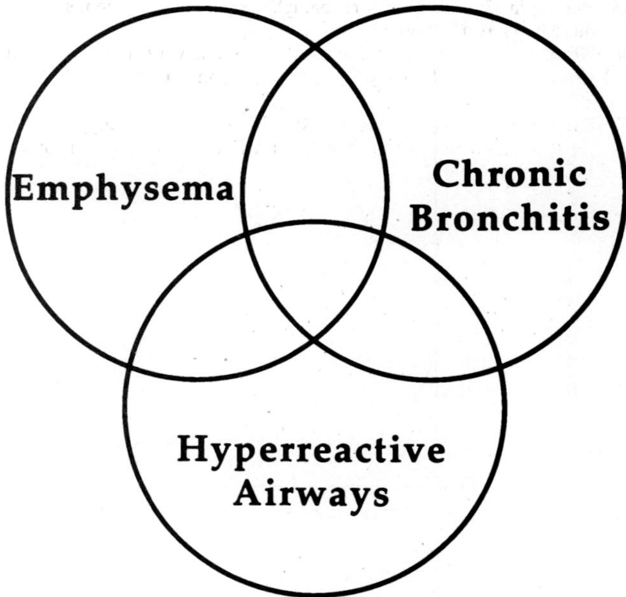

FIGURE 101–1 Patients with chronic obstructive pulmonary disease have any of three disease processes: emphysema, chronic bronchitis, and hyperreactive airways.

death rate for COPD between 1966 and 1986 increased 71 percent, whereas the death rate for coronary heart disease decreased 45 percent during that same period. Rates are increasing among young women and parallel smoking habits. Between 1966 and 1986, death rates increased 7 percent in white men and 12 percent in black men, whereas they increased 41 percent in white women and 43 percent in black women (Fig. 101–2).[7] COPD is a disease of the middle-aged and elderly, with a peak prevalence between 65 and 74 years of age. Women aged 55 to 64 years have a higher prevalence of COPD than age-matched men, but men aged 75 to 84 years have a prevalence of COPD that is 67 percent higher than that of similar-aged women.[8] Women are postulated to have greater adverse effects from smoking than men.[9]

Cigarette smoking has decreased since 1982; 26.5 percent of the adult U.S. population smoke compared with 40.3 percent in 1964.[6] The prevalence in adolescents has not changed since the 1980s but has increased in women.[10] In nonsmoking, healthy individuals from 25 to 35 years of age, the forced expiratory volume at 1 second ($FEV_{1.0}$) decreases approximately 20 to 30 ml/yr and accelerates with age. In patients with COPD, the decline of $FEV_{1.0}$ averages 40 to 80 ml/yr, but 200 ml/yr has been reported.[11]

Risk Factors

Cigarette smoking is the major cause of COPD in the United States for both men and women.[7] COPD develops in approximately 10 to 20 percent of smokers with at least a 20 pack-year history.[5] Other factors may contribute to the development of COPD, such as occupational exposures, environmental exposures, or $alpha_1$-antiprotease deficiency.

Agricultural exposures are suggested as a potential initiator of the inflammatory process in the airways that ultimately lead to chronic airway disease; these include dusts from cereal grains, animal feed, and soils; gases and fumes from such sources as manure and disinfectants; and components of microorganisms, such as endotoxins and fungi. This inflammatory response can lead to fibrotic lesions in the parenchyma and airway walls, inflammatory thickening of airway walls, or emphysema. Dairy, poultry confinement, and swine confinement farmers and tea production workers have an increased incidence of chronic bronchitis. The incidence of COPD increases proportionately with increasing levels of dust exposure. In addition, chronic respiratory effects have been described in grain dust exposure among grain elevator workers. Many dusts can increase mucus production and hypersecretion. Persistent obstruction develops in coal and gold miners, farmers, and grain handlers. Cement, cotton, and cadmium workers have an increased risk of emphysema.[12, 13]

α_1-Antiprotease Deficiency (α_1-Antitrypsin Deficiency)

The most important familial factor associated with COPD, α_1-antiprotease deficiency (α_1-antitrypsin deficiency), was recognized by Laurell and Ericksson in 1963. Inhibition of neutrophil elastase appears to be the primary function of α_1-antiprotease. This antiprotease is transmitted genetically

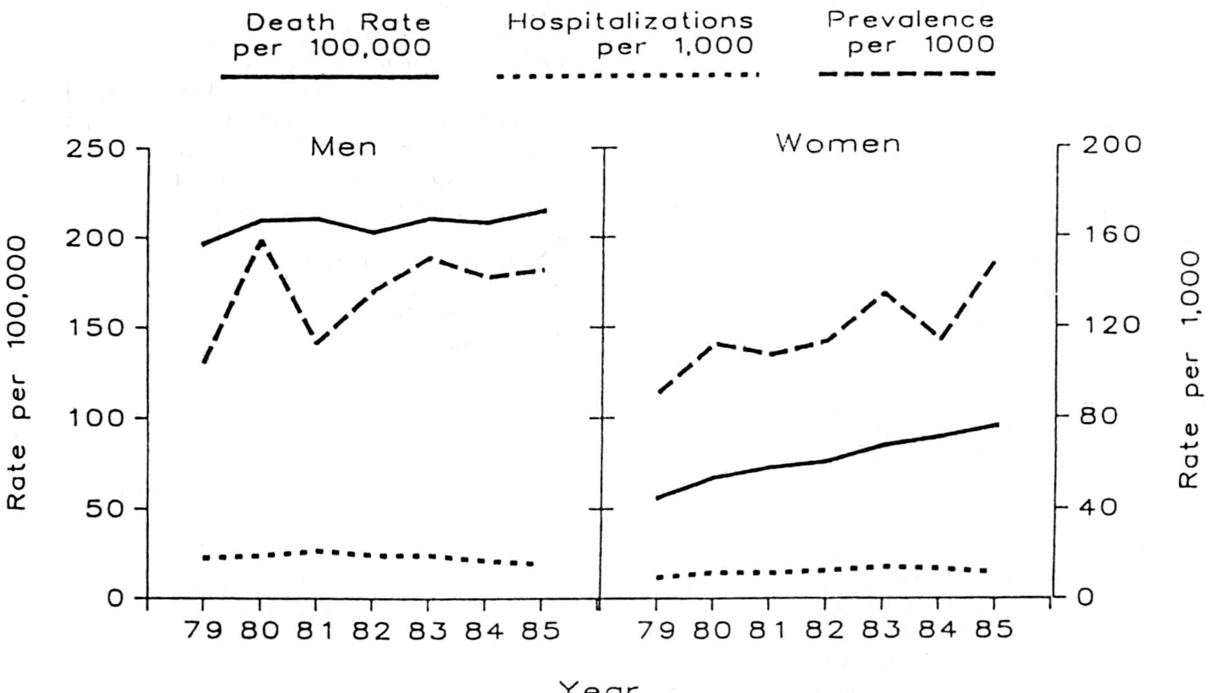

Figure 101–2 Prevalence rates for chronic obstructive pulmonary disease are increasing in women. The prevalence, hospitalization, and mortality rates are given for ages 65 to 74, by sex, in the United States for 1979 to 1985. (From Higgins MW: Chronic airways disease in the United States: trends and determinants. Chest 96:328S–334S, 1989.)

in a codominant fashion. The nomenclature that describes the phenotypes uses the letters F for fast, M for medium, S for slow, and Z for ultraslow in reference to electrophoretic migration speed. The normal phenotype, PiM (Pi indicates protease inhibitor), occurs in more than 90 percent of the population. MS and MZ phenotypes are the next most common. The MS, MZ, and SS phenotypes are only modestly deficient in α_1-antiproteases (about half of the normal serum concentration). Persons with PiMS phenotype may have an increased frequency of airway hyperreactivity. Persons with PiSZ, with an average of 37 percent of the normal serum concentration, rarely develop emphysema. Serum levels of more than 35 percent of normal are thought to provide protection.[14]

Phenotype PiZ is associated with more than 95 percent of the cases of α_1-antiprotease–deficient emphysema. PiZ individuals have about 15 percent of the normal serum concentration of α_1-antiprotease; the remainder consist of PiSZ, Pi null-null, or Pi null-Z phenotypes.[14] The prevalence of α_1-antitrypsin deficiency in America is about 1:3000 people. The Z allele is rare in Asians and African Americans.[14]

Most people with PiZ phenotype eventually become symptomatic with COPD, but considerable variation exists. Smoking has a marked effect on the age at which symptoms develop. Agents in cigarette smoke can oxidize a methionine residue in the reactive center of α_1-antiprotease, inactivating its capacity as an inhibitor. The average smoker of PiZ phenotype has symptoms by age 40, about 15 years earlier than a nonsmoker. The basis for COPD is panacinar emphysema that is often worse in the lower parts of the lungs,[14] unlike the traditional centrilobular emphysema of smokers, which preferentially affects upper lung zones.

PATHOPHYSIOLOGY AND PATHOGENESIS

In COPD, resistance to airflow is increased by conditions inside the lumen, in the wall of the airway, and the peribronchial region. The lumen may be partially occluded by excessive secretions, as occur in chronic bronchitis. Causes in the airway wall include bronchial smooth muscle contraction, hypertrophy of the mucosal glands as in chronic bronchitis, and inflammation and edema of the wall as in bronchitis and asthma. Outside the airway, destruction of lung parenchyma reduces radial traction and consequent narrowing of the airway as in emphysema.[15] The balance between the elastic recoil of the lungs promoting flow and the resistance of the airways limiting flow determines airflow during exhalation.[15, 16]

The major disease of the large airways is chronic bronchitis, which is caused by mucous gland enlargement. Other lesions include inflammation, smooth muscle hyperplasia, cartilage atrophy, and bronchial wall thickening.[16] The hallmark in chronic bronchitis is hypertrophy of mucous glands in the large bronchi and evidence of chronic inflammatory changes in the small airways. Excessive amounts of mucus are found in the airways, and semisolid plugs of mucus may occlude some small bronchi. In addition, the small airways are narrowed and show inflammatory changes, including cellular infiltration and edema of the walls. Granulation tissue is present, and peribronchial fibrosis may develop with an increase in bronchial smooth muscle.[15]

The emphysematous lung shows the loss of alveolar walls with consequent destruction of parts of the capillary bed. The small airways (<2 mm in diameter) are narrowed, tortuous, and reduced in number with thin, atrophied walls.[15] Emphysema is classified as centrilobular or panlobular. Centrilobular emphysema affects respiratory bronchioles in the upper lobes of the lung and is more commonly described in smokers, whereas panlobular emphysema involves lung distal to terminal bronchioles and affects all lung fields but more commonly the lower lobes, as seen in α_1-antiprotease deficiency. In COPD, the severity of emphysema is more significant than the type.[14]

As lung function declines, the alveolar-arterial gradient for oxygen increases due to an abnormal ventilation-perfusion relationship. Hypoxemia and alveolar hypoventilation develops, especially in chronic bronchitis. Alveolar hypoventilation with increased CO_2 retention contributes further to hypoxemia and respiratory acidosis. Hypoxemia and respiratory acidosis promote pulmonary vasoconstriction that imposes an added load on the right ventricle. Ventilation-perfusion inequality leads to hypoxemia with or without CO_2 retention.[15] Both physiologic dead space and physiologic shunt are increased in COPD. The dead space is increased, particularly in emphysema, whereas high values for shunt are especially common in chronic bronchitis.[15]

With exercise, arterial Po_2 (Pao_2) may rise minimally or fall in patients with COPD. The changes depend on the response of ventilation and the cardiac output and the changes in distribution of ventilation and blood flow. In some patients with COPD, the main limiting factor is diminished cardiac output that, in the presence of a ventilation-perfusion inequality, exaggerates any hypoxemia. Hypoxic vasoconstriction reduces the ventilation-perfusion inequality. This local response to a low alveolar Po_2 reduces the blood flow to poorly ventilated regions and minimizes arterial hypoxemia.[15] Although hypoxic vasoconstriction increases Pao_2, it increases pulmonary vascular resistance and pulmonary hypertension and may lead eventually to cor pulmonale.

Patients with CO_2 retention often show higher arterial Pco_2 ($Paco_2$) values on exercise because of limited ventilatory response. The blood flow inequality is caused largely by destruction of portions of the capillary bed, essentially increased dead space. The $Paco_2$ is often normal in early COPD despite their ventilation-perfusion inequality. Any tendency for the $Paco_2$ to rise stimulates the central chemoreceptors to increase ventilation of the alveoli. As COPD progresses, the $Paco_2$ may rise even at rest. Finally, hypercarbia results from an increased work of breathing and CO_2 production and, ultimately, a reduced sensitivity of the respiratory center to CO_2 in some of these patients.[15] The renal tubular cells are very sensitive to changes in $Paco_2$. The increase in $Paco_2$ stimulates proximal tubular reclamation of bicarbonate (HCO_3^-) and distal generation of HCO_3^-. This metabolic alkalosis compensates for the respiratory acidosis chronically.

The abnormalities seen in COPD are explained incompletely by several theories. The protease-antiprotease hypothesis suggests a steady or episodic release of proteolytic enzymes into the lung parenchyma. Normally, plasma protease inhibitors, especially α_1-antiprotease (α_1-antitrypsin), permeates lung tissue and prevents digestion of structural proteins of the lungs. Emphysema results from an augmentation of protease release in the lungs, a reduction in the antiprotease defense within the lungs, or a combination.[14]

Although inflammatory cells are considered the source of proteases, the specific cell has not been found. Proteases released by neutrophils, macrophages, or local cells are considered to be the main cause of lung matrix degradation.[14] The final physiologic consequence is an abnormality in the gas exchange unit of the lung, the *acinus,* as demonstrated in emphysema. The inflammatory cells involved in asthma and COPD are different. In atopic and nonatopic asthma, the inflammatory infiltrate is composed of activated ($CD25^+$) and T helper ($CD4^+$) lymphocytes and activated eosinophils ($EG2^+$) associated with gene expression and secretion of interleukins (IL)-4, IL-5, and IL-10 and the proinflammatory cytokines granulocyte/macrophage colony-stimulating factor and tumor necrosis factor-α. The production of IL-4 and IL-5, but not IL-2 and interferon-γ, is referred to as the *T-helper type 2* (Th2) *phenotype.*[17]

Inflammation occurs in stable and exacerbated COPD. Bronchial mononuclear cells are the predominant cell type with scanty neutrophils in the absence of an exacerbation with infection. In contrast to asthma, relatively few eosinophils are found. In COPD, the mononuclear cells include lymphocytes, plasma cells, and macrophages. The numbers of CD45 (total leukocytes), CD3 (T lymphocytes), CD25 (activated), and VLA-1 (late activation) positive cells and macrophages are increased. An increase in the number of tissue eosinophils compared with that found in normal healthy control subjects is present, but in contrast to asthma, the tissue eosinophils found in COPD do not appear to degranulate.[33] The $CD8^+$ lymphocyte subset is increased in COPD, whereas the increased $CD4^+$ T cell subset is characteristic of mild atopic asthma.[17]

Clinical Presentation

Arbitrarily, patients with COPD have been classified as having chronic bronchitis, emphysema, or airway hyperreactivity. In reality, many patients have a combination of these three or at least more than one disorder, as represented graphically (see Fig. 101–1).

Medical History

History of Present Illness. Usually, symptoms are gradual in onset but progressive. COPD affects middle-aged and older persons except in cases of α_1-antiprotease deficiency as mentioned previously. Cough is the most common symptom in chronic bronchitis. A productive cough in the mornings for at least 3 months per year for a minimum of 2 consecutive years defines chronic bronchitis. Persistent cough correlates inversely with the $FEV_{1.0}$ and is required for diagnosis, although cough correlates poorly with increasing mortality rate.[16]

Dyspnea is another symptom of COPD that occurs initially on exertion but cannot be distinguished from that due to other causes such as congestive heart failure, pulmonary embolism, or pneumonia. The symptom of dyspnea in COPD may reflect expiration flow limitation or inability of the diaphragm to ascend in more severe cases of air trapping. Dyspnea may be associated with cough, wheezing, sputum production, and recurrent respiratory infections.[5]

Family History. A history of emphysema or COPD at an early age in family members is common in cases of α_1-antiprotease deficiency. α_1-Antiprotease deficiency should be suspected and screened in patients who develop severe COPD at a relatively young age (<50 years), have affected siblings or parents, or have smoked sparingly or not at all[1]; when emphysema is predominantly in lower lobes of the lung; or when hepatic cirrhosis occurs without apparent risk factors. A medical history of immunodeficiencies, hereditary abnormalities, or congenital anatomic defects is important in the differential diagnosis of chronic productive cough and recurrent pulmonary infections (Table 101–1).

Social History. A history of cigarette smoking is the most important risk factor[5] for COPD. Particularly in patients with α_1-antiprotease deficiency, smoking will cause premature development of emphysema. Work and environmental exposures might pose additional risk factors (see Risk Factors).

Review of Systems. Awakening with headache or daytime somnolence suggests CO_2 retention as occurs in COPD, particularly with chronic bronchitis. Daytime somnolence may also indicate obstructive sleep apnea as a comorbid condition. In COPD where chronic bronchitis is predominant, an impressive history of cough and sputum production for many years is common. COPD with predominant emphysema includes a long history of exertional dyspnea with minimal cough. Weight loss is more frequent in severe cases of COPD and more common in emphysema. During the late stages of emphysema, appetite is decreased and weight loss occurs due to several factors, including decreased caloric intake and increased work of breathing. Memory loss and decreased attention can be secondary to hypoxemia. Psychiatric problems such as depression and hopelessness are common.

Physical Examination

On physical examination, the best predictor for the presence of COPD is diminished breath sounds.[18–20] However,

TABLE 101–1 Immune, Congenital, and Inherited Causes of Bronchiectasis

Immunodeficiency state	Immunoglobulin (Ig)E subclass deficiency; X-linked agammaglobulinemia; selective IgA, IgM, or IgE deficiency; bare lymphocyte syndrome; chronic granulocytous disease; Nezelof syndrome
Hereditary abnormality	Dyskinetic cilia syndrome, Kartagener's syndrome, α_1-antitrypsin deficiency, cystic fibrosis
Congenital anatomic defect	Williams-Campbell syndrome, Mournier-Kuhn syndrome, pulmonary sequestration, pulmonary artery aneurysm, yellow nail syndrome

a normal chest examination does not exclude mild to moderate COPD, particularly in patients with chronic bronchitis.[20]

Emphysema. In general, the patients with predominant emphysema look asthenic. Tachypnea with a relatively prolonged expiration through pursed lips is common, as is expiration with a grunting sound. On examination of the neck and chest, the use of the accessory muscles of respiration (sternocleidomastoid and intercostal muscles) is common, with lift of the sternum in an anterosuperior direction with each inspiration. The neck veins may distend during expiration and collapse briskly with inspiration. The lower lateral chest wall can be felt to move inward with inspiration. The chest percussion note is hyperresonant, and auscultation of the chest reveals diminished breath sounds. Cardiac dullness is either absent or severely reduced. The absence of a palpable apex beat, retraction of the trachea with inspiration, and upper rib cage involvement often occur due to accessory muscle use.[19–22] Frequently, palpation reveals a sustained forward and downward right ventricular impulse in the subxyphoid region, and a presystolic gallop accentuated during inspiration is commonly auscultated.

Chronic Bronchitis. In patients with COPD where chronic bronchitis is predominant, obesity and cyanosis are frequently seen. Unlike in emphysema, no apparent use of accessory muscles is observed in compensated chronic bronchitis. The chest percussion note is normally resonant, and auscultation reveals coarse rhonchi. A sustained heave along the lower left sternal border indicates right ventricular hypertrophy. In the presence of right ventricular failure, an early diastolic gallop and occasionally a holosystolic murmur can be heard at the left sternal border, and both are accentuated by inspiration. The latter finding indicates functional tricuspid regurgitation that is frequently accompanied by neck vein distention with large v waves and brisk y descents. Peripheral edema suggests overt right ventricle failure. The neurologic examination may demonstrate confusion secondary to hypercapnia or hypoxemia.

Cardiac Considerations in Chronic Obstructive Pulmonary Disease. Increased pressure of the right ventricular afterload causes cor pulmonale with the physical findings discussed earlier and distended neck veins, hepatomegaly, ascites, and leg edema. However, the liver may be palpable without hepatomegaly secondary to hyperinflation and low diaphragms, and the liver span should be considered.

Arrhythmias occur in up to 84 percent of patients with COPD who undergo continuous electrocardiographic monitoring. In patients with stable COPD, approximately 70 percent of the arrhythmias are ventricular in origin. In contrast to patients with stable COPD, patients with acute respiratory failure tend to have a predominance of supraventricular arrhythmias. The supraventricular arrhythmias are especially common in cor pulmonale.[23] Common rhythm disturbances include atrial fibrillation, atrial flutter, paroxysmal atrial or junctional tachycardia, digitalis-induced tachyarrhythmias, premature ventricular contractions, and, less frequently, ventricular tachycardia or fibrillation. Paroxysmal atrial tachycardia with block is an arrhythmia typically associated with digitalis intoxication and frequently occurs in patients with COPD. Multifocal atrial tachycardia (MAT) is a serious supraventricular arrhythmia that often occurs in patients with COPD. Among patients with MAT, 31 to 84 percent have severe COPD and 44 to 55 percent have clinically diagnosed cor pulmonale. Among COPD patients with acute respiratory failure, 17 percent demonstrate MAT. In contrast to other arrhythmias, MAT is not related to the use of digitalis or a manifestation of digitalis toxicity.[23, 24]

Testing

Chest Radiography

Plain chest radiography is not sensitive in mild cases of COPD and is unable to identify a cause for acute exacerbations in many patients.[25] Chest radiography in chronic bronchitis often reveals bronchial wall thickening. In severe cases of chronic bronchitis with airflow obstruction and cor pulmonale, the chest radiograph and computed tomography (CT) scan may show evidence of central pulmonary artery enlargement and cardiomegaly.[26] Increased markings in lower lobes are described in chronic bronchitis.

The radiographic hallmark of emphysema is increased lung volume, flattening of the diaphragm, and focal areas of lucency with vascular attenuation. An enlarged anteroposterior chest diameter ("barrel" chest) and retrosternal clear space, saber-sheath trachea, microcardia, and the presence of bullae are typical (Fig. 101–3). In acute COPD exacerbation, chest radiographs should be taken in all patients to exclude complications such as spontaneous pneumothorax, pneumonia, congestive heart failure, allergic bronchopulmonary aspergillosis, pleural effusion, unsuspected mass, foreign body, or atelectasis.[18]

Computed Tomography

The plain chest radiograph (posteroranterior and lateral) remains the standard in the initial evaluation of patients with COPD. However, the radiographic detection and assessment of emphysema are superior on CT scans compared with chest radiographs.[26] High-resolution CT provides excellent anatomic detail for detecting and characterizing emphysema. The presence and severity of emphysema on CT are known to correlate better with pathologic specimens than with pulmonary function tests. Emphysema appears as areas of low attenuation without definable walls. CT is the most accurate method to detect and evaluate the anatomic severity of emphysema short of postmortem evaluation of the lungs. Regardless, the CT scan may yield false-negative results in mild emphysema.[27] With the diagnosis of emphysema established by a combination of clinical history and pulmonary function tests, the role of CT in the evaluation of emphysema is limited to the evaluation of abnormalities identified initially on chest radiographs, such as potential bronchogenic carcinoma or air-fluid levels within infected bullae.[27] CT scanning with quantitative and anatomic evaluation of emphysema is required in patients undergoing lung volume reduction surgery for severe emphysema.[26]

The role of CT scanning in chronic bronchitis is limited to cases in which other complications are suspected, such as lung carcinoma or bronchiectasis. As in chest radiogra-

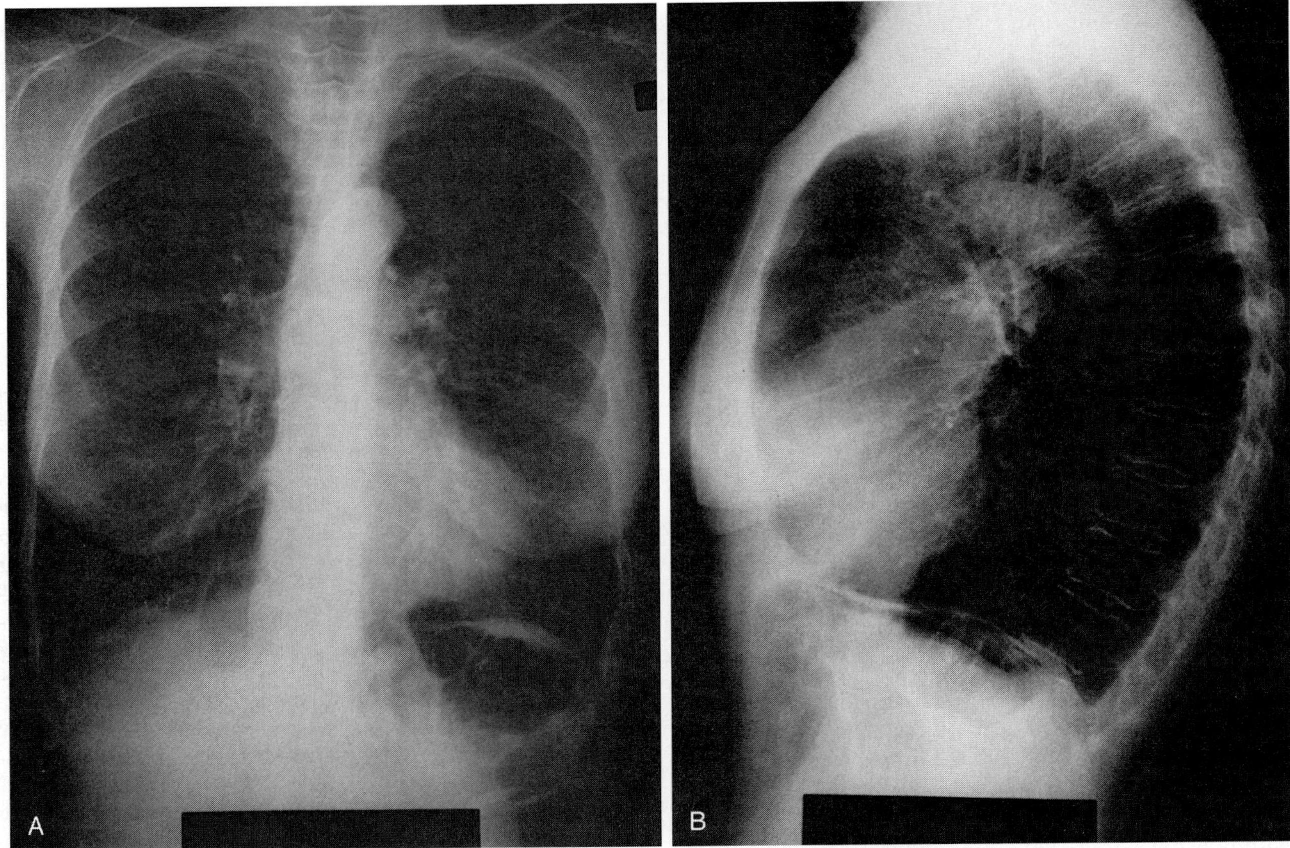

FIGURE 101–3 **A** and **B**, Chest radiographs of a woman with emphysema reveal increased lung volumes and increased retrosternal air space and anteroposterior chest diameter ("barrel chest") and flattened diaphragm.

phy, CT scanning mainly shows bronchial wall thickening.[26] High-resolution CT is also the procedure of choice, after plain chest radiography, for diagnosing bronchiectasis.

Pulmonary Function Testing

In COPD, $FEV_{1.0}$, forced vital capacity (FVC), $FEV_{1.0}$/FVC ratio, maximum midexpiratory flow (FEF 25–75 percent), and maximum expiratory flow at 50 and 75 percent of vital capacity (V_{max} 50 percent and V_{max} 75 percent) are reduced. All of these measurements reflect airway obstruction. The FVC is reduced because the airways close prematurely at an abnormally high lung volume, as reflected by an increased residual volume (RV).[15, 28–30] The flow rate over most of the forced expiration is reduced, and the expiratory time is increased (Fig. 101–4). Dyspnea occurs usually when $FEV_{1.0}$ is less than 60 percent of predicted.[15]

In some patients with COPD, the $FEV_{1.0}$, FVC, and $FEV_{1.0}$/FVC percent may increase significantly after the administration of a bronchodilator aerosol.[15] When using the percent change from the initial value as the criterion for bronchodilator response, at least a 12 percent increase in $FEV_{1.0}$ from the baseline value defines a meaningful response.[28] The failure of expiratory flows to improve after bronchodilator use does not preclude a long-term beneficial response to either bronchodilators or corticosteroids.[1] However, patients who respond to bronchodilators should be treated more aggressively with bronchodilators and possibly with inhaled corticosteroids because this subgroup of patients with COPD may have unsuspected associated asthma features. Thus, the bronchodilator test is a diagnostic test for readily reversible airway dysfunction rather than a therapeutic test.

The total lung capacity (TLC), functional residual capacity (FRC), and RV are typically increased in emphysema. Often, the RV/TLC ratio may exceed 40 percent, with normal typically being less than 30 percent. Striking discrepancies between the FRC determined by the body plethysmograph and the gas dilution techniques (helium equilibration or N_2 washout) are observed; the former is higher by 1 liter or even more. Normally, FRC is 40 to 50 percent of the TLC. The discrepancy reflects the slow test gas equilibration in poorly ventilated areas during gas dilution techniques. In COPD, the increased FRC and RV result from the reduced lung elastic recoil and premature closure of the airways in expiration.[15] Spirometry establishes the diagnosis of COPD but may be normal in chronic bronchitis, where the diagnoses is based on clinical history.[1]

COPD is associated with a reduction in the diffusing capacity for carbon monoxide (DLCO).[1, 28–31] Reduction in the DLCO correlates well with the presence of emphysema. Other causes of decreased DLCO include lung or lobe resection, bronchial obstruction, multiple pulmonary emboli, pulmonary vasculitis, interstitial fibrosis, or anemia.[30] A DLCO below 55 percent of predicted and an $FEV_{1.0}$ of less than 1 L predict desaturation in pulse oximetry during

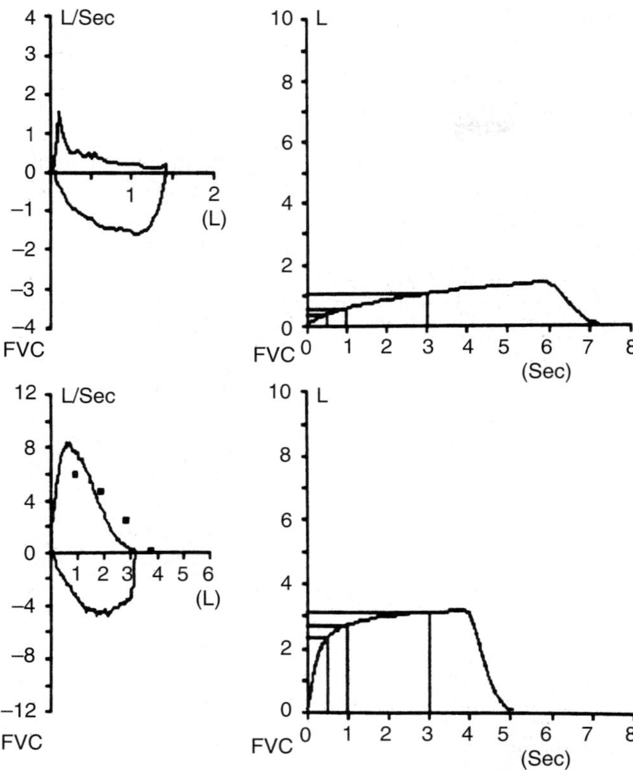

FIGURE 101–4 Expiratory flows are decreased in patients with chronic obstructive pulmonary disease. **Top left,** Flow-volume loop that demonstrates expiratory flow rates (*y* axis) throughout a forced vital capacity (FVC) maneuver (*x* axis) in a patient with chronic obstructive pulmonary disease. **Top right,** Spirogram of the same forced vital capacity maneuver as the flow-volume loop at **left**. Note that the volume (*y* axis) accumulates slowly over time (*s* axis) and never reaches a plateau compared with the normal spirogram in **bottom right**.

exercise. An $FEV_{1.0}$ of less than 1 L has been associated with CO_2 retention and increased mortality rates.[32, 33]

Additional Tests

Blood Tests. Arterial blood oxygenation should be assessed directly by measurement of $Pa{O_2}$ or indirectly by pulse oximetry in all patients with significant airflow limitation at the time of initial evaluation and during symptomatic periods.[18] Determination of $Pa{CO_2}$ is necessary in patients with confusion, cyanosis, and somnolence during the day or who awaken with headache. Secondary polycythemia on a hemoglobin determination suggests chronic hypoxemia and is an indication for oxygen therapy. α_1-Antiprotease deficiency should be suspected in young patients with lower lobe emphysema (30 to 40 years old) or recalcitrant asthma, especially in those with a family history of emphysema, and plasma levels should be measured (see Medical History).[34]

Physiological Tests. The electrocardiogram may demonstrate right atrial enlargement (total increase in P wave amplitude of ≥2.5 mm in lead II) in pulmonary hypertension and right ventricular hypertrophy (small R wave in leads V_1 to V_4) and suggests the need for arterial blood gas analysis.[14] Right-axis deviation and poor R wave progression in V_1 to V_4 may also occur in cor pulmonale. Low voltage in precordial leads is seen in hyperinflated lungs, as occurs in emphysema.

COPD and sleep apnea syndrome may coexist as the *overlap syndrome.* Sleep studies should be considered in patients who have excessive daytime somnolence, snoring with apnea, morning headache, and hypoxemic complications such as cor pulmonale and polycythemia, which may suggest nocturnal hypoxemia even when daytime hypoxemia is absent.[35] The incidence of the overlap syndrome is between 10 and 20 percent of patients with COPD.[35, 36] Patients with COPD and sleep apnea syndrome have an increased risk of developing pulmonary hypertension and cor pulmonale secondary to more severe hypoxemia and hypercapnia compared with patients with only COPD.[35–37] Patients with COPD become more hypoxemic during sleep than during resting wakefulness. Sleep-related hypoxemia is most marked during rapid eye movement (REM) sleep due to hypoventilation, when alveolar ventilation is about 40 percent lower. A normal diminution in central respiratory drive exaggerates REM-related hypoventilation. During REM sleep, hypotonia of postural muscles, including the intercostals and accessory muscles of inspiration, decreases rib cage contribution to ventilation.[35]

DIFFERENTIAL DIAGNOSIS

Differentiating *asthma* from COPD is sometimes difficult. In asthma, airflow obstruction is usually variable over short periods of time and reversible, although an underlying irreversible component may develop when inflammation persists in association with repeated allergen or occupational exposure. In COPD, the airflow limitation is usually persistent and typically deteriorates more rapidly than normal.[17, 38] A hemoglobin adjusted DLCO is normal or increased in asthma compared with COPD and is especially decreased with emphysema.

Bronchiectasis is suspected with a history of copious sputum production, recurrent lung infection, hemoptysis, or radiographic findings of bronchial wall thickening and cystic spaces often with air-fluid levels. Bronchiectasis follows pulmonary infectious diseases such as histoplasmosis, mycobacterial infections, and bacterial pneumonia or noninfectious abnormalities (see Table 101–1). Another form of congenital bronchiectasis, *cystic fibrosis,* is diagnosed with a sweat chloride test, usually at a younger age, and with a family history of cystic fibrosis or pancreatic insufficiency.

During a COPD exacerbation, other processes, such as pneumothorax, pneumonia, myocardial infarction, congestive heart failure, or pulmonary embolism, must be excluded. *Pulmonary embolism* is difficult to diagnose in patients with COPD. It should be suspected in a patient who has an acute exacerbation with right-sided heart failure who fails to respond to the usual therapy with bronchodilators and corticosteroids and develops worsening hypoxemia and dyspnea without evidence of infection and in whom the $Pa{CO_2}$ decreases in the previously hypercapneic patient.[39] Ventilation/perfusion scans are often abnormal in COPD even without pulmonary embolism, making diagnosis more confusing. Spiral CT angiography is the preferred screening test in patients with an underlying cardiorespiratory disorder.[40] Pulmonary angiography is required for definitive diagnosis in cases where screening tests for pulmonary embolism or deep venous thrombosis are equivocal.

NONSURGICAL TREATMENT

Smoking Cessation

Smoking cessation remains the first and most important clinical intervention.[1, 41] $FEV_{1.0}$ improves remarkably in the first year after cessation and continues to improve in subsequent years, although it does not reach a normal nonsmoker level. However, any improvement in $FEV_{1.0}$ has been associated with improvement in the quality of life and survival (see Prognosis). Figure 101–5 compares the cumulative 5-year average decline in $FEV_{1.0}$ in smokers and quitters. Sustained quitters had an overall 5-year decline in $FEV_{1.0}$ of 72 ml, whereas continuing smokers had a decline of 301 ml during the same period.[41] Successful cessation has doubled with use of nicotine chewing gum or nicotine patches (34 versus 21 percent with placebo in the first 6 months[42] and 38 versus 14 percent with psychologic support alone).[43]

Bupropion, an oral antidepressant agent, doubled cessation rates compared with placebo alone, even in patients without a past history of depression, and was superior to nicotine patches alone. A combination of bupropion and nicotine patches may be synergistic.[44] Earlier trials with higher dosages suggested that bupropion increased the risk of seizures. More recent data with the slow-release preparation demonstrate that the risk of seizure is no greater than that found with other antidepressants.[45]

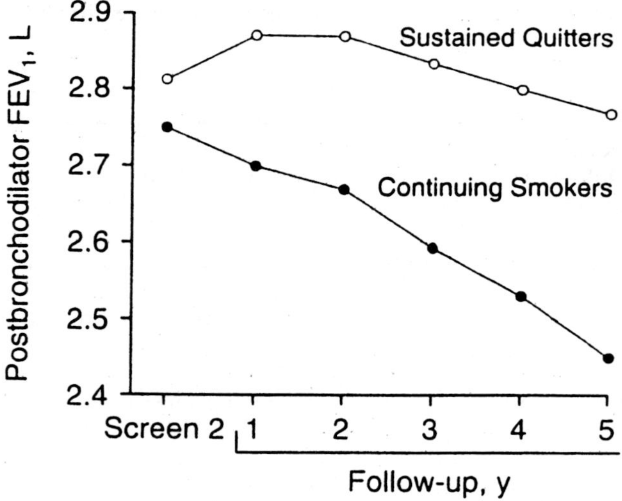

FIGURE 101–5 Mean postbronchodilator forced expiratory volume in 1 second in sustained quitters *(open circles)* declines more slowly than that in continuous smokers *(closed circles)*. (From Anthonisen NR, Connett JE, Kiley JP, et al: Effects of smoking intervention and the use of an inhaled anticholinergic bronchodilator on the rate of decline of FEV. JAMA 272:1497–1505, 1994. Copyright 1994, American Medical Association.)

Vaccination

Annual vaccination against influenza (A and B) has reduced influenza mortality and morbidity rates and is cost effective, especially in high-risk persons with chronic heart, pulmonary, renal, or metabolic disease; chronic anemia; or immunocompromise, and in those older than 65 years.[46] Hypersensitivity reaction to egg protein is a contraindication to the vaccine. The overall protection rate of influenza vaccine is 60 to 80 percent.[1, 47]

Pneumococcal vaccine (purified capsular polysaccharide from 23 pneumococcal serotypes) is also recommended, although its efficacy in debilitated patients with COPD has not been established.[47, 48] It is recommended in persons over 50 years of age and in patients with chronic diseases, including cardiopulmonary disorders. Its efficacy ranges from 67 to 21 percent depending on the population studied.[48] Although it may have a modest efficacy, adverse reactions are rare. Reimmunization is recommended at 6-year intervals; however, this interval between vaccination is controversial.

Inhaled Bronchodilators

Anticholinergic agents antagonize muscarinic receptors, of which at least three are recognized as important in airway control. M1 receptors are localized in parasympathetic ganglia, and blockade of these receptors reduces reflex bronchoconstriction. The bronchoconstrictor action of acetylcholine is mediated entirely by M3 receptors. By contrast, M2 receptors located at cholinergic nerve terminals inhibit the release of acetylcholine, thus acting as autoreceptors that antagonize bronchoconstriction. Nonselective anticholinergics block M1 and M3 receptors, leading to bronchodilatation, due to the relief of intrinsic cholinergic tone and inhibition of cholinergic reflex bronchoconstriction.[49] Ipratropium bromide, a poorly absorbed nonselective anticholinergic, is at least equally effective as beta-adrenergic agonists in COPD and with minimal adverse effects such as dry mouth or tachycardia. One typical trial demonstrated that $FEV_{1.0}$ increased by about 10 percent of baseline values and residual lung volume (air trapping) fell by about 1.0 L (60 percent of baseline value).[50] In patients with COPD, anticholinergic agents are the most potent bronchodilators for maintenance and exacerbation.[50] Ipratropium should be considered as first-line treatment in COPD.

Beta-adrenergic agonists can improve mucociliary clearance and increase $FEV_{1.0}$ and exercise tolerance. Long-acting β_2 agonists, such as salmeterol, benefit patients with COPD[49] but may have side effects, such as tremor, nervousness, and palpitations.[47] The combination of ipratropium and albuterol has demonstrated additive benefit, if not synergy, without increasing side effects.[51–53] These results have been repeated in multiple trials. As an example, the Dey combination trial demonstrated an improved $FEV_{1.0}$ compared with the use of albuterol or ipratropium alone. The combination increased $FEV_{1.0}$ by 24 percent more than with albuterol alone and by 37 percent more than with ipratropium alone.[54] The combination of these two agents in a single metered-dose inhaler (MDI) is available and may improve compliance compared with the use of two MDIs.

The method of bronchodilator delivery, via nebulizer or MDI, has not significantly influenced clinical response. Multiple trials showed that bronchodilator delivery through nebulizer, intermittent positive pressure breathing, or MDI with spacer devices is equally effective in improving dyspnea and bronchodilatation in patients with stable COPD and exacerbations.[55–57] This is also true for bronchodilator delivery in ventilated patients. MDIs are as effective, less costly, more convenient, and associated with less tachycardia compared with nebulizers. To optimize drug delivery, the drug should be delivered via a spacer placed in the inspiratory line within 10 cm proximal to the Y piece of the ventilator. The optimal dose and frequency of administration have yet to be determined. Dosing every 2 to 4 hours is safe and effective for patients with COPD, but hourly dosing may be considered in severe cases. An initial approach to bronchodilator therapy of mechanically ventilated patients with COPD would be to administer no more than 10 puffs of ipratropium and albuterol or equivalent every 2 to 4 hours.[58]

Theophylline

Theophylline is a relatively old drug whose exact mechanism of action in COPD has been debated for decades without resolution. Clearly, theophylline is regarded as a second-line therapy for COPD. Theophylline may be indicated in patients with moderate to severe COPD in whom symptoms are not adequately controlled with optimal doses of inhaled bronchodilators. It may be particularly useful in patients with hypercarbia, although hypercarbic patients more frequently have the significant side effects of theophylline.

Theophylline improves $FEV_{1.0}$, sensation of dyspnea, exercise performance, and sensation of well-being in severe COPD. It significantly improves diaphragmatic contractility, decreases diaphragmatic fatigue, stimulates ventilation centrally, augments the ventilatory response to hypoxia, and reduces end-tidal carbon dioxide. Long-term use increases $FEV_{1.0}$ by 10 to 20 percent and increases right and left ventricular ejection fractions while reducing pulmonary artery pressure significantly. Theophylline also increases mucociliary clearance and has an anti-inflammatory effect.[59–61]

However, theophylline has a narrow therapeutic index with toxicity at levels of 15 μg/ml or higher. Potential drug interactions are summarized in Table 101–2, and pronounced adverse effects include nervousness, tremor and arrhythmias from catecholamine release, and gastrointestinal symptoms. Patients should be selected carefully, the drug should be started at a low dose, serum levels should be measured, and the dose should be increased slowly if a higher blood level is considered necessary. A serum theophylline level of 10 to 15 μg/ml is appropriate, although some recommend blood levels of 8 to 12 μg/ml.[59] Patients should be evaluated for clear improvement in symptoms or peak expiratory flow by home monitoring. If no improvement in peak expiratory flow or symptoms occurs within 4 weeks, the drug should be discontinued.

Corticosteroids

Oral corticosteroids can improve $FEV_{1.0}$ in at least 30 percent of a selected group of patients with COPD and those who respond to bronchodilators during pulmonary function tests are good candidates.[62] An improvement in pulmonary function tests, symptoms, or peak flow should be documented when using oral corticosteroids due to the associated side effects.[62–65] In acute COPD exacerbations, intravenous corticosteroids produced a more rapid improvement of $FEV_{1.0}$ during the first 72 hours of hospital stay compared with those not administered corticosteroids, as shown in Figure 101–6. For patients treated and released from an emergency department, acute corticosteroid admin-

TABLE 101–2 Factors Affecting Theophylline Concentration in Adults

Factor	Decreases Concentration	Increases Concentration	Recommendation
Hypoxia, cor pulmonale, congestive heart failure, cirrhosis		Decreases metabolism	Decrease theophylline dose according to serum levels.
Age		Decreases metabolism	Adjust theophylline dose according to serum levels.
Phenobarbital, phenytoin, carbamazepine	Increases metabolism		Adjust theophylline dose according to serum levels.
Cimetidine		Decreases metabolism	Use alternative H_2 blocker (e.g., famotidine, ranitidine).
Macrolides			
Erythromycin, clarithromycin, azithromycin*		Decreases metabolism	Use alternative antibiotics or adjust theophylline dose.
Quinolones			
Ciprofloxacin, enoxacin, perfloxacin trovafloxacin*		Decreases metabolism	Use alternative antibiotics or adjust theophylline dose or use ofloxacin.
Other Factors			
Rifampin	Increases metabolism		Increase theophylline dose according to serum levels.
Ticlopidine		Decreases metabolism	Decrease theophylline dose according to serum levels.
Smoking	Increases metabolism		Stop smoking or increase theophylline dose.
Fever	Increases metabolism		Fever control

* Insufficient information available to confirm altered theophylline metabolism by this agent.

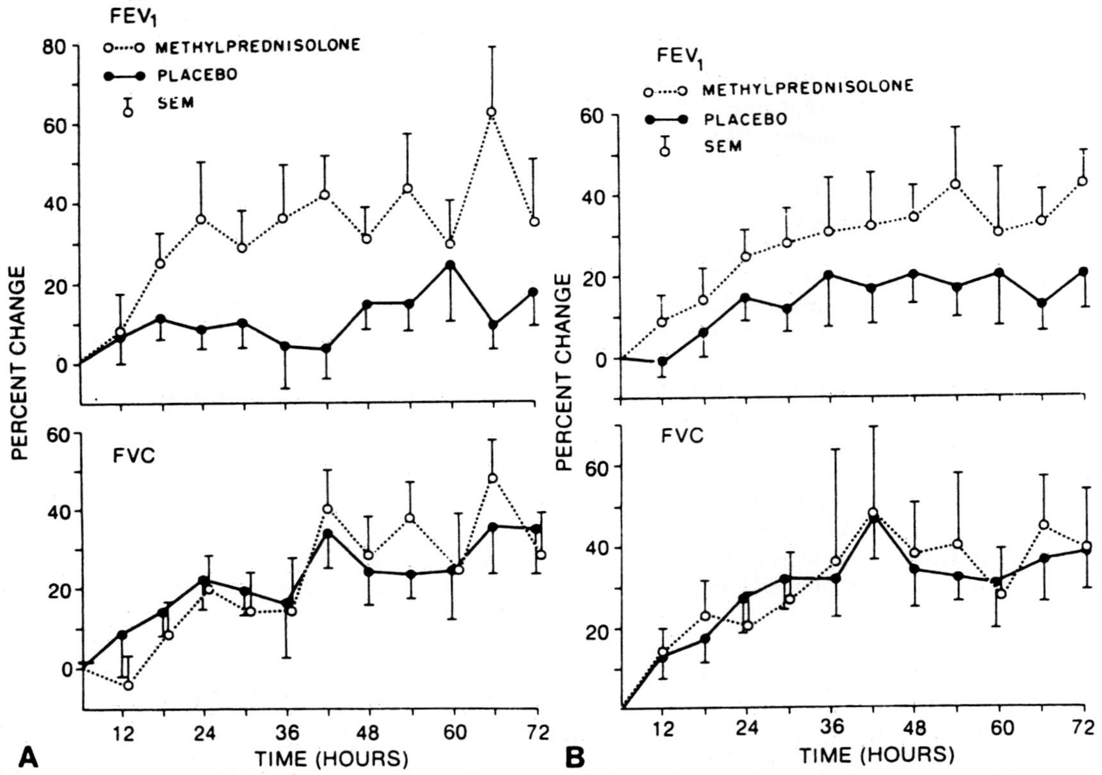

FIGURE 101–6 Patients with chronic obstructive pulmonary disease exacerbations had improved spirometry after methylprednisolone. **A,** Prebronchodilator. **B,** Postbronchodilator. FEV, forced expiratory volume; FVC, forced vital capacity. (**A** and **B,** From Albert RK, Martin TR, Lewis SW: Controlled clinical trial of methylprednisolone in patients with chronic bronchitis and acute respiratory insufficiency. Ann Intern Med 92:753–758, 1980.)

istration significantly decreased the rate of relapse from 33.3 to 8.9 percent in the first 48 hours after discharge.[63, 66] Corticosteroids can be used during infectious exacerbations of COPD if antibiotics are used concommitantly. Chronic inhaled corticosteroids may be useful in patients who have combined COPD and airway hyperreactivity (see Medical History). However, the use of inhaled corticosteroids remains controversial, and trials are in progress to identify those patients who may benefit from them.

Antibiotics

Although the majority of COPD exacerbations are probably viral or noninfectious in origin, antibiotics are routinely prescribed. This habit is imperfect but practical given the time, expense, and uncertainty of laboratory identification of possible infecting agents and is defended in trials. Commonly involved bacterial organisms include *Haemophilus influenzae, Streptococcus pneumoniae, Moraxella catarrhalis,* and *Neisseria* species. Less frequently involved are *Klebsiella* and *Pseudomonas* species. Although still controversial, empiric antibiotic therapy improves peak expiratory flow and decreases or eliminates the symptoms of dyspnea, sputum volume, and purulence.[66–69] Antibiotic therapy in COPD exacerbations has shown a small but statistically and clinically significant improvement in outcome. The choice of antibiotic depends on known susceptibilities when available, epidemiology, costs, side effects, and antibiotic availability. Empiric therapy should be directed toward the most common species but could include amoxicillin, first- or second-generation cephalosporins, fluoroquinolones, doxycycline, trimethoprim-sulfamethoxazole, or the macrolides. Treatment should be continued for 1 or 2 weeks,[67] although regimens of at least 10 days are most common. Dosing of antibiotics once or twice a day increases compliance compared with more frequent regimens.

Amantadine, an antiviral agent, is efficacious for prophylaxis in outbreaks of influenza A and is recommended in nonimmunized high-risk patients (e.g., elderly patients living in a nursing home or elderly patients with comorbid conditions, such as liver failure, heart failure, or immunosuppression) exposed to the virus. Amantadine has a 50 to 90 percent efficacy; side effects include mental status changes, ataxia, tremor, and convulsions, especially in the elderly.[47] Rimantadine, an antiviral derivative of amantadine, appears to be as effective and better tolerated.[70] Ribavarin, a nucleoside analogue that is active against influenzae A and B, is administered via aerosolized solution. This antiviral agent has fewer side effects than amantadine but is expensive compared with other agents.[71]

α_1-Antiprotease Deficiency

The mainstay of treatment in α_1-antiprotease deficiency is to avoid or stop smoking. Specific treatment for this deficiency is available as monthly intravenous infusions of α_1-antitrypsin purified from pooled human plasma to correct the imbalance between α_1-antiprotease and neutrophil elastase. The recommended dose is 250 mg/kg α_1-antiprotease at 28-day intervals.[34] This treatment is recommended in patients with serum levels of α_1-antiprotease of lower than 40 percent. However, even in patients with severe α_1-antiprotease deficiency and emphysema there is only a marginal effect on the rate of decline in $FEV_{1.0}$.[49, 72] Most Z α_1-antiprotease homozygotes would develop only mild lung disease if they abstained from smoking.[72]

Oxygen Therapy

Long-term oxygen therapy prolongs survival in selected patients with COPD.[73, 74] Figures 101–7 and 101–8 show the mortality and survival rates in men and women during oxygen therapy for at least 15 hours daily. After 500 days of follow-up, mortality rates for the group who received oxygen were lower than those in the control group. In men, the mortality rate was 12 percent per year in the treated group compared with 29 percent per year in the control group. In women, the mortality rate was also higher in control subjects than in the oxygen-treated group. Women treated with oxygen survived longer than men treated with oxygen, although only 22 women were included in the study.[73]

Continuous oxygen prolongs survival compared with nocturnal use only (Figs. 101–9 and 101–10). The 12-month mortality rate was 20.6 percent in the nocturnal oxygen therapy group and 11.9 percent in the continuous oxygen therapy group, and the 24-month mortality rates were 40.8 and 22.4 percent, respectively. The overall mortality rate was 31.5 percent for all hypoxic patients within 2 years. Figure 101–10 shows the mortality rate in patients with a $Pa\text{CO}_2$ of 43 mm Hg or higher. Even in these chronically hypercarbic patients with hypoxia, survival was improved with continuous oxygen administration.[74]

Supplemental oxygen is indicated in patients with a $Pa\text{O}_2$ of less than 55 mm Hg or a $Pa\text{O}_2$ of 55 to 59 mm Hg who have cor pulmonale or polycythemia and in patients with oxygen desaturation during exercise, according to current Medicare guidelines. Oxygen improves exercise tolerance, decreases pulmonary hypertension and erythrocytosis, and

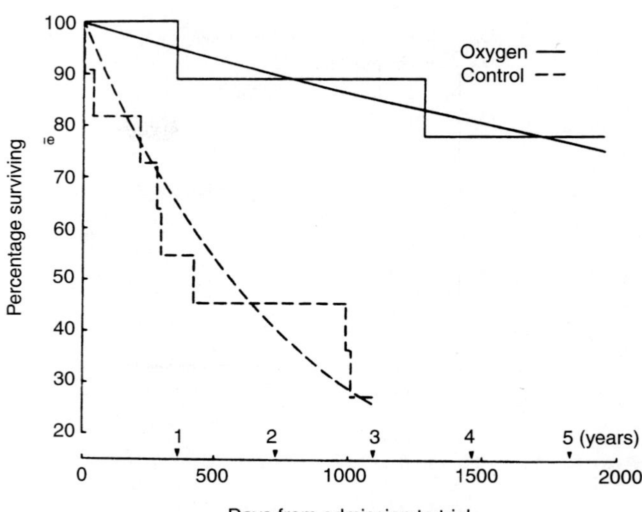

FIGURE 101–8 The mortality of the control group is more than that of the oxygen-treated women from the beginning of the study. (From the Medical Research Council Working Party: Long-term domiciliary oxygen therapy in chronic hypoxic cor pulmonale complicating chronic bronchitis and emphysema. Lancet 1:681–686, 1981.)

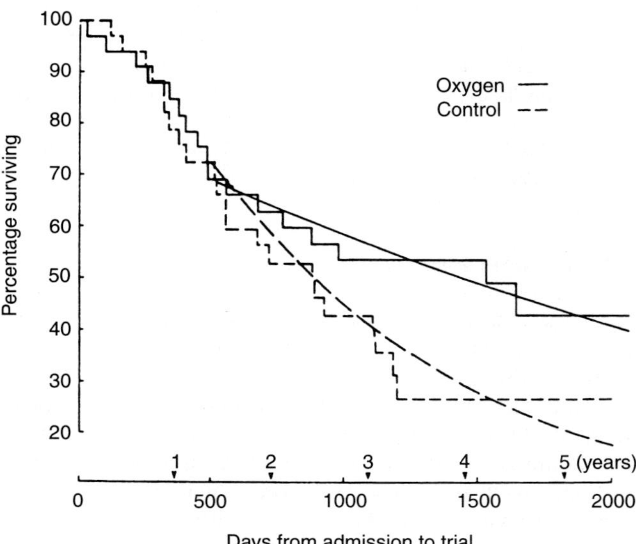

FIGURE 101–7 Mortality in male patients with oxygen therapy was reduced compared with controls after about 500 days. (From the Medical Research Council Working Party: Long-term domiciliary oxygen therapy in chronic hypoxic cor pulmonale complicating chronic bronchitis and emphysema. Lancet 1:681–686, 1981.)

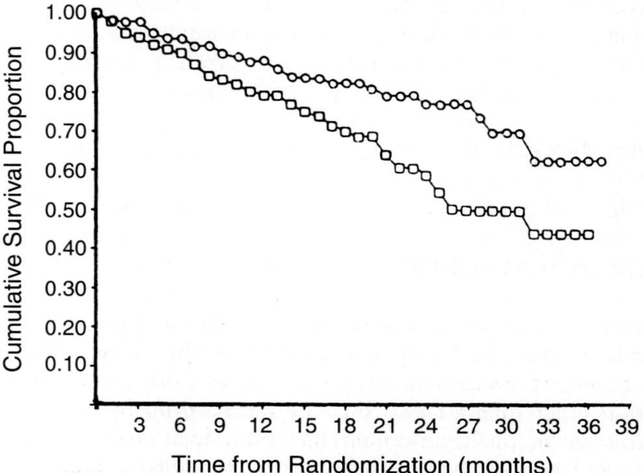

FIGURE 101–9 Overall mortality rates for patients with continuous oxygen therapy is improved compared with those receiving nocturnal oxygen therapy. *Open circles,* continuous oxygen therapy group. *Open squares,* nocturnal oxygen therapy group. (From the Nocturnal Oxygen Therapy Trial Group: Continuous or nocturnal oxygen therapy in hypoxemic chronic obstructive lung disease. Ann Intern Med 93:391–398, 1980.)

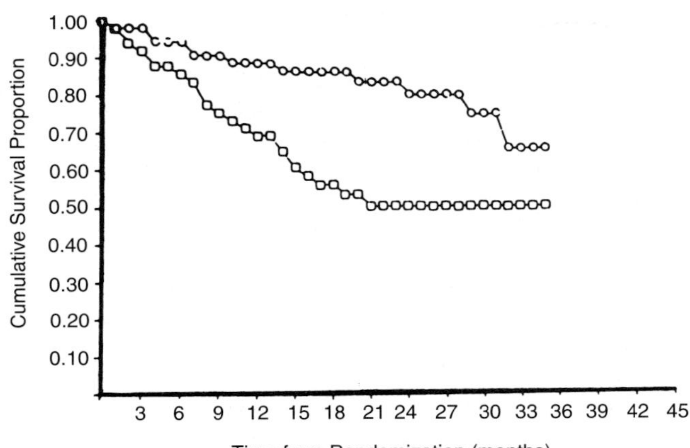

FIGURE 101–10 Survival rates for hypercarbic patients with arterial PCO_2 of more than 43 mm Hg is improved with continuous oxygen therapy. *Open circles,* continuous oxygen therapy group. *Open squares,* nocturnal oxygen therapy group. (From the Nocturnal Oxygen Therapy Trial Group: Continuous or nocturnal oxygen therapy in hypoxemic chronic obstructive lung disease. Ann Intern Med 93:391–398, 1980.)

improves neuropsychologic functions.[73–75] In patients with only nocturnal hypoxemia (arterial saturation <85 percent while sleeping), oxygen therapy at night may be indicated to reach a minimum saturation of approximately 90 percent.[76]

Oxygen does not induce a clinically important increase in $Paco_2$ in patients with stable COPD, even with severe airflow obstruction.[77] However, oxygen therapy may aggravate CO_2 retention during acute respiratory failure in chronically hypercapnic patients. Hypoxemia and acidosis on admission are good indicators to identify patients at the greatest risk for CO_2 narcosis.[78] An inspired oxygen concentration of less than 40 percent is uncommonly associated with a rapidly rising $Paco_2$. Clinically significant improvements in Pao_2 without reaching the ideal Pao_2 goal of 65 mm Hg are possible and avoid disturbances of consciousness. Severe hypoxemia causes death, whereas the disturbances associated with severe CO_2 retention are not usually lethal. In severe hypoxemia, the first priority must be to increase Pao_2.[76] If adequate oxygenation cannot be achieved without progressive hypercapnia, assisted ventilation may be required.

Assisted Ventilation

Patients with severe COPD may require mechanical ventilation after cardiac or general surgery; during an episode of acute respiratory failure secondary to a disease or condition other than COPD, such as sepsis, drug overdose, or trauma; or for acute-on-chronic respiratory failure (COPD exacerbation). The primary objective in intubation and ventilation is to decrease the work of breathing and to rest the respiratory muscles, allowing time for the primary therapies (corticosteroids, bronchodilators, antibiotics, and so on) to take effect.[66, 79] Intubation should be avoided whenever possible without compromising the patient.

Noninvasive modes of ventilation during acute COPD exacerbations have become popular. Negative-pressure ventilation with the use of cuirass shell, tank ("iron lung"), or the plastic Emerson wrap has been successful in patients with chronic respiratory failure due to neuromuscular disease and in patients with central hypoventilation.[79] The role of negative-pressure modes in acute COPD exacerbations is not established.

Noninvasive positive-pressure ventilation (NPPV) has been used in COPD patients during exacerbations and as a bridge from the ventilator to spontaneous breathing.[66, 79] NPPV should not be considered in patients with apnea or agonal respiration, uncontrolled agitation, life-threatening hypoxia, hemodynamic instability, or serious arrythmia or in those with a high risk for aspiration. All of these are indications for endotracheal intubation, as are a falling arterial pH and rising $Paco_2$ secondary to ventilatory failure. A pH of 7.25 or less is generally regarded as significant acidosis, requiring endotracheal intubation.[66, 79]

During positive-pressure ventilation, the lung may not empty completely before the next inspiratory cycle, resulting in end-expiratory lung volumes higher than FRC. Lung volumes may progressively increase. This trapped air volume increases with larger tidal volumes, increased expiratory airflow resistance, and higher lung compliance coupled with a relatively decreased expiratory time. Auto–positive end-expiratory pressure (auto-PEEP) refers to this state of elevated net static recoil pressure of the respiratory system at end expiration that occurs in the dynamically hyperinflated lung.[79] Mechanical ventilation via an endotracheal tube in patients with COPD is more likely to cause dynamic hyperinflation and auto-PEEP than NPPV. Severe auto-PEEP causes volutrauma, pneumothorax, cardiovascular collapse, and an increased work of breathing.

Control of dynamic hyperinflation, or auto-PEEP, is achieved primarily through the facilitation of adequate lung emptying by reducing inspiratory and prolonging expiratory time on the ventilator. A reduction in overall minute ventilation most effectively increases expiratory time; tidal volumes of 5 to 8 ml/kg and rates of 8 to 10 breaths/min are recommended.[79] An inspiratory time shortened by increasing inspiratory flow may increase expiratory time. Sedation and, occasionally, paralysis may be required to reduce the minute ventilation and auto-PEEP, even at the risk of hypercarbia.[66, 79]

Other Considerations

Incentive spirometry is useful before and after major surgery by helping to prevent postoperative atelectasis and perhaps stimulating cough and expectoration. Sustaining maximal deep breaths for 5 to 6 seconds and 5 to 10 sequential breaths should be emphasized and repeated every hour while awake.[80, 81] Incentive spirometry performance correlates with vital capacity (mainly with inspiratory reserve volume), and a sudden decrease in performance may predict pulmonary complication after lobectomy.[82] The use of *intermittent positive-pressure breathing* remains controversial, and no evidence supports home or routine use of this technique to prevent atelectasis[80]; it also has not improved bronchodilator delivery.

Chest percussion and postural drainage with inhaled

bronchodilators may be useful in patients with excessive secretions (30 cc/day or more) or difficult expectoration and in hospital settings with lobar atelectasis secondary to secretions. Otherwise, chest physiotherapy does not improve airflow or gas exchange in stable patients with COPD who produce less than 30 cc/day of sputum.[80, 83]

Nutritional support should be initiated early in patients with COPD and acute respiratory failure. These patients have high incidence of protein-caloric malnutrition.[84] A high carbohydrate load may increase CO_2 production in patients with limited ventilatory reserve with worsening arterial hypercarbia.[85]

Mucolytic use in COPD remains controversial. Iodinated glycerol may improve cough symptoms and well-being and decrease the duration of acute exacerbation (dosage of 60 mg qid) in some studies.[86] Recombinant human deoxyribonuclease (rhDNase) has been shown to reduce sputum viscoelasticity and to improve lung function in patients with cystic fibrosis in the short term but not in COPD. However, long-term efficacy in cystic fibrosis is disappointing.[87]

In patients with secondary polycythemia (hematocrit > 65 percent) due to chronic hypoxemia, *phlebotomy* enhances exercise tolerance, lowers pulmonary artery pressures, and increases the ejection fraction of the right ventricle. The goal of phlebotomy is to maintain a hematocrit below 55 percent.[88] Of course, secondary polycythemia is best treated by avoiding hypoxemia.

Although the benefit of pulmonary *rehabilitation* programs remains controversial, these programs may improve survival and quality-of-life indices, reduce respiratory symptoms, increase the length and intensity of exercise tolerance, and decrease the need for hospitalization. Pulmonary rehabilitation may improve psychological function while reducing anxiety and depression and is associated with increased feelings of hope, control, and self-esteem. As in cardiac rehabilitation, the effects of exercise conditioning disappear rapidly with cessation of exercise.[85]

COPD patients have increased risks of *postoperative pulmonary complications,* with relative risks ranging from 2.7 to 4.7. Smoking is a risk factor for complications. All smokers should stop at least 8 weeks before any operation. Symptoms and airflow obstruction should be aggressively treated before any elective procedure, and elective procedures should be postponed around the time of acute exacerbations of COPD. The combinations of bronchodilators, smoking cessation, corticosteroids, antibiotics, and physical therapy reduce the risk of postoperative pulmonary complications.[89]

Upper abdominal and thoracic surgery carries risks ranging from 10 to 40 percent of postoperative pulmonary complications. Postoperative complications are rare after operations outside the thorax or abdomen. Surgical procedures lasting longer than 3 hours are associated with a higher risk of pulmonary complications. The risk of pulmonary complications in epidural or spinal anesthesia is lower than that with general anesthesia.[89] Postoperative strategies to reduce complications include lung-expansion maneuvers such as deep-breathing exercise, chest percussion, and pain control. Educating patients in advance about preoperative practice of incentive spirometry and cough reduces postoperative complications.[89]

SURGICAL TREATMENT

Lung volume reduction surgery (LVRS), which was first introduced in the 1950s, failed to gain acceptance because of significant operative mortality rates. Although CO_2 laser therapy for the reduction of lung volume was reported in 1991, the report by Cooper and associates[90] of 20 cases in 1995 in which surgical resection was used increased enthusiasm for LVRS. These procedures are still in active research trials but appear to be promising in selected patients with emphysema because perioperative mortality and morbidity rates have decreased.[91] After LVRS, $FEV_{1.0}$ increases to as high as 50 percent, diaphragmatic function is enhanced, the use of accessory muscles is decreased, exercise capacity is improved, and dyspnea is reduced.[91, 92] However, patient selection criteria and surgical technique are not standardized.

Lung transplantation is the other surgical alternative for patients with COPD. Single-lung transplantation is feasible in COPD. Emphysema accounts for about 60 percent of all single-lung transplants in the United States. The cost of the procedure and the lack of an adequate supply of donor lungs remain problematic.[11] Although the quality of life is improved in patients with COPD after single-lung transplantation, life expectancy after transplantation is not increased.

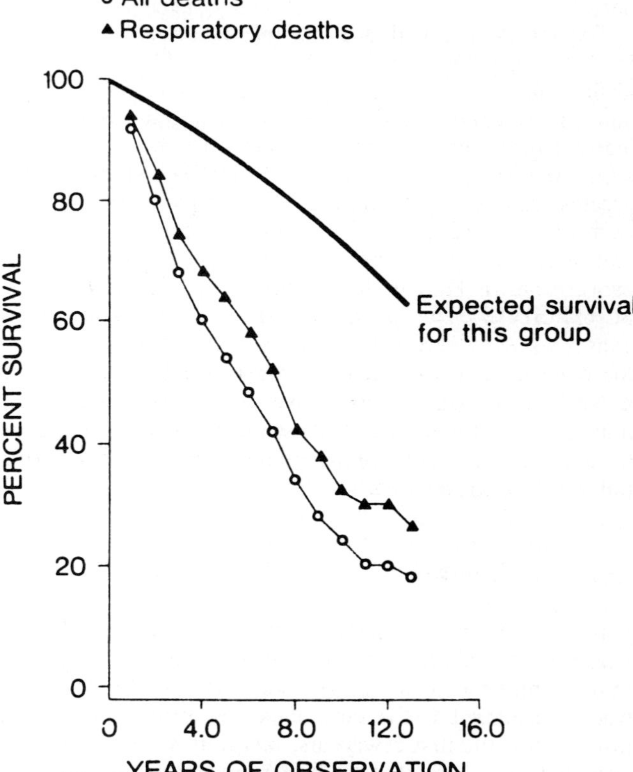

FIGURE 101–11 Survival rates were reduced in 200 patients with chronic respiratory disease compared with expected survival rates for an age-matched general population group. (From Diener CF, Burrows B: Further observations on the course and prognosis of chronic obstructive lung disease. Am Rev Respir Dis 111:719–724, 1975. Official journal of the American Thoracic Society. © American Lung Association.)

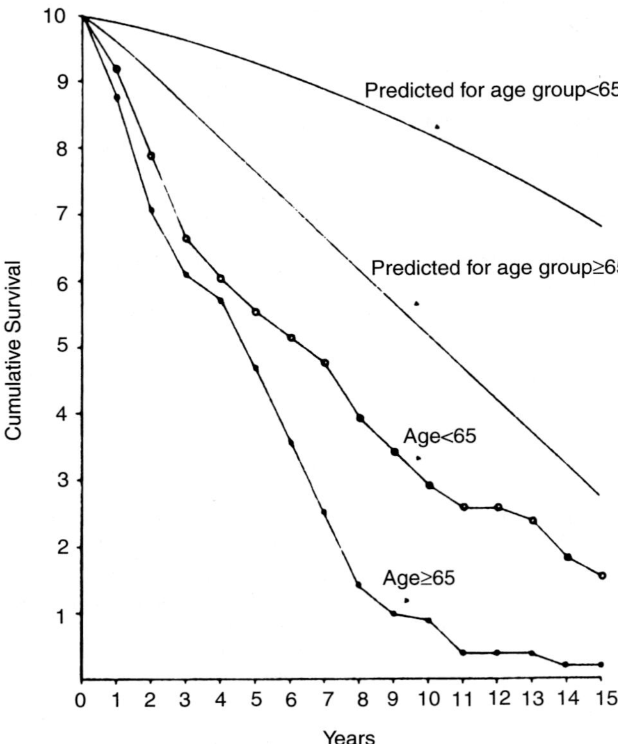

FIGURE 101–12 Survival rates among subjects with chronic obstructive pulmonary disease at least 65 years old or less than 65 years old are reduced compared with the general population. *Curves* indicate the predicted survival rates for a general population of the same age, sex, and smoking habits. *Circles* represent forced expiratory volume in 1 second ($FEV_{1.0}$) of more than 1.25 liters, *squares* represent $FEV_{1.0}$ of at least 0.75 but no more than 1.25 liters, and *triangles* represent $FEV_{1.0}$ of less than 0.75 L. (From Travers GA, Cline MG, Burrows B: Predictors of mortality in chronic obstructive pulmonary disease. Am Rev Respir Dis 119:895–902, 1979.)

PROGNOSIS

Smoking remains the most important negative influence on survival.[11] Because COPD is seen 10 to 40 years after the initiation of smoking, COPD mortality rates will continue to increase even if the entire population stopped smoking today.[10] In patients with COPD, $FEV_{1.0}$ is the single best predictor of mortality, along with older age. In long-term follow-up studies, survival declines with $FEV_{1.0}$. When $FEV_{1.0}$ falls below 1.0 L, death rates approach 10 percent per year.[93–95]

Figure 101–11 shows the 13-year survival rates in 200 patients with COPD compared with expected survival rates for nonsmokers in the same group. Two thirds of deaths were considered to be secondary to chronic respiratory disease. For the first few years, mortality rates in the least impaired group ($FEV_{1.0}$ >1.25 L) did not differ from that expected for a general male population of the same age. However, long-term follow-up showed that mortality rates closely approached those of patients with severe airflow impairment.[95]

In patients at least 65 years old with COPD, survival is predicted by the initial degree of ventilatory impairment (as the fraction of $FEV_{1.0}$ predicted for age). Mortality rates in patients with chronic respiratory disease are markedly increased after 5 years of follow-up compared with predicted survival rates for the general population (Fig. 101–12). Although not as robust as the relationship between declining $FEV_{1.0}$ and survival, hypoxemia and hypercarbia portend a poor prognosis.

In summary, patients with COPD should be educated about their disease and encouraged to participate in smoking cessation programs. Teenagers should be strongly educated to avoid smoking. In patients with COPD and hypoxemia, oxygen improves survival and quality of life. Trials with inhaled corticosteroids in patients with COPD will be available soon, and these agents may improve airflow obstruction with long-term use in selected patients. In the future, chemical and genetic studies will be available to understand and recognize susceptible smokers at risk of developing COPD. LVRS surgery may become a better option for patients with COPD with improved patient selection, operative techniques, and decreased perioperative morbidity and mortality rates.

REFERENCES

1. American Thoracic Society: Standards for the diagnosis and care of patients with chronic obstructive pulmonary disease (COPD) and asthma: chronic obstructive pulmonary disease. Am J Respir Crit Care Med 136:225–238, 1986.
2. Christie RV: Emphysema of the lungs. BMJ 1:105–108, 143–146, 1944.
3. American Thoracic Society: Chronic bronchitis, asthma, and pulmonary emphysema: a statement by the Committee on Diagnostic Standards for Nontuberculosis Respiratory Diseases. Am Rev Respir Dis 85:762–768, 1962.
4. Snider GL, Kleinerman J, Thurlbeck WM, et al: The definition of emphysema. Report of a National Heart, Lung, and Blood Institute, Division of Lung Diseases Workshop, 1985, pp. 182–185.
5. Senior RM, Anthonisen NR: Chronic obstructive pulmonary disease (COPD). Am J Respir Crit Care Med 157:S139–S147, 1998.
6. Monthly Vital Statistics Report 46(suppl), 1996.
7. Higgins MW: Chronic airways disease in the United States: trends and determinants. Chest 96:328S–334S, 1989.
8. Speizer FE: COPD: overview and summary. Am Rev Respir Dis 140:S106–S107, 1989.
9. Xu X, Li B, Wang L: Gender difference in smoking effects on adult pulmonary function. Eur Respir J 7:477–483, 1994.
10. Davis RM, Novotny TE: The epidemiology of cigarette smoking and its impact on chronic obstructive pulmonary disease. Am Rev Respir Dis 140:S82–S84, 1989.
11. Kerstijens HAM, Brand PLP, Postma DS: Risk factors for accelerated decline among patients with chronic obstructive pulmonary disease. Am J Respir Crit Care Med 154:S266–S272, 1996.
12. Becklake MR: Occupational exposures: evidence for a causal association with chronic obstructive pulmonary disease. Am Rev Respir Dis 140:S85–S91, 1989.
13. American Thoracic Society: Respiratory health hazards in agriculture. Am Rev Respir Dis 158:S28–S31, 1998.
14. Cole RB, Nevin NC, Blundell G, et al: Relation of alpha-1-antitrypsin phenotype to the performance of pulmonary function tests and to the prevalence of respiratory illness in a working population. Thorax 31:149–157, 1976.
15. West JB. Obstructive diseases. *In* West JB (ed): Pulmonary Pathophysiology. 2nd ed. pp. 59–80. Baltimore: Williams & Wilkins, 1982.
16. Thurlbeck WM: Pathophysiology of chronic obstructive pulmonary disease. Clin Chest Med 11:389–403, 1990.
17. Jeffrey PK: Structural and inflammatory changes in COPD: a comparison with asthma. Thorax 53:129–136, 1998.
18. Clausen JL: The diagnosis of emphysema, chronic bronchitis, and asthma. Clin Chest Med 11:405–416, 1990.
19. Badgett RG, Tanaka DJ, Hunt DK, et al: Can moderate chronic

obstructive pulmonary disease be diagnosed by historical and physical findings alone? Am J Med 94:188–196, 1993.
20. Pardee NE, Martin CJ, Morgan EH: A test of the practical value of estimating breath sound intensity—breath sounds related to measured ventilatory function. Chest 70:341–344, 1976.
21. Stubbing DG, Mathur PN, Roberts RS, et al: Some physical signs in patients with chronic airflow obstruction. Am Rev Respir Dis 125:549–552, 1982.
22. Pardee NE, Winterbauer RH, Morgan EH: Combinations of four physical signs as indicators of ventilatory abnormality in obstructive pulmonary syndromes. Chest 77:354–358, 1980.
23. Bashear RE: Arrhythmias in patients with chronic obstructive pulmonary disease. Med Clin North Am 68:969–981, 1984.
24. Biggs FD, Lefrak SS, Kleiger RE, et al: Disturbances of rhythm in chronic lung disease. Heart Lung 6:256–261, 1977.
25. Sherman S, Skoney JA, Ravikrishnan KP: Routine chest radiographs in exacerbations of chronic obstructive pulmonary disease. Arch Intern Med 149:2493–2496, 1989.
26. Newell JD: Imaging of airways diseases. Semin Respir Crit Care Med 19:459–468, 1998.
27. Kazerooni EA: Imaging of emphysema and the impact of lung volume reduction surgery. Semin Respir Crit Care Med 19:469–482, 1998.
28. American Thoracic Society: Lung function testing: selection of reference values and interpretative strategies. Am Rev Respir Dis 144:1202–1218, 1991.
29. Burrows B, Strauss RH, Niden AH: Chronic obstructive lung disease, III: interrelationships of pulmonary function data. Am Rev Respir Dis 91:861–868, 1965.
30. Hyatt RE, Scanlon PD, Nakamura M: Diffusing capacity of the lungs. *In* Hyatt RE, Scanlon PD, Nakamura M (eds): Interpretation of Pulmonary Function Tests: A Practical Guide. pp. 41–49. Philadelphia: Lippincott-Raven, 1997.
31. Morrison NJ, Abboud RT, Ramadan F, et al: Comparison of single breath carbon monoxide diffusing capacity and pressure-volume curves in detecting emphysema. Am Rev Respir Dis 139:1179–1187, 1989.
32. Owens GR, Rogers RM, Pennock BE, et al: The diffusing capacity as a predictor of arterial oxygen desaturation during exercise in patients with chronic obstructive pulmonary disease. N Engl J Med 310:1218–1221, 1984.
33. Gilbert R, Keighley J, Chir B, et al: Mechanisms of chronic carbon dioxide retention in patients with obstructive pulmonary disease. Am J Med 38:217–225, 1965.
34. Hubbard RC, Sellers S, Czerski D, et al: Biochemical efficacy and safety of monthly augmentation therapy for alpha 1-antitrypsin deficiency. JAMA 260:1259–1264, 1988.
35. Douglas NJ: Sleep in patients with chronic obstructive pulmonary disease. Clin Chest Med 19:115–125, 1998.
36. Rizzi M, Palma P, Andreoli A, et al: Prevalence and clinical feature of the "overlap syndrome," obstructive sleep apnea (OSA) and chronic obstructive pulmonary disease (COPD), in OSA population. Sleep Breathing 2:69, 1997.
37. Chaouat A, Weitzenblum E, Krieger J, et al: Association of chronic pulmonary disease and sleep apnea syndrome. Am J Respir Crit Care Med 151:82–86, 1995.
38. American Thoracic Society: Standards for the diagnosis and care of patients with chronic obstructive pulmonary disease (COPD) and asthma: chronic obstructive pulmonary disease: pharmacologic therapy. Am J Respir Crit Care Med 136:228–231, 1986.
39. Lippman M, Fein A: Pulmonary embolism in the patient with chronic obstructive pulmonary disease. Chest 39:39–42, 1981.
40. Cross JL, Kemp PM, Walsh CG, et al: A randomized trial of spiral CT and ventilation perfusion scintigraphy for the diagnosis of pulmonary embolism. Clin Radiol 53:177, 1998.
41. Anthonisen NR, Connett JE, Kiley JP, et al: Effects of smoking intervention and the use of an inhaled anticholinergic bronchodilator on the rate of decline of FEV. JAMA 272:1497–1505, 1994.
42. Fiore MC, Kenford SL, Jorenby DE, et al: Two studies of the clinical effectiveness of the nicotine patch with different counseling treatments. Chest 105:524–533, 1994.
43. Raw M, Jarvis MJ, Feyerabend C, et al: Comparison of nicotine chewing-gum and psychological treatments for dependent smokers. BMJ 281:481–482, 1980.
44. Jorenby DE, Leischow SJ, Nides MA: A controlled trial of sustained-release bupropion, a nicotine patch, or both for smoking cessation. N Engl J Med 340:695–691, 1999.
45. Hughes JR, Golstein MG, Hurt RD, et al: Recent advances in the pharmacotherapy of smoking. JAMA 281:72–76, 1999.
46. Riddiough MA, Sisk JE, Bell JC: Influenza vaccination: cost-effectiveness and public policy. JAMA 249:3189–3195, 1983.
47. American Thoracic Society: Standards for the diagnosis and care of patients with chronic obstructive pulmonary disease (COPD) and asthma. Am J Respir Crit Care Med 136:231–234, 1986.
48. Hirschmann JV, Lipsky BA: The pneumococcal vaccine after 15 years of use. Arch Int Med 154:373–377, 1994.
49. Barnes PJ: New therapies for chronic obstructive pulmonary disease. Thorax 53:137–147, 1998.
50. Gross NJ: Anticholinergic agents in COPD. Chest 91:52S–57S, 1987.
51. Combivent Inhalation Aerosol Study Group: In chronic pulmonary obstructive disease, a combination of ipratropium and albuterol is more effective than either agent alone: an 85-day multicenter trial. Chest 105:1411–1419, 1994.
52. Petty TL: The combination of ipratropium and albuterol is more effective than either agent alone. Chest 107:S183–S186, 1995.
53. The Combivent Inhalation Solution Study Group. Routine nebulized ipratropium and albuterol together are better than either alone in COPD. Chest 112:1514–1521, 1997.
54. Gross N, Tashkin D, Miller R, et al: Inhalation by nebulization of albuterol-ipratropium combination (Dey combination) is superior to either agent alone in the treatment of chronic obstructive pulmonary disease. Respiration 65:354–362, 1998.
55. The Intermittent Positive Pressure Breathing Trial Group: Intermittent positive pressure breathing therapy of chronic obstructive pulmonary disease. Ann Intern Med 91:612–620, 1983.
56. Anthonisen NR, Wright EC: IPPB Trial Group: bronchodilator response in chronic obstructive pulmonary disease. Am Rev Respir Dis 133:814–819, 1986.
57. Berry RB, Shinto RA, Wong FH, et al: Nebulizer versus spacer for bronchodilator delivery in patients hospitalized for acute exacerbations of COPD. Chest 96:1241–1246, 1989.
58. Leatherman JW: Mechanical ventilation in obstructive lung disease. Clin Chest Med 17:577–590, 1996.
59. Vassallo R, Lipsky JJ: Theophylline: recent advances in the understanding of its mode of action and uses in clinical practice. Mayo Clin Proc 73:346–354, 1998.
60. Murciano D, Aubier M, Lecocguic Y: Effects of theophylline on diaphragmatic strength and fatigue in patients with chronic obstructive pulmonary disease. N Engl J Med 311:349–353, 1984.
61. Rogers RM, Owens GR, Pennock BE: The pendulum swings again toward a rational use of theophylline. Chest 87:280–282, 1985.
62. Sahn SA: Corticosteroids in chronic bronchitis and pulmonary emphysema. Chest 73:389–396, 1978.
63. Albert RK, Martin TR, Lewis SW: Controlled clinical trial of methylprednisolone in patients with chronic bronchitis and acute respiratory insufficiency. Ann Intern Med 92:753–758, 1980.
64. Shim CS, Williams MH Jr: Aerosol beclomethasone in patients with steroid-responsive chronic obstructive pulmonary disease. Am J Med 78:655–658, 1985.
65. Chung KF: Long-term inhaled corticosteroid therapy in chronic airway obstruction. Eur Respir J 5:913–914, 1992.
66. Madison JM, Irwin RS. Chronic obstructive pulmonary disease. Lancet 352:467–473, 1998.
67. Chodosh S: Treatment of acute exacerbations of chronic bronchitis: state of the art. Am J Med 91:6A–87S, 6A–92S, 1991.
68. Saint S, Bent S, Vittinghoff E, et al: Antibiotics in chronic obstructive pulmonary disease exacerbations. JAMA 273:957–960, 1995.
69. Anthonisen R, Manfreda J, Warren W: Antibiotic therapy in exacerbations of chronic obstructive pulmonary disease. Ann Intern Med 106:196–204, 1987.
70. Prevention and control of influenza: recommendations of the Advisory Committee on Immunization Practices. MMWR 45(RR-5):1–24, 1996.
71. Van Voris LP, Newell PM, Antivirals for the chemoprophylaxis and treatment of influenza. Semin Respir Infect 7:61–70, 1992.
72. Mahadeva R, Thomas DA: Alpha 1-antitrypsin deficiency, cirrhosis and emphysema. Thorax 53:501–505, 1998.
73. Report of the Medical Research Council Working Party: Long term domiciliary oxygen therapy in chronic hypoxic cor pulmonale complicating chronic bronchitis and emphysema. Lancet 1:681–686, 1981.
74. Nocturnal Oxygen Therapy Trial Group. Continuous or nocturnal oxygen therapy in hypoxemic chronic obstructive lung disease. Ann Intern Med 93:391–398, 1980.

75. Anthonisen R: Long-term oxygen therapy. Ann Intern Med 99:519–527, 1983.
76. American Thoracic Society: Standards for the diagnosis and care of patients with chronic obstructive pulmonary disease (COPD) and asthma: O_2 therapy. Am J Respir Crit Care Med 136:235–236, 1986.
77. Goldstein RS, Ramcharan V, Bowes G, et al: Effect of supplemental nocturnal oxygen on gas exchange in patients with severe obstructive lung disease. N Engl J Med 310:425–429, 1984.
78. Bone RC, Pierce AK, Johnson RL Jr: Controlled oxygen administration in acute respiratory failure in chronic obstructive pulmonary disease. Am J Med 65:896–902, 1978.
79. Gladwin MT, Pierson DJ. Mechanical ventilation of the patient with severe chronic obstructive pulmonary disease. Intens Care Med 24:898–910, 1998.
80. American Thoracic Society: Standards for the diagnosis and care of patients with chronic obstructive pulmonary disease (COPD) and asthma: respiratory care modalities. Am J Respir Crit Care Med 136:236–238, 1986.
81. AARC clinical practice guideline. Incentive spirometry. Respir Care 36:1402–1405, 1991.
82. Bastin R, Moraine JJ, Bardocsky G: Incentive spirometry performance: a reliable indicator of pulmonary function in the early postoperative period after lobectomy. Chest 111:559–563, 1997.
83. May DB, Munt PW: Physiologic effects of chest percussion and postural drainage in patients with stable chronic bronchitis. Chest 75:29–32, 1979.
84. Driver AG, McAlevy MT, Smith JL: Nutritional assessment of patients with chronic obstructive pulmonary disease and acute respiratory failure. Chest 82:568–571, 1982.
85. American Thoracic Society: Standards for the diagnosis and care of patients with chronic obstructive pulmonary disease (COPD) and asthma: physical rehabilitation and home care. Am J Respir Crit Care Med 136:239–243, 1986.
86. Petty TL: The National Mycolytic Study: results of a randomized, double-blind, placebo-controlled study of iodinated glycerol in chronic obstructive bronchitis. Chest 97:75–83, 1990.
87. Milla CE: Long term effects of aerosolised rhDNase on pulmonary disease progression in patients with cystic fibrosis. Thorax 53:1014–1017, 1998.
88. Chetty OG, Brown SE, Light RW: Improved exercise tolerance of the polycythemic lung patient following phlebotomy. Am J Med 74:415–420, 1983.
89. Smetana GW: Preoperative pulmonary evaluation. N Engl J Med 340:937–944, 1999.
90. Cooper JD, Trulock EP, Triantafillou AN, et al: Bilateral pneumonectomy (volume reduction) for chronic obstructive pulmonary disease. J Thorac Cardiovasc Surg 109:106–119, 1995.
91. Doyle RL, Mark JBD: Lung volume reduction surgery for the treatment of chronic obstructive pulmonary disease. Adv Intern Med 43:233–252, 1998.
92. Benditt OO, Wood DE, McCool FD, et al: Changes in breathing and ventilatory muscle recruitment patterns induced by lung volume reduction surgery. Am J Respir Crit Care Med 155:279–284, 1997.
93. Burrows B, Earle RH: Course and prognosis of chronic obstructive lung disease. N Engl J Med 280:397–404, 1969.
94. Burrows B, Earle RH: Prediction of survival in patients with chronic airway obstruction. Am Rev Respir Dis 99:865–871, 1969.
95. Diener CF, Burrows B: Further observations on the course and prognosis of chronic obstructive lung disease. Am Rev Respir Dis 111:719–724, 1975.
96. Traver GA, Cline MG, Burrows B: Predictors of mortality in chronic obstructive pulmonary disease. Am Rev Respir Dis 119:895–902, 1979.

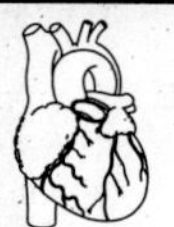

CHAPTER 102

TUMORS OF THE HEART

Robert J. Hall, Hugh A. McAllister, Jr., Denton A. Cooley, and L. Maximilian Buja

SECONDARY TUMORS OF THE HEART
General Considerations
Manifestations
Diagnostic Studies
Treatment
PRIMARY TUMORS OF THE HEART
Cardiac Myxomas
Other Benign Primary Tumors of the Heart
Malignant Primary Tumors of the Heart
TUMORS OF THE PERICARDIUM
Leukemias and Lymphomas

Tumors of the heart are uncommon; moreover, they present in diverse and challenging ways. The heart may be the site of a primary tumor or may be invaded secondarily by malignancies that arise in adjacent or remote organs. In the presence of neoplastic disease, pericardial pain, effusion, tamponade, constriction, rapid increase in heart size, new heart murmurs, electrocardiographic (ECG) changes, atrial or ventricular arrhythmias, atrioventricular (AV) block, and unexplained heart failure are suggestive of secondary invasion of the heart. The triad of obstruction, embolization, and constitutional manifestations characterizes intracavitary tumors, especially myxomas (Table 102–1).

SECONDARY TUMORS OF THE HEART

General Considerations

Metastatic tumors—more frequently carcinomas than sarcomas—that involve the heart, pericardium, or both originate as primaries in some other organ 20 to 40 times more frequently than they originate as primary tumors of the heart (Fig. 102–1).[1, 2] These secondary tumors occur most often in persons beyond the age of 50 years, with an equal incidence in both genders. Cardiac metastases are usually associated with widely disseminated systemic tumor, and their occurrence in patients with malignant tumors has been reported to vary widely (range, 1.5 to 21 percent).[1, 3, 4] All types of malignant disease, including carcinoma, sarcoma, leukemia, and lymphoma, can involve the heart. No malignant tumor, however, has a particular tendency to metastasize to the heart, with the possible exception of malignant melanoma, which involves the myocardium in more than 50 percent of cases.[5] Cardiac metastases are most common with bronchogenic carcinoma[6] and carcinoma of the breast. Metastatic tumors reach the heart by hematogenous spread, lymphatic spread, or direct invasion. Lymphatic spread of tumors occurs particularly frequently with carcinoma of the bronchus and the breast; the proximity of the heart to major mediastinal lymphatic channels seems to explain the high incidence of cardiac metastases from mediastinal tumors.[3]

Manifestations

Involvement of a secondary tumor may be recognized as a pathologic finding without clinical manifestations. More often, however, such involvement *is* symptomatic, and on rare occasions, it may be the first or only expression of a remote primary tumor. Recognition of neoplastic heart disease depends on the physician's awareness of the tumor's probability of occurrence and diverse presentations. Secondary tumors of the heart may involve the pericardium, myocardium, endocardium, valves, and coronary arteries. Direct invasion of the heart through the venae cavae[7] or

TABLE 102–1 General Manifestations of Neoplastic Heart Disease

Pericardial Involvement
Pericarditis, pain
Pericardial effusion
Radiographic enlargement
Arrhythmia, predominantly atrial
Tamponade
Constriction

Myocardial Involvement
Arrhythmias, ventricular and atrial
Electrocardiographic changes
Radiographic enlargement
- Generalized
- Localized

Conduction disturbances and heart block
Congestive heart failure
Coronary involvement
- Angina
- Infarction

Intracavitary Tumor
Cavity obliteration
Valve obstruction and valve damage
Embolic phenomena: systemic, neurologic, coronary
Constitutional manifestations

Hall RJ, Cooley, DA: Neoplastic heart disease. *In* Alexander RW, Schlant RC, Foster V (eds): Hurst's The Heart—Arteries and Veins. 5th ed. pp. 1403–1424. New York: McGraw-Hill, 1982.

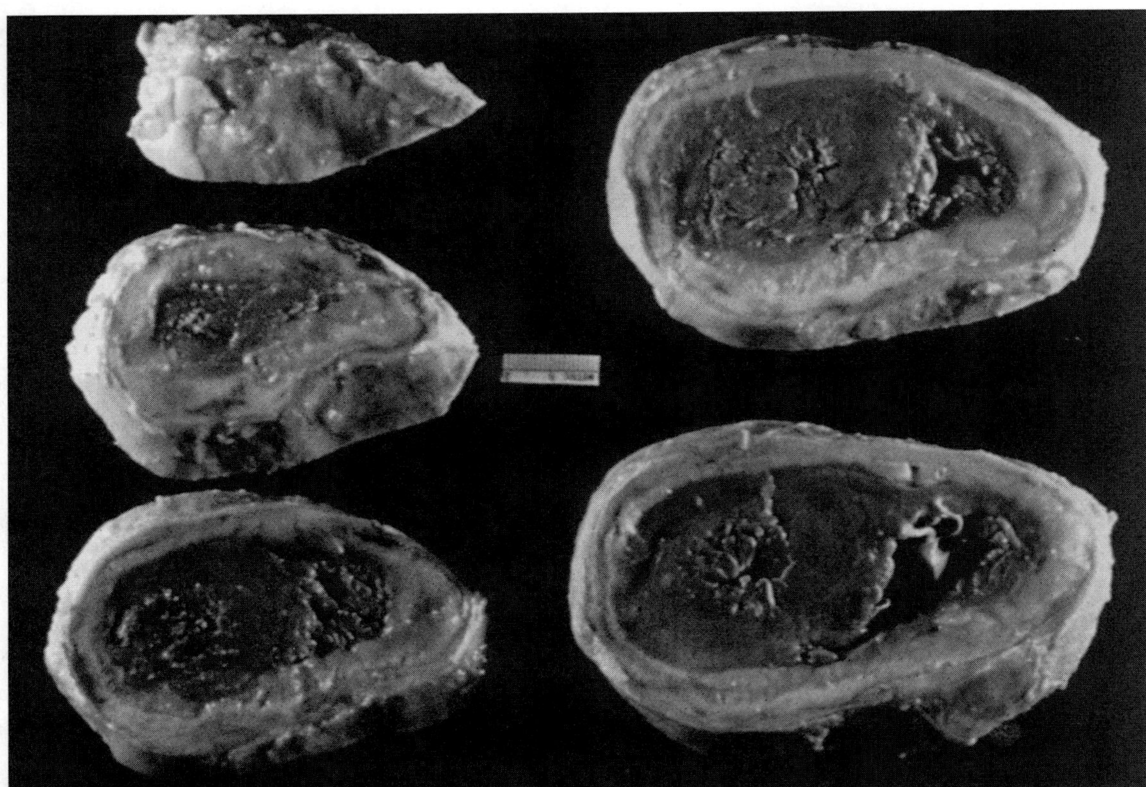

FIGURE 102–1 Metastatic carcinoma of the heart. There is circumferential distribution of the tumor into the pericardial cavity, with infiltration of the epicardium.

pulmonary veins[8] or from an expanding myocardial implant can produce an intracavitary tumor mass resulting in obstruction of blood flow[9] or can cause valvular obstruction.

Depending on the character and location of the cardiac lesion, a variety of manifestations may serve to identify cardiac involvement, especially in a patient with a known malignancy.

Pericardial Involvement

Pericardial involvement is often first manifested by pleuritic chest pain and a pericardial friction rub. Accumulation of fluid—often bloody—within the pericardium may result in progressive cardiac enlargement on roentgenogram, with symptoms and signs of cardiac tamponade, and may be the first manifestation of a cardiac malignancy.[10] Clinically, the jugular venous pressure is increased, the arterial pressure is reduced, and "pulsus paradoxus" may be present. Reduced ECG QRS voltage can be expected. Electrical alternans is generally seen in patients with large effusions and serious tamponade, which usually necessitate prompt pericardiocentesis. The presence of large quantities of pericardial fluid in association with tumor encasing the heart frequently results in persistent cardiac constriction, even after the fluid is withdrawn by pericardiocentesis (see Fig. 102–1).[3]

Myocardial Involvement

Atrial arrhythmias are common, probably because the atrium has less mobility and hence is invaded more often. Atrial flutter and fibrillation are frequent occurrences and are often resistant to conventional therapy. Ventricular extrasystoles and even serious ventricular arrhythmias[11, 12] may accompany a tumor's invasion into the myocardium. Conduction disturbances and complete heart block have been reported.[13] Widespread involvement of muscle by tumor invasion or obstruction of the cardiac lymphatic drainage system may cause congestive heart failure. Myocardial damage and heart failure also may result from some of the chemotherapeutic agents used for patients with neoplastic diseases; combined radiotherapy and chemotherapy may synergistically increase cardiac damage.[14] The ECG abnormalities seen most frequently in patients with neoplastic heart disease are nonspecific changes of the ST segment[15] and the T wave resulting from myocardial or pericardial involvement by the tumor.

Coronary Artery Involvement

In patients with a malignant tumor, angina or myocardial infarction may result from concomitant atherosclerosis,[14] coronary occlusion by tumor embolization,[16] or external coronary compression by the tumor as well as from coronary fibrosis or accelerated atherogenesis in patients who have received radiation to the mediastinum.[14] The ECG pattern of myocardial infarction also can result from massive invasion of the myocardium by a tumor[14] or from a large pericardial effusion.[2, 17]

Intracavitary Tumor

Extensions of tumors such as renal cell carcinoma,[18–20] hepatocellular carcinoma,[21] uterine leiomyomatosis,[22] endometrial sarcoma,[23] and primary leiomyosarcoma of the vena cavae[24–26] along the vena cava and into the right atrium can present as an intracavitary obstructive mass.[27] Intracavitary metastases or an expanding myocardial tumor may progressively obliterate a cardiac chamber[28] or may result in a valvular obstruction and in rare instances produce fever of unknown origin.

Diagnostic Studies

Use of transthoracic (TTE) as well as transesophageal echocardiography (TEE),[19, 29–32] computed tomography (CT),[33–36] and ultrafast CT[35] facilitates identification of pericardial effusion and cardiac masses. Magnetic resonance imaging (MRI) also provides a global view of cardiac anatomy and identifies the location, extent, and attachment site of cardiac tumors.[5, 37–39] Cross-sectional imaging, such as CT and MRI, plays a crucial role in surgical planning for and management of these patients.[40]

The echocardiogram demonstrates features of hemodynamic tamponade: diastolic collapse of the right atrium and ventricle,[41, 42] inferior vena cava plethora with a blunted inspiratory response,[43] and altered inspiratory intracardiac Doppler flow velocities.[44–46]

Pericardiocentesis affords prompt symptomatic relief from pericardial tamponade and often provides a definitive cytologic diagnosis.[30] Ultrasound and fluoroscopic guidance increase the safety of pericardial catheter placement.[47] In some cases, the results of endomyocardial biopsy may contribute to the diagnosis.[19, 48]

Treatment

Malignant pericardial effusion usually recurs rapidly after pericardiocentesis. Depending on the cytologic type and radiosensitivity of the tumor, the treatment of choice is radiation to the cardiac area, with or without systemic chemotherapy.[30, 49] The heart can tolerate 20 to 40 Gy, beyond which the risk of radiation-induced pericardial, myocardial, and valvular[50–52] damage is increased. Patients with malignant pericardial effusions have responded to systemic chemotherapy and to intrapericardial administration of fluorouracil, radioactive gold, nitrogen mustard, and tetracycline.[30, 53] Persistent reaccumulation of fluid may require surgical creation of a "pericardial window."[54, 55] A pericardial pleural communication has also been produced without surgery by inserting a percutaneous balloon catheter into the pericardial sac.[10, 56] Surgical removal of intracavitary obstructing secondary tumors may ameliorate symptoms and prolong survival,[18, 21, 24, 26, 28, 34, 57–59] as may chemotherapy in the occasional patient.[39, 60] MRI, by characterizing the three-dimensional extent and attachment of cardiac tumors, is of particular value in planning a surgical approach aimed at either complete removal or palliative debulking of a tumor mass.[38, 57, 61] TEE has proved to be an effective monitoring device during surgical removal of a cardiac mass.[62] Symptomatic arrhythmias have been controlled using antiarrhythmic therapy.[12]

PRIMARY TUMORS OF THE HEART

Although less common than secondary tumors, primary tumors of the heart are far more challenging to both the physician and the surgeon. These tumors usually present as intracavitary lesions, and more than 75 percent are benign.[63, 64] Current surgical techniques permit removal and potential "cure" in a considerable number of patients with primary tumors.

Primary tumors of the heart and pericardium are rare, occurring with a frequency of 0.001 to 0.28 percent in reported or collected postmortem series.[63] Myxomas, the most common type of primary tumors, constitute nearly 50 percent of all histologically benign tumors of the heart. Table 102–2 presents classification and frequency data collected by the Armed Forces Institute of Pathology for 533 primary tumors and cysts of the heart and pericardium.[65]

Cardiac Myxomas

Intracardiac myxoma is the most frequently occurring benign tumor of the heart. Although most (75 percent) are

TABLE 102–2 Tumors and Cysts of the Heart and Pericardium

Type	n		Percentage	
Benign				
Myxoma	130		24.4	
Lipoma	45		8.4	
Papillary fibroelastoma	42		7.9	
Rhabdomyoma	36		6.8	
Fibroma	17		3.2	
Hemangioma	15		2.8	
Teratoma	14		2.6	
Mesothelioma of the AV node	12		2.3	
Granular cell tumor	3			
Neurofibroma	3			
Lymphangioma	2			
Subtotal		319		59.8
Pericardial cyst	82		15.4	
Bronchogenic cyst	7		1.3	
Subtotal		89		16.4
Malignant				
Angiosarcoma	39		7.3	
Rhabdomyosarcoma	26		4.9	
Mesothelioma	19		3.6	
Fibrosarcoma	14		2.6	
Malignant lymphoma	7		1.3	
Extraskeletal osteosarcoma	5			
Neurogenic sarcoma	4			
Malignant teratoma	4			
Thymoma	4			
Leiomyosarcoma	1			
Liposarcoma	1			
Synovial sarcoma	1			
Subtotal		125		23.5
Total	533		100.00	

Abbreviation: AV, atrioventricular.

From McAllister HA, Fenoglio JJ: Tumors of the Cardiovascular System. Washington, DC: Armed Forces Institute of Pathology, 1978.

located in the left atrium, intracardiac myxomas are also found in the right atrium (18 percent), right ventricle (4 percent), and left ventricle (4 percent).[65] Cardiac myxomas usually originate from the region of the fossa ovalis but may arise from a variety of locations within the atria.[65]

Pathology

Attached to the endocardium by a broad base, myxomas are usually pedunculated, polypoid, and friable, although some may have a smooth, rounded surface. A myxoma appears as a soft, gelatinous, mucoid, usually gray-white mass, often with areas of hemorrhage or thrombosis. Myxomas vary from 1 to 15 cm in diameter, with most measuring 5 to 6 cm.[65] On microscopic examination, the myxoma is composed of an acid mucopolysaccharide myxoid matrix in which polygonal cells (lipidic cells) and occasional blood vessels are embedded. Although myxomas can recur because of incomplete removal[66, 67] and distant growth of embolic myxomatous material has been observed,[66, 68] the existence of a true malignant cardiac myxoma remains doubtful.[63] The occurrence of multiple tumors within the left atrium, bilaterally in each atrium,[69] or simultaneously in the atrium and ventricle[70] is likely the result of multicentric origin rather than metastasis of the tumor.

Clinical Characteristics

Most patients with cardiac myxomas are from 30 to 60 years of age,[71] although myxomas have been discovered in persons of all ages. Children have a higher incidence of ventricular myxomas than adults do.[70, 72] A higher incidence among females has characterized most series.[71] In reported familial occurrences of cardiac myxoma, male patients predominate and tumors are distributed equally on both sides of the heart.[73]

Whereas asymptomatic patients with myxoma have been reported,[70, 74, 75] most present with one or more effects of a triad of constitutional, embolic, and obstructive manifestations.[71] Cardiac myxomas provoke systemic illness (characterized by weight loss, fatigue, fever, anemia [often hemolytic], elevated sedimentation rate, and elevated serum immunoglobulin [Ig] concentration) in 90 percent of patients. The globulin fraction most frequently elevated is IgG, with IgA involved only rarely.[71, 76, 77] Production of interleukin-6 has been related to tumor size, constitutional symptoms, potentiation of metastases, and myocardial infarction with "normal" coronary arteries.[78–83] Less common findings include leukocytosis, erythrocytosis, thrombocytopenia,[84] clubbing, Raynaud's phenomenon, and breast fibroadenomas.[71]

Patients with hemolytic anemia have features of intravascular mechanical destruction, which may be accompanied by pancytopenia. Hemolytic anemia is more likely to occur in patients with calcified myxomas, more commonly in the right atrium. Rarely, an intracavitary myxoma becomes infected[85] and may cause major embolic neurologic events.[86–90]

"Syndrome myxoma" characterizes a subset of patients who have cardiac myxoma associated with pigmented skin lesions and peripheral and endocrine neoplasms.[91–93] These patients, in contrast to those with "sporadic" myxoma, are usually younger, have a high incidence of familial myxoma, and more frequently have multiple and recurrent tumors. A major 17cM locus on chromosome 17q2 that contains the gene for Carney's complex disease has recently been identified.[94]

Systemic tumor embolization occurs in 40 to 50 percent of patients with left atrial myxoma,[71] with tumor fragments or surface clots most commonly embolizing to arteries in the brain, kidneys, and extremities.[95–101] Cutaneous myxoma emboli may manifest as erythematous papules.[102] Rarely does a complete left atrial myxoma become detached and lodge in the aortic bifurcation.[89, 103] Histologic examination of emboli recovered from a peripheral artery at operation can lead to diagnosis of an otherwise unsuspected intracardiac myxoma.[63, 89, 96] Tumor embolization of the central nervous system constitutes about half of all embolic events caused by left atrial myxomas[96, 104]; central nervous system emboli may be the first symptomatic manifestation of a left atrial myxoma[68, 76, 83, 96, 97] and are more common in the left hemisphere. Angiography has revealed *intracranial arterial aneurysms* secondary to myxomatous emboli, and late rupture with intracranial hemorrhage has been reported.[68, 105] Consequently, care must be taken to avoid embolization during surgical removal of an intracardiac myxoma, not only because of the immediate consequences of an embolic phenomena but also because viable metastatic foci may cause symptoms years later.[68] Thus, the patient who has sustained cerebral emboli is not necessarily "cured" even after the primary tumor is surgically removed. Retinal artery embolism can occur with transient[96] or permanent[98] visual impairment. Coronary artery embolism associated with myxoma has been documented both by angiography in living patients and by histology at postmortem study. Occasionally, myocardial infarction is the first manifestation of a myxoma.[63, 95, 99, 106, 107]

Left Atrial Myxoma

Myxomas of the left atrium may obstruct either the mitral or the pulmonary venous orifices[108] and produce symptoms that mimic mitral valve disease. There are frequent episodes of syncope or dizziness, and sudden death may occur. An effect on the severity of any symptom produced by a change in position of the patient is suggestive of myxoma. Constitutional manifestations are common.[71]

On physical examination, the first heart sound is loud and frequently "split," with the second component corresponding to the tumor expulsion from the mitral orifice. The pulmonary component of the second sound is accentuated, and an early diastolic sound, the "tumor plop," usually heard 80 to 120 ms after the aortic closure sound,[71, 109] resembles the sound of an opening snap but is not as sharp and is of a lower frequency. An apical diastolic or systolic murmur or both are present in many patients. The auscultatory findings may vary from time to time or with a change in the patient's position.[71, 109, 110] Features of pulmonary hypertension occur frequently. In contrast to features of the rheumatic mitral valvular disease, left atrial myxoma has a shorter clinical history and persistence of sinus rhythm.

Results of electrocardiography are nonspecific, reflecting hemodynamic alterations similar to those of mitral valvular disease; however, sinus rhythm is generally the rule. The chest roentgenogram reveals left atrial enlargement and the characteristic changes of pulmonary venous congestion and pulmonary hypertension. Calcification may be evident in the tumor even on routine chest x-ray, but this is better appreciated on fluoroscopic examination. The "wrecking-ball" effect of a calcified mobile myxoma may cause destruction of the mitral valve or rupture of the chordae tendineae and may produce severe mitral regurgitation.[110, 111]

IMAGING TECHNIQUES

TTE provides tomographic images of all four cardiac chambers and identifies the size, shape, point of attachment, and motion characteristics of left atrial myxomas.[77, 112] TEE (Fig. 102–2) permits superior imaging of the more posterior cardiac structures[29] and provides high-resolution views of both atria and the atrial septum.[31, 62, 75, 90, 113–115] Left atrial myxomas, especially the point of attachment, are better imaged by TEE (see Fig. 102–2). Visualization of all four chambers permits recognition of multiple tumors[115] or tumors in less common locations. Cine-CT and MRI, both high-resolution imaging techniques, are also useful in the detection and characterization of cardiac masses (Fig. 102–3). Angiography characterizes the tumor's size, location, and mobility[71]; however, echocardiography and other imaging techniques have largely supplanted contrast angiography for imaging of atrial myxomas.[77, 112, 115] Injection of contrast material or passage of a catheter into the chamber containing the myxoma risks embolization of tumor fragments.[100] Coronary angiography can demonstrate a vascular blush in the tumor from branches of the right or left coronary arteries.[116–118] Aneurysms and occlusion of the coronary artery caused by tumor emboli have also been demonstrated by coronary angiography.[95, 99, 117] Because of the reliability of noninvasive imaging, cardiac catheterization appears to be indicated primarily to rule out concomitant coronary artery disease or associated structural heart disease.[117]

DIFFERENTIAL DIAGNOSIS

Left atrial myxomas most often present as, and must be differentiated from, mitral valvular disease. The clinical manifestations are characteristically recent in origin. The symptoms of myxoma may mimic those of a variety of other conditions. Fever, constitutional symptoms, and embolic phenomena mimic infective endocarditis. Muscle pain, skin rash, and Raynaud's phenomenon may simulate peripheral vasculitis.[101, 119, 120] Multiple systemic arterial aneurysms secondary to myxomatous embolization to the cerebral, pulmonary, renal, and muscular arteries have mimicked polyarteritis nodosa.[69, 101] Similarly, coronary artery aneurysmal dilatation and myocardial infarction have been attributed to coronary myxoma embolization.[99] The physician should maintain a high index of clinical suspicion in patients having diverse features, especially when cardiac, embolic, and constitutional manifestations coexist. Echocardiographic imaging of the heart has greatly facilitated the recognition of intracavitary tumors and affords detection in some patients who are asymptomatic.[70, 75]

Myxomas in Other Locations

Right atrial myxomas arise from more diverse sites within the right atrium.[121–124] Producing right atrial obstruction,

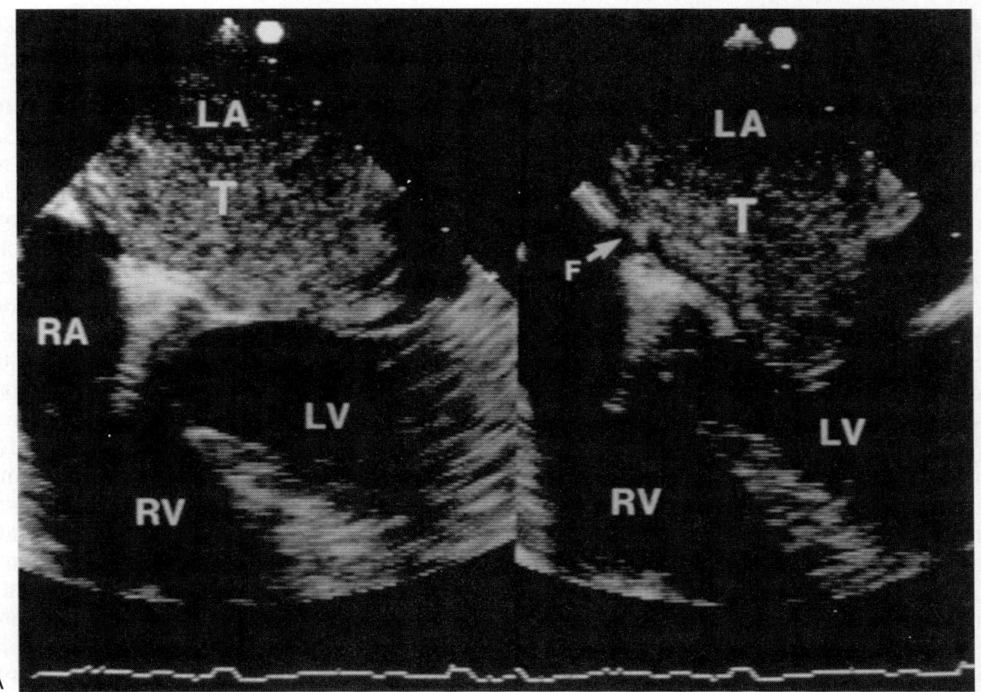

FIGURE 102–2 Transesophageal echocardiogram in the right horizontal plane in a patient with left atrial myxoma. **A,** Systole. **B,** Diastole. F, fossa ovalis; LA, left atrium; LV, left ventricle; RA, right atrium; RV, right ventricle; T, tumor. (**A** and **B,** Courtesy of Susan Wilansky, M.D., Texas Heart Institute and St. Luke's Episcopal Hospital, Houston, Texas.)

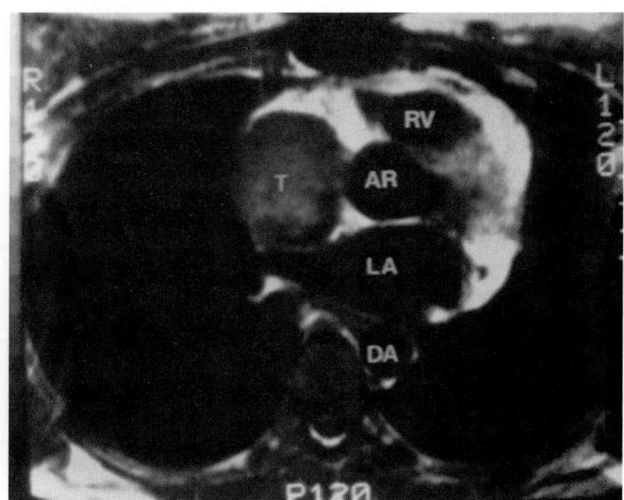

FIGURE 102–3 Right atrial myxoma. Axial T-weighted image through the heart at the level of the root of the aorta shows a homogeneous intermediate signal intensity mass (T) that incompletely fills the right atrium. Note the intrinsic contrast provided by the signal void from surrounding flowing blood. AR, aortic root; DA, descending thoracic aorta; LA, left atrium; RV, right ventricular outflow tract. (Courtesy of Clark L. Carrol, M.D., St. Luke's Episcopal Hospital/Texas Heart Institute and Texas Children's Hospital, Houston, Texas.)

these tumors manifest through low cardiac output and systemic venous hypertension. Elevated venous pressure, hepatomegaly, ascites, and cyanosis[125] are common. The pendular (wrecking-ball) effect of the tumor, especially when calcified, can produce severe tricuspid insufficiency.[110, 126] Pulmonary emboli may be extensive[127, 128]; constitutional symptoms are less common.

On auscultation, a loud, early systolic sound may be heard. This sound occurs as late as 80 ms after the mitral component of the first sound and results from expulsion of the tumor from the right ventricle. A palpable tumor shock may coincide with this sound. A crescendo murmur with inspiratory augmentation preceding the loud tumor expulsion sound is probably caused by early systolic tricuspid regurgitation while the valve is still held open by the tumor.[129] There may be a long diastolic murmur or, more commonly, only a late diastolic rumble, augmented by inspiration, accompanying atrial systole. If major injury to the tricuspid valve occurs, the murmur of tricuspid regurgitation will be present and large V waves will be seen in the jugular venous column. An early diastolic sound may be heard but is less constant than the "tumor plop" that accompanies a left atrial myxoma. The changing quality of the sound and murmurs, their closeness to the ear, and their friction-like quality may mimic a pericardial rub.

Electrocardiography may suggest right atrial enlargement in patients with right atrial myxoma.[124] Low-voltage, right-axis deviation and varying degrees of right bundle branch block have been reported.[130] The chest roentgenogram may reveal some prominence or enlargement of the right atrial shadow and, occasionally, of the right ventricle. Calcification in the tumor may be recognized on plane film or at fluoroscopy and is more common in patients with myxomas of the right atrium.[71]

TTE and TEE provide excellent images of right atrial masses.[19, 29, 74, 75, 77, 131, 132] The latter provides more detail of the tumor and defines the site of attachment.[85, 115] With current noninvasive imaging techniques, catheterization and angiography of the right-sided heart chambers are rarely necessary; these techniques also risk embolization of tumor fragments to the pulmonary arteries.

The clinical features of right atrial myxoma resemble those of rheumatic tricuspid valvular disease, although the latter is always accompanied by significant mitral and, frequently, aortic valve disease. The manifestations of right atrial myxoma have many similarities to those of constrictive pericarditis and Ebstein's anomaly of the tricuspid valve. Tricuspid stenosis and insufficiency are also prominent in carcinoid syndrome, but involvement of the pulmonary valve and other features will distinguish the carcinoid tumor from a right atrial myxoma.

An atrial myxoma may pass through the foramen ovale and may be present in both atria.[85, 133] The tumor is usually dumbbell shaped, with the common stalk attached to the margin of the fossa ovalis.

Myxomas originating from the left ventricle are usually found in younger persons, most often those under 30 years of age.[82, 107] Women are affected three times more often than are men. A short duration of symptoms is also characteristic.[63, 134] Systemic emboli, mostly cerebral,[135] occur in two thirds of the patients, and constitutional symptoms are almost conspicuously absent. Attacks of syncope occur in nearly half of the reviewed cases. Symptoms and physical findings are suggestive of aortic or subaortic obstruction.

Myxomas of the right ventricle result in symptoms and manifestations of right-sided heart failure, syncope, unexplained fever, pulmonary emboli,[136] and a murmur consistent with pulmonary stenosis. A gradient across the right ventricular outlet is characteristic,[137] and the tumor can be visualized angiographically. Echocardiographic imaging, both TTE and TEE, will detect most ventricular myxomas.[115, 138] Transvenous intracardiac biopsy may be helpful in the differential diagnosis of right-sided myxomas.[139–141]

Surgery for Intracavitary Myxoma

Myxomas can be completely removed surgically, and this should be accomplished promptly. For complete removal of a left atrial myxoma, a biatrial approach is employed, excising a full thickness of interatrial septum if the tumor is attached to the region of the fossa ovalis.[57, 142, 143] Left atrial myxomas are commonly attached to the fossa ovalis, and a full thickness of atrial septum should also be resected. If a large portion of the septum is removed, a patch of knitted Dacron cloth should be used for repair. Since fragmentation and embolization of the tumor are an ever-present threat, vigorous palpation and other manipulations of the heart should be avoided until cardiopulmonary bypass is initiated.[68] We usually induce ventricular standstill with cardioplegia solution before manipulating the heart to reduce the possibility of fragmentation of the gelatinous tumor.[71] Either AV valve may require replacement or repair by annuloplasty.[71] Recurrences of atrial myxomas are rare and usually develop within 48 months of initial tumor removal.[67, 144]

Other Benign Primary Tumors of the Heart

The most frequently occurring cardiac tumor in infants and children (more often males)[145] is rhabdomyoma.[63, 146, 147] These tumors usually present early in life with a variety of symptoms including arrhythmias and sudden death. They are occasionally discovered at fetal echocardiography.[148] Rhabdomyomas are usually multiple,[145] most often involve the ventricular myocardium, and project into the cavity or move freely as a pedunculated mass.[149, 150] Associated tuberous sclerosis is present in one third of the patients. Discrete and multiple myocardial hamartomas and rhabdomyomas can cause incessant ventricular tachycardia in infants and have been successfully removed surgically.[57, 142, 145, 151]

Fibromas are usually ventricular and intramural, calcification is common, and most fibromas occur in infants and children.[63, 152] Sudden death has been reported in nearly one third of affected patients, presumably due to involvement of the conduction system, production of arrhythmias, or obstruction of the outflow tract of the left ventricle.[152] Total or partial resection of the tumor, including heart transplantation, has been reported, with excellent probability of long-term survival.[142, 153, 154]

Papillary fibroelastomas arise from the cardiac valves or occasionally from the ventricular endocardium, are most commonly seen in patients over 50 years of age, and traditionally have been seen as a coincidental finding at surgery or postmortem examination.[155] These tumors have multiple papillary fronds attached to the endothelium by a short pedicle (Fig. 102–4). There is a predilection for aortic valve involvement, and fronds of the villous tumor may cause coronary ostial occlusion and lead to angina, myocardial infarction, or sudden death.[63, 156–158] Systemic and cerebral emboli from these lesions also have been reported.[159, 160] Papillary fibroelastomas are being discovered with increasing frequency by echocardiographic (TTE and TEE) imaging of the heart,[161, 162] and successful surgical excision has followed clinical recognition (Fig. 102–5).[155, 159, 163, 164] Calcified fibroelastomas are rare and are identified on fluoroscopy of the heart.[165]

Lipomas may be massive and may occur throughout the heart, including the pericardium. Intramyocardial lipomas are encapsulated and usually small.[63] Tissue characterization by MRI permits preoperative identification of these fatty tumors.[166] Surgical excision of lipomas generally yields excellent long-term results.[142]

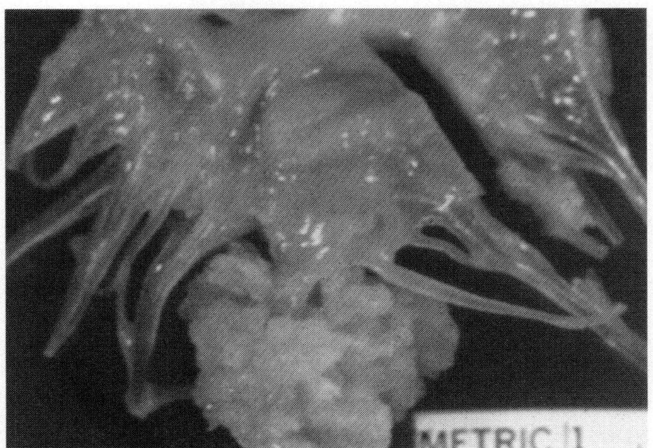

FIGURE 102–4 Fibroelastoma of the mitral valve. This pedunculated lesion is characterized by a cauliflower-like appearance.

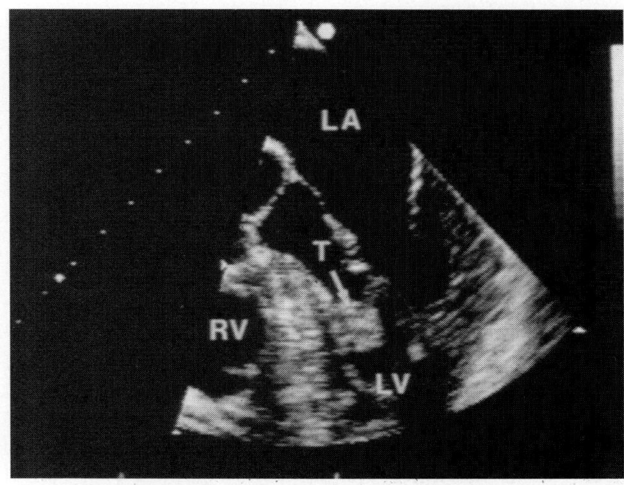

FIGURE 102–5 Transesophageal echocardiogram in the horizontal plane in a patient with papillary fibroelastoma *(arrow)*. LA, left atrium; LV, left ventricle; RV, right ventricle; T, tumor. (Courtesy of Susan Wilansky, M.D., Texas Heart Institute and St. Luke's Episcopal Hospital, Houston, Texas.)

Lipomatous hypertrophy of the atrial septum is a nonencapsulated hyperplasia of adipose tissue and may not represent a true tumor. Varying in size from 2 to 8 cm, the tumescence may bulge into the atrial cavity or superior vena cava orifice[167] and may become a consideration in the differential diagnosis of intracavitary masses. These massive fatty deposits in the atrial septum are associated with large deposits of fat elsewhere in the body and other parts of the heart and are frequently associated with atherosclerotic coronary artery disease.[168] Although at times found coincidentally at postmortem study, lipomatous hypertrophy of the atrial septum can be associated with unexplained supraventricular rhythm and conduction disturbances, recurrent pericardial effusion,[169] and sudden death.[63, 170] Features noted both with TTE (especially from the subcostal approach) and with TEE[171] are distinctive and include atrial septal thickening with a bilobed appearance owing to sparing of the area of the fossa ovalis. CT[172] and MRI provide noninvasive tissue characterization of lipomas, which echocardiography does not provide.[173–176] The diagnosis has been confirmed by percutaneous transvenous biopsy.[177]

Mesothelioma (lymphangioepithelioma)[178] of the AV node is the smallest tumor capable of producing sudden death by causing complete heart block.[63, 178–181] This tumor has been reported in all age groups, from the newborn period to the ninth decade of life, with a strong preponderance in females. These cystic tumors of the AV node[182] most likely originate from either mesothelial or endodermal rests and are always benign.[178, 182, 183] Some immunohistochemical studies have been interpreted to indicate that the tumors have an endodermal origin.[184, 185] The tumor is usually large enough to be recognized grossly at postmortem examination. Most patients with mesothelioma of the AV node have demonstrated partial or complete heart block and Stokes-Adams attacks. Death is often due to complete heart block or ventricular fibrillation. Electrophysiologic study discloses a block proximal to the His bundle.[186] Because complete or partial AV block is the major clinical manifestation of this tumor, the use of a pacemaker to maintain normal ventricular activity appears indicated. Even with cardiac pacing, however, two patients in the Armed Forces Institute of Pathology series developed ventricular fibrillation. It appears that some patients, for reasons that are not clear, do not tolerate electronic pacing safely.[187] Nonetheless, cardiac pacing, coupled with drug therapy to suppress residual AV nodal activity and possible accessory AV pathways, is probably indicated. Chance discovery of a mesothelioma during surgical repair of an atrial septal defect led to successful surgical resection of the tumor.[188]

Paragangliomas (pheochromocytoma, chemodectomas) may rarely be localized within the pericardium.[189] Paragangliomas most commonly occur over the base of the heart in the major region of vagus nerve distribution adjacent to or involving the left atrium.[190] Use of metaiodobenzylguanidine scintigraphy has allowed improved detection of this tumor and localization to the mediastinum.[190] MRI can localize cardiac paragangliomas without the use of contrast material and may provide detailed information to guide surgical excision.[190–192] Surgical resection is difficult, mortality is considerable, and heart transplantation has occasionally been employed.[193, 194]

Malignant Primary Tumors of the Heart

Histologically, almost all primary malignant cardiac tumors are sarcomas, most frequently angiosarcomas,[195] and usually originate in the right atrium or pericardium.[196] One fourth of all angiosarcomas will in part be intracavitary (Fig. 102–6) with valvular obstruction and characteristically will manifest right-sided heart failure and pericardial tamponade with hemorrhagic fluid. Tumor "blush" may be seen at coronary angiography.[197] Surgical resection provides palliative relief.[198]

Rhabdomyosarcoma is the second most frequently occurring primary sarcoma of the heart and, like angiosarcoma, is more common in males. There is no single chamber predilection. Multiple sites are common, and significant obstruction of at least one valve is present in half of the patients.[199, 200] Fibrosarcoma, liposarcoma,[201] primary malignant lymphoma,[202] and occasional sarcomas of other basic cell types constitute the remaining (but infrequently occurring) primary malignant cardiac tumors. Osteosarcoma and malignant fibrous histiocytoma have a predilection for the left atrium.[195, 203–205]

Effective palliation and local control of these tumors can at times be achieved with extensive resection of malignant primary tumors[57, 206–208] and occasionally with heart transplantation,[209] although this approach has been questioned.[210] A right ventricular bypass operation has been employed for symptomatic relief in a patient with a nonresectable right ventricular sarcoma and pulmonary outflow tract obstruction.[211] Echocardiography, MRI, and CT scanning are helpful in diagnosing and planning operative resection of

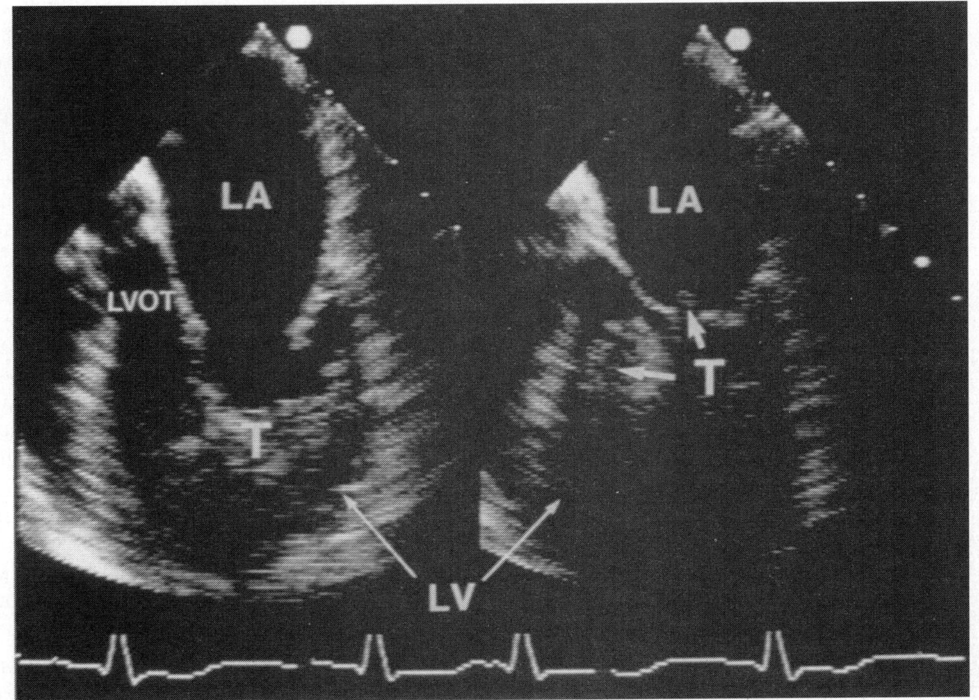

FIGURE 102–6 Transesophageal echocardiogram in the horizontal plane in a patient with angiosarcoma of the left ventricle. **A,** Systole. **B,** Diastole. LA, left atrium; LV, left ventricle; LVOT, left ventricular outflow tract; T, tumor. (**A,** and **B,** Courtesy of Susan Wilansky, M.D., Texas Heart Institute and St. Luke's Episcopal Hospital, Houston, Texas.)

cardiac tumors.[38, 212] Intraoperative echocardiography may be useful to guide surgical resection.[213] Adjuvant chemotherapy and radiation therapy are necessary to improve long-term prognosis; the response to therapy can be assessed by MRI.[39, 195]

TUMORS OF THE PERICARDIUM

Pericardial (mesothelial) cysts are the most commonly occurring benign "tumors" of the pericardium. They are usually found coincidentally on routine radiographic examination of the chest; however, 25 to 30 percent of the patients have chest pain, dyspnea, cough, or paroxysmal tachycardia. Pericardial cysts develop most often in the third or fourth decade of life and occur with equal frequency among men and women.[214, 215] The right costophrenic location is the most common presentation. Echocardiography[29] and CT[215] are most helpful in determining the differential diagnosis. Surgical excision completely relieves symptoms and confirms the diagnosis.[63] Percutaneous aspiration of the cystic contents has been performed as an alternative to surgical resection.[215, 216]

Teratomas are most often extracardiac, yet intrapericardial,[217] and arise and receive their blood supply from the root of the aorta or pulmonary artery through the vasa vasorum. Most are found in infants and children and have a strong preponderance for females.[63] Recurrent, nonbloody pericardial effusion is common in children with this tumor; intrapericardial teratoma is the most likely diagnosis in this setting. Embarrassment of cardiac function results from expansion of the tumor to considerable proportions, at times up to 15 cm in diameter.[218] Surgical excision is the only effective therapy[63] and is curative because the tumor is rarely malignant.[219]

Mesothelioma ranks third in frequency of occurrence among malignant tumors of the heart and pericardium.[65, 220] The clinical manifestations resemble those of pericarditis, constrictive pericardial disease, and vena caval obstruction. Aspiration and histologic examination of the usually bloody pericardial fluid may be diagnostic. Males with mesothelioma outnumber females by a ratio of 2:1, with the peak incidence occurring in the third to fifth decades of life. The prognosis is poor, surgical excision is usually impossible, and treatment with radiation and chemotherapy generally produces only temporary improvement.[221–223]

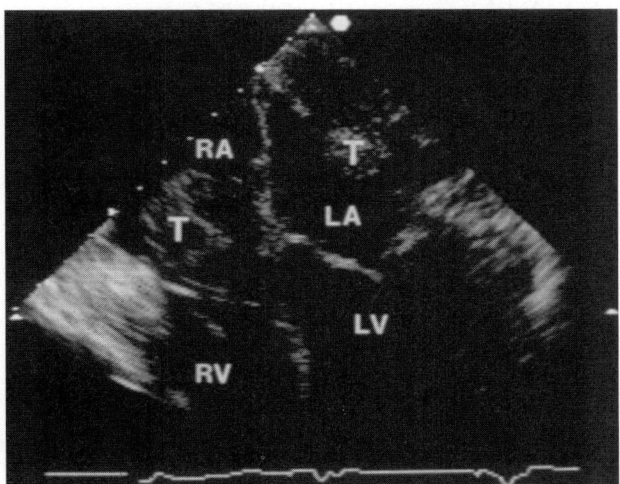

FIGURE 102–7 Transesophageal echocardiogram in the horizontal plane shows extensive lymphoma in both atria. LA, left atrium; LV, left ventricle, RA, right atrium; RV, right ventricle; T, tumor. (Courtesy of Susan Wilansky, M.D., Texas Heart Institute and St. Luke's Episcopal Hospital, Houston, Texas.)

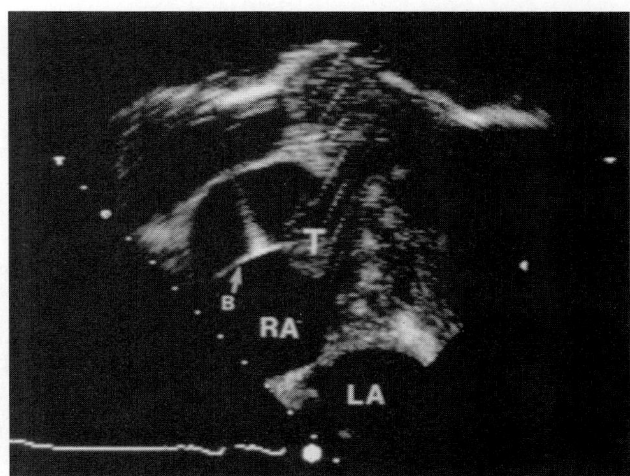

FIGURE 102–8 Transesophageal echocardiogram in the longitudinal plane in a patient with lymphoma. The study was performed during echo-guided biopsy of the mass. B, bioptome; LA, left atrium; RA, right atrium; T, tumor. (Courtesy of Susan Wilansky, M.D., Texas Heart Institute and St. Luke's Episcopal Hospital, Houston, Texas.)

Leukemias and Lymphomas

Leukemic infiltration of the heart is usually found at postmortem study and generally is not suspected before death.[3, 224] Involvement of the heart in patients with malignant lymphoma is common, although it too is infrequently detected before death.[225]

Two varieties of malignancies involving the heart have been described in patients with AIDS: Kaposi's sarcoma and, less commonly, malignant lymphoma.[226–228] Involvement of the heart by Kaposi's sarcoma may be primary or part of a widely disseminated process. The epicardium is a common location, with involvement of the underlying myocardium. Clinical cardiac dysfunction is minimal, although pericardial tamponade, which is potentially fatal, has been reported.[229–232] Lymphomas, usually of high-grade malignant characteristics, occur with increased frequency in patients with AIDS and other immunosuppressed states.[228, 233] Primary and, more commonly, secondary lymphomas involve the heart either as a diffuse infiltrative process or as focal nodules in any layer of the heart. Clinical features may be absent in half of patients. When present, clinical features include cardiomegaly, pericardial effusion, congestive failure, and progressive heart block.[226] Echocardiography is useful for demonstrating pericardial effusion, mass lesions, and wall motion abnormalities (Figs. 102–7 and 102–8). Transvenous biopsy can be useful in making the diagnosis.[234]

REFERENCES

1. Prichard RW: Tumors of the heart: review of the subject and report of one hundred and fifty cases. Arch Pathol 51:98–128, 1951.
2. DeLoach JF, Haynes JW: Secondary tumors of the heart and pericardium: review of the subject and report of one hundred thirty-seven cases. Arch Intern Med 91:224–249, 1953.
3. Kutalek SP, Panidis IP, Kotler MN: Metastatic tumors of the heart detected by two-dimensional echocardiography. Am Heart J 109:343–349, 1985.
4. Abraham KP, Reddy V, Gattuso P: Neoplasms metastatic to the heart: review of 3314 consecutive autopsies. Am J Cardiovasc Pathol 3:195–198, 1990.
5. Mousseaux E, Meunier P, Azancott S: Cardiac metastatic melanoma investigated by magnetic resonance imaging. Magn Reson Imaging 16:91–95, 1998.
6. Weg IL, Mehra S, Azueta V: Cardiac metastasis from adenocarcinoma of the lung. Echocardiographic-pathologic correlation. Am J Med 80:108–112, 1986.
7. Kadir S, Coulam CM: Intracaval extension of renal cell carcinoma. Cardiovasc Intervent Radiol 3:180–183, 1980.
8. Onuigbo WI: Direct extension of cancer between pulmonary veins and the left atrium. Chest 62:444–446, 1972.
9. Labib SB, Schick EC Jr, Isner JM: Obstruction of right ventricular outflow tract caused by intracavitary metastatic disease: analysis of 14 cases. J Am Coll Cardiol 19:1664–1668, 1992.
10. Muir KW, Rodger JC: Cardiac tamponade as the initial presentation of malignancy: is it as rare as previously supposed? Postgrad Med J 70:703–707, 1994.
11. Sheldon R, Isaac D: Metastatic melanoma to the heart presenting with ventricular tachycardia. Chest 99:1296–1298, 1991.
12. Leak D: Amiodarone for control of recurrent ventricular tachycardia secondary to cardiac metastasis. Tex Heart Inst J 25:198–200, 1998.
13. Redwine DB: Complete heart block caused by secondary tumors of the heart. Case report and review of literature. Tex Med 70:59–64, 1974.
14. Kopelson G, Herwig KJ: The etiologies of coronary artery disease in cancer patients. Int J Radiat Oncol Biol Phys 4:895–906, 1978.
15. Hartman RB, Clark PI, Schulman P: Pronounced and prolonged ST segment elevation: a pathognomonic sign of tumor invasion of the heart. Arch Intern Med 142:1917–1919, 1982.
16. Virmani R, Khedekar RR, Robinowitz M: Tumor embolization in coronary artery causing myocardial infarction. Arch Pathol Lab Med 107:243–245, 1983.
17. Salem BI, Schnee M, Leatherman LL: Electrocardiographic pseudo-infarction pattern: appearance with a large posterior pericardial effusion after cardiac surgery. Am J Cardiol 42:681–685, 1978.
18. Shahian DM, Libertino JA, Zinman LN: Resection of cavoatrial renal cell carcinoma employing total circulatory arrest. Arch Surg 125:727–731; discussion 731–732, 1990.
19. Lynch M, Clements SD, Shanewise JS: Right-sided cardiac tumors detected by transesophageal echocardiography and its usefulness in differentiating the benign from the malignant ones. Am J Cardiol 79:781–784, 1997.
20. Chatterjee T, Muller MF, Carrel T: Images in cardiovascular medicine. Renal cell carcinoma with tumor thrombus extending through the inferior vena cava into the right cardiac cavities. Circulation 96:2729–2730, 1997.
21. Fujisaki M, Kurihara E, Kikuchi K: Hepatocellular carcinoma with tumor thrombus extending into the right atrium: report of a successful resection with the use of cardiopulmonary bypass. Surgery 109:214–219, 1991.
22. Garcia FA, Villanueva RA, Narciso FV: Intravenous leiomyomatosis of the uterus and pelvis presenting as a cardiac tumor. Ann Thorac Surg 42(6 suppl):S41–S43, 1986.
23. Philips MR, Bower TC, Orszulak TA: Intracardiac extension of an intracaval sarcoma of endometrial origin. Ann Thorac Surg 59:742–744, 1995.
24. Griffin AS, Sterchi JM: Primary leiomyosarcoma of the inferior vena cava: a case report and review of the literature. J Surg Oncol 34:53–60, 1987.
25. Lupetin AR, Dash N, Beckman I: Leiomyosarcoma of the superior vena cava: diagnosis by cardiac gated MR. Cardiovasc Intervent Radiol 9:103–105, 1986.
26. Rosenthal JT, Colonna JO, Drinkwater DC: Leiomyosarcoma of the vena cava with atrial extension: long-term survival following resection and caval replacement without circulatory arrest. Urology 46:876–878, 1995.
27. Kronzon I, Goodkin GM, Culliford A: Right atrial and right ventricular obstruction by recurrent stromomyoma. J Am Soc Echocardiogr 7:528–533, 1994.
28. Chen RH, Gaos CM, Frazier OH: Complete resection of a right atrial intracavitary metastatic melanoma [see comments]. Ann Thorac Surg 61:1255–1257, 1996.
29. Reeder GS, Khandheria BK, Seward JB: Transesophageal echocardiography and cardiac masses [see comments]. Mayo Clin Proc 66:1101–1109, 1991.
30. Kralstein J, Frishman WH: Malignant pericardial diseases: diagnosis and treatment. Cardiol Clin 5:583–589, 1987.
31. Salcedo EE, Cohen GI, White RD: Cardiac tumors: diagnosis and management. Curr Probl Cardiol 17:73–137, 1992.
32. DeVille JB, Corley D, Jin BS: Assessment of intracardiac masses by transesophageal echocardiography. Tex Heart Inst J 22:134–137, 1995.
33. Gross BH, Glazer GM, Francis IR: CT of intracardiac and intrapericardial masses. AJR 140:903–907, 1983.
34. Watts FB, Jr, Zingas AP, Das L: Computed tomographic diagnosis of an intracardiac metastasis from osteosarcoma. J Comput Tomogr 7:271–272, 1983.
35. Cutrone JA, Georgiou D, Yospur LS: Metastatic spread of cervical carcinoma to the right ventricle and pulmonary arteries: diagnosis by ultrafast computed tomography. Am J Card Imaging 9:275–279, 1995.
36. Barasch E Frazier OH, Silberman H: Left atrial metastasis from hepatocellular carcinoma: a case report. J Am Soc Echocardiogr 7:547–549, 1994.
37. Lund JT, Ehman RL, Julsrud PR: Cardiac masses: assessment by MR imaging. AJR 152:469–473, 1989.
38. Rienmuller R, Tiling R: MR and CT for detection of cardiac tumors. Thorac Cardiovasc Surg 38 (suppl 2):168–172, 1990.
39. Szucs RA, Rehr RB, Yanovich S: Magnetic resonance imaging of cardiac rhabdomyosarcoma. Quantifying the response to chemotherapy. Cancer 67:2066–2070, 1991.
40. Smith DN, Shaffer K, Patz EF: Imaging features of nonmyxomatous primary neoplasms of the heart and pericardium. Clin Imaging 22:15–22, 1998.
41. Levine MJ, Lorell BH, Diver DJ: Implications of echocardiographically assisted diagnosis of pericardial tamponade in contemporary medical patients: detection before hemodynamic embarrassment. J Am Coll Cardiol 17:59–65, 1991.
42. Conrad SA, Byrnes TJ: Diastolic collapse of the left and right ventricles in cardiac tamponade. Am Heart J 115:475–478, 1988.
43. Himelman RB, Kircher B, Rockey DC: Inferior vena cava plethora with blunted respiratory response: a sensitive echocardiographic sign of cardiac tamponade. J Am Coll Cardiol 12:1470–1477, 1988.
44. Hatle LK, Appleton CP, Popp RI: Differentiation of constrictive pericarditis and restrictive cardiomyopathy by Doppler echocardiography [see comments]. Circulation 79:357–370, 1989.
45. Burstow DJ, Oh JK, Bailey KR: Cardiac tamponade: characteristic Doppler observations. Mayo Clin Proc 64:312–324, 1989.
46. Picard MH, Sanfilippo AJ, Newell JB: Quantitative relation between increased intrapericardial pressure and Doppler flow velocities during experimental cardiac tamponade. J Am Coll Cardiol 18:234–242, 1991.
47. Gatenby RA, Hartz WH, Kessler HB: Percutaneous catheter drainage for malignant pericardial effusion. J Vasc Interv Radiol 2:151–155, 1991.
48. Gosalakkal JA, Sugrue DD: Malignant melanoma of the right atrium: antemortem diagnosis by transvenous biopsy. Br Heart J 62:159–160, 1989.
49. Quraishi MA, Costanzi JJ, Hokanson J: The natural history of lung cancer with pericardial metastases. Cancer 51:740–742, 1983.
50. Warda M, Khan A, Massumi A, et al: Radiation-induced valvular dysfunction. J Am Coll Cardiol 2:180–185, 1983.
51. McAllister HA, Hall RJ: Iatrogenic heart disease. *In* Cheng TO (ed): The International Textbook of Cardiology. pp. 871–873. New York: Pergamon, 1986.
52. Stewart JR, Fajardo LF, Gillette SM, Constine LS: Radiation injury to the heart. Int J Radiat Oncol Biol Phys 31:1205–1211, 1995.
53. Shepherd FA, Morgan C, Evans WK: Medical management of ma-

lignant pericardial effusion by tetracycline sclerosis. Am J Cardiol 60:1161–1166, 1987.
54. Appelqvist P, Maamies T, Grohn P: Emergency pericardiotomy as primary diagnostic and therapeutic procedure in malignant pericardial tamponade: report of three cases and review of the literature. J Surg Oncol 21:18–22, 1982.
55. Chan A, Rischin D, Clarke CP: Subxiphoid partial pericardiectomy with or without sclerosant instillation in the treatment of symptomatic pericardial effusions in patients with malignancy. Cancer 68:1021–1025, 1991.
56. Palacios IF, Tuzcu EM, Ziskind AA: Percutaneous balloon pericardial window for patients with malignant pericardial effusion and tamponade [see comments]. Cathet Cardiovasc Diagn 22:244–249, 1991.
57. Murphy MC, Sweeney MS, Putnam JB Jr: Surgical treatment of cardiac tumors: a 25-year experience. Ann Thorac Surg 49:612–617; discussion 617–618, 1990.
58. Poole GV Jr, Meredith JW, Breyer RH: Surgical implications in malignant cardiac disease. Ann Thorac Surg 36:484–491, 1983.
59. Hayashi J, Ohzeki H, Tsuchida S: Surgery for cavoatrial extension of malignant tumors. Thorac Cardiovasc Surg 43:161–164, 1995.
60. Bernet F, Stulz PM, Carrel TP: Long-term remission after resection, chemotherapy, and irradiation of a metastatic myxoma. Ann Thorac Surg 66:1791–1792, 1998.
61. Schrem SS, Colvin SB, Weinreb JC: Metastatic cardiac liposarcoma: diagnosis by transesophageal echocardiography and magnetic resonance imaging. J Am Soc Echocardiogr 3:149–153, 1990.
62. Aru GM, Falchi S, Cardu G, et al: The role of transesophageal echocardiography in the monitoring of cardiac mass removal: a review of 17 cases. J Card Surg 8:554–557, 1993.
63. McAllister HA Jr, Hall RJ, Cooley DA: Primary tumors and cysts of the heart and pericardium. Curr Probl Cardiol 4:1–51, 1999.
64. Burke A, Virmani R: Tumors of the heart and great vessels. *In* Rosai J, Sobin LH (eds): Atlas of Tumor Pathology. l. 3rd Ser. Fasc. 16. p. 231. Washington, DC: Armed Forces Institute of Pathology, 1996.
65. McAllister HA, Fenoglio JJ: Tumors of the Cardiovascular System. Washington, DC: Armed Forces Institute of Pathology, 1978.
66. Read RC, White HJ, Murphy ML: The malignant potentiality of left atrial myxoma. J Thorac Cardiovasc Surg 68:857–868, 1974.
67. Cleveland DC, Westaby S, Karp RB: Treatment of intra-atrial cardiac tumors. JAMA 249:2799–2802, 1983.
68. Desousa AL, Muller J, Campbell R: Atrial myxoma: a review of the neurological complications, metastases, and recurrences. J Neurol Neurosurg Psychiatry 41:1119–1124, 1978.
69. Leonhardt ET, Kullenberg KP: Bilateral atrial myxomas with multiple arterial aneurysms—a syndrome mimicking polyarteritis nodosa. Am J Med 62:792–794, 1977.
70. Morgan DL, Palazola J, Reed W: Left heart myxomas. Am J Cardiol 40:611–614, 1977.
71. Peters MN, Hall RJ, Cooley DA: The clinical syndrome of atrial myxoma. JAMA 230:695–701, 1974.
72. Burech DL, Teske DW, Haynes RE: Right atrial myxoma in a child. Am J Dis Child 131:750–752, 1977.
73. Powers JC, Falkoff M, Heinle RA: Familial cardiac myxoma: emphasis on unusual clinical manifestations. J Thorac Cardiovasc Surg 77:782–788, 1979.
74. Lyons SV, McCord J, Smith S: Asymptomatic giant right atrial myxoma: role of transesophageal echocardiography in management. Am Heart J 121:1555–1558, 1991.
75. Smith ST, Hautamiki K, Lewis JW Jr: Transthoracic and transesophageal echocardiography in the diagnosis and surgical management of right atrial myxoma. Chest 100:575–576, 1991.
76. Glasser SP, Bedynek JL, Hall RJ: Left atrial myxoma. Report of a case including hemodynamic, surgical, histologic and histochemical characteristics. Am J Med 50:113–122, 1971.
77. Fyke FE 3rd, Seqard JB, Edwards WD: Primary cardiac tumors: experience with 30 consecutive patients since the introduction of two-dimensional echocardiography. J Am Coll Cardiol 5:1465–1473, 1985.
78. Soeparwata R, Poem LP, Schmid C: Interleukin-6 plasma levels and tumor size in cardiac myxoma. J Thorac Cardiovasc Surg 112:1675–1677, 1996.
79. Mochizuki Y, Okamura Y, Iida H: Interleukin-6 and "complex" cardiac myxoma. Ann Thorac Surg 66:931–933, 1998.
80. Isobe N, Kanda T, Sakamoto H: Myocardial infarction in myxoma patients with normal coronary arteries. Case reports. Angiology 47:819–823, 1996.
81. Kanda T, Nakajima T, Sakamoto H: An interleukin-6 secreting myxoma in a hypertrophic left ventricle. Chest 105:962–963, 1994.
82. Vaughan CJ, Gallagher M, Murphy MB: Left ventricular myxoma presenting with constitutional symptoms and raised serum interleukin-6 both suppressed by naproxen [letter]. Eur Heart J 18:703, 1997.
83. Wada A, Kanda T, Hayashi R: Cardiac myxoma metastasized to the brain: potential role of endogenous interleukin-6. Cardiology 83:208–211, 1993.
84. Burns ER, Schulman IC, Murphy MJ Jr: Hematologic manifestations and etiology of atrial myxoma. Am J Med Sci 284:17–22, 1982.
85. Kaplan LJ, Weiman DS, Van Decker W: Infected biatrial myxoma: transesophageal echocardiography-guided surgical resection. Ann Thorac Surg 57:487–488; discussion 488–489, 1994.
86. Markel ML, Waller BF, Armstrong WF: Cardiac myxoma. A review. Medicine [Baltimore] 66:114–125, 1987.
87. Rajpal RS, Leibsohn JA, Liekweg WG: Infected left atrial myxoma with bacteremia simulating infective endocarditis. Arch Intern Med 139:1176–1178, 1979.
88. Joseph P, Himmelstein DU, Mahowald JM: Atrial myxoma infected with *Candida:* first survival. Chest 78:340–343, 1980.
89. Schweiger MJ, Hafer JG Jr, Brown R: Spontaneous cure of infected left atrial myxoma following embolization. Am Heart J 99:630–634, 1980.
90. Revankar SG, Clark RA: Infected cardiac myxoma. Case report and literature review. Medicine [Baltimore] 77:337–344, 1998.
91. Scherer K, Muller T, Stolz W: [A case of Carney complex]. Dtsch Med Wochenschr 123:972–976, 1998.
92. Vidaillet HJ Jr, Seward JB, Fyke FE: "Syndrome myxoma": a subset of patients with cardiac myxoma associated with pigmented skin lesions and peripheral and endocrine neoplasms. Br Heart J 57:247–255, 1987.
93. Danoff A, Jormark S, Lorber D: Adrenocortical micronodular dysplasia, cardiac myxomas, lentigines, and spindle cell tumors. Report of a kindred. Arch Intern Med 147:443–448, 1987.
94. Casey M, Mah C, Merliss AD: Identification of a novel genetic locus for familial cardiac myxomas and Carney complex. Circulation 98:2560–2566, 1998.
95. Ztot S, Henry P, Fornes P: [Left atrial myxoma and coronary embolism]. Arch Mal Coeur Vaiss 91:263–266, 1998.
96. Tipton BK, Robertson JT, Robertson JH: Embolism to the central nervous system from cardiac myxoma. Report of two cases. J Neurosurg 47:937–940, 1977.
97. Thompson JR, Simmons CR: Arterial embolus. Manifestation of unsuspected myxoma. JAMA 228:864–865, 1974.
98. Cogan DG, Wray SH: Vascular occlusions in the eye from cardiac myxomas. Am J Ophthalmol 80:396–403, 1975.
99. Tanabe J, Williams RL, Diethrich EB: Left atrial myxoma: association with acute coronary embolization in an 11-year-old boy. Pediatrics 63:778–781, 1979.
100. Pindyck F, Pierce EC 2nd, Baron MG: Embolization of left atrial myxoma after transseptal cardiac cathertization. Am J Cardiol, 1972. 30(5): p. 569–71.
101. Boussen K, Moalla M, Blondeau P: Embolization of cardiac myxomas masquerading as polyarteritis nodosa. J Rheumatol 18:283–285, 1991.
102. Misago N, Tanaka T, Hoshii T: Erythematous papules in a patient with cardiac myxoma: a case report and review of the literature. J Dermatol 22:600–605, 1995.
103. Bradham RR, Gregorie HB Jr, Howell JS: Aortic obstruction from embolizing cardiac myxoma. J S C Med Assoc 75:7–10, 1979.
104. Rafuse PE, Nicolle DA, Hutnik CM: Left atrial myxoma causing ophthalmic artery occlusion. Eye 11:25–29, 1997.
105. Suzuki T, Nagai R, Yamazaki T, et al: Rapid growth of intracranial aneurysms secondary to cardiac myxoma. Neurology 44:570–571, 1994.
106. Cheitlin MD, McAllister HA, de Castro CM: Myocardial infarction without atherosclerosis. JAMA 231:951–959, 1975.
107. Saldanha R, Srikrishna SV, Shetty N: Surgical management of left ventricular myxoma with embolization to the right coronary artery. Tex Heart Inst J 23:230–232, 1996.
108. Stevens LH, Hormuth DA, Schmidt PE: Left atrial myxoma: pulmonary infarction caused by pulmonary venous occlusion. Ann Thorac Surg 43:215–217, 1987.

109. Martinez-Lopez JI: Sounds of the heart in diastole. Am J Cardiol 34:594–601, 1974.
110. Harvey WP: Clinical aspects of cardiac tumors. Am J Cardiol 21:328–343, 1968.
111. Hospital, C.R.o.t.M.G.: Case 42-1973. N Engl J Med 289:853–859, 1973.
112. Pechacek LW, Gonzalez-Camid F, Hall RJ, et al: The echocardiographic spectrum of atrial myxoma: A ten-year experience. Tex Heart Inst J 13:179–195, 1986.
113. Obeid AI, Marvasti M, Parker F: Comparison of transthoracic and transesophageal echocardiography in diagnosis of left atrial myxoma. Am J Cardiol 63:1006–1008, 1989.
114. Mugge A, Daniel WG, Haverich A: Diagnosis of noninfective cardiac mass lesions by two-dimensional echocardiography. Comparison of the transthoracic and transesophageal approaches. Circulation 83:70–78, 1991.
115. Vargas-Barron J, Romero-Cardenas A, Villegas M: Transthoracic and transesophageal echocardiographic diagnosis of myxomas in the four cardiac cavities. Am Heart J 121:931–933, 1991.
116. Rittoo D, Cotter L: Detection of a small left atrial myxoma: value and limitations of four imaging modalities. J Am Soc Echocardiogr 10:874–876, 1997.
117. Chow WH, Chow TC, Tai YT: Angiographic visualization of "tumour vascularity" in atrial myxoma. Eur Heart J 12:79–82, 1991.
118. Van Cleemput J, Daenen W, De Geest H: Coronary angiography in cardiac myxomas: findings in 19 consecutive cases and review of the literature. Cathet Cardiovasc Diagn 29:217–220, 1993.
119. Kaminsky ME, Ehlers KH, Engle MA: Atrial myxoma mimicking a collagen disorder. Chest 75:93–95, 1979.
120. Huston KA, Combs JJ Jr, Lie JR: Left atrial myxoma simulating peripheral vasculitis. Mayo Clin Proc 53:752–756, 1978.
121. Jardine DL, Lamont DL: Right atrial myxoma mistaken for recurrent pulmonary thromboembolism. Heart 78:512–514, 1997.
122. Kuroda H, Nitta K, Ashida Y: Right atrial myxoma originating from the tricuspid valve. J Thorac Cardiovasc Surg 109:1249–1250, 1995.
123. St. John Sutton MG, Mercier LA, Giuliani ER: Atrial myxomas: a review of clinical experience in 40 patients. Mayo Clin Proc 55:371–376, 1980.
124. Roguin N, Amikam S, Riss E: Prolapsing right atrial myxoma: clinical and heamodynamic considerations. Br Heart J 39:577–580, 1977.
125. Meyers SN, Shapiro SE, Barresi V: Right atrial myxoma with right to left shunting and mitral valve prolapse. Am J Med 62:308–314, 1977.
126. Hickie JB, Gibson H, Windsor HM: "The wrecking ball": right atrial myxoma. Med J Aust 2:82–86, 1970.
127. Muroff LR, Johnson PM: Right atrial myxoma presenting as nonresolving pulmonary emboli: case report. J Nucl Med 17:890–892, 1976.
128. Seemann MD, Brenner P: Demonstration of spiral CT scans and reconstructions of a right atrial myxoma with bilateral pulmonary tumor emboli and a coincidental benign mediastinal thymoma. Eur J Med Res 1:515–519, 1996.
129. Massumi R: Bedside diagnosis of right heart myxomas through detection of palpable tumor shocks and audible plops. Am Heart J 105:303–310, 1983.
130. Hospital, C.R.o.t.M.G.: Case 14-1978. N Engl J Med 298:834, 1978.
131. Walker AH, Wilkinson JM, Goiti JJ: Acute bicaval obstruction as a result of intracapsular haemorrhage in a right atrial myxoma: report of a case. Eur J Cardiothorac Surg 11:779–781, 1997.
132. Ohshima H, Kawashima E, Ogawa Y: Demonstration of the inner structure of a right atrial myxoma by transoesophageal echocardiography. Eur Heart J 14:132–134, 1993.
133. Peachell JL, Mullen JC, Bentley MJ: Biatrial myxoma: a rare cardiac tumor. Ann Thorac Surg 65:1768–1769, 1998.
134. Meller J, Teichholz LE, Pichard AD: Left ventricular myxoma: echocardiographic diagnosis and review of the literature. Am J Med 63:816–823, 1977.
135. Abo-Auda WS, Chidambaram BS, Baker K: Ventricular myxoma presenting as acute visual loss. Tenn Med 91:391–392, 1998.
136. Gonzalez A, Altieri PI, Marquez EU: Massive pulmonary embolism associated with a right ventricular myxoma. Am J Med 69:795–798, 1980.
137. Hada Y, Wolfe C, Murray GF: Right ventricular myxoma. Case report and review of phonocardiographic and auscultatory manifestations. Am Heart J 100:871–877, 1980.
138. Nass PC, Neimeyer MG, Brutel de la Riviere A: Left atrial and right ventricular cardiac myxoma. A case report. Eur J Cardiothorac Surg 3:468–470, 1989.
139. Flipse TR, Tazelaar HD, Holmes DR Jr: Diagnosis of malignant cardiac disease by endomyocardial biopsy [see comments]. Mayo Clin Proc 1990. 65:1415–1422.
140. Hammoudeh AJ, Chaaban F, Watson RM: Transesophageal echocardiography–guided transvenous endomyocardial biopsy used to diagnose primary cardiac angiosarcoma. Cathet Cardiovasc Diagn 37:347–349, 1996.
141. Chirillo F, Risica G, Stritoni P: Mobile right atrial mass biopsy guided by biplane transesophageal echocardiography. Int J Card Imaging 11:201–203, 1995.
142. Cooley DA: Surgical management of cardiac tumors. *In* Kapoor AS, Reynolds RD (eds): Cancer and the Heart. p. 126. New York: Springer-Verlag, 1986.
143. Jones DR, Warden HE, Murray GF: Biatrial approach to cardiac myxomas: a 30-year clinical experience [see comments]. Ann Thorac Surg 59:851–855; discussion 855–856, 1995.
144. Bhan A, Mehrotra R, Choudhary SR: Surgical experience with intracardiac myxomas: long-term follow-up. Ann Thorac Surg 66:810–813, 1998.
145. Burke AP, Virmani R: Cardiac rhabdomyoma: a clinicopathologic study. Mod Pathol 4:70–74, 1991.
146. Fenoglio JJ Jr, McAllister HA Jr, Ferrans VJ: Cardiac rhabdomyoma: a clinicopathologic and electron microscopic study. Am J Cardiol 38:241–251, 1976.
147. Abushaban L, Denham B, Duff D: 10 year review of cardiac tumours in childhood [see comments]. Br Heart J 70:166–169, 1993.
148. Holley DG, Martin GR, Brenner JI: Diagnosis and management of fetal cardiac tumors: a multicenter experience and review of published reports [see comments]. J Am Coll Cardiol 26:516–520, 1995.
149. Mahoney L, Schieken RM, Doty D: Cardiac rhabdomyoma simulating pulmonic stenosis. Cathet Cardiovasc Diagn 5:385–388, 1979.
150. Howanitz EP, Teske DW, Qualnan SJ, et al: Pedunculated left ventricular rhabdomyoma. Ann Thorac Surg 41:443–445, 1986.
151. Garson A Jr, Smith RT Jr, Moak JP: Incessant ventricular tachycardia in infants: myocardial hamartomas and surgical cure. J Am Coll Cardiol 10:619–626, 1987.
152. Reul GJ, Howell JF, Rubio PA: Successful partial excision of an intramural fibroma of the left ventricle. Am J Cardiol 36:262–265, 1975.
153. Busch U, Kampmann C, Meyer R: Removal of a giant cardiac fibroma from a 4-year-old child. Tex Heart Inst J 22:261–264, 1995.
154. Valente M, Cocco P, Thiene G: Cardiac fibroma and heart transplantation. J Thorac Cardiovasc Surg 106:1208–1212, 1993.
155. Gorton ME, Soltanzadeh H: Mitral valve fibroelastoma. Ann Thorac Surg 47:605–607, 1989.
156. Israel DH, Sherman W, Ambrose JA: Dynamic coronary ostial obstruction due to papillary fibroelastoma leading to myocardial ischemia and infarction. Am J Cardiol 67:104–105, 1991.
157. Prahlow JA, Barnard JJ: Sudden death due to obstruction of coronary artery ostium by aortic valve papillary fibroelastoma. Am J Forensic Med Pathol 19:162–165, 1998.
158. Deodhar AP, Tometzki AJ, Hudson IN: Aortic valve tumor causing acute myocardial infarction in a child. Ann Thorac Surg 64:1482–1484, 1997.
159. Kasarskis EJ, O'Connor W, Earle G: Embolic stroke from cardiac papillary fibroelastomas. Stroke 19:1171–1173, 1988.
160. Moraes D, Philippides GJ, Shapira OM: Papillary fibroelastoma of the mitral valve with systemic embolization. Circulation 98:1251–1252, 1998.
161. Mayer K, Niederhaeuser U, Jenni R: Images in cardiology. Cardiac papillary fibroelastoma with cerebral and coronary embolic events. Heart 79:307, 1998.
162. al-Mohammad A, Pambakian H, Young C: Fibroelastoma: case report and review of the literature. Heart 79:301–304, 1998.
163. de Virgilio C, Dubrow T, Robertson JM: Detection of multiple cardiac papillary fibroelastomas using transesophageal echocardiography. Ann Thorac Surg 48:119–121, 1989.
164. Wolfe JT 3rd, Finch SJ, Safford RE: Tricuspid valve papillary fibroelastoma: echocardiographic characterization. Ann Thorac Surg1:116–118, 1991.

165. Paelinck B, Vermeersch P, Kockx M: Calcified papillary fibroelastoma of the tricuspid valve. Acta Cardiol 53:165–167, 1998.
166. Tuna IC, Julsrud PR, Click RL: Tissue characterization of an unusual right atrial mass by magnetic resonance imaging. Mayo Clin Proc 66:498–501, 1991.
167. McNamara RF, Taylor AE, Panner BJ: Superior vena caval obstruction by lipomatous hypertrophy of the right atrium. Clin Cardiol 10:609–610, 1987.
168. Shirani J, Roberts WC: Clinical, electrocardiographic and morphologic features of massive fatty deposits ("lipomatous hypertrophy") in the atrial septum. J Am Coll Cardiol 22:226–238, 1993.
169. Tschirkov A, Stegaru B: Lipomatous hypertrophy of interatrial septum presenting as recurring pericardial effusion and mistaken for constrictive pericarditis. Thorac Cardiovasc Surg 27:400–403, 1979.
170. Voigt J, Agdal N: Lipomatous infiltration of the heart. An uncommon cause of sudden, unexpected death in a young man. Arch Pathol Lab Med 106:497–498, 1982.
171. Kindman LA, Wright A, Tye T: Lipomatous hypertrophy of the interatrial septum: characterization by transesophageal and transthoracic echocardiography, magnetic resonance imaging, and computed tomography. J Am Soc Echocardiogr 1:450–454, 1988.
172. Meaney JF, Kazerooni EA, Jamadar DA: CT appearance of lipomatous hypertrophy of the interatrial septum. AJR 168:1081–1084, 1997.
173. Applegate PM, Tajik AJ, Ehman RL: Two-dimensional echocardiographic and magnetic resonance imaging observations in massive lipomatous hypertrophy of the atrial septum. Am J Cardiol 59:489–491, 1987.
174. Fisher MS, Edmonds PR: Lipomatous hypertrophy of the interatrial septum. Diagnosis by magnetic resonance imaging. J Comput Tomogr 12:267–269, 1988.
175. Basso C, Barbazza R, Thiene G: Images in cardiovascular medicine. Lipomatous hypertrophy of the atrial septum. Circulation 97:1423, 1998.
176. Mortele KJ, Mergo PJ, Williams WF: Lipomatous hypertrophy of the atrial septum: diagnosis with fat suppressed MR imaging. J Magn Reson Imaging 8:1172–1174, 1998.
177. Stone GW, O'Kell RT, Good TH: Lipomatous hypertrophy of the interatrial septum: diagnosis by percutaneous transvenous biopsy. Am Heart J 119:406–408, 1990.
178. Manion WC, Nelson WP, Hall RJ: Benign tumor of the heart causing complete heart block. Am Heart J 83:535–542, 1972.
179. Bharati S, Bicoff JP, Fridman JL, et al: Sudden death caused by benign tumor of the atrioventricular node. Arch Intern Med 136:224–228, 1976.
180. Bharati S, Bauernfeind R, Josephson M: Intermittent preexcitation and mesothelioma of the atrioventricular node: a hitherto undescribed entity. J Cardiovasc Electrophysiol 6:823–831, 1995.
181. Burke AP, Anderson PG, Virmani R: Tumor of the atrioventricular nodal region. A clinical and immunohistochemical study. Arch Pathol Lab Med 114:1057–1062, 1990.
182. Fenoglio JJ Jr, Jacobs DW, McAllister HA Jr: Ultrastructure of the mesothelioma of the atrioventricular node. Cancer 40:721–727, 1977.
183. Fine G, Morales AR: Mesothelioma of the atrioventricular node. Arch Pathol 92:402–408, 1971.
184. Linder J, Shelburne JD, Sorge JP: Congenital endodermal heterotopia of the atrioventricular node: evidence for the endodermal origin of so-called mesotheliomas of the atrioventricular node. Hum Pathol 15:1093–1098, 1984.
185. Fine G, Raju U: Congenital polycystic tumor of the atrioventricular node (endodermal heterotopia, mesothelioma): a histogenetic appraisal with evidence for its endodermal origin. Hum Pathol 18:791–795, 1987.
186. Hellemans IM, van Hemel NM, Kooyman CA: Atrioventricular block in childhood caused by mesothelioma. Pacing Clin Electrophysiol 4:216–220, 1981.
187. James TN, Galakhov I: De subitaneis mortibus. XXVI. Fatal electrical instability of the heart associated with benign congenital polycystic tumor of the atrioventricular node. Circulation 56:667–678, 1977.
188. Balasundaram S, Halees SA, Duran C: Mesothelioma of the atrioventricular node: first successful follow-up after excision. Eur Heart J 13:718–719, 1992.
189. Jebara VA, Uva MS, Farge A: Cardiac pheochromocytomas. Ann Thorac Surg 53:356–361, 1992.
190. Hamilton BH, Francis IR, Gross BH: Intrapericardial paragangliomas (pheochromocytomas): imaging features. AJR 168:109–113, 1997.
191. Conti VR, Saydjari R, Amparo EG: Paraganglioma of the heart. The value of magnetic resonance imaging in the preoperative evaluation. Chest 90:604–606, 1986.
192. Saad MF, Frazier OH, Hickey RC: Intrapericardial pheochromocytoma. Am J Med 75:371–376, 1983.
193. Hui G, McAllister HA Jr, Angelini P: Left atrial paraganglioma: report of a case and review of the literature. Am Heart J 113:1230–1234, 1987.
194. Jeevanandam V, Oz MC, Shapiro B: Surgical management of cardiac pheochromocytoma. Resection versus transplantation. Ann Surg 221:415–419, 1995.
195. Burke AP, Cowan D, Virmani R: Primary sarcomas of the heart. Cancer 69:387–395, 1992.
196. Makhoul N, Bode FR: Angiosarcoma of the heart: review of the literature and report of two cases that illustrate the broad spectrum of the disease. Can J Cardiol 11:423–428, 1995.
197. Economides EG, Singh A: Case of tumor neovascularization demonstrated by cardiac catheterization. Cathet Cardiovasc Diagn 43:451–453, 1998.
198. Uchita S, Hata T, Tsushima Y: Primary cardiac angiosarcoma with superior vena caval syndrome: review of surgical resection and interventional management of venous inflow obstruction. Can J Cardiol 14:1283–1285, 1998.
199. Schmaltz AA, Apitz J: Primary rhabdomyosarcoma of the heart. Pediatr Cardiol 2:73–75, 1982.
200. Sholler GF, Hawker RE, Nunn GR: Primary left ventricular rhabdomyosarcoma in a child: noninvasive assessment and successful resection of a rare tumor. J Thorac Cardiovasc Surg 93:465–468, 1987.
201. Cafferty LL, Epstein JI: Primary liposarcoma of the right atrium. Hum Pathol 18:408–410, 1987.
202. Cairns P, Butany J, Fulop J: Cardiac presentation of non-Hodgkin's lymphoma. Arch Pathol Lab Med 111:80–83, 1987.
203. Laya MB, Mailliard JA, Bewtra C: Malignant fibrous histiocytoma of the heart. A case report and review of the literature. Cancer 59:1026–1031, 1987.
204. Wahba A, Liebold A, Birnbaum DE: Recurrent malignant fibrous histiocytoma of the left atrium in a 27-year-old male. Eur J Cardiothorac Surg 7:387–389, 1993.
205. Teramoto N, Hayaski K, Miyatani K: Malignant fibrous histiocytoma of the right ventricle of the heart. Pathol Int 45:315–319, 1995.
206. Dein JR, Frist WH, Stinsen EB: Primary cardiac neoplasms. Early and late results of surgical treatment in 42 patients. J Thorac Cardiovasc Surg 93:502–511, 1987.
207. Putnam JB Jr, Sweeney MS, Colon R: Primary cardiac sarcomas. Ann Thorac Surg 51:906–910, 1991.
208. Takahashi M, Yamamoto S, Saga T: Images in cardiovascular medicine. Endoscopic resection of malignant fibrous histiocytoma in left ventricle. Circulation 98:276–277, 1998.
209. Harlamert HA, Moulton JS, Lewis W: Images in cardiovascular medicine. Primary malignant fibrous histiocytoma of the heart treated with orthotopic heart transplantation. Circulation 97:703–704, 1998.
210. Crespo MG, Pulpon LA, Pradas G: Heart transplantation for cardiac angiosarcoma: should its indication be questioned? J Heart Lung Transplant 12:527–530, 1993.
211. Calderon M, Galvan J, Negri V: Right ventricular bypass for palliation of cardiac sarcoma. Tex Heart Inst J 23:178–179, 1996.
212. Freedberg RS, Kronzon I, Rumancik WM, Liebeskind D: The contribution of magnetic resonance imaging to the evaluation of intracardiac tumors diagnosed by echocardiography. Circulation 77:96–103, 1988.
213. Mora F, Mindich BP, Guarino T: Improved surgical approach to cardiac tumors with intraoperative two-dimensional echocardiography. Chest 91:142–144, 1987.
214. Feigin DS, Fenoglio JJ, McAllister HA Jr: Pericardial cysts. A radiologic-pathologic correlation and review. Radiology 125:15–20, 1977.
215. Stoller JK, Shaw C, Matthay RA: Enlarging, atypically located pericardial cyst. Recent experience and literature review. Chest 89:402–406, 1986.
216. Unverferth DV, Wooley CF: The differential diagnosis of paracar-

diac lesions: pericardial cysts. Cathet Cardiovasc Diagn 5:31–40, 1979.

217. Beghetti M, Prieditis M, Rebeyka IM, Mawson J: Images in cardiovascular medicine. Intrapericardial teratoma. Circulation 97:1523–1524, 1998.
218. Tollens T, Casselman F, Devlieger H: Fetal cardiac tamponade due to an intrapericardial teratoma. Ann Thorac Surg 66:559–560, 1998.
219. MacDonald S, Fay JE, Lynn RB: Intrapericardial teratoma: a continuing challenge. Can J Surg 26:81–82, 1983.
220. Yilling FP, Schlant RC, Hertzler GL: Pericardial mesothelioma. Chest 81:520–523, 1982.
221. Kaul TK, Fields BL, Kahn DR: Primary malignant pericardial mesothelioma: a case report and review. J Cardiovasc Surg [Torino] 35:261–267, 1994.
222. Miyamoto Y, Nakano S, Shimazaki Y: Pericardial mesothelioma presenting as left atrial thrombus in a patient with mitral stenosis. Cardiovasc Surg 4:51–52, 1996.
223. Thomason R, Schlegel W, Lucca M: Primary malignant mesothelioma of the pericardium. Case report and literature review [see comments]. Tex Heart Inst J 21:170–174, 1994.
224. Terry LN Jr, Kligerman MM: Pericardial and myocardial involvement by lymphomas and leukemias. The role of radiotherapy. Cancer 25:1003–1008, 1970.
225. Lynch M, Cobbs W Jr, Miller RL: Massive cardiac involvement by malignant lymphoma. Cardiology 87:566–568, 1996.
226. Acierno LJ: Cardiac complications in acquired immunodeficiency syndrome (AIDS): a review. J Am Coll Cardiol 13:1144–1154, 1989.
227. Lewis W: AIDS: cardiac findings from 115 autopsies. Prog Cardiovasc Dis 32:207–215, 1989.
228. Holladay AO, Siegel RJ, Schwartz DA: Cardiac malignant lymphoma in acquired immune deficiency syndrome. Cancer 70:2203–2207, 1992.
229. Steigman CK, Anderson DW, Macher AM: Fatal cardiac tamponade in acquired immunodeficiency syndrome with epicardial Kaposi's sarcoma. Am Heart J 116:1105–1107, 1988.
230. Aboulafia DM, Bush R, Picozzi VJ: Cardiac tamponade due to primary pericardial lymphoma in a patient with AIDS. Chest 106:1295–1299, 1994.
231. Vijay V, Aloor RK, Yalla SM: Pericardial tamponade from Kaposi's sarcoma: role of early pericardial window. Am Heart J 132:897–899, 1996.
232. Chyu KY, Birnbaum Y, Naqvi T: Echocardiographic detection of Kaposi's sarcoma causing cardiac tamponade in a patient with acquired immunodeficiency syndrome. Clin Cardiol 21:131–133, 1998.
233. Goldfarb A, King CL, Rosenzweig BP: Cardiac lymphoma in the acquired immunodeficiency syndrome. Am Heart J 118:1304–1344, 1989.
234. Andress JD, Polish LB, Clark DM: Transvenous biopsy diagnosis of cardiac lymphoma in an AIDS patient. Am Heart J 118:421–423, 1989.

CHAPTER 103

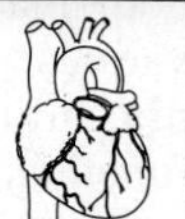

Endocrine Disorders and the Heart

Victor R. Lavis and James T. Willerson

HYPOTHALAMIC-PITUITARY AXIS
SOMATOSTATIN
DEFICIENCY OF GROWTH HORMONE IN ADULTS
ACROMEGALY
Pathophysiology
Clinical Manifestations
Diagnosis
Treatment
ADRENAL INSUFFICIENCY
Pathophysiology
Clinical Manifestations
Diagnosis
Treatment
CUSHING'S SYNDROME
Pathophysiology
Clinical Manifestations
Diagnosis
Treatment
HYPERALDOSTERONISM AND OTHER SYNDROMES OF EXCESSIVE MINERALOCORTICOIDS
Pathophysiology
Clinical Manifestations
Diagnosis
Treatment
DISEASES OF THE ADRENAL MEDULLA: PHEOCHROMOCYTOMA
Pathophysiology
Clinical Manifestations
Diagnosis
Treatment
DIABETES MELLITUS
Pathophysiology
Clinical Manifestations
Diagnosis
Treatment
DISORDERS OF CALCIUM METABOLISM
Pathophysiology
Clinical Manifestations
Diagnosis
Treatment
HYPERTHYROIDISM
Pathophysiology
Clinical Manifestations
Diagnosis
Treatment
HYPOTHYROIDISM
Pathophysiology
Clinical Manifestations
Diagnosis
Treatment
CARCINOID SYNDROME
Pathophysiology
Clinical Manifestations
Diagnosis
Treatment

This chapter provides a review of selected endocrine disorders and their influences on the cardiovascular system.

Hypothalamic-Pituitary Axis

The classic hormones of the anterior pituitary gland can be divided into three classes of related polypeptides: growth hormone (GH) and prolactin, adrenocorticotropin (ACTH) and other peptides derived from the pro-opiomelanocortin precursor, and the glycoprotein hormones thyrotropin (TSH), luteinizing hormone, and follicle-stimulating hormone. ACTH and the glycoproteins have no major cardiovascular effects except those mediated by their respective target organs: the adrenal cortex, the thyroid, and the gonads. There is no known cardiovascular syndrome associated with excessive or deficient prolactin.

Somatostatin

The term *somatostatin* encompasses a family of homologous peptides with multiple endocrine and paracrine actions. The major sources of somatostatins are the brain, the D cells of the pancreatic islets, and the gastrointestinal mucosa. Somatostatin from brain acts via the pituitary portal system to inhibit the secretion of TSH and GH.

In the endocrine pancreas, somatostatin inhibits the secretion of insulin, glucagon, and somatostatin itself. Somatostatin also has diverse inhibitory effects on gastric and pancreatic exocrine secretion and on gastrointestinal activity. Somatostatin receptors, of which there are several molecular species, are widely distributed throughout the body. The various actions of somatostatin appear to be mediated by G_i proteins.

Somatostatin may have a function in cardiac physiology, because it has been reported that cardiac nerves contain somatostatin.[1] However, there has been no description of cardiac symptomatology in states of somatostatin excess. No clinical syndrome of somatostatin deficiency has been recognized.

Deficiency of Growth Hormone in Adults

There is growing recognition of a syndrome of GH deficiency in adults. The clinical features include a loss of lean body mass, increased central adiposity, muscular weakness, various psychologic abnormalities, dyslipidemia, osteopenia, bradycardia, and impaired left ventricular systolic function.[2–4] Perhaps some of the increased cardiovascular mortality rate among adults with hypopituitarism is related to a deficiency of GH.[5, 6] This problem should be suspected in individuals with known hypothalamic-pituitary disease of any cause. For adults, the standard test for the diagnosis of GH deficiency has been the peak response of serum GH to induced hypoglycemia.[7] A synthetic analogue of hypothalamic growth hormone–releasing hormone (GHRH) has become available and shows promise as a diagnostic agent that can avoid the risks of hypoglycemia.[8] A deficiency of GH can be treated with injections of recombinant human GH.

ACROMEGALY

Pathophysiology

Acromegaly is a clinical syndrome caused by excessive circulating GH. It is usually caused by inappropriately high levels of GH secreted by a pituitary adenoma. Rarely, it may be caused by secretion of GHRH by an extrapituitary tumor.[9] Normally, secretion of GH from the anterior pituitary is regulated by the hypothalamic peptides GHRH and somatostatin. There are several molecular variants of circulating GH, of which the relative physiologic significance remains to be elucidated.[10] GH stimulates the production in various tissues of insulin-like growth factor-I (IGF-I, also known as somatomedin C)[11] and, to a lesser extent, IGF-II.[12] These two peptides are structurally homologous to proinsulin.[13] Many of the effects of GH are mediated by the IGFs, especially by IGF-I.[12, 14]

GH, acting directly or via IGFs, has a number of important metabolic effects. Broadly speaking, it promotes net protein anabolism while stimulating lipolysis and ketogenesis. As a result, lipid-derived fuels (i.e., nonesterified fatty acids and ketone bodies) are used for energy by the tissues, including myocardium, that can do so. Amino acids are spared for protein synthesis. When GH is administered on a long-term basis, uptake and catabolism of glucose by muscle and adipose tissue are diminished, leading to insulin resistance and a tendency toward hyperglycemia.[15] Echocardiographic studies indicate that the administration of GH to humans increases heart rate and myocardial contractility.[16]

Clinical Manifestations

The principal manifestations of acromegaly can be classified according to the organ system or systems affected. The growth of bone in adults, in whom the epiphyses are closed, leads to broadening of the hands and feet, with increases in shoe, glove, and ring size. There also is enlargement of the jaw, with dental malocclusion. Hypertrophic bone growth leads to osteoarthritis and nerve entrapment syndromes, which may be major causes of complications. Manifestations of soft tissue growth include thickened, greasy skin; enlargement of abdominal viscera; macroglossia; and goiter. Skin tags are common. An increased incidence of colonic polyps and colon cancer has been reported in patients with acromegaly.[17–19] Metabolic manifestations include hypercalciuria and hyperphosphatemia. Hyperinsulinemia, which is indicative of insulin resistance, is found in most patients. However, clinical evidence of diabetes mellitus occurs in only approximately 10 percent of these individuals.

Acromegaly is a serious disease. Age-specific mortality rates, principally from cardiovascular and respiratory complications, are increased from 1.5- to 3-fold.[19] The principal cardiovascular manifestations of acromegaly are cardiac enlargement, hypertension, premature coronary artery disease (CAD), congestive heart failure (CHF), and arrhythmias.[20–25] Virtually all patients with acromegaly have cardiomegaly, especially older individuals. The increase in cardiac mass, including asymmetric septal hypertrophy, is not directly related to hypertension. Some patients have left ventricular (LV) dilatation and reduction in ejection fraction. At autopsy, local myocardial interstitial fibrosis, lymphocytic infiltration, and small vessel disease of the myocardium[22, 25] have been found in some patients.

Another very common cardiovascular manifestation of acromegaly is systemic arterial hypertension, which occurs in approximately 30 percent of patients,[26] especially those with a longer duration of disease. The hypertension usually responds to medical treatment.[27, 28] In patients with acromegaly, there appears to be reduced activity of the renin-angiotensin-aldosterone axis,[29, 30] confirmed by pressor responses to angiotensin II antagonists,[31] enhanced pressor responsiveness to angiotensin II,[28] and increases in total exchangeable sodium.[30] In addition, intravascular volume expansion occurs in many patients. Each of these alterations may contribute to the development of systemic arterial hypertension.[28] Successful treatment of acromegaly reduces arterial pressure in many hypertensive acromegalic patients.[21, 28]

Premature atherosclerosis occurs in some patients with acromegaly, but its prevalence is not clear. Some patients with acromegaly without evidence of hypertension or atherosclerosis develop cardiomyopathies, as evidenced by cardiomegaly, CHF, and occasional arrhythmias.[22] The CHF may be relatively resistant to conventional medical therapy. Some histologic observations have demonstrated cellular hypertrophy, patchy fibrosis, and myofibrillar degeneration (Fig. 103–1). Autopsy studies of some patients after sudden death have demonstrated degenerative or inflammatory changes in the sinoatrial nerve plexus and the atrioventricular node.[25] Approximately 10 to 20 percent of patients with acromegaly have CHF, and in perhaps 20 percent of these there is no obvious predisposing cause. Diastolic dysfunction is found in some patients with acromegaly in the absence of hypertension or atherosclerosis.[28, 30–35]

Diagnosis

Because GH levels are highly variable, it is important to obtain them under standardized conditions. The most useful diagnostic test involves the oral administration of 75 to 100 g of glucose.[9, 36] In normal individuals, GH levels are

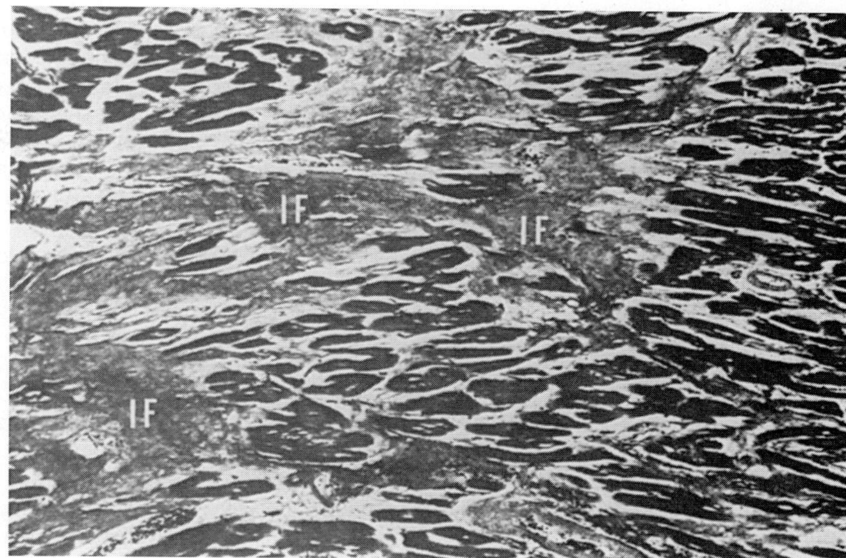

FIGURE 103–1 Histologic appearance of the myocardium from a patient with acromegaly shows hypertrophied fibers and interstitial fibrosis (IF). (Mallory-Heidenhain stain, × 120.) (From Lie JT, Grossman SJ: Pathology of the heart in acromegaly. Am Heart J 100:41, 1980.)

less than 2 ng/ml 90 to 120 minutes after administration of the test dose.[37] Serum IGF-I levels, which correlate well with integrated measurements of GH,[38] are also very helpful in making a diagnosis. In considering the possible diagnosis of acromegaly, it is also important to determine whether there are other alterations in pituitary or hypothalamic function.

Treatment

Most often, the initial treatment for pituitary somatotrophic adenomas is surgery, usually via the transsphenoidal approach.[9, 39] Reported surgical success rates depend on the size of the adenoma and on the stringency of the definition of cure with respect to postoperative GH and IGF-I levels (for a review, see Melmed and associates[39]). Probably at least 40 percent of patients will require some mode of adjunctive therapy. The favored secondary treatment modality is the administration of an analogue of somatostatin, such as octreotide.[39, 40] Treatment with octreotide decreases LV mass in acromegalic patients with cardiac hypertrophy.[41] Octreotide must be injected several times daily; longer-acting analogues of somatostatin are under development. Dopaminergic agonists such as bromocriptine often provide subjective relief of symptoms but do not significantly reduce GH levels in the majority of patients.[9, 39] Pituitary irradiation reduces GH levels slowly over several years, during which cardiovascular disease may progress.[42] In addition, irradiation carries a significant risk of late development of hypopituitarism, as well as brain damage or the development of brain tumors.[35, 39, 42] A survey of a large number of patients showed no increase in mortality rates among those whose post-treatment GH levels were below 2.5 ng/ml,[19] highlighting the importance of reduction of excessive secretion of GH.

Adrenal Insufficiency

Pathophysiology

Adrenal insufficiency occurs when the secretion of adrenal glucocorticoids or mineralocorticoids is less than that needed by the body. Patients can develop adrenal insufficiency for one of several reasons. There may be failure of the pituitary to produce adequate amounts of ACTH or diminished hypothalamic secretion of corticotrophin-releasing hormone (CRH), either as the result of hypothalamic disease or as a consequence of long-term treatment with pharmacologic doses of glucocorticoids. Primary failure of the adrenal cortex may be caused by (1) autoimmune disease associated with the development of anti-adrenal antibodies, sometimes in association with pernicious anemia, autoimmune thyroid disease, type 1 diabetes mellitus, or hypoparathyroidism; (2) destruction of the adrenal cortex by infection, especially tuberculosis, disseminated mycosis, or opportunistic infection such as cytomegalovirus in patients with acquired immunodeficiency syndrome; (3) infarction or hemorrhagic necrosis associated with anticoagulation, the antiphospholipid syndrome, or sepsis, especially meningococcemia; (4) rarely, cancer metastatic to the adrenal glands; or (5) a hereditary defect in organogenesis or the pathway of cortisol synthesis.[43]

Clinical Manifestations

Primary adrenal insufficiency (*Addison's disease*) can occur at any age and affects the two sexes equally.[44] Its major manifestations are weakness, increased skin or mucosal pigmentation, weight loss, anorexia, nausea, vomiting, and hypotension, often with postural hypotension. Hyponatremia, hypochloremia, and hyperkalemia are present in some of these individuals. *Hyponatremia* is caused by the loss of sodium into the urine as the result of aldosterone deficiency, coupled with the inability to excrete free water. *Hyperkalemia* occurs as a result of mineralocorticoid deficiency and reduction in the glomerular filtration rate. *Hypercalcemia,* probably related to volume contraction, may be present. In patients with impaired secretion of ACTH, there usually is adequate secretion of mineralocorticoids by the adrenal zona glomerulosa, which continues to undergo trophic stimulation by circulating angiotensins. Consequently, hyperkalemia is not usually a problem; however, because impaired excretion of free water is a consequence of glucocorticoid deficiency, hyponatremia may occur.

Arterial hypotension is the most common cardiovascular finding in patients with adrenal insufficiency. Syncope occurs in many of these individuals. The heart size is normal or small, pulse volume is reduced, and orthostatic hypotension may be present. Some patients with Addison's disease have mitral valve prolapse, which disappears with appropriate steroid and aldosterone replacement.

Diagnosis

The most convenient screening test for adrenocortical insufficiency is measurement of plasma cortisol after the intravenous injection of cosyntropin, a synthetic preparation of the 1–24 sequence of ACTH.[45, 46] For determination of the cause of adrenocortical insufficiency, there are several useful tests, including measurements of plasma ACTH levels and of plasma cortisol after the prolonged infusion of cosyntropin.[47]

Treatment

Treatment of adrenal insufficiency entails the replacement of glucocorticoids and, if necessary, mineralocorticoids. In previously untreated patients who manifest signs of volume depletion, the vascular compartment should be refilled with intravenous saline. The prompt administration of saline solution is especially important in addisonian crisis, which is characterized by hypotension and cardiovascular collapse. Because myocardial function is usually reduced in this situation, the patient must be carefully monitored during volume resuscitation to avoid pulmonary edema. In acute adrenal insufficiency or in patients experiencing physiologic stress, the dosage of glucocorticoid should be several times the usually daily maintenance dose. For the treatment of acute adrenal crisis, the recommended dose of hydrocortisone is 100 mg IV q6h. Administered in "stress" doses, hydrocortisone, the major natural glucocorticoid, exhibits substantial mineralocorticoid effects.

For maintenance therapy, either hydrocortisone or a less costly short-acting synthetic glucocorticoid, such as prednisone, should be administered orally in physiologic replacement dosage (e.g., 5 to 7.5 mg prednisone qd or hydrocortisone at 15 to 20 mg in the morning and 5 to 10 mg in the afternoon). The usual injectable mineralocorticoid is desoxycorticosterone (DOC), and the oral preparation is fludrocortisone. The replacement dosage for mineralocorticoids should be determined on an individual basis. The usual replacement dosage of fludrocortisone is 0.05 to 0.2 mg qd, together with a liberal intake of dietary sodium.

CUSHING'S SYNDROME

Pathophysiology

Cushing's syndrome results from the actions of excessive circulating glucocorticoids. Its most frequent cause is treatment with pharmacologic doses of glucocorticoids for nonendocrine conditions. Most patients with endogenous Cushing's syndrome have bilateral adrenal hyperplasia with resultant excessive production of glucocorticoids, mineralocorticoids, and androgens. These patients usually have ACTH-producing tumors of the pituitary (Cushing's disease) or ectopic ACTH production (e.g., from lung carcinoma). Approximately 20 percent of cases of endogenous Cushing's syndrome are ACTH independent and are due to either a primary adrenal adenoma or carcinoma. Three times as many women as men have endogenous Cushing's syndrome. Onset usually occurs in the third or fourth decade of life.

Clinical Manifestations

Depending on the cause of Cushing's syndrome, the clinical picture may include the effects of increased androgens, mineralocorticoids, or both and those of glucocorticoids. Major manifestations are truncal obesity, plethora, systolic hypertension, proximal muscle weakness, thinning and fragility of the skin with ecchymoses and purple abdominal striae, hyperglycemia, osteoporosis, psychiatric disturbances, and fatigue.[48] Many patients experience wide swings in mood, ranging from severe depression to frank psychosis or confusion. Frank diabetes mellitus is present in approximately 20 percent of patients. Hyperpigmentation, although uncommon, is a clue to hypersecretion of ACTH from the pituitary. In women with endogenous Cushing's syndrome, hirsutism, a male escutcheon, amenorrhea, and deepening of the voice are due to androgen excess. The major signs of excessive mineralocorticoids are hypertension and hypokalemia (see later).

Cardiovascular. The major cardiovascular abnormality of Cushing's syndrome is arterial hypertension. Possible causes of the hypertension include volume expansion caused by mineralocorticoids and high levels of cortisol and increased production of angiotensin II and vascular hyperreactivity.[49, 50] Unlike patients with essential hypertension, hypertensive patients with Cushing's syndrome of any cause lack the normal nocturnal decline in blood pressure.[51, 52] As the normal diurnal rhythm of pituitary-adrenal secretion is disrupted in Cushing's syndrome, blood pressure may normally be modulated by physiologic fluctuations of circulating adrenal steroids. Hemodynamic, electrocardiographic (ECG), and echocardiographic manifestations are usually associated with systemic arterial hypertension. There may be ECG or echocardiographic evidence of LV hypertrophy, left atrial enlargement, and, on occasion, evidence of diastolic dysfunction. Echocardiographic investigations suggest that asymmetric septal hypertrophy is an almost universal finding in patients with endogenous Cushing's syndrome, whether caused by adrenal adenoma or pituitary hypersecretion of ACTH.[53] Chronic excess production of cortisol may also lead to hyperlipidemia and hypercholesterolemia, which can promote the development of atherosclerosis.[54]

Atrial myxomas and ACTH-independent Cushing's syndrome may coexist in the *Carney complex,* a rare familial syndrome that includes multiple small, pigmented adrenal nodules; spotty cutaneous pigmentation, including lentigines and blue nevi; subcutaneous, mammary, or cardiac myxomas; and other endocrine disorders, such as acromegaly or testicular tumors.[55]

Diagnosis

One milligram of dexamethasone administered late in the evening, with measurement of plasma cortisol between 7AM and 9AM the next morning, serves as a sensitive screening test for endogenous Cushing's syndrome.[56, 57] In normal healthy individuals, serum cortisol levels will be less than 5 μg/dl with this test. Measurement of 24-hour urinary free cortisol serves as an important confirmatory test.[57] False-positive responses may occur with obesity, major depression, treatment with estrogen, or alcoholism, among other conditions. Discrimination of these conditions from true Cushing's syndrome may be aided by measurement of plasma cortisol after suppression of ACTH secretion by low-dose dexamethasone, followed by stimulation with ovine CRH.[58] For discrimination among the several causes of endogenous Cushing's syndrome, various tests are available, including computed tomography (CT) scanning and magnetic resonance imaging (MRI) of the adrenal glands and pituitary and measurement of cortisol levels after the administration of ovine CRH, metyrapone, graded doses of dexamethasone, or a combination.[57, 59] In patients with ACTH-dependent endogenous Cushing's syndrome, the aforementioned techniques may not unequivocally distinguish between pituitary and ectopic sources of ACTH. In this circumstance, determination of ACTH levels in the inferior petrosal sinuses after the administration of ovine CRH has been highly reliable.[59, 60]

Treatment

Treatment of endogenous Cushing's syndrome is dependent on the cause. For Cushing's disease, transsphenoidal pituitary surgery, with or without irradiation, is most frequently used. Surgical removal of the causative tumor should be attempted in patients with adrenal neoplasms and those with ectopic secretion of ACTH. Drugs that inhibit adrenal steroid synthesis are available for inoperable patients.[61, 62]

Treatment of hypertension associated with Cushing's disease is usually performed with agents that block angiotensin II effects, often angiotensin-converting enzyme (ACE) inhibitors. Because hypokalemia is present in some patients with Cushing's syndrome, diuretics must be prescribed with great care. Efforts should be made to replenish potassium, and if a diuretic is used, potassium-sparing diuretics or potassium supplementation in excess of what might be ordinarily required should be considered. In patients with hypokalemia, cardiac glycosides should be used with caution.

HYPERALDOSTERONISM AND OTHER SYNDROMES OF EXCESSIVE MINERALOCORTICOIDS

Pathophysiology

Among patients with systemic arterial hypertension, 2 percent or fewer have primary hyperaldosteronism. Primary hyperaldosteronism is associated with increased secretion of aldosterone, which may arise from an adrenal adenoma or from bilateral adrenal hyperplasia.[63, 64] Patients with functioning adrenal tumors, Cushing's disease (see earlier), ectopic ACTH syndrome, and 11-beta-hydroxylase and 17-alpha-hydroxylase varieties of congenital adrenal hyperplasia can develop a similar syndrome caused by an excess of 11-desoxycorticosterone or other mineralocorticoids.[63, 65, 66] Other conditions that produce a similar syndrome include (1) glucocorticoid-remediable hypertension, caused by the inappropriate production of mineralocorticoids by the adrenal zona fasciculata[67]; (2) the syndrome of apparent mineralocorticoid excess, caused by the action of cortisol on renal mineralocorticoid receptors due to impaired renal inactivation of cortisol[68]; and (3) Liddle's syndrome, due to excessive renal reabsorption of sodium and excretion of potassium caused by mutations in the epithelial sodium channel.[69]

Clinical Manifestations

The major clinical consequences of hyperaldosteronism are systemic arterial hypertension, hypokalemia, and metabolic alkalosis. The most important problem is hypokalemia, because it can predispose to the development of frequent and complex ventricular arrhythmias. ECG signs of hypokalemia include flat T waves, U wave prominence, and prolongation of the QT interval. Polyuria and muscular weakness are other significant consequences of hypokalemia.

Systemic arterial hypertension is rarely severe but may lead to LV hypertrophy and diastolic dysfunction.

Diagnosis

The most useful screening procedure for primary hyperaldosteronism is the identification of hypokalemia in a patient with systemic arterial hypertension, both systolic and diastolic, in the absence of potassium-lowering medications. The diagnosis is confirmed by the demonstration of inappropriately elevated serum or urinary aldosterone levels that fail to suppress during volume expansion.[70–72] Primary hyperaldosteronism can be distinguished from secondary hyperaldosteronism associated with renal vascular disease or with renal or cardiac failure by the measurement of plasma renin activity, which is increased in secondary hyperaldosteronism and reduced in primary hyperaldosteronism.[70–72] It is important to discriminate adrenal adenoma from bilateral hyperplasia as the cause of primary hyperaldosteronism. Several tests have been developed for this purpose, including (1) CT scanning of the adrenal glands; (2) measurement of the precursor steroid, 18-hydroxycorticosterone, which is usually markedly elevated in patients with adenoma; (3) response of plasma aldosterone to standing in the morning, with the level declining in patients with adenoma and rising in patients with hyperplasia; and (4) bilateral adrenal vein catheterization, with determination of ratios of aldosterone to cortisol.[64]

Treatment

Primary hyperaldosteronism can be treated with a competitive inhibitor of mineralocorticoid action, usually spironolactone. Some patients are reluctant to take spironolactone on a long-term basis because it may produce gynecomastia and impotence, especially when doses of more than 200 mg/day are required.[73] Medical therapy provides adequate control of hypokalemia and hypertension in some individuals. However, surgical removal of the aldosterone-producing adenoma is the definitive therapy and is usually recommended for patients in whom there is no strong contraindication. In patients whose primary hyperaldosteronism is caused by bilateral hyperplasia, surgery is not usually effective. Therefore, treatment with spironolactone and other appropriate antihypertensive agents is preferred. Every effort should be made to replace serum potassium.

Diseases of the Adrenal Medulla: Pheochromocytoma

Pathophysiology

Pheochromocytomas are tumors derived from chromaffin cells of the sympathetic nervous system, usually in the adrenal medulla. Their most important secretory products are the catecholamines norepinephrine and epinephrine. Pheochromocytomas that arise outside of the adrenal gland are also called *paragangliomas.* Biochemically and physiologically, the adrenal medulla is an integral part of the sympathetic nervous system.[74] The location of adrenal medullary cells is associated with their ability to form epinephrine, as glucocorticoids secreted from the cortex pass in high concentration directly to the medulla, inducing the synthesis of phenylethanolamine-*N*-methyltransferase, the enzyme that converts norepinephrine into epinephrine. The human adrenal medulla contains approximately 1 mg of catecholamine, mostly epinephrine, per gram of tissue. Catecholamines stimulate glycogenolysis, gluconeogenesis, and lipolysis; inhibit the secretion of insulin; increase systemic vascular resistance; and exert positive inotropic and chronotropic actions on the myocardium.

Fewer than 10 percent of pheochromocytomas are malignant. Most pheochromocytomas are solitary adrenal tumors; 10 percent are bilateral and 10 percent are extra-adrenal. Approximately 5 percent of pheochromocytomas are inherited as part of one of the multiple endocrine neoplasia type II (MEN-II) syndromes, in which bilateral pheochromocytomas and medullary carcinoma of the thyroid coexist. The MEN-IIa syndrome may include hyperparathyroidism,[75] and the MEN-IIb syndrome includes marfanoid habitus and multiple mucosal neuromas of the tongue, lips, gastrointestinal tract, or conjunctivae, usually without parathyroid disease.[76] In these syndromes, bilateral adrenal pheochromocytomas are the rule. Pheochromocytomas may also coexist with the phakomatoses, including multiple neurofibromatoses and von Hippel-Lindau disease (cerebellar or retinal hemangioblastomas, renal and pancreatic tumors).

Clinical Manifestations

Pheochromocytoma is a very rare cause of systemic arterial hypertension in humans, but the morbidity and mortality rates associated with these tumors are significant. These tumors produce paradoxical or sustained hypertension, often with postural hypotension, tachycardia inappropriate to the level of blood pressure, headaches, palpitations, chest pain, arrhythmias, profound sweating, signs of hypermetabolism, glucose intolerance, or hypertension after abdominal trauma or surgery, or a combination. In a patient with hypertension, the coexistence of headache, sweating, and palpitations is highly suggestive of pheochromocytoma.[77]

In patients with pheochromocytoma, systemic arterial hypertension is typically paroxysmal but may be fixed. The episodicity of blood pressure elevation may reflect periodic discharge of catecholamines. Postural hypotension is common, caused by reduction of plasma volume or impairment of sympathetic reflexes.[78, 79]

ECG and echocardiographic manifestations in patients with pheochromocytoma are usually the result of systemic arterial hypertension. ECG signs include evidence of LV hypertrophy, left atrial enlargement, left-axis deviation, nonspecific ST-T wave changes, and ventricular and atrial arrhythmias. Occasionally, the electrocardiogram suggests the presence of myocardial ischemia during attacks of hypertension. The echocardiogram often demonstrates LV hypertrophy with relatively normal LV function. During a hypertensive crisis, the echocardiogram may demonstrate systolic anterior motion of the anterior leaflet of the mitral valve ("SAM pattern") and paradoxical septal motion.[80, 81] The most common cardiovascular causes of death are arrhythmias and the consequences of systemic arterial hypertension, including strokes.

Autopsy studies have demonstrated the presence of myocarditis in about half of patients who die from pheochromocytoma.[82–84] Histologic findings include focal necrosis with infiltration of inflammatory cells, perivascular inflammation, and contraction band necrosis (Fig. 103–2). Scattered areas of fibrosis are also found.

Diagnosis

Hypertensive patients with any of the given clinical problems should be evaluated for pheochromocytoma because detection may be life saving. Two tests are commonly used for diagnosis: measurement of urinary catecholamines, vanillylmandelic acid, and metanephrines and measurement of serum catecholamines.[85] Vanillylmandelic acid and metanephrines are metabolites of catecholamines. In patients with paroxysmal hypertension, it is helpful to collect the urine and blood samples when blood pressure is elevated. The most helpful imaging techniques for localization of pheochromocytoma are CT scanning, MRI, and nuclear scanning with ^{131}I-*meta*iodobenzylguanidine.[77, 86] Scanning with ^{131}I-*meta*iodobenzylguanidine is especially helpful for patients who have already had surgery or who have malignant pheochromocytoma.[86]

Treatment

Specific pharmacologic therapy with an alpha-adrenergic blocker should be initiated as soon as the diagnosis of

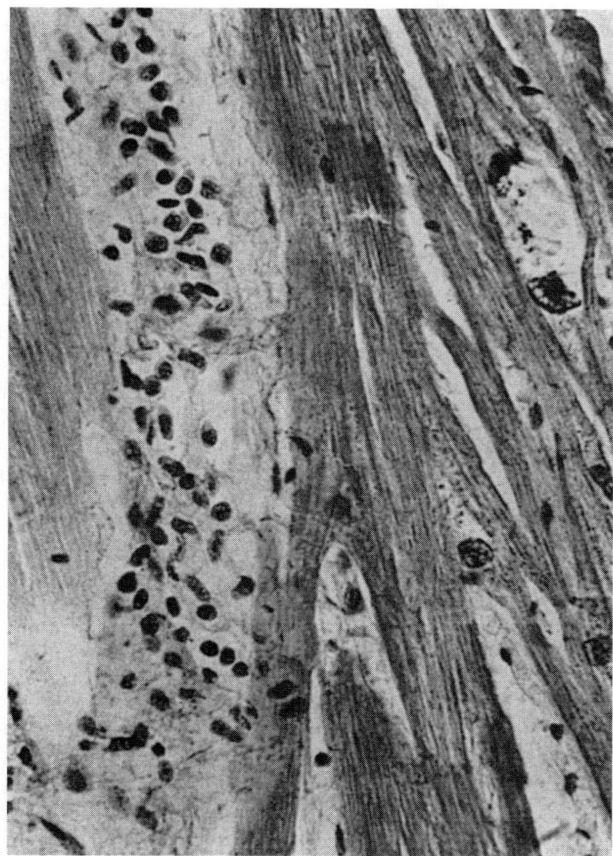

FIGURE 103–2 Histologic appearance of myocardium from a patient with pheochromocytoma shows myocarditis, nuclear degeneration of myocardial fibers, edema, and focal histiocytic infiltration. (H&E, × 285.) (From Van Vliet PD, Burchell HB, Titus JL: Myocarditis associated with pheochromocytoma. N Engl J Med 274:1102, 1966. Copyright © 1966 Massachusetts Medical Society. All rights reserved.)

pheochromocytoma is made. Phenoxybenzamine hydrochloride may be begun at an initial dosage of 10 mg q12h, with the dose being gradually increased every 2 to 3 days until arterial blood pressure is normalized. Other α-adrenergic antagonists can also be used. During treatment with α-adrenergic antagonists, one must be careful to detect postural hypotension associated with hypovolemia.[77, 87] Sodium intake should be liberalized because untreated patients are chronically volume depleted. Adequate control of arterial blood pressure is mandatory before the initiation of any diagnostic or therapeutic procedures, especially surgery to remove the pheochromocytoma. Calcium antagonists may be useful in treating hypertension and reducing catecholamine production resulting from pheochromocytomas.[88]

Beta-receptor–blocking agents may help patients who have significant tachycardia, palpitations, and catecholamine-induced arrhythmias; however, it is important to establish α-adrenergic blockade before commencement of β-receptor blockade. If β-receptor blockade is begun before the establishment of adequate α-receptor blockade, severe hypertension may occur as a result of unopposed α-adrenergic stimulation associated with the increase in circulating catecholamines. Surgical removal of the tumor can be accomplished after adequate α-adrenergic blockade is obtained. The anesthesiologist should be experienced in the management of these patients, with special regard to the treatment of intraoperative tachyarrhythmias. Hypotension after tumor excision should be treated with aggressive volume repletion.

DIABETES MELLITUS

Pathophysiology

Diabetes mellitus is not a single disease but rather is a constellation of metabolic and pathologic abnormalities, with a variety of causes. *Type 1 diabetes* is caused by immunologically mediated destruction of the cells of the pancreatic islets of Langerhans.[89–91] Susceptibility to type 1 diabetes is determined by human leukocyte antigen genotype,[92] with the destructive process being triggered by some environmental event such as viral infection.[91, 93, 94] Patients with type 1 diabetes mellitus may develop other endocrine manifestations of organ-specific autoimmunity, including chronic lymphocytic thyroiditis, Graves' disease, and idiopathic adrenal insufficiency. Type 1 diabetes exhibits a marked predilection for whites and extreme geographic variability of prevalence. Because the peak incidence is during adolescence,[95, 96] type 1 diabetes is also often termed *juvenile diabetes,* although new cases occur throughout life, even into old age. Patients with type 1 diabetes usually eventually develop an absolute deficiency of insulin, so they are prone to develop ketoacidosis unless treated regularly with exogenous insulin.

In the United States, more than 90 percent of patients with diabetes are characterized by strong hereditary predisposition unrelated to human leukocyte antigen type[93, 97] and an association with aging and obesity. This presentation of diabetes has been termed "type 2" but may be etiologically heterogeneous. *Type 2 diabetes* is the most common form of diabetes throughout the world. In the United States, it is the most prevalent form of diabetes among whites of European descent. Its prevalence is greater still among Native Americans, African-Americans and Mexican-Americans. This form of diabetes is not accompanied by any detectable immunologic attack on the pancreas. Because the hyperglycemia is stable and does not lead to metabolic decompensation, type 2 diabetes may be present for a long time before diagnosis. Recent epidemiologic data suggest that the mean duration of type 2 diabetes before diagnosis is 7 to 10 years.

The pathophysiology of type 2 diabetes includes both *insulin resistance* (i.e., impairment of the action of insulin) and *abnormal secretion of insulin,* especially in response to hyperglycemia.[98–104] However, these patients usually have detectable and often substantial circulating insulin levels. Although insulin secretory capability tends to decline over many years, most patients do not require exogenous insulin to prevent metabolic decompensation. Ketoacidosis ordinarily occurs only in the context of a stressful event such as severe infection or infarction of an organ.

The metabolic features of diabetes, which vary in severity among individuals, are those characteristic of inadequacy of insulin action: (1) inadequately restrained catabolism of stored glycogen, triglycerides, and protein; (2) inappropriately increased gluconeogenesis; (3) decreased fractional utilization of circulating glucose by skeletal muscle and adipose tissue; and (4) accelerated ketogenesis in patients with absolute deficiency of insulin. These changes result in hyperglycemia, hyperlipidemia, and in severe cases, net catabolism of protein.

Clinical Manifestations

The major causes of death and disability in patients with diabetes include (1) atherosclerosis, manifested by occlusive coronary, cerebral, and peripheral vascular disease; (2) glomerulosclerosis leading to chronic renal failure; (3) arterial hypertension, which exacerbates cerebral vascular disease, renal insufficiency, and heart failure; (4) congestive heart failure, related to hypertension and ischemic heart disease; (5) peripheral and autonomic neuropathies; (6) proliferative retinopathy, the most common cause of blindness among working-age adults in the United States[105]; and (7) metabolic decompensation, including ketoacidosis and nonketotic hyperosmolar hyperglycemia. Microvascular disease produces widening of basement membranes of capillaries in the retina, conjunctiva, glomerulus, brain, pancreas, and myocardium.[106, 107] The clinical significance of these capillary lesions has not yet been fully elucidated. There is considerable evidence that the control of hyperglycemia and other diabetic metabolic abnormalities can help prevent the ocular, renal, neurologic, and vascular lesions that account for most of the deaths and disabilities among patients with type 1 or 2 diabetes.[108–113]

Type 2 diabetes tends to occur in individuals who are already burdened with various cardiovascular risk factors, including central adiposity; dyslipidemia consisting of elevated levels of triglycerides, low high-density lipoprotein (HDL)-cholesterol and small, dense low-density lipoprotein (LDL)-cholesterol particles; hypertension; and a thrombotic tendency, as indicated by elevated levels of circulating plasminogen activator inhibitor 1.[114, 115]

A number of potentially atherogenic abnormalities of plasma lipoproteins has been observed among diabetic patients. In poorly controlled type 1 diabetes, typically HDL-cholesterol levels are reduced, with mild or no increase in very low-density lipoprotein (VLDL)- and LDL-cholesterol levels. These alterations return to normal when metabolism is normalized with intensive insulin therapy.[116] Rarely, patients with long-standing insulin deficiency may display hyperchylomicronemia,[117] due to the disappearance of lipoprotein lipase, which depends on insulin for its induction.[118] The lipid pattern is different in type 2 diabetes mellitus, which is usually accompanied by obesity. In type 2 diabetes mellitus, one sees elevations in VLDL-cholesterol and triglyceride levels, with reduced HDL-cholesterol levels.[116, 119] Although LDL-cholesterol levels may be elevated or normal, there typically is a shift in their size distribution toward smaller, denser particles, which are believed to be more atherogenic than the LDL of nondiabetic individuals.[120, 121] Control of hyperglycemia can improve the LDL and triglyceride levels but is less effective in raising HDL levels.[116]

Epidemiologic studies show markedly increased cardiovascular mortality rates among persons with diabetes mellitus.[122, 123] CAD, which leads to premature myocardial infarction (MI), is the leading cause of death among adult diabetics.[42] The presence of CAD correlates with the duration of diabetes. In addition, in patients with type 2 diabetes, the level of glycemia is a risk factor for death from cardiovascular disease.[124] Diabetics tend to have larger MIs, a higher incidence of CHF, and higher mortality and morbidity rates associated with the MIs than do nondiabetics.[125–127] Survival after MI is reduced in the diabetic, with mortality rates as high as 25 percent during the first year.[125–127] Patients with diabetes mellitus have a higher incidence of painless MIs than the normal population, with as many as 20 percent of diabetics failing to experience pain during MI. This is the result of the autonomic neuropathy present in many of these patients, who may experience recurrent myocardial ischemia without episodes of angina.[128, 129]

Cardiac autonomic dysfunction exists in many diabetics; this may increase anginal threshold as a consequence of autonomic and sensory neuropathies. In one clinical series, the severity of cardiac dysfunction was related directly to the severity of cardiac autonomic neuropathy.[130–132] Autonomic dysfunction sometimes results in fixed heart rates that respond poorly to physiologic and pharmacologic interventions; this limits the ability of the heart to physiologically adjust cardiac output. Cardiovascular autonomic neuropathy is a strong risk factor for death in patients with diabetes.[133]

In animal models, experimentally induced diabetes results in ventricular dysfunction that may be at least partially corrected by the administration of insulin.[134] In diabetic rats or rabbits, there develops a cardiomyopathy manifested functionally by decreased contractility, with slowing of both contraction and relaxation.[134, 135] These changes can be reversed by chronic treatment of the diabetic animals with insulin.[134, 135] Therefore, in experimental animals, even relatively acute hyperglycemia and insulin deficiency are associated with detectable alterations in ventricular function.

There is an increased risk for the development of CHF in the diabetic patient, as established in the Framingham Heart Study.[127] This increased risk is present even when patients with prior coronary or rheumatic heart disease are excluded and the influences of age, blood pressure, weight, and cholesterol are taken into consideration.[136] This argues for the presence of a diabetic cardiomyopathy. In patients with diabetes and cardiomyopathy, the most common histologic abnormalities are interstitial fibrosis (Fig. 103–3A) and arteriolar hyalinization (Fig. 103–3B).[137–141] Diabetic dogs and humans exhibit diastolic dysfunction associated with interstitial deposition of periodic acid–Schiff–positive glycoproteins (Fig. 103–3C).[142, 143] Noninvasive studies have revealed a variety of abnormalities in diabetic patients, including increased fractional shortening during systole,[144] asynchrony of early diastole,[145] and slowed diastolic filling.[142] These observations suggest that in selected diabetic patients, there is a cardiomyopathy not based on the presence of myocardial ischemia.[146]

The combination of diabetes and hypertension seems to promote the accelerated development of coronary artery

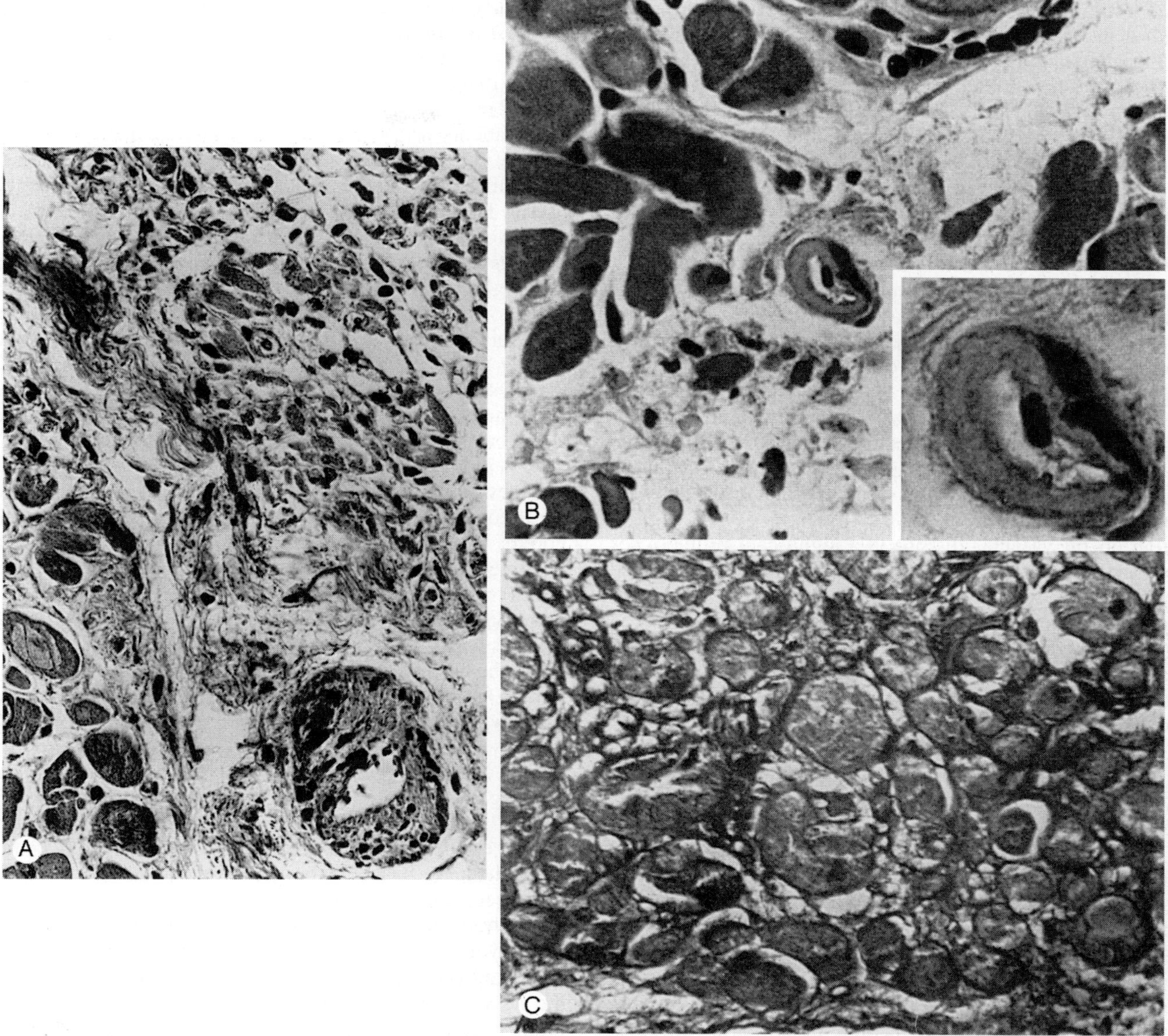

FIGURE 103–3 **A,** Histologic appearance of the myocardium from a patient with diabetes shows arteriolosclerosis and interstitial fibrosis. **B,** Histologic appearance of the myocardium from a patient with diabetes shows hyalinization of a small arteriole. (H&E, × 300.) **Inset,** higher magnification of same arteriole (× 750). **C,** Histologic appearance of myocardium from a patient with diabetes, showing circumferential periodic acid–Schiff–positive material at the periphery of muscle fibers shown in cross section. (PAS stain, × 210.) (**A,** Courtesy of L. Maximilian Buja, M.D. **B,** From Sutherland CG, Fisher BM, Frier BM, et al: Endomyocardial biopsy pathology in insulin-dependent diabetic patients with abnormal ventricular function. Histopathology 14:593, 1989. **C,** From Regan TJ, Lyons MM, Ahmed SS, et al: Evidence of cardiomyopathy in familial diabetes mellitus. J Clin Invest 60:885, 1977.)

disease and cardiomyopathy.[147] Rats with experimental renovascular hypertension and diabetes develop myocardial fibrosis and hypertrophy,[148] as well as microvascular abnormalities.[149] These anatomic lesions are not seen in normotensive diabetic animals.[149–151] Treatment with diltiazem reduces mortality rates in hypertensive diabetic rats, suggesting a pathogenic role for intracellular calcium.[152] Other factors that may contribute to abnormalities in LV function in diabetics include hypertension; increases in GH that develop in patients with difficult-to-control diabetes, which may play a role in the increased collagen deposition in the left ventricles of some diabetics; and an alteration in calcium transport associated with increased sarcolemmal Ca^{2+}-ATPase activity.[153, 154] Increases in sarcolemmal Ca^{2+}-ATPase activity might result in a relative excess of intracellular calcium, contributing to altered diastolic function and injury to heart muscle cells. Some experimental studies have suggested a beneficial effect of the slow calcium channel antagonist verapamil in preventing diabetes-induced myocardial changes in experimental models.[155] Okumura and associates[156] suggested that increased 1,2-diacylglycerol levels with concomitant activation of protein kinase C may play a role in the cardiomyopathy that develops in experimental models. In some experimental models, insulin administration does not correct abnormalities of ventricular function; therefore, the explanation for the development of cardiomyopathy in selected patients with diabetes remains unclear.

In patients with diabetes, cardiovascular disease, hypertension, and nephropathy are closely interrelated. Nephropathy evolves over decades, beginning with glomerular hyperfiltration, followed by the excretion of progressively greater amounts of plasma proteins, and culminating in renal failure.[157] Thickening of mesangial matrix is characteristic of diabetic nephropathy, particularly in the glomerular tuft, where nodular glomerulosclerosis may be found.[158] *Microalbuminuria,* which is defined as consistent excretion of more than 20 μg of albumin/min,[159, 160] predicts cardiovascular mortality rates[161, 162] as well as the development of renal failure.[163–166] Arterial hypertension is also a major risk factor for the development of progressive renal insufficiency.[167–169]

An interesting association with cardiomyopathy is a high prevalence of either septal hypertrophy or CHF in the infants of diabetic mothers.[170] The cardiomyopathy in these infants may be transient and secondary to metabolic problems.

Peripheral vascular disease is a significant problem for patients with diabetes mellitus, sometimes leading to tissue gangrene that requires limb amputation. Small arteries in the feet and below the knee are more likely to be involved in atherosclerosis in patients with diabetes. Cerebral vascular disease and infarction occur more frequently in the diabetic. Renal vasculature may be affected by atherosclerosis in large vessels and by thickening of capillary basement membranes.

Diagnosis

Diabetes mellitus is diagnosed by demonstrating inappropriately high circulating glucose levels. The glycemic criteria for the diagnosis of diabetes were recently revised.[171] For example, fasting plasma glucose levels of higher than 126 mg/dl (7 mmol/L) are considered diagnostic of diabetes. However, the cutoff values should not be interpreted strictly because there is no absolute definition of diabetes. Serum glucose values are continuously distributed in the population,[172] and population studies have disclosed that even among nondiabetic individuals, those with higher levels of glycemia carry greater metabolic and cardiovascular risks.[173, 174] Therefore, the finding of borderline hyperglycemia or impaired glucose tolerance warrants close attention to a patient's cardiovascular risk factors, even if treatment with a hypoglycemic drug is not deemed necessary. The diagnosis of diabetes is strengthened when there is corroborative evidence of diabetic retinopathy, peripheral and coronary vascular disease, peripheral neuropathy, or autonomic dysfunction.

Treatment

The control of blood glucose levels is important for the prevention or retardation of the development of long-term complications of diabetes mellitus.[108, 109] The Diabetes Control and Complications Trial showed that intensive glycemic management of patients with type 1 diabetes substantially reduced the risks of the development or progression of retinopathy, neuropathy, and nephropathy over a period of 3 to 9 years.[110] Studies of patients with type 2 diabetes in Japan and the United Kingdom yielded similar results.[111–113]

In patients with type 1 diabetes mellitus, diet and insulin therapy are critical to management of hyperglycemia. In the future, pancreatic islet transplantation may also be useful. For patients with type 2 diabetes mellitus, diet and regular exercise can improve insulin resistance. Several oral agents, including sulfonylureas,[175, 176] metformin,[177, 178] alpha-glucosidase inhibitors,[179] and thiazolidinediones,[180] alone or in combination, may be effective in lowering glycemia. For reasons unknown, over time there is a continuing decline in pancreatic secretory capability in type 2 diabetes,[181] so treatment with insulin eventually becomes necessary for many patients. Insulin may be administered alone or combined with oral hypoglycemic agents.[181–184]

A randomized, prospective study of patients with type 2 diabetes has shown that intensive treatment of blood pressure reduced complications related to diabetes.[185] It is important to choose antihypertensive drugs carefully. β-Adrenergic–blocking agents reduce complications in patients with type 2 diabetes[186] but entail special risks for patients with type 1 diabetes, especially those attempting strict blood sugar control. In such patients, these drugs, especially the nonselective β-blockers such as propranolol, may impair recovery from hypoglycemia, a situation known as *hypoglycemic unresponsiveness.*[187–190] Regardless of treatment with β-adrenergic–blocking drugs, patients being treated intensively with insulin may have few or no warning signs of hypoglycemia (*hypoglycemic unawareness*),[191, 192] as well as a propensity for hypoglycemic unresponsiveness,[191, 193, 194] adding to the risk for hypoglycemic brain damage. It should be noted that in the patient with preserved hypoglycemic responsiveness, β-blockers will blunt the tachycardia but not the diaphoretic response to hypoglycemia.[188, 190] Furthermore, nonspecific β-blockers may diminish pancreatic secretion of insulin,[195, 196] impair the responsiveness of tissues to insulin,[195, 196] elevate circulating triglyceride levels, and reduce plasma levels of HDL-cholesterol.[195, 197, 198] Care must also be taken with diuretic therapy, which can cause deterioration of insulin resistance in patients with type 2 diabetes mellitus.[199]

Patients with diabetes should be screened for microalbuminuria, defined as consistent excretion of more than 20 μg of albumin/min.[159, 160] Many clinicians consider ACE inhibitors to be the drugs of first choice for the treatment of albuminuria and hypertension in patients with diabetes. ACE inhibitors prevent or retard the progression of diabetic nephropathy,[160, 200] even in normotensive patients. Patients started on ACE inhibitors should be checked for the development of hyperkalemia and deterioration of glomerular filtration.[201]

Among patients with diabetes, hyperlipidemias appear to respond to the same dietary and pharmacologic measures that are appropriate for nondiabetics.[202–204] In patients with type 1 diabetes, excellent blood sugar regulation with insulin can produce normal circulating lipoprotein levels.[205] However, it should be noted that nicotinic acid may exacerbate hyperglycemia by amplifying insulin resistance.[206, 207] In addition, fish oils rich in omega-3 unsaturated fatty acids elevate blood sugar values in patients with type 2 diabetes mellitus, due to inhibition of insulin secretion.[208]

DISORDERS OF CALCIUM METABOLISM

Pathophysiology

Maintenance of the concentration of ionized calcium in extracellular fluid (ECF) within narrow limits is essential for normal neuromuscular excitability and for preservation of skeletal mass. The major hormonal regulator of ECF calcium is parathyroid hormone (PTH), a single-chain polypeptide of 84 amino acids. Its rate of secretion is inversely proportional to the concentration of ionized calcium in ECF, over the physiologic range of calcium values.[209, 210] The relationship between extracellular ionized calcium and secretion of PTH is governed by a calcium-sensing receptor protein that is expressed on the surfaces of parathyroid and renal tubular cells.[211–213] The primary physiologic effect of PTH is to increase the concentration of ionized calcium in ECF. This effect is brought about through augmentation of bone resorption, reduction in the fractional urinary excretion of filtered calcium, and stimulation of phosphaturia. PTH also elevates serum calcium levels by increasing the rate of conversion of 25-hydroxyvitamin D to 1,25-dihydroxyvitamin D, which enhances gastrointestinal absorption of calcium.

PTH has a number of actions on the cardiovascular system, some but not all of which are mediated by hypercalcemia. Administered in vivo or in vitro, PTH produces an increased heart rate and positive inotropic action.[214, 215] These changes are believed to result from entry of calcium into cardiac cells and from increased release of endogenous myocardial norepinephrine. If PTH mediates excessive entry of calcium into cardiac muscle cells, it may also cause necrosis and depressed ventricular function, such as occurs in dystrophic cardiac muscle and in myocardial cells made ischemic followed by reperfusion. In addition, PTH has a direct vasodilatory effect on vascular smooth muscle, although it has not been established whether this is a physiologically relevant action of the hormone.[216]

The major causes of hypercalcemia include primary hyperparathyroidism, secretion of osteolytic factors (e.g., prostaglandins, cytokines, or PTH-related protein[217, 218]) from a variety of neoplasms, and excessive formation of 1,25-dihydroxyvitamin D by the granulomas of sarcoidosis or chronic infections such as tuberculosis.

Primary hyperparathyroidism involves the excessive production of PTH. In many patients, primary hyperparathyroidism is asymptomatic and is discovered as an incidental result of routine laboratory testing. It is most often caused by a solitary parathyroid adenoma. Less frequently, there is generalized parathyroid hyperplasia or carcinoma of the parathyroid gland.[219] The hypercalcemia associated with MEN-I and -II is usually caused by parathyroid hyperplasia. Germline mutations that decrease the sensitivity of the calcium-sensing receptor protein also cause hypercalcemia.[212, 220] Heterozygotes for such mutations have an alteration in the set-point for regulation of PTH secretion,[220a] known as *familial hypocalciuric hypercalcemia*.[212, 220] Secondary hyperparathyroidism, most commonly associated with renal disease, gastrointestinal malabsorption, or a disorder of vitamin D economy, arises from chronic hypocalcemic stimulation of PTH secretion, resulting in hyperplasia of the parathyroid glands.

Hypocalcemia most often arises from renal insufficiency with hyperphosphatemia, inadequate secretion of PTH (*hypoparathyroidism*), cellular resistance to the action of PTH (*pseudohypoparathyroidism*), or some disorder of vitamin D economy. The most important causes of hypoparathyroidism are surgical removal of the glands, usually as the unintended result of operations on the thyroid, and idiopathic hypoparathyroidism, often reflecting immunologically mediated destruction as part of one of the polyglandular autoimmune syndromes.[221] Common problems with vitamin D include dietary deficiency, malabsorption, or some derangement in the multiorgan, multienzyme sequence that produces the final active metabolite, 1,25-dihydroxyvitamin D.

Clinical Manifestations

The typical manifestations of hypercalcemia include polyuria, nocturia, nausea, vomiting, constipation, nonspecific joint and back pains, renal stones, nephrocalcinosis, and renal failure. There is also decreased neuromuscular excitability. In patients with very long-standing or severe hyperparathyroidism, elevation of serum alkaline phosphatase, osteopenia, localized brown tumors of bone, and spontaneous fractures may occur, caused by the effects of PTH on bone. In addition, elevation of urinary cyclic adenosine monophosphate reflects a direct effect of PTH on the kidneys.

Some hypercalcemic patients develop systemic arterial hypertension.[222–224] The precise mechanisms responsible for hypertension in such patients are unclear because the levels of serum calcium are similar in those who are normotensive and those with hypertension. Hypercalcemia may cause deposition of calcium in the renal parenchyma, leading to renal failure and hypertension. Increased serum calcium may also render vascular smooth muscle more sensitive to agents such as angiotensin II and norepinephrine. In patients with hypertension and hyperparathyroidism, the hypertension is not always reversible after surgical correction.[224–226]

Chronic hypercalcemia can lead to ventricular hypertrophy even in the absence of hypertension and to deposition of calcium in the fibrous skeleton of the heart and the valvular tissue and in coronary arteries and myocardial fibers.[227–229] The tendency to extracellular deposition of calcium salts in the heart, lungs, kidneys, and other organs may be estimated by the product of circulating calcium and phosphorus. When the calcium-phosphorus product (each in mg/dl) is greater than 60, there is a risk of metastatic calcification; values over 75 indicate a severe risk. Increases in extracellular calcium lead to subsequent increases in intracellular calcium and may provoke arrhythmias, including fibrillation in isolated cardiac muscle cells.[230] Marked hypercalcemia shortens the QT interval and may lead to ventricular arrhythmias and sudden death in humans.

Hypocalcemia typically produces tetany and other manifestations of neuromuscular hyperexcitability. The ECG effects of hypocalcemia include prolongation of the QT interval and arrhythmias, especially torsades de pointes. In addition, decreases in gastrointestinal motility are often present.

Hypoparathyroidism may cause a dilated cardiomyopathy, presumably secondary to hypocalcemia.[231–234] In these situations, hypomagnesemia and reduced circulating PTH may also contribute.[232, 235]

Diagnosis

Evaluation of a hypercalcemic patient should begin with measurement of the ionized fraction of circulating calcium. If ionized hypercalcemia is confirmed, the next step in differential diagnosis should be determination of PTH dependence through the measurement of intact PTH with a two-site immunoradiometric assay.[236] The combination of hypercalcemia and unequivocally elevated PTH levels most often indicates parathyroid adenoma or hyperplasia. However, one should exclude the diagnosis of familial hypocalciuric hypercalcemia (vide supra).[212] This autosomal dominant condition is characterized by moderate hypercalcemia with some elevation of PTH levels. It has a benign course, usually without renal or osseous complications,[237, 238] and requires no specific treatment. Although the parathyroid glands are usually hyperplastic, parathyroidectomy is of no benefit in familial hypocalciuric hypercalcemia.[237, 238] The keys to diagnosis are the determination of whether other family members are affected and the measurement of urinary calcium excretion. In patients with familial hypocalciuric hypercalcemia, the ratio of calcium to creatinine clearances is less than 0.01.[237, 238]

In a hypocalcemic patient, hypoparathyroidism can be confirmed by the demonstration of inappropriately low serum PTH concentration together with an increased serum phosphorus level. If the PTH level measured with a sensitive two-site assay is not low, another cause of hypocalcemia should be sought.

Treatment

Some patients with asymptomatic primary hyperparathyroidism pursue a relatively benign course, without the development of renal insufficiency, urinary stones, or significant bone disease. However, there is no reliable criterion for prospective identification of this subset of patients.[239, 240] Therefore, if the patient's operative risk is reasonable, surgical removal of the affected parathyroid gland or glands is usually recommended for patients with hyperparathyroidism resulting from parathyroid adenoma or hyperplasia.[239]

If the patient has adequate renal function, the first step in medical treatment of hypercalcemia of any cause should be the restoration of extracellular volume.[241, 242] After volume expansion, intravenous administration of a loop diuretic such as furosemide will promote the excretion of calcium. If these measures do not satisfactorily lower the serum calcium level, several effective drugs are available, including subcutaneous calcitonin, bisphosphonates such as intravenous pamidronate, and intravenous plicamycin (Mithramycin).[242–247] Glucocorticoids are used for the treatment of hypercalcemia caused by excessive circulating 1,25-dihydroxyvitamin D or by some hematologic malignancies.[242, 248] In a patient with hypercalcemia, hypertension should not be treated with a thiazide diuretic, which will promote renal reabsorption of calcium and thereby elevate the serum calcium level.[249, 250]

In patients with hypoparathyroidism, supplementation of calcium is provided by the administration of calcium and vitamin D or one of its metabolites.

HYPERTHYROIDISM

Pathophysiology

Approximately 90 percent of normal thyroid hormone secretion is in the form of thyroxine (T_4), which is thought to be a prohormone. About 99.98 percent of circulating T_4 is bound with high affinity but reversibly to plasma proteins, primarily thyroxine-binding globulin (TBG) and secondarily thyroxine-binding prealbumin. Thyroid hormone action is exerted principally by triiodothyronine (T_3), which is formed by 5′-deiodination of T_4 in the liver and other target tissues. The major actions of T_3 are believed to be mediated via interaction with specific receptors in cell nuclei. T_3 receptors, of which several variants have been described, are members of the steroid receptor superfamily.[251, 252] Initiation of hormonal effects involves a three-way interaction among T_3, T_3 receptors, and specific base sequences of DNA. As a consequence of this binding, alterations occur in gene transcription and protein synthesis, leading to many of the biochemical and metabolic effects observed with thyroid hormone administration.

The net physiologic effect of thyroid hormones on the heart is to increase contractility and heart rate. Increased whole-body oxygen consumption, enhanced cardiac sensitivity to catecholamines, and direct effects of thyroid hormone on the myocardium all may play roles in mediation of these responses. At the cellular level, thyroid hormone increases the activity of plasma membrane Na^+,K^+-ATPase, perhaps via stimulation of synthesis of enzyme subunits. This action results in augmented hydrolysis of *adenosine triphosphate* (ATP) at the site of the sarcolemmal sodium pump, which stimulates cellular oxygen consumption. Thyroid hormone also affects other cellular processes, including transport of glucose and calcium and synthesis of myosin. In addition, treatment with thyroid hormone increases the amount of the mobile cardiac myosin isoenzyme (V_1), whereas the slower V_3 myosin isoform is reduced. Thus, the heart responds to thyroid hormone by enhancing synthesis of a myosin isoenzyme with a rapid ATPase activity.[253–257] The augmented myosin ATPase activity of the hyperthyroid heart appears to contribute to the enhanced contractile response, because the activity of this enzyme regulates the rate of turnover of actin-myosin crossbridge linkages in cardiac muscle. The influence of thyroid hormone on myosin isoenzymes appears to be localized primarily in the ventricles. Hypothyroidism induces opposite effects.[258, 259]

Thyroid hormone also increases peak tension development while shortening the duration of contraction in ventricular muscle. These effects may be related to a more rapid intracellular calcium transit, due to an increase in the number of slow calcium channels with accelerated reuptake of calcium by the sarcoplasmic reticulum.[260–262] Some have suggested that the effects of thyroid hormone on protein synthesis and on myosin isoenzymes in the heart are results of changes in cardiac work rather than direct hormone actions.[263, 264]

Thyrotoxicosis, which is defined as the state of excessive circulating thyroid hormone, can have a variety of causes. The most frequent are (1) production of circulating autoantibodies that activate TSH receptors, producing diffuse toxic goiter (Graves' disease), (2) toxic multinodular goiter or hyperfunctioning solitary thyroid adenoma, (3) subacute thyroiditis, and (4) postpartum and "silent" thyroiditis, probably of autoimmune cause.[265] Less common causes include TSH-secreting adenoma of the pituitary, massive overproduction of chorionic gonadotropin or another low-potency thyroid stimulator in patients with hyperemesis gravidarum or trophoblastic neoplasm,[266, 267] and accidental or purposeful ingestion of thyroid hormone (*thyrotoxicosis factitia*).

The antiarrhythmic drug amiodarone has complex effects on pituitary-thyroid physiology.[268] Patients who receive it are subjected to an immense pharmacologic overload of iodine, which makes up 37 percent of the weight of the drug. Amiodarone is stored in adipose tissue, from which iodide is slowly released into the circulation via slow deiodination.[269, 270] Amiodarone also inhibits both the peripheral and pituitary forms of 5′-deiodinase, the enzymes that convert T_4 to T_3.[270, 271] The normal physiologic response to amiodarone includes elevation of circulating T_4 levels and increases in plasma TSH, which usually return to normal after about 3 months of treatment. In addition, amiodarone may produce hypothyroidism or thyrotoxicosis. In countries such as the United States, with abundant environmental iodine, amiodarone-induced hypothyroidism is more common than thyrotoxicosis.[269] Amiodarone may cause an increase in intrathyroidal Ia–positive T cells, an abnormality found in patients with spontaneous Graves' disease. T cell abnormalities disappear after the discontinuation of amiodarone. Amiodarone may also produce a syndrome of painful inflammatory thyroiditis.[272]

Clinical Manifestations

Patients with hyperthyroidism typically have heat intolerance, warm, moist skin, brittle nails and hair, tremulousness, irritability and emotional lability, increased appetite, weight loss, resting heart rates of more than 90 beats/min, palpitations, muscle weakness, and menstrual abnormalities. On physical examination, a thyrotoxic patient typically has a very active precordium with a right ventricular lift, a palpable pulmonary artery, an enlarged heart, and a systolic ejection murmur. The patient may also have brisk reflexes, a prominent stare, lid lag, a wide pulse pressure, and bounding peripheral pulses. Proptosis and paralyses of extraocular muscles, when they occur, point to Graves' disease as the cause of thyrotoxicosis.

In the young individual, thyrotoxicosis is usually relatively easy to identify, but in elderly patients the typical clinical features may be lacking or far more subtle. Palpable thyroid enlargement or a nodule is present in most patients, but these signs may be absent. The diagnosis of thyrotoxicosis may be delayed or overlooked for long periods of time.

Excessive thyroid hormone causes increases in heart rate, increased cardiac contractility, high cardiac output, increased pulse pressure, shortness of breath with exertion, and generalized weakness.[273–278] Prolonged exposure to even slightly increased amounts of thyroid hormone can lead to cardiac hypertrophy and decreased exercise tolerance.[279] High-output heart failure coexists with thyrotoxicosis in some patients. Cardiac dilatation and hypertrophy, markedly increased cardiac output, and, ultimately, heart failure may develop. The tachycardia observed in hyperthyroidism may be the result of an increased rate of diastolic repolarization and a decreased duration of the action potential in the sinoatrial node cells as a result of exposure to excessive thyroid hormone. The tachycardia may also be a consequence of enhanced cardiac sensitivity to endogenous and exogenous catecholamines resulting from exposure to excess thyroid hormone, although this issue is controversial.[280] Exposure to excessive thyroid hormone increases the number of β-adrenergic receptors without changing their affinity for β-adrenergic agonists, whereas hypothyroidism exerts the opposite effects.[281–283]

Atrial fibrillation with rapid ventricular rate is a particular problem.[276–278] Atrial fibrillation is more common among men than among women with thyrotoxicosis and increases in both sexes with advancing age.[284] Atrial fibrillation occurs in more than 25 percent of thyrotoxic individuals older than 60 years.[284] Even among healthy elderly persons, subclinical hyperthyroidism, manifested only as suppression of TSH levels without thyrotoxic symptoms, entails a threefold increased risk of the development of atrial fibrillation.[285] There is an increased risk for arterial thromboembolism, particularly cerebral thromboembolism, among thyrotoxic patients with atrial fibrillation compared with those in sinus rhythm.[142] The incidence of thromboembolism is highest among patients older than 60 years and in those with preexisting rheumatic or hypertensive heart disease.[284]

Patients with thyrotoxicosis may have angina pectoris, either identified for the first time or aggravated by the increased heart rate, or augmented myocardial contractility with attendant increased myocardial oxygen demand. Most patients with angina and thyrotoxicosis have coronary atherosclerosis, but occasionally the coronary arteries are normal on angiography.[253]

Diagnosis

A measurement of serum TSH below the limits of detection at a reliable laboratory that uses "ultrasensitive" immunoradiometric methodology provides good evidence of thyrotoxicosis. The diagnosis can be confirmed by measurement of circulating thyroid hormones. The serum T_3 level is probably a more reliable index of thyrotoxicosis than is the T_4 level. Due to the frequency with which disease or drugs alter binding of T_4 and T_3 to plasma proteins, one should always obtain an estimate of unbound hormone, such as the free T_4 index, free T_3 index, or T_4 by equilibrium dialysis. If the TSH concentration is low, a high value for one of these indices will confirm the diagnosis of thyrotoxicosis. Measurements of total T_4 and T_3 in the serum may be misleading, because patients with heart disease or other serious illnesses may have decreased peripheral conversion of T_4 to T_3 and decreased plasma protein binding of both hormones.[284] As a result, serum total T_3 concentration and sometimes total T_4 concentration are reduced. Indeed, a normal serum T_3 concentration in a patient with severe cardiac disease suggests that thyrotoxicosis may be present.[284]

Treatment

Management of thyrotoxicosis caused by Graves' disease or toxic nodular goiter is ordinarily begun by treatment with an antithyroid drug, either propylthiouracil or methimazole.[284, 286] These drugs deplete thyroid stores of T_4 and T_3 by inhibiting their synthesis. The antithyroid drug should be administered for several weeks until an euthyroid state is achieved. For patients with severe cardiac manifestations, such as florid CHF, tachyarrhythmia, or unstable angina, more rapid control may be obtained by concurrent treatment with inorganic iodide, which blocks the secretion of thyroid hormones. Methimazole or propylthiouracil should be administered before iodide to prevent conversion of the iodide to thyroid hormone. After a few days, the iodide can be discontinued and the patient can be maintained on an antithyroid drug.

After the patient has been rendered euthyroid with antithyroid drugs, definitive therapy should be undertaken. For patients with Graves' disease and major cardiac problems, thyroidal ablation with radioactive iodine is a preferred definitive therapy.[284] The antithyroid drug may be resumed several days after the administration of radioactive iodine for continued control of symptoms. Ordinarily, several weeks are required for a dose of radioactive iodine to exert its full therapeutic effect. In some patients with Graves' disease, a prolonged course of antithyroid drug together with L-thyroxine may induce spontaneous remission.[287] Surgery is an acceptable alternative therapy for some patients with Graves' disease and often is the preferred form of definitive treatment of toxic nodular goiter. After either radioactive iodine or surgery, hypothyroidism often ensues, eventually requiring treatment with T_4.

Management of amiodarone-induced thyrotoxicosis is an especially vexing problem, for several reasons:

1. Hyperthyroidism can exacerbate the patient's underlying problem with tachyarrhythmias.
2. Antithyroid drugs and ^{131}I are frequently ineffective.
3. The operative risk of thyroidectomy is often high due to underlying ischemic heart disease.
4. Because amiodarone is an antiarrhythmic drug of last resort, its discontinuation may be dangerous. Amiodarone-induced thyrotoxicosis usually appears after months or years of administration of the drug.[288]

There appear to be at least two mechanisms for development of thyrotoxicosis[289]: (1) flooding of iodide into an abnormal gland that has lost its ability to suppress thyroxine production in response to an iodide load; and (2) production of thyroiditis in a previously normal gland. The former variety of amiodarone-induced thyrotoxicosis may be treated with potassium perchlorate together with antithyroid drugs. Patients with amiodarone-induced thyroiditis have been reported to respond to treatment with glucocorticoids.[288]

The management of CHF with thyrotoxicosis includes reducing volume overload with a diuretic, such as intravenous furosemide, and providing control of the heart rate when rapid atrial fibrillation exists. Digoxin or another cardiac glycoside can be administered to slow the rapid ventricular rate, but in the hyperthyroid patient larger doses than usual are often required. This relative resistance is attributed to increased clearance of the digoxin, but it may also be due to the need to inhibit the increased number of Na^+,K^+-ATPase transport units in cardiac muscle. β-Adrenergic blockers such as propranolol help to control heart rate and may be useful, especially in patients without CHF. In the patient with CHF, consideration of using a β-blocker should be carefully reviewed, because such agents may exacerbate heart failure. The decision as to whether to use the agent in a patient with CHF should be based on the extent to which increased heart rate or high-output state is believed to be the cause of the CHF. Esmolol, a rapidly acting β-blocker, can be administered intravenously to allow one to determine potential beneficial or detrimental effects of β-blocking agents in such patients.[290] As an alternative to a β-blocking agent, a slow calcium channel blocker, such as diltiazem or verapamil, can be used to help control heart rate, although the important negative inotropic action of verapamil must be kept in mind.

Treatment of atrial fibrillation in patients with thyrotoxicosis should be directed at controlling the ventricular rate with cardiac glycosides and sometimes with β-blockers or the calcium antagonists diltiazem or verapamil. Successful cardioversion with maintenance of sinus rhythm usually cannot be achieved as long as the thyrotoxicosis continues. Spontaneous reversion of the rhythm to sinus usually occurs within 6 weeks after the return of the euthyroid state, although atrial fibrillation may persist in some older patients. One should consider the use of anticoagulant therapy in a patient with hyperthyroidism and atrial fibrillation. Anticoagulant therapy with warfarin reduces the frequency of embolic events in some patients with atrial fibrillation, but it is associated with an increased risk for hemorrhage. Nevertheless, we recommend anticoagulation for patients with atrial fibrillation and thyrotoxicosis with a dilated heart or heart failure and for those whose rhythm alternates between sinus rhythm and atrial fibrillation.

HYPOTHYROIDISM

Pathophysiology

Hypothyroidism is caused by reduced secretion of T_4, usually as a consequence of destruction of the thyroid gland, often mediated by an autoimmune process, and sometimes after thyroidal surgery or treatment with ^{131}I. Occasionally, hypothyroidism results from decreased secretion of TSH due to pituitary or hypothalamic disease. With secondary hypothyroidism, the signs and symptoms associated with deficiency of other pituitary hormones are often present.

In addition, amiodarone, in common with other organic iodides, inhibits conversion of T_4 to T_3.[271] The drug also interferes with the suppressive actions of T_3 on synthesis and secretion of TSH. These latter actions, exerted at the level of the pituitary, cause increased secretion of TSH.[271]

Clinical Manifestations

Hypothyroidism is twice as common in women as in men. The peak incidence is between the ages of 30 and 60 years. Characteristic symptoms include cold intolerance, dryness of the skin, weakness, impairment of memory and intellectual function, personality change, constipation, hoarseness, menstrual abnormalities, and shortness of breath. Typical physical findings include cold, dry skin; slowed mentation and speech; facial puffiness; and nonpitting edema (myxedema) of the lower extremities. Myxedema reflects a generalized tendency to accumulation of mucopolysaccharide-rich interstitial fluid, which may also be manifested as puffiness of the face and eyes, ascites, pleural or joint effusions, and pericardial effusion (see later). Other classic findings include delayed relaxation of skeletal muscle, as manifested in the Achilles tendon reflex, and the development of a yellowish hue to the skin, resulting from decreased conversion of carotene to vitamin A.

Among hypothyroid patients, exertional dyspnea and easy fatigability are relatively common complaints. Classic cardiovascular physical findings include bradycardia, cardiac enlargement, distant heart sounds, weak arterial pulses, and nonpitting peripheral edema. Less often, there is evidence of CHF. ECG findings include sinus bradycardia, atrioventricular and intraventricular conduction defects, and low voltage.

Hemodynamically, the hypothyroid state is characterized by bradycardia, decreased myocardial contractility, and increased total peripheral resistance.[291] Blood and plasma volumes are reduced, as are stroke volume and cardiac output. Although cardiac enlargement is typical, overt CHF is uncommon.[292–296] When it occurs, CHF is caused by dilated cardiomyopathy.[291] Another important cause of cardiomegaly in hypothyroidism is pericardial effusion, which occurs in up to 30 percent of hypothyroid patients.[291] The effusion is one manifestation of a generalized leakage of protein-rich fluid into interstitial spaces. Cardiac tamponade is unusual but has on occasion been reported as the presenting sign of hypothyroidism.[297]

There are occasional reports of an increased frequency of systemic arterial hypertension in patients with hypothyroidism, although this is not usually seen in patients with severe myxedema.[298, 299] Hypercholesterolemia and hypertriglyceridemia are found in patients with hypothyroidism. Extensive CAD may also be present. Coronary atherosclerosis occurs with twice the frequency in patients with myxedema as in age- and sex-matched control subjects.[300]

Diagnosis

The typical symptoms and physical examination of a patient with hypothyroidism aid in recognition of the condition. However, as is true for hyperthyroidism, in elderly patients some of the classic clinical manifestations of hypothyroidism are subtle or nonexistent.[291] Patients with hypothyroidism may have elevated skeletal muscle enzymes, including creatine kinase, lactic dehydrogenase, and serum glutamic-oxaloacetic transaminase. The mechanisms by which these skeletal muscle enzymes are increased chronically in patients with hypothyroidism is unclear. Measurements of TSH and of serum free T_4 index are the most helpful clinically, with the combination of low serum free T_4 index and increased TSH concentration being diagnostic of hypothyroidism.

Treatment

Patients with hypothyroidism should be treated with T_4.[301] Precipitation or worsening of myocardial ischemia during treatment of hypothyroidism is a clinically important problem.[302] Accordingly, most recommend a low starting dose of T_4, on the order of 0.025 or even 0.012 mg/day, in elderly patients and those predisposed to ischemic heart disease.[301] With such patients, it may be prudent to titrate the dose to less than full replacement levels. For patients at less risk for myocardial ischemia, the starting dose of T_4 may be 0.05 mg/day.[303, 304] The dose may be increased every 4 to 6 weeks until the TSH level is normalized. The usual maintenance dose for adults is about 0.1 to 0.125 mg/day.[303, 304] During this treatment, the patient's cardiovascular condition is monitored carefully, and if there is worsening of angina or marked increases in heart rate or blood pressure, the dose should be reduced to eliminate these effects. In patients with intact pituitary glands, measurement of serum TSH levels provides the most useful marker of the adequacy of replacement therapy.

Treating heart failure in the patient with myxedema is somewhat more complicated than in euthyroid individuals because the patient with myxedema is unusually sensitive to the effects of cardiac glycosides. Patients with unstable or limiting angina and untreated myxedema pose a particularly difficult clinical problem because angina may be exacerbated or an MI may be caused by too vigorous thyroid hormone replacement. One should replace thyroid hormone very carefully in such individuals, with small doses administered as indicated and initial attempts to make the patient comfortable rather than euthyroid. In the patient with extensive CAD and unstable angina, surgical revascularization can be accomplished in association with low-dose thyroid hormone replacement, followed later by full thyroid replacement during the postoperative period. Perioperative morbidity rates are only slightly increased for patients with mild to moderate hypothyroidism.[305, 306] Therefore, necessary cardiovascular surgery need not be postponed until euthyroidism is restored. In the patient with CHF and myxedema without CAD, the careful administration of thyroid hormone in increasing amounts, in association with the use of a diuretic, salt restriction, and digoxin in appropriately small doses, usually leads to the control of CHF in time.

One must be aware of the *euthyroid sick syndrome.*[307–312] Acutely or chronically ill patients often have low serum T_4 and T_3 values without elevation of circulating TSH. The thyroid hormone levels are inversely correlated with survival.[313] The low T_3 values are secondary to decreased extrathyroidal 5′-deiodinase activity, with reduced conversion of T_4 to T_3.[310, 311] The reduced T_4 levels are often related to alterations in protein binding of circulating T_4, causing a decrease in total T_4 but only minimal changes in the level of physiologically active free hormone.[310, 311, 314] There also may be suppression of TSH release due to severe medical illness or drugs such as dopamine. In the euthyroid sick syndrome, the serum TSH is not elevated, which is in contrast with the situation in primary hypothyroidism.[310–312] In difficult cases, further diagnostic discrimination may be obtained through the measurement of serum 3,3,5-triiodothyronine (reverse T_3), the concentration of which typically rises in the euthyroid sick syndrome but declines in hypothyroidism.[310, 311] There is controversy regarding whether individuals with the euthyroid sick syndrome are physiologically hypothyroid, but the administration of T_4 or T_3 does not improve prognosis.[309, 315] A study demonstrated no clinical benefit when T_3 was administered to patients with low circulating T_3 levels accompanying coronary artery bypass graft surgery.[316]

CARCINOID SYNDROME

Carcinoid tumors arise from the neuroendocrine cells of the amine precursor uptake and decarboxylation type in organs derived from the embryonic gut. These tumors can secrete a variety of biologically active substances, including metabolites of serotonin and bradykinin. Release of these substances into the systemic circulation produces the carcinoid syndrome, which includes vasomotor flushes, hypotension, diarrhea, and endocardial thickening, particularly of the right side of the heart, leading to pulmonic stenosis and tricuspid regurgitation.

Pathophysiology

Scattered throughout the organs derived from the embryonic gut are neuroendocrine cells known as *enterochromaffin cells*. These cells, together with other endocrine cells in the thyroid, lung, pancreas, pituitary, and adrenal medulla, constitute the amine precursor uptake and decarboxylation system described by Pearse.[317] Tumors of enterochromaffin cells, which may arise in any of the tissues derived from embryonic entoderm, are known as *carcinoid tumors*. Some carcinoids, especially those arising from the small intestine, stomach, and bronchi, can secrete a wide variety of hormones and other biologically active compounds. Common secretory products of carcinoid tumors are bradykinin, tachykinins, and metabolites of serotonin.[318] In addition, gastric carcinoids typically secrete histamine.[319] Most carcinoid tumors grow slowly and pursue indolent courses. The survival rate is reduced when distant metastases are present.[320]

Clinical Manifestations

The most common clinical elements of the carcinoid syndrome are diarrhea and cutaneous flushes.[320, 321] After years of flushing, patients often develop telangiectases.[322] The appearance of the carcinoid flush may be distinctive for bronchial and gastric carcinoids.[320, 323] Wheezing occurs in a few patients, principally those with bronchial carcinoid. Other endocrine manifestations, such as the ectopic ACTH syndrome, may also be present. It has not been possible to attribute particular symptoms to specific secretory products, with the exception of diarrhea, which appears related to serotonin metabolites. Intestinal and pancreatic carcinoids do not produce the syndrome unless hepatic or systemic metastases are present,[321] presumably reflecting the capability of the liver for first-pass inactivation of their secretory products. The severity of the syndrome is generally correlated with the metastatic tumor burden.[320] Rectal carcinoids do not exhibit evidence of secretory activity and do not produce the syndrome.[320]

One of the striking endocrine manifestations of the carcinoid syndrome involves the heart. It is a matter of controversy whether the cardiac lesions do[320] or do not[324] occur principally in patients with longer-standing, more advanced carcinoid tumors. The typical pathologic lesions are spherical white plaques attached to the luminal surface of the endocardium of the right-sided chambers and of the pulmonic and tricuspid valves, as well as the great veins and coronary sinuses (Fig. 103–4). Carcinoid plaques on the left side of the heart may also be seen at autopsy but are not functionally significant.[325] The predilection for right-sided cardiac lesions presumably reflects inactivation of the responsible hormone or hormones by passage through the lungs. These lesions contain cells embedded in a collagenous stroma, which is rich in glycosaminoglycans but devoid of elastic fibers.[326] The secretory product responsible for development of these lesions may well be serotonin itself. There are correlations between the presence and severity of cardiac valvular lesions and levels of circulating serotonin,[327] as well as excretion of 5-hydroxyindoleacetic acid (5-HIAA).[320] In addition, treatment of obesity with the serotonin reuptake inhibitors fenfluramine and dexfenfluramine has been found to be associated with an increased risk of development of valvular regurgitation, especially of the aortic valve.[328–330] Examination of the affected valves has shown lesions similar to those of the carcinoid syndrome, further strengthening the association between serotonin and valvular disease.[331]

About 20 percent of patients with carcinoid syndrome develop cardiac symptoms.[321] The manifestations of carcinoid heart disease are those typical of pulmonic outflow obstruction, tricuspid regurgitation, or both. Signs and symptoms are those of right ventricular hypertrophy or venous congestion due to tricuspid insufficiency. In long-standing cases, right ventricular failure can occur. The best noninvasive method for diagnosis is two-dimensional echocardiography,[332, 333] although rapid-speed CT scanning and MRI ventriculography should become alternative diagnostic methods in the future.

Diagnosis

For patients with suspected carcinoid syndrome, the diagnosis can best be confirmed through the measurement of excretion of metabolites of serotonin in 24-hour urine collections. For diagnostic purposes, the most important metabolite is 5-HIAA.[320, 321] Because gastric and some bronchial

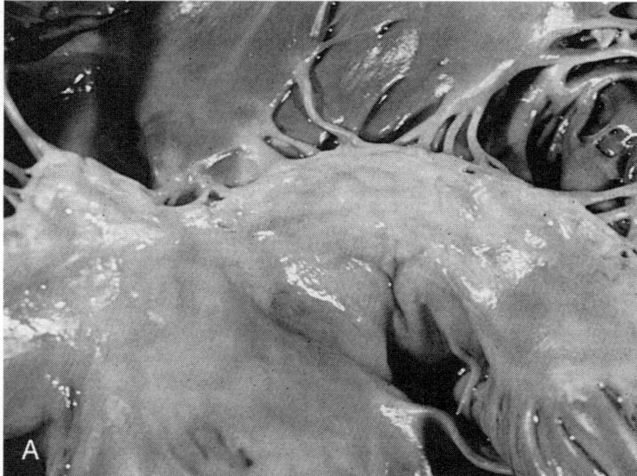

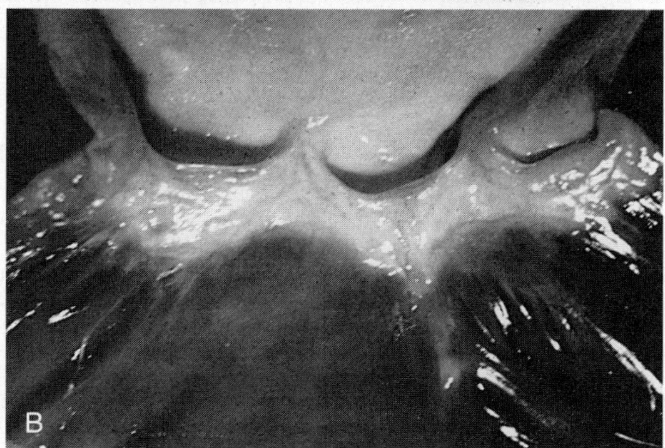

FIGURE 103–4 A, View of the opened tricuspid valve from a patient with carcinoid syndrome shows thickening and contraction of leaflets and chordae tendineae and thickening of the atrial endocardium. **B,** View of the opened pulmonic valve from the same patient shows thickened and retracted cusps and constriction of the valvular ring. (**A** and **B,** Courtesy of L. Maximilian Buja, M.D., from Ferrans VG, Roberts WC: The carcinoid endocardial plaque: An ultrastructural study. Hum Pathol 7:387, 1976.)

carcinoids lack aromatic amino acid decarboxylase,[319, 334] their chief secretory product is 5-hydroxytryptophan rather than serotonin. However, in this situation, urinary 5-HIAA levels are usually elevated anyway due to uptake and decarboxylation of 5-hydroxytryptophan by other tissues.[319, 334]

Treatment

Treatment of carcinoid tumors usually involves surgical removal of accessible tumor, with removal or embolization of hepatic metastases when feasible.[320] In patients with nonresectable tumors, diarrhea can sometimes be controlled with relatively nonspecific serotonin antagonists, such as methysergide maleate or cyproheptadine.[320] In the past, pharmacologic control of flushing was attempted with a variety of agents, including antihistamines, antiserotonins, and inhibitors of prostaglandin synthesis, but the results were often unsatisfactory. An important advance has been the introduction of octreotide, an analogue of somatostatin that controls both diarrhea and flushing.[325] Octreotide must be administered subcutaneously, one to three times daily; longer-acting analogues are under development. Its principal side effects include malabsorption, hypomotility of the gallbladder and formation of gallstones, and mild glucose intolerance. Unfortunately, about 40 percent of patients lose their responsiveness to octreotide after several months of treatment.[320] In general, carcinoid tumors are poorly responsive to standard antineoplastic drugs.[320]

REFERENCES

1. Day SM, Gu J, Polak JM, Bloom SR: Somatostatin in the human heart and comparison with guinea pig and rat heart. Br Heart J 53:153, 1985.
2. DeBoer H, Blok G-J, Van Der Deen EA: Clinical aspects of growth hormone deficiency in adults. Endocr Rev 16:63, 1995.
3. Carroll PV, Christ ER, Bengtsson BA, et al: Growth hormone deficiency in adulthood and the effects of growth hormone replacement: a review. J Clin Endocrinol Metab 83:382, 1998.
4. Sacca L, Cittadinie A, Fazio S: Growth hormone and the heart. Endocr Rev 15:555, 1994.
5. Bates AS, Van't Hoff W, Jones PJ, et al: The effect of hypopituitarism on life expectancy. J Clin Endocrinol Metab 81:1169, 1996.
6. Rosén T, Bengtsson B-Å: Premature mortality due to cardiovascular disease in hypopituitarism. Lancet 336:285, 1990.
7. Shalet SM, Toogood A, Rahim A, et al: The diagnosis of growth hormone deficiency in children and adults. Endocr Rev 19:203, 1998.
8. Aimaretti G, Corneli G, Razzore P, et al: Comparison between insulin-induced hypoglycemia and growth hormone (GH)-releasing hormone + arginine as provocative tests for the diagnosis of GH deficiency in adults. J Clin Endocrinol Metab 83:1615, 1998.
9. Melmed S: Acromegaly. N Engl J Med 322:966, 1990.
10. Baumann G: Growth hormone heterogeneity: genes, isohormones, variants, and binding proteins. Endocr Rev 12:424, 1991.
11. Klapper DG, Svoboda ME, Van Wyk JJ: Sequence analysis of somatomedin-C: confirmation of identity with insulin-like growth factor I. Endocrinology 112:2215, 1983.
12. Underwood LE, Van Wyk JJ: Normal and aberrant growth. *In* Wilson JD, Foster DW (eds): Williams' Textbook of Endocrinology. pp. 1083–1084, 1096–1106. Philadelphia: WB Saunders, 1992.
13. Rinderknecht E, Humbel RE: The amino acid sequence of human insulin-like growth factor I and its structural homology with proinsulin. J Biol Chem 253:2769, 1978.
14. Daughaday WH, Rotwein P: Insulin-like growth factors I and II: peptide, messenger ribonucleic acid and gene structures, serum, and tissue concentrations. Endocr Rev 10:68, 1989.
15. Davidson MB: Effect of growth hormone on carbohydrate and lipid metabolism. Endocr Rev 8:115, 1987.
16. Thuesen L, Christiansen JS, Sorensen JOL, et al: Increased myocardial contractility following growth hormone administration in normal man. Dan Med Bull 35:193, 1988.
17. Ezzat S, Melmed S: Clinical review 18: are patients with acromegaly at increased risk for neoplasia? J Clin Endocrinol Metab 72:245, 1991.
18. Ezzat S, Strom C, Melmed S: Colon polyps in acromegaly. Ann Intern Med 114:754, 1991.
19. Orme SM, McNally RJQ, Cartwright RA, et al: Mortality and cancer incidence in acromegaly: a retrospective cohort study. J Clin Endocrinol Metab 83:2730, 1998.
20. McGuffin WL, Sherman BM, Roth J, et al: Acromegaly and cardiovascular disorders. Ann Intern Med 81:11, 1974.
21. Baldwin A, Cundy T, Butler J, Timmis AD: Progression of cardiovascular disease in acromegalic patients treated by external pituitary irradiation. Acta Endocrinol 108:26, 1985.
22. Lie JT, Grossman SJ: Pathology of the heart in acromegaly. Am Heart J 100:41, 1980.
23. Mather HM, Boyd MJ, Jenkins JS: Heart size and function in acromegaly. Br Heart J 41:697, 1979.
24. Csanady M, Gaspar L, Hogye M, et al: The heart in acromegaly: an echocardiographic study. Int J Cardiol 2:349, 1983.
25. Rossi L, Thiene G, Caregaro L, et al: Dysrhythmias and sudden death in acromegalic heart disease: a clinicopathologic study. Chest 72:495, 1977.

26. Molitch ME: Clinical manifestations of acromegaly. Endocrinol Metab Clin North Am 21:597, 1992.
27. Souadjian JF, Schirger A: Hypertension in acromegaly. Am J Med Sci 254:629, 1967.
28. Moore TJ, Thein-Wai W, Dluhy RG, et al: Abnormal adrenal and vascular responses to angiotensin II and an angiotensin antagonist in acromegaly. J Clin Endocrinol Metab 51:215, 1980.
29. Cain JP, Williams GH, Dluhy RG: Plasma renin activity and aldosterone secretion in patients with acromegaly. J Clin Endocrinol Metab 34:73, 1972.
30. Snow MH, Piercy DA, Robson V, Wilkinson R: An investigation into the pathogenesis of hypertension in acromegaly. Clin Sci Mol Med 53:87, 1977.
31. Ogihara T, Hata T, Maruyama A, et al: Blood pressure to an angiotensin II antagonist in patients with acromegaly. J Clin Endocrinol Metab 48:159, 1979.
32. Hayward RP, Immanuel RW, Nabarro JDN: Acromegalic heart disease: influence of treatment of the acromegaly on the heart. Am J Med 62:41, 1987.
33. Smallridge RC, Rajfer S, Davis K, Schaaf M: Acromegaly and the heart. Am J Med 66:22, 1979.
34. Rodregues EA, Caruana MP, Lahiri A, et al: Subclinical cardiac dysfunction in acromegaly: evidence for a specific disease of heart muscle. Br Heart J 62:185, 1989.
35. Molitch ME: Acromegaly. *In* Collu R, Brown GM, Vanloon GR (eds): Clinical Neuroendocrinology. pp. 189–227. Boston: Blackwell Scientific, 1988.
36. Faglia G, Arosio M, Ambrosi B: Recent advances in diagnosis and treatment of acromegaly. *In* Imura H (ed): The Pituitary Gland. pp. 363–404. New York: Raven, 1985.
37. Stewart PM, Smith S, Seth J, et al: Normal growth hormone response to the 75g oral glucose tolerance test measured by immunoradiometric assay. Ann Clin Biochem 26:205, 1989.
38. Chang-De Moranville BM, Jackson IMD: Diagnosis and endocrine testing in acromegaly. Endocrinol Metab Clin North Am 21:649, 1992.
39. Melmed S, Jackson I, Kleinberg D, et al: Current treatment guidelines for acromegaly. J Clin Endocrinol Metab 83:2646, 1998.
40. Ezzat S, Snyder PJ, Young WF, et al: Octreotide treatment of acromegaly: a randomized multicenter study. Ann Intern Med 117:711, 1992.
41. Lim MJ, Barkan AL, Buda AJ: Rapid reduction of left ventricular hypertrophy in acromegaly after suppression of growth hormone hypersecretion. Ann Intern Med 117:719, 1992.
42. Williams GH, Braunwald E: Endocrine and nutritional disorders and heart disease. *In* Braunwald E (ed): Heart Disease: A Textbook of Cardiovascular Medicine. pp. 1827–1830. Philadelphia: WB Saunders, 1992.
43. Oelkers W: Adrenal insufficiency. N Engl J Med 335:1206, 1996.
44. Knowlton AI, Baer L: Cardiac failure in Addison's disease. Am J Med 74:829, 1983.
45. May ME, Carey RM: Rapid adrenocorticotrophic test in practice. Am J Med 79:679, 1985.
46. Thaler LM, Blevins LS Jr: The low dose (1-μg) adrenocorticotropin stimulation test in the evaluation of patients with suspected central adrenal insufficiency. J Clin Endocrinol Metab 83:2726, 1998.
47. Rose LI, Williams GYH, Jagger PI, Lauler DP: The 48-hour adrenocorticotrophin test for adrenal insufficiency. Ann Intern Med 73:49, 1970.
48. Cushing H: The basophil adenomas of the pituitary body and their clinical manifestations (pituitary basophilism). Bull Johns Hopkins Hosp 50:137, 1932.
49. Saruta V, Suzuki H, Handa M, et al: Multiple factors contribute to the pathogenesis of hypertension in Cushing's syndrome. J Clin Endocrinol Metab 62:275, 1986.
50. Kaplan NM: Cushing's syndrome and congenital adrenal hyperplasia. *In* Kaplan NM (ed): Clinical Hypertension. pp. 422–433. Baltimore: Williams & Wilkins, 1986.
51. Munakata M, Imai Y, Abe K, et al: Involvement of the hypothalamus-pituitary-adrenal axis in the control of circadian blood pressure rhythm. J Hypertens 6(suppl):544, 1988.
52. Piovesan A, Panarelli M, Terzuo M, et al: 24-Hour profiles of blood pressure and heart rate in Cushing's syndrome: relationship between cortisol and cardiovascular rhythmicities. Chronobiol Int 7:263, 1990.
53. Sugihara N, Shimizu M, Kita Y, et al: Characteristics and postoperative courses in Cushing's syndrome. Am J Cardiol 69:1475, 1992.
54. Krieger DT: Physiopathology of Cushing's disease. Endocr Rev 4:22, 1983.
55. Carney JA, Gordon H, Carpenter PC, et al: The complex of myxomas, spotty pigmentation, and endocrine overactivity. Medicine 64:270, 1985.
56. Williams GH, Dluhy RG: Diseases of the adrenal cortex. *In* Wilson J, Braunwald E, Isselbauer KJ (eds): Harrison's Principles of Internal Medicine. 12th ed. pp. 1713–1735. New York: McGraw-Hill, 1991.
57. Kaye TB, Crapo L: The Cushing syndrome: an update in diagnostic tests. Ann Intern Med 112:434, 1990.
58. Yanovski JA, Cutler GB Jr, Chrousos GP, Nieman LK: Corticotropin-releasing hormone stimulation following low-dose dexamethasone administration: a new test to distinguish Cushing's syndrome from pseudo-Cushing's states. JAMA 269:2232, 1993.
59. Loriaux DL, Nieman LK: Corticotropin-releasing hormone testing in pituitary disease. Endocrinol Metab Clin North Am 20:363, 1991.
60. Oldfield EH, Doppman JL, Nieman LK, et al: Petrosal sinus sampling with and without corticotropin-releasing hormone for the differential diagnosis of Cushing's syndrome. N Engl J Med 325:897, 1991.
61. Boggan JE, Tyrrell JB, Wilson CB: Transsphenoidal microsurgical management of Cushing's disease: report of 100 cases. J Neurosurg 59:195, 1983.
62. Nolan PM, Sheeler LR, Hahn JF, Hardy RW Jr: Therapeutic problems with transsphenoidal pituitary surgery for Cushing's disease. Cleve Clin Q 49:199, 1982.
63. White PC: Disorders of aldosterone biosynthesis and action. N Engl J Med 331:250, 1994.
64. Blumenfeld JD, Sealey JE, Schlussel Y, et al: Diagnosis and treatment of primary hyperaldosteronism. Ann Intern Med 121:877, 1994.
65. White PC, Speiser PW: Steroid 11β-hydroxylase deficiency and related disorders. Endocr Metab Clin North Am 23:325, 1994.
66. Kater CE, Biglieri EG: Disorder of steroid 17α-hydroxylase deficiency. Endocr Metab Clin North Am 23:341, 1994.
67. Dluhy RG, Lifton RP: Glucocorticoid-remediable aldosteronism. Endocr Metab Clin North Am 23:285, 1994.
68. Walker BR, Edwards CRW: Licorice-induced hypertension and syndromes of apparent mineralocorticoid excess. Endocr Metab Clin North Am 23:359, 1994.
69. Shimkets RA, Warnock DG, Bositis CM, et al: Liddle's syndrome: heritable human hypertension caused by mutations in the β subunit of the epithelial sodium channel. Cell 79:407, 1994.
70. Kater CE, Biglieri EG, Brust N, et al: Stimulation and suppression of the mineralocorticoid hormones in normal subjects and adrenocortical disorders. Endocr Rev 10:149, 1989.
71. Young WF Jr: Pheochromocytoma and primary aldosteronism: diagnostic approaches. Endocr Metab Clin North Am 26:801, 1997.
72. Bravo EL: Primary aldosteronism. Issues in diagnosis and management. Endocr Metab Clin North Am 23:271, 1994.
73. Rose LI, Underwood RH, Newmark SR, et al: Pathophysiology of spironolactone-induced gynecomastia. Ann Intern Med 87:398, 1977.
74. Wurtman RJ, Axelrod J: Control of enzymatic synthesis of adrenaline in the adrenal medulla by adrenal cortical steroids. J Biol Chem 241:2301, 1966.
75. Steiner AL, Goodman AD, Powers SR: Study of a kindred with pheochromocytoma, medullary carcinoma, hyperparathyroidism and Cushing's disease: multiple endocrine neoplasia, type 2. Medicine 47:371, 1968.
76. Khairi MR, Dexter RM, Burzynski NJ, et al: Mucosal neuroma, pheochromocytoma and medullary thyroid carcinoma: multiple endocrine neoplasia type 3. Medicine 54:89, 1975.
77. Bravo EL, Gifford RW Jr: Current concepts: pheochromocytoma: diagnosis, localization and management. N Engl J Med 311:1298, 1989.
78. Levenson JA, Safar ME, London GM, Simon AC: Haemodynamics in patients with phaeochromocytoma. Clin Sci 58:349, 1980.
79. McManus BM, Fleury TA, Roberts WC: Fatal catecholamine crisis in pheochromocytoma: curable form of cardiac arrest. Am Heart J 102:930, 1981.
80. Cueto L, Arriaga J, Zinser J: Echocardiographic changes in pheochromocytoma. Chest 76:600, 1979.

81. Shub C, Cueto-Garcia L, Sheps SG, et al: Echocardiographic findings in pheochromocytoma. Am J Cardiol 57:971, 1986.
82. Van Vliet PD, Burchell HB, Titus JL: Myocarditis associated with pheochromocytoma. N Engl J Med 274:1102, 1966.
83. Imperato-McGinley J, Gautier T, Ehlers K, et al: Reversibility of catecholamine-induced dilated cardiomyopathy in a child with a pheochromocytoma. N Engl J Med 316:793, 1987.
84. Scott I, Parkes R, Cameron DP: Pheochromocytoma and cardiomyopathy. Med J Aust 148:94, 1988.
85. Manger WM, Gifford RW: Clinical and Experimental Pheochromocytoma. 2nd ed. Chap. 6. Cambridge, MA: Blackwell Scientific, 1996.
86. Maurea S, Cuocolo A, Reynolds JC, et al: Iodine-131-metaiodobenzylguanidine scintigraphy in preoperative and postoperative evaluation of paragangliomas: comparison with CT and MRI. J Nucl Med 34:173, 1993.
87. Landsberg L, Young JB: Catecholamines and adrenal medulla. *In* Wilson JD, Foster DW (eds): Williams' Textbook of Endocrinology. 8th ed. pp. 621–705. Philadelphia: WB Saunders, 1992.
88. Serfas D, Shoback DM, Lorell BH: Phaeochromocytoma and hypertrophic cardiomyopathy: apparent suppression of symptoms and noradrenaline secretion by calcium-channel blockade. Lancet 2:711, 1983.
89. Nerup J, Mandrup-Poulsen T, Molvig J, et al: Mechanisms of pancreatic β-cell destruction in type I diabetes. Diabetes Care 11(suppl 1):16, 1988.
90. Cahill GF Jr, McDevitt HO: Insulin-dependent diabetes mellitus: the initial lesion. N Engl J Med 304:1454, 1981.
91. Atkinson MA, Maclaren NK: The pathogenesis of insulin-dependent diabetes mellitus. N Engl J Med 331:1428, 1994.
92. Todd JA, Bell JI, McDevitt HO: HLA-DQ gene contributes to susceptibility and resistance to insulin-dependent diabetes mellitus. Nature 329:599, 1987.
93. Barnett AH, Eff C, Leslie RDG, Pyke DA: Diabetes in identical twins: a study of 200 pairs. Diabetologia 20:87, 1981.
94. Nerup J, Mandrup-Poulsen T, Molvig J: The HLA-IDDM association: implications for etiology and pathogenesis of IDDM. Diabetes Metab Rev 3:779, 1987.
95. Christau B, Kromann H, Andersen OO, et al: Incidence, seasonal and geographical patterns of juvenile-onset insulin-dependent diabetes mellitus in Denmark. Diabetologia 13:281, 1977.
96. LaPorte RE, Fishbein HA, Drash AL, et al: The Pittsburgh Insulin-Dependent Diabetes Mellitus (IDDM) Registry: the incidence of insulin-dependent diabetes mellitus in Allegheny County, Pennsylvania (1965–1976). Diabetes 30:279, 1981.
97. Newman B, Selby JV, King M-C, et al: Concordance for type 2 (non-insulin-dependent) diabetes mellitus in male twins. Diabetologia 30:763, 1987.
98. Eisenbarth GS, Kahn CR: Etiology and pathogenesis of diabetes mellitus. *In* Becker KL (ed): Principles and Practice of Endocrinology and Metabolism. pp. 1074–1084. Philadelphia: JB Lippincott, 1990.
99. Leahy JL: Natural history of β-cell dysfunction in NIDDM. Diabetes Care 13:992, 1990.
100. DeFronzo RA, Bonadonna RC, Ferrannini E: Pathogenesis of NIDDM: a balanced overview. Diabetes Care 15:318, 1992.
101. Ferrannini E: Insulin resistance *versus* insulin deficiency in non-insulin-dependent diabetes mellitus: problems and prospects. Endocr Rev 19:477, 1998.
102. Gerich JE: The genetic basis of type 2 diabetes mellitus: impaired insulin secretion *versus* impaired insulin sensitivity. Endocr Rev 19:491, 1998.
103. Polonsky KS, Sturis J, Bell GI: Non-insulin-dependent diabetes mellitus: a genetically programmed failure of the beta cell to compensate for insulin resistance. N Engl J Med 334:777, 1996.
104. Taylor SI, Accili D, Imai Y: Insulin resistance or insulin deficiency: which is the primary cause of NIDDM? Diabetes 43:735, 1994.
105. Klein R, Klein BEK, Moss SE: Visual impairment in diabetes. Ophthalmology 91:1, 1984.
106. Williamson JR, Kilo C: Basement membrane physiology and pathophysiology. *In* Alberti KGMM, DeFronzo RA, Keen H, Zimmet P (eds): International Textbook of Diabetes Mellitus. Vol. 2. pp. 1245–1265. New York: John Wiley & Sons, 1992.
107. Factor SM, Okun EM, Minase T: Capillary microaneurysms in the human heart. N Engl J Med 302:384, 1980.
108. Klein R, Klein BEK, Moss SE: The Wisconsin Epidemiological Study of Diabetic Retinopathy: a review. Diabetes Metab Rev 5:559, 1989.
109. Rosenstock J, Raskin P: Diabetes and its complications: blood glucose control vs. genetic susceptibility. Diabetes Metab Rev 4:417, 1988.
110. The Diabetes Control and Complications Trial Research Group: The effect of intensive treatment of diabetes on the development and progression of long-term complications in insulin-dependent diabetes mellitus. N Engl J Med 329:977, 1993.
111. Ohkubo Y, Kishikawa H, Araki E, et al: Intensive insulin therapy prevents the progression of diabetic microvascular complications in Japanese patients with non-insulin-dependent diabetes mellitus: a randomized prospective 6-year study. Diabetes Res Clin Pract 28:103, 1995.
112. UK Prospective Diabetes Study (UKPDS) Group: Intensive blood-glucose control with sulphonylureas or insulin compared with conventional treatment and risk of complications in patients with type 2 diabetes (UKPDS 33). Lancet 352:837, 1998.
113. UK Prospective Diabetes Study (UKPDS) Group: Effect of intensive blood-glucose control with metformin on complications in overweight patients with type 2 diabetes (UKPDS 34). Lancet 352:854, 1998.
114. Stern MP: Diabetes and cardiovascular disease: the "common soil" hypothesis. Diabetes 44:369, 1995.
115. Stern MP: Do non-insulin-dependent diabetes mellitus and cardiovascular disease share common antecedents? Ann Intern Med 124:110, 1996.
116. Dunn FL: Hyperlipidemia in diabetes mellitus. Diabetes Metab Rev 6:47, 1990.
117. Bagdade JD, Bierman EL, Porte D Jr: Diabetic lipemia: a form of acquired fat-induced lipemia. N Engl J Med 276:427, 1967.
118. Taskinen M-R: Lipoprotein lipase in diabetes. Diabetes Metab Rev 3:551, 1987.
119. Garg A, Grundy SM: Treatment of dyslipidemia in non-insulin-dependent diabetes mellitus with lovastatin. Am J Cardiol 62:44J, 1988.
120. Kissebah AH: Low density lipoprotein metabolism in non-insulin-dependent diabetes mellitus. Diabetes Metab Rev 3:619, 1987.
121. Fisher WR: Heterogeneity of plasma low density lipoproteins: manifestations of the physiologic phenomenon in man. Metabolism 32:283, 1983.
122. Haffner SM, Lehto S, Ronnemaa T, et al: Mortality from coronary heart disease in subjects with type 2 diabetes and in nondiabetic subjects with and without prior myocardial infarction. N Engl J Med 339:229, 1998.
123. Gu K, Cowie CC, Harris MI: Mortality in adults with and without diabetes in a national cohort of the U.S. population, 1971–1993. Diabetes Care 21:1138, 1998.
124. Wei M, Gaskill SP, Haffner SM, et al: Effects of diabetes and level of glycemia on all-cause and cardiovascular mortality. Diabetes Care 21:1167, 1998.
125. Stone PH, Muller JE, Hartwell T, et al: The effect of diabetes mellitus on prognosis and serial left ventricular function after acute myocardial infarction: contribution of both coronary disease and diastolic left ventricular dysfunction to the adverse prognosis. J Am Coll Cardiol 14:49, 1989.
126. Herlitz J, Malmberg K, Karlson BW, et al: Mortality and morbidity during a five-year follow-up of diabetics and myocardial infarction. Acta Med Scand 224:31, 1988.
127. Abbott RD, Donahue P, Kannel WB, et al: The impact of diabetes on survival following myocardial infarction in men vs women: the Framingham Study. JAMA 260:3456, 1988.
128. Nesto RW, Phillips RT, Kett KG, et al: Angina and exertional myocardial ischemia in diabetic and nondiabetic patients: assessment by exercise thallium scintigraphy. Ann Intern Med 108:170, 1988.
129. Roy TM, Peterson HR, Snider HL, et al: Autonomic influence on cardiovascular performance in diabetic subjects. Am J Med 87:382, 1989.
130. Ambepityia G, Kopelman PG, Ingram D: Exertional myocardial ischemia in diabetes: a quantitative analysis of anginal perceptual threshold and the influence of autonomic function. J Am Coll Cardiol 15:72, 1990.
131. Zola B, Kahn JK, Juni JE, Vinik AI: Abnormal cardiac function in diabetic patients with autonomic neuropathy in the absence of ischemic heart disease. J Clin Endocrinol Metab 63:208, 1986.

132. Pfeifer MA, Cook D, Brodsky J, et al: Quantitative evaluation of cardiac parasympathetic activity in normal and diabetic man. Diabetes 31:339, 1982.
133. Ewing DJ, Campbell IW, Clarke BF: The natural history of diabetic autonomic neuropathy. Q J Med 49:95, 1980.
134. Fein FS, Strobeck JE, Malhotra A, et al: Reversibility of diabetic cardiomyopathy with insulin in rats. Circ Res 49:1251, 1981.
135. Fein FS, Miller-Green B, Zola B, Sonnenblick EH: Reversibility of diabetic cardiomyopathy with insulin in rabbits. Am J Physiol 250:H108, 1986.
136. Kannel WB, Hjortland M, Castelli WP: Role of diabetes in congestive heart failure: the Framingham Study. Am J Cardiol 34:29, 1974.
137. Zoneraich S: Diabetes and the Heart. Springfield, IL: Charles C Thomas, 1978.
138. Sutherland CG, Fisher BM, Frier BM, et al: Endomyocardial biopsy pathology in insulin-dependent diabetic patients with abnormal ventricular function. Histopathology 14:593, 1989.
139. Rubler S, Dlugash J, Yuceoglu YZ, et al: New type of diabetic cardiomyopathy associated with diabetic glomerulosclerosis. Am J Cardiol 30:595, 1972.
140. Fischer VW, Barner HB, Leskiw ML: Capillary basal laminar thickness in diabetic human myocardium. Diabetes 28:713, 1979.
141. Fisher BM, Gillen G, Lindup GBM, et al: Cardiac function and coronary arteriography in asymptomatic type 1 (insulin-dependent) diabetic patients: evidence for a specific diabetic heart disease. Diabetologia 29:706, 1986.
142. Ruddy TD, Shumak SL, Liu PO, et al: The relationship of cardiac diastolic dysfunction to concurrent hormonal and metabolic states in type I diabetes mellitus. J Clin Endocrinol Metab 66:113, 1988.
143. Regan TJ, Lyons MM, Ahmed SS, et al: Evidence of cardiomyopathy in familial diabetes mellitus. J Clin Invest 60:885, 1977.
144. Thuesen C, Christiansen JS, Mogensen CE, Henningsen P: Cardiac hyperfunction in insulin-dependent diabetic patients developing microvascular complications. Diabetes 37:851, 1988.
145. Sanderson JE, Brown DJ, Rivellese A, Kohner E: Diabetic cardiomyopathy? An echocardiographic study of young diabetics. BMJ 1:404, 1978.
146. Crepaldi G, Nosadini R: Diabetic cardiopathy: is it a real entity? Diabetes Metab Rev 4:273, 1988.
147. Grossman E, Messerli FH: Diabetic and hypertensive heart disease. Ann Intern Med 125:304, 1996.
148. Fein FS, Capasso JM, Aronson RS, et al: Combined renovascular hypertension and diabetes in rats: a new preparation of congestive cardiomyopathy. Circulation 70:318, 1984.
149. Factor SM, Minase T, Cho S, et al: Coronary microvascular abnormalities in the hypertensive-diabetic rat: a primary cause of cardiomyopathy? Am J Pathol 116:9, 1984.
150. Factor SM, Minase T, Bhan R, et al: Hypertensive diabetic cardiomyopathy in the rat: ultrastructural features. Virch Arch [A] 398:305, 1983.
151. Factor SM, Bhan R, Minase T, et al: Hypertensive-diabetic cardiomyopathy in the rat: an experimental model of human disease. Am J Pathol 102:219, 1981.
152. Fein FS, Cho S, Malhotra A, et al: Beneficial effects of diltiazem on the natural history of hypertensive diabetic cardiomyopathy in rats. J Am Coll Cardiol 18:1406, 1991.
153. Schaffer SW, Mozaffari MS, Artman M, et al: Basis for myocardial mechanical defects associated with noninsulin-dependent diabetes. Am J Physiol 256:E25, 1989.
154. Borda E, Pascual J, Wald M, et al: Hypersensitivity to calcium associated with an increased sarcolemmal Ca^{++}ATPase activity in diabetic rat heart. Can J Cardiol 4:97, 1988.
155. Afzal N, Ganguly PK, Dhalla KS, et al: Beneficial effects of verapamil in diabetic cardiomyopathy. Diabetes 37:936, 1988.
156. Okumura K, Akiyama N, Hashimoto H, et al: Alteration of 1,2-diacylglycerol content in myocardium from diabetic rats. Diabetes 37:1168, 1988.
157. Nelson RG, Bennett PH, Beck GJ, et al: Development and progression of renal disease in Pima Indians with non-insulin-dependent diabetes mellitus. N Engl J Med 335:1636, 1996.
158. Mauer SM, Steffes MW, Brown UM: The kidney in diabetes. Am J Med 707:603, 1981.
159. Bennett PH, Haffner S, Kasiske BL, et al: Screening and management of microalbuminuria in patients with diabetes mellitus: recommendations to the Scientific Advisory Board of the National Kidney Foundation from an ad hoc committee of the Council on Diabetes Mellitus of the National Kidney Foundation. Am J Kidney Dis 25:107, 1995.
160. Mogensen CE, Keane WF, Bennett PH, et al: Prevention of diabetic renal disease with special reference to microalbuminuria. Lancet 346:1080, 1995.
161. Messent JWC, Elliott TG, Hill RD, et al: Prognostic significance of microalbuminuria in insulin-dependent diabetes mellitus: a twenty-three year follow-up study. Kidney Int 41:836, 1992.
162. Neil A, Hawkins M, Potok M, et al: A prospective population-based study of microalbuminuria as a predictor of mortality in NIDDM. Diabetes Care 16:996, 1993.
163. Stehouwer CDA, Nauta JJP, Zeldenrust GC, et al: Urinary albumin excretion, cardiovascular disease, and endothelial dysfunction in non-insulin-dependent diabetes mellitus. Lancet 340:319, 1992.
164. Mogensen CE: Microalbuminuria predicts clinical proteinuria and early mortality in maturity-onset diabetes. N Engl J Med 310:356, 1984.
165. Burch-Johnsen K, Kreiner S: Proteinuria: value as predictor of cardiovascular mortality in insulin dependent diabetes mellitus. Br Med J 294:1651, 1987.
166. Jensen T, Burch-Johnsen K, Kofoed-Enevoldsen A, Deckert T: Coronary heart disease in young type I (insulin-dependent) diabetic patients with and without diabetic nephropathy: incidence and risk factors. Diabetologia 30:144, 1987.
167. Parving HH: Impact of blood pressure and antihypertensive treatment on incipient and overt nephropathy, retinopathy, and endothelial permeability in diabetes mellitus. Diabetes Care 14:260, 1991.
168. Rossing P, Hummel E, Smidt UM, Parving HH: Impact of arterial blood pressure and albuminuria on the progression of diabetic nephropathy in IDDM patients. Diabetes 42:715, 1993.
169. Viberti GC, Walker JD: Diabetic nephropathy: etiology and prevention. Diabetes Metab Rev 4:147, 1988.
170. Deorari AK, Saxena A, Singh M, et al: Echocardiographic assessment of infants born to diabetic mothers. Arch Dis Child 64:721, 1989.
171. The Expert Committee on the Diagnosis and Classification of Diabetes Mellitus: Report of the expert committee on the diagnosis and classification of diabetes mellitus. Diabetes Care 20:1183, 1997.
172. Hayner NS, Kjelsberg MO, Epstein EH, Francis T Jr: Carbohydrate tolerance and diabetes in a total community, Tecumseh, Michigan. I. Effects of age, sex, and test conditions on one-hour glucose tolerance in adults. Diabetes 14:413, 1965.
173. Balkau B, Shipley M, Jarrett RJ, et al: High blood glucose concentration is a risk factor for mortality in middle-aged nondiabetic men. Diabetes Care 21:360, 1998.
174. Meigs JB, Nathan DM, Wilson PWF, et al: Metabolic risk factors worsen continuously across the spectrum of nondiabetic glucose tolerance: the Framingham Offspring Study. Ann Intern Med 128:524, 1998.
175. Groop LC: Sulfonylureas in NIDDM. Diabetes Care 15:737, 1992.
176. Melander A, Bitzen P-O, Faber O, Groop L: Sulphonylurea antidiabetic drugs: an update of their clinical pharmacology and rational therapeutic use. Drugs 37:58, 1989.
177. DeFronzo RA, Goodman AM, the Multicenter Metformin Study Group: Efficacy of metformin in patients with non-insulin-dependent diabetes mellitus. N Engl J Med 333:541, 1995.
178. Strumvoli M, Nierjhan N, Perriello G, et al: Metabolic effects of metformin in non-insulin-dependent diabetes mellitus. N Engl J Med 333:550, 1995.
179. Chiasson JL, Josse RG, Hunt JA, et al: The efficacy of acarbose in treatment of patients with non-insulin-dependent diabetes mellitus: a multicenter controlled clinical trial. Ann Intern Med 121:928, 1994.
180. Saltiel AR, Olefsky JM: Thiazolidinediones in the treatment of insulin resistance and type 2 diabetes. Diabetes 45:1661, 1996.
181. U.K. Prospective Diabetes Study Group: U.K. Prospective Diabetes Study 16: overview of 6 years' therapy of type II diabetes: a progressive disease. Diabetes 44:1249, 1995.
182. Turner RC, Holman RR: Insulin use in NIDDM: rationale based on pathophysiology of disease. Diabetes Care 13:1011, 1990.
183. Galloway JA: Treatment of NIDDM with insulin agonists or substitutes. Diabetes Care 13:1209, 1990.
184. Schwartz S, Raskin P, Fonseca V, et al: Effect of troglitazone in insulin-treated patients with type II diabetes mellitus. N Engl J Med 338:861, 1998.

185. UK Prospective Diabetes Study (UKPDS) Group: Tight blood pressure control and risk of macrovascular and microvascular complications of type 2 diabetes: UKPDS 38. BMJ 317:703, 1998.
186. UK Prospective Diabetes Study (UKPDS) Group: Efficacy of atenolol and captopril in reducing risk of macrovascular and microvascular complications in type 2 diabetes: UKPDS 39. BMJ 317:713, 1998.
187. DeFeo P, Bolli G, Perriello G, et al: The adrenergic contribution to glucose counterregulation in type I diabetes mellitus: dependency on A-cell function and mediation through beta$_2$-adrenergic receptors. Diabetes 32:887, 1983.
188. Deacon SP, Barnett D: Comparison of atenolol and propranolol during insulin-induced hypoglycaemia. BMJ 2:272, 1976.
189. Newman RJ: Comparison of propranolol, metoprolol, and acebutolol on insulin-induced hypoglycaemia. BMJ 2:447, 1976.
190. Lager I, Blohme G, Smith U: Effect of cardioselective and nonselective beta-blockade on the hypoglycaemic response in insulin-dependent diabetics. Lancet 1:458, 1979.
191. Gerich JE, Campbell PJ: Overview of counterregulation and its abnormalities in diabetes mellitus and other conditions. Diabetes Metab Rev 4:93, 1988.
192. Clarke WL, Gonder-Frederick LA, Richards FE, Cryer PE: Multifactorial origin of hypoglycemic symptom awareness in IDDM: association with defective glucose counterregulation and better glycemic control. Diabetes 40:680, 1991.
193. Amiel SA, Tamborlane WV, Sacca L, Sherwin RS: Hypoglycemia and glucose counterregulation in normal and insulin-dependent diabetic subjects. Diabetes Metab Rev 4:71, 1988.
194. Lingenfelser T, Renn W, Sommerweck U, et al: Compromised hormonal counterregulation, symptom awareness, and neurophysiological function after recurrent short-term episodes of insulin-induced hypoglycemia in IDDM patients. Diabetes 42:610, 1993.
195. Lithell HOL: Effect of antihypertensive drugs on insulin, glucose, and lipid metabolism. Diabetes Care 14:203, 1991.
196. Pollare T, Lithell H, Selinus H, Berne C: Sensitivity to insulin during treatment with atenolol and metoprolol: a randomized, double blind study of effects on carbohydrate and lipoprotein metabolism in hypertensive patients. BMJ 298:1152, 1989.
197. Stein PP, Black HR: Drug treatment of hypertension in patients with diabetes mellitus. Diabetes Care 14:425, 1991.
198. Weidmann P, Ferrer RC, Sakenhofer H, et al: Serum lipoproteins during treatment with antihypertensive drugs. Drugs 35 (suppl 6):118, 1988.
199. Pollare T, Lithell H, Berne C: A comparison of the effects of hydrochlorothiazide and captopril on glucose and lipid metabolism in patients with hypertension. N Engl J Med 321:868, 1989.
200. Lewis EJ, Unsicker LG, Bain RP, et al: The effect of angiotensin-converting-enzyme inhibition on diabetic nephropathy: the Collaborative Study Group. N Engl J Med 329:1456, 1993.
201. Toto RD: Renal insufficiency due to angiotensin-converting enzyme inhibitors. Miner Electrolyte Metab 20:193, 1994.
202. Garg A, Bonanome A, Grundy SM, et al: Comparison of a high-carbohydrate diet with a high-monounsaturated fat diet in patients with non-insulin-dependent diabetes mellitus. N Engl J Med 319:829, 1988.
203. Garg A, Grundy SM: Diabetic dyslipidemia and its therapy. Diabetes Rev 5:425, 1997.
204. Garg A: Management of dyslipidemia in IDDM patients. Diabetes Care 17:224, 1994.
205. Sosenko JM, Breslow JL, Miettinen OS, Gabbay KH: Hyperglycemia and plasma lipid levels: a prospective study of young insulin-dependent diabetic patients. N Engl J Med 302:650, 1980.
206. Garg A, Grundy SM: Management of dyslipidemia in NIDDM. Diabetes Care 13:153, 1990.
207. Molnar GD, Berge KG, Rosevear JW, et al: The effect of nicotinic acid in diabetes mellitus. Metabolism 13:181, 1964.
208. Glauber J, Wallace P, Griver K, Brechtel G: Adverse metabolic effect of omega-3 fatty acids in non-insulin-dependent diabetes mellitus. Ann Intern Med 108:663, 1988.
209. Pocotte SL, Ehrenstein G, Fitzpatrick LA: Regulation of parathyroid hormone secretion. Endocr Rev 12:291, 1991.
210. Khosla S, Ebeling P, Firek AF, et al: Calcium infusion suggests a "set-point" abnormality of parathyroid gland function in familial benign hypercalcemia and more complex disturbances in primary hyperparathyroidism. J Clin Endocrinol Metab 76:715, 1993.
211. Brown EM, Pollak M, Hebert SC: Sensing of extracellular Ca^{2+} by parathyroid and kidney cells: cloning and characterization of an extracellular Ca^{2+}-sensing receptor. Am J Kidney Dis 25:506, 1995.
212. Brown EM, Pollak M, Seidman CE, et al: Calcium-ion-sensing cell-surface receptors. N Engl J Med 333:234, 1995.
213. Brown EM, Gamba G, Riccardi D, et al: Cloning and characterization of an extracellular Ca^{2+}-sensing receptor from bovine parathyroid. Nature 366:575, 1993.
214. Bogin E, Massry SG, Harary I: Effect of parathyroid hormone on rat heart cells. J Clin Invest 67:1215, 1981.
215. Katoh Y, Klein KL, Kaplan RA, et al: Parathyroid hormone has a positive intropic action in the rat. Endocrinology 109:2252, 1981.
216. Mok LS, Nickols GA, Thompson JC, et al: Parathyroid hormone as a smooth muscle relaxant. Endocr Rev 10:420, 1989.
217. Budayr AA, Nissenson RA, Klein RF, et al: Increased serum levels of a parathyroid hormone-like protein in malignancy-associated hypercalcemia. Ann Intern Med 111:807, 1989.
218. Henderson JE, Shustik C, Kremer R, et al: Circulating concentrations of parathyroid hormone-like peptide in malignancy and in hyperparathyroidism. J Bone Miner Res 5:105, 1990.
219. Aurbach GD, Marx SJ, Spiegel AM: Parathyroid hormone, calcitonin, and the calciferols. *In* Wilson JD, Foster DW (eds): Williams' Textbook of Endocrinology. pp. 1429–1442. Philadelphia: WB Saunders, 1992.
220. Pollak MR, Brown EM, Chou Y-HW, et al: Mutations in the human Ca^{2+}-sensing receptor gene cause familial hypocalciuric hypercalcemia and neonatal severe hyperparathyroidism. Cell 75:1297, 1993.
220a. Khosla S, Ebeling P, Kirek AF, et al: Calcium infusion suggests a "set-point" abnormality of parathyroid gland function in familial benign hypercalcemia and more complex disturbances in primary hyperparathyroidism. J Clin Endocrinol Metab 76:715, 1993.
221. Neufeld M, Maclaren NK, Blizzard RM: Two types of autoimmune Addison's disease associated with different polyglandular autoimmune (PGA) syndromes. Medicine 60:355, 1981.
222. Kleerekoper M, Rao DS, Frame B: Hypercalcemia, hyperparathyroidism and hypertension. Cardiovasc Med 3:1283, 1978.
223. Daniels J, Goodman AD: Hypertension and hyperparathyroidism: inverse relation of serum phosphate level and blood pressure. Am J Med 75:17, 1983.
224. Resnick LM: Calcium, parathyroid disease, and hypertension. Cardiovasc Rev Rep 3:1341, 1982.
225. Diamond TW, Botha JR, Wing J, et al: Parathyroid hypertension: a reversible disorder. Arch Intern Med 146:1709, 1986.
226. Lafferty FW, Hubay CA: Primary hyperparathyroidism: a review of the long-term surgical and nonsurgical morbidities as a basis for a rational approach to treatment. Arch Intern Med 149:789, 1989.
227. Roberts WC, Waller BF: Effect of chronic hypercalcemia on the heart: an analysis of 18 necropsy patients. Am J Med 71:371, 1981.
228. Roberts WC, Waller BF: Chronic hypercalcemia as a risk factor for coronary atherosclerosis. Cardiovasc Rev Rep 4:1275, 1983.
229. Slavich GA, Antonucci F, Sponza E: Primary hyperparathyroidism and angina pectoris. Int J Cardiol 19:266, 1988.
230. Thandroyen FT, Morris AC, Hagler HK, et al: Intracellular calcium transients and arrhythmia in isolated heart cells. Circ Res 69:810, 1991.
231. Huddle KRC: Cardiac dysfunction in primary hypoparathyroidism: a report of 3 cases. South Afr Med J 73:242, 1988.
232. Giles TD, Iteld BJ, Ries KL: The cardiomyopathy of hypoparathyroidism. Chest 79:225, 1981.
233. Rimailho A, Bouchard P, Ahaison G, et al: Improvement of hypocalcemic cardiomyopathy by correction of serum calcium level. Am Heart J 109:611, 1985.
234. Levine SN, Rheams CN: Hypocalcemic heart failure. Am J Med 78:1033, 1985.
235. Csanady M, Forster T, Julesz J: Reversible impairment of myocardial function in hypoparathyroidism causing hypocalcaemia. Br Heart J 63:58, 1990.
236. Nussbaum SR, Zahradnik RJ, Lavigne JR, et al: Highly sensitive two-site immunoradiometric assay of parathyrin and its clinical utility in evaluating patients with hypercalcemia. Clin Chem 33:1364, 1987.
237. Heath H III: Familial (benign) hypocalciuric hypercalcemia: a troublesome mimic of primary hyperparathyroidism. Endocrinol Metab Clin North Am 18:723, 1989.
238. Marx SJ, Attic MF, Levine MA, et al: The hypocalciuric or benign

variant of familial hypercalcemia: clinical and biochemical features in fifteen kindreds. Medicine 6:397, 1981.

239. Consensus Development Conference Panel: Diagnosis and management of asymptomatic primary hyperparathyroidism: Consensus Development Conference statement. Ann Intern Med 114:593, 1991.
240. Scholz DA, Purnell DC: Asymptomatic primary hyperparathyroidism: 10-year prospective study. Mayo Clin Proc 56:473, 1981.
241. Attie MF: Treatment of hypercalcemia. Endocrinol Metab Clin North Am 18:807, 1989.
242. Bilezikian JP: Management of acute hypercalcemia. N Engl J Med 326:1196, 1992.
243. Mundy GR, Wilkinson R, Heath DA: Comparative study of available medical therapy for hypercalcemia of malignancy. Am J Med 74:421, 1983.
244. Perlia CP, Gubisch NJ, Wolter J, et al: Mithramycin treatment of hypercalcemia. Cancer 25:389, 1970.
245. Binstock ML, Mundy GR: Effect of calcitonin and glucocorticoids in combination on the hypercalcemia of malignancy. Ann Intern Med 93:269, 1980.
246. Ralston SH, Gardner MD, Dryburgh FJ, et al: Comparison of aminohydroxypropylidene diphosphonate, mithramycin, and corticosteroids/calcitonin in treatment of cancer-associated hypercalcemia. Lancet 2:907, 1985.
247. Gucalp R, Ritch P, Wiernik PH, et al: Comparative study of pamidronate disodium and etidronate disodium in the treatment of cancer-related hypercalcemia. J Clin Oncol 10:134, 1992.
248. Adams JF: Vitamin D metabolite-mediated hypercalcemia. Endocrinol Metab Clin North Am 18:765, 1989.
249. Sutton RAL: Diuretics and calcium metabolism. Am J Kidney Dis 5:4, 1985.
250. Stier CT Jr, Itskovitz HD: Renal calcium metabolism. Annu Rev Pharmacol Toxicol 26:101, 1986.
251. Evans RM: The steroid and thyroid hormone receptor superfamily. Science 240:889, 1988.
252. Lazar MA: Steroid and thyroid hormone receptors. Endocrinol Metab Clin North Am 20:1, 1991.
253. Glikson M, Freimark D, Leor R, et al: Unstable anginal syndrome and pulmonary oedema due to thyrotoxicosis. Postgrad Med J 67:81, 1991.
254. Gustafson TA, Markham BE, Morkin E: Effects of thyroid hormone on alpha-actin and myosin heavy chain gene expression in cardiac and skeletal muscles of the rat: measurement of mRNA contact using synthetic oligonucleotide probes. Circ Res 59:194, 1986.
255. Litten RZ, Martin BJ, Howe ER, et al: Phosphorylation and adenosine triphosphate activity of myofibrils from thyrotoxic rabbit ears. Circ Res 48:498, 1981.
256. Curfman GD, Crowley RJ, Smith TW: Thyroid-induced alterations in myocardial sodium- and potassium-activated adenosine triphosphatase, monovalent action transport and cardiac glycoside binding. J Clin Invest 59:586, 1977.
257. Samuel JL, Rappaport L, Syrovy I, et al: Differential effect of thyroxine on atrial and ventricular isomyosins in rats. Am J Physiol 250:H333, 1986.
258. Litten RZ III, Martin BJ, Low RB, Alpert NR: Altered myosin isozyme patterns from pressure overloaded and thyrotoxic hypertrophied rabbit hearts. Circ Res 50:856, 1982.
259. Holubarsch C, Goulette RP, Litten R, et al: The economy of isometric force development myosin isoenzyme pattern and myofibrillar ATPase activity in normal and hypothyroid rat myocardium. Circ Res 56:78, 1985.
260. Kim D, Smith TW, Marsh JD: Effect of thyroid hormone on slow calcium channel function in cultured chick ventricular cells. J Clin Invest 80:88, 1987.
261. MacKinnon R, Gwathmey JK, Allen PD, et al: Modulation by the thyroid state of intracellular calcium and contractility in ferret ventricular muscle. Circ Res 63:1080, 1988.
262. Poggesi C, Everets M, Polla B, et al: Influence of thyroid state on mechanical restitution of rat myocardium. Circ Res 60:142, 1987.
263. Klein L, Hong C: Effects of thyroid hormone on cardiac size and myosin content of the heterotopically transplanted rat heart. J Clin Invest 77:1694, 1986.
264. Korecky B, Zak R, Schwartz K, et al: Role of thyroid hormone in regulation of isomyosin composition, contractility, and size of heterotopically isotransplanted rat heart. Circ Res 60:824, 1987.
265. Vargas MT, Briones-Urbana R, Gladman D, et al: Antithyroid microsomal autoantibodies and HLA-DR 5 are associated with postpartum thyroid dysfunction: evidence supporting an autoimmune pathogenesis. J Clin Endocrinol Metab 67:327, 1988.
266. Becks GP, Burrow GN: Thyroid disease and pregnancy. Med Clin North Am 75:121, 1991.
267. Lazarus JH, Othman S: Thyroid disease in relation to pregnancy. Clin Endocrinol 34:91, 1991.
268. Harjai KJ, Licata AA: Effects of amiodarone on thyroid function. Ann Intern Med 126:63, 1997.
269. Martinu E, Safran M, Aghini-Lombardi F, et al: Environmental iodine intake and thyroid dysfunction during chronic amiodarone therapy. Ann Intern Med 101:28, 1984.
270. Trip MD, Wiersinga W, Plomp TA: Incidence, predictability, and pathogenesis of amiodarone-induced thyrotoxicosis and hypothyroidism. Am J Med 91:507, 1991.
271. Burger A, Dinichert D, Nicod P, et al: Effect of amiodarone on serum triiodothyronine, reverse triiodothyronine, thyroxin, and thyrotropin: a drug influencing peripheral metabolism of thyroid hormones. J Clin Invest 58:255, 1976.
272. Roti E, Minelli R, Gardini E, et al: Thyrotoxicosis followed by hypothyroidism in patients treated with amiodarone: a possible consequence of a destructive process in the thyroid. Arch Intern Med 153:886, 1993.
273. DeGroot WJ, Leonard JJ: Hyperthyroidism as a high cardiac output state. Am Heart J 79:265, 1970.
274. Likoff WB, Levin SA: Thyrotoxicosis as the sole cause of heart failure. Am J Med Sci 206:425, 1943.
275. Levin SA, Sturgis CC: Hyperthyroidism masked as heart disease. Boston Med Surg J 190:233, 1924.
276. Sandler G, Wilson GM: The nature and prognosis of heart disease in thyrotoxicosis: a review of 150 patients treated with ^{131}I. Q J Med 28:347, 1959.
277. Summers VK, Surtees SJ: Thyrotoxicosis and heart disease. Acta Med Scand 169:661, 1961.
278. Ikram H: The nature and prognosis of thyrotoxic heart disease. Q J Med 54:19, 1985.
279. Biondi B, Fazio S, Cuocolo A, et al: Impaired cardiac reserve and exercise capacity in patients receiving long-term thyrotropin suppressive therapy with levothyroxine. J Clin Endocrinol Metab 81:4224, 1996.
280. Liggett SB, Shah SD, Cryer PE: Increased fat and skeletal muscle beta-adrenergic receptors but unaltered metabolic and hemodynamic sensitivity to epinephrine in vivo in experimental human thyrotoxicosis. J Clin Invest 83:803, 1993.
281. Hammond HK, White FC, Buxton ILO, et al: Increased myocardial beta-receptors and adrenergic responses in hyperthyroid pigs. Am J Physiol 252:H283, 1987.
282. Brodde OE, Schumann JH, Wagner J: Decreased responsiveness of the adenylate cyclase system in left atria from hypothyroid rats. Mol Pharmacol 17:180, 1980.
283. Whitsett JA, Pollinger J, Matz S: Beta-adrenergic receptors and catecholamine-sensitive adenylate cyclase in developing rat ventricular myocardium: effect of thyroid status. Pediatr Res 16:463, 1982.
284. Woeber KA: Current concepts: thyrotoxicosis and the heart. N Engl J Med 327:94, 1992.
285. Sawin CT, Geller A, Wolf PA, et al: Low serum thyrotropin concentrations as a risk factor for atrial fibrillation in older persons. N Engl J Med 331:1249, 1994.
286. Cooper DS: Antithyroid drugs. N Engl J Med 311:1353, 1984.
287. Hashizume K, Ichikawa K, Sakurai A, et al: Administration of thyroxine in treated Graves' disease. Effects on the level of antibodies to thyroid-stimulating hormone receptors and on the risk and recurrence of hyperthyroidism. N Engl J Med 324:947, 1991.
288. Bartalena L, Brogioni S, Grasso L, et al: Treatment of amiodarone-induced thyrotoxicosis, a difficult challenge: results of a prospective study. J Clin Endocrinol Metab 81:2930, 1996.
289. Bartalena L, Grasso L, Brogioni S, et al: Serum interleukin-6 in amiodarone-induced thyrotoxicosis. J Clin Endocrinol Metab 78:423, 1994.
290. Isley WL, Dahl S, Gibbs H: Use of esmolol in managing a thyrotoxic patient needing emergency surgery. Am J Med 89:122, 1990.
291. Ladenson PW: Recognition and management of cardiovascular disease related to thyroid function. Am J Med 88:638, 1990.
292. Graettinger JS, Muenster JJ, Checchia C: A correlation of clinical and hemodynamic studies in patients with hypothyroidism. J Clin Invest 37:502, 1958.

293. Wieshammer S, Keck FS, Waitzinger J, et al: Left ventricular function at rest and during exercise in acute hypothyroidism. Br Heart J 60:204, 1988.
294. Vora J, O'Malley BP, Petersen S, et al: Reversible abnormalities of myocardial relaxation in hypothyroidism. J Clin Endocrinol Metab 61:269, 1985.
295. McBrion DJ, Hindle W: Myxoedema and heart failure. Lancet 1:1065, 1963.
296. Levey GS, Skelton CL, Epstein SE: Decreased myocardial adenyl cyclase activity in hypothyroidism. J Clin Invest 48:2244, 1969.
297. Zimmerman J, Yahalom J, Bar-On H: Clinical spectrum of pericardial effusion as the presenting feature of hypothyroidism. Am Heart J 106:770, 1983.
298. Streeten DHP, Andersen GH, Howland T, et al: Effects of thyroid function on blood pressure: recognition of hypothyroid hypertension. Hypertension 11:78, 1988.
299. Saito I, Kunihko I, Saruta T: Hypothyroidism as a cause of hypertension. Hypertension 5:112, 1983.
300. Steinberg AD: Myxedema and coronary artery disease: a comparative autopsy study. Ann Intern Med 68:338, 1968.
301. Robuschi G, Safran M, Braverman LE, et al: Hypothyroidism in the elderly. Endocr Rev 8:142, 1987.
302. Keating FR Jr, Parkin TW, Selby JB, Dickinson CS: Treatment of heart disease associated with myxedema. Prog Cardiovasc Dis 3:364, 1960.
303. Fish LH, Schwartz HL, Cavanaugh J, et al: Replacement dose, metabolism and bioavailability of levothyroxine in the treatment of hypothyroidism. N Engl J Med 316:764, 1987.
304. Hennessey JV, Evaul JE, Tseng Y-C, et al: L-Thyroxine dosage: a reevaluation of therapy with contemporary preparations. Ann Intern Med 105:11, 1986.
305. Ladenson PW, Levin AA, Ridgway EC, Daniels GH: Complications of surgery in hypothyroid patients. Am J Med 77:261, 1984.
306. Drucker DJ, Burrow GN: Cardiovascular surgery in the hypothyroid patient. Arch Intern Med 145:1585, 1985.
307. Wehmann RE, Gregerman RI, Burns WH, et al: Suppression of thyrotropin in the low-thyroxine state of severe nonthyroidal illness. N Engl J Med 312:546, 1985.
308. Hamblin PS, Dyer SA, Mohr VS, et al: Relationship between thyrotropin and thyroxine changes during recovery from severe hypothyroxinemia of critical illness. J Clin Endocrinol Metab 62:717, 1986.
309. Brent GA, Hershman JM: Thyroxine therapy in patients with severe nonthyroidal illnesses and low serum thyroxine concentration. J Clin Endocrinol Metab 63:1, 1986.
310. Chopra IJ, Hershman JM, Pardridge WM, Nicoloff JT: Thyroid function in nonthyroidal illnesses. Ann Intern Med 98:946, 1983.
311. Wartofsky L, Burman KD: Alterations in thyroid function in patients with systemic illness: the "euthyroid sick syndrome." Endocr Rev 3:164, 1982.
312. Tibaldi JM, Surks MI: Effects of nonthyroidal illness on thyroid function. Med Clin North Am 69:899, 1985.
313. Kaptein EM, Weiner JM, Robinson WJ, et al: Relationship of altered thyroid hormone indices to survival in nonthyroidal illnesses. Clin Endocrinol 16:565, 1982.
314. Surks MI, Hupart KH, Pan C, Shapiro LE: Normal free thyroxine in critical nonthyroidal illnesses measured by ultrafiltration of undiluted serum and equilibrium dialysis. J Clin Endocrinol Metab 67:1031, 1988.
315. Becker RA, Vaughan GM, Ziegler MG, et al: Hypermetabolic low triiodothyronine syndrome of burn injury. Crit Care Med 10:870, 1982.
316. Klemperer JD, Klein I, Gomez M, et al: Thyroid hormone treatment after coronary-artery bypass surgery. N Engl J Med 333:1522, 1995.
317. Pearse AGE: The cytochemistry and ultrastructure of polypeptide hormone-producing cells of the APUD series and the embryologic, physiologic and pathologic implications of the concept. J Histochem Cytochem 17:303, 1969.
318. Oates JA: The carcinoid syndrome [editorial]. N Engl J Med 315:702, 1986.
319. Oates JA, Sjoerdsma A: A unique syndrome associated with secretion of 5-hydroxytryptophan by metastatic gastric carcinoids. Am J Med 32:333, 1962.
320. Moertel CG: An odyssey in the land of small tumors. J Clin Oncol 5:1503, 1987.
321. Davis Z, Moertel CG, McIlrath DC: The malignant carcinoid syndrome. Surg Gynecol Obstet 137:636, 1973.
322. Sjoerdsma A, Terry LL, Undenfriend S: Malignant carcinoid: a new metabolic disorder. Arch Intern Med 99:1009, 1957.
323. Melmon KL, Sjoerdsma A, Mason DT: Distinctive clinical and therapeutic aspects of the syndrome associated with bronchial carcinoid tumors. Am J Med 39:568, 1965.
324. Ross EM, Roberts WC: The carcinoid syndrome: comparison of 21 necropsy subjects with carcinoid heart disease to 15 necropsy subjects without carcinoid heart disease. Am J Med 79:339, 1985.
325. Kvols LK, Moertel CG, O'Connell MJ, et al: Treatment of the malignant carcinoid syndrome: evaluation of longacting somatostatin analogue. N Engl J Med 315:663, 1986.
326. Ferrans VG, Roberts WC: The carcinoid endocardial plaque: an ultrastructural study. Hum Pathol 7:387, 1976.
327. Robiolio PA, Rigolin VH, Wilson JS, et al: Carcinoid heart disease: correlation of high serotonin levels with valvular abnormalities detected by cardiac catheterization and echocardiography. Circulation 92:790, 1995.
328. Khan MA, Herzog CA, St Peter JV, et al: The prevalence of cardiac valvular insufficiency assessed by transthoracic echocardiography in obese patients treated with appetite-suppressant drugs. N Engl J Med 339:713, 1998.
329. Weissman NJ, Tighe JF Jr, Gottdiener JS, et al: An assessment of heart-valve abnormalities in obese patients taking dexfenfluramine, sustained-release dexfenfluramine, or placebo. N Engl J Med 339:725, 1998.
330. Jick H, Vasilakis C, Weinrauch LA, et al: A population-based study of appetite-suppressant drugs and the risk of cardiac-valve regurgitation. N Engl J Med 339:719, 1998.
331. Connolly HM, Crary JL, McGoon MD, et al: Valvular heart disease associated with fenfluramine-phentermine. N Engl J Med 337:581, 1997.
332. Callahan JA, Wroblewski EM, Reeder GS, et al: Echocardiographic features of carcinoid heart disease. Am J Cardiol 50:762, 1982.
333. Howard RJ, Drobac M, Rider WD, et al: Carcinoid heart disease: diagnosis by two-dimensional echocardiography. Circulation 66:1059, 1982.
334. Sandler M, Scheuer PJ, Watt PJ: 5-Hydroxytryptophan-secreting bronchial carcinoid tumour. Lancet 2:1067, 1961.

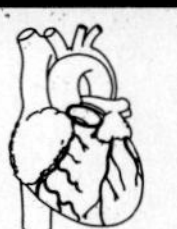

CHAPTER 104

Connective Tissue Diseases and the Heart

Frank C. Arnett and James T. Willerson

CONNECTIVE TISSUE DISEASES
Rheumatoid Arthritis
Systemic Lupus Erythematosus
Scleroderma (Systemic Sclerosis)
Polymyositis and Dermatomyositis
PRIMARY VASCULITIDES
Polyarteritis Nodosum and Variants
Wegener's Granulomatosis
Churg-Strauss Angiitis
Hypersensitivity Angiitis
Giant Cell Arteritis
Takayasu's Arteritis
Kawasaki's Disease
Behçet's Disease
Relapsing Polychondritis
SERONEGATIVE SPONDYLOARTHROPATHIES

The multisystem connective tissue diseases encompass a large number of nosologic entities in which immunologic mechanisms are believed to play central roles in pathogenesis. Each is characterized by distinctive clinical patterns, host susceptibility factors, and in many, serologic markers useful in diagnosis. The heart may be involved in any of these conditions. For each disorder, however, different cardiac structures may be affected, often with unique pathologic lesions, resulting in a variety of clinical cardiovascular sequelae.

Connective Tissue Diseases

Rheumatoid Arthritis

Rheumatoid arthritis (RA) is primarily a chronic progressive polysynovitis of unknown etiology. It leads to progressive joint destruction and disability, as well as to a variety of extra-articular inflammatory lesions (rheumatoid nodules, interstitial lung disease, scleritis, vasculitis, and cardiac lesions) (Fig. 104–1). Immunoglobulin (Ig)M autoantibodies to IgG (rheumatoid factors) are present in the sera and synovia of 80 percent of patients, and immune complexes of anti-IgG/IgG are believed to participate in the articular and extra-articular inflammatory lesions. Genetic predisposition is strongly associated with certain class II major histocompatibility complex (MHC) alleles, especially human leukocyte antigen (HLA)–DR4 and –DR1, which share a specific amino acid sequence in their third hypervariable regions. The severity of joint disease and the occurrence of extra-articular manifestations correlate strongly with high-titer serum rheumatoid factor and homozygosity for the HLA class II susceptibility sequence.[1–4] Paradoxically, methotrexate, the most widely used and effective long-acting therapeutic agent for RA, rarely may induce an accelerated rheumatoid nodulosis syndrome, including many of the cardiac complications described later.[5, 6]

Cardiac structures that may be involved in RA include the pericardium, myocardium, endocardial valves, and coronary arteries[7, 8] (Table 104–1).

Pericardial Disease

Pericardial disease is the most common, with inflammation, granuloma formation, fibrous thickening, and/or small effusions detected in approximately 30 percent of patients during life by echocardiography and in similar frequency at necropsy.[7, 8] However, clinically evident pericarditis with chest pain, fever, and an auscultatory rub is infrequent, occurring in only 2 to 4 percent of patients.[7–9]

Constrictive Pericarditis

Constrictive pericarditis due to pericardial thickening and contracture and/or enlarging effusion is also infrequent but life threatening.[7, 9, 10] The earliest symptoms are usually those of right-sided heart failure with progressive pedal edema and ascites. Later, or when pericardial fluid accumulates rapidly (tamponade), symptoms of left-sided cardiac failure predominate and include dyspnea, orthopnea, and paroxysmal nocturnal dyspnea. Findings on examination include a rapid, weak pulse with paradox, distended jugular veins accentuated during inspiration (Kussmal sign), distant heart sounds, hepatomegaly, and less frequently, a pericardial rub or knock. Clinical suspicion is most important in diagnosis and should lead to a prompt echocardiographic study that, if not definitive, should be followed by cardiac catheterization with pressure studies. In urgent situations in which tamponade is suspected, emergency pericardiocentesis may provide a diagnosis and may be life saving. Rheumatoid pericardial effusions are typically bloody, with elevated white blood cell counts (2000 to 10,000/mm^3), low or absent glucose levels, and low complement levels.[11] Bacterial, mycobacterial, and fungal infections should always be excluded by appropriate stains and cultures of the

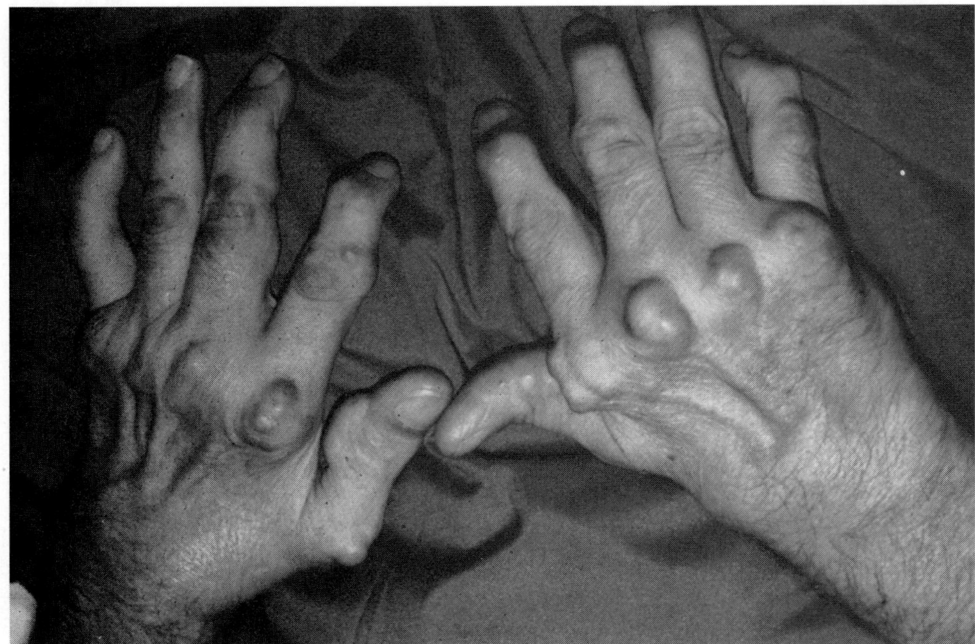

FIGURE 104–1 Rheumatoid arthritis of hands and wrists with symmetric joint swelling, "swan-neck" deformities, and ulnar deviation of the fingers. Multiple subcutaneous (rheumatoid) nodules are also present.

pericardial fluid, as RA patients are often taking corticosteroids or other immunosuppressive drugs.

Relief of cardiac compression and prevention of recurrence are the primary therapeutic goals. Surgical stripping of the pericardium is usually necessary for constrictive pericarditis or compressive pericardial effusions.[9, 12] Before surgery, or when surgery is contraindicated, high doses of oral or IV corticosteroids (60 to 100 mg prednisone equivalent/da), and at times cyclophosphamide (2 mg/kg/da orally or IV), should be given to prevent reaccumulation of fluid.[7, 9] These drugs are not effective for constrictive pericarditis without effusion.

Myocardial Involvement

Myocardial involvement is common at autopsy but is rarely seen clinically.[7, 8] Rheumatoid granulomas have been reported in 3 to 5 percent of cases, and focal nonspecific changes are even more common (Fig. 104–2). Clinical sequelae and treatment depend on the location and extent of myocardial nodulosis. Conduction disturbances may require electrical pacing, and arrhythmias may need appropriate pharmacologic suppression. Heart failure is rare and, if unresponsive to high doses of corticosteroids and cyclophosphamide (see earlier), usually not amenable to other therapies.

Valvular Dysfunction

Valvular dysfunction may also rarely result from rheumatoid nodule deposition.[7] Any of the cardiac valves may be affected, and various degrees of stenosis or regurgitation ensue. A pedunculated, mobile nodule mimicking atrial

TABLE 104–1 Cardiac Manifestations of Rheumatoid Arthritis

Pericardium
Thickening, fibrosis, granulomata, small effusions (30%)
Acute pericarditis (2–4%)
Constrictive pericarditis (rare)
Pericardial tamponade (rare)
Myocardium
Rheumatoid granulomata (rare)
Heart block/conduction disturbances
Arrhythmias
Congestive heart failure
Endocardial Valves
Rheumatoid granulomata (rare)
Valvular stenosis and/or regurgitation
Coronary Arteries
Arteritis (rare)
Myocardial infarction
Global ventricular dysfunction
Arrhythmias

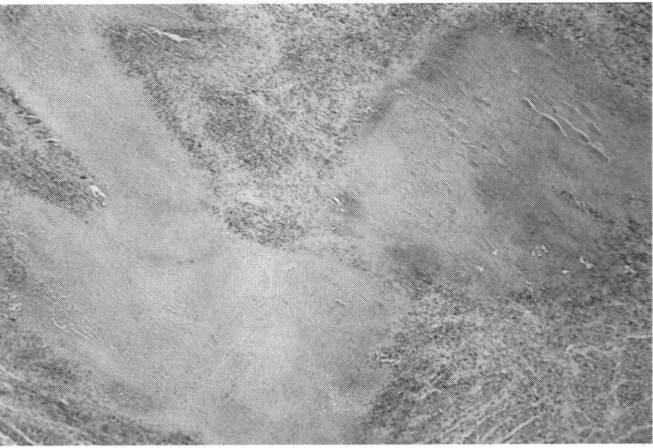

FIGURE 104–2 Histopathology of a typical rheumatoid nodule found in the annulus of the mitral valve at necropsy. Note central zones of necrosis (homogeneous staining material) surrounded by "palisading" histiocytes. (Courtesy of William C. Roberts, M.D., Baylor University Medical Center, Dallas.)

myxoma has been described.[13] Rheumatoid valvular disease is usually mild and rarely requires surgical intervention.

Coronary Vasculitis

Vasculitis of the medium and small coronary arteries is exceedingly rare but may occur within the setting of a generalized systemic vasculitis.[14] Such patients may have frank myocardial infarctions (MIs) or congestive heart failure (CHF) resulting from diffuse myocardial ischemia. Other signs of systemic vasculitis are usually present, including fever, mononeuritis multiplex, ischemic skin, nail, and digital lesions, leukocytosis (often with eosinophilia), and thrombocytosis. Aggressive therapy with high-dose corticosteroids is recommended, usually 80 to 100 mg prednisone equivalent/da (orally or IV and in divided doses), and at times preceded by 3 days each of 1000 mg prednisone equivalent IV (pulse therapy). Consideration should also be given to early initiation of cyclophosphamide (2 mg/kg/da orally or IV) because of the life-threatening nature of this complication. Once cardiac and systemic signs of active vasculitis resolve, prednisone (and later cyclophosphamide) should be tapered slowly over weeks to months with close follow-up of the patient for resurgent signs of vasculitis.

Still's Disease

Still's disease, a systemic disorder, was originally described in children and was subsequently classified, probably erroneously, within the heterogeneous spectrum of juvenile RA.[15, 16] Adult-onset Still's disease is now well recognized. Typical clinical features include high-spiking fever; an evanescent "salmon-colored" rash occurring during times of fever, arthritis, pleurisy, or pericarditis; lymphadenopathy; splenomegaly; and leukocytosis. Serologic testing for rheumatoid factor and antinuclear antibodies (ANA) is typically negative. The disease usually runs a relapsing course over several months and then enters remission without permanent sequelae. However, serious pericardial effusion and/or myocarditis occurs rarely. Serious complications such as cardiac disease require treatment with corticosteroids. Prednisone 60 to 80 mg/da orally or IV and in divided doses should be initiated and continued until cardiac abnormalities resolve or stabilize. Then the daily dose should be tapered over weeks (or months), with frequent monitoring of cardiac signs and symptoms, echocardiograms, and erythrocyte sedimentation rates.

Systemic Lupus Erythematosus

Systemic lupus erythematosus (SLE) is a multisystem autoimmune disease characterized by the potential for inflammatory lesions in many organs (Plate 104–1).[17] The disease may occur in people of any age or race, but young women in the childbearing years are most susceptible, especially blacks and Asians. The etiology of SLE is unknown; however, genetic factors are known to be important, especially hereditary deficiencies of the complement system and certain class II HLA genes (HLA-DR2 and DR3 haplotypes).[17, 18]

Autoantibodies to intracellular nuclear constituents, such as DNA, ribonucleoproteins (e.g., Sm, RNP, Ro, La), and histones, occur characteristically and account for positive ANA tests in more than 95 percent of patients.[17] Autoantibodies to double-stranded DNA and Sm are most disease specific but occur in the minority of patients. Additional autoantibodies are also common, including those to cellular elements (e.g., red blood cells, lymphocytes, platelets, neurons) and plasma components (e.g., IgG, phospholipids). Individual patients with SLE demonstrate their own distinctive profiles of autoantibodies that remain remarkably constant over time. Many of these autoantibodies are associated with and are probably causal for specific clinical manifestations, either via the deposition of antigen-antibody immune complexes or via antibody-mediated tissue damage.

The spectrum of SLE, including its cardiac manifestations and its prognosis, has changed considerably since the early 1960s.[19] With the advent of more sophisticated serologic tests, milder and earlier cases are now recognized. Treatment with corticosteroids and other immunosuppressive agents, as well as more modern antibiotics, antihypertensives, and other drugs, has improved survival from less than 50 percent at 5 years in the 1950s[20] to more than 90 percent at 10 years currently.[21, 22] Concomitantly, the prevalence of lupus carditis has decreased considerably, from being nearly universally present, especially at autopsy, in the precorticosteroid era to 55 percent in 1954, 38 percent in 1971, and 18 percent in 1978.[19] At the same time, there has been an increasing appreciation of premature atherosclerosis as a complication of corticosteroid therapy, nephrotic syndrome, and other factors.[19, 23] In addition, associations or causal relationships have been established between specific autoantibodies and certain cardiac manifestations. Examples include congenital heart block with anti-Ro (SS-A) and La (SS-B) antibodies[24, 25] and valvular disease (Libman-Sacks endocarditis), other cardiac lesions, and intravascular thromboses with antiphospholipid antibodies.[26–28]

Any cardiac structure may be involved in SLE[19, 29–31] (Table 104–2). The presence and extent of pathologic cardiac lesions, however, correlate poorly with clinical manifestations. Acute and/or healed inflammatory lesions scattered focally or diffusely throughout the pericardium, myocardium, valves, and coronary vasculature have been well described, especially in necropsy series. Immunofluorescence studies have demonstrated extensive granular deposits of immunoglobulins and C3 that correlate with the histopathologic changes in these tissues.[32] Therefore, immune complex–mediated injury is believed to be the major cause of lupus carditis rather than autoantibodies that directly target cardiac tissues.[33] In addition, in situ thrombotic events on cardiac valves, other endocardial surfaces, and extracardiac vascular surfaces owing to antiphospholipid antibodies have been recognized more recently as a potential major pathogenetic mechanism.[26–28, 34, 35]

Pericardial Disease

Pericarditis is the most common cardiac complication, occurring in 19 to 48 percent of SLE patients and as the presenting feature in 1 to 2 percent.[19, 29, 30] Clinical features

TABLE 104–2 **Cardiac Complications of Systemic Lupus Erythematosus**

Pericardium
Acute pericarditis
Supraventricular arrhythmias
Pericardial effusions
Pericardial tamponade
Constrictive pericarditis
Myocardium
Myocarditis
Focal inflammatory lesions (immune complexes)
Cardiac "myositis"
Diffuse small vessel thromboses
Endocardium
Libman-Sacks endocarditis
Valvular thickening
Regurgitation and/or stenosis
Intrachamber thrombi
Aortic arch syndrome
Coronary Artery Disease
Premature atherosclerosis
Arteritis
Thrombosis
Other
Pulmonary hypertension
Congenital heart block

include the typical substernal, position-related, pleuritic chest pain, usually confirmed by an auscultatory pericardial rub and typical electrocardiographic changes. Atrial arrhythmias, including flutter and fibrillation, may occur in this setting owing to the close proximity of the sinoatrial node to the pericardium, whereas ventricular ectopy is rare. Echocardiography usually reveals a small pericardial effusion; however, large fluid accumulations with tamponade have been reported (Fig. 104–3A and B). Constrictive pericarditis is rare.[36]

Pericardial fluid associated with SLE shows a mild to moderate inflammatory exudate, occasionally bloody, with white blood cell counts usually in the range of 2000 to 5,000/mm^3, a mildly elevated protein level, and normal glucose levels. LE cells and/or ANAs may be found in the pericardial fluid of seropositive patients but do not discriminate lupus effusions from those with other causes. Complement levels are typically low, and immune complexes have been demonstrated.[19, 37] Pericardiocentesis is rarely necessary for diagnostic purposes, since concomitant pleural effusions exhibiting similar characteristics are usually present and can be aspirated more safely. Prompt removal of pericardial fluid may be life saving when there is tamponade, however, and may be diagnostically necessary when infectious pericarditis is suspected.

The therapy of lupus pericarditis should be dictated by its severity. For mild symptomatic pericarditis, especially without significant pericardial effusion or other serious disease manifestations, indomethacin 75 to 150 mg/da in three divided doses may be effective. Other nonsteroidal anti-inflammatory agents in doses recommended for arthritis may be used alternatively. Most patients, however, require low- to moderate-dose corticosteroids (10 to 40 mg prednisone equivalent/da) to relieve symptoms and/or resolve effusions. Large effusions and/or pericardial tamponade dictates prompt initiation of high doses of intravenous corticosteroids (60 to 100 mg prednisone equivalent in divided doses).

Myocarditis

Myocardial involvement is clinically evident in 8 to 25 percent of reported series.[19] Several pathologic forms have been recognized, including diffuse small vessel obliteration and myocyte destruction, probably as the result of immune complex deposition[19, 38] myocardial cell degeneration and lymphocyte infiltration associated with skeletal myositis, elevated creatine kinase (CK) levels, and anti-nRNP antibodies[39]; and global myocardial ischemia and dysfunction owing to multiple thrombi in small vessels associated with antiphospholipid antibodies.[34, 35]

The earliest clinical manifestations of myocarditis include resting tachycardia, atypical chest discomfort, a gallop rhythm, and nonspecific ST-T wave changes on electrocardiography. More overt signs include cardiomegaly in the absence of pericardial fluid or other causes of cardiac enlargement, CHF, and arrhythmias. Troponin (T and I) levels should be elevated,[40] although there have been no specific studies of lupus myocarditis reported. Echocardiography usually reveals multichamber enlargement, global myocardial dyskinesia, and a reduced ejection fraction. Transendocardial biopsy of the myocardium may be necessary for diagnosis and for determining the type and activity of the disease process.[38] Differential diagnosis should include secondary causes of myocardial dysfunction, such as hypertension, diabetes mellitus, premature atherosclerotic heart disease, and a rare form of vacuolar myocardiopathy associated with chloroquine and other antimalarials used in the treatment of SLE.[41] Active myocarditis requires aggressive corticosteroid therapy along with appropriate measures to control arrhythmias and congestive failure. Prednisone 60 to 100 mg/da in divided doses should be given immediately and the patient's cardiac status monitored closely clinically and by electrocardiography, echocardiography, and levels of CK and troponin T. CHF should be treated as necessary with diuretics, digoxin, nitrates, and/or angiotensin-converting enzyme (ACE) inhibitors. Serious ventricular arrhythmias should be suppressed with appropriate drugs (i.e., lidocaine or procainamide). In fact, although procainamide may induce a lupus-like syndrome, it does not exacerbate idiopathic SLE and can be used safely in such patients. Anticoagulation should also be considered to prevent the formation of mural thrombi, especially when antiphospholipid antibodies, which promote intravascular thrombosis, are present. Once signs of active myocarditis have resolved, prednisone should be tapered slowly over weeks to months with close monitoring (as discussed earlier) for recurrences.

Coronary Artery Disease

Occlusive disease of major coronary arteries with MI has been reported in approximately 4 percent of patients with SLE.[19, 42] Several studies have confirmed a higher than expected rate of MI in women with SLE. Compared with SLE patients without infarctions, these patients tend to be

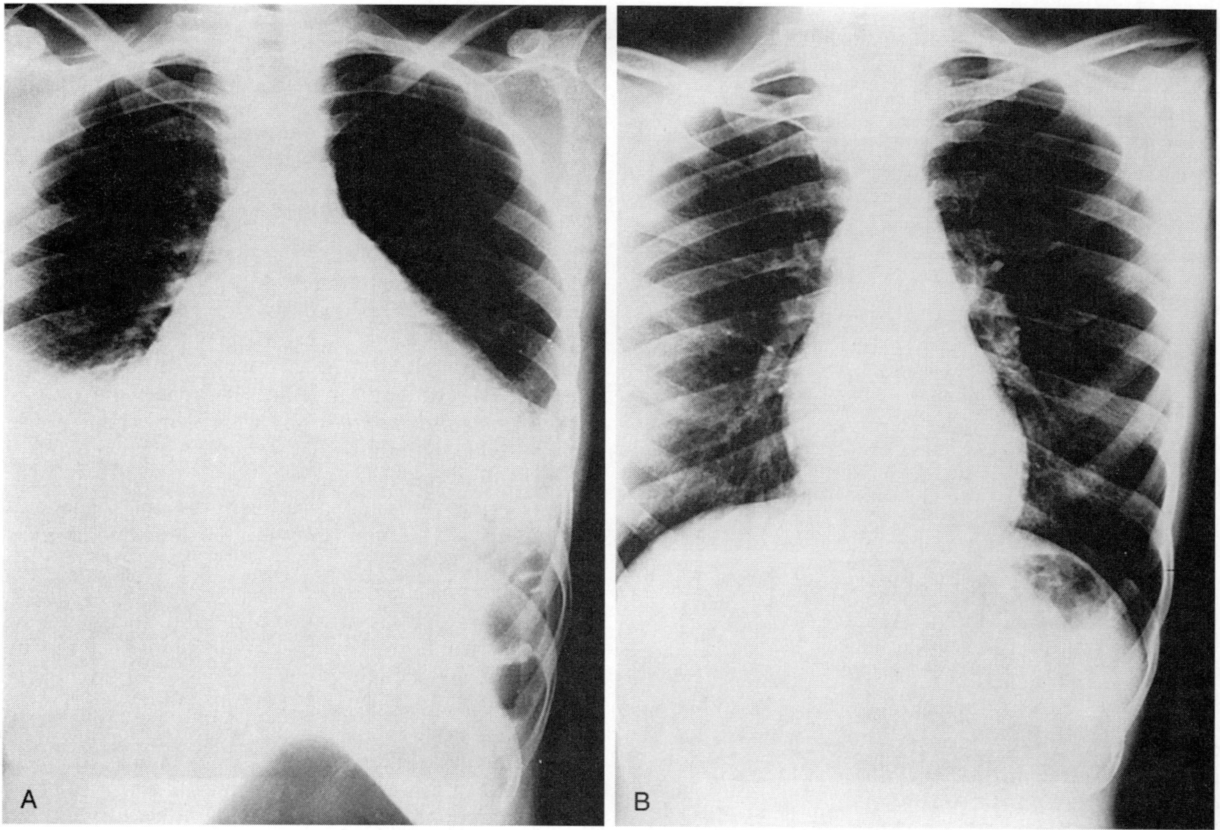

FIGURE 104–3 Chest radiographs of a patient with systemic lupus erythematosus (SLE). **A,** Massive pericardial effusion and bilateral pleural effusions. **B,** Complete resolution of effusions 4 weeks after treatment with corticosteroids.

older and to have a longer duration of disease. There are well-documented cases of MIs occurring in patients in their 20s, often after having had the onset of lupus in childhood.[43, 44] The basis for coronary artery disease in the majority appears to be premature atherosclerosis, possibly as a consequence of acute and chronic vasculitis or as the result of long-term corticosteroid therapy. In some patients, the additional effects of the nephrotic syndrome and/or hypertension may be factors.[23] Previous endothelial cell damage from immune complex disease may be contributory to atheroma formation. Diagnosis and treatment are the same as for usual coronary insufficiency and MI, and all patients receiving corticosteroids should be monitored and treated appropriately for hypercholesterolemia and hypertension.

Coronary artery occlusion resulting from an active vasculitis is rare but has been well documented.[45] It should be suspected when the patient has active signs of lupus, especially vasculitis, affecting other organs. Coronary angiography also may prove helpful diagnostically when a beaded pattern and/or small aneurysms are seen in the coronary artery system. Treatment requires high-dose corticosteroids.

More recently, spontaneous coronary artery thrombosis secondary to the presence of antiphospholipid antibodies has been recognized.[46, 47] In this instance, as in atheromatous disease, the patient may have no other symptoms of active SLE. The presence of a positive lupus anticoagulant with or without a prolonged partial thromboplastin time, a positive test for anticardiolipin antibodies, or a biologic false-positive test for syphilis should raise clinical suspicion of this syndrome. Agents to lyse the coronary thrombus should be given promptly, followed by appropriate anticoagulation.

Valvular Lesions

Valvular involvement in SLE has long been recognized, especially at autopsy; however, it was thought to have little clinical relevance.[19] Libman and Sacks in 1924[48] first described a sterile verrucous endocarditis usually affecting the underside of the mitral leaflets. More recent necropsy studies have found Libman-Sacks endocarditis in approximately 43 percent of lupus patients, with the mitral valve being involved in 24 percent, the aortic valve in 5 percent, the tricuspid valve in 5 percent, and the pulmonic valve in 3 percent.[23, 49] The vegetations appear as small, flat or slightly raised projections adherent to the valve margins, commissures of the leaflets, chordae tendineae, and papillary muscles (Fig. 104–4). Histologically, the vegetations are composed of lymphocytes, plasma cells, fibrous tissue, fibrin, and platelet thrombi, with hematoxylin bodies occasionally observed (Fig. 104–5).[23, 50] Their pathogenesis is believed to arise from fibrin platelet thrombi that subsequently organize on the valve. Ultimately, valvular thickening and fusion of commissures may lead to either valvular regurgitation or stenosis. Although clinical reports most often describe mitral or aortic regurgitation, stenosis of both has been well documented.[51, 52] Occasionally, emboli

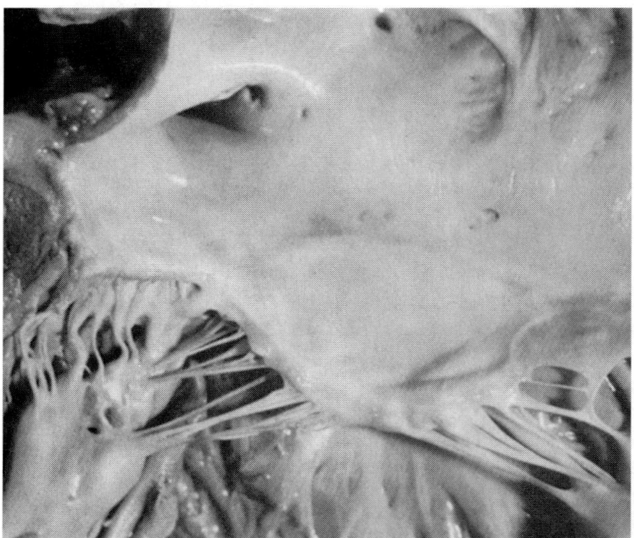

FIGURE 104–4 Necropsy specimen of the left atrium and mitral valve of a patient with SLE. Note focal thickening of the mitral leaflet and chordae tendineae. (From Bulkley BH, Roberts WC: The heart in systemic lupus erythematosus and the changes induced in it by corticosteroid therapy. Circulation 58:243–264, 1975.)

to the coronary or cerebral circulations have been reported.[51]

Transthoracic echocardiographic studies have documented valvular lesions in 18 to 61 percent of patients with SLE.[28, 53] Approximately half of these had verrucous endocarditis and the remainder had rigid and thickened valves showing stenosis, regurgitation, or both. Fifty-four patients with SLE were studied by transesophageal echocardiography.[54] Approximately 50 percent were found to have leaflet thickening, of whom 73 percent had valve regurgitation and 50 percent valve masses. Overall, valve regurgitation was noted in 59 to 64 percent of patients, and it was moderate to severe in one quarter.[54] Over several years of follow-up, almost half of these patients in one study[28] and 22 percent in another,[53] especially those with valvular thickening, required surgical treatment. In addition, a strong association of valvular lesions with circulating antiphospholipid antibodies has been established in several series[26, 27, 55] but not in all.[54, 56] Antiphospholipid antibodies are present in approximately 30 percent of SLE patients when directly measured by anticardiolipin immunoassays and in approximately 7 to 15 percent when detected as a lupus anticoagulant by various coagulation assays.[57–60] A biologic false-positive test for syphilis is another indirect indicator of these autoantibodies. Paradoxically, these antibodies may prolong clotting indices, especially the partial thromboplastin time in vitro (thus the name *lupus anticoagulant*). However, in vivo they promote intravascular clotting. Therefore, patients who have antiphospholipid antibodies may develop spontaneous venous and/or arterial thromboses, including superficial or deep venous clots with pulmonary embolization, cerebrovascular clots with strokes or other neurologic syndromes, digital or extremity ischemia, and a variety of other thrombotic phenomena, including involvement of the cardiac valves. In addition, antiphospholipid antibodies have been associated with recurrent spontaneous abortions, the skin abnormality livedo reticularis (Plate 104–2), and thrombocytopenia.

Other than surgical repair of severely damaged cardiac valves, a therapeutic strategy to prevent valvular damage has not yet been developed.[57] Other thrombotic complications of antiphospholipid antibodies, however, have been shown to be significantly reduced by chronic anticoagulation with warfarin, which maintains the International Normalized Ratio at 3.0.[61] Low-dose aspirin (80 mg/da) probably also has merit in conjunction with warfarin or as the lone prophylactic drug in patients who are found to have antiphospholipid antibodies, but who have had no thrombotic complications. Antimalarials, such as hydroxychloroquine (200 mg/da), may be useful in lowering antiphospholipid antibody levels. Corticosteroids for isolated valvular disease are probably not useful.

A *primary antiphospholipid antibody syndrome* has been described in patients who have clinical thrombotic events associated with positive anticardiolipin antibodies or lupus anticoagulants but who do not have any other features of SLE[62, 63] (Table 104–3). These patients typically have prolonged partial thromboplastin times that are not corrected by the addition of normal plasma. Echocardiographic studies have demonstrated cardiac valvular lesions similar to those of SLE in 36 percent of these patients.[55, 64]

SLE patients, as well as those with primary antiphospho-

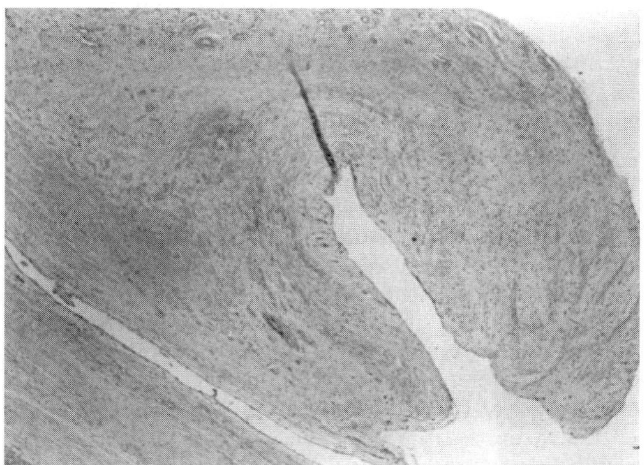

FIGURE 104–5 Histopathology of thickening of the mitral valve leaflet with cellular vascularized fibrous tissue. (From Bulkley BH, Roberts WC: The heart in systemic lupus erythematosus and the changes induced in it by corticosteroid therapy. Circulation 58:243–264, 1975.)

TABLE 104–3 Cardiac Manifestations of Antiphospholipid Antibodies

Verrucous endocarditis (Libman-Sacks)
Embolization to coronaries or extracardiac sites (rare)
Valvular thickening and contracture
Aortic and/or mitral regurgitation and/or stenosis
Coronary vessel thromboses
Myocardial infarction
Global ventricular dysfunction
Mural thrombi (atrial or ventricular)
Aortic arch syndrome

lipid antibody syndrome, may also present with acute coronary artery thromboses and/or global myocardial dysfunction owing to diffuse small vessel clotting.[34, 35] Mural thrombi mimicking atrial myxomata have also been described, as well as the aortic arch syndrome.[65, 66] Therapy should definitely include attempts at clot lysis with thrombolytics, especially early, and anticoagulation, including low-dose aspirin (80 mg/da) and warfarin. Whether corticosteroids are effective is unknown, but in acute situations, these are probably worthy of a trial (60 to 100 mg prednisone/da). Potential benefits in preserving vascular flow must be weighed against deleterious effects on infarct healing; therefore, a corticosteroid trial probably should be brief (1 or 2 days).

Pulmonary Hypertension

Pulmonary hypertension is a rare complication in SLE.[67–69] The majority of patients reported also have had Raynaud's phenomenon and/or other features that suggest overlapping with scleroderma. Similarly, the pathologic findings in small pulmonary arteries are similar to those seen in scleroderma[70, 71] and primary pulmonary hypertension[72] (i.e., that of an obliterative arteropathy characterized by prominent proliferation of the intima) (see Scleroderma).

Congenital Heart Block

The neonatal lupus syndrome (NLE), which includes complete congenital heart block (CCHB) as its most serious manifestation, is a rare disorder that is strongly associated with and probably caused by transplacental passage of maternal autoantibodies to the ribonucleoproteins Ro (SS-A) and La (SS-B).[25, 73, 74] NLE is most commonly manifested as a transient lupus rash in the infant, which disappears at 4 to 6 months' postpartum commensurate with the dissipation of maternal antibodies (Plate 104–3). The majority of anti-Ro/La–positive mothers who bear infants with NLE or CCHB are usually asymptomatic at the time but subsequently develop symptoms of Sjögren's syndrome or, less frequently, SLE.[75] Only a fraction of anti-Ro–positive women produce an abnormal infant, and they almost invariably possess the genetically determined HLA-DR3, DQw2 haplotype. The infants' HLA genes do not appear to be relevant to disease predisposition.[73] Moreover, maternal autoantibodies to certain subspecies of the Ro (52 kD) and La (48 kD) particles increase the likelihood that infants will have the cardiac abnormality.[24] Women who have one child with NLE or CCHD are at high risk (25 percent) for having another affected infant.

Pathologic studies of fetal hearts have shown cellular infiltrates of lymphocytes and plasma cells spread throughout the atrium and ventricle in fetuses that die during the second trimester, whereas calcification and fibrosis have been found in those that die later.[24] In several cases examined, atrial axis discontinuity was apparent, along with replacement of the atrioventricular node by fibrosis or fatty tissue but a normal distal conducting system. Immunofluorescence studies have revealed widespread deposition of immunoglobulins, C3, and fibrin. However, it remains unclear whether the immune reactants contain the anti-Ro and/or -La antibodies.[76–78] Experimental evidence suggests that Ro and/or La antigens may be externally expressed on developing fetal cardiac cells, unlike adult heart tissue, and may serve as targets for direct injury by the autoantibodies.[24, 79]

CCHB appears in the fetus between 18 and 30 weeks of gestation at a time when maternal IgG antibody transfer across the placenta is reaching its peak.[24, 74] Unexpected fetal bradycardia, detected during routine monitoring or at the time of premature labor, is the first sign. The diagnosis is confirmed by fetal electrocardiography, the absence of congenital structural cardiac abnormalities on ultrasonography, and the presence of maternal anti-Ro/La antibodies. When fetal heart block occurs early, death in utero is common; when late, a variable infant is usually delivered, who may at the time or later require a cardiac pacemaker. In addition, the extent of myocardial damage, usually assessed by ultrasonography, provides another element critical to survival. Early detection in utero of an affected but viable fetus provides several potential therapeutic options, including dexamethasone, which crosses the placenta and may suppress cardiac inflammation, and plasmapheresis of the mother to lower anti-Ro/La antibody levels.[80]

Drug-Induced Lupus

A variety of drugs have been reported to cause a lupus-like syndrome and a definite association has been established for a few (Table 104–4). High-dose, long-term procainamide induces a positive ANA in 50 to 75 percent of treated patients, and a lupus-like syndrome occurs in up to 30 percent.[81, 82] Males and females are affected equally in drug-induced lupus. Arthralgias and arthritis are the most common clinical manifestations, followed by pleuropulmonary disease in 33 to 52 percent. Pericarditis occurs in 14 to 18 percent and rarely has been reported to cause tamponade or constriction. Other cardiac complications have not been reported; however, procainamide, like chlorpromazine, may also induce formation of antiphospholipid antibodies.[83] Quinidine less commonly may induce lupus or an arthritis syndrome resembling RA or polymyalgia rheumatica.[84, 85] Renal disease and antibodies to double-stranded DNA are uncommon in drug-induced lupus, and the prognosis in these patients is generally excellent, with the SLE-like illness usually disappearing when the drug is discontinued.

Scleroderma (Systemic Sclerosis)

Scleroderma or systemic sclerosis (SSc) is a chronic multisystem disease characterized by widespread fibrosis and obliterative vascular lesions of the skin and other organs, especially the lungs, heart, kidneys, and gastrointestinal tract.[86] Raynaud's phenomenon occurs in more than 90 percent of cases and is the first symptom in the majority of patients. Typically, skin thickening begins in the distal extremities and progresses centrally, resulting in progressive joint contractures, muscle atrophy, and restricted movement (Plate 104–4). A limited form of the disease is the CREST syndrome (calcinosis, Raynaud's phenomena, esophageal dysmotility, sclerodactyly, and telangiectasia), in which skin and major organ involvement is limited and

TABLE 104–4 Drugs That May Cause Lupus-Like Syndrome

	Frequency of Induction of ANA	Frequency of Induction of Lupus-Like Disease
Definitely Implicated		
Procainamide	50–75%	Up to 30%
Hydralazine	24–54%	2–21%
Isoniazid	20–25%	<1%
Chlorpromazine	20–50%	Uncommon
Methyldopa	14–18%	Uncommon
Quinidine	Rare	Rare
Penicillamine	Rare	Rare
Possibly Implicated		
Diphenylhydantoin		
Phenytoin		
Carbamazepine		
Ethosuxamide		
Trimethadione		
Mephenytoin		
Propythiouracil		
Methimazole		
Practolol		
Atenolol		
Acebutolol		
Propranolol		
Pindolol		
Metoprotal		
Labetalol		
Oxyprenolol		
Captopril		
Sulfasalazine		
Nitrofurantoin		
Lithium		
Levadopa		
Hydrazine		
Phenylzine		
Sulfonamides		
Cimetidine		

Abbreviation: ANA, antinuclear antibody.

the prognosis good (Plate 104–5). Even more localized cutaneous forms of scleroderma include morphea and linear scleroderma, which are not associated with Raynaud's phenomenon or visceral involvement.

Clinical features of SSc often overlap with those of SLE, myositis, and RA, especially in the entity known as *mixed connective tissue disease.*[87] Moreover, SSc in many ways resembles chronic graft-versus-host disease.[88] ANAs are present in 90 percent of patients with SSc, and include some targets that are highly disease specific, such as anticentromere, antitopoisomerase I (Scl-70), and a variety of antinucleolar antibodies.[89, 90] Moreover, different autoantibodies tend to be markers of certain clinical manifestations of SSc. For example, anticentromere antibodies are found in the majority of patients with the CREST syndrome or mild scleroderma and indicate a generally good prognosis (Plate 104–6). Conversely, antitopoisomerase I antibodies correlate with diffuse skin and visceral involvement, especially pulmonary fibrosis, and anti-nRNP and anti-PM-Scl antibodies are associated with complicating myositis. Because of these observations, an immunologic basis for SSc is strongly suspected but poorly understood.[90]

Cardiac involvement in SSc may be caused primarily by the disease itself (myocardial or pericardial scleroderma) or secondarily by pulmonary and/or systemic hypertension.

Myocardial Involvement

The characteristic myocardial lesion of SSc is a patchy fibrosis distributed randomly throughout the right and left ventricles.[70, 86, 91–96] Myocardial fibrosis is frequently found at autopsy, but its actual prevalence in SSc remains unknown (see later). Unlike the fibrosis of coronary atherosclerosis, it does not spare the subendocardial layer and it is not associated with hemosiderin deposition. Ventricular size and weight are usually normal unless pulmonary or systemic hypertension is also present. Myocardial tissue appears to be replaced rather than infiltrated by fibrosis.

The cause of the fibrosis is unknown, but there is considerable evidence suggesting ischemic injury from diseased intramyocardial small arteries and arterioles.[70, 86] The epicardial coronary artery system is normal, unless there is the fortuitous co-occurrence of atherosclerosis. An obliterative vasculopathy of intramyocardial arteries and arterioles, similar to that found in lungs, kidneys, and digital arteries, has been reported in several necropsy studies (Fig. 104–6),[70, 71] but it is not thought by some to adequately explain the degree of myocardial fibrosis. Contraction band necrosis has also been described in postmortem hearts, suggesting that reperfusion injury may cause the fibrosis.[91, 97] This observation first led to the concept of "myocardial Raynaud's phenomenon,"[91] which has subsequently been supported further by the findings of reversible cold-induced abnormalities of myocardial perfusion observed by thallium 201 scintigraphy.[98–100] Transient segmental areas of hypokinesis demonstrated by two-dimensional echocardiography appear to correlate with these lesions. In some studies, these abnormalities appeared to be prevented by the use of nifedipine.[99] The concept of recurrent vasospasm of intramural coronary arteries leading to transient ischemia, reperfusion injury, and subsequent fibrosis is

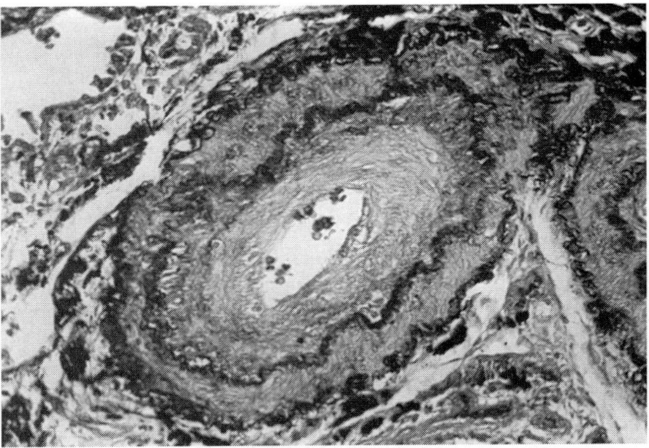

FIGURE 104–6 Photomicrograph of a small pulmonary artery in a patient with scleroderma and rapidly progressive pulmonary hypertension. Note extensive obliterative proliferation of the intima and the lack of inflammatory cells. Similar vascular lesions characterize the digital, cardiac, renal, and other organs involved. (Courtesy of William C. Roberts, M.D., Baylor University Medical Center, Dallas.)

compelling but controversial.[101] Echocardiographic studies suggest impaired relaxation of the left ventricle as a contributing cause to a defective cardiac functional reserve in scleroderma heart disease,[102] as well as correlations between certain echocardiographic patterns and extent of skin involvement and specific autoantibodies.[103] Mast cells that may induce fibrosis after degranulation have been demonstrated in the skin and myocardium of scleroderma patients and may serve as an additional or alternative mechanism through which extensive fibrosis may develop in patients with the disease.[104]

The clinical consequences of myocardial fibrosis are conduction disturbances and/or biventricular CHF. Approximately 50 percent of SSc patients have a normal electrocardiogram and no significant myocardial dysfunction as assessed by radionuclide ventriculography. On the other hand, 58 percent of SSc patients with normal electrocardiograms have been found to have fixed thallium perfusion abnormalities suggesting myocardial fibrosis. Infarction patterns on electrocardiography, especially septal, have been well documented in asymptomatic SSc patients with no evidence of extramural coronary artery disease.

The prevalences of various conduction disturbances in SSc patients have been estimated widely.[96, 105–109] Representative frequencies from electrocardiographic studies are shown in Table 104–5.[86] Most serious are progressive heart block, asystole, and ventricular ectopy, which may lead to syncope or sudden death. Clements and associates[106] demonstrated a correlation of resting electrocardiographic abnormalities and clinical symptoms of palpitations and syncope with significant atrial and ventricular arrhythmias found on 24-hour monitoring. Compared with normal subjects, there is a significant increase in exercise-induced arrhythmias, possibly due to myocardial fibrosis, since arrhythmias correlate with fixed abnormalities of thallium perfusion and rarely occur in SSc patients with normal thallium scans. Patients with the CREST syndrome are less likely to have serious myocardial disease than those with diffuse scleroderma; however, serious ventricular arrhythmias have been documented in CREST patients, as well as myocardial defects of thallium perfusion.[109] Clinically evident myocardial disease in scleroderma is a poor prognostic sign. Heart disease, along with pulmonary and renal failure, is a leading cause of death.[110, 111]

There is no known specific therapy for scleroderma heart disease. Corticosteroids are ineffectual. Whether D-penicillamine, an agent that appears beneficial in scleroderma itself, is effective for the myocardial fibrosis is unknown but is worthy of consideration.[112] Because of the possibility of a vasospastic component to the myocardial disease, nifedipine or other calcium channel blockers both for therapy and as prophylaxis should be considered, as they have proved beneficial in peripheral Raynaud's phenomenon[113] and in preventing cold-induced abnormalities of perfusion observed by thallium scintigraphy.[98–100] Because of their efficacy in scleroderma renal disease, ACE inhibitors may be useful for cardiac scleroderma, especially when the patient has hypertension.[114, 115]

In addition to chronic, fibrotic myocardial disease, an acute inflammatory myocarditis has been reported to occur rarely.[116] These SSc patients typically have accompanying peripheral myositis and elevated MB isoenzyme of creatine kinase (CK-MB) fractions (and probably troponin T levels). CHF and/or conduction disturbances are the primary clinical manifestations. High-dose corticosteroids (60 to 100 mg prednisone equivalent/da in divided doses) appear to be effective in this subset of patients (see recommendations for lupus myocarditis and polymyositis).

TABLE 104–5 Estimated Prevalences of Electrocardiographic Findings in Systemic Sclerosis Based on 436 Cases

Finding	Prevalence
Normal electrocardiogram	56%
PR prolongation	5%
Right bundle branch block	2%
Left bundle branch block	1%
Left anterior fascicular block	5%
Nonspecific conduction abnormality	4%
Second- or third-degree block	1%
Left ventricular hypertrophy	7%
Right ventricular hypertrophy	7%
Low-voltage QRS	5%
Nonspecific T wave abnormality	7%
Atrial ectopy	7%
Ventricular ectopy	5%

Adapted from Follansbee WP, Curtiss EI, Rahko PS, et al: The electrocardiogram in systemic sclerosis (scleroderma). Am J Med 79:183–192, 1985.

Pericardial Involvement

Clinically evident pericarditis in the absence of renal disease occurs in 10 to 15 percent of patients with SSc, and asymptomatic pericardial involvement, including pericardial fibrosis and/or small to moderate effusions, has been found by echocardiography or autopsy in 40 to 60 percent.[86, 117, 118] Acute pericarditis with fever, chest pain, an auscultatory rub, and leukocytosis is unusual. Sudden death, probably from tachyarrhythmias, has been reported in such patients. Chronic pericardial effusions are more common, and tamponade has been reported. Constrictive pericarditis is rare. Large pericardial effusions have been correlated with an impending renal crisis in some studies but not in others.[118] The characteristics of the pericardial fluid have been described in only a few cases. In general, unlike the case in RA or SLE, the fluid is an exudate with only mild inflammatory changes, including low white blood cell counts (4 to 400/mm^3), normal glucose levels, slightly elevated proteins, and no evidence of immune complexes or complement consumption.[119]

Small to moderate pericardial effusions do not require specific therapy. Large effusions usually do not respond to corticosteroids, but acute pericarditis may be responsive. Pericardiocentesis and/or a pericardial window is required for effusions that compromise cardiac function.

Secondary Cardiac Complications

Pulmonary hypertension with right-sided heart failure may develop slowly in patients with progressive pulmonary fibrosis or, more rapidly, in those with a predominantly obliterative vasculopathy of small pulmonary arteries. Indeed, cor pulmonale (right heart failure secondary to lung disease) is the most common cardiac complication of SSc.

The latter form of pulmonary hypertension, without interstitial fibrosis, also tends to occur as a late manifestation of the CREST syndrome (Fig. 104–7).[120] The pulmonary arterial lesions are similar to those in primary pulmonary hypertension, demonstrating prominent intimal proliferation and, at times, a plexiform lesion (see Fig. 104–6).[72, 121] The prognosis for such patients is poor. Recently, intravenous prostacyclin has been shown to reduce pulmonary vascular resistance and to improve outcome when given long term to patients with primary pulmonary hypertension.[122] Similar benefits have been reported in small numbers of scleroderma patients with pulmonary hypertension.[123, 124] Lung transplantation is another consideration, but it is unknown whether similar lesions might develop in the allograft.

Systemic arterial hypertension, typically severe, accompanied by a microangiopathic hemolytic anemia, usually heralds scleroderma renal crisis. Increased systemic renin levels with rapid deterioration of renal function and oliguria occur over days to weeks. Left-sided heart failure is a common consequence. Obliterative arteriolar lesions, similar to those seen elsewhere in SSc (see Fig. 104–6) are found in renal arcuate arteries. Aggressive, prompt lowering of blood pressure, especially with ACE inhibitors, may reverse or stabilize renal failure.[114, 115] Hemodialysis is indicated for those with severe and/or irreversible azotemia. Renal transplantation has been successful in many cases. If chronic rejection of the grafted kidney occurs, it cannot be distinguished histopathologically from recurrent renal scleroderma.

Polymyositis and Dermatomyositis

The idiopathic inflammatory myopathies, polymyositis and dermatomyositis, are characterized by lymphocytic cellular infiltrates and by degeneration and necrosis of proximal skeletal muscles (Fig. 104–8).[125, 126] There is evidence that cell-mediated autoimmunity to skeletal muscle may play an important pathogenetic role; however, the etiology of these orders is unknown. In approximately 10 percent of patients, especially those over the age of 50 years, an underlying malignancy is present, usually a carcinoma. In addition, a similar myositis may accompany the other connective tissue diseases, scleroderma and SLE.

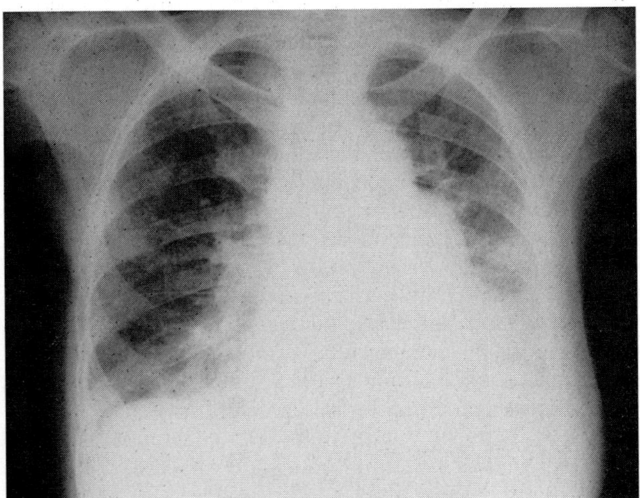

FIGURE 104–7 Chest radiograph of a patient with longstanding CREST (calcinosis, Raynaud's phenomena, esophageal dysmotility, sclerodactyly, and telangiectasia) variant of scleroderma who has developed pulmonary hypertension. Note cardiomegaly with prominence of the pulmonary artery and lack of pulmonary fibrosis. Histopathology of pulmonary vessels of such a patient would appear as in Figure 104–6.

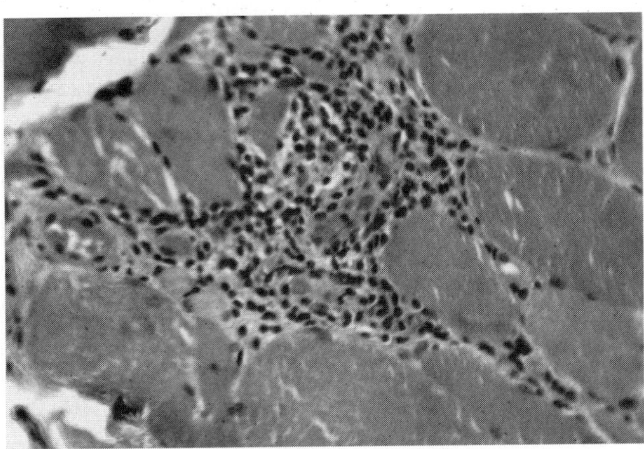

FIGURE 104–8 Photomicrograph of a proximal skeletal muscle of a patient with polymyositis or dermatomyositis. Note round cell infiltration between the muscle bundles. Similar inflammatory lesions may involve the myocardium.

The dominant clinical features are progressive proximal muscle weakness involving the shoulder and pelvic girdles, neck flexors, and the pharyngeal musculature.[125, 126] Distal and respiratory muscle weakness is uncommon except in long-standing and/or untreated disease. CK levels are typically elevated. Electromyography shows a typical myopathic pattern, and biopsy of an affected muscle shows typical histopathologic changes.[125] ANAs are present in 80 to 90 percent of patients, and several specificities (anti-Jo-1, anti-Mi-2) are highly correlated with subsets of these diseases.[127] For example, autoantibodies to tRNA synthetases, such as anti-Jo-1 (his tRNA synthetase) and to other intracellular translation factors, correlate strongly with an inflammatory interstitial lung disease,[128] which over time may lead to cor pulmonale.

Myocardial inflammation, histologically similar to skeletal myositis, may occur. The frequency of cardiac involvement is unknown; however, evidence of myocardial muscle inflammation, as well as small vessel disease, was reported in 30 percent of 20 cases examined at autopsy,[129] although higher frequencies have been reported based on noninvasive cardiac studies.[130–133] The most common clinical manifestations of myocarditis are subtle and nonspecific and include resting tachycardia, atypical chest pain, and nonspecific ST-T wave changes on electrocardiography. Overt CHF, heart block, and arrhythmias have all been reported.[134–137] Myocarditis appears to parallel active skeletal myositis. Serum CK levels are typically elevated. An elevated CK-MB fraction should raise suspicion of myocardial involvement, although an elevated CK-MB fraction may also be the result of regenerating skeletal muscle.[138] Serum troponin T, a more specific indicator of myocardial injury,[40] has been reported to be clinically useful in detecting myocarditis in patients with skeletal myositis.[139, 140] Clinical suspicion of myocarditis raised by examination and electrocardiography should be pursued by studies of troponin T levels and myocardial function, including cardiac ejection fraction. At times, endomyocardial biopsy may be necessary to establish the diagnosis.[141]

Therapy for active myocarditis should be aimed at prompt suppression of the inflammatory response. Corticosteroids in high doses should be given IV and the patient monitored closely. Doses of 60 to 100 mg prednisone equivalent/da in divided doses represents a reasonable starting point, and frequent monitoring of CK and troponin T levels provides the most sensitive measure of response. In patients who are not improving clinically and with falling CK levels, IV "pulses" of up to 1000 mg prednisone equivalents may be necessary. Steroid tapering should begin only after CK and troponin T levels have normalized and should proceed slowly over weeks to months, using the CK and troponin T levels as a guide. If the CK or troponin T levels again begin to rise while the patient remains at a high corticosteroid dose, or if serious steroid side effects are occurring, an immunosuppressive drug, such as methotrexate (15 to 25 mg/wk) or azathioprine (2 mg/kg/da) should be added as a steroid-sparing agent. Arrhythmias, heart failure, and atrioventricular block should be managed in the usual manner.

PRIMARY VASCULITIDES

The primary vasculitides include a group of disorders, each of unknown etiology, characterized primarily by a necrotizing vasculitis.[142, 143] These entities are clinically and serologically distinct from the previously described connective tissue diseases, in which vasculitis may also be a prominent complication, especially in RA and SLE. Moreover, each of the primary vasculitides demonstrates its own distinctive clinical picture of organ involvement, size of vessel affected,[144] host predisposition, and serologic markers. Classification criteria for most have been established.[145–150] However, considerable overlap may occur and may make specific diagnosis impossible. Immune complexes are believed to cause the vascular disease in most cases.[142]

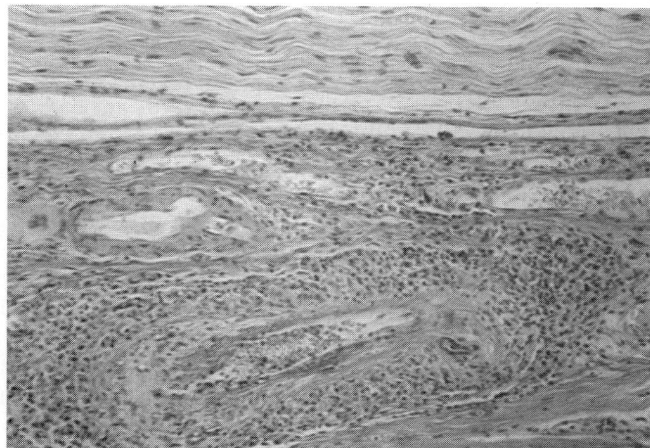

FIGURE 104–9 Histopathology of a medium-sized artery affected by polyarteritis nodosum. Note infiltration and disruption of the vessel wall by inflammatory cells. (From the Clinical Slide Collection on the Rheumatic Diseases, American College of Rheumatology, Atlanta, GA, with permission.)

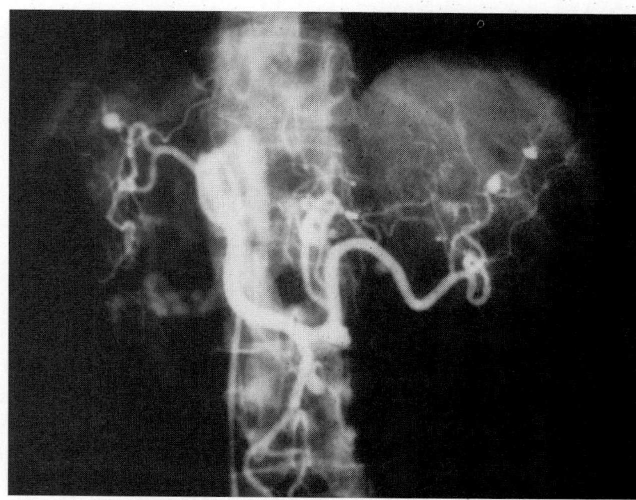

FIGURE 104–10 Celiac angiograph of a patient with polyarteritis nodosum shows multiple aneurysms.

Polyarteritis Nodosum and Variants

Polyarteritis nodosum (PAN) is the classical prototype of a widespread, necrotizing vasculitis.[142, 143, 148] Medium-sized muscular arteries are most prominently involved, usually in a patchy, segmental pattern and often at arterial bifurcations (Fig. 104–9). Small aneurysms may develop and may either rupture or become thrombosed (Fig. 104–10). Less commonly, small arteries, arterioles, and/or veins also may be involved. Necropsy studies in the precorticosteroid era demonstrated myocardial arteritis and infarction in 62 percent of patients, myocardial hypertrophy in 64 percent, and pericarditis in 33 percent.[151]

The typical patient is a middle-aged man. A frank MI, CHF, or pericarditis may be the presenting manifestation of PAN, although other features are usually present, most commonly myalgias, arthralgias, weight loss, peripheral neuropathy, hypertension, or renal insufficiency. Common laboratory abnormalities include low-grade anemia, leukocytosis, thrombocytosis, an elevated erythrocyte sedimentation rate, liver function abnormalities, and in approximately 20 to 30 percent of cases, a positive test for hepatitis B surface antigen.[152] Diagnosis of PAN is based on histopathologic demonstration of necrotizing vasculitis, usually in muscle, sural nerve, or testicular biopsy specimens (see Fig. 104–9), and/or angiographic demonstration of small arterial aneurysms (see Fig. 104–10).[153] ANAs and antineutrophil cytoplasmic antibodies (ANCAs) are typically negative. Treatment with high doses of corticosteroids is mandatory. Prednisone equivalents of 60 to 100 mg/da are usually initially effective, but most patients require the addition of cyclophosphamide (2 mg/kg/da) or azathioprine (2 mg/kg/da).[154, 155] Tapering of prednisone must be accomplished slowly and should be guided by a lack of clinically apparent active vasculitis and laboratory variables (e.g., erythrocyte sedimentation rate, platelet counts, urinary sediment abnormalities). The prognosis for PAN is generally poor; however, if the disease can be controlled early with vigorous therapy, many patients appear to have a self-limited course.[152]

Wegener's Granulomatosis

Wegener's granulomatosis is characterized by a necrotizing granulomatous vasculitis of the upper respiratory tract, lungs, and kidneys.[142, 143, 147, 156] Small and medium-sized arteries and veins are typically involved. ANCAs have been reported in approximately 90 percent of such patients, and frequently, also in microscopic polyarteritis, a similar disease affecting small vessels.[143, 156, 157] Clinical cardiac abnormalities in Wegener's granulomatosis are infrequent. Pericarditis has been reported in 6 percent of patients and myocardial involvement in less than 2 percent.[156, 158] Corticosteroids alone are not effective therapy for Wegener's granulomatosis but should be used initially in doses of 40 to 60 mg prednisone equivalent/da to suppress systemic symptoms. Instead, immunosuppressive agents, especially cyclophosphamide (2 mg/kg/da given orally), should be started promptly, and after several weeks or months prednisone may be tapered and discontinued. After 6 to 12 months, immunosuppressive drugs also can be tapered and discontinued in most patients.[156] The combination of high-dose corticosteroids and cyclosphosphamide is associated with a high risk of infection, especially *P. carinii* pneumonia.[159] Prophylactic therapy with trimethoprim-sulfamethoxasole should be considered in such patients.

Interestingly, several cases of Wegener's granulomatosis have been reported to improve using trimethoprim-sulfamethoxasole alone.[160] A controlled study of trimethoprim 160 mg–sulfamethoxasole 800 mg twice daily versus placebo has been shown to reduce flares of the disease after immunosuppressives have been discontinued in one study,[161] but not in another,[162] which found low-dose methotrexate (0.3 mg/kg/wk) more effective. Useful clinical parameters to follow improvement in Wegener's granulomatosis include sinus and chest x-rays, renal function, and serum ANCA levels. The prognosis has improved considerably with this approach.

Churg-Strauss Angiitis

Churg-Strauss angiitis represents another form of granulomatous vasculitis, primarily affecting the lungs, which occurs in patients with long-standing asthma.[142, 146, 163] Eosinophilia is typically present. Cardiac involvement is similar to that seen in PAN. Corticosteroids in doses similar to those for PAN are recommended. Recently, interferon-alfa has been reported as effective adjunctive therapy.[164]

Hypersensitivity Angiitis

Hypersensitivity angiitis is a common disease of small arteries and veins, usually heralded by a rash. It is classically associated with allergic reactions to drugs, such as sulfonamides, penicillins, and allopurinol.[142, 143, 145] The coronary vasculature may be involved, as well as the pericardium. Treatment includes discontinuation of the offending drug and administration of high-dose corticosteroids (60 to 100 mg prednisone equivalent/da) when there is serious organ involvement.

Giant Cell Arteritis

Giant cell arteritis, also termed temporal, cranial, or granulomatous arteritis, typically affects older persons (above the age of 50 years), most often whites.[149, 165] Medium-sized cranial arteries are affected by a granulomatous inflammation that leads to symptoms of headache, scalp tenderness, jaw claudication, and sudden loss of vision. Some patients also have muscle pain and stiffness around the shoulder and pelvic girdles (polymyalgia rheumatica). Large vessel involvement of the aorta and/or its major branches occurs in 9 to 14 percent of cases, leading to aortic arch syndrome, intermittent claudication, cerebral ischemic attacks, abdominal angina, aortic aneurysm and rupture, and aortic valvular insufficiency.[166, 167] Coronary insufficiency with angina and/or MI has been reported infrequently.[165, 168] The diagnosis should be suspected in any older patient complaining of pain about the head, neck, and/or shoulders. An elevated erythrocyte sedimentation rate is typically found but may occasionally be normal. ANCA is negative. Diagnosis is usually made by biopsy of a temporal artery and/or clinical response to a trial of moderate- to high-dose corticosteroids. Coronary and/or large vessel involvement should be confirmed by appropriate angiographic studies.[166] Corticosteroids in doses adequate to suppress the inflammatory process, usually 50 to 80 mg prednisone equivalent/da, is the initial treatment of choice. Most patients respond to corticosteroids alone, and immunosuppressive agents (e.g., azathioprine, methotrexate, cyclophosphamide) are rarely needed. Useful parameters to follow and guide steroid tapering include the patient's symptoms and the erythrocyte sedimentation rate. If vascular insufficiency of large vessels fails to respond, indicating irreversible arterial obstruction, or if aneurysms continue to enlarge, vascular surgical approaches are indicated.[166]

Takayasu's Arteritis

Also known as pulseless disease, Takayasu's arteritis is another form of granulomatous arteritis affecting the aorta and/or its major branches.[150, 169–171] The disease occurs most commonly in young Asian women but has been reported in all races. HLA-B52 is increased in Japanese patients[172] but not in Americans. CHF due to systemic hypertension is the most common cardiac manifestation. Hypertension occurs in 37 to 50 percent of patients and is caused by renal artery or proximal aortic involvement.[171] Coronary insufficiency or MI may result from aortic involvement at the origin of the coronary system. Coronary arteritis per se is rare. Aortic root dilatation may result in aortic valvular insufficiency. Diagnosis is based on symptoms of aortic arch syndrome, intermittent claudication, and/or cerebral ischemia associated with pulse deficits and/or bruits over large arteries on examination, as well as typical findings on aortic angiography (Fig. 104–11).[171] Treatment entails moderate to high doses of corticosteroids (40 to 60 mg prednisone equivalent/da), occasionally with immunosuppressives[173] and, when necessary, vascular surgical bypass and/or grafting procedures.

Kawasaki's Disease

Kawasaki's disease, also known as mucocutaneous lymph node syndrome, is primarily an acute disease of infants or small children[174, 175] and rarely affects adults.[176] It is characterized by fever, lymphadenopathy, a desquamative skin rash, and mucous membrane lesions (strawberry tongue, urethritis, conjunctivitis). Cardiac involvement occurs in approximately 5 percent of cases and most commonly manifests as coronary artery aneurysms and/or coronary thromboses.[174] Other reported complications include ventricular aneurysms, myocarditis, pericarditis, cardiac tamponade, and CHF. Sudden death attributable to cardiac arrhythmias or MI has been reported in 1.7 percent of cases.[174] Coronary thromboarteritis with aneurysmal dilatation found at autopsy of children dying of Kawasaki's disease is similar to that previously described in infantile polyarteritis.[177] Diagnosis is based on the clinical features of the disease.[175] When clinical examination and/or electrocardiography suggests cardiac involvement, coronary angiography is indicated. Therapy should include high-dose aspirin to prevent coronary thromboses (80 to 100 mg/da in four divided doses or maintenance of a serum salicylate level of 20 to 25 mg/dl), which should be continued for at least 2 months when coronary aneurysms are present. Corticosteroids appear to promote coronary aneurysm formation and are contraindicated. Intravenous gammaglobulin has been reported to be the most effective therapy for Kawasaki's disease, and it may prevent the coronary lesions.[175, 178] The optimal dosing schedule remains controversial. Variously, 400 mg/kg/da for 4 days, 1 g/kg once, and 2 g/kg once have all been reported to abbreviate the acute symptoms and prevent coronary artery aneurysms.

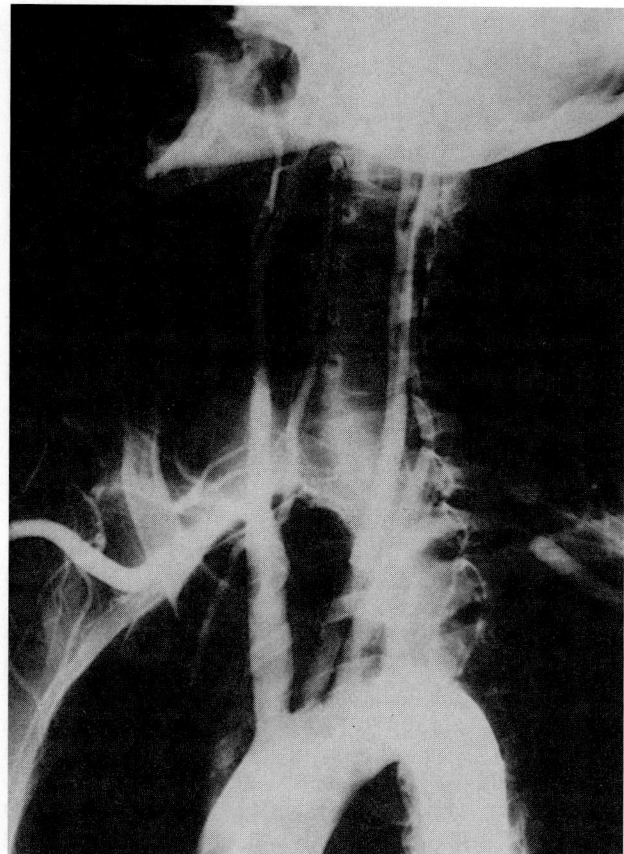

FIGURE 104–11 Arch arteriogram of a patient with Takayasu's arteritis. Note irregularity and/or narrowing of the innominate, right carotid, and left subclavian arteries.

Behçet's Disease

Behçet's disease is characterized by recurrent episodes of oral and genital ulcers and uveitis.[179–181] Other manifestations include recurrent meningoencephalitis, pustulonecrotic skin lesions after trauma (pathergy), arthritis, bowel ulceration, pulmonary artery aneurysms (Hughes-Stovin syndrome),[182] and systemic vasculitis.[179, 180, 183] The disease is most common in young adults of Japanese, Middle Eastern, and Southern European extraction. In these ethnic groups, the histocompatibility antigen HLA-B51 is strikingly increased in patients with Behçet's disease but not in similarly affected Americans or Northern Europeans.[184] The cardiovascular manifestations of Behçet's disease relate to vasculo-occlusive disease, often with aneurysm formation, of small, medium and large vessels, more often veins than arteries.[183, 185] Superficial thrombophlebitis, usually recurrent, is most common, but deep venous occlusion of the superior and inferior vena cavae and of the subclavian, common iliac, femoral, and hepatic veins has been reported. Arterial occlusions of aneurysms of subclavian, renal, carotid, pulmonary, and femoral arteries may also occur. Although coronary vessel involvement should be possible in theory, there is only rare documentation of heart disease per se in this disorder.

Treatment of Behçet's disease begins with corticosteroid therapy, with doses commensurate with the severity of disease.[180] Colchicine[180] and thalidomide[186, 187] have also been reported to be useful. Chlorambucil[188] or azathioprine[189] may be effective in more severe disease, especially with ocular involvement.

Relapsing Polychondritis

Relapsing polychondritis is a rare disorder of unknown etiology in which there is inflammation and destruction of various cartilaginous structures.[190–192] Circulating antibodies to type II collagen have been demonstrated in some patients.[193] Disease onset is usually in middle age, with no differences between the genders. Bilateral auricular chondritis (Plate 104–7) is the most common presenting symptom, followed by laryngotracheal or nasal (saddle nose deformity) involvement, arthritis, fever, or neurosensory hearing loss.[191] A systemic vasculitis affecting medium or large arteries occurs in approximately 15 percent of patients.[191] Cardiovascular complications appear in approximately 24 percent and include most commonly aortic regurgitation, followed by mitral regurgitation, pericarditis, or myocardial ischemia.[190, 191] Aortic or large artery aneurysms with thrombosis or rupture may occur.

Treatment depends on disease severity and organ involvement. Corticosteroids are usually required. Dapsone or immunosuppressive agents may be effective in patients with steroid resistance or intolerance. Cardiac valve replacement may be necessary.[191]

Seronegative Spondyloarthropathies

The seronegative spondyloarthropathies include ankylosing spondylitis, Reiter's disease (reactive arthritis), psoriatic arthritis, and the arthritis associated with the idiopathic inflammatory bowel diseases, ulcerative colitis and Crohn's disease.[194, 195] Although once considered variants of RA, these chronic arthritides are now known to be clinically, epidemiologically, and genetically separate entities. Moreover, rheumatoid factor and ANAs are not present. All are characterized by a sterile inflammatory process affecting spinal and/or peripheral joints, as well as tendon and ligamentous insertions (enthesitis), often leading to bony fusion. In ankylosing spondylitis, the axial skeleton is predominantly involved; joint fusion typically begins first in the sacroiliac joints and then progressively ascends into the lumbar, dorsal, and cervical segments, resulting in a rigid and often deformed spine. Radiographs characteristically show sacroiliitis (Fig. 104–12), "squaring" of vertebrae, and ossification of spinal ligaments between vertebrae (syndesmophytes), giving the appearance of a "bamboo" spine (Fig. 104–13). Reiter's disease and psoriatic arthritis affect primarily peripheral joints, but similar spinal changes, especially sacroiliitis, occur in 20 percent of patients. Peripheral arthritis complicates inflammatory bowel disease in 20 percent and spondylitis in 10 percent of cases. Acute anterior uveitis occurs in approximately 25 percent of patients with a spondyloarthropathy.

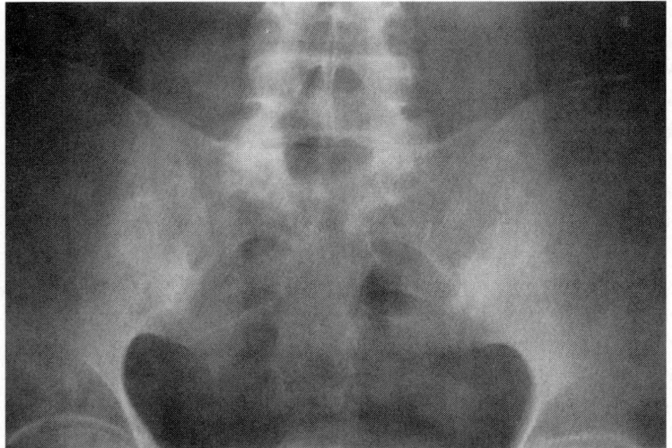

FIGURE 104–12 Pelvic radiograph shows bilateral fusion of the sacroiliac joints (sacroiliitis) in a patient with a spondyloarthropathy.

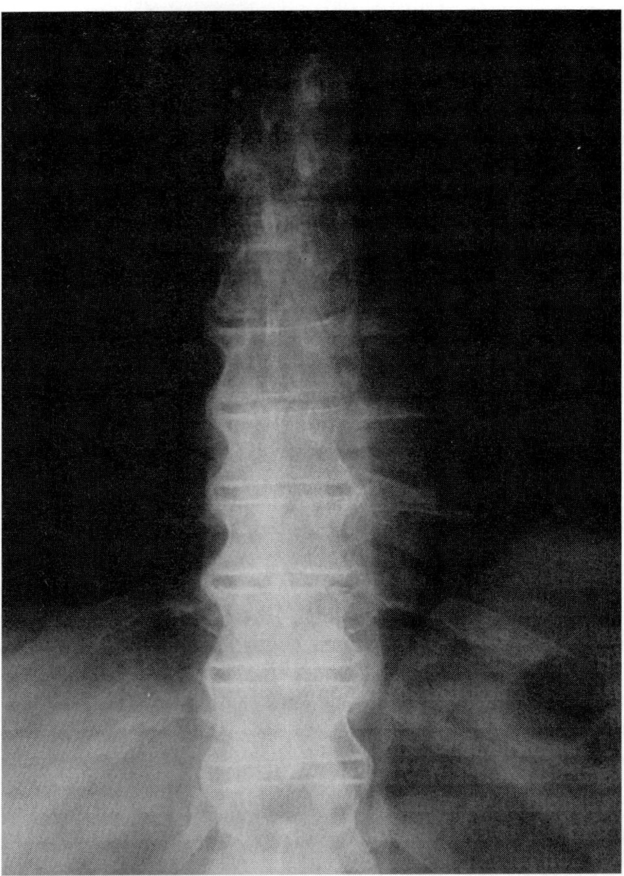

FIGURE 104–13 Thoracolumbar radiograph shows calcified ligaments (syndesmophytes) bridging across intervertebral discs, "bamboo spine," in a patient with ankylosing spondylitis.

The pathogeneses of these diseases are unknown, but there are important clues.[195] The MHC class I antigen HLA-B27, which is present in approximately 6 to 10 percent of the normal white population, is strikingly increased in patients with these diseases (i.e., ankylosing spondylitis [90 percent], Reiter's disease [75 percent], and psoriatic and colitic spondylitis [50 percent]). This finding supports a strong genetic contribution to disease susceptibility and implies a role for MHC class I–restricted cytotoxic T cell responses. The human HLA-B27 gene has been cloned into transgenic rats, and these animals spontaneously develop nearly all the features of the spondyloarthropathies.[196] Venereal infection by *Chlamydia trachomatis* and gastroenteritis caused by *Shigella flexneri, Salmonella, Yersinia,* and *Campylobacter* are known to trigger Reiter's disease (reactive arthritis) (Plate 104–8). Bacterial antigens from each of these triggering organisms can be demonstrated in affected peripheral joints,[197, 198] and circulating bacteria-specific IgA antibodies are typically found in patients who develop reactive arthritis, thus suggesting a persisting mucosal infection.[199–201] Prolonged courses of antibiotics aimed at the triggering microbe appear to shorten the duration of Reiter's disease.[202] The presumptive organism(s) causing ankylosing spondylitis have not been identified; however, gut bacteria are suspected.

A specific cardiac lesion occurs in the spondyloarthropathies and is clinically manifested as aortic regurgitation, atrioventricular or bundle branch conduction defects or, rarely, mitral regurgitation (Fig. 104–14).[203–208] Histopathologically, dilatation and thickening of the walls of the proximal aortic root, especially behind and immediately above the sinus of Valsalva, have been demonstrated, along with thickening and shortening of the aortic valve cusps and the development of a fibrous mass (or bump) below the aortic valve (Fig. 104–15).[203, 209] The thickening is due to adventitial scarring, probably as the result of an inflammatory process. Vasa vasora show surrounding collections of plasma cells and lymphocytes.[203] Mitral regurgitation, although rare, appears to result from similar fibrous thickening at the basal portion of the anterior mitral leaflet and dilatation of the left ventrical (from aortic regurgitation). Bundle branch and complete heart block occurs because of extension of the fibrosing process from the membranous ventricular septum into the muscular septum where it interrupts or destroys conducting fibers in the atrioventricular bundle or proximal bundle branches.[203]

Clinically, approximately 5 percent of patients with ankylosing spondylitis or Reiter's disease have spondylitic heart disease, and it has been rarely reported in psoriatic and colitic spondylitis.[207, 210, 211] The frequency of HLA-B27 approaches 100 percent in reported cases. This complication usually occurs after many years of active arthritis; however, examples of both conduction disturbances, especially first-degree atrioventricular block, and aortic regurgitation have been reported in early disease[212] and even before the appearance of arthritis symptoms.[213] Clinically inapparent aortic involvement may be found by echocardiography. LaBresh and coworkers,[214] using two-dimensional transthoracic echocardiography, demonstrated subaortic fibrous ridging or marked valvular leaflet thickening in 11 of 36 men with ankylosing spondylitis or Reiter's disease but in none of 29 normal age-matched control men. More recently, Arnason and colleagues,[215] using transesophageal echocardiography, detected aortic valve insufficiency in 10 of 29 men with ankylosing spondylitis, as well as the aortic and valvular thickening seen pathologically.

Studies of men who required cardiac pacemakers for complete heart block have noted high frequencies of spondyloarthropathies, often occult, and/or HLA-B27. Bergfeldt and colleagues[216, 217] found clinical or radiographic evidence of spondyloarthropathies in 28 of 223 men (12.5 percent)

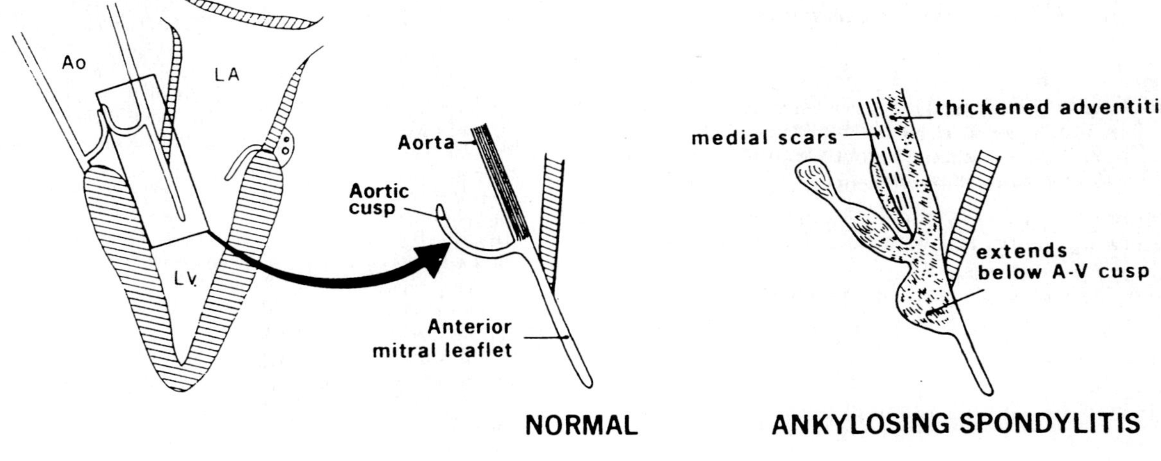

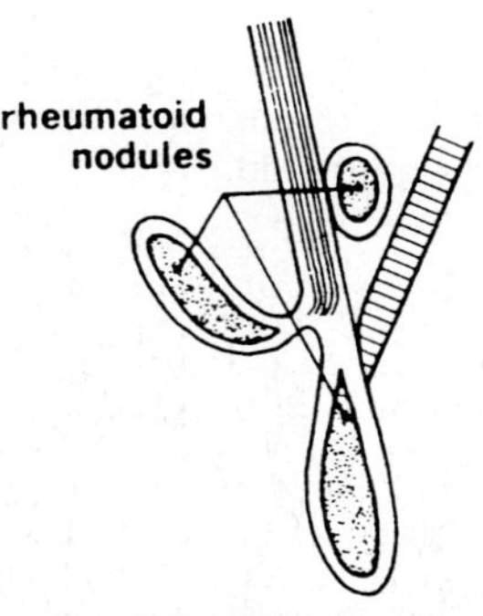

FIGURE 104–14 Schematic representation of the typical cardiac lesions of ankylosing spondylitis contrasted with those of rheumatoid arthritis. Ao, aorta; A-V, atrioventricular; LA, left atrium; LV, left ventricle. (From Bulkley BH, Roberts WC: The heart in systemic lupus erythematosus and the changes induced in it by corticosteroid therapy. Circulation 58:243–264, 1975.)

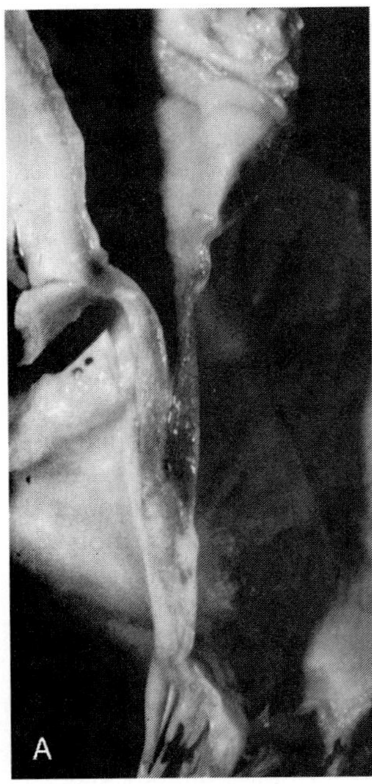

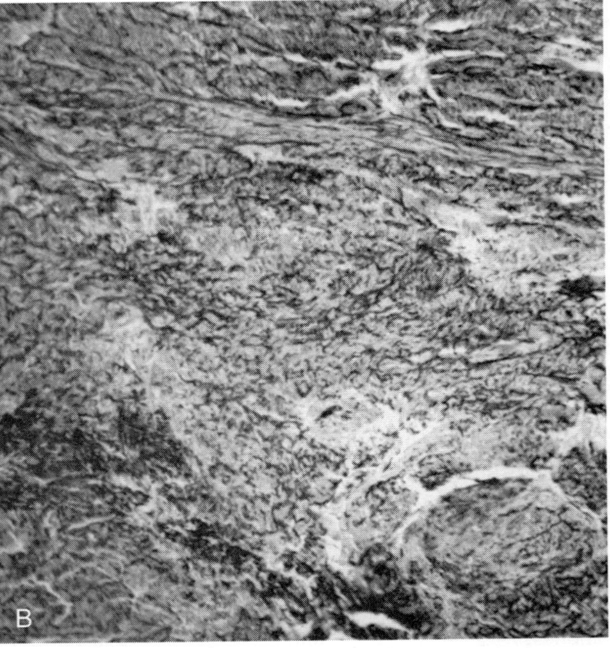

FIGURE 104–15 Necropsy specimens from a patient with ankylosing spondylitis and aortic regurgitation. **A,** Gross section through aortic valve and interventricular septum shows thickening of these structures as in Figure 104–14. **B,** Histopathologic section of same region shows fibrous thickening. (**A** and **B,** Courtesy of William Roberts, M.D., Baylor University Medical Center, Dallas.)

with permanent cardiac pacemakers, 85 percent of whom were HLA-B27–positive. Moreover, among 83 pacemaker recipients who had no clinical or radiographic stigmata of spondylitis, HLA-B27 was present in 17 percent, a significantly higher frequency than in normal controls (6 percent).[218] In another group of 91 patients with lone aortic regurgitation, a B27-associated spondyloarthropathy was found in 15 to 20 percent.[219] Moreover, the combination of lone aortic regurgitation and severe conduction system abnormalities was associated with HLA-B27 in 88 percent of cases.

Aortic regurgitation and, less often, mitral regurgitation progress relatively rapidly, and most patients require prosthetic valve replacement in less than 5 years.[203–205, 209] Patients with complete heart block and other severe conduction disturbances should receive permanent cardiac pacemakers. There is no evidence that anti-inflammatory or immunosuppressive drugs alter the course of spondylitic heart disease.

Rare cardiac features of ankylosing spondylitis and Reiter's disease include reports of pericarditis, myocarditis, global ventricular dysfunction, and giant cell valvulitis.[210, 220–222] A recent comprehensive review of spondylitic heart disease has appeared.[208]

References

1. Arnett FC, Edworthy SM, Bloch DA, et al: The American Rheumatism Association 1987 revised criteria for the classification of rheumatoid arthritis. Arthritis Rheum 31:315–324, 1988.
2. Harris ED Jr: Rheumatoid arthritis. Pathophysiology and implications for therapy. N Engl J Med 322:1277–1289, 1990.
3. Weyand CM, Hicok KC, Conn DL, Goronzy JJ: The influence of HLA-DRB1 genes on disease severity in rheumatoid arthritis. Ann Intern Med 117:801–806, 1992.
4. Feldmann M, Brennan FM, Maini RN: Rheumatoid arthritis. Cell 85:307–310, 1996.
5. Kerstens PJSM, Boerbooms AMT, Jeurissen MEC, et al: Accelerated nodulosis during low dose methotrexate therapy for rheumatoid arthritis. An analysis of ten cases. J Rheumatol 19:867–871, 1991.
6. Williams FM, Cohen PR, Arnett FC: Accelerated cutaneous nodulosis during methotrexate therapy in a patient with rheumatoid arthritis. J Am Acad Dermatol 39:359–362, 1998.
7. Pizzarello RA, Goldberg J: The heart in rheumatoid arthritis. *In* Utsinger PD, Zvaifler NJ, Ehrlich GE (eds): Rheumatoid Arthritis. Etiology, Diagnosis, Management. Philadelphia: JB Lippincott, 1985.
8. Sigal LH, Friedman HD: Rheumatoid pancarditis in a patient with well controlled rheumatoid arthritis. J Rheumatol 16:368–373, 1989.
9. Hara KS, Ballard DJ, Ilstrup DM, et al: Rheumatoid pericarditis: clinical features and survival. Medicine 69:81–91, 1990.
10. Escalante A, Kaufman RL, Quismorio P Jr, Beardmore TD: Cardiac compression in rheumatoid pericarditis. Semin Arthritis Rheum 20:148–163, 1990.
11. Franco AE, Levine HD, Hall AP: Rheumatoid pericarditis: report of 17 cases diagnosed clinically. Ann Intern Med 77:837–844, 1972.
12. John JT Jr, Hough A, Sergent JS: Pericardial disease in rheumatoid arthritis. Am J Med 66:385–390, 1979.
13. Webber MD, Selsky EJ, Roper PA: Identification of a mobile intracardiac rheumatoid nodule mimicking an atrial myxoma. J Am Soc Echocardiogr 8:961–964, 1995.
14. Voyles WF, Searles RP, Bankhurst AD: Myocardial infarction caused by rheumatoid vasculitis. Arthritis Rheum 23:860–863, 1980.
15. Bank I, Marboe CC, Redberg RF, Jacobs J: Myocarditis in adult Still's disease. Arthritis Rheum 28:452–454, 1985.
16. Pouchot J, Sampalis JS, Beaudet F, et al: Adult Still's disease: Manifestations, disease course, and outcome in 62 patients. Medicine 70:118–136, 1991.
17. Hahn BH, Wallace DJ: Dubois Lupus Erythematosus. 5th ed. Baltimore: Williams & Wilkins, 1997.
18. Arnett FC, Reveille JD: The genetics of lupus erythematosus. Rheum Dis Clin N Am 18:865–892, 1992.
19. Stevens MB: Systemic lupus erythematosus and the cardiovascular system. *In* Lahita RG (ed): Systemic Lupus Erythematosus. p 673. New York: John Wiley & Sons, 1987.
20. Harvey AM, Shulman LE, Tumulty PA, et al: Review of the literature and clinical analysis of 138 cases. Medicine 33:219–437, 1954.
21. Hochberg MC, Dorsch CA, Feinglass EJ, Stevens MB: Survivorship in systemic lupus erythematosus. Arthritis Rheum 24:54–59, 1981.
22. Reveille JD, Bartolucci A, Alarcon GS: Prognosis in systemic lupus erythematosus. Arthritis Rheum 33:37–48, 1990.
23. Bulkley BH, Roberts WC: The heart in systemic lupus erythemato-

sus and the changes induced in it by corticosteroid therapy. Am J Med 58:243–264, 1975.

24. Buyon JP: Complete heart block and antibodies to the SSA/Ro-SSB/La antigen systems. Clin Asp Autoimmun 4:8–17, 1990.
25. Scott JS, Maddison PJ, Taylor PV, et al: Connective-tissue disease, antibodies to ribonucleoprotein, and congenital heart block. N Engl J Med 309:209–212, 1983.
26. Straaton KV, Chatham WW, Reveille JD, et al: Clinically significant valvular heart disease in systemic lupus erythematosus. Am J Med 85:645–650, 1988.
27. Leung WH, Wong KL, Lau CP, et al: Association between antiphospholipid antibodies and cardiac abnormalities in patients with systemic lupus erythematosus. Am J Med 89:411–419, 1990.
28. Galve E, Candell-Riera J, Pigrau C, et al: Prevalence, morphologic types, and evolution of cardiac valvular disease in systemic lupus erythematosus. N Engl J Med 319:817–823, 1988.
29. Shearn MA: The heart in systemic lupus erythematosus. Am Heart J 58:452–466, 1959.
30. Hejtmancik MR, Wright JC, Quint R, Jennings FL: The cardiovascular manifestations of systemic lupus erythematosus. Am Heart J 68:119–130, 1964.
31. James TN, Rupe CE, Monto RW: Pathology of the cardiac conduction system in systemic lupus erythematosus. Ann Intern Med 63:402–409, 1965.
32. Bidani AK, Roberts JL, Schwartz MM, Lewis EJ: Immunopathology of cardiac lesions in fatal systemic lupus erythematosus. Am J Med 69:849–858, 1980.
33. Das SK, Cassidy JT: Antiheart antibodies in patients with systemic lupus erythematosus. Am J Med Sci 265:275–280, 1973.
34. Gur H, Keren G, Averbuch M, Levo Y: Severe congestive lupus cardiomyopathy complicated by an intracavitary thrombus: a clinical and echocardiographic followup. J Rheumatol 15:1278–1280, 1988.
35. Kattwinkel N, Villaneuva AG, Labib SB, et al: Myocardial infarction caused by cardiac microvasculopathy in a patient with the primary antiphospholipid syndrome. Ann Intern Med 116:974–976, 1992.
36. Jacobson EJ, Reza MJ: Constrictive pericarditis in systemic lupus erythematosus. Arthritis Rheum 21:972–974, 1978.
37. Hunder GG, Mullen BJ, McDuffie FC: Complement in pericardial fluid of lupus erythematosus. Ann Intern Med 80:453–458, 1974.
38. Berg G, Bodet J, Webb K, et al: Systemic lupus erythematosus presenting as isolated congestive heart failure. J Rheumatol 12:1182–1185, 1985.
39. Borenstein DG, Fye WB, Arnett FC, Stevens MB: The myocarditis of systemic lupus erythematosus. Ann Intern Med 89:619–624, 1978.
40. Adams JE, Bodor GS, Davila-Roman VG: Cardiac troponin I. A marker with high specificity for cardiac injury. Circulation 88:101–106, 1993.
41. Ratliff NB, Estes ME, Myles JL, et al: Diagnosis of chloroquine cardiomyopathy by endomyocardial biopsy. N Engl J Med 316:191–193, 1987.
42. Hosenpud JD, Montanaro A, Hart MV, et al: Myocardial perfusion abnormalities in asymptomatic patients with systemic lupus erythematosus. Am J Med 77:286–292, 1984.
43. Homcy CJ, Liberthson RR, Fallon IT, et al: Ischemic heart disease in systemic lupus erythematosus in the young patient: report of 6 cases. Am J Cardiol 49:478–484, 1982.
44. Spiera H, Rothenberg RR: Myocardial infarction in four young people with SLE. J Rheumatol 10:464–466, 1983.
45. Korbet SM, Schwartz MM, Lewis EJ: Immune complex deposition and coronary vasculitis in systemic lupus erythematosus. Am J Med 77:141–146, 1984.
46. Asherson RA, Mackay IR, Harris EN: Myocardial infarction in a young man with systemic lupus erythematosus, deep vein thrombosis, and antibodies to phospholipid. Br Heart J 56:190–193, 1986.
47. Maaravi Y, Raz E, Gilon D, Rubinow A: Cerebrovascular accident and myocardial infarction associated with anticardiolipin antibodies in a young woman with systemic lupus erythematosus. Ann Rheum Dis 48:853–855, 1989.
48. Libman E, Sacks B: A hitherto underscribed form of valvular and mural endocarditis. Arch Intern Med 33:701–737, 1924.
49. Ropes MW: Systemic Lupus Erythematosus. London: Cambridge University Press, 1976.
50. Shapiro RF, Gample CN, Wiesner KB, et al: Immunopathogenesis of Libman-Sacks endocarditis. Ann Rheum Dis 36:508–516, 1977.
51. Pritzker MR, Ernst JD, Caudill C, et al: Acquired aortic stenosis in systemic lupus erythematosus. Ann Intern Med 93:434–436, 1980.
52. Lerman BB, Thomas LC, Abrams GD, Pitt B: Aortic stenosis associated with systemic lupus erythematosus. Am J Med 72:707–710, 1982.
53. Roldan CA, Shively BK, Crawford MH: An echocardiographic study of valvular heart disease associated with systemic lupus erythematosus. N Engl J Med 335:1424–1430, 1996.
54. Pouchot J, Sampalis JS, Beaudet F, et al: Adult Still's disease: manifestations, disease course, and outcome in 62 patients. Medicine 70:118–136, 1991.
55. Niaz A, Butany J: Antiphospholipid antibody syndrome with involvement of a bioprosthetic heart valve. Can J Cardiol 14:951–954, 1998.
56. Gabrielli F, Alcini E, Prima MA, et al: Cardiac involvement in connective tissue diseases and primary antiphospholipid syndrome: echocardiographic assessment and correlation with antiphospholipid antibodies. Acta Cardiol 51:425–439, 1996.
57. Petri M: The clinical syndrome associated with antiphospholipid antibodies. J Rheumatol 19:505–506, 1992.
58. Love PE, Santoro SA: Antiphospholipid antibodies: anticardiolipin and the lupus anticoagulant in systemic lupus erythematosus (SLE) and in non-SLE disorders. Ann Intern Med 112:682–698, 1990.
59. Roubey RAS: Immunology of the antiphospholipid antibody syndrome. Arthritis Rheum 39:1444–1454, 1996.
60. Asherson RA, Cervera R, Piette JC, et al: Catastrophic antiphospholipid syndrome. Medicine 77:195–207, 1998.
61. Khamashta MA, Cuadrado MJ, Mujic F, et al: The management of thrombosis in the antiphospholipid-antibody syndrome. N Engl J Med 332:993–997, 1995.
62. Asherson RA, Khamashta MA, Ordi-Ros J, et al: The primary antiphospholipid syndrome: major clinical and serological features. Medicine 68:366–374, 1989.
63. Asherson RA: The catastrophic antiphospholipid syndrome. J Rheumatol 19:508–512, 1992.
64. Galve E, Ordi J, Barquinero J, et al: Valvular heart disease in the primary antiphospholipid syndrome. Ann Intern Med 116:293–298, 1992.
65. Leventhal LJ, Borofsky MA, Bergey PD, Schumacher HR Jr: Antiphospholipid antibody syndrome with right atrial thrombosis mimicking an atrial myxoma. Am J Med 87:111–113, 1989.
66. Fereante FM, Myerson GE, Goldman JA: Subclavian artery thrombosis mimicking the aortic arch syndrome in systemic lupus erythematosus. Arthritis Rheum 25:1501–1504, 1982.
67. Nair SS, Askari AD, Popelka CG, Kleinerman JF: Pulmonary hypertension and systemic lupus erythematosus. Arch Intern Med 140:109–111, 1980.
68. Hodson P, Klemp P, Meyers OL: Pulmonary hypertension in systemic lupus erythematosus: a report of four cases. Clin Exp Rheumatol 1:241–245, 1983.
69. Gladman DD, Sternberg L: Pulmonary hypertension in systemic lupus erythematosus. J Rheumatol 12:365–367, 1985.
70. D'Angelo WA, Fries JF, Masi AT, Shulman LE: Pathologic observations in systemic sclerosis (scleroderma). Am J Med 46:428–440, 1969.
71. Norton WL, Nardo JM: Vascular disease in progressive systemic sclerosis (scleroderma). Ann Intern Med 73:317–324, 1970.
72. Rich S, Dantzker DR, Ayres SM, et al: Primary pulmonary hypertension. Ann Intern Med 107:216–223, 1987.
73. Watson RM, Lane AT, Barnett NK, et al: Neonatal lupus erythematosus. Medicine 63:362–378, 1984.
74. Buyon JP, Hiebert R, Copel J, et al: Autoimmune-associated congenital heart block: demographics, mortality, morbidity and recurrence rates obtained from a national neonatal lupus registry. J Am Coll Cardiol 31:1658–1666, 1998.
75. McCune AB, Weston WL, Lee LA: Maternal and fetal outcome in neonatal lupus erythematosus. Ann Intern Med 106:518–523, 1987.
76. Lee LA, Coulter S, Erner S, Chu H: Cardiac immunoglobulin deposition in congenital heart block associated with maternal anti-Ro autoantibodies. Am J Med 83:793–796, 1987.
77. Litsey SE, Noonan JA, O'Connor WN, et al: Maternal connective tissue disease and congenital heart block. N Engl J Med 312:98–100, 1985.
78. Taylor PV, Scott JS, Gerlis LM, et al: Maternal antibodies against fetal cardiac antigens in congenital complete heart block. N Engl J Med 315:667–672, 1986.
79. Viana VS, Garcia S, Nascimento JH, et al: Induction of in vitro

heart block is not restricted to affinity purified anti-52 kDa Ro/SSA antibody from mothers of children with neonatal lupus. Lupus 7:141–147, 1998.

80. Buyon JP, Swersky SH, Fox HE, et al: Intrauterine therapy for presumptive fetal myocarditis with acquired heart block due to systemic lupus erythematosus. Arthritis Rheum 30:44–49, 1987.
81. Harmon CE, Portanova JP: Drug-induced lupus: clinical and serological studies. Clin Rheum Dis 8:121–135, 1982.
82. Hess EV, Mongey AB: Drug-related lupus. Bull Rheum Dis 40:1–8, 1991.
83. Edwards RL, Rick ME, Wakem CJ: Studies on a circulating anticoagulant in procainamide-induced lupus erythematosus. Arch Intern Med 141:1688–1690, 1981.
84. Cohen MG, Kevat S, Prowse MV, Ahern MJ: Two distinct quinidine-induced rheumatic syndromes. Ann Intern Med 108:369–371, 1988.
85. West SG, McMahon M, Portanova JP: Quinidine-induced lupus erythematosus. Ann Intern Med 100:840–842, 1984.
86. Follansbee WP: The cardiovascular manifestations of systemic sclerosis (scleroderma). Curr Probl Cardiol 11:245–298, 1986.
87. Sharp GC, Singsen BH: Mixed connective tissue disease. *In* McCarty DJ (ed): Arthritis and Allied Conditions. p 1080. Philadelphia: Lea & Febiger, 1989.
88. Furst DE, Clements PJ, Graze P, et al: A syndrome resembling progressive systemic sclerosis after bone marrow transplantation. Arthritis Rheum 22:904–910, 1979.
89. Weiner ES, Earnshaw WC, Senecal JL, et al: Clinical associations of anticentromere antibodies and antibodies to topoisomerase I. Arthritis Rheum 31:378–385, 1988.
90. Arnett FC: HLA and autoimmunity in scleroderma (systemic sclerosis). Int Rev Immunol 12:107–128, 1995.
91. Ridolfi RL, Bulkley BH, Hutchins GM: The cardiac conduction system in progressive systemic sclerosis. Am J Med 61:361–366, 1976.
92. Leinwand I, Duryee AW, Richter MN: Scleroderma (based on a study of over 150 cases). Ann Intern Med 41:1003–1041, 1954.
93. Bulkley BH, Ridolfi RL, Salyer WR, Hutchins GM: Myocardial lesions of progressive systemic sclerosis. Circulation 53:483–490, 1976.
94. Sackner MA, Heinz ER, Steinberg AJ: The heart in scleroderma. Am J Cardiol 17:542–559, 1966.
95. Oram S, Stokes W: The heart in scleroderma. Br Heart J 23:243–259, 1961.
96. Deswal A, Follansbee WP: Cardiac involvement in scleroderma. Rheum Dis Clin N Am 22:841–860, 1996.
97. Follansbee WP, Miller TR, Curtiss EI, et al: A controlled clinicopathologic study of myocardial fibrosis in systemic sclerosis (scleroderma). J Rheumatol 17:656–662, 1990.
98. Alexander EL, Firestein GS, Weiss JL, et al: Reversible cold-induced abnormalities in myocardial perfusion and function in systemic sclerosis. Ann Intern Med 105:661–668, 1986.
99. Ellis WW, Baer AN, Robertson RM, et al: Left ventricular dysfunction induced by cold exposure in patients with systemic sclerosis. Am J Med 80:385–392, 1986.
100. Lekakis J, Mavrikakis M, Emmanuel M, et al: Cold-induced coronary Raynaud's phenomenon in patients with systemic sclerosis. Clin Exp Rheumatol 16:135–140, 1998.
101. Follansbee WP, Curtiss EI, Medsger TA Jr, et al: Physiologic abnormalities of cardiac function in progressive systemic sclerosis with diffuse scleroderma. N Engl J Med 310:142–148, 1984.
102. Valentini G, Vitale DF, Giunta A, et al: Diastolic abnormalities in systemic sclerosis: evidence for associated defective cardiac functional reserve. Ann Rheum Dis 55:455–460, 1996.
103. Murata I, Takenaka K, Shinohara S, et al: Diversity of myocardial involvement in systemic sclerosis: an 8-year study of 95 Japanese patients. Am Heart J 135:960–969, 1998.
104. Lichtbroun AS, Sandhaus LM, Giorno RC, et al: Myocardial mast cells in systemic sclerosis: a report of three fatal cases. Am J Med 89:372–376, 1990.
105. Gottdiner JS, Moutsopoulos HM, Decker JL: Echocardiographic identification of cardiac abnormality in scleroderma and related disorders. Am J Med 66:391–398, 1979.
106. Clements PJ, Furst DE, Cabeen W, et al: The relationship of arrhythmias and conduction disturbances to other manifestations of cardiopulmonary disease in progressive systemic sclerosis (PSS). Am J Med 71:38–46, 1981.
107. Roberts NK, Cabeen WR, Moss J, et al: The prevalence of conduction defects and cardiac arrhythmias in progressive systemic sclerosis. Ann Intern Med 94:38–40, 1981.
108. Kostis JB, Seibold JR, Turkevich D, et al: Prognostic importance of cardiac arrhythmias in systemic sclerosis. Am J Med 84:1007–1016, 1988.
109. Follansbee WP, Curtiss EI, Rahko PS, et al: The electrocardiogram in systemic sclerosis (scleroderma). Am J Med 79:183–192, 1985.
110. Altman RD, Medsger TA Jr, Bloch DA, Michel BA: Predictors of survival in systemic sclerosis (scleroderma). Arthritis Rheum 34:403–413, 1991.
111. Nishioka K, Katayama I, Kondo H, et al: Epidemiological analysis of prognosis of 496 Japanese patients with progressive systemic sclerosis (SSc). Scleroderma Research Committee Japan. J Dermatol 23:677–682, 1996.
112. Jiminez SA, Sigal SH: A 15-year prospective study of treatment of rapidly progressive systemic sclerosis with D-penicillamine. J Rheumatol 18:1496–1503, 1991.
113. Coffman JD, Clement DL, Creager MA, et al: International study of ketanserin in Raynaud's phenomenon. Am J Med 87:264–268, 1989.
114. Lopez-Ovejero JA, Saal SD, D'Angelo WA, et al: Reversal of vascular and renal crisis of scleroderma by oral angiotensin-converting-enzyme blockade. N Engl J Med 300:1417–1419, 1979.
115. Whitman HH III, Case DB, Laragh JH, et al: Variable response to oral angiotensin-converting-enzyme blockade in hypertensive scleroderma patients. Arthritis Rheum 25:241–248, 1982.
116. West SG, Killian PJ, Lawless OJ: Association of myositis and myocarditis in progressive systemic sclerosis. Arthritis Rheum 24:662–667, 1981.
117. McWhorter JE, Leroy EC: Pericardial disease in scleroderma (systemic sclerosis). Am J Med 57:566–575, 1974.
118. Smith JW, Clements PJ, Levisman J, et al: Echocardiographic features of progressive systemic sclerosis (PSS). Correlation with hemodynamic and postmortem studies. Am J Med 66:28–33, 1979.
119. Gladman DD, Gordon DA, Urowitz MB, Levy HL: Pericardial fluid analysis in scleroderma (systemic sclerosis). Am J Med 60:1064–1068, 1976.
120. Stupi AM, Steen VD, Owens GR, et al: Pulmonary hypertension in the CREST syndrome variant of systemic sclerosis. Arthritis Rheum 29:515–524, 1986.
121. Mikhail G, Chester AH, Gibbs JS, et al: Role of vasoactive mediators in primary and secondary pulmonary hypertension. Am J Cardiol 15:254–255, 1998.
122. McLaughlin VV, Genthner DE, Panella MM, Rich S: Reduction in pulmonary vascular resistance with long-term epoprostenol (prostacyclin) therapy in primary pulmonary hypertension. N Engl J Med 338:273–277, 1998.
123. Menon N, McAlpine L, Peacock AJ, Madhok R: The acute effects of prostacyclin on pulmonary hemodynamics in patients with pulmonary hypertension secondary to systemic sclerosis. Arthritis Rheum 41:466–499, 1998.
124. Humbert M, Sanchez O, Fartoukh M, et al: Treatment of severe pulmonary hypertension secondary to connective tissue diseases with continuous IV epoprostenol (prostacyclin). Chest 114:80S–82S, 1998.
125. Dalakas MC: Polymyositis, dermatomyositis, and inclusion-body myositis. N Engl J Med 325:1487–1498, 1991.
126. Strongwater SL: Overview and clinical manifestations of inflammatory myositis: polymyositis and dermatomyositis. Mount Sinai J Med 55:435–446, 1988.
127. Reichlin M, Arnett FC: Multiplicity of antibodies in myositis sera. Arthritis Rheum 27:1150–1156, 1984.
128. Friedman AW, Targoff IN, Arnett FC: Interstitial lung disease with autoantibodies against aminoacyl-tRNA synthesases in the absence of clinically apparent myositis. Semin Arthritis Rheum 26:459–467, 1996.
129. Denbow CE, Lie JT, Tancredi RG, Bunch TW: Cardiac involvement in polymyositis. A clinicopathologic study of 20 autopsied patients. Arthritis Rheum 22:1088–1092, 1979.
130. Buchpiguel CA, Roizenblatt S, Lucena-Fernandes MF, et al: Radioisotopic assessment of peripheral and cardiac muscle involvement and dysfunction in polymyositis/dermatomyositis. J Rheumatol 18:1359–1363, 1991.
131. Taylor AJ, Wortham DC, Burge JR, Rogan KM: The heart in polymyositis: a prospective evaluation of 26 patients. Clin Cardiol 16:802–808, 1993.

132. Buchpiguel CA, Roizenblatt S, Pastor EH, et al: Cardiac and skeletal muscle scintigraphy in dermato- and polymyositis: clinical implications. Eur J Nucl Med 23:199–203, 1996.
133. Gonzalez-Lopez L, Gamez-Nava JI, Sanchez L, et al: Cardiac manifestations in dermato-polymyositis. Clin Exp Rheumatol 14:373–379, 1996.
134. Askari AD: Cardiac abnormalities. Clin Rheum Dis 10:31–49, 1984.
135. Tymms KE, Webb J: Dermatopolymyositis and other connective tissue diseases: a review of 105 cases. J Rheumatol 12:1140–1148, 1985.
136. Hochberg MC, Feldman D, Stevens MB: Adult onset polymyositis/dermatomyositis: an analysis of clinical and laboratory features and survival in 76 patients with a review of the literature. Semin Arthritis Rheum 15:168–178, 1986.
137. Tami LF, Bhasin S: Polymorphism of the cardiac manifestations in dermatomyositis. Clin Cardiol 16:260–264, 1993.
138. Larca LJ, Coppola JT, Honig S: Creatine kinase MB isoenzyme in dermatomyositis: a noncardiac source. Ann Intern Med 94:341–343, 1981.
139. Kobayashi S, Tanaka M, Tamura N, et al: Serum cardiac troponin T in polymyositis/dermatomyositis. Lancet 340:726, 1992.
140. Badsha H, Gunes B, Grossman J, Brahn E: Troponin I assessment of cardiac involvement in patients with connective tissue disease and an elevated creatine kinase MB isoform. J Clin Rheumatol 3:131–134, 1997.
141. Weiss J, Shark W, Fishbein M, et al: The use of endomyocardial biopsy in a serious cardiac abnormality associated with polymyositis: a case report. J Rheumatol 9:299–302, 1982.
142. Fauci AS, Haynes BF, Katz P: The spectrum of vasculitis. Ann Intern Med 89:660–676, 1978.
143. Jennette JC, Falk RJ: Small-vessel vasculitis. N Engl J Med 337:1512–1523, 1997.
144. Lie JT, Members and Consultants of the American College of Rheumatology, Subcommittee on Classification of Vasculitis: Illustrated histopathologic classification criteria for selected vasculitis syndromes. Arthritis Rheum 33:1074–1087, 1990.
145. Calabrese LH, Michel BA, Bloch DA, et al: The American College of Rheumatology 1990 criteria for the classification of hypersensitivity vasculitis. Arthritis Rheum 33:1108–1113, 1990.
146. Masi AT, Hunder GG, Lie JT, et al: The American College of Rheumatology 1990 criteria for the classification of Churg-Strauss syndrome (allergic granulomatosis and angiitis). Arthritis Rheum 33:1094–1100, 1990.
147. Leavitt RY, Fauci AS, Bloch DA, et al: The American College of Rheumatology 1990 criteria for the classification of Wegener's granulomatosis. Arthritis Rheum 33:1101–1107, 1990.
148. Lightfoot RW Jr, Michel BA, Bloch DA, et al: The American College of Rheumatology 1990 criteria for the classification of polyarteritis nodosa. Arthritis Rheum 33:1088–1093, 1990.
149. Hunder GG, Bloch DA, Michel BA, et al: The American College of Rheumatology 1990 criteria for the classification of giant cell arteritis. Arthritis Rheum 33:1122–1129, 1990.
150. Arend WP, Michel BA, Bloch DA, et al: The American College of Rheumatology 1990 criteria for the classification of Takayasu arteritis. Arthritis Rheum 33:1129–1134, 1990.
151. Holsinger DR, Osmundson PJ, Edwards JE: The heart in periarteritis nodosa. Circulation 25:610–618, 1962.
152. Sergent JS, Lockshin MD, Christian CL, Gocke DJ: Vasculitis with hepatitis B antigenemia: long-term observations in nine patients. Medicine 55:1–18, 1976.
153. Dahlbert PJ, Lockhart JM, Overholt EL: Diagnostic studies for systemic necrotizing vasculitis. Arch Intern Med 149:161–165, 1989.
154. Fauci AS, Katz P, Haynes BF, Wolff SM: Cyclophosphamide therapy of severe systemic necrotizing vasculitis. N Engl J Med 301:235–238, 1979.
155. Leib ES, Restivo C, Paulus HE: Immunosuppressive and corticosteroid therapy of polyarteritis nodosa. Am J Med 67:941–948, 1979.
156. Hoffman GS, Kerr GS, Leavitt RY, et al: Wegener granulomatosis: an analysis of 158 patients. Ann Intern Med 116:488–498, 1992.
157. Falk RJ, Hogan S, Carey TS, Jennette C, for the Glomerular Disease Collaborative Network: Clinical course of anti-neutrophil cytoplasmic autoantibody–associated glomerulonephritis and systemic vasculitis. Ann Intern Med 113:656–663, 1990.
158. Delevaux I, Hoen B, Selton-Suty C, Canton P: Relapsing congestive cardiomyopathy in Wegener's granulomatosis. Mayo Clin Proc 72:848–850, 1997.
159. Ognibene FP, Shelhamer JH, Hoffman GS, et al: *Pneumocystis carinii* pneumonia: a major complication of immunosuppressive therapy in patients with Wegener's granulomatosis. Am J Respir Crit Care Med 151:795–799, 1995.
160. Spiera H, Lawson W, Weinrauch H: Wegener's granulomatosis treated with sulfamethoxazole-trimethoprim. Arch Intern Med 148:2065–2066, 1988.
161. Stegeman CA, Cohen TJW, deJong PE, Kallenberg CG: Trimethoprim-sulfamethoxazole (co-trimoxazole) for the prevention of relapses of Wegener's granulomatosis. N Engl J Med 335:16–20, 1996.
162. de Groot K, Rein-Keller E, Tatsis E, et al: Therapy for the maintenance of remission in sixty-five patients with generalized Wegener's granulomatosis. Methotrexate versus trimethoprim/sulfamethoxazole. Arthritis Rheum 39:2052–2061, 1996.
163. Lanham JG, Elkon KB, Pusey CD, Hughes GR: Systemic vasculitis with asthma and eosinophilia: a clinical approach to the Churg-Strauss syndrome. Medicine 63:65–80, 1984.
164. Tatsis E, Schnabel A, Gross WL: Interferon-alpha treatment of four patients with the Churg-Strauss syndrome. Ann Intern Med 129:370–374, 1998.
165. Hamilton CR Jr, Shelley WM, Tumulty PA: Giant cell arteritis: including temporal arteritis and polymyalgia rheumatica. Medicine 50:1–27, 1971.
166. Klein RG, Hunder GG, Stanson AW, Sheps SG: Large artery involvement in giant cell (temporal) arteritis. Ann Intern Med 83:806–812, 1975.
167. Klinkhoff AV, Reid GD, Moscovich M: Aortic regurgitation in giant cell arteritis. Arthritis Rheum 28:582–585, 1985.
168. Kay RH, Pooley R, Herman MV: Unsuspected giant cell arteritis diagnosed at open heart surgery. Arch Intern Med 142:1378–1380, 1982.
169. McKusick VA: A form of vascular disease relatively frequent in the Orient. Am Heart J 63:57–64, 1962.
170. Judge RD, Currier RD, Gracie WA, Figley MM: Takayasu's arteritis and the aortic arch syndrome. Am J Med 32:379–392, 1962.
171. Ishikawa K: Natural history and classification of occlusive thromboaortopathy (Takayasu's disease). Circulation 57:27–35, 1978.
172. Isohisa I, Numano F, Maezawa H, Sasazuki T: HLA-Bw52 in Takayasu disease. Tissue Antigens 12:246–248, 1978.
173. Shelhamer JH, Bolkman DJ, Parrillo JE, et al: Takayasu's arteritis and its therapy. Ann Intern Med 103:121–126, 1985.
174. Kawasaki T, Kosaki F, Okawa S, et al: A new infantile acute febrile mucocutaneous lymph node syndrome (MLNS) prevailing in Japan. Pediatrics 54:271–276, 1974.
175. Barron KS: Kawasaki disease in children. Curr Opin Rheumatol 10:29–37, 1998.
176. Milgrom H, Palmer EL, Slovin SF, et al: Kawasaki disease in a healthy young adult. Ann Intern Med 92:467–470, 1980.
177. Glanz S, Bittner SJ, Berman MA, et al: Regression of coronary-artery aneurysms in infantile polyarteritis nodosa. N Engl J Med 294:939–941, 1976.
178. Barron KS, Sher MR, Silverman ED: Intravenous immunoglobulin therapy: magic or black magic? J Rheumatol 19:94–97, 1992.
179. Shimizu T, Ehrlich GE, Inaba G, Hayashi K: Behçet disease. Arthritis Rheum 8:223–260, 1979.
180. James DG: Behçet's disease. Br J Clin Pract 44:364–368, 1990.
181. The International Study Group for Behçet's Disease: Evaluation of diagnostic (classification) criteria in Behçet's disease—towards internationally agreed criteria. Br J Rheumatol 31:299–308, 1992.
182. Durieux P, Bletry O, Huchon G, et al: Multiple pulmonary arterial aneurysms in Behçet's disease and Hughes-Stoven syndrome. Am J Med 71:736–741, 1981.
183. Huong DLT, Wechsler B, Papo T, et al: Arterial lesions in Behçet's disease. A study in 25 patients. J Rheumatol 22:2103–2113, 1995.
184. Ohno S, Ohguchi M, Hirose S, et al: Close association of HLA-Bw51 with Behçet's disease. Arch Ophthalmol 100:1455–1458, 1982.
185. James DG: Recognition of the diverse cardiovascular manifestations in Behçet's disease. Am Heart J 103:457–458, 1982.
186. Hamza MH: Treatment of Behçet's disease with thalidomide. Clin Exp Rheumatol 5:365–371, 1986.
187. Hamuryudan V, Mat C, Saip S, et al: Thalidomide in the treatment of the mucocutaneous lesions of the Behçet syndrome. Ann Intern Med 128:443–450, 1998.

188. O'Duffy JD, Robertson DM, Goldstein NP: Chlorambucil in the treatment of uveitis and meningoencephalitis of Behçet's disease. Am J Med 76:75–84, 1984.
189. Yazici H, Halit P, Barnes CG, et al: A controlled trial of azathioprine in Behçet's syndrome. N Engl J Med 322:281–327, 1990.
190. McAdam LP, O'Hanlan MA, Bluestone R, Pearson CM: Relapsing polychondritis: prospective study of 23 patients and a review of the literature. Medicine 55:193–215, 1976.
191. Michet CJ Jr, McKenna CH, Luthra HS, O'Fallon WM: Relapsing polychondritis: survival and predictive role of early disease manifestations. Ann Intern Med 129:114–122, 1998.
192. Trentham DE, Le CH: Relapsing polychondritis. Ann Intern Med 129:114–122, 1998.
193. Foidart JM, Abe S, Martin GR, et al: Antibodies to type II collagen in relapsing polychondritis. N Engl J Med 299:1203–1207, 1978.
194. Arnett FC: The seronegative spondyloarthropathies. Bull Rheum Dis 37:1–12, 1987.
195. Arnett FC: Seronegative spondyloarthropathies. *In* Dale DC, Federman DD (eds): Scientific American Medicine. pp 1–11. New York: Scientific American, 1998.
196. Hammer RE, Maika SD, Richardson JA, et al: Spontaneous inflammatory disease in transgenic rats expressing HLA-B27 and human beta 2m: an animal model of HLA-B27–associated human disorders. Cell 63:1099–1112, 1990.
197. Rahman MU, Cheema A, Schumacher HR, Hudson AP: Molecular evidence for the presence of chlamydia in the synovium of patients with Reiter's syndrome. Arthritis Rheum 35:521–529, 1992.
198. Granfors K: Do bacterial antigens cause reactive arthritis? Rheum Dis Clin N Am 18:37–48, 1992.
199. Maki-Ikola O, Leirisalo-Repo M, Kantele A, et al: *Salmonella*-specific antibodies in reactive arthritis. J Infect Dis 164:1141–1148, 1991.
200. Maki-Ikola O, Viljanen MD, Tiitinen S, et al: Antibodies to arthritis-associated microbes in inflammatory joint diseases. Rheumatol Int 10:231–234, 1991.
201. Wollenhaupt HJ, Krech T, Schneider C, Zeidler H: Specific serum IgA–antibodies in chlamydial-induced arthritis. Z Rheumatol 88:86–88, 1989.
202. Lauhio A, Leirisalo-Repo M, Lahdevirta J, et al: Double-blind, placebo-controlled study of three-month treatment with lymecycline in reactive arthritis, with special reference to chlamydia arthritis. Arthritis Rheum 34:6–14, 1991.
203. Bulkley BH, Roberts WC: Ankylosing spondylitis and aortic regurgitation. Circulation 48:1014–1027, 1973.
204. Paulus HE, Pearson CM, Pitts W Jr: Aortic insufficiency in five patients with Reiter's syndrome. Am J Med 53:464–472, 1972.
205. Ruppert GB, Lindsay J, Werner FB: Cardiac conduction abnormalities in Reiter's syndrome. Am J Med 73:335–340, 1982.
206. Roberts WC, Hollingsworth JF, Bulkley BH, et al: Combined mitral and aortic regurgitation in ankylosing spondylitis. Am J Med 56:237–242, 1974.
207. Zvaifler NJ, Weintraub AM: Aortitis and aortic insufficiency in the chronic rheumatic disorders: a reappraisal. Arthritis Rheum 6:241–245, 1963.
208. Bergfeldt L: HLA-B27–associated cardiac disease. Ann Intern Med 127:621–629, 1997.
209. Bergfeldt L, Edhag O, Rajs J: HLA-B27 associated heart disease. Am J Med 77:961–967, 1984.
210. Csonka GW: Clinical aspects of Reiter's syndrome. Ann Rheum Dis 38(suppl 1):4–7, 1979.
211. Arnett FC: Incomplete Reiter's syndrome. Clinical comparisons with classical triad. Ann Rheum Dis 38(suppl 1):73–78, 1979.
212. Machado H, Befeler B, Morales AR, Vargas A: Rapidly progressive aortic insufficiency in Reiter's syndrome. Ann Intern Med 81:121–122, 1974.
213. Stewart SR, Robbins DL, Castles JJ: Acute fulminant aortic and mitral insufficiency in ankylosing spondylitis. N Engl J Med 299:1448–1449, 1978.
214. LaBresh KA, Lally EV, Sharma SC, Ho G Jr: Two-dimensional echocardiographic detection of preclinical aortic root abnormalities in rheumatoid variant diseases. Am J Med 78:908–912, 1985.
215. Arnason JA, Patel AK, Rahko PS, Sundstrom WR: Transthoracic and transesophageal echocardiographic evaluation of the aortic root and subvalvular structures in ankylosing spondylitis. J Rheumatol 23:120–123, 1996.
216. Bergfeldt L, Edhag O, Vedin L, Vallin H: Ankylosing spondylitis: an important cause of severe disturbances of the cardiac conduction system. Am J Med 73:187–191, 1982.
217. Bergfeldt L: HLA-B27–associated rheumatic disease with severe cardiac bradyarrhythmias. Am J Med 75:210–215, 1983.
218. Bergfeldt L, Moller E: Complete heart block—another HLA-B27 associated disease manifestation. Tissue Antigens 21:385–390, 1983.
219. Bergfeldt L, Insulander P, Lindblom D, et al: HLA-B27: an important genetic risk factor for lone aortic regurgitation and severe conduction system abnormalities. Am J Med 85:12–18, 1988.
220. Podell TE, Wallace DJ, Fishbein MC, et al: Severe giant cell valvulitis in a patient with Reiter's syndrome. Arthritis Rheum 25:232–234, 1982.
221. Gould BA, Turner J, Keeling DH, et al: Myocardial dysfunction in ankylosing spondylitis. Ann Rheum Dis 51:227–232, 1992.
222. Crowley JJ, Donnelly SM, Tobin M, et al: Doppler echocardiographic evidence of left ventricular diastolic dysfunction in ankylosing spondylitis. Am J Cardiol 71:1337–1340, 1993.

CHAPTER 105

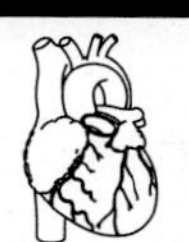

SUBSTANCE ABUSE AND THE HEART

Eric J. Eichhorn and Paul A. Grayburn

COCAINE
History of Cocaine
Pharmacology
Cardiovascular Complications of Cocaine
Effects on the Coronary Circulation
Acute Effects on Peripheral Circulation and Left Ventricular Function
Effect of Cocaine on the Myocardium
Effect of Cocaine on Rhythm Disturbances
Other Cardiovascular Complications of Cocaine Abuse
Treatment of Cardiovascular Complications of Cocaine
ETHANOL
Alcoholic Cardiomyopathy
Pathophysiology of Alcoholic Cardiac Dysfunction
Natural History
Treatment
Alcohol-Related Cardiac Arrhythmias
Effects of Alcohol on Atherosclerosis
Other Effects of Ethanol on the Heart
AMPHETAMINES
MARIJUANA
OTHER CARDIOVASCULAR EFFECTS OF DRUG ABUSE

> "Which is it to-day? I asked. "Morphine or cocaine?" He raised his eyes languidly from the old black-letter volume which he had opened. "It is cocaine," he said; "a seven per cent solution. Would you care to try it?"
>
> Sir Arthur Conan Doyle

Substance abuse was common in Sir Arthur Conan Doyle's time, and it remains a major problem today. The effects of substance abuse on the cardiovascular system can be divided into two broad categories: general effects of substance abuse, such as endocarditis or vasculitis in intravenous drug abusers, and specific cardiovascular toxicity associated with specific drugs. Endocarditis in drug abusers has been discussed in detail in Chapter 18, Infective Endocarditis. Thus, this chapter focuses on cardiovascular manifestations of specific drugs, particularly cocaine and ethanol. Tobacco abuse, which constitutes a major cause of cardiovascular morbidity and mortality owing to premature coronary atherosclerosis, is discussed in Chapter 122, Smoking.

COCAINE

It is estimated that more than 23 million Americans have tried cocaine at least once, and 5 million are current users.[1–4] The cost of cocaine-related hospital admissions exceeds $80 million per year.[4] Cocaine abuse has become a significant socioeconomic burden to our society. Retrospective reviews of hospital records from urban medical centers suggest that 5 to 10 percent of emergency room visits may be due to cardiac complications related to cocaine abuse.[5–7] This represents a substantial monetary and time burden to the health care delivery system. Although the exact incidence of death attributed directly or indirectly to cocaine abuse is not known, it is clear that cardiovascular manifestations of cocaine abuse constitute an important health care issue.

History of Cocaine

The use of cocaine can be traced to South American natives as early as AD 600.[8, 9] Cocaine is an alkaloid and comes from the leaves of the *Erythroxylon coca* plant.[10] These leaves were chewed or sucked for their intoxicating effects by the Indians of Peru and Bolivia. In 1860, the alkaloid was first isolated by Niemann, who noted that it had a bitter taste and produced numbness on the tongue when tasted.[9] In 1880, Von Anrep observed that the skin lost sensation when infiltrated with cocaine.[10] In 1884, Sigmund Freud studied the effects of cocaine and published a report of its use, including using it to wean patients from morphine.[7, 10] In 1884, Hall introduced cocaine as a local anesthetic for dental procedures.[10] The following year, Halsted used it for nerve blocks for surgical procedures.[10]

In the late 1800s, many over-the-counter products—including Coca-Cola, cough syrups, and even some wines[7]—contained small amounts of cocaine. The Harrison Narcotic Act of 1914 classified cocaine as a "narcotic," thus relegating its use to medical purposes only.

Pharmacology

The chemical formula for cocaine is $C_{17}H_{21}NO_4$ (Fig. 105–1), and its chemical name is benzoylmethylecgonine. Cocaine has at least two important properties: (1) it is a local anesthetic with effects on the cellular membrane (by acting on the fast Na^+ channels and decreasing membrane Na^+ permeability), and (2) it augments the effects of catecholamines (norepinephrine and dopamine) through blockade of their reuptake at the synaptic junctions and release of epinephrine and dopamine from the adrenal medulla.[1, 10–13]

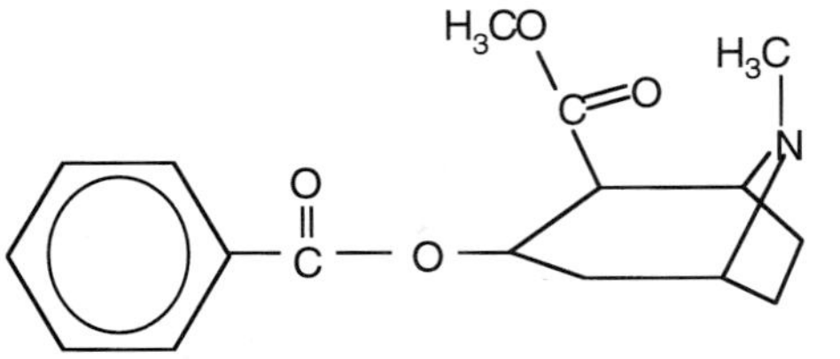

FIGURE 105–1 Chemical structure of cocaine.

Most of the adverse effects of cocaine come from one or both of these properties.

Cocaine is degraded by plasma pseudocholinesterases and, in some animals, by hepatic enzymes.[10] Thus, patients with congenital defects of the pseudocholinesterase system may have marked hypersensitivity to cocaine. Cocaine is degraded to several metabolites, including benzoylecgonine and ethyl methyl ecgonine, which are water soluble and excreted in the urine for 24 to 36 hours after drug use. Other metabolites include ecgonine, norecgonine, and norbenzoylecgonine. Cocaine hydrochloride is a white crystalline powder prepared by dissolving the alkaloid in hydrochloric acid to form a water-soluble salt.[7] The alkaloid, which is known as *free base* or *crack* is soluble in alcohol, acetone, and ether, and it can be manufactured from the hydrochloride by combining it with baking soda. The alkaloid is typically smoked, although it is well absorbed from mucous membranes. The pharmacokinetics of cocaine taken nasally, smoked, and used intravenously are shown in Table 105–1.

Cardiovascular Complications of Cocaine

The first reported cardiovascular complication of cocaine appeared as a case report of prolonged cardiac failure during dental procedures.[14] Further evidence of toxic cardiac effects were noted in studies of cocaine injected into experimental animals.[15–18] However, it was not until 1947 that another report of human myocardial toxicity from cocaine appeared.[19] Since then, numerous reports of the damaging effects of cocaine on the heart have appeared. Because cocaine has multiple and complex effects on the cardiovascular system, we examine its effects on the coronary circulation, peripheral circulation, sympathetic nervous system, and myocardium.

Effects on the Coronary Circulation

Early work in experimental animals has shown that norepinephrine constricts the coronary vasculature.[20] It has only been since the early 1980s that myocardial infarction (MI) and sudden cardiovascular death have been noted in cocaine users.[1, 3, 10, 11, 20–53] The typical profile of a patient who has a cocaine-associated MI is a young male cigarette smoker who is approximately 33 years old.[4, 54] One fourth of these patients have no risk factors for coronary artery disease, and two thirds have a history of cigarette smoking.[7] MI can occur with first-time use or after years of use.[54] In cocaine abusers with MI, ingested doses have ranged from five to six "lines" (approximately 150 mg) to 2 g.[34, 40] The typical cocaine abuser uses 300 to 1000 mg per use.[4] Most patients with cocaine-related MI have angiographically normal coronary arteries with evidence of thrombosis at the time of cardiac catheterization.[7, 32, 54] The mechanism of cocaine-induced ischemia is still being elucidated. However, the pathogenesis of cocaine-induced ischemia must take into account four factors: (1) increased myocardial oxygen demand, (2) cocaine-induced vasoconstriction, (3) endothelial abnormalities that are permissive to vasospasm and/or thrombosis, and (4) promotion and/or acceleration of atherosclerosis by cocaine use.

TABLE 105–1 Effects and Duration of Cocaine Based on Route of Administration

Route	Onset of Action	Peak Effect	Duration
Inhalation (smoking)	3–5 s	1–3 min	5–15 min
Intravenous	10–60 s	3–5 min	20–60 min
Intranasal	1–5 min	15–20 min	60–90 min

Increased Myocardial Oxygen Demand

It has been documented in animals[55, 56] and humans[57] that cocaine acutely raises systemic blood pressure and heart rate, thus increasing myocardial oxygen demand. Effects on heart rate and blood pressure may be masked in anesthetized animals.[56] In addition, these effects may be variable at different cocaine doses.[58] One study in both conscious and anesthetized dogs demonstrated an increase in blood pressure at the lowest dose of cocaine, no change at intermediate doses, and a reduction in pressure at highest doses.[13, 58]

Cocaine-Induced Vasoconstriction

Despite the increase in myocardial oxygen demand, oxygen supply may be severely limited with cocaine abuse. Cocaine has alpha$_1$-adrenergic agonist properties, and its ability to cause coronary vasoconstriction has been established.[1, 22, 25, 26, 54, 57, 59] Such coronary constriction may be blocked in vivo by the alpha-antagonist phentolamine.[57] However, phentolamine does not block the vasoconstrictor actions of cocaine in in vitro denervated models,[54, 60] wherein calcium channel antagonists are able to abolish cocaine-induced vasoconstriction.[60] In such in vitro preparations, cocaine-induced vasoconstriction has been shown to be independent of the endothelium.[54, 60] Thus, cocaine probably exerts its vasoconstrictive effects via three independent mechanisms: (1) direct vasoconstriction, which is calcium channel dependent,[54, 61] (2) indirect vasoconstriction, which is mediated through norepinephrine release by the sympathetic nervous system, and (3) indirect vasoconstriction, which is mediated by other neurohormones such as endothelin-1.[62] The norepinephrine-mediated vasoconstriction can be blocked by phentolamine only in innervated in vivo preparations, thus explaining why in vitro models fail to show an effect of an α-adrenergic antagonist. As direct intracoronary administration of low-dose cocaine in humans (at a dose that does not produce much increase in systemic levels of cocaine) produces no change in coronary sinus blood flow, coronary vascular resistance, or dimensions of the coronary arteries, the major vasoconstrictive effect of cocaine may be mediated by the adrenergic nervous system and not a direct effect.[63]

As cocaine may act in part through an α-adrenergic mechanism, use of a beta-adrenergic blocking agent during a period of myocardial ischemia may result in worsening of coronary vasoconstriction and/or spasm owing to the unopposed α-adrenergic vasoconstriction.[59, 64] Use of a mixed alpha- and beta-blocker, such as labetalol, blunts the increase in rate-pressure product (myocardial oxygen consumption) due to cocaine, but it does not alleviate cocaine-induced coronary arterial vasoconstriction.[65] On the other hand, as compared to pure β-blockers,[64] labetalol did not potentiate coronary vasoconstriction in this study.[65]

Evidence has suggested a second wave of cocaine-induced vasoconstriction approximately 90 minutes after ingestion, a time when the blood concentration of cocaine is low. The mechanism of this effect may be related to increases in cocaine's vasoactive metabolites (benzoylecgonine and ethyl methyl ecgonine).[66]

Previous studies have demonstrated that cigarette smoking by itself causes an increase in myocardial oxygen demand and coronary vasoconstriction.[67] When cigarette smoking is mixed with cocaine use, there is potentiation of cocaine's effect on rate-pressure product increase and on coronary vasoconstriction.[68] Thus, the two agents together synergistically increase myocardial oxygen consumption while reducing myocardial oxygen delivery. Because most cocaine users also smoke cigarettes, there may be additive risk of myocardial ischemia.

Over 9 million subjects who abuse cocaine also simultaneously abuse ethanol.[4] This combination is the most common form of polysubstance abuse seen in emergency rooms and accounts for over 1000 deaths per year.[4] Some data exist to suggest that the combination of alcohol and cocaine increases the risk of drug-induced sudden death 18-fold.[4, 69–71] The reasons for this synergistic deleterious effect is unknown. One study of moderate alcohol administration with low-dose intranasal cocaine demonstrated that alcohol produced very mild potentiation of rate-pressure product at 30 minutes, but not at 60 and 90 minutes.[71] However, ethanol when added to cocaine produced an increase (as opposed to a decrease) in coronary artery diameter. Thus, the combination of ethanol and low-dose cocaine produces an increase in myocardial oxygen demand, but does not produce an inappropriate reduction in myocardial oxygen delivery as cocaine alone does. These data suggest that any increase in sudden death produced by the addition of ethanol to cocaine may be related more to arrhythmic than to ischemic effects.

Both nitroglycerin[72] and verapamil[73] have been shown to ameliorate some of cocaine's harmful effects. Both sublingual nitroglycerin and intravenous verapamil reduced arterial pressure and increased coronary artery dimensions in both diseased and nondiseased segments of coronary artery after cocaine administration.

Endothelial Abnormalities

Direct cocaine-induced vasospasm may not totally explain cocaine-induced ischemia and MI for several reasons. First, a disparate temporal relationship between MI and cocaine ingestion exists in many cases, such that myocardial ischemia may occur long after peak cocaine levels have diminished.[12, 74] Second, two animal studies[55, 75] using higher (street) doses of cocaine and one human study[76] have demonstrated an increase in coronary blood flow with cocaine rather than a decrease, suggesting that cocaine-induced coronary vasoconstriction may be a dose-dependent phenomenon, with low-dose cocaine producing α-adrenergic vasoconstriction and higher doses resulting in resistance vessel vasodilatation owing to increased metabolic needs.[77] Finally, cocaine-mediated vasoconstriction probably requires an underlying endothelial abnormality to produce frank vasospasm and/or thrombosis, although this has been controversial.[78] One study showed that cocaine-induced vasoconstriction was accentuated in regions of atherosclerosis.[79] Thus, dysfunctional endothelium (owing to either accelerated atherosclerosis or intimal proliferation), where production of endothelium-derived relaxing factors (EDRFs) may be impaired, may predispose cocaine abusers to MI.

In a study of 10 long-term cocaine users and 13 control subjects of similar age who had not used cocaine, acetylcholine-mediated vasodilatation in the forearm was impaired in the cocaine subjects.[74] The coronary artery response to acetylcholine infusion was studied in 10 chronic cocaine abusers.[74] In 8 of 10 chronic cocaine abusers with angiographically normal coronary arteries, acetylcholine administration elicited paradoxical vasoconstriction and, in some cases, elicited vasospasm, suggesting dysfunctional endothelium and a deficiency of EDRFs.[74] These data suggest that cocaine users may have impaired endothelium-dependent vasorelaxation. Although it is unclear whether cocaine is directly toxic to endothelial cells or whether this is an indirect effect of periodic hypertension and sheer stress, the decrease in normal endothelial response may be a risk factor in these patients.

In rabbits fed a low-cholesterol diet, endothelial production of prostaglandins is altered by chronic cocaine use, with a disproportionate increase in thromboxane A_2 production compared with prostaglandin F_{1a}.[80] In addition, cocaine has been shown to acutely increase thromboxane A_2 in hypoxic conditions or in the presence of platelet-activating factors.[81] Cocaine has been shown to enhance the response of platelets to thromboxane in an in vitro preparation.[82] These findings suggest that cocaine may actually alter endothelial function, creating a milieu that is permissive for vasoconstriction and/or thrombosis. A lack of EDRF potentiates alpha-vasoconstriction in animals.[83–85] Evidence exists in humans for this same phenomenon. One study shows accentuated vasoconstriction to cocaine administration in regions of atherosclerosis in non–cocaine-abusing patients.[79] Thus, dysfunctional endothelium (owing to either accelerated atherosclerosis or intimal proliferation) may be a predisposing cause for cocaine-induced MI. Alternatively, underlying endothelial abnormalities of any cause may potentiate the vascular effects of cocaine.

Additionally, the presence of intimal proliferation or atherosclerosis and endothelial dysfunction associated with reductions in release of EDRFs may alter the antithrombotic properties of the normal endothelial surface. Such alterations may provide a surface for platelet aggregation and alter local concentrations of such antithrombotic factors as tissue plasminogen activator and thrombomodulin. Indeed, EDRFs have been documented to inhibit platelet aggregation,[86–88] and thromboxane A_2 is known to enhance platelet aggregation.[89] Thus, a deficit of EDRFs and a disproportionate increase in thromboxane A_2 may predispose a cocaine abuser to thrombosis.

The importance of underlying endothelial abnormalities in promoting cocaine-induced MI may explain the relatively low rate of MI among the 5 million chronic cocaine users in this country. For example, Gitter and colleagues[90] studied 101 consecutive cocaine abusers who were admitted to the hospital for chest pain suggestive of myocardial ischemia. MI was ruled out in all subjects by creatine kinase isoenzymes. Thus, whereas cocaine may provoke chest pain owing to increased oxygen demand and coronary vasoconstriction, the development of acute MI is uncommon and probably requires an underlying endothelial abnormality.

Promotion of Atherosclerosis

There is evidence that cocaine may promote the development of atherosclerosis or accelerate the atherosclerotic process. Retrospective autopsy examination of five cocaine abusers who died suddenly revealed intimal proliferation in four of five and thrombus formation in one.[91] In a prospective autopsy examination of 24 cocaine abusers and 14 age- and sex-matched controls, atherosclerosis was not increased in incidence, but was increased in severity.[91] Other retrospective autopsy series have shown a high incidence of premature atherosclerosis in cocaine abusers,[26, 92–94] and cocaine has been demonstrated to accelerate atherosclerosis in cholesterol-fed rabbits.[95]

Acute Effects on Peripheral Circulation and Left Ventricular Function

The effects of cocaine on the peripheral circulation are incompletely understood. It is well known that cocaine causes a modest dose-dependent increase in blood pressure[55, 96] and can even precipitate hypertensive crisis. It has been proposed that this is due to central sympathetic stimulation by cocaine. In support of this concept, the pressor effects of cocaine in dogs can be blocked by anesthesia and by the ganglionic blocker hexamethonium.[56] In addition, single-fiber baroreceptor recordings in the rat aortic arch before and after cocaine administration suggest that cocaine severely depresses baroreceptor afferent discharge, resulting in sympathetic nervous system activation.[97] However, direct nerve recordings in decerebrate cats suggest that cocaine may actually suppress central sympathetic drive, and the site of action may be the hindbrain.[98] Moreover, cocaine's effect on systemic vascular resistance varies from study to study.[55, 96] In one animal study,[96] cocaine did not change systemic vascular resistance in the absence of adrenergic blockade, suggesting that the increase in blood pressure was due to an increase in cardiac output. A study in normal volunteers shows that intranasal cocaine (2 mg/kg) causes a profound increase in central sympathetic outflow to the skeletal muscle bed.[99] However, this is rapidly modulated by the sinoaortic baroreceptors, such that blood pressure increases only modestly. It is tempting to speculate that in the presence of baroreceptor dysfunction, cocaine would cause a dramatic increase in blood pressure that could account for the occasional reports of hypertensive crisis after cocaine abuse. Thus, it appears that although cocaine causes coronary vasoconstriction, it does not cause generalized systemic vasoconstriction when given acutely. Chronic cocaine abuse, however, can cause depletion of dopamine stores, which enhances sensitivity to α-adrenergic vasoconstriction. The effects of cocaine on peripheral vascular tone in chronic cocaine abusers has not been studied.

The acute effects of cocaine on left ventricular contractility have been studied in animals[13, 55, 56, 75, 100–103] and humans.[99] At low concentrations of cocaine ($<10^{-5}$ M), there is an increase in myocardial contractility associated with an increased amplitude and shortened duration of the intracellular calcium transient.[61] At higher doses ($>10^{-4}$ M in vitro and 4 to 10 mg/kg in human studies), cocaine appears to acutely decrease myocardial contractility, as reflected by depression of peak positive dP/dt and global left ventricular ejection fraction, despite an increase in left ventricular end-diastolic pressure. Whereas the fall in left ventricular ejection fraction may in part be due to an increase in afterload, the depression of peak positive dP/dt and studies in more isolated animal preparations[104, 105] suggest that myocardial depression is present. This reduction in contractility is accompanied by a decrease in the amplitude and prolonged time course of the aequorin response in vitro.[61] It has been postulated that this biphasic response to cocaine (increased contractility at low dose and reduced contractility at higher doses) may be due to a catecholamine response at low dose and either blockade of the sodium channels (anesthetic property) at higher doses[105, 106] or decreased calcium sensitivity of the contractile proteins or myofilaments at higher doses.[61, 106–108] In one study,[102] pretreatment with nifedipine, a calcium channel antagonist, protected the heart from myocardial depression and a reduction in coronary blood flow associated with cocaine. However, treatment with nifedipine after cocaine administration did not result in myocardial and coronary protection. Although studies in humans[99] have not shown myocardial depression with acute administration of 2 mg/kg of intranasal cocaine, the doses used have been lower, and such depression may be dose dependent.

Effect of Cocaine on the Myocardium

The two predominant myocardial lesions associated with chronic cocaine abuse are hypertrophy and cardiomyopathy. Brickner and coworkers[109] demonstrated that chronic cocaine abuse is associated with left ventricular hypertrophy in humans. The mechanism whereby this occurs is uncertain, but it may be related to an exaggerated pressor response to sympathetic stimuli. Accordingly, Cigarroa and associates[110] found that chronic cocaine abusers with left ventricular hypertrophy had an elevated peak systolic blood pressure response to treadmill exercise compared with control subjects and cocaine abusers without left ventricular hypertrophy. This finding may be related to cocaine-induced depletion of dopamine stores, leading to hypersensitivity to sympathetic stimuli. In addition, stimulation of adrenergic pathways may result in myocardial growth stimulation, leading to hypertrophic remodeling.[111]

It has long been known that catecholamines can induce myocardial necrosis and dysfunction.[112–114] Additionally, anecdotal and/or necropsy reports of cocaine abusers with myocardial dysfunction[37, 115–117] and myocarditis[3, 24, 118] have been published. There is evidence to suggest that these isolated cases are not unrelated to the cocaine abuse. First, withdrawal of the cocaine can result in temporal improvement in ventricular function in some cases.[115] This improvement is probably not totally explained by a reduction in afterload or blood pressure. Second, other related high-catecholamine conditions, such as pheochromocytoma[119–122] or congestive heart failure,[123–127] can induce or perpetuate myocardial dysfunction. Third, a higher than normal incidence of myocarditis has been found at necropsy in cocaine abusers who die as opposed to an age-matched group of control patients who die of trauma.[118] Finally, other exogenous agents such as amphetamines can induce a potentially reversible cardiomyopathy similar to that seen in cocaine abuse.[128] There is evidence to suggest five separate but related mechanisms for myocardial dysfunction and necrosis: (1) repeated microvascular injury from vasospasm and ischemia, (2) direct toxic effects of catecholamines and/or cocaine on the myocardium, (3) subsensitivity of the contractile mechanism to beta-agonist stimulation owing to β-adrenergic receptor down-regulation, and (4) impurities and other drugs used to "cut" street cocaine may be immunogenic, and (5) change in myocardial phenotype producing dysfunctional contractile proteins.

As mentioned, previous studies have shown that cocaine is a powerful α-adrenergic vasoconstrictor[57] and may cause vasospasm owing to abnormal endothelial function.[74, 80] Chronic administration of cocaine may result in repeated ischemic episodes, leading to myocyte necrosis[3, 22–36] with formation of contraction bands.[129] Additionally, catecholamines are directly toxic to the myocardium,[112–114] and chronic administration of cocaine to rats results in increased levels of norepinephrine in the left ventricle.[130] Finally, street cocaine contains impurities and other agents that may be immunogenic.[118] This may result in inflammation and necrosis within the myocardium and possibly other sites. Ultimately, these mechanisms may be responsible for progressive ventricular dysfunction. Depending on the resulting degree of collagen deposition and fibrosis, varying degrees of ventricular recovery can reasonably be anticipated after cocaine withdrawal.

Effect of Cocaine on Rhythm Disturbances

The effects of cocaine on the action potential resemble those of a type Ia antiarrhythmic agent.[10] Laboratory demonstrations of the effect of cocaine on the myocardium have demonstrated decreased automaticity by depressing phase 0 depolarization[131] and increasing the refractory period.[132, 133] Cocaine is thus felt to inhibit both fast Na^+ channels and repolarizing K^+ but not Ca^{2+} channels. These effects are manifest on the electrocardiogram by a prolongation of the PR, QRS, and QT intervals.[133] By inhibiting sodium influx into cardiac cells, impulse conduction is impaired, creating the substrate for reentrant tachyarrhythmias.[7, 134] Moreover, the inhibition of norepinephrine reuptake by cocaine could potentiate ventricular arrhythmias via a catecholamine effect.[13, 18, 135] Thus, it is not surprising that malignant ventricular arrhythmias have been reported with cocaine abuse.[3, 17, 54, 136–140] Such arrhythmias in the setting of cocaine ingestion appear to require a substrate such as MI, myocarditis, or left ventricular dysfunction.[141] Thus, cocaine-mediated ventricular arrhythmias are probably related to a combination of ventricular dysfunction and catecholamine stimulation that lowers the threshold for inducing ventricular tachycardia and fibrillation. Additionally, as many patients with cocaine abuse have MI and ischemia or myocarditis, ventricular fibrillation may be a sequela of such an acute event. Facilitating conditions for arrhythmias induced by cocaine include hyperpyrexia,[7] seizures,[141] and metabolic acidosis.[142]

Cocaine has also been implicated in supraventricular rhythm disturbances. Cocaine has been noted to unmask Wolff-Parkinson-White syndrome in two cases.[54]

Other Cardiovascular Complications of Cocaine Abuse

Cocaine has been associated with a variety of other cardiovascular complications including hypertensive crisis, aortic rupture,[143–146] vascular thrombosis,[147, 148] stroke,[149–162] and pneumopericardium.[54, 163] In addition, intravenous users are at risk for developing endocarditis (see Ch. 2, Electrocardiography).[164]

Treatment of Cardiovascular Complications of Cocaine

As a majority of MIs attributable to cocaine are due to in situ thrombosis[7, 32, 54] and/or coronary vasospasm,[1, 22, 25, 26, 54, 57–60, 66] rapid-acting nitrates,[72] calcium channel blocking agents,[139, 140] aspirin, and even thrombolytics[165, 166] (should the chest pain and electrocardiographic changes not resolve rapidly with the aforementioned agents) should be considered as initial treatment.

Aspirin should be used to help avoid the formation of thrombi. Aspirin has been shown to improve survival in MI not related to cocaine use[167] and has a good safety profile. Although there are no prospective studies of aspirin in cocaine-related MI, its use appears safe and probably beneficial. The newer platelet inhibitors, such as the glycoprotein IIb/IIIa antagonists, have not been tested in patients with cocaine use and MI, and their higher risk profile make their use uncertain at this time. However, they may be of benefit in some situations. Thrombolytic agents have been shown to improve survival in patients with MI not related to cocaine use.[167] However, aspirin and thrombolytics should be avoided in patients with suspected subarachnoid hemorrhage or at high risk of this complication.

As β-adrenergic blocking agents may potentiate the vasoconstrictive effects of cocaine[64] and may fail to control heart rate in cocaine abusers,[168] they should be avoided. Moreover, if use of a β-adrenergic blocking agent cannot be avoided, a β-blocking agent with α-antagonist properties, such as labetalol, should be used.[169, 170] However, the safety of labetalol in a large series of cocaine users has not been established.

Calcium channel blockers have been shown to attenuate cocaine-induced vasoconstriction[60] and to reduce systemic vascular resistance,[171] and they may prevent malignant arrhythmias[139, 140] in some patients with cocaine-induced ischemia. Although calcium channel blocking agents have no proven benefit in patients with MI unrelated to cocaine use, they have theoretical benefit in cocaine users.

As cocaine increases motor activity, hyperthermia, skeletal muscle injury, and rhabdomyolysis, creatine kinase and the MB isoenzyme of creatine kinase may increase, even in the absence of MI.[166, 172–174] However, the use of troponin I has no cross-reactivity with human skeletal muscle and is more specific for cardiac injury. Thus, troponin I should be used to detect MI.

Benzodiazepines should be used to attenuate the cardiac and central nervous system toxicity of cocaine.[166, 175–177] These agents have anxiolytic effects and reduce blood pressure and heart rate, thereby reducing myocardial oxygen consumption.

Some controversy exists about the use of lidocaine to treat arrhythmias in the presence of cocaine toxicity. As lidocaine and cocaine have sodium channel blocking properties, they may potentiate each other and worsen proarrhythmia or proconvulsant activity.[166]

For patients presenting with cocaine-induced cardiomyopathy, cocaine abstinence may result in progressive improvement.[115] For those cardiomyopathies that do not improve spontaneously, an angiotensin-converting enzyme inhibitor, digitalis, diuretics, and perhaps even a β-adrenergic blocking agent[123, 126] (titrated slowly over several weeks) may be of benefit, although the latter agents have yet to be extensively tested in cocaine-induced cardiomyopathy. Of course, use of a β-adrenergic blocking agent could be used only in patients who remain abstinent.

Rhythm disturbances should probably not be treated with a class Ia agent because QT prolongation may result in torsades de pointes. Instead, the underlying condition (i.e., MI or ischemia, hyperadrenergic state) should be treated as mentioned previously. β-Adrenergic blocking agents may be of value with the understanding that their use could potentiate coronary vasoconstriction.

ETHANOL

Oh many a peer of England brews
Livelier liquor than the Muse,
And malt does more than Milton can
To justify God's ways to man
Ale, man, ale's the stuff to drink
For fellows whom it hurts to think.

Anonymous

Epidemiologic data have shown that nearly 40 percent of the population of the United States consumes alcohol daily and nearly 10 million are chronic alcoholics.[178] Thus, it is not surprising that the cardiovascular effects of alcohol are widespread. The effects of alcohol on the heart fall into three categories: alcoholic cardiomyopathy, arrhythmias, and the beneficial effects of alcohol on the development of atherosclerosis and lipoprotein metabolism.

Alcoholic Cardiomyopathy

The toxic effects of alcohol use have been known for over a century.[179] Alcoholic cardiomyopathy is characterized by features typical of a dilated cardiomyopathy, including chamber dilatation, eccentric hypertrophy, and systolic and diastolic dysfunction.[178, 180, 181] Whereas no clear etiologic mechanism exists for the development of alcoholic cardiomyopathy, it is clear that long-term consumption of alcohol leads to biochemical changes that often precede the development of clinical heart failure symptoms.[182, 183]

Pathophysiology of Alcoholic Cardiac Dysfunction

Alcohol produces both a transient myocardial depression acutely after ingestion and a more chronic alcoholic cardiomyopathy after many years of heavy abuse. The former is reversed within 15 to 30 minutes of hemodialysis.[184] The latter is a more permanent condition.[178, 180, 185] There are at least three basic mechanisms by which alcohol may result in cardiac dysfunction: a direct toxic effect of alcohol or its metabolites, nutritional and vitamin deficiency effects, and toxic effects of alcohol additives, such as cobalt.

Acute Effects of Alcohol on the Myocardium and Circulation

Alcohol has been shown in animals[186] and humans[187–189] to produce a transient depression in myocardial contractility. This depression is more marked in the presence of autonomic blockade.[186, 187, 190] Thus, reflex sympathetic activation, as reflected by a rise in plasma catecholamines and cortisol,[191] may play a role in masking depression of myocardial contractility after alcohol ingestion. Concomitantly with a fall in myocardial contractility, total systemic vascular resistance (a variable related to peripheral small vessel tone) and end-systolic wall stress (which reflects afterload) fall with alcohol ingestion.[188] The fall in afterload and an increase in heart rate[187] help to offset the depression of myocardial contractility and maintain forward output after alcohol ingestion. Left ventricular ejection fraction is depressed at rest after alcohol ingestion, but responds normally to exercise.[187, 190] Alcohol also produces a fall in coronary vascular resistance, but without a change in epicardial vessel dimensions.[192] This suggests that the major effect of alcohol on the coronary circulation is dilatation of the intramyocardial resistance vessels. In addition, as coronary vascular resistance falls, coronary flow increases and arterial-coronary sinus oxygen content difference falls.[192] As alcohol increases extracellular adenosine by inhibiting adenosine uptake via the nucleoside transporter,[193] one might postulate that some of alcohol's actions on the myocardium and coronary circulation may be modulated by adenosine.

Direct Toxic Effects

It is unclear what the direct toxic effects of alcohol are on the heart. Ethanol is metabolized to acetaldehyde after ingestion. It is known that protein synthesis is reduced,[194–196] phospholipid content of membranes is altered,[197] and alterations in fatty acid metabolism[198] are early changes associated with alcohol consumption. Early ultrastructural changes include dilatation of the sarcoplasmic reticulum and the gap junction of the intercalated disk.[199] More chronic ultrastructural changes include myofibrillar degeneration, swollen mitochondria, and cellular edema.[200] End-stage alcoholic cardiomyopathy is characterized by muscle necrosis, inflammation, and fibrosis. These data suggest that the effect of alcohol on the heart may relate to alterations in energy stores, leading to reduced protein synthesis, altered calcium flux across the sarcoplasmic reticulum, and altered membrane content and enzyme activity.[180, 194–196, 201, 202] The latter may result in altered ion transport, especially increased permeability of the muscle cell membrane to sodium. Sodium influx activates magnesium-dependent, sodium-potassium–activated adenosine triphosphatase (ATPase), leading to continued energy requirements. Indeed, ethanol results in an increase in oxygen consumption in the heart.[203] Increased oxygen consumption may be a result of either increased sodium-potassium ATPase activity or decreased myocardial efficiency owing to alterations in substrate utilization with reductions in myocardial efficiency. Reduced myocardial efficiency is characteristic of cardiomyopathic hearts.[126, 204, 205] As cardiac muscle does not possess alcohol dehydrogenase, it cannot metabolize ethanol. Thus, alcohol and its effects may be present in the heart for longer periods of time after ingestion.[180]

The inward flux of sodium ions also results in a stimulation of sodium-calcium exchange in the sarcolemma, producing an increased inward flux of calcium.[178, 206] Although one would postulate that such an effect would result in increased contractility in a manner similar to that for a digitalis compound, such is not the case. It has been postulated that the reason for depressed contractility in the face of increased intracellular calcium concentration may be due to an ability of ethanol to interfere with calcium-troponin binding and/or a reduction in myosin ATPase activity, resulting in a reduced myosin-actin interaction.[207, 208]

Nutritional and Vitamin Deficiencies

As alcohol provides substantial non-nutritive calories, nutritional deficiencies include both malnutrition and vitamin deficiencies, especially thiamine deficiency.[180, 209–213] However, thiamine deficiency cardiomyopathy, beriberi, is characterized by a high-output syndrome rather than a low-output state characteristic of alcohol-induced cardiomyopathy.[209–213] Beriberi often responds dramatically to thiamine administration.

Toxicity of Additives

Two additives to alcohol products, lead and cobalt, have produced cardiomyopathy. In the 1960s, some beer drinkers died of a cardiomyopathy resulting from a cobalt-chloride additive used for foam stabilization.[214–216] These additives are no longer used to produce beer. Lead from stills used to make alcoholic products ("moonshine") has also been implicated in producing a cardiomyopathy.[180, 217]

Other Mechanisms

Finally, hemochromatosis from chronic liver disease due to alcohol exposure can result in a cardiomyopathy.[218–222]

Natural History

Although a clear association between heavy ethanol abuse and cardiomyopathy exists, it is impossible to distinguish alcoholic cardiomyopathy from dilated cardiomyopathy of other causes. Accordingly, the development of congestive heart failure and cardiac chamber dilatation in a patient with a significant drinking history should probably be diagnosed as idiopathic dilated cardiomyopathy. Nevertheless, the natural history of alcoholic cardiomyopathy (idiopathic dilated cardiomyopathy in heavy drinkers) is that symptoms worsen over time with a high mortality if ethanol ingestion persists.[223] In patients who continue to drink, the 3-year mortality is 42 percent.[223] In addition, a small percentage of patients who have a short duration of symptoms and who abstain from drinking will have resolution of their cardiomegaly.[223]

Treatment

The therapy for alcoholic cardiomyopathy is identical to that for any dilated cardiomyopathy, including salt restriction, angiotensin-converting enzyme inhibitors, digoxin, and diuretics. In addition, abstinence from alcohol is essential. Finally, nutritional and vitamin supplements may be necessary in subjects in whom heavy drinking has resulted in malnutrition.

Alcohol-Related Cardiac Arrhythmias

Several forms of cardiac arrhythmias and conduction system abnormalities have been associated with alcohol abuse.[224–228] These include bundle branch blocks,[224] varying degrees of atrioventricular block,[224] supraventricular tachycardias,[225, 226] and ventricular arrhythmias.[227, 228] The term *holiday heart syndrome* was coined by Ettinger and colleagues[225] to describe supraventricular arrhythmias occurring during drinking binges. The most common rhythm disturbance in holiday heart syndrome is atrial fibrillation, although atrial flutter, atrioventricular nodal reentry tachycardia, and frequent atrial premature beats may also occur.[225, 226] These arrhythmias are generally short-lived and can be avoided by abstinence from alcohol. β-Blockers may also be effective in preventing such episodes.

Ventricular arrhythmias, including frequent premature ventricular beats, ventricular tachycardia, and ventricular fibrillation, have been reported after alcohol ingestion in subjects with and without underlying structural heart disease.[226–228] The mechanisms responsible for such potentially lethal arrhythmias are uncertain but may include alcohol-induced heterogeneity of conduction throughout the myocardium,[226] magnesium deficiency,[229, 230] oxygen desaturation owing to sleep apnea,[231] and catecholamine excess during alcohol withdrawal.[232] Several studies suggest an association between alcoholism and sudden death, even in the absence of underlying coronary artery disease.[233–238]

Effects of Alcohol on Atherosclerosis

Despite the fact that chronic alcoholics tend to die suddenly,[239] probably of ventricular arrhythmias, alcohol is known to have beneficial effects on lipoprotein metabolism when consumed in moderate doses. Epidemiologic studies convincingly demonstrate a reduction in the risk of MI among moderate drinkers compared with nondrinkers, even when other risk factors are adjusted.[240–247] This protective effect of alcohol applies only to moderate consumption, as heavy drinkers have an increased risk of coronary heart disease, leading to a so-called J-shaped mortality curve.[248]

The mechanism by which moderate alcohol consumption (1 to 2 drinks per day) protects against coronary artery disease is not fully understood. However, alcohol in moderate doses has been shown to increase levels of high-density lipoprotein and apolipoprotein A-I.[249–256] It is thought that these lipid alterations favor reverse cholesterol transport from the tissues to the liver for metabolism.[257] Importantly, alcoholic liver disease results in loss of these favorable lipid changes.[258] Alcohol also has favorable hemostatic properties, specifically increasing plasma fibrinolytic activity,[259, 260] increasing endothelial plasminogen activator production,[261] and inhibiting platelet aggregation.[262] Recent evidence suggests that regular alcohol consumption may have cardioprotective effects similar to ischemic preconditioning; these may in part be mediated by activation of protein kinase C.[263, 264] Despite the potential beneficial effects of alcohol, it has not yet been shown that increasing alcohol consumption in individual patients can reduce their risk of coronary artery atherosclerosis. Moreover, any potential risk of alcohol on coronary atherosclerosis must be weighed against its potential for abuse, its deleterious side effects, and its potential for exacerbating other conditions, such as hypertension.[265–268]

Other Effects of Ethanol on the Heart

Alcohol consumption has been associated with hypertension independently of age, race, gender, obesity, smoking, salt intake, and educational level.[267–269] The mechanism by which this occurs may be multifactorial, including salt and water retention, a direct pressor effect of alcohol, withdrawal effects, and attenuation of normal baroreflexes.[270, 271] An increase in blood pressure can occur even with mild to moderate daily use.[268] Alcohol has also been implicated as an independent risk factor for left ventricular hypertrophy.[272]

AMPHETAMINES

Amphetamines are noncatecholamine sympathomimetic agents that have been used in the past as nasal decongestants and as treatment for narcolepsy, attention-deficit disorders, and appetite suppression.[273–277] These agents, which are part of the phenylethylamine family, work by releasing norepinephrine from presynaptic nerve endings. They have substantial potential for abuse, and abuse has been reported to lead to several complications including MI, tachycardia, hypertension, arrhythmias, hallucinations, psychosis, convulsions, coma, hyperthermia, rhabdomyolysis, and sudden death.[273–278] Cardiomyopathy has also been reported in patients using amphetamines.[128, 279–282] The etiology of cardiomyopathy in amphetamine abusers is probably similar to that in cocaine abusers.[115–117] Chronic sympathomimetic exposure results in left ventricular dysfunction.[112–114, 119–122] Treatment for these conditions is supportive. Sedation with benzodiazepines and monitoring should be achieved. Rapid external cooling and fluid replacement should be started if the patient is hyperthermic. Whereas β-blocking agents may be considered for the treatment of tachycardia and arrhythmias, the same concern about unopposed alpha stimulation of coronary vasculature should be used in patients with chest pain or MI associated with amphetamine use as in those who abuse cocaine. Thus, labetalol may be the drug of choice for this condition. Blood pressure control may be achieved initially with parenteral agents, such as nitroprusside and nitroglycerin, and oral agents such as labetalol and clonidine. MI should be treated with rapid-acting nitrates, thrombolytic agents, and aspirin. Whereas the use of β-blocking agents in MI has been shown to reduce mortality,[283, 284] it is unknown whether it is beneficial in the setting of amphetamine abuse. If used, labetalol should be the agent of choice, as this agent has α-antagonist properties and should help to minimize the potential problem of unopposed α-vasoconstriction. Cardiomyopathy should be treated with drug abstinence, digoxin, diuretics, and angiotensin-converting enzyme inhibitors. If cardiomyopathy does not resolve, careful institution of β-adrenergic blocking agents may be of benefit in patients who maintain abstinence.[123, 126, 204]

MARIJUANA

Despite widespread use of this agent worldwide, there is very little literature on its effect on the cardiovascular system. Tetrahydrocannabinol is the major byproduct of marijuana smoking. This agent is a powerful antiemetic that is currently used in association with chemotherapy in some special circumstances.[285] Marijuana or cannabis depresses myocardial contractility in patients with angina pectoris[286] and perhaps in those without coronary artery disease.[274, 287] Tetrahydrocannabinol produces bradycardia and hypotension in anesthetized animals,[286] but acutely produces a dose-related tachycardia and an increase in blood pressure in humans who smoke or ingest this agent.[288–290] This effect peaks within 30 minutes of ingestion and persists for over 90 minutes.[290–293] The tachycardia may be mediated by the sympathetic nervous system because it can be abolished by β-adrenergic blockade.[289, 294, 295] However, if the sympathetic nervous system produces these effects, it is unclear why myocardial depression has been noted in some circumstances.[286] Such depression of myocardial performance may be due to enhanced afterload owing to a pressor effect or precipitation of myocardial ischemia. This increase in sympathetic drive can result in electrocardiographic changes.[290, 296]

When tetrahydrocannabinol is taken for long periods of time, the effects on the cardiovascular system are different.[287] Bradycardia, loss of venous tone, and hypotension may develop as a result of decreased sympathetic tone in the peripheral arteries and increased parasympathetic tone.[287, 297–299] Marijuana may modulate the sympathetic nervous system by a dual mechanism.[287] It reduces spontaneous sympathetic efferent activity, and it suppresses inhibitory mechanisms.

Other Cardiovascular Effects of Drug Abuse

Alcohol, cocaine, and amphetamines have been found to have teratogenetic effects on the cardiovascular system of unborn infants.[300, 301] The most common congenital defect associated with alcohol ("fetal alcohol syndrome") is atrial septal defect. Ventricular septal defects, anomalies of the great vessels, and tetralogy of Fallot have also been described.

References

Cocaine

1. Mathias DW: Cocaine-associated myocardial ischemia. Am J Med 81:675–678, 1986.
2. Nicholi AM Jr: The nontherapeutic use of psychoactive drugs: a modern epidemic. N Engl J Med 308:925–933, 1983.
3. Isner JM, Estes NAM III, Thompson PD, et al: Acute cardiac events temporally related to cocaine abuse. N Engl J Med 315:1438–1443, 1986.
4. Pitts WR, Lange RA, Cigarroa JE, Hillis LD: Cocaine-induced myocardial ischemia and infarction: pathophysiology, recognition, and management. Prog Cardiovasc Dis 40:65–76, 1997.
5. Lowenstein DH, Massa SM, Rowbotham MC, et al: Acute neurological and psychiatric complications associated with cocaine abuse. Am J Med 83:841–846, 1987.
6. Brody SL, Slovis CM, Wrenn KD: Cocaine-related medical problems: consecutive series of 233 patients. Am J Med 88:325–331, 1990.
7. Cregler LL: Cocaine: the newest risk factor for cardiovascular disease. Clin Cardiol 14:449–456, 1991.
8. Freud S: Ueber Coca. Centralbl Ther 2:289–314, 1884.
9. Siegel RK: Cocaine smoking. J Psychoactive Drugs 13:271–343, 1982.
10. Ritches JM, Greene NM: Local anesthetics. *In* Gilman AG, Goodman LS, Rall TW, Murad F (eds): The Pharmacological Basis of Therapeutics. 7th ed. pp. 309–310. New York: Macmillan, 1985.
11. Gay GR: Clinical management of acute and chronic cocaine poisoning. Ann Emerg Med 11:562–572, 1982.
12. Nademanee K, Gorelick DA, Josephson MA, et al: Myocardial ischemia during cocaine withdrawal. Ann Intern Med 111:876–880, 1989.
13. Kloner RA, Hale S, Alker K, Rezkalla S: The effects of acute and chronic cocaine use on the heart. Circulation 85:407–419, 1992.
14. Price FW, Leaky AB: Grave and prolonged cardiac failure following the use of cocaine in dental surgery. Lancet 1:797–799, 1911.
15. Watanabe T: Untersuchungen uber die Wirkung der ersten Stanniusschen Ligatur. Z Biol 77:317–331, 1923.
16. Shookhoff C: Zur Kenntnis der Wirkung von Novocain, bez. Cocain auf das Saugetierherz. Z Exp Med 49:110–123, 1926.
17. Mautz FR: Reduction of cardiac irritability by the epicardial and systemic administration of drugs as a protection in cardiac surgery. J Thorac Surg 5:612–628, 1936.
18. Marangoni BA, Burstein CL, Rovenstine EA: Protecting action of procaine against ventricular fibrillation induced by epinephrine during cyclopropane anesthesia. Proc Soc Exp Biol Med 44:594–596, 1940.
19. Young D, Glauber JJ: Electrocardiographic changes resulting from acute cocaine intoxication. Am Heart J 34:272–279, 1947.
20. Vatner SF, Higgins CB, Braunwald E: Effects of norepinephrine on coronary circulation and left ventricular dynamics in the conscious dog. Circ Res 34:812–823, 1974.
21. Gay GR, Sheppard CW, Inaba DS: Cocaine: history, epidemiology, human pharmacology, and treatment. A perspective on a new debut for an old girl. Clin Pharmacol 8:149–178, 1975.
22. Kossowsky WA, Lyon AF: Cocaine and acute myocardial infarction: a probable connection. Chest 86:729–731, 1984.
23. Howard RE, Hueter DC, Davis GJ; Acute myocardial infarction following cocaine abuse in a young woman with normal coronary arteries. JAMA 254:95–96, 1985.
24. Simpson RW, Edwards WD: Pathogenesis of cocaine-induced ischemic heart disease. Arch Pathol Lab Med 110:479–484, 1986.
25. Zimmerman FH, Gustafson GM, Kemp HG: Recurrent myocardial infarction associated with cocaine abuse in a young man with normal coronary arteries: evidence for coronary artery spasm culminating in thrombosis. J Am Coll Cardiol 9:964–968, 1987.
26. Smith HWB, Liberman HA, Brody SL, et al: Acute myocardial infarction temporally related to cocaine use. Clinical, angiographic, and pathophysiologic observations. Ann Intern Med 107:13–18, 1987.
27. Schachne JS, Roberts BH, Thompson PD: Coronary-artery spasm and myocardial infarction associated with cocaine use [letter]. N Engl J Med 310:1665–1666, 1984.
28. Pasternack PF, Colvin SB, Baumann FG: Cocaine-induced angina pectoris and acute myocardial infarction in patients younger than 40 years. Am J Cardiol 55:847, 1985.
29. Cregler LL, Mark H: Relation of acute myocardial infarction to cocaine abuse. Am J Cardiol 56:794–795, 1985.
30. Weiss RJ: Recurrent myocardial infarction caused by cocaine abuse. Am Heart J 111:793, 1986.
31. Coleman DL, Ross TF, Naughton JL: Myocardial ischemia and infarction related to recreational cocaine use. West J Med 136:444–446, 1982.
32. Patel R, Haider B, Ahmed S, Regan TJ: Cocaine related myocardial infarction: high prevalence of occlusive coronary thrombi without significant obstructive atherosclerosis [abstract]. Circulation 78(suppl II):II-436, 1988.
33. Virmani R, Robinowitz M, Smialek JE, Smyth DF: Cardiovascular effects of cocaine: an autopsy study of 40 patients. Am Heart J 115:1068–1076, 1988.
34. Wilkins CE, Matur VS, Ty RC, Hall RJ: Myocardial infarction associated with cocaine abuse. Tex Heart Inst J 12:385–387, 1985.
35. Cregler LL, Mark H: Myocardial infarction associated with cocaine abuse: a case report. Tex Heart Inst J 13:174, 1986.
36. Gould L, Gopalaswamy C, Patel C, Betzu R: Cocaine-induced myocardial infarction. N Y State J Med 85:660–661, 1985.
37. Weiner RS, Lockhart JT, Schwart RG: Dilated cardiomyopathy and cocaine abuse. Report of two cases. Am J Med 81:699–701, 1986.
38. Ring RE, Butman SM: Cocaine and premature myocardial infarction. Drug Ther 57:117–125, 1986.
39. Rod JL, Zucker RP: Acute myocardial infarction shortly after cocaine inhalation. Am J Cardiol 59:161, 1987.
40. Wehbie CS, Vidaillet HJ Jr, Navetta FI, Peter RH: Acute myocardial infarction associated with initial cocaine use. South Med J 80:933–934, 1987.
41. Cantwell JD, Rose RD: Cocaine and cardiovascular events. Phys Sports Med 13:77–82, 1986.
42. Rollinger IM, Belzberg AS, MacDonald IL: Cocaine-induced myocardial infarction. Can Med Assoc J 135:45–46, 1986.
43. Williams MJ, Restieaux NJ, Low CJ: Myocardial infarction in young people with normal coronary arteries. Heart 79:191–194, 1998.
44. Galasko GI: Cocaine, a risk factor for myocardial infarction. J Cardiovasc Risk 4:185–190, 1997.
45. Hoffman RS, Hollander JE: Evaluation of patients with chest pain after cocaine use. Crit Care Clin 13:809–828, 1997.
46. Hollander JE, Vignona L, Burstein J: Predictors of underlying coronary artery disease in cocaine associated myocardial infarction: a meta-analysis of case reports. Vet Hum Toxicol 39:276–280, 1997.
47. Hollander JE: Cocaine-associated myocardial infarction. J R Soc Med 89:443–447, 1996.

48. Hollander JE, Hoffman RS, Gennis P, et al: Cocaine-associated chest pain: one-year follow-up. Acad Emerg Med 2:179–184, 1995.
49. Hollander JE, Todd KH, Green G, et al: Chest pain associated with cocaine: an assessment of prevalence in suburban and urban emergency departments. Ann Emerg Med 26:671–676, 1995.
50. Chakko S, Myerburg RJ: Cardiac complications of cocaine abuse. Clin Cardiol 18:67–72, 1995.
51. Williams MJ, Stewart RA: Serial angiography in cocaine-induced myocardial infarction. Chest 111:822–824, 1997.
52. McLaurin M, Apple FS, Henry TD, Sharkey SW: Cardiac troponin I and T concentrations in patients with cocaine-associated chest pain. Ann Clin Biochem 33:183–186, 1996.
53. Hollander JE, Hoffman RS, Burstein JL, et al: Cocaine-associated myocardial infarction. Mortality and complications. Cocaine-Associated Myocardial Infarction Study Group. Arch Intern Med 155:1081–1086, 1995.
54. Isner JM, Chokshi SK: Cardiovascular complications of cocaine. Curr Probl Cardiol 64:94–123, 1991.
55. Bedotto JB, Lee RW, Lancaster LD, et al: Cocaine and cardiovascular function in dogs: effects on heart and peripheral circulation. J Am Coll Cardiol 11:1337–1342, 1988.
56. Wilkerson RD: Cardiovascular effects of cocaine in conscious dogs: importance of fully functional autonomic and central nervous systems. J Pharmacol Exp Ther 246:466–471, 1988.
57. Lange RA, Cigarroa RG, Yancy CW, et al: Cocaine-induced coronary artery vasoconstriction. N Engl J Med 321:1557–1562, 1989.
58. Schwartz AB, Janzen D, Jones RT, Boyle W: Electrocardiographic and hemodynamic effects of intravenous cocaine in awake and anesthetized dogs. J Electrocardiol 22:159–166, 1989.
59. Vargas R, Gillis RA, Ramwell PW: Propranolol promotes cocaine-induced spasm of porcine coronary artery. J Pharmacol Exp Ther 257:644–646, 1991.
60. Rongione AJ, Steg PG, Gal D, Isner JM: Cocaine causes endothelium-independent vasoconstriction of vascular smooth muscle [abstract]. Circulation 78(suppl II):II-436, 1988.
61. Perreault CL, Hague NL, Ransil BJ, Morgan JP: The effects of cocaine on intracellular Ca^{2+} handling and myofilament Ca^{2+} responsiveness of ferret ventricular myocardium. Br J Pharmacol 101:679–685, 1990.
62. Wilbert-Lampen U, Seliger C, Zilker T, Arendt RM: Cocaine increases the endothelial release of immunoreactive endothelin and its concentrations in human plasma and urine. Reversal by coincubation with s-receptor antagonists. Circulation 98:385–390, 1998.
63. Daniel WC, Lange RA, Landau C, et al: Effects of the intracoronary infusion of cocaine on coronary arterial dimensions and blood flow in humans. Am J Cardiol 78:288–291, 1996.
64. Lange RA, Cigarroa RG, Flores ED, et al: Potentiation of cocaine-induced coronary vasoconstriction by beta-adrenergic blockade. Ann Intern Med 112:897–903, 1990.
65. Boehrer JD, Moliterno DJ, Willard JE, et al: Influence of labetalol on cocaine-induced coronary vasoconstriction in humans. Am J Med 94:608–610, 1993.
66. Brogan WC, Lange RA, Glamann DB, Hillis LD: Prolonged coronary vasoconstriction caused by intranasal cocaine. Ann Intern Med 116:556–561, 1992.
67. Winniford MD, Wheelan KR, Kremers MS, et al: Smoking-induced coronary vasoconstriction in patients with atherosclerotic coronary artery disease: evidence for adrenergically mediated alterations in coronary artery tone. Circulation 73:662–667, 1986.
68. Moliterno DJ, Willard JE, Lange RA, et al: Coronary-artery vasoconstriction induced by cocaine, cigarette smoking, or both. N Engl J Med 330:454–459, 1994.
69. Hearn WL, Flynn DD, Hime GW, et al: Cocaethylene: a unique cocaine metabolite displays high affinity for the dopamine transporter. J Neurochem 56:698–701, 1991.
70. Escobedo LG, Ruttenber AJ, Agocs MM, et al: Emerging patterns of cocaine use and the epidemic of cocaine overdose deaths in Dade County, Florida. Arch Pathol Lab Med 115:900–905, 1991.
71. Pirwitz MJ, Willard JE, Landau C, et al: Influence of cocaine, ethanol, or their combination on epicardial coronary arterial dimensions in humans. Arch Intern Med 155:1186–1191, 1995.
72. Brogan WC III, Lange RA, Kim AS, et al: Alleviation of cocaine-induced coronary vasoconstriction by nitroglycerin. J Am Coll Cardiol 18:581–586, 1991.
73. Negus BH, Willard JE, Hillis LD, et al: Alleviation of cocaine-induced coronary vasoconstriction with intravenous verapamil. Am J Cardiol 73:510–513, 1994.
74. Havranek EP, Nademanee K, Grayburn PA, Eichhorn EJ: Endothelium-dependent vasorelaxation is impaired in cocaine arteriopathy. J Am Coll Cardiol 28:1168–1174, 1996.
75. Fraker TD Jr, Temesy-Armos PN, Brewster PS, Wilkerson RD: Mechanism of cocaine-induced myocardial depression in dogs. Circulation 81:1012–1016, 1990.
76. Majid PA, Cheirif JB, Rokey R, et al: Does cocaine cause coronary vasospasm in chronic cocaine abusers? A study of coronary and systemic hemodynamics. Clin Cardiol 15:253–258, 1992.
77. Mohrman DE, Feigl EO: Competition between sympathetic vasoconstriction and metabolic vasodilation in the canine coronary circulation. Circulation 42:79–86, 1978.
78. Kuhn FE, Gillis RA, Virmani R, et al: Cocaine produces coronary artery vasoconstriction independent of an intact endothelium. Chest 102:581–585, 1992.
79. Flores ED, Lange RA, Cigarroa RG, Hillis LD: Effect of cocaine on coronary artery dimensions in atherosclerotic coronary artery disease: enhanced vasoconstriction at sites of significant stenoses. J Am Coll Cardiol 16:74–79, 1990.
80. Eichhorn EJ, Demian SE, Alvarez LG, et al: Cocaine induced alterations in prostaglandin production in rabbit aorta. J Am Coll Cardiol 19:696–703, 1992.
81. Togna G, Graziani M, Sorrentino C, Caprino L: Prostanoid production in the presence of platelet activation in hypoxic cocaine-treated rats. Haemostasis 26:311–318, 1996.
82. Togna G, Tempesta E, Togna AR, et al: Platelet responsiveness and biosynthesis of thromboxane and prostacyclin in response to in vitro cocaine treatment. Haemostasis 15:100–107, 1985.
83. Alosachie I, Godfraind T: The modulatory role of vascular endothelium in the interaction of agonists and antagonists with α-adrenoceptors in the rat aorta. Br J Pharmacol 95:619–629, 1988.
84. McGrath JC, Monaghan S, Templeton AGB, Wilson VG: Effects of basal and acetylcholine-induced release of endothelium-derived relaxing factor on contraction to α-adrenoceptor agonists in rabbit artery and corresponding veins. Br J Pharmacol 99:77–86, 1990.
85. Demirel E, Hindioglu F, Ercan ZS, Turker RK: Endothelium modulates the effects of α-adrenoceptor agonists in vascular smooth muscle. Gen Pharmacol 20:89–93, 1989.
86. Azuma H, Ishikawa M, Sekizaki S: Endothelium-dependent inhibition of platelet aggregation. Br J Pharmacol 88:411–415, 1986.
87. Furlong B, Henderson AH, Lewis MJ, Smith JA: Endothelium-derived relaxing factor inhibits in vitro platelet aggregation. Br J Pharmacol 90:687–692, 1987.
88. Radomski MW, Palmer RMJ, Moncada S: Comparative pharmacology of endothelium-derived relaxing factor, nitric oxide and prostacyclin in platelets. Br J Pharmacol 92:181–187, 1987.
89. Willerson JT, Hillis LD, Winniford M, Buja LM: Speculation regarding mechanisms responsible for acute ischemic heart disease syndromes. J Am Coll Cardiol 8:245–250, 1986.
90. Gitter MJ, Goldsmith SR, Dunbar DN, Sharkey SW: Cocaine and chest pain: clinical features and outcome of patients hospitalized to rule out myocardial infarction. Ann Intern Med 115:277–282, 1991.
91. Eichhorn EJ, Peacock E, Grayburn PA, et al: Chronic cocaine abuse is associated with accelerated atherosclerosis in human coronary arteries [abstract]. J Am Coll Cardiol 19:105A, 1992.
92. Dressler FA, Malekzadeh S, Roberts WC: Quantitative analysis of amounts of coronary arterial narrowing in cocaine addicts. Am J Cardiol 65:303–308, 1990.
93. Kolodgie FD, Virmani R, Cornhill JF, et al: Increase in atherosclerosis and adventitial mast cells in cocaine abusers: an alternative mechanism of cocaine associated coronary vasospasm and thrombosis. J Am Coll Cardiol 17:1553–1560, 1991.
94. Hollander JE, Shih RD, Hoffman RS, et al: Predictors of coronary artery disease in patients with cocaine-associated myocardial infarction. Cocaine-Associated Myocardial Infarction (CAMI) Study Group: Am J Med 102:158–163, 1997.
95. Kolodgie FD, Virmani R, Cornhill JF, et al: Increase in atherosclerosis and adventitial mast cells in cocaine abusers: an alternative mechanism of cocaine-associated coronary vasospasm and thrombosis. J Am Coll Cardiol 17:1553–1560, 1991.
96. Kuhn FE, Johnson MN, Gillis RA, et al, with the technical assistance of Gold C, Wahlstrom SK: Effect of cocaine on the coronary circulation and systemic hemodynamics in dogs. J Am Coll Cardiol 16:1481–1491, 1990.

97. Andresen MC, Yang M, Nelson SH, Steinsland OS: Cocaine inhibits baroreflex control of blood pressure by actions at arterial baroreceptors. Am J Physiol 258:H1244–H1249, 1990.
98. Raczkowski VFC, Hernandez YM, Erzouki HK, et al: Cocaine acts in the central nervous system to inhibit sympathetic neural activity. J Pharmacol Exp Ther 257:511–519, 1991.
99. Jacobsen TN, Grayburn PA, Snyder RW II, et al: Effects of intranasal cocaine on sympathetic nerve discharge in humans. J Clin Invest 99:628–634, 1997.
100. Shannon RP, Komamura K, Stambler BS, et al: Cocaine causes transient depression followed by sustained increases in myocardial contractility in conscious dogs [abstract]. Circulation 80(suppl III):III-147, 1989.
101. Hale SL, Alker KJ, Rezkalla S, et al: Adverse effects of cocaine on cardiovascular dynamics, myocardial blood flow, and coronary artery diameter in an experimental model. Am Heart J 118:927–933, 1989.
102. Hale SL, Alker KJ, Rezkalla SH, et al: Nifedipine protects the heart from the acute deleterious effects of cocaine if administered before but not after cocaine. Circulation 83:1437–1443, 1991.
103. Abel FL, Wilson SP, Zhao RR, Fennell WH: Cocaine depresses the canine myocardium. Circ Shock 28:309–319, 1989.
104. Morcos NC, Fairhurst AS, Henry WL: Direct but reversible effects of cocaine on the myocardium [abstract]. J Am Coll Cardiol 9:172A, 1988.
105. Woolf JH, Huang L, Ishiguro Y, Morgan JP: Negative inotropic effect of methylecgonidine, a major product of cocaine base pyrolysis, on ferret and human myocardium. J Cardiovasc Pharmacol 30:352–359, 1997.
106. Mouhaffel AH, Madu EC, Satmary WA, Fraker TD: Cardiovascular complications of cocaine. Chest 107:1426–1434, 1995.
107. Egashira K, Morgan KG, Morgan JP: Effects of cocaine on excitation-contraction coupling of aortic smooth muscle from the ferret. J Clin Invest 87:1322–1328, 1991.
108. Perreault CL, Hague NL, Ransil BJ, Morgan JP: The effects of cocaine on intracellular Ca^{2+} handling and myofilament Ca^{2+} responsiveness of ferret ventricular myocardium. Br J Pharmacol 101:679–685, 1990.
109. Brickner ME, Willard JE, Eichhorn EJ, et al: Increased left ventricular mass and wall thickness associated with chronic cocaine abuse. Circulation 84:1130–1135, 1991.
110. Cigarroa CG, Boehrer JD, Brickner ME, et al: Exaggerated pressor response to treadmill exercise in chronic cocaine abusers with left ventricular hypertrophy. Circulation 86:226–231, 1992.
111. Eichhorn EJ, Bristow MR: Medical therapy can improve the biologic properties of the chronically failing heart: a new era in the treatment of heart failure. Circulation 94:2285–2296, 1996.
112. Rona G, Chappel CI, Balazs T, Gaudry R: An infarct-like myocardial lesion and other toxic manifestations produced by isoproterenol in the rat. Arch Pathol 67:443–455, 1958.
113. Mann DL, Kent RL, Parsons B, Cooper G IV: Adrenergic effects on the biology of the adult mammalian cardiocyte. Circulation 85:790–804, 1992.
114. Haft JI: Cardiovascular injury induced by sympathetic catecholamines. Prog Cardiovasc Dis 17:73–85, 1974.
115. Chokshi SK, Moore R, Pandian NG, Isner JM: Reversible cardiomyopathy associated with cocaine intoxication. Ann Intern Med 111:1039–1040, 1989.
116. Duell PB: Chronic cocaine abuse and dilated cardiomyopathy [letter]. Am J Med 83:601, 1987.
117. Bertolet BD, Freund G, Martin CA, et al: Unrecognized left ventricular dysfunction in an apparently healthy cocaine abuse population. Clin Cardiol 13:323–328, 1990.
118. Virmani R, Robinowitz M, Smialek JE, Smyth DF: Cardiovascular effects of cocaine: an autopsy study of 40 patients. Am Heart J 115:1068–1076, 1988.
119. Lam JB, Shub C, Sheps SG: Reversible dilatation of hypertrophied left ventricle in pheochromocytoma: serial two dimensional echocardiographic observations. Am Heart J 109:613–615, 1985.
120. Imperato-McGinley J, Gautier T, Ehlers K, et al: Reversibility of catecholamine-induced dilated cardiomyopathy in a child with a pheochromocytoma. N Engl J Med 316:793–797, 1987.
121. Scully RE, Mark EJ, McNeely WF, McNeely BU: Case records of the Massachusetts General Hospital Case 15-1988. A 26 year-old woman with cardiomyopathy multiple strokes, and an adrenal mass. N Engl J Med 318:970–981, 1988.
122. Velasquez G, D'Souza VJ, Hacksaw BT, et al: Pheochromocytoma and cardiomyopathy. Br J Radiol 57:89–92, 1984.
123. Heilbrunn SM, Shah P, Bristow MR, et al: Increased β-receptor density and improved hemodynamic response to catecholamine stimulation during long-term metoprolol therapy in heart failure from dilated cardiomyopathy. Circulation 79:483–490, 1989.
124. Bristow MR, Port JD, Sandoval AB, et al: β-Adrenergic receptor pathways in the failing human heart. Heart Failure 5:77–90, 1989.
125. Fowler MB, Laser JA, Hopkins GL, et al: Assessment of the β-adrenergic receptor pathway in the intact failing human heart: progressive receptor down-regulation and subsensitivity to agonist response. Circulation 74:1290–1302, 1986.
126. Eichhorn EJ, Bedotto JB, Malloy CR, et al: Effect of beta-adrenergic blockade on myocardial function and energetics in congestive heart failure: improvements in hemodynamic, contractile, and diastolic performance with bucindolol. Circulation 82:473–483, 1990.
127. Eichhorn EJ, McGhie AI, Bedotto JB, et al: Effects of bucindolol on neurohormonal activation in congestive heart failure. Am J Cardiol 67:67–73, 1991.
128. Jacobs LJ: Reversible dilated cardiomyopathy induced by metamphetamine. Clin Cardiol 12:725–727, 1989.
129. Tazelaar HD, Karck SB, Stephens BG, Billingham ME: Cocaine and the heart. Hum Pathol 18:195–199, 1987.
130. Tarizzo V, Rubio MC: Effects of cocaine on several adrenergic system parameters. Gen Pharmacol 16:71–74, 1985.
131. Weidmann S: Effects of calcium ions and local anaesthetics on electrical properties of Purkinje fibres. J Physiol 129:568–582, 1955.
132. Przywara DA, Dambach GE: Direct actions of cocaine on cardiac cellular electrical activity. Circ Res 65:185–192, 1989.
133. Hale SL, Lehmann MH, Kloner RA: Electrocardiographic abnormalities after acute administration of cocaine in the rat. Am J Cardiol 63:1529–1530, 1989.
134. Billman GE: Mechanisms responsible for the cardiotoxic effects of cocaine. FASEB J 4:2469–2475, 1990.
135. Coumel P, Rosengarten MD, Leclercq JF, Attuel P: Role of sympathetic nervous system in nonischemic ventricular arrhythmias. Br Heart J 47:137–147, 1982.
136. Cregler LL, Mark H: Medical complications of cocaine abuse. N Engl J Med 315:1495–1500, 1986.
137. Nanji AA, Filipenko JD: Asystole and ventricular fibrillation associated with cocaine intoxication. Chest 85:132–133, 1984.
138. Benchimol A, Bartall H, Desser KB: Accelerated ventricular rhythm and cocaine abuse. Ann Intern Med 88:519–520, 1978.
139. Billman GE, Hoskins RS: Cocaine-induced ventricular fibrillation: protection afforded by the calcium antagonist verapamil. FASEB J 2:2990–2995, 1988.
140. Billman GE: Effect of calcium channel antagonists on cocaine-induced malignant arrhythmias: protection against ventricular fibrillation. J Pharmacol Exp Ther 266:407–416, 1993.
141. Inoue H, Zipes DP: Cocaine-induced supersensitivity and arrhythmogenesis. J Am Coll Cardiol 11:867–874, 1988.
142. Jonsson S, O'Meara M, Young J: Acute cocaine poisoning: importance of treating seizures and acidosis. Am J Med 75:1061–1064, 1983.
143. Barth CW, Bray M, Roberts WC: Rupture of the ascending aorta during cocaine intoxication. Am J Cardiol 57:496, 1986.
144. Cregler LL: Acute aortic dissection associated with cocaine abuse [letter]. Clin Cardiol 11:806, 1988.
145. Grannis FW Jr, Bryant C, Caffaratti JD, Turner AF: Acute aortic dissection associated with cocaine abuse. Clin Cardiol 11:572–574, 1988.
146. Gadaleta D, Hall MH, Nelson RL: Cocaine-induced acute aortic dissection. Chest 96:1203–1205, 1989.
147. Lisse JR, Davis CP, Thurmond-Anderle M: Cocaine abuse and deep venous thrombosis [letter]. Ann Intern Med 110:571–572, 1989.
148. Wohlman RA: Renal artery thrombosis and embolization associated with intravenous cocaine injection. South Med J 80:928–930, 1987.
149. Mangiardi JR, Daras M, Geller ME, et al: Cocaine-related intracranial hemorrhage. Acta Neurol Scand 77:177–180, 1988.
150. Levine SR, Welch KMA: Cocaine and stroke. Stroke 19:779–783, 1988.
151. Wojak JC, Flamm ES: Intracranial hemorrhage and cocaine use. Stroke 18:712–715, 1987.
152. Nolte KB, Gelman BB: Intracerebral hemorrhage associated with cocaine abuse. Arch Pathol Lab Med 113:812–813, 1989.

153. Bolbe LI, Merkin MD: Cerebral infarction in a user of freebase cocaine ("crack"). Neurology 36:1602–1604, 1986.
154. Lichtenfeld PJ, Rubin DB, Feldman RS: Subarachnoid hemorrhage precipitated by cocaine snorting. Arch Neurol 41:223–224, 1984.
155. Tuchman AJ, Daras M, Zalzal P, Mangiardi J: Intracranial hemorrhage after cocaine abuse. JAMA 257:1175, 1987.
156. Brust JC, Richter RW: Stroke associated with cocaine abuse? N Y State J Med 77:1473–1475, 1977.
157. Seaman ME: Acute cocaine abuse associated with cerebral infarction. Ann Emerg Med 19:34–37, 1990.
158. Caplan LR, Hier DB, Banks G: Current concepts of cerebrovascular disease-stroke: stroke and drug abuse. Stroke 13:869–872, 1982.
159. Klonoff DC, Andrews BT, Obana WG: Stroke associated with cocaine use. Arch Neurol 46:989–993, 1989.
160. Schwartz KA, Cohen JA: Subarachnoid hemorrhage precipitated by cocaine snorting. Arch Neurol 41:705, 1984.
161. Cregler LL, Mark H: Relation of stroke to cocaine abuse. N Y State J Med 87:129–130, 1987.
162. Mody CK, Miller BL, McIntyre HB, et al: Neurologic complications of cocaine abuse. Neurology 38:1189–1193, 1988.
163. Adrouny A, Magnusson P: Pneumopericardium from cocaine inhalation [letter]. N Engl J Med 313:48, 1985.
164. Chambers HF, Morris DL, Tauber MG, Modin G: Cocaine use and the risk for endocarditis in intravenous drug users. Ann Intern Med 106:833–836, 1987.
165. Hollander JE, Burstein JL, Hoffman RS, et al, and the Cocaine Associated Myocardial Infarction (CAMI) Study Group: Cocaine associated myocardial infarction. Clinical safety of thrombolytic therapy. Chest 107:1237–1241, 1995.
166. Hollander JE: The management of cocaine-associated myocardial ischemia. N Engl J Med 333:1267–1272, 1995.
167. ISIS-2 Collaborative Group: Randomised trial of intravenous streptokinase, oral aspirin, both, or neither among 17,187 cases of suspected acute myocardial infarction: ISIS-2. Lancet 2:349–360, 1988.
168. Sand IC, Brody SL, Wrenn KD, Slovis CM: Experience with esmolol for the treatment of cocaine-associated cardiovascular complications. Am J Emerg Med 9:161–163, 1991.
169. Gay GR, Loper KA: The use of labetolol in the management of cocaine crisis. Ann Emerg Med 17:282–283, 1988.
170. Dusenberry SJ, Hicks MJ, Mariani PJ: Labetalol treatment of cocaine toxicity [letter]. Ann Emerg Med 16:235, 1987.
171. Knuepfer MM, Branch CA: Calcium channel antagonists reduce the cocaine-induced decrease in cardiac output in a subset of rats. J Cardiovasc Pharmacol 21:390–396, 1993.
172. Tokarski GF, Paganussi P, Urbanski R, et al: An evaluation of cocaine-induced chest pain. Ann Emerg Med 19:1088–1092, 1990.
173. McLaurin M, Apple FS, Henry TD, Sharkey SW: Cardiac troponin I and T concentrations in patients with cocaine-associated chest pain. Ann Clin Biochem 33:183–186, 1996.
174. Hollander JE, Hoffman RS, Gennis P, et al: Prospective multicenter evaluation of cocaine associated chest pain. Acad Emerg Med 1:330–339, 1994.
175. Guinn MM, Bedford JA, Wilson MC: Antagonism of intravenous cocaine lethality in nonhuman primates. Clin Toxicol 16:499–508, 1980.
176. Catravas JD, Waters IW: Acute cocaine intoxication in the conscious dog: studies on the mechanism of lethality. J Pharmacol Exp Ther 217:350–356, 1981.
177. Catravas JD, Waters IW, Walz MA, Davis WM: Acute cocaine intoxication in the conscious dog: pathophysiologic profile of the acute lethality. Arch Int Pharmacodyn Ther 235:328–340, 1978.

ETHANOL

178. Knochel JP: Cardiovascular effects of alcohol. Ann Intern Med 98:849–854, 1983.
179. Steel G: Heart failure as a result of chronic alcoholism. Med Chron 18:100, 1893.
180. Moushmoush B, Abi-Mansour P: Alcohol and the heart: the long term effects of alcohol on the cardiovascular system. Arch Intern Med 151:36–42, 1991.
181. Mathews EC, Gardin JM, Henry WL, et al: Echocardiographic abnormalities in chronic alcoholics with and without overt congestive heart failure. Am J Cardiol 47:570–578, 1981.
182. Spodick DH, Pigott VM, Chirife R: Preclinical cardiac malfunction in chronic alcoholism: comparison with matched normal controls and with alcoholic cardiomyopathy. N Engl J Med 287:677–680, 1972.
183. Levi GF, Quadri A, Ratti S, Basagni M: Preclinical abnormality of left ventricular function in chronic alcoholics. Br Heart J 39:35–37, 1977.
184. Regan RJ, Ettinger PO, Lyons MM, et al: Ethyl alcohol as a cardiac risk factor. Curr Probl Cardiol 2:1–35, 1977.
185. Alderman LE, Coltart DJ: Alcohol and the heart. Br Med Bull 38:77–80, 1982.
186. Cheng C-P, Shihabi Z, Little C: Acute effects of mildly intoxicating levels of alcohol on left ventricular function in conscious dogs. J Clin Invest 85:1858–1865, 1990.
187. Kelbaek H: Acute effects of alcohol and food intake on cardiac performance. Prog Cardiovasc Dis 32:347–364, 1990.
188. Lang RM, Borow KM, Neumann A, Feldman T: Adverse cardiac effects of acute alcohol ingestion in young adults. Ann Intern Med 102:742–747, 1985.
189. Nixon JV, Klein K, Smucker MW, Raven PB: Effects of acute alcohol ingestion on the left ventricular performance of normal subjects before and after incomplete autonomic blockade. Am J Med Sci 298:161–166, 1989.
190. Kelbaek H, Gjørup T, Hartling OJ, et al: Left ventricular function during alcohol intoxication and autonomic nervous blockade. Am J Cardiol 59:685–688, 1987.
191. Ireland MA, Vandongen R, Davidson L, et al: Acute effects of moderate alcohol consumption on blood pressure and plasma catecholamines. Clin Sci 66:643–648, 1984.
192. Cigarroa RG, Lange RA, Popma JJ, et al: Ethanol-induced coronary vasodilation in patients with and without coronary artery disease. Am Heart J 119:254–259, 1990.
193. Nagy LE, Diamond I, Casso DJ, et al: Ethanol increases extracellular adenosine by inhibiting adenosine uptake via the nucleoside transporter. J Biol Chem 265:1946–1951, 1990.
194. Pachinger OM, Tillmanns H, Mao J, et al: The effects of prolonged administration of ethanol on cardiac metabolism and performance in the dog. J Clin Invest 52:2690–2696, 1973.
195. Schreiber SS, Briden K, Oratz M, Rothschild MA: Ethanol, acetaldehyde, and myocardial protein synthesis. J Clin Invest 51:2820–2826, 1972.
196. Schreiber SS, Reff F, Evans CD, et al: Prolonged feeding of ethanol to the young growing guinea pig, III: effect on the synthesis of the myocardial contractile proteins. Alcoholism 10:531–534, 1986.
197. Reitz RC, Helsabeck E, Mason DP: Effects of chronic alcohol ingestion on the fatty acid composition of the heart. Lipids 8:80–84, 1973.
198. Regan TJ, Khan MI, Ettinger PO, et al: Myocardial function and lipid metabolism in the chronic alcoholic animal. J Clin Invest 54:740–752, 1974.
199. Ettinger PO, Lyons M, Oldewurtel HA, Regan TJ: Cardiac conduction abnormalities produced by chronic alcoholism. Am Heart J 91:66–78, 1976.
200. Urbano-Marquez A, Estruch R, Navarro-Lopez F, et al: The effects of alcoholism on skeletal and cardiac muscle. N Engl J Med 320:409–415, 1989.
201. Katz AM, Freston JW, Messineo FC, Herbette LG: Membrane damage and the pathogenesis of cardiomyopathies. J Mol Cell Cardiol 17(suppl 2):11–20, 1985.
202. Lange LG, Sobel BE: Mitochondrial dysfunction induced by fatty acid ethyl esters, myocardial metabolites of ethanol. J Clin Invest 72:724–731, 1983.
203. Kossler F, Caffier G, Kuchler G: Zur Wirkung homologer *N*-alkanole auf funktionelle Eigenschaften isolierter Skeletmuskeln: I Almung und Kontraktion. Acta Biol Med Germ 30:209–221, 1973.
204. Eichhorn EJ. The paradox of β-adrenergic blockade for the management of congestive heart failure. Am J Med 92:527–538, 1992.
205. Katz A: Cellular mechanisms in congestive heart failure. Am J Cardiol 62:3A–8A, 1988.
206. Blaustein MP: Sodium ions, calcium ions, blood pressure regulation, and hypertension: a reassessment and a hypothesis. Am J Physiol 232:C165–C173, 1977.
207. Rubin E: Alcoholic myopathy in heart and skeletal muscle. N Engl J Med 301:28–33, 1979.
208. Puszkin S, Rubin E: Adenosine diphosphate effect on contractility of human muscle actomyosin: inhibition by ethanol and acetaldehyde. Science 188:1319–1320, 1975.

209. Carson P: Alcoholic cardiac beriberi [editorial]. BMJ 284:1817, 1982.
210. Aalsmeer WC, Wenckebach KF: Herz und Kreislauf, bei der Beriberi Krankheit. Arch Intern Med 16:193–272, 1929.
211. Weiss S, Wilkins RW: Nature of cardiovascular disturbances in nutritional deficiency states (beriberi). Ann Intern Med 11:104–148, 1937.
212. Akbarian M, Yankopoulos NA, Abelmann WH: Hemodynamic studies in beriberi heart disease. Am J Med 41:197–212, 1966.
213. Ayzenberg O, Silber MH, Bortz D: Beriberi heart disease. A case report describing the hemodynamic features. S Afr Med J 68:263–265, 1985.
214. Knieriem HJ, Herbertz G: Electron-microscopic findings and photometric activation: analytical results in experimental cardiac insufficiency caused by cobaltous chloride. Virchows Arch B 2:32–46, 1969.
215. Kasperek K, Siller V, Knieriem HJ: [Neutron activation analysis of cobalt and calcium in experimental cardiac failure caused by cobaltous chloride.] Z Gesamte Exp Med 150:316–324, 1969.
216. Alexander CS: Cobalt-beer cardiomyopathy. A clinical and pathological study of twenty-eight cases. Am J Med 53:395–417, 1972.
217. Asokan SK, Witham AC: Myocardial malfunction of unknown cause. Cardiovasc Clin 4:113–132, 1972.
218. Edwards CQ, Griffen LM, Goldgar D, et al: Prevalence of hemochromatosis among 11,065 presumably healthy blood donors. N Engl J Med 318:1355–1362, 1988.
219. Buja LM, Roberts WC: Iron in the heart. Etiology and clinical significance. Am J Med 51:209–221, 1971.
220. Dabestani A, Child JS, Henze E, et al: Primary hemochromatosis: anatomic and physiologic characteristics of the cardiac ventricles and their response to phlebotomy. Am J Cardiol 54:153–159, 1984.
221. Candell-Riera J, Lu L, Seres L, et al: Cardiac hemochromatosis: beneficial effects of iron removal therapy. An echocardiographic study. Am J Cardiol 52:824–829, 1983.
222. Furth PA, Futterweit W, Gorlin R: Refractory biventricular heart failure in secondary hemochromatosis. Am J Med Sci 290:209–213, 1985.
223. Demakis JG, Proskey A, Rahimtoola SH, et al: The natural course of alcoholic cardiomyopathy. Ann Intern Med 80:293–297, 1974.
224. Ettinger PO, Lyons M, Oldewurtel HA, Regan TJ: Cardiac conduction abnormalities produced by chronic alcoholism. Am Heart J 91:66–78, 1976.
225. Ettinger PO, Wu CF, De La Cruz C Jr, et al: Arrhythmias and the "holiday heart": alcohol-associated cardiac rhythm disorders. Am Heart J 95:555–562, 1978.
226. Greenspon AJ, Schaal SF: The "holiday heart": electrophysiologic studies of alcohol effects in alcoholics. Ann Intern Med 98:135–139, 1983.
227. Greenspon AJ, Stang JM, Lewis RP, Schaal SF: Provocation of ventricular tachycardia after consumption of alcohol. N Engl J Med 301:1049–1050, 1979.
228. Singer K, Lundberg WB: Ventricular arrhythmias associated with ingestion of alcohol. Ann Intern Med 77:247–248, 1972.
229. Iseri LT, Freed J, Bures AR: Magnesium deficiency and cardiac disorders. Ann Intern Med 58:837–846, 1975.
230. Jones JE, Shane SR, Jacobs WH, Flink EB: Magnesium balance in chronic alcoholism. Ann N Y Acad Sci 162:934–936, 1969.
231. Taasan VC, Block AJ, Boysen PG, Wynne JW: Alcohol increases sleep apnea and oxygen desaturation in asymptomatic men. Am J Med 71:240–245, 1981.
232. Talbott GD: Primary alcoholic heart disease. Ann N Y Acad Sci 252:237–242, 1975.
233. Suhonen O, Aromaa A, Reunanen A, Knekt P: Alcohol consumption and sudden coronary death in middle-aged Finnish men. Acta Med Scand 221:335–341, 1987.
234. Gordon T, Kannel WB: Drinking habits and cardiovascular disease: the Framingham study. Am Heart J 105:667–673, 1983.
235. Beard CM, Griffin MR, Offord KP, Edwards WD: Risk factors for sudden unexpected cardiac death in young women in Rochester, Minnesota, 1960 through 1979. Mayo Clin Proc 61:186–191, 1986.
236. Wilhelmsen L, Elmfeldt D, Wedel H: Cause of death in relation to social and alcoholic problems in Swedish men aged 35–44 years. Acta Med Scand 213:263–268, 1983.
237. Kittner SJ, Garcia-Palmieri MR, Costas R Jr, et al: Alcohol and coronary heart disease in Puerto Rico. Am J Epidemiol 117:538–550, 1983.
238. Dyer AR, Stamler J, Paul O, et al: Alcohol consumption, cardiovascular risk factors, and mortality in two Chicago epidemiologic studies. Circulation 56:1067–1074, 1977.
239. Kramer K, Kuller LH, Fisher R: The increasing mortality attributed to cirrhosis and fatty liver in Baltimore (1957–1966). Ann Intern Med 69:273–282, 1968.
240. Yano K, Rhoads GG, Kagan A: Coffee, alcohol, and risk of coronary heart disease among Japanese men living in Hawaii. N Engl J Med 297:405–409, 1977.
241. Barboriak JJ, Rimm AA, Anderson AJ, et al: Coronary artery occlusion and alcohol intake. Br Heart J 39:289–293, 1977.
242. Hennekens CH, Willett W, Rosner B, et al: Effects of beer, wine, and liquor in coronary deaths. JAMA 242:1973–1974, 1979.
243. St Leger AS, Cochrane AL, Moore F: Factors associated with cardiac mortality in developed countries with particular reference to the consumption of wine. Lancet 1:1017–1020, 1979.
244. Kozararevic D, McGee D, Vojvodic N, et al: Frequency of alcohol consumption and morbidity and mortality: the Yugoslavia cardiovascular disease study. Lancet 1:613–616, 1980.
245. Blackwelder WC, Yano K, Rhoads GG, et al: Alcohol and mortality: the Honolulu heart study. Am J Med 68:164–169, 1980.
246. Marmot MG, Rose G, Shipley MJ, Thomas BJ: Alcohol and mortality: a U-shaped curve. Lancet 1:580–583, 1981.
247. Klatsky AL, Friedman GD, Siegelaub AB: Alcohol and mortality: a ten-year Kaiser-Permanente experience. Ann Intern Med 95:139–145, 1981.
248. Wilhelmsen L, Wedel H, Ribblin G: Multivariate analysis of risk factors for coronary heart disease. Circulation 48:950–958, 1973.
249. Castelli WP, Doyle JT, Gordon T, et al: Alcohol and blood lipids: the cooperative lipoprotein phenotyping study. Lancet 2:153–155, 1977.
250. Thornton J, Symes C, Heaton K; Moderate alcohol intake reduces bile cholesterol saturation and raises HDL cholesterol. Lancet 2:819–821, 1983.
251. Hartung GH, Foreyt JP, Mitchell RE, et al: Effect of alcohol intake on high-density lipoprotein cholesterol levels in runners and active men. JAMA 249:747–750, 1983.
252. Crouse JR, Grundy SM: Effects of alcohol on plasma lipoproteins and cholesterol and triglyceride metabolism in man. J Lipid Res 25:486–496, 1984.
253. Moore RD, Pearson TA: Effect of low-dose alcohol versus abstention on apolipoproteins A-I and B. Am J Med 84:884–890, 1988.
254. Burr ML, Fehily AM, Butland BK, et al: Alcohol and high-density lipoprotein cholesterol: a randomized controlled trial. Br J Nutr 56:81–86, 1986.
255. Camargo CA, Williams PT, Vranizan KM, et al: The effect of moderate alcohol intake on serum apolipoproteins A-I and A-II. JAMA 283:2854–2857, 1985.
256. Haskell WL, Camargo C, Williams PT, et al: The effect of cessation and resumption of moderate alcohol intake on serum high-density lipoprotein subfractions: a controlled study. N Engl J Med 310:805–810, 1984.
257. Taskinen MR, Valimaki M, Nikkila EA, et al: High-density lipoprotein subfractions and post heparin plasma lipases in alcoholic men before and after ethanol withdrawal. Metabolism 31:1168–1174, 1982.
258. Okamoto Y, Fujimori Y, Nakano H, Tsujii T: Role of the liver in alcohol-induced alteration of high-density lipoprotein metabolism. J Lab Clin Med 111:482–485, 1988.
259. Meade TW, Chakrabarti R, Haines AP, et al: Characteristics affecting fibrinolytic activity and plasma fibrinogen concentrations. BMJ 1:153–156, 1979.
260. Meade TW, Imeson J, Stirling Y: Effects of changes in smoking and other characteristics of clotting factors and the risk of ischaemic heart disease. Lancet 1:986–988, 1987.
261. Laug EW: Ethyl alcohol enhances plasminogen activator secretion by endothelial cells. JAMA 250:772–776, 1983.
262. Haut MJ, Cowan DH: The effect of ethanol on hemostatic properties of human blood platelets. Am J Med 56:22–33, 1974.
263. Miyamae M, Diamond I, Wiener MW, et al: Regular alcohol consumption mimics cardiac preconditioning by protecting against ischemia-reperfusion injury. Proc Natl Acad Sci U S A 94:3235–3239, 1997.
264. Miyamae M, Rodriguez MM, Camacho SA, et al: Activation of epsilon protein kinase C correlates with a cardioprotective effect of regular ethanol consumption. Proc Natl Acad Sci U S A 95:8262–8267, 1998.

265. Steinberg D, Pearson TA, Kuller LH: Alcohol and atherosclerosis. Ann Intern Med 114:967–976, 1991.
266. Moore RD, Pearson TA: Moderate alcohol consumption and coronary artery disease. Medicine 65:242–267, 1986.
267. Klatsky AL, Friedman GD, Armstron MA: The relationships between alcoholic beverage use and other traits to blood pressure: a new Kaiser-Permanente study. Circulation 73:628–636, 1986.
268. Jackson R, Stewart A, Beaglehole R, Scragg R: Alcohol consumption and blood pressure. Am J Epidemiol 122:1037–1044, 1985.
269. Klatsky AL, Friedman GD, Siegelaub AB, Gerad MJ: Alcohol consumption and blood pressure: Kaiser-Permanente multiphasic health examination data. N Engl J Med 296:1194–1200, 1977.
270. Potter JF, Beevers DG: The possible mechanisms of alcohol associated hypertension. Ann Clin Res 16(suppl 43):97–102, 1984.
271. Abdel-Rahman AA, Wooles WR: Ethanol-induced hypertension involves impairment of baroreceptors. Hypertension 10:67–73, 1987.
272. Manolio TA, Levy D, Garrison RJ, et al: Relation of alcohol intake to left ventricular mass: the Framingham study. J Am Coll Cardiol 17:717–721, 1991.

AMPHETAMINES

273. Chiang W, Goldfrank L: The medical complications of drug abuse. Med J Aust 152:83–88, 1990.
274. Frost DM: Chemical dependency and the heart. S D J Med 44:149–153, 1991.
275. Anderson RJ, Reed WG, Hillis LD, et al: History, epidemiology, and medical complications of nasal inhaler abuse. J Toxicol Clin Toxicol 19:95–107, 1982.
276. Anderson RJ, Garza HR, Garriott JC, Dimaio V: Intravenous propylhexedrine (Benzedrex) abuse and sudden death. Am J Med 67:15–20, 1979.
277. Dowling GP, McDonough ET, Bost RO: Eve and ectasy: a report of five deaths associated with the use of MDEA and MDMA. JAMA 257:1615–1617, 1987.
278. Carson P, Oldroyd K, Phadke K: Myocardial infarction due to amphetamine. BMJ 294:1525–1526, 1987.
279. Call TD, Hartneck J, Dickinson WA, et al: Acute cardiomyopathy secondary to intravenous amphetamine abuse. Ann Intern Med 97:559–560, 1982.
280. Smith HJ, Roche AHG, Jagusch MF, Herdson PB: Cardiomyopathy associated with amphetamine administration. Am Heart J 91:792–797, 1976.
281. Croft CH, Firth BG, Hillis LD: Propylhexedrine induced left ventricular dysfunction. Ann Intern Med 97:560–561, 1982.
282. O'Neill ME, Arnolda LF, Coles DM, Nikolic G: Acute amphetamine cardiomyopathy in a drug addict. Clin Cardiol 6:189–191, 1983.
283. Yusuf S, Peto R, Lewis J, et al: Beta blockade during and after myocardial infarction: an overview of the randomized trials. Prog Cardiovasc Dis 27:335–371, 1985.
284. ISIS-1 (First International Study of Infarct Survival) Collaborative Group: Randomized trial of intravenous atenolol among 16,027 cases of suspected acute myocardial infarction: ISIS-1. Lancet 2:57–66, 1986.

MARIJUANA

285. Johnston LD, O'Malley PM, Bachman JG: Psychotherapeutic, licit, and illicit use of drugs among adolescents. An epidemiological perspective. J Adolesc Health Care 8:36–51, 1987.
286. Prakash R, Aronow WS, Warren M, et al: Effects of marihuana and placebo marihuana smoking on hemodynamics in coronary disease. Clin Pharmacol Ther 18:90–95, 1975.
287. Graham JD: Cannabis and the cardiovascular system. BMJ 1:460–461, 1978.
288. Graham JD, Li DM: Cardiovascular and respiratory effects of cannabis in cat and rat. Br J Pharmacol 49:1–10, 1973.
289. Beaconsfield P, Ginsburg J, Rainsbury R: Marihuana smoking. Cardiovascular effects in man and possible mechanisms. N Engl J Med 287:209–212, 1972.
290. Johnson S, Domino EF: Some cardiovascular effects of marihuana smoking in normal volunteers. Clin Pharmacol Ther 12:762–768, 1971.
291. Paton WD: Pharmacology of marijuana. Annu Rev Pharmacol 15:191–220, 1975.
292. Domino EF, Rennick P, Pearl JH: Dose-effect relations of marijuana smoking on various physiological parameters in experienced male users. Observations on limits of self-titration of intake. Clin Pharmacol Ther 15:514–520, 1974.
293. Kiplinger GF, Manno JE, Rodda BE, Forney RB: Dose-response analysis of the effects of tetrahydrocannabinol in man. Clin Pharmacol Ther 12:650–657, 1971.
294. Perez-Reyes M, Lipton MA, Timmons MC, et al: Pharmacology of orally administered 9-tetrahydrocannabinol. Clin Pharmacol Ther 14:48–55, 1973.
295. Kanakis C, Pouget JM, Rosen KM: The effects of delta-9-tetrahydrocannabinol (cannabis) on cardiac performance with and without beta-blockade. Circulation 53:703–707, 1976.
296. Kochar MS, Hosko MJ: Electrocardiographic effects of marihuana. JAMA 225:25–27, 1973.
297. Hardman HF, Domino EF, Seevers MH: General pharmacological actions of some synthetic tetrahydrocannabinol derivatives. Pharmacol Rev 23:295–315, 1971.
298. Cavero I, Buckley JP, Jandhyala BS: Hemodynamic and myocardial effects of (-)-delta 9-trans-tetrahydrocannabinol in anesthetized dogs. Eur J Pharmacol 24:243–251, 1973.
299. Vollmer RR, Cavero I, Ertel RJ, et al: Role of the central autonomic nervous system in the hypotension and bradycardia induced by (-)-delta 9-trans-tetrahydrocannabinol. J Pharm Pharmacol 26:186–192, 1974.
300. Zierler S: Maternal drugs and congenital heart disease. Obstet Gynecol 65:155–165, 1985.
301. Kennard MJ: Cocaine use during pregnancy: fetal and neonatal effects. J Perinat Neonatal Nurs 3:53–63, 1990.

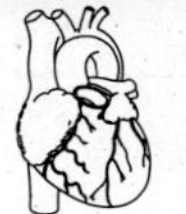

CHAPTER 106

Cardiovascular Involvement in AIDS

Melvin D. Cheitlin and Merle A. Sande

PREVALENCE OF CARDIAC INVOLVEMENT AT AUTOPSY
PREVALENCE OF CARDIOVASCULAR ABNORMALITIES ON ECHOCARDIOGRAPHY
MYOCARDIAL INVOLVEMENT IN HIV-INFECTED PATIENTS
Myocardial Involvement of Known Etiology
Cardiomyopathy in AIDS Patients
Evidence That the HIV Organism Can Cause Cardiomyopathy
Alternative Explanations for Cardiomyopathy in Patients With AIDS
AIDS AND HEALTH CARE WORKERS

From the very beginning of the epidemic of human immunodeficiency virus (HIV) infection, which surfaced in the late 1970s, involvement of the heart was described in autopsies of patients who had died of AIDS. The early reports described Kaposi's sarcoma involving the myocardium and pericardium,[1, 2] often as incidental findings at autopsy. Large series of patients with AIDS described nonbacterial thrombotic endocarditis, a possibly nonspecific finding resulting from the severe cachexia and wasting frequently seen with this disease.[3, 4] Later, larger autopsy series showed frequent evidence of focal pockets of inflammatory cells in the myocardium, at times with incidental findings of fungal or parasitic involvement of the myocardium, but clinical manifestations of this myocardial involvement were unusual. Rarely, severe myocarditis due to toxoplasmosis was seen as a cause of death.

Frequent wall motion abnormalities observed by echocardiography have been described with decreased systolic function, even to the point where the left ventricle is dilated and hypokinetic. Right ventricular dilatation and even right ventricular failure have been described infrequently, probably secondary to pulmonary vascular involvement and cor pulmonale. Other echocardiographic abnormalities, such as mitral valve prolapse, have been described, but these findings may also be related to cachexia and decreased preload, and may therefore be nonspecific.

We are now approaching the end of the second decade of this pandemic. At the beginning of the 21st century, it is predicted that 20 million people around the world will be HIV infected.[5] Even if there were no new infections, this disease and its consequences will be with us until at least 2020. With the introduction of the protease inhibitor drugs, the latent period from infection to the development of AIDS has been extended and the viral burden in the blood markedly reduced. With therapy with a combination of drugs, there is evidence of a decline in morbidity and mortality, even among patients with advanced disease. Palella and colleagues[6] reported a 75 percent reduction in deaths from 35.1 to 8.8/100 person-years among 1255 patients who had at least one $CD4^+$ cell count of fewer than 100 cells/mm^2 before enrollment. However, with these new drugs, new problems have appeared, consisting of metabolic abnormalities with hyperglycemia, hyperlipidemia, and possibly accelerated atherosclerosis.[7]

This chapter examines the evidence for, and the incidence of, clinical cardiovascular involvement and focuses on the possible reasons for the discrepancies between the frequency with which cardiovascular involvement is found by echocardiography and microscopically on examination of the heart and the relative rarity of clinical cardiomyopathy.

Prevalence of Cardiac Involvement at Autopsy

Depending on the series reported in the literature, the incidence of cardiac abnormalities found at autopsy varies from no involvement, when gross cardiac abnormalities alone are considered, to involvement in 70 percent of the cases, when focal lymphocytic infiltration with or without myocyte necrosis is included.[1–4, 8–17] Most patients with "focal myocarditis" have no clinical signs of heart disease, so these collections of cells are incidental findings at autopsy, probably without clinical consequence. Whether the cause of these focal collections of cells is truly a myocarditis due to infection by the HIV organism of the myocardial cell or whether it represents cellular infiltration secondary to myocyte injury caused by some other mechanism (e.g., drugs, "bystander injury," paracrine effects caused by infected macrophages) is unclear. What is certain is that diffuse myocarditis at autopsy is distinctly uncommon and even rare.

When large series of consecutive autopsies performed at centers that provide primary care to AIDS patients are examined, between 5 and 20 percent have cardiovascular lesions of potential clinical importance. At San Francisco General Hospital (SFGH) in a consecutive series of 99 autopsied patients, none had congestive heart failure (CHF)

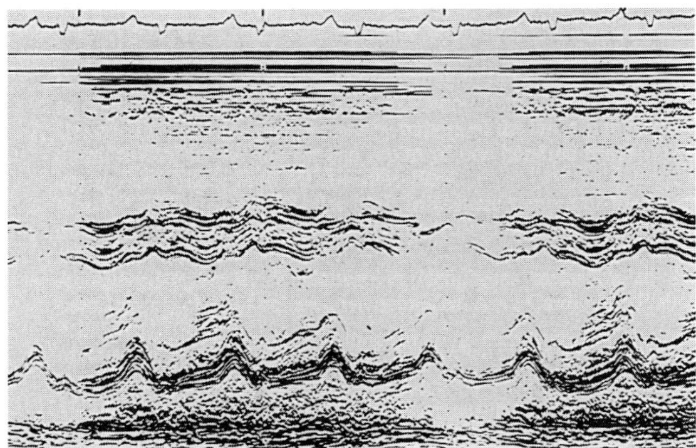

FIGURE 106–1 M-mode echocardiogram in 30-year-old man with AIDS and *Pneumocystis pneumonia.* The right ventricle is enlarged; the left ventricle is normal size. The pulmonary artery pressure is 50/30 mm Hg, the right atrial pressure is 16 mm Hg, and the pulmonary artery wedge pressure is 12 mm Hg. There is a small pericardial effusion.

or cardiomyopathy clinically, nor did any have evidence of a dilated left ventricle at postmortem examination.[17] In other series, patients have been reported with clinical myocarditis, frequently with a known pathogen, such as toxoplasmosis; with pericarditis, frequently without a known pathogen being demonstrated; and with nonbacterial thrombotic endocarditis associated with systemic embolization.[13, 18, 19]

Cardiac involvement by Kaposi's sarcoma is most often clinically silent. Cardiac involvement with lymphoma, often non-Hodgkin's lymphoma, is also much more common in AIDS patients than in non-AIDS patients.[20, 21] On gross autopsy, pericarditis is the most common involvement of the cardiovascular system that has clinical significance.[17] Cor pulmonale and right-sided heart failure are also seen but are distinctly less common (Fig. 106–1).[22]

The cause of death is rarely due to cardiovascular involvement of any kind but rather is respiratory failure and infection.[13, 17, 19] Neoplasms and neurologic involvement are also common causes of death.[12, 14, 23] Of almost 900 autopsied AIDS patients from 15 series in the literature, only 9 (1 percent) had a cause of death that was listed as cardiac.[1–4, 8–15, 17, 19] Of these 9 deaths, 1 patient was taking two known cardiotoxic agents, doxorubicin and interferon; 1 patient had systemic embolization from nonbacterial thrombotic endocarditis; and 2 had toxoplasmic myocarditis. Therefore, 4 of the 9 patients had reasons other than HIV for cardiac involvement. Therefore, only about 0.5 percent of the deaths were possibly attributable only to HIV involvement.

PREVALENCE OF CARDIOVASCULAR ABNORMALITIES ON ECHOCARDIOGRAPHY

Cardiovascular abnormalities observed on echocardiography in patients with HIV infection have been reported in numerous studies, and the prevalence of abnormalities is generally higher than that reported at autopsy. In 1984, Fink and colleagues[24] reported 13 echoes in 15 patients with AIDS, 2 with dilated right ventricles, 3 with left ventricular (LV) hypokinesis, 8 with pericardial effusions, and 3 with tamponade. Most reported studies were not prospective or consecutive series, and only one[25] was stated to be prospective with a longitudinal follow-up and repeat echocardiogram, so that the incidence of abnormalities can be described.

Abnormalities are described in 15 to 60 percent of cases, and the incidence is higher if mitral valve prolapse is included.[26–28] Many of the abnormalities are pericardial effusion or valve-related nonbacterial endocarditis. Infective endocarditis has been seen almost exclusively in intravenous drug–abusing HIV-positive patients (Fig. 106–2). In the four largest series,[27–30] the prevalence of LV hypokinesis varies, from 1.3 percent in 151 HIV-positive patients in the series of Steffen and colleagues[30] to 41 percent in Corallo's series of 102 patients with AIDS.[28] In a more recent echocardiographic series, Akhras and colleagues[31] reported that left ventricular dilatation and/or dysfunction was present in 20 percent of 101 patients with AIDS. They noted that the incidence of most cardiac abnormalities is much higher in patients with AIDS than in those who are just HIV positive.

Hypokinesis can be present without LV dilatation. In most series, the patients with LV hypokinesis had no clinical findings of congestive heart failure. The major exception is the series of Himelman and coworkers,[32] who found echocardiographic abnormalities exclusively in 16 of 25 (64 percent) hospitalized AIDS patients; mitral valve prolapse occurred in only 3 patients (7 percent) of the 45 HIV-positive patients recruited from the outpatient population. The CD4 cell counts were lower in the hospitalized patients (131 ± 186 million/L) than in the ambulatory patients (333 ± 217 million/L). Monsuez and colleagues[29] also noted lower CD4 cell counts in patients with cardiac disease (143 ± 92 million/L) than in those without cardiac disease (294 ± 243 million/L). Levy and associates[27] reported the prevalence of echocardiographic abnormalities

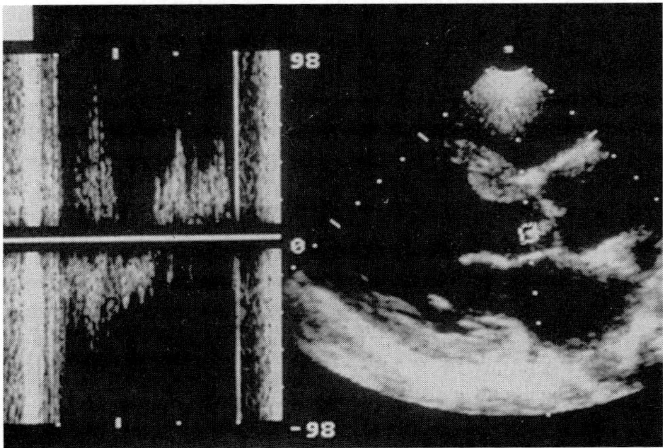

FIGURE 106–2 Two-dimensional echocardiogram and Doppler in a 27-year-old woman with AIDS and a history of intravenous drug abuse (parasternal long-axis view). There is vegetation on the right coronary cusp of the aortic valve. The patient had moderately severe aortic regurgitation.

to be higher with a CD4 lymphocyte count of $100/mm^3$ or less (12 of 22), compared with those with CD4 counts of $100/mm^3$ or more (1 of 14) ($P < 0.01$). These suggest that cardiovascular abnormalities are present in the patients who are the sickest.

Other common abnormalities seen on echocardiography were pericardial effusion, ranging in incidence from 21 percent in Monsuez and associates'[29] series to 44 percent in the series of Akhras and colleagues[31] (Fig. 106–3). The incidence of tamponade varies among different studies: in that of Monsuez and associates,[29] it was 28 percent. In a series of consecutive echocardiograms in 88 AIDS patients at SFGH, pericardial effusion was found in 30 percent. Of 25 patients with pericardial effusion at SFGH, 10 (40 percent) presented with incidental effusions, 10 (40 percent) with pericarditis, and eight (32 percent) with tamponade.

The cause of the pericarditis is not clear. The condition could be related to HIV infection, to an opportunistic infection, or to some other cause. Reynolds and colleagues[33] reported on 14 AIDS patients with pericardial effusion; 10 of the 14 (71 percent) had echocardiographic evidence of tamponade. In 3 of the 14, examination of the fluid revealed the cause: one patient had bacterial infection, one had lymphoma, and one had miliary tuberculosis. Of the 14 patients, 8 (57 percent) had evidence of mycobacterial disease elsewhere. At SFGH, of the 25 patients with clinically important pericardial effusion, 10 required pericardiocentesis, two had pericardial surgical "windows," and three died and underwent autopsy. No cause was found on culture or in examination of the fluid or the tissue in any of the patients.[34]

There are several possible explanations for the differences in frequency with which echocardiographic abnormalities versus autopsy abnormalities are found. Most important is the population from which the study is drawn. The echocardiographic studies are frequently reports of consecutive patients in whom echocardiography was clinically indicated, not of consecutive AIDS patients. At SFGH, in reviewing 88 consecutive echocardiograms performed on AIDS patients, we found cardiovascular abnormalities in 52 patients (59 percent). There was either decreased LV wall motion (nine patients) or LV dilatation with normal wall motion (seven patients), for a total of 16 (18 percent) with LV wall motion abnormalities. There were 21 patients with RV dilatation but normal LV volume and wall motion (24 percent), and 8 others (9 percent) with RV dilatation and tricuspid valve vegetations, presumably resulting from pulmonary disease secondary to tricuspid valve endocarditis. Over the period when the 88 consecutive echocardiograms were performed, presumably obtained for clinical indications, 1171 patients with AIDS were hospitalized at SFGH, so approximately 7.5 percent of those patients underwent echocardiography.

Until recently, the only study attempting to answer the question of how many consecutive HIV-positive patients have cardiovascular abnormalities on echocardiography was a report by Steffen and coworkers.[30] In a prospective study, these authors performed echocardiography on 151 HIV-positive patients, 13 percent of whom were intravenous drug abusers and 74 percent of whom were in Walter Reed stage IV to VI, a classification using CD4 helper cell counts and clinical data indicating advanced HIV disease.[35] Echocardiograms were abnormal in 29 percent. Of these 44 patients with abnormalities, 31 (70 percent) had pericardial effusions, and only 4 of the patients (9 percent) with abnormal echocardiograms exhibited LV dilatation. None of the patients had clinical signs of CHF. The other 13 patients with abnormal echocardiograms had problems that were believed not to be related to HIV disease. Also in this study, HIV patients with associated echocardiographic abnormalities had a significantly lower CD4 lymphocyte count than patients without echocardiographic abnormalities. It is interesting that the mortality rate was the same in the group with normal echocardiograms (34 percent) as in the group with abnormal echocardiograms (41 percent). This was true even in the group with the most advanced clinical disease (Walter Reed stage V and VI), in whom the mortality rate was 44 percent in both the normal and the abnormal echocardiographic group. The incidence of echocardiographic abnormalities therefore appears to depend on the population studied, with the sickest patients and those with a clinical indication for echocardiography having the greatest incidence of echocardiographic abnormalities.

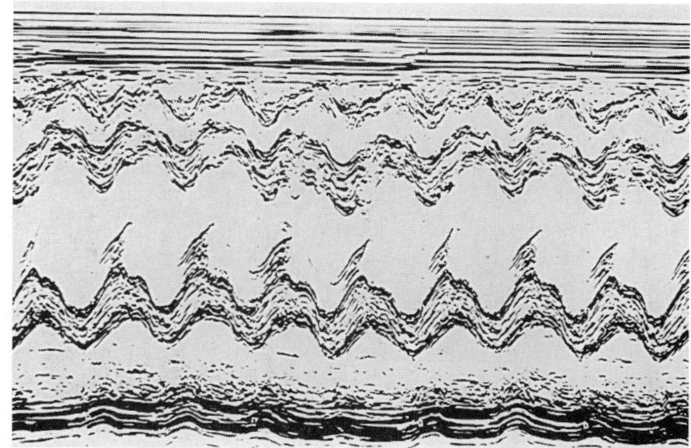

FIGURE 106–3 M-mode echocardiogram in a 47-year-old man with AIDS. There is a large pericardial effusion. The left ventricle is normal.

Akhras and colleagues[31] reported on echocardiograms from 124 consecutive homosexual men who were seropositive for HIV. One hundred one patients had AIDS (group A), and 23 were only HIV positive without overt disease (group B). Doppler echocardiograms were normal in 31 percent of group A patients and in 61 percent of group B patients. Pericardial effusions were present in 44 percent of group A patients and 9 percent of group B patients. LV dilatation and/or dysfunction was present in 20 percent of group A and in none of group B patients. Forty-four of the group A patients had clinical cardiac presentations, with 22 having cardiomegaly with clinical signs of heart failure. Isolated right ventricular dysfunction and dilatation were found in 4 percent of group A patients.

There are four prospective longitudinal echocardiographic studies attempting to document the incidence of cardiomyopathy in HIV patients. Blanchard and colleagues[25] reported on 70 HIV-positive adults prospectively studied with serial echocardiography. There were 50 outpatients, including 44 with AIDS and 6 with AIDS-related complex, and 20 additional patients with asymptomatic HIV infection. All had baseline echocardiographic studies performed when none had symptomatic heart disease. Follow-up studies were performed at 93 months in 52 patients (74 percent) and again at 153 months after baseline studies were performed in 29 patients (41 percent). During the study, 22 patients (44 percent) in the first group and 1 patient (5 percent) in the second group died. Cardiac abnormalities were noted in 26 patients (52 percent) in the first group and in 8 patients (40 percent) in the second group on initial or follow-up studies. An abnormal LV ejection fraction or fractional shortening was seen in 7 patients in the first group; of these, 3 had normal LV function on the later echocardiogram. One patient in the second group had persistent LV dysfunction. Ejection fraction did not change between the baseline and the two follow-up studies in either group. Right-sided cardiac enlargement resolved in 18 patients (44 percent), including 5 of 10 in the first group and 3 of 8 in the second group. Pericardial effusions resolved without intervention in 5 of 12 patients (42 percent) in the first group and in 2 of 4 (50 percent) in the second group. In this study, there was no correlation of CD4 counts with the presence of LV or right ventricular dysfunction. In the patients with pericardial effusion, however, CD4 counts were significantly lower than in those without effusion.

DeCastro and colleagues[36] studied prospectively 136 HIV-positive patients without clinical or echocardiographic evidence of cardiovascular dysfunction on admission. On admission, there were 17 (12.5 percent) without overt disease, 26 (19.1 percent) with AIDS-related complex, and 93 (68.4 percent) with AIDS. Sixty percent of their patients were intravenous drug users. Serial echocardiograms were obtained over a follow-up period of 415 ± 220 days. During the follow-up period, 7 patients, all in the AIDS group, developed clinical and echocardiographic findings of global left ventricular dysfunction, and 6 died of congestive heart failure. In 5 of these patients, an autopsy revealed acute lymphocytic myocarditis in 3, cryptococcal myocarditis in 1, and interstitial edema and fibrosis in 1. In only 1 was LV dysfunction reversible by treatment.

Currie and colleagues[37] reported on an echocardiographic study conducted over 4 years in 296 HIV-infected adults. Thirteen (4 percent) were found to have a dilated cardiomyopathy. These patients had a CD4 cell count of less than 100/mm^2, and median survival in death related to AIDS was 101 days in those with cardiomyopathy, compared with 472 days in those without. Death in the cardiomyopathy patient was most often due to AIDS-related causes rather than to congestive heart failure. Barbaro and colleagues[38] reported on the largest prospective study thus far of 952 asymptomatic HIV-positive patients followed up clinically and with echocardiograms every 6 months. The mean follow-up period was 60 ± 5.3 months. An echocardiographic diagnosis of dilated cardiomyopathy was made in 76 patients (8 percent), with a mean annual rate of 15.9 cases/1000 patients. Myocardial biopsies were performed on all the cardiomyopathy patients, and a histologic diagnosis of myocarditis was made in 83 percent.

Myocardial Involvement in HIV-Infected Patients

Myocardial Involvement of Known Etiology

Two years after AIDS was first described by Gottleib and coworkers,[39] cardiac involvement in AIDS was described by Autran and colleagues,[40] who reported on a Haitian woman with Kaposi's sarcoma involving the heart. Opportunistic organisms have been found in the myocardium, with some, such as *Toxoplasma* and *Cryptococcus,* causing clinical myocarditis, CHF, and death. Usually parasitic or fungal organisms are found in patients dying without clinical evidence of cardiac disease, and their presence in the myocardium is an incidental finding (Figs. 106–4 and 106–5). Recognizing the pathogenic organism that is causing clinical myocarditis is important because therapy is possible. For example, amphotericin B and fluconazole can be used for cryptococcoses,[41] and pyrimethamine and sulfadoxine for *Toxoplasma gondii* myocarditis.[42]

Another way the myocardium can be involved, resulting in clinical cardiac disease, is by neoplasms that are seen in AIDS patients; Kaposi's sarcoma and non-Hodgkin's lymphoma are the most common. Cardiac and pericardial involvement is usually clinically silent and is an incidental finding; occasionally, however, pericarditis due to lymphoma causes tamponade, and a tumor mass may lead to myocardial irritability or may compress the myocardium, causing constrictive pathophysiology with pericardial knock and elevated central venous pressure. Occasionally, an intracavitary tumor mass may cause obstruction to blood flow.

Ioachim and colleagues[43] reported on 21 AIDS patients with cardiac lymphoma, 18 of whom had non-Hodgkin's lymphoma. Most of these are highly aggressive tumors that initially respond to chemotherapy, but long-term prognosis is poor. Gill and colleagues[20] reported on nine AIDS patients with malignant lymphoma. In their series, chest pain resembling acute myocardial infarction was the most common presentation.

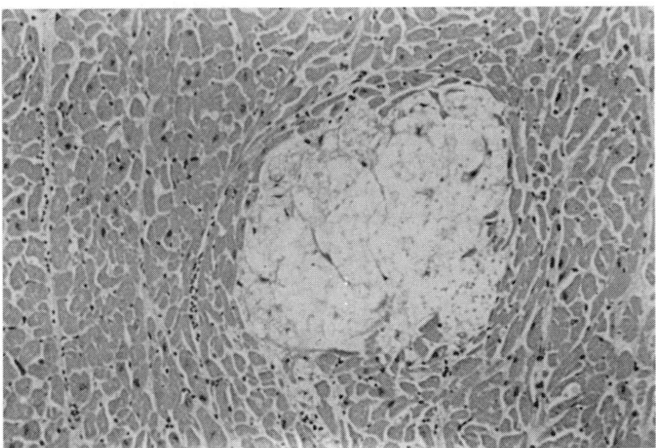

FIGURE 106–4 Myocardial muscle from autopsy in patient with AIDS (medium power) shows cryptococcosis. There is compression of surrounding myocardium but little inflammatory reaction. There was no clinical evidence of cardiac involvement.

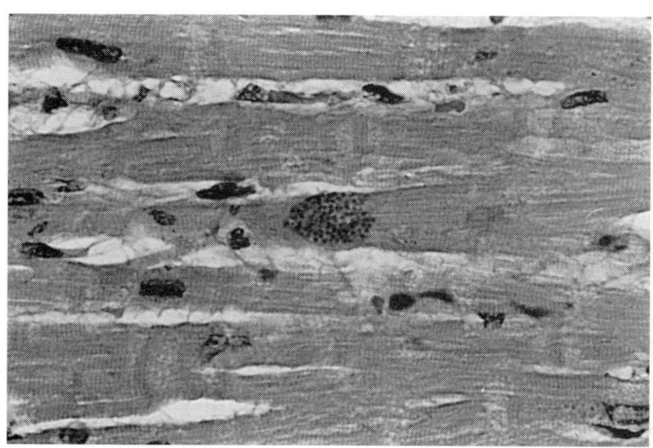

FIGURE 106–5 Myocardial muscle at autopsy from a patient with AIDS (high power) shows a colony of *Toxoplasma gondii*. There was no clinical evidence of cardiac disease.

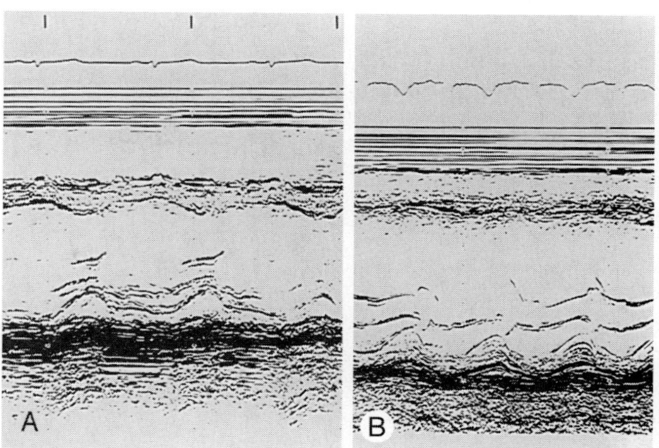

FIGURE 106–6 A, M-mode echocardiogram in a 38-year-old man with AIDS. The left ventricle is normal size (5.3 cm in diastole) with normal function. **B,** M-mode echocardiogram on same patient 18 months later. The left ventricle is enlarged (6.8 cm in diastole), and left ventricular function is decreased.

Cardiomyopathy in AIDS Patients

In 1984, Fink and associates[24] reported on three patients with AIDS and unexplained LV hypokinesis and three patients with pericardial tamponade. Cammarosano and Lewis[4] reported on three patients with nonbacterial thrombotic endocarditis, three with pericarditis, and four with Kaposi's sarcoma. One patient had myocarditis caused by cryptococcosis.

It was not until 1986 that Cohen and coworkers[44] reported on three patients with AIDS with clinical, echocardiographic, and morphologic findings of dilated cardiomyopathy, two of whom had the clinical finding of CHF. At postmortem examination, two of the patients had findings compatible with myocarditis-induced CHF. All patients had focal collections of inflammatory cells, myofibrillar atrophy, and myocardial necrosis.

Reilly and colleagues,[45] pooling cases from the Armed Forces Institute of Pathology and the National Institutes of Health, described 58 consecutive autopsied AIDS patients. Seven (12 percent) had major clinical cardiovascular abnormalities, three had CHF and ventricular tachycardia, one had CHF only, one had LV dysfunction only by echocardiography, one had LV dysfunction followed by sudden death, and one had ventricular tachycardia followed by sudden death. All of these patients had advanced clinical AIDS, and at autopsy, all had focal myocarditis by the Dallas criteria of at least two foci per case and more than five inflammatory cells per high-powered field. Although it was believed that the cause of the clinical cardiac involvement was HIV myocarditis, of the four patients with CHF, two were receiving doxorubicin, 20 mg/m^2 and 100 mg/m^2; two were receiving interferon; and two with LV hypokinesis were receiving interferon, doxorubicin, or interleukin-2. All of these drugs have been shown to produce cardiomyopathy.[32]

Himelman and colleagues[32] described 8 patients with LV dilatation and decreased contractility in 71 patients with AIDS; 4 had CHF (Fig. 106–6). In a large study by Corallo and associates,[28] none of 102 AIDS patients had CHF, even though 41 percent had LV hypokinesis. In Akhras and colleagues'[31] series of 101 AIDS patients, 16 had LV dilatation and low ejection fraction, and 4 had hypokinesis without dilatation. Clinical evidence of congestive heart failure was present in 8 (40 percent) of these.

In autopsy series in the literature, focal myocarditis at autopsy is common, but cardiac causes of death are rare (Figs. 106–7 and 106–8). Of 14 autopsy studies in the literature, 1009 patients with AIDS are reported, with 9 dying of cardiac involvement. One had cryptococcal myocarditis, two had toxoplasmic myocarditis, and five of the nine patients, all with unknown cardiac cause, were reported from one institution.[15] In the largest autopsy series from an institution providing primary care for AIDS patients (rather than a referral center for patients with cardiac disease), Lewis[13] reported on 115 consecutive autopsies in which none of the patients had died of cardiac causes.

Although symptomatic cardiomyopathy in association with HIV-1 infection is unusual and does not appear in consecutive series of patients with HIV infection, individual reports of from one to five cases of patients with LV

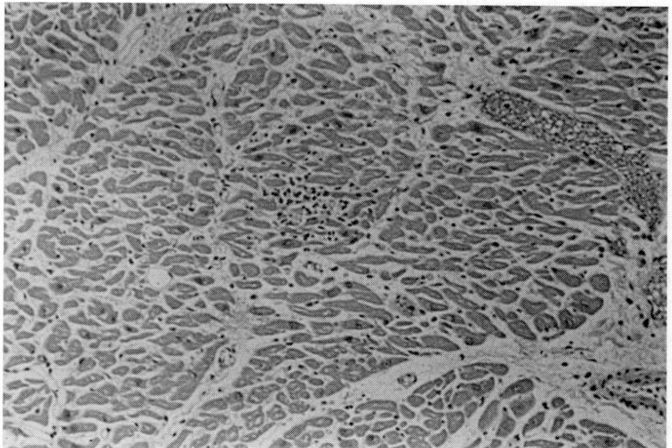

FIGURE 106–7 Myocardial muscle from autopsy in patient with AIDS (high power), with focal area of myocarditis and minimal evidence of myocardial necrosis. This is a focal collection of normal cells with minimal evidence of myocardial cell necrosis. There was no clinical evidence of cardiac involvement.

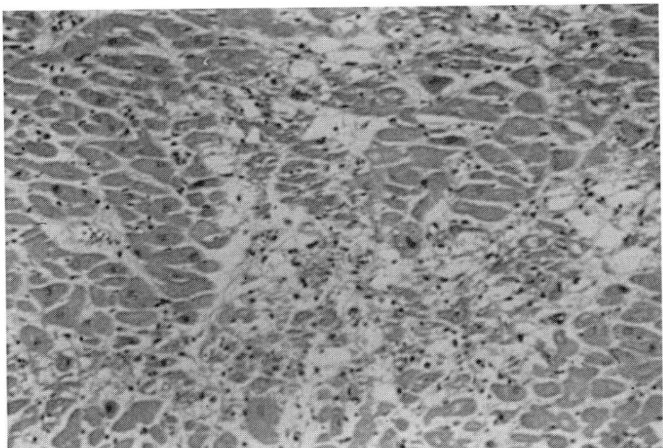

FIGURE 106–8 Myocardial muscle from autopsy in patient with AIDS (high power) shows focal area of myocarditis with round cell infiltration and myocardial cell necrosis. The patient had no clinical evidence of myocardial disease.

dilatation and hypokinesis have been reported often enough that cardiomyopathy associated with AIDS appears to be a definite entity.[36–38, 44–48] This finding could be coincidental because these patients have many other possible explanations for cardiomyopathy. Lending credence to a cause directly related to HIV infection are the reports of cardiomyopathy in children, such as that of 31 pediatric AIDS patients reported on by Lipschultz and colleagues.[49] In this study, 26 percent had decreased LV function on echocardiography, and three died of CHF and one died with sudden death. Although cardiomyopathy is associated with AIDS, the cause of the cardiomyopathy is not apparent.

Evidence That the HIV Organism Can Cause Cardiomyopathy

The most obvious explanation for either focal myocarditis or clinical cardiomyopathy in patients with AIDS is that the HIV organism invades the myocardial cell and causes the myocarditis and later cardiomyopathy. However, the evidence for myocardial invasion by the HIV organism is minimal.

In 1987, Calabrese and associates[50] first reported isolating the HIV organism from myocardium from the right ventricle obtained by biopsy in a patient with a hypokinetic right ventricle and a normal left ventricle. Light microscopy revealed no evidence of myocarditis, but electron microscopy revealed extensive degenerative changes in many myocytes. The cultures from the biopsy did not prove that HIV had invaded the myocardial cell, because blood contamination by the HIV organism could have been the source.

The usual cell membrane receptor for attachment of the HIV organism is the CD4 receptor, which is not present on the myocardial cell. It is possible that there are other receptors or mechanisms by which the virus can enter the myocardial cell. Evidence that the HIV organism can bind to cells by means of receptors other than CD4 has been presented. These cell surface molecules, called CXCR-4 and CCR-5, are receptors for chemokines, a large family of polypeptide chemoattractants that play a role in inflammation and infection. They act as co-receptors for HIV. After the virus binds to CCR-5 or CXCR-4, the gp 41 region of its envelope interacts with a still-undefined domain on the cell membrane, enabling the viral core to enter the cell.[51]

There is some evidence that the virus or a portion of the viral DNA or RNA has been found within the genome of the myocardial cell. Techniques such as in situ hybridization have been used to detect portions of the HIV organism within the nucleus of the myocardial cell, with differing degrees of success. Grody and coworkers[52] reported detecting HIV nucleic acid sequences in cardiac tissue from 6 of 22 patients dying of AIDS. None of the patients had clinical cardiac disease, and all had microscopically normal myocardium. The positive findings were sparse, comprising a few cells per section. With this technique, it cannot be said that the HIV nucleic acid sequences were in the myocardial cells, but they could have been in endothelial cells or even macrophages.

Flomenbaum and coworkers[53] reported one of three hearts from AIDS patients to be positive for HIV-1 DNA sequences without amplification. These authors reported large numbers of proliferating multilamellar membrane bodies in myocytes, which they believed to be an AIDS-specific abnormality. Two other AIDS hearts were positive for HIV-1 DNA after polymerase chain reaction, but, again, the organism could have been outside the myocardial cell. No microscopic myocarditis was seen. Others have also detected viral RNA in situ in myocardial tissue in AIDS patients, but the findings are always sparse and may well not have actually represented involvement of myocardial cells.[54, 55] Most AIDS patients have not had clinical cardiac involvement, and many other reports have been culture negative without any evidence of the viral genome in the myocardial cell.[55–58]

Barbaro and colleagues[38] presented the most convincing evidence so far of HIV virus infection of the myocardial cell. In 63 patients with AIDS and myocarditis on myocardial biopsy, culture of the tissue found coxsackievirus B in 15 patients, cytomegalovirus in 4 patients, and Epstein-Barr virus in 4 patients. A positive hybridization signal was detected in the myocytes of 58 study patients. The staining was sparse, present in 1 to 4 positive cells per section. In 36 of 58 patients with a positive hybridization signal, active myocarditis was documented. However, the positive myocytes were not surrounded by inflammatory cells. Of these 36 patients, 6 were infected with coxsackievirus B, 2 with cytomegalovirus, and 1 with Epstein-Barr virus.

Alternative Explanations for Cardiomyopathy in Patients With AIDS

Opportunistic Infections

Protozoal diseases, such as toxoplasmosis and cryptococcosis, are known to cause myocarditis and even clinical CHF. AIDS patients are subject to infection with other viruses, such as the Epstein-Barr virus and cytomegalovirus, both associated with myocarditis in AIDS.[59, 60] Fungal diseases, such as aspergillosis,[61, 62] and bacterial diseases, such as *Mycobacterium avium intracellulare,*[53] have been described as causing myocarditis.

Viruses are known to cause myocarditis, especially the enterovirus and arbovirus. The most cardiotropic virus is the coxsackie-B virus, and serologic evidence of coxsackievirus B infection has been reported in a fatal case of AIDS-associated cardiomyopathy.[58, 63]

One of the prevalent theories concerning the development of idiopathic cardiomyopathy is that viral myocarditis injures the myocardial cell, precipitating an immunoreaction to the virus, which cross-reacts with the myocardial protein or alters it in such a way that it becomes a foreign antigen, thus initiating complement fixation and myocardial necrosis, leading to inflammatory cell infiltration.[64] Because coxsackievirus B myocardial cell invasion lasts only a few days, by the time cardiomyopathy is seen, the virus is no longer recoverable.

Supporting this concept is a report by Lipschultz and coworkers[65] of a review of 81 children with symptomatic HIV infection. A proportional hazards survival model assessed the impact of coexistent problems on the adverse outcome of CHF, which was present in 12 percent of the patients in a 1.8-year average follow-up period. Thirty patients died during the study interval, 10 with cardiac deaths. HIV encephalopathy was the predictor for cardiopulmonary arrest, and Epstein-Barr viral co-infection, the strongest predictor of CHF.

Immune Cardiomyopathy Precipitated by Myocardial Cell Injury in AIDS

A noninfectious mechanism of myocardial cell injury could lead to cardiomyopathy. In a prospective study, Stimmler and colleagues[66] demonstrated that immunoglobulin G/immunoglobulin M anticardiolipin antibodies were seen in 24 of 26 (92.3 percent) patients with AIDS and in 13 of 14 patients (93 percent) with AIDS-related complex. Mulhall and associates[67] tested 100 male homosexuals and found anticardiolipin antibodies in 57 percent, compared with none of 60 in male heterosexuals. In the homosexuals, anticardiolipin antibodies were evenly distributed among 40 patients with AIDS, 20 with AIDS-related complex, 20 who were HIV positive without disease, as well as in 20 who were HIV negative. None had the thrombocytopenia that is so frequently seen with increased anticardiolipin antibodies in lupus erythematosus. The anticardiolipin antibodies found in this study may be related to the increased incidence of viral infections in gay men, a common stimulus to the development of anticardiolipin antibody, rather than to the HIV infection.

Herskowitz and colleagues[68] identified circulating autoantibodies in four of six AIDS patients with cardiomyopathy, whereas no HIV-positive patient without cardiomyopathy had these antibodies. The cardiac autoantibodies included antimyocin antibodies. These authors performed myocardial biopsies, and with in situ hybridization, genomic probes found no evidence of HIV or other viruses within the cells. Results of enzyme-linked immunospecific assay showed high titers of immunoglobulin G antibody to myosin and to mitochondrial adenine nucleotide. Although this is consistent with the correlation of cardiomyopathy not with HIV but rather with autoimmunity, it is also possible that this was a nonspecific immunoglobulin abnormality, representing activation of a higher gamma polyclonal gammopathy.

Other evidence that an immune-mediated cardiomyopathy is possible is the finding of Fowles and colleagues[69] and of Bolte[70] of defective suppressor cell function in patients with idiopathic cardiomyopathy. In a report by Gu and colleagues,[71] support for an autoimmune mechanism for HIV cardiomyopathy was presented. Twenty-six AIDS patients' hearts and 22 non-AIDS hearts were studied. Sixty percent of the AIDS hearts and 9 percent of the non-AIDS hearts had evidence of myocarditis or cardiomyopathy. Monoclonal antibodies to HIV core proteins P_{17} and P_{24} reacted with certain antigens in the cardiocytes of 38 of 42 AIDS patients and in only 11 of 28 non-AIDS patients. These authors concluded that antibodies raised against HIV react with certain antigenic epitopes in the cardiac muscle, suggesting that the cardiac pathology in AIDS patients is autoimmune in nature and is due to direct HIV infection.

Cytokines as a Possible Cause of Cardiomyopathy

Cytokines, soluble proteins released by immune cells, are biologically active mediators. The cytokinase tumor necrosis factor (TNF) is a 17-kD polypeptide secreted by monocytes and macrophages in the presence of endotoxin and antigens from other microorganisms and is probably the same as cachectin.[72] Injected TNF causes a decrease in ejection fraction and an increase in LV end-systolic and end-diastolic volume. Suffredini and coworkers[73] reported that endotoxin-released TNF depressed LV function independently of its effect on the LV loading conditions. Ho and coworkers[74] explained neuronal cell dysfunction as a result of the cytolytic effect of cytokines released from HIV-infected monocytes. A similar effect could explain myocardial cell dysfunction. Supporting this explanation is the report of Lahdevirta and colleagues[75] of an increased concentration of TNF in patients with advanced HIV-1 infection, consistent with a finding of increased cytokinetic TNF production by peripheral monocytes in patients with AIDS.[76] There is evidence that HIV-infected T cells in AIDS patients are the result of release by abnormal T cells of lymphocytokines that lyse virus-infected cells.[77] It is possible that the rise in cytokines is an epiphenomenon because Levine and associates[78] reported an elevated serum level of TNF in patients with CHF (115 ± 25 units/ml), compared with healthy controls (93 units/ml). Furthermore, the patients with high levels of TNF compared with those with low levels were more cachectic (82 ± 3 percent versus 95 ± 6 percent of ideal body weight).

A report by Herskowitz and colleagues[79] described 35 HIV-positive patients with global LV dysfunction who had undergone endomyocardial biopsy. Cell infiltration, described as active myocarditis or borderline myocarditis, was found in 55 percent of these patients. With myocarditis, the mean ejection fraction was 28 ± 17 percent, versus 48 ± 12 percent for patients without myocarditis. Immunoperoxidase staining revealed CD8 and T lymphocytes to be the predominant cells, and 90 percent of the myocardial biopsy specimens showing myocarditis had intense myocardial expression of major histocompatibility complex class I antigens. The latter suggests that the myocardial inflammatory cells or their secretory products play an important role in the development of markedly depressed LV function associated with the late stage of HIV infection. In a review of the relation of HIV infection and cytokine, Matsuyama and colleagues[80] suggest that AIDS may be a TNF disease.

Change in Ventricular Function Associated With Cachexia

Cachexia results in decreased heart size and probably changes in loading conditions that can affect global ventricular function. In 14 anorexia nervosa patients with cachexia, wall motion abnormalities, as assessed by two-dimensional echocardiography, were found in eight subjects.[81] In animal experiments, starvation has produced decreased LV compliance and decreased peak systolic force associated with myofibrillar atrophy and cardiac interstitial edema.[82] Starvation and protein caloric malnutrition produce a decrease in heart size, myofibrillar atrophy, and interstitial edema.[83, 84] Heart failure is reported, which is especially prominent on refeeding.[85–87]

With myocardial atrophy and loss of cardiac mass, mitral valve prolapse occurs, as well as decreased LV compliance without much change in systolic function.[88] However, decreased compliance can result in decreased preload, which then decreases ejection fraction and stroke volume. This can lead to heart failure precipitated by sodium and water retention, producing an increase in blood volume.[89] Starvation may be associated with hypophosphatemia, which could lead to heart failure. In animal experiments with starvation, there is a marked depletion of cardiac adenosinetriphosphate and a decrease in cardiac stroke work.

Patients with cachexia and starvation can have vitamin deficiency and essential mineral deficiency states. Although it is unlikely that it is a cause of cardiomyopathy in AIDS patients, selenium deficiency has been described, together with reduced cardiac selenium levels.[90] Cardiomyopathy can result from reduced selenium intake, as in the case of Keshan's disease seen in Chinese patients with a diet that is deficient in selenium. One study reported on 10 patients with AIDS and decreased LV fraction shortening on echocardiography who received sodium selenium for 23 days. Six of eight patients showed an improvement in LV fraction shortening.[91]

Drug-Induced Cardiomyopathy

AIDS patients take an enormous variety of prescription and nonprescription drugs, sometimes in addition to recreational drugs. Although some of these drugs are known to produce cardiac toxicity and even cardiomyopathy, the effect of most of the other drugs in immunodeficient patients is not well described. Interleukin-2 and alfa-II interferon[92, 93] have been reported to produce a reversible cardiomyopathy.[46, 94, 95] Chemotherapeutic drugs, such as doxorubicin, can produce cardiomyopathy, as can recreational drugs, such as alcohol and cocaine. Although most patients with AIDS cardiomyopathy have been given doxorubicin in too small a dose to cause cardiomyopathy,[45] it is possible that the dose required to cause cardiomyopathy is smaller in AIDS patients.

Cocaine use has been reported to cause cardiomyopathy as a result of myocarditis, ischemia caused by coronary spasm, acute myocardial infarction caused by coronary spasm, and coronary thrombosis.[96] Approximately one half of the SFGH AIDS study patients have had cocaine exposure. Alcohol abuse is common in this population, and in some, the cardiomyopathy could be caused by alcohol. Other drugs used specifically in AIDS, such as some antiviral agents, might be associated with decreased ventricular function and cardiomyopathy.[97]

One of the most commonly used drugs in AIDS is zidovudine (AZT), a nucleoside analogue that inhibits replication of the HIV virus in vitro, probably by inhibiting the reverse transcriptase enzyme essential to the replication of the retrovirus. No cardiac toxicity was reported in phase I clinical trials, and Richman and colleagues[98] did not demonstrate cardiac toxicity in their studies. Dalakas and coworkers[99] reported a toxic mitochondrial myopathy after 12.8 months of AZT therapy. This coexists with a T cell–mediated inflammatory myopathy restricted to major histocompatibility complex-1 and HLA-A-C antigen and is indistinguishable from the myopathy associated with primary HIV infection with polymyositis in HIV-seronegative patients.[99] The myopathy is characterized by paracrystalloid inclusions in abnormal mitochondria. It is not clear whether this occurs in cardiac muscle.

Herskowitz and colleagues[100] described normalization of abnormal echocardiographic LV systolic function on withdrawal of AZT in AIDS patients with hypokinetic left ventricles. These authors recommended a drug-free period in patients with "AIDS cardiomyopathy."[100] Not supporting the concept that AZT causes cardiac dysfunction is a report by Lipschultz and associates[101] of pediatric AIDS patients studied by echocardiography before and after initiation of AZT. Compared with normal children, children with AIDS demonstrated progressive increases in LV volume and increases in LV mass, but these were not sufficient to maintain normal wall stress. No differences were found between the HIV-infected children who received AZT and those who did not. There was no decrease in contractility in these children, but ventricular performance decreased because of the increased afterload. AZT did not appear to worsen or ameliorate these cardiac abnormalities.

It is apparent that myocarditis secondary to HIV myocardial cell infection is neither the only nor even the most likely explanation for the occasional patient with clinical cardiomyopathy or the more common patient with or without clinical problems but with echocardiographic hypokinesis of a normal or dilated LV. The cause of left ventricular hypokinesis and even clinical congestive heart failure is most likely multifactorial, probably involving viral myocarditis and the effects of cytokines on the myocardial cell.

Metabolic Complications of Antiviral Therapies

With the addition of protease inhibititors to the treatment of HIV infection, it has become apparent that there are several metabolic side effects that have clinical importance. New-onset hyperglycemia, much like type II diabetes mellitus, has occurred as well as worsening of pre-existing diabetes, which has been reported in 1 to 6 percent of people. This problem has occurred with all of the protease inhibitors.[102] The cause of the hyperglycemia is unknown, but its response to the sulfonylureas suggests increased resistance to the peripheral effects of insulin. However, it is not possible to rule out a reduction in insulin secretion.[103] Treatment is similar to that of type II diabetes: diet and oral hypoglycemic drugs.

Disorders of lipid metabolism have also been reported with extreme elevation of triglycerides to more than 1000 mg/dl.[104] These marked elevations have been reported as early as within 2 weeks of initiation of therapy. In the study of ritonavir plus saquinavir, 11 percent of patients developed triglyceride levels greater than 1500 mg/dl. There were no instances of pancreatitis.[105] The mechanism of this disorder of lipid metabolism is unknown. However, there is a 60 percent homology of the catalytic region of the HIV-1 protease to which the drugs bind to two proteins that regulate lipid metabolism: Cytoplasmic retinoic acid binding protein type 1 and low-density lipoprotein receptor–related protein. Binding of the protease inhibitors to CRP would impair hepatic chylomicron uptake and triglyceride clearance.[103] The elevated triglyceride level responds to gemfibrozil.

Finally, an abnormal redistribution of fat from the periphery centrally to the thorax has been reported under various names, the commonest of which is peripheral lipodystrophy. In this syndrome, there are abnormal accumulations of fat in the posterior neck and upper back and abdomen, associated with the initiation of protease inhibitor drugs.[7, 106] There are also elevations in serum cholesterol and triglyceride levels. The abnormal fat redistribution appears to be more in patients taking ritonavir-saquinavir combinations than in those taking indinavir and does not respond to dietary restriction or exercise.

Management of these metabolic problems consists of treatment of the type II diabetes with diet and hypoglycemic drugs. Because the protease inhibitors are such important drugs in the treatment of HIV infection, their value outweighs the problem of the side effects. However, treatment of elevated cholesterol and triglyceride levels is necessary. A potential, if not yet realized, problem is possible interaction between protease inhibitor drugs and 3-hydroxy-3-methylglutanyl coenzyme A reductase drugs, both of which are metabolized by the hepatic cytochrome P-450 system.

The importance of treating these abnormalities is evidenced by the increasing number of reports of premature coronary artery disease in the patients taking protease inhibitor drugs.[107] For this reason, HMG-Co-A-reductase inhibitors should be given to patients with elevated low-density lipoprotein levels together with reduction of other risk factors, such as smoking and hypertension.

AIDS and Health Care Workers

In working with AIDS patients, health care workers have enormous concern about the possibility of contracting the disease. With cardiovascular surgery and cardiopulmonary bypass, concern also exists about the possibility of accelerating the HIV disease. A problem in this era, when attention is increasingly paid to the total cost of health care, is performing expensive procedures at some risk to the health care worker in patients in whom the information gained neither prolongs nor enhances life.

Because almost three quarters of AIDS patients die within 4 years of diagnosis,[108] expensive procedures that lead to morbidity, mortality, and prolonged hospitalization, such as open-heart surgery, are usually not recommended for patients with such a limited life span, unless significant improvement in quality of life is possible. If medically uncontrollable symptoms exist, then invasive procedures that can markedly ameliorate these symptoms can be offered. The best example of such a patient is a 40-year-old man with AIDS who has coronary artery disease with angina pectoris that is unresponsive to intensive medical management. Coronary arteriography is indicated in this situation, and if angioplasty cannot be performed, then the patient should undergo bypass surgery.

Because most patients with AIDS are relatively young, the usual problems that require open-heart surgery are not common. The most common problem at SFGH is that of infective endocarditis and CHF in the intravenous drug abuser. The presence of HIV infection occasions multiple discussions about the risk versus the benefit of valve replacement in these patients. Frater and colleagues[109] reported on 11 HIV-positive patients with endocarditis who underwent valve replacement. Four patients died within 2 months of a resistant, continued sepsis.

Controversy exists as to whether there is acceleration of progression of the disease after cardiopulmonary bypass. Cardiopulmonary bypass produces a temporary depression of phagocytic function and immunoglobulin production.[110] Cardiopulmonary bypass per se in patients without HIV infection causes abnormalities of T4/T8 ratio for up to 6 days after surgery, in contrast to the only temporary depression seen in general surgical procedures not involving cardiopulmonary bypass, after which the T4/T8 ratio returns to normal on the first postoperative day.[111] Acceleration of HIV progression after cardiopulmonary bypass has been reported sporadically. However, there are reports showing no close association between the temporary lymphopenia induced by cardiopulmonary bypass and progression to AIDS.[112] Patients with HIV infection but without opportunistic infections, cancer, or unexplained weight loss can have a prolonged course, especially with CD4 cell counts greater than 200/mm^3 over many years, and should be considered for cardiovascular surgery for the usual indications.

The problem of risk of infection to health care workers has been the focus of a great deal of attention in the literature. The known risk is small, but perceived risk and fear of the disease are great, both among health care workers and among the general public. As of 1992, nearly 100 health care workers in the United States have experienced seroconversion after reported nosocomial exposure. The danger is greatest with exposure to blood, especially with accidental hollow-bore needle sticks from patients with advanced HIV infection and high viral titers.[113] There appears to be little danger from blood splash into the eyes or mouth. In a prospective study at SFGH of 1307 consecutive procedures, accumulated exposure, either parenteral or cutaneous, occurred in 84 procedures (6.4 percent). Parenteral exposure occurred in 1.7 percent. Knowledge of the patient's HIV status before the procedure did not influence the exposure rate, thus refuting the argument that preoperative testing for HIV infection decreases the frequency of accidental exposure to blood.[114]

Several systematic prospective studies of health care workers have looked at thousands of patients and hundreds of exposures to HIV-infected blood. If the results of these studies are combined, the risk of HIV-1 transmission after percutaneous exposure to blood from an HIV-1-infected person is approximately 0.3 percent per exposure (95 percent confidence interval limits 0.13 to 0.7 percent). The risk after mucous membrane or skin exposure is probably substantially smaller.[115]

From these studies of the type of exposure and analysis of risk factors for seroconversion, the importance of the type of exposure (with percutaneous infection being the worst) and the type of fluid (with blood being the worst) becomes apparent. Other important factors to analyze are the concentration of HIV-1 in the fluid, the severity and depth of the exposure, the extent of tissue involved, and other factors, such as the age, temperature, and humidity of the specimen.

The fear of infection among physicians and other health care workers is undeniable, and no matter how small, the risk is clearly evident. However, physicians have a responsibility to treat patients who need their help that stems from the basic philosophic foundation of the healing profession. Like other professions with an even higher apparent personal risk, such as a military personnel, law enforcement officers, and fire fighters, the risk is part of the profession. Although the fear is understandable, it must be managed. Refusal to treat an AIDS patient is not ethical; this position is endorsed by the American College of Physicians and the American Medical Association. The physician, after all, has an ethical imperative and a societal responsibility to care for the sick. The medical profession endorses this responsibility, and the vast majority of physicians agree.

REFERENCES

1. Silver MA, Macher AM, Reichert CM, et al: Cardiac involvement by Kaposi's sarcoma in acquired immune deficiency syndrome (AIDS). Am J Cardiol 53:983, 1984.
2. Hui AN, Koss MN, Meyer PR: Necropsy findings in acquired immunodeficiency syndrome: a comparison of premortem diagnoses with postmortem findings. Hum Pathol 15:670, 1984.
3. Guarda LA, Luna MA, Smith JL Jr, et al: Acquired immune deficiency syndrome: postmortem findings. Am J Clin Pathol 81:549, 1984.
4. Cammarosano C, Lewis W: Cardiac lesions in acquired immune deficiency syndrome (AIDS). J Am Coll Cardiol 5:703, 1985.
5. World Health Organization, Office of Information: Press release. WHO/101. December 10, 1993. Geneva: World Health Organization.
6. Palella FJ Jr, Delaney KH, Moorman AC, et al, and the HIV Outpatient Study Investigators: Declining morbidity and mortality among patients with advanced human immunodeficiency virus infection. N Engl J Med 338:853, 1998.
7. Carr A, Samaras K, Burton S, et al: A syndrome of peripheral lipodystrophy, hyperlipidemia and insulin resistance in patients receiving HIV protease inhibitors. AIDS 12:F51, 1998.
8. Welch K, Finkbeiner W, Alpers CE, et al: Autopsy findings in the acquired immune deficiency syndrome. JAMA 252:1152, 1984.
9. Roldan EO, Moskowitz L, Hensly GT: Pathology of the heart in acquired immunodeficiency syndrome. Arch Pathol Lab Med 111:943, 1987.
10. Wilkes MS, Fortin AH, Felix JC, et al: Value of necropsy in acquired immunodeficiency syndrome. Lancet 2:85, 1988.
11. Baroldi G, Corallo S, Moroni M, et al: Focal lymphocytic myocarditis in acquired immunodeficiency syndrome (AIDS): a correlative morphologic and clinical study in 26 consecutive fatal cases. J Am Coll Cardiol 12:463, 1988.
12. Webb JG, Chan-Yan C, Kiess MC: Cardiac dysfunction associated with the acquired immunodeficiency syndrome (AIDS). Clin Cardiol 11:423, 1988.
13. Lewis W: AIDS: cardiac findings from 115 autopsies. Prog Cardiovasc Dis 32:207, 1989.
14. Miller-Catchpole R, Variakojis D, Anastasi J, et al: The Chicago AIDS Autopsy Study: opportunistic infections, neoplasms, and findings from selected organ systems with a comparison to national data. Mod Pathol 2:277, 1989.
15. Anderson DW, Virmani R, Reilly JM, et al: Prevalent myocarditis at necropsy in the acquired immunodeficiency syndrome. J Am Coll Cardiol 11:792, 1988.
16. Marche C, Trophilme D, Mayorga R, et al: Cardiac involv[e]ment in AIDS: a pathological study, [abstract]. International Conference on AIDS, Stockholm, 4:403, 1988.
17. Magno J, Margaretten W, Cheitlin M: Myocardial involvement in acquired immunodeficiency syndrome: incidence in a large autopsy study [abstract]. Circulation 78:II-459, 1988.
18. Garcia I, Fainstein V, Rios A, et al: Nonbacterial thrombotic endocarditis in a male homosexual with Kaposi's sarcoma. Arch Intern Med 143:1243, 1983.
19. Moskowitz L, Hensley GT, Chan JC, Adams K: Immediate causes of death in acquired immunodeficiency syndrome. Arch Pathol Lab Med 109:735, 1985.
20. Gill PS, Chandraratna PAN, Meyer PR, Levine AM: Malignant lymphoma: cardiac involvement at initial presentation. J Clin Oncol 5:216, 1987.
21. Goldfarb A, King CL, Rosenzweig BP, et al: Cardiac lymphoma in the acquired immunodeficiency syndrome. Am Heart J 118:1340, 1989.
22. Himelman RB, Dohrmann M, Goodman P, et al: Severe pulmonary hypertension and cor pulmonale in the acquired immunodeficiency syndrome. Am J Cardiol 64:1396, 1989.
23. Murray JF, Garay SM, Hopewell PC, et al: Pulmonary complications of the acquired immunodeficiency syndrome: an update. Report of the second National Heart, Lung, and Blood Institute workshop. Am Rev Respir Dis 135:504, 1987.
24. Fink L, Reichek N, St. John Sutton MG: Cardiac abnormalities in acquired immune deficiency syndrome. Am J Cardiol 54:1161, 1984.
25. Blanchard DG, Hagenhoff C, Clow LC, et al: Reversibility of cardiac abnormalities in human immunodeficiency virus (HIV)-infected individuals: a serial echocardiographic study. J Am Coll Cardiol 17:1270, 1991.
26. Kinney EL, Brafman D, Wright RJ II: Echocardiographic findings in patients with acquired immunodeficiency syndrome (AIDS) and AIDS-related complex (ARC). Cathet Cardiovasc Diagn 16:182, 1989.
27. Levy WS, Simon GL, Rios JC, Ross AM: Prevalence of cardiac abnormalities in human immunodeficiency virus infection. Am J Cardiol 63:86, 1989.
28. Corallo S, Mutinelli MR, Moroni M, et al: Echocardiography detects myocardial damage in AIDS: prospective study in 102 patients. Eur Heart J 9:887, 1988.
29. Monsuez JJ, Kinney EL, Vittecoq D, et al: Comparison among acquired immune deficiency syndrome patients with and without clinical evidence of cardiac disease. Am J Cardiol 62:1311, 1988.
30. Steffen HM, Muller R, Schrappe-Bacher M, et al: Prevalence of echocardiographic abnormalities in human immunodeficiency virus 1 infection. Am J Noninvas Cardiol 5:280, 1991.
31. Akhras F, Dubrey S, Gazzard B, Nobel MIM: Emerging patterns of heart disease in HIV infected homosexual subjects with and without opportunistic infections: a prospective colour flow Doppler echocardiography study. Eur Heart J 15:68, 1994.
32. Himelman RB, Chung WS, Chernoff DN, et al: Cardiac manifestations of human immunodeficiency virus infection: a two-dimensional echocardiographic study. J Am Coll Cardiol 13:1030, 1989.

33. Reynolds M, Berger M, Hecht S, et al: Large pericardial effusions associated with the acquired immune deficiency syndrome (AIDS) [abstract]. J Am Coll Cardiol 17:221A, 1991.
34. Galli FC, Cheitlin MD: Pericardial disease in AIDS: frequency of tamponade and therapeutic and diagnostic use of pericardiocentesis [abstract]. J Am Coll Cardiol 19:226A, 1992.
35. Redfield RR, Wright DC, Tramont EC: The Walter Reed staging classification for HTLV-III/LAV infection: special report. N Engl J Med 314:131, 1986.
36. De Castro S, d'Amati G, Gallo P, et al: Frequency of development of acute global left ventricular dysfunction in human immunodeficiency virus infection. J Am Coll Cardiol 24:1018, 1994.
37. Currie PF, Jacobs AJ, Foreman AR, et al: Heart muscle disease related to HIV infections: prognostic implications. BMJ 309:1605, 1994.
38. Barbaro G, DiLorenzo G, Grisorio B, Barbarini G: Incidence of dilated cardiomyopathy and detection of HIV in myocardial cells of HIV-positive patients. Gruppo Italiano per lo Studio Cardiologico Dei Pazienti Affetti da AIDS. N Engl J Med 339:1093, 1998.
39. Gottlieb MS, Schanker HM, Fan PT, et al: *Pneumocystis pneumonia:* Los Angeles. MMWR Morb Mortal Weekly Rep 30:250, 1981.
40. Autran B, Gorin I, Leibowitch M, et al: AIDS in a Haitian woman with cardiac Kaposi's sarcoma and Whipple's disease [letter]. Lancet 1:767, 1983.
41. Kinney EL: Cardiac complications in AIDS: which are significant, which to treat? J Crit Ill 4:49, 1989.
42. Grange F, Kinney EL, Monsuez JJ, et al: Successful therapy for *Toxoplasma gondii* myocarditis in acquired immunodeficiency syndrome. Am Heart J 120:443, 1990.
43. Ioachim HL, Cooper MC, Hellman GC: Lymphomas in men at high risk for acquired immune deficiency syndrome (AIDS): a study of 21 cases. Cancer 56:2831, 1985.
44. Cohen IS, Anderson DW, Virmani R, et al: Congestive cardiomyopathy in association with the acquired immunodeficiency syndrome. N Engl J Med 315:628, 1986.
45. Reilly JM, Cunnion RE, Anderson DW, et al: Frequency of myocarditis, left ventricular dysfunction and ventricular tachycardia in the acquired immune deficiency syndrome. Am J Cardiol 62:789, 1988.
46. Kaminski HJ, Katzman M, Wiest PM, et al: Cardiomyopathy associated with the acquired immune deficiency syndrome. J AIDS 1:105, 1988.
47. Corboy JR, Fink L, Miller WT: Congestive cardiomyopathy in association with AIDS. Radiology 165:139, 1987.
48. Nagoshi MH, Fukuyama O: Cardiac disease associated with the acquired immunodeficiency syndrome: a case report and review of the literature. Hawaii Med J 47:531, 1988.
49. Lipshultz SE, Chanock S, Sanders SP, et al: Cardiovascular manifestations of human immunodeficiency virus infection in infants and children. Am J Cardiol 63:1489, 1989.
50. Calabrese LH, Proffitt MR, Yen-Lieberman B, et al: Congestive cardiomyopathy and illness related to the acquired immunodeficiency syndrome (AIDS) associated with isolation of retrovirus from myocardium. Ann Intern Med 107:691, 1987.
51. Levy JA: Infection by human immunodeficiency virus: CD-4 is not enough. N Engl J Med 335:1528, 1996.
52. Grody WW, Cheng L, Lewis W: Infection of the heart by the human immunodeficiency virus. Am J Cardiol 66:203, 1990.
53. Flomenbaum M, Soeiro R, Udem SA, et al: Proliferative membranopathy and human immunodeficiency virus in AIDS hearts. J AIDS 2:129, 1989.
54. Lipshultz SE, Fox CH, Perez-Atayde AR, et al: Identification of human immunodeficiency virus-1 RNA and DNA in the heart of a child with cardiovascular abnormalities and congenital acquired immune deficiency syndrome: case report. Am J Cardiol 66:246, 1990.
55. Cenacchi G, Re MC, Furlini G, et al: Human immunodeficiency virus type 1 antigen detection in endomyocardial biopsy: an immunomorphological study. Microbiologica 13:145, 1990.
56. Levy WS, Varghese PJ, Anderson DW, et al: Myocarditis diagnosed by endomyocardial biopsy in human immunodeficiency virus infection with cardiac dysfunction. Am J Cardiol 62:658, 1988.
57. Henry K, Dexter D, Sannerud K, et al: Recovery of HIV at autopsy (letter). N Engl J Med 321:1833, 1989.
58. Dittrich H, Chow L, Denaro F, Spector S: Human immunodeficiency virus, coxsackievirus, and cardiomyopathy [letter]. Ann Intern Med 108:308, 1988.
59. Lafont A, Marche C, Wolff M, et al: Myocarditis in acquired immunodeficiency syndrome (AIDS): etiology and progress, abstracted. J Am Coll Cardiol 11:196A, 1988.
60. Stewart JM, Kaul A, Gromisch DS, et al: Symptomatic cardiac dysfunction in children with human immunodeficiency virus infection. Am Heart J 117:140, 1989.
61. Henochowicz S, Mustafa M, Lawrinson WE, et al: Cardiac aspergillosis in acquired immune deficiency syndrome. Am J Cardiol 55:1239, 1985.
62. Cox JN, di Dio F, Pizzolato GP, et al: *Aspergillus* endocarditis and myocarditis in a patient with the acquired immunodeficiency syndrome (AIDS): a review of the literature: case report. Virchows Archiv Pathol Anat Histopathol 417:255, 1990.
63. Patel RC, Frishman WH: Cardiac involvement in HIV infection. Med Clin North Am 80:1493, 1996.
64. Lowry PJ, Thompson RA, Littler WA: Cellular immunity in congestive cardiomyopathy: the normal cellular immune response. Br Heart J 53:394, 1985.
65. Lipshultz SE, Lugmbuhl LM, McIntosh K, Orav EJ: Cardiac morbidity and mortality in children with symptomatic HIV infection [abstract]. Circulation 86:I-362, 1992.
66. Stimmler MM, Quismorio FP Jr, McGehee WG, et al: Anticardiolipin antibodies in acquired immunodeficiency syndrome. Arch Intern Med 149:1833, 1989.
67. Mulhall BP, Naselli G, Whittingham S: Anticardiolipin antibodies in homosexual men: prevalence and lack of association with human immunodeficiency virus (HIV) infection. J Clin Immunol 9:208, 1989.
68. Herskowitz A, Ansari AA, Neumann DA, et al: Cardiomyopathy in acquired immunodeficiency syndrome: evidence for autoimmunity [abstract]. Circulation 80:II-322, 1989.
69. Fowles RE, Bieber CP, Stinson EB: Defective in vitro suppressor cell function in idiopathic congestive cardiomyopathy. Circulation 59:483, 1979.
70. Bolte HD: Immunological defects precursors of myocarditis and dilated cardiomyopathy? J Mol Cell Cardiol 17 [suppl 2]:69, 1985.
71. Gu J, Dische R, Anderson V, et al: Evidence for an autoimmune mechanism of the cardiac pathology in AIDS patients [abstract]. Circulation 86:I-795, 1992.
72. Beutler B, Cerami A: Cachectin and tumour necrosis factor as two sides of the same biological coin: review article. Nature 320:584, 1986.
73. Suffredini AF, Fromm RE, Parker MM, et al: The cardiovascular response of normal humans to the administration of endotoxin. N Engl J Med 321:280, 1989.
74. Ho DD, Pomerantz RJ, Kaplan JC: Pathogenesis of infection with human immunodeficiency virus. N Engl J Med 317:278, 1987.
75. Lahdevirta J, Maury CPJ, Teppo AM, Repo H: Elevated levels of circulating cachectin/tumor necrosis factor in patients with acquired immunodeficiency syndrome. Am J Med 85:289, 1988.
76. Wright SC, Jewett A, Mitsuyasu R, Bonavida B: Spontaneous cytotoxicity and tumor necrosis factor production by peripheral blood monocytes from AIDS patients. J Immunol 141:99, 1988.
77. Ruddle NH: Lymphotoxin production in AIDS. Immunol Today 7:8, 1986.
78. Levine B, Kalman J, Mayer L, et al: Elevated circulating levels of tumor necrosis factor in severe chronic heart failure. N Engl J Med 323:236, 1990.
79. Herskowitz A, Willoughby SB, Beschorner WE, et al: Myocarditis associated with severe left ventricular dysfunction in late stage HIV infection [abstract]. Circulation 86:I-6, 1992.
80. Matsuyama T, Kobayashi N, Yamamoto N: Cytokine and HIV infection: Is AIDS a tumor necrosis factor disease? AIDS 5:1405, 1991.
81. Goldberg SJ, Comerci GD, Feldman L: Cardiac output and regional myocardial contraction in anorexia nervosa. J Adolesc Health Care 9:15, 1988.
82. Abel RM, Grimes JB, Alonso D, et al: Adverse hemodynamic and ultrastructural changes in dog hearts subjected to protein-calorie malnutrition. Am Heart J 97:733, 1979.
83. Smythe PM, Swanepoel A, Campbell JA: The heart in kwashiorkor. Br Med J 1:67, 1962.
84. Garnett ES, Barnard DL, Ford J, et al: Gross fragmentation of cardiac myofibrils after therapeutic starvation for obesity. Lancet 1:914, 1969.
85. Heymsfield SB, Bethel RA, Ansley JD, et al: Cardiac abnormalities

in cachectic patients before and during nutritional repletion. Am Heart J 95:584, 1978.
86. Powers PS: Heart failure during treatment of anorexia nervosa. Am J Psychiatr 139:1167, 1982.
87. Schocken DD, Holloway JD, Powers PS: Weight loss and the heart: effects of anorexia nervosa and starvation. Arch Intern Med 149:877, 1989.
88. Moodie DS: Anorexia and the heart: results of studies to assess effects. Postgrad Med 81:46, 1987.
89. Dworkin BM, Rosenthal WS, Wormser GP, Weiss L: Selenium deficiency in the acquired immunodeficiency syndrome. J Parenter Enter Nutr 10:405, 1986.
90. Dworkin BM, Antonecchia PP, Smith F, et al: Reduced cardiac selenium content in the acquired immunodeficiency syndrome. J Parenter Enter Nutr 13:644, 1989.
91. Zazzo JF, Chalas J, Lafont A, et al: Is nonobstructive cardiomyopathy in AIDS a selenium deficiency–related disease [letter]? J Parenter Enter Nutr 12:537, 1988.
92. Cohen MC, Huberman MS, Nesto RW: Recombinant alpha$_2$ sinterferon–related cardiomyopathy. Am J Med 85:549, 1988.
93. Deyton LR, Walker RE, Kovacs JA, et al: Reversible cardiac dysfunction associated with interferon alfa therapy in AIDS patients with Kaposi's sarcoma. N Engl J Med 321:1246, 1989.
94. Kaul S, Fishbein MC, Siegel RJ: Cardiac manifestations of acquired immune deficiency syndrome: a 1991 update. Am Heart J 122:535, 1991.
95. Sonnenblick M, Rosenmann D, Rosin A: Reversible cardiomyopathy induced by interferon. Br Med J 300:1174, 1990.
96. Chokshi SK, Moore R, Pandian NG, Isner JM: Reversible cardiomyopathy associated with cocaine intoxication. Ann Intern Med 111:1039, 1989.
97. Wharton JM, Demopulos PA, Goldschlager N: Torsade de pointes during administration of pentamidine isethionate. Am J Med 83:571, 1987.
98. Richman DD, Fischl MA, Grieco MH, et al, and the AZT Collaborative Working Group: The toxicity of azidothymidine (AZT) in the treatment of patients with AIDS and AIDS-related complex: a double-blind, placebo-controlled trial. N Engl J Med 317:192, 1987.
99. Dalakas MC, Illa I, Pezeshkpour GH, et al: Mitochondrial myopathy caused by long-term zidovudine therapy. N Engl J Med 322:1098, 1990.
100. Herskowitz A, Bartlett JD, Willoughby SB, et al: Cardiomyopathy associated with antiretroviral therapy in patients with HIV infection: a report of six cases. Ann Intern Med 116:311, 1992.
101. Lipshultz SE, Orav EJ, Sanders SP, et al: Cardiac structure and function in children with human immunodeficiency virus infection treated with zidovudine. N Engl J Med 327:1260, 1992.
102. Eastone JA, Decker CF: New-onset diabetes mellitus associated with the use of protease inhibitor. Ann Intern Med 127:948, 1997.
103. Carr A, Samaras K, Chisholm DJ, Cooper DA: Pathogenesis of HIV-1-protease inhibitor-associated peripheral lipodystrophy, hyperlipidemia, and insulin resistance. Lancet 351:1881, 1998.
104. Danner SA, Carr A, Leonard J, et al: Safety, pharmacokinetics and preliminary efficacy of ritonavir, an inhibitor of HIV-1 protease. N Engl J Med 333:1528, 1995.
105. Cameron DW, et al: Antiretroviral safety and durability of ritonavir (RIT). Saquinavir (SQV) in protease inhibitor-naive patients in year two of follow-up [abstract 388]. *In* Abstracts of the 5th Conference on Ritonavir and opportunistic infections. Chicago, February 1998.
106. Lo JC, Mulligan K, Tai VW, et al: "Buffalo hump" in men with HIV-1 infection. Lancet 351:867, 1998.
107. Henry K, Melroe H, Heubsch J, et al: Severe premature coronary artery disease with protease inhibitors [research letter]. Lancet 351:1328, 1998.
108. Centers for Disease Control: Acquired immunodeficiency syndrome—United States: update. MMWR Morb Mortal Weekly Rep 35:17, 1986.
109. Frater RWM, Sisto D, Condit D: Cardiac surgery in human immunodeficiency virus (HIV) carriers. Eur J Cardiothorac Surg 3:146, 1989.
110. Utley JR: The immune response. *In* Utley JR (ed): Pathophysiology and Techniques of Cardiopulmonary Bypass. Vol. 1. pp. 132–144. Baltimore: Williams & Wilkins, 1982.
111. Pollock R, Ames F, Rubio P, et al: Protracted severe immune dysregulation induced by cardiopulmonary bypass: a predisposing etiologic factor in blood transfusion-related AIDS? J Clin Lab Immunol 22:1, 1987.
112. Lemma M, Vanelli P, Beretta L, et al: Cardiac surgery in HIV positive intravenous drug addicts: influence of cardiopulmonary bypass on the progression to AIDS. Thorac Cardiovasc Surg 40:279, 1992.
113. Cardo DM, Culver DH, Ciesielski CA, et al: A case-control study of HIV seroconversion in health care workers after percutaneous exposure. Centers for Disease Control and Prevention Needlestick Surveillance Group. N Engl J Med 337:1485, 1997.
114. Gerberding JL, Littell C, Tarkington A, et al: Risk of exposure of surgical personnel to patients' blood during surgery at San Francisco General Hospital. N Engl J Med 322:1788, 1990.
115. Henderson DK, Fahey BJ, Willy M, et al: Risk for occupational transmission of human immunodeficiency virus type 1 (HIV-1) associated with clinical exposures: a prospective evaluation. Ann Intern Med 113:740, 1990.

CHAPTER 107

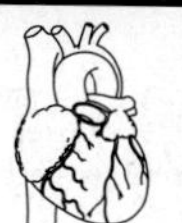

Neuromuscular Disorders and Heart Disease

Joseph Lee, Shilpesh Patel, and James T. Willerson

MYOTONIC DYSTROPHY
FRIEDREICH'S ATAXIA
DUCHENNE'S MUSCULAR DYSTROPHY
BECKER'S MUSCULAR DYSTROPHY
KEARNS-SAYRE SYNDROME
EMERY-DREIFUSS SYNDROME
FACIOSCAPULOHUMERAL MUSCULAR DYSTROPHY
MYOTUBULAR (CENTRONUCLEAR) MYOPATHY
NEMALINE MYOPATHY
OTHER COMBINED SKELETAL MYOPATHIES AND CARDIOMYOPATHIES
Desmin Myopathy
Familial Dilated Cardiomyopathy With Conduction Defect and Muscular Dystrophy

The association between neuromuscular disease and cardiac disorders is a complex one. Cardiac abnormalities are usually manifested as a cardiomyopathy or a disorder of the conduction system. Most of the following neurologic disorders have a known mode of inheritance, and many chromosome locations have been identified. Studies are hindered by the relative infrequency of most of these disorders and the heterogeneity of their phenotypic expression (Table 107–1).

Myotonic Dystrophy

Myotonic dystrophy (Steinert's disease), an autosomal dominant disorder with multisystem manifestations, is the most common inherited form of muscular dystrophy affecting adults. The genetic defect has been localized to chromosome 19 and the protein product identified as a protein kinase with an increased number of cytosine-thymidine-guanine (CTG) repeats in the 3′ untranslated region of the molecule. The gene is strongly expressed in heart muscle.[1] A DNA probe has been developed that directly detects the mutation.[2] The incidence of myotonic dystrophy is estimated to be 10 to 15 cases/100,000 population.[3]

The clinical manifestations are dominated by myotonia, which is a delay of muscle relaxation after contraction and is most evident after a handshake with an affected individual. An early feature is weakness of the neck flexors and atrophy of the masseter, temporal, and sternocleidomastoid muscles (Fig. 107–1). Consequently, patients have a weak cough reflex and incoordination of pharyngeal muscles and are prone to aspiration of oropharyngeal contents.[1] Systemic manifestations include premature frontal baldness, cataracts, atrophy of the gonads, and less commonly, gastrointestinal disorders involving the muscles of the esophagus and the colon.[3]

Autopsy studies have shown that most cardiac pathology resides in the conduction system rather than in the myocardium. Any part of the conduction system can be involved. Reports have shown atrophy, fibrosis, and fatty infiltration of the sinus node, atrioventricular node, His bundle, and bundle branches.[4–6] Electron microscopy studies have shown mitochondrial abnormalities and vacuolation of the sarcoplasmic reticulum.[7] Damage to the latter has been postulated as the explanation for the conduction system abnormalities.[8] Cardiac muscle involvement varies from nonexistent to areas of focal or diffuse fibrosis or fatty infiltration.[9, 10]

Even though neurologic disease is usually the dominant feature, cardiac disease may be the initial cause of presentation.[11] The electrocardiogram (ECG) is abnormal in approximately two thirds of patients and in virtually all patients with clinically severe disease.[12, 13] The most common electrocardiographic abnormalities are prolongation of the PR interval, left anterior fascicular block, and prolongation of the QRS interval (Fig. 107–2). These findings are often associated with sinus bradycardia (in contrast to the sinus tachycardia noted in Duchenne's muscular dystrophy [DMD] and Friedreich's ataxia), premature atrial contractions, atrial fibrillation, and atrial flutter.[13–17] Digitalis is seldom required because of atrioventricular (AV) block. Studies have shown that cardiac disease appears to have a progressive course related to findings on the ECG, with first-degree AV block and left anterior fascicular block being most common in patients with mild-to-moderate disease, and atrial fibrillation and flutter most common in patients with more severe disease.[13, 15] Ventricular conduction defects, such as bundle branch blocks and abnormal axis, occur in approximately 50 percent of patients and may progress from intermittent to sustained.[18] However, H-V interval measurement has been shown to be unable to predict progression of the conduction system disease. Therefore, electrophysiologic studies are recommended only for symptomatic patients.[19] Sudden death occurs and is believed to be due to either high-grade AV block or ventricular tachycardia.[6, 14, 16, 20, 21] One report has shown that in patients with myotonic dystrophy, late potential frequency approaches that of patients with known inducible ventricular tachycardia.[22]

TABLE 107–1 **Manifestations of Neurologic Cardiac Disorders**

Neuromuscular Disorder	Mode of Inheritance	Incidence per 100,000	Age of Onset	Pathology: Cardiac	Pathology: Musculoskeletal	Clinical: Cardiac	Clinical: Musculoskeletal
Myotonic dystrophy	Autosomal dominant	10	3rd–4th decade	Atrophy Interstitial fibrosis and fatty infiltration of the conduction system	Atrophy Interstitial fibrosis and fatty infiltration	AV block Atrial arrhythmias CHF (rare)	Myotonia Atrophy of strap muscles
Friedreich's ataxia	Autosomal recessive	2.0	Child/adolescent	Interstitial fibrosis Myocyte hypertrophy	Normal	Abnormal ECG axis and Q waves Atrial arrhythmias Hypertrophic cardiomyopathy Concentric Asymmetric Dilated cardiomyopathy	Ataxia Kyphoscoliosis
Duchenne's muscular dystrophy	X-linked recessive	2.0	2–5 yr	Myocardial fibrosis in posterobasal LV free wall Degeneration of conducting fibers Noninflammatory arteriopathy	Myofibril necrosis Interstitial accumulation of fat and fibrous tissue	Dysrhythmias ECG abnormalities Dilated and hypertrophic cardiomyopathy	Pseudohypertrophy Proximal limb and neck weakness Contractures Scoliosis and chest cage deformities
Becker's muscular dystrophy	X-linked recessive	0.4	2nd–3rd decade	Focal areas of fatty infiltration and proliferating connective tissue	Same as Duchenne's	Dilated cardiomyopathy	Pseudohypertrophy Proximal limb–girdle weakness and atrophy
Kearns-Sayre syndrome	Maternal, nonmendelian	Rare	Childhood/adolescence	Ragged red fibers	Ragged red fibers Glycogen accumulation Proliferation of abnormal mitochondria	Progressive AV block Dilated cardiomyopathy	Ptosis Ataxia
Emery-Dreifuss syndrome	X-linked recessive Autosomal dominant	Rare	2nd–3rd decade	Focal myocardial fibrosis	Same as Duchenne's	Atrial standstill Progressive conduction block Malignant ventricular arrhythmias Dilated cardiomyopathy	Contractures of elbows, post. cervical muscles, and Achilles tendon Humeroperoneal muscle weakness and atrophy
Facioscapulohumeral muscular dystrophy	Autosomal dominant	0.6	2nd–3rd decade	Unknown	Same as Duchenne's	Atrial abnormalities Conduction delays Atrial fib/flutter	Proximal shoulder and facial weakness and atrophy Lower extremity weakness
Myotubular (centronuclear) myopathy	X-linked recessive	Rare	Variable	Myocardial fibrosis	Hypertrophic fibers with central nuclei	Dilated cardiomyopathy	Respiratory difficulties
Nemaline myopathy	Autosomal dominant with reduced penetrance	Rare	Birth/infancy	Nemaline bodies	Nemaline bodies	Dilated cardiomyopathy	Diffuse muscle weakness and hypotonia

Abbreviations: AV, atrioventricular; CHF, congestive heart failure; ECG, electrocardiographic; fib, fibrillation; LV, left ventricular.

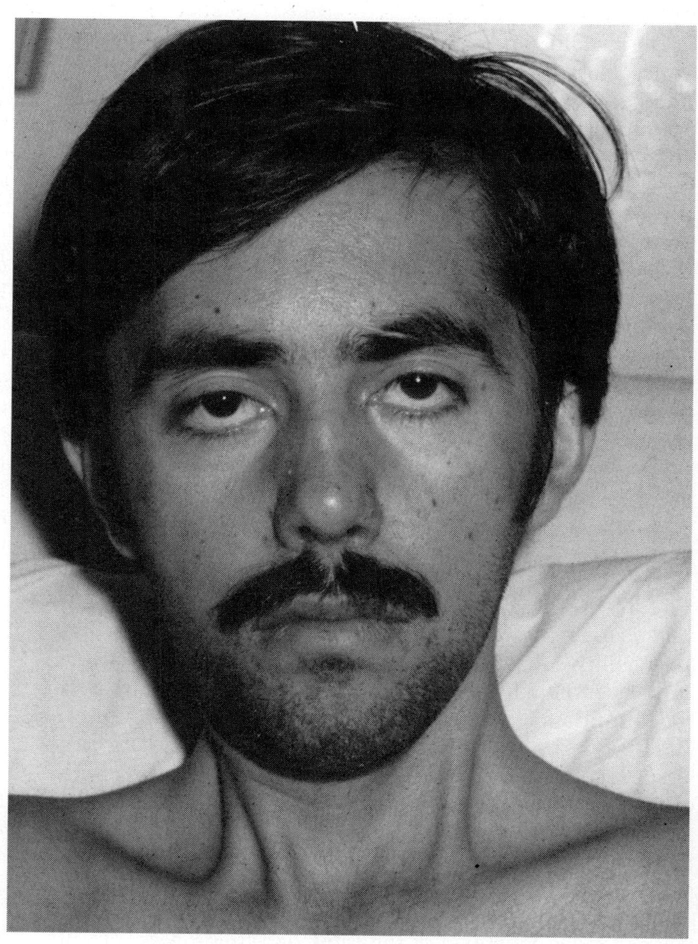

FIGURE 107–1 A 29-year-old man with myotonic dystrophy. The striking feature is the marked atrophy of the sternocleidomastoid muscles. The muscle heads taper and are pencil thin at their clavicular insertions. (Courtesy of Ian Butler, M.D.)

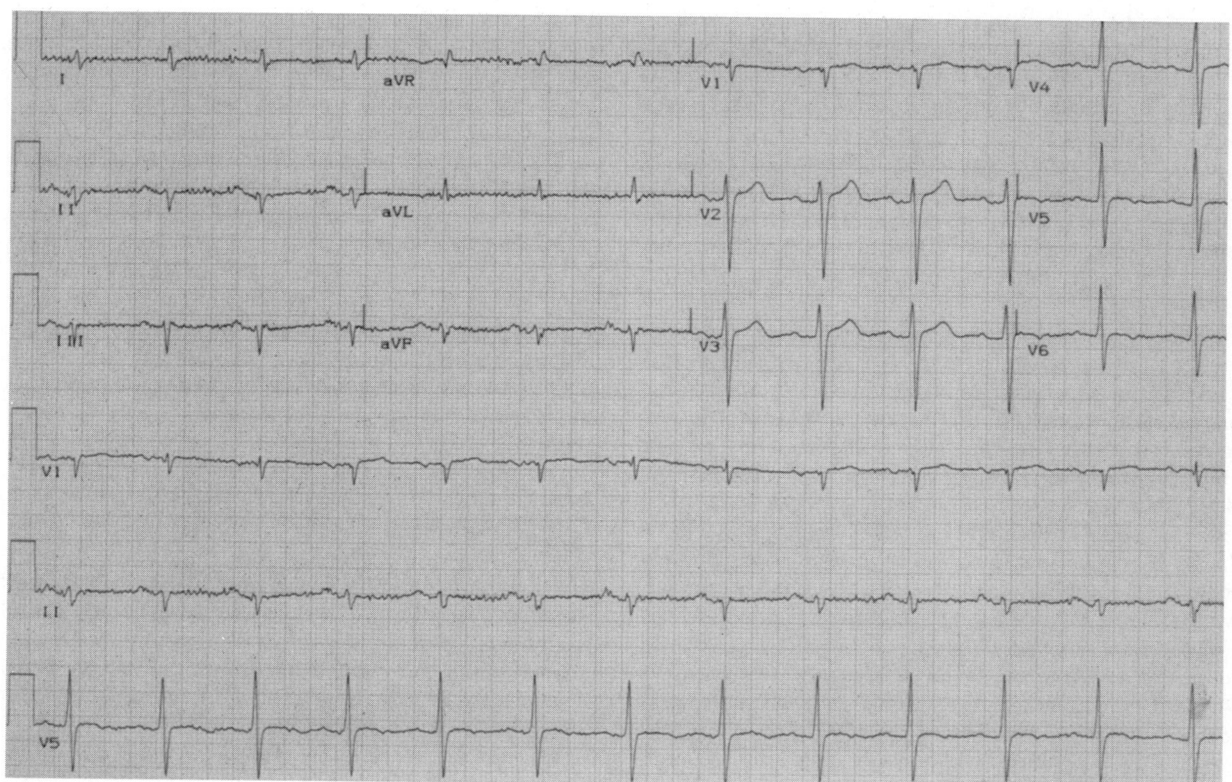

FIGURE 107–2 Electrocardiogram from a 35-year-old man with myotonic dystrophy. Note the left anterior fascicular block, the interventricular conduction delay (QRS, 112 msec), and the first-degree AV block (PR interval, 205 msec).

Heart failure is usually a late manifestation and occurs in less than 10 percent of cases.[6, 8] Electrocardiographic findings of myocardial infarction with normal coronary arteries have been described and are believed to be due to an area of focal necrosis ("pseudoinfarction").[23] Radionuclide ventriculograms have shown depressed ejection fractions in many patients, along with regional wall motion abnormalities, with the apical region being most affected.[24–26] Mitral valve prolapse with an audible midsystolic click has been reported and occurs in approximately one third of patients.[12, 25, 26]

Treatment consists of specific therapy for arrhythmias and congestive heart failure. Advanced heart block can progress to fatal Stokes-Adams attacks unless a pacemaker is inserted.[20] Mitral valve prolapse requires endocarditis prophylaxis.

Friedreich's Ataxia

Friedreich's ataxia is a rare autosomal recessive disease and is one of the progressive hereditary spinocerebellar degenerative disorders. Abnormalities of the cardiac system have been noted since the first description of the disease.[27] The incidence in white populations is approximately 2/100,000. The biochemical defects underlying this disorder have not been identified. However, genetic linkage studies have mapped the gene responsible to chromosome 9.[28]

Friedreich's ataxia is caused by degeneration of the spinocerebellar tracts, the dorsal columns, and the corticospinal tracts. Signs usually begin around puberty and are characterized by ataxia of the trunk and limbs, loss of limb proprioception, pes cavus, hammer toe, extensor plantar responses, and loss of deep tendon reflexes.[29] Kyphoscoliosis develops within a few years of onset and, coupled with weakness of the respiratory muscles, often leads to pulmonary insufficiency and infections. Cardiac involvement has been found in 50 to 90 percent of patients,[30, 31] and with follow-up, the incidence has reached 100 percent.[32] There is no relationship between severity of neurologic disease and cardiac involvement.[30] Many patients succumb to congestive heart failure (CHF) or arrhythmias in middle age, but some patients have a normal life span.[30, 31, 33]

The cardiac histologic changes consistently include diffuse interstitial fibrosis, myocyte hypertrophy, and necrosis.[30, 34, 35] Intimal hyperplasia of intramural coronary arteries has been reported,[36] but no relationship has been shown to account for either regional or global abnormalities in cardiac function as measured by echocardiogram or ECG.[30, 37] Infiltration of the conduction system is believed to be the cause of arrhythmias.

The ECG is abnormal in almost all patients. Sinus tachycardia, a short PR without delta waves, right-axis deviation, left ventricular (LV) hypertrophy, and inferolateral Q waves were noted in a prospective study of 75 patients by Child and colleagues.[30] Abnormally tall R waves were seen in V_1 in 44 percent, and nonspecific ST-T wave changes were noted in 75 percent of patients. Only 8 percent of patients had normal ECGs.[30] Left-axis deviation and repolarization abnormalities have been correlated with concentric LV hypertrophy.[34] Abnormalities on the surface ECG have no correlation with the regional wall motion abnormalities on the ECG. Atrial fibrillation or flutter, supraventricular tachycardia, premature ventricular beats, and ventricular tachycardia have been reported.[38, 39] Atrial dysrhythmias are a marker of ventricular dysfunction and in one study were found in 50 percent of patients before death.[33, 34]

The most common echocardiographic finding in Friedreich's ataxia is concentric LV hypertrophy.[30, 31, 34, 35, 40] Previous reports had noted similarities between the echocardiographic findings of Friedreich's ataxia and those of hypertrophic obstructive cardiomyopathy, leading some to propose that hypertrophic obstructive cardiomyopathy is a characteristic finding in Friedreich's ataxia.[41] However, it has been shown that asymmetric septal hypertrophy occurs much less frequently.[34, 40, 42, 43] The incidence of concentric LV hypertrophy has ranged from 11 percent[30] to 68 percent,[34] and asymmetric septal hypertrophy from 4 percent[17] to 9 percent.[30] Septal myocyte disarray, the histologic marker of genetic hypertrophic cardiomyopathy, has not been consistently found in patients with septal hypertrophy and Friedreich's ataxia.[44, 45] Systolic and diastolic function is usually normal. A less common echocardiographic abnormality seen in Friedreich's ataxia is global hypokinesis, with either normal or increased LV internal dimensions. These patients usually have signs and symptoms of CHF and experience atrial fibrillation or flutter and/or supraventricular tachycardia. Patients with dilated cardiomyopathy usually experience a progressive downhill course in cardiac function, often dying of CHF, arrhythmias, or pulmonary infections.[34] It has been proposed that dilated cardiomyopathy is the end-stage progression of concentric LV hypertrophy.[42] This view has been challenged because of findings at autopsies of minimally dilated LVs with global hypofunction and normal wall thickness in some patients without ventricular hypertrophy on previous echocardiograms.[30] No patients with concentric LV hypertrophy were shown to progress to dilated cardiomyopathy.[34] Some investigators believe that the dilated cardiomyopathy is a fundamentally different type of cardiac involvement that has been designated as "dystrophic."[30] Treatment is nonspecific and consists of treatment of CHF and atrial and ventricular arrhythmias when they occur.

It is not clear why a nonmyopathic disorder with a homogeneous phenotype affects the myocardium in two separate ways. The localization of the gene to chromosome 9 and the identification of the gene and its products should lead to a better understanding of precise pathophysiologic mechanisms.

Duchenne's Muscular Dystrophy

The French neurologist Duchenne first described this form of muscular dystrophy in 1861 as "hypertrophic paraplegia of infancy." Since this original description, much has been learned about the clinical manifestations, biochemical deficiencies, and pathology of this condition. DMD is an X-linked recessive disorder that almost exclusively affects males; females serve as carriers of the genetic abnormality. The incidence is estimated at 20/100,000 male births. The genetic defect is located on the short arm of the X chromosome at the Xp21 site and encodes for the protein dystrophin. The function of dystrophin is at present unclear, but amino acid sequence analysis predicts a rod-shaped protein with structural similarities to the cytoskeletal protein spectrin.[46, 47] Dystrophin is absent from the sarcolemmic membranes of skeletal and cardiac muscle in affected individuals. Quantitative assays for dystrophin and skeletal muscle biopsies can identify female carriers of the genetic defect; this permits more accurate genetic counseling and may assist in prenatal diagnosis of DMD.

The clinical manifestations usually become apparent at 2 to 5 years of age as the young boy begins to walk and becomes active. Typically, the boy appears clumsy in his gait, with frequent falls. He lags behind when playing with his peers. By 5 years of age, obvious motor weakness is evident. The boy must use his hands to climb up himself on getting up from the floor, known as Gowers' maneuver. Pseudohypertrophy, which is replacement of normal muscle by fat and connective tissue, occurs in the gastrocnemius muscle, giving the classic appearance of disproportionally enlarged calves. By the age of 7 to 8 years, contractures of the Achilles tendon and the iliotibial bands result in toe walking and lordotic posture, respectively. The muscle weakness progresses, with a predilection for the neck and proximal limb muscles, resulting in a floppy, unsupported head. As the contractures progress, the boy becomes confined to a wheelchair with severe scoliosis (Fig. 107–3). Respiratory function becomes compromised owing to muscle weakness and chest cage deformities. The average life span is 20 years of age, with cardiac failure (40 percent), respiratory insufficiency (38 percent), and pulmonary infections (8 percent) being the major causes of death.[48]

The cardiac manifestations of DMD include dysrhythmias, abnormal ECGs, and cardiomyopathies of both the dilated (70 percent) and the hypertrophic (26 percent)

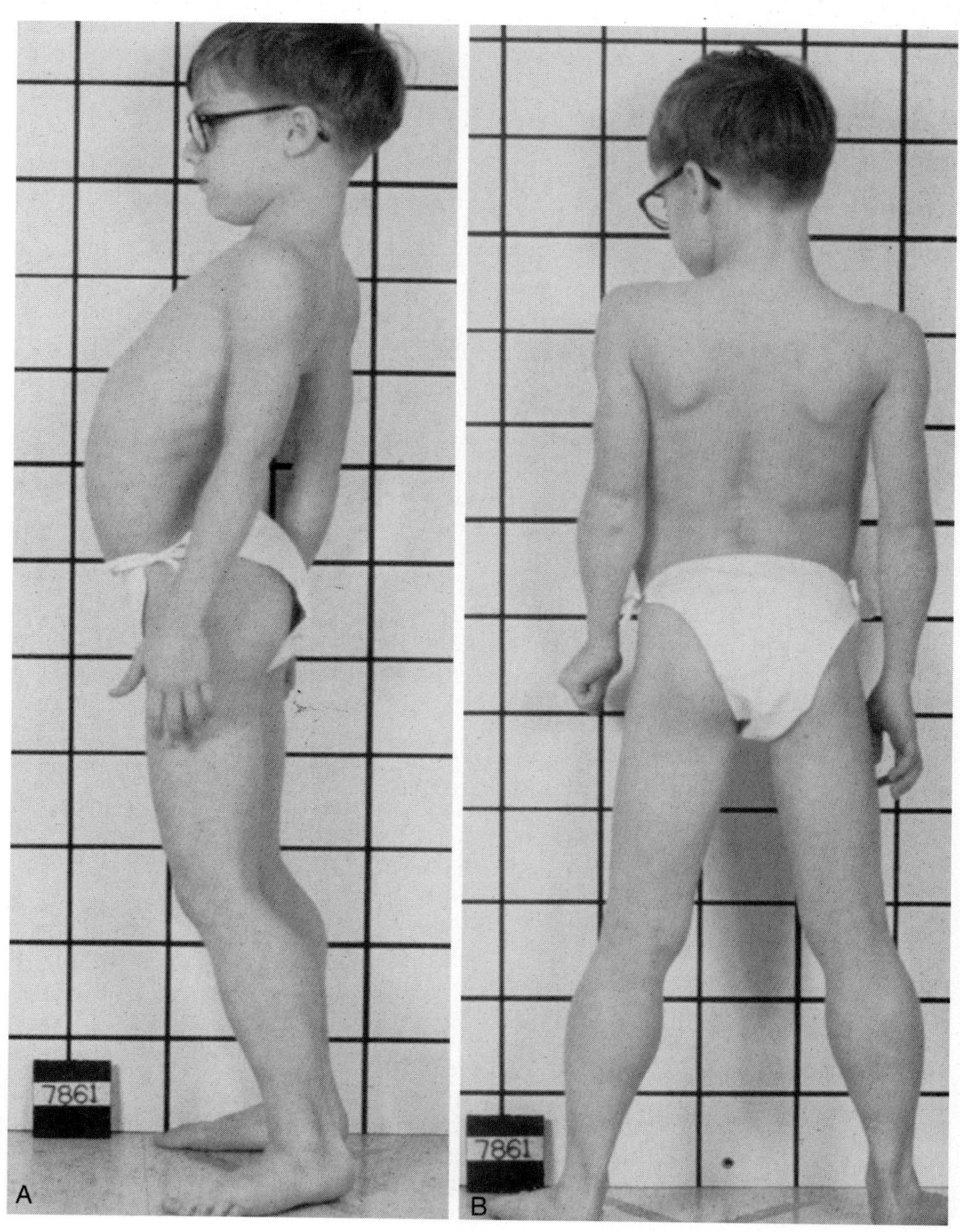

FIGURE 107–3 A and **B,** A 7-year-old boy with Duchenne's muscular dystrophy, demonstrating severe lordosis and pseudohypertrophy of the calves. (**A** and **B,** Courtesy of Ian Butler, M.D.)

TABLE 107–2 Recommendations for Screening of Cardiac Diseases in Duchenne's Muscular Dystrophy

Clinical examination and ECG every 3 mo
Holter monitor, echocardiography, chest and spinal radiograph every 6 mo
Once cardiac involvement is detected, the above examinations should be performed every 3 mo to monitor the patient closely

Abbreviation: ECG, electrocardiogram.

type.[49] The incidence of cardiac involvement is strikingly high, with ECG changes occurring in 60 percent of patients younger than 10 years and detectable cardiomyopathy by echocardiography in virtually every affected individual older than 18 years.[49] Most patients with cardiomyopathies do not demonstrate clinical symptoms of heart failure. The reason for clinically silent heart disease is that the evolution of the cardiomyopathy is slow, allowing the development of more complete compensatory mechanisms. Furthermore, there is a reduced cardiac demand in these relatively immobile patients.[49] Guidelines for screening of cardiac diseases in DMD have been developed[50] (Table 107–2).

The dysrhythmias associated with DMD are inappropriate sinus tachycardia, atrial flutter, premature atrial and ventricular beats, complete heart block, and, rarely, a shifting pacemaker from the sinoatrial to the AV node.[51–55] Ventricular dysrhythmias are uncommon. Degeneration of conduction fibers, along with a noninflammatory occlusive arteriopathy of the sinoatrial and AV nodes, has been reported and may lead to reentry or increased automaticity–induced arrhythmias.[56–58] In addition, dystrophin is absent from the membrane surface of Purkinje cell fibers, and this absence may contribute to conduction abnormalities.[59]

The electrocardiographic abnormalities seen in DMD can be present as early as 2 years of age and are eventually present in more than 95 percent of patients (Fig. 107–4; Table 107–3). These electrocardiographic abnormalities can be explained by the marked focal interstitial and replacement fibrosis that specifically involves the posterobasal wall of the left ventricle and the posterior papillary muscle.[60] The pathologic Q waves are typically deep and narrow (rarely $>$ 0.04 second) and are distinguishable from the Q waves of myocardial infarction, which are usually shallow and broad.[61, 62] Unique patterns of electrocardiographic abnormalities occur frequently in families. Type 1 consists of tall R waves in V_1 and deep Q waves in V_4 and V_6. Type 2 consists of rSR and deep Q waves in V_5 through V_6. This may represent subtle variations in pathology that result from different familial genetic mutations.[61, 63]

LV systolic function deteriorates with age when patients are studied by use of systolic time intervals.[64, 65] Evidence of ventricular failure begins at 10 years of age, worsens precipitously between 14 and 16 years of age, and is uniformly present after 18 years of age.[66, 67] A significant reduction in fractional shortening of the left ventricle is associated with a poor prognosis for survival more than 2 years.[68] Two-dimensional echocardiography is not reliable for evaluating LV systolic function.[69, 70] Thoracic skeletal deformities are common and may alter normal ventricular geometry, making interpretation of echocardiographic measurements difficult. However, echocardiography has dem-

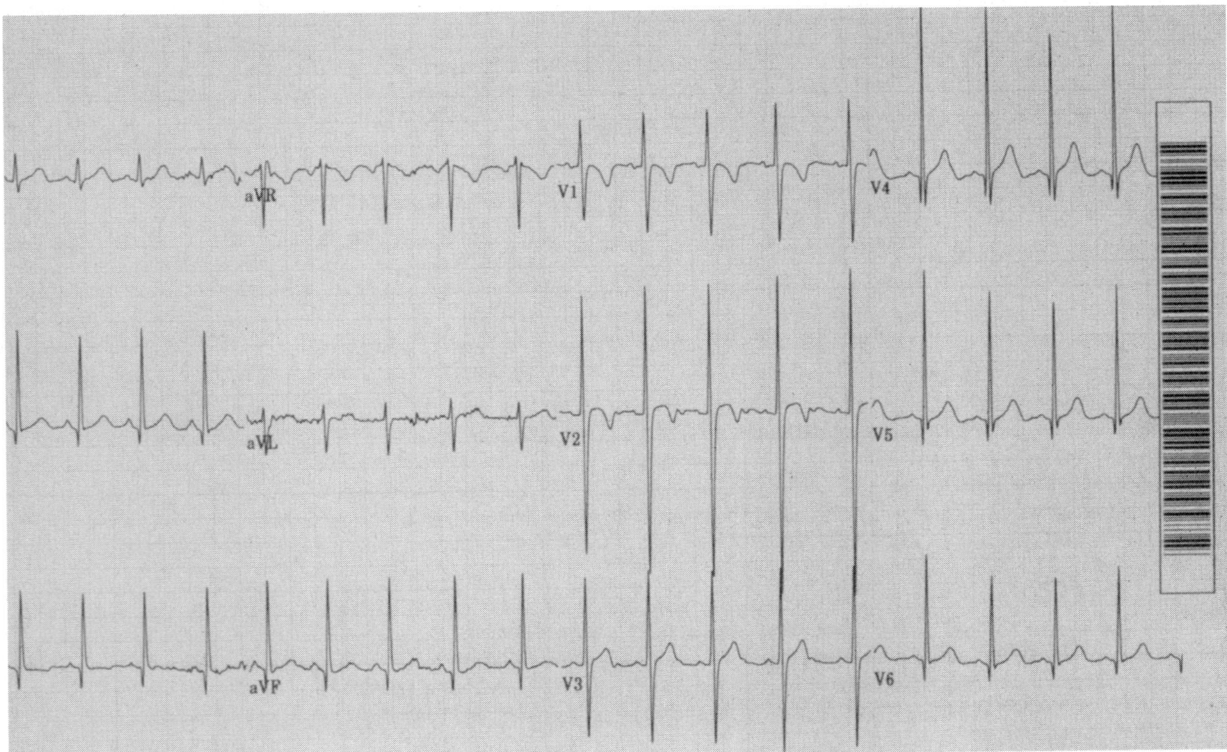

FIGURE 107–4 Electrocardiogram from a 6-year-old boy with Duchenne's muscular dystrophy demonstrates sinus tachycardia, rightward axis, tall R waves in V_1 and V_2, and deep narrow Q waves in the lateral and inferior leads.

TABLE 107–3 Common ECG Abnormalities in Duchenne's Muscular Dystrophy

Tall R wave with high R/S ratio in V_1	64%
Deep narrow Q wave > 4 mm in I, aVL, V_5, V_6	44%
Sinus tachycardia	32%
Right-axis deviation	16%
Short PR interval	6%

Abbreviation: ECG, electrocardiographic.

onstrated an increased incidence of mitral valve prolapse (10 percent), which has been confirmed in autopsy studies.[71, 72] Thallium 201 perfusion studies have revealed decreased blood flow to the posterobasal free wall of the left ventricle, which corresponds to the major pathologic area of fibrosis.[73] Positron emission tomography has shown increased ^{18}F-2, fluorodeoxyglucose, and decreased $^{13}NH_3$ in the posterobasal LV free wall, implying altered metabolic activity in this region.[73] Whether the lack of dystrophin from the myocardial plasma membrane leads to altered transport or metabolic activity is uncertain.

The histopathologic changes studied in DMD are most prominent in the posterobasal LV free wall and the posterior papillary muscle (Fig. 107–5). Light microscopy shows striking replacement of myocardial fibers and connective tissue and extensive interstitial fibrosis[51] (Fig. 107–6). Fibrosis and myofibrillar lysis occurring in the posterior papillary muscle account for the high occurrence of mitral valve prolapse.[72] Degeneration of conducting fibers is seen in the sinoatrial node and the bundle of His. A noninflammatory occlusive arteriopathy affects small arteries (< 1-mm diameter), including nodal arteries, while peculiarly sparing larger vessels.[56] Electron microscopy of the right ventricle in asymptomatic patients shows proliferation of the mitochondria and a striking increase in residual bodies near the perinuclear region. This suggests that a state of extreme metabolic exhaustion exists in the myocardium.[74] Immunoelectron microscopy has localized dystrophin to the cytoplasmic face of the plasma membrane of muscle fibers, reinforcing the hypothesis that DMD is probably the result of plasma membrane instability.[75] Elevated levels of calcium are detected in the muscle cell from the mdx mouse before signs of cell necrosis appear, suggesting that dystrophin plays a role in regulating calcium transport.[76]

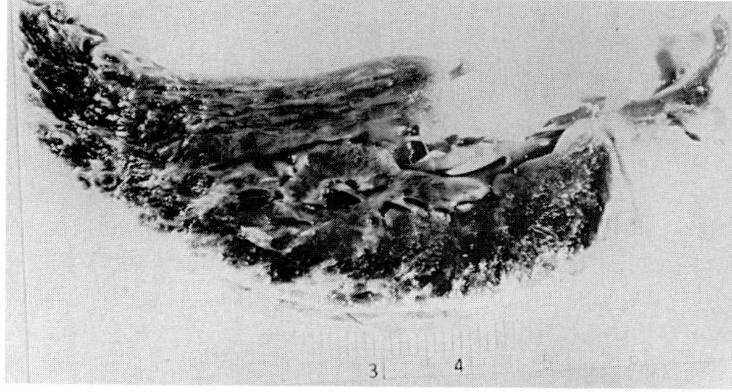

FIGURE 107–5 Heart from a patient with Duchenne's muscular dystrophy. The posterobasal free wall of the left ventricle and the posterior papillary muscle demonstrate focal areas of fibrosis (pale areas). (Courtesy of L. Maximilian Buja, M.D.)

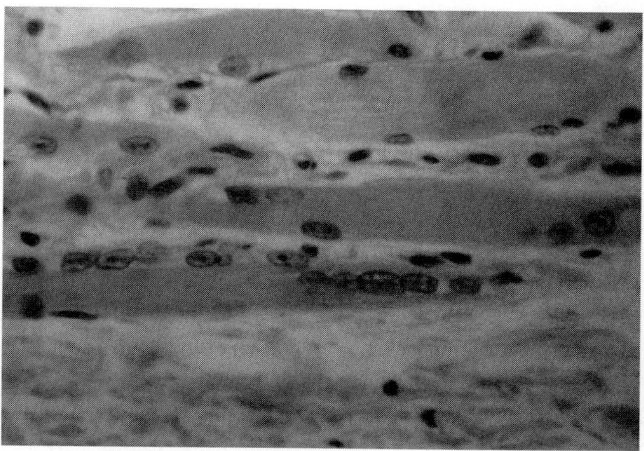

FIGURE 107–6 Muscle biopsy from a patient with Duchenne's muscular dystrophy shows focal areas of interstitial fibrosis and fatty infiltration. (Courtesy of Ian Butler, M.D.)

BECKER'S MUSCULAR DYSTROPHY

Becker's muscular dystrophy (BMD) is an X-linked recessive disorder with an incidence of 4/100,000 male births. This genetic defect involves the short arm of the X chromosome close to that of Duchenne's muscular dystrophy and results in the production of abnormal dystrophin. Unlike DMD, in which muscle biopsies show a complete deficiency of dystrophin, muscle from BMD reveals that dystrophin is present but is abnormal in molecular weight or structure.[47] Quantitative assays for dystrophin can differentiate BMD from DMD.

The musculoskeletal manifestations of BMD tend to be mild, with a late onset and a slow rate of progression. Skeletal muscle weakness becomes apparent at an average age of 11 years, with most patients being able to walk until the age of 30 years.[77–79] Death usually occurs in the fifth decade, often from cardiac causes. Skeletal muscle involvement is similar to that in DMD and includes pseudohypertrophy of the calves, lordosis, and proximal limb-girdle muscle weakness and atrophy.

The cardiac manifestation of BMD (i.e., dilated cardiomyopathy) occurs early and has a rapidly progressive course (Table 107–4). Patients usually maintain a normal level of activity and therefore often manifest symptoms of cardiac failure. Not uncommonly, a young subject pre-

TABLE 107–4 Common ECG Abnormalities in Becker's Muscular Dystrophy

Tall R wave in V_1, V_2
Shallow Q wave in 2, 3, aVF and I, aVL, V_5, V_6
Fascicular blocks
Complete heart blocks

Abbreviation: ECG, electrocardiographic.

sents with symptoms of heart failure, only later to be diagnosed with BMD. The heart is usually globally involved, with dilatation and thinning of all four chambers.[80] Because there is not a severe deformity of the chest cage, echocardiography is useful in demonstrating chamber enlargement.[81] Thallium 201 scanning reveals multiple patchy areas of decreased myocardial uptake in the left ventricle and septum.[80, 82] These regions probably correspond to the islands of proliferating connective tissue and fatty infiltration seen on histopathologic sections of myocardium.

Because the cardiomyopathy is dissociated from the musculoskeletal manifestations, aggressive treatment of heart failure is warranted in these young, otherwise healthy individuals.[81, 83] Standard therapy for CHF is effective, and close follow-up is indicated to monitor the progression of cardiomyopathy. Heart transplantation in young patients with BMD with minimal skeletal muscle involvement has been reported.[84, 85] Studies of these transplanted hearts to determine whether they are affected by a dystrophic process will be informative.

Several cases of BMD have been reported that showed mild or subclinical skeletal muscle involvement with an overt dilated cardiomyopathy.[85a] A group of 28 patients with BMD who had a subclinical or benign myopathy had a thorough cardiologic assessment. Each patient underwent electrocardiography and echocardiographic examinations. Molecular analyses of the dystrophin gene and protein were performed. An unexpectedly high incidence of myocardial involvement was observed among patients affected with subclinical (72 percent) or benign (60 percent) BMD. The cardiac involvement appeared to develop early from the right ventricle. Increases in LV end-diastolic volume and reduction in the ejection fraction appeared to be age related. Severe LV dilation with reduced ejection fraction complicated by life-threatening arrhythmias was present in some of these patients. Contrary to previous reports, which indicated the involvement of 5′ J-end mutations in cardiomyopathies as a result of dystrophin gene alterations, this study showed that despite the apparent concentration of deletions in two regions (5′-end and exons 47 through 49), no general conclusions could be drawn regarding the involvement of specific gene mutations in the development of cardiomyopathy. In these patients, cardiomyopathy was the main clinical feature and complication in patients with subclinical or mild BMD. The cardiac manifestation was characterized by early right ventricular involvement and was later associated with LV impairment. Thus, in mild BMD, myocardial damage may develop, and important cardiomyopathy may be present.

KEARNS-SAYRE SYNDROME

Kearns-Sayre syndrome is one of the mitochondrial myopathies, initially described as a triad consisting of progressive external ophthalmoplegia, pigmentary degeneration of the retina, and heart block.[86] This syndrome is believed to be due to deletions of the mitochondrial DNA.[87] The disease usually presents in late childhood or adolescence, but it has been reported from the age of 7 months to the age of 65 years.[88] Other features include ptosis, torticollis, sensory neural deafness, ataxia, limb weakness, sexual immaturity, short stature, mental retardation, and increased cerebrospinal fluid protein concentration (Fig. 107–7A).

Pathologically, skeletal muscle cells show "ragged red fibers" on Gomori trichrome stain and represent peripheral and intermyofibrillary accumulation of abnormal mitochondria (Fig. 107–7B). On electron microscopy, proliferation of abnormal mitochondria has been noted in cardiac tissue.[89] Extensive changes have been found in the distal portions of the His bundle and proximal bundle branches and are believed to be the reason for the high incidence of AV block.[90] Degenerative myocardial changes have also been noted,[91] as well as no abnormalities.[92] Endomyocardial biopsies have shown mitochondrial abnormalities of myocytes, but the incidence of cardiac muscle disease is less than that of muscle conduction system disease.[89, 93–96]

High-grade heart block is the major manifestation of cardiac involvement in the Kearns-Sayre syndrome. The conduction disturbance is progressive.[90, 92] Patients may present with minimal conduction abnormalities that may progress to bifascicular, trifascicular, and complete AV block (Fig. 107–8A). The course of progression is variable, and progressive heart block from left anterior fascicular block to symptomatic complete heart block over a 7-year period has been documented.[96] His bundle readings in patients who have progressive infranodal block can identify the need for permanent pacemaker insertion. Prophylactic pacemaker insertion has been recommended because sudden death, believed secondary to complete heart block, is not uncommon (Fig. 107–8B).[91] Enhancement of AV nodal conduction has also been noted.[90, 92] Several cases of dilated cardiomyopathy and intractable heart failure have been reported, and myocardial biopsy specimens have shown histologic changes similar to those noted in skeletal muscle.[91, 93, 97] It has been postulated that with a greater awareness of AV conduction disturbances in Kearns-Sayre syndrome and earlier use of demand pacemakers, prolongation of survival occurs, and therefore the cardiomyopathy is given time to develop.[93]

EMERY-DREIFUSS SYNDROME

This rare X-linked recessive muscular dystrophy was originally described by Dreifuss and Hope in 1961 but was more fully characterized, including a description of the cardiac symptoms, by Emery and Dreifuss in 1966.[98] The classic triad described is (1) early contractures of the elbows, posterior cervical muscles, and Achilles tendons; (2) slowly progressive muscle wasting and weakness in a humeroperoneal distribution; and (3) cardiomyopathy and cardiac conduction abnormalities.[99] The genetic defect has been localized by DNA linkage analysis to the Xq27 region of the X chromosome. The identity of the specific gene and protein defect is not known. There is considerable interfamilial variation in Emery-Dreifuss muscular dystrophy (EDMD), with several families fitting an autosomal dominant pattern of inheritance.[99] Although the musculoskeletal manifestations of EDMD are largely benign, with most subjects remaining functionally active to their fifth or sixth decade, the cardiac abnormalities occur early, tend to progress rapidly, and cause significant mortality and even sudden death at young ages.[100]

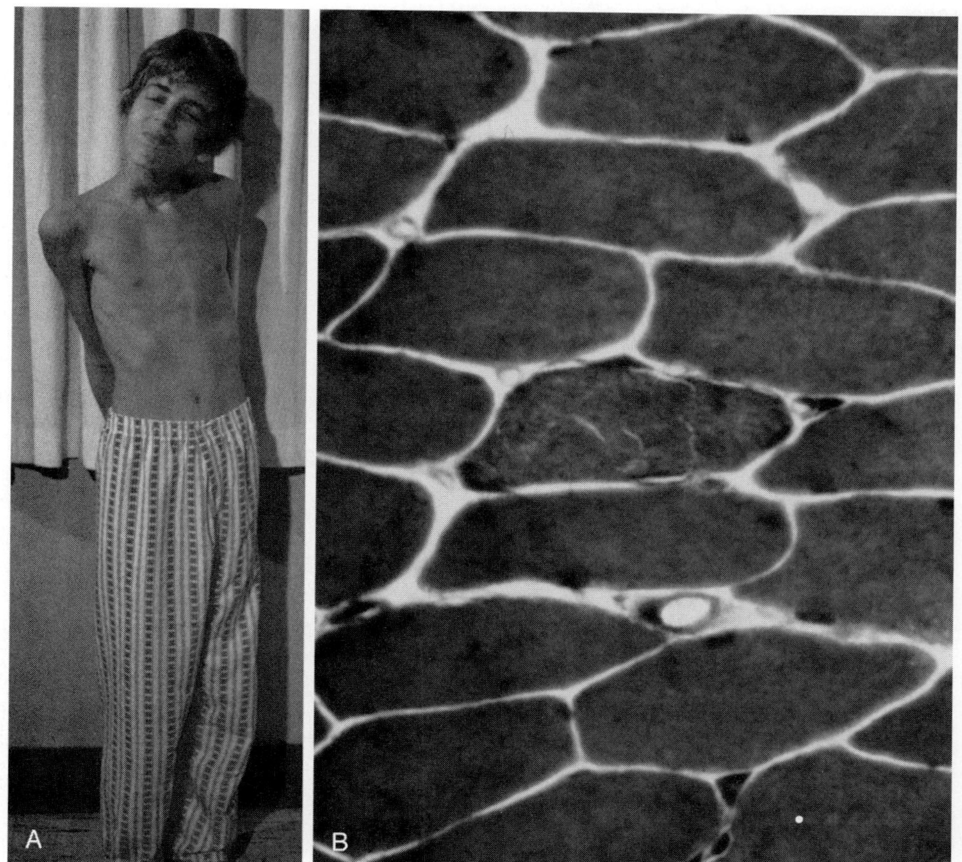

FIGURE 107–7 A, A 13-year-old boy with Kearns-Sayre syndrome. Note the ptosis, torticollis, and mild scoliosis. **B,** Skeletal muscle biopsy from the same patient shows the characteristic "ragged red fibers." (**A** and **B,** Courtesy of Ian Butler, M.D.)

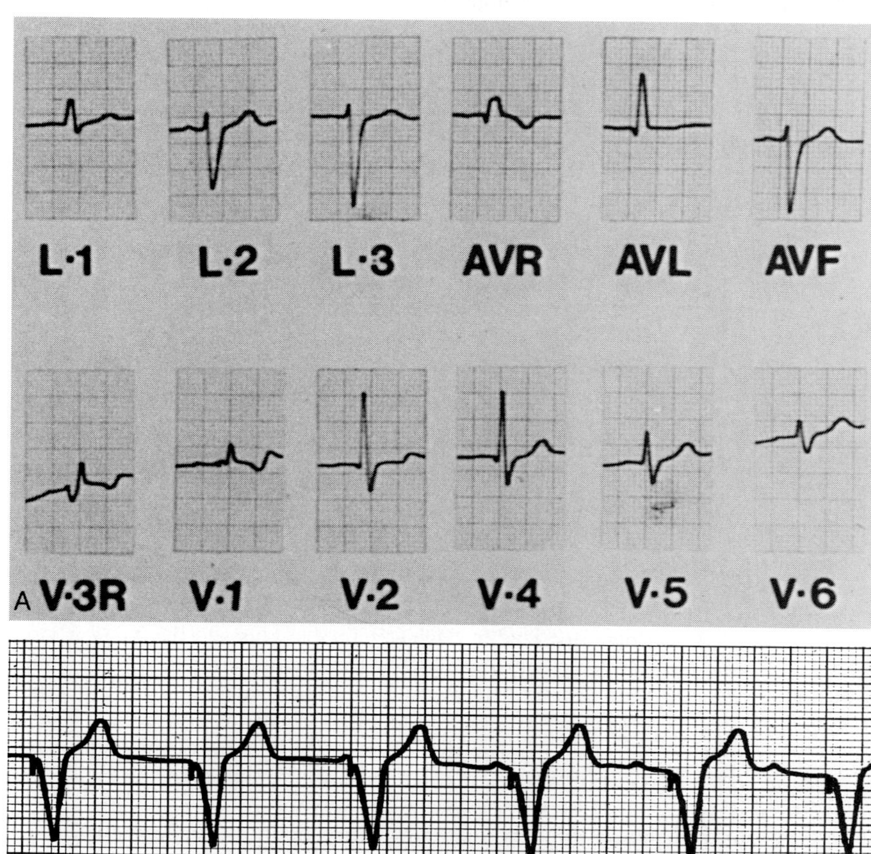

FIGURE 107–8 A, Electrocardiogram from a 16-year-old boy with Kearns-Sayre syndrome. The characteristic findings noted are right bundle branch block, left-axis deviation, and left anterior fascicular block. **B,** One year later, the same patient developed third-degree heart block, and a ventricular pacemaker was inserted. (**A** and **B,** From Butler IJ, Gudoth N: Kearns-Sayre syndrome: a review of a multisystem disorder of children and young adults. Arch Intern Med 136:1290, 1976. Copyright 1976, American Medical Association.)

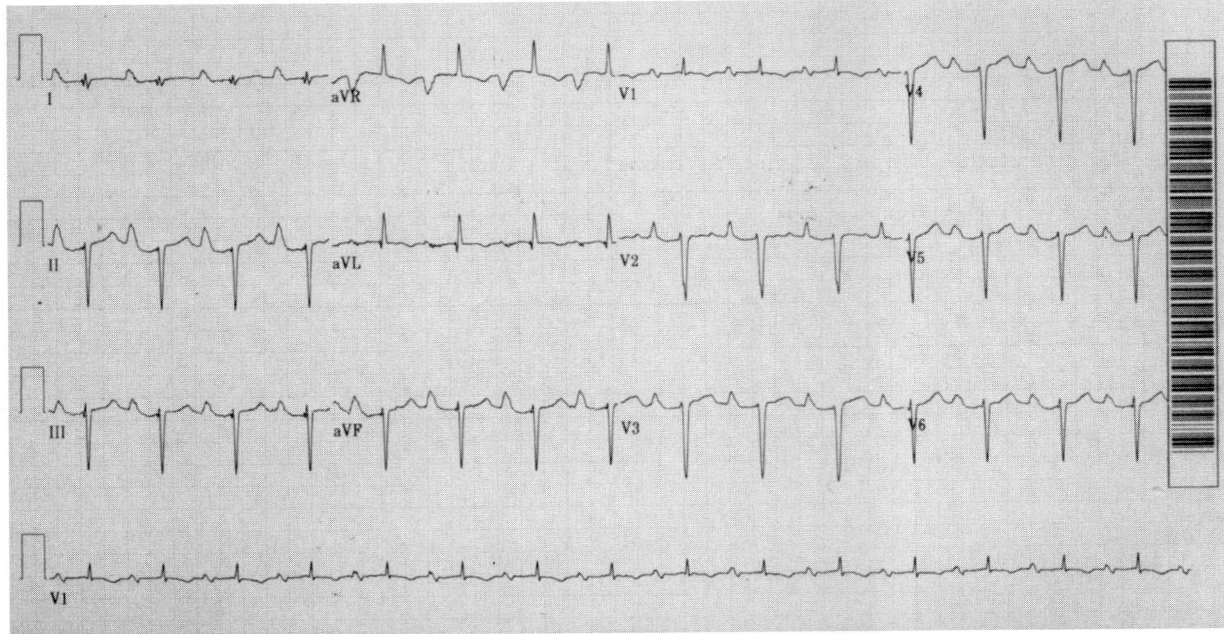

FIGURE 107–9 Electrocardiogram from a 15-year-old boy with Emery-Dreifuss muscular dystrophy demonstrates first-degree atrioventricular block, biatrial abnormality, and loss of R wave amplitude across the entire precordium. A 24-hour Holter monitor showed multiple episodes of nonsustained ventricular tachycardia.

Conduction abnormalities and dilated cardiomyopathy with LV failure are the two types of cardiac disorders that occur in EDMD. First-degree AV block typically presents in the second decade of life (Fig. 107–9).[101] Progression to complete heart block and atrial standstill can result in symptomatic junctional or ventricular escape bradycardias. Permanent atrial paralysis, normally a rare cardiac finding, is frequently seen in EDMD.[102, 103] Ventricular tachyarrhythmias are reported in young patients and may be responsible for the high incidence of sudden death in EDMD.[104] Because arrhythmias tend to be more severe during periods of sleep, 24-hour Holter monitoring is indicated at least annually.[101, 105, 106] Transvenous pacemakers have been prophylactically placed in patients with asymptomatic bradycardia in an attempt to prevent fatal bradyarrhythmias.[104, 107, 108] Prospective, randomized clinical trials studying the effect of pacemakers on survival are needed to clarify the role of such devices in these patients. Prophylactic use of antiarrhythmic agents or automatic implantable cardiac defibrillators may decrease the incidence of sudden death.

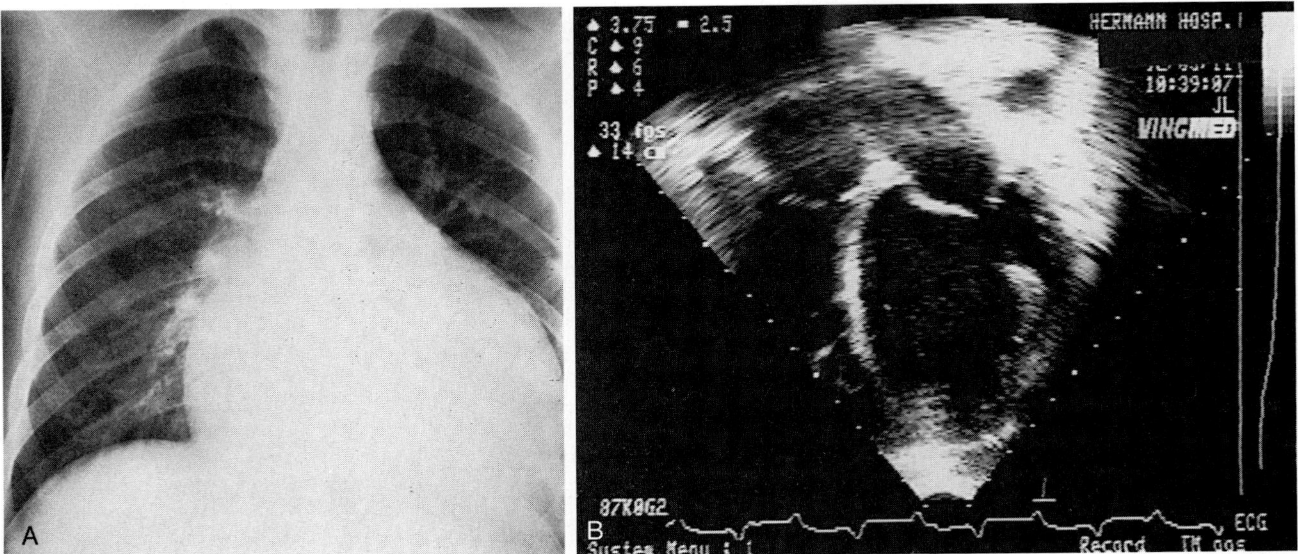

FIGURE 107–10 A, A 17-year-old boy with Emery-Dreifuss muscular dystrophy. Note marked cardiomegaly on posteroanterior chest radiograph. **B,** A two-dimensional echocardiogram of the same patient reveals four-chamber dilatation and a prominent posterior papillary muscle. Doppler studies revealed regurgitation of the mitral and tricuspid valves.

Female carriers appear to develop a late-onset mild conduction disturbance, including first-degree AV block, wandering pacemaker, and intermittent sinus bradycardia.[101]

A rapidly progressive dilated cardiomyopathy has been described, with pronounced mitral and tricuspid regurgitation (Fig. 107–10).[109] Histopathology shows focal myocardial fibrosis and variation in myofiber size.[110, 111] Standard treatment with afterload reduction and diuretics is effective. Cardiac transplantation has been successfully performed in patients with severe cardiomyopathy.[112]

Facioscapulohumeral Muscular Dystrophy

Facioscapulohumeral muscular dystrophy, also known as Landouzy-Dejerine disease, is an autosomal dominant disorder with an incidence of 6 cases/million. Musculoskeletal manifestations appear between 6 and 20 years of age and are slowly progressive. Weakness and atrophy of the proximal shoulder and facial muscles are common. Winging of the scapulae and loose, protruding lips are the more noticeable features that often bring the patient to seek medical attention (Fig. 107–11). Pseudohypertrophy is not common. As the disease progresses, disabling weakness of the lower limbs occurs in 10 to 20 percent of patients.[113]

The most common cardiac finding is left atrial, right atrial, or biatrial P-wave electrocardiographic abnormality in 60 percent of patients. Electrophysiologic studies have demonstrated AV nodal and intranodal conduction delays in 27 percent of patients and easily inducible atrial flutter and fibrillation in most patients.[114, 115] Echocardiographic and Holter monitor studies have not demonstrated cardiac abnormalities. Death from cardiac disease is not common.

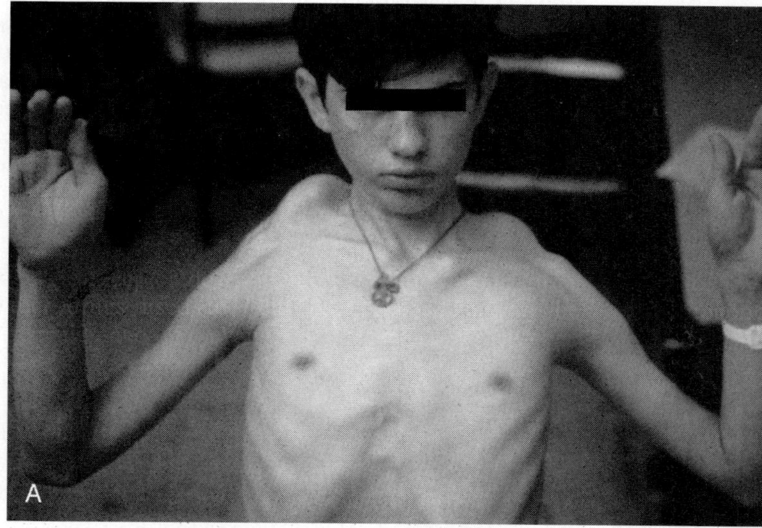

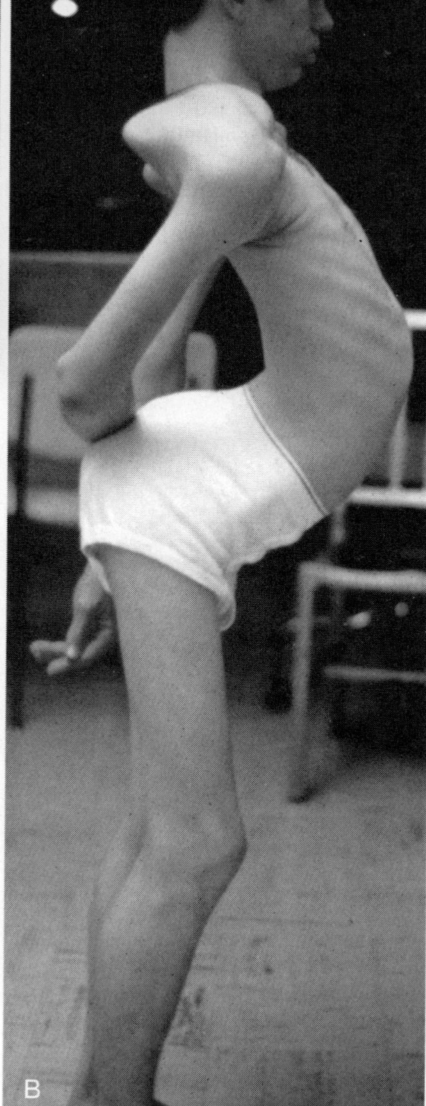

FIGURE 107–11 A and **B,** A 13-year-old boy with facioscapulohumeral muscular dystrophy, showing severe atrophy of proximal shoulder muscles, protruding lips, winging of the scapulae, and deforming lordosis.

MYOTUBULAR (CENTRONUCLEAR) MYOPATHY

Centronuclear myopathy is the most heterogeneous of the congenital myopathies. The clinical picture ranges from severe respiratory difficulty at birth and generalized hypotonia to a late-onset, slowly progressive course.[116] Pathologically, it is characterized by a large portion of hypotrophic muscle fibers, with central (as opposed to peripheral) nuclei and other changes resembling fetal myotubes.[117] One review has shown two types of inheritance, X-linked recessive and autosomal dominant. The former is characterized by a homogeneous clinical picture of respiratory insufficiency and death in the first year, and the latter, by a more benign and prolonged course. The original description of the disease noted myocardial fibrosis and chamber dilation.[117] Verhiest and colleagues[118] described two cases with clinical features similar to those of a dilated cardiomyopathy, and Bethlem and coworkers[119] reported on a 16-year-old girl with CHF, LV enlargement, and hypokinesis on ventriculography. How the myopathy is related to the cardiac disease is not known.

NEMALINE MYOPATHY

Nemaline myopathy is a rare disease characterized by diffuse muscle weakness and hypotonia. It is usually noted at birth or in early infancy. The most severely affected muscles are those of the limb girdle and trunk. Autosomal dominant inheritance with reduced penetrance is believed to be the mode of transmission.[120] Biopsy of skeletal muscles shows small rodlike particles called *nemaline bodies* or *rods* (Fig. 107–12A and B).[121] Nemaline rods have also been found in cardiac muscle and the conduction system, leading investigators to believe that this infiltration may be the cause of arrhythmias and cardiac dysfunction in this disease.[122, 123]

There have been seven reported cases[121, 124–126] of cardiac involvement in patients with nemaline myopathy as adults and at least one reported case in a child.[128] The typical clinical course is the development of a dilated cardiomyopathy and subsequent cardiac failure. Meier and coworkers[122, 123] described a patient with a fatal cardiomyopathy who exhibited nemaline rods in skeletal and cardiac muscle but had no clinical signs of peripheral muscle weakness. Time from onset of symptoms to death was approximately 13 months. Rosenson and associates[126] reported on a 20-year-old man with clinical and histologic proof of skeletal muscle involvement who had a similar clinical course and died 2 years after symptoms of CHF developed. Unfortunately, an autopsy to verify cardiac nemaline rods was not performed. Ishibashi-Veda and coworkers[127] reported the first case of cardiac failure in early infancy, and nemaline rods were verified in both skeletal and cardiac muscle.

One report studied echocardiograms in patients with known nemaline myopathy.[128] All patients had normal wall motion and thickness. The only abnormalities noted were mitral valve prolapse in one patient and a ventricular septal defect in another. Cardiac function on subsequent echos has yet to be reported.

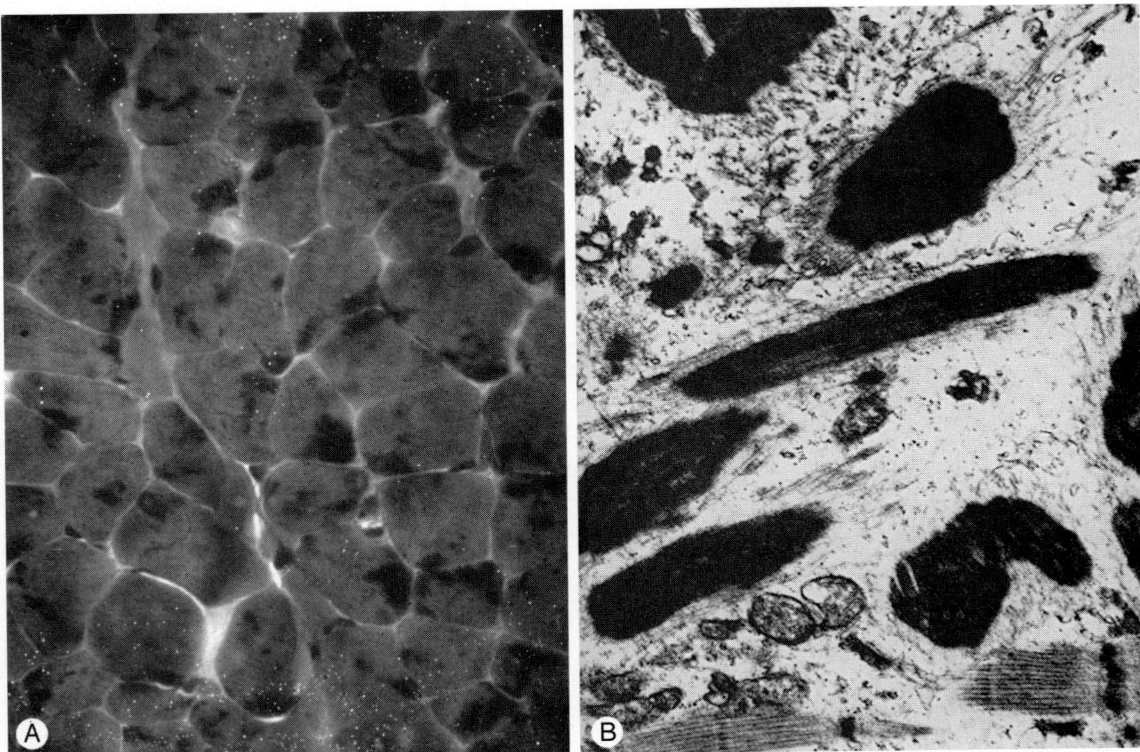

FIGURE 107–12 A, Skeletal muscle biopsy shows numerous nemaline bodies. **B,** Electron micrograph shows nemaline bodies with normal skeletal muscle tissue at the bottom.

Other Combined Skeletal Myopathies and Cardiomyopathies

An apparently new cardioskeletal myopathy has been reported in three unrelated families.[130] Five infants were affected by rapidly progressive generalized muscle weakness, with onset shortly after birth, and dilated cardiomyopathy. All had generalized tremor (clonus) starting in the first week of life. The disease was lethal in all cases between 4 and 6 months. Muscle biopsy, performed in four of the five patients, showed a light microscopic pattern of small type I and normal-sized type II fibers. By electron microscopy, small fibers were affected by myofibrillar disruption and swelling of organelles. Findings in blood and urine suggested a disturbance in energy metabolism, but an extensive search for respiratory chain disorders of mitochondrial fatty acid oxidation in frozen muscle and cultured fibroblasts was negative. The findings support a new progressive autosomal recessive infantile cardioskeletal myopathy in which type I muscle fibers are preferentially affected.

Desmin Myopathy

Desmin myopathy involving cardiac, skeletal, and vascular smooth muscle is a rare idiopathic disorder characterized by abnormal aggregates of desmin-type intermediate filaments; this disorder affects cardiac and skeletal muscle and rarely the intestinal smooth muscle.[131] A 42-year-old woman with atrial fibrillation and progressive restrictive cardiomyopathy has been reported.[131] LV biopsy, cardiac explant, and subsequent autopsy study of skeletal muscle revealed cytoplasmic granulofilamentous inclusions that were continuous with Z lines and were immunoreactive for desmin filaments at both the light immunohistochemical and the electron microscopic level. In addition, microscopic studies showed the presence of characteristic inclusions within the smooth muscle of intramural coronary blood vessels. This may be the first description of desmin inclusions within vascular smooth muscle and underscores the systemic nature of this rare myopathy.

Familial Dilated Cardiomyopathy With Conduction Defect and Muscular Dystrophy

Inherited cardiomyopathies may arise from mutations in genes that are normally expressed in both heart and skeletal muscle and may be accompanied by skeletal muscle weakness.[132] Phenotypically, patients with familial dilated cardiomyopathy (FDC) show enlargement of all four chambers of the heart and have symptoms of congestive heart failure. Inherited cardiomyopathies may also be accompanied by cardiac conduction system defects that affect the atrioventricular node, resulting in bradycardia. Several different chromosomal regions have been linked with the development of autosomal dominant FDC, but the gene defects in these disorders remain unknown. An autosomal dominant disorder involving dilated cardiomyopathy, cardiac conduction-system disease, and adult-onset limb-girdle muscular dystrophy (FDC, conduction disease, and myopathy) has been recently described.[132] Genetic linkage was used to exclude regions of the genome known to be linked to dilated cardiomyopathy and muscular dystrophy phenotypes and to confirm genetic heterogeneity of these disorders. A genomewide scan identified a region on the long arm of chromosome 6 that is significantly associated with the presence of myopathy, identifying familial dilated cardiomyopathy, conduction disease, and myopathy as a genetically distinct disease. Haplotype analysis refined the interval localizing the genetic defect to a 3-cm interval between D6S1705 and D6S1656. This haplotype analysis excluded a number of striated muscle-expressed genes present in this region, including laminin alpha2, laminin alpha4, triadin, and phospholamban.

References

1. Brook JD, McCurrach ME, Harley GH, et al: The molecular basis of myotonic dystrophy: expansion of a trinucleotide (CTG) repeat at the 3′ end of a transcript encoding a protein kinase family member. Cell 68:799, 1992.
2. Shelbourne P, Davies J, Buxton J, et al: Direct diagnosis of myotonic dystrophy with a disease-specific DNA marker. N Engl J Med 328:471, 1993.
3. Harper PS: Myotonic Dystrophy. 2nd ed. Philadelphia: WB Saunders, 1989.
4. Cannon PJ: The heart and lungs in myotonic dystrophy. Am J Med 32:765, 1962.
5. Kennel AJ, Titus JL, Meredith J: Pathologic findings in the atrioventricular conducting system in myotonic dystrophy. Mayo Clin Proc 49:838, 1974.
6. Nguyen HH, Wolfe JT, Holmes DR, et al: Pathology of the cardiac system in myotonic dystrophy. J Am Coll Cardiol 11:662, 1988.
7. Bullock RT, Davis JL, Haara M: Dystrophia myotonica with heart block: a light and electron microscopic study. Arch Pathol 84:130, 1967.
8. Perloff JK: Cardiac involvement in heredofamilial neuromyopathic diseases. Cardiovasc Clin 4:33, 1972.
9. Ludatscher RM, Kerner H, Amikam S, Gelli B: Myotonia dystrophica with heart involvement: an electron microscopic study of skeletal, cardiac and smooth muscle. J Clin Pathol 31:1057, 1978.
10. Motta J, Guilleminault C, Bilingham M, et al: Cardiac abnormalities in myotonic dystrophy: electrophysiologic and histopathologic studies. Am J Med 67:467, 1979.
11. Griggs RC, Davis RJ, Anderson DC, et al: Cardiac conduction in myotonic dystrophy. Am J Med 59:37, 1975.
12. Gottdiener JS, Hawley RJ, Gay JA, et al: Left ventricular relaxation, mitral valve prolapse and intracardiac conduction in myotonic atrophica: assessment by digitized echocardiography and noninvasive His bundle recording. Am Heart J 104:77, 1982.
13. Olofsson D, Forsberg H, Andersson S, et al: Electrocardiographic findings in myotonic dystrophy. Br Heart J 59:47, 1988.
14. Forsberg H, Olofsson B, Gottdiener JS, et al: 24-hour electrocardiographic study in myotonic dystrophy. Cardiology 75:241, 1988.
15. Hawley RJ, Milner MR, Gottdiener JS, Cohen A: Myotonic heart disease: a clinical follow-up. Neurology 41:259, 1991.
16. Hiromasa S, Ikeda T, Kubota K, et al: A family with myotonic dystrophy associated with diffuse cardiac conduction disturbances as demonstrated by His bundle electrocardiography. Am Heart J 111:85, 1986.
17. Florek RC, Triffon DW, Mann DE, et al: Electrocardiographic abnormalities in patients with myotonic dystrophy. West J Med 153:4, 1990.
18. Payne CA, Greenfield JC: Electrocardiographic abnormalities associated with myotonic dystrophy. Am Heart J 65:436, 1963.
19. Prystowsky EN, Pritchett ELC, Roses AD, et al: The natural history of conduction system disease in myotonic muscular dystrophy as determined by serial electrophysiologic studies. Circulation 60:1360, 1979.

20. Petkovich NJ, Dunn M, Reed W: Myotonia dystrophica with AV dissociation and Stokes-Adams attacks. Am Heart J 68:391, 1964.
21. Grigg LE, Chan W, Mond HG, et al: Ventricular tachycardia and sudden death in myotonic dystrophy: clinical electrophysiologic and pathologic features. Am J Cardiol 6:254, 1985.
22. Milner MR, Hawley RJ, Jachim M, et al: Ventricular late potentials in myotonic dystrophy. Ann Intern Med 115:607, 1991.
23. Perloff JK, Stephenson WG, Roberts MK, et al: Cardiac involvement in myotonic muscular dystrophy (Steinert's disease): a prospective study of 25 patients. Am J Cardiol 54:1074, 1984.
24. Hartwig GR, Ran KR, Radoff FM, et al: Radionuclide angiographic analysis of myocardial function in myotonic muscular dystrophy. Neurology 33:657, 1983.
25. Moorman JR, Coleman RE, Packer DL, et al: Cardiac involvement in myotonic muscular dystrophy. Medicine 64:271, 1985.
26. Katz A, Meites I, Bonstein N, et al: Cardiac manifestations of myotonic dystrophy. Funct Neurol 4:355, 1989.
27. Friedreich N: Ueber degenerative Atrophie der spinalen Hinterstrange. Arch Pathol Anat 26:391, 1863.
28. Chamberlain S, Shaw J, Rowland A, et al: Mapping of mutation causing Friedreich's ataxia to human chromosome 9. Nature 334:248, 1988.
29. Harding AE: Friedreich's ataxia: a clinical and genetic study of 90 families with an analysis of early diagnostic criteria and intrafamilial clustering of clinical features. Brain 104:589, 1981.
30. Child JS, Perloff JK, Bach PM, et al: Cardiac involvement in Friedreich's ataxia. J Am Coll Cardiol 7:1370, 1986.
31. Sutton MGS, Olukotun AY, Tagik AJ, et al: Left ventricular function in Friedreich's ataxia: an echocardiographic study. Br Heart J 44:309, 1980.
32. Thoren C: Cardiomyopathy in Friedreich's ataxia (follow-up study of ECG and effects of beta-receptor blockade) [abstract]. Eur J Cardiol 5:282, 1977.
33. Hewer RL: Study of fatal cases of Friedreich's ataxia. BMJ 3:649, 1968.
34. Alboliras ET, Shub P, Gomez MR, et al: Spectrum of cardiac involvement in Friedreich's ataxia: clinical, electrocardiographic and echocardiographic observations. Am J Cardiol 58:518, 1986.
35. Unverferth DV, Schmidt WE, Baker PB, et al: Morphologic and functional characteristics of the heart in Friedreich's ataxia. Am J Med 82:5, 1987.
36. James TN, Fisch C: Observations on the cardiovascular involvement in Friedreich's ataxia. Am Heart J 66:164, 1963.
37. Sanchez-Casis G, Cote M, Barbeau A: Pathology of the heart in Friedreich's ataxia: review of the literature and report of one case. J Can Sci Neurol 3:349, 1976.
38. Harding AE, Hewer RL: The heart disease of Friedreich's ataxia: a clinical and electrocardiographic study of 115 patients, with an analysis of serial electrocardiographic changes in 30 cases. J Med 208:489, 1983.
39. Zimmerman M, Gabathuler J, Adamec R, et al: Unusual manifestations of heart involvement in Friedreich's ataxia. Am Heart J 111:184, 1986.
40. Pentlund B, Sox K: The heart in Friedreich's ataxia. J Neurol Neurosurg Psychiatry 46:1138, 1983.
41. Smith ER, Sangalang VE, Heffernan LP, et al: Hypertrophic cardiomyopathy: the heart disease of Friedreich's ataxia. Am Heart J 94:428, 1977.
42. Gottdiener JS, Hawley RJ, Maron BJ, et al: Characteristics of the cardiac hypertrophy in Friedreich's ataxia. Am Heart J 103:525, 1982.
43. Pasternac A, Drol R, Petitclerc R, et al: Hypertrophic cardiomyopathy in Friedreich's ataxia: symmetric or asymmetric? J Can Sci Neurol 7:379, 1980.
44. Hewer RL: The heart in Friedreich's ataxia. Br Heart J 31:5, 1969.
45. Perloff JK: Pathogenesis of hypertrophic cardiomyopathy. *In* Goodwin JF (ed): Heart Muscle Disease. pp. 7–22. Lancaster, England: MTP, 1985.
46. Koenig M, Monaco AP, Kunkel LM: The complete sequence of dystrophin produces a rod-shaped cytoskeleton protein. Cell 53:219, 1988.
47. Hyser CL: Unraveling the mysteries of Duchenne and Becker muscular dystrophy. Mol Chem Neuropathol 10:15, 1989.
48. Mukoyama M, Kondo K, Hizawa K, et al: Life spans of Duchenne muscular dystrophy patients in the hospital care program in Japan. J Neurol Sci 81:155, 1987.
49. Nigro G, Comi LI, Politano L, et al: The incidence and evolution of cardiomyopathy in Duchenne muscular dystrophy. Int J Cardiol 26:271, 1990.
50. Second International Workshop for the Study of Cardiac and Pulmonary Involvement in X-Linked Muscular Dystrophies. Naples, 1985.
51. Perloff JK, DeLeon AC, O'Doherty D: The cardiomyopathy of progressive muscular dystrophy. Circulation 33:625, 1966.
52. Boaz EP, Lowenberg H: The heart rate in progressive muscular dystrophy. Arch Intern Med 47:376, 1931.
53. Stordtein O: The heart in progressive muscular dystrophy. Exp Med Surg 22:13, 1964.
54. Gailani S, Danowski TS, Fisher DC: Muscular dystrophy. Circulation 17:583, 1958.
55. James TN: Observations of a cardiovascular involvement, including the cardiac conduction system, and progressive muscular dystrophy. Am Heart J 63:48, 1962.
56. Riggs T: Cardiomyopathy and pulmonary embolism in terminal Duchenne's muscular dystrophy. Am Heart J 119:690, 1990.
57. Nomura H, Hizawa K: Histopathological study of the conduction system of the heart in Duchenne progressive muscular dystrophy. Acta Pathol Jpn 32:1027, 1982.
58. Perloff JK, Roberts WC, DeLeon AC, O'Doherty D: The distinctive electrocardiogram of Duchenne's progressive muscular dystrophy. Am J Med 42:179, 1967.
59. Bies RD, Friedman D, Roberts R, et al: Expression and localization of dystrophin in human cardiac Purkinje fibers. Circulation 86:147, 1992.
60. Sanyal SK, Johnson WW, Thapar MK, Pitner SE: An ultrastructural basis for the electrocardiographic alterations associated with Duchenne's progressive muscular dystrophy. Circulation 57:1122, 1978.
61. Fitch CW, Ainger LE: The Frank vector cardiogram in the electrocardiogram in Duchenne muscular dystrophy. Circulation 35:1124, 1967.
62. Shapiro HS, Ribeilima J, Wendt V: Myocardial infarction in progressive muscular dystrophy. Am J Cardiol 14:232, 1964.
63. Slucka C: The electrocardiogram in Duchenne's progressive muscular dystrophy. Circulation 38:933, 1968.
64. Sanyal SK, Tierney RC, Rao PS, et al: Systolic time interval in children with Duchenne progressive muscular dystrophy. Pediatrics 70:958, 1982.
65. Matsuda M, Akatsuka A, Yamaguchi T, et al: Systolic time intervals in patients with progressive muscular dystrophy of the Duchenne type. Jpn Heart J 18:638, 1977.
66. Chenard AA, Becane HM, Tertrain F, et al: Systolic time intervals in Duchenne muscular dystrophy: evaluation of left ventricular performance. Clin Cardiol 11:407, 1988.
67. Utsunomiya T, Mori H, Shibuya N: Long-term observation of cardiac function in Duchenne muscular dystrophy. Jpn Heart J 31:585, 1990.
68. Nagai T: Prognostic evaluation of congestive heart failure in patients with Duchenne muscular dystrophy. Jpn Circ J 35:406, 1989.
69. Kovick RB, Fogelman AM, Abbasi AS, et al: Echocardiographic evaluation of posterior left ventricular wall motion in muscular dystrophy. Circulation 52:447, 1975.
70. Farah MG, Evans EB, Vignos PJ Jr: Echocardiographic evaluation of left ventricular function in Duchenne muscular dystrophy. Am J Med 69:248, 1980.
71. Sanyal SK, Leung RKF, Tierney RC: Mitral valve prolapse in children with Duchenne progressive muscular dystrophy. Pediatrics 63:116, 1979.
72. Sanyal SK, Johnson WW, Dische MR, et al: Dystrophic degeneration of papillary muscle and ventricular myocardium: a basis for mitral valve prolapse in Duchenne muscular dystrophy. Circulation 62:43, 1980.
73. Perloff JK, Henze E, Schelbert HR: Alterations in regional myocardial metabolism, perfusion and wall motion in Duchenne muscular dystrophy studied by radionuclide imaging. Circulation 69:33, 1984.
74. Wakai S, Minami R, Kameda K, et al: Electron microscopic study of the biopsied cardiac muscle in Duchenne muscular dystrophy. J Neurol Sci 84:167, 1988.
75. Watkins SC, Hoffman EP, Slayter HS, et al: Immunoelectron microscopic localization of dystrophin in myofibers. Nature 33:863, 1988.
76. Dunn JF, Radda GK: Total ion content of skeletal and cardiac muscle in the mdx mouse dystrophy: Ca^{2+} is elevated at all ages. J Neurol Sci 103:226, 1991.
77. Adams R, Victor M: Principles of Neurology. 4th ed. New York: McGraw-Hill, 1989.
78. Yazawa M, Ikeda S, Owa M, et al: A family of Becker's progressive

C H A P T E R **108**

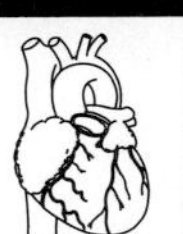

Hematologic Disease and Heart Disease

Martin D. Phillips and James T. Willerson

RED BLOOD CELLS
Anemia
Erythrocytosis
PLATELETS
Thrombocytosis
Platelet Hyperreactivity
DRUG-RELATED HEMATOLOGIC ABNORMALITIES
Heparin-Induced Thrombocytopenia
Quinidine Thrombocytopenia
Other Drug-Related Hematologic Abnormalities
COAGULATION ABNORMALITIES
Coagulopathy of Cardiopulmonary Bypass
Hypercoagulable States
Homocysteine
HEMOCHROMATOSIS
HEREDITARY HEMORRHAGIC TELANGIECTASIA
HEMATOLOGIC MALIGNANCY

Red Blood Cells

Anemia

Severe anemia (i.e., hematocrit generally equal to or less than 27 percent) alters cardiovascular function, leading initially to a marked increase in cardiac output and, with profound anemia, high output heart failure.[1, 2] The patient with profound anemia usually has tachycardia, a hyperactive precordium, wide pulse pressure, bounding peripheral pulses, and a systolic ejection murmur. A third heart sound may also be present. Tissue hypoxia associated with reduced blood viscosity leads to a reduction in systemic vascular resistance and an increase in cardiac output with severe anemia. Prolonged and severe anemia leads to cardiac dilatation and ventricular hypertrophy. Patients with severe and chronic anemia may develop severe cardiovascular decompensation after a period of high output heart failure.

As the oxygen delivery to tissue decreases associated with profound anemia, the hemoglobin-oxygen disassociation curve shifts to the right, resulting in more oxygen being released from hemoglobin. This is due to a number of factors, including an increased red blood cell (RBC) concentration of 2,3-diphosphoglycerate (2,3-DPG), which affects the binding and release of oxygen by hemoglobin. The increased 2,3-DPG displaces the hemoglobin-oxygen disassociation curve to the right, enabling a greater release of oxygen from RBCs at any level of Po_2.

Severe anemia is a particularly important problem in patients with underlying coronary heart disease because the further reduction in oxygen delivery to regions of the myocardium supplied by stenotic coronary arteries may lead to angina and even myocardial infarction. Chronic severe anemia may lead to a dilated cardiomyopathy and conversion from a high output heart failure to a low output state. Thus, to protect cardiovascular function, it is important to elucidate the reasons for anemia and to correct any reversible causes. Cautious transfusion may be critically important acutely in the patient with unstable coronary heart disease syndromes (i.e., unstable angina or myocardial infarction).

The initial approach to anemia should be to determine the underlying cause (Fig. 108–1). Two laboratory tests central to the evaluation are an examination of the peripheral blood smear and a reticulocyte count corrected for the RBC count (absolute reticulocyte count). The blood smear will reveal morphologic abnormalities of the RBCs, which may suggest a cause for the anemia. A low absolute reticulocyte count indicates that the anemia is due to a problem intrinsic to the bone marrow or a lack of precursors such as folic acid, vitamin B_{12}, or iron. On the other hand, an increased absolute reticulocyte count indicates a response to bleeding or hemolysis. A low reticulocyte count and a quickly decreasing hemoglobin concentration suggest ongoing bleeding or hemolysis without an adequate bone marrow response. Causes of bone marrow failure are not discussed here; however, it is always appropriate to evaluate the cause. In the acute setting, if there is cardiovascular compromise, blood transfusion may be needed. Hemolytic anemias present additional problems because they may be ongoing, resistant to transfusion, or in the case of immune hemolytic anemias, difficult to cross-match for transfusion.

Sickle Cell Anemia

Sickle cell anemia is caused by a mutation of the sixth amino acid of the beta-globin chain from glutamic acid to valine, resulting in *hemoglobin S.* This molecule has the capacity to form elongated crystal-like structures known as *tactoids* that impart a crescent or sickle shape to the erythrocyte, particularly in association with decreased tissue oxygen concentration. When RBCs become elongated in vivo, they have a shortened survival time and a tendency to clump, obstructing blood flow. African Americans and Africans develop sickle cell anemia due to a high frequency of the hemoglobin S gene.

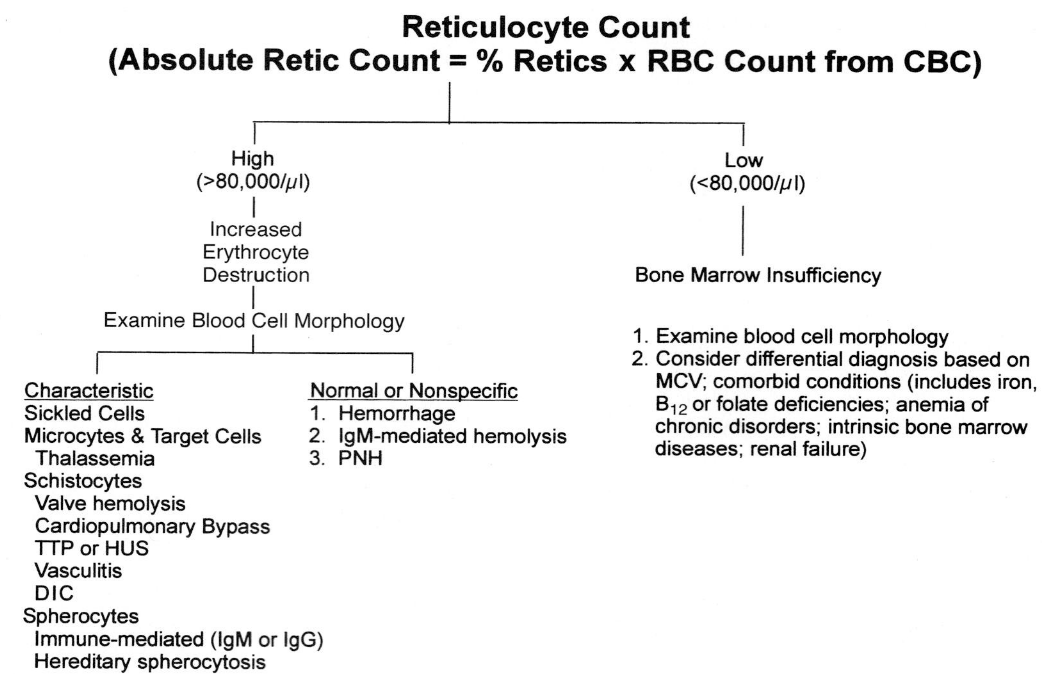

FIGURE 108–1 The diagnosis of anemia may be complex. This algorithm outlines the diagnosis of some of the major causes of anemia relevant to heart disease. CBC, complete blood count; DIC, disseminated intravascular coagulation; HUS, hemolytic-uremic syndrome; Ig, immunoglobulin; MCV, mean corpuscular volume; PNH, paroxysmal nocturnal hemoglobinuria; RBC, red blood cell; TTP, thrombotic thrombocytopenic purpura.

A person heterozygous for hemoglobin S (*sickle trait*) is not usually anemic and rarely has symptoms except at high altitude or in association with the development of marked hypoxemia. Because the hypertonicity and low oxygen tensions encountered in the renal medulla cause local infarctions, isosthenuria and renal papillary necrosis are common by adulthood. However, patients homozygous for hemoglobin S (*sickle cell disease*) often develop painful "crises" at approximately 6 months of age and recurrent symptoms in later years. As with other chronic anemias, the heart enlarges, and cardiac output is increased. However, the tendency for sickle cells to occlude vessels may lead to pulmonary, myocardial, cerebral, and bone infarction or occlusion of a peripheral artery. Pulmonary infarction is a common complication of sickle cell anemia and is usually due to thrombosis in situ.[3, 4] Other common symptoms are chronic impairment of renal function, bone infarction, and susceptibility to infections as a consequence of the autosplenectomy that occurs with repeated infarctions of the spleen. Severe hemolysis is usually found in these patients. Intermittent sickle cell crises characterized by severe muscle aching, bone pain, rhabdomyolysis, severe hemolysis, and fever occur intermittently in these patients. These episodes may be initiated by volume depletion, infection, or electrolyte alterations. Treatment includes bed rest, volume infusion for rehydration, and pain relief with opiates. Transfusion is not routinely indicated. Exchange transfusion is indicated for massive pulmonary infarction (*chest crisis*) or before major surgery.

A promising research direction for the treatment of sickle cell anemia has been the use of drugs to induce fetal hemoglobin synthesis.[5, 6] Hydroxyurea, a drug used for the treatment of thrombocytosis and polycythemia vera, appears to have a therapeutic benefit. After the administration of this drug, an increase in fetal hemoglobin level may occur in association with a marked increase in RBC volume. The potential for the development of neutropenia may be countered by reducing the dose of hydroxyurea. A decrease in the number of vaso-occlusive episodes has been noted in some adult patients treated with this drug.[7] The administration of other agents, such as erythropoietin, together with hydroxyurea may increase fetal hemoglobin production.

The application of gene therapy to sickle cell disease may be possible in the future by the insertion of normal β-globin and regulatory genes into the nucleus of stem cells; this may allow a cure for sickle cell disease.

Thalassemia

Patients with thalassemia usually have a combination of hemolysis and ineffective erythropoiesis. Thalassemias are inherited disorders caused by a decrease in the production of globin chains. The principal types are alpha-thalassemia, in which the α-chain synthesis is absent or reduced, and β-thalassemia, in which the β-chain synthesis is absent or reduced. These abnormalities are more common in persons of Mediterranean ancestry and also occur in African Americans, especially in association with sickle cell trait. They are inherited as autosomal dominant defects. The decreased production of hemoglobin A causes microcytic and hypochromic RBCs. These cells are often target shaped and demonstrate basophilic stippling. After iron deficiency is excluded, the diagnosis of thalassemia is confirmed by quantitative hemoglobin electrophoresis or Southern blot analysis. In patients with thalassemia major, severe anemia usually develops by the second decade of life. The development of congestive heart failure or sudden death associated with arrhythmias often occurs with extensive deposition of iron in many organs, including the heart, in which the atrioventricular node is often involved.[8, 9] Bone marrow transplantation has been used successfully in severe cases and is most effective in childhood before iron deposition has caused organ damage.

Hemolytic

Hemolytic anemias are characterized by the premature destruction of RBCs due to mechanical causes, immune mechanisms, or defects intrinsic to the erythrocyte. Mechanical hemolysis is usually associated with very high fluid shear forces, due to damaged microvasculature; atrioventricular malformations (including atrioventricular shunts); prosthetic heart valves, often in association with paravalvular regurgitation, prosthetic grafts, or patches; severe valvular aortic stenosis; and regurgitant jets such as occur with ruptured sinus of Valsalva aneurysms. These patients generally have evidence of RBC fragmentation, including schistocytes, spur cells, and microspherocytes on their peripheral blood smears (Fig. 108–2). Immune-mediated hemolysis may be due to autoantibodies or alloantibodies directed against RBCs or the use of certain drugs. The RBCs are usually spherocytic. Intrinsic RBC defects include membrane cytoskeleton abnormalities, hemoglobinopathies, or enzyme defects in the pathways that maintain an appropriate reducing intracellular milieu. The erythrocytes may be spherocytic, elliptocytic, "bite" or "blister" cells, or they may contain inclusions of precipitated hemoglobin. As mentioned earlier, patients with sickle cell anemia develop profound hemolysis. In hemolytic anemia, the absolute reticulocyte count is generally increased, anemia is present, and there may be an elevation of serum lactic dehydrogenase (LDH), free hemoglobin in the plasma, a reduction in serum haptoglobin (haptoglobin binds free hemoglobin and may be depleted in the systemic circulation with severe hemolysis), and elevated indirect bilirubin values. The urine dipstick may have a positive blood reaction, with no erythrocytes seen on microscopy. An indication of bone marrow decompensation is a low reticulocyte count with rapidly progressive anemia. The consequences of hemolytic anemia are similar to those of anemia in general and, in severe forms, may lead acutely to a rapid heart rate, wide pulse pressure, and a systolic ejection murmur. The initial development of a high output cardiac state is followed later by the development of ventricular hypertrophy, dilated cardiomyopathy, and a low output state. As is true with other forms of anemia, the sudden development of severe anemia may result in brain or heart injury, including myocardial or cerebral infarction, as a consequence of further exacerbation of tissue hypoxemia.

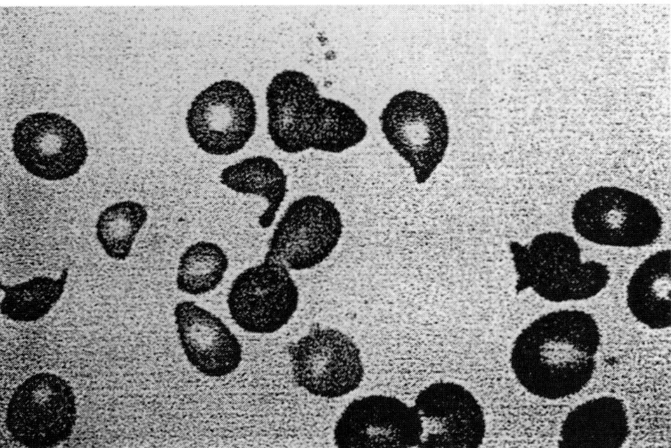

FIGURE 108–2 Examples of schistocytes in the peripheral blood due to leakage around a prosthetic heart valve. The presence of platelets (clumped in this photograph) makes the diagnosis of thrombotic microangiopathy or DIC less likely.

Other causes of the hemolytic anemia important in patients with heart disease include the following.

CARDIOPULMONARY BYPASS

Long cardiopulmonary bypass procedures may be associated with the development of intravascular hemolysis. Lysed RBC ghosts have been shown to be coated with the complement complex C5b-C9.[10] Presumably, the complement pathway is activated as the blood passes through the oxygenator. Although pericardial fluid has been implicated in causing hemolysis, one systematic investigation demonstrated a direct correlation with the quantity of tissue damage and exposure of blood to raw surfaces, unrelated to pericardial fluid per se.[11] Intraoperative blood salvage may also contribute to complement-mediated or mechanical blood cell destruction. Postoperatively, the patient may be anemic with evidence of RBC fragmentation. These problems are generally self-limited after the completion of the extracorporeal circulation. Owing to the presence of free hemoglobin in the plasma, which is nephrotoxic, attention should be given to the renal function. The coagulopathy associated with cardiopulmonary bypass is discussed later.

IMMUNE HEMOLYTIC ANEMIA

Immune hemolytic anemia can occur in several settings and is characterized by reticuloendothelial destruction of antibody-coated erythrocytes. The antibodies may be an isolated autoimmune phenomenon, associated with rheumatic diseases, alloantibodies due to minor transfusion incompatibilities, or secondary to selected drugs. Hydralazine, procainamide, quinidine, and, occasionally, phenytoin may cause a lupus erythematosus–like syndrome, including the development of immune-mediated RBC destruction. The syndrome is also characterized by the development of serositis, including pleural, pericardial, or peritoneal pain; arthralgias; and fever. It is important to identify this cause in the patient with underlying heart disease so a drug leading to a lupus-like syndrome may be discontinued. Most of these patients do not develop renal disease, nor do they have anti–double-stranded DNA antibodies in their sera.

α-Methyldopa causes a positive direct and/or indirect antiglobulin test (formerly known as Coombs test) in up to 10 percent of patients. Only a small minority of these individuals ever develops a hemolytic anemia due to these antibodies.

In immune hemolytic anemia, the direct antiglobulin test is usually positive, except in the case of some drug-induced antibodies that require the presence of a particular metabolite of the offending drug to act as a hapten and allow binding to RBCs. In most cases of drug-induced immune hemolysis, further investigation of the direct antiglobulin test usually demonstrates a "pan-agglutinin," in contrast to autoimmune hemolysis, in which the antibodies are directed against specific RBC antigens.

Because hemolysis due to IgG ("warm antibody") opsonization of erythrocytes is taking place within professional phagocytes, intraerythrocytic contents such as LDH and heme pigments (bilirubin) frequently are not leaked into the circulation. The exception is IgM ("cold antibody") complement-mediated hemolysis, which occurs in the circulation and leads to elevations in plasma LDH and bilirubin. These IgM antibodies may be cold agglutinins after *Mycoplasma* infections, due to major transfusion incompatibility, associated with malignancy, or idiopathic.

The acute treatment of symptomatic anemia can be difficult. The principal elements are the removal of possibly offending drugs, bed rest, adequate hydration, and the administration of folate (1 mg/da) and corticosteroids (usually 60 mg prednisone/da). If the antiglobulin test is positive, the specificity of the antibody and as complete a blood type as possible should be determined. In the case of IgM hemolytic anemia, the patient should be kept warm, and blood and fluids should be prewarmed before administration. The blood bank should be encouraged to participate actively in the patient's care, and least-incompatible blood should be transfused if the clinical situation necessitates transfusion. The reticulocyte count and hemoglobin should be measured at least daily until stability or improvement can be demonstrated.

THROMBOTIC MICROANGIOPATHY

Several related disorders of unknown mechanism are thrombotic thrombocytopenic purpura (TTP), the hemolytic uremic syndrome, and the pregnancy-associated syndrome of hemolysis, elevated liver enzymes, and low platelets (HELLP syndrome). All are characterized by mechanical erythrocyte fragmentation in partially occluded microvasculature (microangiopathic hemolytic anemia) and the formation of platelet thrombi in critical organs. Particularly in thrombocytopenic purpura, a presenting sign may be myocardial ischemia. The combination of mechanical hemolytic anemia with schistocytes, a negative direct antiglobulin test, and thrombocytopenia should raise this concern. The appropriate therapy is daily total plasma exchange transfusion and steroids. Aspirin therapy is controversial.

PAROXYSMAL NOCTURNAL HEMOGLOBINURIA

This disorder has been demonstrated to be due to deficiencies in particular post-translational modifications of certain cell-surface proteins that require phosphoinositol glycan (PIG) anchors.[12] It is a clonal hematopoietic stem cell disorder that results in mild to moderate pancytopenia and frequently in venous or arterial thrombosis. This may occur in unusual locations, such as the hepatic vein (Budd-Chiari syndrome). The blood cells in paroxysmal nocturnal hemoglobinuria are particularly sensitive to complement lysis, especially in an acidic milieu, due to the loss of complement regulatory proteins that require PIG anchors. This is the basis of the classic and definitive test: Ham's test. In many centers, the Ham test is supplanted by flow cytometric analysis of two PIG-anchored molecules: CD55 and CD59. Before cardiovascular surgery is undertaken in an individual with paroxysmal nocturnal hemoglobinuria, exchange transfusion should be considered, because of the activation of complement and other metabolic derangements induced by extracorporeal circulation.

HYPERTHERMIA

Normal RBCs fragment when exposed to a temperature of 49°C in vitro. In some of the hereditary hemolytic anemias, this may occur at temperatures as low as 46°C. Thus, the exposure to severely increased temperatures in the form of cell warmers used to bring transfused RBCs to body temperature before infusion may lead to hemolysis. In rare burn patients or individuals with severe hyperthermia, systemic hemolysis may occur. The blood smear may show characteristic erythrocyte bleb formation, known as *pyropoikilocytosis*.

MECHANICAL TRAUMA

In soldiers undergoing long marches; in joggers running on a hard road, especially under hot and humid conditions; or persons using vibrating machinery, evidence of intravascular RBC destruction may develop as a result of direct trauma to the RBCs in vessels of the hands and feet. Fragmented erythrocytes, elevated plasma LDH and bilirubin levels, and an increased reticulocyte count are expected.

Erythrocytosis

The primary function of RBCs is to deliver oxygen from the lungs to the tissues. Oxygen transport is a complex process that involves several systems, including ventilatory rate and volume, pulmonary diffusing capacity, cardiac output, RBC mass, hemoglobin-oxygen affinity, regional blood flow, and tissue capillary density, as well as the systemic oxygen tension. The maintenance of RBC mass is an important factor. Acute changes in tissue oxygen demand or in systemic oxygen tension are generally met by alterations in ventilatory rate and volume, cardiac output, distribution of blood flow, and hemoglobin-oxygen affinity. Sustained reductions in systemic oxygen concentration cause changes in RBC mass, in plasma volume, and, over a longer period of time, in vascularity at the capillary level. Erythrocytosis (i.e., an increase in hemoglobin, hematocrit, and RBC number) may be a primary bone marrow disorder (*polycythemia vera*) or secondary to sustained tissue hypoxia or an abnormal hemoglobin with a high affinity for oxygen. The secondary forms of erythrocytosis are associated with increased production of *erythropoietin*, a glycoprotein hormone produced primarily in the kidneys in adults that regulates RBC production.[13] Rare tumors produce ectopic erythropoietin. An increase in blood viscosity develops as a consequence of the increase in hematocrit and leads to a paradoxical decrease in tissue oxygenation (Fig. 108–3).

When the physician finds a reproducibly increased hematocrit or hemoglobin level, it is important to identify the causes of the erythrocytosis. An increased RBC mass and normal plasma volume should be documented with an isotope dilution study to distinguish true erythrocytosis from spurious erythrocytosis (*the Gaisbock phenomenon*). The latter is due to a real decrease in plasma volume and a relative increase in hematocrit. It is usually seen in thin, hypertensive, personality "type A" individuals, frequently in association with cigarette smoking. Polycythemia vera may be differentiated from secondary forms of erythrocytosis by splenomegaly, elevated leukocyte or platelet counts, and the absence of any of the factors that may cause a secondary erythrocytosis. Table 108–1 lists selected causes of erythrocytosis.

A serum erythropoietin level may be useful if elevated, indicating ongoing hypoxia. In patients with polycythemia vera or compensated hypoxia, the serum immunoreactive erythropoietin level is either normal or low.[14, 15] An assessment of arterial oxygen tension and arterial oxygen saturation is required in the evaluation of patients with erythrocytosis, because hypoxia may be a correctable factor. An oxygen saturation that is inappropriately low for the measured oxygen tension (PO_2) indicates the presence of methemoglobin, carboxyhemoglobin, or an abnormal hemoglobin variant. In patients with congenital heart disease and right-to-left shunts at the atrial or ventricular level or in association with a patent ductus arteriosus, the hypoxemia is usually not correctable without correction of the shunt. When severe, fixed pulmonary hypertension is present, heart and lung transplantation may be necessary. Hypoxia occurring with chronic lung disease represents a complicated clinical problem, especially when associated with severe emphysema and increases in $P\text{CO}_2$ levels.

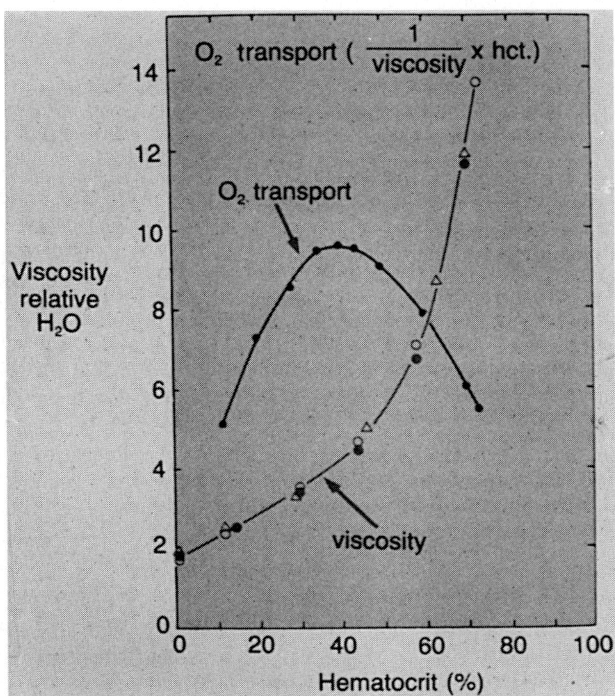

FIGURE 108–3 Viscosity of heparinized normal blood related to hematocrit (hct). (From Williams WJ [ed]: Hematology. 4th ed. New York: McGraw-Hill, 1977. Reproduced with permission of The McGraw-Hill Companies.)

TABLE 108–1 Causes of Erythrocytosis

Dehydration
Hemoconcentration as a result of dehydration, systemic arterial hypertension, or diuretics
Hypoxia
Right-to-left cardiac shunts, such as may occur in selected forms of congenital heart disease, including tetralogy of Fallot, transposition of the great vessels, and pulmonary artery hypertension associated with communications between the systemic and venous circulations
High-altitude pulmonary disease
Sleep apnea
Carbon monoxide intoxication
Hypoventilation
Respiratory center dysfunction
Selected Renal Diseases
Selected Tumors
Androgen Therapy
Myeloproliferative diseases
Polycythemia vera
Primary erythrocytosis
Spurious Erythrocytosis (Gaisbock Phenomenon)

Congenital heart disease with right-to-left shunting is associated with the development of erythrocytosis. Phlebotomy results in a marked increase in serum erythropoietin due to reversal of the compensatory erythrocytosis. The need for and frequency of phlebotomy should be dictated by the patient's symptomatic response or by the serum erythropoietin level as a measure of tissue hypoxia. Some of these patients have a coagulopathy with a low fibrinogen and platelet count.[14] However, even limited phlebotomy is symptomatically beneficial in children with cyanotic congenital heart disease and may improve the coagulopathy.[16, 17] If well tolerated, phlebotomy should be continued until the hematocrit is below 45 percent. Persistently higher levels of hematocrit are associated with reductions in cerebral blood flow. Sustained phlebotomy causes iron deficiency, which helps to control RBC mass and hematocrit. Chemotherapeutic agents are not used for reduction of RBC mass in individuals with cyanotic congenital heart disease.

All patients with erythrocytosis will have an elevated prothrombin time and activated partial thromboplastin time, because the amount of anticoagulant in the test tube is calibrated for a normal ratio of plasma to erythrocytes. Before diagnosing a coagulopathy, the coagulation laboratory must perform a correction for the elevated hematocrit.

PLATELETS

Thrombocytosis

Thrombocytosis may either occur as a consequence of primary thrombocythemia or be secondary to systemic abnormalities, including iron deficiency, severe inflammatory states, and selected malignancies. *Secondary thrombocytosis* is often associated with elevated plasma interleukin-

6 and C-reactive protein levels.[18] *Primary thrombocythemia* is a chronic myeloproliferative disorder characterized by a sustained proliferation of megakaryocytes leading to increased numbers of circulating platelets. Platelet counts in excess of 600,000/mm^3 in association with hyperplasia of bone marrow megakaryocytes, splenomegaly, and a clinical course punctuated by hemorrhagic or thrombotic episodes may occur with this abnormality. This disorder affects primarily middle-aged persons, with the average age at diagnosis being between 50 and 60 years. There is no sexual predilection, although there is a second peak frequency in young women at approximately 30 years of age.

Patients with this entity have been shown to have normal or nearly normal platelet survival times. However, effective platelet production has been estimated to be increased by as much as 10-fold in some patients.

Most clinical problems related to primary thrombocythemia occur with platelet counts in excess of 700,000/mm^3 and include both hemorrhagic and thrombotic episodes.[19, 20] These complications occur most commonly in older patients. However, younger patients may also have thrombotic events, including strokes and myocardial infarction. *Secondary thrombocythemia* rarely causes any hemorrhagic or thrombotic complications. Table 108–2 lists the symptoms identified at the time of diagnosis of patients with markedly elevated platelet counts in a series from Hehlmann and associates.[21] Platelets in patients with primary thrombocythemia are qualitatively abnormal, including increased platelet reactivity.[21, 22]

A thrombopoietin assay may help to distinguish primary and secondary thrombocythemia. Paradoxically, the thrombopoietin level is higher in primary than secondary thrombocythemia. Levels over 500 pg/ml are strongly predictive of a primary process[23]; levels of less than 500 are not indicative. Presumably, the thrombocytosis in secondary thrombocythemia is mediated by inflammatory cytokines to such as interleukin-6.

The clinical manifestations of the marked increase in platelet count vary from patient to patient. Some patients reach medical attention fortuitously as a result of a responsible physician who detected the elevated platelet count during a routine blood cell count. Approximately 13 to 37 percent of patients relate symptoms due to hemorrhagic events, whereas 22 to 84 percent of patients report thromboembolic complications.[21, 22] Symptoms referable to the posterior cerebral circulation are particularly common. Large artery thromboses are known to occur.[24]

Patients may present with angina, myocardial infarction, and cerebrovascular accidents related to extreme increases in platelet counts, often platelet counts in excess of 1 million/mm^3 in both the presence and absence of significant vascular atherosclerosis. The magnitude of the thrombocytosis does not predict a thrombotic or hemorrhagic event.

The use of agents that interfere with platelet aggregation in these patients is a difficult problem. Patients with primary thrombocythemia have a predisposition to hemorrhage that is likely to be potentiated by the use of drugs that interfere with platelet aggregation. Nevertheless, transient ischemic attacks associated with primary thrombocythemia have been reported to respond rapidly to aspirin alone and to aspirin and dipyridamole in combination.[25, 26] Hehlmann and associates[21] reported the treatment of 46 patients with primary thrombocythemia with 250 mg aspirin/day without significant bleeding complications. In patients who have arterial insufficiency syndromes, including transient ischemic attacks, angina pectoris, acute myocardial infarction, ischemia of lower limbs, or compromise of renal function, there is no controversy about the need to lower platelet count and usually to treat with agents that interfere with platelet aggregation. Usually, one attempts to normalize the platelet count or to reach a platelet count at which the patient's symptoms resolve without causing profound anemia or leukopenia associated with the administration of chemotherapeutic agents, including hydroxyurea, busulfan, melphalan, chlorambucil, radioactive phosphorus, and others.[27, 28] At the present time, hydroxyurea (15 mg/kg/day for the first week, followed by a maintenance dose adjusted to maintain an acceptable platelet count but avoid leukopenia) may be the agent of choice. Hydroxyurea lowers platelet count relatively rapidly, and often one can find a dose that keeps the platelet count at a level that avoids occlusive vascular symptoms without causing profound leukopenia. More recently, a new agent, anagrelide, a member of the imidazo-(2,1-b)-quianazolin-2-1 series of com-

TABLE 108–2 Symptoms at Diagnosis of Primary Thrombocythemia

Symptoms	No. of Patients (n = 61)	Percent of Patients
Thromboembolic complications:	51	84
Microcirculation	41	67
Peripheral (tips of fingers and/or toes)	32	53
Gangrene	16	26
Acrocyanosis	16	26
Paresthesias	15	25
Cold tip feeling	5	8
Cerebral	17	28
Dizziness	15	25
Acoustic phenomena	4	7
Disorientation	2	3
Transient ischemic attack	2	3
Epilepsy	1	2
Apoplectic psychosyndrome	1	2
Organic psychosyndrome	1	2
Large vessels	31	51
Arteries	29	48
Lower extremities	18	30
Coronary arteries	11	18
Carotid arteries	3	5
Renal arteries	6	10
Mesenteric arteries	2	3
Subclavian artery	1	2
Veins	4	7
Portal vein	3	5
Splenic vein	3	5
Leg and pelvic veins	2	3
Gastrointestinal hemorrhages	8	13
Other	2	3
Urogenital	2	3
Epistaxis	2	3
Postoperative	2	3
No symptoms	7	12

From Hehlmann R, Jahn M, Baumann B, Kopcke W: Essential thrombocythemia: clinical characteristics and course of 61 cases. CANCER, Vol. 61, No. 12, 1988, pp. 2487–2496. Copyright © 1988 American Cancer Society. Reprinted by permission of Wiley-Liss, Inc., a subsidiary of John Wiley & Sons, Inc.

pounds, has been developed to treat seriously elevated platelet counts associated with vaso-occlusive symptoms.[29] The drug acts primarily by inhibiting megakaryocyte maturation and platelet release.[29] Maintenance therapy of 1 to 4 mg/da has resulted in a reduction in platelet count for prolonged periods of time, and it may be effective in patients who are resistant to hydroxyurea.

A difficult decision is whether patients with primary thrombocythemia in whom the platelet count elevation is detected fortuitously and who are asymptomatic should be treated with agents such as hydroxyurea or anagrelide. Patients with this problem have infrequent but potentially dangerous thromboembolic complications that occur intermittently with intervening long periods of time without life-threatening events. Therefore, in young patients, it may be reasonable to withhold therapy in asymptomatic patients until the development of a clinically significant thrombotic or hemorrhagic event. In older patients likely to have important vaso-occlusive disease, it may be wiser to administer therapy that lowers platelet counts to safer levels.[18, 30]

The probability of a patient with primary thrombocythemia surviving 10 years from the time of detection is estimated as between 64 and 80 percent.[28] Obstetric problems occur frequently, including spontaneous abortions and premature deliveries. When death occurs, it is often due to a thrombotic complication. Transformation to acute myeloid leukemia occurs in less than 2 percent of patients with essential thrombocythemia.

Thrombocytosis is also a complication of polycythemia vera and chronic myelogenous leukemia. In addition to the therapy directed toward the primary disorder, the platelet count should be regulated in the same manner as in essential thrombocytosis.

Platelet Hyperreactivity

Although there is definitive evidence that platelet activation is associated with arterial thrombotic disorders, there are no reliable tests for platelet hyperreactivity in common use.[31] Research is being directed toward two receptors on the platelet surface that are involved in platelet adhesion (glycoprotein [gp] Ib/IX) and aggregation (gp IIb/IIIa). In addition to being targets of therapeutic intervention to prevent arterial thrombosis,[32, 33] multiple genetic polymorphisms of these proteins have been identified.[34, 35] Several studies have demonstrated that one such polymorphism of gp IIb/IIIa, named P_l^{A2} is associated with an increased risk of myocardial infarction and unstable angina and with coronary ischemic syndromes at a younger age than individuals negative for this mutation.[31] However, other studies have failed to show an association. Although a causal relationship has not been proven, the association of genetic markers with platelet hyperreactivity is an active field of investigation.

DRUG-RELATED HEMATOLOGIC ABNORMALITIES

Heparin-Induced Thrombocytopenia

Thrombocytopenia is a rare but important adverse effect of heparin administration, occurring in 1.1 percent of patients receiving porcine and 2.9 percent of patients receiving bovine heparin.[36] A relatively mild thrombocytopenia, with a platelet count usually greater than 100×10^9/L, may occur in the first few days of heparin exposure. A severe, immunologically mediated thrombocytopenia can occur starting 5 to 8 days after the first exposure, or sooner in repeat exposures to heparin, characterized by a rapidly decreasing platelet count due to intravascular platelet clumping. Warkentin and colleagues[37] provides a concise review. The thrombosis of coronary or peripheral arteries is not uncommon, with resultant myocardial infarction or loss of limb or life. Antibodies directed against platelet factor 4 complexed with heparin have been identified.[38] A laboratory test for heparin-induced platelet aggregation is widely available; it is approximately 75 percent sensitive and 100 percent specific. Other tests, including an enzyme-linked immunosorbent assay and platelet serotonin release assay, may be more sensitive but are not widely available. The appropriate course of action if this disorder is suspected is to discontinue all forms of heparin, including subcutaneous prophylactic doses, catheter "flush" solutions, and heparin "locks," because even vanishingly small doses of heparin can sustain the abnormal platelet aggregation. Although the incidence is lower with low-molecular-weight heparin,[39] cross-reactivity with standard heparin is a substantial problem and precludes the use of low-molecular-weight heparin as a substitute once the diagnosis is suspected or established. The therapeutic alternatives are few. Danaproid sodium and recombinant hirudin, or novastatin, direct thrombin inhibitors, may replace heparin.[40, 41] The inhibition of platelet function with aspirin, ticlopidine or anti-IIb/IIIa antibodies (abciximab) is controversial. Inhibition of coagulation with warfarin is not recommended acutely. Experimental drugs such as argatroban may be considered as a last resort. Platelet transfusions are ineffective and contraindicated except to treat hemorrhage. Early recognition and withdrawal of heparin are paramount. The thrombocytopenia usually resolves within 48 hours of the discontinuation of heparin.

Pentosan, an orally administered glycosaminoglycan, has been associated with the heparin-induced thrombocytopenia syndrome.[42]

Quinidine Thrombocytopenia

The thrombocytopenia induced by quinidine is unusual for drug-induced thrombocytopenia because of its severity and duration. Platelet counts as low as 2×10^9/L have been observed and may persist for up to 14 days. Antibodies against numerous platelet antigens have been demonstrated, but gp V is a frequent target.[43] The offending agent may be either the parent quinidine molecule, quinine, or a metabolite.[44]

Other Drug-Related Hematologic Abnormalities

Anemias of varying kinds may be produced by a large number of drugs that are used to treat various cardiovascular abnormalities. Drugs may induce aplastic, hemolytic, and megaloblastic anemias just as they may cause neutropenia, thrombocytopenia, and thrombocytosis. Table 108–3 identifies some of the drugs used to treat cardiovascular problems that lead to hematologic abnormalities.

It is important to consider the role that any drug might play in the development of anemia, leukopenia, or thrombocytopenia in the patient with cardiovascular disease. The correct identification of a drug causing an important hematologic abnormality may lead to correction of that abnormality and avoid some of the consequences of the hematologic problem that would otherwise occur.

COAGULATION ABNORMALITIES

Coagulopathy of Cardiopulmonary Bypass

In addition to hemolysis, cardiopulmonary bypass may have adverse effects on coagulation. There is a platelet defect that is presumed to be due to subthreshold stimulation of the platelets in contact with artificial surfaces that lasts for approximately 24 hours after a procedure.[45] If diffuse oozing of blood is observed despite a normal or nearly normal platelet count, a platelet transfusion may be beneficial. It has been shown that overactivity of the fibrinolytic system, demonstrated by increased levels of fibrin monomer, D-dimer, and tissue plasminogen activator, is associated with clinical blood loss.[46] Studies have demonstrated a beneficial effect of the fibrinolytic inhibitor tranexamic acid on decreasing postoperative blood loss.[47] DDAVP[48] and aprotinin have decreased postoperative blood loss after some difficult surgeries.

The pathogenesis of the platelet and leukocyte dysfunction induced by cardiopulmonary bypass is activation of the complement system via factor XII and kallikrein by the membrane oxygenator.[45, 49] These factors activate the fibrinolytic system in addition to complement, which may explain the observation of enhanced fibrinolysis. Experimentally, an antibody against the C5 component of complement has prevented platelet and leukocyte activation.

Hypothermia below 22°C may cause thrombocytopenia and leukopenia,[50] and the enzymes of the coagulation system do not function optimally at this temperature. Patients should be adequately rewarmed.

The syndrome of "heparin rebound" is thought to be insufficient reversal by protamine of the heparin administered during surgery. The recommended dose of protamine is 1 mg/100 U of heparin administered.[49]

Hypercoagulable States

A consensus has emerged that the hemostatic response is initiated by factor VIIa coming in contact with tissue factor

TABLE 108–3 Hematologic Abnormalities Associated With the Administration of Selected Medications Used to Treat Cardiovascular Problems

Agent	Anemia			Neutropenia
	Aplastic	*Megaloblastic*	*Hemolytic*	
Antiarrhythmic				
Digitoxin	–	–	–	–
Phenytoin	+	+	–	+
Procainamide	–	–	–	+*
Propranolol	–	–	–	+
Quinidine	–	–	+	+
Tocainide	+	–	–	+*
Moricizine	–	–	–	–
Propafenone	–	–	–	+*
Anticoagulant				
Heparin	+†	–	–	–
Phenindione	–	–	–	+
Antihypertensive				
Captopril	+	–	–	+
Glutethimide	+†	–	–	–
Hydralazine	–	–	–	–
Methyldopa	–	–	+	+
Reserpine	–	–	–	–
Diuretic				
Acetazolamide	+	–	–	+
Chlorothiazide	–	–	–	–
Chlorthalidone	–	–	–	+
Diazoxide	–	–	–	–
Ethacrynic acid	–	–	–	+
Hydrochlorothiazide	–	–	–	+
Mercurials	–	–	–	+
Spironolactone	–	–	–	–
Triamterene	–	+	–	–
Vasodilator/inotropic agent				
Amrinone	–	–	–	–

*Pure red cell aplasia.
†Agranulocytosis.
Modified from Rosenthal DS, Braunwald E: Hematological-oncological disorders and heart disease. *In* Braunwald E (ed): Heart Disease. pp. 1742–1766. Philadelphia: WB Saunders, 1992.

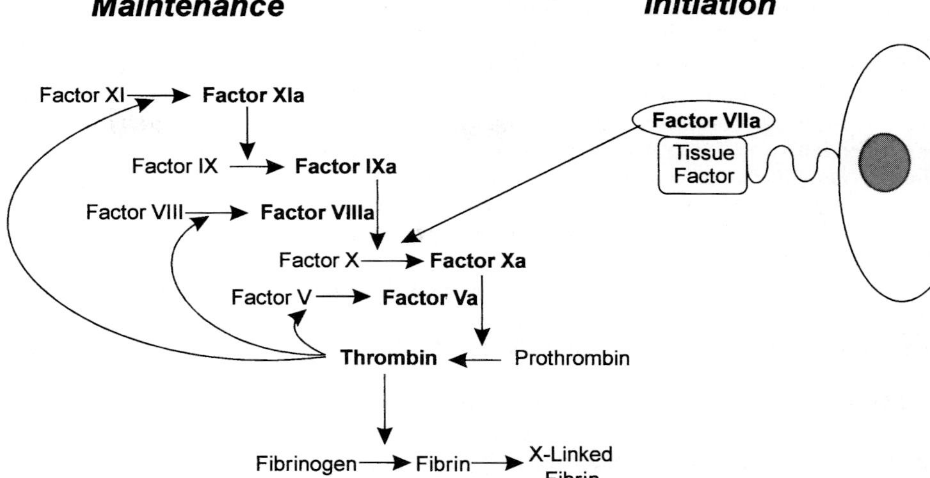

FIGURE 108–4 The revised coagulation cascade. Factor VIIa exposed to tissue factor or exposed subendothelial surfaces or at sites of inflammation activates factors IX and X, which generate a small amount of thrombin from prothrombin. This thrombin, in addition to generating fibrin, feeds back to activate factors XI, VIII, and V to amplify and maintain a coagulation response.

(TF). TF is not normally expressed on tissues that are exposed to flowing blood. However, TF is normally expressed on subendothelial structures, smooth muscle, brain, and activated (but not resting) monocytes (Fig. 108–4). The factor VIIa/TF complex activates factors IX and X to generate thrombin and activate platelets.[51] In addition to cleaving fibrinogen to fibrin, the thrombin that is generated feeds back on factors V and VIII to amplify the coagulation response. This amplification is normally dampened by several natural anticoagulant mechanisms. Deficiencies of these anticoagulants frequently result in abnormal venous thrombosis, with or without pulmonary embolism (Table 108–4). The risk of arterial thrombosis, stroke, and myocardial infarction is not increased by these mutations, although they may interact with traditional risk factors.[52–54]

One such anticoagulant is antithrombin III (ATIII). This plasma protein binds standard heparin (or heparans in vivo) and becomes a potent plasma protease inhibitor, specifically inhibiting thrombin, factor Xa, and factor VIIa. Patients with heterozygous deficiency states are at risk for the development of thrombosis, as are patients with the nephrotic syndrome because ATIII is lost in the urinary protein. A screening test for ATIII deficiency should use a functional assay, because many of the known mutations produced a normal plasma level of ATIII antigen but a

TABLE 108–4 Major Hypercoagulable States

Mechanical Factors	Blood Factors
Prolonged stasis	Antithrombin III deficiency
Congestive heart failure	Protein C or S deficiency
Restrictive garments	Resistance to activated protein C (factor V Leiden)
	Antiphospholipid antibodies (lupus anticoagulant)
	Possibly: heparin cofactor II deficiency excess plasminogen activator inhibitor 1 or histidine-rich glycoprotein
	Prothrombin mutation G20210A
	Hyperhomocysteinemia

decreased functional level. Typically, the age at first thrombosis is 15 to 45 years. Recurrent thrombosis is common. Heparin remains effective for acute treatment, even though the plasma ATIII levels are low. Warfarin is frequently used for life after a thrombosis has occurred. ATIII concentrates are available for replacement therapy at times when full anticoagulation would be dangerous, such as around the time of neurosurgery or parturition.

Protein C and protein S work in combination to proteolytically inactivate factors Va and VIIIa. Both proteins C and S are post-translationally modified by a vitamin K–dependent carboxylase and therefore are lowered in amount by warfarin therapy. Protein S circulates in plasma in a free form and also is bound to the complement protein C4B binding protein. The physiologic significance of the relative amounts of free and bound protein S is controversial. Protein C is an enzyme that can be activated; protein S is a cofactor. The clinical manifestations of heterozygous deficiencies of either are similar to ATIII deficiency. Homozygous deficiencies are rare, severe thrombotic disorders that are frequently manifest as purpura fulminans of the neonate. Protein S may be lost in the urine in the nephrotic syndrome. Protein C should be measured by a functional assay, as described for ATIII. Most protein S mutations result in a decreased plasma concentration; therefore, an antigenic measurement is usually sufficient. The therapy of thrombosis is heparin on an acute basis, followed by warfarin. A protein C concentrate may become commercially available.

A novel mechanism of resistance to activated protein C was described in 1993.[55,56] These authors observed that the plasma of some patients who had personal and family histories of venous thrombosis could not be adequately anticoagulated by the addition of activated protein C in vitro. It was later demonstrated that this phenomenon was due to a mutation in coagulation factor V. The mutated factor Va molecule retains its procoagulant function despite the presence of activated protein C. The mutation causes a substitution of glutamine for arginine at position 506.[57] This mutation is very common, occurring in about 4 percent of the white population. Heterozygosity confers a 7-fold relative lifetime risk of venous thrombosis; homozygosity is associated with a more-than-80-fold risk. Testing is most accurately done by polymerase chain reaction amplification of patient genomic DNA. The mutation results in the loss of an *Mn*lI restriction site. This assay, which is offered by many commercial and research laboratories, is not affected by anticoagulation and reliably distinguishes normal patients, heterozygotes, and homozygotes. A clot (activated partial thromboplastin time)-based assay is available but may be unreliable due to anticoagulant therapy or technical factors.

A very rare mutation of factor V at another activated protein C cleavage site, arginine 306 (*factor V Cambridge*), with a similar phenotype to factor V Leiden has been described.[58]

The syndrome of anti-phospholipid antibodies (lupus anticoagulants) was discussed in Chapter 15, Mitral Valve Disease. The causes of thrombosis in this disorder are still unknown, although the inhibition of binding of the anticoagulant annexin V by anti-phospholipid antibodies has been demonstrated.[59] Intensive anticoagulation to achieve an international normalized ratio (INR) of 3 with warfarin is necessary to prevent recurrence in patients who have experienced thrombosis.[60–62] Aspirin may be of benefit in addition to warfarin or in patients with a detectable anti-phospholipid antibody but no known thrombosis. Other agents, including ticlopidine, Plaquenil, interleukin-3, and thromboxane receptor antagonists, have been of benefit in clinical or experimental settings.[62] These mechanisms combined account for fewer than one third of cases of venous thrombosis. Several other abnormalities have been postulated, but none occur commonly. Deficiency of heparin cofactor II, excess of plasminogen activator inhibitor-1, and histidine-rich glycoprotein have been described in individual case reports. A mutation in thrombomodulin, an endothelial cell-surface cofactor for the generation of activated protein C, was described in one patient, but a physiologic role has not been demonstrated.[63] Purely mechanical factors, including prolonged stasis, congestive heart failure, and sluggish blood flow due to restrictive garments, remain as important risk factors to be avoided.

A recently described mutation in the noncoding 3′ tail of the prothrombin mRNA (G20210A) has been associated with both arterial and venous thrombosis.[64] The mutation is more likely to be found in young patients with thrombotic events,[65, 66] and this abnormality may interact with traditional arterial thrombotic risk factors.[54] Although the mechanism is not clear, this mutation appears to increase plasma prothrombin levels.[67, 68]

Homocysteine

Since the description of premature atherosclerotic vascular disease in individuals with congenital homocystinuria in 1969,[69] there has been an increased recognition of the concentration of plasma homocysteine as an independent cardiovascular disease risk factor in individuals who do not have the severe congenital homocystinuria syndrome.[70] Although many studies have demonstrated an approximately 3-fold relative risk of cardiovascular disease in individuals with a plasma homocysteine level above the upper 5th percentile compared to those below the 90th percentile, a strict cause-and-effect relationship has not been shown. Other studies have not demonstrated a relationship.[71] Many potential mechanisms have been demonstrated in cell culture studies, including enhanced generation of growth factors, increased thromboxane production, antagonism of nitric oxide, inhibition of protein C and thrombomodulin, activation of factor XII, and induction of TF.[72] Homocysteine also increases DNA synthesis in cultured vascular smooth muscle cells via an increase in the synthesis of cyclin A, a component of the growth-regulatory mechanism.[73] A likely factor is the capacity of these sulfur-containing compounds to oxidize lipid moieties. The oxidized forms of lipid molecules have a high atherogenic potential.[74] A common mutation has been identified that is associated with a thermolabile form of methylene tetrahydrofolate reductase (C677T), leading to higher plasma levels of homocysteine,[75] and is associated with an increased risk of cardiovascular disease.[76] An inverse correlation of plasma folate concentration and homocysteine concentration has been established. An increased dietary vitamin intake has the capacity to lower homocysteine levels. This effect may be due to the necessity of vitamins B_6 and B_{12} and folate in the conversion of the essential amino acid methionine to cysteine. It is not clear whether the elevated homocysteine is a cause or an effect of atherosclerosis.[77] Although no study has demonstrated a beneficial effect of pharmacologic lowering of homocysteine levels, some investigators recommend dietary supplementation of vitamin B_6 (10 mg/da), vitamin B_{12} (0.1 mg/da), and folate (1 mg/da).[78–80] The plasma concentration of homocysteine is also increased in a high-fat, high-animal protein diet and in cigarette smokers. The toxic effects of homocysteine may be one of the mechanisms via which these factors are atherogenic.[81] Plasma homocysteine levels increased significantly in some patients after cardiac transplantation, associated with decreased plasma folate levels.[82] These observations may be related to premature atherosclerosis, which can occur after transplantation.

Plasma homocysteine concentration is a weak risk factor for venous thrombosis. A study of 269 patients showed a trend toward an increased risk of venous thrombosis, with plasma homocysteine levels over the 95th percentile, independent of other known risk factors for venous thrombosis. The effect is greatest in older women, and statistical significance was achieved only when women more than 50 years old were included in the analysis.[83] In the rarer syndrome of congenital homozygous homocystinuria, factor V Leiden is strongly associated with both venous and arterial thrombosis of young children, indicating a synergistic effect of these risk factors.[84]

Hemochromatosis

Presumably because of the scarcity of iron in a foraging diet, mammals do not have an efficient mechanism to secrete excess iron. Consequently, individuals with hereditary hemochromatosis who absorb too much dietary iron or individuals with chronic anemia who receive a large transfusional iron load frequently experience iron deposition in several organs, resulting in a characteristic iron overload syndrome. In addition to the heart, the liver, pancreas, pituitary and adrenal glands, and articular cartilages are affected. The cardiac effects of hemochromatosis are discussed in Chapter 5, Nuclear Imaging. Hepatic deposition results in cirrhosis and an increased risk of hepatocellular carcinoma. Pituitary involvement results in decreased gonadotropin secretion and an increased release of adrenocorticotropic hormone, which has homology with β-melanocyte stimulating hormone, causing hyperpigmentation of the skin. The combination of the latter with pancreatic insufficiency is frequently called "bronze diabetes." It may also present as congestive heart failure in a young individual[85] or as conduction abnormalities.[86]

The hereditary form of hemochromatosis is quite common. The prevalence of homozygosity is 3 to 8:1000 in the general population. It is most common in whites. Women are frequently protected from end-organ damage because of menstrual blood loss. Heterozygotes have modestly increased total body iron stores but do not experience organ failure. A candidate gene for hemochromatosis has been located on the short arm of chromosome 6, near the human leukocyte antigen (HLA) genes.[87] The gene product is now called HFE (formerly HLA-8). Although its function is not understood, it is known to associate with the transferrin receptor. HFE knockout mice develop a disease similar to human hemochromatosis. Two intracellular iron transporters (N-ramp 1 and 2) are also being studied.[88] Testing for this disease has been controversial. Serum ferritin alone has been found to be insensitive and nonspecific.[89] The fasting transferrin saturation is very reliable,[90] but the unbound fraction of the serum iron binding capacity may emerge as the most cost-effective screening test.[89, 91] Liver biopsy with iron quantification has a role as a confirmatory test. The treatment of the hereditary form is therapeutic phlebotomy to normalize the serum ferritin. If initiated before organ damage is permanent, it can prevent a catastrophic outcome. In patients with marrow failure or chronic anemia and the need for repeated transfusion, iron chelation therapy is necessary. This is costly and may have side effects.

HEREDITARY HEMORRHAGIC TELANGIECTASIA

Hereditary hemorrhagic telangiectasia ([HHT] Osler-Weber-Rendu syndrome) is a disorder of endothelium that results in multiple telangiectases of the skin and mucous membranes that frequently cause inconvenient and sometimes massive hemorrhage. Organs may also be involved. Large pulmonary telangiectases are of particular relevance because they may result in high-output cardiac failure, right-to-left shunting, and paradoxical embolization. Chronic consumptive coagulopathy is a feature of other vascular malformations but not of HHT. The disorder may be as common as 1:16,500.[92] Cardiac anesthesia is complicated in these patients.[93]

Careful ultrastructural studies of the lesions in HHT has demonstrated that there are direct arteriovenous connections without resistance vessels between the connections.[94] It is thought that the increased venous pressure in lung tissue with little supporting connective tissue may result in the formation of large telangiectatic structures. These may be a nidus for thrombosis or infection that may subsequently embolize to the systemic circulation, or they may be a conduit for small thrombi that arise in the venous circulation to enter the arterial tree. There may be mild to moderate oxygen desaturation due to shunting or, when there are multiple large telangiectases, an increased cardiac output. Other frequent presenting signs are opacities on chest roentgenography, in addition to fine telangiectases of the skin and mucous membranes that cause epistaxis, bloody tears, and gastrointestinal hemorrhage. Iron deficiency is common.

Genetic mutations at three loci have been described that are closely associated with the development of HHT. Two of these mutations are found in families in whom pulmonary arteriovenous malformations are common, and both mutations involve cell surface receptors for transforming growth factor-β (TGF-β). One that maps to 9q33-34 is the TGF-β binding protein endoglin,[95] and the other is a TGF-β II receptor that maps to 3p22.[96] A third, and less common, mutation has been mapped to the long arm of chromosome 12 and is not associated with pulmonary arteriovenous malformations.[96] There appears to be heterogeneity of the specific mutations within these genes.

Treatment is difficult. No single modality has been uniformly effective. Aminocaproic acid or estrogens have had varied efficacy. Skin grafting and laser ablation have been used for cutaneous lesions. Specific lesions can be embolized, but others are likely to recur. The therapy of each patient must be individualized.

HEMATOLOGIC MALIGNANCY

The hematologic malignancies leukemia and lymphoma may have cardiac effects. Pericardial seeding and effusions were discussed in Chapters 64 and 65, Magnetic Resonance Imaging and Pericardial Diseases. They may cause significant anemia and pancytopenia. Myocardial ischemia may be a presenting sign, especially in older individuals. Greatly increased or decreased white blood cell counts or the presence of immature leukocytes on the peripheral blood smear are often diagnostic clues.

Multiple myeloma has been reported to be a very rare cause of high output cardiac failure.[97] Arteriovenous shunting or the elucidation of a cytokine by the malignant plasma cells were suggested mechanisms. There was no evidence of amyloid deposition.[97] The more usual occurrence is the deposition of amyloid, causing an infiltrative cardiomyopathy, as discussed in Chapters 5 and 53, Nuclear Imaging and Restrictive Cardiomyopathy. Many malignancies may cause culture-negative (marantic) endocarditis.[98] This is a difficult diagnostic entity. It may be especially hard to distinguish from subacute bacterial endocarditis.

REFERENCES

1. Datta BN, Silver MD: Cardiomegaly in chronic anemia in rats: an experimental study including ultrastructural, histometric and stereological observations. Lab Invest 2:503, 1975.
2. Baer RW, Vlahakes GJ, Uhling PN, Hoffman IE: Maximum myocardial oxygen transport during anemia and polycythemia in dogs. Am J Physiol 252:H1086, 1987.

3. Gerry JL, Bulkley BH, Hutchins GM: Clinicopathologic analysis of cardiac dysfunction in 52 patients with sickle cell anemia. Am J Cardiol 42:211, 1978.
4. Gaffney JW, Bierman FZ, Donnelly CM: Cardiovascular adaptation to transfusion/chelation therapy of homozygote sickle cell anemia. Am J Cardiol 62:121, 1983.
5. Charache S, Dover G, Smith K: Treatment of sickle cell anemia with 5-azacytidine results in increased fetal hemoglobin production and is associated with nonrandom hypomethylation of DNA around the gamma-delta-beta globin gene complex. Proc Natl Acad Sci U S A 80:4842, 1983.
6. Platt OS, Orkin SH, Dover G: Hydroxyurea enhances hemoglobin production in sickle cell anemia. J Clin Invest 74:652, 1984.
7. Charache S, Terrin ML, Moore RD, et al: Effect of hydroxyurea on the frequency of painful crises in sickle cell anemia. N Engl J Med 332:1317, 1995.
8. Canale C, Terrachini V, Vallebena A: Echocardiographic difference between major and intermediate thalassemia at rest and during isometric effort: yearly follow-up. Clin Cardiol 11:563, 1988.
9. Ehlers S, Levin AR, Klein AA: Natural history, noninvasive cardiac diagnostic studies, and results of cardiac catheterization. *In* Engle MA (ed): Pediatric Cardiovascular Disease: Cardiovascular Clinics II. p. 171. Philadelphia: FA Davis, 1981.
10. Schrier S: Extrinsic nonimmune hemolytic anemia. *In* Hoffman R, Benz EJ Jr (eds): Hematology: Basic Principles and Practice. p. 514. New York: Churchill Livingstone, 1991.
11. Ford EG, Picone AL, Baisden CE: Role of autogenous tissue factors in hemolysis during cardiopulmonary bypass operations. Ann Thorac Surg 55:410, 1993.
12. Yeh ET, Rosse WF: Paroxysmal nocturnal hemoglobinuria and the glycophosphatidyl anchor. J Clin Invest 93:2305, 1994.
13. Spivak JL: Erythrocytosis. *In* Hoffman R, Benz EJ (eds): Hematology: Basic Principles and Practice. p. 319. New York: Churchill Livingstone, 1991.
14. Haga P, Cotes PM, Till JA: Serum immunoreactive erythropoietin in children with cyanotic and acyanotic congenital heart disease. Blood 70:822, 1987.
15. Gidding SS, Stockman JA: Erythopoietin in cyanotic heart disease. Am Heart J 116:128, 1988.
16. Rosenthal A, Nathan DG, Marty AT: Acute hemodynamic effects of red cell volume reduction in polycythemia of cyanotic congenital heart diseases. Circulation 42:297, 1970.
17. Dayton LM, McCullough RE, Scheinhorn DJ: Symptomatic and pulmonary response to acute phlebotomy in secondary polycythemia. Chest 68:790, 1975.
18. Tefferi A, Silverstein MN, Hoagland HC: Primary thrombocythemia [review]. Semin Oncol 22:334, 1995.
19. Hardisty RM, Wolf HH: Haemorrhagic thrombocythaemia: a clinical and laboratory study. Br J Haematol 1:390, 1955.
20. Preston EE: Primary thrombocythaemia. Lancet 1:1021, 1982.
21. Hehlmann R, Jahn M, Baumann B, Kopcke W: Essential thrombocythemia: clinical characteristics and course of 61 cases. Cancer 61:2487, 1988.
22. Buss DH, Stuart JJ, Lipscomb GE: The incidence of thrombotic and hemorrhagic disorders in association with extreme thrombocytosis: an analysis of 129 cases. Am J Hematol 20:36, 1985.
23. Wang JC, Chen C, Novetsky AD, et al: Blood thrombopoietin levels in clonal thrombocytosis and reactive thrombocytosis. Am J Med 104:451, 1998.
24. Johnson M, Gernsheimer T, Johansen K: Essential thrombocytosis: underemphasized cause of large-vessel thrombosis. J Vasc Surg 22:443, 1995.
25. Preston FE, Emmanuel IG, Winfield DA, Malia RG: Essential thrombocythaemia and peripheral gangrene. BMJ 3:548, 1974.
26. Preston FE, Martin JF, Stewart RM, Davies-Jones GA: Thrombocytosis, circulating platelet aggregates and neurological dysfunction. BMJ 2:1561, 1979.
27. Brusamolino E, Canevari A, Salvaneschi L: Efficacy of pipobroman in essential thrombocythemia: a study of 24 patients. Cancer Treat Rep 68:1339, 1984.
28. Hoffman R, Silverstein MN: Primary thrombocythemia. *In* Hoffman R, Benz EJ (eds): Hematology: Basic Principles and Practice. p. 886. New York: Churchill Livingstone, 1991.
29. Silverstein MN, Petitt RM, Solberg LA Jr: Anagrelide: a new drug for treating thrombocytosis. N Engl J Med 318:1292, 1988.
30. Cortelazzo S, Finazzi G, Ruggeri M, et al: Hydroxyurea for patients with essential thrombocythemia and a high risk of thrombosis. N Engl J Med 332:1132, 1995.
31. Weiss EJ, Goldschmidt-Clermont PJ, Schulman SP, et al: The platelet glycoprotein IIIa polymorphism PlA2: an inherited risk factor for coronary thrombotic events [abstract]. Blood 86:1807, 1995.
32. McGhie AI, McNatt J, Ezov N, et al: Abolition of cyclic flow variations in stenosed, endothelium-injured coronary arteries in nonhuman primates with a peptide fragment (VCL) derived from human plasma von Willebrand factor-glycoprotein Ib binding domain. Circulation 90:2976, 1994.
33. Coller BS: Blockade of platelet GPIIb/IIIa receptors as an antithrombotic strategy. Circulation 92:2273, 1995.
34. Lopez JA: The platelet glycoprotein Ib-IX complex. Blood Coagul Fibrinol 5:97, 1994.
35. Newman PJ: Platelet GPIIb/IIIa: molecular variations and alloantigens. Thromb Haemost 66:111, 1991.
36. Chong BH: Heparin-induced thrombocytopenia. Br J Haematol 89:431, 1995.
37. Warkentin TE, Chong BH, Greinacher A: Heparin-induced thrombocytopenia: towards consensus. Thromb Haemost 79:1, 1998.
38. Visentin GP, Ford SE, Scott JP, Aster RH: Antibodies from patients with heparin-induced thrombocytopenia/thrombosis are specific for platelet factor 4 complexed with heparin or bound to endothelial cells. J Clin Invest 93:81, 1994.
39. Warkentin TE, Levine MN, Hirsh J, et al: Heparin-induced thrombocytopenia in patients treated with low-molecular weight heparin or unfractionated heparin. N Engl J Med 332:1330, 1995.
40. Koster A, Kuppe H, Hetzer R, et al: Emergent cardiopulmonary bypass in five patients with heparin-induced thrombocytopenia type II employing recombinant hirudin. Anesthesiology 89:777, 1998.
41. White HD, Ellis CJ, French JK, Aylward P: Hirudin (desirudin) and hirulog (bivalirudin) in acute ischaemic syndromes and the rationale for the Hirulog/Early Reperfusion Occlusion (HERO-2) Study. Aust N Z J Med 28:551, 1998.
42. Rice L, Kennedy D, Veach A: Pentosan induced cerebral sagittal sinus thrombosis: a variant of heparin induced thrombocytopenia. J Urol 160:2148, 1998.
43. Stricker RB, Shuman MA: Quinidine purpura: evidence that glycoprotein V is a target platelet antigen. Blood 67:1377, 1986.
44. Christie DJ, Diaz-Arauzo H, Cook JM: Antibody-mediated platelet destruction by quinine, quinidine, and their metabolites. J Lab Clin Med 112:92, 1988.
45. Colman RW: Hemostatic complications of cardiopulmonary bypass. Am J Hematol 48:267, 1995. Clinical conference.
46. de Haan J, Schonberger J, Haan J, et al: Tissue-type plasminogen activator and fibrin monomers synergistically cause platelet dysfunction during retransfusion of shed blood after cardiopulmonary bypass. J Thorac Cardiovasc Surg 106:1017, 1993.
47. Karski JM, Teasdale SJ, Norman P, et al: Prevention of bleeding after cardiopulmonary bypass with high-dose tranexamic acid: double-blind, randomized clinical trial. J Thorac Cardiovasc Surg 110:835, 1995.
48. Salzman EW, Weinstein MJ, Weintraub RM, et al: Treatment with desmopressin acetate to reduce blood loss after cardiac surgery. N Engl J Med 314:1402, 1986.
49. Woodman RC, Harker LA: Bleeding complications associated with cardiopulmonary bypass. Blood 76:1680, 1990.
50. Shenaq SA, Yawn DH, Saleem A, et al: Effect of profound hypothermia on leukocytes and platelets. Ann Clin Lab Sci 16:130, 1986.
51. Hoffman M, Monroe DM, Oliver JA, Roberts HR: Factors IXa and Xa play distinct roles in tissue factor-dependent initiation of coagulation. Blood 86:1794, 1995.
52. Cushman M, Rosendaal FR, Psaty BM, et al: Factor V Leiden is not a risk factor for arterial vascular disease in the elderly: results from the Cardiovascular Health Study. Thromb Haemost 79:912, 1998.
53. Garg UC, Arnett DK, Evans G, Eckfeldt JH: No association between factor V Leiden mutation and coronary heart disease or carotid intima media thickness: the NHLBI Family Heart Study. Thromb Res 89:289, 1998.
54. Doggen CJ, Cats VM, Bertina RM, Rosendaal FR: Interaction of coagulation defects and cardiovascular risk factors: increased risk of myocardial infarction associated with factor V Leiden or prothrombin 20210A. Circulation 97:1037, 1998.
55. Dahlback B, Carlsson M, Svensson PJ: Familial thrombophilia due

to a previously unrecognized mechanism characterized by poor anticoagulant response to activated protein C: prediction of a cofactor to activated protein C. Proc Natl Acad Sci U S A 90:1004, 1993.
56. Dahlback B: Inherited thrombophilia: resistance to activated protein C as a pathogenic factor of venous thromboembolism. Blood 85:607, 1995.
57. Bertina RM, Koeleman BP, Koster T, et al: Mutation in blood coagulation factor V associated with resistance to activated protein C. Nature 369:64, 1994.
58. Williamson D, Brown K, Luddington R, et al: Factor V Cambridge: a new mutation (Arg306→Thr) associated with resistance to activated protein C. Blood 91:1140, 1998.
59. Rand JH, Wu XX, Andree HA, et al: Antiphospholipid antibodies accelerate plasma coagulation by inhibiting annexin-V binding to phospholipids: a "lupus procoagulant" phenomenon. Blood 92:1652, 1998.
60. Rosove MH, Brewer PM: Antiphospholipid thrombosis: clinical course after the first thrombotic event in 70 patients. Ann Intern Med 117:303, 1992.
61. Khamashta MA, Cuadrado MJ, Mujic F, et al: The management of thrombosis in the antiphospholipid syndrome. N Engl J Med 332:993, 1995.
62. Lockshin MD: Answers to the antiphospholipid-antibody syndrome? N Engl J Med 332:1025, 1995.
63. Ohlin A, Marlar RA: The first mutation identified in the thrombomodulin gene is a 45-year old man presenting with thromboembolic disease. Blood 85:330, 1995.
64. Kapur RK, Mills LA, Spitzer SG, Hultin MB: A prothrombin gene mutation is significantly associated with venous thrombosis. Arterioscler Thromb Vasc Biol 17:2875, 1997.
65. De Stefano V, Chiusolo P, Paciaroni K, et al: Prothrombin G20210A mutant genotype is a risk factor for cerebrovascular ischemic disease in young patients. Blood 91:3562, 1998.
66. Rosendaal FR, Siscovick DS, Schwartz SM, et al: A common prothrombin variant (20210 G to A) increases the risk of myocardial infarction in young women. Blood 90:1747, 1997.
67. Kyrle PA, Mannhalter C, Beguin S, et al: Clinical studies and thrombin generation in patients homozygous or heterozygous for the G20210A mutation in the prothrombin gene. Arterioscler Thromb Vasc Biol 18:1287, 1998.
68. Ferraresi P, Marchetti G, Legnani C, et al: The heterozygous 20210 G/A prothrombin genotype is associated with early venous thrombosis in inherited thrombophilias and is not increased in frequency in artery disease. Arterioscler Thromb Vasc Biol 17:2418, 1997.
69. McCully KS: Vascular pathology of homocysteinemia: implications for the pathogenesis of arteriosclerosis. Am J Pathol 56:111, 1969.
70. Malinow MR: Plasma homocyst(e)ine and arterial occlusive diseases: a mini-review [review]. Clin Chem 41:173, 1995.
71. Folsom AR, Nieto FJ, McGovern PG, et al: Prospective study of coronary heart disease incidence in relation to fasting total homocysteine, related genetic polymorphisms, and B vitamins: the Atherosclerosis Risk in Communities (ARIC) study [see comments]. Circulation 98:204, 1998.
72. Harpel PC, Zhang XX, Borth W: Homocysteine and hemostasis: pathogenetic mechanisms predisposing to thrombosis. J Nutr 126(suppl):1285S, 1996.
73. Tsai J, Wang H, Perrella MA, et al: Induction of cyclin A gene expression by homocysteine in vascular smooth muscle cells. J Clin Invest 97:146, 1996.
74. McCully KS: Homocysteine and vascular disease. Nat Med 2:386, 1996.
75. Frosst P, Blom HJ, Milos R, et al: A candidate genetic risk factor for vascular disease: a common mutation in methylenetetrahydrofolate reductase. Nat Genet 10:111, 1995. Letter.
76. Kluijtmans LA, van den Heuvel LP, Boers GH, et al: Molecular genetic analysis in mild hyperhomocysteinemia: a common mutation in the methylenetetrahydrofolate reductase gene is a genetic risk factor for cardiovascular disease. Am J Hum Genet 58:35, 1996.
77. Kuller LH, Evans RW: Homocysteine, vitamins, and cardiovascular disease [editorial; comment]. Circulation 98:196, 1998.
78. Ubbink JB, van der Merwe A, Vermaak WJ, Delport R: Hyperhomocysteinemia and the response to vitamin supplementation. Clin Invest 71:993, 1993.
79. Verhoef P, Stampfer MJ, Buring JE, et al: Homocysteine metabolism and risk of myocardial infarction: Relation with vitamins B_6, B_{12}, and folate. Am J Epidemiol 143:845, 1996.
80. Chasan-Taber L, Selhub J, Rosenberg IH, et al: A prospective study of folate and vitamin B6 and risk of myocardial infarction in US physicians. J Am Coll Nutr 15:136, 1996.
81. Nygard O, Vollset SE, Refsum H, et al: Total plasma homocysteine and cardiovascular risk profile: the Hordaland Homocysteine Study. JAMA 274:1526, 1995.
82. Berger PB, Jones JD, Olson LJ, et al: Increase in total plasma homocysteine concentration after cardiac transplantation. Mayo Clin Proc 70:125, 1995.
83. den Heijer M, Koster T, Blom HJ, et al: Hyperhomocysteinemia as a risk factor for deep-vein thrombosis. N Engl J Med 334:759, 1996.
84. Mandel H, Brenner B, Berant M, et al: Coexistence of hereditary homocystinuria and factor V Leiden: effect on thrombosis. N Engl J Med 334:763, 1996.
85. Porter J, Cary N, Schofield P: Haemochromatosis presenting as congestive cardiac failure. Br Heart J 73:73, 1995.
86. Wang TL, Chen WJ, Liau CS, Lee YT: Sick sinus syndrome as the early manifestation of cardiac hemochromatosis. J Electrocardiol 27:91, 1994.
87. Bhavsar D, Chen Y, Zheng HD, Drysdale J: Searching for the hemochromatosis grail [review]. Adv Exp Med Biol 356:331, 1994.
88. Andrews NC, Levy JE: Iron is hot: an update on the pathophysiology of hemochromatosis. Blood 92:1845, 1998.
89. Adams PC, Gregor JC, Kertesz AE, Valberg LS: Screening blood donors for hereditary hemochromatosis: decision analysis model based on a 30-year database. Gastroenterology 109:177, 1995.
90. Phatak PD, Cappuccio JD: Management of hereditary hemochromatosis [review]. Blood Rev 8:193, 1994.
91. Kushner JP: Screening for hemochromatosis [editorial]. Gastroenterology 109:315, 1995.
92. Guttmacher AE, McKinnon WC, Upton MD: Hereditary hemorrhagic telangiectasia: a disorder in search of the genetics community. Am J Med Genet 52:252, 1994.
93. Radu C, Reich DL, Tamman R: Anesthetic considerations in a cardiac surgical patient with Osler-Weber-Rendu disease. J Cardiovasc Anesth 6:461, 1992.
94. Braverman IM, Keh A, Jacobson BS: Ultrastructure and three-dimensional organization of the telangiectases of hereditary hemorrhagic telangiectasia. J Invest Dermatol 95:422, 1990.
95. McAllister KA, Grogg KM, Johnson DW, et al: Endoglin, a TGF-beta binding protein of endothelial cells, is the gene for hereditary haemorrhagic telangiectasia type 1. Nat Genet 8:345, 1994.
96. Vincent P, Plauchu H, Hazan J, et al: A third locus for hereditary haemorrhagic telangiectasia maps to chromosome 12q. Hum Mol Genet 4:945, 1995.
97. McBride W, Jackman JD Jr, Gammon RS, Willerson JT: High-output cardiac failure in patients with multiple myeloma. N Engl J Med 319:1651, 1988
98. Williams WJ (ed): Hematology. 4th ed. New York: McGraw-Hill, 1977.

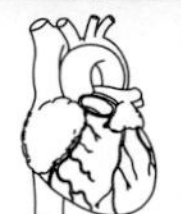

CHAPTER 109

Aging and the Cardiovascular System*

Gary Gerstenblith and Edward G. Lakatta

CARDIOVASCULAR CHANGES WITH AGING
Vascular Structure and Function
Cardiac Structure and Function at Rest
Cardiovascular Function During Exercise
β-Adrenergic Modulation of Cardiovascular Performance
ISCHEMIC HEART DISEASE
Diagnosis
Management
Acute Myocardial Infarction
HYPERTENSION
ARRHYTHMIAS
CONGESTIVE HEART FAILURE

Cardiovascular Changes With Aging

Insofar as atherosclerosis, hypertension, stroke, and heart failure reach epidemic proportions among older members of our society, aging, per se, must be considered to be a major risk factor for these diseases. Quantitative information on age-associated alterations in cardiovascular structure and function in health is essential in order to define and target the specific characteristics of cardiovascular aging that render it a risk factor for these diseases. Such information is also required to differentiate limitations of an elderly individual that relate to disease from those limitations that may fall within expected normal limits. But defining the effects of aging on cardiovascular structure and function is not an easy task because it is difficult to separate aging influences from those of lifestyle (e.g., physical activity, smoking, personality characteristics) and disease. The interactions among these can have a substantial impact on cardiovascular structure and function and can alter the manifestations of "pure" aging effects on the cardiovascular system.

Occult disease and lifestyle changes that occur with aging can cause severe functional impairments. Occult disease is especially pertinent to investigation of age effects on cardiovascular function in humans because coronary atherosclerosis is present in an occult form in at least as great a number of elderly persons as is the overt form of the disease. Regular physical activity affects both the structure and the function of the cardiovascular system. It has been well established in unselected populations that the average daily level of physical activity declines progressively with age. Genetic components of aging, disease, and lifestyle further complicate the picture and, at present, remain largely unknown.

Since the early 1980s, a sustained effort has been applied to characterize the multiple effects of aging in health on cardiovascular structure and function in a single study population, the Baltimore Longitudinal Study on Aging.[1] In these studies, community-dwelling, volunteer participants are rigorously screened to detect both clinical and occult cardiovascular disease and are characterized with respect to lifestyle (e.g., exercise habits) in an attempt to deconvolute the interactions noted previously. Some specific changes in cardiovascular structure and function that occur with advancing age in these healthy humans are identified[1] and summarized later.

Vascular Structure and Function

Ventricular structure and function are in part regulated by the mechanical properties of the vasculature to which the heart is connected, in particular by the peripheral vascular resistance (PVR), arterial impedance, and reflected pulse waves (Fig. 109–1).

Arterial stiffening occurs with aging, even in the absence of clinical hypertension (see Fig. 109–1).[2] This apparently results from changes within the vascular media (among which are an age-associated change in crosslinking of collagen, an increase in the amount of collagen, and changes in the nature of elastin). A substantial remodeling of the intima of conduit vessels, including the fragmentation of the elastic membrane,[3] intimal thickening,[4] cell infiltration, and matrix production,[3] also occurs with aging.[4] However, the relationship of these changes to arterial stiffening is not entirely clear. These anatomic changes are associated with diminished endothelium-mediated vasorelaxation.[5] Even in the absence of clinical hypertension, systolic arterial pressure increases within the clinically "normal" range and is considered to result from the age-associated increase in arterial stiffness (see Fig. 109–1). In populations in whom the increase in arterial stiffness with age is blunted, the arterial pressure increase with age is also blunted. The increased arterial stiffness may not be related strictly to an age-associated change in vascular structure but may also be due in part to increased arterial tonus. There is evidence that baroreceptor activity decreases with age, and this has also been implicated in the general age-associated increase in arterial pressure. In addition, plasma catecholamines increase with aging,[6] which may be a result of exaggerated

*This chapter is in the public domain.

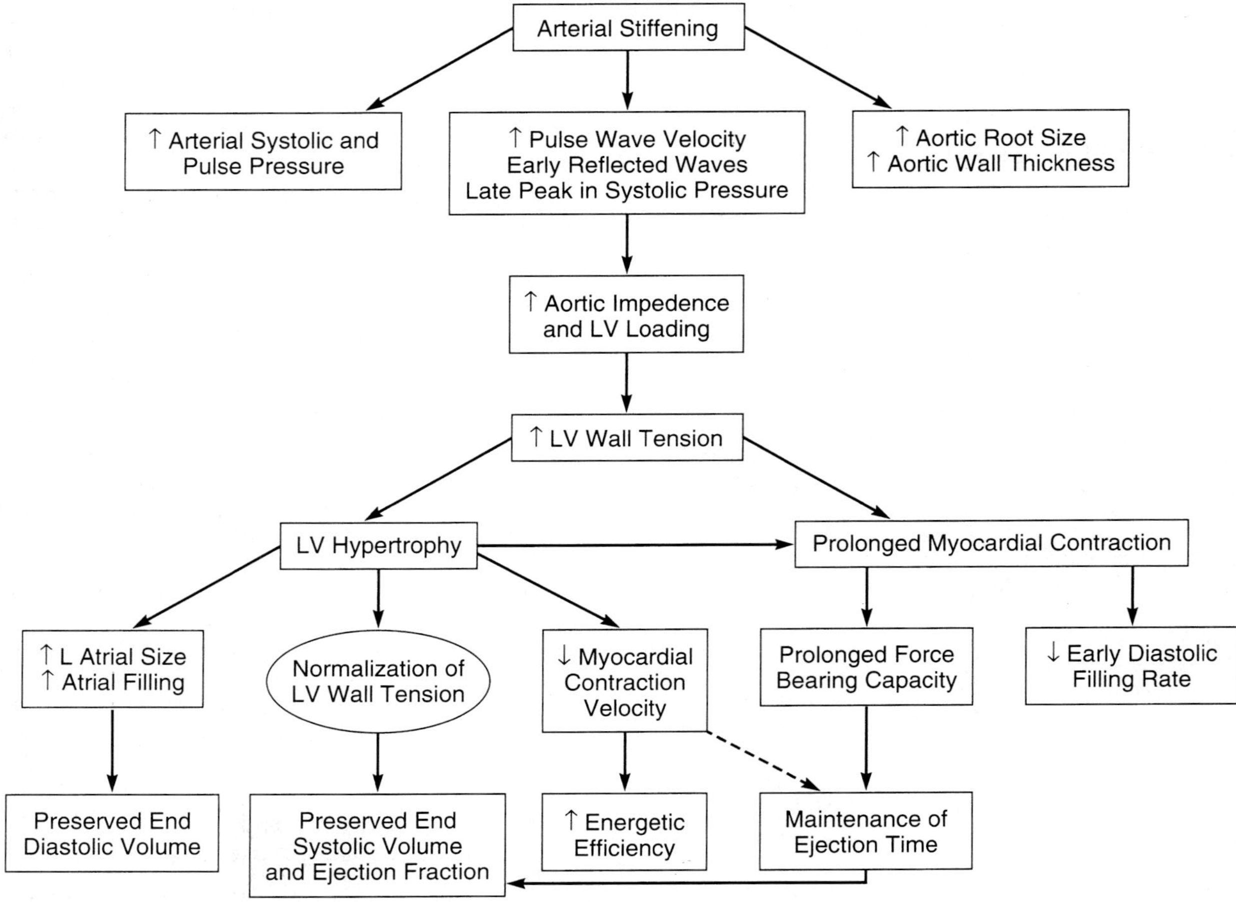

FIGURE 109–1 Cardiac consequences of age-associated increase in central arterial stiffness. L, left; LV, left ventricular.

central nervous system adrenergic flow, possibly associated with blunting of baroreceptor sensitivity. However, elevated plasma catecholamine levels in older individuals are associated with a diminished postsynaptic beta-adrenergic response of the heart and vasculature (see later). It is possible that the diminished postsynaptic response itself could be secondary to exaggerated receptor stimulation and related, in part, to a deficient baroreflex, which leads to inappropriate central nervous system sympathetic flow. Plasma catecholamine levels, however, are not correlated or are inversely correlated with arterial pressure in elderly normotensives and hypertensives.

An increase in PVR accompanies aging in some but not all individuals and may, in part, be secondary to a reduction in skeletal muscle mass with aging,[7, 8] with a concomitant reduction in capillary density. Although the renal blood flow per gram of kidney weight decreases progressively after the fourth decade of life, this occurs in populations in whom cardiac output remains unchanged with aging.[9] Therefore, an increase in renal arterial resistance with aging is not secondary to reduced cardiac output. The nature of this increase in renal vascular resistance is not fully understood.

Arterial stiffness is a major determinant of arterial impedance, which affects the pulsatile ejection of blood from the heart.[10] The aortic impedance is composed of many frequency components. The zero frequency impedance modulus is the PVR, as noted previously. The average of the higher frequency impedance moduli, referred to as the *characteristic aortic impedance,* is the opposition to pulsatile flow. Abnormalities in aortic distensibility, such as those associated with advancing age and clinical hypertension, create a mismatch between ventricular ejection and aortic flow energies, causing the characteristic aortic impedance modulus to increase with age.[10] The increased pulsed-wave velocity, resulting from increased vascular stiffness, causes wave reflection from peripheral sites to the ascending aorta to occur during the ventricular ejection period (see Fig. 109–1). This causes aortic and carotid pressures to continue to increase to a later time during ejection, resulting in an increase in systolic and pulse pressure and a change in the aortic pressure pulse contour of these arteries, which includes a late-occurring peak.[10] Pulsed-wave reflection, in addition to elevating aortic pressure, imposes an additional component to the total vascular load on the left ventricle.[10] Therefore, the total arterial load placed on the left ventricle can be characterized by PVR, characteristic aortic impedance, and pulsed-wave reflection. Although each of these factors changes with age, the extent of change varies dramatically among individuals. Observations indicate that arterial stiffening is reduced in older individuals who regularly engage in vigorous exercise.[1]

Cardiac Structure and Function at Rest

Overall cardiac function in most elderly individuals who do not have clinical or occult disease is adequate to meet the body's pressure and flow requirements at rest. Two cardiac adaptations occur to sustain normal left ventricular (LV) ejection in the presence of the greater arterial stiffness in most older individuals and the increased PVR in some of these individuals (see Fig. 109–1). First, the LV wall thickens modestly, largely owing to an increase in myocyte size. The number of myocytes in the older heart may decrease because of drop-out of some cells.[11] However, the increase in size of the remaining cells in most but not all instances compensates for the cell loss. An increase in the amount of interstitial collagen also occurs. Whereas the LV thickening has been interpreted to result from increased vascular loading of the heart, as indicated previously, a decrease in the efficacy of β-adrenergic modulation of both the heart and the vasculature that occurs with aging,[12] may be implicated in the associated myocardial changes, in part, via a reduction in the heart rate at rest in the sitting position and during routine activities of daily living. In addition, potential age-associated changes in the tissue levels or activities of other growth factors (e.g., angiotensin II, endothelin, transforming growth factor, fibroblast growth factor, or insulin-like growth factor that influence myocardial or vascular cells, or their extracellular matrices, may have a role in the age-associated changes in cardiac structure.

Second, the ability of the myocardium to bear force in late systole is increased and is manifested as a prolongation of the isovolumic relaxation time (see Fig. 109–1). This may be due, at least in part, to a prolongation of the myofilament Ca^{2+} activation that occurs during systole. Studies in animal models indicate that prolonged contractile activation in the aged heart is accomplished by a prolonged cytosolic free Ca^{2+} transient, partly resulting from a reduction in the rate of Ca^{2+} resequestration by Ca^{2+} sinks within the cell.[1] Although the prolonged contractile activation and possibly structural changes in the heart cause the LV early diastolic filling rate to be reduced in healthy elderly humans, an enhanced atrial contribution to ventricular filling maintains the end-diastolic volume at a normal level in most elderly individuals (see Fig. 109–1). In men, a modest cardiac dilatation at end-diastole occurs with aging.[13] The end-systolic volume and ejection fraction at rest are not age-related in healthy men.[13] In healthy men, the supine basal heart rate does not change with aging, but in the sitting position the heart rate decreases slightly with age.[13] However, the resting, sitting cardiac output is not reduced in healthy older men, and stroke volume is preserved. In contrast to men, cardiac output at rest in the sitting position slightly decreases in older versus younger healthy women, as neither end-diastolic nor stroke volume increases with age to compensate for the modest reduction in heart rate.[13] These gender differences appear, in part, to be due to differences in fitness even between sedentary men and women.[13]

Cardiovascular Function During Exercise

Although there is a decrease in the maximal aerobic work capacity in most healthy older individuals, it has become clear that this limitation may not be due solely to limitations of the central circulation. Rather, the limitations of exercise ability in the aged subject are, at least in part, related to peripheral factors that determine oxygen utilization. Peripheral factors that appear to be involved in the age-associated decline in the maximal oxygen consumption, O_2max, include a decline in skeletal muscle mass with aging.[7, 8] Despite this decline, body mass may remain constant because of an increase in body fat, not only subcutaneous but also intraperitoneal and intramuscular.[7, 8] When the O_2max is normalized to muscle mass instead of body weight, the magnitude of the decline associated with aging between 25 and 80 years of age decreases from 60 percent to 14 percent in men and from 50 percent to 8 percent in women.[14] Physical conditioning of older men increases muscle mass and also increases the oxidative capacity per unit of muscle mass.[8]

During high levels of physical exertion, the heart rate is substantially lower in healthy elderly versus younger individuals. The peak rate of LV filling increases in both younger and older subjects during exercise, but a diminished rate of filling of similar magnitude as that observed at rest (i.e., about a 50 percent reduction) is observed in older individuals during exercise.[15] However, cardiac dilatation at end-diastole and end-systole still occurs during vigorous exercise in older relative to younger men. Therefore, healthy older persons do not exhibit a compromised end-diastolic volume due to a "stiff heart," either at rest or during exercise. However, end-diastolic pressure, which has not been measured in healthy older and younger subjects during exercise, may increase with age. During vigorous exercise, the LV stroke volume, which depends on the end-diastolic and end-systolic volumes, is not reduced in healthy elderly subjects.[13] Therefore, in these individuals, the cardiac dilatation at end-diastole outweighs the concomitant age-associated deficiency in end-systolic volume reduction. The maximal cardiac index is only slightly decreased with age in healthy men. In contrast, in older women, stroke volume during exercise is not maintained as well as in older men owing to a relatively smaller end-diastolic volume during exercise in older women than in men.[10] Thus, the maximal cardiac output during vigorous cycle exercise decreases in older women to a greater extent than it does in men because of the reduction in both heart rate and stroke volume in older versus younger women. The inability of healthy older persons of both genders to reduce the LV end-systolic volume during vigorous exercise accounts for a smaller increase in ejection fraction during exercise in these versus younger individuals. Cardiac dilatation and the failure to increase the LV ejection fraction during exercise is more severe in older persons who have silent ischemia (i.e., who do not have signs or symptoms of coronary disease at rest but during exercise have an abnormal electrocardiogram and an abnormal thallium scan) than in those without evidence of coronary disease[16] and is due to a more pronounced inability to reduce the end-systolic volume. The insufficiency in LV end-systolic volume reduction during exercise in healthy older individuals can result from an age-associated decrease in the myocardial contractile reserve or failure of ventricular afterload to sufficiently decrease. The pulsatile determinants of ventricular afterload during exercise have not been characterized with respect to age. The end-systolic volume/systolic blood pressure ratio, an index of myocardial contractility, is not age associated at rest but decreases with age during vigorous exercise.[13] The apparent decrease in LV contractility, as manifested by this index, is more severe in older individuals with silent ischemia than in healthy older individuals.[16] Endurance conditioning in older persons improves the age-associated decline in LV pump function[17] and arterial stiffness;[1] but does not affect the age-associated decline in the maximal heart rate.[17]

β-Adrenergic Modulation of Cardiovascular Performance

The hemodynamic pattern observed in many healthy older persons during exercise (i.e., reduced heart rate and greater cardiac dilatation at end-diastole and end-systole, with maintenance or augmentation of stroke volume) occurs in younger individuals who exercise in the presence of β-adrenergic blockade. Observations show, in fact, that the age-associated differences in heart rate, LV end-diastolic volume, and stroke volume during exercise are abolished when this exercise is performed during β-adrenergic blockade.[18] β-Adrenergic blockade also abolishes the age-associated decrease of the peak filling rate in the sitting position, both at rest and during vigorous exercise.[15] When perspectives from studies that range from measurements of the stress response in intact humans to measurements of subcellular biochemistry in animal models are integrated, a diminished responsiveness to β-adrenergic modulation is among the most notable changes that occur in the cardiovascular system with advancing age (see reference 2 for review). β-Adrenergic modulation of cardiac pacemaker cells accounts, in part, for the increase in heart rate during exercise. Bolus infusions of β-adrenergic agonists cause a diminished heart rate and ejection fraction responses in elderly versus younger subjects.[19] Both the β-adrenergic relaxation of large arteries and the β-adrenergic augmentation of myocardial performance facilitate the ejection of blood from the heart. Therefore, a reduced ability of β-adrenergic stimulation to augment myocardial contractility or to dilate arteries during exercise may be implicated in the alterations in the ventricular ejection pattern observed in some older individuals (i.e., a deficiency of β-adrenergic action could partially account for the relative failure of end-systolic volume to decrease during exercise as much in older individuals as in younger ones). In isolated cardiac muscle and cardiac cells from humans of advanced age, β-adrenergic enhancement of the contraction amplitude is diminished compared with that in younger tissue or cells.[1] Age-associated reductions in the ability of β-adrenergic stimulation to relax arteries and veins in humans and in isolated aortic muscles from senescent animals have also been demonstrated.[12] Mechanisms for age-associated changes in the effectiveness of β-adrenergic stimulation of the myocardium have been demonstrated most extensively in the rat model.[1]

In summary, overall cardiovascular function in most elderly subjects who do not have clinical or occult cardiac disease is adequate to meet the body's requirements for pressure and flow at rest. Age-associated changes in cardiovascular structure and function at rest in healthy community-dwelling volunteers are listed in Table 109–1. The basal supine heart rate is unchanged with aging, but systolic blood pressure becomes moderately increased (even within the clinically normal range). This pressure increase occurs during late systole and is due to early pulsed-wave reflection from the periphery, resulting from an increase in arterial stiffness. To sustain normal LV ejection, the LV wall thickens modestly, largely because of an increase in myocyte size, and the ability of the myocardium to bear force in late systole is increased, due, at least in part, to a prolongation of myofilament Ca^{2+} activation. Although prolonged contractile activation and possibly structural changes in the heart cause the LV early diastolic filling rate to be reduced in healthy elderly humans, an enhanced atrial contribution to ventricular filling prevents a reduction in end-diastolic volume, which is actually mildly increased with age. The end-systolic volume and ejection fraction at rest are not age related.

Age-associated changes in cardiovascular reserve capacity in healthy community-dwelling volunteers are listed in Table 109–2. Although aerobic capacity declines with advancing age in individuals without cardiac disease, the extent to which this can be attributed to a decrement in cardiac reserve is not certain. A substantial part of the age-associated decline in maximal oxygen consumption appears to be due to peripheral factors and, at least in part, can be attributed to an increase in body fat and a decrease in muscle mass with age. Although heart rate is lower in healthy elderly versus younger individuals at high levels of physical work, cardiac dilatation at end-diastole and end-systole occurs in older subjects. Therefore, healthy older subjects do not exhibit a compromised end-diastolic volume due to a "stiff heart," even during exercise. Whereas stroke volume in such individuals is preserved by cardiac dilatation, the increase in ejection fraction with exercise is blunted. This same hemodynamic pattern (i.e., a reduced exercise heart rate and greater cardiac dilatation at end-diastole and end-systole) occurs in subjects of any age who exercise in the presence of β-adrenergic blockade.

TABLE 109–1 Seated Rest: Changes in Cardiac Output Regulations Between 20 and 80 Years of Age in Healthy Humans

Cardiac index*	No Δ
Heart rate	↓ (10%)
Stroke volume	↑ (10%)
Preload	
End-diastolic volume†	↑ (12%)
Early filling	↓
Late filling	↑
Afterload	
Compliance	↓
Reflected waves	↑
Inertance	↑
Peripheral vascular resistance‡	↔
Contractility	No Δ
Ejection fraction	No Δ
Left ventricular mass	↑

*Decreased with age in women.
†Unchanged with age in women.
‡Increased with age in women.

TABLE 109-2 **Exhaustive Upright Exercise: Changes in Aerobic Capacity and Cardiac Regulation Between Ages of 20 and 80 Years in Healthy Men and Women**

Oxygen consumption	↓ (50%)
$(A\text{-}V)O_2$	↓ (25%)
Cardiac index	↓ (25%)
Heart rate	↓ (25%)
Stroke volume	No Δ
Preload	
EDV	↑ (30%)
Afterload	↑
Vascular (PVR)	↑ (30%)
Cardiac (ESV)	↑ (275%)
Cardiac (EDV)	↑ (30%)
Contractility	↓ (60%)
Ejection fraction	↓ (15%)
Plasma catecholamines	↑
Cardiac and vascular responses to β-adrenergic stimulation	↓

Abbreviations: EDV, end-diastolic volume; ESV, end-systolic volume; PVR, peripheral vascular resistance.

Alterations in cardiovascular function that exceed these identified limits for age-associated changes in healthy elderly persons are most likely manifestations of interactions of aging per se, with age-associated changes caused by severe physical deconditioning or the presence of cardiovascular disease, which are, unfortunately, highly prevalent within our population.

Ischemic Heart Disease

Diagnosis

Although the prevalence and severity of autopsy-documented coronary atherosclerosis show a striking increase with age,[20] the diagnosis may be particularly difficult. This is related to the greater likelihood of silent ischemic disease and of atypical presentations of ischemic disease in the older population.[21] A number of factors may be responsible, including a diminished sensation of chest discomfort and the greater incidence of dyspnea as a manifestation of ischemia, rather than the more usual chest discomfort. These may be due to age-associated changes in myocardial diastolic properties and pericardial compliance. In addition, the ability of older individuals to exercise to the point at which ischemic symptoms occur may be decreased because of the increased likelihood of concomitant diseases.

If it is important to know whether or not an older individual has significant coronary atherosclerosis, it is not sufficient to rely on a negative history alone. The cardiac examination is also of limited value. If the patient can exercise on a treadmill, stress testing may be useful. Although specificity tends to decline somewhat as age increases, from 84 percent in those less than 40 years to 70 percent in those over 60 years of age,[22] it is largely reliable, with certain caveats. There is a higher likelihood of baseline ST changes in this population because of the increased incidence of LV hypertrophy, conduction abnormalities, and digitalis intake. In this setting, the predictive accuracy of a positive test is low and a thallium 201 stress test is particularly useful. A second caution is that a negative test has a low predictive accuracy when the patient is unable to exercise to 85 to 90 percent of maximal predicted heart rate. A safe and accurate alternative in patients who cannot exercise sufficiently, or at all, is a pharmacologic test with adenosine, dipyridamole, or dobutamine.[22–25] The accuracy of dipyridamole/thallium 201 scintigraphy is similar in the older and younger populations.[26] Finally, the predictive accuracy of a test depends not only on the degree of ST-segment change but also on the prevalence of disease in the population being examined. Therefore, there is an increased likelihood of a false-negative stress test in an older population with a high pretest probability of disease. The use of cardiac catheterization to diagnose ischemic disease is increasing in the elderly, concomitant with the increasing number and proportion of older individuals who undergo coronary bypass surgery, angioplasty, and valve replacement. Although adverse events themselves—including cerebrovascular and peripheral vascular complications, renal failure, contrast reactions, and disorientation—are the same, the incidence of all of these complications is probably higher in older patients.[27, 28]

Management

The principles of angina management are the same in older and in younger patients. The search for easily reversible factors may be more rewarding in the elderly; therefore, the possibilities of anemia due to occult malignancy, apathetic hyperthyroidism, hypertension, congestive heart failure (CHF), and supraventricular arrhythmias—all of which increase myocardial oxygen demand requirements and decrease supply—should be considered in older patients who present with new-onset or recently progressive anginal symptoms.

The choice of an anti-ischemic regimen for patients without easily reversible precipitating factors is similar in different age groups. If patients continue to experience significant symptoms despite medical therapy, revascularization should be considered. Although early reports indicated an increased incidence of complications of angioplasty in older individuals, mortality rates for both angioplasty and bypass surgery are decreasing in the elderly.[29–31] Perioperative survival after bypass surgery, however, is decreased in older individuals, primarily because of increasing likelihood of coexisting disease, including diabetes, renal and pulmonary insufficiency, and the increased likelihood of advanced coronary disease and impaired LV function.[32] Age is also an important predictor of adverse cerebral outcomes after bypass surgery, including stroke, encephalopathy, confusion, and deterioration of intellectual function.[33] Nevertheless, long-term survival and pain relief compare favorably with those achieved by medical therapy.[34, 35]

Atherosclerosis is progressive, and an important element in its therapy is to identify and treat factors that predispose to accelerated disease. Studies indicate that treatment of hypertension[36, 37] and smoking cessation[38] decrease the rate of cardiac outcomes in older patients. Total cholesterol is associated with increased cardiac mortality in the elderly when the data are adjusted for advanced age, gender, other risk factors, and nutritional status and when first-year events (i.e., those patients with subclinical disease) are excluded.[39] Primary and secondary treatment of hyperlipidemia with 3-hydroxy-3-methylglutaryl coenzyme A (HMG CoA) reductase inhibitors also improve outcomes in older individuals.[40, 41] Although observational studies indicated that estrogen therapy was associated with decreased cardiovascular mortality in postmenopausal women,[42] a large scale randomized intervention study showed no overall effect on myocardial infarction or cardiac death.[43]

Acute Myocardial Infarction

Recognition and treatment of acute myocardial infarction are often more difficult in older persons. In this population, acute infarction more often presents with central nervous system symptoms, hypotension, and dyspnea.[44, 45] The higher mortality and morbidity previously reported in older patients with infarction is present in the placebo arms of randomized trials of thrombolytic therapy,[46, 47] as well as in patients treated with intravenous streptokinase and tissue-type plasminogen activator.[48–50] In addition, complications of myocardial infarction, including CHF, are also increased in older patients. It is unclear whether these adverse outcomes are related to larger infarcts, more advanced coronary disease, decreased ability of uninfarcted muscle to compensate for the infarcted tissue, or altered healing processes in older individuals. Although the use of thrombolytic therapy is associated with significantly decreased mortality in the elderly, it may also be associated with increased hemorrhagic complications, including intracerebral hemorrhage.[51, 52] The official guidelines of the joint American College of Cardiology/American Heart Association Task Force state that thrombolytic therapy in older individuals is acceptable but of uncertain efficacy. This recommendation remains controversial, however, with others arguing that the benefit is clear-cut in this age group.[54] An attractive alternative to thrombolytic therapy is primary angioplasty, which, if performed early in the course of the infarct, is associated with outcomes similar to, or better than, thrombolytic therapy.[55]

Long-term use of the beta-blockers propranolol,[56] metoprolol,[57] and timolol[58] is associated with decreased mortality and reinfarction rates in both older and younger patients. Although the use of aspirin during the postinfarction period has not been specifically addressed in an older population, it is likely that a benefit similar to that observed in the younger population is associated with aspirin intake. Studies from the Medicare database indicate that use of these secondary prevention therapies is relatively low in older individuals, despite their demonstrated benefit.[59, 60] Older patients with apical aneurysm formation should probably receive coumadin. A Netherlands multicenter randomized trial in over 800 patients,[61] in fact, found that administration of oral anticoagulants resulted in significantly lower incidences of recurrent myocardial infarction and death in patients over 60 years of age. The management of complications, including postinfarction ischemia, LV dysfunction, and frequent and complex ventricular arrhythmias after an infarction, is also similar. Revascularization may be beneficial in those with depressed but ischemic myocardium, and the benefit of angiotensin-converting enzyme inhibition therapy in postinfarction patients with extensive damaged myocardium is probably also applicable in the older population.[62] Elderly patients with frequent and/or complex arrhythmias postinfarction do not benefit from class 1C antiarrhythmics[63] but probably benefit from implantable defibrillators to an extent similar to that of the general population.[64]

HYPERTENSION

Hypertension is the most important correctable risk factor for cardiovascular disease in the older population. This is due to both its high prevalence, estimated at up to 40 to 50 percent in those over 65 years of age, and its significant impact on the development of disease.[65] Convincing evidence exists for the effectiveness of therapy in those with even mild diastolic arterial pressure elevations.[36, 66] In older patients with isolated systolic hypertension, treatment with a β-blocker and a diuretic[67] or with a long-acting dihyropyridine calcium antagonist[37] decreased stroke and cardiac event rates.

Initial therapy might be directed to nonpharmacologic maneuvers, including salt and alcohol restriction, weight loss when indicated, and increased physical activity. A randomized trial of reduced sodium intake and weight reduction in those who were obese demonstrated that these benefits were feasible, safe, effective, and additive in elderly hypertensives.[68] There are many agents that can lower blood pressure to a normal value. The sixth report of the Joint National Committee on Prevention, Detection, Evaluation and Treatment of High Blood Pressure[65] emphasizes individualization of drug therapy based primarily on the presence of coexisting diseases and endorses long-acting formulations. In the older patient, coexisting coronary disease, diabetes, CHF, renal impairment, and elevated lipids are more likely to be present. An additional, important and often coexisting factor is LV hypertrophy, which is often associated with diastolic LV dysfunction. Regression of LV mass in this age group is associated with improved relaxation parameters, without compromising systolic function either at rest or during mild, upright bicycle exercise.[69]

ARRHYTHMIAS

There is a significant age-related increase in the incidence and complexity of cardiac arrhythmias.[70–73] This is probably due to age-associated changes in the impulse formation and conduction system that are not related to cardiovascular disease and also to the well-recognized age-associated increase in mitral annular calcification and in hypertensive, vascular, and ischemic disease. Regardless of etiology, both tachycardic and bradycardic arrhythmias have increased hemodynamic significance in older patients because of the increased dependence on diastolic filling time and the atrial contribution to diastolic filling, as well as a decreased ability of the cardiovascular system to compensate for any arrhythmia-induced stress. There are minor changes in the resting electrocardiogram that can probably be attributed to aging per se. These include a decreased incidence of respiratory sinus arrhythmia, an increase in the PR interval, a leftward shift in the QRS axis, and decreased voltage of the R and T waves. These changes are probably related to decreased parasympathetic tone, fibrosis in the conducting system, and increased distance between the heart and the chest wall. Although there is also an age-related increase in LV hypertrophy, myocardial infarction, and more advanced conducting system disease, these are probably related to the presence of silent and/or overt cardiac disease. Ambulatory monitoring is the most valuable and common technique to determine the presence and extent of arrhythmias, their relation to possible cardiac symptoms, and possible adverse prognostic implications. The degree to which arrhythmia in an older patient is considered abnormal, however, is dependent on the frequency and occurrence of similar arrhythmia in older subjects without disease. The incidence of ventricular arrhythmias over a 24-hour period of ambulatory electrocardiographic monitoring in clinically normal older individuals in several studies is presented in Table 109–3.

The evaluation of an older patient with suspected arrhythmias should begin with a detailed history concerning the occurrence of palpitations and near-syncopal and syncopal episodes, particularly the onset and termination, relation to medication, food, position, and alcohol, and the degree of hemodynamic compromise. Because the prognostic significance of ventricular arrhythmias is dependent on the presence of underlying cardiac disease, a history of hypertension and of ischemic or failure symptoms should also be obtained. Symptoms compatible with thyroid disease and anemia, not uncommon conditions that often present with cardiac manifestations in the elderly, should also be sought. The electrocardiogram remains a useful test for evaluation of an arrhythmia. If the arrhythmia is not present during a 12-lead tracing, long-term monitoring can often be helpful, particularly with the use of loop recorders, which can be worn for extended periods and activated to record the rhythm at the time of the event.

Atrial fibrillation is a common arrhythmia in the older age group. The hemodynamic consequences of atrial fibrillation are also more marked in the older population and are due to loss of atrial contribution to LV filling, decreased diastolic time for coronary perfusion, and increased myocardial oxygen demand associated with the higher heart rate. Another significant consequence of atrial fibrillation is the increased likelihood of cerebral and other emboli. The Framingham study[74] reported that the risk of stroke attributed to atrial fibrillation, even after adjusting for the effect of systolic blood pressure, rose from 7.3 percent in those 60 to 69 years of age to 30.8 percent in those aged 80 to 89 years. CHF within the prior 3 months, hypertension, or previous thromboembolism are each significantly and independently associated with an increased risk for stroke in those over 60 years of age.[75]

Several major trials[76–78] have assessed the ability of anticoagulation to prevent thromboembolic complications in older patients with atrial fibrillation. The Copenhagen Atrial Fibrillation, Aspirin, Anticoagulation Study (AFASAK)[79] randomized 1007 patients, with a mean age of 72.8 years, and who had nonrheumatic atrial fibrillation, to warfarin in a dose that resulted in a prothrombin time of 1.5 to 1.9 times control, low-dose aspirin (75 mg/da), and placebo in a 2-year treatment protocol. Thirty-eight percent of the warfarin patients were withdrawn from the study because of refusal to continue, side effects, or noncompliance. The incidence of thromboembolic events did not differ between the aspirin and the placebo groups (20 and 21, respectively) but, in an intention-to-treat analysis, was decreased in the warfarin group to 5, only 1 of which occurred while the patient was receiving sufficient anticoagulation. There was, in addition, a significant decrease in vascular deaths (3 in the warfarin group versus 12 and 13 in the aspirin and the placebo groups, respectively).

The Boston Area Anticoagulation Trial for Atrial Fibrillation[77] randomized 420 patients to low-dose warfarin and placebo and followed them for an average of 2.2 years. The mean ages of the warfarin and the placebo groups were 68.5 and 67.3 years, respectively. It is important to note that the target prothrombin time in the warfarin group was a range of 1.2 to 1.5 times control, that the patients remained within this target range 83 percent of the time, and that only 10 percent of these required premature discontinuation. The warfarin group had an 86 percent decrease in the risk of stroke (from 2.96 percent/yr in the control group to 0.41 percent/yr in the warfarin group, $P = .0022$). There was also a significant decrease in overall deaths (5.97 percent/yr to 2.25 percent/yr, $P = .005$). The frequency of bleeding requiring transfusion or hospitalization did not differ. In sum, it therefore appears reasonable to recommend warfarin to older patients with atrial fibrillation, particularly those with associated CHF or prior myocardial infarction and those who can be monitored closely. In a study of patients with atrial fibrillation and a recent episode of cerebral ischemia, the lowest rates of bleeding and ischemic events occurred at International Normalized Ratio levels of 2.0 to 3.0.[79]

In contrast to the effectiveness of anticoagulation, the safety and efficacy of antiarrhythmic agents in both supraventricular and ventricular arrhythmias is unclear. Although

TABLE 109–3 Incidence of Ventricular Arrhythmias Over a 24-Hr Period of Ambulatory Electrocardiographic Monitoring in Clinically Normal Older Individuals

First Author	Age (yr)	n	Any	Multiform	Couplets	Ventricular Tachycardia
Fleg[70]	60–85	98	80	35	11	4
Wajngarten[71]	70–81	20	76.9	50	19.2	11.6
Ingerslev[72]	>85	22	76	62	19	14
Kantelip[73]	>80	50	96	19	8	2

quinidine treatment is associated with an increased likelihood of maintenance of sinus rhythm, a meta-analysis indicated that it is associated with increased mortality.[80] The increased mortality associated with type 1C agents in the postinfarction period,[60] despite their ability to suppress ventricular arrhythmias on ambulatory monitoring, may also extend to other antiarrhythmic agents, with the possible exception of amiodarone.[81–83] Therefore, no antiarrhythmic agent has been conclusively demonstrated to improve survival in patients with supraventricular and ventricular arrhythmias. Antiarrhythmic therapy should be guided by the extent of associated disability, assessment of proarrhythmic effects, and consideration of additional approaches, including ablation,[84] amiodarone,[83] and the insertion of implantable defibrillators.[64]

Bradycardic arrhythmias are also common in the elderly. In symptomatic patients, it is important to determine whether the symptoms are related to the arrhythmia because older individuals frequently have several reasons for neurologic symptoms. If long-term ambulatory monitoring demonstrates this relationship, pacemakers that allow proper atrial and ventricular sequencing are particularly useful because of the increased dependence on atrial contribution to LV diastolic filling in the elderly. The impact of single- or dual-chamber pacemaker selection on survival in older patients was reported in a study of 36,312 Medicare patients in the United States.[85] The group was randomly chosen and represented 20 percent of those receiving pacemakers over a 3-year period. After adjusting for patient and hospital characteristics, both 1- and 2-year survival were significantly better for those patients who received the dual-chamber model.

Congestive Heart Failure

The incidence and prevalence of CHF are significantly increased with age. CHF is now the most common discharge diagnosis for those over 65 years of age.[86] The high incidence of heart failure is primarily related to the increased likelihood of superimposed ischemic, hypertensive, and degenerative valvular heart disease rather than to myocardial changes associated with aging per se. However, age-related changes in diastolic properties and in the cardiovascular response to β-adrenergic stimulation may result in increased or altered symptomatology in the face of any given stress.

It is important to note that symptoms of CHF in the older population may be due to abnormal diastolic as well as systolic function. The distinction is best made by noninvasive techniques, particularly the echocardiogram. Systolic dysfunction, evidenced by poor ejection and a dilated LV cavity, is commonly seen in the setting of ischemic disease. These patients can best be treated with rest, diuretics, angiotensin-converting enzyme inhibitors, and digitalis. In the enalapril trial of patients in severe heart failure, the average ages of the placebo and the treated groups were 70 and 71 years, respectively.[87] Enalapril therapy was associated with decreased mortality, decreased heart size, and decreased requirement for other medications, as well as with improved New York Heart Association classification. In patients who cannot tolerate angiotensin-converting enzyme inhibitors, the angiotensin-receptor blockers should be considered.[88]

In older patients, CHF symptoms are often due to increased left atrial pressure and may be associated with slowed and delayed LV diastolic relaxation in the presence of normal systolic function. This is often associated with hypertension, with exacerbations occurring at the time of transient ischemic episodes. The echocardiogram shows normal or decreased LV cavity size, normal or enhanced ejection, slowed relaxation, and often, increased wall thickness. Left atrial size may also be increased. Although removal of small amounts of fluid may result in significant immediate improvement, the primary treatment goals include increasing diastolic filling time, maintaining atrial contribution to LV filling, and reducing LV end-diastolic pressure.

Older individuals may particularly benefit from interventions designed to increase education and dietary and medication compliance and that allow early intervention and improved access to health providers. In one report, such an intervention significantly decreased hospitalization rates and improved quality of life.[89]

References

1. Vaitkevicius P, Engel J, Wright J, et al: The age-associated increase in arterial stiffness is attenuated by chronic exercise. Circulation 84:II-29, 1991.
2. Lakatta EG: Cardiovascular regulatory mechanisms in advanced age. Physiol Rev 73:413–467, 1993.
3. Robert L: Aging of the vascular wall and atherogenesis: role of the elastin-laminin receptor. Atherosclerosis 123:169–179, 1996.
4. Nagai Y, Metter EJ, Earley CJ, et al: Increased carotid artery intimal-medical thickness in asymptomatic older subjects with exercise-induced myocardial ischemia. Circulation (in press).
5. Celermajer DS, Sorensen KE, Spiegelhalter DJ, et al: Aging is associated with endothelial dysfunction in healthy men years before the age-related decline in women. J Am Coll Cardiol 24:471–476, 1994.
6. Fleg JL, Tzankoff SP, Lakatta EG: Age-related augmentation of plasma catecholamines during dynamic exercise in healthy males. J Appl Physiol 59:1033, 1985.
7. Borkan GA, Hults DC, Gerzof AF, et al: Age changes in body composition revealed by computed tomography. J Gerontol 38:673, 1983.
8. Meredith CN, Frontera WR, Fisher EC, et al: Peripheral effects of endurance training in young and old subjects. J Appl Physiol 66:2844, 1989.
9. Danziger RS, Tobin JD, Becker LC, et al: The age-associated decline in glomerular filtration in healthy normotensive volunteers: lack of relationship to cardiovascular performance. J Am Geriatr Soc 38:1127, 1990.
10. Nichols WW, O'Rourke MF, Avolio AP, et al: Age-related changes in left ventricular/arterial coupling. *In* Yin FCP (ed): Ventricular Vascular Coupling: Clinical, Physiological, and Engineering Aspects. p. 79. New York: Springer-Verlag, 1987.
11. Olivetti G, Melissari M, Capacco JM, Anversa P: Cardiomyopathy of the aging human heart. Myocyte loss and reactive cellular hypertrophy. Circ Res 68:1560, 1991.
12. Lakatta EG: Deficient neuroendocrine regulation of the cardiovascular system with advancing age in healthy humans [point of view]. Circulation 87:631–636, 1993.
13. Fleg JL, O'Connor FC, Gerstenblith G, et al: Impact of age on the cardiovascular response to dynamic upright exercise in healthy men and women. J Appl Physiol 78:890–900, 1995.
14. Fleg JL, Lakatta EG: Role of muscle loss in the age-associated reduction in VO_{2max}. J Appl Physiol 65:1147, 1988.
15. Fleg J, Schulman SP, Gerstenblith G, et al: Additive effects of age and silent myocardial ischemia on the left ventricular response to upright cycle exercise. J Appl Physiol 75:499–504, 1993.
16. Schulman SP, Lakatta EG, Fleg JL, et al: Age-related decline in left

ventricular filling at rest and exercise. Am J Physiol 263 (Heart Circ Physiol 32):H1932–H1938, 1992.
17. Schulman SP, Fleg JL, Busby-Whitehead J, et al: Continuum of cardiovascular performance across a broad range of fitness levels in healthy older men. Circulation 94:359–367, 1996.
18. Fleg JL, Schulman S, O'Connor F, et al: Effects of acute β-adrenergic receptor blockade on age-associated changes in cardiovascular performance during dynamic exercise. Circulation 90:2333–2341, 1994.
19. Stratton JR, Cerquerira MD, Schwartz RS, et al: Differences in cardiovascular responses to isoproterenol in relation to age and exercise training in healthy men. Circulation 86:504–512, 1992.
20. Elveback L, Lie JT: Continued high incidence of coronary artery disease at autopsy in Olmstead County, Minnesota, 1950–1979. Circulation 70:345, 1984.
21. Mukerji V, Holman A, Alpert M: The clinical description of angina pectoris in the elderly. Am Heart J 117:705, 1989.
22. Hlatky MA, Pryor DB, Harrell FE, et al: Factors affecting sensitivity and specificity of exercise electrocardiography. Am J Med 77:64, 1984.
23. Beller GA: Pharmacologic stress imaging. JAMA 265:633, 1991.
24. Verani MS, Mahmarian JJ, Hixson JB, et al: Diagnosis of coronary artery disease by controlled coronary vasodilation with adenosine and thallium-201 scintigraphy in patients unable to exercise. Circulation 82:80, 1990.
25. Fung AY, Gallagher KP, Buda AJ: The physiologic basis of dobutamine as compared with dipyridamole stress interventions in the assessment of critical coronary stenosis. Circulation 76:943, 1987.
26. Lam JYT, Chaitman BR, Glaenzer M, et al: Safety and diagnostic accuracy of dipyridamole-thallium imaging in the elderly. J Am Coll Cardiol 11:565, 1988.
27. Kennedy JW, Baxley WA, Bunnell IL, et al: Mortality related to cardiac catheterization and angiography. Cathet Cardiovasc Diagn 8:323, 1982.
28. Davis K, Kennedy JW, Kemp HG Jr, et al: Complications of coronary angiography from the Collaborative Study of Coronary Artery Surgery (CASS). Circulation 59:1105, 1979.
29. Jeroudi MO, Kleiman NS, Minor ST, et al: Percutaneous transluminal coronary angioplasty in octogenarians. Ann Intern Med 113:423, 1990.
30. Peterson ED, Jollis JG, Bebchuk DJ, et al: Changes in mortality after myocardial revascularization in the elderly. The National Medicare Experience. Ann Intern Med 121:919, 1994.
31. Thompson RC, Holmes DR, Gersh BJ, et al: Percutaneous transluminal coronary angioplasty in the elderly: early and long-term results. J Am Coll Cardiol 17:1245, 1991.
32. Gersh BJ, Kronmal RA, Schaff HV, et al: Long-term (5 year) results of coronary bypass surgery in patients 65 years old and older. A report from the Coronary Artery Surgery Study. Circulation 68 (suppl II): II-190, 1983.
33. Roach GW, Kanchuger M, Mangano CM, et al: Adverse cerebral outcomes after coronary bypass surgery. N Engl J Med 335:1857, 1996.
34. Gersh BJ, Kronman RA, Schaff HV, et al: Comparison of coronary artery bypass surgery and medical therapy in patients 65 years of age or older. N Engl J Med 313:217, 1985.
35. Mullany CJ, Darling GE, Pluth JR, et al: Early and late results after isolated coronary artery bypass surgery in 159 patients aged 80 years and older. Circulation 82 (suppl IV):IV-229, 1990.
36. European Working Party on High Blood Pressure in the Elderly: Mortality and morbidity results from the European Working Party on High Blood Pressure in the Elderly trial. Lancet 1:1349, 1985.
37. Staessen JA, Fagard R, Thijs L, et al: Randomized double-blind comparison of placebo and active treatment for older patients with isolated systolic hypertension. Lancet 350:757, 1997.
38. LaCroix AZ, Lang J, Scherr P, et al: Smoking and mortality among older men and women in three communities. N Engl J Med 324:1619, 1991.
39. Corti M-C, Guralnik JM, Salaive ME, et al: Clarifying the direct relation between total cholesterol levels and death from coronary heart disease in older persons. Ann Intern Med 126:753, 1997.
40. Lewis SJ, Moye LA, Sacks FM, et al: Effect of pravastatin on cardiovascular events in older patients with myocardial infarction and cholesterol levels in the average range. Results of the Cholesterol and Recurrent Events (CARE) Trial. Ann Intern Med 129:681, 1998.
41. Whitney EJ, Downs JR, Clearfield M, et al: Air Force/Texas coronary atherosclerosis prevention study: extending the benefit of primary prevention to healthy elderly men and women. Circulation 98:I-46, 1998.
42. Stampfer MJ, Colditz GA, Willett WC, et al: Postmenopausal estrogen therapy and cardiovascular disease. Ten year follow-up from the Nurses' Health Study. N Engl J Med 325:756, 1991.
43. Hulley S, Grady D, Bush T, et al: Randomized trial of estrogen plus progestin for secondary prevention of coronary artery disease in postmenopausal women. JAMA 280:605, 1998.
44. Bayer AJ, Chadha JS, Farag RR, Pathy MS: Changing presentation of myocardial infarction with increasing old age. J Am Geriatr Soc 34:263, 1986.
45. Solomon CG, Lee TH, Cook EF, et al: Comparison of clinical presentation of acute myocardial infarction in patients older than 65 years of age to younger patients: the Multicenter Chest Pain Study. Am J Cardiol 63:772, 1989.
46. Gruppo Italiano per lo Studio della Streptochinasi nell'Infarto Miocardico (GISSI): effectiveness of intravenous thrombolytic therapy in acute myocardial infarction. Lancet 1:397, 1986.
47. Wilcox RG, Olsson CG, Skene AM, et al: Trial of tissue plasminogen activator for mortality reduction in acute myocardial infarction. Lancet 2:525, 1988.
48. Aguirre FV, McMahon RP, Mueller H, et al: Impact of age on clinical outcome and postlytic management strategies in patients treated with intravenous thrombolytic therapy. Results from the TIMI II Study. Circulation 90:78, 1994.
49. Maggioni AP, Maseri A, Fresco C, et al: Age-related increase in mortality among patients with first myocardial infarctions treated with thrombolysis. N Engl J Med 329:1442, 1993.
50. Smith SC, Gilpin E, Ahnve S, et al: Outlook after acute myocardial infarction in the very elderly compared with that in patients aged 65 to 75 years. J Am Coll Cardiol 16:784, 1990.
51. Lew AS, Hod H, Cercek B, et al: Mortality and morbidity rates of patients older and younger than 75 years with acute myocardial infarction treated with intravenous streptokinase. Am J Cardiol 59:1, 1987.
52. Anderson JL, Karagounis L, Allen AN, et al: Older age and elevated blood pressure are risk factors for intracerebral hemorrhage after thrombolysis. Am J Cardiol 68:166, 1991.
53. Gunnar RM, Bourdillon PD, Dixon DW, et al, for the ACC/AHA Task Force Subcommittee: guidelines for the early management of patients with acute myocardial infarction. J Am Coll Cardiol 16:249, 1990.
54. Sherry S, Marder V: Mistaken guidelines for thrombolytic therapy of acute myocardial infarction in the elderly. J Am Coll Cardiol 17:1237, 1991.
55. Grines CL, Browne KF, Marco J, et al: A comparison of immediate angioplasty with thrombolytic therapy for acute myocardial infarction. N Engl J Med 328:673, 1993.
56. Beta Blocker Heart Attack Trial Research Group: A randomized trial of propranolol in patients with acute myocardial infarction. I. Mortality results. JAMA 247:1707, 1982.
57. Hjalmarson A, Elmpeldt D, Herlitz J, et al: Effect on mortality of metoprolol in acute myocardial infarction. A double-blind randomized trial. Lancet 2:823, 1981.
58. The Norwegian Multicentre Study Group: Timolol-induced reduction in mortality and reinfarction in patients surviving acute myocardial infarction. N Engl J Med 304:801, 1981.
59. Soumerai SB, McLaughlin TJ, Spiegelman D, et al: Adverse outcomes of underuse of beta-blockers in elderly survivors of acute myocardial infarction. JAMA 277:115, 1997.
60. Krumholz HM, Radford MJ, Ellerback EF, et al: Aspirin for secondary prevention after acute myocardial infarction in the elderly: prescribed use and outcomes. Ann Intern Med 124:292, 1996.
61. Sixty Plus Reinfarction Study Research Group: A double-blind trial to assess long-term oral anticoagulant therapy in elderly patients after myocardial infarction. Lancet 2:990, 1980.
62. Pfeffer MA, Braunwald E, Moye LA, et al: Effect of captopril on mortality and morbidity in patients with left ventricular dysfunction after myocardial infarction. N Engl J Med 327:669, 1992.
63. The Cardiac Arrhythmia Suppression Trial (CAST) Investigators: Preliminary report: effect of encainide and flecainide on mortality in a randomized trial of arrhythmia suppression post myocardial infarction. N Engl J Med 321:406, 1989.
64. Moss AJ, Hall J, Canom DS, et al: Improved survival with an

implanted defibrillator in patients with coronary disease at high risk for ventricular arrhythmia. N Engl J Med 335:1933, 1996.
65. The Sixth Report of the Joint National Committee on Prevention, Detection, Evaluation, and Treatment of High Blood Pressure. NIH Publication No. 98-4080. Bethesda, MD: National Institutes of Health, National Heart, Lung, and Blood Institute, National High Blood Pressure Education Program, 1997.
66. Management Committee of the Australian Therapeutic Trial in Mild Hypertension: treatment of mild hypertension in the elderly. Med J Aust 2:398, 1981.
67. SHEP Cooperative Research Group: Prevention of stroke by antihypertensive drug treatment in older persons with isolated systolic hypertension. JAMA 265:3255, 1991.
68. Whelton PK, Appel LJ, Applegate WB, et al: Sodium reduction and weight loss in the treatment of hypertension in older persons: a randomized controlled trial of nonpharmacologic interventions in the elderly. JAMA 279:839, 1998.
69. Schulman SP, Weiss JL, Becker LC, et al: The effects of antihypertensive therapy on left ventricular mass in elderly patients. N Engl J Med 322:1350, 1990.
70. Fleg JL, Kennedy HL: Cardiac arrhythmias in a healthy elderly population: detection by 24 hour ambulatory electrocardiography. Chest 81:302, 1982.
71. Wajngarten M, Grupi C, Bellotti GM, et al: Frequency and significance of cardiac rhythm disturbances in healthy elderly individuals. J Electrocardiol 23:171, 1990.
72. Ingerslev J, Bjerregaard P: Prevalence and prognostic significance of cardiac arrhythmias detected by ambulatory electrocardiography in subjects 85 years of age. Eur Heart J 7:570, 1986.
73. Kantelip JP, Sage E, Duchene-Marullaz P: Findings on ambulatory electrocardiographic monitoring in subjects older than 80 years. Am J Cardiol 57:398, 1986.
74. Wolf PA, Abbott RD, Kannel WB: Atrial fibrillation: a major contributor to stroke in the elderly. Arch Intern Med 147:1561, 1987.
75. Stroke Prevention in Atrial Fibrillation Investigators: Predictors of thromboembolism in atrial fibrillation: clinical features of patients at risk. Ann Intern Med 116:1, 1992.
76. Petersen P, Godtfredsen J, Boysen G, et al: Placebo-controlled, randomized trial of warfarin and aspirin for prevention of thromboembolic complications in chronic atrial fibrillation. Lancet 1:175, 1989.
77. Boston Area Anticoagulation Trial for Atrial Fibrillation Investigators: the effect of low-dose warfarin on the risk of stroke in patients with nonrheumatic atrial fibrillation. N Engl J Med 323:1505, 1990.
78. Preliminary report of the Stroke Prevention in Atrial Fibrillation Study: special report. N Engl J Med 322:863, 1990.
79. The European Atrial Fibrillation Trial Study Group: Optimal oral anticoagulant therapy in patients with nonrheumatic atrial fibrillation and recent cerebral ischemia. N Engl J Med 333:5, 1995.
80. Coplen SE, Antman EM, Berlin JA, et al: Efficacy and safety of quinidine therapy for maintenance of sinus rhythm after cardioversion. Circulation 82:1106, 1990.
81. Morganroth J, Goin JE: Quinidine-related mortality in the short- to medium-term treatment of ventricular arrhythmias: a meta-analysis. Circulation 84:1977, 1991.
82. Anderson JL: Reassessment of benefit-risk ratio and treatment algorithms for antiarrhythmic drug therapy after the Cardiac Arrhythmia Suppression Trial. J Clin Pharmacol 30:981, 1990.
83. Burkart F, Pfisterer M, Kiowski W, et al: Effect of antiarrhythmic therapy on mortality in survivors of myocardial infarction with asymptomatic complex ventricular arrhythmias: Basel Antiarrhythmic Study of Infarct Survival (BASIS). J Am Coll Cardiol 16:1711, 1990.
84. Epstein LM, Chiesa N, Wong MN, et al: Radiofrequency catheter ablation in the treatment of supraventricular tachycardia in the elderly. J Am Coll Cardiol. 23:1356, 1994.
85. Lamas GA, Pashos CL, Normand S-LT, McNeil B: Permanent pacemaker selection and subsequent survival in elderly Medicare pacemaker recipients. Circulation 91:1063, 1995.
86. Parmley WW: Pathophysiology and current therapy of congestive heart failure. J Am Coll Cardiol 13:771, 1989.
87. The CONSENSUS Trial Study Group: Effects of enalapril on mortality in severe congestive heart failure. N Engl J Med 316:1429, 1987.
88. Pitt B, Segal R, Martinez FA, et al: Randomized trial of losartan versus captopril in patients over 65 with heart failure (Evaluation of Losartan in the Elderly Study, ELITE). Lancet 349:747, 1997.
89. Rich MW, Beckham V, Wittenberg C, et al: A multidisciplinary intervention to prevent the readmission of elderly patients with congestive heart failure. N Engl J Med 333:1190, 1995.

CHAPTER 110

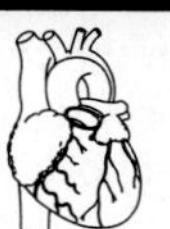

PREGNANCY AND THE HEART

Susan D. Mueller and James T. Willerson

MATERNAL PHYSIOLOGY
Hematologic and Blood Volume Changes
Cardiac Output
Heart Rate
Blood Pressure
Mechanics of a Gravid Uterus
Exercise Response
Hemodynamics of Labor and Delivery
Postpartum Changes
Physiology of Multiple Fetuses
CARDIAC EVALUATION
Cardiac Examination
Noninvasive Testing
Invasive Testing
APPROACH TO CLINICAL PROBLEMS
Signs of Fetal Distress
Hypotension
Cardiac Arrest
Chest Pain
Venous Emergencies
Peripheral Edema and Pulmonary Rales
Fever and Endocarditis
Antibiotic Prophylaxis
Valve Prosthesis
Anticoagulation
RHYTHM DISTURBANCES
Arrhythmias
Sinus Tachycardia
Atrial Flutter or Fibrillation
Supraventricular Tachycardia
Wolff-Parkinson-White Syndrome
Ventricular Arrhythmia
Antiarrhythmic Agents
Heart Block
Cardioversion
Pacemaker
CORONARY ARTERY DISEASE
Risk Factors
Management and Evaluation
HYPERTENSION
Antihypertensive Agents
PULMONARY HYPERTENSION
Primary Pulmonary Hypertension
Secondary Pulmonary Hypertension
AORTIC DISEASE
Aortic Dissection
Marfan's Syndrome
Takayasu's Arteritis
Mycotic Aneurysms
COLLAGEN VASCULAR DISEASE
Systemic Lupus Erythematosus and Anti-Ro Antibody
Dermatomyositis
PERICARDITIS
MYOCARDITIS AND CARDIOMYOPATHY
Myocarditis
Peripartum Cardiomyopathy
Hypertrophic Obstructive Cardiomyopathy or Idiopathic Hypertrophic Subaortic Stenosis
VALVULAR HEART DISEASE
Mitral Valve Prolapse
Acute Rheumatic Fever
Mitral Stenosis
Mitral Regurgitation
Aortic Stenosis
Aortic Regurgitation
Pulmonary Valvular Lesions
Tricuspid Valvular Lesions
CONGENITAL HEART DISEASE
Inheritance
Antibiotic Prophylaxis
Atrial Septal Defect
Ventricular Septal Defect
Patient Ductus Arteriosus
Congenital Aortic Valvular Disease
Coarctation of the Aorta
Tetralogy of Fallot
Ebstein's Anomaly
Eisenmenger's Syndrome
Complex Cyanotic Lesions
CARDIAC SURGERY DURING PREGNANCY
Cardiopulmonary Bypass
Analgesic and Anesthetic Agents
CARDIOVASCULAR DRUGS: PREGNANCY AND LACTATION
Fetal Effects
Lactation
Cardiac Glycosides
Treatment of Arrhythmias
Neonatal Ventricular Tachycardia
Diuretic Agents
Organic Nitrates
Angiotensin-Converting Enzyme Inhibitors
Sodium Nitroprusside
Calcium Channel Antagonists
Beta-Adrenoceptor–Blocking Agents
PREGNANCY AND PATIENTS WITH HEREDITARY LONG QT SYNDROME
OBSTETRIC DRUGS WITH CARDIOVASCULAR EFFECTS

Pregnancy causes dramatic and usually reversible changes in the female cardiovascular system. Maternal heart disease occurs in about 2 percent of pregnancies and is the most important nonobstetric cause of death during pregnancy.[1] During pregnancy, serious disorders may develop that are not presently predictable or preventable, including pulmonary hypertension, peripartum cardiomyopathy, and aortic, carotid, or coronary artery dissection. Unique cardiac and vascular diseases may occur in association with pregnancy, and some more common conditions are associated with a greater risk of complications or death. Underlying cardiovascular or endocrine problems may not allow normal physiologic adaptations, resulting in danger to the mother and fetus.

The dramatic adaptations in cardiac and vascular function during pregnancy that protect the mother from stress include changes in blood pressure, sudden decreases in venous return to the heart, blood loss, and the higher oxygen and workload demands of pregnancy, labor, and delivery. Blood must be pumped through three (or more in the case of multiple conceptions) interconnected circulations: maternal, placental, and fetal. Normally, the blood volume increases by 130 to 150 percent of nonpregnancy values and cardiac output increases by up to 50 percent soon after conception. Uterine arterial blood flow rises to approximately 20 percent cardiac output during pregnancy to meet the needs of the growing fetus. Even after these marked alterations in physiology and anatomy, the maternal system returns to nonpregnancy conditions within weeks after delivery. The physical examination, hemodynamics, exercise response, and respiratory physiology adjust to pregnancy, and findings must be interpreted in the context of the patient's baseline state and the stage of pregnancy.

The fetus and placenta themselves are associated with unique risks to the mother, such as placental vascular thrombosis or ischemia causing pregnancy-induced hypertension and amniotic fluid embolism. Drugs administered to the mother may pose a hazard for the fetus, because some drugs cross the placental barrier. This may be useful in treating fetal cardiac disease, such as arrhythmia, in utero. The ability to perform certain diagnostic tests in the mother is also limited because of concerns about radiation exposure to the fetus.

Severe valvular defects in the mother are best managed by correction before pregnancy. However, surgical repair during pregnancy may be necessary, because fetal mortality rates can exceed 50 percent in women with severe, untreated congenital heart disease.[2] Cardiopulmonary bypass has been successfully performed in pregnant patients since 1958, when Leyse and associates[3] performed the first such procedure. The effects of anesthesia, mechanical ventilation, and hypothermia require special monitoring and management to minimize the risk of fetal death.

Emergencies may occur, including myocardial infarction (MI), aortic dissection, pulmonary or amniotic fluid embolism, and arrhythmias. Evaluation and treatment are a special challenge. Cardiopulmonary resuscitation, when necessary, is performed with standard resuscitative measures, but there are two critical differences. Special efforts must be made to displace the gravid uterus from abdominal vessels that may be compressed, thus lowering cardiac output, and there must be urgent consideration of emergency cesarean section to save the fetus.

The demographics of pregnant women are changing as more women are delaying pregnancy. This may increase the risk for existing atherosclerosis or hypertension in the mother. There is an increased use by women of cocaine, intravenous drugs, alcohol, and cigarettes, which places the cardiovascular system at risk for related diseases. In addition, more women who have undergone corrective surgery for valvular or congenital heart conditions are surviving to puberty and becoming pregnant. Women once believed to be at too high a risk to tolerate pregnancy have safely delivered infants.

MATERNAL PHYSIOLOGY

Pregnancy simulates three simultaneous stressors on the maternal cardiovascular system

1. An internal workload similar to that of endurance exercise
2. An altered vasculature similar to that associated with arteriovenous fistula
3. A hemodynamic state similar to that found with high-output cardiac failure

In response, anatomic changes occur, such as enlargement of the heart, expansion of intravascular volume, and the opening of new vascular beds, which result in alterations in the pattern of blood flow. There may be changes in responsiveness of the vascular beds and of endothelium-derived factors of vasoactive eicosanoids in pregnancy.[4, 5] These changes represent an attempt to meet the increased end-organ demands of the mother and developing fetus for oxygen, nutrients, and waste product removal. In addition, there is a shift of the oxygen hemoglobin dissociation curve that facilitates dissociation and placental transfer of oxygen.[6]

Hematologic and Blood Volume Changes

Normally, hematologic and body water changes occur in response to hormonal and other mediator signals (Fig. 110–1). Estrogen may stimulate sodium reabsorption, and progesterone has a relaxing effect on venous smooth muscle, affecting venomotor tone and elasticity of venous walls. Maternal blood volume is increased by approximately 40 percent at term, with the most rapid increase taking place during the first half of pregnancy. This is initially due to plasma volume increases, followed by an increase in red cell mass (Fig. 110–2).[7, 8] There is an accumulation of sodium (500 to 900 mEq) and total body water (6 to 8 L), most of which is extracellular, due to a reduced colloid osmotic pressure and lower albumin concentrations.[9] An increase in atrial natriuretic factor has been found even in normotensive pregnancies, which rises in the first few days after delivery and promotes fluid diuresis.[10, 11] Despite increased erythropoiesis, hemoglobin, hematocrit, and blood viscosity decrease slightly during pregnancy.[12] Serum levels of several coagulation factors are increased, including fibrinogen and plasminogen, and a slight shortening of the prothrombin time and partial thromboplastin time occurs as pregnancy progresses.[13]

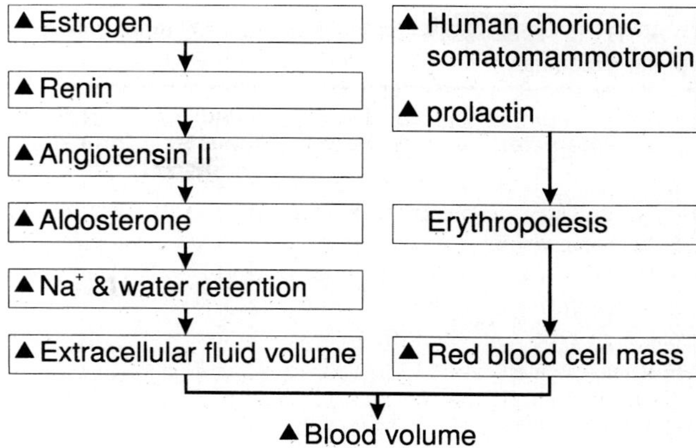

FIGURE 110–1 The mechanisms leading to hypervolemia during pregnancy are multiple, including increased levels of steroid hormones of pregnancy and volume mediators. Plasma renin levels are elevated, and the production of renin is expanded to include the kidneys, uterus, and liver. The placenta may produce growth hormone–like substances, and atrial natriuretic factor is increased in the last trimester of pregnancy in some patients. (From Elkayam U, Gleicher N: Hemodynamics and cardiac function during normal pregnancy and the puerperium. *In* Cardiac Problems in Pregnancy, 2nd ed. pp. 5–24. Copyright © 1990. Reprinted by permission of Wiley-Liss, Inc., a division of John Wiley & Sons, Inc.)

There have been reports of decreases in platelet levels during pregnancy, and platelets may also have a shorter half-life.[14, 15]

Cardiac Output

Cardiac output increases markedly during pregnancy, eventually reaching a level 30 to 50 percent higher than the nonpregnant state. The increase in cardiac output begins around the fifth week of gestation and peaks between the mid-second or third trimester (weeks 20 to 24). Cardiac output is maintained at that level until parturition (see Fig. 110–2). Initially, stroke volume (SV) is the major factor causing the increase in cardiac output, but as pregnancy progresses, an increased heart rate (HR) becomes the more predominant factor (Table 110–1).[16]

Redistribution of the greatly expanded blood volume occurs. Uterine blood flow increases by about 20 percent as the uterine muscle enlarges, and peripheral vascular resistance varies to change in flow patterns (Fig. 110–3). If hypoxia, hypotension, or toxemia occurs, the maternal cardiovascular system is more sensitive to the vasoconstrictive effects of systemic catecholamines.[17, 18]

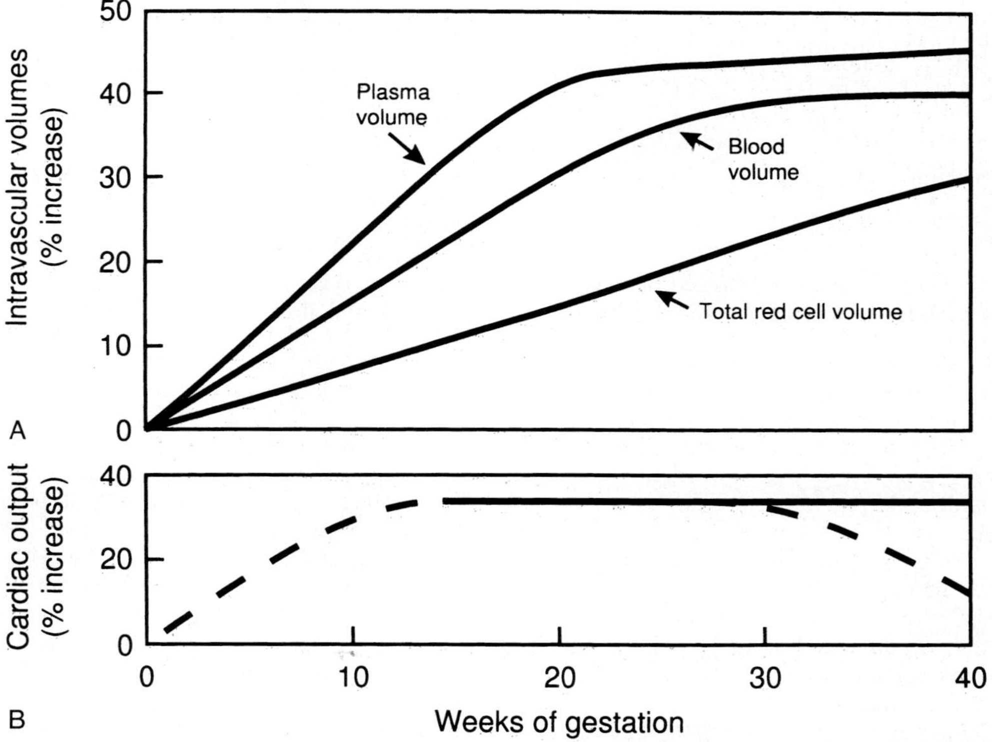

FIGURE 110–2 The timing of the 40 to 50 percent increase in blood volume during pregnancy, peaking at about week 30. **A,** Blood volume rises early in pregnancy owing to an increase in plasma volume, followed by an increase in red blood cell mass. **B,** These increases are shown in relation to the rise in cardiac output, which reaches values of 40 percent above nonpregnant levels by week 20 of pregnancy. *Dashed line* represents the decrease in cardiac output possible due to decreased venous return in the supine position after the 30th week of gestation. (**A** and **B,** From Chatterjee K, Chitlin MD, Karliner J, et al: Cardiology: An Illustrated Text/Reference. Philadelphia: Grower Medical, 1991.)

TABLE 110–1 Cardiocirculatory Changes During Normal Pregnancy

Parameter	1st Trimester	2nd Trimester	3rd Trimester
Blood volume	↑	↑ ↑	↑ ↑ ↑
Cardiac output	↑	↑ ↑ ↑	↑ ↑
Stroke volume	↑	↑ ↑ ↑	↔ or ↓
Heart rate	↑	↑ ↑	↑ ↑ ↑
Systolic blood pressure	↔	↓	↔
Diastolic blood pressure	↓	↓ ↓	↔
Pulse pressure	↑	↑ ↑	↔
Systemic vascular resistance	↓	↓ ↓ ↓	↓ ↓
Oxygen consumption	↔ or ↑	↑ ↑	↑ ↑ ↑
Left ventricular volume	↔	↑	↑
Left ventricular systolic function	↔	↔	↔

Key: ↔, no change compared with nonpregnant level; ↑, small increase; ↑ ↑, moderate increase; ↑ ↑ ↑, large increase; ↓, small decrease; ↓ ↓, moderate decrease; ↓ ↓ ↓, large decrease.

From Elkayam U, Gleicher N: Hemodynamics and cardiac function during normal pregnancy and the puerperium. *In* Cardiac Problems in Pregnancy. 2nd ed. pp. 5–24. Copyright © 1990. Reprinted by permission of Wiley-Liss, Inc., a division of John Wiley & Sons, Inc.

Heart Rate

Heart rate, measured in the sitting, standing, or supine position, increases progressively during pregnancy, peaking and becoming stable during the third trimester, usually by about week 32. There is an average rise of 10 to 20 beats/min, with mean values ranging from 78 to 89 beats/min.[19] By the third trimester, the supine HR is greater than that in the left lateral recumbent position. This increased HR is beneficial in maintaining cardiac output. The SV returns to nonpregnant values near the end of pregnancy.[19] Twin pregnancies lead to an earlier rise in maternal HR, with increases of as much as 40 percent above baseline near term.[20]

Blood Pressure

Blood pressure normally remains unchanged or may even decrease slightly despite the increased cardiac output (Fig. 110–4).[21] Peripheral vascular resistance and blood pressure fall during the second trimester when uteroplacental mass is growing most rapidly. Systemic arterial pressure falls during the first trimester, reaches a low in mid-pregnancy, and returns to normal prepregnancy levels before term. Pulse pressure widens because diastolic blood pressure falls more dramatically than systolic blood pressure.[22] Systemic vasodilatation occurs, probably as a result of increased levels of gestational hormones such as progesterone, circulating prostaglandins, and natriuretic factors that foster relaxation of tubular structures, all in an environment of increased heat production from the developing fetus and an enlarged uterus with a low-resistance circulation.[23, 24]

Mechanics of a Gravid Uterus

Body position substantially affects cardiac output and thus uteroplacental blood flow, particularly in the supine position, during the third trimester.[25] The effect is so significant that a hypotensive pregnant patient should not be left supine. During the second half of pregnancy, the uterus expands beyond the pelvis. Mechanical compression of the iliac veins and arteries and the inferior vena cava against the spine decreases venous return to the heart and results in development of collateral paravertebral circulation to drain the lower extremities (Fig. 110–5).[26] There also is aortoiliac artery compression late in pregnancy that may have significant effects on uteroplacental perfusion, especially during low-flow states.[27] Uterine blood flow is about 3 percent of cardiac output during the first trimester and increases to between 10 and 20 percent by the third trimester.[23] At term, when a supine patient changes position to the lateral recumbent position, a 25 percent increase in cardiac output may occur. A supine hypotensive syndrome may develop due to compression of the inferior vena cava and pelvic veins, which can cause sequestration of up to 30 percent of blood volume.[28] During resuscitation and operative procedures, the supine position should be avoided by placing a wedge or blanket beneath the right hip to rotate the body slightly to the left; this may help maintain uterine blood flow. There also is a mechanical effect on

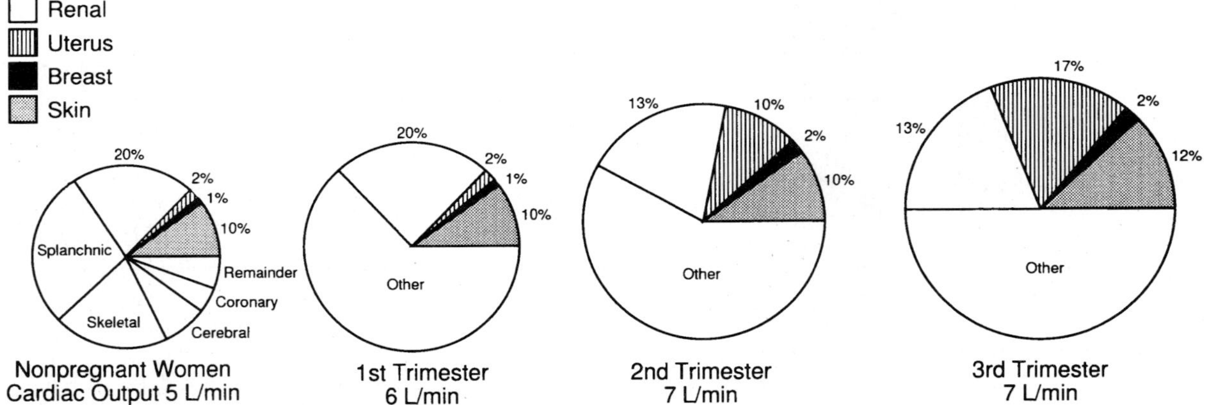

FIGURE 110–3 Percentage of total cardiac output flowing to organs in nonpregnant and pregnant women in each trimester of pregnancy. The increases in blood flow to the skin and breast may be responsible for the malar flush of pregnancy and a mammary souffle heard on auscultation. (From Burrow GN, Ferris T: Medical Complications During Pregnancy. 3rd ed. Philadelphia: WB Saunders, 1988.)

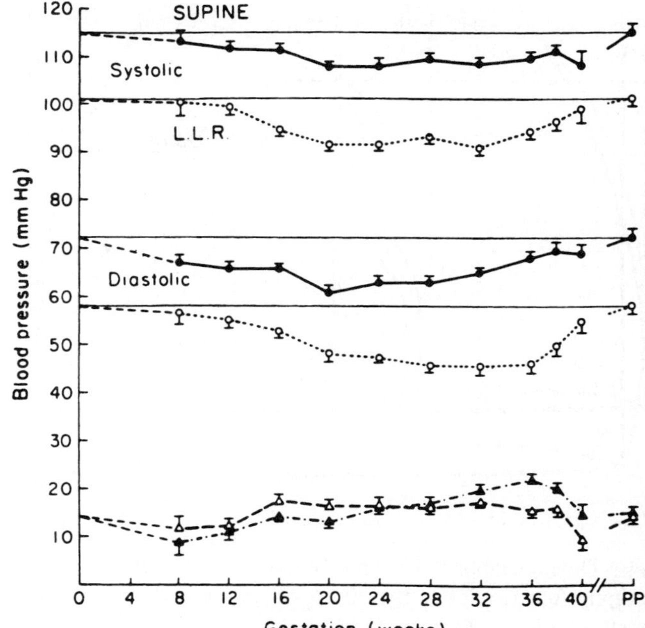

FIGURE 110–4 Systolic and diastolic pressure readings in the supine and left lateral recumbent (LLR) positions from 8 weeks of pregnancy to the postpartum (PP) period. **Bottom,** Systolic pressure readings *(open triangles)* and diastolic pressures *(solid triangles)* when the pregnant woman changes position from the LLR to the supine position. The systolic pressures show a greater change in the first 24 weeks of pregnancy, whereas the diastolic pressures are more dramatically affected after this. (From Creasy RK, Resnik R: Maternal-Fetal Medicine: Principles and Practice, 2nd ed. Philadelphia: WB Saunders, 1989.)

the diaphragm and lungs, with compression of the thoracic cavity causing changes on the chest radiograph and the cardiac examination (Fig. 110–6).[29]

Exercise Response

At rest, the pregnant patient usually has a sinus tachycardia, which helps to maintain the higher cardiac output that occurs at any given workload.[30] There is an increase in maternal oxygen consumption to approximately 20 percent above that of the nonpregnant state.[31] During the third trimester, the effect of the enlarged heart and the gravid uterus in decreasing venous return in certain positions limits the normal SV response to exercise.[32] The maximal cardiac output is reached at lower levels of exercise during pregnancy, and increases in response to exercise are limited as pregnancy progresses.[32]

During the third trimester, normal subjects may experience a 25 percent decrease in uterine blood flow during mild exercise, which may cause fetal hypoxia and episodic bradycardia.[33] Strenuous exercise during pregnancy is not recommended. The usual effect of training is not seen during pregnancy but returns within weeks after delivery (Fig. 110–7).[34]

Hemodynamics of Labor and Delivery

Delivery has been described as a state of physiologic hemorrhage, with an average blood loss of approximately 500

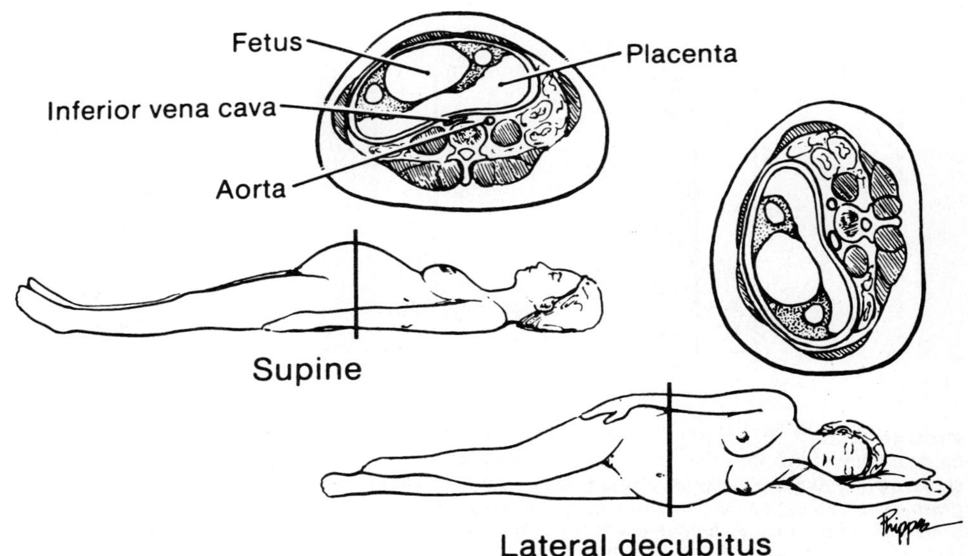

FIGURE 110–5 The gravid uterus may cause compression of abdominal vessels in the supine position. The inferior vena cava may be compressed, decreasing venous return to the heart. Aortic compression may be sufficiently severe to cause a supine hypotensive syndrome and a decrease in uteroplacental perfusion. (From Lee RV, Mezzadri FC: Cardiopulmonary resuscitation of pregnant women. *In* Elkayam U, Gleicher N [eds]: Cardiac Problems in Pregnancy. 2nd ed. pp. 307–319. Copyright © 1990. Reprinted by permission of Wiley-Liss, Inc., a division of John Wiley & Sons, Inc.)

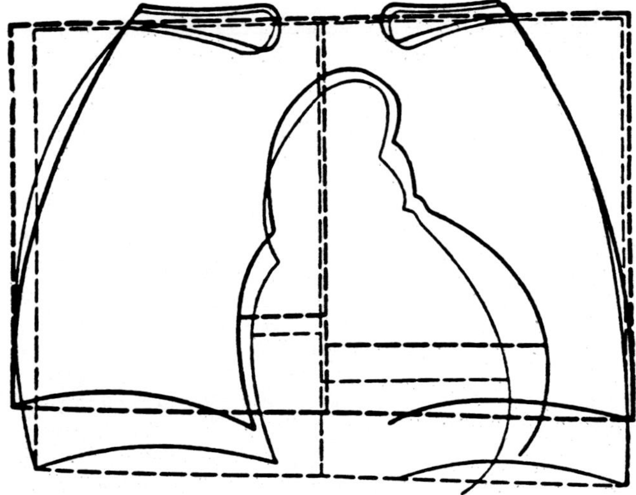

FIGURE 110–6 During pregnancy, there is an elevation of the diaphragm, causing a change in the cardiac outline seen on chest x-ray and on physical findings. The *heavy lines* represent the pregnant state. The *lighter lines* represent the nonpregnant state. (From Klaften E, Palugyay J: Vergleichende Untersuchungen über Lage and Ausdehnung von Herz und Lunge in der Schwanger schaft und im Wochenblatt, Arch Gynaekol 131:347, 1927.)

ml. During labor, HR and blood pressure rise; cardiac output may increase by 30 to 60 percent during uterine contractions, with a cumulative increase between contractions, probably resulting from increased venous return of blood squeezed from the uterus (Table 110–2).[35] The rise in blood pressure is most marked during the second stage of labor. There is an increase in oxygen consumption of up to three times the normal level.

Hemodynamic changes are less pronounced in the left lateral recumbent position and are affected by the type of anesthesia and analgesia used. Caudal and local anesthesia usually do not alter hemodynamic variables and may be safer in patients with heart disease.[36] There is a less dramatic change in patients who deliver by cesarean section, depending on the type of anesthesia used. Marked fluctuations are seen with subarachnoid block anesthesia; smaller

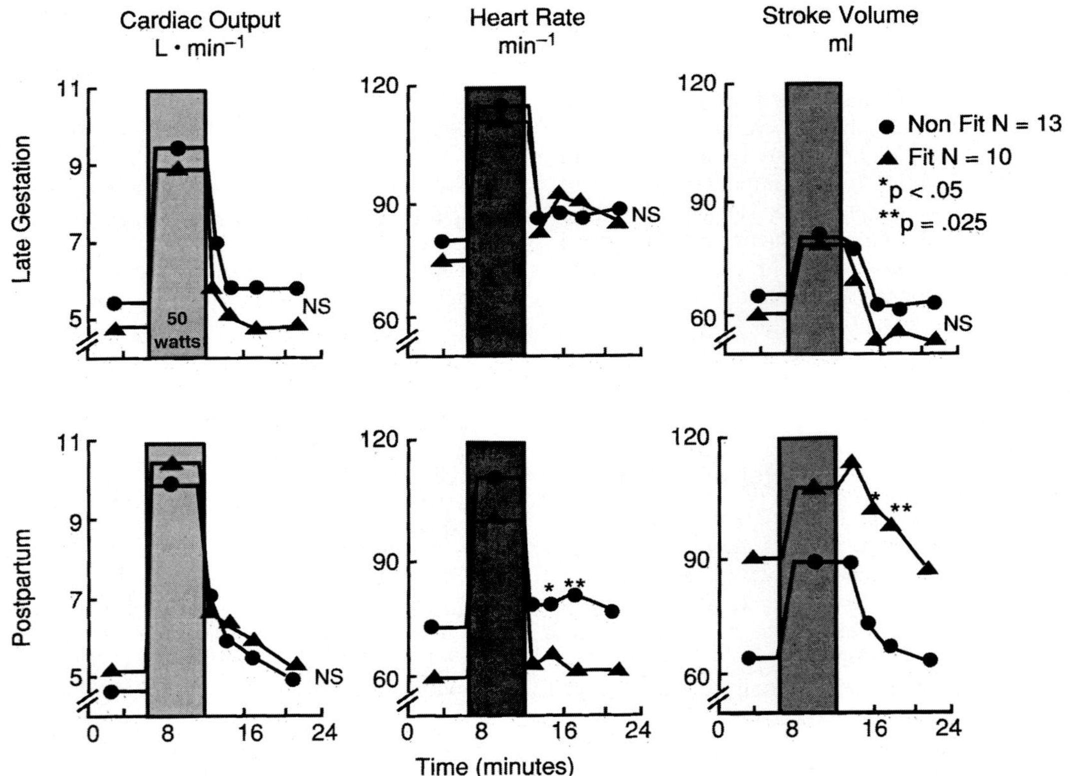

FIGURE 110–7 The usual effect of training is not seen during pregnancy but returns after delivery. This is shown by heart rate, cardiac output, and stroke volume measurements. Nonpregnant, physically trained individuals usually respond to exercise with a greater stroke volume and a smaller increase in heart rate than do untrained individuals. Pregnancy causes an increase in cardiac output at any given level of exercise, and the maximum is reached at lower levels of exercise during pregnancy. Stroke volume response may be limited by a decrease in venous return from vena caval obstruction by the gravid uterus in late gestation. (From Burrow GN, and Ferris T: Medical Complications During Pregnancy. 3rd ed. Philadelphia: WB Saunders, 1988.)

TABLE 110–2 Cardiocirculatory Effects of Uterine Contraction

Parameter	Change	Comments
Blood volume	↑	300–500 ml
Cardiac output	↑	30–60% with cumulative increase between contractions
Heart rate	↑ ↓	Variable responses
Blood pressure	↑	Significant rise of both systolic and diastolic blood pressures, return to baseline between contractions
Peripheral resistance	↔	
Oxygen consumption	↑	Increased gradually to average of 100%

Key: ↑, increase; ↓, decrease; ↔, no significant change.
Hemodynamic effects of uterine contractions are less pronounced in lateral recumbency than in the supine position.
From Elkayam U, Gleicher N: Hemodynamics and cardiac function during normal pregnancy and the puerperium. *In* Cardiac Problems in Pregnancy. 2nd ed. pp. 5–24. Copyright © 1990. Reprinted by permission of Wiley-Liss, Inc., a division of John Wiley & Sons, Inc.

fluctuations occur with thiopental, nitrous oxide, and succinylcholine and with epidural anesthesia without epinephrine.[37–39]

Postpartum Changes

Immediately after delivery, cardiac output may be increased by 60 to 80 percent, depending on the type of anesthesia used, but output decreases soon thereafter. There is an increase in venous return as soon as the fetus is delivered, thus relieving caval compression. Autotransfusion of blood from the uterus into the systemic circulation occurs, increasing cardiac preload. There is a reduction in HR within hours after delivery, causing a decrease in cardiac output. Cardiac output usually falls to prepregnancy levels within 24 hours after delivery but may remain elevated for a few weeks.[35]

Physiology of Multiple Fetuses

More widespread use of fertility agents has raised the incidence of multiple fetuses. The uterus is larger in a multiple pregnancy, causing more mechanical effects, including compression and displacement of thoracic and abdominal contents. There are greater alterations in maternal physiology with multiple fetuses, including a more pronounced increase in HR. The blood volume increases by 50 to 60 percent, or 500 ml more with twin fetuses than in a single pregnancy.[40] The average blood loss is 935 ml with twins, almost 500 ml more than with a single pregnancy.[41] Cardiac output is increased over single pregnancies, whereas the end-diastolic dimensions are approximately the same.[42] During the third trimester, the increased cardiac output is due to increases in HR and SV, whereas in single pregnancy, it is due to HR effects primarily by term. The risk for serious maternal complications is greater because of the increased stress. Pregnancy-induced hypertension is more prevalent and is associated with more frequent complications.

CARDIAC EVALUATION

The normal adaptations to pregnancy lead to subjective symptoms, changes in the physical examination, and altered diagnostic test results that may mimic or mask cardiac disease. Anatomic alterations occur, such as heart enlargement with an increase in left ventricular (LV) end-diastolic volume. Dynamics also change, with a constant variation in preload and afterload. Despite these changes, ejection fraction is not usually changed during pregnancy.[43] Even women with normal pregnancies often have symptoms of fatigue, decreased exercise capacity, palpitations, orthopnea, dyspnea, lightheadedness, and hyperventilation (Table 110–3).[44] It is important to be aware both of the signs and symptoms of normal pregnancy and of those that may herald underlying heart or vascular disease (Table 110–4).

Cardiac Examination

Vasculature

The jugular veins may be distended by an increase in blood volume. Venous vascular beds are more prominent, especially in the lower extremities, even during the first trimester, before caval compression by the enlarged uterus

TABLE 110–3 Cardiac Symptoms and Findings During Normal Pregnancy

Symptoms

Decreased exercise capacity
Tiredness
Dyspnea
Orthopnea
Lightheadedness
Syncope

Physical Findings

Inspection

Hyperventilation
Peripheral edema
Distended neck veins with prominent A and V waves and brisk x and y descents
Capillary pulsation

Precordial Palpation

Brisk, diffuse, and displaced left ventricular impulse
Palpable right ventricular impulse
Palpable pulmonary trunk impulse

Auscultation

Pulmonary rales
Increased first heart sound with exaggerated splitting
Persistent splitting of second heart sound
Early and midsystolic ejection-type murmurs at the lower left sternal edge and/or over the pulmonary area
Continuous murmurs (cervical venous hum, mammary souffle)
Diastolic murmurs

From Elkayam U, Gleicher N: Changes in cardiac findings during normal pregnancy. *In* Cardiac Problems in Pregnancy. 2nd ed. pp. 31–40. Copyright © 1990. Reprinted by permission of Wiley-Liss, Inc., a division of John Wiley & Sons, Inc.

TABLE 110-4 Indicators of Heart Disease During Pregnancy

Symptoms
Severe or progressive dyspnea
Progressive orthopnea
Paroxysmal nocturnal dyspnea
Hemoptysis
Syncope with exertion
Chest pain related to effort or emotion
Signs
Cyanosis
Clubbing
Persistent neck vein distention
A systolic murmur greater than grade I/VI in intensity
Diastolic murmur
Cardiomegaly, general or localized
A split second sound, persisting unchanged during expiration
Criteria for pulmonary hypertension
Left parasternal lift
Loud P_2

From Burrow GN: Medical complications during pregnancy. 3rd ed. Philadelphia: WB Saunders, 1988.

occurs. Venous distensibility increases in the legs, with compliance being highest in the second trimester; this is similar to the effects seen in women who are taking progestin-based oral contraceptives. The antecubital venous pressure remains unchanged (Fig. 110–8). Arterial pulsations are usually full and rapidly collapsing.

Precordium

The precordium is usually active, with a palpable LV impulse that is usually displaced to the left in later pregnancy. A palpable pulmonary artery and right ventricular (RV) impulse are usually present. On auscultation, an increased first sound with exaggerated splitting is sometimes noted. The second heart sound may be increased late in pregnancy and persistently but not fixed split in the left lateral position. Third and fourth heart sounds have been noted in some normal pregnant women but are usually considered abnormal.[45, 46]

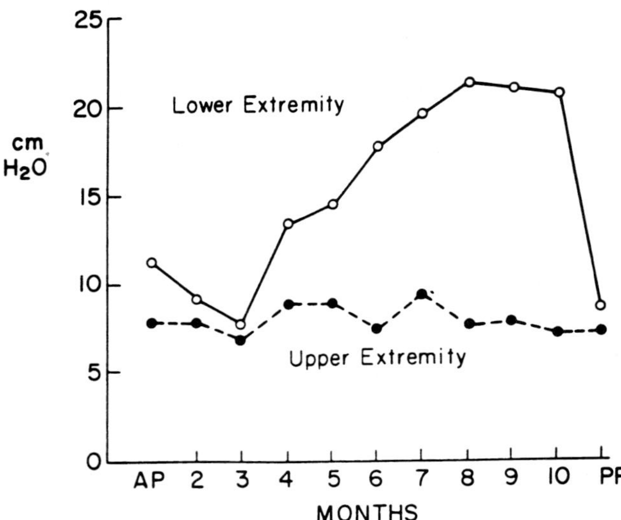

FIGURE 110–8 Upper and lower extremity venous pressures are shown in centimeters of water in relation to months of pregnancy. AP, antepartum measurement; PP, postpregnancy. Venous distensibility in the calf is always greater than that in the forearm, and this widens as pregnancy progresses. (From Creasy RK, Resnik R: Maternal-Fetal Medicine: Principles and Practice. 3rd ed. Philadelphia: WB Saunders, 1989.)

Murmurs

Systolic murmurs are usually innocent and are caused by the hyperkinetic circulation of pregnancy. A systolic murmur occurs in virtually every pregnant woman, beginning late in the first trimester or early in the second trimester, and persists for the duration of the pregnancy. Innocent murmurs are usually grade I to III/VI, soft, and short and have a systolic ejection quality, usually occurring in midsystole. They are commonly heard over the entire precordium. Systolic murmurs should be evaluated further when there is a change in the character of the murmur, an associated fever, accompanying symptoms or signs of congestive heart failure (CHF), or a change in cardiac rhythm and when there is a history of intravenous drug use, rheumatic fever, mitral valve (MV) prolapse, or congenital heart disease.[47]

A cervical venous hum may be heard over the supraclavicular fossa, which usually vanishes with pressure applied by the stethoscope at the site where the venous hum is heard or when the patient assumes the upright position.[45] A "mammary souffle," due to the increased blood flow in mammary vessels, may be detected either as a systolic or a continuous murmur (Fig. 110–9).[48, 49]

Any diastolic murmur should be evaluated to rule out organic disease, even though some soft, medium- to high-pitched diastolic murmurs have been reported in normal pregnancies. Diastolic murmurs may be due to increased flow through the tricuspid or MV or to physiologic dilatation of the pulmonary artery during pregnancy.[50]

Underlying systolic murmurs from aortic or pulmonic stenosis or diastolic murmurs from mitral stenosis may be louder because of the increased blood volume during pregnancy. Murmurs associated with regurgitation across the MV and the aortic valve often decrease in intensity secondary to a reduction in systemic vascular resistance during pregnancy.[45–47] In fact, these murmurs are sometimes inaudible during pregnancy. The increase in intravascular volume may also cause the systolic click and murmur of MV prolapse and the systolic murmur of hypertrophic cardiomyopathy to become softer or inaudible during the late stages of pregnancy.[45–52]

Noninvasive Testing

Electrocardiography

The QRS axis can shift to the left or right during a normal pregnancy. ST segments may show nonspecific ST-T wave abnormalities. Arrhythmias may be detected, and chamber enlargement may be identified.[53]

Chest Radiography

Radiation exposure to the uterus is minimal, but shielding of the pelvic area by a protective lead apron is advised.

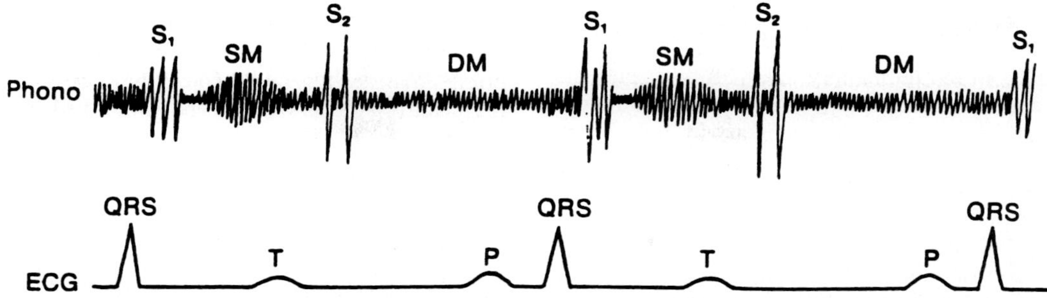

FIGURE 110–9 Phonocardiographic (Phono) and electrocardiographic (ECG) tracings of mammary souffle, a continuous murmur found in 15 percent of pregnant women near term or during lactation. DM, diastolic murmur; SM, systolic murmur. (From Tilkian AG, Conover MB: Understanding Heart Sounds and Murmurs. 2nd ed. Philadelphia: WB Saunders, 1984.)

Chest or abdominal radiographs should be avoided during the first two trimesters.[54] When obtained, a chest radiograph often shows straightening of the left upper cardiac border, an enlarged heart, and prominent lung markings.[55] Pleural effusions may be seen in the first 2 postpartum weeks; however, the effusion is usually small and resorbs.[56]

Two-Dimensional Echocardiography With Doppler

Echocardiography is considered safe for mother and fetus.[57] In the left lateral position, there is an increase in the LV and RV end-diastolic dimensions, resulting from intravascular volume expansion during normal pregnancies.[58] This increased dimension returns to normal after pregnancy. The LV systolic dimension and pressure are usually unchanged, but they may increase slightly. The left and right atria may be slightly dilated. Small pericardial effusions are found in as many as 40 percent of normal women by late pregnancy.[59] Mild tricuspid or pulmonary regurgitation may be detected near term. The tricuspid regurgitation is probably related to right-sided chamber enlargement and relative tricuspid insufficiency. The echocardiogram, however, provides the best and safest means to detect underlying valvular heart disease and determine its severity. Atrial or ventricular septal defects (ASDs and VSDs, respectively) and segmental or global ventricular wall motion abnormalities in the pregnant woman are usually easily detected with echocardiography.

Stress Testing

If coronary artery disease (CAD) is to be screened for or if there is a question of functional capacity or cardiac reserve in the pregnant woman, exercise testing can be performed with bicycle ergometry or treadmill exercise.[60] Fetal bradycardia has been reported with maximal exercise testing; therefore, submaximal exercise testing is usually performed using a low-level exercise protocol with continuous fetal monitoring during testing.[61] Measurement of maximal oxygen consumption during exercise is superior to testing based solely on symptoms.[61] The safety of exercise in the cardiac patient during pregnancy has not been well established, and such testing should be used only for limited cases in which it is vital to learn about low-level and moderate exercise capability, and only with careful monitoring of mother and fetus. Studies in normal women have shown the safety of submaximal maternal exercise with up to approximately 70 percent of maximal aerobic power (maternal HR up to 140 beats/min) for the pregnant patient.[60, 61] However, the presumed diagnostic benefit must outweigh the risk of this testing procedure.

Radionuclide Imaging

The dose of radiopharmaceutical agents used for cardiac imaging that reaches the fetus is calculated to be minimal, but measurements are only approximations and can vary from person to person because of differences in metabolism, placental uptake, and transfer.[62, 63] Therefore, their use should be avoided if possible, particularly during the first half of pregnancy.[64] Other noninvasive techniques, such as echocardiography with low-level stress testing with dobutamine, may be used to establish information related to cardiac function, the presence or absence of intracardiac shunts, and even CAD.

Magnetic Resonance Imaging

Magnetic resonance imaging (MRI) has no associated ionizing radiation exposure and can be used with safety in pregnant women.[65] MRI utilizes information reflected in nuclear magnetic movements to noninvasively determine intervillous blood flow and placental metabolism and transport.[66–68] This technology should be very valuable in determining the efficiency of the cardiovascular pumping system and in evaluating ventricular function and detecting most forms of congenital heart disease in the future.

Invasive Testing

Pulmonary Artery Catheterization

A variety of hemodynamic alterations and stresses are associated with pregnancy that may be challenging to patients with cardiac disease. Stress-producing situations include labor with intense uterine contractions, anesthesia, delivery, surgical procedures, blood loss, and replacement of intravenous fluids, as well as the administration of cardiovascular and obstetric drugs with cardiovascular effects.[69] If there is a possibility of abnormal cardiovascular function during the peripartum period, two-dimensional echocardiography may be useful, but it may be necessary to insert a pulmonary artery catheter to monitor hemodynamic variables.[69] A flow-directed catheter for pressure monitoring can be placed in the pulmonary artery in most patients without the need for fluoroscopy, thus avoiding radiation exposure.[70] Fluoroscopy may be necessary if pulmonary artery catheterization is likely to be difficult, such as in cases of a markedly dilated right heart, severe tricuspid regurgitation, or pulmonary artery hypertension. This must be done with pelvic shielding. Most women with symptomatic cardiac disease during pregnancy should undergo pulmonary artery catheterization during the delivery period. Hemodynamic monitoring of pulmonary capillary wedge and pulmonary artery pressures is usually continued for 24 hours after delivery to ensure hemodynamic stability, because the circulatory changes during the early postpartum period can cause acute hemodynamic deterioration.

Measurements should be interpreted in the context of the normal changes that are expected in pregnancy: a slight fall in systolic arterial blood pressure, a considerable reduction in diastolic pressure, an increase in total blood volume, and reduced peripheral vascular resistance (PVR). Mechanical compression of the inferior vena cava by an enlarged uterus may cause opposite effects.[28, 29, 32] There usually is a decrease in LV filling pressure due to the decreased systemic vascular resistance (SVR). The pulmonary capillary wedge pressure provides an estimate of mean left atrial (LA) and LA end-diastolic pressures.[16, 19, 43] Mixed venous oxygen saturation determination may assist in the detection of an intracardiac shunt.[31, 33]

In some cases, pulmonary artery catheterization is performed on the day before the induction of labor to stabilize the patient's hemodynamic status. Some indications for peripartum pulmonary artery catheterization include New York Heart Association functional class II or higher, documented reduced cardiac output, hemodynamically important mitral or aortic stenosis or pulmonary hypertension, CAD, intractable systemic arterial hypertension, or oliguria unresponsive to fluid challenges.[52, 70] Hemodynamic improvements may be made through pharmaceutical manipulation of HR, SV, pulmonary artery wedge pressure, or SVR with the use of pulmonary artery catheterization to monitor the effect of anesthetic and analgesic agents. Use of this monitoring technique may allow a safer vaginal delivery. Positioning of the patient on her left side may minimize hemodynamic fluctuations secondary to uterine contractions, and the input of these alterations can be measured through pulmonary artery catheterization. Monitoring will ensure that this maneuver does not increase venous return, leading to increased pulmonary pressures and pulmonary edema.

Cardiac Catheterization

Cardiac catheterization is performed only under extreme circumstances, because a relatively high dose of radiation is associated with the procedure. Approximately 500 mrads reach the fetus, even with appropriate pelvic shielding.[54] Therefore, there is a potentially serious effect of ionizing radiation, which is linearly proportional to the absorbed dose; the effects vary according to the stage of fetal development. Fetal malformation is highly unlikely with doses of less than 5 rads.[64] The risk for fetal malformation is highest from weeks 2 to 6 of pregnancy, but risk to brain cells continues up to week 15. Radiation may pose an increased risk for childhood cancer, with the risk being greatest when exposure occurs during the first trimester.

The procedure should be performed through the brachial approach, with appropriate shielding to minimize radiation to the pelvis and abdomen.[71] The techniques of contrast and Doppler echocardiography are used along with cardiac catheterization to reduce the exposure to ionizing radiation. The use of fluoroscopy with cine angiography produces the largest radiation dose; therefore, minimal time exposure should be used to answer specific questions by limitation of the radiation beam to anatomic areas of critical interest.[54]

Approach to Clinical Problems

Signs of Fetal Distress

Maternal cardiovascular disturbances may cause fetal distress. In evaluating or treating pregnant patients, it is imperative to have information about fetal and maternal well being. A fetal monitor can be placed via the cervix on the scalp to allow blood sampling used to evaluate blood gases, pH, and lactic acid concentrations. Fetal HR is traced in relation to uterine contractions during labor with abnormal patterns showing signs of distress (Fig. 110–10)[72]:

1. Baseline undulation (alternation of tachycardia and bradycardia with wide swings)
2. Severe bradycardia (rates $<$ 120 beats/min)
3. Severe tachycardia (rates $>$ 160 beats/min, along with reduced baseline variability)
4. Absent variability (late decelerations or variable decelerations with late recovery)

Hypotension

Most unstable situations are handled by placing the patient in the left lateral decubitus position with fetal monitoring, the administration of oxygen, the maintenance of intravascular volume, and the removal of any agents that may be increasing workload. Hypotensive patients must not be left supine because of potential deleterious mechanical effects (Fig. 110–11; see also Fig. 110–5). If uteroplacental blood flow is reduced due to reduced volume, this must be replaced.[73] In sepsis or low-flow states, there is a greater risk of intravascular coagulopathy because of the enhanced clotting factors associated with pregnancy.[13, 14] There is danger in the administration of fluids because of the reduced colloid oncotic pressure and the resulting greater tendency for capillary leakage and precipitation of pulmonary and peripheral edema.[51]

Cardiac Arrest

The dramatic alterations in physiology render pregnant women more susceptible to and less tolerant of cardiovas-

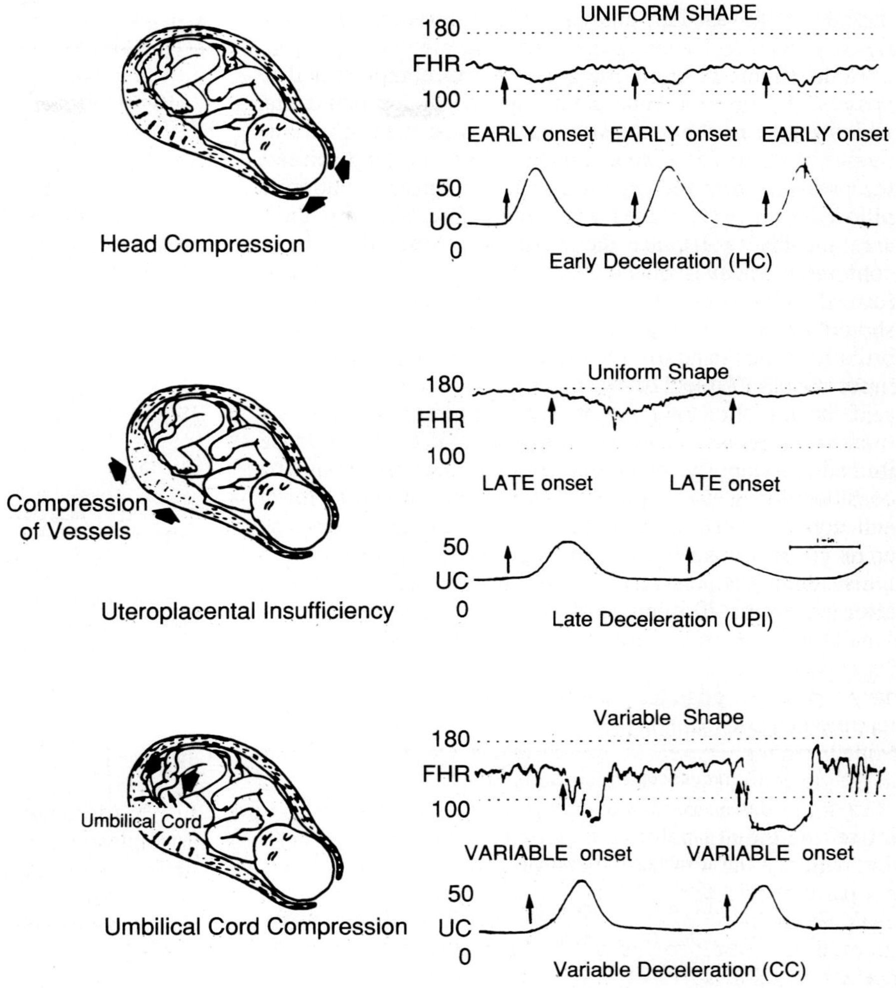

Head Compression
UNIFORM SHAPE
180
FHR
100
EARLY onset EARLY onset EARLY onset
50
UC
0
Early Deceleration (HC)
Compression of Vessels
Uteroplacental Insufficiency
Uniform Shape
180
FHR
100
LATE onset LATE onset
50
UC
0
Late Deceleration (UPI)
Umbilical Cord
Umbilical Cord Compression
Variable Shape
180
FHR
100
VARIABLE onset VARIABLE onset
50
UC
0
Variable Deceleration (CC)

FIGURE 110–10 Fetal heart rate (FHR) deceleration patterns in relation to uterine contractions demonstrate changes seen during decompensation. (From Burrow GN, Ferris T: Medical Complications During Pregnancy. 3rd ed. Philadelphia: WB Saunders, 1988.)

GRAVID UTERUS
Compression of IVC
Compression of Aorta
+
↓Venous Return
Decreased Ventilation
Increased O2 Consumption
Hypotension
↓Cardiac Output
Maternal Hypoxia
↓Uteroplacental Blood Flow
Fetal Acidosis
Maternal Acidemia
Fetal Compromise

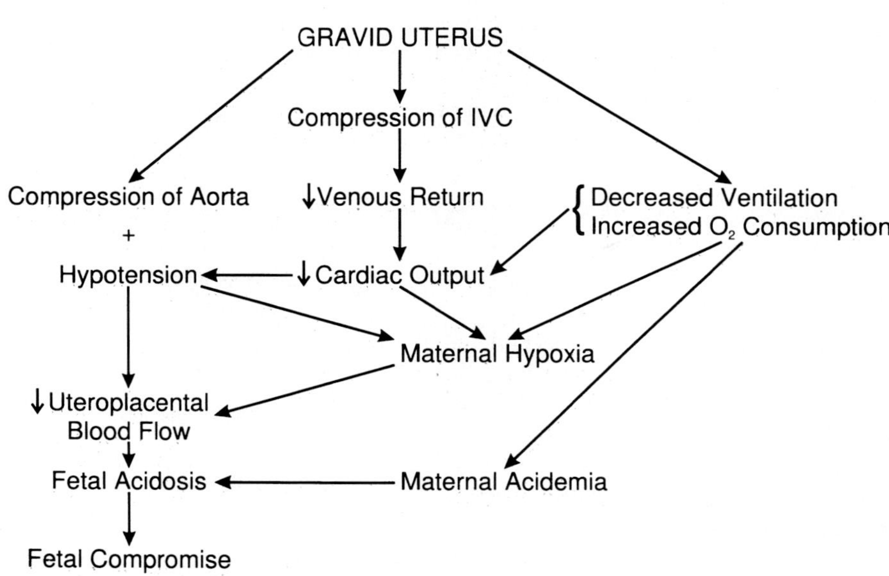

FIGURE 110–11 The effects of pregnancy and the gravid uterus on the response of the cardiovascular system to cardiac arrest and resuscitation. IVC, inferior vena cava. (From Lee RV, Mezzadri FC: Cardiopulmonary resuscitation of pregnant women. *In* Elkayam U, Gleicher N [eds]: Cardiac Problems in Pregnancy. 2nd Ed. pp. 307–319. Copyright © 1990. Reprinted by permission of Wiley-Liss, Inc., a division of John Wiley & Sons, Inc.)

cular insults.[74] Precipitators of cardiac arrest (Table 110–5) include cardiovascular, pulmonary, and obstetric complications, as well as shock, surgery, or drug effects.[73–77]

In the supine position, the gravid uterus compresses iliac vessels, the inferior vena cava, and the abdominal aorta, which may cause hypotension with a reduction in cardiac output of up to 25 percent (see Fig. 110–11). To minimize the pressure from the gravid uterus during resuscitation, a pillow or wedge is placed under the right abdominal flank area and hip to displace the uterus slightly to the left, or continuous manual displacement to the left can be performed by an assistant.[73, 75] Standard resuscitative measures should be used, including defibrillation for ventricular fibrillation and standard pharmacologic therapy, including vasopressors (Table 110–6).[75]

If the initiation of resuscitative measures, fluid restoration, or the release of uterine mass effect does not produce immediate stability, emergent cesarean section should be considered (Fig. 110–12).[76, 77] This decision should be made and delivery performed within 4 to 5 minutes of cardiac arrest to maximize the chances of survival of mother and fetus, although there have been reports of infant survival after more than 20 minutes of arrest.

TABLE 110–5 Causes of Maternal Cardiopulmonary Compromise

Cardiovascular
Decreased Cardiac Output
Arrhythmia
Critical valvular obstruction
Pericardial tamponade
Hypertrophic obstructive cardiomyopathy
Myocardial Dysfunction
Ischemia/infarction
Coronary artery dissection
Peripartum cardiomyopathy
Myocarditis
Congestive heart failure
Trauma: cardiac contusion/perforation
Vascular
Aortic dissection/rupture
Pulmonary
Pulmonary embolism
Amniotic fluid embolism
Pneumothorax
Aspiration pneumonitis
Angioedema
Status asthmaticus
Obstetric Complications
Amniotic fluid embolism
Hemorrhage/hypovolemia
Tocolytic (contraction suppression) therapy
Shock
Hypovolemia
Sepsis
Anaphylaxis
Neurogenic causes
Trauma
Miscellaneous
Drugs: cocaine, poisoning, overdose
Electrolyte imbalance
Anesthetic complications

TABLE 110–6 Resuscitation Strategy for Pregnant Patients

Time (min)	Strategy
0	Initiate cardiopulmonary resuscitation Intubate mother; control pH, P_{CO_2} Monitor fetal studies at least every 60 s
1	If unwitnessed arrest, no maternal response: deliver and continue maternal resuscitation
4	Witnessed arrest, patient past 32 wk, no maternal response: deliver and continue maternal resuscitation Witnessed arrest, patient 24–32 wk, no maternal response: open-chest massage, if no response in 60–90 s: deliver, surfactant for infant as needed, continue maternal resuscitation Witnessed arrest, patient past 24 wk, maternal response: continue life support, deliver for fetal indications
15	Witnessed arrest, patient past 24 wk, viable infant but still requires cardiac massage: deliver, continue maternal resuscitation

From Lee R, Mezzadri FC: Cardiopulmonary resuscitation of pregnant women. *In* Elkayam U, Gleicher N (eds): Cardiac Problems in Pregnancy. 2nd ed. pp. 307–319. Copyright © 1990. Reprinted by permission of Wiley-Liss, Inc., a division of John Wiley & Sons, Inc.

Chest Pain

Chest pain may be caused by cardiovascular, gastrointestinal, pulmonary, or musculoskeletal problems (Table 110–7).[78, 79] Any patient with chest pain not clearly due to gastrointestinal or musculoskeletal problems should be hospitalized with cardiovascular monitoring for evaluation.[78] Creatine kinase (CK) elevations may occur with labor due to intense muscle contractions. Routine electrocardiography (ECG) is used to detect ST-T wave changes. Echocardiography is used to detect MV prolapse and pericardial or valvular disease and can help to determine global or regional ventricular wall motion abnormalities. Evaluation with nuclear perfusion scans is not routinely used because there is a risk of radionuclide exposure to the fetus, but it may be necessary in some patients.[64] Cardiac catheterization is necessary for diagnosis and treatment with balloon angioplasty in patients with severe CAD. MRI had been used safely during pregnancy and can be used to evaluate aortic dissection or aortitis.[67] Transesophageal echocardiography can be used with minimal sedation to detect vegeta-

TABLE 110–7 Causes of Peripartum Chest Pain

Cardiovascular	*Gastrointestinal*
Arrhythmia	Esophagitis
Mitral valve prolapse	Hiatal hernia
Cardiomyopathy	Peptic ulcer
Heart failure	*Lung*
Pericarditis	Pulmonary embolus
Ischemia	Asthma
Aortic dissection	Pulmonary hypertension
Aortitis	Pleuritis
Endocarditis	*Musculoskeletal*
	Rib cage
	Costochondritis

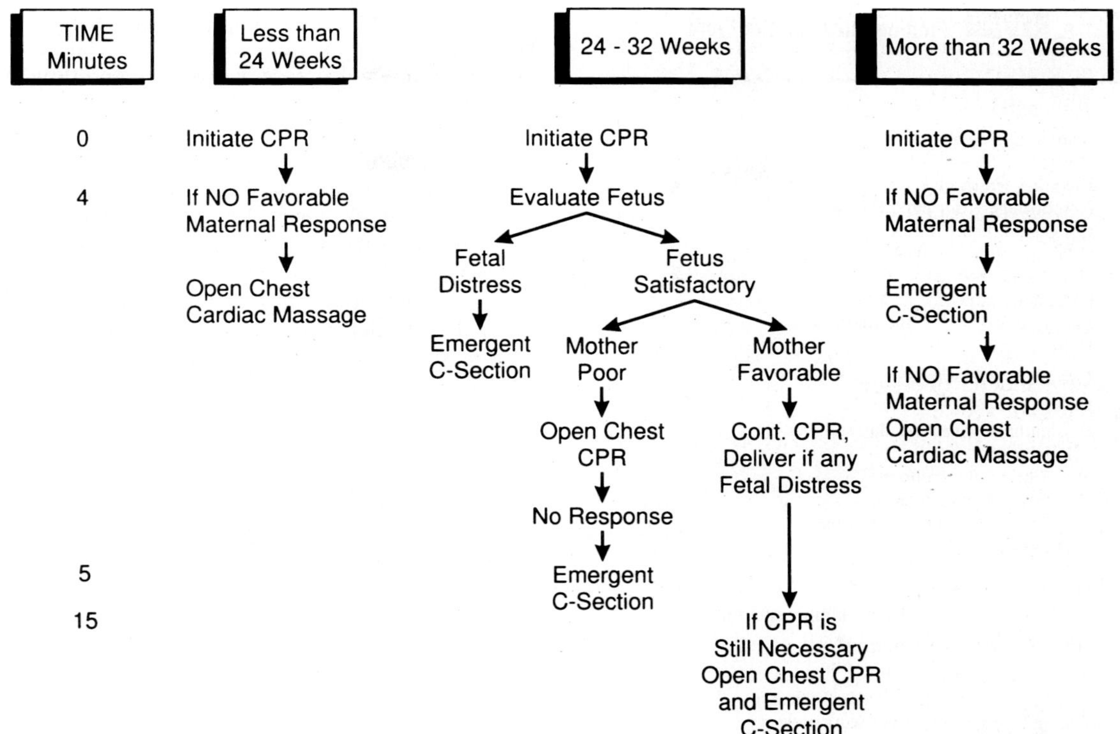

FIGURE 110–12 Approach to consideration of emergent cesarean section (C-section) to salvage the fetus, considered in relation to age of gestation and duration of cardiopulmonary arrest. CPR, cardiopulmonary resuscitation. (From Lee RV, Mezzadri FC: Cardiopulmonary resuscitation of pregnant women. *In* Elkayam U, Gleicher N [eds]: Cardiac Problems in Pregnancy. 2nd ed. pp. 307–319. Copyright © 1990. Reprinted by permission of Wiley-Liss, Inc., a division of John Wiley & Sons, Inc.)

tions or aortic disease. Endocarditis or collagen vascular causes may also be diagnosed through overall assessment, laboratory tests, and cultures.[79] A suspected pulmonary embolus may be confirmed with chest radiography, arterial blood gases, and ECG; the consideration of ventilation-perfusion lung scanning or pulmonary angiography should be determined carefully.

Organic nitrates have been used effectively and safely to help control severe pregnancy-induced hypertension and are commonly used for angina in nonpregnant patients. There are reports of reduced blood pressure with nitrate use causing fetal HR decelerations, bradycardia, and attenuation of spontaneous beat-to-beat variability, probably from a loss of cerebral autoregulation and increased intracranial pressure.[80] Treatment with nitrates may not be free of side effects, so fastidious monitoring of the mother and fetus is required in the event it is used. Further studies are needed to determine fetal safety.[81, 82] Similarly, the safety of calcium antagonists in pregnancy has not been established, but the appropriate use of a slow channel calcium antagonist can be helpful in controlling blood pressure elevation in the pregnant woman.[83–85] Beta-blockers may be the treatment of choice for ischemia during gestation and are also useful in blood pressure control.[86, 87]

Venous Emergencies

Venous thrombosis may occur peripartum or postpartum and can be life threatening when pulmonary thromboembolism results from deep venous thrombosis of the lower extremities or pelvic veins or when amniotic fluid embolism occurs.[88] The veins are distended more than normally due to hormonal and mechanical changes of pregnancy. Septic pelvic thrombophlebitis may occur in association with pelvic infection or complications, predisposing to pulmonary embolus.

Amniotic fluid embolism, caused by a sudden release of amniotic fluid or fetal debris into the maternal venous circulation, is usually lethal. The fetal mortality rate is 40 percent. One half of all patients die within 1 hour of symptom appearance, and survivors usually have neurologic deficits or brain death.[89–92] Clinical findings and symptoms appear suddenly and may be confused with those of pulmonary emboli (Table 110–8).[93, 94] Profound hemodynamic effects occur with a consumptive coagulopathy; most cases occur during labor or vigorous contractions.[93]

Death from pulmonary embolism during pregnancy and the puerperium is still one of the three leading causes of maternal deaths in the United States.[88, 95] Risk factors include prolonged bed rest, operative delivery (vaginal or cesarean), preeclampsia, and congenital hypercoagulability syndromes.[96, 97] Many signs and symptoms of thromboembolic disease are a normal part of pregnancy. The physical examination is not an adequate basis for initiation of therapy; the positive predictive value is as low as 20 percent.[95] Objective tests must be performed, such as impedance plethysmography, duplex ultrasound, Doppler ultrasound, MRI, ventilation-perfusion scanning, or invasive tests with

TABLE 110-8 Findings in Amniotic Fluid Embolism

Symptoms
Sudden dyspnea
Hypotension
Bleeding tendencies
Hemorrhage from puncture sites
Congestive heart failure
Cardiorespiratory arrest
Grand mal seizures
Pulmonary edema
Left ventricular dysfunction/failure
Hemorrhage
Laboratory Findings
Hypoxia
Disseminated intravascular coagulation
Increased
Fibrin split products
Prothrombin time
Partial thromboplastin time
Decreased
Fibrinogen
Thrombocytopenia
Fetal debris in blood from pulmonary artery
Hemodynamic Parameters
↓ Blood pressure
↑ Pulmonary capillary wedge pressure
↓ Left ventricular stroke work index
↓ Systemic vascular resistance
↑ Pulmonary artery pressure
↑ Pulmonary venous resistance
Uterine-Fetal
Uterine atony
Fetal distress

pelvic shielding. False-positive findings on noninvasive testing can be caused by the gravid uterus, so a positive test must be followed by venography.[98] The amount of radiation to the fetus from venography or ventilation-perfusion scanning is small and represents a lower risk than a missed diagnosis.[99] Prophylaxis and treatment must be approached carefully, because anticoagulation measures are associated with teratogenic and other risks for mother and fetus (see later).[100, 101]

Peripheral Edema and Pulmonary Rales

During normal pregnancy, there is marked retention of sodium and water and a decreased interstitial colloid osmotic pressure, which can result in pitting edema of the ankles and legs near term.[9, 51] There is an increase in venous pressure below the level of the uterus due to partial occlusion of the vena cava.[26] This is usually *dependent edema*, which develops during the day and resolves with supine rest. The routine use of drugs to treat dependent edema is not recommended.[9] Occasionally, bibasilar rales may simulate CHF. Rales may be caused by basilar compression of the lungs and atelectasis secondary to enlargement of the uterus and increased abdominal pressure.[44] The jugular veins may appear distended from about the 20th week of pregnancy. Venous pulsations in the neck are usually seen, and the A and V waves are easily definable.

Diuretic agents should be avoided whenever possible because of their potential for adverse fetal effects.[9] These effects include a decrease in uterine blood flow and placental perfusion resulting from decreased blood volume.[102] Teratogenic effects have not been described, but there are reports of jaundice, hyponatremia, bradycardia, and thrombocytopenia with the use of thiazides.[103]

The New York Heart Association functional classification for the assessment of the severity of cardiac disease and prognosis is recommended as a means to estimate symptom limitation in patients in class I or II before pregnancy. Patients who are in class III before pregnancy require special attention and early hospital admission before delivery. Pregnancy is contraindicated for patients in late class III or class IV.[52]

Fever and Endocarditis

Endocarditis should be suspected when a pregnant woman develops fever, a new change in murmur (specifically, a murmur of aortic, mitral, or tricuspid valvular insufficiency), CHF, atrial fibrillation, or a systemic or pulmonary embolus.[104, 105] Symptoms may include weakness, dyspnea, orthopnea, anorexia, nausea, vomiting, myalgia, arthralgia, edema, and pain in the chest, abdomen, or back. Although some of these symptoms may initially be thought to be due to the pregnancy, selected physical findings should raise this as a diagnostic possibility, such as a change in murmur.[106] Risk factors for endocarditis in pregnant women include valvular deformities, MV prolapse, nonbacterial thrombotic vegetations, dilated cardiomyopathies, and intravenous drug use.[107–110] Serial echocardiograms may reveal valvular vegetations, but these must be at least 2 cm in size to be detected on transthoracic echocardiography.[111] Transesophageal echocardiography may detect smaller vegetations. Multiple blood cultures should be obtained before the administration of antibiotics.[112]

The most common organism isolated during pregnancy is *Streptococcus viridans*, but *Staphylococcus* and *Streptococcus* spp. are often found. Any organism capable of causing infective endocarditis in the nonpregnant state can be expected to act as a pathogen during pregnancy. Anaerobes can be cultured from 75 to 95 percent of female genital tracts. In patients with a history of intravenous drug use, *Staphylococcus aureus* is the predominant organism, along with multiple pathogens. In the United States, intravenous drug use has emerged as a major cause of right-sided endocarditis, but in reports from other areas of the world, many patients with right-sided infective endocarditis have a history of septic abortion or puerperal sepsis.[112, 113]

Antibiotic Prophylaxis

Delivery of the fetus and placenta is associated with some risk for bacteremia, but this is relatively low.[110, 114] A large series of women showed a 5 percent incidence of positive blood cultures within 1 hour after delivery. Bacteremia occurs in 10 percent of obstetric patients who develop complications,[110] including pyelonephritis or endoparametritis. Obstetric risk factors for development of endocarditis

TABLE 110-9 **Initial and Subsequent Therapy for Prophylaxis of Infective Endocarditis (Adults)**

	Initially	Subsequently
Dental and upper respiratory tract procedures or surgery		
Regimen A	Aqueous crystalline penicillin Oral penicillin V or erythromycin	Aqueous crystalline penicillin Penicillin V Erythromycin
Regimen B (prosthetic valves)	Ampicillin plus gentamycin or vancomycin	Ampicillin plus gentamycin or gentamycin
Gastrointestinal and genitourinary surgery or instrumentation	Ampicillin plus gentamycin or vancomycin plus gentamycin Amoxicillin	Ampicillin plus gentamycin or vancomycin plus gentamycin Amoxicillin

From Reid CL, Elkayam U, Rahimtoola SH: Infective endocarditis in pregnancy. *In* Elkayam U, Gleicher N (eds): Cardiac Problems in Pregnancy. 2nd ed. pp. 199–214.

include forceps delivery, amniocentesis, prolonged rupture of membranes, and manual removal of the placenta.[110, 114] Patients with prosthetic valves and those with prior episodes of endocarditis are at an increased risk.[110, 115, 116]

The low risk and low cost of antibiotic prophylaxis and the potential seriousness of endocarditis, with mortality rates approaching 30 percent, make antibiotic use appropriate in pregnant patients with valvular heart disease.[114, 117] The regimen suggested by the American Heart Association is used with prophylaxis tailored to the type of procedure being performed and for the presence of prosthetic heart valves (Tables 110–9 and 110–10).

Valve Prosthesis

Tissue valves are occasionally used in women of childbearing age, but these valves deteriorate more rapidly in young individuals (<50 years old) and may require reoperation, because calcification of the valves is common and the incidence even appears to increase during pregnancy.[118–121] Asymptomatic or mildly symptomatic women with one or more functioning prosthetic heart valves can usually tolerate the hemodynamic load of pregnancy.[118] Most problems occur when there is inadequate anticoagulation.[119, 120] If patients are willing to follow a strict regimen of anticoagulation, mechanical valves are preferable because they do not deteriorate as rapidly.[122–124] The risk for thromboembolic events during pregnancy may be reduced through careful adjustment and monitoring of anticoagulation therapy.[123, 124]

In women with prosthetic heart valves, preconception evaluation should include an assessment of the heart and valves, including an evaluation for rhythm abnormalities. Exercise testing before pregnancy may predict the response to an increased hemodynamic load, and echocardiography assists in the evaluation of cardiac structure, function, and anatomy.

Anticoagulation

Anticoagulation may be required during pregnancy for patients with mechanical valve prostheses, venous thrombophlebitis, atrial fibrillation, rheumatic MV disease, enlarged left atrium, intracardiac thrombus, pulmonary embolus, peripartum cardiomyopathy, primary pulmonary hypertension, intracranial thrombosis, or lupus anticoagulant syndrome. Studies have reported favorable outcomes with heparin therapy as opposed to coumadin.[125–127] In many reviews of pregnant patients, it appears that fixed doses of heparin rather than adjusted doses were being used in most cases of thromboembolic events.[128, 129] The incidence of fetal complications significantly increases with anticoagulation; however, adjusted doses of heparin throughout pregnancy, or at least during the first two trimesters, improve fetal outcome.[130–133] This is due to the fact that heparin is a

TABLE 110-10 **Dosages of Antibiotics for Infective Endocarditis Prophylaxis (Adults)**

	Initial Dose*		Subsequent Dose*	
	0.5–1 h	*Preprocedure*	*Dose*	*Frequency*
Penicillin				
Aqueous crystalline	2 million U	IM or IV	1 million U	q6h × 1
Penicillin V	2 g	PO	1 g	q6h × 1
Vancomycin	1 g	IV	1 g	
Erythromycin	1 g	PO	500 mg	q6h × 1
Ampicillin	1–2 g	IV or IM	1–2 g	q8h × 1
Gentamycin	1.5 mg/kg (≤80 mg)	IV or IM	1.5 mg/kg (≤80 mg)	q8h × 1
Amoxicillin	3 g	PO	1.5 g	q6h × 1

*Dosages are for patients with normal renal function and must be modified for dialysis.

From Reid CL, Elkayam U, Rahimtoola SH: Infective endocarditis in pregnancy. *In* Elkayam U, Gleicher N (eds): Cardiac Problems in Pregnancy, 2nd ed. pp. 199–214.

large molecule and does not cross the placenta.[133] Potential complications of long-term heparin include sterile abscesses and hematomas in the abdominal wall, osteoporosis, and thrombocytopenia.[135] The administration of pudendal local anesthesia has the risk of puncturing a blood vessel, with ensuing hemorrhage.

Coumarin derivatives, including coumadin, used during pregnancy are associated with substantial teratogenic risk and a high incidence of fetal wastage from spontaneous abortions, stillbirths, and birth defects, especially when coumadin is given in the first trimester.[135] There may be central nervous system disease, eye defects (e.g., optic nerve atrophy, microphthalmia, and blindness), deafness, congenital heart disease, mental retardation, seizures, scoliosis, spasticity, and microcephaly.[136–138] Death may occur due to intracranial hemorrhage.[138] During the first trimester, *fetal warfarin syndrome* (or *coumarin* or *coumadin embryodystrophy*) has been noted in 5 to 30 percent of newborns. The characteristic findings are nasal bone hypoplasia and epiphyseal stippling, and the nose is depressed, flattened, or ruptured[138–141] (Fig. 110–13). There may be hemorrhage during labor and delivery in the mother and the fetus or neonatal respiratory distress resulting from upper airway obstruction. There are changes in the dose requirements of warfarin as pregnancy progresses.[142] Labor and delivery in a patient on coumadin place the mother and fetus at risk for hemorrhage. The half-life of coumadin is longer in the fetus, so the effects may persist for up to 10 days after its discontinuation.[139, 142]

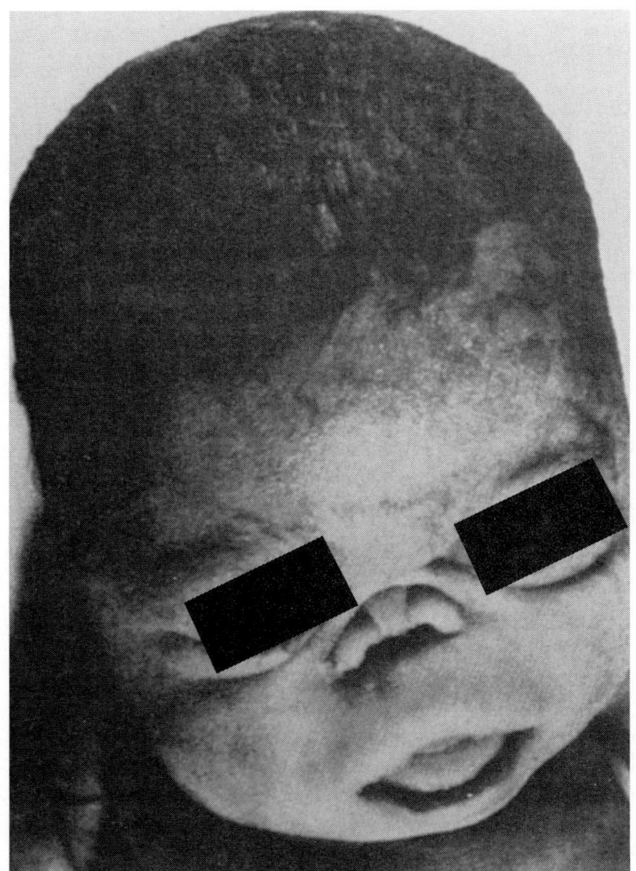

FIGURE 110–13 Newborn with severe nasal deformity. The mother took coumarin throughout her pregnancy because she had a prosthetic heart valve. (From Becker MH: Chondrodysplasia punctata: is maternal warfarin therapy a factor? Am J Dis Child 129:356, 1975. Copyright 1975 American Medical Association.)

If pregnancy is planned, oral anticoagulation should be discontinued and heparin started subcutaneously (Fig. 110–14).[139] If conception occurs while the patient is receiving coumadin, heparin should be instituted immediately after discovery of the pregnancy. Hospitalization for a short time is often advised to establish the required dose of heparin and to teach subcutaneous self-injection. Dosage is adjusted to prolong the activated partial thromboplastin time by 1.5 to 2 times normal values. Alternatively, low molecular weight heparin (1 mg/kg dose) bid may be administered subcutaneously during the first two trimesters of pregnancy. Concentrated heparin is usually administered to the lower abdominal subcutaneous tissue at 12-hour intervals.[134] In order to reduce the risk of bleeding at delivery, subcutaneous heparin should be replaced in the hospital with intravenous heparin at 38 weeks of gestation.[142] Heparin is discontinued at the onset of labor to allow clotting time to normalize before delivery. Heparin is usually continued into early labor when longer labor is anticipated, such as during a first delivery. Epidural anesthesia may increase the risk of bleeding into the epidural or subarachnoid space; pudendal anesthesia may also pose increased risks for bleeding.

Anticoagulation is reinstituted after delivery. The American Academy of Pediatrics considers warfarin to be compatible with breast-feeding. Heparin is not excreted in breast milk and is also compatible.[143, 144]

RHYTHM DISTURBANCES IN PREGNANCY

Arrhythmias

Palpitations and arrhythmias are not uncommon during pregnancy, and treatment is based on maternal and fetal signs of decompensation, annoying associated symptoms, or the presence of underlying heart disease (Fig. 110–15).[146] Studies with the use of Holter monitoring have demonstrated multiple ventricular or atrial premature beats, or both, in approximately 18 percent of pregnant women; their presence does not appear to have any adverse maternal or fetal effect. The increased frequency of arrhythmias may be a result of the adaptive changes in the hemodynamic system that accompany pregnancy, including increased blood volume, venous return, and the end-diastolic volume. With any arrhythmia, the use of stimulants (e.g., drugs, decongestants, cocaine, caffeine, nicotine, alcohol, tea, cola) or agents that might produce electrolyte imbalances should be avoided. There usually is a marked reduction in the number of premature beats after pregnancy.[147–149] The recognition of an arrhythmia is important because it may be an initial manifestation of underlying heart disease. Sustained arrhythmias are relatively uncommon.[146]

Sinus Tachycardia

On average, HR increases by 10 to 20 beats/min during pregnancy.[148, 149] Sinus arrhythmia is common during pregnancy. Because the HR increases by 10 to 15 percent,

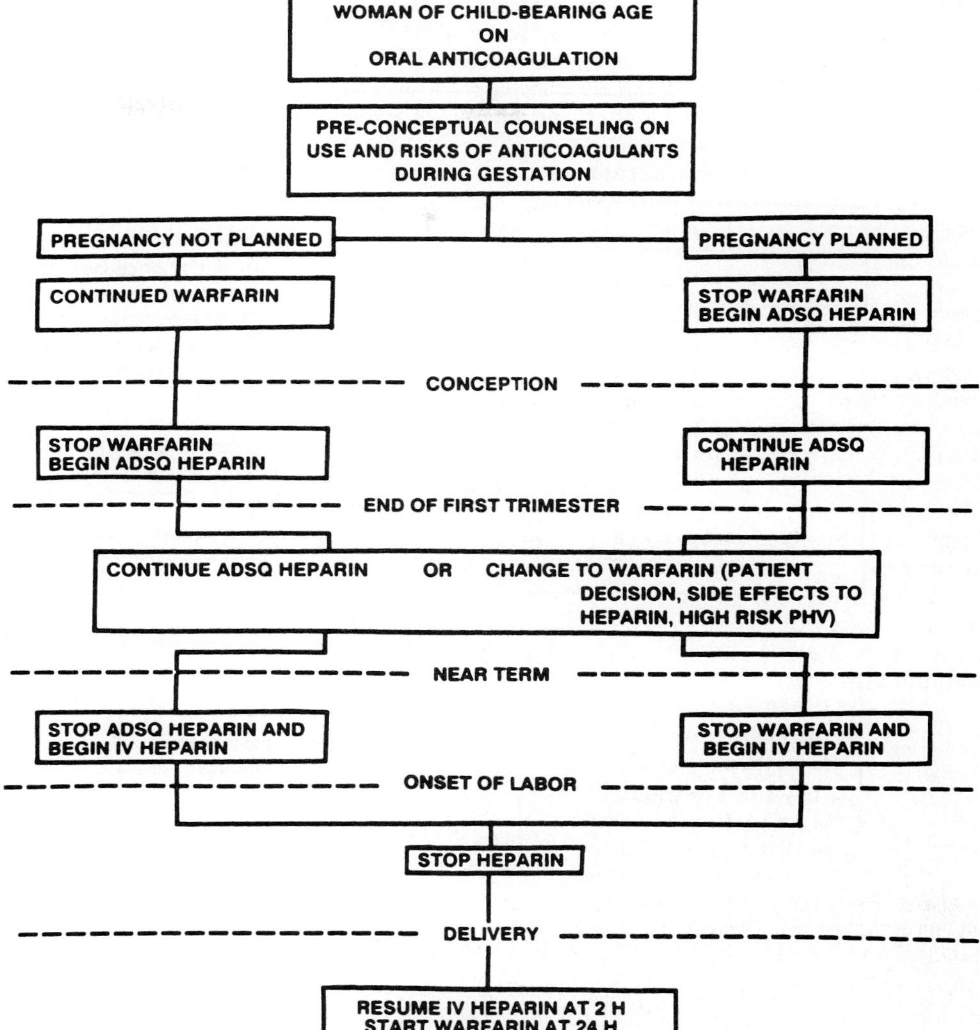

FIGURE 110–14 Algorithm of approach to anticoagulation in women of childbearing age in settings of preconception and planned and unplanned pregnancies and at different stages of pregnancy, labor, and delivery. ADSQ, adjusted dose subcutaneous; IV, intravenous; PHV, prosthetic heart valve. (From McGehee W: Anticoagulation in pregnancy. *In* Elkayam U, Gleicher N [eds]: Cardiac Problems in Pregnancy. 2nd ed. pp. 397–416. Copyright © 1990. Reprinted by permission of Wiley-Liss, Inc., a division of John Wiley & Sons, Inc.)

some women manifest sinus tachycardia during pregnancy. Persistent sinus tachycardia may result from fever, hyperthyroidism, myocardial ischemia, CHF, myocarditis, or metabolic abnormalities. It may also be associated with the use of stimulant drugs.

Atrial Flutter or Fibrillation

Atrial flutter or fibrillation is rare during normal pregnancy and, when present, should lead one to suspect rheumatic MV disease, MV prolapse, thyrotoxicosis, acute pulmonary embolus, or cardiomyopathy.[150] Patients with atrial fibrillation due to rheumatic mitral stenosis have the highest risk of systemic thromboembolism, with an incidence of approximately 16 percent in pregnant patients with rheumatic mitral stenosis and atrial fibrillation.[151, 152] Control of the ventricular rate is usually achieved with digoxin or β-blockers because the safety of calcium channel blockers in pregnancy has not been well established.[153–156] Sinus rhythm may be reestablished with quinidine, procainamide, or electrical cardioversion.[157–163] The decision of whether to use elective cardioversion should be based on the duration of the fibrillation, the size of the left atrium, the presence of symptoms attributable to the atrial flutter/fibrillation, and other factors.[164] Before cardioversion, many patients receive anticoagulation, but the previously discussed risks of anticoagulation make this of greater risk in pregnant patients.[165] The potential risks of this therapy to mother and fetus should be weighed.

Supraventricular Tachycardia

Supraventricular tachycardia is uncommon during pregnancy, with a rate of approximately 3 percent occurring in patients with heart disease.[166] This tachycardia usually is characterized by an atrial rate between 140 to 240 beats/min and narrow QRS complexes and is abrupt in onset and termination.[167]

If the pregnant patient is hemodynamically stable, acute termination can be attempted by vagal stimulation, carotid sinus massage, Valsalva maneuver, or the *diving reflex* (patient immerses face and lips in a pan of cold water).[168]

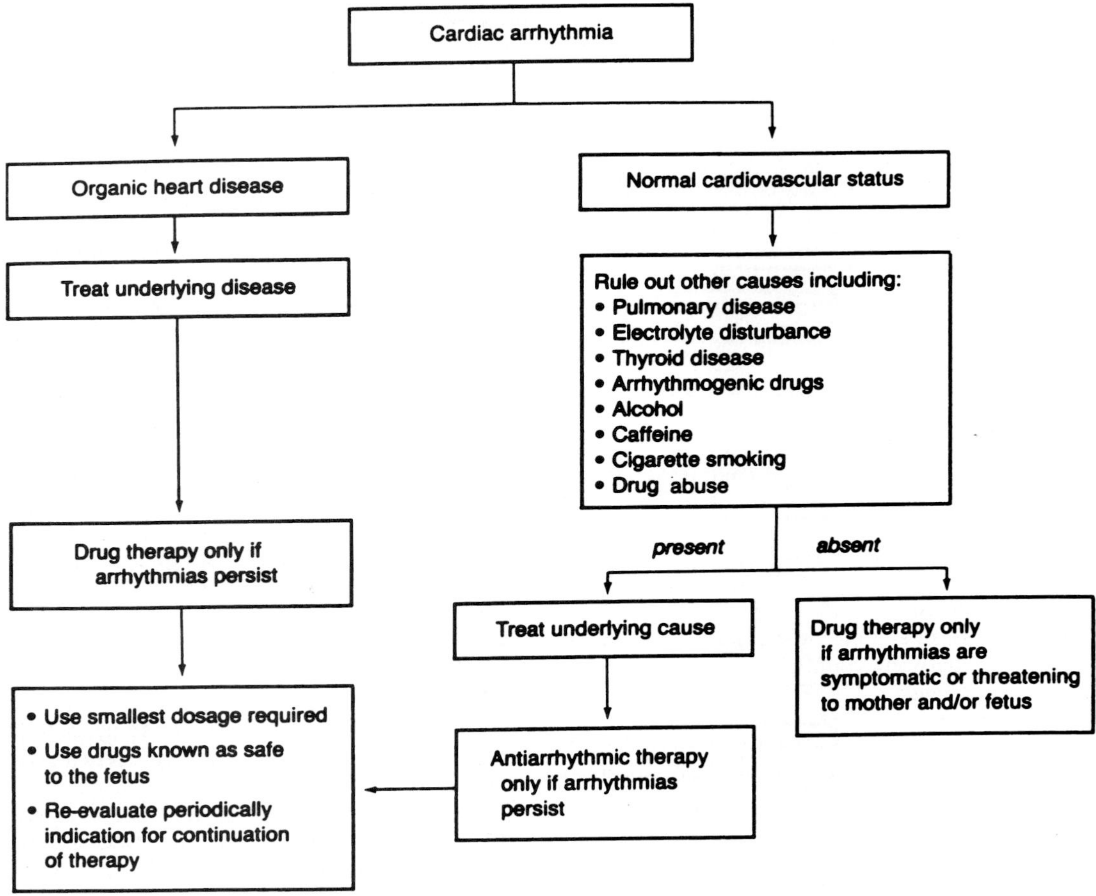

FIGURE 110–15 Algorithm of the approach to arrhythmias that occur during pregnancy. (From Rotmensch HH, Elkayam U, Frishman W: Antiarrhythmic drug therapy during pregnancy. Ann Intern Med 98:487, 1983.)

If vagal stimulation is not effective, intravenous verapamil can be administered as a 5- to 10-mg bolus over 1 to 3 minutes after the patient is placed in a supine position.[167, 168] Intravenous adenosine at 6 to 12 mg may be effective in converting supraventricular tachycardia to normal sinus rhythm during delivery. The dose can be repeated 15 minutes later.[169] Careful monitoring of maternal blood pressure and fetal heart monitoring should be used during drug administration. There may be a hypotensive effect from verapamil, which resolves within 30 minutes of administration. If hypotension develops and is symptomatic, elevation of the legs and volume replacement should be instituted.[168, 170] Because verapamil should not be used in patients with systemic hypotension or CHF, intravenous digoxin can be used as an alternative. Propranolol and procainamide have been used in patients who do not respond to intravenous verapamil, adenosine, digoxin, or combination therapy. Direct-current cardioversion should be used only for tachycardias associated with hypotension or other hemodynamic deterioration and in patients not responsive to other measures. Antiarrhythmic agents are often transferred to the fetus through placental blood flow and should therefore be used with caution.[156, 158, 164, 171–173]

Amiodarone use should be restricted to life-threatening arrhythmias, usually ventricular tachycardia, and should be used only after conventional therapy has failed. Amiodarone has not been shown to have associated teratogenicity, but it may prolong QT intervals and cause bradycardia.[174] Thyroid function should be checked in the mother and the fetus when amiodarone is used, probably on a monthly basis.[175]

Wolff-Parkinson-White Syndrome

The Wolff-Parkinson-White syndrome (WPW) is characterized by an accessory or a preexcitation pathway from atrium to ventricle.[176] Classic electrocardiographic changes are found, including a short PR interval, delta wave, and widened QRS complex. Atrial fibrillation occurs in patients with WPW syndrome; this is a potentially life-threatening arrhythmia, as atrial impulses may be delivered to the ventricle at rates of greater than 280 to 300 beats/min, which can result in hemodynamic deterioration, fibrillation, and death.[177, 178]

It is not known whether pregnancy stimulates patients with WPW syndrome to experience tachyarrhythmias more frequently, but some patients demonstrate these only during pregnancy. The approach to the patient is similar to that for the nonpregnant patient. No diagnostic or therapeutic intervention is recommended for asymptomatic patients. The use of digoxin and verapamil and other agents that preferentially slow atrioventricular (AV) conduction is contraindicated in this disorder. If patients have frequent or severe symptoms with the tachycardia, long-term antiarrhythmic drug therapy may be necessary. Intravenous procainamide or lidocaine may slow impulse conduction though the preexcitation pathway, slowing the HR.[178–180] Direct cardioversion is the preferred mode of therapy when there is hemodynamic compromise in mother or fetus. Cardiac electrophysiologic study and radiofrequency ablation of the preexcitation pathway can be very successful.

Ventricular Arrhythmia

Premature ventricular contractions (PVCs) are common during pregnancy.[181–184] Patients may be asymptomatic or may present with palpitations, skipped beats, or dizziness.[182] Frequent or repetitive PVCs, defined as more than 10 per hour, are uncommon. The presence of PVCs without underlying heart disease does not usually pose a risk for sudden death and is usually not treated.[183, 184] If structural heart disease is present and PVCs occur frequently or if PVCs are complex or changing in morphology, there appears to be a risk to the pregnant patient. CAD is a relatively rare cause of PVCs in pregnancy. Baseline 24-hour electrocardiographic monitoring is performed to quantify the number of PVCs. Echocardiography is performed to identify underlying heart disease. None of the available antiarrhythmic agents are known to be free of serious side effects to the fetus and mother. For a subset of patients who are severely symptomatic or those with LV dysfunction or frequent or repetitive PVCs, treatment may be necessary.[185] Quinidine or procainamide is usually used to treat complex PVCs in women with underlying heart disease, with careful monitoring of serum levels and quantification of the response to these treatments.

Ventricular tachycardia is uncommon during pregnancy and is usually associated with structural heart disease or MV prolapse. Tachycardia can be precipitated by physical exercise, emotional stress, or a change in posture. Physical findings include an intermittent jugular cannon A wave and variable intensity of the first heart sound. If the patient is hemodynamically stable, intravenous procainamide or lidocaine is the recommended drug of choice because both agents are relatively safe and frequently effective.[186–188] In refractory cases, bretylium may be used; however, its safety in human pregnancy has not been well established. Cardioversion is the treatment of choice when there is hemodynamic compromise in the mother or fetus or when there is failure to respond to antiarrhythmic drugs.[189–193]

A complete noninvasive evaluation should be performed to detect underlying heart disease before the institution of long-term therapy. If precipitating factors such as hypoxemia, electrolyte imbalances, drug intoxication, ischemia, or CHF are the causes, these should be treated first before the institution of long-term therapy. β-Adrenergic antagonists may be useful in suppressing ventricular tachycardia that occurs with no apparent heart disease, especially when it is provoked by physical exercise or emotional stress. The safety to mother and fetus has not been well established for newer antiarrhythmic agents.

Antiarrhythmic Agents

Quinidine

Quinidine (Table 110–11) has been used extensively for maternal arrhythmias and occasionally for the treatment of fetal supraventricular tachycardia.[153, 154] This drug is 60 to 80 percent bound to protein, allowing the unbound fraction to be increased because there is hypoalbuminemia in pregnancy. Fetal thrombocytopenia has been reported with quinidine treatment, and there have been reports of spontaneous uterine contractions. Toxic doses may cause premature labor, abortion, or damage to the fetal VIII cranial nerve. The drug is usually considered safe for treatment of maternal and fetal arrhythmias, because side effects are rare in the absence of a prolonged QT interval in the mother. The dose excreted in breast milk is below the recommended pediatric dose and is safe for breast-feeding infants.[160–163]

Procainamide

Transplacental transfer of procainamide occurs; therefore, it has been used during pregnancy to treat fetal supraventricular tachycardia.[153, 154] There have been no reports of teratogenicity; however, with the limited experience of use of this drug, it cannot be recommended for routine use in pregnancy. Although the amount of both procainamide and *N*-acetylprocainamide (NAPA) ingested in breast milk is not expected to produce significant levels, its use in breast-feeding mothers has not been established as safe.[157, 158]

Disopyramide

Disopyramide has been used to treat ventricular and supraventricular arrhythmias without reports of teratogenesis. There are some reports that it induces uterine contractions, and it is excreted in breast milk in concentrations similar to those in plasma. No adverse effects have been seen in infants, but there are insufficient data to recommend it for breast-feeding mothers.[194, 195]

Lidocaine

Lidocaine is used for epidural or local anesthesia and, occasionally, as an antiarrhythmic agent. It crosses the placenta, and elevated levels have been associated with infant central nervous system depression, apnea, seizures, hypotonia, and bradycardia. When fetal acidosis is present, the levels of this drug may be increased, thereby increasing the likelihood of toxicity. There have been no reports of teratogenic effects, and it is thought that lidocaine is safe for use during pregnancy as long as blood levels are kept within safe ranges ($\leq$4 μg/ml).[186–188]

Mexiletine

There are a few reports of mexiletine being used in the treatment of cardiac arrhythmias during pregnancy. This

TABLE 110-11 Guide to the Use of Antiarrhythmic Drugs in Pregnancy

Drug	Route of Administration	Clinical Application	Therapeutic Concentration	Placental Transfer*	Milk/Plasma Ratio	Use in Pregnancy	Comment
Lidocaine	Parenteral	"Choice" in ventricular tachyarrhythmias; digitalis toxicity	2–4 μg/ml	0.5–1.0	?	Safe	Toxic doses and fetal acidosis may cause central nervous system and cardiovascular depression in the neonate
Mexiletine	Oral Parenteral	Termination and prophylaxis in ventricular tachyarrhythmias	0.75–2 μg/ml	1.0	2.0	Probably safe*	
Quinidine	Oral	Paroxysmal atrial tachyarrhythmias,† prophylaxis in atrial and ventricular tachyarrhythmias	2–5 μg/ml	1.0	0.71	Relatively safe	Excessive doses may lead to premature labor, very occasionally neonatal thrombocytopenia
Procainamide	Oral Parenteral	Termination and prophylaxis in atrial and ventricular tachyarrhythmias	4–10 μg/ml (+ NAPA‡ 10–25 μg/ml)	1.3	4.0	Relatively safe	High incidence of maternal antinuclear antibodies and lupus-like syndrome with chronic use
Disopyramide	Oral Parenteral	Atrial and ventricular tachyarrhythmias	3–7 μg/ml	0.4	0.9	Probably safe*	One report documents uterine contractions in association with the drug

Verapamil	Oral Parenteral	Paroxysmal supraventricular tachycardia; rate control in chronic atrial fibrillation	15–30 ng/ml§	0.4	0.23 0.94	Probably safe*	Rapid IV injection may occasionally cause maternal hypotension
Phenytoin	Oral Parenteral	Digitalis toxicity; refractory ventricular tachyarrhythmias	10–18 μg/ml	0.8–1.0	0.18 0.45	Not recommended for chronic use§	High risk of malformations ("fetal hydantoin syndrome"); bleeding disorder
Amiodarone	Oral Parenteral	Treatment and prevention of ventricular and supraventricular tachyarrhythmias	1–2.5 μg/ml	0.1	2.25 10.25	Probably safe‖	Neonatal QT prolongation has been reported
Digoxin	Oral Parenteral	Paroxysmal supraventricular tachyarrhythmias; rate control in chronic atrial fibrillation	1–2 ng/ml	1.0	0.59 0.9	Safe	Adjust dosage when quinidine is given concomitantly
Propranolol	Oral Parenteral	Termination and prophylaxis in atrial and ventricular tachyarrhythmias; rate control in chronic fibrillation	75–100 mg/ml¶	1.27	0.23 1.65	Relatively safe	Chronic administration may be associated with intrauterine growth retardation, premature labor, neonatal hypoglycemia, bradycardia, and respiratory depression

*Umbilical venous/maternal venous concentration ratio.
†Prior digitalization recommended.
‡*N*-Acetylprocainamide.
§Probably safe as acute therapy of digitalis-induced arrhythmia.
‖These drugs have not been studied extensively enough in pregnant patients to establish absolute safety, but no serious adverse effects to the fetus have been reported.
¶Large interindividual variation.
From Rotmensch HH, Pines A, Donchin Y: Antiarrhythmic drugs in pregnancy. *In* Elkayam U, Gleicher N (eds): Cardiac Problems in Pregnancy. 2nd ed. Copyright © 1990. Reprinted by permission of Wiley-Liss, Inc., a division of John Wiley & Sons, Inc.

drug crosses the placenta, and fetal bradycardia, as well as small infants with low APGAR scores or hypoglycemia, has been reported for mothers receiving mexiletine. No teratogenic or long-term adverse effects have been reported. The dose ingested in breast milk appears to be below the therapeutic range, but because of limited information, mexiletine cannot be recommended for use during gestation or lactation.[196]

Amiodarone

Amiodarone has been used for the treatment of maternal and fetal arrhythmias. Side effects have included congenital hypothyroidism with goiter, premature birth, bradycardia, and enlarged fontanelles. It should be used only in refractory cases of ventricular tachyarrhythmias or perhaps in atrial fibrillation, with close monitoring of thyroid function. It is secreted in breast milk in significant quantities, and because its long-term effect on infants is unknown, breast-feeding is not recommended.[174, 175]

Heart Block

First Degree

Transient first-degree AV block has been noted to occur during labor.[197] Isolated first-degree AV block is usually stable. It may be caused by increased vagal tone, myocarditis, acute myocardial ischemia, degenerative conduction system disease, or medications.[198]

Second Degree

Mobitz type I block (*Wenckebach block*) can occur in well-conditioned athletes. It may also develop in the patient who has received too much digoxin and in patients receiving combinations of drugs that slow AV conduction, such as digoxin, verapamil or diltiazem, and/or β-blockers. It also occurs in patients with right CAD and in those with inferior MIs. It is generally stable and requires no treatment in the asymptomatic patient. However, a pacemaker is required if the ventricular rate is slow enough to cause symptoms, especially dizziness or syncope. Mobitz type II or second-degree block is almost always caused by underlying cardiac disease. Pacing, usually including permanent pacing, is recommended in patients with Mobitz type II heart block.[197–200]

Third Degree

Third-degree AV block or complete heart block in the mother is an unstable rhythm and may be associated with syncope and sudden death; therefore, prophylactic pacing is indicated even in asymptomatic patients.[200] Causes of complete heart block during pregnancy include acute myocarditis, calcific valvular aortic stenosis, acute MI or infective endocarditis, degenerative conduction system disease, after surgical correction of VSD, or overdoses of selected cardiac medications (e.g., digoxin, β-blockers, verapamil, or diltiazem).

Idiopathic congenital heart block is the most common cause of complete heart block in the fetus and is often found in infants of mothers with discoid or systemic lupus erythematosus (SLE). Antibodies to a maternal Ro antigen develop, cross the placenta, and bind to similar antigenic structures in fetal conduction tissue, leading to congenital complete heart block, usually with an AV junctional pacemaker. Ordinarily, a pacemaker is required in the teenage years or when patients become symptomatic with increasing physical activity and a relatively fixed HR.[201]

Bundle Branch Blocks

Bundle branch blocks develop in 1 to 2 percent of adult patients; most are more than 40 years old. Pregnant patients with bundle branch block should be evaluated for underlying heart disease. If patients have symptoms of dizziness or syncope, pacing may be required.[202]

Cardioversion

Direct-current cardioversion may be necessary for treatment of maternal tachycardias when they are associated with CHF or hypotension. The safety and efficacy of cardioversion during pregnancy have been well established with energy levels ranging from 10 to 300 J. The only complications reported have been transient fetal arrhythmias, which usually resolve spontaneously immediately after birth. Sedation should be used before elective cardioversion, and ideally, the patient should be fasting to prevent aspiration.[189–192]

Pacemaker

Rate-adaptive pacemakers are necessary in women of childbearing age. The pacemaker is usually placed under the breast to avoid skin irritation and ulceration at the implant site caused by enlargement of the breast and abdomen. Fixed-rate pacemakers pose risks because of their inability to adapt to the changes in HR that are necessary during pregnancy, labor, and delivery. Management of pregnant women with pacemakers should include careful monitoring for signs of CHF or pacemaker dysfunction. At delivery, continuous monitoring should be provided. Rate-responsive pacemakers have been used in women with complete AV block through pregnancy and cesarean section, with no major clinical problems. Function can be monitored on the basis of rate response to submaximal stress testing and daily activities. Prophylaxis for endocarditis with antibiotics should be used when pacemakers are implanted in patients with underlying heart disease.[203–205]

Coronary Artery Disease

MI occurs in fewer than 1 of 10,000 pregnancies, and coronary atherosclerosis is rare in women of childbearing age, apparently due to a protective effect of female hormones.[206] When MI occurs during pregnancy, it may be associated with a high maternal mortality rate, especially during the third trimester or later. Chest pain is common during pregnancy as a symptom of benign disorders, and a low level of suspicion may add to a delay in diagnosis of active CAD.

Risk Factors

Risk factors in women younger than age 50 include high levels of total plasma cholesterol and low-density lipoprotein (LDL) cholesterol, low levels of high-density lipoprotein (HDL) cholesterol, cigarette smoking, diabetes mellitus, hypertension, use of cocaine, toxemia of pregnancy, or a family history of CAD, especially with paternal or maternal history of MI under the age of 55 years.[207–210] Women who smoke or who have used oral contraceptives or drugs (e.g., cocaine) may be at an increased risk for atherosclerosis, coronary artery spasm, and thrombosis.[211–213]

Mechanisms of myocardial ischemia in pregnancy include atherosclerosis, coronary emboli, coronary spasm, and coronary artery dissection.[214, 215] Peripartum acute MI has been found to occur with normal coronary angiographic findings, probably due to spasm or in situ thrombosis.[216, 217] The cause of spasm is not clear, but it has been associated with pregnancy-induced hypertension and, in some instances, with the use of ergot derivatives to suppress lactation.[218]

Coronary artery dissection that occurs immediately postpartum is another relatively common cause of acute MI during the peripartum period.[215–219] Advanced maternal age and parity may predispose to the development of coronary arterial dissection, and most reported cases have occurred in the left anterior descending coronary artery.[219] Collagen vascular disease is another cause of acute MI during pregnancy.[212, 213]

Management and Evaluation

If unstable angina or MI occurs, the patient should be treated in a coronary care unit with a standard medical regimen designed to improve coronary blood flow and to reduce the risk of spasm and thrombosis (usually nitrates, a calcium antagonist, and aspirin). The cardiac workload can be reduced by the use of β-blockers.[220] The long-term safety of organic nitrates and calcium antagonists has not been established, but there are some published data on their use in hypertension, dissections, and arrhythmias. Thrombolytic therapy in the pregnant woman is contraindicated, and we recommend primary angioplasty if an acute anterior Q wave MI develops during the last trimester of pregnancy or soon thereafter. Otherwise, invasive procedures are usually delayed until the conclusion of pregnancy. Evaluation of the patient with chest pain can be performed with echocardiography,[221] serial ECGs, and enzyme measurements. When the patient is stabilized, submaximal exercise testing with two-dimensional echocardiography can be performed to assess the presence of CAD by detecting regional wall motion abnormalities during or immediately after exercise, which could represent myocardial ischemia. A falsely high incidence of abnormal exercise tolerance tests in women has been suggested from exercise ECGs; therefore, some assessment of regional wall motion in the pregnant woman is very helpful.[222–226] A dobutamine stress test with echocardiography might be used to detect CAD through noninvasive methods. If angina cannot be controlled during pregnancy, angioplasty or coronary artery bypass graft surgery can be performed.[227–229] Such procedures should be avoided during the first trimester, if possible, because of the potential effects of ionizing radiation on the fetus.[230]

Delivery imposes an even higher work demand on a compromised heart. Analgesia and supplemental oxygen are used during labor, and the cardiac output is increased by placing the patient in the left lateral decubitus position. Forceps can be used to shorten the second stage of delivery. Cesarean section can be used in patients with active myocardial ischemia or hemodynamic instability who do not respond to medical therapy. Epidural anesthesia may help to reduce hemodynamic fluctuations during labor and may lead to LV unloading due to vasodilatation. If general anesthesia is used, halothane should be avoided in patients with depressed LV systolic function. Continued hemodynamic monitoring is advised for at least 24 hours postpartum.[218–220]

A patient with myocardial ischemia is best managed with an emphasis on reducing cardiovascular stress and careful monitoring during labor and delivery, often with pulmonary artery catheterization.

Hypertension

In measuring the blood pressure of a pregnant woman, measurement in the upper arm in the lateral recumbent position will give falsely low blood pressure readings. Blood pressures are best recorded with the patient in the sitting or the lateral recumbent position. Blood pressure should be measured with the patient in the same position at each visit. Hypertension is defined as a rise in systolic blood pressure of at least 30 mm Hg, or an absolute value of ≥140 mm Hg, or a rise of diastolic pressure of at least 15 mm Hg, or an absolute value of ≥90 mm Hg.[231] The pressure rise is determined from a previously measured baseline value, and pressures must be sustained at a high level on at least two occasions.[232, 233] *Pregnancy-induced hypertension* is a term that includes a wide spectrum of disease severity in hypertensive patients, including preeclampsia, eclampsia, and gestational hypertension (Table 110–12).[234]

Gestational hypertension describes those patients who develop pregnancy-induced hypertension. These patients do not develop other signs and symptoms of preeclampsia. The blood pressure usually returns to normal within 10 days of delivery. There often is a recurrence of pregnancy-induced hypertension after successive pregnancies, and some of these women develop chronic hypertension in later life.[234, 235]

Preeclampsia is defined as the appearance of hypertension after week 20 of gestation, combined with the finding of edema of the hands or face or the development of proteinuria of more than 300 mg during a 24-hour period. Preeclampsia may be mild but is considered severe when *one* of the following conditions exists[236–240]:

1. Blood pressure readings of 160/110 mm Hg on two occasions more than 6 hours apart
2. Proteinuria of 5 g/24 h
3. Oliguria of less than 500 ml of urine during a 24-hour period
4. Cerebral edema
5. Pulmonary edema

Eclampsia describes the presence of convulsions in a woman with preeclampsia if the convulsions are not due

TABLE 110–12 Classification of Hypertension in Pregnancy

Gestational hypertension and/or proteinuria: hypertension and/or proteinuria developing during pregnancy, labor, or the puerperium in a previously normotensive nonproteinuric woman subdivided into
- Gestational hypertension: diastolic blood pressure > 110 once or > 90 twice, 4 h apart
- Gestational proteinuria: >300 mg/24 h or two clean-voided specimens 4 h apart with 2+ reagent strip (1 g/L)
- Gestational proteinuric hypertension (preeclampsia)

Chronic hypertension and chronic renal disease: hypertension and/or proteinuria at the first visit before wk 20 of pregnancy or the presence of chronic hypertension or chronic renal disease diagnosed before, during, or after pregnancy

Unclassified hypertension and/or proteinuria: hypertension and/or proteinuria found either
- At first examination after 20 wk (140 da) in a woman without known chronic hypertension or chronic renal disease

  or
- During pregnancy, labor, or the puerperium when information is insufficient to permit classification is regarded as unclassified during pregnancy and is subdivided into
  - Hypertension (without proteinuria)
  - Proteinuria (without hypertension)
  - Proteinuric hypertension

Eclampsia: the occurrence of generalized convulsions during pregnancy, during labor, or within 7 da of delivery and not caused by epilepsy or other convulsive disorders

From Kaplan NK: Clinical Hypertension. 5th ed. Baltimore: Williams & Wilkins, 1990.

to any other cause. Hypertensive crisis (180/120 mm Hg) can be managed with intravenous hydralazine every 2 to 4 hours or by continuous infusion. Magnesium sulfate, diazoxide, and nitroprusside have also been used (Table 110–13).[241, 242]

Chronic hypertension is a condition in which there is persistence of blood pressures of greater than 140/90 mm Hg before and after pregnancy. Pressures found to be this high during the first 20 weeks of pregnancy are considered a manifestation of chronic systemic arterial hypertension. Usually, women have a low pressure during the first weeks of pregnancy. Preexisting hypertension is associated with an increased incidence and severity of toxemia. Treatment of preexisting hypertension does not decrease this incidence but does reduce complications.

Traditionally, preeclampsia has been thought to represent generalized vasoconstriction, leading to end-organ damage in maternal and fetal tissues.[243, 244] Maternal diastolic blood pressures of greater than 110 mm Hg should be treated promptly, with the goal being to reduce the diastolic pressure to 90 mm Hg. Chronic systemic arterial hypertension may be associated with fetal intrauterine growth retardation, placental abruptio, premature delivery, or superimposed preeclampsia.[245] The fetus should be monitored periodically with ultrasound. Alpha-methyldopa and hydralazine are commonly used during pregnancy because they do not significantly reduce uteroplacental blood flow without a history of fetal anomalies.[246] No randomized trials have been performed to determine the safety of selective β-blockers or calcium channel blockers, but propranolol and atenolol appear to be safe for use throughout pregnancy and may decrease fetal wastage in patients with chronic hypertension.[247, 248] In order to prevent seizures, treatment is usually administered to patients with blood pressures greater than 140/90 mm Hg. Hemorrhage within the central nervous system is the major cause of maternal death from preeclampsia.

Accumulated evidence suggests that preeclampsia may be caused by placental thrombosis, resulting from an early problem with placentation. The renal damage from preeclampsia resembles that caused by immunologic disorders in vascular channels. There appears to be generalized vasospasm, with some increased sensitivity of vascular smooth muscles to pressor substances. It is believed that there is an imbalance in vasoactive eicosanoid production. All of these factors may lead to end-organ hypoperfusion, decreased plasma volume, and hypertension. Placental production of thromboxane A_2 is increased relative to that of prostacyclin in patients with preeclampsia. Aspirin has been used in previous studies to inhibit platelet cyclooxygenase activity[243] and to reduce thromboxane production.[249] Some clinicians use low-dose aspirin in high-risk populations as a prophylactic agent before the onset of clinical symptoms. Data have not conclusively proven the effec-

TABLE 110–13 Drug Treatment of Hypertensive Emergencies

Drug	Onset	Time Course of Action: Maximum	Time Course of Action: Duration	Dosage: IM	Dosage: IV	Interval Between Doses	Mechanism of Action
Hydralazine	10–20 min	20–40 min	3–8 h	10–50 mg	5–25 mg	3–6 h	Direct dilatation of arterioles
Diazoxide	1–2 min	2–3 min	4–12 h	—	50–300 mg	3–10 h	Direct dilatation of arterioles
Trimethaphan camsylate	1–2 min	2–5 min	10 min	—	IV solution 2 g/L; IV infusion rate 1–15 mg/min		Ganglionic blockade
Sodium nitroprusside	0.5–2 min	1–2 min	3–5 min	—	IV solution 0.01 g/L; IV infusion rate 0.2–0.8 mg/min		Direct dilatation of arterioles and veins

From Creasy RK, Resnik R: Maternal-Fetal Medicine: Principles and Practice. 2nd ed. Philadelphia: WB Saunders, 1989.

tiveness of low-dose aspirin or of low-dose aspirin and dipyridamole in the treatment of these patients.[249]

Antihypertensive Agents

The many classes of antihypertensive agents are summarized in Table 110–14 (see also Table 110–113) and in Chapter 80.

The goal of treatment for blood pressure management is the prevention of seizures, central nervous system hemorrhage, pulmonary or cerebral edema, oliguria, renal damage, and fetal compromise, or other cardiovascular catastrophe. Monitoring of patients must include checks for proteinuria, edema, retinal change, cardiac examination findings, bruising tendencies, and deep tendon reflexes. Automated blood pressure recording devices can be used at home for a more comprehensive evaluation of readings. In most cases, adequate data are not available regarding the safety and efficacy of new drugs, especially for some of the new classes, in the fetus and mother (Table 110–15). Therapy is aimed at the prevention of preeclampsia, in some cases with the use of aspirin.

Pulmonary Hypertension

Primary Pulmonary Hypertension

Primary pulmonary hypertension represents a contraindication to pregnancy, as the normal physiologic changes associated with pregnancy and labor pose danger (Table 110–16).[250, 251] Clinical deterioration is common, and maternal death occurs in approximately 40 percent of such patients.[252, 253] Death may occur at any time and cannot be predicted on the basis of the patient's preconception clinical status. Labor and delivery are significant stresses, with death occurring most often during late gestation or in the early postpartum period. If this condition is detected within the first 4 months of pregnancy, interruption of the pregnancy is advised.[254, 255] Symptomatic deterioration usually occurs during the second trimester and is heralded by dyspnea, syncope, chest pain, and RV failure. There is high maternal risk in addition to a high incidence of spontaneous abortions, premature delivery, and neonatal death. Fetal mortality rates are as high as 50 percent.[256]

The increased hemodynamic load on the right ventricle may lead to myocardial ischemia, arrhythmia, or CHF. The presence of a high pulmonary artery pressure and a high pulmonary capillary wedge pressure increases the hemodynamic load on the heart.

If the patient chooses to continue the pregnancy, physical exertion should be restricted to reduce the circulatory load. Elective hospitalization early in pregnancy is recommended to ensure restricted activity and close follow-up.[255] Traditional treatment has included oxygen supplementation, digoxin, and diuretics for symptomatic CHF. Anticoagulation is beneficial in these patients because they are at an increased risk for thromboembolism during pregnancy. Anticoagulation is recommended throughout gestation and at least during the early postpartum period. Investigation into the use of vasodilator therapy, such as calcium channel blockers, has been proposed in nonpregnant patients. Investigations have focused on the possible role of endothelial cells and impairment of the release of endothelium-derived relaxation factor (nitric oxide) in some cases of pregnancy-induced pulmonary hypertension.[255, 256] Treatment has included intranasal nitric oxide or chronic intravenous infusion of prostacyclin.

During labor and delivery, hemodynamic monitoring and blood gas measurements must be obtained. In patients who can tolerate vaginal delivery, spontaneous labor is preferable to induction. Oxygen is administered, and blood loss is immediately replaced. Segmental epidural anesthesia and intrathecal morphine have been used successfully to relieve pain. Because of the RV dysfunction, anesthetics with negative inotropic effects should be avoided. Hemodynamic monitoring should be continued for 48 hours after delivery, and a hospital stay of several days is recommended.[257, 258] Tubal ligation, under local or epidural anesthesia with close cardiac monitoring, is recommended after delivery to prevent future pregnancies.[259]

Secondary Pulmonary Hypertension

Secondary pulmonary hypertension may be a result of chronic thromboembolic pulmonary hypertension or of vascular disease, congenital intracardiac shunts (e.g., VSD, patent ductus arteriosus [PDA], aortopulmonary connection) or, less commonly, ASD leading to a large left-to-right shunt and the development of pulmonary artery hypertension or Eisenmenger's syndrome. If a right-to-left shunt is present, SVR must be maintained throughout labor, delivery, and puerperium. The risks and concerns are the same as for patients with primary pulmonary hypertension.[260]

Aortic Disease

Aortic Dissection

Half of the aortic dissections that develop in women younger than 40 years occur in association with pregnancy. There appears to be a predisposition to this condition during gestation, with more than 200 cases reported during the past 50 years.[261] The incidence increased in women over the age of 30 and in those who have had multiple pregnancies, hypertension, cardiac malformations, coarctation of the aorta, and Marfan's syndrome. Ehlers-Danlos type IV syndrome may also cause acute dissection of the descending thoracic aorta in pregnancy.[262] Dissection most commonly occurs during the third trimester and the peripartum period.[215, 261–263]

Aortography often provides a definitive diagnosis but exposes the fetus to radiation, as does computed tomography. Transesophageal echocardiography and MRI can often detect aortic dissection without radiation exposure.[264–266] Treatment includes the avoidance of systemic arterial pressure elevations during labor and delivery through the use of cesarean section with epidural anesthesia. Hydralazine, orally or intravenously, is the drug of choice for blood pressure reduction in pregnant women with aortic dissec-

TABLE 110-14 **Antihypertensive Drugs in Pregnancy**

Agent	Mechanism of Action	Cardiac Output	Renal Blood Flow	Side Effects	
				Maternal	***Neonatal***
Thiazide	Initial: decreased plasma volume and cardiac output Later: decreased total peripheral resistance	Decreased Unchanged	Decreased Unchanged or increased	Electrolyte depletion, serum uric acid increase, thrombocytopenia, hemorrhagic pancreatitis	Thrombocytopenia
Methyldopa	False neurotransmission, CNS effect	Unchanged	Unchanged	Lethargy, fever, hepatitis, hemolytic anemia, positive Coombs' test result	
Hydralazine	Direct peripheral vasodilatation	Increased	Unchanged or increased	Flushing, headache, tachycardia, palpitations, lupus syndrome	
Prazosin	Direct vasodilator and cardiac effects	Increased or unchanged	Unchanged	Hypotension with first dose; little information on use in pregnancy	
Clonidine	CNS effects	Unchanged or increased	Unchanged	Rebound hypertension; little information on use in pregnancy	
Guanethidine	Impairment of postganglionic adrenergic nerve function	Decreased	Decreased	Postural hypotension	
Propranolol	Beta-adrenergic blockade	Decreased	Decreased	Increased uterine tone with possible decrease in placental perfusion	Depressed respiration
Labetalol	Alpha- and beta-adrenergic blockade	Unchanged	Unchanged	Tremulousness, flushing, headache	See Propranolol
Reserpine	Depletion of norepinephrine from sympathetic nerve endings	Unchanged	Unchanged	Nasal stuffiness, depression, increased sensitivity to seizures	Nasal congestion, increased respiratory tract secretions, cyanosis, anorexia
Ganglionic blockers	Decrease in peripheral resistance through adrenergic blockade	Decreased	Decreased	Marked sensitivity with secondary hypotension	Meconium ileus

Abbreviation: CNS, central nervous system.
From Creasy RK, Resnik R: Maternal-Fetal Medicine: Principles and Practice. 2nd ed. Philadelphia: WB Saunders, 1989.

TABLE 110–15 New Classes of Antihypertensive Drugs

	Adrenergic Agonists			Adrenergic Blockers					
	α	β	$\alpha + \beta$	α	β	Aldomet	Hydralazine	Diazoxide	Digitalis
UPF	↓	No Δ	Low dose primarily β	No Δ	?	± ↓	↑	↓	?–↑
MC	↑	↓	High dose primarily α	↓	No Δ–? ↑	No Δ	No Δ	No Δ	↑

From Kammerer WS, Gross RJ: Medical Consultation: The Internist on Surgical, Obstetric, and Psychiatric Services. 2nd ed. Baltimore: Williams & Wilkins, 1990.

tion, but hypertension can also be treated with a combination of propranolol and nitroprusside (see Table 110–13). Nitroprusside can cause fetal toxicity and should be used only in patients who are refractory to other drugs.[267–274] Patients with known valvular or aortic diseases should undergo surgical repair during the first two trimesters and should be delivered by cesarean section. Patients with acute aortic problems near term are better managed by cesarean section first, followed promptly by treatment of the aortic disease. Successful surgical repair of aortic dissection has been reported in pregnancy.[274, 275]

Marfan's Syndrome

Conception is not advised in women with significant cardiac involvement, including those with asymptomatic dilatation of the aorta. Many of these women have preexisting cardiovascular problems, including aortic regurgitation and dilatation. There is a high incidence of aortic dissection and death among pregnant patients with Marfan's syndrome.[263, 264] More than half of these patients have evidence of mitral or aortic valve abnormalities on auscultation, with 25 percent having detectable aortic regurgitation; the incidence of MV prolapse may be as high as 90 percent in patients with Marfan's syndrome. The incidence of spontaneous abortion is often increased, and because the syndrome is transmitted as an autosomal dominant trait, half of the offspring may be affected. The life span of affected individuals is reduced, and the childbearing years may therefore be limited. For these reasons, preconception counseling should include a discussion of the risks for inheritance of this syndrome and the risks of pregnancy to the mother and fetus.

Some evidence suggests that when the aortic diameter exceeds 40 to 45 mm, there is a higher maternal morbidity and mortality risk during pregnancy from dissection and rupture.[265, 266] The risk is significantly lower in patients with no cardiac complications and a normal aortic diameter. If the patient is already pregnant with an aorta of more than 40 mm in diameter, interruption of the pregnancy should be considered. If a patient elects to continue the pregnancy, all efforts should be focused on reducing pulsatile forces on the aortic wall by limiting physical activity and on a reduction in blood pressure with β-blockers.[272] These maneuvers may reduce the rate of aortic dilatation and the risk of aortic dissection in patients with Marfan's syndrome.[272, 275]

Abdominal delivery by cesarean section may be preferred in women with aortic dilatation and other cardiac complications to avoid the strain of labor. Adequate analgesia should be used, and prophylactic antibiotics are recommended.

TABLE 110–16 High-Risk Maternal Cardiovascular Disorders

Disorder	Maternal Mortality Rate (%)*
Aortic valve disease	10–20
Coarctation of the aorta	5
Eisenmenger's syndrome	30–70
Marfan's syndrome	25–50 (estimated)
Mitral stenosis with atrial fibrillation	14–17
Peripartal cardiomyopathy	15–60
Primary pulmonary hypertension	50
Tetralogy of Fallot	12

*These values, which were compiled from 18 references, represent different study periods and disorders of varying severity; therefore, they must be regarded as approximations.

From Ueland K: Cardiovascular disease complicating pregnancy. Clin Obstet Gynecol 21(2):429–442, 1978.

Takayasu's Arteritis

Takayasu's arteritis is a chronic inflammatory condition of the arteries of unknown origin, which may cause severe stenoses of affected arteries (see Ch. 72).[276] Young women under the age of 30 years are predominantly affected. Pregnancy does not appear to alter the inflammatory activity of this disorder. There is a high prevalence among Asian populations, but this disease is worldwide in origin. Regardless of race, any patient who presents with pulseless hypertensive disease or other features of Takayasu's arteritis for the first time in pregnancy should be evaluated for the presence of aortic regurgitation, hypertension, arterial aneurysms, and retinopathy.[276–283] There is a high risk for pregnancy-induced hypertension in this population. Measurement of blood pressure in the arms may be impossible or unreliable, and lower extremity readings do not allow conclusions to be drawn about perfusion of arteries supplying the upper part of the body and about cerebral perfusion pressure. When the inflammatory process is severe, there have been reports of cerebral hemorrhage, CHF, death, and low-birth-weight infants. If aortic narrowing is present, blood pressure should not be reduced markedly. Invasive monitoring may not be advisable, because arterial catheterization may further injure inflamed vessels.[282]

Glucocorticoids are usually reserved for patients who become pregnant during an acute inflammatory phase of the disease. In general, cytotoxic agents are not advisable during pregnancy. Vaginal delivery is usually tolerated, especially when vacuum extraction or forceps are used to shorten the second stage of labor. General or spinal anesthesia may produce arterial hypotension. Epidural anesthesia should not be used when substantial aortic narrowing is present, due to the fall in blood pressure distal to a narrowed aorta. Prophylactic antibiotics are recommended if aortic regurgitation or vascular stenoses are present. Oral contraceptive use may accelerate the progression of this arteritis and should be avoided during the postpartum period.[276]

Mycotic Aneurysms

Cases of femoral artery mycotic aneurysms have been reported in pregnancy, usually related to the intravenous use of illicit drugs. Pregnancy does not appear to alter the course of this disease, but it does increase the incidence of maternal and fetal complications.[284, 285]

Collagen Vascular Disease

Systemic Lupus Erythematosus and Anti-Ro Antibody

SLE may be associated with myocarditis, pericarditis, or nonbacterial vegetations. If a patient is in remission at the time of conception, there is a 25 percent chance of exacerbation during pregnancy, usually in the last trimester and during the early postpartum period. Rarely is a patient's condition improved with pregnancy.[286–288] Steroids may help to prevent tamponade if pericarditis develops. As noted earlier, a mother with the anti-Ro antibody is more likely to have a baby with congenital complete heart block or endocardial fibrosis. SLE is associated with a high incidence of pregnancy-induced hypertension, often due to lupus nephritis, which sometimes improves with steroid therapy.[289, 290]

Many conventional measures of SLE activity, such as serum complement levels, platelet count, and urinary protein measurement, are invalid during pregnancy. Blood levels of C_3 increase in normal pregnancies. In 75 to 85 percent of patients with stable or decreased C_3, there is worsening of SLE.[291, 292]

The lupus anticoagulant syndrome, with the presence of an antibody to cardiolipin and a risk of developing venous and arterial thromboses, has been reported to be a potential cause of preeclampsia, arthropathies, thrombocytopenia, and prolonged partial thromboplastin time.[293] Patients may present with a history of first-trimester abortions and death in utero during the second and third trimesters. These patients are at a higher risk for bleeding at delivery. There is some evidence that low-dose aspirin and corticosteroids improve outcome. Corticosteroids may also be used during gestation in mothers who have the anti-Ro antibody, in an effort to prevent congenital complete heart block.[294–300]

Dermatomyositis

Dermatomyositis affects women twice as commonly as men and has been reported to develop or worsen during pregnancy.[301] There is a high rate of fetal loss in patients with dermatomyositis or polymyositis, especially when the disease begins during pregnancy.[302] Heart disease can develop from inflammatory lesions of the blood vessels that lead to ischemia or primary involvement of heart muscle itself, resulting in CHF. Some patients develop arrhythmias or heart block. Steroids may be indicated when cardiac problems and other muscle weakness are severe.[303]

Pericarditis

Patients with pericarditis may present with chest pain or heart failure in the peripartum period; maternal deaths have been reported.[304] Dyspnea is a common symptom when the effusion is moderate to large and may result from impaired filling of the ventricles. The dilated pericardium may mechanically compress adjacent structures, causing hoarseness, coughing, and dysphagia. The pregnant patient may incorrectly attribute shortness of breath as being due to pregnancy. Dyspneic patients who have neck vein distention and are hypotensive may deteriorate if they are mistakenly treated with diuretics for presumed CHF without recognition of the presence of a large pericardial effusion.[305, 306] There often is accompanying sharp or stabbing substernal chest pain, which radiates to other areas. The characteristic finding of increased chest pain with the patient in the supine position and partial relief on leaning forward is also found during pregnancy. Upper respiratory symptoms and low-grade fever often precede the onset of chest pain in patients with pericarditis.

The differentiation of a pericardial friction rub may be more difficult during pregnancy, because systolic murmurs and a split first heart sound are common in pregnancy. Pregnant patients with dyspnea, neck vein distention, and chest pain should be fully evaluated. Most cases of pericarditis are self-limited and mild, but the hemodynamic burden of pregnancy and the increased blood volume, together with an associated myocarditis that may accompany pericarditis, may lead to CHF. In the patient with pericarditis, an evaluation for collagen vascular disease should be made, because SLE, rheumatoid arthritis, and scleroderma can cause pericarditis.[307] Idiopathic causes are the most common in pregnancy, but many of these have viral causes such as coxsackievirus, especially after or in association with an upper respiratory infection.[308–311] Lymphadenopathy, myalgias, and a rash may accompany viral pericarditis.[304, 306]

The patient is managed with bed rest, hospitalization, and analgesic medication with aspirin or nonsteroidal agents (e.g., indomethacin) and with monitoring for arrhythmias. Pericardiocentesis can be performed in the pregnant patient via the subxiphoid approach if there is a moderate amount of fluid on the echocardiogram.[312] However, pericardiocentesis should be performed only when there is concern about an infection or a malignancy or when hemodynamic compromise occurs (pericardial tamponade).[304, 306] Surgical intervention may be required for recurrent pericardial tamponade, intractable chest pain, or pyogenic- or neoplastic-related pericarditis. Pericardiectomy is usually effective, and subsequent pregnancies are usually well tolerated.[313] Hemodynamic evaluation is performed via pulmonary artery catheterization with hemodynamic monitoring.[314–316] Cases of idiopathic pericarditis during pregnancy have been reported, usually with uneventful term deliveries. These patients are usually treated with aspirin or indomethacin and, if necessary, steroids for chest pain.

MYOCARDITIS AND CARDIOMYOPATHY

Myocarditis

There is no increase in susceptibility to myocarditis during gestation or the postpartum period.[317] In patients with a previous diagnosis of myocarditis, pregnancy is not advisable because of the chance of residual myocardial dysfunction. Patients who present with an enlarged heart and CHF, arrhythmias, or chest pain may require endomyocardial biopsy to confirm the diagnosis and allow directed treatment with anti-inflammatory agents. Anticoagulation and medical treatment of CHF are also used.[318–321]

Peripartum Cardiomyopathy

Peripartum cardiomyopathy is usually considered an idiopathic primary congestive cardiomyopathy.[322, 323] In 1870, Virchow described a primary heart muscle disease developing in late pregnancy. Women of childbearing age may develop a dilated cardiomyopathy that usually occurs late in the third trimester or the first 3 postpartum months (Fig. 110–16), with a significant decrease in cardiac function (Table 110–17). The incidence in the United States varies between 1:1300 and 1:15,000 pregnancies. There is a higher incidence of 1:100 in certain parts of Africa.[324, 325] The incidence is greater with twin pregnancies, in women who are multiparous, in women over 30 years of age, in black women, and in women in lower socioeconomic groups.

Infant mortality rates are 10 to 30 percent when CHF is present during pregnancy, and maternal mortality rates are 25 to 50 percent within the first few months of the development of this problem. Maternal morbidity and mortality rates of more than 50 percent have been described at 2 to 5 years. The clinical course varies, but approximately 50 percent of patients show complete or nearly complete recovery of cardiac function within the first 6 months postpartum (Fig. 110–17). The remaining 50 percent demonstrate clinical deterioration clinically, persistent LV dysfunction, chronic CHF, or early death, with higher morbidity and mortality rates.[326] In women with enlarged hearts and symptomatic CHF, the risks associated with pregnancy are sufficiently significant to advise the avoidance of subsequent conceptions.[327, 328] If this clinical entity develops during pregnancy, an endomyocardial biopsy sample should be obtained because there is a significant incidence of myocarditis on biopsy of the heart in this form of dilated cardiomyopathy.[329, 330] A diagnosis of peripartum cardiomyopathy depends on excluding other forms of LV dilatation and systolic dysfunction.[331, 332]

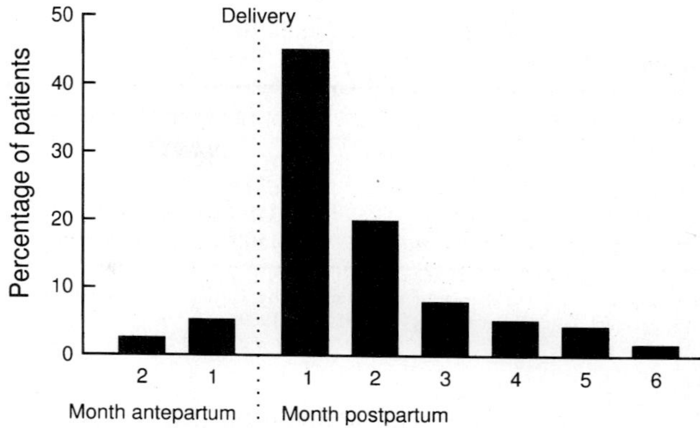

FIGURE 110–16 Onset of peripartum cardiomyopathy in a review of 347 patients as a percentage of patients in the months before and after delivery. The majority of cases occur in the last trimester of pregnancy or first 6 months postpartum. (From Homans DC: Peripartum cardiomyopathy. N Engl J Med 312:1432, 1985. © 1985, Massachusetts Medical Society. All rights reserved.)

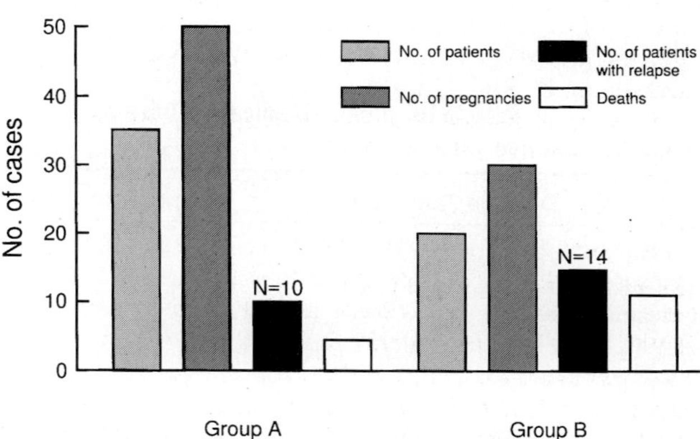

FIGURE 110–17 Number of pregnancies that result in relapse or death in the groups of patients who developed peripartum cardiomyopathy. Group A patients had clinical improvement with normalization of heart size on chest x-ray or left ventricular size and function by echocardiography. Group B patients had persistent cardiomyopathy, left ventricular dysfunction, or both. (From Braunwald E: Heart Disease. 4th ed. Philadelphia: WB Saunders, 1992.)

TABLE 110–17 Left Ventricular Function in Women With Peripartum Cardiomyopathy and Normal Women in the Postpartum Period (Control)*

	PPCM (n = 10)	Control (n = 11)	*P*
EDVI (ml/m²)	95 ± 22	67 ± 9	<.005
ESVI (ml/m²)	66 ± 18	27 ± 5	<.0001
LVWI (g/m²)	139 ± 38	96 ± 8	<.005
EF (%)	29 ± 5	67 ± 5	<.001

Abbreviations: EDVI, end-diastolic volume index; EF, ejection fraction; ESVI, end-systolic volume index; LVWI, left ventricular wall mass index; PPCM, peripartum cardiomyopathy.

*Data expressed as mean ± SD.

From Cole P, Cook F, Plappert T, et al: Longitudinal charges in left ventricular architecture and function in peripartum cardiomyopathy. Am J Cardiol 60:871, 1987. With permission from Excerpta Medica Inc.

TABLE 110–18 Therapeutic Goals for Hemodynamic Intervention

Parameter	Therapeutic Goal
Heart rate	70–100 beats/min
Pulmonary capillary wedge pressure	6–15 mm Hg
Cardiac index	3–5 L/min/m^2
Systemic vascular resistance index	1500–2200 dynes/s/cm^{-5}/m^2

From Lee W, Cotton DB: Peripartum cardiomyopathy: current concepts and clinical management. Clin Obstet Gynecol 32(1):54–67, 1989.

Patients may present with symptoms of CHF, chest pain, palpitations, and, occasionally, peripheral or pulmonary embolization. Physical examination reveals a large heart and often an S_3 and murmurs of mitral or tricuspid regurgitation. The ECG may show changes of LV hypertrophy, ST-T changes, conduction abnormalities, and arrhythmias. Cardiomegaly and pulmonary vascular congestion are seen on chest radiography, occasionally with pleural effusions. Two-dimensional echocardiography characteristically shows four-chamber enlargement, with marked reduction in LV systolic function. Small-to-moderate pericardial effusions may be present, and regurgitation across mitral, tricuspid, or pulmonary valves may be found.[322]

Acute CHF is treated with oxygen, diuretics, inotropic support with digitalis, and "unloading therapy" with vasodilator agents (Tables 110–18 and 110–19). Conservative medical management includes limitation of activity, reduced sodium intake, the use of digoxin, and, in some cases, the use of diuretics. Steroid therapy may be beneficial if an endomyocardial biopsy has confirmed myocarditis.[321] Hydralazine has been used as an afterload-reducing agent and is believed to be safe during pregnancy. Organic nitrates have been used, but experience is limited and hypotension may result, with associated fetal bradycardia. Nitroprusside has been successfully used during pregnancy, but there is evidence in animals of fetal toxicity. Angiotensin-converting enzyme inhibitors (ACEIs) have deleterious effects on blood pressure and renal function in the fetus and are not recommended for use in the antepartum period.[324]

TABLE 110–19 Useful Medication Dosages for Peripartum Cardiomyopathy Patients

	Dosage Regimen	Comments
*Antepartum**		
Furosemide	20–40 mg PO qd to qid	
Hydralazine	20–75 mg PO tid to qid	
Digoxin	0.25–0.37 mg PO qd	
Intrapartum		
Dopamine	2–10 μg/kg/min IV	10 ml/min = 1 μg/kg/min†
Dobutamine	2–10 μg/kg/min IV	20 ml/min = 2 μg/kg/min
		30 ml/min = 3 μg/kg/min

*Use of angiotensin-converting enzyme inhibitors is contraindicated in pregnancy, because of risk of fetal injury and death.

†Drug dosages administered at μg/kg/min may be prepared with the following formula: 1.5 mg × body wt (kg) = total mg drug in 250 ml 5% dextrose in water.

From Lee W, Cotton DB: Peripartum cardiomyopathy: current concepts and clinical management. Clin Obstet Gynecol 32(1):54–67, 1989.

Anticoagulant therapy is recommended, because there is an increased incidence of thrombotic events. The temporary use of an intra-aortic balloon pump may help stabilize patients with severe cardiac decompensation.[333, 334] Cardiac transplantation may be considered after pregnancy in severe cases.[335]

Hypertrophic Obstructive Cardiomyopathy or Idiopathic Hypertrophic Subaortic Stenosis

Hypertrophic obstructive cardiomyopathy is a primary myocardial disease characterized by generalized hypertrophy of the ventricular myocardium, with asymmetric thickening of the upper part of the ventricular septum.[336, 337] There is an increased risk of sudden death of approximately 1 to 3 percent per year with this condition.[338, 339] It is inherited as an autosomal dominant with variable penetrance; therefore, as many as 50 percent of offspring can be affected by this heart lesion.[336–341]

Pregnancy alters the hemodynamics associated with hypertrophic obstructive cardiomyopathy. The increased blood flow of pregnancy may lessen the degree of LV outflow obstruction. Any sudden decrease in venous return due to an obstruction of the inferior vena cava late in pregnancy or to blood loss at delivery may increase the severity of LV outflow tract obstruction. This can be serious when combined with the normal fall in PVR of pregnancy.[338]

The diagnosis may be missed during pregnancy, when systolic murmurs, signs of CHF, and LV hypertrophy may be present normally. An S_4, a systolic thrill along the left lower sternal border and apex, and a more intense murmur in the upright position or during straining maneuvers, such as the Valsalva maneuver, are suggestive of hypertrophic cardiomyopathy with obstruction. Typical symptoms of CHF and sudden death may be the first clinical manifestations of the disease. Physical examination may be normal in some patients who do not have LV outflow tract obstruction. Two-dimensional echocardiography with Doppler is helpful in identifying the presence of LV outflow obstruction and estimating the severity of associated mitral regurgitation. In addition, gated MRI can delineate the severity and extent of asymmetric septal hypertrophy. In a series of patients with hypertrophic cardiomyopathy and pregnancy, there was favorable outcome in the majority of the pregnancies.[341] Fetal outcome does not appear to be affected by maternal hypertrophic cardiomyopathy.

Treatment is indicated if there are symptoms at rest or if there is worsening of the LV obstruction. Medical management during pregnancy should be directed at avoiding sudden volume shifts and maintaining blood volume and venous return to the heart while decreasing the force of myocardial contraction by avoidance of excitement, anxiety, and strenuous activity.[342] If there is evidence of increased obstruction with elevation of LV pressures, volume replacement and vasopressor agents should be used immediately. β-Blockers are the primary medical intervention used in these patients.[343, 344] Calcium channel blockers, such as verapamil, and β-blockers have been used in a few patients to reduce symptoms.[345]

In patients who are symptomatic and known to have LV outflow obstruction, hemodynamic monitoring should be initiated at the onset of labor. Spinal and epidural anesthesia should be avoided in patients with hypertrophic obstructive cardiomyopathy because of the potential to vasodilate and cause hypotension.[346–348] Systemic medication, inhalation analgesia, and paracervical or pudendal blocks are recommended for pain relief during labor and delivery. General anesthesia with potent inhalation agents that are myocardial depressants is recommended for cesarean delivery. There is an increased risk for bacterial endocarditis with the obstructive form of this disease; therefore, prophylactic antibiotics should be administered at delivery.[338] The maintenance of intravascular volume is of utmost importance in labor and delivery, because catecholamine levels may be increased, aggravating this condition. Vaginal delivery is safe in the majority of these patients without increased risk to mother or fetus.[346–348] If symptoms of LV outflow obstruction are present, the second stage of labor can be shortened by the use of forceps or vacuum. Left uterine displacement is advised during labor and delivery to relieve compression on the inferior vena cava and to allow increased venous return to the heart.

At delivery, blood loss, vasodilatation, and sympathetic stimulation from anesthesia should be avoided. Because of the strong vasodilator effect of prostaglandins, they should not be used to stimulate uterine contractions during the peripartum period. Although the safe use of oxytocin has been reported in some patients, it may also have negative effects, and some have recommended the use of ergonovine as a preferred agent for induction of labor in this population. Beta sympathomimetic tocolytic agents may aggravate LV outflow tract obstruction, so magnesium sulfate is preferred for use with premature contractions.

If arrhythmias are present, treatment must be directed at them. Atrial arrhythmias may be found in patients with enlarged left atria and may be associated with thromboembolic complications; anticoagulation therapy should be considered in these patients. Sudden death is most commonly seen during the childbearing years in women with this disorder, but pregnancy does not appear to increase the risk for sudden death. The presence of complex ventricular arrhythmias should be identified with 24-hour electrocardiographic monitoring because they constitute an important prognostic sign.

Valvular Heart Disease

General considerations in any pregnant patient with valvular heart disease should be a determination of the degree of stenosis or regurgitation of the affected valve and chamber sizes, an assessment of the need for anticoagulation, and antibiotic prophylaxis against endocarditis.

Mitral Valve Prolapse

MV prolapse is one of the most common cardiac abnormalities in women. It occurs as a consequence of myxomatous degeneration of the MV leaflets and supporting structures.[349, 350] Other findings or complications include chest pain, arrhythmias or postural hypotension, and mild mitral insufficiency.[351] Most patients are asymptomatic, but the usual symptoms of MV prolapse, such as palpitations, anxiety, fatigue, lightheadedness, and chest pain, may occur during pregnancy.[352] Clicks, murmurs, and symptoms may become less obvious during pregnancy, probably related to the expanded intravascular volume, which may realign the MV complex by increasing LV end-diastolic volume or lengthening the long axis of the left ventricle.[353] Arrhythmias and arterial emboli do not appear to occur more commonly during pregnancy.[354–356] Most patients deliver vaginally, and there does not appear to be a higher incidence of spontaneous abortion or premature delivery.[348, 350]

Studies of pregnant intravenous drug users with systolic murmurs have shown that a large number had MV prolapse or valvular leaflet thickening on echocardiography.

The use of a β-blocker during pregnancy is most likely safe but should be exercised with caution to avoid fetal growth retardation or slowing of the fetal HR. In patients with MV prolapse who are receiving a β-blocker, a trial period off of the medication can be attempted during early gestation.[344] Some patients will require continuation of β-blocking agents during the second half of pregnancy for persistent chest pain or cardiac arrhythmias. An assessment of fetal growth with periodic ultrasound is recommended if β-blockers are used, and they should be discontinued before labor and delivery to reduce fetal effects from the drug.[349]

Progressive mitral regurgitation occurs in approximately 5 percent of patients over many years, especially in those with a murmur of progressive myxomatous degeneration and mitral insufficiency and a mid-systolic click, indicative of MV prolapse. Any patient with MV prolapse and mitral regurgitation or redundant valves or thickened leaflet is at an increased risk for infective endocarditis on the MV and for ruptured chordae tendineae; therefore, antibiotic prophylaxis is recommended.[109] In most patients with uncomplicated MV prolapse who undergo a complicated delivery, antibiotic prophylaxis is given, and it is common in many centers to administer antibiotic prophylaxis for any deliveries in these women.

Acute Rheumatic Fever

This disease may occur initially or recur during pregnancy.[351] Acute rheumatic fever may be associated with carditis or valvular heart disease, leading to CHF, which may be fatal in pregnant women.[357, 358] The incidence of Sydenham's chorea, like rheumatic fever itself, has been reported to be increased in pregnancy. This has been called *chorea gravidarum* and has been reported to cause preterm labor and fetal and maternal death.[359, 360] It is prudent to continue antibiotic prophylaxis against streptococcal infection in pregnant patients with a history of rheumatic fever because rheumatic fever can occur during pregnancy.[361] Treatment usually consists of penicillin, administered as a single intramuscular injection of 1.2 million units of benzathine penicillin or 600,000 units of procaine penicillin IM daily for 10 days. This is followed by continuous prophylaxis as a single monthly injection of 1.2 million units of benzathine penicillin G IM. Oral prophylaxis is less reliable than repository penicillin prophylaxis but can be accomplished with oral sulfadiazine or penicillin.[361, 362]

Chronic rheumatic valvular disease may cause significant valve deformities, increasing morbidity and mortality risks during gestation and the peripartum period. These patients should also receive prophylaxis for endocarditis and should be monitored for hemodynamic changes during labor and delivery, especially in those with severe valvular disease and those who develop symptoms of CHF during pregnancy.[363–365]

Mitral Stenosis

Mitral stenosis resulting from rheumatic fever or streptococcal infections is the most common rheumatic valvular lesion seen during pregnancy.[363, 365, 366] Deterioration may occur in as many as 25 percent of patients due to the increased cardiac output, tachycardia, and fluid retention normally accompanying pregnancy. The maternal death rate is nearly 1 percent, regardless of functional severity (Table 110–20). The rate rises to as high as 5 percent in those with significant functional impairment, and can reach as high as 17 percent in those with atrial fibrillation. Hemodynamic problems occur when flow is obstructed from the left atrium to the left ventricle, causing a reduction in cardiac output and fatigue.

An increased pressure gradient develops across the valve as LV diastolic filling time decreases due to the physiologic increases in HR and cardiac output associated with normal pregnancy. The increased LA pressure and the arrhythmogenic effects of pregnancy may result in atrial flutter or fibrillation, which further accelerates the ventricular rate and elevates LA pressure.[367, 368] During pregnancy, there may be a shift of blood volume, causing sudden decreases in venous return to the heart. If there is significant mitral stenosis, this may cause a decrease in LA pressure and cardiac output. This may explain some of the deaths in women with mitral stenosis who had no prior history of pulmonary congestion before pregnancy.

Elevated LA and pulmonary venous pressures may lead to pulmonary hypertension and dyspnea, orthopnea, or paroxysmal nocturnal dyspnea.[369] Pulmonary congestion symptoms usually worsen beginning at 20th week until term. If such symptoms develop or if mitral stenosis is significant, increases in HR and cardiac output should be minimized by restricting physical activity and by using digoxin or receptor blockade medication, or both, and cautious diuretic therapy. If symptoms worsen during pregnancy, there is an increased risk for arterial embolus, atrial fibrillation, LA thrombus, and right-sided heart failure. If atrial fibrillation develops, the hemodynamic consequences may be significant, including pulmonary edema. Digoxin and sometimes intravenous verapamil are used to slow the ventricular rate. Blood volume can be decreased by restricting salt intake and by careful diuretic use, but there always is the risk of reduced uteroplacental perfusion with diuretics. Thromboembolic complications resulting from the obstructed valve or LA dilatation occur during pregnancy and should be treated promptly with heparin.

Preconception counseling should include an evaluation with echocardiography. If severe mitral stenosis is present, mitral valvuloplasty in a cardiac catheterization laboratory or MV commissurotomy or replacement in an operating room is necessary. An active, asymptomatic woman requires no treatment. During pregnancy, percutaneous balloon mitral valvuloplasty is a good option; alternatively, mitral commissurotomy and even MV replacement have been safely performed in severely symptomatic patients.[370–379] Open heart surgery with valve replacement can be performed in an effort to decrease pulmonary congestion symptoms, but the incidence of fetal death has been reported to be as high as 33 percent. Therefore, closed surgical mitral commissurotomy and balloon mitral valvuloplasty have the best survival rates, with open mitral commissurotomy following closely. The use of closed mitral valvulotomy avoids the fetal complications that may occur with extracorporeal circulation and therefore is preferable to the open surgical technique. During percutaneous balloon valvuloplasty, high radiation exposure and hemodynamic fluctuations may accompany the procedure, with associated risks to the fetus.[364–373]

Labor and Delivery

Labor and delivery may exacerbate the risk for heart failure and death in patients with mitral stenosis. Intravenous fluid administration must be carefully monitored, often along with the hemodynamics using pulmonary artery catheterization. This allows the use of diuretics, digoxin, or β-blockers if LA pressure increases during labor and delivery. Vaginal delivery is allowed in most cases of mitral stenosis unless the valve area is less than 1.5 cm^2 or the patient is symptomatic. Once delivery has occurred, vena caval obstruction from the gravid uterus is relieved, and there is an immediate increase in venous return and pulmonary artery wedge pressure, making hemodynamic monitoring advisable for 24 hours after delivery.[22, 26, 29, 52, 379] Anesthesia is usually epidural for these patients, but there may be an associated fall in pressure, requiring fluid replacement.

TABLE 110–20 **Mortality Rates in Mitral Stenosis**

		Medical Therapy Alone				
	Normal Pregnancy	*NYHA Class I and II*	*Class III*	*Class IV*	Mitral Valvotomy and Valvuloplasty	Mitral Valve Replacement
Maternal mortality (%)	0.03	0.05	4–6	25–40	2–10	5
Fetal mortality (%)	2–4	4–6	30	50	5–25	30–40

Abbreviation: NYHA, New York Heart Association.
From Kammerer WS, Gross RJ: Medical Consultation: The Internist on Surgical, Obstetric, and Psychiatric Services. 2nd ed. Baltimore: Williams & Wilkins, 1990.

Emergency valve replacement may be performed after delivery.[380]

Mitral Regurgitation

This lesion is usually well tolerated during pregnancy because of the decrease in SVR, which reduces afterload.[381] Mitral regurgitation may be due to rheumatic heart disease, myxomatous degeneration, including MV prolapse, ruptured chordae tendineae, papillary muscle dysfunction, endocarditis, or a dilated cardiomyopathy. Symptoms of CHF rarely develop and are treated by restricting activity and fluid. Low-dose diuretics are rarely needed. Arrhythmias can be treated with digoxin. Hydralazine can be used to reduce LV afterload during times of isometric exercise, such as during labor. If mitral regurgitation develops, acute bacterial endocarditis, ruptured chordae tendineae, or papillary muscle dysfunction resulting from an acute MI may be the cause.[52, 381]

Aortic Stenosis

Rheumatic heart disease may have associated aortic valve involvement in approximately 10 percent of pregnant patients with rheumatic valvular heart disease. Bicuspid aortic valves are the most common cause of aortic stenosis in a young woman. Aortic stenosis is uncommon, but when severe, it presents a significant risk to the mother.[382] The maternal mortality rate may be as high as 17 percent.[382] High rates of spontaneous abortion and fetal mortality have been reported. Maternal mortality rates as high as 40 percent have been reported in women undergoing therapeutic abortions, presumably due to hypovolemia and decreased return to the heart. The management of patients who have aortic stenosis due to rheumatic or congenital causes is the same.[383]

Pregnancy can be a particularly serious problem because LV outflow obstruction can jeopardize uterine blood flow and fetal development. The heart is unable to maintain an adequate cardiac output without increasing filling pressure. Any significant fall in venous return may result in a drastic reduction in cardiac output, producing cerebral or myocardial ischemia and decreased peripheral perfusion. Pulmonary venous congestion and dyspnea often occur as LA pressures increase. The LV hypertrophy that accompanies aortic valvular stenosis requires higher LA pressures to fill the thickened ventricle.

Detection of aortic stenosis may be more difficult in pregnant patients because the classic finding of a harsh systolic ejection murmur at the base of the heart radiating to the carotid arteries is similar to the sound of murmurs associated with pregnancy. Exertion may evoke symptoms of fatigue, cerebral insufficiency, syncope, and a decrease in coronary blood flow leading to angina, even if the coronary arteries are normal. Hemodynamic monitoring, fetal monitoring, and antibiotic prophylaxis are necessary during labor and delivery in any patient with aortic stenosis.

All measures should be taken to avoid hypovolemia, and vigorous physical activities should be severely restricted.[52] If symptoms are not controlled by restriction of activity, aortic valve surgery must be considered.[382] In most young women, a commissurotomy or valvuloplasty procedure will produce short-term relief of symptoms, but the risk for recurrent aortic stenosis is high and a definitive procedure is necessary after the pregnancy.[383–387] Even if stenosis is severe, surgery is usually delayed until after pregnancy in the asymptomatic woman. Preconception correction of this lesion is advised to improve the outcome of the fetus and preserve maternal safety.

Aortic Regurgitation

Isolated aortic regurgitation is uncommon in young women during pregnancy, but it is more common than aortic valvular stenosis. It is usually well tolerated and may be the result of a congenital abnormality, often myxomatous degeneration, rheumatic heart disease, endocarditis, systemic arterial hypertension, or systemic vasculitis, such as that occurring with SLE.[388–390] Marfan's syndrome may cause aortic dissection with aortic regurgitation. If aortic regurgitation develops suddenly as a result of endocarditis or aortic root dissection, emergency replacement of the valve may be needed and can be performed even during pregnancy. If pulmonary congestion develops, restriction of activity is important, along with treatment with digitalis, diuretics, and afterload reduction.[52, 388]

Pulmonary Valvular Lesions

Hemodynamically significant abnormalities of the pulmonary valve are uncommon. Almost always, they represent a congenital anomaly that goes unrecognized through childhood. In older series, no maternal deaths were reported with pulmonary stenosis.[388, 389] Primary pulmonary valvular regurgitation is uncommon, but may occur with pulmonary arterial hypertension or surgery for congenital heart disease, such as with tetralogy of Fallot. It is usually well tolerated by both mother and fetus.[388–390]

Tricuspid Valvular Lesions

Tricuspid valvular stenosis is rare in the United States but may be caused by right-sided endocarditis or severe rheumatic heart disease, in which case the aortic valves and MVs are often affected as well. Insufficiency of the tricuspid valve usually does not cause symptoms during pregnancy, and ordinarily no special therapy is indicated.

Congenital Heart Disease

Inheritance

Congenital heart disease is recognized in approximately 0.8 percent of all live births in the United States.[388–390] When one parent has a congenital heart defect, the first child has a 2 to 15 percent chance of having a cardiac

TABLE 110-21 Risk of Congenital Heart Disease in Offspring if One Parent Is Affected

Type of Heart Defect	Risk (%)
Intracardiac Shunts	
Atrial septal defect	3–11
Ventricular septal defect	4–22
Patent ductus arteriosus	4–11
Obstruction to Flow	
Left-sided obstruction*	3–26
Right-sided obstruction	3–22
Complex Abnormalities	
Tetralogy of Fallot	4–15
Ebstein's anomaly	Uncertain
Transposition of the great arteries	Uncertain

The higher number in each range comes from one large series. The incidence in congenital heart disease in the offspring tends to be closer to the lower numbers for most other reported series.
The risk of congenital heart disease in the offspring of women with obstructive lesions is decreased by corrective surgery before pregnancy.
*Includes coarctation, aortic stenosis, discrete subaortic stenosis, and supravalvular stenosis. It does not include idiopathic hypertrophic subaortic stenosis; with this, the child has a 50% chance of having idiopathic hypertrophic subaortic stenosis.
From Chatterjee K, Chitlin MD, Karliner J, et al: Cardiology: An Illustrated Text-Reference. Philadelphia: Gower Medical, 1991.

abnormality (Table 110–21).[388] Congenital heart disease appears to be primarily due to genetic factors, such as chromosomal damage and point mutations. Another 1 to 2 percent of cases are caused by detectable environmental factors, with the most common being maternal rubella during the first trimester of pregnancy. Drugs, alcohol, tobacco, and other factors that decrease uterine blood flow or hinder fetal oxygen supply may also cause congenital heart disease. Severe valvular stenotic lesions may decrease uterine blood flow with risk to the fetus, whereas valvular regurgitation is usually better tolerated. Corrective surgery should be performed before pregnancy if needed, particularly when there is ventricular outflow obstruction. This will improve uterine blood flow and oxygenation to the fetus and may decrease the chance that the child will be born with congenital heart disease. In one series, surgical correction of the LV outflow obstruction before pregnancy resulted in decrease in the fetal mortality rate and halved the incidence of cardiac defects in offspring.[388] Fetal growth and development should be monitored closely in women with cyanosis due to any cardiovascular disorder.

Women with existing congenital heart disease are at an increased morbidity and mortality risk during pregnancy (Tables 110–22 and 110–23). Any lesion associated with pulmonary hypertension has a maternal mortality rate in excess of 50 percent.

Antibiotic Prophylaxis

Official recommendations for antibiotic prophylaxis have not been proposed by the American Heart Association for patients with congenital heart disease who are undergoing uncomplicated vaginal delivery. However, conventional wisdom suggests the administration of antibiotics prophylactically. If the patient has a prosthetic heart valve or a

TABLE 110-22 Cardiovascular Malformations With Frequent Survival to Adult Life, Low Pregnancy Risk

- Septal defects, atrial or ventricular
  - After complete repair
  - With small residual left-to-right shunt
- Tetralogy of Fallot, after repair
  - With or without mild residual valvar insufficiency
- Patent ductus arteriosus, coarctation of the aorta, other malformation after repair
- Bicuspid aortic/pulmonary valve
- Pulmonary stenosis, mild or postoperative

From Wenger NK, Speroff L, Packard B, et al: Cardiovascular Health and Disease in Women. Greenwich, CT: Le Jacq Communications, 1993.

surgically constructed systemic-to-pulmonary shunt at the ventricular level, antibiotic prophylaxis should be administered. The use of antibiotic prophylaxis is not uncommon in many patients with congenital heart disease except in those patients with isolated secundum-type ASDs and those who have undergone a correction of PDA 6 months earlier. The risk of endocarditis may be increased after manual removal of the placenta, so antibiotic prophylaxis is recommended if this is done (see Tables 110–9 and 110–10).[362]

Atrial Septal Defect

The murmur of ASD is frequently discovered during pregnancy, but this defect is usually well tolerated even in patients with a large left-to-right shunt. The systolic ASD murmur, however, is difficult to differentiate from the invariably present similar systolic ejection murmur that develops during pregnancy, and most often, a two-dimensional echocardiogram with Doppler is required to distinguish them. Pulmonary hypertension usually does not occur until the fourth decade of life, along with atrial arrhythmias.[391] Antibiotic prophylaxis is not indicated in patients with secundum-type ASDs. Antibiotics are recommended in patients with ostium primum ASDs and associated cleft MVs to protect against the development of endocarditis on the cleft MV.

Ventricular Septal Defect

Congestive heart failure and arrhythmias have been reported, but usually patients with VSDs tolerate pregnancy

TABLE 110-23 Partial List of Complex Cardiovascular Malformations

- Eisenmenger's syndrome
- Ebstein's, other severe congenital valvar anomalies
- Postoperative cardiovascular malformation with prosthetic valves, implanted pacemakers
- Transposition of the great arteries, after atrial repair (Mustard, other)
- Single ventricle variants, post Fontan repair
- Any defect complicated by major arrhythmia or requiring medication

From Wenger NK, Speroff L, Packard B, et al: Cardiovascular Health and Disease in Women. Greenwich, CT: Le Jacq Communications, 1993.

well. After surgical closure of an uncomplicated VSD, there is no increased risk to pregnancy. There is a report that the risk of congenital heart disease is as high as 22 percent in live-born offspring, with the development of VSDs in 50 percent of them.[388] There may be a transient shunt reversal in patients with pulmonary hypertension, as well as right-to-left shunting with reductions in arterial oxygenation, if there is significant blood loss or anesthetic agents have been used during delivery.[392]

Patent Ductus Arteriosus

PDA is a common congenital defect that occurs in a 2:1 female/male ratio. These defects usually are found and corrected during early childhood, and there usually is a favorable outcome, except in pregnant patients who develop CHF. Patients with CHF require bed rest, diuretics, and digitalis. There have been reports of successful surgical intervention or catheter-induced closure of PDA during pregnancy. These procedures should be reserved for patients with severe CHF unresponsive to medical therapy. During the early postpartum period, women with pulmonary hypertension may develop shunt reversal if they have hypotension; therefore, any blood loss should be corrected immediately with volume replacement or vasopressor agents.[393]

Congenital Aortic Valvular Disease

Bicuspid aortic valves occur in 1 to 2 percent of the population and may cause significant aortic stenosis, with obstruction of the LV outflow tract.[382] The classic murmur can be attributed to the flow-related systolic murmur commonly found in pregnant women, but the presence of an LV impulse, an S_4, or an aortic ejection sound should lead to further evaluation for aortic valvular stenosis.[395] In women who have not had aortic stenosis surgically corrected before pregnancy, there is the potential for worsening, with development of CHF hypotension, angina, and even death. There is a high incidence of cardiac defects in infants of mothers with left heart obstruction.[388]

Patients with severe aortic stenosis with aortic valve areas less than 1 cm^2 ideally should not undergo pregnancy until their valvular heart disease has been surgically corrected. If clinical deterioration occurs after week 22 of gestation and the patient has not responded to medical therapy, surgical intervention may be indicated. Percutaneous balloon valvuloplasty has been performed safely in some of these patients.[395, 396] Other considerations are the same as those discussed in the management of rheumatic fever–related valvular aortic stenosis. However, most patients develop recurrent aortic valvular obstruction within 6 months of the procedure, so percutaneous balloon valvuloplasty should be considered in patients with severe symptoms that are not manageable with medical therapy, with the understanding that it has only a transient beneficial effect and will almost certainly need to be followed at a later date with aortic valve replacement.[397]

Coarctation of the Aorta

If no complications are present, patients with aortic coarctation can safely tolerate pregnancy. Fetal development may be impaired because of decreased uteroplacental blood flow[398, 399] resulting from impeded flow of blood from the left side of the heart. Mortality rates range between 3 and 8 percent, with the majority of deaths occurring before labor and delivery. Deaths may be due to dissection or rupture of the aorta or to associated abnormalities,[388] which may include an aneurysm of the circle of Willis, aortic valvular stenosis (bicuspid aortic valve), PDS, VSD, or MV abnormality. Other complications include systemic arterial hypertension, CHF, and chest pain. There is a higher incidence of congenital heart disease in infants born to mothers with uncorrected coarctation, and fetal mortality rates may be as great as 20 percent. The incidence of congenital heart disease in offspring is approximately 20 percent but appears to diminish by approximately one half if surgical correction is accomplished before pregnancy. Collateral vessels may develop in the mother, which makes cesarean section hazardous. Management includes limitation of physical activity and blood pressure control,[399] but the reduction in blood pressure may lead to compromise in uteroplacental blood flow. Surgical correction of coarctation has been performed during pregnancy with success and may be indicated if uncontrollable systolic arterial hypertension is present or if severe CHF develops.[391]

Tetralogy of Fallot

Tetralogy of Fallot is the most common type of cyanotic congenital heart disease in adults, but most patients with this abnormality have undergone palliative or definitive surgical repair in childhood.[400] The hemodynamic changes of pregnancy may cause clinical deterioration, with an exacerbation of a right-to-left shunt and cyanosis. Poor prognostic signs are a maternal hematocrit of more than 60 percent, arterial oxygen saturation of less 80 percent, RV hypertension, and syncopal episodes. Close monitoring of hemodynamic variables and blood gases is necessary during labor and delivery in patients with this heart lesion who are cyanotic or symptomatic. Surgery to palliate or correct this lesion should be performed before conception because this reduces the risks associated with pregnancy. Reports of this lesion during pregnancy have not been linked to a major risk for death, although there may be a worsening of the clinical condition, sometimes necessitating interruption of the pregnancy.[401] Cardiac defects in infants of these mothers have been reported at rates ranging from 3 to 17 percent. Surgical correction of an incompletely repaired defect is recommended in patients with a residual VSD when the pulmonary-to-systemic flow ratio is 1.51 or greater, in those with RV outflow obstruction causing an increased RV systolic pressure of more than 60 mm Hg, and in those with RV failure due to severe pulmonic valvular regurgitation.

Inhalation analgesia, pudendal, or paracervical block is used for delivery. Epidural block may result in hypotension and shunt reversal and should not be used. A segmental epidural block for the first stage of labor, with pudendal or caudal block for the second stage, has been recommended, along with the use of opiates to control pain.[401, 402]

Ebstein's Anomaly

Several successful pregnancies have been reported in patients with this anomaly. Pregnancy may be complicated by RV failure, infective endocarditis, and paradoxical embolism, with an increase in maternal and fetal complications in cyanotic patients. Labor and delivery in symptomatic or cyanotic patients should include hemodynamic monitoring and efforts to prevent a drop in systemic blood pressure, which can be caused by peripheral vasodilation or blood loss.[403, 404]

Eisenmenger's Syndrome

Patients with Eisenmenger's syndrome have a maternal mortality rate of 38 to 52 percent. There is evidence of poor fetal outcome with this disorder, with a high incidence of premature deliveries, intrauterine growth retardation, and perinatal death.[405–408] Patients with this syndrome should be advised against pregnancy, and early abortion is usually recommended when pregnancy occurs. The management of a pregnant patient with this condition necessitates close follow-up, with restriction of physical activity to minimize hemodynamic burden. There is an increased risk for fatal thromboembolic events, and anticoagulant therapy is indicated for the final 8 to 10 weeks of gestation and for 4 weeks postpartum. Women with signs of premature uterine activity should be hospitalized. Spontaneous labor is preferable to induction. Close monitoring during labor is essential, and patients who are in stable condition may tolerate vaginal delivery. Attempts should be made to shorten the second stage of labor by using forceps or vacuum extraction. Epidural anesthesia may cause peripheral vasodilatation and right-to-left shunting. Local anesthetics can be used to perform an epidural block. Delivery by cesarean section with general anesthesia requires the use of a drug with minimal negative inotropic effects.[394–396]

Complex Cyanotic Anomalies

Disorders such as tricuspid atresia, transposition of the great vessels, truncus arteriosus, and a single ventricle pose a high risk during pregnancy, and pregnancy is therefore not recommended. The rates of maternal morbidity and mortality are significant, and there is a high incidence of fetal wastage and congenital malformations.[408–411]

Cardiac Surgery During Pregnancy

Surgery is avoided during the first trimester because of the risk of teratogenic effects. With fetuses of more than 34 weeks' gestational age, abdominal delivery can be performed at the same time as cardiac surgery if fetal maturity has been confirmed.[412] Cardiopulmonary bypass is not associated with increased maternal mortality rates, but fetal mortality rates may be high as the result of hypothermia, nonpulsatile blood flow, and hypotension. Alterations in the routine use of cardiopulmonary bypass may be necessary to ensure adequate perfusion and oxygenation to both mother and fetus, because there are increased cardiac output and oxygen consumption during pregnancy. Cardiac surgery may be performed for correction of aortic stenosis, valve replacement, aortic aneurysm or dissection, correction of congenital heart disease, or bypass grafting.[413–415] Fetal bradycardia commonly occurs during cardiopulmonary bypass; therefore, continuous fetal monitoring should be provided, with high-risk obstetric consultation available. Episodes of bradycardia are often managed by increasing the flow rate of the cardiopulmonary bypass pump.[416] The fetal HR should be continuously monitored transabdominally by Doppler techniques during the surgery. The fetal HR variability and uterine activity may be useful in evaluating fetal status during anesthesia and the surgical procedure. Fetal tachycardia may result from placental transfer of administered drugs, and fetal bradycardia may be a sign of fetal hypoxia or acidosis, maternal hypothermia, or placental transfer of drugs, such as β-blockers.[417, 418]

Emergency cesarean section during cardiopulmonary bypass should be considered if severe fetal bradycardia occurs. The outcome is usually better if this occurs after 26 weeks of gestation. Other perinatal considerations should include that the increased incidence of fetal congenital heart disease in offspring of mothers with congenital heart disease.[417] At 16 weeks of gestation and later, fetal echocardiography can be performed to determine the status of the fetal heart.

Anesthesia administered during the first trimester has the risk of teratogenicity, primarily when organogenesis is occurring. No specific anesthetic techniques or agents have been found to be superior to others (Tables 110–24 and 110–25).[418] Premature labor and delivery may occur primarily as a result of the disorder that necessitated the surgical procedure and not as a result of the anesthetic agent used. Specific consideration to drugs commonly used during cardiac operations should be given before surgery, such as induction and inhalational agents, narcotics, muscle relaxants, inotropic and vasoactive drugs, β-blockers, vasodilators, calcium channel blockers, antiarrhythmics, anticholinergics, and antibiotics administered perioperatively.

Cardiovascular Drugs: Pregnancy and Lactation

Fetal Effects

Cardiovascular drugs may affect uterine myometrial tone and uteroplacental blood flow (Table 110–26). The fetus may be affected by altered hemodynamics in the mother or from teratogenicity. Placental transfer of drugs can be beneficial for treatment of selected problems in utero.[419, 420] Medication levels in the mother must be monitored, because the levels of some medications may decrease by as much as 40 percent during pregnancy. Although many drugs have a potentially unfavorable effect on a developing

TABLE 110-24 Pharmacologic Effects of Drugs Used for Analgesia and Anesthesia in Obstetrics

Drug	Drug Effects						Concentration (%)	
	CNS*	***CNS†***	***Cardiovascular System***	***Respiratory System***	***Effect on Uterine Contraction***	***Neonate***	***Analgesia***	***Anesthesia***
Inhalation Agents								
N_2O	Analgesia	Anesthesia	SVR ↑, HR ↑, CO ↑ ↓	None	No effect	None	35	60
Halothane	Analgesia	Anesthesia	CO ↓, HR—↓, SVR—, BP ↓	Hypoventilation	Depression	Depression		0.5–0.8
Enflurane	Analgesia	Anesthesia	SVR ↓, BP ↓, CO ↓	Hypoventilation	Depression	Depression	0.5	1
Isoflurane	Analgesia	Anesthesia	SVR ↓, BP ↓, HR ↑, CO—	Hypoventilation	Depression	Depression		
Trichloroethylene								
Methoxyflurane	Analgesia	Anesthesia	No or minimal depression	None	Minimal effect	None/depression	0.4	0.6
Cyclopropane	Analgesia	Anesthesia	HR ↓, CO ↓, BP ↓	None	Minimal effect	None	0.35	0.6
		Anesthesia	Stimulation, arrhythmia	None	Minimal effect	None	3	5
Neuromuscular Blocking Agents	None			Paralysis	No effect	None	**Dosage (mg/kg)**	
Depolarizing			Bradyarrhythmia				1–2	
Succinylcholine								
Nondepolarizing								
Tubocurarine			BP ↓				0.2–0.6	
Pancuronium			BP ↑, HR ↑				0.06–0.1	
Metocurine			Minimal				0.2–0.6	
Vecuronium			Minimal to none				0.05	
Atracurium			Minimal				0.2–0.6	

Abbreviations: BP, blood pressure; CNS, central nervous system; CO, cardiac output; HR, heart rate; SVR, systemic vascular resistance; ↑, increased; ↓, decreased; —, no change.

*Low concentration.

†High concentration.

From Geller E, Rudick V, Niv D: Analgesia and anesthesia during pregnancy. *In* Elkayam U, Gleicher N (eds): Cardiac Problems in Pregnancy. 2nd ed. pp. 283–306. Copyright © 1990. Reprinted by permission of Wiley-Liss, Inc., a division of John Wiley & Sons, Inc.

TABLE 110–25 Pharmacologic Effects of Drugs Used for Analgesia and Anesthesia in Obstetrics

Drug	Drug Effects					Dosage	
	CNS	Cardiovascular System	Respiratory System	Uterine Contraction	Neonate	Sedation/Analgesia (IM, IV)	Anesthesia
Benzodiazepines	Anxiolytic, sedative, hypnotic, amnesic, anticonvulsant	Mild decrease in BP, tachycardia		No effect	Hypothermia, hypotonia, respiratory depression (minimal)		
Diazepam			No effect*			0.05–0.2 mg/kg	0.2–0.6 mg/kg
Lorazepam			No effect*			3–5 mg/kg	
Midazolam			No effect*			0.07–0.08 mg/kg	0.5–0.6 mg/kg
Opioids							
Morphine	Analgesia,* anesthesia†	Postural hypotension, bradycardia	Depression		Marked respiratory depression	0.1–0.15 mg/kg	3 mg/kg
Meperidine	Analgesia, sedation	Postural hypotension, tachycardia	Depression		Respiratory depression	1–1.5 mg/kg	
Pentazocine	Analgesia, sedation	Mild increase in BP, tachycardia	Depression		Respiratory depression	30 mg	
Fentanyl	Analgesia,† anesthesia‡	Bradycardia	Depression		Respiratory depression	1–2 μg/kg	10–100 μg/kg
Induction Agents							
Barbiturates	Sedation, hypnosis	Myocardial depression	Depression	No effect	Depression		3–5 mg/kg
Thiopental							1–2 mg/kg
Methohexital							1–2 mg/kg
Ketamine	Analgesia,* anesthesia‡	Sympathomimetic effect: HR ↑, BP ↑, SVR ↑, CO ↑	Minimal stimulation	Stimulation of uterine contraction	No significant depression‡	0.1–0.3 mg/kg	1–2 mg/kg IV 6–10 mg/kg IM

Abbreviations: BP, blood pressure; CNS, central nervous system; CO, cardiac output; HR, heart rate; SVR, systemic vascular resistance; ↑, Increased; ↓, decreased; —, no change.
*In therapeutic dose.
†Low dose.
‡High dose.
From Geller E, Rudick V, Niv D: Analgesia and anesthesia during pregnancy. *In* Elkayam U, Gleicher N (eds): Cardiac Problems in Pregnancy. 2nd ed. pp. 283–306.

TABLE 110–26 **Effects of α- and β-Adrenergic Receptor Stimulation and Blockade on Maternal-Fetal Physiology**

	Stimulation		Blockade	
	α-Receptor	*β-Receptor*	*α-Receptor*	*β-Receptor*
Fetal heart rate	↔	↑	↔	↔ ↓
Maternal heart rate	↔	↑	↔	↓
Umbilical blood flow	↔	↑	↔	↓
Myometrial activity	↑	↓	↓	↑

Key: ↔, no effect; ↑, increase; ↓, decrease.
From Frishman WH, Chesner M: Use of beta-adrenergic blocking agents in pregnancy. *In* Elkayam U, Gleicher N (eds): Cardiac Problems in Pregnancy. 2nd ed. pp. 351–360.

fetus, when they become necessary, the risk/benefit ratio should be evaluated and the smallest effective dose should be used.

Lactation

Drugs may also be transferred in breast milk to the neonate during lactation. Usually, 1 to 2 percent of a maternal dose of any drug appears in the breast milk. Some drugs are clearly contraindicated during breast-feeding, but in most cases insufficient information is available. If a mother requires medication during lactation, close monitoring of the infant's ingested dose and plasma levels is necessary, along with observation for the adverse effects or toxicity.[153, 154]

Cardiac Glycosides

Digoxin has been used extensively for the treatment of maternal CHF and for supraventricular tachycardias in the mother or fetus. There are no reports of teratogenicity in humans, but excessive doses can be detrimental to the mother and may be lethal to the fetus.[155] Digoxin can be used alone or in combination with a second drug, such as verapamil or quinidine, in the treatment of supraventricular tachycardia or atrial flutter. Pregnancy may be associated with increased levels of digoxin-like substances, especially when systemic arterial hypertension is present, which interfere with the digoxin radioimmunoassay and may cause errors in measurement.[156]

Few adverse effects have been observed in fetuses and mothers who have been receiving digoxin on a long-term basis.[155] The fetal heart has only a limited capacity to bind digoxin during the first half of pregnancy and there is significant maternal protein binding, so only small amounts of digoxin are available to the fetus. In some instances, low birth weights have been reported. This may also be due to the fact that mothers receiving digoxin usually have a shorter duration of pregnancy, with lower birth weights rather than intrauterine growth retardation. The total amount of digoxin ingested daily by an infant who is breast-feeding has been estimated to be approximately 1 percent of the pediatric recommended dose; adverse clinical effects are not usually seen. Digoxin can be continued in breast-feeding mothers.

Treatment of Arrhythmias

The greatest experience with antiarrhythmic drug therapy during pregnancy has been with digoxin, quinidine, and propranolol.[419, 420] However, the choice of antiarrhythmic drugs depends on the specific arrhythmia being treated, the cardiac condition of the patient or fetus, and the known or anticipated actions of the antiarrhythmic drug being considered. For benign arrhythmias, a conservative approach starting initially with preventive measures is appropriate. In the case of more severe or symptomatic arrhythmias, pharmacologic therapy should be begun with drugs that have been proved to be safe to the fetus. Electrical cardioversion of the patient usually may be performed with relative safety for both mother and fetus.

In one study, 25 fetuses with the diagnosis of supraventricular tachycardia were reported from January 1989 to October 1997 among 3117 pregnant women referred for fetal cardiac evaluation.[421] There were 17 fetuses with the diagnosis of supraventricular tachycardia and 8 with atrial flutter. Gestational age ranged from 26 to 40 weeks. Twelve women were hydropic at presentation—6 with supraventricular tachycardia and 6 with atrial flutter. Four fetuses with supraventricular tachycardia showed structural alterations, including 2 with Ebstein's anomaly and 2 with VSDs. Patients were admitted to a fetal cardiology unit for monitoring and treatment. Among 17 fetuses with supraventricular tachycardia, 12 showed a good response to digoxin administration, but this drug was not useful in any of the fetuses with atrial flutter. In 2 women with supraventricular tachycardia and 6 with atrial flutter, the pregnancy was interrupted to perform postnatal cardioversion. The mortality incidence was 3 of 17 fetuses in the supraventricular tachycardia group, including 2 fetuses with Ebstein's anomaly, and 0 of 8 fetuses in the atrial flutter group. In this study, it is apparent that fetal supraventricular tachyarrhythmias are uncommon in the general population of pregnant women. Nevertheless, the fetus may present with severe heart failure and death. Thus, accurate diagnosis and early treatment of these conditions are extremely important. The diagnosis of fetal arrhythmias may be made by using fetal echocardiography; this technique may be used to examine the influence of the arrhythmia on the heart itself. It is generally conceded that digoxin is the treatment of choice for fetal supraventricular tachycardias. However, although maternal administration of digoxin is often effective in treating the fetal supraventricular tachycardia, it may be ineffective on occasion, secondary to poor transplacental drug transfer. Parilla and colleagues[422] treated eight women whose pregnancies were complicated by fetal supraventricular tachycardia and hydrops fetalis; the authors used transplacental therapy or combined maternal and direct fetal intramuscular therapy with digoxin. They described the response to treatment after maternal intravenous administration of digoxin or a combination of fetal intramuscular digoxin and maternal intravenous digoxin for eight hydropic fetuses during nine successful pharmacologic conversions. The maternal intravenous administration of digoxin was performed with standard loading and maintenance protocols. Fetal intramuscular administration of digoxin was accomplished at a dose of 88 μg/kg per 12 to 24 hours to a maximum of three injections in the fetal buttock. Time to onset of the first 2 hours of sinus rhythm, time to onset to more than 90 percent of sinus rhythm, and time to resolution of hydrops fetalis were noted. The mean HR was 257 ± 36 beats/min, and the mean gestational age was 29 ± 4.8 weeks. Fetal supraventricular tachycardia was the result of a reentrant mechanism in all cases. For the three fetuses that underwent successful cardioversion after maternal intravenous administration of digoxin, the time to onset of the first 2 hours of sinus rhythm was 145 ± 114 hours, the time to onset of more than 90 percent sinus rhythm was 176 ± 55 hours, and hydrops fetalis resolved in 41 ± 37 days. In each of the mothers treated in this manner, additional antiarrhythmic drugs were administered to the mother. When treatment was accomplished with fetal intramuscular digoxin administration and maternal intravenous therapy in four fetuses, the time to onset of the first 2 hours of sinus rhythm was 5.5 ± 4 hours, the time to onset of more than 90 percent sinus rhythm was 22 ± 14 hours, and resolution of hydrops fetalis occurred in 25 ± 21 days. In two failed cardioversions, the transplacental treatment alone, the time to onset of the first 2 hours of sinus rhythm was 203 ± 180 hours, and time to onset of more than 90 percent sinus rhythm was 313 ± 270 hours. Once fetal intramuscular therapy was begun in these fetuses, the time to onset for the first 2 hours of sinus rhythm was 17 ± 7 hours, and the time to onset of more than 90 percent sinus rhythm was 60 ± 13 hours. Hydrops fetalis resolved in 45 days in one fetus, whereas the other fetus never had resolution of hydrops despite 100 days of antiarrhythmic therapy. Thus, direct fetal intramuscular injection of digoxin combined with transplacental therapy appears to shorten the time to initial conversion of supraventricular tachycardia and to sustain sinus rhythm in the fetus with SVT complicated by hydrops fetalis.

Fetal tachyarrhythmias may be life-threatening conditions for the fetus. Long-standing tachyarrhythmias may lead to fetal cardiac failure, hydrops, and death. Normalization of the fetal cardiac rhythm leads to resolution of fetal hydrops in most instances. Fetuses with a persistent HR of more than 180 beats/min with a 1:1 AV conduction on M-mode echocardiography are defined as having supraventricular tachycardia. Fetal hydrops is diagnosed if the following signs are seen: pleural or pericardial effusion (or both) or ascites and skin edema (or a combination). Resolution of hydrops often requires 46 weeks after termination of the arrhythmia and usually occurs in the following sequence: diminution of ascites, pleural and pericardial effusions, and disappearance of skin and scalp edema.[423]

Another report suggests that rate-based management of fetal supraventricular tachycardia is important in the successful culmination of a pregnancy. Guntheroth and colleagues[424] evaluated the clinical course of 22 fetuses with supraventricular tachycardia to determine whether HR alone might serve as a basis for conservative management. Hydrops was not encountered with HRs under 230 beats/min in this series of patients. The conditions of all 22 fetuses stabilized without invasive administration of medication. Eighteen were delivered vaginally, and only four were delivered by cesarean section. No fetal or neonatal losses occurred. Regardless of the type of supraventricular tachycardia, reduction in HR in these fetuses to levels preventing or resolving hydrops allowed vaginal term delivery. Digoxin, β-blockers, or verapamil might be used for purposes of reducing HR in the fetus with supraventricular tachycardia.

Neonatal Ventricular Tachycardia

Villain and associates[425] undertook a retrospective study in two fetuses and eight neonates aged 1 to 20 days with ventricular tachycardia. The ventricular tachycardia was persistent in two cases, observed in runs of variable variation in the other eight, and incessant in seven of these latter cases. Only two cases were symptomatic: cardiac failure with shock 16 hours after birth and hydramnios at 16 weeks of gestation. The arrhythmia was monomorphic 9 times out of 10 with fixed (three cases) or variable (seven cases) rates that are greater than 150 beats/min. Intravenous magnesium sulfate in the severe and permanent forms, oral β-blockers to treat ventricular tachycardia associated with acceleration of the sinus rhythm, and oral amiodarone alone or with propranolol in one case were prescribed. Three neonates were not treated either from the outset or after inefficacy of amiodarone. Nine of the patients had their ventricular tachycardias converted to sinus rhythm and were treatment free 12 to 24 months later. The other patient had a slow, well-tolerated ventricular tachycardia. No cause was detected in nine cases. In the remaining patient, there was a metabolic disease of β-oxidation of long-chain fatty acids. These authors concluded that isolated, idiopathic ventricular tachycardia in the neonate usually carries a good prognosis and that relatively simple treatment with β-blockers or amiodarone is usually associated with restoration of sinus rhythm and definitive cure during the first year of life.

Diuretic Agents

Diuretics have been used to manage hypertension, heart failure, and fluid retention and to prevent preeclampsia.[426–434] Their use to prevent or change the perinatal outcome of preeclampsia has not been proved, and they prevent the normal volume expansion of pregnancy. They may have deleterious effects by decreasing placental perfusion due to volume restriction. Their administration does not significantly alter amniotic fluid volume. Furosemide

pointes) postnatally. Propranolol and propafenone successfully controlled the ventricular arrhythmias. Follow-up ECGs and Holter records showed persistent QT prolongation and intermittent episodes of T wave alternans. On propranolol monotherapy, the young child did well and during follow-up was free of ventricular arrhythmias.

Obstetric Drugs With Cardiac Effects

To reduce the incidence of premature delivery, tocolytics, such as terbutaline, are used to stop premature labor.[464–468] These agents may cause maternal tachycardia and are hazardous in patients with mitral stenosis and some other forms of cardiovascular disease.[464–468] Terbutaline should not be used in patients with underlying heart disease or hypertension because it has been associated with maternal pulmonary edema, especially when corticosteroids are used to promote fetal lung maturation. Synthetic oxytocin is preferable to the natural product because it is free of pressor agents. It can be administered to minimize blood loss after delivery, but it should be administered slowly because bolus injection may cause hypotension. Prostaglandins administered in small doses to induce abortion or labor do not usually produce significant hemodynamic effects, but maternal flushing, tachycardia, and hypotension occur when too large a dose is given. Injection of hypertonic solutions into the uterus to produce abortion may result in hypervolemia and, in some cases, hypernatremia, causing intravascular volume overload in the mother.

References

1. McAnulty JH, Metcalfe J, Ueland K: Heart disease and pregnancy. *In* Hurst JW, Schlant RC, Rackley CE, et al (eds): The Heart: Arteries and Veins. 7th ed. pp. 1465–1478. New York: McGraw-Hill Information Services, 1990.
2. Otterson WN, Dunnihoo DR: Cardiac disease. *In* Pauerstein CJ (ed): Clinical Obstetrics. pp. 627–647. New York: John Wiley & Sons, 1987.
3. Leyse R, Ofstun M, Dillard DH, et al: Congenital aortic stenosis in pregnancy, corrected by extracorporeal circulation: offering a viable male infant at term but with anomalies eventuating in his death at four months of age—report of a case. JAMA 176:1009, 1961.
4. Gant NF, Daley GL, Chand S, et al: A study of angiotensin II pressor response throughout primigravid pregnancy. J Clin Invest 52:2682, 1973.
5. Walsh SW, Parisi VM: Eicosanoids and hypertension in pregnancy. *In* Mitchell MD (ed): Eicosanoids in Reproduction. pp. 249–272. Orlando, FL: CRC, 1990.
6. Guyton AC: Textbook of Medical Physiology. 5th ed. Philadelphia: WB Saunders, 1976.
7. Lund CJ, Donovan JC: Blood volume during pregnancy. Am J Obstet Gynecol 98:393, 1967.
8. Chesley LC: Plasma and red cell volumes during pregnancy. Am J Obstet Gynecol 112:440, 1972.
9. Lindheimer MD, Katz AI: Sodium and diuretics in pregnancy. N Engl J Med 288:891, 1973.
10. Cusson JR, Gutkowska J, Rey E, et al: Plasma concentration of atrial natriuretic factor in normal pregnancy. N Engl J Med 313:1230, 1985.
11. Rutherford AJ, Anderson JV, Elder MG, et al: Release of atrial natriuretic peptide during pregnancy and immediate puerperium. Lancet 1:928, 1987.
12. Huisman A, Aarnoudse JG, Heuvelmans JHA, et al: Whole blood viscosity during normal pregnancy. Br J Obstet Gynaecol 94:1143, 1987.
13. Ozanne P, Linderkamp O, Miller FC, et al: Erythrocyte aggregation during normal pregnancy. Am J Obstet Gynecol 147:576, 1983.
14. Pitkin RM, Witte DL: Platelet and leukocyte counts in pregnancy. JAMA 242:2696, 1980.
15. Rakoczi F, Tallian F, Bagdany S, et al: Platelet life-span in normal pregnancy and pre-eclampsia as determined by nonradioisotope technique. Thromb Res 15:553, 1979.
16. Katz R, Karliner JS, Resnik R: Effects of a natural volume overload state (pregnancy) on left ventricular performance in normal human subjects. Circulation 58:434, 1978.
17. Dilts PV, Brinkman CR, Kirschbaum TH, et al: Uterine and systemic hemodynamic interrelationships and their response to hypoxia. Am J Obstet Gynecol 103:138, 1969.
18. Karlsson K: The influence of hypoxia on uterine and maternal placental blood flow, and the effect of alpha-adrenergic blockade. J Perinat Med 2:176, 1974.
19. Metcalfe J, Ueland K: Maternal cardiovascular adjustments to pregnancy. Prog Cardiovasc Dis 16:363, 1974.
20. Rovinsky JJ, Jaffin H: Cardiovascular hemodynamics in pregnancy. III. Cardiac rate, stroke volume, total peripheral resistance, and central blood volume in multiple pregnancy: synthesis of results. Am J Obstet Gynecol 95:787, 1966.
21. Christianson RE: Studies on blood pressure during pregnancy. I. Influence on parity and age. Am J Obstet Gynecol 125:509, 1976.
22. Rovinsky JJ: Blood volume and the hemodynamics of pregnancy. *In* Philipp EE, Parnes J, Newton M (eds): Scientific Foundation of Obstetrics and Gynaecology. pp. 332–340. Philadelphia: FA Davis, 1970.
23. Metcalfe J, Romney SL, Ramsey LH, et al: Estimation of uterine blood flow in normal human pregnancy at term. J Clin Invest 34:1632, 1955.
24. Wood JE: The cardiovascular effects of oral contraceptives. Mod Concepts Cardiovasc Dis 4:37, 1972.
25. Ueland K, Novy MJ, Peterson EN, et al: Maternal cardiovascular dynamics. IV. The influence of gestational age on the maternal cardiovascular response to posture and exercise. Am J Obstet Gynecol 104:856, 1969.
26. Kerr MG, Scott DB, Samuel E: Studies of the inferior vena cava in late pregnancy. BMJ 1:532, 1964.
27. Bieniarz J, Crottongini JJ, Curuchet E, et al: Aortocaval compression by the uterus in late human pregnancy. II. An angiographic study. Am J Obstet Gynecol 100:203, 1968.
28. Howard BK, Goodson JH, Mengert WF: Supine hypotensive syndrome in late pregnancy. Obstet Gynecol 1:371, 1953.
29. Kerr MG: The mechanical effects of the gravid uterus in late pregnancy. J Obstet Gynaecol Br Commonw 72:513, 1965.
30. Artal R, Wiswell R: Exercise in Pregnancy. Baltimore: Williams & Wilkins, 1986.
31. Prowse CM, Galnslar EA: Respiratory and acid-base changes during pregnancy. Anesthesiology 26:381, 1965.
32. Morton MJ, Metcalfe J: Changes in maternal hemodynamics during pregnancy. *In* Artal R, Wiswell R (eds): Exercise in Pregnancy. Baltimore: Williams & Wilkins, 1986.
33. Morris N, Osborn SB, Wright HP, et al: Effective uterine blood flow during exercise in normal and pre-eclamptic pregnancies. Lancet 2:481, 1956.
34. Morton MJ, Paul MS, Campos GR, et al: Exercise dynamics in late gestation: effects of physical training. Am J Obstet Gynecol 152:91, 1985.
35. Adams JG, Alexander AM: Alterations in cardiovascular physiology during labor. Am J Obstet Gynecol 12:542, 1958.
36. Ueland K, Hansen JM: Maternal cardiovascular dynamics. III. Labor and delivery under local and caudal analgesia. Am J Obstet Gynecol 103:8, 1969.
37. Ueland K, Gills RE, Hansen J: Maternal cardiovascular dynamics. I. Cesarean section under subarachnoid block anesthesia. Am J Obstet Gynecol 42:100, 1968.
38. Ueland K, Hansen J, Eng M, et al: Maternal cardiovascular dynamics. V. Cesarean section under thiopental, nitrous oxide and succinyl choline anesthesia. Am J Obstet Gynecol 108:615, 1970.
39. Ueland K, Akamatsu TJ, Eng M, et al: Cardiovascular dynamics. VI. Cesarean section under epidural anesthesia without epinephrine. Am J Obstet Gynecol 114:775, 1972.
40. Veille JC, Morton MJ, Burry KJ: Maternal cardiovascular adaptations to twin pregnancy. Am J Obstet Gynecol 153:261, 1985.

41. Long PA, Oats JN: Preeclampsia in twin pregnancy—severity and pathogenesis. Aust N Z J Obstet Gynaecol 27:1, 1987.
42. Quinley MM, Cruikshank DP: Polyhydramnios and acute renal failure. J Reprod Med 19:92, 1977.
43. Rubler S, Prabodhkumar MD, Pinto ER: Cardiac size and performance during pregnancy estimated with echocardiography. Clin Obstet Gynecol 40:534, 1977.
44. Milne JA, Howie AD, Pack AI: Dyspnea during normal pregnancy. Br J Obstet Gynaecol 85:260, 1978.
45. Cutforth R, MacDonald MB: Heart sounds and murmurs in pregnancy. Am Heart J 71:741, 1966.
46. O'Rourke RA, Ewy GA, Marcus FI: Cardiac auscultation in pregnancy. Med Ann D C 39:92, 1970.
47. Hurst JW, Staton J, Hubbard D: Precordial murmurs during pregnancy and lactation. N Engl J Med 259:515, 1958.
48. Grant RP: A precordial systolic murmur of extracardiac origin during pregnancy. Am Heart J 52:944, 1956.
49. Tabatznik B, Randall TW, Hersch C: The mammary souffle of pregnancy and lactation. Circulation 22:1069, 1960.
50. Perloff JK: The clinical recognition of congenital heart disease. *In* Braunwald E (ed): Heart Disease. 3rd ed. pp. 990–991. Philadelphia: WB Saunders, 1988.
51. Hytten EF, Thomson AM, Taggart N: Total body water in normal pregnancy. J Obstet Gynaecol Br Commonw 73:553, 1966.
52. Sullivan JM, Ramanathan KB: Management of medical problems in pregnancy: severe cardiac disease. N Engl J Med 313:304, 1985.
53. Boyle DM, Lloyd-Jones RL: The electrocardiographic ST segment changes in pregnancy. J Obstet Gynaecol Br Commonw 73:986, 1966.
54. Medical Radiation Exposure of Pregnant and Potentially Pregnant Women: Recommendations of the National Council on Radiation Protection and Measurements. Washington, DC: National Council on Radiation Protection and Measurements, 1977.
55. Turner AF: The chest radiography in pregnancy. Clin Obstet Gynecol 18:65, 1975.
56. Austin JHM: Postpartum pleural effusions? Ann Intern Med 98:555, 1983.
57. Bioeffects Committee of the American Institute of Ultrasound in Medicine. J Ultrasound Med Biol 2:R14, 1983.
58. Laird-Meeter K, VanDeLey G, Bom TH, et al: Cardiocirculatory adjustments during pregnancy: an echocardiographic study. Clin Cardiol 2:328, 1979.
59. Haiat R, Halphen C: Silent pericardial effusion in late pregnancy: a new entity. Cardiovasc Intervent Radiol 7:267, 1984.
60. Ueland K, Novy MJ, Metcalfe J: Cardiorespiratory response to pregnancy and exercise in normal women and patients with heart disease. Am J Obstet Gynecol 115:4, 1973.
61. Carpenter MW, Sady SP, Hoegsberg B, et al: Fetal heart rate response to maternal exertion. JAMA 259:3006, 1988.
62. Graham S, Levin HL, Lilienfield AM, et al: Preconception, intrauterine, and postnatal irradiation as related to leukemia. Natl Cancer Inst Monogr 19:347, 1966.
63. Kereiakes JJ, Rosenstein M: Hand Book of Radiation Doses in Nuclear Medicine and Diagnostic X-Ray. Boca Raton, FL: CRC, 1980.
64. Instrumentation and Monitoring Methods for Radiation Protection: Recommendations of National Council on Radiation Protection and Measurements. Washington, DC: National Council on Radiation Protection and Measurements, 1978.
65. Shellock FG: Biological effects and safety aspects of magnetic resonance imaging. Magn Reson Q 5:243, 1989.
66. Kanal E: An overview of electromagnetic safety considerations associated with magnetic resonance imaging. Ann N Y Acad Sci 649:204, 1992.
67. Mattison DR, Angtuaco T, Miller FC, et al: Magnetic resonance imaging in maternal and fetal medicine. J Perinatol 9:411, 1989.
68. Mattison DR, Kay HH, Miller RK, et al: Magnetic resonance imaging: a noninvasive tool for fetal and placental physiology. Biol Reprod 38:39, 1988.
69. Kirshon B, Lee W, Cotton DB, et al: Indirect blood pressure monitoring in the postpartum patient. Obstet Gynecol 70:799, 1987.
70. Sprung CL, Rackow EC, Civetta J: Direct measurements and derived calculations using the pulmonary artery catheter. *In* Sprung CL (ed): The Pulmonary Artery Catheter: Methodology and Clinical Applications. pp. 105–140. Baltimore: University Park Press, 1983.
71. Grossman W: Pressure measurement. *In* Grossman W (ed): Cardiac Catheterization and Angiography. 3rd ed. pp. 118–134. Philadelphia: Lea & Febiger, 1986.
72. Young BK: The normal and abnormal fetal heart rate. *In* Elkayam U, Gleicher N (eds): Cardiac Problems in Pregnancy. Diagnosis and Management of Maternal and Fetal Disease. 2nd ed. pp. 709–722. New York: Alan R Liss, 1990.
73. Lee RV, Mezzadri FC: Cardiopulmonary resuscitation of pregnant women. *In* Elkayam U, Gleicher N: Cardiac Problems in Pregnancy. 2nd ed. pp. 307–319. New York: Alan R Liss, 1990.
74. Sachs BP, Brown DAJ, Driscoll SG, et al: Maternal mortality in Massachusetts. N Engl J Med 316:667, 1987.
75. American Heart Association: Special resuscitation situations. JAMA 268:2249, 1992.
76. Songster GS, Clark SL: Cardiac arrest in pregnancy: what to do? Contemp Obstet Gynecol 27:141, 1985.
77. Lee RV, Rodgers BD, White LM, et al: Cardiopulmonary resuscitation of pregnant women. Am J Med 81:311, 1986.
78. Sperry KL: Myocardial infarction in pregnancy. J Forens Sci 32:1464, 1987.
79. Ciraulo DA, Markowitz A: Myocardial infarction in pregnancy associated with a coronary artery thrombus. Arch Intern Med 139:1049, 1979.
80. Peng ATC, Gorman RS, Shulman SM, et al: Intravenous nitroglycerin for uterine relaxation in the postpartum patient with retained placenta. Anesthesiology 71:172, 1989.
81. Snyder SW, Wheeler AS, James FM III: The use of nitroglycerin to control severe hypertension of pregnancy during cesarean section. Anesthesiology 51:563, 1979.
82. Wheeler AS, James FM, Greiss FC, et al: Effects of nitroglycerin to control severe hypertension of pregnancy during cesarean section [abstract]. Anesthesiology 51:563, 1979.
83. Wolff F, Breuker KH, Schlensker KH, et al: Prenatal diagnosis and therapy of fetal heart rate anomalies: with a contribution on the placental transfer of verapamil. J Perinat Med 8:230, 1980.
84. Maxwell DJ, Crawford DC, Curry PVM, et al: Obstetric importance, diagnosis, and management of fetal tachycardias. BMJ 297:107, 1988.
85. Klein V, Repke JT: Supraventricular tachycardia in pregnancy: cardioversion with verapamil. Obstet Gynecol 63:165, 1984.
86. Pruyn SC, Phelan JP, Buchanan GC: Long-term propranolol therapy in pregnancy: maternal and fetal outcome. Am J Obstet Gynecol 135:485, 1979.
87. Eliahou HE, Silverberg DS, Reisin E, et al: Propranolol for the treatment of hypertension in pregnancy. Br J Obstet Gynaecol 85:431, 1978.
88. Treffers PE, Huidekoper BL, Weenink GH, et al: Epidemiological observations of thrombo-embolic disease during pregnancy and in the puerperium in 56,022 women. Int J Gynaecol Obstet 21:327, 1983.
89. Clark SL, Cotton DB, Gonile B, et al: Central hemodynamic alterations in amniotic fluid embolism. Am J Obstet Gynecol 158:1124, 1988.
90. Clark SL: Amniotic fluid embolism. Clin Perinatol 13:801, 1986.
91. Plauche WC: Amniotic fluid embolism. Am J Obstet Gynecol 147:982, 1983.
92. Beller FK, Douglas GW, Debrovner CH: The fibrinolytic system in amniotic fluid embolism. Am J Obstet Gynecol 87:48, 1963.
93. Beller FK, Douglas GW, Debrovner CH: The fibrinolytic system in amniotic fluid embolism. Am J Obstet Gynecol 87:48, 1963.
94. Sipes SL, Weiner CP: Venous thromboembolic disease in pregnancy. Semin Perinatol 14:103, 1990.
95. Weiner CP: Thromboembolic disease in the obstetric patient: evaluation, diagnosis, and treatment. *In* Kwaan HC, Samama MM (eds): Clinical Thrombosis. pp. 291–303. Boca Raton, FL: CRC, 1989.
96. Sandler DA, Duncan JS, Ward P, et al: Diagnosis of deep-vein thrombosis: comparison of clinical evaluation, ultrasound, plethysmography, and venoscan with x-ray venogram. Lancet 2:716, 1984.
97. Ginsberg JS, Hirsh J, Bergquist D, et al: Recurrent thromboembolism in pregnancy and puerperium. Am J Obstet Gynecol 160:90, 1989.
98. Hayt DB, Binkert BL: An overview of noninvasive methods of deep vein thrombosis detection. Clin Imaging 14:179, 1990.
99. Ginsberg JS, Hirsh J, Rainbow AJ, et al: Risks to the fetus of radiologic procedures used in the diagnosis of maternal venous thromboembolic disease. Thromb Haemost 61:189, 1989.

100. Howell R, Fidler J, Letsky E, et al: The risks of antenatal subcutaneous heparin prophylaxis: a controlled trial. Br J Obstet Gynaecol 90:1124, 1983.
101. Hull RD, Raskob GE, Hirsh J, et al: Continuous intravenous heparin compared with intermittent subcutaneous heparin in the initial treatment of proximal-vein thrombosis. N Engl J Med 315:1109, 1986.
102. Shoemaker ES, Grant NF, Madden JD, et al: The effect of thiazide diuretics on placental function. Texas Med 69:109, 1973.
103. Rodriquez SU, Leikin SL, Hiller MC: Neonatal thrombocytopenia associated with ante-partum administration of thiazide drugs. N Engl J Med 270:881, 1964.
104. Marcus FI, Ervy GA, O'Rourke RA, et al: The effect of pregnancy on the murmurs of mitral and aortic regurgitation. Circulation 41:795, 1970.
105. Sugrue D, Blake S, MacDonald D: Pregnancy complicated by maternal heart disease at the National Maternity Hospital Dublin, Ireland, 1969 to 1978. Am J Obstet Gynecol 139:1, 1981.
106. Cox SM, Leveno KJ: Pregnancy complicated by bacterial endocarditis. Clin Obstet Gynecol 32:48, 1989.
107. Henderson CE, Terrubile S, Keefe D, et al: Cardiac screening for pregnant intravenous drug abusers. Am J Perinatol 6:397, 1989.
108. Hughes LO, McFadyen IR, Raferty RB: Acute bacterial endocarditis on a normal aortic valve following vaginal delivery. Int J Cardiol 18:261, 1988.
109. MacMahon SW, Roberts JK, Kramer-Fox R, et al: Mitral valve prolapse and infective endocarditis. Am Heart J 113:1291, 1987.
110. Blanco JD, Gibbs RS, Castaneda YS: Bacteremia in obstetrics: clinical course. Obstet Gynecol 58:621, 1981.
111. Mugge A, Daniel WG, Frank G, et al: Echocardiography in infective endocarditis: reassessment of prognostic implications of vegetation size detected by the transthoracic and the transesophageal approach. J Am Coll Cardiol 14:631, 1989.
112. Mandell GL: The laboratory in diagnosis and management. *In* Kaye D (ed): Infective Endocarditis. p. 155. London: University Park Press.
113. Grover A, Anand IS, Varma J, et al: Profile of right-sided endocarditis: an Indian experience. Int J Cardiol 33:83, 1991.
114. Payne DG, Fishburne JI, Rufty AJ, et al: Bacterial endocarditis in pregnancy. Obstet Gynecol 60:247, 1982.
115. Sugrue D, Blake S, Troy P, et al: Antibiotic prophylaxis against infective endocarditis after normal delivery: is it necessary? Br Heart J 44:599, 1980.
116. Ayhan A, Yapar EG, Yuce K, et al: Pregnancy and its complications after cardiac valve replacement. Int J Gynaecol Obstet 35:117, 1991.
117. Shulman ST, Amren DP, Bisno AL, et al: Prevention of bacterial endocarditis [abstract]. Circulation 70:112A, 1984.
118. Norris DC: Management of patients with prosthetic heart valves. Curr Probl Cardiol 7:1, 1982.
119. Born D, Martinez EE, Almeida PA, et al: Pregnancy in patients with prosthetic heart valves: the effect of anticoagulation on mother, fetus, and neonate. Am Heart J 124:413, 1992.
120. Pavankumar P, Venugopal P, Kaul U, et al: Pregnancy in patients with prosthetic cardiac valves: a 10 year experience. Scand J Thorac Cardiovasc Surg 22:11, 1988.
121. Deviri E, Yechezkel M, Levinsky C, et al: Calcification of a porcine valve xenograft during pregnancy: a case report and review of the literature. Thorac Cardiovasc Surg 32:266, 1984.
122. Badduke BR, Jamieson WR, Miyagishima RT, et al: Pregnancy and child rearing in a population with biologic valvular prostheses. J Thorac Cardiovasc Surg 102:179, 1991.
123. Ginsberg JS, Hirsh J: Anticoagulants during pregnancy. Annu Rev Med 40:79, 1989.
124. Wehrmacher WH, Messmore HL: Thromboembolic disease during pregnancy: problems with anticoagulant therapy. Comp Ther 16:31, 1990.
125. Iturbe-Alessio I, Fonseca MCC, Mutchinick O, et al: Risks of anticoagulant therapy in pregnant women with artificial heart valves. N Engl J Med 315:1390, 1986.
126. Chesebro JH, Adams PC, Fuster V: Antithrombotic therapy in patients with valvular heart disease and prosthetic heart valves. J Am Coll Cardiol 8(6 suppl B):41, 1986.
127. Sareli P, England MJ, Berk MR, et al: Maternal and fetal sequelae of anticoagulation during pregnancy in patients with mechanical heart valve prostheses. Am J Cardiol 63:1462, 1989.
128. Gonzalez-Santos JM, Vallejo JL, Rico MJ, et al: Thrombosis of a mechanical valve prosthesis late in pregnancy: case report and review of the literature. Thorac Cardiovasc Surg 34:335, 1986.
129. Weiner CP: Prevention and management of thromboembolic disease during pregnancy. *In* Wenger NK, Speroff L, Packard B (eds): Cardiovascular Health and Disease in Women: Proceedings of an NHLBI Conference. pp. 285–294. Greenwich CT: Le Jacq Communications, 1993.
130. Lee PK, Wang RY, Chow JSF, et al: Combined use of warfarin and adjusted subcutaneous heparin during pregnancy in patients with an artificial heart valve. J Am Coll Cardiol 8:221, 1986.
131. Cohn LH: Anticoagulation in pregnant women with artificial heart valves. N Engl J Med 316:1662, 1987.
132. Elkayam U, Gleicher N: Anticoagulation in pregnant women with artificial heart valves. N Engl J Med 316:1663, 1987.
133. Salazar E, Zajarias A, Gutierrez N, et al: The problem of cardiac valve prosthesis, anticoagulants and pregnancy. Circulation 70:169, 1984.
134. McGehee W: Anticoagulation in pregnancy. *In* Elkayam U, Gleicher N (eds): Cardiac Problems in Pregnancy. 2nd ed. pp. 397–415. New York: Alan R Liss, 1990.
135. Copplestone A, Oscier DG: Heparin-induced thrombocytopenia in pregnancy. Br J Haematol 65:248, 1987.
136. Cotrufo M, De Luca TS, Calabro R, et al: Coumarin anticoagulation during pregnancy in patients with mechanical valve prosthesis. Eur J Cardiothorac Surg 5:300, 1991.
137. Baillie M, Allen ED, Elkington AR: The congenital warfarin syndrome: a case report. Br J Ophthalmol 64:633, 1980.
138. Russo R, Bortolotti U, Schivazappa L, et al: Warfarin treatment during pregnancy: a clinical note. Haemostasis 8:96, 1979.
139. O'Reilly RA: Anticoagulant, antithrombotic, and thrombolytic drugs. *In* Gilman AG, Goodman LS, Gilman A (eds): The Pharmacologic Basis of Therapeutics. 6th ed. pp. 1350–1370. New York: Macmillan, 1980.
140. Normann EK, Stray-Pedersen B: Warfarin-induced fetal diaphragmatic hernia: case report. Br J Obstet Gynaecol 96:729, 1989.
141. Ruthnum P, Tolmie JL: Atypical malformations in an infant exposed to warfarin during the first trimester of pregnancy. Teratology 36:299, 1987.
142. Hall JG, Pauli RM, Wilson KM: Maternal and fetal sequelae of anticoagulation during pregnancy. Am J Med 68:122, 1980.
143. Ibarra-Perez C, Arevalo-Toledo N, Alvarez De La Cadena O, et al: The course of pregnancy in patients with artificial heart valves. Am J Med 61:504, 1976.
144. DeSwiet M, Lewis PJ: Excretion of anticoagulants in human milk. N Engl J Med 297:1471, 1977.
145. Eckstein HB, Jack B: Breast-feeding and anticoagulant therapy. Lancet 1:672, 1970.
146. Rotmensch HH, Rotmensch S, Elkayam U: Management of cardiac arrhythmia during pregnancy. Curr Concepts Drugs 33:623, 1967.
147. Sobotka PA, Mayer JH, Bauernfeind RA, et al: Arrhythmias documented by 24-hr continuous ambulatory electrocardiographic monitoring in young women without apparent heart disease. Am Heart J 101:753, 1981.
148. Szekely P, Snaith L: Paroxysmal tachycardia in pregnancy. Br Heart J 15:195, 1953.
149. Mendelsohn CL: Disorders of the heartbeat during pregnancy. Am J Obstet Gynecol 72:1268, 1956.
150. Olshansky B, Waldo AL: Atrial fibrillation: update on mechanism, diagnosis and management. Mod Concepts Cardiovasc Dis 56:23, 1987.
151. Brand FN, Abbott RD, Kanell WB, et al: Characteristics and prognosis of lone atrial fibrillation. JAMA 254:3449, 1985.
152. Lindsey J Jr, Hurst JW: The clinical features of atrial flutter and their therapeutic implications. Chest 66:114, 1974.
153. Rotmensch HH, Elkayam U, Frishman W: Antiarrhythmic drug therapy during pregnancy. Ann Intern Med 98:487, 1983.
154. Mitani GM, Steinberg I, Lien E, et al: The pharmacokinetics of antiarrhythmic agents in pregnancy and lactation. Clin Pharmacokinet 12:253, 1987.
155. Mitani GM, Harrison EC, Steinberg I, et al: Digitalis glycosides in pregnancy. *In* Elkayam U, Gleicher N (eds): Cardiac Problems in Pregnancy. 2nd ed. pp. 417–428. New York: Alan R Liss, 1990.
156. Valdes R Jr: Endogenous digoxin-like immunoreactive factors: impact on digoxin measurements and potential physiologic implications. Clin Chem 31:1525, 1985.

157. Given BD, Phillippe M, Sanders SP, et al: Procainamide cardioversion of fetal supraventricular tachyarrhythmia. Am J Cardiol 53:1460, 1984.
158. Pittard WB III, Glazier H: Procainamide excretion in human milk. J Pediatr 102:631, 1983.
159. Hill LM, Malkasian GD Jr: The use of quinidine sulfate throughout pregnancy. Obstet Gynecol 54:366, 1979.
161. Cullhed I: Cardioversion during pregnancy: case report. Acta Med Scand 214:169, 1983.
162. Mauer AM, Devaux LO, Lahey ME: Neonatal and maternal thrombocytopenic purpura due to quinidine. Pediatrics 19:84, 1957.
163. Heinonen OP, Slone D, Shapiro S: Birth Defects and Drugs in Pregnancy. Littleton, MA: Publishing Sciences Group, 1977.
164. Merx W, Effert S, Heinrich KW: Heart disease in pregnancy, intra- and postpartum. Z Geburtshilfe Perinatol 178:317, 1974.
165. Byrene Quinn E, Wing AJ: Maintenance of sinus rhythm after DC reversion of atrial fibrillation: a double-blind controlled trial of long acting quinidine b1 sulfate. Br Heart J 32:370, 1970.
166. Hubbard WN, Jenkins BA, Ward DE: Persistent atrial tachycardia in pregnancy. BMJ 287:327, 1983.
167. Vara P, Halminen E: Electrocardiographic examinations during pregnancy and labor. Acta Obstet Gynecol Scand 26:402, 1946.
168. Rotmensch HH, Pines A, Donchin Y: Antiarrhythmic drugs in pregnancy. *In* Elkayam U, Gleicher N (eds): Cardiac Problems in Pregnancy. 2nd ed. pp. 361–380. New York: Alan R Liss, 1990.
169. Propp PA, Broderick K, Pesch D: Adenosine during pregnancy. Ann Emerg Med 21:453, 1992.
170. Wu D, Denes P, Amat-y-Leon F, et al: Clinical, electrocardiographic and electrophysiologic observations in patients with paroxysmal supraventricular tachycardia. Am J Cardiol 41:1045, 1978.
171. Guntheroth WG, Cyr DR, Mack LA, et al: Hydrops from reciprocating atrioventricular tachycardia in a 27-week fetus requiring quinidine for conversion. Obstet Gynecol 66(suppl):29, 1985.
172. Killeen AA, Bowers LD: Fetal supraventricular tachycardia treated with high dose quinidine: toxicity associated with marked elevation of the metabolite 3(S)-3-hydroxyquinidine. Obstet Gynecol 70:445, 1987.
173. Dumesic DA, Silverman NH, Tobias S, et al: Transplacental cardioversion of fetal supraventricular tachycardia with procainamide. N Engl J Med 307:1128, 1982.
174. Foster CJ, Love HG: Amiodarone in pregnancy: case report and review of literature. Int J Cardiol 20:307, 1988.
175. Laurent M, Betremieux P, Biron Y, et al: Neonatal hypothyroidism after treatment by amiodarone during pregnancy. Am J Cardiol 60:942, 1987.
176. Wellens HJJ: Wolff-Parkinson-White syndrome: diagnosis, arrhythmias and identification of the high risk patient. Mod Concepts Cardiovasc Dis 52:53, 1983.
177. Klein GJ, Bashore TM, Sellers TD, et al: Ventricular fibrillation in the Wolff-Parkinson-White syndrome. N Engl J Med 301:1080, 1979.
178. Gleicher N, Meller J, Sandler R, et al: Wolff-Parkinson-White syndrome in pregnancy. Obstet Gynecol 58:748, 1981.
179. Soyka LF: Digoxin: placental transfer, effects on the fetus, and therapeutic use in the newborn. Clin Perinatol 2:23, 1975.
180. McAnulty JH, Metcalfe J, Ueland K: The heart and pregnancy. *In* Hurst JW (ed): The Heart. pp. 1465–1478. New York: McGraw-Hill, 1990.
181. Brodsky MA, Sato AA, Oster PD, et al: Paroxysmal ventricular tachycardia with syncope during pregnancy. Am J Cardiol 58:563, 1986.
182. Akhtar M: Management of ventricular tachyarrhythmias. JAMA 247:671, 1982.
183. Follansbee W, Michelson E, Morganroth J: Nonsustained ventricular tachycardia in ambulatory patients: characteristics and association with sudden cardiac death. Ann Intern Med 92:741, 1980.
184. Pine HL, Fox L, Shook DM: Paroxysmal ventricular tachycardia complicating pregnancy. Am J Cardiol 15:732, 1965.
185. O'Donnell M, Meecham J, Tosson SR, et al: Ventricular fibrillation and reinfarction in pregnancy. Postgrad Med J 63:1095, 1987.
186. Abboud TK, Sarkis F, Blikian A, et al: Lack of adverse neurobehavioral effects of lidocaine [abstract]. Anesthesiology 57:A404, 1982.
187. Bozynski ME, Ruberth LB, Patel JA: Lidocaine toxicity after maternal pudendal anesthesia in a term infant with fetal distress. Am J Perinatol 4:164, 1987.
188. Biehl D, Shnider SM, Levinson S, et al: Placental transfer of lidocaine: effects of fetal acidosis. Anesthesiology 48:409, 1978.
189. Vogel J, Pryor R, Blount S: Direct-current defibrillation during pregnancy. JAMA 193:970, 1965.
190. Schroeder J, Harrison D: Repeated cardioversion during pregnancy. Am J Cardiol 27:445, 1971.
191. Sussman H: Atrial flutter with 1:1 AV conduction successfully treated with DC shock. Dis Chest 49:99, 1966.
192. Curry JJ, Quintana FJ: Myocardial infarction with ventricular fibrillation during pregnancy treated by direct current defibrillation with fetal survival. Chest 58:82, 1970.
193. Finlay AY, Edmunds V: DC cardioversion in pregnancy. Br J Clin Pract 33:88, 1979.
194. Shaxted EJ, Milton PJ: Disopyramide in pregnancy: a case report. Curr Med Res Opin 6:70, 1979.
195. Hopper L, Neuvonen PJ, Korte T: Disopyramide and breast feeding. Br J Clin Pharmacol 21:553, 1986.
196. Lownes HE, Ives TJ: Mexiletine use in pregnancy and lactation. Am J Obstet Gynecol 157:446, 1987.
197. Epstein JR, Altman HE: Heart block in pregnancy. Med Ann DC 20:660, 1951.
198. Rosen KM, Dhingra RC, Loeb H, et al: Chronic heart blocks in adults: clinical and electrophysiologic observations. Arch Intern Med 131:663, 1973.
199. Copeland GD, Stern TN: Wenckebach periods in pregnancy and puerperium. Am Heart J 56:291, 1958.
200. Ginns HM, Holliurake K: Complete heart block in pregnancy treated with an internal pacemaker. Br J Obstet Gynecol 77:710, 1970.
201. Eddy W, Frankenfeld R: Congenital complete heart block in pregnancy. Am J Obstet Gynecol 128:223, 1977.
202. McAnulty JH, Rahimtoola SH, Murphy E, et al: Natural history of "high-risk" bundle branch block. N Engl J Med 307:137, 1982.
203. Schatz JW, Fischer JA, Lee RF, et al: Pacemaker therapy in pregnancy for management of sinus bradycardia-junctional tachycardia syndrome. Chest 65:461, 1974.
204. Abramovici H, Faktor JH, Gonen Y, et al: Maternal permanent bradycardia: pregnancy and delivery. Obstet Gynecol 63:381, 1984.
205. Eraut D, Shaw DB: Sinus bradycardia. Br Heart J 33:742, 1971.
206. Goldman ME, Meller J: Coronary artery disease in pregnancy. *In* Elkayam U, Gleicher N (eds): Cardiac Problems in Pregnancy. 2nd ed. pp. 153–166. New York: Alan R Liss, 1990.
207. Rallings P, Exner T, Abraham R: Coronary artery vasculitis and myocardial infarction associated with antiphospholipid antibodies in a pregnant woman. Aust N Z J Med 19:347, 1989.
208. Welch C, Proudfit W, Sheldon W: Coronary artery in 1000 females less than 50 years of age. Am J Cardiol 35:211, 1975.
209. LaVecchia C, Franceschi S, Decarli A, et al: Risk factors for myocardial infarction in young women. Am J Epidemiol 125:832, 1987.
210. Croft P, Hannaford PC: Risk factors for acute myocardial infarction in women: evidence from the Royal College of General Practitioners Oral Contraception Study. BMJ 298:165, 1989.
211. Hankins DV, Wendel GD, Levenok J, et al: Myocardial infarction during pregnancy: a review. Obstet Gynecol 65:139, 1985.
212. Sasse L, Wagner R, Murray F: Transmural myocardial infarction during pregnancy. Am J Cardiol 35:448, 1975.
213. Movsesian MA, Wray RB: Postpartum myocardial infarction. Br Heart J 62:154, 1989.
214. Muller JE: Prinzmetal's angina: a model for the role of spasm in ischemic heart disease. J Cardiovasc Med 5:19, 1980.
215. Elkayam U, Rose J, Jamison M: Vascular aneurysms and dissections during pregnancy. *In* Elkayam U, Gleicher N (eds): Cardiac Problems in Pregnancy. 2nd ed. pp. 215–230. New York: Alan R Liss, 1990.
216. Raymond R, Lynch J, Underwood D, et al: Myocardial infarction and normal coronary arteriography: a 10-year clinical and risk analysis of 74 infants. J Am Coll Cardiol 11:471, 1988.
217. Sonel A, Erol C, Oral D, et al: Acute myocardial infarction and normal coronary arteries in a pregnant woman. Cardiology 75:218, 1988.
218. Benedetti TJ: Maternal complications of parenteral β-sympathomimetic therapy for premature labor. Am J Obstet Gynecol 145:1, 1983.
219. Shaver P, Carrig T, Baker W: Postpartum coronary artery dissection. Br Heart J 40:83, 1978.
220. Hands ME, Johnson MD, Saltzman DH, et al: The cardiac, obstetric,

and anesthetic management of pregnancy complicated by acute myocardial infarction. J Clin Anesth 2:258, 1990.
221. Corya BC, Rasmussen S, Knebel SB, et al: Echocardiography in acute myocardial infarction. Am J Cardiol 36:1, 1975.
222. Campbell JA: Antenatal radiation hazards. *In* Obstetric Diagnosis by Radiographic, Ultrasonic and Nuclear Methods. pp. 1–4. Baltimore: Williams & Wilkins, 1977.
223. Eaton LW, Weiss JL, Bulkley BH, et al: Regional cardiac dilatation after acute myocardial infarction: recognition by 2-D echocardiography. N Engl J Med 300:57, 1979.
224. Weiss JL, Bulkley BH, Hutchins CM, et al: Two-dimensional echocardiographic recognition of myocardial injury in man: comparison with postmortem studies. Circulation 63:401, 1981.
225. Kagen L, Scheidt S, Butt A: Serum myoglobin in myocardial infarction. Am J Med 62:86, 1977.
226. Adams JQ: Cardiovascular physiology in normal pregnancy: studies with the dye dilution technique. Am J Obstet Gynecol 67:741, 1954.
227. Saxena R, Nolan TE, Von Dohlen T, et al: Postpartum myocardial infarction treated by balloon coronary angioplasty. Obstet Gynecol 79:810, 1992.
228. Cowan NC, DeBelder MA, Rothman MT: Coronary angioplasty in pregnancy. Br Heart J 59:588, 1988.
229. Madjan JF, Walinsky P, Cowchuck JF, et al: Coronary bypass surgery during pregnancy. Am J Cardiol 52:1145, 1983.
230. Levy DL, Warriner RA, Burgess GE: Fetal response to cardiopulmonary bypass. Obstet Gynecol 56:112, 1980.
231. Gallery E, Boyce E, Saunders D, Gyory A: The effect of volume expansion on blood pressure, plasma and extracellular fluid volumes in hypertensive pregnancy. Aust N Z J Obstet Gynecol 20:189, 1980.
232. London G, Safar M, Simon A, et al: Total effective compliance, cardiac output and fluid volumes in essential hypertension. Circulation 57:995, 1978.
233. Smith RU: Cardiovascular alterations in toxemia. Am J Obstet Gynecol 107:979, 1970.
234. Lim YL, Walters WA: Hemodynamics of mild hypertension in pregnancy. Br J Obstet Gynaecol 86:198, 1979.
235. Finnerty FA Jr: Hypertension and pregnancy. Cardiovasc Med 5:559, 1980.
236. Finnerty FA Jr: Toxemia of pregnancy as seen by an internist: an analysis of 1081 patients. Ann Intern Med 44:358, 1956.
237. Freund U, French W, Carlson R, et al: Hemodynamic and metabolic studies of a case of toxemia of pregnancy. Am J Obstet Gynecol 127:206, 1977.
238. Benedetti TJ, Cotton DB, Read JA, et al: Hemodynamic observations in severe preeclampsia using a flow directed pulmonary artery catheter. Am J Obstet Gynecol 136:465, 1980.
239. Rafferty TD, Berkowitz RL: Hemodynamics in patients with severe toxemia during labor and delivery. Am J Obstet Gynecol 138:263, 1980.
240. Lindheimer MD, Katz AI: Hypertension in pregnancy. N Engl J Med 313:675, 1985.
241. Goodlin RC: Severe preeclampsia: another great imitator. Am J Obstet Gynecol 125:747, 1976.
242. Roberts JM: When the hypertensive patient becomes pregnant. Contemp Obstet Gynecol 13:47, 1979.
243. Walsh SW: Preeclampsia, an imbalance in placental prostacyclin and thromboxane production. Am J Obstet Gynecol 152:355, 1985.
244. Gant NF, Chand S, Worley RJ, et al: A clinical test useful for predicting the development of acute hypertension of pregnancy. Am J Obstet Gynecol 120:1, 1974.
245. Gallery ED, Saunders D, Hunyor S, et al: Improvement in fetal growth with treatment of maternal hypertension in pregnancy. Clin Sci Mol Med 55:3593, 1978.
246. Olin P, Maltau JM, Noddeland H, et al: Transcapillary fluid balance in preeclampsia. Br J Obstet Gynaecol 93:235, 1986.
247. Habib A, McCarthy JS: Effects on the neonate of propranolol administered during pregnancy. J Pediatr 91:808, 1971.
248. Sabom M, Curry C, Wise D: Propranolol therapy during pregnancy in a patient with idiopathic hypertrophic subaortic stenosis: is it safe? South Med J 71:328, 1978.
249. Parisi VM: Prevention of pre-eclampsia. *In* Wenger N, Speroff L, Packard B (eds): Cardiovascular Health and Disease in Women. pp. 279–284. Greenwich, CT: Le Jacq Communications, 1993.
250. Elkayam U, Gleicher N: Primary pulmonary hypertension and pregnancy. *In* Elkayam U, Gleicher N (eds): Cardiac Problems in Pregnancy. 2nd ed. pp. 189–198. New York: Alan R Liss, 1990.
251. Takenchi T, Nishii O, Okamura T, et al: Primary pulmonary hypertension in pregnancy. Int J Gynaecol Obstet 26:145, 1988.
252. Slomka F, Salmeron S, Zaetlaoui P, et al: Primary pulmonary hypertension and pregnancy: anesthetic management for delivery. Anesthesiology 69:959, 1988.
253. Gutkind L: Life after transplantations. Transplant Proc 20(suppl 1):1092, 1988.
254. Palvesky HI, Fishman AP: The management of primary pulmonary hypertension. JAMA 265:1014, 1991.
255. Rubin LJ: Primary pulmonary hypertension: practical therapeutic recommendations. Drugs 43:37, 1992.
256. Rich S, Dantzker DR, Ayres SM, et al: Primary pulmonary hypertension: a national prospective study. Ann Intern Med 107:216, 1987.
257. Abboud TK, Raya J, Noueihed R, et al: Intrathecal morphine for relief of labor pain in a parturient with severe pulmonary hypertension. Anesthesiology 59:477, 1983.
258. Dawkins KD, Burke CM, Billingham ME, et al: Primary pulmonary hypertension and pregnancy. Chest 89:383, 1986.
259. Jewett JF, Ober WB: Primary pulmonary hypertension as a cause of maternal death. Am J Obstet Gynecol 71:1335, 1956.
260. Metcalfe J, McAnulty JH, Ueland K: Pulmonary artery hypertension. *In* Heart Disease and Pregnancy: Physiology and Management. 2nd ed. pp. 265–277. Boston: Little, Brown, 1986.
261. Konisbi J, Tatsula N, Kumada K, et al: Dissecting aneurysms during pregnancy and the puerperium. Jpn Circ J 44:726, 1980.
262. Beighton P: Obstetric aspects of the Ehlers-Danlos syndrome. J Obstet Gynaecol Br Commonw 76:97, 1969.
263. Elias S, Berkovitz RL: The Marfan syndrome and pregnancy. Obstet Gynecol 47:358, 1976.
264. Williams GM, Gott VL, Brawley RK, et al: Aortic disease associated with pregnancy. J Vasc Surg 8:470, 1988.
265. Chandrasekaran K, Currie PJ: Transesophageal echocardiography in aortic dissection. J Invasive Cardiol 1:326, 1989.
266. Rosenblum NG, Grossman AR, Mennuti MT, et al: Failure of serial echocardiographic studies to predict aortic dissection in pregnancy patient with Marfan's syndrome. Am J Obstet Gynecol 146:470, 1983.
267. Rigg D, McDonogh A: Use of sodium nitroprusside for deliberate hypotension during pregnancy. Br J Anaesth 53:985, 1981.
268. Dochin Y, Amirav B, Sahar A, et al: Sodium nitroprusside for aneurysm surgery in pregnancy. Br J Anaesth 50:849, 1978.
269. Paul J: Clinical report of the use of sodium nitroprusside in severe pre-eclampsia. Anaesth Intens Care 3:72, 1975.
270. Willoughby JS: Case reports: sodium nitroprusside, pregnancy and multiple intracranial aneurysms. Anaesth Intens Care 12:358, 1984.
271. Stempel JE, O'Grady JP, Morton MJ, et al: Use of sodium nitroprusside in complications of gestational hypertension. Obstet Gynecol 60:533, 1982.
272. Pyeritz RE: Propranolol retards aortic root dilatation in the Marfan syndrome. Circulation 68(suppl III):III-365, 1983.
273. Shoemaker CT, Meyers M: Sodium nitroprusside for control of severe hypertensive disease of pregnancy: a case report and discussion of potential toxicity. Am J Obstet Gynecol 149:171, 1984.
274. Willoughby JS: Review article: sodium nitroprusside, pregnancy and multiple intracranial aneurysms. Anaesth Intens Care 12:351, 1984.
275. Snir E, Levinksy L, Salomon J, et al: Dissecting aortic aneurysm in pregnant women without Marfan disease. Surg Gynecol Obstet 6:167, 1988.
276. Ishikawa K, Matsuura S: Occlusive thromboaortopathy (Takayasu's disease) and pregnancy: clinical course and management of 33 pregnancies and deliveries. Am J Cardiol 50:293, 1982.
277. Wong VCW, Wang RYE, Tse TF: Pregnancy and Takayasu's arteritis. Am J Med 75:597, 1983.
278. Winn HN, Setaro JF, Mazor M: Severe Takayasu's arteritis in pregnancy: the role of central hemodynamic monitoring. Am J Obstet Gynecol 159:1135, 1988.
279. Ask-Upmark E: Case of Takayasu's syndrome accelerated (initiated?) by oral contraceptives. Acta Med Scand 185:119, 1969.
280. Sise MJ, Counihan CM, Shackford SR, et al: The clinical spectrum of Takayasu's arteritis. Surgery 104:905, 1988.
281. Graca LM, Cardoso MC, Machado FS: Takayasu's arteritis and pregnancy: a case of deleterious association. Eur J Obstet Gynecol Reprod Biol 24:347, 1982.
282. Gaida BJ, Gervais HW, Mauer D, et al: Anaesthesiology problems in Takayasu's syndrome. Anaesthetist 40:1, 1991.

283. Jilek D, Dlouhy P, Svoboda J, et al: Takayasu's disease: detection of the early systemic stage of the disease in the pregnant woman. Casopis Lekaru Ceskych 130:20, 1991.
284. Boike GM, Gove N, Dombrowski MP, et al: Mycotic aneurysms in pregnancy. Am J Obstet Gynecol 157:340, 1987.
285. Barrett JM, Van Hooydonk JE, Boehm FH: Pregnancy related rupture of arterial aneurysms. Obstet Gynecol Surv 37:557, 1982.
286. Derksen RH: Systemic lupus erythematosus and pregnancy. Rheumatol Int 40:3, 1991.
287. Varner MW: Autoimmune disorders and pregnancy. Semin Perinatol 15:238, 1991.
288. Godeau P, Piette JC, Frances C, et al: The multiple clinical aspects of lupus. Clin Exp Rheumatol 8(suppl 5):27, 1990.
289. Harvey CJ, Verklen T: Systemic lupus erythematosus: obstetric and neonatal implications. NAACOGS Clin Issue Perinat Womens Health Nurs 1:177, 1990.
290. Lockshin MD: Pregnancy associated with systemic lupus erythematosus. Semin Perinatol 14:130, 1990.
291. Lockshin MD, Qamar T, Levy RA, et al: Pregnancy in systemic lupus erythematosus. Clin Exp Rheumatol 7(suppl 3):195, 1989.
292. James KB, Healy BP: Heart disease arising during or secondary to pregnancy. Cardiovasc Clin 19:81, 1989.
293. Litsey SE, Noonan JA, O'Connor WN, et al: Maternal connective tissue disease and congenital heart block: demonstration of immunoglobulin in cardiac tissue. N Engl J Med 312:98, 1985.
294. Branch DW, Scott JR, Kochenour NK, et al: Obstetric complications associated with the lupus anticoagulant. N Engl J Med 313:1322, 1985.
295. Chua S, Ostman-Smith I, Sellers S, et al: Congenital heart block with hydrops fetalis treated with high-dose dexamethasone: a case report. Eur J Obstet Gynecol Reprod Biol 42:155, 1991.
296. Guzman E, Schulman H, Bracero L, et al: Uterine-umbilical artery Doppler velocimetry in pregnant women with systemic lupus erythematosus. J Ultrasound Med 11:275, 1992.
297. Carroll BA: Obstetric duplex sonography in patients with lupus anticoagulant syndrome. J Ultrasound Med 9:17, 1990.
298. Hughes GRV, Harris NN, Gharavi AE: The anticardiolipin syndrome. J Rheumatol 13:486, 1986.
299. Zulman JI, Tali N, Hoffman GS, et al: Problems associated with the management of pregnancies in patients with systemic lupus erythematosus. J Rheumatol 7:37, 1980.
300. Scott JS: Systemic lupus erythematosus and allied disorders in pregnancy. Clin Obstet Gynecol 6:461, 1979.
301. Tsai A, Lindheimer MD, Lamberg SI: Dermatomyositis complicating pregnancy. Obstet Gynecol 41:570, 1973.
302. Gutierrez G, Dagnino R, Mintz G: Polymyositis/dermatomyositis and pregnancy. Arthritis Rheum 27:291, 1984.
303. Berkowitz RL, Coustan DR, Mochizuki TK: Handbook for Prescribing Medications during Pregnancy. Boston: Little, Brown, 1981.
304. Dullet N, Santora L, Elkayam U: Diseases of the pericardium in pregnancy. *In* Gleicher N, Elkayam U, Galbraith, et al (eds): Principles of Medical Therapy in Pregnancy. pp. 685–689. New York: Plenum Press, 1985.
305. Hollander AG, Crawford JH: Roentgenologic and electrocardiographic changes in the normal heart during pregnancy. Am Heart J 26:364, 1943
306. Probst R, Mier T: Acute pericarditis complicating pregnancy. Obstet Gynecol 22:393, 1963.
307. Elkayam U, Weiss S, Lanidao S: Pericardial effusion and mitral valve involvement in systemic lupus erythematosus. Ann Rheum Dis 36:349, 1977.
308. Krausz Y, Naparstek E, Eliakim M: Idiopathic pericarditis and pregnancy. Aust N Z J Obstet Gynaecol 18:86, 1978.
309. Spodeck DH: Differential diagnosis of acute pericarditis. Prog Cardiovasc Dis 14:192, 1971.
310. Surawicz B, Lassiter KC: Electrocardiogram in pericarditis. Am J Cardiol 26:471, 1970.
311. Burch GE, Sun SC, Colough H, et al: Coxsackie B viral myocarditis and valvulitis identified in routine autopsy specimens by immunofluorescent techniques. Am Heart J 74:13, 1967.
312. Horowitz MS, Schultz CS, Stinson EB, et al: Sensitivity and specificity of echocardiographic diagnosis of pericardial effusion. Circulation 50:239, 1974.
313. Richardson PM, LeRoux BT, Rogers MA, et al: Pericardiectomy in pregnancy. Thorax 25:627, 1970.
314. Blake S, Bonar F, McCarthy C, et al: The effect of posture on cardiac output in late pregnancy complicated by pericardial constriction. Am J Obstet Gynecol 146:865, 1983.
315. Lessing JB, Landan E, Cohen HS, et al: Calcific constrictive pericarditis in pregnancy. J Reprod Med 32:551, 1987.
316. Jaluvka V: On the problem of pregnancy following surgically treated constricted pericarditis. Geburtshilfe Frauenheilkd 29:260, 1969.
317. Aretz HT, Billingham ME, Edwards WD, et al: Myocarditis: a histopathologic definition and classification. Am J Cardiovasc Pathol 1:3, 1986.
318. Farber P, Glasgow L: Viral myocarditis during pregnancy: encephalomyocarditis virus infection in mice. Am Heart J 80:96, 1970.
319. Fujimoto T, Katoh C, Hayakawa H, et al: Two cases of rubella infection with cardiac involvement. Jpn Heart J 20:227, 1979.
320. Pearce J: Heart disease and filterable viruses. Circulation 21:448, 1960
321. Daly K, Richardson PJ, Olsen EGJ, et al: Acute myocarditis: role of histological and virological examination in the diagnosis and assessment of immunosuppressive treatment. Br Heart J 51:30, 1984.
322. Demakis JG, Rahimtoola SH, Sutton GC, et al: Natural course of peripartum cardiomyopathy. Circulation 44:1053, 1971.
323. Midei MC, DeMent SH, Feldman AM, et al: Peripartum myocarditis and cardiomyopathy. Circulation 81:922, 1990.
324. Lee W, Cotton DB: Peripartum cardiomyopathy: current concepts and clinical management. Clin Obstet Gynecol 32:54, 1989.
325. Homans DC: Peripartum cardiomyopathy. N Engl J Med 312:1432, 1985.
326. Melvin K, Richardson P, Olsen E, et al: Peripartum cardiomyopathy due to myocarditis. N Engl J Med 307:731, 1982.
327. St. John Sutton M, Cole P, Saltzman D, et al: Risks of cardiac dysfunction in peripartum cardiomyopathy (PPCM) with subsequent pregnancy. Circulation 80(suppl II):II-320, 1989.
328. Cole P, Cook F, Plappert T, et al: Longitudinal changes in left ventricular architecture and function in peripartum cardiomyopathy. Am J Cardiol 60:871, 1987.
329. O'Connell JB, Costanzo-Nordin R, Subramanian R, et al: Peripartum cardiomyopathy: clinical, hemodynamic, histologic and prognostic characteristics. J Am Coll Cardiol 8:52, 1986.
330. Fenoglio JJ Jr, Ursell PC, Kellogg CF, et al: Diagnosis and classification of myocarditis by endomyocardial biopsy. N Engl J Med 308:12, 1983.
331. Nelson DM, Main E, Crafford W, et al: Peripartum heart failure due to primary pulmonary hypertension. Obstet Gynecol 62:59S, 1983.
332. Carvalho A, Brandao A, Martinez EE, et al: Prognosis in peripartum cardiomyopathy. Am J Cardiol 64:540, 1989.
333. Brantigan CO, Grow JB, Schoonmaker FW: Extended use of intraaortic balloon pumping in peripartum cardiomyopathy. Ann Surg 183:1, 1976.
334. Hovsepian PG, Ganzel B, Sohi GS, et al: Peripartum cardiomyopathy treated with a left ventricular assist device as a bridge to cardiac transplantation. South Med J 82:527, 1989.
335. Frazier OH, Sweeney MS, Radovaneer B, Cooley D: Surgical treatment of heart diseases. *In* Willerson JT (ed): Treatment of Heart Diseases. Vol. 6. pp. 6.3–6.7. New York: Gower Medical, 1992.
336. Shah DM, Sunderji SG: Hypertrophic cardiomyopathy and pregnancy: report of the maternal mortality and review of the literature. Am J Obstet Gynecol Surv 40:444, 1985.
337. Brown AK, Doukas N, Riding WD, et al: Cardiomyopathy and pregnancy. BMJ 29:387, 1967.
338. Kolibash AJ, Ruiz DE, Lewis RP: Idiopathic hypertrophic subaortic stenosis in pregnancy. Ann Intern Med 82:791, 1975.
339. Maron BJ, Roberts WC, Epstein SE: Sudden death in hypertrophic cardiomyopathy: a profile of 78 patients. Circulation 65:1388, 1982.
340. McKenna WJ, Deanfield JF, Faruqui AM, et al: Prognosis in hypertrophic cardiomyopathy: role of age and clinical, electrocardiographic, and hemodynamic features. Am J Cardiol 47:532, 1981.
341. Evans-Jones JC: Hypertrophic cardiomyopathy in pregnancy. J R Soc Med 76:524, 1983.
342. Oakley GDG, McGarry K, Limb DG, et al: Management of pregnancy in patients with hypertrophic cardiomyopathy. BMJ 1:1749, 1979.
343. Sabom MB, Curry RC, Wise DE: Propranolol therapy during pregnancy in a patient with idiopathic hypertrophic subaortic stenosis: is it safe? South Med J 71:328, 1978.

344. Datta S, Kitzmiller JL, Ostheimer GW, et al: Propranolol and parturition. Obstet Gynecol 51:577, 1978.
345. Rosing DR, Idanpaan-Heikkila U, Maron BJ, et al: Use of calcium-channel blocking drugs in hypertrophic cardiomyopathy. Am J Cardiol 55:185B, 1985.
346. Boccio RV, Chung JH, Harrison DM: Anesthetic management of cesarean section in a patient with idiopathic hypertrophic subaortic stenosis. Anesthesiology 65:663, 1986.
347. Loubser P, Suh K, Cohen S: Adverse effects of spinal anesthesia in a patient with idiopathic hypertrophic subaortic stenosis. Anesthesiology 60:228, 1984.
348. Thompson RC, Liberthson RR, Lowenstein E: Perioperative anesthetic risk of noncardiac surgery in hypertrophic obstructive cardiomyopathy. JAMA 254:2419, 1985.
349. Tang LCH, Chang SYW, Wong VCW, et al: Pregnancy in patients with mitral valve prolapse. Int J Gynaecol Obstet 23:217, 1985.
350. Degani S, Abinader EG, Scharf M: Mitral valve prolapse and pregnancy: a review. Obstet Gynecol Surv 44:642, 1989.
351. Piworarska W, Mroczek-Czernecka D: Follow-up of patients with mitral valve prolapse presenting with rhythm disturbances. Ann Clin Res 20:389, 1988.
352. Savage DD, Garrison RJ, Devereux RB, et al: Mitral valve prolapse in the general population. I. Epidemiologic features: the Framingham Study. Am Heart J 106:571, 1983.
353. Rayburn WF, LeMire MS, Bird JL, et al: Mitral valve prolapse: echocardiographic changes during pregnancy. J Reprod Med 32:185, 1987.
354. Artal R, Greenspoon JS, Rutherford S: Transient ischemic attack: a complication of mitral valve prolapse in pregnancy. Obstet Gynecol 71:1028, 1988.
355. Cheng TO: Transient ischemic attack: a complication of mitral valve prolapse in pregnancy. Obstet Gynecol 73:297, 1989.
356. Anzalone N, Landi G: Lacunar infarction in a puerpera with mitral valve prolapse. Ital J Neurol Sci 9:515, 1988.
357. Roess TJ: Acute rheumatic fever with carditis in pregnancy: report of a case and review of the literature. N Engl J Med 258:605, 1958.
358. Ueland K, Metcalfe J: Acute rheumatic fever in pregnancy. Am J Obstet Gynecol 95:586, 1966.
359. Clinch J: Chorea gravidarum. Hosp Med 2:317, 1967.
360. Lewis BV, Parsons M: Chorea gravidarum. Lancet 1:284, 1966.
361. Shulman ST, Amren DP, Bisno AL, et al: Prevention of bacterial endocarditis: a statement for health professions by the Committee on Rheumatic Fever and Infective Endocarditis of the Council of Cardiovascular Disease in the Young [abstract]. Circulation 70:1123A, 1984.
362. Baskin CG, Law S, Wenger NK: Sulfadiazine rheumatic fever prophylaxis during pregnancy: does it increase the risk of kernicterus in the newborn? Cardiology 65:222, 1980.
363. Chesley LC: Severe rheumatic cardiac disease and pregnancy: the ultimate prognosis. Am J Obstet Gynecol 136:552, 1980.
364. Spagnulo M, Pasternack B, Taranta A: Risk of rheumatic-fever recurrences after streptococcal infections: prospective study of clinical and social factors. N Engl J Med 285:641, 1971.
365. Clark SL, Phelan JP, Greenspoon J, et al: Labor and delivery in the presence of mitral stenosis: central hemodynamic observations. Am J Obstet Gynecol 152:984, 1985.
366. Szekely P, Turner R, Snaith L: Pregnancy and the changing pattern of rheumatic heart disease. Br Heart J 35:1293, 1973.
367. Hemmings GT, Whalley DG, O'Connor PH, et al: Invasive monitoring and anesthetic management of a patient with mitral stenosis. Can Anaesth Soc J 34:182, 1987.
368. Gazioglu K, Kaltreider NL, Rosen M, et al: Pulmonary function during pregnancy in normal women and in patients with cardiopulmonary disease. Thorax 25:445, 1970.
369. Schenker JG, Polishuk WZ: Pregnancy following mitral valvotomy: a survey of 182 patients. Obstet Gynecol 32:214, 1968.
370. Palacios IF, Block PC, Wilkins GT, et al: Percutaneous mitral balloon valvotomy during pregnancy in a patient with severe mitral stenosis. Cathet Cardiovasc Diagn 15:109, 1988.
371. El-Maraghy M, Abon Senna I, El-Tehewy F, et al: Mitral valvotomy in pregnancy. Am J Obstet Gynecol 145:708, 1983.
372. Abid A, Abid F, Zargouni N, et al: Closed mitral valvotomy in pregnancy—a study of seven cases. Int J Cardiol 26:319, 1990.
373. Kendrick JM: Open mitral commissurotomy during pregnancy: a case study. J Obstet Gynecol Neonatal Nurs 20:243, 1991.
374. Matorras R, Reque JA, Minquez JA, et al: Commissurotomy and pregnancy: a study of 245 cases. Acta Obstet Gynecol Scand 65:847, 1986.
375. Safian RD, Perman AD, Sachs B, et al: Percutaneous balloon mitral valvuloplasty in a pregnant woman with mitral stenosis. Cathet Cardiovasc Diagn 15:103, 1988.
376. Wallace WA, Harken DE, Ellis LB: Pregnancy following closed mitral valvuloplasty: a long-term study with remarks covering the necessity for careful cardiac management. JAMA 217:297, 1971.
377. Izquierdo LA, Kushnir O, Knieriem K, et al: Effect of mitral valve prosthetic surgery on the outcome of a growth-retarded fetus: a case report. Am J Obstet Gynecol 163:584, 1990.
378. Martin MC, Pernall ML, Borhszak AN, et al: Cesarean section while on cardiac bypass: report of a case. Obstet Gynecol 6:41S, 1981.
379. Ziskind Z, Etchin A, Frenkel Y, et al: Epidural anesthesia with the Trendelenburg position for cesarean section with or without cardiac surgical procedure in patients with severe mitral stenosis: a hemodynamic study. J Cardiothorac Anesth 4:354, 1990.
380. Shah AM, Ikram S, Kulatilake EN, et al: Emergency mitral valve replacement immediately following cesarean section. Eur Heart J 13:847, 1992.
381. Castillo RA, Llado I, Adamsons K: Ruptured chordae tendineae complicating pregnancy: a case report. J Reprod Med 32:137, 1987.
382. Arias F, Pineda J: Aortic stenosis and pregnancy. J Reprod Med 4:229, 1978.
383. Angel JL, Chapman C, Knappel RA, et al: Percutaneous balloon aortic valvuloplasty in pregnancy. Obstet Gynecol 72:438, 1988.
384. Bem-Ami M, Battino S, Rosenfeld T, et al: Aortic valve replacement during pregnancy: a case report and review of the literature. Acta Obstet Gynecol Scand 69:651, 1990.
385. Mooij PN, De Jong PA, Bavinck JH, et al: Aortic valve replacement in the second trimester of pregnancy: a case report. Eur J Obstet Gynecol Reprod Biol 29:347, 1988.
386. Vosa C, Renzulli A, Festa M, et al: Cardiac valve replacement during pregnancy: report of two cases. Ital J Surg Sci 18:175, 1988.
387. Eilen B, Kaiser I, Becker R, et al: Aortic valve replacement in the third trimester of pregnancy. Obstet Gynecol 57:119, 1981.
388. Whittenmore R, Hobbins JC, Engle MA: Pregnancy and its outcome in women with and without surgical treatment of congenital heart disease. Am J Cardiol 50:641, 1982.
389. Canobbio MM: Counseling the adult with congenital heart disease. *In* Roberts WC (ed): Adult Congenital Heart Disease. pp. 733–739. Philadelphia: FA Davis, 1987.
390. Mendelson CL: Cardiac Disease in Pregnancy: Medical Care, Cardiovascular Surgery, and Obstetrical Management as Related to Maternal and Fetal Welfare. Philadelphia: FA Davis, 1960.
391. Espino-Vela J, Alvarado-Toroa A: Natural history of atrial septal defect. Cardiovasc Clin 2:103, 1971.
392. Engle MA, Kline SA, Borer JS: Ventricular septal defect. *In* Roberts WC (ed): Adult Congenital Heart Disease. pp. 803–825. Philadelphia: FA Davis, 1987.
393. Knapp RC, Arditi LI: Pregnancy complicated by patent ductus arteriosus with reversal of flow. NY J Med 67:573, 1967.
394. Shime J, Mocarski EJM, Hastings D, et al: Congenital heart disease in pregnancy: short- and long-term implications. Am J Obstet Gynecol 156:313, 1987.
395. Donzeeau GP, Nguyen A, Touchot B, et al: Acute thrombosis of a St. Jude medical aortic prosthesis in a pregnant woman. Thorac Cardiovasc Surg 33:248, 1985.
396. McFaul PB, Dorman JC, Lamki H, et al: Pregnancy complicated by maternal heart disease: a review of 519 women. Br J Obstet Gynaecol 95:861, 1988.
397. Metcalfe J, McAnulty JH, Ueland K: Heart Disease and Pregnancy: Physiology and Management. Boston: Little, Brown, 1986.
398. Deal K, Wooley CF: Coarctation of the aorta and pregnancy. Ann Intern Med 78:706, 1973.
399. Barash PG, Hobbins JC, Hook R, et al: Management of coarctation of the aorta during pregnancy. J Thorac Cardiovasc Surg 69:781, 1975.
400. Garson H, McNamara DG, Cooley DA: Tetralogy of Fallot in adults. *In* Roberts WC (ed): Congenital Heart Disease in Adults. pp. 493–519. Philadelphia: FA Davis, 1987.
401. Ralstin JH, Dunn M: Pregnancies after surgical correction of tetralogy of Fallot. JAMA 235:2627, 1976.

402. Nora JJ, Nora AH, Wexler P: Hereditary and environmental aspects as they affect the fetus and newborn. Clin Obstet Gynecol 24:851, 1981.
403. Littler WA: Successful pregnancy in a patient with Ebstein's anomaly. Br Heart J 32:711, 1970.
404. Graham TP, Friesinger CG: Complex cyanotic congenital heart disease. *In* Roberts WC (ed): Adult Congenital Heart Disease. pp. 541–566. Philadelphia: FA Davis, 1987.
405. Gleicher N, Midwall J, Hochberger D, et al: Eisenmenger's syndrome and pregnancy. Obstet Gynecol Surv 34:721, 1979.
406. Midwall J, Jaffin H, Herman MV, et al: Shunt flow and pulmonary hemodynamics during labor and delivery in the Eisenmenger's syndrome. Am J Cardiol 42:299, 1978.
407. Rosenberg B, Simon K, Peretz BA, et al: Eisenmenger's syndrome in pregnancy: controlled segmental epidural block for cesarean section. Reg Anaesth 7:131, 1984.
408. Ritsch M, Johansen C, Wennevold A, et al: Tricuspid atresia and pregnancy. Eur J Obstet Gynecol Reprod Biol 31:277, 1989.
409. Hess DB, Hess LW, Heath BJ, et al: Pregnancy after Fontan repair of tricuspid atresia. South Med J 84:532, 1991.
410. Said SA, Veerbeek A, Van Der Weiken LR: Dextrocardia, situs inversus and severe mitral stenosis in a pregnant woman: successful closed commissurotomy. Eur Heart J 12:825, 1991.
411. Stiller RJ, Vintzileos AM, Nochimson DJ, et al: Single ventricle in pregnancy: case report and review of the literature. Obstet Gynecol 64(suppl 3):185, 1984.
412. Zitnik RS, Bradenburg RO, Sheldon R, et al: Pregnancy and open heart surgery. Circulation 39(suppl 1):257, 1969.
413. Bernal JM, Miralles PJ: Cardiac surgery with cardiopulmonary bypass during pregnancy. Obstet Gynecol Surv 41;1, 1986.
414. Becker RM: Intracardiac surgery in pregnant women. Ann Thorac Surg 36:453, 1983.
415. Korsten HH, Van Zundert AA, Mooij PN, et al: Emergency aortic valve replacement in the 24th week of pregnancy. Acta Anaesthesiol Belg 40:201, 1989.
416. Farmakides G, Schulman H, Mohtashemi M, et al: Uterine umbilical velocimetry in open heart surgery. Am J Obstet Gynecol 156:1221, 1987.
417. Abdalla MY, El Din Mostafa E: Contraception after heart surgery. Contraception 45:73, 1992.
418. Mangano DT: Anesthesia for the pregnant cardiac patient. *In* Shnider SM, Levinson G (eds): Anesthesia for Obstetrics. pp. 345–381. Baltimore: Williams & Wilkins, 1986.
419. Lilja H, Karlsson K, Lindecranz K, et al: Treatment of intrauterine supraventricular tachycardia with digoxin and verapamil. J Perinat Med 12:151, 1984.
420. Spinnato JA, Shaver DC, Flinn GS, et al: Fetal supraventricular tachycardia: in utero therapy with digoxin and quinidine. Obstet Gynecol 64:730, 1984.
421. Zielinsky P, Dillenburg RF, de Lima GG, Zimmer LP: Fetal supraventricular tachyarrhythmias: experience of a fetal cardiology referral center. Arq Bras Cardiol 79:337–340, 1998.
422. Parilla BV, Strasburger JF, Socol ML: Fetal supraventricular tachycardia complicated by hydrops fetalis: a role for direct fetal intramuscular therapy. Am J Perinatol 13:483–486, 1996.
423. Petrikovsky B, Schneider E, Ovadia M: Natural history of hydrops resolution in fetuses with tachyarrhythmias diagnosed and treated in utero. Fetal Diagn Ther 11:292–295, 1996.
424. Guntheroth WG, Cyr DR, Shields LE, Nghim HV: Rate-based management of supraventricular tachycardia. J Ultrasound Med 15:453–458, 1996.
425. Villain E, Butera G, Bonnet D, et al: Neonatal ventricular tachycardia. Arch Mal Coeur Vaiss 91:623–629, 1998.
426. Bocci A, Pupita F, Revelli E, et al: The water-salt metabolism in obstetrics and gynecology. Minerva Ginecol 17:103, 1965.
427. Wladimiroff JW: Effect of furosemide on fetal urine production. Br J Obstet Gynaecol 82:221, 1975.
428. Stein WW, Halberstadt E, Gerner R, et al: Effect of furosemide on fetal kidney function. Arch Gynekol 224:114, 1977.
429. Barrett RJ, Rayburn WF, Barr M Jr: Furosemide (Lasix) challenge test in assessing bilateral fetal hydronephrosis. Am J Obstet Gynecol 147:846, 1983.
430. Pulle C: Diuretic therapy in monosymptomatic edema of pregnancy. Minerva Med 56:1622, 1965.
431. DeCecco L: Furosemide in the treatment of edema in pregnancy. Minerva Med 56:1586, 1965.
432. Sibai BM, Grossman RA, Grossman HG: Effects of diuretics on plasma volume in pregnancies with long-term hypertension. Am J Obstet Gynecol 150:831, 1984.
433. Carswell W, Semple PF: The effect of furosemide on uric acid levels in maternal blood, fetal blood and amniotic fluid. J Obstet Gynaecol Br Commonw 81:472, 1974.
434. Jerkner K, Kutti J, Victorin L: Platelet counts in mothers and their newborn infants with respect to antepartum administration of oral diuretics. Acta Med Scand 194:473, 1973.
435. Committee on Drugs, American Academy of Pediatrics: Transfer of drugs and other chemicals into human milk. Pediatrics 84:924, 1989.
436. Cotton DB, Longmire S, Jones MM, et al: Cardiovascular alterations in severe pregnancy-induced hypertension: effects of intravenous nitroglycerin coupled with blood volume expansion. Am J Obstet Gynecol 154:1053, 1986.
437. Broughton Pipkin F, Turner SR, Symonds EM: Possible risk with captopril in pregnancy: some animal data. Lancet 1:1256, 1980.
438. Duminy PC, Burger PT: Fetal abnormality associated with the use of captopril during pregnancy. S Afr Med J 60:805, 1981.
439. Broude AM: Fetal abnormality associated with captopril during pregnancy. S Afr Med J 61:68, 1982.
440. Guignard JP, Burgener F, Calame A: Persistent anuria in a neonate: a side effect of captopril? Int J Pediatr Nephrol 2:133, 1981.
441. Smith AM: Are ACE inhibitors safe in pregnancy? Lancet 2:750, 1989.
442. Kreft-Jais C, Plouin P-F, Tchobroutsky C, et al: Angiotensin-converting enzyme inhibitors during pregnancy: a survey of 22 patients given captopril and nine given enalapril. Br J Obstet Gynaecol 95:420, 1988.
443. Rothberg AD, Lorenz R: Can captopril cause fetal and neonatal renal failure? Pediatr Pharmacol 4:189, 1984.
444. Rosa FW, Bosco LA, Graham CF, et al: Neonatal anuria with maternal angiotensin-converting enzyme inhibition. Obstet Gynecol 74:371, 1989.
445. Millar JA, Wilson PD, Morrison N: Management of severe hypertension in pregnancy by a combined drug regimen including captopril: case report. Aust N Z Med J 96:796, 1983.
446. Boutroy MJ, Vert P, Hurault de Ligny B, et al: Captopril administration in pregnancy impairs fetal angiotensin converting enzyme activity and neonatal adaptation. Lancet 2:935, 1984.
447. Knott PD, Thorpe SS, Lamont CAR: Congenital renal dysgenesis possibly due to captopril. Lancet 1:451, 1989.
448. Devlin RG, Fleiss PM: Captopril in human blood and breast milk. J Clin Pharmacol 21:110, 1981.
449. Postmarketing surveillance for angiotensin-converting enzyme inhibitor use during the first trimester of pregnancy—United States, Canada, and Israel, 1987–1995. MMWR Morb Mort Wkly Rep 46:240–242, 1997.
450. Holbrook RH Jr: Effects of calcium antagonists during pregnancy. Am J Obstet Gynecol 160:1018, 1989.
451. Gilbert RD: Effects of calcium antagonists during pregnancy. Am J Obstet Gynecol 160:1018, 1989. Reply.
452. Read MD, Wellby DE: The use of calcium antagonist (nifedipine) to suppress preterm labour. Br J Obstet Gynaecol 93:933, 1986.
453. Ehrenkranz RA, Ackerman BA, Hulse JD: Nifedipine transfer into human milk. J Pediatr 114:478, 1989.
454. Lindow SW, Davies N, Davey DA, et al: The effect of sublingual nifedipine on uteroplacental blood flow in hypertensive pregnancy. Br J Obstet Gynaecol 95:1276, 1988.
455. Rubin PC: Beta-blockers in pregnancy. N Engl J Med 305:1323, 1981.
456. Ingemarsson I: Cardiovascular complications of terbutaline for premature labor. Am J Obstet Gynecol 142:117, 1982.
457. Strigal R, Pfeiffer U, Aschenbrenner G, et al: Influence of the β-1 selective blocker, metoprolol, on the development of pulmonary edema in tocolytic therapy. Obstet Gynecol 67:537, 1986.
458. Ross MG, Stubblefield PG, Kitzmiller JL: Intravenous terbutaline and simultaneous β-1 blockage for advanced premature labor. Am J Obstet Gynecol 147:897, 1983.
459. Lip GY, Beevers M, Churchill D, et al: Effect of atenolol on birth weight. Am J Cardiol 79:1436, 1997.
460. Frishman WH, Chesner M: Use of beta-adrenergic blocking agents

in pregnancy. *In* Elkayam U, Gleicher N (eds): Cardiac Problems in Pregnancy. 2nd ed. pp. 351–360. New York: Alan R Liss, 1990.

461. Sonesson SE, Fouron JC, Wesslen-Eriksson E, et al: Foetal supraventricular tachycardia treated with sotalol. Acta Paediatr 87:584–587, 1998.
462. Rashba EJ, Zareba W, Moss AJ, et al: Influence of pregnancy on the risk for cardiac events in patients with hereditary long QT syndrome: LQTS Investigators. Circulation 97:451–456, 1998.
463. Mache CJ, Beitzke A, Haidvogl M Jr, et al: Periinatal manifestations of idiopathic long QT syndrome. Pediatr Cardiol 17:118–121, 1996.
464. Burrow GN, Ferris T: Medical Complications During Pregnancy. 3rd ed. Philadelphia: WB Saunders, 1988.
465. Creasy RK, Resnik R: Maternal-Fetal Medicine: Principles and Practice. 2nd ed. Philadelphia: WB Saunders, 1989.
466. Kammerer WS, Gross RJ: Medical Consultation: The Internist on Surgical, Obstetric, and Psychiatric Services. 2nd ed. Baltimore: Williams & Wilkins, 1990.
467. Ueland K: Cardiovascular disease complicating pregnancy. Clin Obstet Gynecol 21:429, 1978.
468. Cunningham FG, MacDonald PC, Gant NF: Williams' Obstetrics. 18th ed. Norwalk, CT: Appleton & Lange, 1989.

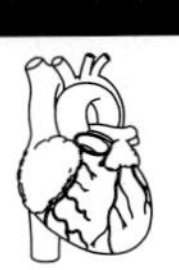

CHAPTER 111

Cardiovascular Changes Associated With Space Flight

Dominick S. D'Aunno

GENERAL EFFECTS
PHYSIOLOGIC ADJUSTMENTS
Fluid Dynamics
Central Venous Pressure Measurements During Simulations
Central Venous Pressure Measurements in Weightlessness
Influence on Myocardial Dynamics
Orthostatic Dysfunction
Alterations in Heart Rate and Blood Pressure
Neurovascular Alteration
Cardiac Conduction
Noninvasive Cardiac Evaluations
Peripheral Vascular Resistance
Cardiac Size
Influence on Organelle Structure and Function
Cardiovascular Recovery
Current Limitations of Cardiovascular Data

The body undergoes many physiologic adaptations in microgravity. Regulatory mechanisms designed to achieve homeostasis at Earth gravity are confronted with an altogether alien environment. Functional and structural alterations are initiated when weightlessness is achieved, unmasking the complexities inherent in maintaining homeostasis on Earth. Once the influence of gravity is lifted, multiple interdependent changes in numerous regulatory systems are observed as new set-points are established.

General Effects

During space flight, astronauts typically demonstrate an increase in height and a tendency to assume the fetal position while at rest.[1] It is thought that the changes in elastic forces in body tissues may be accompanied by changes at the cellular level. Presumably, some of the endocrine and metabolic alterations seen in flight are related to the mechanical effects of weightlessness.[1]

The role of the vestibular system as a gravity receptor is well documented. In weightlessness, this complex system becomes deranged, and a "sensory conflict" exists between the peripheral and central nervous systems. This becomes a major component of space motion sickness, which has affected up to 85 percent of those who have flown in space.[2]

There have been mild disturbances in the sleep patterns of astronauts while in orbit.[3] These usually subside after a few weeks in flight. Of interest is the increase in the rapid eye movement stage of sleep noted early in flight during sleep studies performed on Skylab. This may reflect learning processes as the astronauts begin to adapt to their new environment.[3]

On the basis of information obtained during the Salyut, Mir, and Skylab missions, it is clear that bone and mineral metabolism is substantially affected during exposure to microgravity. Calcium balance becomes increasingly negative throughout the flight, and bone mineral content declines. There is concern regarding the detrimental effects of hypercalcemia, the risk of kidney stone formation resulting from hypercalciuria, the possible effects from calcification of soft tissues, and the increase in fracture potential. Recovery of bone mass may take many months of exposure to normal gravity. There is speculation that an irreversible amount of bone loss will occur at some point, if the duration of exposure to weightlessness is prolonged.[4]

A decrease in red cell mass is associated with space flight, and this may be the result of a transient increase in red cell destruction by the spleen, along with a failure of red cell production to compensate for the losses. Erythropoietin levels become depressed during space flight, but the exact mechanism and the effect on hematopoiesis are still largely unknown.[4] Losses in red cell and hemoglobin mass might also result from a negative-feedback mechanism triggered by the decrease in plasma volume.[5] Simultaneous reduction of plasma volume and red cell mass would result in an almost constant red cell count per unit volume, along with a stable in-flight hematocrit and hemoglobin.[4]

Impairment of the immune system, with a decrease in number and function of T lymphocytes, has been observed during space flight. Decreased cell-mediated immune function has also been noted during space flight; this effect lingers a few weeks after flight before returning to preflight values.[4]

Alterations can also be appreciated at the cellular and nuclear levels. Without a gravitational stimulus, production of the slow-twitch isoform of myosin is down-regulated in muscle fibers.[6] Experiments on cells in cultures studied under microgravity reveal that cell membranes are more susceptible to damage from mechanical stress than in identical conditions under normal Earth gravity (Daniel Feeback, Ph.D., personal communication, 1999).

These highlight a few of the many physiologic changes associated with exposure to weightlessness. The process of adaptation and the precise stimuli that trigger these responses to space flight are still poorly characterized.

PHYSIOLOGIC ADJUSTMENTS

In weightlessness, physiologic systems do not change in isolation. It is the interaction of their modifications and the shifts they impose on each other that provide us the opportunity to obtain new insights and develop a more comprehensive understanding of fundamental homeostatic physiology as a new bodily equilibrium is achieved. This chapter identifies the changes observed in the cardiovascular system as astronauts enter into orbit around Earth (Fig. 111–1).

Human beings spend a great deal of their waking hours in an upright position. To maintain this posture, an efficient system of reflex circulatory mechanisms has evolved to compensate for the hydrostatic pressure generated by gravity. This pressure serves as a stimulus to the autonomic nervous and endocrine systems, which exert control over the cardiovascular system to effect adequate distribution of cardiac output despite positional changes.

Cosmonauts and astronauts have provided anecdotal reports that the onset of weightlessness is accompanied by the feeling of "blood rushing to the head."[7, 8] Subjective sensations of nasal stuffiness and head fullness have also been noted.[9] Photographic evidence clearly demonstrates periorbital puffiness, facial edema, and thickening of the eyelids.[8] Concurrently, the jugular veins and the veins in the temple, scalp, and forehead appear full and distended.[8] The lack of gravity allows the uplifting of the skin on the face, resulting in a fuller appearance. However, fluid shifts play a significant role in these phenomena, especially in regard to venous distention.[10]

Fluid Dynamics

In microgravity, the hydrostatic pressure on the blood columns is lost, and there is a rapid cephalad redistribution of intravascular and extravascular fluids. The alterations in mean intravascular pressure are striking when an astronaut changes from a vertical position on Earth to a weightless posture. Differences from 180 to 90 mm Hg occur on the arterial side of the feet and from 100 to 15 mm Hg on the venous side.[11] The first sequela of such a dramatic change in pressures is redistribution of the intravascular and extravascular fluids. Whereas movement of fluids out of the lower extremities is a transient occurrence in response to postural changes on Earth, in weightlessness this effectively amounts to a permanent displacement.

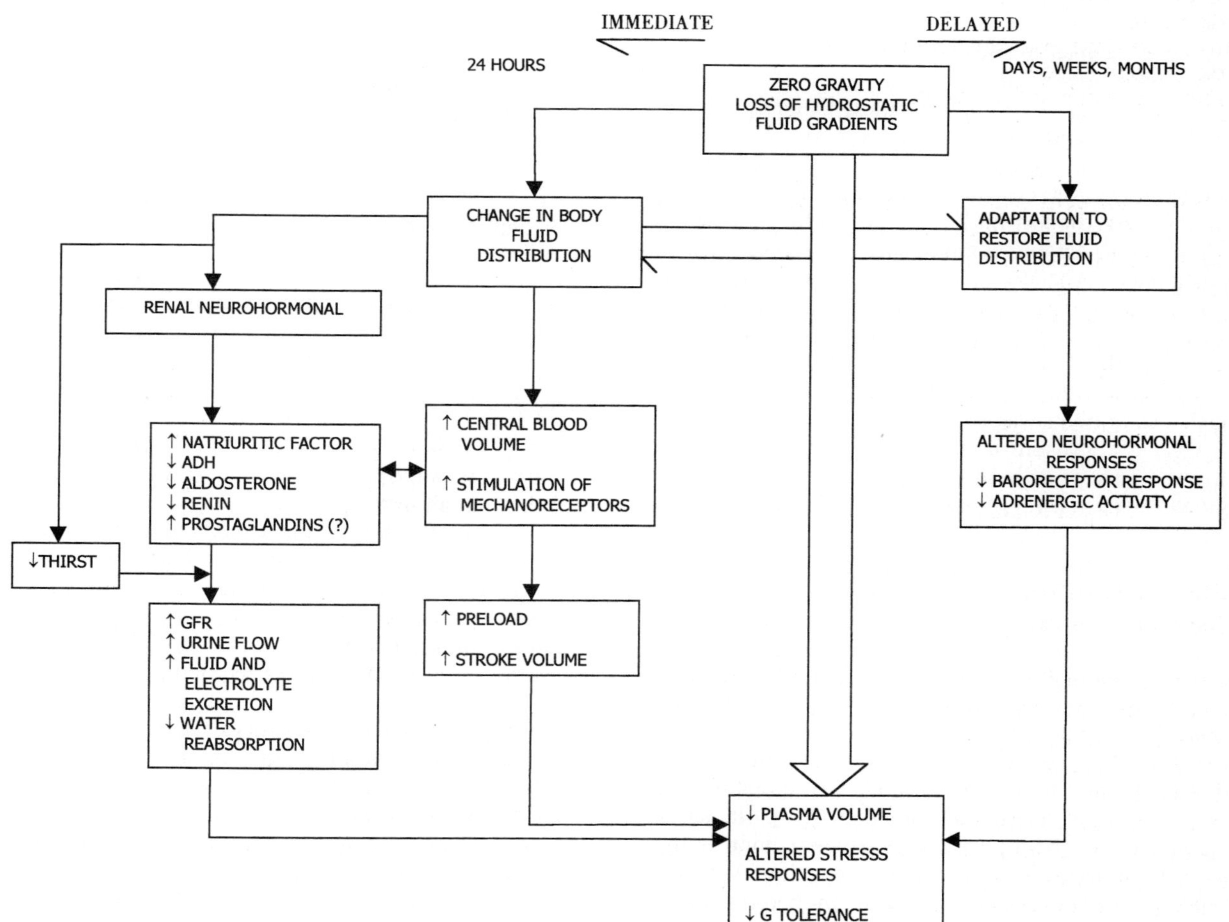

FIGURE 111–1 Suggested cardiovascular response to weightlessness. ADH, antidiuretic hormone; GFR, glomerular filtration rate.

Bed rest studies have investigated fluid shifts with changes in hydrostatic pressures. However, given equal time frames, the volume of fluid shifted from the lower extremities in Earth-normal gravity is much less than that observed in weightlessness.[12] An obvious difference between the horizontal position during a bed rest study on Earth and weightlessness is that some degree of pressure from the abdominal contents is generated by their weight and is relayed to the inferior vena cava. This raises the venous pressure in the lower extremities. In view of the Starling forces, this venous pressure counteracts the tendency for the extravascular fluid to enter the intravascular space. With the advent of weightlessness and the resultant loss of this Starling force, greater volumes of both intravascular and extravascular fluid have the potential for translocation.[13] This may explain, in part, why such larger volumes of fluids are shifted during space flight.[11]

It has been estimated that approximately 1.5 to 2 L of fluid from the lower extremities and an unclear volume from the pelvic region are involved in the redistribution.[14, 15] It is hypothesized that this fluid equilibration serves as a major stimulus for many of the early adaptive changes of the cardiovascular system observed in space flight.[7, 12] As a consequence of the cephalad redistribution of fluid, there is a relative increase in the central intravascular volume. It was once theorized that the acute increase in central volume was accompanied by a concomitant increase in central venous pressure (CVP), and it was this event that initiated acute cardiovascular responses based on reflex adjustments of blood volume. Up until the early 1990s, this paradigm was a widely accepted model and served as the foundation for further investigation and analysis.

The intravascular fluid redistribution is interpreted by the atrial, aortic, and carotid baroreceptors as a volume overload state. The usual compensatory mechanisms are initiated to reduce the central volume toward the set-point appropriate for the normal cardiovascular system on Earth.[16] Although diuresis is usually not observed,[17] a negative water balance occurs as the result of decreased fluid intake and evaporation through the pulmonary system and across the skin (the atmosphere aboard the spacecraft is dry, so insensible water loss may be significant).[18] Studies conducted on shuttle flights STS-61C and STS-26 concluded that total body water decreases by 3.4 percent after 1 to 2 days of exposure to microgravity.[19] Consequently, after a few hours or days, the astronaut reaches a state of appropriate hydration for a weightless environment.

Central Venous Pressure Measurements During Simulations

Ground-based simulations of the physiologic changes similar to those experienced during space flight are bed rest and water immersion studies. Utilizing a 5-degree head-down tilt, bed rest studies have revealed a significant increase in CVP after 30 minutes. The CVP returned to near-normal levels after 90 minutes of head-down tilt.[12] Data from thermoneutral bath immersion studies demonstrate a notable central fluid shift. Initial changes in CVP were similar to those observed during head-down bed rest investigations.[20–22] These data implied an increase in CVP resulting from acute fluid redistribution and led to studies of acute volume and intravascular pressure changes in simulated weightlessness onboard the KC-135 aircraft. The KC-135 performs multiple parabolic flight maneuvers, much like the up and down runs of a roller coaster. These provide 20 to 30 seconds of "weightlessness" followed by periods of up to 2 gravities. It was concluded that the disappearance of hydrostatic gradients during acute weightlessness results in a significant increase in CVP only in subjects who were in the upright position. Subjects who were initially placed in the supine or launch position (lying flat with the legs elevated) demonstrated a paradoxical decrease in CVP with the onset of acute weightlessness.[23] These findings cast doubt on the bed rest study–derived hypothesis that microgravity-induced fluid redistribution results in an increased CVP, which initiates acute cardiovascular adjustments to space flight.[24]

Central Venous Pressure Measurements in Weightlessness

CVP measurements were obtained on two shuttle missions dedicated to space and life sciences. Venous blood pressures of several crew members were obtained with a 19-gauge needle placed in the antecubital vein during flight at 22 hours after launch and on mission days 2 and 7. These values were compared with preflight measurements taken from the same individuals. Despite the physical appearance of a cephalad fluid shift, the venous pressures were at or below preflight supine values.[25] These results directly contradicted the higher CVP values predicted by bed rest studies and upright KC-135 flights. When it is noted that measurements were taken nearly a full day after launch, it is conceivable that adaptation had already taken place. Therefore, the experiment was repeated on a second space flight nearly 2 years later.[26] This time, venous pressures were measured as early as 20 minutes after launch. The results confirmed that the astronauts' in-flight venous pressures were never greater than preflight values. In addition, indirect CVP estimations carried out on shuttle flights in 1986, 1989, and 1990 also showed that at no time during the flight did CVP pressure increase above preflight levels.[18, 27, 28]

The paradoxical observations of a decreased CVP with increased left ventricular (LV) end-diastolic diameter and stroke volume, measured by in-flight echocardiography, have not been explained conclusively. One proposed mechanism to support this observation is that in weightlessness there is an increase in the diastolic compliance of the ventricular myocardium, which results in greater filling at a reduced filling pressure.[29]

Another explanation has focused on the pure biomechanical changes in fluid and body structure dynamics observed in weightlessness. Measurements of intraesophageal pressure changes, CVP changes, and intra-abdominal pressure changes in human subjects flown in parabolic flights onboard the KC-135 aircraft have been performed. These studies have revealed that with acute weightlessness the influence of gravity on the chest wall and intra-abdominal tissues is eliminated and the chest wall expands, resulting in decreased intrathoracic pressure.[30] This would increase cardiac transmural pressure and promote increased cardiac filling at a lower CVP.[23]

In summary, a transient increase in CVP, which was previously believed to serve as a stimulus to the acute cardiovascular adaptations to weightlessness, has not been observed in space flight or during preflight activities. Quite unexpectedly, CVP values were below preflight supine values. Altered fluid dynamics, elimination of gravity-induced hydrostatic pressure, and decreased intrathoracic pressure may explain why an increase in central volume does not result in an increase in CVP in weightlessness.

Influence on Myocardial Dynamics

Cardiac adaptation to microgravity exposure is a complex and poorly understood process. During weightlessness, immediate fluid equilibration results in a relative central volume overload. It has been hypothesized that a subsequent increase in ventricular volume may cause heart failure.[31] Cardiovascular function might also be affected if the myocardium itself deconditions or partially atrophies in a weightless environment. The absence of gravitational force decreases the amount of muscular work performed. The demands on the cardiovascular system are further diminished because there is no hydrostatic gradient to be overcome to effect venous return. As a consequence of muscle atrophy and decreased skeletal muscular activity, baseline cardiac work is reduced. These factors operate to decrease the demands on the cardiovascular system, and therefore on the myocardium itself. As a result, myocardial tissue may in fact decondition because of diminished utilization demands. However, no significant indications of this have been found in astronauts or cosmonauts at rest in space. Echocardiography has determined that circumferential fiber velocity is unchanged and that no significant alterations occur in myocardial mass index or LV wall thickness.[32] Soviet assessment of echocardiographic data likewise supports the finding that there is no significant derangement in contractile parameters.[33] During an 8-month Salyut flight, at rest contractility was shown to be equivalent to preflight levels, and the LV filling to stroke volume ratio, an indicator of contractile function, was constant, suggesting no deterioration in contractility at rest.[34] Therefore, there is strong evidence to support the contention that the myocardium and its ability to contract effectively is not compromised with exposure to weightlessness.

Contractile function during periods of physical stress has also been evaluated in flight.[34] During bouts of exercise on a cycle ergometer, a deficiency in systolic reserves was noted with a subsequent decrease in venous return that was manifest by limited stroke volume and thus cardiac output.[34] To meet the increased cardiac demands associated with intense exercise, the body normally depends on variations in LV capacity, such as diminished end-systolic volume and increased stroke volume. During exercise periods, the cosmonauts were unable to achieve an exercise-induced increase in stroke volume. Heart rate increases were noted but did not reach the levels established during preflight exercise sessions. The overall result suggests an inability to achieve normal cardiac outputs under physical stress, supporting the idea that there is "a deviation of optimal myocardial pump function control."[34] It has been suggested that this dysfunction is not a result of poor LV contractility but rather is caused by hemodynamic resetting and neurovascular alterations, which limit cardiovascular adaptability to exercise. Data collected from missions to date have revealed no significant impairment in mission-oriented cardiovascular performance.[35] However, functional cardiovascular abnormalities have consistently been demonstrated in astronauts during the immediate postflight period,[12] even in missions of only 8 hours' duration.[36] The capacity to perform heavy dynamic leg exercises, viewed as an index of the functional capacity of the cardiovascular system, appears to be preserved in space but is reduced in the upright position post flight.[35] This suggests that the postflight impairment of cardiovascular function is the result of an appropriate adaptation to the altered fluid distribution in microgravity, suddenly rendered inappropriate by return to normal gravity. When an individual returns to the gravity of Earth's surface, reduced plasma volume and neurovascular alterations provide less protection against orthostatic stress.[18] Documented evidence of syncope in astronauts during postflight medical examinations exists.[37] Methods used to quantify orthostatic tolerance include the passive stand test, tilt table testing, and lower-body negative pressure (LBNP).

Orthostatic Dysfunction

Virtually every astronaut displays some degree of orthostatic dysfunction after space flight. The degree of dysfunction on landing day varies significantly among astronauts. Cardiovascular data obtained from astronauts who have flown on missions of short duration (≤16 days) reveal that approximately 75 percent of astronauts demonstrate clinically insignificant, minimal orthostatic dysfunction post flight, whereas 25 percent of postflight astronauts experience presyncopal symptoms when subjected to an upright posture.[38] The subgroup of astronauts who are susceptible to post–space flight orthostatic hypotension exhibits signs and symptoms when orthostatically challenged that are similar to signs and symptoms seen in patients on Earth with orthostatic intolerance caused by autonomic dysfunction.

A landing day presyncopal incident is presented in Figure 111–2. Arterial pressure and heart rate responses during tilt table testing in a patient with adrenergic failure are compared with responses during stand tests performed on a susceptible astronaut before and after space flight. In the top panel, the patient with adrenergic failure had a precipitous fall in both systolic and diastolic pressures during upright tilt. The patient became presyncopal within 2 minutes of tilt testing. In the second panel, the astronaut, who later became presyncopal on landing day, demonstrated normal orthostatic tolerance to upright posture before flight. After space flight, this same astronaut subject became presyncopal with upright posture just after 3 minutes. The adrenergic failure and the postflight astronaut panels bear a striking resemblance. This astronaut had a normal increase in plasma norepinephrine with standing before flight but had no measurable increase in plasma norepinephrine with standing on landing day. All astronauts who became

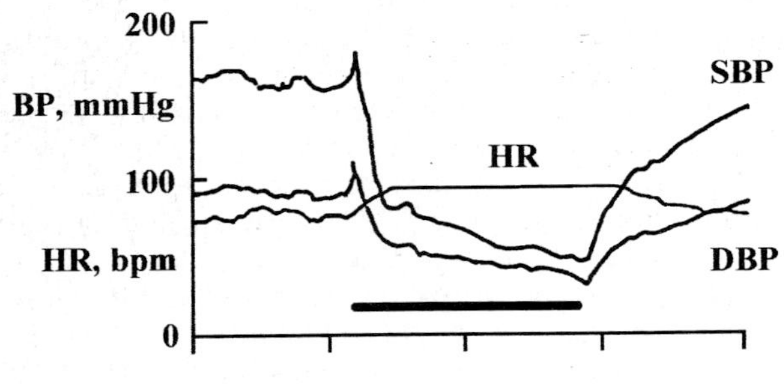

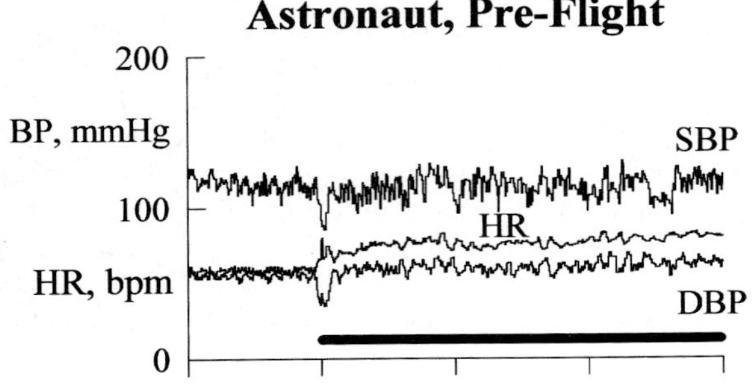

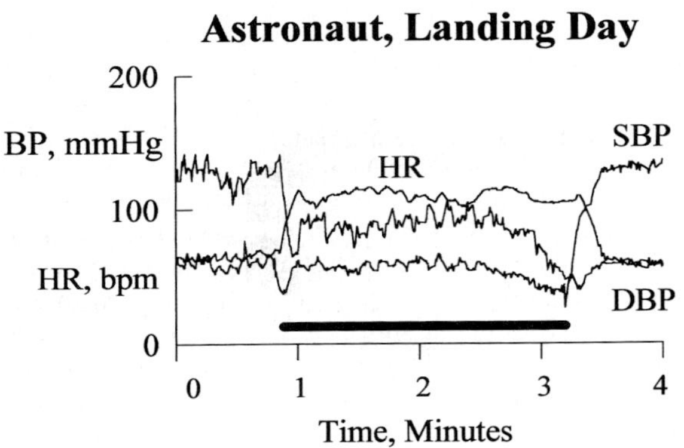

FIGURE 111–2 Original records of beat-to-beat systolic (SBP) and diastolic (DBP) blood pressures (BP) and heart rate (HR) during a tilt test performed on a patient with adrenergic failure **(top)**, a preflight stand test performed on an astronaut **(middle)**, and a stand test performed on the astronaut 2 h after landing **(bottom)**. bpm, beats/min; *horizontal bars,* time in upright posture. (From Fritsch-Yelle JM, Whitson PA, Bondar RL, et al: Subnormal norepinephrine release relates to presyncope in astronauts after spaceflight. J Appl Physiol 81: 2134, 1996.)

presyncopal immediately after flight demonstrated similar patterns of arterial pressure and plasma norepinephrine on landing day. Within 3 days of landing, all of the cardiovascular parameters of the presyncopal astronaut group had returned to preflight status. The space flight–induced autonomic dysfunction in the susceptible astronaut group had resolved spontaneously.[38]

Subnormal increases in plasma norepinephrine with upright posture indicate a functional change in the neurogenic feedback loop, which includes arterial baroreceptors, brain stem, spinal tracts, and sympathetic nerves. Normal supine, but subnormal standing, plasma norepinephrine levels, as observed in the susceptible astronaut group, are also seen in patients with impaired modulation of baroreceptor input.[39] It is suggested that cardiovascular adaptations to microgravity include changes in central modulation of baroreceptor inputs that cause a hypoadrenergic response to orthostatic stress, resulting in presyncope in 25 percent of astronauts returning from space.

A gender-related differential susceptibility to post–space flight orthostatic hypotension has also been described.[38] Of the 25 percent of astronauts that become presyncopal after space flight, 80 percent are female. Many male-female differences in cardiovascular responses have been shown to be estrogen or related, mediated through endothelium-dependent nitric oxide.[40–42] The vasodilatory effects of estrogen may contribute to altered vasoconstrictive responsiveness in women compared with men during orthostatic stress. If women compensate with greater heart rate responses, it may leave them more susceptible than men to orthostatic hypotension in situations in which autonomic function is compromised, for example, after space flight.

Measurements of Orthostatic Tolerance During Space Flight

LBNP is a useful means of assessing orthostatic tolerance because, unlike passive methods, such as tilt table testing and simple stand tests, LBNP can be used in microgravity (Fig. 111–3). Different levels of negative pressure can be applied to the lower portions of the body, resulting in footward displacement of fluids.[43] LBNP can be used to simulate the body's response to exposure to normal gravity while in space and to gauge the degree of cardiovascular deconditioning during space flight and ground-based simulations of weightlessness, such as head-down tilt. LBNP has also been utilized, with a degree of success, as a countermeasure to cardiovascular deconditioning during prolonged bed rest.[44]

LBNP studies have revealed that individuals exposed to bed rest experience cardiovascular deconditioning. This correlates with similar deconditioning noted during space flight. Resting heart rates and orthostatically stressed heart rates (with LBNP) were significantly elevated after just 3 days in flight onboard Skylab.[45] Cardiovascular responses to LBNP continued to show increasing instability, especially during the first 3 weeks of space flight. Evaluation of hemodynamic variables taken during LBNP demonstrates a limited stroke volume response but an enhanced heart rate and cardiac output response.[34] These observations may be a compensatory effort directed toward the maintenance of cerebral perfusion during a state of diminished vascular tone rather than a sequela of a dysfunctional myocardial state.[34] These findings, along with corresponding Soviet data,[46] indicate that in-flight LBNP presents greater stress to the cardiovascular system than the same levels of LBNP before flight. This was attributed to adaptation of the cardiovascular system to the cephalad fluid shift early in flight. An inverse relationship exists between changes in orthostatically stressed heart rates before flight versus after flight, and corresponding changes in blood volume.[37]

Loss of fluid volume is believed to be one of many factors contributing to postflight and in-flight orthostatic intolerance. This has led to a simple countermeasure protocol that helps to protect some crewmembers during reentry

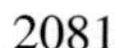

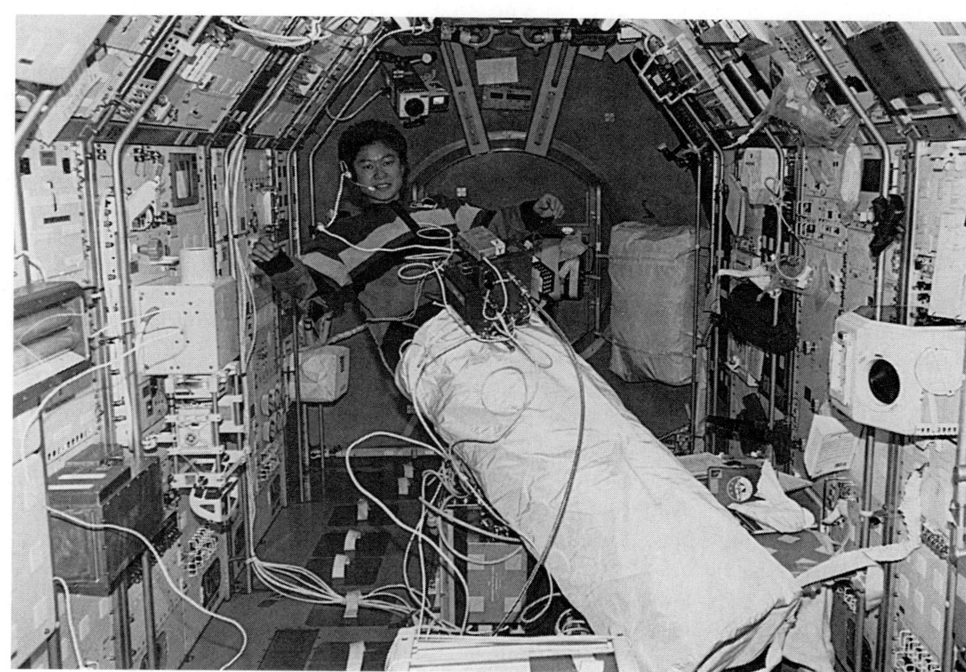

FIGURE 111–3 Astronaut Chiaki Mukai undergoing in-flight lower body negative pressure (LBNP). (From National Aeronautics and Space Administration.)

and immediately after flight to a certain degree. All shuttle astronauts ingest 32 ounces of water or juice and eight 1-g sodium chloride tablets 2 hours before reentry. This produces approximately 1 L of isotonic saline in the stomach. When the use of oral rehydration before reentry is compared with that in astronauts not utilizing the countermeasure, it is evident that saline loading affords a blunted blood pressure and heart rate response to the passive stand test. Before flight, the heart rate in both groups increased on standing from about 55 beats/min to roughly 70 beats/min. After flight, those who did not use the countermeasure showed a significant increase in the resting heart rate to 75 beats/min and a standing heart rate of 110 beats/min.[47] Those who made use of the saline loading countermeasure showed a slight, but not statistically significant, increase in standing heart rate compared with preflight values. A comparison of postflight responses with and without the countermeasure shows that saline loading is associated with a decrease in both resting and stressed heart rates after flight. In addition, mean blood pressure measurements revealed that in those who underwent oral rehydration, there was an increase in mean blood pressure measurements of 2 mm Hg on assumption of the upright position. Bed rest studies have also revealed the usefulness of oral rehydration in providing a minor degree of protection against the loss of tolerance to LBNP by expanding the intravascular volume.[48] Because this protocol seems to be at least partially effective in restoring the preflight cardiovascular state, it has been incorporated into the space shuttle program since 1984.[18]

The effectiveness of the oral rehydration countermeasure varies with flight duration. The cardiovascular index of deconditioning, defined as the change in heart rate minus the change in systolic blood pressure plus the change in diastolic blood pressure,[49] reflects the effectiveness of the countermeasure.[47] For the shortest shuttle flights, there was minimal deconditioning, as measured by the cardiovascular index of deconditioning, in crew members who used the fluid loading countermeasure. However, as flight duration increased, the effectiveness of the countermeasure decreased until, after flights of 4 to 10 days, this index showed no differences between users and nonusers of the fluid loading countermeasure.[18] The degree of orthostatic intolerance is out of proportion to the degree of relative hypovolemia.[50] This has also been noted in prolonged bed rest studies utilizing the oral rehydration protocol and LBNP to assess cardiovascular deconditioning.[12] After simulated weightlessness by head-down bed rest, the correlation between orthostatic hypotension and reduced plasma volume is not compelling,[51] and acute replacement of the lost plasma volume with intravenous saline infusions does not prevent the occurrence of orthostatic dysfunction.[52] Therefore, it appears that the saline loading countermeasure replaces plasma volume, which seems to be a major determinant of orthostatic tolerance only in space flights restricted to short duration. As the time frame of space flight is extended, other cardiovascular and neurologic changes develop that combine with decreased plasma volume, which results in post–space flight orthostatic intolerance.

Alterations in Heart Rate and Blood Pressure

Before flight, when an astronaut goes from supine to standing, the typical increase in heart rate is from about 57 beats/min to roughly 70 beats/min. The heart rate begins to level off about 2 or 3 minutes after the initial increase that follows standing. After flight, a significant rise in the resting heart rate exists, and, in contrast to preflight heart rates, the pulse continues to increase for the duration of the stand test.[18] Mean blood pressure measurements during the stand test are as follows. The preflight response to assuming the upright position is a 6- to 10-mm Hg rise in the mean blood pressure. After flight, the mean blood pressure decreases by 7 mm Hg on assumption of the standing position.[47]

In-flight measurements of heart rate and blood pressure have been performed by use of a modified Holter monitor and automated blood pressure device (Fig. 111–4). In-flight heart rate and diastolic pressures were significantly decreased compared with preflight values. The variability of heart rate and diastolic pressure was also significantly reduced in flight. It has been suggested that these findings may represent in-flight decreases in sympathetic activity and decreased peripheral resistance.[53]

Neurovascular Alteration

Baroreflex Responses

Many studies have investigated autonomic cardiovascular regulation during ground-based simulations and after space flight. Dysregulation of autonomic function is believed to be a major factor in post–space flight orthostatic dysfunction.[50] It is well known that baroreceptors are important in mediating abrupt hemodynamic adjustments to arterial pressure changes.[50] Arterial (carotid) baroreceptor responses have been studied by use of a neck chamber apparatus that can deliver positive or negative pressures to the receptor sites.[54, 55] This device has been used to test the hypothesis that exposure to weightlessness, or simulated weightlessness with bed rest, impairs autonomic regulation of cardiovascular control.[51, 56] Baroreflex impairment develops within 10 days of bed rest and persists for a short time after termination of the test.

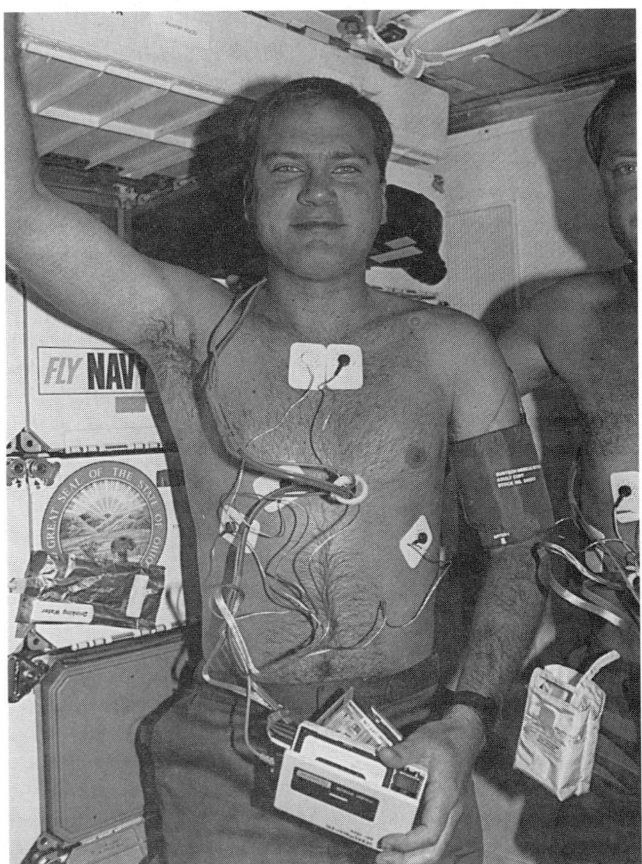

FIGURE 111–4 Astronaut Rick Hiebe wears a modified in-flight Holter monitor and automated blood pressure monitoring device. (From National Aeronautics and Space Administration.)

After space flight, reductions in carotid baroreceptor–cardiac reflex responsiveness were found that significantly correlated with postflight orthostatic intolerance.[57, 58] The following baroreflex parameters were all found to be decreased on landing day: (1) average slopes of R-R intervals to carotid distending pressures, (2) ranges of R-R intervals to carotid distending pressures, and (3) minimal and maximal R-R intervals. These abnormalities persisted 2 days after landing. The operational point, defined as [(R-R intervals at 0 mm Hg neck pressure − minimal R-R intervals)/R-R interval range] × (100 percent), is a measure of the amount of buffering capacity above (hypertensive stimulus) and below (hypotensive stimulus) baseline systolic pressure. Operational points were also found to be significantly reduced on landing day but returned to normal by day 2 after landing.[58]

Valsalva Responses

Postflight changes in arterial pressure and heart rate responses during Valsalva maneuvers have also been studied as an indicator of space flight–induced alterations of autonomic function.[58] Neither systolic nor diastolic pressure increases during phase I were changed after flight. During early phase II, systolic and diastolic pressure reductions were greater immediately after flight and returned to normal by day 3 after landing. Recovery of systolic and diastolic pressure during late phase II were also greater on landing day. Three days after landing, these values were normal. Systolic and diastolic pressure increases between phase III and phase IV were both greater on landing day but not 3 days later. Phase IV systolic and diastolic pressure overshoots were greater on landing day. These had also returned to baseline values 3 days after landing. The ratios of change in R-R intervals to change in systolic pressures were found to be decreased on landing day during the phase II pressure fall and the phase III to phase IV pressure rise. These results suggest a space flight–induced decrease in vagal efferent responsiveness and an increased baroreflex-mediated sympathoexcitation.[58]

The mechanisms underlying the changes in autonomic function are unknown. It is speculated that these alterations may be due to neural plasticity.[59] The term *plasticity* encompasses processes whereby neural mechanisms adapt to environmental changes. The environment of space is unlike that found on Earth, and the autonomic sensory input profiles of astronauts are most likely different under conditions of microgravity. Changes in arterial and venous pressures probably alter arterial and cardiovascular baroreceptor input. In addition, the normal gradient between carotid and aortic pressures in the upright position is no longer present in space. It is conceivable that altered neural inputs from receptors that sense cardiovascular dimensions during exposure to microgravity modify baroreflex mechanisms.[50] Decreased stimulation of receptors may diminish or "blunt" the response curve. It is speculated that up-regulation of adrenergic receptors may take place.[58]

Power Spectral Density Analysis

Arterial pressure is monitored on a beat-by-beat basis by arterial baroreceptors. Continual baroreceptor inputs are modulated by the central nervous system, and appropriate neurohumoral responses are elicited. This constant modulation results in predictable patterns of arterial pressure and heart rate variability that have been well described by spectral analysis techniques, which decompose the heart rate or arterial pressure signals into separate component frequencies. In humans, the major frequencies of interest are the low frequency (0.1 Hz) and the respiratory frequency (0.2 to 0.3 Hz). The low frequency is believed to be modulated by both sympathetic and parasympathetic influences, and the respiratory frequency is thought to be modulated primarily by parasympathetic influences. The total power and the relative power in the different frequencies are used to noninvasively describe autonomic control of heart rate and arterial pressure.

Power spectral density analyses of R-R intervals during supine rest before and after space flight have demonstrated that total power was increased after flight. R-R spectral power in the high-frequency (respiratory) range was not affected by space flight. However, an increase in the R-R spectral power of the low-frequency band was observed after flight. Increases of the ratio of low- to high-frequency R-R interval power was also observed after flight and for 2 days after landing. It has been suggested that this may reflect increased sympathetic-cardiac nerve traffic.[58] The increased levels of circulating norepinephrine found on landing day support this view.[58]

When astronauts return to Earth, standing presents the space flight–adapted central nervous system with autonomic input profiles not present in space, and the altered autonomic response patterns are inappropriate. There are significant alterations in autonomic regulation of cardiovascular function after flight that require up to 2 days to recover. These changes, along with a decreased plasma volume, conspire to decrease orthostatic tolerance in astronauts immediately after flight.

Cardiac Conduction

At the dawn of manned space exploration, there was great concern that weightlessness might induce alterations in the cardiac conduction system. Cardiac dysrhythmias have been noted throughout the United States and Soviet space flight experience.[37] Electrocardiography has been extensively used to study the bioelectric activity of the heart in weightlessness. Minor variations, such as enhanced sinus arrhythmias, minor axis deviations, isolated ectopic beats, and T wave depressions, were noted during the Salyut 6 mission.[33] During the Gemini and the Apollo eras, occasional premature ventricular contractions (PVCs) were seen.[10, 60] During lunar activities, astronauts experienced PVCs, isolated premature atrial contractions, and nonsustained atrial bigeminy. At the time, these arrhythmias were attributed to possible hypokalemia.[61] During the Skylab series, all crewmembers exhibited some form of rhythm disturbance. For most, these were rare PVCs. However, one crew member displayed a five-beat run of ventricular tachycardia during an LBNP testing protocol. Another crew member had periods of wandering supraventricular pacemaker during rest and after exercise. These levels of dysrhythmia were greater while the astronauts were engaged in space flight than during extensive testing on Earth.[62] Data from the shuttle era have revealed evidence of ectopy. While performing an extravehicular activity, one astronaut experienced an episode of sustained ventricular bigeminy. Another crewmember, who showed no prior evidence of any dysrhythmias, demonstrated sustained atrial quadrigeminy during extravehicular activity.[37] Enhanced ventricular ectopy has been documented during reentry of the shuttle.[49] A crew member with a history of occasional PVCs before flight had an eightfold increase in such occurrences at reentry.[49]

The potential for serious cardiac rhythm disturbances is of great concern, and formal studies utilizing 24-hour Holter monitors have been performed to characterize in-flight cardiac conduction abnormalities. One study failed to document an increase in cardiac rhythm disturbances during short-duration shuttle missions (< 14 days)[63] Likewise, a report of cosmonauts onboard the Mir station did not reveal an increase in cardiac arrhythmias for space missions lasting up to 8 months.[64] However, there have been anecdotal reports from the Mir station of serious cardiac dysrhythmias that have adversely affected mission objectives, requiring in-flight activity changes and early termination of missions.[65] A nonsustained, 14-beat run of ventricular tachycardia was reported from routine Holter recordings performed during space flight (Fig. 111–5). This individual had no known history of cardiovascular disease and was asymptomatic.[65]

The mechanism of this episode of ventricular tachycardia is not known. The data appear more consistent with triggered activity initiated by a delayed after-depolarization, or perhaps with increased automaticity rather than reentry. No evidence of ischemia or QT prolongation was noted. Factors that could have initiated such an event might include electrolyte abnormalities, alterations in autonomic function, and perturbations associated with changes in ventricular mass or volume.[65]

The degree to which microgravity and its many variables can be considered arrhythmogenic is not clear. Although nonsustained episodes of ventricular tachycardia, PVCs, and supraventricular ectopy may be seen in normal individuals and have no prognostic importance, this problem warrants further investigation, considering that many fluctuating conditions involved with space flight, such as gravitational loads, electrolyte abnormalities, thermal stress, catecholamine alterations, and autonomic dysregulation have been shown to be important factors in dysrhythmias on Earth.[37]

Noninvasive Cardiac Evaluations

Echocardiography has been used in the American and Soviet space programs to evaluate the effects of space flight

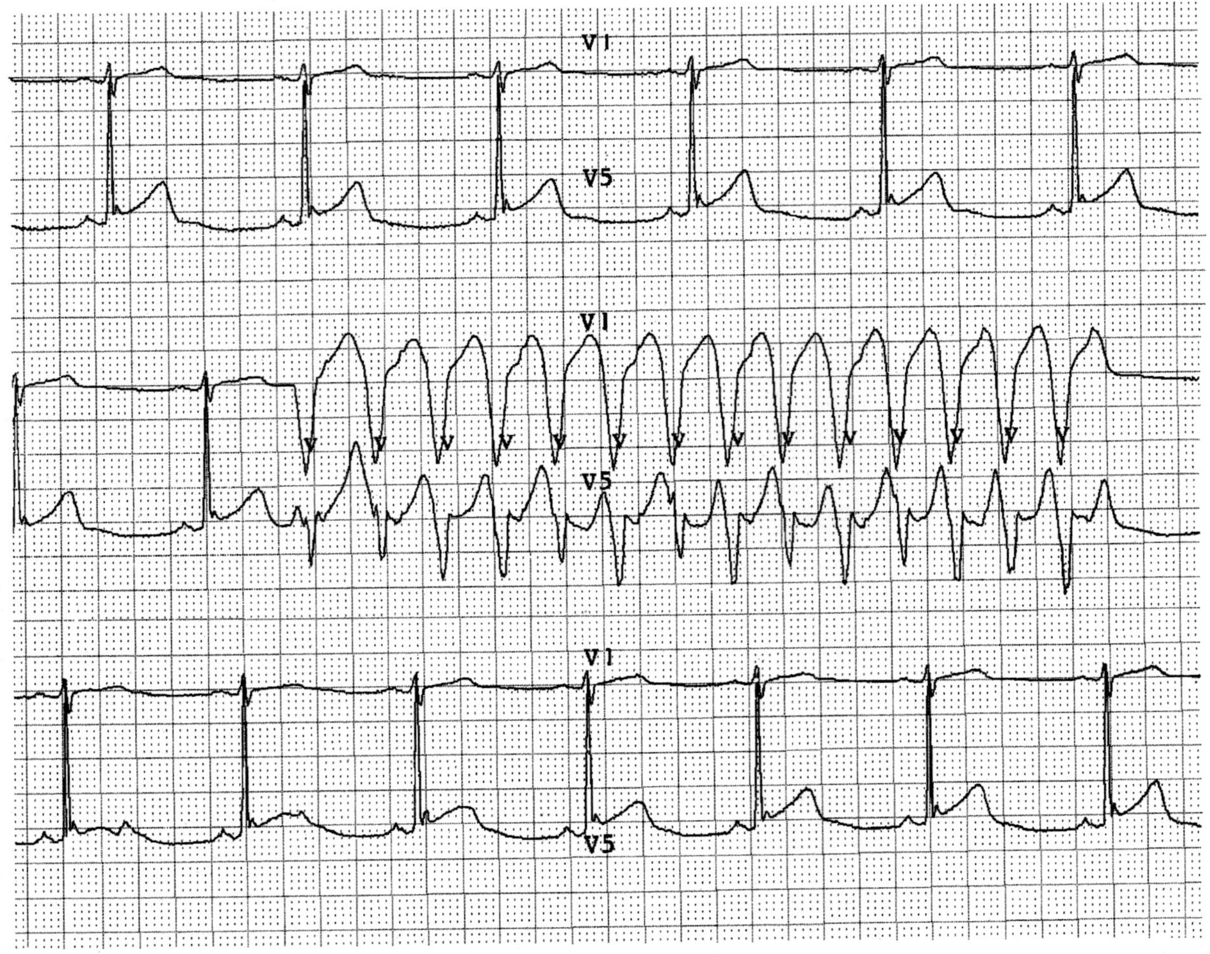

FIGURE 111–5 Nonsustained episode of VT recorded on a two-channel Holter (modified leads V_1 and V_5). The three panels are continuous. Note initiation of event with a late-diastolic premature ventricular complex, as well as electrical alternans during the episode and transient, nonspecific ST-T changes afterward. (Reprinted from American Journal of Cardiology, Vol. 81, Fritsch-Yelle JM, Leuenberger UA, D'Aunno DS, et al, An episode of ventricular tachycardia during long-duration spaceflight, p. 1391, Copyright 1998, with permission from Excerpta Medica Inc.)

on cardiac function (Fig. 111–6).[34, 66, 67] This noninvasive technique has proved reliable and useful for assessing changes in cardiac dimensions, volumes, mass, and performance. Echocardiography has been utilized as an investigative tool to gain insight into the physiologic consequences of weightlessness in several settings, including before, during, and after space flight, as well as during the simulated weightlessness of prolonged bed rest.

On Skylab 4, echocardiograms were obtained before and after flight, during rest, and during LBNP stress, to evaluate LV function. These studies revealed postflight decreases in stroke volume, LV end-diastolic volume, and estimated LV mass. Further analysis concluded that cardiac function and myocardial contractility did not deteriorate, despite decreases in cardiac size and stroke volume.[37] On the Salyut 6 mission, echocardiographic investigations supported these findings.[46] Postflight shuttle data also showed decreases in LV volume index, whereas systolic volume was largely unchanged. The net result was a decrease in stroke volume, but when coupled with the increased heart rate, there was no change in cardiac index.[37] Skylab data revealed an overall decrease in LV mass of 11 percent. The rapid recovery of this mass deficit after flight has led to the hypothesis that this may reflect an alteration in intracellular or interstitial myocardial hydration, yet the precise explanation remains unknown.[68]

On one shuttle mission, two-dimensional M-mode echocardiographic images of the heart were obtained from crew members during their 7-day flight. These data were compared with resting supine values acquired before flight and at selected intervals after flight. Right ventricular dimension was found to be 35 percent lower throughout the period of weightlessness and returned to baseline shortly after flight. LV volume index and LV end-diastolic volume index were 20 percent greater on the first day of flight, and then decreased to 15 percent of preflight values. These changes in ventricular dimensions seem to reflect cephalad fluid shifts noted early in flight. Once a new hemodynamic state is reached, the indices remain below preflight values.[69] Stroke volume closely followed LV end-diastolic volume index measurements. Stroke volume was increased on the first day of weightlessness and decreased to below preflight values for the duration of the mission. After an 85 percent rise in the cardiac index on the first day of flight, values returned to preflight levels for the duration of the mission but were elevated 59 percent during the postflight recovery

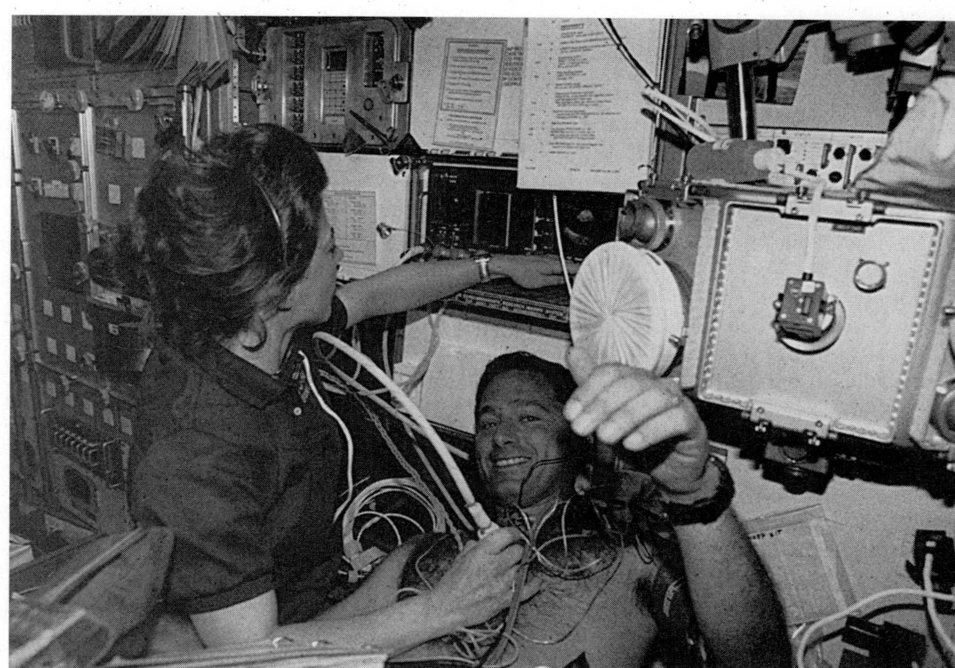

FIGURE 111–6 Astronaut Bonnie Dunbar performs in-flight echocardiography on astronaut Larry DeLucas. (From National Aeronautics and Space Administration.)

period.[69] Recovery to baseline variables from the 7-day flight required a week of reexposure to Earth gravity.[69]

Peripheral Vascular Resistance

During the French-Soviet space flight ARAGATZ onboard the Mir station, echocardiographic investigations revealed that cardiac contractility was not affected by the 25-day mission. At the same time, the total vascular resistance was decreased by 18 percent, which was in agreement with a decrease in local vascular resistance in several areas, such as the brain, kidneys, and lower limbs. On flight day 15, vascular resistance of the brain was 8 percent less than preflight values and decreased to 12 percent by mission day 18. The kidneys, likewise, revealed a decrease in vascular resistance by 10 to 18 percent on flight days 15 and 20. The vascular resistance of the lower extremities showed similar trends. By day 18, resistance was lowered by 8 percent, and this continued to 20 percent less than preflight levels by day 24. Carotid flow was constantly maintained throughout the duration of the flight, whereas cerebral flow was slightly increased as cerebral vascular resistance decreased.[44]

Postflight cardiac output was slightly elevated, along with the heart rate and peripheral blood flow. These variables returned to baseline preflight levels within 7 days. The vascular resistance in cerebral and renal circulations and the total vascular resistance recovered progressively. However, the lower limb vascular resistance showed oscillations during recovery; these were most likely sequelae of vasomotor regulation readaptation associated with extended-duration space flight.[44]

Cardiac Size

The magnitude of variations in LV volume after flight is dependent on preflight LV size and flight duration.[18] Larger heart sizes experienced the greatest decrements, up to 40 percent of their original volumes. Astronauts with smaller heart sizes lost an average of 15 percent. On landing day, both groups demonstrated similar LV end-diastolic volume indexes.[18] In assessing myocardial function, although end-diastolic and stroke volumes were diminished, ejection fraction was not affected.[32, 66] The Soviets have noted an increase in left atrial size after prolonged exposure to weightlessness and attributed these findings to a resetting of the pulmonary hemodynamics secondary to overfilling of the pulmonary vasculature as a result of central fluid shifts.[34]

Influence on Organelle Structure and Function

Abnormalities in mitochondria, sarcoplasmic reticulum, capillaries, and venules of rat myocardium have been observed from Soviet animal experiments after exposure to weightlessness.[31] Decreases in mitochondrial size and myosin adenosine triphosphatase activity in myocardial tissue from rats subjected to microgravity have also been noted. These were directly attributed to underloading of the heart during weightlessness.[70]

Cardiovascular Recovery

Time to recovery of baseline values varies directly with flight duration and indirectly with level of preflight fitness. Soviet data for extended duration flights suggest that return to baseline cardiovascular function is not complete until approximately 4 weeks after flight.[34] Full cardiovascular recovery after flights of shorter duration onboard the shuttle requires approximately 48 hours to 1 week of exposure to normal gravity.[32, 38, 58]

Current Limitations of Cardiovascular Data

Understanding the physiology of the human response to weightlessness optimally requires that the process be observed in its entirety and without outside interference. Knowledge of the mechanisms is paramount to the development of rational and appropriate therapeutic or prophylactic treatments. However, it has been difficult to avoid intervention in studies of the human response to weightlessness because medical personnel are also responsible for ensuring the health, well-being, and optimal performance of those they study. Invariably, this leads to interventions that influence the process of adaptation and inhibit the determination of the mechanisms driving physiologic change.

Other factors also complicate attempts to understand the response to weightlessness and the overall acclimation process in space. To date, a relatively small number of individuals have flown in space. Small sample sizes make it difficult to accurately generalize information obtained from these individuals to a larger population. There have been limited capabilities for scientific biomedical observation owing to operational constraints imposed on most missions. Time is also a limiting factor. More individuals have flown on short-duration missions (<2 weeks), and mission profiles have markedly changed with time and crew complement. As mentioned earlier, prophylactic and therapeutic use of countermeasures, such as those for neurovestibular symptoms, cardiovascular deconditioning, and loss of lean body mass, have obscured some of the effects directly attributable to weightlessness. Despite these limitations, a wealth of biomedical data has been generated that points to definite trends and lends itself to the formation of hypotheses concerning acute responses in zero gravity and subsequent adjustments.[1]

This chapter has examined some of the changes observed in the cardiovascular system when humans are exposed to a weightless environment. Fluid shifts appear to be responsible for acute reflex adjustments, and neurovascular readaptation figures prominently in flights of longer duration. The cardiovascular system seems to adjust quite well to zero gravity after a few weeks, but the response to strenuous exercise appears to be diminished. The major concern for the crewmember is the cardiovascular deconditioning, neurovascular alterations, and orthostatic intolerance experienced on return to gravity.

The arrhythmogenic potential of weightlessness requires further investigation in view of the fact that there is a paucity of information regarding possible mechanisms and predisposing factors. One case of a potentially serious cardiac ventricular arrhythmia has been reported, and numerous accounts of increased ectopy have been described. Although rare, these conduction abnormalities could have serious consequences for the crewmembers and mission objectives.

The possibility of myocardial deconditioning exists. Further analysis must be undertaken to determine the exact mechanisms of change and their relationship to the altered hemodynamics of weightlessness. The role of flight duration as a time-dependent contributor to myocardial and cardiovascular deconditioning must be established. The potential deleterious effects of microgravity on the cardiovascular system and the threat of permanent cardiovascular compromise on return to gravity's domain must also be determined.

The field of space medicine is in its infancy and holds tremendous potential for understanding of the basic physiologic mechanisms of homeostatic regulation. Answers to questions regarding physiologic adaptation hold promise for numerous future therapeutic interventions for disease states on Earth.

References

1. Nicogossian A: Overall physiological response to spaceflight. *In* Nicogossian A, Leach C, Pool S (eds): Space Physiology and Medicine. 2nd ed. p. 150. Philadelphia: Lea & Febiger, 1989.
2. Davis JR, Vanderploeg JM, Santy PA, et al: Space motion sickness during 24 flights of the space shuttle. Aviat Space Environ Med 1988; 59:1185.
3. Parker DE, Reschke MF, Aldrich NG: Performance. *In* Nicogossian A, Leach C, Pool S (eds): Space Physiology and Medicine. 2nd ed. p. 175. Philadelphia: Lea & Febiger, 1989.
4. Leach-Huntoon C, Johnson PC, Cintron NM: Hematology, immunology, endocrinology, and biochemistry. *In* Nicogossion A, Leach C, Pool S (eds): Space Physiology and Medicine. 2nd ed. p. 222. Philadelphia: Lea & Febiger, 1989.
5. Cogli A: Hematological and immunological changes during spaceflight. Acta Astronaut 8:995, 1981.
6. Martin TP, Edgerton VR, Grindland RE: Influence of spaceflight on rat skeletal muscle. J Appl Physiol 65:2318, 1988.
7. Charles J, Bungo M: Cardiovascular physiology in spaceflight. Exp Gerontol 26:163, 1991.
8. Thornton W, Hoffler GW, Rummel JA: Anthropomorphic changes and fluid shifts. *In* Johnson RS, Dietlein LF (eds): Biomedical Results of Skylab. p. 330. Washington, DC: US Government Printing Office, 1977.
9. Gauer OH, Coleman TG, Epstein M, et al: Cardiovascular research. *In* Gauer OH (ed): Life Beyond Earth's Environment: The Biology of Living Organisms in Space. p. 27. Washington, DC: National Academy of Sciences, 1979.
10. Johnson RS, Dietlein LF, Berry CA (eds): Biomedical Results of Apollo, SP-368. Washington, DC: NASA Scientific and Technical Information Office, 1973.
11. Thornton NE, Moore TP, Pool SL: Fluid shifts in weightlessness. Aviat Space Environ Med 58(suppl 9):A86, 1987.
12. Nixon JV, Murray G, Bryant C, et al: Early cardiovascular adaptation to simulated zero gravity. J Appl Physiol 46:541, 1979.
13. Waterfield RL: The effects of posture on the circulating blood volume. J Physiol 72:110, 1931.
14. Moore TP, Thornton WE: Space shuttle flight and postflight fluid shifts measured by leg volume changes. Aviat Space Environ Med 58(suppl 9):A91, 1987.
15. Johnson PC: Fluid volume changes induced by spaceflight. Acta Astronaut 6:1335, 1979.
16. Gauer OH, Henry FP: Neurohormonal control of plasma volume. Int Rev Physiol 9:145, 1976.
17. Leach CS: Fluid control mechanisms in weightlessness. Aviat Space Environ Med 58(suppl 9):A74, 1987.
18. Charles JB, Lathers CM: Cardiovascular adaptation to spaceflight. J Clin Pharmacol 31:1010, 1991.
19. Leach CS, Inners CD, Charles JB: Changes in total body water during spaceflight. J Clin Pharmacol 31:1001, 1991.
20. Aborelius M, Balldin UI, Lilja B, et al: Hemodynamic changes in man during immersion with the head above water. Aerospace Med 43:590, 1972.
21. Begin RM, Epstein M, Sackner MA, et al: Effects of water immersion to the neck on pulmonary circulation and tissue volume in man. J Appl Physiol 40:293, 1976.
22. Echt M, Lange L, Gauer OH: Changes of peripheral venous tone and central transmural venous pressure during immersion in a thermoneutral bath. Pfluegers Arch 352:211, 1974.
23. Pantalos G, Hart S, Mathias J, et al: Central venous, esophageal, and abdominal pressure in humans during parabolic flight. Gravit Space Biol Bull (in press).

24. Norsk P, Foldager N, Bonde-Peterson F, et al: Central venous pressure in humans during short periods of weightlessness. Physiologist 32(suppl 1):S73, 1989.
25. Kirsch KA, Roecker L, Gauer OH, et al: Venous pressures in man during weightlessness. Science 225:218, 1984.
26. Kirsch KA, Haenel F, Roecker L: Venous pressure in microgravity. Naturwissenschafen 73:447, 1986.
27. Sandler H: Things may not be the way they seem. Aviat Space Environ Med 64:247, 1993.
28. Buckey JC, Gaffney FA, Lane LD, et al: Central venous pressure in space. N Engl J Med 328:1853, 1993.
29. Buckey JC, Gaffney FA, Lane LD, et al: Central venous pressure in space. J Appl Physiol 81:19, 1996.
30. Pantalos GM, Sharp MK, Woodruff SJ, et al: The influence of gravity on cardiac performance. Ann Biomed Eng 26:1, 1998.
31. Blomqvist CG: Cardiovascular adaptation to weightlessness. Med Sci Sport Exerc 15:428, 1983.
32. Mulragh SL, Charles JB, Riddle JM, et al: Echocardiographic evaluation of the cardiovascular effects of short-duration spaceflight. J Clin Pharmacol 31:1024, 1991.
33. Vorobyov EI, Gazenko OG, Genn AM, et al: Medical results of Salyut-6 manned spaceflight. Aviat Space Environ Med 54(suppl 1):S31, 1983.
34. Atkov OU, Bednenko VS, Fomina GA: Ultrasound techniques in space medicine. Aviat Space Environ Med 58(suppl 9):A69, 1987.
35. Dietlein LF: Skylab: a beginning. *In* Johnson RS, Dietlein LF (eds): The Proceedings of the Skylab Life Sciences Symposium. p. 795. Houston: NASA, 1975 (Publ. JSC-09275, NASA TMX-58154).
36. Pestov ID, Geratewohl SJ: Weightlessness. *In* Calvin M, Gazenko OG (eds): Ecological and Physiological Basis of Space Biology and Medicine: Foundations of Space Biology and Medicine. Vol. 2. Book 1. p. 305. Washington, DC: US Government Printing Office, 1975 (NASA Publ. SP-374).
37. Bungo MW: The cardiopulmonary system. *In* Nicogossian A, Leach CS, Pool S (eds): Space Physiology and Medicine. 2nd ed. p. 179. Philadelphia: Lea & Febiger, 1989.
38. Fritsch-Yelle JM, Whitson PA, Bondar RL, et al: Subnormal norepinephrine release relates to presyncope in astronauts after spaceflight. J Appl Physiol 81:2134, 1996.
39. Zeigler MG: Postural hypotension. Annu Rev Med 31:239, 1980.
40. Volterrani M, Rosano G, Coats A, et al: Estrogen acutely increases peripheral blood flow in postmenopausal women. Am J Med 99:119, 1995.
41. Williams JK, Adams MR, Herrington DM, et al: Short-term administration of estrogen and vascular responses of atherosclerotic coronary arteries. Cardiol 20:452, 1992.
42. Williams JK, Adams MR, Klopfenstein HS: Estrogen modulates responses of atherosclerotic coronary arteries. Circulation 81:1680, 1990.
43. Wolthius RA, Bergman SA, Nicogossian AE: Physiological effects of locally applied reduced pressure in man. Physiol Rev 54:566, 1974.
44. Arbeillo PH, Gauquelin G, Pottier JM, et al: Results of a 4-week head-down tilt with and without LBNP countermeasure: cardiac and peripheral hemodynamics—comparison with a 25-day spaceflight. Aviat Space Environ Med 63:9, 1992.
45. Johnson RL, Hofflerr GW, Nicogossian AE, et al: Lower body negative pressure: third manned Skylab Mission. *In* Johnson RL, Dietlein LF (eds): Biomedical Results of Skylab. p. 284. Washington, DC: US Government Printing Office, 1977 (NASA Publ. SP-377).
46. Gazenko OG, Genin AM, Yegorov AD: Summary of medical investigation in the U.S.S.R. manned space missions. Acta Astronaut 8:907, 1981.
47. Bungo MW, Charles JB, Johnson PC: Cardiovascular deconditioning during spaceflight and the use of saline as a countermeasure in orthostatic intolerance. Aviat Space Environ Med 56:985, 1985.
48. Hyatt KH, West DA: Reversal of bedrest-induced orthostatic intolerance by lower body negative pressure and saline. Aviat Space Environ Med 48:120, 1977.
49. Bungo MW, Johnson PC: Cardiovascular examinations and observations of deconditioning during the space shuttle orbital flight test program. Aviat Space Environ Med 54:1001, 1983.
50. Eckberg JL, Fritsch JM: Human autonomic responses to actual and simulated weightlessness. J Clin Pharmacol 31:951, 1991.
51. Convertino VA, Doerr DF, Eckberg DL, et al: Head-down bedrest impairs vagal baroreflex responses and provokes orthostatic hypotension. J Appl Physiol 68:1458, 1990.
52. Blomqvist CG, Nixon JV, Johnson RL, et al: Early cardiovascular adaptation to zero gravity simulated by head-down tilt. Acta Astronaut 7:543, 1980.
53. Fritsch-Yelle JM, Charles JB, Jones MM, et al: Microgravity decreases heart rate and arterial pressure in humans. J Appl Physiol 80:910, 1996.
54. Ernsting J, Parry DJ: Some observations on the effects of stimulating the stretch receptors in the carotid artery of man. J Physiol (Lond) 137:45P, 1957.
55. Spenkle JM, Eckburg DL, Goble RL, et al: Device for rapid quantification of human baroreceptor-cardiac reflex responses. J Appl Physiol 60:727, 1986.
56. Eckberg DL, Fritsch JM: Carotid baroreceptor cardiac-vagal reflex responses during 10 days of head-down tilt. Physiologist 33(suppl):S177, 1990.
57. Fritsch-Yelle JM, Charles JB, Bennet BS, et al: Short-duration spaceflight impairs human carotid baroreceptor-cardiac reflex responses. J Appl Physiol 73:664, 1992.
58. Fritsch-Yelle JM, Charles JB, Jones MM, et al: Spaceflight alters autonomic regulation of arterial pressure in humans. J Appl Physiol 77:1776, 1994.
59. Milgram NW, MacLeod CM, Petit TL: Neuroplasticity, learning and memory. *In* Milgram NW, MacLeod CM, Petit TL (eds): Neuroplasticity, Learning and Memory. p. 1. New York: Alan R Liss, 1987.
60. Berry CA, Catterson AD: Pre-Gemini medical predictions vs. Gemini flight results. *In* Gemini Summary Conference. p. 235. February 1 and 2, 1967, Manned Spacecraft Center, Houston, Texas. Washington, DC: US Government Printing Office, 1967 (NASA SP-138).
61. Berry CA: Weightlessness. *In* Parker JF, West URG (eds): Bioastronautic Data Book, p. 349. Washington, DC: US Government Printing Office, 1974 (NASA Publ. SP-30).
62. Bergman SA, Johnson RL, Hoffler GW: Evaluation of the electromechanical properties of the cardiovascular system after prolonged weightlessness. *In* Johnston RS, Dietlein LF (eds): Biomedical Results from Skylab. p. 351. Washington, DC: US Government Printing Office, 1977 (NASA SP-377).
63. Rossum AC, Wood ML, Bishop SL, et al: Evaluation of cardiac rhythm disturbances during extravehicular activity. Am J Cardiol 79:1153, 1997.
64. Goldberger AL, Bungo MW, Baevsky RM, et al: Heart rate dynamics during long-duration spaceflight: report on MIR cosmonauts. Am Heart J 128:202, 1994.
65. Fritsch-Yelle JM, Leuenberger UA, D'Aunno DS, et al: An episode of ventricular tachycardia during long-duration spaceflight. Am J Cardiol 81:1391, 1998.
66. Bungo MW, Goldwater DJ, Popp RL, et al: Echocardiographic evaluation of space shuttle crewmembers. J Appl Physiol 17:863, 1987.
67. Pottier JM, Patat F, Arbeille P, et al: Cardiovascular system and microgravity simulation and inflight results. Acta Astronaut 13:47, 1986.
68. Henry WL, Epstein SE, Griffith JM, et al: Effects of prolonged spaceflight on cardiac function and dimensions. *In* Johnson RS, Dietlein LF (eds): Biomedical Results from Skylab. p. 366. Washington, DC: US Government Printing Office, 1977 (NASA Publ. SP-377).
69. Bungo MW, Charles JR, Riddle J, et al: Echocardiographic investigation of the hemodynamics of weightlessness [abstract]. J Am Coll Cardiol 7:192, 1986.
70. Bonting SL: Space biology research. Trends Biochem Sci 18:265, 1983.

SECTION XI

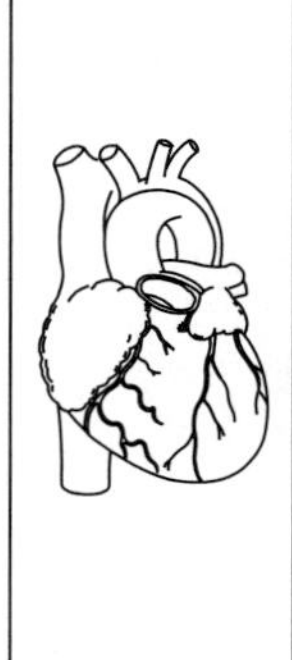

SURGERY AND THE HEART

Evaluation of Patients for Noncardiac Surgery

Anesthesia for Cardiovascular Operations

Intraoperative Hemodynamic Monitoring

CHAPTER 112

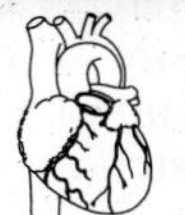

Evaluation of Patients for Noncardiac Surgery

Rajendra H. Mehta and Kim A. Eagle

GENERAL APPROACH
Preoperative Assessment
NONCARDIAC SURGERY FOR THE PATIENT WITH CORONARY ARTERY DISEASE
Preoperative Clinical Assessment
Noninvasive Tests
Invasive Tests
Strategies to Reduce Perioperative Complications
CONGENITAL HEART DISEASE
VALVULAR HEART DISEASE
Mitral Valve Disease
Aortic Valve Disease
CARDIOMYOPATHY
Dilated Cardiomyopathy
Hypertrophic Cardiomyopathy

Internists and cardiologists are often called on to assess patients before noncardiac surgery. With more than 25 million Americans undergoing noncardiac surgical procedures each year, the consultant's role is of considerable magnitude.[1] With technological advances and improvements in surgical techniques, an increasing percentage of morbidity and mortality with surgery is now related to cardiac complications rather than to direct surgical problems.[2] Clinical occult cardiovascular disease often becomes manifest by the stress of noncardiac surgery. About one third of the patients undergoing noncardiac surgery are considered at risk for cardiovascular disease, and about 1.5 million experience in-hospital or long-term complications.[1] This chapter outlines the general approach for preoperative assessment of any patient presenting for noncardiac surgery and reviews specific cardiac conditions, including coronary artery disease (CAD), congenital heart disease, valvular disease, cardiomyopathy, and arrhythmias. It also discusses preoperative, intraoperative, and postoperative management of the patient undergoing noncardiac surgery.

General Approach

Preoperative Assessment

Because the stress of major surgery and anesthesia can affect the circulatory system, it is important to determine the presence of any underlying cardiac disease. This possibility should be considered in all patients who present for surgery. A detailed history is helpful and should include a search for chest pain, shortness of breath, peripheral edema, dizziness, syncope, palpitations, or transient ischemic attacks. The consultant should also determine whether there is a history of congenital heart disease, angina pectoris, myocardial infarction (MI), rheumatic fever, heart murmur, arrhythmias, heart failure, or peripheral vascular disease (including carotid artery disease). A careful review of a patient's medications and allergies is mandatory. The social history should document substance abuse, especially alcohol and cocaine. The need and the urgency of surgery also should be established.

A thorough physical examination is an essential component of the preoperative assessment. The examination should include weight, heart rate, and blood pressure, including a search for postural hypotension. The cardiovascular examination should include a search for jugular venous pulsation, all extremity pulsations, carotid bruits, evidence of cardiomegaly, third heart sound, or murmurs of valvular stenosis or regurgitation.

The history and physical examination should particularly focus on clinical factors that have been shown to correlate with excess perioperative risk of cardiac events, such as prior MI, unstable angina, ventricular tachycardia, congestive heart failure (CHF), and diabetes mellitus. Several studies have established risk indices that include important clinical predictors. These composites of clinical factors can be useful in assessing risk and are discussed in the next section.

It is important to determine the presence of additional comorbid conditions in any patient before surgery is undertaken. This includes anemia, which can reduce cardiac reserve, and renal disease and/or electrolyte imbalances. Diabetes, hypertension, thyrotoxicosis, and myxedema should be well controlled before surgery. Respiratory disease may interfere with proper oxygenation of blood and can prolong the need for postoperative ventilation. Therefore, patients with such diseases may require active pulmonary physiotherapy before surgery. Other important comorbid conditions include a prothrombotic tendency, which can predispose patients to systemic and pulmonary emboli.

Careful consideration and adjustment of medications is also necessary before noncardiac surgery. Patients receiving beta-blockers should not abruptly discontinue their medications. Such an acute withdrawal before surgery can lead to an increase in the risk of myocardial ischemia and infarction.[3] In fact, studies of patients undergoing noncardiac surgery who were taking β-blockers right up to the time of surgery have found no increase in the incidence of hypotension or bradycardia before or after surgery, nor were there intraoperative or postoperative deaths.[4] In fact, several studies suggest that maintaining the patient on perioperative β-blockade can diminish postoperative coronary ischemia and probably MI and cardiac death.[5–9]

It is also important to maintain patients on antihypertensive medications throughout the perioperative period. However, certain agents should generally be stopped before surgery. These include rauwolfia alkaloids, which can potentiate the effect of preoperative medications.[10] It is also advisable to discontinue diuretics 1 day before surgery. Severe diuresis may predispose to hypovolemia, which in turn can predispose to hypotension during anesthesia. Furthermore, hypokalemia associated with diuretic therapy can enhance the effects of digitalis and can increase the risk of digitalis toxicity. The use of digitalis also merits careful consideration.[11, 12] If no clear indication for digitalis, such as atrial fibrillation or heart failure, is discovered, we recommend not administering it during the preoperative period.

Patients receiving oral anticoagulants deserve special consideration because this poses an added risk. When possible, anticoagulants should be discontinued several days before the surgery. Fresh frozen plasma can be used to reverse the prothrombin time, when required. When possible, vitamin K should be avoided. Patients receiving heparin can undergo surgery within hours after it is discontinued. Certain high-risk patients receiving long-term anticoagulation may require hospitalization for conversion from warfarin to intravenous heparin. Examples might include patients who have experienced thromboembolism when the International Normalized Ratio has become subtherapeutic. Another high-risk group is patients with multiple coexisting conditions that make them more susceptible to thromboembolism, such as a ball-in-cage prosthetic mitral valve in combination with chronic atrial fibrillation and/or poor left ventricular (LV) function. Aspirin and newer antiplatelet agents, such as ticlopidine, clopidogrel, and oral platelet receptor antagonists, are usually discontinued at least 4 days before surgery. However, many surgeons may prefer to continue administering the aspirin. In addition, if there is great concern about preoperative coronary risk, then continuation of aspirin may be favored, assuming that surgical bleeding is not likely to be excessive.

The determination of the functional status of a patient is also important. This can be determined by classifying the patient according to the New York Heart Association. Surgical risk is usually proportional to the degree of limitation of cardiac function.[13–17] Functional capacity can also be determined by using the specific activity scale (Table 112–1).[18] It may be important to quantify exercise tolerance in certain subgroups of patients, including cardiac patients, elderly patients, and those undergoing vascular surgery. This issue is addressed subsequently.

TABLE 112-1 **Specific Activity Scale**

Class	Patient Can Perform to Completion
I	Activity requiring ≥ 7 metabolic equivalents (METS) Carry 24 pounds up eight steps Carry objects that weigh 80 pounds Outdooor work (shovel snow, spade soil) Recreation (ski, basketball, squash, handball, jog/walk 5 mph)
II	Activity requiring ≥ 5 (but not ≥ 7) METS Have sexual intercourse without stopping Walk at 4 mph on level ground Outdoor work (garden, rake, weed) Recreation (roller skate, dance fox trot)
III	Activity requiring ≥ 2 (but not ≥ 5) METS Shower/dress without stopping, strip and make bed Walk at 2.5 mph on level ground Outdoor work (clean windows) Recreation (play golf, bowl)
IV	No activity requiring ≥ 2 METS (cannot carry out activities listed above)

Data from Goldman L, Caldera DL, Nussbaum SR, et al: Multifactorial index of cardiac risk in non-cardiac surgical procedures. N Engl J Med 297:845, 1977.

NONCARDIAC SURGERY FOR THE PATIENT WITH CORONARY ARTERY DISEASE

Patients with known or suspected CAD deserve special consideration in the preoperative assessment. More than a million patients who undergo noncardiac surgery each year have CAD,[1] and cardiac events account for more perioperative deaths than any other type of complication.

Preoperative Clinical Assessment

Dripps and colleagues[19] were the first to define a classification scheme that could stratify patients into five classes on the basis of their physical status. In the Dripps–American Society of Anesthesiologists Index (Table 112–2), these classes ranged from normal healthy patients to moribund individuals who were not expected to survive for more than 24 hours.[20] However, the subjective nature of this index prompted investigators to define a more quantitative method for preoperative assessment. To quantify clinical cardiac risk in the preoperative assessment, Goldman and colleagues[21, 22] used a multifactorial approach.

They identified certain clinical features that were independent predictors of cardiac events after noncardiac surgery. These included age greater than 70 years, MI within the 6 months before the surgery, the presence of CHF, aortic valve stenosis, atrial and ventricular arrhythmias, and other variables, as shown in Table 112–3. They used a

TABLE 112-2 **The Dripps–American Society of Anesthesiologists Classification of Physical Status***

1. A normal healthy patient
2. A patient with a mild systemic disease
3. A patient with a severe systemic disease that limits activity but is not incapacitating
4. A patient with an incapacitating systemic disease that is a constant threat to life
5. A moribund patient not expected to survive for 24 hours, with or without operation

**Note:* in the event of emergency operation, precede the number with an E.

Adapted from American Society of Anesthesiologists: New classification of physical status. Anesthesiologist 24:111, 1963.

TABLE 112–3 **The Goldman Multifactorial Cardiac Risk Index**

Criteria	Multivariate Discriminate Function Coefficient	Points
History		
Age 70 yr	0.191	5
MI in previous 6 mo	0.384	10
Physical examination		
S_3 gallop or JVD	0.451	11
Important valvular aortic stenosis	0.119	3
Electrocardiogram		
Rhythm other than sinus or PACs on last preoperative ECG	0.283	7
>5 PVCs/min documented at any time before operation	0.278	7
General status		
$Po_2 < 60$ or $Pco_2 > 50$ mm Hg, K = 3.0 or $HCO_3 < 20$ mEq/L, BUN > 50 or creatinine > 3.0 mg/dl, abnormal SGOT, signs of chronic liver disease, patient bedridden from noncardiac causes	0.132	3
Operation		
Intraperitoneal, intrathoracic, or aortic operation	0.123	3
Emergency operation	0.167	4
Total		53

Abbreviations: BUN, blood urea nitrogen; ECG, electrocardiogram; HCO_3, bicarbonate; JVD, jugular vein distention; K, potassium; MI, myocardial infarction; PAC, premature atrial contraction; Pco_2, partial pressure of carbon dioxide; Po_2, partial pressure of oxygen; PVC, premature ventricular contraction; SGOT, serum glutamic oxaloacetic transaminase.

Adapted from Goldman L, Caldera DL, Nussbaum SR, et al: Multifactorial index of cardiac risk in non-cardiac surgical procedures. N Engl J Med 297:845, 1977.

TABLE 112–5 **The Modified Multifactorial Cardiac Risk Index**

Variables	Points
CAD	
MI within 6 mo	10
MI more than 6 mo	5
Canadian Cardiovascular Society Angina	
Class 3	
Class 4	
Unstable angina within 3 mo	10
Alveolar pulmonary edema	
Within 1 wk	10
Ever	5
Valvular disease	
Suspected critical aortic stenosis	20
Arrhythmias	
Sinus plus atrial premature beats or rhythm other than sinus on last preoperative ECG	5
More than five ventricular premature beats at any time before surgery	5
Poor general medical status*	5
Age over 70 yr	5
Emergency operation	10

Abbreviations: CAD, coronary artery disease; ECG, electrocardiogram; MI, myocardial infarction.

*Oxygen pressure, 60 mm Hg; carbon dioxide pressure, 50 mm Hg; serum potassium, 3.0 mEq/L (3.0 mmol/L); serum bicarbonate, 20 mEq/L (20 mmol/L); serum urea nitrogen, 50 mg/dl (18 mmol/L); serum creatine, 3 mg/dl (260 mmol/L); aspartate aminotransferase abnormal; signs of chronic liver disease; and/or bedridden for noncardiac causes.[19,23]

Adapted from Detsky AS, Abrams HB, McLaughlin JR, et al: Predicting cardiac complications in patients undergoing non-cardiac surgery. J Gen Intern Med 1:211, 1986; and Detsky AS, Abrams HB, Forbath N, et al: Cardiac assessment for patients undergoing non-cardiac surgery: a multifactorial clinical risk index. Arch Intern Med 146:2131, 1986.

stepwise linear discriminant analysis to assign relative weights to each clinical variable. Based on the total score, a preoperative index was derived, consisting of four classes (Table 112–4). There is a stepwise increase in the proportion of patients with cardiac complications with the progression from risk class I to risk class IV on the Goldman index.

Detsky and colleagues[23, 24] modified the Goldman index and improved on its shortcomings. They included a history of advanced angina pectoris within 3 months before surgery, the presence of prior alveolar edema, and the proximity in duration of time of the episode of heart failure to the surgery (Table 112–5). They also simplified the scoring system by converting it into multiples of five. Similar to the Goldman index, a progressively greater risk for cardiac complications was found for increasing scores on this modified index (Table 112–6).

Eagle and colleagues[25, 26] have also documented that a careful clinical evaluation provides important information that helps in both perioperative and long-term risk stratification. They identified five clinical markers that are especially predictive of cardiac events. These include age greater than 70 years, history of diabetes mellitus, history of angina, prior MI, and previous CHF and/or ventricular arrhythmias. The usefulness of these clinical markers has been validated in both vascular and nonvascular groups of patients for perioperative risk stratification.[27, 28] We have defined the usefulness of these clinical markers for long-term risk stratification in the geriatric patient undergoing vascular surgery.[29] These clinical markers should be used in an incremental fashion to classify patients into low-,

TABLE 112–4 **The Goldman Risk Groups**

Risk Group	Patients (n)	Goldman Score	Life-Threatening Complication (Nonfatal)	Cardiac Death
I	537	0–5	4 (0.7%)	1 (0.2%)
II	316	6–12	16 (5%)	5 (2%)
III	130	13–25	15 (12%)	3 (2%)
IV	18	≥26	4 (22%)	

Data from Goldman L, Caldera DL, Nussbaum SR, et al: Multifactorial index of cardiac risk in non-cardiac surgical procedures. N Engl J Med 297:845, 1977.

TABLE 112-6 The Risk Groups for the Modified Multifactorial Cardiac Risk Index*

Risk Class	Total Points	Likelihood Ratios of a Cardiac Event
I	0–15	0.42
II	16–30	3.58
III	>30	14.93

*By using the pretest probability of cardiac complications for each major surgery, the modified Goldman index helps to determine the probability of a cardiac event for each risk score stratum, based on bayesian analysis, by using the likelihood ratios for each stratum.

Adapted from Detsky AS, Abrams HB, McLaughlin JR, et al: Predicting cardiac complications in patients undergoing non-cardiac surgery. J Gen Intern Med 1:211, 1986 and Detsky AS, Abrams HB, Forbath N, et al: Cardiac assessment for patients undergoing non-cardiac surgery: a multifactorial clinical risk index. Arch Intern Med 146:2131, 1986. Copyright 1986, American Medical Association.

moderate-, and high-risk groups (Table 112–7). Patients with none of these clinical markers are in a lower-risk group. Those with one or two markers are in a moderate-risk group, and those with three or more markers are in a high-risk group.

Patients in the low-risk group can usually proceed directly to surgery without further risk stratification. Those in the moderate-risk group are most likely to benefit from further stratification of their cardiac risk by noninvasive testing, for both perioperative and long-term prognosis. Selected patients in the high-risk group may benefit from noninvasive evaluation or, in rare cases, from direct investigation of their coronary anatomy by use of cardiac catheterization.

In summary, the preoperative history and physical examination are extremely important in classifying patients into various clinical risk groups; this facilitates decisions regarding subsequent diagnostic testing and therapy.

Noninvasive Tests

As suggested, noninvasive testing may be very useful for patients defined to be at intermediate or high coronary risk on the basis of clinical evaluation. The goals of noninvasive testing may include determination of the patient's functional capacity, tendency toward inducible myocardial ischemia with stress, history of a previous MI, and LV and valvular function. Of course, the ultimate goal is to acquire knowledge about cardiac dysfunction and ischemic tendencies so that measures can be taken to stabilize these through the perioperative period.

TABLE 112-7 Eagle Index

Clinical Marker	Risk Group Based on Number of Clinical Markers
Age > 70 yr	Low risk (no clinical markers)
Diabetes mellitus	
History of angina	
History of myocardial infarction/ Q wave on ECG	Moderate risk (1 or 2 clinical markers)
Congestive heart failure/ ventricular ectopic activity (requiring treatment)	High risk (3 or more clinical markers)

Abbreviation: ECG, electrocardiogram.

Exercise and Electrocardiographic Stress Testing

Determination of functional capacity has been shown to be extremely useful in identifying patients at greatest risk for perioperative cardiac events. Previous studies have found that patients with poor functional capacity were at increased risk for perioperative cardiac complications.[13–18] For instance, patients unable to achieve 75 to 85 percent of predicted maximal heart rate with treadmill or bicycle exercise had a significantly higher risk for cardiac complications than that of patients who had good functional capacity (Table 112–8). Poor functional capacity appears to be especially predictive of adverse events when it is accompanied by ischemia during or after stress testing. Conversely, patients with demonstrable ischemia but good functional capacity on exercise testing have only a slightly elevated risk of perioperative complications compared with those with both coronary ischemia and poor functional capacity. The negative predictive value of a normal, adequate, electrocardiographic stress test for perioperative MI or death is probably greater than 95 percent. Contrariwise, the positive predictive value is generally 10 to 20 percent.

The overall usefulness of exercise stress testing is limited because a number of patients have nonspecific abnormalities on baseline electrocardiogram (ECG). In this subset of patients with an abnormal baseline ECG, sensitivity may be improved by the addition of myocardial imaging. Furthermore, exercise treadmill testing is often not possible in certain patient subsets. Patients undergoing vascular, orthopedic, or major abdominal or thoracic surgery may not be able to achieve an exercise load sufficient to produce an adequate test. Therefore, exercise electrocardiographic treadmill testing is a useful method for preoperative risk stratification only in the patient who has reasonable functional capacity and an interpretable ECG.

Exercise Treadmill Testing With Thallium Imaging

The combination of exercise treadmill testing and thallium imaging has been found to increase the sensitivity for identifying patients with fixed coronary lesions. Morrow and colleagues[30] showed that patients with thallium redistribution had a twofold greater risk of cardiac events in the perioperative period. The addition of thallium imaging to exercise treadmill testing can help to define the functional importance of coronary ischemia by identifying multiple areas of ischemia or indirect measures of LV dysfunction during ischemia, such as transient ventricular dilatation and increased lung uptake of thallium. However, for patients unable to exercise during the preoperative period, an alternative method for stress testing is needed. For such patients, pharmacologic stress testing is particularly beneficial.

Exercise Echocardiography

Exercise echocardiography is becoming an increasingly popular technique because it is relatively cheaper, is less

TABLE 112-8 **Impact of Poor Functional Capacity on Perioperative Cardiac Risk**

Author	Type of Exercise	Type of Surgery	Patients (n)	Exercise Level Achieved	Incidence of Cardiac Events
Cutler et al[13]	ETT	Peripheral vascular	130	>75% PMHR, no ischemia	0 of 35
				>75% PMHR, with ischemia	6 of 23 (no deaths)
				<75% PMHR, with ischemia	10 of 26 (5 deaths)
McPhail et al[15]	ETT or arm ergometry	Peripheral vascular	101	>85% PMHR	2 of 30
				<85% PMHR	17 of 70
				<85% PMHR, with ischemia	7 of 21
Carliner et al[14]	ETT or bicycle or arm ergometry	Abdominal or thoracic or vascular	200	>5 METS	1 of 92
				<5 METS	5 of 106
Gerson et al[16]	Ex RNA	Abdominal or thoracic	155	HR > 100 and ED > 2 min	4 of 84
				HR < 100 and ED < 2 min	19 of 61
Kopecky et al[17]	Ex RNA	Peripheral vascular	110	>5 METS	0 of 47
				<5 METS	8 of 63

Abbreviations: ECG, electrocardiographic; ED, exercise duration; ETT, exercise treadmill test with ECG monitoring; Ex RNA, exercise radionuclide angiography with ECG monitoring; HR, heart rate; METS, metabolic equivalents; PMHR, predicted maximal heart rate with vigorous exercise.

From Abraham SA, Coles NA, Coley CM, et al: Coronary risk of noncardiac surgery. Prog Cardiovasc Dis 34:205, 1991.

time consuming, and provides valuable information about resting systolic and diastolic LV function, valve function, and presence or absence of pericardial disease compared with exercise thallium testing. Exercise echocardiography appears to be comparable to exercise thallium testing for predicting complications.

Measures of Left Ventricular Function

The potential value of determination of rest and exercise LV ejection fraction has been studied extensively.[31–36] Resting LV ejection fraction of 35 percent or less has been reported to be a predictive factor for subsequent MI.[33, 34] However, patients with severe CAD but without prior MI often have a normal resting LV ejection fraction. Therefore, determination of resting LV ejection fraction has limited sensitivity for predicting perioperative cardiac events. Several studies have suggested that the LV ejection fraction is not predictive of significant perioperative events independent of functional capacity or coronary ischemia.[31–34]

Pharmacologic Stress Testing

DIPYRIDAMOLE-THALLIUM IMAGING

In the past decade, dipyridamole-thallium imaging has been the most widely tested noninvasive strategy for risk stratification before noncardiac surgery. Initially, its usefulness was defined in patients who had poor exercise capacity and/or an uninterpretable ECG. By inhibiting the reuptake of adenosine by the endothelium and red blood cells, dipyridamole causes vasodilatation and an increase in blood flow to both epicardial and subendocardial coronary arteries when these arteries are normal.[37, 38] However, when coronary arteries are diseased, dipyridamole has less capacity to increase perfusion to the myocardium they serve. This leads to an exaggeration of coronary perfusion in normal regions when compared with abnormal zones.[39] This can help to define myocardial regions that are hypoperfused, presumably because of obstructive coronary artery lesions. Boucher and colleagues[40] were the first to define the role of dipyridamole-thallium tests for preoperative risk stratification. They documented that the development of thallium redistribution on preoperative dipyridamole-thallium imaging could be correlated with a higher likelihood of perioperative coronary events after vascular surgery. Subsequent studies have validated these findings.[12, 39–42]

Eagle and colleagues[26] recommended a bayesian approach to the use of dipyridamole-thallium testing before noncardiac surgery. They suggested that the pretest probability was an important factor to consider before a decision is made to perform noninvasive testing and documented this by showing that patients without clinical markers of CAD had an extremely low risk of perioperative cardiac events even when they underwent high-risk surgery, such as vascular surgery.

Several investigators have found that semiquantification of the findings seen on dipyridamole-thallium testing can help further stratify risk for perioperative ischemic events.[43, 44] Patients with multiple thallium abnormalities are at greatest risk for developing perioperative complications. These patients are more likely to have multivessel and/or left main CAD and might benefit from more intensive perioperative medical therapy or even from preoperative coronary revascularization in selected instances.

Initial studies found that reversible thallium defects were predictive of perioperative cardiac events.[23, 40, 42–44] However, subsequent studies have found that fixed thallium defects are predictive of long-term cardiac events.[45, 46] Hendel and colleagues[47] documented that the presence of thallium redistribution was the strongest predictor of perioperative cardiac events. However, fixed thallium defects were the best predictor of long-term cardiac events in their study, which included 360 patients who underwent elective vascular surgery. Subsequently, we have confirmed this in geriatric patients undergoing vascular surgery.[29]

Presumably, fixed defects represent a scar from a previous MI or a severely ischemic myocardium with underlying severe fixed stenosis.[48] The development of ischemic ST segment depression during dipyridamole testing has also been found to be an important predictor of perioperative and late cardiac events.[26] This appears to be similar to the development of ischemic ST segment changes during exercise treadmill testing.

The usefulness of dipyridamole-thallium testing has been defined not only in patients undergoing vascular surgery but also in patients undergoing nonvascular surgery.[28] Dipyridamole-thallium testing appears to have almost equal sensitivity and specificity to that of exercise thallium testing for the identification of fixed coronary lesions, as determined in studies of patients undergoing coronary angiography.[49, 50] It is unclear why several studies have reported very poor sensitivity and specificity for dipyridamole testing for perioperative risk stratification.[51, 52] It is possible that problems with patient selection (routine testing in low-risk patients) or image interpretation may be responsible for these negative reports.

DOBUTAMINE-THALLIUM IMAGING

Dobutamine-thallium imaging has also been found to be useful for preoperative risk stratification at several centers. Preliminary reports suggest that thallium redistribution on preoperative dobutamine-thallium imaging correlated with an increased risk of perioperative events.[53, 54] In addition, normal thallium scans identified a group of patients with a very low risk for subsequent cardiac events.

DIPYRIDAMOLE ECHOCARDIOGRAPHY

Dipyridamole echocardiography is an infrequently used modality in the United States for perioperative risk stratification. Although some reports suggest that the development of wall motion abnormalities identified by echocardiography after high-dose dipyridamole infusion can identify patients with fixed coronary disease who may be at risk for subsequent cardiac events,[55, 56] its usefulness has not been confirmed in other centers. Further study is necessary to determine its sensitivity, specificity, and predictive accuracy compared with dipyridamole-thallium testing.

DOBUTAMINE ECHOCARDIOGRAPHY

Dobutamine echocardiography is increasingly used as a preferred form of pharmacologic stress testing. Segar and colleagues[57] have demonstrated that the development of regional wall motion abnormalities or the loss of myocardial thickening was a sign of an advanced coronary disease, with a sensitivity of nearly 90 percent for identifying a 50 percent or greater stenosis in one or more coronary arteries. Davila-Roman and colleagues[58] screened 93 patients before vascular surgery with dobutamine stress echocardiography. New wall motion abnormalities developed in 23 patients during the test; 19 of these patients underwent subsequent coronary angiography, and 13 underwent coronary revascularization for significant CAD. One of the patients who had undergone coronary revascularization and then subsequently underwent vascular surgery had a perioperative cardiac event. Of 10 patients who did not undergo coronary revascularization, 4 had a postoperative cardiac event, including 2 MIs and 1 death. Patients with postoperative cardiac events tended to have more severe wall motion abnormalities on preoperative testing. No cardiac events occurred in patients who had a negative study result. A normal study result was also found to be associated with fewer cardiac events on long-term follow-up. Other investigators have also identified dobutamine-induced new wall motion abnormalities as a marker for increased risk for perioperative cardiac events.[59–61]

Electrocardiographic Ischemia Monitoring

Raby and colleagues[62] reported that preoperative ischemia identified by Holter monitoring was predictive of postoperative events. In their study of 176 patients undergoing vascular surgery, 18 percent had preoperative ischemia. They reported a sensitivity of 92 percent and a specificity of 88 percent for the identification of postoperative coronary events. Although preoperative ischemia monitoring was found to have an excellent negative predictive value of 99 percent, the positive predictive value was only 38 percent. However, in a study of 474 men referred for elective noncardiac surgery, Mangano and colleagues[63] found preoperative ischemia monitoring to be less than 30 percent sensitive for identifying patients who had perioperative events. They found postoperative ischemia to be the only multivariate correlate of subsequent ischemic events, with a ninefold increase in risk. Intraoperative ischemia was less important than postoperative ischemia for predicting subsequent cardiac events. Raby and colleagues[64] validated these findings, showing a relative risk of 2.7 for developing postoperative cardiac events in patients with intraoperative ischemia and a relative risk of 16 in those with postoperative ischemia. Postoperative ischemia has been found to have a sensitivity of 90 percent for identifying patients who had postoperative cardiac events. Although the sensitivity of ischemia monitoring is very high, the positive predictive value is only 7 percent. Therefore, its use in the clinical setting requires further study. With the increasing use of dobutamine echocardiography and adenosine-thallium testing, this technique is seldom used for preoperative cardiac risk assessment.

Transesophageal Echocardiography

Transesophageal echocardiography allows a clear view of the left ventricle during surgery. Because new wall motion abnormalities of the left ventricle have been found to correlate with ischemia, this has been suggested to be useful for identifying patients experiencing coronary ischemia during surgery. Although preliminary reports suggested that transesophageal echocardiography is sensitive[65–67] for identifying patients at risk for postoperative cardiac complications, others have not confirmed its usefulness. Eisenberg and colleagues[68] reported a poor specificity for this modality of risk stratification. In their study of 332 male veterans undergoing noncardiac surgery, 321 patients did not have a preoperative ischemic event. However, 50 of these patients had intraoperative "ischemia" detected by transesophageal echocardiography. Therefore, the role of this modality for risk stratification of patients undergoing noncardiac surgery is still unclear. Because this technology is both time intensive and costly, its future role for this purpose remains ill defined.

Invasive Tests

Hertzer and colleagues[69] were the first to define the role of preoperative invasive testing. In the 1970s, they performed coronary angiography on all patients before vascular surgery. In their study, the prevalence of severe surgically correctable coronary disease was found to be 25 percent.[70] Subsequently, Eagle and colleagues[26] suggested a cost-effective approach to preoperative risk stratification by selective invasive testing in a small high-risk subset of patients defined by clinical and noninvasive evaluation.

Strategies to Reduce Perioperative Complications

Coronary Revascularization Before Noncardiac Surgery

Hertzer and colleagues[71, 72] showed that patients who underwent coronary artery bypass grafting (CABG) before peripheral vascular surgery had a significantly improved survival at 5 years compared with patients with severe correctable coronary disease who did not undergo CABG (72 percent versus 43 percent, $P = .001$). However, coronary revascularization itself was associated with a substantial periprocedure mortality, and there was no randomized trial of this approach. Nevertheless, the protective role of prior successful CABG has been shown by Foster and colleagues,[73] who studied a cohort of patients with CAD enrolled in the Coronary Artery Surgery Study and who then subsequently required noncardiac surgery. Patients who received medical therapy before noncardiac surgery had a mortality of 2.3 percent. Although the mortality was much lower for those who underwent CABG before noncardiac surgery (0.9 percent), the CABG itself carried a 2.3 percent risk for death. Therefore, the combined overall mortality for coronary revascularization before noncardiac surgery appeared to be equal to if not higher than the mortality of the noncardiac surgery alone without prior coronary revascularization. Eagle and colleagues[74] later reexamined the value of coronary artery bypass surgery on patients undergoing specific noncardiac surgery among the patients enrolled in the Coronary Artery Surgery Study registry. Patients who were not revascularized who underwent high-risk surgery, such as abdominal, vascular, thoracic, and head and neck surgery, each had a combined MI/death rate of greater than 4 percent. In this group of patients, prior CABG was associated with a reduced incidence of postoperative death (1.7 percent versus 3.3 percent, $P = 0.03$) and MI (0.8 percent versus 2.7 percent, $P = 0.002$) as compared with the medical treatment group. Patients undergoing low-risk procedures, such as urologic, orthopedic, breast, and skin operations, had a low mortality of less than 1 percent, regardless of prior revascularization. Prior CABG was also found to be more protective in patients with more severe angina and/or multivessel CAD.[74]

The role of coronary angioplasty for coronary revascularization before noncardiac surgery is even less clear. Several studies have suggested that preoperative coronary revascularization with angioplasty can be safely performed in patients before noncardiac surgery.[75–78] However, none of these studies randomly assigned patients to medical therapy versus percutaneous transluminal coronary angioplasty (PTCA), and therefore, it is not possible to know whether PTCA lowers risk or not. Further studies are needed to clarify this problem. At this time, there is no convincing evidence that coronary angioplasty before noncardiac surgery reduces postoperative risk. Noncardiac surgery should probably be performed several days after PTCA. Arterial remodeling occurs for several days after PTCA, and arterial recoil and acute thrombosis may occur over the first 1 to 2 days after the procedure. On the contrary, delaying surgery beyond 1 to 2 months after PTCA increases the chances of restenosis. Also, because the incidence of coronary restenosis is reduced if it has not occurred within 1 year, patients who are asymptomatic and physically very active between 1 to 5 years after coronary revascularization do not generally require further preoperative risk assessment before noncardiac surgery.

Medical Therapy for Risk Reduction in the Perioperative Period

Several small studies have evaluated the use of perioperative β-blockers in reducing cardiac risk.[5–7] Stone and colleagues[5] gave oral β-blockers 2 hours before the induction of anesthesia in a small randomized trial of patients with mild hypertension. The control group had higher incidence of ischemia than the treatment group (28 percent versus 2 percent). Pasternack and colleagues[6] reported a 3 percent incidence of perioperative MI in patients given perioperative metoprolol as opposed to 18 percent in matched control subjects. In an earlier study, they reported fewer episodes and less total duration of ischemia in patients receiving oral metoprolol before peripheral vascular surgery.[7] More recently, Mangano and colleagues[8] showed that vascular surgery patients randomly assigned to atenolol versus placebo had a reduced cardiac event rate over the first year or two after surgery. Many consider this to be the strongest evidence yet favoring perioperative use of β-blockers, although an accompanying editorial identified several concerns about the baseline differences between the atenolol and placebo groups.[79] Finally, Froehlich and colleagues[9] reported protection against cardiac death after vascular surgery in patients treated with β-blockers in a large observational study. Thus, in patients in whom CAD is strongly suspected, we suggest using β-blockers in the perioperative period, preferably starting at least 12 to 24 hours before the procedure. Few data exist to support the use of calcium channel blockers and nitroglycerin when β-blockers have already been initiated or are contraindicated. Currently, these are recommended for high-risk patients who were previously taking such agents or for those who have active signs of myocardial ischemia without hypotension.

Anesthesia Considerations

The choice of anesthetic agents has not been found to play a significant role in the development of postoperative cardiac complications.[80–83] Because general anesthetics have a negative inotropic action, spinal anesthesia may be preferred for patients with severe LV dysfunction or history of CHF. Pain management in the perioperative period is a crucial part of reducing cardiac risk. Adequate pain control reduces catecholamine surges, which are likely responsible for increase in myocardial oxygen demand, induction of coronary vasospasm, increase in the tendency for plaque rupture, and development of a hypercoagulable state.

Surveillance for Perioperative Myocardial Infarction

Few studies have examined the optimal protocol for the diagnosis of perioperative MI.[84] A strategy using an ECG immediately after surgery and on the first and second day has highest sensitivity, whereas routine measurements of serial creatine kinase-MB had higher false positive rates without increasing the sensitivity. Higher levels of creatine kinase-MB elevation are associated with worse survival.[85] Current recommendation favors monitoring for signs of cardiac dysfunction in patients without evidence of CAD. In patients with known CAD who are undergoing surgical procedures associated with high cardiac risk, ECG at baseline, immediately after surgery, and on the first 2 days after surgery appears to be most cost effective. Measurement of cardiac enzymes should be reserved for patients at high risk and for those who demonstrate clinical, electrocardiographic, or hemodynamic evidence of cardiovascular dysfunction.

Long-Term Risk Stratification and Management

Postoperative patient care involves assessment and treatment of modifiable cardiac risk factors, including hypertension, hyperlipidemia, smoking, obesity, hyperglycemia, and physical inactivity. Patients who sustain a perioperative MI or show evidence of ischemia should be carefully investigated because they have substantial cardiac risk over the subsequent 5 to 10 years. Noninvasive testing to assess LV function and inducible ischemia should be undertaken to identify patients who may benefit from revascularization or optimization of medical therapy.

Overall Approach to Patients With Coronary Artery Disease

An overall strategy for the clinician evaluating a patient with suspected CAD before noncardiac surgery would be as follows. First, the patient should be classified into a clinical risk category on the basis of clinical evaluation alone. As shown in Figure 112–1, patients who do not have clinical markers of risk can be classified into the low-risk category. Such patients do not usually require further risk stratification by noninvasive or invasive strategies. Patients with one or two clinical markers can be classified into the intermediate-risk category. These patients may benefit from further risk stratification by noninvasive means. For these patients, we suggest a noninvasive exercise stress test, which helps to define the patient's functional capacity as well as risk for coronary ischemia during stress. For a patient who is unable to exercise, pharmacologic stress testing is recommended. The selection of the noninvasive pharmacologic stress test should be based on the best available test in the clinician's institution. An attempt should also be made to quantify the degree of ischemia. For example, this can be achieved by determining the number of segments that have reversible defects on thallium images. Patients who have been identified to have severe ischemia at low workloads should be considered for further stratification of their postoperative risk by invasive testing. Coronary angiography should be elected for such patients if they are reasonable candidates for subsequent coronary revascularization.

Patients who have more than two markers by clinical evaluation are classified as high-risk patients. Such patients have a high likelihood of ischemia at low workloads. Therefore, they may or may not benefit from further noninvasive testing. Occasionally, they should proceed directly to invasive testing, provided that they are adequate candidates for coronary revascularization. If not, the best approach may be to cancel surgery or to proceed with a less aggressive procedure when truly elective surgery is under consideration. Coronary angiography for high-risk patients helps define those patients with advanced CAD who require further intervention. This usually includes patients with left main disease or severe triple-vessel disease who should be considered for coronary revascularization before noncardiac surgery. An intra-aortic balloon pump may occasionally be necessary to stabilize the very high-risk patient who is not a candidate for revascularization.

CONGENITAL HEART DISEASE

Patients with congenital heart disease have perioperative issues that deserve special attention. Tikoff and colleagues[86] found that patients with left-to-right cardiac shunts have residual hemodynamic abnormalities even after surgical repair. Others have identified a decreased cardiac output response to exercise in such patients studied after surgery.[87] This includes patients who have undergone surgery for repair of an atrial septal defect, ventricular septal defect, or patent ductus arteriosus. Vigorous treatment of CHF is required for such patients before noncardiac surgery.

Patients who have undergone repair of a left-to-right cardiac shunt and who have pulmonary hypertension are at especially high risk. Those who have a large shunt but only a slight increase in pulmonary artery resistance should undergo cardiac repair before noncardiac surgery. Patients with irreversible pulmonary artery hypertension have an extremely high risk associated with surgery and should not undergo elective procedures unless there is absolutely no alternative. Similarly, patients who have pulmonary-systemic communications should also avoid elective noncardiac surgery because they have poor tolerance to anesthesia.

Patients with prior repair of coarctation of the aorta have a significant frequency of sudden death during follow-up.[88, 89] The causes of death at autopsy included residual cardiac defects with CHF, rupture of a major vessel, dissecting aneurysm, or complications arising from severe atherosclerosis. Such patients also have a high incidence of residual hypertension. Therefore, these patients require close hemodynamic monitoring during the intraoperative and postoperative periods.

Patients with tetralogy of Fallot are also prone to sudden cardiac death. James and colleagues[90] studied the response to bicycle exercise in 43 symptomatic patients an average of 14 years after surgical repair of tetralogy of Fallot. Premature ventricular contractions were recorded in 40

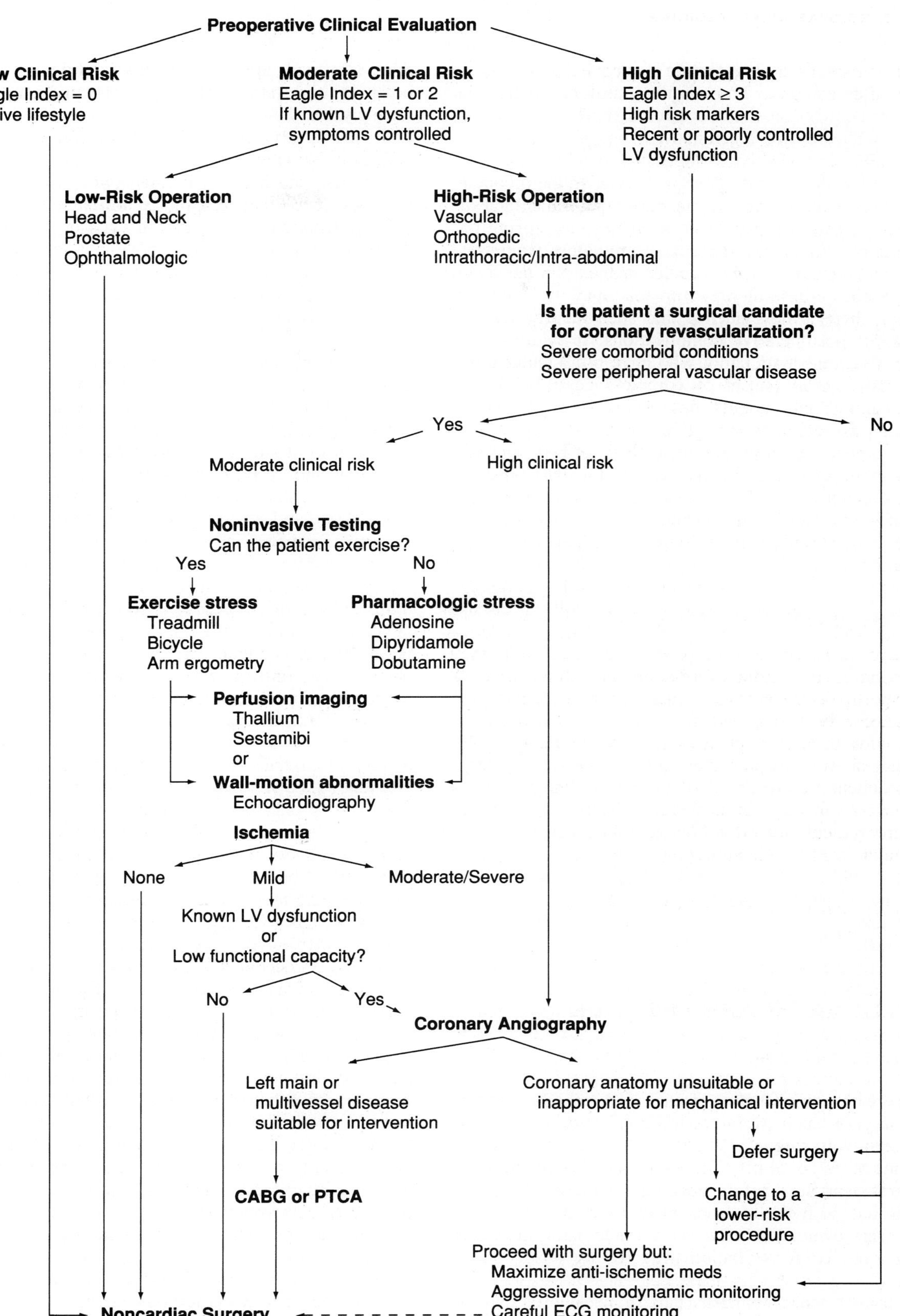

FIGURE 112–1 Suggested algorithm for estimation of preoperative coronary risk of elective or semielective surgery. The most important considerations are the patient's clinical risk profile, the nature of the surgical procedure, and the results of noninvasive testing and/or coronary angiography if indicated. Urgent surgery may preempt risk stratification. High-risk markers: recent myocardial infarction (MI) complicated by angina, congestive heart failure, or positive stress test; unstable or new-onset angina; recent non–Q wave anterior MI; moderate or severe ischemia (redistribution on perfusion imaging in more than one planar view, more than one coronary arterial territory, or four or more myocardial segments, or more severe wall-motion abnormalities on echocardiography). CABG, coronary artery bypass grafting; ECG, electrocardiographic; LV, left ventricular; PTCA, percutaneous transluminal coronary angioplasty.

percent of patients during routine resting ECGs and in 23 percent after exercise. Those with multifocal ventricular premature contractions had occasional short bursts of ventricular tachycardia or bigeminal rhythm. On the basis of these findings, it has been suggested that patients with tetralogy of Fallot should undergo exercise in the preoperative period in an attempt to unmask ventricular tachyarrhythmias. Furthermore, 24-hour Holter monitoring has also been recommended. If frequent premature ventricular contractions or bursts of ventricular tachycardia are found by these modalities, therapy for this may be valuable. However, there is no evidence that such therapy reduces the risk for postoperative complications. In addition, patients with tetralogy of Fallot who have bifascicular block are at risk for late onset of complete heart block and sudden death. Such patients may benefit from His bundle recordings as part of preoperative assessment before noncardiac surgery. Furthermore, the analysis of H-V intervals may help to identify patients at risk for late onset of complete heart block.[91, 92] In patients with evidence of advanced block, temporary pacing may be advised for the perioperative period. Further studies are needed to define the role of preoperative assessment of patients with congenital heart disease who are to undergo noncardiac surgery.

Surgery in patients with cyanotic congenital heart disease with right-to-left shunts poses several unique problems. Because cyanotic patients are prone to polycythemia, they are also prone to thrombus formation. Therefore, diuretics should be avoided for such patients because dehydration may increase the blood viscosity and in turn increase the tendency for thrombosis, particularly cerebral. Patients with a hematocrit value greater than 70 percent should undergo plasmapheresis before noncardiac surgery. Phlebotomy is not advisable in this circumstance, because this can decrease intravascular blood volume and thus increase cyanosis. Patients with a hematocrit value between 55 and 65 percent should receive intravenous fluids starting the night before the surgery.[93] Patients with congenital heart disease should also receive appropriate prophylaxis for bacterial endocarditis.

Valvular Heart Disease

Mitral Valve Disease

Patients with mitral valve disease can usually undergo major surgery, such as intra-abdominal and intrathoracic procedures, with safety.[94] Patients with mitral stenosis who are prone to atrial fibrillation should receive medications to control heart rate before noncardiac surgery. Although digitalis has historically been most used commonly, β-blockers are even more effective for preventing and controlling rapid atrial fibrillation triggered by postoperative stresses.

The use of scopolamine as part of anesthesia may be preferable to atropine because it causes less tachycardia. Patients may benefit from intensive hemodynamic monitoring because they are susceptible to fluid overload.

Patients with mitral regurgitation who are well compensated have little increase in risk during noncardiac surgery. Such patients usually benefit from vasodilators, which reduce afterload, and from inotropic drugs, which reduce heart size and mitral regurgitation. Hemodynamic monitoring may aid in the management of such patients. Patients with mitral valve prolapse need prophylaxis for infective endocarditis. However, they do not generally need any further risk stratification before noncardiac surgery. There is no evidence that treating asymptomatic arrhythmias in such patients has any impact on subsequent outcomes or prognoses.

Aortic Valve Disease

Patients with aortic valve disease who undergo noncardiac surgery have a higher mortality than those with mitral valve disease. Skinner and Pierce[94] found 25 percent mortality among 15 patients who had aortic valve disease and underwent intra-abdominal or intrathoracic procedures. Goldman and colleagues[21] were among the first to document that severe aortic stenosis is a major risk factor for patients undergoing general anesthesia for noncardiac surgery. Therefore, such patients are usually advised to undergo surgical correction of the aortic stenosis before elective noncardiac surgery. However, such patients are often elderly or have severe comorbid conditions. In an attempt to determine the impact of aortic stenosis on prognosis after noncardiac surgery, O'Keefe and colleagues[95] performed a retrospective review of medical records of patients with moderate or severe aortic stenosis who underwent noncardiac surgery at the Mayo Clinic between 1985 and 1987. Severe aortic stenosis was defined as either a peak instantaneous Doppler-derived transvalvular aortic gradient of 4.5 m/sec or more or a calculated aortic valve area of 0.75 cm^2 or less, and moderate aortic stenosis was defined as either a peak instantaneous Doppler-derived aortic gradient of 3.5 to 4.4 m/sec or an aortic valve area of 0.76 to 0.99 cm^2. In 48 patients, 5 experienced significant intraoperative hypotension, but there were no perioperative cardiac deaths. Although this study suggests that selected patients with severe aortic stenosis can safely undergo noncardiac procedures with careful monitoring of anesthesia, others have advocated the use of percutaneous balloon aortic valvuloplasty in patients with critical aortic stenosis who require urgent noncardiac surgery.[96–98]

Symptomatic aortic stenosis in the young patient without any comorbid conditions should prompt aortic valve repair or replacement before noncardiac surgery. However, percutaneous aortic balloon valvuloplasty may be a short-term alternative for critical symptomatic aortic stenosis in elderly patients with comorbidity that either mandates noncardiac surgery and/or precludes aortic valve surgery. For those with asymptomatic aortic valve disease, especially if the patient is physically active, proceeding with surgery is probably safe. A pulmonary artery line for hemodynamic monitoring in such cases is probably helpful to maintain preload and to avoid coronary hypoperfusion, which may accompany systemic hypotension.

Careful consideration is needed in the preoperative management of patients with severe aortic regurgitation to avoid bradycardia because this is poorly tolerated. If possible, this should be prevented with the use of atropine. Like aortic stenosis, such patients are also very sensitive to vasodilatation. A decrease in coronary perfusion can occur, with a drop in aortic diastolic pressure, and this can lead to rapid clinical deterioration.[99] The use of sodium nitroprusside has been recommended in patients with chronic aortic regurgitation. This helps to increase the stroke volume and decrease the LV end-diastolic volume and pressure without changing the heart rate.[99] With the use of vasodilators, it becomes extremely important to monitor the pulmonary capillary wedge pressure to avoid systemic hypotension and to optimize ventricular filling pressures. For the aortic regurgitation, an elevated heart rate from 80 to 100 beats per minute in the intraoperative period is optimal. Continuous electrocardiographic monitoring of precordial leads should often be used to monitor for signs of ischemia in patients with aortic valve disease.

CARDIOMYOPATHY

Dilated Cardiomyopathy

Patients with dilated cardiomyopathy have a dilatation of the left ventricle with a reduced ejection fraction. They usually present with left-sided heart failure, although many have biventricular failure. The use of vasodilators along with positive inotropic agents, such as dobutamine and milrinone, when necessary, can assist in the management of such patients. Inotropic agents should be used extremely cautiously in patients with coexisting CAD, and these patients should be carefully monitored for ischemia and arrhythmias. Monitoring with a pulmonary artery catheter during the intraoperative and postoperative periods is recommended for maintaining optimal preload and avoiding severe CHF in patients with particularly poor ventricular reserve.

Hypertrophic Cardiomyopathy

Patients with hypertrophic obstructive cardiomyopathy do poorly when there is a significant decrease in preload or afterload. β-Blocking agents or calcium channel blockers are often helpful in such patients.[100, 101] Current practice allows once-daily dosing for many of these agents. We recommend that patients continue their usual maintenance dose of these agents during minor surgical procedures. Patients can be switched to shorter-acting preparations before major surgical procedures if it is anticipated that important swings in volume or hemodynamic state are likely.

Patients with hypertrophic cardiomyopathy also do poorly when contractility increases. This can occur during the postoperative period because of a rise in circulating catecholamines resulting from surgical stress or from exogenous adrenergic agents or digitalis. In addition, Thompson and colleagues[102] demonstrated a decreased systemic vascular resistance and increased capacitance when patients with hypertrophic cardiomyopathy received spinal anesthesia.[102] Therefore, it seems logical to avoid spinal anesthesia in favor of general anesthesia in patients with hypertrophic cardiomyopathy who have associated CAD.

REFERENCES

1. Mangano DT: Perioperative cardiac morbidity. Anesthesiology 72:153, 1990.
2. Goldman L: Cardiac risk and complications of noncardiac surgery. Ann Intern Med 98:504, 1983.
3. Miller RR, Olson HG, Amsterdam EA, Mason DT: Propranolol-withdrawal rebound phenomenon: exacerbation of coronary events after abrupt cessation of antianginal therapy. N Engl J Med 293:416, 1975.
4. Kaplan JA, Dunbar RW: Propranolol and surgical anesthesia. Anesth Analg 55:1, 1976.
5. Stone JG, Foex P, Sear JW, et al: Myocardial ischemia in untreated hypertensive patients: effect of a single small oral dose of beta-adrenergic blocking agent. Anesthesiology 68:495, 1988.
6. Pasternack PF, Grossi EA, Baumann FG, et al: Beta blockade to decrease silent myocardial ischemia during peripheral vascular surgery. Am J Surg 158:113, 1989.
7. Pasternack PF, Imparto AM, Baumann FG, et al: The hemodynamics of beta-blockade in patients undergoing abdominal aneurysm repair. Circulation 76(suppl 3):1, 1987.
8. Mangano DT, Layug EL, Wallace A, et al: Effect of atenolol on mortality and cardiovascular morbidity after noncardiac surgery: Multicenter Study of Perioperative Ischemia Research Group. N Engl J Med 335:1713, 1996.
9. Froehlich JB, L'Italien G, Paul S, et al: Improved cardiovascular mortality with perioperative beta-blockade in patients undergoing major vascular surgery. J Am Coll Cardiol 29:219A, 1997.
10. Dundee JW: Iatrogenic disease and anesthesia. BMJ 1:1433, 1958.
11. Likoff W: Indications for preoperative digitalization. *In* Oaks WB, Mayer JH (eds): Pre- and Postoperative Management of the Cardiopulmonary Patient. p. 305–307. New York: Grune & Stratton, 1970.
12. Hillis LD, Cohn PF: Noncardiac surgery in patients with coronary artery disease. Arch Intern Med 138:972, 1978.
13. Cutler BS, Wheeler HB, Paraskos JA, et al: Applicability and interpretation of electrocardiographic stress testing in patients with peripheral vascular disease. Am J Surg 141:501, 1981.
14. Carliner NH, Fisher ML, Plotnick GD, et al: Routine preoperative exercise testing in patients undergoing major non-cardiac surgery. Am J Cardiol 56:51, 1985.
15. McPhail N, Calvin JE, Shariatmadar A, et al: The use of preoperative exercise testing to predict cardiac complications after arterial reconstruction. J Vasc Surg 7:60, 1988.
16. Gerson MC, Hurst JM, Hertzberg VS, et al: Cardiac prognosis in non-cardiac geriatric surgery. Ann Intern Med 103:832, 1985.
17. Kopecky SL, Gibbons RJ, Hollier LH: Preoperative supine exercise radionuclide angiogram predicts perioperative cardiovascular events in vascular surgery, abstracted. J Am Coll Cardiol 7:226A, 1986.
18. Goldman L, Hashimoto B, Cook EF, Loscalzo A: Comparative reproducibility and validity of systems for assessing cardiovascular functional class: advantages of a new specific activity scale. Circulation 64:1227, 1981.
19. Dripps RD, Lamont A, Eckenhoff JE: The role of anesthesia in surgical mortality. JAMA 178:261, 1961.
20. American Society of Anesthesiologists: New classification of physical status. Anesthesiology 24:111, 1963.
21. Goldman L, Caldera DL, Nussbaum SR, et al: Multifactorial index of cardiac risk in non-cardiac surgical procedures. N Engl J Med 297:845, 1977.
22. Goldman L, Caldera DL, Southwick FS, et al: Cardiac risk factors and complications in non-cardiac surgery. Medicine 57:357, 1978.
23. Detsky AS, Abrams HB, McLaughlin JR, et al: Predicting cardiac complications in patients undergoing non-cardiac surgery. J Gen Intern Med 1:211, 1986.
24. Detsky AS, Abrams HB, Forbath N, et al: Cardiac assessment for patients undergoing non-cardiac surgery: a multifactorial clinical risk index. Arch Intern Med 146:2131, 1986.
25. Eagle KA, Singer DE, Brewster DC, et al: Dipyridamole-thallium scanning in patients undergoing vascular surgery. JAMA 257:2185, 1987.
26. Eagle KA, Coley CM, Newell JB, et al: Combining clinical and thallium data optimizes preoperative assessment of cardiac risk before major vascular surgery. Ann Intern Med 110:859, 1989.
27. Lette J, Waters D, Bernier H, et al: Preoperative and long-term cardiac risk assessment: predictive value of 23 clinical descriptures,

7 multivariant scoring systems, and quantitative dipyridamole imaging in 360 patients. Ann Surg 216:192, 1992.
28. Coley CM, Field TS, Abraham SA, et al: Usefulness of dipyridamole-thallium scanning for preoperative evaluation of cardiac risk for non-vascular surgery. Am J Cardiol 69:1280, 1992.
29. Paul SD, L'Italien GJ, Hendel RC, et al: Long-term prognosis after geriatric vascular surgery: does preoperative clinical evaluation and dipyridamole-thallium testing make a difference? [abstract]. Circulation 88:I-11A, 1993.
30. Morrow CE, Schwartz JS, Sutherland DE, et al: Predictive value of thallium stress testing for coronary and cardiovascular events in uremic diabetic patients before renal transplantation. Am J Surg 146:331, 1983.
31. McPhail NV, Ruddy TD, Calvin JE, et al: Comparison of left ventricular function and myocardial perfusion for evaluating perioperative cardiac risk of abdominal aortic surgery. Can J Surg 33:224, 1990.
32. Kazmers A, Cerqueira MD, Zierler RE: The role of preoperative radionuclide ejection fraction in direct abdominal aortic aneurysm repair. J Vasc Surg 8:128, 1988.
33. Franco CD, Goldsmith J, Veith FJ, et al: Resting gated pool ejection fraction: a poor predictor of perioperative myocardial infarction in patients undergoing vascular surgery for infrainguinal bypass grafting. J Vasc Surg 10:656, 1989.
34. Mosley JG, Clarke JMF, Marston A: Assessment of myocardial function before aortic surgery by radionuclide angiocardiography. Br J Surg 72:886, 1985.
35. Pasternack PF, Imparato AM, Riles TS, et al: The value of the radionuclide angiogram in the prediction of perioperative myocardial infarction in patients undergoing lower extremity revascularization procedures. Circulation 72:II-13, 1985.
36. Pasternack PF, Imparato AM, Bear G, et al: The value of radionuclide angiography as a predictor of perioperative myocardial infarction in patients undergoing abdominal aortic aneurysm resection. J Vasc Surg 1:320, 1984.
37. Kubler W, Bretschneider HJ: Competitive inhibition of catalyzed adenosine diffusion as the mechanism of coronary dilating action of pyrimido-pyrimidine derivative. Pflugers Arch 280:141, 1964.
38. Alfonso S, O'Brien GS: Mechanism of enhancement of adenosine action by dipyridamole and lidoflazine in dogs. Arch Int Pharmacodyn Ther 194:181, 1971.
39. Meerdink DJ, Okada RD, Leppo JA: The effect of dipyridamole on transmural blood flow gradients. Chest 96:400, 1989.
40. Boucher CA, Brewster DC, Darling RC, et al: Determination of cardiac risk by dipyridamole-thallium imaging before peripheral vascular surgery. N Engl J Med 312:389, 1985.
41. Leppo J, Plaja J, Gionet M, et al: Non-invasive evaluation of cardiac risk before elective vascular surgery. J Am Coll Cardiol 9:269, 1987.
42. Lette J, Waters D, Lapointe J, et al: Usefulness of the severity and extent of reversible perfusion defects during thallium-dipyridamole imaging for cardiac risk assessment before non-cardiac surgery. Am J Cardiol 64:276, 1989.
43. Levinson JR, Boucher CA, Coley CM, et al: Usefulness of semiquantitative analysis of dipyridamole-thallium-201 redistribution for improving risk stratification before vascular surgery. Am J Cardiol 66:406, 1990.
44. Lane SE, Lewis SM, Pippin JJ, et al: Predictive value of quantitative dipyridamole-thallium scintigraphy in assessing cardiovascular risk after vascular surgery in diabetes mellitus. Am J Cardiol 64:1275, 1989.
45. Daum RM, Cremisi HD, Yeager A, et al: Dipyridamole-thallium imaging for determining perioperative and long-term prognosis in high-risk vascular disease patients. Circulation 77–78 (suppl 2):191, 1988.
46. Cutler BS, Hendel RC, Leppo JA: Dipyridamole-thallium scintigraphy predicts perioperative and long-term survival after major vascular surgery. J Vasc Surg 15:972, 1992.
47. Hendel RC, Whitfield SS, Villegas BJ, et al: Prediction of late cardiac events by dipyridamole-thallium imaging in patients undergoing elective vascular surgery. Am J Cardiol 70:1243, 1992.
48. Dilsizian V, Rocco TP, Freedman NMT, et al: Enhanced detection of ischemic but viable myocardium by the reinjection of thallium after stress-redistribution imaging. N Engl J Med 323:141, 1990.
49. Josephson MA, Brown BG, Hecht HS, et al: Non-invasive detection and localization of coronary stenosis in patients: comparison of resting dipyridamole and exercise thallium-201 myocardial perfusion imaging. Am Heart J 103:1008, 1982.
50. Leppo JA: Dipyridamole-thallium imaging: the lazy man's stress test. J Nucl Med 30:281, 1989.
51. Mangano DT, London MJ, Tubau JF, et al: Dipyridamole-thallium-201 scintigraphy as a perioperative screening test: a reexamination of its predictive potential. Circulation 84:493, 1991.
52. Marwick TH, Underwood DA: Dipyridamole-thallium imaging may not be a reliable screening test for coronary artery disease in patients undergoing vascular surgery. Clin Cardiol 13:14, 1990.
53. Elliott BM, Robison JG, Zellner JL, Hendrix GH: Dobutamine-201 Tl imaging: assessing cardiac risks associated with vascular surgery. Circulation 84:III-54, 1991.
54. Zellner JL, Elliott BM, Robison JG, et al: Preoperative evaluation of cardiac risk using dobutamine-thallium imaging in vascular surgery. Ann Vasc Surg 4:238, 1990.
55. Seveso G, Chiarella F, Previtali M, et al, for the EPIC Study Group: The prognostic value of dipyridamole-echocardiography early after uncomplicated acute myocardial infarction: updated results of the EPIC study [abstract]. J Am Coll Cardiol 19:100A, 1992.
56. Severi S, Michelassi C, Picano E, et al: The prognostic value of dipyridamole-echocardiography, exercise stress electrocardiography, and coronary angiography test in previous myocardial infarction [abstract]. J Am Coll Cardiol 19:100A, 1992.
57. Segar DS, Brown SE, Sawada SG, et al: Dobutamine stress echocardiography: correlation with coronary lesion severity as determined by quantitative angiography. J Am Coll Cardiol 19:1197, 1992.
58. Davila-Roman VG, Waggoner AD, Sicard GA, et al: Dobutamine stress echocardiography predicts surgical outcome in patients with an aortic aneurysm and peripheral vascular disease. J Am Coll Cardiol 21:957, 1993.
59. Langhan EM, Yourkey JR, Franklin DP, et al: Dobutamine stress echocardiography for cardiac risk assessment before aortic surgery. J Vasc Surg 18:905, 1993.
60. Lalka SG, Sawada SG, Dalsing MC, et al: Dobutamine stress echocardiography as a predictor of cardiac events associated with aortic surgery. J Vasc Surg 15:831, 1992.
61. Poldermans D, Rambaldi R, Fioretti PM, et al: Prognostic value of dobutamine-atropine stress echocardiography for peri-operative and late cardiac events in patients scheduled for vascular surgery. Eur Heart J 18(suppl D):D86, 1997.
62. Raby KE, Goldman L, Creager MA, et al: Correlation between preoperative ischemia and major cardiac events after peripheral vascular surgery. N Engl J Med 321:1296, 1989.
63. Mangano DT, Browner WS, Hollenberg M, et al: Association of perioperative myocardial ischemia with cardiac morbidity and mortality in men undergoing non-cardiac surgery. N Engl J Med 323:1781, 1990.
64. Raby KE, Barry J, Creager MA, et al: Detection and significance of intraoperative and postoperative myocardial ischemia and peripheral vascular surgery. JAMA 268:222, 1992.
65. Gewertz BL, Kremser PC, Zarins CK, et al: Transesophageal echocardiographic monitoring of myocardial ischemia during vascular surgery. J Vasc Surg 5:607, 1987.
66. Smith JS, Cahalan MK, Benefiel DJ, et al: Intraoperative detection of myocardial ischemia in high risk patients: electrocardiography versus two dimensional transesophageal echocardiography. Circulation 72:1015, 1985.
67. London MJ, Tubau JF, Wong MG, et al: The "natural history" of segmental wall motion abnormalities detected by intraoperative transesophageal echocardiography: a clinically blinded prospective approach [abstract]. Anesthesiology 69:A7, 1988.
68. Eisenberg MJ, London MJ, Leung JM, et al: Monitoring for myocardial ischemia during non-cardiac surgery: a technology assessment of transesophageal echocardiography and 12-lead electrocardiography. JAMA 68:210, 1992.
69. Hertzer NR, Young JR, Kramer JR, et al: Routine coronary angiography prior to elective aortic reconstruction. Arch Surg 114:1336, 1979.
70. Hertzer NR, Beven EG, Young JR, et al: Coronary artery disease in peripheral vascular patients: a classification of 1,000 coronary angiograms and results of surgical management. Ann Surg 199:223, 1984.
71. Hertzer NR, Young JR, Beven EG, et al: Late results of coronary bypass in patients with peripheral vascular disease: I. Five-year

survival according to age and clinical cardiac status. Cleve Clin J Med 53:133, 1986.

72. Hertzer NR, Young JR, Beven EG, et al: Late results of coronary bypass in patients with peripheral vascular disease. II: five-year survival according to sex, hypertension, and diabetes. Cleve Clin J Med 54:15, 1987.
73. Foster ED, Davis KB, Carpenter JA, et al: Risk of non-cardiac operation in patients with defined coronary disease: the Coronary Artery Surgery Study (CASS) Registry experience. Ann Thorac Surg 41:42, 1986.
74. Eagle KA, Rihal CS, Mickel MC, et al, for CASS Investigators and University of Michigan Heart Care Program: Cardiac risk of noncardiac surgery: influence of coronary artery disease and type of surgery in 3368 operations. Circulation 96:1882, 1997.
75. Huber KC, Evans MA, Bresnahan JF, et al: Outcome of noncardiac operations in patients with severe coronary artery disease successfully treated preoperatively with coronary angioplasty. Mayo Clin Proc 67:15, 1992.
76. Jones SE, Raymond RE, Whitlow PL, Simpfendorfer CC: Using coronary angioplasty as a bridge to major vascular surgery: is it helpful? Circulation 86(suppl I):11A, 1992.
77. Allen JR, Helling TS, Hartzler GO: Operative procedures not involving the heart after percutaneous transluminal coronary angioplasty. Surg Gynecol Obstet 173:285, 1991.
78. Elmore JR, Hallett JW, Gibbons RJ, et al: Myocardial revascularization before abdominal aortic aneurysmorrhaphy: effect of coronary angioplasty. Mayo Clin Proc 68: 637, 1993.
79. Eagle KA, Froehlich JB: Reducing cardiovascular risk in patients undergoing noncardiac surgery [editorial; comment]. N Engl J Med 335:1761, 1996.
80. Cohen MM, Duncan PG, Tate RB: Does anesthesia contribute to operative mortality? JAMA 260:2859, 1988.
81. Leung JM, Goehner P, O'Kelly BF, et al: Isoflurane anesthesia and myocardial ischemia: comparative risk versus sufentanil anesthesia in patients undergoing coronary artery bypass graft surgery. The SPI (Study of Perioperative Ischemia Group). Anesthesiology 74:838, 1991.
82. Baron JF, Bertrand M, Barre E, et al: Combined epidural and general anesthesia versus general anesthesia for abdominal aortic surgery. Anesthesiology 75:611, 1991.
83. Christopherson R, Beattie C, Frank SM, et al: Perioperative morbidity in patients randomised to epidural or general anesthesia for lower extremity vascular surgery: Perioperative Ischemia Randomized Anesthesia Trial Study Group. Anesthesiology 79:422, 1993.
84. Charlson ME, MacKenzie CR, Ales K, et al: Surveillance for post operative myocardial infarction after noncardiac operations. Surg Gynecol Obstet 167:404, 1988.
85. Rettke SR, Shub C, Naessen JM, et al: Significance of mildly elevated creatine kinase (myocardial band) activity after elective abdominal aneurysmectomy. J Cardiovasc Vasc Anesth 56:20, 1991.
86. Tikoff G, Keith TB, Nelson RM, Kuida H: Clinical and hemodynamic observations after closure of large atrial septal defects complicated by heart failure. Am J Cardiol 23:810, 1969.
87. Lueker RD, Vogel JH, Blount SG Jr: Cardiovascular abnormalities following surgery for left to right shunts: observations in atrial septal defects, ventricular septal defects and patent ductus arteriosus. Circulation 40:785, 1969.
88. Maron BJ, Humphries JO, Rowe RD, et al: Prognosis of surgically corrected coarctation of the aorta: a 20-year postoperative appraisal. Circulation 47:119, 1973.
89. Simon AB, Zloto AE: Coarctation of the aorta: longitudinal assessment of operated patients. Circulation 50:456, 1974.
90. James FW, Kaplan S, Schwartz DC, et al: Response to exercise in patients after total surgical correction of tetralogy of Fallot. Circulation 54:671, 1976.
91. Downing JW Jr, Kaplan S, Bove KE: Postsurgical left anterior hemiblock and right bundle branch block. Br Heart J 34:263, 1972.
92. Godman MJ, Roberts NK, Izukawa T: Late postoperative conduction disturbances after repair of ventricular septal defect and tetralogy of Fallot: analysis by His bundle recordings. Circulation 49:214, 1974.
93. Smith RM: Anesthesia for Infants and Children. 3rd ed. St. Louis: CV Mosby, 1968.
94. Skinner JF, Pierce ML: Surgical risk in the cardiac patient. J Chron Dis 17:57, 1964.
95. O'Keefe JH, Shub C, Rettke SR: Risk of noncardiac surgical procedures in patients with aortic stenosis. Mayo Clin Proc 64:400, 1989.
96. Levine MJ, Berman AD, Safian RD, et al: Palliation of valvular aortic stenosis by balloon valvuloplasty as preoperative preparation for noncardiac surgery. Am J Cardiol 62:1309, 1988.
97. Roth RB, Palacios IF, Block PC: Percutaneous aortic balloon valvuloplasty: its role in the management of patients with aortic stenosis requiring major noncardiac surgery. J Am Coll Cardiol 13:1039, 1989.
98. Hayes SN, Holmes DR, Nishimura RA, Reeder GS: Palliative percutaneous aortic balloon valvuloplasty before noncardiac operations and invasive diagnostic procedures. Mayo Clin Proc 64:753, 1989.
99. Bolen JL, Alderman EL: Hemodynamic consequences of afterload reduction in patients with chronic aortic regurgitation. Circulation 53:879, 1976.
100. Bonow RO, Ostrow HG, Rosing DR, et al: Effects of verapamil on left ventricular systolic and diastolic function in patients with hypertrophic cardiomyopathy: pressure volume analysis with a nonimaging scintillation probe. Circulation 68:1062, 1983.
101. Rosing DR, Kent KM, Maron BM, et al: Verapamil therapy: a new approach to the pharmacologic treatment of hypertrophic cardiomyopathy. Circulation 60:1208, 1969.
102. Thompson RC, Liberthson RR, Lowenstein E: Perioperative anesthetic risk of noncardiac surgery in hypertrophic obstructive cardiomyopathy. JAMA 254:2419, 1985.
103. Abraham SA, Coles NA, Coley CM, et al: Coronary risk of noncardiac surgery. Prog Cardiovasc Dis 34:205, 1991.

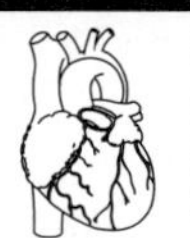

CHAPTER 113

ANESTHESIA FOR CARDIOVASCULAR OPERATIONS

N. Martin Giesecke, and John R. Cooper, Jr.

HISTORY
PREANESTHETIC PREPARATION
Preoperative Assessment
Premedication
Anesthesia Machines and Airway Devices
Intravenous Fluids
Operating Room Environment
Emergency Resuscitation Drugs
ANESTHETIC AGENTS
Characteristics
Uptake and Distribution of Inhaled Anesthetic Agents From the Lungs
Minimum Alveolar Concentration
Opioids
Induction Agents
Muscle Relaxants
MONITORING
Electrocardiography
Blood Pressure
Central Venous Cannulation and Pulmonary Artery Cannulation
Left Atrial Pressure
Electroencephalography
Oxygenation
Clinical Laboratory Studies
Temperature
Urine Output
Intraoperative Echocardiography
CONDUCT OF ANESTHESIA
Induction
Patient Positioning
Maintenance
Coronary Artery Disease
Aortic Stenosis
Aortic Insufficiency
Mitral Stenosis
Mitral Insufficiency
Left Ventricular Aneurysm or Cardiomyopathy
Thoracic or Vascular Operations
Cardiac Transplantation
Transfusion and Blood Conservation
Intraoperative Complications
Cardiopulmonary Bypass
TRANSFER TO CRITICAL CARE UNIT
POSTOPERATIVE CARE
SUMMARY

This chapter provides the practicing cardiologist with an overview of anesthetic management of adult patients who present for cardiac surgery. The management of each patient must, of course, be based on the unique clinical characteristics of the patient, the pathophysiologic mechanisms involved, and the requirements of the surgeon for an expeditious operation. More detailed information can be obtained from selected texts.[1–3]

HISTORY

The origins of cardiovascular anesthesia can be traced to anesthetics given to patients undergoing palliative surgery for congenital cardiovascular disease in the late 1930s and mid-1940s and "closed" valvular surgery in the late 1940s. The era of true "open heart" operations began with John Gibbon's[4] repair of an atrial septal defect by use of cardiopulmonary bypass (CPB) in 1953. Use of CPB was rapidly extended by many surgeons to acquired lesions, with most of these cases being valvular repairs or replacements, until the advent of the coronary artery bypass graft operation (CABG) in the late 1960s.

Anesthetic management of patients for these operations was developed in a highly empirical context because it was based on the clinical experience in a particular institution rather than on rigorous outcome studies. For this reason, significant variations could be found among institutions in the details of anesthetic management for a particular clinical circumstance. Although in some respects, the field has evolved past that point, significant institutional differences may still persist. Details of these techniques can be found in the cited texts. The management techniques discussed here reflect the clinical experience and research at the Texas Heart Institute (THI) and St. Luke's Episcopal Hospital since 1956.

The original anesthetic procedures, agents, and monitoring devices used in the early days of cardiac surgery were primitive by today's standards. Pulse quality and blood pressures could be monitored by the sphygmomanometer, but the continuous electrocardiograph (ECG) was not routinely used until the late 1950s. Direct intra-arterial blood pressure measurement was often not available, and early CPB surgery was performed without it. Interestingly, the electroencephalogram (EEG), still considered a relatively sophisticated monitor, was used as a measure of adequate cerebral perfusion during CPB at several institutions in the 1950s when arterial blood pressures could not be monitored.

Anesthetic agents themselves were limited. In the late 1940s and early 1950s, diethyl ether and cyclopropane (both highly flammable anesthetic gases) and nitrous oxide were available for inhalation, as was sodium thiopental for intravenous use. The presence of the pump oxygenator precluded the use of flammable anesthetic agents, and "balanced" anesthesia was therefore used. This technique employed a combination of drugs, usually an opioid, nitrous oxide, and a muscle relaxant, to achieve analgesia, amnesia, and immobility. This also permitted the use of the cautery, which markedly improved hemostasis. Halothane, the first potent nonflammable inhalational anesthetic agent, was introduced in 1956 and improved management by enabling very high concentrations of oxygen (97 to 99 percent) to be administered. Other advances in techniques and equipment, such as controlled rather than spontaneous ventilation during surgery, better resuscitation drugs, use of postoperative mechanical ventilation, and prolonged use of endotracheal tubes rather than early tracheostomy, gradually came into use.

The introduction in 1969 of a variation of the balanced anesthetic technique—use of oxygen and high-dose intravenous morphine plus muscle relaxation[5]—led to the use of other potent intravenous narcotics, such as fentanyl and its successors, for cardiac anesthesia. This anesthetic technique allowed surgical procedures to be performed on more clinically fragile patients, and it remains in use today.

Preanesthetic Preparation

Preoperative Assessment

The preoperative visit allows a review of pertinent history from the medical record and an interview with the patient covering the medical history, associated diseases, and drug therapy. Medication allergies or adverse responses to antibiotics, local anesthetics, and opioids are specifically noted, as are prior anesthetic experiences, such as nausea, vomiting, prolonged emergence from general anesthesia, difficulty with endotracheal intubation, or rarely, malignant hyperthermia. Specific points of the physical examination are also addressed. These include an airway evaluation aimed at detecting physical characteristics associated with difficult endotracheal intubation, such as prominent, loose, or fragile teeth; presence of dental prostheses; micrognathia; macroglossia; decreased mouth opening; decreased neck mobility; and decreased thyromental distance. Loose or fragile teeth may also become damaged during prolonged intubation, and the patient must be warned of this possibility. Assessment of vascular access, both venous and arterial (i.e., the presence and/or difference of peripheral pulses or blood pressures), is also performed. Laboratory values and invasive and noninvasive cardiac evaluations are reviewed. Perhaps most importantly, this interview affords the anesthesiologist an opportunity to establish a relationship with the patient that may markedly help reduce the patient's anxiety about the anesthetic and the surgery.

Premedication

Despite the calming effect of the preoperative visit, most patients do not desire to be fully alert on arrival at the operating room. Therefore, most anesthesiologists use some form of premedication to further decrease patient anxiety. These medications usually consist of a major tranquilizer and/or an opioid for sedation. Antisialagogues are perhaps not as important as in the past, but they are still useful in view of the fact that attempts at tracheal intubation may cause significant oropharyngeal secretions. Decreasing this secretory response may be especially important with anatomically difficult airways.

Because adults seldom develop reflex bradycardia from surgical stimulation of the vagus nerve, drugs such as atropine, used for both its vagolytic and its antisialagogic effects, are now rarely administered for vagolysis alone. In addition, there is uncertainty about the vagolytic efficacy of intramuscularly administered atropine. Indeed, vagolysis, with its attendant tachycardia, is undesirable in patients with coronary artery disease (CAD). Scopolamine has little vagolytic activity but provides amnestic and antiemetic effects and also decreases salivation; therefore, it is particularly useful in patients with CAD.

In addition to the usual premedication, other drugs can be added in particular circumstances. For example, the obese patient and the patient with gastroesophageal reflux may benefit from the addition of one of the histamine H_2-receptor antagonists (e.g., ranitidine, famotidine), to decrease gastric acidity, and metoclopramide, to improve gastric emptying. Use of these medications may reduce the incidence and/or the morbidity of aspiration of gastric contents during the course of an anesthetic.

Continuation of the patient's routine medications may also be of considerable importance in many cases. This is especially true of beta-blockers. Their discontinuance has been associated with an increased risk of angina and myocardial infarction (MI).[6] Withholding calcium channel blockers has not been associated with an increased risk of angina or MI.[7] Withdrawal of certain antihypertensive agents (especially clonidine) may cause significant rebound hypertension during the postoperative period. Antiarrhythmics are usually continued in patients with ischemia. Additional agents, such as antiparkinsonian, antipsychotic, and antiseizure medications, although they may have possible synergistic effects with anesthetic agents, are usually not discontinued. These medications can be given orally with a small amount of water until an hour or two before surgery. Major anticoagulants, such as warfarin (Coumadin), should be discontinued in elective cases, with conversion to intravenous heparin if anticoagulation is critical. Antiplatelet agents (e.g., dipyridamole, aspirin) may be associated with mild increases in bleeding tendency, but this is usually not significant enough to postpone cardiac surgery. Newer, more potent antiplatelet agents are discussed later. Digitalis, unless used for ventricular rate control, is typically not given on the day of surgery because of the potential for acute swings in potassium levels perioperatively and resultant digitalis toxicity.

Management of diabetic patients is somewhat controversial, but in our experience, those receiving oral agents and stable patients receiving insulin can be easily managed with the usual NPO regimen and withholding of hypoglycemics. "Brittle" insulin-dependent patients may require insulin infusion after being NPO. "Tight" control of blood sugar during cardiac operations is also controversial, being impossible in many cases and unnecessary in most. Nevertheless, there is mounting evidence that persistent hyperglycemia in diabetic patients is associated with a greater likelihood of postoperative wound infection.

For elective cases, the amount of time that a patient must abstain from ingestion of liquids or solids is still considered controversial. Nevertheless, most anesthesiologists recommend a period of at least 4 hours and would probably feel more comfortable with 6 hours. Periods of less than 4 hours, as may be necessary in patients who present for emergency procedures, may call for rapid-sequence induction of anesthesia to decrease the chance of regurgitation and aspiration during induction. Unfortunately, rapid-sequence induction may create problems in certain patients with cardiovascular disease in whom it is desirable to avoid the hypertension and tachycardia that often accompany this technique. Additional pharmacologic intervention with intravenous β-blockers or vasodilators may be necessary during induction of these patients.

Anesthesia Machines and Airway Devices

The modern anesthesia machine allows administration of compressed gases (air, oxygen, and nitrous oxide) from either a central hospital or a local (gas tanks on the anesthesia machine) supply. These machines consist of flowmeters for measuring the amount of gas administered, calibrated vaporizers for the delivery of volatile inhalational anesthetics, a ventilator with monitors, the breathing circuit (which in most cases consists of a circle system with carbon dioxide absorption) and integrated monitors of oxygen level in the anesthetic circuit (oxygen analyzer), patient oxygen saturation (pulse oximeter), and patient expired CO_2 (capnography).[2] Capnography confirms endotracheal intubation and adequate ventilation. It can also give indications of cardiac output, bronchospasm, and air embolism.

Airway devices, in addition to those usually employed (laryngoscopes, endotracheal tubes, face masks, oral and nasal airways), include fiberoptic bronchoscopes and laryngeal masks to assist with difficult intubations, double-lumen endotracheal tubes to allow lung isolation, and injectors to permit transtracheal ventilation if the patient cannot be ventilated by standard means.

Intravenous Fluids

Balanced salt solutions, such as lactated Ringer's solution (with or without dextrose) are the most common intravenous fluids administered during cardiac or vascular surgery. Compensation for relative hypovolemia in hypertensive patients, vasodilatation from anesthetic agents, and use of crystalloid priming solutions with "third spacing" during CPB may require large volumes of fluid to be given. Patients tend to retain this fluid and without diuretics may not experience spontaneous diuresis for 3 to 5 days. In some patients, pulmonary dysfunction or even overt cardiac failure may result. Also, metabolism of lactate tends to produce mild metabolic alkalosis.

Operating Room Environment

Operating room temperature is controlled at levels dictated by the clinical situation. Operating rooms are often kept quite cool to aid in systemic hypothermia and for the comfort of personnel. Significant decreases in patient temperature (to 33° or 34°C) may occur after sternotomy. Because of the large surface area exposed, this heat loss cannot be effectively prevented, even by measures such as heated breathing circuits, warmed intravenous fluids, and thermal mattresses.

Emergency Resuscitation Drugs

As part of the preoperative preparation, anesthesiologists usually prepare the drugs listed in Table 113–1 to be used in case of emergencies, thus significantly shortening the response time. Bolus administration of these drugs rather than infusion is preferred, because an immediate dose-response relationship is generated and a drug's effectiveness or lack thereof can be assessed. Infusions are not routinely prepared, because most patients need bolus administration only. If a sustained effect is desired, an infusion can then be used.

ANESTHETIC AGENTS

Characteristics

The anesthesiologist must consider the various hemodynamic effects of anesthetic agents (Table 113–2) in planning the anesthetic management of a given patient. This choice should take into account the specific pathologic process, the operation itself, and other factors, such as the patient's physical condition and the anesthesiologist's preferences and experience.

Uptake and Distribution of Inhaled Anesthetic Agents From the Lungs

The pharmacologic effects of volatile anesthetics in producing general anesthesia are exerted primarily in the brain and vary with the partial pressure of the drug in cerebral tissues. The partial pressure of the drug in the brain is the same as the partial pressure in the arterial blood because there is no restriction of movement across the blood-brain barrier. Assuming normal circulation, the arterial tension is dependent on, and identical to, the alveolar tension of the agent. Rapid achievement of an alveolar tension constitutes

TABLE 113–1 Resuscitation Drugs*

Medication	Concentration	Usual Dose
Calcium chloride	100 mg/ml	250 mg–1 g
Ephedrine	5 mg/ml	10–20 mg
Epinephrine	10 μg/ml	5–10 μm
Epinephrine	100 μg/ml	100–500 μm
Isoproterenol	20 μg/ml	2–10 μm
Phenylephrine	100 μg/ml	50–100 μm
Trimethaphan	3 mg/ml	3–15 mg

*Atropine, propranolol, labetolol, lidocaine, bretylium, and nitroglycerin are immediately available for bolus infusion but are not placed in syringes.

TABLE 113–2 Characteristics of Anesthetic Agents

Anesthetic Agent	Heart Rate	Myocardial Contractility	Systemic Vascular Resistance
Desflurane	Increase, dose-dependent	Mild decrease, dose-dependent	Mild decrease
Enflurane	No change	Moderate decrease, dose-dependent	Moderate decrease
Halothane	No change	Marked decrease, dose-dependent	Mild decrease
Isoflurane	Increase	Mild decrease, dose-dependent	Mild decrease
Sevoflurane	No change	Mild decrease, dose-dependent	Mild decrease
Nitrous oxide	No change	Mild decrease	Minor increase
Fentanyl	Decrease	None	Minor decrease
Meperidine	Decrease	Minor decrease by metabolites	Minor decrease
Morphine	Decrease	None	Mild decrease
Sufentanil	Decrease	None	Minor decrease

the induction of anesthesia with that particular agent. The rise in alveolar tension directly affects the speed of induction. The rate of rise of the alveolar tension is dependent on factors that affect uptake of the agent from the patient's lungs. These include the patient's alveolar ventilation and cardiac output and the blood solubility of the anesthetic agent. As alveolar ventilation increases, the alveolar concentration of any particular agent increases. Hypoventilation, on the other hand, decreases the rate of rise. Cardiac output affects alveolar tension in the following manner: the higher the cardiac output, the more blood delivered to the alveoli. When more blood is delivered to the alveoli, more anesthetic agent dissolves into that blood and is carried away from the lungs. Therefore, it takes longer for that agent to build a high alveolar tension. Low cardiac output, and therefore less blood passing the alveoli, promotes a rapid rise in alveolar tension, and the patient therefore falls asleep rapidly. Blood solubility also affects the rate of alveolar tension rise. Agents that are relatively insoluble in blood (e.g., nitrous oxide, desflurane) achieve a rapid rise in alveolar tension because little of the agent is lost by being dissolved into the blood itself. Soluble agents, conversely, rapidly dissolve into blood, and the alveolar tension rise is delayed despite the fact that large quantities of the anesthetic may be absorbed into the blood. Awakening after anesthesia reverses the process, and the blood gas solubility determines the awakening time.

Minimum Alveolar Concentration

Minimum alveolar concentration is a term used to indicate inhalational anesthetic potency. It is the amount of anesthetic that will prevent movement in response to a noxious stimulus in 50 percent of patients. The different minimum alveolar concentration values provide the anesthesiologist with the ability to relate the potency of one inhalational anesthetic agent to that of another.

Opioids

The natural (morphine) and the synthetic (meperidine, fentanyl, sufentanil) opioids have profound analgesic properties and are useful in high doses for the maintenance of cardiac patients because of the relatively benign effects of these agents on hemodynamics. They generally produce a mild decrease in heart rate, reduce left ventricular (LV) systolic pressure and end-diastolic volume, have no effect on sympathetic responsiveness, and, most importantly, have little effect on contractility.

Induction Agents

These drugs, given intravenously, provide rapid suppression of consciousness, allowing control of the patient's airway and administration of inhalational agents, which most patients find noxious. They have many hemodynamic effects. Some, such as thiopental and propofol, reduce LV systolic pressure, sympathetic responsiveness, and myocardial contractility. Others, such as the major tranquilizers diazepam and midazolam, have little or no effect on sympathetic responsiveness or myocardial contractility but many cause mild vasodilatation. In the selection of agents, patients with good ventricular function or hypertension are often induced with thiopental, whereas those with poor myocardial function or hypovolemia often receive diazepam or midazolam induction.

Muscle Relaxants

Muscle relaxants are needed to facilitate endotracheal intubation, to aid in surgical exposure, and to prevent patient movement during critical periods during surgery. They can be classified into two different groups. The first group, the depolarizing agents, includes only one clinically used drug: succinylcholine. This agent mimics acetylcholine at the neuromuscular junction, causing a depolarization of the junction, followed by muscle relaxation, through competitive inhibition of acetylcholine. It is commonly used as the initial muscle relaxant or for emergent intubations because the muscle relaxation it provides has the most rapid onset of action. Succinylcholine has other important characteristics, including a very short duration of action and a potential to cause arrhythmias. In certain conditions (e.g., extensive burns, paraplegia, and some other neuromuscular disorders), it may cause hyperkalemia, and its use has been associated with malignant hyperthermia in susceptible patients.

The second group, the nondepolarizing agents, is considerably larger. These agents block the affects of acetylcholine at the neuromuscular junction without also activating the acetylcholine receptor, as does succinylcholine. There are several agents in this group, the prototype being D-tubocurarine. These agents may have various hemodynamic side effects, which are detailed in Table 113–3. In addition, there are considerable variations in the duration of action of these agents. A common muscle relaxant used in cardiac surgery is pancuronium, the atropine-like vagolysis of which counteracts the bradycardia that may result from the

TABLE 113-3 Nondepolarizing Muscle Relaxants

Muscle Relaxant	Hemodynamic Consequences
Atracurium	Hypotension with reflex tachycardia
D-Tubocurarine	Hypotension with reflex tachycardia
Pancuronium	Tachycardia
Vecuronium	None
Doxacurium	None
Mivacurium	Minimal hypotension with reflex tachycardia
Pipecuronium	None

use of large doses of narcotics during anesthetic induction. These agents are all reversible by administration of an anticholinesterase.

MONITORING

Electrocardiography

Electrocardiographic monitoring is now standard practice in all operating rooms. In most programs, continuous dual-lead electrocardiographs are used, commonly leads II and V_5. Lead II is used primarily for detection of arrhythmias and monitoring of the inferior surface of the heart for ischemia; V_5 provides the most sensitive method of monitoring ischemia over the anterior and lateral regions of the heart. Calibration of these leads so that they can be compared with preoperative ECGs is a part of sensible monitoring.

Blood Pressure

Although it is appropriate for many anesthetics to be administered with noninvasive methods of monitoring blood pressure, direct intra-arterial blood pressure monitoring is routine in cardiac surgery. This is most commonly achieved through a catheter inserted into the patient's radial artery, with alternative sites including the ulnar, brachial, femoral, or axillary arteries or the dorsal artery of the foot. The ability to perform continuous beat-to-beat blood pressure monitoring is absolutely essential for any open-heart surgery, except under the most unusual circumstances, and contemporary disposable transducer systems make this very easy to accomplish.

Central Venous Cannulation and Pulmonary Artery Cannulation

Catheterization of the central veins is also a basic technique performed almost universally for cardiovascular surgery. The most common approach is via the subclavian or the internal jugular vein, with occasional use of other sites. The internal jugular vein is preferred by most anesthesiologists because of ease of insertion, accessibility, and a lower incidence of major complications (pneumothorax or arterial puncture with resultant hemothorax). Central venous catheterization affords not only the ability to monitor filling pressures but also a central route for administration of fluids, blood, and vasoactive drugs.

Routine use of the pulmonary artery catheter (PAC) in cardiovascular surgery patients, although widespread, is controversial. Monitoring pulmonary artery pressure and, pulmonary capillary occlusion pressure and obtaining an indication of left-sided filling pressures and volumes appear to be important in patients in whom the ventricular function is disparate, but this is seldom the case in patients undergoing CABG. The use of this catheter has never been documented to specifically improve the outcome of patients who undergo cardiovascular surgical procedures. In addition, on occasion, PAC insertion has been associated with major complications. Nevertheless, some programs consider it a mandatory form of monitoring. The PAC may be useful in certain instances. For example, it allows determination of systemic vascular resistance and permits more rational use of vasodilators in patients requiring an intra-aortic balloon pump. However, as this group of patients makes up only 5 percent of those undergoing cardiac surgery, and because we have consistently been unable to preoperatively predict the patients who would benefit from PAC, we choose not to use this device before surgery in most patients. We believe that its significant risks and cost, without proven benefits, do not justify its routine use.

Left Atrial Pressure

In some centers, measurement of left atrial pressure after cardiac surgery is routine. Physicians in these institutions believe that the use of a left atrial catheter gives immediate indication of left-sided filling pressures and volumes and some indication of myocardial function. Because of the potential for bleeding on removal of the catheter, these devices have not gained wide acceptance. At THI, they are used occasionally in patients who have difficulty being weaned from CPB.

Electroencephalography

The EEG has been used, as mentioned earlier, since the earliest days of cardiac surgery. A large range of devices is now available, including the classical multiple-lead system, computerized spectral arrays or other types of "processed" EEG, and simple bifrontal three-lead monitoring, as is performed at THI. The major purpose of EEG use is, as in the 1950s, for gross monitoring of brain activity, and therefore gross perfusion, during CPB. It is quite sensitive and specific for this purpose. However, because only one region of the brain is monitored with bifrontal EEG, nothing can be determined concerning regional blood flow or occurrence of emboli. Nevertheless, EEG is sensitive to administration of anesthetics, can be used as a crude monitor of anesthetic depth, and permits the monitoring of therapeutic interventions, such as suppression of electroencephalographic activity by thiopental, as when it is administered to patients at risk of cerebral ischemia. It may also provide information during resuscitation as to the adequacy of the measures taken and the need to continue.

Oxygenation

The noninvasive pulse oximeter, a standard monitoring tool for all patients undergoing general or regional anesthesia, affords a quick, usually accurate, indication of arterial oxygen saturation. It may be susceptible to various environmental effects often present in the operating room during cardiovascular surgery. For example, ambient light and electrocautery may diminish the probe's ability to function properly. Peripheral vasoconstriction related to systemic hypothermia or administration of vasopressors may decrease the accuracy of the device or even preclude its use altogether. It cannot be used during CPB.

Clinical Laboratory Studies

A routine requirement for any active cardiovascular surgical program is the ability to obtain accurate, rapid analysis of blood samples for arterial blood gases, electrolytes, hematocrit, hemoglobin, and glucose. Accuracy, of course, is always important, but in this clinical setting, rapidity of analysis is also a requirement. A turnaround time of 10 minutes or less is reasonable for most critical laboratory analyses, including those mentioned earlier.

Intraoperative coagulation monitoring has proved to be an area in need of reliable and rapid laboratory assessment. Expedient monitors, like the activated clotting time, tend to be so nonspecific that they often cannot guide useful therapy. Standard tests, such as prothrombin time, partial thromboplastin time, platelet count, and platelet function assessment, require longer to perform and report, despite advances in measurement machinery. More specific devices, which look at the entire coagulation cascade, have been in use for some time and may be useful in specific cases, but they have not gained wide acceptance.

Temperature

Monitoring of the anesthetized patient's temperature is, of course, standard in all cases. It is particularly important in patients undergoing cardiovascular surgery because of the necessary extremes in temperature to which the patient may be subjected. The standard monitoring site is the nasopharynx because this placement gives the most easily achieved and, best estimate of brain temperature.[8] Rectal or bladder temperatures (core temperatures) may also be used in some institutions. Esophageal temperatures are not usually considered accurate because of the proximity of the esophagus to the aorta, where relatively rapid blood temperature changes may take place, and to the trachea, where air flow may heat or cool the esophageal probe.

Urine Output

Monitoring of urine output is used as an indirect indicator of renal function and cardiac output. The presence of urine flow indicates adequate glomerular perfusion, and absence of flow leads to examination of factors that contribute to adequate cardiac function and output (filling volumes, contractility). No specific urine flow rate is associated with good function, nor is it predictive of postoperative function. In certain patients during CPB, despite good renal perfusion, urine output may fall markedly, presumably owing to lack of pulsatile flow. The specific mechanisms responsible in these patients are obscure, and this fall in urine output is not associated with poor function after surgery. Using modern CPB techniques, the only predictor of poor postoperative renal function is abnormal preoperative renal function.[9]

Intraoperative Echocardiography

Intraoperative echocardiography is considered useful, and in certain cases mandatory, for evaluation of mitral valve repair and for aid in the diagnosis of aortic dissections. Echocardiography can also be used to assess ventricular filling volume, myocardial contractility, and presence of atheromatous plaque in the thoracic aortic. It has also been proposed as a monitor of ischemia by assessing regional wall motion abnormalities via the short-axis view of the left ventricle. However, specific problems with sensitivity and specificity of this mode of monitoring have not been resolved, and this application is controversial.[10]

Anesthesiologists have become involved with operating room echocardiography in many centers. Although questions remain about training and credentialing, our belief is that this process must occur in concert with cardiologists and an appropriate quality assessment program.

Conduct of Anesthesia

Induction

The potent halogenated inhalational agents (halothane, enflurane, isoflurane) have in common the primary actions of depressing myocardial contractility, blocking central sympathetic outflow, and depressing reflexes that are normally active in circulatory compensation (see Table 113–2). It was observed early in the history of cardiovascular anesthesia that patients whose hearts were compensating to generate adequate cardiac output (e.g., mitral valve disease, ventricular aneurysm) tolerated potent inhalational agents poorly because high sympathetic tone was required in the compensation. Potent inhalational agents, even in low doses, reduce myocardial contractility and sympathetic outflow and may result in marked hypotension. For these patients, intravenous opioids supplemented with nitrous oxide, a technique that does not depress contractility or sympathetic outflow, have become the anesthetic of choice.

By contrast, patients with coronary occlusive disease and aortic stenosis usually have normal or near-normal myocardial muscle and are highly reactive to increases in sympathetic tone. These patients experience an inadequate blood supply to a usually nonfailing myocardium and require an anesthetic technique that is directed primarily toward decreasing myocardial oxygen demand. This can be accomplished most simply by potent halogenated inhalational agents, which decrease myocardial work by depressing contractility, blood pressure (afterload), and, at times, heart rate. Other institutions prefer to use high-dose opioids even for these patients, with reliance on vasodilators to decrease preload (pulmonary artery occlusion pressure) and afterload (systemic vascular resistance) while maintaining high contractility and cardiac output. Effective use of the opioid-based technique often requires intraoperative use of a PAC to measure cardiac output and to monitor preload and afterload. Outcome data indicate that neither technique is superior to the other for patients undergoing cardiac surgery.[11] A summary of clinical conditions and anesthetic agent choices is found in Table 113–4.

In evaluating patients preoperatively, indices of LV function, such as ejection fraction and LV end-diastolic pressure, have not proved to be reliable predictors of the response of the ventricle to potent inhalational anesthetics. Patients with CAD and regional hypokinesis with LV ejection fractions estimated as low as 20 to 30 percent often experience hypertension and tachycardia in response to surgical stimulation. During opioid-based anesthesia, they require supplementation with inhalational anesthetics to depress contractility and control hypertension. These patients represent a good example of why flexibility in anesthetic management must be retained. Conversely, some normotensive patients with "good" ventricles are intolerant of inhalational anesthetics and require a change to an opioid technique.

On arrival to the operating room, patients for open-heart surgery are initially monitored with electrocardiography and pulse oximetry while intravenous and intra-arterial catheters are inserted. A calibrated ECG is assessed and compared with the preoperative ECG to permit detection of myocardial ischemia. A printed copy of the initial ECG is retained. If significant ischemia, manifested as ST depression, is found and is not resolved with intravenous β-blockade or nitroglycerin, induction of anesthesia should proceed because ischemia may improve in the face of general anesthesia.

As noted earlier, patients with good myocardial function are induced with thiopental or propofol because the myocardial depressant effects of these agents are generally well tolerated in this population. Those patients with poor cardiac function are usually induced with diazepam or midazolam because these medications do not cause significant myocardial depression. Other agents can also be used. These agents are then supplemented with an opioid, most commonly fentanyl, although sufentanil, morphine, or meperidine may serve equally well in most patients.

TABLE 113–4 Choice of Primary Anesthetic by Disease Based on Myocardial Depression

Narcotic-Based Anesthetic	Halogen-Based Anesthetic
Mitral stenosis or insufficiency	Coronary artery disease
Aortic insufficiency	Aortic stenosis
Ventricular aneurysm	Aortic aneurysm
Coronary artery disease with ventricular failure	Idiopathic hypertrophic subaortic stenosis
Cardiomyopathy	
Constrictive pericarditis	
Cardiac tamponade	

The administration of an opioid at this stage serves three purposes: (1) it speeds induction, (2) it provides "baseline" anesthesia to which inhalational agents can be added if indicated, and (3) it depresses respiration to allow postoperative mechanical ventilation for a desired 4 to 6 hours, which is the case in most open-heart operations. Muscle relaxation, usually provided by pancuronium, is used for intubation. Very often, especially in patients with CAD, β-blockers such as propranolol, esmolol, and metoprolol may have to be given intravenously before administration of pancuronium because of the vagolytic (positive chronotropic) effects of this muscle relaxant, or if the patient's preoperative heart rate is elevated. In other patients with slow or normal heart rates, pancuronium may prevent the undesirable bradycardia that sometimes accompanies larger doses of intravenous opioids. When necessary, an inhalational agent is added at this point to decrease systemic blood pressure before intubation and to attenuate hypertension and tachycardia in response to laryngoscopy. In patients with poor ventricular function, induction may produce immediate hypotension, and intubation may cause a desirable increase in blood pressure. Halogenated inhalational agents are administered after intubation as necessary to control blood pressure, although many patients' pressures decrease as a result of lack of further stimulation until surgical incision. After intubation, insertion of further peripheral and central venous catheters proceeds.

Patient Positioning

At THI, patients are usually placed in a "hands-up" position with anterior displacement and internal rotation of the shoulders by the use of specially designed foam wedges. This position minimizes brachial plexus injury,[12] especially with sternal incisions; a secondary benefit is that continuous access to cannulas and monitoring leads is ensured with the arms positioned in this manner. Brachial plexus injury may also be associated with use of special retractors for harvesting the internal mammary artery.

Maintenance

Problems encountered between intubation and onset of CPB typically relate to the following: an initial lack of surgical stimulation during the time between anesthetic induction and skin incision; abrupt surgical stimulation by skin incision or sternotomy; and manipulation of the heart and great vessels during cannulation of the atrium and aorta. Hypertension and/or hypotension, with or without myocardial ischemia, may occur, requiring measures to be taken by the anesthesiologist. The specific response depends on the clinical situation at the time.

Hypertension is usually treated by increasing anesthetic depth and administration of vasodilators as needed. Tachycardia can also be dealt with by increasing depth of anesthesia and β-blockade. Hypotension is best treated with vasopressors that minimally affect heart rate (e.g., phenylephrine, ephedrine). Myocardial ischemia with hemodynamic aberrations requires correction of the hemodynamics plus treatment of ischemia (e.g., β-blockade, nitroglycerin).

Ischemia occurring with normal hemodynamics is discussed later. If marked myocardial ischemia persists despite therapy, the surgeon must be informed and CPB rapidly instituted.

Coronary Artery Disease

The intraoperative occurrence of myocardial ischemia in CAD patients is of particular concern. From the early days of CABG until the mid-1980s, it was generally believed that most episodes of intraoperative myocardial ischemia were related to hemodynamic aberrations (hypertension, hypotension, tachycardia, or bradycardia) that occurred during surgery. However, pioneering work by Slogoff and Keats[13] showed that although hemodynamic abnormalities could contribute to myocardial ischemia and could, in the worst cases, affect both morbidity and mortality of patients undergoing CABG, there was a significant incidence of myocardial ischemia that was not related to any hemodynamic alteration. This ischemia, which almost certainly corresponds to "silent" ischemia in the awake patient, proved to be a significant marker for morbidity and mortality during coronary artery operations, despite the best anesthetic management. Although most anesthesiologists are convinced that any myocardial ischemia, whether hemodynamically or nonhemodynamically related, should be treated, at the present time it is not known, nor is it apparent from current research, whether treating this nonhemodynamically related ischemia contributes to a significant improvement in morbidity and mortality.

Patients with left main coronary artery stenosis deserve special mention because they appear to be particularly intolerant of significant hypotension. If this occurs, or if such a patient shows ischemic changes on the ECG and does not respond to therapy, then CPB must be used quickly to prevent rapid deterioration.

Aortic Stenosis

As mentioned earlier, patients with aortic stenosis usually have nonfailing myocardiums with the potential for critically decreased coronary blood supply because of the stenosed aortic valve. Anesthetic management is directed at decreasing myocardial oxygen demand. In general, these patients do not tolerate tachycardia well, because of the decrease in myocardial blood supply and the somewhat fixed cardiac output. They are also intolerant of significant hypotension. Typically, their anesthetic management is very similar to that of patients with CAD.

Aortic Insufficiency

Patients with aortic insufficiency may have a failing myocardium, usually have significant volume overload, and classically have a decreased coronary perfusion pressure because of their decreased diastolic pressure. They may tolerate bradycardia poorly because it tends to increase the time for regurgitation to occur. Although decreasing systemic vascular resistance in an attempt to decrease the regurgitant volume might in theory seem to be a good idea, reduction of coronary perfusion pressure would also accompany this type of therapy. Most anesthesiologists choose a technique that tends to avoid bradycardia and maintains afterload within a normal range.

Mitral Stenosis

Patients with mitral stenosis are characterized by volume overload, fixed cardiac output, and usually normal ventricular function. However, they often require a relatively high sympathetic tone to maintain this physiologic state. They tolerate tachycardia and hypovolemia poorly, and techniques that tend to maintain normovolemia and a normal heart rate are therefore used. Patients with mitral stenosis who experience pulmonary edema associated with tachycardia exhibit clinical improvement of their pulmonary edema when given β-blockers to slow the heart rate.

Mitral Insufficiency

Patients with mitral insufficiency are characterized by volume overload of the left side of the heart and may not tolerate bradycardia well. Of note in these patients is the fact that cardiac output can be significantly increased by decreasing afterload. Placement of a PAC, enabling measurement of cardiac output and calculation of systemic vascular resistance and manipulation of that resistance, may be useful for increasing cardiac output.

Left Ventricular Aneurysm or Cardiomyopathy

Patients with LV aneurysm or cardiomyopathy are obviously characterized by a failing myocardium, and anesthetic management is directed toward maintenance of myocardial contractility and cardiac output. Because of volume overload, these patients tend to tolerate vasodilating agents relatively well but may require significant inotropic support, especially after CPB.

Thoracic or Vascular Operations

The principles of anesthetic management for patients undergoing cardiovascular or thoracic surgery is essentially the same as for any cardiac surgery. These patients may have significant, perhaps uncorrectable, cardiac disease, especially coronary artery stenosis. Therefore, management and maintenance are usually directed toward decreasing the incidence of myocardial ischemia, even though critical CAD may not have been previously documented.

Cardiac Transplantation

Patients undergoing cardiac transplantation are managed in a manner similar to those with LV aneurysm or cardiomyopathy. They tend to tolerate general anesthesia relatively well because they typically present in a volume-overloaded state, enabling them to tolerate some degree of vasodilatation caused by anesthetic agents. Anesthetic techniques usually consist of combinations of agents that do not further depress myocardial function during the period before the institution of CPB.

After completion of the transplant procedure, the anesthesiologist's main goal is pharmacologic support of the newly transplanted organ. This usually involves the use of agents that may promote pulmonary vasodilatation, such as dobutamine, milrinone, and isoproterenol, although other agents or multiple drug combinations may be required for successful support of the patient. Although still considered experimental, nitric oxide has proved useful in patients with acute pulmonary hypertensive episodes.[14]

Transfusion and Blood Conservation

Cardiac operations or major vascular noncardiac operations often require transfusion of blood or blood products, at times in large volumes. The anesthesiologist is also often involved in techniques of blood conservation, many of which are quite popular now because of concerns about transfusion of blood products contaminated with infectious agents. Blood conservation methods include the use of bypass suction as much as possible, cell salvaging (especially in noncardiac cases), reinfusion of shed mediastinal blood in cardiac cases, and, in some centers, removal of autologous blood before bypass for transfusion immediately after bypass (this blood may be more useful in the promotion of coagulation, having not been exposed to the extracorporeal circuit). Presurgical autologous blood donation by patients scheduled for cardiovascular surgery has been shown to be of significant impact in reducing banked blood use,[15] but on a cost utilization basis, it is an inefficient practice.[16] In addition, although the practice of predonation by cardiac surgical candidates has been shown to be uneventful in certain situations,[17] because of the anemia that necessarily follows such a donation, the risks must be thoroughly considered for patients with ischemic cardiovascular disease.[18–20]

Another factor of blood conservation involves the increasing use of perioperative antifibrinolytic medications. The synthetic lysine analogs, epsilon aminocaproic acid and tranexamic acid, have been used for the treatment of postcardiopulmonary bypass bleeding since the 1960s and the 1980s, respectively. Aprotinin is a naturally occurring protease inhibitor that is present even in human plasma. In several studies, aprotinin appears more effective than ϵ-aminocaproic acid or tranexamic acid in decreasing postoperative bleeding in the cardiac surgery patient. In the past, antifibrinolytics were used with questionable effect when given only after the diagnosis of postcardiopulmonary bypass bleeding had been made. Although their mechanism of action is still not completely understood, current approaches to therapy with antifibrinolytics involve prophylactic administration before initiation of cardiopulmonary bypass.[21, 22] We tend to use antifibrinolytics only in "redo" surgical procedures because their use in primary operations is of relatively minor benefit (i.e., these patients' need for homologous blood products is minimal). There has been controversy surrounding the use of aprotinin, with some experts believing that there is an increased risk of acute coronary graft failure[23, 24]; others have not found this.[25]

The development of long-acting, potent platelet inhibitors (e.g. ticlopidine, clopidogrel, and abciximab) has allowed clinicians to provide a previously unavailable degree of antithrombolytic therapy to patients at risk for myocardial ischemia.[26–29] Unfortunately, a small percentage of patients who receive these agents in conjunction with coronary angioplasty or stent insertion procedures require emergency surgical intervention. In this subset of patients, prior use of the platelet inhibitor can have profound effects on perioperative hemostasis, especially with abciximab, with the requirement for significant transfusion of blood products.[30–32] Currently, for patients who have received these agents before elective surgery, we measure platelet function before the onset of CPB. A normal prebypass platelet function precludes the need for immediate platelet transfusion after bypass. Those patients presenting for emergent surgery and who have received one of these medications typically receive platelet transfusions at the surgeon's request, as a prophylactic measure. These same patients receive other blood products, as indicated by laboratory studies of coagulation. Shorter-acting platelet inhibitors, such as eptifibatide and tirofiban, may obviate some of these concerns.[33, 34]

Germane to the discussion of transfusion is what constitutes an acceptable hemoglobin and/or hematocrit level in these patients. For patients undergoing CPB, hemodilution is a component of the procedure in almost all cases because of the use of crystalloid primes in the bypass circuit. High postoperative hematocrit values ($\geq$34 percent) have even been shown to be associated with greater risk of Q-wave MI, values worsened LV function and mortality after coronary bypass grafting.[35] In noncardiovascular surgical cases, it has been shown that hemoglobin values greater than 8 mg/dl, as opposed to the long-acknowledged value of 10 mg/dl, are associated with an acceptable postoperative outcome.[12, 36]

Intraoperative Complications

Cardiac arrhythmias are particularly common during open-heart operations, the vast majority being caused by manipulation of the heart. Very often, premature atrial and ventricular contractions or supraventricular tachyarrhythmias occur during cannulation, especially of the right atrium. These usually abate when manipulation ceases. Occasionally, malignant arrhythmias, such as supraventricular tachycardia, atrial fibrillation with a rapid ventricular response, and ventricular tachycardia or fibrillation require cardioversion, with or without pharmacologic therapy.

Hypotension is also common during cardiac operations. It can be caused by decreased cardiac output secondary to manipulation of the heart, blood loss, arrhythmia, myocardial ischemia, mechanical defect of the heart, and, of course, anesthetic drugs. Concerning decreased blood pressure caused by anesthesia, it is natural for blood pressure to fall at that time, as it is natural for the blood pressure to fall when a patient falls asleep in the unanesthetized state.

It is, in fact, necessary for the anesthesiologist to lower blood pressure to permit the operation to take place in most instances. The concept that hemodynamic changes should be restricted, especially in hypertensive patients, to set parameters, (e.g., 20 percent above or below mean preoperative pressure) should be regarded as mythology because it has no scientific basis. Hypotension that occurs with the institution of CPB is almost always secondary to the physical effects of hemodilution and has not been associated with an increased incidence of neurologic complications.[9, 37]

Transient heart block occurs very commonly, especially with certain operations, such as aortic or mitral valve replacement, and also before wash-out of potassium cardioplegia during reperfusion of the heart after any cardiac operation. These transient blocks usually disappear with continued perfusion but may require the use of temporary pharmacologic support or cardiac pacing.

Neurologic complications associated with cardiopulmonary bypass in the absence of low cardiac output syndrome are almost always due to embolic phenomena,[38] especially if a cardiac chamber has been opened or the surgical procedure includes an operation on a calcified left-sided valve. An especially vexing problem is embolization of atheromatous debris from the intima of the aorta, associated with cannulation or aortic cross-clamping or release of the clamp in patients undergoing CABG. Although focal defects are more common with emboli, generalized global neurologic effects may occasionally be seen. Computed tomography or magnetic resonance imaging may be necessary for diagnosis.

Cardiopulmonary Bypass

Anticoagulation

Before placement of cannulae for CPB, patients are anticoagulated with 300 U/kg (or 3 mg/kg) of porcine mucosal heparin. This preparation is used because of the reported lower incidence of heparin-induced thrombocytopenia, and this dosage level, in our experience, produces adequate anticoagulation for at least 1.5 hours of CPB. When CPB times approach 90 minutes, we measure an activated clotting time, and if it is less than 300 seconds, additional heparin can be administered if CPB is expected to continue for a prolonged period. However, we have not found routine monitoring of the activated clotting time to be useful in determining outcome. Achievement of specific activated clotting times (e.g., 400 seconds, 480 seconds), supposedly indicating "adequate" anticoagulation, has not proved useful.[39]

Extracorporeal Circulation

Heparinization allows insertion of aortic and venous cannulae for connection to the extracorporeal circuit. Disposable bubble-type or membrane oxygenators may be used. Membrane oxygenators have the theoretical advantages of causing less destruction to the formed elements of the blood and a lower incidence of gas emboli; consequently, they are currently more popular in clinical use than are bubble-type oxygenators during CPB of 2 hours or less.[40]

The standard prime for the oxygenator is 20 ml/kg of D_5 lactated Ringer's solution, with the intent of causing an approximate 30 percent hemodilution while CPB is ongoing. This produces hematocrit values in the 18 to 30 percent range, which are acceptable for normothermic bypass. If hypothermia is used, lower hematocrit values are preferred, with levels of less than 25 percent desirable if profound hypothermia ($\leq 22°C$) is used.

Hemodilution produces an increased tissue oxygen delivery by improving microcirculatory flow secondary to reduced blood viscosity, an increased transfer of oxygen to red blood cells, reduction of hemolysis and conservation of blood and blood products. There has been a marked decrease in complications associated with CPB because hemodilution was first employed in the early 1960s. Glucose-containing primes are used because the osmotic effect of glucose tends to keep crystalloid solutions intravascularly for longer periods of time, reducing the total amount of crystalloid use during CPB. In addition, glucose also produces an osmotic diuretic effect.[41] Glucose administration results in blood glucose levels of 600 to 900 mg/dl during CPB. These levels are not usually treated (exogenous insulin in normal doses has little effect during CPB) and usually fall to 300 to 400 mg/dl by the end of the operation. Hyperosmolar coma is not associated with this management. Association of high glucose levels with worsened outcome of cerebrovascular accidents, which has been proposed, has not been proved, and in our experience, there is no relation between glucose levels during CPB and neurologic dysfunction. However, this is a controversial point and is the subject of ongoing research at many institutions.

There is a marked variation between institutions and individual surgeons as to what are considered optimal CPB flow rates and perfusion pressures. In general, flow rates of 40 to 60 ml/kg/min and perfusion pressures of 30 to 100 mm Hg are acceptable at THI, although what is judged "best" for individual patients may vary. Perfusion pressures of 50 mm Hg or less have not been associated with an increased incidence of neurologic complications.[9]

Weaning From Cardiopulmonary Bypass

Weaning does not take place, of course, until the coronary blood flow is reestablished, cardioplegia is washed out, and the patient is rewarmed. Easy emergence from bypass is characterized by the following signs: sinus rhythm, heart rate between 60 and 100 beats per minute, no ST segment elevation or depression, and the visible right ventricle contracting with vigor and emptying with each beat. Weaning constitutes a gradual reduction of venous flow to the extracorporeal circuit and therefore a gradual increase in preload to the patient. In essence, this gradual replacement of preload, and hence stretching of the myocardium, once again allows the heart to generate a greater contraction strength (Frank-Starling law of the heart). With the increase in preload and good LV ejection, the venous line is totally occluded, and the patient is off bypass. Additional volume can be easily administered through the arterial line of the bypass circuit. If a patient does not respond to volume infusion with an increase output and the heart distends without increasing contractility, some form of pharmaco-

TABLE 113–5 **Management of Difficult Weaning From Cardiopulmonary Bypass**

Presentation	Possible Diagnosis	Therapy
1. Hypotension		
a. Plus normal contractility, normal heart rate	a. Inadequate preload	a. Volume infusion
b. Plus normal contractility, tachycardia	b. Inadequate preload	b. Volume infusion and/or phenylephrine bolus
c. Plus normal contractility, bradycardia	c. Inadequate preload plus 2 and/or 3	c. Volume infusion and/or phenylephrine bolus or pacemaker
2. Sluggish contraction, wide QRS complex, ST-segment elevation, normal heart rate	a. Air in coronary arteries	a. Increase afterload with phenylephrine
	b. Residual cardioplegia	b. $CaCl_2$, epinephrine, isoproterenol
	c. "Stunned myocardium" (recovering ischemia)	c. Vasopressor infusion
	d. Myocardial infarction	d. Vasopressor infusion, intra-aortic balloon pump
	e. Coronary spasm	e. Papaverine or nitroglycerine into aortic root or coronaries
3. a. Bradycardia or atrioventricular block	a–c. Conduction system damage and/or conditions in 2	a. Pacemaker
b. Plus hypotension		b. Epinephrine bolus
c. Plus normotension or hypertension		c. Isoproterenol bolus

logic and/or mechanical support is necessary to allow separation from bypass. Table 113–5 shows the most common clinical situations and their therapy.

After cardiac decannulation, protamine sulfate is given in order to reverse heparin-induced anticoagulation. Hypotension can result from protamine infusion, usually by one of three mechanisms:

1. Mild hypotension may be related to vasodilatation due to histamine release.
2. An anaphylactic response may occur in patients sensitized to protamine by previous exposure, such as in diabetics using NPH insulin, although the actual incidence is low. The manifestations are usually those of a classic anaphylactic reaction.
3. A third type of reaction, mediated through the heparin-protamine complex with complement activation that causes pulmonary vasoconstriction, has also been rarely reported.

Reactions attributed to protamine but caused by inadequate revascularization in coronary bypass operations may not manifest themselves until heparin is reversed and flow in a borderline bypass graft decreases with improving coagulation state.

Transfer to Critical Care Unit

A patient who is stable at the end of the surgical procedure is transferred to the critical care unit under the supervision of the anesthesiologist. Because significant hemodynamic changes may occur during transport for numerous reasons, some of them obscure, patients are always monitored during this period. Blood pressure monitoring should be considered mandatory, and electrocardiographic monitoring is desirable, although not critical, especially when blood pressure is monitored with a device that shows a continuous waveform.

Postoperative Care

Patients are routinely ventilated for 4 to 6 hours after surgery because most postoperative complications (e.g., bleeding, circulatory failure, arrhythmias, cardiac tamponade) occur during this period. A period of mechanical ventilation excludes respiratory failure factors from the clinical picture in any of these situations, enabling the earlier diagnosis and treatment of circulatory and other problems. Past this point, with a stable patient, there is no added benefit to longer times of mechanical ventilation. With the impact of "managed care" and the desire for relatively rapid progression (i.e. "fast tracking") of patients through their hospitalizations, this point has been embraced by many institutions where overnight ventilation was commonly practiced. Earlier extubation has required a shift away from the high-dose opioid anesthetic techniques that were commonly employed in those hospitals. Fast tracking has been implemented without clinical harm to patients in the short term. It is dependent not only on changing anesthetic techniques but, more importantly, on a shift in attitude of those who provide postoperative care to the patient.[42]

Summary

An overriding principle in our approach to anesthesia is simplicity (i.e., believing that it is just as important not to complicate anesthetic management with therapeutic and diagnostic modalities not known to contribute to successful outcome as it is to use all modalities known to contribute to successful outcome). Using simple techniques, anesthesia can be induced expeditiously, clinical skills and judgment can become highly developed, costs can be reduced, and the anesthesiologist will be less distracted from those aspects of care known to be critical to outcome.

References

1. Kaplan JA, Reich DL, Konstadt SN: Cardiac Anesthesia. 4th ed. Philadelphia: WB Saunders, 1998.
2. Estafanous FG, Barash PG, Reves JG: Cardiac Anesthesia: Principles and Clinical Practice. Philadelphia: JB Lippincott, 1994.
3. Barash PG, Cullen BF, Stoelting RK: Clinical Anesthesia. 3rd ed. Philadelphia: Lippincott-Raven, 1997.
4. Gibbon GH: Application of a mechanical heart and lung apparatus to cardiac surgery. Minn Med 37:171, 1954.

5. Lowenstein E, Hollowell P, Levine LH, et al: Cardiovascular response to large doses of intravenous morphine in man. N Engl J Med 281:1389, 1969.
6. Slogoff S, Keats AS, Ott E: Perioperative propranolol therapy and aortocoronary bypass operation. JAMA 240:1487, 1978.
7. Slogoff S, Keats AS: Does chronic treatment with calcium entry blocking drugs reduce perioperative myocardial ischemia? Anesthesiology 68:676, 1988.
8. Stone JG, Young WL, Smith CR, et al: Do standard monitoring sites reflect true brain temperature when profound hypothermia is rapidly induced and reversed? Anesthesiology 82:344, 1995.
9. Slogoff S, Reul GJ, Keats AS, et al: Role of perfusion pressure and flow in major organ dysfunction after cardiopulmonary bypass. Ann Thorac Surg 50:911, 1990.
10. Cooper JR: Should transesophageal echocardiography routinely be used during coronary artery bypass? Anesth Rev 20:196, 1993.
11. Slogoff S, Keats AS: Randomized trial of primary anesthetic agents in outcome of coronary bypass operations. Anesthesiology 70:179, 1989.
12. Tomlinson DL, Hirsch IA, Kodali SV, Slogoff S: Protecting the brachial plexus during median sternotomy. J Thorac Cardiovasc Surg 94:297, 1987.
13. Slogoff S, Keats AS: Does perioperative myocardial ischemia lead to postoperative myocardial infarction? Anesthesiology 62:107, 1985.
14. Fullerton DA, McIntyre RC Jr: Inhaled nitric oxide: therapeutic applications in cardiothoracic surgery. Ann Thorac Surg 61:1856, 1996.
15. Sandrelli L, Pardini A, Lorusso R, et al: Impact of autologous blood predonation on a comprehensive blood conservation program. Ann Thorac Surg 59:730, 1995.
16. Birkmeyer JD, AuBuchon JP, Littenberg B, et al: Cost effectiveness of preoperative autologous donation in coronary artery bypass grafting. Ann Thorac Surg 57:161, 1994.
17. Kasper SM, Baumann M, Radbruch L, et al: A pilot study of continuous ambulatory electrocardiography in patients donating blood for autologous use in elective coronary artery bypass grafting. Transfusion 37:829, 1997.
18. Kasper SM, Ellering J, Stachwitz P, et al: All adverse events in autologous blood donors with cardiac disease are not necessarily caused by blood donation. Transfusion 38:669, 1998.
19. Goodnough LT, Monk TG: Evolving concepts in autologous blood procurement and transfusion: case reports of perisurgical anemia complicated by myocardial infarction. Am J Med 101:33S, 1996.
20. Van Dyck MJ, Baele PL, Leclercq P, et al: Autologous blood donation before myocardial revascularization: a Holter-electrocardiographic analysis. J Cardiothorac Vasc Anesth 8:162, 1994.
21. Hardy J, Belisle S: Natural and synthetic antifibrinolytics in adult cardiac surgery: efficacy, effectiveness and efficiency. Can J Anaesth 41:1104, 1994.
22. Penta de Peppo A, Pierri MD, Scafuri A: Intraoperative antifibrinolytics and blood-saving techniques in cardiac surgery: a prospective trial of 3 antifibrinolytic drugs. Tex Heart Inst J 22:231, 1995.
23. Cosgrove DM III, Heri B, Lytle BW, et al: Aprotinin therapy for reoperative myocardial revascularization: a placebo-controlled study. Ann Thorac Surg 54:1031, 1992.
24. Alderman EL, Levy JH, Rich JB, et al: Analyses of coronary graft patency after aprotinin use: results from the international multicenter aprotinin graft patency experience (IMAGE) trial. J Thorac Cardiovasc Surg 116:716, 1998.
25. Lemer JH Jr, Stanford W, Bonney SL, et al: Aprotinin for coronary bypass operations: efficacy, safety, and influence on early saphenous vein graft patency. A multicenter, randomized, double-blind, placebo-controlled study. J Thorac Cardiovasc Surg 107:543, 1994.
26. Scrutinio D, Lagioia R, Rizzon P: Ticlopidine treatment for patients with unstable angina at rest: a further analysis of the study of ticlopidine in unstable angina. Eur Heart J 12(suppl G):27, 1991.
27. Schomig A, Neumann FJ, Schuhlen H, et al: A randomized comparison of antiplatelet and anticoagulant therapy after the placement of coronary-artery stents. N Engl J Med 334:1084, 1996.
28. CAPRIE Steering Committee: A randomised, blinded, trial of clopidogrel versus aspirin in patients at risk of ischaemic events (CAPRIE). Lancet 348:1329, 1996.
29. CAPTURE Study Investigators: Randomized placebo-controlled trial of abciximab before and during coronary intervention in refractory unstable angina: the CAPTURE Study. Lancet 349:1429, 1997.
30. Gammie JS, Zenati M, Kormos RL, et al: Abciximab and excessive bleeding in patients undergoing emergency cardiac operations. Ann Thorac Surg 65:465, 1998.
31. Alvarez JM: Emergency coronary bypass grafting for failed percutaneous coronary artery stenting: increased costs and platelet transfusion requirements after the use of abciximab. J Thorac Cardiovasc Surg 115:472, 1998.
32. Juergens CP, Yeung AC, Oesterle SN: Routine platelet transfusion in patients undergoing emergency coronary bypass surgery after receiving abciximab. Am J Cardiol 80:74, 1997.
33. PURSUIT Trial Investigators: Inhibition of platelet glycoprotein IIb/IIIa with eptifibatide in patients with acute coronary syndromes. N Engl J Med 339:436, 1998.
34. PRISM Study Investigators: A comparison of aspirin plus tirofiban with aspirin plus heparin for unstable angina. N Engl J Med 338:1498, 1998.
35. Spiess BD, Ley C, Body SC, et al: Hematocrit value on intensive care unit entry influences the frequency of Q-wave myocardial infarction after coronary artery bypass grafting: the institutions of the multicenter study of perioperative ischemia (McSPI) research group. J Thorac Cardiovasc Surg 116:460, 1998.
36. Carson JL, Poses RM, Spence RK, et al: Severity of anemia and operative mortality and morbidity. Lancet 1:727, 1988.
37. Cooper JR, Slogoff S: Hemodilution and priming solutions for cardiopulmonary bypass. *In* Davis RF, Gravlee GP, Utley Jr (eds): Principles and Practice of Cardiopulmonary Bypass. pp. 124–137. Baltimore: Williams & Wilkins, 1993.
38. Slogoff S, Girgis KZ, Keats AS: Etiologic factors in neuropsychiatric complications associated with cardiopulmonary bypass. Anesth Analg 61:903, 1982.
39. Metz S, Keats AS: Low activated coagulation time during cardiopulmonary bypass does not increase postoperative bleeding. Ann Thorac Surg 49:440, 1990.
40. Clark RE, Beauchamp RA, Magrath RA, et al: Comparison of bubble and membrane oxygenators in short and long perfusions. J Thorac Cardiovasc Surg 78:665, 1979.
41. Metz S, Keats AS: Benefits of glucose-containing priming solution for cardiopulmonary bypass. Anesth Analg 72:428, 1991.
42. Alexander WA, Cooper JR Jr: Preoperative risk stratification identifies low-risk candidates for early extubation after aortocoronary bypass grafting. Tex Heart Inst J 23:267, 1996.

CHAPTER 114

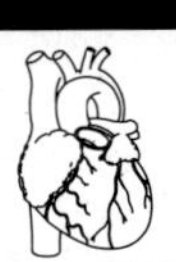

INTRAOPERATIVE HEMODYNAMIC MONITORING

Charles R. Garcia-Rodriguez, Andrew K. Hilton, and Jonathan B. Mark

CARDIOVASCULAR CHANGES DURING ANESTHESIA AND POSITIVE PRESSURE VENTILATION
ELECTROCARDIOGRAPHY
Artifacts and Filters
Lead Configuration
Computerized Electrocardiographic Analysis
ARTERIAL BLOOD PRESSURE MONITORING
Direct Measurement of Arterial Blood Pressure
Components of Direct Blood Pressure Monitoring
Arterial Waveform
Complications of Direct Arterial Pressure Monitoring
Noninvasive Techniques
CENTRAL VENOUS PRESSURE MONITORING
Normal Central Venous Pressure
Complications
PULMONARY ARTERY CATHETERIZATION
Practical Considerations for Insertion
Complications
Pulmonary Artery Wedge Trace
Factors Affecting Data Validity
Predicting Left Ventricular End-Diastolic Volume
Pulmonary Vascular Resistance and Heart Rate
Valvular Disease
Ventilatory Pressure Influences
Ventricular Compliance and Pressure-Volume Relationships
Optimizing Preload
Use of Pulmonary Artery Catheters for Myocardial Ischemia Monitoring
CARDIAC OUTPUT MONITORING
Thermodilution Cardiac Output
Continuous Thermodilution Cardiac Output Measurement
Mixed Venous Oxygen Saturation Measurement
Doppler Ultrasound-Based Cardiac Output (Measurement)
Other Methods of Cardiac Output Measurement
INTRAOPERATIVE TRANSESOPHAGEAL ECHOCARDIOGRAPHY
Indications and Use
Contraindications
Probe Insertion
Complications
Transesophageal Echocardiography and Intraoperative Ischemia
Controversies and Conclusion

As with the practice of medicine through the use of history taking and physical examination, the effective use of supplementary cardiovascular monitoring techniques requires technical skills, an understanding of how the cardiovascular monitors work, and how pathophysiologic states may be recognized with the use of these devices. In the perioperative setting, the use of anesthetic drugs, positive pressure ventilation, and surgical intervention all cause significant cardiovascular changes. Early detection of these changes, before irreversible harm ensues, is the goal of hemodynamic monitoring. Thus, a hierarchy of monitoring methods may be developed, as dictated by individual circumstances. Invasive monitoring places the patient at risk from the associated complications, and in each case the potential benefits must be weighed against this risk. For example, during general anesthesia, the detection of myocardial ischemia using ST-segment with electrocardiographic (ECG) monitoring is clearly superior to clinical examination and is recommended for all patients with risk factors for coronary artery disease. In contrast, pulmonary artery catheter (PAC) monitoring should be reserved for a subset of these patients who have severe cardiovascular instability or who are undergoing extensive surgical procedures.

Historically, anesthesiologists have relied heavily on the clinical assessment of ventilation pattern, pupil size, muscle tone, color, and pulse. Electronic monitors allow physiologic variables not accessible by physical assessment to be measured accurately and displayed and recorded at frequent intervals or even continuously. Monitors are designed to augment rather than to replace clinical skills and thereby improve clinical judgment and diagnosis.

Automated devices that incorporate alarms and data recorders free the clinician from laborious clerical tasks that detract from patient care. Powerful microprocessors have allowed miniaturization of bedside recording devices that can connect to hospital networks for record printing and downloading of data. The creation of standardized anesthesia-related databases allows analysis and comparison of stored information within and between institutions for the purposes of audit and clinical research.

The clinical anesthesiologist has a vital role in cardiovascular monitoring through careful observation and integration of monitored information and sound judgment based on experience and knowledge of individual patient circumstances. Of equal importance, however, when sophisticated monitoring systems fail, the physician must have the medical skills to provide the critical safety net for patients undergoing surgical procedures.

Cardiovascular Changes During Anesthesia and Positive Pressure Ventilation

The induction of general anesthesia attenuates many of the compensatory cardiovascular reflexes, and almost all drugs used to induce general anesthesia are cardiovascular depressants (Table 114–1). As a result, it is normal for blood pressure and cardiac output (CO) to fall after the induction of anesthesia. Most anesthetic agents produce dose-dependent cardiovascular changes. In any individual patient, both preoperative disease and hemodynamic state influence these changes. Significantly exaggerated cardiovascular responses are seen in hypovolemic and hypertensive patients, in whom anesthetic agents abruptly reduce increased sympathetic tone. In addition, patients with "fixed CO" may demonstrate greater cardiovascular depression during general anesthesia because of an inability to increase CO as systemic vascular resistance decreases.

Positive pressure ventilation is required for many operations and may alter all of the determinants of CO, including preload, afterload, heart rate, and contractility. In the absence of hypoxia or hypercapnia, the predominant effects of positive pressure ventilation are mechanical and result from changes in intrathoracic pressure and volume that produce changes in cardiac preload and afterload. During positive pressure inspiration, right atrial pressure (RAP) increases, thereby decreasing right-sided venous return and right ventricular (RV) stroke volume. At the same time, left-sided filling increases as the pulmonary venous blood is propelled from the pulmonary vasculature toward the left atrium, causing left ventricular (LV) stroke volume to increase. In addition, the increased intrathoracic pressure decreases transmural LV pressure, thereby decreasing LV afterload to further aid LV ejection. RV afterload is usually not affected, because the pulmonary circulation is contained within the thorax. These phasic changes in intrathoracic pressure and volume produce disparities between RV and LV output that vary throughout the respiratory cycle. The predominant effect of positive pressure ventilation results from decreasing systemic venous return, producing a form of functional hypovolemia. If large tidal volumes are used in an already hypovolemic patient, venous return can be reduced to a critical level. Thus, the combination of the induction of general anesthesia and the institution of mechanical ventilation often requires rapid intravascular volume expansion and vasoactive drug administration to maintain hemodynamic variables within acceptable limits.

Electrocardiography

In high-risk patients, the perioperative period is associated with a significant incidence of dysrhythmias[1] and ST-segment changes.[2] Intraoperative ECG monitoring is part of routine practice providing the familiar continuous real-time display of one or more standard leads.[3] Modern bedside ECG monitors are able to record a multilead electrocardiogram of diagnostic quality, and computer processing and analysis of the signal aid the detection of ECG changes caused by ischemia or dysrhythmia.

Artifacts and Filters

ECG monitoring artifacts are common in the operating room environment. The loss of electrical contact of electrodes can occur due to inadequate skin preparation, the application of surgical scrub, or tension on ECG leads. Shivering, tremor, movements associated with respiration, or surgery interfere with the electrical signal and may cause a wandering baseline. Equipment commonly used in the operating room may make the electrocardiogram uninterpretable (electrocautery), cause a characteristic regular pattern of interference (cardiopulmonary bypass machines, fluid warming devices), or produce electrical noise at power main frequency (60 Hz in United States, 50 Hz in Europe).

Electronic filtering of the ECG signal is the standard method used to overcome electrical interference. Many

TABLE 114–1 **Cardiovascular Effects of Anesthetic Agents**

	Systemic Vascular Resistance	Heart Rate	Contractility	Right Atrial Pressure
Intravenous induction dose				
Thiopentone	−	+	−	− −
Midazolam	−	NC	NC	NC
Propofol	− −	NC	NC	−
Etomidate	−	+	−	NC
Ketamine	+ +	+ +	−	+ +
Inhalational agents at 1 MAC				
Halothane	NC/−	NC	− −	+
Enflurane	−	+	− −	NC
Isoflurane	− −	+	−	NC

Abbreviations: MAC, minimum alveolar concentration; NC, no change; +, minimal increase; + +, marked increase; −, minimal decrease; − −, marked decrease.

bedside monitors incorporate a *monitor filter mode* that typically has low- and high-frequency filters of 0.5 and 40 Hz, respectively. The low-frequency filter helps to eliminate baseline drift associated with patient movement, and the high-frequency filter reduces electrical noise. However, because the ST segment is a low-frequency component of the electrocardiogram, ST-segment shifts may be exaggerated when a low-frequency filter of 0.5 Hz is used, leading to overdiagnosis of myocardial ischemia.[2, 4] The high-frequency filter may interfere with QRS recognition, causing the J point to be misidentified and ST-segment analysis to be unreliable. A *diagnostic filter mode* available on most bedside ECG monitors has a similar bandwidth (0.05 to 100 Hz) as a 12-lead electrocardiograph. This allows the monitored ECG leads to have the same diagnostic accuracy for detection of ischemia as standard ECG recordings. This diagnostic bandwidth filter should be chosen whenever accurate ST-segment analysis is required.

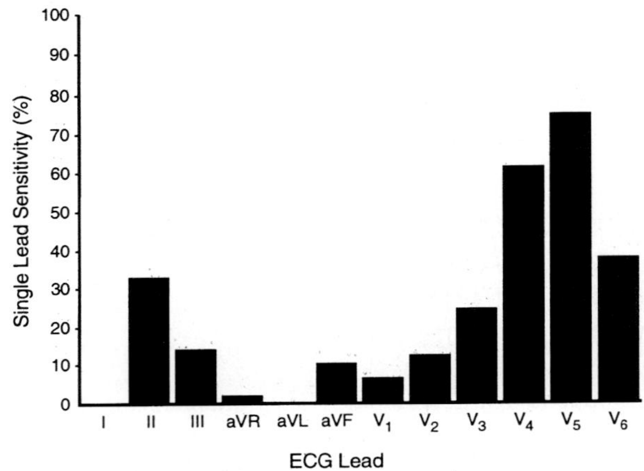

FIGURE 114–1 Single-lead sensitivity for detection of myocardial ischemia in noncardiac surgery patients. Fifty-one episodes of intraoperative ischemia were detected in 25 patients with continuous 12-lead electrocardiography (ECG). Lead sensitivity was calculated by dividing the number of ischemic episodes detected in a single lead by the total number of episodes detected with all 12 leads. Lead V_5 demonstrated the highest single-lead sensitivity (75 percent). Lead II had limited sensitivity (33 percent). The combination of leads II and V_5 increased sensitivity to 80 percent, and the addition of lead V_4 increased sensitivity to 96 percent. (From London MJ, Hollenberg M, Wong MG, et al: Intraoperative myocardial ischemia: localization by continuous 12-lead electrocardiography. Anesthesiology 69[2]:232–241, 1988.)

Lead Configuration

The standard monitoring lead configuration consists of a five-electrode system: four limb leads and one "exploring" unipolar precordial electrode. This configuration allows the monitoring of 7 of 12 standard leads (I, II, III, aVR, aVL, VF, and a single precordial lead). The other precordial leads may be recorded in the operating room by placing the precordial electrode at the standard V_1 through V_6 positions.

The sensitivity of individual ECG leads for the detection of intraoperative myocardial ischemia has been well evaluated. Similar to exercise stress testing, the V_5 lead is the most sensitive, detecting approximately 75 percent of intraoperative ischemic episodes, followed by leads V_4, V_6, and II, which have intermediate sensitivity (Fig. 114–1).[5] The combination of V_5 with another lead (II, III, V_4, or V_6) increases the sensitivity of ischemia detection to 90 percent, with only a small reduction in specificity. Lead II is commonly monitored along with V_5, because it enhances ischemia detection and provides clear evidence of atrial activity, to aid in dysrhythmia detection.[5] Most perioperative ST-segment changes of ischemia are seen as ST-segment depression resulting from subendocardial ischemia. These changes do not localize the area of ischemic myocardium. Less frequently, ST elevation is observed, suggesting transmural ischemia or infarction in the territory subtended by the leads showing these changes.

Monitoring for myocardial ischemia generally focuses on the left ventricle, but RV ischemia may occur in association with inferior myocardial ischemia or infarction due to the common blood supply to these areas of myocardium. With the standard monitored combination of leads II and V_5, RV ischemia may be manifest only as ST elevation in lead II, with or without reciprocal changes of ST depression in lead V_5.[6] Better assessment of RV ischemia is obtained by using right-sided leads such as V_1 or V_4R, the mirror image of the V_4 lead on the right side of the chest.[7, 8]

When a three-electrode ECG monitor is the only one available, it may be modified to allow approximation of standard precordial lead positions. Lead I is selected, the positive exploring electrode (left arm) is located in the precordial V_5 position, and the central negative electrode (right arm) is placed in various positions on the thorax—central subclavicular (CS_5), central manubrial (CM_5), central chest (CC_5), and central back (CB_5) (Fig. 114–2).

To make valid comparisons of ECG morphology throughout the perioperative period, precordial lead position must be kept constant by either leaving the electrode attached or marking the skin. Certain types of surgery or positioning preclude ideal precordial lead selection, such as left-sided thoracotomy. In addition, despite an anatomically correct surface electrode position, ECG morphology and R wave amplitude may be distorted by surgical retraction; movement of the heart within the thorax during prone, sitting, or lateral patient positioning; or positive pressure ventilation. All of these factors confound intraoperative ECG interpretation.

Computerized Electrocardiographic Analysis

Computerized ECG processing was originally developed for exercise stress testing but is routinely incorporated into bedside monitors. It is useful for noise reduction through signal averaging and for automated ST-segment analysis and trending. The latter feature may prove most useful, because most episodes of ischemia in the perioperative period pass undetected when an automated system of analysis and recording is not used.[5, 9] The first step in processing the ECG signal is conversion of the analog signal into a digital format. The voltage range is divided up into a number of discreet measurements that are dependent on the bit size of the microprocessor. Sampling rates typically

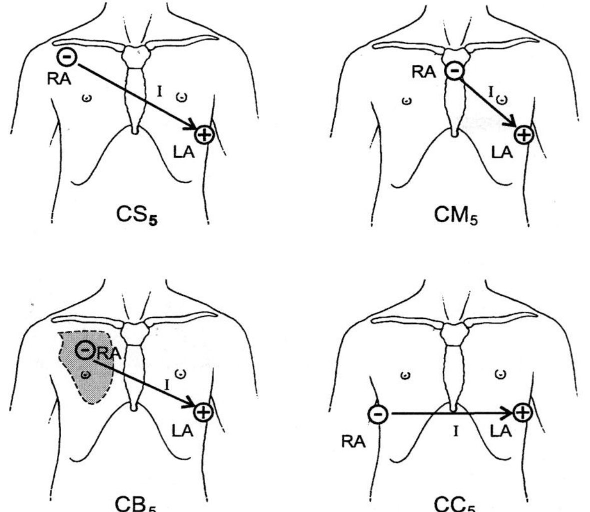

FIGURE 114–2 Modification of the three-electrode bipolar limb lead system to approximate the standard unipolar precordial V_5 position. The positive exploring left arm (LA) electrode is placed in the V_5 position, and the negative central right arm (RA) electrode is placed in the following locations: central subclavicular (CS), central manubrial (CM), central back (CB) overlying the right scapula, and central chest (CC). Lead I is selected on the monitor to create these modified V_5 recordings. (Modified from Mark JB: Atlas of Cardiovascular Monitoring. New York: Churchill Livingstone, 1998.)

in the order of 256 Hz and above result in sampling periods of 4 milliseconds. Low bit size or sampling rate lowers the resolution of the monitor and causes signal distortion due to phase shift of the signal. Using mathematical algorithms, fixed reference fiducial points are identified within the signal, for example the R wave downslope, where there is the most rapid change in signal amplitude. This process allows a baseline QRS complex to be identified and stored as a template with subsequent beats overlaid and averaged. Once the QRS complex or R wave is identified as the fiducial point, the isoelectric baseline and ST-segment measurement points are assigned relative to these. For example, for QRS complex identification, the isoelectric point is chosen 40 milliseconds before QRS onset and the ST segment is measured 60 milliseconds after the J-point. For an algorithm based on R wave identification, the isoelectric point is placed 80 milliseconds before and the ST segment is measured 108 milliseconds after the R wave peak.

Errors may occur when the default setting of the monitor places the isoelectric point or the ST-segment measuring point incorrectly. In cases where there is a short PR interval, the isoelectric point may be placed on the peak of the P wave, producing artifactual ST depression. When a pacing spike is misinterpreted as the R wave peak, both the isoelectric point and the ST segment may be misidentified. Manual adjustment of these points is required in these circumstances.

Computerized interpretation of the electrocardiogram, ST-segment deviation, always requires visual confirmation by the physician. Using these computer-automated ST-segment analysis devices, accurate measurement of ST-segment changes to the nearest 0.01 mV (0.1 mm) is possible, thereby alerting the clinician to small changes before they reach clinical significance. In some monitors, a visual trend line is displayed that represents the summed ST-segment deviations from multiple leads.

In high-risk patients, most intraoperative ST-segment changes occur in the absence of major hemodynamic lability.[10–12] Furthermore, control of hemodynamic variables to within 20 percent of preoperative values does not appear to reduce intraoperative ischemic events.[13, 14] This poor correlation of hemodynamic changes with ischemic ST changes suggests that primarily a reduction in myocardial oxygen supply rather than increased demand is an important mechanism of perioperative ischemia. Hemodynamic control to avoid excessive tachycardia and hypotension is prudent and usually achieved in modern anesthetic practice, but ischemia does still occur. Furthermore, although there are associations between perioperative ischemia and adverse cardiac outcome,[5, 11, 15] ischemic ECG changes in the postoperative period are much more predictive of adverse events than are preoperative or intraoperative ECG changes.[12] It is unclear whether these postoperative ECG changes represent predictive ability or are part of the ischemic event itself. These observations suggest that in patients at high risk for adverse cardiac events, ECG monitoring for myocardial ischemia aided by computerized ECG monitors should be extended into the early postoperative period.[16]

Arterial Blood Pressure Monitoring

Systemic blood pressure represents the necessary driving force, generated by LV contraction for perfusion of the body, and is the major determinant of LV afterload, the workload of the heart. Consequently, reliable, accurate blood pressure measurement is vital in circumstances where rapid change is anticipated, such as intraoperatively and in the critically ill. Standards for intraoperative monitoring require blood pressure measurement at least every 5 minutes,[3] and deviation from desired values is often the major indication for pharmacotherapy. Although it seems intuitive that intraoperative blood pressure lability leads to worse outcome, this has not proved to be the case in clinical practice. This likely results from the rapid detection and early correction of major blood pressure changes during operative procedures.

Direct Measurement of Arterial Blood Pressure

In comparison with noninvasive techniques, direct intra-arterial blood pressure measurement is more costly and requires additional expertise, but it remains the clinical "gold standard" as a safe, accurate, and reliable technique. Arterial cannulation is considered for two major reasons: frequent arterial blood sampling and pressure measurement. During major surgery, arterial blood analysis guides adjustment of pulmonary ventilation and administration of drugs, fluids, and blood products. Systems that have been developed for continuous gas and electrolyte measurement involve the use of either fiberoptic sensors that are placed directly into the artery[17] or an in-line sampling for analysis by ex vivo sensors.

Direct arterial pressure monitoring is considered in any of the following situations[18]:

1. The anticipated hemodynamic change resulting from the operative procedure is sudden or large in magnitude, such as occurs with cardiac or major vascular surgery.
2. Concurrent disease necessitates close hemodynamic observation (e.g., severe aortic stenosis).
3. Pharmacologic or mechanical manipulation of the cardiovascular system is planned (e.g., intra-aortic balloon counterpulsation or deliberate hypotension).
4. Cuff-derived pressures are not obtainable, as in the morbidly obese, the burned patient, or the severely vasoconstricted patient.

Components of Direct Blood Pressure Monitoring

Monitoring systems convert mechanical pressure into an easily quantifiable electrical voltage signal that can be displayed. Mechanical components such as the intravascular catheter, fluid filled tubing, and the electromechanical transducer influence the signal produced, altering displayed waveforms and digital values. Faithful recreation of the arterial pressure waveform requires summation of the first 6 to 10 harmonics derived from Fourier analysis (Fig. 114–3); this is because the arterial waveform contains high-frequency components such as the systolic upstroke and dicrotic notch. For a pulse rate of 120 beats/min (2 Hz), the system dynamic response must be flat to 20 Hz (the 10th harmonic frequency) to avoid waveform distortion. The dynamic response of the catheter/transducer system depends on frictional forces, elasticity, and mass and is characterized by the natural frequency and damping coefficient of the monitoring system. In an ideal system, input and output signals are identical across the whole range of frequencies, but real systems artifactually amplify the output signal when the input frequency approaches the natural resonant frequency of the system. In most catheter/transducer systems, the use of a short length of stiff tubing free of air and clot produces a clinically acceptable natural frequency in excess of 12 Hz.[19]

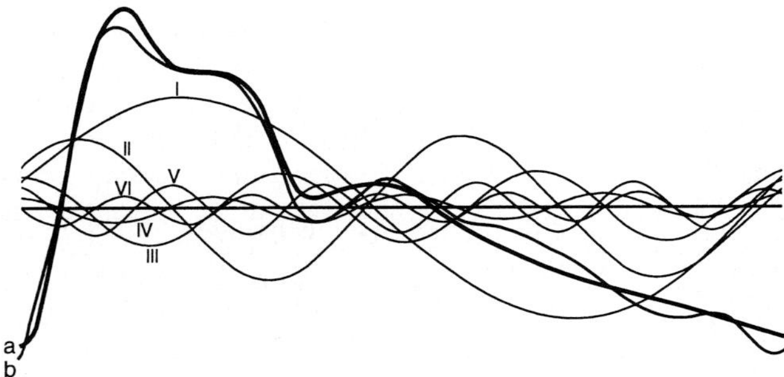

FIGURE 114–3 Mathematical reconstruction of the arterial pressure waveform. Direct recording of carotid artery pressure is shown by the *bold line* (a). A reasonably accurate pressure curve (b) is reconstructed by summation of the first six harmonics, (I, II, III, IV, V, and VI) obtained from a Fourier analysis of the original pressure curve. (From Hansen AT: Pressure measurement in the human organism. Acta Physiol Scand Suppl 19, 1949.)

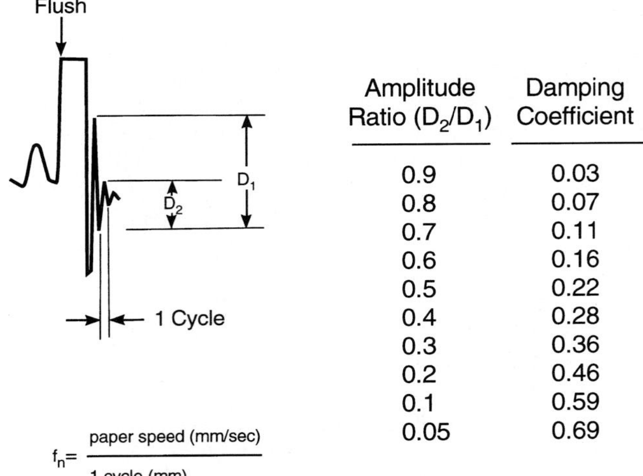

Amplitude Ratio (D_2/D_1)	Damping Coefficient
0.9	0.03
0.8	0.07
0.7	0.11
0.6	0.16
0.5	0.22
0.4	0.28
0.3	0.36
0.2	0.46
0.1	0.59
0.05	0.69

FIGURE 114–4 Fast flush test. The resonant frequency (f_n, Hz) calculated by dividing the paper speed in millimeters per second by the distance in millimeters between successive oscillation peaks. The amplitude ratio between any two successive peaks (D_2/D_1) allows the damping coefficient to be calculated. (From Bedford RF: Invasive blood pressure monitoring. *In* Blitt CD [ed]: Monitoring in Anesthesia and Critical Care Medicine. New York: Churchill Livingstone, 1985, Fig. 5–8.)

The absorption of oscillatory energy by frictional forces is described by use of the system damping coefficient. An underdamped system does not dissipate energy, allows exaggeration of high- and low-pressure values, and produces artifactual peaks in the waveform. Overdamping causes the loss of waveform detail and a narrowed pulse pressure. The introduction of air bubbles to increase system damping is not recommended, as the natural frequency is also lowered, which may paradoxically increase resonance in the system. Optimal damping ensures a flat frequency response beyond the natural frequency but is difficult to achieve.[19] Hence, clinical arterial pressure measurement systems behave as underdamped second-order dynamic systems.[20]

The "fast flush test" performed at the bedside is used to assess the dynamic response of the entire pressure monitoring system (Fig. 114–4).[20, 21] By quickly opening and closing the flush valve, a shock wave is applied to the system, producing a damped oscillation of transducer output. The tighter the oscillation cycles, the higher the natural frequency, and the greater the difference in amplitude of successive oscillations, the more damped the system.

Catheter-tipped transducers circumvent problems of damping and frequency response and can produce very accurate measurements. However, they are much more expensive, and once placed in the artery, they do not allow transducer drift to be assessed through recalibration. Furthermore, issues of transducer level and hydrostatic influences are problems that have not been addressed.[22] Due to these limitations, catheters are not used for routine clinical pressure monitoring.

Modern transducers use semiconductor technology to

etch resistor components of a Wheatstone bridge into the surface of the transducer membrane. A standardized sensitivity of 5 μV/mm Hg allows the exchange of transducers between different monitors. These disposable transducers are highly accurate and incorporate a stiff membrane that produces adequate dynamic range (100 to 500 Hz), and calibration errors and transducer drift are rarely a problem.[23] Although calibration is no longer required, a simple calibration check can be performed by raising the tip of the flushed tubing, exposed to air, above the zeroed transducer. The pressure value displayed should correspond with the pressure exerted by the vertical water column acting on the transducer (note that 10 cm of H_2O pressure equals 7.6 mm Hg).

Perhaps the most common error in pressure measurement occurs when the zeroing stopcock is placed at the wrong level with respect to the patient. This reference level should be established at the outset of the monitoring period and checked repeatedly. Although the mid-axillary line in a supine patient is usually chosen as the phlebostatic axis, a more accurate point for zeroing the transducer is approximately 5 cm posterior to the sternum. Such a reference point obviates the effect of hydrostatic pressures within the heart chambers.[22] Leveling inaccuracies affect all displayed pressures by the same amount, thereby making this a more significant factor for low-pressure systems such as central venous pressure (CVP) or pulmonary artery pressure (PAP) than for systemic arterial pressures.

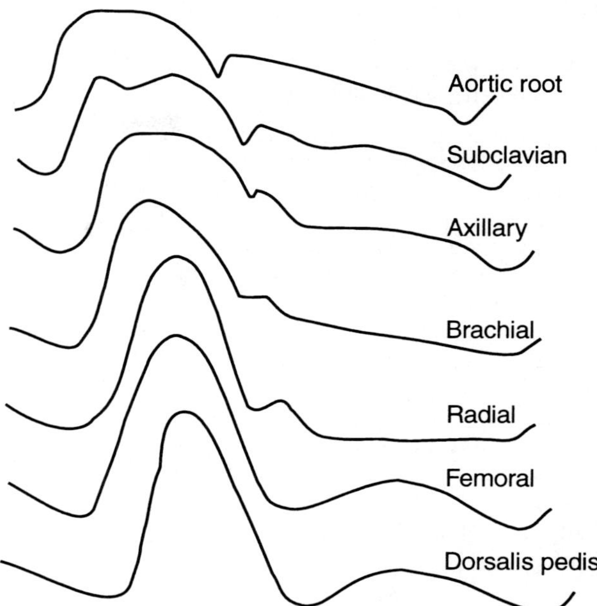

FIGURE 114–5 Pressure wave reflection progressively alters the arterial waveform as it travels from the central aorta to the periphery. Pulse pressure amplification is noted in the peripheral arterial waveforms. (From Bedford RF: Invasive blood pressure monitoring. *In* Blitt CD [ed]: Monitoring in Anesthesia and Critical Care Medicine. New York: Churchill Livingstone, 1985, Fig. 5–3.)

Arterial Waveform

The arterial pressure wave results from the interaction of the forces created by systolic ejection of blood into the vascular tree. The waveform is characterized by a systolic phase—the steep pressure upstroke, peak, and decline until the dicrotic notch—followed by further decline in the diastolic phase. The impedance and compliance of the arterial tree cause pressure wave reflection and resonance, progressively transforming the central aortic waveform shape as it travels to more peripheral sites to produce distal pulse amplification. Other features that distinguish the peripheral arterial waveform from central aortic pressure include a dicrotic notch that is delayed and obscured, a reflected diastolic wave that is more prominent, a systolic peak that is higher, and diastolic nadir that is lower (Fig. 114–5).

Characteristic arterial waveforms are associated with a number of disease states.[24] Pulsus alternans, pulsus bisferiens, pulsus tardus, pulsus paradoxus, and the "spike-and-dome" pattern seen in hypertrophic cardiomyopathy may be discerned in direct recordings of the system arterial blood pressure just as they are often described in the physical examination of the arterial pulses (Fig. 114–6). In addition, other qualitative circulatory inferences can be gleaned from the waveform shape. A short systolic time is associated with high peripheral resistance or hypovolemia, and a slow systolic upstroke is associated with poor myocardial systolic function, especially in the face of high peripheral resistance. One practical application of direct arterial blood pressure monitoring is the quantification of the respiratory variation in systolic blood pressure produced during positive pressure ventilation. Excessive variation of the systolic blood pressure (>15 mm Hg) is highly associated with occult hypovolemia (Fig. 114–7).[25–27]

Complications of Direct Arterial Pressure Monitoring

As with all invasive monitoring techniques, direct arterial pressure monitoring has an associated morbidity rate, but complications are rare in the absence of contributing factors. In a study of 1700 patients undergoing radial artery cannulation, no ischemic complications were demonstrated despite evidence of radial artery occlusion in more than 25 percent of patients, thus demonstrating the value of collateral circulation provided by the ulnar artery.[28] Recanalization and normalization of blood flow usually occurs within 2 weeks.[29] *The Allen test* is designed to evaluate whether ulnar collateral flow is adequate, but its predictive value has been challenged. In many of the reports of ischemic sequelae after cannulation, a normal Allen test preceded the arterial catheterization, and in other cases, uncomplicated arterial cannulation occurs even when the Allen test is abnormal.[28] Overall, the risk of an ischemic complication from peripheral arterial catheterization is less than 0.1 percent.[28, 29] Although serious complications are rare after arterial catheterization, other adverse consequences include infection, fatal hemorrhage, aneurysm formation, arteriovenous fistula, retrograde arterial embolism, and compartment syndrome. Of note, the Australia Incident Monitoring Study, which described 2000 perioperative adverse events, reported a lower incidence of complications related to arterial catheterization than that for either peripheral or central venous cannulation.[30]

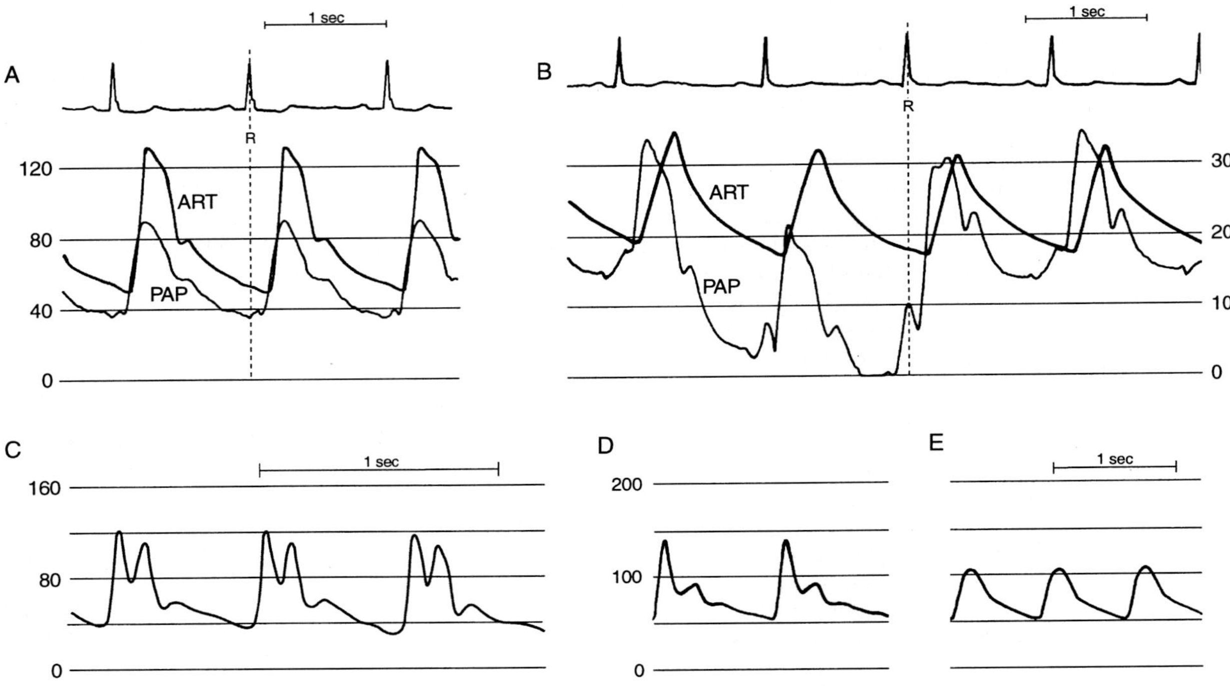

FIGURE 114–6 Characteristic peripheral arterial pressure waveform morphologies associated with pathological conditions. **A,** Normal systemic arterial (ART) and pulmonary artery pressure (PAP) waveforms. **B,** The slurred upstroke and delayed systolic peak of aortic stenosis are apparent in comparison with the normal PAP waveform. **C,** Aortic regurgitation produces a bisferens pulse with a widened pulse pressure. **D,** The spike-and-dome pattern of hypertrophic obstructive cardiomyopathy and the normal waveform **E,** after surgical correction. Pressure scales are in millimeters of mercury. ART scale is on the left, and PAP scale is on the right. (**A–E,** From Mark JB: Cardiovascular monitoring. *In* Miller RD [ed]: Anesthesia. Philadelphia: Churchill Livingstone, 2000.)

Noninvasive Techniques

In 1896, Scipione Riva-Rocci described the first sphygmomanometer as a cuff encircling the arm and a mercury manometer to measure cuff pressure. The standard method for blood pressure measurement involves the use of the inflatable occluding cuff and is based on the work of Korotkoff, who described a series of distinct sounds produced by turbulent flow during cuff deflation. For repetitive clinical monitoring purposes, however, the auscultatory method for blood pressure measurement has a number of limitations. It is highly subjective, labor intensive, and dependent on careful operator technique. Furthermore, reliance on pulsatile blood flow for sound generation leads to underestimation of blood pressure in states of low peripheral blood flow,[18] whereas hardened atherosclerotic vessels require very high cuff pressures and result in falsely high readings.[31]

As a result, for repetitive blood pressure monitoring, automatic oscillotonometers have replaced auscultatory techniques. First described by von Recklinghausen in 1936, oscillometry measures cuff pressure changes caused by arterial pulsations recorded during cuff deflation. The point of maximum cuff pressure fluctuation corresponds to mean arterial pressure, systolic pressure is determined at the point of rapidly increasing oscillations, and diastolic pressure at

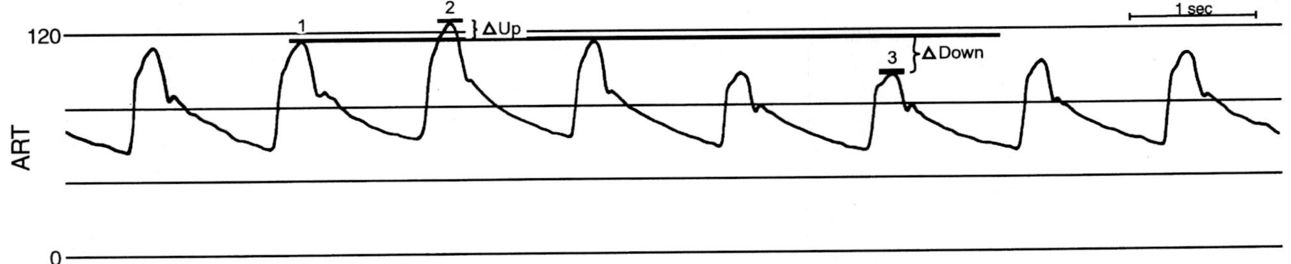

FIGURE 114–7 Systolic pressure variation is the difference between maximal and minimal systolic arterial pressures (ART) recorded over the respiratory cycle. A reference end-expiratory baseline value is identified (116 mm Hg, *solid horizontal line* 1). Total systolic pressure variation is the sum of the early inspiratory systolic pressure increase, termed ΔUp (10.5 mm Hg, line 2), and later decrease in pressure, ΔDown (18.5 mm Hg, line 3) to equal 29 mm Hg. This is much greater than the normal value (5 to 10 mm Hg). The marked increase in total systolic pressure variation and the exaggerated ΔDown component suggests the diagnosis of hypovolemia, despite relatively normal blood pressure and heart rate (52 beats/min). (From Mark JB: Cardiovascular monitoring. *In* Miller RD [ed]: Anesthesia. Philadelphia: Churchill Livingstone, 2000.)

the point of rapidly decreasing oscillations. In general, values for mean and systolic pressure correspond well with direct arterial pressure measured in the radial artery.[32, 33] However, discrepancies between indirect oscillometric and direct arterial pressures may occur under some conditions, with oscillometry tending to overestimate direct arterial pressure during hypotension and to underestimate direct arterial pressure during hypertension.

Although the overall safety of automated blood pressure monitors is underscored by their ubiquitous use in a variety of clinical settings, a number of complications have been reported; these include pain, bruising, limb edema, peripheral neuropathy, thrombophlebitis, and compartment syndrome.[34, 35] Risk is increased by frequent or excessive inflation/deflation cycling occurring when the "stat" measurement mode is used or when repeated cuff inflations occur in an attempt to overcome artifacts caused by tremor, patient movement, or irregular heart rhythm.

Because automated oscillometric blood pressure measurement is intermittent, several techniques have been developed for continuous noninvasive measurement of blood pressure. These include the arterial volume-clamp method with a servo-plethysmomanometer; pulse transit time, using dual oximeters on the ear and finger calibrated by oscillometry[36]; arterial wall displacement[37]; and arterial tonometry using piezoelectric crystals to sense pressure changes transduced through a partially flattened arterial wall.[38] In general, these methods show poor agreement with oscillometry or direct arterial blood pressure measurement and have yet to find widespread clinical use as a substitute for direct arterial pressure monitoring.

Central Venous Pressure Monitoring

Central venous catheterization has been used extensively intraoperatively and in intensive care since the 1950s and continues to expand as new therapeutic indications develop (Table 114–2). Renewed interest in perioperative CVP measurement has gone hand in hand with the continuing debate over the effectiveness of pulmonary artery (PA) catheterization. Understanding the physiologic principles underlying CVP monitoring is essential to derive maximum patient benefit and provides the basis for understanding other waveforms, such as the pulmonary artery wedge pressure (PAWP) and Doppler ultrasound spectral velocity patterns.

TABLE 114–2 Indications for Central Venous Catheterization

- Central pressure monitoring
- Pulmonary artery catheterization and monitoring
- Drug administration
  - Vasoactive drugs
  - Hyperosmolar fluids
  - Chemotherapy agents
  - Prolonged antibiotic therapy
  - Drugs acting primarily on the pulmonary circulation
- Parenteral nutrition
- Rapid fluid infusion
- Temporary transvenous pacing
- Hemodialysis
- Portosystemic shunt insertion
- Aspiration of air emboli
- Inadequate peripheral venous access
- Repeated blood sampling

Normal Central Venous Pressure

CVP reflects the balance among intravascular volume, venous tone, and RV function. CVP is measured in the superior vena cava close to the right atrium and for clinical purposes is assumed to equal RAP.

The direct measurement of CVP is often required in high-risk surgical patients because assessment by physical examination is often inaccurate[39] and further confounded in the operating room by patient positioning, positive pressure ventilation, and the ongoing surgery. In general, a single isolated CVP value provides little information unless it is very high or low. Instead, trends of CVP integrated with changes in other hemodynamic variables prove to be more useful clinically.

It is important to appreciate mechanical events responsible for the characteristic waveform and the relationship with ECG activity. The CVP can be considered to possess three systolic components (C wave, x descent, V wave) and two diastolic components (y descent, A wave). Note that flow from the vena cavae into the right atrium varies inversely with RAP and is maximal during the x and y pressure descents. These pressure-flow relations form the basis for spectral Doppler velocity patterns recorded in the vena cavae or hepatic veins.

Just as careful observation of the arterial pressure waveform provides useful diagnostic information, interpretation of the CVP waveform yields valuable clinical data. The diagnosis and detection of arrhythmias are enhanced by observing acute changes in the CVP waveform. Junctional (atrioventricular nodal) rhythms are common in patients under anesthesia and may cause significant hypotension due to a reduction in CO. The hemodynamic clue to this arrhythmia is the CVP cannon A wave, resulting from atrial contraction against a closed tricuspid valve during ventricular systole. Atrial fibrillation may be recognized in the CVP trace by the absence of an A wave and prominent C-V waves. Effective restoration of atrioventricular synchrony during pacing can be seen in the CVP wave (Fig. 114–8).

RV ischemia can produce systemic arterial hypotension and an elevated CVP displaying a prominent A wave resulting from atrial contraction into a stiff right ventricle. If atrial infarction accompanies RV infarction, the A wave is blunted and CO is significantly depressed.[40] If tricuspid regurgitation is present, a tall, regurgitant C-V wave further increases mean CVP.

Pericardial constriction restricts venous return to the heart and increases CVP. The A and V waves are prominent and the x and y descents are steep, creating an M or a W pattern, similar to RV infarction or other conditions in which RV compliance is reduced. The CVP y descent is halted abruptly as diastolic inflow into the right ventricle is restricted, producing a diastolic pressure plateau (the H wave) and creating a pattern termed *dip-and-plateau* or *square root sign* (Fig. 114–9).

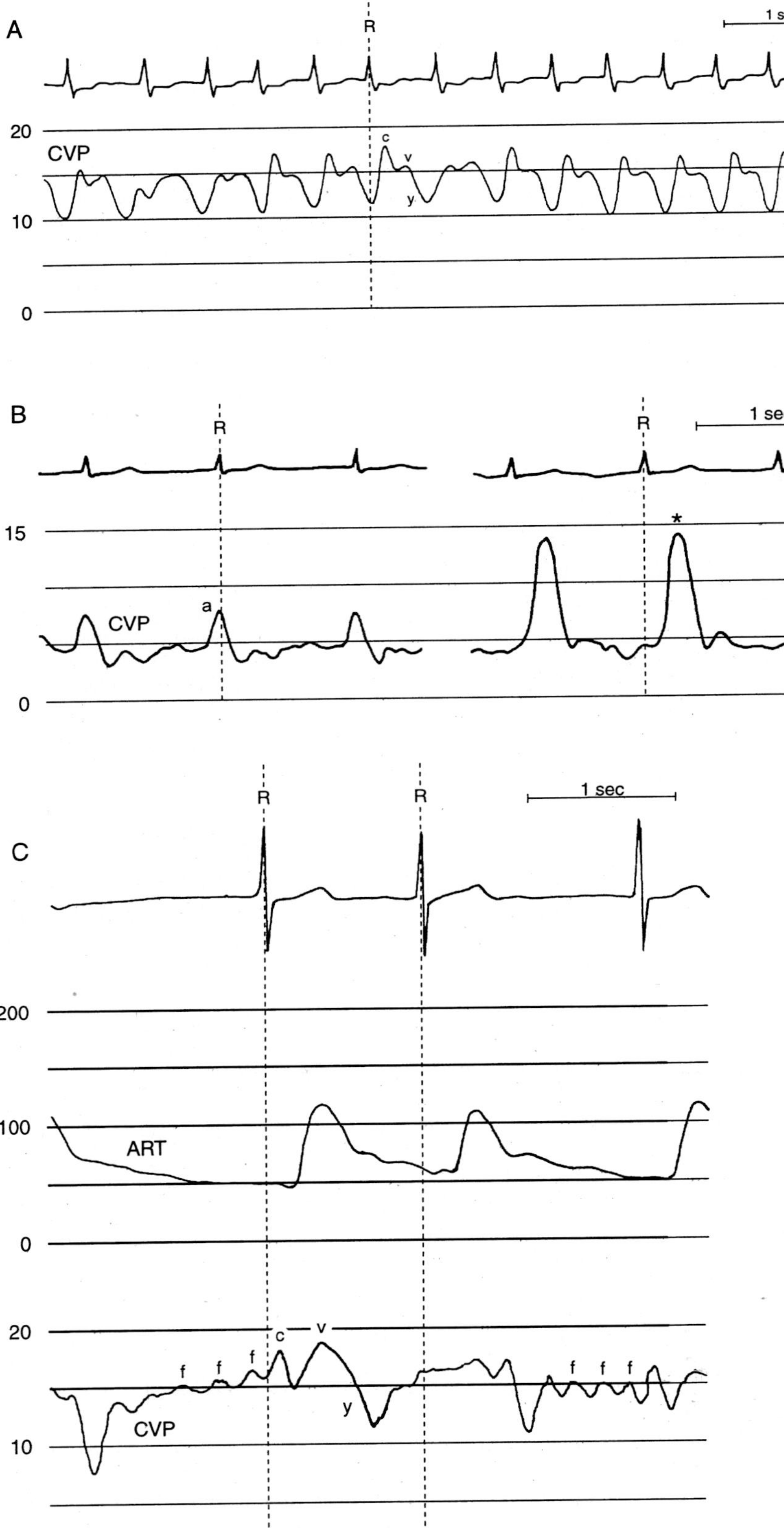

FIGURE 114–8 A, Atrial fibrillation obliterates the central venous pressure (CVP) a wave, augments the c wave, and preserves the v wave and y descent. **B,** Junctional rhythm causes atrial contraction against a closed tricuspid valve to produce tall early systolic cannon A waves (asterisk) that occur after the electrocardiogram R wave **(right).** Compare with sinus rhythm **(left). C,** Fibrillation/flutter (f) waves apparent in the CVP trace aids in diagnosis of the underlying atrial arrhythmia. The CVP c and v waves and the dominant y descent are noted. ART, atrial pressure. (**A–C,** From Mark JB: Cardiovascular Monitoring. *In* Miller RD [ed]: Anesthesia. Philadelphia: WB Saunders, 2000; and Mark JB: Atlas of Cardiovascular Monitoring. New York: Churchill Livingstone, 1998.)

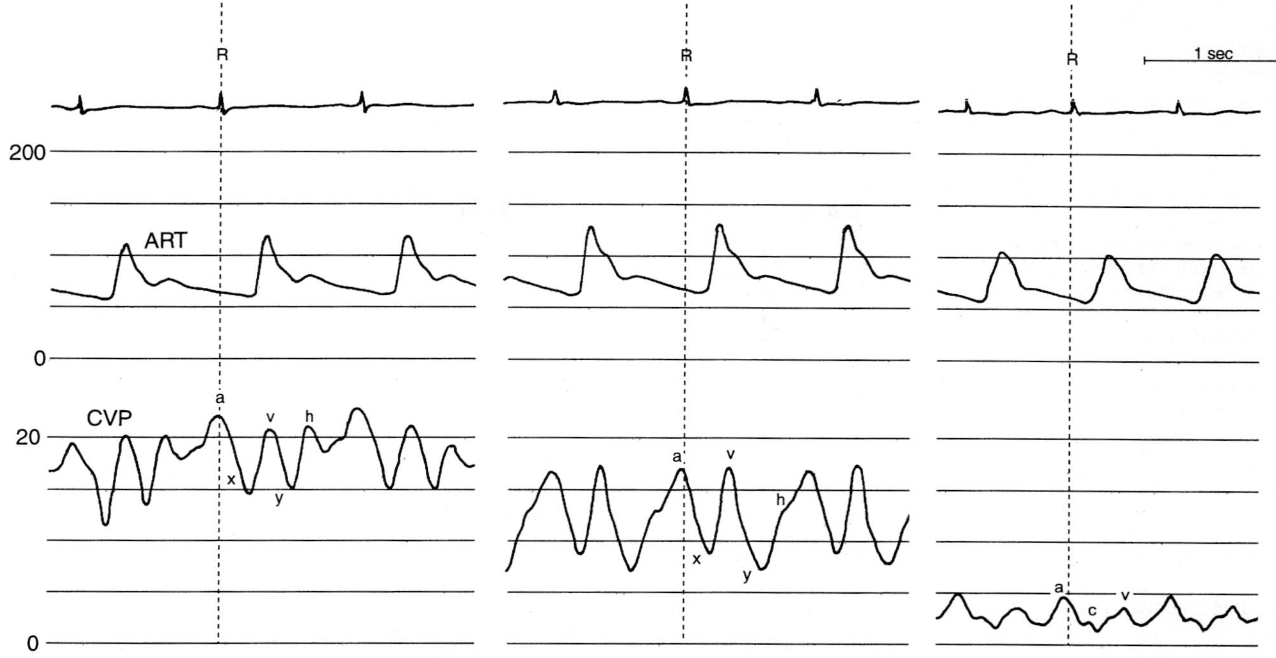

FIGURE 114–9 Pericardial constriction causes increased central venous pressure (CVP) with tall a and v waves, steep x and y descents, and a mid-diastolic plateau (h) wave. Pericardectomy produces resolution of the pathologic CVP waveform. These changes are noted in the progression of panels from **left** to **right.** The steep y descent and h wave pressure plateau are analogous to the "square root sign" seen in the ventricular pressure trace of this condition. The arterial blood pressure (ART) waveform is shown to highlight waveform timing. (Modified from Mark JB: Cardiovascular monitoring. *In* Miller RD [ed]: Anesthesia. Philadelphia: Churchill Livingstone, 2000.)

As in pericardial constriction, the CVP in cardiac tamponade is increased, and there is end-diastolic pressure equalization in all four cardiac chambers. However, in contrast to pericardial constriction, tamponade couples atrial and ventricular volume changes and produces a CVP waveform that is distinguished by the attenuated *y* descent.[41]

Complications

Complications can be divided into those resulting from attempts to gain central vascular access and those resulting from the presence of the CVP catheter in the body (Table 114–3). Serious complications have been described at each vascular access location; arterial puncture is the most common complication. Experienced operators and the use of ultrasound to locate the central vein reduce this risk. If cannulation of the carotid artery occurs, there is a significant risk of hematoma formation compromising airway patency. Controversy exists over whether to remove the catheter from the artery and apply local pressure or whether the catheter should be left in situ and be removed during surgical exploration of the neck and vascular repair. To plan the treatment of complications, vascular surgical consultation should be obtained promptly whenever a large-bore catheter is unintentionally inserted in the carotid or subclavian artery.

PULMONARY ARTERY CATHETERIZATION

Since its introduction into clinical practice in the 1970s for the treatment of patients with acute myocardial infarction,[42] the PAC has been accepted as an important monitoring device for high-risk surgical and critically ill patients. Pulmonary artery catheters allow the measurement of intracardiac pressures, CO, mixed venous hemoglobin saturation, and RV ejection fraction. Along with intracardiac and mixed venous blood samples, these PAC-derived measurements allow the calculation of hemodynamic indices and shunt ratios and provide data that are not obtainable through any other means.[43] However, despite the widespread use of the PAC since the 1970s, controversy concerning its clinical role remains, because PACs have not been shown to result in improved outcome in many of the conditions in which they are used.[44–49]

If PAC monitoring is to have any patient benefit, clinicians who use these catheters must be aware of the methods, indications, and complications of insertion and understand the physiologic and technical principles involved. Only by correctly interpreting and appropriately applying data obtained with continual hemodynamic monitoring will the PAC be fully exploited to provide maximum patient benefit.

Practical Considerations for Insertion

The right internal jugular vein is the most commonly chosen route of central venous access for PAC placement because it affords the most direct path between puncture site and the heart. As the catheter is advanced, the right atrium is encountered at 20 to 25 cm, the right ventricle at 25 to 35 cm, the PA at 35 to 45 cm, and the wedge position at approximately 50 cm.[50] By keeping these estimated dis-

TABLE 114–3 Complications of Central Venous Catheterization

From Gaining Venous Access and Cannulation
Arterial puncture
Hematoma
Hemothorax
Arterial thromboembolism
Arterial cannulation
Airway obstruction
Nerve and brachial plexus injury
Tracheal and laryngeal trauma
Chylothorax
Pneumothorax
Subcutaneous, mediastinal emphysema
Air embolism
Catheter or wire shearing and embolization
From Catheter Presence
Venous thrombosis and thromboembolism
Superior vena cava syndrome
Pulmonary embolism
Infection
Cellulitis
Sepsis
Endocarditis
Arrhythmias
Vascular injury
Arteriovenous fistula
Aortoatrial fistula
Venobronchial fistula
Perforation of superior vena cava, right atrium, right ventricle
Cardiac tamponade
Hydrothorax/hydromediastinum

tances in mind, the clinician can avoid excessive catheter insertion that may lead to catheter coiling or knotting within the heart. The subclavian route of insertion is associated with a higher incidence of pneumothorax, a particularly dangerous complication in patients receiving positive pressure ventilation. From more peripheral sites such as the femoral vein, the PAC may be more difficult to position correctly or adjust intraoperatively when there is limited access to the patient. Because the PAC is balloon tipped and flow guided, patient positioning influences the ease with which it passes through the heart. Head-down positioning aids flotation across the tricuspid valve, and head-up or right-side-down positioning aids flotation across the pulmonic valve.

A large increase in systolic pressure occurs with passage of the PAC from the right atrium to the right ventricle, followed by a diastolic pressure step up that signifies that the catheter has entered the PA. Rather than digital readouts alone, a real-time pressure waveform display is required to identify intravascular catheter tip position. For example, a pressure of 30/10 mm Hg is difficult to interpret and may be recorded from the right ventricle or the PA. Observation of the pressure tracing clarifies the matter because the PA pressure wave has a dicrotic notch with pressure falling steadily from the systolic pressure peak until the next pressure upstroke, whereas the pressure recorded in the right ventricle gradually rises in diastole as the ventricle fills until the onset of systole (Fig. 114–10).

Complications

Complications associated with PA catheterization arise from attempts at venous cannulation, from initial catheter placement and positioning, from the continued presence of the catheter within the body, and from misuse of equipment or misinterpretation of catheter-derived data. The reported frequency of complications varies greatly and is difficult to determine accurately, because most complications are described in case reports or small case series.[51, 52] Minor complications, such as self-limited arrhythmias, occur in up to 50 percent of insertions, but serious life-threatening complications are rare, occurring in 0.1 to 0.5 percent of catheterized patients.[52] A large prospective study of 6245 catheterizations of cardiac and noncardiac surgical patients reported catheter-related serious complications in 0.16 percent and death in 0.016 percent of patients.[53] The authors suggested that the expertise and experience of the attending physician, close supervision of trainees, and attention to detail were factors that minimized complications.

Arrhythmias

Although transient arrhythmias, most commonly premature ventricular contractions (PVCs), frequently accompany passage of the PAC through the heart, complete heart

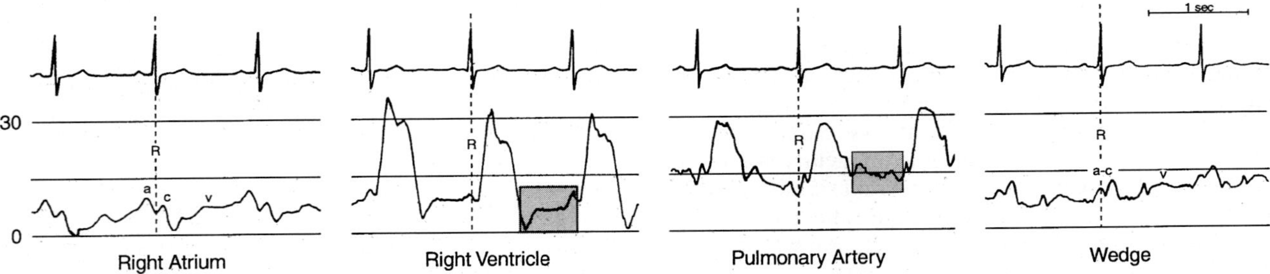

FIGURE 114–10 Characteristic pressure waveforms recorded during passage of a premature atrial contraction. The right atrial pressure trace displays the a, c, and v waves seen in a normal central venous pressure recording. Right ventricular pressure demonstrates the increase in systolic pressure; however, end-diastolic pressure is the same as in the right atrium and is best estimated by the right atrial pressure a wave peak. Increasing right ventricular pressure during diastole in contrast to the decreasing pulmonary artery pressure *(shaded boxes)* helps to differentiate these recordings. Pulmonary artery wedge pressure has a venous pressure morphology similar to that of right atrial pressure, but the a, c, and v waves appear delayed in relation to the electrocardiogram. (From Mark JB: Cardiovascular monitoring. *In* Miller RD [ed]: Anesthesia. Philadelphia: Churchill Livingstone, 2000.)

block, ventricular tachycardia, and ventricular fibrillation have been reported. Shah and associates[53] observed that 68 percent of patients experienced PVCs, with only 3.1 percent requiring treatment. The use of prophylactic lidocaine to suppress catheter-related arrhythmias is of questionable efficacy.[54] Because transient right bundle branch block occurs during catheterization in up to 5 percent of patients,[55–57] complete heart block may be precipitated in patients with preexisting left bundle branch block.[58] However, because this happens rarely,[53, 55] the prophylactic placement of a transvenous pacing wire is not warranted. Instead, transcutaneous pacing should be available or a pacing PAC should be chosen.

Catheter Knotting

Coiling, looping, and knotting of catheters within the heart have been described and are more likely in low-CO states, when the heart chambers are dilated, and when the catheter is advanced to excessive distances.[59, 60] Intracardiac pacing wires or anatomic structures such as chordae tendineae may become entangled in PACs.[61, 62] Catheter knots may be disentangled under fluoroscopic guidance using intravascular snares,[63, 64] or they may be pulled tight and removed with the catheter sheath. If these methods fail or the catheter is entrapped in a cardiac structure, surgical removal is required.

Valvular Damage, Endocarditis, and Thromboembolism

The PAC balloon must be completely deflated before catheter withdrawal to avoid damage to the tricuspid[65] or pulmonary[66] valves. Despite proper catheter management, occult endocardial damage occurs frequently and may result in endocarditis.[67–70] Although bacteremia may produce catheter colonization, catheter-related infection more often results from skin organisms that colonize the introducer sheath.[71] Mermel and colleagues[72] demonstrated a 22 percent incidence of local infection of the introducer sheath but only a 0.7 percent incidence of PAC-associated bacteremia. Scheduled replacement of PACs through new venipuncture sites or over guidewires remains controversial.[73, 74] The risks of infection versus the risks of de novo central venous cannulation must be weighed in the individual patient.[75, 76] The implementation of rigorous infection control techniques will reduce catheter-related infections[77] and should be applied routinely.

Minor thrombi associated with PACs were common but have been markedly reduced by the use of heparin-bonded catheters.[78] Major thromboembolism associated with PAC use remains rare. Although the PAC lumens must always be flushed continuously with a crystalloid solution, the addition of heparin to the flush in an attempt to reduce thrombotic complications has not been shown to be effective and may induce thrombocytopenia.[79]

Pulmonary Vascular Injury

Pulmonary vascular injury is a rare but potentially life-threatening complication of PA catheterization. Pulmonary infarction may result from prolonged balloon inflation or distal catheter migration.[80] Of even greater concern, PA rupture may occur, with an incidence of 0.02 to 2.0 percent and mortality rate of 40 to 70 percent.[81–83] Hemoptysis is the cardinal sign, and advanced age, anticoagulation, and pulmonary hypertension are common, albeit unproved, associations.[82–84]

Treatment focuses on maintaining oxygenation and control of bleeding. Endobronchial intubation with either a single- or double-lumen endotracheal tube allows selective lung ventilation and isolates the bleeding segment.[85] Other treatment involves reversing anticoagulation, antihypertensive therapy to lower PA pressure, and bronchoscopy for endobronchial toilet and identification of the site of bleeding. Although transcatheter embolization with a steel coil[86] or tissue-adhesive occlusive agent[87] may control hemorrhage, surgical lung resection is required when conservative treatment fails[81, 83] or if life-threatening hemothorax develops.[83] Pseudoaneurysm has been reported as a late complication that may require further treatment in patients initially treated conservatively.[81]

Data Interpretation Errors

Perhaps the most common complication of the PAC is an insidious one, the misinterpretation of hemodynamic data. Several investigators have shown a poor level of knowledge among users of PACs, including nurses, physicians, and specialists in critical care medicine.[88–90] A fundamental skill, waveform interpretation, is performed inconsistently even by experienced physicians.[88–91] Clearly, skilled use of the PAC is a basic requirement if catheterization is to have any benefit. These training requirements are well outlined by the American College of Cardiology, American Heart Association, and American Society of Anesthesiologists task forces.[92]

Pulmonary Artery Wedge Trace

When the PAC balloon floats the catheter to a wedged position, a static column of blood connects the catheter tip to a junction point where flow resumes in the pulmonary veins near the left atrium. Because resistance to flow in the pulmonary veins is low, PAWP provides an accurate estimate for pulmonary venous pressure and left atrial pressure (LAP). In addition, the same phasic mechanical events that generate CVP A, C, and V waves create a similar waveform pattern in the LAP and PAWP waveforms. Consequently, the PAWP tracing may be recognized by characteristic A, C, and V waves that reflect a LAP waveform that is slightly delayed and damped by the interposed pulmonary vascular bed. Due to these anatomic factors, the PAWP A wave appears after the ECG R wave, even though it reflects end-diastolic left atrial contraction. PAWP is usually reported as a single mean value for assessment of the hydrostatic back-pressure that influences pulmonary edema formation. As a predictor of LV preload, however, the phasic PAWP recorded at the peak of the A wave provides a better estimate of left ventricular end-diastolic pressure (LVEDP), particularly in patients with LV dysfunction.[93] Although some authors use the term *pulmonary capillary pressure* interchangeably with PAWP (or PA occlusion pressure),

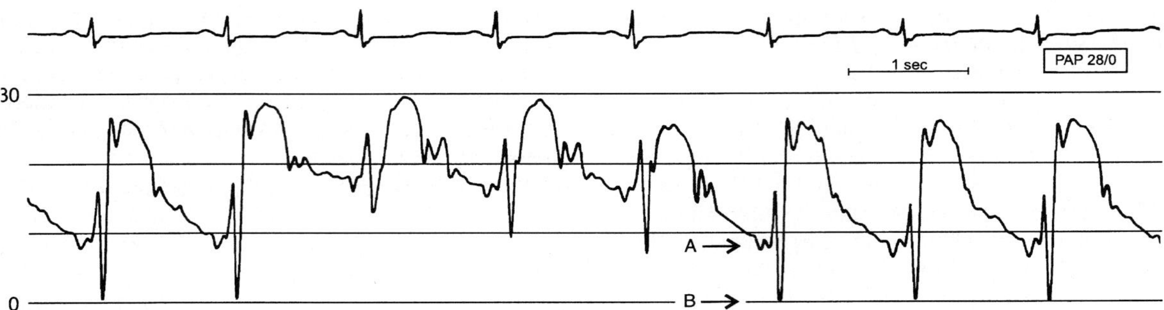

FIGURE 114–11 Artifactual pressure peaks and troughs in the pulmonary artery pressure (PAP) trace appear after the electrocardiogram R wave and result from motion of the premature atrial contraction. The correct value for end-diastolic PAP is 8 mm Hg (A), although the monitor displays an artifactual value of 0 mm Hg (PAP, 28/0 mm Hg, B). (From Mark JB: Cardiovascular monitoring. *In* Miller RD [ed]: Anesthesia. Philadelphia: Churchill Livingstone, 2000.)

capillary pressure is slightly higher than PAWP and may be significantly higher when pulmonary venous pressure is elevated. Pulmonary capillary pressure is different than the wedge pressure and may be derived from the decay curve after PAC balloon inflation.[94, 95]

Factors Affecting Data Validity

Pulmonary Artery Catheter Artifacts

Motion of the PAC induced by cardiac contraction creates artifactual spikes or troughs in the PAP waveform. These catheter fling artifacts are observed often after the ECG R wave when tricuspid valve closure and ventricular contraction set the PAC in motion (Fig. 114–11). Another pressure artifact, termed *overwedging*, is produced when a gradually rising, nonpulsatile pressure is recorded after balloon inflation. This occurs when the catheter tip is forced against the wall of the PA, occluding the PA lumen so that pressure builds from the continuous pressurized flush system. Withdrawing and repositioning the catheter within the PA can ameliorate both of these artifacts.

Catheter Tip Position and Respiratory Influences

West and associates[96] characterized gravity-dependent differences in lung perfusion and ventilation that depending on the relationship of pulmonary arterial pressure (PAP) (Pa), alveolar pressure (PA), and pulmonary venous pressure (Pv). In lung zone 1, PA exceeds both Pa and Pv; in zone 2, PA exceeds Pv but not Pa; and in zone 3, Pa and Pv exceed PA. Consequently, zone 3 conditions must be present in the portion of the lung containing the PAC for the PAWP to provide a valid estimate of LAP (Fig. 114–12). Alveolar rather than intravascular pressures are measured when the catheter tip is located in zone 1 or 2. This may be suspected when the PAWP trace does not have

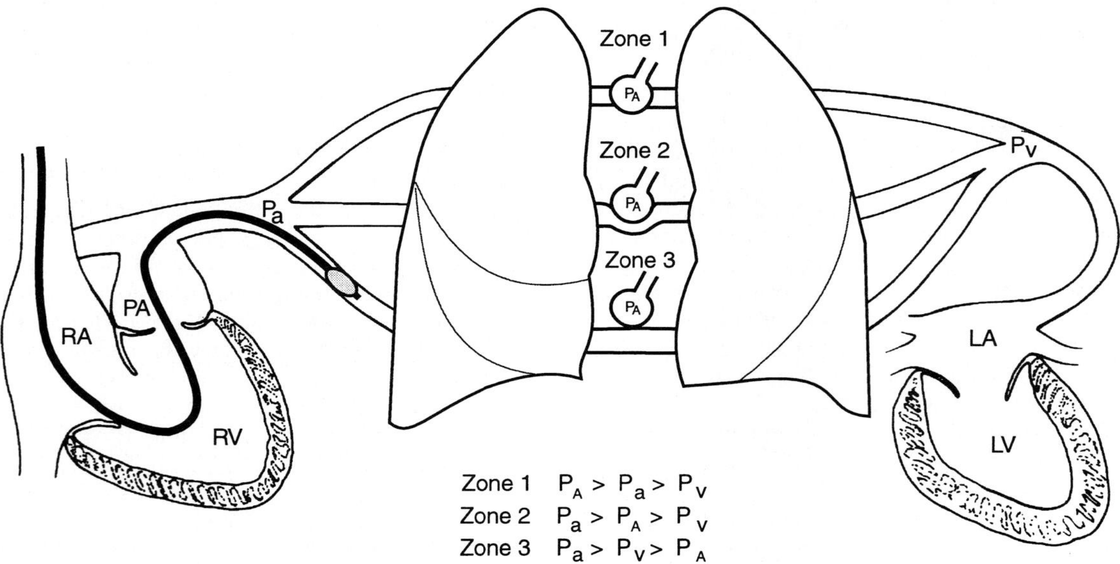

FIGURE 114–12 The pulmonary artery (PA) catheter tip must be wedged in the most dependent part of the lung, zone 3, to measure accurately pulmonary venous (P_V) or left atrial (LA) pressure. When alveolar pressure (P_A) rises above P_V in zone 2 or above pulmonary arterial (P_a) pressure in zone 1, wedge pressure reflects alveolar rather than intravascular pressures. LV, left ventricle; RA, right atrium; RV, right ventricle. (From Mark JB: Cardiovascular monitoring. *In* Miller RD [ed]: Anesthesia. Philadelphia: Churchill Livingstone, 2000.)

characteristic A and V waves and when there is excessive respiratory variation in the trace.

Predicting Left Ventricular End-Diastolic Volume

One of the primary reasons for PAC monitoring is to provide an accurate estimate of LV preload. In clinical practice, LVEDV measurements are not readily available, and pressure surrogates are used as an estimate. In the assessment of LV preload, the further "upstream" from the left ventricle that pressures are measured, the more prone is the estimate to confounding errors (Table 114–4).

Pulmonary Vascular Resistance and Heart Rate

Because normal pulmonary vascular resistance (PVR) is low, pulmonary blood flow ceases at end diastole and pulmonary artery diastolic pressure (PADP) equals LAP. If PVR is elevated, pulmonary blood flow continues throughout the cardiac cycle, and a pressure gradient remains between PA and LA at end diastole. In this case, PADP overestimates downstream LAP or LVEDP, but PAWP remains an accurate estimate for LVEDP because there is no pressure gradient across the static column of blood connecting the wedged catheter tip to the junction point in the pulmonary veins. Pulmonary artery diastolic pressure also overestimates LAP in pulmonary veno-occlusive disease. In this rare condition, PAWP may also overestimate LAP if the site of venous occlusion involves the large pulmonary veins.[97, 98]

When the pulmonary vascular bed is reduced after pneumonectomy or large pulmonary embolus, PAC balloon inflation itself may cause significant obstruction of pulmonary blood flow, reducing LAP while simultaneously increasing PAP.[99] Under these conditions, PAWP measurement artifactually decreases LV preload, so the PAWP value recorded underestimates the true LV filling pressure.

As the duration of diastole shortens with increasing heart rate, the time for flow across the pulmonary bed decreases, producing a diastolic pressure gradient between PAP and LAP similar to that seen in pulmonary hypertension.[100] This effect of tachycardia is greatest when PVR is elevated. Tachycardia may also produce a pressure gradient across the mitral valve, resulting in LAP exceeding LVEDP.

Valvular Disease

When there is significant pulmonary valve regurgitation and RV diastolic pressure is lower than LAP, PAP seeks the lower pressure value at end diastole, and PADP will be lower than LAP and underestimates LVEDP. With aortic valve regurgitation, diastolic filling of the left ventricle occurs as soon as LV pressure falls below aortic root pressure and continues after mitral valve closure. Consequently, PADP, PAWP, and LAP will underestimate LVEDP. With mitral stenosis, a pressure gradient from the left atrium to the left ventricle exists throughout diastole, causing the PAWP and LAP to overestimate LVEDP. Mitral regurgitation produces tall regurgitant C-V waves in the PAWP trace, increasing mean LAP, and the risk of pulmonary edema. Rather than the normal late systolic V wave caused by venous filling of the atrium, the C-V wave begins in early ventricular systole. Mitral regurgitation influences mean PAWP, which in turn overestimates LV filling pressure. LVEDP is lower than mean PAWP and is best estimated by the pressure value recorded before the onset of the C-V wave. Thus, mean PAWP accurately estimates mean LAP in mitral valve disease but overestimates LVEDP. The height of the C-V wave in the PAWP trace has not been found to accurately reflect the severity of mitral regurgitation.[101] The height of the C-V wave depends not only on the volume of regurgitation but also on LA compliance and volume,[102] thus explaining why large C-V waves are often present in acute mitral regurgitation, whereas a similar degree of regurgitation in chronic mitral regurgitation does not produce a tall C-V wave.[103]

TABLE 114–4 **Underestimation and Overestimation of Left Ventricular End-Diastolic Pressure**

Condition	Site of Discrepancy	Cause of Discrepancy
Underestimation		
Decreased left ventricular compliance	Mean LAP < LVEDP	Increased end diastolic A wave
Aortic regurgitation	LAP A wave < LVEDP	Mitral valve closure before end diastole
Pulmonic regurgitation	PADP < LVEDP	Bidirectional runoff for pulmonary artery flow
Right bundle branch block	PADP < LVEDP	Delayed pulmonic valve opening
Decreased pulmonary vascular bed	PAWP < LVEDP	Obstruction of pulmonary blood flow
Overestimation		
Positive end-expiratory pressure	Mean PAWP > mean LAP	Creation of lung zone 1 or 2 or pericardial pressure changes
Pulmonary arterial hypertension	PADP > mean PAWP	Increased pulmonary vascular resistance
Pulmonary veno-occlusive disease	Mean PAWP > mean LAP	Obstruction to flow in large pulmonary veins
Mitral stenosis	Mean LAP > LVEDP	Obstruction to flow across mitral valve
Mitral regurgitation	Mean LAP > LVEDP	Retrograde systolic V wave raises mean atrial pressure
Ventricular septal defect	Mean LAP > LVEDP	Antegrade systolic V wave raises mean atrial pressure
Tachycardia	PADP > mean LAP > LVEDP	Short diastole creates pulmonary vascular and mitral valve gradients

Abbreviations: LAP, left atrial pressure; LVEDP, left ventricular end-diastolic pressure; PADP pulmonary artery diastolic pressure; PAWP, pulmonary artery wedge pressure.
Modified from Mark JB: Atlas of Cardiovascular Monitoring. New York: Churchill Livingstone, 1998.

Ventilatory Pressure Influences

The net distending pressure applied to a cardiac chamber is the pressure of physiologic interest and is best described by transmural pressure. During labored respiration, coughing, Valsalva maneuver, and positive pressure ventilation, a large negative or positive intrapleural pressure change influences intracardiac pressures measured with pressure transducers outside the thorax.[98, 104] The best way to obviate these confounding effects of intrathoracic pressure is to measure intravascular pressures at *end-expiration*. At this point in the respiratory cycle, intrathoracic pressure approximates atmospheric pressure whether the patient is breathing spontaneously or mechanically ventilated. Under these circumstances, central vascular and intracardiac pressures measured at end-expiration will provide the best estimate for transmural pressure. Visual inspection of the waveform display is the most accurate method for identifying end-expiratory pressures. Reliance on digital displays should be avoided, because these are notoriously inaccurate.[105]

Positive end-expiratory pressure (PEEP) influences PAP measurement through its effects on transmural pressure. The degree to which PEEP alters juxtacardiac pressure (and PAWP) depends on pulmonary and chest wall compliance. PEEP usually increases measured PAWP less than one half the value of PEEP applied. Fortunately, high levels of PEEP are required only when pulmonary compliance is markedly reduced, which attenuates the effects of these high airway pressures.[98, 106] Prolonged airway disconnection obviates the effect of PEEP on PAP measurements but may alter venous return and other hemodynamic values and have a deleterious effect on respiratory mechanics and gas exchange. Alternatively, abrupt transient airway disconnection for less than 3 seconds may allow estimation of the influence of high levels of PEEP with a greater margin of safety.[107]

Ventricular Compliance and Pressure-Volume Relationships

Because the pressure-volume relationship of the left ventricle is curvilinear, changes in LVEDP can result from small or large changes in ventricular volume depending on the portion of the compliance curve over which the left ventricle is operating. Conditions causing a marked shift in the compliance curve may result in pressure and volume changing in opposite directions (i.e., increased filling pressure associated with decreased ventricular volume). These physiologic considerations further complicate interpretation of PADP, PAWP, LAP, or LVEDP as measures of LV preload. The ventricular pressure-volume relation is influenced by both intrinsic factors such as wall thickness, chamber size, and passive and active relaxation and extrinsic factors such as pericardial pressure, intrathoracic pressure, and ventricular interdependence.

Optimizing Preload

In view of these considerations, it is not surprising that determining the "optimal" LV filling pressure is a difficult task in many clinical circumstances. One practical approach is to administer a rapid "fluid challenge" (250 ml) over 10 minutes while monitoring the change in PAWP and other hemodynamic variables. Smaller volumes are chosen to decrease the risk of producing pulmonary edema when the baseline PAWP is high or pulmonary capillary injury exists. If the fluid challenge produces a large change in PAWP (>7 mm Hg) or pulmonary edema develops, the left ventricle is operating on the steep portion of its compliance curve. Further fluid administration will worsen pulmonary edema and cause an increase in myocardial oxygen consumption without increasing stroke volume and CO.[98] In contrast, a small increase in PAWP (<3 mm Hg) suggests that the left ventricle is operating on the flat portion of the compliance curve, and further volume administration may be beneficial in improving stroke volume. Once volume status has been optimized and tissue perfusion is still deemed inadequate, stroke volume augmentation will require inotropic support or afterload reduction.

In high-risk surgery, there is considerable evidence that preoperative "optimization" of oxygen delivery with fluids and inotropes to achieve oxygen delivery of more than 600 ml/min/m^2 reduces mortality and morbidity rates and hospital stay.[108–110] This type of treatment, preemptively instituted in the intensive care unit for the treatment of critically ill patients, has been termed *goal-directed therapy*. In contrast to these early interventions, which are PAC guided, delayed hemodynamic resuscitation in critically ill medical and surgical patients with systemic inflammatory response syndrome or severe organ dysfunction has not been shown to lead to improved outcome.[111, 112]

Use of Pulmonary Artery Catheters for Myocardial Ischemia Monitoring

The physiologic changes of myocardial ischemia can be detected with a PAC. Ischemia-induced diastolic dysfunction increases mean PAWP, and the phasic A and V waves become more prominent. Although PADP and PAWP often increase during ischemia, this does not necessarily indicate increased LV preload.[113, 114] Diastolic LV dysfunction, particularly characteristic of demand-induced ischemia, impairs LV relaxation. In these patients, LVEDP may be estimated best by the A wave pressure peak rather than by the mean PAWP. In addition, ischemia may lead to acute mitral valve regurgitation and a tall systolic C-V wave in the wedge trace. Although these changes have been described in patients undergoing surgery, changes in PAWP may be small and difficult to detect clinically. Furthermore, there is no quantitative threshold value for mean PAWP, change in PAWP, or PAWP A or V wave height that is diagnostic of myocardial ischemia. In general, there is poor agreement between ECG, PAC, and echocardiographic indicators of myocardial ischemia when these variables are all monitored simultaneously during surgery.[115, 116] This limits the use of the PAC as a primary monitor for ischemia. Rather, if ischemia is suspected, integration of hemodynamic information from the PAC with other monitored values helps to confirm the diagnosis.

Evidence For and Against Use of the Pulmonary Artery Catheter

Conditions that warrant PAC placement are largely influenced by institutional, geographic,[117] and individual[118] preferences. The widespread dissemination of PAC monitoring occurred before this technology was evaluated rigorously. Studies showing no benefit or worse outcome associated with PAC monitoring[48, 111, 112, 119–124] and studies supporting its use[109, 110, 125–127] provide conflicting evidence.

In the absence of convincing outcome studies, expert panels of the American Society of Anesthesiologists, American Heart Association, and American College of Cardiology have provided practice guidelines that acknowledge these uncertainties but help standardize clinical practice. PAC monitoring must be individualized to each patient based on preoperative cardiac complications; the type, anatomic site, and length of surgery; expected perioperative blood loss, fluid shifts, and physiologic derangement; and patterns of postoperative care.

Pacing Pulmonary Artery Catheters

Multipurpose PACs allow cardiac pacing and intracardiac ECG recording. One device incorporates five outer surface electrodes to allow bipolar atrial, ventricular, or atrioventricular sequential pacing. Although successful pacing is usually achieved intraoperatively in anesthetized patients,[128] these catheters are less reliable in intensive care patients due to the instability of the catheter/endocardium contact. Other PACs have dedicated lumina to accept dedicated ventricular or atrial pacing wires and appear to produce a more secure method of temporary pacing.[129] In a prospective study of 600 cardiac surgical patients, only 18 percent of those receiving a pacing PAC required the pacing capability. Predictors of the need for pacing included sinus node dysfunction/bradydysrhythmias, history of transient complete heart block, aortic stenosis, aortic regurgitation, and cardiac reoperation.[130]

Right Ventricular Ejection Fraction Pulmonary Artery Catheters

Another modification of the PAC allows measurement of right ventricular ejection fraction (RVEF) using a rapid-response thermistor that measures beat-to-beat changes in PA blood temperature.[131] An average residual fraction (RF) of thermal signal with each heartbeat can be determined, from which ejection fraction (EF) can be calculated:

$$EF = 1 - RF_{mean}$$

Because the temperature changes are small, the accurate measurement of RVEF depends on adequate mixing of the thermal bolus and a regular heart rate. Although the monitoring of RVEF per se may have limited value, other derived variables may be more useful clinically; these include stroke volume, right ventricular end-diastolic volume (RVEDV), and RV end-systolic volume. RVEF catheters can aid in the management of RV dysfunction by providing a measure of RVEDV in addition to the traditional pressure surrogates for ventricular preload: CVP and PAWP. Although its efficacy remains unproved, the RVEF PAC might aid in the management of patients with pulmonary hypertension, RV infarction, right coronary disease, and other conditions, such as sepsis and adult respiratory distress syndrome, that require high levels of mechanical ventilation that confound interpretation of cardiac filling pressures.[132]

CARDIAC OUTPUT MONITORING

CO is the total blood flow generated by the heart each minute, and at rest values ranges from 4.0 to 6.5 L/min in the normal adult. Preload, afterload, heart rate, and cardiac contractility determine CO, which is regulated to meet tissue metabolic requirements. As such, CO measurement assesses the status of the circulation as a whole, and when combined with other hemodynamic values, additional derived variables such as pulmonary and systemic vascular resistances can be calculated.

Thermodilution Cardiac Output

Thermodilution CO measurement is based on the indicator dilution method, in which a known amount of substance is injected into the circulation and its concentration is measured over time at a downstream site. When a dye such as indocyanine green is injected as the indicator, continuous withdrawal of arterial blood is required. Recirculation of dye distorts the primary concentration-time curve and produces high background concentrations of dye in the blood.

Thermodilution CO measurement superseded dye dilution when a thermistor incorporated at the PAC tip enabled continuous measurement of blood temperature in the PA. A second thermistor located at the injectate port measures injectate temperature. When a fixed volume of cold injectate is used, the temperature drop measured in the PA is used by the computer to calculate CO based on a modified Stewart-Hamilton equation:

$$CO = \frac{V(T_B - T_I) \cdot K}{\int_0^{\infty} \Delta T_B(t)dt}$$

where V is injectate volume, T_B is blood temperature, T_I is injectate temperature, K is computation constant, and is integral of temperature change over time.

$$\int_0^{\infty} \Delta T_B(t)dt$$

The computation constant (K) adjusts for the specific heat capacity and specific gravity of the injectate and blood, volume of injectate, and size and composition of the PAC.

The average of several measurements performed in rapid succession yields a more accurate CO result than a single measurement alone, and in clinical practice, a 15 percent change in measured CO is usually accepted as significant. The real-time display of the thermodilution curve helps to identify spurious measurements. Although there is reasonable agreement between thermodilution and other methods of CO measurement,[133, 134] technical errors are common and may go unrecognized.[88] Right-sided valvular regurgitation[135] and intracardiac shunts invalidate this method by causing recirculation of the thermal bolus and differences between LV and RV output. If the injectate port is within the PAC introducer sheath, the thermal bolus is not properly delivered to the RA, producing an abnormal thermodilution curve. Additional fluid boluses through peripheral or central venous catheters introduce additional CO measurement errors, depending on the rate, temperature, and timing of the fluid administration.[136]

Proper timing of thermodilution CO measurement during the respiratory cycle is controversial due to the associated changes in RV loading and stroke output. Because the thermodilution CO method measures only the 60 to 70 percent of the thermodilution RV output over several heartbeats, measured CO may vary considerably, depending on the timing of injection of the thermal bolus. Although synchronization of CO measurement at end-inspiration or end-expiration will produce less variation and more reproducibility, a better mean value for CO is obtained by averaging multiple measurements performed throughout the respiratory cycle. This is especially true when large intrathoracic pressure variations occur, such as with positive pressure ventilation.[137]

The use of ice-cold injectate should produce more accurate results than room temperature injectate by increasing the signal-to-noise ratio of the thermal bolus, but several investigators have shown no difference in accuracy between the two methods.[138, 139] Consequently, the simpler, less expensive method applied in most clinical settings involves the use of a 10-ml room temperature injectate. The thermodilution technique is simple to perform repeatedly and quickly, requires only basic clinical skills, obviates the need for repeated blood sampling, and uses a nontoxic, nonrecirculating, and nonaccumulating indicator. For these reasons, thermodilution CO is extensively used as the preferred method in a variety of clinical settings.

Continuous Thermodilution Cardiac Output Measurement

Because heat is the only nonaccumulating indicator, continuous CO measurement methods have focused on modified thermodilution techniques. One method introduces the thermal signal through a PAC that has a blood-warming filament in the right ventricle located 14 to 25 cm from the catheter tip. Thermal damage does not occur because of the brief duration of contact between heating filament and the blood and myocardium, as well as control of filament temperature below 44°C. Continuous thermodilution CO measurement involves the use of a small thermal signal rather than background thermal noise. Computer-controlled algorithms use a stochastic system control filament that switches between on or off states in a random process, with automatic cross-correlation to minimize temperature peaks and enhance signal-to-noise ratio.[140] The displayed CO is updated every 30 seconds and represents an average CO measured over the previous 3 to 6 minutes. Although this averaging delays the response time of continuous thermodilution CO measurement, confounding respiratory influences are attenuated, yielding a more accurate "average" CO.

Compared with other methods of CO measurement, continuous thermodilution CO measurement is reasonably accurate and precise.[141] However, thermal noise contributes a large source of error and is particularly problematic after hypothermic cardiopulmonary bypass.[142] Continuous thermodilution CO measurement should not be considered "real-time" but rather a trend of recent measurements. As such, unlike direct arterial blood pressure monitoring, it is not suitable for identifying acute hemodynamic changes. However, compared with bolus CO measurement performed intermittently every several hours, the continuous CO method provides information earlier and may allow more timely clinical intervention.[141] Because the system is fully automated, it requires less procedural effort than bolus thermodilution CO methods and may decrease the risks of fluid overload, infection, and measurement error.

Mixed Venous Oxygen Saturation Measurement

Mixed venous oxygen saturation measurement provides a method to assess the adequacy of oxygen supply relative to prevailing metabolic demands.[143] Assuming the contribution of dissolved oxygen is negligible, rearrangement of the Fick equation reveals the determinants of mixed venous oxygen saturation:

$$S\text{v}O_2 = S_aO_2 - \left(\frac{\dot{V}O_2}{CO \cdot 1.34 \cdot Hb}\right) \times 100$$

where $S\text{v}O_2$ is mixed venous oxygen saturation (percent), SaO_2 is arterial oxygen saturation (percent), $\dot{V}O_2$ is oxygen consumption (ml O_2/min), Hb is hemoglobin concentration (g/ml), and CO is cardiac output (ml/min) (1.34 ml of oxygen is carried by each gram of hemoglobin).

Mixed venous oxygen saturation thus depends on four factors:

1. Hemoglobin concentration
2. Arterial oxygen saturation
3. CO
4. Oxygen consumption

To the extent that arterial hemoglobin concentration, arterial saturation, and oxygen consumption remain stable, mixed venous oxygen saturation reflects changes in CO.[123]

PACs modified with fiberoptic bundles can measure mixed venous saturation continuously based on the differential absorption of various wavelengths of light by oxyhemoglobin and deoxyhemoglobin. The use of multiple wavelengths of light reduces artifact from vessel wall, PAC thrombus reflection, and circulating optically active compounds such as methylene blue, carboxyhemoglobin, or bilirubin. These catheters may show a drift artifact, requiring recalibration in vivo with a PA blood sample. Combined with thermodilution CO measurement, mixed venous saturation monitoring allows the calculation of other parameters, such as oxygen consumption and delivery. Mixed venous oximetry is safe, convenient, and reliable and provides clinically useful information on the balance between oxygen supply and demand. However, these PAC modifications substantially increase cost, and their use in goal-directed therapy remains controversial. Further study is required to define appropriate indications for their use.[144]

Doppler Ultrasound-Based Cardiac Output (Measurement)

The Doppler principle uses the spectral frequency shift of ultrasound reflected waves from a moving target to calculate the velocity of the target. Doppler-based CO measurement employs high frequency (2–5 MHz) ultrasound reflected from circulating red cells, as described by the Doppler equation.

$$V = \frac{f \cdot c}{2f_0 \cdot \cos\theta}$$

where V is velocity of blood, f is frequency shift, f_0 is ultrasound frequency, θ is the angle between the ultrasound beam vector and velocity vector, and c is velocity of ultrasound in blood (≈1540 m/s).

If the angle of insonation is within 20 of blood flow direction, the error in velocity measurement is less than 6 percent, because cos 20 = 0.94.

Suprasternal positioning of the Doppler probe allowing insonation of the ascending aorta is noninvasive and accurate but labor intensive and requires considerable operator expertise. Signal acquisition cannot be obtained in some patients with short necks, emphysema, or aortic valve disease, and since the probe cannot be fixed in position, this method cannot be used for continuous CO monitoring. Endotracheal tubes and PACs incorporating Doppler probes have been tried with limited success.[145–148] Inaccuracy, poor signal stability, and the need for tracheal intubation or PA catheterization have resulted in poor clinical acceptance.

The esophagus offers a suitable site for probe placement for continuous Doppler CO monitoring. A probe of similar dimensions to an orogastric tube is inserted in the lower esophagus, approximately 35 to 40 cm from the incisors. From this imaging position, the thoracic aorta and esophagus are juxtaposed in parallel, and a reliable Doppler signal may be obtained from the descending aorta. Early esophageal Doppler CO devices were calibrated with CO measurement obtained with suprasternal Doppler[149, 150] and aortic diameter measured with A-mode ultrasound.[149–151] This technique required significant operator expertise and was often inaccurate. Current devices are easier to use because calibration is no longer required and monitors provide a clear auditory and visual display of the spectral Doppler waveform to confirm correct transducer position. With a short period of training, reproducible measurements take less than 5 minutes and are technically easy to acquire.[150, 152] However, the esophageal Doppler technique has generally been limited to tracheally intubated patients.

The area underneath the velocity-time curve is the velocity-time integral and represents the distance traveled by a column of blood with each ventricular ejection. The stroke volume and CO are calculated from this velocity-time integral. In addition, indices of aortic blood flow and the shape of velocity envelope to CO calculation provide information on preload, afterload, and contractility (Fig. 114–13). There are no reports of complications arising from esophageal Doppler monitoring, but care should be taken when esophageal pathology exists or when the patient is anticoagulated. Rather than an actual measurement of CO, Doppler CO monitors provide a reliable and consistent estimate of CO from aortic blood velocity measurement based on the following assumptions:

1. The angle of insonation of blood flow remains constant.

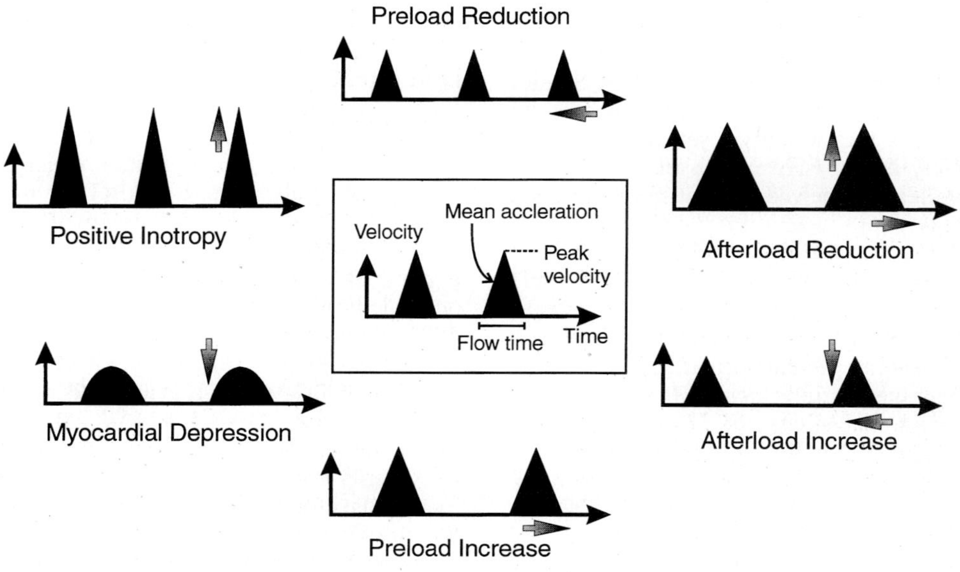

FIGURE 114–13 Spectral Doppler of velocity waveforms recorded using esophageal Doppler cardiac output monitoring. Changes in waveform shape result from alterations in inotropic, preload, and afterload. The Doppler waveform pattern changes in a consistent manner: inotropic changes affect peak velocity and mean acceleration, preload changes affect systolic flow time corrected for heart rate (FT_c), and afterload changes affect FT_c and peak velocity. (Modified from Singer M: Esophageal Doppler monitoring of aortic blood flow: beat-by-beat cardiac output monitoring. Int Anesthesiol Clin 31[3]:99–125, 1993.)

2. The fraction of total CO passing through the descending thoracic aorta remains constant despite changes in CO, preload, afterload, and temperature.
3. The descending thoracic aortic cross-sectional area does not change during systole.

In view of these assumptions, it is not surprising that esophageal Doppler CO measurements show variable agreement with other CO methods. However, the use of Doppler-based CO to monitor trends has proved to be clinically effective for the resuscitation of critically ill and surgical patients. Esophageal Doppler of CO monitoring provides continuous, beat-to-beat assessment of ventricular performance, filling, and systemic vascular resistance, enabling noninvasive optimization of fluid resuscitation.[153] In surgical patients, esophageal Doppler-guided fluid therapy may reduce hospital stay[154–156] by allowing early detection of hypovolemia before other hemodynamic indices change.[157] It is not surprising that Doppler CO monitoring provides an early warning, because reflex tachycardia and vasoconstriction may maintain CO and blood pressure in the presence of occult hypovolemia.

In summary, the esophageal Doppler monitor is safe and reliable and provides unique information on the state of the circulation. It remains to be seen whether large studies will demonstrate efficacy and cost effectiveness and ensure a place for this technique as a routine cardiovascular monitor.[158]

Other Methods of Cardiac Output Measurement

Indicator dilution measurement of CO can be achieved using ionized lithium as an indicator. Lithium chloride is given as a bolus via a central venous catheter, and the dilution curve is measured by a lithium-sensitive electrode, over which arterial blood is drawn at a rate of 4 ml/min during each measurement. Small boluses of lithium (0.15 to 0.3 mmol) allow many measurements each day. Studies indicate that accuracy is high and respiratory influences are obviated because CO is measured over several respiratory cycles. The relatively noninvasive nature and accuracy of this technique have led to renewed interest in dye dilution methods.[159–161]

Another method to measure CO uses Fourier analysis of the arterial pulse wave sensed from direct arterial pressure monitoring or finger probe. Initial calibration of CO against another technique is required. Thoracic bioimpedance measurement of CO is another technique that seems accurate in healthy volunteers but not in critically ill patients.[162, 163] There are few studies that assess the accuracy of these devices in different clinical conditions, and further research is required to develop a useful, real-time, beat-to-beat monitor of CO.

INTRAOPERATIVE TRANSESOPHAGEAL ECHOCARDIOGRAPHY

Intraoperative monitoring of LV function was first described in 1980 using M-mode transesophageal echocardiography (TEE),[164] but expanded rapidly with the advent of two-dimensional sector scanning[165] and the introduction of smaller phased-array transducers.[166] Early intraoperative studies focused predominantly on monitoring global LV function and detecting segmental wall motion abnormalities (SWMAs) indicative of myocardial ischemia. Subsequent technological developments, including biplane and then multiplane transducers, color flow imaging, and other Doppler modalities have provided a plethora of structural and hemodynamic information resulting in a dramatic growth in the use of intraoperative TEE. However, the complexity of the equipment, the breadth of anatomic and physiologic information available, the special demands of the intraoperative environment, and the blurring of the distinction between transesophageal echocardiographic "monitoring" and "diagnosis" have presented new responsibilities and challenges to the clinician who uses this technique in the operating room.[167]

Indications and Use

The indications for intraoperative TEE in both cardiac and noncardiac surgery have grown considerably since it was first introduced as a monitor of LV systolic function (Tables 114–5 and 114–6). In cardiac surgery, TEE has direct applications for the evaluation of structural or functional cardiac defects and for the assessment of both the final result of operation and presence of complications. In noncardiac surgery, TEE can be used to assess the hemodynamic impact of anesthesia and surgery in patients with preexisting heart disease. Furthermore, in both cardiac and noncardiac surgery, urgent transesophageal echocardiographic assessment may aid the diagnosis of sudden, unexpected hemodynamic deterioration.

Intraoperative TEE favorably influences operative outcome in many types of cardiac surgery. In patients undergoing adult valvular surgery[168, 169] and repair of congenital heart defects,[170, 171] compelling evidence suggests that intraoperative TEE improves the outcome in a cost-effective manner.[172] Similar data support the use of TEE in patients with ischemic mitral regurgitation undergoing coronary artery bypass graft surgery (CABG) or mitral valve repair. The routine use of TEE during CABG is more controversial, however, although its use in high-risk patients undergoing CABG seems to be associated with better operative outcome.[173, 174]

Persistent new SWMAs after CABG are more likely to be associated with perioperative myocardial infarction.[175–177] However, it remains uncertain whether further surgery to treat these SWMAs will be beneficial. The interpretation of SWMAs must be made in the context of the severity of the underlying disease process and technical issues related to the perceived success of additional bypass grafting or graft revision. Furthermore, new SWMAs may represent myocardial stunning rather than ischemia. It is hoped that the more widespread use of intraoperative contrast echocardiography will clarify these issues.[178] In patients undergoing noncardiac surgery, it is not clear whether early detection of ischemic SWMAs with the use of TEE allows medical interventions that will decrease the risk of adverse perioperative cardiac events. As a result, in noncardiac surgical patients, transesophageal echocardiographic monitoring is generally reserved for situations in which severe hemodynamic instability requires rapid diagnostic evaluation.

Based on experiences with transesophageal echocardiographic monitoring during CABG surgery,[179] it is probable that TEE has a greater role in guiding intraoperative hemodynamic management than the use of standard monitors, including electrocardiography and PACs.[179, 180] However, due to equipment costs and training requirements for intraoperative TEE, it is unlikely that this technique will supplant standard monitoring in the near future.

Contraindications

Contraindications to the use of intraoperative transesophageal echocardiographic monitoring include those that are standard contraindications in awake patients: oropharyngeal, esophageal, and gastric pathology, particularly obstructive and hemorrhagic lesions. The site of surgery may preclude the use of TEE during, for example, surgery on the upper gastrointestinal tract or upper airway. In addition, constraints imposed by surgical positioning may provide relative contraindications to transesophageal echocardiographic monitoring or may impede or prohibit probe manipulation during surgery. For instance, extreme neck flexion during neurosurgical operations performed with the patient in the sitting position has been associated with postoperative vocal cord paralysis in patients in whom intraoperative transesophageal echocardiographic monitoring was used to detect venous air embolism.[181]

TABLE 114-5 Indications for Transesophageal Echocardiography

Cardiac Surgical Procedure	Evidence	TEE Assessment
Coronary artery bypass graft surgery	Category II	Wall motion/thickening abnormalities Contrast echocardiography
Valve repair	Category I	Extent/mechanism of disease Postbypass valvular function Intracardiac air
Valve replacement	Category II	Prosthetic valvular function postbypass Perivalvular leak Intracardiac air
Thoracic aorta	Category II	Presence/severity for atherosclerosis (site of aortic cross-clamp and possible modification of cardiopulmonary bypass)
	Category I/II	Aortic dissection and its complications
Congenital heart disease	Category I	Confirmation of known abnormalities Diagnosis of unsuspected abnormalities Adequacy of repair Intracardiac air
Placement of monitoring and therapeutic devices	Category III	Pulmonary artery catheter Intra-aortic balloon pump Coronary sinus catheter, venous drainage cannula Endoaortic balloon clamp in minimally invasive surgery
Miscellaneous	Grade I	Myomyectomy (hypertrophic obstructive cardiomypathy) Transmyocardial laser revascularization

Category I: supported by the strongest evidence or expert opinion; TEE is frequently useful in improving clinical outcomes in these settings and is often indicated, depending on individual circumstances. Category II: supported by weaker evidence and expert consensus; TEE may be useful in improving clinical outcomes in these settings, depending on individual circumstances, but appropriate indications are less certain. Category III: little scientific or expert support; TEE is infrequently useful in improving clinical outcomes in these settings, and appropriate indications are uncertain.

American Society of Anesthesiologists/Society of Cardiovascular Anesthesiologists indications for transesophageal echocardiography (TEE) as described in Thys DM, Abel M, Bollen BA: Practice guidelines for perioperative transesophageal echocardiography: a report by the American Society of Anesthesiologists and the Society of Cardiovascular Anesthesiologists Task Force on Transesophageal Echocardiography. Anesthesiology 84:986–1006, 1996.

TABLE 114-6 Indications for Transesophageal Echocardiography During Noncardiac Surgery

Preexisting Cardiac Disease	Evidence	TEE Assessment
Coronary artery disease	Category II	Global LV function Segmental wall motion and thickening Functional mitral regurgitation
Cardiomyopathy	Category II	Ventricular size and function Functional valvular regurgitation (MR, TR) LVOT velocity, SAM and MR (HCM)
Valvular disease	Category II	Severity of regurgitation Impact of loading changes on valvular regurgitation or stenosis Impact of loading changes on ventricular function
Miscellaneous	Category I	Diagnosis of severe intraoperative hemodynamic instability
	Category III	Troubleshooting/confirmation of intracardiac catheters, etc.
	Category III	Monitoring for embolization of air, thrombus, bone marrow Paradoxical embolization

Abbreviations: HCM, hypertrophic cardiomyopathy; LV, left ventricular; LVOT, left ventricle outflow tract; MR, mitral regurgitation; SAM, systolic anterior motion; TEE, transesophageal echocardiography; TR, tricuspid regurgitation.

Category I: supported by the strongest evidence or expert opinion; TEE is frequently useful in improving clinical outcomes in these settings and is often indicated, depending on individual circumstances. Category II: supported by weaker evidence and expert consensus; TEE may be useful in improving clinical outcomes in these settings, depending on individual circumstances, but appropriate indications are less certain. Category III: little scientific or expert support; TEE is infrequently useful in improving clinical outcomes in these settings, and appropriate indications are uncertain.

American Society of Anesthesiologists/Society of Cardiovascular Anesthesiologists indications for TEE as described in Thys DM, Abel M, Bollen BA: Practice guidelines for perioperative transesophageal echocardiography: a report by the American Society of Anesthesiologists and the Society of Cardiovascular Anesthesiologists Task Force on Transesophageal Echocardiography. Anesthesiology 84:986–1006, 1996.

Probe Insertion

The transesophageal echocardiographic probe is placed for intraoperative monitoring after the induction of general anesthesia and tracheal intubation. The introduction of the transesophageal echocardiographic probe is seldom a problem and is rarely associated with significant trauma to the oropharynx. If there are difficulties, the probe can be placed in the anesthetized patient under direct vision with the aid of a laryngoscope.

Complications

Direct complications of TEE are caused by mechanical trauma to the upper gastrointestinal tract and oropharynx, including abrasion, laceration, and perforation. The consequences of transesophageal echocardiographic probe-induced trauma range from minor postoperative pharyngeal discomfort to esophageal perforation,[182] hemorrhagic shock, mediastinitis, or peritonitis.[183–185] Intraoperative TEE theoretically poses a slight increase in these risks because clinicians may attempt more vigorous probe insertion or manipulation in anesthetized patients than in awake patients. However, even though intraoperative TEE is frequently performed in patients who might be considered at increased risk for complications, due to intraoperative hypothermia, anticoagulation, or cardiopulmonary bypass, severe complications appear to be rare events. Indirect complications of intraoperative TEE include bacteremia,[186, 187] airway compromise in small children, and postoperative esophageal dysmotility.[188]

Transesophageal Echocardiography and Intraoperative Ischemia

Since the early 1980s, perioperative myocardial ischemia has been identified repeatedly as a risk factor for adverse postoperative outcome. This association has driven efforts to improve intraoperative monitoring for ischemia and therapies based on its detection. In early investigations, transesophageal echocardiographic monitoring of global and segmental LV function appeared to be the ideal modality for early detection of intraoperative ischemia.[175] These early clinical reports were consistent with experimental evidence showing that acute coronary occlusion produced echocardiographically detectable SWMAs before characteristic ECG changes appeared.[189, 190]

However, both conceptual and practical problems limit TEE as an intraoperative ischemia monitor. Although SWMAs reproducibly occur before ECG changes when ischemia is produced by balloon occlusion of a coronary artery, acute occlusion may not be the appropriate mechanism for the modeling of most intraoperative ischemic events. Also, factors other than myocardial ischemia may be responsible for intraoperative SWMAs; these include conduction abnormalities (e.g., left bundle branch block, ventricular pacing) and abrupt changes in LV preload and afterload as occur after aortic cross-clamping during thoracic or abdominal aortic surgery. Marked increases in RV preload or afterload also may cause septal motion abnormalities that may be misinterpreted as ischemic changes. Furthermore, intraoperative SWMAs often occur in the absence of hemodynamic changes, and this makes it difficult to decide on the appropriate intraoperative medical treatment for these transesophageal echocardiographic changes.[191, 192] In addition, during abdominal aortic surgery, transient SWMAs do not appear to have any immediate postoperative significance.[193] The use of intraoperative TEE to monitor for ischemia is confounded further by the fact that no gold standard exists to validate the transesophageal echocardiographic findings. Most intraoperative studies report only limited concordance between TEE and other

TABLE 114–7 **Transesophageal Echocardiographic Monitoring for Assessment of Ventricular and Valvular Function**

	Two-Dimensional	Color-Flow Doppler	Other
Systolic function			
Global	Fractional area change Fractional volume change		Automatic border detection Color kinesis Fractional shortening (M-mode)
Segmental	Segmental wall motion abnormalities Segmental wall thickening abnormalities		Tissue Doppler
Diastolic function			
General	End-diastolic area/volume	Mitral valve flow (E/A ratio, E deceleration time and slope) Pulmonary venous flow Negative dP/dt (mitral regurgitation)	Isovolumic relaxation time Color M-mode
Pericardial disease	Pericardial constriction, effusion, or localized compression Chamber size Early diastolic RV collapse Late systolic RA collapse	Respiratory variation transvalvular valve flow	
Valvular function			
Regurgitation	Structural abnormalities	Regurgitant jet length, width, and area Regurgitant jet velocity Pressure half-time (AI)	PISA Pulmonary venous (MR) and hepatic venous (TR) Systolic inflow blunting or reversal
Stenosis	Structural abnormalities Valve planimetry	Increased color velocity and variance Peak and mean valve gradients	Continuity equation valve area

Abbreviations: AI, aortic incompetence; MR, mitral regurgitation; PISA, proximal isovelocimetric surface area; RA, right atrial; RV, right ventricular; TR, tricuspid regurgitation.

TABLE 114-8 Transesophageal Echocardiographic Hemodynamic Information

	Two-Dimensional	Color Flow Doppler	Other
Cardiac output/stroke volume	Fractional ventricular volume change	LVOT/RVOT velocity time integral multiplied by respective outflow tract diameter	
LVEDP		Aortic regurgitant jet velocity at end diastole Pulmonary venous flow	
LAP	Left atrial size Motion of interatrial septum		
PAP systolic	Pulmonary artery size RV structure and function	Peak TR jet velocity	
PAP diastolic	RV structure and function		
RAP	Right atrial size Vena caval size, changes with respiration		

Abbreviations: LAP, left atrial pressure; LVEDP, left ventricular end-diastolic pressure; LVOT, left ventricular outflow tract; PAP, pulmonary artery pressure; RAP; right atrial pressure; RV, right ventricular; RVOT, right ventricular outflow tract; TR, tricuspid regurgitation.

ischemia monitors. Of particular concern, there is poor agreement between ECG and transesophageal echocardiographic monitoring for ischemia.[177, 192, 194]

Beyond these conceptual limitations, there are many practical problems with transesophageal echocardiographic monitoring for intraoperative ischemia. Probe positioning must be stable to properly detect SWMAs. Furthermore, interpretation of new SWMAs must be placed in the clinical context that includes the surgical procedure, changes in ventricular loading conditions, conduction abnormalities, and data provided by other monitored variables (electrocardiogram, blood pressure, CVP, PAP, and so on). Accurate, real-time detection of SWMAs in the operating room is difficult. Like most methods of hemodynamic "monitoring," transesophageal echocardiographic monitoring is not truly continuous, because the clinician performing the monitoring must always attend to other clinical responsibilities in the operating room. Technical advances in echocardiography such as "automated border detection" have tried to make transesophageal echocardiographic monitoring more continuous, but these methods require frequent adjustment of gain settings and are disturbed by even slight probe movement.[195]

Controversies and Conclusion

Given the rich diagnostic information provided by TEE, the clinician applying this monitor in the operating room has a tool that provides unique information exceeding the capabilities of traditional intraoperative hemodynamic monitors. Virtually all of the traditional hemodynamic values (e.g., CVP, PAP, and so on) may be estimated with the use of TEE, albeit with some effort and considerable expertise (Tables 114–7 and 114–8). However, the greatest value of intraoperative transesophageal echocardiographic monitoring may be its integration into the traditional monitoring array (with electrocardiography, ECG, PAP, CVP, and so on) in high-risk patients. In this way, intraoperative abnormalities may be detected more easily and confirmed through the examination of multiple hemodynamic variables. For example, subtle ECG abnormalities suggestive of myocardial ischemia may be confirmed by searching for SWMAs on TEE, not only confirming the diagnosis but also refining it by providing anatomic localization of the ischemic myocardium.

References

1. Katz RL, Bigger JT Jr: Cardiac arrhythmias during anesthesia and operation. Anesthesiology 33:193–213, 1970.
2. Slogoff S, Keats AS, David Y, Igo SR: Incidence of perioperative myocardial ischemia detected by different electrocardiographic systems. Anesthesiology 73:1074–1081, 1990.
3. American Society of Anesthesiologists: Standards for Basic Anesthesia Monitoring: ASA Standards, Guidelines and Statements. Park Ridge, IL: American Society of Anesthesiologists, 1993, pp. 4–5.
4. Arbeit SR, Rubin IL, Gross H: Dangers in interpreting the electrocardiogram from the oscilloscope monitor. JAMA 211:453–456, 1970.
5. London MJ, Hollenberg M, Wong MG, et al: Intraoperative myocardial ischemia: localization by continuous 12-lead electrocardiography. Anesthesiology 69:232–421, 1988.
6. Krueger DW, Morrison DA, Buckner JK, et al: Is ST elevation the only electrocardiographic response of the ischemic right ventricle? Am J Cardiol 67:643–645, 1991.
7. Kinch JW, Ryan TJ: Right ventricular infarction. N Engl J Med 330:1211–1217, 1994.
8. Klein HO, Tordjman T, Ninio R, et al: The early recognition of right ventricular infarction: diagnostic accuracy of the electrocardiographic V4R lead. Circulation 67:558–565, 1983.
9. Knight AA, Hollenberg M, London MJ, Mangano DT: Myocardial ischemia in patients awaiting coronary artery bypass grafting. Am Heart J 117:1189–1195, 1989.
10. Knight AA, Hollenberg M, London MJ, et al: Perioperative myocardial ischemia: importance of the preoperative ischemic pattern. Anesthesiology 68:681–688, 1988.
11. Slogoff S, Keats AS: Does perioperative myocardial ischemia lead to postoperative myocardial infarction? Anesthesiology 62:107–114, 1985.
12. Smith H, Nathan H, Harrison M: Failure to predict intraoperative myocardial ischaemia in patients with coronary artery disease. Can J Anaesth 36:539–544, 1989.
13. Leung JM, Goehner P, O'Kelly BF, et al: Isoflurane anesthesia and myocardial ischemia: comparative risk versus sufentanil anesthesia in patients undergoing coronary artery bypass graft surgery: the SPI (Study of Perioperative Ischemia) Research Group. Anesthesiology 74:838–847, 1991.
14. Helman JD, Leung JM, Bellows WH, et al: The risk of myocardial ischemia in patients receiving desflurane versus sufentanil anesthesia for coronary artery bypass graft surgery: the S.P.I. Research Group. Anesthesiology 77:47–62, 1992.
15. Mangano DT, Browner WS, Hollenberg M, et al: Association of perioperative myocardial ischemia with cardiac morbidity and mortality in men undergoing noncardiac surgery: the Study of Perioperative Ischemia Research Group. N Engl J Med 323:1781–1788, 1990.

16. Krucoff MW, Jackson YR, Kehoe MK, Kent KM: Quantitative and qualitative ST segment monitoring during and after percutaneous transluminal coronary angioplasty. Circulation 81:IV-20–IV-26, 1990.
17. Wahr JA, Tremper KK: Continuous intravascular blood gas monitoring. J Cardiothorac Vasc Anesth 8:342–353, 1994.
18. Cohn JN: Blood pressure measurement in shock: mechanism of inaccuracy in auscultatory and palpatory methods. JAMA 199:972–976, 1967.
19. Schwid HA: Frequency response evaluation of radial artery catheter-manometer systems: sinusoidal frequency analysis versus flush method. J Clin Monit 4:181–185, 1988.
20. Gardner RM: Direct blood pressure measurement—dynamic response requirements. Anesthesiology 54:227–236, 1981.
21. Kleinman B, Powell S, Kumar P, Gardner RM: The fast flush test measures the dynamic response of the entire blood pressure monitoring system. Anesthesiology 77:1215–1220, 1992.
22. Courtois M, Fattal PG, Kovacs SJ, et al: Anatomically and physiologically based reference level for measurement of intracardiac pressures. Circulation 92:1994–2000, 1995.
23. Gardner RM: Accuracy and reliability of disposable pressure transducers coupled with modern pressure monitors. Crit Care Med 24:879–882, 1996.
24. O'Rourke MF, Gallagher DE: Pulse wave analysis. J Hypertens Suppl 14:S147–S157, 1996.
25. Coriat P, Vrillon M, Perel A, et al: A comparison of systolic blood pressure variations and echocardiographic estimates of end-diastolic left ventricular size in patients after aortic surgery. Anesth Analg 78:46-53, 1994.
26. Marik PE: The systolic blood pressure variation as an indicator of pulmonary capillary wedge pressure in ventilated patients. Anaesth Intens Care 21:405–408, 1993.
27. Rooke GA, Schwid HA, Shapira Y: The effect of graded hemorrhage and intravascular volume replacement on systolic pressure variation in humans during mechanical and spontaneous ventilation. Anesth Analg 80:925–932, 1995.
28. Slogoff S, Keats AS, Arlund C: On the safety of radial artery cannulation. Anesthesiology 59:42–47, 1983.
29. Mandel MA, Dauchot PJ: Radial artery cannulation in 1,000 patients: precautions and complications. J Hand Surg 2:482–485, 1977.
30. Singleton RJ, Webb RK, Ludbrook GL, Fox MA: The Australian Incident Monitoring Study: problems associated with vascular access: an analysis of 2000 incident reports. Anaesth Intens Care 21:664–669, 1993.
31. Messerli FH, Ventura HO, Amodeo C: Osler's maneuver and pseudohypertension. N Engl J Med 312:1548–1551, 1985.
32. Yelderman M, Ream AK: Indirect measurement of mean blood pressure in the anesthetized patient. Anesthesiology 50:253–256, 1979.
33. Borow KM, Newburger JW: Noninvasive estimation of central aortic pressure using the oscillometric method for analyzing systemic artery pulsatile blood flow: comparative study of indirect systolic, diastolic, and mean brachial artery pressure with simultaneous direct ascending aortic pressure measurements. Am Heart J 103:879–886, 1982.
34. Sutin KM, Longaker MT, Wahlander S, et al: Acute biceps compartment syndrome associated with the use of a noninvasive blood pressure monitor. Anesth Analg 83:1345–1346, 1996.
35. Bickler PE, Schapera A, Bainton CR: Acute radial nerve injury from use of an automatic blood pressure monitor. Anesthesiology 73:186–188, 1990.
36. Young CC, Mark JB, White W, et al: Clinical evaluation of continuous noninvasive blood pressure monitoring: accuracy and tracking capabilities. J Clin Monit 11:245–252, 1995.
37. de Jong JR, Tepaske R, Scheffer GJ, et al: Noninvasive continuous blood pressure measurement: a clinical evaluation of the Cortronic APM 770. J Clin Monit 9:18–24, 1993.
38. Kemmotsu O, Ueda M, Otsuka H, et al: Arterial tonometry for noninvasive, continuous blood pressure monitoring during anesthesia. Anesthesiology 75:333–340, 1991.
39. Bennett D, Boldt J, Brochard L, et al: Expert panel: the use of the pulmonary artery catheter. Intensive Care Med 17:I–VIII, 1991.
40. Goldstein JA, Barzilai B, Rosamond TL, et al: Determinants of hemodynamic compromise with severe right ventricular infarction. Circulation 82:359–368, 1990.
41. Beloucif S, Takata M, Shimada M, Robotham JL: Influence of pericardial constraint on atrioventricular interactions. Am J Physiol 263:H125–H134, 1992.
42. Swan HJ, Ganz W, Forrester J, et al: Catheterization of the heart in man with use of a flow-directed balloon-tipped catheter. N Engl J Med 283:447–451, 1970.
43. Connors AF Jr, McCaffree DR, Gray BA: Evaluation of right-heart catheterization in the critically ill patient without acute myocardial infarction. N Engl J Med 308:263–267, 1983.
44. Tuman KJ, Roizen MF: Outcome assessment and pulmonary artery catheterization: why does the debate continue? Anesth Analg 84:1–4, 1997.
45. Sibbald WJ, Sprung CL: The pulmonary artery catheter: the debate continues. Chest 94:899–901, 1988.
46. Naylor CD, Sibbald WJ, Sprung CL, et al: Pulmonary artery catheterization: can there be an integrated strategy for guideline development and research promotion? JAMA 269:2407–2411, 1993.
47. Robin ED: Death by pulmonary artery flow-directed catheter: time for a moratorium? Chest 92:727–731, 1987.
48. Connors AF Jr, Speroff T, Dawson NV, et al: The effectiveness of right heart catheterization in the initial care of critically ill patients: SUPPORT Investigators. JAMA 276:889–897, 1996.
49. Pulmonary Artery Catheter Consensus Conference: consensus statement. Crit Care Med 25:910–925, 1997.
50. Mark JB: Atlas of Cardiovascular Monitoring. New York: Churchill Livingstone, 1998.
51. Kelso LA: Complications associated with pulmonary artery catheterization. New Horizons 5:259–263, 1997.
52. Practice guidelines for pulmonary artery catheterization: a report by the American Society of Anesthesiologists Task Force on Pulmonary Artery Catheterization. Anesthesiology 78:380–394, 1993.
53. Shah KB, Rao TL, Laughlin S, El-Etr AA: A review of pulmonary artery catheterization in 6,245 patients. Anesthesiology 61:271–275, 1984.
54. Salmenpera M, Peltola K, Rosenberg P: Does prophylactic lidocaine control cardiac arrhythmias associated with pulmonary artery catheterization? Anesthesiology 56:210–212, 1982.
55. Morris D, Mulvihill D, Lew WY: Risk of developing complete heart block during bedside pulmonary artery catheterization in patients with left bundle-branch block. Arch Intern Med 147:2005–2010, 1987.
56. Sprung CL, Elser B, Schein RM, et al: Risk of right bundle branch block and complete heart block during pulmonary artery catheterization. Crit Care Med 17:1–3, 1989.
57. Thomson IR, Dalton BC, Lappas DG, Lowenstein E: Right bundle-branch block and complete heart block caused by the Swan-Ganz catheter. Anesthesiology 51:359–362, 1979.
58. Abernathy WS: Complete heart block caused by the Swan-Ganz catheter. Chest 65:349, 1974.
59. Fibuch EE, Tuohy GF: Intracardiac knotting of a flow-directed balloon-tipped catheter. Anesth Analg 59:217, 1980.
60. Lipp H, O'Donoghue K, Resnekov L: Intracardiac knotting of a flow-directed balloon catheter. N Engl J Med 284:220, 1971.
61. Kranz A, Mundigler G, Bankier A, et al: Knotting of two central venous catheters: a rare complication of pulmonary artery catheterization. Wien Klin Wochens 108:404–406, 1996.
62. Schwartz KV, Garcia FG: Entanglement of Swan-Ganz catheter around an intracardiac structure. JAMA 237:1198–1199, 1977. Letter.
63. Dumesnil JG, Proulx G: A new nonsurgical technique for untying tight knots in flow-directed balloon catheters. Am J Cardiol 53:395–396, 1984.
64. Mond HG, Clark DW, Nesbitt SJ, Schlant RC: A technique for unknotting an intracardiac flow-directed balloon catheter. Chest 67:731–733, 1975.
65. Boscoe MJ, de Lange S: Damage to the tricuspid valve with a Swan-Ganz catheter. BMJ Clin Res 283:346–347, 1981.
66. O'Toole JD, Wurtzbacher JJ, Wearner NE, Jain AC: Pulmonary-valve injury and insufficiency during pulmonary-artery catheterization. N Engl J Med 301:1167–1168, 1979.
67. Bernardin G, Milhaud D, Roger PM, et al: Swan-Ganz catheter-related pulmonary valve infective endocarditis: a case report. Intensive Care Med 20:142–144, 1994.
68. Ehrie M, Morgan AP, Moore FD, O'Connor NE: Endocarditis with the indwelling balloon-tipped pulmonary artery catheter in burn patients. J Trauma 18:664–666, 1978.

69. Greene JF Jr, Fitzwater JE, Clemmer TP: Septic endocarditis and indwelling pulmonary artery catheters. JAMA 233:891–892, 1975.
70. Roush K, Scala-Barnett DM, Donabedian H, Freimer EH: Rupture of a pulmonary artery mycotic aneurysm associated with candidal endocarditis. Am J Med 84:142–144, 1988.
71. Egebo K, Toft P, Jakobsen CJ: Contamination of central venous catheters: the skin insertion wound is a major source of contamination. J Hosp Infect 32:99–104, 1996.
72. Mermel LA, McCormick RD, Springman SR, Maki DG: The pathogenesis and epidemiology of catheter-related infection with pulmonary artery Swan-Ganz catheters: a prospective study utilizing molecular subtyping. Am J Med 91:197S–205S, 1991.
73. Bach A, Bohrer H, Geiss HK: Safety of a guidewire technique for replacement of pulmonary artery catheters. J Cardiothorac Vasc Anesth 6:711–714, 1992.
74. Hagley MT, Martin B, Gast P, Traeger SM. Infectious and mechanical complications of central venous catheters placed by percutaneous venipuncture and over guidewires. Crit Care Med 20:1426–1430, 1992.
75. Cobb DK, High KP, Sawyer RG, et al: A controlled trial of scheduled replacement of central venous and pulmonary-artery catheters. N Engl J Med 327:1062–1068, 1992.
76. Raad I, Umphrey J, Khan A, et al: The duration of placement as a predictor of peripheral and pulmonary arterial catheter infections. J Hosp Infect 23:17–26, 1993.
77. Heard SO, Davis RF, Sherertz RJ, et al: Influence of sterile protective sleeves on the sterility of pulmonary artery catheters. Crit Care Med 15:499–502, 1987.
78. Randolph AG, Cook DJ, Gonzales CA, Andrew M: Benefit of heparin in central venous and pulmonary artery catheters: a meta-analysis of randomized controlled trials. Chest 113:165–171, 1998.
79. Ling E, Warkentin TE: Intraoperative heparin flushes and subsequent acute heparin-induced thrombocytopenia. Anesthesiology 89:1567–1569, 1998.
80. Foote GA, Schabel SI, Hodges M: Pulmonary complications of the flow-directed balloon-tipped catheter. N Engl J Med 290:927–931, 1974.
81. Urschel JD, Myerowitz PD: Catheter-induced pulmonary artery rupture in the setting of cardiopulmonary bypass. Ann Thorac Surg 56:585–589, 1993.
82. Hartmann G, Steib A, Ludes B, Ravanello J: [Perforation of the pulmonary artery following Swan-Ganz catheterization]. Ann Fran Anesth Reanimation 7:486–493, 1988.
83. Kearney TJ, Shabot MM: Pulmonary artery rupture associated with the Swan-Ganz catheter. Chest 108:1349–1352, 1995.
84. Hardy JF, Morissette M, Taillefer J, Vauclair R: Pathophysiology of rupture of the pulmonary artery by pulmonary artery balloon-tipped catheters. Anesth Analg 62:925–930, 1983.
85. Klafta JM, Olson JP: Emergent lung separation for management of pulmonary artery rupture. Anesthesiology 87:1248–1250, 1997.
86. Tayoro J, Dequin PF, Delhommais A, et al: Rupture of pulmonary artery induced by Swan-Ganz catheter: success of coil embolization. Intensive Care Med 23:198–200, 1997.
87. Jondeau G, Lacombe P, Rocha P, et al: Swan-Ganz catheter-induced rupture of the pulmonary artery: successful early management by transcatheter embolization. Cathet Cardiovasc Diagn 19:202–204, 1990.
88. Gnaegi A, Feihl F, Perret C: Intensive care physicians' insufficient knowledge of right-heart catheterization at the bedside: time to act? Crit Care Med 25:213–220, 1997.
89. Iberti TJ, Fischer EP, Leibowitz AB, et al: A multicenter study of physicians' knowledge of the pulmonary artery catheter: Pulmonary Artery Catheter Study Group. JAMA 264:2928–2932, 1990.
90. Iberti TJ, Daily EK, Leibowitz AB, et al: Assessment of critical care nurses' knowledge of the pulmonary artery catheter: the Pulmonary Artery Catheter Study Group. Crit Care Med 22:1674–1678, 1994.
91. Komadina KH, Schenk DA, LaVeau P, et al: Interobserver variability in the interpretation of pulmonary artery catheter pressure tracings. Chest 100:1647–1654, 1991.
92. Roizen MF, Berger DL, Gabel RA, et al: Practice guidelines for pulmonary artery catheterization: a report by the American Society of Anesthesiologists Task Force on Pulmonary Artery Catheterization. Anesthesiology 78:380–394, 1993.
93. Falicov RE, Resnekov L: Relationship of the pulmonary artery end-diastolic pressure to the left ventricular end-diastolic and mean filling pressures in patients with and without left ventricular dysfunction. Circulation 42:65–73, 1970.
94. Collee GG, Lynch KE, Hill RD, Zapol WM: Bedside measurement of pulmonary capillary pressure in patients with acute respiratory failure. Anesthesiology 66:614–620, 1987.
95. Cope DK, Allison RC, Parmentier JL, et al: Measurement of effective pulmonary capillary pressure using the pressure profile after pulmonary artery occlusion. Crit Care Med 14:16–22, 1986.
96. West JB, Dollery CT, Naimark A: Distribution of blood flow in isolated lung: relation to vascular and alveolar pressures. J Appl Physiol 19:713–724, 1964.
97. Wiedemann HP: Wedge pressure in pulmonary veno-occlusive disease. N Engl J Med 315:1233, 1986.
98. O'Quin R, Marini JJ: Pulmonary artery occlusion pressure: clinical physiology, measurement, and interpretation. Am Rev Respir Dis 128:319–326, 1983.
99. Wittnich C, Trudel J, Zidulka A, Chiu RC: Misleading "pulmonary wedge pressure" after pneumonectomy: its importance in postoperative fluid therapy. Ann Thorac Surg 42:192–196, 1986.
100. Enson Y, Wood JA, Mantaras NB, Harvey RM: The influence of heart rate on pulmonary arterial-left ventricular pressure relationships at end-diastole. Circulation 56:533–539, 1977.
101. Snyder RW, Glamann DB, Lange RA, et al: Predictive value of prominent pulmonary arterial wedge V waves in assessing the presence and severity of mitral regurgitation. Am J Cardiol 73:568–570, 1994.
102. Fuchs RM, Heuser RR, Yin FC, Brinker JA: Limitations of pulmonary wedge V waves in diagnosing mitral regurgitation. Am J Cardiol 49:849–854, 1982.
103. Braunwald E, Awe WC: The syndrome of severe mitral regurgitation with normal left atrial pressure. Circulation 27:29–35, 1963.
104. Marini JJ, O'Quin R, Culver BH, Butler J: Estimation of transmural cardiac pressures during ventilation with PEEP. J Appl Physiol Respir Environ Exerc Physiol 53:384–391, 1982.
105. Teplick RS: Measuring central vascular pressures: a surprisingly complex problem. Anesthesiology 67:289–291, 1987. Editorial.
106. Jardin F, Delorme G, Hardy A, et al: Reevaluation of hemodynamic consequences of positive pressure ventilation: emphasis on cyclic right ventricular afterloading by mechanical lung inflation. Anesthesiology 72:966–970, 1990.
107. Pinsky M, Vincent J-L, De Smet J-M: Estimating left ventricular filling pressure during positive end-expiratory pressure in humans. Am Rev Respir Dis 143:25–31, 1991.
108. Wison J, Woods I, Fawcett J, et al: Reducing the risk of major elective surgery: randomised controlled trial of preoperative optimisation of oxygen delivery. BMJ 318:1099–1103, 1999.
109. Shoemaker WC, Appel PL, Kram HB, et al: Prospective trial of supranormal values of survivors as therapeutic goals in high-risk surgical patients. Chest 94:1176–1186, 1988.
110. Boyd O, Grounds RM, Bennett ED: A randomized clinical trial of the effect of deliberate perioperative increase of oxygen delivery on mortality in high-risk surgical patients. JAMA 270:2699–2707, 1993.
111. Gattinoni L, Brazzi L, Pelosi P, et al: A trial of goal-oriented hemodynamic therapy in critically ill patients: SvO2 Collaborative Group. N Engl J Med 333:1025–1032, 1995.
112. Hayes MA, Timmins AC, Yau EH, et al: Elevation of systemic oxygen delivery in the treatment of critically ill patients. N Engl J Med 330:1717–1722, 1994.
113. Dodek A, Kassebaum DG, Bristow JD: Pulmonary edema in coronary-artery disease without cardiomegaly: paradox of the stiff heart. N Engl J Med 286:1347–1350, 1972.
114. Dwyer EM: Left ventricular pressure-volume alterations and regional disorders of contraction during myocardial ischemia induced by atrial pacing. Circulation 42:1111–1122, 1970.
115. Haggmark S, Hohner P, Ostman M, et al: Comparison of hemodynamic, electrocardiographic, mechanical, and metabolic indicators of intraoperative myocardial ischemia in vascular surgical patients with coronary artery disease. Anesthesiology 70:19–25, 1989.
116. van Daele MERM, Sutherland GR, Mitchell MM, et al: Do changes in pulmonary capillary wedge pressure adequately reflect myocardial ischemia during anesthesia: a correlative preoperative hemodynamic, electrocardiographic, and transesophageal echocardiographic study. Circulation 81:865–871, 1990.

117. Knaus WA, Le Gall JR, Wagner DP, et al: A comparison of intensive care in the U.S.A. and France. Lancet 2:642–646, 1982.
118. Vincent JL, Dhainaut JF, Perret C, Suter P: Is the pulmonary artery catheter misused? A European view. Crit Care Med 26:1283–1287, 1998.
119. Bender JS, Smith-Meek MA, Jones CE: Routine pulmonary artery catheterization does not reduce morbidity and mortality of elective vascular surgery: results of a prospective, randomized trial. Ann Surg 226:229–236, discussion 236–237, 1997.
120. Gore JM, Goldberg RJ, Spodick DH, et al: A community-wide assessment of the use of pulmonary artery catheters in patients with acute myocardial infarction. Chest 92:721–727, 1987.
121. Isaacson IJ, Lowdon JD, Berry AJ, et al: The value of pulmonary artery and central venous monitoring in patients undergoing abdominal aortic reconstructive surgery: a comparative study of two selected, randomized groups. J Vasc Surg 12:754–760, 1990.
122. Pearson KS, Gomez MN, Moyers JR, et al: A cost/benefit analysis of randomized invasive monitoring for patients undergoing cardiac surgery. Anesth Analg 69:336–341, 1989.
123. Tuman KJ, Carroll GC, Ivankovich AD: Pitfalls in interpretation of pulmonary artery catheter data. J Cardiothorac Anesth 3:625–641, 1989.
124. Zion MM, Balkin J, Rosenmann D, et al: Use of pulmonary artery catheters in patients with acute myocardial infarction: analysis of experience in 5,841 patients in the SPRINT Registry: SPRINT Study Group. Chest 98:1331–1335, 1990.
125. Berlauk JF, Abrams JH, Gilmour IJ, et al: Preoperative optimization of cardiovascular hemodynamics improves outcome in peripheral vascular surgery: a prospective, randomized clinical trial. Ann Surg 214:289–297, discussion 298–299, 1991.
126. Del Guercio LR: Does pulmonary artery catheter use change outcome? Yes. Crit Care Clin 12:553–557, 1996.
127. Mimoz O, Rauss A, Rekik N, et al: Pulmonary artery catheterization in critically ill patients: a prospective analysis of outcome changes associated with catheter-prompted changes in therapy. Crit Care Med 22:573–579, 1994.
128. Zaidan JR, Freniere S: Use of a pacing pulmonary artery catheter during cardiac surgery. Ann Thorac Surg 35:633–636, 1983.
129. Trankina MF, White RD: Perioperative cardiac pacing using an atrioventricular pacing pulmonary artery catheter. J Cardiothorac Anesth 3:154–162, 1989.
130. Risk SC, Brandon D, D'Ambra MN, et al: Indications for the use of pacing pulmonary artery catheters in cardiac surgery. J Cardiothorac Vasc Anesth 6:275–279, 1992.
131. Vincent JL, Thirion M, Brimioulle S, et al: Thermodilution measurement of right ventricular ejection fraction with a modified pulmonary artery catheter. Intensive Care Med 12:33–38, 1986.
132. Reuse C, Vincent JL, Pinsky MR: Measurements of right ventricular volumes during fluid challenge. Chest 98:1450–1454, 1990.
133. Weisel RD, Berger RL, Hechtman HB: Current concepts measurement of cardiac output by thermodilution. N Engl J Med 292:682–684, 1975.
134. Stetz CW, Miller RG, Kelly GE, Raffin TA: Reliability of the thermodilution method in the determination of cardiac output in clinical practice. Am Rev Respir Dis 126:1001–1004, 1982.
135. Heerdt PM, Pond CG, Blessios GA, Rosenbloom M: Inaccuracy of cardiac output by thermodilution during acute tricuspid regurgitation. Ann Thorac Surg 53:706–708, 1992.
136. Wetzel RC, Latson TW: Major errors in thermodilution cardiac output measurement during rapid volume infusion. Anesthesiology 62:684–687, 1985.
137. Stevens JH, Raffin TA, Mihm FG, et al: Thermodilution cardiac output measurement: effects of the respiratory cycle on its reproducibility. JAMA 253:2240–2242, 1985.
138. Pearl RG, Rosenthal MH, Nielson L, et al: Effect of injectate volume and temperature on thermodilution cardiac output determination. Anesthesiology 64:798–801, 1986.
139. Nelson LD, Anderson HB: Patient selection for iced versus room temperature injectate for thermodilution cardiac output determinations. Crit Care Med 13:182–184, 1985.
140. Yelderman M: Continuous measurement of cardiac output with the use of stochastic system identification techniques. J Clin Monit 6:322–332, 1990.
141. Yelderman M: Continuous cardiac output by thermodilution. Int Anesth Clin 31:127–140, 1993.
142. Bottiger BW, Rauch H, Bohrer H, et al: Continuous versus intermittent cardiac output measurement in cardiac surgical patients undergoing hypothermic cardiopulmonary bypass. J Cardiothorac Vasc Anesth 9:405–411, 1995.
143. Norfleet EA, Watson CB: Continuous mixed venous oxygen saturation measurement: a significant advance in hemodynamic monitoring? J Clin Monit 1:245–258, 1985.
144. Nelson LD: The new pulmonary artery catheters: continuous venous oximetry, right ventricular ejection fraction, and continuous cardiac output. New Horizons 5:251–258, 1997.
145. Segal J, Pearl RG, Ford AJ, et al: Instantaneous and continuous cardiac output obtained with a Doppler pulmonary artery catheter. J Am Coll Cardiol 13:1382, 1989.
146. Segal J, Nassi M, Ford AJ, Schuenemeyer TD: Instantaneous and continuous cardiac output in humans obtained with a Doppler pulmonary artery catheter. J Am Coll Cardiol 16:1398, 1990.
147. Abrams JH, Weber RE, Holmen KD: Continuous cardiac output determination using transtracheal Doppler: initial results in humans. Anesthesiology 71:11–15, 1989.
148. Abrams JH, Weber RE, Holmen KD: Transtracheal Doppler: a new procedure for continuous cardiac output measurement. Anesthesiology 70:134–138, 1989.
149. Mark JB, Steinbrook RA, Gugino LD, et al: Continuous noninvasive monitoring of cardiac output with esophageal Doppler ultrasound during cardiac surgery. Anesth Analg 65:1013–1020, 1986.
150. Freund PR: Transesophageal Doppler scanning versus thermodilution during general anesthesia: an initial comparison of cardiac output techniques. Am J Surg 153:490–494, 1987.
151. Lavandier B, Cathignol D, Muchada R, et al: Noninvasive aortic blood flow measurement using an intraesophageal probe. Ultrasound Med Biol 11:451–460, 1985.
152. Lefrant JY, Bruelle P, Aya AG, et al: Training is required to improve the reliability of esophageal Doppler to measure cardiac output in critically ill patients. Intensive Care Med 24:347–352, 1998.
153. Singer M, Bennett ED: Noninvasive optimization of left ventricular filling using esophageal Doppler. Crit Care Med 19:1132–1137, 1991.
154. Sinclair S, James S, Singer M: Intraoperative intravascular volume optimisation and length of hospital stay after repair of proximal femoral fracture: randomised controlled trial. BMJ 315:909–912, 1997.
155. Mythen MG, Webb AR: Perioperative plasma volume expansion reduces the incidence of gut mucosal hypoperfusion during cardiac surgery. Arch Surg 130:423–429, 1995.
156. Gan TJ, Wakeling H, et al: Interoperative volume expansion guided by esophageal Doppler reduces the incidence of gastric hypoperfusion and may be associated with improved outcome following surgery. Anesthesiology 87:A391, 1997.
157. Hamilton-Davies C, Mythen MG, Salmon JB, et al: Comparison of commonly used clinical indicators of hypovolaemia with gastrointestinal tonometry. Intensive Care Med 23:276–281, 1997.
158. Gan TJ, Arrowsmith JE: The oesophageal Doppler monitor. BMJ 315:893–894, 1997. Editorial.
159. Band DM, Linton RA, O'Brien TK, et al: The shape of indicator dilution curves used for cardiac output measurement in man. J Physiol 498:225–229, 1997.
160. Linton RA, Band DM, Haire KM: A new method of measuring cardiac output in man using lithium dilution. Br J Anaesth 71:262–266, 1993.
161. Linton RA, Linton NW, Band DM: A new method of analysing indicator dilution curves. Cardiovasc Res 30:930–938, 1995.
162. Mattar JA: Noninvasive cardiac output determination by thoracic electrical bioimpedance. Intens Crit Care Dig 7:14–18, 1988.
163. Young JD, McQuillan P: Comparison of thoracic electrical bioimpedance and thermodilution for the measurement of cardiac index in patients with severe sepsis. Br J Anaesth 70:58, 1993.
164. Matsumoto M, Oka Y, Strom J, et al: Application of transesophageal echocardiography to continuous intraoperative monitoring of left ventricular performance. Am J Cardiol 46:95–105, 1980.
165. Hisanaga K, Hisanaga A, Nagata K, Ichie Y: Transesophageal cross-sectional echocardiography. Am Heart J 100:605–609, 1980.
166. Schluter M, Langenstein BA, Polster J, et al: Transoesophageal cross-sectional echocardiography with a phased array transducer system: technique and initial clinical results. Br Heart J 48:67–72, 1982.

167. Hodgins L, Kisslo JA, Mark JB: Perioperative transesophageal echocardiography: the anesthesiologist as cardiac diagnostician. Anesth Analg 80:4–6, 1995. Editorial.
168. Freeman WK, Schaff HV, Khandheria BK, et al: Intraoperative evaluation of mitral valve regurgitation and repair by transesophageal echocardiography: incidence and significance of systolic anterior motion. J Am Coll Cardiol 20:599–609, 1992.
169. Sheikh KH, de Bruijn NP, Rankin JS, et al: The utility of transesophageal echocardiography and Doppler color flow imaging in patients undergoing cardiac valve surgery. J Am Coll Cardiol 15:363–372, 1990.
170. Stevenson JG, Sorensen GK, Gartman DM, et al: Transesophageal echocardiography during repair of congenital cardiac defects: identification of residual problems necessitating reoperation. J Am Soc Echocardiogr 6:356–365, 1993.
171. O'Leary PW, Hagler DJ, Seward JB, et al: Biplane intraoperative transesophageal echocardiography in congenital heart disease. Mayo Clin Proc 70:317–326, 1995.
172. Benson MJ, Cahalan MK: Cost-benefit analysis of transesophageal echocardiography in cardiac surgery. Echocardiography 12:171–183, 1995.
173. Savage RM, Lytle BW, Aronson S, et al: Intraoperative echocardiography is indicated in high-risk coronary artery bypass grafting. Ann Thorac Surg 64:368–373. discussion 373–374, 1997.
174. Sutton DC, Kluger R: Intraoperative transoesophageal echocardiography: impact on adult cardiac surgery. Anaesth Intens Care 26:287–293, 1998.
175. Smith JS, Cahalan MK, Benefiel DJ, et al: Intraoperative detection of myocardial ischemia in high-risk patients: electrocardiography versus two-dimensional transesophageal echocardiography. Circulation 72:1015–1021, 1985.
176. Leung JM, O'Kelly B, Browner WS, et al: Prognostic importance of postbypass regional wall-motion abnormalities in patients undergoing coronary artery bypass graft surgery: SPI Research Group. Anesthesiology 71:16–25, 1989.
177. Comunale ME, Body SC, Ley C, et al: The concordance of intraoperative left ventricular wall-motion abnormalities and electrocardiographic S-T segment changes: association with outcome after coronary revascularization: Multicenter Study of Perioperative Ischemia (McSPI) Research Group. Anesthesiology 88:945–954, 1998.
178. Nanto S, Lim YJ, Masuyama T, et al: Diagnostic performance of myocardial contrast echocardiography for detection of stunned myocardium. J Am Soc Echocardiogr 9:314–319, 1996.
179. Bergquist BD, Bellows WH, Leung JM: Transesophageal echocardiography in myocardial revascularization: II. Influence on intraoperative decision making. Anesth Analg 82:1139–1145, 1996.
180. Mishra M, Chauhan R, Sharma KK, et al: Real-time intraoperative transesophageal echocardiography—how useful? Experience of 5,016 cases. J Cardiothorac Vasc Anesth 12:625–632, 1998.
181. Cucchiara RF, Nugent M, Seward JB, Messick JM: Air embolism in upright neurosurgical patients: detection and localization by two-dimensional transesophageal echocardiography. Anesthesiology 60:353–355, 1984.
182. Spahn DR, Schmid S, Carrel T, et al: Hypopharynx perforation by a transesophageal echocardiography probe. Anesthesiology 82:581–583, 1995.
183. Daniel WG, Erbel R, Kasper W, et al: Safety of transesophageal echocardiography: a multicenter survey of 10,419 examinations. Circulation 83:817–821, 1991.
184. Kharasch ED, Sivarajan M: Gastroesophageal perforation after intraoperative transesophageal echocardiography. Anesthesiology 85:426–428, 1996.
185. Owall A, Stahl L, Settergren G: Incidence of sore throat and patient complaints after intraoperative transesophageal echocardiography during cardiac surgery. J Cardiothorac Vasc Anesth 6:15–16, 1992.
186. Mentec H, Vignon P, Terre S, et al: Frequency of bacteremia associated with transesophageal echocardiography in intensive care unit patients: a prospective study of 139 patients. Crit Care Med 23:1194–1199, 1995.
187. Pongratz G, Henneke KH, von der Grun M, et al: Risk of endocarditis in transesophageal echocardiography. Am Heart J 125:190–193, 1993.
188. Hogue CW Jr, Lappas GD, Creswell LL, et al: Swallowing dysfunction after cardiac operations: associated adverse outcomes and risk factors including intraoperative transesophageal echocardiography. J Thorac Cardiovasc Surg 110:517–522, 1995.
189. Wohlgelernter D, Jaffe CC, Cabin HS, et al: Silent ischemia during coronary occlusion produced by balloon inflation: relation to regional myocardial dysfunction. J Am Coll Cardiol 10:491–498, 1987.
190. Waters DD, Da Luz P, Wyatt HL, et al: Early changes in regional and global left ventricular function induced by graded reductions in regional coronary perfusion. Am J Cardiol 39:537–543, 1977.
191. Leung JM, O'Kelly BF, Mangano DT: Relationship of regional wall motion abnormalities to hemodynamic indices of myocardial oxygen supply and demand in patients undergoing CABG surgery. Anesthesiology 73:802–814, 1990.
192. London MJ, Tubau JF, Wong MG, et al: The "natural history" of segmental wall motion abnormalities in patients undergoing noncardiac surgery: S.P.I. Research Group. Anesthesiology 73:644–655, 1990.
193. Dodds TM, Burns AK, DeRoo DB, et al: Effects of anesthetic technique on myocardial wall motion abnormalities during abdominal aortic surgery. J Cardiothorac Vasc Anesth 11:129–136, 1997.
194. Eisenberg MJ, London MJ, Leung JM, et al: Monitoring for myocardial ischemia during noncardiac surgery: a technology assessment of transesophageal echocardiography and 12-lead electrocardiography: the Study of Perioperative Ischemia Research Group. JAMA 268:210–216, 1992.
195. Cahalan MK, Ionescu P, Melton HE Jr, et al: Automated real-time analysis of intraoperative transesophageal echocardiograms. Anesthesiology 78:477–485, 1993.

SECTION XII

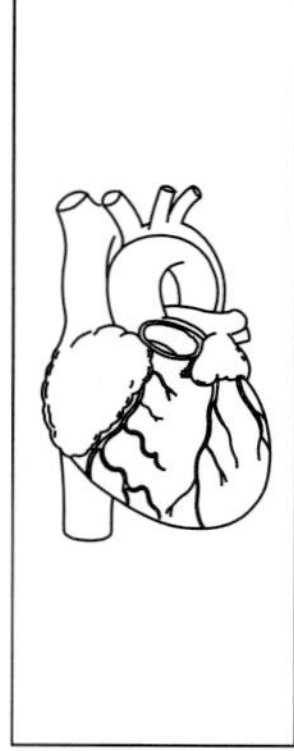

THE GENETIC BASIS FOR CARDIOVASCULAR DISEASE

Classification of Genetic Disorders

Inherited Disorders of Connective Tissue

Muscular Dystrophies Affecting the Heart

Genetic Aspects of Congenital Heart Disease

CHAPTER 115

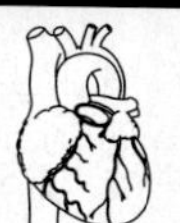

Classification of Genetic Disorders

Dianna Milewicz

CHROMOSOMAL DISORDERS
SINGLE-GENE DISORDERS
MULTIFACTORIAL INHERITANCE

Chromosomal Disorders

Genetic material is packaged within the nucleus of the cell in nuclear material termed *chromatin.* When a cell divides, the genetic material in the nucleus condenses into rod-shaped structures known as *chromosomes.* The total human DNA material is packaged into 46 chromosomes. The 46 chromosomes include 22 pairs of alike, or homologous, chromosomes (homologs) called *autosomes* and two *sex* chromosomes, X and Y. Females have two X chromosomes (XX) and males have an X and a Y chromosome (XY). Each chromosome has a characteristic size and shape that allow the numbering and identification of individual chromosomes.

The study of chromosome structure and inheritance is called *cytogenetics.* Cells for chromosomal analysis must be able to divide in culture, which limits the analysis of human chromosomes to a few cell types. Included in the cells available for study are T lymphocytes collected from the peripheral blood and stimulated to divide with phytohemagglutinin, fibroblasts explanted from skin biopsies and maintained in culture, bone marrow cells, and amniocytes. The chromosomes of a dividing cell are most easily analyzed at the metaphase or the prometaphase stage of mitosis, or cell division. The chromosomes are stained, most typically with Giemsa banding, or G-banding, resulting in a pattern of light and dark bands that is unique for each human chromosome. Approximately 350 to 500 bands are identifiable on the chromosomes using this technique. Morphologically, chromosomes consist of two *chromatids* joined at the *centromere,* or central constriction. The centromere divides the chromosome into the long arm, designated *q,* and the short arm, designated *p* (Fig. 115–1). Chromosomal morphology and staining allow the identification of the 22 homologous chromosomes and the two sex chromosomes (XX or XY), termed a *karyotype* (Fig. 115–2).

Chromosomal disorders occur when there is an excess or deficiency of whole chromosomes or portions of chromosomes. There are many documented numeric and structural abnormalities in chromosomes in the human karyotype, and many of these are associated with cardiovascular disease (Table 115–1).

Aneuploidy is the most common and clinically significant type of chromosomal disorder. Aneuploidy exists when an entire chromosome is missing or when there is an extra chromosome, which means an abnormal number of chromosomes are found on karyotype analysis. Most patients with aneuploidy have trisomy or an extra chromosome (resulting in three homologous chromosomes rather than two). Monosomy, or the loss of an entire chromosome (resulting in only one chromosome of a homologous pair), occurs less often.

Abnormalities of chromosome structure involve chromosomal rearrangement caused by chromosome breakage followed by reconstitution in an abnormal form. Structural rearrangements can involve one or two chromosomes and can retain a complete complement of genetic material

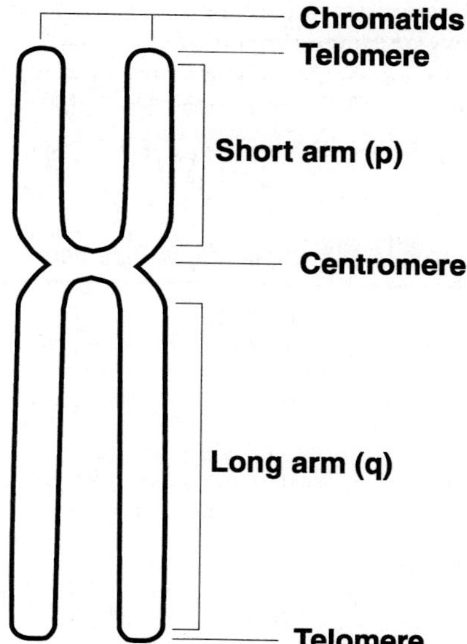

Figure 115–1 Chromosomal structure. Chromosomal structure is based on the position of the *centromere,* which divides the chromosome into a short arm, designated *p,* and a long arm, designated *q.* Pictured here is a *submetacentric* chromosome, in which the centromere is not in the center. Chromosomes can also be *metacentric,* when the centromere is in the center, or *acrocentric,* when the centromere lies near the end of the chromosome. The ends of the chromosome are called the *telomeres. Chromatids* are the two identical strands of a chromosome, connected at the centromere.

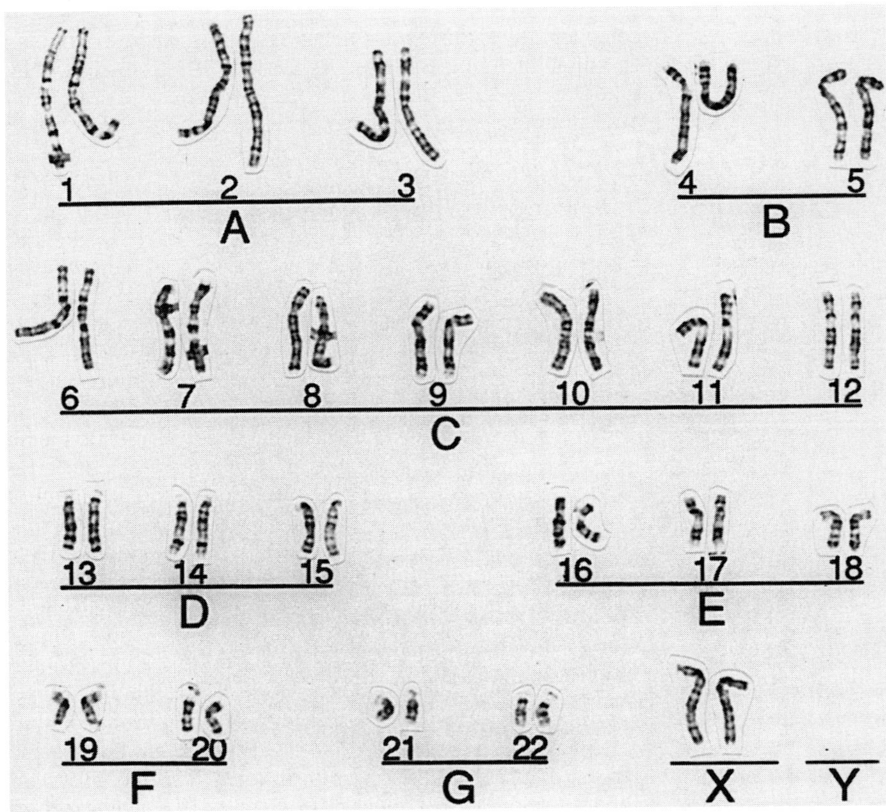

FIGURE 115–2 Human karyotype. Human chromosomes were prepared from a peripheral blood lymphocyte culture arrested in prometaphase and stained by the Giemsa banding method. Chromosomes were then arranged into the 22 pairs of autosomal chromosomes and the pair of sex chromosomes (XX). (Courtesy of Fred Elder, M.D.)

(which usually does not result in a clinical phenotype) or can lead to the loss (deletion) or gain (duplication) of chromosomal material. Typically, duplication, or gain, of portions of human chromosomes is less harmful clinically than is the loss of genetic material.

Contiguous-gene syndromes are disorders caused by microduplications or deletions of chromosomal segments involving genes linked together on the chromosome. Some contiguous-gene syndromes can be recognized by routine cytogenic techniques. Other syndromes are not visible when such techniques are used, so detection requires high-resolution chromosome analysis or studies using fluorescent in situ hybridization. Typically, these syndromes are sporadic, but some of the disorders can be inherited in an autosomal dominant manner.

The major chromosomal disorders associated with car-

TABLE 115-1 Single-Gene Disorders With Major Cardiovascular Features

Name of Disorder	Defective Gene	Prevalence	Inheritance	Chromosomal Localization	Pathology	Cardiovascular Manifestation
Immotile cilia syndrome (Kartagener's syndrome)	Unknown	1:400,000	AR	Unknown	Ciliary immobility	Situs inversus visceral
Long QT syndrome (Romano-Ward syndrome)	Unknown	Unknown	AD	11p15 (30–50% families not linked)	Unknown	Prolonged QT interval, arrhythmias
Jervell-Lange-Nielson syndrome	—	Rare	AR	—	—	Prolonged QT interval, arrhythmias
Tuberous sclerosis	Unknown	1:10,000	AD	9q32–34 16p13	Unknown	Cardiac rhabdomyomata
Hereditary hemorrhagic telangiectasia (Osler-Weber-Rendu disease)	Unknown	—	AD	—	Unknown	Telangiectasias, arteriovenous fistulas, vascular malformations
Adult polycystic kidney disease	Unknown	—	AD	16	Unknown	Berry aneurysms of the cerebral circulation, MVP
Arteriohepatic dysplasia (Alagille's syndrome)	Unknown	Rare	AR	Unknown	Unknown	Peripheral pulmonary artery stenosis

Abbreviations: AD, autosomal dominant; AR, autosomal recessive; MVP, mitral valve prolapse.

diovascular disease lead primarily to congenital heart disease; the disorders and the major defects associated with each syndrome are listed in Table 115–1.

SINGLE-GENE DISORDERS

Single-gene disorders are caused by mutations of specific genes in the human genetic material. Human chromosomes contain an estimated 50,000 to 100,000 genes encoded for a variety of proteins and RNAs that serve specific functions in cells and tissues. These disorders follow the patterns of inheritance originally identified by Mendel in his studies of garden peas (mendelian inheritance). At present, 3300 single-gene disorders that are inherited in a mendelian manner have been identified.[1] A *genetic locus* is a specific location on a chromosome, often used to refer to a certain gene. *Alleles* are alternative forms of a locus or a gene. An individual with two alike alleles at a given gene is *homozygous.* If the alleles are different, the individual is *heterozygous* at the locus.

Changes at a given locus or gene may be benign. *Polymorphic* changes are variations in the genetic material that do not cause disease. In contrast, changes in DNA that do produce disease are termed *mutations.* Mutations in specific genes are the underlying causes of single-gene disorders. Disorders are said to be either autosomal or X-linked, based on the chromosal location of the mutant gene. Autosomal single-gene disorders are caused by mutations in genes on one of the 22 pairs of non–sex chromosomes. X-linked disorders are those caused by mutations on the X chromosome. Dominant conditions are disorders in which a clinical phenotype is expressed in the heterozygous state (that is, the individual has one copy of a mutant gene and one copy of a normal gene). Recessive conditions are disorders that manifest a clinical phenotype in the homozygous state (that is, an individual must have two mutated genes to have the disease).

Autosomal dominant inheritance is expression of a clinical phenotype caused by a heterozygous mutant gene on an autosomal chromosome. As shown in Figure 115–3, the inheritance pattern is vertical (the disorder is passed from one generation to the next generation). Both males and females are affected, although the severity of the disorder can be influenced by the sex of the affected individual. Male-to-male transmission occurs and helps to distinguish autosomal dominant inheritance from X-linked dominant inheritance. An affected individual has a 50 percent chance of passing the condition to any of his or her children. Unaffected family members do not pass the trait on to their children. Of the 3300 identified diseases with Mendelian inheritance, the majority (2470) are inherited in an autosomal dominant fashion.[1]

A number of special characteristics are associated with autosomal dominant inheritance. With classic autosomal dominant inheritance, the affected individual usually has an affected parent, but this is not true in all cases. Sporadic cases (without a family history of the disorder) can arise in dominant disorders through new mutations in the gene, which causes the disorder. The term *variable expression* of a dominant disorder refers to different levels of the clinical expression of a mutated gene. This variability can include the type and severity of symptoms or the variation in the age of onset of a disorder. *Decreased penetrance* of an autosomal dominant condition is the lack of phenotypic expression of a disease in an individual who has inherited the mutated gene that causes the disease. The penetrance of dominant disorders is determined by family or population studies of different disorders and is influenced by the ability of clinical or laboratory studies to detect the phenotype.

In autosomal recessive inheritance, the expression of a clinical phenotype occurs only when an individual has inherited, at a single locus, two genes that are mutated—the affected individual has inherited a mutant gene from both parents (see Fig. 115–3). The parents are heterozygous for the mutant gene and do not have the disease. They are called *carriers.* The inheritance is horizontal rather than

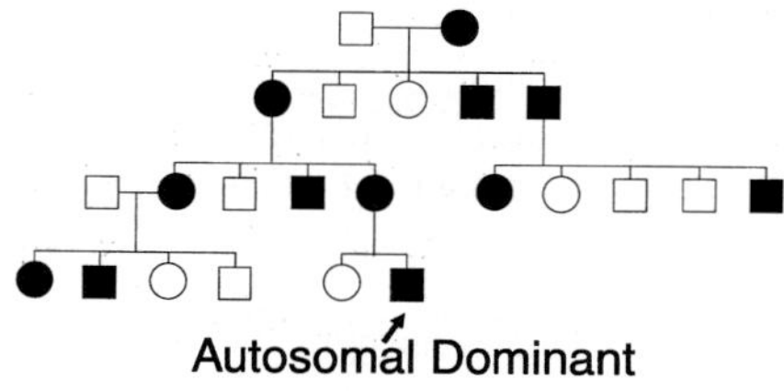

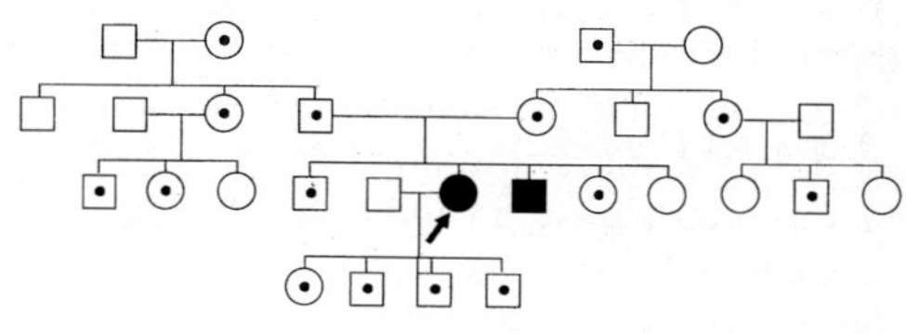

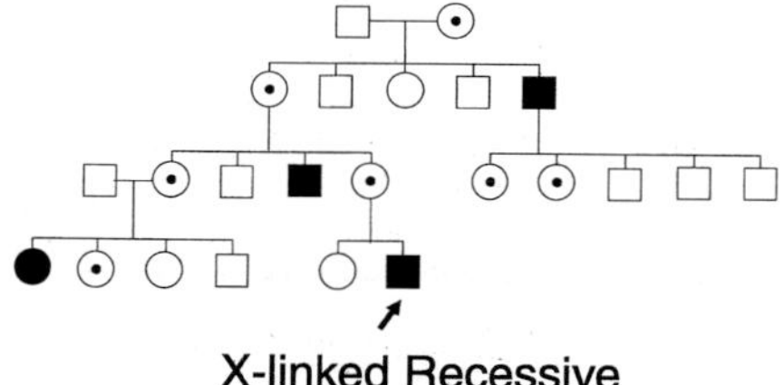

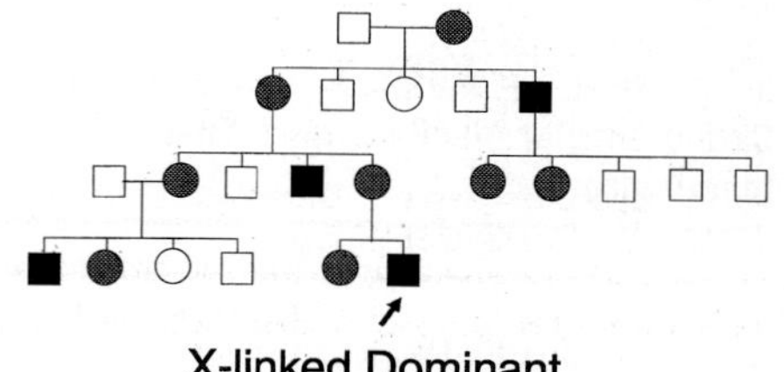

FIGURE 115–3 Mendelian patterns of inheritance. Pedigree patterns for autosomal dominant, autosomal recessive, X-linked recessive, and X-linked dominant patterns of inheritance.

vertical and tends to be limited to siblings within a family. If both parents are carriers of a recessive disorder, they have a 25 percent chance of passing on the disorder to their children. Males and females are equally affected. Consanguinity, or mating between people who are related, can be an underlying cause of the presence of autosomal recessive diseases. Autosomal recessive disorders are often caused by mutations in the genes that encode for enzymes or that transport proteins. Only 647 of the 3300 identified genetic disorders are autosomal recessive.

X-linked disorders are caused by inheritance of a mutant gene found on the X chromosome. Because males have only one X chromosome, X-linked disorders are fully expressed in males. Females have two X chromosomes, and therefore expression of the disease is dependent on whether the mutated gene is dominant or recessive. Diseases that are rarely expressed in females are called X-linked recessive. X-linked recessive disorders are restricted to males, and there is no male-to-male transmission (see Fig. 115–3). Females who carry the mutant gene on one of their X chromosomes rarely express the disease and are therefore carriers. Only 190 of the 3300 identified mendelian disorders are caused by mutant genes on the X chromosome.

X-linked dominant disorders are expressed in both males and females who inherit the X chromosomes with the mutant gene. The pattern of inheritance is vertical, as in autosomal dominant disorders. The distinguishing feature of X-linked dominant disorders is that there is no male-to-male transmission of the condition (see Fig. 115–3).

MULTIFACTORIAL INHERITANCE

Common diseases of adults, such as coronary artery disease, hypertension, diabetes, and schizophrenia, and some congenital malformations, such as club foot, cleft lip, neural tube defects, and pyloric stenosis, demonstrate familial aggregation but are not inherited as a single-gene disorder or a chromosomal abnormality (Table 115–2). Instead, these disorders are multifactorial genetic diseases, indicating that they are caused by the interplay of multiple genes with multiple genetic factors. Multifactorial inheritance is due not to changes in a single gene but to a combination of genetic changes that predispose to or produce the disease. In the most common disorders seen in adults, genetic factors predispose an individual to the disorder, but environmental factors also influence its expression. Although these disorders tend to be familial, no distinct pattern of inheritance can be determined. The risk that family members will develop these disorders cannot be calculated as easily as it can for single-gene disorders, but certain characteristics of multifactorial inheritance help to predict the risk. Recurrence risks represent empiric risk figures and vary among different families, but in general affect only 5 to 10 percent of first-degree relatives. The risk for first-degree relatives is greater than the risk for second-degree relatives. The greater the number of family members affected with the disorder, the greater the risk that other family members will have the disorder. The risk for relatives of an affected patient increases as the frequency of occurrence of the disease in the general population decreases. The more premature the onset of the disease or the more severe the malformation, the greater the recurrence risk for family members. Finally, if the disease is more common in one sex, the risk is higher for relatives of patients of the less susceptible sex. A number of common diseases with cardiovascular manifestations demonstrate multifactorial inheritance. Coronary artery disease (CAD) is a well-studied adult disorder caused by genetic factors in combination with a strong environmental component, and it serves as a model for the manner in which genetic factors influence complex diseases. It is useful to distinguish the existence of heterogeneity within the etiology of this disorder. A small proportion of CAD is caused by single-gene defects such as familial hypercholesterolemia, but the vast majority of cases are multifactorial. Familial aggregation of CAD has been recognized for many years. Many of the initial reports described autosomal dominant inheritance of fatty deposits in the coronary arteries and skin, most probably representing familial hypercholesterolemia.[2–5] Later studies demonstrated a clear familial aggregation of CAD in men who had premature CAD without a clear mode of inheritance.[6] Studies among graduates of Johns Hopkins Medical School demonstrated that CAD was almost four times as common among siblings of individuals with CAD as among siblings of persons without heart disease.[7] Familial aggregations of ischemic heart disease were noted, especially in the families of the female patients, the sex less commonly affected by CAD.[8] Therefore, CAD demonstrates many of the features associated with multifactorial inheritance, including familial aggregation without a clear mode of inheritance and a higher risk for relatives of individuals with premature CAD and relatives of affected females.

A number of genes that predispose to CAD have been identified. A significant contribution to the genetic component of CAD is made by defects in the genes that encode proteins involved in lipoprotein metabolism. A small percentage of myocardial infarcts are caused by single-gene disorders that affect lipoprotein metabolism such as familial hypercholesterolemia. A number of genetic variations or mutations have been identified that affect lipoprotein levels and their metabolism. These include variations in apoE,[9] apoB,[10–12] and Lp(a).[13, 14] Although the genes for proteins that affect lipoprotein metabolism play an important role in predisposing individuals to CAD, future studies will help to define the complex range of genes involved in CAD.

TABLE 115-2 Common Diseases With Cardiovascular Manifestations That Demonstrate Multifactoral Inheritance

Coronary artery disease	Chronic obstructive pulmonary disease
Hypertension	Diabetes mellitus
Congenital heart disease	Obesity

REFERENCES

1. McKusick VA: Mendelian Inheritance in Man. 10th ed. Baltimore: The Johns Hopkins University Press, 1992.
2. Adlersberg D, Parets AD, Boas EP: Genetics of atherosclerosis. Studies of families with xanthoma and unselected patients with coronary artery disease under the age of fifty years. JAMA 141:246, 1949.

3. Muller C: Angina pectoris in hereditary xanthomatosis. Arch Intern Med 64:657–700, 1939.
4. Thannhauser SJ, Magendantz H: The different clinical groups of xanthomatous diseases: a clinical physiological study of 22 cases. Ann Intern Med 11:1662, 1938.
5. Wilkinson CF: Essential familial hypercholesterolemia: cutaneous metabolic and hereditary aspects. Bull N Y Acad Med 26:670, 1950.
6. Yater WM, Traum AH, Brown WG, et al: Coronary artery disease in men eighteen to thirty-nine years of age. Am Heart J 36:334–372, 1948.
7. Thomas CB: The familial occurence of hypertension and coronary artery disease, with observations concerning obesity and diabetes. Ann Intern Med 42:90–127, 1955.
8. Slack J, Evans KA: The increased risk of death from ischaemic heart disease in first-degree relatives of 121 men and 96 women with ischaemic heart disease. J Med Genet 3:239–257, 1966.
9. Davignon J, Gregg RE Sing CF: Apolipoprotein E polymorphism and athersclerosis.
10. Berg K: DNA polymorphism at the apolipoprotein B locus is associated with lipoprotein level. Clin Genet 301:515–520, 1986.
11. Alto-Setala K, Tikkanen MJ, Taskinen MR, et al: Xbal and C/G polymorphisms of the apolipoprotein B gene locus are associated with serum cholesterol and LDL-cholesterol levels in Finland. Arteriosclerosis 74:65–74, 1988.
12. Deeb SS, Failor RA, Brown BG, et al: Association of apolipoprotein B gene variants with plasma apoB and LDL cholesterol levels. Hum Genet 88:463, 1992.
13. Rhoads GG, Dahlen G, Berg K, et al: Lp(a) lipoprotein as a risk factor for myocardial infarction. JAMA 256:2540–2544, 1986.
14. Durrington PN, Hunt L, Ishola M, et al: Apolipoproteins Lp(a), AI, and B and parental history in men with early onset ischaemic heart disease. Lancet 1:1070–1073, 1988.

CHAPTER 116

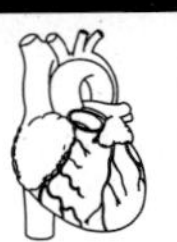

Inherited Disorders of Connective Tissue

Dianna Milewicz

MARFAN'S SYNDROME
Clinical Features
Diagnosis
Genetic Cause of Marfan's Syndrome
EHLERS-DANLOS SYNDROME
Clinical Features
Genetic Causes of Ehlers-Danlos Syndrome Type IV
SUPRAVALVULAR AORTIC STENOSIS
Clinical Features
Genetic Causes of Supravalvular Aortic Stenosis
WILLIAMS' SYNDROME
Clinical Features
Genetic Cause of Williams' Syndrome
PSEUDOXANTHOMA ELASTICUM
Clinical Features
Diagnosis
Genetic Cause of Pseudoxanthoma Elasticum
CUTIS LAXA

This chapter reviews single-gene disorders known or suspected to be the result of mutations in genes that encode for proteins found in the extracellular matrix or connective tissue. Disorders caused by the disruption of connective tissue components by extrinsic factors are addressed elsewhere in this book.

Marfan's Syndrome

Marfan's syndrome is an autosomal dominant disease characterized by pleiotropic manifestations involving the cardiovascular, ocular, and skeletal systems. The disorder affects all races and ethnic groups and has an estimated incidence in the population of 1 in 10,000.[1] The syndrome exhibits marked clinical variability, both among and within families, with essentially complete penetrance. Although Marfan's syndrome is inherited as an autosomal dominant disorder, in approximately one third of cases, individuals have unaffected parents; the syndrome is believed to be caused by germ-line (point) mutations.

Clinical Features

Cardiovascular Manifestations

The most common cardiovascular manifestations are dilatation of the ascending aorta and mitral valve prolapse. Reduced life expectancy in patients with Marfan's syndrome is caused predominantly by cardiovascular complications, of which aortic root dilatation and aortic dissection account for the majority of the deaths.[2] Before the advent of surgical therapy for these cardiovascular complications, the mean life expectancy for patients with Marfan's syndrome was 32 years.

Aortic Root Dilatation

Aortic root dilatation typically begins with dilatation at the sinuses of Valsalva and progresses to involve the proximal ascending aorta.[3–6] The rate of enlargement of the proximal aorta varies widely among individuals, and the enlargement is usually asymptomatic. Therefore, regular assessment of the proximal aorta should be performed annually or more often, depending on the severity of the dilatation and the rate of progression. Transthoracic echocardiography provides precise comparative measurements of aortic root size.[3, 6, 7] Magnetic resonance imaging and transesophageal echocardiography are also useful, particularly in patients with severe thoracic cage abnormalities.[8–10] Aortography is usually limited to studies made before surgery to define the anatomy (Fig. 116–1). Aortic regurgitation commonly occurs as the aorta dilates.[5, 11, 12] The risk for rupture of proximal aorta increases with increasing size of the aortic root. Surgical repair of the proximal aorta is recommended when the aortic root reaches 55 to 60 mm.[2, 13–17] Composite valve graft replacement is achieved by mobilizing buttons of aortic tissue around the coronary arteries for direct nontension anastomosis to the aortic graft.[18] The operative results, particularly since the mid-1980s, have been excellent, with good 5- and 10-year survival.[2, 15, 16, 19] These patients are maintained on anticoagulants and beta-blockers, and routine bacterial prophylaxis is recommended. In addition, routine magnetic resonance imaging of the entire aorta is recommended.[2, 9]

Chronic beta-adrenergic blockade therapy has been proposed as a means of decreasing the stress on the proximal aorta. Although prospective studies supporting the use of such therapy have yet to be published, β-adrenergic blockade is commonly used in patients with Marfan's syndrome. Avoidance of contact sports, strenuous exercise, and isometric exercise is also recommended so as to lower the stress on the proximal aorta.[20]

Aortic Dissection

Some patients with Marfan's syndrome suffer a dissection through the medial wall of the aorta, most often a type I

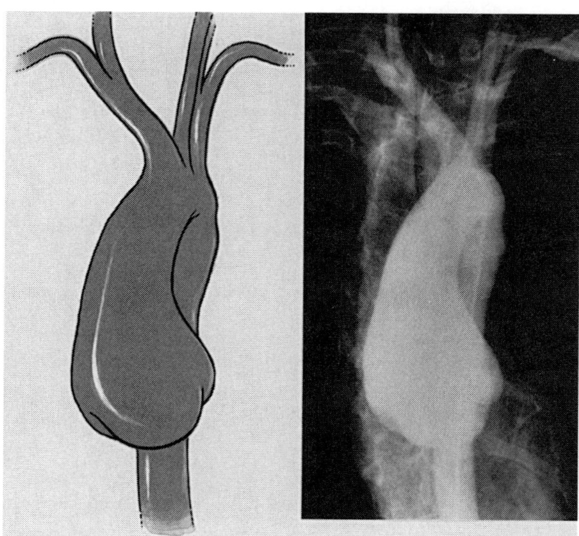

FIGURE 116–1 Illustration and aortogram of an aneurysm of the ascending aorta.

dissection (DeBakey classification), which involves the entire aorta. Less common is type III dissection, which involves the descending thoracic aorta. Dissections involving the ascending aorta can occur in patients who have minimal to no enlargement of the ascending aorta. All forms of dissection are known to occur in the absence of systemic hypertension. Angiography, transesophageal echocardiography, and magnetic resonance imaging are useful techniques for diagnosis of aortic dissection and determination of the extent of an acute dissection. Acute management of an aortic dissection is the same as it is for patients without Marfan's syndrome. Total aortic replacement, which is performed in two stages, is now feasible for patients with chronic type I dissection and fusiform dilatation of the entire aorta.[21]

Mitral Valve Disease

Mitral valve prolapse is present in 70 to 90 percent of patients with Marfan's syndrome.[7, 12, 22] Progression to mitral valve regurgitation occurs in up to half of these patients, but serious mitral regurgitation develops only in approximately one of every eight patients by the third decade of life.[27] In contrast to aortic root dilatation, which is typically asymptomatic, mitral valve prolapse can be associated with chest pain, palpitations, and lightheadedness.[23] It is now feasible to perform a concomitant composite valve graft replacement of the aortic root and a transaortic mitral valve replacement.[23] Echocardiography with Doppler interrogation and color-flow imaging has been the major diagnostic tool for study of the mitral valve.

The incidence of mitral valve prolapse in children with Marfan's syndrome is the same as it is in adults.[7, 24] Children diagnosed with Marfan's syndrome at a young age exhibit more cardiovascular morbidity associated with mitral valve disease (mitral regurgitation) than with aortic root involvement, although aortic root dilatation may appear early in life.[25, 26]

Ocular Complications

Ocular complications related to Marfan's syndrome include ectopia lentis or lens dislocation, myopia, and retinal detachment. The majority of patients are myopic as the result of increased axial globe length.[27] Approximately 60 percent of patients have lens dislocation; the most common direction of displacement is upward and supertemporally. The lens dislocation usually appears at a early age and remains stable. Retinal detachments occur in only a few patients (8 percent).[27]

Skeletal Manifestations

The skeletal manifestations of Marfan's syndrome are the most outwardly striking feature of the disorder and are often the feature that triggers the initial evaluation for possible Marfan's syndrome (Fig. 116–2). Tall stature, due primarily to dolichostenomelia (long, thin legs and arms), is usually present and is reflected in a decreased ratio of upper segment (height minus lower segment) to lower segment (top of pubic ramus to floor) and an arm span that is greater than the height. The reduced upper-to-lower segment ratio can be further exaggerated by scoliosis and kyphosis. Arachnodactyly (long, thin fingers) is also a common feature and can be demonstrated on examination by a positive thumb sign or wrist sign. Also common are scoliosis, loss of thoracic kyphosis (straight back), and chest wall deformities (pectus excavatum or carinatum). Such a patient often has a high-arched palate and crowding of the frontal teeth, joint laxity, and flat feet. Less common are congenital contractures in newborn children with Marfan's syndrome.

Other Manifestations

Another common feature of Marfan's syndrome is striae distensae, or stretch marks, typically located on the pectoral, deltoid, back, or thigh area.[28] Inguinal hernias are also common in patients with Marfan's syndrome.[29] Spontaneous pneumothorax is estimated to occur in up to 11 percent of these patients.[30, 31] Finally, dural ectasia, widening of the lumbosacral spinal canal, is found in 65 percent of patients with Marfan's syndrome.[32, 33]

Diagnosis

The diagnostic criteria for Marfan's syndrome were initially established by an international consortium of clinicians in 1986.[34] These diagnostic criteria were revised in 1997 and are termed the *Ghent criteria* for diagnosing Marfan's syndrome. The diagnosis is based on findings consistent with Marfan's syndrome involving the cardiovascular, skeletal, and ocular systems. The major criteria reflect findings that are more specific for Marfan's syndrome (aortic root dilatation or dissection, lens dislocation, dural ectasia). The minor criteria are findings common in patients with Marfan's syndrome but also common in individuals with other connective tissue disorders and in the general population (Table 116–1).

The diagnosis of Marfan's syndrome may be difficult

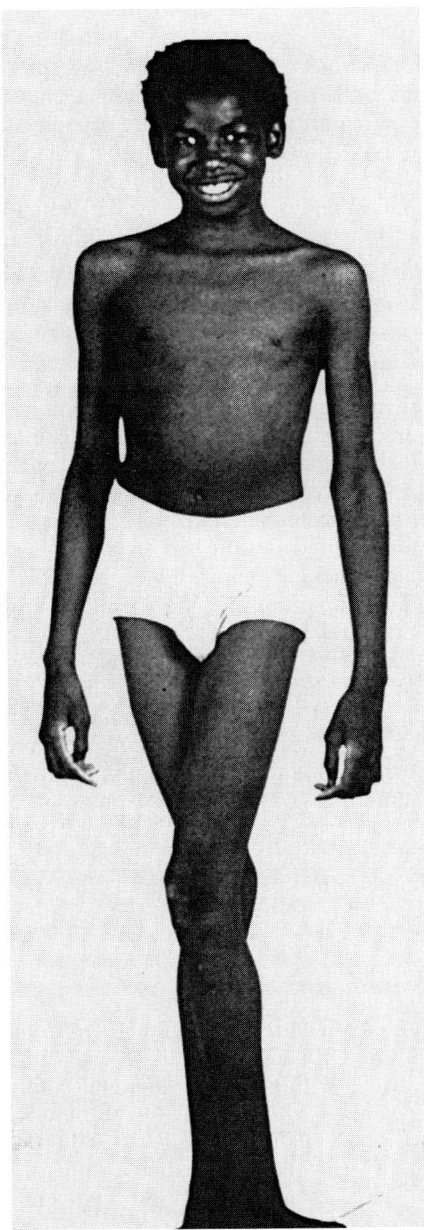

FIGURE 116–2 Skeletal manifestations of Marfan's syndrome: tall stature and long, thin fingers.

because there is no specific laboratory test for the condition. Instead, it is identified by a composite of clinical findings. The diagnostic evaluation for Marfan's syndrome should be performed by physicians experienced with the condition and should include the following:

- A detailed medical and family history
- A complete physical examination
- A thorough eye examination by an ophthalmologist who uses a slit lamp to look for lens dislocation after fully dilating the pupil
- An echocardiogram (a sound-wave picture of the heart) to look for involvement of the cardiovascular system that is often not evident in a physical examination

The criteria for diagnosis are classified according to how specific to Marfan's syndrome the clinical findings are; the major criteria are clinical features that rarely occur in the general population. Minor criteria are features that are present in individuals with Marfan's syndrome but are also commonly present in the general population. The diagnosis requires that at least two of the major manifestations of the condition be present in patients who do not have affected family members. In families in which Marfan's syndrome is known to occur, only one major criterion is required. The major features necessary for the diagnosis include the following:

- Aortic root enlargement (aortic aneurysm)
- Aortic dissection
- Lens dislocation
- Dural ectasia
- The presence of at least four major skeletal features, which include chest wall deformities, long, thin arms and legs (assessed by detailed measurements), and scoliosis greater than 20 degrees

Diagnosis of Marfan's syndrome is a complicated clinical decision that is based on the presence of both minor and major features. For the index case, there must be major criteria in at least two different organ systems and involvement of a third organ system. Alternatively, if a mutation known to cause Marfan's syndrome in others is detected, one major criterion in an organ system and involvement of a second organ system is sufficient for the diagnosis. For the relative of an individual with Marfan's syndrome, there must be a major criterion in an organ system and involvement of a second organ system. Some of the criteria used to diagnosis Marfan's syndrome may arise with age. Therefore, a child may fail to meet the criteria at first but at a later date may have manifestations that definitely meet the criteria. This phenomenon has been termed *emerging Marfan's syndrome.*

Many conditions or syndromes have features in common with Marfan's syndrome and therefore require differentiation. Homocystinuria, an autosomal recessive disorder resulting from a deficiency of cystathionine-synthetase, has many features in common with Marfan's syndrome, including scoliosis, dolichostenomelia, pectus deformity, and lens dislocation. Therefore, any patient suspected of having Marfan's syndrome should undergo a plasma amino acid analysis to document the absence of homocystinuria.

Mitral valve prolapse occurs in an estimated 4 to 7 percent of the general adult population. It can occur as an isolated finding or can be inherited within a family, typically in an autosomal dominant manner.[35–37] Patients with mitral valve prolapse often exhibit thoracic skeletal abnormalities similar to those observed in patients with Marfan's syndrome. These skeletal abnormalities include thoracic kyphosis and pectus deformities.[38] Individuals with skeletal abnormalities and mitral valve prolapse do not meet the diagnostic criteria for Marfan's syndrome. Thoracic aortic aneurysms and aortic dissection can occur in isolated individuals or in familial cases. Aortic dissection with cystic medial necrosis of the aorta has been termed Erheim's disease. A number of case reports in the literature have documented an autosomal dominant inheritance of aortic

TABLE 116-1 **Revised Criteria for Marfan's Syndrome**

System	Major Criteria	Minor Criteria
Skeletal	Presence of at least four of the following manifestations: Pectus carinatum Pectus excavatum requiring surgery Reduced upper segment to lower segment ratio or arm span to height ratio greater than 1.05 Wrist and thumb signs Scoliosis > 20 degrees or spondylolisthesis Reduced extensions at the elbows (<170 degrees) Medial displacement of the medial malleolus, causing pes planus Protrusio acetabulae of any degree (ascertained on radiographs)	Pectus excavatum of moderate severity Joint hypermobility Highly arched palate with crowding of teeth Facial appearance including dolichocephaly, malar hypoplasia, enophthalmos, retrognathia, down-slating palpebral fissures
Ocular	Ectopia lentis (dislocated lens)	Abnormally flat cornea (as measured by keratometry) Increased axial length of globe (as measured by ultrasound) Hypoplastic iris or hypoplastic dilator muscle causing increased miosis
Cardiovascular	Dilatation of the ascending aorta with or without aortic regurgitation and involving at least the sinuses of Valsalva or Dissection of the ascending aorta	Mitral valve prolapse with or without mitral valve regurgitation Dilatation of the main pulmonary artery, in the absence of valvular or peripheral pulmonic stenosis or any other obvious cause, before the age of 40 yr Calcification of the mitral annulus before the age of 40 yr Dilatation or dissection of the descending thoracic or abdominal aorta before the age of 50 yr
Pulmonary	None	Spontaneous pneumothorax Apical blebs (ascertained by chest radiography)
Skin and integument	None	Stretch marks not associated with marked weight changes, pregnancy, or repetitive stress Recurrent incisional hernias
Dura	Lumbosacral dural ectasia by CT or MRI	None
Family/genetic history	Having a parent, child, or sibling who meets these diagnostic criteria independently Presence of a mutation in *FBN1* known to cause Marfan's syndrome Presence of a haplotype around *FBN1*, inherited by descent, known to be associated with unequivocally diagnosed Marfan's syndrome in the family	None

Abbreviations: CT, computed tomography; MRI, magnetic resonance imaging.
From De Paepe A, Devereux RB, Dietz HC, et al: Revised diagnostic criteria for the Marfan syndrome. Am J Med Genet 62:417–426, 1996. Copyright © 1996. Reprinted by permission of Wiley-Liss, Inc., a division of John Wiley & Sons, Inc.

dissection in families without other phenotypic manifestations of Marfan's syndrome.[39–41]

A number of other rare genetic disorders have some features in common with Marfan's syndrome and must therefore be differentiated from Marfan's syndrome. Stickler's syndrome (hereditary arthro-ophthalmopathy) is an autosomal dominant disorder characterized by tall stature, retognathia, midfacial hypoplasia with cleft palate, retinal detachment, and vitreoretinal degeneration. Ehlers-Danlos syndrome type IV is an autosomal dominant disorder associated with skin fragility, skin and joint hypermobility, and arterial and bowel rupture; it is the result of a mutation on the type III collagen gene *COL3A1*. Arterial rupture typically involves large to middle-sized arteries such as the splenic and renal arteries but rarely involves the aorta. Congenital contractural arachnodactyly is an autosomal dominant disorder with skeletal features in common with Marfan's syndrome (e.g., dolichostenomelia, arachnodactyly, scoliosis, pectus deformity), but in addition, these patients have congenital contractures and a crumpled appearance of the pinna ear. These patients do not develop the cardiovascular and ocular problems typical of Marfan's syndrome.

Genetic Cause of Marfan's Syndrome

For many years, it was suspected that the basic defect that causes Marfan's syndrome would lie in a gene that encodes for a protein found in the elastic fiber system. The two major components of the elastic fiber system are an amorphous core, composed of the protein elastin, and closely associated microfibrils (approximately 10 mm in diameter) found on the periphery of the amorphous core (Fig. 116–3).[42–44] In addition, microfibrils not associated with elastin exist in many tissues, including the suspensory ligament of the eye. Although microfibrils are composed of many proteins, the primary protein component is fibrillin-1, a large (350 kd) glycoprotein. The gene for fibrillin *(FBN1)* is large (100 kilobases) and maps to the long arm of chromosome 15 15 (15q15–21).[45–48]

Evidence has clearly established the fibrillin gene

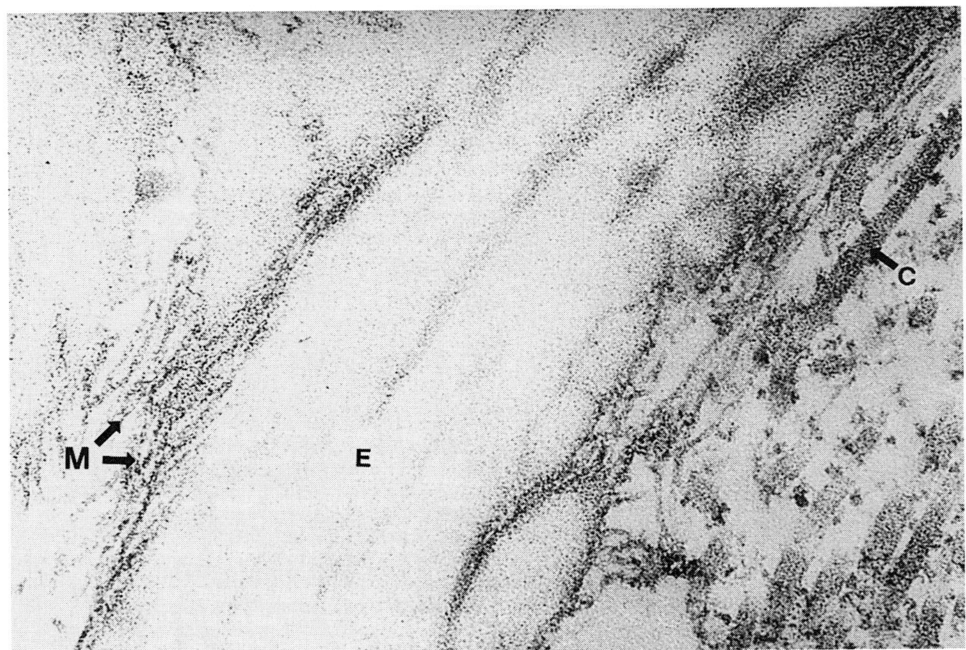

FIGURE 116–3 Electron microscopic examination of microfibrils (M) around the amorphous core of an elastic fiber (E) in human skin. Larger collagen fibers (C) can be seen. (From Milewicz DM: Identification of defects in the fibrillin gene and protein in individuals with the Marfan syndrome and related disorders. Tex Heart J 21:22, 1994.)

(FBN1) on chromosome 15 as the gene that causes Marfan's syndrome if it is defective.[49–52] The disorder segregates in families with polymorphic markers within and close to *FBN1*.[47, 52, 53] There has been no evidence of genetic heterogeneity in families with classic Marfan's syndrome; therefore, only mutations in *FBN1* are responsible for the condition. A number of mutations in *FBN1* have been identified in affected individuals and families.[54–60] Analysis of mutations responsible for Marfan's syndrome indicates that in almost every case the mutations are private—that is, every family or sporadically affected individual has a different mutation. The majority of mutations are missense mutations that alter a single amino acid, but nonsense mutations, small insertions, exon splicing errors, and small intragenic genomic deletions have also been described.[61] All of the mutations are predicted to produce a mutant fibrillin-1 protein, which is critical for the pathogenesis of this disease. The mutant fibrillin-1 protein that is produced is proposed to disrupt microfibril formation even though the other allele is producing a normal fibrillin-1 protein. This is consistent with a "dominant negative" pathogenesis of the mutant allele.

At present, presymptomatic or prenatal diagnosis of Marfan's syndrome can be performed using linkage analysis to identify polymorphic markers within and closely linked to *FBN1* that segregate with the disease in a family. These studies are dependent on the ability to analyze the DNA of a number of individuals in the family to determine the allele that is segregating with the disease. This factor precludes the use of linkage analysis as a diagnostic test in a large number of individuals who are at risk for or are suspected of having Marfan's syndrome. Linkage analysis cannot be used to determine whether an individual has a sporadic case of Marfan's syndrome.

Identification of the causative mutation in *FBN1* that causes Marfan's syndrome in a family or an individual is a formidable task, and at present it can be done only in the research laboratory. Almost every affected family or sporadic individual has its own unique mutation in the *FBN1* gene. There are no identified "hot spots" for mutations in *FBN1,* so the entire coding region of the gene must be screened for the mutations causing the syndrome; clearly, this is both costly and time-consuming, given current techniques.

Familial Thoracic Aortic Aneurysms and Dissections

The majority of patients with thoracic aortic aneurysms and dissections who have cystic medial necrosis on pathologic examination of the aorta do not have Marfan's syndrome or other connective tissue disorders, and the cause of the disease remains unknown. There are reports in the literature of familial aggregation of aortic dissection and aneurysms, but reports prior to the 1960s do not specifically address whether the patients had Marfan's syndrome. Hanley and Jones[62] reported the presence of dissecting aortic aneurysms in two sisters and the son of one of them in the absence of the stigmata of Marfan's syndrome. Opitz[63] described three families with aortic disease due to cystic medial necrosis. Nicod and associates[41] described a family in which nine members over two generations had aortic dissecting aneurysms or aortic dilatation. A recent report describes six families with a dramatic aggregation of thoracic aortic aneurysms and dissections. These families suggest that there is autosomal dominant inheritance of the condition with decreased penetrance and variable expression. In these families, the disease was not linked to *FBN1,* the defective gene in individuals with Marfan's syndrome. The defect causing the autosomal dominant inheritance of thoracic aortic aneurysms and dissections in the absence of features of Marfan's syndrome has not been identified.

A bicuspid aortic valve and coartation of the aorta frequently coexist, suggesting that these malformations result from a single developmental diathesis. McKusick and coworkers[64, 65] added a third component; they suggested that medial necrosis is so commonly encountered in patients with either a bicuspid aortic valve or coarctation as to suggest a common underlying defect. McKusick[64] described two patients with bicuspid aortic valves and ascending aortic dilatation and dissection who had medial necrosis on pathologic examination, and he also described a father and son with both aortic disorders. Families with autosomal dominant inheritance of coarctation of the aorta have been described.[66] Two families with familial aggregation of arterial dissections (both aortic and carotid artery dissections) and bicuspid aortic valves have been described.[67] The familial aggregation of thoracic aortic aneurysms and dissections, bicuspid aortic valve, and coarctation of the aorta, along with medial necrosis, suggests a common cause of these defects of the aorta.[68]

Ehlers-Danlos Syndrome

Ehlers-Danlos syndrome (EDS) (types I through X) comprises a group of heterogeneous disorders that are classified together on the basis of several shared common features: skin hyperextensibility, cutaneous fragility, joint laxity and instability, dystrophic scarring, and easy bruising.[34, 69] There is an increased frequency of mitral valve prolapse in most forms of EDS.[70, 71] The majority of types are inherited in an autosomal dominant manner; the genetic defect is known for only a few.[69]

Clinical Features

The form of EDS with major vascular complications is EDS type IV. EDS type IV is characterized by severe, life-threatening cardiovascular complications, along with gastrointestinal complications. Unlike patients with other forms of EDS, patients with EDS type IV may not have overly extensible skin. Instead, they typically have skin that is thin and translucent, often with a visible venous pattern over the chest, abdomen, and extremities. In addition, EDS type IV patients have a particular facial appearance characterized by thin lips, a thin, delicate nose, and prominent eyes. The hallmark of EDS type IV is the catastrophic internal complications that involve the rupture of arteries, the colon, and the gravid uterus.[72] These complications can occur sequentially in an individual. Spontaneous arterial rupture is more common than aneurysm formation or dissection.[72–75] Vascular complications can occur at almost any arterial site and can result in the formation of an arteriovenous fistula. The most common site of arterial bleeding is the abdominal cavity as the result of the rupture of a visceral vessel or, less commonly, the aorta. Also frequently reported is carotid–cavernous sinus fistula formation, which can result in exophthalmos.[76–78] Although it is not usual, some patients with EDS type IV form abdominal aneurysms.[79, 80] Arterial rupture accounts for most of the deaths of EDS type IV patients, and death typically occurs before 40 years of age.[72, 73] Vascular surgery is commonly complicated by the fact these patients' tissues are extremely friable and do not hold sutures well. Therefore, bleeding should be managed conservatively whenever possible.[73] Angiography is associated with a high rate of complications and should be avoided.[73, 81] Rupture of internal organs primarily of the colon, occurs in these patients. In addition, affected women may experience life-threatening complications during pregnancy, typically near the time of delivery or in the postpartum period. Complications associated with pregnancy include rupture of the gravid uterus, rupture of arteries or internal organs, postpartum hemorrhage, and vaginal lacerations.[82, 83]

Genetic Causes of Ehlers-Danlos Syndrome Type IV

The genetic defect that causes EDS type IV is one or more heterozygous mutations in the gene that encodes for the peptide chains of type III collagen, the *COL3A1* gene found on chromosome 2.[84–89] As a result of the mutation, the connective tissue contains less type III collagen, which plays an important role in maintaining the structural integrity of blood vessels, skin, and internal organs.

A diagnostic test is available to confirm the diagnosis of EDS type IV. This test requires the culture of dermal fibroblasts explanted from a skin biopsy. These cells are metabolically labeled to analyze the synthesis and secretion of type III collagen. In individuals with EDS type IV, this biochemical analysis typically shows abnormal migration and reduced secretion of type III collagen by the cultured dermal fibroblasts.[74, 83] Reduced levels of the amino propeptide of type III collagen are found in the serum of affected individuals, and such a determination has been proposed as a diagnostic test, but it is not currently used.[90]

Supravalvular Aortic Stenosis

Clinical Features

Supravalvular aortic stenosis is an autosomal dominant disorder characterized primarily by the narrowing of the ascending aorta originating at the sinotubular junction just distal to the coronary ostia. The lesion is typically shaped like an hourglass but can also be characterized by diffuse hypoplasia of the entire ascending aorta. Although the lesion is progressive, it is often asymptomatic. Vascular surgery is corrective for symptomatic lesions. The disease can also affect other vascular sites, including the pulmonary arteries and, rarely, the coronary or carotid arteries.

The disorder is inherited in an autosomal dominant manner. Although true penetrance of supravalvular aortic stenosis is uncertain, recent studies indicate that it is close to 100 percent.[91–93] There is extensive variability of expression of the disorder within families; some family members have significant disease that requires surgical repair and others have only minimal disease, with or without peripheral pulmonary artery stenosis.[93] Rarely, an isolated family member exhibits only pulmonary artery stenosis.[94, 95] Sporadic occurrences of the disease do occur, but their cause is unclear. Supravalvular aortic stenosis is a feature of Williams' syndrome (see subsequent section).

Genetic Causes of Supravalvular Aortic Stenosis

A defect in the elastin gene, located on chromosome 7, has been identified as the cause of supravalvular aortic stenosis. Initial linkage studies mapped the disorder to a region of chromosome 7, where the elastin gene is located.[90, 94] Several mutations in the elastin gene have been identified in individuals with supravalvular aortic stenosis.[96] At present, there is no evidence of genetic heterogeneity in this disorder; all cases reported have been linked to the elastin gene.

Williams' Syndrome

Clinical Features

Williams' syndrome is characterized by multiple anomalies that effect the vascular tissue, connective tissue, and tissues of the central nervous system. Features of the disorder include mental retardation (mean IQ of 53 to 58), abnormal facies, growth deficiency, infantile hypercalcemia, hoarse voice, premature aging of the skin, joint laxity, diverticulosis of the bladder and colon, and congenital heart defects, particularly supravalvular aortic stenosis with or without peripheral pulmonary artery stenosis.[97] Williams' syndrome typically occurs sporadically, although there are rare reports of familial cases.[98]

Genetic Cause of Williams' Syndrome

Williams' syndrome is a contiguous-gene syndrome caused by hemizygosity for a chromosomal deletion at 7q11.23 that includes the elastin gene.[98] In all patients reported on, there is complete deletion of one elastin allele, along with segments of the chromosome adjacent to the elastin gene. This deletion is believed to be the cause of the supravalvular aortic stenosis and connective tissue deficiencies in affected individuals. Other, unidentified, genes closely linked to or associated with the elastin gene are believed to be disrupted by the deletion and therefore to be responsible for the mental retardation and infantile hypercalcemia. A detailed physical map and complete BAC/PAC contig of the critical region has been constructed, extending a distance of approximately 2 Mb and delimited by the nondeleted markers *D7S1816* and *D7S489A*.[99] This contig and expressed sequence map will form the basis for the construction of a complete transcription map of the deleted region and will enable genotype-phenotype correlations to be attempted so the genes responsible for the other phenotypic features of Williams' syndrome can be identified.

Pseudoxanthoma Elasticum

Clinical Features

Pseudoxanthoma elasticum (PXE) is an inherited disorder characterized by progressive calcification of elastic fibers in the connective tissue throughout the body.[100, 101] The primary clinical manifestations of the disorder affect the skin, eyes, and cardiovascular system. The estimated prevalence of the disorder is approximately 1 in 100,000.[101]

The skin lesions are pathognomonic for the disorder (Fig. 116–4). Initially, the lesions typically appear at areas of flexure when the affected individual is a teenager. Yellow-orange, papular skin lesions are characteristic. The retinopathy associated with the disorder is characterized by a peau d'orange pigmentation of the retina. Although retinal hemorrhages can occur and typically involve the macula, they rarely lead to total blindness.

The cardiovascular complications are caused primarily by calcification of the elastic media in the arterial system, a process that has been proposed to lead to secondary disruption of the intima and atheromatous plaque formation. Primarily the peripheral arteries are affected, leading to claudication that begins in the third to fourth decade of life. Because the occlusions are slowly progressive, collateral circulation can form and is encouraged by a regular exercise program early in life. The major arteries and the coronary arteries are less commonly involved, but premature coronary artery disease does occur in a few patients with PXE.[102, 103] Strokes, gastrointestinal hemorrhaging, and hypertension are additional clinical features that result from vascular involvement. Mitral valve prolapse and endocardial calcification are observed in some patients with PXE.[104–108]

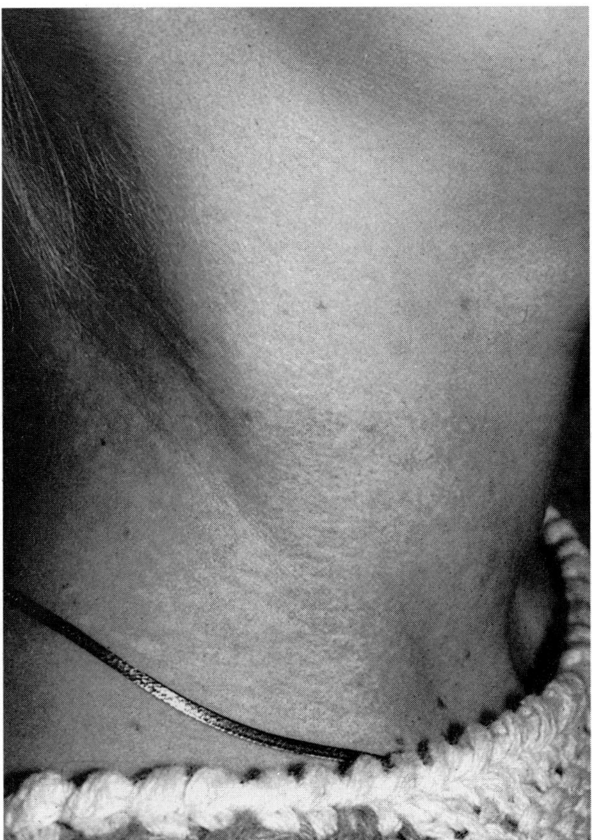

FIGURE 116–4 Skin lesions characteristic of pseudoxanthoma elasticum.

Diagnosis

The precise diagnostic criteria for PXE have not been established.[100] At present, diagnosis is based on the characteristic skin changes and the findings of calcification of elastic fibers on biopsy of affected tissue.[109] Ultrasound has been proposed as a diagnostic test, based on calcification of the vasculature of internal organs.[110]

Genetic Cause of Pseudoxanthoma Elasticum

PXE is usually inherited as an autosomal recessive disorder. However, it can also be inherited in an autosomal dominant manner.[100, 101, 111] Delayed onset of symptoms and variable expression of the disorder make adequate assessment of family members difficult. For unclear reasons, females are more commonly affected than males, with an approximate ratio of 2:1. A genome-wide screen was done of 38 families with two or more affected siblings, using allele-sharing algorithms.[112] This study established that the gene causing PXE is located on chromosome 16p13.1, but the defective gene has not been identified. Both the dominant and the recessive forms of the disease map to this region.

Cutis Laxa

Cutis laxa is a rare connective tissue disorder that can be inherited in an autosomal dominant or recessive manner. The disorder is characterized by genetic heterogeneity and clinical variability. The primary diagnostic feature is loose, hyperextensible skin with decreased elasticity. The redundant skin leads to a premature aged appearance. Other manifestations associated with the skin findings including pulmonary emphysema, bladder divericula, pulmonary artery stenosis, and pyloric stenosis. Some patients with recessively inherited cutis laxa may exhibit tortuous arteries, arterial aneurysms, and fibromuscular renal artery dysplasia.

Histologic examination of the skin reveals marked fragmentation or diminution of elastic fibers. Two groups have report that autosomal dominant cutis laxa is association with mutations in the *ELN* gene.[113, 114] These mutations differ from those observed in patients with supravalvular aortic stenosis, in which the mutations are predicted to lead to haploinsufficiency for *ELN*. The *ELN* mutations reported in patients with cutis laxa predict loss of the functional carboxyl terminus of the tropoelastin molecule.

References

1. Pyeritz RE: The marfan syndrome. *In* Royce PM, Steinmann B (eds): Connective Tissue and its Heritable Disorders. pp. 437–468. New York: Wiley-Liss, 1993.
2. Murdoch JL, Walker BA, Halpern BL, et al: Life expectancy and causes of death in the Marfan syndrome. N Engl J Med 286:804–808, 1972.
3. Child JS, Perloff JK, Kaplan S: The heart of the matter: cardiovascular involvement in Marfan's syndrome. Am Coll Cardiol 14:429–431, 1989.
4. McKusick VA: The cardiovascular aspects of Marfan's syndrome: a heritable disorder of connective tissue. Circulation 11:321–342, 1955.
5. Roberts WC, Honig HS: The spectrum of cardiovascular disease in the Marfan syndrome: a clinico-morphologic study of 18 necropsy patients and comparison to 151 previously reported necropsy patients. Am Heart J 104:115–135, 1982.
6. Marsalese DL, Moodie DS, Vacante M, et al: Marfan's syndrome: natural history and long-term follow-up of cardiovascular involvement. J Am Coll Cardiol 14:422–427, 1989.
7. Brown OR, DeMots H, Kloster FE, et al: Aortic root dilatation and mitral valve prolapse in Marfan's syndrome. Circulation 52:651–657, 1975.
8. Schaefer S, Peshock RM, Malloy CR, et al: Nuclear magnetic resonance imaging in Marfan's syndrome. J Am Coll Cardiol 9:70–74, 1987.
9. Soulen RL, Fishman EK, Pyeritz RE, et al: Marfan syndrome: evaluation with MR imaging versus CT. 1. Radiology 165:697–701, 1987.
10. Simpson IA, de Belder MA, Treasure T, et al: Cardiovascular manifestations of Marfan's syndrome: improved evaluation by transoesophageal echocardiography. Br Heart J 69:104–108, 1993.
11. Lima SD, Lima JAC, Pyeritz RE, Weiss JL: Relation of mitral valve prolapse to left ventricular size in Marfan's syndrome. Ann Thorac Surg 55:739–743, 1985.
12. Hirata K, Triposkiadis F, Sparks E, et al: The Marfan syndrome: cardiovascular physical findings and diagnostic correlates. Am Heart J 3:743–751, 1992.
13. Crawford ES: Marfan's syndrome: broad spectral surgical treatment of cardiovascular manifestations. Ann Surg 198:487–505, 1983.
14. Kouchoukos NT, Wareing TH, Murphy SF, Perillo LB: Sixteen-year experience with aortic root replacement: results of 172 operations. Ann Surg 214:308–318, 1991.
15. Gott VL, Pyeritz RE, Cameron DE, et al: Composite graft repair of Marfan aneurysm of the ascending aorta: results in 100 patients. Ann Thorac Surg 52:38–45, 1991.
16. Gott VL, Pyeritz RE, Magovern GJ, et al: Surgical treatment of aneurysms of the ascending aorta in the Marfan syndrome. N Engl J Med 314:1070–1074, 1986.
17. Treasure T: Elective replacement of the aortic root in Marfan's syndrome. Br Heart J 69:101–103, 1993.
18. Coselli JS, Crawford ES: Technical mini-symposium: composite AVR and graft replacement of the ascending aorta plus coronary ostial reimplantation: How I do it. Sem Thorac Cardiovasc Surg 5:55–62, 1993.
19. Gott V, Greene P, Alejo D, et al: Replacement of the aortic root in patients with Marfan's syndrome. N Engl J Med 340:1307–1313, 1999.
20. Mitchell JH, Blomqvist CG, Haskell WL, et al: Classification of sports. J Am Coll Cardiol 6:1198–1199, 1985.
21. Gouvaras G, Goudevenos J, Adams P: Marfan's syndrome and coarctation: coincidence or association? A case report. J Vasc Dis 41:412–417, 1990.
22. Pyeritz RE, Wappel MA: Mitral valve dysfunction in the Marfan syndrome. Am J Med 74:797–807, 1983.
23. Crawford ES, Coselli JS: Marfan's syndrome: combined composite valve graft replacement of the aortic root and transaortic mitral valve replacement. Ann Thorac Surg 45:296–302, 1988.
24. Morse RP, Rockenmacher S, Pyeritz RE, et al: Diagnosis and management of infantile Marfan syndrome. Pediatrics 86:888–895, 1990.
25. Phornphutkul C, Rosenthal A, Nadas A: Cardiac manifestations of Marfan syndrome in infancy and childhood. Circulation 47:587–597, 1973.
26. Sisk HE, Zahka KG, Pyeritz RE: The Marfan syndrome in early childhood: analysis of 15 patients diagnosed at less than 4 years of age. Am J Cardiol 52:353–358, 1983.
27. Maumenee IH: The eye in the Marfan syndrome. Trans Am Ophthalmol Soc 79:685–733, 1981.
28. Cohen PR, Schneiderman P: Clinical manifestations of the Marfan syndrome. Int J Dermatol 28:291–299, 1989.
29. Pyeritz RE, McKusick VA: The Marfan syndrome: diagnosis and management. N Engl J Med 300:772–777, 1979.

30. Hall JR, Pyeritz RE, Dudgeon DL, Haller JA: Pneumothorax in the Marfan syndrome: prevalence and therapy. Ann Thorac Surg 37:500–504, 1984.
31. Wood JR, Bellamy D, Child AH, Citron KM: Pulmonary disease in patients with Marfan syndrome. Thorax 39:780–784, 1984.
32. Pyeritz RE, Fishman EK, Bernhardt BA, Siegelman SS: Dural ectasia is a common feature of the Marfan syndrome. Am J Hum Genet 43:726–732, 1988.
33. Stern WE: Dural ectasia and the Marfan syndrome. J Neurosurg 69:221–227, 1988.
34. Beighton P, dePaepe A, Danks D, et al: International nosology of heritable disorders of connective tissue, Berlin, 1986. Am J Med Genet 29:581–594, 1988.
35. Devereux RB, Brown WT, Kramer-Fox R, Sachs I. Inheritance of mitral valve prolapse: effect of age and sex on gene expression. Ann Intern Med 97:826–832, 1982.
36. Pader E: The familial incidence of mitral valve prolapse. N Y State J Med 84:395–396, 1984.
37. Devereux RB, Brown WT: Genetics of mitral valve prolapse. Prog Med Genet 5:139–161, 1983.
38. Roman MJ, Devereux RB, Kramer-Fox R, Spitzer MC: Comparison of cardiovascular and skeletal features of primary mitral valve prolapse and Marfan syndrome. Am J Cardiol 63:317–321, 1989.
39. Griffiths GJ, Hayhurst AP, Whitehead R: Dissecting aneurysm of aorta in mother and child. Br Heart J 13:364–368, 1951.
40. Lichtenstein J: Erdheim's cystic medial necrosis in father and son. Birth Defects Orig Art Ser 8:282–283, 1972.
41. Nicod P, Bloor C, Godfrey M, et al: Familial aortic dissecting aneurysm. J Am Coll Cardiol 13:811–819, 1989.
42. Cleary EG, Fanning JC, Prosser I: Possible roles of microfibrils in elastogenesis. Connect Tissue Res 8:161–166, 1981.
43. Goldfischer S, Coltoff-Schiller B, Goldfischer M: Microfibrils, elastic anchoring components of the extracellular matrix, are associated with fibronectin in the zonule of zinn and aorta. Tissue Cell 17:441–450, 1985.
44. Ross R, Bornstein P: The elastic fiber. J Cell Biol 40:366–381, 1969.
45. Corson GM, Chalberg SC, Dietz HC, et al: Fibrillin binds calcium and is coded by cDNAs that reveal a multidomain structure and alternatively spliced exons at the 5′ end. Genomics 17:476–484, 1993.
46. Pereira L, D'Alessio M, Ramirez F, et al: Genomic organization of the sequence coding for fibrillin, the defective gene product in Marfan syndrome. Hum Mol Genet 2:961–968, 1993.
47. Lee B, Godfrey M, Vitale E, et al: Linkage of Marfan syndrome and a phenotypically related disorder to two different fibrillin genes. Nature 352:330–334, 1991.
48. Magenis RE, Maslen CL, Smith L, et al: Localization of the fibrillin gene to chromosome 15, band 15q21.1. Genomics 11:346–351, 1991.
49. Hollister DW, Godfrey M, Sakai LY, Pyeritz RE: Immunohistologic abnormalities of the microfibrillar fiber system in the Marfan syndrome. N Engl J Med 323:152–159, 1990.
50. Milewicz DM, Pyeritz RE, Crawford ES, Byers PH: Marfan syndrome: defective synthesis, secretion and extracellular matrix formation of fibrillin by cultured dermal fibroblasts. J Clin Invest 89:79–86, 1992.
51. Godfrey M, Menashe V, Weleber RG, et al: Cosegregation of elastin-associated microfibrillar abnormalities with the Marfan phenotype in families. Am J Hum Genet 46:661–671, 1990.
52. Dietz HC, Cutting GR, Pyeritz RE, et al. Marfan syndrome caused by a recurrent de novo missense mutation in the fibrillin gene. Nature 352:337–339, 1991.
53. Kainulainen K, Steinmann B, Collins F, et al. Marfan syndrome: no evidence for heterogeneity in different populations, and more precise mapping of the gene. Am J Hum Genet 49:662–667, 1991.
54. Dietz HC, Pyeritz RE, Puffenberger EG, et al: Marfan phenotype variability in a family segregating a missense mutation in the epidermal growth factor-like motif of the fibrillin gene. J Clin Invest 89:1674–1680, 1992.
55. Dietz HC, Saraiva JM, Pyeritz RE, et al: Clustering of fibrillin missense mutations in Marfan syndrome patients at cysteine residues in EGF-like domains. Hum Mutat 1:366–374, 1992.
56. Kainulainen K, Sakai LY, Child A, et al: Two mutations in Marfan syndrome resulting in truncated fibrillin polypeptides. Proc Natl Acad Sci U S A 89:5917–5921, 1992.
57. Godfrey M, Vandemark N, Wang M, et al: Prenatal diagnosis and a donor splice site mutation in fibrillin in a family with Marfan syndrome. Am J Hum Genet 53:472–480, 1993.
58. Hewett DR, Smith R, Sykes BC: A novel fibrillin mutation in the Marfan syndrome which could disrupt calcium binding of the epidermal growth factor-like (EGF) molecule. Hum Mol Genet 2:475–477, 1993.
59. Dietz HC, Valle D, Francomano CA, et al: The skipping of constitutive exons in vivo induced by nonsense mutations. Science 259:680–683, 1993.
60. Dietz HC, McIntosh I, Sakai LY, et al: Four novel *FBN1* mutations: significance for mutant transcript level and EGF-like domain calcium binding in the pathogenesis of Marfan syndrome. Genomics 17:468–475, 1993.
61. Milewicz DM: Identification of defects in the fibrillin gene and protein in individuals with the Marfan syndrome and related disorders. Tex Heart Inst 21:22–29, 1994.
62. Hanley WB, Jones NB: Familial dissecting aortic aneurysm. Br Heart J 29:852–858, 1967.
63. McKusick VA: Mendelian Inheritance in Man. 10th ed. Baltimore: The Johns Hopkins University Press, 1992.
64. McKusick VA: Association of congenital bicuspid aortic valve and Erdheim's cystic medial necrosis. Lancet 6:1026–1027, 1972.
65. McKusick VA, Logue RB, Bahnson HT: Association of aortic valvular disease and cystic medial necrosis of the ascending aorta. Circulation 16:188–194, 1957.
66. Beekman R: Coarctation of the aorta inherited as an autosomal dominant trait. Am J Cardiol 56:818–819, 1985.
67. Schievink WI, Mokir B: Familial aorto-cervicocephalic arterial dissections and congenitally bicuspid aortic valve. Stroke 26:1935–1940, 1999.
68. Lindsay J Jr: Coarctation of the aorta, biscuspid aortic valve and abnormal ascending aortic wall. Am J Cardiol 61:182–184, 1998.
69. Steinmann B, Royce PM, Superti-Furga A: The Ehlers-Danlos syndrome. *In* Royce PM, Steinmann B (eds): Connective Tissue and Its Heritable Disorders. p. 1–5. New York: Wiley-Liss, 1993.
70. Leier CV, Call TD, Fulkerson PK, Wooley CF: The spectrum of cardiac defects in the Ehlers-Danlos syndrome, types I and III. Ann Intern Med 92:171–178, 1980.
71. Jaffe AS, Geltman EM, Rodey GE, Uitto J: Mitral valve prolapse: a consistent manifestation of type IV Ehlers-Danlos syndrome. Circulation 64:121–125, 1981.
72. Pepin MG, Superti-Furga A, Byers PH: Natural history of Ehlers-Danlos syndrome type IV (EDS type IV): review of 137 cases. Am J Hum Genet 51:A44–A44, 1992.
73. Cikrit DF, Miles JH, Silver D: Spontaneous arterial perforation: the Ehlers-Danlos specter. J Vasc Surg 5:248–255, 1987.
74. Pope FM, Naracisi P, Nicholls AC, et al: Clinical presentations of Ehlers-Danlos syndrome type IV. Arch Dis Child 63:1016–1025, 1988.
75. Imahori S, Bannerman RM, Graf CJ, Brennan JC: Ehlers-Danlos syndrome with multiple arterial lesions. Am J Med 47:967–977, 1969.
76. Lach B, Nair SG, Russell NA, Benoit BG: Spontaneous carotid cavernous fistula and multiple arterial dissections in type IV Ehlers-Danlos syndrome. J Neurosurg 66:462–467, 1987.
77. Fox R, Pope FM, Narcisi P, et al: Spontaneous carotid cavernous fistula in Ehlers-Danlos syndrome. J Neurol Neurosurg Psychiatry 51:984–986, 1988.
78. Halbach VV, Higashida RT, Dowd CF, et al: Treatment of carotid-cavernous fistulas associated with Ehlers-Danlos syndrome. Neurosurgery 26:1021–1027, 1990.
79. Kontusaari S, Tromp G, Kuivaneimi H, et al: Inheritance of an RNA splicing mutation in the type III procollagen gene *(COL3A1)* in a family with aortic aneurysms and easy bruisability: phenotypic overlap between familial arterial aneurysms and the Ehlers-Danlos syndrome type IV. Am J Hum Genet 47:112–120, 1990.
80. Kontusaari S, Tromp G, Kuivaniemi J, et al: A mutation in the gene for type III procollagen *(COL3A1)* in a family with aortic aneurysms. J Clin Invest 86:1465–1473, 1993.
81. Sparkman RS: Ehlers-Danlos syndrome type IV: dramatic, deceptive, and deadly. Am J Surg 147:703–704, 1984.
82. Rudd NL, Holbrook KA, Nimrod C, Byers PH: Pregnancy complications in type IV Ehlers-Danlos syndrome. Lancet 1:50–53, 1983.
83. Pope FM, Nicholls AC: Pregnancy and Ehlers-Danlos syndrome type IV. Lancet 1:249–250, 1983.

84. Pope FM, Martin GR, Lichtenstein, JR, et al: Patients with Ehlers-Danlos syndrome type IV lack type III collagen. Proc Natl Acad Sci U S A 72:1314–1316, 1975.
85. Byers PH, Holbrook KA, Barsh GS, et al: Altered secretion of type III procollagen in a form of type IV Ehlers-Danlos syndrome. Lab Invest 44:336–341, 1981.
86. Holbrook KA, Byers PH: Ultrastructural characteristics of the skin in a form of the Ehlers-Danlos syndrome type IV. Storage in the rough endoplasmic reticulum. Lab Invest 44:342–350, 1981.
87. Milewicz DM, Witz AM, Smith ACM, et al: Parental somatic and germ-line mosaicism for a multiexon deletion with unusual end-points in a type III collagen *COL3A1* allele produces Ehlers-Danlos syndrome type IV in the heterozygous offspring. Am J Hum Genet 53:62–70, 1993.
88. Lee B, D'Alessio M, Vissing H, et al: Characterization of a large deletion associated with a polymorphic block of repeated dinucleotides in the type III procollagen gene *(COL3A1)* of a patient with Ehlers-Danlos syndrome type IV. Am J Hum Genet 48:511–517, 1991.
89. Richards AJ, Lloyd JC, Narcisi P, et al: A 27-bp deletion from one allele of the type III collagen gene *(COL3A1)* in a large family with Ehlers-Danlos syndrome type IV. Hum Genet 88:325–330, 1992.
90. Steinmann B, Superti-Furga A, Joller-Jemelka HI, et al: Ehlers-Danlos syndrome type IV: a subset of patients distinguished by low serum levels of the amino-terminal propeptide of type III procollagen. Am J Med Genet 34:68–71, 1989.
91. Olson TM, Michels VV, Lindor NM: Autosomal dominant supravalvular aortic stenosis: localization to chromosome 7. Hum Mol Genet 2:869–873, 1993.
92. Ensing GJ, Schmidt MA, Hagler DJ, et al: Spectrum of findings in a family with nonsyndromic autosomal dominant supravalvular aortic stenosis: a Doppler echocardiographic study. J Am Coll Cardiol 13:413–419, 1989.
93. Schmidt MA, Ensing GJ, Michels VV, et al: Autosomal dominant supravalvular aortic stenosis: large three-generation family. Am J Med Genet 32:384–389, 1989.
94. Lyons RM, Keski-Oja J, Moses HL: Proteolytic activation of latent transforming growth factor-β from fibroblast-conditioned medium. J Cell Biol 106:1659–1665, 1988.
95. Kumar A, Stalker HJ, Williams CA: Concurrence of supravalvular aortic stenosis and peripheral pulmonary stenosis in three generations of a family: a form of arterial dysplasia. Am J Med Genet 45:739–742, 1993.
96. Curran ME, Atkinson DL, Ewart AK, et al: The elastin gene is disrupted by a translocation associated with supravalvular aortic stenosis. Cell 73:159–168, 1993.
97. Morris CA, Leonard CO, Dilts C, Demsey SA: Adults with Williams syndrome. Am J Med Genet 6:102–107, 1990.
98. Ewart AK, Morris CA, Atkinson D, et al: Hemizygosity at the elastin locus in a development disorder, Williams syndrome. Nat Genet 5:11–16, 1993.
99. Hockenhull EL, Carette MJ, Metcalfe K, et al: A complete physical contig and partial transcript map of the Williams syndrome critical region. Genomics 58:138–145, 1999.
100. Christiano AM, Lebwohl MG, Boyd, CD, Uitto J: Workshop on pseudoxanthoma elasticum: molecular biology and pathology of the elastic fibers. J Invest Dermatol 99:660–663, 1992.
101. Neldner KH: Pseudoxanthoma Elasticum. *In* Royce PM, Steinmann B (eds): Connective Tissue and its Inheritable Disorders. Molecular, Genetic and Medical Aspects. pp. 425–436. New York: Wiley-Liss, 1992.
102. Bete JM, Banas JS, Moran J, et al: Coronary artery disease in an 18-year-old girl with pseudoxanthoma elasticum: successful surgical therapy. Am J Cardiol 36:515–520, 1975.
103. Schachner L, Young D: Pseudoxanthoma elasticum with severe cardiovascular disease in a child. Am J Dis Child 127:571–575, 1974.
104. Challenor VF, Conway N, Monro JL: The surgical treatment of restrictive cardiomyopathy in pseudoxanthoma elasticum. Br Heart J 59:266–269, 1988.
105. Navarro-Lopez F, Llorian A. Ferrer-Roca O, Betriu A, Sanz G: Restrictive cardiomyopathy in pseudoxanthoma elasticum. Chest 78:113–115, 1980.
106. Pyertiz RE, Weiss JL, Renie WA, Fine SL. Pseudoxanthoma elasticum and mitral-valve prolapse. N Engl J Med 307:1451–1452, 1975.
107. Lebwohl MG, Distefano D, Prioleau PG, et al: Pseudoxanthoma elasticum and mitral-valve prolapse. N Engl J Med 307:228–231, 1982.
108. Rosenzweig BP, Guarneri E, Kronzon I: Echocardiographic manifestations in a patient with pseudoxanthoma elasticum. Ann Intern Med 119:487–490, 1993.
109. Suarez MJ, Garcia JB, Orense M, et al: Sonographic aspects of pseudoxanthoma elasticum. Pediatr Radiol 21:538–539, 1991.
110. de Paepe A, Vijoen D, Matton M, et al: Pseudoxanthoma elasticum: similar autosomal recessive subtype in Belgian and Afrikaner families. Am J Med Genet 38:16–20, 1991.
111. Greenwald IS, Sternberg PW, Horvitz HR: The lin-12 locus specifies cell fates in Caenorhabditis elegans. Cell 34:435–444, 1983.
112. Struk B, Neldner KH, Rao VH, et al: Mapping of both autosomal recessive and dominant variants of pseudoxanthoma elesticum to chromosome 16p13.1 Hum Mol Genet 11:1823–1828, 1997.
113. Tassbehji M, Metcalfe K, Hurst J, et al: An elastin gene mutation producing abnormal tropoelastin and abnormal elastic fibres in a patient with automosal dominant cutis laxa. Hum Mol Genet 7:1021–1028, 1998.
114. Zhang M, He L, Giro M, et al: Cutis laxa arising from frameshift mutations in exon 30 of the elastin gene (ELN). J Biol Chem 274:981–986, 1999.

C H A P T E R **117**

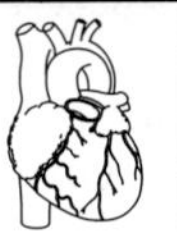

Muscular Dystrophies Affecting the Heart

C. Thomas Caskey

EMERY-DREIFUSS MUSCULAR DYSTROPHY
HYPERTROPHIC CARDIOMYOPATHY
DUCHENNE'S MUSCULAR DYSTROPHY
MYOTONIC DYSTROPHY

The application of molecular genetic analysis to muscular dystrophies affecting the heart has led to the assignment of various diseases to specific regions of the human genome, identification of disease-causing genes, greater understanding of pathogenesis, and more precise methods of diagnosis. Four diseases are selected for discussion here. *Emery-Dreifuss muscular dystrophy* (EMD) has an X-linked recessive and autosomal dominantly inherited form whose genes have recently been discovered. The association of *hypertrophic cardiomyopathy* (HCM) with point mutations in the myosin heavy chain has yielded insight into the pathogenesis of the disease and has led to identification of other candidate genes. Identification of the *Duchenne muscular dystrophy* (DMD) gene provided the first opportunity for multiplex polymerase chain reaction (PCR) amplification for deletion diagnosis, simplifying mutation scanning in this huge gene. Finally, *myotonic dystrophy* (MD) provided a molecular explanation for the clinical observation of anticipation. These four examples illustrate the ability of molecular strategies to identify disease genes and improve diagnosis. It is hoped that understanding of their pathogenesis will subsequently lead to effective therapeutic intervention.

Emery-Dreifuss Muscular Dystrophy

EMD is a rare X-linked recessive disease manifested by early contracture, progressive muscle wasting, and life-threatening cardiomyopathy. The severe cardiovascular manifestation is one of cardiac arrhythmia. Occasional female carriers manifest symptoms, but the major clinical features are found in males. An autosomal form of EMD has also been described.[1, 2]

The molecular defect has been identified by several independent research groups utilizing position cloning, as described in the previous edition of this chapter.[3–5] Following the discovery of the X-linked gene, emerin, an additional phenocopy of heritable type mapped to 1q11-q23, which is inherited as an autosomal dominant trait. Mutations in the lamin A/C gene associated the gene with the disease.[6] Thus, emerin and lamin mutations are the heritable causes of EMD.[5]

Emerin is a 34-kD protein localizing to the nuclear membranes[4] of many cells and bears sequence homology to beta-thymopoietin, another nuclear localizing protein. Lamin A/C can exist as two alternatively spliced forms, A and C, from a single gene.[6] Lamins are members of the intermediate filaments.[7] Immunologic localization places them within the nuclear lamina, thus suggesting they are structural elements of the nuclear envelope. The established interaction of lamin to lamin B receptor, lamin associations proteins and emerin, not only established the EMD phenotype to defects in the nuclear protein complex but also identified other "candidate genes" for involvement in the disease, including other lamins. While many aspects of the pathogenesis are related to these causative gene mutations, the tools for elucidation of the abnormal function and selection of potential therapeutic targets are at hand.

Diagnosis of the two genetic forms of EMD have been achieved by immunohistologic study of biopsies or direct sequencing of mutations. At present, these diagnostic tests should be considered clinical research tools because their validation and standardization are incomplete. Mutations in emerin have been heterogeneous. All mutations lead to loss of the gene product, which is readily confirmed by absence of emerin protein by Western and in situ immunohistology.[4] The molecular diagnosis of lamin defects is more limited in experience but has been achieved by DNA sequence analysis. Both premature chain termination and missense mutations have been observed. Collectively, these lamin mutation data cannot discriminate between haplotype insufficiency and dominant interference by the mutant protein. Immunohistology has failed to discriminate between EMD and control in the family with a 5-amino acid truncation in the carboxyl terminus.[6] More experience is needed with immunologic strategies of lamin diagnosis.

The only current treatment for EMD is support for disability. Because of the extremely common association of cardiac arrhythmia with EMD, pacemaker implantation has been used to prevent sudden deaths.

Hypertrophic Cardiomyopathy

HCM, previously referred to as idiopathic hypertrophic subaortic stenosis, is inherited as an autosomal dominant disease. The clinical manifestations include exertional dyspnea, chest pain, and cardiac arrhythmia leading to sudden death.[8, 9] The sudden demise of young athletes with HCM has received much press and public attention. Symptomatic patients are usually diagnosed by the presence of substantial biventricular hypertrophy detected with two-dimensional echocardiography. At autopsy, the pathologic hallmark of this disease is myocardial hypertrophy with cellular and myofiber disarray.

Genetic linkage studies of selected large pedigrees indicated that a form of HCM was associated with a gene localized to 14q1.[10] These early studies also clearly indicated that these gene loci could not explain all autosomal dominantly inherited cases because the disease in some families segregated independently of the 14q1 genetic marker. Other reports have suggested linkage to chromosomes 16[11] and 18.[12] It is estimated, however, that well over 50 percent of HCM families are associated with the 14q1 locus. Therefore, HCM is a genetically heterogeneous disorder. Furthermore, the disease can arise as a new mutation in some families and can vary in severity from family to family. These confounding clinical features were clarified by identification of the gene causing this disease.

The gene responsible for HCM was identified through a candidate gene study. Recognizing that the beta-cardiac myosin heavy chain mapped to the 14q1 region, Seidman and coworkers[13] investigated this gene as a likely candidate and were proved correct. The Seidman group also showed that missense mutations in the alpha tropomyosin gene cause familial HCM linked to chromosome 15q2, including components of the troponin complex, particularly troponin T. The Seidmans[14] suggested that HCM is a disease of the sarcomere because mutations in the β-myosin heavy chain, α-tropomyosin, and cardiac troponin T may all lead to the same phenotype. The first molecular mutation associated with HCM was a rearrangement between the α- and β-myosin heavy chain genes, giving rise to a hybrid myosin heavy chain.[13] This was quickly followed by many reports identifying point mutations in the β-cardiac myosin heavy chain.[15] The methods by which mutations have been identified vary among laboratories, but all rely consistently on PCR amplification of the gene target from patients, followed by molecular analysis for mutational changes (Fig. 117–1). Peripheral lymphocytes are suitable cell sources to amplify either exons from the nuclear gene or the low level of mRNA transcribed in these cells. Chemical mismatch or ribonuclease A cleavage of mutant and normal mRNA enabled investigators to identify mutations, which were confirmed by DNA sequencing. In one study of 14 families,[16] the identification of 12 different mutations reflected the mutational heterogeneity suggested by the clinical heterogeneity. In three families, identical mutations appeared to arise independently (representing a hot spot for new mutations), whereas in two apparently unrelated Portuguese families, identical genetic markers surrounding the mutation suggested that they were ancestrally related. These studies establish the predominance of new mutations in this disease and explain its heterogeneity. In an extensive comparison of gene mutations to clinical severity, it was suggested that mutations altering the charge of the protein have more severe clinical effects.[17] The correlation, however, was not sufficiently solid to make predictions of phenotype on the basis of mutation studies alone. There are now more than 34 different mutations associated with HCM, all but one being missense mutations. It therefore appears that structural alteration of the β-cardiac myosin heavy chain causes the disease, rather than an absence of the protein. Since HCM has a dominant inheritance pattern, it has been suggested that the mutant protein chain alters configuration of the multiunit protein responsible for the contractibility of muscle.[17]

Using DNA analysis, it is clearly possible to predict a high risk for HCM before the appearance of clinical symptoms. It is also obvious that more study is needed to understand the pathophysiology of the mutant gene. The continued study of families for research purposes immediately raises the question of the value of presymptomatic diagnosis for the expanded family. This is a problem for adult-onset diseases that must be carefully considered before a molecular diagnosis is undertaken. Some have argued that presymptomatic diagnosis would immediately identify young athletes at risk for sudden death. Such risks might be modified by exercise restriction, drugs, or cardiac pacer implants, but these approaches remain unproved at present. Demonstration of an improvement in outcome would provide a strong case for presymptomatic diagnosis. The risk for loss of private health or life insurance coverage must also be considered. A report by the Task Force on Genetic Information and Insurance did not consider presymptomatic diagnosis to be a reason for exclusion or special rating,[18] although this recommendation is not at present accepted by the insurance industry. Although I favor patient knowledge of health risk factors, this is not a universal attitude, and the choice is best left to the informed individual. Presymptomatic diagnosis of HCM is not at present the standard of practice.

DUCHENNE'S MUSCULAR DYSTROPHY

DMD is an X-linked recessive myopathy of childhood, with an incidence of 1 in 3500 male births. The disease is caused by mutations in the dystrophin gene, which contains 76 exons and spans 2.2 megabases. Becker's muscular dystrophy (BMD) results from mutations in the same gene. Since the mid-1990s, there has been a remarkable increase in the understanding of DMD and BMD since the dystrophin gene and its protein product were identified.[19]

The most prominent manifestation of the classic phenotype of DMD is degeneration of skeletal muscle associated with active inflammation. Weakness, beginning during the first 5 years of life, progresses to loss of the ability to walk independently by early in the second decade and death by early in the third decade. Pseudohypertrophy of the calves is often observed. Serum creatinine kinase levels are markedly elevated early in life but decline as muscle mass decreases. DMD also affects cardiac function. Abnormalities are typically detected by electrocardiography (ECG), echocardiography, and Holter monitoring. The primary cardiac dystrophic process causes left ventricular (LV) failure, often complicated by restrictive pulmonary disease. Virtually all male patients over the age of 18 years and some carrier females are affected in this way.

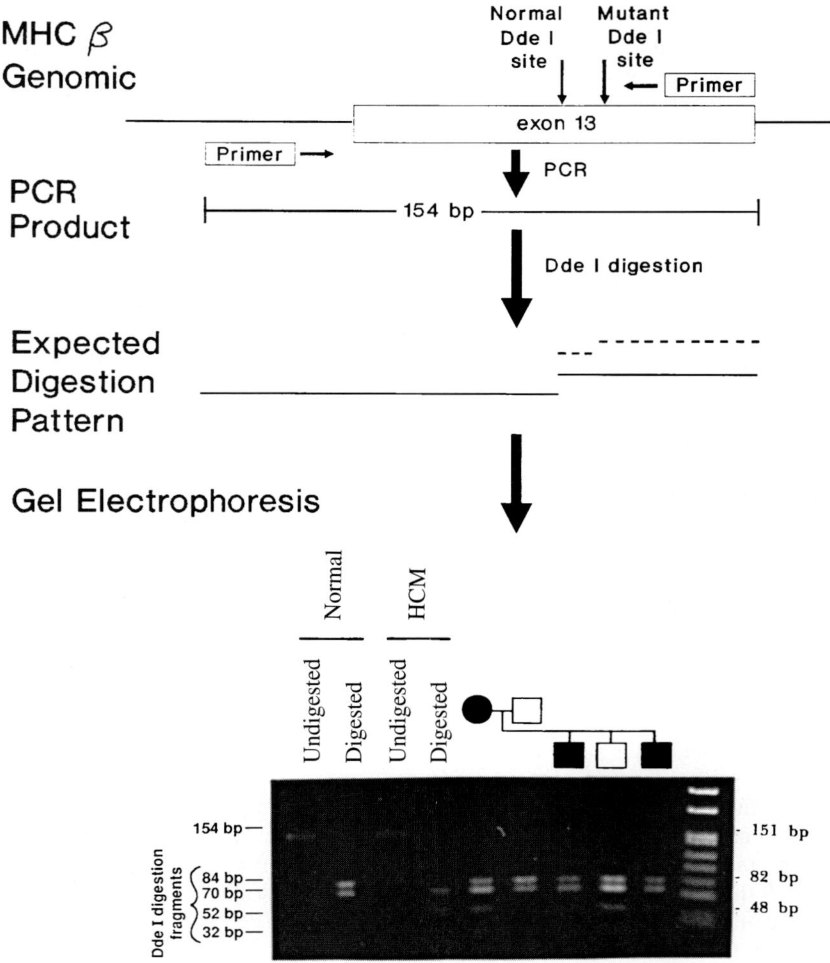

FIGURE 117–1 Diagnosis of a point mutation causing hypertrophic cardiomyopathy (HCM). The relative locations of the normal and mutant *Dde* I restriction sites in exon 13 of the β-cardiac myosin heavy chain (MHC) gene are shown in the upper portion of the figure. The 154–base pair (bp) polymerase chain reaction (PCR) product *(lane 1)* and the relative size of the nucleotide fragments produced after digestion of this product with *Dde* I are also depicted. The lower portion of this figure is a photograph of an ethidium bromide–stained agarose gel illustrating the electrophoretic pattern of the PCR product after digestion with *Dde* I restriction endonuclease. *Lane 2* is wild-type exon 13 DNA digested with *Dde* I and shows two fragments of 84 and 70 bp; *lane 4* is exon 13 DNA from the mutant allele cloned from a patient with HCM digested with *Dde* I and shows three fragments of 70, 52, and 32 bp. Exon 13 PCR product from a normal individual (containing two normal alleles) after digestion with *Dde* I shows two fragments of 84 and 70 bp, and exon 13 PCR product from affected individuals (containing one normal and one mutant allele) shows four fragments of 84, 70, 52, and 32 bp. The individuals in the pedigree are indicated above the appropriate lanes. Size standards are in the extreme right lane. Undigested and digested PCR products from a normal individual and the cloned missense allele are labeled *Normal* and *HCM*, respectively. (Republished with permission of J Clin Invest. From Perryman MB, Yu Q, Marian AJ, et al: Expression of a missense mutation in the messenger RNA for myosin heavy chain in myocardial tissue in hypertrophic cardiomyopathy. J Clin Invest 90:271, 1992; permission conveyed through Copyright Clearance Center, Inc.)

Before the development of molecular diagnostic techniques, muscle histochemistry was the primary means of confirming a clinical diagnosis of DMD. Immunohistochemistry with anti-dystrophin antisera has improved the specificity of the pathologic diagnosis. In addition, dystrophin quantity and size can be assessed by Western blot assay.[21, 22] Early studies revealed an excellent correlation between the absence of dystrophin in patients with DMD and dystrophin of altered size or diminished quantity in patients with BMD who have a milder phenotype.[21, 22] More recent studies demonstrate a spectrum of abnormalities in dystrophin size, quantity, and location in both phenotypes.[23] In addition, the epitope recognized by the antidystrophin antibody can affect whether or not dystrophin protein is detected.[24] Even this level of study may not allow prediction of the phenotype in all cases.

At present, identification of a specific molecular mutation can be achieved in approximately 70 percent of patients with DMD. The majority of DMD-causing mutations described to date are deletions and duplications within the dystrophin gene. Detectable deletion mutations account for approximately 65 percent of affected males[25, 26] and duplications for a further 6 percent.[19, 27] Four out of five cases in which parental origin of a dystrophin duplication could be studied revealed a grandpaternal origin, and in all five cases the duplication originated from a single X chromosome.[19] This is a mechanism not too different from that recently described for factor VIII.

PCR amplification of selected exons, followed by separation of the DNA fragments by gel electrophoresis, is now used routinely for deletion detection. Chamberlain and associates[28] developed a multiplex assay for the simultaneous detection of nine exons that are frequently involved in deletion mutation (Fig. 117–2). The absence of one or more DNA bands defines the location of a gene deletion. This assay, used in combination with a second multiplex assay that amplifies nine additional exons, allows identification of 98 percent of dystrophin gene deletions detectable with Southern analysis.[29] The PCR exon amplification assays are rapid and simple to perform and can reduce the amount of Southern analysis required for mutation detection in DNA diagnostic laboratories.

An alternative molecular method utilizes visual scoring of fluorescently labeled nuclear DNA clones (cosmids) that span the exons most commonly involved in deletions. The technique is referred to as fluorescent in situ hybridization (FISH).[30] The advantage of the technique is speed and direct assay of white blood cells taken from peripheral blood. Quantitation of the fluorescent dots (cosmid probes) observed on each cell using a control DNA probe (centromere) of different fluorescent emission permits cell-to-cell diagnosis for deletions in the DMD gene. Examples of such test results are given in Plate 117–1. The method has superior sensitivity for detection of female carriers. The carrier results indicate one DMD gene present (+FISH) and the second is absent (-FISH). This new approach has the potential to replace carrier detection by all other methods when the mutation event involved is a deletion. The FISH technology is not applicable to point mutations.

In approximately 30 percent of families affected by DMD, no mutation is detected with available DNA diagnostic tests. Carrier detection and prenatal diagnosis are performed with linkage analysis, using informative intragenic and flanking markers to track the chromosome bearing the mutated gene. Small family size, inadequate family member cooperation, and lack of any living affected males may also complicate linkage analysis with genetic markers in families with DMD.[31] Short tandem repeat sequences, which are highly informative length polymorphisms, have proved very useful in linkage analysis.[32–35] Short tandem repeat loci can be easily amplified with PCR and analyzed with polyacrylamide gel electrophoresis. The number of repeats at a particular locus is highly variable from person to person, resulting in reported heterozygote frequencies as high as 90 percent. A high level of heterozygosity allows tracking of genes on individual chromosomes, which greatly facilitates carrier detection and prenatal diagnosis by linkage analysis.

The nonrandom distribution of deletion mutations within the dystrophin gene has been repeatedly demonstrated and was confirmed in a multicenter international study.[36] The reasons for the observed distribution of deletion mutations remain unclear.

Investigators have proposed theories to relate the spectrum of deletion mutations to the spectrum of disease phenotype. The Western blot studies demonstrated absent dystrophin in skeletal muscle from patients with severe disease and a reduced amount or an altered molecular weight of dystrophin in skeletal muscle from patients with milder phenotypes.[21, 22] This observation led to the proposal that deletions that alter the reading frame of the dystrophin mRNA result in the absence of dystrophin and a severe phenotype. The reading frame hypothesis is upheld in 92 percent of cases; severe phenotypes are associated with deletions that cause a frameshift, and milder phenotypes are associated with deletions that do not cause a frameshift.[37] However, the cases that do not support the reading frame hypothesis indicate that this theory alone cannot adequately explain the relationship between deletion mutation and phenotype in all patients. Three additional theories were proposed: (1) differential mRNA splicing could result in the production of an altered size protein despite a frameshift mutation; (2) a new translational start site could occur downstream from a mutation; or (3) a second promoter could exist downstream from a mutation.[38] The use of alternate translational start sites, with or without additional promoters, which would provide a logical explanation for the finding of a milder phenotype associated with a frameshift mutation, has not yet been demonstrated in DMD.

The severity of DMD and the current unavailability of effective therapy have led to extensive use of genetic tests for female carriers, genetic counseling, and prenatal diagnosis. This has enabled families to undertake family planning with an accurate estimate of their genetic risk, which is a remarkable improvement over the era before the discovery of the dystrophin gene. At the moment, most of the families counseled utilize prenatal diagnosis.

There are several well-recognized pitfalls of prenatal diagnosis. Women who bear an affected male with a dystrophin deletion may display gonadal mosaicism, so that analysis of DNA from blood leukocytes appears normal even though the deletion is present in germ cells. This is estimated to occur in 15 percent of isolated DMD cases.[39] When subsequent affected males are born to these mosaic carriers, the mutations are identical to the index cases. This has led to the recommendation that prenatal diagnosis be considered even in cases of apparently new mutations. A second error that has been encountered is the use of linkage analysis for diagnosis in cases mistakenly identified as DMD. This type of error has previously been mentioned in the discussion on Emery-Dreifuss Muscular Dystrophy. A third source of error is the use of linkage analysis in a family whose precise DNA mutation is not known. Since the dystrophin gene is large (2.2 megabases) and mutations can occur in any part of the gene, crossover events during meiosis can separate the short tandem repeat marker from the mutation and thus confound the analysis. Taking all these negative points into account, the improvement in DMD diagnosis is a remarkable success story for molecular genetics.

Since the discovery of the DMD gene defect, immunologic and biochemical studies have shown it to be a critical part of a complex of proteins that span the muscle cell membrane and transmit signals requisite for electromechanical signal transduction.[40] The animo terminus of dystrophin interacts with F-actin and the cysteine with carboxyl terminus interacts with sarcoglycans that, in turn, interact with extracellular laminin only. The identification of these proteins was greatly facilitated by the study of familial childhood dystrophies resembling DMD clinically, but not due to mutations in the dystrophin gene. Whereas

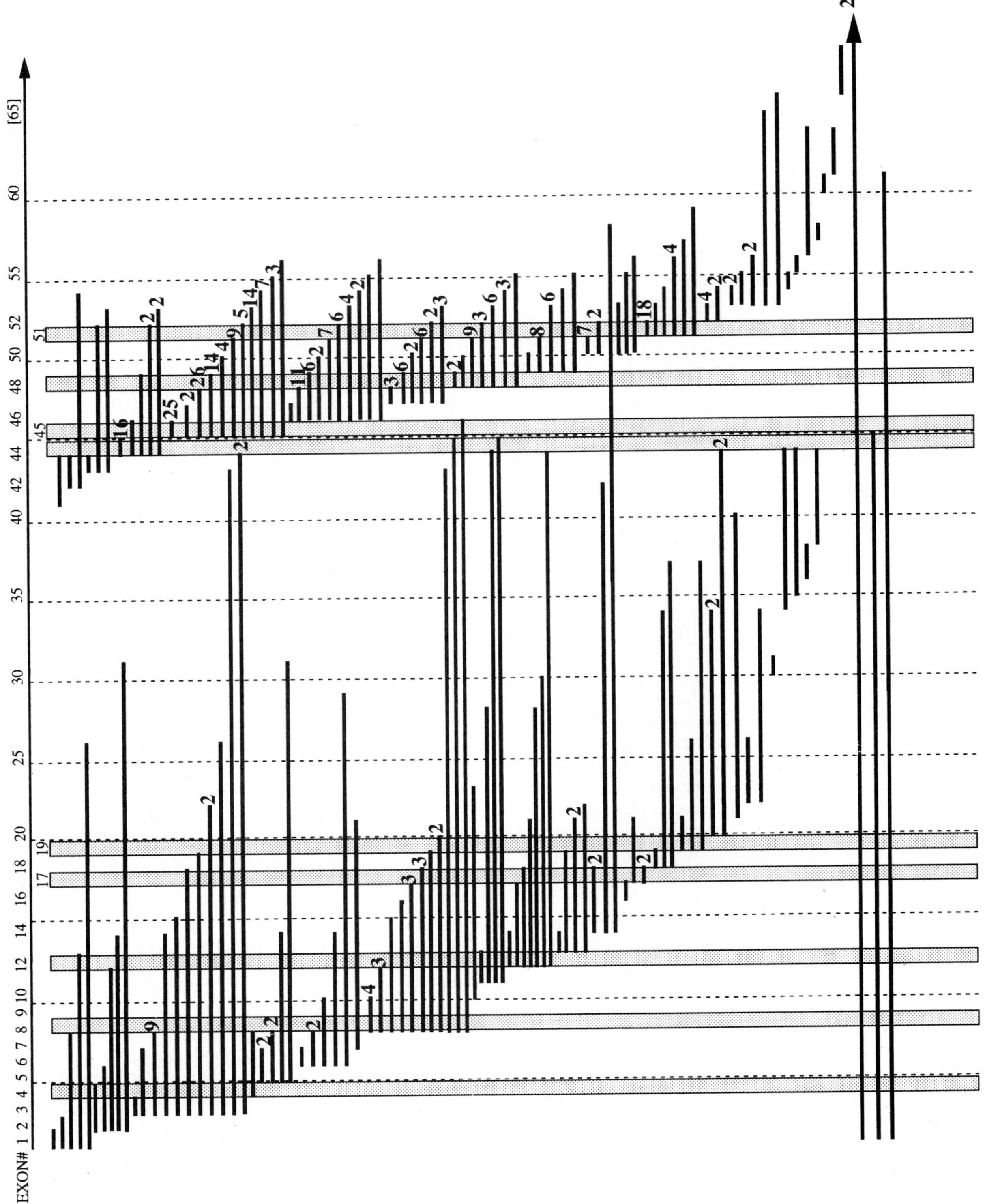

FIGURE 117–2 Comparison of the size and extent of dystrophin gene deletions identified by Southern analysis and polymerase chain reaction (PCR). The location of 416 of the 427 deletions detected in this study is illustrated with respect to exons of the dystrophin gene. Each deletion is represented by a *horizontal line.* Also shown in *vertical shaded bars* are the locations of the nine exons that are amplified by the multiplex PCR. Each deletion that intersects these vertical bars was detected by the multiplex PCR assay. The numbers following a *horizontal line* indicate the number of times each deletion was observed. Two deletions *(arrowheads)* span the entire gene. (From Multicenter Study Group: Diagnosis of Duchenne and Becker muscular dystrophies by polymerase chain reaction. A multicenter study. JAMA 267:2609, 1992. Copyright 1992, American Medical Association.)

the following gene/disease associations are highly informative for understanding the "dystrophin complex," it should be remembered that they represent a minority of the "Duchenne" phenocopies. These additional genetic causes of myopathy are critical to remember in the absence of dystrophin mutation diagnosis.[41]

Merosin is a gene now associated with the autosomal recessively inherited congenital muscular dystrophy.[42] It is the gene defect associated with the Fukuyama syndrome, which mapped to 9q31-33 and was subsequently found to be merosin. In the Asian population, both skeletal muscle and central nervous system (brain structural) anomalies exist. The central nervous system findings are usually identified by white matter anomalies found by computed tomography or magnetic resonance imaging. In Western populations, the features are more specifically associated with the skeletal muscle. Merosin is found in basal laminae of situated muscle and Schwann cells. It binds to the 156-kD dystrophin-associated glycoprotein, alpha-dystroglycan, that is found extracellularly. Absence of merosin disrupts this transcellular link with resulting muscle cell degeneration.

Sarcoglycans (α, β, and γ) are three independently sarcolemma associated proteins that, when defective, lead to clinical myopathies. Campbell was first to report the complex of dystrophin-associated proteins that then became associated with heritable myopathies. The α-dystroglycan binds to the merosin protein discussed previously. The β-sarcoglycan is a transmembrane protein that binds to the carboxyl domain of dystrophin (intracellular).[43, 44] The α-dystroglycan maps to 17q12-q21.[45] It has been found in a French family with autosomal recessive disease and in late-onset limb girdle muscular dystrophy. These mutations are rare (<5 percent of "Duchenne" phenotypes). Rare Tunisian and Japanese patients have been identified as defective in γ-sarcoglycan that also resembles DMD clinically.[46]

The β-sarcoglycan that maps to 4q12 is defective in a group of limb girdle patients and rarely present among a group of patients (1 in 62), such as a female, who clinically presented as DMD. In this case, immunohistology was positive for dystrophin protein but negative for the sarcoglycan complex. Similar findings were observed in the Amish "Duchenne" cases.[47] Additional confirmation of β-sarcoglycan involvement in the complex comes from the study of cardiomyopathic hamsters. These studies led to Straub and Campbell[48] proposing the following structure for the dystrophin-glycoprotein complex (Fig. 117–3).[48]

Therapy for DMD remains difficult. One strategy has been therapy with anti-inflammatory agents, which has the effect of delaying progression of symptoms but has associated steroid side effects.[49, 50] Myoblast transplantation therapy has now been discontinued in clinical trials because of the lack of migration and the short-lived presence of the transplanted cells. Gene replacement therapy is currently the focus of intensive international effort. Minigene versions of the dystrophin gene have clearly corrected the mouse equivalent of DMD.[51, 52] Adenoviral vectors are a promising method for widespread gene delivery, although whether this strategy can affect progression of the disease remains to be seen.[52] A novel concept has been put forward by Davies.[53] She suggests that utrophin, a gene with some similar structural features of dystrophin, can substitute for dystrophin.[53] A strategy to up-regulate utrophin in DMD patients has been put forward and is being investigated at a research level.

Myotonic Dystrophy

MD is the most common adult-onset myopathy (affecting 1 in 5000) and is inherited as an autosomal dominant trait. Clinical manifestations are variable and include progressive muscle weakness, cardiomyopathy, delayed muscle relaxation, cataracts, frontal balding, diabetes mellitus, and male infertility. Remarkably, this disease has the feature of *anticipation*, which is a progressive increase in clinical severity and a decrease in age of onset in successive generations of an affected family. It is not uncommon in a family for an apparently asymptomatic mother to bear a child with severe congenital myopathy associated with profound hypotonia, mental retardation, and death in infancy.

These perplexing clinical features have been partially explained by discovery of the MD gene and the mechanism of mutation.[54–56] Based on our earlier discovery of the expanding triplet repeat mutation causing fragile X mental retardation that explained the anticipation observed in this disorder,[57, 58] we scanned the MD genomic region (determined by the Muscular Dystrophy Association consortium) for other triplet repeats. A triplet repeat in the 3 untranslated region of a protein kinase gene (myotonin protein kinase [DMPK]) identified both the disease gene and the disease-causing mutation (also triplet repeat expansion).[55] The changing character of the GCT triplet repeat in an affected family is shown in Figure 117–3. DMPK is found in many tissues but is expressed at high levels in muscle and brain, which are two of the tissues most associated with symptoms of the disease. It is also clear that a minimum of eight alternately spliced forms are known.[59] It is not yet known how DMPK affects the pathogenesis of MD.

Independent studies have indicated that triplet repeat expansion leads to decreased levels of steady state mRNA in many cell types.[60, 61] As expected, the level of DMPK protein is reduced in the same cells. We presume that the reduction of steady state mRNA is a defect in nuclear RNA processing. This may lead to nuclear trapping of mRNA, which would result in decreased levels of DMPK in the cytoplasm and increased levels in the nucleus. Such possibilities were under active investigation at the time of the previous edition's preparation.

Deduction of DMPK was thought to not fully account for the pleiotropic clinical features because DMPK knockout mice had only mild muscle abnormalities. True models of the disease (triplet repeat knock-ins) at the 3′μT have eluded investigators owing to extreme instability of the repeats and self-elimination by deletion. Success has been achieved using molecular and cell biologic approaches to elucidate the pathology of the CTG repeat expansion. We searched for and identified a CUG binding protein (CUGBP1) that had specificity for single-stranded RNA and sequence and, in binding, regulated the eTNT splicing.[62] Based on the in situ identification of nuclear localization of DMPK transcripts containing expanded CUG repeats, the CUGBP1 binding to these repeats and abnormal splicing of a muscle gene mRNAs, it has not been proposed

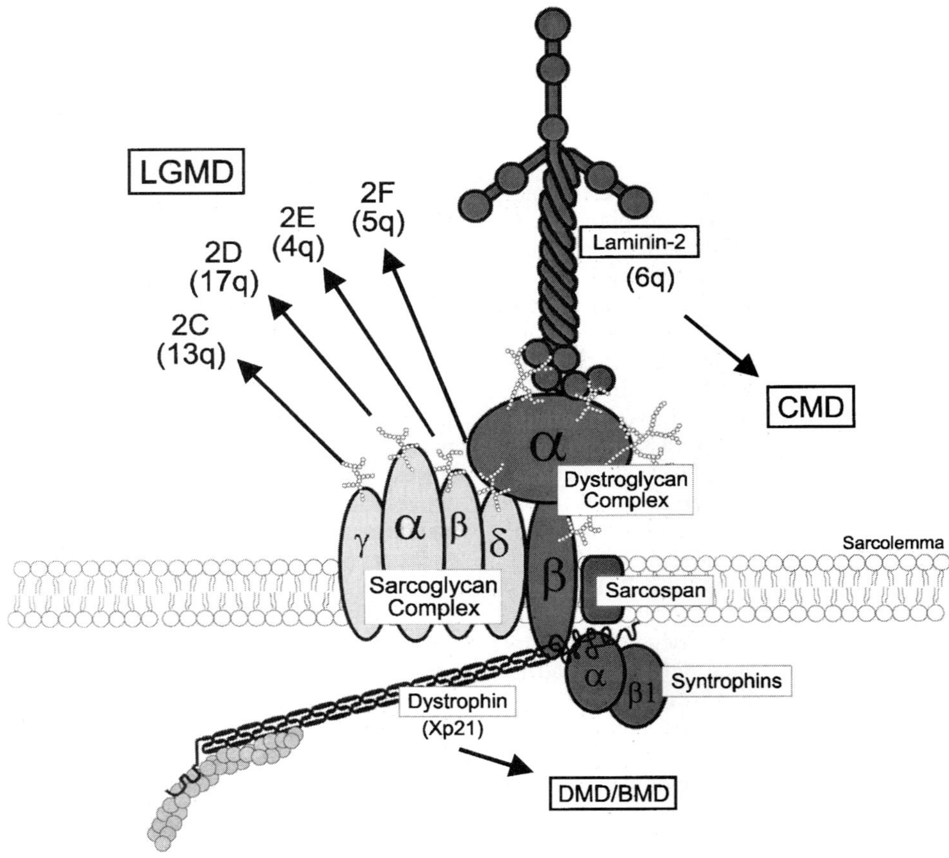

FIGURE 117–3 The composition of the dystrophin glycoprotein complex (DGC) in skeletal muscle. The DGC provides a linkage between the extracellular matrix and the cytoskeleton and is thought to protect the muscle fibers from contraction-induced damage. On the cytoskeletal side, dystrophin binds with its *N*-terminal portion to *F*-actin and with its *C*-terminal portion to β-dystroglycan. β-Dystroglycan in turn, binds α-dystroglycan, which binds to laminin-2 in the extracellular matrix. With the DGC, four single-pass transmembrane proteins called α-, β-, γ-, and δ-sarcoglycan together with sarcospan form a subcomplex at the sarcolemma.
Various forms of muscular dystrophies have been associated with genes encoding several proteins of the DGC. Mutations in the gene encoding for dystrophin cause Duchenne's or the milder form, Becker's muscular dystrophy. Mutations in any of the sarcoglycans cause different forms of autosomal recessive limb-girdle muscular dystrophy and mutations in the gene encoding laminin-2 has been found to be responsible for about 50% of the congenital muscular dystrophies. So far, no mutations in the dystroglycan and the sarcospan gene in humans has been associated with a disease.

that a plethora of cellular and patient abnormalities relates to abnormal splicing.[63] Both insulin and α-tropomyosin mRNA levels are reduced in MD.[64, 65]

It has been proposed that reduced DMPK could have an effect on proteins that undergo phosphorylation. Prime candidates in this consideration have been ion channels, given the frequent cardiac arrhythmias of MD.[66] It is established that DMPK can phosphorylate the beta-subunit of the voltage-dependent Ca^{2+} release channel. That DMPK knockout mice are altered in Ca^{2+} homeostasis supports the concept. Cell culture studies have furthermore shown a voltage-gated sodium channel to be altered by MD. Even more recently, MD regulation of a Cl^- channel has been documented and proposed to be defective in MD.[67] Focus on the phosphorylation of myosin light chain by DMPK has been proposed. Several Rho-binding kinases have homology to DMPK.[68] It has been suggested that the Rho family of small guanosine triphosphate–binding proteins inhibit myosin phosphatase activity and thus influence contractibility. Support for this model is derived from in vitro demonstration of myosin phosphatase by Rho-binding Sec-Thv kinase and genetic studies of *Caenorhabditis elegans* linking DMPK homologous proteins to skeletal muscle organization. It would be satisfying to associate one particular pathologic event to the triplet repeat (CTG) expansion in MD. This would appear unlikely, given our current knowledge that DMPK is involved in a signal transduction pathway via its phosphorylation and effect on other genes transcription by affecting RNA processing (Fig. 117–4).[69] Our studies of humans with the objective of therapy intervention will need to sort out the dominant pathologic target for drug development.

The mechanism of triplet repeat amplification is as yet unresolved. It is clear that both meiotic and mitotic amplification occur. Therefore, increases may be observed in an affected family from generation to generation, as well as within an affected individual at different times (Fig. 117–5). The impact of age-dependent mutation on disease phenotype is unclear.

Molecular studies in yeast of triplet expansion have

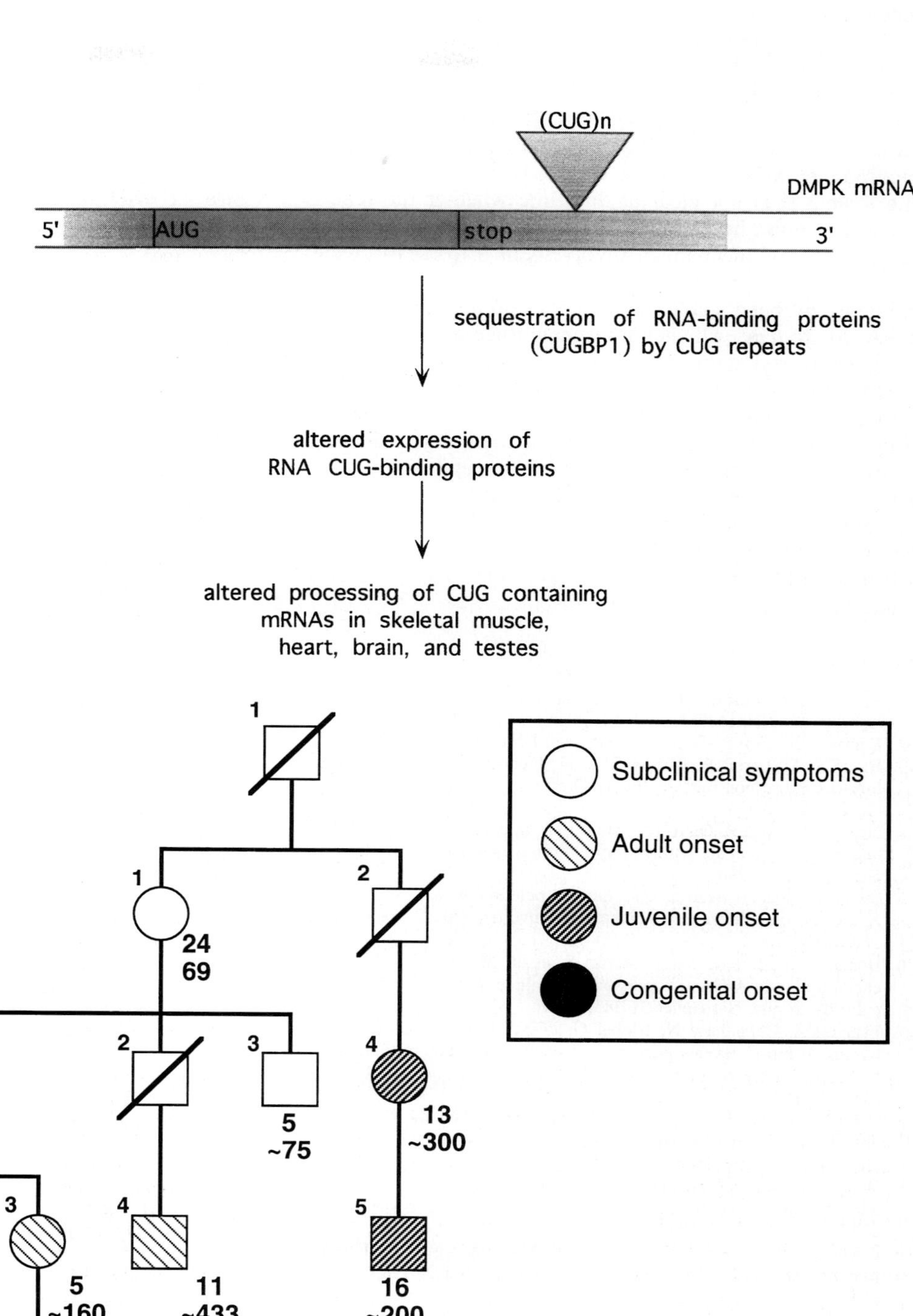

FIGURE 117–4 An RNA model for DM. CTG triplet repeat expansion in the *DMPK* gene is transcribed into CUG repeats in *DMPK* mRNA. CUG triplet repeats are potential binding sites for specific RNA-binding proteins. An increase in the number of RNA-binding sites in DM patients will affect specific RNA-binding proteins, such as CUGBP1. Alteration of the expression of RNA-binding proteins affects the RNA metabolism of several mRNAs and pre-mRNAs containing CUG repeats in the regulatory regions. In agreement with this suggestion, processing of some mRNAs containing CUG repeats in the regulatory regions, such as DMPK, cTnT, and C/EBPβ, are affected in DM patients. The RNA metabolism of other mRNAs in skeletal muscle, brain, heart, and testes could also be altered. Alteration of RNA metabolism in affected tissues might induce the development of clinical symptoms (e.g., myotonia, cardiac abnormalities, mental retardation).

FIGURE 117–5 A five-generation pedigree illustrates GCT triplet repeat expansion as the myotonic dystrophy mutation is passed to successive generations. The numbers below each individual indicate the size of the GCT repeat alleles, in numbers of repeats. The size of the normal allele is indicated above and that of the expanded allele below. The pedigree illustrates how repeat mutations may enlarge dramatically in one generation to cause congenital disease. (From Redman JB, Fenwick RG Jr, Fu YH, et al: Relationship between parental trinucleotide GCT repeat length and severity of myotonic dystrophy in offspring. JAMA 269:1960, 1993. Copyright 1993, American Medical Association.)

documented both deletions and expansions of CTG repeats. The different mutational events relate to the polarity of the repeat with regard to DNA replication. Loop structures can be formed by the single-stranded repeats.[69] If the opposite strand skips the loop, a truncation of the repeat occurs. This is readily shown in a variety of genetic systems. More difficult to show are expansions of the magnitude seen in humans. Presumably they relate to loop formations being incorporated as an expansion when pairing with the opposite strand. It is not clear at this time whether the repeat expansion must be in an expressed gene, reflecting transcription repair mechanism involvement. Efforts to create transgenic mice containing expanded repeats have disappointedly all been stable, thus there is no animal model of expansion to date. All such transgenic mice had the repeats in nonexpressed elements.

Diagnosis of MD is now simplified by DNA analysis of triplet repeat number at the gene locus. The analysis is simple and provides accurate diagnosis in clinically unclear cases, as well as providing options for prenatal diagnosis.[71] The latter application is particularly important because of the anticipation resulting from triplet repeat expansion. An apparently unaffected mother can bear a congenitally affected child with a remarkable amplified triplet repeat. There is no therapy for MD at present.

REFERENCES

1. Emery AEH, Dreifuss FE: Unusual type of benign X-linked muscular dystrophy. J Neurol Neurosurg Psychiatry 29:338, 1966.
2. Emery AEH: Emery-Dreifuss syndrome. J Med Genet 26:637, 1989.
3. Bione S, Maestrini E, Rivella S, et al: Identification of a novel X-linked gene responsible for Emery-Dreifuss muscular dystrophy. Nat Genet 8:323, 1994.
4. Nagano A, Koga R, Ogawa M, et al: Emerin deficiency at the nuclear membrane in patients with Emery-Dreifuss muscular dystrophy. Nat Genet 12:254, 1996.
5. Small K, Iber J, Warren ST: Emerin deletion reveals a common X-chromosome inversion mediated by inverted repeats. Nat Genet 16:96, 1997.
6. Bonne G, DiBarletta MR, Varnous S, et al: Mutations in the gene encoding lamin A/C cause autosomal dominant Emery-Dreifuss muscular dystrophy. Nat Genet 21:285, 1999.
7. Fisher DZ, Chaudhary N, Blobel G: cDNA sequencing of nuclear lamins A and C reveals primary and secondary structural homology to intermediate filament proteins. Proc Natl Acad Sci U S A 83:6450, 1986.
8. Frank S, Braunwald E: Idiopathic hypertrophic subaortic stenosis: clinical analysis of 126 patients with emphasis on the natural history. Circulation 37:759, 1968.
9. Wigle ED, Sasson Z, Henderson MA, et al: Hypertrophic cardiomyopathy: the importance of the site and the extent of hypertrophy. Prog Cardiovasc Dis 28:1, 1985.
10. Jarcho JA, McKenna W, Pare JAP, et al: Mapping a gene for familial hypertrophic cardiomyopathy to chromosome 14ql. N Engl J Med 321:1372, 1989.
11. Ambrosini M, Ferraro M, Reale A: Cytogenetic study in familial hypertrophic cardiomyopathy: identification of a new fragile site on human chromosome 16. Circulation 80 (suppl II): II-458, 1989.
12. Nishi H, Kimura A, Sasaki M, et al: Localization of the gene for hypertrophic cardiomyopathy on chromosome 18q. Circulation 80 (suppl II): II-457, 1989.
13. Tanigawa G, Jarcho JA, Kass S, et al: A molecular basis for familial hypertrophic cardiomyopathy: an alpha/beta cardiac myosin heavy chain hybrid gene. Cell 62:991, 1990.
14. Thierfelder L, Watkins H, MacRae C, et al: Tropomyosin and cardiac troponin T mutations cause familial hypertrophic cardiomyopathy: a disease of the sarcomere. Cell 77:701, 1994.
15. Towbin JA: Molecular genetic aspects of cardiomyopathy. Biochem Med Metab Biol 49:285, 1993.
16. Watkins H, Thierfelder L, Anan R, et al: Independent origin of identical beta cardiac myosin heavy-chain mutations in hypertrophic cardiomyopathy. Am J Hum Genet 53:1180, 1993.
17. Anan R, Greve G, Thierfelder L, et al: Prognostic implications of novel cardiac myosin heavy chain gene mutations that cause familial hypertrophic cardiomyopathy. J Clin Invest 93:280, 1994.
18. NIH/DOE Working Group on Ethical, Legal, and Social Implications of Human Genome Research: Genetic information and health insurance. Report of the Task Force on Genetic Information and Insurance.
19. Hu X, Ray PN, Murphy EG, et al: Duplicational mutation at the Duchenne muscular dystrophy locus: its frequency, distribution, origin, and phenotype/genotype correlation. Am J Hum Genet 46:682, 1990.
20. Clemens PR, Caskey CT: Duchenne muscular dystrophy. Curr Neurol 12:1, 1992.
21. Arahata K, Hoffman EP, Kunkel LM, et al: Dystrophin diagnosis: comparison of dystrophin abnormalities by immunofluorescence and immunoblot analyses. Proc Natl Acad Sci U S A 86:7154, 1989.
22. Hoffman EP, Fischbeck KH, Brown RH, et al: Characterization of dystrophin in muscle-biopsy specimens from patients with Duchenne's or Becker's muscular dystrophy. N Engl J Med 318:1363, 1988.
23. Nicholson LV, Johnson MA, Gardner-Medwin D, et al: Heterogeneity of dystrophin expression in patients with Duchenne and Becker muscular dystrophy. Acta Neuropathol (Berl) 80:239, 1990.
24. Bulman DE, Murphy EG, Zubrzycka-Gaarn EE, et al: Differentiation of Duchenne and Becker muscular dystrophy phenotypes with amino- and carboxy-terminal antisera specific for dystrophin. Am J Hum Genet 48:295, 1991.
25. Koenig M, Hoffman EP, Bertelson CJ, et al: Complete cloning of the Duchenne muscular dystrophy (DMD) cDNA and preliminary genomic organization of the DMD gene in normal and affected individuals. Cell 50:509, 1987.
26. Baumbach LL, Chamberlain JS, Ward PA, et al: Molecular and clinical correlations of deletions leading to Duchenne and Becker muscular dystrophies. Neurology 39:465, 1989.
27. Hu XY, Burghes AH, Bulman DE, et al: Evidence for mutation by unequal sister chromatid exchange in the Duchenne muscular dystrophy gene. Am J Hum Genet 44:855, 1989.
28. Chamberlain JS, Gibbs RA, Ranier JE, et al: Deletion screening of the Duchenne muscular dystrophy locus via multiplex DNA amplification. Nucleic Acids Res 16:11141, 1988.
29. Beggs AH, Koenig M, Boyce FM, Kunkel LM: Detection of 98% of DMD/BMD gene deletions by polymerase chain reaction. Hum Genet 86:45, 1990.
30. Voskova-Goldman A, Peier A, Caskey CT, et al: DMD specific fish probes diagnostically useful in the detection of female carriers of DMD gene deletions. Neurology 48:1633, 1997.
31. Ward PA, Hejtmancik JF, Witkowski JA, et al: Prenatal diagnosis of Duchenne muscular dystrophy: prospective linkage analysis and retrospective dystrophin cDNA analysis. Am J Hum Genet 44:270, 1989.
32. Feener CA, Boyce FM, Kunkel LM: Rapid detection of CA polymorphisms in cloned DNA: application to the 5 region of the dystrophin gene. Am J Hum Genet 48:621, 1991.
33. Oudet C, Heilig R, Mandel JL: An informative polymorphism detectable by polymerase chain reaction at the 3 end of the dystrophin gene. Hum Genet 84:283, 1990.
34. Beggs AH, Kunkel LM: A polymorphic CACA repeat in the 3 untranslated region of dystrophin. Nucleic Acids Res 18:1931, 1990.
35. Clemens PR, Fenwick RG, Chamberlain JS, et al: Carrier detection and prenatal diagnosis in Duchenne and Becker muscular dystrophy families, using dinucleotide repeat polymorphisms. Am J Hum Genet 49:951, 1991.
36. Multicenter Study Group: Diagnosis of Duchenne and Becker muscular dystrophies by polymerase chain reaction. A multicenter study. JAMA 267:2609, 1992.
37. Koenig M, Beggs AH, Moyer M, et al: The molecular basis for Duchenne versus Becker muscular dystrophy: correlation of severity with type of deletion. Am J Hum Genet 45:498, 1989.
38. Malhotra SB, Hart KA, Klamut HJ, et al: Frame-shift deletions in patients with Duchenne and Becker muscular dystrophy. Science 242:755, 1988.
39. Bakker E, Van Broeckhoven C, Bonten EJ, et al: Germline mosaicism and Duchenne muscular dystrophy mutations. Nature 329:554, 1987.
40. Worton R: Muscular dystrophies: diseases of the dystrophin-glycoprotein complex. Science 270:755, 1995.

41. Cox GF, Kunkel LM: Dystrophies and heart disease. Curr Opin Cardiol 12:329, 1997.
42. Sunada Y, Edgar TS, Lotz BP, et al: Merosin-negative congenital muscular dystrophy associated with extensive brain abnormalities. J Neurol 45:2084, 1995.
43. Lim LE, Duclos F, Broux O, et al: β-Sarcoglycan: characterization and role in limb-girdle muscular dystrophy linked to 4q12. Nat Genet 11:257, 1995.
44. Jung D, Yang B, Meyer J, et al: Identification and characterization of the dystrophin anchoring site on β-dystroglycan. J Biol Chem 270:27305, 1995.
45. Duclos F, Straub V, Moore SA, et al: Progressive muscular dystrophy in α-sarcoglycan–deficient mice. J Cell Biol 142:1461, 1998.
46. Noguchi S, McNally EM, Othmane KB, et al: Mutations in the dystrophin-associated protein γ-sarcoglycan in chromosome 13 muscular dystrophy. Science 270:819, 1995.
47. Duclos F, Broux O, Bourg N, et al: β-Sarcoglycan: genomic analysis and identification of a novel missense mutation in the LGMD2E Amish isolate. Neuromuscul Disord 8:30, 1998.
48. Straub V, Campbell KP: Muscular dystrophies and the dystrophin-glycoprotein complex. Curr Opin Neurol 10:168, 1997.
49. Mendell JR, Moxley RT, Griggs RC, et al: Randomized, double-blind six-month trial of prednisone in Duchenne's muscular dystrophy. N Engl J Med 320:1592, 1989.
50. Griggs RC, Moxley RT III, Mendell JR, et al, for the Clinical Investigation of Duchenne Dystrophy Group: Prednisone in Duchenne dystrophy: a randomized, controlled trial defining the time course and dose response. Arch Neurol 48:383, 1991.
51. Lee CC, Pons F, Jones PG, et al: *Mdx* transgenic mouse: restoration of recombinant dystrophin to the dystrophic muscle. Hum Gene Ther 4:273, 1993.
52. Ragot T, Vincent N, Chafey P, et al: Efficient adenovirus-mediated transfer of a human minidystrophin gene to skeletal muscle of *mdx* mice. Nature 361:647, 1993.
53. Tinsley JM, Potter AC, Phelps SR, et al: Amelioration of the dystrophic phenotype of *mdx* mice using a truncated utrophin transgene. Nature 384:349, 1996.
54. Brook JD, McCurrach ME, Harley HG, et al: Molecular basis of myotonic dystrophy: expansion of a trinucleotide (CTG) repeat at the 3 end of a transcript encoding a protein kinase family member. Cell 68:799, 1992.
55. Fu YH, Pizzuti A, Fenwick RG Jr, et al: An unstable triplet repeat in a gene related to myotonic muscular dystrophy. Science 255:1256, 1992.
56. Mahadevan M, Tsilfidis C, Sabourin L, et al: Myotonic dystrophy mutation: an unstable CTG repeat in the 3 untranslated region of the gene. Science 255:1253, 1992.
57. Verkerk AJMH, Pieretti M, Sutcliffe JS, et al: Identification of a gene *(FMR-1)* containing a CGG repeat coincident with a breakpoint cluster region exhibiting length variation in fragile X syndrome. Cell 65:905, 1991.
58. Fu YH, Kuhl DPA, Pizzuti A, et al: Variation of the CGG repeat at the fragile X site results in genetic instability: resolution of the Sherman paradox. Cell 67:1047, 1991.
59. Fu YH, Friedman DL, Richards S, et al: Decreased expression of myotonin-protein kinase messenger RNA and protein in adult form of myotonic dystrophy. Science 260:235, 1993.
60. Mahadevan MS, Amemiya C, Jansen G, et al: Structure and genomic sequence of the myotonic dystrophy (DM kinase) gene. Hum Mol Genet 2:299, 1993.
61. Jansen G, Mahadevan M, Amemiya C, et al: Characterization of the myotonic dystrophy region predicts multiple protein isoform-encoding mRNAs. Nat Genet 1:261, 1992.
62. Timchenko LT, Miller JW, Timchenko NA, et al: Identification of a (CUG)n triplet repeat RNA-binding protein and its expression in myotonic dystrophy. Nucleic Acids Res 24:4407, 1996.
63. Roberts R, Timchenko NA, Miller JW, et al: Altered phosphorylation and intracellular distribution of a (CUG)n in triplet repeat RNA-binding protein in patients with myotonic dystrophy and in myotonic protein kinase knockout mice. Proc Natl Acad Sci U S A 94:13221, 1997.
64. Morrone A, Pegoraro E, Angelinin C, et al: RNA metabolism in myotonic dystrophy: patient muscle shows decreased insulin receptor RNA and protein consistent with abnormal insulin resistance. J Clin Invest 99:1691, 1997.
65. Philips AV, Timchenko LT, Cooper TA: Disruption of splicing regulated by a CUG-binding protein in myotonic dystrophy. Science 280:737, 1998.
66. Timchenko LT, Nastainczyk W, Schneider T, et al: Full-length myotonin protein kinase (72 kDa) displays serine kinase activity. Proc Natl Acad Sci U S A 92:5366, 1995.
67. Benders AAGM, Groenen PJTA, Oerlemans FTJJ, et al: Myotonic dystrophy protein kinase is involved in the modulation of the Ca^{2+} homeostasis in skeletal muscle cells. J Clin Invest 100:1440, 1997.
68. Gong MC, Iizuka K, Nixon G, et al: Role of guanine nucleotide-binding proteins—*ras*-family or trimeric proteins or both—in Ca^{2+} sensitization of smooth muscle. Proc Natl Acad Sci U S A 93:1340, 1996.
69. Timchenko LT, Caskey CT: Triplet repeat disorders: discussion of molecular mechanisms. Cell Mol Life Sci 55:1432, 1999.
70. Schlessinger D, Mandel JL, Monaco AP, et al: Report of the Fourth International Workshop on Human X Chromosome Mapping, 1993. Cytogenet Cell Genet 64:148, 1993.
71. Redman JB, Fenwick RG Jr, Fu YH, et al: Relationship between parental trinucleotide GCT repeat length and severity of myotonic dystrophy in offspring. JAMA 269:1960, 1993.
72. Perryman MB, Yu Q, Marian AJ, et al: Expression of a missense mutation in the messenger RNA for myosin heavy chain in myocardial tissue in hypertrophic cardiomyopathy. J Clin Invest 90:271, 1992.

CHAPTER 118

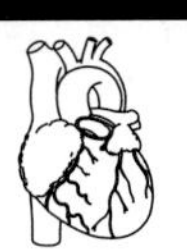

Genetic Aspects of Congenital Heart Disease

Dianna Milewicz

CONGENITAL HEART DISEASE ASSOCIATED WITH CHROMOSOMAL DISORDERS
Down's Syndrome (Trisomy 21)
Turner's Syndrome
DiGeorge's Syndrome, Velocardiofacial Syndrome, and Conotruncal Abnormalities
CONGENITAL HEART DEFECTS DUE TO SINGLE-GENE DEFECTS
Atrial Septal Defects
Holt-Oram Syndrome
Noonan's Syndrome
MULTIFACTORIAL INHERITANCE OF CONGENITAL HEART DISEASE

Congenital heart disease is estimated to affect 4 to 8 of every 1000 live births in the United States.[1] Studies since the early 1970s have focused on defining the genetic factors involved in congenital heart disease, in part to determine its cause and the chances of its recurrence within a family. The general categories of genetic causes involved in congenital heart disease are shown in Table 118–1. Chromosomal disorders are estimated to account for up to 10 percent of congenital heart disease in newborn infants, and this number may increase as new chromosomal disorders are recognized by means of newly developed technology. Single-gene disorders are estimated to account for 5 to 10 percent of congenital heart disease. This category is increasing as more disorders are recognized to follow mendelian patterns of inheritance. The great majority of patients with congenital heart disease are still best explained by multifactorial inheritance—that is, the additive effects of many genes and how they interact with environmental influences. Chapter 1, The History and Physical Examination, reviews the primary environmental and the teratogenic causes of congenital heart disease.

Assessment of a child with congenital heart disease should include a careful examination for associated defects. Extracardiac malformations occur in approximately 25 percent of live-born patients with congenital heart disease, many of whom have an identifiable syndrome.[2] A formal genetic evaluation is warranted, including a karyotype analysis, in patients with congenital heart disease and anomalies involving other systems or abnormal facial appearance (dysmorphic facies). In addition, a careful family history should be obtained to determine whether any other family members have congenital heart disease. Recurrence risks for congenital heart disease in a family are dependent on an initial determination of whether the defect is caused by a single-gene disorder. If the disorder is determined not to be a single-gene disorder, recurrence risks are dependent on the number of family members affected.

Congenital Heart Disease Associated With Chromosomal Disorders

Chromosomal disorders are now estimated to account for 8 to 10 percent of cases of congenital heart disease.[3] The most common chromosomal abnormalities with cardiovascular defects as a feature are shown in Table 118–2. Aneuploidy accounts for the majority of these chromosomal abnormalities. Chromosomal duplications or deletions are less common chromosomal causes of congenital heart disease. A new category of chromosomal anomaly has recently become relevant owing to improved techniques for identifying chromosomal deletions. Fluorescent in situ hybridization has opened the door to the identification of small chromosomal microdeletions that are associated with congenital heart disease (see later section).

Down's Syndrome (Trisomy 21)

Down's syndrome is the most common chromosomal disorder; it is estimated to occur in approximately 1 in 800 births. The risk for having a child with Down's syndrome is dependent on maternal age. The risk is lowest for young women and rises steeply for women over the age of 35 years. Women over the age of 45 years have a 4 percent risk of having a child with Down's syndrome. In the vast majority of Down's syndrome patients there is trisomy of chromosome 21, which results from meiotic nondisjunction

TABLE 118–1 General Categories of Genetic Etiologies of Congenital Heart Disease

Category	Percentage
Chromosomal anomalies	8–10
Single-gene defects	3–5
Multifactorial inheritance	85

TABLE 118-2 Cardiovascular Abnormalities Associated With Selected Chromosomal Abnormalities

Chromosomal Abnormality	Approximate Number of Patients With Cardiovascular Abnormalities (%)	Cardiovascular Abnormalities
Aneuploidy		
+21, Down's syndrome	40	Primarily endocardial cushion defects (60%) but also ASD, VSD, and tetralogy of Fallot
XO, Turner's syndrome	20–40	Coarctation of the aorta, AV stenosis, bicuspid AV, aortic dissection, aortic dilatation
+13, Patau's syndrome	85	VSD, PDA, ASD, dextroversion
+18, Edward's syndrome	>95	VSD and PDA most common; also coarctation of the aorta, ASD, endocardial cushion defect
XXXY	14	PDA, ASD
Deletions		
4p− Wolf-Hirschorn syndrome	40	VSD, ASD, PDA
5p− Cri du chat syndrome	25	VSD, PDA, ASD
13q−	50	VSD
18q−	50	VSD

Abbreviations: ASD, atrial septal defect; AV, aortic valve; PDA, patent ductus arteriosus; VSD, ventricular septal defect.

of the chromosome 21 pair. Approximately 3 percent of cases of Down's syndrome are caused by an extra copy of all or part of chromosome 21 attached to another chromosome (translocation). A very small minority of Down's syndrome cases are caused by mosaicism for trisomy 21, and the phenotype of these patients is usually less severe. Diagnosis is based on karyotype analysis, normally using lymphocytes from a blood sample.

Down's syndrome is usually diagnosed at birth or shortly thereafter based on the characteristic facial features of the syndrome. Other features include various degrees of mental retardation, growth retardation, hypotonia during infancy, and a variety of other anomalies. Congenital heart disease is present in approximately 40 percent of all live neonates with Down's syndrome.[4,5] The heart defects found in children with Down's syndrome include complete atrioventricular canal, ventricular septal defect, partial atrioventricular canal, atrial septal defect, tetralogy of Fallot, and patent ductus arteriosus.[4–7] Complete atrioventricular canal accounts for 60 percent of defects. All of these defects, except for tetralogy of Fallot, have the potential for increased pulmonary blood flow. Patients with Down's syndrome who have congenital heart disease are more predisposed to pulmonary artery hypertension and pulmonary vascular obstructive disease than are chromosomally normal children.[4,8] Therefore, it is advisable to evaluate the cardiac status in Down's syndrome patients at birth. Adults with Down's syndrome have a higher incidence of mitral valve prolapse and aortic regurgitation than do normal adults.[9]

Turner's Syndrome

Turner's syndrome is characterized by a female phenotype with gonadal dysgenesis and sexual immaturity. Affected females are short and have primary amenorrhea in addition to a variety of somatic abnormalities, including webbing of the neck, cubitus valgus, congenital lymphedema, and cardiovascular and renal abnormalities. The incidence of Turner's syndrome is estimated to be 1 in 5000 live female births. Approximately half of the cases of Turner's syndrome result from monosomy of the X chromosome (45,XO). Other cases involve mosaic karyotypes in which only a proportion of the cells are 45,XO and the others are either chromosomally normal or abnormal cells. Diagnosis is based on karyotype analysis, typically using lymphocytes harvested from peripheral blood samples. Barr body analysis on a buccal smear yields false negatives in a significant proportion of these patients and therefore should not be used to diagnose this syndrome.

Coarctation of the aorta is the most common cardiovascular anomaly in patients with Turner's syndrome. Other anomalies include bicuspid aortic valve and aortic valvular stenosis.[10,11] There is also an increased incidence of aortic dissection and dilatation of the ascending aorta in those with Turner's syndrome. These are confined primarily to patients with coarctation of the aorta, bicuspid aortic valve, and systemic hypertension, but they can also occur in the absence of these other defects.[10–14] Dilatation of the ascending aorta has been reported in up to 9 percent of patients with Turner's syndrome.[11] In patients with dissection, the aorta often exhibits pathologic evidence of cystic medial necrosis similar to that found in patients with Marfan's syndrome.

DiGeorge's Syndrome, Velocardiofacial Syndrome, and Conotruncal Abnormalities

DiGeorge's syndrome is a constellation of congenital malformations resulting from abnormalities in the development of the third and fourth brachial arches. The estimated incidence of the disorder is 1 in 20,000. Clinical complications associated with the syndrome include hypoplasia to aplasia of the thymus and parathyroid glands, facial dysmorphism, mental deficiency, and cardiovascular abnormalities.[15–17] The majority of patients with DiGeorge's syndrome come to a physician's attention initially because of cardiovascular abnormalities, typically conotruncal abnormalities that include tetralogy of Fallot, ventricular septal defect, truncus arteriosus, patent ductus ateriosus, and aortic arch anomalies. Most cases of DiGeorge's syndrome are sporadic, although familial cases have been documented.

Before the use of molecular techniques to identify chromosomal deletions, approximately 15 percent of cases of DiGeorge's syndrome were shown to have cytogenetic abnormalities, primarily deletions of 22q11.[18] Studies using fluorescent in situ hybridization have identified deletions in up to 90 percent of cases of DiGeorge's syndrome.[19, 20] The chromosomal deletion is believed to involve more than one gene and is therefore consistent with the classification of DiGeorge's syndrome as a contiguous-gene syndrome.

Velocardiofacial syndrome, or Shprintzen's syndrome, is characterized by overt or submucosal clefting of the palate, developmental delay, small stature, velopharyngeal insufficiency, dysmorphic facies, and congenital heart disease, primarily conotruncal abnormalities, along with a variety of other anomalies.[21] In the past, there was a consensus that DiGeorge's syndrome and velocardiofacial syndrome were etiologically and embryologically related. This was confirmed when it was determined that up to 80 percent of patients with velocardiofacial syndrome have deletions involving defects in the same region of 22q11 that is deleted in DiGeorge's syndrome patients.[19] This suggests that the two disorders represent a spectrum involving defects in the same gene or group of genes.

Some patients with isolated or familial conotruncal cardiac defects have been found to have deletions of 22q11. A study of families with recurrent conotruncal defects demonstrated deletions of 22q11 in five of nine families.[22] In every family, there was phenotypic variation of the cardiac defect; parents having the deletion tended to have milder defects than the children who inherited the deletion. In a study of isolated nonsyndromic conotruncal abnormalities, a significant proportion of patients were found to have 22q11 microdeletions.[23] Among heart defects, 22q11 deletions are found in 50 percent of patients with interruption of the aortic arch, in 30 percent with persistent truncus arteriosus, and in 15 percent with tetralogy of Fallot.[24, 25]

Molecular genetics studies have indicated that a region of 2.0 megabases in length is most commonly deleted in patients with DiGeorge's syndrome and it is termed the *DiGeorge critical region.* The genes have been identified in this region, and studies have implicated one of these genes as the cause of DiGeorge's syndrome.[26–28] A mouse model for DiGeorge's syndrome has been chromosomally engineered, and the mouse model has the same type of cardiovascular abnormalities that are found in patients with the disease.

In summary, deletions involving 22q11 are the causes of a significant number of conotruncal abnormalities associated with two syndromes, DiGeorge's syndrome and velocardiofacial syndrome. In addition, a significant number of isolated patients and families with conotruncal abnormalities have deletions involving the same region of 22q11.

CONGENITAL HEART DEFECTS DUE TO SINGLE-GENE DEFECTS

Single-gene defects caused by mutations in nuclear genes are estimated to be responsible for 3 to 5 percent of congenital heart defects. These single-gene disorders are typically part of a syndrome with multiple phenotypic features. It is important to recognize these mendelian disorders so that the recurrence risk for congenital heart disease can be accurately reported to the family. Table 118–3 is a list of autosomal dominant disorders with congenital heart disease as a major feature. Table 118–4 is a list of metabolic disorders with cardiovascular manifestations.

Atrial Septal Defects

Atrial septal defects (ASDs) can be inherited in an autosomal dominant manner as two separate disorders. The most common disorder is inheritance of ASDs of the secundum type in association with atrioventricular conduction de-

TABLE 118-3 **Mendelian Disorders With Congenital Heart Defects**

Disorder	Descriptive Name	Inheritance	Chromosomal Localization	Congenital Heart Defects
Alagille's syndrome	Arteriohepatic dysplasia	AD	20p11–12	PS
Apert's disease	Acrocephalosyndactyly type I	AD	Unknown	10% of patients PS, VSD, endocardial fibroelastosis
Atrial septal defect (secundum)		AD	8p21	ASD (secundum)
Atrial septal defect with atrioventricular conduction defect		AD	Unknown	ASD (secundum), atrioventricular conduction defect
Carpenter's syndrome	Acrocephalopolysyndactyly	AR	Unknown	PDA, VSD, PS, transposition
Ellis-van Creveld syndrome	Chondroectodermal dysplasia	AR	Unknown	ASD, common atrium
Geleophysic dysplasia		AR	Unknown	LVH, MR, MVP
Holt-Oram syndrome	Heart-hand syndrome	AD	12q2	ASD, VSD
Noonan's syndrome		AD	Unknown	PS, asymmetric septal hypertrophy, ASD, VSD
Shprintzen's syndrome	Velocardiofacial syndrome	AD	22q11	Conotruncal abnormalities
Smith-Lemli-Opitz syndrome		AR	Unknown	Malformations, various types

Abbreviations: AD, autosomal dominant; AR, autosomal recessive; ASD, atrial septal defect; LVH, left ventricular hypertrophy; MR, mitral regurgitation; MVP, mitral valve prolapse; PDA, patent ductus arteriosus; PS, pulmonary stenosis; VSD, ventricular septal defect.

lay.[30–32] The conduction delay rarely progresses to third-degree heart block. If a patient with an ASD is shown to have a prolonged PR interval, a complete family history and evaluation of relatives should be done to determine whether the ASD is due to this inherited disorder.

The second autosomal dominant disorder is the inheritance of an isolated secundum-type ASD.[33] This syndrome has been shown to be genetically heterogeneous with one disease gene mapping to chromosome 5p.[34] The condition is complicated by decreased penetrance and variable expressivity. Identification of ASD or other congenital heart defects in more than one family member should prompt clinical evaluation of all relatives.

Holt-Oram Syndrome

Holt-Oram syndrome is an autosomal dominant disorder characterized by anomalies of the upper limbs and heart. The typical combination is a triphalangeal thumb with a secundum ASD, but there is a great range in the severity of both the heart and the skeletal lesions. The upper limb abnormalities can be unilateral or bilateral and include triphalangeal thumb, foreshortened arms, and phocomelia. Cardiac defects can include single or multiple atrial and ventricular septal defects and disturbances of cardiac rhythm.[35–37] Studies have determined that Holt-Oram syndrome results from mutations in the *TBX5,* T-box gene located at 12q24.1.[38–40] T-box genes encode transcription factors that contain a highly conserved DNA binding motif (T-box). These proteins are believed to play a critical role in tissue specification, morphogenesis, and organogenesis.

Noonan's Syndrome

Noonan's syndrome is an autosomal dominant disorder that shares some phenotypic features with Turner's syndrome.[41, 42] These features include webbing of the neck, congenital lymphedema, short stature, cubitus valgus, and congenital heart disease (although the cardiac lesions are distinct from those seen in patients with Turner's syndrome). Features that are distinct for Noonan's syndrome include deformity of the sternum, mental retardation, hypertelorism, ptosis, cryptorchidism, and the fact that both males and females are affected. The phenotype of Noonan's syndrome is highly variable, and some affected individuals have no clinical problems.

The cardiac lesions associated with Noonan's syndrome vary widely. The most common cardiac abnormality is pulmonary stenosis, which occurs in 50 percent of cases.[18, 41] Asymmetric septal hypertrophy is observed in approximately 20 percent of patients; on histologic examination of the myocardium, it is found to be similar to the myocardial disarray seen with hypertrophic cardiomyopathy.[41, 43] ASDs and ventricular septal defects also occur in patients with Noonan's syndrome. The defective gene that causes Noonan's syndrome has been mapped to 12q22-qter region.[44]

Multifactorial Inheritance of Congenital Heart Disease

After primary genetic factors and chromosomal or single-gene defects have been eliminated as the cause, the majority of cases of congenital heart disease are best explained by multifactorial inheritance. Multifactorial inheritance presumes that a genetic predisposition interacts with an environmental trigger to produce the abnormality. The critical time when these genes are expressed and interact with environmental influences appears to be a narrow period of vulnerability at around 6 weeks of embryonic development.[45]

A number of studies have determined the empirical recurrence risk for families with congenital heart disease, and they are in accordance with the multifactorial model. For a family with one affected child, the empirical recurrence risk for having another child with congenital heart disease is between 1 and 3 percent. This risk increases if a second child has congenital heart disease. The combined data from a number of studies are reflected in Table 118–5.[1, 46]

The empirical recurrence risk for offspring of affected parents indicates a much higher incidence in these offspring.[47] Furthermore, the risk for transmitting a congenital heart defect appears to be two to five times greater if the affected parent is the mother.[48] Table 118–5 documents the suggested recurrence risk for congenital heart disease with either parent affected. The substantially higher risk for recurrence in mothers who are affected has raised the speculation that cytoplasmic inheritance, rather than multifactorial or mendelian modes of inheritance, should be considered in a subset of patients with congenital heart disease.[1, 45, 48]

The empirical risk factors calculated previously employ classification of congenital heart disease on the basis of specific anatomic lesion. More recently, congenital heart disease and recurrence risk have been approached from the viewpoint of disordered embryonic mechanisms. The pathogenic classification, originally proposed by Clark and subsequently modified,[49] includes mesenchymal tissue migration, errors or alterations in cardiac hemodynamics, cell death abnormalities, abnormalities in extracellular matrix, and aberrations in targeted growth.

Although specific cardiac defects are heterogeneous, they can be grouped on the basis of a shared pathogenic mechanism rather than specific anatomic features. Studies indicate that the familial recurrence rates may be greater for certain groups of cardiac defects when they are classified by the type of disordered mechanism.[50–52] In these studies, there is a marked increase in the frequency of congenital heart disease in relatives of probands with abnormal embryonic flow lesions, particularly left-heart blood-flow lesions (e.g., hypoplastic left heart, coarctation, bicuspid aortic valve, patent ductus arteriosus, and type II ventricular septal defect).

Although studies of large populations have defined the empirical risks for recurrence of congenital heart disease, little is known about the genes involved in cardiac develop-

TABLE 118–4 **Metabolic Disorders With Cardiovascular Manifestations**

Name of Disorder	Defective Gene	Prevalence	Inheritance	Chromosomal Localization	Pathology	Cardiovascular Manifestation
Mucopolysaccharidoses						
Hurler's syndrome (MPS IH)	α-L-Iduronidase		AR	4p16.3	Defective degradation of dermatan sulfate and heparin sulfate by lysosomes	HTN, valvular dysfunction, arterial disease
Scheie's syndrome (MPS IS)	α-L-Iduronidase		AR	4p16.3	Defective degradation of dermatan sulfate and heparin sulfate by lysosomes	AI
Hunter's syndrome (MPS II)	Sulfoiduranate sulfate		XLR	Xq26–28	Defective degradation of dermatan sulfate and heparin sulfate	HTN, valvular dysfunction, arterial disease
Morquio's syndrome (mucopolysaccharidosis II)	β-Galactosidase	1:300,000	AR	3p21	Defective degradation of keratan sulfate by lysosomes	Cardiac valvular lesions
Maroteaux-Lamy syndrome (MPS VI)	Aryl sulfatase B	Rare	AR	5q11–13	Defective degradation of dermatan sulfate by lysosomes	Calcified, stenotic aortic valve
Mucolipidoses						
I-cell disease (mucolipidosis II)	N-acetylglucosamine-1-phosphotransferase	Rare	AR	4q21–23	Lysosomal enzymes transport in cells is abnormal Leads to impaired lysosomal function	Cardiomegaly, valvular lesions
Pseudo-Hurler polydystrophy (mucolipidoses III)	N-acetylglucosamine-1-phosphotransferase	Rare	AR	4q21–23	Impaired lysosomal function	Valvular lesions
Sphingolipidoses						
Gaucher's disease type I	Glucocerebrosidase	Rare	AR	1q21	Accumulation of glycosylceramide in lysosomes leads to tissue injury	Pericardial disease
Fabry's disease	α-Galactosidase	1:40,000	X-LD	Xq21–22	Intracellular deposition of glycosphingolipids in lysosomes LV	Valvular dysfunction including MVP, MI, hypertrophy, ECG changes, cerebrovascular involvement, angiokeratoma
Glycogen Storage Diseases						
Type II glycogenosis (Pompe's disease)	Lysosomal acid α-glucosidase	1:175,000	AR	17q23	Intracellular accumulation of glycogen	Cardiomegaly, CHF
Type III glycogenosis	Amylo-1,6-glucosidase	1:125,000	AR	Unknown	Intracellular accumulation of glycogen with shorter outer chains	CHF, sudden death
Acyl-CoA Dehydrogenase Deficiencies						
LCAD deficiency	Long-chain acyl-CoA dehydrogenase	Rare	AR		Impaired oxidation of long-chain fatty acids	Hypertrophic cardiomyopathy, sudden death

Primary Hyperoxaluria						
Primary hyperoxaluria I	Alumine: glyoxylate amino transferase		AR	Unknown	Deposition of calcium oxalate crystals (oxalosis)	Complete atrioventricular block
Primary hyperoxaluria II	D-Glyceric acid dehydrogenase	Rare	AR	Unknown	Deposition of calcium oxalate crystals (oxalosis)	Complete atrioventricular block
Abnormalities of Storage of Sterols Other Than Cholesterol						
Cerebrotendinous xanthomatosis	Hepatic mitochondrial 26-hydroxylase	Rare	AR	Unknown	Block in bile acid synthesis leads to accumulation of cholestanol and cholesterol in tissues	Premature atherosclerosis
Phytosterolemia	Unknown	Rare	AR	—	Increased amounts of phytosterols (plant sterols) in plasma and tissues	Premature atherosclerosis
Disorders of Copper Transport						
Wilson's disease	WD gene	1:50,000	AR	13q14	Failure to incorporate copper into ceruloplasmin and failure to excrete copper into bile leads to toxic accumulation of copper in tissues	Cardiomyopathy
Menkes' disease	MNK gene (copper transporting ATPase enzyme)	1:100,000	XLR	Xp13	Defective intracellular transport leads to deficiency of copper-containing enzymes	Arterial rupture and thrombosis
Homocystinuria	Cystathionine β-synthase*	1:335,000	AR	21q22.3	Accumulation of homocysteine and methionine in plasma	Thromboembolism affecting large and small arteries and veins
Triose-phosphate isomerase deficiency	Triose-phosphate isomerase	Rare	AR	12p13	Deficiency of triose-phosphate isomerase in all tissues	Sudden cardiac death secondary to arrhythmia
Antithrombin deficiency	Antithrombin	1:5000	AD	1q23–25	Lack of inhibition of activated coagulation of the intrinsic system	Deep venous thrombosis, pulmonary embolism
Hereditary orotic aciduria	Uridine-5′-monophosphate synthase	Rare	AR	3q13	Block in UMP biosynthesis	Congenital heart disease
Hemochromatosis	Unknown	1:200–500 (European)	AR	6p21.3	Excessive absorption of iron leads to iron accumulation in tissues	Congestive cardiomyopathy, arrhythmias
Amyloidosis	Prealbumin	1:100,000–million	AD	18q11–12	Extracellular accumulation of plasma prealbumin (transthyretin) as amyloid	Cardiomyopathy, cardiac conduction defects
Zellweger's syndrome	Unknown	Rare	AR	Unknown	Peroxisomes absent or reduced in number leads to defective oxidation and abnormal accumulation of very long chain fatty acids	Patent ductus arteriosus, septal defects
Refsum's disease	Phytanic acid α hydroxylase	Rare	AR	Unknown	Accumulation of phytanic acid in blood and tissues	Nonspecific ECG abnormalities

Abbreviations: AD, autosomal dominant; AI, aortic insufficiency; AR, autosomal recessive; CHF, congestive heart failure; ECG, electrocardiogram; HTN, hypertension; MI, myocardial infarction; MPS, mucopolysaccharidoses; MVP, mitral valve prolapse; UMP, uridine monophosphate; XLR, X-linked recessive.
*Most frequent cause of disorder.

TABLE 118-5 Suggested Recurrence Risks for Congenital Heart Defects Based on the Number of Siblings Affected or the Parent Affected

Defect	Recurrence Risk for Subsequent Children If		Recurrence Risk for Children If	
	One Sibling Affected (%)	*Two Siblings Affected (%)*	*Mother Affected (%)*	*Father Affected (%)*
Ventricular septal defect	3	10	9.5	2.5
Patent ductus	3	10	4	2
Atrial septal defect	2.5	8	6	1.5
Tetralogy of Fallot	2.5	8	2.5	1.5
Pulmonary stenosis	2	6	6.5	2
Coarctation of aorta	2	6	4	2.5
Aortic stenosis	2	6	18	5
Transposition	1.5	5	—	—
Endocardial cushion	2.5	10	14	1
Hypoplastic left heart	3	10	—	—

Adapted from Nora JJ, Berg K, Nora AH: Congenital heart disease: genetics, pp. 53–80. *In* Cardiovascular Diseases, Genetics, Epidemiology and Prevention. New York: Oxford University Press, 1991.

ment that are disrupted to produce cardiac defects. As the defective genes causing single-gene disorders with cardiac malformations are identified, their roles in multifactorial inheritance of congenital heart disease will be able to be determined.

REFERENCES

1. Nora JJ, Nora AH: Cardiovascular Disease: Genetics, Epidemiology and Prevention. pp. 53–80. New York: Oxford University Press, 1991.
2. Greenwood RD, Rosenthal A, Parisi L, et al: Extracardiac abnormalities in infants with congenital heart disease. Pediatrics 55:485, 1997.
3. Nora JJ, Berg A, Nora A: Congenital Heart Disease: Genetics. pp. 53–80. New York: Oxford University Press, 1999.
4. Clark EB: Congenital cardiovascular defects in infants with Down syndrome. Pediatr Rev 11:99–100, 1989.
5. Bhatia S, Verma IC, Shrivastava S: Congenital heart disease in Down syndrome: an echocardiographic study. Indian Pediatr 29:1113–1116, 1992.
6. Ferencz C, Neill CA, Boughman JA, et al: Congenital cardiovascular malformations associated with chromosome abnormalities: an epidemiologic study. J Pediatr 114:79–86, 1989.
7. Khoury MJ, Erickson JD: Improved ascertainment of cardiovascular malformations in infants with Down's syndrome, Atlanta, 1968 through 1989. Am J Epidemiol 136:1457–1464, 1992.
8. Clapp S, Perry BL, Farooki ZA, et al: Down's syndrome, complete atrioventricular canal, and pulmonary vascular obstructive disease [abstract]. J Thorac Cardiovasc Surg 100:115–121, 1990.
9. Goldhaber SZ, Rubin IL, Brown W, et al: Valvular heart disease (aortic regurgitation and mitral valve prolapse) among institutionalized adults with Down's syndrome. Am J Cardiol 57:278–281, 1986.
10. Miller MJ, Geffner ME, Lippe BM, et al: Echocardiography reveals a high incidence of bicuspid aortic valve in Turner syndrome [abstract]. J Pediatr 102:47–50, 1983.
11. Subramaniam PN: Case report: Turner's syndrome and cardiovascular anomalies: a case report and review of the literature. Am J Med Sci 297:260–262, 1989.
12. Rubin K: Aortic dissection and rupture in Turner syndrome [letter]. J Pediatr 122:670, 1993.
13. Lie JT: Aortic dissection in Turner's syndrome. Am Heart J 103:1077–1080, 1982.
14. Lin AE, Lippe BM, Geffner ME, et al: Aortic dilation, dissection, and rupture in patients with Turner syndrome [abstract]. J Pediatr 109:820–826, 1986.
15. Wilson DI, Burn J, Scambler P, Goodship J: DiGeorge syndrome: part of CATCH 22. J Med Genet 30:852–856, 1993.
16. Conley ME, Beckwith JB, Mancer JFK, Tenckhoff L: The spectrum of the DiGeorge syndrome. J Pediatr 94:883–890, 1979.
17. Greenberg F: DiGeorge syndrome: an historical review of clinical and cytogenetic features. J Med Genet 30:803–806, 1993.
18. Greenberg F, Elder FFB, Haffner P, et al: Cytogenetic findings in a prospective series of patients with DiGeorge anomaly. Am J Hum Genet 43:605–611, 1988.
19. Driscoll DA, Salvin J, Sellinger B, et al: Prevalence of 22q11 microdeletions in DiGeorge and velocardiofacial syndromes: implications for genetic counselling and prenatal diagnosis. J Med Genet 30:813–817, 1993.
20. Carey AH, Kelly D, Halford S, et al: Molecular genetic study of the frequency of monosomy 22q11 in DiGeorge syndrome. Am J Hum Genet 51:964–970, 1992.
21. Lipson AH, Yuille D, Angel M, et al: Velocardiofacial (Shprintzen) syndrome: an important syndrome for the dysmorphologist to recognise. J Med Genet 28:596–604, 1991.
22. Wilson DI, Goodship JA, Burn J, et al: Deletions within chromosome 22q11 in familial congenital heart disease. Lancet 340:573–575, 1992.
23. Goldmuntz E, Driscoll D, Budarf ML, et al: Microdeletions of chromosomal region 22q11 in patients with congenital conotruncal cardiac defects [abstract]. J Med Genet 30:807–812, 1993.
24. Goldmuntz E, Clark B, Mitchell L, et al: Frequency of 22q11 deletions in patients with conotruncal defects. J Am Coll Cardiol 32:492–498, 1998.
25. Lewin M, Lindsay E, Jurecic V, et al: A genetic etiology for interruption of the aortic arch type B. Am J Cardiol 80:493–497, 1997.
26. Yamagishi H, Garg V, Matsuoka R, et al: A molecular pathway revealing a genetic basis for human cardiac and craniofacial defects. Science 283:1158–1160, 1999.
27. Novelli G, Amati F, Dallapiccola B: UFD1L and CDC45L: a role in DiGeorge syndrome and related phenotypes? Trends Genet 15:251–253, 1999.
28. Waley R, McKie J, Papapetrou C, et al: Mutations of UFD1L are not responsible for the majority of cases of DiGeorge syndrome/velocardiofacial syndrome without deletion within chromosome 22q11. Am J Hum Genet 65:247–249, 1999.
29. Lindsey E, Botta A, Jurecic V, et al: Congenital heart disease in mice deficient for the DiGeorge syndrome region. Nature 401:379–383, 1999.
30. Bosi G, Sensi A, Calzolari E, Scorrano M: Familial atrial septal defect with prolonged atrioventricular conduction. Am J Med Genet 43:641, 1992.
31. Bizarro RO, Callahan JA, Feldt RH, et al: Familial atrial septal defect with prolonged atrioventricular conduction: a syndrome showing the autosomal dominant pattern of inheritance. Circulation 41:677–683, 1970.
32. Bjornstad G: Secundum type atrial septal defect with prolonged PR interval and autosomal dominant mode of inheritance. Br Heart J 36:1149–1154, 1974.
33. Volti SL, Distefano G, Garozzo R, et al: Autosomal dominant atrial septal defect of ostium secundum type. Ann Genet 34:14–18, 1991.

34. Benson D, Sharkey A, Fatkin D, et al: Reduced penetrance, variable expressivity, and genetic heterogeneity of familial atrial septal defects. Circulation 97:2043–2048, 1998.
35. Basson CT, Cowley GS, Solomon SD, et al: The clinical and genetic spectrum of the Holt-Oram syndrome (heart-hand syndrome). N Engl J Med 330:885–891, 1994.
36. Hurst JA, Hall CM, Baraitser M: The Holt-Oram syndrome. J Med Genet 28:406–410, 1991.
37. Smith AT, Sack GH, Taylor GJ: Holt-Oram syndrome. J Pediatr 95:538–543, 1979.
38. Li Q, Newbury-Ecob R, Terrett J, et al: Holt-Oram syndrome is caused by mutations in *TBX5,* a member of the Brachyury 9T gene family. Nat Genet 1:21–29, 1997.
39. Basson C, Bachinsky D, Lin R, et al: Mutations in human *TBX5* [corrected] cause limb and cardiac malformation in Holt-Oram syndrome. Nat Genet 15:30–35, 1997.
40. Basson C, Huang T, Lin R, et al: Different *TBX5* interactions in heart and limb defined by Holt-Oram syndrome mutations. Genetics 96:2919–2924, 1999.
41. Sharland M, Burch M, McKenna WM, Paton MA: A clinical study of Noonan syndrome. Arch Dis Child 67:178–183, 1992.
42. Sanchez-Cascos A: The Noonan syndrome. Eur Heart J 4:223–229, 1983.
43. Burch M, Mann JM, Sharland M, et al: Myocardial disarray in Noonan syndrome. Br Heart J 68:586–588, 1992.
44. Jamieson C, van der Burgt L, van Reen M, et al: Mapping a gene for Noonan syndrome to the long arm of chromosome 12. Nat Genet 8:357–360, 1994.
45. Nora JJ: Causes of congenital heart diseases: old and new modes, mechanisms, and models. Am Heart J 125:1409–1419, 1993.
46. Nora JJ, Nora AH: Update on counseling the family with a first-degree relative with a congenital heart defect. Am J Med Genet 29:137–142, 1988.
47. Rose V, Gold RJM, Lindsay G, Allen M: A possible increase in the incidence of congenital heart defects among the offspring of affected parents. J Am Coll Cardiol 6:376–382, 1985.
48. Nora JJ, Nora AH: Maternal transmission of congenital heart diseases: new recurrence risk figures and the questions of cytoplasmic inheritance and vulnerability to teratogens. Am J Cardiol 59:459–463, 1987.
49. Clark EB: Mechanisms in the Pathogenesis of Congenital Heart Defects. pp. 3–11. Boston: Martinus-Nijhoff, 1986.
50. Lin AE, Garver KL: Genetic counseling for congenital heart defects. J Pediatr 113:1105–1109, 1988.
51. Ferencz C, Boughman JA, Neill CA, et al: Congenital cardiovascular malformations: questions on inheritance. J Am Coll Cardiol 14:756–763, 1989.
52. Boughman JA, Berg KA, Astemborski JA, et al: Familial risks of congenital heart defect assessed in a population-based epidemiologic study. Am J Med Genet 26:839–849, 1987.

SECTION XIII

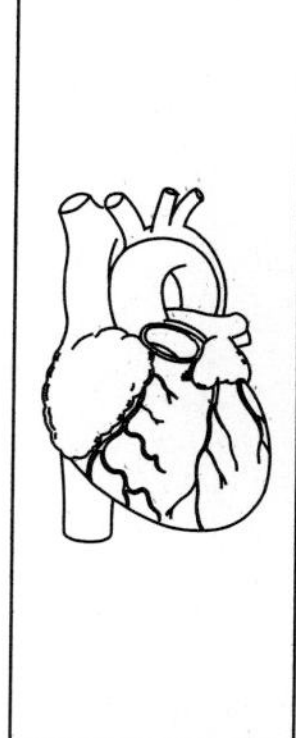

NEWER IMAGING MODALITIES

Rapid-Speed Computed Tomography

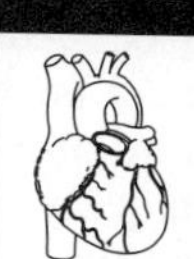

CHAPTER 119

Rapid-Speed Computed Tomography

Matthew J. Budoff and Bruce H. Brundage

TECHNOLOGY AND METHODS
CORONARY ARTERY DISEASE
PERICARDIAL DISEASE
PRIMARY MYOCARDIAL DISEASE
VALVULAR HEART DISEASE
CONGENITAL HEART DISEASE
DISEASE OF THE GREAT VESSELS
CARDIAC TUMORS
CONCLUSION

Ultrafast computed tomography (CT), which is also known as electron beam computed tomography (EBCT), is the least understood of all the cardiovascular imaging techniques. Although the technology has been clinically available since the late 1980s, cardiologists and even radiologists are largely unaware of its capabilities.[1] This chapter reviews the clinical uses of this method and describes some of the potential for even greater use in the near future.

Technology and Methods

The EBCT scanner uses advanced electron beam technology to achieve scan times of 50 milliseconds. Conventional CT scanners, including spiral scanners, rotate the x-ray tube around the patient. They can provide scan times as brief as 300 milliseconds but are still too slow to produce motion artifact–free images of the beating heart.[2] With the EBCT scanner, the patient is positioned inside the x-ray tube, obviating the need to move any part of the scanner during image acquisition. The electron beam is emitted from the cathode, which is several feet superior to the patient's head, and then passes through a magnetic coil, which bends the beam so that it will strike one of four tungsten anode targets. The magnetic coil also steers the beam through an arc of 210 degrees. The x-rays are generated when the electron stream strikes the tungsten anode target and then passes through the patient in a fan-shaped beam and strikes the detector array positioned opposite the anodes. The x-ray attenuation is measured and digitized for standard tomographic reconstruction.

Three imaging protocols are used with the EBCT scanner. They provide the format to evaluate *anatomy, cardiovascular function,* and *blood flow.* The imaging protocol used to study cardiovascular anatomy is called the *volume scanning mode,* and it is similar to scanning protocols used with conventional CT scanners. Single scans are obtained, and then the scanner couch is incremented a preset distance. For noncontrast studies, the table increment is usually the width of the scan slice, so there is no overlap imaging of anatomy. For contrast studies, especially those to be reconstructed three-dimensionally, the table incremention is usually less than the slice width, providing an overlap of information to improve spatial resolution. This scanning mode is used both with and without contrast enhancement and provides high spatial resolution of cardiovascular anatomy. This technique is ideal for an evaluation of the aorta, coronary arteries, and congenital heart disease (see Figs. 119–1, 119–10, and 119–12). Three-dimensional reconstruction can be performed with these volume images. A three-dimensional arteriogram reconstructed from tomographic images has the potential for more complete visualization of the coronary arteries (see Figs. 119–2, 119–3, 119–4, and 119–5).

The *cine scanning protocol* acquires images in 50 milliseconds. Each scan is separated by an 8-millisecond delay, which translates to a scanning rate of 17 scans per second. The scanning period is predetermined by the heart rate. Scans are acquired for the duration of the cardiac cycle. Depending on the heart rate, up to 12 cm of the heart can be imaged in a single scanning period. The acquired images are displayed in a cine loop, making assessment of cardiac and valve motion possible. Blood pool contrast enhancement is achieved by injection of contrast medium boluses via a superficial peripheral vein. The bolus amount for each image acquisition period averages 30 ml.

The *flow mode imaging protocol* acquires a single image gated to the electrocardiogram at a predetermined point in the cardiac cycle (e.g., end diastole [peak of the R wave]). Images can be obtained for every cardiac cycle or multiples thereof. Scanning is initiated before the arrival of a contrast bolus at an area of interest (e.g., left ventricular [LV] myocardium) and is continued until the contrast material has washed in and out of the area. Time-density curves from the region of interest can be created for a quantitative analysis of flow.

Coronary Artery Disease

The association between coronary artery disease (CAD) and coronary calcium (CC) has been known for many years.[3] Comparative anatomic studies have shown that the presence of CC is always indicative of coronary atherosclerosis.[4] Autopsy studies that involved more than 2500 cadaver hearts have demonstrated that the amount of calcium is related to the amount of plaque present.[5–7] EBCT uniquely combines the characteristics of speed and excellent density resolution that have led to a rebirth of interest in the detection of CC as a means of screening asymptomatic populations for coronary atherosclerosis. EBCT can detect very small amounts of CC because of the high temporal resolution that eliminates motion artifact, and CT technology in general is very sensitive in the detection of high-density materials (Fig. 119–1). Moreover, scanning for CC does not require an injection of contrast medium; therefore, a CT technician can perform the study without supervision. The entire procedure takes less than 10 minutes to perform. These features make EBCT an ideal screening test. EBCT studies have demonstrated a linear relationship between coronary calcification and atherosclerotic plaque burden.[8, 9] The ability of EBCT to noninvasively detect and quantify CC has been validated in numerous studies.[10, 11] There is a direct relationship between coronary artery calcium as measured by EBCT and histologic[12, 13] and in vivo intravascular ultrasound[14] measures of atheromatous plaque. Both anatomic and clinical angiographic studies have shown a strong positive correlation between CC and hemodynamically significant stenoses.[15]

Most centers use a calcium score measurement (Agatston method)[10] that takes into account the density and area of the calcification. The score is calculated by multiplying the lesion area by a density factor derived from the maximal Hounsfield unit (HU) within this area. The density factor was assigned in the following manner: 1 for lesions with a maximal density of 130 to 199 HU, 2 for lesions of 200 to 299 HU, 3 for lesions of 300 to 399 HU, and 4 for lesions of more than 400 HU. A total calcium score was determined by summing individual lesion scores from each

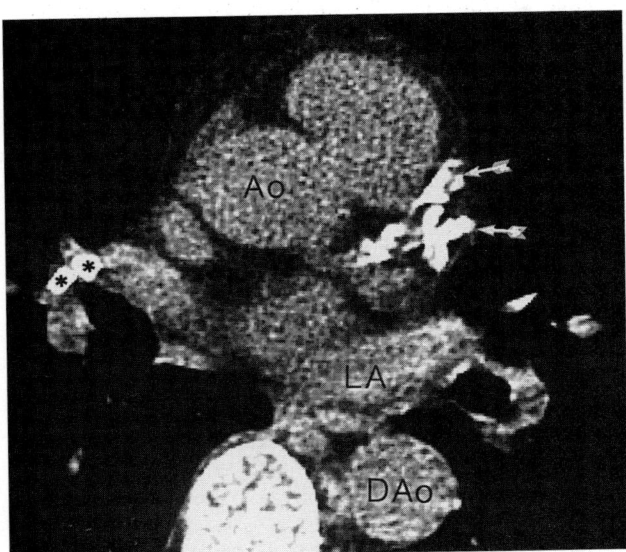

FIGURE 119–1 Calcium in the left anterior descending coronary artery and diagonal branch *(arrows)* is easily identified by ultrafast computed tomography (CT) without contrast enhancement. Ao, aorta; *asterisks,* calcified hilar lymph nodes; DAo, descending aorta; LA, left atrium; PA, pulmonary artery; S, superior vena cava.

of four anatomic sites (left main, left anterior descending, circumflex, and right coronary arteries). Calcium scores have been demonstrated to be more powerful predictors of angiographic stenosis than traditional risk factors[16] or stress testing.[17] Guerci and associates[18] demonstrated a strong correlation between the calcium score and maximum percent luminal coronary stenoses in a small group of asymptomatic patients undergoing diagnostic coronary angiography. Rumberger and colleagues[19] performed an analysis on studies of symptomatic patients and demonstrated that higher calcium scores predict greater degrees of angiographic stenosis. The most powerful and important data for this modality relate to its ability to predict future coronary events in both symptomatic and asymptomatic persons. Detrano and associates[20] examined the prognostic value of EBCT calcium scores for predicting cardiovascular events in 491 patients undergoing cardiac angiography and found a 6-fold event rate increase in patients with calcium scores of higher than 75. Logistic regression that included gender, age, calcium score, and angiographically diseased vessels showed that only EBCT calcium score predicted events. A 19-month follow-up of 1289 asymptomatic patients found a 6.9-fold increase of "hard events" (myocardial infarction and cardiac death) in patients with calcium scores of higher than 50 compared with those with negative or lower scores.[21] Other studies[22, 23] demonstrated odds ratios between 20 and 35.4 for coronary events using various EBCT calcium score thresholds. In one study, patients were 35 times more likely to have a coronary event if the EBCT calcium score was higher than 160. In this study, EBCT was 2- to 8-fold more powerful in predicting cardiac events than were traditional risk factors. Kennedy and colleagues[24] reported that EBCT-detected CC was a stronger predictor of CAD and future events than a sum of all of the traditional risk factors combined. These studies demonstrate that EBCT-detected CC is a very powerful predictor of future events that is unmatched by other screening tests or traditional risk factors.

In the high-resolution volume mode with three-dimensional reconstruction capabilities, EBCT is an emerging technology with the potential to obtain essentially noninvasive coronary angiograms. Because of its unique combination of high spatial and temporal resolution and because image acquisition can be triggered to the electrocardiogram, EBCT is well suited for imaging of the coronary arteries. This modality has been used to visualize native coronary arteries (Fig. 119–2) and bypass grafts (Figs. 119–3 and 119–4). The use of this technique can visualize all bypass grafts (including the left internal mammary artery) with a single contrast injection in a single breathhold. Sensitivities and specificities of up to 98 percent have been reported in comparisons of EBCT images with coronary angiograms.[25] Moshage and associates[26] reported on 27 patients undergoing conventional coronary angiography and EBCT angiography and demonstrated a sensitivity of 88 percent and a specificity of 100 percent for obstructive disease. In reported studies, EBCT angiography provides technically adequate images for evaluation in about 80 to 90 percent of coronary vessels investigated. A study of 28 patients undergoing EBCT and coronary angiography reported an overall accuracy of 90 percent.[27] Achenbach and colleagues[28] reported on 125 cases, with sensitivities

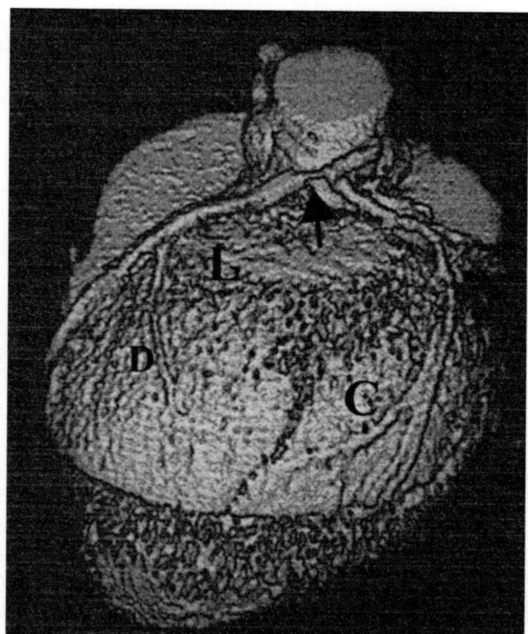

FIGURE 119–2 Three-dimensional reconstruction of a contrast-enhanced electron beam CT study. The left anterior descending coronary artery (L) is seen with a stenosis in the proximal portion *(arrow)*. Multiple diagonal branches (D) are also present. The circumflex and obtuse marginal system (C) is also seen, without stenosis.

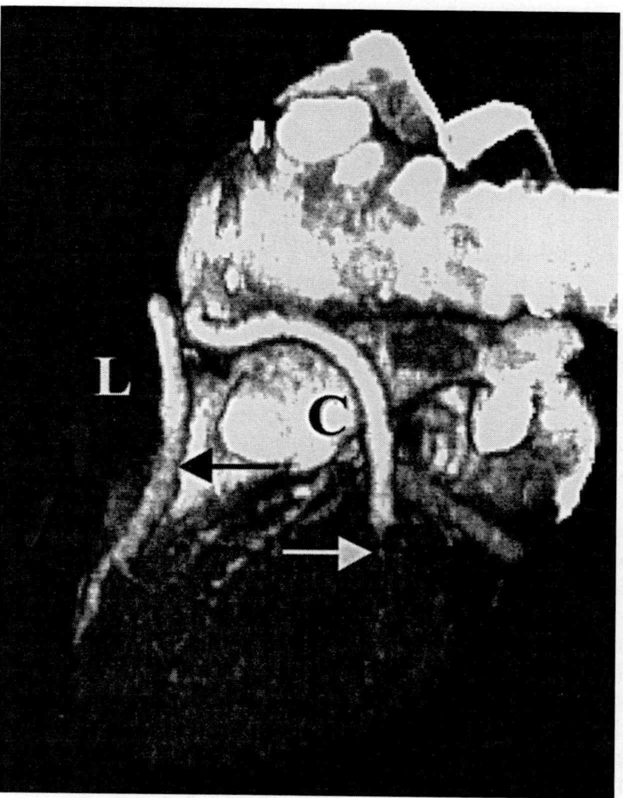

FIGURE 119–4 Three-dimensional reconstruction of two saphenous vein bypass grafts. The graft to the left anterior descending coronary artery (L) has a stenotic midportion *(black arrow)*. The graft to the circumflex distribution (C) reveals a very small obtuse marginal distal to the anastomosis *(white arrow)*.

of 92 percent and specificities of 94 percent. Budoff and associates[29] reported on 52 cases, with an overall accuracy of 87 percent and best visualization of the left main and left anterior descending coronary arteries. With further improvements, EBCT could greatly reduce the cost, complications, and death associated with conventional coronary arteriography.

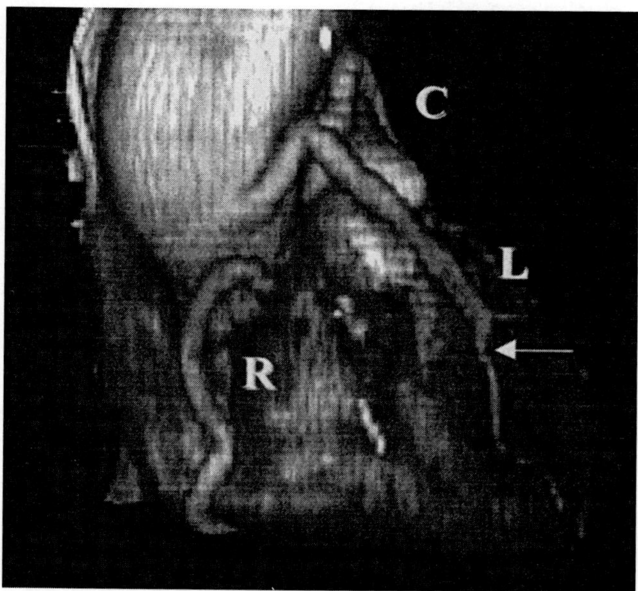

FIGURE 119–3 Three-dimensional reconstruction of a patient with saphenous vein bypass grafts. The native right coronary artery (R) is well seen (without stenosis), as are the bypass grafts to the left anterior descending (L) and circumflex (C) distributions. The anastomotic site of the vein graft into the native anterior descending artery is also seen well *(arrow)*. This modality allows visualization from multiple views in three dimensions.

Douglas Boyd conceived of the ultrafast CT scanner as a tool to evaluate coronary disease, specifically myocardial blood flow.[30] The cine scanning mode is designed to assess cardiac function. The scanning frequency of 17 scans per second is sufficient to study both systolic and diastolic function. The spatial resolution adequately defines the endocardium of both the right and left ventricles, so precise measurement of cardiac volumes and ejection fraction is feasible.[31, 32] Quantitative measurement of wall motion and wall thickening can be made, a feature that is particularly useful for evaluating patients with CAD. Bicycle exercise can be coupled with EBCT scanning to detect exercise-induced ischemia. Both a fall in ejection fraction and the development of a new wall motion abnormality have been shown to be sensitive and specific for the detection of ischemia.[33] Exercise EBCT has also been used to evaluate right ventricular (RV) function in patients with chronic lung disease[34] or obstructive CAD.[35] In a direct comparison study, exercise EBCT may be at least as sensitive and more specific than ^{99m}Tc sestamibi stress testing.[36] Pharmacologic forms of stress testing with dobutamine and dipyridamole infusion is feasible with EBCT, but there is little clinical experience to date.

Rumberger and associates[37] demonstrated the feasibility of evaluating the diastolic performance of the left ventricle.

Diastolic filling variables, such as those measured with blood pool scintigraphy, can be determined with EBCT. Application of this technique may prove useful in detecting subtle changes in LV diastolic function induced by myocardial ischemia.

Except for the complicated and expensive technology of positron emission tomography, there has been no tool for the noninvasive quantitative measurement of myocardial blood flow. Several investigators have demonstrated the potential of EBCT to measure regional myocardial blood flow.[38–40] Simply stated, myocardial blood flow is proportional to the peak iodine concentration in the myocardium after intravenous or intra-arterial injection of an iodinated contrast medium. The technique is accurate for myocardial flows up to 2 ml/min/g. At high flows, rapid washout of iodine from the myocardium before all of the iodine has washed in and extravascular loss of iodine result in the underestimation of myocardial blood flow.[38] Technical factors related to CT scatter and beam hardening may also cause regional inaccuracies.[41] Further research is necessary, but work in progress looks promising for the development of clinically useful methods for accurate quantification of blood flow measurements. Based on the principle that blood flow is proportional to iodine concentration during contrast medium infusion, several investigators have described the use of this technique to detect the presence of myocardial infarction (underperfused or delayed enhancing regions).[42, 43] EBCT could prove very useful in determining infarct size and the effectiveness of reperfusion therapies.

EBCT can provide excellent depiction of ventricular aneurysms and pseudoaneurysms (Fig. 119–5). The three-dimensional aspects of the aneurysm can be determined, and global and regional function can be assessed. Ventricular thrombus can also be easily identified. There is some evidence indicating that EBCT is more sensitive in detecting LV thrombus than transthoracic echocardiography.[44] In addition to its ability to evaluate ventricular function and myocardial blood flow in patients with CAD, EBCT can provide useful information about pericardial and congenital heart disease.

Pericardial Disease

The combination of excellent spatial resolution, tomographic format, and exquisite density differentiation makes EBCT an ideal tool for the diagnosis of pericardial disease. Because the normal pericardium is 1 to 2 mm thick, spatial resolution must be very good for any imaging technique to define this structure. X-ray CT is aided by the fact that epicardial and extrapericardial fat often outline the normal pericardium. Fat, being of very low density, serves as a natural contrast agent (Fig. 119–6). Therefore, minimal pericardial thickening (4 to 5 mm) is well recognized with the use of EBCT. The high density of pericardial calcium makes its detection easy. The three-dimensional representation of anatomy by CT provides the surgeon with precise details of the extent of calcification and the degree of myocardial invasion (Fig. 119–7).

In addition to providing an excellent description of the anatomy of pericardial constriction, EBCT defines the degree of hemodynamic abnormality by describing diastolic filling from ventricular volume measurements every 50 milliseconds throughout diastole.[37] Cine mode images of the right atrium and ventricle can also detect diastolic collapse when pericardial tamponade is present. Enlargement of the superior and inferior vena cavae can be identified when either constriction or tamponade is present. Pericardial effusion is easily detected with EBCT. Occasionally, very small effusions cannot be distinguished from pericardial thickening because the CT densities are similar. However, pericardial fluid, if free in the pericardial space,

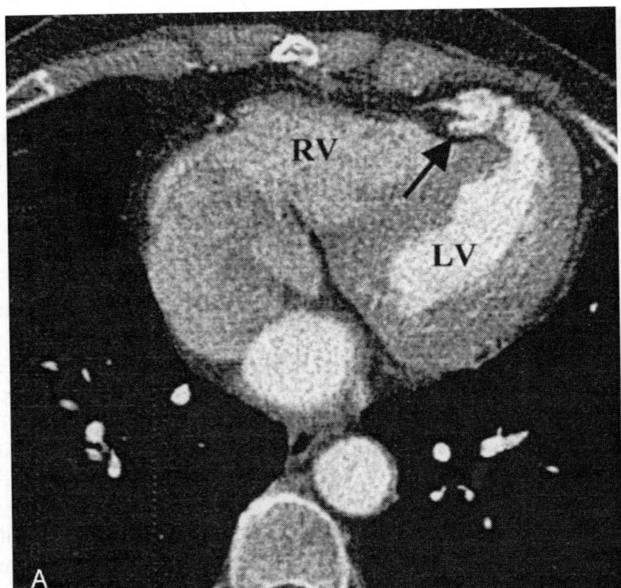

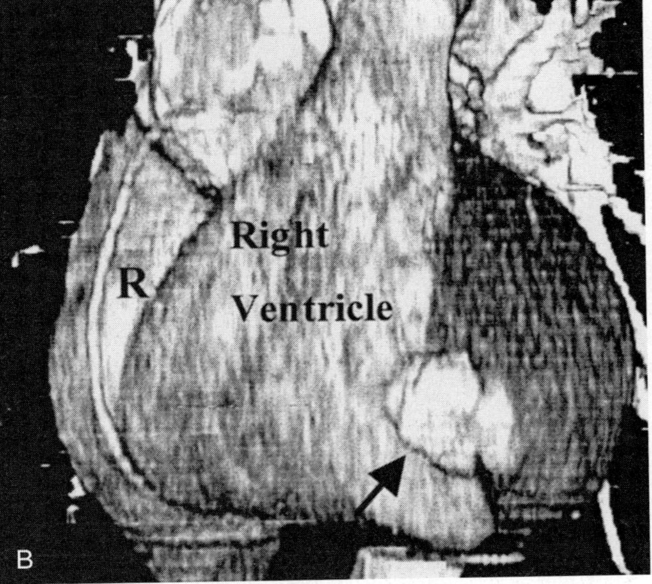

FIGURE 119–5 A patient with possible aneurysm by echocardiography underwent contrast enhanced computer tomography to better define the apex. **A,** Axial two-dimensional image reveals an aneurysm neck and pseudoaneurysm *(arrow)*. RV, right ventricle; LV, left ventricle. **B,** Three-dimensional reconstruction reveals the pseudoaneurysm *(arrow)* and the normal native right coronary artery (R).

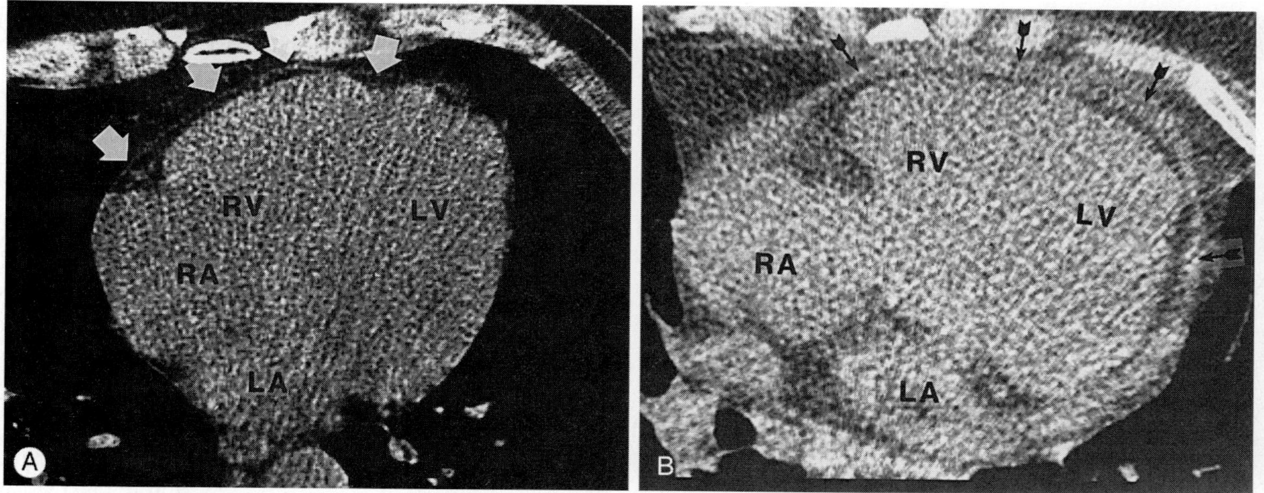

FIGURE 119–6 A, Normal pericardium *(arrows)* is easily identified by ultrafast CT because it is silhouetted between epicardial fat and lung. **B**, Pericardial thickening *(arrows)* is apparent in this ultrafast CT scan of a postoperative heart surgery patient. LA, left atrium; LV, left ventricle; RA, right atrium; RV, right ventricle.

appears as layers, making differentiation from pericardial thickening relatively simple.

EBCT is an excellent diagnostic technique for the evaluation of pericardial cysts and tumors.[45] Because EBCT images the entire thorax and provides clear definition of mediastinal structures, pericardial involvement by metastatic tumors is easily identified. Congenital anomalies, such as absence of the left hemipericardium, are well seen with this modality.[46]

PRIMARY MYOCARDIAL DISEASE

The ability of EBCT to evaluate LV and RV volume and function makes it a useful method for the assessment of primary myocardial disease. Ventricular function can also be evaluated during exercise. Excellent resolution of both endocardial and epicardial borders provides a precise method for determining myocardial muscle volume, which is equivalent to myocardial mass.[47] The various forms of asymmetric hypertrophy typical of hypertrophic cardiomyopathy are clearly evaluated with this technique.[48] Unusual cardiac infections, such as cysticercosis, have also been detected with this imaging technique.

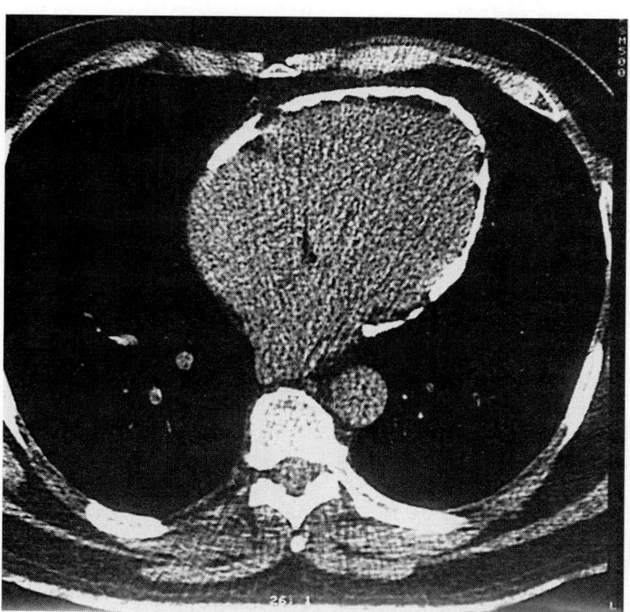

FIGURE 119–7 This densely calcified pericardium is well delineated by ultrafast CT.

VALVULAR HEART DISEASE

EBCT has spatial and temporal resolution that enables the visualization of cardiac valves. Although the simplicity of echocardiography makes it an ideal method for the evaluation of valvular function, EBCT has a role when the results of echocardiography leave unanswered questions. All four cardiac valves can be visualized using the cine mode with contrast medium enhancement. Long-axis views usually provide the best definition of the atrioventricular valves, and short-axis views define the semilunar valves. High-density resolution detects even small amounts of mitral annular and aortic valve calcifications, and valvular and subvalvular apparatus thickening can be well visualized in mitral stenosis (Fig. 119–8). Vegetations resulting from infective endocarditis can be detected with this imaging technique, and associated abnormalities, such as ring or myocardial abscess, can be recognized when other imaging techniques fail.

Quantification of ventricular volume is sometimes useful in the assessment of valvular regurgitation. Regurgitation volume can be accurately determined when only one valve is involved. For example, in a patient with isolated mitral valve regurgitation, LV stroke volume (LV end-diastolic volume minus end-systolic volume) minus RV stroke volume equals regurgitant volume. LV or RV mass can also be measured in an equally precise manner.[31, 47]

There is no method more sensitive than EBCT for the detection of left and right atrial thrombosis (Fig. 119–9).[44]

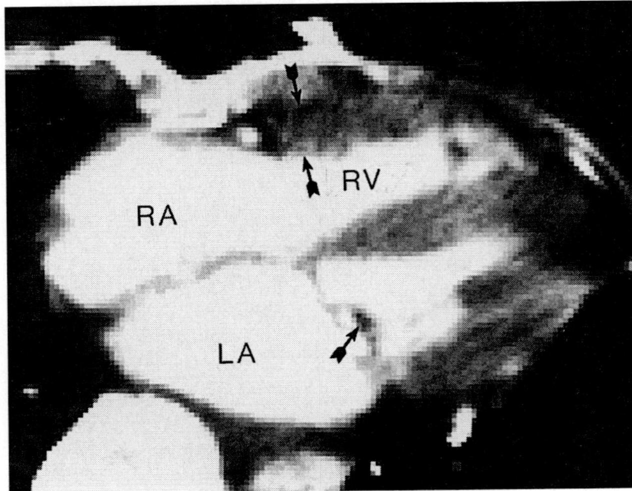

FIGURE 119–8 A single end-systolic frame from a cine CT scan in a patient with mitral stenosis depicts mitral valve thickening *(single arrow),* right ventricular (RV) hypertrophy *(paired arrows),* and right (RA) and left (LA) atrial enlargement.

Although there has been enthusiasm for the use of transesophageal echocardiography, no head-to-head comparison of the two imaging techniques exists for this purpose. Transesophageal echocardiography is clearly more invasive than EBCT for diagnosing this condition. In any event, EBCT is more sensitive than transthoracic echocardiography.[44]

Congenital Heart Disease

EBCT appears to be an ideal technique for the assessment of congenital heart disease. However, relatively little clinical experience has been reported.[49] Considerable experience has been obtained with magnetic resonance imaging.[50] Very similar results have been obtained with EBCT high-resolution scanning. The disadvantages of EBCT are the requirement for the injection of contrast medium and exposure to radiation. The dose for both is acceptably small. EBCT offers advantages over magnetic resonance imaging, including single breathhold to reduce respiratory motion,[51] higher spatial resolution,[52] and reduced slice thickness. An additional advantage of EBCT is the overall study time of 1 to 2 minutes compared with 45 to 90 minutes for magnetic resonance angiography, reducing the time for patients (especially children) to lie perfectly still. EBCT imaging can almost always be completed without the need for sedation. The high-resolution volume mode can provide excellent detail of the anatomic structure of the cardiac chambers and great vessels (Fig. 119–10); see also Figs. 119–1 to 119–4 and 119–6 to 119–9). The flow mode can be used to detect and quantify left-to-right and right-to-left shunts.[53] The cine mode can be used to evaluate RV and LV function, as well as valvular motion. One of the great strengths of EBCT is its capacity to study cardiac anatomy, cardiovascular function, and blood flow during a single study period. EBCT evaluation of congenital heart disease demonstrates the ability to evaluate all aspects of cardiac disease.

Diseases of the Great Vessels

The diagnosis of diseases of the aorta has been well described for conventional x-ray CT. The superior temporal resolution of EBCT significantly improves imaging of the aorta, because motion artifacts are eliminated (Fig. 119–11). EBCT is a superior method for the identification of aortic dissection (Fig. 119–12).[54] The intimal flap is usually well delineated, even in branches of the aorta. In the flow mode, flow can also be assessed in the true and false lumens.

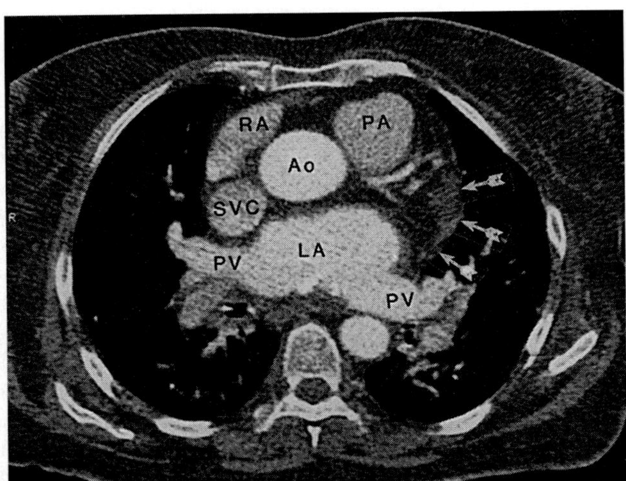

FIGURE 119–9 The left atrial appendage is impacted with thrombus *(arrows)* in this patient with rheumatic mitral valve disease. Note the enlargement of the left atrium (LA) and pulmonary veins (PV). Ao, aorta; PA, pulmonary artery; RA, right atrial appendage; SVC, superior vena cava.

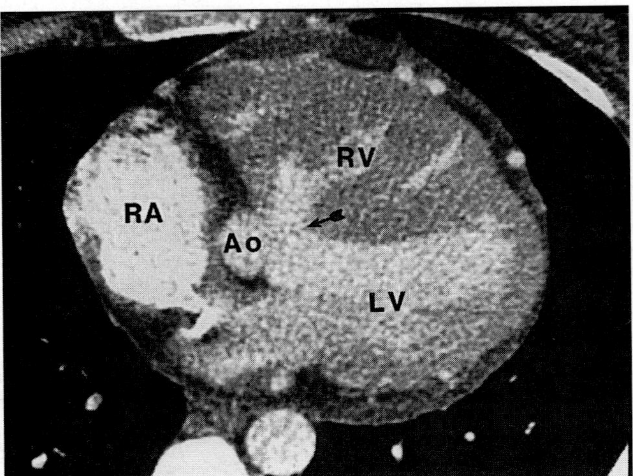

FIGURE 119–10 The ventricular septal defect *(arrow)* in this patient with tetralogy of Fallot is well demonstrated with contrast-enhanced ultrafast CT. Note the severe right ventricular (RV) hypertrophy and the adjacent enlarged coronary arteries. Ao, right aortic sinus of Valsalva; LV, left ventricle; RA, right atrium.

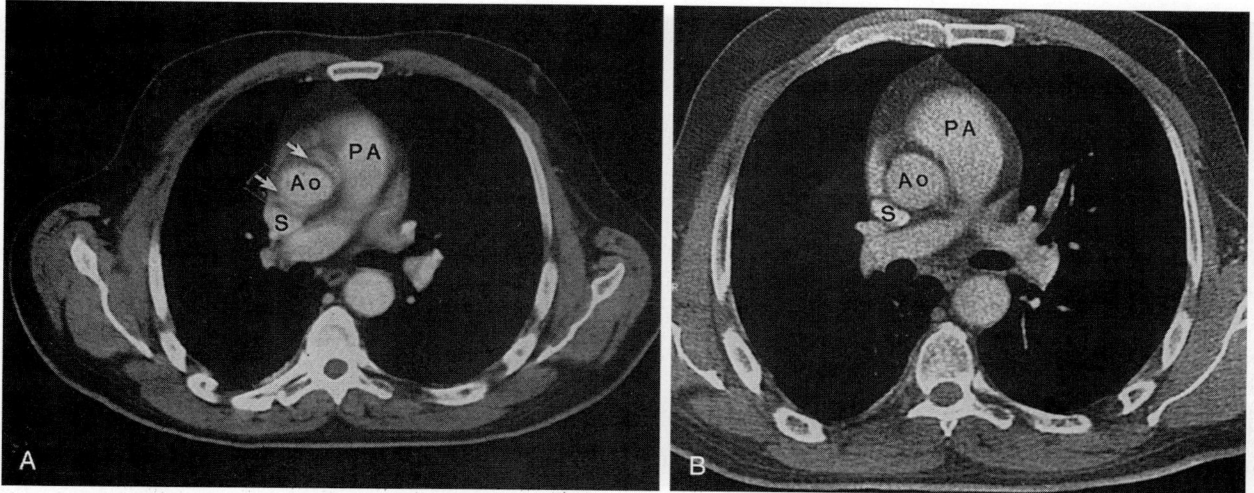

FIGURE 119–11 A, Slow CT scan of the ascending aorta was interpreted as showing a dissection *(arrows)* of the ascending aorta (Ao). PA, pulmonary artery; S, superior vena cava. **B,** Repeat ultrafast CT scan of the same patient 1 day later demonstrates a normal ascending aorta.

EBCT is also an effective method of imaging aortic aneurysms throughout the extent of the aorta. It is particularly useful for imaging ascending aortic aneurysms before and after surgical treatment. Accurate measurements of aortic root diameter can be made easily, and the extent of the aneurysm can be defined. The origin of the coronary arteries is also well visualized (Fig. 119–13). Thrombus within any aortic aneurysm is easily identified on the basis of differences in tissue density during contrast enhancement. Although EBCT cannot define aortic branches as clearly as aortography, it can depict the origin of most major branches. The tomographic format of CT provides excellent definition of the relationship of aortic aneurysms to adjacent structures. Leakage of blood from the aneurysm may be recognizable with contrast enhancement of surrounding tissues. Pericardial tamponade may be detected on the basis of the anatomic and functional changes delineated with volume and cine mode imaging protocols.

EBCT can also be used to image the pulmonary arteries. Large chronic thrombi, presumably resulting from previous embolization, have been successfully detected with this technique (Fig. 119–14).[55] The cross-sectional view of the main and proximal right and left pulmonary arteries provides clear delineation of the proximal extent of the thrombi, which is essential for successful surgical treatment.[56] Research has indicated that EBCT may also be a valid method for the diagnosis of acute pulmonary embolism.[57, 58] EBCT imaging has also been used to define the size of pulmonary arteries in congenital heart disease, information that is essential in planning surgical treatment, especially in pulmonary atresia and truncus arteriosus.[59] Accurate measurement of pulmonary artery size may also be useful in estimating the severity of pulmonary hypertension.[60]

CARDIAC TUMORS

Cardiac tumors are well imaged with EBCT. Myxomas of both atria have been reported with the use of EBCT (Fig.

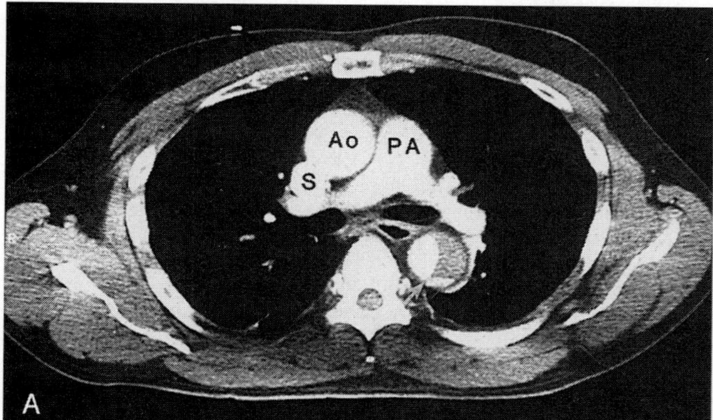

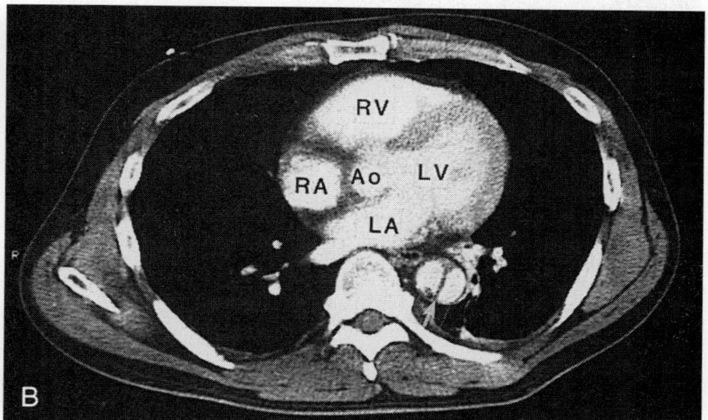

FIGURE 119–12 A, Dissection *(arrow)* of the descending aorta is identified by contrast-enhanced ultrafast CT. At this level, note that a true lumen, false lumen, and thrombus are present. Ao, ascending aorta; PA, pulmonary artery; S, superior vena cava. **B,** More caudad scan of the same patient demonstrates the classic "double-barreled" aorta *(arrow)*. Ao, ascending aorta; LA, left atrium; LV, left ventricle; RA, right atrium; RV, right ventricle.

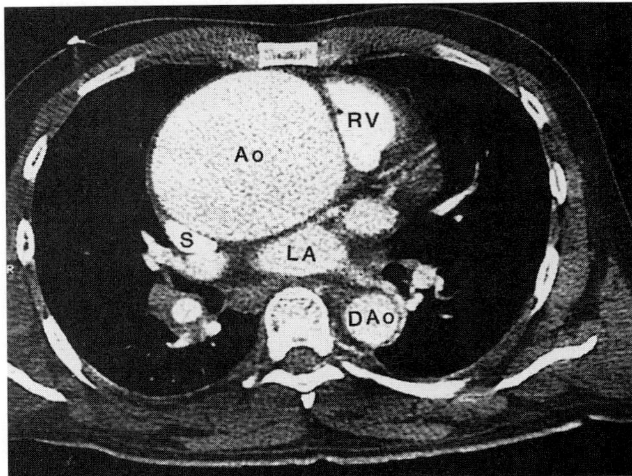

FIGURE 119–13 An 8-cm ascending aortic aneurysm (Ao) is well delineated by ultrafast contrast-enhanced CT. DAo, descending aorta; LA, left atrium; RV, right ventricular outflow tract; S, superior vena cava.

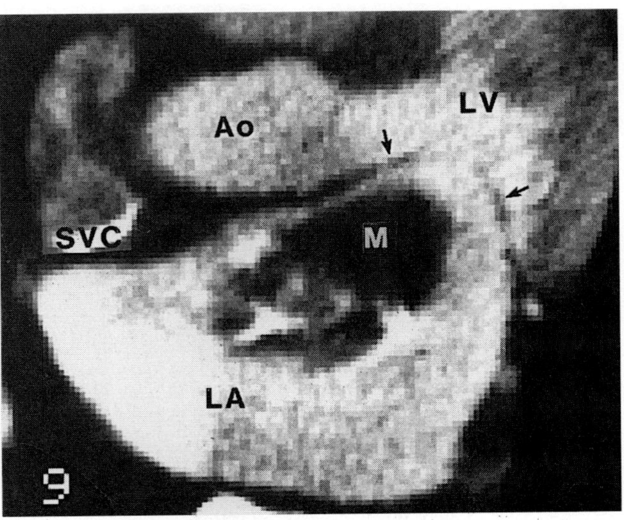

FIGURE 119–15 Single frame from a contrast-enhanced cine CT demonstrates prolapse of a calcified left atrial myxoma (M) into the mitral valve *(arrows)* orifice. Ao, aorta; LA, left atrium; LV, left ventricle; SVC, superior vena cava.

119–15).[61, 62] Although other imaging methods, particularly echocardiography, are more commonly used to evaluate patients with myxoma, the excellent spatial resolution of EBCT and its lack of dependence on an adequate imaging window can provide information that might be missed with transthoracic echocardiography. In one reported example, the origin of right atrial myxoma from the superior vena cava could be determined only with EBCT, and this finding altered the surgical approach to the patient.[62] Other tumors, such as fibropapillomas, intramyocardial fibromas, and metastatic tumors, have also been diagnosed with this technique.[63, 64] The method is particularly good for defining the extent of pericardial involvement by metastatic tumors, and it can be used to determine the functional impact as well.

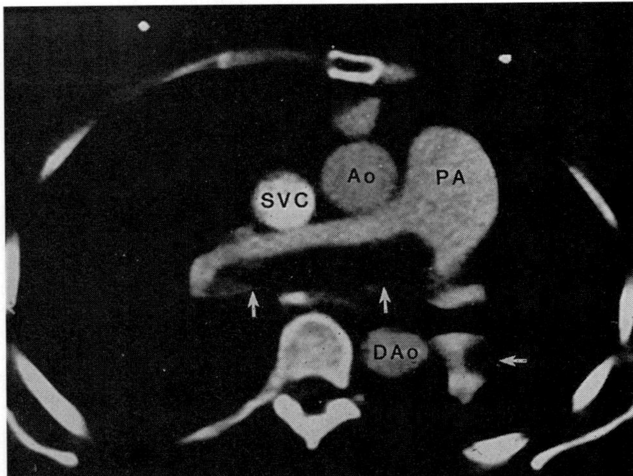

FIGURE 119–14 Large chronic pulmonary embolism *(arrows)* is shown by contrast-enhanced ultrafast CT to involve the proximal right and left pulmonary arteries. Ao, ascending aorta; DAo, descending aorta; PA, pulmonary artery; SVC, superior vena cava.

CONCLUSION

EBCT is an extremely powerful tool for the diagnosis and assessment of virtually every type of cardiovascular disease. The availability of many other imaging modalities and the relatively high cost of EBCT scanners have slowed its adoption for diagnosis by cardiologists, radiologists, and primary caregivers. However, the technology offers some truly unique capabilities, with unmatched prognostic capabilities for cardiac events and noninvasive imaging of the coronary arteries, and clinicians are increasingly using this imaging technique.

REFERENCES

1. Brundage BH, Rich S, Spigos D: Computed tomography of the heart and great vessels: present and future. Ann Intern Med 101:801, 1984.
2. Ritchie CJ, Godwin JD, Crawford CR, et al: Minimum scan speeds for suppression of motion artifacts in CT. Radiology 185:37–42, 1992.
3. Blankenhorn DH: Coronary artery calcification: a review. Am J Med Sci 242:41, 1961.
4. Simons DB, Schwartz RS, Edwards WD, et al: Noninvasive definition of anatomic coronary disease by ultrafast computed tomographic scanning: a quantitative pathologic comparison study. J Am Coll Cardiol 20:1118, 1992.
5. Beadenkopf WG, Daoud AS, Love BM: Calcification in the coronary arteries and its relation of atherosclerosis and myocardial infarction. Am J Roentgenol 92:865–871, 1964.
6. Eggen DA, Strong JP, McGill HC: Coronary calcification: relationship to clinically significant coronary lesions and race, sex and topographic distribution. Circulation 132:948–955, 1965.
7. McCarthy JH, Palmer FJ: Incidence and significance of coronary artery calcification. Br Heart J 36:499–506, 1974.
8. Sangiorgi G, Rumberger JA, Severson A, et al: Arterial calcification and not lumen stenosis is highly correlated with atherosclerotic plaque burden in humans: a histologic study of 723 coronary artery segments using nondecalcifying methodology. J Am Coll Cardiol 31:126–133, 1998.
9. Rumberger JA, Simons DB, Fitzpatrick LA, et al: Coronary artery calcium areas by electron beam computed tomography and coronary atherosclerotic plaque area: a histopathologic correlative study. Circulation 92:2157–2162, 1995.
10. Agatston AS, Janowitz WR, Hilder FJ, et al: Quantitation of coronary

artery calcium using ultrafast computed tomography. J Am Coll Cardiol 15:827, 1990.
11. Wexler L, Brundage BH, Crouse J, et al: Coronary artery calcification: pathophysiology, epidemiology, image methods, and clinical implications: a scientific statement from the American Heart Association. Circulation 94:1175–1192, 1996.
12. Detrano R, Tang W, Kang X, et al: Accurate coronary calcium phosphate mass measurements from electron beam computed tomograms. Am J Card Imaging 9:167–173, 1995.
13. Mautner GC, Mautner SL, Froelich J, et al: Coronary artery calcification: assessment with electron beam CT and histomorphometric correlation. Radiology 192:619–623, 1994.
14. Baumgart D, Schmermund A, Goerge G, et al: Comparison of electron beam computed tomography with intracoronary ultrasound and coronary angiography for detection of coronary atherosclerosis. J Am Coll Cardiol 30:57–64, 1997.
15. Budoff MJ, Georgiou D, Brody A, et al: Ultrafast computed tomography as a diagnostic modality in the detection of coronary artery disease: a multicenter study. Circulation 93:898–904, 1996.
16. Kennedy JM, Shavelle RM, Wang S, et al: Coronary calcium and standard risk factors in symptomatic patients referred for coronary angiography. Am Heart J 135:696–702, 1998.
17. Shavelle DM, Budoff MJ, Lamont DH, et al: Exercise testing and electron beam computed tomography in the evaluation of coronary artery disease. Circulation 96(Suppl I):I-272, 1997.
18. Guerci AD, Spadaro LA, Popma JJ, et al: Relation of coronary calcium score by electron beam computed tomography to arteriographic findings in asymptomatic and symptomatic adults. Am J Cardiol 79:128–133, 1997.
19. Rumberger JA, Sheedy PF, Breen FJ, Schwartz RS: Electron beam CT coronary calcium score cutpoints and severity of associated angiography luminal stenosis. J Am Coll Cardiol 29:1542–1548, 1997.
20. Detrano R, Tzung H, Wang S, et al: Prognostic value of coronary calcification and angiographic stenoses in patients undergoing coronary angiography. J Am Coll Cardiol 27:285–290, 1996.
21. Detrano R, Schwendener C, Doherty T, Secci A: Coronary calcium results predict coronary heart disease deaths in high risk asymptomatic adults. J Am Coll Cardiol 29:128A, 1997.
22. Arad Y, Spadaro LA, Goodman K, et al: Predictive value of electron beam computed tomography of the coronary arteries: 19 month follow-up of 1173 asymptomatic subjects. Circulation 93:1951–1953, 1996.
23. Agatston AS, Janowitz WR, Kaplan GS, et al: Electron beam CT coronary calcium predicts future coronary events. Circulation 94(Suppl I):I-360, 1996.
24. Kennedy JM, Shavelle R, Wong SM, et al: Coronary calcium: the strongest risk factor for coronary artery disease. Am Heart J (in press).
25. Achenbach S, Moshage W, Ropers D, et al: Noninvasive, three-dimensional visualization of coronary artery bypass grafts by electron beam tomography. Am J Cardiol 79:856–861, 1997.
26. Moshage WEL, Achenbach S, Seese B, et al: Coronary artery stenoses: three-dimensional imaging with electrocardiographically triggered, contrast agent-enhanced, electron beam CT. Radiology 196:707–714, 1995.
27. Schmermund A, Rensing BJ, Sheedy PF, et al: Intravenous electron-beam computed tomographic coronary angiography for segmental analysis of coronary artery stenoses. J Am Coll Cardiol 31:1547–1554, 1998.
28. Achenbach S, Moshage W, Ropers D, et al: Comparison of contrast-enhanced electron beam CT and coronary angiography in 125 patients. J Am Coll Cardiol 31:128A, 1998.
29. Budoff MJ, Oudiz RJ, Zalace CP, et al: Intravenous three dimensional coronary angiography using contrast enhanced electron beam computed tomography. J Am Coll Cardiol 29(suppl A):393-A, 1997.
30. Boyd DP, Gould RG, Quinn JR, et al: A proposed dynamic cardiac 3-D densitometer for the early detection and evaluation of heart disease. IEEE Trans Nucl Sci 26:2724, 1979.
31. Reiter SJ, Rumberger JA, Feiring AJ, et al: Precision of right and left ventricular stroke volume measurements by rapid acquisition cine computed tomography. Circulation 74:890, 1986.
32. Rich S, Chomka EV, Stagl R, et al: Determination of left ventricular ejection fraction using ultrafast computed tomography. Am Heart J 112:392, 1986.
33. Roig E, Chomka EV, Castaner A, et al: Exercise ultrafast computed tomography for the detection of coronary artery disease. J Am Coll Cardiol 13:1073, 1989.
34. Himelman RB, Abbott JA, Lee E, et al: Doppler echocardiography and ultrafast cine computed tomography during dynamic exercise in chronic pulmonary disease. Am J Cardiol 64:528, 1989.
35. Mao SS, Budoff MJ, Oudiz RJ, et al: Effect of exercise on left and right ventricular ejection fraction and wall motion. Int J Cardiol 71:23–31, 1999.
36. Budoff MJ, Gillespie R, Georgiou D, et al: Comparison of ultrafast computed tomography and sestamibi in the evaluation of coronary artery disease. Am J Cardiol 81:682–687, 1998.
37. Rumberger JA, Weiss RM, Feiring AJ, et al: Patterns of regional diastolic function in the normal human left ventricle: an ultrafast computed tomographic study. J Am Coll Cardiol 14:119, 1989.
38. Schmermund A: Quantitative evaluation of regional myocardial perfusion using fast x-ray computed tomography. Herz 22:29–39, 1997.
39. Rumberger JA, Bell MR: Measurement of myocardial perfusion and cardiac output using intravenous injection methods by ultrafast (cine) computed tomography. Invest Radiol 27:40–46, 1995.
40. Lui YH, Shu NH, Ritman EL: A fast computed tomographic method for myocardial perfusion. Am J Card Imaging 7:301–308, 1993.
41. Rumberger JA, Bell MR, Feiring JA, et al: Measurement of myocardial perfusion using fast computed tomography. *In* Marcus ML, Schelbert HR, Skorton DJ, Wolf GL (eds): Cardiac Imaging. pp. 688–702. Philadelphia: WB Saunders, 1991.
42. Kramer PH, Goldstein JA, Herfkens RJ, et al: Imaging of acute myocardial infarction in man with contrast-enhanced computed transmission tomography. Am Heart J 108:1514, 1984.
43. Masuda Y, Yoshida H, Morooka N, et al: The usefulness of x-ray computed tomography for the diagnosis of myocardial infarction. Circulation 70:217, 1984.
44. Helgason CM, Chomka E, Louie E, et al: The potential role for ultrafast cardiac computed tomography in patients with stroke. Stroke 20:465, 1989.
45. Stanford W, Rooholamini SA, Galvin JR: Assessment of intracardiac masses and extracardiac abnormalities by ultrafast computed tomography. *In* Marcus ML, Schelbert HR, Skorton DJ, Wolf GL (eds): Cardiac Imaging. p. 703. Philadelphia: WB Saunders, 1991.
46. Stanford W: Computed tomography in the diagnosis of pericardial disease. *In* Brundage BH (ed): Comparative Cardiac Imaging. pp. 451–457. Rockville, MD: Aspen, 1990.
47. Roig E, Georgiou D, Chomka EV, et al: Reproducibility of left ventricular myocardial volume and mass measurements by ultrafast computed tomography. J Am Coll Cardiol 18:990, 1991.
48. Chomka EV, Wolfkiel CJ, Rich S, et al: Ultrafast computed tomography: a new method for the evaluation of hypertrophic cardiomyopathy. Am J Noninvas Cardiol 1:140, 1987.
49. Eldredge WJ: Comprehensive evaluation of congenital heart disease using ultrafast computed tomography. *In* Marcus ML, Schlebert HR, Skorton DJ, Wolf GL (eds): Cardiac Imaging. p. 714. Philadelphia: WB Saunders, 1991.
50. Kersting-Sommerhoff B, Higgins CB: Magnetic resonance of congenital heart disease. *In* Brundage BH (ed): Comparative Cardiac Imaging. pp. 493–502. Rockville, MD: Aspen, 1990.
51. Chernoff DM, Ritchie CJ, Higgins CB: Evaluation of electron beam CT coronary angiography in healthy subjects. AJR 169:93–99, 1997.
52. Duerinckx AJ, Urman MK, Atkinson DJ, et al: Limitations of MR coronary angiography. J Magn Reson Imaging 4:81, 1994.
53. Garrett J, Jaschke W, Aherne T, et al: Quantitation of intracardiac shunts by cine-CT. J Comput Assist Tomogr 12:82, 1988.
54. Rooholamini SA, Stanford W: Ultrafast computed tomography in the diagnosis of aortic aneurysms and dissections. *In* Stanford W, Rumberger J (eds): Ultrafast Computed Tomography in Cardiac Imaging: Principles and Practice. pp. 287–310. Mount Kisco, NY: Futura, 1992.
55. Rich S, Levitsky S, Brundage BH: Pulmonary hypertension from chronic pulmonary thromboembolism. Ann Intern Med 108:425, 1988.
56. Moser KM, Auger WR, Fedullo PF: Chronic major-vessel thromboembolic pulmonary hypertension. Circulation 81:1735, 1990.
57. Galvin JR, Gingrich RD, Hoffman E, et al: Ultrafast computed tomography of the chest. Radiol Clin North Am 32:775–793, 1994.
58. Stanford W, Reiners TJ, Thompson BH, et al: Contrast enhanced thin slice ultrafast computed tomography for the detection of small pulmonary emboli in the pig. Invest Radiol 29:184–187, 1994.

59. Sondheimer HM, Oliphant M, Schneider B, et al: Computerized axial tomography of the chest for visualization of 'absent' pulmonary arteries. Circulation 65:1020, 1982.
60. Kuriyama K, Gamsu G, Stern RG, et al: CT determined pulmonary artery diameters in predicting pulmonary hypertension. Invest Radiol 19:16, 1984.
61. Scholtz TD, Boskis M, Roust L, et al: Noninvasive diagnosis of recurrent familial left atrial myxoma: observations with echocardiography, ultrafast computed tomography, nuclear magnetic resonance imaging and in vitro relaxometry. Am J Card Imaging 3:142, 1989.
62. Seifert P, Chomka EV, Stagl R, et al: Application of the cine computed tomographic scan for precise localization of the origin of an atrial myxoma: surgical implications. Ann Thorac Surg 42:467, 1986.
63. Bertsch MJ, Chomka EV, Brundage BH: Imaging of cardiac tumors. *In* Brundage BH (ed): Comparative Cardiac Imaging. pp. 505–511. Rockville, MD: Aspen, 1990.
64. Stanford W, Rooholamini SA, Glavin JR: Ultrafast computed tomography in the detection of intracardiac masses and pulmonary thromboembolism. *In* Stanford W, Rumberger J (eds): Ultrafast Computed Tomography in Cardiac Imaging: Principles and Practice. p. 235. Mount Kisco, NY: Futura, 1992.

SECTION XIV

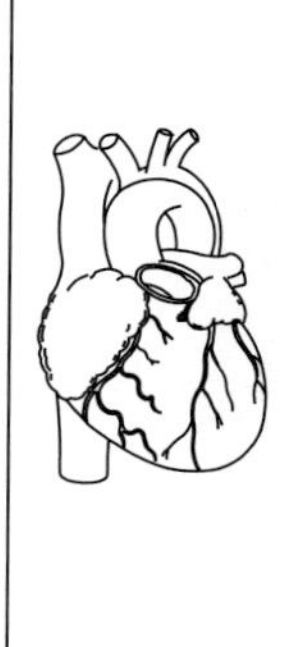

PREVENTIVE CARDIOLOGY

Coronary Risk Factors: An Overview

Exercise

Smoking

Hypertension

Cholesterol Disorders

Obesity

Gene Therapy

Homocysteine and Vascular Disease

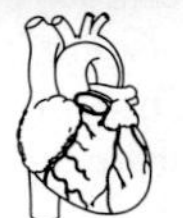

CHAPTER 120

Coronary Risk Factors: An Overview

Donald M. Lloyd-Jones and William B. Kannel

MAGNITUDE OF THE PROBLEM AND SECULAR TRENDS
IMPACT OF THE MAJOR ESTABLISHED RISK FACTORS: RELATIVE, ABSOLUTE, AND ATTRIBUTABLE RISK
Relation of Risk Factors to Specific Cardiovascular Outcomes
Major Established CVD Risk Factors
Atherogenic Living Habits
Other Established Risk Factors
RECENTLY ESTABLISHED RISK FACTORS
White Blood Cell Count
Fibrinogen
Small, Dense LDL
Lipoprotein(a)
Homocysteine and B Vitamins
Hyperinsulinemia/Metabolic Syndrome
POTENTIAL RISK FACTORS UNDER INVESTIGATION
Infection and Inflammation
Iron Excess
RELEVANCE OF RISK FACTORS IN THE ELDERLY
IMPORTANCE OF MULTIVARIATE RISK ASSESSMENT
PREVENTIVE IMPLICATIONS OF RISK FACTOR DETECTION AND CONTROL

A number of risk factors determined by genetic, environmental, dietary, and habitual influences have been firmly established as conferring increased risk for cardiovascular disease (CVD). Support for the "risk factor" concept derives from epidemiologic studies comparing CVD mortality rates among countries and occupational, ethnic, and religious groups. Most important is the evidence that derives from prospective investigations. Since the 1950s, longitudinal prospective epidemiologic studies have been undertaken on tens of thousands of subjects, in a variety of different population samples. These prospective studies are all "observational," not controlled clinical trials; hence, proven causal relationships of individual risk factors to the incidence of CVD cannot be claimed. Because etiology can only be inferred, factors epidemiologically linked to the development of CVD are designated as *risk factors*. In the case of the major established risk factors, controlled trials will not henceforth be pursued because of ethical considerations resulting from the strength of existing epidemiologic evidence.

An epidemiologic association between a proposed risk factor and a disease is likely to be causal if it fulfills the following criteria[1]:

1. Exposure to the proposed risk factor precedes the onset of disease.
2. There is a strong association between exposure and incidence of disease.
3. The association is dose dependent.
4. Exposure is consistently predictive of disease in a variety of populations.
5. The association is independent of other risk factors.
6. The association is biologically and pathogenetically plausible and is supported by animal experiments and clinical investigation.

The major identified CVD risk factors meet most of these criteria. Further support for a causal association between a proposed risk factor and a disease may arise from clinical trials in which modification of the risk factor (by behavioral or therapeutic interventions) is associated with a decreased incidence of the disease.

Absolute risk of disease associated with a given exposure is often expressed as the rate of development of new cases of disease per unit of time (or incidence) in exposed subjects. This proportion may be compared with the proportion among unexposed subjects in a variety of ways. The *relative risk* of disease is the ratio of disease incidence among exposed compared with nonexposed individuals. As such, relative risk measures the strength of the association between exposure and disease, and it may suggest causality, but it gives no indication of the absolute risk of disease. The *attributable risk* of a given exposure describes the fraction of the incidence of disease in a population that can be ascribed to the exposure, assuming a causal relationship exists. The population attributable risk accounts for the proportion of individuals in the population who are exposed, as well as the relative risk. Therefore, attributable risk is a useful concept in determining the public health impact of a given risk factor and in selecting risk factors that should be targeted for prevention programs.[2]

Epidemiologic evidence chiefly describes the evolution of disease in population samples, but the data are also relevant to the occurrence of disease in individuals. Risk factors can be logically categorized into: (1) atherogenic personal attributes (e.g., dyslipidemia); (2) atherogenic living habits (e.g., smoking) or environmental factors that promote them; (3) indicators of active atherogenesis (e.g., leukocytosis); (4) signs of preclinical disease; and (5) host susceptibility to all these influences (e.g., family history). These risk factors can be readily assessed, requiring only ordinary office procedures and simple laboratory tests. By aggregating the risk factors into a composite risk profile, or *global risk assessment,* the joint effect can be estimated and a segment of the asymptomatic population identified who are at high risk for development of coronary artery disease (CAD). An examination of the clinical and public health impact of CVD serves as background for a discussion of the role and interactions of CVD risk factors in the promotion of CVD.

Magnitude of the Problem and Secular Trends

CVD has been the leading cause of death in the United States in every year since 1900, with the exception of 1918.[3] CVD accounts for more deaths each year than the next seven leading causes of death, including cancer, respiratory diseases, accidents, and human immunodeficiency virus infection, combined. In 1995 alone, CVD was the cause of death for over 960,000 men and women.[4] In addition to mortality, CVD contributes significantly to the morbidity of the general population, particularly, but not exclusively, in older individuals. In 1995, CVD was the leading first diagnosis at discharge from acute care hospitals, accounting for nearly 5.9 million inpatient hospitalizations. Currently, approximately 1.1 million Americans suffer a new or recurrent myocardial infarction (MI) yearly.[3] Furthermore, CVD costs the nation hundreds of billions of dollars annually in direct health care expenditures and lost productivity.[5]

Viewed from another perspective, CAD affects more individuals during their life span than any other disease studied to date. The concept of the *lifetime risk* of a given disease provides a useful measure of the absolute burden and public health impact of a disease, as well as indicating an average risk for an individual during his or her lifetime. Lifetime risk estimates account for the age-specific risk of developing a disease and the competing risk of death from another cause before developing the disease of interest. Observations on 7733 subjects over nearly 110,000 person-years of follow-up in the Framingham Heart Study from 1971 to 1996 indicate that the lifetime risk of CAD in this population was 48.6 percent for men (i.e., 1 in 2) and 31.7 percent for women (1 in 3). The lifetime risk up to age 65 years was 20 percent for men and 10 percent for women, indicating significant morbidity even among younger people. Individuals who reached age 70 years free of CAD still had a remaining lifetime risk of 1 in 3 for men and 1 in 4 for women. Thus, there was no age studied beyond which the risk of a first CAD event became minimal.[6]

It is encouraging to note that age-adjusted mortality rates from CVD have been declining steadily since their peak in the mid-to-late 1960s. Available evidence suggests that increasing public awareness of risk factors for CVD, subsequent modifications of lifestyles, and availability of new therapies for primary and secondary prevention of CVD have contributed importantly to this decline. For example, the percentage of the adult population currently smoking cigarettes has decreased dramatically in both whites and blacks, men and women, since 1975. Similarly, the proportion of adults with elevated serum cholesterol (>240 mg/dl) has declined in all segments of the population from the 1960s on. At the same time, however, the number of overweight individuals rose sharply during the 1990s, with implications for increasing prevalence of hypertension and diabetes. In recent years, age-adjusted stroke rates have risen slightly, and the decline in age-adjusted incidence of CAD appears to be leveling off.[5] Data from the Atherosclerosis Risk in Communities Study also indicate that although coronary death has declined, the rate of incident CAD events has remained stable during the 1990s.[7]

The incidence of CAD doubles with each advancing decade of age, and women lag behind men in incidence by 10 years (Fig. 120–1). It is important to recognize, however, that CAD is a more serious threat to women than breast cancer is. Of the various clinical manifestations of atherosclerotic CVD, CAD is the most common and most lethal, equaling all the others combined in incidence.

Impact of the Major Established Risk Factors: Relative, Absolute, and Attributable Risk

Relation of Risk Factors to Specific Cardiovascular Outcomes

The major established risk factors for CVD include dyslipidemia, diabetes mellitus, hypertension, cigarette smoking, male gender, postmenopausal status, and family history of premature CAD. Nontrivial differences exist in the impact of these risk factors on specific cardiovascular events. All the major cardiovascular risk factors contribute importantly to development of CAD, whereas hypertension predominates for stroke and lipid levels play only a small role. For peripheral arterial disease, cigarette smoking and glucose intolerance are most influential. For congestive heart failure, hypertension, left ventricular hypertrophy (LVH), CAD, and diabetes are paramount.[8]

These common risk factors operate in both genders at all ages but with different degrees of influence. Diabetes and a low high-density lipoprotein cholesterol (HDL-C) eliminate the advantage of women over men.[9] Cigarette smoking has a greater influence in men, it is noncumulative, and its impact is reversible after quitting. Fibrinogen is a major independent risk factor for CAD, stroke, and peripheral arterial disease in both genders.[10]

Some risk factors, such as dyslipidemia, impaired glucose tolerance, and fibrinogen, diminish in impact with advancing age. However, decreased risk ratios are offset by a high absolute risk of disease, resulting in a large excess attributable risk. All risk factors are also relevant in the elderly. Isolated systolic hypertension is an important risk factor that is particularly prevalent in older persons. Obesity and weight gain promote all the major atherogenic traits, and physical indolence promotes risk factors and coronary disease at all ages.[10]

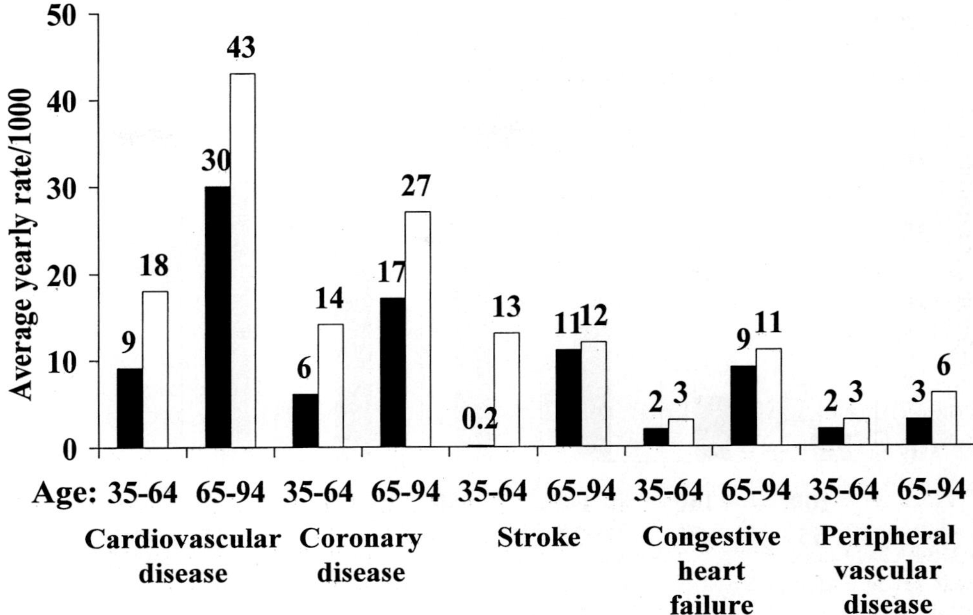

FIGURE 120–1 Incidence of major cardiovascular events by age and gender: Framingham Heart Study, 36-year follow-up. *Black bars,* women; *white bars,* men.

Major Established CVD Risk Factors

Blood Lipids

Evidence incriminating cholesterol in CVD is extensive and unequivocal. Atherosclerosis has been produced in animals by fat-modified diets that raise cholesterol; experimentally induced atheromatous lesions have been found to contain lipid derived from the plasma; CVD cases consistently have higher cholesterol values than persons who remain free of disease; and persons with familial hypercholesterolemia develop premature and extensive CVD. Epidemiologic studies find that CAD mortality parallels the mean serum cholesterol of populations, and prospective epidemiologic studies show that CAD evolves within populations in relation to individual cholesterol values.

The average intake of fat correlates closely with mean levels of cholesterol in population samples around the world. Metabolic studies in humans indicate a predictable joint influence of dietary cholesterol and saturated fat on the serum total and low-density lipoprotein cholesterol (LDL-C).[11, 12] The entire spectrum of atherosclerotic lesions seen in humans has been produced in a variety of experimental animals, including nonhuman primates, by feeding diets enriched with cholesterol and fat to induce hypercholesterolemia. Regression of disease has also been demonstrated after elimination of the offending nutrients.[13]

Therefore, international dietary comparisons, human metabolic investigations, and animal experiments clearly incriminate dietary cholesterol and saturated fat as major contributors to the high serum total cholesterol and LDL-C values characteristic of high CAD-incidence populations.[13] This association is augmented by excessive caloric intake. The nutrients that affect HDL-C are still poorly understood and are under intensive investigation. A high intake of complex carbohydrates is definitely associated with a lower CAD mortality, particularly when the carbohydrate is eaten in place of saturated fat.

The relation of lipids to atherogenesis has evolved from an initial focus on serum total cholesterol to other lipids, then to the lipoproteins that transport them, and is now concerned with the partition of cholesterol into LDL-C and HDL-C components. Current investigation is concerned with the apolipoproteins and the subfractions of high-density lipoprotein (HDL), low-density lipoprotein (LDL), and very low density lipoprotein (VLDL), as well as the impact of small, dense LDL particles. No conclusive epidemiologic data yet exist to demonstrate a unique relationship of apolipoproteins, prostaglandins, or platelet factors to clinical atherosclerotic events. More information is needed on the interaction among blood lipids and homocysteine, fibrinogen, glycosaminoglycans, and prostaglandins that are involved in blood pressure regulation, platelet aggregation, vasospasm, insulin resistance, and smooth muscle proliferation.

CAD develops in relation to the serum total cholesterol in both genders. Within usual cholesterol values of high CVD-incidence countries, there is a strong, graded relationship between the level of total cholesterol and the risk of CAD. Across the spectrum of total cholesterol values, there is a fivefold range of risk with no discernible threshold value below which risk decreases markedly. A serum total cholesterol of 240 mg/dl confers twice the optimal risk of CAD. Populations having long life expectancy and a low CAD incidence have average cholesterol values in the range of 160 to 190 mg/dl.

Lipoprotein cholesterol data from the Framingham Study show that total cholesterol, LDL-C, and HDL-C are all important in determining risk for CAD among individuals aged 45 to 84 years.[11] However, cholesterol-related risk varies widely depending on age, gender, cholesterol lipoprotein fractions, and the burden of other cardiovascular risk factors (Fig. 120–2). The atherogenicity of the serum total cholesterol depends on the relative levels of its LDL-C and HDL-C components. Measurement of these cholesterol lipoprotein fractions is essential after the age of 55 years,

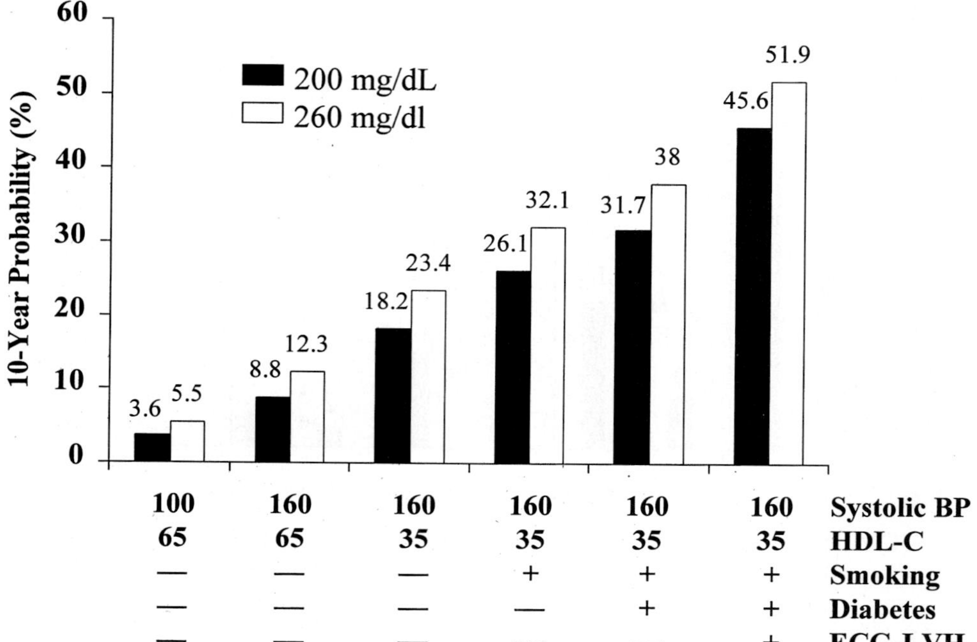

FIGURE 120–2 Predicted probabilities of coronary artery disease (CAD) for total cholesterol of 200 versus 260 mg/dl in men, according to increasing burden of other risk factors. BP, blood pressure; ECG-LVH, electrocardiographic evidence of left ventricular hypertrophy; HDL-C, high-density lipoprotein cholesterol.

when the serum total cholesterol less efficiently identifies candidates for CAD.

The fraction of the serum total cholesterol in LDLs is the atherogenic component, and these effects of LDL-C are well established.[14] LDL-C is responsible for the positive association between the serum total cholesterol and the incidence of CAD. In general, a 10-mg/dl difference in LDL-C is associated with a 5 to 7 percent difference in CAD over 14 years, independent of the other major coronary risk factors. However, for LDL-C, there is a curious strong *inverse* relationship to the incidence of stroke in women, which is significant.

The HDL fraction is *inversely* related to CAD risk, in part reflecting its role in the process of cholesterol removal from the vascular intima.[15] Data from the Framingham Study indicate that whereas LDL-C and HDL-C levels are each independently related to CAD incidence, the protective influence of HDL-C is possibly stronger than the atherogenic influence of LDL-C (Fig. 120–3).[16] For HDL-C, there is also an *inverse* relationship to incidence of stroke, peripheral arterial disease, and congestive heart failure, but the relationship is statistically significant only in the case of heart failure.

To incorporate the effect of HDL-C into a composite

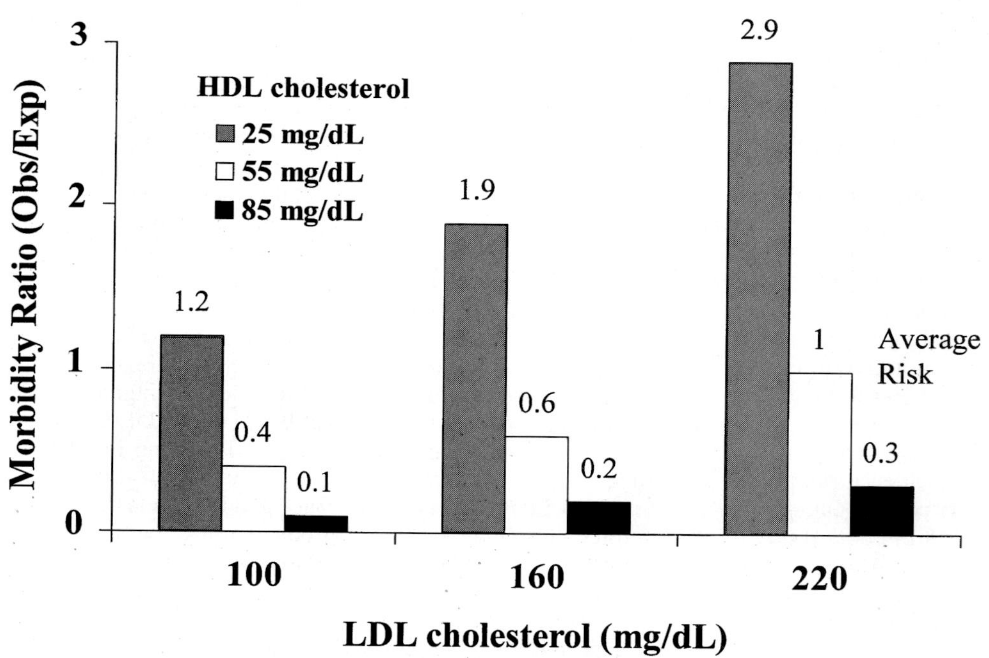

FIGURE 120–3 Relative risk of CAD according to high-density lipoprotein (HDL) and low-density lipoprotein (LDL) cholesterol levels in men 50 to 70 years of age: Framingham Heart Study, 4-year follow-up. Obs/Exp, observed/expected. (From Kannel WB: Lipids, diabetes, and coronary heart disease: insights from the Framingham Study. Am Heart J 110:1100–1107, 1985.)

lipid profile, the use of a ratio of LDL/HDL cholesterol or total cholesterol/HDL-C is recommended. Because of the high correlation between LDL-C and total cholesterol, the latter ratio can serve as a surrogate for the former. As shown in Figure 120–4, increasing the total cholesterol/HDL-C ratio confers increased absolute risk of CAD. In the Framingham Study, this ratio was found to be more efficient at identifying subjects with increased CVD risk than relying on the LDL-C alone, as recommended by the U.S. Expert Panel.[17]

An accurate HDL-C assay is essential because relatively small differences in HDL-C may be associated with large differences in risk of CAD. For example, a 10-mg/dl difference in HDL-C is associated with a 20 percent difference in CAD over 14 years, after adjustment for multiple variables. This estimate is highly significant, emphasizing the benefit of higher HDL-C levels. Low HDL-C is associated with the occurrence of MI in both genders, even at serum cholesterol levels below 200 mg/dl. About 20 percent of MIs after the age of 50 years in the Framingham cohort occurred in persons with low HDL-C (<35 mg/dl). Furthermore, approximately 20 percent of MIs occur in individuals with cholesterol levels in the bottom quartile, and about half of these individuals (10 percent of the total number of MI victims) have simultaneously low HDL-C levels.[11] A review has highlighted this favorable impact of HDL-C on CAD and has found remarkably consistent effects of HDL-C on CAD incidence in men from Framingham, the Lipid Research Clinics Program, the Multiple Risk Factor Intervention Trial (MRFIT), and the British Regional Heart Study.[12]

To date, four large trials aimed at cholesterol-lowering for primary prevention of CAD have been published. Three of the studies[18–20] have included only men with high-risk lipid profiles. The fourth[21] included women and studied patients with average total cholesterol and low HDL-C levels. Each of the studies observed significant reductions in coronary events and/or coronary mortality with cholesterol-lowering therapy, indicating the central role played by lipids in promoting atherogenesis and clinical coronary events.

Analyses from clinical trials show that favorable changes in HDL-C during the course of cholesterol-lowering therapy may help to identify individuals who achieve greater protection from coronary heart disease.[12, 22] Information is also accumulating on the efficacy of preventive measures that lower LDL-C, raise HDL-C, and improve their ratio. Measurement of HDL2 and HDL3 subclasses has not demonstrated any advantage over the total HDL-C as a predictor of CAD, since the levels of these subclasses correlate highly with the total HDL-C. Under investigation is the impact of apolipoprotein-A1 and apolipoprotein-B levels and their importance in determining coronary risk.

Triglycerides as a Risk Factor for CAD

Serum triglyceride values and the VLDLs that transport triglycerides are positively associated with CAD risk in univariate analyses. However, there has been controversy about the existence of an independent contribution to risk of CVD by triglycerides, which was fueled by earlier limitations in measurement of triglycerides and in statistical analysis. Until recently, most prospective studies indicated that the excess risk observed in hypertriglyceridemia was primarily dependent on coexisting low HDL-C values, obesity, and impaired glucose tolerance. Indeed, because the metabolisms of triglycerides and HDL-C are closely linked and there is a strong inverse correlation between their levels, it has been difficult to separate the possible independent effects of triglycerides.[23] The association of CAD with HDL-C levels is uniformly stronger than with triglycerides in the Framingham cohort. However, data from the Lipid Research Clinics[24] and Framingham[25] do indicate a significant impact of triglycerides, after adjustment for HDL-C when log transformations of the lipid levels are used in risk calculations. And in a meta-analysis of 17 population-

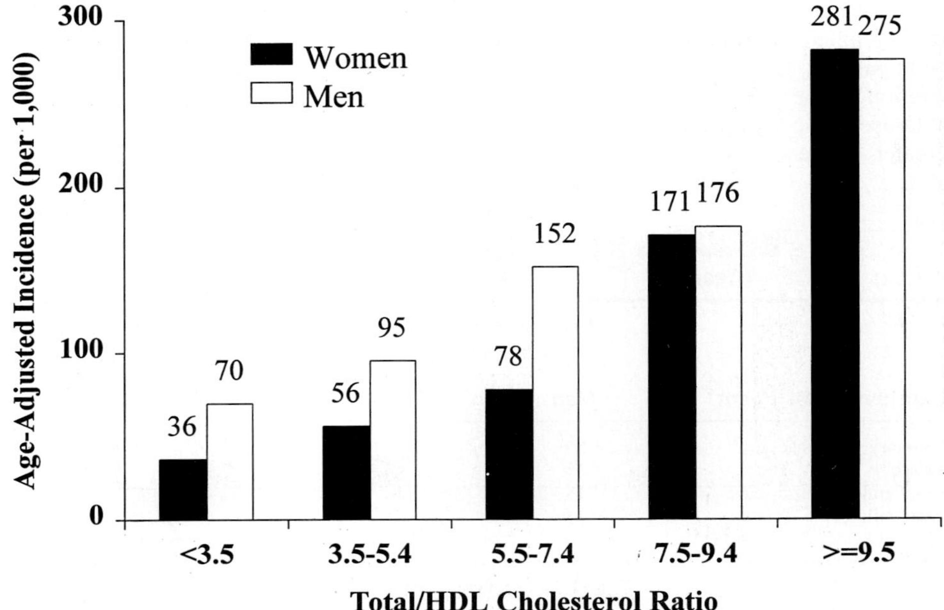

FIGURE 120–4 Incidence of coronary heart disease by total/high-density lipoprotein (HDL) cholesterol ratio among men and women 50 to 90 years of age: Framingham Heart Study, 26-year follow-up.

based prospective studies including more than 57,000 men and women, hypertriglyceridemia was found to be associated with a 30 percent increase in risk of CVD in men and a 75 percent increase in women. The risk remained significantly elevated even after adjustment for HDL-C and other risk factors.[26]

Hypertriglyceridemia is commonly seen in association with other modifiable risk factors, such as diabetes, other atherogenic dyslipidemias, obesity, and hypertension, and the presence of these other factors increases the overall risk of CVD. Therefore, persons with elevated triglyceride levels should be investigated for hyperglycemia, increased LDL-C, depressed HDL-C, insulin resistance, obesity, and alcohol abuse and appropriate countermeasures should be implemented.

Diabetes and Impaired Glucose Tolerance

Although a decline in atherosclerotic CVD morbidity and mortality has been observed in the United States since the 1970s, control and prevention of diabetes have not contributed to this decline. Data from the Third National Health and Nutrition Examination Survey (NHANES III) indicate an increasing prevalence of diabetes and related hyperglycemic disorders, not only in an increasing elderly population but also in specific age groups. Using American Diabetes Association 1997 diagnostic criteria,[27] the prevalence of diagnosed diabetes in 1988 to 1994 was estimated to be 5.1 percent for U.S. adults 20 years of age or older (approximately 10.2 million people). The prevalence of undiagnosed diabetes was 2.7 percent (5.4 million), and the prevalence of impaired fasting glucose was 6.9 percent (13.4 million). Men and women had similar rates of diabetes, but the rates for non-Hispanic blacks and Mexican Americans were 1.6 to 1.9 times the rate for non-Hispanic whites. The prevalence of all diabetes (diagnosed plus undiagnosed) among people 40 to 74 years of age increased from 8.9 percent in 1976 to 1980 to 12.3 percent by 1988 to 1994.[28]

Despite improved diagnostic methods and better treatment for diabetes, physicians continue to encounter a high rate of atherosclerotic cardiovascular events in their diabetic patients. Long-term, prospective epidemiologic investigation of the influence of impaired glucose tolerance on atherosclerotic CVD outcomes indicates a two- to threefold greater incidence in diabetic men and women at all ages. In terms of relative risk, the impact is substantially greater in women, eliminating their advantage over men, and it is most pronounced for stroke and heart failure in women and for peripheral arterial disease in both genders (Table 120–1). However, CAD is the most common and most lethal sequela. Diabetics who have already sustained an MI also have more recurrences and a higher incidence of cardiac failure and LVH.

Adult-onset, hyperinsulinemic, nonketotic diabetes has been shown repeatedly to run in families and to be promoted by obesity. Weight control is the chief preventive measure available for control of diabetes in the general population, and weight loss has been shown to improve glucose tolerance and to reduce insulin resistance. There is every reason to believe that avoidance or control of obesity, particularly of the abdominal (or upper truncal) variety, can delay or possibly avert the onset of diabetes.

There is a clear need for more research to learn why abdominal or upper truncal obesity is more inclined to impair glucose tolerance than generalized obesity. We must also learn more about the precise genetic factors responsible for insulin-resistant diabetes and how fat cells become insulin resistant. Other questions remain as well: Does weight-induced diabetes occur only in those who are genetically predisposed, and is the genetic factor determinative or only permissive? Why does the prevalence of diabetes increase with age?

In the past, fully half of diabetics discovered by screening programs and surveys were previously undetected, suggesting that physicians should periodically check their patients for impaired glucose tolerance, especially when the patients are obese, have dyslipidemia characterized by elevated triglyceride and reduced HDL, or have a positive family history of diabetes. The therapeutic value of identifying new diabetics at an early stage, before symptoms appear, has been questioned, given concerns about labeling asymptomatic individuals with a diagnosis that may affect employability and insurability. However, detection of impaired glucose tolerance can be justified as part of a cardiovascular risk appraisal.

There are two areas of consideration when we contemplate the health benefits of screening for asymptomatic hyperglycemia: diabetes prevention and CVD control. Evidence from long-term studies indicates that persons with transient hyperglycemia or even high-normal values are subject to a high rate of subsequent overt diabetes.[9] This

TABLE 120–1 Risk of Cardiovascular Events in Subjects With Diabetes: Framingham Study, 36-Year Follow-Up, Persons Aged 35–64 Years

Cardiovascular Event	Age-Adjusted Biennial Rate per 1000		Age-Adjusted Risk Ratio		Excess Risk per 1000	
	Men	*Women*	*Men*	*Women*	*Men*	*Women*
Coronary heart disease	39	21	1.5*	2.2†	12	12
Stroke	15	6	2.9†	2.6†	10	4
Peripheral arterial disease	18	18	3.4†	6.4†	13	15
Heart failure	23	21	4.4†	7.8	18	18
All cardiovascular events	76	65	2.2†	3.7†	42	47

*$P < .001$.
†$P < .0001$.

TABLE 120–2 Comparison of Risk Factor Levels: Diabetic Versus Nondiabetic Subjects, Framingham Cohort, 1972 (Age-Adjusted Means)

	Men		Women	
Risk Factor	*Diabetes Present (n = 318)*	*Diabetes Absent (n = 1495)*	*Diabetes Present (n = 328)*	*Diabetes Absent (n = 2178)*
Glucose (mg/dl)	147*	87	134*	86
Systolic BP (mm Hg)	145*	137	149*	140
BMI (kg/m^2)	27.4*	26.0	28.0*	25.4
Hematocrit (%)	48.8*	46.2	43.9	41.9
Uric acid (mg/dl)	5.3*	4.9	4.4*	3.9
LVH (%)	14.5†	7.1	12.4*	5.8
Cigarettes (%)	35.8	43.0	32.3	33.6
Lipids (mg/dl)				
Total cholesterol	223.1	223.4	248.2	248.0
HDL-C	42.1*	46.1	53.0*	57.6
LDL-C	138.2	143.1	155.9	156.0
VLDL-C	37.3*	30.1	33.1*	27.9

Abbreviations: BMI, body mass index; BP, blood pressure; HDL-C, high density lipoprotein cholesterol; LDL-C, low-density lipoprotein cholesterol; LVH, left ventricular hypertrophy; VLDL-C, very low density lipoprotein cholesterol.

*$P < 0.001$.

†$P < 0.01$

From Kannel WB, Wilson PW, Zhang TJ: The epidemiology of impaired glucose tolerance and hypertension. Am Heart J 121:1268–1273, 1991.

risk is magnified when there is coexisting obesity and hypertriglyceridemia. There appears to be justification for screening such high-risk persons as candidates for diabetes who require surveillance and preventive measures to avoid the renal, ophthalmic, and neuropathic consequences of diabetes.

The second area of concern relates to control of atherosclerotic CVD. Most research has concentrated on the impact of overt diabetes, and the influence of lesser degrees of glucose tolerance is debated. However, evidence from the Framingham Study shows that blood glucose values over 130 mg/dl—but below those that previously qualified for a diagnosis of "diabetes"—are associated with an increased risk for atherosclerotic CVD.[22] Data such as these prompted the revision in the American Diabetes Association diagnostic criteria for diabetes.[27] Although the efficacy of blood glucose control in retarding the progression of such cardiovascular sequelae remains to be clarified, there is justification for identifying those patients with impaired glucose tolerance for control of other coexistent cardiovascular risk factors.[29]

Almost all of the diabetics detected in health maintenance or screening programs are of the adult-onset, obesity-related, hyperinsulinemic, keto-resistant variety. The major sequela of such disease is accelerated atherogenesis rather than acute metabolic complications. Diabetics have a higher level of coexisting CVD risk factors, such as hypertension, low HDL-C, high VLDL, small, dense LDL, triglycerides, and obesity (Table 120–2). The risk among diabetics varies considerably depending on their coexisting risk factors (Table 120–3). Since these risk factors appear to operate jointly to promote atherogenesis, there is a distinct possibility that diabetics can reduce their cardiovascular risk by controlling their other risk factors. This is an important consideration, since treatment directed at the hyperglycemia itself has proved disappointing in reducing the atherosclerotic cardiovascular sequelae.[30] Measures taken to improve the overall cardiovascular risk profile of the diabetic patient may prove more successful, but this has not been tested. Hence, persons discovered to have any evidence of impaired glucose tolerance deserve a full evaluation for cardiovascular risk. Protection against cardiovascular sequelae then requires controlling weight, lowering the total cholesterol/HDL-C ratio, controlling blood pressure, and avoiding cigarettes, in addition to reducing blood sugar.

Hypertension

Persistent nonphysiologic elevation of blood pressure is a direct cause of cardiovascular sequelae and premature mortality. Because of its ubiquitous high prevalence throughout the world, its impact on CVD, and the fact that it can be controlled by lifestyle modification and pharmacologic agents, this condition justifies a high priority for detection and treatment. Hypertension has a critical and independent effect on atherogenesis, now its chief lethal sequela. This pathology has replaced accelerated malignant hypertension as the major outcome of uncontrolled hypertension.

TABLE 120–3 Eight-Year Probability of Cardiovascular Events in Diabetics Aged 50 Years, According to Associated Risk Factors: Framingham Study, 26-Year Follow-Up

	Rate per 1000	
Risk Factor	*Men*	*Women*
No risk fractors	54	50
HTN (165 mm Hg)	139	117
HTN + cholesterol (260 mg/dl)	213	159
HTN + cholesterol + cigarettes	193	326
HTN + cholesterol + cigarettes + ECG-LVH	622	323

Abbreviations: ECG-LVH, electrocardiographically demonstrated left ventricular hypertrophy; HTN, hypertension.

TABLE 120–4 **Risk of Cardiovascular Events in Subjects With Hypertension: Framingham Study, 36-Year Follow-Up, Persons Aged 35–64 Years**

	Age-Adjusted Biennial Rate per 1000		Age-Adjusted Risk Ratio		Excess Risk per 1000	
Cardiovascular Event	*Men*	*Women*	*Men*	*Women*	*Men*	*Women*
Coronary heart disease	45	21	2.0	2.2	23	12
Stroke	12	6	3.8	2.6	9	4
Peripheral arterial disease	10	7	2.0	3.7	5	5
Heart failure	14	6	4.0	3.0	10	4
All cardiovascular events	65	35	2.2	2.5	36	21

*All $P < .0001$.

The incidence and prevalence of hypertension tend to rise with age. Hypertension is the most common vascular disease in the United States, affecting nearly 50 million, or approximately one out of every four adults, and it is one of the most powerful contributors to the leading causes of death. It is the chief factor contributing to the 600,000 strokes that occur each year in the United States and is a major factor in the estimated 1.1 million annual coronary events.[3] It is also a major cause of the 50,000 deaths from end-stage renal disease that occurred in the United States in 1996.[31]

Hypertension imposes more than a twofold increased relative risk of CVD compared with age-matched normotensives (Table 120–4). It powerfully and independently predisposes to development of every clinical manifestation of CAD, which is now the most common outcome of hypertension.[32] However, its *relative* impact is greatest for stroke and heart failure. The absolute and relative risk, risk gradients, and attributable risk are at least as great in the elderly as in the young, and its impact is as great in women as in men compared with normotensives.

Risk is proportional to the blood pressure level, without any critical threshold value, and even mild hypertension doubles the risk for CVD. Historically, elevated diastolic blood pressure (DBP) was thought to confer greater risk for cardiovascular events than elevated systolic blood pressure (SBP). However, epidemiologic data suggest that elevated SBP is at least as strong a risk factor as elevated DBP for the development of CVD. Previous reports from the Framingham Heart Study have highlighted the *relative risk* associated with increasing SBP in subjects with isolated systolic hypertension (Fig. 120–5)[33] as well as in those with elevated DBP.[33] Data from nearly 348,000 men free of CHD between the ages of 35 to 57 years, who were screened for the MRFIT study, indicate that the adjusted relative risk of CAD mortality is higher at every stage for SBP than for the same DBP stage. Viewed another way, the relative risk of CAD mortality for subjects in the highest decile compared with those in the lowest decile of SBP was 3.82, as opposed to 2.90 for those in the highest versus lowest decile of DBP. The relative risk for SBP was consistently higher than that for DBP within each decile. When stratified by age, the relative risk of CHD mortality was greater for the top decile of SBP than for the top

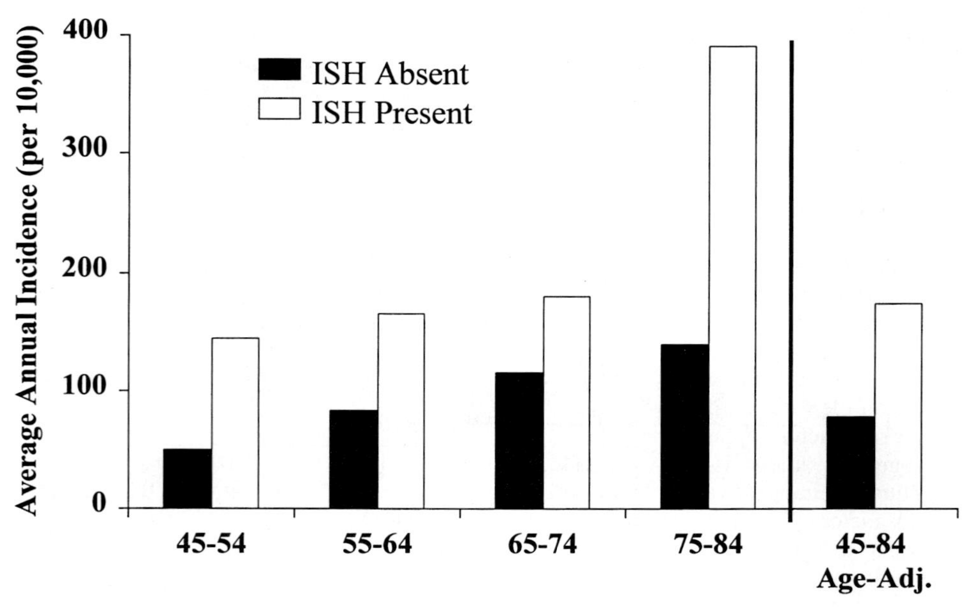

FIGURE 120–5 Incidence of myocardial infarction in men with or without isolated systolic hypertension (ISH), defined as systolic blood pressure ≥ 160 mm Hg and diastolic blood pressure < 95 mm Hg: Framingham Heart Study, 24-year follow-up.

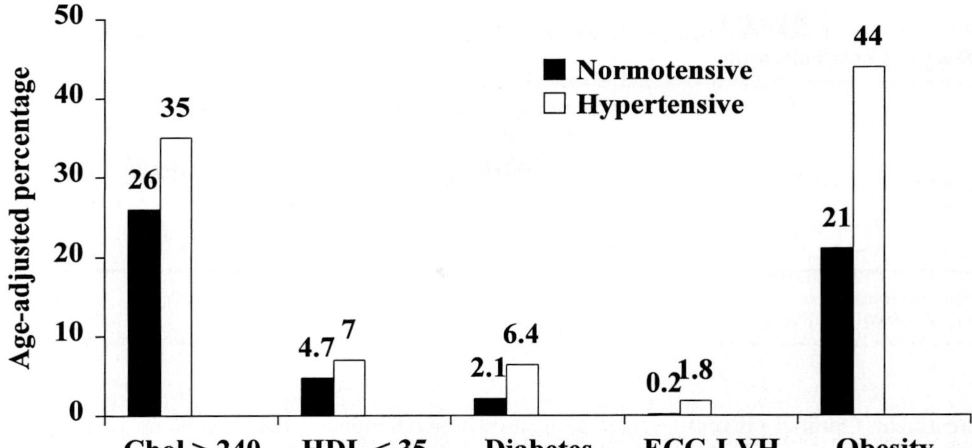

FIGURE 120–6 Prevalence of cardiovascular risk factors by hypertensive status in women aged 35 to 64 years: Framingham Heart Study, 1970–1982. ECG-LVH, electrocardiographic evidence of left ventricular hypertrophy; HDL, high-density lipoprotein.

decile of DBP at every age, except for those aged 35 to 39 years.[34]

In addition, elevated SBP appears to confer a greater *absolute risk* of CVD than does elevated DBP, especially with advancing age. As age increases, mean blood pressure levels tend to rise and the prevalence of hypertension increases. Beyond age 60 years, however, mean DBPs tend to plateau or fall, whereas SBPs continue to increase.[33, 34] Since the majority of CAD events and cardiovascular morbidity occur in older individuals, this trend appears to indicate greater risk conferred by SBP elevation than by DBP elevation. Kannel and coworkers[35] observed that SBP alone predicted the absolute risk of CAD better than did DBP alone. MRFIT data support this finding, with higher age-adjusted rates of CAD mortality for SBP compared with DBP in each blood pressure stage.[34]

Further evidence of the importance of systolic hypertension comes from two clinical trials. The SHEP[36] and SYST-EUR[37] trials were both double-blind, placebo-controlled studies evaluating treatment of isolated systolic hypertension in elderly patients. Both studies demonstrated significant reductions in stroke and other cardiovascular endpoints with active treatment versus placebo.

The risk associated with any degree of hypertension is influenced by the presence of target organ involvement and by the number and level of associated cardiovascular risk factors.[32] More often than in normotensive persons, hypertension occurs in conjunction with other risk factors, such as obesity, hyperlipidemia, and impaired glucose tolerance (Fig. 120–6). The excess cardiovascular risk in hypertensive persons is concentrated in those with an increased LDL-C/HDL-C ratio, impaired glucose tolerance, cigarette smoking, or electrocardiographic (ECG) abnormalities (Fig. 120–7). Therefore, hypertension is best conceptualized as a component of a multivariate CVD risk profile that is the best guide to the urgent need for pharmacologic

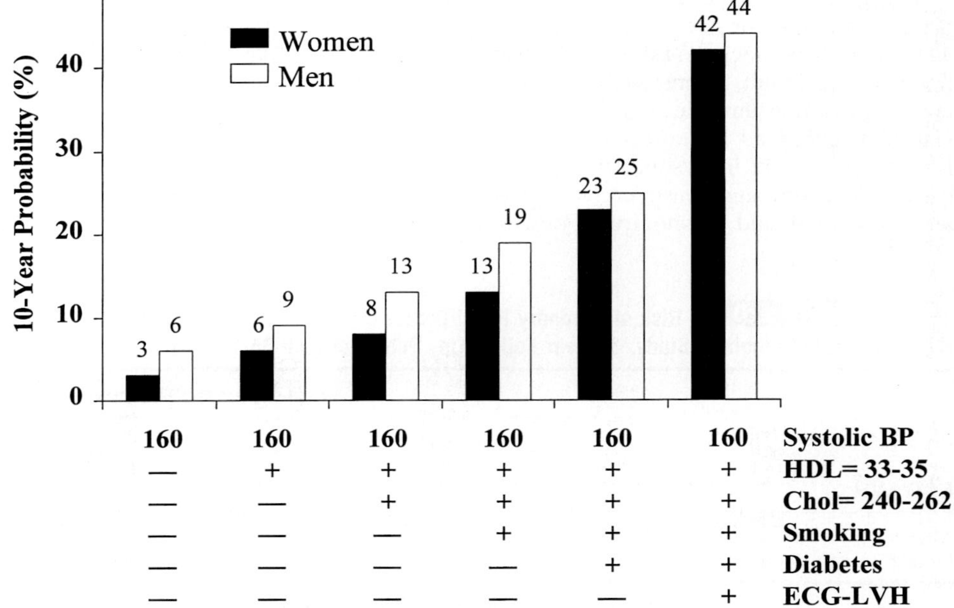

FIGURE 120–7 Predicted probabilities of CAD for men and women with hypertension, according to increasing burden of other risk factors. BP, blood pressure; ECG-LVH, electrocardiographic evidence of left ventricular hypertrophy; HDL, high-density lipoprotein.

TABLE 120–5 **Risk of Cardiovascular Events Imposed by Left Ventricular Hypertrophy, by Age in Each Sex: Framingham Study, 36-Year Follow-Up***

Cardiovascular Event	Age-Adjusted Biennial Rate per 1000		Risk Ratio†		Excess Risk per 1000	
	Men	*Women*	*Men*	*Women*	*Men*	*Women*
35–64	164	135	4.7	7.4	129	117
65–94	234	235	2.8	4.1	151	178

*Cardiovascular events are coronary heart disease, stroke, congestive heart failure, and intermittent claudication.
†All $P < 0.001$.
From Kannel WB, Cobb J: Risk factors in the cohort aged 85 and older. *In* Lewis B, Mancini M, Farinaro E (eds): Current Medical Literature. p. 3, 1992.

treatment. Optimal preventive management of hypertension requires multifactorial treatment to normalize all components of the cardiovascular risk profile before occurrence of target organ involvement. Drug treatment must be used carefully.

The incidence of hypertension continues unabated, despite improved detection and widespread treatment of the general population. In more advanced situations, long-standing hypertension is commonly associated with angina, MI, cardiac failure, renal insufficiency, peripheral vascular disease, retinopathy, stroke, or LVH. The choice of drug therapy for hypertension accompanied by any of these conditions varies and should be individualized for maximal impact on the associated conditions as well as the hypertension itself.[29] Screening for "silent" or unrecognized MIs should be routine, since they occur in marked excess in hypertensive persons.[38]

ECG evidence of LVH is an ominous harbinger of dangerous cardiovascular events and must not be regarded as an incidental accompaniment to hypertension, despite lack of symptoms (Table 120–5). Awaiting evidence of organ damage before treating is unwarranted because the first such evidence is often an MI, stroke, or sudden death. Anatomic and ECG evidence of LVH each independently indicate CAD risk (Table 120–6).

Selection of antihypertensive therapy to prevent coronary disease requires consideration of other factors. Diuretics and some beta-blockers may make management of the lipids more difficult. Agents such as alpha$_1$-blockers, angiotensin-converting enzyme inhibitors, and calcium antagonists that either do not affect or actually improve lipids may be preferable in dyslipidemic patients. For impaired cardiac function, angiotensin-converting enzyme inhibitors and diuretics should be preferred. For associated ischemia, β-blockers are preferable. Therefore, therapy for hypertension must take into consideration associated risk factors, concomitant disease, age, race, and side effect profile. Preceding the use of drug therapy, and concomitant with it, must come weight control, a decreased intake of salt, alcohol, and fat, potassium and magnesium supplementation, and comprehensive risk reduction. Hypertension is, after all, only a single ingredient of the CVD risk profile.

Although the relative risk of CVD sequelae is higher in those with markedly elevated blood pressure, this severe grade of hypertension is rarely seen. Therefore, the bulk of mortality associated with hypertension occurs in patients with mild-to-moderate elevations of blood pressure. Trials of antihypertensive therapy have demonstrated reduction in vascular sequelae, such as stroke, cardiac failure, and renal failure, with less impressive effects on the incidence of CAD events. Meta-analysis of the trial data concerning coronary heart disease has shown significant, but less than anticipated, lowering of coronary morbidity and mortality event rates.[39]

Reasons for the less impressive antihypertensive efficacy against CAD have been postulated. The trials may have been too short in duration to significantly affect atherosclerotic progression, and the sample sizes may have been too small to detect even a sizable reduction in coronary events. Furthermore, no attention was directed to whether the coronary risk profile was improved, and the drugs used are known to have adverse effects on blood lipids and glucose tolerance. There may also have been a predisposition to sudden death associated with some of the antihypertensive therapy used.

Because a large number of persons at risk with mild hypertension must be treated to benefit a few, drug treatment should be targeted at those with a poor cardiovascular

TABLE 120–6 **Risk of Coronary Heart Disease by Electrocardiographic and Roentgenographic Left Ventricular Hypertrophy: Framingham Study, 32-Year Follow-Up, Subjects Aged 35–64 Years**

	Age-Adjusted Biennial Rate per 1000			
	Men: X-Ray LVH		*Women: X-Ray LVH*	
ECG LVH	Absent	Present	Absent	Present
Absent	24	36	10	23
Present	85	100	45	62

Abbreviations: ECG, electrocardiographic; LVH, left ventricular hypertrophy; x-ray, roentgenographic.

risk profile, in which the bulk of candidates for events are concentrated. The criterion for successful intervention against hypertension should be improvement in the entire cardiovascular risk profile rather than reduction of blood pressure alone.

Atherogenic Living Habits

Certain elements of lifestyle greatly influence the incidence of CVD. These elements are typified by unrestrained weight gain, cigarette smoking, and sedentary habits.[10, 13] Type A behavior, characterized by an overdeveloped sense of time urgency, drive, and competitiveness, was noted to predispose to CAD and was shown in the Framingham Study to apply to women as well as to men.[40]

Moderate exercise was found to have a protective effect against CAD in young and old men in the Framingham cohort at any level of other risk factors. It is clearly useful as an adjunct to a comprehensive risk reduction program because it raises HDL-C, helps to lower blood pressure, improves glucose intolerance, and helps to control obesity.[41]

Epidemiologic data from Framingham and elsewhere have shown a protective effect of alcohol intake for CAD.[42] This benefit is not seen with alcohol abuse and is not applicable for stroke, which may be adversely affected. Alcohol raises HDL-C, but this is offset by induced rises in blood pressure and triglycerides with excessive use.

Smoking

The health hazards of smoking have been recognized for more than a century. Some 18 percent of all deaths in the United States in the early 1990s were attributed to cigarette smoking. Currently, cigarette smoking is responsible for nearly 20 percent of cardiovascular morbidity and mortality. Smoking-related illnesses cost the United States approximately $50 billion annually, a large percentage of which is related to CVD.[3]

Cigarette smoking is a powerful risk factor for atherosclerotic CVD. This is not unexpected, since smoking lowers HDL-C, raises fibrinogen, aggregates platelets, decreases the oxygen-carrying capacity of the blood, and causes release of catecholamines, making the myocardium more irritable.[43] These effects can and do precipitate coronary attacks and sudden deaths, particularly in coronary candidates who have other risk factors and a compromised arterial circulation. There is evidence suggesting that the risk for cardiovascular events such as CAD and peripheral arterial disease can be halved in those who quit compared with those who continue to smoke.[43] This benefit is achieved regardless of how long persons have previously smoked. Of the lifestyles that promote CVD, cigarette smoking predominates as the most powerful modifiable risk factor. The risk is related to the amount smoked daily, irrespective of the duration of the habit. The effect is independent of the associated risk factors but greater when these are present, so smoking enhances the risk associated with any risk factor. On quitting, the risk promptly reverts to half that of those who continue to smoke, approximating the risk of nonsmokers, in contrast to effects in non-CVD and overall mortality, for which a residual excess risk remains (Table 120–7). Of the CVDs, only peripheral arterial disease is associated with a residual effect on quitting smoking and an influence of the former amount smoked.

Switching to cigars or a pipe is ineffective because those who continue to smoke will inhale and be exposed to high levels of carbon monoxide and nicotine. The use of filter cigarettes does not reduce risk.

There has been a decline in the prevalence of cigarette smoking since the early 1970s, more pronounced in men than in women. However, those who continue to smoke have not reduced the amount. Men have higher cessation rates than women, as do those who are older and smoke less. Increased alcohol use is associated with a lower quit rate and so is cough, high coffee consumption, and a lower level of education. Filter use was also associated with a higher quit rate.

Persons who quit smoking differ little in their cardiovascular risk factors, except for a greater tendency for diabetics to quit smoking. After quitting, there is a short-term rise in weight in men, which leads to only trivial changes in blood pressure and serum cholesterol. There is a beneficial effect on HDL-C and long-term vital capacity. There are also improvements in oxygen transport, platelet aggregation, and fibrinogen levels.

Three randomized clinical trials of smoking abatement have not demonstrated the reduction in CAD mortality expected from results of observational studies. However, in these trials, too many subjects failed to remain in their assigned categories, and those who switched to pipe and/or cigar smoking were counted as a successful intervention. In addition, there was no objective measure to confirm quitting.

TABLE 120–7 Risk of Death by Cigarette Smoking Status: Framingham Study, Smokers of One Pack per Day for 30 Years

	Age-Adjusted Risk Ratio*			
	Men		*Women*	
Mortality	Continuing Smoker	Former Smoker	Continuing Smoker	Former Smoker
Overall	1.8	1.2	1.8	1.0
Cardiovascular	1.6	1.0	1.8	1.0
Cancer	2.2	1.4	1.6	1.0

*Compared with nonsmokers.

TABLE 120–8 **Weight Fluctuations and Changes in Cardiovascular Risk Factors at Biennial Examinations: Framingham Study**

Risk Factor	Influence of 10-Pound Weight Change on Risk Factor	
	Men	Women
Serum cholesterol (mg/dl)	7.6	5.4
Systolic blood pressure (mm Hg)	4.6	4.2
Blood glucose (mg/dl)	0.6	1.2

TABLE 120–9 **Risk Factor Clustering in Framingham Offspring Study Participants With Elevated Blood Pressure According to Body Mass Index, Subjects Aged 18–74 Years**

Men		Women	
Body Mass Index (kg/m²)	Average Number of Risk Factors	Body Mass Index (kg/m²)	Average Number of Risk Factors
<23.7	1.68 ± 0.91	<20.8	1.80 ± 0.87
23.7–25.5	1.85 ± 0.95	20.8–22.3	2.00 ± 1.02
25.6–27.2	2.06 ± 1.05	22.4–23.9	2.22 ± 1.06
27.3–29.5	2.28 ± 1.09	24.0–26.8	2.20 ± 0.99
≥29.5	2.35 ± 1.08	≥26.8	2.66 ± 1.09

Cessation of smoking is an important aspect of preventive management of survivors of MI or patients with angina pectoris. Many reports have indicated a reduction in fatal reinfarction or sudden death in this secondary prevention population.

There are few drugs or surgical procedures that offer as great a preventive benefit for candidates for cardiovascular events as cessation of cigarette smoking. Because cigarette smoking is such a powerful contributor to cardiovascular, pulmonary, and overall morbidity and mortality and is so highly prevalent and so potentially controllable, it deserves the highest priority among preventive measures against atherosclerotic and pulmonary disease.

Obesity

Weight gain is correlated with worsening of all the major cardiovascular risk factors, and weight loss improves them (Table 120–8). Obesity-related risk factors include hypertension, glucose intolerance, insulin resistance, hypertriglyceridemia, reduced HDL-C, and elevated fibrinogen.[44] Abdominal obesity was confirmed as a particularly atherogenic variety of adiposity because it causes insulin resistance, promoting a cluster of atherogenic risk factors (Fig. 120–8).[45] Largely, but not entirely, as a result of promoted atherogenic risk factors, weight gain is associated with an increased incidence of cardiovascular events.[46]

The long-term relationship between obesity and risk for CVD is strong for both men and women. Multivariate models (including covariates for age, cholesterol, SBP, cigarettes, LVH, and glucose intolerance) indicate in both genders that metropolitan relative weight is significantly associated with the development of CAD and congestive heart failure. In women, metropolitan relative weight is also associated with increased risk for stroke.[46]

The high and increasing prevalence of obesity in affluent countries, its multiple atherogenic concomitants, and its demonstrated association with cardiovascular morbidity and mortality make it a major health hazard. Because of this, a substantial amount of cardiovascular and other disease is attributable to uncontrolled weight gain. Controversy about the relation of body weight to morbidity and mortality has been generated by confounding effects of smoking, coexistent subclinical disease, and short lengths of follow-up. However, long-term follow-up from the Framingham Study of men and women under 50 years of age without other known risk factors did show an association with disease. Obesity is a major contributor to the high prevalence of hypertension, dyslipidemia, and diabetes in the general population. The average number of these risk factors increases with the degree of adiposity (Table 120–9). Weight reduction produces an improvement of all these components of the cardiovascular risk profile.

Body weights exceeding 20 percent above median or "desirable" weights constitute an established hazard to

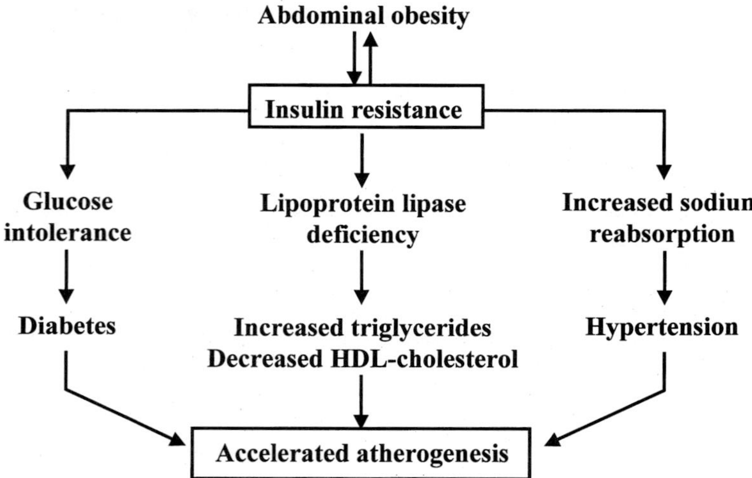

FIGURE 120–8 Pathophysiology of the insulin-resistance syndrome. HDL, high-density lipoprotein.

health. Central or abdominal patterns of obesity appear to have more deleterious metabolic effects. Central obesity has been shown to be related to CHD incidence in several studies.[45, 46] Among men and women in the Framingham Study aged 36 to 68 years, subscapular skinfold was found to be a stronger predictor of 22-year CVD incidence than body mass index in both genders, using logistical models adjusting for multiple risk factors (Table 120–10).

Although there are many unresolved issues, obesity control holds great promise for reducing the risk for many of the leading disabling and lethal illnesses. In some cases, weight control can, in itself, correct hypertension, diabetes, and dyslipidemia, and in other cases, it can reduce the drug dosage needed to treat these conditions. Although the rationale is sound and the potential benefits great, it must be admitted that convincing demonstration of the efficacy of correcting obesity is unlikely to be forthcoming because of the difficulty in achieving sustained weight loss over long periods.

The continued high prevalence of obesity and the ineffectiveness of treatment indicate a need to avoid substantial weight gain and a greater sense of urgency about reversing moderate weight increases. More information is needed about the possible hazards of repeated unsuccessful attempts to lose weight. Further progress in controlling obesity and its metabolic and disease consequences must await further insights into the pathogenesis of the condition and the lifestyles that promote it.

Body weight fluctuation can occur for a variety of reasons, one of which is dieting. Because multiple episodes of weight loss and regain are so common, it is important to examine the health implications of weight cycling. Data from the Western Electric Study[47] indicated that a single cycle of weight gain and loss in men was a positive risk factor for CAD death but not for total mortality. Similarly, data from the Gothenburg Prospective Study[48] revealed that body weight variability at three points in time was a risk factor for subsequent CAD in men and for total mortality in both genders. These results suggest that persons who undergo many or large body weight fluctuations are at greater risk for CAD and mortality than persons with stable body weights. These associations are generally independent of weight-for-height and temporal trends in weight and of a number of cardiovascular risk factors.

Further research is needed to examine independent effects of systematic weight change and weight variability, which will provide a better understanding of the long-term health implications of both voluntary and involuntary weight reduction. Examination of specific methods used for weight reduction may be an important issue for further investigation, which would help to clarify mechanisms by which weight fluctuation may affect health. Preliminary work in this area in animal models has suggested that dietary composition during weight loss/regain cycles may play a key role in the health outcomes.

If dieting is a major component of body weight fluctuation, the public health implications of current weight loss practices must be reexamined. Approximately 50 percent of American women and 25 percent of men are dieting at a given time, mostly without success. The rate of dieting in women is considerably higher than the rate of obesity, so that a great deal of weight fluctuation is occurring in individuals of normal weight. Although it may be premature to make clinical recommendations based on these findings, they do suggest that overweight individuals should be counseled in methods of maintaining weight loss and that relapse prevention must become a more central focus of weight-loss programs.

Other Established Risk Factors

Left Ventricular Hypertrophy

The importance of LVH as a diagnostic and prognostic entity in CVD has gained wide recognition. Noninvasive means are now available for detecting and measuring this condition. Although much has been learned about the precursors, prevalence, incidence, and prognostic outlook for LVH, many unresolved issues remain. Where does beneficial compensatory hypertrophy leave off and detrimental pathologic hypertrophy begin? How much does the ECG pattern of LVH reflect anatomic hypertrophy and how much ischemic myocardial damage? What is the indepen-

TABLE 120–10 Risk of Cardiovascular Events by Measures of Adiposity: Framingham Study, 24-Year Follow-Up, Subjects Aged 35–69 Years

Adiposity Measure	Ratio of 20-Year Age-Adjusted Rate for Q_5/Q_1					
	Coronary Disease		*Stroke*		*CVD*	
	Men	Women	Men	Women	Men	Women
Waist/height	1.6*	1.6*	1.5†	1.2‡	1.4*	1.4*
SSF/BMI	1.5*	1.7†	1.3§	2.4§	1.3†	1.7‡
SSF/TSF	1.6*	2.4*	1.3§	1.3§	1.5*	1.7*
SSF	1.8*	1.8*	1.3§	1.7†	1.4*	1.7†
BMI	1.8*	1.6*	1.2§	1.7†	1.5*	1.7*

Abbreviations: BMI, body mass index; CVD, coronary vascular disease (coronary disease, stroke, heart failure, and peripheral arterial disease); Q_1, lowest quartile; Q_5, highest quartile; SSF, subscapular skinfold; TSF, triceps skinfold.

*$P < .001$.

†$P < .01$.

‡$P < .05$.

§P = not significant.

Reprinted from Journal of Clinical Epidemiology, Vol. 44, Kannel WB, Cupples LA, Ramaswami R, et al, Regional obesity and risk of cardiovascular disease: the Framingham Study, p. 183, Copyright 1991, with permission from Elsevier Science.

dent contribution of electrocardiographically detectable LVH when anatomic hypertrophy is taken into account? How reversible is anatomic and ECG evidence of LVH, and do these parameters respond similarly to lowering of blood pressure and antihypertensive agents? Does regression of ECG and anatomic hypertrophy signify an improved prognosis compared with persistent LVH? Does the appearance of repolarization abnormality in the electrocardiogram with increased voltage indicate ischemic myocardial damage?

LVH has been investigated as a condition predisposing to CVD over 34 years of follow-up in the Framingham Study. Whether present on ECG examination, radiography, or echocardiography, LVH is an ominous harbinger of CVD.[49] It markedly increases the risk for CAD, cardiac failure, stroke, and peripheral arterial disease. This contribution to risk exceeds by threefold that of hypertension, the most common predisposing condition for LVH.

Age, blood pressure, and obesity are the three most common predisposing factors for LVH. Each contributes independently to the occurrence of electrocardiographically detectable LVH. Increases in left ventricular mass on the echocardiogram occur with age, but mostly as a consequence of the increasing prevalence of hypertension, obesity, CAD, and valvular disease with advancing age.

The risk associated with electrocardiographically detectable LVH is particularly great when repolarization abnormality is present along with increased voltage.[49] Electrocardiographically detectable LVH and silent MI are similar in evolution and prognosis. Once overt CAD occurs, electrocardiographically detectable LVH further escalates the risk for cardiovascular events.[50] The ECG evidence of LVH carries a more ominous prognosis than the anatomic evidence signified by radiographic enlargement. Because each independently contributes to risk, it is likely that the ECG and anatomic findings reflect different pathophysiology. Risk is greatest when both are present concomitantly (see Table 120–6).

Weight control and reduction of blood pressure can reduce left ventricular mass. When radiographic LVH reverts to normal, the risk for cardiovascular events is reduced by half that of those that persist (Table 120–11).

The serious prognosis of LVH indicates that it is more than an incidental finding in the course of hypertension and warrants vigorous preventive management. Therefore, when anatomic or ECG evidence of LVH appears, it must be regarded as a grave prognostic sign rather than an innocent compensatory phenomenon.

Family History

CAD tends to cluster in families, particularly among men with early-onset CAD, defined as onset at less than 50 years of age. Established risk factors for CAD, such as SBP, cholesterol, body weight, and cigarette smoking, have also been shown to cluster in families. There has been some question as to whether this is independent of other established risk factors that families tend to share. Therefore, whether or not family history is an independent risk factor remains controversial.

The Framingham Study explored how the impact of a positive family history of CAD varies with early versus late age of CAD onset in the offspring, among men versus women, and for mothers versus fathers dying of CAD. Data from the Framingham Study were analyzed to determine whether a parental history of death from CAD before or after age 65 years was an independent risk factor for CAD of early onset (<60 years) or late onset (≥60 years) among men and women of the cohort.

Parental death due to CAD was associated with a 28 percent increase in the risk for CAD, and the effect was apparently stronger for an early CAD outcome, with adjusted relative risks of 1.5 for early- and 1.2 for late-outcome CAD. The effect of parental CAD death on risk was not entirely mediated by other shared risk factors for CAD. These findings were similar for those with either a mother or a father with CAD, if CAD onset in the offspring occurred before the age of 60 years. For persons with CAD at age 60 years or older, maternal CAD death was a stronger predictor of CAD than was paternal CAD death. The parental history of CAD effects was similar for men and women in the cohort, with adjusted relative risks of 1.3 and 1.2, respectively. However, early age of parental CAD death may account for the association among women (risk ratio RR 1.64), whereas both early and late age of CAD death for either parent was associated with the risk for CAD among men (RR 1.3 and 1.4, respectively).[51] Colditz and associates[52] observed a similar tendency for an association with parental history of MI at 60 years of age or less in a prospective study of CAD in women.

Family history of CAD (parental death from CAD) is therefore a significant independent predictor of CAD when there is control for standard risk factors and length of follow-up. Among men with low risk for CAD by risk factor profile (i.e., nonsmoking, thin, nonhypertensive persons), more than two thirds of those who experience CAD have a positive family history. Therefore, CAD among persons predicted to be at low risk on the basis of standard risk factors may have a substantial genetic component. Although CAD risk can be reduced similarly for persons with a positive or a negative family history of CAD through modification of known risk factors, the residual risk associated with family history is not altered by modification of these factors. Despite an independent effect of family history, the risk for CAD is substantially less for persons with a favorable CAD risk profile, suggesting that preventive measures may be equally effective in persons with a positive family history.

RECENTLY ESTABLISHED RISK FACTORS

More recent additions to the list of CVD risk factors include elevated leukocyte count and fibrinogen levels; small, dense LDL; lipoprotein(a); homocysteine and low levels of certain B vitamins; and hyperinsulinemia.

White Blood Cell Count

Within the normal range of values, a high-normal white blood cell count and fibrinogen both appear to indicate increased risk for CVD and may suggest the presence

TABLE 120–11 **Risk for Cardiovascular Disease Events as a Function of Serial Electrocardiographic Changes**

Serial Electrocardiographic Change	Odds Ratio (95% Confidence Interval)	
	Men	*Women*
*Voltage Change**		
Serial voltage decrease	0.46 (0.26–0.84)	0.56 (0.30–1.04)
No change	1.00	1.00
Serial voltage increase	1.86 (1.14–3.03)	1.61 (0.91–2.84)
	119 events/1138 person-examinations	94 events/914 person-examinations
Repolarization Changes†		
Improved	0.45 (0.20–1.01)	1.19 (0.56–2.49)
No change	1.00	1.00
Worsened	1.89 (1.05–3.40)	2.02 (1.07–3.81)
	108 events/1097 person-examinations	79 events/850 person-examinations

Follow-up interval was from examination n + 1 to examination n + 2.
*Odds ratios for serial voltage changes (between examination n and examination n + 1) reflect adjustment for age and baseline voltage quartile at examination n.
†Odds ratios for serial repolarization changes (between examination n and examination n + 1) reflect adjustment for age and baseline repolarization at examination n.
From Levy D, Salomon M, D'Agostino RB, et al: Prognostic implications of baseline electrocardiographic features and their serial changes in subjects with left ventricular hypertrophy. Circulation 90(4):1786–1793, 1994.

of active, unstable atherosclerotic plaques. There is an inflammatory response to cholesterol and other components of the atheroma in the arterial intima. A high-normal white blood cell count in otherwise healthy persons may indicate such accelerated atherogenesis. A number of prospective epidemiologic studies have shown the incidence of coronary heart disease to be related to the antecedent white blood cell count.[53] In one study, white blood cell counts were obtained from 2794 men and women free of CVD aged 30 to 59 years in the Framingham Offspring Study. The white blood cell count was found to be significantly correlated with other CVD risk factors, most strongly with cigarette smoking. The 12-year age-adjusted incidence of CVD in general and CAD in particular increased progressively in each gender with each tertile increment in white blood cells (Table 120–12). There was an effect of the leukocyte count noted even after controlling for levels of other CVD risk factors. Each standard deviation increment in white blood cell count in men was associated with a 42 percent increment in CAD incidence. There was an apparent interaction with cigarette smoking in men, since the excess risk associated with a high-normal white blood cell count was confined to nonsmokers. Each 1000 increment in white blood cells was associated with a 32 percent increment in CVD in general and a 29 percent increment in CAD in particular.[54] Therefore, the impact of white blood count on risk rivals that of the other major risk factors.

TABLE 120–12 **Risk of Cardiovascular Disease Incidence by White Blood Cell Count: Framingham Offspring, 12-Year Follow-Up, Subjects Aged 30–59 Years**

Tertile of White Blood Cell Count	12-Year Age-Adjusted Rate per 1000	
	*Men**	*Women†*
1 (2600–5400/μl)	52	38
2 (5400–6900/μl)	122	43
3 (6900–14,200/μl)	169	71

*$P < .001$.
†$P < .05$.

Fibrinogen

Even within the usual range of values, fibrinogen has been shown to be another major independent atherogenic risk factor.[55, 56] Significant age-adjusted relationships were noted for CAD, stroke, and peripheral arterial disease in men (Table 120–13). In women, a significant relationship to cardiac failure, but not to stroke, was also noted. CVD, CAD, and all-cause mortality were related to fibrinogen in both genders after age adjustment and after adjustment for the major risk factors. A high-normal fibrinogen value was noted to enhance risk, particularly in hypertensives and cigarette smokers. About half the risk associated with cigarette smoking could be attributed to higher fibrinogen values. A number of prospective studies have now documented excessive cardiovascular events in association with elevated fibrinogen. Each standard deviation increase in fibrinogen is associated with a 1.6-fold increase in CAD incidence, a risk ratio close to that observed for elevated cholesterol.

High-normal and elevated fibrinogen levels may act to increase the risk of CVD by promoting a prothrombotic milieu through increased blood viscosity, increased platelet aggregability, increased fibrin formation, and possibly, through direct infiltration of the vascular wall by fibrinogen. Although it is not entirely clear that fibrinogen bears a causal relationship to CVD, its strong independent association with CVD events makes it at least an important marker of high risk.

Small, Dense LDL

Subclasses of LDL particles have also been studied in relation to the risk of incident CAD. Small, dense LDLs in

TABLE 120-13 Risk of Cardiovascular Events by Tertile of Fibrinogen: Framingham Study, 18-Year Follow-Up, Persons Aged 47–79 Years

	Absolute Risk per 1000 (T_3)		Risk Ratio (T_3/T_1)	
Cardiovascular Event	*Men*	*Women*	*Men*	*Women*
Coronary heart disease	430	296	1.6*	2.6†
Stroke	187	224	1.9‡	2.0‡
Peripheral arterial disease	113	68	1.6‡	1.7§
All cardiovascular events	611	514	1.5†	2.1†

Abbreviations: T_1, lowest tertile of fibrinogen levels; T_3, highest tertile of fibrinogen levels.
*$P < .01$.
†$P < .001$.
‡P = not significant.
§$P < .05$.
Reprinted from Annals of Epidemiology, Vol. 2, Kannel WB, D'Agostino RB, Belanger AJ, Update on fibrinogen as a cardiovascular risk factor, p. 457, Copyright 1992, with permission from Elsevier Science.

particular appear to confer increased risk of CAD.[57, 58] These particles appear to be highly atherogenic owing to their low binding affinity for the LDL receptor, prolonged plasma half-life, avidity for uptake into arterial intima, and susceptibility to oxidation. These types of particles occur at higher levels in patients with combined hyperlipidemia manifesting with high triglyceride and low HDL levels, and in diabetics, and they appear to play an important role in conferring excess risk associated with these conditions.

Lipoprotein(a)

Lipoprotein(a) is an LDL particle containing surface apoprotein(a). The remarkable structural homology between apoprotein(a) and plasminogen has led to speculation that lipoprotein(a) may provide a mechanistic link between atherogenesis and thrombosis. Numerous case-control[59] and several prospective studies have reported an association between lipoprotein(a) levels and all manifestations of CVD in men[60] and women.[61] However, two other prospective studies did not observe an association,[62, 63] possibly due to methodologic issues.

Homocysteine and B Vitamins

In the 1960s, it was noted that patients with inborn errors of metabolism affecting the sulfur-containing amino acids methionine and homocysteine had increased rates of CVD. In the classic example, patients with hereditary homocystinuria, caused by homozygous deficiency of the enzyme cystathionine beta-synthase, were noted to have markedly elevated plasma homocysteine levels and strikingly high rates of premature morbidity and mortality from CVD. This led to intensive investigation into the possible association between elevated levels of homocysteine (hyperhomocysteinemia) in patients without homocystinuria and potential mechanisms of homocysteine-related atherogenesis.

Numerous case-control studies using patients with vascular disease have demonstrated higher levels of homocysteine in affected individuals than in unaffected controls. However, the most compelling evidence of a link between hyperhomocysteinemia and CVD has come from large prospective population studies. Investigators from the Physicians' Health Study reported that elevated levels of homocysteine were a potent independent risk factor for MI, with an apparent threshold for increased risk at homocysteine levels above 15.8 nmol/ml.[64] Other studies have reported increased relative risks for CAD, cerebrovascular disease, and peripheral arterial disease in hyperhomocysteinemia. Boushey and colleagues[65] performed a meta-analysis of 27 studies relating hyperhomocysteinemia to CVD. They reported that the odds ratios for CAD associated with a 5 mmol/L increment in fasting total homocysteine were 1.6 (95 percent CI, 1.4 to 1.7) for men and 1.8 (95 percent CI, 1.4 to 2.3) for women. Hyperhomocysteinemia accounted for an estimated 10 percent of the population-attributable risk of CAD. The odds ratios for cerebrovascular and peripheral arterial disease in men and women combined were 1.5 (95 percent CI, 1.3 to 1.9) and 6.8 (95 percent CI, 2.9 to 15.8), respectively.

Specific mutations in genes coding for enzymes in the metabolic pathways of homocysteine have been characterized and found to occur at high rates in some populations, with differing effects on homocysteine levels and risk for CVD. Currently available evidence suggests that hyperhomocysteinemia has direct cytotoxic effects on the endothelium. In addition, homocysteine appears to have functional prothrombotic effects on endothelium, platelets, and coagulation factors and inhibitory effects on the actions of endogenous anticoagulant and fibrinolytic molecules. However, many of these mechanistic and cellular studies were performed using markedly supraphysiologic doses of homocysteine. Taken together, these data provide evidence for the role of homocysteine as a novel risk factor for CVD. Questions remain as to whether elevated homocysteine concentrations merely reflect the presence of subclinical atherosclerotic or renal disease and thus serve only as a risk marker.

Folate is a substrate and vitamins B_6 and B_{12} are cofactors in the metabolic pathways involving homocysteine. Dietary deficiency and/or low blood levels of these compounds might therefore be expected to elevate homocysteine levels and increase risk for CVD. Various studies have now linked low-normal folate levels and low pyridoxine levels as well as low dietary intakes of these nutrients with both hyperhomocysteinemia and increased risk for CAD, stroke, and peripheral arterial disease.[66] Deficiencies of these nutrients may also act to increase risk of CVD through mechanisms other than homocysteine metabolism. Antioxidant properties and other metabolic effects of these nutrients have been proposed as independent mechanisms by which deficiency may lead to atherosclerosis. A link between low vitamin B_{12} levels and risk of CVD has not been convincingly demonstrated.

Hyperinsulinemia/Metabolic Syndrome

A number of risk factors have been observed to cluster into a metabolic syndrome (alternatively termed the *insulin-resistance syndrome, syndrome X,* or *Reaven's syndrome*[44]) in which insulin resistance and hyperinsulinemia appear to play a central, if not causative, role. The features of this syndrome include truncal obesity, hypertension, hypertriglyceridemia, low HDL, and hyperinsulinemia with or without glucose intolerance or frank diabetes. These patients also tend to have lipid profiles with small, dense LDL particles, postprandial lipemia, and increased plasminogen activator inhibitor-1 levels. In many cases, hyperglycemia is preceded by development of the other risk factors and becomes manifest only late in the development of the syndrome. With the concurrence of these several risk factors in a single individual, the risk for CAD is obviously markedly increased. Because a uniform definition of this syndrome has not been universally adopted, it is difficult to compare clinical and epidemiologic studies attempting to quantify the prevalence of this pattern and the risk in affected individuals. Several studies have reported a relationship between insulin levels and incident CVD in men, after adjustment for other risk factors. Despres and coworkers[67] reported an adjusted odds ratio of 1.6 (95 percent CI, 1.1 to 2.3) for each one standard deviation increase in fasting insulin level among French Canadian men. Pyorala and associates[68] followed 970 men for 22 years and observed a higher incidence of CHD events in those in the highest quintile of plasma insulin level compared with the lower four quintiles. At 5-, 10-, 15-, and 22-year follow-up, the multivariable-adjusted hazard ratios for CHD in the highest quintile were 2.36 (95 percent CI, 1.00 to 5.57), 2.29 (95 percent CI, 1.31 to 4.02), 1.76 (95 percent CI, 1.09 to 2.82), and 1.32 (95 percent CI, 0.89 to 1.97), respectively. Data regarding a relationship between hyperinsulinemia and CVD in women are sparse.

Potential Risk Factors Under Investigation

Infection and Inflammation

There has been increasing interest in the role of inflammation and infectious agents in atherogenesis and risk of clinical CVD events. Histopathologic and molecular studies have clearly demonstrated the important pathophysiologic role played by inflammatory cells and inflammatory mediators such as cytokines. In addition, systemic indicators of subclinical inflammation have been found to be higher in subjects who subsequently develop CVD. For example, Ridker and colleagues[69] observed higher levels of plasma C-reactive protein, an acute-phase reactant, among men in the Physicians' Health Study who developed CHD over the ensuing 8 years, compared with those who remained free of CHD. A similar result was observed among women in the Nurses' Health Study.[70] These higher levels of C-reactive protein were still within the normal range. Interestingly, the risk of CVD was attenuated among men with higher C-reactive protein who were taking aspirin, suggesting that aspirin's salutary effects on reduction of CHD might be mediated in part through an anti-inflammatory mechanism.[69]

One possible mechanism that has been proposed as a link between inflammation and CVD events is chronic endovascular infection. Seroprevalence studies have implicated certain infectious agents as possible contributors to atherogenesis and pathogenesis of acute coronary syndromes. Higher titers of antibodies to *Chlamydia pneumoniae* and cytomegalovirus have been observed in patients with CHD in retrospective case-control studies. Other investigators have noted incorporation of DNA from infectious pathogens among atherosclerotic material retrieved from coronary atherectomy specimens. Secondary prevention trials examining the use of antibiotic therapy directed against chlamydial infection have been undertaken. In one such study, 202 unstable angina patients were randomized to receive either roxithromycin or placebo for 30 days. Over 6 months of follow-up, there was a lower rate of recurrent CHD events among subjects receiving active therapy.[71] These data are intriguing, but further work is needed to understand the potential mechanisms whereby infection may precipitate or promote atherothrombosis and whether treatment is truly effective in reducing events.

Iron Excess

Excess stores of body iron have been proposed as a possible risk factor for CHD. Basic science research has provided interesting data linking increased iron levels with higher potential for atherogenesis through increasing free radical formation and oxidation of lipids. Although these data provide a plausible mechanism for excess body iron stores in atherogenesis, findings from epidemiologic studies have been inconsistent in demonstrating an association. A large epidemiologic study in Finland has consistently implicated excess iron as a risk factor for CHD.[72, 73] However, other reports have not demonstrated any association.[74, 75] One significant problem has been the lack of a universally accepted method of measuring iron status. Further investigation, including basic research and epidemiologic studies, is needed to examine the potential association between iron status and the risk of CVD. At present, the data do not support screening for iron overload as a means to assess risk for CVD; likewise, dietary recommendations for restriction of iron intake are not warranted.

Relevance of Risk Factors in the Elderly

Atherosclerotic CVD is the leading cause of morbidity and mortality in older persons. Among the elderly, the relative risks associated with some of the major risk factors are somewhat attenuated, but this is offset by a higher absolute risk of developing CVD than in younger individuals, owing to advancing age. As discussed previously, even persons who reach age 70 years free of CAD have a high risk of developing it during their remaining life span. The multivariate risk profile predicts CAD as efficiently in the elderly as in younger groups, making it feasible to target higher-risk candidates for risk factor intervention.[76] Hypertension is a dominant risk factor for CVD in the elderly, and isolated systolic hypertension is particularly common and hazardous in this age group.[77] The total cholesterol/HDL-C ratio and triglycerides continue to be relevant in the elderly.[78] Diabetes remains a major risk factor, particularly in women, and the presence of LVH continues to be ominous. Elevated fibrinogen also remains a risk factor even at advanced ages.

Primary prevention clinical trials have shown reductions in CVD endpoints in older populations. Two trials of antihypertensive therapy in older persons with isolated systolic hypertension have been remarkably positive, particularly with respect to stroke prevention.[36, 37] Similarly, subgroup analyses of two large cholesterol-lowering primary prevention trials indicate that the benefit of cholesterol reduction extends to those over age 60 years.[20, 21] Ongoing clinical trials will help determine whether these benefits are observed at even older ages and whether other risk factor modification strategies may benefit the elderly.

Importance of Multivariate Risk Assessment

As is evident from the previous discussion, no single risk factor can adequately predict the occurrence of CVD in an individual. Therefore, an approach of global risk assessment of all CVD risk factors has been recommended to clinicians.[79] To this end, several instruments are now available that can help assess an individual's expected risk of CVD within a given time frame. These instruments have typically been devised from multivariate risk equations derived from large-scale epidemiologic studies.

Optimal risk prediction requires a quantitative synthesis of the various independently contributing risk factors into a composite estimate. For this purpose, multivariate risk functions are employed to quantify the combined effect of these risk factors, with consideration for their interactions.[80] This concept takes into account the multifactorial elements of cardiovascular risk and the continuous gradient of response.

Although categorical assessment of risk by assignment of arbitrary values to designate the point at which a continuous variable, such as blood pressure or blood lipid, is to be considered a risk factor has pragmatic utility, this procedure is not efficient because it tends to overlook those patients at high risk because of multiple marginal abnormalities. Multivariate risk formulations incorporating the major identified risk factors can quantitatively assess risk over a wide range. For office use in assessing risk, scoring systems have been devised based on multiple risk formulations, which provide estimates of risk for various combinations of risk factors at specified ages in each gender (Fig. 120–9).

These risk formulations have been shown to accurately predict disease in a variety of American population samples and in older approximately as well as in young population samples. Addition of other risk factor information adds little to the multivariate risk formulation. For example, the addition of DBP, triglyceride, weight, physical activity, and family history does not enhance the risk estimation, but these factors are important in making decisions regarding implementation of therapy.

Preventive Implications of Risk Factor Detection and Control

CAD is now the most common and most lethal sequela of hypertension, dyslipidemia, glucose intolerance, elevated fibrinogen, and cigarette smoking. These risk factors tend to cluster, and the risk associated with any one is markedly influenced by the others, so that optimal prophylaxis must improve the multivariate risk profile. Therefore, optimal preventive management of hypertension should not impose a penalty of dyslipidemia or glucose intolerance, and more than normalization of the blood pressure is required if CAD is to be prevented. The multivariate risk profile provides the best basis for decisions regarding choice and urgency of treatment.

The total cholesterol/HDL-C ratio is a practical indicator of the joint effect of LDL and HDL entering and leaving the arteries. Optimal lipid-lowering therapy should improve this ratio to a goal of 3.5/total HDL, which corresponds to half the high-average North American risk. For maximal effect, other risk factors should be concomitantly controlled.

Most of the known, highly prevalent risk factors are pharmaceutically modifiable. Impaired glucose tolerance, obesity, low HDL-C, hypertriglyceridemia, and hypertension are metabolically linked and, in combination, are intensely atherogenic. Drug therapy that improves this syndrome should be sought. Thrombogenic tendencies must also be corrected. Increased fibrinogen concentration also tends to occur in association with other risk factors and enhances their impact. The efficacy of pharmaceuticals that lower fibrinogen must therefore be tested. LVH is an ominous harbinger of CAD, cardiac failure, stroke, and sudden death. It can be prevented by early treatment of hypertension, but reversal of LVH may be antihypertensive drug specific. Hygienic measures such as weight control, avoidance of cigarettes, exercise, and modified diet are a useful adjunct to drug therapies. The complex atherosclerotic process affords opportunities for preventive pharmaceutical intervention at each stage in its evolution.

Because of the nature and magnitude of the problem of CAD, it is not prudent to rely on sophisticated innovations in the diagnosis or treatment of symptomatic CAD. Only a preventive approach can make a substantial impact.

Although the final link in the chain of evidence incriminating CAD risk factors remains to be forged for many of the suspected contributors, a number of recommendations seem warranted. In subjects with an ominous cardiovascular risk profile, serious attention to modifiable risk factors is justified. The primary approach should be hygienic.

Step 1

Age		
Years	LDL Pts	Chol Pts
30-34	-1	[-1]
35-39	0	[0]
40-44	1	[1]
45-49	2	[2]
50-54	3	[3]
55-59	4	[4]
60-64	5	[5]
65-69	6	[6]
70-74	7	[7]

Step 2

LDL - C		
(mg/dl)	(mmol/L)	LDL Pts
<100	<2.59	-3
100-129	2.60-3.36	0
130-159	3.37-4.14	0
160-190	4.15-4.92	1
≥190	≥4.92	2

Cholesterol		
(mg/dl)	(mmol/L)	Chol Pts
<160	<4.14	[-3]
160-199	4.15-5.17	[0]
200-239	5.18-6.21	[1]
240-279	6.22-7.24	[2]
≥280	≥7.25	[3]

Step 3

HDL - C			
(mg/dl)	(mmol/L)	LDL Pts	Chol Pts
<35	<0.90	2	[2]
35-44	0.91-1.16	1	[1]
45-49	1.17-1.29	0	[0]
50-59	1.30-1.55	0	[0]
≥60	≥1.56	-1	[-2]

Step 4

Blood Pressure					
Systolic (mm Hg)	Diastolic (mm Hg)				
	<80	80-84	85-89	90-99	≥100
<120	0 [0] pts				
120-129		0 [0] pts			
130-139			1 [1] pts		
140-159				2 [2] pts	
≥160					3 [3] pts

Note: When systolic and diastolic pressures provide different estimates for point scores, use the higher number

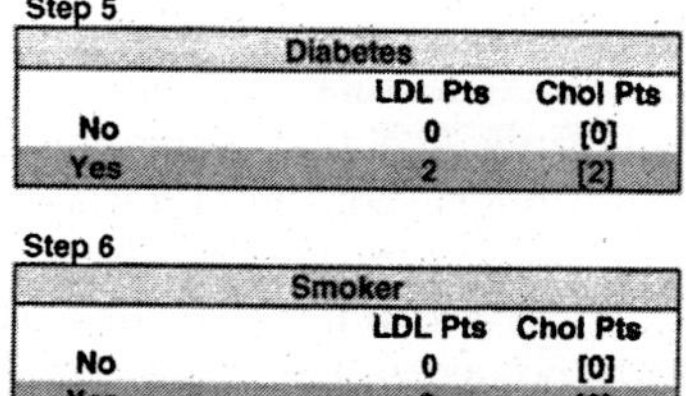

Step 5

Diabetes		
	LDL Pts	Chol Pts
No	0	[0]
Yes	2	[2]

Step 6

Smoker		
	LDL Pts	Chol Pts
No	0	[0]
Yes	2	[2]

A

Step 7 (sum from steps 1-6)

Adding up the points	
Age	______
LDL-C or Chol	______
HDL - C	
Blood Pressure	______
Diabetes	______
Smoker	______
Point total	______

Key	
Color	Relative Risk
green	Very low
white	Low
yellow	Moderate
rose	High
red	Very high

Step 8 (determine CHD risk from point total)

CHD Risk			
LDL Pts Total	10 Yr CHD Risk	Chol Pts Total	10 Yr CHD Risk
<-3	1%		
-2	2%		
-1	2%	[<-1]	[2%]
0	3%	[0]	[3%]
1	4%	[1]	[3%]
2	4%	[2]	[4%]
3	6%	[3]	[5%]
4	7%	[4]	[7%]
5	9%	[5]	[8%]
6	11%	[6]	[10%]
7	14%	[7]	[13%]
8	18%	[8]	[16%]
9	22%	[9]	[20%]
10	27%	[10]	[25%]
11	33%	[11]	[31%]
12	40%	[12]	[37%]
13	47%	[13]	[45%]
≥14	≥56%	[≥14]	[≥53%]

Step 9 (compare to average person your age)

Comparative Risk			
Age (years)	Average 10 Yr CHD Risk	Average 10 Yr Hard* CHD Risk	Low** 10 Yr CHD Risk
30-34	3%	1%	2%
35-39	5%	4%	3%
40-44	7%	4%	4%
45-49	11%	8%	4%
50-54	14%	10%	6%
55-59	16%	13%	7%
60-64	21%	20%	9%
65-69	25%	22%	11%
70-74	30%	25%	14%

* Hard CHD events exclude angina pectoris

** Low risk was calculated for a person the same age, normal blood pressure, LDL-C 100-129 mg/dL or cholesterol 160-199 mg/dL, HDL-C 45 mg/dL for men or 55 mg/dL for women, non-smoker, no diabetes

Risk estimates were derived from the experience of the Framingham Heart Study, a predominantly Caucasian population in Massachusetts, USA

FIGURE 120–9 A and **B,** Coronary heart disease (CHD) score sheets for men and women from the Framingham risk prediction model. The model uses age, total (or fasting low-density lipoprotein [LDL]-) cholesterol, high-density lipoprotein (HDL)-cholesterol, blood pressure, diabetes, and smoking status to estimate risk over a period of 10 years based on men and women 30 to 74 years old at baseline. pts, points. (**A** and **B,** From Wilson PW, D'Agostino RB, Levy D, et al: Prediction of coronary heart disease using risk factor categories. Circulation 97[18]:1837–1847, 1998.)

Illustration continued on following page

In the management of most lipid problems, the focus should be on diet, weight control, and exercise. Because dietary cholesterol and saturated fat have both been shown to raise LDL-C, intake of these nutrients should be reduced. Excessive calories raise both LDL and VLDL and lower HDL, making weight control important. HDL can be raised not only by weight control but by exercising, quitting smoking, increasing fish intake, and moderating use of alcohol. Although some measures taken to reduce LDL occasionally lower HDL as well, the LDL/HDL ratio is usually improved by LDL-lowering regimens. In high-risk coronary candidates unresponsive to hygienic measures, an improvement in the LDL/HDL ratio may be achieved by lipid-lowering drugs. Of these, the statins, fibric acid derivatives, and nicotinic acid also raise HDL.

The atherogenic effects of blood lipids require decades to produce clinical disease, and hence major clinical benefits should not be expected from corrective measures over a

Step 1

Age		
Years	LDL Pts	Chol Pts
30-34	-9	[-9]
35-39	-4	[-4]
40-44	0	[0]
45-49	3	[3]
50-54	6	[6]
55-59	7	[7]
60-64	8	[8]
65-69	8	[8]
70-74	8	[8]

Step 2

LDL - C		
(mg/dl)	(mmol/L)	LDL Pts
<100	<2.59	-2
100-129	2.60-3.36	0
130-159	3.37-4.14	0
160-190	4.15-4.92	2
≥190	≥4.92	2

Cholesterol		
(mg/dl)	(mmol/L)	Chol Pts
<160	<4.14	[-2]
160-199	4.15-5.17	[0]
200-239	5.18-6.21	[1]
240-279	6.22-7.24	[1]
≥280	≥7.25	[3]

Step 3

HDL - C			
(mg/dl)	(mmol/L)	LDL Pts	Chol Pts
<35	<0.90	5	[5]
35-44	0.91-1.16	2	[2]
45-49	1.17-1.29	1	[1]
50-59	1.30-1.55	0	[0]
≥60	≥1.56	-2	[-3]

Step 4

Blood Pressure					
Systolic (mm Hg)	Diastolic (mm Hg) <80	80-84	85-89	90-99	≥100
<120	-3 [-3] pts				
120-129		0 [0] pts			
130-139			0 [0] pts		
140-159				2 [2] pts	
≥160					3 [3] pts

+ Note: When systolic and diastolic pressures provide different estimates for point scores, use the higher number

Step 5

Diabetes		
	LDL Pts	Chol Pts
No	0	[0]
Yes	4	[4]

Step 6

Smoker		
	LDL Pts	Chol Pts
No	0	[0]
Yes	2	[2]

B

(sum from steps 1-6)

Step 7

Adding up the points	
Age	______
LDL-C or Chol	______
HDL - C	______
Blood Pressure	______
Diabetes	______
Smoker	______
Point total	______

Key	
Color	Relative Risk
green	Very low
white	Low
yellow	Moderate
rose	High
red	Very high

(determine CHD risk from point total)

Step 8

CHD Risk			
LDL Pts Total	10 Yr CHD Risk	Chol Pts Total	10 Yr CHD Risk
≤-2	1%	[≤-2]	[1%]
-1	2%	[-1]	[2%]
0	2%	[0]	[2%]
1	2%	[1]	[2%]
2	3%	[2]	[3%]
3	3%	[3]	[3%]
4	4%	[4]	[4%]
5	5%	[5]	[4%]
6	6%	[6]	[5%]
7	7%	[7]	[6%]
8	8%	[8]	[7%]
9	9%	[9]	[8%]
10	11%	[10]	[10%]
11	13%	[11]	[11%]
12	15%	[12]	[13%]
13	17%	[13]	[15%]
14	20%	[14]	[18%]
15	24%	[15]	[20%]
16	27%	[16]	[24%]
≥17	≥32%	[≥17]	[≥27%]

(compare to average person your age)

Step 9

Comparative Risk			
Age (years)	Average 10 Yr CHD Risk	Average 10 Yr Hard* CHD Risk	Low** 10 Yr CHD Risk
30-34	<1%	<1%	<1%
35-39	<1%	<1%	1%
40-44	2%	1%	2%
45-49	5%	2%	3%
50-54	8%	3%	5%
55-59	12%	7%	7%
60-64	12%	8%	8%
65-69	13%	8%	8%
70-74	14%	11%	8%

* Hard CHD events exclude angina pectoris

** Low risk was calculated for a person the same age, normal blood pressure, LDL-C 100-129 mg/dL or cholesterol 160-199 mg/dL, HDL-C 45 mg/dL for men or 55 mg/dL for women, non-smoker, no diabetes

Risk estimates were derived from the experience of the Framingham Heart Study, a predominantly Caucasian population in Massachusetts, USA

FIGURE 120–9 *Continued*

short period of time. The improvement in the lipid profile is typically discernible in a month. Although cellular fat deposits may shrink in weeks, extracellular fat deposits require a year or more to change significantly. Even the mass of fibrous lesions can sometimes be reduced, but this may require 4 or more years of vigorous treatment. Nevertheless, a disproportionate reduction in clinical events has been observed for the rheologically trivial amount of regression induced in the trials. This suggests that treatment may also be stabilizing dangerous lesions.

Control of obesity is one of the chief hygienic measures available to reduce the major cardiovascular risk factors, including hypertension, lipid abnormalities, and hyperglycemia. Obesity is easier to avoid than to correct. A greater sense of urgency is needed concerning correction of modest weight gain, since this often leads insidiously to intractable obesity.

The efficacy of treating diabetes to prevent cardiovascular sequelae has been questioned. It appears more rational to redefine *control* to include normalization of all the multiple metabolic aberrations common to the diabetic state, including the abnormal blood lipids, overweight, and hypertension.

It does not seem wise to rely on physical exercise programs alone to protect against fatal CAD. Physical exercise is best prescribed as one component of a comprehensive program for avoiding CAD. Activities that require movement over a distance seem most valuable. Sustained regular exercise of moderate intensity (50 to 75 percent capacity) for 15 to 30 minutes at least every other day is required to maintain a training effect. However, there is some evidence that lesser levels of exercise may also be beneficial. A vigorous walking program may be more prudent for middle-aged, deconditioned Americans. This will also tend to minimize the considerable orthopedic side effects of vigorous exercise such as jogging.

Because even moderate degrees of hypertension have been shown to double the risk of a coronary event and because the Hypertension Detection and Follow-Up Program has demonstrated the efficacy of treating this mild hypertension, it is especially important to treat this group. However, it can be shown that the bulk of the cardiovascular sequelae in this mild hypertension is concentrated in a small percentage of patients who have other accompanying cardiovascular risk factors and hence a poor cardiovascular profile. It seems best, therefore, to reserve drug treatment for these individuals and to urge hygienic treatment with weight reduction and salt restriction for the remainder of mild hypertensives. The latter must be followed, as hypertension tends to progress and drug treatment may be required at a later stage. Evidence from the Systolic Hypertension Elderly Program and the SYST-EUR trial indicates the efficacy of treating isolated systolic hypertension in the elderly to prevent not only stroke but also CAD.[36, 37]

Despite mandatory warnings on each package that cigarette smoking is hazardous to health, teenagers take up the habit as often as formerly, and teenage girls and younger women are smoking considerably more. Physicians as a group have shown a greater decline in smoking than the general population and can serve as a good role model. However, most are not vigorous or conscientious enough in dispensing this advice or in checking on compliance. They do not always raise the question of smoking in connection with the findings of vascular disease, and do even less so in general health examinations. In addition, most physicians seldom solicit help from the family in getting a patient to quit smoking.

Because of the tenacity of the cigarette habit and the powerful vested interests protecting the tobacco industry, an attempt to develop a "safer" cigarette has been undertaken. The tar and nicotine content has been reduced, largely through the introduction of filter cigarettes. Evidence from Framingham and other studies indicates that this has been of little benefit in reducing the hazard of CVD.

Effective risk factor control will require mobilization of community resources to assist in the endeavor. Such measures should be multidisciplinary and should begin as early in life as possible, when the faulty habits are conditioned and atheromatous lesions are still only in the formative stage. The entire family should be involved in risk factor modification for the high-risk subject. Physicians must develop the preventive skills needed to encourage the behavior modification required. Although the rewards may lie decades in the future, physicians must recognize that such an endeavor will have a greater impact on their patients' ultimate well-being than almost anything else that may be done for their patients.

REFERENCES

1. Hill AB: The environment and disease: association or causation? Proc R Soc Med 58:295, 1965.
2. Hennekens CH, Buring JE: Epidemiology in Medicine. Boston: Little, Brown, 1987.
3. American Heart Association: 1998 Heart and Stroke Statistical Update. Dallas: American Heart Association, 1997.
4. Anderson RN, Kochanek KD, Murphy SL: Report of final mortality statistics, 1995. Monthly Vital Statistics Report. Vol. 45. No. 11. Suppl. 2. Hyattsville, MD: National Center for Health Statistics, 1997.
5. National Heart, Lung, and Blood Institute: Morbidity and Mortality: 1996 Chartbook on Cardiovascular, Lung, and Blood Diseases. Bethesda, MD: National Institutes of Health, Public Health Service, U.S. Department of Health and Human Services, 1996.
6. Lloyd-Jones DM, Larson MG, Beiser A, Levy D: Lifetime risk of developing coronary heart disease. Lancet 353:89–92, 1999.
7. Rosamond WD, Chambless LE, Folsom AR, et al: Trends in the incidence of myocardial infarction and in mortality due to coronary heart disease, 1987 to 1994. N Engl J Med 339:861, 1998.
8. Cupples LA, D'Agostino RB, Kiely D: The Framingham Study. An Epidemiological Investigation of Cardiovascular Disease. Sect. 34. Some Risk Factors Related to the Annual Incidence of Cardiovascular Disease and Death Using Pooled Repeated Biennial Measurements Framingham Heart Study, 30 Year Follow-Up. Bethesda, MD: National Heart, Lung, and Blood Institute, 1987.
9. Kannel WB, McGee DL: Diabetes and glucose tolerance as risk factors for cardiovascular disease: the Framingham Study. Diabetes Care 2:120, 1979.
10. Kannel WB: Bishop lecture. Contribution of the Framingham Study to preventive cardiology. J Am Coll Cardiol 15:206, 1990.
11. Wilson PWF: Importance of lipid fractions for coronary morbidity and mortality. Cholesterol et Prevention Primaire: a qui s'addressent les regimes de prevention cardiovasculaire? 1st ed. pp. 73–80. Paris: CIDIL, 1990.
12. Manson JE, Tosteson H, Ridker PM, et al: The primary prevention of myocardial infarction. N Engl J Med 326:1406, 1992.
13. Report of Inter-Society Commission for Heart Disease Resources: Optimal resources for primary prevention of atherosclerotic diseases. Circulation 70:157A, 1984.
14. Gotto AM Jr, LaRosa JC, Hunninghake D, et al: The cholesterol facts: a summary of the evidence relating dietary fats, serum cholesterol, and coronary heart disease. A joint statement by the American Heart Association and the National Heart, Lung, and Blood Institute. Circulation 81:1721, 1990.
15. Grundy SM, Goodman DS, Rifkind BM, et al: The place of HDL in cholesterol management: a perspective from the National Cholesterol Education Program. Arch Intern Med 149:505, 1989.
16. Kannel WB: Lipids, diabetes, and coronary heart disease: insights from the Framingham Study. Am Heart J 110:1100, 1985.
17. Expert Panel on the Detection, Evaluation, and Treatment of High Blood Cholesterol in Adults: Summary of the Second Report of the National Cholesterol Education Program (NCEP) Expert Panel on the Detection, Evaluation, and Treatment of High Blood Cholesterol in Adults (Adult Treatment Panel II). JAMA 269:3015, 1993.
18. The Lipid Research Clinics Coronary Primary Prevention Trial: Results. I. Reduction in incidence of coronary heart disease. JAMA 251:351, 1984.
19. Frick MH, Elo O, Haapa K, et al: Helsinki Heart Study: primary-prevention trial with gemfibrozil in middle-aged men with dyslipidemia. N Engl J Med 317:1237, 1987.
20. Shepherd J, Cobbe SM, Ford I, et al: Prevention of coronary heart disease with pravastatin in men with hypercholesterolemia. West of Scotland Coronary Prevention Study Group. N Engl J Med 333:1301, 1995.
21. Downs JR, Clearfield M, Weis S, et al: Primary prevention of acute coronary events with lovastatin in men and women with average cholesterol levels: Results of AFCAPS/TexCAPS. Air Force/Texas Coronary Atherosclerosis Prevention Study. JAMA 279:1615, 1998.
22. Wilson PWF, Cupples LA, Kannel WB: Is hyperglycemia associated with cardiovascular disease? the Framingham Study. Am J Med 121:586, 1991.
23. Jeppesen J, Hein HO, Suadicani P, Gyntelberg F: Triglyceride concentration and ischemic heart disease: an eight-year follow-up in the Copenhagen Male Study. Circulation 97:1029, 1998.
24. Criqui MH, Heiss G, Cohen R, et al: Plasma triglyceride level and mortality from coronary heart disease. N Engl J Med 328:1220, 1993.
25. Wilson PWF, Larson MG, Castelli WP: Triglycerides, HDL-cholesterol and coronary artery disease: a Framingham update on their interrelationships. Can J Cardiol 10:105B, 1994.
26. Hokanson JE, Austin MA: Plasma triglyceride level is a risk factor for cardiovascular disease independent of high-density lipoprotein

cholesterol level: a meta-analysis of population-based prospective studies. J Cardiovasc Risk 3:213, 1996.
27. Gavin JR III: Report of the Expert Committee on the Diagnosis and Classification of Diabetes Mellitus. Diabetes Care 20:1183, 1997.
28. Harris MI, Flegal KM, Cowie CC, et al: Prevalence of diabetes, impaired fasting glucose, and impaired glucose tolerance in U.S. adults. The Third National Health and Nutrition Examination Survey, 1988–1994. Diabetes Care 21:518, 1998.
29. Sheps SG: The sixth report of the Joint National Committee on Prevention, Detection, Evaluation, and Treatment of High Blood Pressure. Arch Intern Med 157:2413, 1997.
30. Gaster B, Hirsch IB: The effects of improved glycemic control on complications in type 2 diabetes. Arch Intern Med 158:134, 1998.
31. U.S. Renal Data System: USRDS 1998 Annual Data Report. Bethesda, MD: National Institutes of Health, National Institute of Diabetes and Digestive and Kidney Diseases, 1998.
32. Kannel WB: Influence of multiple risk factors on the hazard of hypertension. J Cardiovasc Pharmacol 16(suppl 5):S53, 1990.
33. Wilson PWF, Kannel WB: Hypertension, other risk factors, and the risk of cardiovascular disease. *In* Laragh JH, Brenner BM (eds): Hypertension: Pathophysiology, Diagnosis, and Management. 2nd ed. p. 99. New York: Raven, 1995.
34. Neaton JD, Kuller L, Stamler J, Wentworth DN: Impact of systolic and diastolic blood pressure on cardiovascular mortality. *In* Laragh JH, Brenner BM (eds): Hypertension: Pathophysiology, Diagnosis, and Management. 2nd ed. p. 127. New York: Raven, 1995.
35. Kannel WB, Gordon T, Schwartz MJ: Systolic versus diastolic blood pressure and risk of coronary heart disease: the Framingham Study. Am J Cardiol 27:335, 1971.
36. SHEP Cooperative Research Group: Prevention of stroke by antihypertensive drug treatment in older persons with isolated systolic hypertension. Final results of the Systolic Hypertension in the Elderly Program (SHEP). JAMA 265:3255, 1991.
37. Staessen JA, Fagard R, Thijs L, et al: Randomised double-blind comparison of placebo and active treatment for older patients with isolated systolic hypertension. The Systolic Hypertension in Europe (SYST-EUR) Trial Investigators. Lancet 350:757, 1997.
38. Kannel WB, Dannenberg AL, Abbott RD: Unrecognized myocardial infarction and hypertension: the Framingham Study. Am Heart J 109:581, 1985.
39. MacMahon S, Peto R, Cutler J, et al: Blood pressure, stroke, and coronary heart disease. Part 1, Prolonged differences in blood pressure: prospective observational studies corrected for the regression dilution bias. Lancet 335:765, 1990.
40. Eaker ED, Haynes SG, Feinleib M: Spouse behavior and coronary heart disease in men: prospective results from the Framingham Heart Study. II. Modification of risk in type A husbands according to the social and psychological status of their wives. Am J Epidemiol 118:23, 1983.
41. Kannel WB, Wilson PWF, Blair SN: Epidemiological assessment of the role of physical activity and fitness in development of cardiovascular disease. Am Heart J 109:876, 1985.
42. Kannel WB: Alcohol and cardiovascular disease. Proc Nutr Soc 47:99, 1988.
43. Kannel WB, McGee DL, Castelli WP: Latest perspectives on cigarette smoking and cardiovascular disease: the Framingham Study. J Cardiac Rehabil 4:267, 1984.
44. Reaven GM: 1988 Banting Lecture. Role of insulin resistance in human disease. Diabetes 37:1595, 1988.
45. Kannel WB, Cupples LA, Ramaswami R, et al: Regional obesity and risk of cardiovascular disease: the Framingham Study. J Clin Epidemiol 44:183, 1991.
46. Higgins MW, Kannel WB, Garrison RJ, et al: Hazards of obesity—the Framingham experience. Acta Med Scand Suppl 723:23, 1988.
47. Hamm PB, Shekelle RB, Stamler J: Large fluctuations in body weight during young adulthood and 25-year risk of coronary death in men. Am J Epidemiol 129:312, 1989.
48. Lissner L, Bengtsson C, Lapidus L, et al: Body weight variability and mortality in the Gothenburg prospective studies of men and women. *In* Bjorntorp P, Rossner S (eds): Obesity in Europe. p. 51. London: Libbey, 1989.
49. Kannel WB, Dannenberg AL, Levy D: Population implications of electrocardiographic left ventricular hypertrophy. Am J Cardiol 60:85I, 1987.
50. Wong ND, Cupples LA, Ostfeld AM, et al: Risk factors for long-term coronary prognosis after initial myocardial infarction: the Framingham Study. Am J Epidemiol 130:469, 1989.
51. Myers RH, Kiely D, Cupples LA, Kannel WB: Parental history is an independent risk factor for coronary artery disease: the Framingham Study. Am Heart J 120:963, 1990.
52. Colditz GA, Stampfer MJ, Willett WC, et al: A prospective study of parental history of myocardial infarction and coronary heart disease in women. Am J Epidemiol 123:48, 1986.
53. Ernst E, Hammerschmidt DE, Bagge U, et al: Leukocytes and the risk of ischemic diseases. JAMA 257:2318, 1987.
54. Kannel WB, Anderson KM, Wilson PWF: White blood cell count and cardiovascular disease. JAMA 267:1253, 1992.
55. Kannel WB, Wolf PA, Castelli WP, D'Agostino RB: Fibrinogen and risk of cardiovascular disease. The Framingham Study. JAMA 258:1183, 1987.
56. Kannel WB, D'Agostino RB, Belanger AJ: Update on fibrinogen as a cardiovascular risk factor. Ann Epidemiol 2:457, 1992.
57. Campos H, Blijlevens E, McNamara JR, et al: LDL particle size distribution. Results from the Framingham Offspring Study. Arterioscler Thromb 12:1410, 1992.
58. Austin MA, Breslow JL, Hennekens CH, et al: Low-density lipoprotein subclass patterns and risk of myocardial infarction. JAMA 260:1917, 1988.
59. Genest J Jr, McNamara JR, Ordovas JM, et al: Lipoprotein cholesterol, apolipoprotein A-I and B and lipoprotein(a) abnormalities in men with premature coronary artery disease. J Am Coll Cardiol 19:792, 1992.
60. Schaefer EJ, Lamon-Fava S, Jenner JL, et al: Lipoprotein(a) levels and risk for coronary heart disease in men: the Lipid Research Clinics Primary Prevention Trial. JAMA 271:999, 1994.
61. Bostom AG, Gagnon DR, Cupples LA, et al: A prospective investigation of elevated lipoprotein(a) detected by electropheresis and cardiovascular disease in women: the Framingham Heart Study. Circulation 90:1688, 1994.
62. Ridker PM, Hennekens CH, Stampfer MJ: A prospective study of lipoprotein(a) and the risk of myocardial infarction. JAMA 270:2195, 1993.
63. Jauhiainen M, Koskinen P, Ehnholm C, et al: Lipoprotein(a) and coronary heart disease risk: a nested case-control study of the Helsinki Heart Study participants. Atherosclerosis 89:59, 1991.
64. Stampfer MJ, Malinow MR, Willett WC, et al: A prospective study of plasma homocysteine and risk of myocardial infarction in US physicians. JAMA 268:877, 1992.
65. Boushey CJ, Beresford SAA, Omenn GS, Motulsky AG: A quantitative assessment of plasma homocysteine as a risk factor for vascular disease. JAMA 274:1049, 1995.
66. Robinson K, Arheart K, Refsum H, et al: Low circulating folate and vitamin B6 concentrations: risk factors for stroke, peripheral vascular disease, and coronary artery disease. Circulation 97:437, 1998.
67. Despres JP, Lamarche B, Mauriege P, et al: Hyperinsulinemia as an independent risk factor for ischemic heart disease. N Engl J Med 334:952, 1996.
68. Pyorala M, Miettinen H, Laakso M, Pyorala K: Hyperinsulinemia predicts coronary heart disease risk in healthy middle-aged men. Circulation 98:398, 1998.
69. Ridker PM, Cushman M, Stampfer MJ, et al: Inflammation, aspirin, and the risk of cardiovascular disease in apparently healthy men. N Engl J Med 336:973, 1997.
70. Ridker PM, Buring JE, Shih J, et al: Prospective study of C-reactive protein and the risk of future cardiovascular events among apparently healthy women. Circulation 98:731, 1998.
71. Gurfinkel E, Bozovich G, Daroca A, et al: Randomised trial of roxithromycin in non–Q-wave coronary syndromes: ROXIS pilot study. Lancet 350:404, 1997.
72. Salonen JT, Nyyssonen K, Korpela H, et al: High stored iron levels are associated with excess risk of myocardial infarction in eastern Finnish men. Circulation 86:803, 1992.
73. Tuomainen TP, Punnonen K, Nyyssonen K, Salonen JT: Association between body iron stores and the risk of acute myocardial infarction in men. Circulation 97:1461, 1998.
74. Sempos CT, Looker AC, Gillum RF, Makuc DM: Body iron stores and the risk of coronary heart disease. N Engl J Med 330:1119, 1994.
75. Corti MC, Guralnik JM, Salive ME, et al: Serum iron level, coronary artery disease, and all-cause mortality in older men and women. Am J Cardiol 79:120, 1997.

76. Harris TB, Cook EF, Kannel WB, Goldman L: Proportional hazards analysis of risk factors for coronary heart disease in individuals aged 65 or older. The Framingham Heart Study. J Am Geriatr Soc 36:1023, 1988.
77. Wilking SV, Belanger AJ, Kannel WB, et al: Determinants of isolated systolic hypertension. JAMA 260:3451, 1988.
78. Wilson PWF, Kannel WB: Hypercholesterolemia and coronary risk in the elderly: the Framingham Study. Am J Geriatr Cardiol 10:52, 1993.
79. Fuster V, Pearson TA: 27th Bethesda Conference. Matching the intensity of risk factor management with the hazard for coronary disease events. J Am Coll Cardiol 27:957, 1996.
80. Wilson PW, D'Agostino RB, Levy D, et al: Prediction of coronary heart disease using risk factor categories. Circulation 97:1837, 1998.

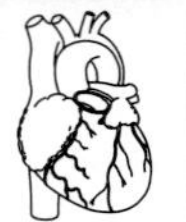

CHAPTER 121

EXERCISE

Benjamin D. Levine, Daniel B. Friedman, C. Gunnar Blomqvist, and Jere H. Mitchell

PRIMARY PREVENTION
SECONDARY PREVENTION
POSSIBLE MECHANISMS FOR THE EFFECT OF EXERCISE TRAINING ON CORONARY HEART DISEASE
Vascular Biology
Exercise Training and Parasympathetic Influences on the Heart
Coagulation
SUMMARY

The response to exercise is now widely used in cardiovascular medicine for such diverse purposes as objective quantification of functional capacity, detection and prognostic evaluation of coronary artery disease (CAD), and determination of the integrity of physiologic systems necessary for control of the circulation and physical work performance.[1] The adaptation to dynamic exercise (i.e., exercise training) leads to increased endurance and aerobic power, and competitive athletes are considered models of optimal physical health. In particular, the case of "Mr. Marathoner" Clarence De Mar, who ran the Boston marathon 34 times up to the age of 66 (and won 7) and who at autopsy in 1955 was reported to have unusually large coronary arteries,[2] promulgated the myth that runners were immune from CAD.[3]

Since the 1950s, extensive literature has developed regarding the benefits and risks of exercise, culminating in the recognition by the American Heart Association[4] and the International Society and Federation of Cardiology[5] that a sedentary lifestyle is an independent and modifiable risk factor for coronary disease. The convincing nature of the sum total of data relating exercise to cardiovascular disease risk led to the first surgeon general's report on this issue.[6] A multinational task force recommended a minimum of 30 minutes of moderate exercise for all able adults on a daily basis.

This chapter explores in detail the role of occupational and recreational exercise in death and complications from CAD. The first section focuses on healthy individuals (primary prevention) and discusses epidemiologic evidence supporting the practice of regular exercise. The second section discusses secondary prevention for patients who already have had some manifestation of CAD such as angina pectoris or myocardial infarction or who have undergone revascularization. Finally, the third section provides a pathophysiologic framework of the possible mechanisms for the beneficial effects of exercise training.

PRIMARY PREVENTION

In the 1950s, Morris and associates[7] first suggested that the rate of CAD was inversely related to the level of physical activity during occupational activities. In the London transportation study, sedentary bus drivers had almost twice the incidence of CAD as conductors who regularly walked up and down the stairs of double-decker busses.[8] In addition, overall death rates, including sudden death, were twice as high in the drivers as in the conductors. Virtually every subsequent study that compared sedentary and active populations has confirmed this protective benefit of regular occupational exercise (Fig. 121–1).[9] Studies in farmers in North Dakota,[10] US postal employees,[11] American railroad workers,[12] and participants of the Health Insurance Plan of New York[13] offer further support to the hypothesis that exercise protects against CAD. However, confounding variables such as obesity, hypertension, and hyperlipidemia made it difficult in the early studies to clearly demonstrate an independent effect of exercise.

Subsequent investigators attempted to control more carefully for other cardiovascular risk factors. Cassel and colleagues[14] examined residents of Evans county in rural Georgia and were able to show that a sedentary occupation was an independent risk factor for CAD.[14] Brunner and associates[15] took advantage of the relatively homogeneous lifestyle of the Kibbutzim of Israel to minimize variability in diet, race, and socioeconomic status; in this population, the sedentary residents still demonstrated two to four times the incidence of CAD as their active counterparts during a 15-year period.

These qualitative observations regarding occupational activity have been extended with quantitative studies by Paffenbarger and associates.[16, 17] These investigators showed that San Francisco longshoremen who performed heavy physical labor, requiring bursts of energy of 5.2 to 7.5 kcal/min (equivalent to brisk walking, slow jogging, or activity such as shoveling snow—1 kcal/min is *roughly* equivalent to 1 MET) with a mean energy expenditure of 1876 kcal above basal requirements per workday, had a 25 percent reduction in CAD rates during 16 years of follow-up compared with workers who were more sedentary (1.5 to 5.0 kcal/min maximal energy requirements during work).

As mechanization and automation have reduced the energy expenditure of many workers on the job, more recent studies have focused on the beneficial effects of *recreational* exercise (Fig. 121–2). In the Multiple Risk Factor Intervention Trial, moderate leisure-time physical activity was associated with a 37 percent reduction in fatal cardiac

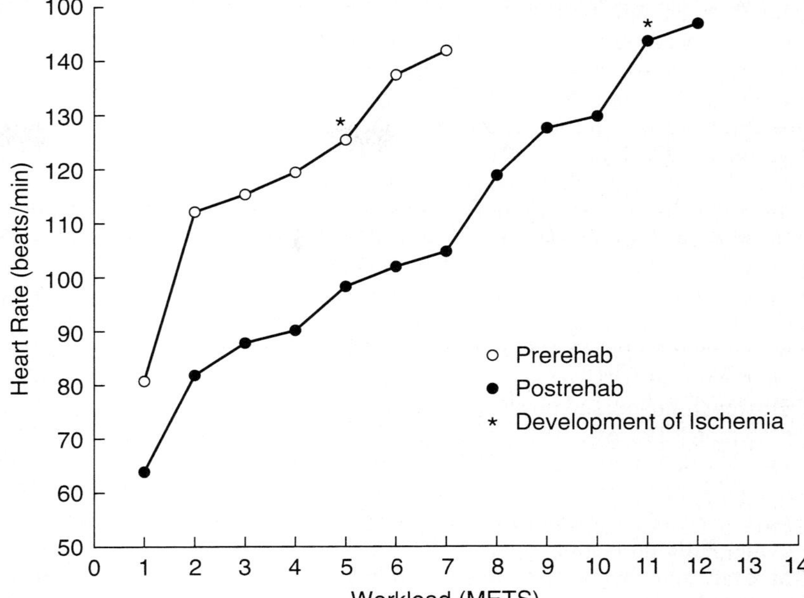

FIGURE 121–1 Change in heart rate during a standard exercise test (Bruce protocol) in a patient with severe coronary artery disease, before *(open circles)* and after *(solid circles)* 12 weeks of cardiac rehabilitation. Ischemia *(asterisk)* manifested by typical angina pectoris and significant ST-segment depression developed at a relatively low workload (5 metabolic equivalents [METS]) before training. After training, ischemia does not develop until very high workloads are achieved (11 METS).

events and sudden deaths and a 30 percent reduction in total deaths compared with a lower level of activity.[18] Both men[18–22] and women[20, 21] appear to benefit from regular vigorous activity or fitness, with a reduction in both cardiovascular and all-cause mortality rates. This protective benefit of exercise may explain a substantial proportion of the difference in cardiovascular mortality seen between rural and urban populations, both by a global reduction in risk factors for CAD in rural populations and an independent effect of exercise.[23]

It is possible that selection bias has contributed to the apparent protective advantage of exercise or fitness in many of these studies of leisure-time activity; that is, naturally robust persons are more likely to exercise or participate in sports than are individuals predisposed to CAD. This question was addressed in a comprehensive investigation of 16,936 Harvard University alumni aged 35 to 72 in which past and present habitual energy expenditure and the risk of myocardial infarction and death were compared.[24] There was a clear reduction in total and cardiovascular mortality rate with regular recreational exercise, regardless of the

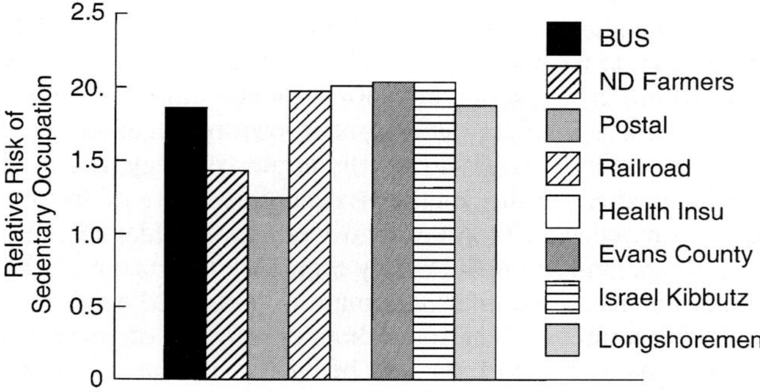

FIGURE 121–2 Summary figure of trials of effect of occupational exercise on cardiovascular death. BUS, London bus drivers; ND, North Dakota.

level of athleticism or sports participation during college. Ex-varsity athletes were at a lower risk of cardiovascular disease only if they continued to exercise later in life, suggesting that exercise itself, rather than a genetic predisposition to fitness, was responsible for the protective effect. This distinction between genetics and habitual exercise was recently confirmed with data from the Finnish Twin Cohort Study,[25] in which nearly 8000 pairs of twins were asked about their exercise habits in 1975 and then followed for 20 years. Among twin pairs who were healthy at the initial examination and discordant for death at follow-up (n = 434), the odds ratio for death was 0.44 among individuals who exercised with vigorous walking at least six times a month compared with those who did not exercise regularly.

More recent follow-up studies of the subjects from the Harvard University alumni study suggests that a significant reduction in cardiovascular mortality can be achieved even if regular exercise is not begun until late in life (age >60).[26] Similar observations have been made from the Honolulu Heart Study, in which 707 older men, age 61 to 81, were followed for 12 years.[27] After adjustment for other risk factors, the mortality rate among men who walked less than 1 mile/da was nearly twice that of men who walked more than 2 miles/da, confirming the beneficial effects of regular physical activity even in the elderly.

It is important to make the distinction between regular exercise and fitness per se. Regular exercise is closely associated with increased physical fitness as reflected by objective measures such as peak work rate on a treadmill or bicycle ergometer or directly measured peak ventilatory oxygen uptake.[28, 29] The strength of the relationship between fitness and cardiovascular disease has generally proved similar to that between physical activity or habitual levels of exercise and mortality.[21, 29–31] Wilhelmsen[30] showed that among 793 healthy Swedes, those with a lower work capacity are more likely to have a myocardial infarction or to die suddenly. In the Lipid Research Clinics Mortality study, 4276 men were followed for an average of 8.5 years after a baseline examination that included a treadmill test.[31] Based on heart rate during stage 2 of the treadmill test and peak exercise capacity, the subjects were divided into quartiles with respect to fitness. They found that the lower quartiles were associated with a greater incidence of cardiovascular death. Blair and colleagues[21] examined physical fitness (maximal treadmill performance) and risk for all-cause and cause-specific mortality rates in 10,224 men and 3120 women. Cardiovascular and all-cause mortality rates declined across higher quintiles of physical fitness in both men and women. These trends remained significant even after adjustment for age, smoking, cholesterol, blood pressure and glucose levels, family history of CAD, and follow-up interval (mean, 8 years).

However, fitness and physical activity are not necessarily synonymous. For example, studies of identical twins have suggested that approximately 40 percent of fitness measures are genetically determined and independent of physical activity.[32] Most importantly, being very fit but sedentary provides little protection against CHD or all-cause death.[33] Moreover, unfit but active men have a lower risk of CHD than do fit, sedentary men.[33] More recently, Blair and colleagues[34] demonstrated that individuals who increased their fitness from one follow-up period to another experienced a decrease in cardiovascular mortality rates by more than 40 percent, providing strong evidence that exercise training as a means of acquiring or maintaining fitness, rather than fitness per se, is the key factor in reducing cardiovascular disease mortality rates.

A critical question regarding the effect of habitual exercise on overall and cardiovascular mortality rates is the "dose" of exercise required to achieve a clinically meaningful reduction.[35] For San Francisco longshoremen, repetitive bouts of high-intensity exercise equivalent to 5.2 to 7.5 kcal/min (roughly equivalent to the second stage of the standard Bruce protocol) during work activities were associated with a reduction in death rates from CAD compared with longshoremen with more moderate levels of exertion (2.4 to 5.0 kcal/min) or compared with sedentary workers (1.5 to 2.0 kcal/min).[17] Thus, for occupational activity, there appears to be a threshold effect at more than 5.0 kcal/min.

For the Harvard University alumni, death rates declined steadily as men increased their energy expenditure during recreational activity from 500 to 2000 kcal/wk (equivalent to walking or running approximately 16 to 18 miles/wk). There was no apparent benefit in terms of cardiovascular mortality rates for those exceeding this level, at least not after the first 10 years of follow-up, but the numbers of subjects who sustained such a high level of activity were small.[24] More extended follow-up, however, has suggested that extreme levels of physical activity (>3500 kcal/wk additional exercise training) may further reduce the incidence of CAD.[26] Of particular note, even a small increase in physical activity, from less than 500 kcal/wk to 500 to 999 kcal/wk was associated with a substantial decrease in total and cardiovascular mortality rates.[24] If physical activity is quantified as distance walked and modeled as a continuous variable, the risk of CHD has been shown in the Honolulu Heart Study to be reduced by 15 percent for every 0.5 mile/da increase in walking distance.[36]

A similar observation has been made with respect to exercise capacity. For both men and women, most of the survival advantage associated with physical fitness can be seen at relatively low levels of exercise capacity; Blair and colleagues[21] have shown that a maximal treadmill work rate equivalent to approximately 10 METS in men and 9 METS in women conferred virtually all the exercise-related protection against cardiovascular disease. These studies suggest that a relatively modest amount of physical activity confers a meaningful reduction in death rates from CAD, and they provide a compelling basis for the recommendation to individuals at high risk for coronary disease to exercise regularly.

A substantial body of evidence thus exists to demonstrate that regular physical exercise is associated with a greater degree of fitness and a reduced incidence of CAD in healthy people.[37] There are several mechanisms by which this protection may be achieved: either by a specific, independent effect of exercise itself (discussed later) or by a reduction in other known risk factors. Exercise may lower blood pressure, decrease the incidence of adult-onset diabetes mellitus, and improve the lipid profile.[6] Persons who are more active also quit smoking with a greater frequency.[38] High levels of high-density lipoprotein (HDL) cholesterol have also been associated with a reduced incidence of CAD,[39] and exercise is associated with higher plasma HDL concentrations.[40, 41] HDL is particularly affected in persons who exercise regularly for periods of several years,[42] primarily by an increase in the half-life of specific subfractions of HDL, most likely HDL-2.[43]

In a series of important studies, Wood and colleagues[44] demonstrated that exercise is as effective as weight loss in terms of improving the lipid profile. Moreover, when exercise and diet are combined, the beneficial effects may be synergistic.[45] They divided 264 moderately obese men and women into three experimental groups: (1) control, (2) those receiving the hypocaloric National Cholesterol Education Program (NCEP) diet, and (3) those receiving the hypocaloric NCEP diet with exercise. Although the diet-only subjects consumed fewer calories, they did not lose as much total body weight or fat weight as did the exercisers. The latter also had a better final abdomen-to-hip circumference ratio, reflecting preferential fat loss around the abdomen. Most importantly, exercise had a favorable effect on the low-density lipoprotein/HDL cholesterol and apolipoprotein B/apolipoprotein A-1 ratios in both men and women. Both ratios have been associated with the development of atherosclerosis.[46] Because a low-fat diet may reduce the HDL cholesterol,[47] exercise may be particularly useful in patients who maintain such a diet. Exercise also lowers triglycerides.[40, 45] This effect occurs even with a single bout of exercise but appears to be cumulative, resulting in a permanent decrease in serum triglycerides.[48]

The effect of exercise on blood pressure control has been somewhat controversial. Blumenthal and associates[49] showed no specific blood pressure–reducing effect of exercise for patients with mild hypertension; their report was from a well designed, large, and randomized trial that included nonobese men and women who were off medications. The study was complicated by the fact that both the exercise and control groups experienced an unexplained significant decrease in blood pressure. However, the subjects with the greatest improvement in aerobic power tended to have the greatest reduction in blood pressure, suggesting that a more rigorous exercise program might result in a more significant reduction in blood pressure.

Other investigations have consistently shown a clear association between exercise and blood pressure reduction.[50–52] However, none of these other studies measured changes in aerobic power or evaluated other possible contributing factors, such as salt intake, weight, and gender. In a carefully controlled study, Gordon and colleagues[53] demonstrated that regular exercise is equivalent in efficacy to diet-induced weight loss for the lowering of blood pressure, with either intervention resulting in a 10 to 11 mm Hg reduction in diastolic blood pressure over 12 weeks. In contrast to the data for exercise and lipid lowering, however, the two interventions together (i.e., diet plus exercise) were neither additive nor synergistic and were not associated with a greater magnitude of blood pressure reduction. In summary, the weight of evidence suggests that regular aerobic exercise contributes to a reduction in blood pressure in mildly hypertensive persons, possibly mediated through changes in skeletal muscle conductance and peripheral resistance.[54] Finally, Blair and associates[55] showed that among 4820 normotensive men and women, the subsequent development of hypertension during the next 1 to 12 years was linked to a lower level of fitness.

The syndrome of abdominal obesity, hyperinsulinemia, and glucose intolerance (which often includes hypertriglyceridemia and hypertension) is associated with a high incidence of CAD.[56] Exercise may improve all components of this high-risk syndrome. Specifically, exercise results in a lower insulin secretion with improved receptor sensitivity.[57] Physical activity can help to produce weight loss, including a reduction in other markers for CAD, such as abdominal obesity. In addition, persons who exercise regularly are less likely to develop non–insulin-dependent diabetes mellitus.[58]

Although exercise confers substantial benefits over time, it is not without risk. The hemodynamic and neuroendocrine responses to an acute bout of exercise raise myocardial oxygen requirements and alter the functional milieu of the myocardium, which may increase the risk of arrhythmias and sudden cardiac death[59] or myocardial infarction.[61, 62] Fortunately, the exercise-related risks for ostensibly healthy individuals are very small.[63, 64] For joggers in the state of Rhode Island, Thompson[65] estimated the risk to be one death per 7620 joggers per year. This risk of dying or triggering a myocardial infarction while exercising is substantially higher for normally sedentary individuals who exercise occasionally than for regular exercisers.[61, 62, 65] Moreover, there is a clear *inverse* dose-response relationship between the frequency of regular exercise and the risk of exercise-induced cardiovascular complications. Thus, the relative risk of triggering a myocardial infarction during or immediately after heavy exercise compared with at other times during the day is only 2.4 for individuals who exercise five or more times per week but increases exponentially to 8.6 (for those who exercise three or four times per week), 19.4 (for those who exercise one or two times per week), and up to 107 for those very sedentary individuals who engage in heavy physical exertion less than one time per week.[61] If the relative risk of dying *during* exercise is compared with the *long-term* health benefits of exercise, the balance of effects still favors regular exercise.[66] Thus, habitual exercisers have a relative risk of dying suddenly *at any time* that is less than half that of sedentary individuals.[60, 66]

Secondary Prevention

Once an individual has experienced the consequences of CAD, attention turns from disease prevention to maximization of functional capacity, minimization of complications, and limit of the progression of disease. This process is generally referred to as secondary prevention, or cardiac rehabilitation.

Cardiac rehabilitation may be broadly defined as the process by which patients with CAD are assisted in achieving their maximal physical capacity and psychosocial wellbeing, usually after a period of acute cardiovascular illness. It is most effective when delivered as an individualized, multifactorial approach that includes education, risk factor modification (including lipid-lowering therapy), and exercise training,[67–70] as first described by Hellerstein and Ford in 1957.[71]

In contrast to the extensive data for apparently healthy persons, studies of the effect of cardiac rehabilitation on death after a myocardial infarction have rarely been of sufficient size to document a prolongation of life from exercise conditioning or rehabilitation services. One important study from Finland did demonstrate a significant reduction in sudden death that was apparent within the first 6 months of the program. The distinguishing feature of this study is that the patients were enrolled very early after their myocardial infarction, within 2 weeks of hospital discharge.[72] This early benefit, manifested by a reduction in mortality rates, suggests an effect of exercise training on altering the propensity for ventricular arrhythmias, possibly through alterations in autonomic tone, as discussed further later.

When the experience of major postinfarction trials are combined in a meta-analysis, the evidence suggests that cardiac rehabilitation significantly reduces cardiovascular mortality rates, including the incidence of sudden death or fatal myocardial infarction, by approximately 25 percent over 3 years,[73, 74] a magnitude equivalent to the beneficial effect of beta-blockade. No difference has been identified, however, for the incidence of recurrent nonfatal myocardial infarction, providing further suggestive evidence that an antiarrhythmic effect of exercise training may be more important than changes in vascular biology or thrombotic potential.

Although the effect of exercise training on mortality rates for patients after a myocardial infarction may still be somewhat debated, exercise conditioning clearly improves the functional capacity of cardiac patients (Fig. 121–3), resulting in an increased maximal oxygen uptake and an increased ischemic threshold.[75] The reduction in resting and exercise heart rate and blood pressure reduces myocardial work during submaximal exercise and allows patients to perform activities of daily living as well as more vigorous activities with fewer symptoms. The mechanism for the improvement in cardiovascular performance, at least initially, is likely due to increases in peripheral skeletal muscle oxygen uptake and utilization.[76] However, when

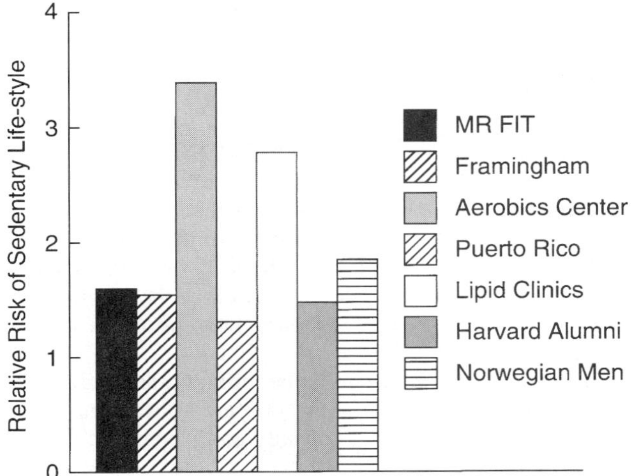

FIGURE 121–3 Summary of trials of the effect of recreational exercise on cardiovascular death. MR FIT, Multiple Risk Factor Intervention Trial.

training is prolonged and intense, even patients with cardiac disease can show improvements in myocardial contractile function.[77] This improvement has been demonstrated in some patients to be associated directly with improvements in myocardial blood flow.[78]

In contrast to the effect of training, prolonged bed rest and inactivity result in a marked reduction in maximal aerobic power.[79] Plasma volume decreases and orthostatic intolerance may ensue after even brief periods of bed rest.[80] This development of "bed rest deconditioning" may cause substantial complications in the acute period after a myocardial infarction by increasing heart rate during submaximal exercise and occasionally resulting in hypotension and reduced coronary perfusion. Its prevention is one of the primary goals of the first phase of cardiac rehabilitation (phase I), which begins as soon as a patient is stable in the hospital after an acute cardiac event (Table 121–1). The focus of this early, in-hospital rehabilitation is assumption of the upright posture and an individualized increase in exercise activity, which together will rapidly reverse the plasma volume shifts that occur with bed rest.[81]

Phase II of cardiac rehabilitation is the short-term, initial outpatient phase of rehabilitation (Table 121–2). An expeditious and orderly transition between phase I and phase II is critical to the success of the rehabilitation process and ensures that patients are properly prepared to respond to the education and training programs. During the acute phase of hospitalization, patients are just beginning to cope with the ramifications of their disease and often have substantial difficulty processing new information.[82] It is during the first few weeks of their outpatient care that they are most open to making significant lifestyle adjustments, and risk factor modification is most likely to be successful. This time period is also a critical one from a medical perspective. The period of the greatest risk for sudden death after a myocardial infarction is the first 3 months after hospitalization,[83] and rehabilitation programs that enroll patients early after a myocardial infarction demonstrate a significant reduction in the rate of sudden death during this high-risk period.[72] This transition period from inpatient to outpatient thus represents a physiologic and psychologic "window of opportunity" for maximizing the benefit of the rehabilitation process. It is also important to emphasize that cardiac rehabilitation and successful changes in lifestyle may be achieved by patients regardless of ethnic group or socioeconomic status.[84]

In addition to education, a major emphasis in phase II rehabilitation is on exercise conditioning. Both static and dynamic exercise training programs are used to increase strength and endurance. When starting the program, an exercise prescription is usually established based principally on a symptom-limited exercise test. The target or training heart rate is usually set at 75 to 85 percent of the measured maximal heart rate, based on the predictable relationship between oxygen uptake and heart rate in normal individuals.[1] Heart rate is thus used as an easily measured estimate of relative exercise intensity. It is important to emphasize that these are only guidelines, which in some patients, such as those with left ventricular dysfunction or who are taking β-blockers or other medications that may affect the heart rate response to exercise, may not accurately reflect exercise intensity. In such cases, the *rating of perceived exertion*, or RPE (Borg scale), may be helpful. This measure rates the perceived effort on a scale from 6 to 20, with 6 to 7 being "very, very light," 19 to 20 being "very, very hard," and 12 to 13 (the optimal training level) being "somewhat hard."[85] This strategy quantifies effort level independently of heart rate level and is scaled based on a physiologic heart rate range in young healthy subjects from 60 at rest to 200 during maximal exercise.[85] This rating system is remarkably consistent within individuals[86] and thus is independent of pharmacologic therapy that may attenuate the normal heart rate response to exercise. Once patients are trained in its use, they can effectively monitor their own exercise intensity at home without the need for sophisticated heart rate–monitoring systems.

TABLE 121–1 Goals of Phase I Cardiac Rehabilitation

- To prevent bed rest deconditioning
- To facilitate rapid recovery of functional capacity
- To shorten duration of cardiac care unit stay and to enable early hospital discharge safely in appropriate patients
- To minimize disability associated with an acute cardiac event and encourage rapid return to work
- To improve communication between health care providers and patients and thus smooth the transition into phase II cardiac rehabilitation and outpatient care

TABLE 121–2 Goals of Phase II Cardiac Rehabilitation

- Supervised exercise training to maximize functional capacity, teach safe exercise practices, and identify patients at risk for complications
- Risk factor modification, including smoking cessation, stress reduction, weight loss, and lowering of cholesterol level
- Education on medications, signs and symptoms of heart disease and its progression, sexual relations, dietary modifications, and activity guidelines

Decisions regarding the optimal training load are complicated in patients with provocable ischemia, for whom the desired training intensity may fall above the ischemic threshold. There is no consensus on how to train patients who have clear provocable ischemia at a low workload and thus are limited by myocardial rather than systemic oxygen transport. Some centers train patients at 75 to 85 percent of directly measured maximal heart rate despite the presence of ischemia in an attempt to maximize the training effect. However, a meaningful training effect can clearly be obtained in patients with or without provocable ischemia through the use of more moderate exercise, at an intensity equivalent to 60 to 75 percent of maximal heart rate.[87] In addition, data from studies in animals suggest that ischemic exercise results in profound and prolonged depression of ventricular contractile function that persists for hours after an exercise bout.[88] Moreover, there is little evidence that myocardial ischemia produces significant adaptive benefits at a cellular or molecular level that might increase the training effect or protect from future episodes of ischemia.[89] In contrast, training above the ischemic threshold is likely to increase the risk of exercise.[90, 91] Training in these patients thus should take place at a heart rate no higher than 10 beats/min below the value at which ischemia develops.[1]

Some caution should also be exercised in patients who have undergone percutaneous revascularization, with or without stent implantation. There is anecdotal evidence that such patients, who have transiently abnormal endothelial function, may be at increased risk for subacute thrombosis due to the high coronary flows associated with exercise training,[92–94] although small controlled trials have failed to document a substantially increased risk, at least with symptom-limited exercise testing.[95] It is probably prudent to wait at least 2 weeks after percutaneous revascularization before engaging in a regular exercise program.[94]

Patients who are at low risk for future events[96] or who have more chronic cardiovascular disease and have not recently sustained an acute cardiac illness may be considered candidates for unmonitored exercise training at home (phase III and phase IV). It has been clearly demonstrated in carefully selected, relatively well educated patients that home-based exercise training and cardiac rehabilitation can be performed safely and with the anticipated training effect.[97]

There is little doubt that vigorous exercise itself is an important risk factor for sudden death, particularly in unfit individuals.[65, 91, 98, 99] This risk is probably outweighed by the overall benefits of habitual exercise.[66] The risk of exercise-induced cardiac arrest is also directly related to the intensity of the exercise.[90] Lower intensity training might therefore theoretically be safer than vigorous exercise, particularly in the unsupervised cardiac patient. In fact, for both men and women, low- to moderate-intensity exercise training at home, at heart rates from 60 to 75 percent maximum, can result in substantial improvements in functional capacity, with an excellent degree of safety and compliance.[87, 100] In addition, as described earlier, even relatively small increases in fitness, equivalent to that obtained in a low- to moderate-intensity training program (with an emphasis on walking or slow jogging), can result in significant decreases in cardiovascular mortality rates.[21] Finally, evidence is accumulating that even patients with stable chronic heart failure (who do not have exercise-induced arrhythmias or ischemia) may safely participate in a program of unmonitored exercise training and experience substantial benefits.[101, 102]

Evidence therefore suggests that when selected properly, some patients may safely undergo unsupervised exercise training that may have important economic ramifications, particularly in communities with scarce resources. It must be emphasized, however, that this approach foregoes the intensive education and risk factor modification that usually take place in a supervised setting.

Possible Mechanisms for the Effect of Exercise Training on Coronary Artery Disease

In addition to the effect of exercise on alteration of known coronary risk factors, exercise training may also induce other adaptations that provide protection against ischemic heart disease. The mechanisms of this protective effect may include anatomic or physiologic changes in the coronary arteries, alterations in autonomic tone, and changes in the coagulation system.

Vascular Biology

The effect of exercise training on the coronary vasculature has been reviewed in detail.[103] Exercise training appears to increase coronary vascular transport capacity, by both structural and functional adaptations, although the results of many studies have varied widely depending on the species studied and training techniques used.[103] Early coronary casting studies in rats suggested that endurance training increases coronary vascularity.[104] These observations have been supported by studies in dogs,[105, 106] and possibly even studies in humans[107–109] demonstrating that epicardial coronary arteries are larger in endurance-trained animals (or humans) than in sedentary animals (or humans). Coronary collateral vessels may also increase with training, particularly if there is underlying arterial narrowing.[110–115]

The role of exercise may be particularly important in modifying the development of atherosclerosis, as demonstrated in a landmark study by Kramsch and colleagues,[116] who studied primates that consumed an atherogenic diet. The experimental group consisted of monkeys who ate a high-fat diet for 2 years, during which they regularly trained on a treadmill. Two control groups ate either a control diet or the atherogenic diet, but they did not exercise. The serum cholesterol level increased to more than 600 mg/dl in all monkeys on the high-fat diet, but the exercising monkeys had significantly lower LDL cholesterol levels and higher HDL cholesterol levels. The exercising monkeys also had substantially reduced overall atherosclerosis incidence, including lesion number, lesion size, and collagen accumulation, although the nature of the vascular lesions produced by this unusual diet may not be representative of the atherosclerotic process in normal humans. Most importantly, the exercising monkeys had significantly larger coronary arteries, with increased absolute coronary luminal diameter, confirming the observations made earlier in dogs by Wyatt and Mitchell.[105]

Although there has been great enthusiasm for the hypothesis that chronic endurance training may increase coronary size and possibly collateral circulation,[103, 115] this hypothesis has been difficult to prove in humans. Anecdotal reports[2] and autopsy studies in British citizens[107] and Masai tribesman[108] suggested that although atherosclerosis may develop in endurance-trained individuals, exercise may enlarge the coronary lumen, preserving normal luminal volume and coronary blood flow. Furthermore, Ehsani and associates[117] provided indirect support for this concept by demonstrating that long-term (12 months), intense training can reduce ischemic ST-segment responses during maximal treadmill exercise in patients with CAD. Other studies have extended these observations to demonstrate that prolonged exercise training can directly reduce the ischemic area at risk, as assessed with radionuclide perfusion imaging.[78]

Haskell and colleagues[118] performed quantitative angiography in a group of ultramarathoners, who compete in races of more than 100 miles. They found that at rest, the combined cross-sectional area of the right, left main, left anterior descending, and circumflex coronary arteries was not larger than a group of control patients with chest pain but angiographically normal coronary arteries. However, the lower myocardial oxygen demand of the athletes during the study may have prevented the investigators from observing a greater coronary diameter.[119]

Of greater importance was the fact that after the infusion of nitroglycerin, an endothelium-independent coronary vasodilator,[120] the total cross-sectional area of the coronary arteries of the runners increased by approximately twice that of the control subjects, demonstrating a significantly greater vasodilator reserve. This increase in maximal flow to cardiac muscle is similar to the increase in maximal conductance of skeletal muscle identified cross-sectionally in endurance athletes[121] and longitudinally with endurance training.[54] Whether this is a structural or functional adaptation, however, is not clear. Substantial evidence has accumulated that exercise training leads to increased vascular responsiveness mediated by increased formation of endothelium-derived relaxation factor (nitric oxide).[122] Maximal conductance in skeletal muscle appears to be associated with a number of other adaptations of the endurance athlete, including eccentric hypertrophy and control of vascular resistance,[123] suggesting that the large vasodilator reserve in both cardiac and skeletal muscle may be closely related.

However, marathon runners clearly do develop and experience the consequences of coronary atherosclerosis.[3] Insights into the pathophysiology of myocardial infarction and acute coronary insufficiency suggest that these acute syndromes occur as a result of sudden rupture into an atherosclerotic plaque, with associated intravascular thrombosis.[124] Whether a plaque ruptures probably depends more on the composition of the plaque (i.e., soft and lipid filled [rupture prone] versus hard and collagenous [rupture resistant]) than on the volume of plaque or degree of stenosis.[125] Thus, although the presence of larger coronary arteries with increased flow reserve might be expected to delay the onset of angina, particularly during exercise, it would not necessarily be expected to reduce the incidence of myocardial infarction. This hypothesis is consistent with the observation that for patients enrolled in cardiac rehabilitation after an acute coronary event, exercise training appears to improve survival primarily by reducing the incidence of sudden death[73] rather than by reducing myocardial infarction.

Exercise Training and Parasympathetic Influences on the Heart

It is becoming widely recognized that autonomic tone, or the balance between sympathetic and parasympathetic efferent neural influences on the heart, plays an important role in the genesis of cardiac arrhythmias.[126, 127] Carotid baroreflex control of heart rate, assessed by measuring the reduction in heart rate induced by infusion of phenylephrine sufficient to raise arterial pressure, was shown by Billman and colleagues[128] to be an important predictor of death after myocardial infarction. Heart rate variability, a more general index of cardiac-vagal tone that is relatively easy to obtain with modern Holter technology, is reduced acutely in acute myocardial infarction[129] and is an important marker for late mortality after myocardial infarction.[130] When used in a multiple regression model designed to identify arrhythmic events (sustained ventricular tachyarrhythmias or arrhythmic death) in survivors of myocardial infarction, depressed heart rate variability was the most powerful independent predictor of life-threatening arrhythmias; when combined with the presence of late potentials on signal-averaged electrocardiography and repetitive ventricular ectopic forms on Holter monitoring, a sensitive (58 percent sensitivity) and surprisingly accurate (33 percent positive predictive accuracy) predictor of arrhythmic events could be identified.[131] These indices were superior to combinations that included left ventricular ejection fraction, exercise electrocardiographic responses, or number of ventricular ectopic beats. When both low heart rate variability and depressed baroreflex sensitivity are present after myocardial infarction, mortality rate is increased by more than 8-fold compared with patients in whom both are well preserved, as demonstrated in the concluded Autonomic Tone and Reflexes After Myocardial Infarction (ATRAMI) trial that involved nearly 1300 patients.[132] Finally, with the use of Holter recording, investigators from the Framingham Heart Study investigated the predictive value of reduced heart rate variability for cardiovascular events in 2501 individuals in this large community-based population.[133] They demonstrated a highly significant increase in risk of nearly 50 percent for every one standard deviation decrement in heart rate variability (determined from the standard deviation of RR intervals).

A number of studies have demonstrated increases in heart rate variability with exercise training, including normal athletes[134, 135] and patients with hypertension[136] or congestive heart failure.[137] Older individuals, who have depressed heart rate variability as a direct effect of aging, may benefit particularly as decreased fitness with age may be at least partially responsible for alterations in autonomic function in this population.[138–140]

Although there are no specific data in humans, animal

studies have confirmed that exercise-induced changes in autonomic control may prevent ventricular fibrillation associated with myocardial ischemia and reduce the risk of sudden death.[141] An elegant awake animal model was developed that confirms this protective effect of increased vagal tone against life-threatening ventricular arrythmias.[142] These studies support the hypothesis that changes in autonomic tone may be an important mechanism for the reduction in sudden death caused by cardiac rehabilitation and exercise training.

Coagulation

With the understanding that most instances of myocardial infarction are caused by acute intravascular thrombosis[124] has come an interest in examining the effect of exercise on the coagulation system. It was recognized in the 18th century that blood from animals that were run to death did not clot.[143] However, data have been somewhat contradictory, and the end result of exercise appears to depend on a fine balance between thrombotic and fibrinolytic promoters and inhibitors that may be modified by the intensity and duration of the exercise and the population being studied.[144–147]

Acutely, high-intensity exercise appears to actually increase concentrations of clotting factors, particularly factor VIII.[148] This increase persists for at least 1 hour and probably does not occur until the level of exercise reaches a sufficiently high intensity (i.e., 95 to 100 percent of maximal oxygen uptake).[149] When high-intensity exercise is sustained over more prolonged periods of time (up to 1 hour), coagulation may be particularly activated, with increased formation of both thrombin and fibrin, possibly due to mechanical stimulation of endothelial cells.[150] Conversely, lower-level exercise induces a 5- to 10-fold increase in plasma fibrinolytic activity that appears to be directly related to the intensity and duration of exercise.[144–151] The mechanism of this increase appears to be via increases in endogenous tissue plasminogen activator activity, which is mediated by circulating epinephrine.[152]

Vigorous exercise has also been shown to reduce the aggregability of platelets,[153] although actual platelet number appears to be increased after exercise, probably through a combination of hemoconcentration and release from spleen, marrow, and lungs.[144]

The effect of chronic exercise or training on the coagulation system is less clear. Training appears to cause primarily a reduction in platelet aggregation,[153] particularly in older patients with cardiovascular disease,[154, 155] and may also reduce plasma fibrinogen concentration.[156]

SUMMARY

Exercise plays a critical role in both the primary and secondary prevention of ischemic heart disease. Epidemiologic investigations show approximately half the incidence of CAD in active compared with sedentary persons. A sedentary lifestyle thus is considered by national and international organizations to be one of the most important modifiable risk factors for cardiovascular complications and death. Fortunately, a moderate level of occupational or recreational activity appears to confer a significant protective effect. Well designed clinical investigations, supported by results from basic animal studies, have demonstrated that this effect is not related to a nonspecific selection bias in favor of already vigorous individuals but rather a direct protective mechanism of exercise. Regular dynamic exercise can improve other known risk factors for CAD, including plasma lipids, glucose intolerance, abdominal obesity, and probably hypertension. However, even when these other risk factors are taken into account, exercise appears to exert an independent protective effect. Once CAD has become manifest, exercise training can clearly improve the functional capacity of patients and reduce overall mortality rates by decreasing the risk of sudden death. These benefits may occur either through direct effects on the coronary arteries, modifications of autonomic control of the circulation, or changes in the blood coagulation system.

REFERENCES

1. Fletcher GF, Froelicher VF, Hartley LH, et al: Exercise standards: a statement for health professionals from the American Heart Association. Circulation 82:2286–2322, 1990.
2. Currens JH, White PD: Half century of running: clinical, physiologic and autopsy findings in the case of Clarence De Mar, "Mr. Marathoner." N Engl J Med 265:988–993, 1961.
3. Noakes TD, Opie LH, Rose AG: Marathon running and immunity to coronary heart disease: fact versus fiction. Clin Sports Med 3:527–543, 1984.
4. Fletcher GF, Blair SN, Blumenthal J, et al: Statement on exercise: benefits and recommendations for physical activity programs for all Americans: a statement for health professionals by the Committee on Exercise and Cardiac Rehabilitation of the Council on Clinical Cardiology, American Heart Association. Circulation 86:340–344, 1992.
5. Bijnen FC, Mosterd WL: Statement of the International Society and Federation of Cardiology, Physical inactivity: a risk factor for coronary heart disease. J Int Soc Fed Card 2:5–6, 1992.
6. U.S. Department of Health and Human Services: Physical Activity and Health: A Report of the Surgeon General. Atlanta: Centers for Disease Control and Prevention, 1996.
7. Morris JN, Crawford MD: Coronary heart disease and physical activity of work: evidence of a national necropsy survey. BMJ 2:1485–1496, 1958.
8. Morris JN, Heady JA, Raffle PAB, et al: Coronary heart disease and physical activity of work. Lancet 2:1111–1120, 1953.
9. Berlin JA, Colditz GA: A meta-analysis of physical activity in the prevention of coronary heart disease. Am J Epidemiol 132:612–628, 1990.
10. Zukel WJ, Lewis RH, Enterline MA, et al: A short term community study of the epidemiology of coronary heart disease: a preliminary report on North Dakota Study. Am J Public Health 49:1630–1639, 1959.
11. Kahn HA: The relationship of reported coronary artery heart disease mortality to physical activity of work. Am J Public Health 53:1058, 1963.
12. Taylor HL, Klepetar E, Keys A, et al: Death rates among physically active and sedentary employees of the railroad industry. Am J Public Health 52:1697–1707, 1962.
13. Shapiro S, Weinblatt E, Frank C, et al: Incidence of coronary artery disease in a population insured for medical care (HIP). Am J Public Health 59:1–101, 1969.
14. Cassel J, Heyden S, Bartel AC, et al: Occupation and physical activity and coronary artery disease. Arch Intern Med 128:920–928, 1971.
15. Brunner D, Manelis G, Modan B, et al: Physical activity at work and the incidence of myocardial infarction, angina pectoris and death due to ischemic heart disease: an epidemiological study in Israeli collective settlements (kibbutzim). J Chron Dis 27:217, 1974.
16. Paffenbarger RS, Laughlin ME, Gima AS, et al: Work activity of

longshoremen as related to death from coronary heart disease and stroke. N Engl J Med 282:1109–1114, 1970.
17. Paffenbarger RS, Hale WE: Work activity and coronary heart mortality. N Engl J Med 292:545–550, 1975.
18. Leon AS, Connett J, Jacobs DR, et al: Leisure-time physical activity levels and risk of coronary heart disease and death: the Multiple Risk Factor Intervention Trial. JAMA 258:2388–2395, 1987.
19. Morris JN, Chave SPW, Adams C, et al: Vigorous exercise in leisure-time and the incidence of coronary heart disease. Lancet 1:333–339, 1973,
20. Kannel WB, Sorlie P: Some health benefits of physical activity: the Framingham Study. Arch Intern Med 139:657–661, 1979.
21. Blair SN, Kohl HW III, Paffenbarger RS, et al: Physical fitness and all-cause mortality: a prospective study of healthy men and women. JAMA 262:2395–2401, 1989.
22. Morris JN, Clayton DG, Everitt MG, et al: Exercise in leisure-time: coronary attack and death rates. Br Heart J 63:325–334, 1993.
23. Garcia-Palmieri MR, Costas R Jr, Cruz-Vidal M, et al: Increased physical activity: a protective factor against heart attacks in Puerto Rico. Am J Cardiol 50:749–755, 1982.
24. Paffenbarger RS, Hyde RT, Wing AL, et al: Physical activity, all-cause mortality and longevity of college alumni. N Engl J Med 314:605, 1986.
25. Kujala UM, Kaprio J, Sarna S, et al: Relation of leisure-time physical activity and mortality: the Finnish twin cohort. JAMA 279:440–444, 1998.
26. Paffenbarger RS Jr, Hyde RT, Wing AL, et al: The association of changes in physical-activity level and other lifestyle characteristics with mortality among men. N Engl J Med 328:538–545, 1993.
27. Hakim AA, Petrovitch H, Burchfiel CM, et al: Effects of walking on mortality among nonsmoking retired men. N Engl J Med 338:94–99, 1998.
28. Astrand PO: Textbook of Work Physiology: Physiological Bases of Exercise. 3rd ed. New York: McGraw-Hill, 1986.
29. Sandvik L, Erikssen J, Thanlow E, et al: Physical fitness as a predictor of mortality among healthy, middle-aged Norwegian men. N Engl J Med 328:533–537, 1993.
30. Wilhelmsen L, Bjure J, Ekstrom-Jodal B, et al: Nine years follow-up of maximal exercise test in a random population sample of middle aged men. Cardiology 69(suppl 2):1–8, 1981.
31. Ekelund L, Haskell WL, Johnson JL, et al: Physical fitness as a predictor of cardiovascular mortality in asymptomatic North American men: the Lipid Research Clinic Mortality Follow-up Study. N Engl J Med 319:1379–1384, 1988.
32. Bouchard C, Lesage R, Lortie G: Aerobic performance in brothers, dizygotic and monozygotic twins. Med Sci Sports Exerc 18:639–646, 1986.
33. Hein HO, Suadiciani P, Gyntelberg F: Physical fitness or physical activity as a predictor of ischemic heart disease? A 17-year follow-up in the Copenhagen Male Study. J Intern Med 232:471–479, 1992.
34. Blair SN, Kohl HW, Barlow CE, et al: Changes in physical fitness and all-cause mortality: a prospective study in healthy and unhealthy men. JAMA 273:1093–1098, 1995.
35. Haskell WL: Health consequences of physical activity: understanding and challenges regarding dose-response. The JB Wolfe Memorial Lecture. Med Sci Sports Exerc 26:649–660, 1994.
36. Hakim AA, Curb JD, Petrovitch H, et al: Effects of walking on coronary heart disease in elderly men. Circulation 100:9–13, 1999.
37. Powell KE, Thompson PD, Caspersen CJ, et al: Physical activity and the incidence of coronary heart disease. Annu Rev Public Health 8:253–287, 1987.
38. Leon AS: Effects of physical activity and fitness on health. *In* Assessing Physical Fitness and Physical Activity in Population-Based Surveys. Hyattsville, MD: US Department of Health and Human Services, National Center for Health Statistics, 1989, DHHS publication no. (PHS) 89-1253.
39. Castelli WP, Doyle JT, Gordon T, et al: HDL cholesterol and other lipids in coronary heart disease: the Cooperative Lipoprotein Phenotyping Study. Circulation 55:767–772, 1977.
40. Leon AS, Haskell WL: The influence of exercise on the concentrations of triglyceride and cholesterol in human plasma. Exerc Sports Sci Rev 12:205–244, 1984.
41. Wood PD, Haskell WL, Klein H, et al: The distribution of plasma lipoproteins in middle aged runners. Metabolism 25:1249–1257, 1976.
42. Rogers MA, Yamamoto C, Hagberg JM, et al: The effects of 7 years of intense exercise training on patients with coronary artery disease. J Am Coll Cardiol 10:321–326, 1987.
43. Herbert PN, Bernier DN, Cullinane EM, et al: High-density lipoprotein metabolism in runners and sedentary men. JAMA 252:1034–1037, 1984.
44. Wood PD, Stefanick ML, Dreon DM, et al: Changes in plasma lipids and lipoproteins in overweight men during weight loss through dieting as compared with exercise. N Engl J Med 319:1173–1179, 1988.
45. Wood PD, Stefanick ML, Williams PT, et al: The effects on plasma lipoproteins of a prudent weight-reducing diet, with or without exercise, in overweight men and women. N Engl J Med 325:461–466, 1991.
46. Naito HK: The association of serum lipids, lipoproteins, and coronary heart disease assessed by coronary arteriography. Ann N Y Acad Sci 454:230–238, 1985.
47. Kraus RM: Regulation of high density lipoprotein levels. Med Clin North Am 66:403–430, 1982.
48. Gyntelber F, Brennan R, Holloszy JO, et al: Plasma triglyceride lowering by exercise despite increase in food intake in patients with type IV hyperlipoproteinemia. Am J Clin Nutr 30:716–720, 1977.
49. Blumenthal JA, Siegal WC, Appelbaum M, et al: Failure of exercise to reduce blood pressure in patients with mild hypertension: results of a randomized controlled trial. JAMA 266:2098–2104, 1991.
50. Martin JE, Dubbert PM, Cushman WC, et al: Controlled trial of aerobic exercise in hypertension. Circulation 81:1560–1567, 1990.
51. Urata H, Tanabe Y, Kiyonaga A, et al: Antihypertensive and volume-depleting effects of mild exercise on essential hypertension. Hypertension 9:245–252, 1987.
52. Duncan JJ, Farr JE, Upton SJ, et al: The effects of aerobic exercise on plasma catecholamines and blood pressure in patients with mild essential hypertension. JAMA 254:2609–2613, 1985.
53. Gordon NF, Scott CB, Levine BD: Comparison of single versus multiple lifestyle interventions: are the antihypertensive effects of exercise training and diet-induced weight loss additive? Am J Cardiol 79:763–767, 1997.
54. Martin WH, Montgomery J, Snell PG, et al: Cardiovascular adaptations to intense swim training in sedentary middle-aged men and women. Circulation 75:323–330, 1987.
55. Blair SN, Goodyear NN, Gibbons LW, et al: Physical fitness and incidence of hypertension in healthy normotensive men and women. JAMA 252:487–490, 1984.
56. Defronzo RA, Ferrannini E: Insulin resistance: a multifactorial syndrome responsible for NIDDM, obesity, hypertension, dyslipidemia, and atherosclerotic cardiovascular disease. Diabetes Care 14:173–194, 1991.
57. King DS, Staten MA, Kohrt WM, et al: Insulin secretory capacity in endurance trained and untrained young men. Am J Physiol 259:E155–E181, 1990.
58. Helmrich SP, Raglend DR, Leung RW, et al: Physical activity and reduced occurrence on non-insulin dependent diabetes mellitus. N Engl J Med 325:147–152, 1991.
59. Myerburg RJ, Kessler KM, Bassett AL, et al: A biological approach to sudden cardiac death: structure, function and cause. Am J Cardiol 63:1512–1516, 1989.
60. Kohl HW, Powell KE, Gordon NF, et al: Physical activity, physical fitness, and sudden cardiac death. Epidemiol Rev 14:37–58, 1992.
61. Mittleman MA, Maclure M, Tofler GH, et al: Triggering of acute myocardial infarction by heavy physical exertion: protection against triggering by regular exertion. N Engl J Med 329:1677–1683, 1993.
62. Willich SN, Lewis M, Lowel H, et al: Physical exertion as a trigger of acute myocardial infarction. N Engl J Med 329:1684–1690, 1993.
63. Gibbons L, Blair SN, Kohl HW, et al: The safety of maximal exercise testing. Circulation 80:846–852, 1990.
64. Levine BD, Zuckerman JH, Cole C: Medical complications of Exercise. *In* Roitman JL (ed): American College of Sports Medicine's Resource Manual: Guidelines for Exercise Testing and Prescription. 3rd ed. pp. 488–498. Baltimore: Williams & Wilkins, 1998.
65. Thompson PD, Funk EJ, Carleton RA, et al: Incidence of death during jogging in Rhode Island from 1975 through 1980. JAMA 247:2525–2538, 1982.
66. Siscovick DS, Weiss NS, Fletcher RH, et al: The incidence of primary cardiac arrest during vigorous exercise. N Engl J Med 311:874–877, 1984.

67. Squires RW, Gau GT, Miller TD, et al: Cardiovascular rehabilitation: status, 1990. Mayo Clin Proc 65:731–755, 1990.
68. Foster C: Exercise training following cardiovascular surgery. Exerc Sports Sci Rev 14:303–323, 1986.
69. Leon AS, Certo C, Comoss P, et al: Scientific evidence of the value of cardiac rehabilitation services with emphasis on patients following myocardial infarction, Section I: exercise conditioning component. J Cardiopulm Rehabil 10:79–87, 1990.
70. Levine BD, Friedman DB, Williams AN: Starting a cardiac rehabilitation program: theory and practice. Cardio 9:26–37, 1992.
71. Hellerstein HK, Ford AB: Rehabilitation of the cardiac patient. JAMA 164:225–231, 1957.
72. Kallio V, Hamalainen H, Hakkila J, et al: Reduction in sudden deaths by a multifactorial intervention programme after acute myocardial infarction. Lancet 2:1081–1094, 1979.
73. Oldridge NB, Guyatt GH, Fischer ME, et al: Cardiac rehabilitation after myocardial infarction, combined experience of randomized clinical trials. JAMA 260:945–950, 1988.
74. O'Connor GT, Buring JE, Yusuf S, et al: An overview of randomized trials of rehabilitation with exercise after myocardial infarction. Circulation 80:234–244, 1989.
75. Mitchell JH: Exercise training in the treatment of coronary heart disease. Adv Intern Med 20:249–272, 1975.
76. Detry J-MR, Rousseay M, Vandenbroucke G, et al: Increased arteriovenous oxygen difference after physical training in coronary heart disease. Circulation 44:109–118, 1971.
77. Ehsani AA, Biello DR, Schultz J, et al: Improvement of left ventricular contractile function by exercise training in patients with coronary artery disease. Circulation 74:350–358, 1986.
78. Belardinelli R, Georgiou D, Ginzton L, et al: Effects of moderate exercise training on thallium uptake and contractile response to low dose dobutamine of dysfunctional myocardium in patients with ischemic cardiomyopathy. Circulation 97:553–561, 1998.
79. Saltin B, Blomqvist CG, Mitchell JH, et al: Response to exercise after bedrest and after training. Circulation 38:1–78, 1968.
80. Gaffney FA, Nixon JV, Karlsson ES, et al: Cardiovascular deconditioning produced by 20 hours of bedrest with head-down tilt (−5°) in middle aged healthy men. Am J Cardiol 56:634–638, 1985.
81. Blomqvist CG, Stone HL: Cardiovascular adjustments to gravitational stress. *In* Shepherd JT, Abboud FM (eds): Handbook of Physiology. Sect. 2, The Cardiovascular System. pp. 1025–1063. Bethesda, MD: American Physiological Society, 1983.
82. Graham LE: Patients' perceptions in the CCU. Am J Nursing 69:1921–1922, 1969.
83. Myerburg RJ, Kessler KM, Castellanos A: Sudden cardiac death: structure, function, and time dependence of risk. Circulation 85(suppl I):I-2–I-10, 1992.
84. Friedman DB, Williams AN, Levine BD: Compliance and efficacy of cardiac rehabilitation and risk factor modification in the medically indigent. Am J Cardiol 79:281–285, 1997.
85. Borg G: Perceived exertion as an indicator of somatic stress. Scand J Rehabil Med 2:92–98, 1970.
86. Chow RJ, Wilmore JH: The regulation of exercise intensity by ratings of perceived exertion. J Card Rehabil 4:382–387, 1984.
87. Gossard D, Haskell WL, DeBusk RF, et al: Effects of low- and high-intensity home-based exercise training on functional capacity in healthy middle-aged men. Am J Cardiol 57:446–449, 1986.
88. Homans DC, Laxson DD, Sublett E, et al: Cumulative deterioration of myocardial function after repeated episodes of exercise-induced ischemia. Am J Physiol H1462–H1471, 1989.
89. Donnely TJ, Sievers RE, Vissern FLJ, et al: Heat shock protein induction in rat hearts: a role for improved myocardial salvage after ischemia and reperfusion? Circulation 85:769–778, 1992.
90. Hossack KF, Hartwig R: Cardiac arrest associated with supervised cardiac rehabilitation. J Card Rehabil 2:402–408, 1982.
91. Cobb LA, Weaver D: Exercise: a risk for sudden death in patients with coronary heart disease. J Am Coll Cardiol 7:215–219, 1986.
92. Sionis D, Glazier JJ, Stammen F, et al: Early exercise testing after successful percutaneous transluminal coronary angioplasty: a word of caution. Am Heart J 123:530–532, 1992.
93. Shah D, Lai P: Acute coronary occlusion during early post-PTCA exercise testing: a rare but avoidable risk. Cathet Cardiovasc Diagn 33:335–339, 1994.
94. Samuels B, Schumann J, Kiat H, et al: Acute stent thrombosis associated with exercise testing after successful percutaneous transluminal coronary angioplasty. Am Heart J 130:1120–1122, 1995.
95. Balady GJ, Leitschuh ML, Jacobs AK, et al: Safely and clinical use of exercise testing one to three days after percutaneous transluminal coronary angioplasty. Am J Cardiol 69:1259–1264, 1992.
96. DeBusk RF, Blomqvist CG, Kouchoukos NT, et al: Identification and treatment of low-risk patients after acute myocardial infarction and coronary-artery bypass graft surgery. N Engl J Med 314:161–166, 1986.
97. Miller NH, Haskell WL, Berra K, et al: Home versus group exercise training for increasing functional capacity after myocardial infarction. Circulation 70:645–649, 1984.
98. Haskell WL: Cardiovascular complications during exercise training of cardiac patients. Circulation 57:920–924, 1978.
99. Van Camp SP, Peterson RA: Cardiovascular complications of outpatient cardiac rehabilitation programs. JAMA 256:1160–1163, 1986.
100. Juneau M, Rogers R, DeBusk RF, et al: Effectiveness of self-monitored, home-based, moderate-intensity exercise training in middle aged men and women. Am J Cardiol 60:66–70, 1987.
101. Coats AJS, Adamopoulos S, Meyer TE, et al: Effects of physical training in chronic heart failure. Lancet 335:63–66, 1990.
102. Hambrecht R, Fiehn E, Weigl C, et al: Regular physical exercise corrects endothelial function and improves exercise capacity in patients with chronic heart failure. Circulation 98:2709–2715, 1998.
103. Laughlin MH, McAllister RM: Exercise training induced coronary vascular adaptation. J Appl Physiol 73:2209–2225, 1992.
104. Tepperman J, Pearlman D: Effects of exercise and anemia on coronary arteries in small animals as revealed by the corrosion-cast technique. Circ Res 9:576–584, 1961.
105. Wyatt HL, Mitchell JH: Influences of physical conditioning and deconditioning on coronary vasculature of dogs. J Appl Physiol 45:619–625, 1978.
106. Bove AA, Dewey JD: Proximal coronary vasomotor reactivity after exercise training in dogs. Circulation 71:620–625, 1985.
107. Prineas Rose GRJ, Mitchell JRA: Myocardial infarction and the intrinsic calibre of coronary arteries. Br Heart J 28:548–552, 1967.
108. Mann GV, Spoerry A, Gran M, et al: Atherosclerosis in the Masai. Am J Epidemiol 96:26–57, 1971.
109. Pellicia A, Spartaro A, Granata M, et al: Coronary arteries in physiological hypertrophy: echocardiographic evidence of increased proximal size in elite athletes. Int J Sports Med 11:120–126, 1990.
110. Eckstein RW: Effect of exercise and coronary artery narrowing on coronary collateral circulation. Circ Res 5:230–235, 1957.
111. Cohen MV, Yipintsoi T, Scheuer J: Coronary collateral stimulation by exercise in dogs with stenotic coronary arteries. J Appl Physiol 52:664–671, 1982.
112. Heaton WH, Marr KC, Capurro N, et al: Beneficial effect of physical training on blood flow to myocardium perfused by chronic collaterals in the exercising dog. Circulation 57:575–581, 1978.
113. Scheel KW, Ingram LA, Wilson JL: Effects of exercise on the coronary and collateral vasculature of beagles with and without coronary occlusion. Circ Res 48:523–530, 1981.
114. Roth DM, White FC, Nichols ML, et al: Effect of long-term exercise on regional myocardial function and coronary collateral development after gradual coronary artery occlusion in pigs. Circulation 82:1778–1789, 1990.
115. Kavanaugh T: Does exercise improve coronary collateralization? A new look at an old belief. Phys Sportsmed 17:96–114, 1989.
116. Kramsch DM, Aspoen AJ, Abramowitz BM: Reduction of coronary atherosclerosis by moderate conditioning exercise in monkeys on an atherogenic diet. N Engl J Med 305:1483–1489, 1981.
117. Ehsani AA, Heath GW, Hagberg JM, et al: Effects of 12 months of intense exercise training on ischemic ST segment depression in patients with coronary artery disease. Circulation 64:1116–1124, 1981.
118. Haskell WL, Sims CS, Myll J, et al: Coronary artery size and dilating capacity in ultra-distance runners. Circulation 87:1076–1081, 1993.
119. Levine BD, Mitchell JH: "Ultra" coronary arteries: bigger and better? Circulation 87:1402–1404, 1993.
120. Vanhoutte PM, Shimokawa H: Endothelium-derived relaxing factor and coronary vasospasm. Circulation 80:1–9, 1989.
121. Snell PG, Martin WH, Buckey JC, et al: Maximal vascular leg conductance in trained and untrained men. J Appl Physiol 62:606–610, 1987.
122. Delp MD: Effects of exercise training on endothelium-dependent peripheral vascular responsiveness. Med Sci Sports Exerc 27:1152–1157, 1995.

123. Levine BD, Buckey JC, Fritsch JM, et al: Physical fitness and cardiovascular regulation: mechanisms of orthostatic intolerance. J Appl Physiol 70:112–122, 1991.
124. Davies MJ, Thomas AC: Plaque fissuring: the cause of acute myocardial infarction, sudden ischaemic death, and crescendo angina. Br Heart J 53:363–373, 1985.
125. Falk E: Why do plaques rupture? Circulation 86(suppl III):III-30–III-42, 1992.
126. Podrid PJ, Fuchs T, Cardinas R: Role of the sympathetic nervous system in the genesis of ventricular arrhythmias. Circulation 82(suppl 2):I-103–I-113, 1990.
127. Schwartz PJ: The autonomic nervous system and sudden death. Eur Heart J 19(suppl F):F72–F80, 1998.
128. Billman GE, Schwartz PJ, Stone HL: Baroreceptor reflex control of heart rate: a predictor of sudden cardiac death. Circulation 66:874–880, 1982.
129. Casolo CG, Stroder P, Signorinin C, et al: Heart rate variability during the acute phase of myocardial infarction. Circulation 85:2073–2079, 1992.
130. Kleiger RE, Miller JP, Bigger JT Jr, et al: Decreased heart rate variability and its association with increased mortality after acute myocardial infarction. Am J Cardiol 59:256–262, 1987.
131. Farrell TG, Bashir Y, Cripps R, et al: Risk stratification for arrhythmic events in postinfarction patients based on heart rate variability, ambulatory electrocardiographic variables and the signal-averaged electrocardiogram. J Am Coll Cardiol 18:687–697, 1991.
132. La Rovere MT, Bigger JT Jr, Marcus FI: Baroreflex sensitivity and heart-rate variability in prediction of total cardiac mortality after myocardial infarction: ATRAMI (Autonomic Tone and Reflexes After Myocardial Infarction) Investigators. Lancet 351:478–484, 1998.
133. Tsuji H, Larson MG, Venditti FJ, et al: Impact of reduced heart rate variability on risk for cardiac events: the Framingham Heart Study. Circulation 94:2850–2855, 1996.
134. Seals DR, Chase PB: Influence of physical training on heart rate variability and baroreflex circulatory control. J Appl Physiol 66:1886–1895, 1989.
135. Shin K, Minamitani H, Onishi S, et al: Autonomic differences between athletes and nonathletes: spectral analysis approach. Med Sci Sports Exerc 29:1482–1490, 1997.
136. Pagain M, Somers V, Furlan R, et al: Changes in autonomic regulation induced by physical training in mild hypertension. Hypertension 12:600–610, 1988.
137. Coats AJ, Adamopoulos S, Radelli A, et al: Controlled trial of physical training in chronic heart failure: exercise performance, hemodynamics, ventilation and autonomic function. Circulation 85:2119–2131, 1992.
138. Bowman AJ, Clayton RH, Murray A, et al: Baroreflex function in sedentary and endurance-trained elderly people. Age Ageing 26:289–294, 1997.
139. Levy WC, Cerqueira MD, Harp GD, et al: Effect of endurance exercise training on heart rate variability at rest in healthy young and older men. Am J Cardiol 82:1236–1241, 1998.
140. Schuit AJ, Van Amelsvoort LGPM, Verheij TC, et al: Exercise training and heart rate variability in older people. Med Sci Sports Exerc 31:816–821, 1999.
141. Billman GE, Schwartz PJ, Stone HL: The effects of daily exercise on susceptibility to sudden cardiac death. Circulation 69:1182–1189, 1984.
142. Vanoli E, DeFerrari GM, Stramba-Badiale M, et al: Vagal stimulation and prevention of sudden death in conscious dogs with a healed myocardial infarction. Circ Res 68:1471–1481, 1991.
143. Hunter J: A Treatise on Blood, Inflammation, and Gunshot Wounds. p. 88. London: 1794.
144. Bourey RE, Santoro SA: Interactions of exercise, coagulation, platelets, and fibrinolysis—a brief review. Med Sci Sports Exerc 20:439–446, 1988.
145. Dufaux B, Order U, Liesen H: Effect of a short maximal physical exercise on coagulation, fibrinolysis, and complement system. Int J Sports Med 12(suppl 1):S38–S42, 1991.
146. Bartsch P, Haeberli A, Straub PW: Blood coagulation after long distance running: antithrombin III prevents fibrin formation. Thromb Haemost 63:430–434, 1990.
147. Weiss C, Seitel G, Bartsch P: Coagulation and fibrinolysis after moderate and very heavy exercise in healthy male subjects. Med Sci Sports Exerc 30:246–251, 1998.
148. Kopitsky RG, Switzer MP, Williams RS, et al: The basis for the increase in factor VIII procoagulant activity during exercise. Thromb Haemost 49:53–57, 1983.
149. Davis GL, Abildgaard CF, Bernauer EM, et al: Fibrinolytic and hemostatic changes during and after maximal exercise in males. J Appl Physiol 40:287–292, 1976.
150. Weiss C, Welsch B, Albert M, et al: Coagulation and thrombomodulin in response to exercise of different type and duration. Med Sci Sports Exerc 30:1205–1210, 1998.
151. Ferguson EW, Barr CF, Bernier LL: Fibrinogenolysis and fibrinolysis with strenuous exercise. J Appl Physiol 47:1157–1161, 1979.
152. Chandler WL, Veith RC, Fellingham GW, et al: Fibrinolytic response during exercise and epinephrine infusion in the same subjects. J Am Coll Cardiol 19:1412–1420, 1992.
153. Rauramaa AJ, Salonen JT, Seppanen K, et al: Inhibition of platelet aggregability by moderate-intensity physical exercise: a randomized clinical trial in overweight men. Circulation 74:939–944, 1986.
154. Williams RS, Eden S, Andersen J: Reduced epinephrine-induced platelet aggregation following cardiac rehabilitation. J Clin Res 1:127–134, 1981.
155. Lehmann M, Hasler K, Bengdalt E, et al: Physical activity and coronary heart disease: sympathetic drive and adrenaline-induced platelet aggregation. Int J Sports Med 7(suppl):34–37, 1986.
156. Stratton JR, Chandler WL, Schwartz RS, et al: Effects of physical conditioning of fibrinolytic variables and fibrinogen in young and old healthy adults. Circulation 83:1692–1697, 1991.

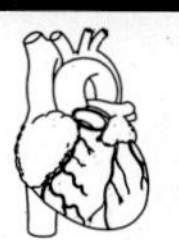

CHAPTER 122

SMOKING

John A. Oates, Craig R. Heim, and Michael D. Winniford

ISCHEMIC HEART DISEASE
Coronary Atherosclerosis
Acute Ischemic Events
Cessation of Smoking
Effect of Smoking: Relation to Other Cardiac Risk Factors
Environmental Tobacco Smoke
Pathophysiology
Coronary Vasospasm
EXTRACARDIAC VASCULAR DISEASE
NICOTINE ADDICTION
PHYSICIAN'S ROLE IN SMOKING CESSATION
SMOKING CESSATION RESULTS

Cigarette smoking is the single most important preventable cause of death in the United States.[1] Approximately 142,000 deaths from cardiovascular disease are attributable to cigarette smoking annually, and smoking significantly increases the risk for myocardial infarction (MI), sudden cardiac death, stroke, peripheral vascular disease, and abdominal aortic aneurysms. Importantly, the risk of cardiac ischemic events is substantially and rapidly reversible on cessation of smoking.

ISCHEMIC HEART DISEASE

The incidence of coronary artery disease (CAD), including sudden cardiac death, is more than doubled in cigarette smokers as a group and is increased fourfold in heavy smokers. There is a dose-response relationship between cigarette smoking and CAD, such that the risk increases with the number of cigarettes smoked daily, the extent of inhalation, and the number of years smoked. Cigarettes lower in tar or nicotine do not confer any protection from ischemic heart disease.

The clearest understanding of smoking-induced ischemic heart disease emerges from the integration of data from epidemiologic and pathophysiologic investigations. In considering the participation of smoking in the etiology of ischemic heart disease, it has been useful to separate the effect of smoking on the development of atherosclerotic stenosis of the coronary arteries from its effects on the process that converts coronary atherosclerosis to acute ischemic events.

The acute cardiac ischemic events all represent an abrupt transition from stable chronic CAD to one of the major consequences of ischemia: unstable angina, MI, and sudden cardiac death. Abundant evidence supports the concept that rupture of a lipid-rich atherosclerotic plaque with attendant thrombus formation is the initiating event in the development of the vast majority of these acute ischemic syndromes (Fig. 122–1).[2, 3]

Coronary Atherosclerosis

Age is a powerful determinant of coronary atherosclerosis, and angiographic studies indicate that the relative risk for coronary stenosis associated with having previously smoked is greatest in the youngest age groups, suggesting an acceleration of the process by smoking. Some of the best evidence is provided by a prospective autopsy study performed in Hawaii[4] and from the study of autopsies on young men who died violently.[5] These studies indicate that there is a strong dose-related association of smoking with atherosclerosis of the abdominal aorta and an association with atherosclerosis of the coronary arteries that is significant but less robust. From these two autopsy studies, as well as from an overview of all of them, one gains the impression that the significant increase in fibrous atherosclerotic plaques and atheroma of the coronary arteries is not of sufficient magnitude to fully account for the greater increase in acute ischemic events that are linked to cigarette smoking.

The finding that the increase in the involvement of the coronary vessels with atherosclerosis is of small magnitude is in agreement with the prospective epidemiologic evidence that stable angina pectoris is increased modestly, if at all, in cigarette smokers over the age of 40 years. In men less than 40 years of age, an increase in stable angina has been detected (twofold), but at 40 years and older the risk is increased only slightly, even after adjusting the incidence of stable angina for the loss of persons at risk owing to acute ischemic events.[6]

Acute Ischemic Events

Prospective epidemiologic studies have consistently demonstrated a substantial increase in the acute coronary ischemic events in individuals who concurrently are smoking.[1] The pernicious effect of cigarette smoking on MI and sudden cardiac death is seen throughout all ages, at least to the age of 70 years, but the increase in risk for a given individual is greatest during middle age. The largest body of prospectively acquired North American data indicate that middle-aged men who smoke have a 10-fold greater risk for sudden cardiac death and a 3.6-fold increase in

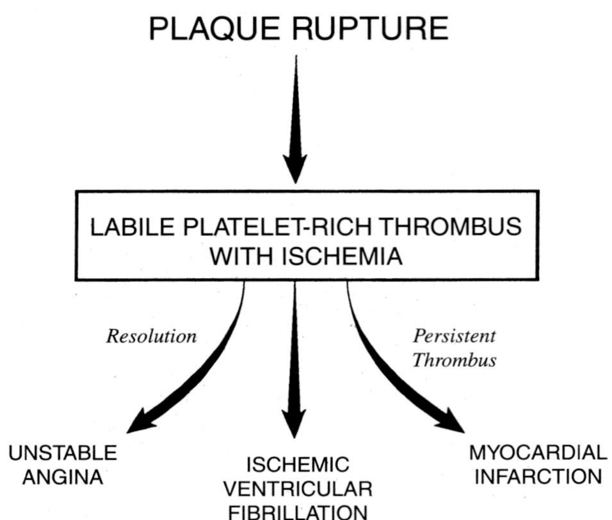

FIGURE 122–1 Initiation of the acute syndromes of myocardial ischemia.

MI (Table 122–1).[7] The risk for sudden cardiac death is disproportionately greater than that for MI, a finding that is replicated to varying degrees in other studies. Of all the coronary risk factors, cigarette smoking is the strongest predictor of sudden cardiac death. The risk for both of these acute ischemic events clearly exceeds that for stable angina.

Although the incidence of coronary deaths in women during middle age is lower, cigarette smoking accounts for about half of these deaths.

Cessation of Smoking

Smoking cessation in individuals without known ischemic heart disease makes an important contribution to reducing the risk for MI.[1, 8–10] The excess risk of MI falls by about 50 percent within the first 2 years after cessation of smoking, consistent with the idea that a substantial component of the risk of acute ischemic events is reversible.

For smokers who already have CAD, cessation is also very effective in reducing the incidence of further acute ischemic events. Survivors of MI have a greater risk of reinfarction if they continue to smoke, as do survivors of sudden cardiac death. For individuals who have angina pectoris or a positive exercise test or who have undergone coronary artery bypass graft surgery, continuing the smoking habit confers a worse prognosis. Cessation of smoking after coronary angioplasty or vascular surgery reduces the rate of restenosis by a third. Therefore, there is a major incentive for smoking cessation in this group of patients. When efforts to achieve cessation are effective, they probably confer a greater benefit than any pharmacologic or surgical intervention.

In economic terms, smoking cessation is a remarkably cost-effective intervention, at least in the short term.[11–13] The total economic burden of smoking-related illness is staggering: approximately $100 billion annually in medical costs and lost wages. It has been estimated that just a 1 percent reduction in smoking prevalence would result in a total savings of $3.2 billion in medical costs alone over a 7-year period.[12]

Effect of Smoking: Relation to Other Cardiac Risk Factors

The risk for CAD imposed by cigarette smoking is magnified by the presence of several other factors that cause ischemic heart disease. Cigarette smoking alone imposes a risk for ischemic heart disease that is independent of other risk factors. However, smoking in conjunction with another risk factor increases the actual rate of ischemic heart disease events to a greater extent than smoking alone. In one large study,[14] smoking increased the 10-year rate of a first CAD event (MI or sudden cardiac death) by 31 per 1000 persons when neither hypercholesterolemia nor hypertension was present. In conjunction with either hypercholesterolemia or hypertension, cigarette smoking increased the rate by 49 per 1000 persons, and when both hypercholesterolemia and hypertension were present the superimposition of smoking increased the rate by 97 per 1000 persons. In women, oral contraceptives enhance the risk imposed by smoking, such that there is a 10-fold increase in the risk of MI in oral contraceptive users who smoke. Therefore, hypercholesterolemia, hypertension, and oral contraceptive use provide an incentive to not smoke or to cease smoking that exceeds the abundant benefit of avoiding this addiction in the rest of the population.

Environmental Tobacco Smoke

There is growing evidence that exposure to environmental tobacco smoke ("passive" smoking) has an adverse effect on cardiovascular health.[15] Pooled results of epidemiologic

TABLE 122–1 Risk of Clinical Manifestations of Coronary Heart Disease in Persons 45–55 Years: Biennial Rate/1000 Person-Years

	Sudden Cardiac Death		Myocardial Infarction		All Coronary-Related Death	
	Men	*Women*	*Men*	*Women*	*Men*	*Women*
Nonsmoker	0.3	0.2	4.2	1.4	1.6	0.5
Smoker	3.2	0.9	15.0	2.0	4.5	1.1
Risk Ratio	10.7	4.5	3.6	1.4	2.8	2.2

studies indicate a 20 percent excess coronary heart disease death rate among nonsmoking spouses of smokers.[16] As many as 40,000 deaths from MI each year may be the result of passive smoking. The mechanisms linking environmental tobacco smoke exposure and cardiovascular disease are probably similar to those for active smoking.[17–21]

Pathophysiology

A review of the mechanisms linking cigarette smoking and ischemic heart disease must consider the fact that whereas smoking accelerates coronary atherosclerosis, it has an even greater effect on the process that abruptly converts atherosclerosis to the acute ischemic events of MI, unstable angina, and sudden cardiac death (see Fig. 122–1). The effect of chronic smoking on the initiation of acute ischemic events appears to be largely reversible, given the substantial and rapid reduction in the incidence of acute ischemic events after smoking cessation. Although there is likely overlap between the mechanisms by which smoking accelerates atherosclerosis and promotes acute ischemic events, it is useful to consider these adverse effects of smoking separately.

Acceleration of Atherosclerosis

As for other risk factors, *vascular endothelial dysfunction* likely plays a central role in the promotion of atherosclerosis in chronic smokers.[22–24] Extensive endothelial abnormalities are present in the umbilical arteries of infants born to smoking mothers, and lesions of endothelial cells, subendothelial damage, and platelet adhesion have been described in vessels of experimental animals exposed to cigarette smoke. Reduced prostacyclin biosynthetic capacity and functional abnormalities of vascular endothelium also result from cigarette smoking. Impaired endothelium-dependent vasodilatation in both forearm and coronary vascular beds has been demonstrated in even young chronic smokers.[24–26] These functional abnormalities may be due to smoking-induced inhibition of nitric oxide release[27, 28] or acceleration of nitric oxide breakdown. Structural endothelial damage may result either from a direct toxic effect of nicotine or other components of cigarette smoke on endothelial cells or from smoking-induced oxidative stress.[24, 29] Smokers have reduced levels of antioxidant vitamins and increased levels of oxidized low-density lipoprotein, a potent inhibitor of endothelial function.[24, 30] Smoking-induced acute and chronic systemic hemodynamic changes may also contribute to vascular endothelial dysfunction. For example, smoking a single cigarette causes an acute rise in systemic blood pressure and heart rate, and chronic smoking results in a persistent elevation in daytime blood pressure.

Smoking is associated with *lipid abnormalities* that may contribute to the development of atherosclerosis.[31, 32] In addition to increased levels of oxidized low-density lipoprotein, smoking produces an increase in very low density lipoprotein and triglycerides and a reduction in high-density lipoprotein levels. Smoking has been shown to increase *monocyte adhesion* to endothelial cells, an important early event in atherosclerosis.[33, 34] Other factors that may contribute to the development of atherosclerosis in smokers include smoking-induced *platelet activation, increased fibrinogen levels,* and *increased blood viscosity.*

Promotion of Acute Ischemic Events

More striking than the effect of smoking on the development of atherosclerosis is the dramatically increased risk of acute ischemic events, including MI and sudden death. Acute systemic and coronary *hemodynamic effects* of smoking are likely to play an important role in the development of these ischemic events. After smoking a single cigarette, systemic arterial pressure, heart rate, and myocardial contractility increase, resulting in a rise in myocardial oxygen demand.[35, 36] Simultaneously, in patients with atherosclerosis, smoking causes acute vasoconstriction of both conduit and resistance coronary vessels, with a fall in coronary blood flow (Fig. 122–2).[36–38] Even in the absence of a hemodynamically significant stenosis, coronary flow may fall by more than 20 percent despite a significant increase in myocardial oxygen demand. In some individuals, smoking causes intense *focal* vasoconstriction or spasm that can lead to myocardial ischemia.[39] These acute hemodynamic effects of smoking in the coronary bed are most likely adrenergically mediated, as they can be prevented by alpha-adrenergic blockade (Fig. 122–3).[40] Adrenergic stimulation has been shown to cause exaggerated coronary vasoconstriction in the setting of endothelial dysfunction.[41, 42] Plasma norepinephrine and epinephrine levels rise acutely after smoking[35]; this catecholamine release may lower arrhythmia threshold and increase the risk of sudden death.

In addition to lowering anginal threshold, repeated episodes of coronary vasoconstriction and elevations of systemic arterial pressure may increase hemodynamic stresses at the site of an atherosclerotic plaque. An increase in shear stress at the site of a vulnerable plaque is considered to be an important cause of plaque rupture.

Smoking has also been shown to exacerbate the cardiovascular effects of cocaine.[43] Both the epicardial coronary constriction and the increase in myocardial oxygen demand caused by cocaine are potentiated by concomitant smoking, perhaps raising the risk of MI and sudden death attributed to cocaine use.

Inhaled *carbon monoxide* in cigarette smoke binds to hemoglobin, reducing oxygen delivery to myocardial cells. Carbon monoxide levels found in smokers have been shown to lower anginal threshold[44, 45] and increase ventricular fibrillation threshold.[46] Carbon monoxide may also have a deleterious effect on vascular endothelial cells.[47]

Coronary thrombosis plays a major role in acute ischemic events, and smoking is associated with several changes in the hemostatic system that lead to a *hypercoagulable state.* These hemostatic changes include an increase in fibrinogen,[48] red cell mass, and blood viscosity, platelet activation with thromboxane A_2 release[49]; and impaired tissue plasminogen activator release from endothelial cells.[50]

Most research on the effects of smoking on the cardiovascular system has focused specifically on nicotine and carbon monoxide, but there are over 4000 other components in cigarette smoke, some of which may also contribute to smoking-induced vascular disease.[51]

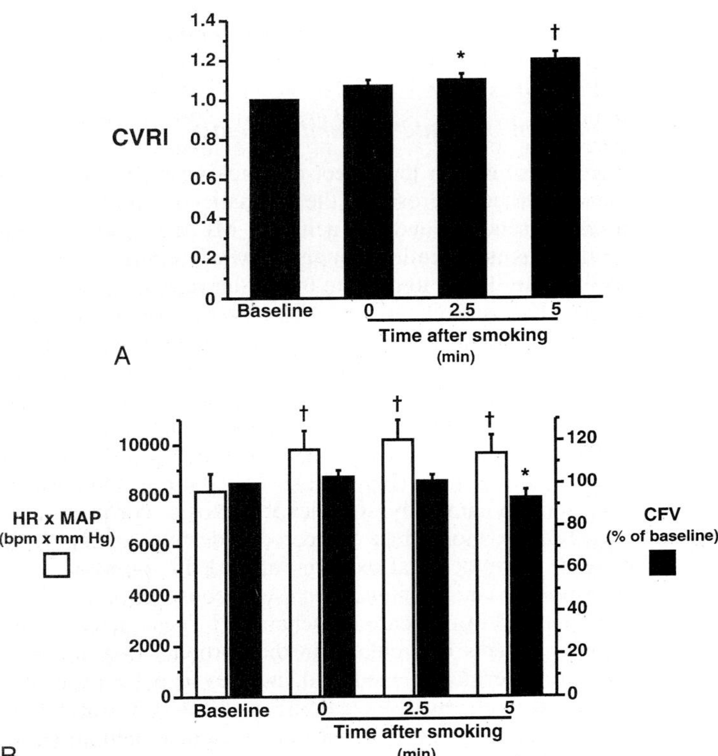

FIGURE 122–2 A, Effect of smoking on heart rate (HR)—mean arterial pressure product (MAP) (a measure of myocardial oxygen demand) and coronary flow velocity (CFV). CFV fell by 7 percent after smoking one cigarette despite an increase in myocardial oxygen demand. **B,** Effect of smoking on coronary vascular resistance index (CVRI). Despite an increase in oxygen demand, coronary resistance rises after smoking. (**A** and **B,** From Quillen JE, Rossen JD, Oskarsson HJ, et al: Acute effect of cigarette smoking on the coronary circulation: constriction of epicardial and resistance vessels. Reprinted with permission from the American College of Cardiology [J Am Coll Cardiol, 1993, 22:642].)

Coronary Vasospasm

A much less common cause of ischemia than plaque rupture, primary coronary vasospasm usually manifests as variant angina but may also cause MI and sudden cardiac death. Coronary vasospasm is strongly associated with cigarette smoking, much more so than with other risk factors.[52]

EXTRACARDIAC VASCULAR DISEASE

Smoking markedly accelerates atherosclerosis in the abdominal aorta, and occlusive disease of its branches is increased as well.[4, 5] Aortic aneurysm, peripheral vascular disease, and renal artery stenosis are increased in smokers. Renovascular hypertension should be strongly suspected in cigarette smokers who have severe hypertension. Cigarette smoking is an independent risk factor in the development of atherosclerosis in the internal pudendal and penile arteries of young impotent men.

Two types of stroke are increased in cigarette smokers.[53] Smoking is a risk factor for cerebral infarction, and the magnitude of risk is a function of the smoking exposure. This occurs in conjunction with an increase in atherosclerosis of the carotid arteries in smokers. Subarachnoid hemorrhage is markedly increased in cigarette smokers, and in women who take oral contraceptives this risk is further enhanced.

NICOTINE ADDICTION

Although psychological and social factors are important determinants of chronic tobacco use, the 1988 Surgeon General's Report[54] emphasized the predominant role of nicotine addiction. The three major conclusions of this report were that cigarettes are addicting, that nicotine is the ingredient that causes the addiction, and that the basis for the addiction is similar to that of drugs such as heroin and cocaine. Nicotine is readily absorbed from tobacco smoke in the lungs and is rapidly transported to the brain, where it acts on neurotransmitter systems. Its many effects on brain function are powerfully reinforcing. Additional features of regular use are tolerance, withdrawal symptoms, and relapse after abstinence. Effective treatment requires multiple behavioral interventions, often combined with pharmacologic therapy.[54]

An appreciation of habitual tobacco use as a form of drug dependence should help physicians to a greater understanding of and empathy for their smoking patients.

PHYSICIAN'S ROLE IN SMOKING CESSATION

Physicians, particularly those who treat patients with cardiovascular disease, can play a very important role in helping patients to stop smoking. Although intensive, organized behavioral programs are more effective than physician interventions, only a small proportion of smokers will enroll in such programs on their own volition. However, 70 percent of all smokers will see a physician during the course of 1 year, making the encounter a timely opportunity for a physician-directed effort. Lack of a long-term relationship with a patient should not hinder the physician's attempt at counseling because it does not decrease the effectiveness or outcome.[55] There are a number of ways in

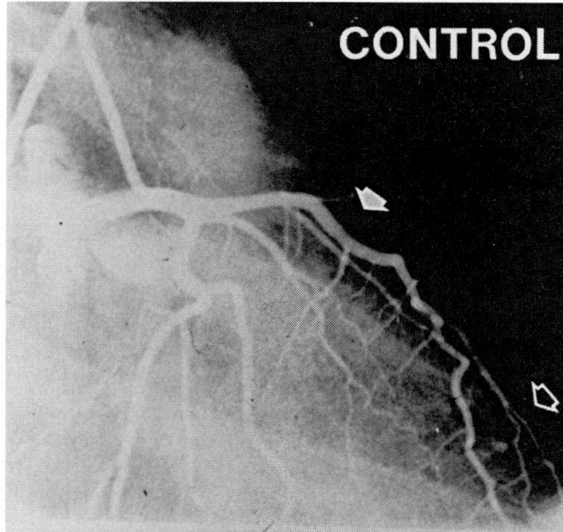

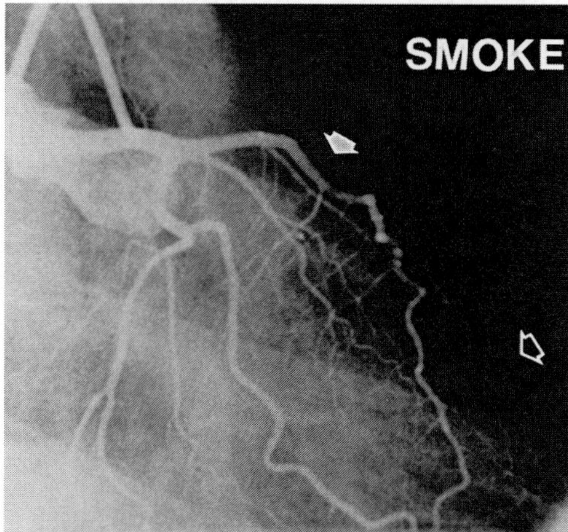

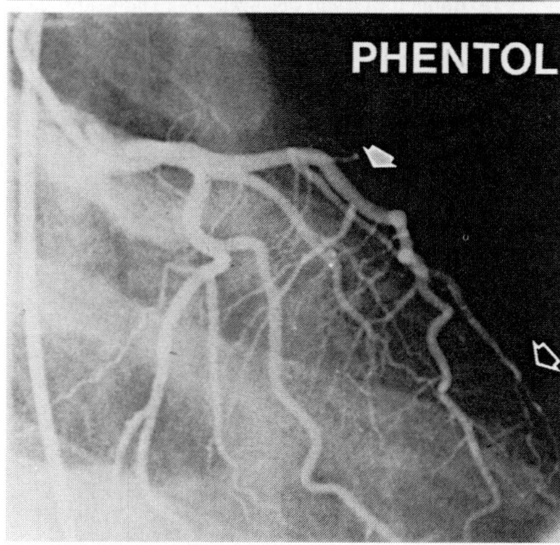

FIGURE 122–3 Reversal of smoking-induced coronary vasoconstriction by phentolamine, an alpha-adrenergic blocker. After smoking a single cigarette (SMOKE), focal constriction is observed in the midportion of the left anterior descending artery *(solid arrows)*, with diffuse narrowing of a diagonal branch *(open arrows)*. Constriction is rapidly reversed by intracoronary phentolamine (PHENTOL).

which physicians can help their patients toward permanent smoking cessation. The Agency for Health Care Policy and Research developed clinical practice guidelines for smoking cessation.[56] All physicians who care for smokers should review these guidelines and develop a consistent approach to smoking cessation.

Physicians should be role models for healthy behaviors, including avoiding tobacco use. Estimates are that only 9 percent of physicians are regular smokers.[57] In addition, physicians' offices and hospitals should be smoke-free environments. Office personnel, including nurses and secretaries, can be trained to participate in smoking interventions, especially by making follow-up phone calls to patients to assess progress and encourage continued abstinence. Office staff can also assist by posting antismoking messages, using chart stickers or other reminders for physicians, maintaining a supply of self-help booklets in examination rooms, and subscribing to waiting room magazines that do not contain tobacco advertisements.[58]

Physicians should take a tobacco use history from all new patients and periodically on return visits. They can be assisted in this effort by their office nurses as part of the check-in process. It has been suggested that this be made a "vital sign."[59] Tobacco use should be recorded on a problem list in the front of the medical record.

Physicians should deliver a strong, unequivocal, and personalized message that the patient should stop smoking. Personalized advice may center on symptoms, the social or economic consequences of smoking, high-risk status for a certain disease, or the recent diagnosis of a definite smoking-related disease.

Beyond the discussion of the risks of smoking and the advice to quit, physicians should discuss the benefits of quitting, reinforce the patient's belief that quitting is possible (self-efficacy), and review potential barriers or obstacles to quitting. The most important step for the physician to take with the patient who is ready is to help set a "quit date." This may be a special day to the patient, such as a birthday, anniversary, or holiday, but will be that day on which the patient stops smoking. Helping patients to plan a quit date increases the likelihood that they will attempt to quit.[60] Changing to a lower-nicotine cigarette and tapering daily consumption may precede the quit day, and nicotine replacement therapy can begin on quit day.

Physicians should offer their patients a booklet that contains tips on quitting and maintaining abstinence. Self-help guides can be ordered in bulk from local units of volunteer organizations such as the American Heart Association or American Lung Association.

The use of nicotine replacement therapy is an effective adjunct to the cessation program. Smoking more than 20 cigarettes per day, smoking within 30 minutes after arising from sleep, finding difficulty in abstaining for long periods in situations where smoking is prohibited, and inhaling are all predictors of nicotine addiction and the need for nicotine replacement. Studies with both the nicotine gum and the nicotine patch have shown higher short-term quit rates than with placebo or no nicotine replacement, and the effectiveness is increased when this therapy is combined with a behavioral program.[61]

Referral to an organized behavioral program may be helpful for those smokers who express interest in such a program. This is unlikely to be effective for smoking patients who are not motivated to participate in an organized program and should not be a first-line recommendation by physicians. In a controlled trial of different physician interventions, of 369 smokers randomized for referral to "stop smoking" classes, only 14 percent investigated the classes and only 5 percent attended.[62]

It has become increasingly clear that continued follow-up is a critical part of an effective smoking cessation effort. This will usually take the form of return visits to the physician, as well as phone calls made by office personnel on a regular basis to assess smoking status, success, obstacles, and problems. In a meta-analysis of treatment programs,[63] success was predicted by multiple contacts with smokers over an extended time using a combination of physician and nonphysician counselors. "Success was not associated with novel or unusual interventions. It was the product of personalized smoking cessation advice and assistance, repeated in different forms by several sources over the longest feasible period."[63]

Smoking Cessation Results

Quitting smoking, whether done by oneself or as part of a program, is best viewed as a dynamic process rather than a discrete event.[64] Physician involvement in the process leads to better outcomes than would otherwise be expected. Simple advice to quit leads to a 1-year abstinence rate of 3 to 5 percent compared with a spontaneous self-quit rate of 0.45 to 1 percent per year.[60, 65] Advice combined with a self-help booklet plus follow-up by phone or letter may increase the success rate to 10 percent. Physician intervention that includes advice, a self-help booklet, counseling, nicotine replacement therapy, and follow-up results in 13 to 18 percent 1-year quit rates.[55]

The cessation rates in formal group intervention programs are usually 20 percent and rarely exceed 30 to 35 percent at 1 year.[66] As previously noted, however, the majority of smokers are not interested in enrolling in such formal programs as the initial approach to cessation.

In patients with underlying CAD, smoking cessation rates tend to be much higher. After an acute MI, simple advice from the primary physician yields success rates of 35 to 45 percent.[67] Nurse-directed intervention programs that begin in the hospital and are continued by telephone after discharge can increase this to 60 percent.[67] In a controlled trial of smokers undergoing coronary arteriography because of a recent or current MI or chest pain, and who were found to have coronary obstruction of at least 50 percent stenosis in one artery, a 57 percent self-reported 1-year cessation rate occurred after an intervention that included a 30-minute inpatient counseling session and an average of four follow-up phone calls delivered by behaviorally trained health educators.[68] Those with MI on admission had 74 percent abstinence at 6 months compared with a 49 percent rate in those who had angina without an MI. In patients undergoing coronary artery bypass graft surgery, cessation rates of 55 percent have been reported with advice alone or after the addition of an intervention delivered by audiovisual aids and written material.[69]

It is apparent that the development of coronary heart disease has a profound effect on subsequent smoking behavior and that aggressive physician intervention at the time of diagnosis can improve on already significant spontaneous cessation rates. These physician interventions do not have to be time consuming and can include the use of nurse reminders, self-help materials, nicotine replacement therapy, and follow-up contacts. Physicians should not become frustrated about perceived low success rates. Patients learn from each quit attempt, and a foundation will be laid for further self-initiated efforts, leading to ultimate success.

References

1. U.S. Department of Health and Human Services: The health consequences of smoking: cardiovascular disease. A report of the Surgeon General. Washington, DC: DHHS Publications, 1983.
2. Oates JA: Aspirin in the prevention of catastrophes of the coronary circulation. *In* Samuelsson B (ed): Advances in Prostaglandin, Thromboxane and Leukotriene Research. p. 57. New York: Raven, 1989.
3. Davies MJ, Thomas A: Thrombosis and acute coronary artery lesions in sudden cardiac ischemic death. N Engl J Med 310:1137, 1984.
4. Reed DM, MacLean CJ, Hayashi T: Predictors of atherosclerosis in the Honolulu Heart Program: I. Biologic, dietary and lifestyle characteristics. Am J Epidemiol 126:214, 1987.
5. The Pathobiological Determinants of Atherosclerosis in Youth Research Group: Relationship of atherosclerosis in young men to serum lipoprotein cholesterol concentrations and smoking. JAMA 265:3018, 1990.
6. Dawber TR: The Framingham Study: The Epidemiology of Atherosclerotic Disease. Cambridge, MA: Harvard University Press, 1980.
7. Kannel WB, McGee DL, Castelli WP: Latest perspectives on cigarette smoking and cardiovascular disease. The Framingham Study. J Cardiac Rehabil 4:267, 1984.
8. Rosenberg L, Kaufman DW, Helmrich SP, et al: The risk of myocardial infarction after quitting smoking in men under 55 years of age. N Engl J Med 313:1511, 1985.
9. Rosenberg L, Palmer JR, Shapiro S: Decline in risk of myocardial infarction among women who stopped smoking. N Engl J Med 322:213, 1990.
10. Cook DG, Shaper AG, Pollock SJ, et al: Giving up smoking and the risk of heart attacks. Lancet 1986; 2:1376.
11. Barendregt JJ, Bonneux L, van der Maas PJ: The health care costs of smoking. N Engl J Med 337:1052, 1997.
12. Lightwood JM, Glantz SA: Short-term economic and health benefits of smoking cessation: myocardial infarction and stroke. Circulation 96:1089, 1997.
13. Cromwell J, Bartosch WJ, Fiore MC, et al: Cost-effectiveness of the clinical practice recommendations in the AHCPR guideline for smoking cessation. Agency for Health Care Policy and Research. JAMA 278:1759, 1997.
14. Relationship of blood pressure, serum cholesterol, smoking habit, relative weight and ECG abnormalities to incidence of major coronary events: final report of the pooling project. The Pooling Project Research Group. J Chronic Dis 31:201, 1978.
15. Kawachi I, Colditz GA, Speizer FE, et al: A prospective study of passive smoking and coronary heart disease. Circulation 95:2374, 1997.
16. Steenland K, Thun M, Lally C, et al: Environmental tobacco smoke and coronary heart disease in the American Cancer Society CPS-II cohort. Circulation 94:622, 1996.
17. Celermajer DS, Adams MR, Clarkson P, et al: Passive smoking and impaired endothelium-dependent arterial dilatation in healthy young adults. N Engl J Med 334:150, 1996.
18. Roberts KA, Rezai AA, Pinkerton KE, et al: Effect of environmental tobacco smoke on LDL accumulation in the artery wall. Circulation 94:2248, 1996.
19. Valkonen M, Kuusi T: Passive smoking induces atherogenic changes in low-density lipoprotein. Circulation 97:2012, 1998.
20. Neufeld EJ, Mietus-Snyder M, Beiser AS, et al: Passive cigarette smoking and reduced HDL cholesterol levels in children with high-risk lipid profiles. Circulation 96:1403, 1997.
21. Hausberg M, Mark AL, Winniford MD, et al: Sympathetic and vascular effects of short-term passive smoke exposure in healthy nonsmokers. Circulation 96:282, 1997.
22. Pitillo MR: Cigarette smoking and endothelial injury: a review. *In* Diana JN (ed): Tobacco Smoking and Atherosclerosis. p. 61. New York: Plenum, 1990.

23. FitzGerald GA, Oates JA, Novak J: Cigarette smoking and hemostatic function. Am Heart J 115:267, 1988.
24. Heitzer T, Yla-Herttuala S, Luoma J, et al: Cigarette smoking potentiates endothelial dysfunction of forearm resistance vessels in patients with hypercholesterolemia. Role of oxidized LDL. Circulation 93:1346, 1996.
25. Campisi R, Czernin J, Schoder H, et al: Effects of long-term smoking on myocardial blood flow, coronary vasomotion, and vasodilator capacity. Circulation 98:119, 1998.
26. Zeiher AM, Drexler H, Wollschlager H, et al: Endothelial dysfunction of the coronary microvasculature is associated with coronary blood flow regulation in patients with early atherosclerosis. Circulation 84:1984, 1991.
27. Campisi R, Czernin J, Schoder H, et al: L-Arginine normalizes coronary vasomotion in long-term smokers. Circulation 99:491, 1999.
28. Kugiyama K, Yasue H, Ohgushi M, et al: Deficiency in nitric oxide bioactivity in epicardial coronary arteries of cigarette smokers. J Am Coll Cardiol 28:1161, 1996.
29. Heitzer T, Just H, Munzel T: Antioxidant vitamin C improves endothelial dysfunction in chronic smokers. Circulation 94:6, 1996.
30. Morrow JD, Frei B, Longmire AW, et al: Increase in circulating products of lipid peroxidation (F2-isoprostanes) in smokers. Smoking as a cause of oxidative damage. N Engl J Med 332:1198, 1995.
31. Duthie GG, Arthur JR, Beattie JA, et al: Cigarette smoking, antioxidants, lipid peroxidation, and coronary heart disease. Ann N Y Acad Sci 686:120, 1993.
32. Craig WY, Palomaki GE, Haddow JE: Cigarette smoking and serum lipid and lipoprotein concentrations: an analysis of published data. BMJ 298:784, 1989.
33. Adams MR, Jessup W, Celermajer DS: Cigarette smoking is associated with increased human monocyte adhesion to endothelial cells: reversibility with oral L-arginine but not vitamin C. J Am Coll Cardiol 29:491, 1997.
34. Weber C, Erl W, Weber K, et al: Increased adhesiveness of isolated monocytes to endothelium is prevented by vitamin C intake in smokers. Circulation 93:1488, 1996.
35. Cryer PE, Haymond MW, Santiago JV, et al: Norepinephrine and epinephrine release and adrenergic mediation of smoking-associated hemodynamic and metabolic events. N Engl J Med 295:573, 1976.
36. Nicod P, Rehr R, Winniford MD, et al: Acute systemic and coronary hemodynamic and serologic responses to cigarette smoking in long-term smokers with atherosclerotic coronary artery disease. J Am Coll Cardiol 4:964, 1984.
37. Czernin J, Sun K, Brunken R, et al: Effect of acute and long-term smoking on myocardial blood flow and flow reserve. Circulation 91:2891, 1995.
38. Quillen JE, Rossen JD, Oskarsson HJ, et al: Acute effect of cigarette smoking on the coronary circulation: constriction of epicardial and resistance vessels. J Am Coll Cardiol 22:642, 1993.
39. Maouad J, Fernandez F, Hebert JL, et al: Cigarette smoking during coronary angiography: diffuse or focal narrowing (spasm) of the coronary arteries in 13 patients with angina at rest and normal coronary angiograms. Cathet Cardiovasc Diagn 12:366, 1986.
40. Winniford MD, Wheelan KR, Kremers MS, et al: Smoking-induced coronary vasoconstriction in patients with atherosclerotic coronary artery disease: evidence for adrenergically mediated alterations in coronary artery tone. Circulation 73:662, 1986.
41. Vita JA, Treasure CB, Yeung AC, et al: Patients with evidence of coronary endothelial dysfunction as assessed by acetylcholine infusion demonstrate marked increase in sensitivity to constrictor effects of catecholamines. Circulation 85:1390, 1992.
42. Zeiher AM, Drexler H, Wollschlaeger H, et al: Coronary vasomotion in response to sympathetic stimulation in humans: importance of the functional integrity of the endothelium. J Am Coll Cardiol 14:1181, 1989.
43. Moliterno DJ, Willard JE, Lange RA, et al: Coronary-artery vasoconstriction induced by cocaine, cigarette smoking, or both. N Engl J Med 330:454, 1994.
44. Allred EN, Bleecker ER, Chaitman BR, et al: Short-term effects of carbon monoxide exposure on the exercise performance of subjects with coronary artery disease. N Engl J Med 321:1426, 1989.
45. Aronow WS: Aggravation of angina pectoris by two percent carboxyhemoglobin. Am Heart J 101:154, 1981.
46. Aronow WS, Stemmer EA, Zweig S: Carbon monoxide and ventricular fibrillation threshold in normal dogs. Arch Environ Health 34:184, 1979.
47. Thom SR, Xu YA, Ischiropoulos H: Vascular endothelial cells generate peroxynitrite in response to carbon monoxide exposure. Chem Res Toxicol 10:1023, 1997.
48. de Maat MP, Pietersma A, Kofflard M, et al: Association of plasma fibrinogen levels with coronary artery disease, smoking and inflammatory markers. Atherosclerosis 121:185, 1996.
49. Benowitz NL, Fitzgerald GA, Wilson M, et al: Nicotine effects on eicosanoid formation and hemostatic function: comparison of transdermal nicotine and cigarette smoking. J Am Coll Cardiol 22:1159, 1993.
50. Newby DE, Wright RA, Labinjoh C, et al: Endothelial dysfunction, impaired endogenous fibrinolysis, and cigarette smoking: a mechanism for arterial thrombosis and myocardial infarction. Circulation 99:1411, 1999.
51. Penn A, Snyder CA: 1,3 Butadiene, a vapor phase component of environmental tobacco smoke, accelerates arteriosclerotic plaque development. Circulation 93:552, 1996.
52. Nobuyoshi M, Abe M, Nosaka H, et al: Statistical analysis of clinical risk factors for coronary artery spasm: identification of the most important determinant. Am Heart J 124:32, 1992.
53. U.S. Department of Health and Human Services: The health consequences of smoking: 25 years of progress. A report of the Surgeon General. Washington, DC: DHHS Publications, 1989.
54. U.S. Department of Health and Human Services: The health consequences of smoking: nicotine addiction. A report of the Surgeon General. Rockville, MD: Office on Smoking and Health, 1988.
55. Ockene JK, Kristeller J, Goldberg R, et al: Increasing the efficacy of physician-delivered smoking interventions: a randomized clinical trial. J Gen Intern Med 6:1, 1991.
56. The Agency for Health Care Policy and Research: Smoking cessation clinical practice guideline. JAMA 275:1270, 1996.
57. Davis RM: Uniting physicians against smoking: the need for a coordinated national strategy. JAMA 259:2900, 1988.
58. Goldsmith MF: More magazines forgo tobacco ads, some by choice, many by chance [news]. JAMA 271:571, 1994.
59. Fiore MC: The new vital sign. Assessing and documenting smoking status. JAMA 266:3183, 1991.
60. Flay BR, Ockene JK, Tager IB: Smoking: epidemiology, cessation, and prevention. Task Force on Research and Education for the Prevention and Control of Respiratory Diseases. Chest 102:277S, 1992.
61. Fiore MC, Jorenby DE, Baker TB, et al: Tobacco dependence and the nicotine patch. Clinical guidelines for effective use. JAMA 268:2687, 1992.
62. Thompson RS, Michnich ME, Friedlander L, et al: Effectiveness of smoking cessation interventions integrated into primary care practice. Med Care 26:62, 1988.
63. Kottke TE, Battista RN, DeFriese GH, et al: Attributes of successful smoking cessation interventions in medical practice. A meta-analysis of 39 controlled trials. JAMA 259:2883, 1988.
64. Cohen S, Lichtenstein E, Prochaska JO, et al: Debunking myths about self-quitting. Evidence from 10 prospective studies of persons who attempt to quit smoking by themselves. Am Psychol 44:1355, 1989.
65. Philips BU Jr, Longoria JM, Calhoun KH, et al: Behavioral prescription writing in smoking cessation counseling: a new use for a familiar tool. South Med J 82:946, 1989.
66. Rigotti NA, Singer DE, Mulley AG Jr, et al: Smoking cessation following admission to a coronary care unit. J Gen Intern Med 6:305, 1991.
67. Taylor CB, Houston-Miller N, Killen JD, et al: Smoking cessation after acute myocardial infarction: effects of a nurse-managed intervention. Ann Intern Med 113:118, 1990.
68. Ockene J, Kristeller JL, Goldberg R, et al: Smoking cessation and severity of disease: the Coronary Artery Smoking Intervention Study. Health Psychol 11:119, 1992.
69. Crouse JR 3rd, Hagaman AP: Smoking cessation in relation to cardiac procedures. Am J Epidemiol 134:699, 1991.

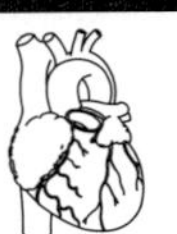

CHAPTER 123

HYPERTENSION

Norman M. Kaplan

ACTION IN THE ABSENCE OF PROOF
OBESITY
SODIUM RESTRICTION
DOUBTS ABOUT SODIUM
POTASSIUM AND OTHER MINERALS
Potassium
Calcium
Magnesium
STRESS
The Stress of Awakening
PHYSICAL ACTIVITY
ALCOHOL
FISH OILS AND OTHER NUTRIENTS
PREVENTION OF INTRAUTERINE GROWTH RETARDATION

Hypertension is clearly associated with three environmental factors—obesity, stress, and sodium—that can be altered in the hope of preventing the development of the disease.[1] The possible ways by which these three factors work to raise the blood pressure are multiple (Fig. 123–1), and there are likely many more than are shown in this already complicated scheme. Because obesity is discussed in Chapter 125, less is said about its putative role than about the other two.

In addition to these three factors, some of many other alterable factors are discussed. The presence of so many possible mechanisms implies that almost all hypertension remains "idiopathic," with an unknown cause. Therefore, this entire discussion is based on potential causes. Evidence that shows associations with these factors and the development of hypertension is fairly strong, but the evidence showing that alteration will permanently prevent hypertension is nonexistent.

This lack of confirmatory evidence does not, however, mean that the potential is not likely to be real. The reasons why confirmation may never be available, include the following:

- Heredity plays a significant role, but there are no definite markers by which to identify the prehypertensive. Without such an unambiguous marker, proof that hypertension has been prevented would be very difficult to obtain.
- Rigorous confirmation of a causal role rather than a coincidental association would require manipulation of the diet, lifestyle, and habits of many thousands of people over perhaps 30 years or longer, the incubation period for hypertension in those who are genetically predestined.
- The monitoring of patient adherence to diet and lifestyle changes would be exceedingly difficult. It takes many 24-hour urine samples to define an individual's usual sodium intake. Stress is not the same in the laboratory as it is in real life, and few agree as to what stress really encompasses.

The effectiveness of any one change might be rather small and incomplete in the absence of simultaneous changes in others as well. Irvine Page proposed a "mosaic" of many pieces to explain hypertension. Figure 123–1 shows only a small number of these pieces in place. For example, a reduction in dietary sodium intake might work in those who are also "high reactors" to stress (Fig. 123–2).[2] In this small but insightful study on young normotensives either with or without a family history of hypertension, those who were 'high reactors' to laboratory stress had a lesser natriuretic response than did those who were low reactors. Therefore, the high reactors would probably be responsive to a reduction in sodium intake as well as to a dampening of their exposure or responsiveness to stress. The others might not respond to either. Considering the difficulty in showing a definite effect on a much easier to define endpoint—death from cardiac cause—with the treatment of almost 50,000 patients with antihypertensive drugs, that are certainly more potent than the dietary and lifestyle changes under consideration,[3] it is easier to see why definitive proof of the ability to prevent hypertension may never be forthcoming.

ACTION IN THE ABSENCE OF PROOF

Absent proof—some say—do nothing. In particular, the call for a population-wide moderate reduction in dietary sodium intake[4] has not been accepted by some experts.[5–8] The hesitation of these experts to advocate what I will attempt to document to be a fairly easy to accomplish and almost certain to be effective preventive maneuver comes in part from a more conservative, scientific hard-nosed attitude that any and all recommendations for change be based on proven benefit. As noted, such proof may be unobtainable, leaving the use of preventive maneuvers in a permanent paralysis. Beyond this somewhat irrational concern, there is another that I consider quite rational: The advocacy of population-wide changes for the potential of prevention must not contain even the seed of adverse effects on even a small part of the population at risk, much less the larger part of the population who are not at risk. Even if more than half of the population will eventually

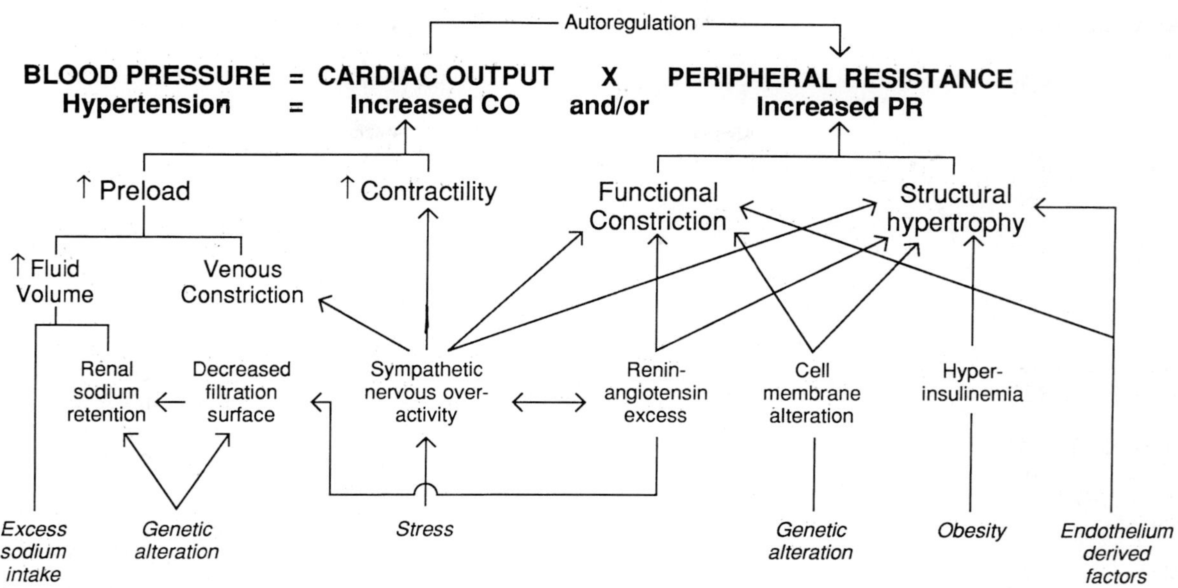

FIGURE 123–1 Some of the factors involved in the control of blood pressure that affect the basic equation: Blood pressure = cardiac output (CO) × peripheral resistance (PR). (From Kaplan, NM: Primary hypertension: pathogenesis. *In* Clinical Hypertension. 7th ed. pp. 41–99. Baltimore: Williams & Wilkins, 1998.)

develop hypertension, if a maneuver such as moderate sodium restriction would harm even 1 percent of the 50 percent who are not susceptible to hypertension, it should not be invoked.

Further coverage of the potential benefits versus risks of moderate sodium restriction will follow. For now, it is sufficient to say that most of the objections against preventive action are strawmen, placed in the field to discourage those who strongly believe that all changes toward a more "natural" lifestyle are desirable.

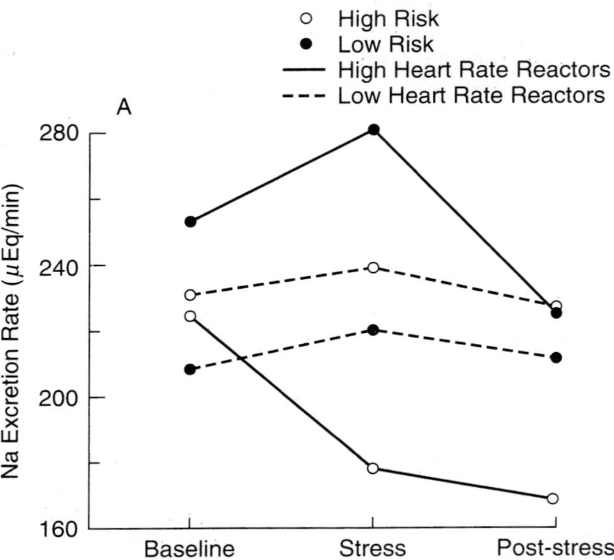

FIGURE 123–2 Rates of sodium excretion during baseline, the stress of competitive mental tasks, and the poststress periods, each of 1-hour duration, in 40 young men. The high-risk subjects had occasional systolic blood pressure above 140 mm Hg or a parental history of hypertension, whereas the low-risk subjects had neither. The high heart rate reactors had mean increases of 13 beats/min during the stress, and the low reactors less than that. (From Light KC, Koepke JP, Obrist PA, Willis PW IV; Psychological stress induces sodium and fluid retention in men at risk for hypertension. Science 220:429, 1983.)

Before beginning a more careful look at specific preventive maneuvers, emphasis should be given to the need for population-wide change. Because there is no way to mark a person as prehypertensive, we cannot use these maneuvers on only the 20 percent or so who are genetically predestined to develop combined systolic and diastolic hypertension or the 50 percent or so who will develop isolated systolic hypertension. Moreover, once hypertension develops, it may be irreversible; even effective reduction in blood pressure to normotensive levels may not remove all of the risks (Fig. 123–3).[9] Therefore, prevention cannot be saved until after blood pressure has been determined to be high, particularly because most hypertensive complications develop in people with blood pressures that are not considered high and in need of treatment. As Geoffrey Rose argued,[10] the prevention of a disease such as hypertension and its major end- result, coronary disease, will certainly require a population-wide approach rather than one focused on only those at obvious high risk. In his words, "The special problems of the few reflect the behavior of the many; and to help the minority, the majority must change."[10]

Nothing more will be said about those risk factors that cannot be altered, including family history, age, gender, and race. Those who are more susceptible because of these may require more preventive care, but this chapter is directed toward alterable factors. In particular, emphasis is given to the probable major benefit to be derived from the prevention of intrauterine growth retardation to protect the most vulnerable part of the population destined to develop hypertension—the poor and deprived.

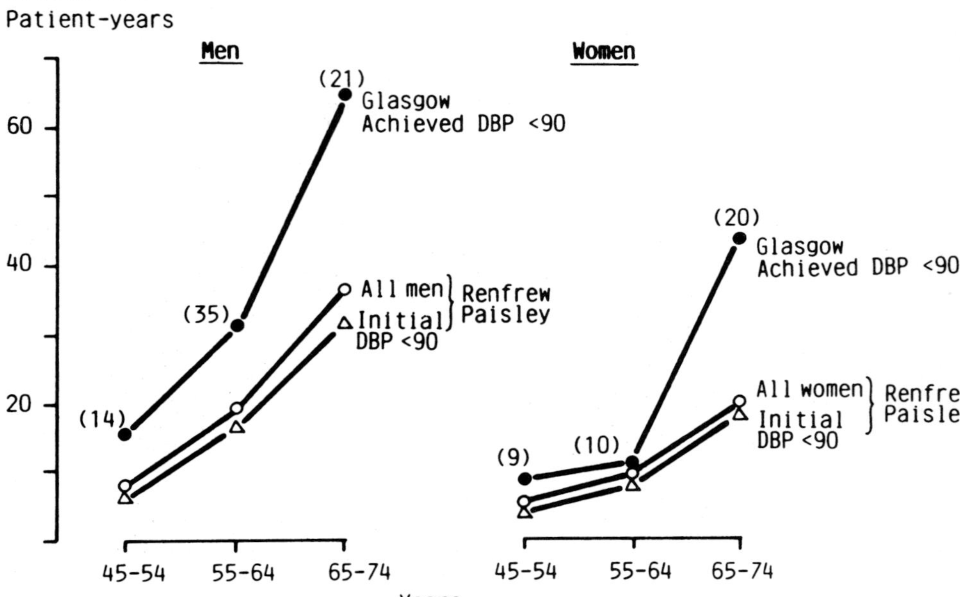

FIGURE 123–3 Age- and sex-specific mortality rates (deaths/1000 patient-yrs) in Glasgow clinic patients whose diastolic blood pressure (DBP) was reduced to less than 90 mm Hg by treatment at their last clinic visit compared with subjects in the Renfrew/Paisley control population. Deaths of the Glasgow clinic patients are given in parentheses. (From Isles CG, Walker LM, Beevers GD, et al: mortality in patients of the Glasgow blood pressure clinic. J Hypertens 4:141, 1986.)

OBESITY

Even though obesity is discussed in Chapter 125, a few words are added here, mainly because, next to cigarette smoking, obesity seems to be the major preventable cause of coronary disease. Although obesity per se is less of a risk factor than others, it is more of a risk factor because of what often accompanies weight gain: a rise in blood pressure, glucose intolerance, dyslipidemias, and physical inactivity. What I called the deadly quartet,[11] but which is better termed the *insulin resistance syndrome,* is common and clearly associated with an increased incidence of coronary disease.

The role of weight gain and obesity in producing hypertension is unequivocal.[12] The effectiveness of weight loss to lower an elevated blood pressure is well documented.[13] Whether the prevention of obesity, particularly in childhood, will protect those who are susceptible to obesity-induced hypertension from developing an elevated blood pressure has not been tested. Nevertheless, the evidence for an independent and impressive prohypertensive effect of weight gain places the prevention of obesity at the top of the recommendations for the prevention of hypertension.

Fortunately, only a modest weight loss may be protective. In the Trials of Hypertension Prevention (TOHP) phase 1,[13] 299 moderately overweight men and women aged 30 through 54 years with diastolic blood pressures between 80 and 89 mm Hg followed a program of reduced calories and increased physical activity during an 18-month period. They lost a mean of 3.83 kg, whereas a matched control group of 239 subjects gained 0.07 kg during that interval. The weight-reduction group had a fall in blood pressure of −5.3/−6.2 mm Hg, a decrease of 2.9/2.3 mm Hg more than was found in the control group (Fig. 123–4). This difference in blood pressure fall translated into a significant difference in the incidence of hypertension defined as diastolic pressures persistently above 90 mm Hg; 13.3 percent of the control group advanced into hypertension, whereas only 6.5 percent of the weight reduction group did so.

SODIUM RESTRICTION

The only other nonpharmacologic intervention that had an impact on the prevention of hypertension in the TOHP study was sodium restriction (see Fig. 123–4). The 305 subjects who were asked to follow a sodium-restricted diet had 55 mmol less sodium in a 24-hour urine collection after 18 months, whereas the 397 control subjects had 11 mmol less per 24 hours. The modest 44 mmol/24-hr difference was associated with a 1.7/0.9 mm Hg lower blood pressure and an 8.6 percent incidence of hypertension compared with an 11.3 percent incidence in the control group.

There is overwhelming evidence that sodium restriction lowers blood pressure in hypertensives, but the effects in normotensives are much less impressive, with reductions of only 1 to 2 mm Hg.[6, 14] These results, often due to very short periods of rigid sodium restriction, do not prove that long-term moderate sodium restriction will not prevent the development of hypertension. Indirect evidence in favor of the potential for such protection comes from a 30-month study of almost 1000 elderly patients whose blood pressure was initially well controlled with the use of one or two antihypertensive drugs and who then discontinued their drug therapy so they could be randomly assigned to one of four regimens: sodium reduction, weight loss, both sodium reduction and weight loss, or nothing (usual care).[15] Despite an average reduction in sodium intake of only 40 mmol/da, the number of patients in the TONE study who remained normotensive during the next 30 months was 38 percent of those on sodium restriction versus 24 percent of those not on sodium restriction.

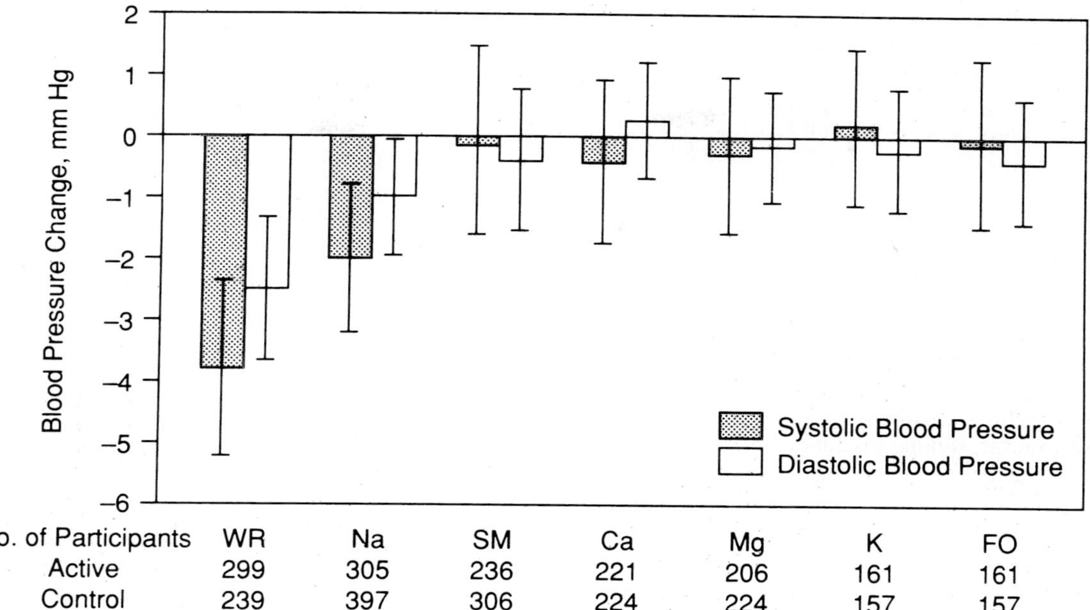

FIGURE 123–4 Net mean changes in systolic and diastolic blood pressure (baseline minus follow-up) with 95 percent confidence intervals. WR, weight reduction; Na, sodium reduction, SM, stress management; Ca, calcium supplementation; Mg, magnesium supplementation; K, potassium supplementation; and FO, fish oil supplementation. (From Trials of Hypertension Prevention Collaborative Research Group: The effects of nonpharmacological interventions on blood pressure of persons with high normal levels: results of the Trials of Hypertension Prevention, Phase I. JAMA 267:1213, 1992. Copyright 1992, American Medical Association.)

Such effects, if applied to the entire population, would produce a very considerable impact on the incidence of hypertension and the development of cardiovascular disease. As noted by Rose,[16] "All the life-saving benefits achieved by current antihypertensive treatment might be equaled by a downward shift of the whole blood pressure distribution by a mere 2–3 mm Hg. The benefits from a mass approach in which everybody received a small benefit may be unexpectedly large."

Confirmation of Rose's prediction has come from Law and associates,[17] who analyzed all of the crossover and randomized controlled trials of dietary sodium restriction published through 1989, consisting of a total of 78, with 18 conducted in normotensive subjects. Although most of these trials were of short duration and involved small numbers of subjects, Law and associates[17] found that in 50- to 59-year-old persons, a decrease in daily sodium intake of 50 mmol for 4 weeks or longer would lower blood pressure by an average of about 5/2 mm Hg. They then estimated the effect of universal reduction of dietary sodium intake by 50 mmol/24 h on death from stroke and coronary disease. The estimate was a 22 percent decrease in the incidence of stroke and a 16 percent decrease in ischemic heart disease, effects that are much more impressive than those found in trials of successful treatment of hypertensive patients (Fig. 123–5).

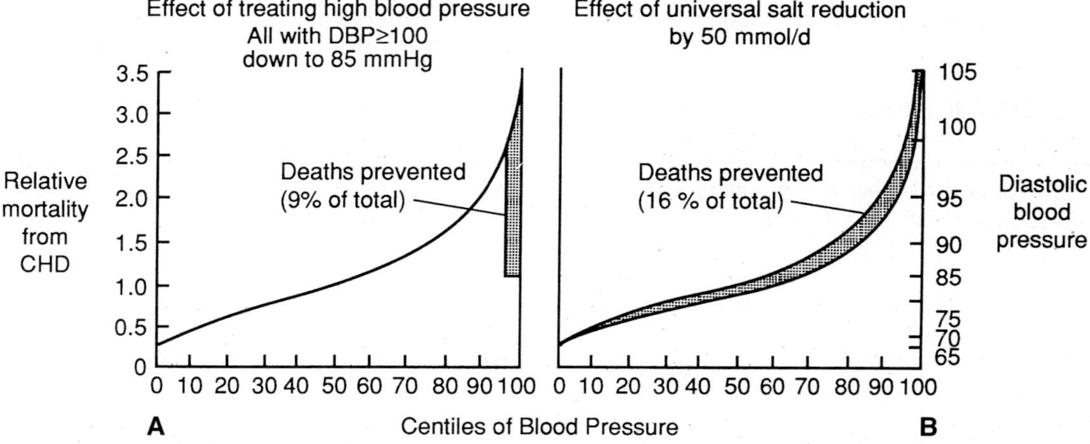

FIGURE 123–5 Frequency distribution of blood pressure in population aged 50 to 59 years shows effects of treatment of high blood pressure **(A)** and universal dietary salt reduction by 50 mmol/24 h **(B)** on mortality rates from stroke and ischemic heart disease. CHD, coronary heart disease. (**A** and **B,** From Law RM, Frost CD, Wald NJ III: Analysis of data from trials of salt reduction. J Am Coll Nutr 10:383, 1991.)

Although the degree of blood pressure fall by Law and associates[17] is about twice that noted in the more carefully controlled, larger, and longer TOPH study,[13] these data all point to a significant potential benefit of universal sodium restriction of only a modest degree. Because daily sodium intake in Western societies averages 150 mmol or more per 24-hour period, a reduction of 50 mmol, about what was accomplished in the TOPH study, would not represent a major overhaul in food intake. Moreover, because more than 75 percent of the sodium in our diets is added during processing rather than at the table or during cooking,[18] a modest reduction in the large amounts of sodium added to most processed foods could help accomplish the desired degree of sodium restriction with little or no need for participation by the individual. Labeling laws implemented in 1993 provide the sodium content of all processed foods and identify the actual percentage of the recommended daily intake of sodium (2.4 g or 110 mmol/da) contained in the product, so that even poorly informed consumers can easily avoid foods with high sodium content. Perhaps those who process food will get the message that foods with high sodium content are not desirable and will continue a trend that has already begun to lower the sodium content of many processed and fast foods.

The need for such population-wide strategies is obvious: In most controlled trials of groups of patients such as TOPH[13] or TONE,[15] it is difficult to reduce sodium intake to much below 120 mmol/24 h even with intensive counseling, repetitive monitoring, and high motivation. It should be much easier to obtain the desired degree of reduction by reducing the nondiscretionary sources of most of the sodium in the diet.

Doubts About Sodium. A few hypertension experts question both the role of sodium excess in the pathogenesis of hypertension and the wisdom of advocating a population-wide strategy of moderate sodium restriction.[5–8] The evidence, although only circumstantial, for a causal role for the high sodium content only recently introduced into the food supply of industrialized societies is so extensive that most are convinced that it is necessary, although not sufficient, part of the pathogenesis of hypertension (Table 123–1). Absolute proof for the role of high sodium intake may never be obtained because it is not possible to manipulate and monitor the sodium intake of thousands of persons almost from birth through midlife and observe the effects, particularly as there is considerable variability in the pressor sensitivity to sodium intake.

TABLE 123–1 Evidence for a Role of Sodium in Primary Hypertension

In multiple populations, the rise in blood pressure with age is directly correlated with increasing levels of sodium intake.

Multiple, scattered groups who consume little sodium (<50 mmol/da) have little or no hypertension. When they consume more sodium, hypertension appears.

Animals that are administered sodium loads, if genetically predisposed, develop hypertension.

Some persons, when administered large sodium loads over short periods of time, develop an increase in vascular resistance and blood pressure.

An increased concentration of sodium is present in the vascular tissue and blood cells of most hypertensives.

Sodium restriction to a level of 60 to 90 mmol/da will lower blood pressure in most persons. The antihypertensive action of diuretics requires an initial natriuresis.

Most studies of the relationships of sodium to hypertension fail to show a significant progressive rise in the prevalence of hypertension with progressively higher levels of sodium intake. The problem is that, with the few exceptions of very primitive societies who ingest almost no sodium and who have almost no hypertension, all industrialized societies are likely beyond the threshold level of sodium intake that is needed for the development of the disease. The situation has been nicely described by Geoffrey Rose[19]:

> There are two kinds of aetiological question: the first seeks the causes of cases and the second seeks the causes of incidence. "Why do some individuals have hypertension?" is a quite different question from "Why do some populations have much hypertension, while in others it is rare?" We were perhaps misled by the example of smoking and lung cancer, which has been taken as a general model for the epidemiological study of causes. It was in fact an exceptional situation, in which there was large heterogeneity of exposure both within and between populations. If everyone in the country had smoked 20 cigarettes a day then clinical, case-control, and cohort studies alike would have led us to conclude that lung cancer was a genetic disease; and in one sense that would have been true, since if everyone is exposed to the necessary external agent then the distribution of cases becomes wholly determined by individual susceptibility.
>
> We reach then this paradox, that the more widespread is a particular environmental hazard, the less it explains the distribution of cases. The cause that is universally present has no influence at all on the distribution of disease, and it may be quite unfindable by the traditional methods of clinical impression and case-control and cohort studies; for these all depend on heterogeneity of exposure.

The evidence outlined in Table 123–1 is, to my mind, sufficient to incriminate sodium and to call for universal restriction in dietary intake. However, respected researchers have advised against a population-wide reduction in sodium intake, calling attention to experiments with rats that had ill effects from various cataclysmic stresses when receiving a minuscule sodium intake.[8, 20] When the designs of the studies are examined, their irrelevancy to the human condition is obvious. As I have written, "So let no one be concerned about the potential harm of moderate restriction of dietary sodium intake. None has been shown in animals, much less in man."[1]

All things considered, a population-wide modest reduction in sodium intake, then, appears to be both fairly easily obtainable and likely to achieve major preventive benefit.

POTASSIUM AND OTHER MINERALS

Before stress, the third of the major environmental factors that could be altered to prevent hypertension, is considered, attention is directed toward potassium and other minerals.

Potassium

As opposed to an excessive sodium intake, some evidence points to an imbalance between too much sodium and too little potassium in the diet as a cause of hypertension. For example, numerous surveys have noted a lower-than-recommended intake of potassium but no greater intake of sodium in poor blacks, particularly in the southern United States, who have a high prevalence of hypertension.[21, 22] The lesser intake of potassium presumably reflects a lower consumption of meats, fruits, and vegetables by those who are poor.

Trials of potassium supplements (40 to 80 mmol/da) have generally shown some lowering of blood pressure in both hypertensives and normotensives on a low-potassium diet.[23, 24] However, no effect of 60 mmol/day of extra potassium for 6 months was noted in the 161 subjects with high-normal blood pressure involved in the TOHP study[13] (see Fig. 123–4). On the other hand, a diet rich in fruits and vegetables, and thereby rich in potassium, provided a substantial fall in blood pressure in a large number of subjects with an initial blood pressure of 131/85 mm Hg.[25]

Calcium

Similar to potassium, dietary intake of calcium has been found to be reduced in black hypertensives in the United States, perhaps related to their higher prevalence of lactase deficiency.[22] However, 1 to 2 g day supplemental calcium has been found to produce little, if any, lowering of blood pressure in normotensive subjects, both in the TOHP study[13] and in multiple other randomized controlled trials involving 835 subjects.[26]

Magnesium

In the TOHP study, 75 mmol/day supplements of magnesium had no effect on blood pressure (see Fig. 123–4), which is in keeping with generally negative findings in both normotensive and hypertensive subjects.[24]

Stress

In many ways, stress-induced activation of the sympathetic nervous system appears to be a likely component of the pathogenetic scheme for hypertension (see Fig. 123–1). Sympathetic nervous hyperactivity may be the pressor mechanism that initially raises the blood pressure intermittently, leading to vascular and cardiac hypertrophy and causing the pressure to remain elevated. The hemodynamic pattern of a high cardiac output and fast pulse (i.e., *hyperkinetic hypertension*), was identified in more than one third of the young borderline hypertensives in the Tecumseh study.[27]

Repetitive stress is the obvious stimulus for sympathetic overactivity, but it has been difficult to prove this. For instance, responses to the acute laboratory stresses used in experimental studies have not been found to correlate with the future development of hypertension.[28] Moreover, the simple awareness of the diagnosis of hypertension has been shown to induce an alerting reaction that provokes higher basal blood catecholamine levels and exaggerated epinephrine and blood pressure responses to mental stress.[29]

Nevertheless, "job strain," quantified and used as a measure of the major source of stress, has been shown to be correlated with the presence of hypertension.[30] The investigators found that hypertensives were more likely to be employed in high-strain jobs, with an odds ratio of 3.1 after adjustment for other possible confounding variables, including age, race, obesity, alcohol and sodium intake, education, and type A behavior pattern. Moreover, in those aged 30 to 40 years with higher levels of job strain, echocardiographically measured left ventricular mass averaged 10.8 g/m^2 more than that in those without job strain.

These data, along with more in both humans and animals,[1] support a role for stress in the pathogenesis of hypertension, likely interacting with multiple other factors to increase vascular resistance[31] (Fig. 123–6). It has not, however, been possible to show that relief of stress as provided through various relaxation methods will prevent hypertension, much less provide more than a placebo effect in lowering the pressure in those with established hypertension, with rare exception.[32] Again, the TOHP study showed what most others have found: Despite the use of four methods of relaxation (slow breathing, progressive muscle relaxation, mental imagery, and stretching) plus techniques to manage stress perceptions, reactions, and situations, the 236 subjects experienced no change in blood pressure (see Fig. 123–4) and no decrease in the incidence of hypertension compared with the control groups during an 18-month follow-up period.[13]

Stress of Awakening

These largely negative results of intervention trials do not negate a causal role for stress and may merely mean that the techniques that are used are inadequate or that it takes much longer to effect a change in the responsiveness to stress.

Activation of the sympathetic nervous system almost certainly plays a role in the increased occurrence of cardiovascular catastrophes in the early morning hours after awakening from sleep. As nicely shown by Panza and associates[33] in their study of 12 normal subjects, significantly higher levels of basal forearm vascular resistance and lower forearm blood flow are present at 7 AM than at 2 or 9 PM (Fig. 123–7). These higher levels of resistance at 7 AM were blunted by the alpha-blocker phentolamine, which had lesser effects at 2 and 9 PM, thereby wiping out the circadian variation in vascular resistance. The nonspecific vasodilator nitroprusside had similar effects at all three times of day, preserving the circadian variation but at a uniformly lower level.

Because there is no way to delete the normal endogenous circadian rhythms or to delay arising from sleep by more than a bit, the sympathetic activation of the early morning hours looms as a significant contributor to an increased risk of cardiovascular diseases at this time. To help prevent these consequences, at least in those who are hypertensive,

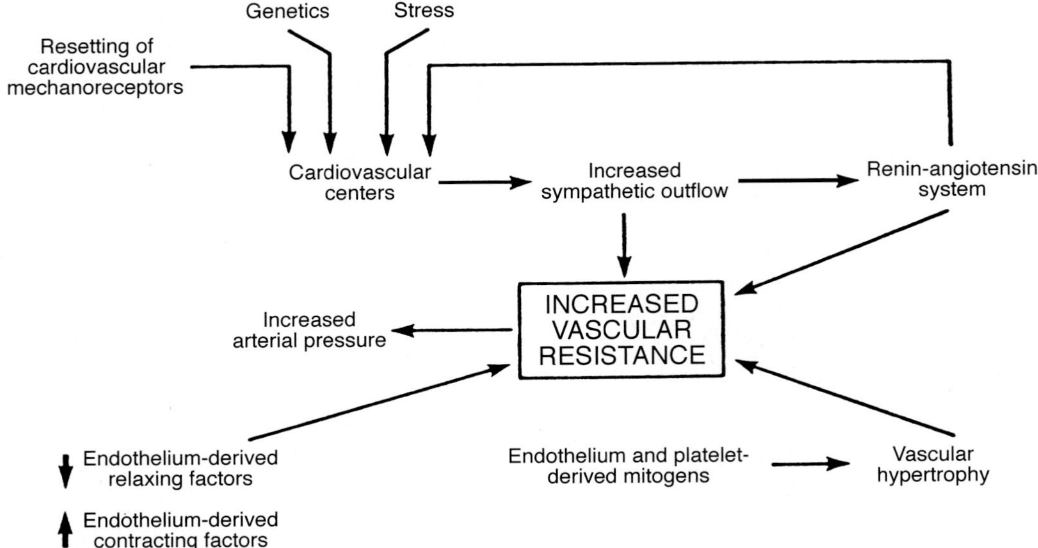

FIGURE 123–6 Indications that an increased sympathetic outflow may be a key factor in primary hypertension. The outflow is increased when arterial baroreceptors are reset so that they exert less inhibition on the vasomotor center. The resetting could be due to genetic changes, either in the endothelial lining of the carotid sinus and aortic arch or at the vasomotor center's or both. The increased sympathetic outflow may be further enhanced by stress. As a consequence of this neurohumoral excitation, the systemic vascular resistance is increased. In addition, the endothelial cells in the resistance blood vessel may secrete less vasodilator and more vasoconstrictor substances, thus compounding the vasoconstriction. Also, mitogens produced in endothelial cells and released from platelets, together with norepinephrine, can cause proliferation of the vascular smooth muscle with a further aggravation of the systemic vasoconstriction. (From Shephard JT: Increased systemic vascular resistance and primary hypertension: the expanding complexity. J Hypertens 8 [suppl 7]:S15, 1990.)

it seems prudent to use antihypertensive agents that maintain effectiveness during the latter part of the night and early morning hours and that block sympathetic activity. Both long-acting α-blockers and β-blockers may serve to soften this susceptibility. In addition, a slow gradual rising from supine to upright rather than a quick jump out of bed may prove to be the better way to face the challenges of the day.

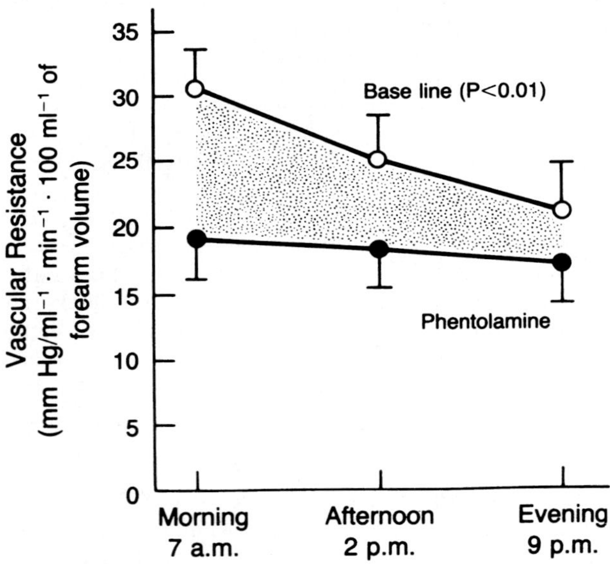

FIGURE 123–7 Mean forearm vascular resistance at three times of the day in 12 healthy subjects. Values shown were obtained at baseline *(open circles)* and after α-sympathetic blockade with the infusion of phentolamine *(solid circles)*. The *stippled areas* indicate the vascular tone contributed by α-sympathetic vasoconstrictor forces, and *vertical bars* indicate standard errors. (From Panza JA, Epstein SE, Quyyumi AA: Circadian variation in muscle tone and its relation to sympathetic vasoconstrictor activity. N Engl J Med 325:986, 1991. Copyright 1991 Massachusetts Medical Society. All rights reserved.)

PHYSICAL ACTIVITY

One way to help overcome stress may be physical activity. Whether that is the way in which physical activity lowers blood pressure, most well-controlled studies do show that regular aerobic exercise will lower blood pressure in hypertensive people,[34] and numerous surveys show a lesser incidence of hypertension in those who are physically fit.[35–37] Because exercise is described in Chapter 121, nothing more is discussed here other than to say that increased physical activity must be one of the most useful and available ways to prevent hypertension and that this protection likely involves a dampening of sympathetic nervous activity.[38]

ALCOHOL

Beyond the major three factors, numerous others that are involved in raising the blood pressure of at least some people may be alterable so primary prevention of hypertension may be possible.

Excessive alcohol consumption certainly serves as a pressor mechanism, responsible for 5 to 10 percent of the hypertension found among men.[39] In the review by MacMahon,[39] about half of all published data indicated that the pressor effect occurred only when average daily consumption is greater than 2 drinks, the equivalent of 1

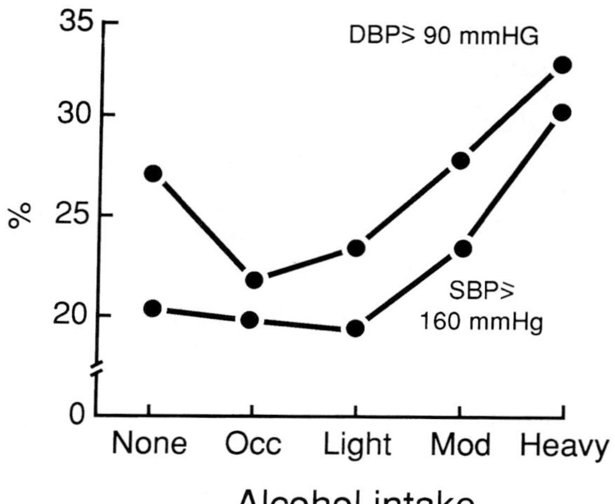

FIGURE 123–8 Age-adjusted prevalence rates of measured systolic and diastolic (SBP and DBP) hypertension by levels of alcohol intake in drinks: occasional (OCC), light (1 or 2 daily), moderate (MOD) (3–6 daily), and heavy (>6 daily). (From Sharper AG, Wannamethee G, Whincup P: Alcohol and blood pressure in middle-aged British men. J Hum Hypertens 2:71, 1988.)

ounce of ethanol. Some have even shown a lower pressure among those who consumed 1 or 2 drinks per day compared with those who drank more[40] (Fig. 123–8). The J-shaped pattern of blood pressure noted in this study of 7735 middle-aged men randomly drawn from general practices in 24 British towns closely fits with the pattern of morbidity and mortality related to alcohol consumption in multiple populations.[41, 42]

There is, then, a need to restrict alcohol consumption to less than 3 usual-sized portions per day in those who drink more than that amount. However, I see no reason to advise abstention unless there are overriding religious or health reasons (e.g., a former alcoholic). Such moderation of alcohol consumption will likely prevent a considerable amount of hypertension while providing the protection from coronary disease that comes from moderate drinking.[41, 42]

FISH OILS AND OTHER NUTRIENTS

The last of the interventions tested in the TOHP study[13] was a daily supplement of 6 g of fish oil containing 3 g of omega-3 fatty acids. During a 6-month interval, no effects on blood pressure (see Fig. 123–4) or on the incidence of hypertension was observed in the 161 ingestors of fish oil compared with the 157 control subjects. These data add to both positive[43] and negative[44] findings and, overall, suggest that little preventive value will likely result from fish oil supplements. Nevertheless, eating more fish may provide protection against heart disease in other ways.[45]

Increased dietary protein has been found in experimental studies to lower blood pressure, but studies in humans remain inconclusive.[46] Antioxidants, including vitamin C, may lower blood pressure,[47] and garlic extract has been shown to be antihypertensive in a few controlled trials.[48] On the other hand, caffeine may raise the pressure acutely, although tolerance to this pressor effect usually develops quickly.[49] Even more impressive data have been collected to document a fall in blood pressure when dyslipidemias are corrected with diet or drugs.[50]

PREVENTION OF INTRAUTERINE GROWTH RETARDATION

The most recently recognized and in many ways the most attainable way to prevent hypertension may be the prevention of intrauterine growth retardation, as manifested by low birth weight for gestational age. As most persistently championed by the English epidemiologist D. J. P. Barker,[51] there is an impressive body of evidence that babies whose intrauterine growth is retarded and who are small at birth are more likely to develop hypertension in adult life. The manner by which this occurs remains uncertain, but a strong argument has been made for a failure of normal fetal kidney development so that fewer nephrons are available, leading to a vicious circle that induces and perpetuates hypertension[52] (Fig. 123–9).

Regardless of the mechanism, small babies become hypertensive adults more frequently than do larger babies. Part of this relationship involves parental hypertension, with hypertensive mothers more likely to give birth to small babies.[53] In addition, mothers who are black and young, who have babies in rapid sequence, and who are poor and unable to eat an adequate diet or receive prenatal care are more likely to have small babies. Obviously, the higher incidence of hypertension and renal damage among African Americans could reflect these characteristics. Effective birth control and adequate prenatal nutrition could

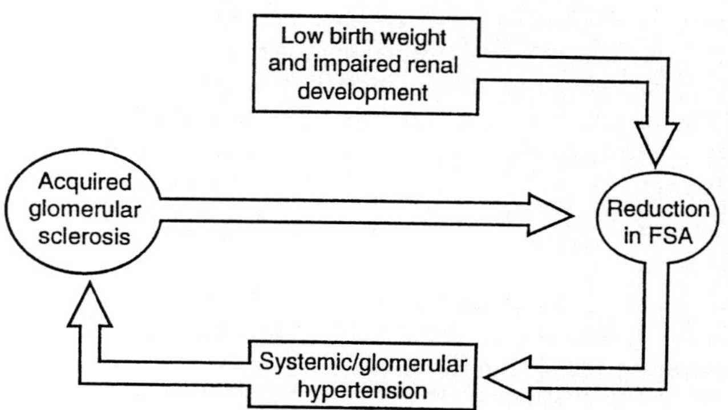

FIGURE 123–9 Diagram of the hypothesis that the risks of developing essential hypertension and progressive renal injury in adult life are increased as a result of congenital oligonephropathy or an inborn deficit of FSA, caused by impaired renal development. Low birth weight, caused by intrauterine growth retardation and/or prematurity, contributes to the oligonephropathy. Systemic and glomerular hypertension in later life results in progressive glomerular sclerosis, further reducing FSA and perpetuating *a vicious circle* that leads, in the extreme, to end-stage renal failure. (From Brenner BM, Chertow GM: Congenital oligonephropathy and the etiology of adult hypertension and progressive renal injury. Am J Kidney Dis 23:171–175, 1994.)

TABLE 123-2 Lifestyle Modifications for Hypertension Prevention and Management

Lose weight if overweight
Limit alcohol intake to no more than 1 oz (30 ml) of ethanol (e.g., 24 oz [720 ml] of beer, 10 oz [300 ml] of wine, or 2 oz [60 ml] of 100-proof whiskey) per day or 0.5 oz (15 ml) of ethanol per day for women and lighterweight people
Increase aerobic physical activity (30 to 45 minutes most days of the week)
Reduce sodium intake to no more than 100 mmol/da (2.4 g of sodium or 6 g of sodium chloride)
Maintain adequate intake of dietary potassium (≈90 mmol/da)
Maintain adequate intake of dietary calcium and magnesium for general health
Stop smoking and reduce intake of dietary saturated fat and cholesterol for overall cardiovascular health

have a major impact if society was willing to provide them.

CONCLUSION

The report of the sixth Joint National Committee provides a summary of lifestyle modifications that have been shown to help manage hypertension and to the potential to prevent its onset (Table 123–2).[54] These seven recommendations seem both appropriate and of great potential value.

As stated earlier, definitive proof of their effectiveness may never be achieved. One of the few relatively long-term trials, which lasted 5 years and involved 201 subjects with high-normal blood pressure at baseline, has shown a decrease in the incidence of hypertension from 19.2 percent among 99 control subjects to 8.8 percent among the 102 who were randomly allocated to a nutritional-hygienic intervention[55] (Table 123–3). The degree of changes in weight, sodium intake, reported alcohol intake, and frequency of physical activity—the interventions that were attempted in this trial—were relatively modest. Nevertheless, the potential shown in this trial for prevention (at best) or delay of onset (at least) of hypertension supports the vigorous pursuit of preventive measures against this disease.

TABLE 123-3 Five-Year Incidence of Hypertension in 201 Young Men and Women With Baseline Blood Pressure Averaging 122/82 mm Hg

	Weight (kg)	Urinary Sodium (mmol/da)	Alcohol Intake (g/da)	Incidence of Hypertension (Diastolic Blood Pressure > 90 mm Hg)
Intervention	−2.0	−41	−9.9	9/102 (8.8%)
Monitor only	+0.8	−11	−7.7	19/99 (19.2%)

Adapted from Stamler R, Stamler J, Gosch FC, et al: Primary prevention of hypertension by nutritional-hygenic means: final report of a randomized, controlled trial. JAMA 262:1801, 1989. Copyright 1989, American Medical Association.

REFERENCES

1. Kaplan NM: Primary hypertension: pathogenesis. *In*: Clinical Hypertension. 7th ed. pp. 41–99. Baltimore: Williams & Wilkins, 1998.
2. Light KC, Koepke JP, Obrist PA, Willis PW IV: Psychological stress induces sodium and fluid retention in men at high risk for hypertension. Science 220:429, 1983.
3. Mulrow CD, Cornell JA, Herrera CR, et al: Hypertension in the elderly. JAMA 272:1932, 1994.
4. Antonios TFT, MacGregor GA: Salt—more adverse effects. Lancet 348:251, 1996.
5. Brown JJ, Lever AF, Robertson JIS, Semple PF: Should dietary sodium be reduced? The sceptics' position. Q J Med 53:427, 1984.
6. Midgley JP, Matthew AG, Greenwood CMT, et al: Effect of reduced dietary sodium on blood pressure. JAMA 275:1590, 1996.
7. Alderman MH, Cohen H, Madhavan S: Dietary sodium intake and mortality: the National Health and Nutrition Examination Survey (NHANES I). Lancet 351:781, 1998.
8. Graudal NA, Galloe AM, Garred P: Effects of sodium restriction on blood pressure, renin, aldosterone, catecholamines, cholesterols and triglyceride. JAMA 279:1383, 1998.
9. Isles CG, Walker LM, Beevers GD, et al: Mortality in patients of the Glasgow Blood Pressure Clinic. J Hypertens 4:141, 1986.
10. Rose G: Preventive cardiology: what lies ahead? Prev Med 19:97, 1990.
11. Kaplan NM: The deadly quartet: upper-body obesity, glucose intolerance, hypertriglyceridemia, and hypertension. Arch Intern Med 149:1514, 1989.
12. Huang Z, Willett WC, Manson JA, et al: Body weight, weight change and risk for hypertension in women. Ann Intern Med 128:81, 1998.
13. Trials of Hypertension Prevention Collaborative Research Group: The effects of nonpharmacologic interventions on blood pressure of persons with high normal levels: results of the Trials of Hypertension Prevention, phase I. JAMA 267:1213, 1992.
14. Cutler JA, Follmann D, Allender PS: Randomized trials of sodium reduction: an overview. Am J Clin Nutr 65(suppl):643S, 1997.
15. Whelton PK, Appel LJ, Espeland MA, et al: Sodium reduction and weight loss in the treatment of hypertension in older persons. JAMA 279:839, 1998.
16. Rose G: Strategy of prevention: lessons from cardiovascular disease. BMJ 282:1847, 1981.
17. Law RM, Frost CD, Wald NJ III: Analysis of data from trials of salt reduction. BMJ 302:819, 1991.
18. Mattes RD, Donnelly D: Relative contributions of dietary sodium sources. J Am Coll Nutr 10:383, 1991.
19. Rose G: Environmental factors and disease: the man-made environment. BMJ 294:963, 1987.
20. Ely DL, Folkow B, Paradise NF: Risks associated with dietary sodium reduction in the spontaneous hypertensive rat model of hypertension. Am J Hypertens 3:650, 1990.
21. National Center for Health Statistics, Carrol MD, Abram S, Dresser CM: Dietary Intake Source Data: United States, 1976–1980. Washington, DC: U.S. Government Printing Office, Vital and Health Statistics, series 11, no. 231, March, 1983. DHHS publication no. (PHS) 83-1681, U.S. Public Health Service.
22. Gerber AM, James SA, Ammerman AS, et al: Socioeconomic status and electrolyte intake in black adults: the Pitt County study. Am J Publ Health 81:1608, 1991.
23. Brancati FL, Appel LJ, Seidler AJ, Whelton PK: Effect of potassium supplementation on blood pressure in African Americans on a low-potassium diet. Arch Intern Med 156:61, 1996.
24. Sacks FM, Willett WC, Smith A, et al: Effect on blood pressure of potassium, calcium and magnesium in women with low habitual intake. Hypertension 31:131, 1998.
25. Appel LJ, Moore TJ, Obarzanek E, et al: A clinical trial of the effects of dietary patterns on blood pressure. N Engl J Med 336:1117, 1997.
26. Allender PS, Cutler JA, Follmann D, et al: Dietary calcium and blood pressure: a meta-analysis of randomized clinical trials. Ann Intern Med 124:825, 1996.
27. Julius S, Krause L, Schork NJ, et al: Hyperkinetic borderline hypertension in Tecumseh, Michigan. J Hypertens 9:77, 1991.
28. Julius S, Jones K, Schork N, et al: Independence of pressure reactivity from pressure levels in Tecumseh, Michigan. Hypertension 17(suppl III):III-12, 1991.
29. Rostrup M, Mundal HH, Westheim A, Eide I: Awareness of high

blood pressure increases arterial plasma catecholamines, platelet noradrenaline and adrenergic responses to mental stress. J Hypertens 9:159, 1991.
30. Schnall PK, Pieper C, Schwartz JE, et al: The relationship between job strain, workplace diastolic blood pressure, and left ventricular mass index. JAMA 263:1929, 1990.
31. Shepherd JT: Increased systemic vascular resistance and primary hypertension: the expanding complexity. J Hypertens 8(suppl 7):S15, 1990.
32. Alexander CN, Schneider RH, Staggers F, et al: Trial of stress reduction for hypertension in older African Americans. Hypertension 28:228, 1996.
33. Panza JA, Epstein SE, Quyyumi AA: Circadian variation in vascular tone and its relation to sympathetic vasoconstrictor activity. N Engl J Med 325:986, 1991.
34. Kokkinos PF, Puneet N, Colleran JA, et al: Effects of regular exercise on blood pressure and left ventricular hypertrophy in African-American men with severe hypertension. N Engl J Med 333:1462, 1995.
35. Paffenbarger RS Jr, Wing AL, Hyde RT, Jung DL: Physical activity and incidence of hypertension in college alumni. Am J Epidemiol 117:245, 1983.
36. Blair SN, Goodyear NN, Gibbons LW, Cooper KH: Physical fitness and incidence of hypertension in healthy normotensive men and women. JAMA 252:487, 1984.
37. Hansen HS, Froberg K, Hyldebrandt N, Nielsen JR: A controlled study of eight months of physical training and reduction of blood pressure in children: the Odense schoolchild study. BMJ 303:682, 1991.
38. Tanaka H, Reiling MJ, Seals DR: Regular walking increases peak limb vasodilatory capacity of older hypertensive humans: implications for arterial structure. J Hypertens 16:432, 1998.
39. MacMahon S: Alcohol consumption and hypertension. Hypertension 9:111, 1987.
40. Shaper AG, Wannamethee G, Whincup P: Alcohol and blood pressure in middle-aged British men. J Hum Hypertens 2:71, 1988.
41. Rimm EB, Klatsky A, Grobbee D, Stampfer MJ: Review of moderate alcohol consumption and reduced risk of coronary heart disease: is the effect due to beer, wine, or spirits? BMJ 312:731, 1996.
42. Thun MJ, Petro R, Lopez AD, et al: Alcohol consumption and mortality among middle-aged and elderly U.S. adults. N Engl J Med 337:1705, 1997.
43. Bonaa KH, Bjerve KS, Straume B, et al: Effect of eicosapentaenoic and docosahexaenoic acids on blood pressure in hypertension: a population-based intervention trial from the Tromso study. N Engl J Med 322:795, 1990.
44. Flaten H, Hostmark AT, Kierulf P, et al: Fish oil concentrate: effects on variables related to cardiovascular disease. Am J Clin Nutr 52:300, 1990.
45. Daviglus ML, Stamler J, Orencia AJ, et al: Fish consumption and the 30-year-old risk of fatal myocardial infarction. N Engl J Med 336:1046, 1997.
46. Obarzanek E, Velletri PA, Cutler JA: Dietary protein and blood pressure. JAMA 275:1598, 1996.
47. Ness AR, Khaw K-T, Bingham S, et al: Vitamin C status and blood pressure. J Hypertens 14:503, 1996.
48. Steiner M, Khan AH, Holbert D, et al: A double-blind crossover study in moderately hypercholesterolemic men that compared the effect of aged garlic and placebo. Am J Clin Nutr 64:866, 1996.
49. Pincomb GA, Lovallo WR, McKey BS, et al: Acute blood pressure elevations with caffeine in men with borderline systemic hypertension. Am J Cardiol 77:270, 1996.
50. Goode GK, Miller JP, Heagerty AM: Hyperlipidemia, hypertension and coronary heart disease. Lancet 345:362, 1995.
51. Barker DJP: Fetal origins of hypertension. J Hypertens 14(suppl 5):S117, 1996.
52. Brenner BM, Chertow GM: Congenital oligonephropathy and the etiology of adult hypertension and progressive renal injury. Am J Kidney Dis 23:171, 1994.
53. Walker BR, McConnachie A, Noon JP, Webb DJ: Contribution of parental blood pressures to association between low birth weight and adult high blood pressure: cross sectional study. BMJ 316:834, 1998.
54. The Sixth Report of the Joint National Committee on Prevention, Detection, Evaluation and Treatment of High Blood Pressure. Arch Intern Med 157:2413, 1997.
55. Stamler R, Stamler J, Gosch FC, et al: Primary prevention of hypertension by nutritional-hygienic means: final report of a randomized, controlled trial. JAMA 262:1801, 1989.

CHAPTER 124

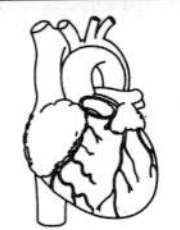

Cholesterol Disorders

Scott M. Grundy

CHOLESTEROL, LIPOPROTEINS, AND CHD
Lipoprotein Metabolism
Relation of LDL to CHD: Concept of Optimal LDL Level
Triglyceride-Rich Lipoproteins and CHD
Relation of Low HDL to CHD
NONDRUG AND DRUG THERAPIES AFFECTING LIPOPROTEIN METABOLISM AND CHD RISK
Nondrug Therapies
Drug Therapies
CHOLESTEROL MANAGEMENT IN PATIENTS WITH CHD (SECONDARY PREVENTION)
Cholesterol-Lowering Therapy in Secondary Prevention
Trials Targeting Atherogenic Dyslipidemia
Estrogen Replacement Therapy in Secondary Prevention
Goals for Therapy in Secondary Prevention
PRIMARY PREVENTION IN PATIENTS WITH CHD RISK EQUIVALENTS
Noncoronary Forms of Clinical Atherosclerotic Disease
Type 2 Diabetes
CHD Risk Equivalency due to Multiple Risk Factors
CHD Risk Equivalency due to Subclinical Atherosclerosis
PRIMARY PREVENTION IN INTERMEDIATE-RISK PATIENTS
Young and Middle-Aged Adults
Elderly Patients
Population Primary Prevention

For many years, cholesterol-lowering therapy was the stepchild of cardiovascular risk reduction. In the 1960s, cigarette smoking was accepted as a major risk factor for both coronary heart disease (CHD) and cancer; this acceptance led to a broad recommendation to the general public to eliminate cigarette smoking as a life habit. In the 1970s, hypertension became accepted as a major risk factor for CHD as well as for stroke. Not only did this acceptance engender clinical recommendations to reduce blood pressure in hypertensive patients, but it also fueled a major effort on the part of the pharmaceutical industry to develop new blood pressure–lowering drugs. Between 1960 and 1980, the acquisition of a large body of epidemiologic and experimental evidence indicated that an elevated serum cholesterol is a major risk for CHD. Nonetheless, several factors stood in the way of applying cholesterol-lowering therapies to reducing CHD risk. For example, for a long time, available cholesterol-lowering drugs were not highly efficacious. During this period, several cholesterol-lowering clinical trials gave ambiguous results.[1, 2] Although a trend toward benefit from therapy was often noted, no single clinical trial gave convincing proof of efficacy of therapy. Importantly, none of the early clinical trials showed a reduction in total mortality resulting from cholesterol-lowering therapy. In fact, some of the trials suggested that reducing serum cholesterol levels with drugs produced unacceptable side effects.[1] Thus, cholesterol-lowering therapy in clinical practice was left in limbo between 1960 and 1985.

A critical change in the cholesterol field occurred with the discovery of 3-hydroxy-3-methylglutaryl coenzyme A (HMG CoA) reductase inhibitors (statins).[3, 4] These agents inhibit the synthesis of cholesterol in the liver and thus increase the expression of low-density lipoprotein (LDL) receptors; the latter response lowers LDL cholesterol levels. The apparent efficacy and safety of statins stimulated the planning and execution of several large controlled clinical trials, of both primary and secondary prevention types. These trials, to be described later, uniformly demonstrated both efficacy and safety of statin therapy. Not only does statin therapy substantially reduce coronary morbidity and mortality, it also significantly lowers total mortality. These clinical trials have now convinced the medical community of the need to control elevated serum cholesterol as part of a strategy of coronary risk reduction.

The purpose of this chapter is to review current concepts of cholesterol management in high-risk patients. Emphasis is given to detection, classification, and therapy in the clinical setting. Highest priority goes to secondary prevention, that is, treatment of patients with established CHD. Next, attention turns to patients who are without CHD but in whom absolute risk for CHD is equivalent to that of patients with CHD. Finally, categories of lower absolute risk are considered.

Cholesterol, Lipoproteins, and CHD

Lipoprotein Metabolism

The essential metabolic pathways of plasma lipid transport have been extensively studied and described.[5] The predominant lipid transported in the circulation is triglyceride. Most of body's triglyceride is, of course, sequestered in adipose tissue. Adipose tissue triglyceride is derived largely from dietary fat that was delivered to adipose tissue by chylomicrons. The triglycerides of chylomicrons are hydrolyzed by lipoprotein lipase, and most of the fatty acids released go directly into adipose tissue, where they are esterified back into triglyceride.

In the fasting state, when plasma insulin levels are low, the activity of hormone-sensitive lipase in adipose tissue is high; triglycerides of adipose tissue are then rapidly hydrolyzed, and the resulting nonesterified fatty acids (NEFAs) are released into plasma. About two thirds of plasma NEFAs enter muscle and are used for fuel energy[6]; much of the remaining NEFAs go to the liver, an organ that uses fatty acids as a major energy source. Approximately one third of NEFAs entering the liver are reesterified into triglyceride; hepatic triglyceride then becomes part of very low density lipoproteins (VLDLs), which are secreted into plasma. When VLDLs arrive at the surface of capillary endothelium, they too interact with lipoprotein lipase and their triglycerides undergo lipolysis.[5] The fatty acids released in this section reenter adipose tissue.

Following hydrolysis of most VLDL triglyceride, VLDL "remnants" are released to the circulation. These remnants are enriched in cholesterol esters. They can either be removed directly by the liver (via LDL receptors) or be transformed into LDLs; the latter conversion occurs through lipolysis of remaining triglycerides and is catalyzed by hepatic triglyceride lipase. LDL is the predominant cholesterol-carrying lipoprotein in serum. Most LDL exits the circulation to the liver after binding to LDL receptors; only small amounts of LDL go to other tissues. Most of serum cholesterol comes ultimately from newly secreted VLDL. The serum concentration of cholesterol, which normally consists mainly of LDL cholesterol, is influenced greatly by the liver's expression of LDL receptors. The synthesis of LDL receptors is tightly regulated. The major factor controlling receptor synthesis is the concentration of cholesterol in liver cells. When hepatic cholesterol rises, synthesis of hepatic LDL receptors is suppressed; conversely, when hepatic cholesterol falls, synthesis of receptors rises.

A large quantity of serum cholesterol also is processed through high-density lipoproteins (HDLs).[7] The first step in this pathway is the formation of nascent HDL, a complex of phospholipids and HDL apolipoproteins. The origins of nascent HDL particles may be multiple; they may derive in part by direct secretion from the liver and gut, or they may form from various products released during lipolysis of chylomicrons and VLDL. Nascent HDL can receive unesterified cholesterol from VLDL, as a byproduct of triglyceride lipolysis, or from the surface cell membranes of peripheral cells. Unesterified cholesterol in HDL is esterified with a fatty acid through the action of a plasma enzyme, lecithin-cholesterol acyltransferase. Newly formed cholesterol esters enter the core of the HDL particles to produce small HDL_3. Further accumulation of unesterified cholesterol, followed by its esterification, gives rise to larger HDL particles, HDL_2. The cholesterol ester of HDL can be transferred either to VLDL, mediated by cholesterol ester transfer protein, or directly into the liver, mediated by scavenger receptor B-1.[8] After loss of cholesterol esters, HDL_2 is reconverted to HDL_3. The process whereby cholesterol passes from peripheral tissues through HDL and back to the liver is called *reverse cholesterol transport*.

Relation of LDL to CHD: Concept of Optimal LDL Level

A large body of evidence indicates that LDL is the major atherogenic lipoprotein. LDL therefore deserves primary consideration for lipid management. An important question must be considered: What is the optimal LDL concentration for minimizing the risk of CHD? The answer to this question appears to lie in the synthesis of several lines of evidence.

Evidence From Basic Science

Abundant basic research points to LDL being an atherogenic agent.[9] LDL cholesterol is the source of most of the cholesterol in atherosclerotic plaques. LDL also appears to be a proinflammatory agent.[9] The "active region" of atherosclerotic plaques contains mainly macrophages[10]; influx of LDL into the arterial wall seemingly "attracts" circulating monocytes and transforms them into active macrophages. According to current concepts, LDL must undergo modification before it can attract and activate macrophages. Candidate modifications of LDL within the intima include oxidation,[11] glycation,[12] and enzymatic degradation.[13] Thus, LDL plays multiple roles in the initiation and maintenance of atherogenesis.

Additional evidence for the atherogenicity of LDL obtains from studies in hypercholesterolemic animals.[14–16] In most animals, atherosclerotic lesions containing lipid-laden cells (macrophages and/or smooth muscle cells) do not develop without some elevation of LDL (or related atherogenic lipoproteins). Studies in experimental animals thus suggest that the lowest possible level of LDL is the optimal level, i.e., "the lower, the better."

Epidemiologic Evidence

Prospective population studies help to quantify the relation between the levels of LDL cholesterol and the incidence of CHD. Earlier studies measured total cholesterol instead of LDL cholesterol; even so, the high correlation between total and LDL cholesterol in populations provides a reasonable estimate of the relation between LDL and CHD. Some of the earlier reports[14–16] suggested a threshold relation between the cholesterol levels and the incidence of CHD. The threshold concentration above which CHD risk appeared to rise was a total cholesterol of about 200 mg/dl, corresponding to an LDL cholesterol of 130 mg/dl. This putative threshold was, however, not confirmed in later and larger prospective studies.[17, 18] The latter showed a continuous relationship between total-cholesterol levels and CHD incidence; the cumulative data from these studies indicated that the risk for CHD declines down to a total cholesterol level of at least 150 mg/dl (corresponding to an LDL cholesterol level of about 100 mg/dl). This relationship is not linear, however, but rather is curvilinear (or log-linear); in other words, the relationship is attenuated at lower LDL levels. Even so, these prospective epidemiologic studies taken as a whole support a level of LDL cholesterol of 100 mg/dl or below as being optimal, that is, associated with the lowest level of risk. These epidemiologic data cannot be discounted when defining the optimal LDL level; they possess two strengths: (1) the studies are consistent across multiple populations, and (2) they contain a very large number of subjects, many more than can be included in clinical trials.

Clinical Trials

Several clinical trials shed light on the relation between LDL cholesterol levels and CHD risk. Some pertinent trials display angiographic endpoints and others, clinical endpoints. The former have tested whether cholesterol-lowering therapy will delay progression or promote regression of coronary lesions.[19] Favorable changes in coronary plaque morphology generally have been observed with cholesterol-lowering therapy; at the same time, major coronary syndromes (myocardial infarction and unstable angina) are strikingly reduced.[19] Several of the angiographic trials employed aggressive cholesterol-lowering therapy and often attained an LDL cholesterol level of 100 mg/dl or below. One study, the Post Coronary Artery Bypass Graft (Post CABG) Trial,[20] specifically compared moderate versus aggressive forms of cholesterol-lowering therapy. Patients in the aggressive therapy arm reached an average LDL cholesterol of below 100 mg/dl; changes in coronary lesions in these patients were more favorable than in patients on moderate therapy, who had an average LDL cholesterol level on treatment of about 130 mg/dl. The results of Post CABG thus support the concept that an LDL cholesterol level of 100 mg/dl or below is optimal.

Clinical trials in which a clinical endpoint is the primary outcome have not been designed specifically to define an optimal LDL cholesterol level. The trials with HMG CoA reductase inhibitors (statins) have documented a definite benefit of LDL lowering. Post hoc analysis of the data from two trials—the Scandinavian Simvastatin Survival Study (4S)[21, 22] and the Cholesterol and Recurrent Events (CARE) trial[23, 24]—attempted to delineate the correlation between LDL cholesterol levels and recurrent coronary morbidity. The CARE analysis[24] supported a threshold relationship; in this trial, no benefit in CHD risk was observed by lowering LDL cholesterol levels to below 125 mg/dl. Post hoc analysis of 4S,[22] on the other hand, suggested a continuous relationship between LDL levels and CHD events down to a concentration of about 100 mg/dl. The latter relationship nonetheless was log-linear, similarly to that noted in prospective epidemiologic studies.[17, 18] Subgroup analysis of the statin trials cannot be taken as the final word on the optimal LDL cholesterol. These trials lack the statistical power to absolutely define the optimal LDL cholesterol. They are much smaller than the large prospective studies and must be considered less powerful. Nonetheless, they are consistent with the concept that the optimal LDL cholesterol is a level of 100 mg/dl or below.

Triglyceride-Rich Lipoproteins and CHD

The triglyceride-rich lipoproteins (TGRLPs) include chylomicrons, VLDLs, and remnant lipoproteins. Both chylomicrons and VLDLs are catabolyzed into cholesterol-rich remnant lipoproteins. Nascent forms of chylomicrons and VLDLs seemingly have little direct atherogenic potential. Nascent lipoproteins are large, cholesterol-poor lipoproteins, and they seemingly filter poorly into the arterial wall. Patients with familial forms of hypertriglyceridemia in which large TGRLPs predominate generally do not suffer from premature CHD.[25] In contrast, the remnants of TGRLPs almost certainly are atherogenic[26]; they are smaller, cholesterol-enriched lipoproteins that can readily filter into the arterial intima. Here they can initiate atherogenesis. Some investigators believe that remnant lipoproteins are even more atherogenic than LDL; even if this is true, however, concentrations of remnants normally are considerably lower than are those for LDL. In most patients with hypertriglyceridemia, however, concentrations of remnants are high; in such patients, elevations in remnant lipoproteins probably contribute significantly to atherogenesis. One condition in which remnants often are elevated is *familial combined hyperlipidemia*; in this disorder, patients typically have elevations of both LDL and VLDL.[27, 28] Another disorder, *familial dysbetalipoproteinemia,*[30] is characterized by a high concentration of a particularly atherogenic form of VLDL remnants called beta-VLDL.

Another way in which elevations in TGRLPs may promote atherogenesis is through modification of other lipoproteins. When TGRLPs are elevated, LDL particles become small and dense. Data support the concept that small, dense LDL particles are more atherogenic than normal-sized LDL.[30, 31] In addition, elevations in TGRLPs reduce the size of HDL particles, which may impair their antiatherogenic potential.[32] Since patients with elevated TGRLPs usually have both small LDL and low HDL, this trio of abnormalities has been called the *lipid triad*, or *atherogenic dyslipidemia.*[33]

Finally, high TGRLP concentrations often denote the presence of the *metabolic syndrome.*[33] This syndrome represents the clustering of four metabolic risk factors in a single person; these risk factor are atherogenic dyslipidemia, elevated blood pressure, glucose intolerance, and a prothrombotic state. The metabolic syndrome usually is accompanied by *insulin resistance,*[34, 35] a condition in which the actions of insulin are impaired. Three major factors underlie insulin resistance: obesity (particularly abdominal obesity), physical inactivity, and genetics.[34, 35] An initiating event leading to insulin resistance may be the overloading of various tissues with lipid.[36, 37] This can result from either an excessive release of NEFAs by adipose tissue (in obese patients) or inadequate utilization of NEFAs by muscle tissue (owing to physical inactivity). Diversion of excess NEFAs to the liver seemingly stimulates the overproduction of multiple factors, leading to atherogenic dyslipidemia, increased hepatic gluconeogenesis, possibly excessive angiotensinogen and its converting enzyme, and prothrombotic factors. These changes probably are responsible for the risk factors accompanying the metabolic syndrome. An elevation of serum TGRLPs can usually be considered a marker for the presence of insulin resistance and the metabolic syndrome.[33, 38] Some of the association between elevated serum triglyceride and CHD risk probably can be explained by the coexistence of elevated TGRLP with other metabolic risk factors.

Relation of Low HDL to CHD

A low level of serum HDL cholesterol correlates strongly with the incidence of CHD in high-risk populations.[39–41] This correlation appears to be related to three factors.[42] First, HDL may be directly antiatherogenic; if so, high levels of HDL may protect against CHD. Various mechanisms have been postulated for this protective action; none has been confirmed unequivocally. Second, a low HDL level commonly reflects the presence of other atherogenic lipoproteins, notably, raised TGRLPs and small, dense LDL. And third, a low HDL, like elevated TGRLPs, is often accompanied by the other nonlipid risk factors of the metabolic syndrome. Although a low HDL level is highly correlated with an increased CHD risk,[39–41] clinical trials have never been carried out to adequately test whether a therapeutic raising of HDL concentrations will significantly reduce risk for CHD.

NONDRUG AND DRUG THERAPIES AFFECTING LIPOPROTEIN METABOLISM AND CHD RISK

Nondrug Therapies

The backbone of risk reduction is the use of nondrug therapies. These therapies are listed in Table 124–1. A regimen to eliminate smoking heads the list of nondrug therapies.[43, 44] For LDL reduction, the aim is to reduce intakes of cholesterol-raising nutrients; these include dietary cholesterol, saturated fatty acids, and *trans* fatty acids.[45, 46] The three major sources of dietary cholesterol are egg yolks, animals fats, and meat. For most people, reduction in intake of egg yolks and animal fats is sufficient; lean meat need not be reduced. Saturated fatty acids are derived from butter fat (whole milk, cheese, ice cream, cream, and butter itself), animal fat (e.g., processed meats and hamburger), and tropical oils (palm oil, palm kernel oil, and coconut oil). *Trans* fatty acids come from butter fat and heavily hydrogenated oils (shortenings and hard margarines). To achieve maximal LDL lowering, current intakes of cholesterol-raising fatty acids should be cut by about half.[45, 46]

The most desirable replacement of cholesterol-raising fatty acids is disputed. Some investigators[47] advocate use of carbohydrates as the replacement in the belief that high-carbohydrate diets promote weight reduction. Others[48, 49] favor unsaturated fatty acids because they do not raise triglycerides or reduce HDL, as do carbohydrates. Among those who favor unsaturated fatty acids, some prefer polyunsaturated fatty acids, whereas others advocate monounsaturated fatty acids. For people who are overweight, it is best to replace cholesterol-raising nutrients with nothing; this will ensure some needed weight loss. The benefits of weight reduction in overweight patients are many.[50] Weight reduction often lowers LDL levels, and it improves other components of the metabolic syndrome: atherogenic dyslipidemia, elevated blood pressure, glucose intolerance, and a prothrombotic state.[45] The metabolic syndrome can also be mitigated by increased physical activity. Although regular exercise may reduce the risk for CHD in multiple ways, beneficial changes in the risk factors of the metabolic syndrome almost certainly make a major contribution.[51]

Dietary adjuncts may further reduce risk (Table 124–2). Among these are the plant stanols; these are derived from plant sitosterols and inhibit cholesterol absorption. An intake of 3 g per day of plant stanols will lower LDL cholesterol levels by 10 to 15 percent.[52, 53] In addition, high intakes of vitamin E (400 IU/da) and vitamin C (500 mg/da) will retard oxidation of LDL[54, 55]; this action may curtail atherogenesis.[11] Epidemiologic studies suggest that high intakes of soluble fiber[56] and moderate intakes of alcohol[57] will reduce the risk for CHD. Several lines of evidence also suggest that omega-3 fatty acids may decrease risk.[58] Therefore, use of these dietary adjuncts can be employed at the discretion and judgment of the physician.

TABLE 124–1 Nondrug Therapies

Therapy	Goal
Smoking cessation	Complete cessation
Reduction in cholesterol-raising fatty acids*	Less than 7% of total energy intake
Reduction in dietary cholesterol	<200 mg/da
Reduction in dietary salt	<2000 mg sodium/da
Elimination of excess body weight	Body mass index < 25 kg/m^2
Increased physical activity	30 min of moderate-intensity exercise/da
Consider adjuncts to dietary therapy (see Table 124–2)	

*Includes dietary saturated fatty acids and *trans* fatty acids.

TABLE 124–2 Dietary Adjuncts

Plant stanols (3 g/da)
High intake of fruits and vegetables (5 servings/da)
Dietary antioxidants
- Vitamin E (400 mg/da)
- Vitamin C (500 mg/da)

Dietary soluble fiber (30 g/da)
Moderate alcohol consumption (1–2 drinks/da)
Omega-3 fatty acids (1–3 g/da)

Drug Therapies

HMG CoA Reductase Inhibitors (Statins)

This class of drugs has emerged as the leader in LDL-lowering drugs.[3, 4] Currently available statins and their standard doses are shown in Table 124–3. At the doses shown, LDL cholesterol levels are reduced in the range of 25 to 35 percent. The statins inhibit cholesterol synthesis in the liver; this action stimulates the synthesis of LDL

TABLE 124–3 Currently Available HMG CoA Reductase Inhibitors (Statins)

Drug	Trade Name	Standard Dose (mg/da)
Lovastatin	Mevacor	40
Pravastatin	Pravachol	40
Simvastatin	Zocor	20
Fluvastatin	Lescol	40
Atorvastatin	Lipitor	10
Cerivastatin	Baycol	0.3

receptors, which effects a lowering of LDL cholesterol levels.[3,4] The statins have been shown to be remarkably safe at standard doses. Rare patients develop myopathy and elevated liver transaminases; both of these abnormalities can be reversed by discontinuation of the drug.

Bile Acid Sequestrants

Available agents in this class include cholestyramine and colestipol.[59] More efficacious sequestrants are currently under development. The sequestrants also increase the synthesis of LDL receptors; this response is achieved by inhibition of absorption of bile acids in the intestine. At tolerable doses, for example, 8 g/da for cholestyramine and 10 g/da for colestipol, LDL cholesterol levels are reduced by 15 to 20 percent. Bile acid sequestrants lower LDL cholesterol levels in an additive manner when combined with statins.[60,61] This combination is useful in patients with very high LDL levels.[60]

Fibric Acids

These drugs have been available for many years. In recent years, it has been learned that their primary action is to activate nuclear receptors called *PPAR-alpha*.[62] This activation elicits a cascade of responses including stimulation of fatty acid oxidation, lipoprotein lipase synthesis, and apolipoprotein AI (apo AI) synthesis. At the same time, synthesis of apolipoprotein CIII (apo CIII) is inhibited. This combination of actions favorably modifies atherogenic dyslipidemia, that is, it lowers plasma triglycerides, transforms small LDLs into normal LDLs, and raises HDL cholesterol levels. Fibrates are valuable for treatment of severe hypertriglyceridemia because they can reduce the risk for acute pancreatitis that accompanies this condition.[63] There is an ongoing dispute whether fibrates will also reduce the risk for CHD in patients with milder forms of hypertriglyceridemia; on the whole, however, a generally favorable trend has been observed.[64,65]

Nicotinic Acid

This agent has long been used to treat elevated serum cholesterol levels. The major action of nicotinic acid, however, is to reduce triglyceride levels. The mechanism of this action is not fully understood. Nicotinic acid inhibits the release of fatty acids by adipose tissue,[66] but the drug appears to modify the formation of lipoproteins in the liver as well. Not only does nicotinic acid reduce triglyceride levels, it also markedly raises HDL levels.[67] The combination of a statin and nicotinic acid is particularly effective for improving *all* the lipoprotein fractions.[68] The drawback of nicotinic acid is that it can be accompanied by a variety of side effects—flushing and itching of the skin, raised glucose and uric acid levels, abnormal liver function tests, and gastrointestinal irritation. About one third of patients who receive nicotinic acid develop side effects that prevent long-term adherence. Crystalline nicotinic acid commonly causes flushing, whereas sustained-release nicotinic acid often produces hepatotoxicity.[59] A new preparation of intermediate-release nicotinic acid, Niaspan, has recently been introduced that minimizes flushing and has a low incidence of hepatotoxicity.[69]

Cholesterol Management in Patients With CHD (Secondary Prevention)

Cholesterol-Lowering Therapy in Secondary Prevention

Patients at greatest risk for developing an acute coronary event (e.g., nonfatal or fatal myocardial infarction) are those who already have established CHD.[59] Prevention of recurrent coronary events is called *secondary prevention*. Previous research has shown that several medical therapies are efficacious in secondary prevention.[70] Most notable among these are smoking cessation, blood pressure control, and use of low-dose aspirin, beta-blockers, and angiotensin-converting enzyme inhibitors. For a long time, a critical question was whether CHD patients would also benefit from cholesterol-lowering therapy. In recent years, this issue has been resolved; the benefits of cholesterol-lowering therapy in secondary prevention have been documented conclusively through controlled clinical trials. These trials fall into three categories: earlier trials, angiographic trials, and statin trials. Each type of trial has provided unique evidence that can be summarized.

Early Secondary Prevention Trials

Several dietary and drug trials of cholesterol-lowering therapy were carried out between 1965 and 1990. Many of the trials gave results suggestive of benefit, although no trial result alone was convincing of both efficacy and safety. However, in 1990, Rossouw and colleagues[71] performed a meta-analysis of secondary prevention trials; the analysis was updated in 1993.[59] It revealed that patients receiving cholesterol-lowering therapy experienced a 15 percent reduction in serum cholesterol levels, a 26 percent decrease in nonfatal myocardial infarction, a 14 percent decline in fatal myocardial infarction, an 11 percent decrease in all cardiovascular deaths, and a 9 percent reduction in total mortality. Noncardiovascular deaths occurring in patients receiving cholesterol-lowering therapy were found not to be increased; this latter finding strongly suggests that reduction of serum cholesterol levels per se carries no serious adverse effects. The meta-analysis of Rossouw and colleagues[71] convinced the National Cholesterol Education Program (NCEP)[59] to place increased emphasis on cholesterol-lowering therapy in patients with established CHD.

Angiographic Trials

A series of trials were designed to determine whether cholesterol-lowering therapy can slow the progression of coronary atherosclerosis or reverse existing coronary lesions. Changes in lesion size were evaluated by coronary angiography. Cholesterol levels were reduced aggressively, usually with multiple drug therapy.[19] These trials demonstrated that lowering of serum cholesterol definitely slows progression of atherosclerosis and commonly induces some regression of coronary lesions. Still, changes in lesion size generally were relatively small and would not be expected to give favorable clinical outcomes. In spite of these small changes, major coronary events in patients receiving cholesterol-lowering therapy actually fell by about one third.[19] This discrepancy between visible changes in coronary plaques and the incidence of major coronary events supported the concept that reducing serum cholesterol stabilizes coronary plaques and reduces the chances of plaque rupture. The findings are consistent with previous pathologic studies that showed that plaque rupture is the primary cause of major coronary events (unstable angina and acute myocardial infarction).[72, 73]

Statin Trials

The efficacy of cholesterol-lowering therapy for secondary prevention has been fully confirmed in three major trials using statins: the Scandinavian Simvastatin Survival Study (4S),[21] Cholesterol and Recurrent Events (CARE),[23] and Long-Term Intervention with Pravastatin in Ischaemic Disease (LIPID).[74] Each trial deserves a brief review.

The 4S trial[21] tested the efficacy and safety of simvastatin in CHD patients having definite hypercholesterolemia. A total of 4444 patients were randomized to simvastatin and placebo for 5.4 years. The primary endpoint was total mortality, and various major coronary events were secondary endpoints. The dose of simvastatin was adjusted to reduce total cholesterol to less than 200 mg/dl. LDL cholesterol concentrations fell on simvastatin therapy by 35 percent. Statin therapy compared with placebo decreased reduced total mortality by 30 percent, major coronary events by 35 percent, coronary revascularization by 37 percent, and coronary mortality by 42 percent. Strokes were also significantly reduced. No serious side effects occurred with simvastatin therapy, nor was noncardiovascular mortality increased.

The CARE study[23] included 4259 patients (14 percent women) with existing CHD. The study was performed in North America and lasted 5 years. Patients at entry had "average" serum cholesterol levels (mean 209 mg/dl). Therapy consisted of pravastatin 40 mg/da versus placebo. On pravastatin therapy, LDL cholesterol concentrations fell from 137 mg/dl to an average of 98 mg/dl. Pravastatin therapy likewise reduced recurrent coronary events by 25 percent, coronary deaths by 24 percent, revascularization procedures by 27 percent, and stroke by 31 percent. Again, no significant side effects of statin therapy were revealed. The CARE trial[23] thus extended the benefits of cholesterol-lowering therapy to CHD patients who have only average cholesterol levels at baseline.

The LIPID trial[74] was performed in Australia and New Zealand. It compared pravastatin 40 mg/da with placebo in 9014 patients with established CHD. Entry criteria and LDL cholesterol levels of LIPID resembled those of the CARE study. Compared with placebo, pravastatin therapy reduced major coronary events by 29 percent, coronary death by 24 percent, revascularization procedures by 24 percent, stroke by 20 percent, and total mortality by 23 percent. All reductions proved to be statistically significant, and no serious side affects were encountered.

Subgroup analysis of these three trials[21, 23, 74] revealed that statin therapy significantly lowered major coronary events in men and women, in older and younger patients, in smokers and nonsmokers, in hypertensive and normotensive patients, and in patients with and without diabetes. Thus, the benefits of statin therapy in secondary prevention appear to extend to most if not all subgroups.

Trials Targeting Atherogenic Dyslipidemia

A persistent question has been whether therapeutic modification of lipoproteins other than LDLs also is efficacious in secondary prevention. The most common abnormality other than elevated LDLs is atherogenic dyslipidemia. Drugs that favorably modify atherogenic dyslipidemia are fibrates and nicotinic acid. Several trials have employed fibrates to test their efficacy in secondary prevention. Some of the earlier trials gave suggestive evidence of benefit. A notable exception was the Coronary Drug Project[75]; this large trial revealed no benefit of clofibrate therapy. Two large secondary prevention trials with fibrates were the Bezafibrate Infarction Prevention (BIP) trial.[65, 76] and the Veterans Affairs HIT.[77] The BIP trial tested bezafibrate in patients with established CHD. According to a preliminary report,[65] the outcome for all participants was negative; bezafibrate therapy did not reduce recurrent rates of major coronary events. On the other hand, in a subgroup of patients with hypertriglyceridemia, bezafibrate treatment seemingly reduced recurrent coronary events.[65] A more positive result has reported preliminary in patients participating in the Veterans Affairs High Density Lipoprotein Intervention Trial (HIT).[77] The fibrate used in this trial was gemfibrozil. The major lipid change on gemfibrozil therapy was a lowering of serum triglycerides; LDL levels were unchanged, and HDL levels rose only slightly compared with placebo. Patients receiving gemfibrozil had a 22 percent reduction in major coronary events. The results of this latter study are impressive and, when combined with previous trial results, suggest a strong trend toward some benefit of fibrate therapy.

Only two secondary prevention trials with nicotinic acid therapy are germane. One arm of the Coronary Drug Project[78] employed nicotinic acid. In this trial, patients who received nicotinic acid experienced a significant reduction in recurrent coronary events. In addition, long-term follow-up of Coronary Drug Project patients treated with nicotinic acid revealed a significant decrease in total mortality. In another study, the Stockholm Ischaemic Heart Disease Study,[79] combination drug therapy with nicotinic acid therapy plus clofibrate gave a significant decrease in recurrent CHD events. Thus, use of nicotinic acid in secondary prevention appears promising, although clinical trial data must be considered to reflect a strong trend and not a definitive result.

Estrogen Replacement Therapy in Secondary Prevention

Observational studies[80] strongly suggest that hormone (estrogen) replacement therapy (HRT) in postmenopausal women with established CHD will reduce risk for recurrent coronary events. These studies led the NCEP to recommend consideration of use of HRT in postmenopausal women with elevated LDL cholesterol. HRT is known to lower LDL levels as well as to raise HDL levels. On the basis of observational studies, many investigators speculated that HRT will reduce risk for coronary events through various mechanisms. These positive trends led to the Heart and Estrogen/progestin Replacement Study (HERS) trial, which was a secondary prevention trial of HRT. The combination of estrogen and progesterone was used as HRT.[81] The results of a trial were a disappointment. For the group as a whole, HRT did not reduce recurrent coronary events nor did it decrease total morbidity. In fact, a trend toward an increase in thrombotic events was noted. In view of the disappointing results of the HERS trial and the favorable results for women in the statin trials, it seems prudent to opt for use of statins over HRT for secondary prevention in postmenopausal women.

Goals for Therapy in Secondary Prevention

The American Heart Association and American College of Cardiology recommend that aggressive medical therapy be employed to reduce risk factors in patients with established CHD.[70] Among these recommendations was a strong endorsement of the NCEP's goal for LDL cholesterol for secondary prevention, namely, a level of 100 mg/dl or below. The NCEP based its goal for LDL cholesterol on evidence that the level of 100 mg/dl or below is optimal for minimizing the risk for CHD. As mentioned before, multiple lines of evidence contributed to this recommendation. To achieve an LDL cholesterol of 100 mg/dl or below, the majority of patients with established CHD will require cholesterol-lowering drugs.[82]

The American Heart Association further recommends that cholesterol-lowering drugs be used routinely for secondary prevention when baseline LDL cholesterol levels are 130 mg/dl or above.[82] Here drug therapy can be initiated without a trial of dietary therapy. In fact, drug treatment can be started when patients are in the hospital for acute coronary syndromes or for coronary procedures. It also can be started on detection of CHD in the outpatient setting. For purposes of cholesterol-lowering therapy, CHD can be defined as a history of stable angina pectoris, acute coronary syndromes (unstable angina or acute myocardial infarction), or coronary procedures (angioplasty or coronary surgery). Although drug therapy takes precedence over dietary therapy, maximal nondrug therapy is indicated for the majority of patients with CHD (see Table 124–2). Smokers should be referred to professional smoking-cessation programs if necessary.[44] The diet should be reduced in saturated fatty acids and cholesterol.[59] Weight reduction in obese and overweight patients will facilitate lowering of serum lipids.[83] A professional nutritionist can often assist in dietary modification. An exercise regimen is usually indicated and is best introduced in a program of cardiac rehabilitation.[84] Supplementing the diet with plant stanols[52, 53] can enhance LDL cholesterol lowering. Other dietary adjuncts may provide further risk reduction (see Table 124–2).

Three questions deserve special consideration for lipid-lowering therapy in secondary prevention: (1) Should patients with baseline LDL cholesterol levels in the range of 100 to 129 mg/dl be started on LDL-lowering drugs? (2) Should patients whose LDL cholesterol levels fall to the range of 100 to 129 mg/dl receive intensified LDL-lowering therapy? and (3) Should CHD patients with atherogenic dyslipidemia receive lipid-lowering drugs that target this form of dyslipidemia? Each question deserves separate attention.

For many CHD patients whose baseline LDL cholesterol levels range from 100 to 129 mg/dl, maximal nondrug therapy, perhaps supplemented by plant stanols (2 to 3 g/da), will achieve an LDL cholesterol level of 100 mg/dl or below. If this approach fails to attain the target of therapy, it can be easily achieved by adding a small dose of statin. Although endpoint data from controlled clinical trials do not provide unequivocal evidence of incremental benefit from use of statins in patients whose baseline levels are in this range, the Post CABG trial[20] strongly supports their use.

If standard doses of statins are employed in CHD patients whose baseline LDL cholesterol levels are 130 mg/dl or higher, about half will fail to reach the target of ≤ 100 mg/dl or below[23, 79]; for those who fail, LDL levels usually will fall to the range of 100 to 129 mg/dl. When this occurs, several options are available. For one, higher doses of statins can be employed to achieve a greater reduction of LDLs. Alternatively, a bile acid sequestrant (or plant stanols) can be added instead of a higher dose of statin. A different approach could be an enhanced mitigation of other risk factors rather than intensification of LDL-lowering therapy. Clinical trials are currently under way to determine more precisely how much incremental benefit can be achieved by reducing LDL cholesterol to below 100 mg/dl.

Many patients with CHD have atherogenic dyslipidemia. In these patients, consideration can be given to combining an LDL-lowering drug with either nicotinic acid or a fibric acid. To date, clinical trials have not been carried out to test the efficacy of combined drug therapy, but the previously mentioned suggestive evidence of benefit from treatment of atherogenic dyslipidemia makes combination therapy attractive. Still, if a fibric acid is used with a statin, the increased risk of myopathy must be taken into account.

Primary Prevention in Patients With CHD Risk Equivalents

Secondary prevention trials of cholesterol-lowering therapy demonstrate the efficiency, safety, and cost-effectiveness of aggressive cholesterol management in CHD patients who are at high risk. The question thus can be raised whether the same benefit will accrue to other patients of similar risk who do not yet manifest clinical CHD. This question raises another, namely, What is the absolute risk for subsequent major coronary events (fatal and nonfatal myocardial infarction) for patients with established CHD? This latter question might be answered by examining the incidence of major coronary events in placebo patients of the CARE[23] and LIPID[79] trials; these patients should be representative of American patients with CHD. For such patients, the projected 10-year risk for major coronary events was about 26 percent. Other reports[85, 86] indicate that the 10-year risk for major coronary events for patients with stable angina pectoris is about 20 percent. Thus, if a patient has a 10-year absolute risk for major coronary events of greater than or equal to 20 percent per 10 years, this patient can be said to have a *CHD risk equivalent.* Such a patient therefore would be a candidate for aggressive LDL-lowering therapy reserved for patients with established CHD.

Noncoronary Forms of Clinical Atherosclerotic Disease

The NCEP's Adult Treatment Panel II (ATP II) report[59] identified three CHD risk equivalents: (1) documented abdominal aortic aneurysm, (2) clinical signs and symptoms of ischemia to the extremities, accompanied by substantial atherosclerosis on angiograms or abnormalities of ankle/brachial pressure ratios or velocities, and (3) substantial carotid atherosclerosis documented by cerebral symptoms (transient ischemic attacks or stroke) accompanied by the demonstration of significant atherosclerosis on sonogram or angiogram. Prospective studies have shown that patients with these forms of atherosclerotic disease carry a risk for coronary morbidity and mortality equal to that of patients with existing CHD.[59] The NCEP thus indicated that patients with these clinical manifestations of noncoronary forms of atherosclerotic disease should undergo the same aggressive LDL-lowering therapy as patients with established CHD. For the American Heart Association,[70] these recommendations include smoking cessation, blood pressure less than 130/85 mm Hg, low-dose aspirin, and LDL cholesterol 100 mg/dl or below. Many patients will require drug therapy to achieve the LDL target. Appropriate nondrug therapies should be used in all patients to maximize risk reduction (see Tables 124–2 and 124–3). If the patient also has atherogenic dyslipidemia (triglyceride > 150 mg/dl and HDL cholesterol < 35 mg/dl), consideration can be given to combining a triglyceride-lowering drug with statin therapy.

Type 2 Diabetes

The concept of CHD risk equivalents can be extended to other high-risk groups, for example, patients with type 2 diabetes. Most authorities now agree that type 2 diabetes in high-risk populations carries an overall risk for CHD morbidity and mortality similar to that of patients with established CHD. Prospective studies[87] show that patients with type 2 diabetes without manifest CHD are at very high risk for developing CHD. Moreover, once these patients develop CHD, their prognosis is much worse than for CHD patients without diabetes.[88, 89] In the United States, high-risk populations in which type 2 diabetes carries a very high risk for CHD include non-Hispanic whites, blacks, Hispanics, and persons of South Asian origin. Thus, patients with type 2 diabetes from these populations deserve the same medical regimen described previously for patients with clinical manifestations of atherosclerotic disease other than CHD.

For patients with type 2 diabetes who do not have established CHD, the following strategy for risk reduction can be recommended: maximal nondrug therapy including complete smoking cessation, blood pressure lowered to less than 130/85 mm Hg, LDL cholesterol lowered to 100 mg/dl or below; and low-dose aspirin. If the patient has atherogenic dyslipidemia (triglyceride > 150 mg/dl and HDL cholesterol < 35 mg/dl), consideration can be given to combining a fibric acid with a statin for combined drug therapy.

CHD Risk Equivalency due to Multiple Risk Factors

Nondiabetic patients without CHD can also be designated as having a risk equivalent to that of CHD patients if their absolute risk for myocardial infarction plus CHD death is greater than or equal to 20 percent in 10 years.[90] At this level of risk, medical therapies in the clinical setting are cost effective. A critical issue is how to assess global absolute risk. The Framingham Heart Study[41] has recently published a risk-assessment tool. It must be noted that its scores were derived largely from whites in Framingham, Massachusetts. However, available data suggest that they also can be applied in the United States to other non-Hispanic whites, blacks, and Hispanics. They probably overestimate risk in Americans of East Asian origin[91] and underestimate risk in South Asians who have immigrated to the United States.[92, 93]

A modified revision of Framingham scoring is given in Table 124–4. Risk scoring, which may lead to lifetime therapies, should not be carried out at the first encounter with the patient. The score for LDL cholesterol should be set after 3 months of maximal dietary therapy (see Table 124–1); the score for blood pressure should be made after 3 months of blood pressure therapy to achieve acceptable control. Goals for risk reduction in patients with multiple risk factors who are found to be at risk equivalent to CHD patients include adoption of maximal nondrug therapy including smoking cessation (see Table 124–1), reduction of blood pressure to less than 130/85 mm Hg, lowering LDL cholesterol to 100 mg/dl or below, and use of low-dose aspirin. Statin therapy will usually be required to achieve the LDL cholesterol target. For patients whose baseline LDL cholesterol levels are in the range of 100 to 129 mg/dl, clinical judgment is required whether to begin cholesterol-lowering drugs. Likewise, when LDL cholesterol falls to the range of 100 to 129 mg/dl on cholesterol-lowering therapy, clinical judgment is required whether to intensify therapy to reach a target of 100 mg/dl or less. If a patient also has atherogenic dyslipidemia (triglyceride > 150 mg/dl and HDL cholesterol < 35 mg/dl), consideration can be given to combining a fibric acid or nicotinic acid with statin therapy.

CHD Risk Equivalency due to Subclinical Atherosclerosis

Many patients will have a 10-year absolute risk according to Framingham scoring (see Table 124–4) in an intermedi-

TABLE 124–4 Scoring for Global Risk Assessment (Modified Framingham Scoring)

Risk Factor	Risk Points: Men	Risk Points: Women
Age (yr)		
40–44	1	0
45–49	2	3
50–54	3	6
55–59	4	7
60+	5	8
*LDL Cholesterol (mg/dl) (on Dietary Therapy)**		
130–159	1	1
160–189	2	2
≥190	3	3
HDL Cholesterol (mg/dl)		
<35	2	5
35–44	1	2
Blood Pressure (mm Hg) (on Treatment)†		
>130/85	2	2
≥140/90	1	1
Baseline Fasting Plasma Glucose (mg/dl)		
110–126	1	2
Current Smoker‡		
No	0	0
Yes	2	2

Adding Up the Points

Age ________ Cholesterol ________
Diabetes ________ HDL Cholesterol ________
Smoker ________ Blood Pressure ________
Total ________

Risk Points	Absolute Risk (Hard CHD) (%): Men	Absolute Risk (Hard CHD) (%): Women
1	2	1
2	2	2
3	3	2
4	5	2
5	6	2
6	7	2
7	9	3
8	13	3
9	16	3
10	20	4
11	25	7
12	30	8
13	35	11
14	45	13
15		15
16		18
17		20

Abbreviations: CHD, coronary heart disease; HDL, high-density lipoprotein; LDL, low-density lipoprotein.
*Patient should be on maximal dietary therapy for 3 months before risk scoring (LDL cholesterol should be average of three values).
†Patient should be on appropriate blood pressure therapy for 3 months before scoring. Blood pressure reading should be the average of three measurements.
‡*Current smoker* means any cigarette smoking in the last year.

ate zone, for example, 10 to 19 percent. These patients could be raised to the category of CHD risk equivalency if they should be found to have advanced coronary atherosclerosis. Although Framingham scoring[41] provides useful information for assessing absolute risk, it must be noted that age becomes the dominant risk factor as people age. This is because age reflects an increasing burden of coronary atherosclerosis, and plaque burden itself becomes a risk factor for major coronary events.[94] Follow-up of patients undergoing coronary angiograms reveals that the likelihood of future coronary events correlates with the severity of coronary atherosclerosis.[95–97] Seemingly, the greater the plaque burden, the greater are the chances that some plaques will be vulnerable and will undergo rupture or erosion, causing an occluding coronary thrombus. Age is correlated with plaque burden and hence is a powerful risk factor in older persons.[94] A better estimate of the risk accompanying a given plaque burden, however, might be obtained if the extent of coronary atherosclerosis could be measured directly. If a patient at intermediate risk is found to have advanced atherosclerotic disease by noninvasive testing, this patient could be moved to a category of CHD risk equivalency. Thus, some patients at intermediate risk are candidates for noninvasive testing for subclinical atherosclerosis.

Several techniques are currently available for estimating the severity of subclinical atherosclerosis. Either these methods can directly identify patients with CHD risk equivalency or the measures can be substituted for age as a risk factor in global risk assessment. These tests include (1) the ankle/brachial blood pressure index (ABI), (2) exercise electrocardiogram (ECG), (3) sonography of the carotid arteries, and (4) electron beam computed tomography (EBCT) of the coronary arteries. Each test and its utility can be described briefly. Also, a strategy for application of these tests in risk assessment is outlined in Figure 124–1.

The ABI is the first test to employ to identify patients with advanced subclinical atherosclerosis. It detects a discrepancy in blood pressures between upper and lower extremities, which usually signifies advanced atherosclerosis in the arteries of the lower extremities. A Doppler ultra-

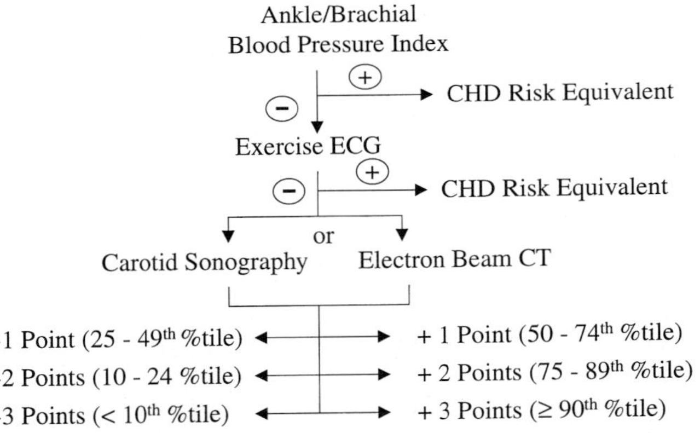

FIGURE 124–1 Strategy for noninvasive assessment of subclinical atherosclerosis. The first test in the sequence is the measurement of the ankle/brachial blood pressure index. If the test is positive, the patient is assigned to the risk of coronary risk equivalency; if negative, the patient proceeds to an exercise electrocardiogram (ECG). If the exercise ECG is abnormal, the patient will enter a regimen appropriate for a coronary heart disease (CHD) risk equivalent; if normal, consideration can be given to either carotid sonography or electron beam computed tomography (CT). The patient's age score (see Table 124–4) is adjusted according to the results of either of these two tests. Points are subtracted from the age score when age- and sex-adjusted scores are less than the 50th percentile, whereas points are added for scores greater than the 50th percentile.

sound velocity detector is employed to obtain an accurate reading of blood pressure. Blood pressure sounds are read in the antecubital fossa and over the posterior tibial and dorsalis pedis arteries. The ABI is determined for each leg. If the ABI is less than 0.90 in either leg, the test is abnormal and indicates advanced atherosclerosis in the peripheral arteries. Prospective studies have found that an abnormal ABI denotes a high risk for future coronary events.[98–102] Thus, an abnormal ABI can count as a CHD risk equivalent. When an abnormal ABI is obtained, further noninvasive testing is unnecessary; the diagnosis of CHD risk equivalency is established (see Fig. 124–1).

If a patient at intermediate risk has a negative ABI, a second level of noninvasive testing is an exercise ECG. The predictive power of this test has been most studied in middle-aged men and probably should be largely restricted to men aged 45 to 75 years. Its utility in men over 75 years and in postmenopausal women is uncertain. As shown in large studies,[103, 104] a "positive" exercise test indicates increased risk for major coronary events. A positive test in middle-age men with risk factors usually signifies the presence of significant coronary atherosclerosis. The predictive power of an abnormal exercise ECG remains high even after correcting for standard risk factors. Currently, exercise ECGs in asymptomatic persons are not recommended to detect "subclinical coronary artery disease" deserving of invasive coronary evaluation.[105] Nonetheless, in middle-aged men with other CHD risk factors, exercise testing could be useful for identifying patients at especially high risk. A positive test probably warrants elevating a patient into the category of CHD risk equivalent. However, a positive test does not justify invasive testing, that is, coronary angiography in the absence of assigned chest pain or proven myocardial dysfunction.

A third level of testing is to estimate coronary plaque burden by noninvasive imaging techniques, with either sonography of the carotid arteries or EBCT of the coronary arteries (see Fig. 124–1). The former method is based on observations that a moderately high correlation exists between the severity of atherosclerosis in carotid and coronary arteries.[106–109] Indeed, measurement of the intimal medial thickness of the carotid arteries by sonography has been reported to predict major coronary events independently of other risk factors.[110, 111] Thus, the finding of a high carotid plaque score adjusted for age and sex could add extra points to age in Framingham scoring (see Table 124–1). Conversely, lower percentiles warrant subtraction of points (see Fig. 124–1). The number of points to add (or subtract) is arbitrary but is consistent with prospective findings.[110, 111]

An alternate third-level test is EBCT. This test has the potential to directly measure coronary plaque burden. EBCT scores for coronary calcium correlate positively with the extent of coronary atherosclerosis, as shown by both autopsy and coronary angiography.[112–117] Some studies[118–120] suggest that estimates of coronary plaque burden by EBCT correlate with risk for major coronary events. If EBCT is used to estimate plaque burden,[94, 121] a conservative approach would be to add more points to the Framingham score for age for scores above the 50th percentile and to subtract them for scores less than the 50th percentile (see Fig. 124–1).

The approach to treatment of risk factors in patients found to be at high risk by combining noninvasive testing with standard risk factors is identical to that described previously for patients having CHD risk equivalents on the basis of multiple CHD risk factors alone.

Primary Prevention in Intermediate-Risk Patients

Young and Middle-Aged Adults

Another category of primary prevention extends to patients at intermediate risk for CHD. Some patients in this category are young adult and middle-age patients who are at risk for developing CHD in the long term, but not in the short term. One definition of intermediate risk could be the presence of any one categorical risk factor (see Table 124–4). If any categorical risk factor is allowed to persist unmodified for many years, cardiovascular complications can occur.[121] For example, many years of cigarette smoking can lead to clinical atherosclerotic disease as well as various types of cancer. Untreated hypertension can produce stroke as well as myocardial infarction. A prolonged hypercholesterolemia alone can promote development of coronary atherosclerosis and lead to myocardial infarction. Thus, an essential axiom of primary prevention is that all categorical risk factors must be treated under medical supervision.[121] In some cases, nondrug therapies will be indicated, whereas in others, drug treatment may be required. Another avenue to intermediate risk is through multiple risk factors. Some of these risk factors may be marginal, and not categorical. If Framingham scoring is carried out and if the 10-year absolute risk is found to be in the range of 10 to 19 percent, this level can be called *intermediate risk.*

Several earlier clinical trials have showed that lipid-lowering therapy will reduce the risk for CHD in primary prevention when patients are at intermediate risk. These trials included the World Health Organization clofibrate trial,[64] the Lipid Research Clinics cholestyramine trial,[122, 123] and the Helsinki Heart Study of gemfibrozil therapy.[65] In spite of a reduction in CHD events in all these trials, total mortality was not reduced by therapy in any of the trials. Consequently, the benefits of cholesterol-lowering therapy were brought into question. One of the limitations of earlier trials was that therapy was not efficacious enough to produce a marked cholesterol lowering. The introduction of statins made it possible to more effectively test the utility of cholesterol lowering in primary prevention. Two major clinical trials have been carried out. The West of Scotland Coronary Prevention Study (WOSCOPS)[124] examined the effects of pravastatin in high-risk patients with hypercholesterolemia. Results of this study were similar to those observed in secondary prevention trials with statins; drug therapy significantly reduced both major coronary events and total mortality. Another primary prevention trial, the Air Force/Texas Coronary Atherosclerosis Prevention Study (AFCAPS/TexCAPS),[125] examined the response to lovastatin therapy in moderate-risk patients with average cholesterol levels. Lovastatin therapy induced a marked decrease in major coronary events (acute myocardial infarction and unstable angina). Baseline risk in the study patients, however, was not high enough to yield a decrease in total mortality. These two primary prevention trials[124, 125] document the efficacy of LDL reduction for decreasing the risk of new-onset CHD. They also provide a wealth of data to compare efficacies of therapy for patients of different risk levels and to calculate cost effectiveness.

The essential goal of risk reduction for patients at intermediate risk is to eliminate the categorical risk factors. This includes counseling of smoking patients in smoking cessation, reducing blood pressure to acceptable levels (<140/90 mm Hg), and decreasing LDL cholesterol concentrations to the desirable range (<130 mg/dl). Maximal nondrug therapies for patients at intermediate risk is indicated as first-line therapy (see Table 124–1). Adjuncts to dietary therapy can be added to nondrug therapies according to clinical judgment of their utility (see Table 124–2). For patients whose LDL cholesterol concentrations are in the range of 130 to 159 mg/dl on maximal nondrug therapy, clinical judgment is required as to whether to add a cholesterol-lowering drug to the regimen. For those patients who are at higher absolute risk, for example, those with a 10-year absolute risk of 15 to 19 percent, a cholesterol-lowering drug may be warranted, as recommended in NCEP guidelines.[59]

Institution of drug treatments to achieve the goals of therapy should not be done "automatically"; it should be done after a careful weighing of the pros and cons. NCEP has particularly introduced caveats for introducing cholesterol-lowering drugs in primary prevention. For example, drug therapy can be delayed in young adults with only mild-to-moderate elevations of LDL cholesterol. Further, the absolute risk in most women with high LDL levels is lower than that of men, and thus, drug therapy should be used more cautiously. In many patients, if the LDL cholesterol can be lowered to within 30 mg/dl of the goal, this may be sufficient.

A second lipid risk factor is atherogenic dyslipidemia. This form of dyslipidemia is a potential target of therapy in primary prevention, but less so than for secondary prevention. Most patients have atherogenic dyslipidemia as a component of the metabolic syndrome. First-line therapy of the metabolic syndrome is weight control and physical activity. Both of the latter will improve the three lipid abnormalities of atherogenic dyslipidemia. Whether to add triglyceride-lowering drugs in the treatment of atherogenic dyslipidemia for the purpose of primary prevention is uncertain. Clinical trials have not been carried out to address this question. If drugs are deemed necessary, the best first choice is probably a statin. The statins reduce atherogenic TGRLPs as well as LDLs. In patients who have persistently high triglyceride or persistently low HDL in spite of statin therapy, a second drug, either nicotinic acid or a fibric acid, can be considered. However, it must be recognized that no clinical trials have ever tested the efficacy of combined drug therapy; also long-term combined therapy may be accompanied by more side effects. Therefore, combined drug therapy should be approached with circumspection in primary prevention.

Elderly Patients

Patients over age 65 years present a special challenge for risk assessment and risk management.[126, 127] Most major coronary events as well as coronary deaths occur after age 65 years. Therefore, primary prevention as well as secondary prevention in older persons is a major issue. Although a growing consensus speaks for aggressive risk-reduction measures in patients with established CHD, more reticence surrounds primary prevention in this age group. Nonetheless, clinical trials support the concept that the benefit from risk factor reduction extends to older age groups. This benefit has been observed for smoking cessation, treatment of hypertension,[128] and cholesterol-lowering therapy.[21, 23, 74, 124, 125] Few would now disagree that physicians should urge older patients to give up the smoking habit, or if necessary, should use drugs to bring blood pressure to near the normal range, even if they do not have manifest CHD. Whether to employ aggressive cholesterol-lowering therapy for primary prevention in older patients is another matter. With demonstration of efficacy of cholesterol-lowering therapy in clinical trials, the major issue essentially becomes who to select for drug therapy. Use of maximal nondrug therapy is reasonable in this age group, but cholesterol-lowering drugs must be used thoughtfully. The major problem with patient selection is the fact that age itself becomes the predominant risk factor in older persons,[94, 121] and the relative risk accompanying elevated serum cholesterol declines with aging.[126, 127]

Noninvasive testing for coronary plaque burden may be particularly valuable in the selection of older patients for cholesterol-lowering drugs. Since a patient's age is such a powerful risk factor, many patients will be classified as having a CHD risk equivalent by Framingham scoring (see Table 124–4). However, since the severity of coronary atherosclerosis varies greatly in the elderly population, noninvasive testing may help to differentiate between those who are truly at high risk, and deserve secondary prevention measures, and those who are at lower risk. Thus, noninvasive testing should be particularly useful for patients over age 65 years (see Fig. 124–1). For example, the ABI can be measured inexpensively on all older people, and if it is abnormal, aggressive therapy with cholesterol-lowering drugs can be instituted. The utility of exercise ECGs to detect myocardial ischemia in elderly patients is uncertain. Even so, it probably can be used in men up to age 75 years, although its reliability in women is uncertain. Carotid B-mode sonography can be used to uncover persons having advanced subclinical atherosclerosis. Likewise, EBCT can look more directly at coronary atherosclerosis. When coronary calcium is measured, the values must be adjusted for age and gender. This is because calcium continues to deposit in established plaques, and coronary calcium scores rise exponentially with age. Thus, patients must be classified according to percentile for age and gender rather than for absolute scores.

It may be prudent to divide the elderly population into two age groups, between 65 and 75 years and over 75 years.[126, 127] A more aggressive approach can be taken for primary prevention in the "younger" elderly (65 to 75 years). The LDL cholesterol targets for primary prevention in the elderly population are still open to question. For patients in the age range of 65 to 75 years, a projected 10-year risk of 15 to 25 percent probably warrants an LDL cholesterol target of 130 mg/dl or below, whereas for a 10-year projection of 25 percent or higher, a target of

100 mg/dl or below may be prudent. Use of low-dose aspirin in older persons at risk for CHD seems warranted, provided there are no contraindications for its use.

Population Primary Prevention

Clinicians can contribute importantly to primary prevention at the population level. The measurement of cholesterol and lipoproteins in all adults provides a powerful tool to educate individual patients who are part of the general public on the dangers of high serum cholesterol. Physician encouragement of their patients to modify risk-associated life habits will amplify other educational messages directed toward the general public. Periodic measurements of serum cholesterol provide physicians with an opportunity to reinforce public health messages. Another reinforcing opportunity is the study of first-degree relatives of patients with elevated LDL cholesterol and other lipid risk factors. The essential message of population primary prevention equates to the use of nondrug therapies (see Table 124–1). The magnitude of benefit that can be achieved by adoption of the measures outlined in Table 124–1 should not be underestimated. The greatest potential for reducing the burden of CHD in the general public resides in population primary prevention.

References

1. Muldoon MF, Manuck SB, Matthews KA: Lowering cholesterol concentrations and mortality: a quantitative review of primary prevention trials. BMJ 301:309–314, 1990.
2. Holme I: An analysis of randomized trials evaluating the effect of cholesterol reduction on total mortality and coronary heart disease incidence. Circulation 82:1916–1924, 1990.
3. Endo A: The discovery and development of HMG CoA reductase inhibitors. J Lipid Res 33:1569–1582, 1992.
4. Grundy SM: HMG-CoA reductase inhibitors for treatment of hypercholesterolemia. N Engl J Med 319:24–33, 1988.
5. Havel RJ, Kane JP: Structure and metabolism of plasma lipoproteins. *In* Scriver CR, Beaudet AL, Sly WS, Valle D (eds): The Metabolic and Molecular Bases of Inherited Diseases. pp. 1841–1851. New York: McGraw-Hill, 1995.
6. Coppack SW, Jensen MD, Miles JM: In vivo regulation of lipolysis in humans. J Lipid Res 35:177–193, 1994.
7. Bruce C, Chouinard RA Jr, Tall AR: Plasma lipid transfer proteins, high-density lipoproteins, and reverse cholesterol transport. Annu Rev Nutr 18:297–330, 1998.
8. Rigotti A, Trigatti B, Babitt J, et al: Scavenger receptor BI—a cell surface receptor for high density lipoprotein. Curr Opin Lipidol 8:181–188, 1997.
9. Navab M, Berliner JA, Watson AD, et al: The yin and yang of oxidation in the development of the fatty streak. Arterioscler Thromb Vasc Biol 16:831–842, 1996.
10. Ross R: Cell biology of atherosclerosis. Annu Rev Physiol 57:791–804, 1995.
11. Heinecke JW: Mechanisms of oxidative damage of low density lipoprotein in human atherosclerosis. Curr Opin Lipidol 8:268–274, 1997.
12. Millican SA, Schultz D, Bagga M, et al: Glucose-modified low density lipoprotein enhances human monocyte chemotaxis. Free Radic Res 28:533–542, 1998.
13. Bhakdi S, Dorweiler B, Kirchmann R, et al: On the pathogenesis of atherosclerosis: enzymatic transformation of human low density lipoprotein to an atherogenic moiety. J Exp Med 182:1959–1971, 1995.
14. Kannel WB, Castelli WP, Gordon T, McNamara PM: Serum cholesterol, lipoproteins, and the risk of coronary heart disease: the Framingham Study. Ann Intern Med 74:1–12, 1971.
15. Relationship of blood pressure, serum cholesterol, smoking habit, relative weight and ECG abnormalities to incidence of major coronary events: final report of the Pooling Project Research Group. J Chronic Dis 31:201–306, 1978.
16. Goldbourt V, Holtzman E, Neufeld HN: Total and high density lipoprotein cholesterol in the serum and risk of mortality: evidence of a threshold effect. BMJ 290:1239–1243, 1985.
17. Stamler J, Wentworth D, Neaton JD: Is the relationship between serum cholesterol and risk of premature death from coronary heart disease continuous and graded? Findings in 356,222 primary screenees of the Multiple Risk Factor Intervention Trial (MRFIT). JAMA 256:2823–2828, 1986.
18. Law MR, Wald NJ, Thompson SG: By how much and how quickly does reduction in serum cholesterol concentration lower risk of ischaemic heart disease? BMJ 308:367–372, 1994.
19. Brown BG, Zhao X-Q, Sacco DE, Albers JJ: Lipid lowering and plaque regression: new insights into prevention of plaque disruption and clinical events in coronary disease. Circulation 87:1781–1791, 1993.
20. The Post Coronary Artery Bypass Graft Trial Investigators: The effect of aggressive lowering of low-density lipoprotein cholesterol levels and low-dose anticoagulation on obstructive changes in saphenous-vein coronary-artery bypass grafts. N Engl J Med 336:153–162, 1997.
21. Scandinavian Simvastatin Survival Study Group: Randomised trial of cholesterol lowering in 4444 patients with coronary heart disease: the Scandinavian Simvastatin Survival Study (4S). Lancet 344:1383–1389, 1994.
22. Pedersen TR, Olsson AG, Faergeman O, et al, for the Scandinavian Simvastatin Survival Study Group: Lipoprotein changes and reduction in the incidence of major coronary heart disease events in the Scandinavian Simvastatin Survival Study (4S). Circulation 97:1453–1460, 1998.
23. Sacks FM, Pfeffer MA, Moye LA, et al, for the Cholesterol and Recurrent Events Trial Investigators: The effect of pravastatin on coronary events after myocardial infarction in patients with average cholesterol levels. N Engl J Med 335:1001–1009, 1996.
24. Sacks FM, Moye LA, Davis BR, et al: Relationship between plasma LDL concentrations during treatment with pravastatin and recurrent coronary events in the Cholesterol and Recurrent Events trial. Circulation 97:1446–1452, 1998.
25. Brunzell JD, Schrott HG, Motulsky AG, Bierman EL: Myocardial infarction in the familial forms of hypertriglyceridemia. Metabolism 3:313–320, 1976.
26. Krauss RM: Atherogenicity of triglyceride-rich lipoproteins. Am J Cardiol 81:13B–17B, 1998.
27. Goldstein JL, Hazzard WR, Schrott HG, et al: Hyperlipidemia in coronary heart disease. I. Lipid levels in 500 survivors of myocardial infarction. J Clin Invest 52:1533–1543, 1973.
28. Goldstein JL, Schortt HG, Hazzard WR, et al: Hyperlipidemia in coronary heart disease. II. Genetic analysis of lipid levels in 176 families and delineation of a new inherited disorder, combined hyperlipidemia. J Clin Invest 52:1544–1568, 1973.
29. Rall SC Jr, Mahley RW: The role of apolipoprotein E genetic variants in lipoprotein disorders. J Intern Med 231:653–659, 1992.
30. Austin MA, Breslow JL, Hennekesn CH, et al: Low-density lipoprotein subclass patterns and risk of myocardial infarction. JAMA 260:1917–1921, 1988.
31. Austin MA, King MC, Vranizan KM, Krauss RM: Atherogenic lipoprotein phenotype. A proposed genetic marker for coronary heart disease risk. Circulation 82:495–506, 1990.
32. Schaefer EJ, McNamara JR, Genest J Jr, Ordovas JM: Clinical significance of hypertriglyceridemia. Semin Thromb Hemost 14:143–148, 1988.
33. Grundy SM: Hypertriglyceridemia, atherogenic dyslipidemia, and the metabolic syndrome. Am J Cardiol 81:18B–25B, 1998.
34. Reaven GM: Insulin resistance and its consequences: non–insulin-dependent diabetes mellitus and coronary heart disease. *In* LeRoith D, Taylor SI, Olefsky JM (eds): Diabetes Mellitus. pp. 509–519. Philadelphia: Lippincott-Raven, 1996.
35. DeFronzo RA, Ferrannini E: Insulin resistance: a multifaceted syndrome responsible for NIDDM, obesity, hypertension, dyslipidemia and atherosclerotic cardiovascular disease. Diabetes Care 14:173–194, 1991.
36. Randle PJ, Priestman DA, Mistry SC, Halsall A: Glucose fatty acid

interactions and the regulation of glucose disposal. J Cell Biochem 55:1–11, 1994.
37. Randle PJ: Regulatory interactions between lipids and carbohydrates: the glucose fatty acid cyle after 35 years. Diabetes Metab Rev 14:263–283, 1998.
38. Mostaza JM, Vega GL, Snell P, Grundy SM: Abnormal metabolism of free fatty acids in hypertriglyceridaemic men: apparent insulin resistance of adipose tissue. J Intern Med 243:265–274, 1998.
39. Miller NE: High-density lipoprotein: a major risk factor for coronary atherosclerosis. Baillieres Clin Endocrinol Metab 1:603–622, 1987.
40. Gordon DJ, Probstfield JL, Garrison RJ, et al: High-density lipoprotein cholesterol and cardiovascular disease. Four prospective American studies. Circulation 79:8–15, 1989.
41. Wilson PWF, D'Agostino RB, Levy D, et al: Prediction of coronary heart disease using risk factor categories. Circulation 97:1837–1847, 1998.
42. Vega GL, Grundy SM: Hypoalphalipoproteinemia (low high-density lipoprotein) as a risk factor for coronary heart disease. Curr Opin Lipidol 7:209–216, 1996.
43. The Surgeon General's 1990 Report on the health benefits of smoking cessation. Executive summary. MMWR Morb Mortal Wkly Rep 39:1–12, 1990.
44. Ockene IS, Miller NH: Cigarette smoking, cardiovascular disease, and stroke. A statement for healthcare professionals from the American Heart Association. Circulation 96:3243–3247, 1998.
45. Grundy SM: Nutrition and diet in the management of hyperlipidemia and atherosclerosis. *In* Shils ME, Olson JA, Shike M, Ross AC (eds): Modern Nutrition in Health and Disease. 9th ed. pp. 1199–1216. Baltimore: Williams & Wilkins, 1999.
46. Grundy SM: The optimal ratio of fat-to-carbohydrate in the diet. Annu Rev Nutr 19:325–341, 1999.
47. Bray GA, Popkin BM: Dietary fat does affect obesity. Am J Clin Nutr 68:1157–1173, 1998.
48. Grundy SM: Comparison of monounsaturated fatty acids and carbohydrates for lowering plasma cholesterol. N Engl J Med 314:745–748, 1986.
49. West CE, Sullivan DR, Katan MB, et al: Boys from populations with high-carbohydrate intake have higher fasting triglyceride levels than boys from populations with high-fat intake. Am J Epidemiol 131:271–282, 1990.
50. Pi-Sunyer FX: A review of long-term studies evaluating the efficacy of weight loss in ameliorating disorders associated with obesity. Clin Ther 18:1006–1035, 1996.
51. Rodriquez BL, Curb JD, Burchfield CM, et al: Physical activity and 23-year incidence of coronary heart disease morbidity and mortality among middle-aged men. The Honolulu Heart Program. Circulation 89:2540–2544, 1994.
52. Miettinen TA, Puska P, Gylling H, et al: Reduction of serum cholesterol with sitostanol-ester margarine in a mildly hypercholesterolemic population. N Engl J Med 333:1308–1312, 1995.
53. Cater NB, Grundy SM: Lowering serum cholesterol with plant sterols and stanols: historical perspectives. *In* Nguyen TT (ed): A Postgraduate Medicine Special Report: New Developments in Dietary Management of High Cholesterol. pp. 6–14. New York: McGraw-Hill, 1998.
54. Jialal I, Grundy SM: Effect of dietary supplementation with alpha-tocopherol on the oxidative modification of low density lipoprotein. J Lipid Res 33:899–906, 1992.
55. Jialal I, Grundy SM: Effect of combined supplementation with alpha-tocopherol, ascorbate, and beta-carotene on low-density lipoprotein oxidation. Circulation 88:2780–2786, 1993.
56. Van Horn L: Fiber, lipids, and coronary heart disease. A statement for healthcare professionals from the Nutrition Committee, American Heart Association. Circulation 95:2701–2704, 1997.
57. Rimm EB, Klatsky A, Grobbee D, Stampfer MJ: Review of moderate alcohol consumption and reduced risk of coronary heart disease: is the effect due to beer, wine, or spirits? BMJ 312:731–736, 1996.
58. Connor SL, Connor WE: Are fish oils beneficial in the prevention and treatment of coronary artery disease? Am J Clin Nutr 66(4 suppl):1020S–1031S, 1997.
59. Expert Panel on Detection, Evaluation, and Treatment of High Blood Cholesterol in Adults: National Cholesterol Education Program: second report of the Expert Panel on Detection, Evaluation, and Treatment of high blood cholesterol (Adult Treatment Panel II). Circulation 89:1329–1445, 1994.
60. Grundy SM, Vega GL, Bilheimer DW: Influence of combined therapy with mevinolin and interruption of bile-acid reabsorption on low density lipoproteins in heterozygous familial hypercholesterolemia. Ann Intern Med 103:339–343, 1985.
61. Vega GL, Grundy SM: Treatment of primary moderate hypercholesterolemia with lovastatin (mevinolin) and colestipol. JAMA 257:33–38, 1987.
62. Fuchart J-C, Duriez P, Staels B: Peroxisome proliferator-activated receptor-alpha activators regulate genes governing lipoprotein metabolism, vascular inflammation, and atherosclerosis. Curr Opin Lipidol 10:245–257, 1999.
63. Zimetbaum P, Frishman WH, Kahn S: Effects of gemfibrozil and other fibric acid derivatives on blood lipids and lipoproteins. J Clin Pharmacol 31:25–37, 1991.
64. Manttari M, Huttunen JK, Koskinen P, et al: Lipoproteins and coronary heart disease in the Helsinki Heart Study. Eur Heart J 11(suppl H):26–31, 1990.
65. Kaplinsky E: The Bezafibrate Infarction Prevention study—preliminary results and implications for treatment. Presented at European Society of Cardiology, Vienna, 1988.
66. Boden G, Chen X, Iqbal N: Acute lowering of plasma fatty acids lowers basal insulin secretion in diabetic and nondiabetic subjects. Diabetes 47:1609–1612, 1998.
67. Vega GL, Grundy SM: Lipoprotein responses to treatment with lovastatin, gemfibrozil, and nicotinic acid in normolipidemic patients with hypoalphalipoproteinemia. Arch Intern Med 154:73–82, 1994.
68. Brown G, Albers JJ, Fisher LD, et al: Regression of coronary artery disease as a result of intensive lipid-lowering therapy in men with high levels of apolipoprotein B. N Engl J Med 323:1289–1298, 1990.
69. Morgan JM, Capuzzi DM, Guyton JR: A new extended-release niacin (Niaspan): efficacy, tolerability, and safety in hypercholesterolemic patients. Am J Cardiol 82:29U–34U, 1998.
70. Smith SC Jr, Blair SN, Criqui MH, et al, for the Secondary Prevention Panel: Preventing heart attack and death in patients with coronary disease. Circulation 92:2–4, 1995.
71. Rossouw JE, Lewis B, Rifkind BM: The value of lowering cholesterol after myocardial infarction. N Engl J Med 323:1112–1119, 1990.
72. Constantinides P: Plaque hemorrhages, their genesis and their role in supraplaque thrombosis and atherogenesis. *In* Glagov S, Newman WP, Schaffer SA (eds): Pathobiology of the Human Atherosclerotic Plaque. pp. 393–411. New York: Springer-Verlag, 1990.
73. Davies MJ: A macro and micro view of coronary vascular insult in ischemic heart disease. Circulation 82(suppl II):II-38–II-46, 1990.
74. The Long-Term Intervention with Pravastatin in Ischaemic Disease (LIPID) Study Group: Prevention of cardiovascular events and death with pravastatin in patients with coronary heart disease and a broad range of initial cholesterol levels. N Engl J Med 339:1349–1357, 1998.
75. Coronary Drug Project Research Group: The coronary drug project: clofibrate and niacin in coronary heart disease. JAMA 231:360–381, 1975.
76. Goldbourt U, Brunner D, Behar S, Reischer-Reiss H: Baseline characteristics of patients participating in the Bezafibrate Infarction Prevention (BIP) study. Eur Heart J 19(suppl H):H42–H47, 1998.
77. Rubins HB, Robins SJ, Collins D: The Veterans Affairs High-Density Lipoprotein Intervention Trial: baseline characteristics of normocholesterolemic men with coronary artery disease and low levels of high-density lipoprotein cholesterol. Veterans Affairs Cooperative Studies Program High-Density Lipoprotein Intervention Trial Study Group. Am J Cardiol 78:572–575, 1996.
78. Clofibrate and niacin in coronary heart disease. JAMA 231:360–381, 1975.
79. Carlson LA, Rosenhamer G: Reduction of mortality in the Stockholm Ischaemic Heart Disease Secondary Prevention Study by combined treatment with clofibrate and nicotinic acid. Acta Med Scand 223:405–418, 1988.
80. Sullivan JM, Vander Zwaag R, Hughes JP: Estrogen replacement and coronary artery disease: effect on survival in postmenopausal women. Arch Intern Med 150:2557–2562, 1990.
81. Hulley S, Grady D, Bush T, et al: Randomized trial of estrogen plus progestin for secondary prevention of coronary heart disease in postmenopausal women. Heart and Estrogen/progestin Replacement Study (HERS) Research Group. JAMA 280:605–613, 1998.

82. Grundy SM, Balady GJ, Criqui MH, et al: When to start cholesterol-lowering therapy in patients with coronary heart disease. A statement for healthcare professionals from the American Heart Association Task Force on Risk Reduction. Circulation 95:1683–1685, 1997.
83. National Institutes of Health: Clinical guidelines on the identification, evaluation, and treatment of overweight and obesity in adults—the evidence report. Obes Res 2:51S–209S, 1998.
84. Fletcher GF, Balady G, Blair SN, et al: Statement on exercise: benefits and recommendations for physical activity programs for all Americans. A statement for health professionals by the Committee on Exercise and Cardiac Rehabilitation of the Council on Clinical Cardiology, American Heart Association. Circulation 94:857–862, 1996.
85. Cleland JG: Can improved quality of care reduce the costs of managing angina pectoris? Eur Heart J 17:A29–A40, 1996.
86. Juul-Moller S, Edvardsson N, Jahnmatz B, et al: Double-blind trial of aspirin in primary prevention of myocardiali infarction in patients with stable chronic angina pectoris. The Swedish Angina Pectoris Aspirin Trial (SAPAT) Group. Lancet 340:1421–1425, 1992.
87. Haffner SM, Lehto S, Ronnemaa T, et al: Mortality from coronary heart disease in subjects with type 2 diabetes and in nondiabetic subjects with and without prior myocardial infarction. N Engl J Med 339:229–234, 1998.
88. Stone PH, Muller JE, Hartwell T, et al: The effect of diabetes mellitus on prognosis and serial left ventricular function after acute myocardial infarction: contribution of both coronary disease and diastolic left ventricular dysfunction to the adverse prognosis. The MILIS Study Group. J Am Coll Cardiol 14:49–57, 1989.
89. Smith JW, Marcus FI, Serokman R: Prognosis of patients with diabetes mellitus after acute myocardial infarction. Am J Cardiol 54:718–721, 1984.
90. Wood D, De Backer G, Faergeman O, et al: Prevention of coronary heart disease in clinical practice. Summary of recommendations of the Second Joint Task Force of European and Other Societies on Coronary Prevention. J Hypertens 16:1407–1414, 1998.
91. Wilson PWF, Abbott RD, D'Agostino RB Jr, et al: Prediction of coronary heart disease in Japanese-American men. Presented at the American Heart Association 71st Scientific Session, November 10, 1998. *In* Abstract Program. p. 437. Dallas, 1998.
92. Williams R, Bhopal R, Hunt K: Coronary risk in a British Punjabi population: a comparative profile of non-biochemical factors. Int J Epidemiol 23:28–37, 1994.
93. Seedat YK, Mayet FG: Risk factors leading to coronary heart disease among the black, Indian and white peoples of Durban. J Hum Hypertens 10(suppl 3):S93–S94, 1996.
94. Grundy SM: 1999. Age as a risk factor: you are as old as your arteries. Am J Cardiol 83:1455–1457, 1999.
95. Ringqvist I, Fisher LD, Mock M, et al: Prognostic value of angiographic indices of coronary artery disease from the Coronary Artery Surgery Study (CASS). J Clin Invest 71:1854–1866, 1983.
96. Emond M, Mock MB, Davis KB, et al: Long-term survival of medically treated patients in the Coronary Artery Surgery Study (CASS) registry. Circulation 90:2645–2657, 1994.
97. Storstein O, Engel I, Erikssen EJ, Thaulow E: Natural history of coronary artery disease studied by coronary arteriography. A seven-year study of 795 patients. Acta Med Scand 210:53–58, 1981.
98. Criqui MH, Coughlin SS, Fronek A: Noninvasively diagnosed peripheral arterial disease as a predictor of mortality: results from a prospective study. Circulation 72:768–773, 1985.
99. Criqui MH, Langer RD, Fronek A, et al: Mortality over a period of 10 years in patients with peripheral arterial disease. N Engl J Med 326:381–386, 1992.
100. McDermott MM, Feinglass J, Slavensky R, Pearce WH: The ankle-brachial index as a predictor of survival in patients with peripheral vascular disease. J Gen Intern Med 9:445–449, 1994.
101. Sikkink CJ, van Asten WN, van't Hof MA, et al: Decreased ankle/brachial indices in relation to morbidity and mortality in patients with peripheral arterial disease. Vasc Med 2:169–173, 1997.
102. Leng GC, Fowkes FG, Lee AJ, et al: Use of ankle brachial pressure index to predict cardiovascular events and death: a cohort study. BMJ 313:1440–1444, 1996.
103. Bruce RA, Fisher LD, Hossack KF: Validation of exercise-enhanced risk assessment of coronary heart disease events: longitudinal changes in incidence in Seattle community practice. J Am Coll Cardiol 5:875–881, 1985.
104. Multiple Risk Factor Intervention Trial Research Group: Exercise electrocardiogram and coronary heart disease mortality in the Multiple Risk Factor Intervention Trial (MRFIT). Am J Cardiol 55:16–24, 1985.
105. Special application: Screening apparently healthy individuals. *In* Froelicher VF, Follansbee WP, Labovitz AJ, Myers J (eds): Exercise and the Heart. pp. 208–229. Boston: Mosby, 1993.
106. Wofford JL, Kahl FR, Howard GR, et al: Relation of extent of extracranial carotid artery atherosclerosis as measured by B-mode ultrasound to the extent of coronary atherosclerosis. Arterioscler Thromb 11:1786–1794, 1991.
107. Crouse JR 3rd: Carotid and coronary atherosclerosis. What are the connections? Postgrad Med 90:175–179, 1991.
108. Crouse JR 3rd, Craven TE, Hagaman AP, Bond MG: Association of coronary disease with segment-specific intimal-medial thickening of the extracranial carotid artery. Circulation 92:1141–1147, 1995.
109. Visona A, Pesavento R, Lusiani L, et al: Intimal medial thickening of common carotid artery as indicator of coronary artery disease. Angiology 47:61–66, 1996.
110. Hodis HN, Mack WJ, LaBree L, et al: The role of carotid arterial intima-media thickness in predicting clinical coronary events. Ann Intern Med 128:262–269, 1998.
111. O'Leary DH, Polak JF, Kronmal RA, et al, for the Cardiovascular Health Study Collaborative Research Group: Carotid-artery intima and medial thickness as a risk factor for myocardial infarction and stroke in older adults. N Engl J Med 340:14–22, 1999.
112. Rumberger JA, Schwartz RS, Simons DB, et al: Relation of coronary calcium determined by electron beam computed tomography and lumen narrowing determined by autopsy. Am J Cardiol 73:1169–1173, 1994.
113. Rumberger JA, Simons DB, Fitzpatrick LA, et al: Coronary artery calcium area by electron-beam computed tomography and coronary atherosclerotic plaque area. A histopathologic correlative study. Circulation 92:2157–2162, 1995.
114. Rumberger JA, Sheedy PF 2nd, Breen JF, et al: Electron beam computed tomography and coronary artery disease: scanning for coronary artery calcification. Mayo Clin Proc 71:369–377, 1996.
115. Budoff MJ, Georgiou D, Brody A, et al: Ultrafast computed tomography as a diagnostic modality in the detection of coronary artery disease: a multicenter study. Circulation 93:898–904, 1996.
116. Guerci AD, Spadaro LA, Popma JJ, et al: Relation of coronary calcium score by electron beam computed tomography to arteriographic findings in asymptomatic and symptomatic adults. Am J Cardiol 79:128–133, 1997.
117. Schmermund A, Baumgart D, Gorge G, et al: Measuring the effect of risk factors on coronary atherosclerosis: coronary calcium score versus angiographic disease severity. J Am Coll Cardiol 31:1267–1273, 1998.
118. Arad Y, Spadara LA, Goodman K, et al: Predictive value of electron beam computed tomography of the coronary arteries. 19-month follow-up of 1173 asymptomatic subjects. Circulation 93:1951–1953, 1996.
119. Guerci AD, Spadaro LA, Goodman KJ, et al: Comparison of electron beam computed tomography scanning and conventional risk factor assessment for the prediction of angiographic coronary artery disease. J Am Coll Cardiol 32:673–679, 1998.
120. Detrano RC, Wong ND, Doherty TM, et al: Coronary calcium does not accurately predict near-term future coronary events in high-risk adults. Circulation 99:2633–2638, 1999.
121. Grundy SM: Primary prevention of coronary heart disease: integrating risk assessment with intervention. Circulation 100:988–998, 1999.
122. Lipid Research Clinics Program: The Lipid Research Clinics Coronary Primary Prevention Trial Results: I. Reduction in the incidence of coronary heart disease. JAMA 251:351–364, 1984.
123. Lipid Research Clinics Program: The Lipid Research Clinics Coronary Primary Prevention Trial Results: II. The relationship of reduction in incidence of coronary heart disease to cholesterol lowering. JAMA 251:365–374, 1984.
124. Shepherd J, Cobbe SM, Ford I, et al: for the West of Scotland Coronary Prevention Study Group: Prevention of coronary heart disease with pravastatin in men with hypercholesterolemia. N Engl J Med 333:1301–1307, 1995.

125. Downs JR, Clearfield M, Whitney E, et al: Primary prevention of acute coronary events with lovastatin in men and women with average cholesterol levels. Results of AFCAPS/TexCAPS. JAMA 279:1615–1622, 1998.
126. Grundy SM: The role of cholesterol management in coronary disease risk reduction in elderly patients. Endocrinol Metab Clin North Am 27:655–675, 1998.
127. Grundy SM, Cleeman J, Rifkind B, Kuller L: Cholesterol lowering in the elderly population. Arch Intern Med 159:1670–1678, 1999.
128. SHEP Cooperative Research Group: Prevention of stroke by antihypertensive drug treatment in older persons with isolated systolic hypertension: final results of the Systolic Hypertension in the Elderly Program (SHEP). JAMA 265:3255–3264, 1991.

CHAPTER 125

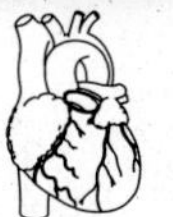

Obesity

James K. Alexander

OBESITY CARDIOMYOPATHY: ANATOMIC CONSIDERATIONS
PATHOPHYSIOLOGY
CLINICAL RECOGNITION
EFFECTS OF WEIGHT LOSS
OBESITY AND HYPERTENSION
OBESITY AND CORONARY HEART DISEASE
EPIDEMIOLOGIC STUDIES
ANATOMIC STUDIES
CORONARY RISK FACTORS
OBESITY AS AN INDEPENDENT RISK FACTOR FOR CORONARY HEART DISEASE
WEIGHT REDUCTION AND CORONARY HEART DISEASE

This chapter is largely devoted to a discussion of the clinical features, pathogenesis, and management of the cardiomyopathy associated with morbid obesity—relating the findings as far as possible to the spectrum of circulatory effects associated with obesity. There follows an update on current concepts regarding the relation between obesity, hypertension, and coronary disease, with some emphasis on preventive aspects.

In any consideration relating to obesity, it is appropriate to note at the outset that an easily obtainable and reliable assessment of the obese state has proved elusive. A variety of indices have been developed utilizing the relationship between body weight, height, and body surface area, including the ponderal index (height/(weight)$^{1/3}$), the quetelet index (weight/height^2 $\times$ 100), the body mass index (weight/height^2), and relative weight (percent predicted "ideal" weight). However, these indices do not differentiate between excess adiposity and increased lean body mass, and when compared with measures of adiposity—such as skinfold thickness, body density, and tritium dilution—they are imprecise, giving rather poor estimates of obesity, useful only at the extremes of distribution.[1, 2] Subjects with a relative weight twice that predicted, or a body mass index of 40 kg/M^2 or greater, have been considered to be morbidly obese. Since these indices have been used in most clinical studies, and since obesity is usually accompanied by an increase in lean body mass, it is not always clear whether the cardiovascular effects observed relate to adipose tissue mass, lean body mass, or both.

Obesity Cardiomyopathy: Anatomic Considerations

In the first postmortem study specifically addressing the relation between heart weight and obesity, Smith and Willius[3] found that the heart weights of 135 obese subjects with an average excess weight of 60 percent (20.5 kg) was greater than that predicted at normal body weight. Subsequent postmortem studies of extremely obese subjects weighing 130 kg or more and free of other cardiac disease demonstrated that the increased cardiac weight is due predominantly to left ventricular hypertrophy.[4–6] Increased epicardial fat and right ventricular hypertrophy are observed in 10 to 20 percent of these cases, with increased left atrial wall thickness in all of those examined for this finding. Isolated right ventricular hypertrophy, that is, cor pulmonale, has not been found.

When the composite data of several studies assessing left ventricular volume and mass by echocardiographic means are tabulated,[7] it is apparent that both volume and mass increase in quasilinear fashion as a function of absolute or relative body weight. Fatty infiltration of the myocardium, although not specific for obesity, is observed in approximately 3 percent of obese subjects at autopsy,[8] sometimes involving the sinus node or infranodal conduction tissue.[9] Echocardiographic appraisal of cardiac anatomy in morbidly obese subjects has demonstrated increased left ventricular mass in 64 to 80 percent, increased left ventricular cavity dimension in left atrial enlargement in 40 percent, and increased left ventricular wall thickness in 56 percent.[10, 11] Duration of obesity correlates positively with left ventricular internal dimension and mass/height index in obese subjects,[12] and these parameters are greater in those with congestive heart failure than in those without.[13]

Pathophysiology

Since much of the data secured in relation to hemodynamics and cardiac function in obesity pertains to very obese subjects, these findings are emphasized, recognizing that applicability to lesser degrees of obesity may be limited.

Adipose tissue oxygen demand at rest, estimated at 1.5 ml/kg/min is relatively modest,[14] but if body adipose tissue mass is large, body oxygen consumption at rest may be increased as much as 50 percent, increasing in direct proportion to body weight.[15] Since the systemic arteriovenous oxygen content difference changes little with weight gain, cardiac output increases in proportion to body oxygen consumption.[16] Similarly, blood volume increases in a quasilinear manner with weight gain, so that parallel increments in cardiac output and blood volume take place.[17–19] Thus, in terms of absolute blood flow, obesity is a high-output state, although cardiac index (cardiac output/body

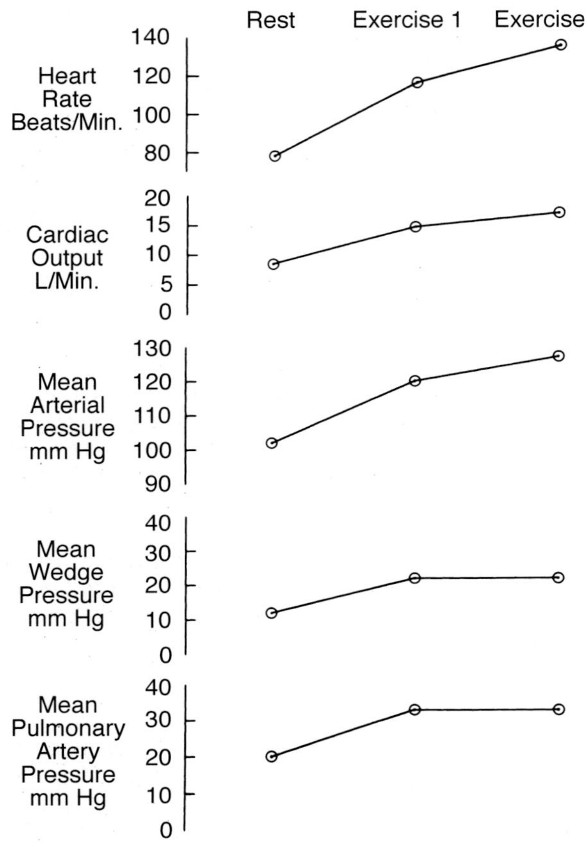

FIGURE 125–1 Hemodynamic data (mean values) secured on right heart catheterization in 22 obese subjects, mean weight 146 ± 4 kg, at rest and during increasing cycle ergometer exercise at two workloads. Note the high cardiac output at rest and the abnormal elevation of mean pulmonary wedge pressure during exercise. (Adapted from Bachman L, Freyschuss U, Hallberg D, Melcher A: Reversibility of cardiovascular changes in extreme obesity. Acta Med Scand 205:367–373, 1979.)

surface area) changes little. Since resting cerebral and renal blood flow are little altered, even in the setting of massive obesity, and increases in splanchnic flow are modest, it appears that the incremental blood flow is largely distributed to adipose tissue.[17] During exercise, the increment in cardiac output as it relates to body oxygen uptake is comparable with that of nonobese subjects.[15]

In very obese subjects, pulmonary hypertension usually develops during exercise, secondary to elevation of left ventricular filling pressure, and in some cases it is present at rest (Fig. 125–1).[18, 21–23] A transpulmonary diastolic pressure gradient (pulmonary artery diastolic to wedge) may also be found in such subjects, secondary to medial hypertrophy of precapillary pulmonary arteries[4, 9] or hypoxic pulmonary vasoconstriction. In some cases, congestive heart failure may evolve over long term, in association with biventricular diastolic pressure elevation, with severe systemic and pulmonary congestion. This circulatory congestive state is characterized by an abnormal elevation of left ventricular filling pressure on exercise or leg raising and a lesser distensibility of the pulmonary vascular bed with increments in total circulating blood volume.[24] Reduction in left ventricular chamber compliance plays a significant role in the pathogenesis of the congestive state.[25]

Impairment of left ventricular diastolic filling, as indicated in echocardiographic study by lowered mean transmitral E/A ratio, prolonged E wave deceleration half-time, and diminished peak filling rate, is usual in morbidly obese subjects, correlating with the percent overweight, left ventricular mass/height index, duration of obesity, and the presence or absence of congestive heart failure.[26] In those patients with diabetes, further worsening of left ventricular diastolic function would take place.[27] Typical circulatory dynamics and left ventricular functional data in a grossly obese subject with circulatory congestion are presented in Table 125–1.[28]

Two separate patterns of left ventricular systolic performance in the setting of marked obesity may be identified by echocardiographic study. By using the ratio of left ventricular wall thickness/end-diastolic chamber radius as an index of wall stress and relating this ratio to a cut-off point for normal ejection fraction, these patterns can be defined. In some such subjects, it has been found that parallel increments in both wall thickness and chamber radius result in maintenance of a normal ratio, with normal wall stress and normal systolic function. In others, the increment in chamber radius is not accompanied by a proportional increment in wall thickness, wall stress is elevated, and systolic function is depressed.[28, 29] "Inadequate" hypertrophic response to volume or pressure overload with chronically elevated wall stress appears to be the basis for this depression of myocardial contractile function.[30] More recently, these findings have been extended to include a more comprehensive appraisal of left ventricular loading conditions in these subjects. Left ventricular frac-

TABLE 125–1 Circulatory Dynamics and Left Ventricular Function in a Very Obese Man with High-Output Circulatory Congestive State*

Vo_2/min (L;STPD)	405
A-Vo_2 (vol %)	3.5
Q (L/min)	11.6
PAP (mm Hg)	52/19
LVP (mm Hg)	135/7
AoP (mm Hg)	135/85
LV max dP/dt (mm Hg/s)	1530
VCF (circum/s)	1.75
EF (%)	78
LVEDV (ml)	215
LVEDC (10^2/mm Hg)	1.6
LVEDWT (cm)	1.4

Abbreviations: AoP, aortic pressure, systolic/diastolic; A-Vo_2, arteriovenous oxygen difference; EF, left ventricular ejection fraction; LV, max dP/dt, maximal rate of left ventricular systolic pressure rise; LVEDC, left ventricular end-diastolic compliance units; LVEDV, left ventricular end-diastolic volume; LVEDWT, left ventricular end-diastolic wall thickness; LVP, left ventricular pressure, systolic/end-diastolic; PAP, pulmonary artery pressure, systolic/diastolic; Q, cardiac output; STPD, standard temperature and pressure, dry; VCF, mean circumferential fiber shortening rate; Vo_2, oxygen consumption.

*This 36-year-old patient weighing 200 kg presented with what appeared to be typical manifestations of congestive heart failure. Note the high cardiac output, pulmonary hypertension without a transpulmonary diastolic pressure gradient, elevated left ventricular filling pressure, and normal indices of left ventricular contractility. Left ventricular diastolic compliance is significantly reduced below the lower normal limit of 2.8 compliance units, and increased left ventricular wall thickness presumably reflects hypertrophy.

Modified from Alexander JK: The cardiomyopathy of obesity. Prog Cardiovasc Dis 27:325–334, 1985.

tional shortening correlates negatively and significantly with left ventricular diastolic dimension, end-systolic wall stress, and systolic blood pressure, as well as ventricular mass.[31]

That some as yet unidentified factor or factors play a role in the genesis of myocardial hypertrophy with morbid normotensive obesity is emphasized by the fact that, in other settings of predominant volume overload, left ventricular wall thickness is less and cavity dimension is greater. Thus, congestive heart failure, when it does occur in morbidly obese subjects, may be associated with a predominance of left ventricular diastolic dysfunction in some cases and both systolic and diastolic dysfunction in others.

Clinical Recognition

The findings on examination of a very obese person presenting in congestive heart failure are not greatly different from those of other etiology, perhaps specific only for the presence of the obesity itself. In general, body weight is in excess of 125 kg. Cyanosis and Cheyne-Stokes respiration are frequently present. Conjunctival suffusion, retinal venous congestion, and papilledema are sometimes observed.[5] Elevated jugular venous pressure may be difficult to confirm owing to cervical adiposity, and carotid pulse volume is usually preserved. Pulmonary rales and pretibial edema are virtually always present. Hepatomegaly and ascites are commonly present, but these are demonstrable with difficulty because of abdominal adiposity. Cardiomegaly is usual, and heart sounds are distant, often with an S_4 gallop. Cardiac murmurs and S_3 gallop are uncommon.

Cardiac rhythm is usually sinus, although atrial fibrillation may develop over the long term.[28] Left ventricular hypertrophy, although marked, is not reflected in the electrocardiogram, possibly because of the considerable soft tissue interposition between heart and electrode. Frequently observed electrocardiographic features include leftward deviation of the QRS axis in the frontal plane, low voltage, right axis deviation, and p pulmonale.[28, 32] Cardiomegaly with evidence of pulmonary vascular congestion are the features on chest roentgenogram. Hypoxemia, often with elevated P_{CO_2} and acidosis, typifies arterial blood gas analysis. Radionuclide gated wall motion study is useful in defining left ventricular systolic performance when satisfactory echocardiographic examination cannot be obtained. Since the circulatory congestive state may evolve in the setting of either preserved or depressed left ventricular systolic function, wall motion study is necessary to differentiate these contingencies.

Rapid weight gain often precedes symptomatic exacerbation in the natural history of the disease. In those with preserved left ventricular systolic function, recurrent episodes of congestion followed by symptomatic improvement may accompany weight gain or loss over as long as 10 to 15 years.[28] Prognosis is probably less favorable in those with depressed systolic function. Mental confusion, disorientation, and somnolence, sometimes proceeding to coma, and presumably reflecting cerebral edema, usually represent preterminal events.[28] However, a predisposition to sudden death is well documented.[33]

Aggressive diuretic therapy is both well tolerated and effective in relief of dyspnea and hypoxemia in patients presenting with pulmonary and systemic congestion. When resistance to intravenous furosemide is encountered, oral hydrochlorothiazide or metolazone given 1 hour before the parenteral injection is often effective. Positive-pressure oxygen therapy should be employed if hypercapnia is present in this setting, and tracheostomy may be necessary. Should systemic hypertension coexist, vasodilator agents will usually reduce both preload and afterload, with salutary effects on left ventricular filling pressure, pulmonary venous pressure, and lung water. Oral and parenteral nitrates have been utilized to advantage, and with accompanying left ventricular systolic dysfunction, angiotensin-converting enzyme inhibitors or angiotensin II receptor antagonists may be employed. Digoxin may be given for control of ventricular rate with atrial flutter or fibrillation, but blood levels relate to lean body mass rather than to body weight in these obese subjects. Thus, use of body weight as a guide to dosage may result in toxicity.[34]

The management of obesity per se remains a complex issue beyond the scope of this treatise. Suffice to say, weight reduction, maintained over long-term, remains the therapeutic goal.

Effects of Weight Loss

Weight loss (135 to 79 kg) 4 months after gastroplasty in morbidly obese subjects results in significant decrements in left ventricular internal dimension and mass when increased pregastroplasty.[11, 35] If achieved over a period of months, body weight decrements in these subjects are accompanied by parallel reductions in resting body oxygen consumption, circulatory blood volume, and cardiac output.[36] Systemic vascular resistance is usually unchanged owing to reduction in blood pressure. Left ventricular end-diastolic volume and pressure at rest tend to fall with weight loss, as do body oxygen consumption, cardiac output, and stroke volume.[8, 35, 36] Oxygen consumption, cardiac output, and stroke volume are less at comparable external workload during exercise. Ventricular function curves based on diastolic pressure and stroke volume may demonstrate improvement[37] or no change.[36] In those subjects with depressed left ventricular fractional shortening and substantial weight loss after gastroplasty (133 to 39 percent overweight), significant increase in shortening fraction at rest (24 to 30 percent) has been demonstrated, accompanied by decrements in ventricular chamber dimension, systolic blood pressure, and end-systolic wall stress.[38] In those with increased mass/height index, improvement in left ventricular diastolic filling was indicated by increased transmitral Doppler E/A ratio and diminished E wave deceleration time.[39] Thus, improvements in diastolic filling at rest with weight loss occur primarily in those subjects with increased left ventricular mass and are accompanied by decreased ventricular mass and improved loading conditions. Comparable elevation of left ventricular filling pressure during exercise before and after weight loss suggests that chamber compliance may not be altered.[36]

Obesity and Hypertension

Epidemiologic studies, largely based on indices relating weight to height, have established a strong association between body bulk and hypertension in children and adolescents, which tends to disappear after middle age.[40–43] There is also a correlation between skinfold thickness and hypertension as well as calculated body fat in young adults, but the majority of obese youngsters are not hypertensive, and some of the most obese are normotensive.[44] Longitudinal studies indicate that those who gain weight most rapidly as they grow older are more likely to become hypertensive.[45, 46] However, the correlation of hypertension with overweight is of a low order.[47, 48] A much better correlation of hypertension with central body fat distribution, as indicated by the waist/hip measurement ratio, has been established.[49, 50]

Although the accuracy of the indirect cuff method in assessment of blood pressure is variable, the presence of hypertension in some obese subjects is well documented.[51–53] Moderately reliable measurements in obese subjects may be achieved using a cuff with a bladder 42 cm in length or longer than the arm diameter.[54, 55]

The mechanisms of obesity-related hypertension appear to differ from those of essential or renovascular hypertension, as evidenced by several observations. There is no correlation of blood volume measurements and renin levels with the level of hypertension in obese subjects.[46] In contrast to the findings in lean hypertensive subjects, systemic vascular resistance is at a lower level, associated with increased cardiac output and pulsed-wave velocity.[56, 57]

Definition of the mechanisms underlying the development of obesity-related hypertension has thus far proved elusive. Review of several proposed hypotheses, including elevated aldosterone levels, enhanced response to pressor agents, and capillary compression by adipocytes, has yielded no firm supporting data.[58] The possibility that hyperinsulinemia is an important factor in the pathogenesis of obesity-related hypertension has received considerable attention. This is a potentially attractive hypothesis, linking the frequent occurrence of insulin resistance and hyperinsulinemia in patients with central obesity to an increased level of sympathetic nervous system activity. Chronic increase in sympathetic activity would then trigger increased cardiac output and peripheral vasoconstriction with insulin-mediated enhancement of renal sodium reabsorption to produce hypertension.[59] Data accumulating from the Normotensive Aging Study in Boston, utilizing 24-hour urinary norepinephrine secretion as an index of sympathetic activity, indicate that urinary norepinephrine increases with body mass index, abdominal girth, and insulin-glucose levels.[60] However, the impact of hyperinsulinemia per se appears blunted by the fact that patients with hyperinsulinemia secondary to pancreatic insulinoma are not hypertensive,[61] chronic intrarenal hyperinsulinemia does not cause hypertension,[62] and peripheral vasoconstriction does not characterize obesity-related hypertension. Further, epidemiologic studies have failed to show a consistent correlation between hypertension and hyperinsulinemia,[63] and long-term insulin resistance in animals does not result in hypertension.[64] Genetic factors may play a role in the failure to demonstrate consistent relationships between insulin resistance and hypertension[65, 66]; however, no association has been found between the neuropeptide-YY1-receptor gene, which increases appetite and blood pressure, and obesity.[67] A binding hypothesis must account for the fact that not all those with upper body obesity are hypertensive, and as many as one third of morbidly obese subjects are normotensive.[68]

Obesity hypertension is associated with increased circulating blood volume and cardiac output as compared with essential hypertension in lean subjects,[56] which comes about as a result of the need for perfusion of adipose tissue.[17] Peripheral vascular resistance, which is reduced in normotensive obese subjects, is inappropriately normal[56] or elevated[69] in hypertensive obese subjects. Cardiac adaptation is characterized by development of eccentric left ventricular hypertrophy.[56, 70] In hypertensive subjects, obesity is the strongest predictor of left atrial enlargement,[71] predisposing to the development of atrial fibrillation.[72]

Although the effect of weight reduction on the incidence of cardiovascular events in obese hypertensives has not been assessed, and estimates of the impact of preventing obesity on hypertension prevalence[73] do not necessarily relate to weight control, weight loss does lead to blood pressure reduction in these subjects. Sustained weight reduction is associated with a decrement in blood pressure in 50 percent or more.[59, 74–76] This decrement tends to take place early, following modest weight loss, often reaching a plateau with further loss of weight.[59–62] The average blood pressure drop over a period of months is generally in the range of 1 to 4 mm Hg systolic and 1 to 2 mm Hg diastolic per kilogram of weight reduction[76–80] with considerable scatter. Some controversy exists as to the relative importance of weight loss per se and of energy intake as the mediator of the hypotensive response.[81, 82] Although dietary regimens in weight reduction generally involve a decrease in sodium intake, blood pressure response to weight loss may occur independent of dietary sodium intake.[83, 84] Hemodynamic changes accompanying blood pressure reduction with weight loss are much the same as those noted previously in patients with cardiomyopathy.[85] Increased glucose tolerance and insulin sensitivity[86–88] with reduced sympathetic tone[59, 88] are additional benefits. Antihypertensive agents may be required over long term for blood pressure control during weight reduction or in its absence. In this setting, a choice other than thiazide diuretics or beta-adrenergic blockers would appear preferable, in view of the potential for those agents to reduce high-density lipoprotein (HDL) cholesterol and glucose tolerance.[89–91]

Obesity and Coronary Heart Disease

The potential impact of obesity in relation to coronary heart disease is significant because of its prevalence in the United States. Taking a body mass index over 27.8 kg/M^2 for men and 27.3 for women (approximately 120 to 125 percent of desirable weight) as indicative of obesity in the National Health and Nutrition Examination Survey, the incidence of obesity increased from 25.4 percent in the period 1976 to 1980 to 33.3 percent in the period 1988 to 1991.[92] In addition, the prevalence of obesity in children and adolescents is 27.1 percent in 6- to 11-year-olds and 21.9 percent in 12- to 18-year-olds.[93] This is noteworthy because about 70 percent of preadolescent obese children remain obese as adults.[94]

Characterization of the relation of obesity to coronary heart disease has included (1) epidemiologic studies relating coronary morbidity and/or mortality to total body or visceral adiposity, (2) anatomic studies examining the relation of adiposity to coronary atheromatous disease, (3) correlation of adiposity with coronary risk factor incidence, and (4) analysis of epidemiologic data with regard to obesity as an independent coronary risk factor.

Epidemiologic Studies

Epidemiologic studies examining the relation of obesity to coronary heart disease mortality and morbidity have, to some extent, yielded conflicting results, owing to failure to control for smoking or preexisting disease, misclassification bias, small cohort size, and/or short-term follow-up.[95] A review of 6 studies involving large cohorts, relatively long follow-up (10 to 16 years), and a focus on coronary disease mortality indicates increased risk with a body mass index greater than 30 kg/M^2 for men and 27 kg/M^2 for women.[96] However, excess total fat mass may have little effect on coronary disease mortality in selected gender, ethnic, social, and racial groups. Furthermore, physical activity may affect coronary disease mortality to a greater extent than does total fat mass. Meta-analysis demonstrates that physical activity has a favorable effect on coronary mortality with or without covariant adjustments for overweight.[97]

A number of epidemiologic studies have emphasized the importance of regional fat distribution as opposed to total body fat mass in relation to the incidence of coronary disease as well as hypertension. Using waist/hip ratio or subscapular skinfold thickness as indices of abdominal visceral (mesenteric and omental) fat, these studies have identified abdominal (central) adiposity as a condition predisposing to coronary heart disease independent of total body fat mass.[98–100] Central obesity is associated with a clustering of coronary risk factors, including dyslipoproteinemia, non–insulin-dependent diabetes mellitus, as well as hypertension and hyperandrogenism.[98, 101, 102] The incidence of these factors increases significantly when the waist/hip ratio is greater than 1.0 in men and 0.8 in women. Pathogenetic mechanisms resulting in expression of these factors with central obesity have been related to "portal" adipose tissue by Bjorntorp.[103] Marked sensitivity of visceral fat depots to lipolytic stimulation results in delivery of large quantities of free fatty acids to the portal vein when these depots are excessive. Excess free fatty acid content in the portal vein is followed by increased hepatic gluconeogenesis, glucose intolerance, production of atherogenic lipoproteins, and decrease in hepatic insulin clearance with hyperinsulinemia and insulin resistance.

Anatomic Studies

Cross-sectional studies examining the extent of coronary atheromatous disease in relation to indices of obesity at autopsy may be subject to the reservation that the nutritional status of the individual may not reflect that which existed during development of the atheromatous lesions. However, a World Health Organization study reported by Montenegro and Solberg[104] is notable in that fatty streaks and raised atheromatous lesions were graded in relation to body weight, trunk length, and thickness of subcutaneous fat in 350 persons from six different geographic and ethnic populations, including accidental deaths. For those whose death was accidental, there was no association between the degree and extent of coronary atheroma and the indices of obesity in the population as a whole or in any of the individual groups. In another World Health Organization study in Europe, the prevalence of coronary stenosis and extent of atheroma were not increased in obese versus thin subjects when hypertensives and diabetics were excluded.[105] In a review of autopsy studies in 1983,[106] there appeared no consistent relation between the presence of adiposity and its degree and the extent of coronary atheromatous disease. Should there be a positive correlation between body fat mass and extent of coronary atheromatous involvement, extensive coronary disease might be anticipated with morbid obesity. Although the series is small, it is noteworthy that little coronary atheromatous disease has been found in postmortem studies of morbidly obese subjects over an age range of 30 to 75 years.[4–6] Two autopsy studies of men dying of accidental or noncoronary disease causes[107, 108] demonstrated a weak correlation between abdominal panniculus thickness and raised coronary atheromatous lesions in whites but not in African Americans. More recently, right coronary atherosclerosis in 1532 young persons dying of external causes has been quantified in relation to body mass index and abdominal panniculus thickness.[109] In men 25 to 34 years old, percentages of fatty streaks and raised atheromatous lesions in the right coronary artery were significantly increased with a body mass index greater than 30, and these values were two to four times higher with abdominal panniculus thickness greater than 17 mm. No correlation was found in women. A number of cross-sectional studies examining the relations between height-weight indices of excess body fat and angiographic severity of coronary disease have shown no correlation,[110, 118] nor have longitudinal studies up to 15[119] and 20[113] years demonstrated any difference in disease progression. In contrast, although the association has not been uniform, several studies have demonstrated a positive correlation between waist/hip ratio or visceral abdominal adipose tissue mass and angiographic severity of coronary disease.[11, 114, 116–118] Thus, even though no allowance was made for risk factors such as dyslipidemia, hypertension, and smoking in most of the anatomic studies, there appears to be no consistent relation between total body fat mass and severity of coronary atheromatous involvement, effectively providing no firm support for the proposition of excess body fat as an independent coronary risk factor (see later). However, at least in one study, anatomic extent of coronary disease was significantly increased in men with body mass index greater than 30 kg/M^2, consonant with findings in epidemiologic studies. On the other hand, the association of coronary disease with abdominal adiposity has been more consistently observed in both anatomic and epidemiologic studies.

Coronary Risk Factors

In addition to hypertension, coronary risk factors associated with obesity include dyslipidemia, diabetes, and hyperuricemia. As body mass index increases, the atherogenic plasma low-density lipoprotein (LDL) cholesterol and triglyceride levels tend to rise, while potentially protective HDL cholesterol levels fall.[120] Correlation of plasma total cholesterol levels with body mass index is significantly less or absent.[121, 122] Correlation between central obesity, as indicated by waist/hip ratio, and atherogenic lipid levels is much stronger and more consistent.[123, 124] Furthermore, central obesity is associated with increased proportions of the small, dense LDL fraction and small very low density lipoprotein, recognized as an atherogenic disorder.[123, 125]

An association of non–insulin-dependent diabetes mellitus with overweight is well documented,[126, 127] with higher incidence as body mass index increases.[122] This condition is characterized by increased insulin levels and insulin resistance. Designation of hyperinsulinemia or insulin resistance as a coronary risk factor remains somewhat controversial. In a review of the subject,[128] it was concluded that there was no firm support for designation of hyperinsulinemia as such. However, a 22-year follow-up study of 970 men 34 to 64 years old, free of cardiovascular disease and diabetes, demonstrated predictability of hyperinsulinemia for coronary heart disease risk to a large extent independent of other coronary risk factors.[129] Although insulin resistance has been proposed as an independent coronary risk factor,[130] there is a metabolic linkage with increased triglyceride and reduced HDL levels.[131] Thus, it is not clear that insulin resistance is in itself atherogenic,[132] and it may be a marker of other hormonal or metabolic abnormalities not adequately assessed by a relation to conventional risk factors.[133] These abnormalities in plasma insulin levels with glucose intolerance and lowered HDL are correlated with truncal obesity but not with total body fat.[134] Non–insulin-dependent diabetes in subjects with central obesity is associated with increased plasma viscosity and fibrinogen levels, also identified as coronary risk factors,[135] but not usually included in multivariate analysis of data in large scale epidemiologic trials.

Gout was identified as a risk factor for coronary heart disease mortality in postmenopausal women in the Chicago Health Association Detection Project in Industry.[136] The association of hyperuricemia and gout in subjects with severe obesity has received little attention in epidemiologic studies.

From a public health standpoint, a consideration of some importance is the tendency to clustering of coronary risk factors in children and adolescents with increased body fat levels (estimated from skinfold measurements) above 25 percent in males and 30 percent in females.[137] A secular trend of increasing obesity, accompanied by increasing risk factor manifestation in such subjects, has been observed since the early 1980s in the Bogalusa Heart Study.[138] Overweight children and adolescents tend to become overweight adults.[139, 140]

Obesity as an Independent Risk Factor for Coronary Heart Disease

Identification of obesity itself as an independent coronary risk factor in epidemiologic studies implies demonstration of a remaining element of risk, presumably due to obesity, when accepted risk factors are accounted for in multivariate analysis. This has proved difficult, to some extent relating to omission of certain obesity-related coronary risk factors in the analyses. As regards weight-height indices and total body fat mass, apart from the Framingham study,[141] three studies have been cited as indicating an independent contribution to coronary risk by obesity itself.[142] The Framingham study has been criticized in that another analysis of the data did not indicate that coronary disease mortality was significantly related to body weight[143] and failure to consider other obesity-related risk factors may have accounted for the result.[144] Of the cited references, the Manitoba Study[145] included only age and blood pressure for analysis beyond obesity, demonstrating a relation to myocardial infarction and sudden death, with no data on coronary heart disease mortality. A later report from Framingham[146] included only smoking in addition to relative weight, reporting total mortality, with no data on coronary disease mortality. In discussing results of the third (Nurses' Health) study,[147] the authors state that inclusion of hypertension, diabetes, and hypercholesterolemia in a separate multivariate analysis attenuated, but did not eliminate, the relation between body mass index and mortality. Thus, in the first two studies, the database did not permit a conclusion regarding independence of obesity (nor was it mentioned by the authors), and in the third study, although not specifically mentioned by the authors, the question was left open. Thoroughgoing meta-analyses of coronary risk factor epidemiologic data with special reference to obesity as appraised by relative weight or weight-height indices were carried out in 1985[148] and 1987.[149] Both analyses failed to demonstrate excess total body fat mass as an independent coronary risk factor. Further, the lack of a reasonably consistent correlation between indices of total fat mass and severity of atheromatous disease as appraised at autopsy or on arteriography emphasizes the disparity between overall fatness by itself and coronary heart disease. The National Cholesterol Education Reports do not list obesity per se, as indicated by relative weight or weight-height indices, as a coronary risk factor.[150] This stance seems consonant with the bulk of evidence currently available.

Excess abdominal adiposity has been proposed as an independent coronary risk factor.[151] However, the metabolic profile of dyslipidemia, diabetes, and hypertriglyceridemia is not consistently found with central obesity, and not all viscerally obese subjects are at increased cardiac risk. Genetic sensitivity to dyslipidemia and diabetes appears to condition the effects of visceral adiposity, thus accounting for the heterogeneous pattern of clinical manifestations.[152] If excess portal adipose tissue does result in a unique effect in relation to coronary disease, and therefore could in some sense be considered an independent risk factor, its effects are not consistent, being significantly modified under different conditions and mediated to the extent that the metabolic profile develops.

In sum, then, it has not been clearly established that either excess total body fat or visceral adiposity can characterize a unique mechanism that directly affects the development or progression of the atheromatous process or its clinical manifestations. Rather, it appears that in both settings the predisposition to coronary disease is mediated by enhancement of a variety of atherogenic factors subject to genetic and environmental conditions.

Weight Reduction and Coronary Heart Disease

Meta-analysis indicates that dieting and weight reduction are correlated with decreases in total cholesterol, LDL, and triglyceride plasma levels and an increase in HDL.[153] The changes in triglyceride and HDL tend to be more consistent than those in total cholesterol or LDL.[154] Similar effects are observed in very obese subjects after gastric bypass or stapling procedures and weight loss.[155, 156] When diabetes and hyperinsulinemia are present, substantial weight reduction is accompanied by enhanced glucose oxidation, diminished insulin levels, and improved insulin sensitivity.[157, 158] Serum uric acid serum levels tend to fall with weight reduction, but there is no correlation between weight change and serum levels.[159]

Although weight loss alters coronary risk factors favorably, its impact on coronary heart disease morbidity and mortality does not seem to be clearly established. In a review of six studies[160] examining the effect of weight loss on longevity, it was concluded that the effect was equivocal. In the British Regional Heart Study, an 80 percent reduction in coronary disease mortality among overweight hypertensive men who achieved normal weight levels was reported, but there was little effect on mortality in nonhypertensive men who lost weight.[161] A 12-year follow-up study of 43,457 overweight (body mass index > 30 kg/M^2) never-smoking U.S. white women aged 40 to 64 years included data on age-adjusted mortality in those with intentional weight loss versus those without weight loss.[162] Cardiovascular mortality was reduced 9 percent in those with obesity-related health conditions and weight loss, but no effect of weight loss was found in those with no preexisting illness. Thus, there appears to be a salutary effect of weight loss and coronary risk factor reduction on mortality in obese subjects with hypertension or coronary heart disease, but a beneficial effect in those without evidence of coronary disease has yet to be demonstrated.

References

1. Keys A, Fidanza F, Karochen MJ, et al: Indices of relative weight and obesity. J Chronic Dis 25:329–343, 1972.
2. Keys A: Overweight, obesity, coronary disease, and mortality. Nutr Rev 38:297–307, 1980.
3. Smith HL, Willius FA: Adiposity of the heart. Arch Intern Med 52:911–931, 1933.
4. Amad KH, Brennan JC, Alexander JK: The cardiac pathology of obesity. Circulation 32:740–745, 1965.
5. Alexander JK, Pettigrove JR: Obesity and congestive heart failure. Geriatrics 22:101–108, 1967.
6. Warnes CA, Roberts WC: The heart in massive (more than 300 pounds or 136 kilograms) obesity. Analysis of 12 patients studied at necropsy. Am J Cardiol 54:1087–1091, 1984.
7. Alexander JK: Cardiac structure and function in obesity. Medicographia 13:9–12, 1990.
8. Carpenter HM: Myocardial fat infiltration. Am Heart J 63:491–496, 1962.
9. James TN, Frame B, Coates EO: De subitaneis mortibus III. Pickwickian syndrome. Circulation 48:1311–1320, 1973.
10. Garcia LC, Laredo E, Aniaga J, et al: Rev Clin Invest 34:235–242, 1982.
11. Alpert MA, Terry BE, Kelly DK: Effect of weight loss on cardiac chamber size, wall thickness and left ventricular function in morbid obesity. Am J Cardiol 55:783–786, 1985.
12. Nakajina T, Fuhoka S, Tokunaga K, et al: Noninvasive study of left ventricular performance in obese patients: influences of duration of obesity. Circulation 71:481–486, 1985.
13. Alpert MA, Terry BE, Mulekar M, et al: Cardiac morphology and left ventricular function in morbidly obese patients with and without congestive heart failure and effect of weight loss. Am J Cardiol 80:736–740, 1997.
14. Nielsen SL: Measurement of blood flow in adipose tissue from the washout of xenon-133 after atraumatic labelling. Acta Physiol Scand 84:187–196, 1972.
15. White RE, Alexander JK: Body oxygen consumption and pulmonary ventilation in obese subjects. J Appl Physiol 20:197–201, 1965.
16. Alexander JK: Obesity and the circulation. Mod Concepts Cardiovasc Dis 32:799–803, 1963.
17. Alexander JK, Dennis DW, Smith WG, et al: Blood volume, cardiac output and distribution of systemic blood flow in extreme obesity. Cardiovasc Res Cent Bull 1:39–44, 1962.
18. Bachman L, Freyschuss U, Hallberg D, Melcher A: Reversibility of cardiovascular changes in extreme obesity. Acta Med Scand 205:367–373, 1979.
19. Messerli FH, Ventura HD, Reisin E, et al: Borderline hypertension and obesity: two prehypertensive states with elevated cardiac output. Circulation 66:55–60, 1982.
20. Alexander JK: Obesity and cardiac performance. Am J Cardiol 14:860–865, 1964.
21. Sugarman HJ, Barn PL, Fairman RP, et al: Hemodynamic dysfunction in obesity hypoventilation syndrome and the effects of treatment with surgically induced weight loss. Ann Surg 207:604–612, 1988.
22. Agarwol N, Shibutani R, Sanfilippo JA, et al: Hemodynamic and respiratory changes in surgery of the morbidly obese. Surgery 92:226–234, 1982.
23. Alaudin-din A, Meterissian S, Lisbona R, et al: Assessment of cardiac function in patients who were morbidly obese. Surgery 108:809–820, 1990.
24. Kaltman AJ, Goldring RM: Role of circulatory congestion in the cardiorespiratory failure of obesity. Am J Med 60:645–653, 1976.
25. Wilcken DE: Left ventricular volume in man: the relation to heart rate and to end-diastolic pressure. Aust Ann Med 17(suppl 3):195–205, 1968.
26. Alpert MA, Lambert CR, Panayiotou H, et al: Relation of duration of morbid obesity to left ventricular mass, systolic function and diastolic filling and effect of weight loss. Am J Cardiol 76:1194–1197, 1995.
27. Shebadeh A, Regan TJ: Cardiac consequences of diabetes mellitus. Clin Cardiol 18:301–305, 1995.
28. Alexander JK: The cardiomyopathy of obesity. Prog Cardiovasc Dis 27:325–334, 1985.
29. Alexander JK, Woodard CB, Quinones MA, et al: Heart failure from obesity. *In* Mancini M, Lewis B, Contaldo F (eds): Medical Complications of Obesity. pp. 179–187. London: Academic, 1978.
30. Ford LE: Heart size. Circ Res 39:297–303, 1976.
31. Alpert MA, Lambert CR, Terry BE, et al: Interrelationship of left ventricular mass, systolic function and diastolic filling in normotensive morbidly obese patients. Int J Obes 19:550–557, 1995.
32. Lillington GA, Anderson MA, Brandenburg RO: The cardiorespiratory syndrome of obesity. Dis Chest 32:1–20, 1957.
33. Duflou J, Virmani R, Robin J, et al: Sudden death as a result of heart disease in morbid obesity. Am Heart J 130:306–313, 1995.
34. Ewy GA, Groves BM, Ball MF, et al: Digoxin metabolism in obesity. Circulation 44:810–814, 1971.
35. Alpert MA, Lambert CA, Terry BE, et al: Effect of weight loss on left ventricular mass in nonhypertensive morbidly obese patients. Am J Cardiol 73:918–921, 1994.
36. Alexander JK, Peterson KL: Cardiovascular effects of weight reduction. Circulation 43:310–318, 1972.
37. Kohli RS, Vetrovec GW, Evans CE, Sugarman H: Improved hemodynamics after surgical weight loss in patients with morbid obesity [abstract]. J Am Coll Cardiol 15:101A, 1990.
38. Alpert MA, Terry BE, Kelly DL: Effect of weight loss on cardiac chamber size, wall thickness, and left ventricular function in morbid obesity. Am J Cardiol 55:783–786, 1985.
39. Alpert MA, Lambert CR, Terry BE, et al: Effect of weight loss on left ventricular filling in obesity. Am J Cardiol 76:1198–1201, 1995.

40. Johnson AL, Cornoni JC, Cassel JC, et al: Influence of race, sex, and weight on blood pressure behavior in young adults. Am J Cardiol 35:523–530, 1975.
41. Voors AW, Webber LS, Frerichs RR, Berenson GS: Body height and body mass as determinants of basal blood pressure in children: the Bogalusa Heart Study. Am J Epidemiol 106:101–108, 1977.
42. Goldring D, Londe S, Sivakoff M, et al: Blood pressure in a high school population. I. Standards for blood pressure and the relation of age, sex, weight, height, and race to blood pressure in children 14 to 18 years of age. J Pediatr 91:884–889, 1977.
43. Shamarin VM, Glazunov IS, Aleksandrov AA, et al: Arterial pressure levels in children aged 12–13 years and their correlations with selected growth indicators. Cor Vasa 22:13–21, 1980.
44. Court JM, Hill GJ, Dunlop M, et al: Hypertension in childhood obesity. Aust Pediatr J 10:296–300, 1974.
45. Hsu PH, Mathewson FAL, Rabkin SW: Blood pressure and body mass index patterns: a longitudinal study. J Chronic Dis 30:93–113, 1977.
46. Rabkin SW, Mathewson FAL, Hsu PH: Relation of body weight to development of ischemic heart disease in a cohort of young North American men after a 26 year observation period: the Manitoba study. Am J Cardiol 39:452–458, 1977.
47. Haynes RB: Is weight loss an effective treatment for hypertension? The evidence against. Can J Physiol Pharmacol 64:825–830, 1986.
48. MacMahon S, Cutlar J, Brittain E, et al: Obesity and hypertension: epidemiological and clinical issues. Eur Heart J 8(suppl B):57–70, 1987.
49. Bjorntorp P: Classification of obese patients and complications related to distribution of surplus fat. Nutrition 6:131–137, 1990.
50. Bjorntorp P: Obesity and adipose tissue distribution as risk factors for the development of disease. A review. Infusionstherapie 17:24–27, 1990.
51. King GE: Errors in clinical measurement of blood pressure in obesity. Clin Sci 32:223–237, 1967.
52. Kvols LK, Rohling BM, Alexander JK: A comparison of intraarterial and cuff blood pressure measurements in very obese subjects. Cardiovasc Res Gen Bull 7:118–123, 1969.
53. Nielsen PE, Jenniche H: The accuracy of auscultatory measurement of arm blood pressure in very obese subjects. Acta Med Scand 195:403–409, 1974.
54. Kirkendall WM, Fenleib M, Freis ED, Mark AL: Recommendations for human blood pressure determinations by sphygmomanometer. Circulation 62:1146A–1155A, 1980.
55. Nielsen PE, Larsey B, Holstein P, et al: Accuracy of auscultatory blood pressure measurements in hypertensive and obese subjects. Hypertension 5:122–127, 1983.
56. Messerli FH, Christie B, DeCarvalho J, et al: Obesity and essential hypertension: hemodynamics, intravascular volume, sodium excretion, and plasma renin activity. Arch Intern Med 141:81–85, 1981.
57. Toto MJJ, Achimastos A, Asmar RG, et al: Pulse wave velocity in patients with obesity and hypertension. Am Heart J 112:136–140, 1986.
58. Alexander JK: Blood pressure and obesity. *In* Matarazzo JD, Weiss SM, Herd JA, Miller NE (eds): Behavioral Health. pp. 877–886. New York: John Wiley & Sons, 1984.
59. Krieger DR, Landsberg L: Mechanisms in obesity-related hypertension: the role of insulin and catecholamines. Am J Hypertens 1:84–90, 1988.
60. Landsberg L: The sympathetic nervous system in obesity-related hypertension. Medicographia 13:27–30, 1991.
61. Tsutsu N, Nunoi K, Kodama T, et al: Lack of association between blood pressure and insulin in patients with insulinoma. J Hypertens 8:479–482, 1990.
62. Hall JE, Brands MW, Mizelle HL, et al: Chronic intrarenal hyperinsulinemia does not cause hypertension. Am J Physiol 260:F663–669, 1991.
63. Maxwell MH, Heber D, Waks AV, et al: Role of insulin and norepinephrine in the hypertension of obesity. Am J Hypertens 7:402–408, 1995.
64. Hall JE, Summers RL, Brands MW, et al: Resistance to the metabolic action of insulin and its role in hypertension. Am J Hypertens 7:772–778, 1994.
65. Landsberg L: Insulin and hypertension. Proc Soc Exp Biol Med 208:315–316, 1995.
66. Mark AL, Anderson EA: Genetic factors determine the blood pressure response to insulin resistance and hyperinsulinemia: a call to refocus the insulin hypothesis of hypertension. Proc Soc Exp Biol Med 208:330–336, 1995.
67. Herzog H, Selbie LA, Zee RYL, et al: Neuropeptide-YY1 receptor gene polymorphism. Cross-sectional analysis in essential hypertension and obesity. Biochem Biophys Res Comm 196:902–906, 1993.
68. Alexander JK, Amad KH, Cole VW: Observations on some clinical features of extreme obesity with particular reference to cardiorespiratory effects. Am J Med 32:512–524, 1962.
69. Ferrannini E: The hemodynamics of obesity: a theoretical analysis. J Hypertens 10:1411–1423, 1992.
70. DeLaMaza MP, Estevez A, Bunout D, et al: Ventricular mass in hypertensive obese subjects. Int J Obes Relat Disord 18:193–197, 1994.
71. Gottdiener JS, Reda DJ, Williams DW, et al: Left atrial size in hypertensive men: influence of obesity, race and age. J Am Coll Cardiol 29:651–658, 1997.
72. Henry W, Morganroth J, Pearlman A, et al: Relation between echocardiographically determined left atrial size and atrial fibrillation. Circulation 53:273–279, 1976.
73. Epstein FH: Estimating the effect of preventing obesity on total mortality and hypertension. Int J Obes 3:163–166, 1979.
74. Rissanen A, Pietinen P, Siljamaki-Ojansuu U, et al: Treatment of hypertension in obese patients: efficacy and feasibility of weight and salt reduction programs. Acta Med Scand 218:149–156, 1985.
75. Reisin E: Weight reduction in the management of hypertension: epidemiologic and mechanistic evidence. Can J Physiol Pharmacol 64:818–824, 1986.
76. Sabotte D, Stunkard AJ: The effects of weight reduction on blood pressure in 301 obese subjects. Arch Intern Med 150:1701–1704, 1990.
77. Cohen N, Glamenbaum W: Obesity and hypertension. Demonstration of a "floor effect." Am J Med 80:177–181, 1986.
78. Novi RF, Porta M, Lamberto M, et al: Reductions of body weight and blood pressure in obese hypertensive patients treated by diet. A retrospective study. Panminerva Med 31:13–15, 1989.
79. Andersen T, Stokholm TH, Nielsen PE: Blood pressure and arm circumference during large weight reduction in normotensive and borderline hypertensive obese patients. J Clin Hypertens 3:547–553, 1987.
80. Staessen J, Fogard R, Amery A: The relationship between body weight and blood pressure. J Hum Hypertens 2:207–217, 1988.
81. Ernsberger P, Nelson DO: Effects of fasting and refeeding on blood pressure are determined by nutritional state, not by body weight change. Am J Hypertens 1:1535–1575, 1988.
82. Weinsier RL, James LD, Darnell BE, et al: Obesity-related hypertension: evaluation of the separate effects of energy restriction and weight reduction on hemodynamic and neuroendocrine status. Am J Med 90:460–468, 1991.
83. Reisen E, Abel R, Modan M, et al: Effect of weight loss without salt restriction on the reduction of blood pressure in overweight hypertensive patients. N Engl J Med 298:1–6, 1978.
84. Tuck ML, Sowers J, Dorafield L, et al: The effect of weight reduction on blood pressure, plasma renin activity, and plasma aldosterone levels in obese patients. N Engl J Med 304:930–934, 1981.
85. Alexander JK: Cardiac effects of weight reduction in obesity hypertension. *In* Messerli FH (ed): The Heart in Hypertension. pp. 427–433. Yorke Medical, 1987.
86. Rocchini AP, Katch V, Schork A, et al: Insulin and blood pressure during weight loss in obese adolescents. Hypertension 10:267–273, 1987.
87. Nobels F, vanGall L, deLeeuw I: Weight reduction with a high protein, low carbohydrate, calorie-restricted diet: effects on blood pressure, glucose and insulin levels. Neth J Med 35:295–302, 1989.
88. Grassi G, Seravalle G, Colombo M, et al: Body weight reduction, sympathetic nerve traffic, and arterial baroreflex in obese normotensive humans. Circulation 97:2037–2042, 1998.
89. Glueck CJ: Nonpharmacologic and pharmacologic alteration of high-density lipoprotein cholesterol: therapeutic approaches to prevention of atherosclerosis. Am Heart J 110:1107–1115, 1985.
90. Feher M: Antihypertensive drugs and the hypertensive diabetic patient. J Hum Hypertens 4:7–9, 1990.
91. Astrup AV: Obesity and diabetes as side-effects of beta-blockers. Ugeskr Laeger 152:2905–2908, 1990.
92. Kuczmarski RJ, Flegal KM, Campbell SM, et al: Increasing preva-

lence of overweight among U.S. adults. The National Health and Nutrition Examination Surveys 1960–1991. JAMA 272:205–211, 1994.
93. Grotmaker SL, Dietz WH, Sobol AM, et al: Increasing pediatric obesity in the United States. Am J Dis Child 141:535–540, 1987.
94. Epstein L: New developments in childhood obesity. *In* Stunkard AI, Wadden TA (eds): Obesity Theory and Therapy. 2nd ed. p. 301. New York: Raven, 1993.
95. Sjostrum LV: Mortality of severely obese subjects. Am J Clin Nutr 55:516S–523S, 1992.
96. Alexander JK: Obesity and coronary heart disease. *In* Alpert MA, Alexander JK (eds): The Heart and Lung in Obesity. Armonk, NY: Futura, 1998.
97. Berlin JA, Colditz GA: A meta-analysis of physical activity in the prevention of coronary heart disease. Am J Epidemiol 132:612–628, 1990.
98. Bjorntorp P: Abdominal fat distribution and disease: an overview of epidemiological data. Ann Med 24:15–18, 1992.
99. Peiris AN, Sothmann MS, Hoffman RG, et al: Adiposity, fat distribution and cardiovascular risk. Ann Intern Med 110:867–872, 1989.
100. Folsom AR, Kaye SA, Sellers TA, et al: Body fat distribution and 5-year risk of death in older women. JAMA 269:483–487, 1993.
101. Despres JP: Abdominal obesity as an important component of insulin-resistance syndrome. Nutrition 9:452–459, 1993.
102. Wild RA: Obesity, lipids, cardiovascular risk, and androgen excess. Am J Med 98:27S–32S, 1995.
103. Bjorntorp P: "Portal" adipose tissue as a generator of risk factors for cardiovascular disease and diabetes. Arteriosclerosis 10:493–496, 1990.
104. Montenegro MR, Solberg LA: Obesity, body weight, body length and atherosclerosis. Lab Invest 18:594–603, 1968.
105. Sternby NH: Atherosclerosis and body build. Bull WHO 53:601–604, 1976.
106. Solberg LA, Strong JP: Risk factors and atherosclerotic lesions: a review of autopsy studies. Arteriosclerosis 3:187–198, 1983.
107. Patel YC, Eggen DA, Strong JP: Obesity, smoking and atherosclerosis: a study of interassociations. Atherosclerosis 36:481–490, 1980.
108. Strong JP, Oalmann MC, Newman WP III, et al: Coronary heart disease in young black and white males in New Orleans: community pathology study. Am Heart J 108:747–759, 1984.
109. McGill HC Jr, McMahan CA, Malcolm GT, et al: Relation of glycohemoglobin and adiposity to atherosclerosis in youth. Arterioscler Thromb Vasc Biol 15:431–440, 1995.
110. Hauner H, Stangl K, Schmatz C, et al: Body fat distribution in men with angiographically confirmed coronary artery disease. Atherosclerosis 85:203–210, 1990.
111. Hartz A, Grubb B, Wild R, et al: The association of waist hip ratio and angiographically determined coronary artery disease. Int J Obes 14:657–665, 1990.
112. Hujamuta K, Toshima H, Koga Y, et al: Relationship between coronary risk factor and arteriographic feature of coronary atherosclerosis. Jpn Circ J 54:442–447, 1990.
113. Reed D, Yano K: Predictors of arteriographically defined coronary stenosis in the Honolulu Heart program. Am J Epidemiol 134:111–122, 1991.
114. Zamboni M, Armellini F, Sheiban I, et al: Relation of body fat distribution in men and degree of coronary narrowings in coronary artery disease. Am J Cardiol 70:1135–1138, 1992.
115. Flynn MA, Cogg MN, Gibney MJ, et al: Indices of obesity and body fat distribution in arteriographically defined coronary artery disease in men. Ir J Med Sci 162:503–509, 1993.
116. Hodgson JM, Wahlquist N, Balazs NDH, Bosall JA: Coronary arteriosclerosis in relation to body fatness and its distribution. Int J Obes Relat Metab Disord 18:41–46, 1994.
117. Clark LT, Karve NM, Rones KT, et al: Obesity, distribution of body fat and coronary disease in black women. Am J Cardiol 73:895–896, 1994.
118. Morricone L, Ferrari M, Enrini R, et al: Angiographically determined coronary artery disease in relation to obesity and body fat distribution. Int J Obes 20(suppl 4):109, 1996.
119. Kramer JR, Matsuda Y, Mulligan JC, et al: Progression of coronary atherosclerosis. Circulation 63:519–526, 1981.
120. Reeder BA, Angel A, Ledoux M, et al: Obesity and its relation to cardiovascular disease risk factors in Canadian adults. Canadian Heart Health Surveys Research Group. Can Med Assoc J 146:2009–2019, 1992.
121. Denke MA, Sempos CT, Grundy SM: Excess body weight: an under-recognized contributor to dyslipidemia in white American women. Arch Intern Med 154:401–410, 1994.
122. Young TK, Gelskey DE: Is non-central obesity metabolically benign? Implications for prevention from a population survey. JAMA 274:1939–1941, 1995.
123. Teny RB, Wood PD, Haskell WL, et al: Regional adiposity pattern in relation to lipids, lipoprotein cholesterol, and lipoprotein subfraction mass in men. J Clin Endocrinol Metab 68:191–199, 1989.
124. Despres JP, Moorjani S, Ferland M, et al: Adipose tissue distribution and plasma lipoprotein levels in obese women: Importance of intra-abdominal fat. Arteriosclerosis 9:203–210, 1989.
125. Superko HR: New aspects of risk factors for the development of atherosclerosis, including small low-density lipoprotein, homocysteine, and lipoprotein(a). Curr Opin Cardiol 10:347–354, 1995.
126. National Institutes of Health Consensus Development Panel: Health implications of obesity. Ann Intern Med 103:1073–1077, 1985.
127. Pi-Sunyer FX: Health implications of obesity. Am J Clin Nutr 53(6 suppl):1595S–1603S, 1991.
128. Wingard DL, Ferrara A, Barrett-Connor EL: Is insulin really a heart disease risk factor? Diabetes Care 18:1299–1304, 1995.
129. Pyorala M, Miattinen H, Laakso M, et al: Hyperinsulinemia predicts coronary heart disease risk in healthy middle-aged men. Circulation 98:398–404, 1998.
130. Despres JP, Lamarche B, Mauriege P, et al: Hyperinsulinemia as an independent risk factor for ischemic heart disease. N Engl J Med 334:952–957, 1996.
131. Laws A, Reaven GM: Evidence for an independent relationship between insulin resistance and fasting plasma HDL-cholesterol, triglyceride and insulin concentrations. J Intern Med 231:25–30, 1992.
132. Stern MP: The insulin resistance syndrome: controversy is dead, long live the controversy! Diabetologia 37:956–958, 1994.
133. Despres JP, Lamarche B, Dagenais GT: Letter to the editor. N Engl J Med 335:977, 1996.
134. Ostlund RE Jr, Staten M, Kohrt WM, et al: The ratio of waist-to-hip circumference, plasma insulin level, and glucose intolerance as independent predictors of the HDL_2 cholesterol level in older adults. N Engl J Med 322:229–234, 1990.
135. Van Gaal L: Body fat mass distribution. Influence on metabolic and atherosclerotic parameters in non-insulin dependent diabetes and obese subjects with and without impaired glucose tolerance. Verb K Acad Geneeskd Belg 51:47–80, 1989.
136. Levine W, Dyer AR, Skekelle RB, et al: Serum uric acid and 11.5 year mortality of middle-aged women. Findings of the Chicago Heart Association detection project in industry. J Clin Epidemiol 42:257–267, 1989.
137. Williams DP, Going SB, Lohman TG, et al: Body fatness and risk for elevated blood pressure, total cholesterol, and serum lipoprotein ratios in children and adolescents. Am J Public Health 82:358–363, 1992.
138. Webber LS, Wattingney WA, Srinivasan AR, et al: Obesity studies in Bogalusa. Am J Med Sci 310(suppl):S53–S61, 1995.
139. Serdula N, Ivery D, Caotes RJ, et al: Do obese children become obese adults? A review of the literature. Prev Med 22:167–177, 1993.
140. Guo SS, Roche AF, Chumlea WC, et al: The predictive value of childhood body mass index values for overweight at age 35. Am J Clin Nutr 59:810–819, 1994.
141. Hubert JW, Feinleib M, McNamara PM, et al: Obesity as an independent risk factor for cardiovascular disease: a 26-year follow-up of participants in the Framingham Heart Study. Circulation 67:968–977, 1983.
142. Eckel RH: Obesity and heart disease: a statement for healthcare professionals from the nutrition committees, American Heart Association. Circulation 96:3248–3250, 1997.
143. Keys A: Longevity of man: relative weight and fatness in middle age. Ann Med 21:163–168, 1989.
144. Sjostrum LV: Mortality of severely obese subjects. Am J Clin Nutr 55:5165–5235, 1992.
145. Rabkin SW, Mathewson FA, Hsu PH: Relation of body weight to development of ischemic heart disease in a cohort of young North Americans after a 26 year observation period: the Manitoba Study. Am J Cardiol 39:452–458, 1977.
146. Garrison RJ, Castelli WP: Weight and thirty-year mortality of men in the Framingham Study. Ann Intern Med 103:1006–1009, 1985.

147. Manson JE, Willett WC, Stampfer MJ, et al: Body weight and mortality among women. N Engl J Med 333:677–685, 1995.
148. Barrett-Connor EL: Obesity, atherosclerosis, and coronary heart disease. Ann Intern Med 103:1010–1019, 1985.
149. Ernsberger P, Haskew P: Rethinking obesity, an alternative view of its health implications. Obes Weight Regul 6:57–137, 1987.
150. The Expert Panel II: Summary of the second report of the National Cholesterol Education Program (NCEP) expert panel on detection, evaluation, and treatment of high blood cholesterol in adults. JAMA 269:3015–3023, 1993.
151. Casassus P, Fontbonne A, Thibult N, et al: Upper body fat distribution: a hyperinsulinemia-independent predictor of coronary heart disease mortality—the Paris Prospective Study. Arterioscler Thromb 12:1387–1392, 1992.
152. Bouchard C, Despres JP, Mauriege P: Genetic and non-genetic determinants of regional fat distribution. Endocr Rev 14:72–93, 1993.
153. Dattilo AM, Kris-Etherton PM: Effects of weight reduction on blood lipids and lipoproteins: a meta-analysis. Am J Clin Nutr 56:320–328, 1992.
154. Margolis S, Dobs AS: Nutritional management of plasma lipid disorders. J Am Coll Nutr 8(suppl):33S–45S, 1989.
155. Gleysteen IJ, Barboriak JI, Sasse EA: Sustained coronary-risk-factor reduction after gastric bypass for morbid obesity. Am J Clin Nutr 51:774–778, 1990.
156. Brolin RE, Kenler HA, Wilson AC, et al: Serum lipids after gastric bypass for morbid obesity. Int J Obes 14:939–950, 1990.
157. Franssila A, Rissanen A, Ekstrand A, et al: Effects of weight loss on substrate oxidation, energy expenditure, and insulin sensitivity in obese individuals. Am J Clin Nutr 55:356–361, 1992.
158. Tochikubo O, Miyajima E, Okabe K, et al: Improvement of multiple coronary risk factors in obese hypertensives by reduction of intra-abdominal fat. Jpn Heart J 35:715–725, 1994.
159. Ashley FW Jr, Kannel WB: Relation of weight changes to changes in atherogenic traits: the Framingham Study. J Chronic Dis 27:103–114, 1974.
160. Williamson DF, Pamuk ER: The association between weight loss and longevity. A review of the evidence. Ann Intern Med 119:731–736, 1993.
161. Wannamethee G, Sharpe AG: Weight change in middle-aged British men: implications for health. Eur J Clin Nutr 44:133–142, 1990.
162. Williams DF, Pamuk E, Thun M, et al: Prospective study of intentional weight loss and mortality in never-smoking overweight U.S. white women aged 40–64 years. Am J Epidemiol 141:1128–1141, 1995.

CHAPTER 126

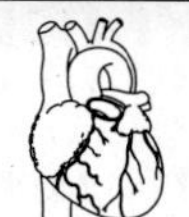

Gene Therapy

Elizabeth G. Nabel and Gary J. Nabel

PRINCIPLES OF GENE THERAPY
VECTOR SYSTEMS
Viral Vectors
Nonviral Vectors
ANIMAL MODELS OF GENE THERAPY
CLINICAL TRIALS
Angiogenesis
CONCLUSIONS AND FUTURE DIRECTIONS

The field of cardiovascular gene therapy has undergone dramatic changes in the past decade.[1, 2] The field began approximately 10 years ago with development of basic techniques for introducing genes into recombinant cells of the vasculature and the heart. Viral and nonviral vectors were designed to facilitate gene transfer and gene expression. Animal models of cardiovascular disease were then developed in order to test vectors and candidate target genes. Within the past 3 years, there has been a rapid expansion of translation of the basic science principles to early-phase human gene therapy trials.[3]

Coincident with the rapid advances in gene transfer, there have been parallel advances in the field of molecular genetics. In the past 15 years, molecular genetic approaches have dramatically changed our understanding of normal cardiovascular function in the pathophysiology of cardiovascular diseases in humans. The cloning of genes important for the development and function of the cardiovascular system has now increased our understanding of cardiovascular physiology and has provided clinician scientists with new tools for assessing risk factors for cardiovascular disease. These advances in molecular cardiology have merged with the development of gene therapy approaches, resulting in new, exciting therapies.

Principles of Gene Therapy

Somatic gene therapy is the introduction of genetic material, RNA or DNA, into a subject's cells as to alter the pattern of gene expression in that cell in order to produce a therapeutic effect.[4] The genetic material used in these approaches includes eukaryotic genes and RNA molecules that encode intercellular, cell surface, and secreted proteins, as well as synthetic oligonucleotides and ribozymes. The principles of gene transfer require that the target gene be cloned and sequenced (Fig. 126–1). The complementary DNA for the gene is ligated into a plasmid expression vector. The expression vector is introduced or transferred into cells in tissue cultured in vitro or into an animal or human being in vivo. Cells are normally resistant to uptake of foreign DNA, and hence, a vector shuttle is required to facilitate transport of the plasmid expression vector into the cell. Within the cytoplasm, the gene vector must avoid degradation by lysosomes so that the recombinant gene is transported to the nucleus. Within the nucleus, the gene can be maintained separate from the cell chromosomes as an episome or it may be integrated into host chromosomes, where it undergoes transcription to messenger RNA and translation to recombinant protein. The recombinant protein can remain intracellular or be secreted, where it has local paracrine effects on surrounding cells or enters the circulation to alter distant tissues.

There are two methods by which genes can be delivered to the cells. Ex vivo gene therapy involves removing cells from the body, genetically modifying them in culture, and returning the genetically modified cells to the body. Ex vivo gene transfer has the advantage of introduction of genetic material into a particular cell type, such as an endothelial cell and a vascular smooth muscle cell, and facilitating analysis of gene expression in that cell type. In vivo gene transfer is the direct introduction of DNA and vector into tissues in the body. In the cardiovascular system, this is accomplished by catheter-mediated gene delivery into endothelial cells and smooth muscle cells or by direct injection into cardiac myocytes. The in vivo gene approach generally results in recombinant gene expression in multiple cell types.

Gene therapy is a relatively new concept in pharmaceutical drug delivery. Traditionally, drug therapy has consisted of delivering proteins or small molecules intravenously to the body to treat a disease. Often, these drugs are given systemically with treatment at a local site. With gene therapy, the recombinant gene is now the drug. An advantage of gene therapy is that the recombinant gene can be introduced locally into the cells or tissue of interest, permitting high local concentration of recombinant protein and minimizing systemic side effects.

Vector Systems

An ideal vector would introduce recombinant genetic material efficiently into a cell, resulting in long-term high-level gene expression. Unfortunately, no such ideal vector exists. Viral and nonviral vectors have been developed, each with unique properties that have application for specific indications (Table 126–1). Several parameters must be considered in the evaluation of a vector, including efficiency of trans-

Principles of Gene Transfer:

1. Gene sequence (cDNA) is inserted into a plasmid expression vector.

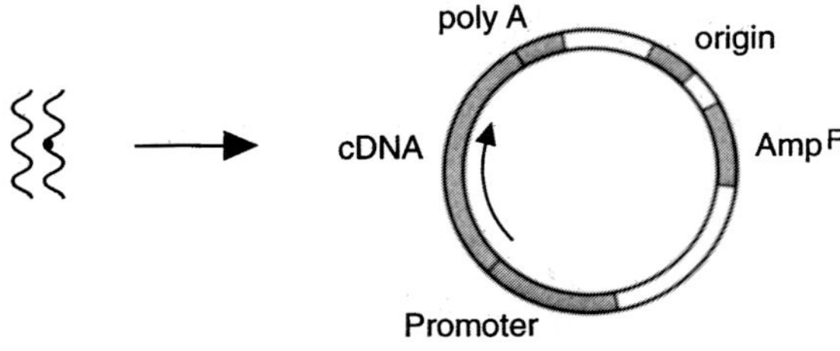

2. Vector is introduced into the host cell.

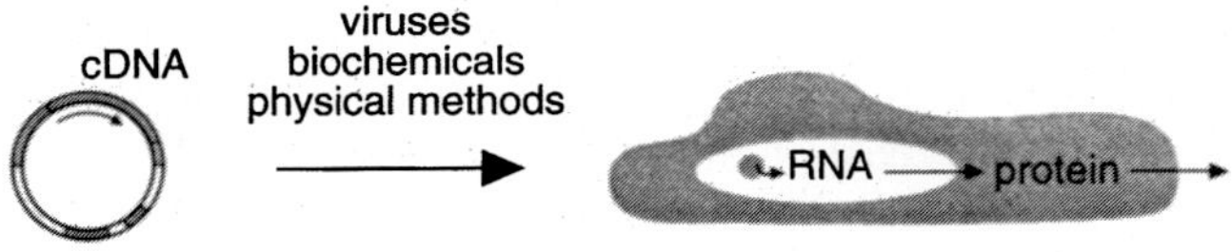

3. Recombinant protein may have intracellular or extracellular effects or may be secreted into the circulation.

FIGURE 126–1 Delivery and expression of recombinant gene. Complementary DNA (cDNA) for gene of interest is ligated into plasmid expression vector. Vector is introduced into host cell alone or with shuttle vector, such as a virus or lipid. Once within cell, recombinant gene is expressed and may exert autocrine or paracrine effects. (From Nabel EG, Pompilli VJ, Plautz GE, Nabel GJ: Gene transfer and vascular disease. Cardiovasc Res 28:445–455, 1994.)

ducing cell types in vitro and in vivo, size and type of genetic material it can introduce, stable transcription and translation of transgenes, and possible immunity against the transgene in vivo.

Viral Vectors

Viral vectors were initially developed because of knowledge gained by virologists on the basic principles of viral entry into human cells. Viruses have adapted themselves to efficiently infect cells and integrate their genes into host chromosomes. The RNA viruses, predominately retroviruses, were first studied. Viruses generally are altered to serve as vectors, such that they do not replicate in the host cell. This phenomenon is termed *replication incompetent.* The viral genes required for viral replication are removed from the virus, and these genes are replaced with transgene sequences. The viral genes necessary to generate infectious particles are supplied in a packaging cell line. Retroviral vectors have been evaluated in many cell types. An advantage of retroviral vectors includes stable integration in host chromosomes. A disadvantage is the requirement for cell replication for retroviral vectors to infect the cell. Because many cardiovascular cells replicate at low indexes, this vector has had limited cardiovascular application.

More recently, a modified form of the human immunodeficiency virus, a lentivirus, has been described. Such lentiviral vectors have the ability to infect nondividing cells and may be applicable to the treatment of vascular diseases.

Adenoviruses are DNA viruses that in wild-type form cause a self-limited respiratory tract infection in human beings. Several properties make adenoviral vectors ideally suited for cardiovascular gene therapy.[5] Adenoviruses infect a wide variety of replicating and nonreplicating cell types in vitro and in vivo. These vectors have been shown to very effectively infect cardiac myocytes after intramyocardial injection or intracoronary infusion.[6, 7] Adenoviral vectors are produced at high titers, allowing efficient transfer in vivo with a small volume of virus. These vectors also have a relatively favorable safety profile. Adenoviral vectors do not integrate into the host genome. However, a disadvantage of adenoviral vectors is that expression of some of the adenoviral proteins results in T- and B-cell immunity.[8–10] This immunity does not preclude their use as vectors and is dependent on the viral titer administered, the route of delivery, and the host tissue. For example, adenoviral gene transfer into the respiratory tract that is associated with greater immunity than gene transfer into blood vessels. Finally, adenoviral vectors can be generated in high titer for human use, and these vectors are now being used in phase I human cardiovascular gene therapy trials.

Adeno-associated virus is a defective human parvovirus, a characteristic that makes it potentially attractive as a gene therapy vector. This virus is normally nonpathogenic in human beings, infects a broad range of cells, and can be prepared in high titers.[11] Adeno-associated virus vectors are difficult to prepare, however, and have not yet been used in human clinical trials. These vectors are currently being studied in a cardiovascular system, and initial reports suggest their use in cardiomyocytes.[12]

Nonviral Vectors

Nonviral vectors were developed in the late 1980s as an alternative to viral vectors.[13] Some scientists were concerned about the potential safety of the introduction of viral vectors in humans. In general, nonviral vectors are less efficient than viral vectors. Two types of nonviral vectors are used in cardiovascular gene therapy, including plasmid DNA and cationic liposomes.

Plasmid DNA has numerous advantages as a gene therapy vector. Plasmids are easy to construct, and they can be produced inexpensively in large quantities. The use of a plasmid expression vector avoids the need for an infectious agent and eliminates the possibly of generalized infection of the host. In arterial gene transfer, plasmid DNA can be encoded on an angioplasty balloon.[14] When the balloon is expanded, the complementary DNA is mechanically introduced into endothelial smooth muscle cells, leading to recombinant gene expression. Plasmid DNA is also commonly used as an injection into skeletal muscle for secretion of recombinant proteins into the circulation. This is being tested now to treat chronic anemias with erythropoietin.[15] In spite of these advantages, plasmid DNA vectors

TABLE 126–1 **Advantages and Disadvantages of Different Vectors for Cardiovascular Gene Therapy**

Vector/Transgene	Advantages	Disadvantages
Retroviruses	Stably integrate into host genome Easily manipulated viral genome No viral gene products; relatively nonimmunogenic Highly efficient transduction of many cell types	Low titers Capacity for insertional mutagenesis In vivo instability Transcriptional shut-off in vivo Require cell proliferation for infection
Adenoviruses	Maintained as an episome Highly efficient transduction of replicating and nonreplicating cells Stable in vivo in absence of immune response High-level transgene expression in vivo Relatively nonpathogenic High titers	Evoke potent host inflammatory and immune responses that eliminate transgene expression and preclude repeated administration Difficult to target to specific cell types Relatively difficult to manipulate viral genome
Adeno-associated virus	Infects replicating and nonreplicating cells Potential for site-specific integration Relatively nonimmunogenic High titers Nonpathogenic in humans	Can accept only small transgenes Difficult to produce in large quantities Does not appear to stably transduce all cell types in vivo Potential for insertional mutagenesis
Plasmid DNA	Easy to manipulate and produce in large quantities Nonpathogenic Relatively nonimmunogenic Does not require an infectious vector Maintained as an episome Can program long-term gene expression in postmitotic cells in vivo	Very low transduction efficiency
Synthetic oligonucleotides	Easy to synthesize in large quantities Relatively high transduction efficiencies if delivered with viral liposomes	Can only reduce or ablate gene expression Large number of nonspecific and nonreproducible biologic effects Cannot target specific cell types Relatively short half-life in vivo
Ribozymes	Can specifically and effectively target messenger RNAs	Can only reduce or ablate gene expression Difficult to deliver to cells in vivo Stability in vivo unclear

From Nabel EG, Leiden JM: Gene transfer approaches for cardiovascular disease. *In* Chian KR (ed): Molecular Basis of Heart Disease. p 86. Philadelphia: WB Saunders, 1998.

have been limited by relatively low efficiencies of transduction in vivo. When injected into tissues, approximately 1 to 2 percent of cells surrounding the injection site are transduced.[16] However, this low transfection efficiency may be sufficient to treat some localized abnormalities and systemic disorders in which low levels of proteins are needed in the plasma.

Cationic liposomes are positively charged lipids that, when combined with plasmid DNA, facilitate entry into cells.[17] Cationic liposomes are positively charged lipids that encapsulate DNA and facilitate uptake into the cell. Numerous cationic liposomes are under development and are promising gene transfer vehicles.[18]

Antisense oligonucleotides are short, chemically synthesized DNA molecules that are designed to be complementary to the coding sequence of the RNA interest in the cell.[19] Antisense oligonucleotides can be introduced into cells by simple diffusion or by liposome-mediated gene transfer. Once inside the cell, the single-stranded oligonucleotides form base pairs with their complimentary RNA and decrease translation of the RNA. Double-stranded synthetic oligonucleotides contain binding sites for specific transcription factors and can be used as "decoys" to ablate the transcription of genes that require these factors for expression.[20] Because oligonucleotides can be synthesized in large quantities and do not require an infectious agent for cell transduction, they are attractive targets for gene therapy. Chemical modification in the backbone of the oligonucleotides can be performed to render them more stable to degradation within a cell. However, oligonucleotides have a short half-life in vivo because of intracellular degradation, and they may be used only in disease conditions in which transient reductions of gene expression are required. Antisense oligonucleotides have been studied in animal models of cardiovascular diseases, where they have been used to disrupt smooth muscle cell proliferation after vascular injury.[21–26] In spite of the initial enthusiasm about the use of oligonucleotides for gene therapy, several features have limited their use. Antisense oligonucleotides can have nonspecific effects to inhibit cell growth that are not sequence specific.[27] Both the oligonucleotide and the chemical contaminants of individual batches of antisense oligonucleotides can have nonspecific cytotoxic effects. Some oligonucleotides affect the expression of multiple genes in addition to the gene against which they were originally designed. This effect often cannot be controlled with the use of scrambled or a mutant oligonucleotide. Thus, in spite of the initial enthusiasm, the use of antisense oligonucleotides for cardiovascular gene therapy will probably be limited by their relatively short half-life and nonspecific effects.

ANIMAL MODELS OF GENE THERAPY

One of the major applications of cardiovascular gene transfer has been the development of animal models of cardiovascular disease. This progress has been made in parallel with the development of animal models made by genetic manipulation, also called *transgenic technology,* in which genes are either overexpressed or knocked out by homologous recombination in mice. The combination of transgenic and gene transfer technology has permitted the development of powerful genetic models of complex cardiovascular diseases.[28]

Transgenic technology has been limited to small animals, such as the mouse, and has been difficult to achieve in larger animal models, which may have more direct relevance to the pathophysiology of cardiovascular diseases. Therefore, gene transfer has been easily adapted to examine the expression and the function of recombinant genes in larger animals, such as the rabbit, dog, and pig. The initial principles of gene transfer in the vasculature were developed by use of ex vivo techniques.[29, 30] In these studies, endothelial or smooth muscle cells were extracted from host blood vessels, genetically modified in culture, and returned to denuded blood vessels in vivo, where recombinant gene expression was monitored. An application of an ex vivo gene transfer is the seeding of vascular prostheses, such as Dacron grafts, with endothelial cells or smooth cells that have been genetically modified to express a recombinant protein. Although these ex vivo approaches in the vasculature were used to establish the principles and feasibility of gene transfer, from a practical perspective, they proved to be complex and cumbersome. They offered little short-term clinical applicability.

Direct in vivo gene transfer has been much more useful in the development of animal models and vascular myocardial diseases.[31] In the vasculature, gene transfer has been used to study growth regulation, angiogenesis, lipoprotein metabolism, and thrombosis. Direct gene transfer to blood vessels by use of catheters (see Fig. 126–2) has been performed in many animal models, including rat,[32–34] rabbit,[35–37] dog,[38–40] pig,[41–43] and sheep[44] with viral and nonviral vectors. The results of many of these catheter-mediated direct gene transfer studies in large animal models have been reviewed elsewhere.[1, 45]

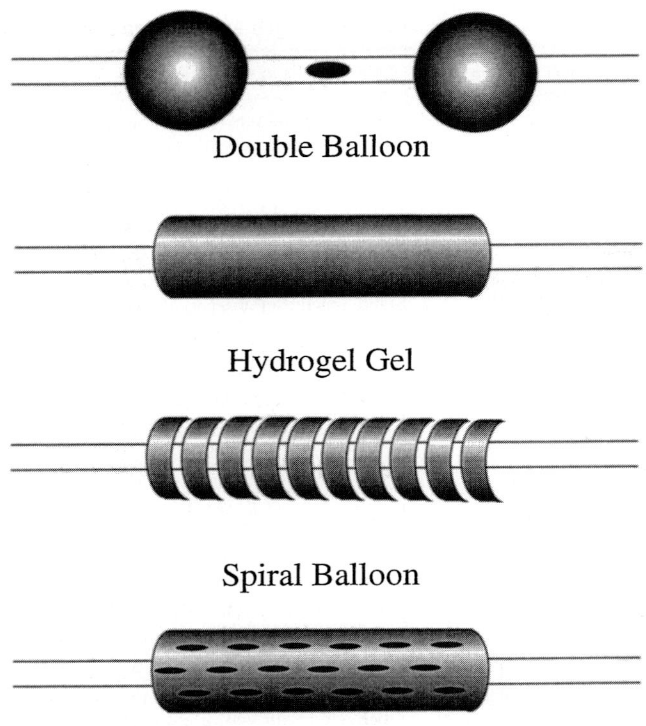

FIGURE 126–2 Gene delivery catheters. Catheters have been developed for catheter-mediated gene delivery, including double balloon, hydrogel gel, spiral balloon, and porous balloon catheters. CABG, coronary artery bypass grafting; PTCA, percutaneous transluminal coronary angioplasty. (From Nabel EG, Nabel GJ: Genetic therapies for cardiovascular disease. *In* Topol EJ [ed]: Textbook of Interventional Cardiology. Philadelphia: WB Saunders, 1998.)

CLINICAL TRIALS

A large number of cardiovascular diseases are potential targets for gene therapy. Most early efforts focused on using gene transfer to correct single-gene recessive disorders, for example, to replace the low-density lipoprotein receptor in hepatocytes from patients with homozygous familial hypercholesterolemia.[46] More recently, investigators have come to understand that gene transfer holds considerable promise for the treatment of more common acquired cardiovascular diseases, such as myocardial ischemia, restenosis, and heart failure. This realization has led to an increase in the number of cardiovascular diseases and patients under investigation with gene transfer technologies (Fig. 126–3). To date, early clinical investigations have focused on angiogenesis and vascular proliferative diseases. It is likely that lessons learned from these trials will be rapidly applied to other cardiovascular disease targets, including plaque rupture, endothelial cell dysfunction, vascular remodeling, heart failure, and transplant atherosclerosis.

Angiogenesis

The field of angiogenesis for myocardial and peripheral ischemia has grown tremendously in the past few years. Several families of growth factors have been identified and tested in animal models. These include the vascular endothelial growth factors (VEGFs). Two isoforms have been studied VEGF[165] and VEGF[121]. The fibroblast growth factors (FGFs) have also been investigated, including FGF-1 and FGF-4. These growth factors have been tested extensively in animal models of myocardial and peripheral ischemia.[40, 46–50]

Several approaches can be taken to introduce recombinant genes or protein into the heart or vasculature. A gene therapy approach involves introduction of recombinant gene into patient cells, and expression of the gene results in continuous production of the protein. Recombinant protein therapy involves the production of the recombinant protein in the laboratory and the administration of the protein to the patient. With this approach, the protein is generally

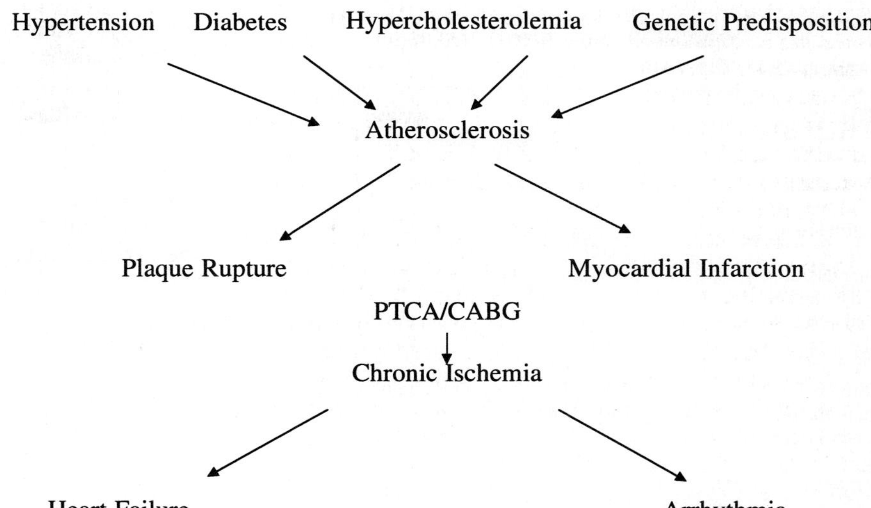

FIGURE 126–3 Targets for genetic therapies in cardiovascular disease.

given once, and the protein is degraded and secreted, resulting in a one-time effect. Oligonucleotide therapy involves the administration of oligonucleotides to cells in a patient, and the oligonucleotides are rapidly degraded, achieving short-term benefits.

There are many phase I clinical trials for myocardial and peripheral angiogenesis that use recombinant angiogenic growth factors (Table 126–2). Both VEGF[165] and VEGF[121] have been studied. These protocols include plasmid DNA injection into skeletal muscle for peripheral angiogenesis, adenovirus-mediated delivery of VEGF[121] to myocardium by intercardiac injection during coronary artery bypass grafting, recombinant VEGF[165] protein therapy for myocardial ischemia, and adenoviral vectors encoding VEGF[121] injected into skeletal muscle to treat peripheral vascular disease. FGF-1 and FGF-4 have also been used in clinical studies both as gene therapy approaches with adenovirus-mediated gene transfer and recombinant protein therapy. These studies have also involved direct cardiac injection during coronary artery bypass grafting and catheter-mediated gene delivery. The results of the phase I studies are now becoming available.[51–55] The delivery of the recombinant gene or protein has been well tolerated. The efficacy of these approaches will need to be evaluated further in phase III randomized, multicenter trials with clinical end points.

Many diseases of the vasculature are characterized by abnormalities in cell proliferation. These diseases are being approached by genetic treatments to inhibit vasculature cell proliferation. Most approaches focus on the regulation of cell proliferation by the cell cycle.[56–59] Numerous target genes have been evaluated in animal models to disrupt progression through G_1 phase of the cell cycle, promote G_1 arrest at the G_1/S transition, or inhibit DNA synthesis in S phase. These approaches have offered promise for inhibition of vascular smooth muscle and macrophage proliferation that occurs after angioplasty in the coronary and femoral artery and for prevention of intimal hyperplasia in venous bypass grafts placed in peripheral or coronary arteries (Table 126–3). Several clinical phase I protocols have been initiated. These include overexpression of VEGF[165] to promote re-endothelialization of injured superficial femoral arteries after angioplasty. The second approach is an ex vivo therapy for peripheral bypass grafts.[60, 61] These venous grafts are incubated with oligonucleotides targeted against the transcription factor E2F. The decoy oligonucleotides disrupt E2F RNA, leading to cell cycle arrest and inhibition of smooth muscle cell hyperplasia in the bypass graft. A third protocol involves the inhibition of smooth muscle cell proliferation in the superficial femoral artery after angioplasty involving thymidine kinase vectors.[43, 62]

Clinical investigators will obtain new information about the delivery, expression, and safety of these recombinant genes from these phase I trials. It is anticipated that this clinical experience will lend itself to the expansion of genetic treatments to other cardiovascular targets (see Table

TABLE 126–2 **Clinical Trials: Angiogenesis**

Factor	Approach	Clinical Setting
VEGF[165]	Gene therapy—plasmid DNA	Direct injection of skeletal muscle—peripheral vascular disease
VEGF[121]	Gene therapy—adenovirus	Intracardiac injection during CABG
VEGF[165]	Recombinant protein therapy	Myocardial ischemia
VEGF[121]	Gene therapy—adenovirus	Direct injection of skeletal muscle—peripheral vascular disease
FGF-1	Recombinant protein therapy	Intracardiac injection during CABG
FGF-4	Gene therapy—adenovirus	Catheter delivery for chronic stable angina
FGF-1	Recombinant protein therapy	Catheter delivery for myocardial ischemia

Abbreviations: CABG, coronary artery bypass grafting; FGF, fibroblast growth factor; VEGF, vascular endothelial growth factor.

TABLE 126-3 **Molecular Therapies for Cardiovascular Diseases**

Therapeutic Target	Candidate Gene
Angiogenesis	VEGF165, VEGF121, FGF-1, FGF-4, FGF-5, NOS
Cell inhibition	p27, p21, NOS, Rb, TK, E2F decoys, other cell cycle inhibitors
Endothelial cell dysfunction	NOS, antioxidants
Plaque rupture	Metalloproteinase inhibitors, leukocyte adhesion molecules, inflammatory inhibitors
Thrombosis	IIb/IIIa inhibitors, TFPI, antithrombin agents
Transplant atheroscleosis	Anti-inflammatory agents, anti–T-cell agents
Heart failure	Beta-adrenergic receptors

Abbreviations: FGF, fibroblast growth factor; TFPI, tissue factor pathway inhibitor; VEGF, vascular endothelial growth factor.

126–3). Candidate targets include thrombosis using overexpression of factors that are antithrombotic, including tissue factor pathway inhibitor. Plaque rupture is another major target that is amenable to catheter-mediated gene delivery. Plaque rupture is a major cause of unstable coronary syndromes and is the result of ongoing inflammation, thrombosis, and matrix deposition within atherosclerotic plaque. This syndrome has been difficult to study because of lack of an appropriate large animal model. Furthermore, many cytokines, growth factors, and coagulation factors contribute to the pathophysiology of plaque rupture. Nonetheless, this is a disease for which further understanding and improved treatments are needed.

Transplant atherosclerosis represents another major candidate for genetic therapies. The major cause of death from cardiac transplantation is progressive coronary atherosclerosis, which is characterized as a diffuse intimal thickening throughout the coronary circulation. Transplant atherosclerosis has also been difficult to study because of a lack of animal models. However, some studies suggest that expression of adenoviral vectors encoding for cell inhibitors, including thymidine kinase, may offer promise as therapies for this disease process.[63]

Heart failure is one of the most common causes of vascular disease. Its morbidity and mortality affect more than 4 million Americans and represent the leading cause of hospitalization of patients over the age of 65. Improvements in pharmacologic therapies have both reduced the mortality and improved the quality of life of patients with heart failure. Advances in programming of gene expression in cardiac myocytes in vivo have generated enthusiasm for developing novel gene- and cell-based therapies for heart failure.[64, 65] Several different gene therapy approaches might be useful for the treatment of heart failure. One approach would be gene therapy to enhance myocardial contractility through the overexpression of beta-adrenergic receptors. A gene transfer approach could also be used to program replication of cardiac myocytes or conversion of fibroblasts to myocytes. Myocyte transplantation has been developed in several animal models and is promising. Although cellular transplantation is a theoretically attractive therapy for heart failure, many hurdles, including a source of cells and the development of a system for delivering these cells throughout the myocardium, must be overcome before this therapy is feasible. In general, gene therapy for heart failure will be limited by a need to develop a system to deliver the recombinant gene profusely throughout the myocardium. This challenge is being addressed through the development of catheters that permit direct injection into the myocardium.

Conclusions and Future Directions

Since the 1980s, remarkable progress has been made in the field of somatic gene therapy. The cloning of human disease related genes has dramatically expanded the number of diseases that can be approached through the use of gene transfer technology. Transgenic and gene targeting approaches have created important new animal models of cardiovascular disease that will be invaluable in developing and testing new genetic treatments.

Despite this progress, important hurdles remain before these advances can be translated into highly effective gene therapies for common cardiovascular diseases. There is a need for better vectors that effectively and efficiently program transgene expression in different cardiovascular cells without invoking immune responses to either the vector or the transgene proteins. Targeted gene expression using cell-specific promoters are being developed. Improved catheters are needed for delivering vectors to the vasculature and the myocardium. Finally, an improved understanding of the pathophysiologic pathways that regulate cardiovascular function in health and disease is needed. The field has developed rapidly, and gene therapy should play an increasingly important role in cardiovascular therapeutics in the future.

References

1. Nabel EG: Gene therapy for cardiovascular disease. Circulation 91:541, 1995.
2. Leiden JM: Gene therapy: promise, pitfalls, and prognosis. N Engl J Med 333:871, 1995.
3. Crystal RG: Transfer of genes to humans: early lessons and obstacles to success. Science 270:404, 1995.
4. Mulligan RC: The basic science of gene therapy. Science 260:926, 1993.
5. Wilson JM: Adenoviruses as gene-delivery vehicles. N Engl J Med 334:1185, 1996.
6. Guzman RJ, Lemarchand P, Crystal RG, et al: Efficient gene transfer in myocardium by direct injection of adenovirus vectors. Circ Res 88:1202, 1993.
7. Barr E, Carroll J, Kalynych A, et al: Efficient catheter-mediated gene transfer into the heart using replication-defective adenovirus. Gene Ther 1:51, 1994.
8. Yang Y, Ertl J, Wilson JM: MHC class 1-restricted cytoxic T lymphocytes to viral antigens destroy hepatocytes in mice infected with E1-deleted recombinant adenoviruses. Immunity 1:433, 1994.
9. Yang Y, Li Q, Ertl HC, et al: Cellular immunity to viral antigens limits E1-deleted adenoviruses for gene therapy. Proc Natl Acad Sci U S A 91:4407, 1994.
10. Tripathy SK, Black HB, Goldwasser E, et al: Immune responses to transgene-encoded proteins limit the stability of gene expression after injection of replication-defective adenovirus vectors. Nat Med 2:545, 1996.

11. Muzyczka N: Use of adeno-associated virus as a general transduction vector for mammalian cells. Curr Top Micobiol Immunol 158:97, 1992.
12. Svensson EC, Marshall DJ, Woodward K, et al: Efficient and stable transduction of cardiomyocytes after intramyocardial injection or intracoronary perfusion with recombinant adeno-associated virus vectors. Circulation 99:201, 1999.
13. Wolff J, Malone R, Williams P, et al: Direct gene transfer into mouse muscle in vivo. Science 247:1465, 1990.
14. Riessen R, Rahimizadeh H, Blessing E, et al: Arterial gene transfer using pure DNA applied directly to a hydrogelcoated angioplasty balloon. Hum Gene Ther 4:749, 1993.
15. Tripathy SK, Svensson EC, Black HB, et al: Long-term expression of erythropoietin in the systemic circulation of mice after intramuscular injection of a plasmid DNA vector. Proc Natl Acad Sci U S A 93:10876, 1996.
16. Acsadi G, Jiao S, Jani A: Direct gene transfer and expression into rat heart in vivo. New Biol 3:71, 1990.
17. Felgner P, Gadek T, Holm M, et al: Lipofection: a highly efficient, lipid-mediated DNA-tranfection procedure. Proc Natl Acad Sci U S A 84:7413, 1987.
18. San H, Yang Z, Pompili V, et al: Safety and short-term toxicity of a novel cationic lipid formulation for human gene therapy. Hum Gene Ther 4:781, 1993.
19. Castanotto D, Rossi JJ, Sarver N, et al: Antisense catalytic RNAs as therapeutic agents. Adv Pharmacol 25:289, 1994.
20. Bielinska A, Shivdasani RA, Zhang LQ, et al: Regulation of gene expression with double-stranded phosphorothioate oligonucleotides. Science 250:997, 1990.
21. Simons M, Edelman ER, DeKeyser J, et al: Anti-sense c-*myb* oligonucleotides inhibit intimal arterial smooth muscle cell accumulation in vivo. Nature 359:67, 1992.
22. Morishita R, Gibbons G, Ellison K, et al: Single intraluminal delivery of antisense cdc2 kinase and proliferating-cell nuclear antigen oligonucleotides results in chronic inhibition of neointimal hyperplasia. Proc Natl Acad Sci U S A 90:8474, 1993.
23. Bennett M, Anglin S, McEwan J, et al: Inhibition of vascular smooth muscle cell proliferation in vitro and in vivo by c-*myc* antisense oligonucleotides. J Clin Invest 93:820, 1994.
24. Shi Y, Fard A, Galeo A, et al: Transcatheter delivery of c-*myc* antisense oligomers reduces neointimal formation in a porcine model of coronary artery balloon injury. Circulation 90:944, 1994.
25. Morishita R, Gibbons GH, Ellison KE, et al: Intimal hyperplasia after vascular injury is inhibited by antisense cdk 2 kinase oligonucleotides. J Clin Invest 93:1458, 1994.
26. Simons M, Edelman E, Rosenberg R: Antisense proliferating cell nuclear antigen oligonucleotides inhibit intimal hyperplasia in a rat carotid artery injury model. J Clin Invest 93:2351, 1994.
27. Epstein SE, Speir E, Finkel T: Do antisense approaches to the problem of restenosis make sense? Circulation 88:1351, 1993.
28. Chien KR: Molecular cardiology in the postmolecular era turning toward complexity. Trends Cardiovasc Med 4:1, 1996.
29. Nabel EG, Plautz FM, Stanley JC, et al: Recombinant gene expression in vivo within endothelial cells of the atrial wall. Science 244:1342, 1989.
30. Wilson J, Birinyi L, Salomon R, et al: Implantation of vascular grafts lined with genetically modified endothelial cells. Science 244:1344, 1989.
31. Nabel E, Plautz G, Nabel G: Site-specific gene expression in vivo by direct gene transfer into the arterial wall. Science 249:1285, 1990.
32. Lee S, Trapnell B, Rade J, et al: In vivo adenoviral vector-mediated gene transfer into balloon-injured rat carotid arteries. Circ Res 73:797, 1993.
33. Chang MW, Barr E, Seltzer J, et al: Cytostatic gene therapy for vascular proliferative disorders using a constitutively active form of retinoblastoma gene product. Science 267:518, 1994.
34. Chang MW, Ohno T, Gordon D, et al: Adenovirus-mediated transfer of the herpes simplex virus thymidine kinase gene inhibits vascular smooth muscle cell proliferation and neointima formation following balloon angioplasty. Mol Med 1:172, 1995.
35. Leclerc G, Gal D, Takeshita S, et al: Percutaneous arterial gene transfer in a rabbit model: efficiency in normal and balloon-dilated atherosclerotic arteries. J Clin Invest 90:936, 1992.
36. Takeshita S, Gal D, Leclerc G, et al: Increased gene expression following liposome-mediated arterial gene transfer associated with intimal smooth muscle cell proliferation: in vitro and in vivo findings in a rabbit model of vascular injury. J Clin Invest 93:652, 1994.
37. Simari R, San H, Rekhter M, et al: Regulation of cellular proliferation and intimal formation following balloon injury in atherosclerotic rabbit arteries. J Clin Invest 98:225, 1996.
38. Lim C, Chapman G, Gammon R, et al: Direct in vivo gene transfer into the coronary and peripheral vasculatures of the intact dog. Circulation 83:2007, 1991.
39. Chapman G, Lim C, Gammon R, et al: Gene transfer into coronary arteries of intact animals with a percutaneous balloon catheter. Circ Res 71:27, 1992.
40. Giordano FJ, Ping P, McKirnan MD, et al: Intracoronary gene transfer of fibroblast growth factor-5 increases blood flow and contractile function in an ischemic region of the heart. Nat Med 2:534, 1996.
41. Nabel E, Yang Z, Liptay S, et al: Recombinant platelet-derived growth factor B gene expression in porcine arteries induces intimal hyperplasia in vivo. J Clin Invest 91:1822, 1993.
42. Nabel EG, Yang ZY, Plautz G, et al: Recombinant fibroblast growth factor-1 promotes intimal hyperplasia and angiogenesis in arteries in vivo. Nature 362:844, 1993.
43. Ohno T, Gordon D, San H, et al: Gene therapy for vascular smooth muscle cell proliferation after arterial injury. Science 265:781, 1994.
44. Lemarchand P, Jones M, Yamada I, et al: In vivo gene transfer and expression in normal uninjured blood vessels using replication-deficient recombinant adenovirus vectors. Circ Res 72:1132, 1993.
45. Nabel E, Leiden JM: Gene transfer approaches for cardiovascular disease. *In* Chien KR (ed): Molecular Basis of Heart Disease. p 86. Philadelphia: WB Saunders, 1999.
46. Grossman M, Raper SE, Kozarsky K, et al: Successful ex vivo gene therapy directed to liver in patient with familial hypercholesterolemia. Nat Genet 6:335, 1994.
47. Pu LQ, Sniderman AD, Brassard R, et al: Enhanced revascularization of the ischemic limb by means of angiogenic therapy. Circulation 88:208, 1993.
48. Unger EF, Banai S, Shou M, et al: Basic fibroblast growth factor enhances myocardial collateral flow in a canine model. Am J Physiol 266:H1588, 1994.
49. Harada K, Grossman W, Friedman M, et al: Basic fibroblast growth factor improves myocardial function in chronically ischemic porcine hearts. J Clin Invest 94:623, 1994.
50. Takeshita S, Weir L, Chen D, et al: Therapeutic angiogenesis following arterial gene transfer of vascular endothelial growth factor in a rabbit model of hindlimb ischemia. Biochem Biophys Res Commun 227:628, 1996.
51. Isner JM, Walsh K, Symes J, et al: Arterial gene therapy for therapeutic angiogenesis in patients with peripheral artery disease. Circulation 91:2687, 1995.
52. Isner JM, Feldman LJ: Gene therapy for arterial disease. Lancet 344:1653, 1994.
53. Baumgartner I, Pieczek A, Manor O, et al: Constitutive expression of phyVEGF165 after intramuscular gene transfer promotes collateral vessel development in patients with critical limb ischemia. Circulation 97:1114, 1998.
54. Losordo DW, Vale PR, Symes JF, et al: Gene therapy for myocardial angiogenesis: initial clinical results with direct myocardial injection of phVEGF165 as sole therapy for myocardial ischemia. Circulation 98:2800, 1998.
55. Schumacher B, Pecher P, von Specht BU, et al: Induction of neoangiogenesis in ischemic myocardium by human growth factors: first clinical results of a new treatment of coronary heart disease. Circulation 97:645, 1998.
56. Braun-Dullaeus RC, Mann MJ, Dzau VJ: Cell cycle progression: new therapeutic target for vascular proliferative disease. Circulation 98:82, 1998.
57. Chang MW, Barr E, Lu M, et al: Adenovirus-mediated over-expression of the cyclin/cyclin-dependent kinase inhibitor p21 inhibits vascular smooth muscle cell proliferation and neointima formation in the rat cartoid artery model of balloon angioplasty. J Clin Invest 96:2260, 1995.
58. Yang Z, Simari R, Perkins N, et al: Role of the p21 cyclin-dependent kinase inhibitor in limiting intimal cell proliferation in response to arterial injury. Proc Natl Acad Sci U S A 93:1905, 1996.
59. von der Leyen HE, Gibbons GH, Morishita R, et al: Gene therapy

inhibiting neointimal vascular lesion: in vivo transfer of endothelial cell nitric oxide synthase gene. Proc Natl Acad Sci U S A 92:1137, 1995.

60. Mann MJ, Gibbons GH, Kernoff RS, et al: Genetic engineering of vein grafts resistant to atherosclerosis. Proc Natl Acad Sci U S A 92:4502, 1995.
61. Morishita R, Gibbons GH, Horiuchi M, et al: A gene therapy strategy using a transcription factor decoy of the E2F binding site inhibits smooth muscle proliferation in vivo. Proc Natl Acad Sci U S A 92:5855, 1995.
62. Guzman RJ, Hirschowitz EA, Brody SL, et al: In vivo suppression of injury-induced vascular smooth muscle cell accumulation using adenovirus-mediated transfer of the herpes simplex virus thymidine kinase gene. Proc Natl Acad Sci U S A 91:10732, 1994.
63. Rekhter MD, Shah N, Simari RD, et al: Graft permeabilization facilitates therapy of transplant arteriosclerosis in a rabbit model. Circulation 98:1335, 1998.
64. Barr E, Leiden JM: Systemic delivery of recombinant proteins by genetically modified myoblasts. Science 254:1507, 1991.
65. Dhawan J, Pabn L, Pavlath G, et al: Systemic delivery of human growth hormone by injection of genetically engineered myoblasts. Science 254:1509, 1991.

CHAPTER 127

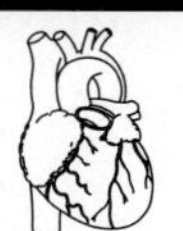

HOMOCYSTEINE AND VASCULAR DISEASE

Ali Moustapha, Ward Casscells, and Killian Robinson

HOMOCYSTEINE METABOLISM
HOMOCYSTEINE SPECIES AND VALUES
DETERMINANTS OF HOMOCYSTEINE
Age
Gender
Genetics
Vitamin Intake
Renal Function
Organ Transplantation
Others
HYPERHOMOCYSTEINEMIA AND VASCULAR DISEASE
Homocysteine and Renal Disease
Homocysteine and Organ Transplantation
Homocysteine and Systemic Lupus Erythematosus
POSSIBLE MECHANISMS OF VASCULAR DAMAGE DUE TO HIGH HOMOCYSTEINE CONCENTRATIONS
THERAPEUTIC STUDIES IN PATIENTS WITH VASCULAR DISEASE AND HOMOCYSTEINE
CONCLUSION

Homocysteine is an intermediate formed during the metabolism of the essential sulfur-containing amino acid methionine. In the rare genetic syndrome of homocystinuria, excessive quantities of homocysteine accumulate in plasma and lead to marked premature atherosclerosis. Milder elevations in homocysteine concentration have been confirmed in multiple cross-sectional and prospective studies to be an independent risk factor for atherosclerotic and atherothrombotic diseases. Increased homocysteine levels can result either from genetic enzyme defects or, more commonly, from acquired deficiencies in folate, vitamin B_{12}, or vitamin B_6. Homocysteine levels are also increased in renal failure patients and organ transplant recipients and may contribute to their increased incidence of atherosclerosis. Mechanisms by which homocysteine may cause vascular damage are not fully understood but include potentially adverse effects on endothelium, platelets, and clotting factors. Supplementation with folic acid either alone or with vitamins B_{12} and B_6 can lower plasma homocysteine level. Several interventional studies to assess the effects of such treatment on clinical outcomes are now in progress.

HOMOCYSTEINE METABOLISM

Homocysteine is the demethylated derivative of the essential sulfur-containing amino acid methionine.[1] The latter is derived from dietary and recycled endogenous proteins and is first converted to *S*-adenosylmethionine, which is an important methyl donor in many transmethylation reactions. *S*-adenosylmethionine is then converted to homocysteine by demethylation and hydrolysis. Homocysteine may either be remethylated to methionine (during relative methionine deficiency) or trans-sulfurated to cystathionine (during relative methionine excess) (Fig. 127–1). There are two remethylation pathways. In one, a methyl group is transferred to homocysteine from 5-methyltetrahydrofolate in a reaction catalyzed by the vitamin B_{12} (cobalamin)–dependent enzyme 5-methyltetrahydrofolate-homocysteine methyltransferase (methionine synthase). In the second remethylation reaction, a methyl group is transferred irreversibly from betaine, or trimethyglycine, to homocysteine. In the trans-sulfuration pathway, homocysteine is first converted to cystathionine in a reaction catalyzed by the vitamin B_6 (pyridoxal 5′-phosphate)–dependent cystathionine beta-synthase. Cystathionine is then transformed to cysteine and other metabolites, which are excreted in the urine. Trans-sulfuration of homocysteine leads also to the formation of glutathione, an abundant and important intracellular buffer that has a major role in the maintenance of a normal intracellular redox potential.

HOMOCYSTEINE SPECIES AND VALUES

In normal subjects, the mean value for plasma homocysteine is about 10 μmol/L, and the 95th percentile is about 16 μmol/L. A level greater than this is often referred to as *hyperhomocysteinemia.* About 80 percent of plasma homocysteine is bound to albumin by a disulfide bridge. Unbound or free homocysteine exists mainly as homocysteine-cysteine or homocysteine-homocysteine (homocystine) disulfides. Truly free homocysteine probably constitutes only 1 to 2 percent of all circulating homocysteine. Total homocysteine describes the sum of all these biochemical homocysteine species and is now often abbreviated to tHcy or homocyst(e)ine (Fig. 127–2). For clarity, the term *homocysteine* is used in this chapter to refer to any of the aforementioned species unless otherwise specified. In some clinical investigations, a methionine loading test is used in which total homocysteine, or one of its species, is measured before and after the administration of methionine.[1, 2] This test has been used in patients who have normal fasting

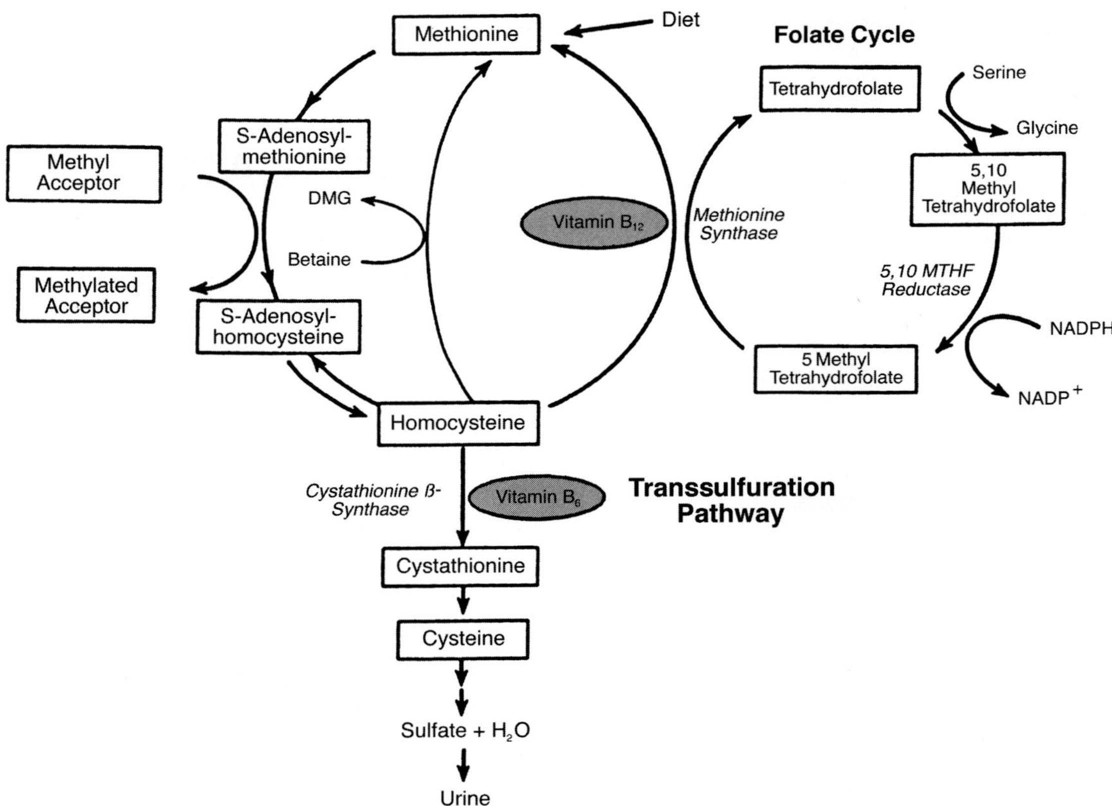

FIGURE 127–1 Metabolic pathways of homocysteine metabolism. (From Mayer EL, Jacobsen DW, Robinson K: Homocysteine and coronary atherosclerosis. Reprinted with permission from the American College of Cardiology. [J Am Coll Cardiol 1996, Vol. 27, pp. 517–527].)

levels but may nevertheless have a latent potential for developing hyperhomocysteinemia. For routine clinical purposes, however, the test has limited use and is time consuming and expensive.

DETERMINANTS OF HOMOCYSTEINE

Determinants of plasma homocysteine include genetic and acquired factors (Table 127–1).

Age

Several studies[3–8] have established a correlation between homocysteine and age. Abnormalities of folate and B vitamins appear to play a major role in the pathogenesis of increased total homocysteine in the elderly.[5, 6] The progressive deterioration in kidney function and age-related decline in cystathionine β-synthase[9, 10] may also provide an additional explanation for the correlation between homocysteine and age.

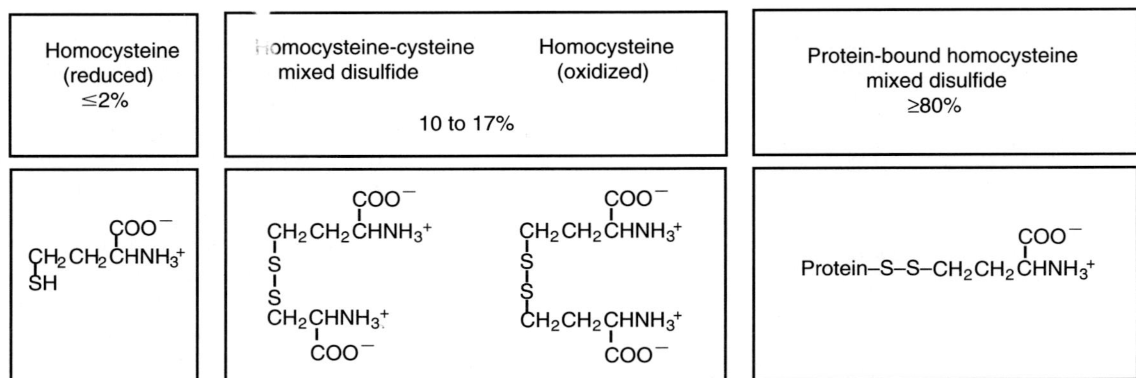

FIGURE 127–2 Forms of homocysteine in plasma. Note that protein-bound homocysteine accounts for 80% of total homocysteine in plasma.

TABLE 127–1 Determinants of Plasma Homocysteine Level

Age
Gender
Inherited
Cystathionine β-synthase absence or deficiency (rare)
Methionine synthase absence or deficiency (rare)
Methylenetetrahydrofolate reductase absence (rare)
Methylenetetrahydrofolate thermolabile variant (common)
Acquired
Folate, vitamin B_{12}, or vitamin B_6 deficiency
Impaired renal function
Psoriasis
Hypothyroidism
Malignancies: acute lymphoblastic leukemia, breast and ovarian carcinomas
Medications: methotrexate, nitrous oxide, phenytoin, carbamazepine, methylxanthines, azathioprine, colestipol, and niacin
Lifestyle habits: low vitamin intake, smoking, coffee intake, sedentary lifestyle

Gender

Homocysteine levels are about 10 percent higher in men than in women, and this may be partly due to the influence of sex hormones.[1–3] The balance of evidence suggests that homocysteine levels increase after menopause.[3, 11–14] The lower levels in premenopausal women may be due to higher estrogen concentrations[12] or to more efficient handling of methionine.[11, 15]

Genetics

Homocystinuria is a rare disease characterized by extremely elevated homocysteine levels. The most common genetic basis is deficiency in cystathionine β-synthase.[16] Other, rare genetic causes of increased homocysteine include absence or deficiency of methylenetetrahydrofolate reductase and methionine synthase.[1, 2] A thermolabile form of methylenetetrahydrofolate reductase is seen more commonly in about 15 percent of the population and may be associated with a higher homocysteine concentration, especially in the presence of low folate levels.[1, 2, 17]

Vitamin Intake

Some studies have underlined the importance of acquired nutritional deficiencies rather than genetic enzyme defects in the pathogenesis of hyperhomocysteinemia in the general population. Homocysteine levels are consistently elevated in patients with vitamin B_{12}[18] and folate deficiencies.[19, 20] Multiple studies have shown that negative correlations exist between levels of plasma homocysteine and those of plasma folate, vitamin B_{12} and vitamin B_6.[1, 2, 5, 6, 21, 22]

Renal Function

Plasma homocysteine concentrations correlate positively with plasma creatinine levels[1, 2, 4, 23] and rise with falling glomerular filtration rate.[1, 2, 24] Several studies have shown that homocysteine levels are elevated in patients with chronic renal failure[25, 26] and can be decreased by dialysis.[25] This elevation in plasma homocysteine level cannot be explained by decreased renal uptake[27] but may be related to impairment of nonrenal, possibly hepatic, metabolism.

Organ Transplantation

Plasma homocysteine concentrations are elevated in patients who have undergone cardiac[28–30] or renal[31] transplantation. Decreased levels of folate and vitamin B_6 impaired renal function, and possibly the antifolate effects of immunosuppressive drugs in these patients may account for this elevation.

Others

Several conditions, including malignancies and psoriasis, may cause high homocysteine levels. Hypothyroidism and various pharmacologic agents may also elevate homocysteine levels (see Table 127–1).

HYPERHOMOCYSTEINEMIA AND VASCULAR DISEASE

The relation between homocysteine and atherosclerosis was first described in patients with homocystinuria.[32] In this autosomal recessive disorder characterized by cystathionine β-synthase deficiency, patients have excessive elevations of plasma homocysteine and usually develop extensive premature vascular disease.[16]

Wilcken and Wilcken[33] were the first to show an association between coronary artery disease and milder elevation of homocysteine. In a case-control study published in 1976, they proved that patients with angiographically proven coronary artery disease had higher postmethionine loading homocysteine mixed disulfide levels than control subjects. Since then, many studies have confirmed the independent association of high homocysteine concentrations with all forms of vascular disease including coronary artery disease, stroke, peripheral vascular disease, and venous thrombosis. Boers and colleagues[34] and Brattström and coworkers[35] showed higher homocysteine levels in patients with peripheral vascular disease and stroke. Clarke and coworkers,[36] using a methionine loading test, showed in 1991 that hyperhomocysteinemia was present in 42 percent of patients with cerebrovascular disease, in 28 percent with peripheral vascular disease, and in 30 percent with coronary artery disease but in none of the control subjects. In addition, the odds ratio for vascular disease in patients with hyperhomocysteinemia was 3.3 after the investigators controlled for conventional risk factors. Aronow and associates[37, 38] showed that a high plasma homocysteine level was associated with a higher prevalence of both coronary artery disease and extracranial carotid artery disease in elderly patients. Similar findings occurred in a study by Selhub and colleagues[39] that involved elderly

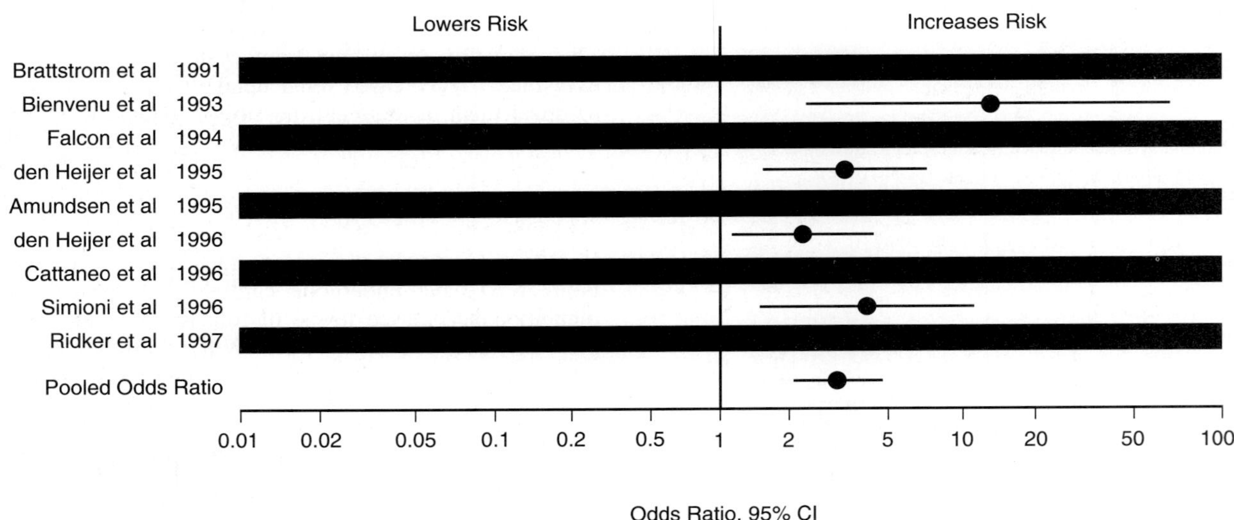

FIGURE 127–3 Risk of venous thromboembolism associated with fasting hyperhomocysteinemia in 9 major studies. The data are presented as odds ratio with 95% confidence intervals on a log scale. (From Ray JG: Meta-analysis of hyperhomocysteinemia as a risk factor for venous thromboembolic disease. Arch Intern Med 158:2105, 1998. Copyright 1998, American Medical Association.)

subjects from the Framingham Heart Study. A large meta-analysis performed by Boushey and associates[40] confirmed these findings and estimated that 10 percent of the risk of coronary artery disease in the general population was attributable to homocysteine. Mild hyperhomocysteinemia was shown to be an independent risk factor for venous thromboembolism in a study performed by den Heijer and colleagues,[41] and a meta-analysis by Ray[42] recently confirmed these findings (Fig. 127–3). These cross-sectional and retrospective studies have been followed up by several prospective investigations, many, but not all, of which have shown that individuals with elevated homocysteine concentrations have a higher incidence of coronary artery disease, stroke, and cardiovascular mortality[43–52] (Table 127–2). Plasma homocysteine level was also independently associated with the progression of peripheral arterial disease in a study by Taylor and colleagues.[53] In a prospective study of 587 patients with documented coronary artery disease, Nygård and coworkers[54] found a strong positive correlation between plasma homocysteine level and overall mortality (Fig. 127–4). Elevated homocysteine level was also associated with isolated systolic hypertension in older patients.[55] One large multicenter study by Graham and coworkers[56] demonstrated that hyperhomocysteinemia augments the effect of other risk factors for atherosclerosis, such as smoking and hypertension.

Homocysteine and Renal Disease

In multiple retrospective[57] and prospective[58, 59] studies of patients with chronic renal failure, higher homocysteine concentrations were associated with an increased risk of atherosclerotic and thrombotic complications, independent of traditional cardiovascular risk factors. Hyperhomocysteinemia was also shown to be an independent risk factor for cardiovascular morbidity and mortality in end-stage renal disease[60] (Fig. 127–5).

TABLE 127–2 Major Prospective and Nested Case-Control Studies of Homocysteine and Atherosclerosis

Authors	Year	N	Population	Vascular Disease	Association
Stampfer et al[43]	92	14,916	Physicians' Health Study	Acute MI or death from CAD	Yes
Eritsland et al[48]	94	610	CABG patients	Graft occlusion	No
Alfthan et al[49]	94	7424	General population	MI or stroke	No
Verhoef et al[50]	94	14,916	Physicians' Health Study	Ischemic stroke	No
Arnesen et al[44]	95	21,826	General population	Coronary heart disease	Yes
Perry et al[45]	95	5661	General population	Stroke	Yes
Chasan-Taber et al[46]	96	14,916	Physicians' Health Study	MI	Yes
Nygård et al[54]	97	587	CAD patients	Mortality	Yes
Evans et al[51]	97	712	General population	Acute MI or death from CAD	No
Wald et al[47]	98	21,520	Physicians' Health Study	Ischemic stroke	Yes
Folsom et al[52]	98	15,792	General population	Coronary heart disease	No

Abbreviations: CABG, coronary artery bypass grafting; CAD, coronary artery disease; MI, myocardial infarction.

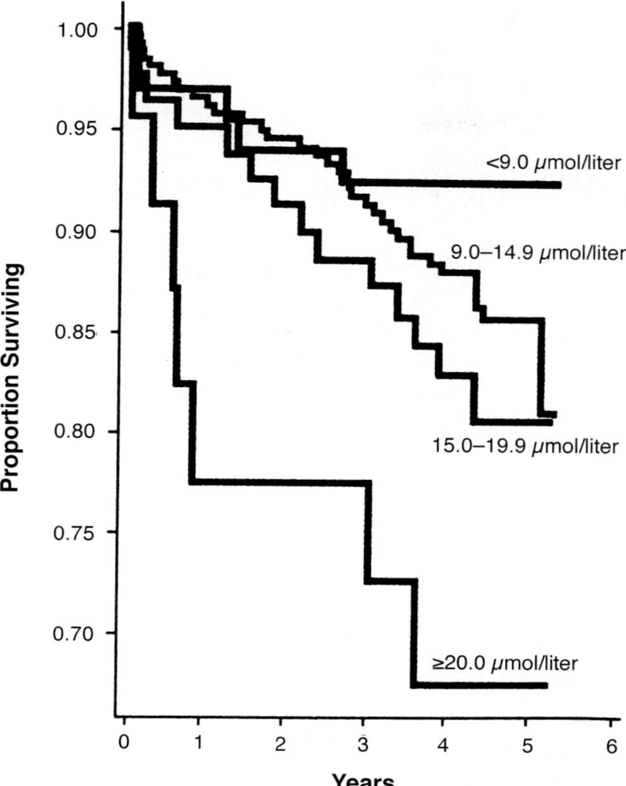

FIGURE 127–4 Estimated survival among patients with coronary artery disease, according to plasma total homocysteine levels. The figure shows estimated survival for 55-year-old male former smokers with three-vessel disease, a left ventricular ejection fraction of 55 percent, a creatinine level of 1.5 mg per deciliter, and a total cholesterol level of 241 mg per deciliter at four different total homocysteine levels. Survival curves have been estimated in a stratified Cox regression analysis. (From Nygård O, Nordrehaug JE, Refsum H, et al: Plasma homocysteine levels and mortality in patients with coronary artery disease. N Engl J Med 337:232, 1997. Copyright © 1997 Massachusetts Medical Society. All rights reserved.)

Homocysteine and Organ Transplantation

Massy and associates[61] showed that hyperhomocysteinemia is more common in kidney transplant recipients with vascular complications than in those without. Similar findings were seen in heart transplant recipients.[30, 62] In a prospective analysis, however, low vitamin B_6 level but not high homocysteine level was shown to be an independent risk factor for cardiovascular events and mortality in heart transplant recipients.[63] More studies are needed to assess the relation between plasma homocysteine level and cardiovascular complications in these populations.

Homocysteine and Systemic Lupus Erythematosus

In a prospective analysis, homocysteine level was shown to be a risk factor for stroke and arterial thrombosis in patients with systemic lupus erythematosus.[64]

Possible Mechanisms of Vascular Damage due to High Homocysteine Concentrations

Although high homocysteine concentrations are associated with atherosclerosis, the possible mechanisms of vascular damage remain unclear. The major focus of current studies is on the endothelium as the primary site of vascular damage with subsequent platelet activation and clotting factor disturbances[1, 2] (Table 127–3).

In vitro studies have shown that homocysteine exerts direct endothelial cytotoxicity.[65, 66] When it is added to plasma, homocysteine is oxidized into homocystine and possibly homocysteine thiolactone, with formation of reactive oxygen species, including hydrogen peroxide and superoxides. This oxidant stress may also play a role in endothelial cell injury before the development of overt vascular damage.[67] Homocysteine may also impair the vasomotor regulatory role of the endothelium. In an in vivo study in monkeys,[68] diet-induced hyperhomocysteinemia was associated with altered endothelium-dependent vascular function, and two studies in humans documented that homocysteine may also be responsible for inhibition of endothelium-dependent flow-mediated dilatation, suggesting inhibition of nitric oxide[69, 70] (Fig. 127–6A). High homocysteine levels may also increase the risk of venous thromboembolism in patients with factor V Leiden mutation.[71] Other potential mechanisms leading to thrombosis or atherosclerosis include increased smooth muscle cell proliferation,[72] oxidation of lipoproteins,[73] decreased platelet survival,[65, 66] increased factor V expression,[74] inactivation of endothelial anticoagulant protein C,[75] and disruption of the processing and secretion of von Willebrand factor.[1, 2]

Therapeutic Studies in Patients With Vascular Disease and Homocysteine

Folic acid lowers homocysteine concentrations. It may be used alone or in combination with vitamin B_{12} and vitamin

TABLE 127–3 Postulated Mechanisms of Homocysteine-Induced Vascular Damage

Effect on endothelium
Oxidative damage to endothelium
Promotion of smooth muscle cell growth
Inhibition of NO release
Reduced synthesis of prostacyclin
Direct cytotoxic injury
Effect on platelet
Promotion of platelet aggregation
Decreased platelet survival
Increased thromboxane A_2 formation
Effect on clotting factors
Decreased antithrombin III activity
Increased activity of factor Xa
Inhibition of t-PA activity
Activation of factor V
Inhibition of protein C
Inhibition of von Willebrand factor

Abbreviations: NO, nitric oxide; t-PA, tissue plasminogen activator.

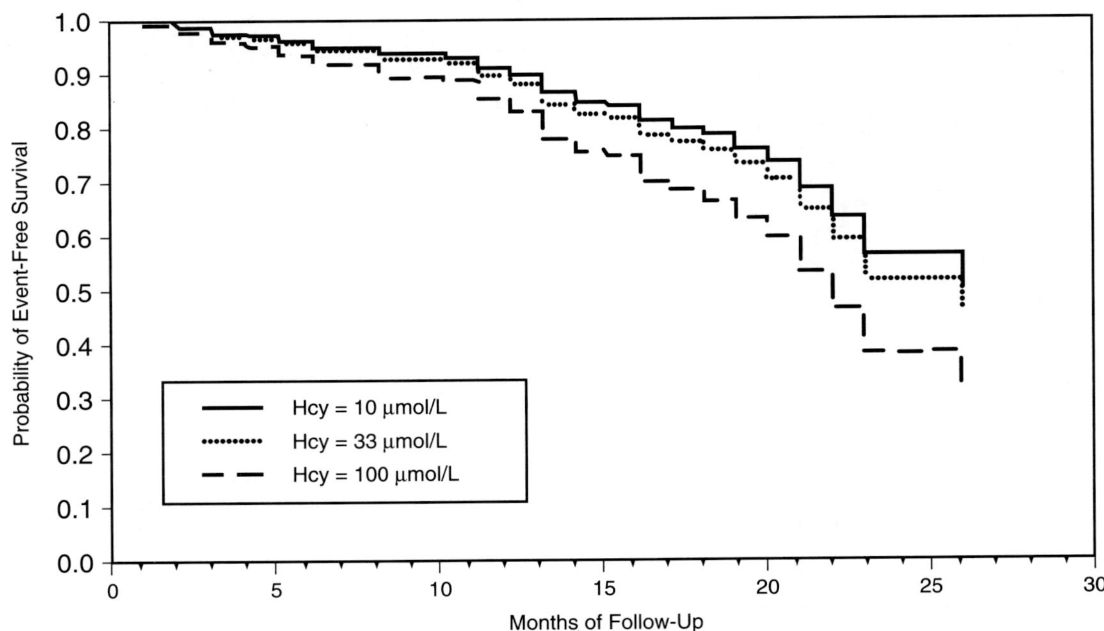

FIGURE 127–5 Probability for event-free survival during the follow-up period for patients with mean homocysteine (Hcy) values of 10, 33 and 100 μmol/L. (From Moustapha A, Naso A, Nahlawi M, et al: Prospective study of hyperhomocysteinemia as an adverse cardiovascular risk factor in end-stage renal disease. Circulation 97[2]:138–141, 1998.)

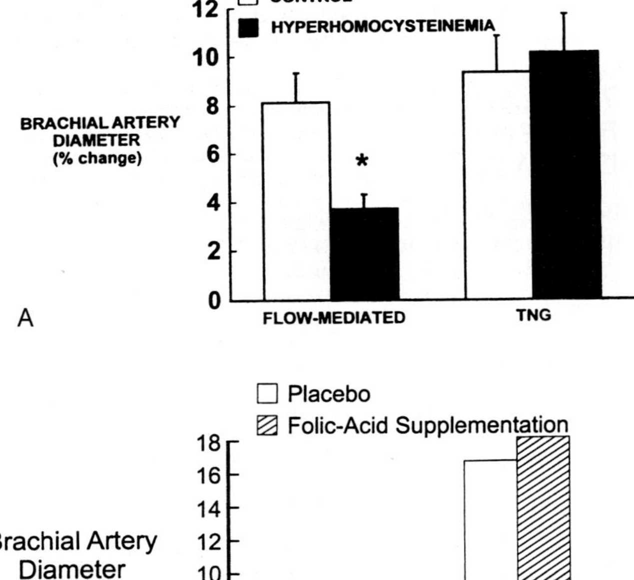

FIGURE 127–6 The effect of **(A)** hyperhomocysteinemia and **(B)** folate supplementation on flow-mediated, endothelium-dependent vasodilation and on trinitroglycerin (TNG)-induced, endothelium-independent vasodilation. (**A,** From Tawakol A, Omland T, Gerhard M, et al: Hyperhomocyst[e]inemia is associated with impaired endothelial-dependent vasodilation in humans. Circulation 95[5]:1119–1121, 1997. **B,** Data from Woo KS, Chook P, Lolin YI, et al: Folic acid supplementation improves arterial endothelial function in hyperhomocysteinemic subjects [abstract]. Circulation 95:I165, 1997.)

B_6. The treatment is rapid and effective, and maximal effects are usually seen after 4 to 6 weeks. The dose and combination of vitamins that should be used remain unclear,[1, 2] but in normal subjects or in patients with vascular disease, the dose may be even less than 1 mg of folic acid daily.[76] Lobo and colleagues[77] used 400 μg of folic acid and reported an effect similar to that seen with 1 and 5 mg. Whether doses lower than 400 μg will confer any benefit requires further investigations.

Folate supplementation has also been explored in other populations with hyperhomocysteinemia. den Heijer and associates[78] showed that a combined vitamin supplementation with 5 mg of folic acid, 0.4 mg of hydroxycobalamin, and 50 mg of pyridoxine effectively reduced homocysteine in patients with venous thrombosis. Patients with renal failure appear to be relatively resistant to folate supplementation. Pharmacologic doses up to 15 mg have been used in this population but have not resulted in normal homocysteine concentrations.[79] Wilcken and coworkers[80] used folic acid in renal transplant recipients and lowered homocysteine concentrations. Similar results were seen in a study by Bostom and associates.[81]

Dietary supplementation with folate may also be effective in lowering homocysteine level. Malinow and coworkers[82] estimated that cereals providing 499 and 665 μg of folic acid daily would decrease plasma homocysteine level by 11 and 14 percent, respectively, in patients with coronary heart disease.

Although folic acid may lower homocysteine concentrations, there is as yet no evidence from randomized trials that this effect improves clinical outcomes. Woo and colleagues[83] showed that folate supplementation ameliorates arterial endothelial function in healthy hyperhomocysteinemic subjects (see Fig. 127–6B). Similar findings were seen with administration of folate and vitamin B_6 in young patients with peripheral arterial disease.[84] Peterson and Spence[85] showed that administration of folate and vitamins B_{12} and B_6 decreases mean carotid plaque area in a group of patients with unexplained atherosclerosis and elevated homocysteine levels. In addition, in the Nurses' Health Study,[86] healthy women in the highest quintile for folate and vitamin B_6 intake had a lesser risk for coronary heart disease than those in the lowest quintile. Controlled intervention studies using folic acid supplements in patients with cardiovascular disease are now in progress to assess the role of vitamin therapy in the treatment of patients with atherosclerosis.[87, 88]

If homocysteine levels are high and no other risk factors for vascular disease are present, vitamin therapy is a reasonable addition to usual treatment. This therapy is innocuous and cheap. In older patients given maintenance doses of folic acid, it is prudent to check vitamin B_{12} level before initiating treatment and perhaps also during follow-up, to ensure that vitamin B_{12} deficiency is not present, because folate therapy could, in theory, mask the neurologic manifestations of B_{12} deficiency.

Conclusion

A high plasma homocysteine concentration is an independent risk factor for cardiovascular diseases. It may account for 10 percent of the incidence of coronary artery disease in the general population and may potentiate the effect of other risk factors for atherosclerosis. The causes for elevated homocysteine concentrations are complex and are likely to be related to suboptimal vitamin status. In the elderly, kidney dysfunction may also play an important role. The mechanisms by which homocysteine may cause vascular damage, if any, remain unclear but may be related to endothelial dysfunction. Vitamin therapy can lower homocysteine levels and may improve the prognosis of patients with atherosclerosis. Intervention studies using vitamin supplements with clinical outcomes as end points are now in progress.

References

1. Refsum H, Ueland PM, Nygård O, et al: Homocysteine and cardiovascular disease. Annu Rev Med 49:31–62, 1998.
2. Mayer EL, Jacobsen DW, Robinson K: Homocysteine and coronary atherosclerosis. J Am Coll Cardiol 27:517–527, 1996.
3. Kang SS, Wong PW, Cook HY, et al: Protein-bound homocyst(e)ine: a possible risk factor for coronary artery disease. J Clin Invest 77:1482–1486, 1986.
4. Brattström L, Lindgren A, Israelsson B, et al: Hyperhomocysteinaemia in stroke: prevalence, cause, and relationships to type of stroke and stroke risk factors. Eur J Clin Invest 22:214–221, 1992.
5. Selhub J, Jacques PF, Wilson PWF, et al: Vitamin status and intake as primary determinants of homocysteinemia in an elderly population. JAMA 270:2693–2698, 1993.
6. Brattström L, Lindgren A, Israelsson B, et al: Homocysteine and cysteine: determinants of plasma levels in middle-aged and elderly subjects. J Intern Med 236:633–641, 1994.
7. Robinson K, Mayer EL, Miller DP, et al: Hyperhomocysteinemia and low pyridoxal phosphate: common and independent reversible risk factors for coronary artery disease. Circulation 92:2825–2830, 1995.
8. Nygård O, Vollset SE, Refsum H, et al: Total plasma homocysteine and cardiovascular risk profile: the Hordaland Homocysteine Study. JAMA 274:1526–1533, 1995.
9. Nordström M, Kjellström T: Age dependency of cystathionine beta-synthase activity in human fibroblasts in homocyst(e)inemia and atherosclerotic vascular disease. Atherosclerosis 94:213–221, 1992.
10. Gartler SM, Hornug SK, Motulsky AG: Effect of chronologic age on induction of cystathionine synthase, uroporphyrinogen I synthase, and glucose-6-phosphate dehydrogenase activities in lymphocytes. Proc Natl Acad Sci U S A 78:1916–1919, 1981.
11. Boers GH, Smals AG, Trijbels FJ, et al: Unique efficiency of methionine metabolism in premenopausal women may protect against vascular disease in the reproductive years. J Clin Invest 72:1971–1976, 1983.
12. Wouters MG, Moorrees MT, van der Mooren MJ, et al: Plasma homocysteine and menopausal status. Eur J Clin Invest 25:801–805, 1995.
13. Brattström LE, Hultberg BL, Hardebo JE: Folic acid responsive postmenopausal homocysteinemia. Metabolism 34:1073–1077, 1985.
14. Dudman NP, Wilcken DE, Wang J, et al: Disordered methionine/homocysteine metabolism in premature vascular disease: its occurrence, cofactor therapy, and enzymology. Arterioscler Thromb 13:1253–1260, 1993.
15. Robinson K, Arheart K, Refsum H, et al: Low circulating folate and vitamin B_6 concentrations: risk factors for stroke, peripheral vascular disease and coronary artery disease. Circulation 97:437–443, 1998.
16. Mudd SH, Skovby F, Levy HL, et al: The natural history of homocystinuria due to cystathionine β-synthase deficiency. Am J Hum Genet 37:1–31, 1985.
17. Kang SS, Passen EL, Ruggie N, et al: Thermolabile defect of methylenetetrahydrofolate reductase in coronary artery disease. Circulation 88:1463–1469, 1993.
18. Brattström L, Israelsson B, Lindgarde F, et al: Higher total plasma homocysteine in vitamin B_{12} deficiency than in heterozygosity for homocystinuria due to cystathionine β-synthase deficiency. Metabolism 37:175–178, 1988.

19. Kang SS, Wong PWK, Norusis M: Homocysteinemia due to folate deficiency. Metabolism 36:458–462, 1987.
20. Stabler SP, Marcell PD, Podell PR, et al: Elevation of total homocysteine in the serum of patients with cobalamin or folate deficiency detected by capillary gas chromatography-mass spectrometry. J Clin Invest 81:466–474, 1988.
21. Ubbink JB, Vermaak WJH, van der Merwe A, et al: Vitamin B_{12}, vitamin B_6, and folate nutritional status in men with hyperhomocysteinemia. Am J Clin Nutr 57:47–53, 1993.
22. Pancharuniti N, Lewis CA, Sauberlich HE, et al: Plasma homocyst(e)ine, folate and vitamin B_{12} concentrations and risk for early-onset coronary artery disease. Am J Clin Nutr 59:940–948, 1994.
23. Andersson A, Brattström L, Israelsson B, et al: Plasma homocysteine before and after methionine loading with regard to age, gender, and menopausal status. Eur J Clin Invest 22:79–87, 1992.
24. Arnadottir M, Hultberg B, Nilsson-Ehle P, et al: The effect of reduced glomerular filtration rate on plasma total homocysteine concentration. Scand J Clin Lab Invest 56:41–46, 1996.
25. Wilcken DEL, Gupta VJ: Sulfur containing amino acids in chronic renal failure with particular reference to homocysteine and cysteine-homocysteine mixed disulfide. Eur J Clin Invest 9:301–307, 1979.
26. Chauveau P, Chadefaux B, Coudé M, et al: Hyperhomocysteinemia, a risk factor for atherosclerosis in chronic uremic patients. Kidney Int 43:S72–77, 1993.
27. van Guldener C, Donker JM, Jakobs C, et al: No net renal homocysteine extraction in fasting humans. Kidney Int 54:166–169, 1998.
28. Ambrosi P, Barlatier A, Habib G, et al: Hyperhomocysteinaemia in heart transplant recipients. Eur Heart J 15:1191–1195, 1994.
29. Berger PB, Jones JD, Olson LJ, et al: Increase in total plasma homocysteine concentration after cardiac transplantation. Mayo Clin Proc 70:125–131, 1995.
30. Gupta A, Moustapha A, Jacobsen DW, et al: High homocysteine, low folate and low vitamin B_6 concentrations, prevalent risk factors for vascular disease in heart transplant recipients. Transplantation 65:544–550, 1998.
31. Arnadottir M, Hultberg B, Vladov V, et al: Hyperhomocysteinemia in cyclosporine-treated renal transplant recipients. Transplantation 61:509–512, 1996.
32. McCully KS: Vascular pathology of homocysteinemia: implications for the pathogenesis of arteriosclerosis. Am J Pathol 56:111–128, 1969.
33. Wilcken DE, Wilcken B: The pathogenesis of coronary artery disease: a possible role for methionine metabolism. J Clin Invest 57:1079–1082, 1976.
34. Boers GH, Smals AG, Trijbels FJ, et al: Heterozygosity for homocystinuria in premature peripheral and cerebral occlusive arterial disease. N Engl J Med 313:709–715, 1985.
35. Brattström L, Israelsson B, Norrving B, et al: Impaired homocysteine metabolism in early-onset cerebral and peripheral occlusive arterial disease: effects of pyridoxine and folic acid treatment. Atherosclerosis 81:51–60, 1990.
36. Clarke R, Daly L, Robinson K, et al: Hyperhomocysteinemia: an independent risk factor for vascular disease. N Engl J Med 324:1149–1155, 1991.
37. Aronow WS, Ahn C, Schoenfeld MR: Association between plasma homocysteine and extracranial carotid arterial disease in older persons. Am J Cardiol 79:1432–1433, 1997.
38. Aronow WS, Ahn C: Association between plasma homocysteine and coronary artery disease in older persons. Am J Cardiol 80:1216–1218, 1997.
39. Selhub J, Jacques PF, Bostom AG, et al: Association between plasma homocysteine concentrations and extracranial carotid-artery stenosis. N Engl J Med 332:286–291, 1995.
40. Boushey CJ, Beresford SA, Omenn GS, et al: A quantitative assessment of plasma homocysteine as a risk factor for vascular disease: probable benefits of increasing folic acid intakes. JAMA 274:1049–1057, 1995.
41. den Heijer M, Koster T, Blom HJ, et al: Hyperhomocysteinemia as a risk factor for deep-vein thrombosis. N Engl J Med 334:759–762, 1996.
42. Ray JG: Meta-analysis of hyperhomocysteinemia as a risk factor for venous thromboembolic disease. Arch Intern Med 158:2101–2106, 1998.
43. Stampfer MJ, Malinow MR, Willett WC, et al: A prospective study of plasma homocyst(e)ine and risk of myocardial infarction in US physicians. JAMA 268:877–881, 1992.
44. Arnesen E, Refsum H, Bonaa KH, et al: Serum total homocysteine and coronary heart disease. Int J Epidemiol 24:704–709, 1995.
45. Perry IJ, Refsum H, Morris RW, et al: Prospective study of serum total homocysteine concentration and risk of stroke in middle-aged British men. Lancet 346:1395–1398, 1995.
46. Chasan-Taber L, Selhub J, Rosenberg IH, et al: A prospective study of folate and vitamin B_6 and risk of myocardial infarction in US physicians. J Am Coll Nutr 15:136–143, 1996.
47. Wald NJ, Watt HC, Law MR, et al: Homocysteine and ischemic heart disease: results of a prospective study with implications regarding prevention. Arch Intern Med 158:862–867, 1998.
48. Eritsland J, Arnesen H, Seljeflot M, et al: Influence of serum lipoprotein(a) and homocyst(e)ine levels on graft patency after coronary artery bypass grafting. Am J Cardiol 74:1099–1102, 1994.
49. Alfthan G, Pekkanen J, Jauhiainen M, et al: Relation of serum homocysteine and lipoprotein(a) concentrations to atherosclerotic disease in a prospective Finnish population based study. Atherosclerosis 106:9–19, 1994.
50. Verhoef P, Hennekens CH, Malinow MR, et al: A prospective study of plasma homocyst(e)ine and risk of ischemic stroke. Stroke 25:1924–1930, 1994.
51. Evans RW, Shaten BJ, Hempel JD, et al: Homocyst(e)ine and risk of cardiovascular disease in the Multiple Risk Factor Intervention Trial. Arterioscler Thromb Vasc Biol 17:1947–1953, 1997.
52. Folsom AR, Nieto FJ, McGovern PG, et al: Prospective study of coronary heart disease incidence in relation to fasting total homocysteine, related genetic polymorphisms, and B vitamins: the Atherosclerosis Risk in Communities (ARIC) study. Circulation 98:204–210, 1998.
53. Taylor LM Jr, DeFrang RD, Harris EJ Jr, et al: The association of elevated plasma homocyst(e)ine with progression of symptomatic peripheral arterial disease. J Vasc Surg 13:128–136, 1991.
54. Nygård O, Nordrehaug JE, Refsum H, et al: Plasma homocysteine levels and mortality in patients with coronary artery disease. N Engl J Med 337:230–236, 1997.
55. Sutton-Tyrrell K, Bostom A, Selhub J, et al: High homocysteine levels are independently related to isolated systolic hypertension in older adults. Circulation 96:1745–1749, 1997.
56. Graham IM, Daly LE, Refsum HM, et al: Plasma homocysteine as a risk factor for vascular disease: the European Concerted Action Project. JAMA 277:1775–1781, 1997.
57. Dennis VW, Robinson K: Homocysteinemia and vascular disease in end-stage renal disease. Kidney Int 57(suppl):S11–17, 1996.
58. Jungers P, Massy ZA, Khoa TN, et al: Incidence and risk factors of atherosclerotic cardiovascular accidents in predialysis chronic renal failure patients: a prospective study. Nephrol Dial Transplant 12:2597–2602, 1997.
59. Jungers P, Chauveau P, Bandin O, et al: Hyperhomocysteinemia is associated with atherosclerotic occlusive arterial accidents in predialysis chronic renal failure patients. Miner Electrolyte Metab 23:170–173, 1997.
60. Moustapha A, Naso A, Nahlawi M, et al: Prospective study of hyperhomocysteinemia as an adverse cardiovascular risk factor in end-stage renal disease. Circulation 97:138–141, 1998.
61. Massy ZA, Chadefaux-Vekemans B, Chevalier A, et al: Hyperhomocysteinaemia: a significant risk factor for cardiovascular disease in renal transplant recipients. Nephrol Dial Transplant 9:1103–1108, 1994.
62. Ambrosi P, Garcon D, Riberi A, et al: Association of mild hyperhomocysteinemia with cardiac graft vascular disease. Atherosclerosis 138:347–350, 1998.
63. Nahlawi M, Naso A, Boparai A, et al: Low vitamin B_6: an independent predictor of cardiovascular morbidity and mortality in heart transplant recipients [abstract]. Circulation 98:I690, 1998.
64. Petri M, Roubenoff R, Dallal GE, et al: Plasma homocysteine as a risk factor for atherothrombotic events in systemic lupus erythematosus. Lancet 348:1120–1124, 1996.
65. Harker LA, Slichter SJ, Scott CR, et al: Homocystinemia: vascular injury and arterial thrombosis. N Engl J Med 291:537–543, 1974.
66. Harker LA, Ross R, Slichter SJ, et al: Homocystine induced arteriosclerosis: the role of endothelial cell injury and platelet response in its genesis. J Clin Invest 58:731–741, 1976.
67. Loscalzo J: The oxidant stress of hyperhomocyst(e)inemia. J Clin Invest 98:5–7, 1996.
68. Lentz SR, Sobey CG, Piegors DJ, et al: Vascular dysfunction in

monkeys with diet-induced hyperhomocyst(e)inemia. J Clin Invest 98:24–29, 1996.
69. Tawakol A, Omland T, Gerhard M, et al: Hyperhomocyst(e)inemia is associated with impaired endothelial-dependent vasodilation in humans. Circulation 95:1119–1121, 1997.
70. Bellamy MF, McDowell IF, Ramsey MW, et al: Hyperhomocysteinemia after an oral methionine load acutely impairs endothelial function in healthy adults. Circulation 98:1848–1852, 1998.
71. Ridker PM, Hennekens CH, Selhub J, et al: Interrelation of hyperhomocyst(e)inemia, factor V Leiden, and risk of future venous thromboembolism. Circulation 95:1777–1782, 1997.
72. Tsai JC, Perrella MA, Yoshizumi M, et al: Promotion of vascular smooth cell growth by homocysteine: a link to atherosclerosis. Proc Natl Acad Sci U S A 91:3369–3373, 1994.
73. Heinecke JW, Rosen H, Susuki LA, et al: The role of sulfur-containing amino acids in superoxide production and modification of low density lipoprotein by arterial smooth muscle cells. J Biol Chem 262:10098–10103, 1987.
74. Rodgers GM, Kane WH: Activation of endogenous factor V by a homocysteine-induced vascular endothelial cell activator. J Clin Invest 77:1909–1916, 1986.
75. Rodgers GM, Conn MT: Homocysteine, an atherogenic stimulus, reduces protein C activation by arterial and venous endothelial cells. Blood 75:895–901, 1990.
76. Homocysteine Lowering Trialists' Collaboration: Lowering blood homocysteine with folic acid based supplements: meta-analysis of randomised trials. BMJ 316:894–898, 1998.
77. Lobo A, Naso A, Arheart K, et al: Reduction of homocysteine levels in coronary artery disease by low-dose folic acid combined with vitamins B_6 and B_{12}. Am J Cardiol 83:821–825, 1999.
78. den Heijer M, Brouwer IA, Bos GM, et al: Vitamin supplementation reduces blood homocysteine levels: a controlled trial in patients with venous thrombosis and healthy volunteers. Arterioscler Thromb Vasc Biol 18:356–361, 1998.
79. Bostom AG, Shemin D, Lapane KL, et al: High dose-B-vitamin treatment of hyperhomocysteinemia in dialysis patients. Kidney Int 49:147–152, 1996.
80. Wilcken DE, Gupta VJ, Betts AK: Homocysteine in the plasma of renal transplant recipients: effects of cofactors for methionine metabolism. Clin Sci 61:743–749, 1981.
81. Bostom AG, Gohh RY, Beaulieu AJ, et al: Treatment of hyperhomocysteinemia in renal transplant recipients. Ann Intern Med 127:1089–1092, 1997.
82. Malinow MR, Duell PB, Hess DL, et al: Reduction of plasma homocyst(e)ine levels by breakfast cereal fortified with folic acid in patients with coronary heart disease. N Engl J Med 338:1009–1015, 1998.
83. Woo KS, Chook P, Lolin YI, et al: Folic acid supplementation improves arterial endothelial function in hyperhomocysteinemic subjects [abstract]. Circulation 95:I165, 1997.
84. van den Berg M, Boers GH, Franken DG, et al: Hyperhomocysteinaemia and endothelial dysfunction in young patients with peripheral arterial occlusive disease. Eur J Clin Invest 25:176–181, 1995.
85. Peterson JC, Spence JD: Vitamins and progression of atherosclerosis in hyperhomocyst(e)inaemia. Lancet 351:263, 1998.
86. Rimm EB, Willett WC, Hu FB, et al: Folate and vitamin B_6 from diet and supplements in relation to risk of coronary heart disease among women. JAMA 279:359–364, 1998.
87. Howard VJ, Chambless LE, Malinow MR, et al: Results of a homocyst(e)ine lowering pilot study in acute stroke patients [abstract]. Stroke 28:234, 1997.
88. Aursnes I: Protocol for a nested case-control study with folic acid in hyperhomocysteinemia [abstract]. Can J Cardiol 13(suppl B):315B, 1997.

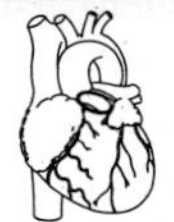

Prosthetic Valve Endocarditis

Charles D. Ericsson

Prosthetic valve endocarditis (PVE) accounts for up to 15 percent of all cases of infective endocarditis.[1] A recent review suggests that early PVE might account for less than 1 percent of all endocarditis.[2] Postoperatively, patients with valve replacements sustain a 3 to 6 percent risk of PVE over 5 years, with the greatest risk occurring between the second and the third month after surgery.[3] Six to 12 months after valve replacement, the risk of PVE is very low (approximately 0.4 percent per year). In defining the need for antibiotic prophylaxis against PVE, risk should be considered to last the lifetime of the patient.

Risk Factors

The type of valve (mechanical versus bioprosthetic) does not influence the overall risk of infection, although risk is somewhat higher either early after mechanical valve replacement or late after bioprosthetic valve replacement.[4] Aging of the bioprosthetic valve is thought to account for the late risk. Rates of PVE do not vary by site of valve replacement (aortic versus mitral). Replacing multiple valves might increase the risk of PVE, but the data are conflicting. Patients undergoing valve replacement to correct structural damage owing to infective endocarditis are at increased risk of developing PVE whether the surgery is done during the acute illness or later after valve healing.

Pathogenesis

The genesis of PVE is substantially the same as native valve endocarditis.[1] The critical features are lack of endothelialization of the native valve annulus and the valve sewing ring that is associated with early risk of endocarditis and repetitive stress owing to leaflet motion and aging of the bioprosthetic valve that probably account for some late-onset endocarditis.

Microbiology

As can be seen in Table A–1, the microbiology of PVE suggests a nosocomial origin of organisms in the first 2 months after valve replacement. Organisms likely acquired through nosocomial bacteremia (e.g., aerobic gram-negative bacilli) drop off in frequency 2 months after valve replacement. Organisms most likely acquired at the time of surgery through intraoperative contamination (e.g., *Staphylococcus* non-*aureus*) finally drop off in frequency 1 year after valve replacement, as does *Staphylococcus aureus,* which could be acquired through either nosocomial blood stream invasion or intraoperative contamination. After 1 year, organisms are distributed more like those causing native valve endocarditis with viridans streptococci leading the list. The exception is that *S.* non-*aureus* remains a relatively common cause of late-onset PVE compared with native valve endocarditis. Invasive infection with formation of perivalvular abscess or partial dehiscence of the prosthetic valve with paravalvular regurgitation is more common when PVE occurs within the first year (59 percent) than later (25 percent).[5]

Clinical Features

The clinical features of PVE are similar to those of infection of native valves. Clinical features range from exceedingly indolent to acute and fulminating. PVE owing to *S. aureus* is usually very severe, with serious central nervous system or cardiac complications occurring in up to 40 percent and mortality rates ranging from as low as 42 percent to as high as 85 percent depending on the series.[6] Invasive disease is suggested by valvular dysfunction, new

TABLE A–1 Microbiology of Prosthetic Valve Endocarditis

	Months After Valve Replacement		
	<2	2–12	>12
Staphylococcus non-*aureus*	++++	++++	++
S. aureus	+++	++	++
Aerobic gram-negative bacilli	++	+	+
Enterococci	+	++	++
Diphtheroids	+	0	+
Fungi	+	+	+
Streptococci	+	+	++++
Fastidious gram-negative coccobacilli	0	0	+
Miscellaneous	+	++	+
Culture-negative	+	++	+

Key: +, 0–10%; ++, 11–20%; +++, 21–30%; ++++, >30%.

electrocardiographic conduction disturbances, fever lasting longer than 9 days despite appropriate antibiotic treatment, and echocardiographic evidence of abscess. Such invasive disease was noted in 64 percent of 116 patients in one series[4] and was most common among infections of aortic valve prostheses occurring within the first year.

DIAGNOSIS

Diagnosing PVE relies heavily on the concept that bacteremia in PVE is continuous. In the absence of prior antibiotic therapy, most blood cultures, regardless of when they were obtained in relation to fever, will be positive. At least three to four blood cultures should be taken from different percutaneous sites. This approach facilitates the recognition of a likely contaminant when only one of many cultures is positive. Unless the patient presents with features of acute bacterial endocarditis or is hemodynamically unstable, antibiotic therapy should ideally be withheld until results of blood cultures clearly indicate the etiologic agent. If a stable patient has already received a short course of antibiotics, the wise approach is to withhold antibiotics until an organism is obtained by culture. Knowing the specific organism remarkably influences the choice and potential toxicity of the antimicrobial regimen.

Generally, the Duke criteria[7] can be applied to diagnosing PVE if the criteria are applied over time and with the use of transesophageal echocardiography to supplement the use of transthoracic echocardiography. Using this approach, the Duke criteria are highly sensitive and specific for PVE with a negative predictive value of 98 to 99 percent.[8] Transesophageal echocardiography is especially helpful in recognition of invasive disease, the absence of which generally allows continued medical management without valve replacement.

THERAPY

The objective of antimicrobial therapy is to eradicate microorganisms from infected vegetations, where there is a dearth of local host defenses, and from the surfaces of foreign material, where polymorphonuclear function is compromised. Cidal therapy is mandated. Use of static regimens is associated with unacceptable relapse rates in endocarditis.

Once an adequate number of cultures have been obtained, stable patients (especially if they were pretreated) can have antibiotics withheld for a few days until a specific organism is isolated. Therapy can then be tailored to the specific isolate. If a patient is clinically unstable, initial empirical therapy can be started with vancomycin plus gentamicin. Vancomycin is preferred because over 80 percent of *S.* non-*aureus* isolated from PVE occurring within the first year after valve replacement are methicillin-resistant, as are up to 30 percent isolated after 1 year.[4, 9] Gentamicin is administered because it is synergistic with vancomycin against both staphylococci and enterococci. Tobramycin should not be substituted for gentamicin because it is not synergistic with all strains of *Enterococcus.* Although data are scant, aminoglycoside antibiotics probably should not be administered as single daily doses when synergy is the goal. Twice or thrice a day regimens are preferred.

If the patient is more than 1-year post valve replacement, HACEK (*Haemophilus* species, *Actinobacillus actinomycetemcomitans, Cardiobacterium hominus, Eikenella corrodens,* and *Kingella* species) organisms occasionally cause PVE. The addition of a third-generation cephalosporin (e.g., ceftriaxone or cefotaxime) to the empirical regimen is reasonable, pending culture results.

When staphylococci cause PVE, the addition of oral rifampin to a regimen of vancomycin or nafcillin plus gentamicin is preferred despite the fact that rifampin in combination with either vancomycin or nafcillin in the test tube is predictably antagonistic. Combinations with rifampin are clinically synergistic because rifampin penetrates better into different compartments of the infection (e.g., intracellularly and into abscesses) and is most effective in helping to eradicate infection on foreign material. The addition of rifampin to a regimen should theoretically be delayed a few days to allow the other agents to lower the concentration of infecting organisms, thereby minimizing the in vivo development of resistance that is so common with rifampin when it is used as a single agent.

Antimicrobial regimens for specific organisms are listed in Table A–2. As a rule, antibiotics are given parenterally and for 6 weeks, although gentamicin is sometimes given

TABLE A–2 Antimicrobial Therapy for Specific Microorganisms Causing Prosthetic Valve Endocarditis

Organism	Antibiotic	Therapy (wk)
Methicillin-sensitive *Staphylococcus aureus*	Nafcillin +	6–8
	Gentamicin +	2
	Rifampin*	6–8
Methicillin-resistant *S. aureus* or non-*aureus*†	Vancomycin +	6–8
	Gentamicin +	2
	Rifampin*	6–8
Penicillin-susceptible streptococci (MIC ≤ 0.1 μg/ml)	Penicillin G or	6
	Ceftriaxone +	6
	Gentamicin	2
	or	
	Vancomycin	6
Enterococci	Penicillin G or	6
	Ampicillin or	6
	Vancomycin +	6
	Gentamicin	6
Penicillin-resistant streptococci	Penicillin G +	6
	Gentamicin	4
HACEK organisms	Ceftriaxone or	6
	Ampicillin +	6
	Gentamicin	4
Diphtheroids	Penicillin G +	6
	Gentamicin or	6
	Vancomycin	6
Candida species	Amphotericin B	6–8 + surgery

Abbreviations: HACEK, *Haemophilus* species, *Actinobacillus actinomycetemcomitans, Cardiobacterium hominus, Eikenella corrodens,* and *Kingella* species; MIC, minimal inhibitory concentration.

*Start rifampin orally after 3–4 days of parenteral antibiotics.

†Some *S.* non-*aureus* are sensitive to nafcillin, but recognition in the laboratory of so-called heteroresistant strains, which might appear sensitive to nafcillin but require vancomycin, is inconsistent. Treating all *S.* non-*aureus* isolates with vancomycin avoids possible misidentification.

for only 2 to 4 weeks to minimize toxicity. Home intravenous antibiotic therapy has been used successfully to treat some patients with PVE. Patients should be stable and have no signs of invasion before therapy is given outside the hospital.[10] The choice of therapy for aerobic gram-negative bacilli depends on results of susceptibility testing; however, a synergistic regimen should be sought. Vancomycin-resistant enterococci are very difficult to treat because no cidal regimen exists. Consultation with an infectious disease expert should be sought.

SURGERY

Up to 40 to 65 percent of patients with PVE require surgery for optimal outcome.[11] In certain settings, the mortality of PVE approaches 100 percent but drops to 10 to 30 percent with appropriate surgery.[1] Some patients with PVE owing to indolent organisms (e.g., viridans streptococci, HACEK organisms, and enterococci) can predictably be managed without surgery, as long as they do not develop indications of invasive disease or other indications for surgery during the course of medical management.[12] Indications for surgery are listed in Table A–3. The timing of surgery is dictated by the hemodynamic status of the patient. Delaying surgery when a patient is hemodynamically unstable does not lead to a better microbiologic outcome and risks irreversible end-organ damage. Length of antibiotic therapy is based on the operative findings. If any evidence of invasion, continued inflammation, or viable organisms exists at the time of surgery, a full course of antibiotics should follow surgery. If PVE is confined to the prosthesis and intraoperative cultures are negative, then the sum of the preoperative and postoperative antibiotics should equal the usual course of antibiotics for the isolated organism.

TABLE A-3 Indications for Cardiac Surgery in Patients With Prosthetic Valve Endocarditis

Organisms
Staphylococcus aureus
Pseudomonas aeruginosa
Candida species and other fungi
Enterococci without bactericidal therapy
Other gram-negative bacilli including *Brucella* and *Coxiella* species
Infection
Paravalvular extension of infection
Persistent bacteremia despite optimal antibiotic therapy
Unexplained, persistent (>9 days) fever in culture-negative prosthetic valve endocarditis
Relapse after optimal therapy
Valve
Unstable prosthesis
Large, hypermobile vegetation (>10 mm)
Consequences of infection
Regurgitant or stenotic valve dysfunction with moderate to severe congestive heart failure

PREVENTION

Prevention of PVE relies on use of antibiotics in the perioperative period. First- or second-generation cephalosporins are reasonable choices for prevention of wound infections; however, data assessing prevention of PVE are lacking. Before dental and other procedures considered at risk for infective endocarditis by the American Heart Association, persons with prosthetic valves should receive prophylactic antibiotics. Vancomycin should be used for prophylaxis if methicillin-resistant *S. aureus* is prevalent in either the hospital performing cardiac surgery or the hospital referring a patient.

Finally, aggressive and effective management of postoperative nosocomial bacteremia is mandatory to prevent early PVE after valve placement or replacement. As a rule, bacteremia that is likely to have arisen from a site of infection other than the prosthetic valve can be treated with choice and duration of antibiotics aimed at the suspected source.[1] If fever or bacteremia does not clear rapidly or evidence suggesting PVE develops during the course of therapy of bacteremia, the duration of therapy should be lengthened to treat presumed PVE.

REFERENCES

1. Karchmer AC: Infections of prosthetic valves and intravascular devices. *In* Mandell GL, Bennett JE, Dolin R (eds): Principles and Practice of Infectious Diseases. Philadelphia: Churchill Livingstone, 2000, pp. 903–917.
2. Dyson C, Barnes RA, Harrison GA: Infective endocarditis: an epidemiological review of 128 episodes. J Infect 38:87–93, 1999.
3. Agnihotri AK, McGiffin DC, Galbraith AJ, et al: The prevalence of infective endocarditis after aortic valve replacement. J Thorac Cardiovasc Surg 110:1708–1724, 1995.
4. Calderwood SB, Swinski LA, Waternaux CM, et al: Risk factors for the development of prosthetic valve endocarditis. Circulation 72:31–37, 1985.
5. Karchmer AW, Gibbons GW: Infections of prosthetic heart valves and vascular grafts. *In* Bisno AL, Waldvogel FA (eds): Infections Associated with Indwelling Devices. Washington, DC: American Society of Microbiology, 1994, pp. 213–249.
6. John MVD, Hibberd PL, Karchmer AW: *Staphylococcus aureus* prosthetic valve endocarditis: optimal management and risk factors for death. Clin Infect Dis 26:1302–1309, 1998.
7. Durack DT, Lukes AS, Bright DK: New criteria for diagnosis of infective endocarditis: utilization of specific echocardiographic findings. Am J Med 96:200–209, 1994.
8. Bayer AS, Bolger AF, Taubert KA, et al: Diagnosis and management of infective endocarditis and its complications. Circulation 98:2936–2948, 1998.
9. Karchmer AW, Archer GL, Dismukes WE: *Staphylococcus epidermidis* causing prosthetic valve endocarditis: microbiologic and clinical observations as guides to therapy. Ann Intern Med 98:447–455, 1983.
10. Huminer D, Bishara J, Pitlik S: Home intravenous antibiotic therapy for patients with infective endocarditis. Eur J Clin Microbiol Infect Dis 18:330–334, 1999.
11. Calderwood SB, Swinski LA, Karchmer AW, et al: Prosthetic valve endocarditis: analysis of factors affecting outcome of therapy. J Thorac Cardiovasc Surg 92:776–783, 1986.
12. Truninger K, Jost CH, Seifert B, et al: Long term follow up of prosthetic valve endocarditis: what characteristics identify patients who were treated successfully with antibiotics alone? Heart 82:714–720, 1999.

INDEX

Page numbers in *italics* refer to figures.
Page numbers followed by t refer to tables.
Page numbers followed by pl refer to color plates.

A wave, 18, *18*
  "cannon," in myocardial infarction, 543, *545*
AAI pacemaker mode, 1770
Abciximab, for unstable angina, 735t, 810–811, 810t–812t
  with thrombolytic agents, TIMI 14 trial of, 771–772
Abdominal aorta, anomalies of, 175
Abdominal aortic aneurysm(s), *1366–1374,* 1366–1376
  anatomic abnormalities in, 1366, *1367–1368,* 1368
  diagnosis of, computed tomography in, *1366*
    digital subtraction angiography in, *1367,* 1374
    magnetic resonance imaging in, *1366*
    physical examination in, 1368
    radiography in, *1368,* 1374
    ultrasonography in, *1367*
  endovascular treatment of, 1432–1435, *1433–1434,* 1434t–1435t
    history of, 1432
    outcome of, 1434–1435
    stent grafts for, 1433–1434, *1433–1434,* 1434t–1435t
  epidemiology of, 1432
  natural history of, 1374
  rupture of, 1368
  sizing of, 1374
  surgical treatment of, *1369–1373,* 1374–1376
    results of, 1375
Abdominal bruit(s), in renal artery disease, 1402
Abdominal disorder(s), *vs.* pulmonary thromboembolism, 1846
ABIOMED total artificial heart, 1235
ABO compatibility, testing for, before heart transplantation, 1219
Abscess(es), pyogenic, *vs.* pulmonary thromboembolism, 1844
  splenic, from infective endocarditis, 416
ACAS (Asymptomatic Carotid Atherosclerosis Study), 1435
Accelerated ventricular rhythm, 1571, *1571*
Accessory pathway(s), concealed, in circus movement tachycardia, 1610, *1611–1612*
    in paroxysmal supraventricular tachycardia, surgical treatment of, 1823–1824
  in preexcitation, 1620, *1620–1621, 1623*
    ablation of, 1630
    long anterograde refractory period in, 1626, *1629*
  radiofrequency catheter ablation of, 1796–1800, *1797–1801*
    and recurrence of conduction, 1799
    complications of, 1799–1800
    in preexcitation, 1630
Accessory pathway(s) *(Continued)*
    localization in, 1796–1797, *1797*
    optimal site for, 1798, *1799–1800*
    procedure for, 1797–1798, *1798*
    success rate of, 1798–1799, *1801*
ACE inhibitor(s). See *Angiotensin-converting enzyme (ACE) inhibitor(s).*
Acebutolol, adverse effects of, 1749–1750
  dosage of, 712t, 1749
  efficacy of, 1749
  electrophysiology of, 1749
  pharmacokinetics of, 1742t–1743t, 1749
^{11}C-Acetate, clearance rates of, and oxidative metabolism, 121–123
Acetoacetate, in myocardial metabolism, 948–949
Acetylcholine, and endothelial dysfunction, in microcirculatory disease, 641
Acetyl-coenzyme A, breakdown of fuels in heart to, *940*
  in fatty acid metabolism, 947, *947*
Acetyl-coenzyme A dehydrogenase, deficiency of, 2174t
Acidosis, lactic, *vs.* pulmonary thromboembolism, 1847
Aciduria, orotic, hereditary, 2175t
ACIP (Asymptomatic Cardiac Ischemia Pilot Investigators) study, 571, 871, *872*
ACME (Angioplasty Compared to Medicine) trial, 795–796, 870–871
Acquired immunodeficiency syndrome (AIDS). See *Human immunodeficiency virus (HIV) infection.*
Acromegaly, 1916–1917, *1917*
  and hypertension, 1507
  clinical features of, 1508, 1916, *1917*
  diagnosis of, 1916–1917
  pathophysiology of, 1916
  treatment of, 1917
Actin, and contractile function, 989t, 990–991, *991,* 1277, *1278*
  interaction with myosin, and ATP, 991–992, *992*
    and left ventricular relaxation, 1003
Actin gene, in hypertrophic cardiomyopathy, 1057–1058
Actinomyces infection(s), and myocarditis, 1110
Action potential, generation of, 1563, *1564*
  in cardiac hypertrophy, 968–970, *969*
  in long QT syndrome, 1657, *1658*
  in sinus node, 1577, *1577*
  of myocardial cells, ventricular differences in, 30
  phases of, 1563, *1565*
Active relaxation, in diastolic dysfunction, 966–967, 967t
Activin, and left-right position of body axis, 923–924
Activity. See also *Exercise.*
Activity *(Continued)*
  and hypertension control, 2240
  and risk of sudden death, 1713
Adaptor, definition of, 917t
Addison's disease. See *Adrenal insufficiency.*
Adenosine, adverse effects of, 1754
  dosage of, 1754
  efficacy of, 1754
  electrophysiology of, 1754
  pharmacokinetics of, 1742t–1743t, 1754
  with SPECT myocardial perfusion imaging, 104
    after myocardial infarction, 674
Adenosine diphosphate (ADP), in myocardial metabolism, 949
Adenosine triphosphate (ATP), and arteriolar vasomotor function, 523
  and calcium pump, of sarcoplasmic reticulum, 997, *997*
  and energy production, 937, *937*
  concentration of, in energy starvation, 999, 999t
  decreased, in myocardial ischemia, *512,* 512–513
  in cardiac hypertrophy, 1010
  in contractile function, 961–962, *962,* 963t
  interaction of, with actin and myosin, 991–992, *992*
Adenovirus(es), as vectors for gene therapy, 2270, 2271t
Adolescent(s). See *Pediatric population.*
ADP. See *Adenosine diphosphate (ADP).*
Adrenal hyperplasia, congenital, and hypertension, 1506, *1507*
Adrenal insufficiency, clinical features of, 1917–1918
  diagnosis of, 1918
  pathophysiology of, 1917
  treatment of, 1918
Adrenomedullin, and circulatory regulation, 1290
Adriamycin. See *Doxorubicin.*
Aerobic capacity, aging and, 2018–2019, 2019t
AFA-SAK (Copenhagen Atrial Fibrillation, Aspirin, Anticoagulation Study), 2021
AFCAPS/TexCAPS (Air Force/Texas Coronary Atherosclerosis Prevention Study), 2253–2254
African trypanosomiasis, 1111
Afterload, ejection fraction and, in aortic stenosis, 331, *331*
Afterload mismatch, and systolic dysfunction, in aortic stenosis, 331–332
Afterloader(s), for delivery of radiotherapy, 832, *833*
Agatston method, for scoring of coronary artery calcification, 2182
Age/aging, and arrhythmias, 2020–2022, 2021t
  and cerebral circulation, 1689
  and circulatory regulation, 1290

Age/aging *(Continued)*
and classification of hypertension, 1514t
and congestive heart failure, 2022
and coronary artery caliber, 615
and diastolic function, 1007
and dilated cardiomyopathy, 1034
and heart failure, 1147–1148
and hypertension, 2020
and outcome of percutaneous mitral balloon valvotomy, 468
and plasma homocysteine levels, 2278, 2279t
and risk of coronary artery disease, 671–673, 672t
and risk of sudden death, 1711, *1712*
and vascular compliance, 1486–1487
cardiovascular changes with, 2015–2019, *2016,* 2018t–1029t
in beta-adrenergic modulation, 2018–2019, 2018t
in cardiac function at rest, 2017
in cardiac function during exercise, 2017–2018
in vascular structure and function, 2015–2016, *2016*
maternal, and Down's syndrome, 2170
of donor heart, and cardiac allograft vasculopathy, 1192, *1193*
Agricultural toxin(s), and chronic obstructive pulmonary disease, 1886
AIDS. See *Human immunodeficiency virus (HIV) infection.*
Air embolism, from coronary angiography, 606
Air Force/Texas Coronary Atherosclerosis Prevention Study (AFCAPS/TexCAPS), 2253–2254
Alanine, metabolism of, 949
Albuterol, for chronic obstructive pulmonary disease, 1892
Alcohol, abuse of, and malnutrition, 1965
incidence of, 1964
with cocaine abuse, 1961
additives in, toxicity of, 1965
and arrhythmias, 1965–1966
and atherosclerosis, 1966
and cardiomyopathy, 1024, 1039–1040, 1964
natural history of, 1965
treatment of, 1965
and contractile function, 1040
and coronary circulation, 1964–1965
and heart failure, 1166
and hypertension, 1498, 2240–2241, *2241*
myocardial effects of, 1964–1965
restriction of, in management of hypertension, 1515–1516
Aldosterone, synthesis of, *1507*
Aldosterone antagonist(s), for heart failure, 1175
Aldosteronism, and hypertension, 1506
monogenic, 1496, 1497t
diagnosis of, 1510
Allen test, 2121
Allergic reaction(s), and dilated cardiomyopathy, 1044
and myocardial disease, 1092–1093
to anesthetics, 608
to contrast agents, 607–608
Allograft(s), aortic, complications of, 323
for aortic valve replacement, 286, *286–288*
for repair of tetralogy of Fallot, 302
with pulmonary atresia, 303, *303*
rejection of. See *Transplantation, heart, rejection of.*
"tolerance" of, 1219
vasculopathy in. See *Cardiac allograft vasculopathy.*
Allorecognition, 1210
Allosteric effect(s), of adenosine triphosphate, in energy starvation, 999
Alpha half-life, 1739
Alpha$_1$-blocker(s), for hypertension, 1520
Alprenolol, dosage of, 712t
Alteplase, and intracranial bleeding, 756, 767, 767t
efficacy of, 768–769, *769*
Amantadine, for influenza prophylaxis, 1894
Ambulatory electrocardiography. See *Holter monitoring.*
Amebiasis, *vs.* pulmonary thromboembolism, 1844
American trypanosomiasis, 1110–1111
Amino acid(s), in myocardial metabolism, 949
Aminorex, and pulmonary hypertension, 1865
Amiodarone, adverse effects of, 1750–1751
and pituitary-thyroid function, 1927
and thyrotoxicosis, 1928
dosage of, 1750
during pregnancy, 2045t, 2046
efficacy of, 1750–1751
electrophysiology of, 1750
for atrial fibrillation, 1637t, 1638
in hypertrophic cardiomyopathy, 1068
for heart failure, 1175
for preexcitation, 1626, 1630t
for prevention of sudden death, 1726
for supraventricular tachycardia, during pregnancy, 2042
pharmacokinetics of, 1742t–1743t, 1750
Amlodipine, dosage of, 713t
for heart failure, 1173
for silent myocardial ischemia, 575
^{13}N-Ammonia, for positron emission tomography, 118
Amniotic fluid embolism, 2037, 2038t
vs. pulmonary thromboembolism, 1847–1848
Amphetamine(s), cardiovascular complications of, 1966
Ampicillin, for infective endocarditis, 407, 407t
Amplatzer ASD occlusion device, 276–277
Amputation, from peripheral vascular disease, rates of, 1404
Amrinone, for heart failure, 1174
Amyloid heart disease, 1082–1086, 1082t, *1083–1087*
classification of, 1082, 1082t
diagnosis of, 1083–1085, *1083–1085*
angiocardiography in, 1085
cardiac catheterization in, 1085, *1085*
computed tomography in, 1085
echocardiography in, 1085, 1139–1141, *1140*
electrocardiography in, 1083, *1084*
endomyocardial biopsy in, 1085
magnetic resonance imaging in, 1085
physical examination in, 1083
radiography in, 1083
radionuclide imaging in, 1085
differential diagnosis of, 1085–1086
pathophysiology of, 1082–1083, *1083*
treatment of, 1086, *1087*
Amyloidosis, 2175t
cardiac, anatomic abnormalities in, 318
pathologic changes in, 1030, 1030pl
Anacrotic pulse, *16,* 16–17, 17t
Anaerobic threshold, in heart failure, *1158*
Anagrelide, for thrombocythemia, 2006–2007
Analog-to-digital converter, in radionuclide imaging, 100
Anemia, 2001–2004, *2002–2003*
cardiovascular manifestations of, 2001
Anemia *(Continued)*
diagnosis of, 2001, *2002*
drugs and, 2007–2008, 2008t
hemolytic, *2003,* 2003–2004
sickle cell, 2001–2002
Anesthesia, cardiovascular response to, 2117, 2117t
for cardiovascular surgery, 2104–2114
administration of maintenance medications before, 2105
agents for, 2106–2108, 2107t–2108t
airway devices for, 2106
hemodynamic monitoring in, 2108–2109
history of, 2104–2105
in aortic insufficiency, 2111
in aortic stenosis, 2111
in cardiac transplantation, 2111–2112
in cardiomyopathy, 2111
in coronary artery disease, 2111
in mitral insufficiency, 2111
in mitral stenosis, 2111
induction of, 2109–2110, 2110t
intravenous fluids for, 2106
maintenance of, 2110–2111
operating room for, 2106
patient positioning for, 2110
postoperative care in, 2114
premedication for, 2105–2106
preoperative assessment and, 2105
resuscitation drugs for, 2106, 2106t
for noncardiac surgery, 2097–2098
obstetric, 2061t–2062t
hemodynamic response to, 2030–2031
hypertrophic cardiomyopathy and, 2055
Anesthetic(s), allergic reactions to, 608
Aneurysm(s), after balloon angioplasty, for aortic coarctation, 266
after myocardial infarction, 554, *555*
aortic. See *Aortic aneurysm(s).*
cardiac, pathologic changes in, 1031–1032, *1032*
from balloon angioplasty, *644*
in polyarteritis nodosum, 1949, *1949*
left ventricular, annular subvalvular, pathologic changes in, 1032
mycotic, from infective endocarditis, 415–416
of coronary artery, *510*
of sinus of Valsalva, 227
echocardiography in, 250–251
ventricular, and cardiomegaly, 10
from myocardial infarction, echocardiography in, 662
in survivors of myocardial infarction, 776
ventricular septal, after closure of ventricular septal defect, 245
ANF (atrial natriuretic factor), in hypertension, 1501, *1501*
Angel wings device, for closure of atrial septal defect, 273, 275, *275*
Angiitis, Churg-Strauss, 1950
hypersensitivity, 1950
Angina, chest pain from, 5, 5t
diagnosis of, electrocardiography in, *44*
physical examination in, 530–531, *531*
during pregnancy, management of, 2047
endorphins and, 570
in aortic stenosis, left ventricular dysfunction and, 331
in thyrotoxicosis, 1927
"ischemic burden" and, 570–571
management of, aging and, 2019–2020
pathology of, 509–511
stable, medical treatment of, 709–721
angiotensin-converting enzyme inhibitors in, 720–721

Angina *(Continued)*
beta-blockers in, 709–711, 711t–712t, *713*
calcium channel blockers in, 711–715, 711t–715t, *714*
clopidrogel in, *717,* 717–718
combination therapy in, 715
nitrates in, 709, *710,* 711t
platelet antagonists in, 715–717, *716,* 717t
risk factor reduction in, 718, *719–720*
vs. angioplasty, 718
pathophysiology of, 528–531, *529–531*
percutaneous transluminal coronary intervention for, 791–799. See also *Percutaneous transluminal coronary intervention (PTCI).*
unstable, antiplatelet agents for, 809–811, 810t–812t, *812*
Braunwald classification of, 724t
coronary artery bypass graft for, 737–738, *738*
directional coronary atherectomy in, 809
glycoprotein IIb/IIIa antagonists for, 730–737, *731–735,* 735t–737t, 810–811, 810t–812t
invasive *vs.* conservative treatment in, 813–815, 814t–815t
medical treatment of, 723–740, 815–816, *816*
algorithm for, *724, 816*
aspirin with heparin in, 723, *725*
CAPTURE study of, 732, *732*
ESSENCE study of, 729–730
low–molecular-weight heparin in, 726–730, *728,* 729t, *730*
platelet antagonists in, 723, *724–725,* 726
platelet glycoprotein IIb/IIIa antagonists in, 730–737, *731–735,* 735t–737t
PRISM study of, 733, 735t–736t
PRISM-PLUS study of, 733–734, *734,* 735t–736t
PURSUIT study of, 732–733, *733,* 735t–736t
TIMI II study of, 729, *730*
natural history of, 696–697
pathophysiology of, 531–532, 738–739
percutaneous transluminal coronary intervention for, 802–816. See also *Percutaneous transluminal coronary intervention (PTCI).*
physical examination in, 532, *533*
prognosis in, 803–804, 804t–805t
troponin and, 813, *813*
risk factors for, 739–740
stenting for, 807–809, 807t–809t, *808*
transluminal extraction atherectomy for, 809
variant (Prinzmetal), medical treatment of, 738, *739*
natural history of, 697–699, *699*
pathophysiology of, 532, 534, *534*
vasospastic. See *Angina, variant (Prinzmetal).*
Angiocardiography, in amyloid heart disease, 1085
in hemochromatosis, 1087
in mitral valve prolapse, 362–363, *363–364*
in restrictive cardiomyopathy, 1080, *1081*
radionuclide, first pass, *106,* 106–107
Angiogenesis, therapeutic. See *Therapeutic angiogenesis.*
vs. arteriogenesis, in development of collateral circulation, 525
Angiography, carbon dioxide digital, in renovascular hypertension, 1429–1430
Angiography *(Continued)*
contrast, in arrhythmogenic right ventricular dysplasia, 1668–1669, *1670*
in cardiac myxoma, 1905
in carotid artery disease, 1401
in renal artery disease, 1403
limitations of, 1460, *1464*
coronary. See *Coronary angiography.*
digital subtraction, in abdominal aortic aneurysms, *1367,* 1374
in pulmonary hypertension, *1876,* 1876–1877
renal, in renovascular hypertension, 1429–1430
Angioplasty, balloon. See *Balloon angioplasty.*
for cardiogenic shock, *1534,* 1534–1535
percutaneous, coronary. See *Percutaneous transluminal coronary angioplasty (PTCA).*
for peripheral vascular disease, of lower extremities, 1413
for renal artery disease, 1404
for subclavian artery occlusive disease, 1440–1441, *1441–1442,* 1441t
SPECT myocardial perfusion imaging after, 675–676
tibioperoneal, 1438–1439, 1439t
Angioplasty balloon dilatation, of atrial septal defect, 280
Angioplasty Compared to Medicine (ACME) trial, 795–796, 870–871
Angiorad Radiation for Restenosis Trial (ARREST), 835–836
Angiorad Radiation Technology for In-Stent Restenosis Trial in Native Coronaries (ARTISTIC), 835
Angiosarcoma, intracavitary, 1908, *1908*
Angiotensin II, and circulatory regulation, 1290
Angiotensin receptor(s), and hypertension, 1500, 1503, *1503*
in cardiac hypertrophy, 964
in myocardial fibrosis, 966
Angiotensin receptor antagonist(s), for heart failure, 1173–1174
diastolic, 1013
for hypertension, 1520
in survivors of acute myocardial infarction, 776
Angiotensin-converting enzyme (ACE) gene, and risk of coronary artery disease, 695
polymorphism of, and hypertension, 1497–1498
Angiotensin-converting enzyme (ACE) inhibitor(s), action of, 1168–1169, 1518–1519
and renal function, 1519, *1519*
during pregnancy, 2065
for heart failure, 1168–1170, *1169,* 1170t
diastolic, 1013
for hypertension, 1517t, 1518–1519, 1519t
for left ventricular hypertrophy, 985
for mitral regurgitation, 353
for myocarditis, 1106
for prevention of sudden death, 1725
for renal artery disease, 1403
for renovascular hypertension, 1524
for ventricular septal defect, in survivors of myocardial infarction, 775
HOPE trial of, 720–721
in aortic dissection, 1383
in diabetic patient, 1924
in survivors of myocardial infarction, 776, *776,* 777t
side effects of, 1519
Anistreplase, antigenicity of, 744
Ankle-brachial index, in peripheral vascular disease, 1406–1407, 1406t, *1407*
in subclinical atherosclerosis, 2252–2253
Ankylosing spondylitis, 1952–1954, *1952–1954*
Annexin, as anticoagulant mechanism, 1319
Annular calcification, radiography of, 71–72
Annular subvalvular left ventricular aneurysm(s), pathologic changes in, 1032
Annuloaortic ectasia, *1388,* 1388–1389
surgical treatment of, 1362
Annuloplasty, for mitral insufficiency, 489–490, *489–490*
Anorexic agent(s), and pulmonary hypertension, 1862, *1863*
valvular disease from, 453
ANPs (atrial natriuretic peptides), in cardiac hypertrophy, 967–968
Anthracycline, and cardiomyopathy, 1024, *1025,* 1041
Antiarrhythmic agent(s), 1739–1755
and anemia, 2008t
and risk of sudden death, 1715
and sinus node dysfunction, 1589
classification of, 1740–1741, 1740t–1741t, *1741*
during pregnancy, 2043–2046, 2044t–2045t, 2063–2064
electrocardiographic effects of, 1742t
for atrial fibrillation, 1636–1638, 1637t
long-term, 1641, *1641–1642*
risks of, 1639–1641, *1640–1641*
for heart failure, 1175
for myocarditis, 1106
for prevention of sudden death, 1725–1727, *1726,* 1730
in arrhythmogenic right ventricular dysplasia, 1673
in older adults, 2022
pharmacokinetics of, 1739–1740, 1742t
states blocked by, 1740t
use dependency of, *1741*
Antiarrhythmics Versus Implantable Defibrillators (AVID) trial, 1069, 1788
Antibiotic(s), and infectious hypothesis in atherosclerosis, 1338
and myocardial hypersensitivity reactions, 1092
for chronic obstructive pulmonary disease, 1894
for endocarditis, in prosthetic valves, 2287–2288, 2287t–2288t
prophylactic, after valvular surgery, 498
during labor and delivery, for infective endocarditis, 2038–2039, 2039t
in patient with congenital heart disease, 2058
for dental procedures, 414t
in rheumatic fever, 397–398, *398*
Antibody(ies), antistreptococcal, in rheumatic fever, 393
for immunosuppressive therapy, 1212–1213
in transplant rejection, 1217–1218
Anticholinergic agent(s), for chronic obstructive pulmonary disease, 1892
Anticoagulant(s), and anemia, 2008t
for heart failure, 1175
for pulmonary hypertension, 1878, 1879–1880
preoperative discontinuation of, 2092
with first-generation thrombolytic agents, 746
Anticoagulant pathway(s), in coagulation system, *1316,* 1318–1319
Anticoagulant protein(s), structure of, 1315–1316, 1317t

Anticoagulation, after valvular surgery, 495, 498
during cardiopulmonary bypass, 2113
during coronary angiography, 602–603
complications of, 608
during pregnancy, 228, 2039–2040, *2040–2041*
for arrhythmias, with syncope, 1703
for embolism prophylaxis, in atrial fibrillation, 1642–1643, 1643t
for pulmonary thromboembolism, 1848
in aortic thromboembolism, 1394
in mitral stenosis, 349
with cardioversion and transesophageal echocardiography, for atrial fibrillation, 1651–1653, *1652,* 1653t
Antidepressant(s), tricyclic, electrocardiographic changes from, 53
Antifibrinolytic agent(s), for intraoperative blood conservation, 2112
Antihypertensive agent(s). See also specific drugs and drug classes.
and autonomic dysfunction, 1554
and prevention of cardiovascular disease, *1512,* 1512–1513, 1513t
and risk of coronary artery disease, 2202
during pregnancy, 2050t–2051t
for diabetic patient, 1924
for left ventricular hypertrophy, 985–986
for renal artery disease, 1403
in aortic dissection, 1383–1384
in heart transplant recipients, 1197
new classes of, 2051t
Anti-idiotypic antibody(ies), in viral myocarditis, 1100–1101
Antilymphocyte antibody, for post-transplantation infection, 1190–1191
Antimyosin imaging, 112, *112–113*
in allograft rejection, 1145
in myocarditis, 1144
Antiphospholipid antibody(ies), hypercoagulable states in, 2010
in systemic lupus erythematosus, 1944, 1944pl, 1944t
Antiplatelet agent(s), for myocardial infarction, with stenting, 823
for peripheral vascular disease, of lower extremities, 1412
for unstable angina, 809–811, 810t–812t, *812*
preoperative discontinuation of, 2092
with thrombolytic agents, 751–752
Antiporter(s), in excitation-contraction coupling, *1281*
α_1-Antiprotease deficiency, and chronic obstructive pulmonary disease, 1886–1887, 1894–1895
Antischkow cell(s), in rheumatic fever, 389
Antistreptococcal antibody(ies), in rheumatic fever, 393
Antitachycardic pacing (ATP), by implantable cardioverter-defibrillator, 1784–1785, *1786*
Antithrombin, as anticoagulant mechanism, 1319
deficiency of, 2175t
Antithrombin III, deficiency of, and hypercoagulable states, 2009, 2009t
α_1-Antitrypsin deficiency, and chronic obstructive pulmonary disease, 1886–1887
Antiviral agent(s), for human immunodeficiency virus infection, and cardiomyopathy, 1980–1981
Anxiety, and chest pain, 6
symptoms of, *vs.* mitral valve prolapse, 376
Aorta, acquired disorders of, 1354, 1355t
anatomy of, 1354, *1355*
Aorta *(Continued)*
aneurysms of. See *Aortic aneurysm(s).*
arteritis in, 1389–1392, 1389t
congenital disorders of, 1354, 1354t
dissecting hematoma of, *vs.* pulmonary thromboembolism, 1845
dissection of. See *Aortic dissection.*
infections of, 1393
layers of, 1354
origin of, in tetralogy of Fallot, 171, *171*
physiology of, 1354
pseudocoarctation of, 1357–1358, *1359*
radiography of, 72
thoracic, magnetic resonance imaging of, 135–136, *135–136*
transposition of, with pulmonary artery, complete, 210, *211*
congenitally corrected, 212, *213–216*
echocardiography in, 249–250
trauma to, 1392
tumors of, 1394
Aortic allograft(s), complications of, 323
Aortic anastomosis, in heart transplantation, *1229,* 1230
Aortic aneurysm(s), abdominal. See *Abdominal aortic aneurysm(s).*
diagnosis of, computed tomography in, electron beam, 2187, *2188*
inflammatory, 1394–1396, *1395*
magnetic resonance imaging in, *134*
thoracic. See *Thoracic aortic aneurysm(s).*
Aortic arch, anomalies of, 174–175, *174–176*
double, 174, *174–175*
left, 174, *174*
right, 174–175, *174–176*
Aortic balloon valvuloplasty, percutaneous, 476–481, *477–480,* 478t–480t. See also *Percutaneous aortic balloon valvuloplasty.*
Aortic coarctation, 156, *157–158,* 1354–1357, *1356–1358*
anatomic abnormalities in, 1354–1355, *1356*
and hypertension, 1506
and pregnancy, 2059
balloon angioplasty for, 265–267
collateral circulation in, 156, *158*
diagnosis of, 194–195, *194–195,* 1357, *1357–1358*
echocardiography in, 248
magnetic resonance imaging in, 136, *136*
natural history of, 1355–1357, *1357–1358*
pathophysiology of, 193–194
pregnancy and, 228
prognosis in, 195
rupture of, 1356
symptoms of, 1356
treatment of, 195
surgical, 295, 299, *299*
types of, *1356*
with bicuspid aortic valve, 1355, *1356,* 2154–2155
Aortic cusp, extension of, with autologous pericardium, 289, *292*
Aortic dilatation, coronary angiography in, 604
Aortic dissection, *1376–1387,* 1376–1388, 1380t, 1384t
classification of, *1377,* 1377–1378
diagnosis of, computed tomography in, *1376,* 1379, 1380t
electron beam, 2187, *2188*
echocardiography in, 454
imaging studies in, 72
initial evaluation in, 1382–1383
magnetic resonance imaging in, *135,* 135–136, *1376,* 1379, 1380t
physical examination in, 1378–1379
radiography in, 1379, 1382, *1382*
Aortic dissection *(Continued)*
transesophageal echocardiography in, 1379, 1380t, *1381*
differential diagnosis of, 1379
during pregnancy, 2049, 2051
etiology of, 1378, *1378,* 1378t
familial, 2154–2155
from aortic coarctation, 156, *157*
from balloon angioplasty, intravascular ultrasonography in, 1457–1458, *1458*
in Marfan's syndrome, 191, *192,* 2150–2151
medical treatment of, 1383–1384, 1384t
pathophysiology of, *1374,* 1374–1375, *1377*
surgical treatment of, 1383–1387, 1384t, *1385–1387*
anesthesia in, 1385
contraindications to, 1384
Dacron graft in, 1384
indications for, 1384t
open technique in, 1384, *1385–1387*
postoperative care in, 1387
results of, 1387
with aortic insufficiency, 1384
with type III dissection, 1384–1385
symptoms of, 1378
with Marfan's syndrome, 1387–1389
Aortic gradient, after percutaneous aortic balloon valvuloplasty, 477–478, 478t
Aortic homograft(s), for repair of tetralogy of Fallot, 302
Aortic impedance, measurement of, 1485, *1486*
Aortic insufficiency, cardiovascular surgery in, anesthesia for, 2111
echocardiography in, 445–446
Aortic jet velocity, in aortic stenosis, 328, *329*
Aortic pressure, central, waveform from, 1486
Aortic regurgitation, 160–161, *161–162,* 191–192, *191–192,* 335–339
diagnosis of, cardiac catheterization in, 429, *430–431,* 431
Doppler echocardiography in, 82–83, *83*
during pregnancy, 2057
from ventricular septal defect, 161, *162*
in ankylosing spondylitis, *1954*
in aortic dissection, 1379
natural history of, in acute form, 338
in chronic form, 338, 338t, *339*
noncardiac surgery in, 2100–2101
pathophysiology of, 335–336, *336*
in acute form, 335–336, *336*
in chronic form, 335, *336*
physical examination in, 336–338, *338*
in acute form, 337–338
in chronic form, 337, *337*
progression of, hemodynamic factors in, *290*
radionuclide studies in, 459–460, *460*
severity of, calculation of, 446, 446pl
survival rates in, *329*
treatment of, 191–192
medical, 338–339
surgical, 286, 289, *290–292*
valve-sparing, 289, *291*
with cusp extension, 289, *292*
with aortic stenosis, 328
Aortic root, dilatation of, in Marfan's syndrome, 454, *454,* 2150, *2151*
Aortic sinus, aneurysms of, congenital, 163, *165*
inappropriate, anomalous coronary artery origin from, 301
Aortic stenosis, 150–151, *150–151,* 180–182, *181–184,* 325–335
and outcome of coronary artery bypass graft, 330
and pregnancy, 2059
aortic valve area in, measurement of, 327–328

Aortic stenosis *(Continued)*
balloon valvuloplasty for, 260–261
calcific, cardiac catheterization in, 427, *428*
cardiovascular surgery in, anesthesia for, 2111
congenital, percutaneous aortic balloon valvuloplasty for, 481
diagnosis of, cardiac catheterization in, 427, *427–430,* 429
Doppler echocardiography in, 81–82, *82,* 326–328
color-flow, 327
morphologic assessment in, 327
echocardiography in, 444–445, 444t, *445*
hemodynamic assessment in, 327–328
physical examination in, 326, *326*
during pregnancy, 2057
in atrial fibrillation, 328
in rheumatic fever, 397
left ventricular dysfunction in, 330–335, *331–334*
and angina, 331
and heart failure, *331,* 331–332
and prognosis with surgery, 334–335
clinical implications of, 332–335, *333–334,* 334t
with low ejection fraction/high gradient, 332, *333*
with low ejection fraction/low cardiac output/low transvalvular gradient, 332–334, *333–334,* 334t
medical treatment of, 330
natural history of, 328–330, *329–330, 331*
noncardiac surgery in, 2100
pathophysiology of, 325–326
severe, 325
severity of, aortic valve resistance and, 335
subvalvular, 182
echocardiography in, 247
supravalvular, 153–154, *154–155,* 182, *184,* 2155–2156
and ventricular outflow tract obstruction, surgical treatment of, 295, *298*
echocardiography in, 247
surgical treatment of, 285–286, *286–289*
valvular, 180–182, *181–183*
course of, 180
diagnosis of, 181–182, *182–183*
echocardiography in, 247–248
pathophysiology of, 180
with aortic regurgitation, cardiac catheterization in, 431
with reduced left ventricular function, 328
with regurgitation, 328
with subaortic stenosis, 328
Aortic thromboembolic disease, 1393–1394
Aortic valve, anatomy of, 149
bicuspid. See *Bicuspid aortic valve.*
quadricuspid, anatomic abnormalities in, 315
Aortic valve area (AVA), calculation of, continuity equation for, 444
in aortic stenosis, 82, *82,* 327–328
cardiac output and, 334t
flow and, 334, *334*
Gorlin equation for, determination of, 427, 429, *429*
nitroprusside and, 335
Aortic valve disease. See also *Aortic regurgitation; Aortic stenosis.*
echocardiography in, *442–445,* 442–446, 443t–444t
Aortic valve replacement, 285–286, *286–289,* 493, *494–497*
for aortic regurgitation, 339
for left ventricular hypertrophy, 986
for rheumatic fever, 397
Aortic valve replacement *(Continued)*
grafts for, 286, *286–288*
percutaneous aortic balloon valvuloplasty as bridge to, 479–480, 479t, *480*
vs. percutaneous aortic balloon valvuloplasty, 481
Aortic valve resistance, and severity of aortic stenosis, 335
Aorticopulmonary window, 220, *221*
Aortitis, anatomic abnormalities in, 317
syphilitic, 1393
Aortography, in aortic regurgitation, 431, *431*
Aortopulmonary collateral artery(ies), in tetralogy of Fallot with pulmonary atresia, 303, *303*
Apo-CIII, and very low-density lipoprotein, 1346
Apoptosis, in cardiac hypertrophy, 960–961
in myocardial ischemia, 513
in myocytes, pathologic changes in, 1031
of vascular cells, modulators of, 1302
Aprotinin, for intraoperative blood conservation, 2112
APSAC, dosage of, 745
side effects of, 767–768
Arachnodactyly, 175–176
Argentine Randomized Trial of Coronary Angioplasty *versus* Bypass Surgery in Multivessel Disease (ERACI), *796,* 797t, 893t, 894
Argyria, *vs.* cyanosis, 13
ARREST (Angiorad Radiation for Restenosis Trial), 835–836
Arrhythmia(s). See also specific type, e.g., *Atrial fibrillation.*
after heart transplantation, 1200
aging and, 2020–2022, 2021t
alcohol and, 1965–1966
and syncope, 1691–1695, 1693t–1694t, *1694*
treatment of, 1703–1704
cocaine and, 1963
congenital, 227
diagnosis of, exercise testing in, 590
during cardiovascular surgery, 2112
during coronary angiography, 608–609
during pregnancy, 2040–2046, *2042,* 2044t–2045t
management of, 228
during pulmonary artery catheterization, 2126–2127
during reperfusion, and risk of sudden death, 1715
during space flight, 2083, *2084*
fetal, 2063–2064
from contrast agents, 608–609
heart rate variability and, 2222–2223
in autonomic dysfunction, 1542
in cardiac hypertrophy, 973
in chronic obstructive pulmonary disease, 1889
in mitral valve prolapse, 364–365, 382–383
in muscular dystrophy, Duchenne's, *1990,* 1990–1991, 1991t
in preexcitation, 1622, *1623–1626,* 1625
in sinus node dysfunction, 1576, 1579–1582, *1581–1582*
progression of, 1588
palpitations in, 7
radiofrequency catheter ablation of. See *Radiofrequency catheter ablation.*
Arrhythmogenic right ventricular dysplasia (ARVD), 1665–1674
anatomic abnormalities in, 1669–1670
and sudden death, 1717–1718, *1718*
classification of, 1665t
diagnosis of, contrast angiography in, 1668–1669, *1670*
Arrhythmogenic right ventricular dysplasia (ARVD) *(Continued)*
echocardiography in, 1667
transesophageal, 1667–1668
electrocardiography in, 1666, *1667–1668*
electrophysiologic studies in, 1669–1670
endomyocardial biopsy in, 1669
magnetic resonance imaging in, 1668, *1669*
radiography in, *1667–1668*
signal averaging in, 1666–1667
familial, 1671
pathogenesis of, 1671
pathology of, 1670–1671, *1672*
risk stratification in, 1674
sudden death from, in young adults, 1671
symptoms of, 1665–1666
treatment of, antiarrhythmic agents in, 1673
heart transplantation in, 1674
implantable cardioverter-defibrillator in, 1673
radiofrequency catheter ablation in, 1673–1674
surgical, 1826–1827, *1826–1829*
with left ventricular involvement, 1672–1673
with myocarditis, 1672–1673
with right precordial ST segment elevation, 1673
Arterial blood gas(es), in pulmonary hypertension, 1866, 1867t
in pulmonary thromboembolism, 1840
Arterial compliance, aging and, 1486–1487
and left ventricular function, 1480
atherosclerosis and, 1488
definition of, 1480, 1491
diabetes mellitus and, 1490
hypertension and, 1488–1490
measurement of, 1483–1487, *1484–1486,* 1484t
direct, 1483–1485, *1484*
indirect, 1484t, *1485–1486,* 1485–1487
smooth muscle relaxation and, 1481–1482, *1482,* 1482t
Arterial disease(s). See also specific type, e.g., *Atherosclerosis.*
degenerative, 1400
dysplastic, 1400
occlusive, thrombolytic therapy for. See *Thrombolytic therapy, for arterial occlusion.*
types of, 1399
Arterial gene therapy, for restenosis, 1421–1422
Arterial pressure. See also *Blood pressure.*
and cerebral blood flow, 1688, *1690*
intraoperative monitoring of, 2119–2123, *2120–2122*
complications of, 2121
direct methods for, 2119–2120, *2120*
noninvasive, 2122–2123
waveform in, *2120–2122,* 2121
space flight and, 2082–2083
"spike-and-dome" configuration of, in cardiomyopathy, hypertrophic, 1130, *1131*
waveforms from, 1482–1483, *1483*
Arterial pulse, abnormalities of, 16–17, *17,* 17t
Arterial switch surgery, echocardiography after, 249–250
takedown of, 306
Arterial trunk, solitary, 171–172, *173*
Arterial wall, layers of, 1275, *1275*
Maxwell model of, 1481, *1481*
zones of, 1480
Arteriogenesis, *vs.* angiogenesis, in development of collateral circulation, 525

Arteriography, in Takayasu's arteritis, 1951, *1951*
pulmonary, in pulmonary thromboembolism, 1841, *1842*
Arteriole(s), coronary, as resistance vessels, 523
Arteriosclerosis, definition of, 1325
Arteriovenous fistula(s), and vascular remodeling, 1304
Gianturco coil occluding device for, 271
pulmonary, 169–170, *170*
systemic, 170
Arteritis, aortic, 1389–1392, 1389t
giant cell, 1391–1392, 1950
Takayasu's, 1950–1951, *1951*. See also *Takayasu's arteritis.*
Artery(ies), physiology of, 1479–1480
and compliance, 1480
stiffness of, aging and, 2015–2016, *2016*
Arthritis, in rheumatic fever, 390
rheumatoid. See *Rheumatoid arthritis.*
Artifact(s), on magnetic resonance imaging, 134, *135*
on pulmonary artery catheterization, 2128, *2128*
on radiography, 65, *66–67*
on SPECT myocardial perfusion imaging, 105
Artificial heart, 1231, 1235. See also *Left ventricular assist device; Mechanical circulatory support.*
ARTISTIC (Angiorad Radiation Technology for In-Stent Restenosis Trial in Native Coronaries), 835
ARVD. See *Arrhythmogenic right ventricular dysplasia (ARVD).*
Ascending aortic aneurysm(s), thoracic, surgical treatment of, *1360–1361*, 1361–1362
Aschoff nodule(s), in rheumatic fever, 388–389, *389*
in rheumatic myocarditis, 1026–1027, *1027*, 1027pl
Ascites, in pericarditis, constrictive, 1262
ASD. See *Atrial septal defect.*
ASDOS (Atrial Septal Defect Occluding System), 276
Ashman's phenomenon, 1569
Aspergillus infection(s), and infective endocarditis, 405
and myocarditis, 1110
Aspirin, and prognosis in unstable angina, 804t–805t
and thrombocythemia, 2006
for atrial fibrillation, in older adults, 2021
for embolism prophylaxis, in atrial fibrillation, 1643, 1643t
for rheumatic fever, 397
in myocardial infarction, cocaine-induced, 1963
mechanism of action of, 716, *716*
prophylactic, in coronary artery disease, 716
side effects of, 717t
with heparin, and mortality, 766t
for unstable angina, 723, *725*
with streptokinase, efficacy of, 745
with thrombolytic agents, 751–753
Asthma, *vs.* pulmonary thromboembolism, 1844
Asymmetric septal hypertrophy. See *Cardiomyopathy, hypertrophic.*
Asymptomatic Cardiac Ischemia Pilot Investigators (ACIP) study, 571, 871, *872*
Asymptomatic Carotid Atherosclerosis Study (ACAS), 1435
Asystolic pause, prolonged, in sinus node dysfunction, 1582
Ataxia, Friedreich's, 1986t, 1988
Atelectasis, rales in, 11
vs. pulmonary thromboembolism, 1844
Atenolol, dosage of, 712t
during pregnancy, 2066
for silent mycocardial ischemia, 575
Atherectomy, burrs for, *790*
devices for, 1440, *1440*
directional coronary, for stable angina, 793–794, 794t
for unstable angina, 809
intravascular ultrasonography during, 1469, 1471, *1471*
for stable angina, 793–794, 794t
high-speed rotational, *790*, 794
transluminal extraction, for unstable angina, 809
Atherogenic dyslipidemia, 2254
studies of, 2249
Atherogenic lifestyle, 2203–2205, 2203t–2205t, *2204*
Atheroma(s), composition of, 1342
Atherosclerosis, acceleration of, smoking and, 2229
aging and, 2019–2020
alcohol and, 1966
and angina, 528, *529*
and peripheral vascular disease, of lower extremities, 1404, *1404–1405*
and renal artery disease, 1402, *1402*
and sinus node dysfunction, 1578
and stroke, 1401, *1401*
and sudden death, 510
and vascular compliance, 1488
and vascular remodeling, 1305–1306
angiographically inapparent, 626
B-mode ultrasonography in, 1446–1451. See also *Ultrasonography, B-mode.*
circulatory dysfunction and, 1295
cocaine and, 1962
compliance of stenosis in, 522
coronary angiography in, 625–638, *627–636*. See also *Coronary angiography, in atherosclerosis.*
definition of, 1325
early events in, 1326–1330, *1327–1329*, 1330t–1332t
in allograft. See *Cardiac allograft vasculopathy.*
in angina pectoris, 509–510
in diabetes mellitus, 1922
in peroneal artery, 1438
in saphenous vein grafts, 516, *517*
treatment of, 879–880, 880t, *881–882*
in tibial artery, 1438
intimal-medial thickness in. See *Intimal-medial thickness (IMT).*
leukocyte-endothelial reactions in, 1330–1331, 1332t
lifestyle promoting, 2203–2205, 2203t–2205t, *2204*
morphology of, 1341–1343
in type I lesions, 1341–1342
in type II lesions, 1342
in type III lesions, 1342
in type IV lesions, 1342
in type V lesions, 1342
in type VI lesions, 1342
in type VII lesions, 1342
in type VIII lesions, 1342–1343
pathogenesis of, *1327–1329*, 1327–1330, 1330t–1331t, 1336–1341, *1339*
infectious hypothesis in, 1336–1338
inflammatory hypothesis in, 1336–1338
lipid hypothesis in, 1338–1341, *1339*
monoclonal hypothesis in, 1336
Atherosclerosis *(Continued)*
response to injury hypothesis in, 1341
pathologic anatomy of, 1325–1326, *1326–1327*
pathophysiology of, 504–505, *504–506*
prevention of, primary, in intermediate-risk patients, 2253–2255
in older adults, 2254–2255
population-based, 2255
progression of, factors affecting, 1325, 2221–2222
renal, progression of, 1428
risk factor(s) for, 1343–1351, 1399–1400
diabetes mellitus as, 1344–1345
hyperlipidemia as, 1345–1348. See also *Hyperlipidemia.*
hypertension as, 1343
obesity as, 1350
physical inactivity as, 1350–1351
psychological stress as, 1351
smoking as, 1343–1344, 2227
thrombosis as, 1348–1350
subclinical, and primary prevention of hyperlipidemia, 2251–2253, *2252*
Atherosclerosis Risk in Communities study, 1344
Atherosclerotic plaque(s), calcification in, intravascular ultrasonography in, *1456*, 1456–1457
composition of, 504, *504*
embolization of, 1394
erosion of, *vs.* rupture, 580–582, *581*
formation of, 504–505, *505*
growth of, 1331–1333, 1333t
in carcinoid syndrome, 1930, *1931*
monitoring of, coronary angiography in, 2248–2249
morphology of, gender and, 584, 584t
intravascular ultrasonography in, 1457–1458, *1458*
pathology of, 1325–1326, *1326–1327*
rupture of, and sudden death, 579–580
and thrombosis, 505, *507–509*, 509
pathologic-angiographic correlation in, 633–634, *633–634*
vs. erosion, 580–582, 580t, *581*
unstable, pathophysiology of, 536–543, *538–542*, 541t, 802–803, *803*
inflammation in, 536, *537–540*
matrix metalloproteinases in, 538–540, 541t
upregulation of integrins in, 536, *537*
upregulation of vascular call adhesion molecules in, 536, *537*
vulnerable, and risk factors for coronary artery disease, in women, 584, 584t
Athlete(s), left ventricular hypertrophy in, 1009–1010
sudden death in, causes of, *1717*
ATP. See *Adenosine triphosphate (ATP).*
ATP (antitachycardic pacing), by implantable cardioverter-defibrillator, 1784–1785, *1786*
Atrial defibrillation, for sinus node dysfunction, 1590–1591
Atrial ectopic rhythm, disturbances of, 1567–1569, *1568–1569*
Atrial escape interval, in dual-chamber pacing, 1768
Atrial fibrillation, *1568*, 1568–1569, 1609, 1632–1645
after repair of secundum atrioseptal defect, 299, *299*
and atrial remodeling, 1633
and embolism, anticoagulation in, 1642–1643, 1643t
and outcome of percutaneous mitral balloon valvotomy, 468–469, 472

Atrial fibrillation *(Continued)*
and Wolff-Parkinson-White syndrome, 1639
aortic stenosis in, 328
central venous pressure in, *2124*
definition of, 1633
diagnosis of, 1633–1636, *1634–1636*
echocardiography in, 1635
electrocardiography in, 1633–1635, *1634–1635*
Holter monitoring in, 1635, *1635*
transesophageal echocardiography in, 1644, 1650–1654
sensitivity of, 1651, *1652*
with cardioversion, and anticoagulation, 1651–1653, *1652,* 1653t
and without anticoagulation, 1653
with fibrillation of less than 48 hours, 1653–1654
during pregnancy, 2041
electrophysiologic basis of, 1818, *1818–1819*
epidemiology of, 1632
etiology of, 1632–1633, 1632t
in hypertrophic cardiomyopathy, 1066, 1068
in older adults, 2021
in preexcitation, 1625, *1625–1626*
in sinus node dysfunction, 1581–1582
in thyrotoxicosis, 1927–1928
natural history of, 1632
pathophysiology of, 1633
post-thoracotomy, 1641–1642
prevention of, 1642
pacemaker therapy in, 1763–1764
radiofrequency catheter ablation of, 1804, 1806, *1806*
treatment of, 1636–1639, 1637t, *1638*
acute, 1636–1639, *1638*
cardioversion in, anticoagulation during, 1643–1644
warfarin before, 1650–1651, 1651t
chronic, 1639
long-term, 1641, *1641–1642*
nonpharmacologic, 1644–1645
risks of, 1639–1641, *1640–1641*
surgical, 1815–1822, *1816–1822*
anatomic-electrophysiologic basis of, 1818–1819, *1818–1820*
contraindications to, 1819
electrophysiologic evaluation before, 1819, 1821
historical aspects of, 1815–1818, *1816–1817*
indications for, 1819
Maze I procedure for, 1818–1819, *1819–1820*
Maze II procedure for, 1821, *1821*
Maze III procedure for, 1821, *1822*
results of, 1821–1822
success of, 1816, 1818
Atrial flutter, 1567–1568, *1608,* 1609. See also *Atrial fibrillation.*
after closure of atrial septal defect, 200, *200–201*
during pregnancy, 2041
electrocardiography in, 1633, *1634*
electrophysiologic basis of, 1818, *1818–1819*
in tricuspid atresia, 185, *186*
left, radiofrequency catheter ablation of, 1804
pathophysiology of, 1633
right common, radiofrequency catheter ablation of, 1801–1804, *1802*
procedure for, 1802–1803, *1802–1803*
recurrence after, 1803–1804
with 2:1 conduction, *1565*
Atrial infarction, electrocardiography in, 34
Atrial muscle, resting membrane potential of, 29
Atrial myxoma, echocardiography in, *88*
Atrial natriuretic factor (ANF), in hypertension, 1501, *1501*
Atrial natriuretic peptides (ANPs), in cardiac hypertrophy, 967–968
Atrial pacing, for sinus node dysfunction, 1590–1591
rapid, secondary pauses after, 1585
Atrial premature beat(s), 1567
Atrial septal defect, 162–163, *163*
and pregnancy, 2058
angioplasty balloon dilatation of, 280
closure of, 271–277, *274–275*
Amplatzer device for, 276–277
Angel Wings device for, 20–21, *20–21,* 273, 275, *275*
ASDOS for, 276
balloon sizing in, 272
CardioSEAL Device for, 273, *274–275*
Clamshell I ASD Occlusion Device for, 271–272
history of, 271
patent ductus arteriosus devices for, 277
patient screening for, 272
principles of, 271–272
Sideris Button Device for, 275–276
technique of, 272–273
echocardiography in, 92, *93,* 239–241, *239–241*
genetic basis of, 927, 2172–2173, 2172t
secundum type, 196–201, *197–201*
clinical features of, *197,* 197–198
echocardiography in, 239, *240*
pathophysiology of, 196–197
prognosis in, 198
treatment of, 198–201, *198–201*
complications of, 200–201, *200–201*
percutaneous repair in, 198–199, *198–199*
sinus venosus, 167, *168*
surgical creation of, with balloon atrial septostomy, 278–279
with anomalies of venous return, 238
with anomalous pulmonary venous connections, 167, *167–168*
Atrial Septal Defect Occluding System (ASDOS), 276
Atrial septostomy, balloon, 278–279
Blade, 279–280
Atrial tachycardia, 1606–1609, *1607–1608*
automatic, surgical treatment of, 1824, *1825*
multifocal, 1569, *1569*
paroxysmal, *1607*
permanent, 1606, *1608*
radiofrequency catheter ablation of, 1804, *1805–1806*
Atrial valvular angle lesion(s), 158, *160*
Atrioseptal defect, anomalies of, echocardiography in, *239–241,* 239–242
secundum, surgical treatment of, 299, *299*
Atrioventricular block, 1572–1575, *1574–1575,* 1574t
and syncope, 1692
bilateral bundle branch, 1574t, 1574–1575
carotid sinus massage in, *1601*
classification of, 1597–1598, *1598,* 1598t
complete, 1573–1574, 1596, *1597, 1600*
pacemaker therapy for, 1759
paroxysmal, *1603–1604*
congenital, pacemaker therapy for, 1762
during pregnancy, 2046
exercise-induced, pacemaker therapy for, 1762
Atrioventricular block *(Continued)*
first-degree, 1572–1573
in Emery-Dreifuss syndrome, 1994, *1994*
pacemaker therapy for, 1762
in sinus node dysfunction, and prognosis, 1587–1588
Mobitz I, 1573
Mobitz II, 1573, *1599*
second-degree, 1573, *1599*
pacemaker therapy for, 1759, 1760t–1761t, 1762
syncope in, 8
Wenckebach, 1573, *1599*
during pregnancy, 2046
Atrioventricular canal, 209–210
Atrioventricular conduction system, blood supply to, *1596*
disturbances of, electrocardiography in, 1597, *1599–1600*
Atrioventricular delay, rate-adapted, 1769
Atrioventricular dissociation, heart sounds in, 1677
importance of, 1677–1679
jugular venous pulse in, 1677
systolic blood pressure in, 1679
Atrioventricular interval, in pacemaker therapy, 1767
Atrioventricular junction, accelerated rhythm in, 1570, 1610
ectopic rhythms of, 1569–1670
radiofrequency catheter ablation of, 1806–1807
Atrioventricular nodal artery, anatomy of, and coronary angiography, 611
Atrioventricular nodal reentrant tachycardia, radiofrequency catheter ablation of, 1800–1801, *1801–1802*
slow pathway procedure for, 1800–1801, *1802*
surgical treatment of, 1824
Atrioventricular nodal tachycardia, 1609–1610, *1609–1610*
Atrioventricular node, ectopic rhythms of, 1569–1570
mesothelioma of, 1907–1908
resting membrane potential of, 29
Atrioventricular pressure gradient, in mitral stenosis, 347, *347–348*
Atrioventricular septal defect, surgical treatment of, 299–300, *300*
Atrioventricular sequential pacing, by implantable cardioverter-defibrillator, 1783–1784, *1784*
Atrioventricular valve, anatomy of, 147
Atrioventricular valvular regurgitation, 190–191
Atrium, left. See *Left atrium.*
remodeling of, atrial fibrillation and, 1633
right. See *Right atrium.*
single, 203–204
Augmentation index, 1486–1487
Auricularis, in mitral valve, 372
microscopic anatomy of, 355, *355*
Auscultation, *20–21,* 20–27, 22t–26t, *24, 27*
after exercise, 21
in mitral valve prolapse, 359–360, *359–360,* 376, *377,* 378
in myocardial infarction, 543, 547–548, *547–549*
of clicks, 22, 23t, *24*
of first heart sound, *21,* 21–22, 22t
of gallop sounds, 20, *20,* 22, 24, 27
of murmurs, 22, *24*
of second heart sound, *21,* 21–22
sequence in, 20–21
technique of, 20–21

Austin Flint murmur, in aortic regurgitation, 337
Autoantibody(ies), in systemic lupus erythematosus, 1941
Autograft(s), pulmonary, for aortic stenosis, 286, *289*
Autoimmune disorder(s), and dilated cardiomyopathy, 1045–1046
Automated edge detection system(s), for quantification of coronary artery stenosis, 628
Automatic atrial tachycardia(s), surgical treatment of, 1824, *1825*
Automatic implantable cardioverter-defibrillator(s). See *Implantable cardioverter-defibrillator(s).*
Automatic mode switching, in pacemaker therapy, 1773
Automaticity, in cardiac hypertrophy, 973
  myogenic, 523
Autonomic dysfunction, acute *vs.* subacute, 1550–1551
  and risk of sudden death, 1715
  and syncope, 1691, 1692t
    diagnosis of, 1698–1699
    neurally mediated, 1553, *1554*
  chronic, 1551, *1551*
  classification of, 1537, 1539t
  clinical feature(s) of, 1537–1543, *1540–1542,* 1541t, 1543t
    arrhythmias as, 1542
    hypertension as, 1542, *1542*
    hypotension as, 1537–1541, *1540–1541,* 1541t
    noncardiac, 1543, 1543t
    vascular, 1542–1543
  diagnosis of, 1543–1550, 1543t–1544t, *1544–1549*
    carotid sinus massage in, 1545, *1548*
    clonidine challenge test in, 1545, *1549*
    plasma catecholamines in, 1545, *1548–1549*
    sympathetic microneurography in, 1545, 1550, *1550*
    tilt test in, 1544–1545, *1547*
    24-hour monitoring in, 1544–1545, *1545–1548*
    Valsalva maneuver in, 1544, *1544*
  drugs causing, 1554
  etiology of, non-neurogenic, 1544t
  exercise and, 1545, *1547*
  food intake and, 1545, *1547*
  heart transplantation and, 1550, *1551*
  in diabetes mellitus, 1922
  in postural tachycardia syndrome, 1553
  localized, 1550
  mitral valve prolapse and, 365–366, 383
  primary, 1550–1551, *1551*
  secondary, 1551–1553
    from diabetes mellitus, 1551–1552
    from familial amyloid polyneuropathy, 1552
    from Riley-Day syndrome, 1551
    from spinal cord injury, 1552–1553, 1552t, *1553*
  space flight and, 2082
  toxins causing, 1554
Autonomic failure syndrome(s), chronic, 1551, *1551*
Autonomic nervous system, control of sinus node by, 1583–1584
  in circulatory regulation, 1288
  physiology of, 1537, *1538*
Auto-positive end-expiratory pressure (auto-PEEP), for chronic obstructive pulmonary disease, 1896
Autosomal dominant inheritance, 2147
Autosomal recessive inheritance, 2147–2148
AV. See *Atrioventricular* entries.
AVA. See *Aortic valve area (AVA).*
AVID (Antiarrhythmics Versus Implantable Defibrillators) trial, 1069, 1788
AVSD. See *Atrioventricular septal defect.*
Azathioprine, action of, 1212, *1213*
  dosage of, 1214t
  for myocarditis, 1106–1108, *1107,* 1107t
Azimilide, adverse effects of, 1753
  dosage of, 1753
  efficacy of, 1753
  electrophysiology of, 1753
  for atrial fibrillation, 1637t
  pharmacokinetics of, 1753
Azonemal, definition of, 917t
Azotemia, prerenal, from diuretic therapy, 1167
AZT. See *Zidovudine.*
Azygos vein, continuity with inferior vena cava, 169, *169*

Back-projection, in radionuclide imaging, 101, *101*
Bacteremia, *vs.* pulmonary thromboembolism, 1846
Bacterial infection(s), and pericarditis, 1246
  aortic, 1393
Bacterial myocarditis, 1109
"Ballerina foot" deformity, in mitral valve prolapse, 363, *363,* 380, *380*
Balloon(s), for delivery of radiotherapy, 832, 835, *835*
Balloon angioplasty, abrupt closure after, 869, 875
  and intimal hyperplasia, 875
  aneurysms from, *644*
  devices for, *790*
  dissection from, intravascular ultrasonography in, 1457–1458, *1458*
  efficacy of, type of lesion and, 869, 869t
  for aortic coarctation, 265–267
  for obstruction of great vessels, 262–264
  for pulmonary artery stenosis, 264, *265*
  for pulmonary venous stenosis, 267
  for superior vena caval obstruction, 267
  for unstable angina, 807–809, *808–809,* 809t
  history of, 257, 790
  in systemic veins, 267
  mechanism of action in, 791, *791*
  natural history of, 875
  restenosis after, interventions affecting, 808
  results of, 263
  vs. directional coronary atherectomy, for stable angina, 793–794, 794t
  vs. medical therapy, for stable angina, 795–796
  vs. stenting, for stable angina, 792, 793t
  with stenting, for stable angina, outcome of, 794, 795t
Balloon atrial septostomy, 278–279
Balloon flotation catheter(s), for cardiac catheterization, in pulmonary hypertension, 1874
Balloon valvotomy, percutaneous, for rheumatic mitral stenosis, *464–473,* 464–476, 466t, 469t–470t. See also *Percutaneous mitral balloon valvotomy.*
Balloon valvuloplasty, 434
  for aortic stenosis, 260–261
  for mitral stenosis, 261–262, 434–435
  for pulmonary stenosis, 189, 435–436
    double-balloon technique in, 259, *259*
    results of, 259–260
  for tricuspid stenosis, 262
Balloon valvuloplasty *(Continued)*
  for valvular stenosis, pulmonary, 258–260, *259*
  history of, 257
  percutaneous aortic, 476–481, *477–480,* 478t–480t. See also *Percutaneous aortic balloon valvuloplasty.*
  percutaneous tricuspid, 481–482
  pulmonary, 463–464, 464t
Balloon-expandable stent(s), 792
  for peripheral arterial disease, 1441, *1442*
  placement of, intravascular ultrasonography in, 1467–1469, *1468,* 1469t
"Bamboo spine," in ankylosing spondylitis, 1952, *1952*
BARI (Bypass Angioplasty Revascularization Investigation), 796, 797t, *798*
Barium swallow, 419
Barlow's syndrome. See *Mitral valve prolapse.*
"Barrel chest," in chronic obstructive pulmonary disease, 1889, *1890*
Barth's syndrome, and dilated cardiomyopathy, 1039
Basel Antiarrhythmic Study of Infarct Survival (BASIS) trial, 1726
Basic-helix-loop-helix (bHLH), definition of, 917t
BASIS (Basel Antiarrhythmic Study of Infarct Survival) trial, 1726
Basket device, for removal of foreign bodies, 281
Battery(ies), for implantable cardioverter-defibrillators, 1780
Bayes' theorem, 671
Becker's muscular dystrophy, 1986t, 1991–1992, 1991t
  genetic basis of, *2164*
  in familial dilated cardiomyopathy, 1039
Bed rest, recommendations for, history of, 893, 894t
  vs. cardiac rehabilitation, 895
Behçet's disease, 1951
Belgium Netherlands Stent (Benestent II) trial, 807, 808t, 876
Benznidazole, for Chagas' disease, 1044, 1111
Benzodiazepine(s), in obstetric analgesia, 2062t
Bepridil, dosage of, 713t
Beri-beri heart disease, 1090–1091, 1091t
Bernheim effect, in aortic stenosis, 325
Bernoulli equation, 79–80, 422
  for calculation of intravalvular pressure gradients, 441–442
Beta half-life, of drugs, 1740
Beta radiation, *vs.* gamma radiation, for restenosis, 831
Beta-adrenergic modulation, of cardiovascular performance, aging and, 2018–2019, 2018t
Beta-adrenergic receptor(s), sensitivity to, and hypertension, 1499
Beta-blocker(s), and cardiac rehabilitation, 901–902
  before noncardiac surgery, 2097
  cardioprotective effect of, 1518
  contraindications to, 712t
  during pregnancy, 2050t, 2066
  for atrial fibrillation, 1636, 1637t
  for cardiovascular complications of cocaine abuse, 1963–1964
  for heart failure, 1170–1171, *1171*
  for hypertension, 1517t, 1518
    in heart transplant recipients, 1197
  for hypertrophic cardiomyopathy, 1068
  for long QT syndrome, 1661, 1704
  for mitral valve prolapse, during pregnancy, 2055

Beta-blocker(s) *(Continued)*
for myocarditis, 1106
for pheochromocytoma, 1921
for prevention of sudden death, *1724,* 1724–1725
for stable angina, 709–711, 711t–712t, *713*
combination therapy with, 715
for syncope, 1702
in aortic dissection, 1382–1383
in survivors of myocardial infarction, 772–773, *772–774*
mechanism of action for, *713*
nonspecific *vs.* selective, 711
side effects of, 711, 711t, 1518
Beta-Cath, *834,* 835
Beta-hydroxybutyrate, in myocardial metabolism, 948–949
Betapace. See *Sotalol.*
Bezafibrate Coronary Atherosclerosis Intervention trial, 1346
Bezold-Jarisch reflex, injection of contrast agents and, 601
Biatrial enlargement, electrocardiography in, 34
Bicuspid aortic valve, 150, *150–151*
anatomic abnormalities in, 315, 315pl
and aortic regurgitation, 160, *161*
and aortic stenosis, 180, *181,* 285, *286,* 427, *427*
and pregnancy, 2059
aortic coarctation in, *195*
echocardiography in, 91, *91,* 247–248, *248*
transesophageal, *442*
leaflet mobility in, 443, *444*
with aortic coarctation, 1355, *1356,* 2154–2155
Bicycle ergometry, for exercise testing, 586–587
Bifascicular block, electrocardiography in, 41–42
pacemaker therapy for, 1760t, 1762
Bigeminal pulse, 16
Bigenic, definition of, 917t
Biglycan, in eroded atherosclerotic plaques, 581
Bile acid sequestrant(s), 2248
Billowing mitral valve. See *Mitral valve prolapse.*
Biomedicus left ventricular assist device, 852, *852*
Biopsy, endomyocardial. See *Endomyocardial biopsy.*
lung, in pulmonary hypertension, 1877
Bioptome(s), for removal of foreign bodies, 281
Bisferious pulse, *16,* 16–17
Bisoprolol, for heart failure, 1170–1171
Bite(s), snake, and myocardial disease, 1092
Biventricular hypertrophy, electrocardiography in, 35–36, *36*
Blade atrial septostomy, 279–280
Blalock-Taussig anastomosis, for L-transposition, 212
for tetralogy of Fallot, 218, *219*
for tricuspid atresia, with pulmonary stenosis, 187
Blanking period(s), in pacemaker therapy, 1768
Bleeding, from thrombolytic agents, 766–768, 767t–768t
intracerebral, after myocardial infarction, fibrinolytic agents and, 756
from aortic coarctation, 1356–1357
Blood, viscosity of, in erythrocytosis, 2004–2005, *2005*
Blood flow, coronary. See *Coronary blood flow.*
Blood gas(es), arterial, in pulmonary hypertension, 1866, 1867t
in pulmonary thromboembolism, 1840
Blood loss, acute, *vs.* pulmonary thromboembolism, 1847
Blood pressure, 24-hour monitoring of, in autonomic dysfunction, 1544–1545, *1545–1548*
arterial, intraoperative monitoring of, 2119–2123, *2120–2122*
complications of, 2121
direct methods for, 2119–2121, *2120*
noninvasive, 2122–2123
waveform in, *2120–2122,* 2121
during exercise testing, 587
during pregnancy, 2028, *2029*
in differential diagnosis of supraventricular tachycardia, 1613t
measurement of, 14–16, *15,* 15t–16t, 1509
monitoring of, during cardiovascular surgery, 2108
segmental, in lower extremities, 1407
space flight and, 2081–2082, *2082*
systolic, in atrioventricular dissociation, 1679
Blood pressure screening, and recommendations for follow-up, 1513–1514, 1514t
Blood vessel(s), compliance of, adventitia and, 1275
injury to, and vascular remodeling, *1300,* 1301
layers of, 1275, *1275*
pressure-volume relationships in, 1481, *1481*
structure of, 1480–1481
Blood volume, during pregnancy, 2026–2027, *2027*
B-mode ultrasonography. See *Ultrasonography, B-mode.*
BMPs (bone morphogenetic proteins), and cardiogenesis, 922–923
Body fat, distribution of, and risk for atherosclerosis, 1350
Body size, and coronary artery caliber, 615
Body temperature, monitoring of, during cardiovascular surgery, 2109
Body weight, indices of, 2259
variability in, and risk of coronary artery disease, 2205
Bolus lacing, for thrombolytic therapy, 1427
Bone morphogenetic proteins (BMPs), and cardiogenesis, 922–923
Border zone, in myocardial infarction, 514
Borrelia burgdorferi infection, and myocarditis, 1098, 1109–1110
Bovine pericardial valve(s), complications of, 323
Brachial artery, radiofrequency signal of, 1483, *1484*
Brachytherapy, delivery systems for, 832, *832–835,* 835
endovascular, for peripheral vascular disease, 1441–1443, *1442,* 1442t
Bradycardia, in spinal cord injury, 1552–1553, 1552t, *1553*
sinus, 1564–1566
treatment of, pacemaker therapy in, 1590
Bradycardia-tachycardia syndrome, in sinus node dysfunction, 1581, *1582*
Brain death, and cardiac allograft vasculopathy, 1196
Braunwald classification, in percutaneous transluminal coronary intervention, 804, 804t, *806*
of unstable angina, 724t
Breastfeeding, cardiovascular drugs and, 2053
Bretylium, adverse effects of, 1751–1752
dosage of, 1751
efficacy of, 1751
electrophysiology of, 1751
pharmacokinetics of, 1742t–1743t, 1751
Brevibloc. See *Esmolol.*
Brockenbrough's sign, 182
"Bronchial" artery(ies), in pseudotruncus arteriosus, 219, *220*
Bronchial "cuffing," 72, *73*
Bronchiectasis, *vs.* chronic obstructive pulmonary disease, 1891
Bronchitis, chronic. See also *Chronic obstructive pulmonary disease (COPD).*
definition of, 1885
diagnosis of, physical examination in, 1889
pathophysiology of, 1887
Bronchodilator(s), for chronic obstructive pulmonary disease, 1892–1893
"Bronze diabetes," 1087
Brown-Dodge method, of quantification of coronary artery stenosis, 628
Brugada's syndrome, 38–39, *39*
and sudden death, 1720–1721
Bruit(s), abdominal, in renal artery disease, 1402
Bucindolol, for heart failure, 1171
Buerger's disease, 1400
Bundle branch block, 1598–1604, *1601–1604,* 1604t
alternating, *1603*
and prognosis in coronary artery disease, 702t
bilateral, 1574–1575, 1574t
chronic, 1602–1604, *1603–1604,* 1604t
during pregnancy, 2046
heart rate during, and diagnosis of supraventricular tachycardia, 1611, *1614–1615*
in myocardial infarction, 41–42, 1598–1602, *1601*
treatment of, 1600, 1602
in survivors of myocardial infarction, 778–779
left, *1574–1575,* 1575
electrocardiography in, 36–37, *37*
in myocardial infarction, 548–549
in wide QRS tachycardia, 1679, *1680*
incomplete, 37
left ventricular hypertrophy in, electrocardiography and, 36
prognosis in, 39–40
with ventricular tachycardia, *1686*
right, 1575, *1575*
after closure of ventricular septal defect, 205, *206*
electrocardiography in, 37–39, *38–39*
in arrhythmogenic right ventricular dysplasia, *1667–1668*
incomplete, electrocardiography in, 39
prognosis in, 39–40
with supraventricular tachycardia, *1684*
with ventricular tachycardia, *1685*
Bundle branch reentry ventricular tachycardia, radiofrequency catheter ablation of, 1809, *1811–1812*
Bypass Angioplasty Revascularization Investigation (BARI), 796, 797t, *798*
Bypass tract(s), in preexcitation, 42

c7E3, and natural history of myocardial infarction, 702
c7E3 Fab Antiplatelet Therapy in Unstable Refractory Angina (CAPTURE) Study, 732, *732*

Ca^{2+}-ATPase, in cardiac hypertrophy, 963
in sarcoplasmic reticulum, and cardiac hypertrophy, 983
CABG. See *Coronary artery bypass graft (CABG).*
CABG-PATCH (Coronary Artery Bypass Graft–Implantable Cardioverter Defibrillator Study), 1788t
CABRI (Coronary Angioplasty *versus* Bypass Revascularization Investigation), *796,* 797t, 873t, 874
Cachexia, and cardiomyopathy, in human immunodeficiency virus infection, 1980
CAD. See *Coronary artery disease.*
CAFS (conotruncal anomaly face syndrome), genetic basis of, 925–926
Calan. See *Verapamil.*
Calcification, in aortic stenosis, 326, 427, *428*
in atherosclerotic plaques, 1342
intravascular ultrasonography in, *1456,* 1456–1457, 1464
in constrictive pericarditis, 1263, *1263–1265*
in mitral valve prolapse, *361, 378–379*
of coronary arteries, in angina, 530–531, *531*
in atherosclerosis, 626
scoring of, 2182, *2182*
of porcine prosthetic valves, *322,* 323
Calcineurin inhibitor(s), action of, 1212, *1213*
and hypertension, 1197
and nephrotoxicity, 1197–1198
and neurotoxicity, 1198–1199
dosage of, 1214t
Calcium, and contractile function, 962, *962,* 963t
and excitation-contraction coupling, 992–993, 992t, *993,* 998–999
cytoplasmic, regulation of, 1282, *1283*
cytosolic levels of, and myocardial ischemia, 1008
dietary, and hypertension, 1498
control of, 2239
handling of, in aortic stenosis, 332
metabolism of, disorders of, 1925–1926
response of contractile proteins to, 991–992, *992*
retention of, in sarcoplasmic reticulum, 998
transport of, in myocytes, *965*
uptake of, and left ventricular relaxation, 1003–1004
Calcium antagonist(s), and natural history of variant angina, 697–699, *699*
for heart failure, 1168, 1173
for hypertension, 1517t, 1519–1520
safety of, 1520
Calcium channel(s), in plasma membrane, and excitation-contraction coupling, 994
Calcium channel blocker(s), chemical structure of, *714*
dosage of, 713t
during pregnancy, 2065–2066
for atrial fibrillation, 1636, 1637t
for diastolic heart failure, 1012
for dilated cardiomyopathy, 1049
for hypertrophic cardiomyopathy, 1068
for myocardial fibrosis, in scleroderma, 1947
for pulmonary hypertension, 1878–1879, *1879–1880*
for stable angina, 711–715, 711t–715t, *714*
combination therapy with, 715
indications for, 715t
mechanism of action for, *714*
side effects of, 715, 715t
Calcium current, in cardiac hypertrophy, 971
Calcium pump, and excitation-contraction coupling, 1281, *1281*
Calcium pump *(Continued)*
in plasma membrane, 994
in sarcoplasmic reticulum, 996–998, *997–998*
Calcium sign, in aortic dissection, 1382, *1382*
Calcium transient, in cardiac hypertrophy, 971–972
in systolic dysfunction, 964, *965*
Caldesmon, and vascular smooth muscle contraction, 1281
Calgary Study, 1730
Caliper(s), for quantification of coronary artery stenosis, 628
Calponin, and vascular smooth muscle contraction, 1281
Canadian Amiodarone Myocardial Infarction Arrhythmia Trial (CAMIAT), 1751
Canadian Amlodipine/Atenolol In Silent Ischemia (CASIS) study, 573
Canadian Implantable Defibrillator Study (CIDS), 1731t, 1732, 1788, 1788t
Candesartan, for heart failure, 1174
Candidal infection(s), and myocarditis, 1110
"Cannon" A wave(s), 18, *18*
in myocardial infarction, 543, *545*
CAPRI trial, of cardiac rehabilitation, 900
CAPRIE (Clopidogrel *versus* Aspirin in Patients at Risk for Ischaemic Events) trial, 717, *717,* 1412
Captopril, for heart failure, 1170t
for hypertension, 1518
Captopril test, in renovascular hypertension, 1510
CAPTURE (c7E3 Fab Antiplatelet Therapy in Unstable Refractory Angina) Study, 732, *732*
Carbohydrate(s), in myocardial metabolism, 942–943, *943*
CarboMedics bileaflet valve, 486
Carbon dioxide digital angiography, in renovascular hypertension, 1429–1430
Carbon monoxide, and myocardial ischemia, smoking's effect on, 2229
Carcinoid heart disease, 1093
anatomic abnormalities in, 318, 318pl
Carcinoid syndrome, clinical features of, 1930, *1931*
diagnosis of, 1930–1931
pathophysiology of, 1930
treatment of, 1931
Cardiac. See also *Heart* entries.
Cardiac actin gene, in hypertrophic cardiomyopathy, 1057–1058, *1062*
Cardiac allograft vasculopathy, 1191–1197, *1192–1195,* 1218
clinical features of, 1191–1192
diagnosis of, 1193–1194, *1194–1195*
angiography in, 642–643, *642–643*
intravascular ultrasonography in, 1464, *1466*
etiology of, 1195–1196
incidence of, 1191, *1192*
pathology of, 1194–1195
prevention of, gene therapy in, 1197, 1220
prognosis in, 1191
risk factors for, 1192–1193, *1193*
treatment of, 1196–1197
gene therapy in, 2274
Cardiac aneurysm(s), pathologic changes in, 1031–1032, *1032*
Cardiac arrest, during pregnancy, 2034–2036, 2036t, *2037*
Cardiac Arrest Study Hamburg (CASH), 1731–1732, 1731t, 1788
Cardiac Arrest Study in Seattle: Conventional Versus Amiodarone Drug Evaluation Trial (CASCADE), 1730
Cardiac catheterization, collaboration with surgeon in, 282
contrast agents for, advances in, 419
during closure of atrial septal defect, 272
during pregnancy, 2034
financial issues in, 282
for hemodynamic assessment, 1125–1126
history of, 257
in amyloid heart disease, 1085, *1085*
in aortic regurgitation, 429, *430–431,* 431
with aortic stenosis, 431
in aortic stenosis, 427, *427–430,* 429
in cardiac tamponade, 1255–1256
in cardiomyopathy, dilated, 1048, 1126, *1126*
hypertrophic, 224, *226,* 1127–1132, *1129–1132*
restrictive, 1080, *1081,* 1126–1127, 1126t–1127t, *1127–1129*
in endomyocardial biopsy, 1132–1133
in L-transposition, 212
in mitral regurgitation, 354, 424–426, *425–426*
with mitral stenosis, 426–427
in mitral stenosis, 419–424, *420–423,* 423t
transseptal technique of, 423–424
in mitral valve prolapse, 362–363, *363–364,* 380, *380–381*
in pericarditis, constrictive, 1263–1265, *1265*
in pseudotruncus arteriosus, 219–220
in pulmonary hypertension, 1873–1875, *1874*
risks of, 1874–1875
technical considerations in, 1874
in pulmonary stenosis, 189
in pulmonary valve disease, 432, *432*
in risk stratification for sudden death, 1723
in tetralogy of Fallot, 214
in tricuspid atresia, 185, 187
in tricuspid insufficiency, 432
in tricuspid stenosis, 432, *433*
interventional, 257–282. See also specific procedure, e.g., *Balloon angioplasty.*
laboratory for, layout of, 595
of prosthetic valves, 432–434, 433t–434t, *434*
technical aspects of, 419
therapeutic, for valvular disease, 434
with closure of atrial septal defect, 199–200
Cardiac chamber(s), abnormal communication between, *196–209,* 196–210, 196t
and atrial septal defect, 196–201, *197–201.* See also *Atrial septal defect.*
and coronary sinus fistula, 204
and endocardial cushion defect, 209–210
and partial anomalous pulmonary venous connection, 204, *204*
and patent ductus arteriosus, 208–209, *208–209*
and septum primum defect, 201, *202–203,* 203
and single atrium, 203–204
and sinus venosus defect, 204
and ventricular septal defect, 204–208, *206–207*
Cardiac conduction, disorders of. See *Conduction disorder(s).*
Cardiac depressant(s), for heart failure, 1166
Cardiac dilatation, electrophysiologic consequences of, 972
Cardiac failure, biologic markers of, 973–974
Cardiac glycoside(s), during pregnancy, 2063
for amyloid heart disease, 1086
for pulmonary hypertension, 1878
Cardiac hypertrophy, 955–974

Cardiac hypertrophy *(Continued)*
and diastolic function, 1009–1011
animal models of, 967t
as physiologic adaptation, 955, 979
cell death in, 960–961
cell division and, 960
clinical features of, 983–985, *984*
definition of, 979
eccentric, 980, *980*
electrophysiologic aspect(s) of, 968–973, *969–970*
action potential as, 968–970, *969*
arrhythmias as, 973
genetic expression and, 972–973
inward current as, 971–972
outward current as, *970,* 970–971
resting potential as, 968–970
endocrine function of heart and, 967–968
genetic factors in, 982
growth signals in, 957–960
DNA targets and, 958–959
permanent changes in gene expression and, 959–960
sensors and, 958
transduction systems and, 958
transgenic technology and, 959
transient changes in gene expression and, 959
myocardial adaptation to, 956–957, 956t–957t
biologic processes in, 956, 956t
energy metabolism and, 956–957, 957t
natural history of, 985
pathologic changes in, 1022, *1022*
pathophysiology of, 979–983, *980–983,* 980t
genetic factors in, 982
myocyte functional alterations in, 983, *983*
signal transduction in, 981–982, *982*
patterns of, 979–981, *980–981,* 980t
progression to heart failure, 983, *983*
transcription factors in cardiogenesis and, 927–928
treatment of, 985–986
Cardiac myosin binding protein C gene, in hypertrophic cardiomyopathy, 1057, *1062*
Cardiac neurosis, 6
Cardiac output, after percutaneous mitral balloon valvotomy, *467*
and aortic valve area, 334t
during pregnancy, 2027, *2028,* 2028t
and organ distribution, *2028*
in mitral stenosis, 423
monitoring of, 2131–2134, *2133*
Doppler ultrasonography in, *2133,* 2133–2134
mixed venous oxygen saturation in, 2132–2133
thermodilution in, 2131–2132
Cardiac pseudoaneurysm(s), pathologic changes in, 1032
Cardiac rehabilitation, 893–908
after coronary artery bypass graft, 903
after percutaneous transluminal coronary angioplasty, 903
and exercise capacity, 900–901
and mortality, 898t
and return to work, 898t, 904
beta-blockers and, 901–902
center-based, 907
circuit training in, 897
compliance with, 902
complications of, 899–900
cost efficacy of, documentation of, 907
definition of, 896
early studies of, 895–896
Cardiac rehabilitation *(Continued)*
economic issues in, 904–905
efficacy of, 2219–2221, *2220,* 2220t
animal studies of, 895
prediction of, 904
exercise testing in. See *Exercise testing.*
expanded utilization of, 906
future of, 905–908
documentation of benefits and, 907
early patient contact and, 905–906
for underserved populations, 906
increased physician awareness and, 906
new models in, 905, 907–908
patient diversity and, 906
health risk appraisal model of, 908
home-based, 907–908
in older adults, 903
intervention studies of, 897, 898t, 899
meta-analysis of, 899
left ventricular dysfunction and, 902
PERFEXT study of, 900–901, *901,* 903
prescription for, 896–897
programs for, assessment of, by Joint Commission of Accreditation of Healthcare Organizations (JCAHO), 904–905
right ventricular dysfunction and, 902–903
volunteer community model of, 908
vs. bed rest, 893, 894t, 895
with risk factor modification, 904
Cardiac relaxation, 1001–1013
and early diastolic filling, 1004–1005, *1006*
and myocardial load, 1004
diastolic dysfunction and, 1001–1002, *1002.* See also *Diastolic dysfunction.*
left ventricular, 1002–1004
Cardiac reserve, aging and, 2018, 2018t
Cardiac sarcoidosis, 1113–1114
Cardiac shunt(s), echocardiography in, 92, *92–93*
Cardiac silhouette, expiration and, *70*
normal, *66*
pathology affecting, 71
Cardiac surgery. See also specific procedure.
anesthesia for. See *Anesthesia, for cardiovascular surgery.*
during pregnancy, 2060, 2061t–2062t
Cardiac tamponade, and pericardial effusion, 1250
and shock, 1530
diagnosis of, cardiac catheterization in, 1255–1256
echocardiography in, 661–662, *661–662,* 1253–1255, *1254*
electrocardiography in, 1255
physical examination in, 1251–1253, *1252*
radiography in, 1255
in myocardial infarction, 555–556
pathophysiology of, 1251
and characteristics differing from constrictive pericarditis, 1259–1261, *1259–1261*
and common characteristics with constrictive pericarditis, 1258–1259
pericardiocentesis in, 1257–1258
hemodynamic assessment after, 1256–1257, *1257*
treatment of, 1257–1258
vs. pulmonary thromboembolism, 1845
Cardiac tissue, ablation of, percutaneous transcatheter, for sinus node dysfunction, 1591
Cardiac transplantation. See *Transplantation, heart.*
Cardiac tumor(s), 1901–1909
clinical features of, 1901, 1901t
diagnosis of, computed tomography in, electron beam, 2187–2188, *2188*
Cardiac tumor(s) *(Continued)*
in human immunodeficiency virus infection, 1909
lymphomatous, 1909, *1909*
magnetic resonance imaging of, 136–137
pericardial, 1909, *1909*
primary, 1903–1909, 1903t, *1905–1908*
fibroma, 1906
lipoma, 1907
malignant, *1908,* 1908–1909
mesothelioma of atrioventricular node, 1907–1908
myxoma, 1903–1906, *1905–1906.* See also *Myxoma, cardiac.*
papillary fibroelastoma, 1906, *1906*
rhabdomyoma, 1906
secondary, 1901–1903, *1902*
clinical features of, 1901–1903
in coronary arteries, 1902
intracavitary, 1903
myocardial, 1902
pericardial, 1902
diagnosis of, 1903
sites of origin in, 1901, *1902*
treatment of, 1903
Cardiac valve(s), radiography of, *71*
replacement of. See also *Prosthetic valve(s).*
for infective endocarditis, 410–412, *411,* 411t
Cardiofacial syndrome(s), genetic basis of, 925–926
Cardiogenesis, and postnatal heart, 927–929
early, extrinsic signals for, 922–923
genetic basis of, 915–918
in *Drosophila, 916,* 917
tinman and, 919, 922
in knockout mice, 918, 929
left-right position in, 923–924
looping morphogenesis in, 923–924
myocyte proliferation in, 924–925
postmitotic phenotype in, 928–929
stages in, *916*
terminology related to, 917t
transcription factor(s) in, 918–922
and postnatal cardiac hypertrophy, 927–928
evolutionary conservation of, 922
GATA, 920
HAND, 920
Iroquois-related homeobox gene 4 as, 919–920
myocyte enhancer factor–2 as, 918–919
NK-2 homeodomain proteins as, 919
serum response factor as, 921
T-box as, 922
transcriptional enhancer factor–1 as, 921
Cardiogenic shock. See *Shock, cardiogenic.*
Cardiomegaly, differential diagnosis of, 9–10, 9t
Cardiomyopathy, alcoholic, 1024, 1964
natural history of, 1965
treatment of, 1965
and sudden death, 1718–1719
anthracycline and, 1024, *1025,* 1041
cardiovascular surgery in, anesthesia for, 2111
classification of, 1125, 1125t
cocaine and, 1962–1963
dilated, 1034–1049
acquired, 1045
alcoholic, 1039–1040
anatomic abnormalities in, 1036–1037, *1037,* 1037t
autoimmune, 1045–1046
cocaine and, 1040
definition of, 1034

Cardiomyopathy *(Continued)*
diagnosis of, 1046–1048, *1047*
cardiac catheterization in, 1126, *1126*
echocardiography in, 84, *85,* 86, 1138–1139, *1138–1139*
laboratory studies in, 1046–1047
physical examination in, 1046
radiography in, 1047
diastolic function in, 1011–1012
epidemiology of, 1034
etiology of, 1034, 1035t, *1038*
familial, 1038–1039, 1038t
autosomal dominant, 1039
autosomal recessive, 1039
in Barth's syndrome, 1039
in Becker's muscular dystrophy, 1039
in Duchenne's muscular dystrophy, 1039
with conduction defects and muscular dystrophy, 1997
X-linked, 1039
hypersensitivity, 1044
idiopathic, 1038
in Emery-Dreifuss syndrome, *1994,* 1995
in Kawasaki's disease, 1044–1045
in nemaline myopathy, 1996
in rheumatoid arthritis, 1044
in scleroderma, 1044
in systemic lupus erythematosus, 1044
inflammation-induced, 1041–1045, 1041t–1042t
from HIV, 1043
from viral infections, 1041–1043, 1041t–1042t
myocarditis and, 1105
natural history of, 1034–1036, *1035,* 1035t
noncardiac surgery in, 2102
obesity and, 1045
pathologic changes in, 1023–1024, *1024–1025*
pathophysiology of, 1036, *1036*
peripartum, 1045
radionuclide imaging in, 1143
tachycardia and, 1045
treatment of, 1048–1049, 1049t
pacemaker therapy in, 1764
vs. ischemic cardiomyopathy, 1036
familial, 175
hemodynamic assessment in, 1125–1126
hypertrophic, 224, *225–226,* 226, 1055–1069
and risk of sudden death, 1716–1717, *1717*
diagnosis of, 1061–1065, *1062–1064*
cardiac catheterization in, 1127–1132, *1129–1132*
echocardiography in, 86, *87,* 1063–1065, *1064, 1135–1137,* 1135–1138
electrocardiography in, 1062–1063, *1063*
electrophysiologic studies in, 1065
history in, 1061–1062, *1062*
physical examination in, 1062
radiography in, 1062
radionuclide imaging in, 1143–1144
during pregnancy, 2054–2055
from subaortic stenosis, 151, *152*
genetic basis of, 2160–2161, *2162*
genetic studies in, 1065
natural history of, 1065–1066, *1066*
noncardiac surgery in, 2102
obstructive *vs.* nonobstructive, 1060
pathogenesis of, 1055–1061, *1056,* 1056t
dominant negative *vs.* haploinsufficiency in, 1059–1060

Cardiomyopathy *(Continued)*
genetic linkage analysis in, 1055, *1056,* 1056t
HCM disease genes in, 1055–1058, *1056,* 1056t
left ventricular systolic function in, 1060–1061, *1061*
murine models of, 1059
sarcomere structure and, 1058–1059
pathologic changes in, 1022–1023, *1023*
Q wave in, 49, *50*
treatment of, 1066–1069, *1067*
in asymptomatic patient, *1067,* 1067–1068
in genotype-positive, phenotype-negative patient, 1067, *1067*
in mildly symptomatic patient, *1067,* 1067–1068
pacemaker therapy in, 1069, 1763
pharmacologic, 1068
surgical, 1068–1069
with atrial fibrillation, 1068
vs. amyloid heart disease, 1085
in diabetes mellitus, 1922–1924
in human immunodeficiency virus infection, *1976–1978,* 1976–1981
antiviral agents and, 1980–1981
cachexia and, 1980
cytokines in, 1979–1980
drugs and, 1980
from direct involvement of HIV organism, 1978
from opportunistic infections, *1976–1977,* 1976–1979
myocardial cellular injury in, 1979
in muscular dystrophy, Becker's, 1992
infantile, 1024
ischemic, *vs.* dilated cardiomyopathy, 1036
magnetic resonance imaging in, 139, *140*
nonischemic, surgical treatment of, 1826
obesity and, 2259
peripartal, 1024
peripartum, 1114, *2053,* 2053–2054, 2053t–2054t
restrictive, 1075–1088
and amyloid heart disease. See *Amyloid heart disease.*
and heart failure, 1149–1150
cardiac catheterization in, 1126–1127, 1126t–1127t, *1127–1129*
definition of, 1075
diagnosis of, 1077–1082, *1078–1081*
angiocardiography in, 1080, *1081*
cardiac catheterization in, 1080, *1081*
echocardiography in, 1079–1080, *1079–1080*
electrocardiography in, 1079
history in, 1077–1078
Holter monitoring in, 1081
physical examination in, 1077–1078, *1078*
radiography in, 1078–1079, *1079*
radionuclide imaging in, 1081–1082
echocardiography in, 86, *86,* 1139–1141, *1140*
eosinophilia in, 1075–1077, *1076–1077,* 1076t
etiology of, 1126t
pathologic changes in, 1024–1025
pathophysiology of, 1075
radionuclide imaging in, 1144, 1144t, *1145*
stages of, 1076
treatment of, 1082
vs. constrictive pericarditis, 90, 1127t, 1266–1267

Cardiomyopathy *(Continued)*
vs. radiation-induced heart disease, 1088–1089
toxic, 1024, *1025*
Cardiomyoplasty, 1235–1236
Cardioplegia, during coronary artery bypass grafting, 839, 841
Cardiopulmonary bypass, and coagulopathy, 2008
and hemolysis, 2003
anticoagulation during, 2113
complications of, 839
during pregnancy, 2060
during valvular surgery, 486, *487*
extracorporeal circulation for, 2113
weaning from, 2113–2114, 2114t
Cardiopulmonary resuscitation (CPR), during cardiac rehabilitation, rates of, 900
during pregnancy, 2026, 2036t
Cardioquin. See *Quinidine.*
CardioSEAL Device, for closure of atrial septal defect, 273, *274–275*
Cardiothoracic ratio, and prognosis in heart failure, 1159
Cardiovascular performance, beta-adrenergic modulation of, aging and, 2018–2019, 2018t
Cardiovascular reflex(es), in circulatory regulation, 1288–1289, *1289*
Cardioversion, during pregnancy, 2946
for atrial fibrillation, 1637–1639
anticoagulation during, 1643–1644
warfarin before, 1650–1651, 1651t
with transesophageal echocardiography, cost-effectiveness of, 1653
without anticoagulation, 1653
restoration of sinus rhythm after, failure of, 1582
Carditis, in rheumatic fever, 390–391
Cardizem. See *Diltiazem.*
CARE (Cholesterol and Recurrent Events) trial, 541, *542,* 1340–1341
Carney complex, 1918
Carnitine deficiency, and myocardial disease, 1091
Carnitine palmitoyl transferase, in fatty acid oxidation, 947–948
Carotid angioplasty, 1436–1437
Carotid artery, B-mode ultrasonography of, 1446–1451. See also *Ultrasonography, B-mode.*
intimal-medial thickness of, and symptomatic vascular disease, 1450–1451, *1451*
measurement of, 1447
reproducibility of, 1447, 1448t
validity of, 1447–1448
normal *vs.* abnormal, 1448–1451, 1448t, *1449–1451,* 1450t
progression of, 1449–1450, *1450,* 1450t
risk factors and, 1449
Carotid artery disease, *1401,* 1401–1402
cerebral embolization in, prevention of, 1437–1438
clinical features of, 1401
diagnosis of, 1401
epidemiology of, 1435
natural history of, 1401–1402
treatment of, 1402
atherectomy in, devices for, 1440, *1440*
carotid angioplasty in, 1436–1437
endarterectomy in, 1435–1436
gene therapy in, 1440
radiation therapy in, 1440–1441
stents in, 1440
tibioperoneal angioplasty in, 1439, 1439t

Carotid endarterectomy, 1435–1436
restenosis after, 1436
Carotid pulse, contour of, in aortic stenosis, 326, *326*
palpation of, 16, *16*
Carotid sinus hypersensitivity, 1553
pacemaker therapy for, 1763
Carotid sinus massage, in atrioventricular block, *1601*
in autonomic dysfunction, 1545, *1548*
in supraventricular tachycardia, 1611, 1613t
Carotid sinus syndrome, pacemaker therapy for, 1702, 1761t
pathophysiology of, 1691
Carotid upstroke, assessment of, 16–17, *17*
Carvallo sign, *345*
Carvedilol, for heart failure, 1170–1171
CASCADE (Cardiac Arrest Study in Seattle: Conventional Versus Amiodarone Drug Evaluation Trial), 1730
CASH (Cardiac Arrest Study Hamburg), 1731–1732, 1731t, 1788
CASIS (Canadian Amlodipine/Atenolol In Silent Ischemia) study, 573
CASS. See *Coronary Artery Surgery Study (CASS).*
Catalytic domain, in coagulation system, 1316, 1318
Catecholamine(s), and atrial fibrillation, 1609
in cardiac hypertrophy, 968
plasma, in autonomic dysfunction, 1545, *1548–1549*
polymorphic ventricular tachycardia sensitive to, and sudden death, 1721
urinary, in pheochromocytoma, 1511
Catheter(s), and coronary vasospasm, 640
balloon flotation, for cardiac catheterization, in pulmonary hypertension, 1874
for coronary angiography, 598–599, *598–599*
for delivery of gene therapy, 2272, *2272*
for delivery of radiotherapy, 832, *833–835*
for directional coronary atherectomy, 793
for intravascular ultrasonography, 1454, *1455*
high-frequency, 1473
injury from, 607
Park blade septostomy, 279
position of, for radiofrequency ablation of accessory pathways, *1798*
for radiofrequency ablation of atrioventricular nodal reentrant tachycardia, *1802*
for radiofrequency ablation of right common atrial flutter, 1802, *1802*
Swan-Ganz, use of, 558, *559*
Catheter ablation. See *Radiofrequency catheter ablation.*
Catheter fulguration, of His bundle, 1815–1816
Cationic liposome(s), as vectors for gene therapy, 2271
CCHB (complete congenital heart block), 1945
cdks (cyclin-dependent kinases), and postmitotic phenotype, 928
Ceftriaxone, for infective endocarditis, penicillin-susceptible, 406, 406t
Cell(s), division of, and cardiac hypertrophy, 960
electrical activity in, 968–969, *969*
metabolic pathways in, 938, *939*
Cell death, in cardiac hypertrophy, 960–961
Cellular immunity, in viral myocarditis, *1099,* 1099–1100
Central aortic pressure, waveform from, 1486
Central nervous system, disorders of, electrocardiography in, 55–56, *57*
from infective endocarditis, 416
Central nervous system (CNS), and pain threshold, 570
Central obesity, and coronary artery disease, 2264
Central vein(s), cannulation of, for hemodynamic monitoring, 2108
Central venous pressure, in atrial fibrillation, *2124*
in constrictive pericarditis, 2123, *2125*
intraoperative monitoring of, 2123–2125, 2123t, *2124–2125,* 2126t
complications of, 2125, 2126t
space flight and, 2078–2079
Cerebral circulation, physiology of, 1688–1690, *1690*
Cerebral hemorrhage, from aortic coarctation, 1356–1357
Cerebral hypoperfusion, symptoms of, 1540, *1541,* 1541t
Cerebral hypoxia, and syncope, 1689
Cerebral protection device(s), 1438
Cerebroside(s), myocardial accumulation of, in Gaucher's disease, 1090
Cerebrotendinosus xanthomatosis, 2175t
Cerebrovascular accident. See *Stroke.*
Cerebrovascular arteriole(s), vasoconstriction of, in syncope, 1691
Cerebrovascular disease, and syncope, 1695–1696
Cesarean section, emergency, cardiovascular indications for, 2036, *2037*
Chagas' disease, and dilated cardiomyopathy, 1043–1044
and myocarditis, 1110–1111
Characteristic impedance, definition of, 1491
Chemotherapy, and myocardial disease, 1092–1093
for amyloidosis, 1086, *1087*
Chest pain, differential diagnosis of, 3, 5–6, 5t
during pregnancy, 2036–2037, 2036t
in angina pectoris, 5, 5t
in anxiety, 6
in aortic dissection, 1378
in arrhythmogenic right ventricular dysplasia, 1666
in myocardial infarction, 5–6, 543
in pericarditis, 6
acute, 1268
in pulmonary hypertension, 1864, 1864t
in pulmonary thromboembolism, 1836
in unstable angina, 531
in variant angina, 532
noncardiac, 6
Chest physiotherapy, for chronic obstructive pulmonary disease, 1896–1897
Chest radiography. See *Radiography.*
CHF. See *Congestive heart failure (CHF).*
CHF-STAT (Survival Trial of Antiarrhythmic Therapy in Congestive Heart Failure), 1727
Child(ren). See *Pediatric population.*
Childbirth, antibiotic prophylaxis during, for infective endocarditis, 2038–2039, 2039t
hemodynamic response to, 2029–2031, 2031t
mitral stenosis and, 2056–2057
Chimeric antibody(ies), for immunosuppressive therapy, 1213
Chlamydial infection(s), and atherosclerosis, 1337–1338
Cholelithiasis, after heart transplantation, 1200
Cholesterol, embolization of, 1394
in atherosclerotic plaques, *1326*
serum, and prognosis in coronary artery disease, 718, *719*
and risk of coronary artery disease, 2194–2197, *2196–2197*
Cholesterol *(Continued)*
elevated. See *Hyperlipidemia.*
management of, nondrug therapies in, 2247, 2247t
pharmacologic, 2247–2248, 2247t
Cholesterol and Recurrent Events (CARE) trial, 541, *542,* 1340–1341
Cholesterol Lowering Atherosclerosis Study (CLAS), 1346, 1409
Cholesterol pericarditis, 1242, *1242*
Chordae tendinae, rupture of, from mitral valve prolapse, 189–190
in mitral regurgitation, 158, *159*
prognosis in, 560
Chorea, Sydenham's, in rheumatic fever, 391, *392*
Chromosomal disorder(s), and congenital heart disease, 2170–2172, 2171t
classification of, *2145–2146,* 2145–2147, 2146t
Chromosome(s), structure of, 2145, *2145*
Chronaxy, 1766
Chronic obstructive pulmonary disease (COPD), 1885–1898
and sleep apnea syndrome, 1891
and treatment of hypertension, 1522t, 1523
α_1-antitrypsin deficiency and, 1886–1887
definition of, 1885, *1885*
diagnosis of, 1888–1891, 1888t, *1890–1891*
computed tomography in, 1889–1890
electrocardiography in, 1891
history in, 1888, 1888t
laboratory studies in, 1891
physical examination in, 1888–1889
pulmonary function tests in, 1890–1891, *1891*
radiography in, 1889, *1890*
differential diagnosis of, 1891–1892
pathophysiology of, 1887–1888
prevalence of, 1885–1886, *1886*
prognosis in, *1897–1898,* 1898
risk factors for, 1886
treatment of, *1892–1896,* 1892–1897, 1893t
antibiotics in, 1894
bronchodilators in, 1892–1893
corticosteroids in, 1893–1894, *1894*
mechanical ventilation in, 1896
oxygen therapy in, 1895–1896, *1895–1896*
smoking cessation in, 1892, *1892*
surgical, 1897
theophylline in, 1893, 1893t
Chronic renal failure, and pericarditis, 1247
Chronotropic imcompetence, pacemaker therapy for, 1759
Churg-Strauss syndrome, 1075, 1950
Chylomicron(s), and hyperlipidemia, 1345
Chylopericardium, 1247
CIDS (Canadian Implantable Defibrillator Study), 1731t, 1732, 1788, 1788t
Cigarette smoking. See *Smoking.*
Cilostazol, for claudication, 1411
Cineangiography, equipment for, 594
in mitral valve prolapse, *361, 378–379, 381*
Circuit training, in cardiac rehabilitation, 897
Circulation, cerebral, physiology of, 1688–1690, *1690*
cocaine and, 1962
collateral. See *Collateral circulation.*
coronary. See *Coronary circulation.*
fetal, 196
regulation of, 1286–1291, *1287, 1289*
aging and, 1290
autonomic nervous systems in, 1288
cardiovascular reflexes in, 1288–1289, *1289*

Circulation *(Continued)*
exercise in, 1290
hormones in, 1290
local factors in, 1286–1288, *1287*
mental stress in, 1290
neurotransmitter–endothelial cell interactions in, 1289–1290
neurotransmitters in, 1288
nitroxidergic nerves in, 1289
orthostatic stress in, 1290–1291
vascular remodeling in, 1299–1307. See also *Vascular remodeling.*
Circulatory dysfunction, 1290–1295, *1291–1292*
and atherosclerosis, 1295
and vasovagal syncope, 1290–1291
diabetes and, 1292
gene transfer for, 1295
heart failure and, 1294, *1294*
hypercholesterolemia and, 1294
hypertension and, 1292–1294
obesity and, 1292, *1293–1294*
smoking and, 1292
Circumflex artery(ies), bypass surgery on, *840, 845,* 846
collateral pathways to, 637
left, absent, coronary angiography in, 621
anatomy of, and coronary angiography, 610
and left anterior descending artery, separate origins from left sinus of Valsalva, 619, 621, *621–622*
origin from right coronary sinus, angiography in, 619, *619–621*
Circus movement tachycardia, 1610, *1611–1612*
in preexcitation, 1622, *1623–1624,* 1625
treatment of, 1626, *1629,* 1630, 1630t
Cirrhosis, *vs.* constrictive pericarditis, 1266
Clamshell I ASD Occlusion Device, 271–272
CLAS (Cholesterol Lowering Atherosclerosis Study), 1346, 1409
Class A artery(ies), 524
Class B artery(ies), 524
Claudication, exercise training for, *1410,* 1410–1411
medical treatment of, 1409–1412
Click(s), 22, 23t, *24*
in mitral valve prolapse, 351, 359–360, *359–360,* 376, *377*
of prosthetic valves, 27, *27*
Clonidine, during pregnancy, 2050t
for hypertension, 1520
Clonidine challenge test, in autonomic dysfunction, 1545, *1549*
Clonidine suppression test, in pheochromocytoma, 1511
Clopidogrel, for peripheral vascular disease, of lower extremities, 1412
for stable angina, *717,* 717–718
Clopidogrel *versus* Aspirin in Patients at Risk for Ischaemic Events (CAPRIE) trial, 717, *717,* 1412
Clot-selective thrombolytic agent(s), 743
90-minute patency rate of, 744–745, 744t
development of, 742
first-generation *vs.* second-generation, 743–745, 744t
safety of, 755–757, 756t
Clubbing, differential diagnosis of, 13
in patent ductus arteriosus, 209, *209*
pathogenesis of, 14
CMV (cytomegalovirus) infection, after heart transplantation, prevention of, 1190–1191
c-myc oncogene, in aortic regurgitation, 336
CNS. See *Central nervous system (CNS).*
Coactivator(s), definition of, 917t
Coagulation cascade, 2009, *2009*
tissue factor in, 726, *728*
Coagulation factor(s), in variant angina, 534, *534*
properties of, 1317t
Coagulation system, 1315–1319, *1316,* 1317t
anticoagulant pathways in, *1316,* 1318–1319
catalytic domain in, 1316, 1318
contrast agents and, 601–602
epidermal growth factor domain in, 1316
exercise and, 2223
Kringle domain in, 1316
procoagulant pathways in, *1316,* 1318
propeptide/carboxyglutamic acid–rich domain in, 1315–1316
pseudosubstrates in, 1318
signal peptide in, 1315
Coagulopathy, cardiopulmonary bypass and, 2008
with hypercoagulable states, 2008–2010, *2009,* 2009t
Coanda effect, 450
Coarctation of aorta. See *Aortic coarctation.*
Cocaine, abuse of, socioeconomic impact of, 1959
with alcohol abuse, 1961
and arrhythmias, 1963
and atherosclerosis, 1962
and cardiomyopathy, 1962–1963
and coronary circulation, 1960–1962
and dilated cardiomyopathy, 1040
and endothelial dysfunction, 1961–1962
and left ventricular function, 1962
and left ventricular hypertrophy, 1962–1963
and myocardial infarction, 779, 1960–1961
and myocardial oxygen consumption, 1960
and myocarditis, 1963
and peripheral circulation, 1962
and vasoconstriction, 1960–1962
cardiovascular complications of, treatment of, 1963–1964
chemical structure of, *1960*
history of, 1959
pharmacology of, 1959–1960, *1960,* 1960t
Coincidence counting, in positron emission tomography, 113
Cold, and angina, 529
Colitis, ischemic, after repair of abdominal aortic aneurysm, 1375
Collagen, in arterial wall, 1480
Collagen vascular disease(s), anatomic abnormalities in, 315–318, *316–318,* 316pl
during pregnancy, 2052
lesions resembling, 317–318, *317–318*
pericarditis in, 1241–1242, 1247
Collateral artery(ies), aortopulmonary, in tetralogy of Fallot with pulmonary atresia, 303, *303*
Collateral circulation, anatomy of, 504
coronary, 525–526
coronary angiography of, 637–638
development of, in therapeutic angiogenesis, *1418,* 1418–1419
in aortic coarctation, 156, *158,* 194
Collateral vessel(s), closure of, 270–271
Collimator(s), function of, 100, *100*
Color-flow Doppler echocardiography, in aortic stenosis, 327
in assessment of mitral regurgitation severity, 353
principles of, 442
Commissurotomy, for mitral stenosis, 486, *487–488*
history of, and outcome of percutaneous mitral balloon valvotomy, 468, 472
Commissurotomy *(Continued)*
outcome of, *vs.* percutaneous mitral balloon valvotomy, 474–475
Complete congenital heart block (CCHB), 1945
Compliance, arterial. See *Arterial compliance.*
Compton radiation "fog," 65, *67*
Computed tomography (CT), electron beam, 2181–2188
in angina, 530
in atherosclerosis, with calcification, 626
in cardiac tumors, 2187–2188, *2188*
in congenital heart disease, 2186, *2186*
in coronary artery disease, 2181–2184, *2182–2184*
in great vessel disease, 2186–2187, *2187–2188*
in myocardial disease, 2185
in pericardial disease, 2184–2185, *2185*
in subclinical atherosclerosis, 2253
in valvular disease, 2185–2186, *2186*
principles of, 2181
scanning protocol for, 2181
with exercise, 2183
in abdominal aortic aneurysms, *1366*
in amyloid heart disease, 1085
in aortic dissection, *1376,* 1379, 1380t
in carotid artery disease, 1401
in chronic obstructive pulmonary disease, 1889–1890
in hemochromatosis, 1088
in inflammatory aortic aneurysms, 1395–1396
in pericarditis, constrictive, 1263, *1264*
in pulmonary hypertension, 1873
in thoracic aortic aneurysm, 1358, *1359*
spiral, in abdominal aortic aneurysms, for predicting outcome of endovascular treatment, 1432
in pulmonary thromboembolism, 1841, *1841*
in renovascular hypertension, 1430
Concealed accessory pathway(s). See *Accessory pathway(s), concealed.*
Concentric left ventricular hypertrophy, 979–980, 980t, *981*
Concentric remodeling, in left ventricular hypertrophy, 980, 980t, *981*
Conduction delay, intraventricular, electrocardiography in, 42
Conduction disorder(s). See also *Heart block; specific disorder(s).*
and prognosis in sinus node dysfunction, 1587–1588
and syncope, 1692
intraventricular, electrocardiography in, 36–42, *37–43*
myocardial, from infective endocarditis, 413
with familial dilated cardiomyopathy, and muscular dystrophy, 1997
Conduction system, space flight and, 2083, *2084*
Conduit(s), complications of, 323
Congenital aortic sinus aneurysm, 163
Congenital heart disease, and arrhythmias, 227
and pregnancy, 228–229
and truncus arteriosus, 220–221, *221–222*
chromosomal disorders and, 2170–2172, 2171t
classification of, 180
combination anomalies in, 170–172, *171–173*
complex, 210–220, *211–222*
and double-outlet right ventricle, 212, 214, *216–217*
and D-transposition, 210, *211*

Congenital heart disease *(Continued)*
and L-transposition, 212, *213–214*
and pulmonary atresia with ventricular septal defect, 219–220, *220*
and tetralogy of Fallot, 214, *217–219,* 218–219
echocardiography in, 92–94, *93–94,* 251
with cyanosis, 210–220, *211–222*
surgical treatment of, 302–303, *303*
without cyanosis, 210
coronary angiography in, 616–625, *616–625*
benign, 617–621, *618–622,* 618t
incidence of, 617, 617t
with adverse outcomes, 621–624, *623–624*
diagnosis of, computed tomography in, electron beam, 2186, *2186*
during pregnancy, 2057–2060, 2058t. See also *Pregnancy, congenital heart disease and.*
echocardiography in, 91–94, *91–94*
from single-gene defects, 2172–2173, 2172t–2175t
genetic basis of, 925–927
incidence of, on coronary angiography, 617, 617t
inheritance of, 2057–2058, 2058t
mendelian, 2172t
magnetic resonance imaging in, 137–138, *137–138*
natural history of, 179–180, 285
noncardiac surgery in, 2098, 2100
presentations in, 237
radionuclide studies in, for quantification of shunts, *461,* 461–462
recurrence risk of, affected siblings and, 2176t
surgical treatment of, 285–308. See also specific disease *and* specific procedure.
heart-lung transplantation in, 306, *307–308,* 308
syndromes with, 175–176, *176*
treatment of, 257–282. See also specific disorder.
history of, 257–258
valvular, 180–193, *181–193*
and aortic regurgitation, 191–192, *191–192*
and aortic stenosis, 180–182, *181–184*
and atrioventricular valvular regurgitation, 190–191
and mitral stenosis, 184
and mitral valve prolapse, 189–190
and mitral valve regurgitation, 191
and pulmonary stenosis, 187–189, *188–190*
and pulmonary valve regurgitation, 192
and tricuspid atresia, 185, *185–187,* 187
and tricuspid stenosis, 184
echocardiography in, 91–92, *91–92*
valvular obstruction in, 150–156, *150–156*
with abnormal aortic/arterial branching, 172–175, *173–176*
with abnormal communications, 161–163, *163–165,* 163–170, *166–170*
closure of, 269–271
distal to atrioventricular valves, 163, *164–165*
of coronary artery with cardiac chamber or thoracic vessel, 164, *166*
of great arteries, 164, 167
proximal to atrioventricular valves, 161–164, *164*
pulmonary venous, 167–168, *167–168*
systemic venous, 168–169, *169–170*
with aortic coarctation, 156, *157–158*
Congenital heart disease *(Continued)*
with multifactorial inheritance, 2173–2176, 2176t
Congestive heart failure (CHF), and circulatory dysfunction, 1294, *1294*
and treatment of hypertension, 1522, 1522t
cardiac enlargement in, 9, 9t
definition of, 1148
diagnosis of, exercise testing in, 1157, *1158*
diastolic dysfunction and, 1001. See also *Diastolic dysfunction.*
doxorubicin and, 1092–1093
in older adults, 2022
in survivors of myocardial infarction, angiotensin-converting enzyme inhibitors for, 776, *776,* 777t
in thyrotoxicosis, 1928
left-sided, dyspnea in, 4
pleural effusion in, 12, 12t
treatment of, diuretics in, 1166–1167, 1166t
with resistant edema, 1178
vs. pulmonary thromboembolism, 1845
Connective tissue disorder(s), 1939–1949, *1940–1948,* 2150–2157
anatomic abnormalities in, 319–320
in myxomatous degeneration, 319–320, *319–320*
and cutis laxa, 2157
and dermatomyositis, *1948,* 1948–1949
and Ehlers-Danlos syndrome, 2155
and Marfan's syndrome, 2150–2155, *2151–2152,* 2153t, *2154.* See also *Marfan's syndrome.*
and polymyositis, *1948,* 1948–1949
and pseudoxanthoma elasticum, *2156,* 2156–2157
and pulmonary hypertension, 1865
and rheumatoid arthritis, 1939–1941, *1940,* 1940t. See also *Rheumatoid arthritis.*
and scleroderma, 1945–1948, *1946,* 1947t, *1948.* See also *Scleroderma.*
and supravalvular aortic stenosis, 2155–2156
and systemic lupus erythematosus, 1941–1945, *1943–1944,* 1944t, 1946t. See also *Systemic lupus erythematosus (SLE).*
and Williams' syndrome, 2156
with mitral valve prolapse, 357, 375
Conotruncal abnormality(ies), 2171–2172
Conotruncal anomaly face syndrome (CAFS), genetic basis of, 925–926
Constrictive pericarditis. See *Pericarditis, constrictive.*
Contiguous-gene syndrome(s), 2146
Continuity equation, for calculation of aortic valve area, 444
Continuous-wave Doppler waveform examination, in peripheral vascular disease, of lower extremities, 1408
Contraceptive(s), and hypertension, 1507–1508
Contractile function, aging and, 2017
alcohol and, 1040, 1964
and systolic dysfunction, 961–963, *962,* 963t
biochemical mechanisms in, 1277–1281, *1278, 1280*
contractile proteins and, 1277–1279, *1278*
crossbridge hypothesis of, 1058
excitation-contraction coupling and. See *Excitation-contraction coupling.*
in aortic stenosis, 332–333
marijuana and, 1966–1967
proteins and, 989–991, 989t, *990–991*
reversibility of, oxidative metabolism and, 121–123, *122*
space flight and, 2079
Contractile protein(s), 989t, 990–991, *990–991,* 1277–1279, *1278*
Contractile protein(s) *(Continued)*
interactions among, 991–992, *992*
response to calcium, 991–992, *992*
Contractility, and myocardial oxygen consumption, 521–522
Contrast agent(s), advances in, 419
arrhythmias from, 608–609
for coronary angiography, 600–602, *600–602*
injection of, 602, *602*
for positron emission tomography, 118
physiologic effects of, *601,* 601–602
toxicity of, 607–608
Contrast angiography. See *Angiography, contrast.*
Contrast echocardiography, of atrial septal defect, 240
Contrast venography, in pulmonary thromboembolism, 1843
Cook deflector wire, for removal of foreign bodies, 281
COPD. See *Chronic obstructive pulmonary disease (COPD).*
Copenhagen Atrial Fibrillation, Aspirin, Anticoagulation Study (AFA-SAK), 2021
Copenhagen Male Study, 1346
Copper, transport of, disorders of, 2175t
Cor pulmonale, in pulmonary thromboembolism, 1836
Cor triatriatum, echocardiography in, 242–243
Cornell voltage criteria, for diagnosis of left ventricular hypertrophy, 35
Coronary angiography, 592–645
after myocardial infarction, indications for, 895
anatomic considerations in, 609–611
anticoagulation during, 602–603
before noncardiac surgery, 2096–2097
calculation of infarct/risk area in, 616, *616*
cannulation of coronary ostium in, 599, *599*
catheters for, 598–599, *598–599*
complication(s) of, 605–609, 605t
allergic, 607–608
from anesthetics, 608
from anticoagulation, 608
from arrhythmias, 608–609
from cannulation, 605–607
from contrast agents, 607–608
hemodynamic, 609
incidence of, 605t
myocardial infarction as, 607
neurologic, 606
peripheral vascular, 605–606
contrast agents for, 600–602, *600–602*
injection of, 602, *602*
coronary artery dimensions and, 614–616, *614–616,* 614t. See also *Coronary artery(ies), dimensions of.*
epicardial coronary artery tone during, nitroglycerin and, 603
equipment for, 592–596, *593, 595*
digital processors and, 594
fluoroscopic display units and, 594
for image resolution, 594–595
image intensifiers and, 593–594
in cineangiography, 594
physical layout of, 595
X-ray generators and, 592–593
history of, 860
in abnormal left ventricular function, 604
in aortic dilatation, 604
in atherosclerosis, 625–638, *627–636*
for hemodynamic assessment, limitations of, 632–633
for physiologic assessment, 629–633, *630–632*
limitations of, 632

Coronary angiography *(Continued)*
of coronary flow reserve, 629–631, *631–632*
of fractional flow reserve, 631–632
for visual assessment, 626–627, *627*
insensitivity of, 626
quantitative, 627–629
automated edge detection systems for, 628
Brown-Dodge method of, 628
caliper method of, 628
problems with, 629
videodensitometry for, 628–629
with calcification, 626
with compensatory dilatation, 625–626
with diabetes mellitus, 626
in cardiac allograft vasculopathy, 1193
in cardiomyopathy, dilated, 1126
in congenital anomalies, 616–625, *616–625*
benign, 617–621, *618–622,* 618t
incidence of, 617, 617t
with adverse outcomes, 621–624, *623–624*
in coronary arterial fistulas, 624–625, *625*
in coronary artery aneurysms, 643–644, *644*
in coronary embolism, 645
in coronary vasospasm, 638–640, *639–640*
in heart failure, 604
in left main coronary artery stenosis, 603–604
in microcirculatory coronary disease, 641–642
in mitral regurgitation, 354
in mitral valve prolapse, 380, *380–381*
in monitoring atherosclerotic plaques, 2248–2249
in myocardial infarction, 633–637, *633–637*
pathologic correlation with, 633–634, *633–634*
thrombolysis with, 634, *635*
with angiographically normal arteries, 641
with reocclusion, 636–637
in radiation-induced coronary artery disease, 642
in shock, 604
in spontaneous coronary artery dissection, *640,* 640–641
in total anomalous pulmonary venous connection, 222, 224
in vasculitis, 643
magnetic resonance. See *Magnetic resonance angiography (MRA).*
of bypass grafts, *599,* 599–600
of collateral circulation, 637–638
of left coronary artery, *612*
of right coronary artery, *613*
outpatient, 604–605
patient preparation for, 596–597
personnel for, 596
quantitative, *vs.* PET myocardial perfusion imaging, 681–682, *682*
radiation safety during, 595, *595*
technical history of, 595
vascular access for, 597–598
views in, *611–613,* 611–614
Coronary Angioplasty *versus* Bypass Revascularization Investigation (CABRI), *796,* 797t, 873t, 874
Coronary arterial fistula(s), 227
angiography in, 624–625, *625*
surgical treatment of, 301–302
Coronary arteriography, in angina pectoris, 6
Coronary arteriole(s), as resistance vessels, 523
Coronary artery(ies), anatomy of, 149–150, *503,* 503–504
and infarct/risk area, 616, *616*
Coronary artery(ies) *(Continued)*
aneurysms of, coronary angiography in, 643–644, *644*
anomalous origin of, 138, *138*
above sinotubular ridge, coronary angiography in, 621
and risk of sudden death, 1716
from posterior sinus of Valsalva, coronary angiography in, 621
from pulmonary artery, 624, *624*
surgical treatment of, 301–302, *302*
with proximal interarterial or septal course, 621–624, *623*
calcification of, 72
in angina, 530–531, *531*
in atherosclerosis, 626
circumflex. See *Circumflex artery(ies).*
compensatory dilatation of, in atherosclerosis, 625–626
congenital anomalies of, 226–227
echocardiography in, 250
contrast angiography of, in arrhythmogenic right ventricular dysplasia, 1669
dimensions of, 614–616, *614–616,* 614t
age and, 615
body size and, 615
coronary dominance and, 614, *615*
gender and, 615
normal, 614, *614,* 614t
vasomotor tone and, 615–616
dissection of, 509, *509,* 509pl
dominance of, 172
and coronary angiography, 611
and coronary artery caliber, 614, *615*
ectopic, 172, *173*
embryology of, 616–617, *617*
epicardial, 522
fistulas of, 164, *166*
intravascular imaging of, 667
left, anatomy of, 503, *503*
anomalous origin from pulmonary artery, 301, *302*
normal, coronary angiography of, *612*
stenosis of, coronary angiography in, 603–604
left anterior descending, anatomy of, and coronary angiography, 610
and left circumflex artery, separate origins from left sinus of Valsalva, 619, 621, *621–622*
bypass surgery on, *840,* 843–846, *845*
minimally invasive, 852, *853–854,* 854
with sequential grafts, 846, 851, *851*
collateral pathways to, 637
fusiform aneurysm of, *644*
muscular bridges at, 618, *618*
stenosis of, echocardiography in, 667
left circumflex, and coronary angiography, 610
left main, anatomy of, and coronary angiography, 609–610
atresia of, 624
mycotic aneurysm of, *510*
origin of, from pulmonary artery, 172, 174, *174*
polyarteritis nodosa of, *510*
ramus intermedius branch of, anatomy of, and coronary angiography, 610
right, anatomy of, 503, *503*
and coronary angiography, 610
bypass surgery on, *840–844,* 843
collateral pathways to, 637
normal, coronary angiography of, *613*
single, coronary angiography in, 623
size of, exercise and, 2222
spasm of, coronary angiography in, 638–640, *639–640*
Coronary artery(ies) *(Continued)*
from coronary angiography, 606–607
in unstable angina, 532, *533*
in variant angina, 532, *533,* 534
medical treatment of, 738, *739*
Coronary artery bypass graft (CABG), anatomic considerations in, *840,* 841
and mortality, 861, *862*
angiography of, *599,* 599–600
before noncardiac surgery, 2097
cardiac rehabilitation after, 903
clinical trial(s) of, 861–866, *862–868,* 862t
Coronary Artery Surgery Study in, 862t, 864
European Cooperative Surgery Study in, 862t, 864, *865–866*
meta-analysis of, 864, 866
summary of, 867–869
Veterans Affairs Cooperative Study Trial in, 861–864, 862t, *863*
complications of, 839
conduit for, 846, *847–850*
conventional technique of, *841–845,* 841–846
coronary sinus cannulation in, 841, *841*
internal mammary artery vein graft in, 846, *847–850*
and recurrent disease, 867, *867–868*
radial artery graft in, 846
saphenous vein graft in, *842,* 843, 846, 865–866, 866t
using circumflex artery, *840, 845,* 846
using left anterior descending artery, *840,* 843–846, *845*
with sequential grafts, 846, 851, *851*
using right coronary artery, *840–844,* 843
electron beam computed tomography of, 2182, *2183*
for myocardial infarction, outcome of, *87,* 877–878, 878t
for stable angina, *vs.* percutaneous transluminal coronary angioplasty, 796, *796,* 797t, 798, *798*
for unstable angina, 737–738, *738*
history of, 839, 860–861
in older adults, 2019
in patient with human immunodeficiency virus infection, 1981
indications for, 839
minimally invasive, 852–856, *853–854*
advantages of, 854, 856
disadvantages of, 854, 856
technique of, 852, *853–854,* 854
using left anterior descending artery, 852, *853–854,* 854
myocardial preservation during, 839, 841
nonrandomized data on, 877, *878*
outcome of, with aortic stenosis, 330
patency of, assessment of, magnetic resonance imaging in, 140, 140t, *141*
pathologic changes in, 516, *517*
preoperative evaluation in, *840,* 841
reoperation after, 851, 880, *881–882*
sequential, 846, 851, *851*
vs. percutaneous transluminal coronary angioplasty, clinical trials of, 871–874, 873t
BARI, 873t, 874
CABRI, 873t, 874
Emory Angioplasty *versus* Surgery trial, 872, 873t
ERACI, 873t, 874
German Angioplasty Bypass Investigation, 872, 873t, 874
Randomized Intervention Treatment of Angina trial, 872, 873

Coronary artery bypass graft (CABG) *(Continued)*
Toulouse Trial, 873t, 874
warm, 841
with ventricular assist device, 851–852, *852*
Coronary Artery Bypass Graft–Implantable Cardioverter Defibrillator (CABG-Patch) Trial, 1279, 1728t, 1788t
Coronary artery disease, aging and, 2019–2020
anatomic abnormalities in, 503–518
and acute myocardial infarction, 511–512
and angina pectoris, 509–511
and coronary atherosclerosis, 504–505, *504–506.* See also *Atherosclerosis.*
and coronary circulation, *503,* 503–504
and coronary thrombosis, 505–509, *507–508*
and infarct development, 513–514, *514–515*
and myocardial ischemia, *512,* 512–513
and myocardial modulation, 516–518
and nonatherosclerotic coronary vascular disease, 509, *509–510,* 511t
and reperfusion, 514–515
and sinus node dysfunction, 1578
and sudden death, 509–511
risk of, 1715–1716
and treatment of hypertension, 1522, 1522t
cardiovascular surgery in, anesthesia for, 2111
classification of, 528t
diagnosis of, computed tomography in, electron beam, 2181–2184, *2182–2184*
echocardiography in, 88–90, *89,* 666–667, *667*
magnetic resonance imaging in, 139–140, *141*
radionuclide ventriculography in, 676
SPECT myocardial perfusion imaging in, 671–673, 672t
disability from, 893–894
during pregnancy, 2046–2047
epidemiology of, 2194, *2195*
exercise testing in, 588–589
from metastatic cardiac tumors, 1902
genetic basis of, 2148
in allograft. See *Cardiac allograft vasculopathy.*
in systemic lupus erythematosus, 1942–1943
in women, demographics of, 582, 582t
risk factors for, 579
and mechanism of death, 583–584, 583t–584t
and plaque morphology, 582
multivariate risk assessment in, 2210, *2211–2212*
natural history of, 691–704
left ventricular dysfunction and, 695–696, *696–698*
risk factors and, 691–695, *692–695*
noncardiac surgery in, and reduction of perioperative complications, 2097–2098, *2099*
anesthesia for, 2097–2098
invasive studies before, 2096–2097
noninvasive studies before, 2094–2096, 2095t
preoperative evaluation for, 2092–2094, 2092t–2094t
risk stratification for, 2098, *2099*
pathogenesis of, *507*
pathophysiology of, *530*
percutaneous transluminal coronary angioplasty for. See *Percutaneous transluminal coronary angioplasty (PTCA).*
Coronary artery disease *(Continued)*
prevention of, exercise for, 2216–2223. See also *Exercise.*
probability of, age and, 671–673, 672t
gender and, 671–673, 672t
prognosis in, electrocardiography and, 702–703, 702t
exercise testing and, 589, *589,* 589t
radionuclide ventriculography and, 703–704, *704,* 704t
radionuclide ventriculography in, *676,* 676–677
SPECT myocardial perfusion imaging in, 673
protective effects of aspirin in, 716
quantification of, 627–629
radiation-induced, coronary angiography in, 642
radiotherapy and, 831
right, SPECT myocardial perfusion imaging of, *104*
risk factor(s) for, 2193–2213, 2194–2203, *2196–2197,* 2198t–2200t, *2200–2201*
absolute *vs.* relative, 2193
and primary prevention of hyperlipidemia, 2250–2253, *2252,* 2252t
and risk factors for sudden death, 1713–1714, 1713t, *1714*
and specific outcomes, 2194
antihypertensive therapy and, *1512,* 1512–1513, 1513t
blood lipids as, 2194–2197, *2196–2197*
detection of, preventive implications of, 2210–2213
diabetes mellitus as, 2198–2199, 2198t–2199t
epidemiologic criteria for, 2193
established, 2205–2206, 2207t
family history as, 2206
hypertension as, 1511, *1511,* 2199–2203, *2200–2201,* 2200t, 2202t. See also *Hypertension.*
in older adults, 2209–2210
left ventricular hypertrophy as, 2205–2206, 2207t
low HDL level as, 2246–2247
modified Framingham scoring of, 2252t
obesity as, *2204,* 2204–2205, 2204t–2205t. See also *Obesity.*
potential, 2209
recently established, 2206–2209, 2207t–2208t
electrocardiography serial changes as, 2207t
fibrinogen as, 2207, 2208t
homocysteine as, 2208–2209
insulin-resistance syndrome as, 2209
lipoproteins as, 2208
small, dense LDL as, 2207–2208
vitamin B as, 2208–2209
white blood cell count as, 2206–2207, 2207t
second-hand smoke as, 2228–2229
sedentary lifestyle as, 2216–2217, *2217*
smoking as, 2203–2204, 2204t. See also *Smoking.*
trends in, 2194, *2195*
triglyceride-rich lipoproteins as, 2246
triglycerides as, 2197–2198
severity of, and outcome of thrombolytic therapy, 762
and prognosis in variant angina, 698–699
number of affected vessels and, 860, *860–862*
smoking and, 2227–2230, 2228t, *2231*
surgical treatment of, anatomic considerations in, *840,* 841
Coronary artery disease *(Continued)*
coronary artery bypass graft in, 839–856. See also *Coronary artery bypass graft (CABG).*
endarterectomy in, *855,* 856
transmyocardial laser revascularization in, 856
therapeutic angiogenesis for, 1422–1424, *1423*
weight loss and, 2265
Coronary artery dissection, spontaneous, coronary angiography in, *640,* 640–641
Coronary Artery Surgery Study (CASS), 862t, 864
and effect of left ventricular dysfunction on coronary artery disease, 695, *696*
Coronary artery thrombosis, and Q wave myocardial infarction, 534–536, *535*
Coronary atherosclerosis. See *Atherosclerosis.*
Coronary balloon(s), *790*
Coronary blood flow, after injection of contrast agents, 601, *601*
and degree of stenosis, on angiography, 627, *627*
epicardial coronary arteries and, 522
grading of, 636
myocardial oxygen consumption and, 521–522
velocity of, measurement of, *631*
Coronary circulation, *503,* 503–504
alcohol and, 1964–1965
cocaine and, 1960–1962
collateral, 525–526
coronary steal and, 526
determinants of, 521–526
dual regulation of, 632
embryology of, 616–617, *617*
endothelium-dependent vasodilatation and, 524
left ventricular hypertrophy and, 526
normal, left ventricular wall segments and, 659, *660*
resistance vessels and, 522–524
Coronary embolism, angiography in, 645
Coronary flow reserve, 113–118, *114–118*
absolute *vs.* relative, 116–117, *117*
and percent diameter stenosis, 117–118, *118*
assessment of, coronary angiography in, 629–631, *631–632*
mechanisms of, 114, *115,* 116
severity of stenosis and, 114, *115*
Coronary microcirculation, 632
diseases of, angiography in, 641–642
Coronary ostia, anatomy of, 609
cannulation of, 599, *599*
Coronary resistance vessel(s), 522–524
Coronary sinus(es), cannulation of, in coronary artery bypass graft, 841, *841*
echocardiography of, 238
fistulas of, 204
right, origin of left circumflex artery from, 619, *619–621*
Coronary steal, 526
Coronary thrombosis, pathophysiology of, 505, *507–509,* 509
Coronary trunk(s), orientation of, and coronary angiography, 609
Coronary turgor, and diastolic function, 1007
Coronary vascular resistance, smoking and, *2231*
Coronary vasculitis, in rheumatoid arthritis, 1941
Coronary vasospasm, smoking and, 2230
Coronary vein(s), anatomy of, 150
Corrected sinus node recovery time (CSRT), *1584,* 1584–1585

Corridor procedure, for atrial fibrillation, 1816
Corticosteroid(s), action of, 1212, *1213*
  and obesity, 1199
  and osteoporosis, 1199
  for adrenal insufficiency, 1918
  for chronic obstructive pulmonary disease, 1893–1894, *1894*
  for giant cell arteritis, 1392
  for immunosuppresive therapy, 1214
  for polyarteritis nodosum, 1949–1950
  for polymyositis, 1949
  for rheumatic fever, 397
  for systemic lupus erythematosus, with myocarditis, 1942
    with pericarditis, 1942
  for transplant rejection, 1217
Cortisol, synthesis of, *1507*
Corvert. See *Ibutilide.*
Cough, angiotensin-converting enzyme inhibitors and, 1170
  differential diagnosis of, 6
  in pulmonary thromboembolism, 1837
  syncope from, 8–9
Counter storage, in pacemakers, 1774, *1774–1775*
Coxsackievirus B3 (CVB3), and myocarditis, 1098–1099
Coxsackievirus infection(s), *vs.* pulmonary thromboembolism, 1844
CPR. See *Cardiopulmonary resuscitation (CPR).*
C-reactive protein, and atherosclerosis, 1337
  and risk of myocardial infarction, 536, *539, 542*
Creatine kinase-MB, in myocardial infarction, 549, *553*
  in myocarditis, 1103
CREST syndrome, 1946, 1946pl, 1947–1948, *1948*
Critical stenosis, 525
Crossbridge cycling, in vascular smooth muscle, light chain phosphorylation and, 1279, *1280*
Crossbridge hypothesis, of contractile function, 1058
Cross-matching, before transplantation, 1219
Crosstalk, in pacemaker, 1777
Cryosurgery, for ablation of atrioventricular nodal reentrant tachycardia, 1824
Cryptococcosis, and cardiomyopathy, in human immunodeficiency virus infection, 1976, *1976,* 1978–1979
CSRT (corrected sinus node recovery time), *1584,* 1584–1585
CTLA-4 immunoglobulin, 1213
CUGBP1, in myotonic dystrophy, 2165–2166, *2167*
Cushing's syndrome, and hypertension, 1506
  clinical features of, 1918–1919
  diagnosis of, 1919
  pathophysiology of, 1918
  treatment of, 1919
Cutis laxa, 2157
CVB3 (coxsackievirus B3), and myocarditis, 1098–1099
Cyanosis, central, 12–14, 12t
  differential diagnosis of, 12–13, 12t
  in pulmonary thromboembolism, 1836
  peripheral, 12t, 13–14
Cyanotic heart disease, pregnancy and, 2060
  surgical treatment of, 302–303, *303*
Cyclic adenosine monophosphate (cAMP), and calcium pump, of sarcoplasmic reticulum, 997–998, *998*
Cyclin-dependent kinases (cdks), and postmitotic phenotype, 928
Cyclooxygenase, activity of, aspirin and, 716
Cyclophosphamide, and myocardial disease, 1092–1093
Cyclosporine, action of, 1212, *1213*
  and hypertension, 1508
  and nephrotoxicity, 1197–1198
  and neurotoxicity, 1198–1199
  and post-transplantation hypertension, 1197
  dosage of, 1214t
  for myocarditis, 1106–1108, *1107,* 1107t
Cyst(s), pericardial, 1242
  and cardiomegaly, 10
Cystic medial disease, and annuloaortic ectasia, 1388
  aortic, and aortic regurgitation, 429, *430*
Cytokine(s), and myocyte proliferation, in cardiogenesis, 925
  in cardiac hypertrophy, 968
  in cardiomyopathy, from human immunodeficiency virus infection, 1979–1980
  in endothelial injury, and atherosclerosis, 1330t
  in heart failure, 1154
  in myocarditis, from human immunodeficiency virus infection, 1109
  in viral myocarditis, 1101
  produced by endothelium, 1332t
  release of, and restenosis, 1306
  secretion of, in T cell activation, 1211
Cytokine inhibitor(s), for heart failure, 1176
Cytokine-release syndrome, 1212
Cytomegalovirus (CMV) infection, after heart transplantation, prevention of, 1190–1191
Cytoskeleton, in systolic dysfunction, 965
Cytotoxic lymphocyte(s), in animal models of viral myocarditis, 1100

Dacron graft(s), for peripheral vascular disease, of lower extremities, 1412
  for repair of aortic dissection, 1384
Dacron patch angioplasty, for aortic coarctation, 299, *299*
DAD (delayed after-depolarization), 1563
Dallas criteria, for diagnosis of myocarditis, 1042, 1042t, 1096
Dalteparin, for unstable angina, 726, 728, *728*
Das Angel Wings device, for closure of atrial septal defect, 198–199, *198–199,* 273, 275, *275*
Daunorubicin, and dilated cardiomyopathy, 1041
DDD pacemaker mode, 1770–1771
DDI pacemaker mode, 1771
Decapentaplegic (dpp), and cardiogenesis, 922
Deceleration trauma, aortic, 1392
Decorin, in eroded atherosclerotic plaques, 581
Defibrillation, atrial, for sinus node dysfunction, 1590–1591
Defibrillation threshold, for implantable cardioverter-defibrillator, 1785–1787
Defibrillator in Acute Myocardial Infarction Trial (DINAMIT), 1788t
Defibrillator in Nonischemic Cardiomyopathy Treatment Evaluation (DEFINITE), 1788t
Dehydration, during reentry from space flight, 2080–2081
Delayed after-depolarization (DAD), 1563
Delivery, antibiotic prophylaxis during, for infective endocarditis, 2038–2039, 2039t
  hemodynamic response to, 2029–2031, 2031t
Demand ischemia, *vs.* supply ischemia, 1008
Dental procedure(s), prophylactic antibiotics for, 414t–415t
Depolarization, abnormal, in arrhythmogenic right ventricular dysplasia, 1666, *1667–1668*
Depolarization *(Continued)*
  dyssynchronous, and heart failure, 1150
  ion activity during, 1–2
Depolarizing agent(s), for cardiovascular surgery, 2107–2108, 2108t
Dermatomyositis, *1948,* 1948–1949
  during pregnancy, 2052
Descending aortic aneurysm(s), thoracic, surgical treatment of, 1362–1364, *1365*
Desferroxamine, for hemochromatosis, 1088
Desmin myopathy, 1997
Desmopressin, for postural hypotension, 1556, 1558
Dexamethazone suppression test, in Cushing's syndrome, 1919
Dexfenfluramine, and pulmonary hypertension, 1862, *1863*
dHAND, and cardiogenesis, 920
  in cardiofacial syndromes, 926
Diabetes Control and Complications trial, 1345
Diabetes mellitus, 1921–1925, *1923*
  and atherosclerosis, 1344–1345
  and circulatory dysfunction, 1292
  and coronary artery disease, in women, 579
    risk of, 2198–2199, 2198t–2199t
  and outcome of PTCA, 759, 874–875
  and primary prevention of hyperlipidemia, 2251
  and vascular compliance, 1490
  atherosclerosis in, 626
  autonomic dysfunction in, 1551–1552
  cardiovascular surgery in, premedication for, 2105–2106
  classification of, 1921
  clinical features of, 1922–1924, *1923*
  diagnosis of, 1924
  obesity and, 2264
  pathophysiology of, 1921–1922
  protease inhibitors and, 1980–1981
  silent myocardial ischemia in, 571
  treatment of, 1924–1925
  with unstable angina, percutaneous transluminal coronary intervention in, 811, *812*
Diastole, stages of, 1001
Diastolic blood pressure, measurement of, 14
Diastolic chamber distensibility, 1002
Diastolic clicks, 22, 23t, *24*
Diastolic dysfunction, biologic determinant(s) of, 966–967, 967t
    active relaxation as, 966–967, 967t
  heart failure from, treatment of, 1012–1013
  in aortic stenosis, 331, *331*
  in heart failure, 1151
  left ventricular filling patterns in, 1005, *1006*
Diastolic filling, early, cardiac relaxation and, 1004–1005, *1006*
  in mitral stenosis, 421–422, *422*
Diastolic function, aging and, 1007
  cardiac hypertrophy and, 1009–1011
  during pregnancy, 1005
  extrinsic factors affecting, 1005–1007
  in dilated cardiomyopathy, 1011–1012
  left ventricular, in hypertrophic cardiomyopathy, 1060–1061, *1061*
  myocardial ischemia and, 1007–1009, *1009*
  on radionuclide ventriculography, 109, *109*
Diastolic gradient, in mitral stenosis, 422, *422–423*
Diastolic heart disease, 1075
Diastolic injury current, 43
Diastolic murmur(s), 26t
Diastolic pressure gradient, flow rate and, 347, *348*
Diastolic pulmonary artery pressure, in pulmonary hypertension, 1870

Diastolic rumble, in mitral stenosis, 348
"Diastolic suction," 1005
Diet, calcium in, and hypertension, 1498
control of, 2239
cholesterol in. See *Cholesterol.*
for diabetes mellitus, 1924
magnesium in, and hypertension, control of, 2239
potassium in, and hypertension, 1498
control of, 2239
sodium in, and hypertension, 1498
in "high reactors" to stress, *2235*
restriction of, and hypertension, control of, 2236–2238, *2237,* 2238t
sodium-restricted, for heart failure, 1165
for hypertension, 1515, *1515*
with exercise, and risk of coronary artery disease, 2218
Diffusing capacity for carbon monoxide (DLCO), in chronic obstructive pulmonary disease, 1890–1891
DIG (Digitalis Investigation Group) trial, 1049
DiGeorge's syndrome, 2171–2172
Digital processor(s), for coronary angiography, 594
Digital subtraction angiography, in abdominal aortic aneurysms, *1367,* 1374
Digitalis, electrocardiographic changes from, 53
for atrial fibrillation, 1636
for dilated cardiomyopathy, 1049
for heart failure, 1174
for mitral regurgitation, 352
for preexcitation, *1629*
for viral dilated cardiomyopathy, 1043
Digitalis Investigation Group (DIG) trial, 1049
Digoxin, adverse effects of, 1755
dosage of, 1754–1755
during pregnancy, 2045t, 2063–2064
efficacy of, 1755
electrophysiology of, 1754
for atrial fibrillation, 1637t
for heart failure, 1168, 1174
diastolic, 1012
pharmacokinetics of, 1742t–1743t, 1754
Dihydropyridine(s), for hypertension, 1517t, 1519–1520
Dilated cardiomyopathy. See *Cardiomyopathy, dilated.*
Diltiazem, adverse effects of, 1754
dosage of, 712t, 1754
efficacy of, 1754
electrophysiology of, 1754
for atrial fibrillation, 1637, 1637t
for preexcitation, *1629*
for pulmonary hypertension, 1878–1879, *1879–1880*
for silent myocardial ischemia, 575
mechanism of action for, 715
pharmacokinetics of, 1742t–1743t
D-Dimer, plasma levels of, in pulmonary thromboembolism, 1840
DINAMIT (Defibrillator in Acute Myocardial Infarction Trial), 1788t
Diphtheria, and myocarditis, 1109
Dipyridamole, with ^{201}thallium imaging, before noncardiac surgery, 2095–2096
in dilated cardiomyopathy, 1143
with echocardiography, before noncardiac surgery, 2096
with SPECT myocardial perfusion imaging, 103
after myocardial infarction, 674
Directional coronary atherectomy, for stable angina, 793–794, 794t
intravascular ultrasonography during, 1469, 1471, *1471*
Disopyramide, adverse effects of, 1745
dosage of, 1745
during pregnancy, 2043, 2044t
efficacy of, 1745
electrocardiographic changes from, 53
for atrial fibrillation, 1637t
for hypertrophic cardiomyopathy, 1068
pharmacokinetics of, 1742t–1743t, 1745
use dependency of, *1741*
Disseminated intravascular coagulation, *vs.* pulmonary thromboembolism, 1847
Distensibility, definition of, 1491
Diuretic(s), and anemia, 2008t
and hypokalemia, 1517–1518
and potassium monitoring, 1166–1167
and prerenal azotemia, 1167
during pregnancy, 2064–2065
for heart failure, 1166–1167, 1166t
for hypertension, 1516–1518
action of, 1516–1517
loop, 1517t
potassium-sparing, 1516, 1517t
thiazide, 1516, 1517t
during pregnancy, 2050t
for pulmonary hypertension, 1878
preoperative discontinuation of, 2092
DLCO (diffusing capacity for carbon monoxide), in chronic obstructive pulmonary disease, 1890–1891
DMPK gene, in myotonic dystrophy, 2165–2166, *2167*
DNA target(s), as growth signals, in cardiac hypertrophy, 958–959
Dobutamine, and arterial compliance, in heart failure, 1491
for acute heart failure, 1178
for cardiogenic shock, 1531–1532
for heart failure, 1168
with echocardiography, before noncardiac surgery, 2096
Dobutamine stress echocardiography. See *Echocardiography, dobutamine stress.*
Dobutamine-thallium imaging, before noncardiac surgery, 2096
Dofetilide, adverse effects of, 1753
dosage of, 1753
efficacy of, 1753
electrophysiology of, 1753
for atrial fibrillation, 1637t
pharmacokinetics of, 1753
Dolichostenomelia, in Marfan's syndrome, 2151
Donor heart, age of, and cardiac allograft vasculopathy, 1192, *1193*
Dopamine, during SPECT myocardial perfusion imaging, 104
for cardiogenic shock, 1531–1532
for heart failure, 1168
Doppler echocardiography. See *Echocardiography, Doppler.*
Doppler exercise stress testing, in peripheral vascular disease, of lower extremities, 1407–1408
Doppler flow wire, in cardiac allograft vasculopathy, 1194
Doppler phenomenon, 441
Doppler tissue imaging (DTI), in constrictive pericarditis, *vs.* restrictive cardiomyopathy, 90
of left ventricular diastolic function, 79
L-DOPS (L-threo-dihydroxyphenylserine), for postural hypotension, *1557,* 1558
Double aortic arch, 174, *174–175*
Double-balloon valvuloplasty, for mitral stenosis, 261–262, 465, *465*
for pulmonary stenosis, 259, *259,* 436
Double-inlet ventricle, surgical treatment of, 306
Double-outlet right ventricle, 212, 214, *216–217*
echocardiography in, 93
Down's syndrome, 176, 2170–2171
Doxazosin, for hypertension, 1520
Doxorubicin, and congestive heart failure, 1092–1093
and dilated cardiomyopathy, 1041
toxicity of, 679
dpp (decapentaplegic), and cardiogenesis, 922
Dressler's syndrome, 1269
Dripps–American Society of Anesthesiology, classification of physical status by, 2092, 2092t
Drop attack(s), 1696
Drosophila, cardiogenesis in, *916,* 917
tinman and, 919, 922
Drug(s). See also specific drug(s) and classes of drug(s).
alpha half-life of, 1739
and autonomic dysfunction, 1539t
and hematologic abnormalities, 2007–2008, 2008t
and hypertension, 1508
and long QT syndrome, 1659, 1659t, 1693, 1694t
and myocarditis, 1097t
and pericardial disease, 1247
and risk of sudden death, 1715
and sinus node dysfunction, 1578
and systemic lupus erythematosus, 1945, 1946t
beta half-life of, 1740
clearance of, 1739
electrocardiographic changes from, 53
palpitations from, 7
Drug abuse. See *Substance abuse.*
Dry pericarditis. See *Pericarditis, acute.*
DTI. See *Doppler tissue imaging (DTI).*
D-transposition, 210, *211*
Duchenne's muscular dystrophy. See *Muscular dystrophy, Duchenne's.*
Duct-Occlud Device, for patent ductus arteriosus, 269
Duke criteria, for diagnosis of infective endocarditis, 402–403, 403t
Duke Treadmill Score, *589*
Duplex ultrasonography. See *Ultrasonography, duplex.*
Dura mater prosthetic valve(s), complications of, 323
Duteplase, and intracranial bleeding, 756, 767, 767t
DVI pacemaker mode, 1771
Dynamic exercise, *vs.* isometric exercise, 897
Dysautonomia. See *Autonomic dysfunction.*
Dyslipidemia. See also *Hyperlipidemia.*
and natural history of coronary artery disease, 693–694, *694–695*
atherogenic, 2254
studies of, 2249
Dyspnea, differential diagnosis of, 4–5, 4t
in arrhythmogenic right ventricular dysplasia, 1666
in chronic obstructive pulmonary disease, 1888
in heart failure, 1155
in pulmonary hypertension, 1862–1864, 1864t
in pulmonary thromboembolism, 1836
paroxysmal nocturnal, 5
Dystrophin, and muscular dystrophy, 1039
in muscular dystrophy, Duchenne's, 2162–2163, *2164*

Dystrophin glycoprotein complex (DGC), in myotonic dystrophy, *2166*

EAD. See *Early afterdepolarization (EAD).*
Eagle Index, for surgical risk stratification, 2093–2094, 2094t
Early afterdepolarization (EAD), 1563
  in arrhythmogenic right ventricular dysplasia, 1671
  in torsades de pointes, 1659–1660
Early repolarization, electrocardiography in, 53, *54*
EAST (Emory Angioplasty *versus* Surgery Trial), *796,* 797t, 872, 873t
EBCT. See *Computed tomography (CT), electron beam.*
EBDA (effective balloon dilating area), and outcome of percutaneous mitral balloon valvotomy, 468
Ebstein's anomaly, 160, *161,* 184, 192–193, *193*
  clinical features of, 192–193, *193*
  echocardiography in, 91, 243–245, *244*
  pathophysiology of, 192
  pregnancy and, 2060
  surgical treatment of, 289, *295*
  treatment of, 193
  with tricuspid stenosis, 156
  Wolff-Parkinson-White syndrome in, surgical treatment of, 1823
Eccentric hypertrophy, 980, *980*
ECG. See *Electrocardiography.*
Echo dropout, in atrial septal defect, 240
  in ventricular septal defect, 244
Echocardiographic score, after percutaneous mitral balloon valvotomy, *471,* 471–472
  and outcome of percutaneous mitral balloon valvotomy, 468, 469t
Echocardiography, 76–94
  advances in, 76
  after percutaneous mitral balloon valvotomy, 474
  contrast, of atrial septal defect, 240
  dobutamine stress, 89–90
    after myocardial infarction, for detection of viable myocardium, 664–665
    exercise and, in silent myocardial ischemia, 574
    in infarct-related artery patency, 665
    in myocardial ischemia, 666
    safety of, 666
  Doppler, color-flow, in aortic stenosis, 327
      in assessment of mitral regurgitation severity, 353
      principles of, 442
    continuous-wave, 441
    during pregnancy, 2033
    for assessment of hemodynamic function, 79–80
    in aortic regurgitation, 82–83, *83*
    in aortic stenosis, 81–82, *82,* 326–328, 444–445, *445*
      color-flow, 327
      morphologic assessment in, 327
    in assessment of mitral regurgitation severity, 353–354
    in atrial septal defect, 241
    in cor triatriatum, 243
    in dilated cardiomyopathy, 1048
    in flow and shunt quantification, 241
    in infective endocarditis, 84, *85*
    in mitral regurgitation, 81
    in mitral stenosis, 80–81, *80–81*
    in mitral valve prolapse, 81, *81*
    in patent ductus arteriosus, 250

Echocardiography *(Continued)*
    in pericarditis, constrictive, *vs.* restrictive cardiomyopathy, 1267
    in pulmonary hypertension, 1870, *1871,* 1871t
    in restrictive cardiomyopathy, 1079–1080, *1080*
    in right ventricular outflow obstruction, 249
    in valvular heart disease, 80–83, *80–83*
    in ventricular septal defect, 244–245, *245*
    of left ventricular outflow tract gradient, in hypertrophic cardiomyopathy, 1136–1137, *1137*
    of prosthetic valves, 83, *84*
    pulsed-wave, 441
    technique of, 440–442, *441*
  during cardiovascular surgery, 2109
  during space flight, 2083–2085, *2085*
  history of, 76
  in amyloid heart disease, 1085, 1139–1141, *1140*
  in anomalies of atrial septum, *239–241,* 239–242
  in anomalies of venous return, *238,* 238–239
  in anomalies of ventricular inflow, 242–244, *244*
  in aortic coarctation, 248
  in aortic dissection, 454
  in aortic insufficiency, 445–446
  in aortic regurgitation, 337, *338*
  in aortic stenosis, 444–445, 444t, *445*
  in aortic valve disease, *442–445,* 442–446, 443t–444t
  in arrhythmogenic right ventricular dysplasia, 1667
  in assessment of left ventricular diastolic function, 79
  in assessment of left ventricular function, 445–446
  in assessment of left ventricular mass, 78–79
  in atrial fibrillation, 1635
  in atrial myxoma, *88*
  in atrial septal defect, 239–241, *239–241*
    secundum type, 197–198
  in bicuspid aortic valve, 247–248, *248*
  in cardiac shunts, 92, *92–93*
  in cardiac tamponade, 1253–1255, *1254*
  in cardiac tumors, 1903
  in cardiomyopathy, 84, *85–87,* 86
    dilated, 84, *85,* 86, 1138–1139, *1138–1139*
    hypertrophic, 224, 1063–1065, *1064, 1135–1137,* 1135–1138
    hypertrophic obstructive, 86, *87*
    restrictive, 86, *86,* 1139–1141, *1140*
  in concurrent valvular disease, 445
  in congenital heart disease, 91–94, *91–94*
    complex, 92–94, *93–94,* 251
    valvular, 91–92, *91–92*
  in coronary artery disease, 88–90, *89,* 659–667, 666–667, *667*
  in Ebstein's anomaly, 243–245, *244*
  in endocardial cushion defect, 247, *247*
  in flail mitral valve leaflet, 450, *450,* 450pl
  in Friedreich's ataxia, 1988
  in heart failure, 1156
  in hemochromatosis, 1087, 1141
  in human immunodeficiency virus infection, *1974–1975,* 1974–1976, 1977, *1977*
  in identification of source of pulmonary embolism, 86, *88–89*
  in infective endocarditis, 403–404, *404,* 404t, *454,* 454–455
    and indications for surgical treatment, 410–411, 411t, *1851*
  in left ventricular outflow obstruction, 247–248, *248*

Echocardiography *(Continued)*
  in L-transposition, 212
  in Marfan's syndrome, 453–454, *454*
  in mitral regurgitation, *450,* 450–451, 450pl
  in mitral stenosis, 243, *447–449,* 447–450, 448t
    for treatment planning, *449,* 449–450
  in mitral valve disease, 446–451, *447–450,* 447t–448t, 450pl
  in mitral valve prolapse, 361–362, *362,* 379–380, *379–380, 447,* 451
  in myocardial infarction, 88, *89,* 554–555, *555–556*
    for detection of complications, *661–663,* 661–664
    for detection of viable myocardium, 664–665
  in myocarditis, 1103–1104
  in patent ductus arteriosus, 250
  in patent foramen ovale, 241–242
  in patient evaluation for mitral valve repair, 451, 451pl
  in pericardial effusion, *90,* 90–91, *1248,* 1249–1250
  in pericarditis, acute, 1269
    constrictive, 1263
  in pheochromocytoma, 1920
  in *Pneumocystis carinii* pneumonia, *1974*
  in pulmonary hypertension, 452–453
  in pulmonary stenosis, 453
  in pulmonary thromboembolism, 1841, *1841*
  in regional wall motion abnormalities, 659, *660*
  in restrictive cardiomyopathy, 1079–1080, *1079–1080*
  in rheumatic fever, 393, *394*
  in right ventricular outflow obstruction, 248–249
  in risk stratification for sudden death, 1722
  in sarcoidosis, 1141
  in tetralogy of Fallot, 214, 246–247
  in transplant rejection, 1218
  in transposition of great arteries, 249–250
  in tricuspid regurgitation, 451–452, *452*
  in tricuspid stenosis, 451
  in ventricular septal defect, 244–246, *245*
  intraoperative, for detection of myocardial infarction/ischemia, 666
  intrauterine, 251
  M-mode, 76
    after aortic valve replacement, *288*
    in left ventricular hypertrophy, 984, *984*
    in mitral valve prolapse, 378–380
    in pulmonary hypertension, 1868–1869
  of prosthetic valves, 453, 453pl
  scanning windows for, 76, *77–78,* 78
  stress, for risk stratification in coronary artery disease, 88–90
  technique of, 76, *77–78,* 78
  three-dimensional, 76
  transesophageal. See *Transesophageal echocardiography (TEE).*
  transthoracic, in aortic dissection, 1380t
    in infective endocarditis, 404
  two-dimensional, in dilated cardiomyopathy, 1048
    in myocardial infarction, for diagnosis, 660–661
      for prognosis, 661
    in myocardial ischemia, 660
    in pulmonary hypertension, 1869
    intravascular, 667
    technique of, 440, *441*
Eclampsia, 1507, 2047–2048, 2048t
ECM. See *Extracellular matrix (ECM).*
ECSS (European Coronary Surgery Study), 862t, 864, *865–866*

Ectopia lentis, in Marfan's syndrome, 2151
Ectopic impulse, in myocardial infarction, 543
Edema, differential diagnosis of, 11
peripheral, during pregnancy, 2038
Effective balloon dilating area (EBDA), and outcome of percutaneous mitral balloon valvotomy, 468
Effective valve area, in prosthetic valves, 433t, 434
Effector response(s), in heart transplant rejection, 1211–1212
Efferent pathway(s), in neurally mediated syncope, 1691
Efficacy and Safety of Subcutaneous Enoxaparin in Non–Q Wave Coronary Events (ESSENCE) trial, 729–730
EGF (epidermal growth factor) domain, in coagulation system, 1316
eHAND, and cardiogenesis, 920
Ehlers-Danlos syndrome, 2155
anatomic abnormalities in, 319
vs. Marfan's syndrome, 2153
Einthoven triangle, *32*
Eisenmenger's syndrome, hemoptysis in, 7
pregnancy and, 2060
pulmonary artery hypertrophy in, *222*
ventricular septal defect in, *207,* 207–208
and pulmonary hypertension, 1857, *1858*
Ejection fraction, after myocardial infarction, thrombolytic therapy and, 754, 754t
afterload and, in aortic stenosis, 331, *331*
and indications for management of mitral valve prolapse, 384
and natural history of coronary artery disease, 696, *698*
and prognosis in heart failure, 1159
in aortic stenosis, left ventricular dysfunction and, *333–334,* 333–335
in mitral regurgitation, 426
Ejection sound(s), in aortic stenosis, valvular, 180–181
Ejection time, heart rate and, in aortic stenosis, 429, *430*
Elastic modulus, definition of, 1491
Elastin, in arterial wall, 1480
Elderly patient(s). See *Older adult(s).*
Electrical activity, cellular, 968–969, *969*
Electrical alternans, 53–54
Electrocardiographic gating, in magnetic resonance imaging, 134
Electrocardiography, 29–59
ambulatory. See *Holter monitoring.*
and prognosis in coronary artery disease, 702–703, 702t
and prognosis in silent myocardial ischemia, 574
determination of QRS axis in, *32,* 32–33
drugs affecting, 53
during cardiovascular surgery, 2108
during exercise testing, 587–588, *588*
during pregnancy, 2032
exercise stress. See *Exercise stress electrocardiography.*
for preoperative ischemia monitoring, 2096
in amyloid heart disease, 1083, *1084*
in angina, *44,* 530
in aortic stenosis, valvular, 181, *183*
in arrhythmogenic right ventricular dysplasia, 1666, *1667–1668*
in atrial fibrillation, *1568,* 1633–1635, *1634–1635*
in atrial flutter, *1565, 1608,* 1609, 1633, *1634*
in atrial infarction, 34
in atrial tachycardia, 1606, *1607–1608*
in atrioventricular conduction disturbances, 1597, *1599–1600*

Electrocardiography *(Continued)*
in beri-beri heart disease, 1091
in biatrial enlargement, 34
in bifascicular block, 41–42
in biventricular hypertrophy, 35–36, *36*
in bradycardia-tachycardia syndrome, 1581, *1582*
in bundle branch block, 1574–1575, *1574–1575,* 1574t
in cardiac tamponade, 1255
in cardiac transplantation, 58, *59*
in cardiomyopathy, dilated, 1047, *1047*
hypertrophic, 224, *225,* 1062–1063, *1063*
restrictive, 1079
in chronic obstructive pulmonary disease, 1891
in early repolarization, 53, *54*
in Ebstein's anomaly, *193*
in electrolyte abnormalities, 50–53, *51–52*
in Emery-Dreifuss syndrome, 1994, *1994*
in fascicular block, 40–41, *40–41*
in Friedreich's ataxia, 1988
in heart failure, 1157
in hemochromatosis, 1087
in hypothermia, 56, 58, *58*
in intraventricular conduction delay, 42
in Kearns-Sayre syndrome, 1992, *1993*
in left atrial enlargement, *33,* 33–34
in left bundle branch block, 36–37, *37*
in left ventricular hypertrophy, 34–35, *35*
with conduction disorders, 36
in long QT syndrome, 1660, *1660*
in L-transposition, 212, *215–216*
in mitral valve prolapse, 360–361, 378, *381*
in multifocal atrial tachycardia, *1569*
in muscular dystrophy, Becker's, 1991–1992, 1991t
Duchenne's, 1990, *1990,* 1991t
in myocardial infarction, 44, *45–47,* 46, 548–549, *550–553*
anterior, 48
inferior, 48, *49*
localization of, 47–48
non–Q wave, 48–49
old, 46–47
posterolateral, 48, *49*
Q wave, *535*
in myocardial ischemia, 42–44, *44–45*
in myocarditis, 55, 1103–1104
in myotonic dystrophy, 1985, *1987*
in pericarditis, 55, *56*
acute, 1268, *1269*
constrictive, 1262
vs. restrictive cardiomyopathy, 1266–1267
in pheochromocytoma, 1920
in preexcitation, 42, *42–43,* 1620–1622, *1621–1622*
in pulmonary hypertension, 1867, *1868,* 1868t
in pulmonary stenosis, valvular, 188–189, *189–190*
in pulmonary thromboembolism, 55, *57,* 1837, 1840, 1840t, *1841–1842,* 1842
in right atrial enlargement, 34, *34*
in right bundle branch block, incomplete, 39
in right ventricular hypertrophy, *33–34,* 35
in risk stratification for sudden death, 1722
in scleroderma, 1947, 1947t
in septum primum, 201, *202–203*
in sinus node dysfunction, 1583
in tetralogy of Fallot, 214
in transplant rejection, 1218
in tricuspid atresia, 185, *185–186*
in trifascicular block, 41–42
in unstable angina, 532

Electrocardiography *(Continued)*
in variant angina, 532, *533*
in ventricular septal defect, 205, *206*
in ventricular tachycardia, *1571*
in wide QRS tachycardia, *1678,* 1679–1687, *1682–1686*
in Wolff-Parkinson-White syndrome, 42, *42–43*
interpretation of, 58–59
intraoperative, 2117–2119, *2118–2119*
artifacts in, 2117–2118
computerized analysis of, 2118–2119
electronic filtering in, 2117–2118
lead configuration for, 2118, *2118–2119*
leads for, 30
placement of, 54–55
Mason-Likar modification of, 586
P wave in, 30–31, *31.* See also *P wave.*
PR segment in, 31
principles of, 1–2
QRS complex in, 31. See also *QRS complex.*
QT interval in, 32. See also *QT interval.*
signal-averaged, 30
in dilated cardiomyopathy, 1047, *1047*
in evaluation of syncope, 1698
in risk stratification for sudden death, 1723
ST-T wave in, 31. See also *ST-T wave.*
twelve-lead, 30
U wave in, 32. See also *U wave.*
ventricular gradient in, 32
waveform sequence in, 30–31, *31*
Electrochemical gradient, in excitation-contraction coupling, *1281,* 1281–1282
Electrode(s), for pacemakers, 1765–1766
placement of, for twelve-lead electrocardiography, 30
Electroencephalography, during cardiovascular surgery, 2108
Electrolyte abnormality(ies), and myocardial disease, 1091–1092
and risk of sudden death, 1715
electrocardiography in, 50–53, *51–52*
in adrenal insufficiency, 1917
Electromechanical dissocation, during myocardial rupture, 556–557
Electron beam computed tomography. See *Computed tomography (CT), electron beam*
Electronic appliance(s), interference with pacemakers by, 1778
Electrophysiologic study(ies), before surgery for atrial fibrillation, 1819, 1821
in arrhythmogenic right ventricular dysplasia, 1669–1670
in evaluation of syncope, 1698
with tilt table testing, 1699–1700
in hypertrophic cardiomyopathy, 1065
in risk stratification for sudden death, 1723
in sinus node dysfunction, *1584,* 1584–1587, *1586*
Electrophysiologic Study *vs.* Electrocardiographic Monitoring (ESVEM) study, 1730
ELITE II (Evaluation of Losartan in the Elderly) trial, 1174
Embolectomy, pulmonary, 1850
Embolism, amniotic fluid, *vs.* pulmonary thromboembolism, 1847–1848
aortic, 1393–1394
cerebral, in carotid artery disease, prevention of, 1437–1438
coronary, angiography in, 645
fat, *vs.* pulmonary thromboembolism, 1847
from cardiac myxoma, 1904
from coronary angiography, 606

Embolism *(Continued)*
from infective endocarditis, 413–415, *414*
in sinus node dysfunction, 1576
mitral valve prolapse and, 381–382
pulmonary. See *Pulmonary thromboembolism.*
sources of, 1400
systemic, from mitral valve prolapse, 364
tumor, *vs.* pulmonary thromboembolism, 1847
venous air, *vs.* pulmonary thromboembolism, 1847
Emerin, in Emery-Dreifuss muscular dystrophy, 2160
Emery-Dreifuss muscular dystrophy, 2160
Emery-Dreifuss syndrome, 1986t, 1992–1995, *1994*
genetic basis of, 1992
EMIAT (European Myocardial Infarct Amiodarone Trial), 1726
Emory Angioplasty *versus* Surgery Trial (EAST), *796,* 797t, 872, 873t
Emphysema. See also *Chronic obstructive pulmonary disease (COPD).*
definition of, 1885
diagnosis of, physical examination in, 1889
pathophysiology of, 1887
Employment, return to, cardiac rehabilitation and, 898t, 904
Enalapril, for heart failure, *1169,* 1170t, *1172*
Encainide, use dependency of, *1741*
Encephalopathy, hypertensive, 1524
Endarterectomy, *855,* 856
carotid, 1435–1436
restenosis after, 1436
Endoaneurysmorrhaphy, for repair of transverse aortic aneurysms, *1364*
Endocardial cushion defect(s), 209–210
echocardiography of, 247, *247*
Endocardial fibroelastosis, congenital, pathologic changes in, 1031
Endocardial friction lesion(s), in mitral valve prolapse, 356, *356–357,* 362, *362*
left ventricular, in mitral valve prolapse, 373, *373*
Endocardial ventriculotomy, for ischemic ventricular tachycardia, 1830
Endocarditis, from pulmonary artery catheterization, 2127
in prosthetic valves, 2286–2288, 2286t–2288t
clinical features of, 2286–2287
diagnosis of, 2287
microbiology of, 2286, 2286t
pathogenesis of, 2286
prevention of, 2288
risk factors for, 2286t
treatment of, 2287–2288, 2287t–2288t
in rheumatic fever, 391, *394*
in systemic lupus erythematosus, 1943–1944, *1944*
infective. See *Infective endocarditis.*
nonbacterial thrombotic, 401
Endocarditis parietalis fibroplastica, 1075
Endocardium, mural, pathologic changes in, 1031
Endocrine disorder(s), 1915–1931. See also specific disorder, e.g., *Diabetes mellitus.*
anatomic abnormalities in, 318–319, *318–319*
and syncope, 1695–1696
pathologic changes in, 1030
Endomyocardial biopsy, 1021–1022
cardiac catheterization in, 1132–1133
in amyloid heart disease, 1085
in arrhythmogenic right ventricular dysplasia, 1669
Endomyocardial biopsy *(Continued)*
in dilated cardiomyopathy, 1048
in hemochromatosis, 1087–1088
in myocarditis, 1104–1105, 1104t
in radiation-induced heart disease, 1088
in transplant rejection, 1027–1028, *1028–1029,* 1028t
acute, 1217
indications for, 1133
Endomyocardial fibrosis, and restrictive cardiomyopathy, 1075. See also *Cardiomyopathy, restrictive.*
vs. amyloid heart disease, 1085
with eosinophilia, anatomic abnormalities in, 317–318, *318,* 318pl
Endorphin(s), and angina, 570
Endothelial cell(s), antithrombotic products of, 1330t
as procoagulant mechanism, 1318
functions of, 1330t
interactions with neurotransmitters, and circulatory regulation, 1289–1290
procoagulant products of, 1330t
surface of, assembly of fibrinolytic components at, *1313,* 1313–1314
Endothelin, release of, and hypertension, 1503, *1503*
in heart failure, 1154
Endothelin inhibitor(s), for heart failure, 1176
Endothelium, and arterial function, 1481
and vasodilatation, 524
as sensor for mechanical overload, 958
cytokines produced by, 1332t
dysfunction of, and hypertension, 1502–1503, *1503,* 1511–1512, *1512*
pulmonary, 1859–1860, *1860*
and microcirculatory disease, 641, 681
cocaine and, 1961–1962
injury to, in atherogenesis, *1327–1329,* 1327–1330, 1330t–1331t
in myocardial infarction, 536
interaction with leukocytes, in atherogenesis, 1330–1331, 1332t
release of hormones by, in heart failure, 1154
release of vasoactive substances by, 1276, *1276*
Endothelium-derived contracting factor(s), and circulatory regulation, 1288
Endothelium-derived growth factor(s), and vascular remodeling, 1301, 1301t
Endothelium-derived relaxing factor(s), and circulatory regulation, 1286–1288, *1287*
Endovascular brachytherapy, for peripheral vascular disease, 1441–1443, *1442,* 1442t
End-systolic volume, and prognosis in myocardial infarction, 677
in mitral regurgitation, 460
left ventricular, and prognosis in myocardial infarction, 561, *561*
Energy, consumption and provision of, by heart muscle, 937–938, *937–938*
depletion of, 999, 999t
metabolism of, and myocardial adaptation to cardiac hypertrophy, 956–957, 957t
in systolic dysfunction, 961
production of, adenosine triphosphate and, 937, *937*
transfer of, 938
metabolic pathways in, 938–939, *940*
Energy correction factor, in radionuclide imaging, 100
Energy starvation, 999, 999t
eNOS (enzyme nitric oxide synthase), 524
and vascular remodeling, 1304
eNOS (enzyme nitric oxide synthase) gene transfer, for circulatory dysfunction, 1295
Enoxaparin, for non–Q wave myocardial infarction, 729–730
for unstable angina, 729–730
Enterochromaffin cell(s), in carcinoid syndrome, 1930
Enterococcal endocarditis, 407, 407t
Enzyme(s), serum, in myocardial infarction, 549, *553,* 553–554
Enzyme nitric oxide synthase (eNOS), 524
and vascular remodeling, 1304
Enzyme nitric oxide synthase (eNOS) gene transfer, for circulatory dysfunction, 1295
Eosinophilia, endomyocardial fibrosis with, anatomic abnormalities in, 317–318, *318,* 318pl
in restrictive cardiomyopathy, 1075–1077, *1076–1077,* 1076t
Eosinophilic myocarditis, 1113, *1113*
causes of, 1025t
Ephedrine, for postural hypotension, 1556
EPIC (Evaluation of IIb/IIIa Platelet Receptor antagonist 7E3 in Preventing Ischemic Complications) trial, 823
Epicardial cell(s), "spike-and-dome" configuration in, in Brugada's syndrome, 1721
Epicardial coronary artery(ies), 522
Epidermal growth factor (EGF) domain, in coagulation system, 1316
EPILOG (Evaluation of PTCA to Improve Long-term Outcome by c7E3 GP IIb/IIIa Receptor Blockade) study, 735, 735t, 810, 811t
Epinephrine, release of, and hypertension, 1498–1499, *1499*
EPISTENT (Evaluation of Platelet IIb/IIIa Inhibitor for Stenting) trial, 734, 735t, 807, 812t
Epoprostenol, for pulmonary hypertension, 1879, *1880*
Epsilon-aminocaproic acid, for intraoperative blood conservation, 2112
Epsilon wave, in arrhythmogenic right ventricular dysplasia, 1666, *1667,* 1717, *1718*
Eptifibatide, for unstable angina, 732–733, *733,* 735t–736t, 810
with tissue plasminogen activator, Impact-AMI study of, 771
ERACI (Argentine Randomized Trial of Coronary Angioplasty *versus* Bypass Surgery in Multivessel Disease), *796,* 797t, 893t, 894
Erdheim's cystic medial necrosis, 1362
Erdheim's disease, 2152
Ergonovine, for assessment of coronary vasospasm, 638–639, *639–640*
Erythema marginatum, in rheumatic fever, 391, *392*
Erythrocyte(s), disorders of, 2001–2005, *2002–2005,* 2005t. See also *Anemia; Erythrocytosis.*
Erythrocytosis, 2004–2005, *2005,* 2005t
Esmolol, adverse effects of, 1750
dosage of, 712t, 1750
efficacy of, 1750
electrophysiology of, 1750
for atrial fibrillation, 1636, 1637t
pharmacokinetics of, 1742t–1743t, 1750
Esophageal procedure(s), antibiotic prophylaxis for, 415t
ESSENCE (Efficacy and Safety of Subcutaneous Enoxaparin in Non–Q Wave Coronary Events) trial, 729–730
Essential hypertension. See *Hypertension, essential.*

Estrogen, and circulatory regulation, 1290
Estrogen replacement therapy, in secondary prevention of hyperlipidemia, 2249–2250
Ethanol. See *Alcohol.*
Ethmozine. See *Moricizine.*
Ethnicity, and natural history of coronary artery disease, 694–695
European Coronary Surgery Study (ECSS), 862t, 864, *865–866*
European Myocardial Infarct Amiodarone Trial (EMIAT), 1726
Euthyroid sick syndrome, 1929–1930
Evaluation of IIb/IIIa Platelet Receptor antagonist 7E3 in Preventing Ischemic Complications (EPIC) trial, 823
Evaluation of Losartan in the Elderly (ELITE II) trial, 1174
Evaluation of Platelet IIb/IIIa Inhibitor for Stenting (EPISTENT) trial, 734, 735t, 807, 812t
Evaluation of PTCA to Improve Long-term Outcome by c7E3 GP IIb/IIIa Receptor Blockade (EPILOG) study, 735, 735t, 810, 811t
Event recorder(s), for evaluation of syncope, 1697–1698
EVSEM (Electrophysiologic Study *vs.* Electrocardiographic Monitoring) study, 1730
Excitation-contraction coupling, 992–998, 992t, *993, 995–998, 1281–1284,* 1281–1285
  calcium and, 992–993, 992t, *993*
  calcium flux during, *993,* 998–999
  cytoplasmic calcium levels and, 1282, *1283*
  dyad in, 995, *995*
  electrochemical gradient, *1281,* 1281–1282
  G proteins in, 1283, *1283*
  guanosine triphosphate–binding proteins in, *1284,* 1284–1285
  in systolic dysfunction, 964
  mitogen-activated protein kinases in, 1285
  phosphoinositide pathway in, *1283*
  plasma membrane in, 993–995
    calcium channels of, 994
    calcium pump of, 994
    sodium pump and, 995
    sodium-calcium exchanger and, 994–995
    sodium-hydrogen exchange and, 995
  sarcoplasmic reticulum in, 996–998, *996–998*
    calcium pump of, 996–998, *997–998*
    calcium release channels of, 996, *996*
  signal transduction in, 1282–1285, *1284*
  structures participating in, 992t, *993*
  tyrosine kinases in, 1284, *1284*
Exercise, and autonomic dysfunction, 1545, *1547*
  and blood pressure control, 2218–2219
  and circulatory regulation, 1290
  and coagulation, 2223
  and parasympathetic influences on heart, 2222–2223
  and postural hypotension, 1554, *1555*
  and pulmonary capillary wedge pressure, in heart failure, 1150, *1150*
  and risk for atherosclerosis, 1350–1351
  and vascular remodeling, 1303–1304
  auscultation after, 21
  beta-blockers and, 901–902
  cardiovascular function during, aging and, 2017–2018
  during SPECT myocardial perfusion imaging, 103
  dynamic *vs.* isometric, 897
  for peripheral vascular disease, of lower extremities, *1410,* 1410–1411
Exercise *(Continued)*
  for prevention of coronary artery disease, mechanisms in, 2221–2223
    primary, 2216–2219, *2217*
    secondary, 2219–2221, *2220,* 2220t
  in heart failure, 1166
  in management of hypertension, 1516
  in Wolff-Parkinson-White syndrome, 1625–1626, *1628*
  prescription for, 896–897
  protective effect of, 2216–2218
  rate-adaptive pacemaker therapy during, 1771–1772
  response to, during pregnancy, 2029, *2030*
  risks of, 2219
  vascular effects of, 2221–2222
  vs. fitness, 2217–2218
Exercise capacity, and prognosis in heart failure, 1159
  cardiac rehabilitation and, 900–901
Exercise electron beam computed tomography, 2183
Exercise intolerance, in peripheral vascular disease, of lower extremities, 1406
Exercise radionuclide ventriculography, 107, 109
  and prognosis in myocardial infarction, 677–678, *678*
  in coronary artery disease, for diagnosis, 676
Exercise stress echocardiography, before noncardiac surgery, 2094–2095
  in myocardial ischemia, 665–666, 665t
Exercise stress electrocardiography, and prognosis in coronary artery disease, 703
  and prognosis in subclinical atherosclerosis, 2253
    in older adults, 2254
  in atrial fibrillation, 1636, *1636*
Exercise testing, 586–590
  after myocardial infarction, 589–590, *590*
  and eligibility for transplantation, 1187
  and Holter monitoring, 572–573
  before hospital discharge, 896
  before noncardiac surgery, 2094, 2095t
  before revascularization, 590
  bicycle ergometry for, 586–587
  contraindications to, 586–587, 586t
  during pregnancy, 2033
  economic issues in, 904–905
  electrocardiography during, 587–588, *588*
  false-positive results of, 589
  in coronary artery disease, 588–589
    in European Cooperative Surgery Study, *865–866*
  in diagnosis of arrhythmias, 590
  in evaluation of syncope, 1698
  in heart failure, 1157, *1158*
  in peripheral arterial disease, 590
  in peripheral vascular disease, of lower extremities, 1407–1408
  in pulmonary hypertension, 1873
  in risk stratification for sudden death, 1722–1723
  in silent myocardial ischemia, 571–572
  in sinus node dysfunction, 1583
  in valvular disease, 590
  indications for, 586–587, 587t
  interpretation of, 587–588, *588*
  postexercise period of, 587
  prognostic use of, 589, *589,* 589t
  treadmill for, 587
Expiration, on radiography, *70*
Expiratory flow, in chronic obstructive pulmonary disease, 1890, *1891*
Extracardiac conduit(s), for repair of tetralogy of Fallot, 302
Extracellular matrix (ECM), in eroded atherosclerotic plaques, 581
Extracorporeal circulation, for cardiopulmonary bypass, 2113
Extrasystole, ventricular, 1570–1571

Fabry's disease, 1090, 2174t
  anatomic abnormalities in, 319
  pathologic changes in, 1029, 1029pl
"Facies mitralis," 348
Facioscapulohumeral muscular dystrophy, 1986t, *1995,* 1995–1996
Fainting. See *Syncope.*
False aneurysm(s). See *Pseudoaneurysm(s).*
Familial amyloid polyneuropathy, and autonomic dysfunction, 1552
Familial dysautonomia, 1551
FANA (fluorescent antinuclear antibody) test, in pulmonary hypertension, 1866
Fascicular block, electrocardiography in, 40–41, *40–41*
"Fast flush test," 2120, *2120*
Fat embolism, *vs.* pulmonary thromboembolism, 1847
Fatigue, in pulmonary hypertension, 1864, 1864t
Fatty acid(s), as fuel for respiration, 940, *940*
  in myocardial metabolism, 946–948, *947*
  metabolism of, defective, 948
Fatty streak(s), in atherosclerosis, 1325–1326
FDG ([^{18}F]-fluorodeoxyglucose), as tracer of metabolic pathways, 940–942, *941–942*
Felodipine, dosage of, 713t
  for hypertension, clinical trials of, 1343
Femoral artery, cannulation of, for coronary angiography, 597–598
  pseudoaneurysms of, from coronary angiography, 606
Femoropopliteal graft(s), for peripheral vascular disease, of lower extremities, 1412
Fenestrated Fontan procedure, umbrella devices for, 278
Fenfluramine, and pulmonary hypertension, 1862, *1863*
  valvular disease from, 453
Fetal alcohol syndrome, 1967
Fetal circulation, 196
Fetal distress, 2034, *2035*
Fetal warfarin syndrome, 2040, *2040*
Fetal wastage, congenital heart disease and, 228–229
Fetus(es), arrhythmias in, 2063–2064
  cardiac drugs affecting, 228
  echocardiography in, 251
  multiple, cardiovascular impact of, 2031
Fever, during pregnancy, 2038
  in pulmonary thromboembolism, 1837
FGF (fibroblast growth factor), and myocyte proliferation, in cardiogenesis, 924–925
  and vascular remodeling, 1302–1303
Fibric acid(s), for hyperlipidemia, 2248
Fibrillin gene, and Marfan's syndrome, 2153–2154
Fibrinogen, and atherosclerosis, 1349
  and coronary artery disease, risk of, 2207, 2208t
  smoking and, 1344
Fibrinolytic agent(s), 743
Fibrinolytic system, 1311–1315, *1312, 1314*
  components of, assembly at endothelial cell surface, *1313,* 1313–1314
  in pulmonary hypertension, 1861–1862
  pathophysiologic aspects of, 1315
  plasminogen activator inhibitor and, 1313

Fibrinolytic system *(Continued)*
plasminogen activators and, 1311–1312
regulation of, 1312–1313
structure of, 1311, *1312*
Fibrin-specific thrombolytic agent(s), 743
Fibroblast growth factor (FGF), and myocyte proliferation, in cardiogenesis, 924–925
and vascular remodeling, 1302–1303
Fibroelastoma, echocardiography in, *88*
papillary, 1907, *1907*
Fibroelastosis, endocardial, congenital, pathologic changes in, 1031
Fibroma, cardiac, 1907
Fibromuscular dysplasia, renovascular hypertension and, 1428, 1505–1506
revascularization for, 1430
Fibrosa, microscopic anatomy of, *355,* 355–356
Fick principle, in measurement of cardiac output, in mitral stenosis, 423
Figure-eight configuration, in total anomalous pulmonary venous connection, 222, *223*
Filament(s), in myocytes, 1276–1277, *1277–1278*
First pass radionuclide angiocardiography, *106,* 106–107
Fish oil, and hypertension control, 2241
Fitness, *vs.* exercise, 2217–2218
FK-506. See *Tacrolimus.*
Flail mitral valve leaflet, echocardiography in, 450, *450,* 450pl
"Flash" pulmonary edema, 1178
Flecainide, adverse effects of, 1747
dosage of, 1747
efficacy of, 1747
electrophysiology of, 1747
for atrial fibrillation, 1637t, 1638
risks of, 1640, *1640*
pharmacokinetics of, 1742t–1743t, 1747
Flectin, and left-right position of body axis, 923
Floppy valve, anatomic abnormalities in, 319–320, *319–320*
Flosequinan, for heart failure, 1173
Flow metabolism imaging, and cardiac risk, *682,* 683, *684*
Flow velocity curve, transmitral valve, 1004–1005
Fludrocortisone, for postural hypotension, 1556
Fluid balance, weightlessness and, 2077–2078
Fluorescent antinuclear antibody (FANA) test, in pulmonary hypertension, 1866
^{18}F-Fluorodeoxyglucose (FDG), as tracer of metabolic pathways, 940–942, *941–942*
Fluoroscopic display unit(s), for coronary angiography, 594
Fluvastatin, for hyperlipidemia, clinical trials of, 1339–1340
Foam cell(s), in atherosclerotic plaques, *1326*
Folic acid, and plasma homocysteine levels, 2281, *2282,* 2283
Fontan procedure, fenestrated, for tricuspid atresia, 306
umbrella devices for, 278
for tricuspid atresia, with pulmonary stenosis, 187
Food intake, and autonomic dysfunction, 1545, *1547*
Foramen ovale, anatomy of, 147, *148*
Forceps, vascular retrieval, 281
Foreign body(ies), transcatheter removal of, 280–281
Fosinopril, for heart failure, 1170t
Fossa ovalis, 162–163
anatomy of, 147, *148*
Fourier phase analysis, on radionuclide ventriculography, 110
Fractional flow reserve, assessment of, coronary angiography in, 631–632
Fragmin during Instability in Coronary Artery Disease Study (FRISC), 726, *728,* 729t, 814–815, 815t
Framingham Heart Study, 1338
of coronary artery disease risk factors. See *Coronary artery disease, risk factor(s) for.*
of sudden death, 1710
of syncope, 1700
Friction rub, pleural, in pulmonary thromboembolism, 1837
Friedreich's ataxia, 1986t, 1988
Friedreich's sign, 19
FRISC (Fragmin during Instability in Coronary Artery Disease Study), 726, *728,* 729t, 814–815, 815t
Functional murmur(s), 22
Fungal endocarditis, 409
anatomic abnormalities in, 321
Fungal infection(s), and myocarditis, 1097t, 1110
Furosemide, for congestive heart failure, 1166, 1166t
Fusion beat(s), ventricular, in wide QRS tachycardia, 1679, *1682*

G protein(s), in excitation-contraction coupling, 1283, *1283*
GABI (German Angioplasty Bypass Investigation), *796,* 797t, 872, 873t, 874
Gain-of-function, definition of, 917t
Gallop(s), auscultation of, 20, 22, 24, 27
differential diagnosis of, 10–11
summation, 27
Gallstone(s), after heart transplantation, 1200
Gamma camera(s), single-crystal, for radionuclide imaging, 99–100, *100*
Gamma radiation, *vs.* beta radiation, for restenosis, 830–831
GAMMA-ONE trial, 835
Gamma-variate curve(s), for quantification of shunts, in congenital heart disease, 461, *461*
Ganciclovir, for post-transplantation infection, 1190–1191
Ganglionectomy, left cervicothoracic sympathetic, for long QT syndrome, 1704
Ganglionic blocker(s), during pregnancy, 2050t
Gastrointestinal disorder(s), chest pain in, 6
Gastrointestinal procedure(s), antibiotic prophylaxis for, 414t, 416t
Gastrulation, definition of, 917t
GATA transcription factor(s), in cardiogenesis, 920, 959
and postnatal cardiac hypertrophy, 928
Gated-equilibrium radionuclide ventriculography, 107, *107–108,* 107pl
Gaucher's disease, 1090, 2174t
pathologic changes in, 1030
Gender, and coronary artery caliber, 615
and dilated cardiomyopathy, 1034
and left ventricular hypertrophy, 1010
and natural history of coronary artery disease, 692–693, *693*
and plaque morphology, 584, 584t
and plasma homocysteine levels, 2279, 2279t
and risk of coronary artery disease, 671–673, 672t
and risk of sudden death, *1712,* 1713
Gene expression, changes in, and cardiac hypertrophy, 959–960
Gene therapy, 2269–2274
Gene therapy *(Continued)*
animal models of, 2271–2272, *2272*
arterial, for restenosis, 1421–1422
clinical trials of, 2272–2274, *2273,* 2273t–2274t
for angiogenesis, 2272–2274, 2273t–2274t
delivery catheters for, 2272, *2272*
ex vivo *vs.* in vivo, 2269
for carotid artery disease, 1440
for muscular dystrophy, Duchenne's, 2165
for myocardial modulation, 516, 518
for prevention of allograft vasculopathy, 1197, 1220
for tibioperoneal occlusion, 1440
future of, 2274
principles of, 2269, *2270*
transgenic technology in, 2272
vector systems for, 2269–2271, *2270,* 2271t
with vascular endothelial growth factor gene, 1419–1420, *1420*
clinical trials of, 1420–1421, *1421*
Gene transfer, for circulatory dysfunction, 1295
Genetic disorder(s), cardiac manifestations of, 224
classification of, 2145–2148
chromosomal, *2145–2146,* 2145–2147, 2146t
modes of inheritance in, *2147,* 2147–2148, 2148t
single-gene, with cardiovascular features, 2146t, *2147,* 2147–2148, 2172–2173, 2172t–2175t
X-linked, 2148
Genetic linkage analysis, in hypertrophic cardiomyopathy, 1055, *1056,* 1056t
Genetic polymorphism(s), and risk of coronary artery disease, 695
Genetic testing, in hypertrophic cardiomyopathy, 1065–1066
Genitourinary tract procedure(s), antibiotic prophylaxis for, 414t, 416t
Gentamicin, for infective endocarditis, penicillin-susceptible, 405–406, 406t–407t
staphylococcal, 407–408, 408t–409t
German Angioplasty Bypass Investigation (GABI), *796,* 797t, 872, 873t, 874
GESICA (Gruppo de Estudio de la Sobrevida en la Insuficiencia Cardiaca en Argentina) trial, 1726
Ghent criteria, 2151, 2153t
Giant cell arteritis, 1391–1392, 1950
Giant cell myocarditis, 1093, 1112–1113, *1113*
Gianturco coil occlusion device, for abnormal vascular communications, 271
for patent ductus arteriosus, 268–269, *270*
Gianturco-Grifka vascular occlusion device, for patent ductus arteriosus, 269
GISSI-2 (Gruppo Italiano per lo Studio Della Sopravvivenza Nell'Infarto Miocardico) database, 692, 693t
Glenn procedure, for tricuspid atresia, with pulmonary stenosis, 187
Global Utilization of Streptokinase and Tissue Plasminogen Activator for Occluded Arteries (GUSTO-I) study. See under *GUSTO.*
Glossopharyngeal neuralgia, and syncope, 9
Glucose, as fuel for respiration, 940, *940*
metabolism of, glycogen and, 944–945
glycolysis and, 945
pyruvate and, 943, *943,* 945–946, *946*
regulatory sites of, 943–946, *944, 946*
phosphorylation of, 943–944, *944*
serum, in diabetes mellitus, 1924

Glucose metabolism, and myocardial blood flow, imaging of, positron emission tomography in, 123–124, *123–124*
Glucose tolerance, impaired, and risk of coronary artery disease, 2198–2199, 2198t–2199t
Glucose transporter(s) (GLUT), 943–944, *944*
GLUT (glucose transporters), 943–944, *944*
Glycogen, and glucose metabolism, 944–945
Glycogen storage disease(s), 2174t
pathologic changes in, 1028–1031, 1029pl–1030pl, *1030*
Glycolysis, and glucose metabolism, 945
Glycoprotein IIb/IIIa antagonist(s), and natural history of myocardial infarction, 702
for unstable angina, 730–737, *731–735,* 735t–737t, 810–811, 810t–812t
with interventional therapies, 734–737, *735,* 737t
with thrombolytic therapy, 771–772, *772*
Glycoprotein IIb/IIIa receptor(s), expression of, 730, *731,* 732
Goldman Multifactorial Cardiac Risk Index, 2093t
Goodpasture's syndrome, *vs.* pulmonary thromboembolism, 1846
Goose-neck deformity, in ostium primum, *203*
Gorlin equation, for determination of aortic valve area, 427, 429, *429*
for determination of mitral valve area, 422, *422,* 474
Gout, after heart transplantation, 1200
anatomic abnormalities in, 319, *319*
Gradient-echo magnetic resonance imaging, 134, *134*
Graft(s). See also *Coronary artery bypass graft (CABG).*
Dacron, for peripheral vascular disease, of lower extremities, 1412
for repair of aortic dissection, 1384
Grampian Region Early Antistreplase Trial (GREAT), of prehospital thrombolytic therapy, 757–758
Granulomatosis, Wegener's, 1950
anatomic abnormalities in, 317
vs. pulmonary thromboembolism, 1846
Granulomatous infection(s), *vs.* pulmonary thromboembolism, 1844
Granulomatous myocarditis, causes of, 1025t
Granulomatous pericarditis, 1242, 1242pl
Gray gelatinous lesion(s), in atherosclerosis, 1325
GREAT (Grampian Region Early Antistreplase Trial), of prehospital thrombolytic therapy, 757–758
Great artery(ies), abnormal communications between, 161–163, *163–165*
distal to atrioventricular valves, 163, *164–165*
proximal to atrioventricular valves, 163–164, *164*
transposition of, 164
corrected, 164, 167
echocardiography in, 93, *94,* 249–250
surgical treatment of, 303, *304–305,* 306
Great vein(s), malpositions of, 221–224, *223*
and partial anomalous pulmonary venous connection, 221–222
and total anomalous pulmonary venous connection, 222, *223,* 224
Great vessel(s). See also *Aorta.*
abnormal communication between, *196–209,* 196–210, 196t
diseases of, electron beam computed tomography in, 2186–2187, *2187–2188*
magnetic resonance imaging of, 135–136, *135–136*
Great vessel(s) *(Continued)*
obstruction of, 193–196, *194–195*
aortic coarctation and, 193–195, *194–195*
balloon angioplasty for, 262–264
inferior vena cava obstruction and, 195–196
pulmonary artery stenosis and, 195
superior vena cava obstruction and, 195
transposition of, complete, 210, *211*
congenitally corrected, 212, *213–216*
"Ground-glass" appearance, in restrictive cardiomyopathy, 86, *86*
Growth factor(s), and vascular remodeling, 1301, 1301t
release of, and restenosis, 1306
Growth hormone, deficiency of, 1915–1916
excessive, and acromegaly, 1916
for dilated cardiomyopathy, 1049
Growth promoter(s), vascular, 1301–1302
Growth signal(s), in cardiac hypertrophy, 957–960
DNA targets and, 958–959
permanent changes in gene expression and, 959–960
sensors and, 958
transduction systems and, 958
transgenic technology and, 959
transient changes in gene expression and, 959
Gruppo de Estudio de la Sobrevida en la Insuficiencia Cardiaca en Argentina (GESICA) trial, 1726
Gruppo Italiano per lo Studio della Sopravvivenza nell'Infarto Miocardico (GISSI-2) database, 692, 693t
GTP (guanosine triphosphate)-binding protein(s), in excitation-contraction coupling, *1284,* 1284–1285
Guanethidine, during pregnancy, 2050t
Guanosine triphosphate (GTP)-binding protein(s), in excitation-contraction coupling, *1284,* 1284–1285
Guide wire traversal test, before thrombolytic therapy, 1427
Gunshot wound(s), and aortic trauma, 1392
GUSTO (Global Utilization of Streptokinase and Tissue Plasminogen Activator for Occluded Arteries) study, 691, *692,* 693t, *701*
of myocardial infarction, 821–822, *822*
of unstable angina, 804

H wave, *17,* 19
HACEK microorganism(s), and infective endocarditis, 408, 409t
"Hammocking," holosystolic, in mitral valve prolapse, 362, 379
HAND transcription factor(s), in cardiogenesis, 920
Hand-heart syndrome(s), genetic basis of, 926
HCM disease gene(s), in hypertrophic cardiomyopathy, 1055–1058, *1056,* 1056t
HDL. See *High-density lipoprotein (HDL).*
Health care worker(s), human immunodeficiency virus infection and, 1981–1982
Health risk appraisal model, for cardiac rehabilitation, 908
Heart. See also *Cardiac* entries.
anatomy of, *147–149,* 147–150
at rest, aging and, 2017
cellular electrical activity in, 968–969, *969*
development of. See *Cardiogenesis.*
embryogenesis of, transcription factors in, 918
Heart *(Continued)*
endocrine function of, and cardiac hypertrophy, 967–968
"nutrition" of, 939–940
radiography of. See *Radiography.*
size of, radiographic assessment of, *68,* 71
space flight and, 2085
Heart block, after heart transplantation, 1200
bilateral bundle branch, 1574t, 1574–1575
complete, 1573–1574
congenital, in systemic lupus erythematosus, 1945
during cardiovascular surgery, 2113
during pregnancy, 2046
first-degree, 1572–1573
in Kearns-Sayre syndrome, 1992, *1993*
in survivors of myocardial infarction, 778
Mobitz I, 1573
Mobitz II, 1573
second-degree, 1573
Wenckebach, 1573
Heart failure, acute, 1178
advanced, surgical treatment of, 1224–1236
cardiomyoplasty in, 1235–1236
heart transplantation in, 1224–1231, *1226–1232.* See also *Transplantation, heart, in advanced heart failure.*
mechanical circulatory support in, *1231–1234,* 1231–1235
history of, 1231, *1231*
left ventricular assist device in, 1231–1235, *1233–1234*
partial left ventriculectomy in, 1236
after myocardial infarction, 1177, *1177*
and circulatory dysfunction, 1294, *1294*
and vascular compliance, 1490–1491
classification of, 1158–1159, 1159t
clinical course of, 1161
clinical features of, 1147, *1147*
congestive. See *Congestive heart failure (CHF).*
coronary angiography in, 604
cough in, 6
definition of, *1147,* 1147–1148
diagnosis of, 1154–1158, *1156–1158*
echocardiography in, 1156
electrocardiography in, 1157
exercise testing in, 1157, *1158*
history in, 1155
laboratory studies in, 1158
magnetic resonance imaging in, 1156
physical examination in, of venous pressure, 1155, *1156*
pulmonary, 1155–1156
radiography in, 1156, *1157*
venous pressure in, 1155, *1156*
etiology of, 1148–1150, 1149t
from diastolic dysfunction, treatment of, 1012–1013
from infective endocarditis, *410–411,* 410–412, 411t
growing prevalence of, 1147–1148
hyponatremia and, 1178–1179
in aortic stenosis, left ventricular dysfunction and, *331,* 331–332
in older adults, 1177
left ventricular dysfunction and, 1177–1178
malabsorption in, 1179
pathophysiology of, 1150–1154, *1150–1154,* 1150t, 1152t
cytokines in, 1154
diastolic dysfunction in, 1151
endothelial activity in, 1154
feedback loops in, 1154, *1154*
fiber slippage in, 1151–1152

Heart failure *(Continued)*
infarct expansion in, 1151
left ventricular dysfunction in, 1150, *1150*
myocyte lengthening in, 1151
myocyte thickening in, 1151
natriuretic peptides in, 1154
neurohumoral activation in, 1152, *1152*
renin-angiotensin-aldosterone system activation in, 1153, *1153*
sympathetic nervous system activation in, 1152–1153
systolic dysfunction in, 1150–1151, 1150t
vasopressin in, 1153–1154
ventricular remodeling in, 1151, 1152t
prognosis in, 1159–1161, *1160*
cardiac enlargement and, 1159
ejection fraction and, 1159
exercise capacity and, 1159
hyponatremia and, 1161
plasma norepinephrine and, *1160,* 1160–1161
ventricular arrhythmias and, 1159–1160
progression to, from cardiac hypertrophy, 983, *983*
severity of, assessment of, 1158–1159, 1159t
sudden death in, 1161
systemic symptoms of, 1179
treatment of, aldosterone antagonists in, 1175
amlodipine in, 1173
angiotensin receptor blockers in, 1173–1174
angiotensin-converting enzyme inhibitors in, 1168–1170, *1169,* 1170t
antiarrhythmic agents in, 1175
anticoagulants in, 1175
beta-blockers in, 1170–1171, *1171*
calcium antagonists in, 1173
cardiac depressants in, 1166
digitalis in, 1174
digoxin in, 1174
diuretics in, 1166–1167, 1166t
exercise in, 1166
experimental, 1176–1177
gene therapy in, 2274
goals of, 1165
immunization in, 1166
inotropic agents in, 1168, 1174–1175
isosorbide dinitrate with hydralazine in, 1171–1173, *1172*
mibefradil in, 1173
nitrates in, 1173
salt restriction in, 1165
smoking cessation in, 1166
surgical, 1175–1176
symptomatic, 1165–1168, 1166t
vasodilators in, 1167–1168
weight loss in, 1165
Heart murmurs. See *Murmur(s).*
Heart muscle, consumption and provision of energy by, 937–938, *937–938*
Heart Outcomes Prevention Evaluation (HOPE) trial, 720–721
Heart rate, and ejection time, in aortic stenosis, 429, *430*
and myocardial oxygen consumption, 522
during bundle branch block, and diagnosis of supraventricular tachycardia, 1611, *1614–1615*
during exercise testing, 587
during pregnancy, 2028, 2028t
fetal, monitoring of, 2034, *2035*
intrinsic, assessment of, in sinus node dysfunction, 1583–1584
measurement of, pulmonary artery catheterization in, 2129
Heart rate *(Continued)*
smoking and, *2230*
space flight and, 2081–2082, *2082*
variability of, and arrhythmias, 2222–2223
and risk of sudden death, 1723
Heart size, in mitral stenosis, 420, *420*
Heart sound(s), first, *21,* 21–22, 22t
fourth, 11, *20,* 27
from prosthetic disc valves, 27, *27*
in amyloid heart disease, 1083
in angina, 530
in aortic regurgitation, 337
in atrial septal defect, 197
in atrioventricular dissociation, 1677
in cardiac myxoma, left atrial, 1904
right atrial, 1906
in cardiogenic shock, 1531
in cardiomyopathy, dilated, 1046
hypertrophic, 1062
restrictive, 1078, *1078*
in Ebstein's anomaly, 192
in heart failure, 1156
in mitral regurgitation, 351
in mitral stenosis, 348, *349*
in myocardial infarction, 543, *544,* 547–548, *547–549*
in pericarditis, constrictive, 1262
in pulmonary regurgitation, 343
in tricuspid stenosis, 344
palpation of, 19–20
second, *21,* 21–22
splitting of, *21*
third, 10–11, *20,* 22, 24
Heart transplantation. See *Transplantation, heart.*
Heart-hand syndrome, 176
Heart-lung transplantation. See *Transplantation, heart-lung.*
HeartMate left ventricular assist device, 1231–1235, *1233–1234*
explant procedure for, 1232, 1235
features of, 1232
implant procedure for, 1232, *1233–1234*
indications for, 1232
Heat, in energy metabolism, and myocardial adaptation to cardiac hypertrophy, 957, 957t
Heat stroke, cardiac complications of, 1093
Hedgehog protein, and cardiogenesis, 922
Helicobacter pylori, and atherosclerosis, 1338
Helsinki Heart Study, 1337
Hematologic disorder(s), drugs and, 2007–2008, 2008t
vs. pulmonary thromboembolism, 1847
Hematologic malignancy, 2011
Hemizygous, definition of, 917t
Hemochromatosis, 1086–1089, 2010–2011, 2175t
diagnosis of, 1087–1088
echocardiography in, 1141
pathologic changes in, 1030, 1030pl
pathophysiology of, 1086–1087
treatment of, 1088
Hemodilution, during cardiopulmonary bypass, 2113
Hemodynamic assessment, after pericardiocentesis, in cardiac tamponade, 1256–1257, *1257*
in cardiogenic shock, 1530
in cardiomyopathy, 1125–1126
Hemodynamic monitoring, during cardiovascular surgery, 2108–2109
intraoperative, 2116–2137
electrocardiography for, 2117–2119, *2118–2119*
for cardiac output monitoring, 2131–2134, *2133*
Hemodynamic monitoring *(Continued)*
of arterial blood pressure, 2119–2123, *2120–2122*
complications of, 2121
direct methods for, 2119–2121, *2120*
noninvasive, 2122–2123
waveform in, *2120–2122,* 2121
of central venous pressure, 2123–2125, 2123t, *2124–2125,* 2126t
pulmonary artery catheterization in, 2125–2131, *2126–2128,* 2129t. See also *Pulmonary artery(ies), catheterization of.*
transesophageal echocardiography for, 2134–2137, 2135t–2137t
Hemoglobinuria, paroxysmal nocturnal, 2004
Hemolytic anemia, *2003,* 2003–2004
Hemoptysis, differential diagnosis of, 6–7, 7t
in pulmonary hypertension, 1864
in pulmonary thromboembolism, 1837
Hemorrhage, from aortic coarctation, 1356–1357
in thrombocythemia, 2006
Hemorrhagic telangiectasia, hereditary, 2011
Hemosiderosis, pathologic changes in, 1030, 1030pl
Heparin, and prognosis in unstable angina, 804t–805t
and thrombocytopenia, 2007
during coronary angiography, 602–603
during pregnancy, 2039–2040, *2041*
for pulmonary thromboembolism, 1848
low-molecular-weight, for pulmonary thromboembolism, 1848
for unstable angina, 726–730, *728,* 729t, *730*
with aspirin, for unstable angina, 723, *725*
with thrombolytic agents, and mortality, 764–766, 764t–766t
efficacy of, 749, 750t–751t, 751, *752*
with tissue plasminogen activator, and natural history of myocardial infarction, 701
Heparin rebound, 603
Hereditary hemorrhagic telangectasia, 2011
HERG mutation(s), in long QT syndrome, 1658–1659
Heterokaryon, definition of, 917t
Hexabrix (ioxaglate), chemical structure of, *600,* 601
Hexaxial reference system, *32,* 32–33
5-HIAA (5-hydroxyindoleacetic acid), in carcinoid syndrome, 1930–1931
Hibernation, myocardial. See *Myocardial hibernation.*
High-density lipoprotein (HDL), and hyperlipidemia, 1347–1348
and risk of coronary artery disease, 2195–2197, *2196–2197*
low levels of, and coronary artery disease, 2246–2247
metabolism of, 2245
HIRA gene, in cardiofacial syndromes, 926
Hirsutism, immunosuppression and, 1199
His bundle, catheter fulguration of, 1815–1816
Histogram storage, in pacemakers, 1774, *1774–1775*
History, 3–13, 4t–12t. See also under specific disease.
HIV. See *Human immunodeficiency virus (HIV) infection.*
HLA. See *Human leukocyte antigen (HLA).*
HLA-B27 gene, in spondyloarthropathy, 1952–1954
HMG CoA reductase inhibitor(s), 2247–2248, 2247t
Hoarseness, in pulmonary hypertension, 1864

Holiday heart syndrome, 1965
Holodiastolic rumble, in mitral stenosis, 348–349
Holosystolic "hammocking," in mitral valve prolapse, 362, 379
Holosystolic murmur, 22, *24*
in mitral regurgitation, 351
in ventricular septal defect, 205
Holter monitoring, and exercise testing, 572–573
and myocardial perfusion imaging, 573–574
and sinus node dysfunction, 1583
during space flight, 2081–2082, *2082*
in atrial fibrillation, 1635, *1635*
in cardiomyopathy, dilated, 1047
restrictive, 1081
in differential diagnosis of palpitations, 8
in risk stratification for sudden death, 1723
in silent myocardial ischemia, 572
and prognosis, 574–575
results of, and prognosis in coronary artery disease, 703, 703t
Holt-Oram syndrome, 176, 2172t, 2173
Homeobox, definition of, 917t
Homeodomain, definition of, 917t
Homocysteine, and risk of coronary artery disease, 2208–2209
levels of, and atherosclerosis, 1349
metabolism of, 2277, *2278*
plasma levels of, 2277–2278
age and, 2278, 2279t
cardiovascular disease and, 2010
elevated, and vascular disease, 2279–2281, *2280–2282,* 2280t–2281t
folic acid and, 2281, *2282,* 2283
gender and, 2279, 2279t
renal function and, 2279–2280, *2282*
systemic lupus erythematosus and, 2281
transplantation and, 2279, 2281
vitamin deficiency and, 2279, 2279t
species of, 2277–2278, *2278*
Homocystinuria, 2175t
Homograft(s). See *Allograft(s); Transplantation.*
Homologous combination, definition of, 917t
HOPE (Heart Outcomes Prevention Evaluation) trial, 720–721
Horizontal steal, in SPECT myocardial perfusion imaging, 101
Hormone(s), in endothelial injury, and atherosclerosis, 1330t
Horner's syndrome, 1379
HOT (Hypertension Optimal Treatment) trial, 1343
Hourglass supravalvular aortic stenosis, 153–154, *154–155*
Human immunodeficiency virus (HIV) infection, and dilated cardiomyopathy, 1043
and health care workers, 1981–1982
and myocarditis, 1108–1109
and pericarditis, 1246
cardiac tumors in, 1909
cardiomyopathy in, *1976–1978,* 1976–1981
cardiovascular complications of, evidence of at autopsy, 1973–1974, *1974*
historical perspective on, 1973
echocardiography in, *1974–1975,* 1974–1976
epidemiology of, 1973
Human karyotype, *2146*
Human leukocyte antigen (HLA), in dilated cardiomyopathy, 1045–1046
in rheumatic fever, 387
typing of, before transplantation, 1219
Humoral immunity, in cardiac allograft vasculopathy, 1193
Humoral immunity *(Continued)*
in viral myocarditis, 1100–1101
Hunter's syndrome, 2174t
Hurler's syndrome, 2174t
anatomic abnormalities in, *318,* 318–319
Hydralazine, with isosorbide dinitrate, for heart failure, 1171–1173, *1172*
Hydrochlorothiazide, for congestive heart failure, 1166, 1166t
5-Hydroxyindoleacetic acid (5-HIAA), in carcinoid syndrome, 1930–1931
11β-Hydroxysteroid dehydrogenase, and monogenic hypertension, 1496–1497, 1497t
Hydroxyurea, for sickle cell disease, 2002
for thrombocythemia, 2006
Hyperaldosteronism, clinical features of, 1919
diagnosis of, 1919
pathophysiology of, 1919
treatment of, 1920
Hypercalcemia, 1925–1926
electrocardiography in, 52–53
Hypercapnia, and pulmonary hypertension, 1859t
Hypercholesterolemia, and circulatory dysfunction, 1294
and natural history of coronary artery disease, 693–694, *694–695*
Hypercoagulable state(s), 2008–2010, *2009,* 2009t
Hyperemic response, in coronary artery stenosis, angiographic assessment of, 629–631, *631–632*
Hyperhomocysteinemia, and vascular disease, 2279–2281, *2280–2282,* 2280t
Hyperinsulinemia, and hypertension, 1502
Hyperkalemia, electrocardiography in, 50, *51,* 52
Hyperlipidemia, and cardiac allograft vasculopathy, 1192
and coronary artery disease, in women, 579
and treatment of hypertension, 1522t, 1523
epidemiology of, 1338, *1339*
genetic basis of, 1338–1339
in atherosclerosis, 1338–1341, *1339*
lipoproteins and, 1348
high-density, 1347–1348
low-density, 1346–1347
very low-density, 1345–1346
management of, nondrug therapies in, 2247, 2247t
pharmacologic, 2247–2248, 2247t
prevention of, primary, in patient with CHD risk equivalents, 2250–2253, *2252,* 2252t
secondary, 2248–2250
angiographic trials of, 2248–2249
early trials of, 2248
estrogen replacement therapy in, 2249–2250
goals of, 2250
statin trials of, 2249
trials of atherogenic dyslipidemia in, 2249
statin trials in, 1339–1341
Hyperlipoproteinemia, pathologic changes in, 1030
type II, anatomic abnormalities in, 319
Hyperoxaluria, 2175t
Hyperparathyroidism, 1925–1926
and hypertension, 1507
Hyperpolarizing factor, and endothelium-dependent vasodilatation, 524
Hypersensitivity angiitis, 1950
Hypersensitivity reaction(s), and dilated cardiomyopathy, 1044
Hypersensitivity reaction(s) *(Continued)*
and myocardial disease, 1092–1093
Hypertension, after cardiac transplantation, 1197
and cerebral circulation, 1689
and circulatory dysfunction, 1292–1294
and coronary artery disease, in women, 579
risk of, 2199–2203, *2200–2201,* 2200t, 2202t
and pain threshold, 569
and vascular compliance, 1488–1490
and vascular remodeling, *1300,* 1301, 1305
autonomic dysfunction and, 1542, *1542*
classification of, age and, 1514t
control of, alcohol and, 2240–2241, *2241*
calcium and, 2239
fish oil and, 2241
lifestyle modification and, 2242t
magnesium and, 2239
morning sympathetic activation and, 2239–2240, *2240*
multifactorial approach to, 2234, *2235*
nutrition and, 2241
obesity and, 2236, *2237*
population-based approach to, 2234–2235, *2236*
potassium and, 2239
prevention of intrauterine growth retardation and, *2241,* 2241–2242
sodium restriction and, 2236–2238, *2237,* 2238t
stress management and, 2239–2240, *2240*
definition of, 1513–1514, 1513t–1514t
diagnosis of, 1508–1511, 1509t–1510t
history in, 1508
laboratory work-up in, 1509, 1509t
physical examination in, 1508–1509
during pregnancy, 1514–1515, 2047–2049, 2048t–2051t
and eclampsia, 2047–2048, 2048t
and preeclampsia, 2047
chronic, 2048
classification of, 2048t
gestational, 2047
treatment of, 2049, 2050t–2051t
endothelial dysfunction and, 1511–1512, *1512*
essential, pathophysiology of, 1497–1505, *1499–1504*
alcohol in, 1498
atrial natriuretic factor in, 1501, *1501*
calcium intake in, 1498
decreased activity of vasodilating systems in, *1500–1501,* 1500–1502
endothelial dysfunction in, 1502–1503, *1503*
familial predisposition in, 1497–1498
hyperinsulinemia in, 1502
increased activity of vasoconstrictor systems in, 1498–1500, *1499–1500*
ionic membrane abnormalities in, *1504,* 1504–1505
kallikrein-kinin system in, *1500,* 1500–1501
obesity in, 1498
physical inactivity in, 1498
potassium intake in, 1498
prostaglandins in, *1501,* 1501–1502
psychological stress in, 1498
renal sodium retention in, 1502, *1502*
renin-angiotension system in, 1498–1500, *1500*
signal transduction abnormalities in, 1503–1504, *1503–1504*
sodium intake in, 1498
sympathetic nervous system in, 1498–1499, *1499*

Hypertension *(Continued)*
vascular structure in, 1505
iatrogenic, 1508
in acromegaly, 1916
in aortic coarctation, 194
in arms, 194
in Cushing's syndrome, 1918
in diabetes mellitus, 1922–1923
and atherosclerosis, 1344
in hypercalcemia, 1925
in older adults, 2020
in pediatric population, 1514, 1514t
malignant, 1515
monogenic, pathophysiology of, 1496–1497, 1497t
natural history of, *1511–1512,* 1511–1515, 1513t–1514t
antihypertensive agents and, *1512,* 1512–1513, 1513t
definition of disease and, 1513–1514, 1513t–1514t
pathologic consequences and, 1511–1512, *1511–1512*
pathophysiology of, obesity in, 1350, 2261–2262
prevention of, 2213
pulmonary. See *Pulmonary hypertension.*
refractory, treatment of, 1523–1524
renovascular, 1428–1431, *1430–1431*
and fibromuscular dysplasia, 1428, 1505–1506
carbon dioxide digital angiography in, 1429–1430
diagnosis of, 1509–1510, 1510t
natural history of, 1428
pathophysiology of, 1505–1506
prevalence of, 1428
renal angiography in, 1429–1430
scintigraphy in, 1429
screening for, 1429
treatment of, 1524
secondary, diagnosis of, 1509–1511, 1510t
pathophysiology of, 1505–1508, *1507*
acromegaly in, 1507
aldosteronism in, 1506
aortic coarctation in, 1506
congenital hyperplasia in, 1506, *1507*
Cushing's syndrome in, 1506
during pregnancy, 1507
hyperparathyroidism in, 1507
obstructive sleep apnea in, 1507
oral contraceptives in, 1507–1508
pheochromocytoma in, 1506
renal disease in, 1505
thyroid disease in, 1506–1507
treatment of, *1515–1521,* 1515–1524, 1517t, 1522t
alcohol restriction in, 1515–1516
chronic obstructive pulmonary disease and, 1522t, 1523
congestive heart failure and, 1522, 1522t
coronary artery disease and, 1522, 1522t
during pregnancy, 1523
exercise in, 1516
hyperlipidemia and, 1522t, 1523
in older adults, 1523
left ventricular hypertrophy and, 1522, 1522t
peripheral vascular disease and, 1522t, 1523
pharmacologic, *1516,* 1516–1521, 1517t, *1519*
$alpha_1$-blockers in, 1520
alpha-methyldopa in, 1520
angiotensin II antagonists in, 1520
angiotensin-converting enzyme inhibitors in, 1517t, 1518–1519, *1519*

Hypertension *(Continued)*
beta-blockers in, 1517t, 1518
calcium antagonists in, 1517t, 1519–1520
clonidine in, 1520
combination therapy in, 1521–1522
dihydropyridine in, 1517t, 1519–1520
diuretics in, 1516–1518
monotherapy in, *1516*
sequential, 1521, *1521*
reserpine in, 1520
vasodilators in, 1517t, 1520–1521
refractory, 1523–1524
renal failure and, 1522–1523, 1522t
sodium restriction in, 1515, *1515*
stroke and, 1522t, 1523
weight loss in, 1515, *1516*
Hypertension Optimal Treatment (HOT) trial, 1343
Hypertensive crisis, treatment of, 1524
Hyperthermia, and hemolytic anemia, 2004
cardiac complications of, 1093
Hyperthyroidism, clinical features of, 1927
diagnosis of, 1927–1928
mitral valve prolapse with, 358, 375
pathophysiology of, 1926–1927
treatment of, 1928
Hypertrophic cardiomyopathy. See *Cardiomyopathy, hypertrophic.*
Hypertrophic subaortic stenosis, carotid pulses in, *17*
Hypocalcemia, 1925–1926
and myocardial disease, 1091–1092
Hypoglycemia, in diabetes mellitus, 1924
Hypokalemia, diuretics and, 1517–1518
electrocardiography in, 52, *52*
in aldosteronism, 1510
in hyperaldosteronism, 1919
Hypolipidemic agent(s), and recurrence of myocardial infarction, 541, *542*
for stable angina, *vs.* angioplasty, 718
Hypomagnesemia, and myocardial disease, 1092
Hyponatremia, and prognosis in heart failure, 1161
heart failure and, 1178–1179
Hypoparathyroidism, 1925–1926
Hypophosphatemia, and myocardial disease, 1092
Hypotension, after repair of thoracic aortic aneurysms, 1364
during cardiovascular surgery, 2112
during pregnancy, 2034
from angiotensin-converting enzyme inhibitors, 1170
in adrenal insufficiency, 1918
in pulmonary thromboembolism, 1836
orthostatic, and syncope, 8, 1691, 1692t
treatment of, 1702–1703
autonomic dysfunction and, 1537–1541, *1540–1541,* 1541t
causes of, 15–16, 16t
in Parkinson's disease, 1558, 1558t
management of, 1554–1558, 1554t–1558t, *1555, 1557*
nonpharmacologic, 1554, *1555,* 1556t
pharmacologic, 1556, 1556t, *1557,* 1558
precipitators of, 1541t
thrombolytic therapy and, 768
Hypothalamic-pituitary axis, 1915
Hypothermia, cardiac complications of, 1093–1094, 1094t
electrocardiography in, 56, 58, *58*
Hypothyroidism, clinical features of, 1929
diagnosis of, 1929

Hypothyroidism *(Continued)*
pathophysiology of, 1928–1929
treatment of, 1929–1930
Hypovolemic shock, 1529
in myocardial infarction, treatment of, 1532
Hypoxia, and cerebral circulation, 1688–1689, *1690*
and pulmonary hypertension, 1859t
in erythrocytosis, 2005, 2005t
Hysteresis, *1772,* 1772–1773
Hysteria, and syncope, 9

IABP. See *Intra-aortic balloon pump (IABP).*
Ibutilide, adverse effects of, 1752
dosage of, 1752
efficacy of, 1752
electrophysiology of, 1752
for atrial fibrillation, 1637
pharmacokinetics of, 1752
ICAM. See *Intracellular adhesion molecule(s) (ICAM).*
ICD(s). See *Implantable cardioverter-defibrillator(s).*
I-cell disease, 2174t
Idioventricular tachycardia, *1571,* 1571–1572
IgG. See *Immunoglobulin G (IgG).*
IL-6 (interleukin-6), and myocyte proliferation, in cardiogenesis, 925
Image intensifier(s), for coronary angiography, 593–594
Image resolution, in coronary angiography, 594–595
Imdur. See *Isosorbide mononitrate.*
Immune disorder(s), pericarditis in, 1247
Immune function, evaluation of, before heart transplantation, 1219
Immune hemolytic anemia, 2003–2004
Immune response, in rheumatic fever, 386–387
Immunity, cellular, in viral myocarditis, *1099,* 1099–1100
humoral, in cardiac allograft vasculopathy, 1193
in viral myocarditis, 1100–1101
Immunization, against streptococcal infections, 398
in heart failure, 1166
Immunoglobulin(s), CTLA-4, 1213
Immunoglobulin G (IgG), for myocarditis, 1108
Immunomodulation, for dilated cardiomyopathy, 1049
Immunosuppressive therapy, 1212–1214, *1213,* 1214t
advances in, 1224
and hirsutism, 1199
and infection, after heart transplantation, 1189–1191, *1191*
and malignancy, 1198, *1198*
and nephrotoxicity, 1197–1198
and neurotoxicity, 1198–1199
and pregnancy, 1200
biologic agents for, 1212–1213
for dilated cardiomyopathy, 1049
for giant cell myocarditis, 1112–1113
for myocarditis, 1106–1108, *1107,* 1107t
for viral dilated cardiomyopathy, 1043
for Wegener's granulomatosis, 1950
future of, 1219–1220
in transplantation for advanced heart failure, 1225
pharmacologic agents for, 1212, *1213*
physical agents for, 1213–1214
standard protocol for, 1214, 1214t
Impact-AMI Study, 771
IMPACT-II (Integrilin to Minimize Platelet Aggregation and Coronary Thrombosis) study, 810

Impedance, definition of, 1491
Implantable cardioverter-defibrillator(s), 1779–1790, *1780–1786,* 1789t
atrioventricular sequential pacing by, 1783–1784, *1784*
clinical trials of, 1787–1790, 1788t–1789t
components of, 1780
cost-effectiveness of, 1790
defibrillation threshold for, 1785–1787
detection by, 1781–1784, *1784*
development of, 1779–1780, *1780–1782*
diagnostic storage by, 1785, *1785–1786*
for atrial fibrillation, 1645
for heart failure, 1175
for long QT syndrome, 1662
for prevention of sudden death, 1727–1730, 1728t, 1731–1732, 1731t, *1732*
for ventricular fibrillation, 1784
for ventricular tachycardia, 1784–1785
future developments in, 1790
implantation of, 1779–1780, *1780–1782*
in arrhythmogenic right ventricular dysplasia, 1673
in hypertrophic cardiomyopathy, 1069
indications for, 1788–1789, 1789t
magnet response by, 1787
malfunction of, 1787
pacing by, 1785, *1786*
primary prevention of sudden death by, 1789–1790
secondary prevention of sudden death by, 1787–1788, 1788t–1789t
sensing by, 1780–1781, *1783*
waveforms of, *1781*
Impulse formation, disorders of, 1563
Impulse propagation, disorders of, 1564
IMT. See *Intimal-medial thickness (IMT).*
Inactivity, and hypertension, 1498
Incentive spirometry, for chronic obstructive pulmonary disease, 1896
"Incisional tachycardia," radiofrequency catheter ablation of, 1804
Inducible nitric oxide synthase (INOS), in viral myocarditis, 1101
Infantile cardiomyopathy, 1024
Infarct(s), expansion of, 35
echocardiography in, 662–663
in heart failure, 1151
extension of, 562
in survivors of myocardial infarction, 777–778, 777t
extent of, thrombolytic therapy and, 763–764
location of, and natural history, 699, *700,* 700t
morphologic features of, 513, *515*
progression of, 534–536, *535*
determinants of, 513–514, *514–515*
remodeling of, in survivors of myocardial infarction, 778
severity of, 894–895, 894t
size of, estimation of, 557
thrombolytic therapy and, 754
Infarct imaging, 110–113, *111–113*
antimyosin antibody, 112, *112–113*
recent developments in, 112–113
technetium-labeled agents for, 110–112, *111*
Infarct-avid imaging, in myocardial infarction, 554
Infarction, myocardial. See *Myocardial infarction.*
pulmonary. See *Pulmonary infarction.*
Infarct-related artery patency, dobutamine stress echocardiography in, 665
Infarct/risk area, calculation of, 616, *616*
Infection(s). See also specific type, e.g., *Viral infection(s).*
Infection(s) *(Continued)*
after heart transplantation, *1189,* 1189–1191, *1191*
diagnosis of, 1190
incidence of, 1190, *1191*
prevention of, 1190–1191
and atherosclerosis, 1336–1338
and risk of coronary artery disease, 2209
from pacemaker implantation, 1775
vs. pulmonary thromboembolism, 1846
Infective endocarditis, 401–416
after valvular surgery, 498
anatomic abnormalities in, 320–321
and aortic regurgitation, 160, *161*
clinical features of, 402
complication(s) of, *410–413,* 410–416, 411t, 414t
cardiac, *410–412,* 410–413, 411t
embolic, 413–415, *414*
in central nervous system, 416
mycotic aneurysms as, 415–416
myocardial conduction defects as, 413
perivalvular extension as, 413
splenic abscess as, 416
diagnosis of, 402–405, 403t–404t, *404*
Duke criteria for, 402–403, 403t
echocardiography in, 403–404, *404,* 404t
laboratory studies in, 402–403, 403t
physical examination in, 402
with negative blood cultures, 404–405
during pregnancy, 2038–2039, 2039t
echocardiography in, 84, *85, 454,* 454–455
epidemiology of, 401
etiology of, microorganisms in, 405, 405t
from mitral valve prolapse, 364
in human immunodeficiency virus infection, 1974, *1974*
medical treatment of, 405–410, 406t–409t
in enterococcal infections, 407, 407t
in fungal infections, 409
in gram-negative infections, 408–409
in HACEK infections, 408, 409t
in penicillin-susceptible streptococcal infections, 405–407, 406t–407t
in staphylococcal infections, 407–408, 408t–409t
with negative blood cultures, 409–410
metastatic, 416
mitral valve prolapse and, 381
natural history of, 401
pathophysiology of, 401
prevention of, 414t–416t, 416
recurrence of, *412,* 412–413
risk factors for, 401, 404t
sites affected by, 401
surgical treatment of, echocardiographic indications for, 410–411, *411,* 411t
Inferior vena cava, anatomy of, 147
anomalous connections of, 168
continuity with azygos vein, 169, *169*
dimensions of, in estimation of right atrial pressure, 1871, *1872*
interruption of, 169, *169*
interruption of blood flow through, for pulmonary thromboembolism, 1850
obstruction of, 195–196
Inflammation, and atherosclerosis, 1336–1338
and dilated cardiomyopathy, 1041–1045, 1041t–1042t
and risk of coronary artery disease, 2209
in chronic obstructive pulmonary disease, 1888
in unstable atherosclerotic plaques, 536, *537–540*
Inflammatory aortic aneurysm(s), 1394–1396, *1395*
Inhalation anesthetic(s), minimum alveolar concentration of, 2107
obstetric, 2061t
uptake of, 2106–2107
Inheritance, autosomal recessive, 2147–2148
mendelian, 2147, *2147*
multifactorial, 2148, 2148t
congenital heart disease with, 2173–2176, 2176t
Innocent murmur(s), 22
INOS (inducible nitric oxide synthase), in viral myocarditis, 1101
Inotropic agent(s), for cardiogenic shock, 1532
for heart failure, 1168, 1174–1175
Inoue technique, for percutaneous mitral balloon valvuloplasty, 465, *466*
vs. double-balloon technique, 473–474
Input impedance, definition of, 1491
Insertional mutagenesis, definition of, 917t
Inspiration, degree of, on radiography, 67, 69, *70*
Insulin, and circulatory regulation, 1290
for diabetes mellitus, 1924
overproduction of, and hypertension, 1502
Insulin-like growth factor, and circulatory regulation, 1290
Insulin-resistance syndrome, and risk of coronary artery disease, 2209
pathophysiology of, *2204*
Integra stent, with carotid endarterectomy, 1437
Integrilin. See *Eptifibatide.*
Integrilin to Minimize Platelet Aggregation and Coronary Thrombosis (IMPACT-II) study, 810
Integrin(s), and platelet adhesion, 730
in leukocyte-endothelial interaction, and atherosclerosis, 1330–1331
upregulation of, in unstable atherosclerotic plaques, 536, *537*
Interatrial septal defect, 196, 196t
Interchordal hooding, in mitral valve prolapse, 373, *373*
Interleukin(s), in viral myocarditis, 1101
Interleukin-1 (IL-1), and vascular remodeling, 1301–1302
Interleukin-6 (IL-6), and myocyte proliferation, in cardiogenesis, 925
International Society of Heart and Lung Transplantation (ISHLT), histopathologic grading of rejection by, 1216, *1216,* 1216t
Interventricular pressure gradient, in ventricular septal defect, on echocardiography, 245, *245*
Interventricular septum, rupture of, in myocardial infarction, 547, *548*
vascular supply to, and coronary angiography, 611
Intestinal lipodystrophy, 1090
Intimal hyperplasia, after stenting, 876
and restenosis, 827, *829*
balloon angioplasty and, 875
in cardiac allograft vasculopathy, 1194–1196
intravascular ultrasonography in, *1456*
physiology of, *1300*
Intimal-medial thickness (IMT), of carotid artery, and symptomatic vascular disease, 1450–1451, *1451*
measurement of, 1446
reproducibility of, 1447, 1448t
validity of, 1447–1448
normal *vs.* abnormal, 1448–1451, 1448t, *1449–1451,* 1450t
progression of, 1449–1450, *1450,* 1450t
risk factors and, 1449
Intra-aortic balloon pump (IABP), for cardiogenic shock, 1532–1533, *1533*

Intra-aortic balloon pump (IABP) *(Continued)*
physiologic effects of, *727*
Intracellular adhesion molecule(s) (ICAM), in leukocyte-endothelial interaction, and atherosclerosis, 1330–1331, 1332t
Intracranial bleeding, after myocardial infarction, fibrinolytic agents and, 756
from thrombolytic agents, 766–768, 767t–768t
Intrapericardial pressure, in cardiac tamponade, 1251
in constrictive pericarditis, *vs.* cardiac tamponade, 1260
Intrauterine echocardiography, 251
Intrauterine growth retardation, prevention of, and hypertension control, *2241,* 2241–2242
Intravalvular implantation, for mitral insufficiency, 493
Intravalvular pressure gradient, calculation of, Bernoulli equation for, 441–442
Intravascular echocardiography, 667
Intravascular ultrasonography. See *Ultrasonography, intravascular.*
Intravascular volume, during pregnancy, 228
Intravenous pyelography, in renovascular hypertension, 1429
Intraventricular conduction delay, electrocardiography in, 42
Intrinsic heart rate (IHR), assessment of, in sinus node dysfunction, 1583–1584
Inward current, in cardiac hypertrophy, 971–972
Iodine, for hyperthyroidism, 1928
in radiographic contrast agents, 600, *600*
Ion(s), activity of, during depolarization and repolarization, 1–2
Ion channel(s), drugs blocking, 1659, 1659t
genetic mutations of, in long QT syndrome, 1657–1659, 1657t, *1658*
Ionic membrane(s), abnormalities of, and hypertension, *1504,* 1504–1505
Ioxaglate (Hexabrix), chemical structure of, *600,* 601
IP_3, in excitation-contraction coupling, 1282
Ipratropium bromide, for chronic obstructive pulmonary disease, 1892
Iriquois-related homeobox gene 4 (IRX4), in cardiogenesis, 919–920
IRIS (Isostent for Restenosis Intervention Study Isostents) trial, 836
Iron deposition disease. See *Hemochromatosis.*
Iron excess, and risk of coronary artery disease, 2209
IRX4 (Iriquois-related homeobox gene 4), in cardiogenesis, 919–920
"Ischemic burden," and angina, 570–571
Ischemic colitis, after repair of abdominal aortic aneurysms, 1375
Ischemic heart disease. See *Coronary artery disease.*
ISDN. See *Isosorbide dinitrate.*
ISHLT (International Society of Heart and Lung Transplantation), histopathologic grading of rejection by, 1216, *1216,* 1216t
Isometric exercise, *vs.* dynamic exercise, 897
Isoptin. See *Verapamil.*
Isordil. See *Isosorbide dinitrate.*
Isosorbide dinitrate, dosage of, 711t
for silent myocardial ischemia, 575
with hydralazine, for heart failure, 1171–1173, *1172*
Isosorbide mononitrate, dosage of, 711t
Isostent for Restenosis Intervention Study Isostents (IRIS) trial, 836
Isradipine, dosage of, 713t

IVUS. See *Ultrasonography, intravascular.*

J point, in early repolarization, 53, *54*
J wave, in hypothermia, 56, *58*
Janeway lesion(s), in infective endocarditis, 402
Jarvik artificial heart, 1231, 1235
Jaundice, from pulmonary thromboembolism, 1837
Jervell and Lange-Nielsen syndrome, and long QT syndronme, 1659, 1694
surgical treatment of, 1828–1829
Jet(s), in mitral regurgitation, color flow imaging of, 353
Joint Commission on Accreditation of Healthcare Organizations (JCAHO), assessment of cardiac rehabilitation programs by, 904–905
Jones criteria, for diagnosis of rheumatic fever, 390t
Judkins curve catheter, 598–599, *598–599*
Jugular venous pressure, and right atrial pressure, 1870–1871
elevated, causes of, 18t
in cardiac tamponade, 1251, *1252*
in heart failure, 1155
in pericarditis, constrictive, 1262, *1262*
Jugular venous pulse, in atrioventricular dissociation, 1677
in myocardial infarction, *545–546*
in restrictive cardiomyopathy, 1078
palpation of, *17–18,* 17–19, 18t
Juxtacrine, definition of, 917t

Kallikrein-kinin system, and hypertension, *1500,* 1500–1501
Kaposi's sarcoma, cardiac, 1909
Kartagener's syndrome, genetic basis of, 926–927
Karyotype, human, *2146*
K^+_{ATP} channel(s), and arteriolar vasomotor function, 523
Kawasaki's disease, 1951
and dilated cardiomyopathy, 1044–1045
and myocarditis, 1112
coronary angiography in, 643
Kearns-Sayre syndrome, 1986t, 1992, *1993*
Kerley B line(s), 72, 420
Ketone body(ies), in myocardial metabolism, 948–949
Kidney(s). See also *Renal* entries.
sodium retention by, and hypertension, 1502, *1502*
Knife wound(s), and aortic trauma, 1392
Knockout mice, cardiogenesis in, 918, 929
Korotkoff sounds, 14
Kringle domain, in coagulation system, 1316
Kussmaul sign, in constrictive pericarditis, 1260
KVLQT1 mutation(s), in long QT syndrome, 1658, *1694*
Kwashiorkor, 1091

Labetalol, dosage of, 712t
during pregnancy, 2050t, 2066
in aortic dissection, 1383
Labor, anesthesia during. See *Anesthesia, obstetric.*
antibiotic prophylaxis during, for infective endocarditis, 2038–2039, 2039t
hemodynamic response to, 2029–2031, 2031t
mitral stenosis and, 2056–2057

Lactation, cardiovascular drugs and, 2053
Lactic acidosis, *vs.* pulmonary thromboembolism, 1847
Lactic dehydrogenase (LDH), in myocardial infarction, 553, *553*
Lambert-Beer law, 628
Lamifiban, and natural history of myocardial infarction, 702
for unstable angina, 736t
with thrombolytic agents, Paradigm trial of, 771
Lamoteplase, efficacy of, 822
Landouzy-Dejerine disease. See *Facioscapulohumeral muscular dystrophy.*
Lanoxin. See *Digoxin.*
Laser revascularization, transmyocardial, 856
LCAD deficiency, 2174t
LCAS (Lipoprotein and Coronary Atherosclerosis Study), 1339
LDH. See *Lactic dehydrogenase (LDH).*
LDL. See *Low-density lipoprotein (LDL).*
Le Compte operation, 303, *305,* 306
Lead(s), for implantable cardioverter-defibrillators, *1781*
for intraoperative electrocardiography, configuration of, 2118, *2118–2119*
for pacemakers, 1765–1766, *1766*
Lead fixation device(s), for pacemaker leads, 1765–1766
Leaflet(s), fibrosis of, in mitral valve prolapse, 356, *356*
mobility of, in aortic stenosis, 443, *443–444*
prolapse of, 363, *364*
thickening of, in mitral valve prolapse, 362, *362*
Left anterior descending artery. See *Coronary artery(ies), left anterior descending.*
Left atrial anastomosis, in heart transplantation, *1226–1228,* 1230
Left atrial function, in mitral stenosis, 347–348
Left atrial isolation procedure, for atrial fibrillation, 1815, *1816–1817*
Left atrial pressure, in mitral regurgitation, 350, *350*
monitoring of, during cardiovascular surgery, 2108
Left atrium, anatomy of, 148, *148*
angle lesions of, in mitral valve prolapse, 374, *374*
anomalous connection of superior vena cava with, 168–169
connection with vena cava, 169, *170*
dilatation of, radiographic assessment of, 71
drainage of right superior vena cava to, 238
enlargement of, electrocardiography in, *33,* 33–34
in mitral regurgitation, 424, *425*
in mitral stenosis, 420, *420–421*
myxoma of, 1904–1905, *1905–1906*
Left bundle branch block. See *Bundle branch block, left.*
Left cervicothoracic sympathetic ganglionectomy, for long QT syndrome, 1704
Left heart, sympathetic denervation of, for long QT syndrome, 1662
Left heart filling pressure, elevated, and pulmonary hypertension, 1857, 1857t
Left stellectomy, for long QT syndrome, 1662
Left ventricle, aneurysms of, annular subvalvular, pathologic changes in, 1032
cardiovascular surgery in, anesthesia for, 2111
circulation to, *503,* 503–504
diastolic function of, on echocardiography, 79

Left ventricle *(Continued)*
diastolic pressure in, in aortic regurgitation, 336, *337*
in mitral regurgitation, 425, *425*
dilatation of, in cardiomyopathy, 1138, *1138–1139*
endocardial friction lesions of, in mitral valve prolapse, 373, *373*
fibrosis in, in mitral valve prolapse, 373, *373*
filling patterns of, in diastolic dysfunction, 1005, *1006*
filling rates of, aging and, 1007
myxoma of, 1906
pressure recordings in, in aortic stenosis, 427, *428*
pressure-volume relationships in, 1001–1002, *1002*
in amyloid heart disease, 1085, *1085*
in aortic regurgitation, 336, *336*
myocardial ischemia and, 1008, *1009*
pseudoaneurysms of, and shock, 1530
magnetic resonance imaging in, 138, *139*
reduction surgery on, for heart failure, 1176
relaxation of, 1002–1004
remodeling of, in dilated cardiomyopathy, 1037, 1037t
in myocardial infarction, 562
restraint devices for, in heart failure, 1176–1177
size of, on echocardiography, 78–79
stroke volume of, radionuclide studies of, 459
wall segments of, and normal coronary circulation, 659, *660*
Left ventricular assist device, for cardiogenic shock, 1533
HeartMate, 1231–1235, *1233–1234*
history of, 1231
results with, 1235
without transplantation, 1235
Left ventricular diastolic function, in hypertrophic cardiomyopathy, 1060–1061, *1061*
Left ventricular dysfunction, and cardiac rehabilitation, 902
and heart failure, 1148–1149, 1149t, 1177–1178
and natural history of coronary artery disease, 695–696, *696–698*
and risk of sudden death, 1714, *1714*
in aortic stenosis, 330–335, *331–334*
and angina, 331
and heart failure, 331–332, *332*
and prognosis with surgery, 334–335
clinical implications of, 332–335, *333–334,* 334t
with low ejection fraction/high gradient, 332, *333*
with low ejection fraction/low cardiac output/low transvalvular gradient, 332–334, *333–334,* 334t
in arrhythmogenic right ventricular dysplasia, 1669
in heart failure, 1150, *1150*
in mitral regurgitation, 366
in muscular dystrophy, Duchenne's, 1990–1991
Left ventricular ejection fraction (LVEF), and natural history of coronary artery disease, 696, *698*
and prognosis in mitral regurgitation, 352, *352*
and prognosis in myocardial infarction, 677, *677*
angiotensin-converting enzyme inhibitors and, 721
Left ventricular ejection fraction (LVEF) *(Continued)*
in mitral regurgitation, 460
in myocarditis, 1105
treatment and, 1107, 1107t
on first pass radionuclide angiocardiography, 106, *106*
on radionuclide ventriculography, 109
Left ventricular end-diastolic volume (LVEDV), assessment of, 79–80
in heart failure, 1155
prediction of, pulmonary artery catheterization in, 2129, 2129t
Left ventricular end-systolic volume (LVESV), and prognosis in myocardial infarction, 561, *561*
during exercise, aging and, 2017
Left ventricular function, abnormal, coronary angiography in, 604
and prognosis in myocardial infarction, 677–679, *679*
arterial compliance and, 1480
assessment of, before noncardiac surgery, 2095
echocardiography in, 445–446
cocaine and, 1962
during silent myocardial ischemia, 571
in hypertrophic cardiomyopathy, echocardiography in, 1137–1138
in obesity, 2260–2261, 2260t
in peripartum cardiomyopathy, 2053t
on gated-equilibrium radionuclide ventriculography, 107, *107*
reduced, in aortic stenosis, 328
Left ventricular hypertrophy, and coronary artery disease, risk of, 2205–2206, 2207t
and coronary circulation, 526
and diastolic function, 1009–1011
and treatment of hypertension, 1522, 1522t
augmentation of, 986
clinical features of, 983–985, *984*
cocaine and, 1962–1963
concentric, 979–980, 980t, *981*
electrocardiography in, 34–35, *35*
with conduction disorders, 36
gender and, 1010
in aortic stenosis, 325
in athletes, 1009–1010
in hypertension, and risk of coronary artery disease, 2202, 2202t
in hypertrophic cardiomyopathy, 1064, *1064*
natural history of, 985
pathologic changes in, 1022, *1022*
pathophysiology of, signal transduction in, 981–982, *982*
patterns of, 979–981, *980–981,* 980t
treatment of, 985–986
Left ventricular impulse, palpation of, 19
Left ventricular outflow, obstruction of, echocardiography in, 247–248, *248*
Left ventricular outflow tract, anatomy of, 149, *149*
obstruction of, from subaortic stenosis, 151, *153*
from supravalvular aortic stenosis, 153–154, *154–155*
surgical treatment of, 295, *296–298*
Left ventricular outflow tract gradient, Doppler echocardiography of, in hypertrophic cardiomyopathy, 1136–1137, *1137*
Left ventricular pressure, in cardiomyopathy, dilated, 1126, *1126*
hypertrophic, 1130, *1131*
restrictive, *1127, 1129*
in mitral regurgitation, 350, *350*
Left ventricular reduction surgery, 1236
Left ventricular systolic function (LVSF), assessment of, 79–80
magnetic resonance imaging in, 138, *138*
in cardiomyopathy, hypertrophic, 1060–1061, *1061, 1130*
Left ventriculectomy, partial, 1236
Left ventriculography, in mitral stenosis, 424
Left-right axis malformation(s), genetic basis of, 926–927
Lenegre's disease, and sudden death, 1721
Lens(es), dislocation of, in Marfan's syndrome, 2151
Leptospirosis, and myocarditis, 1110
Leukemia, cardiac infiltration of, 1909
cardiovascular complications of, 2011
Leukocyte(s), interaction with endothelium, in atherogenesis, 1330–1331, 1332t
Levine's sign, 5
Lev's disease, and sudden death, 1721
Libman-Sacks vegetation, on echocardiography, *87*
Licorice, and hypertension, 1508
Liddle's syndrome, and monogenic hypertension, 1497
Lidocaine, adverse effects of, 1746
dosage of, 1746
during pregnancy, 2043, 2044t
efficacy of, 1746
electrophysiology of, 1745–1746
pharmacokinetics of, 1742t–1743t, 1746
use dependency of, *1741*
Life change(s), and risk of sudden death, 1713
Lifestyle, and hypertension control, 2242t
atherogenic, 2203–2205, 2203t–2205t, *2204*
Light chain phosphorylation, and crossbridge cycling in vascular smooth muscle, 1279, *1280*
Lipid hypothesis, in atherosclerosis, 1338–1341, *1339*
Lipid Research Clinics Cholestyramine trial, 2253
Lipodystrophy, intestinal, 1090
peripheral, protease inhibitors and, 1981
Lipoma, cardiac, 1907
Lipoprotein(s), and hyperlipidemia, 1348
and risk of coronary artery disease, 2208
high-density. See *High-density lipoprotein (HDL).*
low-density. See *Low-density lipoprotein (LDL).*
metabolism of, 2244–2245
triglyceride-rich, and coronary artery disease, 2246
Lipoprotein and Coronary Atherosclerosis Study (LCAS), 1339
Lisinopril, for heart failure, 1170t
Lithium, electrocardiographic changes from, 53
Liver disease, and pulmonary hypertension, 1865
Loeffler's eosinophilic endomyocardial disease, 1075
Long QT syndrome(s), 1656–1662
acquired, 1693
and sudden cardiac death, 1719–1720, 1719t–1720t
and syncope, 1693–1695, 1693t–1694t
congenital, 1693–1694
diagnosis of, criteria for, 1661, 1661t, 1704, 1719t
electrocardiography in, 1660, *1660*
physical examination in, 1660
during pregnancy, 2066–2067
etiology of, 54, 54t
genetic mutations in, *1694,* 1694–1695
natural history of, 1660–1661, 1661t
pathophysiology of, 1656–1660, 1657t, *1658,* 1659t

Long QT syndrome(s) *(Continued)*
animal models in, 1660
competing hypotheses on, 1656
drugs in, 1659, 1659t, 1693, 1694t
genetic basis in, 1657–1659, 1657t, *1658*
historical perspective on, 1656
Jervell and Lange-Nielsen syndrome in, 1659, 1694
torsades de pointes in, 1659–1660
syncope in, natural history of, 1701
treatment of, 1661–1662, 1704–1705
surgical, 1828–1829
Loop diuretic(s), for congestive heart failure, 1166, 1166t
for hypertension, 1517t
Looping morphogenesis, in cardiogenesis, 923–924
Lordosis, in facioscapulohumeral muscular dystrophy, *1995*
Losartan, for heart failure, 1174
for hypertension, 1520
for prevention of sudden death, 1725
Lovastatin, for hyperlipidemia, clinical trials of, 1340
Lovosimendan, for heart failure, 1168
Low-density lipoprotein (LDL), and atherosclerosis, 1295, 1305–1306, 1331
and coronary artery disease, natural history of, 693–694, *694–695*
prognosis in, 718, *719*
risk of, 2195–2197, *2196,* 2245–2246
and recurrence of myocardial infarction, hypolipidemic agents and, 541, *542*
metabolism of, 2245
optimal level of, 2245–2246
small/dense, and risk of coronary artery disease, 2207–2208
Lower body negative pressure, in space flight, 2080, *2081*
Lower extremity(ies), peripheral vascular disease of, *1404–1410,* 1404–1413, 1405t–1406t, 1409t, 1411t. See also *Peripheral vascular disease, of lower extremities.*
Low–molecular-weight heparin, for pulmonary thromboembolism, 1848
for unstable angina, 726–730, *728,* 729t, *730*
LQTS mutation(s), and long QT syndrome, 1694
L-transposition, 212, *213–216*
echocardiography in, 249–250
Lung(s). See also *Pulmonary* entries.
biopsy of, in pulmonary hypertension, 1877
magnetic resonance angiography of, 136, *137*
transplantation of, for chronic obstructive pulmonary disease, 1897
volume reduction surgery of, for chronic obstructive pulmonary disease, 1897
Lupus erythematosus valvulitis, anatomic abnormalities in, 316–317, 317pl
LVAD. See *Left ventricular assist device.*
LVEF. See *Left ventricular ejection fraction (LVEF).*
LVESV. See *Left ventricular end-systolic volume (LVESV).*
LVH. See *Left ventricular hypertrophy.*
LVOT. See *Left ventricular outflow tract.*
LVSF. See *Left ventricular systolic function (LVSF).*
Lyme disease, and myocarditis, 1098, 1109–1110
Lymphocytic myocarditis, 1024t, 1025, *1026–1027*
animal models of, 1100
Lymphoma, atrial, 1909, *1909*
Lymphoma *(Continued)*
cardiovascular complications of, 2011
Lymphoproliferative disorder(s), in transplant recipients, 1198

MACH-I (Mortality Assessment in Congestive Heart Failure) trial, 1173
Macrophage(s), accumulation of, in atherogenesis, *1328,* 1330t, 1342
in ruptured atherosclerotic plaques, 580, *581*
Macro-reentrant circuit(s), in atrial fibrillation, 1818, *1819*
MADIT (Multicenter Automatic Defibrillator Implantation Trial), 1069, 1727, *1728,* 1728t, 1751, 1788t, 1789
MADS, definition of, 917t
Magnesium, in diet, and hypertension, control of, 2239
transport of, in myocardial ischemia, 512, *512*
Magnet pacemaker mode, 1771
Magnetic resonance angiography (MRA), in coronary artery disease, 139–140, *141*
in renovascular hypertension, 1429
pulmonary, 136, *137*
Magnetic resonance imaging (MRI), artifacts on, 134, *135*
clinical applications of, 133, 133t
contraindications to, 134–135
during pregnancy, 2033
electrocardiographic gating in, 134
future of, 140
gradient-echo, 134, *134*
in abdominal aortic aneurysms, *1366*
in amyloid heart disease, 1085
in aortic dissection, *135,* 135–136, *1376,* 1379, 1380t
in arrhythmogenic right ventricular dysplasia, 1668, *1669*
in assessment of patency of coronary artery bypass graft, 140, 140t, *141*
in cardiac myxoma, 1905, *1906*
in cardiac patient, special considerations for, 134–135, *134–135*
in cardiomyopathy, 139, *140*
in carotid artery disease, 1401
in congenital heart disease, 137–138, *137–138*
in heart failure, 1156
in hemochromatosis, 1088
in inflammatory aortic aneurysms, 1395–1396
in left ventricular pseudoaneurysm, 138, *139*
in myocarditis, 139, 1104
in pericarditis, constrictive, 1263, *1265*
in pulmonary embolism, 136, *137*
in pulmonary hypertension, 1872–1873
in renal artery disease, 1403
in right ventricular dysplasia, 139, *140*
of cardiac tumors, 136–137
of great vessels, 135–136, *135–136*
of pericardium, *137,* 138
of thoracic aorta, 135–136, *135–136*
of ventricular volume, 138–139, *138–139*
principles of, 133–134, *134*
spin-echo, 133, *134*
Mahaim fiber(s), supraventricular arrhythmias from, surgical treatment of, 1824–1825
Major histocompatibility complex (MHC), in allorecognition, 1210
in viral myocarditis, 1100
Malabsorption, in heart failure, 1179
Maladie de Roger, 205, *206*
Malignancy. See also *Cardiac tumor(s).*
and pericardial effusion, 1250
Malignancy *(Continued)*
immunosuppression and, 1198, *1198*
radiotherapy and, 831–832
Malignant hypertension, 1515
Malnutrition, alcohol abuse and, 1965
and myocardial disease, 1090–1091, 1091t
Malonyl coenzyme A, in fatty acid oxidation, 947–948
Mammary artery(ies), internal, for coronary artery bypass graft, 846, *847–850*
recurrent disease in, 867, *867–868*
"Mammary souffle," 2032, *2033*
MAPK (mitogen-activated protein kinase), in excitation-contraction coupling, 1285
pathway for, in cardiac hypertrophy, 958, 982
Marasmus, 1091
Marfan's syndrome, 175–176, 2150–2155, *2151–2152,* 2153t, *2154*
anatomic abnormalities in, 319
and pregnancy, 2051
annuloaortic ectasia with, 1388
aortic dissection with, 1387–1389
aortic regurgitation in, 191, *192*
clinical features of, 2150–2151, *2151–2152*
diagnosis of, 2151–2153, 2153t
echocardiography in, 453–454, *454*
genetic basis of, 2153–2155, *2154*
Marijuana, cardiovascular complications of, 1966–1967
Maroteaux-Lamy syndrome, 2174t
Mason-Likar modification, of electrocardiography, 586
MASS (Medicine, Angioplasty or Surgery Study), 796, 871, *872*
Matrix metalloproteinases (MMPs), in atherosclerotic plaques, 538–540, 541t
Maze I procedure, for atrial fibrillation, 1645, 1818–1819, *1819–1820*
Maze II procedure, for atrial fibrillation, 1821, *1821*
Maze III procedure, for atrial fibrillation, 1821, *1822*
McCallum's patch, in rheumatic fever, 390
MDC (Metoprolol in Dilated Cardiomyopathy) trial, 1725
Mechanical circulatory support, history of, 1231
in advanced heart failure, *1231–1234,* 1231–1235
Mechanical ventilation, for chronic obstructive pulmonary disease, 1896
Mechanosensing, endothelium in, 958
Mediastinum, radiation to, complications of, 318
Medication(s). See *Drug(s).*
Medicine, Angioplasty or Surgery Study (MASS), 796, 871, *872*
MEDICORP cerebral protection device, 1438
MEF2 (myocyte enhancer factor–2), in cardiogenesis, 918–919
Membranous subaortic stenosis, 151, 153, *153*
"Memory" T wave(s), 53
Mendelian inheritance, 2147, *2147*
in congenital heart disease, 2172t
Menkes' disease, 2175t
MERIT-HF (Mortality Effect of Metoprolol in Patients with Heart Failure) trial, 1725
Merosin, in muscular dystrophy, Duchenne's, 2165
Mesothelial hyperplasia, 1243
Mesothelioma, of atrioventricular node, 1907–1908
pericardial, 1242–1243
Metabolic disorder(s), anatomic abnormalities in, 318–319, *318–319,* 818pl

Metabolic disorder(s) *(Continued)*
and myocardial disease, 1090–1092, 1091t
and pericardial disease, 1247
and syncope, 1695–1696
vs. pulmonary thromboembolism, 1847
with cardiovascular manifestations, 2174t–2175t
Metabolism, control of, *vs.* regulation, 939
pathways for, cellular, 938, *939*
in energy transfer, 938–939, *940*
tracing of, 940–942, *941–942*
Metazoal infection(s), and myocarditis, 1112
Methicillin, *Staphylococcus aureus* susceptible to, 407–408, 408t–409t
Methimazole, for hyperthyroidism, 1928
Methyldopa, during pregnancy, 2050t
α-Methyldopa, for hypertension, 1520
Metolazone, for congestive heart failure, 1166, 1166t
Metoprolol, dosage of, 712t
during pregnancy, 2066
for heart failure, 1170–1171, *1171*
for prevention of sudden death, *1724,* 1724–1725
for silent myocardial ischemia, 575
in survivors of myocardial infarction, 772, *772*
Metoprolol in Acute Myocardial Infarction (MIAMI) study, 1724
Metoprolol in Dilated Cardiomyopathy (MDC) trial, 1725
Mexiletine, adverse effects of, 1747
dosage of, 1746
during pregnancy, 2043, 2044t, 2046
efficacy of, 1746–1747
electrophysiology of, 1746
for long QT syndrome, 1657
pharmacokinetics of, 1742t–1743t, 1746
MHC. See *Major histocompatibility complex (MHC).*
MI. See *Myocardial infarction.*
Mibefradil, for heart failure, 1173
MICABG. See *Minimally invasive coronary artery bypass graft (MICABG).*
Mice, knockout, cardiogenesis in, 918, 929
Microangiopathy, thrombotic, 2004
Microcirculation, coronary, 632
angiography of, 641–642
endothelial dysfunction and, 641, 681
Microtubule(s), in systolic dysfunction, 964
Microvena snare loop, 281
Micturition, and syncope, 9, 1691
Midodrine, for postural hypotension, 1556
Midsystolic buckling, in mitral valve prolapse, 361–362, 379
Midsystolic click(s), *24*
Milrinone, for heart failure, 1168, 1174
Minimally invasive coronary artery bypass graft (MICABG), 852–856, *853–854*
advantages of, 854, 856
disadvantages of, 854, 856
technique of, 852, *853–854,* 854
Minimum alveolar concentration, of inhalation anesthetics, 2107
Minoxidil, and left ventricular hypertrophy, 985
for heart failure, 1173
Missile wound(s), and aortic trauma, 1392
MITI (Myocardial Infarction Triage and Intervention) study, of prehospital thrombolytic therapy, 757–758
Mitogen-activated protein kinase (MAPK), in excitation-contraction coupling, 1285
pathway for, in cardiac hypertrophy, 958, 982
Mitral commissurotomy, percutaneous mitral balloon valvotomy after, 468
Mitral flail leaflet(s), and prognosis in mitral regurgitation, 352, *353*
Mitral gradient, after percutaneous mitral balloon valvotomy, *467*
Mitral insufficiency, cardiovascular surgery in, anesthesia for, 2111
holosystolic murmur in, *24*
in atrial septal defect, 197
in survivors of myocardial infarction, 775
surgical treatment of, *489–492,* 489–493
intravalvular implantation in, 493
repair techniques for, 489–490, *489–490*
replacement techniques for, 490–493, *491–492*
Mitral leaflet(s), anatomy of, 149, *149*
Mitral regurgitation, 158, *159–160,* 191, 350–353, *350–353*
after percutaneous mitral balloon valvotomy, 469
diagnosis of, angiography in, 354
cardiac catheterization in, 354, 424–426, *425–426*
Doppler echocardiography in, 81
echocardiography in, *450,* 450–451, 450pl
physical examination in, 351
radionuclide studies in, 460–461
during pregnancy, 2057
ejection fraction in, 426
from mitral valve prolapse, 363
in cardiomyopathy, dilated, echocardiography in, 1139
hypertrophic, 224, *225,* 1132, *1132*
echocardiography in, 1137, *1137*
restrictive, 1078
left ventricular dysfunction in, 366
mitral valve prolapse and, 380–381
natural history of, 351–352, *352–353*
noncardiac surgery in, 2100
papillary muscle rupture and, 663, *663,* 663pl
pathophysiology of, *350,* 350–351
severity of, assessment of, 353–354, 450–451
survival rates in, *329*
treatment of, medical, 352–353
surgical, 289, *293–294*
with mitral stenosis, cardiac catheterization in, 426–427
Mitral stenosis, 154–156, *156,* 184, *347–349,* 347–350
cardiac output in, 423
diagnosis of, cardiac catheterization in, 419–424, *420–423,* 423t
computed tomography in, electron beam, *2186*
Doppler echocardiography in, 80–81, *80–81*
echocardiography in, 243, *447–449,* 447–450, 448t
electrocardiography in, *33*
physical examination in, 348–349, *349*
diastolic filling period in, 421–422, *422*
diastolic gradient in, 422, *422–423*
during pregnancy, 2056–2057, 2056t
echocardiography in, for treatment planning, *449,* 449–450
hemoptysis in, 7
in rheumatic fever, 397
left ventriculography in, 424
natural history of, 349
pathophysiology of, 347–348, *347–348*
pulmonary artery wedge pressure in, 421, *422*
pulmonary vascular resistance in, 423
rheumatic, percutaneous mitral balloon valvotomy for, *464–473,* 464–476, 466t, 469t–470t. See also *Percutaneous mitral balloon valvotomy.*
Mitral stenosis *(Continued)*
severity of, assessment of, 448–449, 448t
treatment of, balloon valvuloplasty in, 261–262, 434–435
cardiovascular surgery in, anesthesia for, 2111
medical, 349–350
surgical, 289, *294,* 486–489, *487–488*
Mitral valve, anatomy of, *148,* 149, 372, *372,* 446–447, *447*
calcification of, and outcome of percutaneous mitral balloon valvotomy, 468, 472
in mitral stenosis, 421, *421*
congenital anomalies of, echocardiography in, *91,* 92
floppy, anatomic abnormalities in, 319–320, *319–320*
gross anatomy of, 355, *355*
Hurler's syndrome in, *318*
microscopic anatomy of, *355,* 355–356
repair of, in mitral valve prolapse, 366
patient evaluation for, echocardiography in, 451, 451pl
replacement of, 490–493, *491–492*
rheumatic valvulitis of, *316*
rheumatoid disease of, 317
surgical procedures on, 486–493, *488–492*
for mitral insufficiency, *489–492,* 489–493
for mitral stenosis, 486–489, *487–488*
systolic anterior motion of, in cardiomyopathy, hypertrophic, 1135, *1136*
Whipple's disease in, *317*
Mitral valve area, determination of, errors in, 423, 423t
Gorlin equation for, 422, *422,* 474
Mitral valve disease. See also *Mitral regurgitation; Mitral stenosis; Mitral valve prolapse.*
echocardiography in, 446–451, *447–450,* 447t–448t, 450pl
Mitral valve prolapse, 158, *159–160,* 354–366
and arrhythmias, 382–383
and autonomic dysfunction, 383
and embolism, 381–382
and infective endocarditis, 381
and mitral regurgitation, 380–381
and stroke, 381–382
and sudden death, 382–383
associated abnormalities in, 375
clinical features of, 358–360, *359–360,* 375–378, *377*
on physical examination, 359–360, *359–360,* 376, *377,* 378
complication(s) of, 363–366
arrhythmias as, 364–365
autonomic dysfunction as, 365–366
infective endocarditis as, 364
mitral regurgitation as, 363
systemic embolism as, 364
course of, 189–190
definition of, 355
diagnosis of, 190
angiocardiography in, 362–363, *363–364*
angiography in, 380, *380–381*
cardiac catheterization in, 362–363, *363–364,* 380, *380–381*
cineangiography in, *361, 378–379, 381*
echocardiography in, 361–362, *362,* 378–380, *379–380, 447,* 451
Doppler, 81, *81*
electrocardiography in, 360–361, 378, *381*
during pregnancy, 2055
epidemiology of, 357, 374–375
genetic factors in, 357, 373
historical perspective on, 354–355, 371

Mitral valve prolapse *(Continued)*
hyperthyroidism with, 358
in Marfan's syndrome, 2151, 2153
in muscular dystrophy, Duchenne's, 1991, *1991*
management of, 366, 383–384
nomenclature in, 355, 371–372
noncardiac surgery in, 2100
pathology of, 356–357, *356–358,* 373–374, *373–375*
pathophysiology of, 189
prognosis in, 366, 383
secondary, 358, 372
skeletal disorders with, 357
symptoms of, 358–359, 375–376
treatment of, 190
surgical, *293*
vs. panic disorder, 358, 376
with connective tissue disorders, 357
Mitral valve replacement, for rheumatic fever, 397
Mitral valvuloplasty, 434–435
Mixed venous oxygen saturation, measurement of, 2132–2133
MMF. See *Mycophenolate mofetil (MMF).*
M-mode echocardiography. See *Echocardiography, M-mode.*
MMPs. See *Matrix metalloproteinases (MMPs).*
Mobitz I atrioventricular block, 1573
Mobitz II atrioventricular block, 1573
Modified Multifactorial Cardiac Risk Index, 2093t–2094t
Mönckeberg's medial calcific sclerosis, 1325
Monoclonal hypothesis, in atherosclerosis, 1336
Monocyte(s), accumulation of, in atherogenesis, 1327, *1327,* 1330t
Mononuclear cell(s), in myocardium, 1026t
Moricizine, adverse effects of, 1748–1749
dosage of, 1748
efficacy of, 1748
electrophysiology of, 1748
for prevention of sudden death, 1726
pharmacokinetics of, 1742t–1743t, 1748
Morphology discrimination algorithm(s), for implantable cardioverter-defibrillators, 1784, *1784*
Morquio's syndrome, 2174t
Mortality Assessment in Congestive Heart Failure (MACH-I) trial, 1173
Mortality Effect of Metoprolol in Patients with Heart Failure (MERIT-HF) trial, 1725
Moxonidine, for heart failure, 1176
MRA. See *Magnetic resonance angiography (MRA).*
MRFIT (Multiple Risk Factor Intervention Trial), 1338
MRI. See *Magnetic resonance imaging (MRI).*
MTT (Myocarditis Treatment Trial), 1107, *1107*
Mucocutaneous lymph node syndrome, 1951. See also *Kawasaki's disease.*
Mucolipidosis, 2174t
Mucolytic(s), for chronic obstructive pulmonary disease, 1897
Mucopolysaccharide(s), deposition of, in mitral valve prolapse, 374, *375*
Mucopolysaccharidosis, 2174t
anatomic abnormalities in, *318,* 318–319
pathologic changes in, 1029
Müller sign, 337
Multicenter Automatic Defibrillator Implantation Trial (MADIT), 1069, 1727, *1728,* 1728t, 1751, 1788t, 1789
Multicenter Unsustained Tachycardia (MUSTI) Trial, 1728t, 1729, 1788t
Multifocal atrial tachycardia, 1569, *1569*
Multiple risk Factor Intervention Trial (MRFIT), 1338
Mural endocardium, pathologic changes in, 1031
Mural thrombus, from myocardial infarction, echocardiography in, 663, *663*
Murmur(s), 22, *24*
continuous, 26t
diastolic, 26t
in aortic regurgitation, 337–338
differential diagnosis of, 10, 10t
during pregnancy, 2032, *2033*
holosystolic, 22, *24*
in mitral regurgitation, 351
in mitral valve prolapse, 360
in ventricular septal defect, 205, *548*
in aortic coarctation, *1356*
in aortic dissection, 1379
in aortic stenosis, 326, *326*
valvular, 180–181
in hypertrophic cardiomyopathy, 224
in infective endocarditis, 402
in mitral stenosis, 349
in mitral valve prolapse, 376, *377,* 378
in myocardial infarction, 543, 547–548, *547–549*
in pulmonary stenosis, valvular, 188
in tricuspid regurgitation, 344, *345*
in tricuspid stenosis, 344
systolic, 22, *24,* 25t
in mitral valve prolapse, 360
Muscle relaxant(s), for cardiovascular surgery, 2107–2108, 2108t
Muscular bridge(s), coronary angiography in, 617–619, *618,* 618t
Muscular dystrophy, Becker's, 1991–1992, 1991t
genetic basis of, *2164*
in familial dilated cardiomyopathy, 1039
Duchenne's, 1988–1991, *1989–1991,* 1990t–1991t
cardiac complications of, 1989–1991, *1990–1991,* 1990t–1991t
clinical features of, 1989, *1989*
genetic basis of, 1989, 2161–2165, *2164*
in familial dilated cardiomyopathy, 1039
myocardial changes in, 1030
prenatal diagnosis of, 2163
Emery-Dreifuss, 2160
facioscapulohumeral, *1995,* 1995–1996
in familial dilated cardiomyopathy, with conduction defects, 1997
Muscular subaortic stenosis, 151, *152*
MUSIC criteria, for stent expansion, 1469t
Musset sign, 337
Mustard procedure, 249
takedown of, 306
MUSTI (Multicenter Unsustained Tachycardia) Trial, 1728t, 1729, 1788t
Mutagenesis, insertional, definition of, 917t
Mycophenolate mofetil (MMF), action of, 1212, *1213*
for cardiac allograft vasculopathy, 1196
Mycotic aneurysm(s), during pregnancy, 2052
from infective endocarditis, 415–416
of coronary artery, *510*
Mycotic infection(s), and myocarditis, 1110
Myocardial biopsy. See *Endomyocardial biopsy.*
Myocardial blood flow, and oxygen consumption, 122, *122*
electron beam computed tomography of, 2184
transmural distribution of, 525
Myocardial bridge(s), and risk of sudden death, 1716
Myocardial bridge(s) *(Continued)*
coronary angiography in, 617–619, *618,* 618t
Myocardial cell(s), action potentials of, ventricular differences in, 30
ultrastructure of, *990*
Myocardial contractility. See *Contractile function.*
Myocardial disease, allergic, 1092–1093
from metastatic cardiac tumors, 1902
in diabetes mellitus, 1922, *1923*
in rheumatoid arthritis, 1940, *1940*
metabolic disorders and, 1090–1092, 1091t
primary, electron beam computed tomography in, 2185
Myocardial fibrosis, and diastolic dysfunction, 966
and diastolic function, 1006
in acromegaly, 1916, *1917*
in scleroderma, *1946,* 1946–1947, 1947t
interstitial, 1022
pathologic changes in, 1022
replacement, 1022
Myocardial hibernation, 515, 548
and heart failure, 1149
metabolic identification of, positron emission tomography for, 119
Myocardial infarction, acute, electrocardiography in, 44, *45–47,* 46
amphetamines and, 1966
and cardiogenic shock, 1530
and pericarditis, 1247
and risk of sudden death, 1715–1716
anterior, electrocardiography in, 48
bundle branch block in, 41–42, 1598–1602, *1601*
treatment of, 1600, 1602
cardiac rehabilitation after. See *Cardiac rehabilitation.*
chest pain in, 5–6
cocaine and, 779, 1960–1961
complicated, classification as, 894, 894t
complication(s) of, 511–512
echocardiography in, *661–663,* 661–664
infarct expansion as, 662–663
mural thrombus as, 663, *663*
papillary muscle rupture as, 663, *663,* 663pl
pericardial effusion as, 661–662, *661–662*
ventricular aneurysm as, 662
ventricular pseudoaneurysm as, 664, 664pl
ventricular septal defect as, 664
ventricular wall rupture as, 664
coronary angiography after, indications for, 895
coronary angiography in, 633–637, *633–637*
pathologic correlation with, 633–634, *633–634*
with reocclusion, 636–637
detection of viable myocardium after, echocardiography in, 664–665
diagnosis of, 543–557, *543–558*
auscultation in, 543, 547–548, *547–549*
criteria for, 47
echocardiography in, 88, *89,* 660–661
electrocardiography in, 548–549, *550–553*
history in, 543
non–Q wave, risk factors for, 739–740
old, electrocardiography in, 46–47
palpation in, 543, *544–546*
pathology of, 511–512, 511pl
pathophysiology of, 534–536, *535, 537,* 821
physical examination in, 543, *544*
scintigraphy in, 554–557, *554–558*

Myocardial infarction *(Continued)*
serum enzymes in, 549, *553,* 553–554
differential diagnosis of, 557
disability from, 893–894
during cardiac rehabilitation, rates of, 900
during noncardiac surgery, monitoring for, 2098
during pregnancy, 2046–2047
ejection fraction after, thrombolytic therapy and, 754, 754t
estimation of infarct size in, 557
exercise testing after, 589–590, *590*
from coronary angiography, 607
from infective endocarditis, 413
heart failure after, 1177, *1177*
hibernation in, 548
hospital discharge after, psychological impact of, 893
hypovolemic shock in, treatment of, 1532
imaging of infarct in, 110–113, *111–113*
antimyosin antibody, 112, *112–113*
recent developments in, 112–113
in angiographically normal coronary arteries, 641
in diabetes mellitus, 1922
in older adults, 2020
infarct in. See *Infarct(s).*
inferior, electrocardiography in, 48, *49*
intraoperative, echocardiography in, 666
localization of, 47–48
modulation of, advances in, 516, 518
natural history of, infarct location and, 699, *700,* 700t
prophylactic percutaneous transluminal coronary angioplasty and, 700–701
thrombolytic therapy and, 699–702, *701*
non–Q wave, 534, *535.* See also *Angina, unstable.*
electrocardiography in, 48–49
medical treatment of, 723–740
algorithm for, *724*
aspirin with heparin in, 723, *725*
ESSENCE study of, 729–730
low–molecular-weight heparin in, 726–730, *728,* 729t, *730*
platelet antagonists in, 723, *725,* 726
platelet glycoprotein IIb/IIIa antagonist(s), 730–737, *731–735,* 735t–737t
PRISM-PLUS study of, 733–734, *734,* 735t–736t
thrombolytic therapy in, 760
TIMI II study of, 729, *730*
pathophysiology of, 738–739
percutaneous transluminal coronary intervention for, 802–816. See also *Percutaneous transluminal coronary intervention (PTCI).*
outcome of, preconditioning and, 514
posterolateral, electrocardiography in, 48, *49*
prognosis in, 560–562, 560t, *561–562*
C-reactive protein levels and, 536, *539, 542*
echocardiography and, 661
radionuclide ventriculography and, 677–678, *677–679*
thrombolytic agents and, 821, *821*
troponin levels and, 538, *540*
Q wave, 37
coronary thrombosis and, 534–536, *535*
diagnosis of, 548–549, *550–553*
treatment of, 742–779
thrombolytic therapy in, 742–771. See also *Thrombolytic therapy.*
recurrence of, low-density lipoproteins and, 541, *542*

Myocardial infarction *(Continued)*
risk factors for, smoking cessation and, 2228
risk stratification in, 894–896, 894t
"silent," 543
SPECT myocardial perfusion imaging after, 673–675, *674*
subendocardial, pathology of, 511
survivors of, heart failure in, 1148
prevention of recurrence in, 779
treatment of, *772–776,* 772–779, 777t
algorithm for, *774*
angiotensin-converting enzyme inhibitors in, 776, *776,* 777t
beta-blockers in, 772–773, *772–774*
bundle branch block and, 778–779
cardiogenic shock and, 773
heart block and, 778
infarct expansion and, 778
infarct extension and, 777–778, 777t
mitral insufficiency and, 775
pericarditis and, 776–777
pseudoaneurysms and, 776
recurrent ischemia and, 779
right ventricular infarct and, 773–774, *775*
ventricular aneurysms and, 775–776
ventricular septal defect and, 774–775
treatment of, algorithm for, 769–771, *770*
antiplatelet agents in, with stenting, 823
coronary artery bypass graft in. See *Coronary artery bypass graft (CABG).*
pacemaker therapy in, 1762–1763. See also *Pacemaker therapy.*
percutaneous transluminal coronary angioplasty in. See also *Percutaneous transluminal coronary angioplasty (PTCA).*
vs. stenting, 823, *823*
vs. thrombolytic agents, 822–823, *823*
with cardiogenic shock, 824
with thrombolytic agents, 823–824
percutaneous transluminal coronary intervention for, *821–823,* 821–824
surgical. See *Coronary artery bypass graft (CABG).*
thrombolytic therapy in, 742–771. See also *Thrombolytic therapy.*
prehospital, 824
ventricular function in, evaluation of, 557–560, *559*
ventricular tachycardia after, radiofrequency catheter ablation of, 1808–1809, *1810–1812*
vs. pulmonary thromboembolism, 1845
without atherosclerosis, 511t
Myocardial Infarction Triage and Intervention (MITI) study, of prehospital thrombolytic therapy, 757–758
Myocardial ischemia, acute, initiation of, *2228*
smoking and, 2227–2229, 2228t, *2230–2231*
amount of, and angina, 570–571
and diastolic function, 1007–1009, *1009*
and heart failure, 1149
and left ventricular dysfunction, in aortic stenosis, 332
demand *vs.* supply, 1008
diagnosis of, echocardiography in, 660
electrocardiography in, 42–44, *44–45*
exercise stress echocardiography in, 665–666, 665t
in hypertrophic cardiomyopathy, 1061
intraoperative, detection of, transesophageal echocardiography in, 2136–2137
echocardiography in, 666
monitoring of, pulmonary artery catheterization in, 2130–2131

Myocardial ischemia *(Continued)*
pathogenesis of, *512,* 512–513
pathologic changes in, 1031
prognosis in, 574–575
recurrent, in survivors of myocardial infarction, 779
silent, 569–576
altered pain perception and, 569–570
exercise testing in, 571–572
historical perspective on, 569
Holter monitoring in, 572
in diabetes mellitus, 571
left ventricular function in, 571
psychological aspects of, 570
suppression of, results of, 575–576
triglycerides and, 1346
with syncope, treatment of, 1705
without atherosclerosis, 511t
Myocardial load, abnormal, and heart failure, 1149
and cardiac relaxation, 1004
Myocardial necrosis, in myocardial infarction, 534, *535*
pathologic changes in, 1031
progression of, 513
Myocardial oxygen consumption, 521–522
and exercise prescription, 896
cocaine and, 1960
contractility and, 521–522
heart rate and, 522
rate-pressure product and, 522
systolic wall tension and, 521
Myocardial perfusion imaging, PET, 116, *116*
SPECT, 101–105, 102pl, *104–105.* See also *SPECT myocardial perfusion imaging.*
Myocardial Raynaud's phenomenon, 1946
Myocardial steal, 101
Myocardial stunning, 515, 548
and heart failure, 1149
metabolic identification of, positron emission tomography for, 119
stunning in, 548
Myocardial viability, as state of reversible contractile dysfunction at rest, 119
assessment of, positron emission tomography for, *120–124,* 120–125, 121t
and contractile function after revascularization, *124,* 125
and imaging of blood flow and glucose metabolism, 123–124, *123–124*
oxidative metabolism in, 121–123, *122*
water-perfusable tissue index in, *120,* 120–121, 121t
positron-emitting radiopharmaceuticals for, 119–120
Myocarditis, 1096–1114
bacterial, 1109
etiology of, 1098
classification of, 1096
clinical features of, 1102–1103
cocaine and, 1963
diagnosis of, 1102–1105, 1104t
Dallas criteria for, 1042, 1042t, 1096
echocardiography in, 1103–1104
electrocardiography in, 55, 1103–1104
endomyocardial biopsy in, 1104–1105, 1104t
laboratory studies in, 1103
magnetic resonance imaging in, 139, 1104
physical examination in, 1103
radionuclide imaging in, 1144–1145
scintigraphy in, 1103–1104
during pregnancy, 2053
eosinophilic, 1113, *1113*
causes of, 1025t
epidemiology of, 1096–1098

- Myocarditis *(Continued)*
  - etiology of, 1096–1098, 1096t–1097t
  - from human immunodeficiency virus, 1108–1109
  - fungal, 1097t, 1110
  - giant cell, 1093, 1112–1113, *1113*
  - granulomatous, causes of, 1025t
  - historical perspective on, 1096
  - in Fabry's disease, 1090
  - in Kawasaki's disease, 1112
  - in polymyositis, 1948–1949
  - in rheumatic fever, 391
  - in systemic lupus erythematosus, 1942
  - in Whipple's disease, 1090
  - lymphocytic, 1024t, 1025, *1026–1027*
  - metazoal, 1112
  - natural history of, 1105
  - neonatal, 1103
  - neutrophilic, causes of, 1026t
  - pathologic changes in, 1024t–1026t, 1025–1026, *1026*
  - peripartum, 1114
  - protozoal, 1110–1112
  - rheumatic, 1026–1027, *1027,* 1027pl
  - rickettsial, 1110
  - spirochetal, 1109–1110
  - toxic, 1097t
  - treatment of, 1106–1108, *1107,* 1107t
    - conventional, 1106
    - immunosuppression in, 1106–1108, *1107,* 1107t
    - supportive, 1106
    - transplantation in, 1108
  - viral, etiology of, 1096t–1097t, 1097–1098
    - pathophysiology of, 1098–1102, *1099, 1102*
      - animal models of, 1098–1099
        - significance of, 1101–1102, *1102*
      - cellular immunity in, *1099,* 1099–1100
      - cytokines in, 1101
      - humoral immunity in, 1100–1101
  - with arrhythmogenic right ventricular dysplasia, 1672–1673
- Myocarditis Treatment Trial (MTT), 1107, *1107*
- Myocardium, and adaptation to cardiac hypertrophy, 956–957, 956t–957t
  - biologic processes in, 956, 956t
  - energy metabolism and, 956–957, 957t
  - biopsy of. See *Endomyocardial biopsy.*
  - contractility of. See *Contractile function.*
  - intrinsic stiffness of, and diastolic dysfunction, 966
  - iron deposits in, in hemochromatosis, 1086
  - metabolism of, adenosine diphosphate in, 949
    - amino acids in, 949
    - and contractile function, 936–937, *936–937*
    - carbohydrates in, 942–943, *943*
    - energy transfer in, 938
    - fatty acids in, 946–948, *947*
    - gene expression and, 937, *937*
    - glucose in, regulatory sites of, 943–946, *944, 946*
    - ketone bodies in, 948–949
    - nutrition and, 939–940
    - pyruvate in, 943, *943,* 945–946, *946*
    - stages of, 939, *940*
    - substrate competition and, 940, *941*
    - tracing pathways for, 940–942, *941–942*
  - mitochondrial volume in, and oxygen consumption, 938, *938*
  - mononuclear cells in, 1026t
  - preservation of, during coronary artery bypass grafting, 839, 841
- Myocardium *(Continued)*
  - reversibly dysfunctional, on positron emission tomography, 119
  - risk zone in, 514, *514*
  - rupture of, and electromechanical dissociation, 556–557
  - space flight and, 2079
- Myocyte(s), abnormalities of, in dilated cardiomyopathy, 1037, *1037*
  - apoptosis in, pathologic changes in, 1031
  - calcium transport in, *965*
  - growth of, stimuli for, 981
  - hypertrophy of, and cardiac hypertrophy, 979
  - lengthening of, in heart failure, 1151
  - proliferation of, in cardiogenesis, 924–925
  - subcellular structure of, 1276–1277, *1277*
  - thickening of, in heart failure, 1151
  - transplantation of, for heart failure, 2274
- Myocyte abnormality hypothesis, in long QT syndrome, 1656
- Myocyte enhancer factor-2 (MEF2), in cardiogenesis, 918–919
- MyoD, and cardiac hypertrophy, 958–959
- MyoD family, definition of, 917t
- Myofibrillar lysis, in cardiac hypertrophy, 1022
- Myogenic automaticity, 523
- Myoglobin, serum, in myocardial infarction, 549, *553*
- Myopia, in Marfan's syndrome, 2151
- Myosin, and contractile function, 989–990, *990,* 1277, *1278*
  - interaction with actin, and left ventricular relaxation, 1003
  - interaction with actin and ATP, 991–992, *992*
- α-Myosin, and contractile function, 962–963, 963t
- Myosin-binding protein C, and contractile function, 1058
- Myosin essential light chain gene, in hypertrophic cardiomyopathy, 1057
- β-Myosin heavy chain, in hypertrophic cardiomyopathy, 2162, *2162*
- β-Myosin heavy chain gene, in hypertrophic cardiomyopathy, *1056,* 1056–1058, 1056t, *1062*
- Myosin mutation(s), in hypertrophic cardiomyopathy, and prognosis, 1716–1717
- Myosin regulatory light chain gene, in hypertrophic cardiomyopathy, 1057
- Myotomy-myectomy, for hypertrophic cardiomyopathy, 1068–1069
- Myotonic dystrophy, 1985–1988, 1986t, *1987*
  - cardiovascular complications of, 1985
  - clinical features of, 1985, *1987,* 2165
  - electrocardiography in, 1985, *1987*
  - genetic basis of, 1985, 2165–2168, *2167*
- Myotubular myopathy, 1986t, 1996
- Myxoma, atrial, echocardiography in, *88*
  - cardiac, 1903–1906, *1905–1906*
    - clinical features of, 1904
    - intracavitary, surgical treatment of, 1906
    - left atrial, 1904–1905, *1905–1906*
      - electron beam computed tomography in, *2188*
    - left ventricular, 1906
    - pathology of, 1904
    - right atrial, 1905–1906
- Myxomatous degeneration, anatomic abnormalities in, 319–320, *319–320*
- Myxomatous mitral valve. See *Mitral valve prolapse.*

- Na^+/Ca^{2+} exchanger, current from, in cardiac hypertrophy, 971
- Na^+/Ca^{2+} exchanger *(Continued)*
  - in diastolic dysfunction, 1012
  - in left ventricular relaxation, 1003
- Nadolol, dosage of, 712t
- Nafcillin, for infective endocarditis, staphylococcal, 407–408, 408t–409t
- Na^+,K^+-ATPase, in cardiac hypertrophy, 963
- NASCET (North American Symptomatic Carotid Endarterectomy Trial), 1435
- NASPE/BPEG code, for pacemakers, 1758–1759, 1758t
- National Exercise and Heart Disease Project (NEHPD), 897
- Natriuretic peptide(s), for heart failure, 1154, 1168
- Natural killer cell(s), in viral myocarditis, 1100
- "Negative contrast," in atrial septal defect, 240, *241*
  - in ventricular septal defect, 245
- Nemaline myopathy, 1986t, 1996, *1996*
- Neointimal fibrous proliferation, and angina, 528, *529*
- Neonatal lupus syndrome, 1945
- Neonatal myocarditis, 1103
- Neonatal ventricular tachycardia, 2064
- Nephropathy, in diabetes mellitus, 1924
- Nephrotoxicity, immunosuppression and, 1197–1198
- Neurogenic repolarization abnormality(ies), 55–56, *57*
- Neurohumoral system, activation of, in heart failure, 1152, *1152*
- Neurologic disorder(s), *vs.* pulmonary thromboembolism, 1846
- Neurologic study(ies), in evaluation of syncope, 1700
- Neuromuscular blocking agent(s), in obstetric anesthesia, 2061t
- Neuromuscular disorder(s), 1985–1997
  - Becker's muscular dystrophy and, 1991–1992, 1991t
  - Duchenne's muscular dystrophy and, 1988–1991, *1989–1991,* 1990t–1991t
  - Emery-Dreifuss syndrome and, 1992–1995, *1994*
  - facioscapulohumeral muscular dystrophy and, *1995,* 1995–1996
  - Friedreich's ataxia and, 1988
  - Kearns-Sayre syndrome and, 1992, *1993*
  - myotonic dystrophy and, 1985–1988, *1987*
  - myotubular myopathy and, 1996
  - nemaline myopathy and, 1996, *1996*
- Neurotoxicity, immunosuppression and, 1198–1199
- Neurotransmitter(s), in circulatory regulation, 1288
  - interactions with endothelial cells, and circulatory regulation, 1289–1290
- Neutrophil(s), activation of, in arrhythmogenic right ventricular dysplasia, 1671
- Neutrophilic myocarditis, causes of, 1026t
- New York Heart Association, functional classification system of, and eligibility for transplantation, 1187
- NFAT transcription factor(s), in cardiogenesis, and postnatal cardiac hypertrophy, 928
- Nicardipine, dosage of, 713t
- Nicotine, addiction to, 2230
- Nicotine replacement therapy, 2231
- Nicotinic acid, for hyperlipidemia, 2248
- Niemann-Pick disease, pathologic changes in, 1030
- Nifedipine, dosage of, 712t
  - during pregnancy, 2065–2066
  - for hypertensive crisis, 1524
  - for pulmonary hypertension, 1878–1879, *1879–1880*

Nifedipine *(Continued)*
mechanism of action for, 715
Nifurtimox, for Chagas' disease, 1044, 1111
Nimodipine, dosage of, 713t
Nisoldipine, dosage of, 713t
Nitinol stent(s), for balloon angioplasty, 264
Nitinol-polyester device, for closure of atrial septal defect, 198–199, *198–199*
Nitrate(s), chemical structure of, *710*
dosage of, 711t
during pregnancy, 2065
for chest pain, during pregnancy, 2037
for heart failure, 1173
for stable angina, 709, *710,* 711t
Nitric oxide, and circulatory regulation, 1286–1287, *1287*
and endothelium-dependent vasodilatation, 524
release of, and hypertension, 1502–1503, *1503*
in heart failure, 1154
Nitric oxide synthase, in cardiac hypertrophy, 968
Nitroglycerin, and epicardial coronary artery tone, during coronary angiography, 603
and smooth muscle relaxation, and arterial compliance, 1481–1482, *1482*
dosage of, 711t
for heart failure, 1167
mechanism of action for, *710*
Nitroprusside, and aortic valve area, 335
and arterial compliance, in heart failure, 1491
during pregnancy, 2065
for acute heart failure, 1178
for heart failure, 1167
for hypertensive crisis, 1524
in aortic dissection, 1383
Nitroxidergic nerve(s), and circulatory regulation, 1289
NK-2 homeodomain protein(s), in cardiogenesis, 919
NKX2-5 mutation(s), in atrial septal defect, 927
NODAL gene, in left-right axis malformation, 926–927
Nonbacterial thrombotic endocarditis, 401
Nonejection systolic click(s), in mitral valve prolapse, 376, *377*
Noninvasive positive-pressure ventilation, for chronic obstructive pulmonary disease, 1896
Non–Q wave myocardial infarction, 48–49
Nonsteroidal anti-inflammatory drug(s) (NSAIDs), for acute pericarditis, 1269
Noonan's syndrome, 2172t, 2173
Norepinephrine, excretion of, mitral valve prolapse and, 365–366
plasma, and prognosis in heart failure, *1160,* 1160–1161
during orthostatic stress, from space flight, 2080
release of, and hypertension, 1498–1499, *1499*
Norepinephrine inhibitor(s), for heart failure, 1176
Norpace. See *Disopyramide.*
North American Symptomatic Carotid Endarterectomy Trial (NASCET), 1435
NSAID(s). See *Nonsteroidal anti-inflammatory drug(s) (NSAIDs).*
Nuclear factor$_{KB}$, factors activating, 1332t
Nuclear imaging. See *Radionuclide imaging.*
Nutrition, and myocardial metabolism, 939–940
Nutritional support, in chronic obstructive pulmonary disease, 1897
Obesity, and atherosclerosis, 1350
and cardiomyopathy, 2259
and cardiovascular effects of weight loss, 2261
and circulatory dysfunction, 1292, *1293–1294*
and coronary artery disease, 2262–2265
anatomic studies of, 2263
as independent risk factor, 2264–2265
epidemiologic studies of, 2263
in women, 579
risk factors for, 2263–2264
risk of, *2204,* 2204–2205, 2204t–2205t
and dilated cardiomyopathy, 1045
and hypertension, 1350, 1498, 2236, *2237,* 2261–2262
control of, 2212–2213
corticosteroids and, 1199
diagnosis of, 2261
indices of, 2259
pathophysiology of, 2259–2261, *2260,* 2260t
left ventricular function in, 2260–2261, 2260t
pulmonary hypertension in, 2260, *2260*
Obstructive shock, 1530
Obstructive sleep apnea, and hypertension, 1507
chronic obstructive pulmonary disease and, 1891
Occupation(s), sedentary, and risk of coronary artery disease, 2216, *2217*
Ochronosis, anatomic abnormalities in, 318, 318pl
Ocreotide, for acromegaly, 1917
for postural hypotension, 1556
Oculoplethysmography, in carotid artery disease, 1401
OKT-3, action of, 1212
for transplant rejection, 1217
Older adult(s), arrhythmias in, 2020–2022, 2021t
atherosclerosis prevention in, 2254–2255
cardiac rehabilitation in, 903
coronary artery bypass graft in, 2019
coronary artery disease risk factors in, 2209–2210
heart failure in, 1177
hypertension in, 2020
treatment of, 1523
myocardial infarction in, 2020
percutaneous mitral balloon valvotomy in, results of, 472
percutaneous transluminal coronary angioplasty in, 2019
percutaneous transluminal coronary intervention in, for unstable angina, 811, 813, 813t
Oligonucleotide(s), as vectors for gene therapy, 2271, 2271t
On-line Mendelian Inheritance in Man (OMIM), 917t, 925–926
Onset algorithm(s), for implantable cardioverter-defibrillators, 1782–1783
Opioid(s), for cardiovascular surgery, 2107
for obstetric analgesia, 2062t
Opportunistic infection(s), in human immunodeficiency virus infection, and cardiomyopathy, *1976–1977,* 1976–1979
Oral contraceptive(s), and hypertension, 1507–1508
Orotic aciduria, hereditary, 2175t
Orthopnea, 5
Orthostatic hypotension. See *Hypotension, orthostatic.*
Orthostatic intolerance, 1553
Orthostatic stress, and circulatory regulation, 1290–1291
Orthostatic stress *(Continued)*
space flight and, 2079–2081, *2080–2081*
Ortner's syndrome, in pulmonary hypertension, 1864
Osborne wave, 1094, *1094*
in hypothermia, 56, *58*
Oscillometry, 2122–2123
Osler node(s), in infective endocarditis, 402
Osler-Weber-Rendu syndrome, 224
Osteogenesis imperfecta, anatomic abnormalities in, 319
Osteoporosis, corticosteroids and, 1199
Ostium primum, 201, *202–203,* 203
clinical features of, 203, *203*
natural history of, 201, 203
pathophysiology of, 201, *202–203*
prognosis in, 203
treatment of, 203
Output amplifier(s), in pacemakers, 1764
Outward current, in cardiac hypertrophy, *970,* 971–972
Overdrive atrial pacing study(ies), in sinus node dysfunction, *1584,* 1584–1585
Oxalosis, pathologic changes in, 1030, 1030pl
Oxidative metabolism, and reversibility of contractile function, 121–123, *122*
Oximetry, transcutaneous, in peripheral vascular disease, of lower extremities, 1408–1409
Oxprenolol, dosage of, 712t
Oxygen consumption, in obesity, 2259–2260
mitochondrial volume in myocardium and, 938, *938*
myocardial. See *Myocardial oxygen consumption.*
myocardial blood flow and, 122, *122*
peak, and eligibility for transplantation, 1187
ventilatory, and exercise prescription, 896
Oxygen saturation, in total anomalous pulmonary venous connection, 222
Oxygen therapy, for chronic obstructive pulmonary disease, 1895–1896, *1895–1896*
for pulmonary hypertension, 1878
Oxygenation, monitoring of, during cardiovascular surgery, 2109
Oxytocin, cardiovascular effects of, 2067

P mitrale, *33,* 33–34
P pulmonale, electrocardiography in, 34, *34*
P wave, 30–31, *31*
abnormalities of, *33,* 33–34
in atrial flutter, 1633, *1634*
in atrial premature beats, 1567
in atrioventricular junctional ectopic rhythm, 1570
in atrioventricular nodal tachycardia, 1609–1610, *1609–1610*
in cardiac transplantation, 58, *59*
in multifocal atrial tachycardia, 1569, *1569*
in supraventricular tachycardia, 1606, *1607*
in tricuspid atresia, 185, *186*
P450 enzyme(s), and drug metabolism, 1739–1740
Pacemaker(s), diagnostic applications of, *1773–1774,* 1773–1775
electrical interference with, 1778
electrodes for, 1765–1766
function codes for, 1590t
leads for, 1765–1766, *1766*
malfunction of, *1776–1777,* 1776–1778
modes for, 1769–1771, 1770t
monitoring system function of, 1774–1775
NASPE/BPEG code for, 1758–1759, 1758t
programming of, 1774, *1774–1775*

Pacemaker(s) *(Continued)*
pulse generators for, 1764–1765
storage capabilities of, 1774, *1774–1775*
tachycardia mediated by, 1777
timing intervals for, 1767–1769, *1768–1769*
Pacemaker cell(s), in sinus node, 1577, *1577*
Pacemaker inhibition, failure of, 1777
Pacemaker syndrome, 1771
Pacemaker therapy, atrial, 1590–1591
atrioventricular interval in, 1767
automatic mode switching in, 1773
blanking periods in, 1768
complications of, procedure-related, 1775–1776
dual-chamber, modes for, 1770–1771, 1770t
timing intervals in, 1767–1768, *1768–1769*
during pregnancy, 2046
follow-up in, 1778–1779, 1778t
for arrhythmias, with syncope, 1703
for atrial fibrillation, 1644–1645
for carotid sinus syndrome, 1702
for heart failure, 1176
for hypertrophic cardiomyopathy, 1069
for long QT syndrome, 1661–1662
for sinus node dysfunction, 1589–1590, 1590t
for syncope, vasovagal, 1702
history of, 1758
hysteresis in, *1772,* 1772–1773
indications for, 1590, 1759–1764, 1760t–1761t
ACC/AHIA guidelines for, 1760t–1761t
classification of, 1762t
in atrial fibrillation, 1763–1764
in atrioventricular block, 1759, 1760t–1761t, 1762
in bifascicular block, 1760t, 1762
in cardiomyopathy, dilated, 1764
hypertrophic, 1763
in carotid sinus hypersensitivity, 1763
in chronotropic incompetence, 1759
in myocardial infarction, 1762–1763
in neurally mediated syncope, 1763
in sinus node dysfunction, 1759, 1760t
in trifascicular block, 1760t, 1762
pacing thresholds for, 1766–1767
prophylactic, for bundle branch block, 1602
rate-adaptive, 1771–1772
rate-drop response in, 1773
sensing in, 1767
single-chamber, modes for, 1769–1770
timing intervals in, 1767, *1768–1769*
total atrial refractory period in, 1768
upper-rate behavior in, 1768–1769
Pacing threshold(s), 1766–1767
PACT (Plasminogen Activator Compatibility Trial), 759–760
PAI (plasminogen activator inhibitor), production of, and atherosclerosis, 1349
regulation of, 1313
PAIMS (Plasminogen Activator Italian Multicenter Study), 763–764
Pain, in chest. See *Chest pain.*
perception of, and silent ischemia, 569–570
Pain threshold, central nervous system processing and, 570
Pallor, in autonomic dysfunction, 1542–1543
Palmaz balloon expandable stent, 263–264
Palpation, precordial, in mitral valve prolapse, 359
Palpitation(s), differential diagnosis of, 7–8, 7t
in arrhythmogenic right ventricular dysplasia, 1665–1666
PAMI (Primary Angioplasty in Myocardial Infarction) trial, 822, *823*
Panel reactive antibody (PRA) screening, before transplantation, 1219
for transplant rejection, 1215, 1218
Panic disorder, *vs.* mitral valve prolapse, 358, 376
Papillary fibroelastoma, 1907, *1907*
Papillary muscle, energy metabolism in, and myocardial adaptation to cardiac hypertrophy, 957, 957t
rupture of, and mitral regurgitation, 663, *663,* 663pl
prognosis in, 560
Papillary muscle dysfunction, in myocardial infarction, 543
Parachute mitral valve, 154–155
mitral stenosis from, surgical treatment of, 289, *294*
Paracrine, definition of, 917t
Paradigm trial, 771
Paradoxical pulse, 15, *15*
Paradoxical splitting, *21,* 22t
Paraganglioma, 1920
cardiac, 1908
PARAGON study, 735t–736t
Paraplegia, after repair of abdominal aortic aneurysms, 1375
from descending aortic aneurysms, 1362
Parasitic infection(s), and pericarditis, 1241
Parasympathetic nervous system, physiology of, 1537, *1538*
Parasystolic ventricular tachycardia, 1571
Parathyroid hormone, and calcium regulation, 1925
Paravalvular obstruction, 150–156, *150–156*
PARIS (Peripheral Artery Radiation Investigational Study), 1443
Park blade septostomy catheter, 279
Parkinson's disease, orthostatic hypotension in, 1558, 1558t
Paroxysmal nocturnal dyspnea, 5
Paroxysmal nocturnal hemoglobinuria, 2004
Paroxysmal supraventricular tachycardia (PSVT), 1567
surgical treatment of, 1823–1824
Patch angioplasty, for aortic coarctation, 299, *299*
Patent ductus arteriosus, 208–209, *208–209*
and pregnancy, 2059
clinical features of, 209, *209*
echocardiography in, 250
large, 208–209, *208–209*
low-pressure, 208
prognosis in, 208–209
treatment of, 267–269, *270*
Gianturco coil occluding device in, 268–269, *270*
Gianturco-Grifka vascular occluding device in, 269
Rashkind occluding device in, 268
surgical, 300–301
Patent foramen ovale, 163
echocardiography in, 241–242
PAV. See *Percutaneous aortic balloon valvuloplasty.*
PAWP. See *Pulmonary artery wedge pressure.*
PCR. See *Polymerase chain reaction (PCR).*
PDGF (platelet-derived growth factor), and vascular remodeling, 1301, 1303
Peak oxygen consumption (V_{O_2}), and eligibility for transplantation, 1187
Peak systolic gradient, and severity of pulmonary stenosis, 258
Pediatric population, hypertension in, 1514, 1514t
sinus node dysfunction in, 1578
T wave in, 53
Penetrating artery(ies), 524
Penicillin, for infective endocarditis, 405–407, 406t–407t
Pentoxifylline, for claudication, 1411
PercuSurge guide wire, 1438
Percutaneous angioplasty, for peripheral vascular disease, of lower extremities, 1413
for renal artery disease, 1404
for renal artery stenosis, 1431–1432, *1431*
for subclavian artery occlusive disease, 1441–1442, *1441–1442,* 1441t
Percutaneous aortic balloon valvuloplasty, 476–481, *477–480,* 478t–480t
antegrade technique of, 476–477
as bridge to aortic valve replacement, 479–480, 479t, *480*
complications of, 478
for cardiogenic shock, 480–481, 480t
for congenital aortic stenosis, 481
immediate results of, 477–478, 478t
indications for, 481
long-term follow-up after, 478–479, *478–479*
mechanism of, 477
retrograde technique of, 476, *477*
vs. aortic valve replacement, 481
Percutaneous mitral balloon valvotomy, complications of, 469–470, 469t
during pregnancy, 475
follow-up after, *470–473,* 470–476, 470t
double-balloon *vs.* Inoue technique, 473–474
echocardiographic score in, *471,* 471–472
echocardiography in, 474
in older patient, 472
in optimal candidates, 473, *473*
in patients with atrial fibrillation, 472
in patients with calcified mitral valves, 472
in patients with pulmonary hypertension, 472–473
in patients with surgical commissurotomy, 472
in patients with tricuspid regurgitation, 473
vs. surgical commissurotomy, 474–475
for rheumatic mitral stenosis, *464–473,* 464–476, 466t, 469t–470t
immediate outcome of, 466–467, 466t, *467*
mechanism of, 465–466
outcome of, factors predicting, 467–469
patient selection for, 464
technique of, 464–465, *465–466*
antegrade double-balloon, 465, *465*
vs. Inoue, 473–474
Inoue, 465, *466*
Percutaneous pulmonary balloon valvuloplasty, 463–464, 464t
Percutaneous transcatheter cardiac tissue ablation, for sinus node dysfunction, 1591
Percutaneous transluminal coronary angioplasty (PTCA), before noncardiac surgery, 2097
cardiac rehabilitation after, 903
for cardiac allograft vasculopathy, 1196
for myocardial infarction, 879
vs. stenting, 823, *823*
vs. thrombolytic agents, 822–823, *823*
with thrombolytic agents, 823–824, 879
for saphenous vein graft disease, 880, 880t
for stable angina, *vs.* coronary artery bypass graft, 796, *796,* 797t, 798, *798*
vs. medical therapy, 795–796
history of, 790

- Percutaneous transluminal coronary angioplasty (PTCA) *(Continued)*
  - in older adults, 2019
  - nonrandomized data on, 877, *878*
  - outcome of, in diabetic patients, 759, 874–875
  - pathology of, 516, *516–517*
  - prophylactic, and natural history of myocardial infarction, 700–701
  - *vs.* coronary artery bypass graft, clinical trial(s) of, BARI, 873t, 874
    - CABRI, 873t, 874
    - Emory Angioplasty *versus* Surgery, 872, 873t
    - ERACI, 873t, 874
    - German Angioplasty Bypass Investigation, 872, 874
    - Randomized Intervention Treatment of Angina, 872
    - Toulouse, 873t, 874
  - *vs.* coronary atery bypass graft, clinical trials of, 871–874, 873t
  - *vs.* hypolipidemic agents, for stable angina, 718
  - *vs.* medical therapy, clinical trials of, 870–871, *872*
  - *vs.* thrombolytic therapy, *758,* 758–760
- Percutaneous transluminal coronary intervention (PTCI), Braunwald classification in, 804, 804t, *806*
  - devices for, *790*
  - diabetes mellitus and, 874–875
  - for myocardial infarction, *821–823,* 821–824
    - with cardiogenic shock, 824
  - for stable angina, atherectomy in, 793–794, 794t
    - combined modalities of, 794, 795t
    - long-term results of, 795
    - patient selection for, 794–798, *796, 797t, 798*
      - in multivessel disease, 796, *796,* 797t, 798, *798*
      - in one-vessel disease, 795–796
      - in stable angina, 794–795
    - restenosis after, 798t–799t, 799
    - stents in, 791–792, 792t–793t. See also *Stent(s).*
  - for unstable angina, 802–816
    - balloon angioplasty in, 807–809, *808–809,* 809t
    - diabetes and, 811, *812*
    - future of, 816
    - in older adults, 811, 813, 813t
    - medical treatment of, 815–816, 815t, *816*
    - rationale for, 806–807
    - risk stratification in, 804, *805–807,* 805t, 806
    - stenting in, 807–809, 807t–809t, *808*
  - history of, 869–870
  - nonrandomized data on, 877, *878*
  - types of, 790
- Percutaneous transluminal renal angioplasty (PTRA), 1430, *1430*
- Percutaneous tricuspid balloon valvuloplasty, 481–482
- PERfusion, PERformance Exercise Trial (PERFEXT), 900–901, *901,* 903
- Peribronchial "cuffing," 72, *73*
- Pericardial constraint, and diastolic function, 1005–1006
- Pericardial cyst(s), 1242
  - and cardiomegaly, 10
- Pericardial disease, anatomic abnormalities in, 1241–1243, *1242*
  - degenerative, 1246
  - diagnosis of, computed tomography in, electron beam, 2184–2185, *2185*
- Pericardial disease *(Continued)*
    - missed, 1245
  - drug-induced, 1247
  - etiology of, 1246–1247
    - diversity of, 1245
  - from metastatic cardiac tumors, 1902
  - idiopathic, 1246
  - in rheumatoid arthritis, 1939, 1940t
  - in scleroderma, 1947
  - in systemic lupus erythematosus, 1941–1942, *1943*
  - metabolic, 1247
  - neoplastic, 1247
  - radiation-induced, 1247
  - traumatic, 1247
- Pericardial effusion, 1247–1251, *1248*
  - cardiomegaly in, 9–10
  - diagnosis of, 1247–1250, *1248*
    - echocardiography in, *90,* 90–91, *1248,* 1249–1250
    - magnetic resonance imaging in, 137
    - pericardioscopy in, 1250
    - physical examination in, 1247–1249
    - radiography in, 1249
    - scintigraphy in, 1249
  - etiology of, 1250
  - in myocardial infarction, echocardiography in, 661–662, *661–662*
- Pericardial fluid, cytologic analysis of, 1241
  - examination of, 1250–1251
- Pericardial friction rub, 1268
  - in myocardial infarction, 548
- Pericardial knock, 1262
- Pericardial prosthetic valve(s), bovine, complications of, 323
- Pericardial tumor(s), 1242–1243, 1909, *1909*
- Pericardiectomy, for recurrent pericarditis, 1270
- Pericardiocentesis, 1250–1251
  - for cardiac tumors, secondary, 1903
  - in cardiac tamponade, 1257–1258
    - hemodynamic assessment after, 1256–1257, *1257*
  - in constrictive pericarditis, with rheumatoid arthritis, 1939–1940
- Pericardioscopy, in pericardial effusion, 1250
- Pericarditis, acute, 1267–1269, *1269*
    - clinical course of, 1269
    - diagnosis of, echocardiography in, 1269
      - electrocardiography in, 1268, *1269*
      - laboratory studies in, 1268–1269
      - physical examination in, 1268
      - radiography in, 1269
    - etiology of, 1268
    - pathology of, 1268
    - symptoms of, 1268
  - acute fibrinous. See *Pericarditis, acute.*
  - anatomic abnormalities in, 1241–1242, 1241pl, *1242*
  - bacterial, 1246
  - chest pain in, 6
  - cholesterol levels in, 1242, *1242*
  - chronic effusive, 1251
  - constrictive, 1258–1267, *1259–1265*
    - central venous pressure in, 2123, *2125*
    - diagnosis of, 1265–1266
      - cardiac catheterization in, 1263–1265, *1265*
      - computed tomography in, 1263, *1264*
      - echocardiography in, 1263
        - *vs.* restrictive cardiomyopathy, 1267
      - electrocardiography in, 1262
        - *vs.* restrictive cardiomyopathy, 1266–1267
      - laboratory studies in, 1262
      - magnetic resonance imaging in, 1263, *1265*
- Pericarditis *(Continued)*
      - physical examination in, 1261–1262, *1262*
      - radiography in, 1262–1263, *1263–1264*
        - *vs.* restrictive cardiomyopathy, 1267
    - etiology of, 1261
    - history in, 1261
    - in rheumatoid arthritis, 1939–1940
    - pathophysiology of, 1258–1261, *1259–1260*
      - and characteristics differing from cardiac tamponade, 1259–1261, *1259–1261*
      - and common characteristics with cardiac tamponade, 1258–1259
    - *vs.* cirrhosis, 1266
    - *vs.* restrictive cardiomyopathy, 90, 1127t, 1266–1267
  - diagnosis of, electrocardiography in, 55, *56*
  - during pregnancy, 2052–2053
  - granulomatous, 1242, 1242pl
  - in collagen vascular disease, 1241–1242, 1247
  - in human immunodeficiency virus infection, 1975, *1975*
  - in infective endocarditis, 413
  - in rheumatic fever, *388,* 391, *394*
  - in survivors of myocardial infarction, 776–777
  - myocardial infarction and, 1247
  - recurrent, 1269–1270
  - rheumatoid, 1242, *1242*
  - tuberculous, 1241, 1261
  - viral, 1246
  - *vs.* pulmonary thromboembolism, 1845
- Pericardium, autologous, for aortic cusp extension, 289, *292*
    - for repair of supravalvular aortic stenosis, *298*
  - magnetic resonance imaging of, 137, *137*
- Peripartum cardiomyopathy, 1024, 1045, *2053,* 2053–2054, 2053t–2054t
- Peripartum myocarditis, 1114
- Peripheral airways disease, definition of, 1885
- Peripheral arterial disease, exercise testing in, 590
- Peripheral Artery Radiation Investigational Study (PARIS), 1443
- Peripheral edema, differential diagnosis of, 11
  - during pregnancy, 2038
- Peripheral lipodystrophy, protease inhibitors and, 1981
- Peripheral vascular disease, 1399–1413
  - and treatment of hypertension, 1522t, 1523
  - atherosclerosis and, 1399–1400. See also *Atherosclerosis.*
  - dysplastic, 1400
  - embolism and, 1400
  - in diabetes mellitus, 1924
  - of carotid artery, *1401,* 1401–1402
  - of lower extremities, *1404–1410,* 1404–1413, 1405t–1406t, 1409t, 1411t
    - atherosclerosis and, 1404, *1404–1405*
    - diagnosis of, 1405–1409, 1406t, *1407*
      - ankle-brachial index in, 1406–1407, 1406t, *1407*
      - continuous-wave Doppler waveform examination in, 1408
      - contrast angiography in, 1409
      - duplex ultrasonography in, 1408
      - exercise Doppler stress test in, 1407–1408
      - history in, 1405–1406
      - noninvasive vascular studies in, 1406, 1406t
      - physical examination in, 1405–1406

Peripheral vascular disease *(Continued)*
pulse volume recording in, 1408
segmental pressure measurements in, 1407
transcutaneous oximetry in, 1408–1409
indications for referral in, 1411, 1411t
natural history of, 1404–1405, *1405,* 1405t
treatment of, 1409–1413, 1409t, *1410,* 1411t
exercise training in, *1410,* 1410–1411
goals of, 1409t
medical, 1409–1412, 1409t
percutaneous angioplasty in, 1413
surgical, 1412–1413
radiotherapy for, 1442–1443, *1442,* 1443t
renal artery, *1402,* 1402–1403
thrombosis and, 1400
vasculitis and, 1400
vasospastic disease and, 1400
Peripheral vascular resistance, aging and, 2016
during space flight, 2085
hypertension and, 1488
Peritonitis, *vs.* pulmonary thromboembolism, 1846
Peroneal artery, atherosclerosis in, 1438
Persistent common arterioventricular canal, 163
with tetralogy of Fallot, 175, *176*
Persistent left superior vena cava, 168
Perth Coronary Register Study, 691, 693t
PET. See *Positron emission tomography (PET).*
PET myocardial perfusion imaging, 116, *116,* 679–685, *681–685*
clinical applications of, 679–680, *680,* 680pl
economic issues in, 682
flow metabolism patterns in, and cardiac risk, *682,* 683, *684*
revascularization and, 683–684, *685–686*
future developments in, 685
new concepts in, 680–681, *681–682*
therapeutic guidelines from, 681–682
vs. quantitative coronary angiography, 681–682, *682*
vs. SPECT imaging, 105
Phenothiazine(s), electrocardiographic changes from, 53
Phenoxybenzamine hydrochloride, for pheochromocytoma, 1921
Phentermine, valvular disease from, 453
Phenytoin, during pregnancy, 2045t
pharmacokinetics of, 1742t–1743t
Pheochromocytoma, and hypertension, 1506
clinical features of, 1920, *1921*
diagnosis of, 1510–1511, 1920
pathophysiology of, 1920
plasma catecholamines in, 1545, *1549*
treatment of, 1920–1921
vs. pulmonary thromboembolism, 1847
Phlebotomy, for erythrocytosis, 2005
for hemochromatosis, 1088
Phonocardiography, in mitral valve prolapse, *377*
in myocardial infarction, *547*
Phosphoinositide pathway, in excitation-contraction coupling, *1283*
Phospholipid(s), degradation of, in myocardial ischemia, 513
Phosphorylation potential, 999
Photomultiplier(s), for radionuclide imaging, 99
Photopheresis, for cardiac allograft vasculopathy, 1196
for immunosuppressive therapy, 1213
Physical activity. See *Activity; Exercise.*
Physical examination, 13–27, *15–27,* 15t–17t, 23t–26t
auscultation in, *20–21,* 20–27, 22t–26t, *24, 27.* See also *Auscultation.*
blood pressure measurement in, 14–16, *15,* 15t–16t
inspection in, 13–14
of precordium, 19–20
palpation of pulse in, arterial, 16–17, *16–17,* 17t
jugular venous, *17–18,* 17–19, 18t
Physical fitness, *vs.* exercise, 2217–2218
Physicians' Health Study, 1337
Phytosterolemia, 2175t
Pigmentation, 13
Pimobendan, for heart failure, 1174
Pindolol, dosage of, 712t
PIOPED (Prospective Investigation of Pulmonary Embolism Diagnosis), 1840
PISA. See *Proximal isovelocity acceleration (PISA) echocardiography.*
Pituitary gland, anterior, hormones of, 1915
radiotherapy to, for acromegaly, 1917
Pitx2, and left-right position of body axis, 924
Planar acquisition mode, 100
Plaque(s). See *Atherosclerotic plaque(s).*
Plasma membrane, in excitation-contraction coupling, 993–995
calcium channels and, 994
calcium pump and, 994
sodium pump and, 995
sodium-calcium exchange and, 994–995
sodium-hydrogen exchange and, 995
Plasma norepinephrine (PNE), and prognosis in heart failure, *1160,* 1160–1161
Plasma renin activity, in heart failure, 1153, *1153,* 1158
in renal artery disease, 1402
in renovascular hypertension, 1429, 1510
Plasmapheresis, for immunosuppressive therapy, 1213–1214
Plasmid expression vector(s), for gene therapy, 2269–2271, *2270,* 2271t
Plasminogen, activation of, by clot-selective thrombolytic agents, 743–744, 748–749, *749*
Plasminogen activator(s), and fibrinolysis, 1311
production of, regulation of, 1312–1313
protein structure of, 1311–1312
Plasminogen Activator Compatibility Trial (PACT), 759–760
Plasminogen activator inhibitor (PAI), production of, and atherosclerosis, 1349
regulation of, 1313
Plasminogen Activator Italian Multicenter Study (PAIMS), 763–764
Plasminogen steal, 748
Platelet(s), activation of, *731*
and restenosis, 1306, 1306t
and thrombosis, 1349
adhesion of, in pulmonary hypertension, 1861–1862
in unstable angina, 531
disorders of, 2005–2007, 2006t
hyperreactivity of, 2007
Platelet antagonist(s), for intraoperative blood conservation, 2112
for stable angina, 715–717, *716,* 717t
for unstable angina, 723, *724–725,* 726
Platelet Glycoprotein IIb/IIIa in Unstable Angina Receptor Suppression Using Integrin Therapy (PURSUIT) study, 732–733, *733,* 735t, 811, 812t
Platelet Receptor Inhibition in Ischemic Syndrome Management in Patients Limited by Unstable Signs and Symptoms (PRISM-PLUS) study, 733–734, *734,* 810
Platelet Receptor Inhibition in Ischemic Syndrome Management (PRISM) study, 733, 735t–736t, 811
Platelet-derived growth factor (PDGF), and vascular remodeling, 1301, 1303
Plethysmography, in peripheral vascular disease, of lower extremities, 1407
Pleural effusion, differential diagnosis of, 11–12, 12t
in pericarditis, constrictive, 1262
Pleural friction rub, in pulmonary thromboembolism, 1837
PN (protease nexin), as anticoagulant mechanism, 1319
PNE (plasma norepinephrine), and prognosis in heart failure, *1160,* 1160–1161
Pneumococcal infection(s), and pericarditis, 1246
Pneumocystis carinii pneumonia, echocardiography in, *1974*
Pneumonia, *vs.* pulmonary thromboembolism, 1843–1844
Polar map(s), from SPECT myocardial perfusion imaging, 104–105, *104–105*
Polyarteritis nodosa, *1949,* 1949–1950
of coronary arteries, *510*
Polychondritis, relapsing, 1951–1952, 1952pl
Polymerase chain reaction (PCR), in diagnosis of viral myocarditis, 1042
in muscular dystrophy, Duchenne's, *2164*
Polymorphic ventricular tachycardia, 1572
Polymyositis, *1948,* 1948–1949
Polyneuropathy, familial amyloid, and autonomic dysfunction, 1552
Pompe's disease, 2174t
Porcine prosthetic valve(s), complications of, *322,* 322–323
Positive end-expiratory pressure (PEEP), and pulmonary artery catheterization, 2130
Positive pressure ventilation, cardiovascular response to, 2117
Positron emission tomography (PET), 113–125, *114–124*
contrast agents for, 118
for assessment of myocardial viability, 119–125, *120–124,* 121t
and contractile function after revascularization, *124,* 125
blood flow and glucose metabolism in, 123–124, *123–124*
oxidative metabolism in, 121–123, *122*
water-perfusable tissue index in, *120,* 120–121, 121t
for identification of reversibly dysfunctional myocardium, 119
for metabolic identification of myocardial hibernation and stunning, 119
for myocardial perfusion imaging. See *PET myocardial perfusion imaging.*
of coronary flow reserve, 113–118, *114–118*
absolute *vs.* relative, 116–117, *117*
and percent diameter stenosis, 117–118, *118*
mechanisms of, 114, *115,* 116
severity of stenosis and, 114, *115,* 116
principles of, 113
Positron-emitting tracer(s), of metabolic pathways, 941, *941*
Postmicturition syncope, 1691
Postural hypotension. See *Hypotension, orthostatic.*
Postural tachycardia syndrome, 1541, 1553
Posture, and radiography, *70*
Postventricular atrial refractory period, in dual-chamber pacing, 1768
Potassium, dietary, and hypertension, 1498

Potassium *(Continued)*
control of, 2239
monitoring of, during diuretic therapy, 1166–1167
transport of, in myocardial ischemia, 512, *512*
Potassium channel(s), in smooth muscle cell function, and pulmonary hypertension, 1860–1861, *1861*
Potassium channel gene(s), expression of, and cardiac hypertrophy, 972
Potassium channel opener(s), for long QT syndrome, 1705
Potassium current, diminished, in long QT syndrome, 1657–1659, *1658*
Potassium-sparing diuretic(s), for hypertension, 1516, 1517t
Power spectral density analysis, after space flight, 2083
PR interval, in atrioventricular block, *1599*
first-degree, 1572
PR segment, 31
PRA (panel reactive antibody) screening, before transplantation, 1219
for transplant rejection, 1215, 1218
PRAISE (Prospective Randomized Amlodipine Survival Evaluation Study Group), 1173
Pravastatin, and prognosis in coronary artery disease, *719*
and risk of coronary artery disease, *695*
for hyperlipidemia, clinical trials of, 1339
Prazosin, during pregnancy, 2050t
for heart failure, 1173
for hypertension, 1520
Preconditioning, and outcome of myocardial infarction, 514
Precordial palpation, in mitral valve prolapse, 359
Precordium, examination of, 19–20
Prednisone, for myocarditis, 1106–1108, *1107,* 1107t
for recurrent pericarditis, 1270
Preeclampsia, 1507, 2047
Preexcitation, 1620–1631
accessory pathways in, 1620, *1620–1621, 1623*
ablation of, 1630
long anterograde refractory period in, 1626, *1629*
atrial fibrillation in, 1625, *1625–1626*
circus movement tachycardia in, 1622, *1623–1624,* 1625
electrocardiography in, 42, *42–43,* 1620–1622, *1621–1622*
exercise in, 1625–1626, *1628*
incidence of, 1622
intermittent, 1625, *1627*
low-risk, diagnosis of, 1625–1626, *1627–1629*
nomenclature in, 1621t
pathophysiology of, *1620*
treatment of, 1626, *1629,* 1630, 1630t
in patient with arrhythmias, 1630
in patient without arrhythmias, 1630–1631
Pregnancy, after heart transplantation, 1199–1200
and prosthetic valves, 2039
anticoagulation during, 2039–2040, *2040–2041*
aortic dissection during, 2049, 2051
aortic regurgitation during, 2057
arrhythmias during, 2040–2046, *2042,* 2044t–2045t
atrial fibrillation, 2041
atrial flutter, 2041
sinus tachycardia, 2040–2041

Pregnancy *(Continued)*
supraventricular tachycardia, 2041–2042
bundle branch block during, 2046
cardiac arrest during, 2034–2036, 2036t, *2037*
cardiac evaluation during, 2031–2034, 2031t–2032t, *2032–2033*
echocardiographic, 2033
electrocardiographic, 2032
of murmurs, 2032, *2033*
precordial, 2032
radiographic, 2032–2033
vascular, 2031–2032, *2032*
with cardiac catheterization, 2034
with exercise testing, 2033
with magnetic resonance imaging, 2033
with pulmonary artery catheterization, 2033–2034
with radionuclide imaging, 2033
cardiac output during, 2027, *2028,* 2028t
cardiac surgery during, 2060, 2061t–2062t
cardiomyopathy during, hypertrophic, 2054–2055
peripartum, *2053,* 2053–2054, 2053t–2054t
cardiopulmonary resuscitation during, 2026, 2036t
cardiovascular drug(s) during, 2060–2066, 2063t
alpha/beta-adrenergic stimulation/blockade and, 2063t
angiotensin-converting enzyme inhibitors, 2065
antiarrhythmic, 2043–2046, 2044t–2045t, 2063–2064
beta-blockers, 2066
calcium channel blockers, 2065–2066
cardiac glycosides, 2063
diuretics, 2064–2065
fetal effects of, 2060–2063, 2063t
nitrates, 2065
nitroprusside, 2065
cardioversion during, 2946
chest pain during, 2036–2037, 2036t
collagen vascular disease during, 2052
congenital heart disease and, 228–229, 2057–2060, 2058t
and antibiotic prophylaxis, 2058
aortic coarctation as, 2059
aortic valvular, 2059
atrial septal defect as, 2058
cyanotic, 2060
Ebstein's anomaly as, 2060
Eisenmenger's syndrome as, 2060
patent ductus arteriosus as, 2059
tetralogy of Fallot as, 2059–2060
ventricular septal defect as, 2058–2059
coronary artery disease during, 2046–2047
dermatomyositis during, 2052
diastolic function during, 1005
fetal distress during, 2034, *2035*
fever during, 2038
heart block during, 2046
heart rate during, 2028, 2028t
high-risk cardiac disorders and, 2051t
hypertension during, 1507, 1514–1515, 2047–2049, 2048t–2051t
and eclampsia, 2047–2048, 2048t
and preeclampsia, 2047
chronic, 2048
classification of, 2048t
gestational, 2047
treatment of, 1523, 2049, 2050t–2051t
hypotension during, 2034
infective endocarditis during, 2038–2039, 2039t

Pregnancy *(Continued)*
long QT syndrome during, 2066–2067
Marfan's syndrome and, 2051
mycotic aneurysms during, 2052
myocardial infarction during, 2046–2047
myocarditis during, 2053
pacemaker therapy during, 2046
percutaneous mitral balloon valvotomy during, 475
pericarditis during, 2052–2053
peripheral edema during, 2038
physiology of, 2026–2031, *2027–2030,* 2028t, 2031t
and exercise response, 2029, *2030*
blood volume and, 2026–2027, *2027*
during labor and delivery, 2029–2031, 2031t
during postpartum period, 2031
gravid uterus and, 2028–2029, *2029–2030*
hematologic changes and, 2026–2027, *2027*
with multiple fetuses, 2031
pulmonary hypertension during, 2049, 2051t
pulmonary thromboembolism during, 2037–2038
rales during, 2038
rheumatic fever during, 2055–2056
systemic lupus erythematosus during, 2052
Takayasu's arteritis during, 2051–2052
valvular disease during, 2055–2057, 2056t
venous emergencies during, 2037–2038, 2038t
ventricular arrhythmias during, 2043
Wolff-Parkinson-White syndrome during, 2042–2043
Premature ventricular contractions (PVCs), during pregnancy, 2043
Preoperative evaluation, for noncardiac surgery, and maintenance medications, 2092
approach to, 2091–2092, 2092t
coronary artery disease and, 2092–2094, 2092t–2094t. See also *Coronary artery disease, noncardiac surgery in.*
history in, 2091t
Prerenal azotemia, from diuretic therapy, 1167
Pressure gradient(s), in aortic valve, calculation of, *445*
in mitral stenosis, 448, *448*
in prosthetic valves, 453
Pressure-volume relationship(s), pulmonary artery catheterization and, 2130
PREVENT (Proliferation Reduction with Vascular Energy Trial), 836
Primary Angioplasty in Myocardial Infarction (PAMI) trial, 822, *823*
Primary antiphospholipid antibody syndrome, 1944
Primary autonomic failure syndrome, 1550–1551, *1551*
Prinzmetal angina. See *Angina, variant (Prinzmetal).*
PRISM (Platelet Receptor Inhibition in Ischemic Syndrome Management) study, 733, 735t–736t, 811
PRISM-PLUS (Platelet Receptor Inhibition in Ischemic Syndrome Management in Patients Limited by Unstable Signs and Symptoms) study, , *733–734, 734,* 810
Procainamide, adverse effects of, 1745
and systemic lupus erythematosus, 1945, 1946t
during pregnancy, 2043, 2044t
efficacy of, 1745
electrocardiographic changes from, 53

Procainamide *(Continued)*
electrophysiology of, 1744
for atrial fibrillation, 1637, 1637t
for preexcitation, *1629*
inotropic potential of, 1744t, 1745
pharmacokinetics of, 1742t–1743t, 1744–1745
Procoagulant mechanism(s), in coagulation system, 1318
Procoagulant pathway(s), in coagulation system, *1316*
Procoagulant protein(s), abnormalities of, in pulmonary hypertension, 1866
structure of, 1315–1316, 1317t
Proliferation Reduction with Vascular Energy Trial (PREVENT), 836
Promoter(s), definition of, 917t
Pronestyl. See *Procainamide.*
Propafenone, adverse effects of, 1748
dosage of, 1748
efficacy of, 1748
electrophysiology of, 1748
for atrial fibrillation, 1637t
pharmacokinetics of, 1742t–1743t, 1748
Propeptide/carboxyglutamic acid–rich domain, in coagulation system, 1315–1316
Propranolol, adverse effects of, 1749
dosage of, 712t, 1749
during pregnancy, 2045t, 2050t, 2066
efficacy of, 1749
electrophysiology of, 1749
for atrial fibrillation, 1636, 1637t
for prevention of sudden death, 1724, *1724*
in aortic dissection, 1382
in survivors of myocardial infarction, *773*
pharmacokinetics of, 1742t–1743t, 1749
Propylthiouracil, for hyperthyroidism, 1928
Prospective Investigation of Pulmonary Embolism Diagnosis (PIOPED), 1840
Prostacyclin, and endothelium-dependent vasodilatation, 524
for pulmonary hypertension, 1879I
synthesis of, aspirin and, *716*
Prostaglandin(s), and hypertension, *1501,* 1501–1502
cardiovascular effects of, 2067
Prosthesis, for tetralogy of Fallot, 246–247
Prosthetic valve(s), and pregnancy, 2039
catheterization of, 432–434, 433t–434t, *434*
choice of, 486
complications of, *321–322,* 321–323
with all valve types, *321,* 321–322
with bioprosthetic valves, 322–323
with rigid-framed valves, 322
disproportion of, 322
Doppler echocardiography of, 83, *84*
echocardiography of, 453, 453pl
endocarditis in, 2286–2288, 2286t–2288t
clinical features of, 2286–2287
diagnosis of, 2287
microbiology of, 2286, 2286t
pathogenesis of, 2286
prevention of, 2288
risk factors for, 2286
treatment of, 2287–2288, 2287t–2288t
for aortic stenosis, 286, *286–288*
heart sounds from, 27, *27*
infective endocarditis with, treatment of, 409t
pressure gradients in, 433, 433t
types of, 321
Protamine, after heparin administration, 603
allergic reactions to, 608
Protease inhibitor(s), metabolic complications of, 1980–1981
Protease nexin (PN), as anticoagulant mechanism, 1319
Protein(s), anticoagulant, structure of, 1315–1316, 1317t
contractile, 989t, 990–991, *990–991,* 1277–1279, *1278*
interactions among, 991–992, *992*
C-reactive, and atherosclerosis, 1337
and prognosis in myocardial infarction, 536, *539, 542*
NK-2 homeodomain, in cardiogenesis, 919
procoagulant, abnormalities of, in pulmonary hypertension, 1866
structure of, 1315–1316, 1317t
Protein C, in hypercoagulable states, 2009
Protein kinase C, and production of tissue-type plasminogen activator, 1312–1313
Protein S, in hypercoagulable states, 2009
Protodiastolic gallop, 22, 24
Protozoal infection(s), and myocarditis, 1110–1112
Proximal aorta, anomalies of, 250–251
Proximal isovelocity acceleration (PISA) echocardiography, in mitral stenosis, 80–81
Proximal isovelocity surface area, in assessment of mitral regurgitation severity, 353
"Pruned tree" appearance, of pulmonary arteries, in atrial septal defect, 197, *197*
Pseudoaneurysm(s), after myocardial infarction, 555, *558*
cardiac, pathologic changes in, 1032
femoral artery, from coronary angiography, 606
in survivors of myocardial infarction, 776
left ventricular, and shock, 1530
magnetic resonance imaging in, 138, *139*
radiotherapy and, 831
Pseudocoarctation, of aorta, 1357–1358, *1359*
Pseudofusion, 1776, *1777*
Pseudo-Hurler polydystrophy, 2174t
Pseudosubstrate(s), in coagulation system, 1318
Pseudotruncus arteriosus, 219–220, *220*
Pseudoxanthoma elasticum, *2156,* 2156–2157
Psoriatic arthritis, 1952
PSVT. See *Paroxysmal supraventricular tachycardia (PSVT).*
Psychiatric disorder(s), syncope in, 1705
vs. pulmonary thromboembolism, 1846
Psychological stress, and hypertension, 1498
and regulation of circulation, 1290
and risk of atherosclerosis, 1351
and risk of sudden death, 1713
"high reactors" to, and hypertension, dietary sodium and, *2235*
PTCA. See *Percutaneous transluminal coronary angioplasty (PTCA).*
PTCI. See *Percutaneous transluminal coronary intervention (PTCI).*
PTE. See *Pulmonary thromboembolism.*
PTRA. See *Percutaneous transluminal renal angioplasty (PTRA).*
Pulmonary. See also *Lung(s).*
Pulmonary arteriography, in pulmonary thromboembolism, 1841, *1842*
Pulmonary arteriovenous fistula(s), 169–170, *170*
Pulmonary artery(ies), agenesis of, *vs.* pulmonary thromboembolism, 1845
anomalous origin of coronary artery from, 227
anomalous origin of left coronary artery from, 301, *302*
catheterization of, 2108, 2125–2131, *2126–2128,* 2129t
and prediction of left ventricular end-diastolic volume, 2129, 2129t
Pulmonary artery(ies) *(Continued)*
complications of, 2126–2127
data interpretation errors in, 2127
during pregnancy, 2033–2034
for measurement of heart rate, 2129
for measurement of pulmonary vascular resistance, 2129
for measurement of right ventricular ejection fraction, 2131
for monitoring and pacing, 2131
for myocardial ischemia monitoring, 2130–2131
in valvular disease, 2129
pressure-volume relationships and, 2130
technical aspects of, 2125–2126, *2126*
validity of data from, *2128,* 2128–2129
ventilatory pressure influences on, 2130
ventricular compliance and, 2130
wedge trace in, 2127–2128, *2128*
compliance of, in pulmonary hypertension, 1872–1873
enlargement of, in mitral stenosis, 420, *420*
injury to, from catheterization, 2127
origin of, *173*
from coronary artery, 172, 174, *174,* 624, *624*
"pruned tree" appearance of, in atrial septal defect, 197, *197*
transposition with aorta, complete, 210, *211*
congenitally corrected, 212, *213–216*
echocardiography in, 249–250
Pulmonary artery pressure, diastolic, in pulmonary hypertension, 1870
elevation of. See *Pulmonary hypertension.*
Pulmonary artery wedge pressure, after pericardiocentesis, 1256
in mitral regurgitation, *425,* 425–426
in mitral stenosis, 421, *422*
in pericarditis, constrictive, 1263–1264, *1265*
Pulmonary atresia, tetralogy of Fallot with, *172*
surgical treatment of, 303, *303*
with ventricular septal defect, 219–220, *220*
Pulmonary autograft(s), for aortic stenosis, 286, *289*
Pulmonary capillary wedge pressure, exercise and, in heart failure, 1150, *1150*
Pulmonary disease, chest pain in, 6
cough in, 6
dyspnea in, 4, 4t
hemoptysis in, 7
obstructive, *vs.* pulmonary thromboembolism, 1844
Pulmonary edema, "flash," 1178
radiography in, 72, *73–74,* 74
rales in, 11
Pulmonary embolectomy, 1850
Pulmonary fibrosis, and pulmonary hypertension, 1865
Pulmonary function test(s), in chronic obstructive pulmonary disease, 1890–1891, *1891*
in pulmonary hypertension, 1867, 1867t
Pulmonary homograft(s), for repair of tetralogy of Fallot, 302
Pulmonary hypertension, 1856–1881
and outcome of percutaneous mitral balloon valvotomy, 472–473
arterial, radiography in, 74, *75*
definition of, 1856
diagnosis of, 1862–1867, 1864t, 1867t
angiography in, *1876,* 1876–1877
cardiac catheterization in, 1873–1875, *1874*
computed tomography in, 1873

Pulmonary hypertension *(Continued)*
diastolic pulmonary artery pressure in, 1870
echocardiography in, 452–453
Doppler, 1870, *1871,* 1871t
M-mode, 1868–1869
two-dimensional, 1869
electrocardiography in, 1867, *1868,* 1868t
exercise testing in, 1873
history in, 1862–1864, 1864t
laboratory studies in, 1866–1867, 1867t
lung biopsy in, 1877
magnetic resonance imaging in, 1872–1873
physical examination in, 1865–1866
physiologic measurements in, 1869t, 1871t
radiography in, 1867–1868
radionuclide imaging in, *1875,* 1875–1876
review of systems in, 1864–1865
right atrial pressure in, 1870–1871, *1871–1872*
during pregnancy, 2049, 2051t
in atrial septal defect, 162, *163,* 196–198
in obesity, 2260, *2260*
in systemic lupus erythematosus, 1945
management of, 1877–1881, *1879–1880*
anticoagulants in, 1878, 1880
cardiac glycosides in, 1878
diuretics in, 1878
heart-lung transplantation for, 306
oxygen therapy in, 1878
surgical, 1880–1881
vasodilators in, 1878–1880, *1879–1880*
natural history of, 1881
pathophysiology of, 1857–1862, 1857t–1859t, *1859–1863*
elevated left heart filling pressure in, 1857, 1857t
hyperkinetic, 1857–1858, *1858*
obstructive/obliterative, 1858–1862, 1858t–1859t, *1859–1863*
anorexic agents in, 1862, *1863*
endothelial cells in, 1859–1860, *1860*
fibrinolysis in, 1861–1862
smooth muscle cells in, 1860–1861, *1861*
prevalence of, 1856
prognosis in, 1881
venous, radiography in, 72, *72–74,* 74
Pulmonary infarction, radiographic features of, 1837, *1838–1839*
Pulmonary insufficiency, and pulmonary hypertension, 1866
Pulmonary regurgitation, 161
clinical features of, 343–344
low-pressure, 343
Pulmonary rehabilitation, for chronic obstructive pulmonary disease, 1897
Pulmonary stenosis, 154, *155,* 187–189, *188–190*
arterial, 195
balloon angioplasty for, 264, *265*
balloon angioplasty for, 262–264
balloon valvuloplasty for, 258–260, *259,* 435–436
double-balloon technique in, 259, *259*
results of, 259–260
echocardiography in, 453
in tetralogy of Fallot, 214, 218
percutaneous balloon valvuloplasty for, 463–464, 464t
severity of, peak systolic gradient and, 258
subpulmonary, 189
valvular, 187–189, *188–190*
diagnosis of, 188–189, *188–190*
Pulmonary stenosis *(Continued)*
echocardiography in, 249
prognosis in, 189
surgical treatment of, 289, 295
syndromes associated with, 187, *188*
treatment of, 189
venous, balloon angioplasty for, 267
with tricuspid atresia, treatment of, 187
Pulmonary thromboembolism, and dyspnea, 4
and shock, 1530
clinical features of, 1835–1837, *1837*
with infarction, 1837, *1837*
without infarction, 1836–1837
diagnosis of, 1840–1843, *1841–1842*
echocardiography in, 1841, *1841*
electrocardiography in, 55, *57,* 1837, 1840, 1840t, *1841–1842, 1842*
laboratory studies in, 1840
magnetic resonance imaging in, 136, *137*
pulmonary arteriography in, 1841, *1842*
radiography in, 74–75
venous ultrasonography in, 1843
ventilation/perfusion lung scan in, 1840, *1841*
differential diagnosis of, 1843–1848, 1843t
vs. abdominal disorders, 1846
vs. abscess, 1844
vs. amebiasis, 1844
vs. amniotic fluid embolism, 1847–1848
vs. asthma, 1844
vs. atelectasis, 1844
vs. cardiac tamponade, 1845
vs. congestive heart failure, 1845
vs. coxsackievirus infection, 1844
vs. dissecting aortic hematoma, 1845
vs. fat embolism, 1847
vs. granulomatous infection, 1844
vs. hematologic disorders, 1847
vs. infections, 1846
vs. metabolic disorders, 1847
vs. myocardial infarction, 1845
vs. neoplasm, 1844
vs. neurologic disorders, 1846
vs. obstructive pulmonary disease, 1844
vs. pericarditis, 1845
vs. pneumonia, 1843–1844
vs. psychiatric disorders, 1846
vs. pulmonary artery agenesis, 1845
vs. renal disease, 1846–1847
vs. right-sided intracavitary cardiac lesions, 1845–1846
vs. systemic lupus erythematosus, 1844–1845
vs. tuberculosis, 1844
vs. tumor embolism, 1848
vs. venous air embolism, 1848
during pregnancy, 2037–2038
factors predisposing to, 1835
hyperhomocysteinemia and, 2280, *2280*
prevention of, 1848, 1849t
prognosis in, 1850–1851
radiographic features of, 1837, *1838–1839*
sources of, 1835, *1836,* 1836pl
identification of, echocardiography in, 86, *88–89*
treatment of, 1848–1850, 1849t–1850t
anticoagulation in, 1848
embolectomy in, 1850
interruption of blood flow through inferior vena cava in, 1850
thrombolytic therapy in, 1848–1849, 1850t
vs. chronic obstructive pulmonary disease, 1891
Pulmonary valve(s), anatomy of, 148, *148*
dysplastic, 315
Pulmonary valve(s) *(Continued)*
quadricuspid, anatomic abnormalities in, 315
Pulmonary valve disease, acquired, natural history of, 344
pathophysiology of, 343
treatment of, 346
cardiac catheterization in, 432, *432*
Pulmonary valve regurgitation, 192
Pulmonary vascular disease, and suitability for heart-lung transplantation, 306
Pulmonary vascular resistance, in mitral stenosis, 348, 423
in pulmonary hypertension, 1869t, 1871t
measurement of, pulmonary artery catheterization in, 2129
Pulmonary vein(s), anomalous, *137*
surgical treatment of, 300, *300*
anomalous connections of, 167–168, *167–168*
partial anomalous connection between, 204, *204,* 221–222
total anomalous connection in, 222, *223,* 224
Pulmonary venous velocity, in assessment of mitral regurgitation severity, 353
Pulmonary vessel(s), radiography of, 68–69, *70,* 72–75, *72–75*
Pulsatile pressure, changes in, and arterial compliance, 1483, *1484,* 1485
Pulse, anacrotic, *16,* 16–17, 17t
arterial, abnormalities of, 16–17, *17,* 17t
assessment of, before coronary angiography, 596
configuration of, 16–17, *16–17,* 17t
in aortic regurgitation, 337
in mitral regurgitation, 351
jugular venous, palpation of, *17–18,* 17–19, 18t
Pulse contour analysis, for measurement of arterial compliance, 1484t, 1486, *1486*
Pulse generator(s), for pacemakers, 1764–1765
Pulse height analyzer(s), for radionuclide imaging, 99
Pulse pressure, abnormal, causes of, 15, 15t
Pulse volume recording, in peripheral vascular disease of lower extremities, 1408
Pulse wave velocity, definition of, 1491
for measurement of arterial compliance, 1484t, 1485
in hypertension, 1490
Pulsed spray, for thrombolytic therapy, 1427
Pulsus alternans, 16, *16*
in myocardial infarction, 543, *544*
Pulsus lentus, in aortic stenosis, 326, *326*
Pulsus paradoxus, 15, *15*
in cardiac tamponade, 1252
"Pumpkin" heart, in Ebstein's anomaly, 193, *193*
Purkinje fibers, resting membrane potential of, 29
PURSUIT (Platelet Glycoprotein IIb/IIIa in Unstable Angina Receptor Suppression Using Integrin Therapy) study, 732–733, *733,* 735t, 811, 812t
PVCs. See *Premature ventricular contractions (PVCs).*
PVR. See *Pulmonary vascular resistance.*
Pyelography, intravenous, in renovascular hypertension, 1429
Pyogenic abscess(es), *vs.* pulmonary thromboembolism, 1844
Pyruvate, and glucose metabolism, 943, *943,* 945–946, *946*

Q wave, during tachycardia, 1687

Q wave *(Continued)*
in amyloid heart disease, *1084*
in left bundle branch block, and myocardial infarction, 37
in myocardial infarction, 534–536, *535*
electrocardiography in, 548–549, *550–553*
inferior, 48, *49*
in old myocardial infarction, 46–47
in pulmonary embolism, 55, *57*
noninfarction, 49–50, *50*
QRS axis, determination of, *32,* 32–33
in frontal plane, in wide QRS tachycardia, 1683, *1683*
QRS complex, 31
in atrial fibrillation, *1634,* 1635
in atrioventricular block, Mobitz I, 1573
Mobitz II, 1573
in fascicular block, 40
in supraventricular tachycardia, 1606, *1607,* 1611, *1614*
in ventricular extrasystole, 1570
in ventricular tachycardia, 1571
in Wolff-Parkinson-White syndrome, *1634,* 1635
pseudofusion, 1776, *1777*
QT interval, 32
after injection of contrast agents, 601
in torsades de pointes, 1572
Quadricuspid aortic valve, anatomic abnormalities in, 315
Quadricuspid pulmonary valve, anatomic abnormalities in, 315
"Quadruple cadence," in Ebstein's anomaly, 192
Quinaglute. See *Quinidine.*
Quincke sign, 337
Quinidine, adverse effects of, 1744t
and syncope, 1640
and thrombocytopenia, 2007
and torsade de pointes, 1720
dosage of, 1742
drug interactions with, 1741, 1741t
during pregnancy, 2043, 2044t–2045t
efficacy of, 1742, 1744
electrocardiographic changes from, 53
electrophysiology of, 1742
for atrial fibrillation, 1637–1638, 1637t
risks of, 1640, *1641*
for preexcitation, *1629*
in older adults, 2022
inotropic potential of, 1741, 1741t
pharmacokinetics of, 1742, 1742t–1743t
Quinopril, for heart failure, 1170t

R wave, in myocardial infarction, posterolateral, 48
Race, and risk of sudden death, *1712,* 1713
Radial artery, for coronary artery bypass graft, 846
Radial pulse, palpation of, 16
RADIANT trial, 836
Radiation, and coronary artery disease, coronary angiography in, 642
Radiation "fog," 65, *67*
Radiation safety, 830–831
during coronary angiography, 595, *595*
Radiation therapy. See *Radiotherapy.*
Radiocontrast agent(s), for SPECT myocardial perfusion imaging, 101–102, 102pl
Radiofrequency catheter ablation, for arrhythmias, with syncope, 1703
for atrial fibrillation, 1644
history of, 1796
in arrhythmogenic right ventricular dysplasia, 1673–1674
Radiofrequency catheter ablation *(Continued)*
of accessory pathways, 1796–1800, *1797–1801*
and recurrence of conduction, 1799
complications of, 1799–1800
in preexcitation, 1630
localization in, 1796–1797, *1797*
optimal site for, 1798, *1799–1800*
procedure for, 1797–1798, *1798*
success rate of, 1798–1799, *1801*
of arrhythmias, indications for, 1796t
of atrial fibrillation, 1804, 1806, *1806*
of atrial tachycardia, 1804, *1805–1806*
of atrioventricular junction, 1806–1807
of atrioventricular nodal reentrant tachycardia, 1800–1801, *1801–1802*
slow pathway procedure for, 1800–1801, *1802*
of "incisional tachycardia," 1804
of left atrial flutter, 1804
of right atrial common flutter, 1801–1804, *1802*
procedure for, 1802–1803, *1802–1803*
recurrence after, 1803–1804
of ventricular tachycardia, 1807–1809, *1807–1812*
bundle branch reentry, 1809
failure of, *1810*
idiopathic, 1807–1808, *1807–1810*
postinfarction, 1808–1809, *1810–1812*
Radiofrequency pulse(s), in magnetic resonance imaging, 133–134
Radiofrequency signal, in intravascular ultrasonography, *1457*
of brachial artery, 1483, *1484*
Radiograph(s), assessment of, 69, 71
Radiography, artifacts on, 65, *66–67*
benefits of, 65
degree of inspiration and, 67, 69, *70*
during pregnancy, 2032–2033
image clarity in, 65, *66*
in abdominal aortic aneurysms, *1368,* 1374
in amyloid heart disease, 1083
in aortic coarctation, *194,* 1357, *1357–1358*
in aortic dissection, 1379, 1382, *1382*
in aortic pseudocoarctation, 1358, *1359*
in aortic stenosis, supravalvular, *184*
valvular, 181, *182*
in aortic trauma, 1392
in arrhythmogenic right ventricular dysplasia, *1667–1668*
in atrial septal defect, secundum type, 197, *197*
in cardiac tamponade, 1255
in chronic obstructive pulmonary disease, 1889, *1890*
in dilated cardiomyopathy, 1047
in heart failure, 1156, *1157*
in hemochromatosis, 1087
in hypertrophic cardiomyopathy, 1062
in L transposition, 212, *213–214*
in patent ductus arteriosus, 209, *209*
in pericardial effusion, 1249
in pericarditis, acute, 1269
constrictive, 1262–1263, *1263–1264*
vs. restrictive cardiomyopathy, 1267
in pseudotruncus arteriosus, 219, *220*
in pulmonary arterial hypertension, 74, *75*
in pulmonary edema, 72, *73–74,* 74
in pulmonary embolism, 74–75
in pulmonary hypertension, 1867–1868
in pulmonary stenosis, valvular, 188, *188–189*
in pulmonary thromboembolism, 1837, *1838–1839*
in pulmonary venous hypertension, 72, *72–74,* 74
Radiography *(Continued)*
in restrictive cardiomyopathy, 1078–1079, *1079*
in systemic lupus erythematosus, 1942, *1943*
in tetralogy of Fallot, 214, *217*
in thoracic aortic aneurysms, 1358, *1359*
in total anomalous pulmonary venous connection, 222, *223*
in tricuspid atresia, *185*
of pulmonary vessels, 68–69, *70,* 72–75, *72–75*
overexposure in, 65, *66*
posture and, *70*
principles of, 65–69, *68–70*
views in, 65, *66,* 67, *68*
Radionuclide angiocardiography, first pass, *106,* 106–107
Radionuclide imaging, 99–125. See also *Positron emission tomography (PET); Scintigraphy; SPECT myocardial perfusion imaging; Ventriculography.*
acquisition modes for, 100–101, *101,* 101pl
planar, 100
tomographic, 100
during pregnancy, 2033
in allograft rejection, 1145
in amyloid heart disease, 1085
in cardiomyopathy, dilated, 1048, 1143
hypertrophic, 1143–1144
restrictive, 1081–1082, 1144, 1144t, *1145*
in congenital heart disease, for quantification of shunts, *461,* 461–462
in myocarditis, 1144–1145
in pulmonary hypertension, *1875,* 1875–1876
in renal artery disease, 1402
in risk stratification for sudden death, 1723
in valvular regurgitation, 459–461, *460*
aortic, 459–460, *460*
mitral, 460–461
infarct, 110–113, *111–113*
physical principles of, 99–101, *100*
positron emission tomography in, 113–125, *114–124*
single-crystal gamma camera for, 99–100, *100*
SPECT myocardial perfusion imaging in, 101–105, 102pl, *104–105*
ventriculography in, 105–110, *106–109*
Radionuclide ventriculography, 105–110, *106–109*
after myocardial infarction, 677–678, *677–679*
analysis of, *109,* 109–110
exercise, 107, 109
first pass radionuclide angiocardiography in, *106,* 106–107
gated-equilibrium, 107, *107–108,* 107pl
in coronary artery disease, for assessment of prognosis, *676,* 676–677
for diagnosis, 676
in tetralogy of Fallot, *218*
in valvular disease, 459
in ventricular septal defect, 205, *206*
results of, and prognosis in coronary artery disease, 703–704, *704,* 704t
Radiopharmaceutical(s), positron-emitting, for assessment of myocardial viability, 119–120
Radiotherapy, and coronary artery disease, 831
and heart disease, 1088–1089
and malignancy, 831–832
and pericardial disease, 1247
and pericarditis, constrictive, 1261
and pseudoaneurysms, 831
delivery system(s) for, 832, *832–835,* 835

Radiotherapy *(Continued)*
balloons as, 832, 835, *835*
beta-emitting stents as, 835, *836*
catheter-based, 832, *833–835*
for benign proliferative disorders, 827
for cardiac tumors, secondary, 1903
for carotid artery disease, 1440–1441
for peripheral vascular disease, 1442–1443, *1442,* 1443t
for restenosis, animal models of, 827–828, *828*
clinical trials of, 828, *829,* 830, 835–836
future of, 836
gamma *vs.* beta, 830–831
long-term consequences of, 831–832
mediastinal, complications of, 318
pituitary, for acromegaly, 1917
"Ragged red fiber(s)," in Kearns-Sayre syndrome, 1992, *1993*
Rales, 11
during pregnancy, 2038
Ramipril, for heart failure, 1170t
vascular protective effects of, 720–721
Randomized Intervention Treatment of Angina (RITA) trial, 796, *796,* 797t, 870–871, 872, 873t
Rapamycin, action of, 1212, *1213*
for cardiac allograft vasculopathy, 1196
Rapeseed oil, and pulmonary hypertension, 1865
Rapid-speed computed tomography. See *Computed tomography (CT), electron beam.*
Rash, in rheumatic fever, 391, *392*
Rashkind patent ductus arteriosus occluding device, 268
use of in ventricular septal defect, 277
Rastelli operation, 303, *304*
Rate-adapted atrioventricular delay, 1769
Rate-adaptive pacemaker therapy, 1771–1772
Rate-drop response, in pacemaker therapy, 1773
Rate-pressure product, and myocardial oxygen consumption, 522
Raynaud's phenomenon, and pulmonary hypertension, 1864t, 1865
in autonomic dysfunction, 1543
myocardial, 1946
Rb, and postmitotic phenotype, 928–929
Reactive hyperemic response, in coronary artery stenosis, angiographic assessment of, 629–631, *631–632*
Reaven's syndrome, and risk of coronary artery disease, 2209
Recanalization, rapidity of, and mortality, 762
thrombolytic therapy for, 748–749, *749*
and mortality, 754–755, *755–756,* 755t
clinical trials of, 762–763, 763t
Red blood cell(s), disorders of, 2001–2005, *2002–2005,* 2005t. See also *Anemia; Erythrocytosis.*
Red blood cell mass, space flight and, 2067
Redel Duct-Occlud Device, for patent ductus arteriosus, 269
Redirection entre ventriculaire (REV) operation, 303, *305,* 306
Reduced energy direct-current ablation, in arrhythmogenic right ventricular dysplasia, 1673–1674
Reendothelialization, after balloon injury, 1422
Reentrant mechanism(s), in arrhythmogenic right ventricular dysplasia, 1671
Reentry, and arrhythmias, in cardiac hypertrophy, 973
and atrial fibrillation, 1633
Reentry circuit, in ventricular tachycardia, radiofrequency catheter ablation of, 1808, *1810–1812*
Refsum's disease, 2175t
REGRESS (Regression Growth Evaluation Statin Study), 1339
Rehabilitation. See *Cardiac rehabilitation.*
Rehydration, during reentry from space flight, 2080–2081
Reinfarction, thrombolytic agents and, 746
Reiter's disease, 1952–1954
Relapsing polychondritis, 1951–1952, 1952pl
"Relaxation filling period," 1005
Remodeling, atrial, atrial fibrillation and, 1633
definition of, 955
Renal angiography, in renovascular hypertension, 1429–1430
Renal artery disease, *1402,* 1402–1403
atherosclerosis and, 1402, *1402*
diagnosis of, 1402–1403
treatment of, 1403–1404
Renal artery stenosis, percutaneous angioplasty for, 1431–1432, *1431*
revascularization for, 1431
stents for, 1431–1432, *1431*
Renal atherosclerosis, progression of, 1428
Renal disease, and hypertension, 1505
diagnosis of, 1511
vs. pulmonary thromboembolism, 1846–1847
Renal failure, and treatment of hypertension, 1522–1523, 1522t
chronic, and pericarditis, 1247
Renal function, and plasma homocysteine levels, 2279–2280, *2282*
angiotensin-converting enzyme inhibitors and, 1170, 1519, *1519*
contrast agents and, 607
Renin-angiotensin system, and hypertension, 1498–1500, *1500*
Renin-angiotensin-aldosterone system, in cardiac hypertrophy, 968
in heart failure, 1153, *1153*
Renovascular hypertension. See *Hypertension, renovascular.*
Reperfusion, arrhythmias during, and risk of sudden death, 1715
outcome of, 514–515
Replication incompetence, 2270
Repolarization, abnormal, in arrhythmogenic right ventricular dysplasia, 1666, *1667–1668*
early, electrocardiography in, 53, *54*
ion activity during, 1–2
Reserpine, during pregnancy, 2050t
for hypertension, 1517t, 1520
Resistance vessel(s), 522–524
Respiration, fuels for, 940, *941*
Respiratory disorder(s), parenchymatous, *vs.* pulmonary thromboembolism, 1843–1844
Respiratory tract procedure(s), antibiotic prophylaxis for, 414t–415t
Response to injury hypothesis, in atherogenesis, *1327–1329,* 1327–1330, 1330t–1331t, 1341
Restenosis, after balloon angioplasty, interventions affecting, 808
after carotid endarterectomy, 1436
after percutaneous transluminal coronary intervention, 798t–799t, 799
after stenting, 876
intravascular ultrasonography in, 1469, *1470–1471*
arterial gene therapy for, 1421–1422
intimal hyperplasia and, 827, *829*
phases of, 1306–1307, 1306t
radiotherapy for, 827–836. See also *Radiotherapy.*
recoil and remodeling in, 827
Resting membrane potential, 1–2
generation of, 1563, *1564*
in cardiac hypertrophy, 968–970
Restrictive cardiomyopathy. See *Cardiomyopathy, restrictive.*
Resuscitation, during cardiovascular surgery, drugs for, 2106, 2106t
Reteplase, efficacy of, 822
Reticulocyte count, in anemia, 2001
Retransplantation, 1200
Retrograde conduction, concealed, during supraventricular tachycardia, 1679, *1680–1681*
Retrovirus(es), as vectors for gene therapy, 2270, 2271t
definition of, 917t
REV (redirection entre ventriculaire) operation, 303, *305,* 306
Revascularization. See also *Coronary artery bypass graft (CABG); Percutaneous transluminal coronary angioplasty (PTCA).*
and flow metabolism outcomes, 683–684, *684–685*
assessment of, SPECT myocardial perfusion imaging in, 675–676
before noncardiac surgery, 2097
detection of viable myocardium after, echocardiography in, 664–665
exercise testing before, 590
for cardiogenic shock, *1534,* 1534–1535
for fibromuscular dysplasia, 1430
for renal artery stenosis, 1431
history of, 859–861, *860–862,* 862t
in renal artery disease, 1404
indications for, 880, 882t–883t
nonrandomized data on, 877, *878*
recovery of contracile function after, PET assessment of, *124,* 125
survival after, 684–685
transmyocardial laser, 856
Rhabdomyoma, cardiac, 1907
Rhabdomyosarcoma, cardiac, 1908
Rheobase, 1766
Rheumatic fever, 386–398
and mitral stenosis, 347, *347*
and myocarditis, 1098
clinical features of, 390–393, 390t–391t, *392*
cardiac, 390–391, 391t
dermatologic, 391, *392,* 393
in joints, 390
diagnosis of, echocardiography in, 393–394, *394*
Jones criteria in, 390t
laboratory studies in, 393
differential diagnosis of, 393
during pregnancy, 2055–2056
epidemiology of, 387–388, *387–388*
historical perspective on, 386
mortality in, 394–395, *396*
natural history of, 394–397, *395–396*
pathogenesis of, 386–387
pathology of, 388–390, *388–390*
treatment of, 397–398, 398t
Rheumatic myocarditis, 1026–1027, *1027,* 1027pl
Rheumatic valvulitis, anatomic abnormalities in, 315–316, 315pl–316pl, 316, *316, 317,* 317pl
computed tomography in, electron beam, *2186*
Rheumatoid arthritis, 1939–1941, *1940,* 1940t
and dilated cardiomyopathy, 1044
coronary vasculitis in, 1941
myocardial disease in, 1940, *1940*
pathophysiology of, 1939

Rheumatoid arthritis *(Continued)*
pericardial disease in, 1939, 1940t
pericarditis in, 1242, *1242*
constrictive, 1939–1940
Still's disease in, 1941
valvular disease in, 1940–1941
Rib(s), notching of, in aortic coarctation, 1357, *1357*
Ribozyme(s), as vectors for gene therapy, 2271, 2271t
definition of, 917t
Rickettsial myocarditis, 1110
Right atrial anastomosis, in heart transplantation, *1227, 1229,* 1230
Right atrial isolation, for automatic atrial tachycardia, 1824, *1825*
Right atrial pressure, after pericardiocentesis, 1256–1257
in cardiomyopathy, restrictive, *1128*
in heart failure, 1155
in pericarditis, constrictive, 1263, *1265*
vs. cardiac tamponade, 1260, *1260*
in pulmonary hypertension, 1870–1871, *1871–1872*
in tricuspid regurgitation, 452
Right atrium, anatomy of, 147, *147*
compression of, in cardiac tamponade, 1253
enlargement of, electrocardiography in, 34, *34*
in restrictive cardiomyopathy, 1080, *1081*
myxoma of, 1905–1906
Right heart, catheterization of, in cardiac tamponade, 1255–1256
Right ventricle, anatomy of, 147–148, *148*
collapse of, in cardiac tamponade, 1253, *1254*
in myocardial infarction, *661–662*
contrast angiography of, in arrhythmogenic right ventricular dysplasia, 1668–1669, *1670*
diastolic pressure in, in cardiac tamponade, 1253
dilatation of, in cardiomyopathy, 1138, *1138–1139*
disconnection procedure in, for arrhythmogenic right ventricular dysplasia, 1827, *1828–1829*
double-outlet, 212, 214, *216–217*
echocardiography in, 93
dysplasia of, 226
arrhythmogenic, 1665–1674
infarction of, and cardiogenic shock, treatment of, 1533–1534
treatment of, 773–774, *775*
myocardial infarction in, echocardiography in, 661
stroke volume of, radionuclide studies of, 459
volume overload in, in atrial septal defect, 239, *239*
Right ventricular dysfunction, and cardiac rehabilitation, 902–903
in cardiomyopathy, dilated, 1143
Right ventricular dysplasia, magnetic resonance imaging in, 139, *140*
Right ventricular ejection fraction, in mitral regurgitation, 461
measurement of, pulmonary artery catheterization in, 2131
Right ventricular failure, after heart transplantation, 1187
Right ventricular hypertrophy, electrocardiography in, *33–34,* 35
from secundum atrioseptal defect, 299, *299*
in pulmonary hypertension, 1867, *1868,* 1869
Right ventricular impulse, palpation of, 19
Right ventricular outflow, obstruction of, echocardiography in, 248–249
Right ventricular outflow tract, tachycardia in, in arrhythmogenic right ventricular dysplasia, 1673
Right ventricular pressure, in cardiomyopathy, restrictive, *1127*
Right ventricular systolic function (RVSF), assessment of, magnetic resonance imaging in, 139
Right ventricular systolic pressure (RVSP), assessment of, 80
in tricuspid regurgitation, 452, *452*
Rigid-framed valve(s), complications of, 322
types of, 321
Riley-Day syndrome, 1551
Rimantadine, for influenza prophylaxis, 1894
Risk zone, in myocardial infarction, 514, *514*
RITA (Randomized Intervention Treatment of Angina) trial, 796, *796,* 870–871, 872, 873t
Romano-Ward syndrome, surgical treatment of, 1828–1829
Romhilt-Estes point score system, for diagnosis of left ventricular hypertrophy, 35
"Rosettes," in pulmonary edema, 72, *74*
Rotablator, *790,* 794
Rotational ablation device(s), for atherectomy, 1439–1440, *1440*
Roth spot(s), in infective endocarditis, 402
RS interval, in wide QRS tachycardia, 1687
^{82}Rubidium, for positron emission tomography, 118
"Runaway pacemaker," 1777
RVSF. See *Right ventricular systolic function (RVSF).*
RVSP. See *Right ventricular systolic pressure (RVSP).*
Rythmol. See *Propafenone.*

SA. See *Sinoatrial* entries.
SACT (sinoatrial conduction time), in sinus node dysfunction, 1585–1586, *1586*
"Safety pacing," 1777
"Sail sound," in Ebstein's anomaly, 192
Salicylate(s), for rheumatic fever, 397
Saphenous vein graft(s), *842,* 843, 846, 865–866, 866t
electron beam computed tomography of, *2183*
pathologic changes in, 516, *517*
recurrent disease in, 866–867, 867t
treatment of, 879–880, 880t, *881–882*
Sarcoglycans, in muscular dystrophy, Duchenne's, 2165
Sarcoidosis, cardiac, 1113–1114
echocardiography in, 1141
Sarcomere(s), dysfunction of, and cardiac remodeling, 1059
physiology of, 1058–1059
shortening of, in heart failure, 1150
Sarcoplasmic reticulum (SR), Ca^{2+}-ATPase in, and cardiac hypertrophy, 983
calcium retention in, 998
in excitation-contraction coupling, 996–998, *996–998*
calcium pump of, 996–998, *997–998*
calcium release channels of, 996, *996*
Sarns/3M total artificial heart, 1235
Saturation step-up, in shunting, 1125–1126
SAVE (Survival And Ventricular Enlargement) trial, *1177*
Scandinavian Simvastatin Survival Study, 541, *542,* 718, *719*
Scheie's syndrome, 2174t
SCID (severe combined immunodeficiency) mice, viral myocarditis in, 1100
Scimitar syndrome, 167, 204, *204*
surgical treatment of, 300, *300*
Scintigraphy, for estimation of infarct size, 557, *559*
in myocardial infarction, 554–557, *554–558*
for assessment of prognosis, 703–704, *704,* 704t
in myocarditis, 1103–1104
in pericardial effusion, 1249
in renovascular hypertension, 1429, 1510
in silent myocardial ischemia, 573, 573t
and prognosis, 575
ventilation-perfusion, in pulmonary embolism, 74–75
Scintillation counter(s), 99
Scleroderma, 1945–1948, *1946,* 1947t, *1948*
and dilated cardiomyopathy, 1044
clinical features of, 1945–1946, 1946pl
myocardial fibrosis in, *1946,* 1946–1947, 1947t
pericardial disease in, 1947
Scoliosis, in Duchenne's muscular dystrophy, 1989, *1989*
Scripps Coronary Radiation to Inhibit Proliferation Post-Stenting (SCRIPPS) trial, 828, *829,* 830
Second window of protection, 514–515
Secondary Prevention Reinfarction Israeli Nifedipine Trial (SPRINT), 692, 693t
Second-hand smoke, and risk of coronary artery disease, 2228–2229
Sectral. See *Acebutolol.*
Secundum atrioseptal defect, surgical treatment of, 299, *299*
Sedentary occupation(s), and risk of coronary artery disease, 2216, *2217*
Segmental pressure measurement, in peripheral vascular disease of lower extremities, 1407
Segmental wall motion abnormality(ies), intraoperative detection of, transesophageal echocardiography in, 2134, 2136–2137
Seizure(s), immunosuppression and, 1199
vs. syncope, 9
Seldane. See *Terfenadine.*
Selectin(s), in leukocyte-endothelial interaction, and atherosclerosis, 1330, 1332t
Selenium deficiency, and myocardial disease, 1091
Self-expanding stent(s), 792
Semilunar valve, dysplastic, 315
Senning procedure, takedown of, 306
Sense amplifier(s), in pacemakers, 1764
Sensing, in pacemaker therapy, 1767
"Sensory conflict," in weightlessness, 2076
Sepsis, from arterial cannulation, 606
Septal fascicular block, electrocardiography in, 40–41
Septal hypertrophy, asymmetric. See *Cardiomyopathy, hypertrophic.*
Septal tricuspid leaflet, displacement of, in Ebstein's anomaly, 243–244, *244*
Septic shock, 1529
Septum primum defect, 201, *202–203,* 203
clinical features of, 203, *203*
natural history of, 201, 203
pathophysiology of, 201, *202–203*
prognosis in, 203
treatment of, 203
SERCA-2, expression of, and cardiac hypertrophy, 1010

SERCA-2 *(Continued)*
in diastolic dysfunction, 1011–1012
Seronegative spondyloarthropathy, 1952–1954, *1952–1954*
Serum response factor (SRF), in cardiogenesis, 921
Sestamibi, for SPECT myocardial perfusion imaging, 102
Severe combined immunodeficiency (SCID) mice, viral myocarditis in, 1100
Shock, cardiogenic, 1530–1535, *1533–1534*
diagnosis of, 1531
etiology of, 1530
hemodynamic assessment in, 1530
in myocardial infarction, 543, *544*
incidence of, 1530–1531
mortality from, 1530–1531
pathophysiology of, 1530
percutaneous aortic balloon valvuloplasty for, 480–481, 480t
predictors of, 1530–1531
treatment of, 773, 1531–1535, *1533–1534*
angioplasty in, *1534,* 1534–1535
dobutamine in, 1532
dopamine in, 1531–1532
history of, 1531
intra-aortic balloon pump for, 1532–1533, *1533*
left ventricular assist devices for, 1533
with right ventricular infarction, 1533–1534
with myocardial infarction, percutaneous transluminal coronary intervention for, 824
causes of, 1529, 1529t
coronary angiography in, 604
hypovolemic, 1529
in myocardial infarction, treatment of, 1532
obstructive, 1530
septic, 1529
Shone's syndrome, 91, 155, *156,* 184
Shoshin beri-beri, 1091
Shprintzen's syndrome, 2172
Shunt(s), flow in, echocardiography of, 241, 246
in congenital heart disease, quantification of, radionuclide studies in, *461,* 461–462
left-to-right, after percutaneous mitral balloon valvotomy, 470
atrial, 196t
in patent ductus arteriosus, 208, *208*
saturation step-up in, 1125–1126
right-to-left, in atrial septal defect, 240
in patent foramen ovale, 242
in pulmonary stenosis, 154
saturation step-up in, 1125–1126
Sicilian Gambit classification, of antiarrhythmic drugs, 1741t
Sick sinus syndrome. See *Sinus node, dysfunction of.*
Sickle cell disease, 2001–2002
vs. pulmonary thromboembolism, 1847
Sideris Button Device, for closure of atrial septal defect, 275–276
Signal averaged electrocardiography, in evaluation of syncope, 1698
Signal averaging, in arrhythmogenic right ventricular dysplasia, 1666–1667
Signal peptide, in coagulation system, 1315
Signal pulse, in radionuclide imaging, 100
Signal transduction, in excitation-contraction coupling, 1282–1285, *1284*
in left ventricular hypertrophy, 981–982, *982*
Signal-averaged electrocardiography, 30
in dilated cardiomyopathy, 1047, *1047*
Signal-averaged electrocardiography *(Continued)*
in risk stratification for sudden death, 1723
Silent ischemia. See *Myocardial ischemia, silent.*
Simvastatin, and prognosis in coronary artery disease, 718, *719*
Single atrium, 203–204
Single-crystal gamma camera(s), for radionuclide imaging, 99–100, *100*
Sinoatrial block, 1566–1567
Sinoatrial conduction time (SACT), in sinus node dysfunction, 1585–1586, *1586*
Sinoatrial disease. See *Sinus node, dysfunction of.*
Sinoatrial exit block, in sinus node dysfunction, 1580–1581, *1581*
Sinoatrial node, resting membrane potential of, 29
Sinotubular ridge, anomalous coronary artery origin above, coronary angiography in, 621
Sinus arrest, 1566–1567
in sinus node dysfunction, 1577, *1578,* 1580
Sinus bradycardia, 1564–1566
in sinus node dysfunction, 1580
Sinus node, action potentials in, 1577, *1577*
arrhythmias of, 1564
autonomic control of, 1583–1584
dysfunction of, and syncope, 1692
arrhythmias in, 1576, 1579–1582, *1581–1582*
diagnosis of, 1579, 1582–1587, *1584, 1586*
electrocardiography in, 1583
electrophysiologic studies in, *1584, 1584–1587, 1586*
exercise testing in, 1583
Holter monitoring in, 1583
intrinsic heart rate in, 1583–1584
embolism in, 1576
etiology of, 1576
extrinsic, 1578–1579
in pediatric population, 1578
intrinsic, 1578
mortality from, 1587
natural history of, 1587–1588
pathophysiology of, *1577–1578,* 1577–1579
sinus pause/arrest in, 1577, *1578*
symptoms of, 1576, 1579
treatment of, 1588–1591, 1590t
pacemaker therapy in, 1759, 1760t
pacing in, 1589–1590, 1590t
pharmacologic, 1589
effective refractory period of, 1586
pacemaker cells in, activity of, 1577, *1577*
Sinus node artery, anatomy of, and coronary angiography, 610
Sinus node recovery time (SNRT), *1584,* 1584–1585
Sinus node reentrant tachycardia, in sinus node dysfunction, 1582
Sinus of Valsalva, aneurysms of, 227
echocardiography in, 250–251
left, anomalous origin of coronary arteries from, 622, *623*
posterior, anomalous origin of coronary arteries from, 621
right, anomalous origin of left anterior descending artery from, 622–623
anomalous origin of left coronary artery from, 623, *623*
Sinus pause, 1566–1567
in sinus node dysfunction, 1577, *1578,* 1580
Sinus rhythm, restoration of, failure of, 1582
Sinus tachycardia, 1566
during pregnancy, 2040–2041
in sinus node dysfunction, 1579–1580
Sinus venosus defect(s), 204
atrial septal, 167, *168*
Sirolimus. See *Rapamycin.*
Situs ambiguus, heart-lung transplantation for, 306, *307–308,* 308
Situs inversus, genetic basis of, 926–927
heart-lung transplantation for, 306, *306–307,* 308
Skeletal disorder(s), in Marfan's syndrome, 2151, *2151*
with mitral valve prolapse, 357, 375
Skin lesion(s), in pseudoxanthoma elasticum, 2156, *2156*
in rheumatic fever, 391, *392,* 393
in secondary hypertension, 1508
SLE. See *Systemic lupus erythematosus (SLE).*
Sleep apnea, chronic obstructive pulmonary disease and, 1891
Smoke, second-hand, and risk of coronary artery disease, 2228–2229
Smoking, and atherosclerosis, 1343–1344
and chronic obstructive pulmonary disease, 1886, 1888
and circulatory dysfunction, 1292
and claudication, 1409
and coronary artery disease, 2227–2230, *2228–2231,* 2228t
acute ischemic events in, 2227–2229, 2228t, *2230–2231*
atherosclerosis, 2227
in women, 579
pathophysiology of, 2229, *2230–2231*
risk of, 2203–2204, 2203t
and coronary vascular resistance, *2231*
and coronary vasospasm, 2230
and heart rate, *2230*
and myocardial oxygen consumption, cocaine and, 1961
and natural history of coronary artery disease, 691–692
and nicotine addiction, 2230
Smoking cessation, and risk of myocardial infarction, 2228
classes for, 2232
for chronic obstructive pulmonary disease, 1892, *1892,* 1898
for heart failure, 1166
physician's role in, 2230–2232
results of, 2232
Smooth muscle, relaxation of, and arterial compliance, 1481–1482, *1482,* 1482t
Smooth muscle cell(s), abnormalities of, in pulmonary hypertension, 1860–1861, *1861*
proliferation of, in atherogenesis, 1327–1328, *1328–1329,* 1333t
Snake bite(s), and myocardial disease, 1092
Snare technique, for placement of Gianturco coil patent ductus arteriosus occluding device, 269, *270*
for removal of foreign bodies, 280–281
SNERP (sinus node effective refractory period), 1586
"Snowman" configuration, in total anomalous pulmonary venous connection, 222, *223*
SNRT (sinus node recovery time), *1584,* 1584–1585
Sodium, dietary, and hypertension, 1498
in "high reactors" to stress, *2235*
restriction of, and hypertension, control of, 2236–2238, *2237,* 2238t
in heart failure, 1165
in hypertension, 1515, *1515*

Sodium *(Continued)*
renal retention of, and hypertension, 1502, *1502*
transport of, in myocardial ischemia, 512, *512*
Sodium channel(s), during depolarization, 30
Sodium current, augmented, in long QT syndrome, 1657
Sodium-calcium exchanger, of plasma membrane, and excitation-contraction coupling, 994–995
Sodium-hydrogen antiport, abnormalities of, in hypertension, 1505
Sodium-hydrogen exchanger, in excitation-contraction coupling, *1281,* 1282
of plasma membrane, and excitation-contraction coupling, 995
Sodium-lithium countertransport, abnormalities of, in hypertension, 1504
Sodium-potassium pump, in excitation-contraction coupling, *1281*
Sodium-potassium-ATPase, abnormalities of, in hypertension, 1504, *1504*
Sokolow-Lyon criteria, for diagnosis of left ventricular hypertrophy, 35
Solitary arterial trunk, 171–172, *173*
SOLVD trial, 776
Somatostatin(s), properties of, 1915
Sotalol, adverse effects of, 1752
dosage of, 712t, 1752
during pregnancy, 2066
efficacy of, 1752
electrophysiology of, 1752
for atrial fibrillation, 1637t
for prevention of sudden death, 1727
pharmacokinetics of, 1742t–1743t, 1752
Space flight, and blood pressure, 2081–2082, *2082*
and central venous pressure, 2078–2079
and conduction system, 2083, *2084*
and heart rate, 2081–2082, *2082*
and myocardial dynamics, 2079
and organelle structure, 2085
and orthostatic dysfunction, 2079–2081, *2080–2081*
and red cell mass, 2067
baroreflex response to, 2082
cardiac evaluation during, noninvasive, 2083–2085, *2085*
cardiovascular recovery after, 2085
cardiovascular response to, 2077, *2077*
data limitations of, 2086
Valsalva response to, 2082
Specific Activity Scale, 2092t
SPECT myocardial perfusion imaging, 101–105, 102pl, *104–105*
accuracy of, 671
analysis of images from, 104–105, *104–105,* 104pl
artifacts on, 105
contrast agents for, 101–102, 102pl
dopamine during, 104
exercise during, 103
for assessment of revascularization, 675–676
future developments in, 685
Holter monitoring and, 573–574
in coronary artery disease, for assessment of prognosis, 673
for diagnosis, 671–673, 672t
for evaluation after myocardial infarction, 673–675, *674*
physical principles of, 101
preoperative, 675
sensitivity and specificity of, 671–673, 672t
sympathomimetics during, 104
vasodilators during, 103–104

SPECT myocardial perfusion imaging *(Continued)*
vs. PET perfusion imaging, 105
Sphingolipidosis, 2174t
"Spike-and-dome" configuration, in epicardial cells, in Brugada's syndrome, 1721
of arterial pressure, in cardiomyopathy, hypertrophic, 1130, *1131*
Spinal cord, protection of, during repair of descending aortic aneurysms, 1362, 1364, *1365*
Spinal cord injury, and autonomic dysfunction, 1552–1553, 1552t, *1553*
Spin-echo magnetic resonance imaging (MRI), 133, *134*
Spiral computed tomography. See *Computed tomography (CT), spiral.*
Spirochetal infection(s), and myocarditis, 1109–1110
Spironolactone, for heart failure, 1175
for hyperaldosteronism, 1920
Splenic abscess, from infective endocarditis, 416
Splitting, of heart sounds, *21,* 22t
Spondyloarthropathy, seronegative, 1952–1954, *1952–1954*
Spongiosa, in mitral valve, 372
in mitral valve prolapse, 357, *358*
microscopic anatomy of, *355,* 356
SPRINT (Secondary Prevention Reinfarction Israeli Nifedipine Trial), 692, 693t
SR. See *Sarcoplasmic reticulum (SR).*
SRF (serum response factor), in cardiogenesis, 921
St. Jude Medical bileaflet valve, 486
St. Jude prosthetic valve, pressure gradients in, 433t, *434*
ST segment, drugs affecting, 53
during exercise testing, 588, *588*
in acute myocardial infarction, 44, *45–46,* 46
in myocardial infarction, *551–552*
in myocardial ischemia, 43, *44–45*
in pericarditis, 55, *56*
in silent myocardial ischemia, 571–573
right precordial, elevation of, in arrhythmogenic right ventricular dysplasia, 1673
Stability algorithm(s), for implantable cardioverter-defibrillators, 1782–1783
Stannous pyrophosphate, ^{99}Tc, for infarct imaging, 110–112, *111*
Staphylococcus, and infective endocarditis, 405, 405t, 408
Staphylococcus aureus, methicillin-susceptible, and infective endocarditis, 407–408, 408t–409t
Starvation, and myocardial disease, 1091, 1091t
Statin drug(s), for allograft vasculopathy prophylaxis, 1192
for hyperlipidemia, 1339–1341, 2247–2248, 2247t
primary prevention of, 1340
secondary prevention of, 1340–1341, 2249
Stedicor. See *Azimilide.*
Steinert's disease. See *Myotonic dystrophy.*
Stellectomy, left, for long QT syndrome, 1662
Stem cell transplantation, for amyloidosis, 1086, *1087*
Stent(s), balloon-expandable, 792
clinical uses of, 792, 792t–793t
efficacy of, 875–877
for abdominal aortic aneurysms, 1433–1434, *1433–1434,* 1434t–1435t
for aortic coarctation, 266

Stent(s) *(Continued)*
for balloon angioplasty, 263–264
for cardiac allograft vasculopathy, 1196
for myocardial infarction, *vs.* percutaneous transluminal coronary angioplasty, 823, *823*
with antiplatelet agents, 823
for renal artery stenosis, 1431, *1431*
for stable angina, 791–792, 792t–793t
efficacy of, 792–793, 792t–793t
vs. balloon angioplasty, 792, 793t
for subclavian artery occlusive disease, 1441, 1441t, *1442*
for systemic venous obstruction, 267
for tibioperoneal occlusion, 1440
for unstable angina, 807–809, 807t–809t, *808*
history of, 791
placement of, intravascular ultrasonography during, 1467–1469, *1468,* 1469t
radioactive, 835, *836*
rationale for, 791–792
restenosis in, radiotherapy for, 828, *829,* 830
self-expanding, 792
with balloon angioplasty, for stable angina, outcome of, 794, 795t
with carotid endarterectomy, 1436–1437
Stent Restenosis Study (STRESS), 876
Stented xenograft(s), for aortic stenosis, 286, *286*
Sternal angle of Louis, 17–18
Sternocleidomastoid muscle(s), atrophy of, in myotonic dystrophy, *1987*
Steroid-eluting electrode(s), for pacemakers, 1765
Stethoscope, use of, 20
Stickler's syndrome, *vs.* Marfan's syndrome, 2153
Still's disease, in rheumatoid arthritis, 1941
Sting(s), and myocardial disease, 1092
Storage disease(s), pathologic changes in, 1028–1031, 1029pl–1030pl, *1030*
Strain, definition of, 1491
Streptococcal infection(s), and infective endocarditis, 405, 405t
and myocarditis, 1109
and rheumatic fever, 386–387
vaccine for, 398
Streptococcus, penicillin-susceptible, antibiotics for, 405–407, 406t–407t
Streptokinase, and intracranial bleeding, 766–768, 767t–768t
and mortality, *vs.* t-PA, 755t
and natural history of myocardial infarction, 699–702, *701*
antigenicity of, 744
dosage of, 745
efficacy of, 745–746, 747t, 754t
for arterial occlusive disease, 1426–1427
dosage of, 1427
mechanism of action for, 745
side effects of, 767–768
Stress, and hypertension, 1498, 2239–2240, *2240*
and regulation of circulation, 1290
and risk of atherosclerosis, 1351
definition of, 1491
"high reactors" to, and hypertension, dietary sodium and, *2235*
STRESS (Stent Restenosis Study), 876
Stress echocardiography, dobutamine. See *Echocardiography, dobutamine stress.*
exercise, in myocardial ischemia, 665–666, 665t
for risk stratification in coronary artery disease, 88–90

Stress echocardiography *(Continued)*
pharmacologic, in myocardial ischemia, 666
Stroke, *1400,* 1401–1402
and treatment of hypertension, 1522t, 1523
atherosclerosis and, 1401, *1401*
clinical features of, 1401
diagnosis of, 1401
mitral valve prolapse and, 190, 364, 381–382
natural history of, 1401–1402
risk of, antihypertensive therapy and, *1512,* 1512–1513, 1513t
hypertension and, 1511, *1511*
treatment of, 1402
Stroke volume, ventricular, radionuclide studies of, 459
ST-T wave, 31
abnormalities of, 50
in hypokalemia, 52, *52*
Stunning, myocardial. See *Myocardial stunning.*
Subaortic stenosis, 151–153, *152–153*
after repair of atrioventricular septal defect, 300
and ventricular outflow tract obstruction, surgical treatment of, 295, *296–298*
aortic stenosis with, 328
hypertrophic, carotid pulses in, *17*
during pregnancy, 2054–2055
idiopathic hypertrophic. See *Cardiomyopathy, hypertrophic.*
membranous, 151, 153, *153*
muscular, 151, *152*
tunnel, 153
Subarachnoid hemorrhage, electrocardiography in, 55, *57*
Subclavian artery(ies), in collateral circulation, in aortic coarctation, 156, *158*
occlusion of, 1441–1442, *1441–1442,* 1441t
right, anomalous origin of, 174, *174*
Subclavian steal syndrome, 9
and syncope, 1695
Subcutaneous nodule(s), in rheumatic fever, 391, *392*
Subpulmonary stenosis, 189
Substance abuse, and infective endocarditis, 408
Substance P, and endothelial dysfunction, in microcirculatory disease, 641
Subvalvular aortic stenosis. See *Aortic stenosis, subvalvular.*
Succinylcholine, for cardiovascular surgery, 2107
Sudden Cardiac Death in Heart Failure trial, 1728t, 1729–1730
Sudden death, 1710–1732
atherosclerotic plaque rupture and, 579–580
definition of, 1710
epidemiology of, 1710, *1711*
from arrhythmias, in mitral valve prolapse, 364–365
from hypertrophic cardiomyopathy, 224
in aortic stenosis, 328
in arrhythmogenic right ventricular dysplasia, histologic basis of, 1671
in young adults, 1671
in athletes, causes of, *1717*
in heart failure, 1161
in hypertrophic cardiomyopathy, 1066
prevention of, 1069
in long QT syndrome, 1660–1661
in women, epidemiology of, 579
mitral valve prolapse and, 382–383
pathology of, 509–511
pathophysiology of, 1721–1722
prevention of, 1724–1732

Sudden death *(Continued)*
angiotensin receptor antagonists in, 1725
angiotensin-converting enzyme inhibitors in, 1725
antiarrhythmic agents in, 1725, 1730
implantable cardioverter-defibrillator in, 1727–1730, 1728t, 1731–1732, 1731t, *1732*
pharmacologic, *1724, 1724–1727, 1726*
primary, implantable cardioverter-defibrillator in, 1789–1790
secondary, 1730–1732, 1731t, *1732*
risk factor(s) for, 1711–1714, *1712, 1713t, 1714*
activity as, 1713
age as, 1711, *1712*
and risk factors for coronary artery disease, 1713–1714, 1713t, *1714*
arrhythmogenic right ventricular dysplasia as, 1717–1718, *1718*
Brugada's syndrome as, 1720–1721
coronary artery anomalies as, 1716
coronary artery disease as, 1715–1716
dilated cardiomyopathy as, 1718–1719
hypertrophic cardiomyopathy as, 1716–1717, *1717*
Lenegre's disease as, 1721
Lev's disease as, 1721
long QT syndrome as, 1719–1720, 1719t–1720t
myocardial infarction as, 1715–1716
psychological, 1713
race as, *1712,* 1713
time and, 1710–1711, *1712*
transient, 1715
valvular heart disease as, 1718
ventricular fibrillation as, 1721–1722
ventricular tachycardia as, 1721–1722
Wolff-Parkinson-White syndrome as, 1720
risk stratification for, 1722–1724
cardiac catheterization in, 1723
echocardiography in, 1722
electrocardiography in, 1722
electrophysiologic studies in, 1723–1724
exercise testing in, 1722–1723
heart rate variability in, 1723
Holter monitoring in, 1723
radionuclide imaging in, 1723
signal-averaged electrocardiography in, 1723
secondary prevention of, by implantable cardioverter-defibrillators, 1787–1788, 1788t–1789t
Summation gallop, 11, 27
Superior vena cava, anatomy of, 147
anomalous connections of, 168–169
left, persistent, echocardiography in, 238, *238*
obstruction of, 195
balloon angioplasty for, 267
pressure in, in cardiac tamponade, *1252*
right, drainage to left atrium, 238
Supine position, during pregnancy, 2028–2029, *2029*
Supply ischemia, *vs.* demand ischemia, 1008
Supravalvular aortic stenosis, 153–154, *154–155,* 182, *184,* 2155–2156
and ventricular outflow tract obstruction, surgical treatment of, 295, *298*
echocardiography in, 247
Supraventricular arrhythmia(s), from Mahaim fibers, surgical treatment of, 1824–1825
Supraventricular tachycardia, 1606–1618. See also *Atrial fibrillation; Atrial flutter; Atrial tachycardia.*
circus movement, 1610, *1611–1612*

Supraventricular tachycardia *(Continued)*
classification of, 1606, 1606t, *1607*
differential diagnosis of, 1611–1618, *1614–1618*
blood pressure in, 1613t
carotid sinus massage in, 1611, 1613t
electrical alternans of QRS complex in, 1611, *1614*
heart rate during bundle branch block in, 1611, *1614–1615*
mode of initiation in, 1611, *1615–1617,* 1618
mode of termination in, *1617,* 1618
steps in, 1618, *1618*
during pregnancy, 2041–2042
fetal, 2063–2064
palpitations in, 7
radiofrequency catheter ablation of, 1796–1807, *1797–1806.* See also *Radiofrequency catheter ablation.*
treatment of, 1703–1704
wide QRS tachycardia during, *1678–1681,* 1679
with right bundle branch block, *1684*
Surgical Control of Hyperlipidemia study, 1409
Survival And Ventricular Enlargement (SAVE) trial, *1177*
Survival with Oral d-Sotalol (SWORD) trial, 1727
Swan-Ganz catheter, use of, 558, *559*
"Swan-neck" deformity, in rheumatoid arthritis, *1940*
SWORD (Survival with Oral d-Sotalol) trial, 1727
Sydenham's chorea, in rheumatic fever, 391, *392*
Sympathetic imbalance hypothesis, in long QT syndrome, 1656
Sympathetic microneurography, in autonomic dysfunction, 1545, 1550, *1550*
Sympathetic nervous system, activation of, in heart failure, 1152–1153
in morning, and hypertension control, 2239–2240, *2240*
obesity and, 1292, *1293–1294*
and hypertension, 1498–1499, *1499*
physiology of, 1537, *1538*
Sympathetic outflow, regulation of, 1288
Sympathomimetic agent(s), during SPECT myocardial perfusion imaging, 104
for postural hypotension, 1556
Syncope, 1688–1706
cerebral circulatory physiology and, 1688–1690, *1690*
classification of, 1688, 1689t
definition of, 1688
diagnosis of, 1696–1700, *1697*
autonomic function testing in, 1698–1699
initial evaluation in, 1696–1697, *1697*
invasive electrophysiologic studies in, 1698
neurologic studies in, 1700
noninvasive studies in, 1697–1698
differential diagnosis of, 8–9, 8t
economic impact of, 1705
epidemiology of, 1700–1701
etiology of, 1688, 1689t
from arrhythmias, treatment of, 1703–1704
from cough, 8–9
from myocardial ischemia, treatment of, 1705
from orthostatic hypotension, treatment of, 1702–1703
in aortic stenosis, 325
in orthostatic hypotension, 8

Syncope *(Continued)*
in psychiatric disorders, 1705
in pulmonary hypertension, 1864, 1864t
natural history of, 1700–1701
in long QT syndrome, 1701
in neurally mediated syndromes, 1701
with cardiovascular etiology, 1701
neurally mediated, 1553, *1554*
pacemaker therapy for, 1763
pathophysiology of, 1690–1696, 1690t–1694t, *1694*
cardiovascular, 1690–1695, 1690t–1694t, *1694*
arrhythmias and, 1691–1695, 1693t–1694t, *1694*
mechanical, 1695
neurally mediated syndromes and, 1690–1691, 1690t
cerebrovascular, 1695–1696
metabolic, 1695–1696
quinidine and, 1640
treatment of, in neurally mediated syndromes, 1702
vasovagal, 8, 1290–1291, 1540–1541, 1553, *1554*
treatment of, 1702
"Syndrome myxoma," 1904
Syndrome X, and risk of coronary artery disease, 2209
Syntenic, definition of, 917t
Syphilis, cardiovascular, 1393
Systemic lupus erythematosus (SLE), 1941–1945, 1942t, *1943–1944,* 1946t
and dilated cardiomyopathy, 1044
antiphospholipid antibodies in, 1944, 1944pl, 1944t
autoantibody profiles in, 1941
clinical features of, 1941, 1942t
congenital heart block in, 1945
coronary angiography in, 643
coronary artery disease in, 1942–1943
drug-induced, 1945, 1946t
during pregnancy, 2052
myocarditis in, 1942
pericardial disease in, 1941–1942, *1943*
plasma homocysteine levels and, 2281
pulmonary hypertension in, 1945
valvular disease in, 1943–1945, *1944,* 1944t
vs. pulmonary thromboembolism, 1844–1845
Systemic sclerosis. See *Scleroderma.*
Systemic vein(s), balloon angioplasty in, 267
Systolic anterior motion, of mitral valve, in cardiomyopathy, hypertrophic, 1135, *1136*
Systolic blood pressure, measurement of, 14
Systolic click, 22, 23t, *24*
in mitral valve prolapse, 359–360, *359–360*
nonejection, in mitral valve prolapse, 376, *377*
Systolic dysfunction, biologic determinant(s) of, 961–964, *962,* 963t, *965*
calcium transient as, 964, *965*
contractile apparatus as, 961–963, *962,* 963t
cytoskeleton as, 965
energy metabolism as, 961
excitation-contraction coupling as, 964
membrane proteins as, 963–964
in aortic stenosis, 331–332
in heart failure, 1150–1151, 1150t
Systolic ejection murmur(s), 22, *24,* 25t
Systolic function, left ventricular, in hypertrophic cardiomyopathy, 1060–1061, *1061*
Systolic wall tension, and myocardial oxygen consumption, 521
T cell(s), activation of, in heart transplant rejection, 1210–1211, *1211*
in ruptured atherosclerotic plaques, 580–581
T wave, abnormalities of, 50
in hyperkalemia, 50, *51*
in left bundle branch block, *38*
in myocardial infarction, 548–549, *553*
in pericarditis, 55, *56*
in right bundle branch block, 38, *39*
juvenile, 53
"memory," 53
Tachyarrhythmia(s), and syncope, 1692–1693
diagnosis of, pacemaker therapy in, *1773,* 1773–1774
palpitations in, 7, 7t
Tachycardia, and dilated cardiomyopathy, 1045
atrioventricular nodal reentrant, surgical treatment of, 1824
circus movement. See *Circus movement tachycardia.*
idioventricular, *1571,* 1571–1572
in pulmonary thromboembolism, 1836
in thyrotoxicosis, 1927
paroxysmal supraventricular, 1567
polymorphic ventricular, 1572
Q wave during, 1687
radiofrequency catheter ablation of, 1796–1809. See also *Radiofrequency catheter ablation.*
sinus, 1566
during pregnancy, 2040–2041
in sinus node dysfunction, 1579–1580
sinus node reentrant, in sinus node dysfunction, 1582
supraventricular. See *Supraventricular tachycardia.*
ventricular. See *Ventricular tachycardia.*
Tacrolimus, action of, 1212, *1213*
and nephrotoxicity, 1197–1198
and neurotoxicity, 1198–1199
and post-transplantation hypertension, 1197
dosage of, 1214t
Takayasu's arteritis, 1389–1391, *1390,* 1390t, 1950–1951, *1951*
and pregnancy, 2051–2052
classification of, 1389, *1390*
diagnosis of, 1389, 1390t, 1391
etiology of, 1389
natural history of, 1391
treatment of, 1391
Tambocor. See *Flecainide.*
Tangier disease, 1347–1348
Taurine deficiency, and myocardial disease, 1091
T-box, in cardiogenesis, 922
Teboroxime, for SPECT myocardial perfusion imaging, 102
^{99m}Technetium-labeled agent(s), for infarct imaging, 110–112, *111,* 625
for SPECT myocardial perfusion imaging, 102–103, 102pl
^{99m}Technetium-labeled glucarate, for infarct imaging, 112–113
^{99m}Technetium-pyrophosphate, for infarct imaging, 110–112, *111*
TEE. See *Transesophageal echocardiography (TEE).*
Telangiectasia, hemorrhagic, hereditary, 2011
Tembid. See *Isosorbide dinitrate.*
Temperature, body, monitoring of, during cardiovascular surgery, 2109
in unstable atherosclerotic plaques, 536, *538*
Temporal arteritis, 1391–1392
Terazosin, for hypertension, 1520
Terbutaline, cardiovascular effects of, 2067
Terfenadine, and long QT syndrome, 1659
Tetralogy of Fallot, 170–171, *171–172,* 214, *217–219,* 218–219
clinical features of, 214, *217–219*
computed tomography in, electron beam, *2186*
echocardiography in, 92, *93,* 246–247
pathophysiology of, 214
pregnancy and, 2059–2060
prognosis in, 218, *219*
surgical treatment of, 302–303
syncope in, 8
treatment of, 218
with persistent common arterioventricular canal, 175, *176*
with pulmonary atresia, surgical treatment of, 303, *303*
Tetrofosmin, for SPECT myocardial perfusion imaging, 102–103
Texas Heart Institute, grading system for allograft rejection, 1027–1028, 1028t
TFPI inhibitor, as anticoagulant mechanism, 1318–1319
TGF-β1 (tumor growth factor–β1), and vascular remodeling, 1303
Thalassemia, 2002–2003
Thallium 201 imaging, before noncardiac surgery, 2094
in dilated cardiomyopathy, 1143
in myocardial infarction, 554, *555*
in pulmonary hypertension, 1875–1876
in silent myocardial ischemia, 573
SPECT myocardial perfusion, 101–102, 102pl. See also *SPECT myocardial perfusion imaging.*
Theophylline, for chronic obstructive pulmonary disease, 1893, 1893t
Therapeutic angiogenesis, for carotid artery disease, 1440
for coronary artery disease, 1422–1424, *1423*
gene therapy for, 2272–2274, 2273t–2274t
principles of, *1417–1418,* 1418–1419
vascular endothelial growth factor gene therapy in, 1419–1420, *1420*
clinical trials of, 1420–1421, *1421*
Thermodilution, for measurement of cardiac output, 2131–2132
Thermodynamics, laws of, and energy transfer, 938
Thiamine deficiency, alcohol and, 1965
and myocardial disease, 1090–1091, 1091t
Thiazide diuretic(s), and pregnancy, 2050t
for hypertension, 1516, 1517t
Thoracic aorta, magnetic resonance imaging of, 135–136, *135–136*
Thoracic aortic aneurysm(s), 1359–1365, *1359–1365*
diagnosis of, 1358, *1359*
familial, 2154–2155
natural history of, 1361
surgical treatment of, *1360–1365,* 1361–1365
postoperative management in, 1364
results of, 1364
with annuloaortic ectasia, 1362
with ascending thoracic lesions, *1360–1361,* 1360–1362
with descending thoracic lesions, 1362–1364, *1365*
with transverse arch lesions, 1362, *1363–1364*
Thoracic vessel(s), communication of coronary artery with, 164, *166*
Thoracotomy, atrial fibrillation after, 1641–1642
"Three" sign, in aortic coarctation, 194, *195*

Three-dimensional intravascular ultrasonography, 1473, *1474*
L-Threo-dihydroxyphenylserine (L-DOPS), for postural hypotension, *1557,* 1558
Thrills, palpation of, 17, 20
Thrombi, in prosthetic valves, 321, *321*
Thrombin antagonist(s), for unstable angina, 723, 726
Thrombocythemia, 2005–2007, 2006t
Thrombocytopenia, heparin and, 2007
  quinidine and, 2007
Thrombocytosis, 2005–2007, 2006t
Thromboembolism, and pulmonary hypertension, 1865
  aortic, 1393–1394
  from pulmonary artery catheterization, 2127
  in sinus node dysfunction, 1588
  pulmonary. See *Pulmonary thromboembolism.*
Thromboendarterectomy, for pulmonary hypertension, 1880–1881
Thrombolytic agent(s), and prognosis in myocardial infarction, 821, *821*
  and reinfarction, 746
  classification of, 742–743
  clot-selective, 743
    development of, 742
    first-generation *vs.* second-generation, 743–745, 744t
    90-minute patency rate of, 744–745, 744t
    safety of, 755–757, 756t
  comparative biochemical properties of, 768, *768*
  dosage of, 748–749, *749*
  efficacy of, 768–769, *769*
    plateau of, 821–822, *822*
  fibrin-selective, 743
  fibrin-specific, 743
  first-generation, 746–746
    anticoagulants with, 746
    efficacy of, 745–746
    mechanism of action for, 745
    vs. second-generation, 762–763, 763t
  for myocardial infarction, prehospital, 824
    vs. percutaneous transluminal coronary angioplasty, 822–823, *823*
    with percutaneous transluminal coronary angioplasty, 823–824, 879
  pharmacokinetics of, 748
  second-generation, 746–748, *747,* 747t
    efficacy of, 746, *747,* 747t, 748
Thrombolytic therapy, algorithm for, 769–771, *770*
  and ejection fraction, after myocardial infarction, 754, 754t
  and infarct size, 754
  and mortality, 761–762, 764–766, 764t–766t
  and natural history of myocardial infarction, 699–702, *701*
  and ventricular function, 761
    and extent of infarction, 763–764
  anticipated developments in, 757
  clinical studies of, 762–763, 763t
  conjunctive, 749–753, 750t–753t, *752*
    importance of, 760–761
  contraindications to, 767t
  economic issues in, 760
  failure of, 770–771
  for arterial occlusion, 1426–1428, 1428t
    administration method for, 1427
    dosage of, 1427
    outcome of, predictors of, 1428t
    patient selection in, 1427–1428
    rationale for, 1426
  for non–Q wave myocardial infarction, 760
  for pulmonary thromboembolism, 1849–1850, 1850t
Thrombolytic therapy *(Continued)*
  for tibioperoneal occlusion, 1439–1440
  guide wire traversal test before, 1427
  in prehospital period, 757–758
  interpretation of endpoints in, 761
  recanalization with, and mortality, 754–755, *755–756,* 755t
  safety of, 766–768, 767t–768t
  severity of coronary artery disease and, 762
  vs. PTCA, *758,* 758–760
  with glycoprotein IIb/IIIa antagonist(s), 771–772, *772*
    Paradigm trial of, 771
    TIMI 14 trial of, 771–772
Thrombomodulin, as anticoagulant mechanism, 1319
Thrombosis, and atherosclerosis, 1348–1350
  and instability of atherosclerotic plaques, 802–803, *803*
  and myocardial infarction, 511
  and shock, 1530
  aortic, 1393–1394
  etiology of, 1400
  in atherosclerotic plaque erosion, 581–582
  in cardiomyopathy, dilated, 1139
  in unstable angina, 531
  intraluminal, intravascular ultrasonography in, 1465–1466, *1467*
  mural, from myocardial infarction, echocardiography in, 663, *663*
  pathophysiology of, 505, *507–509,* 509
  vascular endothelial cell function and, 1311–1319. See also *Coagulation system; Fibrinolytic system.*
Thrombosis in Myocardial Infarction IIIB (TIMI IIIB) study, 814, 814t
Thrombosis in Myocardial Infarction (TIMI-I) study, of thrombolytic therapy, complications of, 756, 756t
  of tissue plasminogen activator, 746
Thrombosis in Myocardial Infarction (TIMI) trial, for grading of coronary blood flow, 636
Thrombotic endocarditis, nonbacterial, 401
Thrombotic microangiopathy, 2004
Thrombotic thrombocytopenic purpura, anatomic abnormalities in, 317
Thromboxane A_2, synthesis of, aspirin and, *716*
Thyroid disease, and hypertension, 1506–1507
Thyroid hormone(s), for hypothyroidism, 1929–1930
  interaction of, 1926–1927
Thyrotoxicosis, 1927–1928
Thyroxine, for hypothyroidism, 1929–1930
Tibial artery, atherosclerosis in, 1438
Tibioperoneal angioplasty, 1439, 1439t
Tibioperoneal occlusion, atherectomy for, devices for, 1439–1440, *1440*
  stents for, 1440
  thrombolytic therapy for, 1439–1440
Ticlopidine, chemical structure of, *717*
  for peripheral vascular disease, of lower extremities, 1412
Tikosyn. See *Dofetilide.*
Tilt table testing, in autonomic dysfunction, 1544–1545, *1547*
  in syncope, 1699
    vasovagal, *1540*
    with electrophysiologic studies, 1699–1700
Time-activity curve(s), for quantification of shunts, first pass radionuclide angiocardiography in, *106,* 106–107
  in congenital heart disease, 461, *461*
  on radionuclide ventriculography, *109,* 109–110
TIMI 14 (Thrombosis in Myocardial Infarction 14) study, 771–772
TIMI II (Thrombosis in Myocardial Infarction II) study, 729, *730*
  of thrombolytic therapy, complications of, 756, 756t
  of tissue plasminogen activator, 746
TIMI IIB (Thrombosis in Myocardial Infarction IIB) study, 742
TIMI IIIB (Thrombosis in Myocardial Infarction IIIB) study, 814, 814t
Timolol, dosage of, 712t
  for survivors of myocardial infarction, *773*
TIMP(s). See *Tissue inhibitors of metalloproteinases (TIMPs).*
Tinman, and cardiogenesis, in *Drosophila,* 919, 922
Tirofiban, for unstable angina, 733–734, *734,* 736t
Tissue factor, as procoagulant mechanism, 1318
  in coagulation cascade, 726, *728*
  in variant angina, 534, *534*
Tissue inhibitors of metalloproteinases (TIMPs), in unstable atherosclerotic plaques, 539–541, 541t
Tissue plasminogen activator (t-PA), 90-minute patency rate of, 744–745, 744t
  activation of, regulation of, *1313,* 1313–1314
  allergic reactions to, 767–768
  and fibrinolysis, 1311
  and intracranial bleeding, 766–768, 767t–768t
  and mortality, 764–766, 764t–766t
    vs. streptokinase/urokinase, 755t
  and natural history of myocardial infarction, 699–702, *701*
  anticipated developments in, 757
  defective production of, and fibrinolysis, 1315
  development of, 746
  dosage of, 748–749, *749*
  efficacy of, 746, *747,* 747t, 748
    vs. reteplase, 822
  for arterial occlusive disease, 1426–1427
    dosage of, 1427
  pharmacokinetics of, 748
  production of, regulation of, 1312–1313
  studies of, 753–754, 754t
  vs. PTCA, *758,* 758–760
  with conjunctive and adjunctive agents, 752–753
  with heparin, 752–753
  with Integrilin, Impact-AMI study of, 771
Tobacco. See *Smoking.*
Tocainide, adverse effects of, 1746
  dosage of, 1746
  efficacy of, 1746
  electrophysiology of, 1746
  pharmacokinetics of, 1742t–1743t, 1746
Tocolytic(s), cardiovascular effects of, 2067
Tomographic acquisition mode, 100–101, *101,* 101pl
Tonocard. See *Tocainide.*
Toprol, dosage of, 712t
Toricelli equation, 422
Torsades de pointes, 1572
  in arrhythmogenic right ventricular dysplasia, histologic basis of, 1671
  in long QT syndrome, 1659–1660
    surgical treatment of, 1828–1829
  quinidine and, 1720
Total artificial heart(s), 1231, 1235
Total atrial refractory period, in pacemaker therapy, 1768

Total cholesterol (TC), and coronary artery disease, in women, 583, 583t
Total coronary area, 614, 614t
Totipotent, definition of, 917t
Toulouse Trial, 873t, 874
Toxic cardiomyopathy, 1024, *1025*
Toxic myocarditis, 1097t
Toxin(s), agricultural, and chronic obstructive pulmonary disease, 1886
and autonomic dysfunction, 1539t, 1554
and risk of sudden death, 1715
Toxoplasmosis, and cardiomyopathy, in human immunodeficiency virus infection, 1976, *1977,* 1978–1979
and myocarditis, 1098, 1111–1112
t-PA. See *Tissue plasminogen activator (t-PA).*
TRACE (Trandolapril Cardiac Evaluation) study, 1725
Trandolapril Cardiac Evaluation (TRACE) study, 1725
Transcription factor(s), definition of, 917t
in cardiogenesis, 918–922
and postnatal cardiac hypertrophy, 927–928
evolutionary conservation of, 922
Transcriptional enhancer factor–1 (TEF-1) family, in cardiogenesis, 921
Transcutaneous oximetry, in peripheral vascular disease, of lower extremities, 1408–1409
Transduction systems, in cardiac hypertrophy, 958
Transesophageal echocardiography (TEE), advantages of, 237
before noncardiac surgery, 2096
during closure of atrial septal defect, 272
in aortic dissection, 1379, 1380t, *1381*
in aortic regurgitation, 82–83, *83*
in aortic stenosis, 81–82, *82*
in arrhythmogenic right ventricular dysplasia, 1667–1668
in atrial fibrillation, 1644, 1650–1654. See also *Atrial fibrillation, diagnosis of, transesophageal echocardiography in.*
in atrial septal defect, 240–241, *240–241*
in bicuspid aortic valve, 248, *248*
in cardiac myxoma, 1905, *1905*
in cor triatriatum, 243
in coronary artery disease, 88–90, *89*
in infective endocarditis, 84, *85,* 404, 411, *411,* 454, *454*
in mitral stenosis, 449, *449*
in mitral valve prolapse, 362, *362,* 380, *380*
in patent foramen ovale, 242
in pulmonary embolism, 86, *88*
intraoperative, 2134–2137, 2135t–2137t
complications of, 2136
contraindications to, 2135
for detection of ischemia, 2136–2137
in mitral valve prolapse, *293*
indications for, 2134–2135, 2135t–2136t
probe insertion for, 2135–2136
range of data from, 2136t–2137t, 2137
of bicuspid aortic valve, *442*
of prosthetic valves, 83, *84*
Transfusion(s), during cardiovascular surgery, 2112
Transgene(s), definition of, 917t
Transgenic technology, in gene therapy, 2272
Transient outward current, in cardiac hypertrophy, *970,* 971–972
Transluminal extraction atherectomy, for unstable angina, 809
Transmitral valve flow velocity curve, 1004–1005
Transmyocardial laser revascularization, 856
Transplantation, and plasma homocysteine levels, 2279, 2281
heart, allocation system for, 1185–1187, *1186*
and autonomic dysfunction, 1550, *1551*
anesthesia for, 2111–2112
arteriopathy after, angiography in, 642–643, *642–643*
complication(s) of, arrhythmias as, 1200
cardiac allograft vasculopathy as, 1191–1197, *1192–1195.* See also *Cardiac allograft vasculopathy.*
gout as, 1200
heart block as, 1200
hypertension as, 1197
long-term, 1187
malignancy as, 1198, *1198*
nephrotoxicity as, 1197–1198
neurotoxicity as, 1198–1199
obesity as, 1199
surgical, 1187
coronary angiography after, 604
donor availability for, 1185, *1186*
electrocardiography in, 58, *59*
for arrhythmogenic right ventricular dysplasia, 1674
for myocarditis, 1108
for peripartum myocarditis, 1114
future of, 1200–1201
history of, 1224
immunologic evaluation before, 1219
in advanced heart failure, 1224–1231, *1226–1232*
donor/recipient selection for, 1224
early postoperative management in, 1230
heterotopic technique in, 1225, *1228–1230,* 1230
immunosuppressive therapy for, 1225
orthotopic technique in, 1225, *1226–1227*
results of, 1230–1231
infection after, *1189,* 1189–1191, *1191*
diagnosis of, 1190
incidence of, 1190, *1191*
prevention of, 1190–1191
myocardial bridges after, 619
patient selection for, 1185–1187, *1186*
pregnancy after, 1199–1200
rejection of, *1188,* 1188–1189
acute, 1216–1217
allorecognition in, 1210
antibody-mediated, 1217–1218
chronic. See *Cardiac allograft vasculopathy.*
diagnosis of, 1188–1189
effector responses in, 1211–1212
future therapy for, 1219–1220
histopathology of, 1214–1215, *1216,* 1216t
hyperacute, 1215–1216
immunosuppressive therapy for. See *Immunosuppressive therapy.*
incidence of, 1188, *1188,* 1214, *1215*
myocardial biopsy in, 1027–1028, *1028–1029,* 1028t
noninvasive testing for, 1218–1219
pathogenesis of, 1210
radionuclide imaging in, 1145
risk factors for, 1188
T cell activation in, 1210–1211, *1211*
types of, 1214, 1215t
retransplantation after, 1200
survival after, 1185, *1186*
heart-lung, for congenital heart disease, 306, *307–308,* 308
Transplantation *(Continued)*
for pulmonary hypertension, 1881
lung, for chronic obstructive pulmonary disease, 1897
myocyte, for heart failure, 2274
stem cell, for amyloidosis, 1086, *1087*
Transposon, definition of, 917t
Transseptal double-balloon valvuloplasty, for mitral stenosis, 261–262
Transthoracic echocardiography (TTE), in aortic dissection, 1380t
in infective endocarditis, 404
Transvalvular gradient, low, in aortic stenosis, left ventricular dysfunction and, 333–334, *334,* 334t
Transverse aortic arch, aneurysms of, surgical treatment of, 1362, *1363–1364*
Trauma. See specific location, e.g., *Aorta.*
Treadmill exercise testing, 587
Triangle of Koch, and radiofrequency catheter ablation of atrioventricular nodal reentrant tachycardia, 1800, *1801*
Triaxial reference system, *32,* 32–33
Tricuspid atresia, 156, 185, *185–187,* 187
surgical treatment of, 306
with pulmonary stenosis, treatment of, 187
Tricuspid balloon valvuloplasty, percutaneous, 481–482
Tricuspid insufficiency, diagnosis of, cardiac catheterization in, 432
V wave in, and myocardial infarction, 543, *546*
Tricuspid leaflet, septal, displacement of, in Ebstein's anomaly, 243–244, *244*
Tricuspid regurgitation, 160, *160–161*
and outcome of percutaneous mitral balloon valvotomy, 473
and pulmonary hypertension, 1866
clinical features of, 344, *345*
diagnosis of, echocardiography in, 451–452, *452*
etiology of, 343
in cardiomyopathy, dilated, echocardiography in, 1139
jugular venous pulse in, *18*
natural history of, 344
Tricuspid stenosis, 156
balloon valvuloplasty for, 262
clinical features of, 343–344, *344*
congenital, 184
diagnosis of, cardiac catheterization in, 432, *433*
echocardiography in, 451
in rheumatic fever, 397
natural history of, 344
Tricuspid valve, repair of, 289, *295*
surgical procedures on, 493
Tricuspid valve disease, acquired, clinical features of, 344, *345*
pathophysiology of, 343
treatment of, 346
Tricyclic antidepressant(s), electrocardiographic changes from, 53
Trifascicular block, electrocardiography in, 41–42
pacemaker therapy for, 1760t, 1762
Trigger impulse, in radionuclide imaging, 100
Triggered activity, and impulse formation disorders, 1563
Triglyceride(s), and myocardial ischemia, 1346
and risk of coronary artery disease, 2197–2198
deposits of, diseases found in, 1030
in myocardial metabolism, 946–948, *947*
protease inhibitors and, 1981
Triglyceride-rich lipoprotein(s), and coronary artery disease, 2246

Trisomy 21, 2170–2171
Tropical endomyocardial fibrosis. See *Cardiomyopathy, restrictive.*
Tropomyosin, and contractile function, 991, *992,* 1277, *1278*
α-Tropomyosin gene, in hypertrophic cardiomyopathy, 1057
Troponin, and contractile function, 991, *991–992*
  and prognosis in unstable angina, 805t, 813, *813*
  serum levels of, and prognosis in myocardial infarction, 538, *540,* 553–554
Troponin I gene, in hypertrophic cardiomyopathy, 1057
Troponin T gene, in hypertrophic cardiomyopathy, 1057, *1062*
  murine models of, 1059
Truncus arteriosus, 220–221, *221–222*
  type IV, 171
Trypanosoma cruzi, and dilated cardiomyopathy, 1043–1044
  and myocarditis, 1110–1111
Trypanosomiasis, African, 1111
  American, 1110–1111
TTE. See *Transthoracic echocardiography (TTE).*
T-tubule(s), in plasma membrane, 993
Tube drift correction, in radionuclide imaging, 100
Tuberculosis, *vs.* pulmonary thromboembolism, 1844
Tuberculous pericarditis, 1241, 1261
Tumor growth factor–β (TGF-β), and cardiogenesis, 923
Tumor growth factor–β1 (TGF-β1), and vascular remodeling, 1303
Tumor necrosis factor–α (TNF-α), in cardiac hypertrophy, 968
  inhibitors of, for heart failure, 1176
"Tumor plop," 11, 1904
Tunnel subaortic stenosis, 153
Turner's syndrome, 176, 2171
  clinical features of, 14
  with aortic coarctation, 1357
Twelve-lead electrocardiography, 30
Type A personality, and risk of atherosclerosis, 1351
Tyrosine kinase(s), in excitation-contraction coupling, 1284, *1284*

U wave, 32
  factors affecting, 54
  in hypokalemia, 52, *52*
Uhl's anomaly, 226
  in arrhythmogenic right ventricular dysplasia, 1673
Uhl's syndrome, surgical treatment of, 1828
Ulceration index, 634–636, *636*
Ultrafast computed tomography. See *Computed tomography (CT), electron beam.*
Ultrasonography. See also *Echocardiography.*
  B-mode, 1446–1451
    for definition of arterial dimensions, 1451
    in atherosclerosis, advantages of, 1446
      for measurement of intimal-medial thickness, 1447–1448. See also *Intimal-medial thickness (IMT).*
    principles of, 1446–1447, *1447*
  Doppler, in monitoring of cardiac output, *2133,* 2133–2134
  duplex, in carotid artery disease, 1401
    in peripheral vascular disease, of lower extremities, 1408
    in renal artery disease, 1402
Ultrasonography *(Continued)*
    in renovascular hypertension, 1429
  in abdominal aortic aneurysms, *1367*
  intravascular, 1454–1459
    catheters for, 1454, *1455*
      high-frequency, 1473
    clinical trials of, 1472t
    diagnostic applications of, 1463–1466, 1463t, *1464–1467*
      in ambiguous lesions, 1464, *1465*
      in calcification, 1464
      in cardiac allograft vasculopathy, 1464, *1466*
      in intraluminal thrombosis, 1465–1466, *1467*
      in restenosis, 1469, *1470–1471*
    early studies of, 1461–1462, 1462t
    expanded clinical applications of, 1473
    for in vivo assessment of plaque morphology, 1457–1458, *1458*
    for measurement of arterial lumen, 1456
    future of, 1471, 1473, *1474*
    guidelines for, 1462–1463, 1462t–1463t
    history of, 1460–1461
    in calcified atherosclerotic plaque, *1456,* 1456–1457
    in cardiac allograft vasculopathy, 1194, *1194–1195*
    interpretation of, 1454–1456, *1456–1457*
    interventional, 1466–1471, *1468–1471,* 1468t
      during directional atherectomy, 1469, 1471, *1471*
      during procedure, 1467–1471, *1468–1471,* 1469t
      during stent placement, 1467–1469, *1468,* 1469t
      prior to procedure, 1466–1468
    intracardiac, 1473
    principles of, 1454, *1455*
    raw radiofrequency signal in, *1457*
    sensitivity and specificity of, 1461
    three-dimensional, 1473, *1474*
    vessel patterns in, 1461, 1462t
  venous, in pulmonary thromboembolism, 1843
Umbrella occlusion device(s), for closure of vascular communications, 278
Unicuspid aortic stenosis, 150–151, *151*
United Network for Organ Sharing (UNOS), 1185–1186, *1186*
University Diabetes Group program, 1345
"Unloading therapy," for peripartum cardiomyopathy, 2054, 2054t
UNOS (United Network for Organ Sharing), 1185–1186, *1186*
u-PA. See *Urokinase-type plasminogen activator (u-PA).*
Upper tracking rate, in dual-chamber pacing, 1768
Upper-rate behavior, in pacemaker therapy, 1768–1769
"Upward creep," during SPECT myocardial perfusion imaging, 105
Uremia, *vs.* pulmonary thromboembolism, 1846–1847
Urine output, monitoring of, during cardiovascular surgery, 2109
Urography, rapid-sequence, in renal artery disease, 1402
Urokinase, and mortality, *vs.* t-PA, 755t
  for arterial occlusive disease, 1426–1427
    dosage of, 1427
  mechanism of action for, 745
Urokinase-type plasminogen activator (u-PA), activation of, regulation of, *1313,* 1313–1314
Urokinase-type plasminogen activator (u-PA) *(Continued)*
  and fibrinolysis, 1311
  protein structure of, 1311–1312
Uterus, gravid, physiology of, 2028–2029, *2029–2030*

V wave, 19
  in tricuspid insufficiency, and myocardial infarction, 543, *546*
VACA (Valvuloplasty and Angioplasty of Congenital Anomalies), 258
Vaccination, against streptococcal infections, 398
Vagal maneuver(s), for preexcitation, 1626, *1629,* 1630t
Valsalva maneuver, in autonomic dysfunction, 1544, *1544*
Valsalva response, space flight and, 2082
Valsartan, for heart failure, 1174
Valvular aortic stenosis, 180–182, *181–183.* See also *Aortic stenosis, valvular.*
Valvular disease, anatomic abnormalities in, 315–323
    in collagen vascular disease, 315–318, *316–318*
    in congenital disorders, 315. See also *Congenital heart disease* and specific disorder.
    in endocrine disorders, 318–319, *318–319*
    in infective endocarditis, 320–321
    in metabolic disorders, 318–319, *318–319,* 318pl
    in myxomatous degeneration, 319–320, *319–320*
    in prosthetic valves, *321–322,* 321–323
  and sudden death, 1718
  cardiac catheterization in, therapeutic, 434
  concurrent, echocardiography in, 445
  congenital. See *Congenital heart disease, valvular.*
  diagnosis of, computed tomography in, electron beam, 2185–2186, *2186*
    radionuclide studies in, 459–462, *460–461*
      of aorta, 459–460, *460*
      of mitral valve, 460–461
  Doppler echocardiography in, 80–83, *80–83*
  during pregnancy, 2055–2057, 2056t
  exercise testing in, 590
  from anorectic agents, 453
  in carcinoid syndrome, 1930, *1931*
  in rheumatoid arthritis, 1940–1941
  in systemic lupus erythematosus, 1943–1945, *1944,* 1944t
  noncardiac surgery in, 2100
  surgical treatment of, 485–498. See also specific procedure *and* specific disease.
    cardiopulmonary bypass during, 486, *487*
    completion of, 493, 495
    complications of, 498
    history of, 485
    postoperative care in, 495, 498
    suture technique in, 486
    traditional *vs.* minimally invasive, 485
    valve repair *vs.* replacement in, 485–486
Valvular obstruction, 150–156, *150–156*
Valvular pulmonary stenosis, 187–189, *188–190*
Valvular regurgitation, 158–161, *159–162*
  aortic, 160–161, *161–162*
  mitral, 158, *159–160*
  pulmonary, 161
  tricuspid, 160, *160–161*
Valvulitis, in rheumatic fever, 389, *390*
  lupus erythematosus, anatomic abnormalities in, 316–317, 317pl

Valvulitis *(Continued)*
rheumatic, anatomic abnormalities in, 315–316, 315pl–316pl, *316*
rheumatoid, anatomic abnormalities in, 316, *317,* 317pl
Valvuloplasty, balloon. See *Balloon valvuloplasty.*
Valvuloplasty and Angioplasty of Congenital Anomalies (VACA), 258
Vancomycin, enterococci resistant to, 407
for infective endocarditis, 407–408, 408t–409t
penicillin-susceptible, 406t–407t, 407
VANQWISH (Veterans Affairs Non–Q Wave Infarction Strategies in Hospital) trial, 814, 814t
Variant angina. See *Angina, variant (Prinzmetal).*
Vascular access, for coronary angiography, 597–598
Vascular cell(s), apoptosis of, modulators of, 1302
Vascular cell adhesion molecule (VCAM), upregulation of, in unstable atherosclerotic plaques, 536, *537*
Vascular communication(s), abnormal, closure of, 269–271
umbrella devices for, 278
Vascular compliance. See also *Arterial compliance.*
abnormalities of, 1487–1491
from aging, 1487–1488
from atherosclerosis, 1488
from diabetes mellitus, 1490
from heart failure, 1490–1491
from hypertension, 1488–1490
definition of, 1491
factors affecting, 1479
Vascular disease, hyperhomocysteinemia and, 2279–2281, *2280–2282,* 2280t–2281t
Vascular endothelial cell(s), and thrombosis, 1311–1319. See also *Coagulation system; Fibrinolytic system.*
Vascular endothelial growth factor (VEGF), for angiogenesis, 2272–2273, 2273t
in angiogenesis, 1417–1418
in arterial gene therapy, 1421–1422
in therapeutic angiogenesis, 1419–1420, *1420*
clinical trials of, 1420–1421, *1421*
for coronary artery disease, 1422–1424, *1423*
Vascular remodeling, flow-related, 1304
growth promoters in, 1301–1302
growth-regulating vasoactive substances and, 1302–1303
pathologic, 1304–1307, 1306t
in atherosclerosis, 1305–1306
in hypertension, 1305
in restenosis, 1306–1307, 1306t
physiologic, 1303–1304
physiology of, 1299–1303, *1300,* 1301t
types of, *1300*
vasodilatation and, 1304
Vascular retrieval forceps, 281
Vascular smooth muscle, crossbridge cycling in, light chain phosphorylation and, 1279, *1280*
electrochemical gradient in, *1281,* 1281–1282
latch state in, 1279
types of, 1275
Vascular smooth muscle cell(s), phenotype of, hypertension and, 1489
replication of, and restenosis, 1306–1307, 1306t
Vascular surgery, SPECT myocardial perfusion imaging before, 675
Vascular system, development of, 1417–1418
exercise and, 2221–2222
Vascular tone, modulating factors in, 1299, *1300*
Vascular waterfall, 525
Vasculitis, 1400
coronary, in rheumatoid arthritis, 1941
coronary angiography in, 643
necrotizing, pathology of, *510*
primary, *1949,* 1949–1952, *1951*
and Behçet's disease, 1951
and Churg-Strauss angiitis, 1950
and giant cell arteritis, 1950
and hypersensitivity angiitis, 1950
and Kawasaki's disease, 1951
and polyarteritis nodosum, *1949,* 1949–1952
and relapsing polychondritis, 1951–1952, 1952pl
and Takayasu's arteritis, 1950–1951, *1951*
and Wegener's granulomatosis, 1950
Vasculogenesis, 1417–1418
Vasculopathy, in transplanted heart. See *Cardiac allograft vasculopathy.*
Vasoactive substance(s), endothelial release of, 1276, *1276*
growth-regulating, and vascular remodeling, 1302–1303
Vasoconstriction, cocaine and, 1960–1962
in obstructive pulmonary hypertension, 1858–1859, 1858t–1859t, *1859*
Vasoconstrictor system(s), increased activity of, and hypertension, 1498–1500, *1499–1500*
Vasodilatation, adenosine and, 523
and vascular remodeling, 1304
endothelium-dependent, 524
nitrates and, 709, *710*
Vasodilating system(s), decreased activity of, and hypertension, *1500–1501,* 1500–1502
Vasodilator(s), during SPECT myocardial perfusion imaging, 103–104
for cardiogenic shock, in myocardial infarction, 1532
for claudication, 1411
for heart failure, 1167–1168
for hypertension, 1517t, 1520–1521
for mitral regurgitation, 352–353
for pulmonary hypertension, 1878–1880, *1879–1880*
Vasomotor tone, and quantification of coronary artery stenosis, 629
in transplanted heart, 642
variations in, and coronary artery caliber, 615–616
Vasopressin, in heart failure, 1153–1154
Vasospasm, coronary. See *Coronary artery(ies), spasm of.*
Vasospastic angina. See *Angina, variant (Prinzmetal).*
Vasospastic disease, 1400
Vasovagal reaction(s), during cardiac catheterization, in pulmonary hypertension, 1874–1875
Vasovagal syncope, 8, 1290–1291, 1540–1541, 1553, *1554*
tilt test in, *1540*
Vaughan-Williams classification, of antiarrhythmic agents, 1740t
VCAM. See *Vascular cell adhesion molecule (VCAM).*
VDD pacemaker mode, 1771
Vector system(s), for gene therapy, 2269–2271, *2270,* 2271t
Vectorcardiography, 30
Vegetation(s), in infective endocarditis, and embolism, 414–416
and indications for surgical treatment, 410–411, *411,* 411t
VEGF. See *Vascular endothelial growth factor (VEGF).*
Velocardiofacial syndrome, 2171–2172
genetic basis of, 925–926
Vena cava, connection with left atrium, 169, *170*
inferior. See *Inferior vena cava.*
radiography of, 67–68, *68*
superior. See *Superior vena cava.*
Venography, contrast, in pulmonary thromboembolism, 1843
Venous air embolism, *vs.* pulmonary thromboembolism, 1847
Venous disease(s), types of, 1399
Venous hum, 19
Venous pressure, during pregnancy, 2031–2032, *2032*
in cardiac tamponade, 1252, *1252*
in heart failure, 1155, *1156*
Venous pulse, jugular, palpation of, *17–18,* 17–19, 18t
Venous return, anomalies of, echocardiography in, *238,* 238–239
Venous thrombosis, during pregnancy, 2037–2038, 2038t
Venous ultrasonography, in pulmonary thromboembolism, 1843
Ventilation, mechanical, for chronic obstructive pulmonary disease, 1896
positive pressure, cardiovascular response to, 2117
Ventilation/perfusion scintigraphy, in pulmonary embolism, 74–75
in pulmonary hypertension, 1875, *1875*
in pulmonary thromboembolism, 1840, *1841*
Ventilatory oxygen consumption, and exercise prescription, 896
Ventricle(s), left. See *Left ventricle.*
double-inlet, surgical treatment of, 306
inversion of, 212, *213–216*
pressure-volume relationship in, *332*
in amyloid heart disease, 1085, *1085*
right. See *Right ventricle.*
Ventricular activation time, 31
Ventricular aneurysm(s), and cardiomegaly, 10
computed tomography of, electron beam, 2184, *2184*
from myocardial infarction, echocardiography in, 662
in survivors of myocardial infarction, 776–776
Ventricular arrhythmia(s), 1570–1575, *1571*
alcohol and, 1965–1966
and prognosis in heart failure, 1159–1160
atrioventricular block as, 1572–1575, *1574–1575,* 1574t. See also *Atrioventricular block.*
bedside evaluation of, 1572
cocaine and, 1963
during pregnancy, 2043
extrasystolic, 1570–1571
histologic basis of, 1671, *1672*
in myocarditis, 1103
in older adults, 2021, 2021t
tachycardia as, 1571, *1571*
polymorphic, 1572
Ventricular assist device(s), warm heart surgery with, 851–852, *852*
Ventricular compliance, pulmonary artery catheterization and, 2130
Ventricular diastolic pressure, in constrictive pericarditis, *vs.* cardiac tamponade, 1259, *1259*

Ventricular dysfunction, after myl
infarction, 1177
definition of, 1148
Ventricular ectopy, and risk of sueath,
1714
Ventricular extrasysole, 1570–157
Ventricular fibrillation, idiopathicudden
death, 1721–1722
implantable cardioverter-defibri for,
1784
in Wolff-Parkinson-White syndı1625,
1626
Ventricular fibrillation zone, detec', by
implantable cardioverter-defibr,
1782, *1783*
Ventricular filling, impaired, differ
diagnosis of, 1266
in restrictive cardiomyopathy,
in constrictive pericarditis, *vs.* catam-
ponade, 1259, *1259*
Ventricular function, and extent of tion,
thrombolytic therapy and, 763
evaluation of, in myocardial infa, 557–
560, *559*
in myocardial infarction, and pro, 561
intraoperative monitoring of, tranhageal
echocardiography in, 2136t
left. See *Left ventricular function.*
regional, on radionuclide ventricuphy,
110
thrombolytic therapy and, 761
Ventricular fusion beat(s), in wide Q
tachycardia, 1679, *1682*
Ventricular gradient, 32
Ventricular inflow, anomalies of,
echocardiography in, 242–244,
Ventricular interaction, 1005
in constrictive pericarditis and carcam-
ponade, 1259, 1264
Ventricular muscle, resting membranential
of, 29
Ventricular outflow tract, obstruction
surgical treatment of, 295, *296–2*
Ventricular premature beat(s), 1570–1
Ventricular pseudoaneurysm(s), from
myocardial infarction, 664, 664pl
Ventricular remodeling, in heart failur51,
1152t
Ventricular septal aneurysm(s), after cle of
ventricular septal defect, 245
Ventricular septal defect, 163, *164,* 2048,
206–207
after myocardial infarction, *556*
prognosis in, 560
and aortic regurgitation, 161, *162*
surgical treatment of, 289, *290*
and pregnancy, 2058–2059
closure of, 277–278
echocardiography in, 92, *92,* 244–2445
from myocardial infarction, echocardra-
phy in, 664
in Eisenmenger's syndrome, and pulmary
hypertension, 1857, *1858*
in holosystolic murmur, *548*
in survivors of myocardial infarctin, 4–
775
in tetralogy of Fallot, echocardiogph in,
246
large, 205, *206,* 207
membranous, 205
pathophysiology of, 204–205
small, 205, *206*
surgical treatment of, 300
with Eisenmenger's complex, *207,*07–208
with pulmonary atresia, 219–220, *0*
with transposition of great arteriesurgical
treatment of, 303, *305,* 306

Ventricular tachycardia, 1571, *1571*
and risk of sudden death, 1714
atrioventricular dissociation in, 1677
during space flight, 2083, *2084*
idiopathic, *1683*
and sudden death, 1721–1722
surgical treatment of, 1825, *1826*
implantable cardioverter-defibrillators for,
1784–1785
ischemic, surgical treatment of, 1829–1830
neonatal, 2064
radiofrequency catheter ablation of, 1807–
1809, *1807–1812*
failure of, *1810*
idiopathic, 1807–1808, *1807–1810*
postinfarction, 1808–1809, *1810–1812*
with left bundle branch block, *1686*
with right bundle branch block, *1685*
Ventricular tachycardia zone, detection of, by
implantable cardioverter-defibrillator,
1782–1784, *1783*
Ventricular volume, assessment of, magnetic
resonance imaging in, 138–139, *138–139*
on radionuclide ventriculography, 109
Ventricular wall, rupture of, echocardiography
in, 664
Ventricularis, in mitral valve, 372
microscopic anatomy of, *355,* 356
Ventriculectomy, right, for arrhythmogenic
right ventricular dysplasia, 1827,
1828–1829
Ventriculography, radionuclide. See
Radionuclide ventriculography.
Ventriculotomy, endocardial, for ischemic
ventricular tachycardia, 1830
Verapamil, adverse effects of, 1753–1754
dosage of, 712t, 1753
during pregnancy, 2045t, 2065
efficacy of, 1753
electrophysiology of, 1753
for atrial fibrillation, 1636, 1637t
for hypertension, 1519–1520
for hypertrophic cardiomyopathy, 1068
for preexcitation, *1629*
for supraventricular tachycardia, during pregnancy, 2042
for unstable angina, *739*
mechanism of action for, 715
pharmacokinetics of, 1742t–1743t, 1753
Verrucae, in rheumatic fever, 389, *390*
Verrucous endocarditis of Libman and Sacks.
See *Lupus erythematosus valvulitis.*
Vertebrobasilar transient ischemic attacks, and
syncope, 9
Vertical steal, in SPECT myocardial perfusion
imaging, 101
Very low-density lipoprotein (VLDL), and
hyperlipidemia, 1345–1346
Veterans Affairs Cooperative Study Trial,
861–864, 862t, *863*
Veterans Affairs Non–Q Wave Infarction
Strategies in Hospital (VANQWISH) trial,
814, 814t
Veterans Affairs Vasodilator Heart Failure Trial
(V-HeFT), *1169, 1172*
V-HeFT (Veterans Affairs Vasodilator Heart
Failure Trial), *1169, 1172*
Video display unit(s), for coronary
angiography, 594
Videodensitometry, for quantification of
coronary artery stenosis, 628–629
Viral infection(s), and dilated cardiomyopathy,
1041–1043, 1041t–1042t
and myocarditis. See *Myocarditis, viral.*
and pericarditis, 1241, 1246
Viral vector(s), for gene therapy, 2270–2271,
2271t

Visceral obesity, and coronary artery disease,
2264
Vitamin B, and risk of coronary artery disease,
2208–2209
Vitamin deficiency, and plasma homocysteine
levels, 2279, 2279t
Vitamin E, with angiotensin-converting
enzyme inhibitors, HOPE trial of,
720–721
VLDL. See *Very low-density lipoprotein (VLDL).*
Vo_2 (peak oxygen consumption), and eligibility
for transplantation, 1187
Volume depletion, and shock, 1529
Volume expander(s), for syncope, from
orthostatic hypotension, 1703
Volume overload, and heart failure, 1149
Volunteer community model, for cardiac
rehabilitation, 908
von Willebrand factor, abnormalities of, in
pulmonary hypertension, 1861–1862
VOO pacemaker mode, 1770
VSD. See *Ventricular septal defect.*
VVI pacemaker mode, 1769
VVT pacemaker mode, 1769

Wall motion, abnormalities of,
echocardiography in, 659, *660*
Wall tension, definition of, 1491
Wallstent, with carotid endarterectomy, 1437
Warfarin, during pregnancy, 2040, *2040*
for atrial fibrillation, in older adults, 2021
for embolism prophylaxis, in atrial fibrilla-
tion, 1642–1643, 1643t
for pulmonary thromboembolism, 1848
Washington Radiation for Instant Restenosis
(WRIST) trial, 835
Wasp sting(s), and myocardial disease, 1092
Water-perfusable tissue index, in assessment of
myocardial viability, *120,* 120–121, 121t
Wedge angiography, in pulmonary
hypertension, 1876–1877
Wegener's granulomatosis, 1950
anatomic abnormalities in, 317
vs. pulmonary thromboembolism, 1846
Weight. See *Body weight.*
Weight cycling, and risk of coronary artery
disease, 2205
Weight loss, and coronary artery disease, 2265
cardiovascular effects of, 2261
in management of heart failure, 1165
in management of hypertension, 1515, *1516*
Weight training, in cardiac rehabilitation, 897
Weightlessness. See also *Space flight.*
and bone mineral content, 2076
and fluid dynamics, 2077–2078
cardiovascular response to, 2077, *2077*
data limitations of, 2086
"sensory conflict" in, 2076
Wenckebach atrioventricular block, 1573, *1599*
during pregnancy, 2046
Wenckebach interval, 1768, *1770*
West of Scotland Coronary Prevention Study
(WOSCOPS), 2253
Westmark sign, 74
Whipple's disease, 1090
anatomic abnormalities in, 317, *317*
White blood cell count, and coronary artery
disease, risk of, 2206–2207, 2207t
Whole-body autoregulation, and hypertension,
1502
Wide QRS tachycardia, atrioventricular
dissociation in, 1679, *1682*
during supraventricular tachycardia, *1678–1681,* 1679

Wide QRS tachycardia *(Continued)*
concealed retrograde conduction in, 1679, *1680–1681*
phase 3 block in, *1678,* 1679
electrocardiography in, *1678,* 1679–1687, *1682–1686*
and bundle branch block–shaped complexes, 1683–1687, *1684–1686*
and concordant pattern in precordial leads, 1683, *1684*
and QRS axis in frontal plane, 1683, *1683*
limitations of, 1686t
etiology of, 1677, *1678*
Williams' syndrome, 182, 2156
Wilson's disease, 2175t
Windkessel effect, 1479, 1486
Window hypothesis, 46–47
Wingless protein, and cardiogenesis, 922
Wolff-Parkinson-White syndrome, and sudden death, 1720
atrial fibrillation and, 1639
during pregnancy, 2042–2043
Wolff-Parkinson-White syndrome *(Continued)*
electrocardiography in, 42, *42–43*
exercise in, 1625–1626, *1628*
surgical treatment of, 1822–1823
tachycardia in, 1625, *1625*
ventricular fibrillation in, 1625, *1626*
Women, atherosclerotic plaque rupture in, *vs.* erosion, 580–582, 580t, *581*
coronary artery disease in, demographics of, 582, 582t
risk factors for, 579
and mechanism of death, 583–584, 583t–584t
and plaque morphology, 582
sudden death in, epidemiology of, 579
Wood unit(s), 423
World Health Organization clofibrate trial, 2253
WOSCOPS (West of Scotland Coronary Prevention Study), 2253
WRIST (Washington Radiation for Instant Restenosis) trial, 835

X descent,
Xenograft(ted, for aortic stenosis, 286, *286*
X-ray gene), for coronary angiography, 592–5
Xylocaine *idocaine.*

Y descent,
in cardiponade, 1251–1252, *1252*

Z pulse, inuclide imaging, 100
Zellwegerdrome, 2175t
Zic3 genetus inversus, 926
Zidovudirdiac toxicity of, 1980
z$Paco_2$, irnic obstructive pulmonary disea87
Zymogenerties of, 1317t

ISBN 0-443-07000-8